SEVENTH EDITION

TEXTBOOK OF THERAPEUTICS
DRUG AND DISEASE MANAGEMENT

Editors

Eric T. Herfindal, Pharm.D., M.P.H.
Professor Emeritus
School of Pharmacy
University of California
San Francisco, California

Dick R. Gourley, Pharm.D.
Dean, College of Pharmacy
Professor of Pharmacy Practice and Pharmacoeconomics
University of Tennessee College of Pharmacy
Memphis, Tennessee

Consulting Editors

Kimberly A. Bergstrom / Richard A. Helms / Joan E. Kapusnik-Uner / Shalini Lynch
David J. Quan / Nathan Rawls / Timothy H. Self

LIPPINCOTT WILLIAMS & WILKINS
A **Wolters Kluwer** Company
Philadelphia • Baltimore • New York • London
Buenos Aires • Hong Kong • Sydney • Tokyo

Editor: Daniel Limmer
Managing Editor: Matthew J. Hauber
Marketing Manager: Anne E.P. Smith
Production Editor: Shannon T. Benner
Development Editor: Daniel V. Edson

351 West Camden Street
Baltimore, MD 21201-2436 USA

530 Walnut Street
Philadelphia, PA 19106-3621 USA

The publisher is not responsible (as a matter of product liability, negligence, or otherwise) for any injury resulting from any material contained herein. This publication contains information relating to general principles of medical care which should not be construed as specific instructions for individual patients. Manufacturers' product information and package inserts should be reviewed for current information, including contraindications, dosages, and precautions.

Printed in the United States of America

Library of Congress Cataloging-in-Publication Data

Textbook of therapeutics: drug and disease management / editors, Eric T. Herfindal, Dick R. Gourley; consulting editors, Kimberly Bergstrom ... [et al.].– 7th ed.
p. ; cm.
Includes bibliographical references and index.
ISBN 0-7817-2414-7
1. Chemotherapy. 2. Therapeutics. I. Herfindal, Eric T. II. Gourley, D.R.H., 1922-
[DNLM: 1. Drug Therapy. WB 330 T3555 2000]
RM262 .C5 2000
615.5′8–dc21

00-037061

The publishers have made every effort to trace the copyright holders for borrowed material. If they have inadvertently overlooked any, they will be pleased to make the necessary arrangements at the first opportunity.

To purchase additional copies of this book, call our customer service department at **(800) 638-3030** or fax orders to **(301) 824-7390.** International customers should call **(301) 714-2324.**

01 02 03 04
2 3 4 5 6 7 8 9 10

Consulting Editors

Kimberly A. Bergstrom, Pharm.D.
Vice President
Your Doctor, Inc.
Berkeley, California

Richard A. Helms, Pharm.D., BCNSP
Professor and Chair
Department of Clinical Pharmacy
University of Tennessee College of Pharmacy
Memphis, Tennessee

Joan E. Kapusnik-Uner, Pharm.D.
Senior Knowledge Engineer
First Data Bank–The Hearst Corp.
San Bruno, California

Shalini Lynch, Pharm.D.
Drug Experience Associate
Medical and Safety Services
Alza Corporation
Palo Alto, California

David J. Quan, Pharm.D.
Assistant Clinical Professor
Department of Clinical Pharmacy
School of Pharmacy
University of California, San Francisco
Clinical Pharmacist
Department of Pharmaceutical Services
UCSF Medical Center
San Francisco, California

Nathan Rawls, Pharm.D.
Associate Professor of Pharmacy Practice and Pharmacoeconomics
University of Tennessee College of Pharmacy
Clinical Specialist
Veterans Affairs Medical Center
Memphis, Tennessee

Timothy H. Self, Pharm.D.
Professor of Clinical Pharmacy
Department of Clinical Pharmacy
University of Tennessee College of Pharmacy
Memphis, Tennessee

Contributors

David S. Adler, Pharm.D.
UCSD Anticoagulation Clinic and VA San Diego Anticoagulation Clinic
Professor
Department of Clinical Pharmacy
School of Pharmacy
University of California, San Francisco
San Francisco, California

Shawn R. Akkerman, Pharm.D., BCPS
Assistant Director
Clinical Pharmaceutical Research Program
Emory Healthcare
Decatur, Georgia

Brian K. Alldredge, Pharm.D.
Professor of Clinical Pharmacy and Clinical Professor of Neurology
Departments of Clinical Pharmacy and Neurology
School of Pharmacy
University of California, San Francisco
San Francisco, California

Betsy Althaus, Pharm.D.
Assistant Clinical Professor
Department of Clinical Pharmacy
School of Pharmacy
University of California, San Francisco
San Francisco, California

Ann B. Amerson, Pharm.D.
Professor
Department of Pharmacy Practice and Science
University of Kentucky College of Pharmacy
Lexington, Kentucky

Kristan Marie Augustin, Pharm.D., BCOP
Clinical Pharmacy Specialist, Blood and Marrow Transplantation
Division of Pharmacy
University of Texas M.D. Anderson Cancer Center
Houston, Texas

Lisa M. Avery, Pharm.D.
Clinical Pharmacist
St. Joseph's Hospital
Princeton, New Jersey

Carol Balmer, Pharm.D.
Associate Professor
University of Colorado School of Pharmacy
Denver, Colorado

Jeffrey N. Baldwin, Pharm.D., FAPhA, FASHP
Associate Professor of Pharmacy Practice and Pediatrics
University of Nebraska Medical Center
Omaha, Nebraska

Joseph A. Barone, Pharm.D., FCCP
Associate Professor and Chair
Department of Pharmacy Practice and Administration
Rutgers University College of Pharmacy
Piscataway, New Jersey

Elizabeth A. Beltz, Pharm.D.
Clinical Pharmacy Specialist MICU/Pulmonary and Adjunct Assistant Professor
University of Iowa College of Pharmacy
Department of Pharmaceutical Care
University of Iowa Hospitals and Clinics
Iowa City, Iowa

Rosemary R. Berardi, Pharm.D., FASHP
Professor of Pharmacy, College of Pharmacy
Clinical Pharmacist, Gastroenterology
Department of Pharmacy, University of Michigan Health System
University of Michigan
Ann Arbor, Michigan

Kimberly A. Bergstrom, Pharm.D.
Vice President
Your Doctor, Inc.
Berkeley, California

Paul M. Beringer, Pharm.D., BCPS
Assistant Professor
Department of Clinical Pharmacy
University of Southern California
Los Angeles, California

Kathryn Blake, Pharm.D.
Clinical Research Scientist
Clinical Pediatric Pharmacology
The Nemours Children's Clinic
Jacksonville, Florida

Sybelle A. Blakey, Pharm.D., BCPS
Clinical Assistant Professor
Department of Pharmacy Practice
Mercer University Southern School of Pharmacy
Atlanta, Georgia

Bradley A. Boucher, Pharm.D., FCCP, BCPS
Professor
Department of Clinical Pharmacy
University of Tennessee College of Pharmacy
Memphis, Tennessee

Eric G. Boyce, Pharm.D.
Professor of Clinical Pharmacy
Philadelphia College of Pharmacy
University of the Sciences in Philadelphia
Philadelphia, Pennsylvania

Ronald L. Braden, Pharm.D.
Clinical Pharmacy Specialist, Critical Care
Veterans Administration Medical Center
Associate Professor
University of Tennessee College of Pharmacy
Memphis, Tennessee

J. Richard Brown, Pharm.D., BCPS, FASHP
Professor
University of Tennessee College of Pharmacy
Clinical Pharmacy Specialist
Veterans Administration Medical Center
Memphis, Tennessee

Rex O. Brown, Pharm.D., BCNSP, FCCP
Professor and Vice-Chair
Department of Clinical Pharmacy
University of Tennessee College of Pharmacy
Memphis, Tennessee

Howard A. Burris III, M.D.
Director of Drug Development
The Sarah Cannon Cancer Centers
Nashville, Tennessee

R. Keith Campbell, R.Ph., B.Pharm., M.B.A.
Associate Dean and Professor of Pharmacy
College of Pharmacy
Washington State University
Pallman, Washington

Patricia L. Canales, Pharm.D., BCPP
Assistant Professor
Department of Pharmacy Practice
Auburn University School of Pharmacy
Tuscaloosa Veterans Administration Medical Center
Tuscaloosa, Alabama

Jannet M. Carmichael, Pharm.D., BCPS, FCCP
Clinical Pharmacy Coordinator
Department of Pharmacy
VA Medical Center
Associate Professor of Medicine
Department of Internal Medicine
University of Nevada
Reno, Nevada

Marshall Cates, Pharm.D., BCPP
Assistant Professor
Department of Pharmacy Practice
Samford University McWhorter School of Pharmacy
Birmingham, Alabama

Dawn M. Chandler-Toufieli, Pharm.D.
Assistant Professor of Clinical Pharmacy
Massachusetts College of Pharmacy and Allied Health Sciences
Boston, Massachusetts

Jennie T. Chang, Pharm.D.
Clinical Research Fellow
University of California, San Francisco/Coulter Pharmaceutical
Palo Alto, California

Ziba Gorji Chang, Pharm.D.
Community Pharmacy Practice Resident
Virginia Commonwealth University School of Pharmacy
Richmond, Virginia

Judy L. Chase, Pharm.D.
Clinical Pharmacy Specialist
University of Texas M.D. Anderson Cancer Center
Houston, Texas

Jack J. Chen, Pharm.D., BCPS
Assistant Professor of Pharmacy Practice
Western University of Health Sciences College of Pharmacy
Pomona, California

Cinda L. Christensen, Pharm.D.
Clinical Specialist in Infectious Diseases
Department of Pharmaceutical Services
University of California, Davis Medical Center
Sacramento, California
Assistant Clinical Professor
School of Pharmacy
University of California, San Francisco
San Francisco, California

Bruce D. Clayton, B.S., Pharm.D., R.Ph.
Professor of Pharmacy Practice and Associate Dean
Butler University College of Pharmacy and Health Sciences
Indianapolis, Indiana

Unamarie Clibon, Pharm.D., MD
Practicing Physician
Texas Cancer Care
Arlington, Texas

G. Dennis Clifton, Pharm.D., FCCP
Professor and Chair
Department of Pharmacy Practice
Washington State University and The Heart Institute of Spokane
Spokane, Washington

Stephen C. Cooke, Pharm.D.
Assistant Professor
Department of Pharmacy Practice and Pharmacoeconomics
University of Tennessee College of Pharmacy
Director of Pharmacy Services
Memphis Mental Health Institute
Memphis, Tennessee

Carlos C. da Camara, Pharm.D., BCPS
Assistant Professor
Department of Pharmacy Practice
Campbell University School of Pharmacy
Cary, North Carolina

Martha G. Danielson, Pharm.D.
Pharmacy Clinical Research Specialist, Pediatrics
Division of Pharmacy
University of Texas M.D. Anderson Cancer Center
Houston, Texas

Dena Behm Dillon, Pharm.D.
Clinical Pharmacy Specialist, Infectious Diseases
Department of Pharmaceutical Care
University of Iowa Hospitals and Clinics
Iowa City, Iowa

Betty J. Dong, Pharm.D.
Professor
Departments of Clinical Pharmacy and Family and Community Medicine
School of Pharmacy
University of California, San Francisco
San Francisco, California

Vicky Dudas, Pharm.D.
Assistant Clinical Professor
Department of Clinical Pharmacy
School of Pharmacy
University of California, San Francisco
San Francisco, California

Kirsten M. Duncan, Pharm.D.
Clinical Pharmacy Consultant
Assistant Clinical Professor
Department of Clinical Pharmacy
School of Pharmacy
University of California, San Francisco
San Francisco, California

James C. Eoff III, Pharm.D.
Executive Associate Dean and Professor
Department of Pharmacy Practice and Pharmacoeconomics
University of Tennessee College of Pharmacy
Memphis, Tennessee

Erika J. Ernst, Pharm.D.
Assistant Professor
University of Iowa College of Pharmacy
Iowa City, Iowa

William E. Evans, Pharm.D.
Professor of Clinical Pharmacy and Pediatrics
First Tennessee Chair of Excellence
Departments of Clinical Pharmacy and Pediatrics
University of Tennessee and St. Jude Children's Research Hospital
Memphis, Tennessee

Rebecca S. Finley, Pharm.D., M.S.
Professor of Pharmacy Practice and Chair
Department of Pharmacy Practice and Pharmacy Administration
Philadelphia College of Pharmacy
Philadelphia, Pennsylvania

Clarence L. Fortner, M.S.
Director, Scientific Affairs
North American Market Region
Pharmacia & Upjohn
Bel Air, Maryland

Stephan Foster, Pharm.D.
Associate Professor
Department of Pharmacy Practice and Pharmacoeconomics
University of Tennessee College of Pharmacy
Memphis, Tennessee

Carla B. Frye, Pharm.D., BCPS, R.Ph.
Associate Professor of Pharmacy Practice
Butler University College of Pharmacy and Health Sciences
Indianapolis, Indiana

Darlene F. Fujimoto, Pharm.D.
Assistant Clinical Professor
Department of Family Medicine
University of California, Irvine
Orange, California

Stephen H. Fuller, Pharm.D.
Associate Professor
Department of Pharmacy Practice
Campbell University School of Pharmacy
Cary, North Carolina

Marie E. Gardner, Pharm.D.
Associate Professor
Department of Pharmacy Practice
University of Arizona College of Pharmacy
Tucson, Arizona

Christa M. George, Pharm.D., BCPS
Assistant Professor
Department of Pharmacy Practice and Pharmacoeconomics
University of Tennessee College of Pharmacy
Memphis, Tennessee

Mark A. Gill, Pharm.D.
Professor
Department of Pharmacy Practice
University of Southern California School of Pharmacy
Los Angeles, California

Tracey L. Goldsmith, Pharm.D.
Clinical Manager
Department of Pharmacy
Hermann Hospital
Houston, Texas

Edgar R. Gonzalez, Pharm.D., FASHP
Clinical Liaison
Commonwealth Health Benefits, Inc.
Richmond, Virginia

Greta K. Gourley, M.S.N., Ph.D., Pharm.D.
Associate Professor
Department of Pharmacy Practice and Pharmacoeconomics
University of Tennessee College of Pharmacy
Memphis, Tennessee

Emily B. Hak, Pharm.D., BCNSP
Associate Professor
Department of Clinical Pharmacy
University of Tennessee College of Pharmacy
Memphis, Tennessee

Lawrence J. Hak, Pharm.D., BCPS, BCNSP
Professor
Department of Clinical Pharmacy
University of Tennessee College of Pharmacy
Memphis, Tennessee

Scott D. Hanes, Pharm.D., BCPS
Assistant Professor
Department of Clinical Pharmacy
University of Tennessee College of Pharmacy
Memphis, Tennessee

Thomas C. Hardin, Pharm.D., BCPS, FCCP
Clinical Coordinator
Pharmacy Services
Audie L. Murphy Memorial Veterans Hospital
San Antonio, Texas

Mary F. Hebert, Pharm.D.
Associate Professor
University of Washington School of Pharmacy
Seattle, Washington

Richard A. Helms, Pharm.D., BCNSP
Professor and Chair
Department of Clinical Pharmacy
University of Tennessee College of Pharmacy
Memphis, Tennessee

Robert P. Henderson, Pharm.D., FASHP, FCCP, BCPS
Professor and Vice Chair, Clinical Pharmacy Specialist
Department of Pharmacy Practice
Samford University McWhorter School of Pharmacy
Birmingham, Alabama

Evelyn R. Hermes-DeSantis, Pharm.D., PCPS
Clinical Assistant Professor
Department of Pharmacy Practice and Administration
Rutgers University College of Pharmacy
Piscataway, New Jersey

Katherine C. Herndon, Pharm.D., BCPS
Assistant Professor
Department of Pharmacy Practice
Samford University McWhorter School of Pharmacy
Birmingham, Alabama

Richard N. Herrier, Pharm.D.
Assistant Professor
Department of Pharmacy Practice
University of Arizona College of Pharmacy
Tucson, Arizona

Anne M. Hoffmeister, Pharm.D.
Fellow in Critical Care Pharmacotherapy
Department of Pharmacy Practice and Pharmacy Administration
University of the Sciences Philadelphia College of Pharmacy
Philadelphia, Pennsylvania

Valerie W. Hogue, Pharm.D., CDE
Associate Professor
Clinical and Administrative Pharmacy Sciences
Howard University School of Pharmacy
Washington, D.C.

John M. Holbrook, Ph.D.
Professor
Department of Pharmaceutical Sciences
Mercer University Southern School of Pharmacy
Atlanta, Georgia

James M. Holt, Pharm.D.
Assistant Professor
Department of Pharmacy
Veterans Administration Medical Center
Memphis, Tennessee

Collin A. Hovinga, Pharm.D.
Pediatric Pharmacotherapy Fellow
Department of Clinical Pharmacy
University of Tennessee College of Pharmacy
Memphis, Tennessee

Jason L. Iltz, Pharm.D.
Assistant Professor of Pharmacy Practice
Washington State University at Spokane College of Pharmacy
Spokane, Washington

Heather J. Johnson, Pharm.D.
Assistant Professor
Department of Pharmacy Practice
University of Pittsburgh Medical Center
Pittsburgh, Pennsylvania

Jannifer L. Johnson, Pharm.D.
Medical Science Liaison
Science Oriented Solutions
Decatur, Georgia

Suzanne Fields Jones, Pharm.D.
Associate Director of Drug Development
The Sarah Cannon Cancer Center
Nashville, Tennessee

Barbara S. Kannewurf, Pharm.D.
Clinical Pharmacist
Cardiology Clinical Institution
University of Washington Medical Center
Seattle, Washington

Steven R. Kayser, Pharm.D.
Director
Anticoagulation Clinic
Clinical Professor of Pharmacy
Department of Clinical Pharmacy
School of Pharmacy
University of California, San Francisco
San Francisco, California

Daniel T. Kennedy, Pharm.D., BCPS
Assistant Professor
Department of Pharmacy
Virginia Commonwealth University School of Pharmacy
Richmond, Virginia

Wendy Klein-Schwartz, Pharm.D.
Associate Professor
Department of Pharmacy Practice
University of Maryland School of Pharmacy
Baltimore, Maryland

Susannah E. Koontz, Pharm.D.
Clinical Practice Specialist, Pediatric Hematology/Oncology
Division of Pharmacy
University of Texas M.D. Anderson Cancer Center
Houston, Texas

Amy Galpin Krauss, Pharm.D., BCPS
Clinical Pharmacy Specialist
Methodist Hospitals of Memphis
Memphis, Tennessee

S. Casey Laizure, Pharm.D.
Associate Professor
Department of Clinical Pharmacy
University of Tennessee College of Pharmacy
Memphis, Tennessee

Roger D. Lander, Pharm.D., FASHP, FCCP, BCPS
Professor and Chair
Department of Pharmacy Practice
Samford University McWhorter School of Pharmacy
Birmingham, Alabama

Christy R. Lawrence, Pharm.D.
Clinical Pharmacist
Department of Army
Fort Campbell, Kentucky

Robert H. Levin, Pharm.D.
Professor of Clinical Pharmacy and Pediatrics
School of Pharmacy
University of California
UCSF Program Director
San Francisco General Hospital
San Francisco, California

Bobby L. Lobo, Pharm.D., BCPS
Associate Professor
Department of Pharmacy Practice and Pharmacoeconomics
University of Tennessee College of Pharmacy
Clinical Pharmacists
Methodist Hospital
Memphis, Tennessee

Richard D. Lozano, R.Ph.
Clinical Practitioner
Department of Pharmacy
University of Texas M.D. Anderson Cancer Center
Houston, Texas

Janet A. Lyle, Pharm.D., FCSHP
Clinical Oncology Pharmacist
Department of Pharmacy
Alta Bates Medical Center
Berkeley, California

Pierre A. Maloley, Pharm.D.
Clinical Liaison, Medical Affairs
Roche Laboratories
Associate Professor
Pharmacy Practice, Internal Medicine
University of Nebraska Medical Center
Omaha, Nebraska

Margaret Malone, Ph.D., BCNSP, FCCP
Professor
Department of Pharmacy Practice
Albany College of Pharmacy
Albany, New York

Delbert L. Mandl, Pharm.D.
Assistant Professor
Department of Pharmacy Practice
Washington State University
Spokane, Washington

Hewitt W. Matthews, Ph.D.
Dean and Hood-Meyer Professor
Department of Pharmaceutical Sciences
Mercer University School of Pharmacy
Atlanta, Georgia

Gary R. Matzke, Pharm.D., FCCP
Professor of Pharmacy Practice
Department of Pharmacy and Therapeutics
University of Pittsburgh School of Pharmacy
Pittsburgh, Pennsylvania

Monique Mayo, Pharm.D.
Clinical Pharmacist Consultant
San Diego, California

Diane Nykamp McCarter, Pharm.D.
Professor
Department of Pharmacy Practice
Mercer University Southern School of Pharmacy
Atlanta, Georgia

Maureen P. McColl, Pharm.D.
Clinical Pharmacy Specialist
Clinical Pharmacy Department
University Hospital
Stony Brook, New York

John N. McCormick, Pharm.D.
Clinical Pharmacy Specialist
St. Jude Children's Research Hospital
Memphis, Tennessee

William J. McIntyre, Pharm.D.
Assistant Professor
Department of Pharmacy Practice
University of Arkansas for Medical Science College of Pharmacy
Little Rock, Arkansas

Constance McKenzie, Pharm.D.
Assistant Professor and Director
Drug Information Center
Campbell University
Buies Creek, North Carolina

Gail W. McSweeney, Pharm.D.
Clinical Pharmacy Consultant
San Francisco, California

Helen Meldrum, Ed.D.
Associate Professor
Social and Administrative Sciences
Massachusetts College of Pharmacy and Health Sciences
Boston, Massachusetts

Laura Boehnke Michaud, Pharm.D., BCOP
Clinical Pharmacy Specialist
Division of Pharmacy
University of Texas M.D. Anderson Cancer Center
Houston, Texas

Susan W. Miller, Pharm.D., FASCP, CGP
Professor
Department of Pharmacy Practice
Mercer University Southern School of Pharmacy
Atlanta, Georgia

Jay F. Mouser, Pharm.D., BCNSP
Assistant Professor
OSU College of Pharmacy
Portland Campus
Oregon Health Sciences University
Portland, Oregon

Alan H. Mutnick, Pharm.D., FASHP
Senior Assistant Director, Clinical Practice
Department of Pharmaceutical Care
University of Iowa Hospitals and Clinics
Iowa City, Iowa

David E. Nix, Pharm.D.
Associate Professor Pharmacy Practice
University of Arizona College of Pharmacy
Tucson, Arizona

Paul E. Nolan Jr., Pharm.D.
Associate Professor
University of Arizona College of Pharmacy
Tucson, Arizona

Gary M. Oderda, Pharm.D., M.P.H.
Professor
Department of Pharmacy Practice
University of Utah College of Pharmacy
Salt Lake City, Utah

Gary Ogawa, Pharm.D.
Program Coordinator
iKnowMed, Inc.
Berkeley, California

Neeta Bahal O'Mara, Pharm.D.
Assistant Professor of Pharmacy Practice
School of Pharmacy
Butler University
Indianapolis, Indiana

Michael A. Oszko, Pharm.D., BCPS
Associate Professor
Department of Pharmacy Practice, School of Pharmacy
Department of Family Medicine, School of Medicine
University of Kansas
Kansas City, Kansas

Shirley M. Palmer, Pharm.D.
Assistant Professor Pharmacy Practice
Medical College of Virginia School of Pharmacy
Richmond, Virginia

Beth Logsdon Pangle, Pharm.D., BCNSP
Pediatric Clinical Specialist
Department of Pharmacy
Cook Children's Medical Center
Fort Worth, Texas

Louise Parent-Stevens, Pharm.D., BCPS
Clinical Assistant Professor
Department of Pharmacy Practice
University of Illinois at Chicago College of Pharmacy
Chicago, Illinois

Dina K. Patel, Pharm.D.
Clinical Pharmacy Specialist
Department of Pharmacy
University of Texas M.D. Anderson Cancer Center
Houston, Texas

Constance M. Pfeiffer, Pharm.D., BCPS, BCOP
Clinical Assistant Professor
Department of Pharmacy Practice and Administration
Rutgers University College of Pharmacy
Piscataway, New Jersey

Stephanie J. Phelps, Pharm.D.
Professor
Department of Clinical Pharmacy
University of Tennessee College of Pharmacy
Memphis, Tennessee

Jerry R. Phipps Jr., Pharm.D.
Drug Information Resident
University of Tennessee College of Pharmacy
Memphis, Tennessee

Ronnie D. Raspberry, M.D.
Chief of Dermatology Section
Medical Service
VA Medical Center
Memphis, Tennessee

Christopher Rathbun, Pharm.D., BCPS
Associate Professor
Department of Pharmacy Practice
University of Oklahoma Health Sciences Center College of Pharmacy
Oklahoma City, Oklahoma

Nathan Rawls, Pharm.D.
Associate Professor
Department of Pharmacy Practice and Pharmacoeconomics
University of Tennessee College of Pharmacy
Clinical Specialist
Veteran Affairs Medical Center
Memphis, Tennessee

Lori A. Reisner, Pharm.D.
Associate Clinical Professor
Department of Clinical Pharmacy
University of California, San Francisco
San Francisco, California

Beth H. Resman-Targoff, Pharm.D.
Clinical Associate Professor
Department of Pharmacy Practice
University of Oklahoma College of Pharmacy
Oklahoma City, Oklahoma

Ted L. Rice, M.S., BCPS
Associate Professor
University of Pittsburgh School of Pharmacy
Pittsburgh, Pennsylvania

Daniel C. Robinson, Pharm.D.
Associate Professor and Chair
Department of Pharmacy Practice
University of Southern California School of Pharmacy
Los Angeles, California

Marjorie D. Robinson, Pharm.D.
Assistant Professor
Department of Pharmacy Practice
Nova Southeastern University
Ft. Lauderdale, Florida

Ronald J. Ruggiero, Pharm.D.
Clinical Professor
Clinical Pharmacy and Obstetrics, Gynecology and Reproductive Sciences
School of Pharmacy
The Medical Center at the University of California, San Francisco
San Francisco, California

R. Michelle Sanders, Pharm.D., BCNSP
Assistant Professor
Pharmaceutical Department
St. Jude Children's Research Hospital
Memphis, Tennessee

Debbie Scholtz, Pharm.D., BCPS, CDE
Assistant Professor
Department of Pharmacy Practice and Pharmacoeconomics
University of Tennessee College of Pharmacy
Memphis, Tennessee

Charles F. Seifert, Pharm.D., FCCP, BCPS
Professor of Pharmacy Practice and Regional Dean for Lubbock Programs
School of Pharmacy
Texas Tech University Health Sciences Center
Lubbock, Texas

Stephen M. Setter, Pharm.D.
Assistant Professor of Pharmacy Practice
Washington State University College of Pharmacy
Spokane, Washington

Sam K. Shimomura, Pharm.D.
Professor
Department of Clinical Pharmacy
Western University of Health Sciences College of Pharmacy
Pomona, California

Stephen D. Silberstein, M.D.
Professor of Neurology and Director, Jefferson Headache Center
Department of Neurology
Thomas Jefferson University
Philadelphia, Pennsylvania

Renu F. Singh, Pharm.D.
Assistant Clinical Professor
Department of Pharmacy Practice
Wayne State University College of Pharmacy and Allied Health
Detroit, Michigan

Ralph E. Small, Pharm.D.
Professor of Pharmacy and Medicine
Virginia Commonwealth University
Medical College of Virginia Campus
Richmond, Virginia

Sharon D. Solomon, M.D.
Resident in Ophthalmology
Department of Ophthalmology
University of California, San Francisco
San Francisco, California

Mary M. Sotirhos, Pharm.D.
Clinical Pharmacy Department
Pinnacle Health Enterprises
Rutgers University
North Brunswick, New Jersey

Kevin M. Sowinski, Pharm.D., BCPS
Assistant Professor
Department of Pharmacy Practice
Purdue University School of Pharmacy and Pharmacal Sciences
Indianapolis, Indiana

Robert J. Stagg, Pharm.D.
Senior Director, Clinical Research
Department of Clinical Research
Coulter Pharmaceutical
South San Francisco, California

Gregory V. Stajich, Pharm.D.
Associate Professor of Pharmacy Practice
Mercer University Southern School of Pharmacy
Atlanta, Georgia

Robert C. Stevens, Pharm.D., FCCP, BCPS
Associate Professor
Department of Clinical Pharmacy
University of Tennessee College of Pharmacy
Memphis, Tennessee

Glen L. Stimmel, Pharm.D., FCCP
Professor of Clinical Pharmacy and Psychiatry
University of Southern California Schools of Pharmacy
and Medicine
Los Angeles, California

Janice L. Stumpf, Pharm.D.
Clinical Pharmacist and Clinical Assistant Professor
Department of Pharmacy Services
University of Michigan Health System and College of Pharmacy
Ann Arbor, Michigan

David S. Tatro, Pharm.D.
Drug Information Consultant
San Carlos, California

Mary E. Teresi, Pharm.D.
Director, Clinical Research
Department of Pediatrics
University of Iowa College of Medicine
Iowa City, Iowa

Paula A. Thompson, M.S., Pharm.D., BCPS
Assistant Professor
Samford University McWhorter School of Pharmacy
Birmingham, Alabama

Camille W. Thornton, Pharm.D.
Assistant Professor
Department of Pharmacy Practice and Pharmacoeconomics
University of Tennessee College of Pharmacy
Memphis, Tennessee

Karen J. Tietze, Pharm.D.
Professor
Department of Pharmacy Practice and Pharmacy Administration
University of the Sciences Philadelphia College of Pharmacy
Philadelphia, Pennsylvania

Theodore G. Tong, Pharm.D.
Professor of Pharmacy Practice, Pharmacology and Toxicology,
Public Health
Associate Dean for Academic Affairs
University of Arizona College of Pharmacy
Tucson, Arizona

Kevin A. Townsend, Pharm.D., BCPS
Clinical Education Consultant
Pfizer, Inc.
Clinical Assistant Professor of Pharmacy
University of Michigan Health System and College of Pharmacy
Ann Arbor, Michigan

VanAnh Trinh, Pharm.D.
Clinical Pharmacist
Department of Pharmacy
University of Texas M.D. Anderson Cancer Center
Houston, Texas

J. Edwin Underwood Jr., Pharm.D.
Associate Professor
Samford University McWhorter School of Pharmacy
Birmingham, Alabama

Jeanne H. Van Tyle, Pharm.D.
Professor
Butler University College of Pharmacy
Indianapolis, Indiana

Mary L. Wagner, M.S., Pharm.D.
Associate Professor
Department of Pharmacy Practice and Administration
Rutgers University College of Pharmacy
Piscataway, New Jersey

Jeffrey J. Weber, Pharm.D., BCPS
Clinical Specialist, Pharmacy
Department of Pharmacy Services
Bryan LGH Medical Center
East Campus
Lincoln, Nebraska

Robert T. Weibert, Pharm.D.
Clinical Professor
Department of Clinical Pharmacy
UCSD School of Pharmacy
San Diego, California

Barbara G. Wells, Pharm.D.
Professor and Dean
Idaho State University College of Pharmacy
Pocatello, Idaho

Gina R. Westfall, Pharm.D.
Post-Doctoral Research Fellow
Pharmacy Practice, Internal Medicine
University of Nebraska Medical Center
Omaha, Nebraska

E. Ashley Whigham, Pharm.D.
Ambulatory Resident
University of Tennessee College of Pharmacy
Memphis, Tennessee

Amy L. Whitaker, Pharm.D.
Clinical Instructor
Virginia Commonwealth University
Medical College of Virginia Campus
Richmond, Virginia

John R. White Jr., Pharm.D.
Associate Professor
Department of Pharmacy Practice
Washington State University
Pullman, Washington

Michael Z. Wincor, Pharm.D., BCPP
Associate Professor
Clinical Pharmacy Psychiatry and the Behavioral Sciences
University of Southern California Schools of Pharmacy and Medicine
Los Angeles, California

Annie Wong-Beringer, Pharm.D.
Associate Professor of Pharmacy Practice
Western University of Health Sciences
Pomona, California
Infectious Diseases Specialist
Department of Pharmacy
Huntington Memorial Hospital
Huntington Beach, California

J. Douglas Wurtzbacher, Pharm.D., Ph.D.
Assistant Professor
Department of Pharmacy Practice and Pharmacoeconomics
University of Tennessee College of Pharmacy
Memphis, Tennessee

Yuri Yanishevski, M.Sc.
Research Fellow
Departments of Clinical Pharmacy and Pediatrics
University of Tennessee and St. Jude Children's Research Hospital
Memphis, Tennessee

Winnie M. Yu, Pharm.D.
Assistant Professor
Department of Pharmacy and Therapeutics
University of Pittsburg School of Pharmacy
Pittsburg, Pennsylvania

Dawn G. Zarembski, Pharm.D.
Assistant Professor
Department of Pharmacy Practice
Midwestern University Chicago College of Pharmacy
Downers Grove, Illinois

Caroline S. Zeind, Pharm.D.
Assistant Professor
Department of Pharmacy Practice
Massachusetts College of Pharmacy Health Sciences
Boston, Massachusetts

Preface

In the quarter century since the publication of the first edition of this textbook, healthcare has undergone revolutionary changes, none more dramatic than in the area of therapeutics. Witness the advent of biotechnology, gene therapy, pharmacogenomics, and pharmacokinetics. The fact that the first edition of the book required 500 pages to cover the major therapeutic modalities available in 1974 and that this edition is 2000+ pages speaks to the explosion in the availability of therapeutic alternatives.

Healthcare costs have increased at a rate far in excess of other areas of the economy (per capita cost of $387 in 1972, $3,098 in 1992, and $5,712 by end of 1999). A healthcare system that encouraged high levels of utilization, discouraged cost-consciousness, and created tolerance for inefficiency was ripe for revolutionary change. Initially, managed care was the embodiment of that change. It is arguable whether managed care achieved the goals it was intended to achieve. Aggressive utilization controls by managed care organizations have resulted in consumer and provider dissatisfaction of unprecedented proportions. Anti-managed care legislation, malpractice litigation, and a powerful consumer backlash have all contributed to a strong national movement to once again change the healthcare system.

What are we going to try this time? What will be the American healthcare system of the new millennium? We have learned some valuable lessons in the past 25 years: 1. The appropriate use of pharmaceuticals can significantly reduce suffering and increase the quality and length of life; 2. New technologies, including pharmaceuticals, have brought improvements in quality at substantial increases in the cost of treating an episode of illness; 3. An aging population will continue to require increasing medical services; 4. Uninsured patients consume an increasing share of healthcare resources (43.4 million patients/16.1% of the population in 1997); 5. 20% of those who access the healthcare system incur 80% of the expense; 6. Managing costs by arbitrarily denying access to care is not a viable strategy. Regardless of how we decide to pay for healthcare, we believe that the principles of disease management should be an integral component of the healthcare system.

By using the scientific, economic, and human strategies of disease management as outlined in this book, we will go a long way toward achieving the goal of optimal and rational medical care affordable by a society that places a strong emphasis on health and wellness. *Disease management* is the process of caring for patients using standardized treatment strategies that ensure appropriate utilization and high quality care across the continuum (The Disease Management Strategies Research Study & Resource Guide, published by NMHCC, 1998). Disease management is a highly effective strategy in controlling healthcare costs and improving outcomes. It focuses on chronic, costly disease states with high co-morbidity as well as acute, catastrophic episodes of care. By basing therapeutic decisions on scientific and clinical evidence clearly delineated in treatment algorithms and protocols, bias is reduced and the arbitrary and heavy-handed managed care strategies that have failed in the past can be eliminated.

As disease management has matured as a concept, so have the requirements of a textbook that attempts to provide student and practitioner with sufficient information organized in a useful and logical way. For this edition, we have made extensive changes in format to enhance readability and to highlight certain areas we think are critical, such as treatment goals, pharmacoeconomic considerations, psychosocial issues, and key points in each chapter.

Editorial Team for the Textbook

We are pleased to have the assistance of seven consulting editors. These colleagues bring a breadth of experience in practice, education, and research to the editorial team of the textbook and casebook. The editors, consulting editors, and staff have worked together to redesign the structure of the books, as well as providing editorial review throughout the editorial process. The consulting editors for the textbook are Drs. Kim Bergstrom, Richard Helms, Joan Kapusnik-Uner, Shalini Lynch, David Quan, Nathan Rawls, and Timothy Self. The editorial assistant for the textbook is Karin Ingram, who has provided continuity among the editors, consulting editors, and authors, as well as the editorial staff at Lippincott Williams & Wilkins. Without her organization, attention to detail, and persistence, this textbook could not have been completed. We owe her our gratitude for a job well done!

Editorial Team for the Casebook

The casebook for the seventh edition has been redesigned by the new editors, Drs. Greta Gourley and James Holt. It is divided into sections based on the textbook. The cases refer the student/practitioner to specific chapters in the textbook for further information to assist them in resolving the cases. All cases have a consistent format and are categorized as Level 1, 2, or 3 based on their degree of therapeutic difficulty. Case questions are based on identifiable educational objectives from the Universal Set of Educational Objectives presented in Section 1 of the casebook. All cases have disease management questions, and most cases have questions relating to psychosocial issues, pharmacoeconomics, and key points from the textbook. The consulting editors for the casebook are Drs. Camille Thornton, J. Douglas Wurtzbacher, and Caroline Zeind. The editorial assistant for the casebook is Kelli Beard, who has been the liaison between the editors, consulting editors, case contributors, and editorial staff at Lippincott Williams & Wilkins. Our gratitude to her for a job well done!

Acknowledgments

We would like to express our appreciation to our colleagues at Lippincott Williams & Wilkins for being flexible and responsive to our needs as editors. We would also like to acknowledge our colleagues and translators in Japan who translated the fourth and sixth editions of the textbook and casebook into Japanese. Our appreciation to Dr. Hiroshi Fukuchi and his colleagues for making the Japanese edition a reality. Over the seven editions of the textbook we owe many individuals who have served as authors, consulting editors, and editors our gratitude for joining us in making this an outstanding textbook.

However, in order to sustain an effort of this magnitude for over 25 years, we also relied on the support of our families. They have provided the support and encouragement to make this textbook a reality. Patt Herfindal and Greta Gourley have always been supportive of our efforts and provided the encouragement to continue the textbook. Our love and thanks to them!

E.T.H. and D.R.G.

Contents

CHAPTER 1

CLINICAL PHARMACODYNAMICS

S. Casey Laizure, Yuri Yanishevski, and William E. Evans

Clinical pharmacokinetics is the application of pharmacokinetic principles in a patient care setting. Probably the most difficult aspect of clinical pharmacokinetics is understanding the full potential and practical limitations of using specific pharmacokinetic models of drug disposition to attain target concentrations based on only one or two measured serum drug concentrations (SDCs). Although a good understanding of common pharmacokinetic models (e.g., first-order elimination and Michaelis–Menten kinetics) is crucial, the competent clinician will have knowledge of not only the mathematics of these models, but also the principles, assumptions, and potential errors underlying their clinical application. Furthermore, a broad therapeutic knowledge is also necessary because measured SDCs must be interpreted with respect to the patient's clinical condition and the pharmacodynamics of the therapeutic agent. This chapter presents a pragmatic approach to clinical pharmacokinetics, focusing on the use of measured SDCs for the adjustment of patient drug therapy. Therapeutic issues are covered in later chapters.

BASIC PHARMACOKINETIC PARAMETERS

The often ephemeral understanding of the three basic pharmacokinetic parameters of the one-compartment open model, volume of distribution (V), clearance (Cl), and half-life ($t_{1/2}$) resides in the esoteric nature of their definitions and the difficulty of trying to build a foundation of basic concepts from terms that seem to contradict deduction. For example, a drug that distributes in a volume greater than the human body and a clearance that defines a volume of blood from which all drug is removed have no apparent connection to physiologic variables or how drugs are actually handled by the body. This is not an attempt to refute the traditional definitions but an attempt to focus on the more pragmatic mathematical meanings and interrelationships of the three basic pharmacokinetic parameters and how alterations in these parameters affect the steady-state concentration after chronic dosing.

Volume of Distribution

V is a proportionality constant that equates the SDC to the total amount of drug in the body.[1] This concept is depicted in Figure 1.1. In this example, the concentration of drug is measured only in the water phase, analogous to the measurement of drug in blood (serum or plasma) of patients. The following examples are thus analogous to the common practice of measuring drug in serum and calculating the V based on the one-compartment open model, with the assumption of homogeneous distribution of drug throughout the body equivalent to the measured serum concentration.

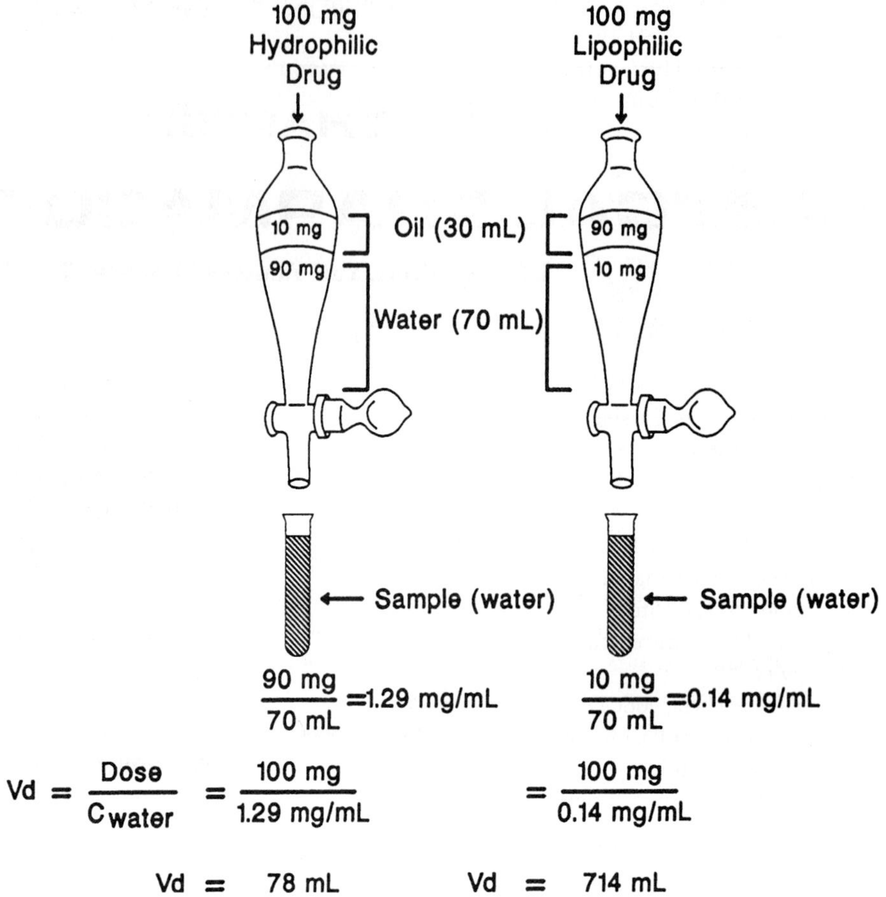

Figure 1.1. Apparent volume of distribution. The hydrophilic (water-soluble) drug distributes mainly (90%) in the water compartment (measured fluid), and the apparent volume of distribution is similar to the actual volume of the water phase (78 mL versus 70 mL). In contrast, the lipophilic (oil-soluble) drug distributes primarily (90%) into the oil compartment (which is not measured, analogous to tissue in patients), and the calculated volume is 714 mL. Obviously, the lipophilic drug did not actually distribute into 714 mL because the flask is only 100 mL, but this is the *apparent* volume needed to account for all 100 mg of drug in the flask assuming a uniform concentration equivalent to that measured in the water phase, C_{water} (i.e., 0.14 mg/mL × 714 mL = 100 mg).

When drug is added to the flask, it partitions between the oil and water, depending on its lipophilicity. Hydrophilic compounds tend to remain in the water phase, and lipophilic compounds distribute more extensively into the oil phase. The *apparent* volume of distribution of drug in the flask is determined by measuring the concentration of drug in the water phase (drug in oil phase does not contribute to measured concentration in water phase) and determining the volume that would be required to account for all the drug put in the flask. In this example, 100 mg of a hydrophilic drug is put in one flask, with 90 mg distributing into the water and 10 mg into the oil. The measured concentration of hydrophilic drug in water is the total amount of drug in the water phase divided by the volume of water (i.e., 90 mg/70 mL = 1.29 mg/mL). Thus, to account for all the drug in the flask if it existed at the concentration measured in the water phase, one would divide 100 mg by 1.29 mg/mL to obtain 78 mL (apparent volume of distribution). The apparent volume is close to the volume of water in the flask because the hydrophilic drug distributes primarily into the water phase. In contrast, when 100 mg of a lipophilic drug is put into the other flask, 90 mg distributes into the oil phase and only 10 mg remains in the water phase. The measured concentration of lipophilic drug in the water is the total amount of drug in the water phase divided by the volume of water (i.e., 10 mg/70 mL = 0.14 mg/mL). Thus, to account for all the drug in the flask, assuming it existed at the concentration measured in the water phase, one would divide 100 mg by 0.14 mg/mL to obtain 714 mL (apparent volume of distribution). The apparent volume is much greater than the actual volume of the container because most of the drug has distributed outside the water phase. Hence, the apparent volume is a function of the amount of drug put in the flask (or body) and the measured concentration of drug in the water phase (or serum) and is unrelated to any physical volume.

As can be appreciated from this discussion, V has no physiologic basis, and thus it does not relate to volume of serum, blood, or total body water. Theoretically, if V is determined experimentally from multiple SDCs after a single dose of a drug and the calculated V equals the volume of serum in the patient's body, then all the drug must be in the patient's serum, assuming a uniform concentration. When V is greater than the serum volume, this simply means that to equate the SDC with the total amount of drug in the body, a value greater than the serum volume is required. A V greater than the serum volume indicates that some portion of the drug is located outside the serum. Although it is common to speculate on where a drug distributes based on its V, technically such speculation is not valid. If a drug has a V of 0.7 L/kg, it might be tempting to assume that the drug distributes in total body water because total body water is approximately

70% of total body weight. However, V could just as easily be elevated because of distribution or binding to some other body tissue. The fact that V is 0.7 L/kg indicates only that the drug distributes outside the serum. Determining where the drug goes when it leaves the serum compartment requires data other than just V.

Assuming a one-compartment model and a single dose (X_0) of a drug with first-order elimination (rate constant k), the total amount of the drug remaining ($X_{(t)}$) in the body after some time interval (t) can be converted to serum concentration ($C_{(t)}$) by dividing both sides of the following equation by V:

$$X_{(t)} = X_0 e^{-kt} \tag{1.1}$$

$$\frac{X_{(t)}}{V} = \frac{X_0 e^{-kt}}{V} \tag{1.2}$$

$$C_{(t)} = C_0 e^{-kt} \tag{1.3}$$

For a specific drug, if the V of the drug and an SDC are known, then the total amount of drug in the patient's body can be estimated. For example, if the measured SDC of theophylline is 12 mg/L and the V is 35 L, then the total amount of drug in the body can be estimated as follows:

$$\text{Amount} = (\text{SDC})(V) = (12\ \text{mg/L})(35\ \text{L}) = 420\ \text{mg} \tag{1.4}$$

This same equation can also be used to calculate the loading dosage necessary to achieve a specific peak SDC after a single dose. *Amount* in this case refers to the amount of the loading dose. Thus, the same equation can be used to calculate the loading dosage necessary to achieve an initial theophylline SDC of 15 mg/L in a patient with a V of 35 L.

$$\text{Loading dosage} = (\text{SDC}_{\text{target}})(V) = (15\ \text{mg/L})(35\ \text{L}) = 525\ \text{mg} \tag{1.5}$$

This equation assumes that the SDC of theophylline before the loading dose was given is zero. Patients with drug already in their body may need only a partial loading dose (e.g., a patient in status epilepticus with a phenytoin SDC of 5 mg/L). If the desired target SDC is 20 mg/L, then a loading dosage that will raise the SDC from 5 to 20 mg/L is needed. The following equation takes into account drug present in the patient:

$$\text{Loading dosage} = \frac{(\text{SDC}_{\text{target}} - \text{SDC}_{\text{observed}})(V)}{(S)(F)} = \frac{(20\ \text{mg/L} - 5\ \text{mg/L})(70\ \text{L})}{(0.92)(1.0)} = 1141\ \text{mg} \tag{1.6}$$

where $\text{SDC}_{\text{observed}}$ is the SDC before the partial loading dose is given, S is the fraction of active drug by weight in the salt formulation (parenteral phenytoin is phenytoin sodium, which is 92% phenytoin), and F is the bioavailability ($F = 1$ for intravenous [IV] administration). This latter equation is appropriate for calculating a partial or full loading dosage for most drugs given by the parenteral or oral route, when the V is known.

Clearance

Cl is a proportionality constant that relates the rate of drug elimination to the SDC.[1] Cl should not be equated with drug elimination rate because Cl is a flow rate measured in units of volume per time (e.g., milliliters per minute). However, if the Cl of a drug is known, then the rate of drug elimination can be calculated by multiplying the Cl by the SDC (assuming first-order drug elimination).

$$\text{Rate of drug elimination} = (\text{SDC})(\text{Cl}) \tag{1.7}$$

The rate of drug elimination applies only to the SDC used in the calculation. If a different SDC value is used, a different rate of drug elimination is calculated. Thus, the rate of drug elimination is constantly changing and directly proportional to the change in the SDC for a first-order process (i.e., as the SDC increases, the rate of drug elimination increases proportionately).

If a patient receives a drug by a constant IV infusion, intermittent IV infusion, or oral dosing at regular intervals, the steady-state SDC is determined by the dosage and the Cl. The steady-state SDC occurs when the rate of drug in (i.e., dosage rate) is equivalent to the rate of drug out (i.e., rate of drug elimination). The SDC at which the rate in equals the rate out is determined solely by the Cl and dosage.

Case Study 1

L.L. presents to the emergency room diaphoretic and complaining of sharp substernal chest pain radiating to the left shoulder. The patient is admitted to rule out a myocardial infarction. L.L.'s physician begins a constant IV infusion of an antiarrhythmic drug at a rate of 4 mg/minute. The following kinetic parameters are estimated from measured SDCs in this patient. Estimate the steady-state concentration that will occur with this dosage.

$t_{1/2}$	1.5 hr
V	130 L
Cl	1 L/min

The steady-state SDC is reached when administration rate of the drug equals the rate of drug elimination (Equation 1.7) from the serum. Multiplying the SDC by the Cl gives the rate of drug elimination. The volume term, L, cancels out, leaving the units as milligrams per minute. These are the same units as for the administration rate. When the SDC reaches 4 mg/L, the rate of drug elimination equals the rate of drug administration (4 mg/minute) and thus steady state is achieved.

SDC	Cl	Rate of Drug Elimination
1 mg/L ×	1 L/min =	1 mg/min
2 mg/L ×	1 L/min =	2 mg/min
3 mg/L ×	1 L/min =	3 mg/min
4 mg/L ×	1 L/min =	4 mg/min (steady state)

The steady-state SDC achieved with a constant IV infusion is calculated using the following equation:

$$C_{SS} = \frac{ko}{Cl} \tag{1.8}$$

where C_{SS} is the steady-state SDC and ko equals the rate of drug administration. For a drug given by IV intermittent infusion or oral dosing, the mean steady-state SDC that will be achieved can be calculated using the following equation:

$$\overline{C}_{SS} = \frac{(F)(D)}{(Cl)(\tau)} \tag{1.9}$$

where $\overline{C}_{SS}$ is the mean steady-state SDC, F is the bioavailability, D is the dosage, Cl is the clearance, and τ is the dosing interval. Note that the mean steady-state concentration is defined as follows:

$$\overline{C}_{SS} = \frac{AUC_{\tau}}{\tau} \tag{1.10}$$

where AUC_{τ} is the area under the concentration–time curve for a single dosing interval and τ is the time duration of the dosing interval. The $\overline{C}_{SS}$ calculated from this equation is *not* equivalent to taking the average of the peak and trough from a dosing interval.

Half-Life

The half-life ($t_{1/2}$) is the time required for the serum concentration to decrease by one-half.[1] It is a transformation of the elimination rate constant to a form more easily interpreted. Do not confuse k or $t_{1/2}$ with the rate of drug elimination (Equation 1.7). The parameter k is a mathematical variable that defines a constant exponential rate of change; it can be estimated from two measured SDCs (e.g., a measured peak and trough) drawn within the same dosing interval. Assuming a one-compartment model with first-order elimination, k is estimated by plotting the natural log (ln) of the concentration versus time and determining the slope of the line passing through the peak and trough. The calculated slope will be equal to $-k$. The k may be calculated by taking the natural log of the quotient of the peak divided by the trough and dividing by the time interval between the peak and trough. This solution to k can be derived from the standard calculation for the slope of a line from two points:

$$k = -m = -\left[\frac{(\ln SDC_{trough} - \ln SDC_{peak})}{(T_{trough} - T_{peak})}\right] = -\left[\frac{\ln\left(\frac{SDC_{trough}}{SDC_{peak}}\right)}{(T_{trough} - T_{peak})}\right] \tag{1.11}$$

$$k = \frac{\ln\left(\frac{SDC_{peak}}{SDC_{trough}}\right)}{(T_{trough} - T_{peak})} \tag{1.12}$$

where m is the slope of the line of a semilog plot of the natural log of the SDCs versus time. The SDC_{peak} and SDC_{trough} are Y values, and the T_{trough} and T_{peak} are the corresponding times at which the trough and peak were collected, or the X values. Clinically, Equation 1.12 is used to calculate k. Obviously, there are limitations in estimating the slope of a line from only two measured SDCs: Any error in the measured SDC or the time of collection will create an error in the estimate of k (or $t_{1/2}$).

Case Study 2

G.W. is a 55-year-old woman receiving gentamicin 80 mg every 8 hours. A peak SDC of 5.2 μg/mL is drawn 30 minutes after the end of a 30-minute infusion and a trough SDC of 1.7 μg/mL is drawn 7 hours after the end of the infusion. Calculate the half-life of gentamicin in this patient:

$$k = \frac{\ln\left(\frac{5.2\ \mu g/mL}{1.7\ \mu g/mL}\right)}{(7.5\ hr - 1.0\ hr)} = 0.172\ hr^{-1} \tag{1.13}$$

To compute the half-life from k, k is divided into the ln 2 (i.e., 0.693).

$$t_{1/2} = \frac{\ln 2}{k} = \frac{0.693}{k} = \frac{0.693}{0.172\ hr^{-1}} = 4.0\ hr \tag{1.14}$$

A measured peak and trough concentration allows an estimation of $t_{1/2}$. Half-life provides information about specific aspects of the drug's disposition, such as how long it will take to reach steady state once maintenance dosing is started and how long it will take for "all" the drug to be eliminated from the body once dosing is stopped (usually considered five half-lives). Also, once the k and an SDC are known, three calculations will aid in the individualization of a patient's dosing regimen: extrapolation, back-extrapolation, and determination of the time required for the concentration to decrease to some specified SDC. These functions are derived by solving for the appropriate variable in the following equation:

$$C_{(t)} = C_0 e^{-kt} \tag{1.15}$$

where $C_{(t)}$ is the concentration after t time has elapsed, C_0 is a measured SDC, k is the elimination rate constant, and t is some specified time interval. In the previous gentamicin example ($SDC_{peak} = 5.2$ μg/mL, $SDC_{trough} = 1.7$ μg/mL, $k = 0.172\ hour^{-1}$, $\tau = 8$ hours), Equation 1.15 can be used to calculate the C_{min}, defined as the theoretical SDC at the end of the dosing interval (extrapolation); the C_{max}, defined as the theoretical SDC at the instant the infusion is complete (back-extrapolation); and the time interval required for the concentration to fall from the C_{max} to some lower SDC (e.g., 0.5 μg/mL).

1. The concentration at the end of the dosing interval is calculated by extrapolating from the SDC_{peak} to the end of

the dosing interval (time interval equals 7, or 8 hours − 1 hour) using Equation 1.15.

$$C_{(t)} = C_0 e^{-kt} = (5.2\ \mu g/mL)e^{(-0.172\ hr^{-1})(7.0\ hr)} = 1.5\ \mu g/mL \quad (1.16)$$

2. Equation 1.15 can be rearranged to back-extrapolate, or determine the concentration that occurred at some earlier time. The theoretical peak concentration, C_{max}, which occurs at the instant the infusion is complete, is determined by back-extrapolating from the SDC_{peak} to the time the infusion ended (30 minutes).

$$C_{(t)} = \frac{C_0}{e^{-kt}} = \frac{5.2\ \mu g/mL}{e^{(-0.172\ hr^{-1})(0.5\ hr)}} = 5.7\ \mu g/mL \quad (1.17)$$

3. The time interval for the concentration to drop from 5.7 µg/mL (C_{max}) to 0.5 µg/mL is determined by solving for t in Equation 1.15.

$$t = \frac{\ln\left(\frac{C_o}{C_{(t)}}\right)}{k} = \frac{\ln\left(\frac{5.7\ \mu g/mL}{0.5\ \mu g/mL}\right)}{0.172\ hr^{-1}} = 14.1\ hr \quad (1.18)$$

The three pharmacokinetic parameters, Cl, V, and $t_{1/2}$, define specific characteristics of drug disposition. Table 1.1 summarizes the clinical utility of each pharmacokinetic parameter.

Table 1.1 ▪ Clinical Utility of the Three Basic Pharmacokinetic Parameters of the One-Compartment Open Model

Parameter	Use	Equation
Volume of distribution, V (units: volume, e.g., L)	Determine a loading dosage	1.6
	Determine amount of drug in body	1.4
	Make qualitative assessment of distribution of drug in the body	
Clearance, Cl (units: volume/time, e.g., L/hour)	Determine the steady-state concentration that will be achieved from a specific maintenance dosage	1.8 and 1.9
Elimination rate constant, k (units: reciprocal time, e.g., hour $^{-1}$)	Determine how long it will take to reach steady state once maintenance dosing started, or how long it will take for the concentration to drop from some specified concentration to some lower concentration	$5 \times t_{1/2}$
Half-life, $t_{1/2}$ (units: time, e.g., hours)		1.16

The three basic pharmacokinetic parameters of first-order elimination are clearance, volume, and half-life. These parameters have specific, well-defined clinical utility.

RELATIONSHIP BETWEEN HALF-LIFE, CLEARANCE, VOLUME, AND STEADY-STATE CONCENTRATION

Cl and V are independent pharmacokinetic parameters. This means Cl may change without affecting V, and V may change without affecting Cl. Half-life is a dependent function whose value depends on Cl and V. If half-life changes, then Cl or V must have changed. An often inappropriately applied equation is:

$$Cl = (k)(V) \quad (1.19)$$

which often is interpreted to mean a dependence of Cl on V. A mathematical equation can be algebraically rearranged in many ways, but it should not be deduced that one parameter is dependent on another simply because of the way the equation is written. For example, if an experiment demonstrates that an increase in blood pressure (BP) correlates with increasing age and a linear regression of BP (dependent variable) as a function of age (independent variable) is performed, an equation for estimating BP from age is derived:

$$BP = (Age)(m) + b \quad (1.20)$$

where m is the slope of the regression line and b is the intercept. Equation 1.20 could be rearranged algebraically to give the following equation:

$$Age = \frac{BP - b}{m} \quad (1.21)$$

It is absurd to conclude from this equation that decreasing a patient's BP will decrease the patient's age. Thus, an equation does not necessarily define the relationships between the variables in the equation. This same situation exists for $Cl = kV$. The form of the equation that correctly reflects the relationship between the parameters is:

$$k = \frac{Cl}{V} \quad (1.22)$$

Cl and V are the primary pharmacokinetic parameters that determine drug disposition. Cl can be thought of as representing the sum of all drug elimination processes in the body, and V represents the distribution of drug. The steady-state concentration of a drug achieved after constant IV infusion or the mean steady-state concentration achieved after multiple oral or multiple intermittent IV infusions depends on Cl only (Equations 1.8 and 1.9, respectively). Changes in V have no effect on the steady-state or mean steady-state concentration. Intuitively it may seem that, for example, because a decrease in V will mean that the same amount of drug is distributed in a smaller volume, the concentration must increase. However, the basic principle, which states that Cl and V are independent, would be violated because the only way the steady-state concentration could increase is for the Cl to decrease

(Equations 1.8 and 1.9). The question then arises as to exactly what effect changes in V have on drug disposition. Case Study 1, involving an antiarrhythmic, can be used to illustrate the consequence of a decrease in V.

Application to Case Study 1

The patient is admitted to the hospital with chest pain. Subsequent clinical examination and laboratory data confirm a myocardial infarction (MI) complicated by congestive heart failure (CHF). The patient's condition improves over the next 2 days and the IV antiarrhythmic is discontinued and an oral antiarrhythmic is prescribed. Two days later the patient again develops runs of ventricular tachycardia despite adequate oral antiarrhythmic therapy. The patient is put back on a continuous IV infusion of the same antiarrhythmic as before. However, the patient's CHF has responded to therapy, which has led to a diuresis of edematous fluid. The antiarrhythmic is distributed into total body water, with the result that the V of the antiarrhythmic has decreased by one-third. Clearance has remained unchanged. Describe how the drug disposition from the start of the 4-mg/minute IV infusion to steady state will be altered.

The Cl and V before CHF resolution and after are as follows:

	Before Treatment	After Treatment
Cl	1 L/min	1 L/min
V	130 L	87 L

The rate of drug elimination can be calculated by taking the present SDC and multiplying by the Cl (Equation 1.7). Although the V has decreased, at an SDC of 4 mg/L and a Cl of 1 L/minute, the rate of drug elimination will be 4 mg/minute (4 mg/minute = 4 mg/L × 1 L/minute). No matter how V changes the rate of drug elimination at an SDC of 4 mg/L will always be 4 mg/minute as long as the Cl remains unchanged. On the other hand, k is a dependent function, and it will change with changes in Cl and V. How k changes and what effect it has on drug disposition is more easily interpreted if k is expressed as $t_{1/2}$. Because $k = \text{Cl}/V$ (Equation 1.22) and $k = 0.693/t_{1/2}$, then

$$\frac{0.693}{t_{1/2}} = \frac{\text{Cl}}{V} \qquad (1.23)$$

Solving for $t_{1/2}$ gives the following:

$$t_{1/2} = \frac{0.693\ V}{\text{Cl}} \qquad (1.24)$$

This equation can be used to calculate the change in half-life when the V decreases from 130 to 87 L.

$$t_{1/2\,130\text{L}} = \frac{(0.693)(130\text{ L})}{1\text{ L/min}} = 90\text{ min} \qquad (1.25)$$

$$t_{1/2\,87\text{L}} = \frac{(0.693)(87\text{ L})}{1\text{ L/min}} = 60\text{ min} \qquad (1.26)$$

Table 1.2 ▪ The Effect of Changes in Clearance and Volume on Half-Life and Steady-State Concentration

Independent Parameters		**Dependent Parameters**	
Clearance	Volume	Half-Life	C_{SS}
↑	⇆	↓	↓
↓	⇆	↑	↑
⇆	↑	↑	⇆
⇆	↓	↓	⇆
↑	↑	?	↓
↑	↓	↓	↓
↓	↑	↑	↑
↓	↓	?	↑

Clearance and volume are independent parameters whose values determine the elimination rate constant (or half-life) of drug from the serum and the steady-state concentration achieved after maintenance dosing. The half-life is affected by both the clearance (inversely proportional) and volume (directly proportional), as expressed in Equation 1.23. The steady-state concentration is affected only by the clearance, as shown in Equations 1.8 and 1.9. The "?" in this table indicates that the effect on half-life cannot be determined without knowing the specific changes in Cl and V.

The decrease in V results in a decrease in the $t_{1/2}$ with no change in the steady-state concentration. The time to reach steady-state will decrease from 7.5 hours (1.5 hours × 5) to 5.0 hours (1.0 hours × 5), but the steady-state concentration achieved will be unchanged. Table 1.2 gives the relative changes in $t_{1/2}$ and C_{SS} that occur when Cl and V change.

In the case of multiple IV intermittent infusions or oral dosing, the C_{SS} in Table 1.2 refers to the mean C_{SS}, as defined in Equation 1.10. Although it is true that changes in V do not alter the mean C_{SS}, perturbations in V do affect the peak and trough concentrations within the dosing interval. Figure 1.2 compares changes in Cl and V for an IV constant infusion and an IV intermittent infusion. As Figure 1.2*B* illustrates, a decrease in V for intermittent IV infusions leads to greater fluctuations between the peak and trough concentrations. It is foreseeable that the increased fluctuation between the peak and trough could result in transient toxicities associated with high peaks or periods of subtherapeutic concentrations associated with low troughs. The actual impact of alterations in V depends on the degree of change in V and the pharmacodynamic characteristics of the therapeutic agent in question.

USING SERUM DRUG CONCENTRATIONS TO OPTIMIZE DRUG THERAPY

Rationale for Therapeutic Drug Monitoring

Routine clinical monitoring using SDCs is reserved for therapeutic agents that have a defined therapeutic range and a low therapeutic index. A defined therapeutic range is characterized by both an upper and a lower limit, where exceeding the upper limit is associated with a high probability of unacceptable toxicity and falling short of the lower limit is associated with a low probability of achieving a significant clinical therapeutic benefit. A low therapeutic index indicates that the serum concentrations necessary to achieve the therapeutic effect are close to serum concentrations that result in significant clinical toxicity. The implication is that dosing patients based on population-averaged pharmacokinetic parameters results in an unacceptable incidence of therapeutic failures or clinical toxicity directly attributable to low or high serum concentrations, respectively. The therapeutic ranges given in Table 1.3 are by no means corroborated by unequivocal evidence, and much controversy surrounds the use of therapeutic ranges for which there are few, if any, well-controlled pharmacodynamic studies. However, these ranges are generally accepted as a good starting point for therapy and represent the current standards of practice.

A therapeutic range must not be used as the primary determinant of a patient's drug regimen. It would be inappropriate to consider achievement of a specific serum concentration as the clinical endpoint of therapy. The endpoint of therapy is always defined by a clinical response. If the clinical response is achieved when the SDC is outside the commonly stated therapeutic range, the patient's clinical condition rather than the SDC should take precedence. For example, if a patient taking digoxin for chronic atrial fibrillation did not respond when the steady-state trough SDC ($SDC_{SS\text{-}trough}$) was below 2.0 ng/mL but is now responding with an $SDC_{SS\text{-}trough}$ of 2.3 ng/mL (therapeutic range 0.8–2.0 ng/mL), as evidenced by an acceptable ventricular response and no drug toxicity, then this should be considered a clinically acceptable digoxin concentration, with no need to change the dosage regimen.

Only a limited number of therapeutic agents are routinely monitored and doses adjusted by use of SDCs (Table 1.3). The methods by which dosing adjustments based on SDCs are made include the following:

- Collection of steady-state peak and trough SDCs after multiple intermittent IV infusions and application standard one-compartment model
- Collection of a single SDC at steady state during a constant IV infusion
- Collection of a single trough SDC concentration at steady state during multiple oral dosing
- Collection of two SDCs at two different steady-state concentrations achieved while on two different dosages of a drug exhibiting Michaelis–Menten kinetics

One-Compartment Pharmacokinetic Model (Intermittent Intravenous Infusions)

The method, first applied to aminoglycoside dosing in burn patients by Sawchuk and Zaske,[2] uses standard equations of the one-compartment pharmacokinetic

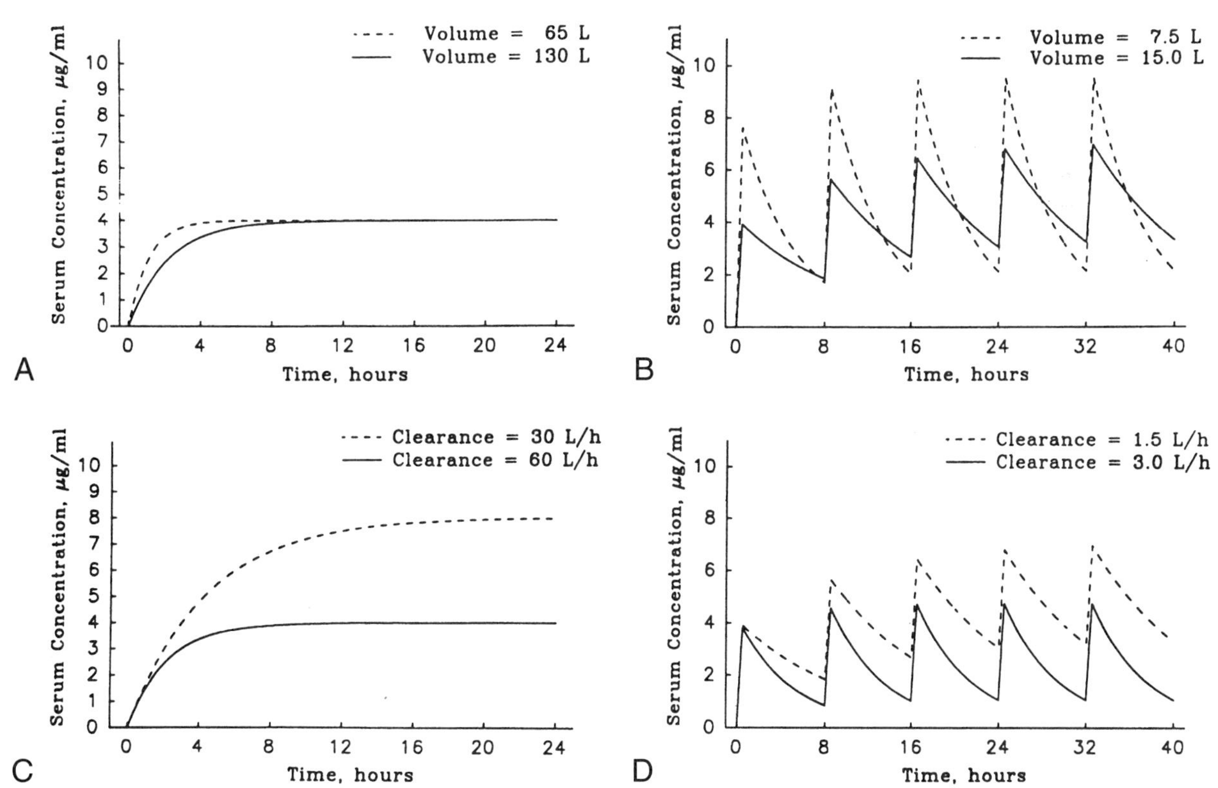

Figure 1.2. Effect of clearance and volume changes on the concentration–time profile of a continuous and intermittent intravenous (IV) drug infusion. **A** and **B,** IV constant infusion and IV intermittent infusion, respectively. The *dashed line* represents the change in the concentration–time plot if volume is decreased by one-half with no change in clearance. For both **A** and **B,** time to reach steady state is decreased. For **A,** steady-state concentration is unchanged. For **B,** mean steady-state concentration is unchanged, but the peak is higher and the trough lower. **C** and **D,** IV constant infusion and IV intermittent infusion, respectively. The *dashed line* represents the change in the concentration–time plot if clearance decreases by one-half with no change in volume. Time to reach steady state is increased and steady-state concentration is doubled.

model and can be used for dosage adjustment for any drug that fulfills the following criteria:

- Drug disposition can be adequately described by a one-compartment model.
- The serum drug concentrations are drawn after steady state has been achieved.
- Drug is given by an intermittent intravenous infusion.
- Sufficient SDCs are available (minimum, one peak and one trough).

The first criterion should not be misconstrued to imply that the pharmacokinetic disposition must be monoexponential. The aminoglycosides are known to exhibit multicompartmental disposition, as does vancomycin, which may also be adjusted by this method. Multicompartment disposition does not preclude using one-compartment pharmacokinetic equations. However, if the drug's disposition is complicated by a significant distribution phase or other multicompartment nature, then the clinical relevance of this simplification must be understood. The caveat to using one-compartment equations for dosage adjustment of drugs exhibiting multicompartment disposition is the need to recognize the possible errors involved. In this method, the distribution phase of a two-compartment drug such as vancomycin is ignored. This means that the predicted peak concentration is lower than the actual peak concentration and indirectly implies that the actual peak during the distribution phase is not clinically important. Also, if a one-compartment model is assumed for a drug like vancomycin, then the peak concentration must not be collected in the distribution phase because this will result in unacceptable error in the calculation of V and k (Fig. 1.3).

The application of one-compartment equations to aminoglycoside dosing adjustment as described by Sawchuk and Zaske is often viewed as excessively complicated. However, a better description would be that this method is lengthy because the actual step-by-step process is straightforward.

Step 1. Find out the amount and times of doses given to the patient and the values and times of the measured SDCs.
Step 2. Calculate elimination rate constant (half-life) from peak and trough.
Step 3. Determine C_{max} (concentration at instant the infusion is completed).
Step 4. Determine C_{min} (concentration at the end of the dosing interval).
Step 5. Calculate volume of distribution.
Step 6. Determine target peak and trough desired for patient's therapy.
Step 7. Calculate τ.
Step 8. Calculate dosage.
Step 9. Calculate theoretical peak and trough that will be achieved from the dosage and τ recommended.

Table 1.3 ▪ Drugs Commonly Monitored in the Clinical Setting

Drug	Therapeutic Range	Half-Life (hr)	Volume (L/kg)	Clearance	SDC Type	Disposition	References
Digoxin	0.8–2.0 ng/mL	41	7.0	180 mL/min/1.73 m^2	$C_{SS\text{-}trough}$	Two-compt.	9,10
Theophylline	5–20 μg/mL	8	0.5	0.65 mL/min/kg	$C_{SS\text{-}trough}$	Two-compt.	11
Lidocaine	1.5–5.0 μg/mL	2	1.2	15.6 mL/min/kg	C_{SS}	Two-compt.	12–14
Procainamide	4–12 μg/mL	3.3	2.0	8.6 mL/min/kg	$C_{SS\text{-}trough}$	Two-compt.	15
Lithium[a]	0.6–1.4 mEq/L	21	0.8	10–40 mL/min	$C_{SS\text{-}12hr}$	Two-compt.	16,17
Quinidine	2–5 μg/mL	7	2.5	4.5 mL/min/kg	$C_{SS\text{-}trough}$	Two-compt.	18,19
Gentamicin[b]	5–10 μg/mL peak <2 μg/mL trough	2	0.21	–	Peak and trough	One-compt.	20,21
Tobramycin[b]	5–10 μg/mL peak <2 μg/mL trough	2.1	0.27	–	Peak and trough	One-compt.	20
Amikacin[b]	20–30 μg/mL peak <5 μg/mL trough	2.2	0.25	–	Peak and trough	One-compt.	21
Carbamazepine[c]	4–12 μg/mL	12.3	1.0	0.91 mL/min/kg	$C_{SS\text{-}trough}$	–	22,23
Phenobarbital	15–40 μg/mL	100	0.58	2.5 mL/min/m^2	$C_{SS\text{-}trough}$	Two-compt.	23,24
Phenytoin	10–20 μg/mL	N/A	0.7	N/A	$C_{SS\text{-}trough}$	Nonlinear	25
Valproic acid	50–100 μg/mL	13	0.24	4–6 mL/min/m^2	$C_{SS\text{-}trough}$	Two-compt.	23,26
Vancomycin	25–40 μg/mL peak 5–15 μg/mL trough	7	0.72	1.2 mL/min/kg	Peak and trough	Two-compt.	27,28

This table covers only the most commonly monitored drugs. The stated therapeutic ranges and the pharmacokinetic parameters are for patients with normal hepatic and renal function and have significant variability, as reported in the literature.

compt., compartment; *N/A*, not applicable.

[a]Lithium clearance averages 20% of creatinine clearance.

[b]Aminoglycoside clearance depends on renal function. Half-life given assumes young patient with normal renal function.

[c]Carbamazepine parameter values after autoinduction.

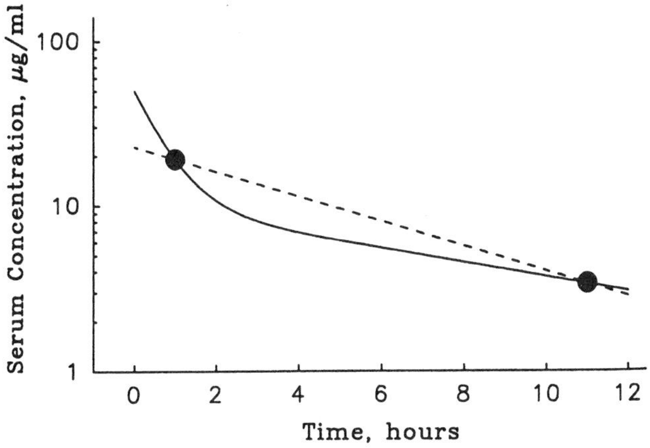

Figure 1.3. Consequence of sampling in the distribution phase and applying one-compartment pharmacokinetic equation. *Dashed line:* error incurred if the Sawchuk–Zaske equations are used to adjust dosage for a drug that exhibits two-compartment disposition and the peak serum concentration is collected in the distribution phase. The steeper slope calculated when the peak collected in the α phase results in an overestimation of the terminal elimination rate constant, *k* (the estimated $t_{1/2}$ is shorter than the actual $t_{1/2}$). The high peak and overestimated *k* both contribute to underestimation of the volume. The larger the elevation of the peak, the greater the underestimation of the dosage and τ, leading to low peaks and high troughs.

Case Study 3

Patient J.L. is a 55-year-old woman with a suspected nosocomial pneumonia. Gentamicin 100 mg given as a 30-minute infusion every 8 hours is started. Peak and trough serum drug concentrations are drawn around the third dose. The actual times of the doses and measured SDCs are as follows:

Time	
0810	Dose 1: 100 mg IV infusion over 30 min
1550	Dose 2: 100 mg IV infusion over 30 min
2355	Dose 3: 100 mg IV infusion over 30 min
2245	SDC 1: 1.8 μg/mL
0115	SDC 2: 5.1 μg/mL

For nosocomial pneumonia, a peak concentration of 8.0 μg/mL and a trough around 1.0 μg/mL is desired. Calculate the dosage and τ that will achieve the desired peak and trough concentrations in this patient.

Step 1

Timeline

0810	1550	2245	2355	0115
Dose 1	Dose 2	SDC 1	Dose 3	SDC 2

It is common practice to draw a trough and peak around the third aminoglycoside dose, as depicted on this timeline, so that the trough SDC is collected near the end of the second dosing interval, then the third dose is given and a peak SDC is collected 30 minutes after the end of a 30-minute infusion. Because the trough and peak are collected during different dosing intervals, the time intervals between the peak and trough SDCs and the start of their respective dosing infusions are determined. Obtaining the trough and peak in this fashion is common practice. However, this method is not optimal, and good arguments can be made to collect the peak and trough within the same dosing interval. The rationale for collecting the peak and trough around the third dose is that it is more efficient and generally considered adequate.

	Value	Time from Start of Last Infusion to the SDC
SDC 1 (trough)	1.8 μg/mL	1550 → 2245 = 6:55 (6.92 hr)
SDC 2 (peak)	5.1 μg/mL	2355 → 0115 = 1:20 (1.33 hr)

Step 2

Because the SDCs are collected under steady-state conditions, they are treated as if they were collected within the same dosing interval. The time interval just calculated is based on the theory that at steady state, dosing regimens are superimposable, so that 6.92 hours after the start of each dosing infusion, the SDC will be 1.8 μg/mL, and 1.33 hours after the start of the dosing infusion, the SDC will be 5.1 μg/mL. Therefore, the time required for the concentration to decrease from 5.1 μg/mL to 1.8 μg/mL will be the time difference between the two intervals, or 5.59 hours (6.92 hours – 1.33 hours). If a semilog graph of the natural log of the SDCs and the time intervals were constructed, the elimination rate constant (*k*) would be defined as the negative slope of the line, or the *k* and $t_{1/2}$ may be calculated mathematically, as previously discussed (Equations 1.12 and 1.14):

$$k = \frac{\ln\left(\dfrac{SDC_{peak}}{SDC_{trough}}\right)}{(T_{trough} - T_{peak})} = \frac{\ln\left(\dfrac{5.1\ \mu g/mL}{1.8\ \mu g/mL}\right)}{(6.92\ hr - 1.33\ hr)} = 0.186\ hr^{-1} \quad (1.27)$$

$$t_{1/2} = \frac{\ln 2}{k} = \frac{0.693}{0.186\ hr^{-1}} = 3.7\ hr \quad (1.28)$$

where SDC_{trough} and SDC_{peak} are the measured trough and peak concentrations and T_{trough} and T_{peak} are the time intervals calculated in Step 1. Do not confuse the time interval with the clock time the peak and trough were collected.

Step 3

The C_{max}, which is the theoretical peak concentration within the dosing interval occurring at the instant the infusion is complete, is calculated by back-extrapolation from the SDC_{peak} to the end of the infusion:

$$C_{max} = \frac{SDC_{peak}}{e^{(-k)(T_{peak} - T_{infusion})}} = \frac{5.1\ \mu g/mL}{e^{(-0.186\ hr^{-1})(1.33\ hr - 0.5\ hr)}} = 5.96\ \mu g/mL \quad (1.29)$$

where T_{peak} is the time interval from the start of the dosing infusion to the time the peak was collected and $T_{infusion}$ is the length of the infusion.

Step 4

The C_{min}, which is the theoretical trough concentration within the dosing interval occurring at the end of the dosing interval, is calculated by extrapolating from C_{max} to the end of the dosing interval. The τ used in this equation is the scheduled dosing interval.

$$C_{min} = C_{max} e^{(-k)(\tau - T_{infusion})} \quad (1.30)$$

$$C_{min} = 5.96\ \mu g/mL\ e^{(-0.186\ hr^{-1})(8\ hr - 0.5\ hr)} = 1.5\ \mu g/mL \quad (1.31)$$

Step 5

The calculation of V uses the C_{max} and C_{min} previously calculated.

$$V = \frac{\text{Dosage}\ (1 - e^{-kT_{infusion}})}{(T_{infusion})(k)[C_{max} - (C_{min} e^{-kT_{infusion}})]} \quad (1.32)$$

$$V = \frac{100\ mg\ (1 - e^{(-0.186\ hr^{-1})(0.5\ hr)})}{(0.5\ hr)\ (0.186\ hr^{-1})(5.9\ mg/L - 1.5\ mg/L\ e^{(-0.186\ hr^{-1})(0.5\ hr)})} = 21\ L \quad (1.33)$$

Step 6

The target peak and trough are 8.0 μg/mL and 1.0 μg/mL, respectively.

Step 7

A new dosing interval is calculated based on the desired steady-state peak and trough concentrations and the k calculated in Step 2.

$$\tau = \frac{\ln\left(\frac{C_{max\text{-}target}}{C_{min\text{-}target}}\right)}{k} + T_{infusion} \quad (1.34)$$

$$\tau = \frac{\ln\left(\frac{8.0\ \mu g/mL}{1.0\ \mu g/mL}\right)}{0.186\ hr^{-1}} + 0.5\ hr = 11.7\ hr \quad (1.35)$$

Step 8

The new τ calculated in Step 7 is rounded to a convenient dosing interval (12 hours) and used along with the calculated k from Step 2 and calculated V from Step 5 to determine a new dosage to achieve the desired peak and trough (Step 6).

$$\text{Dosage} = (T_{infusion})(k)(V)(C_{max\text{-}target})\left(\frac{1 - e^{-k\tau}}{1 - e^{-kT_{infusion}}}\right) \quad (1.36)$$

$$\text{Dosage} = (0.5\ hr)(0.186\ hr^{-1})(21\ L)(8.0\ mg/L) \times \left(\frac{1 - e^{(-0.186\ hr^{-1})(12\ hr)}}{1 - e^{(-0.186\ hr^{-1})(0.5\ hr)}}\right) = 158\ mg \quad (1.37)$$

For convenience the dosage could be rounded to 150 mg.

Step 9

Both the τ and the dosage have been rounded to convenient values (recommendation is 150 mg every 12 hours); therefore, the theoretical peak and trough SDC at steady state will be slightly different from the target values predicted in Step 6.

$$C_{max\text{-}SS} = \frac{ko(1 - e^{-kT_{infusion}})}{(k)(V)(1 - e^{-k\tau})} \quad (1.38)$$

$$C_{max\text{-}SS} = \frac{(160\ mg)(1 - e^{(-0.186\ hr^{-1})(0.5\ hr)})}{(0.186\ hr^{-1})(21\ L)(1 - e^{(-0.186\ hr^{-1})(12\ hr)})} = 8.1\ mg/L \quad (1.39)$$

$$C_{min\text{-}SS} = C_{max\text{-}SS} e^{(-k)(\tau - T_{infusion})} \quad (1.40)$$

$$C_{min\text{-}SS} = 8.1\ mg/L\ e^{(-0.186\ hr^{-1})(12\ hr - 0.5\ hr)} = 0.95\ mg/L \quad (1.41)$$

Note that $C_{max\text{-}SS}$ and $C_{min\text{-}SS}$ are the concentrations occurring at the instant the infusion is complete and the end of the scheduled dosing interval, respectively. If the predicted clinical peak (30 minutes postinfusion) and trough (30 minutes preinfusion) are desired, they may be calculated by extrapolating 0.5 hour from the C_{max} and back-extrapolating 0.5 hour from the C_{min}, respectively. In recent years, once-daily dosing of aminoglycosides has become increasingly popular.[1a] When using the once-daily method, the peak concentration is not measured; thus, the technique of aminoglycoside dosing adjustment described previously cannot be used. However, the trough concentration must be measured to ensure that it is very low to undetectable. Each dose is now like a loading dose, and the objective is to make sure that the aminoglycoside is not accumulating between doses. If accumulation occurs, the dosing interval most likely needs to be extended; it is unlikely that the dose needs to be reduced.

Constant Intravenous Infusions

Two drugs commonly are given by a continuous intravenous infusion: lidocaine and theophylline. The most appropriate time to draw an SDC is after steady-state conditions have been achieved (five times the $t_{1/2}$). A steady-state C_{SS} allows the calculation of Cl, which in turn allows the determination of what dosage must be given to achieve a specific target steady-state concentration (refer to Table 1.1 and Equation 1.8).

Case Study 4

Patient K.N. has received several boluses of lidocaine, and a continuous IV infusion at a rate of 2 mg/minute has been started. Ten hours after the start of the infusion, an SDC is collected. K.N. has responded well to the lidocaine infusion but is still having occasional brief runs of premature ventricular contractions. The SDC reported by the laboratory is 2.7 μg/mL. His physician wants to increase the infusion rate enough to achieve a steady-state concentration of 4.0 μg/mL. Calculate a new administration rate to achieve the desired steady-state concentration.

Equation 1.8 could be used to solve for clearance, and then using the calculated Cl and target C_{SS} a new *ko* could be calculated. However, this type of problem can also be solved more simply without determining the Cl directly. First recognize that the ratio of the administration rate, *ko*, to the C_{SS} must be constant if the Cl is unchanged.

$$\text{Cl} = \frac{ko}{C_{SS}} \quad (1.42)$$

$$\frac{ko}{\text{SDC}_{SS}} = \frac{ko_{\text{new}}}{C_{\text{SS-target}}} \quad (1.43)$$

Thus, for any infusion rate, the *ko* divided by the C_{SS} must equal the Cl. Given a known infusion rate (*ko*) and a measured steady-state SDC (SDC_{SS}), a new infusion rate (ko_{new}) can be computed that will achieve a new target steady-state concentration ($C_{\text{SS-target}}$):

$$ko_{\text{new}} = \frac{(ko)(C_{\text{SS-target}})}{\text{SDC}_{SS}} \quad (1.44)$$

where *ko* is the administration rate of the IV continuous infusion that achieved the measured steady-state concentration (SDC_{SS}), ko_{new} is the new administration rate, and $C_{\text{SS-target}}$ is the new estimated SDC achieved when ko_{new} reaches steady-state conditions. Thus, for K.N. the new administration rate is calculated as follows:

$$\frac{2.0 \text{ mg/min}}{2.7 \text{ mg/L}} = \frac{ko_{\text{new}}}{4.0 \text{ mg/L}} \quad (1.45)$$

$$ko_{\text{new}} = \frac{(2.0 \text{ mg/min})(4.0 \text{ mg/L})}{2.7 \text{ mg/L}} = 2.96 \text{ mg/min} \approx 3.0 \text{ mg/min} \quad (1.46)$$

This is an easy and quick method of adjusting a continuous IV infusion based on a steady-state SDC determination. However, it is important to remember the assumptions underlying this process: The measured SDC is a steady-state concentration, the drug is eliminated by a first-order process, and Cl has not changed.

If an SDC is collected before steady-state conditions have been achieved, then its usefulness for dosage adjustment is much more limited because the Cl cannot be calculated from an SDC that is not a steady-state concentration. It is possible to glean some information from a non–steady-state SDC, although the necessity of using a population-based rather than individualized pharmacokinetic parameter makes specific dosage estimations much less reliable. The non–steady-state SDC can be interpreted only by assuming a value for the $t_{1/2}$. The $t_{1/2}$ is needed to estimate how close to steady-state conditions the SDC was drawn.

Case Study 5

Patient D.E. is a 33-year-old nonsmoking woman who has been on a theophylline constant IV infusion at a rate of 35 mg/hour for 12 hours. A theophylline SDC drawn at this time (12 hours after the start of the infusion) is 16.2 μg/mL. Decide whether the administration rate should be changed.

The real question being asked is what the serum concentration of theophylline will be at steady state. To answer this question, the population value for $t_{1/2}$ will be assumed (Table 1.3, $t_{1/2} = 8$ hours). Remember that the $t_{1/2}$ determines how long it takes to reach steady state (Table 1.1). Usually this is considered five times the $t_{1/2}$, so steady state would be achieved at 40 hours into the constant IV infusion. At 12 hours into the infusion the SDC is between 50% (one $t_{1/2}$, 8 hours) and 75% (two $t_{1/2}$, 16 hours) of the steady-state concentration. The estimated fraction of the steady-state concentration the SDC at 12 hours represents is determined as follows:

$$\text{Fraction of } C_{SS} = 1 - e^{-kt} = 1 - e^{(-0.087 \text{ hr}^{-1})(12 \text{ hr})} = 0.65 \quad (1.47)$$

So at 12 hours into the infusion the SDC has accumulated to a concentration of about 65% what it will be when it reaches steady state. To calculate the predicted concentration that will be achieved if the infusion is continued at the same rate to steady-state conditions, the SDC is divided by the fraction of C_{SS}:

$$C_{SS} = \frac{\text{SDC}_{(t)}}{1 - e^{-kt}} = \frac{16.2 \ \mu\text{g/mL}}{1 - e^{(-0.087 \text{ hr}^{-1})(12 \text{ hr})}} = 25 \ \mu\text{g/mL} \quad (1.48)$$

where $\text{SDC}_{(t)}$ is the measured SDC at time *t*, and *t* is the time interval from the start of the IV infusion to collection of the sample. Thus, it would be prudent to reduce the administration rate to avoid accumulation of drug to concentrations associated with theophylline toxicity. The rate could be adjusted using Equation 1.44, assuming the SDC_{SS} achieved at an administration rate of 35 mg/hour will be 25 μg/mL.

When applying the first-order pharmacokinetic equations to measured peak and trough SDCs or adjusting a constant IV infusion based on a single measured steady-state SDC, patient-specific pharmacokinetic parameters are estimated from the SDCs. In Case Study 5 it is impossible to determine any patient-specific pharmacokinetic parameters, so a population-based pharmacokinetic parameter must be used. This reduces the probability that our predicted steady-state concentration will be accurate; however, it is the best estimate that can be made from the available data.

Multiple Oral Dosing

The majority of therapeutic agents monitored by collection of SDCs are drugs given by mouth. For such drugs, the Cl cannot be estimated based on a single measured SDC, as with a constant IV infusion, nor can the first-order pharmacokinetic equations be applied to a measured peak and trough concentration. The amount of drug absorbed after oral administration (F) and the time of the C_{max} (T_{max}) are highly variable, which makes estimation of patient-specific pharmacokinetic parameters such as Cl and V infeasible. In this situation, a measured steady-state trough concentration ($SDC_{SS\text{-}trough}$) is used for dosage adjustment. For a drug that exhibits first-order elimination, dosage adjustment is based on an equation analogous to Equation 1.43:

$$\frac{\text{Dosage}}{SDC_{SS\text{-}trough}} = \frac{\text{Dosage}_{new}}{C_{SS\text{-}trough}} \quad (1.49)$$

where $SDC_{SS\text{-}trough}$ is the measured SDC corresponding to Dosage, and Dosage_{new} is a new dosage predicted to produce a target steady-state concentration of $C_{SS\text{-}trough}$. The measured SDC is assumed to be a steady-state concentration, the drug is assumed to be eliminated by a first-order process, and the Cl is assumed to remain constant. In addition, Equation 1.49 also assumes that bioavailability (F) and the absorption rate (ka) remain constant and the τ has not been changed.

Case Study 6

Patient E.T. is a 55-year-old man who has been on 0.125 mg oral digoxin daily for the past month. E.T.'s physician wants the digoxin SDC to attain a concentration of 1.6 ng/mL. An SDC drawn this morning was reported by the clinical chemistry laboratory as 0.8 ng/mL. The physician requests your assistance in adjusting E.T.'s regimen to achieve the target concentration of 1.6 ng/mL. Using Equation 1.49, you can make a recommendation quickly.

$$\frac{0.125\text{ mg}}{0.8\text{ ng/mL}} = \frac{\text{Dosage}_{new}}{1.6\text{ ng/mL}} \quad (1.50)$$

$$\text{Dosage}_{new} = \frac{(0.125\text{ ng/mL})(1.6\text{ ng/mL})}{0.8\text{ ng/mL}} = 0.25\text{ mg} \quad (1.51)$$

Thus, if the dosage is increased to 0.25 mg every day, then the serum concentration should increase to 1.6 ng/mL. Caution should be exercised in applying this equation because of the number of assumptions necessary for the estimation to remain valid. Additionally, nothing is known about the peak concentration achieved within the dosing interval. If peak concentrations are unrelated to clinical efficacy and toxicity (digoxin), or if the half-life of the drug is extremely long so that there is very little fluctuation between the peak and trough concentrations within a dosing interval (phenobarbital, phenytoin, lithium), then this assumption is reasonable. However, if the peak concentration is clinically important and $t_{1/2}$ is short relative to the dosing interval (theophylline, procainamide, carbamazepine, valproic acid), then careful consideration must be given to the possibility of high peak concentrations when increasing the dosage based on measured trough SDCs.

Case Study 7

Patient F.N. is an outpatient taking a generic brand of carbamazepine 400 mg every 8 hours. A measured steady-state trough concentration taken early this afternoon (7 hours after the last dose) was 6.3 μg/mL. The patient is complaining of transient headache, dizziness, and diplopia with an onset about 30 minutes after taking each dose and persisting for about 30 minutes to 1 hour. F.N. has been on this dosing schedule for the past month; before this F.N. was taking 300 mg every 8 hours. However, on this lower dosage the patient was having approximately two grand mal seizure episodes per month. The patient has not experienced any seizures on the higher dosing regimen.

In F.N. the peak concentration achieved is unknown, although the side effects experienced shortly after each dose suggest that the peak concentration after each dose is causing transiently toxic concentrations. This indicates a need to reduce the dosage, but a lower dosage may not control F.N.'s seizures. In fact, reducing the patient's dosage may not be appropriate in this circumstance, given the past history of seizure activity while on 300 mg every 8 hours. Instead, the same daily dosage of carbamazepine (1200 mg) could be given, but the dosing interval reduced from 8 to 6 hours. This will reduce the peak concentration and increase the trough concentration, thereby reducing the fluctuation between the highest and lowest concentration within the dosing interval. The mean steady-state concentration should remain unchanged because the total daily dosage has not changed. Ideally, the peak concentration will be reduced enough to ameliorate the transient concentration-dependent toxicities F.N. is experiencing.

Michaelis–Menten Kinetics (Phenytoin)

The pharmacokinetic parameters Cl and $t_{1/2}$ and the methods of dosage adjustments discussed up to this point apply only to drugs that are eliminated by a first-order process. The individualization of phenytoin dosing in patients cannot be done with any of the three methods previously described because phenytoin obeys Michaelis–Menten kinetics (MMK).[3] The most significant clinical implication of MMK is that disproportionate changes in steady-state SDC occur with changes in dosage. Whereas the ratio between the dosage and C_{SS} is constant (as long as Cl remains constant) for first-order elimination processes such that any change in dosage is followed by a proportional change in the C_{SS}, for MMK the ratio of dosage to C_{SS} decreases with increasing dosage (Cl decreases as dosage increases). Note that V was not included in our list of pharmacokinetic parameters that are not applicable to MMK. This is because MMK pertains to the elimination of drug from the body, not the distribution of drug in the body. V is not related (independent of Cl) to the elimination mechanisms of drug from the body, and the relationship of V to total amount of drug in the body remains valid for drugs that obey MMK.

The best way to understand the concepts and clinical implications of MMK is to compare it with first-order elimination. For MMK, the elimination rate of drug from the body is described by the following equation:

$$\text{Rate of drug elimination} = \frac{(V_{max})(C)}{K_m + C} \quad (1.52)$$

where C is the serum concentration (in milligrams per liter), V_{max} is the maximum rate of drug elimination (in milligrams per day), and K_m is the serum concentration at which the elimination rate is equal to one-half the maximum rate. Compare this equation with Equation 1.7, the calculation of the rate of drug elimination for a drug that obeys first-order kinetics. The most important parameter determining the clinical significance of MMK is K_m. If the normal therapeutic concentrations are much less than the K_m, then Equation 1.52 simplifies to a first-order process (Equation 1.7). As the serum concentration approaches Km, drug elimination becomes nonlinear and Equation 1.52 cannot be simplified to Equation 1.7. All drugs eliminated by liver metabolism must have some K_m and V_{max}, but fortunately the majority of drugs have K_m values that are much greater than the normal therapeutic concentrations, so for the majority of drugs, first-order elimination can be assumed.

Table 1.4 compares the average values for K_m and V_{max} of phenytoin with those of a hypothetical drug for which

Table 1.4 ▪ Michaelis–Menten Kinetics: Dependence of Nonlinear Elimination on K_m

SDC (mg/L)	K_m (mg/L)	V_{max} (mg/day)	Rate of Drug Elimination (mg/day)	Clearance (L/day)
Drug A				
1	7	600	75	75
5			250	50
10			353	35
15			409	27
20			444	22
Drug B				
1	300	600	2	2.0
5			10	2.0
10			19	1.9
15			28	1.9
20			38	1.9

Drug A is representative of K_m and V_{max} values within the normal range expected for phenytoin. Drug B is a hypothetical drug whose V_{max} is identical to Drug A, but for which the K_m is much greater. The rate of drug elimination is calculated using Equation 1.52. The clearance is calculated by dividing the rate of drug elimination (milligrams per day) by the SDC (milligrams per liter), which is an algebraic rearrangement of Equation 1.7. Drug B behaves in a first-order manner (clearance remains approximately constant), demonstrating that the most important parameter determining nonlinear disposition in the therapeutic range is K_m. If for Drug A and Drug B the V_{max} were doubled to 1200 mg/day, then the rate of drug elimination would be doubled and the clearance would be doubled, but Drug A would still be nonlinear and Drug B would still follow first-order kinetics.

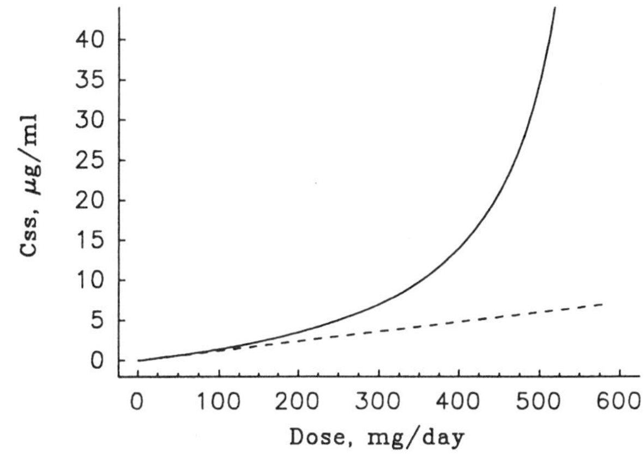

Figure 1.4. The relationship between steady-state concentration and dose for a drug that demonstrates Michaelis–Menten kinetics in the normal therapeutic concentration range (K_m = 7 mg/L; V_{max} = 600 mg/day). At low plasma concentrations (Cp), the drug obeys first-order elimination ($Cp << K_m$); as concentration approaches and exceeds K_m, there is a disproportionate increase in steady-state concentration when dosage is increased. When serum concentration is much greater than K_m, elimination approaches zero-order elimination. Zero order is characterized by an infinitely increasing serum concentration, so steady-state concentrations will never occur.

K_m is much greater than the normal serum concentrations (approximates first-order elimination). Note that the Cl of phenytoin decreases as the serum concentration increases. Do not equate a decreasing Cl with a decreasing rate of drug elimination; the rate of drug elimination increases with increasing serum concentration for drugs that obey MMK, but the increase in drug elimination is not proportional to the increase in dosage. This concept of a decreasing clearance with increasing serum concentration has two very important implications for dosage adjustment. An elimination rate constant, k, cannot be defined. Because Cl decreases as serum concentration increases, the k decreases as the serum concentration increases (Equation 1.22); thus, it is not possible to extrapolate or back-extrapolate if two SDCs are known because the semilog plot of drug elimination is not linear. Also, the ratio between a dosage and its C_{SS} decreases as the dosage increases. Again, this can be deduced by noting that the Cl decreases with increasing serum concentration and examining the effect of decreasing the Cl on Equations 1.8 and 1.9 (Fig. 1.4).

Several methods have been proposed for adjusting phenytoin dosage based on steady-state SDCs. These methods require two steady-state concentrations determined from SDCs collected while the patient is on two different maintenance dosages. The algebraic method derived by solving two simultaneous equations[4] is best because it allows the new dosage to be estimated without the need for graphing. Thus,

$$K_m = \frac{\text{Dosage}_2 - \text{Dosage}_1}{\dfrac{\text{Dosage}_1}{C_{SS_1}} - \dfrac{\text{Dosage}_2}{C_{SS_2}}} \quad (1.53)$$

where Dosage_1 and Dosage_2 are two different dosages of phenytoin in milligrams per day and C_{SS1} and C_{SS2} are their respective steady-state concentrations. The K_m is calculated first and then used in the calculation of the V_{max}.

$$V_{max} = \text{Dosage}_1 + \left(K_m \times \frac{\text{Dosage}_1}{C_{SS_1}} \right) \quad (1.54)$$

Case Study 8

Patient C.W. has a long-standing seizure disorder controlled with phenytoin 600 mg/day. However, at this dosage the patient experienced an unacceptable level of side effects, the most debilitating of which was ataxia. The steady-state concentration while the patient was on this regimen was 26 μg/mL. C.W. had been on 300 mg/day before the increase to 600 mg/day; however, on the lower dosage, which produced a steady-state concentration of 6 μg/mL, the patient experienced approximately one grand mal seizure episode per month. The patient's physician had hoped that the increase to 600 mg/day would produce a steady-state concentration around 16 μg/mL and result in good seizure control without unacceptable side effects. Recommend a dosage to achieve a steady-state concentration of 16 μg/mL.

To estimate the dosage required to achieve the target steady-state concentration of 16 μg/mL, use Equations 1.53 and 1.54 to calculate the K_m and V_{max}, and then use these values to estimate a new dosage.

$$K_m = \frac{300\ \text{mg/day} - 600\ \text{mg/day}}{\frac{600\ \text{mg/day}}{26\ \text{mg/L}} - \frac{300\ \text{mg/day}}{6\ \text{mg/L}}} = 11\ \text{mg/L} \quad (1.55)$$

$$V_{max} = 600\ \text{mg/day} + \left(11\ \text{mg/L} \times \frac{600\ \text{mg/day}}{26\ \text{mg/L}} \right) = 850\ \text{mg/day} \quad (1.56)$$

The estimates of K_m and V_{max} are used to calculate a new maintenance dosage to achieve a C_{SS} of 16 μg/mL using the following equations:

$$\text{Dosage} = \frac{V_{max}}{1 + \frac{K_m}{C_{SS}}} \quad (1.57)$$

$$\text{Dosage} = \frac{850\ \text{mg/day}}{1 + \frac{11\ \text{mg/L}}{16\ \text{mg/L}}} = 500\ \text{mg/day} \quad (1.58)$$

Three assumptions when applying this method are:

- Both SDCs were collected under steady-state conditions.
- The same dosage form (must be same brand-name product) was administered.
- Protein binding remains constant.

These assumptions must be followed strictly to avoid excessive error in the new dosage estimation. The clinical utility of this method is limited by the requirement for two SDCs collected while the patient is on two different steady-state dosing regimens. In an inpatient setting it is unlikely that two SDCs on two different steady-state dosing regimens will be available. This method is most likely to be used in an epilepsy clinic for the adjustment of phenytoin in ambulatory patients, which introduces a fourth assumption: 100% patient compliance.

PHYSIOLOGIC VARIABLES AFFECTING DRUG CLEARANCE

Hepatic Drug Elimination

The disposition of drugs eliminated primarily by hepatic metabolism can be affected by alterations in protein binding, liver enzymes, and liver blood flow. It is important to understand the mechanism by which changes in protein binding, liver enzymes, or liver blood flow can affect drug disposition to predict when such changes may be of clinical importance in a specific patient. The compartmental mathematical models are inadequate for this purpose because they describe changes in total drug concentration using hybrid parameters that have no direct correlation to the physiologic processes responsible for drug elimination. To evaluate changes in these determinants of hepatic drug clearance, a model that includes these as parameters and defines their mathematical relationship to clearance can be used. One such model is the venous equilibrium model (VEM). The VEM is an attempt to construct a pharmacokinetic model for drug clearance using model parameters that correspond to specific physiologic determinants of drug elimination.

For drugs cleared predominantly by hepatic metabolic processes (phenytoin, phenobarbital, theophylline, valproic acid, carbamazepine), the Cl of the drug from the body is approximately equivalent to the hepatic drug clearance. In these cases, drug elimination is the difference between the amount of drug entering the liver and the amount of drug exiting the liver, as illustrated in Figure 1.5. C_{in} is the concentration of drug in the blood entering

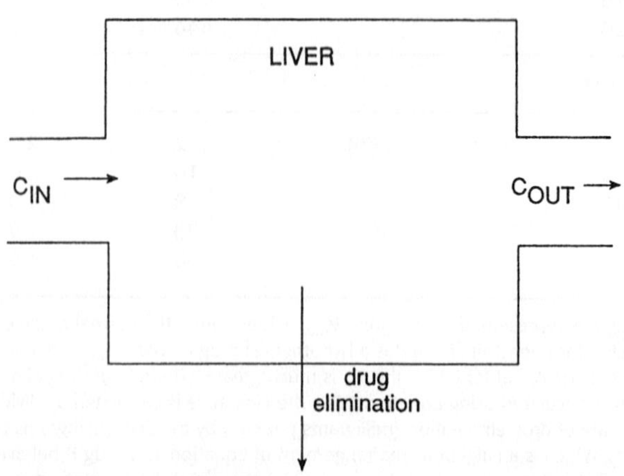

Figure 1.5. Venous equilibrium model of hepatic drug elimination. A hepatically eliminated drug enters the liver, where it is metabolized. The difference between C_{in} and C_{out} represents the amount of drug eliminated from the blood as it passes through the liver. From this simple scheme, the concept of organ clearance is illustrated and used to explain the derivation of Equations 1.59 and 1.60.

the liver, C_{out} is the concentration of drug in the blood exiting the liver, and the arrows represent the flow of blood through the liver. Thus, the rate of drug elimination would be described by the following equation:

$$\text{Rate of drug elimination} = Q(C_{in}) - Q(C_{out}) \quad (1.59)$$

where Q equals the liver blood flow (approximately 1.5 L/minute in humans), and C_{in} and C_{out} are as previously defined. Because blood flow into the liver must be equivalent to blood flow out of the liver (it is within a closed system), Equation 1.59 simplifies to $Q(C_{in} - C_{out})$. This is the rate of drug eliminated by the liver (in milligrams per minute). Dividing this by the rate of drug entering the liver gives a unitless parameter known as the extraction ratio (ER).

$$ER = \frac{Q(C_{in} - C_{out})}{Q(C_{in})} = \frac{C_{in} - C_{out}}{C_{in}} \quad (1.60)$$

The ER is an indicator of the efficiency of the processes responsible (e.g., metabolism) for eliminating drug from the blood as it passes through the liver. The ER can range from 0 to 1. An ER of 1 means 100% of the drug entering the liver is eliminated, and an ER of 0 means none of the drug entering the liver is eliminated. The hepatic clearance (Cl_H) of a drug is the liver blood flow multiplied by the ER, Cl_H equals Q(ER). The ER as defined in Equation 1.60 assumes that the drug is not bound to any proteins in the blood. When protein binding is considered, the ER is best described by the following equation[5,6]:

$$ER = \frac{(f_U)(Cl_{int})}{Q + (f_U)(Cl_{int})} \quad (1.61)$$

where f_U is the fraction of the total drug in the blood that is unbound, Q is the liver blood flow, and Cl_{int} is the intrinsic clearance of free drug. The Cl_{int} is the theoretical value for clearance of the drug by the liver if it is not protein bound, and it is an indication of the liver's enzymatic capacity to eliminate a drug if access is not impeded by protein binding or liver blood flow.

High-Clearance Drugs

A high-clearance drug is one that has an extraction ratio greater than or equal to 0.7. For the purpose of qualitative prediction of the effect of changes in f_U, Cl_{int}, and Q on $C_{SS\text{-}total}$ and $C_{SS\text{-}free}$, the extraction ratio is assumed to be 1.0. Thus, the Cl of the drug simplifies to Cl_H equals Q, which means that the clearance depends on the rate of presentation of drug to the liver (i.e., the liver blood flow). For a high-extraction (high-E) drug given by the IV route, alterations in protein binding and enzyme induction or inhibition have no effect on the clearance of drug by the liver. The elimination of drug by the liver is so efficient that a protein-bound drug is stripped from its protein-binding sites and metabolized. Concomitant administration of drugs that inhibit or induce hepatic enzymes has no effect because drug clearance depends only on Q and induction and inhibition affect Cl_{int}, which is not a determinant of drug clearance for high-E drugs. Although protein-binding changes do not alter clearance of a high-E drug, it may alter the relationship between total drug concentration and therapeutic and toxic effects (i.e., the therapeutic range).

The free drug in the blood is the pharmacologically active portion of drug. Drug molecules bound to proteins usually are considered pharmacologically inactive because the steric interference of the protein molecule inhibits binding of the drug molecule to the active receptor site, and protein-bound drug cannot easily diffuse from the blood compartment to the site of action. Thus, the therapeutic effect is more closely related to the free drug concentration than to the total drug concentration. The use of total concentration is strictly for purposes of feasibility; in fact, the underlying assumption is that the interindividual and intraindividual variability in protein binding (or f_U) is small. In the case of a high-E drug, a change in protein binding secondary to displacement from protein-binding sites (increase in f_U) or an increase in protein-binding receptor sites (decrease in f_U) causes the free concentration of drug to increase or decrease, respectively, with no change in the total drug concentration, thus altering the relationship between total concentration and therapeutic or toxic effects. Such alterations in f_U can lead to changes in the therapeutic range, which is based on total SDC.

Low-Clearance Drugs

A low-clearance drug is one for which hepatic elimination is restricted by the enzymatic capacity of the liver rather than the liver blood flow. In this case, the clearance depends on both the intrinsic free clearance of drug by the liver, Cl_{int}, and the free fraction of drug in the blood, f_U, such that Cl_H equals $f_U Cl_{int}$. Alterations in liver blood flow, Q, have no effect on clearance of a low-extraction (low-E) drug as the rate of presentation of drug to the liver exceeds the ability of liver to eliminate the drug. Decreased protein binding results in an increase in hepatic clearance, and an increase in protein binding causes a decrease in hepatic clearance; enzyme induction increases hepatic clearance and enzyme inhibition decreases hepatic clearance. Changes in f_U are particularly important because of the alteration in the total concentration–response relationship (i.e., therapeutic range).

Case Study 9

Patient E.W. is a 55-year-old man with a long-standing seizure disorder currently taking phenytoin 200 mg twice a day; he has maintained good seizure control with phenytoin levels around 18 μg/mL. He had been on phenytoin 300 mg/day for the past 2 years but the dosage was increased recently because his phenytoin level decreased to 12 μg/mL. Six months ago E.W. was diagnosed with prostate cancer. The patient's prognosis remains good despite a weight loss of 35 pounds over the last 6 months. Today E.W. comes to the clinic with nystagmus upon lateral gaze and mild ataxia. A stat phenytoin is reported as 19 μg/mL. The only other clinically significant laboratory value is a low albumin, 2.9 g/dL. E.W.'s physician says levels from past visits have been as high and even higher without any signs or symptoms of toxicity, and requests your expertise in speculating on the reason for this patient's apparent phenytoin toxicity.

Phenytoin is a highly protein bound (90%), hepatically eliminated, low-E drug. The major plasma protein to which phenytoin binds is albumin. The effect of a low albumin is fewer protein-binding sites in the plasma, which results in an increase in the f_U. Normally, phenytoin is 90% protein bound ($f_U = 0.10$), which is equivalent to a free phenytoin therapeutic range of 1.0 to 2.0 μg/mL. In the case of E.W., this would be equivalent to a free phenytoin concentration of 1.9 μg/mL. However, because f_U is increased via a reduced number of albumin protein-binding sites in the plasma, the proportion of the measured total concentration that is free drug is increased, such that the free concentration is more than 10% of the measured total concentration. A formula has been proposed for estimating the free concentration based on the degree of hypoalbuminemia[7]:

$$C_{\text{free}} = \frac{(\text{SDC}_{\text{total}})(0.1)}{(0.2)(\text{Alb}) + 0.1} \tag{1.62}$$

where C_{free} is the estimated free concentration of phenytoin in the blood, $\text{SDC}_{\text{total}}$ is the measured SDC, and Alb is the serum albumin in milligrams per deciliter. For E.W., the estimated free concentration would be

$$C_{\text{free}} = \frac{(19\ \mu\text{g/mL})(0.1)}{(0.2)(2.9) + 0.1} = 2.8\ \mu\text{g/mL} \tag{1.63}$$

This estimate of the free phenytoin concentration would be equivalent to a total serum concentration of 28 μg/mL if the patient had a normal serum albumin. The f_U has increased from the presumed normal of 0.1 to 0.15:

$$f_U = \frac{C_{\text{free}}}{C_{\text{total}}} = \frac{2.8\ \mu\text{g/mL}}{19\ \mu\text{g/mL}} = 0.15 \tag{1.64}$$

demonstrating that small increases in the f_U can have a significant effect on the relationship between the total measured phenytoin serum concentration and free serum concentration. In the case of E.W., the phenytoin dosage should not have been increased from 300 mg/day to 400 mg/day. Phenytoin is a low-E drug that is bound to albumin. Decreased albumin results in an increase in f_u. Increasing f_u causes C_{SStotal} to decrease, but C_{SSfree} remains unchanged. This means the measured phenytoin concentration will decrease, which in the case of E.W. led to an increase in his phenytoin dosage. However, the dosage should not have been increased because the free phenytoin concentration would not change.

The perturbations in drug disposition for high- and low-E drugs that are hepatically eliminated are summarized in Table 1.5. Protein-binding changes affect the f_U, alterations in intrinsic metabolic capacity through enzyme induction or inhibition affect the Cl_{int}, and changes in blood flow secondary to hemodynamic instability are represented by changes in Q. This table describes only VEM predictions for high-E drugs given IV (lidocaine) and low-E drugs given by the IV or oral route (phenytoin, phenobarbital, valproic acid, carbamazepine, theophylline). For drugs with intermediate extraction ratios (between 0.3 to 0.7), simplification of these equations results in poor approximations, and because the parameters of the VEM are impractical to determine clinically, this physiologic model is not useful.

Renal Drug Elimination

The renal route of drug elimination is important for digoxin, procainamide, lithium, gentamicin, amikacin, tobramycin, and vancomycin. Unlike hepatic drug elimination, which cannot be assessed quantitatively, renal

Table 1.5 ▪ The Venous Equilibrium Model: The Effect of Changes in Q, f_U, and Cl_{int} on Steady-State Free and Total Drug Concentration

Independent Parameters			Dependent Parameters	
Q	f_U	Cl_{int}	$C_{\text{SS-total}}$	$C_{\text{SS-free}}$
High-Clearance Drug (IV only)				
↑	⇆	⇆	↓	↓
↓	⇆	⇆	↑	↑
⇆	↑	⇆	⇆	↑
⇆	↓	⇆	⇆	↓
⇆	⇆	↑	⇆	⇆
⇆	⇆	↓	⇆	⇆
Low Clearance Drug (IV or oral)				
↑	⇆	⇆	⇆	⇆
↓	⇆	⇆	⇆	⇆
⇆	↑	⇆	↓	⇆
⇆	↓	⇆	↑	⇆
⇆	⇆	↑	↓	↓
⇆	⇆	↓	↑	↑

The parameters of the venous equilibrium model are liver blood flow (Q), fraction of drug unbound in the blood (f_U), and the free intrinsic clearance (Cl_{int}). These three parameters determine the total steady-state concentration ($C_{\text{SS-total}}$) and the free or unbound steady-state concentration ($C_{\text{SS-free}}$) of drug in the blood. For a high-extraction drug (IV route), $C_{\text{SS-total}}$ and $C_{\text{SS-free}}$ are equally affected by changes in Q, with f_U remaining constant; changes in f_U are directly related to $C_{\text{SS-free}}$ but do not affect $C_{\text{SS-total}}$. Changes in Cl_{int} secondary to enzyme induction or inhibition do not affect $C_{\text{SS-total}}$ or $C_{\text{SS-free}}$. For a low-clearance drug, changes in Q do not affect $C_{\text{SS-total}}$ or $C_{\text{SS-free}}$; changes in f_U are inversely related to changes in $C_{\text{SS-total}}$ but do not affect $C_{\text{SS-free}}$. Alterations in Cl_{int} affect an inversely related change in $C_{\text{SS-total}}$ and $C_{\text{SS-free}}$ equally (f_U is unchanged). For a high-extraction drug given IV or a low-extraction drug given IV or orally, changes in f_U alter the relationship between total serum drug concentration and free serum drug concentration at steady state. This can result in a significant alteration in the relationship between total serum drug concentration at steady state and the therapeutic and toxic effects (i.e., a change in the therapeutic range; see Case Study 9).

function can be estimated from a measured 24-hour urinary creatinine or from a measured serum creatinine using the Cockcroft–Gault equation[8]:

$$\text{CrCl} = \frac{(140 - \text{Age})(\text{Weight})}{(72)(\text{Scr})} \quad (1.65)$$

where CrCl is the estimated creatinine clearance in milliliters per minute, age is in years, weight is in kilograms and refers to the lean body weight, and SCr is the serum creatinine in milligrams per deciliter. Equation 1.65 is an estimation of creatinine clearance in male patients based on serum creatinine. If the patient is female, then the same calculation is performed, but the answer is multiplied by 0.85. The estimated creatinine clearance is an indication of the patient's kidney function and correlates with the renal elimination of drugs. Assessment of a patient's renal function is particularly important for the initial maintenance dosing of drugs with significant renal elimination. Once measured SDCs are available, the patient's drug therapy can be individualized based on these SDCs, and serum creatinine determinations are used in assessing the stability of renal function rather than adjusting dosages. Various dosing nomograms have been developed based on the patient's estimated renal function and are summarized in Table 1.6.

PHARMACODYNAMICS

The clinical utility of pharmacokinetic modeling is limited by the fact that it only provides predictions about the SDC achieved when a patient is given a certain dosage of drug (i.e., it is a model of the dose–concentration relationship). However, even in patients in whom identical SDCs occur, there usually is a significant difference in response. The purpose of pharmacodynamic modeling is to describe and predict this variability of response (i.e., it is a model of the concentration–effect relationship). When pharmacokinetic and pharmacodynamic modeling are combined, they provide a powerful tool for quantifying the clinical effects of drugs. For example, it is known that older adults are more sensitive to the opiate agonistic effects of morphine. This increased sensitivity could caused by either differences in the SDC achieved in younger and older patients given the same dosage (in milligrams per kilogram) or by differences in the clinical effects achieved in the older and younger patients with identical SDCs. The former is evaluated by comparing their pharmacokinetic parameters (Cl, V, and $t_{1/2}$), and the latter is evaluated by comparing their pharmacodynamic parameters (E_{max} and EC_{50}).

The most common pharmacodynamic model fit to concentration–effect data is the sigmoid E_{max} model[33]:

$$E = \frac{E_{max} \times C^n}{EC_{50}^n + C^n} \quad (1.66)$$

where E is a measured clinical effect, E_{max} is the maximum response possible, C is the SDC that caused E, EC_{50} is the SDC at which the measured effect is at one-half of E_{max}, and n determines the sigmoidal shape of the concentration–effect relationship. Conducting a pharmacodynamic analysis involves measuring a clinical effect such as BP and determining the plasma concentration at the time the BP measurement is made. Then BP is plotted against the SDC. The E_{max}, EC_{50}, and n are estimated by a computer program that determines the values of these parameters that give the best fit between the predicted effect, determined by solving Equation 1.66, and the actual observed effect.

Table 1.6 ▪ Maintenance Dosing Estimation for Drugs Eliminated Primarily by the Kidney

Drug	Nomogram		References
Digoxin	$Cl_{digoxin} = 1.07 \times CrCl + 28$		29
Aminoglycosides	Sarubbi–Hull nomogram		30,31
Vancomycin	University of Alabama Hospital Vancomycin dosing nomogram[a]		32
	Loading dosage = 15–20 mg/kg TBW		
	Maintenance dosage = 12–15 mg/kg TBW to be given each interval as determined from CrCl		
	CrCl	**Dosing Interval**	
	<10	[b]	
	10–15	96	
	16–25	72	
	26–35	48	
	36–40	36	
	41–50	30	
	51–65	24	
	66–85	18	
	86–120	12	
	>120	8	
Lithium	None: SDCs should be monitored carefully when initiating therapy in patients with renal insufficiency.		17,33
Procainamide	None: NAPA SDCs should be monitored in patients with renal insufficiency.		15

Drugs with significant renal elimination (Table 1.3) should have an initial maintenance dosage estimate based on the patient's renal function. For most drugs that fall into this category, there are many published nomograms, of which one is listed here.

CrCl, creatinine clearance based on a stable creatinine (if patient > 60 years old and serum creatinine < 1.0, use serum creatinine of 1.0); *TBW*, total body weight; *SDC*, serum drug concentration; *NAPA*, *N*-acetylprocainamide.

[a]Reproduced with permission from University of Alabama Drug Resource Center.

[b]For dosing in patients with CrCl < 10, use measured SDCs.

Tolerance and Sensitivity

The relationship between concentration and effect for a specific drug action often changes over time, causing either a reduction (tolerance) or increase (sensitization) in the drug's effects. How a drug's effects change over time can significantly alter patient response. A classic example is the dosing of nitroglycerin sustained-release preparations for angina. Around-the-clock dosing results in tolerance to the beneficial effects of nitroglycerin for anginal pain. This tolerance can be avoided by having the patient take the medication only while awake. The nitrate-free interval that occurs during sleep reduces the development of tolerance. Such changes in the concentration–effect relationship are evaluated by plotting the SDC for a drug against an effect measured at the time of the SDC determination. The occurrence of tolerance and sensitization is determined from the hysteresis of the concentration–effect plot (Fig. 1.6).

PHARMACOKINETICS SOFTWARE OVERVIEW

Software applications have been developed to facilitate pharmacokinetic modeling in the patient care and research environment. Major features of the available software packages are summarized in Table 1.7. A software search should begin with a complete assessment of the prospective user's clinical methods and patient populations. Careful review of the literature on available programs and product demonstrations is recommended. The clinicians responsible for providing pharmacokinetic consultations should be thoroughly trained to use the programs and must understand the underlying pharmacokinetic principles and limitations.

CONCLUSION

An SDC cannot be interpreted without a clinical assessment of the patient, including the disease state being treated, the clinical condition of the patient, a complete drug dosing history, the exact time the SDC was collected, pertinent laboratory data, and assessment of concomitant drug therapy (Table 1.8). Collection of this information is difficult and the clinical pharmacist must be

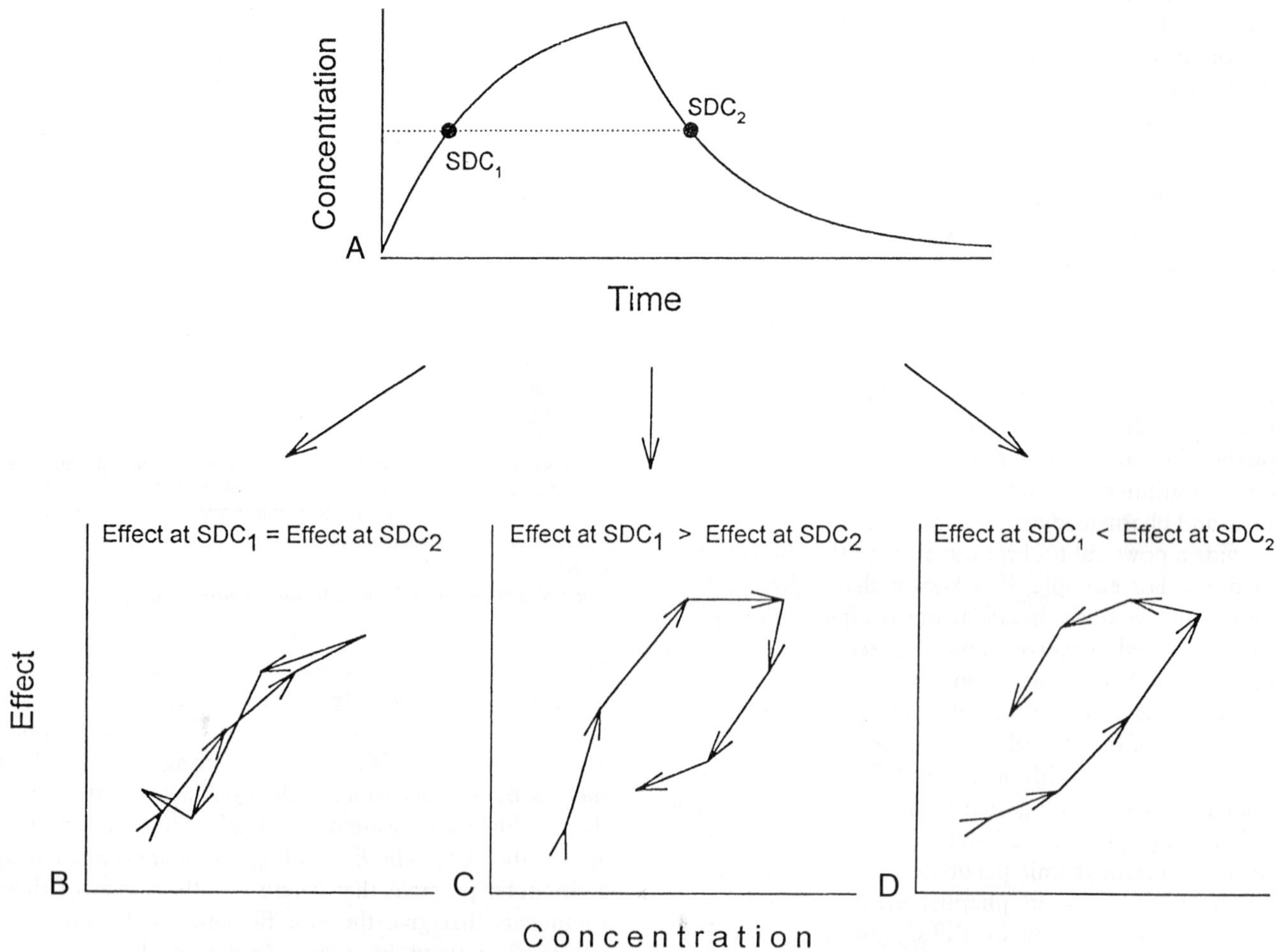

Figure 1.6. Tolerance and sensitivity. **A,** Concentration–time profile after a single dose of drug with SDC$_1$ and SDC$_2$. If a response is measured at two time points, the concentration–effect relationship can be compared between the two points (typically this is done for many points). If the response at SDC$_1$ equals the response at SDC$_2$, neither tolerance nor sensitization occurs (**B,** no hysteresis). If the response at SDC$_1$ is greater than the response at SDC$_2$, tolerance occurs (**C,** clockwise hysteresis). If the response at SDC$_1$ is less than SDC$_2$, sensitization occurs (**D,** counterclockwise hysteresis).

Table 1.7 ▪ Selected Pharmacokinetic Modeling Software

Program	Brief Description	Reference
Abbottbase PK System	Clinical software for Bayesian PK analysis of several widely used drugs.	34
ACSL BioMed	Comprehensive tool designed to simulate clinical trials of drugs.	35
ADAPT II	A set of programs for simulation, parameter estimation, and sample schedule design.	36
BIOPAK	Statistical analysis package for bioavailability/bioequivalence studies.	37
Kinetica	The software offers a wide range of built-in analyses in Windows 95/NT environment.	38
ModelMaker	Powerful and intuitive Windows simulation package for scientists and engineers.	39
Nonlin	Nonlinear regression analysis with extensive PK and PD models (mainframe, DOS, and Windows versions)	40
NONMEM	Nonlinear mixed-effects modeling of individual and population PK data.	41
PKAnalyst	An extension of RSTRIP for Windows, has more than 20 built-in PK models.	42
POP3CM	A visual compartmental population analysis program for a three-compartment model.	43
Practical Pharmacokinetics	Designed for teaching and practice of clinical PK. It guides clinicians in dosage adjustment of more than 400 drugs.	44
RADKinetics	Program for dosage adjustment of gentamicin and vancomycin.	45
SAAM II	A Windows program for PK/PD and enzyme kinetic studies. Allows visual model design.	46
SCIENTIST Pharmacokinetic Library	A set of PK models that can be used to analyze experimental data using MicroMath's SCIENTIST.	47
Simkin	Clinical PK software for most commonly monitored drugs.	48
USC*PACK	Collection of many modules for clinical and research PK analyses.	49

PK, pharmacokinetic; *PD,* pharmacodynamic.

Table 1.8 ▪ Information Necessary for Clinical Interpretation of Measured Serum Drug Concentrations (SDCs)

Drug monitored	Dosage Route of administration History: length of time on this drug and length of time on present dosing regimen
Measured SDC	Exact time measured SDC collected Time interval between administration of last dose and collection of SDC Reason for SDC determination
Patient information	Demographics: age, sex, weight, height History of present illness Past medical history Laboratory data: serum creatinine, liver function tests, any other abnormal lab values Pertinent clinical parameters: heart rate, blood pressure, temperature, chest x-ray, nutritional status, mental status
Other drug therapy	Drug–drug interactions Drug–disease interactions Drug–food interactions

The information needed to assess a patient's drug therapy is highly variable and depends on the drug and clinical circumstances. This table is a basic starting point.

prepared to perform a hands-on assessment and to talk to the patient, physician, nurse, or other health care provider. This cannot be overemphasized because it is not the application of pharmacokinetic theory or therapeutic knowledge but the quality of the information for assessment that often determines the quality of the clinical recommendation.

This chapter provides practical knowledge for the application of principles to therapeutic drug monitoring, and it should be viewed as the starting point toward acquiring the skills and knowledge needed to become a competent clinical pharmacist.

KEY POINTS

- The volume of distribution determines the loading dosage.
- The dosage and clearance determine the steady-state concentration.
- The half-life determines the time to reach steady state and the time for "all" drug to be eliminated from the body.
- If the half-life changes, it is because clearance or volume changed.
- The dosage of a drug divided by the steady-state concentration equals the clearance.
- If a drug obeys first-order pharmacokinetics, then a simple ratio of dosage to steady-state concentration can be used to estimate a new dosage as long as the clearance has not changed.
- Phenytoin is an example of a drug that obeys Michaelis–Menten rather than first-order pharmacokinetics. In this case, as plasma concentration increases, the clearance decreases and the half-life gets longer.

- The venous equilibrium model is useful for the prediction of drug interactions for hepatically eliminated drugs.
- Pharmacodynamics is an attempt to correlate the plasma concentration of a drug to its therapeutic or toxic effects.
- Pharmacokinetic software is widely available to assist in the application of pharmacokinetic and pharmacodynamic principles in both research and patient care.
- Drug concentrations must be interpreted with due consideration of therapeutic principles and the patient's clinical condition.

REFERENCES

1. Gibaldi M, Perrier D. Pharmacokinetics. 2nd ed. New York: Marcel Dekker, 1982.

1a. Preston SL, Briceland LL. Single daily dosing of aminoglycosides. Pharmacotherapy 15:297–316, 1995.

2. Sawchuk RJ, Zaske DE. Pharmacokinetics of dosing regimens which utilize multiple intravenous infusions: gentamicin in burn patients. J Pharmacokinet Biopharm 4:183–195, 1976.
3. Martin E, Tozer TN, Sheiner LB, et al. The clinical pharmacokinetics of phenytoin. J Pharmacokinet Biopharm 5:579, 1977.
4. Mullen WM. Optimal phenytoin therapy: a new technique for individualizing dosage. Clin Pharmacol Ther 23:228–232, 1978.
5. Wilkinson GR, Shand DG. A physiologic approach to hepatic drug clearance. Clin Pharmacol Ther 18:377, 1975.
6. Shand DG, Cotham RH, Wilkinson GR. Perfusion-limited effects of plasma drug binding on hepatic drug extraction. Life Sci 19:125, 1976.
7. Sheiner LB, Tozer TN. Clinical pharmacokinetics: the use of plasma concentrations of drugs. In: Melmon KL, Morrelli HF, eds. Clinical pharmacology: basic principles in therapeutics. New York: Macmillan, 1978:71–109.
8. Cockcroft D, Gault M. Prediction of creatinine clearance from serum creatinine. Nephron 16:31–34, 1976.
9. Keys PW. Digoxin. In: Evans WE, Schentag JJ, Jusko WJ, eds. Applied pharmacokinetics. Spokane, WA: Applied Therapeutics Inc., 1980:319.
10. Reuning RH, Garaets DR. Digoxin. In: Evans WE, Schentag JJ, Jusko WJ, eds. Applied pharmacokinetics. 2nd ed. Spokane, WA: Applied Therapeutics Inc., 1986:570.
11. Hendeles L, Massanari M, Weinberger M. Theophylline. In: Evans WE, Schentag JJ, Jusko WJ, eds. Applied pharmacokinetics. 2nd ed. Spokane, WA: Applied Therapeutics Inc., 1986:698.
12. Benowitz NL, Meister W. Clinical pharmacokinetics of lignocaine. Clin Pharmacokinet 3:177–201, 1978.
13. Rowland M, Thomson PD, Guichard A, et al. Disposition of lignocaine in normal subjects. Ann NY Acad Sci 179:383–398, 1971.
14. Pieper JA, Rodman JH. Lidocaine. In: Evans WE, Schentag JJ, Jusko WJ, eds. Applied pharmacokinetics. 2nd ed. Spokane, WA: Applied Therapeutics Inc., 1986:639.
15. Coyle JD, Lima JJ. Procainamide. In: Evans WE, Schentag JJ, Jusko WJ, eds. Applied pharmacokinetics. 2nd ed. Spokane, WA: Applied Therapeutics Inc., 1986:698.
16. Nielsen-Kudsk F, Amdisen A. Analysis of the pharmacokinetics of lithium in man. Eur J Clin Pharmacol 16:271–277, 1979.
17. Amdisen A, Carson SW. Lithium. In: Evans WE, Schentag JJ, Jusko WJ, eds. Applied pharmacokinetics. 2nd ed. Spokane, WA: Applied Therapeutics Inc., 1986:698.
18. Ochs HR, Grub EE, Greenblatt DJ, et al. Intravenous quinidine: pharmacokinetic properties and effects on left ventricular performance in humans. Am Heart J 99:468–475, 1980.
19. Ueda CT. Quinidine. In: Evans WE, Schentag JJ, Jusko WJ, eds. Applied pharmacokinetics. 2nd ed. Spokane, WA: Applied Therapeutics Inc., 1986:712.
20. Schentag JJ. Aminoglycosides. In: Evans WE, Schentag JJ, Jusko WJ, eds. Applied pharmacokinetics. Spokane, WA: Applied Therapeutics Inc., 1980:174.
21. Zaske D. Aminoglycosides. In: Evans WE, Schentag JJ, Jusko WJ, eds. Applied pharmacokinetics. 2nd ed. Spokane, WA: Applied Therapeutics Inc., 1986:331.
22. Bertilsson L, Tomson T. Clinical pharmacokinetics and pharmacological effects of carbamazepine and carbamazepine-10,11-epoxide. Clin Pharmacokinet 11:177–198, 1986.
23. Levy RH, Wilensky AJ, Friel PN. Other antiepileptic drugs. In: Evans WE, Schentag JJ, Jusko WJ, eds. Applied pharmacokinetics. 2nd ed. Spokane, WA: Applied Therapeutics Inc., 1986:540.
24. Wilensky AJ, Friel PN, Levy RH, et al. Kinetics of phenobarbital in normal subjects and epileptic patients. Eur J Clin Pharmacol 23:87–92, 1982.
25. Winter ME, Tozer TN. Phenytoin. In: Evans WE, Schentag JJ, Jusko WJ, eds. Applied pharmacokinetics. 2nd ed. Spokane, WA: Applied Therapeutics Inc., 1986:493.
26. Klotz U, Antonin KH. Pharmacokinetics and bioavailability of sodium valproate. Clin Pharmacol Ther 21:736–743, 1977.
27. Matzke GR, McGory RW, Halstenson CE, et al. Pharmacokinetics of vancomycin inpatients with various degrees of renal function. Antimicrob Agents Chemother 25:433–437, 1984.
28. Matzke GR. Vancomycin. In: Evans WE, Schentag JJ, Jusko WJ, eds. Applied pharmacokinetics. 2nd ed. Spokane, WA: Applied Therapeutics Inc., 1986:399.
29. Dobbs SM, Mawer GE, Rodgers EM, et al. Can digoxin dose requirements be predicted? Br J Clin Pharmacol 3:231–237, 1976.
30. Hull JH, Sarubbi FA. Gentamicin serum concentrations: pharmacokinetic predictions. Ann Intern Med 85:183–189, 1976.
31. Sarubbi FA, Hull JH. Amikacin serum concentrations: prediction of levels and dosage guidelines. Ann Intern Med 89:612–618, 1978.
32. Como JA, Farringer JA. Vancomycin dosing recommendations. Drug Inf Bull 22:5, 1988.
33. DeVane CL: Fundamentals of monitoring psychoactive drug therapy. Baltimore: Williams & Wilkins, 1990.
34. Abbottbase PK System by Abbott Laboratories, Inc., Abbott Park, IL.
35. ACSL BioMed, MGA Software, 200 Baker Ave., Concord, MA 01742.
36. D'Argenio DZ, Schumitzky A. ADAPT II user's guide, biomedical simulation resource. Los Angeles: USC, 1997.
37. BIOPAK by Scientific Consulting, 5625 Dillard Rd., Suite 215, Cary, NC 27511.
38. Kinetica by InnaPhase, http://www.innaphase.com.
39. ModelMaker by Cherwell Scientific Publishing, http://www.cherwell.com.
40. Pharsight, Palo Alto, CA.
41. Beal SL, Sheiner LB. NONMEM users guide. San Francisco: NONMEM Project Group, UCSF.
42. PKAnalyst by MicroMath, http://www.micromath.com.
43. Lindstrom MJ, Bates DM. Nonlinear mixed effects models for repeated measures data. Biometrics 46:673–687, 1990.
44. Practical Pharmacokinetics by ClinPharm International, New Orleans, LA 70184-4008.
45. RADKinetics by RADSoft, P.O. Box 64, Irwin, IA 51446.
46. SAAM II by SAAM Institute, 4530 Union Bay Place NE, Suite 212, Seattle, WA 98105.
47. SCIENTIST Pharmacokinetic Library by MicroMath, http://www.micromath.com.
48. Simkin, 1035 NW 57th Street, Gainesville, FL 32605.
49. Jelliffe R, Schumitzky A, Van Guilder M, et al. User manual for version 10.7 of the USC*PACK collection of PC programs. Los Angeles: Laboratory of Applied Pharmacokinetics, University of Southern California School of Medicine, 1995.

CHAPTER 2

ADVERSE DRUG REACTIONS AND DRUG-INDUCED DISEASES

Joseph A. Barone and Evelyn R. Hermes-DeSantis

TREATMENT GOALS: ADVERSE DRUG REACTIONS

- Identify potential risk factors for the development of adverse drug reactions and drug-induced diseases.
- Recognize the elements of a preventable adverse drug reaction.
- Participate in national and, when appropriate, institutional reporting systems.
- Implement early recognition and prevention programs.

BACKGROUND

Adverse drug reactions (ADRs) contribute to overall health care costs by increasing morbidity, and even mortality in severe cases.[1] A meta-analysis of prospective ADR studies estimates the ADR fatality rate to be 0.32%, resulting in 106,000 deaths in 1994, placing it as the fourth leading cause of death in the United States after heart disease, cancer, and stroke.[2] The Joint Commission on Accreditation of Healthcare Organizations (JCAHO) and the Food and Drug Administration (FDA) place a high priority on the recognition and reporting of ADRs by health care professionals to improve the quality of life of patients receiving drug therapy.

To demonstrate the impact of ADRs on the cost of health care, one can use the number of hospital admissions that are drug related. Approximately 5% of reported hospitalizations are a result of an ADR, and the incidence has not changed over the past 30 years.[2,3] Many ADRs are acute and necessitate expensive emergency room care. Drug classes often involved in ADR-related admissions include antibiotics, anticoagulants, anticonvulsants, cardiovascular agents, respiratory drugs, and pain medications.[3,4] ADRs can also occur in hospitalized patients and may increase length of stay and necessitate medical and pharmacologic interventions. It is estimated that 11% of hospitalized patients experience an ADR, with 2.1% considered serious.[2]

DEFINITION

There is discussion regarding the terms *ADR, side effect,* and *drug allergy.* The World Health Organization (WHO) endorses an ADR definition that many health care practitioners have also adopted: "any response to a drug which is noxious and unintended, and which occurs at doses used in man for prophylaxis, diagnosis, or treatment."[5] An ADR may therefore include an exaggerated drug response, an unwanted effect on an organ system different from that being treated, an allergic or hypersensitivity reaction, an idiosyncratic reaction, or a drug interaction that causes an increased or diminished response.[6] A side effect and a drug allergy are both types of ADRs. A side effect, also called a type A reaction, is an example of a dose-related, predictable reaction to a drug.[1,7]

It is typically accepted that a side effect of a drug is known to occur in a given percentage of the population and has been observed with regular frequency. A side effect is also expected based on the pharmacologic activity of the agent. A drug allergy is an example of a non–dose-related, unpredictable adverse effect to a drug and is also called a type B reaction. Other type B reactions include idiosyncratic, immunologic, carcinogenic, and teratogenic effects.[1] Some side effects that are not drug allergies are inappropriately classified as such. For example, nausea secondary to narcotic use is not immunologically mediated and should not be considered an allergy; however, an anaphylactic reaction to penicillin is an adverse reaction that should be categorized as a true allergic reaction.[8] Unfortunately, reactions reported to health care professionals by patients or caregivers during the course of history taking often are mislabeled as allergies. This mislabeled diagnosis is often perpetuated throughout the patient's medical record. If not corrected, it may result in inadequate medical care in future circumstances.

ADRs must be further classified in terms of severity, causality, and preventability. Most institutions and community providers follow published algorithms that assist in this task.[9–11] Preventable ADRs should be a focus of any ADR reporting system in both ambulatory care and hospital settings. Most preventable ADRs involve administration of drugs or related compounds to which documented allergies exist, drugs affecting coagulation, drugs requiring therapeutic drug monitoring, and drug dosages not adjusted for renal impairment.[11] By identifying trends, risk factors, and circumstances that contribute to a preventable ADR, practitioners can implement programs to decrease its occurrence.[12,13] Refer to Table 2.1 for severity definitions and Table 2.2 for preventable reactions.

REPORTING

National ADR Reporting System

The FDA requirements on ADR reporting vary depending on the source of the report. Pharmaceutical manufacturers are legally required to report all ADRs to the FDA. However, the manufacturers do not fulfill this reporting requirement through information submission alone. The manufacturers must also use the reported data to verify the reaction and analyze additional reports for trends.[14–16] Although clinicians are viewed as critical in monitoring drugs for safety issues after approval, participation in the monitoring structure is voluntary. It is important to note that hospitals are under a federal mandate to report problems with medical devices.[17]

The question of what constitutes a reportable ADR can be answered by examining the FDA's definition of an ADR and the types of reactions the FDA is most interested in reviewing. With the increasing speed of some drug approvals, the FDA has become increasingly dependent on postmarketing surveillance to monitor reactions involving new chemical entities. Thus, any reaction to a new drug (e.g., a drug on the market 3 years or less), whether or not it is included in the product labeling and regardless of its severity, should be reported. The FDA places particular emphasis on unexpected and serious reactions. Reactions of these types should be reported for any medication, not only those that are newly approved.[18,19] Because of the complex nature of adverse event reporting for drugs, biologicals, and devices, the FDA launched the MedWatch program in 1993 (Fig. 2.1). The goals of the MedWatch Program are to simplify the reporting process, clarify what should be reported to the FDA, enhance awareness of serious adverse drug or device reactions, and provide feedback to health care providers about issues related to product safety. The MedWatch system should be used to report cases involving death; life-threatening hazards; hospitalization (admission or prolongation); disability; birth defects, miscarriages, stillbirths, or birth with disease; the need for medical or surgical treatment to prevent impairment; or any combination of the above. It is not necessary to show a direct causal relationship.[20] The FDA also oversees ADR reporting for biological agents (e.g., vaccines) as well as devices, and any reaction to these agents or products should be reported as well.

To simplify the reporting process, MedWatch uses one telephone number so that health care practitioners can report events efficiently and do not have to identify a

Table 2.1 ▪ Severity Definitions

Severity	Definition
Minor	No antidote, therapy, or prolongation of hospitalization
Moderate	A change in drug therapy, specific treatment, or an increased hospitalization by at least 1 day
Severe	Potentially life threatening, caused permanent damage or required intensive medical care
Lethal	Directly or indirectly contributed to the death of the patient

Source: Anonymous. ASHP Guidelines on adverse drug reaction monitoring and reporting. Am J Hosp Pharm 49:336–337, 1989.

Table 2.2 ▪ Elements of a Preventable Adverse Drug Reaction

Inappropriate drug use based on the patient's clinical condition
Inappropriate dosage, route, or frequency of administration based on patient-specific variables (e.g., age, weight, underlying disease)
Omission of appropriate laboratory monitoring, including therapeutic drug monitoring
Previous allergy or drug reaction history
Known drug–drug interaction
Known administration technique error (e.g., rapid vancomycin administration leading to red man syndrome)

Source: Schumock GT, Thornton JP. Focusing on preventability of adverse drug reactions. Clin Pharmacol Ther 30:239–245, 1992.

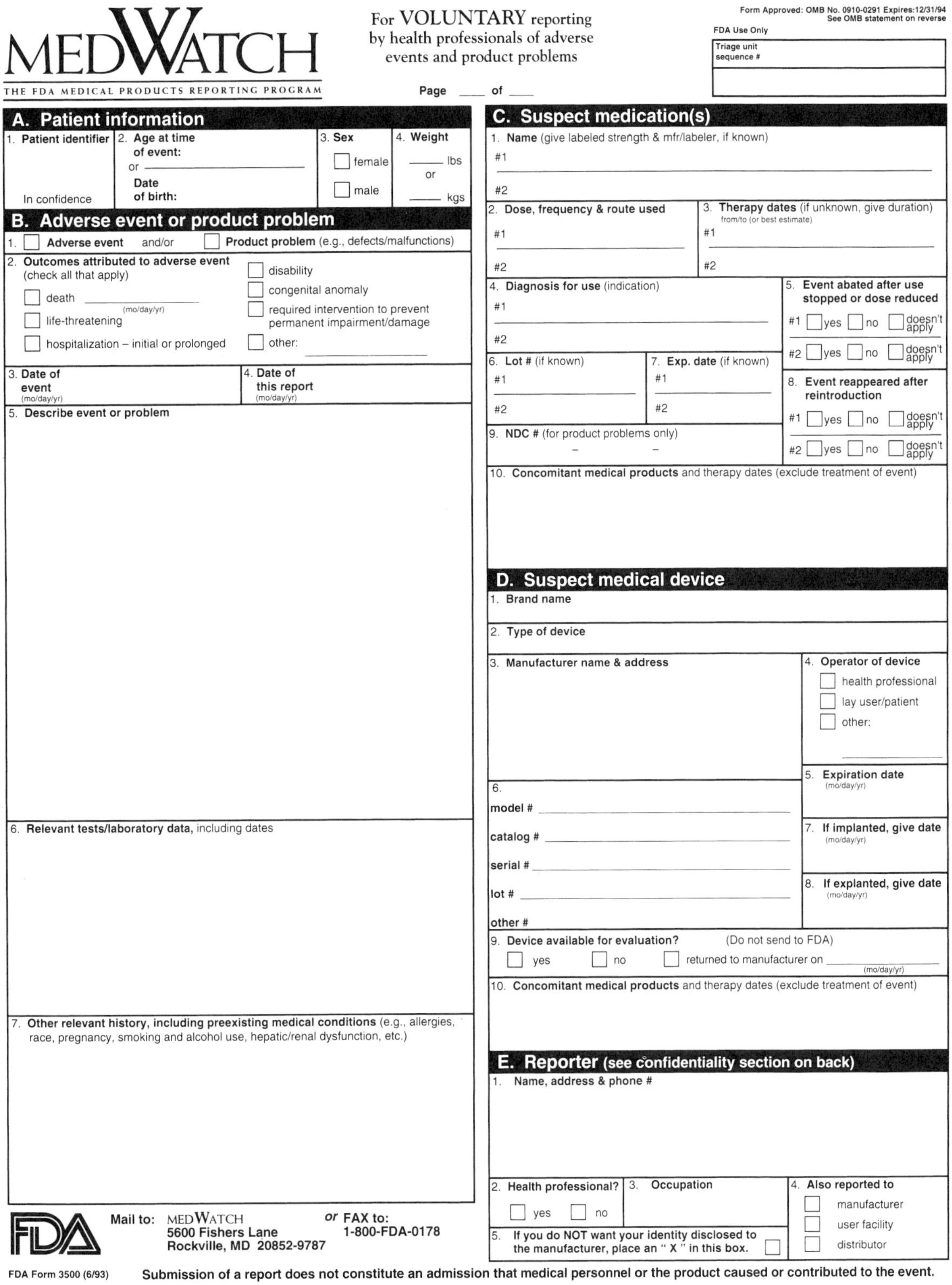

MEDWATCH
THE FDA MEDICAL PRODUCTS REPORTING PROGRAM

For VOLUNTARY reporting by health professionals of adverse events and product problems

Page ___ of ___

Form Approved: OMB No. 0910-0291 Expires:12/31/94
See OMB statement on reverse

FDA Use Only

Triage unit sequence #

A. Patient information

1. Patient identifier — In confidence
2. Age at time of event: or Date of birth:
3. Sex — female / male
4. Weight — ___ lbs or ___ kgs

B. Adverse event or product problem

1. Adverse event and/or Product problem (e.g., defects/malfunctions)
2. Outcomes attributed to adverse event (check all that apply)
   - death ___ (mo/day/yr)
   - life-threatening
   - hospitalization – initial or prolonged
   - disability
   - congenital anomaly
   - required intervention to prevent permanent impairment/damage
   - other: ___
3. Date of event (mo/day/yr)
4. Date of this report (mo/day/yr)
5. Describe event or problem
6. Relevant tests/laboratory data, including dates
7. Other relevant history, including preexisting medical conditions (e.g., allergies, race, pregnancy, smoking and alcohol use, hepatic/renal dysfunction, etc.)

C. Suspect medication(s)

1. Name (give labeled strength & mfr/labeler, if known) #1 #2
2. Dose, frequency & route used #1 #2
3. Therapy dates (if unknown, give duration) from/to (or best estimate) #1 #2
4. Diagnosis for use (indication) #1 #2
5. Event abated after use stopped or dose reduced — #1 yes no doesn't apply; #2 yes no doesn't apply
6. Lot # (if known) #1 #2
7. Exp. date (if known) #1 #2
8. Event reappeared after reintroduction — #1 yes no doesn't apply; #2 yes no doesn't apply
9. NDC # (for product problems only) – –
10. Concomitant medical products and therapy dates (exclude treatment of event)

D. Suspect medical device

1. Brand name
2. Type of device
3. Manufacturer name & address
4. Operator of device — health professional / lay user/patient / other:
5. Expiration date (mo/day/yr)
6. model # / catalog # / serial # / lot # / other #
7. If implanted, give date (mo/day/yr)
8. If explanted, give date (mo/day/yr)
9. Device available for evaluation? (Do not send to FDA) — yes / no / returned to manufacturer on ___ (mo/day/yr)
10. Concomitant medical products and therapy dates (exclude treatment of event)

E. Reporter (see confidentiality section on back)

1. Name, address & phone #
2. Health professional? — yes / no
3. Occupation
4. Also reported to — manufacturer / user facility / distributor
5. If you do NOT want your identity disclosed to the manufacturer, place an " X " in this box.

FDA

Mail to: MEDWATCH
5600 Fishers Lane
Rockville, MD 20852-9787

or FAX to:
1-800-FDA-0178

FDA Form 3500 (6/93)

Submission of a report does not constitute an admission that medical personnel or the product caused or contributed to the event.

Figure 2.1. MedWatch form for reporting adverse drug reactions.

particular department to call (e.g., devices, drugs, or biologicals). Methods for submitting information to the FDA via MedWatch are as follows: by using a prepaid U.S. mail reporting form (FDA 3500), by calling 1-800-FDA-1088, by facsimile transmission to 1-800-FDA-0178, and via Internet on the FDA Web site (www.fda.gov/medwatch).

As part of the MedWatch system, there is a specific monitoring system for special nutritional products. The Special Nutritional Adverse Event Monitoring System was established in 1993 and was instituted as a searchable

ADVICE ABOUT VOLUNTARY REPORTING

Report experiences with:
- medications (drugs or biologics)
- medical devices (including in-vitro diagnostics)
- special nutritional products (dietary supplements, medical foods, infant formulas)
- other products regulated by FDA

Report SERIOUS adverse events. An event is serious when the patient outcome is:
- death
- life-threatening (real risk of dying)
- hospitalization (initial or prolonged)
- disability (significant, persistent or permanent)
- congenital anomaly
- required intervention to prevent permanent impairment or damage

Report even if:
- you're not certain the product caused the event
- you don't have all the details

Report product problems – quality, performance or safety concerns such as:
- suspected contamination
- questionable stability
- defective components
- poor packaging or labeling

How to report:
- just fill in the sections that apply to your report
- use section C for all products except medical devices
- attach additional blank pages if needed
- use a separate form for each patient
- report either to FDA or the manufacturer (or both)

Important numbers:
- 1-800-FDA-0178 to FAX report
- 1-800-FDA-7737 to report by modem
- 1-800-FDA-1088 for more information or to report quality problems
- 1-800-822-7967 for a VAERS form for vaccines

If your report involves a serious adverse event with a device and it occurred in a facility outside a doctor's office, that facility may be legally required to report to FDA and/or the manufacturer. Please notify the person in that facility who would handle such reporting.

Confidentiality: The patient's identity is held in strict confidence by FDA and protected to the fullest extent of the law. The reporter's identity may be shared with the manufacturer unless requested otherwise. However, FDA will not disclose the reporter's identity in response to a request from the public, pursuant to the Freedom of Information Act.

The public reporting burden for this collection of information has been estimated to average 30 minutes per response, including the time for reviewing instructions, searching existing data sources, gathering and maintaining the data needed, and completing and reviewing the collection of information. Send your comments regarding this burden estimate or any other aspect of this collection of information, including suggestions for reducing this burden to:

Reports Clearance Officer, PHS
Hubert H. Humphrey Building,
Room 721-B
200 Independence Avenue, S.W.
Washington, DC 20201
ATTN: PRA

and to:
Office of Management and Budget
Paperwork Reduction Project
(0910-0230)
Washington, DC 20503

Please do NOT return this form to either of these addresses.

FDA Form 3500-back **Please Use Address Provided Below – Just Fold In Thirds, Tape and Mail**

Department of Health and Human Services
Public Health Service
Food and Drug Administration
Rockville, MD 20857

Official Business
Penalty for Private Use $300

NO POSTAGE NECESSARY IF MAILED IN THE UNITED STATES OR APO/FPO

BUSINESS REPLY MAIL
FIRST CLASS MAIL PERMIT NO. 946 ROCKVILLE, MD

POSTAGE WILL BE PAID BY FOOD AND DRUG ADMINISTRATION

MEDWATCH
The FDA Medical Products Reporting Program
Food and Drug Administration
5600 Fishers Lane
Rockville, MD 20852-9787

Figure 2.1 *(continued)*

database on the FDA Web site in May 1998. Reports on this site are from the MedWatch System.[21]

Adverse events associated with vaccines must be reported by vaccine manufacturers and health care practitioners to the Department of Health and Human Services (DHHS), as legislated by the National Childhood Vaccine Injury Act of 1986. The DHHS, in conjunction with the FDA and the Centers for Disease Control and Prevention (CDC), developed the Vaccine Adverse Event Reporting System (VAERS). The system is the MedWatch equivalent for vaccines. VAERS receives about 10,000 reports per year, of which 15% are serious.[22]

Health Care Organization-Based Reporting Systems

The JCAHO, an independent health care accrediting body, places a great deal of emphasis on ADR reporting and analysis. In addition, the FDA recognizes that hospitals play an important role in postmarketing surveillance.[20,23,24] Although adverse reaction monitoring is a shared responsibility of medical, pharmacy, and nursing personnel, it often becomes the obligation of the pharmacy department to develop, initiate, and manage the ADR reporting system. This function is carried out under the auspices of the Pharmacy and Therapeutics Committee.[17]

Most effective ADR programs contain four fundamental components: a definition of an ADR that clearly describes reportable ADRs; a concurrent method of monitoring and reporting adverse drug events; a system for reviewing and evaluating ADRs for severity, causality, probability, and preventability; and a system for using the results of the ADR program to improve patient care. The Pharmacy and Therapeutics Committee should review each of these components. Several types of reporting systems have been described in the literature and include voluntary programs using standardized reporting forms,[25] computerized alerts of tracer and antidote drugs and abnormal laboratory parameters,[26] and review of medical records based on coding of adverse events.[27] Pharmacy and Therapeutics Committee approval of any ADR program should be obtained before implementation because the JCAHO requires hospitals and health care organizations to follow written procedures in reporting ADRs.[24]

Outpatient-Based Reporting Systems

Health care is moving more to the ambulatory care setting; detecting ADRs in this arena is important. Postmarketing surveillance continues to detect clusters of ADRs and develop ADR profiles of newly released drugs. In addition, a move toward changing the status of medications from prescription to over-the-counter (OTC) will require all health care professionals to increase their questioning of total medication use when obtaining patient histories. OTCs are not innocuous agents, and the burden should be placed on the ambulatory care professionals to monitor patients for ADRs associated with nonprescription medications.

Pharmacovigilance

Safety profiles are an important aspect of a drug submission that must be reviewed before FDA approval of a new molecular entity. However, generating sufficient numbers to detect rare and serious ADRs is difficult. Even phase III trials may not enroll enough patients or be carried out over a long enough period of time to detect a rare ADR that may occur in fewer than 1 in 1000 patients.[1,28–30] In addition to the small numbers of subjects in clinical trials as compared to the general population that will use the drug, clinical trials often do not include patient populations that may be at a higher risk of developing an ADR. Such populations include older adults and children.

Once a drug is approved, it will quickly be used in thousands of patients with concomitant diseases and medications. This is why there is a high level of probability that within the first year of marketing a new drug, previously unidentified ADRs and drug interactions will become apparent.[1] If a problem is identified from these spontaneous reports, the FDA has several options to protect the public, including letters or safety alerts to health professionals, labeling changes, epidemiologic studies, postmarketing surveillance, inspection of manufacturer's practices, or product withdrawal.[20] Examples of these occurrences are plentiful. Felbamate was approved for treating tonic–clonic seizures in 1993 and within 6 months was implicated in numerous cases of aplastic anemia. Troglitazone, an oral antidiabetic agent marketed in 1997, required labeling changes regarding hepatic dysfunction and relevant patient monitoring within the first year.[31] Mibefradil, a calcium channel blocker, was approved August 1997, and within 6 months serious drug interactions were identified. Following that, numerous other drugs were found to interact with mibefradil, leading to its voluntary withdrawal in June 1998.[32] Bromfenac, a nonsteroidal anti-inflammatory drug (NSAID), was approved in July 1997; after reports of severe liver dysfunction, a black box warning was placed in the labeling in February 1998. Because of continued reports of toxicity and death, the drug was voluntarily withdrawn in June 1998.[33] Most recently, tolcapone, an antiparkinson agent approved in August 1997, has been given revised labeling concerning severe hepatotoxicity and death, as well as a black box warning in November 1998.[34] Sildenafil has also required revised labeling to reflect concerns about increased cardiovascular events associated with the use of the drug in patients with underlying cardiovascular or cerebrovascular disease.[35]

VARIABLES AFFECTING ADR INCIDENCE AND SEVERITY

Certain variables predispose individuals to develop ADRs. These variables can be patient or drug focused. In terms of patient variables, age, underlying disorder (including metabolic dysfunction), and genetic factors may influence the likelihood of developing an ADR. Efforts are being undertaken to increase the inclusion of particular subgroups of the population in clinical trials. Drug variables that also may affect the incidence of adverse reactions are the route of administration, product formulation, and duration of therapy.

Patient Variables

Older Adults

ADRs in older adults are serious clinical problems. In a study by Mannesse and colleagues, 42% of hospitalized older adults (70 years or older) evaluated in the study had one or more ADRs and 24% had severe reactions. There was a significant correlation between severe ADRs and a fall before admission, gastrointestinal (GI) bleeding or hematuria, and the use of three or more drugs. Older adults are better able to identify and correlate mild ADRs with drug therapy than more serious ADRs.[36]

Because both hepatic and renal function decline with age, older adults are subject to changes in metabolism that affect the clearance of drugs and active metabolites.[37] Decreased hepatic blood flow can lead to an increased bioavailability of active metabolites and ultimately increased serum concentrations of certain drugs with high first-pass clearance characteristics. Drugs that do not undergo high hepatic clearance may be affected by decreased microsomal enzyme activity, especially of the phase I metabolism type. The result is a decreased metabolism in general, which again leads to increased serum concentrations.[38,39]

The decline in renal function is more readily apparent in older adults. A decline in glomerular filtration rates (GFR) of approximately 35% is not uncommon.[40] The GFR may be low despite a normal serum creatinine, which can be misleading. For drugs that are excreted unchanged in the urine, dosages should be adjusted and carefully monitored to avoid excessive serum drug concentrations.

Age-related changes in metabolism and clearance should be correlated to the therapeutic index of the drug being used. Clinicians should be especially concerned with agents having a narrow therapeutic index and should monitor drug concentrations if appropriate (as with digoxin, quinidine, theophylline, and phenytoin). Even with agents that have a high therapeutic index, clinicians should exercise appropriate caution in monitoring patients.[38]

Neonates

Neonates experience ADRs through primary and secondary exposures. Several reasons for these ADRs include placental transfer of drugs, which results in exposure in utero; a lack of information on drug use in neonates; altered drug disposition, metabolism, and excretion profiles; multiple drug administration; and exposure through breast milk.[41–43] As a further complication, many neonates are born in critical condition with multiple-organ compromise. Neonates are also susceptible to developing adverse reactions though percutaneous absorption of environmental agents that are not meant for therapeutic use (e.g., antiseptics containing phenol, alcohol, and other disinfectants).

The pediatric population, and neonates specifically, are at an increased risk of ADRs affecting short- and long-term growth and development. Neurodevelopmental ADRs are of particular concern because of the susceptibility of the central nervous system (CNS). Psychoactive drugs can cause significant defects (e.g., sleep disturbances, hyperactivity and irritability, and behavioral disturbances). Drugs can also affect somatic development. Some examples in the literature include tetracycline's effect on tooth enamel and phenytoin-induced gingival hyperplasia. Adverse neurodevelopmental and somatic outcomes are difficult to predict because of insufficient studies and interindividual variability.[43]

Drug metabolism and excretion are crucial components of successful drug therapy in neonates. The neonate is not born with full capacity to process exogenous substrates. For example, the hepatic glucuronyl transferase system can take up to 4 weeks postpartum to become fully functional. Gray baby syndrome can develop if agents dependent on the glucuronyl transferase pathway (e.g., chloramphenicol) are administered to neonates. Specific dosage adjustments are required.[44] The demethylation and hydroxylation pathways necessary for theophylline metabolism may take a year to develop fully.[45] A full-term newborn has approximately 33% of the GFR of an adult. Kidney function continues to improve rapidly, and by the time a child is approximately 9 to 12 months of age, the kidney function is equivalent to that of an adult. Until the organ systems have a chance to develop, neonates and infants are at a higher risk of developing ADRs because of the immaturity of their organs. (See Chapter 96, Pediatric and Neonatal Therapy.)[2]

Patients with Human Immunodeficiency Virus

The incidence of ADRs in patients infected with the human immunodeficiency virus (HIV) appears to be higher than that in the general population.[46–48] Severe immunosuppression, development of drug-specific antibodies, and impaired capacity to clear drugs and unchanged metabolites result in an increased sensitivity to drug toxicity. In most cases, the drug reactions are not life threatening, but they often lead to suboptimal changes in therapy, which may limit the number of effective treatment plans. A classic example of increased hypersensitivity in patients infected with HIV is illustrated by the use of trimethoprim–sulfamethoxazole (TMP/SMX). In a study conducted at San Francisco General Hospital, 83% (29 of 35 patients) experienced some level of toxicity to TMP/SMX as they were being treated for *Pneumocystis carinii* pneumonia (PCP).[49] This figure is much higher than was reported in a group of hospitalized patients with no known HIV history (2 to 8%; Table 2.3).[50]

Because of the current practice of treating HIV with combination drug therapy, the clinician must remember that the patient may be at risk for additive drug toxicity and drug–drug interactions, all of which are superimposed on the underlying disease.[51]

Genetics

The rates of metabolism and elimination of various substances may be influenced by genetic factors (e.g., G-6PD deficiency resulting in drug-induced hemolytic anemia; acetylator status and drug-induced systemic lupus erythematosus [SLE]).[52] It has been reported that some

Table 2.3 ▪ Combined Rates of Hypersensitivity Reactions in Patients with the Human Immunodeficiency Virus

Drug	Rate of Occurrence
Amoxicillin	17–40%
Amphotericin B	4–15
Antituberculosis medication	3–20
Ciprofloxacin	5.7
Clindamycin and pyrimethamine	21–33
Trimethoprim–sulfamethoxazole	37–69
Fluconazole	6–13
Pentamidine	5–15
Sulfadiazine–pyrimethamine	13–34

Source: Harb GE, Jacobson MA. Human immunodeficiency virus (HIV) infection: does it increase susceptibility to adverse drug reactions? Drug Saf 9:1–8, 1993.

degree of polymorphism is present in up to 50% of the enzyme systems involved in drug metabolism. Enzyme systems that have been evaluated include acetylation, oxidation, and hydroxylation. Some phenotypes can be predicted from a single blood sample by available genotyping methods.[53] In many cases, however, screening tests for genetically susceptible patients often are not easily performed and clinical decisions must be based on the available epidemiologic data.

Drug Variables

Route of Administration

The route of administration and drug formulation are variables associated with the likelihood of developing an ADR.[54] Intravenous administration may be associated with side effects local to the site of injection, such as phlebitis and extravasation, as well as with systemic adverse effects secondary to rapid increases in drug–blood concentrations and accelerated clinical response. Oral administration, which is generally associated with decreased bioavailability, may be associated with somewhat milder adverse effects.[53] Variability in absorption of oral agents subsequent to drug–drug or drug–food interactions can also change side effect profiles. Local adverse effects, such as irritation to GI mucosa, may also result from oral administration. Topically applied medications can also cause systemic toxicity (e.g., ophthalmic β-blockers).

Product Formulation

Product formulations that alter the extent and the rate of absorption may also affect the incidence of ADRs. Sustained-release products may avoid the potential for adverse effects from excessive peaks and inadequate troughs associated with immediate-release products. For example, sustained-release antihypertensive agents produce more consistent serum drug concentration and, therefore, fewer potentially suboptimal trough periods and lower peak concentrations that may be associated with lightheadedness and other side effects.[53] Flushing secondary to niacin has been a major contributor to noncompliance and therefore therapeutic failures with this agent. The sustained-release product, which avoids the peak serum concentrations of the immediate-release preparations, is associated with a decreased incidence of flushing. However, sustained-release niacin products have been implicated in causing hepatic dysfunction.[55]

Duration of Therapy

The duration of therapy may also be a causative factor in ADRs. For example, in patients greater than 60 years of age, an increased duration of therapy with NSAIDs was associated with an increased risk of upper GI toxicity.[56] Meperidine's active metabolite, normeperidine, accumulates in patients with renal dysfunction and may result in seizure activity. This is most likely to occur with chronic administration rather than with single-dose or intermittent therapy.[57]

DRUG-INDUCED DISEASES

Disease state management, the collective management of all aspects of a patient's disease, is rapidly becoming the standard practice in health care. ADR monitoring and management should be part of this process. It is impossible to consider the desired outcomes of drug therapy without taking into account potential adverse consequences of treatment. The remaining sections of this chapter focus on major organ systems most commonly associated with adverse pharmacologic reactions. The reader will be referred to other chapters in this book that describe in detail the mechanisms of specific drug-induced diseases.

Hypersensitivity Reactions

Many drug reactions are often erroneously called hypersensitivity or allergic reactions.[58,59] True hypersensitivity reactions are immunologically mediated through a series of reproducible steps. The four classic hypersensitivity reactions are outlined in Table 2.4.[60]

Type I hypersensitivity reactions are most often associated with β-lactam antibiotics, which include penicillins and cephalosporins.[61] Although allergic reactions to penicillin have been reported to occur in 0.7 to 8% of the general population, anaphylaxis occurs in only 0.01% of identified treatment courses. The true immunochemistry of the penicillin reaction has been characterized, and cross-sensitivity to cephalosporins has been postulated based on chemical structure and similarities, typically a four-membered β-lactam ring. Hypersensitivity reactions that are mediated by immunoglobulin E show clinical cross-reactivity between penicillins and cephalosporins in approximately 5% of patients.[62] Imipenem (a carbapenem antibiotic) has a bicyclic nucleus and is associated with cross-reactivity in approximately 50% of penicillin-allergic patients.[63] Meropenem (a new carbapenem antibiotic) also cross-reacts in penicillin allergy.[64] Aztreonam, a monocy-

Table 2.4 ▪ Classic Hypersensitivity Reactions

Type	Antibody	Mechanism	Examples and Causative Agents
I	IgE	Anaphylactic Antigen–antibody reaction on mast cells leading to histamine, leukotriene, platelet-activating factor release	True systemic anaphylactic reaction Penicillin and cephalosporins Classic example of the hapten hypothesis
II	IgG IgM	Cytotoxic Antigen-specific antibodies directed against antigens on cell surface	Hemolytic anemia Penicillin and quinine are examples of causative agents
III	IgG IgM	Complex mediated Immune complexes interact with antibodies	Serum sickness Penicillin, cephalosporins, isoniazid, phenytoin, etc.
IV	T cells	Delayed hypersensitivity Generally takes more than 12 hr to develop Antigen interacts directly with sensitized T cells	Typically seen with topical therapies rather than systemic Characterized clinically by rash that worsens on subsequent or repetitive administration

Source: Lachmann PJ, Peters DK, eds. Clinical aspects of immunology. 4th ed. Boston: Blackwell Scientific, 1982.
Ig, immunoglobulin.

clic β-lactam antibiotic, is poorly immunogenic. β-Lactam–allergic patients have been given aztreonam and have not demonstrated any clinical signs of cross-sensitivity. Structural differences may therefore be a significant determinant in the incidence of hypersensitivity reactions.

Hypersensitivity reactions may manifest as acute urticaria, rhinitis, bronchial asthma, and angioedema. Depending on the severity of the reaction, there may also be peripheral circulatory collapse; therefore, immediate medical care should be sought. The offending agent should be removed. Epinephrine should be administered and repeated every 15 to 20 minutes as needed, up to three doses. Oxygen should be administered if available. Because the patient may be experiencing vascular collapse, fluid therapy should be initiated as needed to maintain blood pressure. If the patient is unresponsive to fluid replacement, a pressor agent infusion may be needed. β-Agonists, diphenhydramine, and a steroid should also be administered after the emergent situation is controlled.

Hepatotoxicity

Drug-induced hepatotoxicity has been associated with more than 800 drugs. Hepatotoxicity can be difficult to diagnose because correlation to a specific drug may be difficult and injury can present acutely or after prolonged drug administration.[65] The severity of drug-induced hepatotoxicity can range from mild alteration in liver function tests to hepatic failure. Table 2.5 lists some of the risk factors associated with hepatotoxic reactions. Using acetaminophen as an example, chronic ethanol ingestion can induce the cytochrome P-450 enzyme systems and deplete glutathione stores. Patients with chronic ethanol ingestion may be at an increased risk for liver toxicity following therapeutic dosages of acetaminophen.[66,67]

Acute liver injury can be cytotoxic or cholestatic. Cytotoxic injury involves direct injury to the hepatocytes with necrosis that can be localized or diffuse throughout the liver. Aminotransferase concentrations can be elevated to up to 500 times the normal concentrations. Prominent signs and symptoms include fatigue, anorexia, nausea, and jaundice. Drug-induced cytotoxic injury can progress to fulminant hepatic failure. Acetaminophen, isoniazid, methyldopa, and phenytoin have been associated with direct cytotoxic reactions that have led to mortality rates of 10% or higher.[68,69]

Cholestatic injury results in a characteristic decrease in bile flow. Hepatic injury of this type leads to jaundice and pruritus, and aminotransferase concentrations are only moderately elevated. Cholestatic hepatic injury has a

Table 2.5 ▪ Risk Factors Associated with Hepatotoxic Reactions

Factor	Example
Age	
Adults > children	Isoniazid, halothane
Older adults > others	Nonsteroidal anti-inflammatory drugs
Children > adults	Valproic acid, aspirin
Sex	
Female > male	Methyldopa, drug-induced chronic active hepatitis
Drugs	
Alcohol, phenobarbital	Can induce cytochrome P-450 system and enhance the toxicity of agents converted to active metabolites
Disease	
AIDS	Increased susceptibility to hepatotoxic effects of sulfamethoxazole–trimethoprim
Diabetes	Enhances toxicity of carbon tetrachloride
Hyperthyroidism	Enhances toxicity of carbon tetrachloride
Arthritis	Active rheumatoid arthritis, rheumatic fever, and systemic lupus erythematosus enhance the hepatic effects of aspirin

Source: Zimmerman HJ. Hepatotoxicity. Dis Mon 39:675–787, 1993.

Table 2.6 ▪ Drugs Implicated in Causing Chronic Active Hepatitis

Dantrolene
Diclofenac
Isoniazid
Nitrofurantoin
Methyldopa
Papaverine

Source: Zimmerman HJ. Hepatotoxicity. Dis Mon 39:675–787, 1993.

much better prognosis than does cytotoxic injury, with a mortality rate of less than 1%.[68]

Chronic liver damage consists of a group of disorders including chronic hepatitis, steatosis, pseudoalcoholic liver disease, granulomatous disease, and cirrhosis. Chronic lesions can result from continued or repeated exposure to hepatotoxic agents. Table 2.6 lists a number of drugs that have been implicated in causing chronic active hepatitis.[68]

Most cases of drug-induced hepatotoxicity involve the transformation of the parent drug to an active intermediate that may be inherently toxic or evoke an immune response. Some drugs implicated in hepatic injury include anesthetic agents (e.g., halothane), chlorpromazine, anticonvulsants (e.g., phenytoin and valproic acid), NSAIDs, and allopurinol. Herbal products and teas have also been implicated in several cases of severe hepatotoxicity.[70] The specific hepatotoxicity profiles associated with each of these agents are beyond the scope of this chapter. Health care practitioners should be aware that a plethora of agents could cause hepatotoxicity and that careful history taking is crucial in a patient who presents with nonspecific symptoms.[68]

Pancreatitis

Pancreatitis can be characterized as either acute or chronic. A literature review by Underwood and Frye[71] described that a large number of medications can cause acute pancreatitis, whereas few cause chronic pancreatitis. Clinical symptoms of pancreatitis include acute abdominal pain and increased blood and urine pancreatic enzyme concentrations. Morphologic changes in the pancreas itself are minor or absent. Based on a system originally developed by Mallory and Kern,[72] implicated drugs can be classified into three categories (Table 2.7). Table 2.8 summarizes the agents that have been shown to have a definite association with pancreatitis.[71–73]

Nephrotoxicity

Drug-induced nephrotoxicity depends on the concentration of drug presented to the kidney and the biochemical or physiologic effects of the drug on the tissue.[74] Factors that influence the concentration of given drugs in the kidney include mechanisms for the transport of drugs across the tubular epithelium, the rate of water versus drug reabsorption, plasma protein binding, and rate of urine

Table 2.7 ▪ Drug-Induced Pancreatitis

Criteria for Drug-Induced Pancreatitis

Pancreatitis developed during treatment with the drug.
Pancreatitis disappeared upon withdrawal of the drug.
Pancreatitis recurred upon rechallenge.

Elements of Classification

Definite	Literature report met all three criteria.
Probable	Literature reports did not meet all three criteria, but an association was thought to exist.
Doubtful	Published evidence was either inadequate or contradictory.

Source: Mallory A, Kern F. Drug-induced pancreatitis: a critical review. Gastroenterology 78:813–820, 1980.

Table 2.8 ▪ Examples of Drugs Suspected in Drug-Induced Pancreatitis

Drug	Comments
Asparaginase	Frequently reported to cause pancreatitis. Possible direct cytotoxic effect.
Azathioprine	Mechanism of injury unknown but thought to be related to the immunosuppressive effects of azathioprine.
Didanosine	Pancreatitis detected in 3–23% of patients in clinical reports. Dosages higher than 10 mg/kg/day are more likely to cause pancreatitis.
Estrogens	Estrogen use is known to cause hyperlipidemia, a risk factor for pancreatitis development.
Furosemide	Suggested direct toxic effect. A similar outcome was observed upon bumetanide administration.
Mercaptopurine	Mechanism may be Type II or Type IV hypersensitivity reaction.
Pentamidine	Mechanism may be direct toxic effect. Toxicity may be related to cumulative dosage. Also often administered after exposure to sulfonamides.
Sulfonamides	Pancreatitis accompanied by fever, chills, pruritus, and rash. Possible allergic reaction.
Sulindac	Most reports received through the voluntary reporting system. Strong correlation with rechallenge.
Tetracyclines	Occurred primarily in patients with preexisting liver disease.
Thiazides	Among the first class of drugs to be associated with pancreatitis. Possible direct toxic effect or electrolyte abnormalities (e.g., hypercalcemia).
Valproic acid	Can occur within normal dosages of the drug. Has occurred in children. Possible direct toxic effect or idiosyncratic reaction.

Source: Underwood TW, Frye CB. Drug-induced pancreatitis. Clin Pharm 12:440–448, 1993. Mallory A, Kern F. Drug-induced pancreatitis: a critical review. Gastroenterology 78:813–820, 1980. Wilmink T, Fric TW. Drug induced pancreatitis. Drug Saf 14:406–423, 1996.

flow. Some of the drugs most commonly associated with nephrotoxicity include the aminoglycosides, amphotericin B, cisplatin, cyclosporine, and NSAIDs.[75–79]

Four types of lesions are used to describe drug-induced kidney damage: acute tubular necrosis (ATN), acute tubulointerstitial disease (ATID), chronic tubulointerstitial disease (CTID), and glomerulonephritis (GN). A list of drugs associated with each of these lesions is provided in Table 2.9. A complete discussion of drug-induced nephrotoxicity can be found in Chapters 21 and 22.

From an ADR reporting system standpoint, drug-induced nephrotoxicity should be monitored closely because the majority of these ADRs are preventable. For example, underlying renal dysfunction necessitates a dosage adjustment of many drugs. Compromise to the nephron can be avoided by carefully monitoring drug concentrations and altering drug dosages accordingly.

Hematologic Disorders

Drug-induced hematologic disorders encompass a wide variety of disorders, only some of which are mechanistically understood. The reader is referred to the chapters in this book describing anemias, where aplastic anemia, agranulocytosis, hemolytic anemia, megaloblastic anemia, and thrombocytopenia are discussed. All of these hematologic disorders have been associated with ADRs.

Cardiovascular Effects

The scope of this topic is much larger than can be covered in a chapter focusing on ADRs. The reader is referred to the chapters in this book that discuss cardiovascular disorders and critical care issues. Cardiovascular adverse reactions require specific management.

ADRs involving the cardiovascular system are not specifically limited to agents used to treat cardiovascular disease. For example, bronchodilator therapy and sympathomimetic effects of various cough and cold remedies may negatively affect cardiac rate and rhythm regulation. Many antiarrhythmic agents may also be proarrhythmic.[80,81] Tricyclic antidepressants, in an overdose situation, cause electrocardiographic changes that can be life-threatening.[82] In addition to certain cardiac medications, bradycardia can also be induced by agents such as carbamazepine, methyldopa, and H_2 antagonists.[83–85] Some agents used in chemotherapy regimens, such as the anthracyclines, have a dose-limiting side effect of causing congestive cardiomyopathy.[86] Additionally, some diuretics and β-blockers may adversely affect lipid risk profiles, the clinical outcome of which remains to be elucidated.[87] In addition to the known risk of primary pulmonary hypertension,[88] more recently there have been concerns with valvular abnormalities associated with appetite-suppressant drugs,[89] leading to the withdrawal from the market of dexfenfluramine and fenfluramine. Careful monitoring of patients for cardiovascular ADRs is crucial because the potential for negative sequelae is enormous.

Pulmonary Effects

Pulmonary injury secondary to pharmacologic treatment has been associated with more than 150 medications.[90–92] Table 2.10 lists agents known to cause pulmonary disease. Four mechanisms of drug-induced pulmonary disease have been described: direct cytotoxic effect on alveolar endo-

Table 2.9 ▪ Drugs Associated with Nephrotoxicity

Acute Tubular Necrosis	**Glomerulonephritis**
Antibiotics:	Allopurinol
Aminoglycosides	Ampicillin
Amphotericin B	Captopril
Cephalosporins	Cyclophosphamide
Quinolones	Daunorubicin
Nitrofurantoin	Gold
Sulfonamides	Heroin
Tetracycline (outdated)	Mercury
Pentamidine	Methicillin
Radiocontrast media	NSAIDs
Miscellaneous agents:	Penicillamine
Acetaminophen	Penicillin
Carbamazepine	Rifampin
Cisplatin	Sulfonamides
Cyclosporine	Thiazides
Mephenytoin	Trimethadione
Quinine	**Chronic Tubulointerstitial Disease**
Quinidine	Acetaminophen
Tacrolimus	Aspirin
Diazepam	Lithium
Barbiturates	Methyl-CCNU
Codeine	Phenacetin
Ethanol	NSAIDs
Lovastatin	Cyclosporine
Ifosfamide	Tacrolimus
Mithramycin	**Miscellaneous Mechanisms**
Foscarnet	Prerenal azotemia
IVIG	NSAIDs
Hydralazine	**Renal Tubular Acidosis and Concentration Defects**
Methotrexate	Lithium
Methoxyflurane	Amphotericin B
Streptozocin	**Postrenal Obstruction**
Acute Tubulointerstitial Disease	Methysergide
Penicillins	Acyclovir
Other antibiotics:	Methotrexate
Cephalosporins	Ergotamine
Rifampin	Sulfonamides
Sulfonamides	Hydralazine
Ciprofloxacin	Methyldopa
NSAIDs	Pindolol
Miscellaneous:	Atenolol
Allopurinol	
Cytosine arabinoside	
Interferon	
Azathioprine	
Captopril	
Cimetidine	
Clofibrate	
Furosemide	
Phenytoin	
Thiazides	

Source: References 75–79.
NSAIDs, nonsteroidal anti-inflammatory drugs.

Table 2.10 ▪ Agents Known to Cause Pulmonary Disease

Cardiovascular	Anti-inflammatory	Chemotherapy
Amiodarone	Aspirin	Azathioprine
Angiotensin-converting enzyme inhibitors	Gold	Bleomycin
Anticoagulants	Methotrexate	Busulfan
β-Blockers	Nonsteroidal anti-inflammatory drugs	Chlorambucil
Dipyridamole	Penicillamine	Cyclophosphamide
Tocainide	**Miscellaneous**	Etoposide
Antibiotics	Bromocriptine	Melphalan
Amphotericin B	Dantrolene	Mitomycin
Nitrofurantoin	Oral contraceptives	Nitrosourea
Sulfasalazine	Hydrochlorothiazide	Procarbazine
Sulfonamides	Tricyclic antidepressants	Vinblastine
Pentamidine		Ifosfamide

Source: Rosenow EC III. Drug-induced pulmonary disease. Dis Mon 5:258–310, 1994.

thelial cells, deposition of phospholipid within the alveolar macrophages, oxidized injury by drugs, and immune-mediated injury (e.g., drug-induced SLE).[93]

Bronchospasm can occur commonly as a drug-induced effect. This ADR has been identified with all of the β-blockers and is reversible within 1 to 7 days of discontinuation. Symptoms include a dry, unproductive cough.[93] β-Blockade can precipitate asthmatic attacks. Even a cardioselective agent, such as atenolol or metoprolol, may precipitate bronchospasms and should be avoided in asthmatic patients if possible.[94] Aggravation of chronic obstructive pulmonary disease with subsequent death has been reported secondary to topical timolol because the drug can be systemically absorbed.[95] Angiotensin-converting enzyme (ACE) inhibitors cause cough in approximately 15% of the population, with a 2:1 ratio of women to men. Aspirin administration can also lead to bronchospasm in approximately 4 to 20% of all patients with asthma.[96] The pathogenesis is thought to be related to cyclooxygenase inhibition and subsequent destabilization of mast cells and bronchial smooth muscle constriction.[97] All NSAIDs, which inhibit cyclooxygenase, can also produce this reaction, and the degree of cross-reactivity is related to the degree of cyclooxygenase inhibition. These patients may also have increased levels of cysteinyl leukotrienes and increased airway reactivity to these agents. There is supporting information that 5-lipoxygenase inhibitors may improve pulmonary function in these patients.[98]

Noncardiogenic pulmonary edema can develop secondary to narcotic use, as cases have been reported with heroin, methadone, and propoxyphene administration. The mechanism of this reaction is unclear but could be related to a direct toxic effect on the alveolar–capillary membrane. Other possible mechanisms include hypoxemia, CNS effects resulting in a neurogenic pulmonary edema, and immunologic activation. The pulmonary edema generally improves within 24 to 48 hours and radiologic clearing results after approximately 2 to 4 days.[99]

Sexual Dysfunction

Normal sexual function is mediated by various physiologic mechanisms including neurogenic, psychogenic, vascular, and hormonal factors. These functions are coordinated by the hypothalamus, limbic system, and cerebral cortex. It is expected, then, that medications interfering with any of these systems may also interfere with sexual function.[100]

Sexual dysfunction is often associated with antihypertensive and antipsychotic medications. Antihypertensive agents are reported to be associated with sexual dysfunction more than any other type of drug. However, the majority of associations between antihypertensive therapy and sexual dysfunction are from case reports.[101] Thiazide diuretics, peripheral and central sympatholytics, and β-blockers have all been associated with a decline in sexual function. The adverse events include impotence, loss of libido, ejaculatory failure, and anorgasmia. Calcium channel blockers and ACE inhibitors appear to have a lower potential for causing sexual dysfunction.[102] Combination therapy appears to be associated with a higher incidence of sexual dysfunction than monotherapy.

Antipsychotic or antidepressant medications are also associated with a variety of effects on sexual function (e.g., impotence, priapism, anorgasmia, and diminished libido); however, ejaculatory failure is the most frequently reported.[102,103] All classes of antidepressants have been associated with some degree of sexual dysfunction.[104] These agents may impair sexual function through anticholinergic and sympatholytic activity, through effects on neurotransmitters or hormonal secretion (e.g., increased serum prolactin concentrations secondary to amoxapine), or by causing sedation.[102]

It is important to realize that the disease states for which these medications are prescribed may independently be associated with an alteration in normal sexual function. For example, sexual dysfunction has been shown to occur frequently (up to 17%) in untreated hypertensive men.[105] Hypertensive diabetics have an even higher incidence of impotence (25 to 60%).[106] With regard to the psychiatric population, impotence in untreated patients can be as high as 70% and varies with the particular diagnosis. The high incidence of sexual dysfunction associated with these disease states is an important consideration when evaluating the relationship of drug administration to an alteration in sexual function, and baseline data on sexual function before the institution of therapy may be helpful in differentiating disease and drug effects.

Additional medications that have been associated with sexual dysfunction, although less often than the aforementioned agents, are the H_2 antagonists (e.g., cimetidine, ranitidine, famotidine, and nizatidine), anticonvulsants (e.g., carbamazepine, phenytoin, phenobarbital, and primidone), antiarrhythmic agents (amiloride, disopyramide, and digoxin), NSAIDs (e.g., indomethacin and naproxen), benzodiazepines (e.g., alprazolam, diazepam, and lorazepam), baclofen, bromocriptine, clofibrate, ketoconazole, metoclopramide, and opioids when used chronically.[102]

PHARMACOECONOMICS

Drug-related morbidity and mortality costs $30 to $136 billion annually in the United States,[1,107] making it one of the more costly diseases.[107] It has been estimated that in hospitalized patients, ADRs increase length of stay by approximately 2 days and increase hospital cost by $2000.[1] The cost of drug-related morbidity and mortality in nursing facilities alone has been estimated to be $7.6 billion.[108] It has also been estimated that consultant pharmacy services may decrease this cost by 47%.[108]

CONCLUSION

ADRs are an important cause of morbidity and mortality. Drug-induced disease is common in certain patient populations, such as older adults, newborns, HIV-infected patients, and patients with impaired hepatic or renal function. Many ADRs are both reversible and preventable. Because they are reversible, early identification and treatment are of great importance. The preventable nature of adverse reactions is the motivation for current reporting programs. It is through reporting that high-risk patient populations are identified so that certain medications can be avoided. The monitoring programs currently in place rely on voluntary reporting from health care professionals and mandatory reporting from pharmaceutical manufacturers. The increased complexity of drug therapy requires increased vigilance on the part of health care practitioners. In many cases the pharmacist is in a unique position to safeguard the patient from preventable ADRs.

KEY POINTS

- ADRs significantly increase patient morbidity and mortality.
- Recognition and reporting of ADRs is a high priority of the JCAHO and the FDA.
- An ADR is any response to a drug that is noxious and unintended and occurs at normal dosages.
- ADRs must be classified in terms of severity, causality, and preventability.
- MedWatch is the FDA reporting system for ADRs.
- Patient variables that influence the likelihood of developing an ADR include age, underlying disorder, and genetic factors.
- Drug classes frequently involved in ADRs include antibiotics, anticoagulants, anticonvulsants, cardiovascular agents, respiratory, and pain medications.
- Many drug reactions are erroneously called hypersensitivity or allergic reactions.
- Virtually every organ system in the body can be affected by an ADR.

REFERENCES

1. Holland EG, De Gruy FA. Drug-induced disorders. Am Fam Physician 56:1781–1788, 1997.
2. Lazarou J, Pomeranz BH, Corey PN. Incidence of adverse drug reactions in hospitalized patients. A meta-analysis of prospective studies. JAMA 279:1200–1205, 1998.
3. Einarson TR. Drug-related hospital admissions. Ann Pharmacother 27:832–840, 1993.
4. Prince BS, Goetz CM, Rihn TL, et al. Drug-related emergency department visits and hospital admissions. Am J Hosp Pharm 49:1696–1700, 1992.
5. Karch FE, Lasagna L. Adverse drug reactions: a critical review. JAMA 234:1236–1241, 1975.
6. Fincham JE. An overview of adverse drug reactions. Am Pharm NS31:47–52, 1991.
7. Berkow R, ed. The Merck manual of diagnosis and therapy. 16th ed. Rahway, NJ: Merck Research Laboratories, 1992:2642–2644.
8. Anderson JA. Allergic reactions to drugs and biological agents. JAMA 268:2845–2857, 1992.
9. Anonymous. ASHP guidelines on adverse drug reaction monitoring and reporting. Am J Hosp Pharm 46:336–337, 1989.
10. Naranjo CA, Busto U, Sellers EM, et al. A method for estimating the probability of adverse drug reactions. Clin Pharmacol Ther 30:239–245, 1981.
11. Pearson TF, Pittman DG, Longley JM, et al. Factors associated with preventable adverse drug reactions. Am J Hosp Pharm 51:2268–2272, 1994.
12. Burnum JF. Preventability of adverse drug reactions [Letter]. Ann Intern Med 85:80, 1976.
13. Melmon KL. Preventable drug reactions - causes and cures. N Engl J Med 284:1361–1368, 1971.
14. Faich GA. National adverse drug reaction reporting: 1984–1989. Arch Intern Med 151:1645–1647, 1991.
15. Rossi AC, Knapp DE. Discovery of new adverse drug reactions. A review of the Food and Drug Administration's spontaneous reporting system. JAMA 252:1030–1033, 1984.
16. McQueen K. ADR monitoring: rationale, impact and cost issues. Calif J Hosp Pharm 2:5–7, 1990.
17. Goldman SA, Kennedy DL. MedWatch: FDA's medical products reporting program. A joint effort toward improved public health. Postgrad Med 103:13–16, 1998.
18. Edlavitch SA. Adverse drug event reporting. Improving the low US reporting rates [Editorial]. Arch Intern Med 148:1499–1503, 1998.
19. Baum C, Anello C. The spontaneous reporting system in the United States. In: Strom BL, ed. Pharmacoepidemiology. New York: Churchill Livingstone, 1989:107–118.
20. White GG, Love L. The MedWatch program. Clin Toxicol 36:145–149, 1998.
21. The special nutritional adverse event monitoring system. 1998, Nov 17 [cited Dec 1, 1998]. Available from http://www.fda.gov.
22. Ellenberg SS, Chen RT. The complicated task of monitoring vaccine safety. Public Health Rep 112:10–20, 1997.
23. Johnson JM. Contributing to drug safety [Editorial]. Am J Hosp Pharm 47:1280, 1990.
24. Hoffman RP. Adverse drug reaction revisited - JCAHO. Hosp Pharm 23:685–686, 1988.
25. Seeger JD, Kong SX, Shumock GT. Characteristics associated with ability to prevent adverse drug reactions in hospitalized patients. Pharmacotherapy 18:1284–1289, 1998.
26. Raschkle RA, Gollihare B, Wunderlich TA, et al. A computer alert system to prevent injury from adverse drug events. Development and evaluation in a community teaching hospital. JAMA 280:1317–1320, 1998.
27. Corr K, Stoller R. Adverse drug event reporting at Veterans Affairs facilities. Am J Health Syst Pharm 53:314–315, 1996.
28. Stang PE, Fox JL. Adverse drug events and the Freedom of Information Act: an apple in Eden. Ann Pharmacother 26:238–243, 1992.

29. Edwards IR, Biriell C. Harmonisation in pharmacovigilance. Drug Saf 10:93–102, 1994.
30. Auriche M, Loupi E. Does proof of causality ever exist in pharmacovigilance? Drug Saf 9:230–235, 1993.
31. Sigmund W. Dear Healthcare Professional Letter: Rezulin. 1997. December 1 [cited Dec 1, 1998]. Available from http://www.FDA.gov/medwatch/safety/1997/rezul3.html.
32. Roche Laboratories announces withdrawal of Posicor from the market. FDA Talk Paper 1998, Jun 8 [cited Dec 1, 1998]. Available from http://www.fda.gov/bbs/topics/ANSWERS/ANS00876.html.
33. Wyeth-Ayerst Laboratories announces the withdrawal of Duract from the market. FDA Talk Paper 1998, Jun 22 [cited Dec 1, 1998] Available from http://www.fda.gov/bbs/topics/ANSWERS/ANS00879.html.
34. Ellison RH. Written communication. Nov. 17, 1998. Roche Laboratories. Nutley, NJ.
35. Postmarketing safety of sildenafil citrate (Viagra). [cited Dec 1, 1998] Available from http://www.fda.gov/cder/consumerinfo/viagra/safety3.html.
36. Mannesse CK, Derkx FHM, de Ridder MAJ, et al. Adverse drug reactions in elderly patients as contributing factor for hospital admission: cross sectional study. BMJ 315:1057–1058, 1997.
37. French EH. ADRs and metabolic changes in the elderly. US Pharmacist 5:H1–H28, 1994.
38. Greenblatt DJ, Sellers EM, Shader RI. Drug disposition in old age. N Engl J Med 306:1081–1088, 1982.
39. Brawn LA, Castleden CM. Adverse drug reactions: an overview of special considerations in the management of the elderly patient. Drug Saf 5:421–435, 1990.
40. Rowe JW, Andres R, Tobin JP, et al. The effects of age on creatinine clearance in man: a cross sectional and longitudinal study. J Gerontol 31:155–163, 1976.
41. Knight M. Adverse drug reaction in neonates. J Clin Pharmacol 34:128–135, 1994.
42. Toddywalla VS, Patel SB, Betrabet SS, et al. Can chronic maternal drug therapy alter the nursing infant's hepatic drug metabolizing enzyme pattern? J Clin Pharmacol 35:1025–1029, 1995.
43. Gupta A, Waldhauser LK. Adverse drug reactions from birth to early childhood. Pediatr Clin North Am 44:79–92, 1997.
44. Kapusnik-Uner JE, Sande MA, Chambers HF. Tetracyclines, chloramphenicol, erythromycin, and miscellaneous antibacterial agents. In: Hardman JG, Gilman AG, Limbird LE, eds. Goodman and Gilman's the pharmacological basis of therapeutics. New York: McGraw-Hill, 1996:1123–1154.
45. Hendeles L, Jenkins J, Temple R. Revised FDA labeling guideline for theophylline oral dosage forms. Pharmacotherapy 15:409–427, 1995.
46. Bayard PJ, Berger TG, Jacobson MA. Drug hypersensitivity reactions and human immunodeficiency virus disease. J Acquir Immune Defic Syndr 5:1237–1257, 1992.
47. Peters BS, Carlin E, Weston RJ, et al. Adverse effects of drugs used in the management of opportunistic infections associated with HIV infection. Drug Saf 10:439–454, 1994.
48. Harb GE, Jacobson M. Human immunodeficiency virus (HIV) infection. Does it increase susceptibility to adverse drug reactions? Drug Saf 9:1–8, 1993.
49. Gordin FM, Simon GL, Wofsy CB, et al. Adverse reactions to trimethoprim–sulfamethoxazole in patients with the acquired immunodeficiency syndrome. Ann Intern Med 100:495–499, 1984.
50. Jick H. Adverse reactions to trimethoprim–sulfamethoxazole in hospitalized patients. Rev Infect Dis 4:426–428, 1982.
51. Anonymous. Drugs for HIV infection. Med Lett Drugs Ther 39:111–116, 1997.
52. Goedde HW. Ethnic differences in reactions to drugs and other xenobiotics: outlooks of a geneticist. In: Kalow W, Goedde HS, Agerwal DP, eds. Ethnic differences in reactions to drugs and xenobiotics. New York: Alan R. Liss, 1986.
53. Benetz LZ, Kroetz DL, Sheiner LB. Pharmacokinetics. The dynamics of drug absorption, distribution, and elimination. In: Hardman JG, Gilman AG, Limbird LE, eds. Goodman and Gilman's the pharmacological basis of therapeutics. New York: McGraw-Hill, 1996:3–28.
54. Florence AT, Jani PU. Novel oral drug formulation. Their potential in modulating adverse effects. Drug Saf 10:233–266, 1994.
55. Witztum JL. Drugs used in the treatment of hyperlipoproteinemias. In: Hardman JG, Gilman AG, Limbird LE, eds. Goodman and Gilman's the pharmacological basis of therapeutics. New York: McGraw-Hill, 1996:875–897.
56. Carson JL, Willett LR. Toxicity of nonsteroidal anti-inflammatory drugs: an overview of the epidemiological evidence. Drugs 46(suppl 1):243–248, 1993.
57. Meperidine. In: McEvoy GK, ed. AHFS drug information. Bethesda, MD: American Society of Health-System Pharmacists, 1998.
58. Preston SL, Briceland LL, Lesar TS. Accuracy of penicillin allergy reporting. Am J Hosp Pharm 51:79–84, 1994.
59. Lin RY. A perspective on penicillin allergy. Arch Intern Med 152:930–937, 1992.
60. Lachmann PJ, Peters DK, eds. Clinical aspects of immunology, 4th ed. Boston: Blackwell Scientific, 1982.
61. Kishiyama JL, Adelman DC. The cross-reactivity and immunology of beta-lactam antibiotics. Drug Saf 10:318–327, 1994.
62. Thompson JW, Jacobs RF. Adverse effects of newer cephalosporins. An update. Drug Saf 9:132–142, 1993.
63. Saxon A, Adelman DC, Patel A, et al. Imipenem cross-reactivity with penicillin in humans. J Allergy Clin Immunol 82:213–217, 1988.
64. Package insert. Merrem (Meropenem). Zeneca. Wilmington, DE, 1998.
65. Døssing M, Sonne J. Drug-induced hepatic disorders. Incidence, management and avoidance. Drug Saf 9:441–449, 1993.
66. Maddrey WC. Hepatic effects of acetaminophen: enhanced toxicity in alcoholics. J Clin Gastroenterol 9:180–185, 1987.
67. Anker AL, Smilkstein MJ. Acetaminophen. Concepts and controversies. Emerg Med Clin North Am 12:335–349, 1994.
68. Zimmerman HJ. Hepatotoxicity. Dis Mon 39:675–787, 1993.
69. Lee WM. Drug-induced hepatotoxicity. N Engl J Med 333:1118–1127, 1995.
70. Larrey D, Vial T, Pauwels A, et al. Hepatitis after germander *(teucrium chamaedrys)* administration: another instance of herbal medicine hepatotoxicity. Ann Intern Med 117:129–132, 1992.
71. Underwood TW, Frye CB. Drug-induced pancreatitis. Clin Pharm 12:440–448, 1993.
72. Mallory A, Kern F. Drug-induced pancreatitis: a critical review. Gastroenterology 78:813–820, 1980.
73. Wilmink T, Fric TW. Drug-induced pancreatitis. Drug Saf 14:406–423, 1996.
74. Walker RJ, Duggin GG. Drug nephrotoxicity. Annu Rev Pharmacol Toxicol 28:331–345, 1988.
75. Schlondorff D. Renal complications of nonsteroidal anti-inflammatory drugs. Kidney Int 44:643–653, 1993.
76. Clive DM, Stoff JS. Renal syndromes associated with nonsteroidal antiinflammatory drugs. N Engl J Med 310:563–572, 1984.
77. Whelton A, Hamilton CW. Nonsteroidal anti-inflammatory drugs: effects on kidney function. J Clin Pharmacol 31:588–598, 1991.
78. Humes HD. Aminoglycoside nephrotoxicity. Kidney Int 33:900–911, 1988.
79. Choudhury D, Ahmed Z. Drug induced nephrotoxicity. Med Clin North Am 81:705–717, 1997.
80. CAST (Cardiac Arrhythmia Suppression Trial) Investigators. Preliminary report: effect of encainide or flecainide on mortality in a randomized trial of arrhythmia suppression after myocardial infarction. N Engl J Med 321:406–412, 1989.
81. Roden DM. Risks and benefits of antiarrhythmic therapy. N Engl J Med 331:785–791, 1994.
82. Pellinen TJ, Farkkilae M, Keikrila J, et al. Electrocardiographic and clinical factors of tricyclic antidepressant intoxication. Ann Clin Res 19:12, 1987.
83. Benassi E, Bo G, Cocito L, et al. Carbamazepine and cardiac conduction disturbances. Ann Neurol 22:280–281, 1987.
84. Rosen B, Ovsyshcher IA, Zimlichman R. Complete atrioventricular block induced by methyldopa. PACE Pacing Clin Electrophysiol 11:1555–1558, 1988.
85. Hart A. Cardiac arrest associated with ranitidine. BMJ 299:519, 1989.
86. Rhoden W, Hasleton P, Brooks N. Anthracyclines and the heart. Br Heart J 70:499–502, 1993.
87. Henkin Y, Como JA, Oberman A. Secondary dyslipidemia. Inadvertent effects of drugs in clinical practice. JAMA 267:961–968, 1992.
88. Abenhaim A, Moride Y, Brenot F, et al. Appetite-suppressant drugs and the risk of primary pulmonary hypertension. N Engl J Med 335:609–619, 1996.
89. Khan MA, Herzog CA, St Peter JV, et al. The prevalence of cardiac valvular insufficiency assessed by transthoracic echocardiography in obese patients treated with appetite-suppressant drugs. N Engl J Med 339:713–718, 1998.
90. Rosenow EC, Myers JL, Swensen SJ, et al. Drug-induced pulmonary disease: an update. Chest 102:239–250, 1992.
91. Gregory AS, Grippi MA. The clinical diagnosis of drug-induced pulmonary disorders. J Thorac Imaging 6:8–18, 1991.
92. Goodwin SD, Glenny RW. Nonsteroidal anti-inflammatory drug-associated pulmonary infiltrates with eosinophilia. Review of literature and Food and Drug Administration adverse drug reaction reporting. Arch Intern Med 152:1521–1524, 1992.
93. Rosenow EC. Drug-induced pulmonary disease. Dis Mon 5:258–310, 1994.
94. Hoffman BB, Lefkowitz RJ. Catecholamines, sympathomimetic drugs, and adrenergic receptor antagonists. In: Hardman JG, Gilman AG, Limbird LE,

eds. Goodman and Gilman's the pharmacological basis of therapeutics. New York: McGraw-Hill, 1996:199–248.

95. Dunn TL, Gerber MJ, Shen AS, et al. The effect of topical ophthalmic instillation of timolol and betaxolol on lung function in asthmatic subjects. Am Rev Respir Dis 133:264–268, 1986.
96. Settipane GA. Aspirin and allergic disease: a review. Am J Med 74(suppl 6a):102–109, 1983.
97. Szczeklik A, Grylewski RJ. Asthma and anti-inflammatory drugs. Mechanisms and clinical patterns. Drugs 25:533–543, 1983.
98. Holgate ST, Bradding P, Sampson AP. Leukotriene antagonists and synthesis inhibitors: new directions in asthma therapy. J Allergy Clin Immunol 98:1–13, 1996
99. Cooper JAD, White DA, Matthay RA. Drug-induced pulmonary disease. Part 2: noncytotoxic drugs. Am Rev Respir Dis 133:488–505, 1986.
100. Smith PJ, Talbert RL. Sexual dysfunction with antihypertensive and antipsychotic agents. Clin Pharm 5:373–384, 1986.
101. Prisant LM, Carr AA, Bottini PB, et al. Sexual dysfunction with antihypertensive drugs. Arch Intern Med 154:730–736, 1994.
102. Anonymous. Drugs that cause sexual dysfunction: an update. Med Lett Drugs Ther 34:73–78, 1992.
103. Deamer RL, Thompson JF. The role of medications in geriatric sexual function. Clin Geriatr Med 7:95–110, 1991.
104. Woodrum ST, Brown CS. Management of SSRI-induced sexual dysfunction. Ann Pharmacother 32:1209–1215, 1998.
105. Bulpitt CJ, Dollery CT, Carne S. Change in symptoms of hypertensive patients after referral to hospital clinic. Br Heart J 38:121–128, 1976.
106. Buvat J, Lamaire A, Buvat-Herbaut M, et al. Comparative investigations in 26 impotent and 26 nonimpotent diabetic patients. J Urol 133:34–38, 1985.
107. Johnson JA, Bootman JL. Drug-related morbidity and mortality. A cost-of-illness model. Arch Intern Med 155:1949–1956, 1995.
108. Bootman JL, Harrison DL, Cox E. The health care cost of drug-related morbidity and mortality in nursing facilities. Arch Intern Med 157:2089–2096, 1997.

CHAPTER 3

DRUG INTERACTIONS

David S. Tatro

DEFINITION

A drug interaction can be defined as the modification of the effects of one drug (i.e., the object drug) by the prior or concomitant administration of another (i.e., the precipitant drug).[1] Adverse drug interactions can cause a loss in therapeutic effect, toxicity, or unexpected increases in pharmacologic activity. The basic definition of a drug interaction should focus on patient outcomes that are of potential clinical importance, not on additive or beneficial effects occurring with simultaneous drug administration. Thus, one should be seeking a response that is greater than the sum of the independent actions of the drugs (i.e., potentiation) or an action that is less than expected (i.e., antagonism).

This chapter does not consider physical or chemical interactions (i.e., intravenous incompatibilities) or beneficial interactions (i.e., clinically useful or intended interactions such as coadministration of probenecid and penicillin).

The goal of this chapter is to review drug interactions in a context that will allow application of this knowledge to patient care. Clinically important examples are used to assist the reader in the detection, assessment, and prevention of drug interactions. Drug and patient factors that increase the risk of occurrence of a drug interaction are presented. Limitations of the drug interaction literature are reviewed.

At the conclusion of this chapter, the reader should be able to

- Define a drug interaction
- Describe the mechanisms by which drug interactions occur, including the distinction between pharmacokinetic and pharmacodynamic interactions
- Differentiate between enzyme substrates, inducers, and inhibitors
- Provide examples of drug interactions caused by enzyme induction or inhibition and demonstrate how to avoid or manage these interactions
- Discuss the limitations of available drug interaction literature
- Identify characteristics most likely to predispose patients to the risk of the occurrence of a clinically important drug interaction
- Identify general strategies for the management or avoidance of drug interactions

EPIDEMIOLOGY

In a study involving 9900 patients with 83,200 drug exposures, 234 (6.5%) of 3600 adverse drug reactions were attributed to drug interactions.[2] The incidence of potential drug interactions has been observed to be 17% in surgical patients, 22% in patients on medical wards, 19% in nursing home patients, and 23% in outpatient clinics.[3–6] In a prospective study involving 2422 patients, 113 patients were taking potentially interacting drugs; however, only 7 patients developed clinical evidence of a drug interaction (0.3% of the total number of patients).[7] This does not preclude the more common occurrence of certain clinically important drug interactions.[8]

Knowledge of drug interactions may allow early recognition and prevention of adverse consequences. The most comprehensive understanding of clinically important drug interactions can be achieved by combining knowledge of the mechanisms with the recognition of high-risk patients and the identification of drugs with a narrow therapeutic index.[9]

MECHANISMS

Understanding the pharmacology of a drug and the mechanism by which a drug may interact can assist in prediction or early recognition of a drug interaction. In a drug interaction, the drug for which the effect is altered (either increased or decreased) is called the object drug, and the drug that induces the interaction is the precipitant drug.

Drug interactions often are characterized as being either pharmacokinetic or pharmacodynamic. Pharmacokinetic interactions influence the disposition of a drug in the body and involve the effects of one drug on the absorption, distribution, metabolism, and excretion of another. Because of large interpatient and intrapatient variability in drug disposition, pharmacokinetic interactions seldom produce serious clinical consequences. Although the percentage of patients who experience serious effects of these drug interactions is small, there are numerous examples of these interactions resulting in devastating consequences. Pharmacokinetic interactions often are associated with changes in plasma drug concentrations, and, when feasible, observing the clinical status of the patient and monitoring serum drug concentrations may provide useful information about potential interactions. Pharmacodynamic interactions are related to the pharmacologic activity of the interacting drugs. This category is the most common mechanism by which drugs interact. Mechanisms of pharmacodynamic interactions include synergism, antagonism, altered cellular transport, and effects on receptor sites.

Pharmacokinetic Interactions

Pharmacokinetic interactions are characterized by changes in the kinetics of the object drug, including absorption, distribution, metabolism, and excretion.

Altered Gastrointestinal Absorption

Changes in drug absorption from the gastrointestinal (GI) tract can result from various mechanisms, including altered pH, altered bacterial flora, formation of drug chelates or complexes, drug-induced mucosal damage, and altered GI motility. These changes may produce a decrease or increase in drug absorption. The former is the most common. Interactions affecting absorption often require the simultaneous presence of both drugs in the stomach; therefore, separating the administration times of the two agents by at least 2 hours often prevents these interactions. Drug interactions affecting the absorption rate of a drug are most clinically important when the drug has a short half-life or when a rapid peak plasma concentration is needed to achieve a therapeutic effect.[9] In the latter instance, a decrease in the rate of absorption of the object drug may produce subtherapeutic concentrations. Unless the bioavailability of a drug is altered, interactions changing the absorption rate of a drug with a long half-life usually are of little clinical consequence. Cancer patients receiving chemotherapy may experience drug-induced mucosal damage, decreasing the bioavailability of poorly absorbed medications.[9]

Altered pH

The nonionized form of a drug is more lipid soluble and more readily absorbed from the GI tract into the systemic circulation than the ionized form. Most drugs are weak acids or bases. Therefore, acidic drugs that have dissolved tend to be absorbed in the upper portion of the GI tract, where they are in an acidic medium. The opposite is true of weak bases. Drugs such as antacids that increase the gastric pH may delay the absorption of certain drugs (e.g., ketoconazole).

CLINICAL CONSIDERATION. Clinically important interactions occurring by this mechanism are rare. This interaction may be avoided by adjusting the administration times of the two agents. Separating the administration times of each agent by at least 2 hours often prevents these interactions.

CLINICALLY IMPORTANT EXAMPLES. Administering antacids (e.g., sodium bicarbonate) with ketoconazole may decrease the absorption of the antifungal agent by reducing tablet dissolution.[10,11] If antacids are administered during ketoconazole therapy, the antacid should be given at least 2 hours after the antifungal agent.[10] In addition to antacids, H_2-antagonists may reduce ketoconazole tablet dissolution.[12]

Altered Intestinal Bacterial Flora

Antibiotic administration may decrease the number of bacteria in the GI tract. The greatest numbers of bacteria are found in the large intestine. Some drugs have been shown to be affected by changes in the intestinal flora.[13]

CLINICAL CONSIDERATIONS. This mechanism of interaction appears to be rare. Drug interactions resulting from changes in the intestinal bacterial flora tend to involve drugs that are incompletely absorbed from the upper GI tract or undergo enterohepatic recirculation.[13] The onset and reversal of this interaction are delayed, requiring up to several weeks. Thus, adjusting the administration times of the two drugs would not alter interactions occurring by this mechanism.

CLINICALLY IMPORTANT EXAMPLE. In approximately 10% of the patients receiving digoxin, 40% or more of an orally administered dose of the drug is metabolized by GI flora to inactive digoxin reduction products.[10,14,15] Clarithromycin and erythromycin appear to reverse this process by altering GI bacteria, allowing more digoxin to be absorbed. Digoxin toxicity may occur.[15–17] The effects of this interaction may persist for weeks to months after erythromycin is discontinued.

Complexation or Chelation

Certain drugs (e.g., tetracycline) can combine with other drugs (e.g., iron preparations) or food (e.g., milk) in the GI tract to form poorly absorbed complexes.

CLINICAL CONSIDERATIONS. Although different mechanisms may cause changes in the absorption of the object drug from the GI tract, clinically important interactions are uncommon. Administering the object drug in the absence of the precipitant will minimize the occurrence of this interaction. Therefore, it may be necessary to lengthen the interval between administration of the two drugs by as much as possible, preferably by 2 to 4 hours.

Clinically Important Examples. Administering an aluminum–magnesium hydroxide antacid with ciprofloxacin may drastically decrease the absorption of the antibiotic by about 85%, resulting in a decrease in the pharmacologic effect.[10] If antacids are administered during ciprofloxacin therapy, the antacid should be given at least 6 hours before or 2 hours after the antibiotic dose. Magnesium and aluminum cations in the buffers in didanosine tablets decrease GI absorption of ciprofloxacin by forming a chelate with the antibiotic.[18] Tetracycline forms an insoluble chelate with iron salts, decreasing absorption and serum levels of both drugs.[10] The anti-infective response may be decreased. A similar mechanism has been proposed for the decreased absorption of ciprofloxacin and norfloxacin that occurs when coadministering sucralfate and antacids.[19–21] The binding resin cholestyramine decreases the absorption of exogenously administered thyroid by binding thyroid hormone in the GI tract.[21] Other agents that can interfere with drug absorption by binding to the object drug or by forming complexes or chelates with the object drug include activated charcoal, antacids, colestipol, and various polyvalent cations (e.g., iron salts).

Drug-Induced Mucosal Damage

Drugs that damage the GI mucosa may reduce the absorption of certain drugs.[9,22]

Clinical Considerations. Antineoplastic agents are most commonly implicated. This mechanism remains to be confirmed.

Clinically Important Example. Reduced GI absorption of certain digoxin preparations has been attributed to alterations in the intestinal mucosa induced by chemotherapy regimens (e.g., cyclophosphamide, vincristine, procarbazine, plus prednisone).[23,24] The effects of this interaction appear to be minimized by administering digoxin capsules or digitoxin.[24,25]

Altered Motility

Increased absorption can occur when the drug is retained at the site of optimal absorption for a prolonged period of time. Because of the large absorptive area of the small intestine, it is the primary site of drug absorption from the GI tract. Changes in GI motility may increase or decrease absorption. Increasing GI motility may decrease absorption by reducing the amount of time that an orally administered drug is in contact with the absorbing surface.[22] A decrease in bioavailability may result from slowing dissolution or delaying gastric emptying.

Clinical Considerations. Clinically important interactions caused by this mechanism are rare. Interactions occurring as a result of altered GI motility result from systemically administering the precipitant drug. Therefore, separating the administration times of the interacting drugs would not prevent this interaction.

Clinically Important Examples. The increase in cyclosporine absorption that occurs when concurrently administering metoclopramide has been attributed to an increase in stomach emptying time. This may result in an increase in the immunologic and toxic effects of cyclosporine.[26] Conversely, by increasing GI motility, metoclopramide may decrease the absorption of orally administered digoxin.[27] This interaction may not occur with digoxin formulations that have high bioavailability (e.g., digoxin capsules or elixir).[28] Anticholinergic drugs are an example of a class of drugs that slow GI transit time.

Displaced Protein Binding

Many drugs are reversibly bound to plasma proteins. Concurrently administering more than one drug bound to the same protein fraction may displace either agent from its binding site, increasing the free concentration of the displaced drug. The drug with the highest affinity (i.e., association constant) for the binding site will displace the drug with the lower association constant.[13] After displacement from the protein-binding site, there is immediate redistribution to the tissues. Subsequently, there is a compensatory increase in metabolism or excretion, resulting in a steady-state free plasma concentration similar to the level that existed before the displacement.[22,29] Drugs bound to plasma protein are pharmacologically inactive because they are not available to extravascular receptor sites. In addition, the bound form is not available for metabolism or excretion. Thus, once the object drug is displaced from the protein-binding site, not only is more drug free to exert its pharmacologic action, but additional drug becomes available for metabolism, excretion, and redistribution to other tissues. The absolute concentration of unbound drug is called the free concentration, and the fraction of the total concentration of unbound drug is the free fraction.[13] The total plasma concentration of drug is the sum of the bound form and the free (unbound) drug. When drug is released from plasma protein, the increase in free drug concentration that occurs is transient. As the free fraction increases, it becomes available for metabolism, and the total drug concentration decreases. Because drugs that are highly bound to plasma protein tend to remain in the vascular space, the volume of distribution of these drugs often is small.[13] An equilibrium is maintained between the free drug in the circulation and the protein-bound drug, and as the drug is metabolized and excreted, the agent is released from its protein-binding site. The fact that one drug displaces another is not sufficient to predict the pharmacologic outcome of a potential interaction. The overall pharmacologic effect of protein displacement usually is minimal. Clinically important interactions may result from protein displacement if displacement is accompanied by enzyme inhibition or if the displaced drug has a small apparent volume of distribution, narrow therapeutic index, and rapid onset of action.[9]

Plasma proteins act as a storage site or reservoir, limiting extravascular distribution. Examples of protein-binding sites are listed in Table 3.1.[13]

The systemic clearance of certain drugs (e.g., lidocaine, propranolol) is independent of protein binding. Because both the bound and unbound forms of these drugs are removed from the plasma, their clearance is determined by hepatic blood flow. Thus, changes in protein binding do not affect the clearance of these drugs.

Clinical Considerations. Clinically important drug interactions involving displacement from protein binding are uncommon because once the object drug is displaced from plasma protein, it is rapidly cleared from the body.[8] Important interactions occur when displacement is accompanied by enzyme inhibition, as occurs when coadministering warfarin and phenylbutazone. In addition, a protein displacement interaction may be clinically important if the displaced drug has a small apparent volume of distribution, narrow therapeutic index, and rapid onset of action.[9]

Clinical Examples. Examples of drugs that are highly protein bound include phenytoin (90%), tolbutamide (96%), and warfarin (99%).[8] Common precipitant drugs include sulfonamides (e.g., sulfisoxazole), aspirin, and phenylbutazone.[8,29] The metabolite of chloral hydrate, trichloroacetic acid, displaces warfarin from its protein-binding site, increasing the hypoprothrombinemic effect of warfarin.[30,31] However, the effect is slight and transient. By continually administering both drugs, the free warfarin levels return to the concentrations that existed before the interaction. Although phenylbutazone displaces warfarin from plasma protein, it also inhibits the metabolism of the more potent S (–) warfarin enantiomorph, increasing the anticoagulant response to warfarin.[32,33]

Altered Metabolism

The effects of one drug on the metabolism of a second are well documented. Concurrently administering one drug with another may lead to an increase or decrease in the metabolic rate. These modifications may affect the intensity and duration of activity. The major site of drug metabolism is the liver; however, other tissues, including white blood cells, skin, lung, and GI tract, are involved in drug metabolism. Drug-metabolizing enzymes primarily convert lipophilic drugs into water-soluble metabolites, which may be excreted more readily. Drug metabolism may be divided into two types: Phase I, which includes hydroxylation, oxidation, and reduction, and Phase II, which includes glucuronide, glycine, and sulfate conjugation. Phase II metabolism often is preceded by Phase I, preparing the drug for conjugation.[34] The major hepatic enzyme system consists of the microsomal P-450 mixed-function oxygenases; however, there are numerous forms of cytochrome P-450 (CYP).[9] It is estimated that there are between 20 and 200 different CYP human genes.[34] According to the current classification, the entire group represents a superfamily consisting of families (designated by an arabic or roman numeral) and subfamilies (designated by a capital letter) based on the similarity of the amino acid sequences of the encoded P-450 isozyme protein.[34,35] The individual gene is designated by an arabic numeral.[34,35] Of the CYP genes that have been identified, families CYP1 (or CYPI), CYP2, CYP3, and CYP4 are involved with drug metabolism.[34] Numerous drugs have been identified as substrates for the metabolism by subfamilies of these CYP enzymes (Table 3.2).[10,34–57] However, it is not known which CYP isozyme is responsible for oxidation of most drugs. Over the past 15 years, the CYP2D6 isozyme has been the most extensively studied. This enzyme is not present in 5 to 10% of Caucasians, who have been designated as poor metabolizers. More than one isozyme may be involved in the metabolism of a drug (e.g., propafenone). Furthermore, a drug may act as a competitive inhibitor of one isozyme while being metabolized by another.[34] For example, quinidine inhibits the CYP2D6 isozyme but is metabolized (i.e., oxidized) by CYP3A4. Drug interactions involving this enzyme system occur only if both drugs bind to the active site of the same form of the enzyme. Because of interpatient and intrapatient variability, it is difficult to anticipate the clinical importance of potential interactions that occur by alterations in metabolism.

Increased Metabolism (Enzyme Induction)

This interaction mechanism results from increased production of drug-metabolizing enzymes (i.e., enzyme-binding sites) and involves primarily Phase I metabolism.[13] Because protein synthesis is involved, this interaction typically has a slow onset and may require up to 3 weeks before the maximum effect is observed. Although the precipitant drug usually induces the enzymes that enhance the metabolism of the object drug, some drugs (e.g., carbamazepine) increase their own metabolism. When the drug responsible for enzyme induction (i.e., the precipitant drug) is discontinued, the process reverses. However, reversal of enzyme induction often is a slower process than the onset. As the number of enzymes decreases, the serum concentration of the object drug gradually increases if the dosage is not decreased. Thus, for example, in patients

Table 3.1 ▪ Drug Protein-Binding Sites

Binding Site	Drug
Plasma protein	
Albumin	Warfarin
α-1-acid glycoprotein	Amitriptyline Disopyramide Lidocaine Propranolol
Lipoprotein	Cyclosporine
Transcortin	Corticosteroids
Tissue	
Sodium–potassium adenosine triphosphatase	Digoxin

Table 3.2 ▪ Drugs Identified as Being Substrates for CYP Isozymes

CYP Enzyme	Substrate
1A2	Acetaminophen
	Caffeine
	Clozapine (major)
	Cyclobenzaprine
	Diazepam (?)
	Fluvoxamine
	Haloperidol
	Isotretinoin
	Methadone
	Mexiletine (minor)
	Mirtazepine
	Naproxen
	Olanzapine
	Ondansetron
	Phenacetin
	Propafenone
	Propranolol
	Riluzole
	Ritonavir
	Ropivacaine
	Tacrine
	Tamoxifen
	TCAs (demethylation)
	Amitriptyline
	Clomipramine
	Desipramine
	Imipramine
	Nortriptyline
	Testosterone
	Theophylline (major)
	Verapamil
	R-warfarin
	Zileuton
	Zolpidem
2A6	Ritonavir
	Tamoxifen
2B6	Cyclophosphamide
	Ifosfamide
	Tamoxifen
2C8	Benzphetamine
	Diazepam
	Diclofenac
	Isotretinoin
	Omeprazole
	Paclitaxel (major)
	Retinoic acid
	Tolbutamide
2C9	Barbiturates
	Hexobarbital
	Mephobarbital
	Carvedilol
	Dapsone
	Diclofenac
	Dronabinol
	Fluoxetine
	Flurbiprofen
	Glimepiride
	Ibuprofen
	Indomethacin
	Losartan
	Mefenamic acid
	Mephenytoin
2C9 *(continued)*	Mirtazepine
	Montelukast
	Naproxen
	Phenytoin
	Piroxicam
	Ritonavir
	Suprofen (?)
	TCAs
	Amitriptyline
	Imipramine
	Terbinafine
	Tetrahydrocannabinol
	Tolbutamide
	Torsemide
	S-warfarin
	Zafirlukast
	Zileuton
2C18	Naproxen
	Piroxicam
	Retinoic acid
	S-tetrahydrocannabinol
	S-warfarin
2C19	Carisoprodol
	Citalopram
	Desmethyldiazepam
	Diazepam
	Divalproex sodium
	Hexobarbital
	Lansoprazole
	Mephenytoin
	S-mephenytoin
	Omeprazole
	Propranolol
	Ritonavir
	TCAs
	Clomipramine
	Imipramine
	Valproic acid
2D6	Carvedilol
	Chloroquine (possible)
	Chlorpromazine
	Clozapine (?)
	Codeine
	Cyclobenzaprine
	Debrisoquin
	Delavirdine
	Dexfenfluramine
	Dextromethorphan
	Dolasetron
	Donepezil
	Encainide
	Flecainide
	Fluoxetine
	Fluphenazine
	Halofantrine (?)
	Haloperidol
	Hydrocodone
	Hydroxyamphetamine
	Labetalol
	Maprotiline
	Methamphetamine
	Metoprolol

(continued)

Table 3.2 *(continued)*

CYP Enzyme	Substrate
2D6 *(continued)*	Mexiletine (major)
	Mirtazepine
	Morphine
	Olanzapine (minor)
	Ondansetron
	Oxamniquine
	Oxycodone
	Paroxetine
	Pentazocine
	Perphenazine
	Phenformin
	Primaquine (possible)
	Propafenone
	Propoxyphene
	Propranolol (minor)
	Risperidone
	Ritonavir
	Ropivacaine
	Selegiline
	Sertraline
	Sparteine
	Tamoxifen
	TCAs (hydroxylation)
	Amitriptyline
	Clomipramine
	Desipramine
	Imipramine
	Nortriptyline
	Thioridazine
	Timolol
	Tolterodine (major)
	Tramadol
	Trazodone
	Trimipramine
	Venlafaxine
	Zolpidem
2E1	Acetaminophen
	Chlorzoxazone
	Dapsone
	Enflurane
	Ethanol (minor)
	Halothane
	Isoflurane
	Isoniazid
	Methoxyflurane
	Ondansetron
	Ritonavir
	Sevoflurane
	Tamoxifen
	Theophylline
3A3	Erythromycin
	Midazolam
3A4	Acetaminophen
	Alfentanil
	Alprazolam
	Amiodarone
	Amlodipine
	Astemizole
	Atorvastatin
	Benzphetamine
	Bromocriptine
	Busulfan
3A4 *(continued)*	Carbamazepine
	Cerivastatin
	Chlorpromazine
	Cisapride
	Citalopram
	Clarithromycin
	Clindamycin
	Clonazepam
	Cocaine
	Codeine
	Cyclobenzaprine
	Cyclophosphamide
	Cyclosporine
	Dapsone
	Delavirdine
	Dexamethasone
	Dextromethorphan
	Diazepam
	Diltiazem
	Disopyramide
	Dolasetron
	Donepezil
	Doxorubicin
	Dronabinol
	Erythromycin
	Ethinyl estradiol
	Ethosuximide
	Etoposide
	Felodipine
	Fentanyl
	Granisetron
	Halofantrine
	Hydrocortisone
	Ifosfamide
	Indinavir
	Isradipine
	Itraconazole (?)
	Ketoconazole
	Lansoprazole
	Lidocaine
	Loratadine
	Losartan
	Lovastatin
	Mibefradil
	Miconazole
	Midazolam
	Mifepristone
	Mirtazepine
	Montelukast
	Navelbine
	Nefazodone
	Nelfinavir
	Nevirapine
	Nicardipine
	Nifedipine
	Nimodipine
	Nisoldipine
	Nitrendipine
	Omeprazole
	Ondansetron
	Paclitaxel (minor)
	Pimozide

(continued)

Table 3.2 *(continued)*

CYP Enzyme	Substrate	CYP Enzyme	Substrate
3A4 *(continued)*	Pravastatin	3A4 *(continued)*	Tretinoin
	Progesterone		Triazolam
	Propafenone		Troglitazone
	Quinidine		Troleandomycin
	Quinine		Venlafaxine
	Ritonavir		Verapamil
	Salmeterol		Vinblastine
	Saquinavir		Vincristine
	Sertraline		R-warfarin (?)
	Simvastatin		Yohimbe
	Sufentanil		Zileuton
	Tacrolimus		Zolpidem (major)
	Tamoxifen	3A5–7	Ethinyl estradiol
	TCAs (demethylation)		Lovastatin (3A5)
	Amitriptyline		Midazolam (3A5)
	Clomipramine		Nifedipine (3A5)
	Imipramine		Quinidine
	Teniposide		Terfenadine
	Terfenadine		Testosterone
	Testosterone		Triazolam
	Theophylline (minor)		Vinblastine
	Tiagabine		Vincristine
	Tolterodine		

Source: References 10, 34–57.
CYP, cytochrome P-450; *TCAs,* tricyclic antidepressants.

receiving warfarin and phenytoin concurrently, bleeding could occur if the enzyme inducer, phenytoin, is discontinued without an adjustment in the anticoagulant dosage.

Clinical Considerations. This mechanism of interaction has a slow onset because protein synthesis is involved and may take up to several weeks before the maximum effect is seen. If an interaction occurs, the serum levels of the object drug may be reduced, producing a decrease in therapeutic activity. To compensate for this interaction, when practical, monitor serum drug concentrations and observe the patient for loss of therapeutic effects. Often, it is necessary to increase the dosage of the object drug or select a noninteracting alternative. When a patient is stabilized on both drugs, if the precipitant drug is discontinued or the dosage is decreased, serum levels of the object drug may increase and toxicity could occur. Dissipation of the effects of the interaction after discontinuation of the precipitant drug is also slow. Once again, patients should be monitored for changes in clinical response.

Clinically Important Examples. Phenytoin increases the hepatic metabolism of mexiletine, producing a decrease in steady-state plasma mexiletine levels and a reduction in efficacy.[58] Similarly, theophylline and phenytoin appear to increase the metabolism of each other. When both drugs are administered concomitantly, serum drug concentrations may decrease and loss of seizure control or an exacerbation of pulmonary symptoms may result.[10] Other drugs that induce hepatic enzymes are listed in Table 3.3.[10,40–42,47,48,51,53,55,56]

Decreased Metabolism (Enzyme Inhibition)

As occurs with enzyme induction, enzyme inhibition usually involves the liver and results from competition between the precipitant and object drugs for binding sites on the enzyme. However, because this mechanism involves direct competition, the onset of interactions is more rapid than with enzyme induction, often occurring within hours. Unless the precipitant drug has a long half-life, enzyme inhibition generally reaches a maximum effect within 24 hours.[59] Less commonly, a noncompetitive mechanism, which suspends the metabolic activity of an enzyme, may be involved.[13] Drug interactions involving enzyme inhibition often result in clinical effects that are protracted or intensified as the object drug reaches a steady-state plasma concentration. The enzymes involved most often are monooxygenase enzymes.[9] When metabolism of the object drug is inhibited, new steady-state plasma levels are achieved in approximately five half-lives. However, the inhibitory effect of the precipitant drug on the metabolism of the object drug is usually maximal within three half-lives. Upon discontinuing the enzyme-inhibiting drug (i.e., precipitant drug), plasma concentrations of the object drug decrease, resulting in loss of efficacy unless appropriate action is taken. The time frame for reversal of the interaction depends on the half-life of the object drug but usually occurs within 24 hours. As with most pharmacokinetic interactions, enzyme inhibition appears to be dose-related, with higher dosages producing greater inhibition.

Clinical Considerations. Enzyme inhibition is one of the most common mechanisms of drug interactions. The

Table 3.3 ▪ Drugs That Induce CYP Isozymes

CYP Enzyme	Inducer
1A2	Charcoal broiling Cigarette smoke Omeprazole Phenobarbital Primidone Rifampin
2B6	Phenobarbital Phenytoin Primidone
2C8	Phenobarbital Primidone
2C9	Carbamazepine Ethanol Phenytoin Rifampin
2C19	Rifampin
2D6	Not induced by common inducers
2E1	Ethanol Isoniazid
3A4	Carbamazepine Glucocorticoids Dexamethasone Prednisone Phenobarbital Phenylbutazone Phenytoin Primidone Rifabutin Rifampin Sulfinpyrazone Troglitazone (?)
3A5–7	Phenobarbital Phenytoin Primidone Rifampin

Source: References 10, 40–42, 47, 48, 51, 53, 55, 56.
CYP, cytochrome P-450.

onset and reversal of this interaction often occur within 24 hours. This interaction usually produces an increase in serum drug concentration, resulting in a possible augmentation of both the pharmacologic and adverse effects of the object drug. Clinically important interactions are most common with drugs that have a narrow therapeutic index and when the plasma concentration is near the upper end of the therapeutic range. When a hepatic microsomal enzyme–inducing drug (e.g., carbamazepine) is administered with an enzyme inhibitor (e.g., verapamil), the effect of the inhibitor appears to predominate and the effect of the inducer is attenuated. Stereospecific drug interactions involving warfarin metabolism are most clinically important when the greatest effect occurs with the more potent S(–) enantiomer.[8]

Clinically Important Examples. Erythromycin and other macrolide antibiotics can inhibit the metabolism of astemizole and terfenadine, increasing the serum concentrations of the antihistamines as well as the risk of life-threatening cardiotoxicity.[10] Omeprazole appears to inhibit the oxidative metabolism of diazepam, resulting in increased serum concentrations of the benzodiazepine and producing an increase the pharmacologic effect.[60] Similarly, isoniazid inhibits the hepatic metabolism of phenytoin, producing an increase in serum phenytoin concentrations and a corresponding increase in the pharmacologic and toxic effects of the drug.[61,62] Phenytoin toxicity appears to be most significant in patients who are slow acetylators of isoniazid.[62] Other drugs that inhibit metabolic enzymes are listed in Table 3.4.[10,35–38,40–42,47–57,63]

First-Pass Metabolism

Some drugs are metabolized extensively during the first pass through the wall of the GI tract and liver.[9,22] In this instance, small amounts of a drug reach the systemic circulation (e.g., 10% of an orally administered dose of propranolol). Thus, drugs that increase or decrease liver blood flow may have profound effects on the bioavailability of the object drug. In addition, drugs with a high first-pass metabolism tend to compete for metabolic enzyme sites, enhancing each other's bioavailability.[22] In other instances, oral bioavailability may be decreased by increased first-pass metabolism in the presence of enzyme induction.

Clinical Considerations. The object drug must be given orally. A clinically important interaction will be seen when the precipitant drug is an enzyme inducer or inhibitor.

Clinically Important Examples. Propafenone increases plasma concentrations of both metoprolol and propranolol by decreasing first-pass metabolism and reducing systemic clearance. Propafenone and the β-blockers are metabolized by the hepatic CYP oxidase system (i.e., CYP2D6), and propafenone appears to inhibit metoprolol and propranolol metabolism.[64,65] The pharmacologic and adverse effects of these β-blockers may be increased. Rifampin lowers serum verapamil levels by increasing first-pass hepatic metabolism of verapamil.[66,67] In addition, rifampin appears to induce the hepatic microsomal enzymes (CYP1A2 and CYP3A4) responsible for the metabolism of verapamil.

Renal Excretion

The renal excretion of one drug may be increased or decreased by coadministering another drug. Most lipid-soluble drugs are metabolized by the liver to inactive, water-soluble metabolites before renal excretion. Various mechanisms may be involved with interactions affecting renal elimination, including competition for active tubular secretion and pH-dependent renal tubular transport.

Active Tubular Secretion

Active tubular secretion of drug molecules occurs in the proximal portion of the renal tubule. In order for the drug to pass from the systemic circulation to the tubular lumen, the drug is transported, by combining with a protein, through the basolateral and brush border membranes.

Although each protein has a unique affinity for an anion or cation, drugs that use a similar system for transport appear to interact by competitive inhibition of transport proteins.[13] Saturation of the transport system by the precipitant drug may decrease the tubular secretion of the object drug.

Clinical Considerations. Interactions resulting from this mechanism tend to occur rapidly. Plasma concentrations of the object drug may be increased, producing an increase in therapeutic and toxic effects.

Clinically Important Examples. Cyclosporine may decrease etoposide renal clearance by inhibiting drug transport in the brush border of the proximal renal tubule, increasing serum etoposide concentrations and the risk of toxicity.[68] Probenecid appears to impair the tubular secretion of methotrexate. Methotrexate serum concentrations have shown a threefold to fourfold increase when concurrently administering probenecid.[69] Quinidine reduces the renal and biliary clearance of digoxin by 30 to 40%, increasing serum digoxin concentrations in approximately 90% of the patients receiving both drugs.[10,70]

Passive Tubular Reabsorption

The excretion and reabsorption of many drugs from the renal tubules occur by passive diffusion, which is regulated by the concentration and lipid solubility of the drug on both sides of the cell membrane.[13] Nonionized drug molecules are preferentially reabsorbed over ionized drugs, with the ratio determined by the pH and pKa of the drug.[13] Although strongly acidic and basic drugs tend to be ionized in the usual range of urinary pH (i.e., 5 to 8), the degree of ionization of weak acids and bases varies with the pH of the urine. Therefore, an increased amount of weakly acidic drug is reabsorbed from an acidic urine, whereas basic drugs are excreted. The opposite is true in an alkaline urine.[1]

Clinical Considerations. Interference with renal elimination may be clinically important if the fraction of unmetabolized drug is large and if the drug has a narrow therapeutic index (e.g., thiazide diuretics decrease renal lithium clearance, producing toxicity).

Clinically Important Examples. Administering sodium bicarbonate, 245 mEq over 5 hours, has been reported to

Table 3.4 ▪ Drugs That Inhibit CYP Isozymes

CYP Enzyme	Inhibitor
1A2	Anastrazole
	Cimetidine
	Ciprofloxacin
	Diethyldithiocarbamate
	Enoxacin
	Erythromycin
	Fluvoxamine
	Grapefruit juice (?)
	Mexiletine
	Mibefradil
	Mirtazepine (weak)
	Norfloxacin
	Propranolol
	Ritonavir
	Tacrine
2A6	Diethyldithiocarbamate
	Ketoconazole
	Methoxsalen
	Miconazole
	Pilocarpine
	Ritonavir
2B6	Diethyldithiocarbamate
	Orphenadrine
2C8	Anastrazole
	Diethyldithiocarbamate
	Omeprazole
2C9	Amiodarone (2C9)
	Anastrazole
	Chloramphenicol
	Cimetidine
	Diclofenac
	Disulfiram
	Fluconazole
	Fluoxetine
	Flurbiprofen
2C9 *(continued)*	Fluvastatin
	Fluvoxamine
	Ketoprofen
	Metronidazole
	Miconazole
	Phenylbutazone
	Ritonavir
	Sulfonamides
	Sulfadiazine
	Sulfamethizole
	Sulfamethoxazole
	Sulfinpyrazone
	Trimethoprim
	Troglitazone
	Zafirlukast
2C18	Cimetidine
2C19	Felbamate
	Fluoxetine
	Fluvoxamine
	Omeprazole
	Ritonavir
	Tolbutamide
	Topiramate (?)
	Tranylcypromine
	Troglitazone
2D6	Amiodarone
	Chloroquine
	Cimetidine
	Codeine
	Delavirdine
	Dextropropoxyphene
	Doxorubicin
	Fluoxetine
	Fluphenazine
	Fluvoxamine

(continued)

Table 3.4 *(continued)*

CYP Enzyme	Inhibitor
2D6 *(continued)*	Haloperidol
	Lomustine
	Methadone
	Mibefradil
	Mirtazepine (weak)
	Norfluoxetine
	Norfluvoxamine
	Paroxetine
	Perphenazine
	Primaquine
	Propafenone
	Propranolol
	Quinidine
	Ranitidine
	Ritonavir
	Sertraline (suspected)
	Thioridazine
	Venlafaxine
	Vinblastine
	Vinorelbine
	Yohimbe
2E1	Diethyldithiocarbamate
	Disulfiram
	Ritonavir
3A3	Cimetidine
	Nefazodone (suspected)
	Ranitidine
3A4	Anastrazole
	Cimetidine
	Clarithromycin
	Clotrimazole
	Danazol
	Delavirdine
	Diethyldithiocarbamate
3A4 *(continued)*	Diltiazem
	Erythromycin
	Fluconazole
	Fluoxetine
	Fluvoxamine
	Grapefruit juice
	Indinavir
	Itraconazole
	Ketoconazole
	Metronidazole
	Mibefradil
	Miconazole
	Mirtazepine (weak)
	Nefazodone
	Nelfinavir
	Nevirapine
	Norfloxacin
	Norfluoxetine
	Paroxetine
	Propranolol
	Quinidine
	Quinine
	Ranitidine
	Ritonavir
	Saquinavir
	Sertraline
	Troglitazone
	Troleandomycin
	Zafirlukast
3A5–7	Clotrimazole
	Ketoconazole
	Metronidazole
	Miconazole
	Troleandomycin

Source: References 10, 35–38, 40–42, 47–57, 63.
CYP, cytochrome P-450.

increase renal lithium clearance, possibly decreasing the clinical effectiveness of lithium.[71] Chronic antacid therapy with a magnesium and aluminum hydroxide combination has been associated with increased salicylate clearance and a 30 to 70% decrease in serum salicylate levels.[10]

Pharmacodynamic Interactions

In contrast to pharmacokinetic interactions, pharmacodynamic interactions have not been amply studied or reported. Pharmacodynamic interactions involve changes in the response of the patient to a drug combination without alterations in the serum concentration or pharmacokinetics of the object drug. Because pharmacologic responses to a drug may be difficult to assess, pharmacodynamic studies are difficult to perform.[13] Investigations are further complicated because pharmacokinetic and pharmacodynamic drug interactions may occur simultaneously. Because pharmacodynamic interactions often involve drugs with similar or opposing pharmacologic activity, many of these interactions can be anticipated by an understanding of the pharmacology of each of the drugs.[1] Often, observing patients for changes in their clinical condition and making the appropriate dosage adjustment corrects the situation.

Synergistic and Antagonistic Effects

When a drug interaction involves synergistic or antagonistic effects, the therapeutic or toxic effects of two concurrently administered agents are greater or less, respectively, than the sum or the difference of their individual activity. These interactions often involve drugs acting on the same organ system (e.g., central nervous system) or site.

Clinical Considerations. Synergism is probably the most common mechanism by which drug interactions occur.

Clinically Important Examples. Propranolol and verapamil have synergistic or additive cardiovascular effects.[10] Both drugs have direct negative inotropic and chronotropic effects. In the management of hypertension and

Table 3.5 ▪ Drugs with a Narrow Therapeutic Index

Aminoglycoside antibiotics
Cyclosporine
Digoxin
Hypoglycemic agents
Lidocaine
Lithium
Phenytoin
Procainamide
Theophylline
Tricyclic antidepressants
Warfarin

Source: References 8, 9.

unstable angina, concurrently administering propranolol and verapamil is acceptable and generally effective; however, serious adverse cardiovascular effects may occur.[10] Propranolol does not affect verapamil kinetics, and verapamil has only minimal effects on propranolol concentration. The pharmacologic and toxic effects of propranolol and verapamil may be enhanced in some patients. Aminoglycosides have been reported to stabilize the postjunctional membrane and impair prejunctional calcium influx and acetylcholine output, thereby potentiating the neuromuscular effects of succinylcholine.[10]

The pharmacologic effects of fluoxetine may be reversed by concurrently administering cyproheptadine. Fluoxetine has serotonergic activity, and cyproheptadine is a serotonin antagonist.[72] The capacity of warfarin to interfere with the activation of the vitamin K–dependent clotting factors is reversed by vitamin K administration, allowing possible thrombus formation.

Altered Transport System and Effects at Receptor Sites

These drug interactions involve interference with physiologic transport systems, limiting the access of certain drugs into cells.

Clinical Considerations. The serum concentration of the drugs is unchanged unless a pharmacokinetic interaction occurs simultaneously.

Clinically Important Examples. Both phenothiazines (e.g., chlorpromazine) and tricyclic antidepressants (e.g., amitriptyline) inhibit the neuronal uptake of guanethidine, preventing the antihypertensive activity of guanethidine.[10]

RISK FACTORS

High-Risk Drugs

Drugs having the highest risk of being involved in a clinically important drug interaction often have a narrow therapeutic index, a steep dose–response curve, and potent pharmacologic effects.[1,7,9] When a drug has a narrow therapeutic index, the toxic dosage may be only slightly more than the therapeutic dosage. Similarly, when a drug has a steep dose–response curve, a small change in dosage may result in a large increase in clinical effect. Therefore, a small increase in the serum concentration of drugs with these characteristics may produce an exaggerated pharmacologic response or toxicity. Patients receiving drugs with a narrow therapeutic index should be monitored routinely for possible drug interactions. Examples of drugs with a narrow therapeutic index are listed in Table 3.5.[8,9] Conversely, a slight decrease in the plasma concentration of drugs with a steep dose–response curve may result in loss of therapeutic effects; examples include corticosteroids, carbamazepine, quinidine, oral contraceptives, and rifampin.[9] Drugs with a wider therapeutic index are less likely to be involved in clinically important interactions.

High-Risk Patients

Drug interactions that would be of minor clinical importance in most patients with less severe forms of a disease could cause significant exacerbation of the clinical condition in patients with more severe forms of the disease (Table 3.6).[9] Loss of therapeutic activity can be particularly important in situations that could result in an unwanted outcome (e.g., pregnancy), or where a serious pathologic condition is being suppressed (e.g., connective tissue disorder or a malignancy).[9] Because the risk of experiencing a drug interaction increases with the number of drugs a patient receives, severely ill patients or older adults who are taking multiple drugs may also be at an increased risk for drug interactions.[9] Additionally, patients being treated for certain diseases appear to be at an increased risk of experiencing a drug interaction because of the drug therapy prescribed for their disorders (Table 3.6).[13,73]

Table 3.6 ▪ Causes of Increased Risk of Drug Interactions

Severity of the Disease State Being Treated
Aplastic anemia
Asthma
Cardiac arrhythmia
Diabetes
Epilepsy
Hepatic precoma
Hypothyroidism
Drug Interaction Potential of Therapy
Cardiovascular disease
Connective tissue disorders
Gastrointestinal disease
Infection
Metabolic disorders
Psychiatric illness
Respiratory ailments
Seizure disorders

Source: References 9, 13, 73.

ONSET OF DRUG INTERACTIONS

There is considerable variation in the time of onset of drug interactions, ranging from seconds to weeks.[13] Knowledge of the onset can assist in minimizing the adverse effects associated with interactions by enabling the clinician to select the most appropriate monitoring parameters. Interactions that occur when administering the first dose or within 24 hours of administering the precipitant drug may require immediate attention. Because protein synthesis is involved in enzyme induction, it may be 2 weeks or more before the full potential for a clinically important interaction is evident. Thus, an interaction would not be expected to occur by this mechanism in a patient receiving 1 or 2 days of treatment with an enzyme-inducing drug.[13] Conversely, enzyme inhibition results from competition between two drugs for the same enzyme site and may occur rapidly after administering precipitant drug. Patients should be monitored for changes in their clinical status soon after initiation of an interacting combination.

The time of onset of an interaction may be affected by the half-lives of the respective drugs. When the precipitant drug has a long half-life, it may take several days for plasma concentrations to reach steady state, delaying the onset of the interaction. The half-life of the object drug may also influence the onset of the interaction. Drug interactions occurring by similar mechanisms may have a more rapid onset when the object drug has a shorter half-life because new steady-state plasma levels are achieved sooner. For example, cimetidine inhibits the metabolism of warfarin and theophylline. The latter drug has a considerably shorter half-life than the former. Therefore, a clinically important interaction may occur within 1 day of adding cimetidine to the drug regimen of a patient stabilized on theophylline but may take a week or longer in a patient receiving warfarin.

The mechanism by which a drug interaction occurs can influence the onset of clinical effects. When relevant, the effect of the mechanism on the onset of an interaction was described in the clinical considerations section for the specific mechanism of interaction.

PREVENTION

Many drug interactions can be avoided if adequate precautions are taken. Monitoring therapy and making appropriate adjustments in the drug regimen may circumvent a potentially serious drug interaction. Patients receiving drugs with a narrow therapeutic index should be monitored routinely for possible drug interactions. These drug interactions may be life threatening or have serious clinical consequences. Hospitalized patients often are given warfarin with an interacting agent without the occurrence of clinical consequences. In the hospital setting, patients' prothrombin times are monitored daily and appropriate adjustments are made in the warfarin dosage whether or not a potential drug interaction is suspected. No symptoms of an interaction are observed. However, in order to avoid possible bleeding or the risk of exacerbating the condition being treated, adjustments in the warfarin dosage are necessary if the interacting drug is stopped after the patient is discharged from the hospital.

DRUG INTERACTION RESOURCES AND THEIR LIMITATIONS

It is not surprising that administering one drug may modify the action of another drug given simultaneously. Whenever a patient receives multiple-drug therapy, the possibility of a drug–drug interaction exists. In addition, as the number of drugs a patient receives increases, so does the potential for a drug interaction. Fortunately, the interactions with the greatest clinical importance are uncommon.

Pharmacists and physicians cannot be aware of all possible drug interactions. However, over the past three decades, drug interactions have received considerable attention. The medical literature is replete with anecdotal case reports, controlled clinical trials, and review articles on this subject. In addition, new interactions are being reported constantly. Comprehensive textbooks have been written on drug interactions, detailing the clinical effects, mechanisms, and management of potential drug interactions.[10,13] Computer systems for storage and retrieval of drug interaction information and for patient monitoring have been developed.[74,75] Other available sources of drug interaction information include meetings, continuing education programs, professional seminars, and the Internet. Even the manufacturer's package brochure contains a section describing known and suspected drug interactions.

However, it is often difficult to interpret the relevance of drug interaction data because they are derived from animal or in vitro studies, investigations involving healthy volunteers given a single dose of a drug, and anecdotal case reports.[9] In addition, studies may illustrate and emphasize pharmacokinetic findings without demonstrating clinically important changes in patient outcome.

When evaluating drug interaction literature, it is important to be aware of the type of documentation supporting the proposed interaction (i.e., case report, animal study, controlled study). For a controlled study, one must evaluate the study design, including sample size, route of administration, duration of therapy, and type of subjects (e.g., healthy volunteers versus clinical patients).

The following problems can be associated with using the medical literature to determine clinical importance.[10,13,76]

Use of Animal Studies

It may not be possible to extrapolate interactions based on animal studies to humans. Animals often receive much higher dosages by weight than would be administered to humans.

Anecdotal Case Reports

Drug interactions based on a single case report require additional controlled studies to verify their clinical importance. One must rule out other explanations for the observed event (e.g., natural progression of the disease being treated). However, well-documented case reports often give rise to controlled trials.

Healthy Volunteers

Results of studies involving healthy volunteers or a small number of patients may not allow adequate evaluation of a potential interaction. Some pharmacokinetic interactions may be determined to occur by statistical analysis in normal, healthy volunteers (usually young adults) but may not be clinically important when observed in patients. In other instances, healthy volunteers may not exhibit an interaction that is observed in patients, particularly older adults. For example, the ability of erythromycin to reduce warfarin clearance is more pronounced in patients than in healthy subjects.

Magnitude of Effect

A study may fail to identify or accurately describe a potential drug interaction based on the magnitude of the effect of that interaction. Factors that may interfere with assessing the degree of effect are as follows:

- Order of administration: Treatment with the object drug is started after the patient is stabilized on the precipitant drug. No interaction may be observed in this instance until the precipitant drug is discontinued. Thus, in a patient receiving chronic cimetidine treatment before the initiation of warfarin therapy, no interaction would be observed. However, if cimetidine is discontinued after the warfarin dosage is stabilized, a higher dosage of anticoagulant may be required. Clinically important interactions are more likely to occur when the precipitant drug is added to the regimen of a patient stabilized on the object drug.
- Duration of treatment: An interaction with a delayed onset may not be observed if the study is not conducted for an adequate period of time. Neurotoxicity that occurs when concurrently administering lithium and carbamazepine may be observed only after the drug combination is given for several days.
- Adequate dosage: Most drug interactions are dose related. Larger dosages of the precipitant drug tend to produce greater effects in the object drug. If an adequate dosage of the drug is not administered, one may fail to observe an interaction. Thus, although high-dose salicylates (e.g., more than 3 g/day aspirin) antagonize the uricosuric action of probenecid, occasional low dosages do not.
- Dosage form: It is necessary to consider the effects of food on theophylline absorption on an individual product basis, for example. Although food can be ingested with many theophylline preparations without the occurrence of an interaction, *Theo-24* taken less than 1 hour before a high-fat meal may increase in both theophylline absorption and peak serum levels.
- Presence of multiple drugs: In a preliminary investigation, the presence of propylene glycol in intravenous nitroglycerin preparations was reported to interfere with the anticoagulant effect of heparin. Subsequent studies have demonstrated the effect on heparin to be caused by the nitroglycerin.

Extrapolation to Chemically or Pharmacologically Related Drugs

Based on pharmacokinetic (e.g., elimination) or pharmacodynamic differences, not all members of a drug class interact in the same manner. Cimetidine inhibits the hepatic microsomal enzymes involved in the metabolism of diazepam; however, famotidine does not appear to affect diazepam metabolism. In addition, cimetidine does not alter oxazepam metabolism.

Use of Mean Values

For drug interactions that occur in a small number of patients, no statistically significant difference in response may be observed between the control group and the study group. However, if one analyzes the results for individual subjects, there may be a clinically important change in a small number of patients. For example, some patients exhibit a fivefold increase in serum digoxin concentrations when concurrently administering quinidine, but in others the effect is minimal.

Variability in Patient Response

In well-controlled drug interaction studies, it is not unusual to find a wide variation in the response of patients to the same drug regimen. Thus, whereas one patient may experience a life-threatening reaction, a second patient may not experience any adverse effects. Often it is not possible to explain these differences; however, the following factors account for some of the variability.

- Age: Very young children and older adults may be at increased risk of experiencing drug interactions. Studies indicate that older adults receive approximately 25% of all prescription drugs dispensed. In addition, this age group extensively uses over-the-counter medications. Furthermore, older adults may have other chronic diseases or decreased renal or hepatic function, necessitating careful monitoring of drug therapy. However, irrespective of age, drug therapy should be closely monitored in any patient with decreased organ function. Drug interactions involving enzyme induction may occur less often in older adults.[77]
- Genetic factors: Certain drug interactions may be more important in some patients because of genetic factors. For example, the toxicity resulting from the inhibitory effect of isoniazid on phenytoin metabolism appears to be more important in slow acetylators of isoniazid than in those who metabolize the drug more rapidly.
- Disease states: Diseases such as impaired renal function, hepatic dysfunction, and hypoalbuminemia may adversely influence the response to drugs used concurrently. In addition, patients with certain disease states, including cardiovascular, connective tissue, GI, infectious, lipid, psychiatric, respiratory, or seizure disorders, may be at a higher risk of experiencing moderate to severe drug interactions.[13] This may be related either to changes in drug disposition as a result

of the disease or, more commonly, to the types of drugs used in treating the disease.

- Alcohol consumption: Acute alcohol intolerance (disulfiram reaction) may occur in patients consuming alcohol while taking other drugs, including cefazolin, cefmetazole, cefoperazone, and cefotetan.
- Smoking: Smoking has been shown to increase the activity of drug-metabolizing enzymes in the liver.[78] Smoking stimulates the metabolism of theophylline and mexiletine. Compared to nonsmokers, smokers may require larger dosages of these drugs in order to maintain therapeutic serum levels. In addition, administering an enzyme-inducing drug may not have as significant an effect on the object drug as might occur in a nonsmoking patient receiving the same drug combination. There is evidence indicating that the effects of administering multiple enzyme-inducing drugs to the same patient are less than additive.[79]

CONCLUSION

It is helpful to understand the clinical importance of potentially interacting drug combinations. Although one does not want the choice of therapy to be detrimental to the patient, it is equally important not to deprive a patient of worthwhile treatment by overreacting to a potential interaction that lacks clinical importance or that can be circumvented easily.

KEY POINTS

- Most interacting drug combinations can be administered concurrently if the patient is monitored appropriately and corresponding adjustments are made in the drug dosage, dosing interval, or route of administration.
- Understanding the mechanisms by which drugs interact and having a knowledge of those drugs and of patients at increased risk of experiencing potentially important drug interactions will allow one to anticipate and prevent clinical problems.
- Careful attention should be given to interactions involving drugs that have a narrow therapeutic index (e.g., cyclosporine, digoxin, phenytoin, theophylline, warfarin).
- When a patient's clinical condition changes unexpectedly, all drug treatment should be reviewed.
- When possible, a suspected interaction should be placed in clinical perspective, and one should be prepared to offer recommendations for minimizing possible consequences.
- Factors that help minimize the occurrence of drug interactions include being aware of over-the-counter drugs, dietary supplements, and nutritional products that the patient is taking; avoiding unnecessary therapy; observing the patient for unexpected changes in clinical response; and monitoring serum drug levels, particularly for drugs with a narrow therapeutic index.
- The importance of educating patients about potential drug interactions that may be associated with their treatment regimens should not be overlooked. Patient knowledge of unexpected reactions that could occur when coadministering other prescription and over-the-counter drugs could lead to the early detection or prevention of possibly important drug interactions.

REFERENCES

1. Berkow R, ed. The Merck manual of diagnosis and therapy. 16th ed. Whitehouse Station, New Jersey: Merck Sharp & Dohme Research Laboratories, 1992:2634–2640.
2. Boston Collaborative Drug Surveillance Program. Adverse drug interactions. JAMA 220:1238–1239, 1972.
3. Durrence CW, DiPiro JT, May JR, et al. Potential drug interactions in surgical patients. Am J Hosp Pharm 42:1553–1555, 1985.
4. Borda IT, Slone D, Jick H. Assessment of adverse reactions within a drug surveillance program. JAMA 205:645–647, 1968.
5. Blaschke TF, Cohen SN, Tatro DS. Drug–drug interactions and aging. In: Jarvik LF, Greenblatt DJ, Harman D, eds. Clinical pharmacology in the aged patient. New York: Raven 16:11–26, 1981.
6. Stanaszek WF, Franklin CE. Survey of potential drug interaction incidence in an outpatient clinic population. Hosp Pharm 13:255–263, 1978.
7. Puckett WH, Visconti JA. An epidemiological study of the clinical significance of drug–drug interactions in a private community hospital. Am J Hosp Pharm 28:247-253, 1971.
8. Aronson JK, Grahame-Smith DG. Adverse drug interactions. BMJ 282:288–291, 1981.
9. McInnes GT, Brodie MJ. Drug interactions that matter: a critical reappraisal. Drugs 36:83–110, 1988.
10. Tatro DS, ed. Drug interaction facts. St. Louis: Facts and Comparisons, 2000.
11. Van Der Meer JWM, Keuning JJ, Scheijgrond HW, et al. The influence of gastric acidity on the bio-availability of ketoconazole. J Antimicrob Chemother 6:552–554, 1980.
12. Piscitelli SC, Goss TF, Wilton JH, et al. Effects of ranitidine and sucralfate on ketoconazole bioavailability. Antimicrob Agents Chemother. 35:1765–1771, 1991.
13. Hansten PD. Drug interactions analysis and management. St. Louis: Facts and Comparisons, 2000.
14. Lindenbaum J, Rund DG, Butler VP, et al. Inactivation of digoxin by the gut flora: reversal by antibiotic therapy. N Engl J Med 305:789–794, 1981.
15. Morton MR, Cooper JW. Erythromycin-induced digoxin toxicity. Ann Pharmacother 23:668–670, 1989.
16. Guerriero SE, Ehrenpreis E, Gallagher KL. Two cases of clarithromycin-induced digoxin toxicity. Pharmacotherapy 17:1035–1037, 1997.
17. Midoneck SR, Etingin OR. Clarithromycin-related toxic effects of digoxin. N Engl J Med 333:1505, 1995.
18. Sahai J, Gallicano K, Oliveras L, et al. Cations in the didanosine tablet reduce ciprofloxacin bioavailability. Clin Pharmacol Ther 53:292–297, 1993.
19. Parpia SH, Nix DE, Hejmanowski LG, et al. Sucralfate reduces the gastrointestinal absorption of norfloxacin. Antimicrob Agents Chemother 33:99–102, 1989.
20. Nix DE, Watson WA, Handy L, et al. The effect of sucralfate pretreatment on the pharmacokinetics of ciprofloxacin. Pharmacotherapy 9:377–380, 1989.
21. Garrelts JC, Godley PJ, Peterie JD, et al. Sucralfate significantly reduces ciprofloxacin concentrations in serum. Antimicrob Agents Chemother 34;931–933, 1990.
22. Brodie MJ, Feely J. Adverse drug interactions. BMJ 296:845–849, 1988.
23. Kuhlman J, Zilly W, Wilke J. Effects of cytotoxic drugs on plasma level and renal excretion of beta-acetyldigoxin. Clin Pharmacol Ther 30:518–527, 1981.
24. Kuhlman J, Wilke J, Rietbrock N. Cytostatic drugs are without significant effect on digitoxin plasma level and renal excretion. Clin Pharmacol Ther 32:646–651, 1982.
25. Bjornsson TD, Huang AT, Roth P, et al. Effects of high-dose cancer chemotherapy on the absorption of digoxin in two different formulations. Clin Pharmacol Ther 39:25–28, 1986.
26. Wadhwa NK, Schroeder TJ, O'Flaherty E, et al. The effect of oral metoclopramide on the absorption of cyclosporine. Transplant Proc 19:1730–1733, 1987.
27. Manninen V, Melin J, Apajalahti A, et al. Altered absorption of digoxin in patients given propantheline and metoclopramide. Lancet 1:398–399, 1973.
28. Johnson BF, Bustrack JA, Urbach DR, et al. Effect of metoclopramide on digoxin absorption from tablets and capsules. Clin Pharmacol Ther 36:724–730, 1984.

29. Rolan PE. Plasma protein binding displacement interaction: why are they still regarded as clinically important? Br J Clin Pharmacol 37:125–128, 1994.
30. Boston Collaborative Drug Surveillance Program. Interaction between chloral hydrate and warfarin. N Engl J Med 286:53–55, 1972.
31. Udall JA. Warfarin-chloral hydrate interaction: pharmacological activity and clinical significance. Ann Intern Med 81:341–344, 1974.
32. Banfield C, O'Reilly R, Chan E, et al. Phenylbutazone–warfarin interaction in man: further stereochemical and metabolic considerations. Br J Clin Pharmacol 16:669–675, 1983.
33. O'Reilly RA, Trager WF, Motley CH, et al. Stereoselective interaction of phenylbutazone with [$^{12}C/^{13}C$]warfarin pseudoracemates in man. J Clin Invest 65:746–753, 1980.
34. Brosen K. Recent developments in hepatic drug oxidation: implications for clinical pharmacokinetics. Clin Pharmacokinet 18:220–239, 1990.
35. Gonzalez FJ, Idle JR. Pharmacogenetic phenotyping and genotyping: present status and future potential. Clin Pharmacokinet 26:59–70, 1994.
36. Murray M. P-450 enzymes: inhibition mechanisms, genetic regulation and effects of liver disease. Clin Pharmacokinet 23:132–146, 1992.
37. Tucker GT. The rational selection of drug interaction studies: implications of recent advances in drug metabolism. Int J Clin Pharmacol Ther Toxicol 30:550–553, 1992.
38. van Harten J. Clinical pharmacokinetics of selective serotonin reuptake inhibitors. Clin Pharmacokinet 24:203–220, 1993.
39. Andersson T. Omeprazole drug interaction studies. Clin Pharmacokinet 21:195–212, 1991.
40. Tatro DS. Cytochrome P-450 enzyme drug interactions. Drug Newsletter 14:59–60, 1995.
41. Mullen WJ, North DS, Weiss MA. Pharmaceuticals and the cytochrome P-450 isoenzymes: a tool for decision making. Pharm Practice News 25:20–24, 1998.
42. Miners JO, Birkett DJ. Cytochrome P-4502C9: an enzyme of major importance in human drug metabolism. Br J Clin Pharmacol 45:525–538, 1998.
43. Gantmacher J, Mills-Bomford J, Williams T. Interaction between warfarin and oral terbinafine. BMJ 317:205, 1998.
44. Michalets EL. Clinically significant cytochrome P-450 drug interactions: author's reply. Pharmacotherapy 18:892–893, 1998.
45. Bailey DG, Arnold MO, Spence JD. Grapefruit juice–drug interactions. Br J Clin Pharmacol 46:101–110, 1998.
46. Nakajima M, Kobayashi K, Shimada N, et al. Involvement of CYP 1A2 in mexiletine metabolism. Br J Clin Pharmacol 46:55–62, 1998.
47. Jefferson JW. Drug interactions: friend or foe? J Clin Psychiatry 59 (suppl 4):37–47, 1998.
48. Michalets EL. Update: clinically significant cytochrome P-450 drug interactions. Pharmacotherapy 18:84–112, 1998.
49. Nemeroff CB, De Vane CL, Pollock BG. Newer antidepressants and the cytochrome P-450 system. Am J Psychiatry 153:311–320, 1996.
50. Bertz RJ, Granneman GR. Use of in vitro and in vivo data to estimate the likelihood of metabolic pharmacokinetic interactions. Clin Pharmacokinet 32:210–258, 1997.
51. Goldberg RJ. The P-450 system. Arch Fam Med 5:406–412, 1996.
52. Teteishi T, Graham SG, Krivoruk Y, et al. Omeprazole does not affect measured CYP3A4 activity using the erythromycin breath test. Br J Clin Pharmacol 40:411–412, 1995.
53. Spatzenegger M, Jaeger W. Clinical importance of hepatic cytochrome P-450 in drug metabolism. Drug Metab Rev 27:397–417, 1995.
54. Halliday RC, Jones BC, Smith DA, et al. An investigation of the interaction between halofantrine, CYP2D6 and CYP3A4: studies with human liver microsomes and heterologous enzyme expression systems. Br J Clin Pharmacol 40:369–378, 1995.
55. Kroemer HK, Fromm MF, Eichelbaum M. Stereoselectivity in drug metabolism and action: effects of enzyme inhibition and induction. Ther Drug Monit 18:388–392, 1996.
56. Thummel KE, Wilkinson GR. In vitro and in vivo drug interactions involving human cytochrome CYP3A. Annu Rev Pharmacol Toxicol 38:389–430, 1998.
57. Preskorn SH. Clinically relevant pharmacology of selective serotonin reuptake inhibitors. Clin Pharmacokinetic 32 (suppl 1):1–21, 1997.
58. Begg EJ, Chinwah PM, Webb C, et al. Enhanced metabolism of mexiletine after phenytoin administration. Br J Clin Pharmacol 14:219–223, 1982.
59. Dossing M, Pilsgaard H, Rasmussen B, et al. Time course of phenobarbital and cimetidine mediated changes in hepatic drug metabolism. Eur J Clin Pharmacol 25:215–222, 1983.
60. Gugler R, Jensen JC. Omeprazole inhibits oxidative drug metabolism. Gastroenterology 89:1235–1241, 1985.
61. Murray FJ. Outbreak of unexpected reactions among epileptics taking isoniazid. Am Rev Respir Dis 86:729–732, 1962.
62. Brennan RW, Dehejia H, Kutt H, et al. Diphenylhydantoin intoxication attendant to slow inactivation of isoniazid. Neurology 20:687–693, 1970.
63. Humphries TJ. Clinical implications of drug interactions with the cytochrome P-450 enzyme system associated with omeprazole. Dig Dis Sci 36:1665–1669, 1991.
64. Wagner F, Kalusche D, Trenk D, et al. Drug interaction between propafenone and metoprolol. Br J Clin Pharmacol 24:213–220, 1987.
65. Kowey PR, Kirsten EB, Fu CHJ, et al. Interaction between propranolol and propafenone in healthy volunteers. J Clin Pharmacol 29:512–517, 1989.
66. Mooy J, Bohm R, van Kemenade J, et al. The influence of antituberculosis drugs on plasma level of verapamil. Eur J Clin Pharmacol 32:107–109, 1987.
67. Barbarash RA, Bauman JL, Fischer JH, et al. Near-total reduction in verapamil bioavailability by rifampin: electrocardiographic correlates. Chest 94:954–959, 1988.
68. Lum BL, Kaubisch S, Yahanda AM, et al. Alteration of etoposide pharmacokinetics and pharmacodynamics by cyclosporine in a Phase I trial of modulate multidrug resistance. J Clin Oncol 10:1635–1642, 1992.
69. Aherne GW, Piall E, Marks V, et al. Prolongation and enhancement of serum methotrexate concentrations by probenecid. BMJ 1:1097–1099, 1978.
70. Hedman A, Angelin B, Arvidsson A, et al. Interactions in the renal and biliary elimination of digoxin: stereoselective differences between quinine and quinidine. Clin Pharmacol Ther 47:20–26, 1990.
71. Thomsen K, Schou M. Renal lithium excretion in man. Am J Physiol 215:823–827, 1968.
72. Feder R. Reversal of antidepressant activity of fluoxetine by cyproheptadine in three patients. J Clin Psychiatry 52:163–164, 1991.
73. Tatro DS. Drugs interfering with control of the diabetic patient: hypoglycemic drug–drug interactions. Rev Drug Interact 1:3–34, 1974.
74. Tatro DS, Briggs RL, Chavez-Pardo R, et al. Detection and prevention of drug interactions utilizing an online computer system. Drug Info J 9:10–17, 1975.
75. Tatro DS, Briggs RL, Chavez-Pardo R, et al. Online drug interaction surveillance. Am J Hosp Pharm 32:417–420, 1975.
76. Tatro DS. Understanding drug interactions. Facts and Comparisons. Drug Newsletter 7:57–59, 1988.
77. Salem SAM, Rajjayabun P, Shepherd AMM, et al. Reduced induction of drug metabolism in the elderly. Age Ageing 7:68, 1978.
78. Tatro DS. Effects of smoking on drug therapy. Facts and Comparisons. Drug Newsletter 13:49–51, 1994.
79. Perucca E, Hedges A, Makki A, et al. A comparative study of the relative enzyme-inducing properties of anticonvulsant drugs in epileptic patients. Br J Clin Pharmacol 18:401–410, 1984.

CHAPTER 4
CLINICAL TOXICOLOGY

Wendy Klein-Schwartz and Gary M. Oderda

Clinical toxicology deals with the assessment and medical treatment of patients exposed acutely or chronically to potentially harmful agents. Because of the diverse nature of the substances involved in poisonings and the wide range of clinical manifestations and their treatment, optimal management of the poisoned patient is achieved through an interdisciplinary approach to patient care. Expertise provided by physicians, nurses, pharmacists, social workers, and paraprofessionals contributes greatly to the care of these patients.

BACKGROUND

Poisoning is a serious problem in the United States today. The American Association of Poison Control Centers (AAPCC) Toxic Exposure Surveillance System (TESS) reported 2,241,082 human poison exposures in 1998.[1] This figure does not reflect the actual number reported to poison centers nationally because reporting is voluntary. Although it is difficult to be certain of the true magnitude of the problem, it is estimated that each year 2.4 to 4.6 million poison exposure cases occur nationally, with accidental poisoning accounting for 9027 deaths in 1995.[1,2]

Poisoning is a common type of pediatric injury. Children's natural curiosity can have disastrous consequences: 53% of poisonings occur in children less than 6 years old.[1] Most childhood poisonings are unintentional and result from ingestion. The most common substances involved in poison exposures in children less than 6 years old are drugs, personal care products, cleaning substances, and plants. The drugs most commonly involved are analgesics and antipyretics, cough and cold products, topical preparations, antimicrobials, vitamins, and gastrointestinal (GI) preparations. Fortunately, many poison exposures in children result in minimal toxicity and can be managed outside a health care facility.

For poison exposures reported to poison centers, 7.1% occur in children between 6 and 12 years old and 7.1% occur in adolescents between 13 and 19 years.[1] Poisonings in adolescents and adults are more often intentional and generally are responsible for more significant morbidity and mortality than those in children. Whereas 92% of exposures in children 6 to 12 years old are unintentional, only 54% are unintentional in adolescents. Approximately 33% of poisonings reported to poison centers involve adults over 19 years old, and 72% of these exposures are unintentional.[1] Unintentional exposures can result from therapeutic errors, product misuse, and environmental and occupational exposures. Intentional exposures include suicide attempts, substance abuse, and drug misuse. Unintentional exposures are common in older adults, in part because of the large number of medications many older adults take as well as physiologic and psychological changes associated with aging.[3]

ROLE AND STATUS OF POISON CENTERS

The first poison center was established in Chicago in 1953. Today, poison centers exist in most major U.S. metropolitan areas. Regional poison centers can more efficiently and effectively provide information to a large population or geographic area. A region may be defined as a major metropolitan area, a portion of a large state, an entire state, or several states. In some more populous states such as

Florida, Texas, and California, systems of regional poison centers exist. Regional centers often handle 15,000 or more human exposure calls each year. Regional poison centers handle large numbers of cases, allowing staff to develop expertise. Poison centers receive calls relating to drugs, chemicals, household products, personal care products, plants, animal toxins, fish toxins, food poisoning, and other toxins. Approximately 43% of calls involve exposures to drugs. The majority of calls to the poison center come from the public and can be managed in a non–health care facility.

A regional poison center provides telephone information 24 hours a day, using comprehensive information sources and management protocols, and has access to regional treatment facilities for patient referral and transport. Additional components include a regional system for providing poisoning care, public and health professional education programs, and a regional data collection and reporting system.

Clinical pharmacists or nurses often are administratively responsible for operating the center and providing professional input into the treatment of the poisoned patient. Specialists in poison information, usually pharmacists or nurses, are responsible for providing primary telephone consultations.

The AAPCC has criteria for poison centers and certifies centers meeting these standards. In 1994, there were 87 poison centers in the United States.[4] In 1999, there were 60 poison centers certified by the AAPCC. Poison centers (both certified and noncertified) reporting cases to the AAPCC served 95.3% of the U.S. population in 1998.

Poison centers provide cost savings by managing many poison exposures at the site and preventing unnecessary visits to health care facilities. A benefit–cost analysis found that poison centers reduced the number of patients who were medically treated but not hospitalized by 24% and the number of hospitalizations by 12%.[5] For every dollar spent on poison center services, almost $8 in savings is realized. A study found that the average cost per successful outcome with poison center services was approximately half of that without the services of a regional poison center.[6]

Despite the important public health function of poison centers and their cost savings, many poison centers have been faced with unstable or declining funding since the early 1990s. This funding crisis has resulted in several regional poison centers closing or being threatened with closure. A congressional hearing to address the problem was held in March 1994; although the hearing increased awareness of the funding problems, no specific action resulted. An analysis of potential economies of scale performed by researchers at the Center for Health Policy Research at the George Washington University Medical Center in 1997 recommended a partially integrated system of poison centers linked through a single 800 number. In 1999 federal funding for a single national toll-free telephone number and a national education campaign to promote the number and poison prevention was approved. Bills allocating federal money to stabilize funding of regional poison control centers are being considered. The future of these bills and poison center funding is yet to be determined.

Poison information and drug information centers differ in several respects. Poison centers provide services both to professionals and to the general public, whereas some drug information centers provide information only to health professionals. The volume of calls to poison centers usually is higher than for drug information centers. Rapid retrieval of information is necessary in poison centers because of the potential emergency nature of calls. Therefore, the information sources used for handling the majority of cases are mainly secondary resources. The assessment and recommendations are provided during the initial call to the center. As a result, the depth of literature evaluation performed in a poison center is less than that in a drug information center.

POISON PREVENTION

Strategies for injury prevention include education, engineering and technology, and enforcement (legislation and regulation). A major component of poison center activity is poison prevention education. Poison prevention education often is targeted to parents and caretakers of young children, with emphasis on poison prevention and treatment strategies. Although poison prevention activities may decrease the number of pediatric exposures and minimize the severity of childhood intoxications, these efforts generally have little impact on intentional poisonings in adults.

Technologic advances with a major impact on childhood poisonings include child-resistant closures (CRCs) and child-resistant blister packs. Legislation and regulations about warning labels and CRCs have played key roles in the decline of serious poisonings in children. Child-resistant packaging of many household products and prescription drugs was mandated by the Poison Prevention Packaging Act in 1970. This act has resulted in a 65% decline in ingestions of products packaged in CRCs.[7] The decline in aspirin poisoning dramatically demonstrates the impact of CRCs. Forty years ago aspirin was the leading cause of unintentional poisonings and poisoning deaths in children under 5 years old. There has been a progressive decline in both aspirin ingestion and deaths since the mid-1960s.[8] In 1997, ingestion of aspirin alone in children under 6 years old accounted for 0.39% of exposures in this age group reported to poison centers.[1] Although other factors may have contributed to this decline, including greater public awareness of the dangers of aspirin and increasing use of acetaminophen, the CRC packaging requirements for aspirin-containing products are considered the major factor.

Pharmacists play a critical role in enforcing drug packaging legislation and regulations. All prescription drugs should be dispensed in CRCs unless specifically excluded by law. Recent regulations require CRCs on mouthwashes containing more than 5% ethanol and child-resistant blister packaging and warning labels on iron products with 30 mg or more of iron. If a patient requests a non-CRC, the pharmacist should warn the patient to store the container properly to avoid an unintentional poisoning. Older adults who request non-CRCs may not have young children of their own, but many have grandchildren who come to visit.

Pharmacists should promote poison prevention by distributing educational materials and syrup of ipecac. Parents should be cautioned to contact their poison center, physician, or pharmacist before giving the ipecac so that the situation can be evaluated to determine the appropriateness of administering an emetic. If syrup of ipecac is indicated, the health professional can review dosing with the caller, follow up to determine whether the person has vomited, and provide additional instructions about the side effects of ipecac or symptoms to watch for that might indicate the need for additional evaluation and treatment. If ipecac is not indicated, the health professional can discourage its use and recommend other treatment if necessary. Use of activated charcoal outside of health care facilities is not routinely recommended because of difficulty with administration; however, some poison centers are investigating the feasibility of recommending it at home.[9]

ANALYSIS OF A POISONING SITUATION: TYPES OF QUESTIONS ASKED

In some poisoning calls, the caller does not volunteer enough information initially for the pharmacist to assess the situation. The fact that an overdose has occurred is not always obvious. Occasionally a poisoning situation can be uncovered only by persistent questioning. Inquiries relating to tablet identification or other general information may involve a poisoning, and this information can be elicited by determining why the caller needs the information.

In addition, poisoning should be considered in the differential diagnosis whenever there is an abrupt onset of illness with multiple organ system involvement, especially if the patient is a child under 5 years old or has a history of a previous ingestion.[10]

When a poisoning is suspected, the following information must be obtained to analyze the situation (Fig. 4.1):

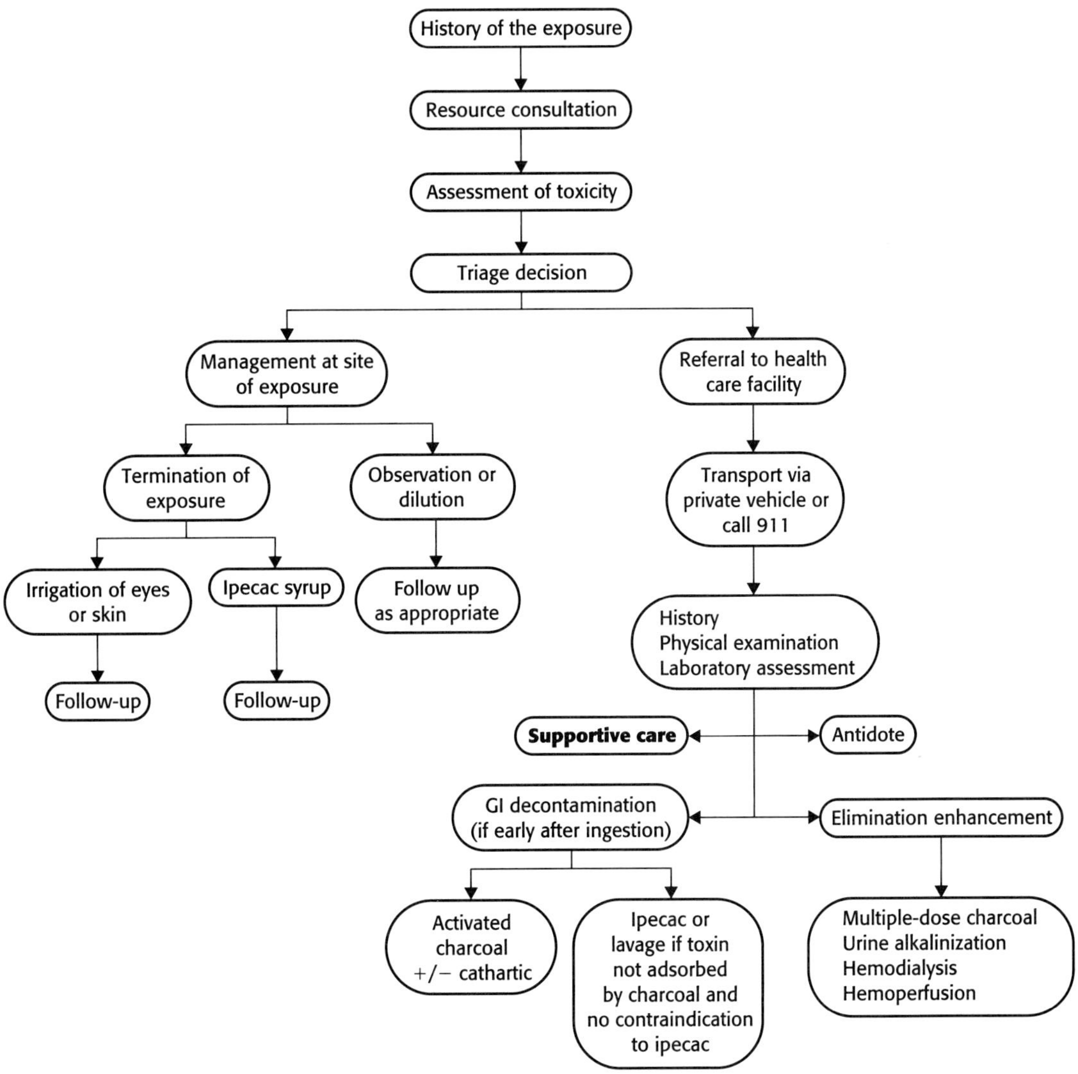

Figure 4.1. Algorithm for assessment and treatment of a poison exposure.

- Substance. This information should include ingredients and their percentages. Examples of situations in which the substance involved may be unknown include patients who are unable to give a history (e.g., patient is comatose) or who ingest tablets or capsules from an unmarked container or who ingest an unidentified plant.
- Amount. If an accurate determination of the amount ingested is impossible and the product is potentially toxic, one must assume that a potentially toxic amount was ingested or that the total amount originally in the container was ingested. In intentional exposures, the patient's report of the amount ingested should be considered suspect.
- Time since exposure. By knowing about the onset and duration of action of the substance, one can determine whether the symptoms are consistent with the history of the amount ingested and the time since exposure. In addition, treatment recommendations, such as whether to empty the stomach, may be influenced by the length of time since ingestion.
- Symptoms. Determine whether symptoms are consistent with the substance involved; if not, determine what other substances or medical conditions may be responsible for these symptoms. Severe signs and symptoms, such as respiratory and cardiovascular collapse, necessitate immediate treatment. Some treatment modalities are contraindicated when certain signs or symptoms are present (e.g., emetics in the comatose patient).
- Patient's age and weight. These are important considerations in determining the toxicity of the substance and dosing antidotes.
- Past medical history and prior therapy. The patient's medical history may influence the treatment or severity of the intoxication. Some home remedies may complicate therapy, whereas other prior treatments may influence subsequent recommendations.

INFORMATION SOURCES

After the poisoning history and the patient's current clinical status are obtained, appropriate information sources are consulted. The major toxicology information sources are secondary sources designed to allow rapid retrieval of toxicity and management information. The primary literature should be consulted in some cases.

The following references are strictly toxicology-oriented and do not include other important references, such as pharmacology or drug interaction texts that are available in both pharmacies and poison centers.

Poisindex[R] (B. Rumack, ed. Englewood, CO: Micromedex, new edition published four times yearly) is a computerized database with information on most commercial products and other agents, including biologicals such as plants and venomous animals. It is usually available either as a compact disk (CD-ROM) system or a multiuser intranet system. The editorial board is made up of people actively involved with poisoning and poison centers throughout the United States. For each product, the manufacturer's name, the type of product, ingredients, percentages (if available), and tablet imprint (if applicable) are listed. Specific toxicity information also may be included. For all agents the user is referred to the appropriate managements. Managements are preceded by overviews that contain summaries of emergency treatment and toxicity information, eliminating the need to scan many screens of information initially. The overview is followed by the complete management, which includes information on available forms, pharmacology, clinical effects, kinetics, range of toxicity, laboratory (e.g., blood levels), treatment, and major references. The major advantages of this system are ease of use; storage of a large amount of data in a small space; timeliness; detailed management protocols; information on drugs, chemicals, household products, food poisoning, mushrooms, snakes, and drug imprint codes; and cross-referenced product information. It is an essential resource for poison centers and is also useful for other health care providers.

Toxicology of the Eye, 4th ed. (W. M. Grant and J. S. Schuman. Springfield, IL: Charles C. Thomas, 1993) is an excellent resource on the effects of various agents upon contact with the eye as well as agents that produce ocular toxicity systemically. This is evident in this two-volume set's subtitle, *Effects on the Eyes and Visual System from Chemicals, Drugs, Metals & Minerals, Plants, Toxins & Venoms; also Systemic Side Effects from Eye Medications.* Specific human information is discussed where available. A separate treatment section is included.

Patty's Industrial Hygiene and Toxicology, 3rd ed. (G. D. Clayton and F. E. Clayton, eds. New York: Wiley, 1981) is a series published in three volumes. Volume 1 discusses general principles, Volume 2A, 2B, and 2C specific toxicology information, and Volume 3 industrial hygiene practice. Poison centers find Volume 2A, 2B, and 2C the most useful. Both chronic and acute exposures to industrial chemicals are described. For each chemical, information such as the following is provided: source, use, and industrial exposure; physical and chemical properties; determination in the atmosphere; physiologic response; hygiene standard of permissible exposure; flammability; and odor and warning properties.

Ellenhorn's Medical Toxicology: Diagnosis and Treatment of Human Poisoning, 2nd ed. (M. J. Ellenhorn, S. Schonwald, G. Ordog, and J. Wasserberger. Baltimore: Williams & Wilkins, 1997), *Clinical Management of Poisoning and Drug Overdose*, 3rd ed. (L. M. Haddad, M. W. Shannon, and J. F. Winchester, eds. Philadelphia: W.B. Saunders, 1998), and *Goldfrank's Toxicology Emergencies*, 6th ed. (L. R. Goldfrank, N. E. Flomenbaum, N. A. Lewin, et al., eds. Norwalk, CT: Appleton & Lange, 1998) are textbooks of clinical toxicology that provide reviews of poisoning by drugs, chemicals, and biologicals including clinical manifestations of toxicity, mechanism of toxicity, pharmacokinetics and toxicokinetics, diagnostic evaluation, and management. Tables and algorithms enhance the presentation of material.

Hazardous Materials Toxicology: Clinical Principles of Environmental Health (J. B. Sullivan and G. R. Krieger. Baltimore: Williams & Wilkins, 1992) begins by discussing general principles of hazardous material toxicology. It then moves into regulatory, health, and safety aspects of hazardous materials and emergency medical response and hazardous materials. Specific information on toxic materials is provided in two ways. Section IV describes toxic hazards by industrial site. For example, chemical hazards in the tire and rubber manufacturing industry are covered. The remaining section covers specific toxins. This text is an excellent reference for those concerned with occupational and environmental exposures.

Proctor and Hughes' Chemical Hazards of the Workplace, 3rd ed. (G. J. Hathaway, N. H. Proctor, J. P. Hughes, et al. New York: Van Nostrand Reinhold, 1991) has introductory chapters that deal with general toxicologic concepts. The majority of the book consists of short monographs on 542 chemicals most likely to be encountered in the workplace. It is well referenced and an excellent source of information on common and obscure chemicals found in the workplace.

Disposition of Toxic Drugs and Chemicals in Man, 5th ed. (R. C. Baselt. Foster City, CA: Chemical Toxicology Institute, 2000) provides a summary of current information on toxic drugs and chemicals in the human body. Each monograph includes the structure, occurrence and usage, blood concentrations, metabolism and excretion, toxicity, analysis, and references. This reference is very useful for interpreting laboratory findings in patients or from postmortem toxicologic analysis.

Handbook of Pesticide Toxicology (W. J. Hayes and E. R. Laws. San Diego, CA: Academic Press, 1991) is a three-volume set. Volume 1 provides general principles of pesticide toxicology. Volumes 2 and 3 provide information on specific pesticides including identity, properties and use, toxicity to laboratory animals, and toxicity to humans. The sections on toxicity to humans include experimental exposure, accidental and intentional poisoning, use experience, laboratory findings, pathology, and treatment of poisoning.

Poisoning and Drug Overdose, 3rd ed. (Kent Olson, ed. Norwalk, CT: Appleton & Lange, 1999) is a compact, portable handbook. Each section is in outline form; many sections include figures and tables. Section 1 provides comprehensive evaluation and treatment. Section 2 is on the diagnosis and treatment of specific poisons and drugs. Each monograph provides information on mechanism of toxicity, toxic dosage, clinical presentation, diagnosis, and treatment. Section 3 reviews therapeutic drugs and antidotes discussed in Sections 1 and 2. Section 4 describes environmental and occupational toxicology.

SUPPORTIVE CARE

Supportive care is the most important part of treating the seriously intoxicated patient. Close attention to airway, breathing, level of consciousness, and blood pressure is critical. Although some clinical toxicologists may argue about the value of some GI decontamination procedures or disagree over the specific indications for extracorporeal removal of toxins, there is no disagreement about the value of supportive care. In serious intoxications, supportive care sustains the patient while the toxin is being detoxified by liver metabolism or renal elimination.

All patients with central nervous system (CNS) depression should be given naloxone (0.4 to 2.0 mg) in case altered mental status is the result of opioid intoxication. Naloxone rapidly reverses CNS depression from opioids and helps identify certain substances responsible for the intoxication but has no serious consequences if given to patients without opioid intoxication. Blood glucose should be assessed rapidly by fingerstick glucometer and intravenous dextrose (50 mL D50W [50% dextrose in water]) administered for hypoglycemia. If blood glucose cannot be measured immediately, glucose should be administered anyway to rule out hypoglycemia. Flumazenil, the benzodiazepine antagonist, is not routinely recommended in overdose cases because of potential adverse consequences, including seizures and dysrhythmias in patients with coingestants.

Airway and breathing should be assessed immediately. If respirations are compromised, the patient should be intubated and placed on a ventilator. Intravenous diazepam or lorazepam is first-line therapy for seizures. Hypotension is treated initially with intravenous fluids. If blood pressure remains low, vasopressors such as dopamine or norepinephrine should be administered. A patient with an overdose of potentially cardiotoxic agents or unknown agents should be on a cardiac monitor. Fluid and electrolyte status should be monitored and intravenous fluids adjusted accordingly.

The need for supportive care and the level of supportive care required depend on the toxin and the patient. Similarly, the time period during which supportive care is needed varies among patients. Decisions about extubation and discontinuing vasopressors are based on continued assessment of the patient's level of consciousness and blood pressure.

DECREASING ABSORPTION

The toxic potential of an ingestion can be decreased by minimizing GI absorption. Emptying the stomach, administering an adsorbent, and inducing catharsis are potential treatments that should be considered when a toxic dosage has been ingested. Ideally, GI decontamination should be performed within an hour of ingestion, and for most substances benefit is minimal by 4 hours. Examples of drugs for which GI decontamination may be warranted up to 12 hours after ingestion include salicylates, which delay gastric emptying; anticholinergics, which decrease GI motility; and phenytoin, which is slowly and erratically absorbed from the GI tract.

Activated charcoal has become the primary treatment modality in the emergency department (ED) for preventing absorption from the GI tract. The use of ipecac syrup or gastric lavage is limited to patients who have taken agents not adsorbed by activated charcoal. The major role of ipecac syrup is for use in the home to treat ingestions with the potential for mild toxicity. The use of ipecac syrup has decreased from 13.4% of all exposures reported to TESS in 1983 to 1.2% of all exposures in 1998, whereas use of activated charcoal increased from 4.0% of all exposures in 1983 to 6.8% of all exposures in 1998.[1] Some of the decrease in ipecac syrup use may be attributable to a decrease in the percentage of children included in the TESS system. In 1983 64% of all reported exposures were in children less than 6 years old, as compared with 53% in 1998.[1]

Comparison of Gastrointestinal Decontamination Modalities: Ipecac and Lavage

Early studies suggested that ipecac was more effective than lavage.[11,12] In many studies comparing emesis and lavage, the size of the lavage tube is not mentioned or it is smaller than is currently recommended. Tubes with small lumens, such as Levine tubes, cannot remove large particles of tablets, whole tablets, or groups of tablets clumped together. Lavage with a large Ewald tube, 28 to 36 Fr or larger, should more efficiently empty the stomach. A recent volunteer study using a crossover design compared ipecac with lavage with a 40-Fr tube in 19 adults using a technetium-99m marker and found that ipecac recovered 54.1% whereas lavage recovered 35.5%.[13] In contrast, ED-based studies using large lavage tubes suggest that lavage is superior.[14,15] Potential methodologic biases in these studies leave this issue unresolved.[16] Of concern is the fact that even with large lavage tubes, patients have residual intragastric solids after lavage.[17,18] Another important consideration is that the percentage return with either emesis or lavage is low.[19–21]

When gastric emptying is warranted (i.e., home management, ingestion of an agent not adsorbed by activated charcoal), ipecac-induced emesis should be the procedure of first choice in children. When emetics are contraindicated, lavage is preferred. Lavage should be considered in adults who are treated early after the ingestion of substances with high inherent toxicity (e.g., cyclic antidepressants). Ipecac syrup should not be administered to patients who will be receiving activated charcoal because of the risk of aspirating vomited charcoal.

Comparison of Gastrointestinal Decontamination Modalities: Activated Charcoal Versus Other Modalities

Several human volunteer studies comparing ipecac or lavage with activated charcoal have found activated charcoal superior.[22–24] For example, a crossover study using 5 g ampicillin as the test drug found activated charcoal and cathartic most effective, preventing absorption of 57%, followed by ipecac (38%) and gastric lavage (32%).[24]

ED-based studies in overdosed patients have been performed with the goal of determining whether any of these procedures affect patient outcome. Problems inherent with these studies include difficulty enrolling sufficient numbers of patients, the wide variety of substances in different combinations and at varying dosages, and varying times after ingestion of arrival at EDs. Very few data are available in children. A prospective, randomized, unblinded trial comparing charcoal alone with ipecac plus charcoal in 70 children found a statistically significantly longer time in the ED before receiving charcoal, higher proportion of patients who vomited charcoal, and longer duration of time discharged patients spend in the ED in the ipecac plus charcoal group as compared with the charcoal-only group.[25] There was no difference in the proportion of children admitted or the proportion who improved in the ED between groups, but this may have been related to insufficient power to detect a difference because of the small number of patients.

A prospective randomized study of ipecac or lavage plus activated charcoal and a cathartic compared with activated charcoal and a cathartic in 592 acute oral drug overdose cases found no difference in the number of hospital days, number of days in the intensive care unit (ICU), clinical deterioration, and morbidity and mortality between the two groups.[26] Lavage improved outcome if performed in obtunded patients within 1 hour of ingestion. Critics of the study argue that the possibility of type II error exists (the failure to prove a benefit for gastric emptying does not mean that no benefit exists).[27] In addition, the seven sickest patients were assigned to the lavage group in a nonrandom manner, and patients were excluded if they took agents not adsorbed by charcoal.[27] Both maneuvers biased the study against showing a benefit for gastric emptying. A study in 876 patients, which was designed to replicate the preceding study, found no difference between any of the groups in any of the outcome measures.[28] These investigators recommended against using gastric emptying procedures in adults after acute overdose even if they present with toxicity within 1 hour.

In another prospective study, patients with a symptomatic overdose were randomly assigned to receive either gastric emptying or activated charcoal, whereas asymptomatic patients were just observed or were given activated charcoal.[29] Activated charcoal provided no benefit in asymptomatic patients, and gastric emptying in symptomatic patients did not improve outcome and increased the likelihood of aspiration pneumonitis. A possible bias toward nonemptying exists because the population had limited toxicity and because patients who took agents not well adsorbed by charcoal or with delayed toxicity were excluded.[27] Albertson et al.[30] also found a higher risk of aspiration in patients receiving ipecac syrup and activated charcoal than in patients receiving activated charcoal alone in a study of 200 overdosed patients. There was no difference in the percentage hospitalized, the percentage admitted to an ICU, or the number of hospital or ICU days, but there was a difference in the mean time the patients spent in the ED (mean of 6.8 hours in the ipecac and charcoal group and 6 hours in the activated charcoal–only group).

A comparison of three methods of GI decontamination (activated charcoal alone, saline lavage with activated charcoal, and activated charcoal with saline lavage and activated charcoal) in 51 patients presenting to an ED with tricyclic antidepressant overdose demonstrated no statistically significant differences in clinical effects or outcome measures.[31] However, a trend toward decreased length of stay, ICU time, and mechanical ventilation time in the group treated with activated charcoal, saline lavage, and activated charcoal was noted. The clinical significance of this trend is tentative because this group may have had less neurologic impairment on initial presentation. A concern with finding no difference between the groups was the low power (ranging from 11 to 40% depending on the group) to detect 24-hour differences in clinical outcome measures.

The American Academy of Clinical Toxicology and the European Association of Poison Centers and Clinical Toxicologists recently published a series of position statements on GI decontamination questioning the utility of GI decontamination, especially gastric emptying. The following summarizes key points from those position statements:

- There is no evidence from clinical studies that ipecac improves the outcome of poisoned patients, and its routine administration in the ED should be abandoned.[32]
- There is no certain evidence that gastric lavage improves clinical outcome, it may cause significant morbidity, and it should not be considered unless the patient has ingested a potentially life-threatening amount of a poison and the procedure can be undertaken within 60 minutes of ingestion.[33]
- Administering activated charcoal may be considered if a patient has ingested a potentially toxic amount of a poison (which is known to be adsorbed to charcoal) up to 1 hour previously; there are insufficient data to support or exclude its use more than 1 hour after ingestion.[34]
- Experimental data conflict regarding the use of cathartics in combination with activated charcoal. Based on the available data, the routine use of a cathartic in combination with activated charcoal is not endorsed. If a cathartic is used, it should be limited to a single dose to minimize adverse effects.[35]

Overall, these data suggest a limited role for gastric emptying. The majority of patients treated in a health care facility can be treated with activated charcoal alone. GI decontamination with activated charcoal appears to be as effective as or superior to gastric emptying with ipecac or lavage. Ipecac syrup's role is primarily for children with toxic ingestions for whom treatment in a health care facility is considered unnecessary.

Syrup of Ipecac

Syrup of ipecac acts locally on the GI tract and centrally through stimulation of the chemoreceptor trigger zone and the vomiting center. Emetics are absolutely contraindicated in the following situations:

- Patients with significant CNS depression manifested by severe lethargy, loss of the gag reflex, or unconsciousness. The risk of aspiration of the vomitus into the lungs, a potentially severe complication, is significant.
- Patients who are seizing or in whom seizures are imminent. Aspiration is a significant risk.
- Patients who have ingested a caustic substance. Strong acids and bases may produce severe burns of the mucous membranes of the mouth and esophagus. During emesis, these tissues will be reexposed to the caustic, and further damage may occur. In addition, the force of vomiting may cause perforation of the damaged esophagus.
- Patients who have ingested hydrocarbons (e.g., kerosene, gasoline). Aspiration risk is high because of their low viscosity, low surface tension, and high volatility. When aliphatic hydrocarbons are ingested, emptying the stomach is unnecessary because absorption from the GI tract does not appear to be responsible for toxicity. Ingestions of aromatic hydrocarbons, halogenated hydrocarbons, or potentially dangerous chemicals such as pesticides in a hydrocarbon solvent may necessitate GI decontamination under medical supervision, and activated charcoal is preferred.

Syrup of ipecac is available without a prescription in 15- and 30-mL containers. Syrup of ipecac is almost 100% effective in producing emesis when dosed appropriately.[36] Although the use of ipecac syrup at home in children under 1 year old has been questioned, several studies have demonstrated that ipecac syrup is effective at inducing vomiting and safe in this age group.[37–39] However, it is not recommended in infants less that 6 months old.

Vomiting usually occurs about 18 minutes after a 15- to 30-mL dose is administered.[36] The dosage of ipecac syrup is 10 mL in children under 1 year old, 15 mL in older children, and 30 mL in adolescents and adults. After ipecac, at least 4 to 6 oz of water in children and 12 to 16 oz in adults is recommended. Although milk has been shown to delay vomiting from syrup of ipecac in adult volunteers,[40] another study failed to demonstrate a delay in clinical situations involving children.[41] If vomiting does not occur in 15 to 20 minutes, the initial dosage may be repeated one time. If vomiting still does not occur, the decision to lavage or administer activated charcoal in a health care facility would be based primarily on the patient's condition and the potential danger of the ingested agent.

Ipecac should be given as soon after the ingestion as possible. Saincher et al.[42] evaluated the efficacy of ipecac after an ingestion of 3900 mg acetaminophen in human volunteers using a four-limbed randomized crossover design of control and ipecac at 5, 30, and 60 minutes after ingestion. Bioavailability was 67% lower than in controls when ipecac was given at 5 minutes (statistically significant), 11% at 30 minutes, and 21% at 60 minutes. By analyzing poison center data, Bond[43] concluded that home use of ipecac syrup was safe and effective in reducing the need for pediatric ED visits. Increased use of ipecac syrup explained 45% of the variation in rates of ED referral among poison centers. Outcomes among home-treated patients were good. Home use of ipecac syrup allowed more cost-effective management of childhood poisoning.

The most common side effects of therapeutic dosages of ipecac are diarrhea and mild drowsiness. The adverse effects in children 6 to 11 months and 12 to 35 months of age who were given ipecac syrup for a potentially toxic ingestion are summarized in Table 4.1.[37]

Table 4.1 ▪ Development of Side Effects Possibly Related to Ipecac Administration

	Patients with Side Effect (%)	
Side Effect	**6–11 mo**	**12–35 mo**
Diarrhea	25.7	25.8
Drowsiness	19.0	19.5
Irritability and hyperactivity	5.7	2.6
Coughing and choking	2.9	3.6
Diaphoresis and flushing	1.0	0.0
Fever	4.8	0.7

Source: Reference 37.

Protracted vomiting (persistent vomiting for more than 3 hours after the initial episode) was seen in 4.2% of all patients. This is of concern because persistent vomiting may delay the administration of activated charcoal. Therefore, ipecac should not be given to patients who will be receiving activated charcoal.

Toxic reactions to large dosages of ipecac syrup or inadvertent use of the fluid extract of ipecac, which is 14 times stronger than ipecac syrup, have been reported. The most common complications are GI and cardiovascular. In large dosages, ipecac is a cardiotoxin and has been shown to cause reversible depression of T waves, bradycardia, atrial fibrillation, and hypotension. Death has been reported after ingestion of as little as 10 mL of the fluid extract in a 4-year-old child.[44] A 14-month-old child died after a therapeutic dose of ipecac syrup, but death was attributed to an anatomic defect.[45] A fatal intracerebral hemorrhage was reported in an 84-year-old woman given ipecac syrup and activated charcoal after ingesting a nontoxic amount of boric acid.[46] Fatalities have also been reported in adults with bulimia or anorexia nervosa who ingest large amounts of ipecac chronically to lose weight.[47]

Gastric Lavage

Gastric lavage has very limited clinical application. It may be considered for overdoses where the substance is not adsorbed by activated charcoal. Gastric lavage is a procedure in which a tube is inserted into the stomach through the nose or the mouth. The patient should be in the left lateral decubitus position with the head forward and down. The contents of the stomach are first aspirated through this tube. Fluid is then instilled into the tube, allowed to mix with gastric contents, and then removed via the same tube. The process is repeated until the gastric washings are clear. Three lavage methods were found to remove 80 to 85% of a technetium-99m diethylenetriaminepentaacetic acid marker when the procedure was begun 5 minutes after the marker was administered.[48] With the use of a double-syringe method, lavage was completed in less than half the time, about 3 minutes, as compared with other methods.

Lavage may be performed in comatose patients. The patient's airway should be protected by prior insertion of a cuffed endotracheal tube to prevent aspiration. Patients with seizures may undergo lavage once seizures have been controlled. Lavage is contraindicated in caustic ingestions because the lavage tube may produce additional esophageal and gastric damage as it is inserted. Initial management of a caustic ingestion is limited to dilution with milk or water followed by an evaluation of the extent and degree of burns.

The size of the lavage tube is one of the most important factors determining the effectiveness with which the stomach is emptied. Optimally, a 36-Fr (12 mm, or about 0.5 inch in diameter) or larger Ewald or Lavacuator tube should be used by the oral route in adults. Nasogastric tubes usually are smaller and therefore less effective. Smaller tubes (16 to 18 Fr) are used in children, markedly limiting the effectiveness of the procedure.

The lavage solution usually is tap water or a normal saline solution. In children, however, it is safer to use normal saline instead of water because of the child's limited tolerance for electrolyte-free solutions. Water intoxication, tonic–clonic seizures, and coma can result from a 5% increase in body water from absorption of electrolyte-free solutions. Each wash is approximately 200 to 300 mL in adults or 10 mL/kg (usually 50 to 100 mL) in children. The procedure usually requires several liters of fluid in adults.

Activated Charcoal

Activated charcoal is an odorless, tasteless, fine black powder that is an effective nonspecific adsorbent of a wide variety of drugs and chemicals. Two characteristics are necessary for activated charcoal to be effective: small particle size with large surface area and low mineral content (vegetable origin). For these reasons, charcoal tablets are ineffective. Activated charcoal products with higher surface areas have been developed.[49] Activated charcoal has been shown to be ineffective for cyanide, ethanol, methanol, caustic alkalis, and mineral acids.[50]

The dosage of charcoal is approximately 10 times the amount of the ingested agent. Because this dosage does not take into account tablet excipients or food that may bind to the charcoal, which decreases its adsorptive capacity, it is a good idea to give an excess of charcoal. The usual dosages of activated charcoal are 1 g/kg or 60 to 100 g in adults and 15 to 30 g in children. One measuring tablespoonful of activated charcoal contains 5 to 6 g. If commercially packaged charcoal products are not used, the pharmacy should prepackage weighed charcoal because the density of charcoal products may vary. Activated charcoal should be stored in tightly sealed glass or metal containers. Prolonged exposure to vapors of the atmosphere decreases adsorptive capability. Activated charcoal is mixed with water to the consistency of a slurry and is administered either orally or by lavage tube. Charcoal does not mix well with water and must be shaken vigorously.

This usually is not a problem with commercially packaged products, which contain sorbitol or a suspending agent.

Activated charcoal particle size is important in determining the amount of adsorption. Roberts et al.[51] compared the effectiveness of low-surface-area charcoal (LSA, Liquichar, 950 m^2/g) and high-surface-area charcoal (HSA, CharcoAid 2000, 2,000 m^2/g) in human volunteers ingesting 50 mg/kg of acetaminophen. The 4-hour plasma acetaminophen levels were 44 to 85% lower in the HSA charcoal than in the LSA charcoal group. A statistically significantly lower area under the curve was also seen with HSA charcoal than with LSA charcoal. In addition, all subjects felt that the HSA charcoal product was less gritty and more palatable.

Because time is important in determining the efficacy of gastric decontamination, prehospital administration should be encouraged. Wax and Cobaugh,[52] in a review of prehospital charts of patients who were transported to an ED, showed that GI decontamination was done in 3 of 361 patients (2%), all of whom received ipecac. Follow-up data at a single hospital showed that 30 of 43 (70%) patients who might have been suitable candidates for activated charcoal received it in the ED. Median time to administration of activated charcoal in the ED was 82 minutes, a significant delay compared to starting it in the field. In a similar study, Crockett et al.[53] performed a retrospective review of emergency medical service run sheets and ED records of poisoned patients in two hospitals. Patients who met prehospital criteria for administration of activated charcoal were divided into two groups: those who received prehospital activated charcoal and those who did not. All patients who did not receive prehospital activated charcoal were given activated charcoal in the ED. The average time for prehospital activated charcoal administration was 5 minutes after first encounter with the paramedics, as compared with 51.4 minutes for those receiving it in the ED. Further study is needed before use of activated charcoal in the home can be recommended because poor palatability may compromise ability to administer it.

Saline and Hyperosmotic Cathartics

Cathartics are used in conjunction with activated charcoal to further decrease the absorption of the ingested agent from the GI tract. By speeding the travel of gastric contents, cathartics decrease the likelihood of absorption. A study in rats demonstrated that sodium sulfate enhanced the effect of activated charcoal in preventing the absorption of the drugs tested.[54] There are no clinical studies to document the efficacy of cathartics in overdose, and studies in human volunteers have shown conflicting findings. Two studies in human volunteers found that cathartics had no effect on aspirin absorption when used with activated charcoal.[55,56] A study using sorbitol as the cathartic demonstrated that activated charcoal and sorbitol resulted in significantly lower aspirin absorption than did activated charcoal alone.[57] An additional effect of cathartics has been demonstrated when the ingested agent is a sustained-release product.[58]

Saline cathartics, such as magnesium sulfate and magnesium citrate, or hyperosmotic cathartics, such as sorbitol, are the agents of choice. Irritant cathartics, such as aloes or cascara, and oil-based cathartics, such as castor oil, are not recommended.

Magnesium sulfate is administered orally in approximately a 10% concentration at 250 mg/kg or 15 to 20 g in an adult. Magnesium sulfate is available as Epsom's salts or as a sterile 10 or 50% solution. Magnesium citrate is used in a dosage of 200 mL in adolescents and adults or 5 mL/kg in children. The adult sorbitol dosage usually is 1 to 3 g/kg as a 35 to 70% solution, and the children's dosage is 1 to 1.5 g/kg as a 35% solution. Cathartics are administered orally or via lavage tube. If charcoal has been administered, the appearance of a charcoal stool indicates that the charcoal (and perhaps the toxic agent) has passed through the GI tract. A study in human volunteers demonstrated that sorbitol enhanced GI transit of charcoal to a greater extent than did magnesium citrate or magnesium sulfate.[59] The onset time of sorbitol is most rapid, followed by magnesium citrate and then magnesium sulfate. Sorbitol produces a higher number of stools in children than do other agents.[60] These cathartics generally are considered safe. However, the patient's hydration and electrolyte balance should be monitored, especially if repeated doses of the cathartic are administered. Magnesium-containing cathartics should not be used in patients with decreased renal function because absorbed magnesium may accumulate and produce toxicity. Hypermagnesemia has been reported after a single 17.5-g dose of magnesium citrate in a 77-year-old woman with theophylline toxicity and poor renal function.[61]

ENHANCING ELIMINATION

If a poison has been absorbed in potentially dangerous quantities, multiple-dose activated charcoal, alteration of urine pH, hemodialysis, and hemoperfusion can be considered. These procedures are not warranted in the majority of poisoned patients and must not replace supportive care.

Multiple-Dose Activated Charcoal

Elimination via the GI tract can be augmented for drugs that are secreted into the stomach or undergo biliary secretion. The use of multiple doses of activated charcoal has also been called GI dialysis. Multiple doses of activated charcoal are recommended for acute or chronic intoxications with dapsone, phenobarbital, and theophylline and for acute intoxications with phenytoin. The excretion half-life for theophylline has been reported to decrease between 50 and 75% after multiple doses of activated charcoal.[62,63] A randomized trial in patients with phenobarbital overdose demonstrated a shorter phenobarbital half-life in the multiple-dose than in the single-dose charcoal group but found no differences in the time course or patient outcome.[64] With the cyclic antidepressants, which undergo enterohepatic recirculation, the effectiveness of multiple-dose charcoal has not been demonstrated convincingly, and it is not recommended.[65–68] Conflicting evidence has been presented for salicylates. Most recently, Mayer et al.[69] showed that multiple-dose charcoal did not enhance excretion of salicylates in human volunteers.

In a porcine model, Chyka et al.[70] found that the characteristics of drugs that enhanced elimination with multiple-dose activated charcoal include a prolonged distributive phase, nonrestrictive protein binding, a small volume of distribution, a long half-life, and a low intrinsic clearance. A review of studies on multiple-dose charcoal found that increased clearance from multiple-dose charcoal has been demonstrated for only a few drugs, and improved outcome has not been demonstrated for any drugs.[71] Aspiration of charcoal and charcoal-induced bowel obstruction are potential complications. A 39-year-old woman on methadone maintenance therapy administered multiple doses of activated charcoal for an amitriptyline overdose developed a 4-cm perforation in the sigmoid colon and a 120-g obstructing charcoal mass.[72]

In multiple-dose activated charcoal regimens, activated charcoal is administered every 4 to 6 hours. A cathartic is administered with the first dose but generally is not administered with subsequent doses. When multiple doses of cathartics have been administered, fluid and electrolyte problems, including hypernatremia and hypermagnesemia, have been reported.[67,73–76]

A 55-year-old salicylate-poisoned patient inadvertently received 30 g magnesium sulfate every 6 hours for four doses, 120 cc 70% sorbitol for two doses, and an activated charcoal preparation containing 70% sorbitol for four doses.[77] She developed an acute abdomen and died. Postmortem revealed a profoundly dilated bowel containing fluid and activated charcoal, with a perforation at the hepatic flexure. This case illustrates that when multiple doses of activated charcoal are given, it is essential that an activated charcoal preparation that does not contain a cathartic be available.

Alteration of Urine pH

Alteration of urine pH to increase the amount of drug in the ionized form and thereby decrease tubular reabsorption has a very limited role in treating most poisoned patients. Despite the theoretical advantages of removing the drug from the body more quickly, no controlled trials have documented changes in patient outcome.

Urine alkalinization increases the renal elimination of phenobarbital (not short-acting barbiturates, such as pentobarbital and secobarbital) and salicylate. Sodium bicarbonate is administered (usually in adults 88 mEq is added to the first liter of intravenous fluid; in children 2 mEq/kg is added to initial intravenous fluids and infused over 1 hour, with subsequent doses of 1 to 2 mEq/kg as needed, with a goal of a urine pH of 7.0 to 8.0). An alkaline urine may be difficult to achieve in severely salicylate-poisoned children and is not recommended by some clinicians in this subset of patients.[78]

Urine acidification increases the renal elimination of amphetamines, phencyclidine, and strychnine; however, it is no longer recommended. Overdoses with these drugs, especially phencyclidine, can produce muscle injury, resulting in rhabdomyolysis and myoglobinuria; in the presence of an acidic urine, myoglobin can precipitate in the tubules, leading to acute renal failure.

Dialysis and Hemoperfusion

In the severely intoxicated patient, hemodialysis or hemoperfusion may be considered to rapidly remove certain toxins from the blood. Hemodialysis removes drugs from the blood by diffusion across a synthetic semipermeable membrane. The dialysate is replaced, continuously or intermittently, with a fresh solution of carefully defined composition. This specialized technique is not available at all hospitals.

The use of dialysis in poisoning cases is limited. The ingested agent must be dialyzable, distributed in or rapidly equilibrated with plasma water, and removed at a rate significantly higher than by normal metabolism and renal excretion. The fact that a drug is dialyzable does not mean that dialysis is indicated.

Dialysis may be considered in patients who are severely intoxicated with a dialyzable drug and are not responding to conservative therapy. Dialysis may be indicated for severe intoxications with ethanol, isopropanol, methanol, ethylene glycol, lithium, phenobarbital, theophylline, and salicylates. Two toxins for which dialysis may be indicated before significant toxicity develops are methanol and ethylene glycol ingestion. Both alcohols are metabolized to compounds more toxic than the parent compound. Methanol is metabolized to formaldehyde and formic acid; ethylene glycol is metabolized to glycoaldehyde, glycolate, glyoxylate, and oxalic acid. If the methanol and ethylene glycol can be removed by dialysis before metabolism, toxicity is minimized.

Hemoperfusion involves pumping blood from the patient through a cartridge containing coated activated charcoal or uncoated activated charcoal in a fixed-bed system. To be effective, not only must the toxin be adsorbed by the material in the column, but the amount removed by hemoperfusion must significantly reduce the total body burden of the ingested agent. For some drugs that are effectively adsorbed, such as the cyclic antidepressants, a large volume of distribution results in a small proportion of the total body burden being eliminated, even if the blood is completely cleared of the drug after passing through the column. Hemoperfusion has been found to be extremely effective for removing theophylline, producing a marked drop in blood levels and a rapid improvement in clinical picture.[79] Potential complications include bleeding, destruction of blood cells (including a significant drop in the platelet count immediately after the procedure), removal of plasma proteins, and hypothermia.[80]

As with dialysis, hemoperfusion should be limited to severely intoxicated patients who have ingested a drug removed by hemoperfusion and are not responding to conservative therapy. In most situations, aggressive supportive care should be adequate to maintain the patient until his or her body is able to detoxify and eliminate the toxin.

SYSTEMIC ANTIDOTES

Although systemic antidotes are available for only a few commonly ingested agents, they may be lifesaving in some intoxications. Early administration of emergency antidotes may be necessary to stabilize the critically ill patient. Antidotes act by a variety of mechanisms to antagonize the effects of a systemically absorbed toxin. Some examples of different mechanisms include reversal of the toxin's action at the receptor (e.g., naloxone for opioids, flumazenil for benzodiazepines, atropine and pralidoxime for organophosphate pesticides), chelation to enhance removal from the body (e.g., deferoxamine for iron), detoxification of the toxic substances or toxic metabolite (*N*-acetylcysteine for acetaminophen), or prevention of metabolism to toxic metabolites (e.g., ethanol or fomepizole for ethylene glycol).

Antidotes can play an important role in treating the poisoned patient but do not replace supportive care and other previously described treatment modalities. If an antidote is available for a particular intoxicant, specific indications should be considered before its use to ensure maximum benefit with minimal adverse effects.

Table 4.2 is a list of major systemic antidotes. Naloxone, deferoxamine, digoxin immune Fab, and *N*-acetylcysteine are also discussed in this section.

Naloxone

Naloxone is one of the most commonly used antidotes because it is used as both a diagnostic and a therapeutic agent in patients presenting with altered mental status. Because naloxone has no opiate agonist activity, administration to patients in whom the coma is not opiate-induced produces no adverse effects. Considered the drug of choice for initial reversal of opioid overdose, naloxone is a pure opiate antagonist without opiate agonist properties. Naloxone competes with opioids at the μ, κ, δ, and σ receptors. Reversal of respiratory depression results from naloxone's action at the μ_2 receptor.

Naloxone reverses CNS and respiratory depression. As a result of naloxone's short half-life of 1 hour, its duration of action is short. Naloxone's antagonistic effects can be as short as 30 minutes but may last as long as 4 hours. The duration of action of naloxone often is shorter than the duration of action of the ingested opioid, especially with methadone and diphenoxylate. It is very important that these patients be monitored closely for reemergence of CNS and respiratory depression so that naloxone boluses can be readministered or a naloxone infusion started.

Naloxone antagonizes naturally occurring and synthetic opiates, including heroin, morphine, codeine, meperidine, propoxyphene, pentazocine, diphenoxylate, and dextromethorphan. For some opiates, particularly propoxyphene and pentazocine, larger than usual dosages of naloxone are needed. If given at a high enough dosage, naloxone rapidly reverses any opiate-induced symptoms.

The usual adult dosage is 0.4 to 2 mg intravenously. Dosages of 0.1 mg/kg or 0.4 to 2 mg have been recommended in children. If no response is seen, the dosage should be repeated. At least 10 mg naloxone should be administered before opiates are ruled out as the cause of toxicity. A continuous infusion of naloxone can be considered after the initial bolus dose of naloxone reverses the opiate effects if long-acting agents such as methadone or diphenoxylate are involved, poorly antagonized agents such as propoxyphene or pentazocine have been taken, large dosages of naloxone are needed to reverse the initial opiate effects, or the naloxone must be repeated frequently to reverse recurring opiate effects. The naloxone bolus sufficient to reverse the respiratory depression is administered. The infusion is initiated at two-thirds of the naloxone bolus dose per hour.[81] At 15 minutes after initiation of the infusion, half of the bolus dose should be readministered. The infusion rate is titrated based on the patient's response. If the patient becomes symptomatic at a given infusion rate, symptoms should again be reversed with a naloxone bolus and the infusion rate should be increased. In adults, the naloxone concentration in D5W (5% dextrose in water) usually is adjusted to deliver the required dosage in 100 mL of solution per hour.

An alternative to using a naloxone infusion is the long-acting opioid antagonist nalmefene.[82] With a half-life of 8 hours, nalmefene's prolonged duration of action, ease of administration, and safety may prove beneficial. Patients are less likely to experience resedation than with naloxone. The intravenous dosage of nalmefene is 0.5 to 1 mg.

Naloxone is considered a very safe drug. Isolated case reports of adverse reactions generally have occurred in perioperative patients. The most common adverse effect is precipitation of opiate withdrawal. Opioid-dependent patients may experience vomiting, abdominal pain, diaphoresis, piloerection, and agitation after reversal of opiate effects by naloxone. The opioid withdrawal symptoms are not life-threatening and resolve without specific treatment. To avoid the possibility of opiate withdrawal, some clinicians start with lower naloxone dosages (0.4 mg) and then rapidly titrate up as needed.

Deferoxamine

Deferoxamine is a chelating agent that binds with ferric iron. The iron–deferoxamine complex (ferrioxamine) is less toxic and more easily excreted by the kidneys than iron alone. Ferrioxamine produces an orange- to red-brown urine in some patients. The presence of a color change indicates that free iron was present and chelated. However,

Table 4.2 ▪ Major Systemic Antidotes

Antidote	Poison	Usual Dosage and Route	Comments
N-Acetylcysteine	Acetaminophen	140 mg/kg orally as a loading dose, then 70 mg/kg every 4 hr for a total of 17 maintenance doses.	Dilute 20% solution 1:3 and administer as 5% solution. Most effective when initiated within 10 hr. Intravenous use not approved in U.S.
Atropine	Carbamate insecticides Organophosphate insecticides Other anticholinesterases	Test dose of 2 mg IV in an adult and 0.05 mg/kg in a child up to 2 mg; anticholinergic symptoms are seen only if poisoning is not present. Doses are repeated as needed (up to 2000 mg/day in severe cases), with the end point being cessation of secretions.	In severe organophosphate ingestions it is usually given in combination with pralidoxime.
British anti-Lewisite (dimercaprol; BAL)	Arsenic, gold, mercury, lead	Given by deep IM injection. Dosage variable depending on the agent being chelated and severity of intoxication. Usually 3–5 mg/kg/dose.	Contraindicated in iron, cadmium, or selenium because complex is toxic. For lead, used in combination with other agents.
Calcium	Calcium channel blockers	Adult: Calcium chloride (10%) 1 g IV over 5 min; may be repeated.	Monitor serum calcium if more than one dose is administered; produces positive inotropic effect; less effective for atrioventricular block or hypotension; less useful in massive intoxications.
Cyanide antidote kit (amyl nitrite, sodium nitrite, sodium thiosulfate)	Cyanide	Amyl nitrite: breathe 30 sec of each 60 sec until sodium nitrite is ready. Use a new ampule every 3 min. For adults 300 mg sodium nitrite (10 mL) usually is given IV, over at least 5 min, followed by 12.5 g sodium thiosulfate IV. If symptoms persist, one-half this dosage of sodium nitrite is repeated. The dosage of sodium nitrite for children depends on the hemoglobin level and is included in the package literature. Children are given 1.65 mg/kg sodium thiosulfate.	Overzealous administration of sodium nitrite especially in children can produce severe methemoglobinemia.
Deferoxamine	Iron	15 mg/kg/hr IV (see text).	Indications: serum iron ≥63 µmol/L (350 µg/dL) and symptomatic or ≥90 µmol/L (500 µg/dL) regardless of symptoms. Orange-red urine indicates the presence of the deferoxamine–iron chelate; urine color change is not always present.
Digoxin immune Fab	Digoxin Digitoxin	Administered IV. Dosage = body load (mg)/0.5 (mg bound/vial). See package insert for dosing. Tables based on amount ingested or serum digoxin levels.	Indicated in severe cases unresponsive to standard antiarrhythmics (see text). Total serum digoxin level increases dramatically after administration, but the digoxin is bound to the Fab fragment and is not toxic.
Diphenhydramine	Phenothiazine-induced extrapyramidal symptoms	Adults: 50 mg IV. Children: 1–2 mg/kg up to a total of 50 mg IV.	

(continued)

Table 4.2 *(continued)*

Antidote	Poison	Usual Dosage and Route	Comments
Disodium-Ethylenediaminetetraacetic acid (calcium EDTA)	Lead, some other heavy metals	75 mg/kg/day IV or IM given in 3–6 divided doses for up to 5 days. May repeat course after at least 2 days.	May produce renal tubular necrosis. If decreased renal function is present, dialysis may be needed to remove chelate.
Ethanol	Ethylene glycol, methanol	Ethanol is given to maintain a 22 mmol/L (100 mg/dL) blood level. Loading dose (oral) is 0.8 mL/kg 95% ethanol given over 30 min followed by an average maintenance dosage of 0.15 mL/kg/hr PO. Loading dose (IV) of 10% ethanol is 7.6 mL/kg IV over 30–60 min followed by an average maintenance dosage of 1.4 mL/kg/hr IV. Monitor blood levels of ethanol and adjust accordingly.	Chronic drinkers may need higher dosages and nondrinkers may require lower dosages. Dosage must be increased if dialysis is used. Glucose usually is administered simultaneously.
Flumazenil	Benzodiazepines	Initial dosage 0.2 mg IV. If adequate consciousness not obtained in 30 sec, inject another 0.3 mg IV over 30 sec. Further doses of 0.5 mg may be administered IV at 1-min intervals to a maximum total dosage of 3 mg. Most patients respond to 1–3 mg.	Contraindicated in patients who have taken tricyclic antidepressants or have been given benzodiazepines to treat a life-threatening condition. Seizures may occur if patients have benzodiazepine dependence.
Fomepizole	Ethylene glycol	Administer as slow intravenous infusion over 30 min. Loading dose of 15 mg/kg followed by 10 mg/kg every 12 hr for 4 doses; then 15 mg/kg every 12 hr until ethylene glycol level is <20 mg/dL.	Increase dosing to every 4 hr during dialysis. Probably also effective for methanol but not yet approved for this indication.
Glucagon	β-Blockers	50–150 μg/kg IV bolus initially (5–10 mg in adults); 2–5 mg/hr as needed.	Increases myocardial contractility.
Methylene blue	Nitrates and nitrites	0.2 mL/kg IV of a 1% solution over 5 min.	Reverses methemoglobinemia.
Naloxone	Opiates	0.1 mg/kg/dose IV in children; 0.4–2 mg in adults (see text).	Should be given several times if no effect before opiates are ruled out as the cause of symptoms. Short duration of action.
Oxygen	Carbon monoxide	Inhalation.	Consider hyperbaric oxygen.
D-Penicillamine	Copper, gold, mercury, lead, arsenic	Children 20–100 mg/kg/day (depends on the metal being chelated). Adults: 1–1.5 g/day.	Avoid in patients with penicillin allergy. Inhibits enzymes that are pyridoxal dependent, so pyridoxine usually is given concurrently (10–25 mg/day).
Physostigmine	Anticholinergics	Children: 0.5 mg slow IV. If no response and no cholinergic symptoms, give 0.5 mg every 5 min until a response is seen or 2 mg is reached. Repeat lowest effective trial dosage if severe symptoms recur. Adults: 1–2 mg slow IV. May repeat up to 4 mg total if no response and no cholinergic symptoms. 1–4 mg may be needed for severe symptoms.	Short duration of action. Atropine should be available to reverse any cholinergic effects. Must be given slowly. Of limited usefulness. Avoid when cyclic antidepressants may be involved or in patients with cardiac conduction defects.

(continued)

Table 4.2 *(continued)*

Antidote	Poison	Usual Dosage and Route	Comments
Pralidoxime	Organophosphates, severe carbamate ingestions, but not carbaryl	Adults: 1 g IV over 2 min. Children: 25–50 mg/kg slow IV. Either dose may be repeated every 8–12 hr as needed.	Given in combination with atropine. Little benefit if administered more than 36 hr after poisoning.
Pyridoxine	Isoniazid, monomethylhydrazine mushrooms	1 g pyridoxine IV per g of isonicotinic acid hydrazide ingested at a rate of 1 g every 2–3 min. If amount is unknown, administer 5 g. May be repeated.	Indicated for management of seizures and correction of acidosis.
Sodium bicarbonate	Tricyclic antidepressants	1–2 mEq/kg IV bolus, then IV drip to maintain serum pH of 7.5.	For cardiac arrhythmias, conduction disturbances, and hypotension.
Succimer (DSMA)	Lead	Children: 10 mg/kg every 8 hr for 5 days.	Monitor liver function at least weekly.
Vitamin K_1	Oral anticoagulants (e.g., warfarin, brodifacoum)	Oral: 5–10 mg/day for warfarin and 10–25 mg/day for long-acting agents; dosages of 100–125 mg daily and higher have been needed. Intravenous infusion preferable in severe cases at a rate of not more than 1 mg/min.	May need weeks to months of therapy depending on dosage and type of anticoagulant ingested.

the absence of a urine color change does not rule out iron poisoning.

Deferoxamine should be given in iron intoxications with serum iron levels of 90 µmol/L (500 µg/dL) or greater. Deferoxamine should be considered for patients with levels of 63 to 90 µmol/L (350 to 500 µg/dL) who are symptomatic. In symptomatic iron-intoxicated patients whose clinical presentation is serious (severe vomiting, coma, hypotension, metabolic acidosis) deferoxamine should be administered before serum iron level results are available.

Deferoxamine is given intravenously at a rate of 15 mg/kg/hour. Hypotension may occur at higher infusion rates. Higher infusion rates have been used in severe iron poisonings.[83] If hypotension develops, the infusion rate should be decreased or fluids and vasopressors administered to support blood pressure. According to the package insert, the maximum recommended daily dosage is 6 g, although there is no evidence to support this limitation and patients have been treated with higher dosages without adverse effects. Deferoxamine infusion can be discontinued when clinical toxicity resolves, serum iron level is normal, abdominal film for iron tablets is negative, and urine color returns to normal.

The most common adverse reactions to deferoxamine include generalized erythema, urticaria, and hypotension. Deferoxamine acts as a siderophore for *Yersinia enterocolitica;* the virulence of the *Yersinia* increases and sepsis can occur. The association of deferoxamine therapy with the development of adult respiratory distress syndrome (ARDS) is controversial. Four patients treated with 15 mg/kg/hour deferoxamine for 65 to 92 hours developed ARDS.[84] A further review of treated patients revealed that pulmonary toxicity was of concern only in patients treated with deferoxamine for more than 24 hours. However, iron poisoning also is associated with ARDS, and it has not be determined whether the deferoxamine or iron poisoning itself is responsible for this complication.

Digoxin Immune Fab

Digoxin-specific antibodies or digoxin immune Fab (Digibind) can be lifesaving in digitalis glycoside poisoning.[85] Digoxin immune Fab was used in the management of 296 (10.0%) of the 2972 cardiac glycoside ingestions reported to the AAPCC TESS database in 1998.[1] Digoxin immune Fab has a high binding affinity for digoxin that is greater than digoxin's affinity for the sodium–potassium ATPase. Although digoxin immune Fab binds digitoxin, its affinity for digitoxin is approximately one-tenth its affinity for digoxin. Digoxin immune Fab is produced by immunizing sheep with digoxin coupled as a hapten to an immunogenic protein carrier, which produces antibodies to digoxin. The antibodies are cleaved and the digoxin-specific Fab fragments are isolated and purified. The Fab fragment is one-third the size of the original IgG antibody. The advantages of this smaller size include a larger volume of distribution, the ability to be excreted renally, and less immunogenicity.

Digoxin immune Fab should be considered in life-threatening digoxin or digitoxin poisoning from acute overdose or chronic intoxication. Although serum concentrations of digoxin may be helpful in evaluating digoxin-poisoned patients, determination of whether digoxin immune Fab should be used is based on the patient's clinical condition. Digoxin immune Fab is indicated in patients with life-threatening arrhythmias (e.g., ventricular arrhythmias), conduction defects or progressive brady-arrhythmias (e.g., severe sinus bradycardia), third-degree heart block, or severe hyperkalemia (usually more than 5.0 mEq/L) resistant to treatment. Life-threatening digitalis toxicity was reversed in 21 of 26 patients in one series and 52 of 56 patients in another series with digoxin immune Fab administration.[85,86] The failures were the result of inadequate supply of digoxin immune Fab ($n = 2$), refractory low cardiac output ($n = 5$), anoxic CNS damage ($n = 1$), or multiple-drug overdose with uncertain diagnosis of digitalis toxicity ($n = 1$). The multicenter trial of 148 patients treated with digoxin immune Fab demonstrated response in 133 (90%) patients, with resolution in 119 and improvement in 14 patients.[87] There was no response in 15 (10%) patients. A postmarketing surveillance study in 745 patients found complete or partial resolution in 74%, with no response or uncertain response in the remaining 26%.[87] A multicenter study of digoxin immune Fab in children found resolution of digitalis toxicity in 27 of 29 patients (93%), with 3 children receiving more than one dose.[88] These investigators suggested that children at highest risk for digoxin toxicity are those with an ingestion of 0.3 mg/kg, who have underlying heart disease or a serum digoxin concentration of 6.4 nmol/L (5.0 ng/mL) or more.

Each vial of digoxin immune Fab contains 38 mg, which binds 0.5 mg of digoxin. Once reconstituted with sterile water for injection, the product can be stored in a refrigerator for up to 4 hours. Digoxin immune Fab usually is given as an intravenous infusion over 30 minutes in normal saline but may be given as a bolus injection if cardiac arrest is imminent. The dosage can be determined from the amount of digoxin or digitoxin ingested in acute poisonings or by the serum level in chronic intoxications. In general, the number of vials required equals the body load (in milligrams) of digoxin divided by 0.5 (digoxin bound per vial). Tables to determine the dosage in children and adults based on the amount ingested or the serum concentration are included in the product package insert. The total serum digoxin level increases markedly after administration of digoxin immune Fab, but the digoxin is bound to the Fab fragment and is not toxic. In patients with renal failure, elimination of the digoxin–Fab complex is slow, and some patients may develop a rebound in free digoxin concentrations.

Allergic reactions are rare, but skin testing is recommended for patients with a known allergy to sheep proteins or previous treatment with digoxin immune Fab. Serum potassium levels, which are elevated in acute digoxin intoxication, drop after digoxin immune Fab reverses toxicity. This occurs because patients with digoxin poisoning have a potassium deficit as a result of the loss of intracellular potassium to the extracellular space and subsequent renal elimination. A potential complication of digoxin immune Fab is heart failure in patients with intrinsically poor cardiac function who depend on digoxin's inotropic effect.

N-Acetylcysteine

In 1998, 111,454 acetaminophen exposures were reported to the AAPCC TESS, of which 50,043 were treated in a health care facility.[1] *N*-Acetylcysteine was used in the management of 11,127 of these cases. The major toxic effect of acetaminophen overdose is hepatic necrosis, which results from saturation of the enzymes in the nontoxic sulfate and glucuronide conjugation pathways and increased formation of the toxic metabolite by the cytochrome P-450 mixed function oxidase system. Glutathione, which detoxifies the toxic metabolite under normal conditions, is depleted in overdose situations. The protective effect of *N*-acetylcysteine relates to its activity as a glutathione substitute or precursor or to its enhancement of the activity of the sulfate conjugation pathway.

N-Acetylcysteine therapy should be initiated in adults with a history of ingesting 7.5 g or more of acetaminophen, in children with 200 mg/kg or more of acetaminophen, or in any patient in whom the amount ingested is unknown. *N*-Acetylcysteine therapy can be initiated up to 24 hours after ingestion but is most effective if started early. A study of 2540 patients with acetaminophen overdoses treated with oral *N*-acetylcysteine found that *N*-acetylcysteine therapy is most efficacious if initiated within 8 hours of the ingestion but that an effect on liver enzyme elevations could be demonstrated up to 24 hours after ingestion.[89] A better survival rate and fewer complications have been demonstrated after late administration of *N*-acetylcysteine in patients with acetaminophen-induced hepatic failure.[90] A plasma acetaminophen concentration at 4 or more hours after ingestion should be obtained and interpreted using the modified Matthew–Rumack nomogram (Fig. 4.2) to determine whether to continue *N*-acetylcysteine therapy. The nomogram, a semilogarithmic plot of plasma acetaminophen level and time, has two lines that define the plasma acetaminophen level as no hepatic toxicity (below the lower line), possible hepatic toxicity (between the two lines), and probable hepatic toxicity (above the upper line). A 4-hour plasma acetaminophen concentration of 992 μmol/L (150 μg/mL) is considered possibly hepatotoxic. A plasma acetaminophen concentration that falls at or above the lower line is an indication for the full course of *N*-acetylcysteine even if the level subsequently falls below the lower line. If the initial plasma acetaminophen concentration is below the lower line, *N*-acetylcysteine is not necessary. For patients overdosing on extended-release acetaminophen, the manufacturer recommends treating with *N*-acetylcysteine if the first plasma acetaminophen level is at or above the line. If the first plasma acetaminophen level is below the line, the level should be repeated 4 to 6 hours after the first level and the patient treated with *N*-acetylcysteine if the second level is at or above the line.

N-Acetylcysteine is approved for use in the United States in an oral dosing regimen consisting of a loading dose of 140 mg/kg followed by 17 maintenance doses of 70 mg/kg every 4 hours (total dosage of 1330 mg/kg/68 hours). Available in a 10 or 20% concentration, the solution should be diluted to a 5% solution before the patient drinks it or it is administered down a nasogastric tube. The main side effects of *N*-acetylcysteine are nausea and vomiting. Patients may have difficulty retaining

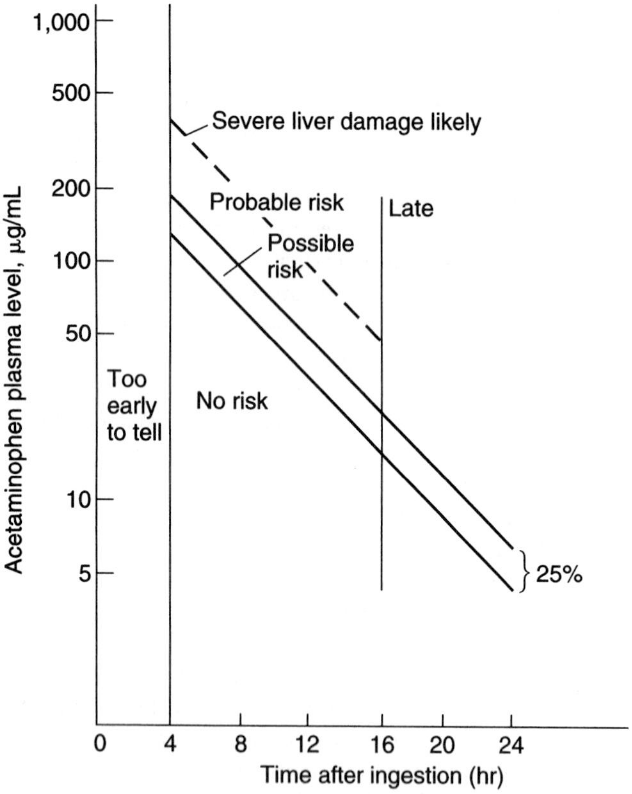

Figure 4.2. Matthew–Rumack nomogram for acetaminophen poisoning. Plasma levels drawn before 4 hours may not represent peak levels. The nomogram should be used for single acute ingestions only. (Adapted with permission from Arch Intern Med 141:380–385, 1981. Copyright 1981.)

N-acetylcysteine, which should be readministered if the patient vomits within 1 hour of the dose. Although concomitant administration of activated charcoal may result in some decrease in *N*-acetylcysteine bioavailability, which can be overcome by administering more *N*-acetylcysteine, it is not necessary to alter the dosage because the currently recommended loading dose is considered more than enough to prevent toxicity.[91,92]

Although the approved route of administration is oral in the United States, *N*-acetylcysteine is administered intravenously in most other countries. There are theoretical advantages for both oral *N*-acetylcysteine when intrahepatic levels are higher and for intravenous *N*-acetylcysteine when blood levels are higher. The oral regimen is associated with fewer adverse effects than the intravenous route. The most common adverse effects after oral administration are nausea, vomiting, and diarrhea. The intravenous route has been reported to cause hypotension and allergic reactions including rash, urticaria, bronchospasm, angioedema, and anaphylactoid reaction. These adverse events occur less often if the dose is diluted and administered slowly over 1 hour.[93]

In Europe and Canada, the intravenous dosing regimen for *N*-acetylcysteine consists of 300 mg/kg over a 20-hour period. A 48-hour intravenous regimen (total dosage 980 mg/kg/48 hours) was found to be superior to the 20-hour course but less effective than the 72-hour oral regimen in high-risk patients with delayed presentation (16 to 24 hours).[93] High-risk patients were those with markedly elevated plasma acetaminophen concentrations. All three regimens demonstrated similar efficacy when started within 8 to 10 hours of the overdose, but the longer oral course was more efficacious than the shorter intravenous courses in patients with treatment delay of more than 16 hours after ingestion. Presumably the important factor here is the duration of treatment, not the route by which treatment is administered. Studies are being conducted at the Oregon Poison Center and the Central Texas Poison Center investigating the efficacy of discontinuing *N*-acetylcysteine approximately 36 hours after ingestion of acetaminophen in patients with negative plasma acetaminophen levels and normal aspartate aminotransferase concentrations at that time. Until those studies are complete, patients should be treated with the standard oral 18-dose regimen.

KEY POINTS

- Clinical toxicology provides a challenging opportunity for pharmacist involvement in patient care. To effectively function as an information resource, it is essential to follow new developments in this growing field.
- Treatment of the poisoned patient may involve providing supportive care, terminating the exposure, hastening excretion of the toxin, and administering antidotes.
- Thorough patient evaluation and application of these general treatment principles to the specific poisoning situation are essential for definitive treatment.
- Although poison exposures occur more commonly in children under 6 years of age, more serious poisonings often occur in adolescents and adults.
- Poison centers improve poisoning outcomes and reduce health care costs.
- Pharmacists play a critical role in enforcing legislation and regulations related to drug packaging with CRCs.
- Poisoning should be considered in the differential diagnosis whenever there is an abrupt onset of illness with multiple organ system involvement, especially if the patient is under 5 years old or has a history of a previous ingestion.
- The major toxicology resources are secondary sources designed to allow rapid retrieval of toxicity and management information.
- Supportive care is the most important component of treating the seriously intoxicated patient.
- Minimizing absorption of the toxin from the GI tract is most effective if performed early, ideally within the first hour after ingestion.
- Ipecac syrup is no longer used routinely in EDs unless the toxin is not adsorbed by activated charcoal. Ipecac syrup still plays a role in home management of less serious intoxications in children.

- Numerous studies have demonstrated that activated charcoal is as effective as or more effective than other GI decontamination modalities. Therefore, activated charcoal is considered the primary method of preventing absorption in ED-treated patients.
- Enhancing elimination from the body by multiple-dose activated charcoal, urine alkalinization, hemodialysis, or hemoperfusion may be considered for some toxins.
- Antidotes can be lifesaving in some intoxications, and it is important that pharmacists be familiar with their specific indications, dosing and administration, and potential adverse effects.

REFERENCES

1. Litovitz TL, Klein-Schwartz W, Caravati EM, et al. 1998 annual report of the American Association of Poison Control Centers Toxic Exposure Surveillance System. Am J Emerg Med 17:435–487, 1999.
2. Vital Statistics of the United States. Mortality. CDC Wonder (http://wonder.cdc.gov).
3. Klein-Schwartz W, Oderda GM, Booze L. Poisoning in the elderly. J Am Geriatr Soc 31:195, 1983.
4. Litovitz TL, Kearney TE, Holm K, et al. Poison control centers: is there an antidote for budget cuts? Am J Emerg Med 12:585–599, 1994.
5. Miller T, Lestina DC. Costs of poisoning in the United States and savings from poison control centers: a benefit–cost analysis. Ann Emerg Med 29:239–245, 1997.
6. Harrison DL, Draugalis JR, Slack MK, et al. Cost–effectiveness of regional poison control centers. Arch Intern Med 156:2601–2608, 1996.
7. Centers for Disease Control. Unintentional poisoning among young children. MMWR 32:117–118, 1983.
8. Done AK. Aspirin overdosage: incidence, diagnosis and management. Pediatrics 62(Suppl):890, 1978.
9. Spiller HA, Rodgers GC. Prospective evaluation of administration of activated charcoal (AC) in the home [abstract]. J Toxicol Clin Toxicol 35:483, 1997.
10. Mofenson HC, Greensher J. The unknown poison. Pediatrics 54:336, 1974.
11. Boxer L, Anderson FP, Rowe DS. Comparison of ipecac-induced emesis with gastric lavage in the treatment of acute salicylate ingestion. J Pediatr 74:800, 1969.
12. Goldstein L. Emesis vs. lavage for drug ingestion. JAMA 208:2162, 1969.
13. Young WF, Bivins HG. Evaluation of gastric emptying using radionuclides: gastric lavage versus ipecac-induced emesis. Ann Emerg Med 22:1423–1427, 1993.
14. Auerbach PS, Osterloh J, Braun O, et al. Efficacy of gastric emptying: gastric lavage versus emesis induced with ipecac. Ann Emerg Med 15:692, 1986.
15. Tandberg D, Diven BG, McLeod JW. Ipecac-induced emesis versus gastric lavage: a controlled study in normal adults. Am J Emerg Med 4:205, 1986.
16. Litovitz TL. Emesis versus lavage for poisoning victims. Am J Emerg Med 4:294, 1986.
17. Suetta JP, Aminton DN. Residual gastric content after gastric lavage and ipecacuanha-induced emesis in self-poisoned patients. J R Soc Med 84:35–38, 1991.
18. Suetta JP, Marsh S, Gaunt ME, et al. Gastric emptying procedures in the self-poisoned patients, are we forcing gastric contents beyond the pylorus? J R Soc Med 84:274–276, 1991.
19. Corby D, Decker W, Moran M, et al. Clinical comparison of pharmacologic emetics in children. Pediatrics 42:361, 1968.
20. Arnold FJ Jr, Hodges JF Jr, Barta RA Jr. Evaluation of the efficacy of lavage and induced emesis in treatment of salicylate poisoning. Pediatrics 23:286, 1959.
21. Corby D, Lisciandro R, Lehman R, et al. The efficacy of methods used to evacuate the stomach after acute ingestions. Pediatrics 40:871, 1967.
22. Curtis RA, Barone J, Giacona N. Efficacy of ipecac and activated charcoal/cathartic. Prevention of salicylate absorption in a simulated overdose. Arch Intern Med 144:48, 1994.
23. Neuvonen PJ, Vartiainen M, Tokola O. Comparison of activated charcoal and ipecac syrup in prevention of drug absorption. Eur J Clin Pharmacol 24:557, 1983.
24. Tenenbein M, Cohen S, Sitar OS. Efficacy of ipecac, induced emesis, orogastric lavage and activated charcoal for drug overdose. Ann Emerg Med 16:838–841, 1987.
25. Kornberg AE, Dolgin J. Pediatric ingestions: charcoal alone versus ipecac and charcoal. Ann Emerg Med 20:648–651, 1991.
26. Kulig K, Bar-Or D, Cantrill SV, et al. Management of acutely poisoned patients without gastric emptying. Ann Emerg Med 14:562, 1985.
27. Perrone J, Hoffman RS, Goldfrank LR. Special considerations in gastrointestinal decontaminations. Concepts and controversies in toxicology. Emerg Med Clin North Am 12:285–299, 1994.
28. Pond SM, Lewis-Driver DJ, Williams GM, et al. Gastric emptying in acute overdosage: a prospective randomized controlled trial. Med J Aust 163:345–349, 1995.
29. Merigian KS, Woodward M, Hedges JR, et al. Prospective evaluation of gastric emptying in the self-poisoned patient. Am J Emerg Med 8:479–483, 1990.
30. Albertson TE, Derlet RW, Foulke GE, et al. Superiority of activated charcoal alone compared with ipecac and activated charcoal in the treatment of acute toxic ingestions. Ann Emerg Med 18:56–59, 1989.
31. Bosse GM, Barefoot JA, Pfeifer MP, et al. Comparison of three methods of gut decontamination in tricyclic antidepressant overdose. J Emerg Med 13:203–209, 1995.
32. American Academy of Clinical Toxicology; European Association of Poisons Centres and Clinical Toxicologists. Position statement: ipecac syrup. J Toxicol Clin Toxicol 35:699–709, 1997.
33. American Academy of Clinical Toxicology; European Association of Poisons Centres and Clinical Toxicologists. Position statement: gastric lavage. J Toxicol Clin Toxicol 35:711–719, 1997.
34. American Academy of Clinical Toxicology; European Association of Poisons Centres and Clinical Toxicologists. Position statement: single-dose activated charcoal. J Toxicol Clin Toxicol 35:721–741, 1997.
35. American Academy of Clinical Toxicology; European Association of Poisons Centres and Clinical Toxicologists. Position statement: cathartics. J Toxicol Clin Toxicol 35:743–752, 1997.
36. Robertson W. Syrup of ipecac: a slow or fast emetic? Am J Dis Child 103:136, 1962.
37. Litovitz TL, Klein-Schwartz W, Oderda GM, et al. Safety and efficacy of ipecac administration in children younger than one year of age. Pediatrics 76:761, 1985.
38. McCray EA, Bonfiglio JF, Sigell LT. Home administration of syrup of ipecac to infants. Drug Intell Clin Pharm 18:792, 1984.
39. Gaudreault P, McCormick MA, Lacouture PG, et al. Poisoning exposures and use of ipecac in children less than 1 year old. Ann Emerg Med 15:808, 1986.
40. Varipapa RJ, Oderda GM. Effect of milk on ipecac induced emesis. N Engl J Med 296:112, 1977.
41. Klein-Schwartz W, Litovitz TL, Oderda GM, et al. The effect of milk on ipecac-induced emesis. J Toxicol Clin Toxicol 29:505–511, 1991.
42. Saincher A, Sitar DS, Tenenbein M. Efficacy of ipecac during the first hour after drug ingestion in human volunteers. Clin Toxicol 35:600–615, 1997.
43. Bond GR. Home use of syrup of ipecac is associated with a reduction in pediatric emergency department visits. Ann Emerg Med 25:338–341, 1995.
44. Bates B, Grunwaldt E. Ipecac poisoning. Am J Dis Child 103:1, 1962.
45. Robertson WO. Syrup of ipecac associated fatality: a case report. Vet Hum Toxicol 21:87, 1979.
46. Klein-Schwartz W, Gorman RL, Oderda GM, et al. Ipecac use in the elderly: the unanswered question. Ann Emerg Med 13:1152, 1984.
47. Adler AG, Walinsky P, Krall RA, et al. Death resulting from ipecac syrup. JAMA 243:1927, 1980.
48. Shrestha M, George J, Chin MJ, et al. A comparison of three gastric lavage methods using the radionuclide gastric emptying study. J Emerg Med 14:413–418, 1996.
49. Cooney DO. A "superactive" charcoal for antidotal use in poisonings. Clin Toxicol 11:387, 1977.
50. Picchioni AL. Charcoal and saline laxatives for treatment of poison ingestion. Vet Hum Toxicol 21:132, 1979.
51. Roberts JR, Greely EJ, Schoffstall JM. Advantage of high-surface area charcoal in a human acetaminophen ingestion model. Acad Emerg Med 4:167–174, 1997.
52. Wax PM, Cobaugh DJ. Prehospital gastrointestinal decontamination of toxic ingestions: a missed opportunity. Am J Emerg Med 16:114–116, 1998.
53. Crockett RC, Krishel SJ, Manoguerra A, et al. Prehospital use of activated charcoal: a pilot study. J Emerg Med 14:335–338, 1995.
54. Chin L, Picchioni AL. Charcoal and saline laxatives for treatment of poison ingestion. Vet Hum Toxicol 21:132, 1979.
55. Sketris IS, Mowry JB, Czajka PA, et al. Saline catharsis: effect on aspirin bioavailability in combination with activated charcoal. J Clin Pharmacol 22:59, 1982.
56. Easom JM, Caraccio TR, Lovejoy FH. Evaluation of activated charcoal and

magnesium citrate in the prevention of aspirin absorption in humans. Clin Pharm 1:154, 1982.
57. Krenzelok EP, Heller MB. Comparison of activated charcoal and activated charcoal with sorbitol in human volunteers [abstract]. Vet Hum Toxicol 28:498, 1986.
58. Goldberg MJ, Spector R, Park GD, et al. The effect of sorbitol and activated charcoal on serum theophylline concentrations after slow-release theophylline. Clin Pharmacol Ther 41:108, 1987.
59. Krenzelok EP, Keller R, Stewart RD. Gastrointestinal transit times of cathartics combined with charcoal. Ann Emerg Med 14:1152, 1985.
60. James LP, Nichols MH, King WD. A comparison of cathartics in pediatric ingestions. Pediatrics 96:235–238, 1995.
61. Weber WA, Santiago R. Hypermagnesemia: a potential complication during treatment of theophylline intoxication with oral activated charcoal and magnesium-containing cathartics. Chest 95:56, 1989.
62. Berlinger WG, Spector R, Goldberg MJ, et al. Enhancement of theophylline clearance by oral activated charcoal. Clin Pharmacol Ther 33:351, 1983.
63. Ohning BL, Reed MD, Blumer JL. Continuous nasogastric administration of activated charcoal for the treatment of theophylline intoxication. Pediatr Pharmacol 5:241, 1986.
64. Pond SM, Olson KR, Osterloh JD, et al. Randomized study of the treatment of phenobarbital overdose with repeated doses of activated charcoal. JAMA 251:3104, 1984.
65. Goldberg MJ, Park GD, Spector R, et al. Lack of effect of oral activated charcoal on imipramine clearance. Clin Pharmacol Ther 38:350–353, 1985.
66. Karkkainen S, Neuvonen PJ. Pharmacokinetics of amitriptyline influenced by oral charcoal and urine pH. Int J Clin Pharmacol Ther Toxicol 24:326–332, 1986.
67. Scheinin M, Virtanen R, Iisalo E. Effect of single and repeated doses of activated charcoal on the pharmacokinetics of doxepin. Int J Clin Pharmacol Ther Toxicol 23:38–42, 1985.
68. Swartz CM, Sherman A. The treatment of tricyclic antidepressant overdose with repeated charcoal. J Clin Pyschophapharmacol 4:336–340, 1984.
69. Mayer AL, Sitar DS, Tennenbein M. Multiple-dose charcoal and whole bowel irrigation do not increase clearance of absorbed salicylate. Arch Intern Med 152:393–396, 1992.
70. Chyka PA, Holley JE, Mandrell TD, et al. Correlation of drug pharmacokinetics and effectiveness of multiple dose activated charcoal therapy. Ann Emerg Med 25:356–362, 1995.
71. Tennenbein M. Multiple doses of activated charcoal: time for reappraisal? Ann Emerg Med 20:529–531, 1991.
72. Gomez HF, Brent JA, Munoz DC, et al. Charcoal stercolith with intestinal perforation in a patient treated for amitriptyline ingestion. J Emerg Med 12:57–60, 1994.
73. Caldwell JW, Nowa AJ, Dehaass DD. Hypernatremia associated with cathartics in overdose management. West J Med 147:593–596, 1987.
74. Garrelts JC, Watson WA, Sweet DE, et al. Magnesium toxicity secondary to catharsis during management of theophylline poisoning. Am J Emerg Med 7:34–37, 1989.
75. Grean J, Woolf A. Hypermagnesemia associated with catharsis in a salicylate-intoxicated patient with anorexia nervosa. Ann Emerg Med 8:200–203, 1989.
76. McCord MM. Toxicity of sorbitol-charcoal suspension. J Pediatr 111:307–308, 1987.
77. Brent J, Kulig K, Rumack BH. Iatrogenic death from sorbitol and magnesium sulfate during treatment for salicylism [abstract]. Vet Hum Toxicol 31:334, 1989.
78. Elenbaas RM. Critical review of forced alkaline diuresis in acute salicylism. Crit Care Q 4:89, 1982.
79. Russo M. Management of theophylline intoxication with charcoal-column hemoperfusion. N Engl J Med 300:24, 1979.
80. Pond S, Rosenberg J, Benowitz NL, et al. Pharmacokinetics of hemoperfusion for drug overdose. Clin Pharmacokinet 4:329, 1979.
81. Goldfrank L, Weisman RS, Errick JK, et al. A dosing nomogram for continuous infusion of intravenous naloxone. Ann Emerg Med 15:566–570, 1986.
82. Kaplan JL, Marx JA. Effectiveness and safety of intravenous nalmefene for emergency department patients with suspected narcotic overdose: a pilot study. Ann Emerg Med 22:187–190, 1993.
83. Boehnert M, Lacouture PG, Guttmacher A, et al. Massive iron overdose treated with high-dose deferoxamine infusion [abstract]. Vet Hum Toxicol 27:291, 1985.
84. Tenenbein M, Kowalski S, Sienko A, et al. Pulmonary toxic effects of continuous desferrioxamine administration in acute iron poisoning. Lancet 339(8795):699–701, 1992.
85. Smith TW, Butler VP, Habert E, et al. Treatment of life-threatening digitalis intoxication with digoxin-specific Fab antibody fragments. Experience in 26 cases. N Engl J Med 307:1357, 1982.
86. Wenger TL, Butler VP, Haber E, et al. Treatment of 63 severely digitalis-toxic patients with digoxin-specific antibody fragments. J Am Coll Cardiol 5:118A–123A, 1985.
87. Smith TW. Review of clinical experience with digoxin immune Fab. Am J Emerg Med 9:1–5, 1991.
88. Woolf AD, Wenger T, Smith TW, et al. The use of digoxin-specific Fab fragments for severe digitalis intoxication in children. N Engl J Med 326:1739–1744, 1992.
89. Smilkstein MJ, Knapp GL, Kulig KW, et al. Efficacy of oral *N*-acetylcysteine in the treatment of acetaminophen overdose. Analysis of the national multicenter study (1976 to 1985). N Engl J Med 319:1557, 1998.
90. Keays R, Harrison PM, Wendon JA, et al. Intravenous acetylcysteine is paracetamol induced fulminant hepatic necrosis: a prospective controlled trial. BMJ 303(6809):1026–1029, 1991.
91. Ekin BR, Ford DC, Thompson MIB, et al. The effect of activated charcoal on *N*-acetylcysteine absorption in normal subjects. Am J Emerg Med 5:483, 1987.
92. Chamberlain JM, Gorman RL, Oderda GM, et al. The use of activated charcoal in a simulated poisoning with acetaminophen: a new loading dose for *N*-acetylcysteine. Ann Emerg Med 22:1398–1402, 1993.
93. Smilkstein MJ, Bronstein AC, Linden C, et al. Acetaminophen overdose: a 48 hour intravenous *N*-acetylcysteine treatment protocol. Ann Emerg Med 20(10):1058–1063, 1991.

CHAPTER 5

CLINICAL LABORATORY TESTS AND INTERPRETATION

Charles F. Seifert and Beth H. Resman-Targoff

Patient assessment should be based on information obtained through laboratory data and a good history and physical examination. If the laboratory data are not consistent with the history and physical examination, the results should be suspect and the tests repeated. Several steps are involved in the collection, evaluation, and reporting of laboratory data. These multiple steps may result in an increased chance of error. Therapeutic and management decisions may be based on a misleading laboratory value. Examples of errors of this type include estimations of creatinine clearances based on non–steady-state serum creatinine (SCr) values, or a normal hematocrit (Hct) in a dehydrated patient, or the evaluation of total phenytoin concentrations in hypoalbuminemic patients. This chapter reviews routinely encountered laboratory tests not thoroughly covered in other parts of this text, including their regulation, critical ranges, clinical application, and drug interference. Sodium, potassium, chloride, carbon dioxide content, calcium, magnesium, phosphate, and urinalysis are thoroughly covered in the chapters on fluid and electrolytes, acid-base disorders, and renal diseases.

DEFINITION

Laboratory test abnormalities are values outside the normal range for a population. True abnormalities are reproducible and usually are associated with signs and symptoms consistent with a disease state. Laboratory test abnormalities are not in themselves diseases, but increases or decreases in values are associated with various diseases. Abnormal values may be caused by drugs, including spurious interference, side effects, or therapeutic effects. Diseases associated with laboratory tests discussed include renal and liver dysfunction, diabetes mellitus, hyperuricemia or gout, myocardial infarction (MI), pancreatitis, malnutrition, malignancies, inflammatory diseases, anemia, blood dyscrasias, infections, and bleeding or clotting disorders.

TREATMENT GOALS: LABORATORY TESTS

- Laboratory test values generally are not treated.
- Treatment goals depend on the specific disease causing the laboratory test abnormality and usually are focused on modifying the underlying disease process rather than on changing the lab test value.
- An example of a laboratory test goal includes treating hyperuricemia in a patient with gout, where the goal may be to decrease the uric acid value to between 5 and 6 mg/dL. Another is the use of warfarin to treat a patient with deep venous thrombosis; the dosing goal is an international normalized ratio of 2.0 to 3.0.

GENERAL PRINCIPLES

Specimen Collection

Blood and urine are the most common body fluids used for analytic purposes. Phlebotomists should be familiar with the test being performed, know the appropriate container for collection, and know how the collection procedure may affect the results. Verification that computer-printed labels match requisitions at the nurses' station and the patient's wristband is essential. Specimens should not be drawn until the patient's identity is confirmed. Proper techniques help avoid hemolysis and bacterial contamination. Particular attention should be paid to tests in which timing is important (e.g., in relation to ingestion of food or drugs). Special precautions are necessary for blood cultures and specimens obtained from indwelling catheters, especially central venous access catheters. Strict urine collection procedures must be followed to ensure valid results. A freshly obtained urine specimen is crucial when testing for bilirubin, red blood cells, and white blood cells because these undergo decomposition if left standing at room temperature. Unpreserved urine specimens are also predisposed to microbial overgrowth at room temperature. A good rule for all specimens is to deliver them to the laboratory within 1 hour of collection or refrigerate them. Proper techniques for performing each method of collection can be found in Henry's *Clinical Diagnosis and Management by Laboratory Methods*[1] or other textbooks on laboratory methods.

Methods of Analysis

Several methods are available in the clinical laboratory to assay desired substances in body fluids. Two commonly used techniques are chromatography and immunoassays. The type of compound to be measured determines which assay is used. Certain methods are used for qualitative measurements and others for quantitative measurements. Qualitative measurements detect only whether the substance is present, not the quantity of substance. A urine toxicology screen is an example of a qualitative test in which knowing whether a substance is present usually is more important than knowing its amount. Sensitivity and specificity are important aspects of a clinical laboratory test. Sensitivity is commonly defined as the lowest detectable value of a substance, and specificity is the ability to differentiate the substance of interest in the presence of other interfering substances. Sensitivity and specificity are calculated by the following formulas:

$$\text{Sensitivity} = \text{True positives}/(\text{True positives} + \text{False negatives}) \times 100$$

$$\text{Specificity} = \text{True negatives}/(\text{True negatives} + \text{False positives}) \times 100$$

Ideally, sensitivity and specificity should each be at least 95%. Most clinical laboratories have strict performance criteria for their assay techniques. These criteria vary widely between institutions and can greatly affect the interpretation of individual patient results. Most clinical laboratories use the most accurate method with the best automation at a reasonable cost. For each individual clinical laboratory, particular attention to accuracy, precision, and quality control are essential for reliable, reproducible results.[2]

Reference Values

Normal ranges are provided as a guideline, but individual laboratory results may vary considerably. Values outside the quoted normal range may be considered abnormal but not clinically important, whereas certain values in the normal range with a particular disease state are actually abnormal (e.g., normal hemoglobin in a patient with chronic obstructive airway disease). Laboratories may evaluate substances with different assays of varying degrees of precision. Certain tests are time dependent, and the time at which the sample is drawn is crucial in determining whether the patient sample is truly within the reference range. This is especially true for most serum drug concentrations. Most normal reference ranges quoted in this chapter are reproduced with permission from Young.[3]

Drug Interference

Medications affect laboratory test results in two major ways. A drug's intrinsic pharmacokinetic, pharmacologic, or toxicologic properties may alter the formation, regulation, release, or elimination of the substance being tested (e.g., hydrochlorothiazide blocks the tubular secretion of uric acid, exogenous insulin affects serum glucose, and toxic acetaminophen concentration affects serum transaminases). Medications may also directly interfere with the assay used to detect the substance (e.g., ascorbic acid causes false-negative results with urine glucose by the glucose oxidase method). For each laboratory test discussed, this chapter includes a brief section on common medications that affect the test results.

Système Internationale d'Unités

The conversion of measurements of body fluid substances to a molar concentration unit is based on the fact that substances in the body interact on a molar basis. It also standardizes units internationally. Several societies, including the American Medical Association and the American College of Physicians and their official journals (*JAMA* and *Annals of Internal Medicine*), have adopted Système Internationale (SI) units as their sole reference standard. Other journals still accept both sets of units. Reference laboratories in most hospitals and most clinicians in the United States have not accepted this change willingly and still use the older reference standards. For each laboratory test in this chapter, both SI units and conventional units with a conversion factor (CF) are given. To convert from conventional units to SI units, multiply the results in conventional units by the CF.

SPECIFIC LABORATORY TESTS

Serum Creatinine

(SI units: males, 50 to 110 μmol/L; females, 10 μmol/L lower [males, 0.6 to 1.2 mg/dL; females, 0.1 mg/dL lower]; CF = 88.40)

Creatinine is an amino acid formed as a waste product of creatine, an important energy storage substance in muscle metabolism. Creatinine is an anhydride of creatine and is not used in the body.[4] Formation of creatinine is fairly constant, with about 1.6 to 1.7% of creatine transformed to creatinine each 24 hours (Fig. 5.1). This in turn depends on the total muscle content of creatine and creatine phosphate. Factors that affect creatine levels, such as diet, fever, and muscle damage, do not readily influence SCr level. The SCr concentration is also fairly constant, and urinary excretion is the result of glomerular filtration and proximal tubular secretion. The SCr level is a more reliable indicator of renal function than the blood urea nitrogen (BUN).

SCr concentration increases in the presence of impaired renal function. Because up to 50% of renal function is lost before the SCr level becomes abnormally elevated, it is not a good indicator of early renal dysfunction. Even with its pitfalls, creatinine clearance based on 24-hour urinary excretion of creatinine is the most reliable readily available clinical test to evaluate glomerular filtration. Several methods exist for the rapid estimation of creatinine clearance based on the patient's age, ideal body weight, and SCr level. The methods are discussed in more detail in Chapters 21 and 22, Acute and Chronic Renal Diseases, and Chapter 1, Clinical Pharmacodynamics. A steady-state SCr level is necessary for an accurate estimation. Certain methods are more inaccurate in older adults and in patients with decreased muscle mass.[5]

Drugs that may cause an elevated SCr level by interfering with tubular secretion of creatinine are cephalosporins, cimetidine, salicylates, and trimethoprim. Drugs such as acetohexamide, ascorbic acid, flucytosine, levodopa, lidocaine, methyldopa, *p*-aminohippurate, and phenolsulfonphthalein may cause increases by interfering with the analytical method of SCr determination.[6]

Blood Urea Nitrogen

(SI units, 3.0 to 6.5 mmol/L [8 to 18 mg/dL]; CF = 0.357)

Urea is the predominant end product of protein and amino acid catabolism and is made in the liver through the urea cycle. It is the main nonprotein nitrogen (NPN) constituent in the blood. Other NPN substances include amino acids, uric acid, creatinine, and ammonia. Total NPN determinations are no longer used clinically. Urea is distributed to all intracellular and extracellular fluids and is freely diffusible across most cell membranes.[4] Urea is excreted mostly by the kidneys, with only small amounts excreted in sweat and in the intestines.

When there is a large increase of nonprotein compounds such as urea in the blood, azotemia is present. Azotemia can be categorized as prerenal, renal, and postrenal. Prerenal azotemia is the result of inadequate perfusion of kidneys with otherwise normal renal function. Causes of prerenal azotemia include dehydration, decreased blood

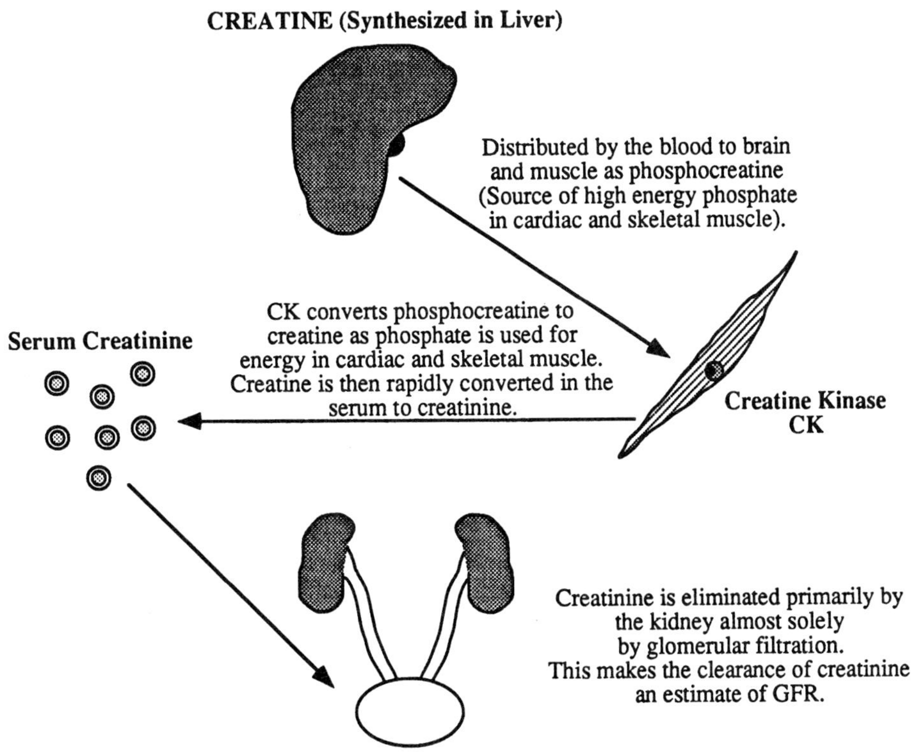

CREATINE (Synthesized in Liver)
Distributed by the blood to brain and muscle as phosphocreatine (Source of high energy phosphate in cardiac and skeletal muscle).
CK converts phosphocreatine to creatine as phosphate is used for energy in cardiac and skeletal muscle. Creatine is then rapidly converted in the serum to creatinine.
Serum Creatinine
Creatine Kinase CK
Creatinine is eliminated primarily by the kidney almost solely by glomerular filtration. This makes the clearance of creatinine an estimate of GFR.

Figure 5.1. Creatinine production. *GFR*, glomerular filtration rate.

volume, shock, and heart failure. Renal azotemia is decreased glomerular filtration as a result of acute or chronic renal disease, including glomerulonephritis, interstitial nephritis, and tubular necrosis. Postrenal azotemia is most commonly the result of urinary tract obstruction. The extreme form of azotemia, known as uremia, is a constellation of symptoms resulting from severe elevations in BUN (35.7 to 71.4 mmol/L) and other substances not adequately cleared by the kidney. Uremic symptoms include acidosis, water and electrolyte imbalance, nausea, vomiting, and neuropsychiatric changes including stupor or deep coma.[4] Agents noted for causing acute interstitial nephritis usually accompanied with an allergic reaction include allopurinol, cephalosporins, penicillins, nonsteroidal anti-inflammatory agents, and phenytoin.[6] Common agents that may cause acute tubular necrosis include aminoglycosides, amphotericin B, angiotensin-converting enzyme (ACE) inhibitors, carboplatin, cisplatin, cyclosporine, diuretics, gold salts, ifosfamide, intravenous contrast media, lithium, pentamidine, tacrolimus, tetracyclines, and vancomycin.[7] Agents that may increase the risk of urolithiasis include allopurinol, calcium salts, carbonic anhydrase inhibitors, indinavir, and triamterene.[7] Nephrolithiasis occurs in 1 to 3% of patients on a lamivudine–zidovudine combination but may occur in up to 12% with the addition of indinavir.[8,9]

BUN can be used as an estimate of renal function. As with creatinine levels, a clinically important elevation is not observed until glomerular filtration is decreased by at least 50%. A decreased BUN usually is not clinically significant, but a few conditions may cause a significant decrease. These include poor nutrition, high fluid intake, and severe liver disease where urea synthesis is decreased. Drugs that may increase BUN by methodologic interference are chloral hydrate, chloramphenicol, ammonium salts, acetohexamide, and sulfonylureas; those that decrease BUN include chloramphenicol and streptomycin.[6]

BUN and SCr concentrations may be evaluated simultaneously. To yield more information than either alone, the BUN is divided by the SCr. This is called the BUN:creatinine ratio; the normal ratio ranges from 40:1 to 60:1. Table 5.1 indicates clinical causes of elevated BUN and SCr with elevated or normal BUN:creatinine ratios.

Table 5.1 ▪ BUN: Creatinine Ratio in Clinical Conditions with Elevated BUN and Serum Creatinine

≥60 : 1	Prerenal azotemia (e.g., heart failure, dehydration) Postrenal azotemia (e.g., obstructive uropathy) Impaired renal function plus excess protein intake or tissue breakdown Drugs such as tetracycline and glucocorticosteroids
<60 : 1	Prerenal azotemia in hepatic cirrhosis Renal dialysis Renal failure in muscular patients Decreased urea production (e.g. low protein intake, severe diarrhea, or vomiting)

Table 5.2 ▪ Classification of Hyperglycemia

- Primary
  - Insulin-dependent diabetes mellitus
  - Non–insulin-dependent diabetes mellitus
- Secondary
  - Hyperglycemia resulting from disease of the pancreas
    - Inflammation
      - Acute pancreatitis (rare)
      - Chronic pancreatitis
      - Pancreatitis caused by mumps
      - ? Cell damage caused by coxsackievirus B_4 infection
      - ? Autotimmunine disease
    - Pancreatectomy
    - Pancreatic infiltration
      - Hemochromatosis
      - Tumors
    - Trauma to pancreas (rare)
  - Hyperglycemia related to other major endocrine diseases
    - Acromegaly
    - Cushing's syndrome
    - Thyrotoxicosis
    - Pheochromocytoma
    - Hyperaldosteronism
    - Glucagonoma
    - Somatostatinoma
  - Hyperglycemia caused by drugs
    - Corticosteroids, acetazolamide, thiazide diuretics, and β-agonists
    - Pentamidine (late), tacrolimus, and protease inhibitors
  - Hyperglycemia related to other major disease states
    - Chronic renal failure
    - Chronic liver disease
    - Infection
  - Miscellaneous hyperglycemia
    - Pregnancy
    - Related to insulin receptor antibodies (acanthosis nigricans)

Plasma Glucose

(Fasting SI units, 3.9 to 6.1 mmol/L [70 to 110 mg/dL]; however, normal ranges depend on the method; CF = 0.05551)

Laboratory determinations of glucose level usually are performed on venous plasma specimens. Whole blood determinations are used only for capillary blood used in fingerstick devices. Serum and plasma glucose concentrations are identical and are 10 to 15% higher than whole blood measurements. Glucose is a clinically important carbohydrate, along with fructose and galactose. Disorders of carbohydrate metabolism, such as diabetes, are evaluated in part by measurement of plasma glucose either in the fasting state or after suppression or stimulation. The blood glucose concentration is regulated within narrow limits by hormones produced by the pancreas and through other mechanisms mediated by the adrenergic and cholinergic nervous systems.[10] Glucose is a major source of energy for brain, muscle, and fat. The brain is the only tissue that does not require insulin for glucose use. If glucose is not available exogenously (fasting state), the body, through hormonal mechanisms (counterregulatory hormones: glucagon, epinephrine, cortisol, and somatostatin), will form its own glucose by tissue and hepatic gluconeogenesis and hepatic glycogenolysis. Glucose is therefore carefully regulated by glucagon and insulin secretion, which compensates for food ingestion and fasting states. (Refer to Chapter 19, Diabetes Mellitus, for a detailed discussion of carbohydrate metabolism in normal and diabetic patients.)

Methods for clinical determination of glucose are either chemical or enzymatic. Chemical analysis is based on the reducing properties of glucose and uses a color change reaction that is measured spectrophotometrically. The enzymatic method is based on the reaction of glucose and glucose oxidase. This is a very specific method and generally is inexpensive. Ascorbic acid can interfere with this method and result in decreased values.

Elevated plasma glucose concentrations, or hyperglycemia, can be caused by a number of syndromes and diseases. The classification of hyperglycemia is shown in Table 5.2.[7,10] A fasting plasma glucose of 7.7 mmol/L (140 mg/dL) or greater is considered abnormal.

Hypoglycemia is a syndrome of low plasma glucose with related symptoms. In adults, an overnight fasting plasma glucose below 2.5 mmol/L (45 mg/dL) is considered abnormal and above 3.0 mmol/L (55 mg/dL) is considered the lower limit of normal. In neonates, less than 1.9 mmol/L (35 mg/dL) is abnormal and in infants and children less than 2.5 mmol/L (45 mg/L) is abnormal. Table 5.3 shows the classification of common causes of hypoglycemia.[7,10]

Uric Acid

(SI units, 120 to 420 μmol/L [2.0 to 7.0 mg/dL]; CF = 59.48; see Chapter 33, Gout and Hyperuricemia)

Table 5.3 ▪ Classification of Common Causes of Hypoglycemia

- No anatomic lesion present
  - Fasting plasma glucose normal
    - Reactive hypoglycemia
      - Functional hypoglycemia
      - Alimentary hypoglycemia
      - Diabetic and impaired glucose tolerance
  - Fasting plasma glucose low
    - Drug-induced hypoglycemia
      - Oral hypoglycemic agents
      - ACE inhibitors
      - Insulin
      - Ethanol
      - Salicylates (late in overdose)
      - Pentamidine (early in therapy)
      - Combinations of the above
  - Factitious: fasting glucose normal or low
- Anatomic lesion present
  - Insulinoma
  - Extrapancreatic neoplasms
  - Adrenocortical insufficiency
  - Hypopituitarism
  - Massive liver disease

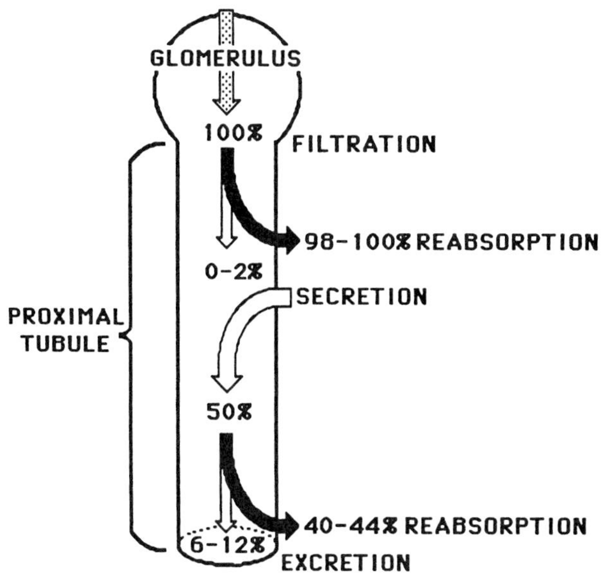

Figure 5.2. Uric acid excretion.

Uric acid is the end product of purine metabolism. The major rate-limiting step in the synthesis of uric acid is the intracellular concentration of 5-phosphoribosyl-1-pyrophosphate (PRPP). Uric acid serves no biologic function. Approximately two-thirds of uric acid is excreted by the kidneys and one-third through the gastrointestinal tract. Assuming that the uric acid filtered through the glomerulus equals 100%, 98 to 100% of this glomerular filtrate is reabsorbed in the proximal portion of the proximal convoluted tubule (Fig. 5.2).[11] Fifty percent of the original amount is secreted into the distal portion of the proximal convoluted tubule, but 40 to 44% is subsequently reabsorbed, and 6 to 12% of the original glomerular filtrate eventually excreted.

Hyperuricemia is caused by either an overproduction of uric acid (increased destruction of nucleoproteins, high-protein diet, or inborn enzymatic defects) or an underexcretion (renal defect). Because the serum is saturated with urate at a concentration of 420 μmol/L (7 mg/dL), as serum urate concentrations exceed this saturation point, monosodium urate crystals deposit in and around the joints and cartilage and in the kidneys, sometimes eliciting the disease known as gout. As urinary pH increases, the solubility of uric acid increases; decreasing urinary pH may precipitate urate nephrolithiasis in patients with high urine uric acid concentrations. Asymptomatic hyperuricemia is classified as an elevated serum uric acid without symptoms of acute gouty arthritis.[11] With increasing uric acid levels, there is an increased risk of developing acute gout. There is a 2.0 to 4.1% 5-year cumulative incidence of gouty arthritis in men with serum urate levels ranging from 416 to 529 μmol/L (7.0 to 8.9 mg/dL) as compared with a 5-year cumulative incidence of 0.5 to 0.6% with serum urate levels of 410 μmol/L (6.9 mg/dL) or less. The incidence of gouty arthritis increases tremendously as urate levels rise above 535 μmol/L (9.0 mg/dL). The 5-year cumulative incidence for men with serum urate levels of 535 to 589 μmol/L (9.0 to 9.9 mg/dL) and 595 μmol/L (10.0 mg/dL) or more was 19.8% and 30.5%, respectively.[12] After one attack of gout, a patient may never have another or may have a recurrence 3 to 42 years later (mean = 11.4 years).[12]

Agents that have a cytotoxic effect, causing an increased turnover of nucleic acids, may increase uric acid concentrations (e.g., antimetabolite and chemotherapeutic agents used to treat neoplastic diseases, such as methotrexate, busulfan, vincristine, prednisone, and azathioprine).[6] Agents that decrease the renal clearance or block tubular secretion may cause a substantial elevation in serum urate concentrations (e.g., thiazide and loop diuretics, pyrazinamide, and ethambutol).[6,13] Diuretic-induced hyperuricemia accounts for 95% of acute attacks of gout in women over 60 years of age and 56% of men.[14] Some agents, such as salicylates, probenecid, sulfinpyrazone, and phenylbutazone, inhibit the tubular secretion of urate at low dosages, but at high dosages also inhibit tubular reabsorption, inducing a marked uricosuric effect.[4] Tacrolimus and cyclosporine may cause hyperuricemia in more than 3% of patients through an unknown mechanism.[15] Allopurinol therapeutically lowers serum uric acid by inhibiting xanthine oxidase (an enzyme that converts xanthine to uric acid in purine metabolism), and uricosuric agents such as probenecid are also used therapeutically to lower serum uric acid by blocking proximal tubular reabsorption. Ascorbic acid, caffeine, glucose, levodopa, methyldopa, and theophylline may interfere with the analytical technique and cause falsely high results.[4,6]

Enzymes

Enzymes are located in all body tissues and are responsible for the organic catalytic conversion of chemicals throughout the body. When enzymatically active cells are lysed or destroyed, certain enzymes are released into the serum. These enzymes are measured to assess which tissue is damaged. Only active cells release high quantities of enzymes in the serum. The more acute and extensive tissue injury is, the greater the rise in enzymes released from that tissue. Chronic smoldering damage causes moderate release of similar enzymes, with patterns usually different from those in acute injury.

Isoenzymes are proteins with different amino acid sequences, arising primarily from different tissues, which have the same enzymatic action. Clinically, these isoenzyme fractions are used to determine which tissue is damaged, and through their particular patterns, clinical diagnoses are made. Isoenzymes usually are separated by gel electrophoresis. For example, creatine kinase (CK) has two enzymatic subunits: MM and BB. BB is found predominantly in brain and travels very rapidly to the anode, whereas MM, which is found predominantly in skeletal muscle, moves very slowly toward the anode.[16] Even though the two isoenzymes have the same enzymatic activity, they are of different sizes and electronegativity and predominate in different tissues.

Enzymatic units are determined on a micromolar catalytic basis. One international unit (IU) is the amount of enzyme that catalyzes the conversion of 1 μmol substrate per minute. The SI unit for enzymatic activity is known as the katal (kat). One katal is equal to 1 mol catalyzed per second.[16] One μkat is equal to 1 μmol substrate catalyzed per second; therefore, 1 μkat = 60 IU.

Creatine Kinase

(SI units, 0 to 2.16 μkat/L [0 to 130 IU/L]; however, normal ranges vary considerably with method; CF = 0.01667)

CK, formerly known as creatine phosphokinase, catalyzes the conversion of phosphocreatine to creatine, releasing high-energy phosphate to skeletal and cardiac muscle (Fig. 5.1). Creatine is an unstable molecule and is converted very rapidly to creatinine. CK is a dimer consisting of two subunits: M and B. Brain tissue yields approximately 90% BB (CK_1) and 10% MM (CK_3), cardiac tissue yields approximately 40% MB (CK_2) and 60% MM, and normal serum contains virtually 100% MM, as does skeletal muscle. Clinical conditions causing elevated serum CK involve primarily skeletal muscle or cardiac tissue. The brain fraction is almost never observed in serum, even after a cerebrovascular accident, because the enzyme does not readily cross the blood–brain barrier.[16]

Almost any damage to skeletal muscle will cause an elevation in serum CK. Severe acute rhabdomyolysis secondary to trauma, prolonged coma, or overdoses of various drugs may cause dramatic rises of CK, ranging from 167 to 1670 μkat/L (10,000 to 100,000 IU/L).[17] Other conditions damaging skeletal muscle such as progressive muscular dystrophy, polymyositis or dermatomyositis, delirium tremens, seizures, or hypothyroidism may cause significant elevations in CK.

CK serum concentrations begin to rise approximately 4 to 8 hours after the acute myocardial injury, peak at 12 to 24 hours, and may persist throughout the initial 72 hours.[18] An MB fraction greater than 6% of the total is indicative of myocardial injury.[19] Several studies have shown that patients with a history of angina compatible with acute MI in whom total peak CK serum concentrations were normal but MB isoenzyme fractions were greater than 6% of the total had true acute microinfarctions.[20–22]

Intramuscular injections of medications may cause a variable elevation in CK of 2 to 6 times the normal concentration. These elevations return to normal within 48 hours after cessation of the injections. CK rises in more than 50% of patients receiving countershock or defibrillation but usually returns to normal in 48 to 72 hours.[6] Several medications have been reported to cause rhabdomyolysis in therapeutic and overdose situations, including opiates, cocaine, phencyclidine, amphetamines, theophylline, antihistamines, fibric acid derivatives, barbiturates, aminocaproic acid, certain antibiotics, chloroquine, colchicine, corticosteroids, and vincristine.[17] Patients receiving therapeutic dosages of neuroleptics may rarely experience the neuroleptic malignant syndrome, which may cause severe elevations in CK.[23] Lovastatin has also been reported to cause severe rhabdomyolysis alone (0.5%) or in combination with gemfibrozil (5%), niacin, cyclosporine (as high as 30%), and erythromycin.[24]

Lactate Dehydrogenase

(SI units, 1.6 to 3.17 μkat/L [100 to 190 IU/L]; CF = 0.01667)

Lactate dehydrogenase (LDH) catalyzes the conversion of pyruvate to lactate anaerobically to generate adenosine triphosphate.[25] LDH is in high concentrations in cardiac and skeletal muscle, liver, kidney, lung parenchyma, and erythrocytes (Ercs). It is essential to analyze the sample promptly, and it must be hemolysis-free for an accurate LDH measurement. LDH can be separated into five distinct components. The five LDH isoenzymes all have approximately the same molecular weight but different charges. LDH_5 has the greatest mobility and LDH_1 the least. Table 5.4 lists the LDH isoenzymes and their relative activity in each tissue.[16]

Serum LDH almost always is elevated after an acute MI. The serum LDH begins to rise 10 to 12 hours after the acute event, reaching a peak in 48 to 72 hours, with prolonged elevation for up to 14 days.[6] Increased serum LDH level, with LDH_1 greater than LDH_2 (flipped enzymes), occurs in acute MI in approximately 80% of patients, but also occurs in acute renal infarction, pernicious anemia, and hemolysis.[6] In a large MI with biventricular failure, LDH_5 levels may also be elevated because of liver congestion.

LDH_5 may be markedly elevated in hepatitis and may also be elevated in other hepatic disorders. LDH elevations may occur 50% of the time with malignant tumors, usually with a nonspecific isoenzyme pattern. LDH is elevated in approximately 60% of patients with lymphomas and 90% of patients with leukemias. Marked elevations of LDH_5 levels are seen in patients with skeletal muscle damage, extensive burns, and trauma. Pulmonary embolus and infarction may cause elevations in LDH_2 and LDH_3; if cor pulmonale is present, LDH_5 also rises. In nephrotic syndrome, LDH_4 and LDH_5 rise, but in nephritis and renal infarction LDH_1 and LDH_2 rise. All forms of hemolysis, including sickle cell crisis and drug-induced hemolysis, cause elevations in LDH_1 and LDH_2.[26,27]

All drugs causing damage to these tissues cause elevations in LDH. Hepatotoxic agents and agents inducing hemolysis increase serum LDH concentrations.[27,28]

Troponins

(Troponin I [cTnI] SI units, 0.7 to 1.5 μg/L [0.7 to 1.5 ng/mL]; CF = 1.0)

Troponin is a complex of three proteins: troponin T, troponin C, and troponin I.[16] Each troponin has its own specific function in the regulation of myosin and actin in the contractile process. cTnI is very sensitive and specific for myocardial tissue. After acute myocardial injury, cTnI starts to rise approximately 2 hours after myocardial damage (2 to 6 hours faster than CK-MB), with peak elevations occurring at about 24 to 36 hours. There is a 13-fold greater concentration of cTnI than CK-MB in the heart, and cTnI is at least as sensitive for the clinical detection of cardiac injury as CK-MB.[29] cTnI is much more specific than CK-MB for cardiac tissue and is not elevated after endurance exercise or in skeletal muscle injury, chronic muscle disease, hypothyroidism, or chronic renal failure, or in postoperative patients without myocardial injury.[29,30] Elevations of cTnI greater than 2.0 μg/L is indicative of acute myocardial injury.[29–31] Unlike CK-MB, cTnI can also detect acute myocardial injury for up to 12 days without the lack of specificity and necessary

Table 5.4 ▪ Lactate Dehydrogenase Isoenzyme Nomenclature

Nomenclature of Isoenzyme Starting with Most Anodic	Composition: Proportion of Monomers[a] in Each Isoenzyme	Relative Content[b] of Isoenzyme					
		Myocardium	Liver	Skeletal Muscle	Brain	Kidney	Red Blood Cells
1	HHHH	++++	±	±	++	+	+++
2	HHHM	++++	±	±	++	+	+++
3	HHMM	+	+	+	++	++	+
4	HMMM	±	++	++	++	++	±
5	MMMM	±	++++	++++	±	++	±

Source: Pincus MR, Zimmerman HJ, Henry JB. Clinical enzymology. In: Henry JB, ed. Clinical diagnosis and management by laboratory methods. 19th ed. Philadelphia: WB Saunders Company, 1996:283.

[a]Monomer H (myocardial). Monomer M (skeletal muscle).

[b]Content graded from ±, which represents almost no activity, to ++++, which represents high activity.

isoenzyme separation of LDH.[31] Hamm et al.[32] studied two troponin I levels at least 4 hours apart and at least 6 hours after the onset of pain in 773 consecutive emergency room patients who had acute chest pain for less than 12 hours without ST segment elevation. Troponin I was positive in all 47 patients with evolving MI. The cardiac event rate in patients with negative troponin I during 30 days of follow-up was only 0.3%. Several authors recommend cTnI as the gold standard serologic test to quickly diagnose acute myocardial injury and have developed protocols for its use in this diagnosis.[29,30]

Aspartate Aminotransferase

(SI units, 0 to 0.58 μkat/L [0 to 35 IU/L]; CF = 0.01667)

Aspartate aminotransferase (AST), formerly known as serum glutamic oxaloacetic transaminase (SGOT), is one of several transaminases responsible for transfer of amino groups in gluconeogenesis. AST is responsible for transferring an amino group from aspartate to α,β-glutaric acid, forming glutamate and oxaloacetate.[25] The highest concentrations of AST are in cardiac and hepatic tissues.

AST usually appears within 8 hours after myocardial injury, peaks in 24 hours, and returns to baseline in 4 to 6 days.[6] AST rises in virtually all types of hepatic diseases. Its peak concentration and ratio to other enzymes reflect the type of hepatic damage. These differences are discussed later, in the discussion of hyperbilirubinemia.

Several medications may cause elevations in AST levels through either direct hepatocellular damage or cholestasis.[7,28,33,34] Cholinergic drugs and opioids cause elevation of transaminases through spasm of the sphincter of Oddi.[35] Several agents (commonly isoniazid and rifampin) may cause transient elevations in transaminase levels.[28,36,37] Initially, dye-binding techniques were used to assay for transaminases, which accounted for several drug interferences including isoniazid, but with newer ultraviolet techniques, there is very little interaction with the assay.[35]

Alanine Aminotransferase

(SI units, 0 to 0.58 μkat/L [0 to 35 IU/L]; CF = 0.01667)

Alanine aminotransferase (ALT), formerly known as serum glutamate pyruvate transaminase (SGPT), transfers an amino group from alanine to α-ketoglutarate, forming glutamate and pyruvate.[25] ALT is very specific for hepatic tissue and is almost always absent in acute MI. It is much more sensitive to hepatic damage, and levels rise faster and higher than those of AST in most types of hepatocellular damage.

γ-Glutamyl Transferase

(SI units, 0 to 0.50 μkat/L [0-30 IU/L]; CF = 0.01667)

γ-Glutamyl transferase (GGT) catalyzes the transfer of a γ-glutamyl group from one peptide to another.[25] The kidneys, liver, and pancreas contain large quantities of GGT. Several isoenzymes of GGT have been isolated, but to date no clinical utility for them has been found.[16]

The elevation of GGT parallels that of alkaline phosphatase (ALP) and rises higher in cholestatic and obstructive diseases than in acute hepatocellular diseases. It is always elevated in acute pancreatitis, and its rise is faster and greater than that of ALP in obstructive jaundice. GGT is the most sensitive biochemical indicator of alcohol exposure because elevation exceeds that of other commonly monitored liver enzymes. In alcoholic hepatitis, GGT is usually the enzyme that rises fastest and has the highest peaks. Agents such as phenytoin and phenobarbital that induce the cytochrome P-450 enzyme system may cause elevations in GGT.[6]

Phosphatases

Phosphatases are primarily responsible for catalyzing cleavage of monophosphate esters and may be acid or alkaline.[25] Acid phosphatases have optimal enzymatic activity at a pH of 5, and ALP has an optimal enzymatic activity at a pH of 9.[16] Acid phosphatase (SI units, 0 to 90 μkat/L [0 to 5.5 IU/L]; CF = 16.67) is found primarily in prostate, Ercs, and platelets. Approximately 60 to 75% of men with prostate cancer have elevated acid phosphatase concentrations.[6]

ALP (SI units, 0.5 to 2.0 μkat/L [30 to 120 IU/L]; CF = 0.01667) is found in most tissues but is derived predominantly from hepatic, osseous, and intestinal cells.[6] The placenta produces high concentrations of ALP in the third trimester as a result of high fetal osteoblastic activity. Children in the active growth phase produce ALP at two to five times adult rates. The osseous and hepatic isoenzymes of ALP can be readily identified in electrophoretic patterns of serum.[38]

ALP is elevated in most disorders of bone involving osteoblastic activity. Metastatic disease to bone may cause substantial elevations in ALP levels. ALP is also elevated in acute fractures, hyperparathyroidism, osteogenic sarcoma, and Paget's disease.[16]

ALP is secreted into bile, and an elevation may be the first clue to intrahepatic or extrahepatic cholestasis.[19,39] The diagnosis of intrahepatic or extrahepatic disease cannot be delineated by the peak height of the serum ALP concentration.[39] When biliary obstruction is complete, ALP serum concentrations are almost always three to eight times normal, whereas with incomplete obstruction, concentrations are only two to three times normal.[40]

Amylase

(SI units, 0 to 2.17 μkat/L [0 to 70 Somogyi units/dL; 0 to 130 IU/L]; Somogyi to IU CF = 1.85, Somogyi to SI units CF = 0.031, IU to SI units CF = 0.01667)

Amylase enzymatically cleaves large polysaccharides into oligosaccharides and monosaccharides in the gastrointestinal tract through salivary and pancreatic secretions. Amylase is present as α-, β-, and γ-amylase, but only α-amylase is of clinical interest. Amylase is present in a variety of human tissues including the pancreas, salivary glands, muscle, adipose tissue, kidney, brain, lung, fallopian tubes, intestine, spleen, and heart.[41] Normal serum amylase is composed of approximately 40% pancreatic isoenzyme (P-type isoamylase) and 60% salivary isoenzyme (S-type isoamylase).[42] This percentage changes with age so that after age 70, P-type isoamylase makes up only 20% of total serum amylase.[41]

Serum amylase concentrations rise within 6 to 48 hours after the onset of acute pancreatitis in more than 80% of patients.[42] Values greater than four times the upper limit of normal are highly suggestive of the diagnosis.[41] This is a sensitive measure of acute pancreatitis, but it is not highly specific because several other conditions may present with acute abdominal pain and elevated serum amylase levels, including biliary colic, perforated peptic ulcer, and mesenteric infarction.[42] In acute pancreatitis, the urinary clearance of amylase increases, possibly because of altered renal tubular function. A urinary amylase:creatinine ratio greater than 0.04 suggests acute pancreatitis; however, this method is unreliable because elevated ratios may also be seen with other conditions, such as burns, renal insufficiency, and ketoacidosis.[41,42] The usefulness of isoenzyme separation is limited because other intestinal sources also account for P-type isoamylase. Patients with acute alcoholic pancreatitis have normal serum amylase levels approximately 30% of the time.[42]

Parotitis and mumps cause elevations of S-type isoamylase. Chronic alcohol consumption may also increase S-type isoamylase. This is an important consideration because alcohol is the most common cause of acute pancreatitis. Macroamylase is a circulating complex of normal amylase bound to immunoglobulin G (IgG) or IgA.[41] Analysis of macroamylase reveals variable amounts of both P-type and S-type isoamylase. Macroamylasemia is an acquired benign condition that must be separated from other causes of hyperamylasemia.

Medications that cause spasm of the sphincter of Oddi, such as narcotics and cholinergic agents, may cause elevations in serum amylase.[6] Agents definitely associated with causing pancreatitis include 5-aminosalicylic acid, azathioprine, didanosine, estrogens, furosemide, 6-mercaptopurine, methyldopa, metronidazole, pentamidine, sulfonamides, sulindac, tetracycline, thiazide diuretics, and valproic acid.[43] Certain pancreatic enzyme preparations contain amylase and lipase, which may elevate serum amylase and lipase values.[6]

Lipase

(SI units, 0 to 2.66 μkat/L [0 to 0.6 Cherry–Crandal units/mL, 0 to 160 IU/L]; Cherry–Crandal to IU CF = 278, Cherry–Crandal to SI units CF = 4.63)

Lipase hydrolyzes glycerol esters of long-chain fatty acids at the 1 and 3 positions, producing β-monoglyceride and 2 mol free fatty acid. Serum lipase should not be confused with lipoprotein lipase because these are entirely different enzymes. Lipase is located in the stomach, intestine, leukocytes, fat cells, and milk, but predominates in the pancreas.[41] Serum lipase concentrations usually are elevated in patients with acute pancreatitis and are more predictive than amylase.[41,42] Serum lipase increases at approximately the same time as amylase in acute pancreatitis, but elevations may persist for much longer than serum amylase (7 to 10 days).[41] Serum lipase concentrations may also be elevated in other acute abdominal illnesses.[42] Medications that may elevate serum lipase concentrations are very similar to those that elevate serum amylase.

Bilirubin

(SI units: Total, 2 to 18 μmol/L; Direct, 0 to 4 μmol/L [Total, 0.1 to 1.0 mg/dL; Direct, 0 to 0.2 mg/dL]; CF = 17.10)

Bilirubin is a metabolic byproduct of the lysis of Ercs by the reticuloendothelial system (RES; Fig. 5.3). The RES catabolizes hemoglobin into free iron, globin, and biliverdin, which is rapidly converted to bilirubin. Unconjugated bilirubin is poorly soluble in serum, so it is transported to the liver bound to albumin. This unconjugated form is also known as indirect or prehepatic bilirubin. In the liver, glucuronyl transferase conjugates bilirubin with two molecules of glucuronic acid, forming bilirubin diglucuronide.[40] This form of bilirubin is highly soluble in serum and is known as direct or hepatic bilirubin. Direct bilirubin is transported through the biliary tree with bile acids and stored in the gallbladder as bile. When bile is released during the digestive process, intestinal bacteria convert bilirubin into several compounds, collectively called bilinogen. An estimated 10% of bilinogen is reabsorbed from the intestine into the bloodstream and resecreted by the liver. Small amounts of bilinogen are then excreted in the urine (urobilinogen), accounting for the urine's straw color. However, most bilinogen is directly eliminated in the feces (stercobilinogen), accounting for their characteristic dark brown color. Small portions of bilinogen are converted to bilins by intestinal flora, which are also eliminated in the feces. The presence of bilirubin in the urine implies direct bilirubin because indirect bilirubin is bound to serum albumin, which normally should not be filtered by the glomerulus.[39] δ-bilirubin is a protein-bound pigment that may falsely raise total bilirubin measurements during hepatobiliary disease. Agents that may interfere with the bilirubin assay include ascorbic acid, dextran, intravenous contrast agents, propranolol, and rifampin.[7]

Causes of hyperbilirubinemia can be classified into three broad categories: prehepatic (hemolysis), hepatic (defective removal of bilirubin from the blood or defective conjugation), and posthepatic (obstruction of the extrahepatic biliary tree), also called cholestatic or obstructive.[40] As serum bilirubin concentrations rise above approximately 34 μmol/L, classic scleral icterus and jaundice

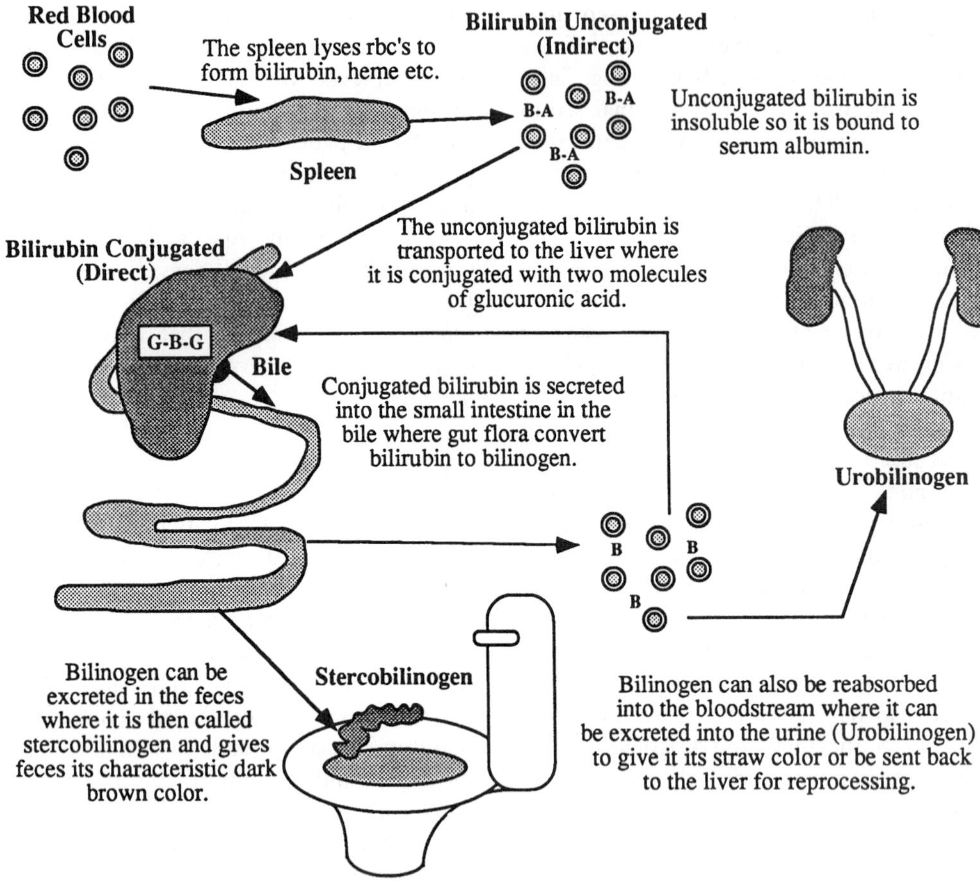

Figure 5.3. Bilirubin formation, metabolism, and excretion. *RBCs,* red blood cells.

Table 5.5 ▪ Usual Enzymatic Patterns in Hyperbilirubinemia

	Fecal Bilinogen	Urine Bilirubin	Direct Bili (% total)	AST	ALT	ALP	GGT	LDH
Hemolysis	↑	–	<20%	nl	nl	nl	nl	↑↑↑ $LDH_1 > LDH_2$
Hepatocellular damage (viral or toxin)	↓	+	>40%	↑↑↑↑	↑↑↑↑↑	↑↑	↑↑	↑↑ LDH_5
Alcoholic hepatitis	↓	+	<30%	↑↑	↑	↑	↑↑↑	nl
Obstructive or cholestatic jaundice	↓	+	>50%	↑	↑	↑↑↑	↑↑↑	↑ LDH_5
Alcoholic cirrhosis	nl	±	<30%	↑↑ nl (25%)	↑ nl (50%)	↑	↑	nl

AST, aspartate aminotransferase; *ALT,* alanine aminotransferase; *ALP,* alkaline phosphatase; *GGT,* γ-glutamyl transferase; *LDH,* lactate dehydrogenase; *nl,* normal; ↑, increased; ↓, decreased.

develop. Table 5.5 summarizes the enzymatic patterns of the common causes of hyperbilirubinemia.

Hemolytic jaundice results from the rapid destruction of Ercs overwhelming the ability of the liver to process excess bilirubin. Tissue hematomas or collection of blood in body cavities may increase the serum bilirubin. Severe sepsis or malignancy-induced disseminated intravascular coagulation, sickle cell crisis, or certain medications may induce hemolytic anemia. Drug-induced hemolytic anemia may be immune mediated[27] (methyldopa, penicillins, cephalosporins, quinidine, ibuprofen, and triamterene), hemoglobin oxidation mediated[44] (dapsone, antimalarials, sulfonamides, aspirin, nitrates, methylene blue, and ascorbic acid), megaloblastic mediated[45] (antineoplastics, anticonvulsants, and alcohol), or sideroblastic mediated with bone marrow suppression[46] (chloramphenicol, alcohol, lead, and antituberculous agents).

Hepatocellular injury from viral hepatitis, alcoholic hepatitis, toxin-mediated hepatitis, or cirrhosis may elevate serum bilirubin concentrations. Viral hepatitis usually causes elevations in direct bilirubin levels. Viral hepatitis may cause extreme elevations in transaminases (167 to 334 μkat/L, 10,000 to 20,000 IU/L), with ALT levels usually greater than those of AST. Medications commonly reported to cause direct hepatocellular damage include acetaminophen, amiodarone, amsacrine, halothane, indinavir, irinotecan, tetracycline, troglitazone, valproic acid, isoniazid, rifampin, methyldopa, labetalol, and tacrine.[7,28,33,34] Drug-induced hepatocellular damage may be indistinguishable from acute viral hepatitis. Alcoholic hepatitis presents in patients with acute or chronic alcohol ingestion. Transaminase elevations are only a fraction of those seen in viral or toxin-induced hepatitis. AST concentration usually is greater than ALT, but GGT levels may be markedly elevated by the effects of alcohol on GGT release.

Patients with obstructive jaundice usually present with light clay-colored stools and dark cola-colored urine because of reabsorption of conjugated bilirubin from the biliary ducts, with redistribution to the urine and lack of bilinogen in the stool. The lack of bile acids in the gastrointestinal tract because of obstruction may cause steatorrhea. Transaminase levels usually are only mildly elevated unless severe obstruction occurs, causing hepatocellular damage. ALP and GGT concentrations usually are quite high. The most common cause of biliary obstruction is choledocholithiasis (gallstones) obstructing the common bile duct. Obese, middle-aged women are highly predisposed to choledocholithiasis; however, it may occur in both sexes at any age. Other causes of obstructive jaundice include carcinoma of the head of the pancreas, pancreatitis, or other neoplastic invasion of the papilla of Vater. Cholestatic changes may be caused by an intrahepatic defect of the transport of bilirubin into hepatic canaliculi.[40] Cholestatic jaundice closely resembles posthepatic biliary obstruction, except the stools are only somewhat lighter than normal because there is less exclusion of bilirubin from the duodenum. Common medications that induce obstructive or cholestatic jaundice include C-17 alkyl steroids, estrogens, chlorpromazine, and erythromycin estolate. Other medications may cause a mixed picture of hepatic injury through an atypical (phenytoin) or granulomatous (quinidine, allopurinol) pattern.[28]

Common pitfalls in the application of liver function tests to determine the cause of hyperbilirubinemia include dependence on single tests rather than patterns of abnormality; normal results, implying no disease (in cirrhosis, 25% of patients have normal AST and 50% of patients have normal ALT); abnormal liver function tests, suggesting only liver disease; failure to recognize hepatocellular disease with low transaminase and high ALP levels, or failure to recognize cholestasis or obstruction with high transaminase and low ALP levels; or failure to repeat tests that did not correlate with clinical results.[40]

Serum Proteins

Total Protein

(SI units, 60 to 80 g/L [6.0 to 8.0 g/dL]; CF = 10)

Serum proteins are separated by serum protein electrophoresis into prealbumin, albumin, and globulin fractions.

Prealbumin

(SI units, 1.5 to 3.6 g/L [0.15 to 0.36 g/dL]; CF = 10)

Prealbumin makes up a very small percentage of total protein (less than 1%) and is not widely used for clinical management. Prealbumin contains retinol binding protein, which plays a role in the transport and metabolism of vitamin A.[47] Prealbumin is exquisitely sensitive to nutritional intake and has a short half-life in the circulation.[47] Measurements of prealbumin therefore have clinical utility as a marker for nutritional status.[47]

Albumin

(SI units, 40 to 60 g/L [4.0 to 6.0 g/dL]; CF = 10)

Albumin is by far the most abundant serum protein. Albumin is synthesized in the liver and accounts for up to 65% of total protein. Albumin has three major functions: controlling oncotic pressure in the plasma, transporting amino acids synthesized in the liver to other tissues, and transporting poorly soluble organic and inorganic ligands.[47]

Albumin accounts for 80% of the oncotic pressure of the plasma. Capillary hemodynamics are controlled by four major forces, including intravascular oncotic pressure, interstitial oncotic pressure, capillary hydrostatic pressure, and interstitial hydrostatic pressure (Fig. 5.4). Intravascular oncotic pressure and interstitial hydrostatic pressure are the forces holding fluid in the intravascular space, and capillary hydrostatic pressure and interstitial oncotic pressure force fluid into tissue spaces. Normally, intravascular oncotic pressure overrides capillary hydrostatic pressure, creating a net hemodynamic flow into the vasculature. These forces may be disrupted, causing local edema, ascites, or anasarca. Malnutrition, malignancy, severe trauma, or burns cause a net catabolic state, decreasing serum albumin and oncotic pressure. In hepatic cirrhosis, there is decreased synthesis of albumin and increased portal capillary pressure, resulting in ascites. In severe sepsis, toxin-mediated increases in capillary permeability allow intravascular albumin to escape into the interstitial tissues, accounting for increases in interstitial oncotic pressure. Nephrotic syndrome and protein-losing enteropathies cause increased losses of serum albumin, resulting in anasarca. Congestive heart failure alters pulmonary capillary hydrostatic pressure, resulting in pulmonary edema. Table 5.6 summarizes changes in capillary hemodynamics resulting from various disease states. Dehydration and hemodilution may increase or decrease serum albumin concentrations, respectively.

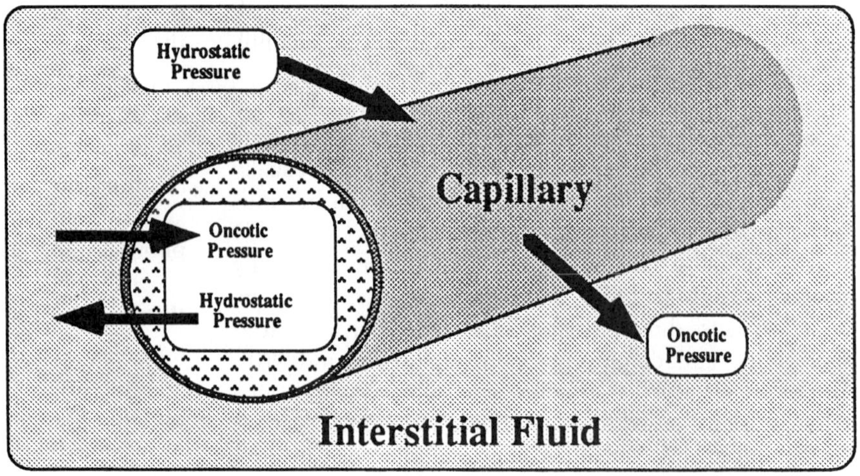

Figure 5.4. Capillary hemodynamic forces.

Table 5.6 ▪ Common Disease States Resulting in Altered Capillary Hemodynamics

Disease	Mechanism	Serum Albumin	Capillary Hydrostatic Pressure	Interstitial Oncotic Pressure
Malnutrition	Decreased protein synthesis; increased protein catabolism	↓↓↓	nl	nl
Malignancy	Increased protein catabolism	↓↓	nl, ↑ Tumor compression	nl
Burns	Increased protein catabolism; altered skin capillary permeability	↓↓↓	nl	↑↑, skin
Hepatic cirrhosis	Decreased albumin synthesis; increased portal capillary hydrostatic pressure	↓↓↓	↑↑↑, portal	nl, ↑
Sepsis	Toxin-altered capillary permeability	↓↓↓	nl	↑↑↑
Congestive heart failure	Increased pulmonary and systemic capillary hydrostatic pressure caused by biventricular failure	nl, ↓ Malnutrition caused by cardiac cachexia	↑↑↑, pulmonary or systemic	nl
Nephrotic syndrome	Loss of albumin into the urine caused by glomerular damage and leakage	↓↓↓	nl	nl

nl, normal; ↓, decreased; ↑, increased.

Albumin acts as a carrier protein for both organic and inorganic molecules, which may bind ionically or covalently.[47,48] Several common medications that are highly insoluble in serum bind more than 90% to albumin, including phenytoin, salicylates, phenylbutazone, first-generation sulfonylureas, valproic acid, warfarin, and certain sulfonamides.[48] Because free drug is thought to be the active portion, changes in serum albumin concentrations may have a large influence on drug distribution and pharmacologic effect.[49]

Globulin

(SI units, 20 to 40 g/L [2.0 to 4.0 g/dL]; CF = 10)

The globulin fraction makes up one-third of total protein and has four major components: α_1, α_2, β, and γ.[47] Important proteins located in the α_1 zone are α_1-antitrypsin, which is a scavenger enzyme for lysosomal proteases, and α_1 acid glycoprotein (AAG). Young patients with homozygous α_1-antitrypsin deficiency develop severe pulmonary emphysema caused by protein lysis by elastase. AAG is an acute-phase reactant that acts as a carrier protein for certain poorly soluble medications. AAG is elevated transiently in a variety of clinical conditions, including burns, chronic pain, enzyme induction, rheumatoid arthritis, morbid obesity, MI, malignancy, surgery, and trauma. Several common medications bind to AAG, including amitriptyline, chlorpromazine, dipyridamole, disopyramide, erythromycin, imipramine, lidocaine, meperidine, methadone, nortriptyline, propranolol, and quinidine.[48] The transient elevations in AAG levels during the previously mentioned conditions may cause important changes in the binding and pharmacologic effect of these medications.

The α_2 portion consists primarily of α_2-macroglobulin, haptoglobin, and ceruloplasmin. α_2-Macroglobulin is another major protease inhibitor, haptoglobin is a carrier protein for hemoglobin, and ceruloplasmin is a copper-binding protein. The β portion is composed of low-density lipoprotein (LDL), transferrin, C_3, and fibrinogen.[47] LDL is the major transport protein for cholesterol to tissues, transferrin transports ferric iron stores to bone marrow for erythropoiesis, C_3 is a major component of the complement system, and fibrinogen is a coagulation precursor for fibrin. The γ-globulin portion is composed of antibody immunoglobulins IgA, IgE, IgG, and IgM. IgA is responsible for surface immunity, IgE binds to mast cells and is responsible for hypersensitivity reactions, IgM is responsible for initial humoral immunity, and IgG is responsible for sustained humoral immunity.[47] The primary disorder associated with hypergammaglobulinemia is multiple myeloma.

Complete Blood Count with Differential

The complete blood count (CBC) provides information about the Ercs, leukocytes, and platelets. The number of parameters provided with a CBC depends on the type of machine used for the analysis. Any other desired tests may be ordered separately.

In the normal adult, blood cells are made predominantly in the bone marrow of the sternum, skull, ribs, vertebrae, and pelvis and the proximal ends of the long bones (humerus and femur).[50] The pathways of hematopoiesis from the pluripotential stem cell and the relationship between the different cell lines are shown in Figure 5.5.[51]

Erythrocytes

(Males, 4.3 to 5.9 × 10^{12}/L [4.3 to 5.9 × $10^6/mm^3$]; females, 3.5 to 5.0 ×10^{12}/L [3.5 to 5.0 ×$10^6/mm^3$]; CF = 1)

The main functions of Ercs, or red blood cells, are to carry oxygen from the lungs to the tissues and transport carbon dioxide back to the lungs. Anemia occurs when the hemoglobin, Hct, or Erc count is below the normal range.[52] This can be a result of impaired Erc production, increased Erc destruction, or blood loss. The extent of anemia generally is described by the hemoglobin or Hct values. The red blood cell indices may be used to further characterize the anemia by cell morphology or color.[53] Normal-sized Ercs are called normocytes, small ones are microcytes, and large Ercs are macrocytes. If there is abnormal variation in size, the patient is said to have anisocytosis, which is a feature of most anemias. Those with normal amounts of hemoglobin are said to be normochromic, those with low hemoglobin are hypochromic, and those with increased hemoglobin are hyperchromic. Abnormally shaped cells are poikilocytes.[52] *Polycythemia* means "many blood cells" but usually refers to an increased red blood cell mass or an elevated Hct value.[53]

Red cell production is regulated by tissue oxygenation. Tissues receive inadequate oxygen if there is an insufficient supply in inspired air, impaired oxygen transport from the alveoli into the bloodstream, inadequate hemoglobin to carry oxygen, abnormal blood flow, or a failure of hemoglobin to release bound oxygen at tissue sites.[54] This can occur in diseases such as anemia, in cardiac or pulmonary disease, or with decreased oxygen tension in the air, such as at high altitudes.[51] Smokers tend to have a stimulation of Erc production.[55] Hypoxia or decreased oxygenation stimulates the production of erythropoietin, with over 85% being produced by the kidneys. A small amount of erythropoietin is produced elsewhere, probably by the liver. Erythropoietin stimulates and accelerates all aspects of Erc production and release.[50] Erythropoietin

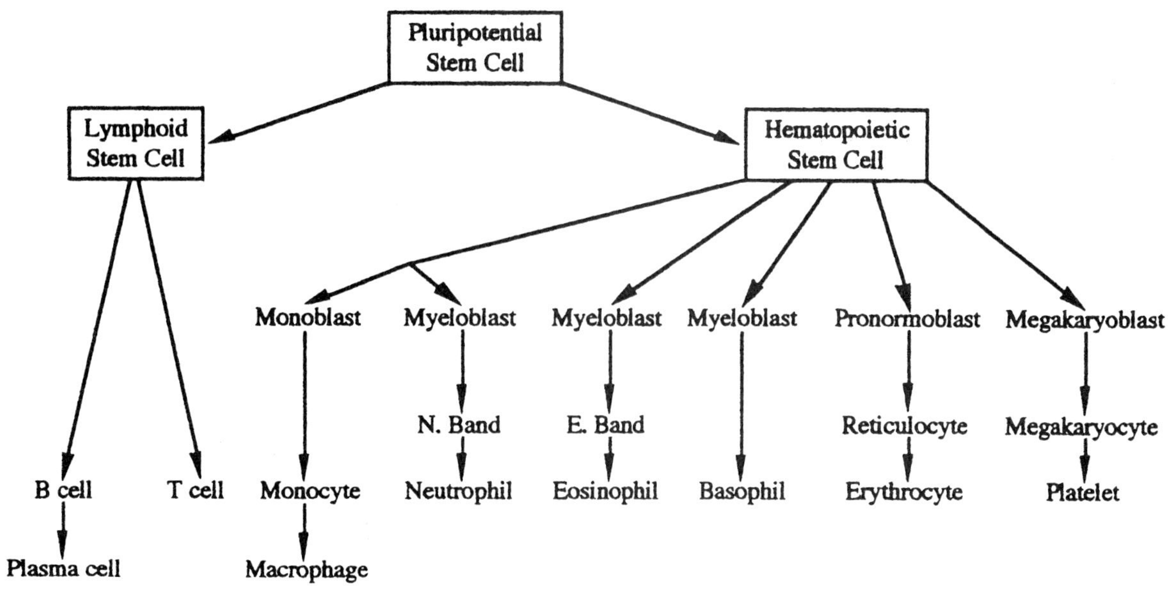

Figure 5.5. Hematopoiesis.

increases in most anemias, but its production and effects may be impaired in those associated with chronic diseases.[56] If tissue oxygen concentrations are perceived as inadequate, Erc production continues, regardless of the Erc count or hemoglobin concentration, resulting in a secondary or reactive polycythemia.[55]

The life span of Ercs in circulation is 120 days. They are removed by the RES.[51] This includes phagocytic cells in circulation and in the spleen, liver, lymph nodes, bone marrow, lungs, and other tissues.[50] With an abnormally large spleen, there is increased destruction of normal cells. The spleen may be enlarged in conditions such as liver disease, congestive heart failure, leukemias, lymphomas, or protozoal infections.[54] There can be accelerated destruction of Ercs by a normal spleen when they contain abnormal hemoglobin or have abnormal membranes or enzymes. Increased destruction can also occur with abnormal physical, chemical, microbiologic, or immunologic conditions.[53]

Hemolysis is the disruption of the mature Erc membrane and release of hemoglobin before the end of the usual life span. It can take place in the spleen (or other RES organs) or vasculature. This accelerated destruction of cells can occur in response to physical trauma or massive exertion; severe burns; infections such as malaria, mycoplasmal pneumonia, or mononucleosis; or toxic insults such as *Clostridium* infections or brown recluse spider bites. Hemolysis can also occur with drugs and chemicals such as arsine gas or copper salts. With oxidizing drugs such as nitrites or nitrates, methemoglobin can be formed and lead to severe cases of Erc destruction.[53,54]

Destruction of Ercs may be mediated by antibodies. Various types of antibody-mediated hemolysis are associated with drugs. Penicillins and cephalosporins can bind to Erc membranes and stimulate production of IgG antibodies and hemolysis. Cephalosporins can also change Erc membranes, leading to binding of immunoglobulins. Methyldopa can directly induce a positive antiglobulin reaction and hemolysis. The Ercs may also be destroyed as "innocent bystanders". Drug–antibody complexes can settle on the surface of Ercs and attract complement, which hemolyzes the cells. This has been reported with interferons, quinine, quinidine, *p*-aminosalicylic acid, phenacetin, rifampin, antihistamines, chlorpromazine, sulfonylureas, sulfonamides, and insecticides.[7,53]

Patients with chronic diseases such as infections, kidney or liver disease, various endocrine disorders, rheumatoid arthritis, or neoplasms often have anemia. Aplastic anemia involves a pancytopenia or a depression of Ercs, neutrophils, and platelets. About 11 to 20% of cases can be attributed to drug or chemical exposure and about 6% to infectious hepatitis.[53] It can occur secondary to infections; neoplasms; radiation; drugs such as chloramphenicol, ticlopidine, gold salts, indomethacin, sulfonamides, thioamides, anticonvulsants, or antineoplastic drugs; or chemicals such as benzene or chlordane.[7,53,57] Reports of aplastic anemia with felbamate led the U.S. Food and Drug Administration to recommend that patients be withdrawn from that drug.[58] About 70% of cases are primary or idiopathic, in which there is no known predisposing cause. Patients with aplastic anemia may later develop acute leukemia or myelodysplastic syndrome.[53] Polycythemia vera is a myeloproliferative syndrome in which there is a spontaneous increase in Ercs. The predominant picture is one of Erc proliferation, but other elements of the blood are also hyperactive. It most commonly presents between 50 and 60 years of age but can occur at any age. Thrombosis and hemorrhage are common complications.[59]

Hemoglobin

(Males, 8.45 to 10.65 mmol/L or 136 to 172 g/L [13.6 to 17.2 g/dL]; females, 7.45 to 9.30 mmol/L or 120 to 150 g/L [12.0 to 15.0 g/dL]; CF = 0.6206 for mmol/L and 10 for g/L)

Hemoglobin, the primary component of Ercs, transports oxygen and carbon dioxide.[52] Hemoglobinopathies occur when genes code for abnormal amino acid sequences. The most common abnormal hemoglobin is sickle hemoglobin. Thalassemias are characterized by decreased synthesis of globin chains.[60]

The preferred assay for hemoglobin is the cyanmethemoglobin method. Errors in venipuncture technique can lead to hemoconcentration, which results in falsely elevated values for hemoglobin and cell counts. The difference in the normal range between men and women is thought to result mainly from androgen stimulation of erythropoiesis on the marrow. Estrogen probably has a slight suppressive effect on Erc production.[52] Menstrual blood loss is also a contributing factor.[54] In older men, the hemoglobin tends to fall. This occurs to a lesser extent in women, who may even have a slight increase in the value. As a result, there is a less than 0.62 mmol/L (1 g/dL) sex difference in hemoglobin in older people. There is a diurnal variation of approximately 8 to 9% in hemoglobin concentrations, with the highest value in the morning and the lowest in the evening.[52] Hemoglobin values are approximately 0.62 mmol/L (1 g/dL) lower in blacks than in whites. Some attribute this to a higher incidence of iron deficiency anemia in blacks.[61]

Hematocrit

(Males, 0.39 to 0.49 [39 to 49%]; females, 0.33 to 0.43 [33 to 43%]; CF = 0.01)

The Hct is the ratio of the volume of Ercs to that of whole blood or the packed Erc volume.[52] It increases when more fluid is lost than Ercs and dehydration occurs, as is seen in patients with vomiting, diarrhea, burns, or prolonged fever or those taking diuretics. An inappropriate polycythemia occurs with renal cancer, hepatomas, pheochromocytomas, or adrenal adenomas in which there is elevated erythropoietin and Hct.[53,62] The Hct is unreliable for patient assessment immediately after blood loss or transfusion.[52]

Reticulocytes

(10 to 75×10^9/L [10,000 to 75,000 mm^{-3}]; CF = 0.001; or 0.001 to 0.024 [0.1 to 2.4% Ercs]; CF = 0.01)

Reticulocytes are immature Ercs. Generally, the absolute reticulocyte count is more useful than the percentage of Ercs. Reticulocytes provide an estimate of Erc production; however, as the Hct drops, increasingly immature reticulocytes are released into the blood. These cells take longer to mature in circulation, as shown here:

Hct (%)	Reticulocyte	Maturation Time (days)
0.40–0.45	(40–45)	1.0
0.35–0.39	(35–39)	1.5
0.25–0.34	(25–34)	2.0
0.15–0.24	(15–24)	2.5
<0.15	(<15)	3.0

To estimate Erc production accurately in response to anemia, a correction factor must be used to account for this longer maturation time and avoid overestimating the erythropoietic response. The reticulocyte production index (RPI) can be calculated as follows:

$$\text{RPI} = (\text{Reticulocyte count/Normal reticulocyte count} \times \text{Patient's Hct/Normal Hct}) \div \text{Maturation time}$$

In general, an RPI greater than 3 represents an adequate response to anemia and an RPI less than 2 indicates an inadequate increase in Erc production.[51,63] The reticulocytes are most markedly increased in patients with hemolysis or acute blood loss; they also increase when iron or vitamin B_{12} is administered to a deficient patient. If the reticulocyte count is normal but the hemoglobin low, there is an inadequate response to anemia, as may be seen in iron deficiency. If the reticulocyte count is elevated but the hemoglobin is normal, there is probably some destruction or loss of Ercs occurring, and the body is appropriately compensating for the loss.[54]

Erythrocyte Indices

The size and hemoglobin content of Ercs can be quantified by the Erc indices.

The mean corpuscular volume (MCV) is the average volume of Ercs. It can be measured by machines or calculated by the formula MCV = Hct/Ercs.[52] The normal range is 76 to 100 fL in SI units (a femtoliter is 10^{-15} liter), or 76 to 100 μm^3.[3] The MCV is decreased in microcytic anemia and elevated in macrocytic anemia. Young Ercsand reticulocytes are larger than mature cells, so when there is rapid Erc production, the MCV increases. This type of macrocytosis can be observed in compensated hemolytic conditions or when a patient is recovering from acute blood loss. Megaloblastic changes can occur when DNA production is impaired but RNA production is normal. This causes nuclear maturation to lag behind cytoplasmic maturation. This change occurs in all cells but is most dramatic and can be most easily diagnosed in Erc precursors. The most common causes of megaloblastosis are deficiencies of vitamin B_{12} or folic acid, which are required for DNA synthesis.[53] Drugs that interfere with DNA synthesis by blocking folate metabolism (e.g., methotrexate, trimethoprim, or triamterene), interfering with vitamin B_{12} absorption (e.g., colchicine or cholestyramine), or inhibiting purine synthesis (e.g., azathioprine or 6-mercaptopurine), pyrimidine synthesis (e.g., 5-fluorouracil), or deoxyribonucleotide synthesis (e.g., cytarabine or hydroxyurea) may also cause megaloblastosis.[53,64] It may also result from drugs that decrease folate absorption, such as oral contraceptives, phenytoin, phenobarbital, and primidone.[53] Excessive alcohol intake is associated with macrocytosis caused by poor nutrition, impaired folic acid absorption and metabolism, and direct toxic effects on developing erythroblasts. Macrocytic anemia also can be associated with hypothyroidism, multiple myeloma, myelodysplastic syndromes, and enzyme defects, as in Lesch–Nyhan syndrome.[53,64] A microcytic anemia is associated with iron deficiency anemia, thalassemias, sideroblastic anemia, and sometimes anemia of chronic disease.[53]

The mean corpuscular hemoglobin (MCH) is the weight of the hemoglobin in the average red blood cell. It is calculated by MCH = Hb/Ercs.[52] The normal range is 27 to 33 pg.[3] In microcytic anemia it is decreased, and in macrocytic anemia, increased.[52] Hypochromic cells are associated with iron deficiency anemia, thalassemias, sideroblastic anemia, and sometimes anemia of chronic disease.[53]

The mean corpuscular hemoglobin concentration (MCHC) is the average concentration of hemoglobin in a given volume of packed Ercs and is described by MCHC = Hb/Hct.[52] The normal range is 330 to 370 g/L in SI units, or 33 to 37 g/dL (CF = 10).[3] In microcytic anemia it is decreased. In macrocytic anemia, it may be normal or decreased. In hypochromic anemias, both the MCH and MCHC are decreased.[52] The red cell distribution width (RDW) quantifies the extent of variation in the size of Ercs. The reference value is 11.5 to 14.5. It may be calculated by RDW = (Standard deviation of Erc size)/MCV.[6]

Erythrocyte Sedimentation Rate

(Males, 0 to 20 mm/hour; females, 0 to 30 mm/hour, Westergren technique)

The Erc sedimentation rate (ESR) is the rate of fall from the top of a column of Ercs in anticoagulated blood over a given period of time. It is directly proportional to the weight of the cell aggregates and inversely proportional tothe surface area and the plasma viscosity. Microcytes settle more slowly than macrocytes. The ESR generally increases in anemia and decreases if there are abnormal or irregularly shaped Ercs. The ESR gradually increases with age and modestly increases during pregnancy. The ESR is used mainly as an indicator of active inflammatory diseases (e.g., rheumatoid arthritis), chronic infection (e.g., tuberculosis, hepatitis, subacute bacterial endocarditis), collagen disease, or neoplastic disease (e.g., multiple myeloma) and may be used to monitor the disease course. It is particularly useful in the diagnosis and monitoring of temporal arteritis and polymyalgia rheumatica. The Westergren technique is widely used as the standard for determining ESR. Alternatives are the Wintrobe method and the zeta sedimentation ratio.[52,63]

Leukocytes

(3.2 to $9.8 \times 10^9/L$ [3200 to 9800 mm^{-3}]; CF = 0.001)

Laboratories commonly report six types of leukocytes or white blood cells found in the peripheral blood: neutrophils, bands, lymphocytes, monocytes, eosinophils, and basophils. Less mature or abnormal forms may be observed in certain disease states. The differential white count indicates the fraction of the total leukocyte count that is accounted for by each type (addition of the differentials should total 1.00). The leukocyte and differential counts can change within minutes to hours of stimulation.[54] Cigarette smokers have a higher average leukocyte count. It is about 30% higher in heavy smokers who inhale, with an increase in neutrophils, lymphocytes, and monocytes. In leukocytosis, the total leukocyte count is elevated. Exercise can lead to a leukocytosis with an increase in neutrophils caused by shifting of cells and lymphocyte drainage into blood.[52] The leukocyte count tends to be lower in blacks than in whites.[61]

The leukocyte count or the differential count may be abnormal in patients with sepsis. However, this is not always the case, and normal values do not rule out an infection. False results may occur with hemorrhage, hemolysis, trauma, diabetic ketoacidosis, and sickle cell crisis. The differential often is abnormal after surgery.[61]

Leukemias are malignant diseases characterized by abnormal leukocytes, which may be greatly increased in number (although they may also be decreased). A massive increase in leukocytes as a systemic response to various conditions (e.g., tuberculosis, severe burns, eclampsia, hemolysis, hemorrhage) is called a leukemoid reaction because the hematologic picture strongly resembles that seen in chronic leukemia. Different white blood cell lines may predominate, depending on the cause.[65]

Granulocytes

Granulocytes are leukocytes with granules in their cytoplasm. They develop from the same precursor cell as monocytes in the bone marrow (Fig. 5.5). Their synthesis is stimulated by the hormone colony-stimulating factor for granulocytes (G-CSF) and granulocytes and monocytes (GM-CSF). Unlike Ercs, granulocytes retain their nuclei. Cells remain in the maturation and storage pool in the marrow for about 8 days.[51] The cells can be released within minutes of a stimulus.[54] Granulocytes usually spend less than a day in circulating blood. Their primary site of activity is in tissues.[51] There are three main types of granulocytes: neutrophils (including bands), eosinophils, and basophils.[54]

NEUTROPHILS. (1.8 to $7.8 \times 10^9/L$ [1800 to 7800 mm^{-3}]; CF = 0.001)

In normal adults, about 56% of leukocytes are neutrophils, also called polymorphonuclear (meaning many forms of nuclei) leukocytes (PMNs), polys, segmented neutrophilic granulocytes, or segs. The lower limit of the normal range is $1.8 \times 10^9/L$ (1800 mm^{-3}) for white adults and $1.1 \times 10^9/L$ (1100 mm^{-3}) for black adults. There is some diurnal variation in neutrophils, with highest values in the afternoon and lowest in the morning. The nuclei of neutrophils have two to five lobes connected by thin filaments.[52] Their cytoplasm is packed with enzyme-containing granules that react with both acidic and basic stains.[54] Bands or stabs are the immature form of neutrophils.[51] They have thicker strands connecting their nuclear lobes or U-shaped nuclei that look like curved bands. Band neutrophils normally average 3% of leukocytes. A shift to the left means that there is an increase in the number of bands and immature neutrophils in the blood.[52] The term is derived from a time when the differential was reported on a grid that listed the immature forms on the left and the mature neutrophils on the right.[54] When tissue is damaged or foreign material enters the body, substances are released that stimulate neutrophils to move to that area. This is called chemotaxis. Chemotaxis can be abnormal in some diseases, such as Hodgkin's disease, cirrhosis, rheumatoid arthritis, and diabetes mellitus. The neutrophils then phagocytize and enzymatically destroy microorganisms and other materials at the site.[54]

The neutrophils must attach to the particles before they can engulf them. This attachment is enhanced by the presence of antibodies or complement coating the surface of the particles. It is decreased by exposure to alcohol, aspirin, prednisone, or nonsteroidal anti-inflammatory drugs.[54] This action of neutrophils is important in host defense against infection, but when enzymes are released outside the cell, it may also play a part in causing tissue damage to the host in other diseases. Neutrophils are stored in the bone marrow and in the marginal granulocyte pool along the vessel walls or in capillary beds.[51] In response to stress, they can be released from these sites into the circulating pool, resulting in neutrophilia. In an acute infection, the neutrophils leave the circulation and migrate into the tissues. Production of neutrophils also increases, in which case more immature forms are seen. If supply cannot keep up with demand, neutropenia may occur. Toxic suppression of the bone marrow may also be involved in this process.[65]

An increase in neutrophils is associated with some infections (especially bacterial), various inflammatory diseases (e.g., rheumatoid arthritis, vasculitis), tissue necrosis (e.g., MI or burns), metabolic disorders (e.g., uremia, diabetic ketoacidosis, thyroid storm), and tumors. Endogenous or exogenous adrenal corticosteroids cause lymphocytes and eosinophils to disappear from circulation within 4 to 8 hours, with circulating granulocytes increasing because they are released from the marrow storage pool.[54,65] Prolonged use of corticosteroids can lead to chronic neutrophilia by decreasing the rate at which neutrophils leave circulation.[65] Epinephrine can cause granulocytosis within minutes and probably is the mediator of neutrophilic leukocytosis associated with physiologic stimuli such as exercise, emotional stress, or exposure to extreme temperatures. Other drugs that can stimulate neutrophilia include lithium, histamine, heparin, digitalis, and many toxins, venoms, and heavy metals (e.g., lead, mercury).[54,65]

Neutropenia is a result of impaired production, increased destruction, or altered distribution of neutrophils. It occurs when the absolute neutrophil count (ANC) is below the normal range and is associated with certain bacterial (e.g., typhoid, tularemia, brucellosis), viral (e.g., measles, rubella), and protozoal (e.g., malaria) infections or an overwhelming infection of any kind. This can occur when demand exceeds supply and neutrophils leave circulation and migrate to tissues faster than they can be replaced by the bone marrow. It can be caused by drugs interfering with DNA synthesis (e.g., tacrolimus, pentamidine, lamivudine, zidovudine, phenothiazines, anticonvulsants, antibiotics, sulfonamides), idiosyncratic drug reactions (e.g., chloramphenicol, gold salts, antithyroid drugs, indomethacin, quinidine), or treatment with cytotoxic drugs or radiation.[7] There can be increased destruction of neutrophils through immunologic mechanisms in patients receiving drugs such as aminopyrine, phenylbutazone, or sulfapyridine.[65] Neutropenia is also seen with hypersplenism caused by liver or storage diseases, some collagen vascular diseases (e.g., lupus erythematosus), and folic acid or vitamin B_{12} deficiency.[6,54]

A more severe form of neutropenia is agranulocytosis, in which the granulocytes suddenly disappear. Often other blood elements are also affected.[65] Agranulocytosis can occur as a complication of drug therapy (e.g., clozapine and ticlopidine).[7,66] The ANC is calculated by multiplying the total leukocyte count by the sum of the percentage of mature neutrophils (segs) plus the percentage of immature neutrophils (bands): ANC = Total leukocytes × (% segs + % bands).[6] When the neutrophil count is below 1.0×10^9/L (1000 mm^{-3}), there is an increased risk of infection, and when it is less than 0.5×10^9/L (500 mm^{-3}), this risk is even higher.[65]

Eosinophils. (0 to 0.45×10^9/L [0 to 450 mm^{-3}]; CF = 0.001)

Eosinophils are structurally similar to neutrophils, but their cytoplasm contains larger round or oval granules that contain enzymes and have a strong affinity for acid (red) stains. Their nuclei usually contain two connected segments. Eosinophils normally average 3% of leukocytes. The count is higher in patients with allergic conditions.[52] Eosinophils are capable of phagocytosis but are not bactericidal. They modulate activities associated with immunologically mediated inflammation and can damage the larvae of some helminth parasites. Eosinophils are elevated in allergic diseases (e.g., asthma, hay fever), parasitic infections (e.g., trichinosis), infectious diseases (e.g., scarlet fever), certain skin disorders (e.g., atopic dermatitis, eczema, pemphigus), neoplastic diseases, collagen vascular diseases, adrenal cortical hypofunction, ulcerative colitis, and hypereosinophilic syndromes.[54,65] Eosinophilia may also be associated with drug use (e.g., pilocarpine, digitalis, sulfonamides). Eosinophils are low during acute stress or other conditions with elevated epinephrine secretion or elevated levels of adrenal corticosteroids and in acute inflammatory states.[65]

Basophils. (0 to 0.2×10^9/L [0 to 200 mm^{-3}]; CF = 0.001) Basophils look similar to neutrophils except that their nuclei are less segmented and their cytoplasmic granules are larger and have a strong affinity for basic (blue) stains. They average about 0.5% of total leukocytes.[52] They show diurnal variation, with levels highest during the night and lowest in the morning.[65] Tissue basophils are called mast cells. Both basophils and mast cells have IgE receptors on their cell membranes. They react with antigens and cause release of histamine, slow-reacting substance of anaphylaxis, and other substances from the basophil granules, producing immediate hypersensitivity reactions.[51] Basophils may be elevated in allergic reactions, myeloproliferative disorders, chronic hemolytic anemia, and hypothyroidism and after splenectomy. They may be low with chronic corticosteroid therapy, acute infection, or stress, or in patients with hyperthyroidism.[65]

Lymphocytes

(1.0 to 4.8×10^9/L [1000 to 4800 mm^{-3}]; CF = 0.001)

Lymphocytes are mononuclear cells without cytoplasmic granules. They average 34% of leukocytes in adults.[52] They may form plasma cells, which are not normally present in blood. Plasma cells may be found in patients with neoplasms (e.g., multiple myeloma), viral or chronic infections, allergic states, and other conditions with increased γ-globulin concentrations.[65] Lymphocytes and plasma cells are important for the immune defenses of the body. Normally, the majority of circulating lymphocytes are T cells, which are responsible for cell-mediated immunity including delayed hypersensitivity, graft rejection, graft-versus-host reactions, defense against intracellular organisms, and probably defense against neoplasms. They have a life span of months to years. They are named for the thymus gland, where they differentiate.[51]

B-lymphocytes account for 10 to 20% of circulating lymphocytes and are responsible for humoral immunity. They are named for the bursa of Fabricius, where they develop in birds. In humans, the bursal equivalent is thought to be in fetal liver and bone marrow, with further differentiation occurring in secondary lymphoid organs. These organs, important for postnatal lymphocyte production, include the spleen, lymph nodes, and intestine-associated lymphoid tissue. B-cells have a life span of days and can differentiate into antibody-producing plasma cells.[51]

There are also null or unmarked (non-T, non-B) lymphocytes that cannot be classified. Although lymphocytes can be found in circulation, they concentrate mainly in the lymph nodes, spleen, mucosa of alimentary and respiratory tracts, bone marrow, liver, skin, and chronically inflamed tissue.[54,65]

Changes in the proportion of lymphocytes in the total leukocyte count usually reflect changes in numbers of granulocytes.[54] An absolute or relative increase in lymphocytes occurs with some viral or other infections (e.g., tuberculosis, infectious mononucleosis, cytomegalovirus, pertussis, toxoplasmosis, hepatitis, mumps, chickenpox), thyrotoxicosis, Addison's disease, inflammatory bowel disease, vasculitis, and hypersensitivity reactions to drugs (e.g., phenytoin, para-aminosalicylic acid).[6,65] When the number of lymphocytes is decreased abnormally (lymphocytopenia) or function is impaired, the patient suffers from immunodeficiency. This can be an inherited disorder or may be associated with immunodeficiency syndromes (e.g., acquired immune deficiency syndrome).[65] Lymphopenia may occur with diseases such as congestive heart failure, renal failure, miliary tuberculosis, myasthenia gravis, systemic lupus erythematosus, or defects of lymphatic circulation.[6] Lymphocytopenia can also occur after irradiation or administration of antineoplastic drugs or with high concentrations of adrenocortical hormones. Lymphocyte dysfunction may be observed with chronic lymphocytic leukemia, multiple myeloma, Hodgkin's disease, sarcoidosis, leprosy, malnutrition, or terminal malignancy.[65]

Monocytes

(0 to 0.8×10^9/L [0 to 800 mm^{-3}]; CF = 0.001)

Monocytes are the largest cells in normal blood, with a diameter two to three times that of Ercs. They have a single nucleus that is partly lobulated and may appear round, oval, or horseshoe-shaped. Their cytoplasm contains fine granules. Monocytes average 4% of leukocytes.[52] After circulating briefly, they enter the tissues, transform into the larger macrophages, and remain there for several months. Macrophages are capable of motility, phagocytosis, killing microorganisms and malignant cells, and interactions with the immune system. They synthesize and secrete many biologically active molecules. They have important functions in host defense and control of hematopoiesis. They remove old or defective blood cells in the marrow and inhaled particles in the lungs.[51] Monocytes are elevated in some infectious diseases (e.g., mycotic, rickettsial, protozoal, viral infections; tuberculosis, subacute bacterial endocarditis), leukemias, lymphomas, sarcoidosis, inflammatory bowel disease, and collagen vascular diseases.[6,65] The circulating monocytes and tissue macrophages together compose the mononuclear phagocyte system or RES.[51]

Platelets

(130 to 400×10^9/L [130 to $400 \times 10^3/mm^3$]; CF = 1)

Platelets maintain the integrity of blood vessels and play a key role in hemostasis. The precursors of platelets are megakaryocytes (Fig. 5.5). Their proliferation and maturation are controlled by megakaryocyte colony-stimulating factor (Meg-CSF) and thrombopoietin. Normally, about two-thirds of platelets are in circulation and one-third in the spleen. When the spleen is enlarged, however, up to 90% may be sequestered there. In patients without a spleen, all are in circulation. Platelets circulate for about 8 to 11 days.[51]

Platelets are removed from circulation by the mononuclear phagocytic system.[51] Antibodies may also destroy platelets. They may be directed against the platelets, or the platelets may be destroyed when an immune complex attaches to them. Immune destruction of platelets may occur with exposure to drugs such as amrinone, carbamazepine, quinine, quinidine, gold salts, sulfonamides, or heparin.[7,67]

Thrombocytopenia, a low number of circulating platelets, can occur as a congenital or acquired disorder. It may result from decreased production, abnormal distribution or dilution, or increased destruction of platelets. These may be associated with factors such as neoplasms; immune processes; infections; exposure to drugs, chemicals, or toxins; or an enlarged spleen and may be combined with abnormalities of other blood elements, as in aplastic anemia. Thrombocytosis, an elevated number of circulating platelets, can be part of a reactive process or myeloproliferative disorder.[67] Half of patients with an otherwise unexplained increase in platelets are found to have a malignancy.[6]

Platelets are activated at times of vascular injury by exposure to substances such as collagen and thrombin. They adhere to exposed surfaces and aggregate in the presence of calcium. They release adenosine diphosphate (ADP), which promotes further aggregation. When platelets are activated, glycoprotein IIb/IIIa receptors on their membranes undergo conformational changes that allow binding of fibrinogen and von Willebrand factor. This leads to cross-linkage of platelets and platelet plug formation.[67,68] Aggregation is also stimulated by thromboxane A_2 from platelets and inhibited by prostacyclin (prostaglandin I_2) from vascular endothelium. Both are products of platelet arachidonic acid metabolism mediated by cyclooxygenase (Fig. 5.6).[69] Platelets also release various substances that activate or allow progression of the clotting cascade. These actions lead to the formation of thrombi. Overall platelet function may be assessed by the bleeding time. Various in vitro techniques using activator substances may also be used to assess platelet aggregation. Platelet contraction within thrombi is responsible for clot retraction.[67]

If the count is 20 to 50×10^9/L (20 to $50 \times 10^3/mm^3$), the patient is at a high risk for minor spontaneous bleeding and bleeding after surgery, and if it is less than 20×10^9/L ($20 \times 10^3/mm^3$), the patient is at risk for more serious bleeding.[6] Platelet function is impaired in various diseases such as uremia, myeloproliferative or lymphoproliferative disorders, myeloma, systemic lupus erythematosus, chronic immunologic thrombocytopenic purpura, or dis-

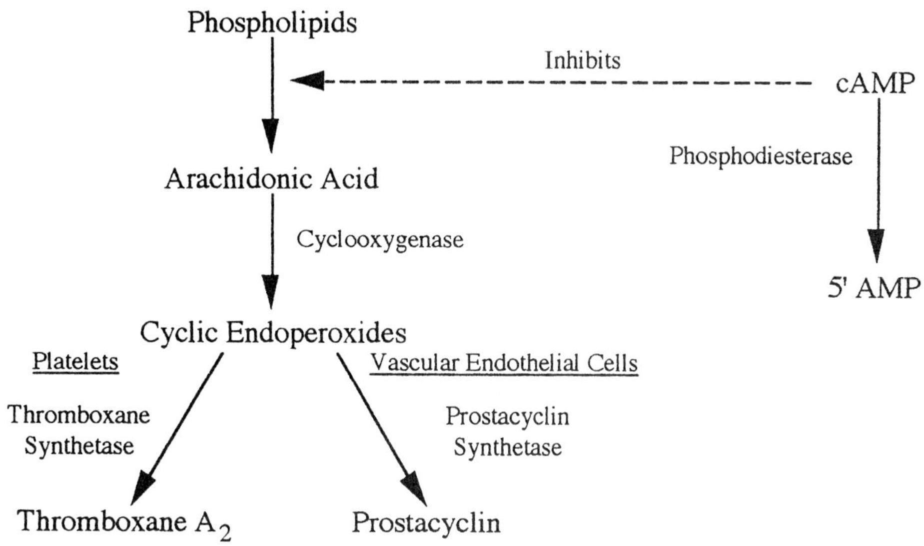

Figure 5.6. Arachidonic acid pathway. *AMP,* adenosine monophosphate; *cAMP,* cyclic adenosine monophosphate.

seminated intravascular coagulation. Numerous drugs can also interfere with platelet function. Most affect the arachidonic pathway shown in Figure 5.6. Aspirin irreversibly acetylates platelet cyclooxygenase, thus inhibiting aggregation for the life of the platelet by decreasing formation of thromboxane A_2. This effect is observed for up to 10 days after ingestion of aspirin. Most other nonsteroidal anti-inflammatory drugs also affect platelet cyclooxygenase, but it is a reversible effect observed only while the drug is present. Other drugs inhibit platelet effects by activating adenylate cyclase (e.g., prostaglandins) or inhibiting phosphodiesterase (e.g., dipyridamole), both of which result in increased cyclic AMP.[67] Ticlopidine and clopidogrel are drugs that inhibit ADP-induced platelet aggregation. Abciximab, a monoclonal antibody, is a platelet glycoprotein IIb/IIIa receptor antagonist.[68] Examples of additional drugs that may inhibit aggregation include dextran, antimicrobial agents (e.g., penicillins, cephalosporins), psychotropics (e.g., imipramine, chlorpromazine), clofibrate, and β-adrenergic blocking agents (e.g., propranolol). Synthesis of platelets is inhibited by flucytosine, zidovudine, interferons, and numerous antineoplastic agents.[7] Ethanol can inhibit both synthesis and function of platelets.[67]

Coagulation Tests

Clotting Cascade

The clotting cascade involves the progressive activation of clotting factors, resulting in a stable fibrin clot. Platelets and other substances help or accelerate this progression. A simplified diagram of the traditional clotting cascade is shown in Figure 5.7. The process is actually much more complex, with additional clotting factor interactions not shown. The clotting factors are identified by Roman numerals, although they also have other names. Each factor must be activated before it can activate other factors in the sequence. The active forms of most factors are serine proteases, except V and VIII, which act as cofactors. Factors II, VII, IX, and X require vitamin K for their synthesis. The main source of phospholipid is platelets. Ionized calcium is required for some of the steps to proceed. The intrinsic pathway is initiated by contact activation (e.g., by exposure to damaged vascular endothelium). The extrinsic pathway is stimulated by factors released from damaged tissue. The two pathways come together at factor X to form the common pathway.[70]

Different tests are used to assess the body's ability to form a clot by evaluating the function of different parts of the clotting cascade. They can also be used to monitor anticoagulant drug therapy. For most coagulation tests, the blood is centrifuged to remove platelets. Citrate is added to bind calcium and thus prevent the cascade from progressing. Patients with defective or deficient clotting factors can experience bleeding. This may be a congenital disorder such as hemophilia, in which there is a deficiency of factor VIII or IX, an acquired disorder such as the impaired factor synthesis seen in liver disease, vitamin K deficiency, or an effect of drugs.[70]

Activated Partial Thromboplastin Time

(25 to 38 seconds)

The activated partial thromboplastin time (aPTT) is used to assess the integrity of the intrinsic and common coagulation pathways. It is performed by adding a contact activating agent (e.g., kaolin, ellagic acid, or celite), phospholipid, and calcium to citrated plasma, then measuring the time required for a clot to form. It will be prolonged if there is a deficiency of factor XII, XI, IX, VIII, X, V, II, fibrinogen, prekallikrein, or high-molecular-weight kininogen, or if an inhibitor of one of those is present.[70] It is not affected by abnormal factor VII or XIII.

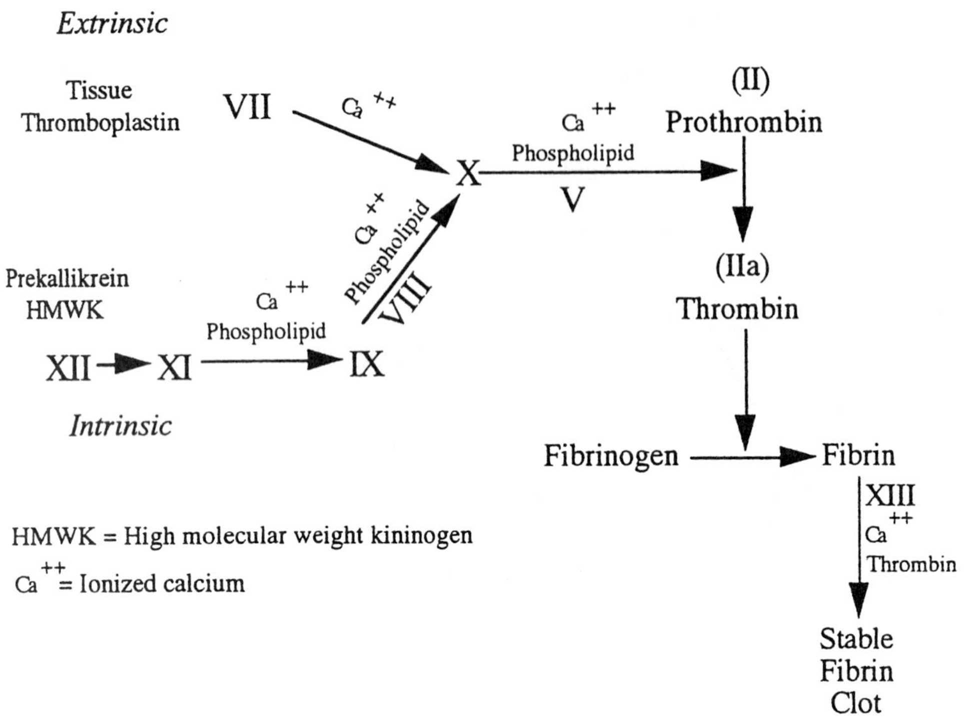

Figure 5.7. Clotting cascade.

The aPTT usually is prolonged when the concentration of the clotting factors is less than 30% of normal.[6] It is also abnormal in patients with a lupus-like anticoagulant and sometimes in those with liver failure because many clotting factors are synthesized in the liver. It may be shortened in an active coagulopathy. It is the most common test used to monitor unfractionated heparin therapy, and it can be prolonged in the presence of thrombolytic drugs or coumarin derivatives.[70]

Prothrombin Time

(11 to 16 seconds)

The prothrombin time (PT) is used to evaluate the extrinsic and common pathways. Tissue thromboplastin (e.g., brain, lung, or placenta extract or human recombinant tissue factor with phospholipid) and calcium are added to citrated plasma, and the time to clot formation is measured.[71,72] The PT is prolonged if there is a deficiency of factor VII, X, V, or II, or fibrinogen, (concentrations less than 30% of normal) or the presence of an inhibitor to one of those factors. It is not affected by abnormal factor VIII or IX.[6,70] For standardization of test results, the PT is expressed as the International Normalized Ratio (INR). This is calculated by the formula $INR = PT\ ratio^{(ISI)}$, where PT ratio is the ratio of patient's PT:mean control PT and ISI is the International Sensitivity Index, which relates an individual batch of thromboplastin to the World Health Organization international reference preparation.[71] The PT is prolonged in liver disease, in patients with a vitamin K deficiency, and in disseminated intravascular coagulation. It is used to monitor coumarin (e.g., warfarin) treatment, but may be prolonged by the presence of heparin or a thrombolytic drug.[70] An extensive discussion of drugs that affect the clotting tests is found in Chapter 44, Thromboembolic Disease.

Thrombin Time

(17 to 25 seconds)

The thrombin time (TT) is used to assess the body's ability to convert fibrinogen to fibrin. Thrombin is added to citrated plasma, and the time for clotting is measured. The thrombin time is prolonged if there is a deficiency or abnormality of fibrinogen, or if heparin or fibrin–fibrinogen degradation products are present.[70] It can also be prolonged in patients with uremia or high concentrations of monoclonal immunoglobulins (e.g., myeloma or macroglobulinemia).[6] It may also be used in monitoring thrombolytic therapy (e.g., streptokinase or urokinase).[71]

Bleeding Time

(120 to 480 seconds)

The bleeding time may be used as a screening test to assess platelet function, but it is imprecise. It is performed by making a uniform incision on the arm while a blood pressure cuff on the upper arm is inflated to maintain a constant pressure of 40 mm Hg. Blood that beads up is removed by filter paper, with care taken not to touch the wound and disturb platelet plugs. The blood is removed to prevent fibrin from forming and stopping the bleeding. The endpoint of the test is when there is no longer a spot on the filter paper after blotting. The test is prolonged when there is platelet dysfunction, when the number of platelets is less than 100 $\times 10^9$/L (100 $\times 10^3$/mm^3), or when a platelet-inhibiting drug is present. It also is prolonged in patients with uremia or von Willebrand's disease.[67] If the bleeding time is shorter than expected, many young, active platelets may be present.[54]

D-Dimer

(<200 ng/mL)

D-Dimer fragments are produced when a fibrin clot is lysed. Their presence provides evidence of a physiologic response to intravascular fibrin formation. In the presence of decreased platelets, prolonged aPTT, PT, TT, and increased fibrin degradation products, a positive D-dimer is highly predictive of disseminated intravascular coagulation in patients at risk. A D-dimer assay may be used as a screening test for venous thrombosis. The plasma D-dimer enzyme-linked immunosorbent assay (ELISA) is very sensitive for pulmonary embolism (PE), and is abnormal in more than 90% of patients with PE. A normal D-dimer value provides more than 90% assurance that a patient does not have a PE. However, the test lacks specificity and may also be elevated in patients with other diseases, such as MI, pneumonia, heart failure, cancer, sickle cell disease, or recent surgery.[73,74]

IMPROVING OUTCOMES

Several studies have been done to evaluate the effects of various strategies to alter clinician practice involving diagnostic test ordering. Oxman et al.[75] reviewed 102 trials of interventions to improve professional practice. Of these 102 trials, 12 involved attempts to alter physician behavior with regard to test ordering. The following types of interventions were included in the evaluation: educational materials, conferences, outreach visits, local opinion leaders, patient-mediated interventions, audit and feedback, reminders, marketing, multifaceted interventions, and local consensus processes. Oxman et al. concluded that there was no ideal strategy for altering physician behavior regarding test ordering. A wide range of interventions exists that, if used appropriately based on the best evidence available, could lead to dramatic improvements in the care of patients. Other chapters in this textbook discuss various strategies to improve the diagnosis and management of individual disease states. Outcome evaluations are reviewed based on these strategies. Appropriate clinical laboratory test ordering, monitoring, and interpretation are an important component of these strategies to improve patient outcomes.

CONCLUSION

This chapter has reviewed commonly encountered clinical laboratory tests including SCr, BUN, plasma glucose, uric acid, enzymes, bilirubin, serum proteins, clotting tests, and CBC with differential. Reliable measurements are an integral component of treating any patient. Laboratory test values that do not correlate with a patient's clinical picture should be repeated. Reference values should be used from the given clinical laboratory in which the test was performed. Critical or treatment values for a given test in a clinical situation should be considered, rather than just normal or abnormal values. Drugs may alter a particular laboratory test, and medication histories and administration profiles should be reviewed thoroughly for potential drug causes of these alterations. Clinical laboratory tests are a major component of diagnosing and treating patients. Understanding their regulation, critical ranges, clinical applications, and limitations is vital.

KEY POINTS

- Laboratory test values that do not correlate with a patient's clinical picture should be repeated.
- Reference values should be used from the given clinical laboratory in which the test was performed.
- Critical or treatment values for a given test in a clinical situation should be considered rather than just normal or abnormal values.
- Drugs may alter a particular laboratory test, and medication histories and administration profiles should be reviewed thoroughly for potential drug causes of these alterations.
- The more acute and extensive tissue injury is, the greater the rise in enzymes released from that tissue. Chronic smoldering damage causes moderate release of similar enzymes, with patterns usually different from those in acute injury.
- Azotemia is a rise in BUN and can be categorized as prerenal (inadequate renal perfusion), renal (decreased glomerular filtration), and postrenal (urinary tract obstruction). To yield more information about the category of renal dysfunction, the BUN is divided by the SCr (BUN:creatinine ratio); the normal ratio ranges from 40:1 to 60:1 (SI units).
- cTnI, CK, AST, and LDH are the enzymes that rise after an acute MI. cTnI and CK are the first to rise, but CK falls to normal values within 72 hours. LDH is slower to rise but can stay elevated, like cTnI, for up to 10 to 14 days.
- Causes of hyperbilirubinemia can be classified into three broad categories: prehepatic (hemolysis), hepatic (defective removal of bilirubin from the blood or defective conjugation), and posthepatic (obstruction of the extrahepatic biliary tree), also called cholestatic or obstructive.
- Common pitfalls in the use of liver function tests to assess the causes of hyperbilirubinemia include dependence on single tests rather than patterns of abnormality; normal results, implying no disease (AST is normal in 25% of patients with cirrhosis and ALT is normal in 50%); abnormal liver function tests, suggesting only

liver disease; or failure to recognize hepatocellular disease with low transaminase and high ALP levels; or failure to recognize cholestasis or obstruction with high transaminase and low ALP levels.

- Albumin has three major functions: controlling oncotic pressure in the plasma, transporting amino acids synthesized in the liver to other tissues, and transporting poorly soluble organic and inorganic ligands.
- The main function of Ercs, or red blood cells, is to carry oxygen from the lungs to the tissues and transport carbon dioxide back to the lungs. Anemia occurs when the hemoglobin or Hct is below the normal range. This can be a result of impaired Erc production, increased Erc destruction, or blood loss.
- Laboratories commonly report six types of leukocytes or white blood cells found in the peripheral blood: neutrophils, bands, lymphocytes, monocytes, eosinophils, and basophils. The differential white count indicates the fraction of the total leukocyte count that is accounted for by each type (addition of the differentials should total 1.00). A shift to the left means an increase in the number of bands and immature neutrophils in the blood.
- Neutropenia is a result of impaired production, increased destruction, or altered distribution of neutrophils. It occurs when the ANC is below normal. When the neutrophil count is below 1.0×10^9/L, there is an increased risk of infection, and when it is less than 0.5×10^9/L, this risk is even higher.
- Thrombocytopenia, a reduced number of circulating platelets, can occur as a result of decreased production, abnormal distribution or dilution, or increased destruction of platelets. If the count is 20 to 50×10^9/L, the patient is at a high risk for minor spontaneous bleeding and bleeding after surgery, and if it is less than 20×10^9/L, the patient is at risk for more serious bleeding.
- The aPTT is the most common test used to monitor unfractionated heparin therapy, and the PT, expressed as the INR, is used to monitor coumarin treatment.

REFERENCES

1. Henry JB, Kurec AS. The clinical laboratory: organization, purposes, and practice. In: Henry JB, ed. Clinical diagnosis and management by laboratory methods. 19th ed. Philadelphia: WB Saunders, 1996:3–39.
2. Pincus MR. Interpreting laboratory results: reference values and decision making. In: Henry JB, ed. Clinical diagnosis and management by laboratory methods. 19th ed. Philadelphia: WB Saunders, 1996:74–91.
3. Young DS. Implementation of SI units for clinical laboratory data. Style specifications and conversion tables. Ann Intern Med 106:114–129, 1987.
4. Woo J, Henry JB. Metabolic intermediates and inorganic ions. In: Henry JB, ed. Clinical diagnosis and management by laboratory methods. 19th ed. Philadelphia: WB Saunders, 1996:162–193.
5. Smith CL, Hampton EM. Using estimated creatinine clearance for individualizing drug therapy: a reassessment. DICP Ann Pharmacother 24:1185–1190, 1990.
6. Wallach J. Interpretation of diagnostic tests. 6th ed. Boston, MA: Little, Brown, 1996.
7. Gelman CR, Rumack BH, Hess AJ. DRUGDEX®System. 96th ed. Englewood, CO: MICROMEDEX, Inc.
8. Hammer SM, Squires KE, Hughes MD, et al. A controlled trial of two nucleoside analogues plus indinavir in persons with human immunodeficiency virus infection and CD4 cell counts of 200 per cubic millimeter or less. N Engl J Med 337:725–733, 1997.
9. Gulick RM, Mellors JW, Havlir D, et al. Treatment with indinavir, zidovudine, and lamivudine in adults with human immunodeficiency virus infection and prior antiretroviral therapy. N Engl J Med 337:734–739, 1997.
10. Threatte GA, Henry JB. Carbohydrates. In: Henry JB, ed. Clinical diagnosis and management by laboratory methods. 19th ed. Philadelphia: WB Saunders, 1996:194–207.
11. Stanaszek WF, Seifert CF. Arthritis in the elderly: presentation, treatment and monitoring aspects. J Ger Drug Ther 3:5–89, 1989.
12. Campion EW, Clynn RJ, DeLabry LO. Asymptomatic hyperuricemia. Risks and consequences in the normative aging study. Am J Med 82:421–426, 1987.
13. Steele MA, Des Prez RM. The role of pyrazinamide in tuberculosis chemotherapy. Chest 94:845–850, 1988.
14. Borg EJT, Rasker JJ. Gout in the elderly. A separate entity? Ann Rheum Dis 46:72–76, 1987.
15. Van Thiel DH, Iqbal M, Jain A, et al. Gastrointestinal and metabolic problems associated with immunosuppression with either CyA of FK 506 in liver transplantation. Transplant Proc 22 (Suppl 1):37–40, 1990.
16. Pincus MR, Zimmerman HJ, Henry JB. Clinical enzymology. In: Henry JB, ed. Clinical diagnosis and management by laboratory methods. 19th ed. Philadelphia: WB Saunders, 1996:268–295.
17. Koppel C. Clinical features, pathogenesis and management of drug-induced rhabdomyolysis. Med Toxicol Adv Drug Exp 4:108–126, 1989.
18. Zeller FP, Bauman JL. Current concepts in clinical therapeutics: acute myocardial infarction. Clin Pharm 5:553–572, 1986.
19. Young LY, Holland EG. Interpretation of clinical laboratory tests. In: Young LY, Koda-Kimble MA, eds. Applied therapeutics: the clinical use of drugs. 6th ed. Vancouver, WA: Applied Therapeutics, Inc., 1995:4-1–4-20.
20. Hong RA, Licht JD, Wei JY, et al. Elevated CK-MB with normal total creatine kinase in suspected myocardial infarction: associated clinical findings and early prognosis. Am Heart J 111:1041–1047, 1986.
21. Lee TH, Weisberg MC, Cook F, et al. Evaluation of creatine kinase and creatine kinase-MB for diagnosing myocardial infarction. Clinical impact in the emergency room. Arch Intern Med 147:115–121, 1987.
22. Yusuf S, Collins R, Lin L, et al. Significance of elevated MB isoenzyme with normal creatine kinase in acute myocardial infarction. Am J Cardiol 59:245–250, 1987.
23. Pearlman CA. Neuroleptic malignant syndrome: a review of the literature. J Clin Psychopharmacol 6:257–273, 1986.
24. Henwood JM, Heel RC. Lovastatin. A preliminary review of its pharmacodynamic properties and therapeutic use in hyperlipidaemia. Drugs 36:429–454, 1988.
25. Montgomery R, Dryer RL, Conway TW, et al. Biochemistry. A case-oriented approach. 2nd ed. St Louis: Mosby, 1977.
26. Diggs LW. Sickle cell crises. Am J Clin Pathol 44:1–19, 1965.
27. Petz LD. Drug-induced immune haemolytic anaemia. Clin Haematol 9:455–483, 1980.
28. Kaplowitz N, Aw TY, Simon FR, et al. Drug-induced hepatotoxicity. Ann Intern Med 104:826–839, 1986.
29. Keffer JH. The cardiac profile and proposed practice guideline for acute ischemic heart disease. Am J Clin Pathol 107:398–409, 1997.
30. Jaffe AS. In search of specificity: the troponins. ACC Curr J Rev 3:29-33, 1995.
31. Alexander RW, Pratt CM, Roberts R. Diagnosis and management of patients with acute myocardial infarction. In: Alexander RW, Schlant RC, Fulter V, eds. Hurst's the heart, arteries and veins. 7th ed. New York: McGraw-Hill, 1998:1345–1433.
32. Hamm CW, Goldmann BU, Heeschen C, et al. Emergency room triage of patients with acute chest pain by means of rapid testing for cardiac troponin T or troponin I. N Engl J Med 337:1648–1653, 1997.
33. Clark JA, Zimmerman HJ, Tanner LA. Labetalol hepatotoxicity. Ann Intern Med 113:210–213, 1990.
34. Davis KL, Thal LJ, Gamzu ER, et al. A double-blind, placebo-controlled multicenter study of tacrine for Alzheimer's disease. N Engl J Med 327:1253–1259, 1992.
35. Sher PP. Drug interferences with clinical laboratory tests. Drugs 24:24–63, 1982.
36. Girling DJ. The hepatic toxicity of antituberculosis regimens containing isoniazid, rifampicin, and pyrazinamide. Tubercle 59:13–32, 1978.
37. Mitchell JR, Zimmerman HJ, Ishak KG, et al. Isoniazid liver injury: clinical spectrum, pathology, and probable pathogenesis. Ann Intern Med 84:181–192, 1976.

38. Moss DW. Diagnostic aspects of alkaline phosphatase and its isoenzymes. Clin Biochem 20:225–230, 1987.
39. Chopra S, Griffin PH. Laboratory tests and diagnostic procedures in evaluation of liver disease. Am J Med 79:221–230, 1985.
40. Pincus MR, Zimmerman HJ, Henry JB. Assessment of liver function. In: Henry JB, ed. Clinical diagnosis and management by laboratory methods. 19th ed. Philadelphia: WB Saunders, 1996:253–267.
41. Kao YS, Liu FJF, Alexander DR. Laboratory diagnosis of gastrointestinal tract and exocrine pancreatic disorders. In: Henry JB, ed. Clinical diagnosis and management by laboratory methods. 19th ed. Philadelphia: WB Saunders, 1996:515–548.
42. Geokas MC, Baltaxe HA, Banks PA, et al. Acute pancreatitis. Ann Intern Med 103:86–100, 1985.
43. Berardi RR, Henderson LM. Pancreatitis. In: Dipiro JT, Talbert RL, Yee GC, et al, eds. Pharmacotherapy: a pathophysiologic approach. 3rd ed. Stamford, CT: Appleton & Lange, 1997:815–828.
44. Gordon-Smith EC. Drug-induced oxidative haemolysis. Clin Haematol 9:557–586, 1980.
45. Scott JM, Weir DG. Drug-induced megaloblastic change. Clin Haematol 9:587–619, 1980.
46. Yunis AA, Salem Z. Drug-induced mitochondrial damage and sideroblastic change. Clin Haematol 9:607–619, 1980.
47. McPherson RA. Specific proteins. In: Henry JB, ed. Clinical diagnosis and management by laboratory methods. 19th ed. Philadelphia: WB Saunders, 1996:237–252.
48. MacKichan JJ. Influence of protein binding and use of unbound (free) drug concentrations. In: Evans WE, Schentag JJ, Jusko WJ, eds. Applied pharmacokinetics principles of therapeutic drug monitoring. 3rd ed. Vancouver, WA: Applied Therapeutics, Inc., 1992:5-1–5-48.
49. Zini R, Riant P, Barre J, et al. Disease-induced variations in plasma protein levels. Implications for drug dosage regimens (Part I). Clin Pharmacokinet 19:147–159, 1990.
50. Schwabbauer M. Normal erythrocyte production, physiology, and destruction. In: Stiene-Martin EA, Lotspeich-Steininger CA, Koepke JA, eds. Clinical hematology: principles, procedures, correlations. 2nd ed. Philadelphia: Lippincott, 1998:57–72.
51. Hutchison RE, Davey FR. Hematopoiesis. In: Henry JB, ed. Clinical diagnosis and management by laboratory methods. 19th ed. Philadelphia: WB Saunders, 1996:594–616.
52. Morris MW, Davey FR. Basic examination of blood. In: Henry JB, ed. Clinical diagnosis and management by laboratory methods. 19th ed. Philadelphia: WB Saunders, 1996:549–593.
53. Elghetany MT, Davey FR. Erythrocytic disorders. In: Henry JB, ed. Clinical diagnosis and management by laboratory methods. 19th ed. Philadelphia: WB Saunders, 1996:617–663.
54. Sacher RA, McPherson RA. Widmann's clinical interpretation of laboratory tests. 10th ed. Philadelphia: FA Davis, 1991:1–6.
55. Knapp DD. Introduction to erythrocyte abnormalities. In: Stiene-Martin EA, Lotspeich-Steininger CA, Koepke JA, eds. Clinical hematology: principles, procedures, correlations. 2nd ed. Philadelphia: Lippincott, 1998: 125–138.
56. Koss W. Anemias of abnormal iron metabolism and hemochromatosis. In: Stiene-Martin EA, Lotspeich-Steininger CA, Koepke JA, eds. Clinical hematology: principles, procedures, correlations. 2nd ed. Philadelphia: Lippincott, 1998:175–191.
57. Behrens JA. Anemias of bone marrow failure and systemic disorders. In: Stiene-Martin EA, Lotspeich-Steininger CA, Koepke JA, eds. Clinical hematology: principles, procedures, correlations. 2nd ed. Philadelphia: Lippincott, 1998:139–154.
58. Anonymous. Recommendation for the immediate withdrawal of patients from treatment with Felbatol (felbamate). FDA Med Bull 24(2):5, 1994.
59. Pereira IT. Chronic myeloproliferative disorders. In: Stiene-Martin EA, Lotspeich-Steininger CA, Koepke JA, eds. Clinical hematology: principles, procedures, correlations. 2nd ed. Philadelphia: Lippincott, 1998:455–472.
60. Safko R. Anemias of abnormal globin development: hemoglobinopathies. In: Stiene-Martin EA, Lotspeich-Steininger CA, Koepke JA, eds. Clinical hematology: principles, procedures, correlations. 2nd ed. Philadelphia: Lippincott, 1998:192–216.
61. Shapiro MF, Greenfield S. The complete blood count and leukocyte differential count. An approach to their rational application. Ann Intern Med 106:65–74, 1987.
62. McGuire MJ, Spivak JL. Erythrocytosis and polycythemia. In: Spivak JL, Eichner ER, eds. The fundamentals of clinical hematology. 3rd ed. Baltimore: Johns Hopkins University Press, 1993:117–128.
63. Riedinger TM, Rodak BF. Quantitative laboratory evaluation of erythrocytes. In: Stiene-Martin EA, Lotspeich-Steininger CA, Koepke JA, eds. Clinical hematology: principles, procedures, correlations. 2nd ed. Philadelphia: Lippincott, 1998:106–124.
64. Eichner ER. Macrocytic anemia. In: Spivak JL, Eichner ER, eds. The fundamentals of clinical hematology. 3rd ed. Baltimore: Johns Hopkins University Press, 1993:27–46.
65. Davey FR, Hutchison RE. Leukocytic disorders. In: Henry JB, ed. Clinical diagnosis and management by laboratory methods. 19th ed. Philadelphia: WB Saunders, 1996:664–700.
66. Alvir JMJ, Lieberman JA, Safferman AZ, et al. Clozapine-induced agranulocytosis: incidence and risk factors in the United States. N Engl J Med 329:162–167, 1993.
67. Miller JL. Blood platelets. In: Henry JB, ed. Clinical diagnosis and management by laboratory methods. 19th ed. Philadelphia: WB Saunders, 1996:701–718.
68. Ferguson JJ, Waly HM, Wilson JM. Fundamentals of coagulation andglycoprotein IIb/IIIa receptor inhibition. Am Heart J 135:S35–S42, 1998.
69. Siegel JE, Peterson P. Laboratory monitoring of anticoagulant therapy. In: Stiene-Martin EA, Lotspeich-Steininger CA, Koepke JA, eds. Clinical hematology: principles, procedures, correlations. 2nd ed. Philadelphia: Lippincott, 1998:682–688.
70. Miller JL. Blood coagulation and fibrinolysis. In: Henry JB, ed. Clinical diagnosis and management by laboratory methods. 19th ed. Philadelphia: WB Saunders, 1996:719–747.
71. Hirsh J, Dalen JE, Deykin D, et al. Oral anticoagulants: mechanism of action, clinical effectiveness, and optimal therapeutic range. Chest 108 (suppl):231S–246S, 1995.
72. Hirsh J, Poller L. The international normalized ratio: a guide to understanding and correcting its problems. Arch Intern Med 154:282–288, 1994.
73. Ens GE. Laboratory evaluation of fibrinolysis. In: Stiene-Martin EA, Lotspeich-Steininger CA, Koepke JA, eds. Clinical hematology: principles, procedures, correlations. 2nd ed. Philadelphia: Lippincott, 1998: 650–656.
74. Goldhaber SZ. Pulmonary embolism. N Engl J Med 1576:93–104, 1998.
75. Oxman AD, Thomson MA, Davis DA, et al. No magic bullets: a systemic review of 102 trials of interventions to improve professional practice. Can Med Assoc J 153:1423–1431, 1995.

CHAPTER 6

RACIAL, ETHNIC, AND GENDER DIFFERENCES IN RESPONSE TO DRUGS

H. W. Matthews and Jannifer Johnson

For a growing number of drugs, the percentage of patients who react differently or adversely is determined by their racial and ethnic background and gender differences. The adage that "one size does not fit all" illustrates the increasingly recognized fact that racial, ethnic, and gender differences must be taken into account in prescribing drug therapy. Factors that affect drug response based on racial, ethnic, and gender differences fall into three major categories: environmental, cultural (psychosocial), and genetic. The major drugs and classes that show varying effects among racial, ethnic, and gender groups are the antipsychotics, benzodiazepines, antidepressants, cardiovascular agents and antihypertensives, atropine, analgesics, antidiabetic agents, and alcohol. Even though therapeutic response, metabolism, and side effects may differ with various medicines with racial, ethnic, and gender differences, clinical significance often is not established. This chapter focuses primarily on the effects of racial, ethnic, and gender differences on drug responses.

TREATMENT GOALS: APPROACHING RACIAL, ETHNIC, AND GENDER DIFFERENCES IN RESPONSE TO DRUGS

- Consider factors affecting drug response in different racial, ethnic, and gender groups.
- Identify drugs that show genetic polymorphism in drug metabolism.
- List the incidence of poor or slow metabolizers in different racial groups.
- Identify the incidence of slow acetylators in some racial and ethnic groups.
- Predict racial and ethnic differences in response to antihypertensive agents, psychotropic agents, and certain miscellaneous agents.
- Consider gender-related differences in pharmacokinetic properties; however, the clinical significance of these differences has not been clearly established.
- Be aware of possible gender differences in response to psychotropic agents.

FACTORS AFFECTING DRUG RESPONSE

Environmental

Environmental factors may have significant influences on drug response, metabolism, disposition, and excretion. Some of these factors are shown in Table 6.1. It is well known that ethnic variations in diet may play a major role in the absorption, and therefore plasma levels, of a drug. Studies comparing the metabolism of antipyrine between Asian Indians and Indian immigrants in England revealed that as immigrants adopted the lifestyle and dietary habits of the British, their drug metabolism became more rapid.[1] Similar findings were observed among Sudanese and Western Africans.[2,3] Cigarette smoking and heavy drinking, are known to activate liver enzymes, thus increasing drug metabolism.[4] Pregnancy, stress, diurnal rhythms, and fever may operate independently or simultaneously in the same person, thus affecting in different ways and to different degrees the processes of drug absorption, distribution, biotransformation, and excretion.

Table 6.1 ▪ Factors Affecting Drug Responses in Different Racial, Ethnic, and Gender Groups

Environmental	Cultural (psychosocial)
Chronic alcohol ingestion	Attitudes
Multiple disease states	Beliefs
Diet	Family influence
Fever	Therapy expectations
Cigarette smoking	Genetic
Pregnancy	Pharmacogenetics
Stress	Genetic polymorphism
Diurnal rhythms	

Cultural (Psychosocial)

Drug efficacy and compliance are affected by cultural or psychosocial factors such as beliefs, attitudes, therapy expectations, communication skills, and family influences. Noncompliance with medication regimens is a major problem in the treatment of chronic medical conditions. Contrasting cultural beliefs across ethnic groups can affect medication compliance and hence drug effectiveness. For example, Kinzie et al.[5] report that 61% of depressed medicated refugee patients from Southeast Asia showed no evidence of tricyclic antidepressants (TCAs) in the blood, although they were all adequately treated with TCA dosages. The majority of these patients reported not taking the prescribed TCAs and pretended to comply with medication regimens for a number of reasons. In a South African study involving a long-term regimen of oral phenothiazines among black, white, and colored patients, rates of compliance varied between 33% for black, 50% for colored, and 75% for white patients.[6]

Expectations of medications also play an important role in patient compliance. Clinicians working with refugees and other Asian populations report that these patients typically expect medicines from the Western culture to work quickly, to have a high potential for severe side effects, and to be effective only for the control of the "superficial" manifestations, not underlying conditions of the diseases.[7] The investigators concluded that Asian refugees, unless carefully counseled, often have difficulty appreciating the need for maintenance therapy in most psychiatric conditions.[7]

Pharmacogenetics

Pharmacogenetics is the study of genetically determined variations in drug response.[8] In healthy individuals, genetically controlled differences in the way individuals metabolize (i.e., oxidize and acetylate) drugs are major determinants of racial and ethnic differences in response to medicines. Genetic polymorphisms (multiple forms of enzymes governing drug metabolism) account for interindividual differences in their ability to metabolize drugs that are controlled by a single gene. The focus of this discussion is on pharmacogenetic metabolism related to the cytochrome P-450 (CYP) enzymes catalyzing the biotransformation of debrisoquine (debrisoquin hydroxylase, known as CYP2D6) and mephenytoin (mephenytoin hydroxylase, known as CYP2C19) and the acetylation polymorphisms (Table 6.2).[8,9] These are the most important clinical polymorphisms because many drugs are metabolized by their pathways.

Debrisoquine Polymorphism

Debrisoquine is an antihypertensive agent that was found to exhibit a genetic polymorphism in its oxidated metabolism.[10] Two distinct phenotypes were observed in the population with a urinary ratio of debrisoquine to its main 4-hydroxy metabolite. Those who were deficient in their ability to oxidize the substrate are called poor metabolizers (PMs), whereas extensive metabolizers (EMs) biotransform a substantial amount of the drug to its metabolite.

The importance of debrisoquine polymorphic oxidation lies in the fact that more than 30 commonly prescribed medications are metabolized by this pathway.[11] Drugs metabolized by this pathway include antidepressants, anticonvulsants, antipsychotics, opioids, antiarrhythmics, and β-blockers (Table 6.2). PMs and EMs may experience problems when being treated with these agents. PMs do not metabolize the drugs in question well and often develop elevated plasma concentrations, leading to adverse effects. However, EMs do not respond to recommended dosages because drug concentrations are too low.[8] The prevalence of the PM phenotype in all ethnic groups studied ranges between 2 and 10%, with no or very few PMs among Asians (Table 6.3).[12]

Mephenytoin Polymorphism

The polymorphism of mephenytoin hydroxylation varies according to racial and ethnic differences. Drug categories affected by mephenytoin polymorphism include antidepressants and antianxiety agents (Table 6.2). The incidence of PMs is 2 to 5% among Caucasians and 15 to 20% in

Table 6.2 ▪ Some Drugs That Show Genetic Polymorphism in Drug Metabolism

Debrisoquine Polymorphism	Acetylation Polymorphism	Mephenytoin Polymorphism
Amitriptyline	Clonazepam	Diazepam
Imipramine	Nitrazepam	Imipramine
Clomipramine	Hydralazine	Mephobarbital
Nortriptyline	Procainamide	Hexobarbital
Chlorpromazine	Isoniazid	Omeprazole
Haloperidol	Caffeine	
Labetalol	Phenelzine	
Metoprolol		
Timolol		
Propranolol		

Source: Relling MV, Evans WE. Genetic polymorphisms of drug metabolism. In: Evans WE, Schentag JJ, Josko WJ, et al., eds. Applied pharmacokinetics: principles of therapeutic drug monitoring. 3rd ed. Vancouver, WA: Applied Therapeutics, 1992; and Meyer UA. Drugs in special patient groups: clinical importance of genetics in drug effects. In: Melman KL, Morrelli HF, Hoffman BB, et al., eds. Melman and Morrelli clinical pharmacology: basic principles in therapeutics. 3rd ed. New York: McGraw-Hill, 1992:875–894.

Table 6.3 ▪ Incidence of Poor or Slow Metabolizers in Different Racial Groups

Metabolic Polymorphism	Drug Examples	Poor or Slow Metabolizers (%) Caucasian	Asian
Debrisoquine	Desipramine Amitriptyline Haloperidol Metoprolol Phenacetin	5–10	<1
Acetylation	Caffeine Hydralazine Procainamide Isoniazid	50	7–22
Mephenytoin	Diazepam Imipramine	2–5	15–20

Source: Levy RA. Ethnic and racial differences in response to medicines. Preserving individualized therapy in managed pharmaceutical programs. Reston, VA: National Pharmaceutical Council, 1993:1–42; and Nakamura K, Goto F, Ray WA, et al. Interethnic differences in genetic polymorphism of debrisoquine and mephenytoin hydroxylation between Japanese and Caucasian populations. Clin Pharmacol Ther 38:402–408, 1985.

Table 6.4 ▪ Incidence of Slow Acetylators in Some Racial and Ethnic Groups

Group	Slow Acetylators (%)
Caucasians	50
American Blacks	50
Japanese	10
Canadian Eskimo	5
Egyptians	80–90
Moroccans	80–90
Chinese	15

Source: Nakamura K, Goto F, Ray WA, et al. Interethnic differences in genetic polymorphism of debrisoquine and mephenytoin hydroxylation between Japanese and Caucasian populations. Clin Pharmacol Ther 38:402–408, 1985.

Japanese, and no PMs were found among Panamanian Cuna Amerindians (Table 6.3).[13,14] A study in an unmedicated population of older adults showed a higher incidence of slow metabolizers among African Americans (18.5%) than among Caucasians (4.1%).[15] It was not determined whether these differences resulted from genetic or environmental factors.

Acetylation Polymorphism

Polymorphic *N*-acetylation was first studied when serum concentrations of isoniazid showed substantial interindividual variability.[16] Patients were classified as slow acetylators (SA) and rapid acetylators (RA) according to their ability to metabolize isoniazid. American and European Caucasians and American Blacks have approximately equal numbers of SAs and RAs, whereas in Japanese and Canadian Eskimo subjects, the percentage of RAs is high and SAs is low (Table 6.4).[17] Commonly prescribed medications metabolized by this pathway include procainamide, hydralazine, phenelzine, and clonazepam (Table 6.2).

DRUG RESPONSE TO RACIAL AND ETHNIC DIFFERENCES

The drug categories that have been studied the most and shown to be most clinically significant in their actions with regard to racial and ethnic differences are cardiovascular (antihypertensives) and central nervous system agents (psychotropics).

Variations in Effects of Cardiovascular Drugs

Antihypertensive Agents

Essential hypertension is considered to be a multifactorial disorder. Recent studies have identified characteristics that may help predict the efficacy of monotherapy in controlling this disease. These characteristics include physiologic factors, such as sodium sensitivity, plasma renin activity, and sympathetic nervous system activity, as well as demographic environmental factors.[18] These characteristics of individual patients are important considerations in antihypertensive drug selection because of the increasing numbers and classes of antihypertensive agents and the difference in response among ethnic and racial groups.

Although all antihypertensive agents can be effective in the general population, in specific racial and ethnic racial groups some are more predictable than others and some require different dosages for an equivalent effect (Table 6.5).

Diuretics

The pathophysiology of hypertension in a large segment of the black population is characterized by enhanced sodium retention and expanded plasma volume. Diuretics are useful as monotherapy and in combination with other agents in the treatment of hypertension in black patients. Diuretics are effective in this racial group because they reduce plasma volume and intracellular sodium concentrations. The reduction in blood pressure with diuretics results from a decrease in total peripheral resistance that is related to a decreased sensitivity of the vascular wall to pressor substances and possibly to stimulation of the prostacyclin and kallikrein–kinin vasodilator systems.[19]

Monotherapy with diuretics tends to cause a greater reduction in blood pressure in black than in white hypertensives. Studies by the Veterans Administration[20] documented an average decrease in blood pressure in hypertensive black men of approximately 20/13 mm Hg, as opposed to an average decrease of 15/11 mm Hg in white men, despite a lower dosage of diuretic in the black men.

β-Blockers

The Veterans Administration Cooperative Study Group on Antihypertensive Agents[21] showed that fewer black than white subjects reached their blood pressure goals while taking β-blockers. It has also been shown that differences in plasma renin activity are believed to underlie many of the cross-racial and ethnic differences in response to β-blockers. A greater proportion of white people than black people have elevated plasma renin activity, thus requiring lower therapeutic dosages of a β-blocker. The

Table 6.5 ▪ Racial and Ethnic Differences in Response to Antihypertensive Agents

Comparison Groups	Drug Class or Agent	Clinical Response	References
African American and Caucasian	Calcium channel blockers	African Americans respond to monotherapy as well as Caucasians.	19
Asian American and Caucasian	Calcium channel blockers	Asian Americans experience more side effects.	34
African American and Caucasian	β-Blockers	African Americans respond less than Caucasians; no difference if diuretic is added.	20,30
African American and Caucasian	Propranolol	African Americans have a higher renal clearance.	27
Chinese and Caucasian	Propranolol	Chinese are twice as sensitive to the effects on blood pressure.	31
African American and Caucasian	Diuretics	African Americans respond better.	19,20
African American and Caucasian	Labetalol (combined α- and β-blocker)	African Americans respond the same as Caucasians.	28
African American and Caucasian	ACE inhibitors	Monotherapy more effective in Caucasians; no difference if diuretic is added.	32
Asian American and Caucasian	ACE inhibitors	Asian Americans experience more side effects.	34

reasons for these differences may be differences in renal physiology, which may be genetically determined. For example, the renin–angiotensin system is more often suppressed relative to sodium intake and excretion in blacks than in whites.[22] It has been shown that 36 to 62% of black hypertensive patients have suppressed plasma renin activities, as compared to 19 to 55% of white hypertensive patients.[23] Even in normotensive patients, plasma renin activity is lower in Blacks than in Whites.[24,25] Therefore, β-blockers, which are believed to work in part by lowering plasma renin, would be less effective in Blacks, who already have lowered renin levels. Even though Blacks tend to fall into the low-renin category, with a volume-dependent, salt-sensitive type of hypertension, subgroups within the black population do respond to β-blockers.

Pharmacokinetic and pharmacodynamic factors may also explain the difference in response to β-blockers. Racial differences in affinity for the lymphocyte β-receptor may explain documented differences in response. For example, a study by Johnson[26] showed that the affinity of the β-receptor for propranolol was greater in white than in black patients.[26] Another study concluded that black patients may be less responsive to the effects of β-blockers than whites because of observed higher renal clearance of propranolol.[27]

Evidence exists that Blacks may even respond differently to different β-blockers. For example, labetalol (a combined α–β-blocker), unlike propranolol, is equally effective in controlling blood pressure in black and white patients.[28] It was also shown that bisoprolol produced significant decreases in both systolic and diastolic blood pressure in black patients, and there also was a trend for atenolol to decrease blood pressure.[29] Also, Blacks respond to β-blockers in combination with diuretics as well as Whites do.[20,30] Therefore, pharmacotherapy with β-blockers must be specifically directed toward the individual patient.

Chinese also seem to exhibit altered sensitivity to β-blockers, but conversely to that of black Americans. A study involving the pharmacokinetics and pharmacodynamics of propranolol compared men of Chinese descent and white American men.[31] The Chinese men exhibited 200% higher sensitivity to the effect of propranolol on blood pressure and heart rate than Caucasians. The investigators concluded that the higher sensitivity to β-blockers may result from the β-receptor–mediated suppression of plasma renin activity, and this greater sensitivity to plasma renin activity suppression in Chinese men may partially explain their greater sensitivity to the hypotensive effects of propranolol.

Angiotensin-Converting Enzyme Inhibitors

Angiotensin-converting enzyme (ACE) inhibitors act through a renin-dependent mechanism. Therefore, the major determinant in response to ACE inhibitors in hypertensive patients is their renin activity. Patients with high plasma renin show much greater response to the antihypertensive effects of ACE inhibitors than do low-renin patients. Therefore, one would generally expect ACE inhibitors to be less effective in black than in white patients. This difference was observed with captopril and enalapril; however, when the diuretic hydrochlorothiazide was added, the racial difference in response was eliminated.[32]

Calcium Channel Blockers

The hypotensive effect of calcium channel blockers as monotherapy in black patients is comparable to that observed in white patients and significantly greater than that observed in black patients treated with β-blockers or ACE inhibitors.[19] Blacks, older adults, and low-renin hypertensive patients tend to have an enhanced calcium influx–dependent vasoconstriction.[33] This may explain, in part, the excellent antihypertensive effectiveness of monotherapy with calcium channel blockers in black patients.

Comparison of hypertension management in Asian American patients with white patients, using either calcium channel blockers or ACE inhibitors, showed that dosage reduction and the experience of side effects were all significantly more common in Asian patients than in white patients.[34] This finding points out the need for additional studies on the outcome of hypertension management in Asian American patients.

In summary, the low-renin profile, salt retention, expanded plasma volume, and increased intracellular concentrations of sodium and calcium found in many black hypertensive patients may provide the pathophysiologic basis for the significant differences observed in response to antihypertensive agents. When used as monotherapy to treat black hypertensive patients, diuretics and calcium channel blockers tend to produce a greater reduction in blood pressure than do β-blockers and ACE inhibitors.

Variation in Effects of Central Nervous System Drugs

Psychotropic Agents

Racial and ethnic differences must be considered in decisions about the use of psychotropic drugs (Table 6.6). Growing evidence seems to indicate that the pharmacodynamic and pharmacokinetic influences of these agents differ between races, and these differences can affect clinical outcome.

Antipsychotic Agents

Comparisons of antipsychotic activity among different racial groups reveal both similarities and potentially important differences (Table 6.6). Blacks, Caucasians, and Hispanics do not differ in their pharmacokinetics or dosage requirements of antipsychotic drugs; however, Asians seem to have a lower threshold than Whites for both the therapeutic and adverse effects of these agents.[35] Increased absorption, reduced hepatic hydroxylation, and pharmacodynamic factors all play a role in dosage differences.[36] Midha et al.[37] and Jann et al.[38] reported that Chinese patients showed higher haloperidol plasma concentrations than in Caucasians, Hispanics, and Blacks. Lam et al.[39] showed intrahepatic and interethnic variability among Blacks, Caucasians, Chinese, and Mexican Americans in reduced haloperidol:haloperidol ratios; compared with the other three ethnic groups, the Chinese patients had the lowest ratio.[39] Additionally, the haloperidol dosage required for the black and white groups was significantly greater than that required for the Chinese group to achieve comparable plasma levels. This observation that Asian patients require lower dosages than do other groups is strengthened by pharmacokinetic studies that report higher plasma or serum drug concentrations in Asian patients, even when weight and body surface area are controlled.[38] Additionally, other investigators have reported that lower antipsychotic dosages are required in Asian populations than in Caucasians.[40–42] Cultural, environmental, and genetic factors may all be involved in this difference in dosage requirement.[1] Therefore, it seems prudent to use lower than usual initial dosages of antipsychotic drugs in the treatment of Asian patients.

It should be noted that the use of antipsychotics in Blacks is more common than in other racial groups.[43] This may be explained, in part, by the fact that black patients generally receive more severe diagnoses, such as schizophrenia rather than an anxiety or mood disorder.[44] Perhaps for similar reasons, Blacks tend to receive substantially higher dosages of antipsychotics. This may also result from the stereotype that Blacks are more difficult to treat and less compliant.[43]

Table 6.6 ▪ Racial and Ethnic Differences in Response to Psychotropic Agents

Comparison Groups	Drug Class or Agent	Clinical Response	References
Chinese, African American, Hispanic, and Caucasian	Haloperidol	Chinese showed higher plasma concentrations.	49
Asian and Caucasian	Antipsychotics	Lower dosages are required in Asian population.	51–53
African American and Caucasian	Chlorpromazine	African Americans showed more rapid improvement.	56
African American and Caucasian	Nortriptyline	African Americans had steady-state plasma concentrations that were 50% higher.	58
African American and Caucasian	Imipramine	African Americans showed more rapid improvement.	56
Hispanic and Caucasian	Antidepressants	Hispanics appeared to experience more overall side effects.	60
Asian and Caucasian	Antidepressants	Asians achieved significantly higher plasma concentrations and had lower clearance rates.	63
Chinese, Caucasian, and Hispanic	Antidepressants	Chinese and Hispanics require lower dosages; side effects greater in Hispanics than Caucasians.	22
Asian and Caucasian	Alprazolam	Asians exhibit higher serum concentrations, lower clearance, and longer half-lives.	53
Chinese and Caucasian	Diazepam	Chinese showed smaller volumes of distribution and higher mean serum concentrations.	64
Asian and Caucasian	Diazepam	Caucasians showed higher clearance rates.	1

Raskin and Cook[45] studied the effects of chlorpromazine and imipramine in black and white inpatients. In general, black patients showed greater clinical improvement than white patients on measured psychiatric illnesses, irrespective of treatment. However, these differences were more apparent early in treatment, at 1 week as compared to 2 or 3 weeks. Significant differences were found in drug effects when comparing black men and women. Chlorpromazine was more efficacious for treating black women, and black men were therapeutically more responsive to imipramine. Methodologic concerns include an overrepresentation of patients with the diagnosis of schizophrenia among African Americans (especially men) and the fact that black patients were much younger and significantly more educationally and economically disadvantaged than their white counterparts.

Lieberman et al.[46] observed a genetically determined increased risk of agranulocytosis during clozapine therapy in about 20% of Ashkenazi Jewish patients. This adverse reaction developed only in about 1% of chronic schizophrenic patients. The investigators used human leukocyte antigen typing to identify the haplotype (a cluster of genes that are involved in immune recognition and autoimmunity) that is associated with the development of clozapine-induced agranulocytosis.

Antidepressant Agents

There is not much published information about differences in antidepressant pharmacology among African American, Caucasian, Hispanic, and Asian patients. Additional controlled pharmacokinetic and pharmacodynamic studies with these classes of drugs must be carried out before clinical applications of TCAs in different racial groups can be made.

General findings seem to indicate that for a given dosage of TCAs, African American patients show higher blood levels and faster therapeutic response than Caucasians. Also, black patients tend to manifest a greater degree of toxic effects than white patients.[43] An often cited study by Ziegler and Biggs[47] reports that steady-state plasma levels of nortriptyline in patients treated with equal oral dosages were 50% higher in black patients than in white patients.[47] It should be noted, however, that the study has been criticized for improper correction of plasma concentrations on the basis of weight.[48] Also, the investigators did not use a fixed-dose protocol or clearly outline diagnostic criteria or description of gender distribution.[43]

Although many studies indicate that Hispanic and Asian patients require lower dosages of TCAs, the results are inconsistent. Hispanic patients also appear to experience more overall side effects with antidepressants than Caucasians; however, a single-dose study comparing plasma nortriptyline levels and clearance rates in healthy Hispanic and Caucasian volunteers failed to demonstrate any major differences between the two groups.[49,50]

Survey data collected from multiple Asian countries indicate that both imipramine and amitriptyline are used in much lower dosage ranges than is typical in the United States.[51] Additionally, single-dose pharmacokinetic studies indicate that Asians achieve significantly higher plasma concentrations of TCAs and have lower clearance rates than do Caucasians.[52] However, it should be noted that some of the research did not adjust for patient weight.[52] Therefore, the role of racial and ethnic differences in response to antidepressants remains unclear because of limited, and sometimes conflicting, data.

Antianxiety Agents

A single-dose pharmacokinetic study using alprazolam showed that Asians manifested significantly higher plasma concentrations, lower clearance, and longer half-lives than did Caucasians.[53] Lin et al.[54] showed that the clearance rate of diazepam was higher in Caucasians, suggesting that diazepam is metabolized at a significantly higher rate in Caucasians than Asians. Another study showed that healthy male Chinese subjects showed smaller volumes of distribution and higher mean serum concentrations than their white counterparts.[53] Pharmacokinetic differences in the metabolism of these benzodiazepines may result from the fact that there is a higher incidence of PMs among Asians (e.g., Japanese) than among Caucasians.[1]

Based on the data observed, it is suggested that Asian psychiatric patients require smaller initial and maintenance dosages of benzodiazepines (i.e., alprazolam and diazepam) for similar clinical effects than do Caucasian patients.[54]

Bipolar Agents

There is little evidence for claims of racial and ethnic differences in response to lithium. However, one study reports that African Americans have a significantly longer plasma half-life of lithium than do Caucasians and Chinese.[55] It has also been reported that Japanese patients require lower dosages of lithium and respond to lower plasma lithium levels than their U.S. counterparts for the treatment of bipolar illness.[56] Honda and Suzuki[57] report that Caucasians in the United States have higher lithium clearances and larger volumes of distribution than do Japanese.

In summary, Asians in general need lower dosages and exhibit adverse effects at lower dosages than do Whites when given psychotropic drugs. Hispanics tend to require less antidepressant medication and report more adverse effects at lower dosages than Whites. Blacks, in general, respond better than Whites to antidepressants, have higher plasma levels, and show a greater degree of adverse effects.

Miscellaneous Agents

Analgesics

Racial and ethnic differences have been demonstrated for the metabolism of codeine. Wood and Zhou[12] showed that Chinese patients were less able to metabolize codeine than Caucasian patients. Another study comparing Swedish Caucasian and Chinese subjects revealed that the excretion of unchanged codeine was significantly higher in Chinese subjects than in Swedish Caucasians.[58] The clinical consequences of these differences in the pharmacokinetics of codeine must be considered in establishing dosing levels for the treatment of pain.

Mucklow et al.[59] observed racial and ethnic differences in the metabolism of paracetamol (acetaminophen). Asian immigrants had lower acetaminophen clearance and longer half-life than did Caucasians. It has also been observed that the mean combined recovery of paracetamol metabolites in Caucasians was twice that observed in Ghanaians and Kenyan Blacks.[30] These findings were attributed to a lower level of microsomal oxidation in Africans and Asians.

Interethnic differences were found to exist in the disposition of and response to morphine between Chinese and white subjects.[60] Chinese subjects had a significantly higher clearance of morphine than did white subjects. The higher clearance was caused by a higher glucuronidation to morphine-3-glucuronide and morphine-6-glucuronide. In contrast, Chinese subjects were less sensitive than white subjects to the respiratory and vasodepressant effects but not to the nausea-producing effects of morphine.

In an open trial of low-dose buprenorphine in treating methadone withdrawal, four Caucasian responders required 1 to 2 hours to respond, whereas the two African-American responders required only 10 to 20 minutes.[61] This finding suggests that there are racial differences in the metabolism of buprenorphine.

Alcohol

North American Indians, Chinese, and Japanese show a faster rate of alcohol metabolism (i.e., conversion to the aldehyde) and less tolerance than Caucasians.[62] Asians of Mongoloid heritage, American Indians, Japanese, and Chinese show more symptoms of intoxication after alcohol use than Caucasians and are much more sensitive to its adverse effects, including facial flushing, palpitations, and tachycardia. Facial flushing occurs in 45 to 85% of Asians and 3 to 29% of Caucasians.[63] The flushing is caused by the accumulation of acetaldehyde due to an unusual less active liver aldehyde dehydrogenase.[30,63] An atypical alcohol dehydrogenase that has higher alcohol metabolism is present in 85 to 90% of Asians and may also contribute to increased blood levels of acetaldehyde.[63]

Jewish men and women have one of the lowest percentages of severe alcohol-related problems of any group. One reason proposed is that Jewish men may have an increased sensitivity to low dosages of alcohol. This internal checkpoint might lead Jewish men to avoid high intake of alcoholic beverages.[64]

Atropine

In 1921 Paskind[65] reported that initial bradycardia, attributed to central vagal stimulation before peripheral cholinergic blockade after parenteral administration of atropine does not occur in African Americans at dosages that cause bradycardia in Caucasians. Similar results were reported in a study from South Africa.[66] However, the black patients were more susceptible to the late bradycardia effect, which occurs about 1 hour after administration. They also observed that the tachycardia effect was significantly more pronounced in African Blacks than in Whites.[66]

Zhou and Wood[67] report that healthy Chinese subjects showed a greater increase in heart rate than Caucasians after receiving intravenous atropine. There was no difference in the bradycardia effect that occurred in both groups.

Table 6.7 ▪ Gender Differences in Pharmacokinetic Properties

Parameter	Observation
Absorption	Generally, absorption is lower in women.
Volume of distribution	Volume of distribution of lipophilic drugs is higher and volume of distribution of hydrophilic drugs is lower in women.
Protein binding	No clinically significant difference.
Elimination half-life	Longer in women than in men.
Renal elimination	Renal clearance via tubular secretion but not by glomerular filtration may be lower in women.

Source: Reference 70.

DRUG RESPONSE TO GENDER DIFFERENCES

Gender is a factor that can often lead to interindividual differences in the metabolism of drugs.[68] Studies done to assess sex differences in drug metabolism are inconclusive because confounding factors such as menstrual cycle, pregnancy, lactation, menopause, and the use of oral contraceptives often were not taken into consideration.[69,70] In studies where gender differences in metabolism and pharmacokinetics exist, women generally tend to have lower absorption rates than men (Table 6.7).

In general, drugs that are metabolized by hepatic oxidation have lower metabolic clearance and longer elimination half-lives in women who are on oral contraceptives than in those who are not.[69] The clinical significance of gender-related differences in the pharmacokinetic properties of some drugs has not been clearly established. Giudicelli and Tillement[68] conclude that it is unnecessary to change dosage or frequency of administration of a drug based on gender-related differences in metabolism.

Physiologic differences between the sexes in hormone and enzyme levels and basal metabolism influence the metabolism of various drugs.[71] For example, gender differences in muscle mass, disposition of muscle tissue, and vascular resistance could cause variation in response to intramuscular injections. Gender differences in gastric motility, secretion, and metabolic rate may influence plasma levels of orally administered drugs. However, it must be pointed out that the clinical significance of these influencing factors has not been established.

Variations in Effects of Cardiovascular Drugs

Treatment of mild to moderate hypertension in young and middle-aged women produces more adverse effects from antihypertensive agents than in men.[72] In a study using a controlled-release form of verapamil, the mean plasma concentration was higher in women than in men.[73] Men and women may respond differently to anticoagulant therapy. A study showed that the use of anticoagulant agents in women resulted in no significant improvement in reinfarction mortality.[74] This same study reported that women given thrombolytic agents had a lower reduction in mortality than did men.

Variation in Effects of Central Nervous System Drugs

Psychotropic Agents

Gender differences in drug therapy probably have been studied the most with the psychotropic agents (Table 6.8). This could result in part from the observation that women have higher admission rates than men for mental disorders and a greater severity of symptoms.[75,76]

Antipsychotic Agents

There are conflicting reports of gender differences in response to antipsychotic agents. Pinals et al.[77] concluded that there were no significant gender differences in response to antipsychotic drugs; however, another study demonstrated that women had greater improvement than men in response to agents such as pimozide and chlorpromazine.[78,79] In one study, male schizophrenic patients required less medication than female patients.[80] Another study showed that male schizophrenic patients generally require less medication, at lower dosages, and have a more favorable outcome of psychotropic therapy than female patients.[81] However, findings from Yonkers et al.[79] indicate that women seem to experience greater efficacy with antipsychotic agents and a greater likelihood of adverse reactions. Xie et al.[70] suggest that women may require a lower dosage of antipsychotic agents than men.

Antidepressant Agents

Despite the prevalence of depression in women, data on gender and response to antidepressants are sparse. Also, data on gender differences in TCA therapy are conflicting.[82]

Studies of imipramine seem to indicate a preferential response in men.[83,84] Risch et al.[85] report that depressed women are less responsive to imipramine than are bipolar women, unipolar men, or bipolar men.

Davidson and Pelton[86] report that depressed women who suffered from panic attacks responded better to monoamine oxidase inhibitors than men. However, the report also indicated that depressed men with panic attacks responded better to TCAs than women.

Antianxiety Agents

Most of the literature on gender differences related to benzodiazepines focuses primarily on pharmacokinetics. In a review by Yonkers et al.[79] it seems as though benzodiazepines that undergo conjugation are eliminated more slowly in women. The clearance of oxazepam, temazepam, and chlordiazepoxide has been reported to be lower in women than men.[87,88] The clearance of alprazolam, diazepam, and demethyldiazepam, which undergo oxidative metabolism, has been shown to be higher in women than men.[89,90] The clearance of nitrazepam, bromazepam, triazolam, and lorazepam, which undergo reduction, has not been found to be influenced by gender.[91–94]

Miscellaneous Agents: Analgesics

In order to determine whether gender differences are associated with κ-opioid agonism, the analgesic efficacy of two other predominantly κ-opioid analgesics, nalbuphine and butorphanol, was compared in men and women who underwent surgery for removal of third molar teeth. Both nalbuphine and butorphanol produced significantly greater analgesia in women than in men. This observation may result from a difference in κ-opioid–activated endogenous pain-modulating circuits.[95]

A lysine salt of aspirin was absorbed more quickly in women than in men (mean absorption times of 16.4 and 21.3 minutes, respectively, although the bioavailability,

Table 6.8 ▪ Gender Differences in Response to Psychotropic Agents

Drug Class or Agent	Clinical Response	References
Chlorpromazine	Women show greater improvement in response.	78,79
Monoamine oxidase inhibitors	Depressed women with panic attacks respond better.	85
Tricyclic antidepressants	Depressed men with panic attacks respond better.	85
Imipramine	Men respond better than women.	83,84
Imipramine	Depressed women are less responsive than unipolar and bipolar men.	85
Oxazepam, temazepam	Women eliminate more slowly than men.	87,88
Alprazolam, diazepam	Renal clearance is higher in women.	89,90
Triazolam, lorazepam	Renal clearance is the same in men and women.	91,94

54%, was the same in both groups). In contrast, after intramuscular administration, aspirin was absorbed more slowly in women than men (mean absorption time of 97 and 53 minutes, respectively) but again the bioavailability, 89%, was the same in both groups.[96]

After acute cocaine administration, women reported greater "nervousness" but not a "high" and did not differ from men on cardiovascular indices. On a "nervousness" scale, the peak effects were twice as great in the women and, during the 45 minutes after cocaine use, these levels decreased only 18%, compared to a 60% decrease in men.[97]

CONCLUSION

The premise that a drug will act identically in people of different races, ethnic groups, genders, or cultures has been challenged and found to be flawed. Therefore, racial, ethnic, and gender representation in clinical trials must be broadened. For a growing number of drugs, the percentage of patients who react differently or adversely is determined by their racial and ethnic background as well as by gender. The study of racial, ethnic, and gender differences in response to medicines has been limited primarily to a few classes of drugs; however, future studies probably will yield significant data about these differences in the action of many additional drugs.

Formulary development and management represent a strategic attempt to control drug therapy costs. However, the formulary must not be so restrictive that it ignores the fact that patients in specific groups metabolize drugs differently, have different clinical responses, and experience different side effects. Therefore, racial, ethnic, and gender differences require us to balance control of drug cost with the need for individualized therapy.

KEY POINTS

- Therapeutic response, metabolism, and side effects may differ with various medicines because of racial, ethnic, and gender differences.
- Genetically controlled differences in the way individuals metabolize drugs are major determinants of racial and ethnic differences in response to medicines.
- Drug categories that have been shown to be most clinically significant in their actions with regard to racial and ethnic differences are cardiovascular and central nervous system agents.
- When used as monotherapy to treat black hypertensive patients, diuretics and calcium channel blockers tend to produce a greater reduction in blood pressure than β-blockers and ACE inhibitors.
- Asians in general need lower dosages of psychotropic drugs and exhibit adverse effects at lower dosages than do Whites.
- Hispanics tend to require less antidepressant medication and report more adverse effects at lower dosages than do Whites.
- Blacks, in general, respond better than Whites to antidepressants, have higher plasma levels, and show a greater degree of adverse effects.
- North American Indians and Chinese and Japanese patients show a faster rate of alcohol metabolism (i.e., conversion to the aldehyde) and less tolerance than do Caucasians.
- The clinical significance of gender-related differences in the pharmacokinetic properties of some drugs has not been clearly established.
- In studies where gender differences in metabolism and pharmacokinetics exist, women generally tend to have lower absorption, greater volume of distribution of lipophilic drugs, no differences in protein binding, longer half-lives, and possibly lower renal clearance than men.
- Physiologic differences between men and women in hormone and enzyme levels and basal metabolism influence the metabolism of various drugs.
- Gender differences in drug therapy have been studied the most in the psychotropic agents.
- In general, women show greater improvement in response to antipsychotic agents and a greater likelihood of adverse reactions than men. However, women seem to be less responsive to imipramine than men.

REFERENCES

1. Lin KM, Poland RE, Lesser IM. Ethnicity and psychopharmacology. Cult Med Psychiatry 10(2):151–165, 1986.
2. Branch RA, Salih SY, Homeida M. Racial differences in drug metabolizing ability: a study with antipyrine in the Sudan. Clin Pharmacol Ther 24:283–286, 1978.
3. Fraser HS, Mucklow JC, Bulpitt CJ, et al. Environmental effects on antipyrine half-life in man. Clin Pharmacol Ther 22:799–808, 1977.
4. Robinson R. Individualization of drug therapy: considering ethnic differences. Consult Pharm 5(6):328–334, 1990.
5. Kinzie JD, Leung P, Boehnlein JK, et al. Antidepressant blood levels in southeast Asians. Clinical and cultural implications. J Nerv Ment Dis 175:480–485, 1987.
6. Gillis LS, Trollip D, Jakoet A, et al. Noncompliance with psychotropic medication. S Afr Med J 72:602–606, 1987.
7. Lin KM, Shen WW. Pharmacotherapy for southeast Asian psychiatric patients. J Nerv Ment Dis 179(6):346–350, 1991.
8. Meyer UA. Drugs in special patient groups: clinical importance of genetics in drug effects. In: Melman KL, Morrelli HF, Hoffman BB, et al., eds. Melman and Morrelli clinical pharmacology: basic principles in therapeutics. 3rd ed. New York: McGraw-Hill, 1992:875–894.
9. Relling MV, Evans WE. Genetic polymorphisms of drug metabolism. In: Evans WE, Schentag JJ, Jusko WJ, et al., eds. Applied pharmacokinetics: principles of therapeutic drug monitoring. 3rd ed. Vancouver, WA: Applied Therapeutics, Inc., 1992:1–32.
10. Mahgoub A, Idle JR, Dring LG, et al. Polymorphic hydroxylation of debrisoquine in man. Lancet 2:584–586, 1977.
11. Evans WE, Relling MV, Rahman A, et al. Genetic basis for a lower prevalence of deficient CYP2D6 oxidative drug metabolism phenotypes in black Americans. J Clin Invest 91:2150–2154, 1993.
12. Wood AJ, Zhou HH. Ethnic differences in drug disposition and responsiveness. Clin Pharmacokinet 20:350–373, 1991.
13. Levy RA. Ethnic and racial differences in response to medicines. Preserving individualized therapy in managed pharmaceutical programs. Reston, VA: National Pharmaceutical Council, 1993:1–42.
14. Nakamura K, Goto F, Ray WA, et al. Interethnic differences in genetic polymorphism of debrisoquine and mephenytoin hydroxylation between Japanese and Caucasian populations. Clin Pharmacol Ther 38:402–408, 1985.
15. Pollock BG, Perel JM, Kirshner M, et al. *S*-mephenytoin 4-hydroxylation in older Americans. Eur J Clin Pharmacol 40:609–611, 1991.

16. Mitchell RS, Bell JC. Clinical implications of isoniazid blood levels in pulmonary tuberculosis. N Engl J Med 257:1066–1071, 1957.
17. Weber WW, Hein DW. *N*-acetylation pharmacogenetics. Pharmacol Rev 37:25–79, 1985.
18. Weinberger MH. Racial differences in antihypertensive therapy: evidence and implications. Cardiovasc Drugs Ther 4:379–382, 1990.
19. Hall WD. Pathophysiology of hypertension in blacks. Am J Hypertens 3(12):366S–371S, 1991.
20. Veterans Administration Cooperative Study Group on Antihypertensive Agents. Comparison of propranolol and hydrochlorothiazide for the initial treatment of hypertension: I. Results of short-term titration with emphasis on racial differences in response. JAMA 248:1996–2003, 1982.
21. Veterans Administration Cooperative Study Group on Antihypertensive Agents. Racial differences in response to low-dose captopril are abolished by the addition of hydrochlorothiazide. Br J Clin Pharmacol 14:97S–101S, 1982.
22. Gillum RF. Pathophysiology of hypertension in blacks and whites. Hypertension 1(5):468–475, 1979.
23. Wisenbaugh PE, Garst JB, Hull C, et al. Renin, aldosterone, sodium and hypertension. Am J Med 52(2):175–186, 1972.
24. Levy SB, Lilley JJ, Frigon RP, et al. Urinary kallikrein and plasma renin activity as determinants of renal blood flow. The influence of race and dietary sodium intake. J Clin Invest 60(1):129–138, 1977.
25. Luft FC, Grim CE, Higgins JT Jr, et al. Differences in response to sodium administration in normotensive white and black subjects. J Lab Clin Med 90(3):555–562, 1977.
26. Johnson JA. Racial differences in lymphocyte beta-receptor sensitivity to propranolol. Life Sci 53(4):297–304, 1993.
27. Johnson JA, Burlew BS. Racial differences in propranolol pharmacokinetics. Clin Pharmacol Ther 51:495–500, 1992.
28. Oster G, Huse DM, Delea TE, et al. Cost effectiveness of labetalol and propranolol in the treatment of hypertension among blacks. J Natl Med Assoc 79:1049–1055, 1987.
29. Neutel JM, Smith DH, Ram CV, et al. Comparison of bisoprolol with atenolol for systemic hypertension in four population groups (young, old, black and nonblack) using ambulatory blood pressure monitoring. Am J Cardiol 72:41–46, 1993.
30. Kitler ME. Clinical trials and transethnic pharmacology. Drug Saf (5):378–391, 1994.
31. Zhou H, Koshakji RP, Silberstein DJ, et al. Altered sensitivity to and clearance of propranolol in men of Chinese descent as compared with American whites. N Engl J Med 320:565–570, 1989.
32. 1988 report of the Joint National Committee on Detection, Evaluation, and Treatment of High Blood Pressure. Arch Intern Med 148:1023–1038, 1988.
33. Buhler FR. Antihypertensive treatment according to age, plasma renin and race. Drugs 35:495–503, 1988.
34. Hui KK, Pasic J. Outcome of hypertension management in Asian Americans. Arch Intern Med 157(12):1345–1348, 1997.
35. Bond WS. Ethnicity and psychotropic drugs. Clin Pharm 10:467–470, 1991.
36. Jann MW, Grimsley SR. Pharmacogenetics of agents on the central nervous system. J Pharm Pract 6(1):2–16, 1993.
37. Midha KK, Chakraborty BS, Ganes DA, et al. Intersubject variation in the pharmacokinetics of haloperidol and reduced haloperidol. J Clin Psychopharmacol 9:98–104, 1989.
38. Jann MW, Chang WH, Lam YW, et al. Comparison of haloperidol and reduced haloperidol plasma levels in four different ethnic populations. Prog Neuropsychopharmacol Biol Psychiatry 16:193–202, 1992.
39. Lam YW, Jann MW, Chang WH, et al. Intra- and interethnic variability in reduced haloperidol to haloperidol ratios. J Clin Pharmacol 35:128–136, 1995.
40. Lin KM, Finder E. Neuroleptic dosage for Asians. Am J Psychiatry 140:490–491, 1983.
41. Potkin SG, Shen Y, Pardes H, et al. Haloperidol concentrations elevated in Chinese patients. Psychiatry Res 12:167–172, 1984.
42. Lin KM, Lau JK, Smith R, et al. Comparison of alprazolam plasma levels in normal Asian and Caucasian male volunteers. Psychopharmacology 96:365–369, 1988.
43. Strickland TL, Ranganath V, Lin KM, et al. Psychopharmacologic considerations in the treatment of black American populations. Psychopharmacol Bull 27(4):441–448, 1991.
44. Bell CC, Mehta H. Misdiagnosis of black patients with manic depressive illness: second in a series. J Natl Med Assoc 73:101–107, 1981.
45. Raskin A, Cook TH. Antidepressants in black and white inpatients. Arch Gen Psychiatry 32:643–649, 1975.
46. Lieberman JA, Yunis J, Egea E, et al. HLA-B38, DR4, DQw3 and clozapine-induced agranulocytosis in Jewish patients with schizophrenia. Arch Gen Psychiatry 47:945–948, 1990.
47. Ziegler VE, Biggs JT. Tricyclic plasma levels: effects of age, race, sex, and smoking. JAMA 238(20):2167–2169, 1977.
48. Rifkin A, Klein DF, Quitkin F. Possible effect of race on tricyclic plasma levels [letter]. JAMA 239:1845–1846, 1978.
49. Mendoza R, Smith MW, Poland RE, et al. Ethnic psychopharmacology: the Hispanic and Native American perspective. Psychopharmacol Bull 27(4):449–461, 1991.
50. Gaviria M, Gil AA, Javaid JI. Nortriptyline kinetics in Hispanic and Anglo subjects. J Clin Psychopharmacol 6:227–231, 1986.
51. Yamashita I, Asano Y. Tricyclic antidepressants: therapeutic plasma level. Psychopharmacol Bull 15:40–41, 1979.
52. Rudorfer MV, Lane EA, Chang WH, et al. Desipramine pharmacokinetics in Chinese and Caucasian volunteers. Br J Clin Pharmacol 17:433–440, 1984.
53. Kumana CR, Lauder IJ, Chan M, et al. Differences in diazepam pharmacokinetics in Chinese and white Caucasians: relation to body lipid stores. Eur J Clin Pharmacol 32:211–215, 1987.
54. Lin KM, Poland RE, Smith MW, et al. Pharmacokinetic and other related factors affecting psychotropic responses in Asians. Psychopharmacol Bull 27(4):427–439, 1991.
55. Chang SS, Pandey GN, Zhang MY, et al. Racial differences in plasma and RBC lithium levels. Paper presented at the American Psychiatric Association, Los Angeles, CA. Continuing Medical Education Syllabus and Scientific Proceedings, 1984:239–240.
56. Takahashi R. Lithium treatment in affective disorders: therapeutic plasma level. Psychopharmacol Bull 15(4):32–35, 1979.
57. Honda Y, Suzuki T. Transcultural pharmacokinetic study on Li concentration in plasma and saliva. Psychopharmacol Bull 15(4):37–39, 1979.
58. Yue QY, Svensson JO, Alm C, et al. Interindividual and interethnic differences in the demethylation and glucuronidation of codeine. Br J Clin Pharmacol 28:629–637, 1989.
59. Mucklow JC, Fraser HS, Bulpitt CJ, et al. Environmental factors affecting paracetamol metabolism in London factory and office workers. Br J Clin Pharmacol 10:67–74, 1980.
60. Zhou HH, Sheller JR, Nu H, et al. Ethnic differences in response to morphine. Clin Pharmacol Ther 54(5):507–513, 1993.
61. Banys P, Clark HW, Tusel DJ, et al. An open trial of low dose buprenorphine in treating methadone withdrawal. J Subst Abuse Treat 11(1):9–15, 1994.
62. Kalow W. Ethnic differences in drug metabolism. Clin Pharmacokinet 7:373–400, 1982.
63. Chan AW. Racial differences in alcohol sensitivity. Alcohol 21(1):93–104, 1986.
64. Monteiro MG, Klein JL, Schuckit MA. High levels of sensitivity to alcohol in young adult Jewish men: a pilot study. J Stud Alcohol 52:464–469, 1991.
65. Paskind HA. Some differences in response to atropine in white and colored races. J Lab Clin Med 7:104–108, 1921.
66. Meyer EC, Sommers DK, Schoeman HS. The effect of atropine on heart-rate: a comparison between two ethnic groups. Br J Clin Pharmacol 25:776–777, 1988.
67. Zhou HH, Wood AJ. Atropine produces a greater increase in heart rate in Chinese than Caucasians [Abstract]. Clin Res 38:7A, 1990.
68. Giudicelli JF, Tillement JP. Influences of sex on drug kinetics in man. Clin Pharmacokinet 2:157–166, 1977.
69. Bonate PL. Gender-related differences in xenobiotic metabolism. J Clin Pharmacol 31:684–690, 1991.
70. Xie CX, Piecoro LT, Wermeling DP. Gender-related considerations in clinical pharmacology and drug therapeutics. Crit Care Nurs Clin North Am 9(4):459–468, 1997.
71. Proksch RA, Lamy PP. Sex variation and drug therapy. Drug Intell Clin Pharm 11:398–406, 1977.
72. Shapiro AP, Rytan GH. Hypertension in women: differences and implications. In: Eaka E, Packard B, Wenger N, et al., eds. Coronary heart disease in women: reviewing the evidence, identifying the needs. New York: Haymarket Doyma, 1987:172.
73. Gupta S, Atkinson L, Tu T, et al. Age and gender-related changes in stereoselective pharmacokinetics and pharmacodynamics of verapamil and norverapamil. Br J Clin Pharmacol 40:325–331, 1995.
74. Rice-Wray E. An assessment of long-term anticoagulant administration after cardiac infarction. Second report of the working party on anticoagulant therapy in coronary thrombosis to the medical research council. BMJ 2:837–843, 1964.
75. Kramer M. Cross-national study of diagnosis of the mental disorders: origins of the problem. Am J Psychiatry 125(suppl 10):1–11, 1969.
76. Weich MJ. Behavioral differences between groups of acutely psychotic (schizophrenic) males and females. Psychiatr Q 42(1):107–122, 1968.

77. Pinals DA, Malhotra AK, Missar CD, et al. Lack of gender differences in neuroleptic response in patients with schizophrenia. Schizophr Res 22:215–222, 1996.
78. Chouinard G, Annable L. Pimozide in the treatment of newly admitted schizophrenic patients. Psychopharmacology 76:13–19, 1982.
79. Yonkers KA, Kando JC, Cole JO, et al. Gender differences in pharmacokinetics and pharmacodynamics of psychotropic medication. Am J Psychiatry 149(5): 587–595, 1992.
80. Taylor MA, Levine R. Influence of sex of hospitalized schizophrenics on therapeutic dosage levels of neuroleptics. Dis Nerv Syst 32(2):131–134, 1971.
81. Demer HC, Bird EG. Chlorpromazine in the treatment of mental illness. IV Final results with analysis of data on 1,523 patients. Am J Psychiatry 113:972–978, 1957.
82. Dawkins K. Gender differences in psychiatry: epidemiology and drug response. CNS Drugs 3(5):393–407, 1995.
83. Perel JM, Irani F, Hurwic M, et al. Tricyclic antidepressants: relationships among pharmacokinetics, metabolism, and clinical outcomes. In: Garattini S, ed. Depressive disorders. Stuttgart: FK Schattauer, 1978:325–336.
84. Prange A. Discussion. (Published discussion following a paper by Feighner et al.) Am J Psychiatry 128:1230–1238, 1972.
85. Risch SC, Huey LY, Janowsky DS. Plasma levels of tricyclic antidepressants and clinical efficacy: review of the literature. Part II. J Clin Psychiatry 40:58–69, 1979.
86. Davidson J, Pelton S. Forms of atypical depression and their response to antidepressant drugs. Psychiatry Res 17:87–95, 1986.
87. Divoll M, Greenblatt DJ, Harmatz JS, et al. Effect of age and gender on disposition of temazepam. J Pharm Sci 10:1104–1107, 1981.
88. Greenblatt DJ, Divoll MK, Abernethy DR, et al. Age and gender effects on chlordiazepoxide kinetics: relation to antipyrine disposition. Pharmacology 38:327–334, 1989.
89. Allen MD, Greenblatt DJ, Harmatz JS, et al. Desmethyldiazepam kinetics in the elderly after oral prazepam. Clin Pharmacol Ther 28:196–202, 1980.
90. Kristjansson F, Thorsteinsson SB. Disposition of alprazolam in human volunteers: differences between genders. Acta Pharm Nord 3:249–250, 1991.
91. Divoll M, Greenblatt DJ. Effect of age and sex on lorazepam protein binding. J Pharm Pharmacol 34:122–123, 1982.
92. Jochemsen R, van der Graaff M, Boeijinga JK, et al. Influence of sex, menstrual cycle and oral contraceptives on the disposition of nitrazepam. Br J Clin Pharmacol 13:319–324, 1982.
93. Ochs HR, Greenblatt DJ, Friedman H, et al. Bromazepam pharmacokinetics: influence of age, gender, oral contraceptives, cimetidine and propranolol. Clin Pharmacol Ther 41:562–570, 1987.
94. Smith RB, Divoll M, Gillespie WR, et al. Effect of subject age and gender on the pharmacokinetics of oral triazolam and temazepam. J Clin Psychopharmacol 3:172–176, 1983.
95. Gear RW, Miaskowski C, Gordon NC, et al. Kappa-opioids produce significantly greater analgesia in women than in men. Nat Med 2(11):1248–1250, 1996.
96. Aarons L, Hopkins K, Rowland M, et al. Route of administration and sex differences in the pharmacokinetics of aspirin, administered as its lysine salt. Pharm Res 6:660–666, 1989.
97. Kosten TR, Kosten TA, McDougle C, et al. Gender differences in response to intranasal cocaine administration to humans. Biol Psychiatry 39:147–148, 1996.

CHAPTER 7

BIOTECHNOLOGY

Kimberly Bergstrom and Monique Mayo

Since October 1982, when the first recombinant human insulin was approved by the U.S. Food and Drug Administration (FDA), an additional 50 medicines and vaccines have been developed and approved by companies involved in biotechnology. The race to complete the mapping of our genetic makeup has yielded exciting breakthroughs in our understanding of important disease processes, which we are beginning to address at the genetic and chromosomal levels. This chapter focuses on the impact of biotechnology on our understanding of the immune system and the products that have resulted from that understanding. Additionally, it touches on products that have recently been developed to fight malignancies, genetic and cardiovascular diseases, and infectious diseases.

Although major advances in our understanding of the immune system have occurred in the last decade, much remains to be learned. Undoubtedly the acquired immune deficiency syndrome (AIDS) epidemic has been responsible for the increased focus on the immune system. This attention has yielded virtually daily breakthroughs that are exposing new pieces of a very complex and important puzzle. It is clear that many diseases, including cancer, infections, and genetic diseases, are influenced by the immune system.

The primary function of the immune system is to defend the host from foreign substances. The immune system must first recognize the foreign substance as nonself and then destroy or neutralize it.[1] The immune system has two functional divisions of defense against foreign substances: specific and nonspecific.

NONSPECIFIC IMMUNE RESPONSE

The nonspecific (innate) immune response is stimulated the first time a foreign substance (antigen) enters the host.[1] Components of the nonspecific response perform functions that provide both physical and biochemical defenses.[2] The skin, the mucous membranes, and the cilia of the respiratory tract provide physical defenses. The biochemical defenses include the process of inflammation, release of lysozyme, and the initiation of the complement cascade.[2] Inflammation is a complex series of events that occur when tissue is injured. Vasoactive substances such as histamine are released, stimulating neutrophil and macrophage migration to the area of tissue injury to ingest (phagocytose) the antigen that is responsible.[2]

Complement is set in motion by the recognition of either an antigen–antibody complex or bacteria or viruses. The cascading effect of activated complement stimulates biologic activities, including chemotaxis of monocytes, neutrophils, basophils, and eosinophils; the release of hydrolytic enzymes; and ultimately the destruction or inactivation of the invading antigen.[2] Lysozyme (a bactericidal substance) is also released from nasal mucosa, saliva, and tears in high concentrations in response to bacterial invasion.

Nonspecific cellular components of the innate system include granulocytes (neutrophils, 60 to 70% of white blood cell counts [WBCs]; basophils, less than 1% of WBCs; eosinophils, 1 to 3% of WBCs) and mononuclear phagocytes (monocytes and macrophages). Eosinophils ingest immune complexes (antigen–antibody complexes) and clear parasitic organisms.[2] Basophils help to mediate immune responses by releasing substances such as histamine in response to antigen–antibody complexes. Macrophages and neutrophils are primarily responsible for the ingestion of particles, a process called phagocytosis.

Phagocytosis is an important component of the nonspecific immune response. Macrophages (phagocytes) envelop the antigen and expose it to internal enzymes that degrade and inactivate it. The antigen is completely digested by degradative enzymes or it appears on the surface of the macrophage, where T lymphocytes (from the specific immune system) can recognize the antigen and react to it.[3]

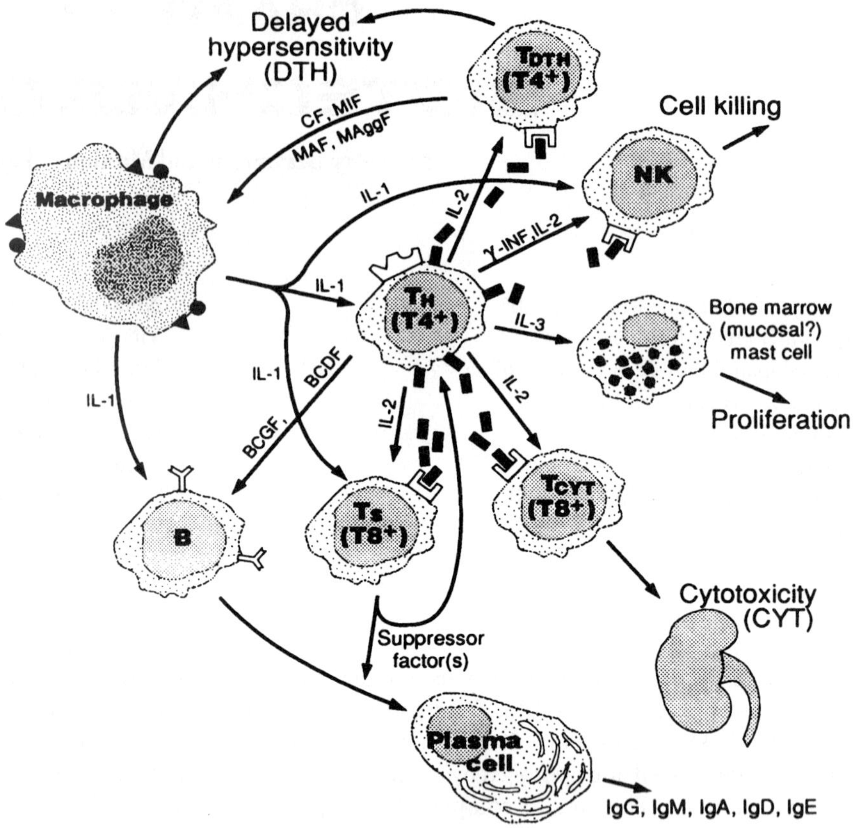

Figure 7.1. Cellular events of cell-mediated immunity and response. *B,* basophil; T_H, T helper cells; T_S, T suppressor cells; T_{CYT}, cytotoxic T cells; T_{DTH}, T cells-delayed type hypersensitivity. (From Bellanti JA, Rocklin RE. Cell-mediated immune reactions. In: Immunology III. Philadelphia: WB Saunders, 1985:181, with permission.)

SPECIFIC IMMUNE RESPONSE

The specific immune system recognizes and eliminates antigens with specialized and sophisticated cells, primarily macrophages and T and B lymphocytes. T lymphocytes are primarily responsible for cell-mediated immunity, delayed hypersensitivity, transplant rejection, and tumor surveillance (Fig. 7.1). B lymphocytes are responsible for humoral, or antibody-mediated, immunity.

There are four types of T lymphocytes: helper T cells, suppressor T cells, cytotoxic T cells, and memory T cells. Helper T cells regulate the cell-mediated response to antigens. When macrophages of the nonspecific immune system present antigen to the helper T cells, a series of events is set into motion: The helper T cells release interleukin-2 (IL-2) and interferon-γ (IFN-γ), which in turn stimulate other helper T cells and NK T cells, respectively. IL-2 also stimulates cytotoxic T cells, which attack the antigen-presenting cells, causing cellular lysis and death by boring holes through the cell membrane and releasing lysing enzymes.[2]

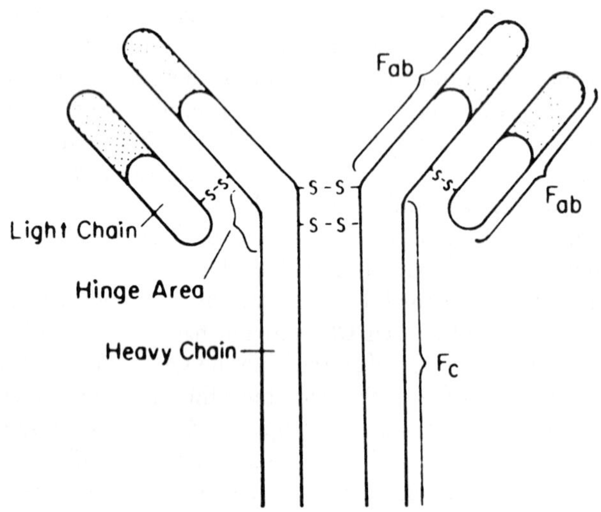

Figure 7.2. Basic structure of an antibody. *Fc,* crystallizable fragment; *Fab,* fragment of antigen binding; *S-S,* disulfide bond. (From Campion J. A basic review of the immune system. US Pharmacist 15[8]:19–26, 1990, with permission.)

Suppressor T cells have the opposite effect on cells. They act on cytotoxic cells and plasma cells to inhibit their proliferation and the production of antibodies. Suppressor T cells play a critical role in the development of tolerance, which is particularly important in cases of autoimmune disease or some types of drug therapy.

Memory T cells are integrally involved in delayed hypersensitivity reactions. They secrete macrophage chemotactic factor, which stimulates chemotaxis of monocytes and macrophages to the antigen contact site, and macrophage inhibitory factor, which helps to keep macrophages in the area. The delayed hypersensitivity reaction occurs 24 to 48 hours after initial contact because of the time required to accumulate these cells.

B lymphocytes are responsible for antibody-mediated or humoral immunity. Each mature B lymphocyte carries on its surface an antibody that is specific for one particular antigen.[1] If a mature B lymphocyte comes in contact with its specific antigen, it is stimulated to differentiate into an

Table 7.1 ▪ Characteristics of the Five Classes of Human Immunoglobulins

	Immunoglobulin Class				
Variable	**IgG**	**IgM**	**IgA**	**IgE**	**IgD**
Heavy chain	γ	μ	α	ϵ	δ
Subclasses	γ 1, 2, 3, 4	μ 1, 2	α 1, 2	None	None
Extra chains	None	Joining	Joining and secretory	None	None
Serum concentration (mg/100 mL)	1000	100	250	0.01	3
Plasma half-life (days)	21	5	6	2	3
Molecular weight	150,000	900,000 (polymer)	350,000 (polymer)	190,000	180,000
Major function	Primary or secondary response	Primary response	Secretory response	Allergic response	Membrane receptor (?)

Reprinted with permission from Tami JA, Parr M, Thompson JS. The immune system. Am S Hosp Pharm 43:2495, 1986.

antibody-producing cell called a plasma cell. Plasma cells that encounter helper T cells may differentiate further into memory cells, which have a long life span. Upon future encounters with that specific antigen, memory cells can more quickly mount a heightened immune response.[1] Antibody production is the primary responsibility of the B lymphocyte.

Antibodies are made up of four polypeptide chains (two light chains and two heavy chains). The basic structure of an antibody is Y-shaped (Fig. 7.2). The top portion binds to a specific antigen and is known as the fragment of antigen binding (Fab) portion. The base of the antibody, called the crystallizable fragment (Fc), is the portion that determines the biologic function of the antibody, such as complement activation and opsonization.[2] Opsonization is the ability of antibodies to increase their adherence to foreign antigens to facilitate phagocytosis. Antibodies generally are divided into five distinct immunoglobulin (Ig) classes: IgG, IgM, IgA, IgE, and IgD. Each class of antibody has its own specific function and response to antigen (Table 7.1).

A third type of lymphoid cells that are important to the specific immune system are killer cells and natural killer (NK) cells. Killer cells recognize and destroy antigen bound to antibodies (antibody-dependent cell-mediated cytotoxicity). NK cells also have the ability to recognize and destroy tumors and other foreign antigens. This cytotoxicity is independent of antibody–antigen binding.

Antibody-dependent cell-mediated cytotoxicity requires the orchestration of many substances, including lymphokines, monokines, colony-stimulating factors (CSFs), and interleukins to communicate between cells and to elicit the checks and balances of the immune system. In the absence of a normally functioning immune system, the host is susceptible to infection, tumors, and eventually death.

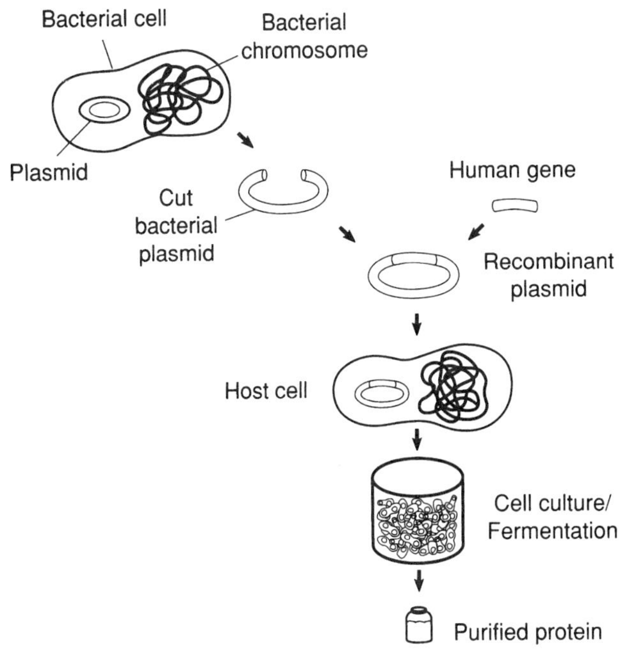

Figure 7.3. Summary of the steps typically involved in the formation of a recombinant DNA molecule. (From An introduction to pharmaceutical biotechnology. Regents of the University of Wisconsin System, 1990, with permission.)

RECOMBINANT DNA TECHNOLOGY

Many cellular mediators of the immune system can now be produced in clinically useful quantities by recombinant DNA technology. With this technology, the natural genetic processes that take place in mammalian, bacterial, and yeast cells can be manipulated to produce human proteins, such as erythropoietin (EPO), in large enough quantities to be useful in the treatment of human disease.

Recombinant DNA technology entails isolating the gene (i.e., a specific segment of DNA) that contains the genetic code for a desired protein and inserting it into a cell that can reproduce that protein rapidly. The result is large quantities of the desired protein.

Yeast cells, *Escherichia coli* bacteria, and mammalian cells (Chinese hamster ovary cells, human myeloma cells) are used most commonly to reproduce human proteins. These cell types are used because they can be genetically manipulated easily and quickly, they multiply and divide rapidly, and they provide large quantities of protein.[4]

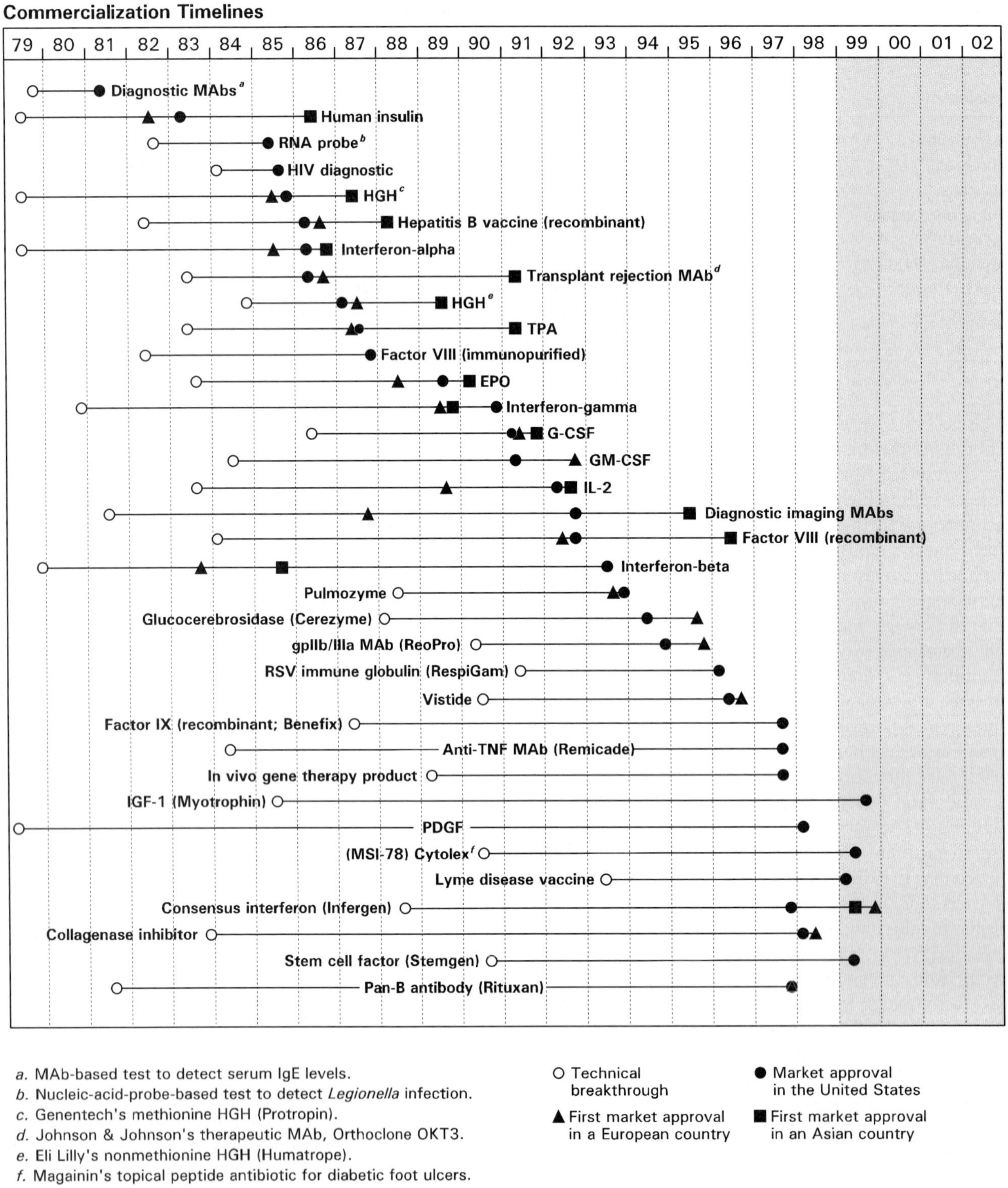

Figure 7.4. Commercialization timelines for biomedical products. (From Vivian Lee and Associates and Decision Resources, Inc. 1998 Update: commercialization timelines for biomedical products. SPECTRUM pharmaceutical industry dynamics portfolio, December 1998, with permission.)

E. coli cells are genetically simple and well-understood cell types, which makes them ideal host cells for recombinant DNA molecules. However, they cannot perform some of the more complicated processes of fine-tuning proteins, such as glycosylation, that the more advanced mammalian cells can perform. If glycosylation is not necessary, as with interferons, *E. coli* is a less expensive and simpler choice for a host cell.[4]

Commercialization Timelines (continued)

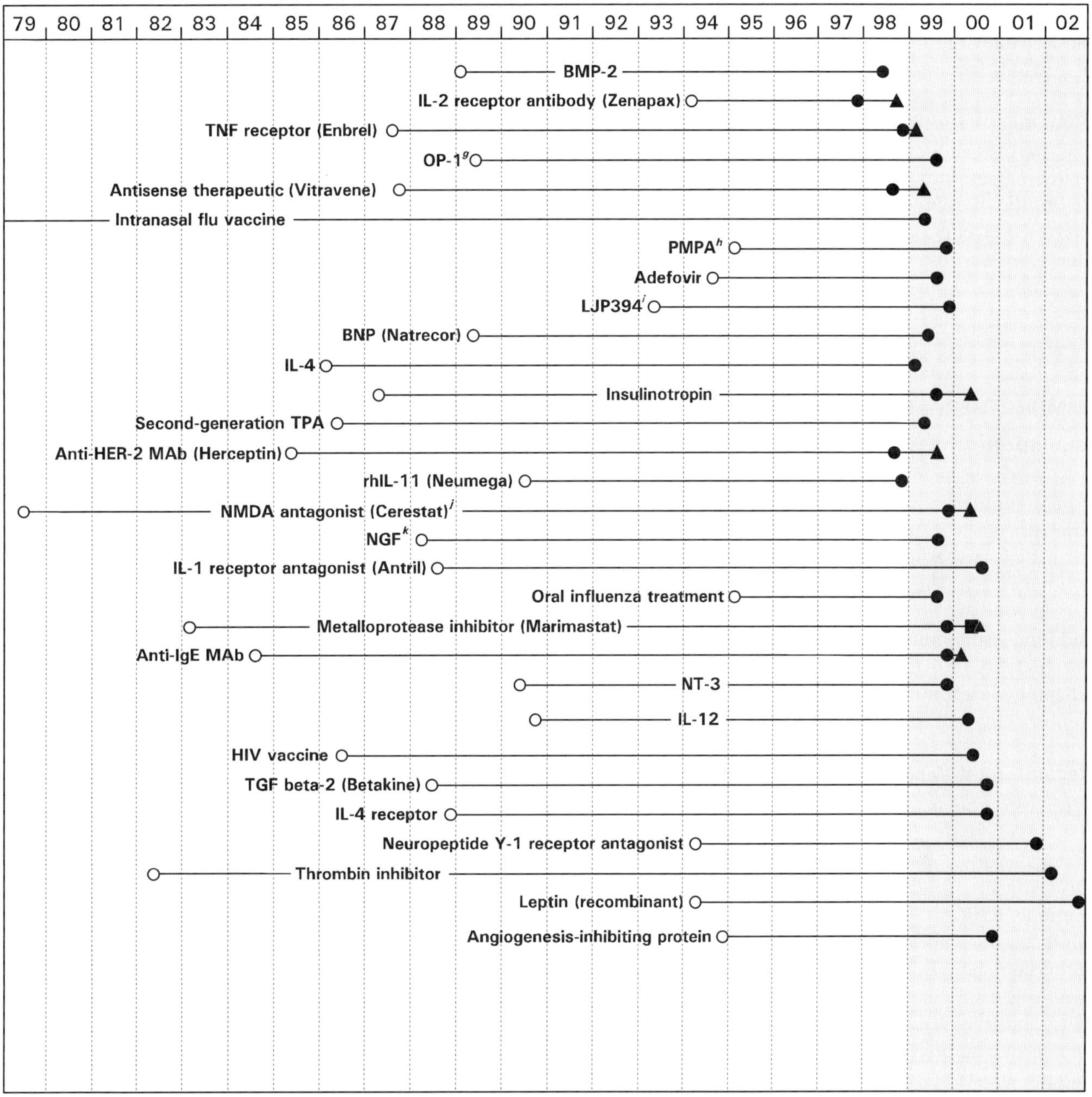

g. Creative Biomolecules' osteogenic protein for treatment of osteoporosis.
h. Gilead Sciences' reverse transcriptase inhibitor.
i. La Jolla Pharmaceutical's anti-dSDNA antibody drug for lupus.
j. Cambridge NeuroScience's NMDA receptor antagonist for stroke.
k. Genentech's nerve growth factor.

Figure 7.4 *(continued)*

To produce a specific protein, the corresponding gene from the DNA strand must be isolated. A gene can be isolated easily if the amino acid sequence of the desired protein is known. If not, a DNA probe may be used to isolate the specific gene. The desired gene is then cut precisely from the DNA molecule by restriction enzymes.

The isolated gene is then inserted into the host cell, with a plasmid, to produce the desired protein (Fig. 7.3). A plasmid is a circular strand of DNA that can replicate freely inside a host cell. Plasmids are found in *E. coli*, where they are isolated and cut open.[4] The human gene is then spliced to the plasmid by DNA ligase to form the recombinant DNA molecule. The DNA molecule is inserted into the host cell through a process called transformation (the uptake of foreign DNA into a cell).[4] As host cell division and replication take place, the plasmid-containing human gene is also replicated. The host cell replicates into millions of genetically identical cells capable of producing the desired protein. The protein is secreted, harvested, purified, and formulated into the final commercial product.[4]

Among the commercially available pharmaceuticals that have been developed through recombinant DNA technology are human insulin, human growth hormone, IFN-α, IFN-β, IFN-γ, tissue plasminogen activator, hepatitis B (HB) vaccine, and hematopoietic growth factors (granulocyte colony-stimulating factor [G-CSF], granulocyte–macrophage colony-stimulating factor [GM-CSF], EPO). Many more, including a number of new monoclonal antibodies, are described in Figure 7.4.

IMMUNOTHERAPEUTICS

Immunization

When an antigen enters an organism, the specific immune system stimulates antibody production against that specific antigen. It retains memory of that antigen exposure, so that upon reexposure to the antigen, it can mount a rapid and complete immune response. Active immunization uses this basic principle to help develop a complete and long-lasting immunity to certain diseases by exposing the body to a harmless portion of the antigen. (See Chapter 65, Immunizations) for a more complete discussion of active and passive immunization.

Recombinant Vaccines

With recombinant DNA technology, a vaccine that is devoid of both pathogenic potential and extraneous material can be produced. The discovery that plasmid DNA can be directly transfected into animals to elicit an immune response has opened up a new and exciting approach for producing vaccines.[5] Recombinant DNA technology has also made it possible to develop vaccines from organisms that are difficult to grow, such as cancer cells and the AIDS virus. Currently, two genetically engineered vaccines are licensed for human use: the HB vaccine and the Lyme disease vaccine.[5] The HB vaccine was developed by incorporating the gene that encodes the HB surface antigen polypeptide into a plasmid and cloning it in yeast, *E. coli,* and mammalian cells. The ability of the recombinant HB vaccine to confer immunity is similar to that of the plasma-derived vaccine.

The Lyme disease vaccine (LYMErix) was approved by the FDA in December 1998 and is the second recombinant vaccine to become licensed for human use. Lyme disease is caused by infection with the bacteria *Borrelia burgdorferi,* which is carried by ticks that transmit the infection from animals to humans. The Lyme disease bacteria can affect the joints, tendons, heart, or nervous system, resulting in arthritis, heart abnormalities, and paralysis of one or both sides of the face. This genetically engineered vaccine contains an outer surface protein of *B. burgdorferi* called OspA. The vaccine works by stimulating antibodies that specifically target this outer surface protein. When the tick begins sucking a vaccinated person's blood, it ingests these antibodies, which then neutralize the bacteria inside the tick, thereby preventing transmission of the bacteria to the host.

Recombinant vaccines are substantially more costly to produce than conventional vaccines, and they must be purified to a much higher standard than previously required of older, conventional vaccines. Because of the expense of manufacturing genetically engineered vaccines for human use, it is unlikely that recombinant vaccines will be developed to replace existing licensed human vaccines that have proven safety and efficacy.[5] In addition, several safety issues surround the use of recombinant vaccines in humans. These include the ability of the plasmid to integrate itself into the genome of a cell, the ability of the plasmid to induce immunologic tolerance, and the risk of the plasmid to induce an autoimmune response to the host cell's DNA.[5] In anticipation of further clinical trials in humans using recombinant vaccines, the FDA has issued a set of guidelines that should be considered when plasmid DNA is prepared for vaccine studies in humans.[6]

Biologic Response Modifiers

Cytokines are responsible for the growth and differentiation of the cells of the immune system (Fig. 7.5). Cytokines that are products of monocytes and macrophages are called monokines; those derived from lymphocytes are called lymphokines. Cytokines have a broad range of overlapping immunologic, inflammatory, and physiologic properties. The cytokines that have been produced through recombinant DNA technology are broadly called biologic-response modifiers. They include interleukins, CSFs, and interferons. These immunomodulators may be specific (e.g., target identifiable tumor antigens) or nonspecific (alter the response and function of the immune system against a stimulus without reference to a specific antigen).

Interleukins

The interleukins have been called the hormones of the immune system. They are the molecular mediators of immune system cells and induce replication and differentiation of those cells and activate the expression of certain functions. At least 14 different interleukins have been identified, each with its own cell targets and functions. Some interleukins have been cloned through recombinant DNA technology and are undergoing clinical trials to determine their clinical usefulness. Currently two interleukins, IL-2 and IL-11, have been approved by the FDA for clinical use. IL-2 is approved for use in the treatment of metastatic renal cell carcinoma and metastatic malignant melanoma. IL-11 is approved for the prevention of chemotherapy-induced thrombocytopenia in patients with nonmyeloid malignancies.

IL-1

IL-1 is a potent hematopoietic agent that also has effects on other organ systems. It is actually two distinct

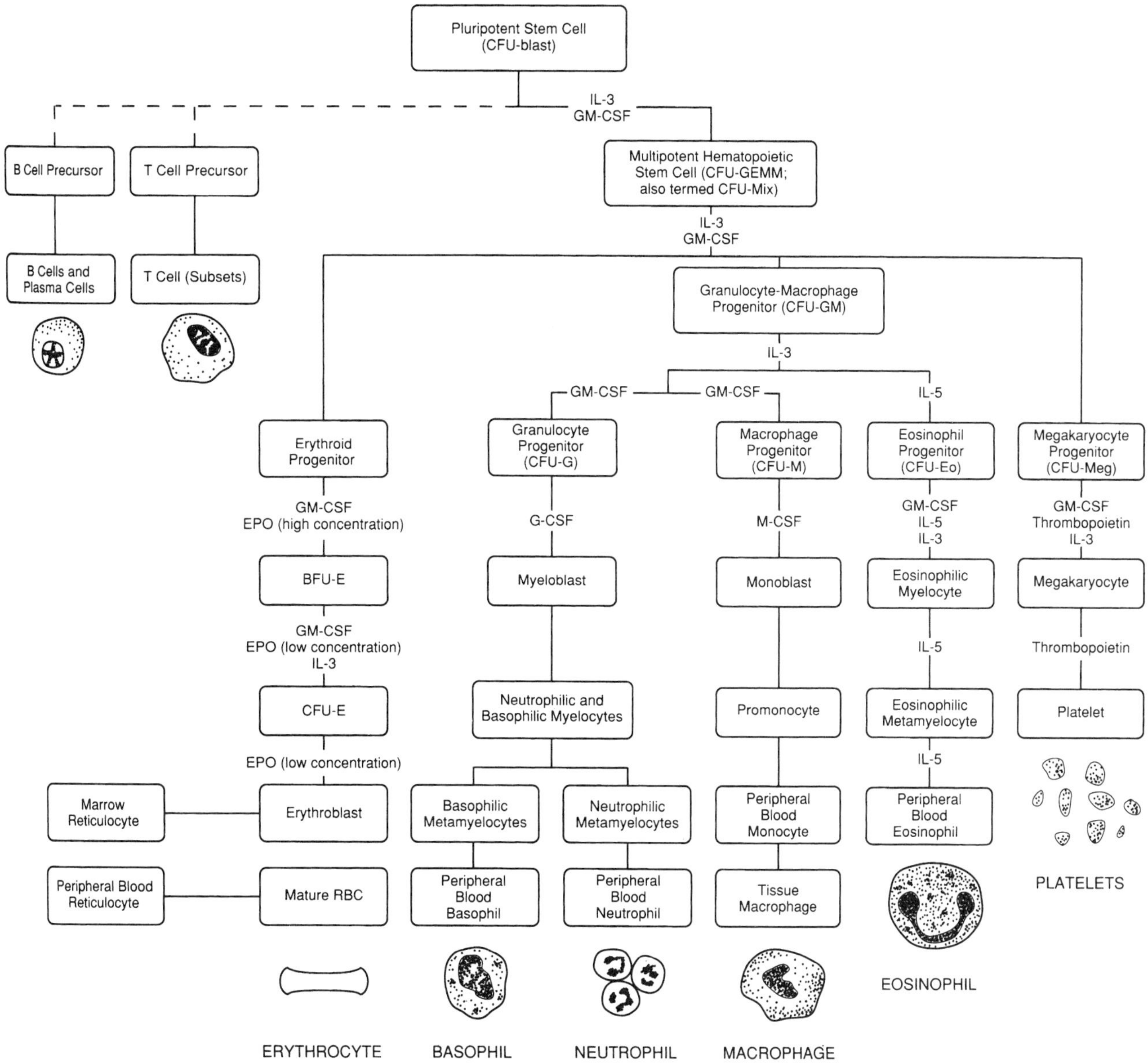

Figure 7.5. Differentiation of the hematopoietic stem cell from the pluripotent form to the highly differentiated macrophages, lymphocytes, erythrocytes, and granulocytes and growth factors responsible for their differentiation. (From Shriner DA. Colony-stimulating factors: clinical trials in humans. Highlights on Antineoplastic Drugs 8:6–14, 1990, with permission.)

molecules: IL-1α, and IL-1β. Although IL-1α and IL-1β are structurally different molecules with only 45% homology at the nucleotide level and 26% homology at the peptide level, they have virtually identical biologic effects.[7] IL-1 is produced by a number of cells, including mononuclear phagocytes, fibroblasts, NK cells, and T lymphocytes.[8,9] The in vitro hematologic effects of IL-1 include the activation of T cells, GM-CSF, G-CSF, macrophage CSF (M-CSF), interleukins 2, 3, 4, 5, and 6, and IFN-γ. In vivo, IL-1 plays an important role as a regulator of hematopoiesis by inducing a variety of hematopoietically active cytokines and by synergizing with these cytokines to amplify the hematopoietic response.[10] In humans, IL-1 has undergone phase I and II testing for the treatment of cytopenias caused by standard chemotherapy as well as high-dose chemotherapy with stem cell transplantation.[10] Clinical studies show that in patients undergoing autologous bone marrow transplantation, IL-1 decreases the length of time to neutrophil recovery. It is thought that a shorter time to neutrophil recovery may correlate with a decreased incidence of infection after bone marrow transplantation.[10] Other studies have demonstrated that IL-1 can increase the leukocyte and platelet counts in patients with solid tumors.[11] The most commonly observed side effects with IL-1 include fever with rigors or chills, tachycardia, headaches, myalgia, erythema and phlebitis at the injection site, transient hypertension, and hypotension at higher dosages.[11]

IL-2

IL-2 was the first of the interleukins to receive FDA approval, with an initial indication as a treatment for metastatic renal cell carcinoma. More recently, IL-2 has been approved for the treatment of metastatic malignant melanoma. Also known as T-cell growth factor, IL-2 has been shown to increase the proliferation of a subset of T lymphocytes called lymphocyte-activated killer (LAK) cells, which lyse a broad range of tumor targets. In patients with metastatic renal cell carcinoma, IL-2 has an objective response rate of 20%, with 5% of patients achieving a complete response. Response duration varies but can be prolonged (more than 12 months), with some patients remaining in complete remission for more than 60 months.[12] IL-2 given in combination with LAK cells has shown similar clinical results. The combination of IL-2 and LAK cells is called adoptive immunotherapy, which means the transfer of active immunologic reagents (LAK cells stimulated by IL-2) to a tumor-bearing host. The goal of adoptive immunotherapy is to have the tumor-targeted immunologic agents destroy the tumor specifically.[12]

In metastatic malignant melanoma, IL-2 monotherapy has shown an objective response of 16%, with 6% of patients achieving a complete response. The median duration of response was 9 months.[13] The FDA-recommended dosing schedule for both renal cell carcinoma and metastatic melanoma is 6×10^5 IU/kg given intravenously as a 15-minute bolus every 8 hours for up to 14 doses.[12] After 9 days of rest, the schedule is repeated for another 14 doses to a maximum of 28 doses per course, as tolerated. The major drawback to IL-2 therapy is its toxicity. Patients treated with the original IL-2 regimens required intensive care, and in clinical trials the treatment was associated with mortality rates of 1 to 6%. IL-2 can produce a severe capillary leak syndrome that leads to fluid retention, prerenal azotemia, respiratory distress, and interstitial edema. A great deal of effort has been expended in managing and limiting the side effects of IL-2 treatment. More recently developed regimens with moderate and low dosages and subcutaneous rather than intravenous administration have resulted in better tolerability.[12]

IL-3

IL-3 has been called multi-CSF because of its ability to stimulate the proliferation and activity of every member of the hematopoietic cell line.[8] In vitro, IL-3 acts directly on progenitor stem cells to amplify their response to more lineage-specific factors (G-CSF, M-CSF, and EPO), resulting in erythroid, granulocytic, monocytic, and megakaryocytic proliferation. In clinical studies, IL-3 has shown stimulatory effects on leukocytes, neutrophils, eosinophils, monocytes, reticulocytes, and platelets. Clinical trials with IL-3 have focused on its use after bone marrow transplantation, after combination chemotherapy, as a peripheral blood progenitor mobilizing agent for patients who are to undergo autologous stem cell transplantation, and as a sequential agent in combination with GM-CSF or G-CSF.[10] Overall, these studies suggest that in selected clinical settings, IL-3 can modestly accelerate platelet recovery and may reduce some of the complications and costs of prolonged thrombocytopenia. However, most of the beneficial effects on platelet recovery have been noted at higher dosages, which have been associated with profound side effects.[14] The role of IL-3 in combination with G-CSF or GM-CSF after cytotoxic chemotherapy has not been established. However, clinical trials show that these agents given in combination may act synergistically and result in significantly higher numbers of progenitor cells in the peripheral blood than when either agent is used alone.[15]

IL-4

IL-4 is a pleiotropic cytokine that was first identified in 1982 as a B-cell growth factor.[16] IL-4 affects a wide variety of cell types, including B and T lymphocytes, NK cells, LAK cells, monocytes and macrophages, mast cells, eosinophils, basophils and fibroblasts, and endothelial cells. In vitro, IL-4 has been shown to inhibit the growth of cells from malignant melanoma, breast carcinoma, ovarian carcinoma, mesothelioma, neurofibrosarcoma, and renal cell carcinoma.[10] A number of ongoing clinical trials are evaluating IL-4 for the treatment of solid tumors. However, myocardial toxicity, gastric mucosal injury, and acantholytic dermatosis have been reported after its administration. The incidence and severity of these side effects correlate strongly with both the dosage and duration of administration.[17]

IL-5

IL-5 is derived from a T-cell subset and is known as T-cell replacing factor, B-cell growth factor, and eosinophil-differentiating factor.[18] IL-5 acts primarily on B cells to stimulate the production of IgA. Because it is responsible for inducing a secretory response to gastrointestinal or respiratory pathogens, IL-5 may play an important role in mucosal immunity, one of the first defense mechanisms of the nonspecific immune system. IL-5 has also been shown to induce eosinophilic differentiation of acute myeloid leukemia (AML) blasts, suggesting the presence of specific IL-5 receptors on AML cells.[19]

IL-6

IL-6 is an inflammatory cytokine synthesized by blood monocytes, granulocytes, blood vessel endothelial cells, smooth muscle cells, connective tissue fibroblasts, chondrocytes of the cartilage, osteoblasts, keratinocytes of the skin, mesangial cells of the kidney, brain astrocytes, microglial cells, pituitary cells, and stromal endometrium cells.[20] IL-6 plays an important role in the defense mechanisms of the body, including immune response, hematopoiesis, and acute phase reactions.[15] A number of phase I and II clinical trials have been conducted with IL-6 to evaluate its effect on platelet counts in patients undergoing chemotherapy or radiation therapy. The results of the studies have been mixed. Side effects reported with IL-6 include fevers, myalgias, and fatigue at nearly all dosages. IL-6 has also been found to be essential for the survival and growth of multiple myeloma cells, which express specific receptors for this cytokine.[21] In addition to the hematologic and immune effects of IL-6, it has a number of endocrine and metabolic actions. IL-6 is a potent stimulator of the hypothalamic–pituitary–adrenal axis, and it stimulates the secretion of growth hormone, inhibits thyroid-stimulating hormone secretion, and decreases serum lipid concentrations.[22]

IL-7

IL-7 is produced by bone marrow stromal cells and has growth-promoting and possibly differentiating effects on pre-B cells and immature thymocytes. In vitro, IL-7 has been shown to have a proliferative effect on T cells and LAK cells and stimulate tumoricidal activity in monocytes and macrophages. In vivo studies in mice show an increase in B-cell precursors, numbers of immature and mature B cells, and numbers of CD8+ and CD4+ cells in the spleen; however, the effects on myeloid progenitors have not been consistent.[23]

IL-8

IL-8 is a cytokine with potent and specific neutrophil activation and chemoattractant properties. It has been detected in the circulation during septic shock and endotoxemia and after administering IL-1α.[24] IL-8 and its receptors have attracted considerable attention as targets for drug development for a number of human inflammatory diseases. Ischemia–reperfusion injury, adult respiratory distress syndrome, and certain forms of glomerulonephritis and dermatitis are all disease states in which neutrophil activation has been implicated in the disease process.[25]

IL-10

IL-10, originally named cytokine synthesis inhibitor factor, is produced by type 2 helper cells, monocytes and macrophages, and B lymphocytes.[26] In vitro, IL-10 is thought to play a role in the negative feedback system that inhibits synthesis of proinflammatory cytokines and CSFs. Because IL-10 can downregulate the production of inflammatory cytokines in activated macrophages, T cells, neutrophils, and eosinophils, it can cause immunosuppression. Preclinical studies suggest that IL-10 may be useful in a number of clinical settings in which proinflammatory cytokines are overexpressed, such as chronic inflammation, autoimmune disease, transplant rejection, graft versus host disease, and sepsis.[27,28]

IL-11

IL-11 is the second interleukin to receive FDA approval. IL-11 is indicated for the secondary prevention (i.e., in patients who have experienced thrombocytopenia in a prior course of chemotherapy) of chemotherapy-induced thrombocytopenia and for the reduction of the need for platelet transfusions in patients with nonmyeloid malignancies. Commonly, patients who are receiving chemotherapy develop thrombocytopenia in addition to neutropenia and anemia. Platelet transfusions may be required to decrease the risk of bleeding. Platelet transfusions, though safe, carry the risk of infectious disease transmission, just as other blood products do. In addition, transfusions often must be repeated frequently and can cause delays in administering chemotherapy. IL-11 is a unique thrombopoietic growth factor produced by the bone marrow stromal cells. It causes the proliferation of hematopoietic stem cells and megakaryocytic progenitors and induces megakaryocytic maturation.[29] Two randomized, double-blind, placebo-controlled clinical trials have evaluated the efficacy of IL-11 in the prevention of thrombocytopenia after single or repeated sequential cycles of various chemotherapy regimens. The first clinical trial was performed in patients with solid tumors or lymphoma who had received a prophylactic platelet transfusion for severe thrombocytopenia during their previous chemotherapy cycles. This study found that at 50 μg/kg daily (given subcutaneously), IL-11 allowed a significant number of these patients to avoid platelet transfusions during a subsequent chemotherapy cycle.[30] The second clinical trial was done in patients with advanced breast cancer who were undergoing dose-intensive chemotherapy with cyclophosphamide plus doxorubicin. This group of patients had not previously experienced severe chemotherapy-induced thrombocytopenia. This study concluded that administering IL-11 significantly reduced the platelet transfusion requirement for these patients and allowed maintenance of the planned dosage over repeated cycles.[29] Adverse reactions reported with IL-11 include edema (59%), tachycardia (20%), palpitations (14%), atrial fibrillation or flutter (12%), dyspnea (48%), and pleural effusions (10%).[13] The recommended dosage of IL-11 is 50 μg/kg given once daily as a subcutaneous injection. IL-11 should be initiated 6 to 24 hours after the completion of chemotherapy and continued until postnadir platelet counts are greater than 50,000 cells/μL. Treatment should be continued for no more than 21 days and should be discontinued at least 2 days before the next planned cycle of chemotherapy.[13]

IL-12

IL-12 is a heterodimeric cytokine, which makes it unique among the known interleukins. The IL-12 protein consists of two disulfide-bonded subunits encoded by two distinct genes. IL-12 has been shown in vitro to exert a number of immunoenhancing effects on the activities of NK cells, LAK cells, and T lymphocytes, induce IFN-γ production from peripheral blood lymphocytes (PBLs), and augment the lytic activity of PBLs against a variety of targets.[31,32] Given the role of IL-12 in the initiation of cell-mediated immunity, there is interest in the use of this cytokine for prophylaxis and treatment of infectious diseases.[33] In addition, IL-12 may play a key role in stimulating host T-cell mediated antitumor activities. Clinical trials are under way to evaluate the efficacy of IL-12 as an antineoplastic agent in the management of renal cell carcinoma, melanoma, breast cancer, and other cancers.[11]

IL-13

IL-13 is produced by activated T cells and shares many biologic activities with IL-4.[18]

IL-14

IL-14 is a B-cell growth factor secreted by T cells and some malignant B cells. IL-14 has been shown to induce B-cell proliferation, inhibit Ig secretion, and selectively expand some B-cell subpopulations. Although little is known about the physiologic role of this cytokine, IL-14 has been detected in patients with aggressive B-cell non-Hodgkin's lymphoma.[18]

It has been proposed that the production of IL-14 may play a significant role in the rapid proliferation of aggressive non-Hodgkin's lymphoma. Interrupting this pathway could be a useful goal of therapy for patients who are resistant to conventional chemotherapy.[34]

IL-17

IL-17 is produced primarily by peripheral blood T cells.[18] In vitro studies show that IL-17 causes the differentiation of bone marrow stem cells into the neutrophil cell line. Additionally, IL-17 has been shown to induce the production of G-CSF and GM-CSF. It is not yet clear whether the differentiation of stem cells into neutrophils is a direct or indirect effect of IL-17.[35]

Colony-Stimulating Factors

The CSFs (GM-CSF, G-CSF, M-CSF, stem cell factor [SCF], and EPO) are the most promising of the cytokines because of their broad range of clinical applications.[36] These glycoproteins have been cloned through DNA technology, and four (GM-CSF, G-CSF, SCF, and EPO) have been approved by the FDA for clinical use. CSFs help to regulate the growth and differentiation of hematopoietic cells. There are two main CSF classes. Class 1 CSFs such as SCF and GM-CSF act at the partially committed stem cell level to cause differentiation and proliferation of multiple cell lines (monocytes, granulocytes, eosinophils, etc.). Class 2 CSFs such as G-CSF, M-CSF, and EPO act on already differentiated cell lines to stimulate proliferation of more specific cell types.[37]

Granulocyte–Macrophage Colony-Stimulating Factor

GM-CSF supports the expansion of both monocytic and granulocytic cell lines and also cell lines containing myeloid, erythroid, and megakaryocytic cells when combined with EPO. GM-CSF received FDA approval for use in bone marrow transplantation (BMT) on the basis of a pivotal randomized, placebo-controlled, multicenter trial of 128 patients. Patients receiving high-dose chemotherapy and autologous bone marrow transplants for lymphoid malignancies were randomized to receive placebo or 250 μg/m^2/day of GM-CSF administered as a 2-hour infusion for 21 days after transplant. The patients receiving GM-CSF experienced a neutrophil recovery 7 days earlier than the placebo-treated group (19 versus 26 days). It was also noted that days of hospitalization, days of antibiotic use, and the incidence of documented infection were lower in the GM-CSF treated group. In addition to its indication for accelerating myeloid recovery in patients with lymphoid cancers undergoing autologous bone marrow transplantation, it has received FDA approval for use in patients who have BMT failure or engraftment delay in both the allogeneic and the autologous setting. In the setting of peripheral stem cell transplantation, GM-CSF has also received approval to help mobilize peripheral blood progenitor cells for transplant as well as for use after peripheral cell transplantation.

GM-CSF has been used to accelerate myeloid recovery in patients undergoing chemotherapy for AML.[38–40] In one uncontrolled trial, GM-CSF reduced the median recovery time of neutrophils by 4 days in patients receiving 6-thioguanine, standard-dose cytarabine, and daunorubicin and by 9 days in patients receiving high-dose cytarabine and mitoxantrone.[39] In a larger, randomized, placebo-controlled trial, 124 patients undergoing induction and consolidation therapy for acute myelogenous leukemia were randomized to receive GM-CSF or placebo on day 11 if a day 10 bone marrow sample was aplastic. The median time to recover an absolute neutrophil count of 500/μL or more was 11 days in the GM-CSF group and 14 days in the placebo group ($p = 0.01$). The median survival time was 325 days in the GM-CSF group and 135 days in the placebo group ($p = 0.035$). GM-CSF is being studied in a variety of clinical areas to reduce the incidence and severity of mucositis, stomatitis, and diarrhea in patients undergoing chemotherapy treatment, to reduce fungal infections in patients with cancer and patients, to promote wound healing, and as an HB adjuvant. The most commonly reported adverse effects of GM-CSF include injection site reactions, slight temperature elevations after injection, bone pain, and myalgias.

Granulocyte Colony-Stimulating Factor

G-CSF is a cell-lineage–specific CSF that stimulates granulocyte progenitor cells to differentiate into granulocytes. G-CSF received FDA approval following a phase III trial in which 211 patients were randomized to receive 200 μg/m^2 of G-CSF or placebo after chemotherapy with cyclophosphamide, doxorubicin, and etoposide. G-CSF reduced the duration of neutropenia from 6 days to 3 days in the first cycle as well as the incidence of febrile neutropenia (57 versus 28% in cycle 1), the length of first cycle hospital stay, and the days of intravenous antibiotic use.[40] Additional studies consistently show a significantly shorter duration of leukopenia than in placebo controls.[41–43] Small studies of G-CSF show reductions in infection, mucositis, and fever and greater adherence to scheduled chemotherapy regimens.[42,44] G-CSF has also received approval to reduce the duration of neutropenia and neutropenia-related clinical sequelae in patients with nonmyeloid malignancies who are undergoing myeloablative chemotherapy followed by marrow transplantation. It has also received approval to reduce the incidence and duration of sequelae of neutropenia (e.g., fever, infection, and oropharyngeal ulcers) in symptomatic patients with congenital neutropenia, cyclic neutropenia, or idiopathic neutropenia. G-CSF has also been approved for use in patients who fail to engraft after receiving an autologous bone marrow transplant and for mobilization of autologous peripheral blood progenitor cells after chemotherapy.

The American Society of Clinical Oncology (ASCO) recently published CSF guidelines with a principal goal of creating a useful, practical document that would help clinicians improve patient outcomes and medical practice. The guidelines state that in consideration of both efficacy and cost-modeling analyses, the primary administration of CSFs should be used as a prophylactic measure only when the chemotherapy being administered is expected to have an incidence of febrile neutropenia more than 40% of the time. However, some high-risk patients, including those with bone marrow compromise, preexisting neutropenia, substantial irradiation of the pelvic area, history of recurrent febrile neutropenia during previous chemotherapy exposure, and open wounds, would benefit from treatment with CSFs even when a less myelosuppressive chemotherapy regimen is used. The guidelines recommend that CSFs not be used in patients who are neutropenic but afebrile, in patients undergoing CSF priming, or in patients with myelodysplastic syndromes, or to treat febrile neutropenic patients unless they are high-risk patients such as those with pneumonia, hypotension, multiorgan dysfunction, or fungal infections.[45]

Macrophage Colony-Stimulating Factor

Macrophage colony-stimulating factor (M-CSF), also called CSF-1, selectively stimulates the proliferation and differentiation of the macrophage cell line. It has been studied in the treatment of cancer in patients with invasive fungal infections after bone marrow transplant. Forty-six patients received M-CSF at dosages ranging from 100 to 2000 $\mu g/m^2$/day. The M-CSF did not affect monocyte, neutrophil, or lymphocyte counts. There was a significant difference in survival in patients who received M-CSF compared with historical controls who received antifungal agents (27 versus 5%). However, the difference resulted entirely from better survival in patients with a Karnofsky score greater than 20% with invasive candidiasis. Thrombocytopenia was the dose-limiting toxicity seen in 11 of the 46 patients. M-CSF is currently approved only in Japan.

Stem Cell Growth Factor

The newest stem cell growth factor, rHuSCF (Stemgen), was approved by the FDA in the fall of 1998 to help mobilize peripheral blood progenitor cells for the support of high-dose chemotherapy and autologous stem cell transplants. When used in combination with G-CSF, SCF stimulates production of stem cells harvested before high-dose chemotherapy and then reinfused back into the patient to help establish a new population of blood cells. It is often difficult to collect enough peripheral blood stem cells in order to allow a safe transplantation procedure. rHuSCF works by stimulating the release of stem cells from the bone marrow into the peripheral blood.

In a randomized clinical trial in more than 200 patients with breast cancer undergoing stem cell transplantation, patients received either SCF in combination with G-CSF or G-CSF alone. Treatment with the combination of growth factors resulted in greater stem cell collections and a greater proportion of patients (63%) reaching their target number of stem cells when compared with G-CSF alone (47%). Other studies support the efficacy of SCF in patients with lymphoma and multiple myeloma. The most common side effects reported with SCF include mild to moderate injection site reactions (81%) and systemic allergic reactions (3 to 4%).[46]

Erythropoietin

Erythropoietin (EPO) is the primary regulator of red blood cell production and thus is an important cytokine for the erythroid cell line. Recombinant human EPO-α (rHEPO) is approved for use in the treatment of anemia associated with chronic renal failure in patients on dialysis and predialysis patients, severe anemia associated with zidovudine (AZT) therapy in AIDS, anemic patients scheduled to undergo elective noncardiac, nonvascular surgery, and anemia in patients with cancer receiving chemotherapy.

EPO was the first recombinant stimulating factor to be approved for use in humans, and many trials have confirmed its benefit in transfusion-dependent patients. The use of EPO in anemia in patients with renal failure and AIDS is discussed in Chapter 14, Other Anemias, and Chapter 76, Human Immunodeficiency Virus (HIV) Infection–Antiretroviral Therapy; it is important to be aware of the studies of its use in treating the anemia of patients undergoing cancer chemotherapy. In double-blind trials involving 124 patients with cancer-induced anemia, 132 patients receiving a cisplatin-containing regimen, and 157 patients receiving other chemotherapy not containing cisplatin, the mean weekly hematocrit level in EPO-treated patients in all three treatment groups increased from 28.6 to 32.1%. The mean weekly hematocrit level for the placebo-treated group remained essentially unchanged over the same time period (28.4 to 28.8%). The transfusion requirements during the second and third months of therapy for EPO-treated patients were less than for placebo patients, although the difference did not reach statistical significance.[40]

The common adverse effects associated with EPO therapy generally are mild and include hypertension, rash, headache, arthralgias, and nausea and vomiting. A rapid rise in red blood cell count caused by EPO administration can also result in severe hypertension, thrombosis, and seizures.

Interferons

The interferons are a group of naturally occurring glycoproteins produced by a variety of cell types in response to viral, antigenic, or mitogenic stimuli. They were originally discovered in 1957 when Isaacs and Lindenmann observed that virus-infected cells produced a protein that rendered them resistant to other viruses.[47] In addition to their antiviral action, interferons affect a number of vital cellular and body functions, including hormone stimulation, immunity, metabolism, and tumor development.

Interferons have been categorized into two classes: type 1 (IFN-α, IFN-β, and IFN-θ) and type 2 (IFN-γ). Many cell types in response to many different factors, including infectious agents, produce the type 1 interferons. The type 2 interferons are produced only by T lymphocytes and NK cells stimulated by antigens or mitogens and IL-2.[48] Whereas naturally occurring interferons are glycosylated, recombinant interferons produced in *E. coli* are not. However, activity does not seem to be diminished by their unglycosylated state. Whereas IFN-α and IFN-β are similar in structure, cell receptor site interactions, and biologic effects, IFN-γ interacts at a different receptor site, has a different structure, and appears to have greater antitumor, immunomodulatory, and cytolytic effects.[49]

To date, IFN-α has been approved for use in the treatment of chronic viral hepatitis B and C, condyloma acuminata, hairy cell leukemia, AIDS-related Kaposi's sarcoma, follicular non-Hodgkin's lymphoma, chronic malignant melanoma, and Philadelphia chromosome positive chronic myelogenous leukemia (CML). IFN-β has been approved for use in ambulatory patients with relapsing–remitting multiple sclerosis to reduce the frequency of clinical exacerbations of the disease. IFN-γ is approved by the FDA to reduce the frequency and severity of serious infections associated with chronic granulomatous disease.

IFN-α

IFN-α was the first of the interferons to be approved for clinical use. It has been widely used as first-line or adjuvant treatment for several other solid tumors and hematologic malignancies. Hairy cell leukemia was the first malignancy against which IFN-α was found to have significant activity. Although up to 90% of patients respond to IFN-α treatment, up to 50% relapse within a short period of time. Studies show that continuous treatment with IFN-α leads to a long-term survival up to 6 years in 82% of patients when dosages of 2×10^6 U/m^2 are used.[50]

In the early 1980s, IFN-α was recognized as an effective agent in the treatment of CML. The mechanism of action of interferon in CML is not completely understood. CML is caused by a specific chromosomal abnormality, the Philadelphia chromosome. It is thought that IFN-α not only is antiproliferative to normal and leukemic stem cells, but may suppress the oncogene responsible for the Philadelphia chromosomal translocation, thus restoring normal adherence to marrow stromal cells, preventing their premature release into the peripheral blood. By selectively repressing the Philadelphia-positive stem cells, IFN-α encourages the repopulation of the bone marrow with normal Philadelphia-negative stem cells.

Two studies, one by the Cancer and Leukemia Group B (CALGB) and another by the Italian Cooperative Study Group on Chronic Myeloid Leukemia, both confirm the efficacy of IFN-α in the management of chronic phase CML. In the CALGB trial, 107 patients received IFN-α at a dosage of 5 MU/m^2 daily (given subcutaneously) until progression of disease; 59% of patients achieved at least a partial remission for a median of 52 months, and a complete cytogenetic response (complete disappearance of all Philadelphia-positive cytology) was achieved in 14 patients (13%).[51] In the Italian study, the dosages of interferon used were lower than the CALGB trial, 3 MU daily for the first 2 weeks, 6 MU daily for the second 2 weeks, and 9 MU daily thereafter. In this study, 322 patients were randomized to either IFN-α (218 patients) or conventional-dose hydroxyurea (104 patients). Complete cytogenetic responses occurred in 8% of IFN-α patients and none occurred in the hydroxyurea group. The time to progression to an accelerated or blast crisis phase was longer in the IFN-α group (median more than 72 months) than the hydroxyurea group (median 45 months), $p < 0.001$, and overall survival was longer with IFN-α than with hydroxyurea (72 versus 45 months, $p = 0.002$).[52] Interferon has clearly shown a survival benefit over conventional treatment for patients with CML.

In solid tumors, IFN-α's efficacy has been clinically documented in malignant melanoma, metastatic renal cell carcinoma, bladder cancer, and AIDS-related Kaposi's sarcoma. Since 1978, more than 12 phase II trials have documented the antitumor activity of IFN-α against malignant melanoma. Response rates of up to 16% have been reported. In a phase III, randomized, controlled trial of 287 patients with deep primary tumors or regional lymph node involvement, adjuvant IFN-α was compared with observation alone in patients who had previously undergone surgical removal of their primary tumor. Dosages of 20 MU/m^2 daily (given intravenously) for 1 month followed by 10 MU/m^2 three times weekly (subcutaneously) for 48 weeks resulted in a median relapse-free survival significantly greater in the IFN-α group (1.7 versus 0.98 years) and an overall median survival of 3.82 versus 2.78 years for the control group.[53] This was the first trial in almost 20 years to show that an adjuvant agent could alter the natural progression of malignant melanoma.

IFN-α has been studied in the treatment of renal cell cancer, and response rates of 10 to 15% have been reported (2% complete response rates). When IFN-α is combined with IL-2, response rates of 38% have been noted.[48] The role of sequential IFN-α followed by IFN-γ is also being studied. IFN-α has also been studied in breast cancer, ovarian cancer, colorectal cancer, and superficial bladder cancer. Although response rates of only 5 to 10% have been seen in breast cancer and ovarian cancer, three trials in colorectal cancer combining 5 fluorouracil (5FU) and IFN-α have produced response rates of 26 to 63%, and trials in superficial bladder cancer have produced response rates of 43%.[54] These encouraging results have led to other trials of gastrointestinal malignancies with this combination of products. In a review of IFN-α, Spiegel[55] reports the incidence of adverse effects in 1403 patients (Table 7.2).

IFN-β

IFN-β was approved in 1994 for the treatment of exacerbating–remitting ambulatory multiple sclerosis patients based on the results of a multicenter, randomized, double-blind, placebo-controlled trial. In that trial, IFN-β resulted in fewer exacerbations, fewer severe exacerbations, and less progression of T2 signal abnormalities seen on yearly magnetic resonance imaging scans.[56]

In both solid and hematologic malignancies, IFN-β has shown modest results overall. Its activity against renal cell, melanoma, and colorectal cancers, as well as its activity in hairy cell leukemia, CML, or non-Hodgkin's lymphoma does not seem to offer any advantage over IFN-α.[49] The best clinical responses to IFN-β have been seen in Kaposi's sarcoma,[57] with a 40 to 50% response rate, and glioma brain tumors, where a 10 to 20% response rate has been reported.[49]

IFN-γ

IFN-γ has been FDA approved to reduce infectious complications in patients with chronic granulomatous disease, an inherited immunodeficiency syndrome. A study of 128 patients who received either IFN-γ or placebo (subcutaneously three times a week for 1 year) had two study endpoints. The first was the time to serious infection (defined as a clinical event leading to hospitalization and parenteral antibiotic administration), and the second was the number of serious infections, length of hospitalization, and effect on existing infection. After 1 year, 77% of patients treated with IFN-γ were infection-free, compared to 30% in the placebo-treated group. There were 50% fewer serious infections in the IFN-γ group (compared with placebo).

The toxicities of IFN-γ appear to be similar to those of IFN-α and IFN-β, although headaches appear to be more severe and may be dose-limiting. IFN-γ has also been shown to increase serum triglyceride levels by inhibiting lipoprotein lipase.

Table 7.2 ▪ Incidence of Adverse Experiences with Interferon-α

	All Patients (n = 1403)	
Adverse Effects	**Any Severity (%)**	**Grades III, IV (%)**
Flulike symptoms	96	37
Nausea/vomiting	42	5
Other gastrointestinal symptoms	24	2
Central nervous system	33	7
Cardiovascular	12	2
Skin	13	1
Respiratory	6	1
Alopecia	6	<1
Weight loss	5	1
Hepatic	<1	0

Reprinted with permission from Spiegel RJ. The alpha interferons: clinical overview. Semin Oncol 14:1–12, 1987.

Monoclonal Antibodies

The most diverse and best studied of the biologicals, the monoclonal antibodies, have met recent commercial success with far-reaching therapeutic applicability in cancers, transplantation rejection, drug toxicities, Crohn's disease, rheumatoid arthritis, and other diseases. The clinical applications of monoclonal antibodies for diagnostic imaging are also extensive, particularly for cancer, infectious diseases, and heart disease. This has led to the FDA approval of monoclonal imaging agents to detect the presence, location, and extent of myocardial necrosis in acute ischemic heart disease and the detection of colorectal, ovarian, and prostate cancer. Although the theoretical applications seem endless, the practical applications have been somewhat slow in developing, partly because of the difficulties inherent in monoclonal antibody production.

Monoclonal antibody production begins with the identification of the B lymphocyte responsible for the production of a specific antibody to a specific antigen.[58] Antigen to which the desired antibody will respond is first injected into a mouse (Fig. 7.6). The antigen stimulates B lymphocytes (the precursor of the antibody-secreting plasma cell) to produce a specific antibody against that antigen. B lymphocytes are then recovered from the spleen of the mouse. Only a few of the B lymphocytes recovered from the mouse spleen actually secrete the desired antibody. The B lymphocytes are then mixed with myeloma cells (a cell line that can live forever in culture) in polyethylene glycol, resulting in the membranes of the two cell types being fused together.

The technique of fusing myeloma cells and B lymphocytes, developed by Kohler and Milstein in the mid-1970s, results in a hybridoma. The hybridomas are grown for several weeks. Enzyme-linked immunoabsorbent assay (ELISA) or radioimmunoassay (RIA) methods then are used to select the appropriate antibody-secreting hybridoma. The target antigen is chemically bound to the bottom of the testing tray in wells, and the hybridoma cells are added to each of the wells. Antibodies produced inside the wells that are specific for the target antigen bind to the antigen at the bottom of the wells. Radioactive or enzyme-labeled secondary antibodies that are specific for the primary antibodies are then added to the wells, and the mixture is incubated and rewashed. The wells that show radioactivity or a color reaction due to the enzyme are

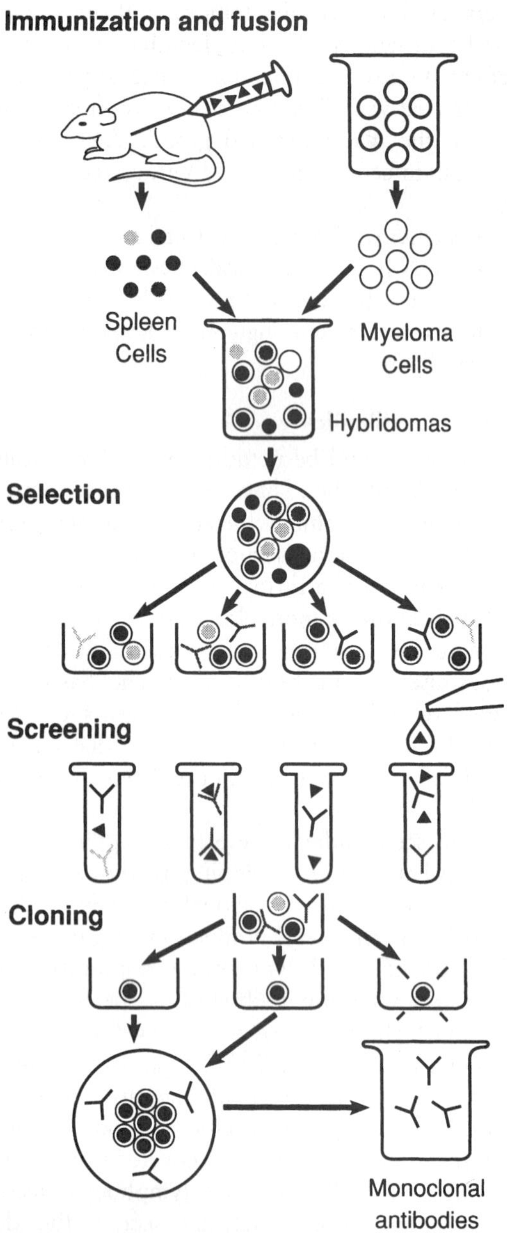

Figure 7.6. Summary of the steps involved in the production of monoclonal antibodies. (From Chisolm R. On the trail of the magic bullet. High Technology Business 3:57–63, 1983, with permission.)

those that contain the desired antibody. Once identified, the hybridomas containing the desired antibody can be cloned.

Monoclonal antibodies exert their killing effect on cells in three primary ways. The first is through antibody-dependent cell-mediated cytotoxicity. As with the rest of the immune system, when an antibody attaches to an antigen, effector cells such as monocytes, macrophages, granulocytes, and some lymphocytes bind to the constant region (Fc) of the antibody and cause enzymatic puncture of the antigenic cell membrane, ultimately resulting in cell death.

A second mechanism of monoclonal antibody action is to target molecules on the cell surface that are critical to that cell's growth or differentiation. For example, monoclonal antibodies have been prepared against a growth factor receptor HER-2-neu, found overabundantly on the cell surface of up to one-third of patients with breast cancer. The HER-2-neu antibody, when combined with chemotherapy, improves the duration of treatment response and overall survival in women with metastatic breast cancer. A third method of killing is through complement-mediated cytotoxicity. Monoclonal antibodies, primarily IgM, invoke the release of complement, which sets off the complement cascade to mediate cell destruction.

Researchers have also been able to augment the effectiveness of monoclonal antibodies by conjugating them with radioisotopes, toxins, chemotherapeutic agents, and drug-filled liposomes (Fig. 7.7). Radioconjugates used in the treatment of malignancies have been successful because they do not have to enter the cells to induce a killing effect. Instead, they can exert their energy over several cells (the field effect). Nearby healthy tissue, especially in areas in which the conjugate may be detained, such as the liver and spleen, may be injured.[59] A radioconjugate monoclonal ^{131}I anti-B1 antibody that targets the CD20 antigen on the cell surface of B cells will soon be on the market for the treatment of low-grade non-Hodgkin's lymphoma. Monoclonal antibodies fused with all or part of plant or bacterial toxins are called immunoconjugates. Monoclonal antibodies conjugated with ricin-A, a plant toxin, have been used to treat melanoma, lymphoma, rheumatoid arthritis, and leukemia.

Antineoplastic monoclonal antibody conjugates are also being used to deliver antineoplastics to specific areas of the body. This helps to improve the therapeutic:toxic ratio of systemic chemotherapy. Antineoplastic conjugates have been tried in colorectal, breast, and ovarian cancers and in malignant melanoma and glioma. Researchers have

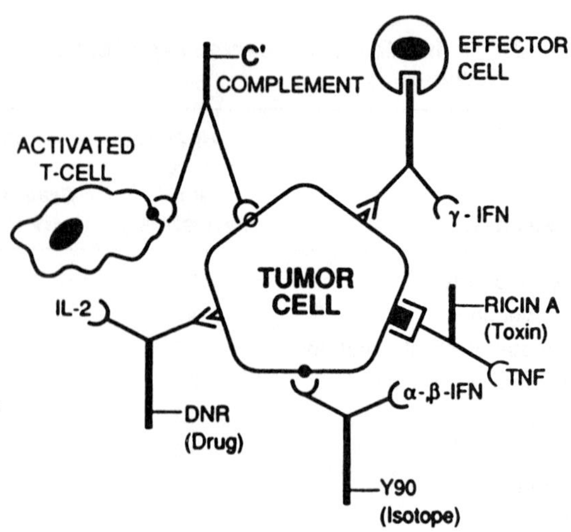

Figure 7.7. Various uses of monoclonal antibodies. *C'*, complement; *DNR*, daunorubicin; *IFN*, interferon; *IL-2*, interleukin-2; *TNF*, tumor necrosis factor. (From Dillman R. Monoclonal antibodies for treating cancer. Ann Intern Med 111:592–603, 1989, with permission.)

developed a doxorubicin-conjugated monoclonal antibody yielding a drug that is 10 times more cytotoxic than doxorubicin alone. Liposome-carrying drugs conjugated to monoclonal antibodies also show promise. The liposomes concentrate the drug in cells of the reticuloendothelial system, liver, and spleen and thus reduce drug uptake to other critical organs, such as the heart, kidneys, and gastrointestinal tract. Liposome-containing doxorubicin and daunorubicin have been developed to reduce the cardiotoxic potential of these drugs. They are both indicated for treatment of HIV-related Kaposi's sarcoma.

Another advance in the mechanistic development of monoclonal antibodies is the engineering of bispecific monoclonal antibodies, which can be bidirected to both a tumor cell and an effector cell such as a monocyte or lymphocyte.[60] Bispecific monoclonal antibodies can bind two different antigenic determinants simultaneously to bring effector cells into close contact with tumor cells for improved cellular cytotoxicity. These monoclonal antibodies have been developed by cross-linking hybridomas. Antibodies directed against the CD3T-cell receptor subunit of cytotoxic T cells help to trigger the effector function once it is brought into contact with the tumor cell. These bispecific antibodies have been tested in clinical trials against Hodgkin's lymphoma and look very promising.

Genetically engineered monoclonal antibody fragments directed to site-specific antigens have also been developed. The rationale for developing these fragments is based on their greater ability to gain access to tumors because of their smaller size and more rapid clearance from the circulation.[60] Digoxin-specific Fab antibody fragments are commercially available for the treatment of digitalis toxicity. The digoxin antibody fragments bind specifically to unbound (free) digoxin in the intravascular space, preventing and reversing the glycoside's toxic effect. The Fab has advantages over the intact antibody in that it causes less immunogenicity because it lacks the antigenic Fc and is cleared from the circulation more rapidly.

Eternacept (Enbrel), a dimeric fusion protein consisting of tumor necrosis factor (TNF) receptor linked to the Fc portion of human IgG1 antibody, has been FDA approved for the management of rheumatoid arthritis in patients in whom disease-modifying antirheumatic drugs had failed. Eternacept is a soluble, free-floating molecule that binds to TNF to block its binding to cell surface TNF receptors. By blocking TNF binding to cell surfaces, it prevents the inflammatory response processes of rheumatoid arthritis.[61]

Monoclonal Antibodies in Transplantation

Muromonab-CD3 (Orthoclone OKT3, Ortho) is the only commercially available monoclonal antibody for the treatment of acute renal, cardiac, and hepatic allograft rejection. It has also been used prophylactically to prevent acute rejection. Muromonab-CD3 is a murine (mouse) IgG monoclonal antibody that directs its action against the CD3 molecule present on the surface of thymocytes and mature T-lymphocytes. CD3 forms a complex with the T-cell antigen receptor (TCR) to induce T-cell function (activation and proliferation) and activation of cytotoxic cells that contribute to graft versus host disease. It has been shown in vivo that administering this antibody results in the coating of circulatory T cells and their subsequent disappearance from the circulation. By interfering with the CD3, muromonab-CD3 does not allow the complex to form, rendering the T cells inactive.

In the first controlled trial in 123 patients with acute rejection of cadaver transplants, the rejection reversal rate was 94% with muromonab-CD3, compared to 75% with high-dose steroids. The 1-year graft survival rate was also higher with muromonab CD3 (62%) than with high-dose steroids (45%).[60]

Side effects of muromonab-CD3 include pyrexia, dyspnea, headache, nausea, vomiting, and diarrhea. These effects generally begin within 1 hour of administering the first dose of the drug and diminish over the next several hours. On days 2 through 5 of treatment, pruritus, rash, aseptic meningitis, and altered mental status have been reported to occur. The side effects are probably caused by muromonab-CD3–induced increases in TNF and IL-2.

Patients can also develop human antimouse antibodies (HAMA) to the monoclonal antibody, which can lead to an abrogated therapeutic response. In general, most patients can undergo two to three courses of muromonab-CD3 without developing a decreased response.

Two additional humanized monoclonal antibodies have been FDA approved for the prevention of acute organ rejection in patients receiving renal transplants. Daclizumab (Zenapax) was approved in 1997 in adult and pediatric patients, and basiliximab (Simulect) was approved in 1998. Because these agents are humanized monoclonal antibodies, they do not produce the HAMA response seen with muromonab-CD3.

Monoclonal Antibodies in Cancer Treatment

The initial studies involving monoclonal antibodies in the treatment of cancers involved primarily hematologic malignancies. More than 25 trials in 135 patients resulted in complete remission in approximately 5% of patients, partial response in 16%, and minor response in an additional 17% of patients.[60]

Most patients treated in these studies had refractory disease and compromised immune systems, making it difficult for them to respond to immunotherapy. Additionally, these earlier studies were done with mouse monoclonal antibodies, leading to a significant HAMA response that limited the duration of treatment. Other problems identified in these earlier trials included heterogeneous antigens expressed on the surface of tumor cells; immune complex formation between free, circulating antigens and monoclonal antibodies; disappearance or modulation of antigens on the tumor cell surface; and the short half-life of the mouse monoclonal in the human circulation.

With these problems identified, researchers set out to minimize these problems, achieve site-specific delivery of monoclonals to the tumor cells with minimal disruption to normal tissue, and produce a more stable monoclonal conjugate, resulting in a longer half-life of the monoclonal antibody.[60]

The first monoclonal antibody approved for cancer treatment was rituximab (Rituxan). Rituximab was approved in early 1998 for the treatment of refractory or recurrent low-grade (follicular) non-Hodgkin's lymphoma. Rituximab is a chimeric anti-CD20 monoclonal antibody that targets CD20 antigens, which are expressed on more than 90% of both normal and malignant B cells and are required for cell cycle initiation and differentiation. When rituximab binds to the CD20 antigen on the cells surface, it induces both complement-mediated and antibody-dependent cellular cytotoxicity, which results in cell death.

The phase III pivotal trial evaluated 166 patients with low-grade follicular lymphoma that was recurrent or resistant to chemotherapy.[62] Rituximab at a dosage of 375 mg/m^2 weekly for 4 weeks yielded overall response rates of 50% (6% complete responses and 44% partial responses) in 151 evaluable patients. The mean time to progression was not reached at more than 9 months. Side effects were mostly mild and included fever, chills, nausea, and headache. More recently, in Europe, eight fatal cases of a severe cytokine release syndrome have accompanied initial doses of rituximab.[63] Severe cytokine release syndrome usually manifests within 1 or 2 hours of the first infusion of the drug and is characterized by severe dyspnea, bronchospasm, or hypoxia with or without fever, chills, rigors, urticaria, and angioedema. The FDA is considering a boxed label warning in the package insert to alert physicians to this rare but fatal reaction.

Trastuzumab (Herceptin), the first monoclonal antibody used in the treatment of advanced breast cancer, was approved in September 1998 for the treatment of women with metastatic breast cancer whose tumors overexpress the epidermal growth factor receptor 2 protein-HER2. Because of a genetic alteration in the HER2 gene, approximately one-third of all breast cancer tumors overexpress HER2 on the cell surface. Trastuzumab, a mouse monoclonal engineered to closely resemble a human antibody, binds to the HER2 receptors on the cell surface of the tumor cells and through this binding mechanism inhibits tumor cell growth.

Trastuzumab has been studied in clinical trials in combination with chemotherapy. In a randomized, controlled clinical trial, 469 patients with HER2 overexpressing metastatic breast cancer were randomized to trastuzumab plus chemotherapy or chemotherapy alone. In this trial, patients who received trastuzumab combination therapy had a median time to disease progression of 7.2 months, compared to 4.5 months for those receiving chemotherapy alone. Additionally, the 1-year survival rate for the trastuzumab combination arm was 79%, compared to 68% for chemotherapy alone.[64] Trastuzumab was also studied alone in women who had relapsed after chemotherapy for metastatic disease. The overall response rate was 14% (3% complete responses) and the median response time was 9 months. The biggest risk of using trastuzumab is its potential for causing a weakening of the heart muscle, leading to congestive heart failure. This side effect was most pronounced when trastuzumab was used in combination with doxorubin and cyclophosphamide. Therefore, trastuzumab is not approved for use with that combination of chemotherapy drugs. Other side effects include neutropenia, anemia, abdominal pain, and diarrhea. Also, fever, nausea, vomiting, pain, weakness, and headache can occur with about one-half of all first infusions of the drug.[65]

Other recent studies of monoclonal antibodies used to treat malignancies have focused on the use of immunoconjugates, radioconjugates, and chemotherapy conjugates. Iodine ^{131}I tositumomab is a monoclonal antibody conjugated with the radioisotope ^{131}I. This anti-CD20 monoclonal antibody targets CD20 antigens on the cell surface of B lymphocytes. Therefore, it has the same immunotoxic effect as rituximab with the added benefit of a radioisotope that can be delivered directly to the tumor. It is expected that the FDA will approve ^{131}I tositumomab (Bexxar) in mid 2000.[66]

Monoclonal Antibodies in Cardiovascular Therapeutics

In 1994 the FDA approved abciximab (ReoPro, Centocor B.V. and Eli Lilly) for the prevention of acute ischemic complications in patients with percutaneous transluminal coronary angioplasty (PTCA) who were at high risk for abrupt closure of the treated vessel. Abciximab is the Fab of the chimeric human–murine monoclonal antibody 7E3, with antiplatelet activity designed to reduce arterial thrombus formation after PTCA. It acts by binding to an adhesion receptor involved in platelet aggregation and preventing the binding of fibrinogen, von Willebrand factor, and other adhesive molecules to receptor sites on activated platelets.[67]

Abciximab was studied in a multicenter, double-blind, placebo-controlled trial in 2099 patients who were at high risk for abrupt closure of the treated coronary vessel. The primary endpoint was the occurrence of any of the following events within 30 days of PTCA: death, myocardial infarction, or the need for urgent intervention for recurrent ischemia. There was a 4.5% lower incidence of the primary endpoint in the monoclonal antibody treated group than in the placebo group. This difference was statistically significant.[67] Its indications for use have since been widened to include the reduction of acute blood clot complications for all patients undergoing any coronary intervention and the treatment of unstable angina not responding to conventional medical therapy when percutaneous coronary intervention is planned within 24 hours. Additionally, it has recently shown long-term mortality benefit when used in combination with stents compared with stenting alone.

Abciximab is associated with a greater frequency of major bleeding complications, which limits its use in patients who are at high risk for bleeding. It has also been shown to cause allergic reactions (anaphylaxis), thrombocytopenia, hypotension (mostly caused by bleeding complications), anemia, pleural effusions, pain at the injection site, and peripheral edema.[67]

Monoclonal Antibodies in Gastrointestinal Therapeutics

In 1999, the FDA approved the first monoclonal antibody for the treatment of Crohn's disease. Infliximab (Remicade) is a part-human, part-mouse antibody that acts by binding to TNF-α, thereby reducing its production and the associated intestinal inflammation seen with Crohn's disease. Infliximab is also the only drug approved for fistulizing Crohn's disease. In a randomized, double-blind, placebo-controlled dose ranging study, 108 patients with moderate to severe active Crohn's disease were randomized to receive a single intravenous dose of placebo or 5, 10, or 20 mg/kg infliximab.[68] The primary endpoint of the study was a reduction in the Crohn's disease activity index (CDAI) at week 4. Secondary endpoints included the proportion of patients who were in clinical remission at week 4 (CDAI less than 150) and clinical response over time. Sixteen percent of the placebo patients achieved a clinical response compared to 82% of the patients receiving 5 mg/kg infliximab ($p < 0.001$), and 48% of patients receiving 5 mg/kg infliximab were in clinical remission at week 4, compared to only 4% of placebo-treated patients.

Patients with fistulizing Crohn's disease of at least 3 months' duration were also studied. Ninety-four patients received three doses of placebo or 5 or 10 mg/kg infliximab at weeks 0, 2, and 6 and were followed for up to 26 weeks. Again the primary endpoint was the proportion of patients experiencing a clinical response, defined as a reduction of 50% or more in the number of draining fistulas upon gentle compression without an increase in other medications or surgery for Crohn's disease. Of placebo-treated patients, 26% achieved a clinical response, compared to 68% of patients in the 5 mg/kg infliximab-treated group ($p = 0.002$).[69] Long-term treatment studies are under way to determine the safety and efficacy of infliximab beyond the established number of doses for Crohn's disease and fistulizing Crohn' disease.

GENE THERAPY

The underlying cause of many human diseases can be traced to genetic abnormalities. Whether the abnormality is the lack of a receptor, a defective feedback loop, or the overproduction or underproduction of some pharmacologically active substance, many times the cause is a defect in the genetic code. Traditional therapeutic approaches focus on providing the missing substance or blocking the action of a substance that is overproduced or to which the body is overly sensitive. The aim of gene therapy is to correct the underlying defect in the genetic code.

Gene therapy involves the introduction of foreign genetic material into selected cells in the body to treat disease. It has been made possible by developing effective ways to transfer DNA into mammalian cells and by advances in recombinant DNA technologies.[70] Current approaches in gene therapy do not involve reproductive germ cells (i.e., ovum and spermatozoan). Because gene therapy is performed only on nonreproductive cells, its therapeutic effects are not passed on to future generations.

Genetic material can be introduced into mammalian cells by viral and nonviral vectors. Nonviral vectors used in gene transfer consist primarily of liposomes and molecular conjugates.[71] Viral vectors most commonly used in gene transfer include adenoviruses and retroviruses. The major difference between retroviruses and adenoviruses is that retroviruses permanently introduce genes into the chromosomes of infected cells and adenoviruses do not.[72] Currently, about 60% of all approved gene therapy trials use retroviral vectors, 20% use nonviral delivery systems, 10% use adenoviral vectors, and the remainder use other types of viral vectors.[73]

Nonviral Vectors

Nonviral vectors are primarily synthetic vectors such as liposomes and molecular conjugates. Liposomes, when combined with DNA of any size, can form a lipid–DNA complex capable of delivering genes to many cell types.[71] However, liposomes cannot target specific cell types, so gene transfer occurs primarily in cells that are near the site of administration.[71] Molecular conjugates consisting of protein or synthetic ligands can be coupled with DNA to form a protein–DNA complex. This type of gene delivery system can target different cell types because ligands are target–cell specific.[71]

Viral Vectors

Adenoviral Vectors

Adenoviral vectors are DNA viruses that can infect both dividing and nondividing cells. To construct adenoviral vectors, a portion of the viral genome called the E1 region is deleted.[74] This creates space for the therapeutic gene to be inserted, and it renders the virus incapable of self-replication, which prevents viral spread.[75] Adenoviral vectors are efficient in transferring genes into most tissues; unfortunately, gene expression lasts for only a short time (5 to 10 days postinfection).[76] Enthusiasm for adenoviral vectors has been tempered by the discovery that a significant immune response can be produced by the host against the transduced cells.[75] Recently, the first true phase I gene therapy clinical trials with an adenovirus vector began. Healthy volunteers were injected intradermally with adenoviral vectors to determine the exact type of immunologic response that occurs.[75]

Retroviral Vectors

Retroviruses are the most commonly used vectors for ex vivo gene transfer (Fig. 7.8).[77] This ex vivo approach has been favored for early trials because it is technically less complicated and the modified cells can be monitored and controlled before they are given to a patient. One of the primary advantages of retroviral vectors is their ability to

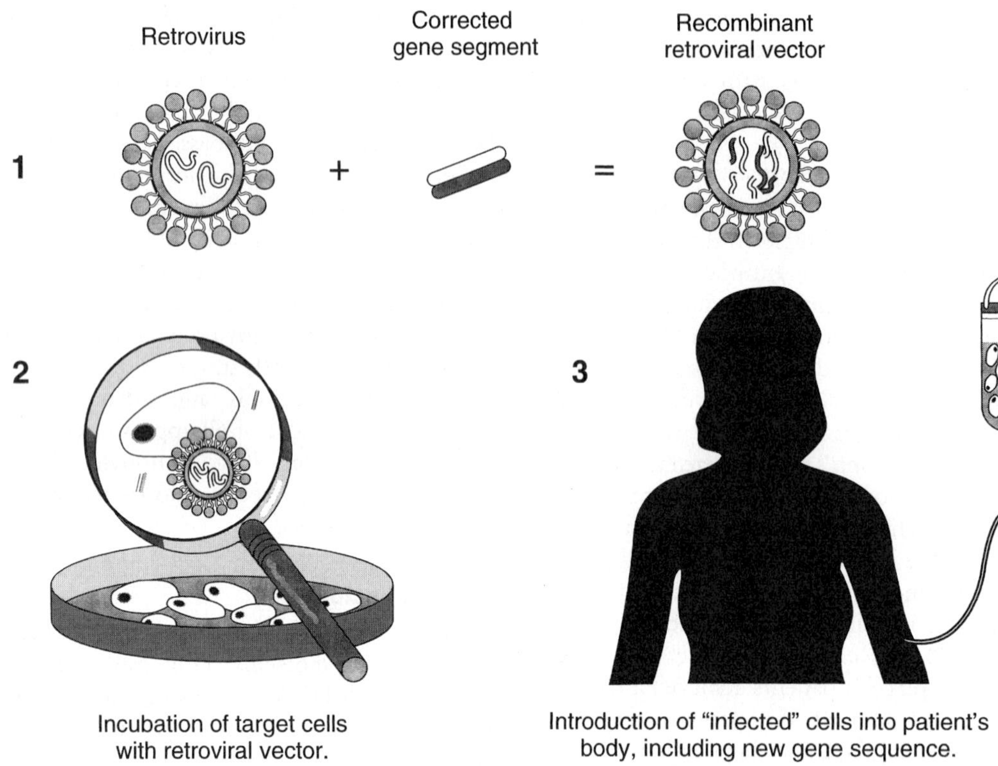
Retrovirus
Corrected gene segment
Recombinant retroviral vector
1
+
=
2
3
Incubation of target cells with retroviral vector.
Introduction of "infected" cells into patient's body, including new gene sequence.

Figure 7.8. Ex vivo gene transfer process. **1.** The retrovirus is altered through recombinant DNA technology to add the gene sequence that is to be delivered to the patient. **2.** The retroviral vector is incubated with the target cells, and the desired gene is inserted into the target cells. **3.** The target cells with the desired gene are infused into the patient.

integrate in a stable manner into the host genome, which provides the possibility of long-term gene expression. In addition, retroviruses do not elicit an immune response in the host, as adenoviral vectors do. The main disadvantages of retroviral vectors are that their titers are too low for efficient in vivo gene transfer. Additionally, theoretical safety concerns surround the use of retroviral gene delivery. There is a risk of generating replication competent retroviruses (RCR) (i.e., retroviruses that can replicate in the host to cause viral infections) and the risk of inducing insertional mutations through the random integration of the provirus into the host genome.[78]

Manufacture of Viral Vectors

Pharmaceutical companies face significant issues when determining how to manufacture mass quantities of gene therapy. Good manufacturing practice and quality control procedures, as required by the FDA, are difficult to ensure when working with biologic systems such as viral vectors. With retroviral vectors, the primary safety concern is that an RCR could arise during the manufacturing process. This issue has been analyzed extensively by the National Institutes of Health (NIH) Recombinant DNA Advisory Committee and the FDA. The two groups concluded that with the current FDA-required quality control procedures, it is highly unlikely that a patient would ever receive sufficient RCR to produce a retroviremia or malignancy. However, the manufacturing and testing process that ensures this degree of safety is complex and costly.[73] As a result, it could take several years and millions of dollars for a pharmaceutical company to develop an efficient manufacturing system that could produce safe and effective gene therapy vectors on a large scale.[73] Although viral gene delivery systems are considered an efficient form of gene delivery, two factors suggest that nonviral gene delivery systems will be preferred: safety and ease of manufacturing. A synthetic gene delivery system would eliminate the danger of producing a recombinant RCR or other toxicity that could occur with the use of biologically active viral particles.[73]

Ethical Considerations in Gene Therapy

Gene therapy for the treatment of serious disease is widely accepted as ethically appropriate when performed in the context of a clinical trial. Because side effects from gene therapy protocols have been minimal, there is the risk that genetic engineering may be used for nontherapeutic purposes (i.e., cosmetic purposes). The first Gene Therapy Policy Conference organized by the NIH Recombinant DNA Advisory Committee addressed this issue in September 1997. They discussed a case in which a U.S. biotechnology company had developed the technology for transferring genes into hair follicle cells. The company began searching for genes that promote hair growth, with the clinical objective of reversing chemotherapy-induced alopecia in cancer patients. However, once a product is licensed for a specific indication, it can be prescribed by physicians for off-label use. The committee concluded that the FDA would need to use a careful risk to benefit analysis when evaluating gene therapy products that would take into account the extensive off-label use that can occur with any product.[73]

Although genetic cloning is not considered gene therapy, a recent trial has attracted considerable attention. In February 1997, scientists in Scotland published an article in *Nature* that described the successful breeding of cloned sheep. An udder cell from a 6-year-old adult sheep was cultured in vitro and the nucleus of this cell was transferred to an enucleated egg, which was then implanted into a surrogate mother. This process led to the birth of a healthy lamb, Dolly, which was genetically identical to the sheep from which the udder cell was taken. This work demonstrated that the process responsible for the normal differentiation of cells could be overcome by nuclear transfer of a differentiated cell into an enucleated egg.[79] Dolly is the first mammal to develop from a cell that was derived from adult tissue. This experiment has attracted worldwide attention and has led to speculation about the possibility of cloning humans.[79] Because scientific advances are occurring rapidly, moral and ethical issues must be taken into consideration.

Clinical Applications of Gene Therapy

Inhibition of Oncogene Expression

Oncogenes, or tumor-promoting genes, have been implicated in a number of cancers. Oncogenes cause uncontrolled cell growth when mutated or overexpressed, so neutralization of these genes could reverse the malignant phenotype.[78] Methods to replace or deactivate overexpressed tumor-promoting genes have been pursued by a number of researchers. The most common method is to introduce antisense RNA into the cell to stop expression of the oncogene. More recent efforts have included both antisense RNA to stop the activity of the tumor-promoting oncogene and a mutant antisense resistant oncogene with the desired activity. This method is theorized to inhibit the expression of the endogenous oncogene, and the "corrected" oncogene restores regulated DNA synthesis.[80]

Introduction of Tumor Suppressor Genes

Tumor suppressor genes, such as p53, are responsible for maintaining normal cell replication. A malfunctioning or missing tumor suppressor gene results in the uncontrolled proliferation of certain malignancies. By introducing a suppressor gene, it may be possible to reverse the malignant potential of the tumor cells.[80] A phase I clinical trial was completed in which lung tumors were injected with a p53 retrovirus. The treatment was nontoxic and suppressed tumor growth in six of nine patients.[81] Mutant or absent p53 status has also been shown to be associated with resistance to radiation therapy and to apoptosis-inducing chemotherapy.[81] The combination of p53 gene transduction with radiation or chemotherapy has resulted in local tumor control that is superior to either therapy alone and is currently under investigation in clinical trials.[81]

Suicide Gene Therapy

Because retroviral DNA is incorporated into rapidly dividing cancer cells more rapidly than normal cells, it is possible to preferentially introduce genetic material into cancer cells. By introducing genes that make the tumor susceptible to substances that will not normally harm cells or cause them to metabolize harmless substances into toxic substances, tumor cells can be killed preferentially. An example of a common suicide gene is the herpes simplex thymidine kinase gene, which is currently being used in a large phase III trial for patients with glioblastoma multiforme. Nucleoside analogs such as acyclovir and ganciclovir bind to this gene product but not to endogenous thymidine kinase. Another example is the *E. coli* cytosine deaminase *(cd)* gene. This gene, which is not present in normal mammalian cells, causes the cell to metabolize 5-fluorocytosine, a nontoxic substance, into 5-fluorouracil, which is toxic to cells. If this gene is inserted into cancer cells, they become susceptible to a substance that will not harm normal cells.[80,82] A number of clinical trials are evaluating the role of suicide gene therapy for the treatment of brain tumors, ovarian cancer, and malignant mesothelioma.[78]

Immunomodulatory Gene Therapy

Introducing tumor-killing cytokines into tumor cells can enhance the host immune response. This can be accomplished in vivo, where the genes for cytokine production are introduced into the tumor, or in vitro, where the cytokine gene is introduced into the tumor cells in culture and the tumor cells are then reinfused into the patient. In a number of preclinical cancer models, injection with tumor cells expressing cytokines such as IL-2, GM-CSF, or IFN-γ can generate cellular immunologic activity against tumors and in many cases can cure or significantly control the growth of established local or metastatic tumors.[81] A combined cytokine and costimulatory molecule vaccination shows promise as a way to increase the efficiency of tumor vaccines.[81] The most widely studied costimulatory molecule, B7, binds to the CD28 receptor on T cells and enhances T-cell activation. Transfection of B7 alone into tumor cells inhibits tumor growth through immunologic activity.[81] Covaccination of B7 with IL-2 markedly enhances this activity and may define future approaches to the improvement of vaccination strategies.[81] Another gene therapy approach is to enhance the tumor-killing ability of tumor-infiltrating lymphocytes (TIL) by inserting the gene for TNF into harvested TIL cells and then reinfusing them. This localizes the therapeutic effect of TNF and limits systemic exposure.[83]

Clinical Trials

Therapeutic trials of gene therapy have been undertaken in cancer, genetic diseases, and infectious diseases. Genetic diseases that have been targeted include severe combined immune deficiency (SCID), Gaucher's disease, Franconia's anemia, cystic fibrosis, and hypercholesterolemia.[72] To date the only infectious disease targeted by gene therapy has been AIDS. More than 300 clinical protocols have been approved worldwide and more than 3000 patients have carried genetically engineered cells. One phase III and several phase II clinical trials are under way, with the remainder of the clinical studies being smaller phase I or II trials.

Cancer

The first human trial of gene therapy conducted in the United States began in May 1989 and was designed not as a direct therapeutic trial but as a method of marking cells critical to the treatment of cancer. The trial used a retroviral vector to genetically mark TILs in patients with cancer.[70] In TIL therapy, which is used for metastatic melanoma and renal cell carcinoma, part of the tumor is removed, and the lymphoid cells that had successfully infiltrated the tumor are harvested. These TIL cells are then cultured with IL-2 to stimulate growth. The large numbers of TIL cells are then reinfused into the patient. The TIL cells were marked by inserting the genetic code for the bacterial antibiotic resistance gene neomycin phosphotransferase, and it became possible to track them.[80]

A phase III trial currently under way in more than 40 centers in North America and Europe, is scheduled to enroll 250 patients who have the diagnosis of glioblastoma multiforme, a malignant brain tumor. The goal of this trial is to insert a gene capable of directing cell killing to the tumor cells while protecting the normal brain cells. In the case of glioblastoma multiforme, the only dividing cells in the area of a brain tumor are tumor cells and the vascular endothelial cells which supply blood to the tumor. Because retroviral vectors transduce only into dividing cells, only tumor cells and tumor blood vessel cells would be targeted. Retroviral vectors are being modified to carry the herpes simplex thymidine kinase gene. This gene can add a phosphate group to nonphosphorylated nucleosides, whereas the endogenous human thymidine kinase cannot. Thus, when an abnormal nucleoside, such as the drug ganciclovir, is given to a patient, only the cells that express the herpes simplex thymidine kinase gene will phosphorylate the drug, incorporate it into their DNA, and be killed. In the clinical trial, the retroviral vectors carrying the herpes simplex thymidine kinase gene are injected into the patients in the area of residual tumor after surgical resection. After 7 days, the patients are treated with ganciclovir. Results of this clinical trial are not yet available.[73] Several phase II trials are evaluating gene therapy vectors as vaccines for the treatment of metastatic malignant melanoma and for head and neck squamous cell carcinoma.[73]

Genetic Diseases

In September 1990, a therapeutic trial designed to treat adenosine deaminase (ADA) deficiency in children with SCID was initiated.[70] The protocol called for the isolation of peripheral lymphocytes from an ADA-deficient patient. The human ADA gene was then introduced into the lymphocytes with a retroviral vector in vitro. The modified lymphocytes were multiplied and then reintroduced into two young girls. The patients were re-treated at 6- to 8-week intervals.[70] Today, both girls are doing well and continue to lead essentially normal lives. They both continue to receive polyethylene glycol-ADA (PEG-ADA). Both girls have gene-engineered T lymphocytes in their circulation after more than 7 years; however, no definitive conclusion can be drawn about the roles of PEG-ADA and gene therapy in their excellent clinical course.[73]

Familial hypercholesterolemia, a disease characterized by extraordinarily high levels of cholesterol, has also been treated with gene therapy. The disease is caused by defective or absent receptors for low-density lipoprotein (LDL). The gene therapy protocol calls for a portion of the patient's liver to be removed. The hepatocytes obtained from the liver then undergo retroviral-mediated gene transfer of the LDL receptor genes. The altered liver cells are then returned to the patient's liver via a catheter.[70,84] Initial results have been encouraging. with the first patient tolerating the procedure well and showing evidence of engraftment and an improvement in LDL:HDL ratio from 10:13 pretreatment to 5:8 posttreatment.[85]

CONCLUSION

A thorough knowledge of the immune system is a prerequisite to the understanding of many human diseases. With new knowledge about the regulation of the immune system, coupled with the powerful tools offered by recombinant DNA technology, a new era in the diagnosis and treatment of many diseases that have eluded effective intervention is beginning.

KEY POINTS

- Our understanding of recombinant DNA technology and gene therapy is fundamentally changing the way we will treat diseases in the future.
- Biotechnology products are being produced at a remarkably rapid pace and are providing new therapies for some diseases that previously had no treatment (Table 7.3).
- Gene therapy can offer a cure for many previously incurable diseases if the techniques for its production are refined and safety concerns are addressed.
- Pharmacists must have a working knowledge of the immune system, of new methods of drug delivery, and of the different biotechnologically produced therapeutic products that will be the drugs of the future.

Table 7.3 ▪ Biotechnology Products in the Marketplace

Therapeutic Category	Product (Trade Name), Company	Application	Approval Date
Autoimmune disorders	Recombinant interferon-β1B (Betaseron), Berlex Labs/Chiron	Relapsing, remitting multiple sclerosis	1993
	Recombinant interferon-β1B (Avonex), Biogen	Relapsing forms of multiple sclerosis	1996
Blood disorders	Human antihemophilic factor (Alphanate), Alpha Therapeutic Corp.	Treatment of hemophilia A or acquired factor VII deficiency	1997
	Human coagulation factor IX (virus-filtered) (AlphaNine SD), Alpha Therapeutic Corp.	To prevent and control bleeding in patients with factor IX deficiency caused by hemophilia B	1996
	Coagulation factor IX (recombinant) (BeneFix), Genetics Institute	Treatment of hemophilia B	1997
	Recombinant antihemophilic factor (Bioclate, Helixate), Centeon	Blood-clotting factor VIII for the treatment of hemophilia A	2/93 1994
	(Kogenate), Bayer		1989
	(Recombinate), Baxter Healthcare (Genetics Institute)		1986
	Epoetin-α (Epogen), Amgen	Treatment of anemia associated with chronic renal failure and anemia in AZT-treated HIV-infected patients	1989, 12/90 (AZT indication only)
	Epoetin-α (Procrit), Ortho Biotech	Anemia in patients on cancer chemotherapy	1993
		Use in anemic patients scheduled to undergo elective noncardiac, nonvascular surgery	2/96
	Immune globulin (Venoglobulin-S), Alpha Therapeutic Corp.	Primary immunodeficiency	1995
		Idiopathic thrombocytopenic purpura	1/91
		Kawasaki disease	1/91
	Granulocyte–macrophage colony-stimulating factor (Leukine), Immunex	Neutrophil recovery after autologous and allogeneic BMT	1991, 11/95
		Treatment of neutropenia after induction chemotherapy in older patients with acute myeloid leukemia	1995
		Mobilization of peripheral progenitor cells for peripheral stem cell transplant	2/95
	Granulocyte colony-stimulating factor (Neupogen), Amgen	Chemotherapy-induced neutropenia	1994
		BMT accompanied by neutropenia	2/94
		Severe chronic neutropenia	1995
		Autologous BMT engraftment or failure	2/95
		Mobilization of autologous peripheral blood progenitor cells after chemotherapy	1991
	Interleukin-11 (Neumega), Genetics Institute	Prevention of severe chemotherapy-induced thrombocytopenia	1/97
Cancer	Liposomal daunorubicin (DaunoXome), NeXstar Pharmaceuticals Inc.	Treatment for HIV-related Kaposi's sarcoma	1996
	Pegylated liposomal doxorubicin hydrochloride (Doxil STEALTH), SEQUUS Pharmaceuticals Inc.	Second-line therapy for Kaposi's sarcoma in patients with AIDS (liposomal drug delivery)	1/95
	Interferon-α (Intron A), Schering-Plough	Hairy cell leukemia	1986
		AIDS-related Kaposi's sarcoma	1/88
		Malignant melanoma	1992
	(Roferon-A), Hoffmann-La Roche Inc.	Follicular lymphoma with chemotherapy	1997
	2-CDA (Leustatin), Ortho Biotech	Hairy cell leukemia	1993
	Pegasparginase (Oncaspar), Enzon/Rhone-Poulenc Rorer	Pegylated asparaginase for the treatment of acute lymphoblastic leukemia	1994
	Porfimer sodium (Photofrin), Ligand Pharmaceuticals	Palliative treatment of totally and partially obstructing cancers of esophagus	1/95
	Interleukin-2 (Proleukin), Chiron	Treatment of renal carcinoma	1992
		Treatment of metastatic melanoma	1998
	Rituximab (Rituxan), IDEC Pharmaceuticals/Genentech	Relapsed or refractory low-grade or follicular CD20-positive B-cell non-Hodgkin's lymphoma	1/97
Cardiovascular disorders	Tissue plasminogen activator (Activase) Genentech	Treatment of acute myocardial infarction	1/87, 10/96
		Treatment of acute massive pulmonary embolism	1990
	(Retavase), Centocor, Inc.	Treatment of acute ischemic stroke within 3 hr of onset	1996

(continued)

Table 7.3 *(continued)*

Therapeutic Category	Product (Trade Name), Company	Application	Approval Date
	Human albumin (Albutein), Alpha Therapeutic Corp.	Treatment of hypovolemic shock Use in cardiopulmonary bypass procedures	1986
	Abciximab (ReoPro), Centocor, Inc./Eli Lilly	Reduce acute blood clot–related complications in high-risk PTCA patients Reduce acute blood clot–related complications for all patients undergoing any coronary intervention Treatment of unstable angina not responding to convention treatment when PTCA is planned within 24 hr	2/94 2/97
Endocrine disorders	Recombinant insulin (Humalog), Eli Lilly (Humulin-human), Eli-Lilly (Novolin-human), Novo Nordisk	Treatment of diabetes	1996 1982 1982
	Repaglinide (Prandin), Novo Nordisk	Antidiabetic agent for the treatment of type 2 diabetes	2/97
Genetic disorders	Growth hormone (BioTroin), Biotech General (Protropin), Genentech (Norditropin), Novo Nordisk	Growth hormone deficiency in children	1995 1985 1997
	(Geref), Serono labs (GenoTropin), Pharmacia and Upjohn	Growth hormone deficiency in children and adults	1995 1997
	(Humatrope), Eli Lilly	Somatotropin deficiency syndrome in adults	1996
	Somatropin rDNA (Nutropin/Nutropin AQ), Genentech	Growth hormone deficiency in children and adults Growth failure associated with chronic renal insufficiency before kidney transplantation Short stature associated with Turner syndrome	1993, 1/94 1996 2/96
	Dornase, α recombinant (Pulmozyme), Genentech	Mild to moderate cystic fibrosis Advanced cystic fibrosis	2/93 2/96
	Ceredase, Genzyme	Treatment of type I Gaucher's disease	1991
Infectious diseases	Liposomal amphotericin B (Abelcet), The Liposome Company (AmBisome), NeXstar Pharmaceuticals Inc. (AMPHOTEC), SEQUUS Pharmaceuticals	Treatment of invasive fungal infections in patients who are refractory to or intolerant of conventional amphotericin B Second-line treatment of invasive aspergillosis infections	1/95 1997 1/96
	Interferon-α (Infergen)	Hepatitis C	1997
	Immune globulin enriched in antibodies against respiratory syncytial virus (Respi-Gam), MedImmune, Inc.	Prevention of respiratory synctytial virus in infants under 2 with bronchopulmonary dysplasia or history of prematurity	1996
Immune function disorders	Interferon-γ1b (Actimmune), Genentech	Treatment of chronic granulomatous disease	2/90
	Adenosine deaminase (Adagen), Enzon	Treatment of severe combined immunodeficiency disease	1990
Reproductive disorders	Follicle-stimulating hormone (Follistim), Organon Inc. (Fertinex), Serono Labs	Recombinant hormone for treatment of infertility	1997 1996
	Follitropin-α (Gonal-F)	Functional infertility not caused by primary ovarian failure	1997
Transplant	CMV immune globulin (CytoGam), MedImmune Inc.	Prevention of cytomegalovirus in patients undergoing kidney transplant	1990
	Muromonab-CD-3 (Orthoclone OKT3), Ortho Biotech	Reversal of acute kidney, heart, and liver transplant rejection	1986
	Daclizumab (Zenapax), Hoffmann-La Roche Basiliximab (Simulect), Novartis Pharmaceutical Corp.	Humanized monoclonal antibody for the prevention of kidney transplant rejection	2/97 1998
Vaccines	Recombinant hepatitis B vaccine (Recombivax-HB), Merck (Engerix-B), SmithKline Beecham	Hepatitis B vaccine for adolescents and high-risk infants/adults/dialysis/pediatrics	1987 1989 1993 1989
Other	Platelet-derived growth factor becaplermin (Regranex-Gel), Ortho-McNeil/Chiron	Treatment of diabetic foot ulcers	2/97

AZT, azidothymidine; *HIV*, human immunodeficiency virus; *BMT, bone marrow transplantation; AIDS*, acquired immune deficiency syndrome; *PTCA*, percutaneous transluminal coronary angioplasty.

REFERENCES

1. Tami JA, Parr M, Thompson J. The immune system. Am J Hosp Pharm 43:2483–2493, 1986.
2. Koeller J, Tami J. Concepts in immunology and immunotherapeutics. Bethesda, MD: ASHP Publications, 1990.
3. Campion J. A basic review of the immune system. US Pharmacist 15(8):19–26, 1990.
4. An introduction to pharmaceutical biotechnology. Regents of the University of Wisconsin System, 1990.
5. Dertzbaugh MT. Genetically engineered vaccines: a review. Plasmid 39:100–113, 1998.
6. Butler VA. Points to consider on plasmid DNA vaccines for preventive infectious disease indications. Docket no. 96N-0400. Rockville, MD: Food and Drug Administration, 1996.
7. Johnson CS. Interleukin-1: therapeutic potential for solid tumors. Cancer Invest 11(5):600–608, 1993.
8. Staren E, Essner R, Economou JS. Overview of biological response modifiers. Semin Surg Oncol 5:379–384, 1989.
9. Kirkpatrick C. Biological response modifiers. Interferons, interleukins, and transfer factor. Ann Allergy 62:170–176, 1989.
10. Vose JM, Armitage JO. Clinical applications of hematopoietic growth factors. J Clin Oncol 13(4):1023–1035, 1995.
11. Maini A, Morse PD, Wang CY, et al. New developments in the use of cytokines for cancer therapy. Anticancer Res 17:3803–3808, 1997.
12. Whittington R, Faulds D. Interleukin-2, a review of its pharmacological properties and therapeutic use in patients with cancer. Drugs 46:446–514, 1993.
13. Oprelvekin (IL-11; Neumega) package insert, Genetics Institute, 1998.
14. Kaushansky K. The thrombocytopenia of cancer: prospects for effective cytokine therapy. Hematol Oncol Clin North Am 10(2):431–455, 1996.
15. Newland AC. Is interleukin 3 active in anticancer drug-induced thrombocytopenia? Cancer Chemother Pharmacol 38(Suppl):S83–S38, 1996.
16. Puri RK, Siegel JP. Interleukin-4 and cancer therapy. Cancer Invest 11:473–486, 1993.
17. Leach MW, Snyder EA, Sinha DP, et al. Safety evaluation of recombinant human interleukin-4. Clin Immunol Immunopathol 83(1):8–11, 1997.
18. Cohen MC, Cohen S. Cytokine function: a study in biologic diversity. Am J Clin Pathol 105:589–598, 1996.
19. Baumann MA, Paul CC, Grace MJ. Effects of interleukin-5 on acute myeloid leukemias. Am J Hematol 39:269–274, 1992.
20. Bauer J, Herrman F. Interleukin-6 in clinical medicine. Ann Hematol 62:203–210, 1991.
21. Bataille R, Harousseau JL. Multiple myeloma. N Engl J Med 336(23):1657–1664, 1997.
22. Papanicolaou DA, Wilder RL, Manolagas SC, et al. The pathophysiologic roles of interleukin-6 in human disease. Ann Intern Med 128:127–137, 1998.
23. Appasamy PM. Interleukin-7: biology and potential clinical applications. Cancer Invest 11:487–499, 1993.
24. Van Zee KJ, Fischer E, Hawes AS, et al. Effects of intravenous IL-8 administration in nonhuman primates. J Immunol 148:1746–1752, 1992.
25. Murphy PM. Neutrophil receptors for interleukin-8 and related CXC chemokines. Semin Hematol 34(4):311–318, 1997.
26. Cortes J, Kurzrock R. Interleukin-10 in non-Hodgkin's lymphoma. Leuk Lymphoma 26(3–4):251–259, 1997.
27. Geissler K. Current status of clinical development of interleukin-10. Curr Opin Hematol 3(3):203–208, 1996.
28. De Vries JE. Immunosuppressive and anti-inflammatory properties of interleukin. Ann Med 27(5):537–541, 1995.
29. Isaacs C, Roberg NJ, Bailey FA, et al. Randomized placebo-controlled study of recombinant human interleukin-11 to prevent chemotherapy-induced thrombocytopenia in patients with breast cancer receiving dose-intensive cyclophosphamide and doxorubicin. J Clin Oncol 15(11):3368–3377, 1997.
30. Tepler I, Elias L, Smith JW, et al. A randomized placebo-controlled trial of recombinant human interleukin-11 in cancer patients with severe thrombocytopenia due to chemotherapy. Blood87(9):3607–3614, 1996.
31. Gately MK. Interleukin-12: a recently discovered cytokine with potential for enhancing cell-mediated immune responses to tumors. Cancer Invest 11:500–506, 1993.
32. Tahara H, Lotze MT. Antitumor effects of interleukin-12: applications for the immunotherapy and gene therapy of cancer. Gene Ther 2:96–106, 1995.
33. Romani L, Puccetti P, Bistoni F. Interleukin-12 in infectious diseases. Clin Microbiol Rev 10(4):611–636, 1997.
34. Ford R, Tamayo A, Martin B, et al. Identification of B-cell growth factors in effusion fluids from patients with aggressive B-cell lymphomas. Blood 86(1):283–293, 1995.
35. Spriggs, MK. Interleukin-17 and its receptor. J Clin Immunol17(5):366–369, 1997.
36. Gabrilove J. Introduction and overview of hematopoietic growth factors. Semin Hematol 26:1–4, 1989.
37. Yee GC. Focus on GM-CSF and G-CSF: promising biotherapeutics for use in hematology and oncology. Hosp Formul 25:943–948, 1990.
38. Bettelheim P, Muhm M, Valent P, et al. GM-CSF in combination with cytotoxic chemotherapy in AML patients. Bone Marrow Transplant 1:127–130, 1990.
39. Buechner T, Hiddemann W, Koenigsmann M, et al. Recombinant human GM-CSF following chemotherapy in high-risk AML. Bone Marrow Transplant 1:131–133, 1990.
40. Vose JM, Armitage JO. Clinical applications of hematopoietic growth factors. J Clin Oncol 13(4):1023–1035, 1995.
41. Moore M. Hematopoietic growth factors in cancer. Cancer 65:836–844, 1990.
42. Appelbaum FR. The clinical use of hematopoietic growth factors. Semin Hematol 26:7–14, 1989.
43. Morstyn G, Lieschke G, Sheridan W, et al. Clinical experience with recombinant human granulocyte colony-stimulating factor and granulocyte macrophage colony-stimulating factor. Semin Hematol 26:9–13, 1989.
44. Glaspy J, Golde D. Clinical applications of the myeloid growth factors. Semin Hematol 26:14–17, 1989.
45. American Society of Clinical Oncology. Recommendations for the use of hematopoietic colony-stimulating factors: evidence-based, clinical practice guidelines. J Clin Oncol 12:2471–2508, 1994.
46. Sopall EJ, Wheeler CA, Turnet SA, et al. A randomized phase 3 study of PBPC mobilization by stem cell factor (SCF, STEMGEN) and Filgrastim in patients with high-risk breast cancer [Abstract #2629]. Blood 90(10, Suppl 1), 1997.
47. Tyring SK. Interferons: biochemistry and mechanisms of action. Am J Obstet Gynecol 172:1350–1353, 1995.
48. Agarwala S, Kirkwood J. Interferons in the therapy of solid tumors. Oncology 51:129–136, 1994.
49. McManus BC. Clinical use of biologic response modifiers in cancer treatment. Ann Pharmacother 24:761–767, 1990.
50. Takaku F. Clinical application of cytokines for cancer treatment. Oncology 51:123–128, 1994.
51. Ozer H, George SL, Schiffer CA, et al. Prolonged subcutaneous administration of recombinant alpha 2b interferon in patients with previously untreated Philadelphia chromosome-positive chronic-phase chronic myelogenous leukemia: effect on remission duration and survival: Cancer and Leukemia Group B Study 8583. Blood 82(9):2975–2984, 1993.
52. Tura S, Baccarani M, Zuffa E, et al. Interferon alpha 2a as compared with conventional chemotherapy for the treatment of chronic myeloid leukemia. N Engl J Med 330:820–825, 1994.
53. Kirkwood JM, Strawderman MH, Ernstoff MS, et al. Interferon alfa-2b adjuvant therapy of high-risk resected cutaneous melanoma: the Eastern Cooperative Oncology Group Trial EST 1684. J Clin Oncol 14:7–17, 1996.
54. Urabe A. Interferons for the treatment of hematological malignancies. Oncology 51:137–141, 1994.
55. Spiegel RJ. The alpha interferons: clinical overview. Semin Oncol 14:1–12, 1987.
56. Weinstock-Guttman B, Ransohoff RM, Kinkel RP, et al. The interferons: biological effects, mechanisms of action and use in multiple sclerosis. Ann Neurol 37:7–13, 1995.
57. Triozzi P, Rinehart J. The role of IFN-beta in cancer therapy. Cancer Surv 8:799–807, 1989.
58. Vaickus L. Antitumor antibodies as therapeutic reagents. Pharmacol ther 15(12):143–161, 1990.
59. Dillman RO. Monoclonal antibodies for treating cancer. Ann Intern Med 111:592–603, 1989.
60. Reisfeld RA. Monoclonal antibodies in cancer immunotherapy. Clin Lab Med 12(2):201–216, 1992.
61. ENBREL package insert, Immunex Corporation and Wyeth-Ayerst Laboratories, 1998.
62. McLaughlin P, Cabanillas AJ, Grillo-Lopez A. IDEC-C2B8 anti CD20 antibody: final report on a phase III pivotal trial in patients with relapsed low-grade or follicular lymphoma. Blood 88:90a, 1996.
63. Roche Rituximab Warnings Strengthened in European labeling. Health News Daily via NewsEdge Corporation. December 1, 1998.
64. Slamon D, Leyland-Jones B, Shak S, et al. Addition of Herceptin (humanized anti-HER2 antibody) to first line chemotherapy for HER2 overexpressing metastatic breast cancer (HER2+/MBC) markedly increases anti-cancer activity: a randomized, multi-national controlled phase III trial. Proc ASCO 377(17): 98a, 1998.

65. Herceptin package insert, Genentech, 1998.
66. Tang K, Harp DR. Bexxar phase II/III enrollment complete: BLA submission on schedule for 4Q 1998. BT Alex Brown Research, 1998.
67. ReoPro package insert. Centocor, Eli Lilly & Company, 1995.
68. Targan SR, Hanauer SR, van Deventer SJH, et al. A short-term study of chimeric monoclonal antibody cA2 to tumor necrosis factor alpha for Crohn's disease. N Engl J Med 337(15):1029–1035, 1997.
69. Remicade package insert, Centocor, 1998.
70. Tolstoshev P. Gene therapy, concepts, current trials and future direction. Annu Rev Pharmacol 32:573–596, 1993.
71. Roth JA, Cristiano RJ. Gene therapy for cancer: what have we done and where are we going? J Natl Cancer Inst 89(1):21–39, 1997.
72. Kerr WG, Mule JJ. Gene therapy: current status and future prospects. J Leukemia Biol 56:210–214, 1994.
73. Anderson WF. Human gene therapy. Nature 392(Suppl):25–30, 1998.
74. Weichselbaum RR, Kufe D. Gene therapy of cancer. Lancet 349(Suppl II):10–12, 1997.
75. Kay MA, Liu D, Hoogerbrugge PM. Gene therapy. Proc Natl Acad Sci USA 94:12744–12746, 1997.
76. Verma IM, Somia N. Gene therapy: promises, problems and prospects. Nature 389:239–242, 1997.
77. Blattner WA. Retroviruses that cause human disease. In: Wyngaarden JB, Smith LH, Bennett JC. Cecil textbook of medicine. 19th ed. Philadelphia: WB Saunders, 1992:1845.
78. Hwu, P, Rosenberg SA. Gene therapy of cancer. In: DeVita VT. Cancer: principles & practice of oncology. 5th ed. Philadelphia: Lippincott-Raven, 1997:3005.
79. Wilmut I, Schnieke AE, McWhir J, et al. Viable offspring derived from fetal and adult mammalian cells. Nature 385:810–813, 1997.
80. Tolaza EM, Economou JS. Gene therapy of cancer. In: Haskell CM. Cancer treatment. 4th ed. Philadelphia: WB Saunders, 1995:305.
81. Hall SJ, Chen S, Woo SL. Gene therapy '97: the promise and reality of cancer gene therapy. Am J Hum Genet 1:785–790, 1997.
82. Rosenberg SA. Immunotherapy and gene therapy of cancer. Cancer Res 51(Suppl):5074s–5079s, 1991.
83. Culver KW. Clinical applications of gene therapy for cancer. Clin Chem 40:510–512, 1994.
84. Ledley FD. Hepatic gene therapy: present and future. Hepatology 18:1263–1273, 1993.
85. Grossman M, Raper SE, Kozarsky K, et al. Successful ex-vivo gene therapy directed to liver in a patient with familial hypercholesterolaemia. Nat Genet 6(4):335–341, 1994.

CHAPTER 8

PATIENT COMMUNICATION IN CLINICAL PHARMACY PRACTICE

Marie E. Gardner, Richard N. Herrier, and Helen Meldrum

DEFINITION

Patient communication in clinical practice is defined as the dialog between a pharmacist and patient for the purpose of obtaining information needed to assess patient status, provide patient education, and support the patient's attempts to comply with the therapeutic regimen.

TREATMENT GOALS: PATIENT COMMUNICATION

- Obtain an accurate medication history.
- Evaluate new symptoms.
- Verify patient understanding of key information about disease and treatment.
- Assess the status of chronic diseases.
- Identify and address factors that may reduce compliance.
- Verify existing patient compliance practices.

INTRODUCTION

The health care professions are founded on strong technical and people skills. Although all health professionals are well versed in the technical aspects of their profession, most are not as skilled in interpersonal communication. In contemporary clinical practice, good communication skills are critical to achieving optimal patient outcomes. The goal of this chapter is to briefly summarize some of the skills required to provide high-quality patient consultation and education. These techniques are very important in improving outcomes for the patient and for increasing practitioners' satisfaction with their professional roles. Although this is a broad topic, the focus of this chapter is limited to a review of essential communication skills, clinical interviewing and medication history guidelines, symptom assessment, basic medication consultation skills, and strategies for interviewing to improve compliance and monitor clinical progress.

In this era of technological wonders, clear, direct, and sensitive communication between people seems to be in short supply. Extensive research on customer service and patient education shows that when providers communicate well, patients are more likely to comply with treatment plans and are less likely to complain or entertain thoughts of legal retribution because of perceived mistreatment. Additionally, Bolton[1] states that 80% of professionals who fail at their jobs do so because of poor human relations skills. Humanistic psychologist Carl Rogers[2] concludes that people seek counseling because of poor communication with others in their lives. Effective interpersonal communication may be the most important skill we can develop. To function as professionals, pharmacists must not only maintain an open attitude of ongoing learning about human relations, but also master the specific skills of questioning, empathic response, responsible language use, assertiveness, and conflict management.

SKILLS IN ASKING QUESTIONS

Most people are not very conscious about the types of questions they ask. Questions can be organized on a continuum from highly open to restricted to leading. Closed questions narrow the patient's options and evoke minimal recall levels of information instead of thoughtful elaborated responses. Table 8.1 shows examples.

When seeking information from most patients, it is best to begin with open-ended questions. These start with *who, what, where, when,* and *how*. Such questions allow the patient to answer in any number of ways. For example, a question such as "How have you been feeling since starting this new medication?" can elicit a response that the patient is feeling better (and is happy with the medication) or that side effects are present (and presumably the patient is unhappy with the medication). This type of question is preferred over "Are you feeling better?" and "The medicine hasn't made you sick, has it?" In medication history interviews and consultations, the use of open-ended questions is of paramount importance.

It is important to remember that not all open questions are equally effective. "Why didn't you finish your antibiotic?" implies strong criticism and will provoke a defensive reaction from the patient. In most cases, when trying to elicit the patient's reasoning, it is better to start with a universal statement and move to an open question (e.g., "Most people don't realize how important it is to finish an antibiotic because an infection can appear to be gone but actually be lingering. What has been your experience in trying to take antibiotics?"). Although many pharmacists fear that this approach will consume too much time, when quick questions are asked in ways that produce defensiveness, patients learn to hide the real and truthful answers because they do not trust their health care providers.

What Is Empathic Responding and Why Is It Essential?

Many pharmacists have had no coursework in basic counseling and communication skills. Providers often are fearful that they won't know what to do if the patient has a deeply emotional reaction. "I'm sorry" sounds empty and inadequate in the face of such feeling. However, empathic communication is a key skill that helps patients open up and share their concerns. Specifically, empathic communication means using reflective responding, a type of active listening that reflects the thought or feeling of the speaker's communication. Practitioners fear opening up Pandora's box by encouraging patients to elaborate on issues that they might not otherwise discuss in a direct fashion. However, if pharmacists do not use this essential skill, patients may conclude that the provider is not interested or that the discussion is bothersome or too time-consuming. Extensive research links empathic communication to patient satisfaction, improved diagnostic assessment, less litigation, and better outcomes.[3–5]

Sometimes, the professional demeanor of pharmacists appears to be cultivated to protect the provider from his or her own discomfort. Unfortunately, such a demeanor prevents genuine communication with the patient. Every provider has heard mentors and colleagues say, "Don't let it get to you." On some level, this advice could be translated as "Don't have feelings about the patient." Without use of empathy skills, which include reflective responding, effective paraphrasing, summarizing, and using words that mirror the patient's thoughts and feelings, providers often report feeling overwhelmed by their patients' or coworkers' emotional reactions, with no idea about how to handle the situation.

Effective empathy skills help patients feel safe in discussing their concerns with providers. When trust is established, the patient is more likely to reveal clinically relevant data. Much of the theory on empathic facilitation is based on the work of Carl Rogers.[2,6] Rogers and colleagues came to believe that three conditions were necessary for the maintenance of mental health: congruence (patients would not need to develop a protective facade), unconditional positive regard (patients would feel warmth, interest, respect, and fondness from their providers), and nonjudgmental understanding (patients benefit most when they feel that they can share their perceptions, which will be accepted as valid without feedback that communicates approval or disapproval).

Because these conditions often are lacking, most people express their feelings indirectly. Indirect messages are hard to decode, and the listener's interpretation of the speaker's message generally goes unspoken. Indirect communication is one reason why needs and expectations often are not met.

This indirect expression of concerns is replicated in patients' patterns of questions about medications. For instance, they may present secondary concerns ("What if I forget to take this with food?") that mask a deeper concern ("What if this makes me sicker?"). The presentation of peripheral concerns may test the provider. If the provider heedlessly launches into a lecture about how to remember to take the medicine at mealtime, then he or she is missing the deeper meaning. Given this response, the patient may be afraid to ask whether the medicine will cause illness because such a question could be interpreted as an insult to the pharmacist who is providing the medicine. Reflective responding reduces the emotional charge present during medication counseling. With the emotional tone decreased, the patient is able to process the information in

Table 8.1 ▪ Open- and Closed-Ended Questions

Very open	How have you been feeling since starting this new medication?
Open	What exactly has changed since you have started taking this medication?
Moderately open	Of the drugs we have tried, which do you think works best for you?
Highly closed	You're not having any side effects, are you?

Table 8.2 ▪ Possible Responses to Emotional Content in Patient Consultation

Judgmental response	"Of course this is the right medication. I wouldn't question the doctor on this."
Diverting response	"Oh, yes. When is your next appointment with the doctor?"
Advise giving	"I'd give this a good try if I were you."
Questioning/probing	"What did you see the doctor about?"
Reflective responding	"You sound concerned about taking this."

a more conscious manner.[7] Patients who are upset may need repeated demonstrations of empathy to relax to the point that information can be exchanged. Often, it is easier to learn about this type of reflective listening by examining what is *not* an empathic response. For instance, if the patient says to the pharmacist, "Do you think I'm getting the right medicine?" a variety of responses are possible. Table 8.2 shows examples of responses.

Judgmental responses imply judgment against what the patient is saying, diverting responses change the subject, advice giving moves to problem solving before the real concern is even known, and questioning seeks to probe the issue but neglects the emotional tone. All four of these responses avoid an open, nonjudgmental discussion of what is really bothering the patient. A fifth type of response, the reflecting or empathic response, attempts to open the discussion of the problem as perceived by the patient.

Making a reflective response initially is difficult for some pharmacists because most of us have not been taught these skills. Reflective responding attempts to reflect in words what the patient is saying or feeling. The reflection may be based on the content or thought expressed by the patient or the feelings associated with it, which are often not expressed overtly. Reflecting responses are especially useful when the patient is demonstrating emotions. Angry looks, pounding fists, averted eye contact, and head drooping all convey certain emotional states. Hesitating gestures or remarks such as "Well, I *guess* I could try it" all suggest concerns that must be brought to light gently. The first step in reflective responding is to identify and label the emotional state. The four basic emotional states are *mad, sad, glad,* and *afraid.* During patient consultation, observe nonverbal signs or verbal cues (e.g., hesitating words) that suggest one of the four feeling states. The second step is to put the word describing the feeling state into a sentence. Some basic structures for sentences include "Sounds like you're frustrated by that," "That would be frustrating," and "I can see that you're frustrated by it." Remarks such as these let patients know that you are listening and truly attempting to understand their concerns. Patients and their concerns remain the focus of the encounter. It is important to remember that skills in empathy do not come naturally. Rubin, Judd, and Conine[8] showed that untrained allied health students could not recognize what constitutes an empathic response. If health care providers do not master the skill of expressing empathy, communication will remain controlled by and centered on the practitioner. Patients are more likely to feel empowered and retain a sense of personal control if they can express their feelings in an atmosphere of acceptance.[9]

Responsible Language Use

In everyday discussion it is all too easy to blame other people for negative feelings or to pretend that emotions and thoughts are not important. The goal of communicators is to take responsibility for their messages and analyze them for suggestions of blame or denial. Pharmacists have high visibility as part of the interdisciplinary medical team, and each member of the team is responsible for analyzing breakdowns in communication and assessing their own roles in causing and solving the problem. Particularly when one is offering advice or making a complaint, or when there is a conflict of views, careless language choices can create a destructive communication climate. For example, when working with a patient who is noncompliant with an asthma control regimen, the pharmacist could say, "You are trying to overuse your medication now to make up for not using it correctly when you should have known better" (blaming) or "Oh, well, I guess as long as your attacks aren't too serious" (denial). Responsible language is the appropriate alternative. For example, the pharmacist could say, "I'm concerned about your having three more asthma attacks this month than last. Let's look at how you have been using the medication." Responsible language incorporates a statement of concern citing specifics of the case and a statement or question about what to do next. Notice that the pharmacist's comment neither places blame nor denies that a potentially serious situation exists. It focuses on the problem (more frequent attacks) as perceived by the pharmacist and proposes a joint effort to solve the problem. The skills of responsible ownership of language and specificity come together when we attempt to send assertive messages.

Assertiveness

With patients and coworkers alike, pharmacists must sometimes set limits on behavior that is too demanding, inappropriate, or uncompromising. For example, a consultant pharmacist to a nursing home recently had a case in which a 26-year-old drug-dependent man was admitted for total parenteral nutrition after a bout of alcoholic pancreatitis. The pharmacist was present at the nursing station and had to deal with his constant demands for intravenous narcotics, which were not clinically indicated. The pharmacist decided to use the CLEAR system, an acronym for the steps in formulating an assertive message.[10]

Clear description: "This is the fifth time this hour you have asked for morphine."

Listen: "I'm ready to listen if something new has come up."

Emotional reaction: "I'm finding it difficult to get my work done with the disruptions."

Assert: "I need you to not keep asking."

Results expected: "If you can do this for us, we will be able to work with you more during the time that you are here" or "... we will be able to respond more quickly when you really need us."

This assertive message incorporates the elements of a specific description of the problem behavior, a sharing of feelings that the behavior provokes, and a description of the consequences if the behavior does not stop. Sending clear, responsible messages is usually enough to help patients understand what kind of problems such behavior creates.

Conflict Management

When faced with an emotionally charged situation, most professionals try to avoid the other person, become too passive and accommodating, give in to the urge to fight in a competitive fashion, or compromise their needs prematurely. It is difficult to lower the emotional temperature of an interpersonal conflict so that the two parties can collaborate effectively. The assertiveness and empathy skills discussed previously are helpful in situations when used with appropriate timing and with sensitivity to the setting. Additionally, pharmacists have the option of deflection, which is a strategy of partial agreement. For example, it is more effective to say to a nurse, "You've got a good point. It would be great if we had more technicians; then we could get special orders up to you much faster" than to aggressively be defensive in the face of accusations about slow response.

Also, some of the criticism directed at the pharmacy is very vague. "You guys have got to get your act together" is a typical annoying criticism to which it is too easy to respond in kind. Instead, a strategy of inquiry is needed. A question such as "What is it exactly that makes it hard for you to do your job?" can go a long way toward eliciting useful information. When colleagues provide the information, empathic responding can address their concerns. As a last resort, if tempers are running too high, defer further discussion until after a cool-down period.

With improved skills of empathic and reflective responding, assertiveness, deflection, and inquiry, a strategy of deferral rarely is needed. Using an appropriate combination of these conflict management skills will keep difficult situations from escalating. Additional case studies on conflict resolution in pharmacy practice can be found in other sources.[10]

CLINICAL INTERVIEWING SKILLS

Many of the skills discussed in the previous section apply to clinical interviewing and medication consultation processes. This section discusses clinical interviewing skills as they relate to pharmacy practice. The term *interviewing* here means "bringing into view" the patient's problems and associated issues. The skills associated with interviewing can be applied to a highly structured, complete assessment of medication use or to a brief conversation with the patient about an adverse drug reaction. Each of these is discussed in more detail in this section.

Medication History

A thorough, detailed, up-to-date medication history provides the necessary background for consultation with the patient. Pharmacists have the most knowledge about patients' medication use patterns and outcomes. This allows them to communicate effectively with patients and medical providers on matters of drug therapy. Obtaining a detailed history of medication use entails more than giving the patient a form to complete. Knowledge of what history content to obtain and which process skills to use is fundamental to providing good pharmaceutical care in this area. Research shows that skills in medication history interviewing are improved with training on specific techniques.[11,12] The following is a step-by-step guide to conducting a comprehensive medication history.

Opening the Interview

The first of the core skills is opening the interview. Depending on the setting, the interview may have been requested, or perhaps this is a service offered to all patients. Greet the patient warmly. Identify yourself to the patient. Verify the patient's identity and that of others (e.g., caregivers) who are present. Caregivers may be needed to assist in clarifying information. On the other hand, if the patient is alert and oriented and can give valid information, address your remarks to the patient. State the purpose of the interview and relate it to expected outcomes for the patient. For example, you might start by saying, "Mrs. Smith, Dr. Welch asked me to speak with you about your medications so we can get a complete picture of what medications you are taking and how they are working."

Setting the Stage for Good Communication

Let the patient know about how long the interview will take to determine whether the interview can be completed at that time. Arrange furniture to allow face-to-face communication at eye level. Sit 2 to 4 feet from the patient, if possible. One study showed patients perceived pharmacists who used these nonverbal skills as more available to them, thus facilitating good rapport and better information exchange.[13] Maintain good nonverbal communication throughout the interview: lean slightly forward and maintain an open body posture and good eye contact. These skills are associated with patient satisfaction with care.[4]

Control the Flow of Information

The pharmacist must maintain the direction of the interview without appearing brusque or asking questions in an authoritarian style. Using appropriate questioning skills and having a structured framework are imperative to obtaining complete information in a manner that facilitates dialog while allowing the pharmacist to maintain control. Begin by asking the patient, "Tell me about the medications you are currently taking." Use open-ended, broad questions to start data gathering and proceed to closed-ended and forced-choice questions for discriminating details. Recall that open-ended questions start with *who, what, where, when, why,* and *how.* These questions cannot be answered with a *yes* or *no*. If the patient answers inappropriately, the pharmacist should suspect some barrier to communication, such as language differences, hearing difficulties, or diminished mental capacity. After obtaining information about the current medications, ask about past medication usage, allergies and adverse reactions, and lifestyle. Use as many open-ended questions as possible, minimizing the use of closed-ended questions. For example, ask "What medications for diabetes have you taken in the past?" rather than "Have you ever taken tolazamide? Or glipizide?" It may be necessary to ask such specific questions, but they should not be used to start discussion of past medications because they limit the patient's responses and do elicit other information. However, such questions are helpful if the patient admits to taking medication but can't recall the name. Using a closed-ended statement such as "Have you ever taken tolazamide?" at that time is appropriate. It can also be very helpful to ask such questions at the very end of an interview in which you may be asked to help select therapy. If you are planning to suggest a specific medication for the patient, ask the patient whether he or she has ever taken it. Patients with chronic conditions often have taken numerous medications, with both good and disastrous results. It is not uncommon for the patients to forget their past medications, only to recall having had a particular one when asked directly. The patient may then respond that he or she has taken the medication in question and that it did not help or caused a problem. This will change your recommendation.

After obtaining a block of related information, such as present medications, give a brief summary or paraphrase of pertinent points (e.g., "Mrs. Smith, you've told me you currently take hydrochlorothiazide and digoxin for your heart, and you used to take potassium, but you're not on it now and you're concerned that you need it. Is that correct?"). Between subsections of the history, use transitional statements to let the patient know that you are asking about a different type of information. After making the preceding statement, the pharmacist might say, "Now I'd like to ask about any allergies or reactions to medications you've had." Again, open the discussion with an open-ended statement such as "Tell me about your allergies." Keep using open-ended statements such as "What other reactions have you had?" to obtain further information. When clarification is needed, it is often necessary to use closed-ended questions. For example, the pharmacist might say, "You mentioned being allergic to 'mycin' but can't recall the name of the medication. Could it be erythromycin?"

The pharmacist needs to keep control of the interview to maximize effort while being efficient. When a long interview is expected, invariably the dialog strays from the topic at hand. The patient may ramble or ask a lot of questions or want to discuss matters not related to drug therapy. The pharmacist must keep the framework of questioning in mind, know what must be asked, and politely defer topics that are not germane to the drug history. Look for openings to bring the subject into focus (e.g., "Mr. Jones, you've been telling me how unpleasant it is to be in the hospital and I'd like to focus on how this medicine can help you stay out of the hospital."). When it is necessary to interrupt, address the patient by name and simply state your need to ask a certain question. Remember that the goal is not to have a social conversation with the patient but to obtain the medication history.

Obtain Complete Information

Table 8.3 shows a suggested order of content for a complete medication history. Begin by asking for information about the current prescribed medications. A broad opening question allows the patient to list all the medications currently prescribed. For each medication, ask specifically for the purpose, dosage, duration of use, some assessment of how the drug is working, and any problems the patient perceived. For medications taken as needed, question the patient to determine the amount used per day and per dose. Also, it is important to know what symptoms

Table 8.3 ▪ Content Items for a Comprehensive Medication History

Major Category of Information	Specific Areas to Probe
Current prescribed medications	Drug name Purpose Dosage Duration Beneficial effects Adverse effects
Current nonprescription medications	Drug name Purpose or symptoms treated Dosage and frequency of use Duration Assessment of effects
Past medication usage	Drug name Purpose Time period of use Reason for discontinuation
Drug allergies and adverse reactions	Drug name Date of reaction Type and severity of reaction
Lifestyle factors	Herbal remedies used Nicotine usage Alcohol usage Illicit drug usage Dietary habits Occupation Stressors

or in what context the patient uses the as-needed medications. Be attentive to vague responses. For example, a patient may state that he uses the β-agonist inhaler "only when I really need it." Question specifically how much the patient uses and how many times per day. Similarly, when the patient's responses include words such as *sometimes, not often,* or *occasionally,* probe for more specifics and document amounts of medications used.

After asking about prescribed routine and as-needed medications, ask about nonprescription medications used regularly. Because patients may not perceive vitamins or cold products as medications, it may be necessary to specifically ask, "What medications do you take for a cold? For stomach problems? For a headache?" Another approach is to query the patient using an approach similar to the review of systems used by physicians. Begin by asking about medications used for disorders of the head, eyes, ears, nose, and throat. Next, ask about products for respiratory, gastrointestinal, genitourinary, and skin conditions. When the patient mentions using any medication, ask specifically about the amounts used, duration of use, and outcome of treatment. Ask about herbal remedies and alternative treatments and obtain sufficient detail. This section of the patient's medication history usually is the longest but it is the most important. When it is done properly, the pharmacist will have a complete history of the medications currently being used by the patient.

Past medication usage is the next large block of data to be obtained. Ask about the medications previously used to treat the patient's clinical conditions. This is important because the pharmacist would not want to recommend medications that were ineffective or caused adverse reactions. It is useful to ask, "Why was that medication stopped?" or "Who stopped that medication?" It is helpful to know whether the physician advised stopping the medication or whether the patient made the decision alone. Before proceeding to the next history section, summarize significant points in past drug history to allow the patient to clarify information or add data.

Obtain complete information on drug sensitivities. Remember that many patients think of any adverse reaction as an "allergy," so it is important to clearly define the nature of the drug reaction. Begin with an open-ended statement such as "Tell me about any drug allergies or bad reactions you've had from medications." Ask for details of the reaction (when it occurred, what exactly happened) to provide a clear picture.

Last, ask about lifestyle issues that may affect drug therapy. These include dietary habits, tobacco and alcohol consumption, and illicit drug use. Because nicotine and alcohol are a factor in response to many drug therapies, it is important to quantify their intake, even though it may be uncomfortable for the pharmacist to do so. A useful suggestion is to open the discussion with a statement describing the importance of that information to you (e.g., "Mr. Smith, I'd like to ask about your intake of alcohol and tobacco because these can affect the way your medicines work. How much alcohol do you drink?"). Specify the amount and type of alcohol used. Note whether the patient smokes and how much. If he or she has stopped, it may be useful to know when. You may need to assess other factors related to specific disorders (e.g. stressors for patients with heart or ulcer disease or environment for the patient with asthma).

Closing the Interview

When you believe you have obtained all the vital information, it is time to close the interview. Begin with a brief summary of only the most important points, not every specific detail. Note any concerns that you or the patient has about the medications and review recommendations for resolution of problems. Ask the patient to verify agreement on the issues and tell the patient what to expect next. Ask the patient whether there is anything he or she wants to add and whether he or she has any other questions. If not, the interview is ended. Here is an example of a good closure: "Mr. Smith, we've talked about your heart and diabetes medications, and you mentioned some 'weak spells,' which I think may be caused by one of your medications. You're concerned about them, too. I am going to discuss them with your doctor. Is there anything else you would like to add or discuss?"

Symptom-Based Interview

During an interview, at a bedside visit, over the telephone, or at the prescription counter, the patient may mention symptoms that could be related to drug therapy. Knowing how to explore the patient's symptoms and evaluate their relationship to a disease or its treatment is a key component of the pharmacist's assessment skills. The first step is to get the patient to reveal more information about the symptom. An introductory statement such as "Tell me about that" will get the patient to provide more detail. The key symptom questions are used to explore the symptom. The following specific, open-ended questions seek specifics that help define whether the symptom is related to drug therapy.[14,15] Depending on the patient's response to your statement, it may not be necessary to ask all six questions.

Onset/timing: When did you notice this? When did it start?

Duration: How long have you had this problem?

Context: Under what circumstances does this symptom appear?

Quality: What does it feel like?

Treatment: What makes it better? What have you been doing about it?

Associated symptoms: What other symptoms are you having?

Insufficient recognition and symptom probing is common, especially among inexperienced pharmacists. Without proper symptom probing, pharmacists can jump to erroneous conclusions that the symptom is caused by a disease state or recommend a treatment without knowing the real cause. For example, a patient taking a nonsteroidal anti-inflammatory drug (NSAID) complains of fatigue. The pharmacist may simply recommend a vitamin to help fatigue. However, the patient's responses to the key symptom questions could reveal that the fatigue started soon after the medication and that the patient has gastric distress and has tried vitamins without success. These answers suggest a different cause for the fatigue.

The key symptom questions are important also when there is a tendency to attribute every symptom to a medication, as patients may be inclined to do. For instance, a pharmacy student reviewed the chart of a patient with bipolar illness, seizures, and Parkinsonism. The patient was on several medications, including carbamazepine and carbidopa/levodopa. The patient complained of blurred vision and insomnia, which the student believed were caused by the medications. When the patient was interviewed using the questioning technique just described, she indicated that she had blurred vision only out of the left eye, and that she had insomnia "since the day I was born." Answers to further questions suggested that her symptoms probably were not related to her drug therapy.

Knowledge of each drug's side effect profile and the disease state symptoms is essential in determining whether the symptom is a drug-related adverse effect. Onset of the symptom is very important to ascertain. If the symptom began or worsened after starting a new medication, then it is more likely that the problem is drug related.

Students and new practitioners often are confused about what to do once the symptom has been explored. Determining the seriousness of the problem can be difficult. It is helpful to ask yourself, "What is the worst thing that can happen in this case?" "If this is an adverse reaction to the medication, what will happen if the medication is continued? What will happen to the patient (and disease process) if the medication is stopped?" Easily discernible side effects, such as dizziness from an antihypertensive, are managed by practical suggestions without need to discontinue drug therapy. Even so, the patient may elect to stop taking the medication and the pharmacist must think ahead and advise the patient accordingly. More serious toxicities necessitate calling the patient's physician or advising the patient to discuss the problem with the physician as soon as possible. The most important aspect of addressing symptoms is to obtain enough information to make an informed clinical judgment.

BASIC MEDICATION CONSULTATION

Consultation on medication use is one of the pharmacist's most important activities, whether in a community pharmacy, clinic, or institutional site. Consultation on new medications is mandated by the Omnibus Budget Reconciliation Act of 1990, and most states require counseling for all patients on either new or both new and refill prescriptions.[16,17] The traditional method of consultation involved providing information: The pharmacist "told" and the patient "listened." There was little true dialog because the pharmacist often asked closed-ended questions such as "Do you understand?" "Do you have any questions?" As noted previously, such closed-ended questions tend to restrict the flow of information. When the pharmacist merely provides information, there is no opportunity to ascertain what the patient knows or thinks about the medication.

The pharmacist–patient consultation techniques developed by the Indian Health Service three decades ago and further refined in collaboration with colleagues around the country teach an interactive method of consultation that seeks to verify what the patient knows about using the medication and fill in the gaps with only the most basic information when needed.[18] Research shows that people forget 90% of what they hear within 60 minutes of hearing it.[1] Any counseling technique that is based on the pharmacist speaking most of the time will be ineffective in promoting patient understanding because patients almost immediately forget what they hear. If the patient is an active participant in the process, he or she will learn more. Engaging patient participation in the exchange entails the use of specific, open-ended questions that seek to determine what the patient already knows about the medication; then the practitioner provides new information to the patient and summarizes at the end of the consultation.

Basic Medication Consultation Skills: The Prime Question Technique

The interactive technique for consulting on medications consists of two sets of open-ended questions. One set is for a new prescription (prime questions), and the other is for refill prescription consultation (show-and-tell questions), as shown in Table 8.4. Using these questions makes counseling an interactive process that engages the patient, thereby making him or her an active participant. The questions provide an organized approach to ascertain what the patient already knows about the medication. Such a systematic approach is associated with improved recall of prescription instructions.[19] The pharmacist can praise the patient for information correctly recalled, clarify points misunderstood, and add new information when needed. It spares the pharmacist from repeating information already known by the patient, which is an inefficient use of time. The steps in the consultation process are described in detail here.

Open the Consultation

When the prescription is ready and the patient is called for counseling, establish rapport by introducing yourself by name and stating the purpose of the consultation. Verify the patient's identity by asking for identification or at least asking, "And you are?" after you identify yourself. If the

Table 8.4 ▪ Medication Consultation Skills

Prime Questions for New Prescriptions	Related Probes
What did your doctor tell you the medication is for?	What were you told the medication is for? What symptom is it supposed to help? What is it supposed to do?
How did your doctor tell you to take the medication?	How were you told to take the medication? How much? How often? What does three times a day mean to you? What did your doctor say to do when you miss a dose?
What did your doctor tell you to expect?	What were you told to expect? What good effects are you supposed to notice? What bad effects did the doctor say to watch for? What should you do if a bad reaction occurs?

Show-and-Tell Questions for Refill Prescriptions	Related Probes
What are you taking this medication for? How do you take it? What kind of problems are you having with this medication?	How is your medication working? How many of these did you take yesterday? What bad effects have you noticed from taking this medication?

patient does not speak English, has difficulty hearing, or otherwise cannot answer, you must overcome this barrier before discussing the medication.

If time and help permit and a private space is available, suggest that the consultation be conducted there and move to that area. This will be important for patients who have hearing problems or those wanting extra privacy. Sit facing the patient, and maintain the appropriate interpersonal distance (1.5 to 2 feet) during the consultation.

Conduct the Counseling Session

Begin by asking the prime questions if the prescription is a new one or the show-and-tell questions for a refill prescription. If the patient is able to tell you what the medication is for, you may choose to probe further or move to the next question. Probing further may be helpful when the patient answers in broad or vague terms. An example would be the patient receiving a β-blocker who tells you the medication is for "my heart." You may want to ask in an open-ended fashion, "What is it supposed to do for your heart?" Avoid asking "Is it for chest pains?" or similar closed-ended questions because you may alarm the patient by your suggestions and you might waste time if multiple questions are needed. If the patient does not know what the medication is for or asks, "Don't you know?" you should then ask why he or she visited the physician. The patient may describe symptoms of a condition known to be treatable with the medication in question. If so, indicate which symptoms the medication will help. If the patient is totally unaware, a referral back to the physician is indicated, lest the pharmacist judge in error the indication for the medication.

After verifying that the patient knows what the medication is for, ask the second prime question. Often, patients are unaware of the dosage instructions or say, "It's on the label, isn't it?" Be aware of the optimal dosing instructions; the patient may respond correctly "twice a day," but you may need to advise on exact timing or indicate whether to take the drug with meals. Other questions to include under the second prime question are how long to take the medication, exactly how much or how often to take as-needed medications, what to do when a dose is missed, and how to store the medication. When possible, rather than providing facts, ask the patient, "What did the doctor say about how long to take this medication?" or "What will you do if you miss a dose?" Remember, asking a question of the patient prompts his or her attention, whereas talking at the patient is passive and the patient may not listen as well. Think of the counseling session as an opportunity to find out what the patient knows rather than a place to showcase your knowledge. Keep the information you provide brief and to the point, limited to filling in the gaps and providing extra knowledge needed to ensure proper medication use.

After reviewing information about how to take the medication, proceed to the third prime question. Most often, patients have been told nothing about side effects or even beneficial effects. If the patient's answer notes expected beneficial effects, follow up by asking, "What side effects were you warned about?" to determine his or her knowledge of potential side effects. Other questions subsumed under the third prime question relate to how the patient will know whether the medication is working, what precautions to take while taking the medication, and what to do if the medication doesn't work.

If the patient is unaware of adverse drug effects, mention the main or most serious adverse effects and what to do if they occur. Research shows that patients want information about their medications, especially adverse effects, and that providing such information does not lead to the development of those reactions in most cases.[20–23] Recent work on communicating about risk, in this case risk of drug reactions, suggests a four-quadrant model in which each quadrant requires specific communication skills.[24] The quadrants are shown having a combination of either high or low probability of occurrence with high or low magnitude. An example of high probability and high magnitude would be the common and severe toxicities of cancer chemotherapy. Use empathic communication in discussing the risks of therapy in this case. High probability and low magnitude is exemplified by gastric complaints from erythromycin. Many commonly prescribed medications have common, bothersome, but not serious side effects. Useful communication skills include providing information about how the medication will work, why it is a good therapy, and how to manage expected side effects. In the third quadrant, where there is low probability but high magnitude (e.g., stroke with an oral contraceptive), careful assessment of the patient's perceptions about the possible side effects is needed. Be aware of how the patient's perceptions may differ from your own. When discussing serious potential adverse effects, some patients may hear "This is unlikely to happen" and tune out the specifics about the toxicity. Therefore, ask the patient for feedback on the discussion of toxicity. In the fourth case, the low probability and low magnitude of risk may be associated with a perception that the medication may have little value to the patient. Again, heavy-handed tactics to convince, scare, or otherwise threaten the patient are not effective. Questioning patients to determine their view of the possible benefits of taking the medication is needed. Follow with comments to match the patient's assessment. For example, when a patient says, "Well, I could get an allergic reaction from this," the issue of the adverse effect is first and foremost in her mind, whereas the pharmacist may think, "I've never seen anyone allergic to this." Respond to, but don't minimize, the patient's concern. Rather than trying to convince the patient that no one becomes allergic to it, the pharmacist could say "Yes, that's possible. Which do you think is worse: putting up with the pain or taking a chance on the medication?" This brings into the open the discussion of the risks and benefits of treatment. If the pharmacist can effectively explain the potential benefits, the patient may decide to try the medication. At times, the authors have found it useful to contract with the patient (e.g., "Mr. Jones, we've discussed both the good and bad about taking this medicine, and I know you still have concerns about side effects. I really think this medicine is best for you. Would you be willing to try it for a week and I will check in with you after a few days to see how things are going?" More often than not, the anticipated adverse effects do not appear.

Using effective consultation skills to address adverse reactions sets the stage for better patient compliance. However, the mere act of taking a medication when one is not used to doing so poses a problem for compliance. After asking the prime questions, use a universal statement to address compliance. A universal statement describes the situation for a group, then narrows down to focus on the individual (e.g., "Mrs. Green, a lot of patients have trouble fitting a time for taking medications into their daily schedule. What problems do you foresee in taking this?" It may be necessary to probe daily habits and suggest a way to tie taking medication into a particular activity. For instance, if the patient always makes coffee in the morning, having the medication nearby may be a sufficient reminder to promote compliance. A partnership approach is an effective way to address compliance issues.

Close the Consultation

Most consultations are a combination of the patient knowing some information and the pharmacist providing additional information as the prime questions are reviewed. For this reason, it is important to close the consultation with the final verification. Think of the final verification as asking the patient to play back everything he or she has learned to check that the information is complete and accurate. Say to the patient, "Just to make sure I didn't leave anything out, please go over with me how you are going to use the medication." Although the language seems bulky, if the question were phrased "Just to make sure you've got this . . ." the patient may feel embarrassed if he or she does not recall important facts. At this point, the patient should describe correct use of the medication. Any errors can be corrected and any omissions clarified. Then, ask the patient whether there is anything else he or she needs and offer help as needed.

A similar process is used for refill prescriptions. The show-and-tell questions verify patient understanding of proper use of chronic medications or medications that the patient has used in the past. The pharmacist begins the process by showing the medication to the patient (i.e., opening the bottle and displaying the contents). Then the patient tells the pharmacist how he or she uses the medication by answering the questions shown in Table 8.5. Note that the doctor is omitted as a reference because the patient should have been counseled properly before this and should have all the information needed for proper medication usage. The show-and-tell technique allows the pharmacist to detect problems with compliance or unwanted drug effects. If the patient answers the second question (how the medication is taken) incorrectly, the patient may be noncompliant or the physician may have changed the dosage. The pharmacist must further define the reason for the discrepancy. The second show-and-tell question also allows the pharmacist to ask the patient to demonstrate use of an inhaler or injectable or how to measure liquid doses to ensure proper usage.

Some pharmacists have difficulty asking the third question (on side effects), fearing that they may arouse suspicion in the patient. However, research discounts this notion. If potential adverse effects were discussed when the patient was counseled initially, it seems natural, and certainly relevant, to ask the patient about adverse effects at the refill visit. If new symptoms are present, explore this further using the key symptom questions. Clinical judg-

Table 8.5 ▪ Steps in the Recognize, Identify, and Manage Model for Compliance Counseling

Step	Example
Recognize potential noncompliance	
For objective signs, use a supportive compliance probe.	"I noticed that this refill was due 3 weeks ago."
For subjective signs, use a reflecting response.	"It sounds like you're unsure about taking this medication."
Identify cause of noncompliance and manage problem	
Knowledge deficits	Provide verbal and written information and verify patient's understanding.
Practical impediments (complicated dosing schedule, adverse reaction, forgetfulness)	Simplify dosing regimen, use medication boxes, obtain history about adverse reactions, and manage appropriately.
Attitudinal barriers	Maintain nonjudgmental attitude, use empathy, use open-ended and universal statements.

ment will dictate whether the problem is medication related and how it should be managed.

Barriers to the Consultation

The clinical skills just described are easily applied when there are few or no barriers in communication between patient and pharmacist. In reality, there are often obstacles to overcome in the environment or within the pharmacist or patient. Examples of problems in the pharmacy environment include lack of privacy, interruptions, high workload, and insufficient staff. Barriers within the pharmacist include lack of desire or skills to adequately counsel patients, stereotyping patients and problems, and personal stress. A detailed analysis of these barriers is beyond the scope of this discussion but can be found elsewhere.[18] Barriers that the patient brings to the encounter are discussed here.

The structured approach for obtaining a medication history and for medication counseling can be likened to knowing the road on which one is traveling. Unforeseen events happen on every path. During the clinical encounter, unforeseen issues may arise at any time. Just as one must remove or negotiate around obstacles on the highway, the pharmacist must recognize and manage barriers during the encounter if the consultation is to reach the desired end. Patient-related barriers can be categorized into two types: functional and emotional. Functional barriers include problems with hearing and vision, which make it difficult for the patient to absorb information during the consultation. Language barriers and illiteracy are formidable obstacles to proper consultation. Recognizing these usually is not difficult because the signs of poor vision are easy to observe. Likewise, language problems become apparent early in the consultation. Strategies specific to each barrier are needed. For instance, moving to a quiet area, repeating information, and asking feedback of the patient are important when hearing is a problem. Giving clear verbal instructions and using large-type print materials are helpful when the patient has vision difficulties. Using translators and picture diagrams and involving English-speaking caregivers are important when language problems exist. Many functional barriers are permanent. Emotional barriers may be long-standing if mental illness is involved; however, many emotional barriers are transitory but have a profound impact on the consultation.

Emotional barriers are common in everyday interactions, including pharmacist–patient communication. When improperly handled, they contribute to further aggravation, break down communication, and thus inhibit effective consultation. Patients may directly or indirectly express anger, hostility, sadness, depression, fear, anxiety, and embarrassment during consultation with the pharmacist. They may also give the attitude of a "know-it-all," be suspicious of medications, or seem unmotivated or uninterested. Some of these barriers are momentary, such as the frustration experienced when the prescription can't be filled because the medication is unavailable. The patient with a chronic pain syndrome may have a varying interest level because he or she is uncomfortable or in pain. The attitude of the patient who "knows" all about his or her medications probably will not change in time. This patient needs understanding and a nonjudgmental attitude to maintain an open dialog for consultation.

Emotional barriers can be difficult to discern. Most patients will not say, "I'm angry and frustrated about feeling so ill" or "I'm upset that my doctor didn't spend that much time with me." Instead, their feelings surface in statements such as "I don't know why it takes all day to put a few pills in the bottle!" and "I don't know why I have to take this stupid medicine." Unfortunately, we usually respond to the content of the message (e.g., "I'll have this ready for you as soon as I can") and in doing so overlook the opportunity to respond to the issues behind the statement, which affect the encounter and, more importantly, the patient's decision to comply with therapy. At the beginning of this chapter, several nonverbal and verbal clues were mentioned that suggest different emotional tones (e.g., pounding fists associated with anger). It takes patience and practice to listen *beyond* the words. The first step is to notice these nonverbal and verbal clues, identify the feeling state they represent, and respond with a reflecting or empathic statement. To the patient in the second example, the pharmacist might say, "Sounds like you've been frustrated with other things you've tried," rather than "This is a good medicine, Joe, and I really think it will help." Recall that a statement such as this can occur at any time in the consultation and that this barrier of frustration should be dealt with before the consultation is closed. Embarrassment is a factor when vaginal preparations, condom use, and similar topics are the subject of the consultation. Again, observe for signs of embarrassment, such as averted gaze or fidgeting, and respond with "This can be hard to talk about, but we need to discuss it." Be matter-of-fact, move to a private space, and speak in a normal tone of voice to alleviate the embarrassment. Additional strategies can be found in other references.[25]

Once these barriers are removed, consultation can proceed, with both parties devoting attention to the primary issues of drug therapy and usage rather than to any interpersonal difficulties. These skills are also applicable during the medication history interview and discussion of medication compliance, which is covered in the next section.

PSYCHOSOCIAL ASPECTS

Psychosocial factors play an important role in all pharmacist–patient interactions. Success or failure of patient care depends on the recognition of these factors, several of which are discussed in some depth here. Patient health beliefs, both cultural and noncultural, influence their interpretation of pharmacist communication and the appropriateness and accuracy of patient responses. Using open-ended questions helps the pharmacist elicit culture-specific beliefs and advise patients whose English skills are insufficient to enable effective communication. Secondly, patient readiness to comply with a therapeutic regimen and receptivity to education efforts varies according to psychological, emotional, and cultural factors that accompany the diagnosis of an acute or chronic disease. These important issues must be addressed to achieve effective patient education and compliance. Finally, compliance with therapeutic regimens in chronic disease requires significant long-term behavioral changes. Pharmacists must recognize that these changes are difficult to initiate and to maintain over time. To improve compliance, pharmacists must demonstrate their understanding of the inherent difficulty of change and use an empathic, caring approach.

COMPLIANCE AND DISEASE MONITORING

The pharmacist's role in monitoring and managing medication use is most vital in the case of patients requiring chronic drug therapy, especially with diseases that are asymptomatic. Many factors contribute to the pharmacist's success in ensuring beneficial outcomes. Among them are practice site, pharmacist competence, support of administration, and breadth of responsibilities, including prescriptive authority. Hatoum and Akhras[26] have documented extensively the value of pharmacists' contributions to ambulatory care sites such as community group practices and the patient's home. The Indian Health Service has provided a full range of pharmaceutical care services to its patients for more than three decades. Besides the traditional dispensing role, Indian Health Service pharmacists offer private consultations to all patients and have prescriptive authority for refilling chronic medications based on their assessment of the patient's needs.[27,28] Some pharmacists have been educated to provide primary care as pharmacist practitioners, and this movement has spread to other practice sites. Currently, several states have passed regulations that allow pharmacists to prescribe.[15] Whether the practice is a sophisticated one or more typical of contemporary community pharmacy, providing pharmaceutical care to patients requiring chronic drug therapy can have significant positive outcomes. To effectively provide long-term pharmaceutical care, several important factors must be considered.

Whose Disease Is It, Anyway?

One of the most common misperceptions held by health professionals regarding chronic disease is that the professional manages the disease. Nothing could be further from the truth, and this medical myth is probably one of the major contributors to compliance problems among patients with chronic diseases. In the traditional model, health professionals perceive their roles to be in diagnosing, treating, and managing disease. As drug therapy managers, clinical pharmacists focus on blood levels, pharmacokinetic dosage calculations, and drug interactions. Guided by this focus on technical aspects of patient care, health professionals often get frustrated and angry when patients don't follow instructions or, despite the provider's best efforts, achieve only partially satisfactory results. In reality, the only time the health professional manages the treatment is during an office visit or institutionalization in a hospital or long-term care facility. Most of the time, the patient controls the treatment of his or her disease, especially those that require continuous medication. Failure to recognize this basic truth creates considerable tension in patient–provider relationships, provider frustration and anger, poor communication, negative provider attitudes toward individual patients, poor patient outcomes, patient distrust of providers, and legal consequences that contribute to rising health care costs.[29–32]

One author strongly suggests that noncompliance in diabetes mellitus is caused largely by the failure of providers to recognize that their goal is not treating the disease but helping the patient treat the disease.[33] That contention is supported by current medical literature that links good communication and a partnership style of provider–patient relationship to increased satisfaction, increased compliance, and better patient outcomes.[4,31,32]

To be successful in helping patients achieve good outcomes, the pharmacist must eschew the traditional medical myth about who manages the disease and adopt a partnership approach, acting as a facilitator. Remember that it is the *patient's* disease; the provider's job is to help the patient manage it.

Go Slow and Use Interactive Techniques

Patients can absorb only a limited amount of new information at each encounter. Too many times, in an attempt to do a thorough job, health professionals inadvertently overwhelm the patient with information at or near the time of diagnosis or treatment initiation. A patient's active listening abilities last less than a minute during a monolog; therefore, he or she retains only a few pieces of information from a prolonged discussion and may miss key facts. In addition, a large volume of technical information may confuse or frighten patients, leading to the poor outcomes that educational efforts are intended to prevent.[34]

Successful patient educators do two things: give patients information in small, manageable increments and actively involve the patient in the educational process by creating an interactive dialog and using other hands-on approaches that are consistent with adult learning principles.[34] For the pharmacist, at the time of the initial prescription, this means verifying that the patient understands how to take the medicine and is aware of its most common side effects. For example, with hydrochlorothiazide 25 mg daily for hypertension, the pharmacist should verify that the patient knows what it's for, knows to take it once daily in the morning, understands that it takes a while before any changes in blood pressure occur, and knows that he or she will notice increased urination during the first week that should lessen after that. Discussions about diet, exercise, and related issues can wait until later visits. Giving the patient a handout on hypertension and diuretics would be appropriate and can lead to questions and subsequent educational efforts.

Set the Stage for Future Encounters

Many providers initially explain to patients how they are going to monitor them for disease control and progression so that patients view subsequent questions, lab tests, and examinations as a normal part of their care. However, few providers follow a similar process regarding compliance. Therefore, without previous explanations, provider questions about compliance are likely to be associated with parent-type sanctions from the provider. To avoid this "punishment," patients may avoid disclosing compliance problems when asked. Providers can prevent this common problem by remembering who ultimately manages the disease and using specific strategies during the initial patient contact. Explain that compliance is very important to successful outcomes but that you know how hard it is to remember to take medication every day. Tell the patient that you expect that he or she will be like most patients and experience some difficulties remembering to take the medication. Ask patients to keep track of those instances, if possible, and explain that you will be asking them at each visit about what kinds of problems they have had with the medicine (the third show-and-tell question). This can easily be done in association with explanations about how the progress of the disease will be monitored.

Monitoring and Education at Return Visits

Organizing an effective approach to evaluating and educating patients with chronic disease at return visits may be problematic in a busy practice setting. One simple way to look at all patients returning for follow-up of a chronic disease is to assess the three *C*s: *control, complications,* and *compliance.* The first *C* refers to control of the chronic disease. To evaluate the control, objective findings such as blood pressure and range of motion can be coupled with subjective findings from the consultation, such as reports of dizziness, nocturnal voiding, and morning stiffness. The second *C* refers to complications caused by both disease progression and drug effects. A combination of subjective findings from the patient interview and objective findings from the health record or patient profile, physical findings during examination, and pertinent lab and other test results can be used to evaluate the presence of potential complications quickly. For example, a patient with hypertension, diabetes mellitus, and osteoarthritis who takes captopril, chlorpropamide, and ibuprofen can be asked about the presence of cough, difficulty sleeping, and poor exercise tolerance. These questions are intended primarily to detect congestive heart failure or renal failure caused by hypertension or diabetes, but they also will help detect drug-related problems such as cough caused by the angiotensin-converting enzyme (ACE) inhibitor and renal effects from the ibuprofen. Checking recent lab values for creatinine, electrolytes, and blood glucose will help detect diabetes, hypertension- or NSAID-induced renal impairment, excessive chlorpropamide dosage, and ACE inhibitor hyperkalemia.

The third *C* relates to compliance problems. The pharmacist's actions can be broken up into three steps: Recognize potential compliance problems, identify probable causes, and manage the problem with specific steps. This recognize, identify, and manage (RIM) model is an easy way to enhance patient compliance.[35] In this model (Table 8.5), subjective and objective findings are used to detect potential compliance problems. The provider reviews the health record or drug profile for objective evidence of potential compliance problems before talking with the patient. During profile review, three items should alert the pharmacist to potential compliance problems. The first, and most common, is a discrepancy between the number of doses that should have been taken and the number of doses dispensed. Second, incomplete refill requests (e.g., only one or two out of more chronic medications due at the same time) raise suspicion for noncompliance. Third is the prescribing of a new medication that may be taken to offset adverse effects from another medication, if the effect is unrecognized as such. Many times, patients present to the medical provider with a new complaint. If the provider doesn't make the connection between the new symptom and the side effect, it may eventually result in compliance or therapeutic problems. If a patient on ACE inhibitors has a new or repeat prescription for cough suppressants or antibiotics for bronchitis, the pharmacist should suspect ACE inhibitor–induced cough. In extreme cases, patients may stop the needed drug and continue with the drug used to treat the side effects, which is unnecessary and could pose risks.

Care must be given in interpreting these signs. Positive findings during profile or chart review call for further exploration before a definite compliance problem can be ascertained. In some cases there are rational explanations for the objective findings. The patient may be getting refills at another location, or the doctor may have told the patient to change the dosage schedule or to stop the drug altogether.

When the profile suggests noncompliance, the best approach is to begin consultation using the show-and-tell technique for refill prescriptions. The patient may provide clues to confirm the pharmacist's suspicions. If not, the pharmacist must initiate a more direct approach using a supportive compliance probe. This is a specific type of statement in which the pharmacist uses "I" language, describes specifically what he or she sees, and asks a question to probe the discrepancy (e.g., "I noticed when I reviewed your profile that you hadn't had your prednisone refilled in about 2 weeks. I was concerned that there might have been some changes that I'm not aware of." This combination of "I noticed" and "I'm concerned" can be very effective in getting a dialog started in a nonthreatening manner. Another useful approach is the universal statement (e.g., "Most of my patients have problems remembering to take every dose of their medication. What kinds of problems are you having?"). Open the discussion of compliance problems with nonthreatening language and there is a greater likelihood that the patient will disclose the problems.

During the consultation, the patient may provide the pharmacist with clues to compliance problems not revealed by patient record review. Indeed, patients may refill their medications on time but actually take only some of the doses. Patients who tell the pharmacist that they are taking their medication differently than prescribed provide a strong indication of a potential compliance problem. Some may be quite obvious, such as when the patient asks, "Why do I have to keep taking this medicine?" This is a red flag because it seems fairly obvious that the patient does not want to take the prescription. However, many statements are more subtle. Examples of these vague clues, called pink flags, include "My doctor says I should take it," "My doctor wants me to take it," or "I'm supposed to be taking it." These statements usually are made in response to the first two show-and-tell questions. Other pink flags are more closely associated with the third question, such as when a long pause occurs during the patient's reply, which may indicate potential problems. For example, "What kinds of problems are you having with the medication?" may prompt the following pink flag responses: "Well, none, really" or a hesitation before saying, "No, none." Reflecting responses are appropriate (e.g., "Seems like you're not too sure about taking that" or "Sounds like you think there may be a problem."). These open the dialog in a nonthreatening manner and focus on the patient's perceptions or suggestion that a problem exists.

Patients may ask, "Does this medicine have any side effects? What kind of side effects does this have? Is this anything like (specific drug)?" More often than not, pharmacists simply answer the question without really listening to the underlying concern. An appropriate response would be "Why do you ask?" especially if the patient looks hesitant or the intonation of the question suggests doubt about taking the medication. Often, when the authors use this question, patients disclose that a relative had it or something like it, or the media reports problems with it. These indirect experiences create enough doubt that the patient wavers about taking the medication. Obviously, if the pharmacist does not recognize these pink flags, the consultation will be in vain because the patient will leave without having the underlying doubt resolved. Therefore, it is crucial to develop keen active listening skills to identify the presence of the pink flags and use reflecting responses to probe the problem. During the show-and-tell questioning, patients may disclose symptoms that may indicate an adverse drug effect. This is sometimes a reason for premature discontinuation of treatment or for skipping doses. When this appears to be the case, use of the key symptom questions will help identify the exact nature of the problem. Resolution of the problem will be dictated by clinical urgency.

Once the presence of the compliance problem has been confirmed, further use of reflecting and other responses can identify the nature of the problem. Compliance problems can be categorized in three groups. The first is a knowledge deficit. In these cases, patients have insufficient information, lack skills, or have misinformation that prevents compliance. Examples are a patient who put contraceptive jelly on toast and the patient who was never shown or has forgotten how to use an inhaler. The second group involves practical impediments or barriers, such as complex drug regimens involving multiple drugs or different dosage schedules, difficulty in developing routines that facilitate medication compliance, difficulty in opening containers, or insufficient mental aptitude to comply. The final category is attitudinal barriers. Among the most difficult to identify and manage, these include patient beliefs about health, disease, or treatment that are inconsistent with the prescribed regimen. These may reflect differences in cultural beliefs.[36–38] Perceived severity of risk in relation to the perceived benefit of treatment plays a large role in determining patient compliance.[38] Other factors, such as the patient's desire to be in control and the belief that he or she can successfully implement the recommended treatment, also strongly influence compliance.[34] Finally, the most prevalent and potentially the most difficult belief differences to overcome are patients' lay theories.[38] Common lay theories held by patients include "You need to give your body a rest from medicine or it will become immune to it," "You only need to take medicine when you feel sick, not when you feel OK," or "If one dose is good, then two must be better."

Once the specific cause is identified, a specific strategy to manage that problem can be attempted. Most knowledge and skill deficiencies can be corrected with education or training. Practical impediments respond well to specific measures such as simplifying regimens, use of easy-open containers, and the aid of a spouse or caregiver. Attitudinal issues tend to be the most complex and difficult to solve. Even lay theories, which seem to be easily debunked, are extremely difficult to overcome because the nature of lay theories makes them highly resistant to change. Again, it takes practice, careful listening, repeated conversations, and a supportive climate to help patients acknowledge these barriers. They will only do so when they feel that the pharmacist will not denigrate them or argue against their beliefs. Partnership language and gentle confrontation on the facts are indicated. Over time, repeated efforts to enlighten may change the patient's view.

CONCLUSION

Contemporary pharmacy practice is changing rapidly. Pharmaceutical care, which focuses on the patient's outcomes of drug therapy, is the founding principle for practitioners. New systems for pharmaceutical care delivery are appearing almost daily. From the pioneering work done by the Indian Health Service, which uses pharmacists across the spectrum of care, model clinical pharmacy practices that incorporate their principles into community pharmacies are evolving.[39–41] Whether one practices in a community, hospital, or other setting, the delivery of high-quality pharmaceutical care involves the skills and techniques discussed in this chapter, as well as others that support the pharmacist–patient interaction. As direct patient contact and responsibility for drug therapy outcomes become the main tasks for the pharmacist, the skills of interpersonal communication, medication history interview and consultation, and compliance monitoring and enhancement become the tools of the trade. The consistent application of a high degree of interpersonal and clinical skill by the pharmacist will lead to optimal outcomes for the patient.

KEY POINTS

- Patient communication skills are essential tools for successful clinical practice.
- Successful pharmacist–patient communication requires the creation of a dialog, active involvement of the patient in the interview or education process, good pharmacist listening skills, and pharmacist feedback to verify correct interpretation of patient information and emotions.
- Effective interviewing begins with broad open-ended questions and consists largely of focused open-ended questions. Closed-ended questions should be limited to clarifying patient responses and verifying the absence of important clinical information not elicited by open-ended questions.
- The primary goal of patient education activities, such as patient consultation, is to verify patient understanding of key points.
- During patient consultation and education, the pharmacist must identify and deal with informational deficiencies, patient emotions, and functional limitations to ensure that patients understand and can carry out therapeutic recommendations.
- It is important for the pharmacist to remember that her or his job is to help the patient achieve optimal results from treatment, not ensure them.
- Patients can absorb only limited amounts of information at one time. Therefore, give information gradually so patients do not become overwhelmed.
- When evaluating the status of patients with chronic diseases, focus attention on three important aspects: control of the disease, compliance with therapeutic regimens, and the presence of complications caused by the disease state or drug therapy.
- During all types of pharmacist–patient communication, listen carefully to the patient's responses. Many times they contain subtle clues that can lead the pharmacist to the correct assessment or reveal unspoken concerns or emotions that may interfere with education and compliance.

REFERENCES

1. Bolton R. People skills. New York: Simon & Schuster, 1979.
2. Rogers C. On becoming a person. Boston: Houghton Mifflin, 1961.
3. McWhinney I. The need for a transformed clinical method. In: Steward M, Roter D, eds. Communicating with medical patients. Thousand Oaks, CA: Sage, 1989:25–40.
4. Roter D, Hall J. Doctors talking with patients, patients talking with doctors. New York: Auburn House, 1992.
5. Henbest R, Steward M. Patient-centeredness in the consultation, 2: does it really make a difference? In: Family practice. New York: Oxford Press, 1980.
6. Lickhart W. Rogers' necessary and sufficient conditions revisited. Br J Guid Counsel 12:113–123, 1984.
7. Barrett-Lennard GT. The empathy cycle: refinement of a nuclear concept. J Counsel Psychol 28(2):91–100, 1981.
8. Rubin FL, Judd MM, Conine TA. Empathy: can it be learned and retained? Phys Ther 57:644–647, 1977.
9. Kalisch B. What is empathy? Am J Nurs 73:1541–1552, 1973.
10. Meldrum H. Interpersonal communication in pharmaceutical care. New York: Pharmaceutical Products Press, 1994.
11. Gardner ME, Burpeau-DiGregorio MY. Objective assessment of pharmacy students' interviewing skills. Am J Pharm Educ 49:137–144, 1985.
12. Gardner ME, McGhan WF. Objective assessment of interviewing skills: a comparison of two history types. Am J Pharm Educ 50:165–169, 1986.
13. Ranelli PL. The utility of nonverbal communication in the profession of pharmacy. Soc Sci Med 13A:733–736, 1979.
14. Billings JA, Stoeckle JD. The clinical encounter. Chicago: Year Book Medical Publishers, 1989.
15. Boyce RW, Herrier RN. Obtaining and using patient data. Am Pharm NS31:65–71, 1991.
16. Meade V. OBRA '90: how has pharmacy reacted? Am Pharm NS35:12–16, 1995.

17. Pugh CB. PreOBRA '90 Medicaid survey: how community pharmacy practice is changing. Am Pharm NS35:17–23, 1995.
18. Boyce RW, Herrier RN, Gardner ME. Pharmacist–patient consultation program, unit 1: an interactive approach to verify patient understanding. New York: Pfizer, Inc., 1991.
19. Gardner ME, Hurd PD, Slack MK. Effect of information organization on recall of medication instructions. J Clin Pharm Ther 14:1–7, 1989.
20. Morris LA, Grossman R, Barkdoll GL, et al. A survey of patient sources of prescription drug information. AJPH 74(10):1161–1162, 1984.
21. Lamb GC. Can physicians warn patients of potential side effects without fear of causing those side effects? Arch Intern Med 154:2753–2756, 1994.
22. Howland JS, Baker MG, Poe T. Does patient education cause side effects? J Fam Pract 31(1):62–64, 1980.
23. Gardner ME, Rulien N, McGhan WF, et al. A study of perceived importance of medication information provided in a health maintenance organization setting. Drug Intell Clin Pharm 22:596–598, 1988.
24. Meldrum H, Hardy M. Challenges in communication about risk. Proceedings of the conference, United States Pharmacopeial Convention, Rockville, MD, 1995:36–49.
25. Pharmacist–patient consultation program, unit 2: counseling patients in challenging situations. New York: Pfizer, Inc., 1993.
26. Hatoum HT, Akhras K. 1993 Bibliography: a 32-year literature review on the value and acceptance of ambulatory care provided by pharmacists. Ann Pharmacother 27:1106–1119, 1993.
27. Church RM. Pharmacy practice in the Indian Health Service. Am J Hosp Pharm 44:771–775, 1987.
28. Herrier RN, Boyce RW, Apgar DA. Pharmacist-managed patient care services and prescriptive authority in the U.S. Public Health Service. Hosp Form 25:67–80, 1990.
29. Beckman HB, Markakis KM, Suchman AL, et al. The doctor patient relationship and malpractice: lessons from plaintiff depositions. Arch Intern Med 154: 1365–1370, 1994.
30. Anderson LA, Zimmerman MA. Patient and physician perceptions of their relationship and patient satisfaction: a study in chronic disease management. Patient Educ Counsel 20:27–36, 1993.
31. DiMatteo MR. The physician–patient relationship: effects on quality of health care. Clin Obstet Gynecol 37:149–161, 1994.
32. Viinamake H. The patient–doctor relationship and metabolic control in patients with type I (insulin dependent) diabetes mellitus. Int J Psychiatry Med 23:265–274, 1993.
33. Anderson RM. Is the problem of noncompliance all in our heads? Diabetes Educ 11:31–34, 1985.
34. Herrier RN, Boyce RW. Compliance with prescribed drug regimens. In: Bressler R, Katz M, eds. Geriatric pharmacology. New York: McGraw-Hill, 1993:63–77.
35. Pharmacist–patient consultation program, unit 3: counseling to enhance compliance. New York: Pfizer, Inc., 1985.
36. Eraker SA, Kirscht JP, Becker MH. Understanding and improving patient compliance. Ann Intern Med 100:258–268, 1984.
37. Becker MH. Patient adherence to prescribed therapies. Med Care 23:539–555, 1985.
38. Leventhal H. The role of theory in the study of adherence to treatment and doctor patient interactions. Med Care 23:556–563, 1985.
39. Meade V. Adapting to providing pharmaceutical care. Am Pharm NS34:37–42, 1994.
40. Meade V. Pharmacist in Richmond launches pharmaceutical care program. Am Pharm NS34:43–45, 1994.
41. Meade V. Helping pharmacists provide disease-based pharmaceutical care. Am Pharm NS35:45–48, 1995.

CHAPTER 9

FLUID AND ELECTROLYTE THERAPY AND ACID-BASE BALANCE

Gail W. McSweeney

The body maintains its internal liquid environment by balancing the amounts, volume, and composition of water, electrolytes, proteins, acids, and bases. Body weight is approximately 60% water, and within this water are dissolved or suspended the elements and formed substances needed to generate energy, maintain and manufacture body components, metabolize nutrients and drugs, and eliminate waste. It is important to remember that changes in body water, salts, and pH are not diseases but rather deviations from the environmental conditions within which the body can function normally and protect and repair itself. Metabolic processes can continue only within very narrow limits of size, composition, and pH of body fluid. Any effort to normalize the amount, composition, distribution, and pH of body fluids, whether by internal homeostatic processes or by externally applied therapeutic measures, is aimed at restoring and maintaining an environment in which body functions can proceed normally.

PHYSIOLOGY OF BODY WATER BALANCE

Body water is divided into three compartments: intracellular, interstitial, and vascular.[1–3] The interstitial and vascular compartments taken together are called the extracellular fluid (ECF). In the nonobese, well-conditioned 70-kg man, water inside the cells (intracellular fluid, ICF) makes up 40 to 45% (30 L) of body weight. Interstitial water, that between cells, accounts for 11 to 15% (10 L) and vascular water (that inside the walls of the blood vessels) is approximately 5% (3.5 L). The actual amount of body water varies slightly according to age, sex, and body muscle and fat content; when estimating body water in an individual patient, the contribution of these factors must be taken into consideration. At birth, the newborn is approximately 75% water; the slight weight loss seen after birth is actually water loss from evaporation as the infant adjusts to an air environment. By the end of the first year of life, the infant's total body water (TBW) is about 60%. At maturity, men usually have a water content of 60%; the TBW of women of the same age, height, and weight is estimated to be about 5% less because of their smaller amount of muscle mass. Obese people are less than 60% water by weight because fat has negligible intracellular water; the absolute decrease in percentage of TBW is a function of the degree of obesity. For practical purposes, TBW in obese patients is estimated using ideal rather than actual body weight and not factoring in the negligible amount of water contained in fat. The TBW of older adults usually is below 60% because of their lower muscle mass resulting from lower levels of exercise and endogenous anabolic hormones.

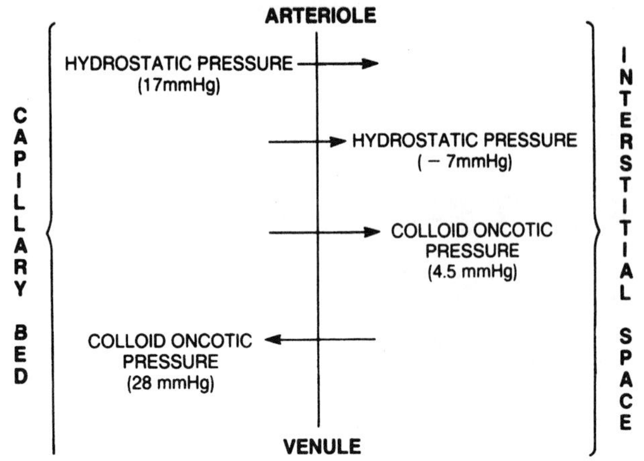

Figure 9.1. Forces regulating water movement in the extracellular fluid.

Body water is constantly being circulated between the three body compartments, with the connection occurring at the capillary level. Under stable conditions, the volume of each compartment remains constant, but there is a continuous interchange of individual molecules across the water-permeable cell membranes. This exchange is regulated by the difference in hydrostatic and protein (oncotic) pressures on the arteriole and venule side of the capillaries. At the heart level, cardiac output and arterial tone determine the intravascular or blood hydrostatic pressure. At the arteriole side of the capillary, this hydrostatic pressure is approximately 17 mm Hg and pushes solute-free water out into the interstitial or third space. Proteins, primarily albumin, and negative hydrostatic pressure in the third space simultaneously pull water from the vascular space into the third space. The combined effect of these two processes accounts for the movement of water out of the vascular space. On the venule side of the capillary bed, intravascular oncotic pressure pulls 95% of the extruded water back into the vascular space; the remaining 5% is returned by the action of the lymphatic collecting system (Fig. 9.1).

The volumes of the three compartments remain normal only as long as the described hydrostatic and oncotic forces remain normal relative to each other. In assessing the appropriateness of body water content, it is crucial to evaluate not only the total volume but also its distribution among the three body spaces. Dehydration is the state in which the volume of fluid is low in all three compartments. Hypovolemia is a state in which the intravascular volume is low, but this term does not describe or quantify the volumes of the interstitial and intracellular spaces. TBW overload means only that TBW is greater than 60%; this term does not describe specifically the volume of any individual compartment. When the phrase *TBW overload* is used, the actual distribution of volume in each compartment must be known before an appropriate therapeutic intervention can be determined. For example, fluid accumulates in the interstitial space if blood (hydrostatic) pressure is normal but oncotic pressure is low; the resulting clinical condition is called edema. With low albumin levels, the volume of the third space gradually expands at the expense of the vascular space. In the most severe cases, death results from too low circulating blood volume (hypovolemia) in the presence of interstitial space overload (edema) and TBW greater than 60%. In this situation, more fluid must be given to support the circulating vascular volume, even though the edema will worsen and the TBW continue to rise. Only correction of the underlying disequilibrium between the hydrostatic and oncotic pressures, by raising the low albumin or lowering the blood pressure, will normalize the volumes of the three fluid compartments.

PHYSIOLOGY OF BODY SOLUTE BALANCE

Osmotic pressure keeps the volume of the three body fluid compartments constant; only solute-free water moves freely across cell membranes. The concentration of dissolved ions (electrolytes) in each compartment creates the osmotic pressure that holds water in each space. These ions and their distribution are listed in Table 9.1. The normal serum osmolality (osmotic concentration) is 280 to 300 mmol/kg (280 to 300 mOsm/L). Sodium and chloride are the main ions in the ECF, and potassium and phosphate are those of the ICF. Other ions are present, but they are at concentrations too low to contribute significantly to the osmotic gradient. Other important osmotically active substances are glucose, urea, phospholipids, cholesterol, and neutral fats. A molecule of glucose has one-eighteenth and urea has one-third the osmotic strength of an atom of an electrolyte. Osmolality is determined by all the particles mentioned, but the nonelectrolytes contribute little unless their values are abnormally high; the effective osmolality is very close to twice the serum sodium in the ECF and twice the potassium in the ICF (Table 9.1).

The equation used to determine osmolality is as follows:

$$\text{Osmolality (mmol/kg)} = 2 \times \text{Sodium (mmol/L)} + \text{Glucose (mmol/L)}/18 + \text{Urea (mmol/L)}/3$$

Body processes function best within a serum osmolality of 280 to 300 mmol/kg, so the kidneys attempt to maintain

Table 9.1 ▪ Approximate Composition of Body Fluid (mmol/L)

	Plasma (total = 300)	Interstitium (total = 304)	Cell (total = 300)
Na	141.0	144.0	16.0
K	4.0	4.0	150.0
Ca	2.5	2.5	–
Mg	2.0	2.0	34.0
Cl	100.0	114.0	–
HCO_3	25.0	30.0	10.0
PO_4/SO_4	1.0	1.5	50.0
Protein/acid	25.0	6.0	40.0

this value and increase glucose and urea excretion when their concentrations rise above normal; if this is not possible or sufficient, they increase sodium excretion. In the physiologic sense, the need (biologic priority) to maintain a normal osmolality is greater than the need to maintain a normal body sodium.

When the concentration of ions in any compartment changes, water migrates across cell membranes to reestablish osmotic equilibrium. If the serum sodium rises, the osmolality of the vascular space is momentarily higher than that of the interstitial and intracellular spaces. Water moves from these two areas to dilute the vascular space until the correct relative osmolalities of all three compartments are reestablished. The result is a decrease in the size of the interstitial and intracellular spaces and an increase in the volume of the vascular space. If the serum sodium falls, the opposite happens and the size of the interstitial and intracellular compartments increases.

MAINTENANCE FLUID AND ELECTROLYTE NEEDS

Salt and water balance in the body is maintained by the equilibrium between oral intake of fluid and electrolytes, evaporation of solute-free water across the skin and lungs, and controlled renal excretion of water and electrolytes. The amount of water that evaporates (insensible loss) is a function of body surface area and respiratory rate. In a 70-kg man, the amount is approximately 1 L/day and remains constant. The kidneys increase or decrease their electrolyte and fluid output by the action of antidiuretic hormone (ADH) and aldosterone; this activity compensates for daily variations in oral fluid and electrolyte intake. ADH regulates the amount of water reabsorbed in the distal tubule of the kidney by assessing the osmolality of the ECF. If the osmolality of the ECF is higher than normal, ADH is released and water is reabsorbed in the renal tubules; if the osmolality is low, the converse is true. Another name for ADH is vasopressin. It increases vascular tone and causes constriction of blood vessels, especially those leading to the kidneys. Aldosterone increases sodium reabsorption, and release of this hormone is stimulated by a low circulating blood volume and a low total body sodium. These two hormones, along with stimulation of thirst centers in the brain, enable the body to maintain TBW and sodium within 1% of normal over wide variations in daily intake. In the case of an extremely low circulating plasma volume, ADH and aldosterone acting together can cause the kidneys to reabsorb essentially all salt and water. This is the mechanism for acute tubular necrosis and renal failure seen in hypovolemic shock. Renal failure from this cause can be reversed if the vascular volume is restored before permanent injury to the kidneys occurs.

The amount of water and electrolytes needed to replace insensible loss, maintain adequate perfusion of the body cell mass, and result in a urine output sufficient to excrete metabolic waste varies according to body size in a nonlinear way. This is because the change in body surface area relative to body mass as size increases is not linear. The first 10 kg of body weight needs 100 mL/kg, the next 10 kg needs 50 mL/kg, and each kilogram beyond 20 needs 20 mL/kg. A 50-kg man has a water need of 2100 mL/day; this is derived from 1000 mL for his first 10 kg of weight, 500 mL for the next 10 kg, and 600 mL for the remaining 30 kg. Calculation of water needs in children follows the same rule: A 15-kg child needs 1250 mL/day. Remember to use ideal weight in obese patients. Insensible loss of free water increases in febrile patients; a patient needs an extra 10% of the calculated need for water for each 1°C elevation in body temperature.

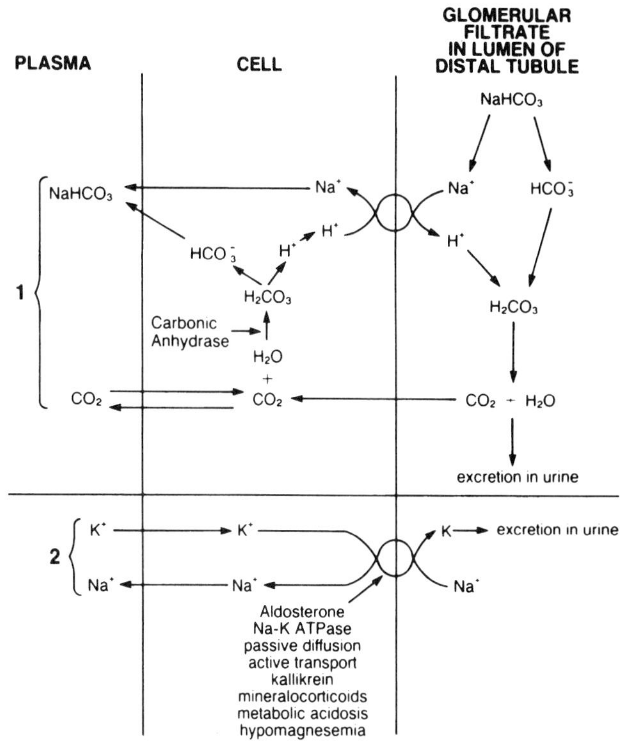

Figure 9.2. Mechanisms of Na-K exchange in the distal renal tubule.

The amounts of electrolytes needed to maintain normal total body levels vary because the kidneys adjust excretion constantly. This adjustment is centered around increasing or decreasing sodium excretion to maintain a normal circulating vascular volume and composition. When necessary, the kidney can reduce sodium loss to zero by increasing potassium and hydrogen excretion (Fig. 9.2). For practical purposes, the amounts of electrolytes needed to maintain homeostasis without stimulating inordinate amounts of ADH and aldosterone are linearly related to the water needs. The values used to determine daily maintenance fluid and electrolyte needs are listed in Table 9.2. Oral or intravenous replacement of maintenance needs should always include sodium and potassium. Deficiencies of the other electrolytes develop more slowly, and they are not always given during short-term therapy. For a 50-kg woman with normal TBW and electrolytes, an appropriate maintenance intravenous solution is 5% dextrose,

Table 9.2 ▪ Maintenance Needs per 24 Hours

Water	
0–10 kg	100 mL/kg
10–20 kg	50 mL/kg
>20 kg	20 mL/kg
Electrolytes	
Na	3 mmol (3 mEq)/100 mL H_2O need
K	2 mmol (2 mEq)/100 mL H_2O need
Cl	2 mmol (2 mEq)/100 mL H_2O need
Ca	0.05–0.1 mmol (0.1–0.2 mEq)/kg
Mg	0.05 mmol (0.1 mEq)/kg
PO_4	0.1 mmol (2.8 mg)/kg

Use ideal body weight in obese patients.

0.2% saline (D5 1/4NS) with potassium chloride 20 mmol/L infused at approximately 85 mL/hour. This provides 2040 mL fluid, 79 mmol sodium, and 41 mmol potassium; these amounts approximate those calculated using Table 9.2. This patient also receives 120 mmol chloride; cations must be given with an equal number of anions to maintain electrical neutrality, but giving excess chloride ions almost never causes hyperchloremia in patients with adequate renal function. Acetate salts of sodium and potassium are available and can be used if chloride anions must be avoided. Acetate is converted to bicarbonate in the body. Bicarbonate salts can be added directly to intravenous solutions, but they raise the pH of the product and may cause precipitation of electrolytes or drugs.

DISORDERS OF BODY WATER AND SOLUTE

Sodium

Serum sodium is the major determinant of intravascular volume because it is the osmotically active substance in greatest concentration in the compartment.[4–14] Abnormalities in salt and water intake or excretion alter sodium concentration. This will affect the interstitial volume because its major osmotic substance is also sodium, and the two compartments are in equilibrium with each other.

The usual serum sodium concentration is 135 to 147 mmol/L (135 to 147 mEq/L). Levels above or below this are called hypernatremia or hyponatremia, respectively. The terms refer only to concentration and do not indicate whether the abnormality is the result of increases or decreases in the total amounts of sodium, water, or both in the body.

Hypernatremia

Hypernatremia is almost always the result of a free water deficit. An elevated total body sodium can result from an excessive intake of salt but is almost impossible to achieve if renal function is adequate. Clinically important symptoms of hypernatremia generally do not appear until the serum level is greater than 160 mmol/L and are the result of central nervous system (CNS) dehydration (Table 9.3). Any treatment to correct an altered serum or total body sodium value should not be so rapid and aggressive as to create new CNS problems; equilibration across the blood–brain barrier is slower than across other semipermeable membranes in the body, and rapid changes can cause seizures. The treatment for hypernatremia depends on whether the cause is too little water or too much sodium. Hypernatremia from water loss indicates a decrease in TBW, not just in intravascular volume. Because the concentration of osmotically active substances across the three compartments is always in equilibrium, the interstitial sodium concentration and the intracellular potassium concentration are as elevated as the intravascular sodium. Calculating the amount of free water needed to correct the

Table 9.3 ▪ Symptoms and Causes of Hypernatremia and Hyponatremia

Hypernatremia	Hyponatremia
Serum level > 147 mmol/L (147 mEq/L)	Serum level < 135 mmol/L (135 mEq/L)
Causes	
Decreased water intake	Low-sodium diet with diuretics
Fever	Diuretics
Excessive salt intake	Congestive heart failure
Diabetes insipidus	Cirrhosis
Hyperventilation	Replacement of body secretion loss with electrolyte-free solutions
	Adrenal insufficiency
	Osmotic diuresis
	Syndrome of inappropriate secretion of antidiuretic hormone
Signs and Symptoms	
Thirst	Apathy or agitation
Dry mucous membranes	Fatigue
Decreased skin turgor	Anorexia or nausea
Acute weight loss	Headache
Confusion	Muscle cramps
Hallucinations	Tachycardia
Intracranial hemorrhage	Oliguria or anuria
Coma	Confusion
	Seizures
	Coma
	Shock
Treatment of Hypernatremia	
Water deficit (L) = [1 − (140/Measured Na)] × Weight (kg) × 0.6	
Treatment of Hyponatremia	
Dilution: Sodium and water restriction	
Depletion: Sodium deficit (mmol) = (140 − Measured Na) × Weight (kg) × 0.6	

concentrations of all electrolyte values and return the volumes of all three compartments to normal involves the use of the following equation:

$$\text{Water deficit (L)} = [1 - 140/\text{Measured serum sodium (mmol/L)}] \times \text{Body weight (kg)} \times 0.6$$

The deficit is replaced with electrolyte-free oral or intravenous solutions, such as 5% dextrose in water (D5W), given over 18 to 24 hours in addition to calculated maintenance fluid and electrolyte needs.

If hypernatremia is the result of an actual increase in the amount of sodium in the body, treatment is directed at removal of sodium from the body and involves the use of diuretics and D5W to increase renal elimination while maintaining a normal TBW.

Hyponatremia

Hyponatremia is a serum sodium concentration less than 135 mmol/L, but clinically important symptoms usually do not appear until the level is below 120 mmol/L and are the result of CNS water intoxication (Table 9.3). As with hypernatremia, the cause must be determined before treatment begins. Hyponatremia can result from dilution or depletion or be factitious. Dilutional hyponatremia is a condition in which the total body sodium is actually high but TBW is increased to a greater degree; the result is a low serum sodium concentration. It occurs in conditions such as cirrhosis and congestive heart failure, when effective cardiac output reaching the kidneys is diminished. This, along with the low sodium concentration, is a stimulus for ADH and aldosterone secretion. The result is further salt and water retention, and affected patients usually are edematous because of the attendant increase in the interstitial fluid compartment size. Diuretics are not a treatment and may be contraindicated because they will exacerbate the hyponatremia by causing sodium excretion that exceeds water elimination. Salt and water restriction, bed rest (to increase venous return to the heart), and correction of the primary disorder are the initial treatments. However, these measures must not be so aggressive as to compromise intravascular volume or further decrease renal blood flow.

Hyponatremia from depletion is a true decrease in the total body sodium, with or without a water deficit. It most commonly results from gastrointestinal (GI) losses from vomiting, excessive diuretic therapy, adrenal insufficiency, and replacement of losses from perspiration with electrolyte-free fluid. Patients show signs of dehydration (dry mucous membranes, skin tenting, lethargy) and, in extreme cases, hypovolemia. The amount of sodium needed to replace the total body deficit is calculated with the following equation:

$$\text{Sodium deficit (mmol)} = [140 - \text{Measured serum sodium (mmol/L)}] \times \text{Body weight (kg)} \times 0.6$$

Appropriate solutions to replace the sodium deficit are 0.9% saline (154 mmol sodium and chloride per liter) or 3% saline (513 mmol sodium and chloride per liter) given in addition to daily maintenance fluids and electrolytes. Because hyponatremia usually does not occur acutely, the deficit may be replaced over several days to avoid intravascular volume overload, seizures, pulmonary edema, or congestive heart failure.

Factitious hyponatremia results from accumulation of osmotically active substances, such as glucose and lipids, in the intravascular space. Sodium is diluted as water moves from the interstitial to the vascular space to normalize the osmotic pressure. The degree of hyponatremia usually is mild. Serum sodium falls only 1.6 mmol/L for every 5.3-mmol/L (100-mg/dL) increase in blood glucose, and treatment consists of correcting the underlying disorder.

Alterations in Fluid Compartment Integrity

Trauma, tissue ischemia, endotoxemia, hypoalbuminemia, and decreased cardiac output result in hypovolemia by damaging capillary membranes or disrupting the hydrostatic and oncotic forces governing fluid movement across them. The symptoms of hypovolemia are tachycardia, low central venous pressure (CVP), low pulmonary capillary wedge pressure, and decreased urine output. Blood pressure is not a good measure of this condition because increases in sympathetic tone can maintain the blood pressure near normal in the presence of a greatly decreased circulating volume.

In the cases of trauma, ischemia, and endotoxemia, capillary pore size increases (capillary leak syndrome); water, solute, and plasma proteins, primarily albumin, flow into the interstitial (third) space. This leak can be localized to an area of injury or ischemia (surgery, trauma) or generalized throughout the body (endotoxemic shock from Gram-negative sepsis). The amount of fluid lost from the intravascular space varies with the degree of injury but can result in hypovolemia severe enough to cause cardiovascular collapse and death if the circulating volume is not maintained. Treatment consists of correcting the underlying disorder to normalize capillary permeability while replacing the lost intravascular fluid with a solution of the same composition. Blood has no role in this therapy because the formed elements of the intravascular fluid are not being lost to the third space. The two categories of replacement solutions are crystalloid and colloid. *Crystalloid* is a general term for an aqueous solution containing electrolytes. Normal (0.9%) saline and lactated Ringer's (LR) solution are most commonly used for treating hypovolemia because they are isotonic with the ECF and are most effective in maintaining the circulating volume. *Colloid* is a general term for a solution containing plasma proteins or other colloidal molecules; three types are available. Plasma protein fraction (PPF) is approximately 85% albumin and 15% globulin; it is available as a 5% solution. Albumin is available as a 5 or 25% solution and hetastarch as a 6% solution. Hetastarch is a mixture of ethoxylated amylopectin molecules having an average molecular weight of 450,000 Da; they exert the same hemodynamic effect as albumin. It is not extracted from pooled human plasma and is much less expensive than PPF or albumin. All three products also contain 130 to 160 mmol sodium and chloride per liter. The use of colloid infusions remains controversial. Although some albumin does move into the third space when capillary pore size increases, it is much less than the amount of salt and water that leaks out; serum protein levels do not fall quickly or appreciably. Colloid temporarily decreases the rate at which fluid migrates into the third space but may exacerbate hypovolemia 24 to 36 hours later as it moves into the interstitial space and begins to draw fluid there. Unless the actual serum albumin is below the level needed to maintain the capillary venule oncotic pressure gradient (20 to 25 g/L) or aggressive crystalloid therapy is not restoring intravascular volume, the routine use of colloid solutions is not recommended.

During the treatment of hypovolemia, the rate of fluid administration into the vascular space must meet or exceed the rate of loss to maintain tissue perfusion and can exceed 1 L/hour in extreme cases. Urine output should be kept at a minimum of 0.5 mL/kg/hour, the level at which a circulating volume sufficient to perfuse body tissues is present. Normalization of heart rate and CVP also are indicators of normal intravascular volume and can be monitored along with urine output. During resuscitation, the rate of fluid administration is adjusted hourly to maintain an adequate intravascular volume. It is important to remember that although edema can appear in some patients during this process, it is the capillary leak that is causing the edema, not the resuscitation process. When healing begins, this extra fluid and solute are returned to the vascular compartment and excreted. Diuretics have no role in correcting edema caused by capillary leak syndromes, and their use can further deplete the intravascular volume.

Hypoalbuminemia without a concurrent capillary leak can result in hypovolemia with edema. Capillary venule oncotic pressure is low, and fluid that moved into the interstitial space on the arterial side of the capillary bed is not returned to the vascular system. Treatment for this condition consists of intravenous albumin in sufficient amounts to normalize the arteriovenous capillary oncotic pressure. Edema resolves only if this can be accomplished.

Hypovolemia caused by a decreased cardiac output (congestive heart failure, cardiomyopathy, myocardial infarction) cannot be corrected by giving fluids. In these conditions, hypovolemia exists on the arterial side of the heart because of pump failure; the venous side of the circulatory system may be overloaded and the patient may be edematous. Treatment options are confined to agents that improve cardiac output, such as inotropes.

If hypovolemia is the result of blood loss, then whole blood or packed red blood cells with normal saline (NS) or LR is indicated to reestablish the hematocrit above 0.25 g/L (25%) with a normal circulating volume.

Losses of Body Water and Solute

In prolonged vomiting, diarrhea, or losses through perforations in organs or the GI tract leading to the skin (fistulas), water and solute are lost from the body. The compositions of these fluids depend on the area affected and are listed in Table 9.4. When the exact origin of the fluid is not known, laboratory analysis helps in selecting an appropriate replacement solution. This analysis often is necessary in the case of enterocutaneous fistula (communication between the GI tract and the skin). Because such fistulas can make circuitous tracts through the body before reaching the skin, the organ nearest the exit site is not necessarily the one from which the fluid is draining. Diarrhea is most often of distal small bowel or colonic origin, but in cases of secretory diarrhea, such as in giardiasis or acquired immunodeficiency syndrome, the fluid may arise from the duodenum or jejunum. In all cases of abnormal loss, the fluid composition should be determined. Appropriate replacement solutions, in addition to maintenance needs, are given at a rate to restore and maintain normal body water and solute.

Table 9.4 ▪ Approximate Concentrations of Body Secretions (mmol/L and mEq/L)

	Na	K	Cl	HCO_3
Saliva	10	25	10	15
Stomach	60	10	85	–
Bile	150	5	100	40
Pancreas	140	5	80	120
Small bowel	110	5	105	30
Terminal ileum	117	5	105	–
Sweat	45	5	60	–
Cerebrospinal fluid	140	3	130	–

ACID-BASE BALANCE

For physiologic processes to occur at a normal rate, body pH must remain within a narrow range.[1,15–23] Although it varies slightly among body compartments (the ICF has a pH of approximately 6.9 and some subcellular components, such as the mitochondria, have usual levels even lower), normal total body acid-base balance is assumed to be present when the arterial pH is between 7.35 and 7.45.

Cellular metabolism, energy generation, and protein metabolism add large amounts of acid to the body daily. It is predominantly in the form of carbon dioxide (CO_2), but some hydrogen ions and weak organic and inorganic nonvolatile acids also are generated. Almost no alkaline substances result from metabolic processes, so body acid-base homeostatic mechanisms exclusively buffer or eliminate acids. Hemoglobin, proteins, and phosphate buffer only nonvolatile acids. The amount of acid they can buffer cannot be changed because the amounts of them in the body are fixed; no adjustment can be made if the amount of acid in the body increases. These three systems contribute little to the total buffering capacity of the body and are not discussed in detail here.

The bicarbonate–carbonic acid system buffers carbon dioxide and can adjust quickly to changes in the daily acid load. It keeps body pH in the normal range by maintaining the correct ratio between the concentrations of bicarbonate (HCO_3) and carbonic acid (H_2CO_3) in the blood. This relationship is described by the Henderson–Hasselbach equation:

$$pH = pK_{carbonic\ acid} + \log (HCO_3/H_2CO_3)$$

When the HCO_3/H_2CO_3 (24 mmol/1.2 mmol) concentrations are at a ratio of 20:1, the pH is 7.4 because the pK of carbonic acid is 6.1 and the log of 24/1.2 is 1.3. Carbonic acid concentrations are not obtained in the patient care setting; the value reported by clinical laboratories is the partial pressure of CO_2 (pCO_2). A 40-mm Hg pCO_2 corresponds to a H_2CO_3 concentration of 1.2 mmol. The pCO_2 is maintained within the normal range because CO_2 generated by cellular metabolism is continuously diffused and eliminated across the lungs. The capacity of the lungs to excrete CO_2 is so great it is saturated only in cases of severe pulmonary disease.

The kidneys are responsible for maintaining the serum HCO_3 within the normal range by reabsorbing bicarbonate ions from the glomerular filtrate and by generating new HCO_3 ions in renal tubular cells. This generation is accomplished by the action of the enzyme carbonic anhydrase on carbon dioxide and water to form carbonic acid. Carbonic acid quickly dissociates into H and HCO_3; the hydrogen ion is secreted into the urine and the bicarbonate transported from the renal tubular cells into the vascular system. The capacity of this reaction to generate new HCO_3 is not saturated unless renal function is severely compromised (Fig. 9.2).

Acid-base disturbances begin as carbon dioxide or bicarbonate serum concentration changes. If the problem originates with carbon dioxide, the resultant change in pH is said to be of respiratory origin; if it begins with bicarbonate, the change is said to be of metabolic origin. A plasma pH below 7.35 is called acidosis and can be of respiratory or metabolic origin; a plasma pH above 7.45 is called alkalosis and is also of respiratory or metabolic origin. When plasma pH goes outside the normal range, the lungs and the kidneys begin processes that act to compensate and normalize the pH value. It cannot be overemphasized that it is the ratio between carbon dioxide and bicarbonate, not the absolute numbers, that determines pH. The body has a greater physiologic need (biologic priority) to have a plasma pH between 7.35 and 7.45 than it does to have "normal" levels of pCO_2 and HCO_3. When the respiratory center in the medulla oblongata perceives a change in pH, it causes the lungs to adjust the pCO_2 by increasing or decreasing the respiratory rate. Although it occurs quickly, this process can completely correct the pH only when the change in HCO_3 concentration is minor; it is limited by how fast or slow a person can breathe in and out and by the capacity of the intracellular hemoglobin and phosphate buffering systems. The kidneys, by increasing or decreasing the plasma HCO_3, may take several days to fully compensate and normalize a pH altered by a change in CO_2 concentration, but they have a much greater total buffering capacity.

A high plasma HCO_3 is not synonymous with metabolic alkalosis; it also is seen in compensated respiratory acidosis. A change in one value is the appropriate physiologic response to a change in the other because the result is a normal pH. No attempt, other than determining and correcting the primary problem, should be made to correct an individual abnormal laboratory value. The only exceptions are when the plasma pH is above 7.6 or below 7.1. It is appropriate in these circumstances to give bicarbonate or hydrochloric acid to normalize the pH of the body without regard to the cause of the disturbance because death may be imminent.

PRIMARY ACID-BASE DISTURBANCES

Metabolic Acidosis

Metabolic acidosis is the condition in which the plasma pH is below 7.35 as a result of a low bicarbonate concentration in the blood. A low serum HCO_3 results from losses from the body, decreased renal regeneration of HCO_3, or increased amounts of acid added to the body by ingestion or metabolic processes. As the bicarbonate concentration falls, the lungs attempt to lower the pCO_2 and maintain a normal pH by increasing the depth and rate of respiration (Kussmaul breathing). The symptoms of metabolic acidosis occur in the cardiopulmonary system or CNS but usually are not clinically important at a pH greater than 7.1 (Table 9.5).

The number of positively charged ions in the body must always equal the number negatively charged. In the plasma, this electrical neutrality is achieved with dissolved electrolytes and proteins in the following relationship:

$$Na^+ = Cl^- + HCO_3^- + \text{Unmeasured anions}$$

Unmeasured anions consist of plasma proteins and small amounts of other negatively charged substances, such as SO_4 and PO_4, not measured by the tests usually done by clinical laboratories. The usual amounts of these anions in the blood have a combined ionic strength of 8 to 16 mmol/L (8 to 16 mEq/L); this value is called the anion gap and rarely changes. Assuming that Na remains con-

Table 9.5 ▪ Metabolic Acidosis (pH < 7.35, HCO_3 < 22 mmol (22 mEq)/L)

Causes	Signs and Symptoms
Ketoacidosis	Kussmaul breathing
Renal failure	Hyperkalemia
Hypoxia or anoxia	Ventricular arrhythmias
Diarrhea	Lethargy
Salicylates	Stupor
Methanol	Coma
Chloride loading	

Treatment (pH at or below 7.1)

HCO_3 deficit (mmol and mEq) = (24 − Measured HCO_3) × Weight (kg) × 0.5

stant, a change in the number of any one of the anions necessitates a change in one or both of the others to maintain electrical neutrality. Because the number of unmeasured anions is fixed, the Cl and HCO_3 are alterable. With the addition of acid (Cl), the fall in the HCO_3 actually is an appropriate compensatory response to maintain the electrical neutrality of the blood (a condition with an even higher biologic priority than maintenance of a normal pH). Metabolic acidosis occurs when the HCO_3 goes down and the HCO_3/CO_2 ratio becomes abnormal.

Metabolic acidosis is divided into non–anion gap and positive anion gap varieties. In non–anion gap acidosis, the number of unmeasured anions is the same as usual, so the decreased serum bicarbonate level is secondary to chloride loading, an actual loss of bicarbonate from the body, or decreased bicarbonate generation. In positive anion gap acidosis, the number of unmeasured anions has increased and the HCO_3 has dropped to maintain electrical neutrality. The cause of a positive anion gap acidosis is the contribution of nonvolatile acids to the blood. This can result from abnormal metabolic processes, such as diabetic ketoacidosis and hypoxia, or in poisonings by substances that dissociate at physiologic plasma pH. Salicylate and methanol overdoses commonly cause this particular kind of metabolic acidosis. It is important to make the distinction between these two types of metabolic acidosis before determining or beginning any treatment regimen.

Treatment of Non–Anion Gap Metabolic Acidosis

Loss of bicarbonate (prolonged diarrhea, upper GI fistulas), inability to generate bicarbonate (renal failure), or chloride loading (NS infusions, NaCl overdoses) are the three causes of this type of metabolic acidosis. Treatment consists of correcting the underlying cause and replacing the bicarbonate deficit. Except in cases of renal failure or profound and continuing GI losses, the kidneys generate sufficient bicarbonate and normalize the pH when the cause of the acidosis has been corrected. Acute HCO_3 replacement is done only when the plasma pH is at or below 7.1 or the patient is exhibiting life-threatening symptoms of acidosis. The amount of the bicarbonate deficit can be determined by use of the following equation:

$$HCO_3 \text{ deficit (mmol)} = [24 - \text{Measured } HCO_3 \text{ (mmol/L)}] \times \text{Body weight (kg)} \times 0.5$$

The volume of distribution of HCO_3 is estimated to be 10% less than the TBW, so the factor used is 0.5 rather than 0.6. One-half of the calculated dosage is given (this amount usually changes the pH by 0.2). The goal of emergency bicarbonate replacement therapy is to correct existing cardiac or CNS disturbances by achieving a plasma pH at or above 7.2. Because the onset of acidosis usually is gradual, the CNS has slowly equilibrated to a low pH. Rapidly changing the plasma pH relative to the CNS pH can cause seizures and death because CNS pH normalization lags behind. As the plasma pH normalizes over hours or days by renal bicarbonate generation, the CNS pH equilibrates at a rate tolerable to the patient and complications are avoided. The additional risks of inducing alkalosis or hypernatremia by administering sodium bicarbonate often outweigh any benefit of quickly normalizing the pH.

Non–anion gap acidosis in renal failure is the result of the reduced ability of damaged kidneys to generate bicarbonate. It is usually chronic and mild and most patients are asymptomatic. Renal failure severe enough to cause significant acidosis almost always necessitates hemodialysis; the composition of the dialysate is modified to improve serum HCO_3 concentrations and pH.

In cases of diarrheal or fistula outputs that exceed the ability of the kidneys to generate HCO_3, it is necessary to give bicarbonate. This usually is done with sodium or potassium acetate rather than bicarbonate salts, for reasons stated previously, but sodium bicarbonate can be used. The composition of the fluid being lost should be determined by laboratory analysis. The amount of base given should be enough to correct the initial deficit with continuing therapy in quantities sufficient to match daily losses.

Positive Anion Gap Metabolic Acidosis

Positive anion gap acidosis is the result of a rise in the number of unmeasured anions (nonvolatile acids) in the plasma with a resultant drop in HCO_3 concentration. These acids can be the byproducts of metabolic processes seen in diabetes and prolonged starvation (ketosis), anaerobic carbohydrate metabolism, and accumulation of ingested acids (salicylate and methanol poisoning) or acids normally produced in the body that cannot be eliminated, as is the case in renal failure.

During intracellular hypoglycemia, fat becomes the sole substrate for energy generation. This quickly results in the production of ketone bodies. In diabetes, the cause of the low intracellular glucose is a lack of insulin, which prevents glucose transport from the blood into cells. In starvation, a total absence of glucose from the body forces a change to fat metabolism. Ketone bodies dissociate and contribute hydrogen ions and the anion β-hydroxybutyrate. In cases of tissue hypoxia, insufficient oxygen to support the action of the Krebs cycle results in the activation of an alternative pathway for energy generation, the Cori cycle. Its metabolic byproduct is lactic acid; H ions and lactate accumulate after dissociation and acidosis results.

The treatment for anion gap acidosis always is correction of the underlying problem. Intravenous insulin is given in the case of diabetes; in lactic acidosis, restoring an appropriate circulating volume or plasma oxygen-carrying capacity is indicated; in poisoning, hemodialysis or gastric lavage may be needed to remove toxic substances from the body. To reiterate, HCO_3 is given only if the pH is at or below 7.1 or if there are clinically important symptoms of acidosis.

Metabolic Alkalosis

Metabolic alkalosis is defined as a plasma pH above 7.45 caused by a high bicarbonate concentration in the blood.

Table 9.6 ▪ Metabolic Alkalosis (pH > 7.45, HCO_3 > 28 mmol (28 mEq)/L)

Causes	Signs and Symptoms
Liver failure	Cheyne–Stokes breathing
Diuretics	Hypokalemia
Nasogastric suction	Muscle cramping
Hyponatremia	Seizures
Hyperaldosteronism	
Corticosteroids	
Treatment (pH at or above 7.6)	
HCl deficit (mmol and mEq) = (103 – Measured Cl) × Weight (kg) × 0.2	

The anion gap is never affected by this condition. As the HCO_3 rises, the lungs compensate by lowering the depth and rate of respiration (Cheyne–Stokes breathing) in an effort to increase the pCO_2 and thereby normalize the plasma pH. Important symptoms associated with alkalosis generally do not appear at a pH below 7.6 (Table 9.6).

The most common causes of metabolic alkalosis are loss of chloride ion (nasogastric suction, loop diuretics, mineralocorticoid excess), ECF depletion, and hepatic failure. Diuretics and mineralocorticoids stimulate exchange of hydrogen and potassium ions for sodium in the renal tubules; this induces both hypokalemia and alkalosis (Fig. 9.2). Diuretics cause volume depletion and hyponatremia, which further stimulate H and K loss. Volume depletion itself leads to alkalosis because of the increased concentration of HCO_3 molecules in a reduced plasma space; this condition is called contraction alkalosis. Because the body generates almost no basic substances during metabolism and base ingestion is uncommon, alkalosis from other causes is rare.

Treatment of Metabolic Alkalosis

Metabolic alkalosis as the result of sodium and chloride loss accompanying volume contraction is called saline responsive. Replacing sodium stops aldosterone-stimulated exchange of H for Na in the renal tubules, and replacing chloride ions stops the generation of HCO_3 needed to maintain electrical neutrality. Volume expansion reduces the HCO_3 concentration in the vascular space. NS is the treatment of choice in this condition because it is slightly higher in sodium (154 mmol/L) and much higher in chloride (154 mmol/L) than the ECF. An amount of this solution that will restore the TBW deficit should normalize body sodium and chloride. Some patients with metabolic alkalosis present with TBW overload and may not be able to tolerate a sodium load. The alkalosis can be treated with an infusion of hydrochloric acid or arginine hydrochloride. HCl is preferred because severe hepatic dysfunction usually is the cause of alkalosis in these patients, and administering arginine can precipitate hepatic coma. The dosage of HCl to replace the hydrogen and chloride deficits can be determined by the use of the following equation:

$$\text{HCl (mmol)} = [103 - \text{Measured Cl (mmol/L)}] \times \text{Body weight (kg)} \times 0.2$$

The volume of distribution of chloride is 33% of TBW, so the multiplication factor is 0.2. Giving one-half the HCl deficit over 12 to 24 hours should lower the plasma pH by 0.2 and not cause a significant CNS pH gradient. Hydrochloric acid solutions for intravenous use are not commercially available; extemporaneous compounding of a 0.1 to 0.2 N solution (10 to 20 mmol HCl/L) is necessary. Infusion into a central venous catheter rather than a peripheral intravenous line is recommended to reduce the risk of phlebitis.

Metabolic alkalosis can be the result of hypokalemia secondary to ICF/ECF exchange of hydrogen for potassium ions and from mineralocorticoid excess. These types of alkalosis are saline resistant, and treatment consists of potassium replacement. Alkalosis caused by decreased aldosterone degradation (secondary hyperaldosteronism) seen in severe hepatic disease may respond to the aldosterone antagonist spironolactone. Patients with mineralocorticoid-producing tumors of the adrenal or pituitary glands need therapy with aminoglutethimide or surgery.

Respiratory Acidosis

Respiratory acidosis is a plasma pH lower than 7.35 as the result of a pCO_2 higher than 40 mm Hg. The hemoglobin-buffering system is activated in acute respiratory acidosis and sequesters hydrogen ions inside red blood cells. However, it is a weak system and can raise the HCO_3 by only 1 mmol/L for every 10-mm Hg rise in pCO_2. To completely correct the plasma pH, a 5-mmol/L rise in HCO_3 is needed for every 10-mm Hg rise in pCO_2. It is the slow generation of HCO_3 in the kidney that eventually raises the plasma HCO_3 enough to compensate for the respiratory acidosis and normalize the pH.

Because the CO_2 excretion capacity of normal lungs is always greater than metabolic production, respiratory acidosis occurs only as a result of severe pulmonary disease (Table 9.7).

Table 9.7 ▪ Respiratory Acidosis (pH < 7.35, pCO_2 > 40 mm Hg)

Causes	Signs and Symptoms
Emphysema	Anxiety
Airway obstruction	Disorientation
Bronchoconstriction	Vasodilation
Pneumonia	Increased cardiac output
Respiratory depression	Coma
Treatment	
Bronchodilators, antibiotics, respiratory support	

Treatment of Respiratory Acidosis

Treatment always consists of correcting the underlying pulmonary disorder and may include antibiotics, bronchodilators, and steroids. Intubation and mechanical ventilation may be needed if respiratory depression accompanies the acidosis. Rapid correction of the pH should be avoided, and bicarbonate is indicated only if plasma pH is at or below 7.1. Chronic respiratory acidosis with emphysema and chronic obstructive pulmonary disease (COPD) develops slowly and is rarely severe enough to necessitate treatment. The stimulus for respiration in these patients may still be an elevated CO_2, but many have adapted to hypoxia as the respiratory drive; lowering the pCO_2 and raising the pO_2 acutely is not recommended because apnea can result.

Respiratory Alkalosis

Respiratory alkalosis is a pCO_2 lower than 40 mm Hg, causing a plasma pH higher than 7.45. The defense against this type of alkalosis is the movement of hydrogen ions (intracellular H_2PO_4 goes to HPO_4) to the vascular space. The phosphate buffering system, like hemoglobin, is small in capacity and cannot normalize the pH in severe respiratory alkalosis; it can only lower the HCO_3 by 3.5 mmol/L for every 10-mm Hg drop in pCO_2 (Table 9.8).

Treatment of Respiratory Alkalosis

Voluntary hyperventilation, mechanical ventilation, and rapid breathing caused by hypoxemia lower the pCO_2; correcting the disorder involves normalizing the pCO_2 by raising the CO_2 concentration of inspired air. This can be done by increasing the concentration of inspired CO_2 delivered by a ventilator or by having the patient rebreathe his or her own expired air from a bag placed loosely over the nose and mouth.

Compensatory Responses to Acid-Base Disturbances

All primary acid-base disturbances engender a compensatory response; for example, metabolic acidosis results in a drop in pCO_2 (compensating respiratory alkalosis). It can be difficult to determine the primary disturbance if the plasma pH has been returned to normal. It is also possible for two primary acid-base problems to occur together; the only exception is that respiratory acidosis and respiratory alkalosis cannot occur simultaneously. Correct diagnosis of the patient's diseases and a medication history are essential to establish the causes of an acid-base disorder and initiate treatment. No simple calculation using the arterial blood gases and serum electrolyte levels will suffice, given the complexity of the body's buffering and compensatory mechanisms. Excellent nomograms (Fig. 9.3) exist to help the clinician determine the constituents of an acid-base disturbance. This determination, combined with the history, guides treatment decisions.

Table 9.8 ▪ Respiratory Alkalosis (pH > 7.45, pCO_2 < 40 mm Hg)

Causes	Signs and Symptoms
Hyperventilation	Confusion
Respiratory stimulants	Tetany
Hypoxemia	Syncope
Treatment	
Rebreathing CO_2	

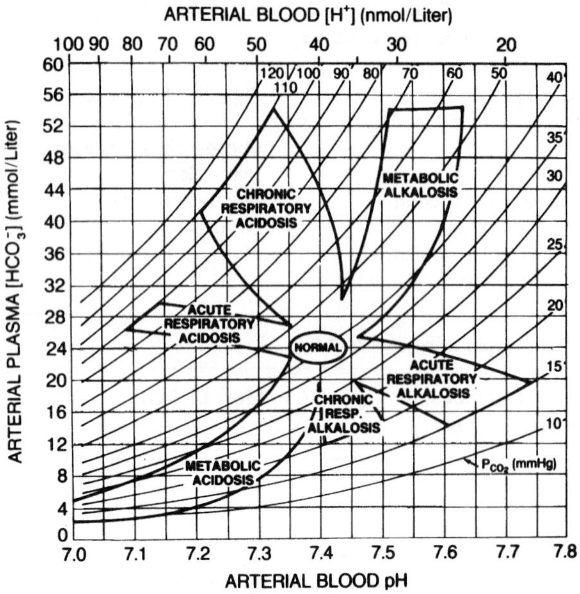

Figure 9.3. Acid-base nomogram. (Reprinted from Cogan MG, Rector FC. Acid-base disorders. In: Brenner BM, Rector FC, eds. The kidney. 3rd ed. Philadelphia: WB Saunders, 1986:457–518.)

ELECTROLYTES

The major electrolytes in the body are sodium, chloride, bicarbonate, potassium, calcium, magnesium, and phosphate. Normal serum levels are listed in Table 9.1. Sodium is linked to TBW; maintenance of normal levels and correction of abnormalities were discussed earlier. The role of chloride in the body is as an osmotic substance and the major anion in the ECF; it has no innate physiologic function. Bicarbonate is linked to the acid-base homeostatic system and was also discussed earlier. The physiologic functions of the remaining electrolytes are to maintain membrane potentials for nerve conduction and muscle contraction (potassium, calcium, and magnesium), to generate the energy needed to maintain these potentials and to do the work of body functions and movement (phosphorus), and to maintain the strength of the bone mass (calcium and phosphorus). The main reservoirs of these ions are the intracellular space and bone. Serum levels fall slowly when intake goes down because numerous hormonal and homeostatic mechanisms exist to keep serum levels within the normal range. The serum concentrations of these electrolytes are low relative to sodium and to their own intracellular concentrations, but it is their intravascular concentrations that control physiologic activities. Serum levels must be kept within a narrow range or serious difficulties, such as arrhythmias, seizures, and tetany, will result.

Potassium

The amount of potassium in the vascular space accounts for only 0.4% of the total amount in the body.[24–28] The normal serum concentration ranges from 3.5 to 5.0 mmol/L (3.5 to 5 mEq/L), and its major functions are in impulse transmission, cardiac contractility, and aldosterone secretion. The major route of potassium excretion is the kidney. Elimination can increase when intake is high, but the kidneys have no way to conserve potassium; a deficiency state develops rapidly if intake drops. Hyponatremia also causes potassium loss via renal exchange processes that are discussed in the Sodium section (Fig. 9.2).

Serum levels of potassium do not completely depend on the relationship between intake and output and sodium homeostasis. The large intracellular pool of potassium can be a source of ions to support the intravascular concentration; when a low serum level finally develops, it usually represents not just a low circulating amount of potassium but also an acquired intracellular deficit that can approach several hundred millimoles. Changes in acid-base status alter the distribution of potassium ions in the body. In acidosis, potassium is exchanged across cell membranes with hydrogen ions as the body attempts to hide and buffer protons (acid) in the intracellular space; this will help maintain a normal pH. The converse is true in alkalosis. The serum potassium rises (acidosis) or falls (alkalosis) by 0.6 mmol/L for every 0.1 change in pH from the value of 7.4.

Hyperkalemia

High serum potassium can be a true medical emergency and almost always manifests itself initially by the sudden appearance of cardiac arrhythmias. This most often occurs at serum levels above 6 mmol/L. The symptoms and causes of hyperkalemia are listed in Table 9.9. Actual total body potassium can be high, normal, or (occasionally) low; it is the intravascular concentration that effects physiologic activities and causes the cardiac disorders. The life-threatening potential of the cardiac abnormality determines the type, complexity, and sequence of treatment given. Any exogenous sources of potassium such as IV fluids or drugs containing potassium should be discontinued immediately.

Measures used to correct hyperkalemia act by normalizing neuromuscular membrane potential, shifting ions back into the intracellular space, or removing potassium from the body. Membrane potential and, therefore, the strength of muscular contraction are determined by the relative concentrations of potassium, calcium, and magnesium at the cell membrane. If the potassium-induced arrhythmia is life-threatening, 2.5 to 5 mmol (5 to 10 mEq) calcium is given over several minutes to temporarily correct the potassium–calcium ratio and eliminate the cardiac problem. If necessary to maintain good cardiac function until measures that permanently normalize the serum potassium take effect, a constant infusion of intravenous calcium at a rate determined by simultaneous electrocardiographic (ECG) monitoring is indicated. Calcium gluconate (2.3 mmol/g) or calcium chloride (6.8 mmol/g) is used, but therapy cannot continue for long periods because hypercalcemia will become a problem.

A different treatment approach is to shift potassium ions from the vascular to the intracellular space. Sodium

Table 9.9 ▪ Symptoms and Causes of Hyperkalemia and Hypokalemia

Hyperkalemia	Hypokalemia
Serum level > 5 mmol/L (5 mEq/L)	Serum level < 3.5 mmol/L (3.5 mEq/L)
Causes	
Renal failure	Amphotericin B
Acidosis	Diuretics
Crush injury	Diarrhea
Red cell hemolysis	Decreased intake
Potassium-sparing diuretics	Corticosteroids
Excess ingestion of potassium (salt substitutes)	Renal tubular acidosis
Adrenal insufficiency	Alkalosis
Hypoaldosteronism	Vomiting
	Fanconi's syndrome
	Hyperaldosteronism
	Licorice
Signs and Symptoms	
Electrocardiographic findings	Electrocardiographic findings
Peaked T waves	Flat or inverted T waves
Depressed ST segment	Depressed ST segment
Disappearance of P wave	Muscle weakness
Widened QRS complex	Diminished reflexes
Muscle weakness	Paralysis
Paresthesias	Weak pulse
Gastrointestinal hypermotility	Ileus
Flaccid paralysis	Depression
	Confusion
	Hypotension
Treatment of Hyperkalemia	
Calcium (as chloride or gluconate salt) 2–5 mmol over 5–10 min	
Na bicarbonate 50 mmol over 2–3 min	
Regular insulin 10 U in 50 g dextrose over 5–10 min	
Sodium polystyrene sulfonate resin 30–60 g in 20% sorbitol orally or rectally	
Hemodialysis or peritoneal dialysis	
Treatment of Hypokalemia	
KCl 10 mmol/hr × 4 doses, check serum K, repeat as necessary	

bicarbonate administration produces a temporary alkalosis and lower serum potassium by 0.6 mmol/L for every 0.1 elevation in pH. This therapy, like calcium infusion, cannot be continued for long periods because sodium overload and metabolic alkalosis will result. Fifty-milliliter vials and preloaded syringes of 8.4% (1 mmol/mL) and 500-mL containers of 5% (0.6 mmol/mL) sodium bicarbonate are commercially available; 4.2% (0.5 mmol/mL) preloaded syringes are available for pediatric or neonatal use.

Glucose and insulin infusions are another treatment option. Potassium ions move with glucose across cell membranes in the presence of insulin. A ratio of 2 to 3 g glucose per unit of insulin is needed to maintain a normal blood glucose level during this process; 25 to 30 U regular insulin per liter of 10% dextrose solution and 10 U in 50 mL 50% dextrose are the commonly administered solutions. This is a temporary solution, like calcium and sodium bicarbonate administration, because potassium ions are not removed from the body. However, it does allow treatment to continue without significant complication for long periods of time.

Two therapies remove potassium from the body but act slowly. Although they should be initiated as soon as possible, they will not correct cardiac arrhythmias in a timely fashion and cannot be considered acute treatments for hyperkalemia. The cationic–anionic exchange resin sodium polystyrene sulfonate (SPS), given orally or rectally, binds potassium to itself by exchange with sodium in the GI tract; 1 g SPS removes 1 mmol potassium and adds 2 to 3 mmol sodium. The resin is very constipating, so it is given with sorbitol, an osmotic cathartic, and water to prevent fecal impaction. The oral route is preferred over rectal administration because the contact time with the GI mucosa is longer. The initial dosage is 30 to 60 g resin in 20% sorbitol (commercial preparations are available) and can be repeated every 1 to 2 hours if the serum potassium level remains high. Sodium overload can occur, so monitoring for congestive heart failure, edema, and pulmonary edema is necessary in patients at risk of developing these problems. Patients will complain about therapy because the resin has the consistency of sand and a very unpleasant taste. As a last resort in treating hyperkalemia, peritoneal or hemodialysis can be used to remove potassium from the body. This procedure is very invasive and should be used only if the patient's condition is life-threatening and other treatment methods have or will fail.

Hypokalemia

Hypokalemia can also be a cardiac medical emergency, with rhythm disturbances appearing at serum levels below 3 mmol/L. Fortunately, the patient may exhibit muscle weakness and malaise before ECG changes appear. The symptoms and causes of hypokalemia are listed in Table 9.9. Correction of underlying diseases or discontinuation of drug therapy contributing to hypokalemia is a basic part of the initial treatment.

Hypokalemia secondary to hyponatremia is almost always accompanied by hypochloremic alkalosis as the renal conservation of sodium causes secretion of potassium and hydrogen ions (Fig. 9.2). For every 3 mmol sodium reabsorbed, 2 mmol potassium and 1 mmol hydrogen are lost in the urine. The hydrogen ion needed for the exchange with sodium is generated from the action of carbonic anhydrase on water and carbon dioxide. Carbonic acid in renal tubular cells dissociates into hydrogen and bicarbonate; hydrogen ion is secreted into the urine and bicarbonate is resorbed into the blood. When enough bicarbonate ions accumulate in serum, alkalosis results. Any concomitant hyponatremia and alkalosis must be corrected for hypokalemia treatment to be successful. The chloride salt of potassium is the treatment of choice because alkalosis must be corrected. As chloride loading proceeds, bicarbonate excretion by the kidneys increases, generation decreases, and alkalosis resolves. If a nonchloride salt of potassium is given, renal excretion and intracellular shifting of potassium will continue and the hypokalemia will not correct (Fig. 9.2).

An intracellular deficit of potassium almost always precedes and accompanies an intravascular deficit; large amounts of potassium will be needed before the total body and serum levels normalize. Oral or intravenously administered potassium shifts slowly into the ICF to correct that deficit, so the rate of potassium chloride infusion must not be so rapid as to cause interim hyperkalemia. Under most conditions, intravenous potassium chloride at 10 mmol/hour will not cause hyperkalemia in a patient with a serum level below 3.5 mmol/L, and 30 to 40 mmol given over 3 to 4 hours in D5W or NS is the most common rate of potassium replacement. The serum potassium is checked 1 to 2 hours later and the treatment repeated until the level is 3.8 to 4.0 mmol/L. In patients with profound hypokalemia and continuing potassium wasting, such as those with renal tubular acidosis from amphotericin B therapy, replacing the potassium deficit can entail very large dosages. In these instances, 20 to 50 mmol/hour may be needed; a central line is always necessary because infusion into a peripheral vein at a rate greater than 10 mmol/hour almost always causes intolerable pain and phlebitis at the infusion site.

Oral administration of potassium chloride can correct hypokalemia, but many patients experience considerable GI irritation and vomiting when given more than 20 mmol/dose or 60 mmol/day. They often refuse therapy because of the bad taste of oral solutions. Wax matrix tablets have greater patient acceptance than liquid potassium, but the problem of gastric irritation remains. Attempts to replace large potassium deficits by mouth often are unsuccessful, and simultaneous IV replacement may be needed.

Chloride

Chloride is the major anion in the ECF, but it has no inherent physiologic function.[4,18] It usually goes up or down in synchronous fashion with total body sodium, but a change in chloride concentration causes an acid-base disturbance. Because electrical neutrality must be maintained and the concentration of unmeasured ions is fixed, there will be an immediate change in the serum bicarbonate concentration. The effect will be metabolic acidosis or alkalosis depending on the resultant increase or decrease in the bicarbonate:pCO_2 ratio.

The disorders of body chloride result from its loss from the body (vomiting, diuretics), hypernatremia, chloride loading (saline infusion), or changes in acid-base balance. In acidosis and alkalosis, the change in the serum chloride concentration is almost always a compensatory response to an initial change in the bicarbonate value. In this instance, the serum chloride will not normalize, nor should there be an effort made to normalize it by giving or withholding chloride until the cause of the acid-base abnormality is identified and corrected. When this occurs, the chloride concentration normalizes naturally via renal homeostatic mechanisms.

Hyperchloremia

A serum level greater than 105 mmol/L is considered abnormal. Because it is the result of metabolic acidosis, hypernatremia, or chloride loading, treatment is aimed at correcting the underlying disorder. The composition of oral or intravenous fluids should be determined and adjustments made if they appear to be the cause of the problem. Changing a NS infusion to an LR or 0.45% saline infusion or replacing sodium chloride with sodium acetate may solve the problem. If the cause of the hyperchloremia is metabolic acidosis or respiratory alkalosis, correcting these disturbances is the only treatment. When hypernatremia caused by overingestion of sodium chloride is the cause, treatment is free water replacement and diuresis; in hypernatremia caused by water loss, the treatment is electrolyte-free water replacement (see Sodium).

Hypochloremia

A serum chloride below 95 mmol/L is considered hypochloremia. Because the ECF chloride changes with ECF sodium, hyponatremia causes hypochloremia. This is an appropriate compensatory mechanism to maintain electrical neutrality, and the chloride normalizes with correction of the ECF sodium concentration.

The most common causes of hypochloremia are nasogastric suction, vomiting, and diuretic therapy. Large amounts of chloride and acid are lost with stomach fluid, so therapy consists of replacing the volume of the NG aspirate or vomiting with high-chloride solutions such as NS or LR. Diuretics cause hypochloremia by mechanisms discussed in the Hyponatremia section. Therapy consists of liberalizing sodium chloride intake, reducing the diuretic dosage, and correcting symptomatic hyponatremia and hypokalemia with saline and potassium chloride solutions.

Calcium

The major repository of calcium in the body is bone; only 1% of the total amount in the body is in the fluid spaces.[29–38] The normal serum concentration is 2.2 to 2.6 mmol/L (8.8 to 10.3 mg/dL), but only 50% is available to exert its physiologic effect; the other 50% is bound to albumin and other proteins. Serum calcium concentration does not fluctuate as a direct result of daily intake and excretion of the ion. The synchronous activity of parathyroid hormone, vitamin D, and calcitonin regulates GI absorption, renal excretion, and skeletal deposition or resorption of calcium and determines the serum calcium. There is also an inverse relationship between serum calcium and phosphate; if one goes up or down, the other changes in the opposite direction to maintain their equilibrium.

Calcium has a variety of specific physiologic functions in the body. It is essential to neuromuscular conduction because it stabilizes cell membrane permeability and excitability, and it inhibits some enzymes in the Krebs cycle, stimulates gastrin, reduces renal blood flow, and is active in the blood coagulation cascade as factor IV. The normal range is narrow, and some laboratories still measure total serum calcium, not just the active ionized 50%. This presents a problem in determining the physiologically active amount of the ion in the serum. Because 50% is protein bound, primarily to albumin, a low serum albumin results in a low total serum calcium concentration; this does not necessarily mean there is a low ionized level. For each 10-g/L decrease in the serum albumin concentration, total serum calcium decreases 0.02 mmol/L. For example, a patient with an albumin of 20 g/L has a reported total calcium of 1.95 mmol/L; although the value is below normal, it does not represent a low ionized (free) level. Mathematically correcting the albumin to a normal of 40 gm/L raises the total calcium to 2.4 mmol/L. It can be assumed from this correction that the free calcium is normal and physiologic hypocalcemia is not present. The formula for this calculation is as follows:

$$[(40 - \text{Reported serum albumin}) \times 0.2] + \text{Reported serum calcium} = \text{Corrected serum calcium}$$

When the ionized calcium is reported, this correction need not be made.

Acid-base disturbances affect the ionized:bound calcium ratio but not total serum calcium. Some hydrogen ions circulate in the blood bound to albumin. In acidosis, more hydrogen ions are bound to albumin as the body attempts to buffer acid and normalize the plasma pH; this displaces calcium ions from their binding sites, and the amount of free calcium in the blood rises. The converse is true in alkalosis. For each 0.1 change in pH, the ionized calcium changes 0.42 mmol/L in the opposite direction.

Hypercalcemia

Hypercalcemia is defined as a corrected total serum calcium above 2.6 mmol/L (10.3 mg/dL) or an ionized value above 1.15 mmol/L. The symptoms and causes are listed in Table 9.10. Any sources of exogenous calcium should be discontinued immediately. It is important to note that the mental aberrations seen with hypercalcemia can be profound and not always related in a linear fashion to the degree of hypercalcemia. Any evaluation of an apparently mentally ill or comatose patient should include a serum calcium level.

Table 9.10 ▪ Symptoms and Causes of Hypercalcemia and Hypocalcemia

Hypercalcemia	Hypocalcemia
Serum level > 2.6 mmol/L (total, corrected) (10.3 mg/dL) 1.2 mmol/L (ionized) (2.3 mEq/L)	Serum level < 2.2 mmol/L (total, corrected) (8.8 mg/dL) 1.0 mmol/L (ionized) (2.0 mEq/L)
Causes	
Bone neoplasms	Renal failure
Hyperparathyroidism	Hypoparathyroidism
Hypervitaminosis D	Vitamin D deficiency
Prolonged immobilization	Diuretics
Sarcoidosis	Mithramycin
Paget's disease	Transfusion with citrated blood
Acidosis	Lithium
Idiopathic hypercalcemia	Adrenal insufficiency
Alkalosis of infancy	Pancreatitis
Hypervitaminosis A	Hyperphosphatemia
Aluminum osteodystrophy	Colchicine
	Hypomagnesemia
	Fluoride poisoning
Signs and Symptoms	
Muscle weakness	Numbness or tingling of fingertips or around mouth
Anorexia	Fatigue
Lethargy	Nausea
Depression	Hyperactive reflexes
Psychosis	Chvostek's sign
Stupor	Trousseau's sign
Coma	Tetany
	Lethargy
	Depression
	Psychosis
	Stupor
	Coma
Treatment of Hypercalcemia	
Normal saline and furosemide, calcitonin, etidronate, pamidronate, mithramycin, phosphate, steroids	
Treatment of Hypocalcemia	
Calcium (chloride or gluconate) IV 2–5 mmol (5–10 mEq) over 15–30 min or calcium carbonate PO 2–10 g daily	

The therapies for hypercalcemia involve shifting ions back into the bone or removing calcium from the body. The removal therapies are given first because they work faster and are generally more effective in an acute situation. Loop diuretics, such as furosemide and bumetanide, increase renal calcium excretion in addition to their better-known effects on sodium and chloride elimination. The initial furosemide dosage is 1 mg/kg; it is given with an amount of NS that will maintain a normal body water and sodium when a urine output of 200 to 500 mL/hour is achieved. Potassium must also be added to this therapy to prevent hypokalemia from the action of the loop diuretic. This washout therapy may need to be continued for extended periods if the cause of the hypercalcemia is severe or abnormally large amounts of calcium continue to appear in the vascular compartment.

Treatments that shift calcium back into bone are slow and may become ineffective because of tachyphylaxis. Parenteral calcitonin is used because it rapidly increases bone uptake of calcium; although the effect is rapid, it is of short duration, and tachyphylaxis develops within days. The initial parenteral dosage for treating hypercalcemia is 4 IU/kg salmon calcitonin given every 12 hours by subcutaneous or intramuscular injection; after 2 days, this can be increased to a maximum dosage of 8 IU/kg given every 6 hours, but additional hypocalcemic effect usually does not result. Intranasal calcitonin is effective in treating established osteoporosis in women who cannot take hormone replacement therapy but is not useful in managing acute or chronic hypercalcemia. Etidronate disodium is a bisphosphonate that inhibits osteoclastic bone resorption by binding hydroxyapatite. Initial treatment is with 7.5 mg/kg/day given intravenously once daily for 3 days. The infusion time must be at least 2 hours to avoid proximal renal tubular damage (seen in patients with preexisting renal disease) and the theoretical risk of transient hypocalcemia. Once the serum calcium has been controlled, oral therapy with 20 mg/kg/day can be given if the hypercalcemia is expected to recur (e.g., bone metastases in patients with cancer). Pamidronate disodium appears to be more effective than etidronate in treating hypercalcemia and offers the advantages of quicker onset and longer duration of action without the disadvantage of inhibiting bone mineralization at high dosages. It is dosed at 60 to 90 mg given intravenously over at least 2 hours. The treatment can be repeated as often as every 7 days if necessary. Calcitonin in combination with bisphosphonates is used in the acute management of hypercalcemia.

Steroids, such as prednisone, are useful in managing chronic mild hypercalcemia. The initial prednisone dosage varies between 15 and 100 mg/day, with an onset of action of 3 to 10 days. Steroids work by antagonizing activation of vitamin D in the liver and reducing bone resorption; for these reasons, they are not effective in hypercalcemia secondary to hyperparathyroidism. Oral phosphate is not a treatment option in this type of hypercalcemia. Because the ordinarily reciprocal relationship between serum calcium and phosphate levels has not been sustained, the amount by which the serum calcium falls when phosphate concentration rises usually is small. The risk of soft tissue calcification by calcium–phosphorus complexes often exceeds the benefit of this therapy. If raising the serum phosphate results in a calcium–phosphate product (multiply serum calcium [in mg/dL] and phosphate [in mg/dL] to get this value) exceeds 50, precipitation can occur. In the rare instances when hypophosphatemia is the cause of hypercalcemia, administering 30 to 100 mmol/day (1 to 3 g) of phosphorus should solve the problem. Sodium phosphate replacement products are available; Phospho-Soda solution contains 25 mmol (800 mg) phosphate/5 mL, Neutra-Phos capsules contain 8 mmol (250 mg) phosphate, and the solution contains 32 mmol (1 g) phosphate/300 mL. These products also contain considerable amounts of sodium as the obligate cation, so they must be used with caution.

An effective but potentially toxic therapy for hypercalcemia is mithramycin; it is indicated only when other therapies fail. Mithramycin is a cancer chemotherapeutic agent that acts by inhibiting DNA-dependent bone osteoclast RNA synthesis. This will slow or stop bone resorption. The initial dosage is 25 μg/kg daily up to a weekly maximum of 150 μg/kg. The onset of action is 12 to 48 hours and the duration 3 to 7 days. Although these dosages are considerably smaller than those used in cancer treatment, the risk of hematologic and GI toxicity remains.

Hypocalcemia

Hypocalcemia is defined as a corrected serum level below 2.20 mmol/L (8.8 mg/dL) or an ionized level below 1 mmol/L. The symptoms and causes are listed in Table 9.10. Acute treatment involves intravenous calcium. The chloride salt contains 6.8 mmol/g (13.5 mEq calcium/g) and the gluconate and gluceptate salts 2.3 mmol/g (4.6 mEq calcium/g). The initial dosage is 2.5 to 5 mmol calcium followed by an infusion of 0.075 to 0.1 mmol calcium/kg/hour. Calcium level, blood pressure, and ECG should be monitored during this process to evaluate cardiac function and avoid hypercalcemia. Patients whose symptoms of hypocalcemia do not resolve with calcium replacement should be evaluated for hypomagnesemia because the abnormalities can mimic each other and often appear together.

Treatment of chronic hypocalcemia is directed at correcting the underlying cause. Most often the cause of chronic hypocalcemia is a low level of biologically active vitamin D. This appears in advanced hepatic or renal disease because of decreased transformation of cholecalciferol (D_3) by these organs to the active form, 1,25-dihydroxycholecalciferol (1,25-DHC). The serum level of calcium will not normalize until the level of 1,25-DHC is normal. Therapy usually involves calcium and vitamin D supplementation. Ergocalciferol (D_2) in a dosage of 1.25 to 5 mg (50,000 to 200,000 IU/day) or dihydrotachysterol (DHT) in a dosage of 0.25 to 1 mg/day (equivalent to 30,000 to 120,000 IU of D_2) is used. The onset of action can be several weeks and the effect prolonged because of the long half-life of vitamin D. Activated forms of vitamin D must be given if renal or hepatic transformation of ergocalciferol and dihydrotachysterol is absent or unreliable. 25-Hydroxycholecalciferol (calcifediol) in dosages of 50 to 100 μg/day or 1,25-DHC (calcitriol) in dosages of 0.25 to 1 μg/day are available. The active forms of vitamin D have an onset of action of 3 to 7 days and are preferred because their shorter half-lives reduce the risk of prolonged hypercalcemia. Calcium supplementation with 25 to 100 mmol/d (1 to 4 g) elemental calcium is begun simultaneously. Several salts of calcium are available for oral therapy, but calcium carbonate contains the highest amount of elemental calcium, 10.2 mmol (400 mg) per 1000 mg calcium carbonate. Calcium lactate is 1.5 mmol (60 mg) per 300 mg, calcium gluceptate contains 2.2 mmol (80 mg) per 1000 mg, and calcium gluconate 2.3 mmol (90 mg) per 1000 mg. Calcium carbonate is the preferred preparation because the number of tablets the patient must take is lower than with the other salts. Liquid calcium carbonate and calcium gluceptate are available for use in patients with achlorhydria or those receiving H_2 antagonist therapy because tablet dissolution in the GI tract may be incomplete without gastric acid. When hypocalcemia is caused by hypoparathyroidism, parathyroid hormone replacement is indicated and is the only therapy that raises the serum calcium.

Magnesium

The average adult body contains approximately 1000 mmol (2000 mEq) magnesium, 99% of which is in bone and the intracellular compartment.[39,40] Of the 1% remaining in the vascular space, 25% is bound to proteins; it is the ionized 75% that exerts the physiologic effect. Serum magnesium is maintained in the normal range of 0.8 to 1.2 mmol/L (1.6 to 2.4 mEq/L) by efficient renal conservation and excretion mechanisms and the ability to draw on the intracellular space for replacement ions when intake falls. In conjunction with calcium and potassium, magnesium regulates neuromuscular excitability and conduction on the cell membrane; it also has a role in parathyroid hormone release. Deviations from a normal serum magnesium rarely appear as an isolated problem. Most often, calcium, potassium, and phosphate levels also are abnormal, indicating a generalized abnormality in the solute concentration of the intracellular compartment. This pattern of electrolyte disturbances is most commonly seen in prolonged starvation.

Hypermagnesemia

Hypermagnesemia is defined as a serum level above 1.2 mmol/L (2.4 mEq/L), but serious symptoms usually do not occur until the level is above 2.4. The symptoms and causes of hypermagnesemia are listed in Table 9.11. Because large loads of magnesium can be excreted easily by the kidneys, hypermagnesemia is rarely seen without attendant severe renal dysfunction. Magnesium-containing antacids are often a contributing factor in this situation. All sources of exogenous magnesium should be discontinued.

The treatments for an elevated magnesium involve eliminating it from the body or shifting it back into the intracellular space. Glucose and insulin can be used for brief periods of time, as in the treatment of hyperkalemia, but the only effective means of removing it from the body are peritoneal and hemodialysis.

Table 9.11 ▪ Symptoms and Causes of Hypermagnesemia and Hypomagnesemia

Hypermagnesemia	Hypomagnesemia
Serum level > 1.2 mmol/L (2.4 mEq/L)	Serum level < 0.8 mmol/L (1.6 mEq/L)
Causes	
Renal failure Hyperparathyroidism Hypoaldosteronism Adrenal insufficiency Lithium	Amphotericin B Cis-platinum Diuretics Diarrhea Hypervitaminosis D Vitamin D deficiency Vomiting Hyperaldosteronism Aminoglycosides
Signs and Symptoms	
Weakness Nausea or vomiting Hypotension Respiratory depression Coma	Tremor Hyperactive reflexes Confusion Seizures
Treatment of Hypermagnesemia	
Dextrose and insulin, hemodialysis	
Treatment of Hypomagnesemia	
Magnesium SO_4 IV 0.15–0.25 mmol/kg/day Magnesium oxide 300–600 mg PO (6.25 mmol Mg) BID–TID	

Hypomagnesemia

Hypomagnesemia is defined as a serum level below 0.8 mmol/L (1.6 mEq/L); symptoms can appear at levels below 0.6. The symptoms and causes of hypomagnesemia are found in Table 9.11. Hypomagnesemia usually appears with hypokalemia, hypocalcemia, and hypophosphatemia. Levels of these electrolytes should be measured when low levels of magnesium are found. There is almost always a large deficit when serum levels fall; the total body deficit of magnesium may be as much as 25 mmol at this point. Therapy is with the sulfate or oxide salts of magnesium. The available product for intravenous administration is magnesium sulfate; each gram of the 50% solution contains 4 mmol (8 mEq) magnesium. The initial dosage is 0.25 mmol/kg/day if the serum level is less than 0.6 mmol/L and 0.15 mmol/kg/day if it is between 0.7 and 1.2. This amount should be given over 1 to 4 hours and the serum level checked 1 to 2 hours later. The delay before measuring the serum concentration gives time for intracellular shifting; as is the case with potassium, an exact replacement dosage cannot be determined from the serum level alone. The oral replacement of large deficits can be difficult. Magnesium is a saline cathartic, and the large dosages needed for replacement may produce diarrhea. When this route of administration is chosen, up to 20 mmol/day given in divided doses usually is tolerated. Magnesium oxide capsules are most commonly given (6.2 mmol/250 mg MgO) because of convenience for the patient, but solutions of magnesium sulfate are also available.

Phosphorus

Of the total body phosphate, 99.99% is contained in bone and the intracellular space.[41,42] The normal serum level is 0.8 to 1.6 mmol/L (2.5 to 5 mg/dL). The equilibrium between serum calcium (reciprocal with phosphate), intracellular stores, parathyroid hormone, vitamin D, renal conservation and excretion mechanisms, and oral intake maintains a normal serum level. The specific physiologic function of phosphate in the body is to form high-energy phosphate bonds of adenosine diphosphate and triphos-

Table 9.12 ▪ Symptoms and Causes of Hyperphosphatemia and Hypophosphatemia

Hyperphosphatemia	Hypophosphatemia
Serum level > 1.6 mmol/L (5.0 mg/dL)	Serum level < 0.8 mmol/L (2.5 mg/dL)
Causes	
Renal failure Hypoparathyroidism	Aluminum antacids Prolonged starvation Nutritional depletion Diuretics Vitamin D deficiency Hyperaldosteronism Corticosteroids Alkalosis Renal tubular defects Syndrome of inappropriate secretion of antidiuretic hormone
Signs and Symptoms	
Renal osteodystrophy Ca–PO_4 complex deposition in soft tissue	Muscle weakness Bone pain Paresthesias Irritability Respiratory insufficiency Hemolytic anemia Rhabdomyolysis Proximal muscle atrophy Cardiomyopathy Seizures Coma
Treatment of Hyperphosphatemia	
Dextrose and insulin, hemodialysis	
Treatment of Hypophosphatemia	
Na or K phosphate IV or PO 0.05–0.6 mmol PO_4/kg/day	

phate in glycolysis (anaerobic metabolism) and in the Krebs cycle. Another important function of phosphate, as 2,3-diphosphoglycerate, is to facilitate the release of oxygen from hemoglobin.

Hyperphosphatemia

Hyperphosphatemia is defined as a serum level above 1.6 mmol/L and almost always results from decreased excretion in the presence of severe renal dysfunction. Symptoms and causes of hyperphosphatemia are listed in Table 9.12. The major risk of hyperphosphatemia, and the reason it is most commonly corrected, is the hypocalcemia it reciprocally causes; a high phosphate level alone does not have significant negative physiologic consequences. Any patient with an elevated phosphate level needs a serum calcium check because the physiologic disturbances from an abnormal calcium level are serious. The only available treatments for hyperphosphatemia are reducing phosphorus intake and decreasing its absorption from the GI tract by precipitating it with aluminum-containing antacids and with glucose–insulin infusions. Peritoneal dialysis or hemodialysis is used to lower serum phosphate levels when hypocalcemia is a problem, but they are not very efficient or effective therapies.

Hypophosphatemia

Hypophosphatemia is defined as a serum level below 0.8 mmol/L, but symptoms rarely appear if it is above 0.3; the abnormality usually is the result of starvation and appears with simultaneous deficits in other intracellular ions. Symptoms and causes are listed in Table 9.12. Therapy consists of replacement with the sodium or potassium salts of phosphate. Repletion must be slow because calcium–phosphate precipitation in soft tissue can result if therapy is so aggressive that there is no time for a drop in circulating calcium ions. The initial phosphate dosage is 0.3 to 0.6 mmol/kg/day if the serum level is below 0.3 and 0.2 to 0.3 mmol/kg/day if it is between 0.4 and 0.8. Therapy should be given over at least 6 hours to allow for equilibration into the intracellular space, where the majority of the body deficit occurs; the serum level is checked 3 to 4 hours after the end of the infusion. Oral replacement can be given with sodium phosphate solution or capsules in divided doses (refer to the section on hypercalcemia for phosphate content of available products).

KEY POINTS

- Identifying and correcting disorders of fluids, electrolytes, and acid-base balance can be difficult. The body's internal environment is constantly changing, adjusting to and correcting for internal and external forces that disturb homeostasis. Normal serum levels of electrolytes do not always reflect normal body water or pH status; abnormal values may be appropriate compensatory responses to maintain homeostasis, and treatment consists of finding and correcting the primary disturbance. Normal body functions continue only within narrow ranges of ionic composition, pH, and intravascular volume and pressure.
- When evaluating any patient, establishing and maintaining a hemodynamic status sufficient to perfuse and oxygenate cells is the first priority and must be done quickly.
- With the exception of exsanguination (acute, massive blood loss), changes in fluids, electrolytes, and pH usually occur slowly, and some compensatory mechanisms operate.
- Correcting an isolated abnormal laboratory value without regard to its cause and contribution to overall patient status will further complicate the patient's condition without any benefit.
- Any therapy chosen must be given in a way and at a rate that reestablishes and supports homeostasis without causing treatment-induced (iatrogenic) complications.

REFERENCES

1. Brenner BM, Levine SA, eds. The kidney. 5th ed. Philadelphia: WB Saunders, 1995.
2. Various. Fluid and electrolyte therapy. Pediatr Clin North Am 37(2):241–504, 1990.
3. Cohn SH, Vaswani A. Changes in body chemical composition with age measured by total-body neutron activation. Metabolism 25:85, 1976.
4. Votey SR, Peters AL, Hoffman JR. Disorders of water metabolism: hyponatremia and hypernatremia. Emerg Med Clin North Am 7(4):749–769, 1989.
5. Feig PU, McCurdy DK. The hypertonic state. N Engl J Med 297:1444–1454, 1977.
6. Zarinetchi F, Berl T. Evaluation and management of severe hyponatremia. Adv Intern Med 41:251–283, 1996.
7. Kovacs L, Robertson GL. Syndrome of inappropriate anti-diuresis. Endocrinol Metab Clin North Am 21(4):859–875, 1992.
8. Chan TY. Drug-induced syndrome of inappropriate secretion of anti-diuretic hormone. Causes, diagnosis and treatment. Drugs Aging 11(1):27–44, 1997.
9. Faber MD, Kupin WL, Heilig CW, et al. Common fluid and electrolyte and acid-base problems in the intensive care unit: selected problems. Semin Nephrol 14(1):8–22, 1994.
10. Harris BH, Gelfand JA. The immune response to trauma. Semin Pediatr Surg 4(2):77–82, 1995.
11. Field M, Rao M. Intestinal electrolyte transport and diarrheal disease, part 1. N Engl J Med 321:800–806, 1989.
12. Field M, Rao M. Intestinal electrolyte transport and diarrheal disease, part 2. N Engl J Med 321:879–883, 1989.
13. Choi PT, Yip G, Quinonez LG, et al. Colloids vs crystalloids in fluid resuscitation: a systematic review. Crit Care Med 27(1):200–210, 1999.
14. Roberts JS, Bratton SL. Colloid volume expanders. Problems, pitfalls and possibilities. Drugs 55(5):621–630, 1998.
15. Hyneck ML. Simple acid-base disorders. Am J Hosp Pharm 42:1992–2006, 1985.
16. Gluck SL. Acid-base. Lancet 352(9126):474–479, 1998.
17. Rutecki GW, Whittier FC. An approach to clinical acid-base problem solving. Compr Ther 24(11–12):553–559, 1998.
18. McLaughlin M, Kassirer J. Rational treatment of acid-base disorders. Drugs 39(6):841–855, 1990.
19. Fulop M. Flow diagrams for the diagnosis of acid-base disorders. J Emerg Med 16(1):97–109, 1998.
20. Adroque HJ, Madias NE. Changes in plasma potassium concentration during acute acid-base disturbances. Am J Med 71:456, 1981.
21. Weber JN. Treatment of metabolic alkalosis with intravenous administration of hydrochloric acid. CSHP Voice 13:1–3, 1986.
22. Adrogue HJ, Madias NE. Management of life-threatening acid-base disorders. First of two parts. N Engl J Med 338(1):26–34, 1998.

23. Adroque HJ, Madias NE. Management of life-threatening acid-base disorders. second of two parts. N Engl J Med 338(2):107–111, 1998.
24. Brater DC. Serum electrolyte abnormalities caused by drugs. Prog Drug Res 30:9–69, 1986.
25. Stanszek WF. Current approaches to management of potassium deficiency. Drug Intell Clin Pharm 19:176, 1985.
26. Clark BA, Brown BS. Potassium homeostasis and hyperkalemic syndromes. Endocrinol Metab Clin North Am 24(3):573–591, 1995.
27. Perazella MA, Mahnansmith RL. Hyperkalemia in the elderly: drugs exacerbate impaired potassium homeostasis. J Gen Intern Med 12(10):646–656, 1997.
28. Gennari FJ. Hypokalemia. N Engl J Med 339(7):451–458, 1997.
29. Pederson KO. The effect of bicarbonate, CO_2 and pH on serum calcium fractions. Scand J Clin Lab Invest 27:147, 1979.
30. Bushinsky DA, Monk RD. Calcium. Lancet 352(9124):306–311, 1998.
31. Tohme JF, Bilezikian JP. Hypocalcemic emergencies. Endocrinol Metab Clin North Am 22(2):363–375, 1993.
32. Gucalp R, Ritch P, Wiernik PH, et al. Comparative study of pamidronate disodium and etidronate disodium in the treatment of cancer-related hypercalcemia. J Clin Oncol 10(1):134–142, 1992.
33. Boden SD, Kaplan FS. Calcium homeostasis. Orthop Clin North Am 21(1):31–42, 1990.
34. Bordier P. The effect of $1(OH)D_3$ and $1,25\ (OH)_2D_3$ on the bone of patients with renal osteodystrophy. Am J Med 64:101–107, 1978.
35. Kanis J. Vitamin D metabolism and its clinical application. J Bone Joint Surg 64B:542–557, 1982.
36. Siminoski K, Josse RG. Prevention and management of osteoporosis: consensus statements of the Scientific Advisory Board of the Osteoporosis Society of Canada. 9. Calcitonin in the treatment of osteoporosis. CMAJ 1;155(7):962–965, 1996.
37. Pun KK, Chan LWL. Analgesic effect of intranasal salmon calcitonin in the treatment of osteoporotic vertebral fractures. Clin Ther 2:205–208, 1989.
38. Sekima M, Takami H. Combination of calcitonin and pamidronate for emergency treatment of malignant hypercalcemia. Oncol Rep 5(1):197–199, 1998.
39. Abbott LG, Rude RK. Clinical manifestations of magnesium deficiency. Miner Electrolyte Metab 19(4–5):314–322, 1993.
40. Rude RK. Magnesium metabolism and deficiency. Endocrinol Metab Clin North Am 22(2):377–395, 1993.
41. Chernow B, Rainey TG. Iatrogenic hyperphosphatemia: a metabolic consideration in critical care medicine. Crit Care Med 9:772, 1981.
42. Clark CL, Sacks GS, Dickerson RN, et al. Treatment of hypophosphatemia in patients receiving specialized nutrition support using a graduated scheme: results from a prospective clinical trial. Crit Care Med 23(9):1504–1511, 1995.

CHAPTER 10

GENERAL NUTRITION

Margaret Malone

Clinicians practicing in an institutional or community setting should be familiar with general nutritional guidelines. These practitioners have an ideal opportunity to provide nutritional and health promotion advice to the public. In this chapter, general and population-specific nutritional recommendations are addressed. The reader is referred to the chapters pertaining to particular disease states for additional information.

An increasing prevalence of obesity in the United States has led to a renewed effort to modify the food intake of the population by providing information in the media. In addition, data about specific nutritional supplements such as folic acid and calcium have been promoted. Improving the health of the nation through diet and behavior modification is a challenge for all health professionals.

TREATMENT GOALS: GENERAL NUTRITION

- Improve understanding of the principles of a healthful diet.
- Understand the health risks associated with obesity.
- Recognize the importance of regular exercise.
- Ensure adequate folic acid intake in women of childbearing age.
- Be familiar with nutritional recommendations for high-risk groups, including patients with diabetes mellitus and hypertension and older adults.
- Educate patients about the benefits of adequate fiber and calcium intake.
- Provide appropriate advice to consumers about vitamin, antioxidant, and nutritional supplements.

PSYCHOSOCIAL ASPECTS OF GENERAL NUTRITION

One of the most challenging aspects of improving the nation's health is that those who are at the greatest risk, especially those on a low income, have the least access to health care and information. Written information, including leaflets available in health care settings and in grocery stores, may be largely ignored or unread. This may be because of the higher cost and perceived inconvenience of preparing meals rich in fruits and vegetables compared to less expensive, high-fat fast foods. Another problem may be that people are unable or unwilling to read the information provided. Using audiovisual techniques or the Internet may make the information more appealing. Targeting schools would help to instill better dietary habits at an early age. Finally, the cost of supplements is often expensive and may not be affordable by those most likely to benefit.

GENERAL NUTRITION GUIDELINES

The following section describes the current recommendations for healthful eating and dietary guidelines. These guidelines differ from the reference values for intakes of essential nutrients to maintain health, known as the dietary reference intakes (DRIs), which vary with age, gender, and other factors. DRIs are reference values that include the estimated average requirement (EAR), the recommended dietary allowance (RDA), the adequate intake (AI), and the tolerable upper intake level (UL).[1–3] Each of these components addresses a specific criterion for adequacy. The EAR is the intake that meets the needs for a particular

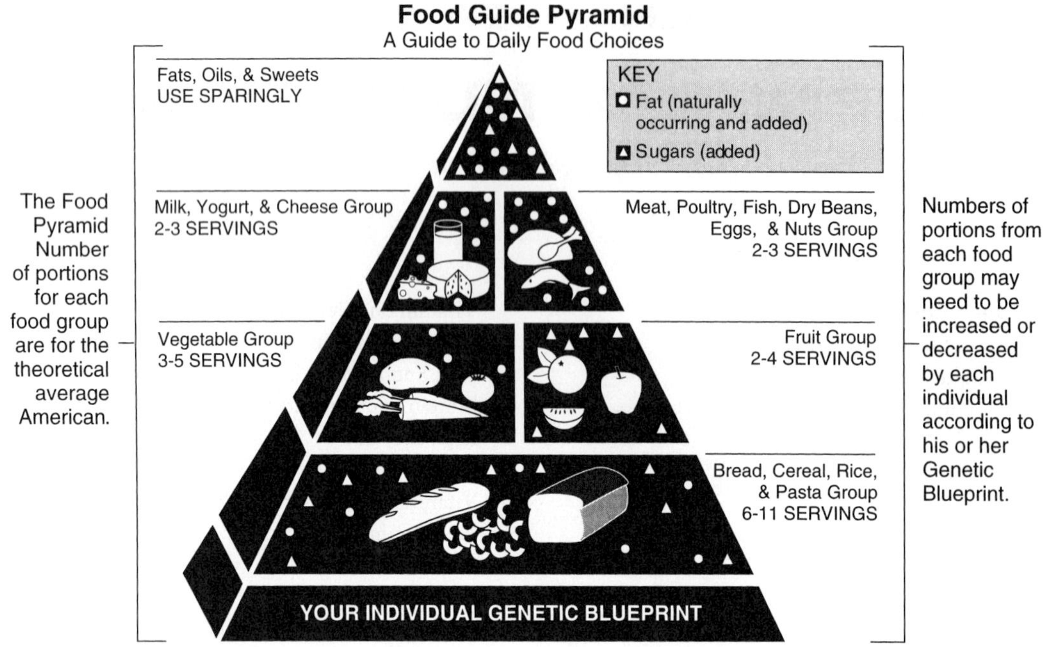

Figure 10.1. The U.S. food guide pyramid, modified to take genetic variability into account. (Reprinted with permission from Victor Herbert, copyright 1992.)

Table 10.1 ▪ U.S. Dietary Guidelines for Adults

Eat a variety of foods.
Maintain a healthy weight.
Choose a diet low in fat (<30% total daily calories), saturated fat (<10% of daily fat calories), and cholesterol (<300 mg/day).
Eat plenty of fruits, vegetables, and whole-grain products.
Use sugars in moderation.
Use salt and sodium in moderation.
If you drink alcoholic beverages, do so in moderation.

nutrient of 50% of the people within the defined group. The RDA is the intake that meets the nutrient needs of 97 to 98% of the people within the group and is intended to be applied to healthy people. The AI is the average observed intake that appears to sustain a defined nutritional state, such as normal levels of circulating proteins. The UL represents the maximum intake of a nutrient that is unlikely to pose a risk for almost all (98%) people. In contrast, dietary guidelines and health policy recommendations are designed to promote the selection of foods to achieve a nutritionally adequate diet and include recommendations on nonnutrients such as fiber and advice about fat and cholesterol intake.

A healthful diet should follow three simple rules: moderation, variety, and balance. Advice on dietary selection from the basic food groups has been incorporated into a food guide pyramid by the U.S. Departments of Agriculture and of Health and Human Services (Fig. 10.1).[4] Individual diets are modified to take into account genetic variability. The general dietary guidelines that health care practitioners should advocate are presented in Table 10.1.[5,6] Normal healthy people require 25 to 30 kcal/kg/day, with 30% or less of the caloric intake coming from fat. Protein intake should be between 0.8 and 1.0 g/kg/day.

In line with other Western countries and the World Health Organization, the definitions of overweight, preobese and obese have been updated. Overweight is defined as a body mass index (BMI) higher than 25 kg/m^2, preobese as a BMI 25.0 to 29.9 kg/m^2, and obese as a BMI higher than 30 kg/m^2.[7] Based on these definitions, the crude prevalence rate of overweight and obesity was 55% during the period 1988 to 1994. This reinforces the need for all health care professionals to take part in health promotion strategies, including those directed at improved eating and exercise behaviors.

People who are obese, especially those with central adiposity, are at a high risk for the development of comorbid conditions such as diabetes mellitus and cardiovascular disease. Diet and exercise are the mainstay of any weight loss program. The goals of weight loss and management are to prevent further weight gain, reduce body weight, and maintain a lower body weight over the long term.[8] For overweight patients (BMI 27 to 35), a decrease of 300 to 500 kcal/day should result in a desired weight loss of 10% from baseline in 6 months. More obese patients (BMI higher than 35) should reduce their calorie intake by 500 to 1000 kcal/day to achieve the same effect. Total fat intake should be 30% or less of the daily energy intake. Patients should be encouraged to exercise. Typical activities might including walking or swimming at a slow pace for 30 minutes three times a week. The goal would be to exercise at a level of moderate intensity at least 45 minutes per day most days of the week. Pharmacotherapy for obesity is addressed elsewhere in this book.

POPULATION-SPECIFIC NUTRITIONAL CONSIDERATIONS

The populations and indications outlined in the following section require particular attention because of their special needs and new data about nutritional needs.

Pregnancy

Folic Acid Requirements

Several studies provide supportive evidence for the role of folic acid in the prevention of neural tube defects. Folate supplements during pregnancy have long been recommended as prophylaxis against megaloblastic anemia in the third trimester. When used for prevention of neural tube defects, folate levels must be adequate in the first 4 weeks after conception, before neural tube closure.[9] Because many women do not realize they are pregnant until after this time, difficulties arise in establishing the most appropriate method of supplementation. The U.S. Public Health Service advises women of childbearing age to ensure that they have a daily folate intake of at least 400 μg per day and that women with a previous baby with neural tube defect take at least 4 mg/day as a supplement. Three possible approaches to increasing folic acid intake include increasing public awareness by health promotion campaigns, fortifying foods, particularly cereals, and recommending the use of supplements in women of childbearing age. Fortification of enriched cereal grains at 1.4 mg/kg grain was initiated recently.[10] Based on estimates of usual intake of these foods and bioavailability of folate, this would increase folate intake by around 100 μg per day.[11] Such food fortification has raised controversy about the inadequacy of the level of supplementation[12] and potential adverse effects caused by the possible masking of pernicious anemia (especially in older adults), antagonism of anticonvulsant therapy if ingested in large doses, hypersensitivity reactions to folate, and interference with zinc nutriture.[13,14] Promotion of folate supplements to women at high risk has been criticized because they must be taken in the periconceptual period and made available to those who might benefit most, such as economically disadvantaged women with limited access to health care.

Iron Requirements

The use of iron supplements for all pregnant women has also been questioned. Although many women develop anemia during pregnancy, for the majority it is clinically insignificant and iron stores return to baseline values postpartum without intervention. Iron therapy commonly causes gastrointestinal disturbance, including nausea, vomiting, diarrhea, and constipation, thereby exacerbating problems often associated with pregnancy. In practice, iron therapy should be prescribed or recommended only in the presence of clinically significant iron deficiency anemia.

Diabetes Mellitus

Recommendations for Dietary Intake and Fat Consumption

The current American Diabetes Association nutrition guidelines for diabetic patients are similar to the current health promotion recommendations for the general population.[15] Obese patients are encouraged to lose weight and limit their total caloric intake, especially their intake of saturated fat. Polyunsaturated fats or, ideally, monounsaturated fats are to be used in place of saturated fats. The composition of atherosclerotic plaques closely mirrors dietary fat intake, which has also been demonstrated for adipose tissue.[16] Because polyunsaturated fatty acids are easily oxidized, this may lead to an increase rather than a decrease in cardiovascular disease. Monounsaturated fatty acids may be preferred because they resist such oxidation. They appear to have no adverse effects on serum low-density lipoprotein (LDL) cholesterol in contrast to high-carbohydrate diets, which may adversely affect triglycerides, very-low-density lipoproteins, and high-density lipoproteins.[17] Trans-fatty acids are produced when vegetable oils are heated, which alters their texture and melting point and produces partially hydrogenated fat, often contained in vegetable shortening and margarine. These fatty acids appear to adversely affect blood cholesterol by elevating levels of LDL and lipoprotein Lp(a), each of which is believed to be atherogenic. The effects of trans-fatty acids on blood cholesterol are intermediate between those of saturated and unsaturated fats.[18]

Recommendations for Carbohydrate Intake

The concern that absorption of simple sugars is more rapid than the absorption from complex carbohydrates and therefore detrimental to the diabetic patient may be unfounded. However, data from nondiabetic patients with a high risk of cardiovascular disease demonstrate that a low glycemic diet is beneficial in improving insulin sensitivity.[19] Control over total energy intake is more important. The guidelines suggest that alternative sweeteners such as honey, corn syrup, fruit juice, sugar alcohols, or molasses have no advantage over sucrose in terms of limiting calorie intake or improving diabetic control.

Recommendations for Protein Intake

The guidelines have moved away from defining the diet in terms of percentages of nutrients, except for protein, which is recommended to be between 10 and 20% of the daily intake. Protein restriction in the diabetic population remains controversial. Diabetic nephropathy, which is present in 35% of insulin-dependent diabetic patients and 5 to 10% of patients with non–insulin-dependent diabetes mellitus, may be reduced by protein restriction in the early phase of the incipient nephropathic process.[20] However, in a large study with a mean follow-up period of 2.2 years, 840 patients with various chronic renal diseases were randomized to different dietary protein intakes. In this study, 555 patients with moderate renal impairment (glomerular filtration rate [GFR] of 25 to 55 mL/minute) showed only limited benefit. This was manifest as a slower decline in renal function 4 months after receiving a low-protein diet (0.58 g protein/kg/day) than in patients receiving a protein intake of 1.3 g/kg/day. Of 255 patients with more severe renal impairment (GFR 13 to 24 mL/minute) randomized to receive either a low-protein diet or a very-low-protein diet (0.28 g/kg/day), no significant slowing in the progression of renal disease was observed.[21] Others have proposed that protein restriction in diabetic patients may lead to protein malnutrition. It has been suggested that they may have increased catabolism, leading to higher rather than lower requirements than in the normal population.

Patients with High Blood Pressure

The Joint National Committee made several recommendations about lifestyle changes and dietary modification in the Sixth Report on the Prevention, Detection, Evaluation and Treatment of High Blood Pressure (JNC VI).[22] The guidelines are consistent with advice for a general healthful diet and lifestyle in normal healthy people. These include weight loss if overweight, increased exercise, moderate or no alcohol intake, smoking cessation, and limited intake of fat, especially saturated fat and cholesterol. Although reducing fat intake should have beneficial effects in those with dyslipidemia and reduce energy intake overall, no direct data suggest a beneficial effect on blood pressure of reduced fat intake. Similarly studies that have evaluated reduced protein intake or varying proportions of carbohydrate intake have shown minimal effect on blood pressure. Specific recommendations were made regarding sodium, potassium, calcium, and magnesium intake.[22]

Certain populations, including African Americans, older adults, and patients with hypertension or diabetes, are more sensitive to changes in dietary sodium intake. The majority of sodium consumed in an average U.S. diet comes from processed foods. The average consumption is estimated to be around 150 mmol/day (2.4 g sodium, 6 g sodium chloride). By reducing the intake of these foods, it should be possible to achieve a desired intake of 100 mmol sodium per day. A higher potassium intake than is generally achieved currently, around 90 mmol/day, was recommended. This level of intake may be beneficial in reducing blood pressure in patients with hypertension and may protect against the development of high blood pressure. Ideally, the increased potassium intake should be obtained from increased consumption of fruits and vegetables rather than from supplements, salt substitutes, or potassium-sparing diuretics. Lower calcium and magnesium intake seems to be associated with a higher prevalence of hypertension. However, the committee did not recommend the use of calcium or magnesium supplements to reduce blood pressure.

Geriatric Population

Early in the next century, 20% of Americans will be over the age of 65 years. Malnutrition in older adults is a recognized problem caused by a variety of factors (Table 10.2). Polypharmacy is common in this population because many older adults take both prescribed and over-the-counter (OTC) medications for chronic illness. For this reason, clinicians should be aware of the potential for drug–nutrient interactions that may lead to deficiency of a particular nutrient or generalized weight loss caused by inadequate food intake associated with medication use.[23]

Nutrition Screening Initiative

Recognition of the problem of malnutrition in older adults led to a national collaborative approach in which a lifestyle screening tool, the Nutrition Screening Initiative Checklist, was developed to identify older adults at risk for low nutrient intake.[24] The best predictors of perceived poor health were taking three or more drugs per day and having changed one's diet because of illness. Lack of money, eating fewer than two meals per day, and not eating many fruits or vegetables were the strongest predictors of inadequate nutrient intake.

Alterations in Nutrient Requirements Associated with Aging

Digestion and absorption of most macronutrients, such as protein, carbohydrate, and fat, are qualitatively unaffected by aging. Although these functions are somewhat reduced, the capacity of the gastrointestinal tract is sufficient for this reduction not to be significant.[25] A more controversial area is the proposed alteration in micronutrient requirements for people over 50 years. There is evidence that B_{12} absorption may be impaired in older adults by atrophic gastritis and achlorhydria, which may be present in 30 to

Table 10.2 ▪ Possible Causes of Malnutrition in Older Adults

Decreased intake
Problems with chewing and swallowing
Poor dentition
Dementia
Depression, causing decreased interest in food
Social isolation
Lack of mobility, causing difficulty with shopping
Poverty
Decreased absorption
Bowel surgery
Malabsorption syndromes (e.g., lactose intolerance, atrophic gastritis)
Increased requirements
Infection
Inflammation
Trauma
Drug therapy
Drug–nutrient interactions
Gastrointestinal side effects of medications (e.g., nausea, vomiting, diarrhea, constipation)
Alterations in taste perception
Difficulty swallowing caused by dry mouth
Central nervous system effects

40% of this population. Recent recommendations suggest that those over 50 years should meet their DRI for vitamin B_{12} by consuming foods fortified with B_{12} or take a dietary supplement.[3] Elevated homocysteine levels associated with subclinical B_{12}, B_6, and folate deficiency may be implicated in vascular disease and neuropsychiatric disorders, including presenile dementia.[26–28]

Older adults also are known to have lower levels of the active form of vitamin D, 1,25-dihydroxyvitamin D_3. This may result from a combination of factors, including low-level exposure to sunlight, reduced intake of dairy products, and decreased synthesis of active vitamin D by the kidney after parathyroid hormone stimulation. It has been proposed that the current recommended intake for vitamin D is too low to maintain bone health and that in older adults not exposed to sunlight, administration of a low-dose supplement (10 μg/day) is warranted. However, clinicians should review at least annually the supplements being consumed by their patients, especially the fat-soluble vitamins. Hypercalcemia and hypercalciuria associated with the inadvertent intake of 1200 IU per day of vitamin D have been reported.[29] It has also been suggested that the current recommendations for vitamin A intake in older adults are too high. This may be a result of increased absorption from the gastrointestinal tract or decreased clearance in the liver of retinyl esters from chylomicron remnants, and it may result in hepatotoxicity.[30]

In older adults having a dietary intake of less than 125 mg/day of vitamin C, the incidence of cataracts was reported to be four times higher than in those receiving 500 mg/day.[31,32] However, a dietary intake of 100 to 200 mg/day vitamin C appears to be sufficient to saturate body stores. Vitamin E supplementation in short-term studies (3 months) has been shown to improve immune function in older adults, but no long-term benefit from chronic supplementation has been demonstrated.[33]

Studies suggest that in people older than 85 years,[34] exercise is important in maintaining or improving muscle strength, whereas the use of a multinutrient supplement in those with a nutritionally adequate diet provided no additional benefit.[35]

RECOMMENDATIONS FOR SPECIFIC NUTRIENTS

This section addresses some of the issues and controversies related to particular nutrients and the proposed therapeutic benefits associated with their intake.

Dietary Fiber

The average daily intake of dietary fiber in most adults is around 11 g per day. However, current recommendations for normal healthy people suggest that the intake should be 10 to 17 g/1000 kcal, or 20 to 35 grams per day. The majority of people find this level of fiber intake to be unpalatable. Some common problems with fiber intake, such as abdominal distension and gas, can be reduced by gradually stepping up intake over a period of 4 to 6 weeks. Evidence that fiber interferes with drug absorption is limited. This interference may be more important for drugs with a narrow therapeutic index, such as digoxin and warfarin. Absorption of calcium, magnesium, zinc, and iron may be reduced. This is likely to be clinically significant only in those with other predisposing risk factors for malabsorption.[36,37]

Dietary fiber may be defined as water insoluble (e.g., the cellulosic polysaccharides lignin and cellulose) or water soluble (noncellulosic polysaccharides including pectins, gums, and mucilages). Each type of fiber has different effects on gastrointestinal motility and function. Soluble fibers are fermented by colonic microflora mainly in the cecum to short-chain fatty acids (acetic, propionic, and butyric acids). These are important fuels for the colonic enterocyte and promote water and electrolyte absorption. Soluble fibers have been shown to delay gastric emptying and slow small intestinal transit time. This can be useful in reducing postprandial blood glucose concentrations, for example, in patients with dumping syndrome. The ability of the viscous gel matrix formed from soluble fibers such as guar gum, oat bran, and psyllium to bind bile acids and cholesterol may explain their cholesterol-lowering properties. Insoluble fibers are less susceptible to degradation, and because of their water-retaining properties they increase fecal bulk, leading to decreased colonic transit time and stimulation of the defecation reflex.

Calcium Supplements and Osteoporosis

Osteoporosis is characterized by a reduction in bone mineral density. The majority of white women are at risk of sustaining osteoporosis-related fractures, especially of the wrist, hip, and spine. There is wide intraindividual variation in bone mineral density because it is influenced by many dietary and lifestyle factors. To minimize fracture risk, young women should have regular menses, consume a nutritionally adequate diet, perform regular physical activity, consume only a moderate amount of alcohol, if any, and refrain from smoking. The DRI for calcium for adolescents or young adults between 11 and 24 years is 1200 to 1500 mg/day.[38] The DRI is 1000 mg/day for men between 25 and 65 years and women 25 to 50 years (or up to 65 years if taking estrogens). Because estrogen has a recognized protective effect, postmenopausal women should seriously consider estrogen replacement therapy.[39] In the absence of estrogen replacement, calcium intake should be 1.5 g/day.[40] Aloia et al.[41] report a prospective controlled randomized study in which early postmenopausal women received 400 IU vitamin D daily and either placebo, 1700 mg calcium per day in divided doses or 1700 mg calcium and hormone replacement therapy. They conclude that although it is less effective than calcium with hormonal replacement therapy, calcium alone significantly retards bone loss and improves calcium balance. Calcium supplementation has also been reported to be of value in reducing the risk of hip fractures and other nonvertebral fractures in healthy, older (mean age 84 years), ambulatory women.[42]

In this study, participants were randomized to receive placebo or 1200 mg elemental calcium (as tricalcium phosphate) and 800 IU (20 μg)/day vitamin D_3 (cholecalciferol) for an 18-month period.[42] As discussed earlier, an adequate vitamin D intake in addition to calcium supplements is important, particularly in those who are confined to their homes or have limited exposure to sunlight.[43]

Optimum calcium intake is best obtained from dietary sources, but in practice an intake of 1200 to 1500 mg/day is difficult to achieve without supplements. Particular attention should be paid to vegetarians because 70% of dietary calcium comes from dairy products in the U.S. population. Lactovegetarians have not been found to differ from omnivores in their risk for osteoporosis. However, vegans should be encouraged to take supplements, calcium-fortified juices, or soy milk to meet the DRI.[44] The solubility of different calcium salts is not a major determinant of absorbability, but absorption is greater if the supplements are taken with protein, lactose, vitamin D, and acidic foods and in divided doses.[45] Absorption is decreased by oxalate-containing foods such as cocoa, spinach, kale, unpolished rice, wheat bran, and alkaline foods. Numerous calcium supplements are available as OTC products that vary in their elemental calcium content and salt form (Table 10.3). Before advising patients to take regular calcium supplements, clinicians must ensure that there are no contraindications or drug interactions. Constipation is a common complaint of patients taking chronic calcium therapy of 2400 mg/day. Calcium supplementation may cause problems with renal stone formation, arrhythmias, or milk alkali syndrome if renal function is compromised or dosages are excessive (more than 60 g/day). The UL is 2.5 g/day.[3]

Some authors suggest that osteoporosis may be caused in part by a long-term acid load imposed by the diet that is partially buffered by bases derived from bone. If this is demonstrated in larger, longer-term studies, supplementation of the diet with potassium bicarbonate may be beneficial in reducing osteoporosis.[46]

Sodium Intake for the General Population

The general recommendation for all people, including those who are normotensive, to reduce sodium intake has been called into question. The proposed benefits of a reduction in sodium intake are a reduction in blood pressure and a consequent decline in the number of strokes and myocardial infarctions. Some authors have proposed that potential negative effects are associated with decreased sodium intake, including an increase in circulating renin and aldosterone, suggesting activation of the renin–angiotensin–aldosterone system.[47] Data from the most recent meta-analysis of the effects of sodium restriction on blood pressure, renin, aldosterone, catecholamines, cholesterols, and triglyceride are controversial.[47] Based on these data, a mean daily reduction of 160 mmol sodium/day for 7 days decreased blood pressure by only 1.2/0.3 mm Hg in normotensive subjects, which would not justify the advice to reduce salt intake. In hypertensive subjects, a mean daily sodium reduction of 118 mmol/day for 28 days reduced blood pressure by 3.9/1.9 mm Hg, suggesting that reduced salt intake in this group is a useful adjunctive therapy. Data from a large randomized, controlled trial of nonpharmacologic interventions in older adults support this recommendation of reduced salt intake and weight loss as a reasonable, effective nonpharmacologic therapy in 60- to 80-year-olds.[48] Data from several large studies, including the Dietary Approaches to Stop Hypertension trial, suggest that the dietary guidelines outlined in Table 10.1 are appropriate advice for improved lifestyle.[49,50]

Vitamin Supplements

Every year millions of consumers spend billions of dollars on multivitamin, mineral, and other dietary supplements available in pharmacies and health food stores or ordered via mail or the Internet. Approximately 25% of all U.S. adults use vitamin supplements daily and up to 50% use them less regularly. Pharmacists have been criticized for promoting supplements or at least passively advising consumers about the appropriate use of vitamin, mineral, and nutritional supplements.[51] The majority of vitamin and mineral supplements contain the recommended daily intake and do not pose a direct hazard to health, although they are rarely indicated for adequately nourished people. However, certain groups, such as older adults, pregnant or lactating women, strict vegetarians, and those on very-low-calorie diets may benefit. Specific vitamin products are marketed to meet the special needs of these groups. The vitamin content of some of these products is presented in Table 10.4. Compared to the standard or

Table 10.3 ▪ Elemental Calcium Content of Common Supplements

Calcium Salt	Percentage	Amount (mEq/g)	Examples
Calcium glubionate	6.5	3.3	1.8 g (115 mg Ca)/5 mL
Calcium gluconate	9.3	4.6	500-mg tablet = 45 mg Ca
Calcium lactate	13	9.2	325-mg tablet = 42.3 mg Ca
Calcium citrate	21	12	950-mg tablet = 200 mg Ca
Calcium carbonate	40	20	500-mg tablet = 200 mg Ca
Calcium acetate	25	12.6	667-mg tablet = 169 mg Ca

Table 10.4 ▪ Content of Common Multivitamin Preparations Formulated for Specific Adult Groups

Type	A (IU)	D (IU)	E (IU)	B_1 (mg)	B_2 (mg)	B_3 (mg)	B_5 (mg)	B_6 (mg)	B_{12} (μg)	C (mg)	Folic acid (μg)	Biotin acid (μg)	Iron (mg)	Ca^{2+} (mg)
General purpose	5000	400	30	2.25	2.6	20	10	3	9	90	400	45	27	–
Women	5000	400	30	1.5	1.7	20	10	2	6	60	400	–	27	450[a]
Men	5000	400	45	2.25	2.55	20	10	3	9	200	400	–	–	–
55+	6000	400	60	4.5	3.4	20	20	6	25	120	400	–	–	200[a]
55–65[b]	5000	400	45	1.5	1.7	20	10	3	25	60	400	–	4	200[a]
65+[b]	6000	400	45	1.5	1.7	20	10	3	25	60	200	–	3	80
Stress	0	0	30	10	10	100	20	5	12	500	400	–	–	–
Pregnancy	8000	400	30	1.7	2	20	–	4	8	60	800	–	60	–
				Thiamine	Riboflavin	Niacin	Pantothenic acid	Pyridoxine	Cobalamin					

[a]Also contains zinc 15 mg.
[b]Also contains multiple trace elements.

general multivitamin formulation, those designed for older adults have additional vitamin A and E and commonly contain multiple trace elements. Vitamins for pregnancy often contain calcium and zinc. Vitamins designed for women contain calcium and those designed for men have additional vitamin E and C. Prenatal vitamins contain extra vitamin A, folic acid, and iron. Some formulations (stress formula) contain megadoses of vitamins[52] and increased intakes of antioxidants[53] and are promoted to people with human immunodeficiency virus infection.

Megadose vitamin therapy from supplementation is defined as treatment with one or more vitamins in amounts 10 or more times the DRI. Vitamins are essential nutrients for which the human body has a minimum requirement, and exceeding that requirement is unlikely to provide additional benefit and may do harm. Although they are readily excreted, megadoses of water-soluble vitamins may lead to toxicity.

Ergogenic Aids and Nutritional Supplements in Sports Medicine

Ergogenic aids in the form of sports and exercise nutritional supplements are promoted as enhancing athletic performance. The nutritional supplement market directed at amateur and professional athletes has been estimated to amount to billions of dollars. Some are suggested to promote weight loss or alter body composition by increasing lean body mass.[54] Multivitamin and mineral supplements for the most part are promoted to enhance metabolic efficiency. Although a balanced diet should be adequate to provide most athletes' needs, nutritional supplements often are used in an attempt to gain a competitive advantage.[55] These products are widely promoted by advertisement campaigns in body-building magazines, health clubs, and fitness centers and their widespread availability through mail order, the Internet, and retail stores.

Marketing claims commonly are based on extrapolation of data from animal models, in vitro data, or epidemiologic studies.[56] The majority of the studies that involve evaluation of ergogenic aids are flawed. Design problems include inadequate sample size, lack of appropriate control groups or control of nutrient intake, poorly designed training programs, and lack of proper analytical measures and control for possible placebo effects. Such deficiencies in study design make it difficult or impossible to draw definitive conclusions.

Protein Supplements

Under normal circumstances, dietary protein provides the amino acids needed for energy production and muscle protein synthesis. There is a constant turnover of protein in the body, resulting in a daily loss of nitrogen in the form of urea and amino acids. When protein intake is excessive, there is increased formation of urea, which is excreted in urine and sweat, and enhanced gluconeogenesis, or conversion of the carbon skeleton, to fat and glycogen stores. The increase in the use of protein for energy during exercise is small. Only during strenuous endurance training has it been shown that athletes require more protein, accounting for 5 to 10% of energy production. The amount of excess protein in the average American diet usually is more than enough to cover this increase. Studies in long-distance runners document that protein requirements are elevated 50 to 100% above the RDI during the first month of increased workload. Therefore, approximately 1.2 to 1.4 g/kg/day should result in a positive nitrogen balance. It is unclear whether high protein intakes actually improve endurance.[57] The effect of protein loading on muscle mass and strength is less defined, and additional research is necessary before conclusions can be made. Although protein intake can be enhanced by increasing overall food intake, particularly that of high-protein foods, this may lead to an unwanted increase in caloric intake. For this reason, protein supplements in the form of protein hydrolysates and food-grade L-amino acids have become popular among body builders. Nevertheless, there is no documented improvement in performance or muscle size or strength associated with the use of these supplements in normally nourished people.

Arginine

Arginine is an amino acid known to have an effect on several physiologic functions important to exercise metabolism. Most notable is the increase in growth hormone concentrations observed after oral administration of L-ornithine, a precursor of arginine. However, the effects of an acute rise in growth hormone on lean body mass and fat stores are unknown. The rate of creatine production, an energy source for muscle tissue, has been shown to increase with arginine supplementation, but the small increase in creatine level may not be enough to affect exercise performance. Arginine supplementation at 2 to 10 g/day as an ergogenic agent appears promising, but definitive conclusions are speculative until additional research is performed.

Carnitine

L-Carnitine is a nonessential amino acid synthesized in vivo from methionine and lysine. Its principal metabolic function is the transport of long-chain fatty acids into the mitochondria, where they are oxidized.[58] L-Carnitine is particularly important in skeletal muscle and the myocardium, which obtain their primary energy source from fatty acid oxidation. Several studies have been conducted in athletes to evaluate the effect of carnitine on performance and metabolic function, but results have been inconsistent. Poor study design is a factor.[59] At present, L-carnitine supplementation does not appear to be warranted in this setting.

Vitamins and Minerals

Exercise has been shown to increase the need for certain vitamins and minerals, especially water-soluble vitamins.

However, studies in endurance athletes have observed that they typically consume up to three times the average person's nutrient intake, from a variety of foods. Based on these findings, it has been extrapolated that their vitamin intake is concurrently increased and should be adequate.[60]

High doses of vitamins may be taken to target specific functions; for example, vitamin B_6 has been promoted for relief of premenstrual symptoms, menopausal symptoms, and depression. Although this practice is often assumed to be safe, harmful effects may occur. It has been reported that over a 2- to 40-month period, severe sensory nervous system dysfunction was seen in subjects self-dosing with 2 to 6 g of vitamin B_6 supplementation.[61] The dysfunction was not always reversed when the supplementation ceased.

Chromium

Chromium has been generally recognized for its ability to facilitate the insulin–tissue interaction, thereby decreasing the amount of insulin needed for glucose uptake by the tissues. In addition, chromium picolinate supplementation has been found to decrease serum cholesterol concentrations.[62] Chromium is therefore promoted as an ergogenic aid that will enhance metabolism, increase muscle, and decrease body fat. The amount of chromium in a typical U.S. diet is less than the estimated AI of 50 to 200 μg/d. The benefits of chromium supplementation on athletic performance have not been documented. It should be noted that there have been several case reports of chromium toxicity, manifested primarily as renal dysfunction, thrombocytopenia, and toxic hepatitis associated with excessive intake of OTC products.[62]

Inosine

Inosine is used to synthesize adenosine nucleotides and is a precursor for the synthesis of adenosine triphosphate (ATP). ATP is the immediate energy source for muscle contraction. As a supplement, inosine is promoted as an energy enhancer and an aid to endurance, recuperation, and strength. The proposed mechanism is by promoting vasodilation and oxygen availability to muscles by increasing 2,3-diphosphoglycerate (2,3-DPG) in red blood cells. The lack of these effects has been described, with no increases in 2,3-DPG in red blood cells and no changes in time to exhaustion or treadmill performance.[63] Excess inosine is not converted to adenosine nucleotidase, but is metabolized by the enzyme xanthine oxidase to uric acid, contributing to gout in susceptible people. Xanthine oxidase is present in muscle tissue and generates free radicals, which are associated with fatigue during exercise. For these reasons, inosine supplementation may be more detrimental than helpful for the enhancement of athletic performance.[54]

In summary, there is little evidence to support the use of nutritional ergogenic supplements to enhance athletic performance. Although short-term use of these supplements is unlikely to be harmful, when the opportunity arises health practitioners should educate athletes and their coaches about basic nutritional concepts and the role of diet over unproven supplements.

Antioxidant Nutrients

Antioxidant nutrients (β-carotene, vitamin E, vitamin C, and selenium) have been proposed to have a role in the prevention of cancer and cardiovascular disease. Support for this hypothesis comes primarily from animal studies and epidemiologic data. In cardiovascular disease, antioxidants may limit the oxidation of LDL cholesterol which is then taken up by macrophages to form foam cells characteristic of early atherogenic disease. In cancer, it has been suggested that antioxidants act via a scavenging mechanism to prevent DNA damage by free radicals.

Prevention of Cardiovascular Disease

Two large-scale studies, the Nurses Health Study[64] and the Health Professionals Follow Up Study,[65] reported an inverse association between higher vitamin E (α-tocopherol) consumption and cardiovascular risk. The reduction in risk was apparent only after 2 to 4 years of taking supplements. However, in both groups the risk reduction was confined to a subgroup taking supplements. The maximum reduction in men was seen in those taking 100 to 249 IU per day. The authors suggest that the lack of benefit seen with dietary vitamin E intake alone is consistent with experimental evidence that resistance of LDL cholesterol to oxidation is achieved only at levels of vitamin E that are 10 to 100 times the DRI. In the same study, no reduction in cardiovascular risk was associated with high intakes of vitamin C. Because vitamin C is a water-soluble vitamin, it has been proposed that it is less likely to be effective as an antioxidant because of inadequate penetration of the LDL cholesterol core. β-Carotene intake was associated with a decreased risk of cardiovascular disease in former and current smokers but not in those who had never smoked.[65]

A secondary prevention study, the Cambridge Heart Antioxidant Study (CHAOS), found that high doses of vitamin E, 400 or 800 IU/day, were associated with a 77% decrease in the incidence of nonfatal myocardial infarction. There was no significant effect on cardiovascular death or total mortality.[66] In a subgroup analysis, 156 men who had undergone coronary artery bypass grafting were randomly assigned to either colestipol–niacin or placebo. Both groups received a cholesterol-lowering diet. Patients had repeat angiography after 2 years to determine the extent of previously observed lesions. Men who had a supplementary intake of 100 IU or more of vitamin E were found to have less disease progression than those with an intake less than 100 IU per day.[67]

Currently available data do not support the use of β-carotene as an antioxidant supplement. There appear to be no significant benefits in primary or secondary prevention of ischemic heart disease, and there may be possible adverse effects.[68] Although the data are limited, there does appear to be some supporting evidence for a beneficial effect of vitamin E supplements.

Prevention of Cancer

Data about the protective role of antioxidants in carcinogenesis and treatment of a variety of tumor types are conflicting. Many studies that suggest potential benefit are based on animal models or epidemiologic data showing lower levels of β-carotene, vitamins E and C, or selenium in patients with cancer than in healthy controls.[69]

The Finnish Alpha Tocopherol, Beta Carotene (ATBC) Cancer Prevention Study evaluated the effect of vitamin E and β-carotene on the incidence of lung cancer in male smokers.[70] The study involved 29,000 middle-aged male smokers randomly assigned to receive dietary supplementation with β-carotene (20 mg per day), α-tocopherol (50 mg per day), both, or placebo. Patients who received β-carotene had a higher incidence of lung cancer. Although those who received α-tocopherol had no significant difference in the incidence of lung cancer, there were fewer cases of prostate cancer. In the α-tocopherol group there was an increased number of hemorrhagic strokes. These findings were somewhat unexpected when compared with previous data. Possible explanations are that these findings may have been due to chance, the dosage of vitamin E was too low to affect tumor development, or, because the median duration of the study was 6 years, it was too short to provide protection against a carcinogenic process that may have been initiated decades earlier. As a secondary finding, the ATBC group concluded that there were no significant benefits of α-tocopherol at the dosage used or of β-carotene for secondary prevention of cardiovascular disease.[71]

Two other primary prevention studies, the Physicians' Health Study[72] and the Beta-Carotene and Retinol Efficacy Trial (CARET),[73] have been published. In the first of these, 22,071 male physicians aged 40 to 84 years were enrolled in a randomized, double-blind, placebo-controlled trial of β-carotene 50 mg on alternate days or placebo. There were no significant effects in the overall incidence of malignant neoplasm, cardiovascular disease, or mortality between the groups. In the CARET study, 18,314 smokers, former smokers, and workers exposed to asbestos were randomly assigned to receive 30 mg β-carotene and 25,000 IU retinol (as retinyl palmitate) per day or placebo. After an average of 4 years of supplements, the CARET study was discontinued 21 months earlier than planned because of a significant increase in the relative risk of lung cancer (1.28, confidence interval [CI] 1.04 to 1.57, $p = 0.02$) in the active treatment group.

Vitamin C has an antioxidant role at levels normally obtained from the diet; however, larger dosages (more than 500 mg/day) achieved with supplements may be harmful. In this situation, vitamin C may act as a pro-oxidant, particularly in the presence of iron. A number of studies suggest that vitamin C plays a role in wound healing, the immune response, protection from cancer, cataract prevention, and cholesterol metabolism. However, large intervention studies are also needed before supplements can be recommended.[74]

It is tempting to recommend antioxidant supplements on the basis of possible beneficial effects and relative lack of toxicity.[75,76] This may be most pertinent in patients with risk factors for cardiovascular disease and cancer. However, with the possible exception of vitamin E, a better strategy would be to recommend a diet rich in fruits and vegetables, as outlined in Table 10.1.

CONCLUSION

Clinicians in all settings should take the opportunity to participate in preventive health care by promoting healthful diet, exercise, and lifestyle changes to individual patients. Knowledge of the literature about specific patient groups should enable the pharmacist to make appropriate recommendations and provide improved pharmaceutical care.

KEY POINTS

- Advocate the principles of a healthful diet rich in fruits and vegetables and low in saturated fat.
- Encourage achievement and maintenance of an appropriate body weight through dietary modification and exercise.
- Ensure that women of childbearing age have a folic acid intake of at least 400 µg per day.
- Pay attention to the special nutritional needs of high-risk groups, including patients with diabetes mellitus and hypertension and older adults.
- Be familiar with various types of fiber and proposed health benefits of a high-fiber diet.
- Encourage optimal calcium intake to reduce the risk of osteoporosis.
- Be aware of the often unsubstantiated claims for nutritional supplements, especially in the areas of sports medicine and immune enhancement.
- Understand the risks and benefits associated with antioxidant nutrients in the prevention of cardiovascular disease and cancer.

REFERENCES

1. Food and Nutrition Board, Institute of Medicine. Dietary reference intakes. Nutr Rev 55(9):319–326, 1997.
2. Food and Nutrition Board, Institute of Medicine. Use of dietary reference intakes. Nutr Rev 55(9):327–331, 1997.
3. Yates AA, Schlicker SA, Suitor CW. Dietary reference intakes: the new basis for recommendations for calcium and related nutrients, B vitamins, and choline. J Am Diet Assoc 98:699–706,1998.
4. USDA's food guide pyramid. Home and Garden Bulletin no. 249. Washington, DC: US Department of Agriculture, 1992.
5. Dietary Guidelines for Americans. USDA Home and Garden Bulletin no. 232. 3rd ed. Washington, DC: Government Printing Office (1990-272-930), 1990.

6. Healthy people 2000: national health promotion and disease prevention objectives. DHHS Publication no. (PHS) 91-50212. Washington, DC: U.S. Department of Health and Human Services, 1990.
7. Flegal KM, Carroll MD, Kuczmarski RJ, et al. Overweight and obesity in the United States: prevalence and trends, 1960–1994. Int J Obes 22:39–47, 1998.
8. Expert panel on the identification, evaluation and treatment of overweight and obesity in adults. Executive summary of the clinical guidelines on the identification, evaluation, and treatment of overweight and obesity in adults. Arch Intern Med 158:1855–1867, 1998.
9. Czeizel AE, Dudas I. Prevention of the first occurrence of neural tube defects by periconceptional vitamin supplementation. N Engl J Med 327:1832–1835, 1992.
10. US Department of Health and Human Services, Food and Drug Administration. Food standards: amendment of the standards of identity for enriched grain products to require addition of folic acid. Federal Register 61:8781–8807, 1996.
11. Gregory JF. Bioavailability of folate. Eur J Clin Nutr 51(Suppl):554–559, 1997.
12. Daly S, Mills JL, Molloy AM, et al. Minimum effective dose of folic acid for food fortification to prevent neural tube defects. Lancet 350:1666–1669, 1997.
13. Wald NJ, Bower C. Folic acid, pernicious anaemia and prevention of neural tube defects. Lancet 343:307, 1994.
14. Campbell NRC. How safe are folic acid supplements? Arch Intern Med 156:1638–1644, 1996.
15. American Dietetic Association. Nutrition recommendations and principles for people with diabetes mellitus. Diabetes Care 18(1):16–19, 1995.
16. Felton CV, Crook D, Davies MJ, et al. Dietary polyunsaturated fatty acids and composition of human aortic plaques. Lancet 344:1195–1196, 1994.
17. Kwiterovich PO. The effect of dietary fat, antioxidants, and pro-oxidants on blood lipids, lipoproteins, and atherosclerosis. J Am Diet Assoc 97(Suppl):S31–S41, 1997.
18. Position paper on trans fatty acids. Am J Clin Nutr 63:663–670, 1996.
19. Frost G, Leeds A, Trew G, et al. Insulin sensitivity in women at risk of coronary heart disease and effect of a low glycemic diet. Metabolism 47(10):1245–1251, 1998.
20. Carella MJ, Gossain VV, Rovner DR. Early diabetic nephropathy. Emerging treatment options. Arch Intern Med 154(6):625–630, 1994.
21. Klahr S, Levey AS, Beck GJ, et al. The effect of dietary protein restriction and blood pressure control on the progression of renal disease. Modification of Diet in Renal Disease Study Group. N Engl J Med 330(13):877–884, 1994.
22. Joint National Committee on Detection, Evaluation and Treatment of high blood pressure. The Sixth Report of the Joint National Committee on Prevention, Detection, Evaluation and Treatment of High Blood Pressure (JNC VI). Arch Intern Med 157:2413–2446, 1997.
23. Varma RN. Risk for drug induced malnutrition is unchecked in elderly patients in nursing homes. J Am Diet Assoc 94:192–194, 1994.
24. Posner BM, Jette AM, Smith KW, et al. Nutrition and health risks in the elderly: the Nutrition Screening Initiative. Am J Public Health 83:972–978, 1993.
25. Lovat LB. Age related changes in gut physiology and nutritional status. Gut 38:306–309, 1996.
26. Welch GN, Loscalzo J. Homocysteine and atherothrombosis. N Engl J Med 338:1042–1050,1998.
27. Rimm EB, Willett WC, Hu FB, et al. Folate and vitamin B_6 from diet and supplements in relation to risk of coronary heart disease among women. JAMA 279:359–364, 1998.
28. Robinson K, Arheart K, Refsum H, et al. Low circulating folate and vitamin B_6 concentrations risk factors for stroke, peripheral vascular disease and coronary artery disease. Circulation 97:437–443, 1998.
29. Adams JS, Lee G. Gains in bone mineral density with resolution of vitamin D intoxication. Ann Intern Med 127:203–206, 1997.
30. Russell RM, Suter PM. Vitamin requirements of elderly people: an update. Am J Clin Nutr 58:4–14, 1993.
31. Jacques PF, Chylack LT. Epidemiologic evidence of a role for the antioxidant vitamins and carotenoids in cataract prevention. Am J Clin Nutr 53:352S–355S, 1991.
32. Kneckt P, Heliovaara M, Rissanen A, et al. Serum antioxidant vitamins and risk of cataract. BMJ 305:1392–1394, 1992.
33. Russell RM. Micronutrient requirements of the elderly. Nutr Rev 50:463–466, 1992.
34. Campion EW. The oldest old. N Engl J Med 330:1819–1820, 1994.
35. Fiatarone MA, O Neill EF, Doyle Ryan N, et al. Exercise training and nutritional supplementation for physical frailty in very elderly people. N Engl J Med 330:1769–1775, 1994.
36. Hunt R, Fedorak R, Frohlich J, et al. Therapeutic role of dietary fibre. Can Fam Physician 39:897–910, 1993.
37. Koruda MJ. Dietary fiber and gastrointestinal disease. Surg Gynecol Obstetr 177:209–214, 1993.
38. NIH Consensus Development Panel on Optimal Calcium Intake. JAMA 272:1942–1948, 1994.
39. Wardlow GM. Putting osteoporosis into perspective. J Am Diet Assoc 93:1000–1006, 1993.
40. Recker RR. Current therapy for osteoporosis. J Clin Endocrinol Metab 76:14–16, 1993.
41. Aloia JF, Vaswani A, Yeh JK, et al. Calcium supplementation with and without hormone replacement therapy to prevent postmenopausal bone loss. Ann Intern Med 120:97–103, 1994.
42. Chapuy MC, Arlot ME, Duboeuf F, et al. Vitamin D_3 and calcium to prevent hip fractures in elderly women. N Engl J Med 327:1637–1642, 1992.
43. Thomas MK, Lloyd-Jones DM, Thadhani RI, et al. Hypovitaminosis D in medical inpatients. N Engl J Med 338:777–783, 1998.
44. Weaver CM, Plawecki KL. Dietary calcium: adequacy of a vegetarian diet. Am J Clin Nutr 59:1238S–1241S, 1994.
45. Recker RR. Prevention of osteoporosis: calcium nutrition. Osteoporosis Int 3(Suppl 1):163–165, 1993.
46. Sebastian A, Harris ST, Ottaway JH, et al. Improved mineral balance and skeletal metabolism in postmenopausal women treated with potassium bicarbonate. N Engl J Med 330:1776–1781, 1994.
47. Graudal NA, Galloe AM, Garred P. Effects of sodium restriction on blood pressure, renin, aldosterone, catecholamines, cholesterols and triglyceride. JAMA 279:1383–1391, 1998.
48. Whelton PK, Appel LJ, Espeland MA, et al. Sodium reduction and weight loss in the treatment of hypertension in older persons. JAMA 279:839–846, 1998.
49. Stamler J. Setting the TONE for ending the hypertension epidemic. JAMA 279:878–879, 1998.
50. Antonios TFT, MacGregor GA. Salt-more adverse effects. Lancet 348:250–251, 1996.
51. O'Donnell JT. Nutrition fraud: vitamins and obesity–pharmacists' responsibilities. J Pharm Pract 1:131–149, 1988.
52. Bauernfeind JC. Nutrification of foods. In: Shils ME, Olson JA, Shike M. Modern nutrition in health and disease. 8th ed. Philadelphia: Lea & Febiger, 1994.
53. Kotler DP. Antioxidant therapy and HIV infection: 1998. Am J Clin Nutr 67:7–9, 1998.
54. Rosenbloom C, Millard-Stafford M, Lathrop J. Contemporary ergogenic aids used by strength/power athletes. J Am Diet Assoc 92:1264–1266, 1992.
55. Williams MH. Nutritional ergogenics: help or hype? J Am Diet Assoc 92:1213–1214, 1992.
56. Grunewald KK, Bailey RS. Commercially marketed supplements for bodybuilding athletes. Sports Med 15:90–103, 1993.
57. Bucci LR. Nutrients as ergogenic aids for sports and exercise. Boca Raton, FL: CRC, 1990;52:14–18.
58. Boehm KA, Helms RA, Christensen ML, et al. Carnitine: a review for the pharmacy clinician. Hosp Pharm 28:843, 847–850, 1993.
59. Walter JH. L-Carnitine. Arch Dis Child 74:475–478, 1996.
60. Singh A, Pelletier PA, Deuster PA. Dietary requirements for ultra endurance exercise. Sports Med 18(5):301–308, 1994.
61. Anonymous. Still time for rational debate about vitamin B_6 [editorial]. Lancet 351:1523, 1998.
62. Cerulli J, Grabe DW, Gauthier I, et al. Chromium picolinate toxicity. Ann Pharmacother 32:428–431, 1998.
63. Williams MH, Kreider RB, Hunter DW, et al. Effect of inosine supplementation on 3-mile treadmill run performance on Vo_2 peak. Med Sci Sports Exerc 22:517–522, 1990.
64. Stampfer MJ, Hennekens CH, Manson JE, et al. Vitamin E consumption and the risk of coronary disease in women. N Engl J Med 328:1444–1449, 1993.
65. Rimm EB, Stampfer MJ, Ascerio A, et al. Vitamin E consumption and the risk of coronary heart disease in men. N Engl J Med 328:1450–1456, 1993.
66. Stephens NG, Parsons A, Schofield PM, et al. Randomised controlled trial of vitamin E in patients with coronary disease: Cambridge Heart Antioxidant Study (CHAOS). Lancet 347:781–786, 1996.
67. Hodis HN, Mack WJ, LaBree L, et al. Serial coronary angiographic evidence that antioxidant vitamin intake reduces progression of coronary artery sclerosis. JAMA 273:1849–1854, 1995.
68. Stephens N. Antioxidant therapy for ischemic heart disease: where do we stand? Lancet 349:1710–1711, 1997.
69. Ozols RF. Chemoprevention of cancer. Curr Probl Cancer 18:1–69, 1994.

70. The ATBC Cancer Prevention Study Group. The effect of vitamin E and beta carotene on the incidence of lung cancer and other cancers in male smokers. N Engl J Med 330:1029–1035, 1994.
71. Rapola JM, Virtamo J, Ripatti S, et al. Randomised trial of alpha tocopherol and beta carotene supplements on incidence of major coronary events in men with previous myocardial infarction. Lancet 349:1715–1720, 1997.
72. Hennekens CH, Buring JE, Manson JE, et al. Lack of effect of long term supplementation with beta carotene on the incidence of malignant neoplasms and cardiovascular disease. N Engl J Med 334:1145–1149, 1996.
73. Omenn GS, Goodman GE, Thornquist MD, et al. Effects of a combination of beta carotene and vitamin A on lung cancer and cardiovascular disease. N Engl J Med 334:1150–1155, 1996.
74. Gershoff SN. Vitamin C: new roles, new requirements? Nutr Rev 51:313–326, 1993.
75. Garewal HS, Diplock AT. How "safe" are antioxidant vitamins? Drug Saf 1391:8–14, 1995.
76. Meyers DG, Maloley PA, Weeks D. Safety of antioxidant vitamins. Arch Intern Med 156:925–935, 1996.

CHAPTER 11

VITAMINS AND MINERALS

Diane Nykamp McCarter and John Holbrook

For several decades, the relationships between dietary insufficiencies and the occurrence of diseases such as scurvy, pellagra, and beriberi have been well known. More recently, researchers have discovered a relationship between the maintenance of an optimal state of health and good nutritional practices. Proper nourishment improves the ability to learn, concentrate, participate in physical activities, and resist or overcome injury and disease. It is also critical to the prevention and management of heart disease, diabetes, hypertension, obesity, and other disorders.

The literature (both technical and lay) abounds with information about the use of nutrients to prevent or treat disorders. The public has become more concerned with nutrition, especially how good nutrition relates to self-care and wellness. The public is also concerned with the amount of food they consume and the use of nutritional supplements. Controversy remains as to whether the U.S. Food and Drug Administration (FDA) has regulatory authority over vitamin supplement manufacturers who make unsubstantiated claims about the effectiveness of their products in the treatment or prevention of disease.

This chapter focuses on the basic nutrients that the body needs.

TREATMENT GOALS: VITAMINS AND MINERALS

- Encourage patients to develop good nutritional practices that will promote wellness and prevent disease.
- Enhance the patient's ability to recognize and treat nutrient deficiencies or toxicity.
- Maintain an optimal state of health in patients with special needs caused by medical conditions or use of medications, which alter nutritional status.
- Foster awareness that optimal nutritional intake, not supplements, is the most appropriate and cost-effective way to obtain vitamins and minerals.

Table 11.1 ▪ Recommended Dietary Allowances

Patient Parameters						Fat-Soluble Vitamins				Water-Soluble Vitamins							Minerals						
Age (yr) or Condition	Weight[a] (kg)	Weight[a] (lb)	Height[a] (cm)	Height[a] (in)	Protein (g)	Vitamin A (μg RE)[b]	Vitamin D (IU)[c]	Vitamin E (IU)[d]	Vitamin K (μg)	Ascorbic Acid (C, mg)	Thiamine (B_1, mg)	Riboflavin (B_2, mg)	Niacin (B_3, mg)	Pyridoxine (B_4, mg)	Folate (μg)	Cyanocobalamin (B_{12}, μg)	Calcium (mg)	Phosphorus (mg)	Magnesium (mg)	Iron (mg)	Zinc (mg)	Iodine (μg)	Selenium (μg)
Infants																							
0.0–0.5	6	13	60	24	13	375	300	4	5	30	0.3	0.4	5	0.3	25	0.3	400	300	40	6	5	40	10
0.5–1	9	20	71	28	14	375	400	6	10	35	0.4	0.5	6	0.6	35	0.5	600	500	60	10	5	50	15
Children																							
1–3	13	29	90	35	16	400	400	9	15	40	0.7	0.8	9	1	50	0.7	800	800	80	10	10	70	20
4–6	20	44	112	44	24	500	400	10	20	45	0.9	1.1	12	1.1	75	1	800	800	120	10	10	90	20
7–10	28	62	132	52	28	700	400	10	30	45	1	1.2	13	1.4	100	1.4	800	800	170	10	10	120	30
Males																							
11–14	45	99	157	62	45	1000	400	15	45	50	1.3	1.5	17	1.7	150	2	1200	1200	270	12	15	150	40
15–18	66	145	176	69	59	1000	400	15	65	60	1.5	1.8	20	2	200	2	1200	1200	400	12	15	150	50
19–24	72	160	177	70	58	1000	400	15	70	60	1.5	1.7	19	2	200	2	1200	1200	350	10	15	150	70
25–50	79	174	176	70	63	1000	200	15	80	60	1.5	1.7	19	2	200	2	800	800	350	10	15	150	70
51+	77	170	173	68	63	1000	200	15	80	60	1.2	14	15	2	200	2	800	800	350	10	15	150	70
Females																							
11–14	46	101	157	62	46	800	400	12	45	50	1.1	1.3	15	1.4	150	2	1200	1200	280	15	12	150	45
15–18	55	120	163	64	44	800	400	12	55	60	1.1	1.3	15	1.5	180	2	1200	1200	300	15	12	150	50
19–24	58	128	164	65	46	800	400	12	60	60	1.1	1.3	15	1.6	180	2	1200	1200	280	15	12	150	55
25–50	63	138	153	64	50	800	200	12	65	60	1.1	1.3	15	1.6	180	2	800	800	280	15	12	150	55
51+	65	143	160	63	50	800	200	12	65	60	1	1.2	13	1.6	180	2	800	800	280	10	12	150	55
Pregnant					60	800	400	15	65	70	1.5	1.6	17	2.2	400	2.2	1200	1200	320	30	15	175	65
Lactating																							
First 6 mo					65	1300	400	18	65	95	1.6	1.8	20	2.1	280	2.6	1200	1200	355	15	19	200	75
Second 6 mo					62	1200	400	16	65	90	1.6	1.7	20	2.1	260	2.6	1200	1200	340	15	16	200	75

Source: Reprinted with permission from Recommended dietary allowances. 10th ed. Washington, DC: National Academy Press, 1989.

The allowances, expressed as average daily intakes over time, are intended to provide for individual variations among most normal persons as they live in the United States under usual environmental stresses. Diets should be based on a variety of common foods in order to provide other nutrients for which human requirements have been less well defined.

[a] Weights and heights of reference adults are actual medians for the U.S. population of the designated age, as reported by NHANES II. The median weights and heights of those under 19 years of age were taken from Hamill PV et al. Am J Clin Nutr 32:607, 1979. The use of these figures does not imply that the height-to-weight ratios are ideal.

[b] Retinol equivalents: 1 retinol equivalent = 1 μg retinol or 6 μg β-carotene.

[c] As cholecalciferol 10 μg cholecalciferol = 400 IU of vitamin D.

[d] α-Tocopherol equivalents 1 mg d-α-tocopherol = α-TE = 1.49 IU.

Vitamins

Vitamins are non–energy-producing organic substances that are essential in small amounts for the maintenance of normal metabolic functions. They are categorized into two groups: the fat-soluble vitamins (A, D, E, and K) and the water-soluble vitamins (B complex and C). All vitamins, with the exception of D, K, and biotin, must be supplied completely from dietary sources.[1,2] The majority of vitamins are obtained from plant and animal sources, with the exceptions of vitamin K and biotin, which are produced by microorganisms in the intestinal tract, and vitamin D, which is synthesized from cholesterol in the skin. The amount of vitamin K synthesized is sufficient to meet the body's needs, but some dietary supplementation of biotin usually is required. The amount of vitamin D produced in the skin may or may not be sufficient to meet the body's needs because its synthesis depends on exposure to ultraviolet light.

VITAMIN REQUIREMENTS

Reference values for nutrient requirements for the American population are undergoing close scrutiny, and a number of recommendations for change are expected to occur. In keeping with the Nutrition Labeling and Education Act of 1990, terminology has been changed in an effort to convey nutrition label information in a way that enables people to observe and comprehend the information readily and to understand its significance in the context of a total daily diet. The term *Recommended Dietary Allowance* (RDA) has been replaced with *Dietary Reference Intake* (DRI) to reflect an increasing understanding of the need for nutrient intake that is adequate to prevent deficiency diseases and promote optimal health. The new terminology includes the following:

- Daily Value (DV): A dietary reference value to help consumers use food label information to plan a healthful overall diet. These values have been in use since 1994 and describe the percentage of the daily value for each nutrient that a serving of a food provides. DVs must be prominently displayed on every food label. Two sets of reference values are used to determine DVs:
  1. Daily Reference Values (DRVs): A set of dietary references that apply to fat, saturated fat, cholesterol, carbohydrate, protein, fiber, sodium, and potassium. DRVs are used for nutrients for which no set of standards previously existed. The DRVs for cholesterol, sodium, and potassium, which do not contribute calories to the diet, remain the same regardless of the caloric intake.
  2. DRIs: A set of dietary references for essential vitamins and minerals and, in selected age groups, protein. The term *DRI* replaces the term *RDA*. The RDA values have remained the same for the time being (except for protein), although these values are being examined closely and recommendations for changes are expected. DRIs are based on three types of reference values: the RDA, Estimated Average Requirement (EAR), and Tolerable Upper Intake Level (UL). DRIs reflect a shift in emphasis from preventing deficiency diseases to decreasing the risk of chronic disease through improved nutritional intake.
- Recommended Dietary Allowances (RDAs): A set of estimated nutrient allowances established by the National Academy of Science that is updated periodically to reflect current scientific knowledge.[3] RDAs should not be confused with U.S. Recommended Daily Allowances, which are set by the FDA and are based on current Recommended Dietary Allowances. One of the reasons for changing the terminology from *RDA* to *DRI* is to avoid confusion.
- UL (also called maximum upper limits, or MULs): The maximum level of daily nutrient intake that is unlikely to pose risks of adverse health effects to almost all of the people in the group for whom it is designated.
- EAR: The intake value estimated to meet the requirement defined by a specified indicator of adequacy in 50% of an age- and gender-specific group.
- Adequate Intake (AI): Values used when sufficient evidence is not available to estimate an average intake requirement or RDA. AIs indicate an average intake that appears to sustain a desired indicator of health, such as calcium in bone. The term *AI* will replace the older term *Estimated Safe and Adequate Daily Dietary Intake* (ESADDI).[4–7] Table 11.1 lists the 1989 vitamin and mineral RDA values. Table 11.2 lists the updated RDA values for the newly created age subgroup of 19 to 22 years. This subgroup was created to recognize the higher nutritional requirements in this group of the population.

Table 11.2 ▪ New RDAs for Adults Between Ages 19 and 22

Nutrient	Men	Women
Protein	44 g	56 g
Vitamin A	800 μg	1000 μg
Vitamin D	7.5 μg (300 IU)	7.5 μg (300 IU)
Vitamin E	8 mg	10 mg
Vitamin C	60 mg	60 mg
Thiamin (B_1)	1.1 mg	1.5 mg
Riboflavin	1.3 mg	1.7 mg
Niacin	14 mg	19 mg
Vitamin B_6	2 μg	2.2 μg
Folacin	400 μg	400 μg
Vitamin B_{12}	3 μg	3 μg
Pantothenic acid	4–7 mg	4–7 mg
Biotin	100–200 μg	100–200 μg
Calcium	1000 mg	1000 mg
Phosphorus	800 mg	800 mg
Magnesium	300 mg	350 mg
Iron	10 mg	18 mg
Zinc	15 mg	15 mg
Iodine	150 μg	150 μg
Fluoride	1.5–4 mg	1.5–4 mg
Selenium	50–200 μg	50–200 μg

VITAMIN STABILITY

In general, fat-soluble vitamins are not destroyed during cooking. However, water-soluble vitamins are easily dissolved in cooking water and may be destroyed through heating. Ascorbic acid (vitamin C) suffers the greatest loss in nutritive value through cooking. Riboflavin is only sparingly water soluble and is not removed as quickly (when cooked in water) as the other water-soluble vitamins. When meats are broiled or roasted, thiamine losses are 25% or less. Constant low-temperature cooking improves palatability of meat but decreases the nutritive value. Wilting of vegetables or dehydration of most foods results in considerable nutrient loss. Improper storage or dicing and cutting of fruits and vegetables before cooking in water also can result in vitamin loss. Fruits and vegetables should be consumed raw or cooked in a minimum amount of liquid to help retain their maximum vitamin content. Other vitamin-conserving cooking methods include steaming, microwaving, and stir frying.[8] Steaming or microwaving is especially beneficial for vegetables containing thiamine, riboflavin, pyridoxine, folic acid, and ascorbic acid. Microwave cooking requires a shorter cooking time and less water and generally results in greater retention of heat-labile nutrients.[9]

Fat-Soluble Vitamins

Vitamins A, D, E, and K are classified as fat-soluble vitamins. Their absorption is facilitated by bile salts or dietary fat, and they are stored in moderate amounts in the body. Vitamins A and D function like hormones, interacting with specific intracellular receptors in their target tissues. Toxicity associated with the fat-soluble vitamins can occur because fat-soluble vitamins can be stored with other lipids in fatty tissues and can accumulate. The characteristics of fat-soluble vitamins are listed in Table 11.3.

VITAMIN A

Functions of Vitamin A

Vitamin A is essential for vision, dental development, and growth and reproduction. Vitamin A is also necessary for the synthesis of hydrocortisone and the regulation and differentiation of epithelial tissue. The integrity of the mucous membranes of the eyes, skin, mouth, gastrointestinal tract, and genitourinary tract is maintained by this vitamin, which is required for the production of mucus.[10]

Properties of Vitamin A

Vitamin A includes three natural compounds found in animal sources (retinol, retinal, and retinoic acid) and three provitamins found in plants (α-, β-, and γ-carotene). Retinol apparently is responsible for the actions of the vitamin in the reproductive process and retinal is the functional compound of the visual cycle. Retinoic acid, the active form of vitamin A, is associated with growth and cell differentiation. Retinoic acid cannot replace retinal in the visual cycle and is not able to support reproduction.[11] β-Carotene, the most abundant plant source, does not possess inherent vitamin A activity but yields retinol after absorption and metabolism. One international unit (IU) of vitamin A is equal to 0.3 μg retinol or 0.6 μg β-carotene. Large amounts of β-carotene can be ingested over a long period of time without development of toxic effects (other than skin pigmentation) because only 20 to 30% of a dose is absorbed from the gastrointestinal tract, and it is metabolized at a rate of approximately 50 to 60% of normal dietary intake.[12] When the dietary intake of retinol is in the range of the recommended dietary allowance, the majority is absorbed; however, excess amounts ingested in the diet are excreted.

Vitamin A Deficiency

There is now evidence that β-carotene has important functions other than being the precursor of vitamin A and therefore should be ingested in amounts greater than needed to meet the vitamin A requirements. Vitamin A deficiency usually is caused by fat malabsorption syndromes or malnutrition. Deficiency produces a variety of symptoms that include nyctalopia (night blindness), diminished production of corticosteroids, xerophthalmia (drying of the cornea), keratinization of the skin, growth failure, and fetal malformations. Vitamin A deficiency can impair resistance to infections by breaking down mucous membranes.[13]

Vitamin A Toxicity

Acute and chronic vitamin A toxicity are well-recognized conditions in adults. Acute poisoning may occur after a single dose greater than 1,000,000 IU. Chronic toxicity is determined mainly by the dosage and duration of therapy. Usually a dosage of more than 100,000 IU daily for several months causes hypervitaminosis A.[14] Prolonged daily use of vitamin A in dosages of 25,000 IU or more may result in hypervitaminosis resembling a cirrhosis-like liver syndrome. Symptoms of chronic use of vitamin A include fatigue, vomiting, cheilosis, dizziness, nausea, and irritability, followed by generalized skin desquamation. Pruritus, dry, scaly skin, bone pain, changes in hair and nail texture, increased cerebrospinal fluid pressure, and hypercalcemia may also occur. Concern about an excess intake of vitamin A during pregnancy has increased in recent years because of its structural and metabolic relationship to other vitamin A analogs (retinoids), especially 13-*cis*-retinoic acid (isotretinoin), which is teratogenic. A daily dosage lower than 10,000 IU is not thought to be teratogenic.[15]

Table 11.3 ▪ Summary of Fat-Soluble Vitamins

Vitamin	Function	Deficiency	Large Dosages	Therapeutic Uses	Sources
Vitamin A Retinol Retinal Retinoic acid β-carotene	Growth Vision Dental development Reproduction Hydrocortisone synthesis Epithelial tissue differentiation Mucous membrane maintenance	Nyctalopia Xerophthalmia Faulty bone and tooth development Keratinization Fetal malformation Decreased production of cortical steroids Impaired resistance to infection	Acute Fatigue Cheilitis Dizziness Nausea and vomiting Irritability Desquamation Chronic Hypercalcemia Dry, scaly skin Bone pain Changes in hair and nail texture Increased cerebrospinal pressure Pruritus	Dermatology Oncology	Liver Milk Butter and margarine Dark-green, leafy vegetables Carrots Sweet potatoes
Vitamin D Ergocalciferol (D_2) Cholecalciferol (D_3)	Bone mineralization Maintenance of normal neuromuscular activity Maintenance of serum calcium and phosphorus levels	Associated with inadequate calcium and phosphorus Rickets (children) Osteomalacia (adults) Secondary hyperparathyroidism	Hypercalcemia (weakness anorexia, vomiting, diarrhea, polydipsia, polyuria, and mental changes) Constipation Proteinuria Vague aches Metallic or bad taste Renal failure Hypertension	Renal osteodystrophy Hypoparathyroidism	Sunlight Butter Egg yolk Fatty fish Liver Fortified milk and bread
Vitamin E *dl*-α-tocopherol (1 mg = 1.49 IU)	Antioxidant: maintains integrity of cell membrane Enhances vitamin A uptake Inhibition of prostaglandin production Cofactor in steroid metabolism Related to action of selenium	Neurologic syndrome (ataxia, muscle weakness, nystagmus, loss of touch or pain) Anemia in premature infants Hemolysis of red blood	Increase the effects of oral anticoagulants	Intermittent claudication Retrolental fibroplasia	Wheat germ oil Nuts Green, leafy vegetables
Vitamin K Phylloquinone (K_1) Menaquinone (K_2) Analog: Menadione (K_3)	Coagulation Formulation of prothrombin and other clotting proteins	Prolonged clotting time Deficiency symptoms can be produced by coumarin anticoagulants and antibiotic therapy	Vomiting Toxicity can be induced by water-soluble analog Neonatal jaundice Dietary supplements can block effect of oral anticoagulant	Coagulation disorders Anticoagulant-induced prothrombin deficiency	Green leaves (spinach, cabbage) Liver Synthesis in intestine by bacteria Cheese, egg yolk

Source: Williams SR, ed. Nutrition and diet therapy. St. Louis: Mosby, 1997; Sizer FS, Whitney EN, eds. Hamilton & Whitney's nurition: concepts and controversies. 6th ed. St. Paul: West Publishing, 1994; Weigley ES, Mueller DH, Robinson CH, eds. Robinson's basic nutrition and diet therapy. 8th ed. Columbus, OH: Merrill, 1997.

Therapeutic Uses of Vitamin A

Vitamin A analogs (retinoids) have been developed to improve the therapeutic index of vitamin A. Isotretinoin, etretinate, and acitretin were developed as less toxic and more effective agents. However, they have caused embryopathy.[15] Retinoids have had a major impact on the practice of dermatology[16] and are under investigation for the possible effect of decreasing the risk of cancer[17–19] and reducing the rate of infections.[20] There remains controversy about the relationship between an above-average β-carotene intake and a lowered incidence of cancer and cardiovascular disease, especially when β-carotene is used in combination with vitamins E and C.[21–23]

Until further research is conducted, advice to vitamin A users is understandably conservative. Dosages higher than 10,000 IU should not be recommended and consumers should rely on dietary intake of foods containing β-carotene.[24,25] Excess use of retinol supplements may cause serious adverse reactions; however, increasing the dietary intake of retinol by eating more green and yellow vegetables may be beneficial and avoid toxicity. No definitive statement can be made at this time about the use of vitamin A in wound healing, although recent studies have reported that vitamin A promotes wound healing.

VITAMIN D

Functions of Vitamin D

Vitamin D is considered a hormone rather than a vitamin, although it is not a natural hormone. Vitamin D, in conjunction with parathyroid hormone (PTH) and calcitonin, is needed for calcium and phosphate metabolism. This in turn supports normal mineralization of bone and neuromuscular activity.

Dietary Reference Intakes for Vitamin D

DRIs have been established for both men and women: ages 25 to 50, 5 μg; 51 to 70, 10 μg; and 71 and older, 15 μg.

Properties of Vitamin D

Vitamin D refers to both D_2 (calciferol, ergocalciferol) and D_3 (cholecalciferol). D_2 and D_3 occur naturally and are equipotent. Either may supply the body's daily requirements. These forms have an onset of action time of 10 to 24 hours and may be stored in the body for prolonged periods.

Ninety percent of dietary vitamin D is absorbed from the small intestine. Vitamin D_3 may be absorbed more rapidly and completely than vitamin D_2.

The supply of vitamin D depends on ultraviolet light radiation for conversion of plant ergosterol to vitamin D_2 or for conversion of skin 7-dehydrocholesterol to vitamin D_3. Dietary intake of vitamin D is unnecessary in people who spend adequate amounts of time in sun (5 to 15 minutes exposure of face, neck, and arms per day). The new vitamin D DRIs are estimated to provide enough vitamin D even for people with limited sun exposure. Vitamins D_2 and D_3 require activation (hydroxylation) by both the liver and the kidney. Vitamin D_3 is absorbed into the circulation and converted by hepatic microsomal enzymes to 25-hydroxycholecalciferol, which in turn is hydroxylated in the kidney to its active metabolite, 1,25-dihydroxycholecalciferol (calcitriol). Calcitriol has pharmacologic activity that lasts from 3 to 5 days. The production rate of calcitriol is closely regulated by plasma calcium and PTH. PTH mobilizes calcium from bone to maintain normal calcium concentrations, whereas vitamin D promotes bone mineralization.[26]

Dihydrotachysterol (DHT) is a synthetic vitamin D analog activated in the liver that does not require renal hydroxylation. DHT has a rapid onset of action (2 hours), a shorter half-life, and a greater effect on mineralization of bone salts than does vitamin D.

Vitamin D Deficiency

Vitamin D deficiency may be induced by renal and hepatic disease, malabsorption syndromes, short bowel syndrome, hypoparathyroidism, and long-term anticonvulsant therapy. Vitamin D deficiency results in inadequate absorption of calcium and phosphorus from the intestinal tract. A deficiency of these minerals leads to faulty mineralization of bone and teeth, resulting in rickets in children and osteomalacia in adults. Also, increased PTH secretion is caused by a decreased serum calcium level, resulting in secondary hyperparathyroidism.

Vitamin D Toxicity

Large dosages of vitamin D (50,000 IU or more per day) may result in toxicity, although tolerance to vitamin D varies widely. Initial manifestations of toxicity result from hypercalcemia and include weakness, anorexia, vomiting, diarrhea, polydipsia, polyuria, mental changes, and proteinuria. Prolonged hypercalcemia may result in calcification of soft tissue, including the heart, blood vessels, renal tubules, and lungs. Death can result from cardiovascular or renal failure.

Therapeutic Uses of Vitamin D

A vitamin D–resistant state exists in chronic renal failure. Renal osteodystrophy is characterized by a decreased ability of the kidney to convert 25-hydroxycholecalciferol to 1,25-dihydroxycholecalciferol. Active vitamin D (calcitriol) or dihydrotachysterol must be supplemented to lower the concentrations of PTH and raise the plasma calcium concentration to allow bone formation. Vitamin D supplementation is also needed in hypoparathyroidism, which is characterized by hypocalcemia and hyperphosphatemia. Generally, if a patient has an inadequate diet and little exposure to sunlight, a vitamin D supplement may be appropriate.

An anticonvulsant-induced hypocalcemia is thought to be caused by induction of the hepatic microsomal P-450 enzyme system and is treated with vitamin D, 25-hydroxycholecalciferol, and possibly calcium. Combination therapy is required because vitamin D obtained from the diet, supplements, or sun exposure is converted to inactive metabolites with prolonged anticonvulsant use.

VITAMIN E

Functions of Vitamin E

Many of the actions of vitamin E are related to its antioxidant properties. Vitamin E stabilizes the lipid portion of the cell membrane by preventing oxidation of polyunsaturated phospholipids, thereby maintaining the integrity of the cell membrane. Other functions of vitamin E include enhancement of vitamin A use, inhibition of prostaglandin production, and stimulation of an essential cofactor in steroid metabolism.

Properties of Vitamin E

α-Tocopherol is the most active and abundant form of vitamin E, occurring naturally in substances such as wheat germ oil. Vitamin E is 20 to 40% absorbed from the gastrointestinal tract and is distributed to all tissues via the lymphatic system.

Vitamin E Deficiency

Vitamin E deficiency occurs primarily in premature infants and in patients with severe malabsorptive disease, such as cystic fibrosis. The neurologic syndrome of ataxia, muscle weakness, nystagmus, and loss of the senses of touch and pain have been attributed to vitamin E deficiency.[27,28]

Vitamin E Toxicity

Current literature includes little evidence that vitamin E produces any harmful effects. A daily intake of 200 to 600 mg (1 IU = 0.6 mg d-α-tocopherol) appears to be innocuous in most people. The most commonly recurring complaint with large dosages (300 to 3200 IU/day) is gastrointestinal upset (nausea, flatulence, or diarrhea), weakness, or fatigue.[29] Large dosages of vitamin E may increase the risk of hemorrhagic stroke, and intravenous use has been associated with infant death.[30] Although vitamin E has been reported to increase the effects of oral anticoagulants, this interaction remains controversial.[31,32]

Therapeutic Uses of Vitamin E

Vitamin E is reported to be beneficial in the treatment or prevention of a wide range of conditions. Vitamin E has been shown to protect from cancers[33–38] of the prostate, stomach, esophagus, and lung. Vitamin E is also being investigated for its role in reducing the risk of heart disease in part by decreasing lipid peroxidation and reducing platelet adhesiveness.[39–49] It is also thought that vitamin E may improve immune function.[50–52]

Parenteral administration of vitamin E appears to be effective in preventing retrolental fibroplasia, hemolysis, and pulmonary oxygen toxicity in premature infants.[53]

Scientists now believe that vitamin E acts with selenium as a cellular antioxidant, protecting cell membranes from peroxidase damage. However, there is no scientific basis for vitamin E supplementation in a host of conditions, including infertility, arthritis, angina, muscular dystrophy, diabetes, premenstrual syndrome, nocturnal leg cramps, and in the enhancement of athletic performance.

VITAMIN K

Functions of Vitamin K

The only rational use of vitamin K is for the correction of bleeding tendencies caused by its deficiency. Such a deficiency is unlikely to occur because of intestinal bacterial synthesis of the vitamin. For this reason, there are no dietary recommended allowances.

Properties of Vitamin K

Vitamin K is essential for the hepatic synthesis of prothrombin and other clotting proteins. Vitamin K compounds are chemically called quinones and include phylloquinone (K_1) and menaquinone (K_2), which are synthesized by intestinal flora, and menadione (K_3), the water-soluble analog.

Vitamin K Deficiency

Vitamin K deficiency, clinically resulting in hemorrhage, may result from destruction of intestinal flora associated with antibiotic use and especially with prolonged poor dietary intake, as may be seen during hospitalization. The role of antibiotics, especially select second- and third-generation cephalosporins, in producing hypoprothrombinemia is thought to result from a common structural side chain that inhibits a vitamin K–dependent step in the synthesis of prothrombin in the liver. When these antibiotics are used, prothrombin time should be monitored, and in many instances a prophylactic dose of vitamin K is given.[54] Aspirin and other salicylates can also induce hypoprothrombinemia. Also, large amounts of vitamins A and E, mineral oil, and bile acid sequestrants interfere with absorption of vitamin K.[55] Advanced liver damage, when caused by cancer and cirrhosis, results in a deficiency of clotting factors that cannot be alleviated by administering vitamin K. However, increased prothrombin time as a result of vitamin K deficiency responds to supplementation.

Infants are unable to synthesize vitamin K because they have sterile intestinal tracts at birth. A single prophylactic dose of vitamin K (0.5 to 1 mg intramuscularly or subcutaneously) should be given to infants to protect them until synthesis begins and to supplement dietary intake. Phylloquinone (phytonadione) is the agent of choice to prevent bleeding tendencies,[56] but caution must be exercised with intravenous use.

Vitamin K Toxicity

Vitamin K is nontoxic, even in massive dosages. Too rapid an intravenous injection of phylloquinone may result in flushing and cause a sense of constriction in the chest. Menadione in dosages of more than 10 mg parenterally may produce hemolysis, hyperbilirubinemia, and kernicterus in premature newborns.

Water-Soluble Vitamins

The B complex vitamins and vitamin C are the water-soluble vitamins. The B complex includes thiamine, riboflavin, nicotinic acid, pyridoxine, pantothenic acid, biotin, folic acid, and cyanocobalamin.

Water-soluble vitamins act as cofactors for specific enzyme systems in the body. Many water-soluble vitamins are not active until phosphorylation occurs after ingestion (thiamine, riboflavin, niacin, and pyridoxine) or until coupled to specific nucleotides (riboflavin, niacin).

Water-soluble vitamins are stored only to a limited extent, so a daily supply is desirable. When excessive amounts are ingested, the unneeded portion generally is excreted. However, even water-soluble vitamins can be toxic, especially when large amounts are ingested for prolonged periods.

Certain conditions or situations may cause depletion of water-soluble vitamins and result in the appearance of deficiency symptoms. These include fever (which may accelerate vitamin metabolism), the stress of injury or surgery, and hyperthyroidism. Deficiencies of water-soluble vitamins may begin as a depletion of body stores without evidence of clinical symptoms such as abnormal laboratory indices. Initial clinical symptoms include loss of appetite, weight loss, headache, apathy, insomnia, or excitability. In severe deficiency states, specific clinical syndromes such as beriberi or pellagra occur. Characteristics of the water-soluble vitamins are listed in Table 11.4.

THIAMINE

The principal role of thiamine (B_1) is as a coenzyme in the form of thiamine pyrophosphate, which plays a vital role in the intermediate metabolism of carbohydrates in decarboxylation (removal of carbon dioxide) and transketolation (transfer of carbon units), such as the conversion of pyruvic acid into acetyl-coA and the synthesis of acetylcholine. Individual requirements for thiamine are related to metabolic rate and are greatest when carbohydrates are the primary source of calories. Thiamine is also necessary for the transmission of nerve impulses.

Thiamine deficiency results in beriberi, characterized by peripheral neuritis. The symptoms of peripheral neuritis include sensory disturbances in the extremities, loss of muscle strength, muscle wasting (dry beriberi), edema (wet beriberi), tachycardia, and an enlarged heart.

In the United States, the most common cause of thiamine deficiency is excessive alcohol intake, which is often associated with poor dietary habits, decreased absorption of nutrients, and decreased activation of thiamine pyrophosphate. The Wernicke–Korsakoff syndrome, characterized by paralysis of eye muscles and nystagmus and associated with excess alcohol intake, is caused primarily by a thiamine deficiency.[57]

RIBOFLAVIN

Riboflavin (vitamin B_2) is converted to two coenzymes, flavin mononucleotide (FMN) and flavin adenine dinucleotide (FAD), which are required for normal tissue respiration. Riboflavin is also required for activation of pyridoxine. Under normal conditions, riboflavin, like all B vitamins, is readily absorbed from the gastrointestinal tract, specifically the duodenum. Dietary sources of riboflavin include milk and dairy products, meats, and green, leafy vegetables. Large dosages may cause yellow discoloration of urine.

A deficiency of riboflavin, as with inadequate dietary intake, malabsorption syndromes, or high alcohol consumption, leads to singular stomatitis, cheilosis, corneal vascularization, or dermatoses.

NIACIN

Niacin (vitamin B_3) is a component of the coenzymes nicotinamide adenine dinucleotide (NAD) and nicotinamide adenine dinucleotide phosphate (NADP). These two coenzymes are important in the oxidation-reduction reactions essential for tissue respiration. Niacin (nicotinic acid) is essential for conversion of food to energy, fat synthesis, growth, and healthy skin. Niacin may be converted in the body to niacinamide (nicotinamide), but either form can be used by the body.

Both excessive intake of alcohol and protein-calorie malnutrition may lead to the niacin deficiency state known as pellagra, with initial symptoms of an erythematous eruption resembling sunburn. Later, the three *D*s of dermatitis, diarrhea, and dementia occur, followed by death if the deficiency is not corrected.

Niacin (but not niacinamide) is a peripheral vasodilator. It causes the release of histamine, resulting in a transient flushing of the skin and a tingling sensation, dizziness, nausea, gastrointestinal upset, and activation of peptic ulcer disease. The flushing sensation generally begins 20 minutes after ingestion and lasts 30 to 60 minutes. After 3 to 6 weeks of therapy, the flushing side effect usually decreases markedly.[58] The adverse effects of niacin may be diminished by increasing the dosage slowly (100 mg, three times a day each week), administering with food or milk, or administering 60 minutes after a 325-mg dose of aspirin.

Niacin is also effective in lowering total cholesterol and low-density lipoprotein (LDL) levels while increasing high-density lipoprotein (HDL) levels. Niacin is used in the treatment of lipid disorders, with initial dosages of 50 to 100 mg twice daily for the first week, gradually increasing over a period of 1 month to 3 g per day. Niacin should be taken with food and should not be taken in conjunction with alcohol or hot drinks. Consumption of alcohol or hot beverages increases the amount of flushing. Niacin is available at a low cost, but

Table 11.4 ▪ Water-Soluble Vitamins

Vitamin	Function	Deficiency	Large Dosages	Sources
Thiamine Vitamin B_1	Carbohydrate metabolism Normal growth Nervous system function Acetylcholine synthesis	Beriberi Peripheral neuritis Loss of memory Depression Muscle wasting Edema Tachycardia Enlarged heart	Nontoxic even in very large dosages of 100–500 mg parenterally	Milk Pork Liver Nuts Whole grains Enriched flour and cereals
Riboflavin Vitamin B_2 Flavin mononucleotide Flavin adenine dinucleotide	Building and maintaining body tissues	Cheilosis Glossitis Seborrheic dermatitis Burning and itching eyes Achlorhydria	No toxicity	Milk Eggs Meat Liver Green, leafy vegetables
Niacin Nicotinic acid Nicotinamide	Conversion of food to energy Tissue respiration Fat synthesis Growth Healthy skin	Pellagra Erythematous eruptions Dermatitis Diarrhea Dementia	Transient flushing of skin and tingling sensation (vasodilation) Dizziness Nausea Gastrointestinal upset Peptic ulcer disease Liver toxicity Hyperuricemia Glucose intolerance Lower serum lipids with 3–6 g cholesterol and triglycerides	Lean meats Fish Whole grains Green vegetables
Pyridoxine Vitamin B_6 Pyridones: Pyridixine Pyridoxamine Pyridoxal	Amino acid transformation Metabolism of tryptophan to serotonin Modify action of steroid hormones	Seborrheic-like skin Glossitis Stomatitis Peripheral neuropathy Anemia Drugs: hydralazine, penicillamine, isoniazid, cycloserine, and estrogen	Peripheral sensory neuropathy Ataxia	Wheat Corn Meat Potatoes
Ascorbic acid (Vitamin C)	Synthesis of collagen, important for wound healing and reducing stress of injury and infection Synthesis of epinephrine from adrenal glands Conversion of folic acid to folinic acid Iron absorption	Defect in collagen formation: poor wound healing, aching joints, increased susceptibility to infection, weakened cartilage and capillary walls Scurvy	Possible kidney stones Diarrhea with 4–15 g/day Gout Lower serum cholesterol Rebound scurvy Increased absorption of iron Interference with oral anticoagulants Treatment of pressure sores Impaired bacterial activity	Citrus fruits Tomatoes Leafy vegetables Melons
Pantothenic acid	Carbohydrate metabolism Gluconeogenesis Synthesis and degradation of fatty acids Sterol synthesis Steroid hormone synthesis Porphyrin synthesis	Usually seen only with severe, multiple B-complex deficits	Essentially nontoxic in humans	Meat Poultry Fish Cereals Fruits and vegetables Milk
Biotin	Carbohydrate metabolism Fat metabolism	Seborrheic dermatitis Algesia	Essentially nontoxic in humans	Liver Egg yolk Synthesized by intestinal bacteria
Folic acid	Red blood cell maturation Interrelated with B_{12}	Megaloblastic anemia In pregnancy, neural tube defects in offspring	Essentially nontoxic in humans	Liver Green, leafy vegetables
Cobalamin B_{12}	DNA synthesis Red blood cell formation	Pernicious anemia Peripheral neuropathy Macrocytic anemia	Essentially nontoxic in humans	Liver, meat, milk, eggs, cheese

Source: Marcus R, Coulston AM. Water-soluble vitamins. In Hardman JG, Limbird LE, Molinoff PB, et al., eds. Goodman & Gilman's the pharmacological basis of therapeutics. 9th ed. New York: McGraw-Hill, 1996; Cataldo CB, DeBruyne LK, Whitney EN, eds. Nutrition and diet therapy. 3rd ed. St. Paul: West Publishing, 1992; Siaer FS, Whitney EN, eds. Hamilton & Whitney's nutrition: concepts and controversies. 6th ed. St. Paul: West Publishing, 1994. Weigley ES, Mueller DH, Robinson CH, eds. Robinson's basic nutrition and diet therapy. 8th ed. Columbus, OH: Merrill, 1997.

it is not free of serious side effects. (See Chapter 20, Hyperlipidemia.) Niacin may cause reversible hepatitis, intolerable gastrointestinal disturbances, glucose intolerance, and hyperuricemia. Fasting blood glucose levels, liver function values, and uric acid levels should be monitored during chronic therapy.[59,60]

Sustained-release niacin formulations have been used in the treatment of hyperlipidemia because it was thought that the gradual absorption of niacin would minimize adverse reactions and increase compliance. However, the most serious side effect of hepatotoxicity appears to be dose related with both oral dosage forms (immediate release and extended release). When liver enzymes exceed three times the upper limit of normal, niacin should be discontinued. A decrease in dosage of 50% is needed with the use of extended-release formulations. The maximum dosage of extended release niacin is 2 g. Additionally, certain extended-release products have been linked to fulminant hepatitis.[59]

PYRIDOXINE

Vitamin B_6 consists of a group of related compounds known as the pyridines, which include pyridoxine, pyridoxamine, and pyridoxal. The pyridines are converted to the active form of vitamin B_6, pyridoxal phosphate, in the gastrointestinal tract.

Pyridoxal phosphate is a coenzyme involved in the metabolism of protein, carbohydrates, and fat. In protein metabolism, vitamin B_6 participates in the decarboxylation of amino acids and the conversion of tryptophan to niacin or serotonin. Pyridoxine may also modify the actions of steroid hormones by interacting with steroid receptor complexes.[61]

Vitamin B_6 deficiency caused by dietary restrictions is seldom seen in adults, although a deficiency in the alcoholic population may be as high as 30%. Symptoms of pyridoxine deficiency include seborrhealike skin lesions on the face, glossitis, stomatitis, peripheral neuropathy, and anemia. Drug-induced deficiencies have been observed with vitamin B_6 antagonists such as hydralazine, penicillamine, isoniazid, cycloserine, and estrogen. Pyridoxine has been reported to decrease phenobarbital and phenytoin serum levels when daily doses of 200 mg are administered for 4 weeks. Pyridoxine antagonizes the therapeutic action of levodopa by facilitating the conversion of levodopa to dopamine outside the central nervous system. Patients treated with levodopa should avoid supplemental B_6. Concurrent B_6 use does not adversely affect the levodopa–carbidopa combination because carbidopa is a peripheral dopa decarboxylase inhibitor.

Large dosages of 0.2 to 6 g/day for 2 months to 3 years may result in toxic symptoms of peripheral sensory neuropathies, with associated ataxia and numbness and clumsiness of the hands and feet.[62,63]

Pyridoxine supplementation has been reported to be beneficial in decreasing depression with concurrent oral contraceptive therapy, reducing carpel tunnel syndrome pain, and alleviating premenstrual syndrome (PMS) symptoms. Although clinical trials do not support pyridoxine therapy for PMS, it is used and should be limited to a dosage of 100 mg daily to prevent sensory neuropathies.[64,65]

VITAMIN C (ASCORBIC ACID)

Ascorbic acid is involved in a variety of metabolic functions, including direct stimulation of peptide synthesis and hydroxylation of proline and lysine in collagen formation, epinephrine synthesis, and conversion of folic acid to folinic acid. Vitamin C also facilitates the gastrointestinal absorption of iron. The adrenal cortex, leukocytes, and platelets contain high concentrations of vitamin C. The amount found in the leukocytes is less susceptible to depletion than that present in plasma.[66] Ascorbic acid deficiency results in defective collagen synthesis, joint pain, anemia, poor wound healing, and increased susceptibility to infection. The severe form of vitamin C deficiency is called scurvy. The clinical findings in patients with scurvy include ecchymoses, petechial hemorrhages, easy bruising, loosening of the teeth secondary to gum inflammation, muscle weakness, and joint pains. Plasma levels of vitamin C may be low in cigarette smokers and women taking oral contraceptives.[67,68]

Large daily doses of 1 to 3 g ascorbic acid may result in formation of kidney stones because of excessive excretion of oxalate produced by the metabolism of ascorbic acid.[69] Severe diarrhea and precipitation of gout as the result of excretion of uric acid in predisposed people may also occur.[70]

Rebound scurvy may be seen in both infants and adults after cessation of the use of megadoses of vitamin C.[71] An infant born to a mother taking large amounts of vitamin C can metabolize the vitamin at a more rapid rate than normal. Adults who abruptly stop high-dose therapy experience loosened teeth and bleeding gums. In both instances, an increased rate of vitamin C elimination results in a relative deficiency when large quantities are no longer available. Therefore, patients should be advised to taper the dosage of vitamin C instead of suddenly discontinuing therapy.

Other adverse effects that have been reported with intake of megadoses of vitamin C include absorption of excessive amounts of iron, uricosuria with resultant stone formation, gastrointestinal disturbances, interference with anticoagulants, cell damage, and impaired bactericidal activity of leukocytes.

Ingestion of 1 to 3 g vitamin C has been advocated by Linus Pauling as a protective factor against the common cold.[72] Some studies show a decrease in frequency and severity of symptoms of the common cold[73,74] or an enhanced resistance to upper respiratory infections.[75] Others have found this not to be true.[76,77] The value of vitamin C in prevention of the common cold or as a cure for cancer remains unsubstantiated by randomized, well-designed, double-blind clinical studies.[78]

Vitamin C and other antioxidants have been associated with protection against cataract formation and macular degeneration.[78]

PANTOTHENIC ACID

Pantothenic acid, a constituent of coenzyme A, is needed for enzyme-catalyzed reactions such as the metabolism of carbohydrates, gluconeogenesis, synthesis and metabolism of fatty acids, and synthesis of sterols, steroid hormones, and porphyrins. Because pantothenic acid is widely distributed in the diet, a deficiency is rare and would be expected to occur only in a malnourished person.

BIOTIN

Biotin is important in carbohydrate and fat metabolism. Biotin is available from a wide variety of foods and is also synthesized by bacteria in the intestinal tract. A deficiency is rare but may result from inadequate synthesis. Exfoliative dermatitis is the primary deficiency symptom. Infants who are deficient in biotin because of malabsorption syndromes exhibit the symptoms of Leiner's disease. These infants should be treated with an intravenous form of biotin that is available as an investigational drug.

VITAMIN B_{12}

Vitamin B_{12} participates as a coenzyme in DNA synthesis, cell reproduction, red blood cell (RBC) formation, and nerve maintenance. It may also be needed for the incorporation of folic acid into cells.

Vitamin B_{12} also occurs in several forms designated as cobalamins. Commercially available cyanocobalamin is the most stable form.

Intrinsic factor is secreted by parietal cells in the stomach and regulates the amount of vitamin B_{12} absorbed in the terminal ileum. Because vitamin B_{12} is so well conserved by the body through enterohepatic recycling, signs of deficiency may not be seen for 3 to 5 years after absorption has ceased.[79] Because cyanocobalamin is important in cell production, the signs and symptoms of deficiency are manifested in organ systems with rapidly replicating cells. A deficiency results in megaloblastic anemia, characterized by mature red blood cells that lack oxygen-carrying capacity. Megaloblastic anemia may also occur after surgical removal of the body or fundus of the stomach, which contains parietal cells that secrete intrinsic factor, or removal of part of the ileum, where absorption of the vitamin occurs. Pernicious anemia, a genetic disorder, occurs when intrinsic factor is not produced and, consequently, vitamin B_{12} is not absorbed. In pernicious anemia, mature RBCs are not produced because of a lack of DNA synthesis. The characteristic symptoms of the disorder include pallor, anorexia, dyspnea, prolonged bleeding time, weight loss, glossitis, and neurologic disturbances including depression and unsteady gait (see Chapters 12 and 13).

A vitamin B_{12} deficiency may exist in older adults without the classic laboratory, hematologic, or clinical manifestations. This vitamin B_{12} deficiency appears to be caused by an inability to absorb protein-bound vitamin B_{12}. It is manifested in neurologic and psychiatric abnormalities without the classic hematologic abnormalities. Older adults with a serum B_{12} level of less than 200 pg/mL should be treated initially with 1 μg/day B_{12} until serum B_{12} exceeds 300 pg/mL or with B_{12} intramuscularly (100 μg/day for 2 weeks, then 1000 μg/month for life) if serum B_{12} does not exceed 300 pg/mL.[80] Vitamin B_{12} is available as a tablet, a solution for intramuscular injection, and an intranasal gel. The gel is reported by the manufacturer to have greater bioavailability than oral tablets and is easier to administer than an intramuscular injection.

Cyanocobalamin has no therapeutic value beyond that of correcting deficiencies. The use of vitamin B_{12} to boost energy is not supported by the literature.

FOLIC ACID

Folic acid is functionally related to cyanocobalamin because both are essential for DNA synthesis. Folic acid is also important in cell reproduction, including RBC formation and protein synthesis.

Folacin is the term for folic acid (pteroylglutamic acid). Approximately 25% of the folacin found in food is in the active (tetrahydrofolic acid) form and is readily absorbed and stored in the liver. Ascorbic acid prevents its oxidation.

The usual causes of folic acid deficiency are similar to those previously discussed with other B vitamins. In addition, a deficiency may occur during pregnancy, causing birth defects such as neural tube defects (spina bifida and anencephaly). Women of childbearing age should have an intake of at least 0.4 mg folic acid daily to reduce the risk of fetal neural tube defects.[81,82] As of January 1998, the FDA has required all cereal and grain products to be fortified with folic acid at a concentration that on average provides an additional 0.1 mg folic acid.[83–85] Fortification of food products with folic acid is also being investigated as a way to reduce the risk of heart disease by reducing blood levels of homocysteine.[86]

Deficiencies can also occur with oral contraceptive use, in older adults as the result of a poor diet, and in infants whose formulas lack folic acid or vitamin C. A folic acid deficiency can also occur with anticonvulsants such as phenytoin or primidone. These agents lower serum folate by inhibiting deconjugase enzymes in the gastrointestinal tract. The anemia that results from folic acid is characterized by a reduction in the number of RBCs, the release of large nucleated cells (macrocytic, megaloblastic), low hemoglobin levels with a high color content in RBCs, and lowered leukocyte and platelet counts.

Folic acid therapy corrects the anemia associated with vitamin B_{12} deficiency, but it does not prevent or correct neurologic disturbances associated with vitamin B_{12} deficiency (see Chapter 13).

Minerals

Minerals are inorganic substances that are classified as either macronutrients or micronutrients. Macronutrients are required in daily amounts of 100 mg or more, whereas micronutrients are required in amounts of less than 100 mg daily. A summary of essential minerals is included in Table 11.5. Other minerals are found widely in nature and in the human body, but their functions are uncertain, and many are considered contaminants. With all minerals, a narrow therapeutic index exists between general requirements and toxic levels.

Sources of minerals vary according to the composition of the soil in which they are found. In regions where the soil has been depleted of minerals, the population may experience deficiencies. Deficiencies may result from chronic ingestion of highly refined foods (flour and cereals) unless they have been fortified with the minerals lost during processing. Whole-grain foods are preferred to refined foods because of their higher content of zinc, copper, iron, pyridoxine, pantothenic acid, biotin, folic acid, and vitamin E.

In this section, emphasis is placed on a discussion of calcium, iron, and zinc because of their well-understood functions. Table 11.6 lists the new DRIs for calcium, magnesium, fluoride, and phosphorus. Table 11.7 lists the interactions that involve minerals.

CALCIUM

Calcium is essential for the functional integrity of the nervous and muscular systems, for normal cardiac function, for conversion of prothrombin into thrombin, and as the major mineral component of bone.

Table 11.5 ▪ Summary of Minerals

Mineral	Physiologic Functions	Deficiency	Clinical Applications
Chlorine (chloride), major anion of extracellular fluid	Required for fluid–electrolyte balance, acid–base balance, gastric acidity	Deficiency of chloride alone rare	Losses in GI disorders, vomiting, diarrhea, and GI tract damage
Chromium	Favors normal glucose tolerance	Impaired glucose clearance, peripheral neuropathy, ataxia	Required for normal glucose use; role in management of diabetes controversial; required for carbohydrate and lipid metabolism; lowers serum cholesterol and LDL, increases HDL
Cobalt	Integral part of B_{12}	Pernicious anemia	Excess leads to polycythemia
Copper 30% absorbed from diet inversely related to zinc, essential for proper iron use	Synthesis of melanin, collagen, hemoglobin, and connective tissue	Decreased red blood cell production and poor wound healing	Menke's kinky hair syndrome, absorption disorder, toxicity, Wilson' disease
Fluoride	Contributes to structure of teeth and soft tissues	Dental caries	May be useful in osteoporosis, toxicity, fluorosis, mottled enamel
Iodine	Thyroxine and tri-iodothyronine synthesis	Creatinism, goiter, myxedema	Regulation of basal metabolic rate growth, reproduction, cellular metabolism
Magnesium 25–65% absorbed primarily in small intestine. Efficiently absorbed and highly conserved. A person on a high-magnesium diet absorbs only about 1/4 of the intake but on a low magnesium diet more than 3/4 of the intake is absorbed.	Nerve cell function enzyme activator, skeleton synthesis	Occurs in alcoholics, diabetics, and with malabsorption syndrome (symptoms: tremor, spasm, irritability, lack of coordination, convulsions) Excretion enhanced by mineralocorticoids, hypercalcemia, phosphate depletion, and alcohol ingestion	Uses in therapy include intravenous magnesium sulfate as anticonvulsant, electrolyte replenisher, uterine relaxant; magnesium gluconate for oral supplementation; magnesium citrate or sulfate as laxative; magnesium carbonate, oxide, hydroxide, or trisilicate as antacid Hypermagnesemia rare except in renal failure; excess may cause diarrhea

(continued)

Table 11.5 *(continued)*

Mineral	Physiologic Functions	Deficiency	Clinical Applications
Manganese Substitute for magnesium in some reactions	Cofactor for enzyme systems involved in bone formation; required for formation of mucopolysaccharides	Not observed in humans	
Molybdenum	Cofactor for xanthine oxidase	Not observed in humans	
Phosphorus 70% absorbed by jejunum, maintained by renal resorption; normal plasma concentration, 3.0 mg/dL to 4.5 mg/dL	Skeletal synthesis, component of vitamins and essential for coenzyme formation, contributes to structure of teeth and soft tissue	Occurs with prolonged excessive use of alcohol or nonabsorbable antacids, prolonged vomiting, liver disease, hyperparathyroidism	Dibasic calcium phosphate used orally; hyperphosphatemia associated with chronic renal disease, hypoparathyroidism, tetany
Potassium Major cation of intracellular fluid; normal range, 3.5–5.0 mEq/L, 3–4.5 mg/dL	Required for fluid–electrolyte balance, acid–base balance, muscle activity, carbohydrate metabolism, protein synthesis	Produces sore, weak, or painful muscles	Losses occur in GI disorders and diarrhea; used in treatment of diabetic acidosis; required for fluid balance
Selenium 90% absorbed	Acts synergistically with vitamin E to protect cell membranes from oxidative damage	Thigh tenderness, deficiency due to total parenteral nutrition, malnutrition	Incidence of cancer may result from low intake of selenium; marginal deficiency when soil content is low
Sodium Major cation of extracellular fluid; normal range, 136–145 mEq/L, under hormonal control of aldosterone	Required for fluid balance, acid–base balance, cell permeability, normal muscle irritability	Losses occur in GI disorders and diarrhea; weakness, mental confusion, nausea, lethargy, and muscle cramping may result	Fluid balance, blood pressure, membrane permeability, neuromuscular function may be altered by depletion or retention
Sulfur Obtained from protein	Structure of skin and cartilage, component of vitamins, important coenzyme formation		

Source: Williams SR, ed. Nutrition and diet therapy. 8th ed. St. Louis: Mosby, 1997: 223–224; Weigley ES, Mueller DH, Robinson CH, eds. Robinson's basic nutrition and diet therapy. 8th ed. Columbus, OH: Merrill, 1997:208–209.

GI, gastrointestinal; *LDL,* low-density lipoprotein; *HDL,* high-density lipoprotein.

Table 11.6 ▪ New Dietary Reference Intakes

			Fluoride		Phosphorus			
Age and Sex	Calcium	Magnesium	AI	UL	AI	EAR	RDA	UL
0–6 mo			0.1 mg	0.7 mg	100 mg			
6–12 mo			0.5 mg	0.9 mg	275 mg			
1–3 yr			0.7 mg	1.3 mg		380 mg	460 mg	3 g
4–8 yr			1.1 mg	2.2 mg		405 mg	500 mg	3 g
9–13 yr	1300 mg		2.0 mg	10 mg		1055 mg	1250 mg	4 g
Boys 14–18 yr	1300 mg		3.2 mg	10 mg		1055 mg	1250 mg	4 g
Girls 14–18 yr	1300 mg		2.9 mg	10 mg		1055 mg	1250 mg	4 g
Men ≥19 yr	1000 mg >50 yr, 1200 mg	420 mg	3.8 mg	10 mg		580 mg	700 mg	19–70 yr, 4 g >70 yr, 3 g
Women ≥19 yr	1000 mg >50 yr, 1200 g[a]	310 mg	3.1 mg	10 mg				19–70 yr, 4 g >70 yr, 3 g
Pregnant and lactating women 14–18 yr			2.9 mg	10 mg		580 mg	700 mg	
Pregnant and lactating women 19–50 yr			3.1 mg	10 mg		580 mg	700 mg	

AI, adequate intake; *UL,* tolerable upper intake level; *EAR,* estimated average requirement; *RDA,* recommended dietary allowance.

[a]Dietary reference intake for postmenopausal women is 1500 mg; UL for calcium intake is 2.5 g.

Table 11.7 ▪ Mineral Interactions

Mineral	Drug or Agent	Interaction or Effect
Calcium	β-Blockers	Decreased β-blocker absorption
	Calcium channel blockers	Possible reduction in efficacy of calcium channel blocker
	Corticosteroids	Decreased calcium absorption
	Fiber	Decreased calcium absorption
	Iron	Decreased iron absorption
	Oxalic acid (found in rhubarb and spinach)	Decreased calcium absorption
	Phenytoin	Decreased phenytoin absorption
	Phosphorus (found in dairy products)	Decreased calcium absorption
	Phytic acid (found in bran and cereals)	Decreased calcium absoprtion
	Quinidine	Decreased quinidine renal excretion and increased pharmacologic effects
	Salicylates	Increased salicylic acid renal excretion and decreased pharmacologic effects
	Tetracycline	Decreased serum tetracycline levels
	Thiazide diuretics	Increased calcium absorption
	Vitamin D	Increased calcium absorption
Copper	Penicillamine	Copper deficiency
Iodine	Lithium	Additive or synergistic effect in inhibiting thyroid function
Iron	Antacids	Decreased iron absorption
	Ascorbic acid	200 mg ascorbic acid per 30 mg iron increases iron absorption
	Caffeine	Decreased iron absorption
	Dairy products	Decreased iron absorption
	Oxalic acid (found in rhubarb and spinach)	Decreased iron absorption
	Phosphorus (found in dairy products)	Decreased iron absorption
	Phytic acid (found in bran and cereals)	Decreased iron absorption
Magnesium	Alcohol	Decreased magnesium absorption
	Calcium	Decreased magnesium absorption
	Diuretics	Increased magnesium absorption
	Phosphorus	Decreased magnesium absorption
Phosphorus	Antacids (Al or Mg)	Decreased phosphorus absorption
	Calcium	Decreased phosphorus absorption
	Iron	Decreased phosphorus absorption
Zinc	Alcohol	Decreased serum zinc levels
	Bran or dairy products	Decreased zinc absorption
	Copper	An excess of either may cause decreased absorption of the other
	Diuretics	Increased zinc excretion
	Penicillamine	Zinc deficiency
	Phytic acid	Decreased zinc absorption
	Phosphorus	Decreased zinc absorption
	Tetracycline	Decreased tetracycline absorption

Of total body calcium, 99% is found in bone and 1% is present in serum. Of the calcium found in serum, 45% is bound to plasma proteins. The calcium in bone serves as a reservoir to maintain normal plasma calcium levels.[87] The interaction of PTH, vitamin D, and calcitonin is responsible for maintaining a normal calcium level of 2.12 to 2.62 mmol/L (8.5 to 10.5 mg/dL).

Calcium absorption occurs in the small intestine at a steady rate of 30% of intake, increasing to approximately 50% during growth periods, pregnancy, and lactation.

Hypocalcemia usually occurs when the plasma calcium level falls below 8 mg/dL. An exception occurs when plasma protein concentration is low. In this case, calcium is reported as less than normal. Chronic, excessive intake of calcium causes adverse effects that range from minor to life threatening and are clearly dose related. In a healthy person, 1 to 2 g calcium per day is unlikely to cause problems. However, possible adverse effects include nausea, bloating, constipation (which may be prevented by increased fiber and water consumption), and flatulence (especially with oral intake of calcium carbonate).[88] Symptoms of hypercalcemia generally occur with ingestion of more than 4 to 5 g/day.[89] Signs and symptoms of hypercalcemia include nausea, vomiting, anorexia, headache, muscle weakness, depression, apathy, fatigue, hypertension, nervousness, insomnia, and urolithiasis.[90,91]

Calcium supplements are suggested for prevention or control of osteoporosis,[92,93] hypertension,[94,95] and colon cancer,[96] but the only confirmed use is for correction of dietary deficiency. Of commercially available supplements, calcium carbonate (oyster shell) provides the greatest amount of elemental calcium (40%). Taking calcium carbonate with food increases its absorption. Calcium absorption is impaired in patients with achlorhydria (especially geriatric patients). Calcium citrate (21% elemental calcium) has been shown to have better solubility and absorption, particularly in patients with impaired acid secretion. Absorption of calcium decreases with age.[97,98]

Two natural sources of calcium, bone meal and dolomite, should be avoided because of the risk of lead contamination. The risk of contamination is especially great for pregnant or lactating women, infants, children, and possibly older adults.

IRON

Iron is essential in the functioning of all biologic systems. It is essential for oxygen transport as a constituent of hemoglobin and myoglobin and is also found in a number of enzymes such as cytochromes, catalases, and oxidases.

Iron in the body is either functional or stored. Functional iron is found in hemoglobin and myoglobin, whereas stored iron is found in association with transferrin, ferritin, and hemosiderin. The storage sites of ferritin and hemosiderin are the liver, spleen, and bone marrow.

Dietary iron absorption is highly variable, ranging from 2 to 40% depending on the type and source. Heme iron and nonheme iron are the two forms of dietary iron. Heme iron is obtained from animal protein sources and is 15 to 35% absorbed.[99] Meat may facilitate the absorption of heme iron by stimulating production of gastric acid. Nonheme iron constitutes most dietary iron found in grain products, vegetables, and dairy products and has an absorption rate of 2 to 20%. A healthy person absorbs approximately 10% of dietary iron. Iron absorption may increase to 20% if iron stores are low or iron requirements are high, as in menstruation, pregnancy, or growth stages. In the presence of iron deficiency anemia, absorption becomes more efficient to help meet the body's needs.[100] Absorption of nonheme iron is influenced by the levels of iron stores and by concomitantly consumed dietary components. A factor such as availability of ascorbic acid may increase the bioavailability of nonheme iron.

Iron deficiency is a recognized nutritional deficiency in the United States. Iron deficiency usually occurs in high-risk groups that include infants, children, adolescents, women of childbearing age, frequent blood donors, and chronic aspirin users. Iron deficiency in these groups usually is treated or prevented with supplements. (See Chapter 13.)

ZINC

Zinc is important in the growth and maintenance of healthy skin and in the development and continued functioning of the male sex organs. It is also necessary for the synthesis of DNA, RNA,[101] and connective tissue and bone. It is necessary for normal sense of taste, increased oxygen-carrying capacity in normal and sickle RBCs, spermatogenesis, ova formation, and the mobilization and transport of vitamin A from the liver. Zinc also assists in immune function and affects behavior and learning performance.[102–103]

Ten to 40% of dietary zinc is absorbed from the small intestine. The absorption of zinc appears to be associated with nutritional status and may also be influenced by a zinc-binding ligand secreted by the pancreas. Zinc absorption is inhibited by the formation of insoluble complexes with other nutrients such as phytate (found in cereals), calcium, vitamin D, protein, and fiber. Excessive copper or iron intake competes with zinc to interfere with absorption. Zinc salts (acetate and sulfate) appear to have the highest degree of bioavailability.[104] Zinc sulfate can be irritating to the gastrointestinal tract.

Zinc deficiency related to increased urinary excretion may be associated with surgery, diabetes, fever, alcohol consumption, and therapy with corticosteroids, estrogens, and thiazide diuretics. Clinical manifestations of zinc deficiency include loss of taste (hypogeusia) or smell, dermatitis, macular degeneration, and poor wound healing.[104] Acrodermatitis enteropathica is the deficiency syndrome resulting from human genetic deficiency.

Zinc therapy in dosages of 220 mg two or three times daily may be of value in facilitating wound healing and treating hypogeusia in zinc-deficient patients. Zinc gluconate lozenges may reduce the duration of cold symptoms.[105–107]

Reported signs of zinc toxicity in humans include anorexia, nausea, lethargy, dizziness, and diarrhea. Vomiting may occur after ingestion of more than a 2-g dose.

CHROMIUM

Chromium is a trace mineral needed for appropriate glucose use, lipid metabolism, and insulin receptor sensitivity.[108] It has been reported to be beneficial in the treatment of type II diabetes. One study[109] sponsored by the U.S. Department of Agriculture reports that administering 500 µg chromium two times per day resulted in a decrease in 2-hour and fasting glucose and insulin levels and decreased total plasma cholesterol levels. At this same dosage, chromium supplementation for 2 months was found to significantly improve glycosylated hemoglobin (HbA1c) values, an indication of how well glucose is metabolized.[110]

The adequate intake for chromium is 50 to 200 µg. It is found in nature as a component of glucose tolerance factor in whole grain products, mushrooms, liver, brewer's yeast, raw sugar, beets, honey, grapes, raisins, and clams. Considering its wide occurrence, it would be expected that attaining an adequate chromium intake would not be difficult; however, it has been proposed that 90% of American diets are deficient in chromium.[111] Chromium deficiency symptoms include hyperglycemia, glucosuria, peripheral neuropathy, and ataxia, some of the same symptoms associated with diabetes.

Chromium supplementation has been used as an adjunct to obesity treatment because of its ability to increase insulin sensitivity, lower plasma glucose levels, and improve lean body mass. However, some concerns have been raised about the potential for accumulation and toxicity. A model developed by Stearns et al.[111] predicts that chromium (III) may accumulate in human tissues to levels at which DNA damage has been observed in animals and in vitro. However, animal studies support the view that chromium is virtually nontoxic even at dosages 2000 times greater than dosages used in humans.[112] Since chromium supplementation has increased, several cases of toxicity resulting in renal failure have been reported.[113]

SELENIUM

Selenium, an antioxidant, is a component of the enzyme glutathione peroxidase, thought to deactivate lipid peroxidases, which are strong oxidizing agents that cause cell injury. The relationship between dietary selenium intake and cancer incidence is being investigated. Limited epidemiologic evidence suggests that the risk of certain types of cancer and stroke[114] are inversely related to selenium intake. Because of the potential for toxicity, unsupervised use of selenium for cancer prevention should be discouraged. Selenium is being used (although claims remain unfounded) in heart disease, arthritis, heavy metal poisoning, sexual dysfunction, and aging. Selenium toxicity includes loss of hair, brittle fingernails, fatigue, irritability, and garlic odor or breath. Selenium deficiency rarely occurs in humans and supplementation generally is not recommended.

PSYCHOSOCIAL ISSUES

Several psychosocial issues are important, especially as they relate to socioeconomic status, cultural beliefs, and consumer fads.

- Vitamins are not energy sources. They function as coenzymes or enzymes in biochemical processes in which energy is produced during the metabolism of carbohydrates, lipids, and protein.
- Vitamin and mineral supplements can never be considered substitutes for adequate dietary intake.
- There is little or no advantage to using vitamins from natural sources rather than those produced synthetically. The primary difference between natural and synthetic vitamins is their cost.
- Vitamin deficiencies are most common in older adults because of inadequate dietary intake and physiologic changes associated with aging.
- Use of vitamin or mineral supplements does not enhance one's ability to cope with stress unless one is deficient in B complex vitamins.
- No current research shows definitively that vitamin or mineral supplements improve athletic skill, enhance sexual performance, or prevent aging except when a deficiency is present.
- Vitamins are not cure-alls. They are capable only of preventing diseases caused by deficiency.

Conclusion

Vitamins are organic compounds that are essential for the body's biochemical processes. Vitamins, or their precursors, must be obtained through the diet because they generally are not manufactured by the body or under certain circumstances are produced in insufficient amounts. A positive relationship exists between the maintenance of optimal health and an optimal diet. Vitamin supplementation should not be a substitute for a well-balanced diet. For the normal population, the recommended number of daily servings from the five basic food groups (meats, vegetables, fruits, dairy products, and grains) provide the needed recommended dietary allowances. However, certain groups in the general population with high metabolic requirements, malabsorption syndromes, inadequate dietary intake, or stress require additional nutrients.

The fat-soluble vitamins A, D, E, and K are stored in the body for months. Therefore, fat-soluble vitamin toxicity is related to accumulation of vitamins in fatty tissues. The water-soluble vitamins, vitamin B complex and C, have very small reserves maintained in the body, and a daily supply is desired. Water-soluble vitamins usually are nontoxic but can cause adverse effects when they are ingested for prolonged periods in excessive quantities.

Minerals are inorganic substances. Several of these elements, particularly calcium, iron, and zinc, are important catalysts in various enzymatic activities or play a role in hormonal metabolism. The importance of these elements must not be overlooked while investigators attempt to understand the nutritional importance of other minerals.

Consumers often have questions about compounds that are not considered "true" or "real" vitamins. To protect the consumer's health and finances, health care practitioners must be knowledgeable and provide the necessary information about vitaminlike substances.

KEY POINTS

- Daily values are nutrient references that have replaced the RDAs on food product labels.
- Consumers should rely on an adequate dietary intake of food rather than on nutrient supplementation.
- Attention should be focused on vitamin E research and its therapeutic use on reducing the risk of cancer and heart disease and enhancing immune response.
- Niacin remains a successful treatment for the management of hypercholesterolemia as long as ongoing supervision and instructions are provided by a qualified health care provider.

- Minerals are important to good health, but the consumer must be cautioned that with all minerals, the therapeutic index between general requirements and toxic levels is narrow.

REFERENCES

1. Anonymous. Federal Register 44:16139, 1979.
2. American Dietetic Association. Position paper: vitamin and mineral supplementation. J Am Diet Assoc 96:73–77, 1996.
3. Anonymous. Food and Drug Administration Drug Bulletin 13:27, 1983.
4. Kennedy E, Meyers L, Layden W. The 1996 dietary guidelines for Americans: an overview. J Am Diet Assoc 96:234–237, 1996.
5. Standing Committee on the Scientific Evaluation of Dietary Reference Intakes, Food & Nutrition on Board, Institute of Medicine. Dietary reference intakes (DRIs) for calcium, phosphorus, magnesium, vitamin D, and fluoride. Washington, DC: National Academy Press, 1997.
6. Kurtzwell P. The new food label: better information for special diets. FDA Consumer 29:19–25, 1995.
7. Anonymous. Dietary reference intakes. Nutr Rev 55(9):319–326, 1997.
8. Sizer FS, Whitney EN, eds. Hamilton & Whitney's nutrition: concepts and controversies. 6th ed. St Paul: West Publishing, 1994:550–553.
9. Boyle MA, Zyla G. Personal nutrition. 3rd ed. New York: West Publishing, 1996:213–215.
10. Williams SR, ed. Nutrition & diet therapy. 8th ed. St. Louis: Mosby, 1997:160–166.
11. Hathack JN, Hattan DG, Jenkins MY, et al. Evaluation of vitamin A toxicity. Am J Clin Nutr 52:183–202, 1990.
12. Sirling HF, Laing SC, Barr DG. Hypercarotenemia and vitamin A overdosage from proprietary baby food. Lancet 1:1089, 1986.
13. Sommer A, Djunaedi E, Loeden AA, et al. Impact of vitamin A supplementation on childhood mortality. Lancet 1:1169–1173, 1986.
14. Rothman KJ, Moore LL, Singer MR, et al. Teratogenicity of high vitamin A intake. N Engl J Med 333(21):1369–1373, 1995.
15. Lammer EJ, Chen DT, Hoar RM, et al. Retinoic acid embryopathy. N Engl J Med 313:837–841, 1985.
16. Orfanos CE, Zouboulis CC. Current use and future potential role of retinoids in dermatology. Drugs 53(3):358–388, 1997.
17. deKlerk NH, Musk AW, Ambrosini GL, et al. Vitamin A and cancer prevention II: comparison of the effects of retinol and beta-carotene. Int J Cancer 75(3):362–367, 1998.
18. DiGiovanna JJ. Retinoids for the future: oncology. J Am Acad Dermatol 27:S34–S37, 1992.
19. Patterson RE, White E, Kristal AR, et al. Vitamin supplements and cancer risk: the epidemiologic evidence. Cancer Causes Control 8(5):786–802, 1997.
20. Coutsodis A, Bobat RA, Coovadia HM, et al. The effects of vitamin A supplementation on the morbidity of children born to HIV-infected women. Am J Public Health 85(8):1076–1081, 1995.
21. Hennekens CH, Buring JE, Manson JE, et al. Lack of effect of long-term supplementation with beta carotene on the incidence of malignant neoplasms and cardiovascular disease. N Engl J Med 334:1145–1149, 1996.
22. Omenn GS, Goodman GE, Thornquist MD, et al. Effects of a combination of beta carotene and vitamin A on lung cancer and cardiovascular disease. N Engl J Med 334:1150–1155, 1996.
23. Rowe PM. β-Carotene takes a collective beating. Lancet 347:249–252, 1996.
24. Woodall AA, Jack CI, Jackson MJ. Caution with beta-carotene supplements. Lancet 347:967–968, 1996.
25. Rautalahti M, Virtamo J, Haukka J. The effect of alpha-tocopherol and beta-carotene supplementation on COPD symptoms. Am J Respir Crit Care Med 156(5):1447–1452, 1997.
26. Haussler MR, Haussler CA, Jurutka PA. The vitamin D hormone and its nuclear receptor: molecular actions and disease states. J Endocrinol (154S): S57–73, 1997.
27. Cavalier L, Ouahchi K, Kayden HJ, et al. Ataxia with isolated vitamin E: heterogeneity of mutations and phenotypic variability in a large number of families. Am J Hum Genet 62(2):301–310, 1998.
28. Sokol RJ, Butler-Simon N, Conner C, et al. Multicenter trial of *d*-alpha-tocopheryl polyethylene glycol 1000 succinate for treatment of vitamin E in children with chronic cholestasis. Gastroenterology 104 (6):1727–1735, 1993.
29. Bendich A, Machlin LJ. Safety of oral intake of vitamin E. Am J Clin Nutr 48:612–619, 1988.
30. Mino M. Clinical uses and abuses of vitamin E in children. Proc Soc Exp Biol Med 200(2):266–270, 1992.
31. Bendrich A, Machlin LJ. Safety of oral intake of vitamin E. Am J Clin Nutr 48:612–619, 1988.
32. Kim JM, White RH. Effect of vitamin E on the anticoagulant response to warfarin. Am J Cardiol 77:545–546, 1996.
33. Smigel K. Vitamin E reduces prostate cancer rates in Finnish trials: U.S. considers follow-up. J Natl Cancer Inst 90(6):416–417, 1998.
34. Patterson RE, While E, Kristal AR, et al. Vitamin supplements and cancer risk: the epidemiologic evidence. Cancer Causes Control 8:786–802, 1997.
35. Bonn D. Vitamin E may reduce prostate-cancer incidence. Lancet 315(9107): 961, 1998.
36. Heinonen OP, Albanes D, Virtamo J, et al. Prostate cancer and supplementation with alpha-tocopherol and beta carotene: incidence and mortality in a controlled trial. J Natl Cancer Inst 90(6):440–446, 1998.
37. Macready N. Vitamins associated with lower colon-cancer risk. Lancet 350(9089):1452, 1997.
38. Virtamo J, Rapola JM, Ripatti S, et al. Effect of vitamin E and beta carotene on the incidence of primary nonfatal myocardial infarction and fatal coronary heart disease. Arch Intern Med 158(6):668–675, 1998.
39. Stephen NG, Parsons A, Schofield PM, et al. Randomized controlled trial of vitamin E in patients with coronary disease: Cambridge Heart Antioxidant Study (CHAOS). Lancet 347(9004):781–786, 1996.
40. Calzada C, Bruckdorfer KR, Rice-Evans CA. The influence of antioxidant nutrients on platelet function in healthy volunteers. Atherosclerosis 128(1): 97–105, 1997.
41. Losonczy KG, Harris TB, Havlik RJ. Vitamin E and vitamin C supplement use and risk of all-cause and coronary heart disease mortality in older persons: the established populations for epidemiologic studies of the elderly. Am J Clin Nutr 64(2):190–196, 1996.
42. Hodis HN, Mack WJ, LaBree L. Serial coronary angiographic evidence that antioxidant vitamin intake reduces progression of coronary artery atherosclerosis. JAMA 273(23):1949–1954, 1995.
43. Rimm EB, Stampfer MJ. The use of antioxidants in preventive cardiology. Curr Opin Cardiol 12(2):188–194, 1997.
44. Stampfer MJ, Rimm EB. Epidemiologic evidence for vitamin E in prevention of cardiovascular disease. Am J Clin Nutr 62(Suppl 6):1365S–1369S, 1995.
45. Stampfer MJ, Hennekens CH, Manson JE, et al. Vitamin E consumption and the risk of coronary disease in women. N Engl J Med 328(20):1444–1449, 1993.
46. Rimm EB, Stampfer MJ, Ascherio A, et al. Vitamin E consumption and the risk of coronary heart disease in men. N Engl J Med 328(20):1450–1456, 1993.
47. Jialal I, Govett C. The nutritional management of coronary artery disease. Compr Ther 20(9):495–499, 1994.
48. Jialal I, Fuller CJ, Huet BA. The effect of alpha-tocopherol supplementation on LDL oxidation. A dose-response study. Arterioscler Thromb Vasc Biol 15(2):190–198, 1995.
49. Ferraro J. Vitamin E improves immunity in elderly patients. RN 60(9):17–18, 1997.
50. Meydani SN, Beharka AA. Recent developments in vitamin E and immune response. Nutr Review 56(1):S49–S58, 1998.
51. Beharka A, Redican S, Leka L, et al. Vitamin E status and immune function. Methods Enzymol 282:247–263, 1997.
52. Meydani SN, Meydani M, Blumberg JB, et al. Vitamin E supplementation and in vivo immune response in healthy elderly subjects. A randomized controlled trial. JAMA 277(17):1380–1386, 1997.
53. Bell EF. History of vitamin E in infant nutrition. Am J Clin Nutr 46:183–186, 1987.
54. Breen GP, St Peter WL. Hypoprothrombinemia associated with cefmetazole. Ann Pharmacother 31(2):180–184, 1997.
55. Weigley ES, Mueller DH, Robinson CH, eds. Robinson's basic nutrition and diet therapy. 8th ed. Columbus, OH: Merrill, 1997:175.
56. Marcus R, Coulston AM. Fat soluble vitamins. In: Hardman JG, Limbird LE, eds. Goodman & Gilman's the pharmacological basis of therapeutics. 9th ed. New York: McGraw-Hill, 1996:1584.
57. Hoyumpa AM. Mechanisms of thiamine in chronic alcoholism. Am J Clin Nutr 33:2750, 1980.
58. Marcus R, Coulston AM. Water-soluble vitamins. The vitamin B complex ascorbic and ascorbic acid. In: Hardman JG, Limbird LE, Molinoff PB, et al., eds. Goodman & Gilman's the pharmacological basis of therapeutics. 9th ed. New York: McGraw-Hill, 1996:889–891.
59. Anonymous. ASHP therapeutic position statement on the safe use of niacin in the management of dyslipidemias. Am J Health Syst Pharm 54(24):2815–2819, 1997.

60. Knodel LC. Niacin: innocuous vitamin, but potentially toxic drug. Toxic Subst J 13(4):313–316, 1994.
61. Marcus R, Coultston AM. Water-soluble vitamins. The vitamin B complex and ascorbic acid. In: Hardman JG, Limbird LE, eds. Goodman & Gilman's the pharmacological basis of therapeutics. 9th ed. 9. New York: McGraw-Hill, 1996:1561–1563.
62. Schaumburg H, Kaplan J, Windebank A, et al. Sensory neuropathy with low dose pyridoxine abuse. A new megavitamin syndrome. N Engl J Med 310:445–448, 1983.
63. Parry G, Bredesen DE. Sensory neuropathy with low-dose pyridoxine. Neurology 35:1466, 1985.
64. Nader S. Premenstrual syndrome. Tailoring treatment to symptoms. Postgrad Med 90(1):173–180, 1991.
65. Mortola JF. A risk-benefit appraisal of drugs used in the management of premenstrual syndrome. Drug Saf 10(2):160–169, 1994.
66. Levine M, Cantilena CC, Dhariwal KR. In situ kinetics and ascorbic acid requirements. World Rev Nutr Diet 72:114–127, 1993.
67. Kallner AB, Hartmann D, Hornig DH. On the requirements of ascorbic acid in man: steady-state turnover and body pool in smokers. Am J Clin Nutr 34:1347–1355, 1981.
68. Rivers JM. Oral contraceptives and ascorbic acid. Am J Clin Nutr 28:550–554, 1975.
69. Schmidt KH, Hagmaier V, Horning DH, et al. Urinary oxalate excretion after large intakes of ascorbic acid in man. Am J Clin Nutr 34:305–311, 1981.
70. Stein HB, Hasan A, Fox IH. Ascorbic acid-induced uricosuria: a consequence of megavitamin therapy. Ann Intern Med 84:385–388, 1976.
71. Marcus R, Coulston AM. Water-soluble vitamins. In: Hardman JG, Limbird LE, eds. Goodman & Gilman's the pharmacological basis of therapeutics. 9th ed. New York: McGraw-Hill, 1996:1568–1571.
72. Pauling L. Vitamin C and the common cold. San Francisco: WH Freeman, 1970:39–52, 83–88.
73. Baird IM, Hughes RE, Wilson HK, et al. The effects of ascorbic acid and flavonoids on the occurrence of symptoms normally associated with a common cold. Am J Clin Nutr 32:1686–1690, 1979.
74. Schwartz J, Weiss ST. Dietary factors and chronic respiratory symptoms. Am J Epidemiol 132:67–76, 1990.
75. Peters EM, Goetzsche JM, Grobbelaar B, et al. Vitamin C supplementation reduces the incidence of postrace symptoms of upper-respiratory-tract infection in ultramarathon runners. Am J Clin Nutr 57:170–174, 1993.
76. Hemila H. Vitamin C supplementation and the common cold: was Linus Pauling right or wrong. Int J Vitam Nutr Res 67(5):329–335, 1997.
77. Mossad SB. Treatment of the common cold. BMJ 317(7150):33–36, 1998.
78. Gershoff SN. Vitamin C (ascorbic acid): new roles, new requirements? Nutr Rev 51:313–326, 1993.
79. Cataldo CB, DeBruyne LK, Whitney EN, eds. Nutrition and diet therapy. 3rd ed. St Paul: West Publishing, 1992:133.
80. McRae TD, Freedman ML. Why vitamin B_{12} deficiency should be treated aggressively. Geriatrics 44(11):70–79, 1989.
81. Willett WC. Folic acid and neural tube defect: can't we come to a closure? Am J Public Health 82:666–668, 1992.
82. Anonymous. Use of folic acid–containing supplements among women of childbearing ages: United States, 1997. MMWR Morb Mortal Wkly Rep 47(7):131–435, 1998.
83. Anonymous. Food standards: amendment of the standards of identity for enriched grain products to require addition of folic acid (21 CFR 136, 137, and 139). Federal Register 58(197):5305–5312, 1993.
84. Anonymous. Recommendations for the use of folic acid to reduce the number of cases of spina bifida and other neural tube defects. MMWR Morb Mortal Wkly Rep 41(RR-14):1–7, 1992.
85. Anonymous Food labeling health claims and label statements: folate and neural tube defects. Federal Register 58(197):53254–53295, 1993.
86. Milinow MR, Duell PB, Hess DL, et al. Reduction of plasma homocysteine levels by breakfast cereal fortified with folic acid in patients with coronary heart disease. N Engl J Med 338:1009–1015, 1998.
87. Marcus R. Agents affecting calcification: calcium parathyroid hormone, calcitonin, vitamin D, and other compounds. In: Hardman JG, Limbird LE, eds. Goodman & Gilman's the pharmacological basis of therapeutics. 9th ed. New York: McGraw-Hill, 1996:1520–1521.
88. Leverson DI, Bockman RS. A review of calcium preparations. Nutr Rev 52(7):221–232, 1994.
89. Beall DP, Scofield RH. Milk-alkali syndrome associated with calcium carbonate consumption. Report of 7 patients with parathyroid hormone levels and an estimate of prevalence among patients hospitalized with hypercalcemia. Medicine 74(20):89–96, 1995.
90. Bullimore DW, Miloszewski KJ. Raised parathyroid hormone levels in the milk alkali syndrome: an appropriate response? Postgrad Med 63(743):789–792, 1987.
91. French JK, Holdaway, IM Williams LC. Milk alkali syndrome following over-the-counter antacid self-medication. N Z Med J 99(801):322–323, 1986.
92. Kleerekoper M. Detecting osteoporosis. Beyond the history and physical examination. Posgrad Med 103(4):45–47, 51–52, 62–63, 1998.
93. Morii H, Kanis JA. Osteoporosis update 1997. Osteoporos Int 7(Suppl 3):S1–S5, 1997.
94. McCarron DA, Oparil S, Resnik LM, et al. Comprehensive nutrition plan improves cardiovascular risk factors in hypertension. Am J Hypertens 11(1):31–40, 1998.
95. McCarron DA. Importance of dietary calcium in hypertension (letter). J Am Coll Nutr 17(1):97–99, 1998.
96. Lipkin M, Newmark H. Calcium and the prevention of colon cancer. J Cell Biochem Suppl 22:65–73, 1995.
97. Barger-Lux MJ, Heaney RP, Lanspa SJ. An investigation of sources of variation in calcium absorption efficacy. J Clin Endocrinol Metab 80:406–411, 1995.
98. Nicar MJ, Pak CYC. Calcium bioavailability from calcium carbonate and calcium citrate. J Clin Endocrinol Metab 61:391–393, 1985.
99. Monsen ER. Iron nutrition and absorption: dietary factors which impact iron bioavailability. J Am Diet Assoc 88(7):786–790, 1990.
100. Bridges KR, Bunn HF. Anemias. In: Fauci AS, Braunwald E, Isselbacher KJ, et al., eds. Harrison's principles of internal medicine. 14th ed. New York: McGraw-Hill, 1994:639–640.
101. Weigley ES, Mueller DH, Robinson CH, eds. Robinson's basic nutrition and diet therapy. 8th ed. Columbus, OH: Merrill, 1997:202–203.
102. Chandra RK. Nutrition and the immune system: an introduction. Am J Clin Nutr 66(2):460S–463S, 1997.
103. Whitney EN, Cataldo CB, DeBruyne LK, et al., eds. Nutrition for health and health care. St. Paul: West Publishing, 1996:194–196.
104. Prasad AS. Discovery of human zinc and studies in an experimental human model. Am J Clin Nutr 53:403–412, 1991.
105. Garland ML, Hagmeyer KO. The role of zinc lozenges in treatment of common cold. Ann Pharmacother 32:63–69, 1998.
106. Anonymous. Zinc lozenges reduce the duration of cold symptoms. Nutr Rev 55(3):82–85, 1997.
107. Mossad SB, Mackin ML, Medendork SV, et al. Zinc gluconate lozenges for treating the common cold: a randomized, placebo-controlled, double-blind study. Ann Intern Med 125:81–88, 1996.
108. Whitney EN, Cataldo CB, DeBruyne LK, et al., eds. Nutrition for health and health care. St. Paul: West Publishing, 1996:199–200.
109. Anderson RA. Chromium as an essential nutrient for humans. Regul Toxicol Pharmacol 26:S35–S41, 1997.
110. Anderson RA, Cheng N, Bryden NA, et al. Elevated intakes of supplemental chromium improve glucose and insulin variables in individuals with type 2 diabetes. Diabetes 46(11):1786–1791, 1997.
111. Stearns DM, Belbruno JJ, Wetterhahn KE. A prediction of chromium (III) accumulation in humans from chromium dietary supplements. FASEB J 9(15):1650–1657, 1975.
112. Anderson RA, Bryden NA, Polansky MM. Lack of toxicity in chromium chloride and chromium picolinate in rate. J Am Coll Nutr 16(3):273–279, 1997.
113. Larsen Joanne MS, RD. Ask the Dietician. Hopkins Technology, LLC, June 4, 1998.
114. Mark SD, Wang W, Fraumen JF Jr., et al. Do nutritional supplements lower the risk of stroke or hypertension? Epidemiology 9(1):9–15, 1998.

CHAPTER 12

PARENTERAL AND ENTERAL NUTRITION IN ADULT PATIENTS

Rex O. Brown

Specialized nutrition support includes parenteral nutrition (PN) and enteral nutrition (EN). EN has been used for hundreds of years, but PN is a fairly new treatment. In 1968, Dudrick et al.[1] reported that growth and development could be sustained with long-term PN in an infant who could not be fed via the gastrointestinal tract. Most practitioners consider this the beginning of modern clinical nutrition. In the last 35 years, many advances have been made to allow safe and efficacious PN and EN delivery.

Since the original report by Dudrick et al.,[1] the prevalence and complications of malnutrition have become more widely appreciated. A practical way to assess malnutrition in patients is to include weight change, dietary intake, gastrointestinal symptoms, and functional capacity in the history and assess muscle and fat loss during the physical examination.[2] Despite the increased awareness of malnutrition and its negative effects, undernutrition goes undetected in many patients, and many are undertreated.[3]

PN and EN are powerful and expensive medical therapies. Their potential complications have led to the development of nutrition support teams that work to make specialized nutrition support safe and efficacious. Traditionally, the nutrition support team has included a physician, pharmacist, nurse, and dietitian. The physician usually directs the nutrition support team. Surgeons, gastroenterologists, and intensivists most commonly serve as nutrition support team physicians. The pharmacist's role has ranged from providing a properly compounded PN formulation to directing the team. Most commonly, the pharmacist assists in prescribing the nutrient formulation, monitors the patient for metabolic complications, educates other practitioners about compatibilities and drug–nutrient interactions, and assists the health care system in developing a cost-effective formulary of nutrition products. In some health care systems, the pharmacist directs or coordinates the nutrition support team, with complete or nearly complete responsibility for PN and EN prescribing, compounding, and delivery. Nurses have also directed nutrition support teams, but traditionally their role has been limited to intravenous catheter insertion and site care, nasogastric tube placement, and selection of nutrition support products. These products include central line insertion kits, dressing trays, parenteral and enteral pumps, and multilumen catheters. Nurses also monitor patients receiving PN or EN for mechanical, infectious, and metabolic complications. Registered dietitians perform nutritional or metabolic assessments, establish caloric and protein goals, monitor patients receiving PN or EN, and document calorie counts from PN, EN, and oral intake. The roles of the disciplines overlap, depending on staffing and training/experience of each member. Many practitioners serve on the nutrition support team on a part-time basis.

TREATMENT GOALS: PARENTERAL AND ENTERAL NUTRITION IN ADULT PATIENTS

- Improve nutritional status in patients with undernutrition.
- Maintain nutritional status in patients who have adequate nutritional stores and need PN or EN.
- Achieve appropriate fluid, electrolyte, trace element, and vitamin balance in patients needing PN or EN.
- Promote wound healing in patients who have had major gastrointestinal surgery or been subjected to thermal injury.
- Improve the quality of life in patients who need PN or EN.

NUTRITIONAL ASSESSMENT

Nutritional assessment evaluates a patient's nutritional status and can be used to detect and quantitate malnutrition in a variety of diseases. The ideal nutritional assessment includes measurement of body cell mass. Body cell mass includes fat-free tissue such as skeletal muscle, smooth muscle, and solid organs. Unfortunately, it is difficult to measure this body compartment using standard nutritional assessment methods. In one study of seriously ill hospitalized adults, a depressed body mass index (below the 15th percentile) was associated with a significant increase in hospital mortality.[4] Body mass index is calculated by dividing body weight in kilograms by height in meters squared. These data suggest that severe undernutrition in hospitalized patients increases mortality. Interestingly, a slightly depressed body weight in healthy middle-aged women may actually improve mortality.[5] In a 16-year longitudinal study of female registered nurses, all-cause mortality increased substantially as body mass index increased. Women who maintained their weight at least 15% below the U.S. average did not demonstrate an increase in mortality.[5] It is important to note that the former study compared severe undernutrition to slightly depressed nutritional status and normal nutritional status in the acute care setting, and the latter study evaluated different weight groups of healthy women over time.

Nutritional assessment has traditionally been divided into four parts: history and physical examination, anthropometric measurement, biochemical assessment of serum proteins, and evaluation of immune status.

History and Physical Examination

The history and physical examination should be used to screen for patients who require a more thorough assessment. A history of unintentional weight loss, either chronic or acute, usually is a sign of suboptimal nutritional intake or altered metabolism. Chronic disease, gastrointestinal disease, certain social factors, and an abnormal metabolic state may be risk factors for developing malnutrition (Table 12.1). Physical signs suggesting malnutrition include edema, decubitus ulcers, muscle wasting, poor wound healing, and glossitis. Comprehensive history and physical examination can be used to categorize patients with documented unintentional weight loss, chronic disease, or physical signs as described.

Table 12.1 ▪ Risk Factors for Undernutrition That Can Be Detected in a Patient History and Physical Examination

Chronic disease	Social factors
Renal failure	Alcohol abuse
Liver failure	Drug abuse
Chronic obstructive pulmonary disease	Abnormal metabolic state
Congestive heart failure	Cancer
Diabetes	Sepsis
Gastrointestinal disease	Trauma or thermal injury
Peptic ulcer disease	
Inflammatory bowel disease	
Pancreatitis	
Short bowel syndrome	

The alternative to a complete nutritional assessment is to use clinical judgment during the patient history and physical. Detsky et al.[2] suggest asking a short series of questions that include information about weight loss over the previous 6 months, recent dietary intake in relation to usual patterns, presence of significant gastrointestinal symptoms, and functional capacity. This technique, called subjective global assessment, is easier and less expensive than a comprehensive nutritional assessment.

Anthropometric Measurements

Anthropometric measurements are used to assess fat and somatic protein stores. Somatic protein stores include skeletal muscle and visceral organs. Subcutaneous fat often is assessed by a series of measurements with a skinfold caliper. The most popular sites for skinfold measurement are the triceps, subscapular, and calf areas. The sum of the triceps and calf skin folds (in millimeters) can be used to determine percentage body fat:

$$\text{Males (\% body fat)} = 0.735\ (\text{triceps SF} + \text{calf SF}) + 1$$

$$\text{Females (\% body fat)} = 0.610\ (\text{triceps SF} + \text{calf SF}) + 5.1$$

This method is attractive because it is noninvasive and inexpensive. The assessment of skinfold measurements can be erroneous if a patient has edema, the equipment is not standardized, or multiple observers are used. Also, some patients may have very little subcutaneous fat and be in excellent physical condition (e.g., athletes such as runners or body builders).

The somatic protein compartment may be assessed indirectly by using the body mass index. Arm muscle area and midarm muscle circumference have been used in the past to assess somatic protein but are rarely used now.

Biochemical Assessment of Serum Proteins

Serum concentrations of several constitutive proteins have been used initially and serially during specialized nutrition support intervention. Unfortunately, factors such as metabolic stress, hydration status, and hepatic function influence these serum concentration measurements. Although these serum markers lack sensitivity and specificity, some of them are very good prognostic indicators of patient outcome and therefore continue to be the subject of intense study. Albumin, transferrin, and prealbumin are the constitutive proteins used most often. Other serum proteins are being studied, but their role in nutritional assessment has not been determined.

Albumin is a protein with a half-life of 21 days and a large body pool compared with those of other secretory proteins. The normal serum concentration of albumin is 35 to 50 g/L (3.5 to 5.0 g/dL) in adults. A decrease in the serum concentration of albumin suggests inadequate protein intake, especially when the serum concentration is chronically depressed. Bed rest, overhydration, and transcapillary escape secondary to metabolic stress such as sepsis can depress the serum concentration of albumin. Regardless of the cause, a depressed serum albumin concentration is associated with higher hospital morbidity and mortality. Because factors other than nutrition can lower the serum concentration of albumin, the use of it as a nutritional marker must be interpreted cautiously. However, its use as a prognostic indicator cannot be ignored.

Transferrin is a secretory protein with a half-life of 8 days that acts as a carrier for iron. It has a much smaller body pool than albumin, and its normal serum concentration is 2 to 3.5 g/L (200 to 350 mg/dL). Because transferrin has a smaller body pool and shorter half-life than albumin, it is much more sensitive to protein calorie deprivation or nutritional repletion. Therefore, it is used often in serial monitoring of patients receiving specialized nutrition support. Serum transferrin concentrations are attractive because they respond to nutritional repletion quickly (e.g., with weekly monitoring), are easy to measure, and are becoming available in many institutions. Iron deficiency anemia increases the transferrin serum concentration, whereas injury and sepsis depress it.

Prealbumin, also called thyroxine-binding prealbumin and transthyretin, has a normal serum concentration of 0.15 to 0.4 g/L (15 to 40 mg/dL). It is the major carrier protein for thyroxine and retinol-binding protein and has a half-life of 2 days. Because of the short half-life and small body pool, prealbumin is sensitive to nutritional deprivation and repletion. Many health care systems have added this laboratory test because it is inexpensive and easy to perform. The serum concentration of prealbumin rises during nutrition support, even when the nitrogen balance remains negative. The correlation between improvement in nitrogen balance and increase in serum prealbumin concentration is highly significant. Acutely stressful events such as trauma or sepsis are known to depress serum prealbumin concentration, and chronic renal failure elevates it.

Retinol-binding protein, fibronectin, and insulinlike growth factor I have all been studied for their role in documenting nutritional repletion. Retinol-binding protein serum concentration is influenced by vitamin A status and the glomerular filtration rate. Its short half-life of 12 hours may make it too sensitive to nutritional deprivation or intake. Fibronectin is a glycoprotein nonspecific opsonin. It has a half-life of about 24 hours and is synthesized by the liver. Although fibronectin appears to respond positively during nutrition support, many other factors can alter its serum concentration (e.g., sepsis, trauma, shock). Insulinlike growth factor I is a growth hormone–dependent protein with broad anabolic activity. The concentration correlates very well with nitrogen balance and increases during nutritional repletion.[7]

Evaluation of Immune Status

The relationship between malnutrition, depressed immune status, and infection has been appreciated for years. Immune stores (total lymphocyte count, TLC) and immune function (cell-mediated immunity) sometimes are assessed in patients who need specialized nutrition. Immune stores usually are assessed by determination of the TLC, which includes predominantly thymus-derived lymphocytes (T cells). The TLC is calculated from the product of peripheral white blood cell (WBC) count and the percentage of lymphocytes.

$$\text{TLC (in cells/L or cells/mm}^3\text{)} = \text{WBC (in cells/L or cells/mm}^3\text{)} \times \text{\% lymphocytes/100}$$

A TLC greater than 2×10^9/L (2000/mm^3) suggests adequate immune stores in adult patients.

Immune function can be assessed by measuring the response to common antigens through skin testing. Antigens that have been used in this procedure include *Candida albicans*, mumps, streptokinase and streptodornase, tetanus, and *Trichophyton*. Most patients who have intact immune function respond to both *Candida* and mumps skin tests; therefore, these are most commonly used. A positive test result is skin induration of an area 5 mm or larger at the site of application within 24 to 48 hours. Older adults may react slowly and not demonstrate a positive response until 72 hours after application. Many other factors, such as drug therapy (e.g., steroids, histamine antagonists, anesthetic agents) and certain disease states (e.g., cancer), can interfere with the body's cell-mediated immunity, which severely limits the usefulness of these tests in the clinical setting.

Bioelectrical Impedance

A promising method for assessment of lean body mass or body cell mass is bioelectric impedance analysis (BIA).[8] This noninvasive technique is based on the premise that lean tissue is an excellent electrical conductor because of its high water and electrolyte composition. When a high-frequency alternating current is passed through the human body, electrical impedance can be measured with electrodes positioned on the wrist and ankle of a subject. Impedance measurements are translated into electric reactance and resistance values that can be used to derive body composition parameters including lean body mass, body cell mass, body fat, and total body water. Although further validation of this technique is needed before widespread use can be recommended, BIA is a safe, inexpensive, and reproducible method for evaluating body composition, especially in the outpatient setting.

Types of Malnutrition

Marasmus is a form of undernutrition that results from chronic protein and calorie deprivation. Patients with this disorder are easy to identify because they have considerable wasting of somatic protein and fat. Their serum protein concentrations and immune status often are normal. This disorder is seen in patients who suffer from chronic disease and ingest a suboptimal amount of nutrition over a long period of time. Table 12.2 compares the various types of malnutrition.

Kwashiorkor is classified as protein deficiency. Patients with kwashiorkor typically have adequate or excess caloric stores, as evidenced by sufficient body fat (Table 12.2). Patients with kwashiorkor have depressed serum concentrations of constitutive proteins and often have depressed immune function. The most common cause of this disorder is severe metabolic stress (e.g., trauma, sepsis, thermal injury). Kwashiorkor often is difficult to diagnose at the bedside because these patients appear to be well-nourished or overnourished.

Combined kwashiorkor and marasmus results when a patient with marasmus is subjected to metabolic stress. These patients have deficits in all categories of the nutritional assessment and have the highest risk for hospital morbidity and mortality (Table 12.2).

Patients with excess body weight secondary to fat are classified as obese if they are more than 20% above their ideal body weight. Obesity is a type of malnutrition that usually results from prolonged caloric intake beyond what is needed or used. If subjected to metabolic stress, these patients can quickly develop kwashiorkor.

Because no single nutritional assessment marker effectively identifies all patients at nutritional risk and because many nonnutritional factors affect the currently used tests, investigators continue to evaluate new nutritional assessment methods. Some of the methods currently under investigation include underwater weighing, muscle strength testing, magnetic resonance imaging, neutron activation analysis, and radioisotope analysis. Some of these methods are too expensive or invasive for general clinical use; however, BIA shows particular promise.

TOTAL CALORIE AND PROTEIN REQUIREMENTS

After completion of the nutritional assessment in a patient who is going to receive specialized nutrition support, the total calorie and protein goals must be determined. There is controversy among nutritional support practitioners on whether nonprotein calories and protein should be separated when determining calorie goals.[9] Most of the original research in this area in the 1970s emphasized nonprotein calories in determining nutrition requirements, especially with PN. More recently, practitioners have been dosing nutritional support using total calories, which includes the protein component. All EN products are marketed in total calories (i.e., 1 kcal/mL), so total calorie dosing is the only practical method using this nutrition intervention. By using total calories with PN, the practitioner would be using a similar method of dosing for both PN and EN. The nutritional goals are different for each patient, based on the nutritional assessment results, the reason for initiating nutrition support, and the patient's size.

Total Calories

The patient's total caloric requirement may be predicted by several different methods. The degree of metabolic stress and chronic disease also help determine energy requirements. The most widely used method is the calculation of the basal energy expenditure (BEE) using the Harris–Benedict equations developed in 1919.[10] The BEE was developed by measuring oxygen consumption using direct calorimetry in 239 healthy male and female subjects. The two equations use the patient's sex, weight, height, and age.

$$\text{Males: BEE (kcal/day)} = 66.4730 + 13.7516\ \text{Weight (kg)} + 5.0033\ \text{Height (cm)} - 6.7550\ \text{Age (yr)}$$

$$\text{Females: BEE (kcal/day)} = 655.0950 + 9.5630\ \text{Weight (kg)} + 1.8496\ \text{Height (cm)} - 4.6756\ \text{Age (yr)}$$

BEE reflects the number of kilocalories expended during a 24-hour period in a fasting subject at bedrest in a dimly lit room.

Table 12.2 ▪ Types of Malnutrition

Characteristic	Marasmus	Kwashiorkor	Combined Kwashiorkor and Marasmus	Obesity
Weight for height	↓	Normal or ↑	↓	↑
Fat stores	↓	↑	↓	↑
Somatic protein stores	↓	Normal or ↑	↓	↑
Immune function	Normal	↓	↓	Normal
Serum protein concentrations	Normal	↓	↓	Normal

Several nomograms and stress factor calculations can be used to estimate the resting energy expenditure (REE) of a patient with certain clinical conditions (e.g., injury). Unfortunately, when patients have multiple conditions, the estimates far exceed the actual REE in most patients. Therefore, use of these nomograms and stress factors should be abandoned. As more knowledge of the effects of disease states on caloric needs has been appreciated, there has been a gradual reduction in total calorie estimates to sustain health.[11] A total calorie dosage 10 to 20% above the BEE should be adequate for most patients. Patients with severe trauma, major burns, or sepsis may require up to 50% more calories than the calculated BEE.

Some investigators have even challenged the use of the BEE equations because other calculated equations such as the World Health Organization (WHO) equations have proved superior across many patient populations.[12] These equations were based on measurements from approximately 11,000 people.

$$\text{Men (18–30 yr): EE} = 64.4 \times \text{Weight (kg)} - 113 \times \text{Height (m)} + 3000$$

$$\text{Men (30–60 yr): EE} = 19.2 \times \text{Weight (kg)} + 66.9 \times \text{Height (m)} + 3769$$

$$\text{Women (18–30 yr): EE} = 55.6 \times \text{Weight (kg)} + 1397.4 \times \text{Height (m)} + 146$$

$$\text{Women (30–60 yr): EE} = 36.4 \times \text{Weight (kg)} - 104.6 \times \text{Height (m)} + 3619$$

Energy expenditure (EE) in these equations is calculated in kilojoules per day. By dividing kilojoules by 4.1, one can calculate kilocalories per day.

In certain circumstances, the information required to calculate caloric needs using the BEE or WHO equations may not be available, so an alternative method is used to determine the total calorie requirements. If the patient's weight is known, an estimated total calorie goal may be calculated. A range of 25 to 35 kcal/kg/day is generally accepted for most patients. A total caloric goal of 25 kcal/kg/day would be used for an elective surgical patient who is otherwise healthy, whereas a patient with sepsis or trauma would require at least 35 kcal/kg/day. A severely burned patient may require as much as 40 kcal/kg/day initially.

Patients who are older or have an abnormal body size create a particular problem when dosing total calories by body weight. For example, infusing calories to an obese patient at 35 kcal/kg/day will result in overfeeding and potential exacerbation of the obesity. Most practitioners would use an adjusted weight (e.g., ideal body weight + 0.25 [actual body weight − ideal body weight]) for total calorie and protein dosing. Undernourished patients should always be dosed on actual body weight, never ideal body weight. Dosing of energy in children and neonates is discussed in Chapter 97. Because of gradual loss of body cell mass over time, older adults require a lower dosage of energy based on body weight (e.g., 25 kcal/kg/day). It may be most prudent to determine energy dosages in older adults using the BEE formulas because age is a factor in the equations.

Table 12.3 ▪ Protein Requirements for Adults

Condition	Protein Dosage (g/kg/day)
Maintenance	1.0
Mild stress	1.2
Moderate stress or repletion	1.5
Severe stress	2.0

When available, indirect calorimetry is an ideal way to measure a patient's REE. This involves using a metabolic cart and measuring the concentration of oxygen consumed (VO_2) and carbon dioxide produced (VCO_2) over time.[13] After measuring VO_2 and VCO_2, the complete Weir formula can be used to calculate the patient's REE.[14]

$$\text{REE} = (3.941\ VO_2 + 1.106\ VCO_2)1.44 - 2.14\ \text{UUN}$$

REE is in kilocalories per day, VO_2 is in milliliters per minute, VCO_2 is in milliliters per minute, and UUN is urinary urea nitrogen in grams per 24 hours. If a 24-hour urine sample is obtained the same day indirect calorimetry is performed, the nitrogen data are used in the calculation. The difference in the REE obtained from the complete Weir formula and the abbreviated Weir equation (without the UUN term) is less than 2%.[14] Thus, a 24-hour urine specimen is not required for each REE determination by indirect calorimetry. Many practitioners add 10 to 30% to the measured REE to allow for movement and patient interventions during the day.

Protein

Protein requirements depend on many factors. In health, the Recommended Dietary Allowance (RDA) for protein for an adult person is 0.8 g/kg/day. In hospitals, patients generally are stressed and thus may require higher dosages of protein. Depending on the patient's clinical status, the protein requirement may range from 0.6 to 2.2 g/kg/day. As metabolic stress increases, the protein required to maintain adequate protein stores increases. An elective operative procedure such as cholecystectomy results in mild stress and a modest increase in protein requirements (Table 12.3). Patients with infections have a moderate degree of stress, and those with traumatic injury or sepsis may be severely stressed.[15] Severe thermal injury may require protein dosages greater than 2 g/kg/day in selected situations.

Each patient should be monitored closely to determine whether the desired response is achieved (e.g., nutritional repletion, wound healing). During periods of metabolic stress, protein turnover is markedly increased, and urinary excretion of urea nitrogen is elevated, which can lead to rapid erosion of the body cell mass if adequate protein is not administered. The gold standard to measure protein nutriture is nitrogen balance, with the obvious goal of achieving nitrogen equilibrium or a positive balance. This measurement is obtained by subtracting nitrogen output from nitrogen input during a 24-hour period (Table 12.4). Nitrogen input is calculated by dividing protein intake for 24 hours by 6.25 (protein is approximately 16% nitrogen). Nitrogen output is calculated by adding 4 g to the grams of urea nitrogen excreted in the urine during a 24-hour period. The 4 g represents nonmeasurable nitrogen losses such as stool, skin, and nonurea nitrogen losses in the urine. A nitrogen balance of 2 to 6 g/day suggests adequate intake of total calories and protein. A nitrogen balance between –2 and 2 g/day suggests that nitrogen equilibrium has been attained. A nitrogen balance below –2 g/day suggests that more protein or more total calories are needed.

PARENTERAL NUTRITION

PN should be reserved for patients who need specialized nutrition support and do not have a functional or accessible gastrointestinal tract. With the multitude of available PN products, the practitioner needs sound guidelines to provide this therapy in a safe and efficacious way. Practice guidelines and standards developed by the American Society for Parenteral and Enteral Nutrition[16,17] are summarized in Table 12.5. This group has also prepared guidelines for the use of PN and EN in adults with cancer, acquired immune deficiency syndrome, liver failure, renal failure, pancreatitis, respiratory failure, inflammatory bowel disease, short-bowel syndrome, intestinal pseudo-obstruction, critical illness, pregnancy, neurologic impairment, and old age.[18]

Table 12.4 ▪ Nitrogen Balance Calculation

$\text{Nitrogen balance} = N_{in} - N_{out}$

$N_{in} = \text{Protein intake (g)}/6.25$

$N_{out} = [\text{UUN (g/L)} \times \text{24-hr urine volume (L)}] + 4\text{ g}$

Table 12.5 ▪ Parenteral Nutrition Practice Guidelines

Patients who cannot receive enteral nutrition who already are or can become undernourished are candidates for parenteral nutrition.

Peripheral parenteral nutrition may be used in selected patients for up to 2 weeks, especially when central vein parenteral nutrition is not feasible.

Use central vein parenteral nutrition when parenteral nutrition will be needed for more than 2 weeks, peripheral venous access is compromised, nutritional requirements are large, or fluid restriction is necessary.

Patients should be monitored by health care professionals trained to detect the infectious, mechanical, metabolic, and nutritional complications of intravenous feeding. Treat abnormalities promptly.

The indications for home parenteral nutrition are the same as for hospital parenteral nutrition.

Patients receiving home parenteral nutrition should be reevaluated periodically for the potential benefits of this therapy.

Source: Guidelines for use of parenteral and enteral nutrition in adult and pediatric patients. JPEN J Parenter Enteral Nutr 17:9SA–11SA, 1993.

Types of Parenteral Nutrition

PN may be given via a central or peripheral vein. Although central PN is more commonly used, peripheral PN is used by some institutions in certain patients.[19]

Peripheral PN can be used as a sole source of nutrition or as an adjunct to an oral or enteral diet. Generally, 900 mOsm/L is the maximum osmolality tolerated by peripheral veins. A solution of 600 mOsm/L is better tolerated and may lower the risk of phlebitis. The electrolytes added to PN formulations contribute substantially to the osmolality of the PN solution (e.g., NaCl 50 mEq/L contributes 100 mOsm to each liter of solution). Subtherapeutic dosages of heparin or hydrocortisone or concurrent infusion of fat emulsion with peripheral PN have been used to decrease the risk of phlebitis. Peripheral PN is intended to be used for short periods of time (e.g., 5 to 7 days) as adjunctive therapy. A formulation with a final protein concentration of 3 to 5% and a dextrose concentration of 5 to 10% is commonly used for this type of therapy. It is extremely difficult to meet a patient's nutritional requirements because of the large volumes of fluid required. Also, peripheral PN has not demonstrated a significant benefit over the infusion of crystalloid, which makes this therapy questionable.[20]

Most patients receive PN via a central vein. The superior vena cava is used most often after percutaneous catheterization of the subclavian, internal, or external jugular vein. The catheter may be placed in the operating room or at the patient's bedside using sterile technique and radiographic verification. A double- or triple-lumen catheter is used most often because patients who require PN often receive other intravenous medications or blood products. This provides access for the additional intravenous infusions without interrupting the administration of PN. When the catheter tip is placed into the superior vena cava, concentrated substrates may be infused because of the high rate of blood flow in this vein. Thus, required nutrients may be delivered in small volumes without causing thrombophlebitis. This method is particularly effective in patients who have large energy and protein requirements or who need fluid restriction. If the catheter is properly cared for, it can be used indefinitely.

Parenteral Nutrition Formula Components

Protein

The initial protein products used in PN formulations were hydrolysates of naturally occurring proteins (fibrin, casein). Today, commercially available forms of parenteral protein are provided as crystalline amino acids. If protein

Table 12.6 ▪ Parenteral Amino Acid Categories and Product Examples

Patient Category	Product Examples
Standard	Aminosyn II, FreAmine III, Travasol
Fluid-restricted	Novamine 15%, Aminosyn-II 15%, Clinasol 15%
Liver failure	HepatAmine, Hepatasol
Renal failure	Aminosyn RF, NephrAmine, RenAmin, Aminess
Metabolic stress	FreAmine HBC, Branchamin, Aminosyn-HBC

is oxidized for energy, it yields 4 kcal/g. Patients undergoing severe metabolic stress may need large dosages of protein and use it as a preferential calorie source.

Currently marketed amino acid products in the United States are provided as standard or modified amino acids. Standard amino acid products are used for patients with normal organ function and normal nutritional needs. Modified amino acid formulations are marketed for patients with hepatic failure, renal failure, fluid restriction, or metabolic stress. Currently available amino acid products for PN are listed in Table 12.6.

The standard amino acid formulas are composed of physiologic mixtures of essential and nonessential amino acids. Although these products are commercially available in several concentrations, many institutions are now stocking only the 10% or 15% concentrations because lower concentrations can be made easily by adding sterile water via an automated compounder. These products are marketed with or without maintenance electrolytes.

Patients with severe liver failure develop many metabolic abnormalities, including disturbances in electrolyte and amino acid homeostasis. Some of these patients develop hepatic encephalopathy associated with decreased concentrations of branched-chain amino acids (BCAA) and elevated concentrations of aromatic amino acids (AAA) and methionine. The BCAAs include leucine, isoleucine, and valine, and the AAAs are phenylalanine, tyrosine, and tryptophan. In the absence of encephalopathy, patients with liver failure who require PN may be maintained on standard amino acids. However, when hepatic encephalopathy is severe, the modified amino acid formula for hepatic failure may be used. Generally, patients should meet one of the following criteria to receive the modified amino acid: hepatic encephalopathy grade 2 or higher or hepatic encephalopathy associated with PN formulations containing standard amino acid solutions in dosages needed for nutritional support. The modified amino acid formula contains high concentration of BCAAs and low concentrations of AAAs and methionine. Although normalization of the amino acid profile has been shown with this product, an improvement in overall patient outcome has not been demonstrated uniformly in clinical trials. One randomized clinical trial[21] found a decrease in hepatic encephalopathy scores and a lower prevalence of mortality in patients receiving this formulation, but another study[22] failed to show any difference in encephalopathy scores and mortality with this product.

Patients with severe renal failure also have several metabolic changes, including electrolyte alterations and protein intolerance. In patients who are not being dialyzed, daily protein dosage should be restricted to 0.6 to 0.8 g/kg/day. Patients with acute renal failure who are undergoing hemodialysis may be given 1.0 to 1.2 g protein/kg/day, and patients undergoing peritoneal dialysis may receive 1.2 to 1.5 g protein/kg/day. Patients receiving continuous arterial venous hemodialysis may receive protein dosages of 1.2 to 2 g/kg/day if clinically indicated. Modified amino acids for renal failure, which contain primarily essential amino acids, are more expensive than standard amino acids and have not demonstrated clinical benefit over standard amino acids.[23,24] Thus, patients with severe renal failure should be given standard amino acids as part of PN.

Some critically ill patients who need PN are markedly fluid overloaded. In these patients, it is usually beneficial to use the smallest possible volume to deliver PN. Commercially available 15% amino acid products can be used to concentrate the PN formula in patients with overhydration or edema. A theoretical disadvantage to using a 15% amino acid solution for PN is that they contain a lower percentage of BCAAs secondary to solubility problems. This may not be a clinically important difference in adults but would be a critical issue in infants and children requiring PN.

Patients who are highly stressed have altered energy and protein metabolism. These patients take up BCAAs into skeletal muscle for energy. This has led to development of modified amino acid products with enhanced concentrations of BCAAs. These products have been proposed to stimulate protein synthesis, decrease protein catabolism, and act as a preferential fuel source. The many clinical trials using amino acids with an enhanced BCAA content have produced equivocal results. Some suggest that patients receiving these modified amino acids have lower skeletal muscle catabolism and enhanced protein synthesis.[25] In contrast,other studies have found a lack of clinical benefit when BCAA-enriched solutions were compared with standard amino acids.[26] Given the expense of the products and the equivocal results of clinical trials, careful evaluation is needed before these products are used.

Carbohydrates

The nonprotein energy source in PN solutions may be carbohydrate only or a combination of carbohydrate and fat. The carbohydrate component of the nutrient solutions usually is dextrose. Other carbohydrates such as xylitol, fructose, and sorbitol have been studied but have not gained wide acceptance in the United States. Each gram of hydrated dextrose provides 3.4 kcal. Dextrose stock solutions of 5 to 70% are available for use in PN solutions. Many institutions purchase only the 70% dextrose solution because dilutions can be made using an automated compounder and sterile water.

Generally, dextrose infusion should not exceed 5 mg/kg/minute (25 kcal/kg/day) during PN.[27] This appears to be the maximum rate of glucose oxidation by the human body. Rates higher than 5 mg/kg/minute can be associated with lipogenesis, increased carbon dioxide production, and hepatic steatosis. Many clinicians use dextrose dosages of 3 to 4 mg/kg/minute (15 to 20 kcal/kg/day) in PN formulations, especially in glucose-intolerant patients.

An advisory group of nutrition support pharmacists has prepared an excellent report on safe practices for prescribing, labeling, and compounding PN formulations.[28] Information about PN stability, compatibility, and filtration is also included in this report. Dosage ranges for dextrose and total calories in adults, children, and neonates receiving PN are included in this report.[28] Overfeeding patients with dextrose via PN continues to be a problem in acute care institutions, especially academic medical centers where there are many inexperienced prescribers.[29] In one study, hyperglycemia was noted in 49% of patients given more than 5 mg/kg/minute dextrose, compared to 11% and 0% in patients given 4 5 mg/kg/minute and less than 4 mg/kg/minute, respectively.[30]

Fat

The first intravenous fat emulsion product introduced in the United States contained cottonseed oil, but it was removed from the U.S. market in 1965 because of severe adverse reactions. Today, commercially available fat emulsions contain soybean oil or combinations of soybean and safflower oils. Fat emulsions should be given as part of a patient's PN regimen to prevent essential fatty acid deficiency or provide calories. Essential fatty acid deficiency has both biochemical and clinical signs. Biochemical evidence usually becomes apparent within 1 to 3 weeks after fat-free PN is started. Biochemical evidence includes high serum concentrations of saturated fatty acids, low concentrations of essential fatty acids, and a triene:tetraene ratio greater than 0.4. Clinical evidence of essential fatty acid deficiency usually does not appear until several weeks of fat-free PN has been given. Manifestations of essential fatty acid deficiency include thrombocytopenia, delayed wound healing, fatty liver, alopecia, and dry, thick, desquamating skin.

Intravenous fat emulsions provide a concentrated source of calories (9 kcal/g fat) and can correct or prevent essential fatty acid deficiency. Absolute contraindications to the administration of fat emulsions include pathologic hyperlipidemia, lipoid nephrosis, severe egg allergy, and acute pancreatitis associated with hyperlipidemia. Patients with acute pancreatitis who do not have hyperlipidemia may receive intravenous fat emulsions. Fat emulsions should be used cautiously in patients with severe liver disease, acute respiratory distress syndrome, or blood coagulation disorders. Most clinicians recommend administering no more than 30% of the total calories as fat, with the remainder being given as carbohydrate and protein. The usual adult daily dosage of fat is 0.5 to 1 g/kg/day, with a maximum dosage of 2.5 g/kg/day; however, the maximum dosage is rarely used in clinical practice. Table 12.7 lists commercially available fat emulsions, which are composed of either soybean or soybean and safflower oil mixtures and are generally called long-chain triglycerides. Fat emulsion products are marketed in concentrations of 10% (1.1 kcal/mL), 20% (2.0 kcal/mL), and 30% (3.0 kcal/mL). The 30% product is not approved for direct infusion into patients in the United States, but only for preparation of total nutrient admixtures (TNAs). The 10% and 20% products can be infused at a maximum rate of 125 mL/hr and 60 mL/hr respectively; however, they are rarely given that fast. Currently, most clinicians infuse the daily dosage of fat over a 24-hour period as a continuous infusion or as a component of a TNA. The lipid emulsions contain varying amounts of the essential fatty acids, egg yolk phospholipid as an emulsifying agent, and glycerin, which makes the products isotonic.

Table 12.7 ▪ Intravenous Fat Emulsion Products

Product	Lipid Source	Linoleic Acid (%)	Linolenic Acid (%)
Intralipid	100% soybean	50	9
Liposyn II	50% soybean/50% safflower	65.8	4.2
Liposyn III	100% soybean	54.5	8.3

If administered in the recommended dosages, intravenous fat emulsions are very safe. Most side effects are caused by excessive dosages of fat emulsions or excessive rates of infusion. Adverse reactions include nausea and vomiting, headache, fever, chills, chest or back pain, and irritation at the infusion site. Reactions that may be associated with long-term use include hepatomegaly, jaundice, splenomegaly, and thrombocytopenia.

The ability of intravenous fat emulsions to modify immune function is controversial. Because of the complexity associated with induction and control of the immune system, fat emulsions may alter different components of the immune response. Some studies suggest that intravenous fat emulsions impair the bactericidal and migratory functions of polymorphonuclear cells and decrease bacterial clearance by the mononuclear phagocyte system. Biochemical mediators derived from the Ω-6 family of fatty acids may induce inflammation and immunosuppression, whereas metabolic end products from the Ω-3 fatty acids may produce opposite effects. One clinical study in trauma patients suggests greater morbidity, mechanical ventilation, and hospital stay in patients receiving intravenous fat emulsion as part of PN than in a similar group receiving PN without fat.[31] It is not clear whether the fat in the control group or the higher calorie content was responsible for the difference in clinical outcome. This type of study must be confirmed.

Other types of fats can also have unique and potent effects on the immune system. Medium-chain triglycerides may have fewer immunosuppressive properties, be more rapidly available, and provide more energy than traditional intravenous fat emulsions.[32] Currently, fat emulsion products are being developed that contain different fatty acid profiles, designed for better use of fat. Fat emulsions containing medium-chain triglycerides, Ω-3 fatty acids, short-chain triglycerides, or carnitine may become available after clinical trials are completed. These new products probably will be marketed as a physical mixture of the different triglycerides (e.g., long-chain triglyceride, 25%, and medium-chain triglyceride, 75%) or as a structured triglyceride. A structured triglyceride has different fatty acids attached to the glycerol backbone in distinct proportions (e.g., two medium-chain fatty acids and one long-chain fatty acid on each glycerol).

Electrolytes

Electrolytes in maintenance or therapeutic dosages must be added to the PN each day to maintain electrolyte homeostasis (Table 12.8). Requirements for individual electrolytes vary, depending on many factors in a patient's clinical course.[28] Electrolyte imbalance may result from insufficient intake or extraordinary losses. Patients may have large renal or extrarenal losses of electrolytes and fluid. Extrarenal electrolyte losses may include losses from diarrhea, vomiting, fistulas, or nasogastric suctioning. In addition, various pharmacotherapeutic interventions may decrease or increase individual electrolyte requirements. For example, sodium ticarcillin administration delivers a substantial amount of sodium to the patient and causes renal potassium wasting. Amphotericin B therapy increases magnesium and potassium renal losses. Relative electrolyte deficiencies may develop as a result of intracellular shifts of electrolytes from the extracellular fluid compartments. For instance, intracellular shifts of potassium occur during metabolic alkalosis because intracellular hydrogen ions are exchanged for extracellular potassium ions. Also, refeeding chronically starved patients results in an intracellular shift of potassium, phosphorus, and magnesium.[33]

Electrolytes are available as single- or multiple-entity products. Once the phosphorus dosage has been determined and added, the remaining cations are given as chloride or acetate salts. Patients with metabolic acidosis should have the majority of electrolytes added as acetate salts, whereas patients with metabolic alkalosis should have most salts added as chloride.

Table 12.8 ▪ Adult Electrolyte Concentrations Used in Parenteral Nutrition Solutions for Patients with Normal Electrolyte Concentrations and Normal Organ Function

Sodium chloride	30 mEq/L
Sodium phosphate	15 mmol/L
Potassium acetate	40 mEq/L
Calcium gluconate	5 mEq/L
Magnesium sulfate	12 mEq/L

Table 12.9 ▪ Recommended Adult Intravenous Dosages of Vitamins

Vitamin	Daily Intravenous Dosage
Fat-soluble vitamins	
A	3300 IU[a]
D	200 IU
E	10 IU
Water-soluble vitamins	
B_1 (thiamine)	3 mg
B_2 (riboflavin)	3.6 mg
B_3 (pantothenic acid)	15 mg
B_5 (niacin)	40 mg
B_6 (pyridoxine)	4 mg
B_{12} (cyanocobalamin)	5 μg
C (ascorbic acid)	100 mg
Folic acid	400 μg
Biotin	60 μg

[a]International units.

Vitamins and Trace Elements

Vitamins are an essential component of a patient's daily PN regimen because they are necessary for normal metabolism and cellular function. Four fat-soluble and nine water-soluble vitamins are recognized as essential. The American Medical Association Nutrition Advisory Group established guidelines for daily parenteral administration of vitamins during PN.[34] The suggested amounts for 12 of the vitamins are shown in Table 12.9. These 12 vitamins are available in the suggested amounts from a few commercial manufacturers as a multiple-entity product that is added to the PN solutions daily. Vitamin K usually is not included in commercially available multivitamin adult formulations to avoid complications in patients receiving warfarin. Patients not receiving anticoagulants may receive vitamin K as phytonadione 0.5 to 1 mg/day or 5 to 10 mg/week during PN. Many vitamins are available as single-entity products that can be used for patients with documented vitamin deficiencies. The United States experienced two prolonged periods of parenteral multivitamin shortage during the 1990s that necessitated rationing. When these products are not available for daily use, thiamine (50 mg 3 times per week), pyridoxine (5 to 10 mg/day), folic acid (0.4 to 1 mg/day), niacin (40 to 50/mg/day if available), and ascorbic acid (100 mg/day) should be given as single-entity products in PN. Vitamin B_{12} should be given monthly (100 μg.) if the multiple-entity products are not available for daily use in PN.

Trace elements are also a necessary part of a daily PN solution. Trace elements are metabolic cofactors essential to the proper function of several enzyme systems in the body. Suggested amounts for zinc, copper, chromium, manganese, and selenium are listed in Table 12.10.[28] Zinc

Table 12.10 • Recommended Adult Intravenous Dosages of Trace Elements

Element	Daily Intravenous Dosage
Zinc[a]	2.5–5 mg
Copper	0.3–0.5 mg
Chromium[b]	10–15 μg
Manganese	60–100 μg
Selenium	20–60 μg

Source: Reference 28.

[a]Acute catabolic state, additional 2.0 mg.

[b]Intestinal losses, increase daily dosage to 20 μg.

requirements increase in metabolic stress or with large gastrointestinal losses. Zinc, chromium, and selenium are excreted by the kidneys, and manganese and copper are excreted through the biliary tract. Therefore, for patients with cholestatic liver disease, copper and manganese should be limited in or withheld from the PN solution. The trace elements are available as single- or multiple-entity products for admixture into PN formulations. Parenteral guidelines for molybdenum and iodine have not been established; however, these trace elements are available commercially.

Total Nutrient Admixtures

In the past, PN formulations consisted of an admixture of dextrose and protein (two-in-one), and intravenous fat was being added to these solutions at some institutions. The intravenous admixture of dextrose, amino acids, and fat emulsion is known as a TNA. Intravenous fat is a water-in-oil emulsion stabilized by the anionic emulsifier egg yolk phospholipid. When properly prepared, the TNA is stable for at least 48 hours.

The use of TNAs has several advantages over two-in-one formulations. It may decrease the risk of infection because fewer central-line manipulations are involved. It also decreases the time spent in PN administration. In addition, lipids mixed with dextrose and amino acids do not support bacterial growth as well as the fat emulsion alone. Giving the fat emulsion slowly and continuously over a 24-hour period improves oxidation of the lipids and reduces the potential for immunosuppression by long-chain triglycerides.

Despite these advantages, there are some concerns about TNAs. It is not possible to detect particulate matter in a TNA. Also, because the fat particles are fairly large, the TNA cannot be filtered with a 0.22-μm filter. Also, it is difficult to know the particle size before the emulsion cracks. Furthermore, only a few medications are known to be compatible with and can be added to the TNAs. Drugs that are known to be compatible include cimetidine, ranitidine, famotidine, heparin, and insulin. There is also greater potential for waste using this method because most pharmacies prepare one bag for each 24-hour period.

TNA must be prepared carefully to ensure stability.[28] Creaming and coalescence of the fat emulsion result when electrolytes are added directly to it. The anionic emulsifier in the fat emulsion may be adversely affected by divalent cations and acidifying agents. Therefore, dosages of divalent cations that may be added to the TNA are limited. Adding these electrolytes beyond the recommended amounts neutralizes the negative potential at the surface of the emulsion and causes the admixture to coalesce.

Prescribing and Labeling

The National Advisory Group on Standards and Practice Guidelines for Parenteral Nutrition addressed the prescribing and labeling of PN formulations.[28] The group suggests that all PN formulation labels be standardized to show the amounts of macronutrients, electrolytes, micronutrients, and medications given per day. For health care systems that prescribe by amounts per liter, the daily amount should be listed first, followed by the amount per liter in parentheses. Templates of standardized labels for adult and pediatric PN appear in Figures 12.1 and 12.2, respectively. When intravenous fat emulsion is infused as a separate entity, a label listing product, strength, volume, grams per kilogram, and grams is proposed (Fig. 12.3). This proposed standardization should be particularly useful as patients are transferred across health care system environments (i.e., hospital, extended care facility, clinic, home). The group also proposed that pharmacist-to-pharmacist communication take place to ensure accurate transfer of the PN prescription.[28]

Complications of Parenteral Nutrition

The complications of PN may be divided into three broad categories: infectious, technical, and metabolic. Catheter-related sepsis, the most common infectious complication, may occur as a result of contamination during line placement or poor catheter care. Catheter sepsis can be minimized with a strict protocol for line insertion and catheter care. Many institutions have nutrition support nurses who assist in line placement and perform the central catheter dressing changes.

Technical complications, such as pneumothorax, hydrothorax, and arterial puncture, may occur during placement of the catheter. Proper training and careful technique minimize the chance of these technical complications.

Several metabolic complications may occur. Fluid overload may occur because patients receiving PN often require several other intravenous fluids. Metabolic acidosis and metabolic alkalosis often occur in patients who receive PN. Metabolic complications related to the carbohydrate component of PN include hyperglycemia, hyperosmolar coma, and adverse effects of overfeeding. Hyperglycemia usually is identified through frequent monitoring of serum glucose concentrations. This complication may be managed by adding insulin to the PN formulation, decreasing the dextrose concentration, or decreasing the infusion rate.

Institution/Pharmacy Name, Address, and Pharmacy Phone Number

Name	Dosing weight	Location
Administration date/time		Expiration date/time
Base formula	Amount/day	(Amount/L)
Dextrose	g	(g/L)
Amino acids[a]	g	(g/L)
Lipid[a]	g	(g/L)
Electrolytes		
Sodium chloride	mEq	(mEq/L)
Sodium acetate	mEq	(mEq/L)
Potassium chloride	mEq	(mEq/L)
Potassium acetate	mEq	(mEq/L)
Potassium phosphate	mmol of P	(mmol/L)
	(mEq of K)	(mEq/L)
Sodium phosphate	mmol of P	(mmol/L)
	(mEq of Na)	(mEq/L)
Calcium gluconate	mEq	(mEq/L)
Magnesium sulfate	mEq	(mEq/L)
Vitamins, trace elements, and medications		
Multiple vitamins[a]	mL	
Multiple trace elements[a]	mL	
Insulin	IU	(U/L)
H_2 antagonists[a]	mg	

Rate ______ mL/hr   Volume ______ mL   Infuse over 24 hr

Admixture contains ______ mL plus ______ mL overfill.

Central Line Use Only

[a]Specify product name.

Figure 12.1. Standard PN label template for adults. (Reprinted with permission from JPEN J Parenter Enteral Nutr 22:52, 1998.)

Carbohydrate overfeeding may cause excess carbon dioxide production, leading to respiratory acidosis, elevated liver function test results, and hepatic steatosis. These problems usually can be avoided with a dextrose infusion rate of 5 mg/kg/minute (25 kcal/kg/day) or less. Disorders may occur with nearly all electrolytes. Malnourished patients who begin PN often experience hypokalemia and hypophosphatemia secondary to the intracellular shift of those ions, induced by dextrose. Vitamin and trace element disorders may also occur (e.g., vitamin A toxicity during PN in patients with renal failure and low serum zinc concentrations in severe metabolic stress). The dosages of these micronutrients may be adjusted to alleviate metabolic complications.

Monitoring of Patients Receiving Parenteral Nutrition

Because many metabolic complications may occur in patients receiving PN, patients should be monitored. Table 12.11 lists some guidelines for monitoring patients receiving PN.

Drug Compatibility Considerations in Parenteral Nutrition

When the PN formulation is used as a drug vehicle, the overall amount of fluid administered and the number of intravenous line manipulations decrease. Patients who are fluid restricted, receive home PN, or have limited venous access may benefit from receiving their medications in the PN formulation.

Drugs that are added to the PN formulation must be physically and chemically stable in it. It is not wise to add a drug to these formulations when frequent dosage changes are anticipated. When no dosage changes are anticipated, pharmacodynamic actions are consistent with continuous delivery, and the drug is physically compatible, addition to the PN formulation is reasonable. Amino acid concentration, solution pH, and ambient room temperature all may affect the stability of the drug added to a PN formulation. Also, drugs added to the PN formulation may have an adverse effect on selected nutrients. Heparin, regular human insulin, and most histamine-2 receptor antagonists are compatible in TNAs. Iron dextran, metoclopramide, human albumin, theophylline, heparin, regular human insulin, and histamine-2 receptor antagonists are compatible in two-in-one PN formulations.

Numerous studies have been conducted on calcium and phosphorus compatibility in PN formulations. Many factors can contribute to calcium phosphate precipitation, such as the relative amounts of calcium and phosphorus additives, pH of the PN formulation, concentration of the amino acid solution, and mixing process used for prepara-

Institution/Pharmacy Name, Address, and Pharmacy Phone Number

Name	Dosing weight	Location
Administration date/time		Expiration date/time
Base formula	Amount/kg/day	Amount/day
Dextrose	g/kg	g
Amino acids[a]	g/kg	g
Electrolytes		
Sodium chloride[b]	mEq/kg	mEq
Sodium acetatc[b]	mEq/kg	mEq
Potassium chloride[b]	mEq/kg	mEq
Potassium acetate[b]	mEq/kg	mEq
Potassium phosphate[b]	mmol of P/kg	mmol of P
	(mEq of K)/kg	(mEq of K)
Sodium phosphate[b]	mmol of P/kg	mmol of P
	(mEq of Na)/kg	(mEq of Na)
Calcium gluconate	mEq/kg	mEq
Magnesium sulfate	mEq/kg	mEq
Vitamins, trace elements, and medications		
Multiple vitamins[a]	mL/kg	mL
Multiple trace elements[a]	mL/kg	mL
L-cysteine	mg/g protein	mg
H_2 antagonists[a]	mg/kg	mg
Rate ______ mL/hr	Volume ______ mL	Infuse over 24 hr

Admixture contains ______ mL plus ______ mL overfill.

Central Line Use Only

[a]Specify product name.

[b]Because the admixture usually contains multiple sources of sodium, potassium, chloride, acetate, and phosphorus, the amount of each electrolyte per kilogram provided by the PN admixture is determined by adding the amount of electrolyte provided by each salt.

Figure 12.2. Standard PN label template for neonates and children. (Reprinted with permission from JPEN J Parenter Enteral Nutr 22:52, 1998.)

Institution/Pharmacy Name, Address, and Pharmacy Phone Number

Name	Dosing weight	Location	
Administration date/time		Expiration date/time	
	Volume	Amount/kg/day	Amount/day
Intravenous fat emulsion (%)	______ mL	g/kg	g

Infusion rate ______ mL/hr Infuse over ______ hr

Contains overfill; discard any unused volume after 24 hr.

For peripheral or central line administration

Figure 12.3. Standard intravenous fat emulsion label template for adults, neonates, and children. (Reprinted with permission from JPEN J Parenter Enteral Nutr 22:52, 1998.)

Table 12.11 ▪ Guidelines for Monitoring Patients Receiving Parenteral Nutrition

Fingersticks for glucose every 6 hr. If >300 mg/dL, draw stat samples for serum glucose and potassium.
Measure total fluid intake and output daily.
Weigh patient at least once per week.
Use sliding scale with regular human insulin.
Draw samples for prealbumin or transferrin tests each week.
Draw samples for comprehensive metabolic panel at least once a week, basic metabolic panel daily in the intensive care unit.[a]
Draw samples for magnesium and phosphorus determinations at least twice per week.
Collect 24-hr urine for nitrogen balance determination each week in new patients and patients who have not attained nitrogen equilibrium.

[a]Frequency of laboratory measurements is dictated by severity of the patient's illness.

Table 12.12 ▪ Summary of Recommendations for Extemporaneous Compounding and Filtration of Parenteral Nutrition Admixtures

Optimize additive sequence and validate as safe and efficacious.
Review manual methods of compounding regularly and when contracts with macronutrient manufacturers change.
Manufacturers of automated compounders should provide an additive sequence that ensures safety.
Visually inspect all compounded parenteral nutrition formulations for particulate contamination or formation and phase separation when intravenous fat has been added.
Use a filter when infusing central or peripheral parenteral nutrition admixtures. Standards of practice vary, but a 1.2-μm air-eliminating filter for lipid-containing admixtures and a 0.22-μm air-eliminating filter for non–lipid-containing admixtures are recommended.
Administer parenteral nutrition admixtures within the following time frames: If stored at room temperature, start the infusion within 24 hr after mixing; if refrigerated, start the infusion within 24 hr of rewarming.
If symptoms of acute respiratory distress, pulmonary embolus, or interstitial pneumonitis develop, stop the infusion immediately and check thoroughly for precipitates. Institute appropriate medical interventions.

Source: Reference 28.

tion of PN admixtures. A safety alert published by the Food and Drug Administration (FDA) cautions that improper preparation of TNAs with automated compounding systems may result in calcium phosphate precipitates. Life-threatening hazards such as microvascular pulmonary emboli and subacute interstitial pneumonitis have been linked to calcium phosphate precipitates from improperly prepared PN formulations. Recommendations for proper compounding of TNAs have been suggested by the National Advisory Group on Standards and Practice Guidelines for Parenteral Nutrition (Table 12.12). Generally, solutions with amino acid concentrations greater than 2.5% and a pH less than 6.0 favor solubility of calcium and phosphorus. Some studies report incompatibilities between therapeutic dosages of iron and fat. Human albumin is reported to be compatible in most two-in-one solutions and TNAs by some manufacturers (e.g., Abbott). There are few data on albumin compatibility with TNAs by other manufacturers. Whenever a question of compatibility arises, it is best to obtain information from a recent text on intravenous admixtures. If no data exist on a particular combination, the safest approach is to not add the medication to the PN formulation.

ENTERAL NUTRITION

The use of EN dates back to the ancient Egyptians, who used nutritional enemas to preserve health. EN by tube has been mentioned and used since that time, but only during the last 25 years has it been used extensively in acute and chronic care settings. Most practitioners believe that if the gastrointestinal tract is functional and accessible, it should be used for the delivery of specialized nutrition support. The development of new feeding tubes, modern administration equipment, surgically placed enterostomies, and sophisticated enteral formulas have greatly improved this method. Enteral feeding by tube is thought to preserve the gastrointestinal mass and possibly prevent gastrointestinal translocation of bacteria and endotoxin, which has been associated with sepsis and multiple-organ dysfunction syndrome. Consequently, practitioners in specialized nutrition support are making extraordinary efforts to deliver enteral nutrients to critically ill patients.

Table 12.13 ▪ Summary of American Society for Parenteral and Enteral Nutrition Guidelines for Enteral Nutrition

Use enteral nutrition by tube feeding in patients who are or will become undernourished and in whom oral feedings are inadequate.
Obtain access to the gastrointestinal tract in the most natural and least invasive manner.
During the administration of enteral nutrition, patients should be monitored by trained health care professionals knowledgeable in the potential pulmonary, mechanical, gastrointestinal, and metabolic complications of enteral tube feeding.
Candidates for home enteral nutrition should be evaluated by a multidisciplinary team of health care professionals.

Source: Reference 35.

The American Society for Parenteral and Enteral Nutrition has published practice guidelines for the rational use of EN.[35] A summary of these recommendations appears in Table 12.13. EN should not be used when the gastrointestinal tract is not functional (e.g., postoperative ileus) or when enteral nutrients are undesirable (e.g., severe acute pancreatitis).

Types of Enteral Feeding Delivery

There are many ways to deliver enteral nutrients into the gastrointestinal tract, and EN can be delivered safely and efficaciously in most patients as either short- or long-term therapy (Fig. 12.4).

Nasogastric or nasoduodenal feeding tubes are used for patients who need enteral access for a short time (e.g., a few weeks). These soft, small-bore tubes have virtually replaced the large nasogastric tube, which is now used only for nasogastric suction. These tubes, made of polyurethane or silicone, have several advantages over the large nasogastric tubes. Most of them have a weighted tip, which facilitates transpyloric passage of the tube into the small bowel. Irritation to the nose, pharynx, and esophagus is less likely when these smaller tubes are used. Also, patients may eat food and swallow without difficulty when the softer tubes are used. These tubes usually are packaged with a stylet, which aids in proper placement during intubation.

A surgical gastrostomy provides enteral access for long-term EN therapy (months to years). The nutrients are

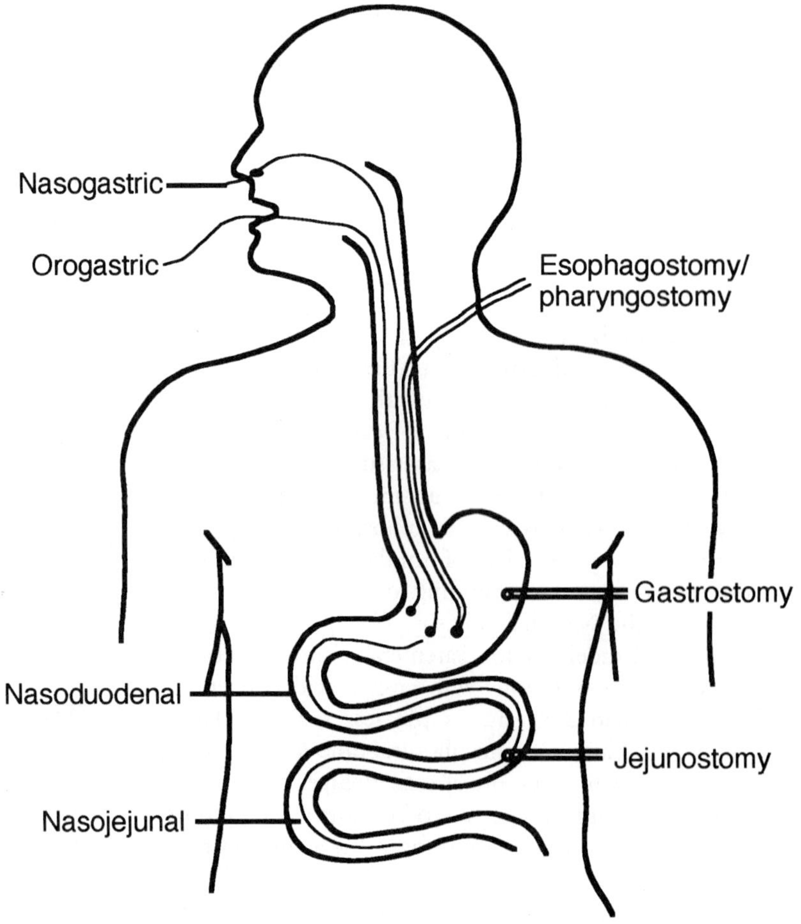

Figure 12.4. Enteral nutrition access sites. Enteral access can be obtained at bedside or in a surgical suite. Nasogastric and orogastric feeding tubes usually are placed at bedside. Placement of nasoduodenal or nasojejunal tubes usually requires fluoroscopy or esophagogastroduodenoscopy. Percutaneous endoscopic gastrostomy tubes may be placed under local anesthesia at bedside or in an endoscopy suite. Open gastrostomy or jejunostomy requires an operative procedure.

Table 12.14 ▪ Enteral Formula Categories with Examples of Commonly Used Products

Isotonic tube feeding	Isocal, Osmolite, Nutren
Oral supplement	Ensure, Ensure Plus, Sustacal
Fluid-restricted tube feeding	Two Cal-HN, Isocal-HCN
Chemically defined tube feeding	Vital-HN, Criticare-HN, Vivonex-TEN
Fiber-containing standard tube feeding	Ultracal, Jevity
Low-protein, low-electrolyte, or electrolyte-free tube feeding[a]	Travasorb-Renal, Supena, Nepro
Modified protein, electrolyte-free, or restricted tube feeding[b]	HepaticAid, Nutrihep
Low-carbohydrate, high-fat tube feeding[c]	Pulmocare, Glucerna, Respilor, Oxepa, Nutrivent, Choice DM
High-protein tube feeding	Traumacal
High-protein, fiber-containing tube feeding[d]	Promote with fiber, Replete with fiber, Isosource VHN
Immune-enhancing diet	Impact, Perative, ImmunAid
Protein module	Promod, Promix-RD
Fat module	Microlipid
Carbohydrate module	Polycose

[a]Used occasionally in acute renal failure, chronic renal dysfunction, and chronic renal failure.
[b]Used in liver failure with hepatic encephalopathy.
[c]Used occasionally in respiratory failure or diabetes.
[d]Used occasionally in trauma or sepsis.

infused directly into the stomach via the gastrostomy tube, bypassing the mouth, pharynx, and esophagus. The Stamm gastrostomy and percutaneous endoscopic gastrostomy (PEG) are the two most common types for long-term use. The Stamm gastrostomy usually is done by a general surgeon in the operating room using general anesthesia. PEGs are done by general surgeons or gastroenterologists in a surgical suite or at the bedside, using local anesthesia.

Jejunostomies for EN are done for both short-term and long-term access.[36] A tube jejunostomy is placed during laparotomy and can be used for long-term enteral access. This type of jejunostomy is particularly effective in a patient who has severe, chronic gastroparesis (e.g., some diabetic patients). The chance of aspiration of nutrients is low because both the pyloric and the lower esophageal sphincter protect the airway when feedings are delivered into the jejunum. The transgastric jejunostomy is also placed surgically at the time of laparotomy, but this is used for short-term enteral access. When supplemental enteral feedings are no longer needed and the patient is taking adequate nutrients by mouth, the transgastric jejunostomy can be removed at the bedside without surgical intervention.

Enteral Nutrition Products

Currently, more than 200 enteral products are marketed in the United States. Most health care systems that administer these products develop formularies by creating several categories and stocking one product in each one. Table 12.14 lists 14 categories of enteral formulas and some examples in each category. Patients with normal fluid requirements, normal nutritional needs, and normal electrolyte status usually can be treated with isotonic, nutritionally complete formulas. Several institutions use products with added dietary fiber as their standard enteral formula presumably for improved gastrointestinal tolerance. Patients who are eating part of their diet orally often can take 8 to 32 oz of an oral enteral supplement. This obviates placement of an enteral feeding tube. Fluid-restricted enteral formulas are reserved for patients who have a problem with overhydration and edema (e.g., congestive heart failure). These products are extremely low in free water and can be dangerous when given to a patient who does not need severe fluid restriction. When gastrointestinal digestive capabilities are compromised, a chemically defined enteral formula often is used because most of the nutrients are in elemental or predigested form. Several products are marketed for patients with renal failure, liver failure, respiratory failure, diabetes, compromised immune function, and severe metabolic stress. These products are more expensive than standard enteral formulas. When a patient's specific needs cannot be met with commercially available enteral formulas, specific macronutrients (carbohydrate, fat, protein) can be added to these formulas to meet special needs. Several of these formulas are listed in Table 12.14.

Administration of Enteral Feedings

There are three ways to administer enteral feeding to institutionalized or home-bound patients: continuous, intermittent, and bolus. Continuous feeding, used preferentially in the institutionalized patient, involves an enteral pump that infuses the formula at a constant rate. The advantages of this method are less risk of aspiration, less nursing time, decreased gastrointestinal distension, and decreased diarrhea. Continuous feeding is more sophisticated and more expensive than the other methods. Intermittent feeding is used in the home setting and in some extended-care facilities. The desired volume of formula (usually 240 to 480 mL) is infused over a short period of time (e.g., 1 hour) several times each day. Bolus feeding consists of rapid administration of the desired volume of formula into the patient's ostomy tube. This method is used most often in the home-bound or nursing home patient who has a gastrostomy tube in place. When bolus feedings are administered into the stomach, the risk of aspiration, gastric distension, and diarrhea is higher. However, the bolus method is the simplest way to administer enteral nutrients, making it attractive in the home setting. In general, bolus feedings should not be given via jejunostomy.

EN usually is started at a slow rate and increased gradually to the desired goal. Most adults can tolerate an initial rate of 25 to 50 mL/hour. The isotonic formulas often can be started at 50 mL/hour, and the more concentrated formulas (2 kcal/mL) are started at 25 mL/hour. Patients who are slowly regaining bowel function should be started at a slower rate (e.g., 25 mL/hr or less). Many institutions increase the infusion rate of the EN formula by 25 mL/hour/day when gastrointestinal tolerance and fluid and electrolyte status are acceptable. This enables most patients to achieve the desired rate within 3 to 4 days. Little evidence supports dilution of hyperosmolar formulas to enhance gastrointestinal tolerance. In fact, in one study, patients who received an undiluted hyperosmolar enteral formula received more calories and protein without any increase in gastrointestinal side effects than groups receiving diluted hyperosmolar formulas or isotonic formulas.[37] Therefore, the use of diluted enteral formulas (e.g., half-strength) should be abandoned.

Complications of Enteral Nutrition

EN complications can be divided into four categories: pulmonary, gastrointestinal, mechanical, and metabolic.[38] Aspiration of EN formula into the lungs is a serious complication of this type of therapy. It occurs in the patient who has developed vomiting or impaired gastric emptying. This serious complication often results in pneumonia, requiring mechanical ventilation in an intensive care unit. Frequent examination of the abdomen and meticulous checking of gastric residuals aspirated through the feeding tube may help to assess the risk of aspiration. Prokinetic drugs such as metoclopramide, cisapride, and erythromycin have been used with some success in patients who have poor gastric emptying of EN formulas. Diabetic patients and patients with septic processes are particularly prone to delayed gastric emptying.

Gastrointestinal complications include vomiting and diarrhea. Vomiting usually can be prevented by increasing the enteral feeding rate slowly, as described earlier, and checking the patient's abdomen often. Most institutions elevate the head of the patient's bed at least 30° in gastric-fed patients. Diarrhea is a common problem in patients who receive EN; however, its cause often is elusive. Patients whose enteral nutrient rate is decreased by one-half often demonstrate decreased diarrhea.[39] The rate may then be gradually increased to the desired goal, as tolerated. Suggested causes of diarrhea in association with enteral tube feeding include antibiotic administration, hypoalbuminemia, hyperosmolar formulas, lactase deficiency, and lack of a nutrition support team. The authors of an excellent report carefully examined diarrhea in tube-fed patients and found hyperosmolar drug solutions containing sorbitol (e.g., theophylline) to be the most likely cause.[40] Therefore, all drugs administered via the gastrointestinal tract should be inspected in patients who have diarrhea associated with EN. Some patients demonstrate decreased stool volume and frequency when they are switched from a standard enteral formula to a chemically defined formula. Pharmacologic agents such as kaolin pectin may be helpful as first-line pharmacotherapy. Diarrhea associated with EN has also been treated successfully with banana flakes.[41] Loperamide and diphenoxylate should be used as a last resort in treating diarrhea. A severe gastrointestinal complication of EN via jejunostomy is pneumatosis intestinalis with bowel infarction and necrosis. This has occurred in up to 5% of patients receiving EN by this route. It appears that this is a complication of critically ill patients who are hemodynamically unstable (e.g., patients with hypotension and tachycardia who are receiving intravenous pressor agents) and fed via jejunostomy.[42] Therefore, regular abdominal examinations of patients receiving feedings by this route and stopping EN during periods of instability are prudent measures.

Mechanical complications occur in a feeding tube that has become kinked or occluded. A kinked tube can be withdrawn slowly until it straightens out. This should be done without the enteral formula infusing. Slow irrigation of the tube lumen with warm water administered by a 30-mL syringe opens some occluded feeding tubes. Cranberry juice, cola syrup, and pancreatic enzymes in water have also been used with some success. Some practitioners have decreased tube occlusion by using a pancreatic enzyme flush prophylactically.[43] Occasionally, the stylet can be passed back into the lumen of the tube. This may remove or break up any concretion. This should be done by a physician and only in tubes that do not let the stylet exit through a side port.

Virtually all metabolic complications that happen with PN can occur with EN. Hyperglycemia usually is not as severe with EN because the nutrients are being infused into the gastrointestinal tract rather than into a large vein. Some institutions in which the pharmacy department prepares and dispenses the enteral formulas have programs that allow the addition of electrolytes (e.g., KCl, Fleet Phosphosoda) to help treat or prevent metabolic complications.

Monitoring the Patient Receiving Enteral Nutrition

Patients who receive EN should be monitored frequently to ensure safety and efficacy. Many complications can be averted with meticulous patient monitoring. Some monitoring guidelines are listed in Table 12.15.

Table 12.15 ▪ Monitoring Patients Receiving Enteral Nutrition

Raise head of bed to at least 30° at all times.
Check gastric residuals every 6 hr. If >150 mL, replace residual and hold feedings for 4 hr and recheck; if <150 mL, restart, or if still >150 mL, hold feedings.
Fingerstick for glucose every 6 hr and regular human insulin to scale. If >300 mg/dL, draw stat serum glucose and potassium samples.
Draw samples for comprehensive metabolic panel, phosphorus, total CO_2, and magnesium determination as needed.[a]
Draw basic metabolic panel daily in the intensive care unit.
Draw sample for prealbumin or transferrin determination each week.
Collect 24-hr urine for nitrogen balance each week.

[a]Frequency of laboratory measurements is dictated by severity of the patient's illness.

Drug Compatibility Considerations in Enteral Nutrition

In many patients receiving EN, the feeding tube may be the only way to administer drugs.[44] Therefore, any incompatibilities between drug and enteral formula or tube are of paramount importance. Phenytoin and warfarin have been reported to be altered by EN administration. Patients who receive both phenytoin (300 mg/day as the suspension) and EN are reported to have subtherapeutic serum concentrations of drug.[45] Interestingly, there does not appear to be a problem when this drug is administered to normal subjects who take concomitant oral enteral supplements or nasogastric tube feedings.[46,47] It is unclear what effect the difference in subjects (patients versus normal subjects) has on this interaction. Difficulty has been reported in attaining a therapeutic international normalized ratio with warfarin administration during concurrent enteral feeding. Initially this problem was thought to be caused by the high vitamin K content of some commercially available enteral formulas. Manufacturers have decreased the vitamin K content of most enteral formulas over the last 15 years; however, the problem with warfarin and enteral formulas still exists. One study demonstrated lower recovery of warfarin mixed with an enteral formula than when mixed with distilled water.[48]

HOME CARE

Home Nutrition Therapy

Although most hospitalized patients receiving PN or EN can return to an oral diet before discharge, some require continued specialized nutrition support at home. The hospital nutrition support team members usually work with an assigned home health care company. The team devises a specialized nutrition support prescription that will meet the patient's fluid and nutritional requirements with an administration schedule that is compatible with the patient's lifestyle. PN or EN formulations often are given as a nocturnal continuous drip over an 8- to 18-hour period. This allows patients to work or participate in other activities during the day. However, some patients receiving EN prefer periodic bolus feedings during the day. The home health pharmacy will compound the EN or PN formulation and provide the patient with the necessary equipment for its administration. Approximately 2 to 5 days before hospital discharge, clinicians from the home health agency or nutrition support team will begin training the patient and family to administer the nutrition regimen. The patient and family are also trained to detect adverse effects that may occur during administration. In addition, the home health agency works with the patient's physician, nurse, and pharmacist to ensure that the patient is monitored between office visits.

Specialized nutrition support in the home is costly, yet it is much more economical than keeping the patient hospitalized. Examples of patients who may require home PN are those with extensive small bowel resection (short bowel syndrome), chronic enteritis from radiation therapy, or severe Crohn's disease. These patients receive PN via a permanent, centrally placed catheter (e.g., Hickman catheter, implanted port). Patients who receive home EN can absorb nutrients via the gastrointestinal tract but are unable to consume adequate nutrients by mouth. Examples of those who receive home EN include patients with severe ulcerative colitis, colon cancer, cerebral trauma, or head and neck cancer. The administration route chosen for enteral feeding depends on the patient's diagnosis and the estimated duration of EN. Surgical gastrostomy or jejunostomy is often used in these patients. Home nutrition programs have improved the quality of life for many patients who require these therapies and have allowed many to return to nearly normal lifestyles.

PHARMACOKINETIC AND PHARMACODYNAMIC CONSIDERATIONS

Altered disposition of drugs has been demonstrated with both malnutrition and changes in macronutrient intake.[49] Much of this research has been performed in animals, but more clinical studies in patients are being conducted. In general, the systemic clearance of many drugs is significantly lower in undernourished patients than in well-nourished patients. Some drugs demonstrate higher clearance when given concurrently with aggressive dosages of macronutrients (e.g., protein). Clearances of theophylline in children[50] and gentamicin in normal adult subjects[51] increased significantly when they were given with high-protein diets. This finding may be clinically important because there is a trend to give higher dosages of protein to patients who need specialized nutrition support, especially in the critical care setting.

CONCLUSION

Many questions in specialized nutrition support remain to be answered through basic and clinical research.[52] Nutrition support team members should be as involved in EN as in PN. Many patients, especially those hospitalized in the intensive care unit, are receiving EN as a sole source of nutrition or in combination with PN. By focusing on only the PN component, the nutrition support team can miss an opportunity to improve patient care. EN is associated with pulmonary, mechanical, gastrointestinal, and metabolic complications that can be prevented or treated efficiently when patients are monitored closely. There is an association between the use of EN in critical illness and the development of morbidity. Clearly, patients receiving EN have significantly fewer cases of pneumonia and abdominal abscesses than patients receiving PN. Most of this work has been done in trauma patients. It would be unfortunate if nutrition support team members were not involved with this therapy as more data become available. More patients are likely to receive EN and fewer to receive PN over the next few years.

KEY POINTS

- The pharmacist's role on the nutrition support team may include directing, monitoring patients for metabolic complications, educating other practitioners and patients, compounding parenteral and enteral formulations, assuming responsibility for development of a cost-effective nutrition formulary, and providing information about compatibilities and drug–nutrient interactions.
- Nutritional assessment involves measuring the body cell mass, fat mass, and constitutive proteins in the blood. A thorough nutritional assessment will help determine whether the patient needs to gain, maintain, or lose weight.
- Subjective global assessment is an excellent way to determine the nutritional status of a patient. This is usually done during the history and physical examination.
- The Harris–Benedict equations for BEE and the WHO equations both appear to be adequate for estimating total calorie goals in unstressed adult patients.
- The REE of adult patients can be assessed most accurately using indirect calorimetry.
- Peripheral vein PN should be used for only about 1 week because of frequent vein rotation.
- Central vein PN should always be used when calorie and energy needs are high, therapy will be given for an extended period of time, or fluid restriction is needed.
- The dextrose dosage during PN should never exceed 5 mg/kg/minute.
- TNAs may result in fewer catheter site infections, less nursing administration and pharmacy preparation time, and lower cost than a 2-in-1 PN delivery system.
- Enteral formulations often are given via nasogastric tube, nasoenteric tube, gastrostomy, or jejunostomy.
- Enteral formulations may be administered as a continuous infusion, intermittent infusion, or bolus.
- Changing to an enteral formulation with fiber and eliminating sorbitol from liquid medications are two effective interventions to treat EN-associated diarrhea.
- Home PN and EN programs continue to grow because administering this therapy at home is much cheaper than prolonging hospitalization.

REFERENCES

1. Dudrick SJ, Wilmore DW, Vars HM, et al. Long-term parenteral nutrition with growth, development, and positive nitrogen balance. Surgery 64:134–142, 1968.
2. Detsky AS, Smalley PS, Chana J. Is this patient malnourished? JAMA 271:54–58, 1994.
3. Wilson MG, Vaswani S, Liu D, et al. Prevalence and causes of undernutrition in medical outpatients. Am J Med 104:56–63, 1998.
4. Galanos AN, Pieper CF, Kussin PS, et al. Relationships of body mass index to subsequent mortality among seriously ill hospitalized patients. Crit Care Med 25:1962–1968, 1997.
5. Manson JE, Willett WC, Stampfer MJ, et al. Body weight and mortality among women. N Engl J Med 333:677–685, 1995.
6. Baker, JP, Detsky AS, Wesson DE, et al. Nutritional assessment: a comparison of clinical judgment and objective measurements. N Engl J Med 306:969–972, 1982.
7. Donahue SP, Phillips LS. Response of IGHF-1 to nutritional support in malnourished hospital patients: a possible indicator of short-term changes in nutritional status. Am J Clin Nutr 50:962–969, 1989.
8. Brodie D, Moscrip V, Hutcheon R. Body composition measurement: a review of hydrodensitometry, anthropometry, and impedance methods. Nutrition 14:296–310, 1998.
9. Miles JM. Should protein be included in calorie calculations for a TPN prescription? Yes protein should be included. Nutr Clin Pract 11:204–205, 1996.
10. Harris JA, Benedict FC. A biometric study of basal metabolism. Pub. no. 279. Washington, DC: Carnegie Institute of Washington, 1919.
11. Elia M. Changing concepts of nutrient requirements in disease: implications for artificial nutritional support. Lancet 345:1279–1284, 1995.
12. Garrel DR, Jobin N, DeJonge LH. Should we still use the Harris and Benedict equations? Nutr Clin Pract 11:99–103, 1996.
13. McClave SA, Snider HL. Use of indirect calorimetry in clinical nutrition. Nutr Clin Pract 7:207–221, 1992.
14. Weir JB de V. New methods for calculating metabolic rate with special reference to protein metabolism. J Physiol (Lond) 109:1–9, 1949.
15. Shaw JHF, Wildbore M, Wolfe RR. Whole body protein kinetics in severely septic patients: the response to glucose infusion and total parenteral nutrition. Ann Surg 205:288–294, 1987.
16. Anonymous. Parenteral nutrition. JPEN J Parenter Enteral Nutr 17(Suppl):9SA–11SA, 1993.
17. Anonymous. Standards for nutrition support: hospitalized patients. Nutr Clin Pract 10:208–219, 1995.
18. Anonymous. Nutrition support for adults with specific diseases and conditions. JPEN J Parenter Enteral Nutr 17(Suppl):12SA–26SA, 1993.
19. Everitt NJ, McMahon MJ. Peripheral venous nutrition. Nutrition 10:49–57, 1994.
20. Doglietto GB, Gallitelli L, Pacelli F, et al. Protein-sparing therapy after major abdominal surgery. Lack of clinical effects. Ann Surg 223:357–362, 1996.
21. Cerra FB, Cheung NK, Fischer JF, et al. Disease-specific amino acid infusion (F080) in hepatic encephalopathy: a prospective, mixed double-blind, controlled trial. JPEN J Parenter Enteral Nutr 9:288–295, 1985.
22. Michel H, Bories P, Aubin JP, et al. Treatment of acute hepatic encephalopathy in cirrhotics with a branched-chain amino acids versus a conventional amino acids mixture. Liver 5:282–289, 1985.
23. Feinstein EI, Blumenkrantz MJ, Healy M, et al. Clinical and metabolic responses to parenteral nutrition in acute renal failure. Medicine 60:124–137, 1981.
24. Mirtallo JM, Schneider PS, Marko, et al. A comparison of essential and general amino acid infusions in the nutritional support of patients with compromised renal function. JPEN J Parenter Enteral Nutr 6:109–113, 1982.
25. Garcia-de-Lorenzo A, Ortiz-Leyba C, Palnas M, et al. Parenteral administration of different amounts of branch-chain amino acids in septic patients: clinical and metabolic aspects. Crit Care Med 25:418–424, 1997.
26. von Meyenfeldt MF, Soeters PB, Vente JP, et al. Effect of branched chain amino acid enrichment of total parenteral nutrition on nitrogen sparing and clinical outcome of sepsis and trauma. A prospective randomized double-blind trial. Br J Surg 77:924–929, 1990.

27. Burke JF, Wolfe RR, MuDancy CJ, et al. Glucose requirements following burn injury: parameters of optimal glucose infusion and possible hepatic and respiratory abnormalities following excessive glucose intake. Ann Surg 190:275–285, 1979.
28. National Advisory Group on Standards and Practice Guidelines for Parenteral Nutrition. Safe practices for parenteral nutrition formulations. JPEN J Parenter Enteral Nutr 22:49–66, 1998.
29. Schloerb PR, Henning JF. Patterns and problems of adult total parenteral nutrition use in U.S. academic medical centers. Arch Surg 133:7–12, 1998.
30. Rosmarin DK, Wardlaw GM, Mirtallo J. Hyperglycemia associated with high, continuous infusion rates of total parenteral nutrition dextrose. Nutr Clin Pract 11:151–156, 1996.
31. Battistella FD, Wildergren JT, Anderson JT, et al. A prospective, randomized trial of intravenous fat emulsion administration in trauma victims requiring total parenteral nutrition. J Trauma 43:52–58, 1997.
32. Hyltander A, Sandstrom R, Lundholm K. Metabolic effects of structured triglycerides in humans. Nutr Clin Pract 10:91–97, 1995.
33. Solomon SM, Kirby DF. The refeeding syndrome: a review. JPEN J Parenter Enteral Nutr 14:90–97, 1990.
34. Anonymous. Multivitamin preparations for parenteral use: a statement by the Nutrition Advisory Group. JPEN J Parenter Enteral Nutr 3:253–262, 1979.
35. Anonymous. Enteral nutrition. JPEN J Parenter Enteral Nutr 17(Suppl):8SA–9SA, 1993.
36. Sarr MG, Mayo S. Needle catheter jejunostomy: an unappreciated and misunderstood advance in the care of patients after major abdominal operations. Mayo Clin Proc 63:565–572, 1988.
37. Keohane PP, Attrill H, Love M, et al. Relation between osmolality of diet and gastrointestinal side effects in enteral nutrition. BMJ 288:678–680, 1984.
38. Cabre E, Gassull MA. Complications of enteral feeding. Nutrition 9:1–9, 1993.
39. Heimburger DC, Sockwell DG, Geels WJ. Diarrhea with enteral feeding: prospective reappraisal of putative causes. Nutrition 10:392–396, 1994.
40. Edes TE, Walk BE, Austin JL. Diarrhea in tube-fed patients: feeding formula not necessarily the cause. Am J Med 88:91–93, 1990.
41. Emery EA, Ahmad S, Koethe JD, et al. Banana flakes control diarrhea in enterally fed patients. Nutr Clin Pract 12:72–75, 1997.
42. Delany HM, Lindine P. The pros and cons of needle catheter jejunostomy. Nutrition 4:119–124, 1988.
43. Sriram K, Jayanthi V, Lakshimi RG, et al. Prophylactic locking of enteral feeding tubes with pancreatic enzymes. JPEN J Parenter Enteral Nutr 21:353–356, 1997.
44. Beckwith MC, Barton RG, Graves C. A guide to drug therapy in patients with enteral feeding tubes: dosage form selection and administration methods. Hosp Pharm 32:57–64, 1997.
45. Bauer LA. Interference of oral phenytoin absorption by continuous nasogastric feedings. Neurology 32:570–572, 1982.
46. Nishimura LY, Armstrong EP, Plezia PM, et al. Influence of enteral feedings on phenytoin sodium absorption from capsules. Drug Intell Clin Pharm 22:130–133, 1988.
47. Doak KK, Haas CE, Dunningan KJ, et al. Bioavailability of phenytoin acid and phenytoin sodium with enteral feedings. Pharmacotherapy 18:637–45, 1998.
48. Kuhn TA, Garnett WR, Wells BK, et al. Recovery of warfarin from an enteral nutrient formula. Am J Hosp Pharm 46:1395–1399, 1989.
49. Anderson KE. Influences of diet and nutrition on clinical pharmacokinetics. Clin Pharmacokinet 14:325–346, 1988.
50. Feldman CH, Hutchinson VE, Sher TH, et al. Interaction between nutrition and theophylline metabolism in children. Ther Drug Monit 4:69–76, 1982.
51. Dickson CJ, Schwartzman MS, Bertino JS. Factors affecting aminoglycoside disposition: effects of circadian rhythm and dietary protein intake on gentamicin pharmacokinetics. Clin Pharmacol Ther 39:325–328, 1986.
52. Klein S, Kinney J, Jeejeebhoy K, et al. Nutrition support in clinical practice: review of published data and recommendations for future research directions. Am J Clin Nutr 66:683–706, 1997.

CHAPTER 13

IRON DEFICIENCY AND MEGALOBLASTIC ANEMIAS

Mary E. Teresi

Overview

DEFINITION

Anemia is a hematologic condition in which there is quantitative deficiency of circulating hemoglobin (Hb), often accompanied by a reduced number of red blood cells (erythrocytes). Causes of anemia are blood loss, impaired erythropoiesis, and abnormal erythrocyte destruction. Nutritional deficiencies (iron, cobalamin [B_{12}], folate) are the most common cause of anemia throughout the world.[1,2]

Erythropoiesis is a controlled physiologic process. In response to changes in tissue oxygen availability, the kidney regulates production and release of erythropoietin, which stimulates the bone marrow to produce and release red blood cells. Erythrocytes originate from pluripotent stem cells in the bone marrow and undergo multiple steps of differentiation and maturation. Early stages of red cell production consist of large cells with immature nuclei (pronormoblasts and basophilic normoblasts). As cells mature, Hb is incorporated, the nucleus is extruded, and cell size decreases. Various nutrients are needed for normal erythropoiesis. Lack of B_{12} or folate can interfere with cell maturation, resulting in the release of megaloblasts (erythroid precursors with immature nuclei). Iron deficiency interferes with Hb production and incorporation into the maturing cells, which continue to divide, resulting in the release of smaller cells (microcytic).

TREATMENT GOALS: ANEMIAS

- Identify patients at risk for developing nutritional anemias.
- Prevent nutritional deficiencies and anemia.
- Treat nutritional deficiency and/or anemia by providing the appropriate nutrient.
- Document and confirm the deficiency state as the cause of the anemia.
- Identify and, when possible, rectify the pathologic state responsible for the deficiency.
- Develop therapeutic monitoring plans.
- Optimize patient compliance with treatment plan by minimizing treatment side effects, costs, and inconvenience.
- Prevent long-term sequelae.

PATHOPHYSIOLOGY

Anemia, which has many causes, is not a single disease entity but a sign of disease. Regardless of the cause, anemia is associated with a reduction in circulating Hb because of reduced numbers of erythrocytes or less Hb per erythrocyte.

The number of erythrocytes in normal people varies with age, sex, and atmospheric pressure. People who live at high altitudes have more erythrocytes to compensate for the reduced oxygen in the air. At sea level, the average normal man has 5.5×10^{12} erythrocytes/L ($5.5 \times 10^6/mm^3$). The erythrocytes occupy 47% of the blood, and this value is called the packed cell volume or hematocrit (Hct). The normal ranges for red blood cell measurements (Hb, Hct) vary with age and laboratory, but in general, values that are more then 2 standard deviations (SD) below the mean warrant further investigation.[1] Blood from healthy men contains approximately 9.9 mmol/L (16 g/dL) Hb. All these parameters are lower for healthy women. Values for neonates, which show no sex differences, are higher at birth, but after several weeks they decrease to below those of women. Thereafter the values rise gradually, and at puberty sex differences appear (Table 13.1).

The physiologic result of low circulating Hb is the reduced capacity for blood to carry oxygen. Consequently, less oxygen is available to tissues, including those of the heart, brain, and muscles, leading to the clinical manifestations of anemia.

CLINICAL PRESENTATION AND DIAGNOSIS

Regardless of the cause of anemia, the clinical features depend on the rate of development and the compensatory ability of the cardiovascular and pulmonary system to adjust to tissue hypoxia. Lower Hb levels often are tolerated with minimal symptoms if the anemia develops slowly and the body is able to compensate.

Signs and Symptoms

Overt signs of anemia are listed in Table 13.2. Cardiomegaly and high-output heart failure also are possible in severe cases.

Although the symptoms of anemia are distinctive, they can also be manifestations of other disorders, such as cancer or an inflammatory process. A comprehensive history and physical examination are important in the assessment of the anemic patient. More specifically, dietary habits, drug histories, surgical procedures, and occupation should be documented. Close questioning about blood loss, menses, gastrointestinal symptoms, and history of pregnancy provides useful information.

In addition, vitamin deficiencies may cause other symptoms before overt anemia develops. As noted in Table 13.2, neurologic or oral changes may occur with B_{12} deficiency and may precede anemia.

Table 13.1 ▪ Normal Hematologic Values by Age

	Mean Hb (−2 SD)		Mean Hct (−2 SD)	
Age	Conventional (g/dL)	SI (mmol/L)	Conventional (g/dL)	SI (mmol/L)
1–3 days	18.0 (14.0)	11.2 (8.7)	54 (42)	0.54 (0.42)
6 mo–2 yr	12.0 (10.5)	7.4 (6.5)	36 (32)	0.36 (0.32)
12–18 yr				
Male	14.5 (13.0)	9.0 (8.1)	43 (38)	0.43 (0.38)
Female	14.0 (12.0)	8.7 (7.5)	41 (36)	0.41 (0.36)
Adult				
Male	15.5 (13.5)	9.6 (8.4)	47 (40)	0.47 (0.40)
Female	14.0 (12.0)	8.7 (7.5)	41 (36)	0.41 (0.36)

Source: Reference 1.

Table 13.2 ▪ Signs and Symptoms of Anemia and Vitamin Deficiency

Anemia in General	Iron Deficiency	Vitamin B_{12} Deficiency
Fatigue	Developmental delays	Peripheral neuropathy
Pallor	Behavioral disturbances	"Strange" feeling in extremities
Dyspnea	Altered central nervous system development	Loss of hand coordination
Light-headedness	Impaired work capacity	Deterioration in handwriting
Dizziness	Preterm delivery	Tingling of extremities
Palpitations	Delivery of low-birthweight baby	Loss of proprioception
Increased heart rate		Depression
Chest pain		Psychosis
Loss of concentration		Spinal cord degeneration
		Sore tongue or mouth

Source: References 1–5, 18, 27, 35, 55.

Diagnosis

A detailed medical and medication history along with hematologic and biochemical tests, including a full blood screen, are essential for identifying the type of anemia and in many cases directing the treatment. As the nutritional anemias progress in stages (normal, negative nutrient balance, nutrient depletion, nutrient deficiency, anemia), monitoring early indicators of depletion may prevent the progression to overt anemia. Risk factors for certain vitamin deficiencies (Table 13.3) and reported symptoms (Table 13.2) often suggest the possible cause of anemia or alert the physician to the potential for anemia.

Hematologic Tests

Hematologic tests (Table 13.4) are less expensive and more available than biochemical tests and provide information on the characteristics of the red blood cells. A full blood screen provides information on Hb and Hct levels as well as cell size and color.

Many aspects of the cellular elements of blood can be quantified by automated blood analyzers, including blood Hb concentration, cell counts, and the mean corpuscular volume (MCV). From these primary measurements, the Hct, mean corpuscular hemoglobin (MCH), and the mean corpuscular hemoglobin concentration (MCHC) are calculated automatically. MCV, MCH, and MCHC are collectively known as the erythrocyte indices. The MCV correlates with cell size (smaller cells take up less volume) and is particularly valuable in differentiating microcytic anemias, which have a reduced MCV (less than 80 fL), from macrocytic anemias, which have a greater than normal MCV (more than 100 fL). However, the MCV may appear normal in combination anemias, where the microcytic cells of iron deficiency are counterbalanced by the macrocytic cells of a B_{12} or folate deficiency. In this instance, a peripheral blood smear can aid in identifying the existence of a mixed anemia. The MCH and MCHC provide information on cell color (lower Hb, less color). Hypochromic anemias such as iron deficiency anemia have a low MCHC, indicating lower-than-normal Hb concentrations. Another parameter, the red blood cell distribution width (RDW), expressed as the coefficient of variation of the volume of distribution width, indicates the variation in erythrocyte size in a blood sample. A characteristic of iron deficiency anemia is an increased RDW, reflecting the anisocytosis seen in blood smears.

Other hematologic investigations include reticulocyte counts, differential white cell count, platelet count, and microscopic examination of peripheral blood smears and bone marrow aspirates. The normal life span of an erythrocyte is 120 days. As old erythrocytes are removed from the circulation by reticuloendothelial cells, they are replaced by young erythrocytes from the bone marrow. These immature cells, called reticulocytes, make up 1 to 1.5% of the total erythrocyte population in a normal person. Because reticulocytes are a young population of red blood cells, they are an important marker of bone marrow activity. Reticulocytosis, an increase in reticulocyte numbers, indicates increased bone marrow activity. Transient reticulocytosis often occurs in response to iron, B_{12}, or folic acid therapy for the respective deficiency states.

Biochemical Tests

Biochemical tests (Table 13.4) for assessing anemias include measurement of serum vitamin concentrations (iron, B_{12}, folate), transport proteins (transferrin, transcobalamin II [TCII]), saturation of protein-binding sites

Table 13.3 ▪ High-Risk Populations for Development of Nutritional Anemias

Population	Predisposing Factors	Type of Anemia
Children[3,16]	Growth, poor diet	Iron deficiency
Teenagers[3]	Growth, diet, menstruation	Iron deficiency
Women[3,16]	Menstruation, diet	Iron deficiency
Pregnant women[3,16]	Fetal needs, diet	Iron, folate deficiency
Older adults[4,70,71]	Achlorhydria	Iron, B_{12} deficiency
	Diet	Iron, B_{12}, folate deficiency
	Underlying disease	Iron, B_{12}, folate deficiency
	Organ function	Iron, B_{12}, folate deficiency
	Drug-induced	Iron, B_{12}, folate deficiency
Alcoholics[69]	Diet	Iron, folate deficiency
	Liver or gastrointestinal disease	Iron, B_{12}, folate deficiency
Patients with human immunodeficiency virus[4,72,73]	Achlorhydria	Iron, B_{12} deficiency
	Diet	Iron, B_{12}, folate deficiency
	Drug-induced	B_{12}, folate deficiency

Table 13.4 ▪ Selected Hematologic and Biochemical Parameters

Component	Specimen		Representative Reference Range: Conventional	Representative Reference Range: SI
Hematocrit	B	M	45–52%	0.45–0.52
		F	37–48%	0.37–0.48
Hemoglobin	B	M	13–18 g/dL	8.1–11.2 mmol/L
		F	12–16 g/dL	7.4–9.9 mmol/L
Erythrocyte count	B		4.2–5.9 × 10^6/mm	4.2–5.9 × 10^6/mm
Reticulocyte count	B		0.5–1.5% erythrocytes	
Mean corpuscular volume	Ery			80–94 fmol
Mean corpuscular hemoglobin	Ery		27–32 pg	1.7–2.0 fmol
Mean corpuscular hemoglobin concentration	Ery		32–36 g/dL	19–22.8 mmol/L
Red cell distribution width	Ery		11.5–14.5%	
Iron	S	M	80–200 μg/dL	14–35 μmol/L
		F	60–190 μg/dL	11–29 μmol/L
Transferrin	S		170–370 mg/dL	1.7–3.7 g/L
Total iron-binding capacity	S		250–410 g/mL	45–72 μmol/L
Transferrin saturation	S		20–55%	
Transferrin receptors	S			2.8–8.5 mg/L
Ferritin	S	M > F	1.5–30.0 μg/dL	15–300 μg/L
Zinc protoporphyrin	S		<70 μg/dL red cell	<80 μmol/mol heme
Folate (as pteroglutamic acid)				
Normal	S		2–10 ng/mL	4–22 nmol/L
Borderline	S		1–1.9 ng/mL	2.5–4 nmol/L
	Ery		150–800 ng/mL	
Vitamin B_{12}	S		200–1000 pg/mL	150–750 pmol/L
Methylmalonic acid (mean ± 3 SD)	S			53–376 nmol/L
Homocysteine (mean ± 3 SD)	S			4.1–21.3 μmol/L
Holo-transcobalamin II	P			Mean for control group +2 SD

Source: References 1, 6, 7, 9, 10.

B, whole blood; *M,* male; *F,* female; *Ery,* erythrocyte; *S,* serum.

Table 13.5 ▪ Selected Laboratory Characteristics of the Nutritional Anemias

Type	Mean Corpuscular Volume	Red Blood Cell Distribution Width	Peripheral Smear	Additional Investigations
Iron deficiency	L[a]	H	Hypochromic, microcytic	↓ Iron, ↓ ferritin, ↑ transferrin, ↑ zinc protoporphyrin, ↑ TfR
Vitamin B_{12} deficiency[b]	H	H	Macrocytic	↓ S-vitamin B_{12}, ↑ methylmalonic acid, ↑ homocysteine, ↑ intrinsic factor antibodies
Folate deficiency	H	H	Macrocytic	↓ S-folate,[c] ↓ erythrocyte folate
Chronic disease	L	H	Hypochromic, normocytic	↓ Iron, ↓ transferrin, nl TfR
	N	N	Normochromic, normocytic	nl TfR
Blood loss	N	N	Normochromic, normocytic	Clinical evidence, occult blood loss

L, low; *H,* high; *TfR,* transferrin receptors; *nl,* normal.

[a]Normal in early iron deficiency.

[b]Includes pernicious anemia.

[c]Varies with diet.

(transferrin saturation), and storage amounts (ferritin). More specific tests also can be used: serum transferrin receptors (TfR), erythrocyte zinc protoporphyrin (ZPP) concentration (iron deficiency), homocysteine (Hcy) and methylmalonic acid (MMA) serum concentrations (B_{12} and folate deficiencies), and antibodies to intrinsic factor (IF) or parietal cells (B_{12}).[3–12]

Selected laboratory characteristics of iron deficiency anemia and megaloblastic anemias are summarized in Table 13.5. Generally, diagnosis of a nutritional anemia depends on an accurate and complete medical, drug, and symptom history and assessment of multiple laboratory and biochemical tests rather than a single result.

TREATMENT

Treating nutritional anemia involves identifying and correcting the cause if possible, replenishing deficient nutrients, and alleviating symptoms. This may involve restoring missing nutrients, restoring blood volume by transfusions, or treating the cause by medical or surgical methods. Inadequate dietary intake of nutrients often is a cause of nutritional deficiencies that may lead to anemia. Dietary counseling and follow-up may be sufficient for some patients, but many need supplementation. Careful assessment of the patient's drug history may help identify possible pharmacotherapeutic agents that affect nutrient status or red blood cells directly. Some deficiencies may necessitate long-term or lifelong therapy, and patients must be counseled and monitored appropriately.

Iron Deficiency Anemia

Iron deficiency occurs when the body iron is insufficient for the normal formation of Hb, iron-containing enzymes, and other functional iron compounds such as myoglobin and those of the cytochrome system. Iron deficiency can be classified according to its severity (Table 13.6): normal stores, negative iron balance, iron store depletion (low serum ferritin), decreased serum iron (low serum iron, increased total iron-binding capacity [TIBC]), and anemia (reduced Hb with microcytic, hypochromic erythrocytes).[3] Erythrocytes of patients with mild, early-stage iron deficiency often appear to be normal in color and size (i.e., normochromic, normocytic).

Other conditions with low MCV and MCHC, such as thalassemia and anemia of chronic disease, generally can be differentiated from iron deficiency anemia by assessment of various laboratory values (Table 13.6).

PHYSIOLOGIC IMPORTANCE OF IRON

Iron is an essential element for many physiologic processes, including erythropoiesis, tissue respiration, and several enzyme-catalyzed reactions.[1] The average adult body contains 3 to 5 g elemental iron, distributed into two major components: functional iron and storage.[1,3] Functional iron exists predominantly as Hb (1.5 to 3 g) in circulating erythrocytes, with lesser amounts in myoglobin and tissue enzymes.

Hb is the oxygen-binding protein in erythrocytes of vertebrates; it transports oxygen absorbed from the lungs to the tissues. Each Hb molecule consists of a globin surrounded by four heme groups, which contain all the iron. Globin consists of linked pairs of polypeptide chains. Fetal Hb has two α- and two γ-globin chains. In normal erythrocyte development, the γ-chains are replaced by β-chains, and a normal human adult has two α- and two β-chains. The composition of these chains differs in patients with genetically determined disorders such as thalassemia and sickle cell anemia. (See Chapter 14, Other Anemias.)

Hb forms an unstable, reversible bond with oxygen, allowing oxygen release at lower oxygen tension, as is encountered in the tissues. In iron deficiency anemia and other chronic anemias, Hb has a reduced affinity for oxygen. This allows oxygen to transfer more readily from the erythrocytes to the tissues. Myoglobin, a hemoprotein in muscle, accepts oxygen from Hb in the peripheries and acts as an oxygen store in muscle. If oxygen supply is limited, myoglobin releases its oxygen to cytochrome oxidase, the terminal enzyme in the mitochondrial respiratory chain, which has a higher affinity for oxygen than myoglobin and so allows oxidative phosphorylation to occur.

Table 13.6 ▪ Laboratory Values in Various Stages of Iron Deficiency

Stage	Serum Ferritin (μg/L)	Serum Iron	Total Iron-Binding Capacity	Zinc Protoporphyrin	Transferrin Saturation (%)	Transferrin Receptors	Hemoglobin
Normal	>15	nl	nl	nl	>16	nl	nl
Negative balance	>15	nl	nl	nl	>16	nl	nl
Iron store depletion	<15	nl	nl	nl	>16	nl	nl
Iron deficiency	<15	↓	nl	↑	<16	↑	nl
Iron deficiency anemia	<15	↓	↑	↑	<16	↑	↓
Anemia of chronic disease	↓, ↑ or nl	nl	nl or ↓	↑	nl or ↓	nl	↓
Thalassemia	nl or ↑	nl	nl	nl	nl	nl	↓

Source: References 1, 3, 10, 18.
nl, normal.

Transferrin, a β-globulin synthesized by the liver, is a specific iron-binding protein in blood that transports iron through the plasma and extravascular spaces. Each molecule of transferrin can bind two molecules of iron in the ferric state. In normal circumstances, it is only 30 to 50% saturated. The ability of transferrin to bind iron is called the iron-binding capacity. TIBC, which reflects serum transferrin concentrations, is a well-recognized value in the investigation of anemias. It represents the amount of iron that can bind to transferrin to give 100% saturation of the binding sites. The TIBC is high in iron deficiency and low in iron overload. Most cells obtain their iron from transferrin. In the case of reticulocytes and developing erythrocytes in the bone marrow, most of the iron taken up is used for Hb synthesis.

Storage iron (0.3 to 1.5 g), in the form of ferritin and hemosiderin, which is located mainly in the parenchymal cells of the liver and the reticuloendothelial cells of the bone marrow, spleen, and liver, replenishes functional iron. Iron stores account for one-third of body iron in healthy men. Iron stores are more variable and are generally lower in children and women of childbearing potential. Low iron stores are an early sign of iron deficiency and may help differentiate between iron deficiency anemia and other causes of anemia (Table 13.6).

Iron Needs

Body iron usually is kept constant by a delicate balance between the amounts lost and absorbed. There is no physiologic mechanism for excreting iron in humans. Consequently, there is only a limited ability to compensate for excessive loss or absorption of iron. Iron balance is a conservative system, and in the normal adult, even if iron intake is negligible, it takes at least 2 to 3 years to develop iron deficiency.

Iron needs are determined by total losses from the body. Daily iron needs vary according to age and sex (Table 13.7). Total daily iron loss amounts to 1 mg/day in men. Iron losses in women of childbearing potential are higher than those in men because of menstruation and pregnancy. Iron is lost from the gastrointestinal tract by sloughing of iron-containing mucosal cells and extravasation of erythrocytes, by skin exfoliation, and by shedding of urinary tract epithelial cells. Iron loss through sweat is minimal, so manual laborers working in hot conditions are not at risk.

Blood loss in menstruating women varies, but if it exceeds 80 mL, it can lead to iron deficiency. Average iron losses through menstruation are about 0.3 to 0.5 mg/day. Menstrual iron losses are lower in women taking oral contraceptives and higher in those using an intrauterine device.[1,3]

Iron needs increase to 3 to 4 mg/day during pregnancy to account for obligatory losses, the expanded maternal erythrocyte mass that occurs in pregnancy, and the placenta and fetus. Iron needs are greatest in the second and third trimester, when the highest fetal erythrocyte needs occur. Some of the iron incorporated in the expanded maternal erythrocyte mass returns to the iron pool after pregnancy, but peripartum blood loss partly nullifies this contribution. Because menstruation does not start until several weeks after delivery, iron losses are reduced. However, breastfeeding offsets some of the gain.[1,3]

The need for iron is high in the first year of life and throughout childhood because of rapid growth and erythropoiesis during this period. Normal full-term infants need to absorb a minimum of 0.3 mg of iron daily in the first year of life. Premature infants can need up 1 mg/day. Children's iron needs increase with age (Table 13.7).

Iron Absorption

Iron absorption is regulated by iron needs and body stores. When iron stores are low or depleted, a higher proportion of available iron is absorbed. Absorption decreases when the stores are replete. The serum ferritin concentration, which reflects body iron stores, is inversely related to iron absorption. However, this feedback process can be overwhelmed when large amounts of iron are presented for

Table 13.7 ▪ Recommended Daily Allowances for Iron, Folic Acid, and Vitamin B_{12}

Category	Age (yr)	Iron (mg)	Age (yr)	Folic Acid (μg)	Age	Vitamin B_{12} (μg)
Infants	0–0.5	6	0–0.5	25	0–0.5	0.3
	0.5–1	10	0.5–1	35	0.5–1	0.5
Children	1–10	10	1–3	50	1–3	0.7
			4–6	75	4–6	1
			7–10	100	7–10	1.4
Boys and men	11–18	12	11–14	150	11+	2
	19+	10	15+	200		
Girls and women	11–50	15	11–14	200	11+	2
	51+	10	15+	180		
Pregnant women		30		400		2.2
Lactating women		15		260–280		2.6

Source: Values determined by the Food and Nutrition Board of the National Research Council. Recommended daily allowances provide adequate nutrition in most healthy people under usual environmental stresses and are not minimum needs.

absorption (e.g., in iron overdosing or toxicity cases).[1] In some clinical states such as primary hemochromatosis, thalassemia, and sideroblastic anemia, iron absorption remains normal and even elevated despite increased iron stores.

The iron content of food and its bioavailability determine whether the diet can meet physiologic needs. Dietary iron is present as two major pools: heme iron and nonheme iron. Heme iron, found only in meats, is two to three times more absorbable than nonheme iron, found in plant-based and iron-fortified foods. Ingested heme compounds and organic nonheme iron complexes are broken down in the acid environment of the stomach to ferric ions and heme molecules, respectively. The stomach's acidity promotes reduction of iron from the ferric state to the ferrous state, which is better absorbed. Patients with achlorhydria secondary to age or gastrectomy tend to absorb nonheme iron poorly.[1,3,13–15]

Iron is absorbed primarily in the upper duodenum. The iron-absorptive capacity is limited by the rate at which iron is transferred from the intestinal lumen to the plasma. The reduced (ferrous) iron binds to specific sites on the lumen and is actively carried across the intestinal membrane. Iron absorbed by these cells is incorporated into an iron carrier pool, most of which is deposited as ferritin or used by the mitochondria for enzyme synthesis. It is then lost by sloughing during the usual intestinal cell turnover. A smaller proportion of the iron from the carrier pool is transferred to the plasma, where the ferric form binds tightly to transferrin.

A number of factors can inhibit or promote iron absorption (Table 13.8). Foods that can reduce iron absorption by forming less-soluble complexes include coffee, tea, milk and milk products, eggs, whole-grain breads and cereals, and any food containing bicarbonates, carbonates, oxalates, or phosphates. Commercial processing or enhancers can improve absorption from food in some cases. Enhancers of nonheme iron absorption are food acids such as citric, lactic, or ascorbic acids and meats.[3,13–15] Ascorbic acid, the most powerful promoter, has a dose-related effect on nonheme iron absorption. In its presence, ferric iron is converted to the ferrous state, maintaining iron solubility in the alkaline environment of the duodenum and upper jejunum. Ascorbic acid also forms an alkaline-stable chelate with ferric chloride in the stomach. Meat, itself a rich source of iron, promotes absorption of nonheme iron. Quantitatively, 1 g meat enhances nonheme iron absorption to about the same extent as 1 mg of ascorbic acid. Citric acid, a common food additive and a less powerful promoter of iron absorption, has an additive effect to ascorbic acid.

Table 13.8 ▪ Factors Associated with Iron Absorption

Factor	Associations
Promoting absorption Inorganic iron	Ionic iron, particularly in the ferrous form, is better absorbed than ferric iron and organically bound iron.
Ascorbic acid	Ascorbic acid helps to convert ferric iron to ferrous iron.
Acid	Gastric hydrochloric acid promotes the release and conversion of dietary iron to the ferrous form.
Chelates	Iron chelated to low-molecular-weight substances such as sugars (fructose and sucrose), amino acids, and succinate facilitates iron binding to the intestinal mucosa.
Clinical states	Iron deficiency, increased erythropoiesis, pregnancy, anoxia, and pyridoxine deficiency promote absorption.
Reducing absorption Alkaline	Alkaline pancreatic secretions containing phosphate probably convert iron to insoluble ferric hydroxide; antacids.
Dietary	Dietary phosphates and phytates in cereals and tannins in tea probably complex iron.
Clinical states	Chronic diarrhea, steatorrhea, adequate iron stores, decreased erythropoiesis, and acute or chronic inflammation reduce absorption.

EPIDEMIOLOGY

Occurrence

Iron deficiency, estimated to occur in more than 2.5 billion people throughout the world, is the most common cause of nutritional anemia.[3,16–18] Data from the third Nutritional Health and Nutrition Examination Survey (NHANES III) in the United States indicated that the incidence of iron deficiency was highest for toddlers aged 1 to 2 years (9%), adolescent girls (9%), and women of childbearing potential (11%), with iron deficiency anemia occurring in 3%, 2%, and 5%, respectively. This corresponds to approximately 240,000 toddlers and 3.3 million women having iron deficiency anemia. For women of childbearing potential, iron deficiency was more common in minorities, people with lower incomes, and multiparous women. Iron deficiency occurred in less than 1% of men and adolescent boys between 12 and 50 years of age and in 4% of men 70 years and older.[19]

Etiology

The primary causes of iron deficiency are listed in Table 13.9. Blood loss from any body site is the major cause of iron deficiency in men and nonmenstruating women and girls. Bleeding may be occult or overt. A common site of blood loss is the gastrointestinal tract. If bleeding is not obvious, a test for occult blood in the stool may give the first indication of blood loss. Common sources of blood loss in the gastrointestinal tract are peptic ulcers and esophageal varices. Nonsteroidal anti-inflammatory agents such as aspirin and indomethacin often are responsible for gastrointestinal bleeding, especially if taken with warfarin. In the absence of upper gastrointestinal symptoms,

Table 13.9 ▪ Factors Associated with Iron Deficiency

Factor	Association
Dietary	Starvation, poverty, vegetarianism, religious practice, food fads
Blood loss	
Women and girls	Menstruation, postmenopausal bleeding, pregnancy
General	Esophageal varices, peptic ulcer, drug-induced gastritis, carcinomas of stomach and colon, ulcerative colitis, hemorrhoids, renal or bladder lesions (hematuria), hookworm infestation, other organ bleeding (hemoptysis), frequent blood donation, athletic training, widespread bleeding disorders
Malabsorption	Celiac disease (gluten-induced enteropathy), partial and total gastrectomy, chronic inflammation
Increased requirements	Rapid growth (as in childhood and adolescence), pregnancy

investigations should be directed to the lower gastrointestinal tract. Bleeding hemorrhoids rarely result in anemia, but neoplasms are a common cause of bleeding, particularly in older adults. The incidence of colon cancer, which can cause bleeding, increases 40-fold between ages 40 and 80. Other causes of gastrointestinal blood loss include hookworm infestation, Meckel's diverticulum, and ulcerative colitis. Hookworm is a major cause of iron deficiency anemia in tropical areas.

Iron deficiency has also been noted in athletes, particularly adolescent girls, marathon runners, and other endurance athletes. Up to 50% of adolescent female athletes demonstrate some degree of iron depletion, but anemia is uncommon. Blood loss is believed to result from ischemia of the gastrointestinal tract because blood is shunted to muscles during prolonged exercise. Marathon runners can lose at least 3 mg iron daily for several days after a marathon race. Another short-term anemia related to sports is the dilutional anemia that can result from plasma volume expansion in the early weeks of conditioning.[20,21]

Poor nutrition, defective intake, and decreased assimilation of iron rarely cause iron deficiency in people living in Western countries. Iron deficiency caused by inadequate dietary iron intake is predominantly a problem of infants, children, and pregnant women, whose daily needs are higher. In some populations, where the diet is mainly of vegetable origin with little meat, women are likely to suffer from nutritional iron deficiency. Iron malabsorption may occasionally cause iron deficiency, although it is rarely an important cause unless iron stores are low or there are other contributing factors such as blood loss, pregnancy, or poor nutrition. The two most common conditions in which iron absorption is a problem are gluten enteropathy (celiac disease) and gastrectomy. Other conditions associated with iron deficiency anemia include pernicious anemia,[22,23] pica syndrome,[24] and chronic inflammatory disease such as rheumatoid arthritis.[1,2]

CLINICAL PRESENTATION AND DIAGNOSIS

Signs and Symptoms

Iron deficiency precedes the manifestations of anemia. Most people with iron deficiency have minimal anemia and are asymptomatic.[25] Progression to iron deficiency anemia is often insidious, although mildly lowered Hb concentrations generally decrease work capacity. The development of symptoms depends on the rate of iron loss and the body's ability to compensate. Symptoms generally become evident when the blood Hb concentration falls below 6.2 mmol/L (10.0 g/dL), although some patients remain asymptomatic even with Hb concentrations of 4.3 mmol/L (7.0 g/dL).

The usual signs and symptoms of iron deficiency anemia are often present (Table 13.2). Other problems caused by the gross epithelial changes associated with chronic iron deficiency include brittle or spoon-shaped nails, angular stomatitis, atrophic tongue, and pharyngeal and esophageal webs causing dysphagia and atrophic gastric mucosa. Iron deficiency, in addition to its hematologic effects, may also be associated with diverse problems such as impaired work performance;[2,3] low birthweight, prematurity, and increased perinatal mortality;[2,3] and impaired psychomotor behavior, cognitive function, and central nervous system development in infants and young children.[18,26,27]

A common symptom of iron deficiency anemia is pica, a condition in which the person craves unusual substances that generally have nutritional value. Pagophagia, or habitual ice eating, is a common form of pica in some communities. Other people consume earth and particles of clay cooking pots. Such ingestions have led to metabolic problems, including heavy metal poisoning.[24]

Diagnosis

Most cases of iron deficiency anemia are identified on the basis of a medical history, full blood count, and peripheral smears.[1–3,9] In iron deficiency anemia, hematologic changes are evident only after all body iron stores have been depleted and there is insufficient iron to maintain normal erythrocyte morphology and mass (Table 13.6). Blood Hb concentrations and erythrocyte numbers are normal in mild cases. Serum ferritin is the first parameter to change with iron deficiency. As the deficiency worsens, the MCV and erythrocyte count decrease markedly, the RDW increases, and eventually, the Hb decreases. When Hb concentrations are 4.4 mmol/L (7.0 g/dL) or less for women or 5.6 mmol/L (9.0 g/dL) or less for men, microscopic examination of peripheral blood smears shows hypochromia and poikilocytosis.

Although the ultimate proof of iron deficiency is the absence of stainable iron in bone marrow aspirates, this procedure is not used routinely because it is painful and expensive. Peripherally, the proportion of reticulocytes usually is normal, but transient increases may follow acute hemorrhage or treatment with iron. The white cell count and platelets generally are normal.

Serum ferritin concentration is an early and specific indicator of body iron stores and is very useful in distinguishing iron deficiency from other causes of microcytic anemia. Ferritin concentrations fall in iron deficiency states but increase abnormally in iron storage conditions. Serum ferritin concentrations of less than 15 μg/L (normal, 15 to 300 μg/L) generally are diagnostic for iron deficiency in adults (Table 13.6). However, interpretation of ferritin levels entails consideration of other patient factors, such as coexisting inflammatory processes, liver disease, or malignancy. Ferritin is an acute phase reactant to inflammatory diseases such as rheumatoid arthritis or acute infection. In these diseases, serum ferritin concentrations increase, with the lower level of normal increasing to 50 μg/L. Patients with levels between 12 μg/L and 50 μg/L should be investigated further for iron deficiency anemia. An abnormal release of ferritin from hepatocytes can also occur with acute hepatic necrosis or inflammation. To rule out iron deficiency anemia in patients with an inflammatory disease or liver disease, especially hepatitis, other tests, such as ZPP or serum TfR concentration, which are not affected by these underlying processes, should be used.

Final heme synthesis involves the incorporation of iron into the protoporphyrin ring. When iron is insufficient to support heme production, zinc is incorporated into the protoporphyrin and ZPP is produced instead of heme. Serum concentrations of ZPP, which measure the amount of protoporphyrin not incorporated into heme, increase when insufficient iron is available for Hb synthesis. A concentration of more than 80 μmol/mol heme indicates iron deficiency. This measurement has less daily variability than serum iron concentration or transferrin saturation and is an earlier indicator of iron-deficient erythropoiesis than anemia. However, it is not as early an indicator of deficiency as serum ferritin. Because it correlates with deficiency at the tissue level, some advocate its use before or concurrently with serum ferritin.[3,9,18] In assessing ZPP values, one must be aware that other conditions in which iron support for erythropoiesis is insufficient (lead poisoning, myelodysplastic syndromes, anemia of chronic disease) also result in increased ZPP concentrations.

Serum TfR measurement reflects the number of transferrin receptors on immature red cells and is an indication of bone marrow erythropoiesis. Whereas ferritin is an early indicator of iron deficiency, TfR measurement provides information on the later stages of iron deficiency, increasing only after iron stores are depleted.

However, it is not affected by inflammatory processes, and it is useful in differentiating iron deficiency from anemia caused by chronic disease, infection, or inflammation.[9,10,25,28,29] Use of the TfR:serum ferritin ratio has been advocated for earlier and more sensitive detection of iron deficiency.[28,29]

Serum iron levels and the TIBC are other traditional measures for evaluating iron deficiency. However, these are less sensitive and more variable than ferritin determinations and often are normal in the early stages of iron deficiency. A low serum iron with a high TIBC level generally is characteristic of iron deficiency. Normal to low serum iron levels with a normal or low TIBC is associated with anemias of chronic disease. In thalassemia, hemoglobinopathies, and sideroblastic anemia, serum iron levels are normal or high. Transferrin saturation, another indicator of body iron stores, is below 16% in most cases of iron deficiency anemia. Transferrin saturation levels below 5% are found only in iron deficiency. However, there is considerable overlap with anemias of chronic disease.

Assessment of the predictive values of some of these tests in patients without evidence of inflammatory disease showed that bone marrow examination and serum ferritin were 100% predictive in patients with iron depletion, iron deficiency (insufficient for erythropoiesis), and iron deficiency anemia. The ZPP values were normal (0% predictive value) with iron depletion but 100% predictive in patients with iron deficiency or iron deficiency anemia. Transferrin saturation had 0% predictive value for iron depletion, 71% for iron deficiency, 78% for mild iron deficiency anemia, and 96% for severe iron deficiency anemia. Hb concentrations were not predictive until anemia developed (100% for mild or severe anemia), and MCV was 22% predictive for mild and 100% predictive for severe anemia.[25]

Which tests are used to assess iron status depends on the patient's history and condition, the goal of the evaluation (early detection of iron depletion versus assessment of the existence or cause of an anemia), and laboratory equipment available. To check for anemia, Hb or Hct may be assessed, with other tests ordered if anemia is found. Monitoring iron depletion to prevent anemia includes using tests with sensitivity for the earlier stages of iron deficiency. Many clinicians use the ferritin test as the first-line test of iron status because it is an early indicator of iron store depletion. However, concurrent inflammatory or infectious processes or neoplasms reduce its reliability. Therefore, multiple tests often are used to assess iron status.

In the absence of a specialized hematology facility, a tentative diagnosis of iron deficiency can be made by giving a trial of iron therapy and monitoring Hb concentrations and reticulocyte counts. Significant reticulocytosis occurs 7 to 10 days after the start of treatment, and the Hb concentrations increase at a rate of 1.2 mmol/L/day (2 g/L/day) over 3 to 4 weeks. Inflammatory disease may retard reticulocytosis.

PREVENTION

Prevention is accomplished by identifying high-risk patients (Table 13.3) and correcting iron deficiencies before anemia develops. Management is directed toward identifying and treating the underlying cause of the iron deficiency and correcting the iron deficiency through diet or supplementation.

Dietary Manipulation

The primary prevention of iron deficiency, and hence anemia, should occur through dietary manipulation. For overall prevention of iron deficiency, food fortification has been recommended, especially in developing countries where diets do not contain iron-rich foods such as red meat.[30,31] Targeted fortification for infants through formula and commercial cereals and for schoolchildren through meal programs has been successful in developed countries. Widespread fortification of foods in the United States may account for the lower incidence of iron deficiency anemia in women of childbearing potential. However, even with fortification, iron deficiency and iron deficiency anemia still occur.[19,31] When dietary iron supplementation is not possible or adequate, oral supplementation should be initiated.

The U.S. Centers for Disease Control (CDC) recently published guidelines for preventing iron deficiency in high-risk groups.[3] In infants, the CDC recommends the following:

- Breastfeeding for 4 to 6 months after birth
- Use of 1 mg/kg/day of iron from supplemental foods or iron drops when breastfeeding is stopped
- Use of only iron-fortified infant formula as a substitute for breast milk
- Use of 2- to 4-mg/kg/day of iron drops (max 15 mg/day) for preterm or low-birthweight infants starting at 1 month and continuing until 12 months after birth
- Introduction of iron-fortified infant cereal at age 4 to 6 months (two or more servings should meet iron needs)

For adolescent girls and nonpregnant women of childbearing potential, iron-rich foods and foods that enhance iron absorption should be encouraged. For pregnant women, the CDC recommends starting oral low-dose (30 mg/day) iron supplementation at the first prenatal visit.[3]

Generally, iron stores become depleted by 4 months of age in term infants unless an adequate exogenous supply of iron is provided. Although breast milk is thought to provide enough iron to prevent deficiency, a study done in Argentina demonstrated a 27.8% incidence of iron deficiency anemia in children breastfed for 6 months and a 7.1% incidence in children who received formula.[32] This indicates the need for caution in relying solely on breast milk to meet iron needs through 6 months of age in all children. Maternal diet and amount of breast milk consumed may affect the amount of iron provided to the infant.

The iron content of infant formulas continues to be evaluated to ascertain the optimal amount of iron to prevent iron deficiency anemia. Lower iron concentrations (2.3 mg/L versus 12.7 mg/L and 3.0 mg/L versus 5 mg/L) in healthy, non–iron-deficient, term infants were as efficacious as higher concentrations in preventing iron deficiency anemia.[33,34] However, in a high-risk group of infants, an iron concentration of 12.8 mg/L was found to be superior to 1.1 mg/L in maintaining iron status (preventing iron deficiency) and psychomotor development.[35] This enforces the need to monitor therapy to ensure appropriate response and dosing.

Providing supplemental iron to other high-risk groups, such as children with inadequate dietary intake, women of childbearing potential, and pregnant women, continues to be recommended, but the optimal dosage and schedule are debated.[3,16,17,36,37] Anemic and nonanemic children 3 to 6 years of age who received 6 mg/kg elemental iron either daily, twice weekly, or weekly had similar hematologic response after 3 months of therapy. In the children with anemia, all three regimens reversed the anemia and replenished ferritin levels. The incidence of side effects was dramatically different between the dosing groups: 35.4%, 7.4%, and 0% for daily, twice weekly, and weekly administration, respectively, in children with anemia at the start of the study and 39.7%, 6.6%, and 5.7%, respectively, in the nonanemic children. The major complaints were anorexia, nausea, abdominal discomfort, constipation, and diarrhea.[38] This study, and other clinical trials in preschool-age children, adolescent girls, and pregnant women, have demonstrated that weekly iron supplementation provides similar efficacy with fewer side effects than daily iron therapy for the prevention and possible treatment of iron deficiency.[16,17,36] However, the design limitations of many of these studies have lessened the value of the results.[37]

Iron supplementation during pregnancy is controversial. Treatment can be geared toward prevention of iron deficiency anemia, prevention of iron store depletion, or avoidance of a negative iron balance. The CDC recommends universal treatment with 30 mg iron/day during pregnancy to prevent iron deficiency.[3] This can be done using a prescribed multivitamin and iron preparation or over-the-counter iron preparations. However, because iron can cause side effects and potentially affect absorption of other nutrients, selective supplementation only for women at risk of iron deficiency anemia also has been advocated.[16] The recommended dosages and schedules of iron supplements also vary from 30 to 240 mg/day to 60 mg once a week.[3,16] The higher dosages may be needed in populations in which the prepregnancy anemia rate is high because the women are more likely to have depleted iron stores before becoming pregnant. Patient tolerance and compliance with the iron regimen must be assessed. If patients are not able to tolerate daily supplementation, reducing the daily dosage or dosing on a weekly schedule are other options.

Screening for Iron Deficiency

The CDC recommends assessing infants for risk of iron deficiency and screening (Hb and/or Hct) those who are at risk (preterm, low birthweight, low-iron diet) at 9 to 12 months and at 15 to 18 months of age. In addition, the CDC recommends screening all nonpregnant girls starting in adolescence and continuing every 5 to 10 years throughout their childbearing years. Women with high risk factors (poor diet, excessive menstrual bleeding, chronic blood loss) should be screened annually. In pregnant women, Hb should be measured at the first prenatal visit to assess the need for iron replacement therapy or prophylaxis.[3]

TREATMENT

Although dietary improvements may reduce the risk of iron deficiency, the poor absorption of iron from foods limits the usefulness of dietary therapy in correcting an existing deficiency. Therefore, iron deficiency generally is corrected with oral or parenteral iron. Because indiscriminate iron administration can delay the diagnosis of underlying causes, a workup should be completed before therapy is initiated. Most iron therapy is given by the oral route, with few situations justifying the use of parenteral iron. With appropriate therapy, the Hb levels improve within a few weeks, and the patient feels better. Adequate iron must be supplied in the early stages of treatment to optimize the response.

Pharmacotherapy

Oral Iron Therapy

Oral iron supplementation is safer, more convenient, and less expensive than parenteral therapy. Oral iron preparations are salt forms, which vary in elemental iron content, cost, and effectiveness. Iron absorption from ferrous salts is considered better than that from ferric salts.

The dosage of the iron product is based on the elemental iron content. Generally, 30 to 40 mg elemental iron is used to treat iron deficiency states. These numbers are derived from calculating the maximum rate of Hb regeneration:

$$0.25 \text{ g Hb/100 mL blood/day} \times 5000 \text{ mL blood} \times 3.4 \text{ mg Fe/1 g Hb} = 40 \text{ mg Fe/day}$$

Because only 10 to 20% of iron is absorbed, 200 to 400 mg iron would result in absorption of 40 mg elemental iron. Ferrous sulfate tablets contain only 20% elemental iron (60 mg Fe/300-mg tablet). Therefore, 1000 to 2000 mg ferrous sulfate would result in absorption of 40 mg elemental iron (200 mg/20% or 400 mg/20%). This accounts for the standard dosing of ferrous sulfate at 300 mg three times a day (180 mg elemental iron per day). When switching from one form of iron to another, care must be taken in calculating the dosages of different salts needed to provide equivalent elemental iron quantities (Table 13.10). Maximum absorption occurs if iron is taken before or between meals.

The most common side effects of oral iron therapy are epigastric distress, abdominal cramping, nausea, diarrhea, and constipation caused by gastric irritation. The reported incidence of these side effects ranges from 15 to 46% with daily dosing.[1,16,39] These side effects appear to be dose related. Options for minimizing these side effects include reducing the daily dosage, taking the iron with food (at the expense of lower absorption), or changing to once-a-week dosing.[16,39] Use of enteric-coated products to minimize gastrointestinal effects is not recommended because the coating prevents dissolution in the stomach, thus minimizing iron absorption.[1,14] Iron therapy can also cause the stools to appear black, and patients should be educated about differences between iron stool changes and those associated with gastrointestinal bleeding.

Iron absorption may be reduced in patients with reduced gastric acid production or prior gastrointestinal surgeries. When an inability to absorb iron is suspected, an oral iron absorption test should be administered. This consists of administering an oral bolus dose of 325 mg ferrous sulfate (65 mg elemental iron) and measuring the

Table 13.10 ▪ Common Oral Iron Preparations

Proprietary Name	Active Ingredient	Elemental Iron	Iron (%)
Tablets			
Ferrous sulfate USP (generic)	Ferrous sulfate	60 mg/300 mg tablet 65 mg/325 mg tablet	20
Feosol	Ferrous sulfate, dried	65 mg/325 mg tablet	32
Ferrous gluconate USP (generic)	Ferrous gluconate	34 mg/300 mg tablet	12
Fergon	Ferrous gluconate	37 mg/320 mg tablet	
Ferrous fumarate	Ferrous fumarate	66 mg/200 mg tablet	33
Nephro-Fer	Ferrous fumarate	115 mg/350 mg tablet	
Liquids			
Feosol elixir	Ferrous sulfate	8.8 mg/mL	20
Fer-In-Sol syrup	Ferrous sulfate	3.6 mg/mL	
Fer-In-Sol drops	Ferrous sulfate	25 mg/mL	
Fer-Iron drops	Ferrous sulfate	25 mg/mL	
Fergon elixir	Ferrous gluconate	6.8 mg/mL	12
Feostat suspension	Ferrous fumarate	6.6 mg/mL	33
Feostat drops	Ferrous fumarate	25 mg/mL	

Source: Reference 74.
USP, U.S. Pharmacopeia.

serum iron level 2 and 4 hours later. The serum iron level should rise by 21 to 23 μmol/L (115 to 128 μg/dL). Failure to attain this response generally indicates decreased absorption.[14] Antacids, histamine-2 blockers, and proton pump inhibitors may also decrease iron absorption. A careful medication history should be obtained to check for potential drug interactions before an absorption test or parenteral therapy is initiated.

Parenteral Iron Therapy

Although the efficacy of parenteral iron therapy is similar to that of oral therapy, the potential for serious side effects limits its use. Indications for parenteral iron therapy include severe iron malabsorption, noncompliance with oral iron therapy, severe intolerance to oral therapy that cannot be controlled by altering the dosage or form of oral iron, and excessive iron loss or erythropoiesis such as that seen in patients on renal dialysis receiving erythropoietin.[14,15]

Iron dextran, a complex of ferric hydroxide and dextran, is the only parenteral iron preparation available in the United States. It is available in 2-mL single-dose amber vials that contain 50 mg elemental iron per milliliter.

The amount of parenteral iron needed to replenish iron stores and restore Hb levels in patients with iron deficiency anemia can be approximated using the following formula:[14,15]

$$\text{Dosage (mg)} = 0.3 \times \text{Body weight (lb)} \times [100 - (\text{Hb (g/dL)} \times 100/14.8)]$$

The formula can be modified to use kilograms instead of pounds:

$$\text{Dosage (mg)} = 0.66 \times \text{Body weight (kg)} \times [100 - (\text{Hb (g/dL)} \times 100/14.8)]$$

The iron dosage calculated is divided by 50 (50 mg iron/mL) to provide the volume of iron dextran injection needed. Therefore, a 160-pound (73-kg) man with a Hb level of 10 g/dL would need approximately 1560 mg iron or 31 mL iron dextran:

$$1557 \text{ mg} = 0.3 \times 160 \text{ lb} \times [100 - (10 \text{ g/dL} \times 100/14.8)]$$

$$1557 \text{ mg}/50 \text{ mg/mL} = 31 \text{ mL}$$

For children weighing less than 15 kg, a normal mean Hb of 12 g/L is used in place of 14.8 g/dL in this equation.[15]

These formulas do not take into account active blood loss. To determine the iron replacement dosage in these patients, one assumes that 1 mL of normochromic, normocytic erythrocytes contains 1 mg elemental iron:

$$\text{Dosage (mg)} = 1 \text{ mg iron/mL blood} \times \text{Blood loss (mL)} \times \text{Hct}$$

Therefore, a patient with blood loss of 250 mL and a Hct of 23% would need approximately 57.5 mg (1.2 mL) iron dextran. An alternative method is giving periodic injections until the Hb level has returned to a desired level. For each 1% increase in hemoglobin desired for a 70-kg adult, 1 mL iron dextran (50 mg) is needed. Maximum daily dosages for children are 0.5 mL for those weighing less than 4 kg, 1 mL for those 4 to 10 kg, and 2 mL for those weighing more than 10 kg.

Parenteral iron is administered by deep intramuscular injection into the upper quadrant of the buttock or intravenously, either as a bolus or a total-dose infusion (TDI). Regardless of the parental form used, a test dose of 25 mg (0.5 mL) should be administered before therapy is initiated to determine potential reactions. The test dose should be administered in the same manner (intramuscularly or intravenously) as the intended therapy, and patients should be monitored for an hour before receiving the full daily dose. Most adverse reactions occur during or shortly after the test dose and range from mild, transient reactions to life-threatening, anaphylactic reactions. The mild, transient reactions include dyspnea, headache, nausea, vomiting, flushing, itching, urticaria, fever, hives, and pain in the chest, abdomen, or back. These less serious side effects can be treated with nonsteroidal anti-inflammatory drugs. Anaphylactic reactions generally are characterized by sudden onset of respiratory difficulty or cardiovascular collapse. A reaction to the test dose warrants standard therapy for anaphylaxis, including epinephrine, diphenhydramine hydrochloride, and corticosteroids. These medications should be readily available during the administration of iron dextran. It is important to note that not all anaphylactic reactions are elicited by the test dose, and a severe reaction could occur during administration of the therapeutic dose even though the test dose was uneventful. Systemic reactions may also occur 1 to 2 days after parenteral iron therapy. These include lymphadenopathy, myalgias, arthralgias, and back pain.[14,15]

The incidence of adverse events is about 26%, but most are mild, transient reactions. Anaphylaxis occurs in about 2 to 5% of patients. The incidence of adverse events is higher in patients with rheumatoid arthritis (flare in symptoms or severe anaphylactic reaction), other collagen vascular disease, or infection and in patients receiving large iron dosages.[14,15] Parenteral iron therapy should be used cautiously in these patients, and premedication with methylprednisolone may be warranted.

If the intramuscular route is selected, a Z-track technique is recommended for administration. This technique involves moving the subcutaneous tissue over the injection site laterally before injecting the needle. After the iron is administered, the tissue is slowly released as the needle is removed, covering the needle track. This minimizes leakage through the needle track and skin staining. This technique is painful, and necrotic skin ulcerations have occurred after multiple intramuscular injections of iron dextran.[15] Another limitation of intramuscular therapy is that only 2 mL (100 mg) iron can be delivered per injection, and the manufacturer recommends that the total daily dosage not exceed 100 mg/day. Therefore, 160-lb man who needs 1560 mg iron would need 15 to 16 injections. For multiple injections, the buttock site should be alternated.

Intravenous iron dextran use prevents skeletal muscle deposition and local tissue reactions. However, this route results in a 10% incidence of serious adverse effects, including anaphylactic and other allergic reactions. The dosage can be delivered via multiple small bolus dose injections or by a continuous TDI. The bolus injections are given by slow intravenous push (50 mg/minutes or less), and as with the intramuscular injections, the dosage should not exceed 2 mL (100 mg) per injection and the total daily dosage should not exceed 100 mg.

The TDI method offers the advantages of providing the full therapeutic dosage, minimizing patient discomfort, and increasing convenience and compliance. Although TDI does not have FDA approval, it is commonly used in practice.[1,14,15] For TDI, the total dosage of iron dextran is diluted in 250 to 1000 mL of normal saline or 5% dextrose solution and administered over 4 to 6 hours. Local phlebitis is less likely to occur if normal saline is used as the diluent rather than dextrose. In addition, slower infusion rates may minimize irritation.

Contraindications to Iron Therapy

Iron preparations should not be used in conditions such as hemochromatosis and hemosiderosis, which already signify iron overload. In thalassemia and anemic conditions with chronic inflammatory disease such as rheumatoid arthritis, iron is contraindicated because these conditions have normal to high iron stores because of impaired use of iron. Care must be exercised in giving iron to alcoholic patients because elevated iron store, with or without hemochromatosis, can occur in this group. Patients with alcoholic liver disease such as cirrhosis generally do not suffer from hemochromatosis, but those with marked increases in iron deposition and body stores are likely to have genetically determined hemochromatosis. Iron should be used carefully in enteritis, diverticulitis, colitis, and ulcerative colitis because of local effects. Patients receiving repeated blood transfusions generally become iron overloaded because of the high erythrocyte iron content.

Iron Toxicity

Iron toxicity can be either acute, such as in overdose and accidental poisoning, or chronic, as in overload that occurs in hemochromatosis, hemosiderosis, and thalassemia. An iron-overloaded person usually has more than 4 g body iron. Iron, which is ordinarily stored in reticuloendothelial cells, is deposited as ferritin and hemosiderin into hepatocytes of the liver and eventually other tissues and organs. Hemochromatosis is associated with severe iron overload. Recently, noninvasive methods such as computed tomography and magnetic resonance imaging have been used to determine hepatic iron content.

The pathogenesis of iron overload is associated with increased mucosal iron absorption, the parenteral administration of iron as blood transfusions, or injections of therapeutic iron preparations. Diet is unlikely to cause iron overload unless other factors or problems are present. Normal people absorb the usual amounts of iron, even when the dietary iron load is increased 5 to 10 times. Amounts of 300 to 500 mg/day can be tolerated, although there are some exceptions. Worldwide, alcohol consumption is considered a common cause of iron overload. Another potential cause of iron overload is the controversial practice in some developed countries of fortifying food with iron. Although this addition may be useful for women, it may lead to a grossly excessive iron intake by men. The prevalence of hemochromatosis is 0.5%, which is higher than that of iron deficiency in men. Indiscriminate use of iron supplements can be harmful. Intrinsic metabolic abnormalities may account for increased iron absorption from the small intestine. Such abnormalities occur in primary idiopathic hemochromatosis (hereditary hemochromatosis) and in some anemias.

Iron overload secondary to anemias can be divided into two classes: that in patients with hypoplastic bone marrow, where the main source of iron is blood transfusion (e.g., aplastic anemia) and that in patients with hyperplastic bone marrow, where the iron excess results from increased iron absorption secondary to ineffective erythropoiesis (e.g., thalassemia major, sideroblastic anemia, and some hemolytic anemias). Treatment of transfusional iron overload generally consists of chelation therapy, such as deferoxamine.[40]

Monitoring Iron Deficiency Therapy

The primary objective is to reverse the anemia. Response to iron therapy generally is evident within the first week by reticulocytosis. Hb should also increase, although the rate of increase depends on the severity of the anemia, whether the cause of iron depletion (blood loss, increased needs) has resolved, and the usual range for an individual. The rate of increase for a man with a usual blood Hb of 10 mmol/L (16.0 g/dL) is faster than that for a pregnant woman who would normally have a blood Hb of about 6.5 mmol/L (10.5 g/dL). Serial blood hemoglobin measurements generally indicate an increase of 0.02 to 0.9 mmol/L per day (0.03 to 0.14 g/dL/day). However, for practical purposes, most patients are not reevaluated until after 3 or 4 weeks of oral therapy. Anemia is corrected within about 6 weeks. A rapid recovery generally indicates that the cause of iron loss is no longer present. Poor responders should be evaluated to ensure adequacy of the dosage to meet the patient's iron needs, patient compliance, potential sources of iron loss (bleeding), and potential drug interactions.

A second objective in instituting iron therapy is to replenish iron stores. Generally this is a nonurgent phase of treatment that takes about 4 to 6 months to accomplish. Serum ferritin concentration and iron saturation can be used as guides for this stage of therapy. Some patients need long-term iron therapy because of blood loss or malabsorption problems. Iron dosages for these patients should be adjusted to the losses. Periodic serum ferritin determinations should be used as a guide to the patient's iron status.

Megaloblastic Anemias

Megaloblastic anemia is a subclass of the macrocytic anemias. Nonmegaloblastic macrocytic anemias (those not resulting from disorders of DNA synthesis) are caused primarily by alcoholism, liver disease, and hypothyroidism. Megaloblastic anemia is characterized by a lowered blood Hb mass because of reduced erythropoiesis secondary to defective DNA synthesis in the developing erythroid cells of the bone marrow. Deficiencies of vitamin B_{12} or folate are the major causes of megaloblastic anemia, followed by drug-induced interference, either direct or indirect, with DNA synthesis or nutritional status.

Reduced availability or absence of one-carbon-unit coenzymes, such as methylcobalamin (active B_{12}) or formyltetrahydrofolic acid (active folic acid), results in impaired DNA synthesis in developing erythroid cells. These cells do not divide normally, and fewer large but well-hemoglobinized cells (megaloblasts) form in the bone marrow. The resulting megaloblasts are characterized by an abnormal nucleus because of greater cytoplasmic (rather than nuclear) maturity. Cells released into the circulation are larger than normal (macrocytic) and generally normochromic. Morphologic changes observed in the peripheral smear include macroovalocyte erythrocytes and multilobed neutrophilic granulocytes. These erythrocytes have a reduced life span.

In addition to the erythroid changes, similar effects on other hemopoietic cell lines in the bone marrow can lead to leukopenia, thrombocytopenia, or pancytopenia. Other rapidly dividing tissue can also be affected, particularly the mucosal epithelium of the gastrointestinal tract.[5,41,42]

It is important to distinguish anemia caused by B_{12} from folate deficiency in order to optimize treatment. A positive response (correction of anemia) to folate therapy does not confirm that folate deficiency was the cause of the anemia because folate supplementation can correct anemia caused by B_{12} deficiency. If this situation occurs, the B_{12} deficiency continues and the neurologic and gastrointestinal effects of B_{12} deficiency may develop.[5,43,44]

Vitamin B_{12} Deficiency Anemia

Like iron deficiency, B_{12} deficiency anemia is preceded by various stages of B_{12} depletion (Table 13.11).[45,46] Because the liver B_{12} stores are large (2 to 5 mg), B_{12} deficiency develops over many years, and the onset of symptoms tends to be gradual. In addition to affecting erythropoiesis, B_{12} deficiency results in neurologic and gastrointestinal manifestations (Table 13.2).

These symptoms do not appear to correlate with the development of anemia and often occur without evidence of hematologic affects of B_{12} deficiency. More importantly, the neurologic damage is progressive and, if untreated, can be permanent.

PHYSIOLOGIC IMPORTANCE OF VITAMIN B_{12}

Vitamin B_{12}, also known as cobalamin (Cbl), occurs in both synthetic and biologically active forms. It is a cobalt-containing vitamin that cannot be synthesized by mammalian tissue. Therefore, it must be obtained through dietary intake or supplementation. Some bacterial synthesis of B_{12} occurs in the large bowel and the cecum, but there is no absorption at these sites.

B_{12} is an essential cofactor for three known enzymatic reactions: conversion of methylmalonyl-Co A to succinyl-Co A, a critical step in propionate metabolism; methylation of Hcy to methionine by methionine synthetase; and interconversion of leucine and β-leucine by leucine 2,3-aminomutase.[4] B_{12} deficiency inhibits the activity of these enzymes, resulting in increases in metabolites such as MMA and Hcy. Some speculate that excess of 2-MMA (part of the conversion of methylmalonyl-Co A to succinyl-Co A) may be associated with the neurologic symptoms of B_{12} deficiency.[47]

Table 13.11 ▪ Stages of Vitamin B_{12} Deficiency

Stage	B_{12} Concentration	Mean Corpuscular Volume	Hemoglobin	Signs and Symptoms
Normal	Normal	Normal	Normal	None
Negative balance	Normal	Normal	Normal	None
Depletion of stores	Slight decrease	Normal	Normal	Possible
B_{12} deficient erythropoiesis	Moderate decrease	Increased	Normal	Possible
B_{12} deficiency anemia	Severe decrease	Increased	Decreased	Probable

Source: Modified from Goodman KI, Salt WV. Vitamin deficiency: important new concepts in recognition. Postgrad Med 88:147–158, 1990.

Vitamin B_{12} Needs

The daily requirement for humans is 0.5 to 1.0 μg. The average diet in the United States supplies 5 to 15 μg/day, but there is a wide variation. Some unusual diets, such as vegan, macrobiotic, or weight-reduction diets that drastically restrict food selection, may not meet the minimum daily needs. The total body stores amount to 2 to 5 mg, mainly in the liver. Thus, B_{12} deficiency takes years to develop.[42,45]

Vitamin B_{12} Absorption and Metabolism

Vitamin B_{12}, particularly at the usual low levels in foods, is well absorbed from the gastrointestinal tract by an orderly sequence of events involving three different binding proteins: R-proteins, IF, and TCII.[4,48,49] The R-proteins, a group of high-affinity, B_{12}-binding glycoproteins, are produced predominantly by leukocytes and are present in a variety of biologic secretions, including gastric fluid, plasma, saliva, tears, milk, and bile. Their function is not fully understood. Extravascular R-proteins, also known as cobalophilins, are the first binding proteins encountered by B_{12} as it is released from food in saliva and gastric juices. Although cobalamin can bind to R-proteins or IF, at the low gastric pH, binding to gastric R-proteins is favored. The relative binding of the vitamin also depends on the dosage and the amounts of R-protein and IF secreted. The cobalamin remains bound to R-proteins in the upper small intestine until pancreatic proteases such as trypsin partially degrade the complex, releasing B_{12}, which then binds to IF. IF, a specific B_{12}-binding glycoprotein, is synthesized and secreted by the parietal cells of the stomach. IF secretion parallels hydrochloric acid secretion. IF functions as a chaperone for B_{12} once it is freed from the cobalophilins. The IF–B_{12} complex, which is highly resistant to proteolysis, passes down the small intestine to the distal ileum, where it attaches to specific receptors on the luminal side of the mucosal cells (enterocytes). The attachment is not energy dependent, but extracellular calcium and a pH higher than 5.4 are needed. IF is released at the cell surface, and the vitamin is taken up by the enterocyte. Approximately 4 hours later, B_{12} exits the cells, bound to transcobalamin. The majority (approximately 80%) of B_{12} in the circulation is bound to transcobalamin I (TCI), an intravascular R-protein (also called haptocorrin). However, haptocorrins are not responsible for delivering B_{12} to peripheral tissues. TCII is the functional binding protein that delivers B_{12} to the tissues. Patients with TCII deficiency may have normal serum B_{12} concentrations because binding to TCI compensates for lowered TCII proteins. However, features of severe B_{12} deficiency occur because the TCI–B_{12} complex does not deliver the vitamin to the tissues.

Another mechanism for B_{12} absorption involves diffusion and not IF. This mechanism is biologically important only when large amounts are ingested and generally provides only small quantities of the vitamin. However, this mechanism is being explored as a potential method of providing oral B_{12} therapy to people with low levels of IF (pernicious anemia).

The daily cellular needs for B_{12} are low, and much of that ingested is stored in the liver. Vitamin B_{12} is conserved in the body by enterohepatic recycling. Biliary excretion of B_{12} is much higher than excretion in urine or feces. Vitamin B_{12} and its analogs in bile are excreted bound to biliary R-protein. When the complex comes into contact with pancreatic enzymes in the upper small intestine, B_{12} and its analogs are released because of biliary R-protein degradation. Only B_{12} binds to fresh IF; the analogs are excreted in the feces. As well as being the major route of B_{12} analog excretion, bile may play a role in enhancing B_{12} absorption. When the diet contains little or no B_{12}, as may be the case for strict vegans, biliary cobalamin is conserved to the extent that clinical deficiency may take up to 20 years to develop. When malabsorption occurs, as in pernicious anemia, endogenous and dietary B_{12} are lost and deficiency develops within 3 to 6 years. This accounts for the slow and insidious course of pernicious anemia.

EPIDEMIOLOGY

Occurrence

B_{12} deficiency becomes increasingly prevalent with advancing age. In people over age 65, the incidence ranges from 5 to 40.5% depending on the criteria used to define deficiency.[11,46,48,50,51] Blacks tend to have higher B_{12} concentrations than do whites, and it is unclear whether using standard normal range values to assess B_{12} status underrecognizes mild B_{12} deficiency in this population.[48] Metabolic evidence (deoxyuridine suppression, MMA, and Hcy tests) of B_{12} deficiency is present in approximately 50 to 75% of people with low B_{12} concentrations, despite the absence of clinical signs or symptoms of deficiency.[51] This means that B_{12} is deficient at the cellular (bone marrow and other tissues) level. Anemia is a later finding of B_{12} deficiency, so the deficiency often is diagnosed and treated before anemia develops.

Etiology

Populations at high risk for B_{12} deficiency are listed in Table 13.3. Causes of B_{12} deficiency include inadequate intake, malabsorption, B_{12} degradation, and inadequate B_{12} use (Table 13.12). In developed countries, dietary causes are rare and may be important only in vegans (strict vegetarians who do not consume foods of animal origin, including milk, cheese, and eggs), breastfed babies of vegan mothers, and people living in countries where poor nutrition is widespread. Most cases of deficiency are secondary to malabsorption associated with pernicious anemia, gastric lesions, gastrectomy, achlorhydria, and a number of small bowel disorders.[4,17,42,46,51,52] Inadequate B_{12} use results from drug interactions, congenital or acquired enzyme deficiencies, and abnormal B_{12} binding proteins.

Table 13.12 ▪ Causes of Vitamin B_{12} and Folic Acid Deficiencies

Vitamin B_{12} deficiency	
Dietary	Inadequate intake
Malabsorption	Inadequate production of intrinsic factor, competition for B_{12}, disorders of terminal ileum, drugs
Impaired transport	Transcobalamin II deficiency
Folic acid deficiency	
Dietary	Inadequate intake, unbalanced diet, excessive cooking
Malabsorption	Intestinal mucosal changes
Increased requirements	Pregnancy, infancy, malignancy, increased hematopoiesis
Impaired metabolism	Drugs, enzyme deficiencies

Pernicious Anemia

Pernicious anemia, defined as B_{12} malabsorption caused by the loss of gastric IF secretion, is thought to be the most common cause of B_{12} deficiency. The term *pernicious* is used because the anemia is insidious and progressive (Table 13.11). Current evidence suggests that pernicious anemia is caused by an autoimmune reaction against gastric parietal cells. Most patients have increased levels of circulating antibodies, particularly those directed against antiparietal cells and IF.[4,8]

The incidence of pernicious anemia is about 1% in the general population, with most cases occurring in people over 60 years of age. There is a distinctive racial and geographic distribution, with pernicious anemia more common in temperate regions such as North America and northern Europe than in tropical countries. Juvenile pernicious anemia is less common. These patients often develop clinical features of B_{12} deficiency during the second decade of life. Inherited conditions leading to pernicious anemia in infancy or early childhood may be caused by a lack of IF or the production of abnormal IF by an otherwise normal stomach.[26,46,48,51]

Gastric Disorders

Gastric disorders, most commonly gastrectomy, are the second most common cause of vitamin B_{12} malabsorption. Complete gastrectomy results in an absolute deficiency of IF, and megaloblastic anemia develops 3 to 6 years after surgery unless supplementation is given. Partial gastrectomy is a variable cause of B_{12} deficiency. Deficiency is also possible if sufficient gastric mucosa has been destroyed by ingestion of corrosive chemicals, by tumors, or by chronic gastritis.

Even when the diet is adequate, some stomach abnormalities prevent the release of the vitamin from foods. These include atrophic gastritis, achlorhydria, vagotomy, partial gastrectomy, and the use of H_2-receptor antagonists.

Intestinal Problems

Small intestine disorders are the third most common cause of B_{12} deficiency. Abnormal situations leading to malabsorption range from impaired transfer of the vitamin from R-protein to competition for luminal B_{12} or a low pH in the ileum.

B_{12} malabsorption also occurs in the Zollinger–Ellison syndrome if the associated hypersecretion of gastric acid is left uncontrolled. The associated lowering of pH in the duodenum inactivates pancreatic proteolytic enzymes.

Surgical resection or bypass of the ileum also increases the likelihood of malabsorption. Most patients who have lost more than 5 cm of distal ileum have abnormal Schilling test results. Even in the presence of IF, B_{12} malabsorption occurs in conditions such as tropical sprue, Crohn's disease, celiac disease, lymphomas, and Whipple's disease, in which alteration or destruction of the ileal absorptive surface occurs. In the recessive disorder, Imerslund–Grasbeck's disease, selective B_{12} malabsorption through a poorly understood mechanism, occurs in association with proteinuria.

Bacterial overgrowth, particularly by *Bacteroides* and coliforms, in blind loops or diverticula results in B_{12} malabsorption. Absorption returns to normal when patients are given tetracycline, lincomycin, or metronidazole. The mechanism of B_{12} uptake by bacteria is unclear. Most intestinal bacteria avidly absorb the unbound vitamin, but only small amounts are taken up when it is bound to IF. Parasitic infections, such as tapeworm *Diphyllobothrium latum* (from eating undercooked freshwater fish) or *Giardia lamblia,* also cause B_{12} deficiency.

Drug-Induced Vitamin B_{12} Deficiency

Drug-induced B_{12} deficiency has been associated with a number of pharmacotherapeutic agents. Colchicine, *p*-aminosalicylic acid, neomycin, H_2-receptor blockers, proton pump inhibitors, and biguanide hypoglycemic agents decrease absorption of B_{12}.[4,46,52–54] Agents that reduce B_{12} absorption in the ileum include ethanol and cholestyramine. Nitrous oxide oxidizes the central cobalt atom, which inhibits its ability to function as a cofactor in the methionine synthase reaction,[4] thus affecting cells of the bone marrow, nervous system, and other tissues. Use of nitrous oxide in patients over 60 years of age or with other potential risk factors for B_{12} deficiency should be avoided.[4,5,52]

CLINICAL PRESENTATION AND DIAGNOSIS

Signs and Symptoms

Clinical manifestations reflect abnormalities of the blood, gastrointestinal tract, and nervous system (Table 13.2). In severe cases the peripheral blood film exhibits severe macrocytic anemia, leukopenia with hypersegmentation of the polymorphonuclear cells, and thrombocytopenia. Nonspecific symptoms related to anemia include apathy, weakness, fatigue, palpitations, and breathlessness. The mucous membranes usually are pale, and in Caucasians the skin is pale and yellow-tinted because of the anemia and the mild jaundice of ineffective erythropoiesis.

Gastrointestinal tract or neurologic changes may occur in the absence of hematologic changes. Sore tongue is the most common oral complaint. Glossitis, burning of the mouth, and a beefy red tongue are other manifestations. Other gastrointestinal symptoms include diarrhea, gas, heartburn, nausea, and vague abdominal pain.[4,5,42,55]

Neurologic manifestations include peripheral neuropathies, degeneration of the spinal cord, and altered mental states.[4,5,42,43,46,51,55] B_{12} deficiency results in distinct changes in the nervous system, beginning with demyelination of nerves. These changes often are progressive, and if the deficiency is not corrected, they can be irreversible. Peripheral nerve damage results in symmetric paresthesias (numbness and tingling of the extremities) and reduction of pain and temperature sensation. The most serious problem, subacute degeneration of the spinal cord, is associated with loss of position and vibration sense, resulting in ataxia and weakness. Lateral column disruption leads to weakness and spasticity, exemplified by myoclonus, hyperreflexia, and a positive Babinski's sign. If the condition remains untreated, instability of gait and virtual paralysis result.

Psychiatric manifestations include impaired mentation, delirium, paranoia, psychosis, irritability, depression, and personality changes.[4–5,42,43,46,51,55]

Diagnosis

Early diagnosis of B_{12} deficiency relies on identifying risk factors for deficiency (Table 13.3), obtaining a complete medical, dietary, and medication history, and assessing appropriate clinical laboratory tests. The goal is to prevent development of anemia or neurologic symptoms by earlier recognition and treatment of B_{12} deficiency.

Measurement of plasma B_{12} concentrations is simple and inexpensive and is considered the standard test for diagnosing B_{12} deficiency.[4,41,48,49,56] Limitations of the test include the inability to distinguish total from metabolically active B_{12} (bound to TCII, or holo-TC), discrepancies between concentrations and symptoms, and reference ranges that may not be applicable to all patients, such as blacks and older adults.[4,46,48,49] For example, people with TCII deficiency could have a normal B_{12} concentration but be B_{12} deficient at the tissue level because of a lack of the transport protein. Measurement of holo-TC would overcome this problem and be a better measure of actual B_{12} available to the tissues. However, limited assay availability has hindered clinical use of this test. Another alternative is measurement of TCII saturation, which decreases early in B_{12} deficiency. However, because only small amounts of B_{12} are bound to TCII, low levels of detection are needed, which results in increased variability, thus limiting its clinical usefulness.

"Normal" B_{12} concentrations also occur despite an actual B_{12} deficiency in liver disease, myeloproliferative disorders, and nitrous oxide anesthesia.[4,41,56] Cutoff points for normal B_{12} concentrations also vary, and symptoms do not always occur with low values. Recent studies have documented that asymptomatic patients with low B_{12} concentrations have metabolic abnormalities strongly suggestive of B_{12} deficiency at the cellular level, which reverse with B_{12} treatment.[4,6,11,50,51] Therefore, in patients with B_{12} concentrations in the low normal range (whether they are symptomatic or not), additional tests, such as biochemical assessment of metabolite production (MMA and Hcy), should be conducted.

Functional deficiency of B_{12} inhibits reactions converting MMA to succinyl-Co A and Hcy to methionine, resulting in accumulation of MMA and Hcy (Fig. 13.1). Marked elevation of these serum metabolites (more than 3 SD increase from the mean) occurs in more than 95% of patients with B_{12} deficiency.[7] Because folate deficiency can also result in accumulation of Hcy, MMA is considered more specific for B_{12} deficiency. However, MMA also increases in renal disease, so renal function should be assessed when MMA is measured. Disadvantages of using metabolite concentrations are cost and access, which have limited their clinical use.[4,6,7,47,49,51,56]

Once B_{12} deficiency is noted, assessment of the cause (malabsorption versus other) guides treatment selection. Anti–gastric parietal cell or anti-IF antibodies (IFAs) can be measured to provide information about a patient's ability to absorb B_{12}. Anti–gastric parietal cell antibodies often are found in patients with gastritis not affecting B_{12} absorption and thus are not diagnostically sensitive or specific for assessing B_{12} absorption.[8,56] However, IFAs rarely occur without B_{12} malabsorption and are found in 50 to 75% of patients with pernicious anemia.[8,41,56] The British Committee for Standards in Haematology guidelines state that detection of IFAs eliminates the need for absorption tests (e.g., Schilling test) in most patients.[56]

A Schilling test (with or without IF) is an alternative method of assessing B_{12} malabsorption.[4,41,45,48,49,56] Several types of Schilling tests are available. The standard test is divided into three stages. In stage I, an oral dose (1 μg for adults, 0.5 to 1 μg for children) of ^{57}Co-labeled B_{12} is given, followed by a 1-mg intramuscular dose of unlabeled B_{12}. The large intramuscular dose saturates B_{12}-binding proteins in the blood. Consequently, there are fewer binding sites for ^{57}Co-labeled B_{12}, and a substantial proportion is excreted in the urine. Urine is collected over 24 hours and the amount of labeled B_{12} measured. B_{12} absorption is considered to be impaired if less than 10% of the label is excreted in the urine. If less than 5% is excreted, the diagnosis is consistent with pernicious anemia.

Stage II of the test distinguishes between the possible causes of the malabsorption (e.g., pernicious anemia, lack of ileal absorptive sites, or bacterial overgrowth proximal to the terminal ileum). The same procedure is followed as in stage I except that IF is given with the radiolabeled B_{12}. If the B_{12} deficiency is caused by lack of IF (pernicious

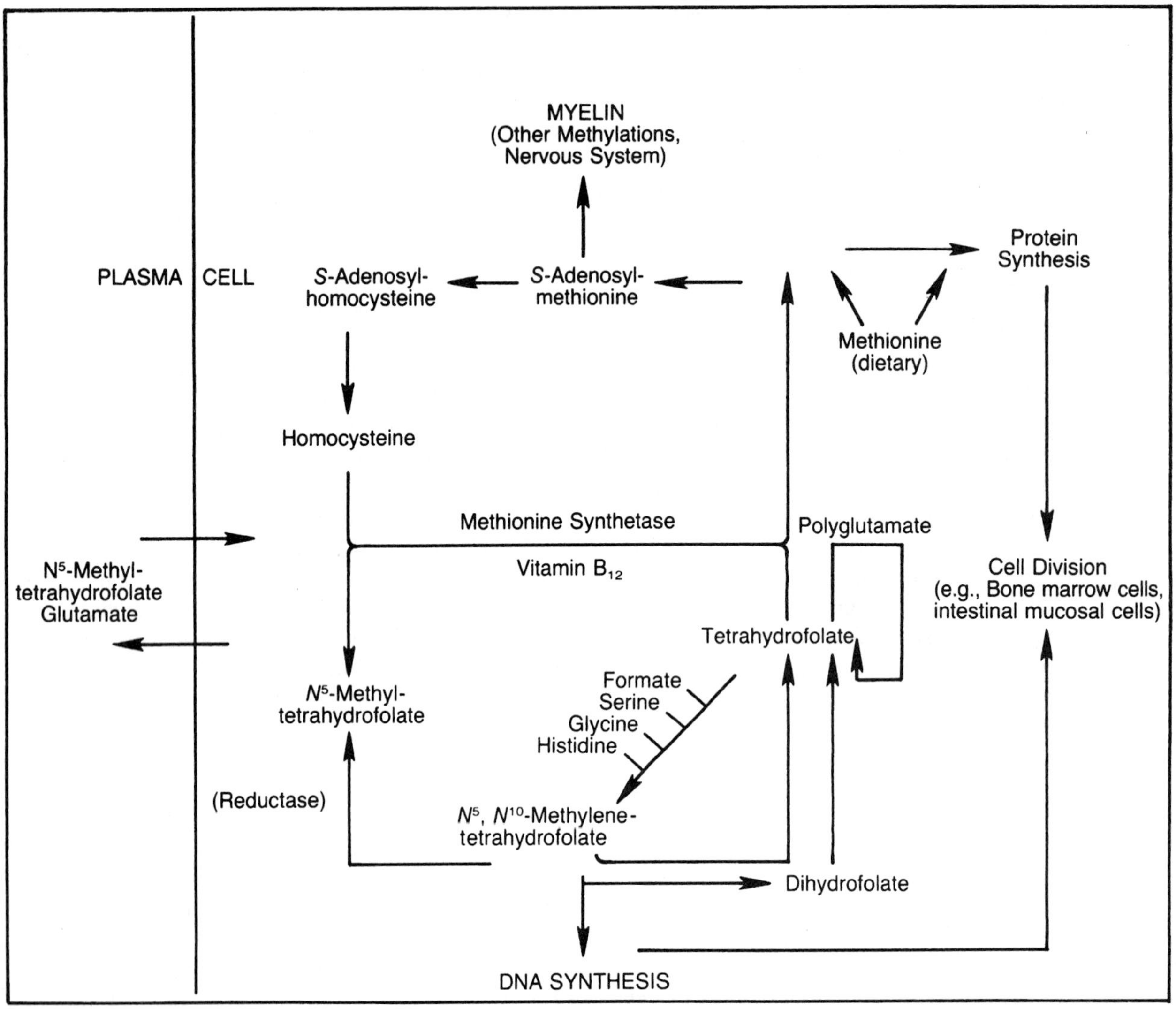

Figure 13.1. Normal vitamin B_{12} and folate metabolism in mammalian cells.

Table 13.13 ▪ Summary of Schilling Test Results in Vitamin B_{12} Deficiency

Condition	Stage I	Stage II	Stage III
Normal	Normal		
Inadequate diet	Normal		
Pernicious anemia	Low	Normal	
Bacterial overgrowth	Low	Low	Normal
Ileal defect	Low	Low	Low

anemia), stage I should be abnormal and stage II should be normal. If both stages are abnormal, an ileal disorder, bacterial overgrowth, pancreatic disorders, or fish tapeworm infestation may be causing B_{12} malabsorption. Stage III of the test, which involves giving the patient antibiotics (usually tetracycline 250 mg orally four times a day for 10 to 14 days) and then repeating the stage I test, checks for possible bacterial overgrowth (Table 13.13).

The Schilling test depends on renal function and a complete 24-hr urine collection. Decreased renal function and incomplete urine collection lead to inaccurate results. In addition, H_2-antagonists and proton pump inhibitors may cause falsely abnormal results by preventing the degradation of R-protein and decreasing the secretion of endogenous IF. Conditions that reduce hydrochloric acid production (H_2-antagonists) and other situations in which acid and IF secretion are reduced (achlorhydria, complete or partial gastrectomy) can give falsely normal Schilling test results. The problem is that the aqueous, crystalline B_{12} used in the test differs in bioavailability from the usually food-bound vitamin that must be released to participate in the uptake process. A modified Schilling test (protein bound absorption test [PBAT]) using protein-bound B_{12} more closely resembles the physiologic state.[4]

Use of the Schilling test may decrease as other tests become available to assess B_{12} absorption that are less expensive, do not expose patients to radiation, and do not entail 24 hours of sample collection.[4,48,49,56]

Anemia is a late presentation of B_{12} deficiency (Table 13.11) that may be avoided with early detection and correction of B_{12} depletion. Hematologic tests, such as a blood smear and the red cell indices, help differentiate the cause of anemia. Macrocytosis (MCV greater than 100 fL) often occurs with B_{12} deficiency, but its also occurs with other conditions, such as liver disease, myxedema, acute myelogenous leukemia, acquired sideroblastic anemia, aplastic anemia, hemolytic anemia, posthemorrhagic states, and splenectomy. Evaluating the smear for megaloblastic changes, such as neutrophil hypersegmentation and oval-shaped erythrocytes, generally differentiates a B_{12} or folate deficiency from other causes. If iron deficiency occurs along with B_{12} deficiency, the MCV may appear normal, but the blood smear should show both megaloblastic and microcytic cells.[21,41,42,46,56]

Less commonly used tests include thymidine uptake (deoxyuridine suppression test [dUST]) by bone marrow cells, food cobalamin absorption, erythropoietin measurement, and gastrin and pepsinogen analysis.[4,49,56] Folate concentrations also are generally assessed to rule out a concurrent folate deficiency.

TREATMENT

Management includes identifying B_{12} deficiency early (before anemia or neurologic symptoms develop), correcting the cause of the deficiency if possible, replenishing depleted stores, and if necessary, administering maintenance B_{12} therapy. Once anemia or other symptoms develop, the aim of treatment is to reverse the symptoms (achieve hematologic remission, reverse or retard nervous system complications, and eliminate gastrointestinal symptoms) and replenish B_{12} stores.

Treatment options include dietary changes and supplemental B_{12} given orally, intranasally, or parenterally.

Dietary adjustments may be warranted in patients with poor or restricted diets. Dietary sources of B_{12} include fresh liver (the richest source), eggs, meat, kidney, milk, dairy products, fish, and shellfish. However, dietary changes provide little benefit for patients with malabsorption states such as pernicious anemia.

Pharmacotherapy

Oral Vitamin B_{12} Therapy

When B_{12} absorption is normal but there is dietary deficiency (e.g., strict vegetarian or restricted diets), oral B_{12} therapy is the preferred route. In the presence of adequate absorption, the usual oral dosage of B_{12} supplementation is 1 to 10 μg/day. Oral B_{12} therapy may also be used to treat some drug-induced B_{12} deficiencies (e.g., nitrous oxide).[5] Oral cyanocobalamin is well absorbed, with peak serum concentrations being reached 8 to 12 hours after ingestion.

A debated area is use of oral B_{12} therapy in patients with impaired absorption (e.g., pernicious anemia, complete or partial gastrectomy).[4,46] Because approximately 1% of an oral dose of B_{12} can be absorbed by a nonspecific, non–IF-dependent process, large oral dosages may provide sufficient B_{12} to correct the deficiency, replenish stores, and resolve symptoms. In a randomized controlled trial in 33 patients with B_{12} deficiency, 2 mg oral cyanocobalamin taken daily for 120 days was compared with 1 mg given intramuscularly on days 1, 3, 7, 10, 14, 21, 30, 60, and 90. The oral therapy resulted in significantly higher serum B_{12} concentrations and lower serum MMA concentrations than intramuscular therapy.[57] Symptoms of B_{12} deficiency resolved in both groups, but the incidence of anemia at baseline was low. In another study, eight patients with megaloblastic anemia were treated with daily oral dosages of 1.5 mg of either cyanocobalamin ($n = 3$), hydroxy-cobalamin ($n = 4$), or methylcobalamin ($n = 1$) for 1 year. After 3 or 4 days of therapy, patients reported increased appetite, alertness, and well-being. Reticulocytosis occurred after a few days, with peak effect by the end of the first week of therapy. B_{12} concentrations returned to normal range in a median of 14.5 days, and Hb rose to above 6.2 mmol/L (10 g/dL; normal range 7.5 to 11.2 mmol/L, or 12 to 18 g/dL) in a median of 34.4 days. The responses were similar to those reported after intramuscular administration, although the hematologic response appeared to be slightly slower.[58] Other reports also support the use of oral therapy.[59,60] The dosing of the oral product is important. Dosages of less than 150 μg generally do not restore B_{12} and Hb concentrations, and dosages between 250 and 500 μg may be affected by variable absorption, resulting in erratic responses. Therefore, in patients with malabsorption, B_{12} dosages should be 1000 μg or higher to produce favorable long-term results.[61] Concerns with oral therapy are the potential for erratic absorption, poor compliance, and subsequent development of neurologic symptoms. Patient evaluation and monitoring for compliance and therapeutic response should whether long-term oral therapy is optimal for each patient.

Parenteral Vitamin B_{12} Therapy

A number of different parenteral B_{12} treatment plans exist (Table 13.14), but no controlled treatment studies were found in the literature to support the regimens.[48] Because of the safety of these agents, dosages of 100 to 1000 μg of B_{12} can be given. Dosages under 15 μg generally are insufficient to completely correct the later stages of B_{12} deficiency. All regimens use more frequent dosing initially to correct the deficiency, followed by injections every 1 to 3 months, based on the patient's response, for life.

Proponents for the higher (more than 1000 μg) dosage argue that lower (less than 300 μg) dosages sometimes are insufficient to maintain serum concentrations within the normal range because B_{12} needs vary (1.5 to 10 μg/day) and there is a wide intrasubject response to replacement

Table 13.14 ▪ Summary of Various Parenteral B_{12} Regimens

Dosage	Frequency	References
100 μg	Daily for 1 wk, then every other day for 7 doses, then every month for life	75
100 μg	Every week, then	71
1000 μg	Every 1–3 mo for life	
500–1000 μg	Daily for 1 wk, then weekly for 1 mo, then monthly for life	42,45
1000 μg	Every week ×4, then every month for life	46
1000 μg	On days 1, 3, 7, 10, 14, 21, 30, then monthly for life	5,57

dosages.[46] In addition, few problems have been reported with parenteral B_{12}, with any extra B_{12} (beyond the daily needs) being excreted, largely unchanged, in the urine. That the excess B_{12} is eliminated is an argument for use of the lower dose; it is less wasteful and should meet the needs of most patients. B_{12} generally is administered intramuscularly, although deep subcutaneous injection also can be used. Peak serum concentrations after intramuscular injection are reached in about 1 hour. The half-life of the parenteral B_{12} is about 6 days; its half-life in the liver is 400 days. With impaired liver or kidney function, more frequent dosing is necessary.

Two synthetic forms of B_{12} are available: cyanocobalamin and hydroxocobalamin. After intramuscular administration, cyanocobalamin appears to be excreted more rapidly than hydroxocobalamin, which is more highly protein bound. Therefore, hydroxocobalamin may allow less frequent dosing (every 3 months) during maintenance therapy.[4] Indications for both of these agents are similar, although hydroxocobalamin may be preferred for treating B_{12} deficiencies because optic neuropathies may worsen with cyanocobalamin administration.

The synthetic B_{12} products are well tolerated, and allergic reactions are rare. Medical attention should be sought if a rash or wheezing develops. Although anaphylactic reactions can occur after parenteral administration, they are rare. An intradermal test dose is recommended for patients with a history of suspected allergic reactions to B_{12}. No adverse effects have been documented when the normal daily needs for these agents are administered during pregnancy. B_{12} crosses the placenta, and at birth the neonatal level can be two to five times that of the mother. Injections containing benzyl alcohol should not be used in neonates or immature infants because of possible toxicity from the preservative. B_{12} is excreted in breast milk, and no problems have been reported for humans taking the normal daily allowances. No geriatric problems have been reported.[46]

Intranasal Vitamin B_{12} Therapy

A more recent development in B_{12} therapy is intranasal administration.[46] Currently, an intranasal gel (400 μg cyanocobalamin) is available in the United States, with recommended dosing of three times a week.[62] Because the experience with the gel is limited, it is generally used in patients who refuse or cannot tolerate parenteral therapy and do not respond to oral treatment. A recent report documents the efficacy of a metered-dose nasal spray of hydroxocobalamin (750 μg per puff) in treating six patients with documented B_{12} deficiency.[63] One puff was administered in each nostril on days 0, 14, and 21. B_{12} concentrations increased significantly 1 hour after the dose. However, most of the concentrations fell below the normal range before the next dose. The spray was well tolerated, with no reports of nasal irritation or sensitivity. This study supports further investigation into the dosing and efficacy of this product.

Monitoring Vitamin B_{12} Deficiency Therapy

Response varies depending on the stage (Table 13.11) of B_{12} deficiency being treated. In the later stages, reticulocytosis occurs rapidly, with a maximum reticulocyte count seen 4 to 7 days after treatment starts. The neutrophil count also increases by this time, although the hypersegmented polymorphonuclear neutrophils persist for several weeks. Hb concentrations gradually increase over the first 2 months of therapy. Macrocytosis may persist for several months after treatment is started because of the long half-life of erythrocytes.[42,59] Serum iron concentrations may decrease because the accelerated erythropoiesis requires more Hb production. Some patients may need supplemental iron. If iron stores become depleted, the hematologic response to B_{12} therapy could be delayed.[22,23] The rapid erythropoiesis may also cause hypokalemia. Serum potassium concentrations should be monitored during the first 48 hours of treatment in patients who have cardiac disease (especially those on potassium-depleting diuretics) or other risk factors for significant potassium depletion.

Oral and gastrointestinal symptoms generally resolve within the first 3 days of therapy, and patients report an overall feeling of well-being.[5,55] Reversal of neurologic manifestations and dementia takes several weeks. Most resolve by 6 months of B_{12} therapy, although maximum benefit may take as long as 1.5 years. However, some patients have incomplete responses, which is thought to depend on the duration of the neurologic problem before treatment.[5,42] Serum B_{12} concentrations increase to within the normal range, and metabolite concentrations (MMA and Hcy) decrease to within the normal range, generally within the first month of therapy.[57]

Patients not responding to therapy may need a dosage adjustment (higher dosage), a change in dosing form (oral to intramuscular), and evaluation for drug interactions, drug-induced bone marrow effects, and other medical problems.

Folate Deficiency

Like B_{12} deficiency, folate deficiency occurs in stages, with depletion of stores leading to deficiency that can result in megaloblastic anemia and other hematologic abnormalities (thrombocytopenia, leukopenia).[64] Treating a B_{12} deficiency megaloblastic anemia with folic acid may correct the anemia but does not correct the B_{12} deficiency or prevent the development of neurologic changes. Therefore, it is important to determine the cause of a megaloblastic anemia before initiating therapy.

Folate also is critical in early pregnancy for fetal neural tube development.[65] To reduce the incidence of neural tube defects, since January 1998 the FDA has required enriched grains to be fortified with folic acid at a concentration that provides, on average, 100 μg per day.[66] In addition, the role of folate deficiency is being evaluated in heart disease, stroke, and peripheral arterial disease. Increased Hcy concentrations appear to correlate with the occurrence of these diseases, and because folate replenishment reduces Hcy concentrations, some have speculated that folate may have an important role in preventing or treating these diseases.[64,67,68,76]

PHYSIOLOGIC IMPORTANCE OF FOLATE

Reduced forms of folate (tetrahydrofolate) are cofactors for transformylation reactions in the biosynthesis of purines and thymidylates of nucleic acids. In folate deficiency, reduced thymidylate synthesis leads to defective DNA synthesis, resulting in megaloblast formation and bone marrow suppression. Folate is also involved in the methylation cycle and is essential in providing methyl groups for a wide range of cellular methyltransferases. In particular, folate is needed in Hcy metabolism (Fig. 13.1), which accumulates in folate deficiency.[7,64,65,67]

Folate Needs

Folate needs depend on metabolic and cell turnover rates. In general, the minimum daily requirement is 50 to 100 μg/day.[42,64] In pregnancy, an additional 400 μg/day is recommended.[43,66] More than 2% is degraded daily, so a continuous dietary supply is essential. The average amount stored in the body is 5 to 10 mg, one-half of which is found in the liver. With folate depletion, deficiency leading to anemia generally occurs within 6 months.

Folate Absorption and Metabolism

Folate is a water-soluble vitamin found in many plant and animal foods. Dietary sources are primarily polyglutamates, which must be converted to the monoglutamate form for absorption. This process often is impaired in malabsorption syndromes, such as sprue. The percentage of dietary folate absorbed depends on the source, with liver, yeast, and egg yolk having high absorption; only 10% of most other dietary sources is absorbed. Active absorption of dietary folate occurs mainly in the proximal part of the small intestine. Synthetic folate (folic acid) is already in the monoglutamate form and has greater stability and better absorption (almost twice the bioavailability) than dietary folate.[64,65] Folic acid from pharmaceutical products is almost completely absorbed in the upper duodenum, even in the presence of malabsorption.

The principal circulating form of folic acid, *N*-5-methyltetrahydrofolate, is extensively bound to plasma proteins. There is no specific transport protein. Some enterohepatic cycling of folic acid occurs, although significant amounts are not reabsorbed from the bile.

Amounts of folic acid beyond the daily needs are excreted almost entirely as metabolites by the kidney.

EPIDEMIOLOGY

Inadequate diet, alcoholism, and pregnancy are the most common causes of folate deficiency. Other causes include increased requirements, malabsorption, enhanced metabolism, and interference in the metabolism or clearance by other pharmacotherapeutic agents.

Malnutrition is often a significant cause of folate deficiency. Folate-rich foods include raw spinach, broccoli, cauliflower, peanuts, and peas. Folate is highly susceptible to cooking or processing. Heating foods (microwaving or boiling) decreases the amount of folate available by up to 50%. People at risk of inadequate folate intake include alcoholics whose main caloric intake is in the form of ethanol, narcotic addicts who have a poor diet, older adults who often do not feel like eating or who eat commercially prepared foods, institutionalized people who have no control over their diet, adolescents who may skip meals and eat junk foods, and pregnant women who have increased needs that often are not met by dietary intake.[42,43,56,64]

In alcoholics, the incidence of folate deficiency has been reported to be as high as 60%.[69] Poor diet and altered absorption are the primary causes.

During pregnancy, a large increase in nucleic acid synthesis is associated with growth of the fetus, placenta, and uterus and with the increased maternal erythrocyte mass. Folate needs may triple during pregnancy, and if supplements are not taken, particularly in the last trimester, megaloblastic anemia may develop in the mother. In addition, folate is essential for fetal neural tube development, and supplementation in the periconceptional period has been shown to reduce the occurrence of neural tube defects.[43,65] Worldwide, folate deficiency occurs in up to one-third of pregnancies. In the United States, the incidence is about 4%, but it increases up to eightfold with multiple gestations, teenage pregnancies, and closely spaced pregnancies.[64]

Folate needs increase during malignancy, increased erythropoiesis, and conditions causing rapid cell turnover. Folate deficiency is very common in myeloproliferative disorders such as chronic myeloid leukemia and myelofibrosis, often leading to thrombocytopenia or anemia. The increased folate needs in chronic hemolytic anemia, exfoliative dermatitis, generalized psoriasis, or extensive burns can also lead to folate deficiency. In these cases, adequate supplementation is needed. Anemia is more likely to occur if several contributing factors are present.

Various drugs can affect folate absorption, metabolism, and use (Table 13.15). Folate supplementation generally is not necessary during short courses of these drugs (e.g., oral sulfonamide antibiotics). However, chronic or high-dose therapy may necessitate folate supplementation to prevent deficiency. Methotrexate, a folate antagonist, binds to dihydrofolate reductase and prevents reduction of folate to its active intracellular form. When high dosages of methotrexate are given (e.g., in cancer treatment protocols), bone marrow suppression and mucositis generally occur unless leucovorin, a reduced form of folate, is coadministered. It should be noted that supplemental folate may alter the central nervous system effect of phenytoin, and patients may need an increase in phenytoin dosage to maintain efficacy.

CLINICAL PRESENTATION AND DIAGNOSIS

Signs and Symptoms

Signs and symptoms of folate deficiency are similar to those of other anemias (Table 13.2). In addition, megaloblastosis, glossitis, diarrhea, and weight loss may occur.

Diagnosis

As with B_{12} deficiency, early diagnosis and prevention of anemia depend on identification and treatment of high-risk patients (Table 13.3). Serum or erythrocyte folate concentrations may be determined to assess folate status (Table 13.4). Within 5 weeks of inadequate folate intake, the serum folate declines to the subnormal range, whereas the erythrocyte folate concentration does not decline until about 3 months.[41] However, serum folate measurement has the disadvantage of being sensitive to dynamic changes in folate metabolism, such as reflecting folate absorbed from a recent meal. Therefore, serum concentrations fluctuate from day to day, closely reflecting dietary intake. Falsely normal values can be obtained if folate-rich foods are consumed within a few days before evaluation. Erythrocyte folate concentration reflects tissue status and is felt to be a better indicator of depletion.[41,56]

Increased plasma Hcy concentration is another indicator of folate deficiency.[7] This biochemical marker may also be increased by B_{12} deficiency and with decreased renal function. Both of these conditions should be concurrently evaluated when this test is used.

In the later stages of folate deficiency, a blood smear and hematologic evaluation often show macrocytosis with megaloblastosis. Megaloblastosis must be interpreted in light of B_{12} status because of similar findings in B_{12} deficiency. Both erythrocyte folate and serum B_{12} concentrations should be measured.[64] Anemia occurs only when tissue levels are depleted, so a normal serum folate concentration does not exclude deficiency. The diagnosis of megaloblastic anemia caused by folate deficiency entails a demonstration of reduced folate tissue levels, as reflected by erythrocyte folate concentrations.

Table 13.15 • Drug-Induced Folate Deficiency

Reduced absorption	
	Ethanol
	Metformin
	Cholestyramine
	Sulfasalazine
	Sulfamethoxazole
	Oral contraceptives
	Some anticonvulsants
Altered metabolism	
	Some anticonvulsants
	Methotrexate
	Trimethoprim
	Triamterene
	Pentamidine
	Alcohol

Source: References 41, 64.

TREATMENT

The primary prevention of folate deficiency, and hence anemia, should occur through dietary manipulation or oral supplementation.

Pharmacotherapy

Women planning to become pregnant should take at least 400 μg/day, to prevent fetal neural tube defects. Because many pregnancies are not planned, the FDA has mandated food fortification to enhance the daily folate intake in all women by 100 μg/day.[66] There are two concerns with this approach. One is that the increase in folate intake could mask a B_{12} deficiency by "correcting" the anemia.[76] However, one would hope to detect a B_{12} deficiency before anemia develops. Also, folate dosages of 1 mg or more generally are needed to produce and maintain a remission in a B_{12} deficiency anemia.[43] The other concern is that the folate amount is too low and does not provide enough to prevent neural tube defects.[66] Therefore, 400 μg folic acid daily is still recommended for pregnant women and women who are trying to become pregnant.[64,66] This dosage will also minimize the chance of the women developing folate-deficiency anemia during the latter part of the pregnancy, when folate needs increase. Dosages less than 1 mg are available in numerous over-the-counter preparations.

Folate deficiency usually is treated with oral folic acid 1 mg daily.[77] This dosage is available only by prescription. Parenteral administration is indicated when oral administration is unacceptable (preoperatively, postoperatively, or if nausea or vomiting is a problem) or not possible (malabsorption syndromes or after gastric resection). Available parenteral formulations contain 5 mg/mL and may be given intramuscularly, subcutaneously, or intravenously.[77]

The duration of therapy depends on the underlying cause. Replacement therapy should be continued until the underlying problem has been corrected. If this is impossible, lifelong therapy is needed. B_{12} studies should also be undertaken in people requiring long-term folate supplementation. Long-term therapy may be needed in chronic hemolytic states, myelofibrosis, and refractory malabsorption. Postgastrectomy states, prolonged stress or infection, chronic fever, and persistent diarrhea may also increase needs.

Monitoring Folate Deficiency Therapy

In anemic patients, treatment response can be monitored by following the reticulocyte count, which peaks 5 to 8 days after treatment begins. Hematologic findings (Hb, MCV) should be normal in about 2 months. Measuring erythrocyte folate levels for several months during the treatment can confirm replenishment of tissue stores. For patients with deficiency without anemia, folate stores are replenished in about 3 weeks.[42]

KEY POINTS

- Nutritional anemias may be prevented by early identification of at-risk patients, monitoring for vitamin deficiency, and providing supplementation or replacement therapy.
- Pregnant women, young children, and older adults are prone to nutritional anemias and should be monitored for potential deficiencies of iron, B_{12}, and folate.
- Nutritional deficiencies develop in stages, with anemia occurring at the final stage. Other hematologic and biochemical changes occur earlier in the deficiency, allowing diagnosis to be made before anemia develops.
- If anemia does result, it usually can be treated simply and effectively, although determining and correcting the primary cause of anemia can be difficult.
- Where possible, dietary manipulation should be used as a maintenance strategy. In some cases, particularly with pernicious anemia, lifelong therapy is necessary.
- Iron deficiency is common during pregnancy and early childhood, and the CDC recommends supplementation in both groups.
- Based on elemental iron content and absorption, the usual dosage of ferrous sulfate to treat iron deficiency is 300 mg taken three times a day.
- If parenteral iron therapy is needed, the TDI method offers the advantage of fewer office visits, needlesticks, and local side effects than intramuscular or bolus intravenous dosing.
- Oral B_{12} therapy (dosages greater than 1 mg per day) may be used to treat B_{12} deficiencies, even those caused by malabsorption (pernicious anemia).
- Maintenance B_{12} therapy generally is 1 mg intramuscularly every 1 to 3 months or 1 mg orally daily.
- Gastrointestinal and neurologic symptoms of B_{12} deficiency can develop before anemia.
- Pregnant women and women planning to become pregnant should take supplemental folic acid (400 μg per day).
- Because 1 mg folic acid per day can reverse the anemia associated with B_{12} deficiency but does not prevent the neurologic symptoms, the cause of a megaloblastic anemia should be determined before therapy is initiated.
- For patients who need long-term vitamin supplementation, compliance should be monitored because patients may discontinue use once symptoms improve.
- Response to therapy generally occurs within the first week (reticulocytosis), although correction of the anemia may take 2 to 3 months.

REFERENCES

1. Massey AC. Microcytic anemia. Differential diagnosis and management of iron deficiency anemia. Med Clin North Am 76:549–566, 1992.
2. Brown RG. Determining the cause of anemia. General approach, with emphasis on microcytic hypochromic anemias. Postgrad Med 89(6):161–170, 1991.
3. Anonymous. Recommendations to prevent and control iron deficiency in the United States. Centers for Disease Control and Prevention. MMWR Morb Mortal Wkly Rep 47(RR-3):1–29, 1998.
4. Markle HV. Cobalamin. Crit Rev Clin Lab Sci 33(4):247–356, 1996.
5. Schilling RF. Vitamin B_{12} deficiency: underdiagnosed, overtreated? Hosp Pract 30:47–54, 1995.
6. Metz J, Bell AH, Flicker L, et al. The significance of subnormal serum B_{12} concentration in older people: a case control study. J Am Geriatr Soc 44:1355–1361, 1996.
7. Savage DG, Lindenbaum J, Stabler SP, et al. Sensitivity of serum methylmalonic acid and total homocysteine determinations for diagnosing cobalamin and folate deficiencies. Am J Med 96:239–246, 1994.
8. Carmel R. Reassessment of the relative prevalences of antibodies to gastric parietal cell and to intrinsic factor in patients with pernicious anemia: influence of patient age and race. Clin Exp Immunol 89:74–77, 1992.
9. Worwood M. The laboratory assessment of iron status: an update. Clin Chim Acta 259:3–23, 1997.
10. Ahluwalia N. Diagnostic utility of serum transferrin receptors measurement in assessing iron status. Nutr Rev 56(5):133–141, 1998.
11. Lindenbaum J, Rosenberg IH, Wilson PWF, et al. Prevalence of cobalamin deficiency in the Framingham elderly population. Am J Clin Nutr 60:2–11, 1994.
12. Phekoo K, Williams Y, Schey SA, et al. Folate assays: Serum or red cell? J R Coll Physicians Lond 31(3):291–295, 1997.
13. Layrisse M, Garcia-Casal MN. Strategies for the prevention of iron deficiency through foods in the household. Nutr Rev 55(6):223–239, 1997.
14. Swain RA, Kaplan B, Montgomery E. Iron deficiency anemia. When is parental therapy warranted? Postgrad Med 100(5):181–193, 1996.
15. Kumph VJ. Parenteral iron supplementation. Nutr Clin Pract 11:139–146, 1996.
16. Viteri FE. Iron supplementation for the control of iron deficiency in populations at risk. Nutr Rev 55(6):195–209, 1997.
17. Stephenson LS. Possible new developments in community control of iron-deficiency anemia. Nutr Rev 53(2):23–30, 1995.
18. de Andraco I, Castillo M, Walter T. Psychomotor development and behavior in iron-deficient anemic infants. Nutr Rev 55(4):125–132, 1997.
19. Looker AC, Dallman PR, Carroll MD, et al. Prevalence of iron deficiency in the United States. JAMA 277:973–976, 1997.

20. Beddall A. Anemias. Practitioner 234:714–715, 1992.
21. Rowland TW. Iron deficiency in the young athlete. Pediatr Clin North Am 37:1153–1163, 1990.
22. Demiroglu H, Dundar S. Pernicious anemia patients should be screened for iron deficiency during follow-up. N Z Med J 110:147–148, 1997.
23. Hash RB, Sargent MA, Katner H. Anemia secondary to combined deficiencies of iron and cobalamin. Arch Fam Med 5:585–588, 1996.
24. Sayetta RB. Pica: an overview. Am Fam Physician 33(5):181–185, 1986.
25. Hastka J, Lasserre J-J, Schwarzbeck A, et al. Laboratory tests of iron status: Correlation or common sense? Clin Chem 42(5):718–724, 1996.
26. Roncagliolo M, Garrido M, Walter T, et al. Evidence of altered central nervous system development in infants with iron deficiency anemia at 6 mo: delayed maturation of auditory brainstem responses. Am J Clin Nutr 68:683–690, 1998.
27. Lozoff B, Jimenez E, Wolf AW. Long-term developmental outcome of infants with iron deficiency. N Engl J Med 325:687–694, 1991.
28. Punnonen K, Irjala K, Rajamaki A. Serum transferrin receptor and its ratio to serum ferritin in the diagnosis of iron deficiency. Blood 89(3):1052–1057, 1997.
29. Skikne BS. Circulating transferrin receptor assay: coming of age. Clin Chem 44(1):7–9, 1998.
30. Hurrell RF. Preventing iron deficiency through food fortification. Nutr Rev 55(6):210–222, 1997.
31. Hallberg L, Hulten L, Gramatkovski E. Iron absorption from the whole diet in men: how effective is the regulation of iron absorption? Am J Clin Nutr 66:347–356, 1997.
32. Calvo EB, Galindo AC, Aspres NB. Iron status in exclusively breast-fed infants. Pediatrics 90(3):375–379, 1992.
33. Walter T, Pino P, Pizarro F, et al. Prevention of iron deficiency anemia: Comparison of high- and low-iron formulas in term healthy infants after six months of life. J Pediatr 132:635–640, 1998.
34. Haschke F, Vanura H, Male C, et al. Iron nutrition and growth of breast- and formula-fed infants during the first 9 months of life. J Pediatr Gastroenterol Nutr 16:151–156, 1993.
35. Moffatt MEK, Longstaffe S, Besant J, et al. Prevention of iron deficiency and psychomotor decline in high-risk infants through use of iron-fortified infant formula: a randomized clinical trial. J Pediatr 125:527–534, 1994.
36. Beard JL. Weekly iron intervention: the case for intermittent iron supplementation. Am J Clin Nutr 68:209–212, 1998.
37. Hallberg L. Combating iron deficiency: daily administration of iron is far superior to weekly administration. Am J Clin Nutr 68:213–217, 1998.
38. Lui XN, Kang J, Zhao L, et al. Intermittent iron supplementation in Chinese preschool children is efficient and safe. Food Nutr Bull 16:139–146, 1995.
39. Harju E. Clinical pharmacokinetics of iron preparations. Clin Pharmacokinet 17(2):69–89, 1989.
40. Cohen A. Treatment of transfusional iron overload. Am J Pediatr Hematol Oncol 12:4–8, 1990.
41. Colon-Otero G, Menke D, Hook CC. A practical approach to the differential diagnosis and evaluation of the adult patient with macrocytic anemia. Med Clin North Am 76(3):581–597, 1992.
42. Davenport J. Macrocytic anemia. Am Fam Physician 53(1):155–162, 1996.
43. Bower C, Wald NJ. Vitamin B_{12} deficiency and the fortification of food with folic acid. Eur J Clin Nutr 49:787–793, 1995.
44. Dickinson CJ. Does folic acid harm people with vitamin B_{12} deficiency? Q J Med 88:357–364, 1995.
45. Goodman KI, Salt WB. Vitamin B_{12} deficiency. Important new concepts in recognition. Postgrad Med 88(3):147–158, 1990.
46. Swain R. An update of vitamin B_{12} metabolism and deficiency states. J Fam Pract 41:595–600, 1995.
47. Allen RH, Stabler SP, Savage DG, et al. Elevation of 2-methylcitric acid I and II levels in serum, urine, and cerebrospinal fluid of patients with cobalamin deficiency. Metabolism 42:978–988, 1993.
48. Delva MD. Vitamin B_{12} replacement. To B_{12} or not to B_{12}? Can Fam Physician 43:917–922, 1997.
49. Nexo E, Hansen M, Rasmussen K, et al. How to diagnose cobalamin deficiency. Scand J Clin Lab Invest 54(Suppl 219):61–76, 1994.
50. Stott DJ, Langhorne P, Hendry A, et al. Prevalence and haemopoietic effects of low serum vitamin B_{12} levels in geriatric medical patients. Br J Nutr 78:57–63, 1997.
51. Carmel R. Cobalamin, the stomach, and aging. Am J Clin Nutr 66:750–759, 1997.
52. Brigden ML. A systematic approach to macrocytosis. Sorting out the causes. Postgrad Med 97(5):171–186, 1995.
53. Marcuard SP, Albernaz L, Khazanie PG. Omeprazole therapy causes malabsorption of cyanocobalamin (vitamin B_{12}). Ann Intern Med 120:211–215, 1994.
54. Termanini B, Gibril F, Sutliff VE, et al. Effect of long-term gastric acid suppressive therapy on serum vitamin B_{12} levels in patients with Zollinger-Ellison syndrome. Am J Med 104:422–430, 1998.
55. Field EA, Speechley JA, Rugman FR, et al. Oral signs and symptoms in patients with undiagnosed vitamin B_{12} deficiency. J Oral Pathol Med 24:468–470, 1995.
56. Amos RJ, Dawson DW, Fish DI, et al. Guidelines on the investigation and diagnosis of cobalamin and folate deficiencies. A publication of the British Committee for Standards in Haematology. Clin Lab Haematol 16:101–115, 1994.
57. Kuzminski AM, Del Giacco EJ, Allen RH, et al. Effective treatment of cobalamin deficiency with oral cobalamin. Blood 92(4):1191–1198, 1998.
58. Kondo H. Haematological effects of oral cobalamin preparations on patients with megaloblastic anemia. Acta Haematol 99:200–205, 1998.
59. Altay C, Cetin M. Oral treatment in selective vitamin B_{12} malabsorption. J Pediatr Hematol Oncol 19(3):245–246, 1997.
60. Lederle FA. Oral cobalamin for pernicious anemia: medicine's best kept secret? JAMA 265:94–95, 1991.
61. Elia M. Oral or parenteral therapy for B_{12} deficiency. Lancet 352:1721–1722, 1998.
62. Romeo VD, Sileno A, Wenig DN. Intranasal cyanocobalamin [letter]. JAMA 268:1268–1269, 1992.
63. Slot WB, Merkus FWHM, Van Deventer SJH, et al. Normalization of plasma vitamin B_{12} concentration by intranasal hydroxocobalamin in vitamin B_{12}-deficient patients. Gastroenterology 113:430–433, 1997.
64. Swain RA, St Clair L. The role of folic acid in deficiency states and prevention of disease. J Fam Pract 44(2):138–144, 1997.
65. Eskes TKAB. Folates and the fetus. Eur J Obstet Gynecol Reprod Biol 71:105–111, 1997.
66. Oakley GP. Eat right and take a multivitamin. N Engl J Med 338(15):1060–1061, 1998.
67. Folsom AR, Nieto J, McGovern PG, et al. Prospective study of coronary heart disease incidence in relation to fasting total homocysteine, related genetic polymorphisms, and B vitamins. The Atherosclerosis Risk in Communities (ARIC) Study. Circulation 98:204–210, 1998.
68. Malinow MR, Duell PB, Hess DL, et al. Reduction of plasma homocyst(e)ine levels by breakfast cereal fortified with folic acid in patients with coronary heart disease. N Engl J Med 338:1009–1015, 1998.
69. Gloria L, Cravo M, Camilo ME, et al. Nutritional deficiencies in chronic alcoholics: relationship to dietary intake and alcohol consumption. Am J Gastroenterol 92(3):485–489, 1997.
70. Quinn K, Basu TK. Folate and vitamin B_{12} status of the elderly. Eur J Clin Nutr 50:340–342, 1996.
71. Mansouri A, Lipschitz DA. Anemia in the elderly patient. Med Clin North Am 76(3):619–630, 1992.
72. Rule SAJ, Hooker M, Costello C, et al. Serum vitamin B_{12} and transcobalamin levels in early HIV disease. Am J Hematol 47:167–171, 1994.
73. Paltiel O, Falutz J, Veilleux M, et al. Clinical correlates of subnormal vitamin B_{12} levels in patients with the human immunodeficiency virus. Am J Hematol 49:318–322, 1995.
74. Anonymous. United States Pharmacopeial Convention Inc: iron supplements (systemic) in USP DI. Drug information for the health care professional. 19th ed. Rockville, MD: United States Pharmacopeial Convention, 1999: 1774–1785.
75. Anonymous. United States Pharmacopeial Convention Inc: vitamin B_{12} (Systemic) in USP DI. Drug information for the health care professional. 19th ed. Rockville, MD: United States Pharmacopeial Convention, 1999: 2962–2965.
76. Tucker KL, Mahnken B, Wilson PWF, et al. Folic acid fortification of the food supply. Potential benefits and risks for the elderly population. JAMA 276(23):1879–1885, 1996.
77. Anonymous. United States Pharmacopeial Convention Inc: folic acid (systemic) in USP DI. Drug information for the health care professional. 19th ed. Rockville, MD: United States Pharmacopeial Convention, 1999: 1517–1520.

CHAPTER 14

OTHER ANEMIAS

Janice L. Stumpf and Kevin A. Townsend

Although the clinical features of anemias resulting from many causes are often similar, treatment modalities and prognosis are quite distinct. In this chapter, a variety of anemias are discussed, including the anemias of chronic disease and renal failure, aplastic anemia, sickle cell anemia, thalassemia, and hemolytic anemia.

TREATMENT GOALS: OTHER ANEMIAS

- Improve the anemia of chronic disease by treating the infectious, inflammatory, or neoplastic underlying condition.
- Increase hematocrit concentrations toward normal values in patients with anemia of renal failure by administering recombinant human erythropoietin while maintaining iron stores.
- Remove the causative agent in patients who develop aplastic anemia and provide supportive care with transfusions and antibiotic therapy as well as definitive therapy with immunosuppressive agents or bone marrow transplantation.
- Prevent the adverse consequences of sickle cell anemia by providing transfusions, vaccinations, and prophylactic antibiotics as indicated; provide effective treatment for painful vasoocclusive crises, infections, and other complications; and treat the disorder itself with hydroxyurea or bone marrow transplantation.
- Correct the anemia and suppress the ineffective erythropoiesis of β-thalassemia major by providing regular blood transfusions.
- Avoid blood transfusion–associated iron overload by administering concomitant iron chelation therapy.
- Manage hemolytic anemia by identifying and controlling etiologic factors and providing appropriate supportive care.

Anemia of Chronic Disease

The anemia of chronic disease is a mild, often asymptomatic condition that occurs in conjunction with a variety of infectious, inflammatory, and neoplastic disorders. The anemia develops 1 to 2 months after the onset of diseases such as chronic osteomyelitis, tuberculosis, rheumatoid arthritis, systemic lupus erythematosus, vasculitides, and carcinomas including Hodgkin's disease and solid tumors. Although renal insufficiency also is a chronic disease, the associated anemia manifests differently and therefore is discussed separately.

PATHOPHYSIOLOGY

The common pathology of anemia of chronic disease appears to be a defect in iron transport from the reticuloendothelial system (RES), hepatocytes, and intestinal epithelial cells to the plasma and erythroid precursor cells.[1] In addition, a moderate shortening of red blood cell (RBC) life span may be noted that is unaccompanied by increased erythrocyte production. In fact, erythropoietin concentrations may be low relative to the measured hematocrit.

Although the reasons for these abnormalities are not known, it has been suggested that the cytokine interleukin-1 may be the primary mediator of the pathology of anemia of chronic disease.[1,2] Interleukin-1 stimulates the elaboration of high concentrations of lactoferrin from leukocytes at sites of inflammation. This protein preferentially binds iron and prevents its mobilization to the plasma. Macrophages then take up the iron–lactoferrin complex, resulting in accumulation of iron in the cells of the RES. Alternatively, interleukin-1 may induce the synthesis of ferritin, allowing increased iron storage and restricting the amount of iron available to the bone marrow. Other cytokines, including tumor necrosis factor and interferon, may also have a role in suppressing erythropoiesis.[2]

CLINICAL PRESENTATION AND DIAGNOSIS

Because it is associated with many diseases and a unifying pathogenesis has not been elucidated, anemia of chronic disease remains a diagnosis of exclusion. The erythrocytes typically are normochromic and normocytic, but may be microcytic. The hematocrit concentration rarely falls below 30%; if it does, other causes of anemia should be investigated thoroughly. The reticulocyte count is low or within normal limits and serum iron levels and iron binding protein saturation are low. However, in contrast to the picture of iron deficiency anemia, ferritin levels are elevated in the anemia of chronic disease. Anemia caused by iron deficiency as a sole diagnosis or in conjunction with the anemia of chronic disease is unlikely if the serum ferritin concentration exceeds 50 μg/L.[1] These and other manifestations, including elevations in haptoglobin and fibrinogen levels and erythrocyte sedimentation rate, are known collectively as the acute phase reaction, a response to inflammation that may persist with chronic conditions.

TREATMENT

Because the anemia of chronic disease generally is mild, no specific therapy is necessary in most cases. The degree of anemia correlates well with the severity of the associated disease state, and reversal of the underlying disorder corrects the anemia. However, if the patient becomes symptomatic, blood transfusions may be beneficial. Iron replacement regimens have been attempted, but have been uniformly ineffective and may place the patient at risk of iron toxicity. The anemia of chronic disease has responded to therapy with recombinant human erythropoietin; however, the role of this agent in the clinical setting has not been established.[1,2]

Anemia of Renal Failure

The anemia that complicates end-stage renal disease generally is more severe than that associated with other chronic diseases. The severity of the anemia appears to correlate with the extent of the uremia, but not with the cause of the underlying renal disease. Most patients with serum creatinine concentrations higher than 310 μmol/L (3.5 mg/dL) and 97% of those on maintenance dialysis are affected. The cells are normochromic and normocytic but often are irregular in shape. Although hematocrit levels may fall to 20 to 30% or less, not all patients become symptomatic. This tolerance of such low hematocrit concentrations may be explained by the compensatory reduction in oxygen–hemoglobin affinity, allowing improved delivery of oxygen to the tissues. Despite this adaptation, an estimated 25% of patients receiving dialysis needed treatment with blood transfusions before the widespread use of recombinant erythropoietin.[3] In addition to the commonly known symptoms of anemia (e.g., fatigue, increasing angina and shortness of breath), vague complaints of generalized coldness, anorexia, insomnia and depression, which were not associated with anemia until recently, may be improved with adequate therapy.

PATHOPHYSIOLOGY

The anemia of renal failure is a multifactorial process but is primarily the result of reduced secretion of erythropoietin by the diseased kidneys. This hormone stimulates the proliferation and maturation of erythrocytes and is released when the availability of oxygen to the organs is diminished. Although to some extent synthesized extrarenally in the liver, serum erythropoietin concentrations in uremic patients are markedly lower than those measured in patients with similar degrees of anemia and normal renal function.

Other factors that contribute to the anemia are the accumulation of inhibitors of erythropoiesis, reduced RBC life span, and chronic blood loss.[3] In support of the presence of suppressive substances, erythropoietin-induced stimulation of erythroid progenitors is blunted in vitro by uremic serum. In addition, while erythropoietin levels remain stable, the anemia improves after dialysis, perhaps indicating removal of these substances. Parathyroid hormone and the polyamine spermine have been implicated in reducing marrow responsiveness to erythropoietin; however, data are conflicting and the identity of the inhibitory substances remains unknown.

Erythrocyte survival also decreases to an average of one-half of normal in uremia due to a mild, chronic hemolysis. The cause of the red cell destruction is unclear; however, hypersplenism or increases in erythrocyte fragility induced by parathyroid hormone may contribute. This abnormality may not be corrected by dialysis, yet also does not appear to be a defect in the red cells. A similar reduction in erythrocyte life span is noted after transfusion of blood products from nonuremic donors to patients with renal failure.

Chronic blood loss both from a gastrointestinal source and during hemodialysis may also contribute to the anemia. Because of defects in platelet function, uremic patients have an elevated risk of bleeding; occult blood loss is reported in more than 20% of patients receiving dialysis.[4] An estimated 2 g of iron is lost annually during hemodialysis, increasing the likelihood of a concurrent iron deficiency anemia. In addition, the intestinal absorption of iron may be compromised by the chronic use of iron-chelating antacids. Other factors that may aggravate the anemia of end-stage renal disease include folic acid deficiency caused by losses to the dialysate, the accumulation of the fat-soluble vitamin A, aluminum toxicity caused by long-term hemodialysis and the use of aluminum-containing phosphate binders, and osteitis fibrosa, a complication of hyperparathyroidism in which myelofibrosis reduces viable erythroid cellular mass.

TREATMENT

Before the initiation of therapy aimed at the primary abnormality, other potential causes of anemia should be identified and addressed. Iron and folate supplementation should be provided as necessary, and blood loss and the use of aluminum-containing antacids should be minimized whenever possible. The treatment for acute symptoms of hypoxia consists of the transfusion of RBCs. However, although transfusions may readily correct the anemia, they carry the risk of hypersensitivity reactions and the transmission of viral hepatitis. In addition, bone marrow suppression and iron overload necessitating deferoxamine therapy may occur after multiple, chronic transfusions.

Androgens

Traditionally, the use of androgens has been recommended for treating anemia in selected patients with end-stage renal disease. These agents stimulate the synthesis of erythropoietin and/or the production of RBCs in the bone marrow. However, they are not universally effective and rarely fully correct the anemia. Elevations in hematocrit concentrations of 5% or more compared to baseline were documented in 50% of patients able to tolerate the drugs in a 6-month controlled cross-over trial.[4] Therapy with the injectable formulations nandrolone decanoate and testosterone enanthate resulted in significantly greater improvements in hematocrit levels than the two oral androgens studied, fluoxymesterone and oxymetholone. Transfusion needs were not reduced during androgen therapy. Patients with lower pretreatment hematocrit concentrations, bilateral nephrectomies, or intact parathyroid glands had poorer response rates. Based on these results and the propensity for virilization effects such as hirsutism, changes in external genitalia, amenorrhea, acne, and voice deepening, the usefulness of androgens for this indication is limited. Injectable androgens are recommended over oral agents, and nandrolone decanoate is preferred in female patients because of its greater ratio of anabolic to androgenic activities. Nandrolone decanoate and testosterone enanthate are administered as weekly intramuscular injections of 1.5 to 2.5 mg/kg and 4 to 7 mg/kg, respectively. If an adequate response is not achieved after a 6-month trial, the agent should be discontinued. Therapy with oral androgens (fluoxymesterone 10 to 30 mg daily) may then be attempted. However, in addition to the adverse effects associated with the injectable agents, the oral androgens may induce liver dysfunction and hepatic cancer.

Recombinant Human Erythropoietin

Advances in recombinant technology have made possible the production of human erythropoietin (epoetin alfa, epoetin), a peptide whose 166–amino acid structure is identical to that of the native hormone. The availability of epoetin has revolutionized the therapy of anemia associated with end-stage renal disease and all but eliminated the use of androgen therapy.

In a multicenter study of the efficacy of epoetin, intravenous doses of 150 or 300 U/kg were administered to 333 anemic patients three times weekly after hemodialysis.[5] Target hematocrit concentrations of 35% or a 6% above baseline were achieved in more than 97% of patients within 12 weeks. In addition, the need for routine red cell transfusions was eliminated within 2 months. Quality of life was enhanced as evidenced by increased energy and activity levels, cold tolerance, and appetite. A median dosage of 75 U/kg maintained these effects. Lack of response in the remaining patients was attributed to other causes of anemia, such as myelofibrosis and blood loss.

Patients with end-stage renal disease with hematocrit levels under 30% or requiring blood transfusions may be considered candidates for epoetin treatment. Although it was once commonly given as intravenous bolus doses of 50 to 100 U/kg three times weekly after hemodialysis, subcutaneous administration of epoetin is preferred and has been used successfully in predialysis and continuous ambulatory peritoneal dialysis (CAPD) populations as well. The bioavailability of epoetin after subcutaneous administration is approximately 48% (range, 14.5 to 96.5%); however, lower, more sustained plasma concentrations are achieved through slow release from the subcutaneous depot.[6] The elimination half-life after subcutaneous injection is approximately 28 hours, whereas that after intravenous administration ranges from 4 to 11 hours. Similar efficacy has been provided by the subcutaneous route with epoetin dosages 23 to 52% lower than those of the intravenous route. An initial subcutaneous regimen of 25 to 50 U/kg two or three times weekly is recommended.[6,7] Alternatively, once-weekly subcutaneous injections of epoetin also are effective yet require the same total dosage as intravenous therapy. Intraperitoneal administration generally is impractical because of the high dosages needed to produce plasma concentrations comparable to those achieved by subcutaneous or intravenous administration.[6,7]

Dose-dependent rises in hematocrit and reticulocyte counts are seen after 2 to 6 weeks of therapy.[8] Hematocrit concentrations should be determined weekly; if the hematocrit has not increased to target range or by more than 3 percentage points after 4 weeks of therapy, the dosage should be adjusted upward.[7] Once a hematocrit of 30% is attained, the dosage should be reduced by 50% and titrated every 4 weeks to maintain hematocrit concentrations of 33 to 38%.[6] It should be noted that this goal hematocrit level remains controversial in that it provides only partial correction of the anemia.[7,9] Preliminary data suggest that normalization of hematocrit concentrations from 33 to 42% may result in significant improvements in physiologic and quality of life measures without compromising patient safety.[9]

Adverse effects associated with epoetin therapy include myalgias, headache, flank pain, hypertension, and seizures. In addition, local reactions, such as burning, pain, and irritation, have been reported after subcutaneous injection. Increases in blood pressure appear to be a hemodynamic consequence of the rising hematocrit. As the anemia is corrected, compensatory vasodilation decreases and peripheral vascular resistance and blood pressure increase. Blood pressure elevations necessitate the institution or upward adjustment of antihypertensive medications in 30 to 40% of patients within 6 months of epoetin initiation.[10] Seizures may accompany uncontrolled hypertension. Therefore, close monitoring and control of blood pressure levels are essential.

Increases in predialysis concentrations of serum creatinine, potassium, and phosphate have also been documented. The reduced effectiveness of dialysis noted with higher hematocrit levels and increased dietary intake may account for these changes. In addition, clotting of arteriovenous access sites has occurred in up to 14% of epoetin-treated patients. In contrast, in another report, the incidence of graft thrombosis was no greater than that of a historical control hemodialysis population not receiving epoetin.[6]

During the acute erythroid response, iron may be used more rapidly than it is released to transferrin from the RES. A functional and an absolute iron deficiency may therefore develop, which may compromise further response to epoetin. Patients with pretreatment iron overload have experienced beneficial 39% reductions in serum ferritin levels within 6 months. Ferritin levels and transferrin saturation should be determined at baseline and monthly until the goal hematocrit is achieved; iron stores should be measured at 2- to 3-month intervals thereafter. If the ferritin concentration or transferrin saturation falls below 100 μg/L or 20%, respectively, intravenous or oral iron supplementation should be initiated.[6,7]

Epoetin allows clinicians to correct the anemia of renal disease on a long-term basis in both dialysis and predialysis patients. The high response rate indicates that the predominant cause of the anemia is erythropoietin deficiency. Other pathogenetic mechanisms, such as the presence of inhibitors of erythropoiesis, may also be operative, yet may be overwhelmed clinically by excessive exogenous erythropoietin. The high cost of epoetin should be considered in the context of savings resulting from reductions in other interventions. Routine blood transfusions, androgen therapy, and hospitalizations due to complications of these modalities may be eliminated completely. In addition, improvements in quality of life parameters may lead to greater rehabilitation potential and a return to productive lives for more patients with end-stage renal disease.

Aplastic Anemia

Aplastic anemia is distinguished by hypocellularity of the bone marrow and subsequent pancytopenia that is unrelated to malignancy or myeloproliferative disease. The characteristic anemia, neutropenia, and thrombocytopenia result from failure of the pluripotential stem cell due to congenital or acquired processes. Although the causative mechanisms remain unknown, advances in therapy have greatly improved the overall prognosis.

EPIDEMIOLOGY

The annual incidence of aplastic anemia in United States is estimated to be two to five cases per million population.[11] The prevalence of disease is higher in Korea and Japan, perhaps reflecting increased exposure to viral hepatitis and environmental toxins. Two peaks are evident in the distribution of ages of onset: Approximately 25% of those affected are younger than 15 years, and 50 to 70% are over 40 years of age.

Although many causes have been identified, up to 70% of cases of aplastic anemia are classified as idiopathic. Myelosuppression is a component of several congenital diseases but is more commonly acquired after exposure to drugs, chemicals, ionizing radiation, or viruses (Table 14.1).

Bone marrow suppression resulting from drugs or chemicals is often dose and duration dependent and may result from direct or immune-mediated stem cell toxicity. Chloramphenicol is the best-documented cause of drug-induced aplastic anemia. Reversible erythroid suppression is noted in approximately 50% of those receiving more than 1 week of high-dose systemic therapy but has been reported after even ophthalmic administration of the antibiotic. In contrast, rare idiosyncratic marrow suppression manifesting weeks to months after exposure is also associated with chloramphenicol. Before the availability of bone marrow transplantation (BMT) and alternative treatments, this reaction was fatal in 90% of cases, often within 1 year of clinical presentation.

Aplastic anemia may also arise concurrently with or after viral infection. Hepatitis, most often non-A, non-B (including hepatitis C), precedes up to 5% of cases of aplastic anemia; however, the severity of the infection does not predict the subsequent development of bone marrow suppression. Myelosuppression usually is noted within 6 months of the onset of hepatitis.

Table 14.1 ▪ Causes of Aplastic Anemia

- Acquired
  - Drugs and chemicals
    - Acetazolamide
    - Anticonvulsants
      - Carbamazepine
      - Felbamate
      - Phenytoin
      - Primidone
    - Arsenic
    - Benzene
    - Cancer chemotherapy
    - Chloramphenicol
    - Chlorpromazine
    - Ethanol
    - Gold salts
    - Insecticides
    - Phenylbutazone
    - Quinacrine hydrochloride
    - Sulfa drugs
    - Ticlopidine
  - Viral
    - Cytomegalovirus
    - Epstein-Barr virus
    - Hepatitis
    - Herpes varicella zoster
    - Human immunodeficiency virus
    - Influenza
    - Parvovirus
    - Rubella
  - Other
    - Eosinophilic fasciitis
    - Ionizing radiation
    - Mycobacterial infection
    - Paroxysmal nocturnal hemoglobinuria
    - Pregnancy
    - Thymoma
    - Transfusional graft versus host disease
- Congenital
  - Amegakaryocytic thrombocytopenia
  - Dubowitz syndrome
  - Dyskeratosis congenita
  - Familial aplastic anemia
  - Fanconi's anemia
  - Shwachman–Diamond syndrome

PATHOPHYSIOLOGY

In normal hematopoiesis, three cell lines originate from the pluripotential stem cell, producing erythrocytes, granulocytes, and platelets. Both cellular and humoral factors regulate the stem cells to maintain a balance between self-replication and differentiation into particular cell types. Aplastic anemia develops when hematopoiesis is interrupted because of deficient or defective stem cells. In addition to reduced numbers of progenitor cells, suggested pathophysiologic mechanisms include immune-mediated suppression of stem cell function, disturbances in the bone marrow microenvironment, and alterations in the cellular or humoral interactions that normally sustain hematopoiesis.[12–14] Research with a variety of treatment modalities supports immune-mediated destruction of marrow cells as the most likely cause of the majority of cases of acquired aplastic anemia.

CLINICAL PRESENTATION AND DIAGNOSIS

Stem cell dysfunction may be incomplete and result in unequal effects on each cell type. Therefore, the earliest clinical signs are determined by the cell line affected to the greatest degree. Often, features of a mild anemia, such as pallor and fatigue, are reported initially and may be more pronounced if accompanied by bleeding due to thrombocytopenia. Ecchymoses and petechiae also indicate a low platelet count. Less commonly, infection caused by the underlying neutropenia is the presenting manifestation of aplastic anemia. Signs of infection such as fever should be monitored closely as the neutropenia progresses because inflammation may not be apparent.

Decreased numbers of morphologically normal cells are observed in the peripheral blood. The erythrocytes are normochromic and normocytic or slightly macrocytic. The corrected reticulocyte count is markedly reduced, as is the absolute granulocyte count. Bone marrow biopsy reveals extensive areas of hypocellularity interspersed with small patches of hematopoietic cells.

TREATMENT

Treating patients with aplastic anemia includes removal of potential causative agents, supportive care, and the restoration of normal hematopoiesis with pharmacologic therapy or BMT.[13,14] In mild cases, supportive care should be provided in anticipation of spontaneous recovery. Blood transfusions, preferably leukocyte-depleted products, should be reserved for patients with symptomatic anemia to delay sensitization to alloantigens. Blood products from family members should not be used in candidates for marrow transplantation because of the development of antibodies to histocompatibility antigens of the donor, increasing the risk of graft rejection. Overall, nontransfused patients fare better after BMT than their transfused counterparts.

Antiplatelet antibodies that reduce platelet function and life span also develop after 1 to 2 months of repeated transfusions. Patients often become refractory to subsequent transfusions, although a dose–response relationship has not been established. Platelets should be administered to maintain a platelet count higher than 20×10^9/L (20,000/mL) and to treat active bleeding.

Because of the risk of hematoma, intramuscular injections should be avoided whenever possible in patients with thrombocytopenia, as should aspirin, nonsteroidal anti-inflammatory drugs, and other agents with antiplatelet properties. Menses should be suppressed hormonally to prevent menorrhagia in female patients with aplastic anemia.

Prompt recognition and treatment of infection is vital in the patient with aplastic anemia and severe neutropenia. Broad-spectrum antibiotics should be initiated in any patient with fever of unknown origin. If a pathogen is not identified and the patient continues to be febrile after 48 to 72 hours of treatment, empiric antifungal therapy with amphotericin B should be considered.

Bone Marrow Transplantation

BMT has become the treatment of choice for severe aplastic anemia, with greatest success achieved in younger patients undergoing the procedure soon after diagnosis (Table 14.2).[12–14] Initially, a donor who is human lymphocyte antigen (HLA) compatible must be identified. There is a 25% chance that a sibling will be HLA identical. Graft rejection may develop because of minor antigenic differences between donor and recipient marrow and previous sensitization by blood transfusions. Therefore, a course of immunosuppressive therapy is administered before transplantation. Historically, this conditioning regimen consisted of intravenous cyclophosphamide (50 mg/kg daily for 4 days) combined with total body or total lymphoid irradiation. Alternatively, regimens of cyclophosphamide and cyclosporine with or without antithymocyte globulin (ATG) have been used.[12–14] These protocols have reduced graft rejection to 3 to 5% in some series.[13,14] Two to six weeks after intravenous infusion of marrow cells, the donor cells have engrafted, and blood cells begin to be produced.

The interval between transplantation and the return of hematopoiesis and normal immune function poses the greatest threat to the patient. Supportive care should include isolation in a sterile environment, transfusions of blood products as needed, and close monitoring for signs of infection. Prophylactic antifungal therapy and bowel sterilization with nonabsorbable oral antibiotics may be undertaken in attempts to reduce the incidence of systemic infections. Interstitial pneumonitis may complicate transplantation within the first 3 months and occurs in approximately 18% of patients with aplastic anemia. In more than 39% of cases, cytomegalovirus is implicated and is associated with a mortality rate of more than 70%.[15] Infection with *Aspergillus, Candida, Pneumocystis carinii,* herpes simplex virus, and herpes varicella zoster virus has also been reported. Trimethoprim–sulfamethoxazole and acyclovir prophylaxis often are administered to inhibit

Table 14.2 ▪ Considerations in the Selection of Therapy for Aplastic Anemia

	Bone Marrow Transplantation	Immunosuppression
Age	≤ 20 yr	> 40 yr
Human lymphocyte antigen–matched sibling	Yes	No
Absolute neutrophil count	< 200/mL	> 200/mL
Blood product transfusions	None or minimal	–

activation of *Pneumocystis* and herpes viruses, respectively. In addition, the use of immune globulin to prevent cytomegalovirus activation is advocated at some centers.

Acute graft-versus-host-disease (GVHD), in which donor lymphocytes attack the host tissue, occurs in 30 to 60% of patients within 2 months after transplantation despite prophylactic immunosuppression.[13] Regimens of methotrexate or cyclosporine alone or in combination are used to prevent GVHD;[14] the addition of prednisone may further improve outcome.[13] Initial presenting signs of acute GVHD include skin rash and diarrhea. Elevations in liver function tests and severe immunodeficiency may also develop. Once established, GVHD may be managed with ATG, prednisone, or cyclosporine, with response rates of 30 to 50%.[13]

Chronic GVHD manifests as a serious complication more than 3 months after transplantation in approximately 20% of surviving patients.[14] The reaction is similar to that of a systemic autoimmune disease (e.g., systemic lupus erythematosus) with skin, gastrointestinal, hepatic, lymphoid, lung, and ophthalmic involvement. After treatment regimens of prednisone and cyclosporine or azathioprine, 80% of afflicted patients recover.[13] The risk of acquiring and severity of GVHD are directly correlated to patient age. Therefore, most transplantations are performed in patients under age 40.

Immunosuppression

Immunosuppressive therapy generally is reserved for older patients with aplastic anemia or those without an HLA-matched marrow donor. A variety of agents, both alone and in combination, have been used to treat the disease, including ATG, antilymphocyte globulin (ALG), corticosteroids, and cyclosporine.[12–14]

ATG and ALG are prepared in animals and react against human thymocytes and lymphocytes, respectively. The mechanism by which these agents positively affect aplastic anemia is unknown, but they presumably inactivate cytotoxic lymphocytes responsible for suppression of hematopoiesis. In addition, proliferation and differentiation of hematopoietic progenitors may be stimulated. The overall efficacy of ATG and ALG is difficult to assess from current research because of variations in preparations, treatment protocols, and severity of illness in the study populations. However, response rates of 30 to 75% have been reported.[12]

In a typical treatment protocol, a test dose is administered and, in the absence of anaphylaxis, is followed by a total ATG or ALG dosage of 100 to 160 mg/kg divided over 4 to 10 days, with each dose infused intravenously over 4 to 12 hours.[12,14] Response is usually observed within 1 to 3 months after therapy. A second course may be effective in those in whom initial therapy fails and in the 25 to 30% of patients who relapse.

Adverse effects of ATG and ALG include fever, chills, rash, headache, and hypotension. Serum sickness, manifesting with fever, rash, and arthralgias, may be evident 1 to 2 weeks after therapy; however, symptoms may be alleviated by concurrent corticosteroid therapy. Transient reductions in white blood cell and platelet counts are also reported. Hematologic complications, such as myelodysplasia, leukemia, and paroxysmal nocturnal hemoglobinuria, develop in 30 to 50% of patients, with the prevalence increasing with time.

Data regarding the usefulness of high-dose methylprednisolone in conjunction with ATG and ALG are conflicting.[14] Methylprednisolone 1 mg/kg/day often is added to the regimen to control antiserum-induced toxicities. The efficacy of high-dose corticosteroids alone for treating aplastic anemia has not been demonstrated conclusively.

Immunosuppression with cyclosporine alone has yielded response rates similar to those of ATG.[12–14] Effects usually are observed after 2 to 10 weeks of treatment. Long-term maintenance therapy with cyclosporine often is needed, increasing the risk of renal toxicity and other adverse effects. In a controlled study, the addition of cyclosporine to the combination of ALG and methylprednisolone increased the rate of complete or partial remission from 39 to 65% at 3 months.[11] This intensive immunosuppression resulted in more rapid and complete responses as well as fewer relapses compared with ALG plus corticosteroid therapy alone.

Androgens

Androgens once were widely used to treat aplastic anemia because of their stimulatory effects on hematopoiesis (predominantly red cell production). However, in patients with severe disease, oral oxymetholone and intramuscular nandrolone decanoate produced responses similar to those produced by supportive care alone. In addition, androgens do not potentiate the effects of ATG or ALG therapy. Although androgens have no apparent role in the management of severe forms of the disease, those with mild aplastic anemia or Fanconi's anemia not amenable to marrow transplantation may benefit from treatment. Initial responses are detected after 3 to 6 months of therapy; however, adverse effects such as virilization and hepatotoxicity may limit the prolonged courses needed to achieve effects in all cell lines.

Hematopoietic Growth Factors

Hematopoietic growth factors stimulate the proliferation of progenitor cells and thus may have applications to many hypoplastic disorders.[12,16,17] Although recombinant human granulocyte colony-stimulating factor (G-CSF, filgrastim) and granulocyte–macrophage colony-stimulating factor (GM-CSF, sargramostim) have been the most extensively studied, interleukins (IL-1, IL-3, IL-6) and epoetin have also been used for aplastic anemia. Both intravenous and subcutaneous G-CSF and GM-CSF to patients with aplastic anemia have produced marked elevations in leukocyte counts, primarily through increases in neutrophils. Trilineage responses with improvements in red cell and platelet counts are rare; adding epoetin to the regimen may increase RBC counts and reduce transfusion needs in some patients. In general, response is inversely related to the severity of disease, and the effects do not persist after G-CSF or GM-CSF discontinuation. Although data are limited, transient but inconsistent increases in leukocyte, platelet, and reticulocyte counts have also been demonstrated after therapy with interleukins.[16]

Because growth factors do not correct the underlying stem cell disorder, these agents should be used only in conjunction with definitive therapies for aplastic anemia (i.e., immunosuppression or BMT). Adding G-CSF as supportive therapy has improved survival by reducing mortality caused by infection.[17] Large-scale prospective clinical studies in aplastic anemia populations are necessary to determine optimal protocols for therapy with recombinant hematopoietic growth factors in combination with other treatment modalities.

PROGNOSIS

With supportive care alone, 80% of patients with severe aplastic anemia (Table 14.3) die within 1 to 2 years, with median survival of 6 months.[11–13] Advances in BMT and immunosuppressive therapy have dramatically improved this outcome. Long-term disease-free survival after transplantation ranges from 63 to 92%.[12,14] Survival rates following immunosuppressive therapy are equivalent or superior to those of transplantation, with best outcomes in patients over 20 years of age with absolute neutrophil counts higher than 200/mL.[13,14]

Table 14.3 ▪ Criteria for the Diagnosis of Severe Aplastic Anemia

Peripheral blood counts	Two or three of the following: Neutrophils $< 0.5 \times 10^9$/L Platelets $< 20 \times 10^9$/L Reticulocytes < 0.01
Bone marrow biopsy	One of the following: Severe hypocellularity (< 25% normal) Moderate hypocellularity (25 to 50% normal) with < 30% of residual cells being hematopoietic

Source: References 12, 13.

Sickle Cell Anemia

The term *sickle cell disease* encompasses a variety of hemoglobinopathies, including sickle cell anemia, sickle hemoglobin C (SC) disease, and sickle cell thalassemia. Although the clinical presentation of these disorders is often similar, the manifestations of sickle cell anemia are more severe and are therefore the focus of the following discussion.

EPIDEMIOLOGY

The Hb S gene confers protection against *Plasmodium falciparum* infection in infancy. Therefore, populations residing in or originating from areas where malaria is endemic have the highest frequency of the AS and SS genotypes. The distribution of sickle disease is no longer restricted to Africa, Saudi Arabia, and India; however, areas of concentration remain. Up to 25% of people in West Africa possess the Hb S gene. Among African Americans in the United States, 0.17% have sickle cell anemia, whereas 8% have the sickle trait.[18]

PATHOPHYSIOLOGY

The hemoglobin molecule is a tetramer comprised of four polypeptides linked to iron-carrying heme groups. More than 600 different types of hemoglobin have been distinguished, including hemoglobins A_1, A_2, C, F, and S. Only three variants are considered to be normal: hemoglobin A_1 (Hb A_1), hemoglobin A_2 (Hb A_2), and fetal hemoglobin (Hb F). Fetal hemoglobin accounts for 70 to 80% of the hemoglobin in the red cells of newborns. A gradual conversion occurs until the eighth postnatal month, when the normal adult pattern of 95 to 98% Hb A_1, less than 3.5% Hb A_2, and less than 2% Hb F is represented.[19]

The Hb A_1 tetramer consists of two pairs of globin chains, α and β, which have distinct primary structures. Sickle cell anemia is a homozygous condition that results from the substitution of valine for glutamic acid in both of the β-chains. Because each parent contributes a single β-chain gene, the heterozygous genotype AS is also possible and is expressed as the sickle cell trait phenotype.

Deoxygenation in the capillaries induces rapid polymerization of the sickling hemoglobin, Hb S, and results in formation of helical strands of parallel fibers.[20] The elongated, crescent-shaped cells characteristic of sickle cell anemia are thereby produced. The affected erythrocytes are rigid and unable to pass through the microvasculature, leading to vasoocclusion with subsequent painful ischemia and chronic organ damage. In general, the sickling is reversible upon reexposure to oxygen; however, repeated sickling episodes eventually damage the cell membrane. The sickled conformation is sustained and the cells subject to hemolysis and removal by the liver or spleen.

The rate of Hb S polymerization depends on its concentration in the erythrocyte. The copolymerization of Hb S with Hb F inhibits further polymer growth; intracellular

Hb F concentrations are inversely correlated with disease severity.

CLINICAL PRESENTATION AND DIAGNOSIS

Signs and Symptoms

Sickle cell anemia presents with constitutional, hematologic, and vasoocclusive manifestations (Table 14.4) late in the first postnatal year, after levels of the protective fetal hemoglobin have diminished. Skeletal growth and sexual maturation are impaired, although catch-up growth is apparent by adulthood.

Because of recurrent microinfarcts, the spleen is initially enlarged and then completely fibrosed by 6 years of age. This functional autosplenectomy and defects in other host defenses greatly increase the likelihood of infection, especially with *Streptococcus pneumoniae* and *Hemophilus influenzae.*

Table 14.4 ▪ Complications of Sickle Cell Anemia

- Constitutional
  - Impaired growth and development
  - Increased risk of infection
    - Meningitis
    - Osteomyelitis
    - Pneumonia
    - Pyelonephritis
    - Septicemia
- Hematologic
  - Hemolytic anemia
  - Aplastic crises
  - Splenic sequestration crises
- Vasoocclusive
  - Cardiovascular
    - Cardiac enlargement
    - Systolic murmur
  - Gastrointestinal
    - Autosplenectomy
    - Gallstones/cholecystitis
    - Hepatic crises/right upper quadrant syndrome
    - Hepatic insufficiency
    - Intrahepatic cholelithiasis
  - Genitourinary
    - Hematuria
    - Impotence
    - Priapism
    - Renal insufficiency
  - Neurologic
    - Cerebral thrombosis
    - Intracerebral hemorrhage
    - Seizures
    - Subarachnoid hemorrhage
  - Ocular
    - Retinopathy
    - Secondary glaucoma
  - Painful crises
  - Pulmonary
    - Acute chest syndrome
    - Chronic obstructive disease
    - Infarction
  - Skin and Skeletal
    - Arthropathy
    - Aseptic necrosis
    - Dactylitis
    - Leg ulcers

Hemolysis accompanied by inadequate erythropoiesis results in a normochromic, normocytic anemia, with hematocrit levels ranging from 18% to 30%. The chronic anemia leads to a hyperdynamic circulatory system and subsequent cardiac hypertrophy and systolic ejection murmurs. The anemia is aggravated during aplastic crises, when erythropoiesis is further suppressed by acute infection or folate deficiency.

Painful vasoocclusive crises produced by sludging of sickled cells in the microcirculation are the most common reason for hospitalization. The frequency and severity of painful crises vary greatly between individuals. In one review of more than 12,200 pain episodes, approximately 5% of patients with sickle cell anemia had 3 to 10 pain episodes each year, whereas another 39% did not experience pain.[21] The episodes are sudden and last for an average of 4 to 6 days. Pain is most often reported in the long bones, spine, pelvis, chest, and abdomen and must be differentiated from infection and other acute processes. Factors that may precipitate vasoocclusive crises include acidosis, heat or exercise (dehydration), cold (vasoconstriction), infection, stress, menses, and high altitudes.

Recurrent sickling and subsequent infarction produce chronic damage to many organ systems. Hematuria and an inability to concentrate urine progress in some patients to renal failure. Neurologic complications such as cerebrovascular accidents and seizures develop in 6 to 12% of patients, with a recurrence rate of 60 to 90%. Acute chest syndrome, manifesting with pleuritic chest pain, dyspnea, and pulmonary infiltrates, may eventually result in pulmonary fibrosis and chronic obstructive disease. Intrahepatic fibrosis is also reported. Impotence may occur, usually after multiple episodes of priapism.

In addition to indices of anemia, laboratory abnormalities include elevations in platelet count and leukocytosis caused by demargination of granulocytes from vessel walls into the circulation. Irreversibly sickled cells are seen in the blood smear.

Individuals with sickle cell trait generally are asymptomatic, although sickling manifestations may occur at extreme levels of hypoxia or acidosis. Transient hematuria, renal papillary necrosis, pulmonary embolism, and splenic infarction have been rarely associated with the AS phenotype. Life expectancy is normal in those with the sickle trait. In contrast, although 85 to 90% of patients with sickle cell anemia may now survive to the age of 20 years, median ages at death for males and females are 42 and 48 years, respectively.[19]

Diagnosis

Sickle cell diseases are diagnosed by hemoglobin electrophoresis, which reveals the types and proportion of hemoglobins present.[18,19] This rapid, inexpensive screening test establishes the patient's genotype, enabling appropriate genetic counseling and education. If both parents have the AS genotype, there is a 1 in 4 chance that their child will have homozygous SS disease. Prenatal diagnosis is also possible. Genotyping may be performed in the first trimester of pregnancy using fetal cells obtained by amniocentesis or chorionic villus sampling.

TREATMENT

Management of Major Complications

Anemia

Physiologic adaptations such as low Hb S–oxygen affinity allow patients with sickle cell anemia to tolerate relatively low hematocrit levels. Therefore, therapy is supportive, with blood transfusions reserved for acute, symptomatic exacerbations in the anemia. High folate utilization arising from continuously elevated red cell production may lead to folate deficiency and induce an aplastic crisis. Folate supplementation (1 mg orally daily) is recommended to maintain adequate stores. Aplastic crises may also develop from viral (most commonly, human parvovirus B19) infections, necessitating prompt diagnosis and treatment. Recovery of erythropoiesis generally occurs within 5 to 10 days, as the underlying infection resolves.

Infection

Bacterial infection is the leading cause of death in patients with sickle cell anemia. Therefore, a thorough search for an infectious source should be undertaken in any patient presenting with a painful crisis and fever.

Pneumonia may be treated empirically with parenteral cefuroxime because its spectrum of activity includes the most likely pathogens, *S. pneumoniae* and *H. influenzae*. If a clinical response is not apparent after 24 to 48 hours, infection with *Mycoplasma pneumoniae* should be suspected and erythromycin or azithromycin added to the antibiotic regimen. Meningitis occurs 200 to 300 times more frequently in children with sickle cell anemia, with *Pneumococci* being isolated in approximately 80% of cases.

Children older than 2 years should be immunized with polyvalent pneumococcal vaccine and a booster dose given after 3 to 5 years to children younger than 10 years at the time of revaccination. Although a 50% reduction in the incidence of pneumococcal infection has been demonstrated after immunization, the vaccine protects against a limited number of pneumococcal serotypes. Prophylactic oral penicillin for patients with sickle cell disease reduces the incidence of pneumococcal septicemia by 84%.[22] Therefore, oral penicillin VK 125 mg should be given twice daily, beginning at the age of 2 to 3 months. The dosage should be increased to 250 mg twice daily at 3 years of age and therapy continued at least to the age of 5 years.[18,19] *H. influenzae* vaccination and other routine immunizations should also be provided.

Salmonella species are isolated in up to 80% of patients with sickle cell disease and osteomyelitis. A 4- to 6-week course of treatment with ampicillin or a cephalosporin is needed. Leg ulcers should receive local care and be monitored closely for potential progression to osteomyelitis.

Painful Crises

The goals of therapy for painful vasoocclusive crises are to provide supportive care and effective analgesia while eliminating potential precipitating factors. Vigorous enteral or parenteral hydration should be initiated and oxygen administered if hypoxia from pulmonary involvement is evident. Both nonnarcotic and narcotic analgesics are used, depending on the severity of pain.

Those with mild to moderately painful crises should be treated as outpatients. Oral hydration with 3 to 4 L (150 mL/kg for children) of fluid daily should be encouraged and pain treated with acetaminophen, aspirin, or nonsteroidal anti-inflammatory drugs.[18] Pain unresponsive to these agents may be controlled by codeine or oxycodone, as single agents or in combination with acetaminophen. In addition, the efficacy of the parenteral nonsteroidal anti-inflammatory drug ketorolac in treating painful crises has been reported.[23]

Inpatient treatment with parenteral hydration and narcotic analgesics is necessary for severe painful crises. Scheduled, around-the-clock narcotic administration is preferred over as-needed regimens. The pain–anxiety cycle is thereby diminished and relief often is achieved with lower total dosages. Oral narcotic protocols have been used but are not universally accepted by patients, especially if nausea and vomiting are present. Frequent intramuscular or subcutaneous injections cause local pain and promote abscesses and subsequent infection. In addition, drug absorption may be erratic. Peak effects associated with intravenous bolus administration may lead to excessive central nervous system depression. Continuous intravenous infusions are ideal for initial therapy because a dosage range may be specified, allowing safe titration to pain control. Success with patient-controlled analgesia (PCA) has also been reported, and patients with severe, refractory pain may experience relief with epidural analgesia.[18,23]

Because narcotics have similar effects at equianalgesic dosages, various regimens alleviate symptoms. Agents with mixed agonist–antagonist properties (e.g., pentazocine, buprenorphine) are not recommended for patients with histories of outpatient narcotic use because withdrawal may be precipitated. Although widely used, meperidine should be avoided because its metabolite, normeperidine, accumulates after repeated high doses and may induce seizures, especially in the presence of renal insufficiency or underlying neurologic disease. The short duration of action of meperidine (2 to 4 hours) also makes administration less practical. Morphine sulfate is the narcotic of choice. In patients unable to tolerate morphine because of nausea, vomiting, or pruritus, hydromorphone may be substituted. Adjuvant therapy with promethazine or hydroxyzine may promote analgesia and reduce narcotic requirements; however, adverse effects also may be potentiated. Recently, the efficacy of intravenous methylprednisolone in significantly reducing the duration of narcotic treatment was demonstrated in a study of 36 children and adolescents.[24]

Analgesic dosages must be individualized and based on the degree of outpatient narcotic use and previous inpatient needs. Tolerance to narcotic analgesic effects after chronic administration may dramatically increase parenteral needs. Although patients may appear manipulative and exhibit drug-seeking behavior, adequate analgesia should be provided; placebos should not be given.

A continuous intravenous infusion of morphine (100 mg/100 mL 5% dextrose) at a rate of 0.05 to 0.10 mg/kg/hour may be used for the first 24 to 48 hours. Alternatively, 0.10 to 0.15 mg/kg morphine may be administered as an intravenous bolus every 3 to 4 hours. In one protocol, a morphine loading dose of 0.05 mg/kg is followed by PCA pump delivery of maximum dosages of 0.06 to 0.1 mg/kg/hour, with a 4-hour lockout limit of 0.2 to 0.3 mg/kg. In addition, the pump can be programmed to infuse low-dose morphine 0.02 mg/kg/hour intravenously.[18] Adverse effects such as respiratory depression, oversedation, and blood pressure reductions should be monitored and the dosage decreased if indicated.

As the pain subsides, the continuous infusion should be discontinued and the total daily morphine dosage divided into 4 to 6 intravenous bolus doses. The dosage should be tapered by 20 to 30% daily while the interval is maintained. Once the daily intravenous dosage is 50% of that initially needed, conversion to an equianalgesic dosage of an oral narcotic can be made.

Because of the addictive potential, chronic oral narcotic use should be discouraged, although some believe that severe painful crises may be aborted by early treatment. Unfortunately, many patients become both psychologically and physically dependent on these agents. Continuity of care and communication between health care providers is therefore essential to eliminate the possibility of multiple sources of narcotic prescriptions. Psychosocial support and nonpharmacologic coping techniques, such as relaxation therapy, behavior modification, and self-hypnosis, should be explored thoroughly.

Management of the Sickle Cell Disease

Transfusion Therapy

Partial exchange transfusions, in which more than 50% of the patient's erythrocytes are replaced by donor red cells, prevent vasoocclusive crises. Hypertransfusion until the hematocrit level has doubled temporarily halts erythroid Hb S production and also inhibits sickling. Because of the inherent risks of hepatitis transmission and iron overload, however, transfusions generally are reserved for the management of acute complications and, chronically, for indications such as prevention of strokes in children at high risk (Table 14.5).[25]

Table 14.5 ▪ Indications for Transfusion in Patients with Sickle Cell Anemia

Management of acute complications
Acute chest syndrome
Anemia exacerbation
Aplastic crises
Cerebrovascular accidents
Priapism
Splenic sequestration crises
Prophylaxis
Preoperative
Chronic transfusion therapy
Cerebrovascular accident prevention
Pregnancy
Refractory pain
Recurrent acute chest syndrome

Table 14.6 ▪ Agents Studied for the Treatment of Sickle Cell Anemia

5-Azacytidine	Medroxyprogesterone
Butyrate	Nifedipine
Cetiedil	Papaverine
Clotrimazole	Pentoxifylline
Cytarabine	Piracetam
Desmopressin	Sodium cyanate
Dextran	Ticlopidine
Epoetin alfa	Urea
Hydergine	Valproic acid
Hydroxyurea	Zinc sulfate
Isoxsuprine	

Pharmacologic Management

Many pharmacologic modalities have been directed against the sickling abnormality (Table 14.6); until recently, these therapies have yielded minimal clinical benefit, in part because of limiting adverse effects. Inhibitors of Hb S polymerization, such as sodium cyanate and urea, are not dependably effective; in addition, sodium cyanate is associated with neurologic toxicity. Cetiedil, desmopressin, and clotrimazole alter fluid and electrolyte transport across the red cell membrane. These agents functionally decrease intracellular Hb S concentrations and thereby reduce the polymerization rate. Pentoxifylline may prevent vasoocclusive crises by increasing red cell deformability and decreasing blood viscosity. These effects improve blood flow through the microvasculature in peripheral vascular occlusive diseases; however, further studies are needed to establish the role of pentoxifylline in sickle cell anemia.

Increasing production of the protective fetal hemoglobin is another approach to therapy. The antineoplastics 5-azacitidine and cytarabine enhance Hb F production; however, bone marrow suppression produced by these agents is problematic and long-term efficacy is uncertain. More promising are the results of clinical studies of hydroxyurea.[26,27] After treatment with hydroxyurea, the proportion of Hb F and the number of cells containing Hb F increase, resulting in prolonged red cell survival. In addition, reductions in neutrophil counts, increases in RBC water content and the deformability of sickled cells, and alterations in erythrocyte–endothelial adhesiveness may contribute to its efficacy. Clinical response, including a 50% reduction in the frequency of painful crises and hospitalizations for sickling complications, was demonstrated in 299 patients enrolled in a multicenter placebo-controlled, double-blind study.[27]

Hydroxyurea is approved by the U.S. Food and Drug Administration for adults with recurrent moderate or severe painful crises (i.e., three or more episodes per year).[28] Experience with hydroxyurea in infants and children is limited but encouraging.[23] Initial adult dosages of 15 mg/kg once daily may be increased by 5 mg/kg every 12 weeks to a maximum daily dosage of 35 mg/kg. Reversible, dose-dependent myelosuppression and the potential for carcinogenic effects of long-term therapy underscore the importance of close monitoring. Discontinuation of the drug should be considered if Hb F levels fail to increase after 3 to 6 months at maximum tolerated dosages. Data regarding the benefit of epoetin in conjunction with hydroxyurea are conflicting;[29,30] however, studies of hydroxyurea with other agents with differing mechanisms of action are under way.

Bone Marrow Transplantation

BMT can cure sickle cell anemia.[31,32] Survival and successful engraftment rates of 91% and 73%, respectively, were noted after a median of 24 months' follow-up in 22 children with symptomatic disease.[31] Optimal candidates for BMT are younger (less than 16 years) patients with an HLA-matched sibling and high risk of severe morbidity (e.g., history of cerebrovascular accident, recurrent acute chest syndrome, debilitating pain) who have been minimally transfused and have no significant disease-associated organ damage. Because the clinical course of sickle cell anemia is quite variable and symptoms may not be apparent for months to years after birth, it remains unclear how best to identify patients who would benefit most from this procedure. The risks of transplantation must be carefully considered in light of reduced morbidity noted with improved management of complications and advances in antisickling drug therapy. In the future, genetic engineering may cure the disease by transferring normal hemoglobin genes into patients with sickle cell anemia.

Thalassemias

The thalassemias are a group of hereditary disorders of hemoglobin synthesis characterized by impaired production of one or more of the normal polypeptide chains of globin. Any of the four polypeptides (α, β, γ, δ) that occur in normal hemoglobin may be involved. However, the most prevalent thalassemia syndromes are those that involve diminished or absent synthesis of the α- or β-globin chains of HbA_1.[33–35]

EPIDEMIOLOGY

The thalassemia syndromes are collectively one of the most common genetic disorders in humans. An estimated 190 million people throughout the world carry a hemoglobinopathy gene, and more than half of these are thalassemia genes.[36] Populations that are most affected include Asian, African, Eastern Indian, and Mediterranean.[34,37] Because the geographic distribution of this disorder is similar to that of malaria, it is thought that certain types of thalassemia may offer protection from *Plasmodium falciparum* infection.[33,35] The incidence of α-thalassemia is more common in Southeast Asia, China, and certain areas of Africa, and β-thalassemia syndromes are concentrated in Mediterranean countries such as Greece and Italy. In North America, β-thalassemia is found primarily in people of Greek, Italian, and African ancestry. Genetic analysis studies indicate that approximately 30% of black Americans are silent carriers of α-thalassemia.[34]

Because of their similar geographic distributions, coinheritance of sickle cell anemia with thalassemia is not uncommon. Detailed discussion of various sickle cell–thalassemia syndromes can be found elsewhere.[34]

PATHOPHYSIOLOGY

The imbalance in polypeptide chain production secondary to impaired synthesis of the α- or β-chain of globin accounts for the pathogenesis of all the clinically severe thalassemia syndromes. Reduced production of the normal $\alpha_2\beta_2$ tetramer of Hb A_1 results in the production of smaller erythrocytes with a low hemoglobin content. The synthesis and accumulation of excess normal globin chains within the red cell lead to the formation of unstable aggregates, which may precipitate and cause cell membrane damage. These deformed cells undergo premature destruction either in the bone marrow (extravascular hemolysis) or the peripheral circulation (intravascular hemolysis).[33,38] Chronic hemolysis is a primary complication of the clinically significant α- and β-thalassemia syndromes (e.g., Hb H disease and β-thalassemia major).

The ineffective erythropoiesis and microcytic, hypochromic anemia described earlier are associated with a compensatory increase in the absorption of dietary iron. This may contribute to the iron overload that often results from blood transfusion therapy. There is also an increase in erythropoietic activity in the bone marrow and in extramedullary sites (i.e., liver, spleen, and lymph nodes). In severe forms of thalassemia (e.g., β-thalassemia major), excessive erythropoiesis causes significant bone marrow hypertrophy, growth retardation, lymphadenopathy, and hepatosplenomegaly.[33,38] Bone marrow expansion in untreated patients leads to skeletal deformities and fragility.

α-Thalassemia

PATHOPHYSIOLOGY

Four genes are involved in the production of α-globin chains, with one pair occurring on each DNA strand (αα/αα). The most common forms of α-thalassemia result from deletion of one or more of these genes. Excess production of β- and γ-chains results in the formation of unstable and nonfunctional γ_4 (hemoglobin Bart's) and β_4 (hemoglobin H) tetramers.[33] Four α-thalassemia syndromes have been identified (Table 14.7).

The deletion of a single α-gene is classified as a silent carrier state and is the most common gene abnormality in the world. Up to 2% Hb Bart's can be isolated in cord blood of these people at birth. Hb Bart's disappears within the first year of life. Fortunately, there are virtually no clinical manifestations of the silent carrier state, and laboratory values such as hemoglobin concentration and mean corpuscular volume (MCV) usually are within normal limits.[39,40] These people do not need treatment.

The deletion of two α-genes is classified as α-thalassemia trait or α-thalassemia minor. The most common genotype for this disorder is a homozygous α gene deletion (-α/-α). Patients with α-thalassemia trait experience a mild microcytic, hypochromic anemia without hemolysis.[39,40] In Southeast Asians, however, both α-gene deletions often occur on the same chromosome (–/αα). This genotype is associated with a more pronounced microcytosis (MCV 70 ti 80 fL, or 70 to 80 μm^3) and mild hemolysis. In α-thalassemia trait, Hb Bart's (γ_4) makes up 2 to 10% of hemoglobin in cord blood and disappears within the first year of life.[34] Hemoglobin concentrations of adults with α-thalassemia trait usually are normal or only slightly decreased.[39,40] Not surprisingly, this disorder often is identified in patients by chance during routine laboratory blood tests. Because most patients are asymptomatic, treatment is seldom warranted.

Another α-thalassemia syndrome, more common in Asian populations, is Hb H disease. This disorder is associated with the deletion of three of the four α-genes (–/-α). As mentioned, hemoglobin H is an unstable tetramer of β-globin chains (β_4) formed when a marked reduction of α-globin production yields a substantial surplus of β-globin chains. This hemoglobin variant constitutes 5 to 30% of total circulating hemoglobin in affected adults. In patients with Hb H disease, Hb Bart's represents 10 to 40% of the hemoglobin pool at birth and is found in trace amounts during adulthood.[34] The unstable β_4 containing Hb H gradually undergoes oxidation and precipitates within the cell. These deformed cells are removed and hemolyzed primarily by the spleen.

Clinical manifestations associated with Hb H disease include microcytosis, mild to moderate chronic hemolytic anemia, mild jaundice, and splenomegaly.[40] Enlargement of the spleen results from both the trapping of deformed red cells and extramedullary erythropoiesis in that organ. In most patients, Hb H disease is not severe enough to impair routine activities, interfere with reproductive function, or reduce longevity.[40] However, circumstances such as infection, pregnancy, or exposure to oxidant drugs can precipitate severe exacerbations of the hemolytic anemia.

In certain patients with Hb H disease, especially those with severe splenomegaly, splenectomy often is beneficial in reducing symptoms and slowing the rate of hemolysis. In rare instances, patients with severe forms of Hb H disease are blood transfusion dependent.[40]

Deletion of all four α-genes is classified as Hb Bart's hydrops fetalis and is incompatible with life.[33,40] An affected fetus will be prematurely stillborn in the second or third trimester or will expire within hours after birth. Hemoglobin in an affected fetus will be more than 80% Hb Bart's. Physical findings include massive edema

Table 14.7 ▪ Comparison of α-Thalassemia Syndromes

Syndrome	Genotypes	Typical Hemoglobin Concentration (g/L)	RBC Morphology	Clinical Manifestations
Silent carrier	-α/αα	150	Normal	None
α-Thalassemia trait	-α/-α or --/αα	120–130	Microcytic	Mild anemia
Hb H disease	--/-α	60–100	Microcytic; deformed	Chronic hemolysis; splenomegaly
Hydrops fetalis	--/--	–	Nucleated RBC	Intrauterine or neonatal death

(hydrops), ascites, and hepatomegaly, and peripheral blood examination reveals immature nucleated erythrocytes (erythroblasts), target cells, reticulocytosis, and hypochromia.

CLINICAL PRESENTATION AND DIAGNOSIS

Physicians can diagnose severe forms of α-thalassemia by demonstrating the presence of Hb Bart's or Hb H. After treatment with an oxidant dye such as brilliant cresyl blue, microscopic evaluation of erythrocytes of affected patients reveals precipitated globin aggregates (inclusions).[39] Diagnosis of milder forms may be done through a DNA electrophoretic analysis technique known as Southern blotting.[39,40] Because most α-thalassemia syndromes are associated with a benign clinical course, prenatal diagnosis usually is not critical. An exception occurs when couples are at risk of a hydrops pregnancy (e.g., Southeast Asian or Chinese ancestry or prior α-thalassemic hydrops pregnancy). Prenatal diagnosis of the fetus involves gene mapping of DNA acquired by chorionic villus sampling (first trimester) or amniocentesis (second trimester).[40] A positive diagnosis of Hb Bart's hydrops fetalis allows the option of early termination of the pregnancy, which may protect the health of the mother by preventing toxemia and peripartum hemorrhage.[33]

β-Thalassemia

PATHOPHYSIOLOGY

In contrast to α-thalassemia, where gene deletion is the mechanism, β-thalassemia syndromes usually result from faulty mRNA transcription of the β-gene.[34] Excess α-chains accumulate and cause membrane damage in RBC precursors. This process leads to the premature destruction of the cells in the bone marrow or peripheral blood.[33,39] Because α- and δ-chain production usually is unaffected, increased levels of Hb A_2 ($\alpha_2\delta_2$) are common to most of the β-thalassemias. More than 150 genetic mutations are associated with β-thalassemia. However, patients can be classified as either heterozygous or homozygous for the β-gene. Further distinction is then made based on clinical manifestations and severity (i.e., phenotype) of the syndrome (Table 14.8).

Heterozygous β-thalassemia is much less severe than homozygous forms of the disease. Patients either have a clinically undetectable disorder (β-thalassemia minima) or one that results in only mild anemia (β-thalassemia minor or β-thalassemia trait). In general, patients with β-thalassemia minima are asymptomatic, have laboratory blood values (i.e., hemoglobin concentration and MCV) within normal limits, and need no treatment. Definitive diagnosis can be made by measuring the relative synthetic rates of β- and α-chains.[34,39]

Patients with β-thalassemia minor usually have a mild hypochromic, microcytic anemia. Hemoglobin concentration in these patients generally is not less than 100 g/L. Microcytosis is more pronounced, with MCV values of approximately 60 fL (60 μm^3). Clinical manifestations such as splenomegaly and hyperplastic marrow usually are absent. Nutritional deficiencies, infection, and pregnancy may exacerbate anemia in patients with β-thalassemia minor. However, because these people are predisposed to iron overload because of enhanced absorption of dietary iron, long-term iron supplementation and routine blood transfusions during pregnancy should be avoided, if possible. Medical care for these patients should also involve genetic counseling.[34] Screening patients for β-thalassemia minor often is done through quantification of Hb A_2. Ranges of Hb A_2 levels in normal patients and those with β-thalassemia minor are 2 to 3% and 3.5 to 8%, respectively.[34]

Homozygous forms of β-thalassemia can be classified as either β-thalassemia intermedia or β-thalassemia major. The intermedia form is associated with moderate anemia

Table 14.8 ▪ Comparison of β-Thalassemia Syndromes

Syndrome	Typical Hemoglobin Concentration (g/L)	Clinical Manifestations	Conventional Treatment
Heterozygous			
Minima	Normal	None	None
Minor (trait)	> 100	Mild anemia	Genetic/medical counseling
Homozygous			
Intermedia	70–100	Moderate to severe anemia; impaired growth and splenomegaly in severe cases	Intermittent blood transfusion and chelation therapy
Major	20–70	Severe anemia, abnormal skeletal growth, splenomegaly, iron overload complications	Chronic blood transfusion and chelation therapy

and may necessitate intermittent treatment with blood transfusions. Hemoglobin concentrations in patients with β-thalassemia intermedia usually range from 70 to 100 g/L. In contrast, β-thalassemia major (Cooley's anemia) is associated with severe anemia and necessitates intensive chronic treatment. Hemoglobin concentration and MCV in these patients usually range from 20 to 70 g/L and 50 to 60 fL (50 to 60 μm^3), respectively.[34,41]

CLINICAL PRESENTATION AND DIAGNOSIS

Excessive erythropoiesis (secondary to severe anemia) in the bone marrow and extramedullary sites is a primary complication of untreated β-thalassemia major. Bone marrow hypertrophy with subsequent abnormal skeletal growth usually develops in children from the second year of life through 10 years of age. Abnormal skeletal changes are most apparent in the craniofacial bones and include maxillary overgrowth, protrusion of teeth, and separation of orbits. Cortical thinning of weight-bearing bones may lead to recurrent fractures in these patients. Fortunately, skeletal abnormalities are almost completely prevented if adequate blood transfusion therapy is initiated early in life. Excessive extramedullary erythropoiesis leads to significant lymphadenopathy and hepatosplenomegaly.[36]

Red cell damage and subsequent chronic hemolysis that occur in β-thalassemia major are caused by precipitated intracellular aggregates of excess α-chains. Removal of these deformed red cells by the spleen contributes to splenomegaly that, if uncorrected by splenectomy, can significantly increase blood transfusion needs. Chronic hemolysis also is associated with gallstone formation, which is present in 70% of thalassemic children over 15 years of age.[36,41]

TREATMENT

Conventional treatment for most patients with β-thalassemia major continues to be supportive therapy with chronic blood transfusion and iron chelation regimens. The main goal of this approach is to prevent or reduce major complications of the disease. Experience with BMT in thalassemic patients has progressed substantially, and this approach offers a curative treatment for a small portion of patients. Research in gene therapy is ongoing and may eventually provide a more widely available cure of clinically significant thalassemias.

Transfusion and Chelation

The primary approach to treatment for patients with β-thalassemia major is chronic blood transfusions in conjunction with intensive iron chelation therapy. The goals of transfusion and chelation therapy are to suppress excessive erythropoiesis, prevent anemia, and minimize or prevent the accumulation of toxic amounts of excess iron.

An appropriate transfusion regimen is critically important in accomplishing these goals.[42] Transfusion protocols designed to achieve pretransfusion hemoglobin concentrations of 95 g/L or less have been shown to result in a lower transfusion need and better control of total body iron accumulation compared with more aggressive (supertransfusion) regimens designed to maintain higher pretransfusion hemoglobin concentrations.[42] Transfusion protocols vary between institutions, and different types of patients have different needs. However, typical transfusion programs involve transfusing patients every 3 to 4 weeks on an outpatient basis. Longer intervals between transfusions (i.e., every 5 to 6 weeks) have been shown to increase iron accumulation and should be avoided. The adequacy of a given transfusion regimen is best evaluated by monitoring a patient's growth rate and serum hemoglobin concentrations.[36,41,43,44]

Important complications associated with chronic blood transfusions include sensitization reactions, viral infection, and iron overload. Febrile and urticarial reactions to packed red blood cells (PRBCs) caused by sensitization to leukocyte surface antigens may occur. However, the incidence of these reactions has been greatly reduced through improved typing and matching techniques. Many institutions administer leukocyte-depleted RBC products to thalassemic patients in order to avoid this complication.[36,41,44] A more hazardous problem of chronic blood transfusions is viral infection. Careful screening of donors and donated blood products has reduced the risk of human immunodeficiency virus (HIV) transmission to less than 1 per 150,000 units transfused. Hepatitis B may be prevented through proper vaccination of uninfected thalassemic patients who are initiating or being maintained on chronic transfusion programs. Hepatitis C transmission remains a common threat to transfused patients, with an incidence of about 5%.[36,41] Donor screening for hepatitis C has reduced the risk of transmission of this disease. Patients who become infected with hepatitis C are at risk for liver failure and hepatocellular carcinoma.[42] The use of interferon-α is a treatment option for patients with hepatitis C. However, in thalassemic patients infected with the virus, the effectiveness of antiviral therapy is higher in patients with lower total body iron accumulations. Therefore, optimal iron chelation takes on greater importance in this patient population.[42]

The primary cause of morbidity and mortality in patients with β-thalassemia major who receive adequate transfusion therapy is iron overload associated with the intensive administration of blood products. Each unit of PRBCs (450 mL) contains 200 to 250 mg elemental iron. By 12 years of age, a properly transfused thalassemic probably has received more than 50 g of iron. The normal iron content of the body is 2 g, and there is no natural mechanism by which excess amounts are excreted. Iron overload and subsequent toxicity occur when the capacity of the storage proteins (ferritin and hemosiderin) and the transport protein (transferrin) is exceeded. The molecular mechanism of toxicity is thought to be intracellular and circulatory accumulation of excess unbound iron, which acts as a catalyst in Haber–Weiss and Fenton reactions.

This produces reactive oxygen radicals that oxidize membrane lipids and damage cellular components.[36,41,44]

The clinical effects of iron overload on normal growth, the liver, endocrine function, and the heart are most pronounced. Growth impairment in children with β-thalassemia major probably is multifactorial and may involve hypogonadism, impaired growth hormone system, hyposecretion of adrenal androgen, and impaired cartilage growth.[42] With respect to effects on the liver, hepatic fibrosis often develops in transfused thalassemic children during the first decade of life, and older patients often have histologic evidence of cirrhosis. Hepatic iron accumulation may occur after only 2 years of transfusion therapy and can lead to the rapid development of portal fibrosis. Mild prolongations of clotting time often are observed. Liver disease remains a common cause of death in patients with β-thalassemia major.[42] Diabetes mellitus secondary to the effects of hemochromatosis on the pancreas may occur and can be managed by standard insulin replacement therapy. The manifestations of iron overload on the heart include pericarditis, atrial and ventricular arrhythmias, and congestive heart failure. Cardiomegaly secondary to hypoxia usually is not significant in adequately transfused patients. In underchelated patients, cardiac dysfunction is the primary cause of death.[36,41,42] For all of these reasons, chronic iron chelation therapy must accompany standard blood transfusion regimens.

The only agent currently available for chelating and removing excess iron is deferoxamine, a trihydroxamic acid produced by *Streptomyces pilosus*.[42] Parenterally administered deferoxamine penetrates cell membranes and combines with free intracellular iron to form the complex ferrioxamine. Liver parenchymal cells are a large source of chelatable iron. Ferrioxamine is then transported extracellularly and is readily excreted in the urine and bile. The general goal of treatment with deferoxamine is to control total body iron and, if possible, create a negative iron balance in which the amount of iron removed exceeds the amount of iron administered during transfusions.[36,41,42,44] Adequate chelation therapy with deferoxamine in patients with thalassemia major has been shown to decrease the risks of iron overload, such as diabetes and cardiac disease, and improve survival.[43,45]

One component of iron chelation therapy that plays an important role in initiation and dosage adjustment decisions is the assessment of total body iron. Hepatic iron concentration may be the most quantitative indicator of total body iron.[42] Several methods to accomplish this have been described. Body iron burden has been measured indirectly through the measurement of serum ferritin, 24-hour deferoxamine-induced urinary iron excretion, computed tomography, and magnetic resonance imaging (MRI). Of these methods, measurement of serum ferritin is the most commonly used technique to assess body iron. However, because serum ferritin is an acute phase reactant, its concentrations may fluctuate independently of total body iron with conditions such as fever, acute infection, chronic inflammation, and hepatic damage. For this reason, serum ferritin alone may be an inaccurate assessment of body iron in certain patients.[42] Measurement of urinary iron excretion induced by deferoxamine is of limited value because of the poor correlation between urinary iron concentration and hepatic iron concentration. The amount of iron excreted in the urine depends on several factors, including body iron load, deferoxamine dosage, and erythropoiesis rate. The use of MRI may play a role in detecting the presence of iron within cardiac tissue. However, this technique is not currently useful for making quantitative estimates of iron load.

Total body iron may be assessed through liver biopsy and the subsequent measurement of hepatic tissue iron concentration. This method is the most sensitive and specific approach for determining total body iron in patients with thalassemia.[42]

In clinical practice, the initiation of chelation therapy often is based on serial serum ferritin measurements during regular blood transfusions. Alternatively, liver biopsy to determine hepatic iron concentrations may be a more accurate indicator for the initiation of deferoxamine. Many patients are initiated on chelation therapy after approximately 1 year of regular blood transfusions.[42] Chelation therapy usually is initiated in transfusion-dependent patients by 3 to 4 years of age. Because of poor oral absorption, deferoxamine must be given parenterally. The subcutaneous route generally is considered to achieve the best balance between safety and efficacy for promoting iron removal in thalassemic patients. Because of its short half-life (5 to 10 minutes), deferoxamine usually is administered by continuous infusion to maximize exposure time between the drug and excess iron. Typical deferoxamine dosing regimens are 40 to 50 mg/kg/day infused subcutaneously over 8 to 12 hours, 5 to 7 days a week. Treatment usually is administered with a portable infusion pump while the patient is sleeping. One approach to deferoxamine iron chelation therapy is summarized in Table 14.9. The clinical benefits of regular transfusion and chelation therapy initiated at an early age include a reduced risk of complications from iron-induced organ damage (e.g., cardiac disease and impaired glucose tolerance) and a reduced risk of early death.[43,45]

Intravenous deferoxamine dosing regimens (50 to 80 mg/kg/day) have also been shown to be safe and efficacious.[46] Continuous intravenous ambulatory deferoxamine therapy may be appropriate for patients with greatly elevated hepatic iron concentrations who are at increased risk for complications and early death from iron overload. Because rapid intravenous infusion may cause hypotension, the rate of administration should not exceed 15 mg/kg/hour.[44,47]

Monitoring total body iron burden and chelation therapy efficacy should include the measurement of

Table 14.9 ▪ Guidelines for Iron Chelation with Deferoxamine

Time Course	Assessment Interval	HIC (mg/g)	DFO Regimen
Baseline[a]	Yearly	< 3.2 mg/g	No DFO; recheck in 6 mo
		≥ 3.2 mg/g	25 mg/kg/night × 5 nights/wk
Before age 5	Yearly	< 3.2 mg/g	Stop DFO; recheck in 6 mo
		3.2–6.9 mg/g	25 mg/kg/night × 5 nights/wk
		≥ 7 mg/g	35 mg/kg/night × 6 or 7 nights/wk
Ages 5–10	Every 18 mo	< 3.2 mg/g	Stop DFO; recheck in 6 mo
		3.2–6.9 mg/g	40 mg/kg/night × 5 nights/wk
		7–14.9 mg/g	40 mg/kg/night × 6 or 7 nights/wk
		≥ 15 mg/g	40–50 mg/kg/night × 7 nights/wk
After age 10	Every 18 mo	< 3.2 mg/g	Stop DFO; recheck in 6 mo
		3.2–6.9 mg/g	40 mg/kg/night × 5 nights/wk
		7–14.9 mg/g	40 mg/kg/night × 6 or 7 nights/wk
		≥ 15 mg/g	50 mg/kg/night × 7 nights/wk

Source: Reference 42.

HIC, hepatic iron concentration from liver biopsy (milligrams iron per gram dry weight of liver biopsy); *DFO,* deferoxamine.

[a]After 1 year of regular transfusions.

hepatic iron concentrations, serum ferritin concentrations (normal, 18 to 300 μg/L), and possibly urinary iron excretion. Chelation therapy with deferoxamine designed to maintain hepatic iron concentrations of 0.2 to 1.6 mg iron per gram of liver tissue (dry weight) has been shown to reduce the risk of complications from iron overload. However, this approach has also been associated with an increased risk of adverse drug effects. In contrast, maintaining hepatic iron concentrations higher than 15 mg iron per gram of liver (dry weight) results in a lower risk of drug toxicity but an increased risk of cardiac disease and early mortality secondary to iron overload.[42] Therefore, some authors suggest a target reference range of 3.2 to 7 mg iron per gram of liver (dry weight). Maintaining a serum ferritin value of less than 2500 ng/mL has been correlated with an excellent prognosis for prolonged survival without cardiac disease.[45] As previously discussed, urinary iron excretion depends on many factors and may not correlate reliably with the efficacy of iron chelation therapy.[36,44,48]

In most patients, deferoxamine used in typical chelation regimen dosages is a safe drug. Common side effects of subcutaneous infusion include local irritation and urticaria at the injection site, diarrhea, leg cramps, tachycardia, and abdominal discomfort. Some reports associate deferoxamine with a variety of adverse visual and auditory effects. The mechanism of this toxicity is not well understood. Patients on deferoxamine should receive regular vision and hearing evaluations. Other serious adverse effects reported with deferoxamine include changes in renal function and pulmonary toxicity.[42] Patients with lower iron burdens and patients receiving high dosages of deferoxamine (more than 50 mg/kg) are likely to be at greater risk for toxicity.[41,42,47]

Because of the inconvenience, high cost, and frequent noncompliance with parenteral deferoxamine therapy, research efforts have focused on the development of a safe, effective, and inexpensive oral medication for iron chelation. The most promising compounds to date are those of the hydroxypyridine family. One agent of this class, deferiprone, has shown efficacy similar to that of subcutaneous deferoxamine.[49] However, a recent report evaluating the use of deferiprone in 19 patients with thalassemia major demonstrated this agent to be associated with an inadequate control of total body iron and potential worsening of hepatic fibrosis.[50] More controlled clinical evaluation of these agents may be necessary to better understand their potential role in the management of thalassemia.

Patients with β-thalassemia intermedia often are not blood transfusion dependent. However, in severe forms of this syndrome, ineffective erythropoiesis and anemia are sometimes significant enough to inhibit growth and development and lead to skeletal fragility and injury. In these cases, patients with β-thalassemia intermedia should be treated with intermittent courses of transfusion and chelation therapy.[41,42]

Ascorbic Acid Supplementation

Ascorbic acid supplementation may enhance iron removal during chelation therapy in some thalassemic patients by increasing the iron pool that is available for deferoxamine to bind with.[42] However, some evidence exists that this process may also increase iron-induced formation of cytotoxic oxygen free radicals. One recommended approach is to check tissue ascorbic acid concentrations in patients with diminished response to deferoxamine. Patients with low levels may be supplemented with 100 mg ascorbic acid 30 minutes to 1 hour before receiving deferoxamine.[42]

Splenectomy

Because of increased erythropoietic activity and trapping of red cells by the spleen, patients with β-thalassemia major develop splenomegaly. Proper transfusion therapy may slow the process, but gradual enlargement of the spleen usually occurs. In patients who receive chronic transfusion therapy, splenomegaly is associated with increased transfusion needs to maintain an adequate hemoglobin concentration. Administering greater volumes of blood products increases the amount of iron a patient receives and makes successful chelation more difficult. Therefore, when blood transfusion needs exceed 200 mL/kg/year, splenectomy is indicated. After spleen removal, transfusion needs will decrease substantially. Because splenectomized patients, especially young children, are predisposed to certain bacterial infections, splenectomy should be avoided until the age of 4 or 5 years. Furthermore, all splenectomized patients should be vaccinated against pneumococcus, meningococcus, and *Haemophilus influenzae* at the earliest appropriate age.[36,41,44]

Bone Marrow Transplantation

Since the initial successful case in 1982, considerable experience has been gained with BMT in patients with β-thalassemia major. Survival and disease-free survival rates in a group of 139 patients receiving BMT for thalassemia were 73% and 58%, respectively.[51] A later series of 89 patients aged 1 to 15 years demonstrated survival and rejection-free survival rates of 92% and 85%, respectively.[52] Therefore, if an HLA-compatible donor exists, BMT offers thalassemic patients a reasonable chance for cure. The risk of graft failure and mortality associated with BMT varies among different institutions and different patients and must be weighed against the high rate of survival and the good quality of life that is associated with conventional transfusion and chelation therapy for at least the first two decades. Thalassemic patients with the highest chances for rejection-free survival after BMT are those who are young, well chelated, and in good clinical condition.[51,52]

FUTURE THERAPIES

Another technique that has shown some success in treating patients with β-thalassemia major is to reduce transfusion needs by increasing Hb F synthesis.[53–56] Agents that have been investigated as clinical stimulators of Hb F synthesis include hydroxyurea, butyrate, and azacitidine. The adverse effects (i.e., bone marrow suppression and mutagenicity) and unknown long-term efficacy of these agents have limited their use in treating thalassemia.

Gene therapy also holds great potential as a definitive cure for patients with severe forms of thalassemia.[57] Current limitations in the use of this therapy to treat thalassemia include inefficient gene expression and regulation.

PROGNOSIS

Before the implementation of adequate transfusion and chelation programs, children with β-thalassemia major suffered from skeletal deformities, growth and development retardation, progressive enlargement of the liver and spleen, congestive heart failure, and recurrent infections. More than 80% of these patients died within the first 5 years of life. The widespread use of regular transfusion programs and effective chelation therapy has led to a significant improvement in the quality and duration of life for thalassemic patients. BMT is a currently available therapy that provides a chance for a cure of the disease in a small portion of patients.

PREVENTION

Prevention of β-thalassemia major is another effective approach. Multifaceted programs involving education, genetic counseling, and prenatal diagnosis have led to a significant reduction in the incidence of this disease in certain areas.[33] In Sardinia, for example, such a program was associated with a 95% reduction in the incidence of β-thalassemia major over a 16-year period.[58] Inexpensive and simple DNA analysis techniques can provide a safe and accurate diagnosis at 8 to 14 weeks' gestation.[41]

Hemolytic Anemias

Hemolytic anemias are caused by an increased rate of RBC destruction. The anemia is of greatest clinical concern when the rate of RBC destruction exceeds that of erythropoiesis. The hemolytic process may occur chronically or manifest as an acute episode depending on the cause. Acute hemolysis generally is a more clinically threatening event. Many anemias have a hemolytic component because of the production of defective or damaged RBCs (e.g., megaloblastic anemias, thalassemias, sickle cell anemia).[59] Because there are many causes of hemolytic anemia, this section focuses on those that are amenable to specific medical treatment and those that are drug-induced.

EPIDEMIOLOGY

The incidence of hereditary spherocytosis and hereditary elliptocytosis in the United States is approximately 220 and 400 per million, respectively. Glucose-6-phosphate dehydrogenase (G6PD) deficiency is the most common inherited erythrocyte enzyme disorder worldwide, affecting almost 200 million people, but not all patients with G6PD deficiency are significantly predisposed to oxidative hemolysis.[34,60]

The majority of acquired hemolytic anemias are idiopathic. Many are caused by immune reactions, collagen vascular disease, or malignancy. Drugs are the causative agents in less than 10% of cases. Hemolytic anemias can be categorized as either inherited or acquired disorders. Inherited hemolytic anemias include defective globin synthesis, erythrocyte membrane defects, and erythrocyte enzyme deficiencies. Acquired hemolytic disorders are caused by an extrinsic event and do not involve a genetic component. Typically, the acquired hemolytic anemias are either immune-mediated, caused by physical stress on the red cell, or induced by certain infections (Table 14.10).

Table 14.10 ▪ Classification of Common Hemolytic Anemias

Inherited
- Globin synthesis defect
  - Sickle cell anemia
  - Thalassemia
  - Unstable hemoglobin disease
- Erythrocyte membrane defect
  - Hereditary spherocytosis
  - Hereditary elliptocytosis
  - Hereditary stomatocytosis
- Erythrocyte enzyme defect
  - Hexose monophosphate shunt defect (e.g., glucose-6-phosphate dehydrogenase)
  - Glycolytic (Embden–Meyerhof) enzyme defect (e.g., pyruvate kinase)
  - Other enzyme defect (e.g., adenylate kinase)

Acquired
- Immune mediated
  - Warm reacting antibody (immunoglobulin G)
    - Primary (idiopathic)
    - Secondary (e.g., collagen vascular disease, lymphoproliferative disorders)
    - Drug-induced
  - Cold agglutinin disease (immunoglobulin M)
    - Acute (e.g., mycoplasma pneumonia, infectious mononucleosis)
    - Chronic (e.g., lymphoid neoplasms, idiopathic)
  - Paroxysmal nocturnal hemoglobinuria
  - Transfusion reactions
  - Hemolytic disease of newborns
- Microangiopathic and traumatic
  - Disseminated intravascular coagulation
  - Hemolytic uremic syndrome
  - Thrombotic thrombocytopenic purpura
  - Prosthetic or diseased heart valves
- Infection
- Exogenous substances
- Other
  - Liver disease
  - Hypophosphatemia

PATHOPHYSIOLOGY

The average RBC life span is 120 days. During severe hemolytic episodes this can be as low as 5 days. RBCs are hemolyzed within the circulation (intravascular hemolysis) or taken up by the RES and destroyed (extravascular hemolysis). Intravascular hemolysis may be caused by trauma to the RBC, complement fixation to the RBC (immune mediated), or exposure to exogenous substances. Under normal circumstances, however, most RBC catabolism is performed extravascularly by the RES in the liver and spleen. Specific drug-induced mechanisms of RBC hemolysis are discussed later in the context of G6PD deficiency and immune-mediated hemolysis.

After lysis of the RBC, hemoglobin is released into the blood, where it is bound by the plasma protein haptoglobin. Free heme molecules are bound by the plasma protein hemopexin. The hemoglobin–haptoglobin complex is cleared rapidly from the circulation by the RES, and the heme component is metabolized to unconjugated (indirect) bilirubin. In the liver, this is linked with glucuronic acid forming conjugated (direct) bilirubin, which passes from the bile duct into the intestine. Fecal bacteria then metabolize conjugated bilirubin to urobilinogen, which is excreted primarily in the feces. Iron from heme catabolism is stored as ferritin or hemosiderin.[59,61]

During hemolysis, if the haptoglobin-binding capacity is exceeded, unbound hemoglobin levels increase, resulting in hemoglobinemia. In this case, free hemoglobin is filtered through the glomerulus and usually is reabsorbed by the proximal tubules. In severe intravascular hemolysis, the reabsorptive capacity is exceeded, causing hemoglobinuria. Also during severe intravascular hemolysis, some heme molecules in the circulation are transferred from hemopexin to albumin, forming methemalbumin. When the liver's conjugating capacity is exceeded during moderate or severe hemolysis, unconjugated (indirect) bilirubin serum levels increase.[59]

CLINICAL PRESENTATION AND DIAGNOSIS

The primary diagnostic features of hemolytic anemia are a marked reticulocytosis and jaundice (including scleral icterus) caused by hyperbilirubinemia. A corrected reticulocyte count greater than 2.5% is a typical response to hemolysis. The severity of the anemia may also be judged by the extent to which the hematocrit is decreased. The enzyme lactate dehydrogenase is released from the RBC during hemolysis, and plasma levels may be elevated. Red cell membranes may sustain incomplete damage, resulting in the formation of spherocyte-shaped erythrocytes. These cells have an increased susceptibility to splenic removal.[61] Splenomegaly usually is present in cases of chronic hemolysis. A summary of important findings in hemolytic anemia is presented in Table 14.11.

With respect to immune-mediated hemolysis, diagnostic evaluation includes the direct antiglobulin test (DAT,

Table 14.11 ▪ Common Diagnostic Features of Hemolytic Anemia

	Moderate Hemolysis	Severe Hemolysis
Physical findings		
Jaundice	+	+
Hemoglobinuria	0	+
Laboratory indices: plasma/serum		
Reticulocytosis	+	++
Plasma hemoglobin	+	++
Red blood cell hemoglobin	Low	Low
Hematocrit	Low	Low
Bilirubin (unconjugated)	+	++
Haptoglobin	Low	Low or absent
Hemopexin	Normal or low	Low or absent
Methemalbumin	0	+
Lactate dehydrogenase	+ (Variable)	++ (Variable)
Laboratory indices: urine		
Hemoglobin	0	+
Hemosiderin	0	+

or Coomb's test), which detects the presence of IgG or C3 (complement) on the RBC surface. Patients may have positive DAT results without hemolysis (up to 15% of hospitalized patients). Therefore, this result must be correlated with other clinical evidence of a hemolytic process. The indirect antiglobulin test (IAT, or indirect Coomb's test) detects the presence of antibodies against RBCs in the serum rather than on the surface of the RBC itself. This test is most commonly used in blood banks for antibody screening and cross matching blood for transfusion.[61] During oxidative hemolytic anemias, denatured hemoglobin precipitates within the RBC, forming Heinz bodies, which are visible during microscopic examination. Heinz bodies are removed rapidly by the spleen, creating "bite" cells, which are erythrocytes that appear to have a bite of cytoplasm removed.[60]

Inherited Hemolytic Anemia: G6PD Deficiency

Hereditary spherocytosis, elliptocytosis, and stomatocytosis are all genetic disorders inherited in an autosomal dominant fashion and are associated with altered RBC morphology. Hemolysis and clinical sequelae tend to be more pronounced with hereditary spherocytosis than with the other two. Splenectomy usually corrects anemia in these patients. Supplemental folic acid therapy (1 mg daily) also is recommended.[59]

The most prevalent inherited RBC enzyme defect is G6PD deficiency, a sex-linked (X-chromosome) disorder.

EPIDEMIOLOGY

Affected female patients are predominantly heterozygous and have both normal and G6PD-deficient RBCs. They are fairly resistant to RBC hemolysis. However, men and homozygous women have predominantly G6PD-deficient RBCs and are predisposed to more severe hemolytic episodes. Cultural distribution of this disorder is similar to that of thalassemia, occurring often in Blacks and people of Mediterranean cultures. The "A–" variant of G6PD is found primarily in Blacks. Enzyme activity in these patients is 8 to 20% of normal. In the United States, approximately 13% of black males and 3% of black females are affected. The Mediterranean-type variant of G6PD has 0% to 4% of normal enzyme activity. Consequently, these patients are generally at greater risk of developing hemolytic anemia and the associated clinical manifestations are more pronounced.[60]

PATHOPHYSIOLOGY

The G6PD enzyme, in conjunction with glutathione and nicotinamide adenine dinucleotide phosphate, acts as a protective antioxidant for RBCs against external oxidative stresses (Fig. 14.1). In the presence of G6PD deficiency, oxidative stresses on the RBC such as drugs, infection, or acidosis can lead to denaturation of the globin chains. Denatured globin precipitates intracellularly onto the cell membrane as Heinz bodies, and premature hemolysis occurs.[60,62] This type of disorder is often called oxidative hemolysis.

Many drugs and substances have been associated with hemolytic anemia in G6PD-deficient patients. However, the list of agents for which there is strong evidence of an association is small (Table 14.12).[60,62] A patient's susceptibility to the oxidative stress of a particular drug varies according to several factors. The type of G6PD genetic variant present (i.e., type A– or Mediterranean-type) is a major determinant. Other factors include patient age, other sources of oxidant stress, dosage of an offending drug, and patient metabolism and elimination of an offending drug. During hemolytic episodes in susceptible patients, signs and symptoms usually develop within 2 to 3 days of drug initiation. The hemolysis is primarily intravascular and generally results in pronounced hemoglobinuria.

TREATMENT

Withdrawal or avoidance of any potentially oxidant drugs or other substances is the most important component of

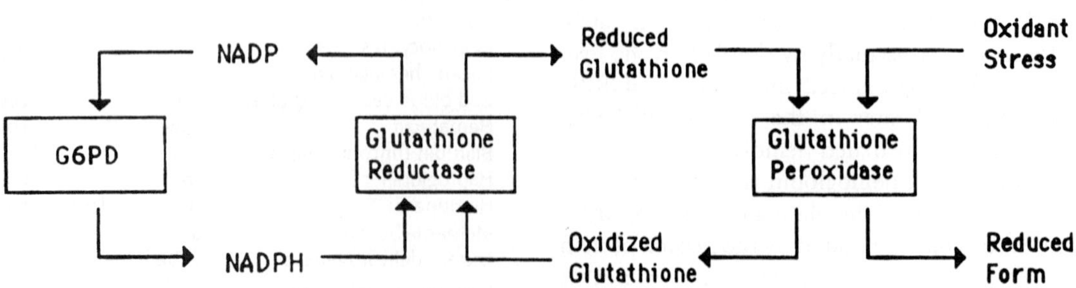

Figure 14.1. Antioxidant mechanism of G6PD. *NADP,* nicotinamide adenine dinucleotide phosphate; *NADPH,* nicotinamide adenine dinucleotide phosphate, reduced form.

Table 14.12 ▪ Drugs and Substances Associated with Hemolytic Anemia in G6PD Deficiency

Primaquine	Sulfapyridine
Nalidixic acid	Phenazopyridine
Ciprofloxacin	Dapsone
Nitrofurantoin	Methylene blue
Sulfacetamide	Naphthalene (mothballs)
Sulfamethoxazole	Fava beans

treatment. In patients with A– variant G6PD deficiency, hemolysis usually is mild and self-limited, and therapy is seldom needed. In patients with Mediterranean-type deficiency experiencing severe hemolysis, blood transfusions may occasionally be warranted in symptomatic patients. Folic acid supplementation should be given for 2 to 3 weeks after an acute hemolytic episode and may be necessary for extended periods in patients with chronic hemolysis. In patients who develop severe hemolytic anemia with hemoglobinuria, intravenous hydration to maintain adequate urine output may be necessary to prevent acute renal failure.[60,62]

The primary approach when caring for patients who have documented G6PD deficiency or those who may be at risk (e.g., family history, ethnic background) is prevention. Several factors should be considered before such patients are given a potentially hemolyzing drug, including patient age, renal function, type of G6PD variant that may be present, availability of alternative drugs, and severity of primary illness. A specific quantitative assay of G6PD is available for screening patients who may be deficient.[62]

Acquired Hemolytic Anemia: Autoimmune Hemolysis

Acquired hemolytic anemias are made up of a diverse group of disorders (Table 14.10). Microangiopathic hemolytic anemias including disseminated intravascular coagulation, hemolytic uremic syndrome, and thrombotic thrombocytopenic purpura generally are caused by alterations such as fibrin deposition or narrowing of the microvasculature. Therapy for these disorders involves treating the underlying disease. Acquired hemolytic anemias secondary to RBC trauma occur in up to 10% of patients with prosthetic or diseased heart valves because of pressure gradient stresses placed on the RBC membrane. Beneficial treatment in these patients includes correcting iron deficiency and limiting exertion. Valve replacement may be necessary when less invasive measures fail.

Autoimmune hemolytic anemia results from the binding of complement or anti-RBC antibodies to the red cell membrane in affected patients. These disorders may be classified according to the temperature at which the antibodies have the greatest affinity for and interaction with red cells.

Cold Agglutinin Hemolytic Anemia

PATHOPHYSIOLOGY

Cold agglutinin disorders involve the binding of IgM antibodies to RBCs at low temperatures (4°C). This agglutination process is reversed quickly during warming. Most cold agglutinins do not appreciably shorten RBC survival. Acute cold agglutinin disease often is associated with mycoplasma pneumonia or infectious mononucleosis. Hemolysis typically begins 5 to 10 days after recovery from the infection and is mild and self-limited. Chronic cold agglutinin disease often occurs spontaneously in older adults, especially those with lymphoproliferative disorders, and results in poor peripheral circulation.

TREATMENT

Treating cold agglutinin disease involves preventing exposure to cold environments, folic acid supplementation, blood transfusions (if necessary), and treating any underlying diseases. Occasionally patients may respond to plasmapheresis or cytotoxic agents such as cyclophosphamide or chlorambucil. Splenectomy and corticosteroids are of questionable value.[59,61]

Warm Autoimmune Hemolytic Anemia

PATHOPHYSIOLOGY

Warm reacting antibodies have the greatest affinity for red cells at room temperature (37°C) and usually are of the IgG or occasionally IgA type. The mechanism of hemolysis involves the attachment and subsequent destruction of IgG-coated erythrocytes to receptors on macrophages in the RES. This process occurs primarily in the spleen. This type of immunohemolytic anemia may be idiopathic, secondary to an underlying disease that affects the immune system (e.g., chronic lymphocytic leukemia, non-Hodgkin's lymphoma, or systemic lupus erythematosus), or secondary to certain drugs. Many of these patients have a chronic mild anemia and splenomegaly, but clinical presentation varies widely. This disorder is more common in adults and in women. The presence of IgG autoantibodies is detected by a positive DAT.[59,61]

TREATMENT

Before patients with immunohemolytic anemia are treated, drugs that have been associated with this condition should be excluded as the cause. Therapy should be based on the severity of the anemia. Patients with mild hemolysis usually do not need therapy. When hemolysis is clinically significant, corticosteroid therapy usually is effective and blood transfusions may be needed. The mechanism of steroid action in immunohemolytic anemia is thought to involve a reduction in the clearance of IgG-coated RBCs from the circulation by interference with macrophage receptor function or phagocytosis. Typically, prednisone is administered in a dosage of 1 to 2 mg/kg/day and continued until hemoglobin levels have normalized. Hemoglobin concentration usually begins to increase within 3 to 4 days after prednisone is initiated. Once hemoglobin has returned to baseline, prednisone therapy is tapered slowly over several months. Approximately 60 to 70% of patients treated in this manner have a sustained suppression of hemolysis. However, more than 80% of these patients relapse as steroids are tapered or after they are withdrawn. Intravenous immune globulin (IVIG) is less effective in treating warm autoimmune hemolytic anemia, producing transient remission in only 40% of patients. Splenectomy benefits 50 to 60% of patients who relapse or fail to respond to corticosteroids. In patients who are refractory to steroids and splenectomy (about 10% of cases), alternative therapies for consideration include immunosuppressive agents (e.g., cyclophosphamide or azathioprine), danazol, IVIG, and cyclosporine. Corticosteroids may also be reinstituted and maintained indefinitely at the lowest effective dosage. Patients who undergo splenectomy should receive vaccination against pneumococcus, meningococcus, and *H. influenzae* approximately 2 weeks before surgery. Cross matching patients with immunohemolytic anemia for blood transfusions is difficult because the antibody that is present often reacts with all normal donor cells.[59,61]

Drug-Induced Immunohemolytic Anemias

Examples of drugs associated with immunohemolytic anemias are listed in Table 14.13. There are three proposed mechanisms by which drugs can initiate this condition:

- Autoimmune (methyldopa type): Up to 10% of patients receiving methyldopa in daily dosages of 2 g develop a positive DAT. Only a small percentage of these patients (1% or less) develop an extravascular hemolysis. The patient's RBCs are coated with IgG but not complement. The mechanism of this condition is not well understood but may involve the inhibition of suppressor T cells. If hemolysis occurs, it gradually subsides over a period of weeks after drug discontinuation, but the patient's DAT may remain positive for more than a year.[59,61]

Table 14.13 ▪ Examples of Drugs Associated with Immunohemolytic Anemia

Autoimmune (methyldopa type)	Drug Adsorption (hapten type)	Immune Complex Adsorption (innocent bystander type)
Methyldopa	Penicillins	Quinidine
Levodopa	Cephalosporins	Quinine
Mefenamic acid	Tetracycline	Phenacetin
Cimetidine		Acetaminophen
Procainamide		

- Drug adsorption (hapten type): In patients receiving large dosages of penicillins (e.g., 15 to 20 million units per day) or cephalosporins, the drug nonspecifically adsorbs to the RBC membrane, forming a hapten complex. Antibodies are then formed against this complex, resulting in extravascular hemolysis within 7 to 14 days after initiation of the drug. The DAT is positive for IgG during therapy. Hemolysis subsides quickly after the drug is withdrawn.[59,61]
- Immune complex adsorption (innocent bystander type): In this rare type of drug-induced immunohemolytic anemia, the offending agent binds to plasma proteins and induces the production of IgM antibodies. A drug–antibody complex forms that adheres nonspecifically to the red cell membrane. Complement (C3) is activated and irreversibly fixes to the membrane surface. The drug–antibody complex dissociates from the RBC, and only C3 is detected by a DAT. The hemolytic process usually occurs intravascularly and may be associated with hemoglobinemia, hemoglobinuria, and acute renal failure.[59,61]

A fourth type of process may result from the administration of high-dose cephalosporins. In this case, the drug binds to the red cell membrane, causing it to be modified, which results in the nonspecific adsorption of serum proteins. This process is not immune mediated, nor does hemolysis occur.

KEY POINTS

- Anemia is a reduction in the concentration of viable erythrocytes or hemoglobin in the circulation resulting in a reduced oxygen-carrying capacity of blood.
- There are several basic mechanisms by which anemia may occur, including impaired or absent erythropoiesis (e.g., anemia of chronic disease, aplastic anemia, anemia of renal failure), impaired hemoglobin synthesis (e.g., sickle cell anemia, thalassemia), and premature red cell destruction (e.g., hemolytic anemia). These mechanisms may coexist.
- Diseases or conditions that are often the primary cause of anemia include chronic infection or inflammation, neoplastic diseases, renal disease, exposure to certain pathogens or chemicals, exposure to certain drugs, inherited abnormalities, and autoimmune processes.

- Anemia has many potential causes and is actually a symptom of an underlying condition. Treatment should focus not only on correcting the anemia and its associated symptoms but also on identifying and correcting underlying causes, when possible.
- Anemia of chronic disease generally is mild and associated with infectious, inflammatory, and neoplastic disorders.
- There is no specific therapy for the anemia of chronic disease; rather, the anemia remits with successful management of the underlying condition.
- Although there are many potential pathogenetic mechanisms, the anemia of renal failure probably is caused by the deficiency of the hormone erythropoietin.
- Definitive management of the anemia of renal failure consists of supplementation with recombinant human erythropoietin to increase hematocrit concentrations toward normal values while maintaining iron stores.
- Aplastic anemia is caused by a defect or deficiency of the pluripotential stem cell, resulting in anemia, agranulocytosis, and thrombocytopenia.
- Management of aplastic anemia includes removal of the causative agent when possible, supportive care with transfusions and antibiotic therapy, and, depending on patient-specific factors, immunosuppressive therapy or BMT.
- Sickle cell anemia is a genetic disorder whose manifestations are highly variable but may include vasoocclusive crises, cerebrovascular accidents, aplastic crises, splenic dysfunction and associated infectious complications, and recurrent, debilitating pain.
- In addition to managing complications, definitive therapy for sickle cell anemia may now include hydroxyurea or BMT.
- The thalassemias are a group of hereditary disorders of hemoglobin synthesis characterized by impaired production of one or more of the normal polypeptide chains of globin.
- Chronic hemolysis is a primary complication of the clinically significant α- and β-thalassemia syndromes.
- Clinical manifestations of untreated β-thalassemia major include bone marrow hypertrophy, skeletal deformities and fragility, growth retardation, lymphadenopathy, and hepatosplenomegaly.
- Standard therapy of β-thalassemia major includes regular blood transfusions to correct anemia and suppress ineffective erythropoiesis along with iron chelation therapy to avoid the systemic toxicities of iron overload associated with transfusions.
- Other potential therapies for treating patients with β-thalassemia major include hemoglobin switching (i.e., stimulation of fetal hemoglobin production) and BMT.
- Hemolytic anemias, which may occur as an acute episode or chronic condition and may take place intravascularly or extravascularly, have many different causes but generally occur when the rate of RBC destruction exceeds that of erythropoiesis.
- Many types of anemias have a hemolytic component (e.g., megaloblastic anemias, thalassemias, sickle cell anemia) caused by the production of defective or damaged RBCs.
- Management of hemolytic anemia should focus on controlling etiologic factors.

REFERENCES

1. Sears DA. Anemia of chronic disease. Med Clin North Am 76:567–579, 1992.
2. Means RT. Pathogenesis of the anemia of chronic disease: a cytokine-mediated anemia. Stem Cells 13:32–37, 1995.
3. Erslev AJ, Besarab A. Erythropoietin in the pathogenesis and treatment of the anemia of chronic renal failure. Kidney Int 51:622–630, 1997.
4. Neff MS, Goldberg J, Slifkin RF, et al. A comparison of androgens for anemia in patients on hemodialysis. N Engl J Med 304:871–875, 1981.
5. Eschbach JW, Abdulhadi MH, Browne JK, et al. Recombinant human erythropoietin in anemic patients with end-stage renal disease. Ann Intern Med 111:992–1000, 1989.
6. Zachee P. Controversies in selection of epoetin dosages. Drugs 49:536–547, 1995.
7. Gahl GM, Eckardt KU. Erythropoietin 1997: a brief update. Perit Dial Int 17(Suppl 2):S84–S90, 1997.
8. Eschbach JW, Egrie JC, Downing MR, et al. Correction of the anemia of end-stage renal disease with recombinant human erythropoietin. N Engl J Med 316:73–78, 1987.
9. Eschbach JW. Erythropoietin: the promise and the facts. Kidney Int 45(Suppl 44):570–576, 1994.
10. Maschio G. Erythropoietin and systemic hypertension. Nephrol Dial Transplant 10(Suppl 2):4–79, 1995.
11. Bjorkholm M. Aplastic anaemia: pathogenetic mechanisms and treatment with special reference to immunomodulation. J Intern Med 231:575–582, 1992.
12. Guinan EC. Clinical aspects of aplastic anemia. Hematol Oncol Clin North Am 11:1025–1044, 1997.
13. Stewart FM. Hypoplastic/aplastic anemia. Role of bone marrow transplantation. Med Clin North Am 76:683–697, 1992.
14. Young NS, Barrett AJ. The treatment of severe acquired aplastic anemia. Blood 85:3367–3377, 1995.
15. Weiner RS, Dicke KA. Risk factors for interstitial pneumonitis following allogeneic bone marrow transplantation for severe aplastic anemia: a preliminary report. Transplant Proc 19:2639–2642, 1987.
16. Kojima S. Use of hematopoietic growth factors for treatment of aplastic anemia. Bone Marrow Transplant 18(Suppl 3):S36–S38, 1996.
17. Bacigalupo A, Broccia G, Corda G. Antilymphocyte globulin, cyclosporine, and granulocyte colony stimulating factor in patients with acquired severe aplastic anemia (SAA): a pilot of the EBMT SAA working party. Blood 85:1348–1353, 1995.
18. National Institutes of Health National Heart, Lung, and Blood Institute. Management and therapy of sickle cell disease. National Institute of Health publication no. 96-2117, 1995.
19. Lane PA. Sickle cell disease. Pediatr Clin North Am 43:639–664, 1996.
20. Bunn HF. Pathogenesis and treatment of sickle cell disease. N Engl J Med 337:762–769, 1997.
21. Platt OS, Thorington BD, Brambilla DJ, et al. Pain in sickle cell disease: rates and risk factors. N Engl J Med 325:11–16, 1991.
22. Gaston MH, Verter JI, Woods G, et al. Prophylaxis with oral penicillin in children with sickle cell anemia. N Engl J Med 314:1593–1599, 1986.
23. Reed W, Vichinsky EP. New considerations in the treatment of sickle cell disease. Annu Rev Med 49:461–474, 1998.
24. Griffin TC, McIntire D, Buchanan GR. High-dose intravenous methylprednisolone therapy for pain in children and adolescents with sickle cell disease. N Engl J Med 330:733–737, 1994.
25. Adams RJ, McKie VC, Hsu L, et al. Prevention of first stroke by transfusions in children with sickle cell anemia and abnormal results on transcranial Doppler ultrasonography. N Engl J Med 339:5–11, 1998.
26. Rodgers GP, Dover GJ, Noguchi CT, et al. Hematologic responses of patients

with sickle cell disease to treatment with hydroxyurea. N Engl J Med 322: 1037–1045, 1990.
27. Charache S, Terrin ML, Moore RD, et al. Effect of hydroxyurea on the frequency of painful crises in sickle cell anemia. N Engl J Med 332:1317–1322, 1995.
28. Droxia package insert. Princeton, NJ: Bristol-Myers Squibb, 1998.
29. Goldberg MA, Brugnara C, Dover GJ, et al. Treatment of sickle cell anemia with hydroxyurea and erythropoietin. N Engl J Med 323:366–372, 1990.
30. Rodgers GP, Dover GJ, Uyesaka N, et al. Augmentation by erythropoietin of the fetal-hemoglobin response to hydroxyurea in sickle cell disease. N Engl J Med 328:73–80, 1993.
31. Walters MC, Patience M, Leisenring W, et al. Bone marrow transplantation for sickle cell disease. N Engl J Med 335:369–376, 1996.
32. Vermylen C, Cornu G. Bone marrow transplantation for sickle cell disease. Am J Pediatr Hematol Oncol 16:18–21, 1994.
33. Weatherall DJ. The thalassemias. BMJ 314:1675–1678, 1997.
34. Jandl JH. Blood: textbook of hematology. Boston: Little, Brown, 1987.
35. Steinberg MH. Thalassemia: molecular pathology and management. Am J Med Sci 296:308–321, 1988.
36. Wonke B. Prospects of β-thalassemia major. Indian Pediatr 24:969–975, 1987.
37. Huisman TH. Frequencies of common β-thalassemia alleles among different populations: variability in clinical severity. Br J Haematol 75:454–457, 1990.
38. Festa RS. Modern management of thalassemia. Pediatr Ann 14:597–606, 1985.
39. Beutler E. Disorders of hemoglobin. In: Fauci AS, Braunwald E, Isselbacher KJ, et al. Harrison's principles of internal medicine. 14th ed. New York: McGraw-Hill, 1998:650–652.
40. Liebhaber SA. α-Thalassemia. Hemoglobin 13:685–721, 1989.
41. Fosburg MT, Nathan DG. Treatment of Cooley's anemia. Blood 76:435–444, 1990.
42. Oliveri NF, Brittenham GM. Iron-chelating therapy and the treatment of thalassemia. Blood 89:739–761, 1997.
43. Brittenham GM, Griffith PM, Nienhuis AW, et al. Efficacy of deferoxamine in preventing complications of iron overload in patients with thalassemia major. N Engl J Med 331:567–573, 1994.
44. Lerner N. Medical management of β-thalassemia. Prog Clin Biol Res 309:14–22, 1989.
45. Olivieri NF, Nathan DG, MacMillan JH, et al. Survival in medically treated patients with homozygous β-thalassemia. N Engl J Med 331:574–578, 1994.
46. Olivieri NF, Berriman AM, Tyler BJ, et al. Reduction in tissue iron stores with a new regimen of continuous ambulatory intravenous deferoxamine. Am J Hematol 41:61–63, 1992.
47. Cohen A. Current status of iron chelation therapy with deferoxamine. Semin Hematol 27:86–90, 1990.
48. Pippard MJ. Iron overload and iron chelation therapy in thalassemia and sickle cell haemoglobinopathies. Acta Haematol 78:206–211, 1987.
49. Olivieri NF, Koren G, Matsui D, et al. Reduction of tissue iron stores and normalization of serum ferritin during treatment with the oral iron chelator L1 in thalassemia intermedia. Blood 79:2741–2748, 1992.
50. Olivieri NF, Brittenham GM, McLaren CE, et al. Long-term safety and effectiveness of iron-chelation therapy with deferiprone for thalassemia major. N Engl J Med 339:417–423,1998.
51. Barrett AJ, Lucarelli G, Gale RP, et al. Bone marrow transplantation for thalassemia: a preliminary report from the international bone marrow transplant registry. Prog Clin Biol Res 309:173–185, 1989.
52. Lucarelli G, Galimberti M, Polchi P, et al. Marrow transplantation in patients with thalassemia responsive to iron chelation therapy. N Engl J Med 329:840–844, 1993.
53. Stamatoyannopoulos JA, Nienhuis AW. Therapeutic approaches to hemoglobin switching in treatment of hemoglobinopathies. Annu Rev Med 43:497–521, 1992.
54. Lowrey CH, Nienhuis AW. Treatment with azacitidine of patients with end-stage β-thalassemia. N Engl J Med 329:845–848, 1993.
55. Dover GJ. Hemoglobin switching protocols in thalassemia: experience with sodium phenylbutyrate and hydroxyurea. Ann N Y Acad Sci 850:80–86, 1998.
56. Loukopoulos D, Voskaridou E, Stamoulakatou A, et al. Hydroxyurea therapy in thalassemia. Ann N Y Acad Sci 850:120–128, 1998.
57. Steinberg MH. Prospects of gene therapy for hemoglobinopathies. Am J Med Sci 302:298–303, 1991.
58. Higgs DR. The thalassemia syndromes. Q J Med 86:559–564, 1993.
59. Tabbara IA. Hemolytic anemias: diagnosis and management. Med Clin North Am 76:649–668, 1992.
60. Beutler E. G6PD deficiency. Blood 84:3613–3636, 1994.
61. Winkelstein A, Kiss JE. Immunohematologic disorders. JAMA 278:1982–1992, 1997.
62. Mehta AB. Glucose-6-phosphate dehydrogenase deficiency. Postgrad Med J 70:871–877, 1994.

CHAPTER 15

COAGULATION DISORDERS

E. Ashley Whigham and Camille W. Thornton

Hemostasis

Hemostasis is the body's ability to maintain blood in its fluid state while it is within the vasculature and minimize blood loss by promoting clotting when the blood is outside of the vasculature. For this to occur there must be coordination of blood vessels, platelets, coagulation factors, natural inhibitors, and the fibrinolytic proteins existing in an overlapping system of checks and balances.[1] Normal hemostasis requires three responses: the vascular response, formation of a platelet plug, and formation of a fibrin clot. At the same time, naturally occurring anticoagulant proteins inhibit the action of clotting factors in an attempt to control thrombosis, fibrinolysis, and inflammation. The fibrinolytic system also dissolves and removes excess fibrin deposits to preserve vascular patency.

THE VASCULATURE

The main role of the vasculature is to prevent bleeding. Normal intact vascular endothelium repels platelets and red blood cells (RBCs) and secretes substances to inhibit clotting. The initial vascular response to trauma is vasoconstriction, which shunts blood away from the damaged area. Traumatic disruption of the vessel endothelial lining triggers formation, binding, and/or activation of various substances. Trauma also exposes substrates that facilitate attachment and formation of the platelet plug, which is the primary hemostatic mechanism. The secondary hemostatic mechanism controls the formation of a fibrin clot via the ordered interaction of a series of tissue and blood components or factors. Primary and secondary hemostasis operates simultaneously. During this time, inhibitor systems also operate to prevent propagation of the clot, and fibrinolysis is activated for eventual removal of the clot.

PLATELET PATHOPHYSIOLOGY

Platelets play a dominant role in the spontaneous prevention of blood loss from damaged blood vessels. Immedi-

Table 15.1 ▪ Characteristics of Coagulation

Factor	Synonym(s)	Plasma Half-Life (hr)	Plasma Concentration (mg/dL)	Coagulation Pathway (E, I, C)	Biochemical Group
Procoagulants					
I	Fibrinogen	100–150	200–400	C	
II	Prothrombin, prethrombin	50–80	10	C	Vitamin K-dependent
III	Tissue factor, tissue thromboplastin		0	E	
IV	Calcium ion		9–10	E, I, C	
V	Proaccelerin, labile factor	24	1	C	
VII	Proconvertin, SPCA, stable factor	6	0.05	E	Vitamin K-dependent
VIII	Antihemophilic factor (AHF) Antihemophilic globulin Antihemophilic factor A Platelet cofactor I	12	0.01	I	
vWf	von Willebrand factor	24	1		
IX	Christmas factor Antihemophilic factor B Plasma thromboplastin component Platelet cofactor II	24	0.3	I	Vitamin K-dependent
X	Stuart-Prower factor	25–60	1	C	Vitamin K-dependent
XI	Plasma thromboplastin antecedent Antihemophilic factor C	40–80	0.5	I	Contact factor
XII	Hageman factor	50–70	3	I	Contact factor
XIII	Fibrin stabilizing factor	150	1–2	C	
Prekallikrein	Fletcher factor	35	5	I	Contact factor
High-molecular-weight kininogen	Contact activation factor	150	6	I	Contact factor
Inhibitors/fibrinolysis					
Antithrombin III		24–36	18–30	I	Vitamin K-dependent
Protein C		16	0.4	I, C	Vitamin K-dependent
Protein S		42	2.3	I, C	Vitamin K-dependent
Plasminogen		48	20–40	C	

Sources: References 1, 3.

E, Extrinsic; *I,* intrinsic; *C,* common; *SPCA,* serum prothrombin conversion accelerator.

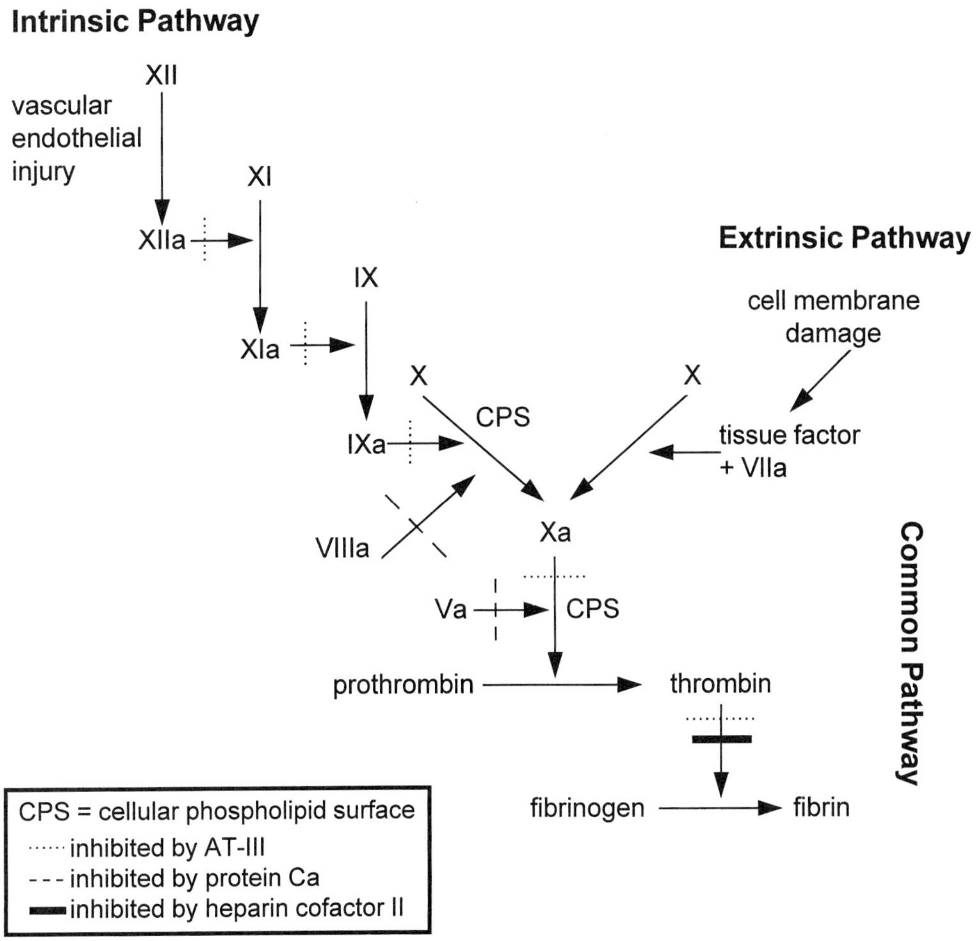

Figure 15.1. Components and inhibitors of the intrinsic, extrinsic, and common coagulation pathways.

ately after tissue injury, platelets clump together to form a primary hemostatic plug through a series of overlapping phases, which stops blood flow while maintaining vascular integrity. These phases include adhesion, aggregation, secretion, and elaboration of procoagulant activity. This series of steps ultimately results in the formation of a permanent insoluble fibrin clot that is essential for long-term hemostasis.

Platelets are fragments of megakaryocytes, which are large stem cells that are formed in the bone marrow. The normal platelet concentration is 150,000 to 400,000/mm^3 of blood, and production appears to be directly proportional to demand. This allows for the repair of minor ruptures that occur routinely in everyday life. After formation and release from the bone marrow, approximately 25 to 35% of platelets are found in the spleen and the remainder in the circulation. The average lifespan of a platelet is 7 to 10 days, and younger platelets are more physiologically active than older ones.[2]

COAGULATION AND FIBRINOLYSIS

The nomenclature and characteristics of the factors that are involved in the coagulation cascade are summarized in Table 15.1. The Roman numeral designations for clotting factors generally correspond to their order of discovery. Many clotting factors fall into one of two major groups, based on their biochemical properties. Factors XI, XII, prekallikrein, and high-molecular-weight kininogen are known as contact activation factors because they initiate the contact phase of the coagulation pathway. Factors II, VII, IX, and X are vitamin K-dependent coagulation factors synthesized by the liver. Vitamin K is an essential cofactor for hepatic carboxylation of glutamic acid residues. The *t*-carboxyglutamic acid residues allow the calcium binding that is essential for normal clotting activity. Vitamin K-deficient persons continue to produce factors II, VII, IX, and X, but in inactive forms. Factor III (tissue factor) is found in many tissues; factor IV (calcium) comes from diet and bone. Hepatic biosynthesis provides the other factors listed in Table 15.1.[3]

The coagulation cascade comprises reaction complexes, each including an enzyme, a substrate, and a reaction accelerator. The numerous steps amplify the activation process, which ensures a rapid response at sites of injury. The product of these reactions is the potent enzyme thrombin, which is formed by the catalytic action of factor Xa (activated factor X) on prothrombin (Fig. 15.1). There are two classic pathways that lead to the generation of factor Xa, called the extrinsic and intrinsic pathways.

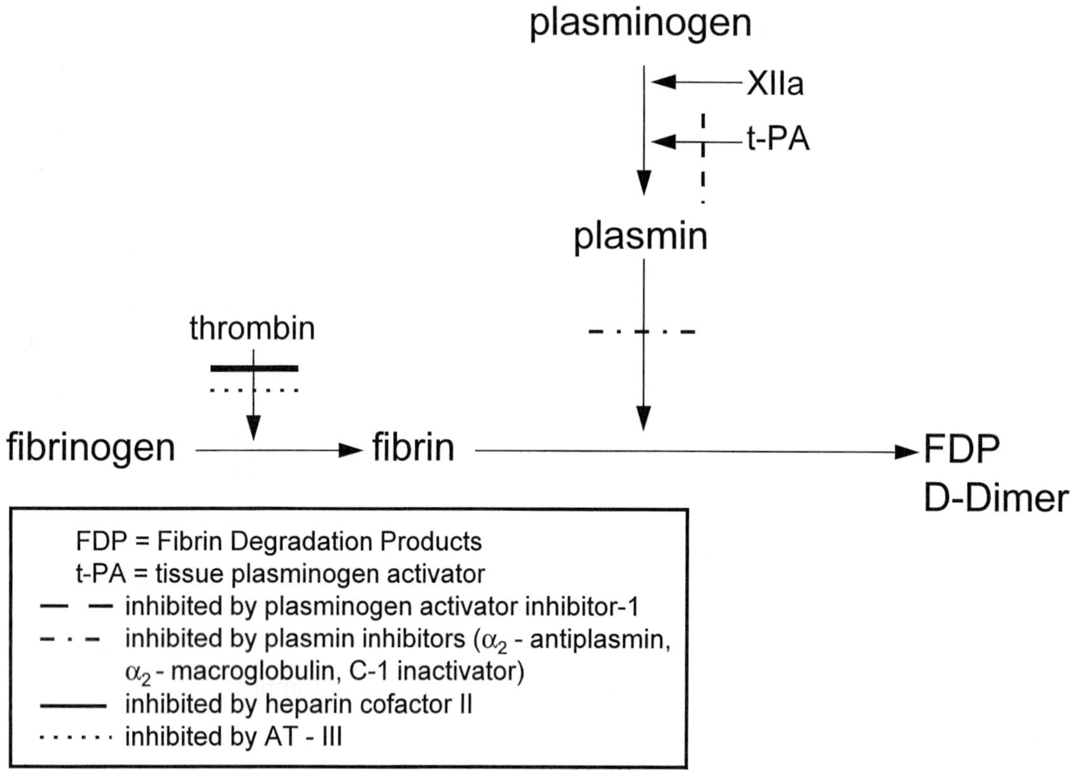

Figure 15.2. Components of fibrin formation and degradation.

The extrinsic coagulation pathway is so designated because it is activated by tissue factor, which is not a normal component of the blood. The rate-limiting step in thrombin formation via the extrinsic pathway is the amount of tissue factor released at the site of injury.

The intrinsic pathway comprises a system in which all components are normal blood constituents (hence the name "intrinsic"). In this pathway, components from each reaction form the enzyme for the next. It is initiated when contact of blood with an abnormal surface (e.g., collagen fibers exposed in the subendothelial layer of traumatized blood vessels) activates factor XII (left path, Fig. 15.1).

The intrinsic and extrinsic pathways differ in how factor X is activated. Once factor Xa is formed, the common pathway is activated (Fig. 15.1, lower center path). Thrombin also activates platelets. The platelets and attached fibrin clot act as a plug to minimize further blood loss.

After the fibrin clot is formed, fibrinolysis is initiated to remove the clot and restore blood flow. Fibrinolysis is mediated by the enzyme plasmin. Plasmin circulates in the inactive form of plasminogen. Tissue plasminogen activators (t-PAs) that are present in endothelial cells and other tissues activate plasminogen to form plasmin, which in turn cleaves fibrin into fibrin degradation products (FDPs) (Fig. 15.2).

The intact vessel endothelium and natural anticoagulants continuously maintain normal blood flow. Disruption of endothelial integrity or release of tissue factor after injury activates both the platelet and coagulation systems, resulting in an insoluble fibrin clot that limits further bleeding. Fibrinolysis is then activated, which results in vascular patency by breaking down the fibrin clot. Abnormalities in these systems may occur at virtually any step and may result in bleeding or coagulation disorders.

Platelet Disorders

Thrombocytopenia

Thrombocytopenia is defined as a decrease in the number of blood platelets and is one of the most common causes of abnormal bleeding. A platelet count less than $100,000/mm^3$ is considered mild thrombocytopenia and causes few symptoms. Counts less than $50,000/mm^3$ constitute moderate thrombocytopenia and are associated with some bleeding potential. In severe thrombocytopenia (counts less than 10,000 to $20,000/mm^3$), spontaneous life-threatening bleeding can occur. At platelet counts less than $100,000/mm^3$ the bleeding time becomes progressively longer. However, it is important to note that the actual risk for bleeding depends on both the number of platelets available and how well they function.

Thrombocytopenia has many causes, which should be distinguished to optimize the therapeutic approach. A decrease in the platelet count may occur from (1) a decrease in production, (2) altered distribution (sequestration), or (3) increased destruction of platelets.

A decrease in platelet production may occur from conditions that either alter normal formation of platelets (thrombopoiesis) or decrease the number of marrow megakaryocytes. Examples include marrow injury (e.g., myelosuppressive drugs, chemicals, radiation, or viral infections such as rubella, cytomegalovirus, Epstein-Barr virus, and human immunodeficiency virus), marrow failure (e.g., aplastic anemia and hereditary disorders), or marrow replacement (e.g., leukemia, tumor metastases and fibrosis). Ineffective thrombopoiesis caused by severe vitamin B_{12} or folate deficiency is characterized by a normal or increased number of megakaryocytes in the bone marrow associated with inadequate availability of platelets in the circulation. All of these disorders may be successfully treated with platelet transfusions.

Altered distribution of platelets can result from any disorder that causes splenomegaly (e.g., alcoholic liver disease, congestive heart failure, lymphomas, sickle cell disease, and myeloproliferative diseases). In this situation the actual number of total body platelets is normal, but their distribution in the body is altered.

Increased destruction of platelets can result from increased platelet utilization and from immunologic and nonimmunologic mechanisms. Disseminated intravascular coagulation (DIC) is an example of a condition that causes increased platelet consumption. Immunologic causes of thrombocytopenia include drug-induced immune thrombocytopenia (e.g., quinidine, quinine, gold, and heparin), autoantibody production (e.g., systemic lupus erythematosus (SLE) and autoimmune thrombocytopenic purpura), and autoantibody-produced thrombocytopenia (e.g., placental transfer and history of multiple transfusions).

Massive blood loss may result in dilutional thrombocytopenia when treated with large amounts of fluids having few or no platelets. Other miscellaneous causes of thrombocytopenia are thrombotic thrombocytopenic purpura (TTP), prosthetic heart valves, extracorporeal perfusion, hemodialysis, and snake envenomation.

The symptoms of thrombocytopenia include symmetric petechiae and purpura on the extremities and trunk, mild to moderate bleeding of mucosal surfaces (oropharynx, nose, and the gastrointestinal, pulmonary, and genitourinary systems), and easy or spontaneous bleeding.

TREATMENT GOALS: THROMBOCYTOPENIA

- Identify and correct underlying medical or surgical conditions where possible.
- Discontinue known drug therapies that cause thrombocytopenia.
- Initiate drug therapies that ameliorate or arrest thrombocytopenia.
- Administer coagulation factors and platelets where indicated.
- Offer supportive care for the associated signs and symptoms.

Autoimmune Thrombocytopenic Purpura

Autoimmune thrombocytopenic purpura (AITP) is characterized by decreased numbers of circulating platelets, normal or increased numbers of megakaryocytes in the bone marrow, and clinical signs and symptoms related to the low platelet count. Most cases of AITP involve shortened platelet survival due to immune-mediated platelet destruction by antiplatelet autoantibodies of the immunoglobulin (Ig) G or IgM subtypes.

EPIDEMIOLOGY

Clinically, AITP is divided into acute and chronic forms. The acute form most commonly occurs in young, previously healthy children 2 to 8 years of age and affects both sexes equally. The onset in 80% of patients is seen several weeks after an acute viral infection, most often an upper respiratory infection but also varicella, rubeola, or rubella. The syndrome had also been seen after immunizations. Approximately 80% of patients will have a complete remission within several weeks to months, regardless of therapy. The annual incidence of the acute form is approximately 4 : 100,000 children, although many times AITP remains undiagnosed because of its transient and self-limiting nature. The chronic form occurs more often in women between 20 and 40 years of age, with a female:male ratio of 3 : 1.[4–6] It has an insidious onset and a lower rate of acute bleeding; in some cases the chronic form is detected as an incidental finding. It is sometimes associated with another underlying disease (e.g., SLE, other autoimmune disorders, chronic lymphocytic leukemia, or lymphoma)[4,6] and is not usually preceded by a viral infection. Chronic AITP undergoes remissions and exacerbations, persisting for more than 6 months and often for years. Only about 20% of patients will have a spontaneous remission, regardless of therapy. Although the exact incidence is unknown, chronic AITP is a relatively common hematologic disorder.

Human immunodeficiency virus (HIV)-associated thrombocytopenia is one of the most common hematologic complications of the infection, although it is not considered an acquired immunodeficiency syndrome (AIDS)-defining illness. Thrombocytopenia in patients with HIV infection resembles AITP in clinical and laboratory presentation. Patients have normal to increased numbers of megakaryocytes without evidence of splenomegaly.

CLINICAL PRESENTATION AND DIAGNOSIS

Signs and Symptoms

Acute AITP is characterized by an abrupt onset, whereas onset of the chronic form is insidious. In most patients the physical examination is remarkable only for the hemorrhagic abnormalities associated with the low platelet count. Small punctate red macules (petechiae) and a dark red-purple discoloration of the skin reflecting larger areas of hemorrhage (purpura) are the classic signs of AITP. These can occur anywhere on the external surface of the skin as well as internally, the gastrointestinal tract being the most common internal site. Bleeding of the nasal, oropharyngeal, and vaginal mucosa; easy bruising with ecchymoses; conjunctival hemorrhage; epistaxis; and menorrhagia are common. Hematuria, retinal hemorrhage, and joint bleeding are less common. Splenomegaly is absent. Central nervous system (CNS) bleeding is seen in approximately 1% of patients. Intracranial hemorrhage occurs early in the acute form of AITP and is most common in patients with platelet counts less than 20,000/mm^3. It is considered the most serious risk with AITP, owing to its associated high morbidity and mortality. Manifestations include altered mental status and headache.

Patients with chronic AITP usually have a higher platelet count compared to those with the acute form. Minor skin and mucous membrane bleeding may be the sole manifestations, and some patients are asymptomatic.

Diagnosis

The diagnosis is usually a process of eliminating other disorders that also cause thrombocytopenia. This is especially true for children with signs and symptoms of acute AITP. The differential diagnosis of AITP includes a wide array of hematologic diseases including leukemia, marrow hypoplasia, DIC, aplastic anemia, TTP, and lymphoma. Nonhematologic causes of thrombocytopenia include systemic infection, thyroid disease, tuberculosis, and autoimmune diseases such as SLE. HIV infection should be considered as a possible diagnosis for patients who fit into high-risk categories. Drug-induced thrombocytopenia should also be excluded, and any drug that is capable of causing thrombocytopenia should be discontinued (Table 15.2). Splenomegaly, adenopathy, fever, and malaise are uncommon in acute AITP and may suggest other disorders when present.

Laboratory testing reveals isolated thrombocytopenia, unless bleeding has been sufficient to cause anemia. A complete blood examination shows a decreased number of platelets with an elevated mean platelet volume and platelet distribution width. On peripheral smear, the platelets are larger in size and appear to be less mature than normal. Thrombocytopenia in acute AITP may be severe (platelet count 10,000 to 20,000/mm^3), whereas patients with chronic AITP generally have higher counts (30,000 to 75,000/mm^3). Bleeding time is prolonged in proportion to the degree of thrombocytopenia. Of interest, the bleeding time for a given platelet count is shorter than that for thrombocytopenia caused by decreased platelet production, because the circulating platelets are young and "superactive." This accounts for the lack of bleeding symptoms in some patients despite severe thrombocytopenia. The prothrombin time (PT), activated partial thromboplastin time (aPTT), and erythrocyte sedimentation rate usually remain normal. Almost all patients have normal hemoglobin, hematocrit, and RBC indices, although chronic gastrointestinal hemorrhage or menorrhagia may occasionally cause iron deficiency anemia. Bone marrow examination shows normal or increased numbers of immature megakaryocytes.

Table 15.2 ▪ Drugs That Cause Thrombocytopenia

Amrinone (8)[a]	Ethanol (7)
Anti-inflammatory agents (1, 2, 3)	Estrogens (7)
Aspirin	Furosemide (1, 5)
Fenoprofen	Gold salts (2)
Indomethacin	Heparin (2)
Phenylbutazone	Histamine H_2 antagonists (8)
Piroxicam	Cimetidine
Tolmetin	Ranitidine
β-Blockers (3, 4, 8)	Methyldopa (2)
Alprenolol	Penicillins (3, 5, 8)
Oxprenolol	Ampicillin
Propranolol	Carbenicillin
Carbamazepine (2, 8)	Methicillin
Clofibrate (3)	Penicillin G
Cytotoxic agents (7)	Ticarcillin
Busulfan	Penicillamine (2, 8)
Cytarabine	Phenytoin (2)
Daunorubicin	Quinidine (2)
Flucytosine	Quinine (2)
Fluorouricin	Rifampin (8)
Mechlorethamine	Sulfinpyrazone (1, 4)
Mercaptopurine	Thiazide diuretics (8)
Methotrexate	Chlorothiazide
Mithramycin	Hydrochlorothiazide
Mitomycin	Tocainide (8)
Dextran (4, 8)	Trimethoprim (8)
Digitoxin (2)	Valproic acid (2)
Dipyridamole (3, 5, 6)	

[a]Numbers in parentheses indicate confirmed and suspected mechanisms of thrombocytopenia: 1, Inhibits cyclo-oxygenase; 2, Drug-induced immune; 3, Inhibits aggregation; 4, Inhibits adhesion; 5, Inhibits release reaction; 6, Inhibits phosphodiesterase; 7, Myelosuppression; 8, Mechanism not documented.

TREATMENT

The major goals in the treatment of AITP are to decrease the risk of hemorrhage and to obtain complete remission of the disease. Traditionally, these goals are met either by suppressing the production of antiplatelet antibodies or by inhibiting platelet phagocytosis. Supportive measures to reduce the risk of bleeding include restriction of physical activity and avoidance of drugs that alter platelet activity and should be implemented for all patients. For patients with chronic AITP secondary to another disorder, treatment of the underlying disease will benefit the AITP.

Acute Autoimmune Thrombocytopenic Purpura

More than 80% of patients with acute AITP will have a complete spontaneous recovery within a few weeks to months of the disease onset, irrespective of which (if any) treatment is given.[2,5] Considerable controversy exists regarding the decision to treat the disease or simply let it run its course. Intracranial hemorrhage is the primary concern of clinicians who prefer early treatment. Others choose not to treat because of adverse effects, cost, the low frequency of CNS bleeding, and the self-limiting nature of the disease. Some clinicians base the decision to treat on the platelet count, electing to treat when the count is less than 20,000/mm^3. Other factors in the treatment decision include days of hospitalization, the potential for outpatient treatment, and parental concern regarding intracranial hemorrhage and administration of blood products. Recent studies documenting a more rapid platelet response in treated compared to untreated patients,[7] coupled with the known early occurrence of CNS bleeding, provide evidence favoring early treatment.

The goal of treatment is to rapidly increase the platelet count to a hemostatically safe level.[8] For many years, prednisone was considered the drug of choice for treating acute AITP. Hypothesized mechanisms of action include a prolongation of platelet lifespan by suppressing reticuloendothelial system phagocytosis, inhibition of platelet-associated immunoglobulin production, and enhancement of bone marrow platelet production.[9] At the traditional dose of 1 to 2 mg/kg/day, the onset of action is about 72 hours, with a return to normal platelet counts within 1 to 2 weeks in approximately 60 to 70% of patients.[10] In some patients it may take up to 4 weeks to see a maximal response. After a response is documented over 4 to 8 weeks, the dose is tapered; then the drug is discontinued. A problem with the traditional doses is the discordance between the timing of drug effect and the maximal risk for CNS bleeding. Studies of higher doses (4 mg/kg/day) show a more rapid response[7,8,11]; however, the optimal corticosteroid dose and route of administration have not been established. Adverse effects are minimal at low doses, whereas higher doses have been associated with weight gain, epigastric discomfort, glycosuria, and behavioral changes to name a few.[9,11]

Intravenous high-dose immune globulins (IVIGs) were discovered by serendipity to have efficacy in acute AITP.[12] IVIG has many simultaneous effects on platelet function, which occur through inhibition of Fc receptor-mediated platelet binding in the reticuloendothelial system. IVIG alters T- and B-cell numbers and function. It also produces a reduction in platelet-associated immunoglobulins, which is seen within 3 days. Another possible effect is an alteration in secretion and binding of interleukins. The total dose of IVIG to be administered is 2 g/kg, given as either 0.4 g/kg/day for 5 days or 1 g/kg/day for 2 days. This usually results in a response in 1 to 3 days, with about 80% of patients showing a platelet count greater than 50,000/mm^3 at 72 hours after treatment. If the effect is not sustained, repeat doses may be given. Adverse effects of IVIG include nausea, vomiting, headache, and fever, which seem to occur more often (50 to 60%) in patients who receive the total dose over 2 days.[7,8] However, these symptoms usually abate after about 1 day and are readily managed with acetaminophen. The long-term response to IVIG, assessed as maintenance of a platelet count greater than 20,000/mm^3 with no subsequent bleeding, is about 62%.[12]

Short-course high-dose IVIG therapy may also be of value when a temporary but rapid rise in platelet count is necessary (e.g., for surgery or during exposure to stressors such as infection). In children with severe bleeding and/or a high risk of intracranial hemorrhage, corticosteroids and IVIG may be given concomitantly. This combination has been shown to increase the platelet count more rapidly than either drug alone.[6,9,12]

Small- and medium-scale comparative studies of IVIG and prednisone, sometimes with a "no-treatment" cohort, have yielded several interesting findings:

- Both IVIG and prednisone (4 mg/kg/day, tapered over 21 days) caused fewer days of thrombocytopenia (20,000/mm^3) compared to no treatment. The use of IVIG produced a significantly faster increase of platelet count greater than 50,000/mm^3 than prednisone alone.[7]
- A trial comparing IVIG doses of 1 g/kg for 2 days and 0.8 g/kg once yielded similar responses as measured by days of thrombocytopenia and days to reach a "safer" platelet count (50,000/mm^3).[8]
- An early pilot study suggested that patients who had a rapid response to IVIG had a better long-term prognosis compared to those with a slow response.[13]

The decision whether to use prednisone or IVIG as initial therapy requires consideration of many factors. IVIG may be preferable because it has a more rapid onset of action compared to traditional doses of prednisone; however, higher prednisone doses may yield comparable onset of action. Some investigators prefer IVIG, with the belief that it may have a disease-modifying role.[9] Some practitioners consider prednisone to be the "gold standard" and favor its use because of familiarity with the drug. Much lower cost and concern regarding administration of blood products also favor prednisone, although a shortened hospital stay with IVIG may offset some of the cost. Additional studies are clearly necessary to clarify this clinical decision.

Anti-D (WinRho) is a Rh_o (D) immune globulin made from freeze-dried γ-globulin (IgG) fraction, which contains antibodies to Rh_o (D). It is indicated for the treatment of nonsplenectomized, Rh_o (D)-positive children with chronic or acute ITP, adults with chronic ITP, and children and adults with ITP secondary to HIV infection. Patients should be treated with an initial dose of 50 μg/kg as a single injection. If the patient's hemoglobin level is less than 10 g/dL, the dose should be reduced to 25 to 40 μg/kg to minimize the risk of increasing the severity of anemia. If a subsequent dose is required to elevate platelet counts, a dose of 25 to 60 μg/kg is recommended. Once a response to therapy is seen, the maintenance dose is 25 to 60 μg/kg, which should be individualized depending on the patient's platelet and hemoglobin levels.[14]

Splenectomy is avoided for treatment of children because of the risk of postsplenectomy sepsis. This is particularly true for children younger than 6 years of age and immunosuppressed patients, who have the highest risk of overwhelming postsplenectomy infection. If splenectomy is contemplated, pneumococcal and *Haemophilus influenzae* immunizations should be given before the surgery.

Chronic Autoimmune Thrombocytopenic Purpura

Chronic AITP is primarily a disease of adults, but approximately 10 to 20% of children with acute AITP have a poor response to treatment, and their AITP will evolve into the chronic form. Therapy for chronic AITP is usually begun with 1 mg/kg/day of prednisone, although 2 mg/kg/day has been used in severe cases. A positive response should be seen in 3 to 7 days, although 2 to 4 weeks may be needed for maximal response.[9] Once the platelet count is greater than 100,000/mm^3, the dose of prednisone should be tapered slowly and reduced to the lowest effective dose, preferably on an alternate-day schedule. If no response is observed after 3 to 4 weeks, alternative treatment should be instituted. If a therapeutic response is obtained, and the patient can tolerate the drug, prednisone is given on a long-term basis, because the disease is recurrent and spontaneous remission is uncommon. The initial response rate to steroid therapy may be as high as 50 to 80%, but in fewer than 20% of patients will be able to receive long-term corticosteroid therapy, owing to relapse or adverse reactions.[9,15]

In patients whose disease is refractory to steroid treatment, who are unable to tolerate long-term treatment, or who have a life-threatening hemorrhage, splenectomy is usually considered next. Postulated mechanisms for efficacy include a reduction in the phagocytosis of antibody-coated platelets and a reduction of platelet-associated antibody production. It is important that the operative procedure include a search for and removal of all accessory splenic tissues. Corticosteroids or IVIG are often given before surgery to boost the platelet count and reduce the risk of perioperative bleeding. Polyvalent pneumococcal vaccine should be administered preoperatively. Some clinicians also advocate daily oral penicillin therapy for several years after surgery.[2] A complete remission of AITP has been reported in up to 80% of patients after splenectomy.[2,15,16] Platelet kinetic studies may be performed to assess the degree of splenic sequestration; this may assist in the decision to perform splenectomy. In one study, a platelet count greater than 120,000/mm^3 at the time of discharge, age less than 30 years, preoperative corticosteroid dependence, and splenic sequestration (measured preoperatively) were associated with a more favorable response to splenectomy.[15]

The role of IVIG in treating chronic AITP is limited by its short duration of action. Although 90% of patients have a brisk increase in platelet count, this effect usually lasts less than 3 weeks, with only about 10% of patients achieving a long-term remission. Repeated infusions usually give equivalent response rates. However, maintenance therapy with IVIG is not cost-effective. IVIG is therefore generally reserved for patients who have symptomatic bleeding or to prepare the patient for surgery or other invasive procedures.

The treatment of patients who are refractory to corticosteroids and splenectomy is problematic. Immunosuppressive therapy is usually considered next. Azathioprine, cyclophosphamide, and the vinca alkaloids (vincristine and vinblastine) are the most commonly used agents. Azathioprine is believed to interfere with the response of T-cells to antigenic challenge, with an additional more generalized reduction in T-helper activity. It is given in a dose of 1 to 3 mg/kg/day (or 100 to 200 mg/day); the dose is reduced if the patient becomes leukopenic.[10] It is usually given in conjunction with steroids and may have a steroid-sparing effect for some patients. Approximately one-half of patients show an adequate platelet response over several months. The long-term response is approximately 40% at one year and 32% at two or more years.[9] Side effects are usually less serious than with cyclophosphamide, bone marrow suppression being the most important. Azathioprine is considered the safest agent for long-term therapy.

Cyclophosphamide is given in an oral dose of 2 to 3 mg/kg/m^2 daily or 600 to 1000 mg/m^2 intravenously every 3 to 4 weeks.[9] Improvement is usually seen in 2 to 6 weeks, with a maximum response in platelet count seen in 8 weeks. Treatment is continued for 4 to 6 weeks after an adequate platelet count is achieved. Studies demonstrating complete remission in 30 to 40% of patients are an advantage with cyclophosphamide. Unfortunately, side effects, including bone marrow suppression, hemorrhagic cystitis, and bladder fibrosis, may limit its use.

Vinca alkaloids have been reported to be beneficial in more than 50% of patients who are refractory to steroids and splenectomy. Vincristine (0.25 mg/kg to a maximum dose of 2 mg) and vinblastine (0.125 mg/kg to a maximum dose of 10 mg) are given intravenously every 2 to 6 weeks.[9] Response occurs more rapidly than with azathioprine or cyclophosphamide, but relapses usually occur in 3 to 4 weeks. These agents are believed to decrease the rate of destruction of platelets by inhibiting phagocytosis and decreasing antibody levels.[4] Vincristine may also bind selectively to platelet tubulin, such that when the antibody-coated platelet is phagocytosed, the macrophages are poisoned. Vincristine and vinblastine have been loaded onto platelets in an attempt to deliver them selectively to macrophages that are responsible for platelet destruction, but this is not commonly done because of its impracticality and lack of advantage over conventional administration. The incidence of side effects is relatively high with the vinca alkaloids. Vincristine may cause transient malaise, fever after injection, temporary jaw pain, alopecia, and a variety of neuropathies. Leukopenia, abdominal pain, and headache are associated with vinblastine.

Danazol, an anabolic steroid, is thought to decrease phagocytosis of platelets by decreasing the number of phagocytic cell IgG Fc-receptors.[4] Doses are usually between 400 to 800 mg/day initially, then tapered to 50 to 200 mg daily. Clinical response is normally seen within 8 weeks. Side effect frequency is low and includes virilization, fibrinolysis, and hepatic dysfunction. Danazol is contraindicated during pregnancy.

Intravenous anti-Rh(D) immunoglobulin has been used with moderate success in the treatment of autoimmune thrombocytopenic purpura and in a few cases of refractory HIV-associated thrombocytopenia. The mechanism of action appears to be inhibition of reticuloendothelial system function; however, it does not appear to be effective in Rh-negative or splenectomized patients.[9,10]

Other therapies that have been studied in limited numbers of patients include colchicine, high-dose ascorbic acid, cyclosporine, interferon-α, and anti-Fc receptor monoclonal antibodies. Plasma transfusion and plasma exchange (plasmapheresis) may have some merit, especially in life-threatening emergencies, but for chronic AITP they are of little value.

Although spontaneous complete remission of chronic AITP is unusual, the long-term prognosis is usually favorable. Most patients will have stable, mild-to-moderate thrombocytopenia. The objective of therapy in chronic AITP is to keep the patient hemostatically safe (i.e., platelet counts higher than 30,000 to 50,000/mm^3), not necessarily to obtain a complete remission. A review of the literature on patients with refractory disease showed a median death rate of 5.1%, caused either by uncontrolled bleeding or by complications of the therapy. High-risk groups included patients with a history of bleeding, those with the concomitant presence of other bleeding disorders, and those older than 60 years of age.[15]

Human Immunodeficiency Virus–Associated Thrombocytopenia

Patients with this syndrome are generally treated only when the thrombocytopenia is symptomatic. One approach is to control the underlying disease via the use of zidovudine or other antiretroviral agents. This treatment is based on the hypothesis that HIV-associated thrombocytopenia is caused by a direct effect of the virus on the bone marrow and/or immune system. Zidovudine doses of 200 mg every 6 hours have yielded an increase in the platelet count over 2 to 6 weeks.[4]

Most studies of corticosteroids in HIV-associated thrombocytopenia have reported a moderate to excellent initial response but a return to pretreatment values when the dose is reduced. The high rate of steroid-induced adverse effects, the low rate of sustained response, and the possibility of opportunistic infections must all be considered before corticosteroid therapy is used in treating patients with HIV-associated thrombocytopenia.

The use of IVIG in the treatment of HIV-associated thrombocytopenia shows a high initial response rate, ranging from 70 to 100%.[17,18] Because it does not increase susceptibility to opportunistic infections, IVIG therapy may be the treatment of choice for HIV-associated thrombocytopenia. However, the effect is usually only transient.

The efficacy of splenectomy in patients with HIV-associated thrombocytopenia is not well established. The literature reports effects ranging from increased platelet counts in 80% of patients receiving corticosteroids plus splenectomy[2,6] to no response.[4] Splenectomy, like corticosteroid therapy, may increase the susceptibility to opportunistic infections in patients with HIV-induced thrombocytopenia and may also increase the risk of progression to AIDS.

The prognosis for HIV-associated thrombocytopenia is poor because of the underlying illness.

Thrombotic Thrombocytopenic Purpura

Thrombotic thrombocytopenic purpura (TT) is an uncommon but devastating disorder of multiorgan involvement. The original triad of clinical characteristics consisting of thrombocytopenia, microangiopathic hemolytic anemia (hemolysis secondary to RBC fragmentation), and neurologic abnormalities has been expanded to a pentad with the addition of fever and renal dysfunction. Extensive widespread occlusion by platelets and hyaline material in the capillaries and arterioles (but not the venules) of nearly all organs is the hallmark of the disease and is responsible for the high mortality.

EPIDEMIOLOGY

Despite many theories about the exact cause of TTP, the primary cause remains puzzling. Immunologic abnormalities have been suspected because of the hemolytic anemia and thrombocytopenic purpura associated with the disease and because TTP has occurred in other diseases of an immune nature, such as SLE, scleroderma, Sjögren's syndrome, and rheumatoid arthritis.

Precipitating factors may be found in as many as 70% of patients.[19] Bacterial or viral infection is the most common (including HIV infection at any stage), occurring in up to 40% of patients. Pregnancy is the comorbid condition in 10 to 25%, with the disease occurring either antepartum or postpartum. Other precipitating conditions include postoperative status, myocardial infarction, lymphoma, carcinoma, bee stings, and dog bites. Drugs such as penicillins, sulfonamides, cyclosporine A, penicillamine, oral contraceptives, iodine, ticlopidine, mitomycin, cisplatinum, and bleomycin have also been implicated.

Although TTP has been reported in all age groups, ranging from infants to the very old, it occurs most commonly between the ages of 30 and 40. It is found in both sexes, with most studies showing a slightly higher occurrence in females (female:male 3:2).[19] Most patients have previously enjoyed good health. The overall incidence in the population is not known but is believed to be small.

PATHOPHYSIOLOGY

The pathogenesis of TTP is unknown. Many believe that the diffuse microvascular thrombi are caused by abnormal platelet aggregation, adhesion, and release on the microarterial endothelial surfaces, without activation of the coagulation cascade.[2,19] The numerous defects in patients with TTP suggest that more than one factor plays a role in its pathogenesis. Evidence suggests that mechanisms may include the following[19,20]:

- Absent fibrinolytic activity in the area of microvascular thrombi but normal activity in the circulating blood.
- Prostacyclin deficiency or diminished release. Prostacyclin causes vasodilation and is a natural inhibitor of platelet aggregation and adhesion. The lack of this factor would therefore favor vasoconstriction and platelet aggregation. Increased destruction and altered binding of prostacyclin have also been postulated.
- An unknown substance that precipitates platelet aggregation may be present in the blood.
- An unknown substance that prevents platelet aggregation may be lacking.
- A defect in the production of plasma von Willebrand factor may cause the formation of abnormal large multimer fragments.

CLINICAL PRESENTATION AND DIAGNOSIS

Signs and Symptoms

Presenting signs and symptoms of TTP are variable and nonspecific, including complaints of malaise, weakness, fatigue, abdominal pain, nausea and vomiting, arthralgia, fever, and hemorrhage. Neurologic symptoms such as headache, syncope, vertigo, ataxia, aphasia, behavioral or mental status changes, and seizures are the most frequent complaints. Signs of hemorrhage, including petechiae and purpura, are the next most commonly seen. Target organ dysfunction may also be seen in the eyes, heart, and lungs. It is important to remember that not all patients will have symptoms in each of these categories.

Diagnosis

TTP should be suspected in patients who have the symptoms mentioned above. Biopsy findings of subendothelial and intraluminal occlusive accumulation in arterioles and capillaries of fragmented platelets and fibrin deposits can usually confirm the diagnosis. Hematologic, neurologic, renal, cardiovascular, gastrointestinal, and pulmonary abnormalities all appear to be secondary to occlusion in the microcirculation. Severe microangiopathic hemolytic anemia associated with negative Coombs test results is seen in the majority of patients. Bilirubin and lactate dehydrogenase levels are markedly elevated owing to RBC hemolysis. The hemoglobin concentration averages 8 to 9 g/dL. Peripheral blood smears reveal odd-shaped fragmented and nucleated RBCs, with an abundance of reticulocytes. Severe thrombocytopenia is invariably present, with platelet counts usually below 30,000 to 50,000/mm^3 and bone marrow biopsies showing large numbers of megakaryocytes. The coagulation screen is normal except for mild elevations in fibrin degradation products in up to 70% of patients[19]; this is a useful parameter for distinguishing TTP from DIC. Renal involvement is present in 40% of patients,[4] with laboratory tests showing proteinuria, microscopic hematuria, and elevated blood urea nitrogen (BUN) and serum creatinine levels.

TREATMENT

In the past, TTP was almost uniformly fatal; but in the last 20 years, researchers have had remarkable success in devising treatment strategies. Therapies include plasma infusion or exchange, corticosteroids, splenectomy, and antiplatelet, immunosuppressive, and cytotoxic agents. Success is unpredictable, each approach showing some benefit in certain patients but little benefit in others. The individual effectiveness of each modality is not known, because several or all are commonly administered simultaneously.

Plasmapheresis (exchange transfusion with fresh frozen plasma (FFP)) is the treatment of choice for TTP, producing a response rate near 80%.[2] When this procedure is not available, infusions of FFP are started, although this yields a lower overall response rate. The therapeutic rationale for plasmapheresis is to remove toxic substances and immune complexes and/or to replace deficient factor(s) that are responsible for the inhibition of platelet aggregation or stimulation of prostacyclin. The fact that improvement is seen in some patients with plasma infusion alone suggests a deficiency of an unknown factor. Plasmapheresis has been associated with a higher response rate and lower mortality than plasma infusion, although it is technically more difficult and expensive. It should be initiated as soon as possible, with a single plasma volume exchange daily until clinical manifestations improve and the platelet count exceeds 150,000/mm^3 for 2 to 3 days.[4,19] Plasma exchange is then gradually replaced by plasma infusion. Adverse effects of plasma therapy include hypersensitivity reactions, acute infection, hepatitis, and volume overload (seen primarily with plasma infusion). Patients with a poor response to plasmapheresis with fresh frozen plasma may benefit from the substitution of cryosupernatant as the replacement solution.[19,20]

Corticosteroids have an unknown benefit but are almost universally used, in part because the differential diagnosis often includes vasculitis or other steroid-responsive diseases. Prednisone is begun at 1 to 1.5 mg/kg/day (or its equivalent), in conjunction with other therapeutic modalities.[4,19,20] The dose is then slowly tapered. Corticosteroids alone are not generally effective in treating the acute disease but may be useful in combination with other therapies. They are also used (alone or in combination) to reduce the remission rate and treat relapses.

Antiplatelet agents such as aspirin and dipyridamole are commonly administered in the acute phase. However, in some patients they may worsen bleeding without providing a beneficial effect.[2,4] After remission is achieved, maintenance doses of aspirin and dipyridamole may be given for prevention of relapse. The antiplatelet agent ticlopidine should not be used, because it has been implicated as a causative factor in some cases of TTP. Infusions of prostacyclin have been administered, because deficiencies of this vasodilator and platelet aggregation inhibitor have been observed in patients with TTP. The effectiveness of this modality has been questionable, and its use is restricted to patients whose disease is unresponsive to other treatments. Sulfinpyrazone and dextran are also reserved for patients with refractory disease.

Splenectomy is reserved for patients who show no response to other therapies and those who cannot be weaned off plasma therapy. It has also been shown to reduce the relapse rate. Vincristine may be given in severe cases at a dosage of 2 mg weekly.[19,20] IVIG has shown a variable effect and is used only in patients with refractory disease.

Platelet transfusions have been shown to worsen the microvascular occlusion and are therefore not given.[2,19,20] Because TTP is a disease of the platelets, heparin has no beneficial effect and can even be harmful by increasing the risk of bleeding.

Supportive care for the associated symptoms should be provided. Hemodialysis may be necessary for patients with severe renal failure.

Relapses of TTP are generally milder in severity than the initial presentation. They are treated with plasma infusion (plasmapheresis is reserved for severe cases) or aspirin and dipyridamole combined with corticosteroids. To prevent relapse, aspirin, dipyridamole, and steroids may also be given as prophylaxis to patients with severe infections, to patients after surgery, and to women during subsequent pregnancies. Splenectomy is another useful measure for preventing relapses. Patient education is important to facilitate prompt evaluation and treatment of relapses.

PROGNOSIS

Before 1965, TTP was considered an infrequent, complicated, progressive, and nearly always fatal disease. Without treatment, TTP remains a fatal disorder in 80 to 90% of patients. Fortunately, with advances in the understanding and treatment of the disease, up to 70 to 80% of patients can now be expected to survive with appropriate treatment, most with few or no sequelae.[19,20] Early intervention minimizes the risk of long-term neurologic or renal sequelae.

The improved survival rate has resulted in larger numbers of patients with relapsed or chronic disease. Approximately 15 to 50% of patients who survive after TTP will have a relapse.[2,19] Relapses are usually milder than the initial disease. They occur at intervals of months or years, and the patient is relatively healthy in the interim periods.

Platelet Function Disorders

Disorders of platelet function may cause bleeding or thrombosis independent of the platelet count. Congenital disorders of platelet function are rare and encompass defects in any of the four previously described actions. Acquired platelet function disorders are common, are often associated with clinically significant bleeding, and may be caused by medical conditions as well as by a variety of drugs.

Uremia is a commonly encountered medical condition that is associated with a variety of platelet function defects. Almost all uremic patients have prolonged bleeding times and abnormal in vitro platelet function,[21] with a correlation between the bleeding time prolongation and the degree of renal insufficiency. The abnormalities are thought to be caused by unknown substances that are present in uremic plasma, because most defects abate with dialysis or improved renal function. Most patients experience bleeding, but this is rarely a cause of serious morbidity.

Cardiac bypass induces a platelet function disorder that is caused by factors related to the bypass procedure itself. Most defects correct spontaneously after completion of the bypass. Other conditions that are associated with abnormalities in platelet function include liver disease, dysproteinemias (e.g., multiple myeloma or macroglobulinemia), and myeloproliferative disorders.

The management of patients with platelet function disorders consists of both supportive care and administration of specific agents to improve platelet function. Supportive measures include avoidance of situations that are associated with a high risk of bleeding and medications that alter platelet function or numbers (Table 15.2). The underlying disorder should be corrected or treated when possible. Platelet transfusions are useful for patients after bypass surgery, but are otherwise avoided unless bleeding is life threatening. For uremic patients with bleeding, desmopressin or conjugated estrogens will correct the bleeding time and slow clinical bleeding.[21] Oral contraceptives may be given to reduce menorrhagia.

Drug-Induced Platelet Disorders

The pharmacist must recognize drugs that adversely affect platelets. Avoidance of their use entirely or close monitoring of platelet counts and function may be necessary for certain patients. Familiarity with these agents also facilitates assessment of drugs as potential causative factors in patients with platelet abnormalities. Although many drugs affect platelet activity adversely, the literature must be evaluated carefully before an "antiplatelet" label is placed on a therapeutic agent that only rarely produces clinically significant manifestations.

Drug-induced platelet disorders include those that alter platelet function and those that cause thrombocytopenia. Drug-induced disorders of platelet function are further subdivided (in descending order of prevalence) into drug interference with (1) platelet membranes or membrane receptor sites, (2) prostaglandin biosynthetic pathways, (3) phosphodiesterase activity, and (4) unknown mechanisms.[22] Either decreased production or increased destruction of platelets may cause drug-induced thrombocytopenia. Table 15.2 lists commonly implicated drugs and their proposed mechanisms of action.

Aspirin is by far the most common and well-documented cause of drug-induced platelet dysfunction. This is mediated by aspirin-induced abnormalities on both platelets and endothelial cells. At the platelet level, aspirin irreversibly acetylates cyclooxygenase. This reduces platelet synthesis of cyclic endoperoxides and thromboxane A_2, resulting in loss of thromboxane A_2-mediated platelet stimulation and vasoconstriction. Platelets cannot regenerate cyclooxygenase; therefore, the effect of aspirin on thromboxane A_2 is irreversible. In contrast, endothelial cells can synthesize new cyclooxygenase; therefore, prostacyclin synthesis resumes after the aspirin is metabolized. The net effect of aspirin reflects its action on the platelets and endothelial cells. The irreversible loss of platelet cyclooxygenase often dominates, with a reduction in platelet stimulation. The peak effect of a single dose occurs in 2 to 4 hours, but because aspirin's effect on platelets is irreversible, its pharmacodynamic activity may last up to 10 days or the lifespan of the platelet. When aspirin is administered to a normal person, bleeding time is prolonged by a factor of 1.5 to 2,[21] but significant bleeding is uncommon. Aspirin may be associated with clinically significant hemorrhage when the hemostatic system is stressed (e.g., surgery or other invasive procedure), such as in older adults, patients with hemophilia, patients with coexisting thrombocytopenia or other bleeding risk (e.g., peptic ulcer disease), patients taking other drugs with antiplatelet effect, or patients undergoing neurologic or ophthalmic surgery. It should also be avoided late in pregnancy.

Other nonsteroidal anti-inflammatory agents such as indomethacin, ibuprofen, naproxen, piroxicam, and ketorolac also prevent thromboxane A_2 generation by inhibiting platelet cyclooxygenase.[21,22] With these drugs the platelet effect is reversible, occurring only while the drug is present in the circulation. The bleeding time is only slightly prolonged, and the effects abate as the drug is cleared from the plasma.

Dipyridamole is sometimes used therapeutically for its antithrombotic activity, usually in combination with aspirin. The mode of action is believed to be prevention of cyclic adenosine monophosphate (AMP) breakdown by inhibition of phosphodiesterase activity. Increased platelet cyclic AMP levels inhibit platelet aggregation and release. Unlike aspirin, dipyridamole does not alter bleeding time or platelet survival.

Ticlopidine-induced antiplatelet effects occur via a mechanism that is not well established. Ticlopidine induces a thrombasthenic-like state without altering the expression of platelet membrane receptors. This may occur via inhibition of common signal transduction pathways in platelets. The drug prolongs bleeding time; however, severe hemorrhage is not a prominent side effect.[21]

Penicillin and related compounds prolong bleeding time and occasionally have clinically important effects on platelet function. These effects are mediated by an interaction with platelet membrane receptors that reduces responsiveness to stimulation by adenosine diphosphate (ADP) and epinephrine and decreases platelet aggregation.[21] Platelet dysfunction begins several days after initiation and abates several days after discontinuation of the drug. High-dose carbenicillin is the prototype example of a drug that produces this effect. Similar effects have been seen with penicillin G, ampicillin, ticarcillin, piperacillin, methicillin, and nafcillin. Cephalosporins may also alter platelet function, although this effect is not as well documented, and the clinical relevance is not well established. Significant bleeding is uncommon unless the patient has other risk factors such as renal failure or ulcer disease.

Dextran, a partially hydrolyzed polymer of glucose, is used as a plasma volume expander in patients with certain types of shock, impaired renal function, and other conditions in which improved circulation is desirable. It also prolongs bleeding time, impairs fibrin polymerization, decreases blood viscosity, and alters platelet function. For these reasons, dextran is sometimes used in the prophylaxis of venous thrombosis and pulmonary thromboembolism. The mechanism of the antiplatelet activity is not known but may involve inhibition of platelet aggregation and reduced platelet agonist activity. Dextran should be used with caution in treating patients with coexisting thrombocytopenia.

Alcohol impairs platelet function and primary hemostasis. Large quantities of ethanol can inhibit prostaglandin endoperoxide synthesis and decrease thromboxane A_2 production, thereby causing a decrease in platelet aggregation and release. Alcohol ingestion may also directly suppress bone marrow thrombocyte production. Alcoholism can decrease ADP storage pools and platelet agonist (ADP and epinephrine) activity. Moreover, alcoholism is associated with other factors that may cause platelet dysfunction. Alcohol-mediated platelet dysfunction can occur in the absence of liver disease and is reversible; the platelet count returns to baseline 7 to 21 days after discontinuation.[4]

Drug-induced immune thrombocytopenia is a relatively uncommon platelet disorder that is caused by a number of drugs. Two mechanisms have been postulated:

- Formation of an immunoglobulin-drug immune complex that attaches to and destroys the platelet, via either accelerated reticuloendothelial system phagocytosis or complement-associated intravascular lysis. In this scenario the platelet is considered an "innocent bystander."
- Binding of the drug to the platelet membrane, creating a hapten that induces a structural change, ultimately resulting in the formation of antiplatelet antibodies.

Drug-induced immune thrombocytopenia is more common in adults, is not dose-related, and is associated with antibody persistence for many years. The clinical presentation of petechiae, purpura, and mucous membrane bleeding is similar to that for the chronic form of autoimmune thrombocytopenia. However, its rapid onset (6 to 12 hours after reexposure), the severity of both symptoms and thrombocytopenia (commonly less than 10,000/mm^3), and the rapid sustained recovery after the drug is terminated are distinguishing features of the drug-induced form.[2,23] The primary management is discontinuation of the drug. Platelet destruction generally abates in 3 to 7 days but may persist for weeks to months after drug discontinuation in some patients. High-dose IVIG or a short course of corticosteroids may be given to shorten the recovery period.[23] Plasmapheresis may be used for critically ill patients. Drug-induced immune thrombocytopenia has been best documented with heparin, gold, quinidine, and quinine (which may be used therapeutically or found in soft drinks and street drugs). Other common drugs that cause this syndrome are listed in Table 15.2.

Heparin is the most common cause of drug-induced thrombocytopenia, with an overall incidence of 3 to 5% with intravenous therapy[23,24] and with fewer than 3% of patients developing platelet counts less than 100,000/mm^3. The incidence is much lower with subcutaneous administration, yet this syndrome has been seen after the use of the small doses used in heparin flushes or even in patients with heparin-coated intravenous catheters. Thrombocytopenia is more common with bovine-derived heparin (versus porcine). Heparin causes two types of platelet disorders, type I and type II.

In type I, a mild gradual thrombocytopenia develops over the first few days of treatment. Platelet counts rarely fall below 100,000/mm^3. The thrombocytopenia usually resolves spontaneously, even with continued heparin therapy. It is not dose-dependent and is thought to be caused by an induced platelet proaggregant effect that results in enhanced sequestration and destruction.[25] Most patients are asymptomatic, and treatment is not indicated.

Type II is much less common, appearing after 5 to 14 days of therapy (unless the patient has been previously exposed). Characteristics include platelet counts of 60,000 to 100,000/mm^3 that remain low until the drug is discontinued. After heparin is stopped, platelet counts return to normal values in 5 to 7 days. A common hypothesis proposes the formation of a platelet-associated IgG that reacts with heparin, forming a heparin-antibody immune complex. This complex binds to platelet Fc receptors, which causes in vivo platelet activation and aggregation.[25] The resultant "paradoxical" thrombosis may be arterial (more common) or venous, may occur at multiple sites, and in some cases is devastating. Concomitant with the onset of thrombocytopenia, extensive arterial or venous thrombosis with limb ischemia or gangrene, myocardial infarction, stroke, recurrent pulmonary embolism (PE), and skin necrosis have been observed.

Treatment of type I consists of monitoring the platelet count every 2 to 3 days. In type II, heparin should be immediately discontinued, and alternative anticoagulants such as dextran, aspirin, danaparoid, lepirudin, thrombolytics, and/or warfarin should be initiated. Platelet counts should return to normal a few days after discontinuation.[23] Unfortunately, thrombectomy or limb amputation may be necessary in some patients with type II disease, and mortality may be as high as 30%. A high in vitro cross-reaction rate has been reported with various low-molecular-weight heparins (LMWHs).[25] These should therefore also be avoided unless a lack of cross-reactivity has been demonstrated.

Danaparoid, which is a heparinoid compound, is related to LMWH.[26] Advantages associated with this drug include its in vitro inhibition of platelet activation by heparin-induced thrombocytopenia (HIT)-IgG and its ability to reduce thrombin generation in vivo by inhibiting factor Xa. However, it has been associated with a 10% in vitro cross-reactivity and less than 5% in vivo cross-reactivity. Currently, danaparoid is the alternate anticoagulant about which the most experience has been reported. Treatment of HIT with danaparoid should include a loading dose of a 2250 U intravenous bolus followed by 400 U/hr every 4 hours, then 300 U/hr every 4 hours, and then a maintenance dose of 150 to 200 U/hr to maintain anti-factor Xa levels between 0.5 and 0.8 U/mL.[27] Lepirudin is another treatment option for HIT. It inactivates fibrin clot-bound and soluble thrombin. Because its chemical structure is different from that of the heparins, no platelet aggregation cross-reactivity occurs between the agents. Lepirudin has been found to trigger the formation of IgG antihirudin antibodies in approximately 50% of patients with HIT who receive it for longer than 5 days. Also, in patients with renal failure, there is a high risk associated with bleeding due to drug accumulation because it is renally metabolized and excreted.[26] One advantage for using lepirudin is the ability to monitor its effect through aPTTs. The loading dose is a 0.4 mg/kg IV bolus followed by a maintenance dose of 0.15 mg/kg/hr IV. Adjustments should be made to the maintenance dose to maintain an aPTT of 1.5 to 3.0 times normal.[27]

Cytotoxic agents can cause thrombocytopenia because of their myelosuppressive action on the hematopoietic system. In contrast to other forms of drug-induced thrombocytopenia, which affect mature platelets in the circulation, antineoplastic agents cause a dose-dependent reduction in bone marrow platelet precursors. Precursors of all three cell lines (white blood cells [WBC], RBC, and thrombocyte) are suppressed, the onset and severity being related to the lifespan of existing cells. In this regard, thrombocytopenia is intermediate, occurring gradually over 7 to 10 days.[28] Host factors such as age, nutritional status, and preexisting bone marrow compromise affect the severity and symptoms. Drugs that may cause significant bone marrow suppression include cytarabine, the nitrosoureas, busulfan, methotrexate, cyclophosphamide, and mercaptopurine.[4,23] Busulfan may cause a severe prolonged thrombocytopenia due to an irreversible reduction in the number of marrow stem cells. Vincristine is an exception and may even stimulate thrombopoiesis.[23,29] The primary management consists of prophylactic platelet transfusions when the counts fall below 10,000 to 20,000/mm^3, single-donor platelets being preferable because of a lower incidence of alloimmunization.[28] When possible, chemotherapeutic regimens should be tailored to avoid the simultaneous administration of drugs that are known to cause this effect. A new therapeutic approach is the administration of interleukins; several have megakaryocyte stimulating properties. One of these is interleukin-11 (IL-11), which causes the proliferation of hematopoietic stem cells and megakaryocyte progenitors to occur. It is also able to induce megakaryocytic maturation. Doses of 25 to 75 μg/kg/day have been found to ameliorate chemotherapy-induced thrombocytopenia in women who have stage 3 or 4 breast cancer. IL-11 was also found to decrease the number of platelet transfusions in patients with various cancer diagnoses undergoing chemotherapy with different regimens.[30]

Cocaine may also have a toxic effect on megakaryocytes, causing oropharyngeal and mucous membrane bleeding with platelet counts less than 10,000/mm^3.[4] This effect is unrelated to the route of administration. Bone marrow aspiration demonstrates a reduced number of megakaryocytes, without involvement of the WBC and RBC cell lines. The platelet count generally increases over 2 to 3 weeks after discontinuation of the drug.

Disseminated Intravascular Coagulation

DIC is an intermediary syndrome caused by a second coexisting disease. The activating conditions encompass a broad spectrum of unrelated events (Table 15.3). Infection is the most common associated disorder, meningococcemia being the prototype. The precipitating conditions share as a common feature: a breakdown of the intricate balance between coagulation and fibrinolysis, the systems that maintain blood in a fluid state within the vasculature. In DIC, simultaneous in vivo activation of the coagulation and fibrinolytic systems results in both thrombosis and hemorrhage. The clinical manifestations of DIC are highly variable and depend on the underlying disease process and the relative balance between coagulation and fibrinolysis in the individual patient.

Although the activating disease states are variable, once initiated, DIC results in the same pathophysiologic sequence: (1) In vivo activation of the coagulation system resulting in intravascular thrombin generation, (2) intravascular fibrin clot formation with end-organ ischemia, (3) activation of the fibrinolytic systems, and (4) depletion of blood coagulation proteins and platelets. The stronger the triggering process and the longer the process continues, the more severe the associated DIC.

PATHOPHYSIOLOGY

In Vivo Activation of the Coagulation System

The triggering event for DIC is the release of procoagulant material into the circulation due to either vascular endothelial or tissue injury. The smooth layer lining the vascular endothelium normally repels clotting factors and platelets. Exposure to toxins or inflammatory mediators

Table 15.3 ▪ Conditions Associated with Disseminated Intravascular Coagulation

Acute (Fulminant)		

Infection
  Bacterial
    Gram-negative (endotoxin)
    Gram-positive (muco-polysaccharides)
  Viral
    Cytomegalovirus
    Hepatitis
    Varicella
    Human immunodeficiency virus (HIV)
  Rickettsial
    Rocky mountain spotted fever
  Others (mycoplasmal, chlamydial, fungal, mycobacterial, protozoal)
Obstetric accidents
  Amniotic fluid embolism
  Placental abruption
  Retained fetus syndrome
  Eclampsia
  Abortion
	Tissue injury
	  Burns
	  Crush injuries and tissue necrosis
	  Multiple trauma
	  Head trauma
	  Extensive surgery
	Malignancy
	  Leukemia
	    Acute promyelocytic (M-3)
	    Acute myelomonocytic (M-4)
	  Most metastatic solid tumors
	  Others (pheochromocytoma, myeloma, neuroblastoma, sarcoma, histiocytosis X, polycythemia vera)
	  Chemotherapy for leukemia (massive blast cell lysis)
	Intravascular hemolysis
	  Hemolytic transfusion reaction
	  Minor hemolysis
	  Massive transfusion
		Acute liver disease
		  Obstructive jaundice
		  Acute hepatic failure
		Prosthetic devices
		  LeVeen or Denver shunt
		  Aortic balloon assist device
		Cardiovascular
		  Postcardiac arrest
		  Aortic aneurysm
		  Giant hemangiomas
		  Acute myocardial infarction
		  Peripheral vascular disorders
		Pulmonary
		  Adult respiratory distress syndrome (ARDS)
		  Pulmonary embolism or infarction
		  Hyaline membrane disease
		Miscellaneous
		  Snake bite envenomation
		  Hyperthermia or hypothermia
		  Heat stroke
		  Aspirin or organic solvent poisoning

Chronic (Low Grade)		

Malignancy
  Leukemia
  Most metastatic solid tumors
Cardiovascular disease
  Aortic aneurysm
  Giant hemangioma
	Collagen vascular disorders
	  Systemic lupus erythematosus
	  Rheumatoid arthritis
	  Sjögren's syndrome
	  Dermatomyositis
	Renal vascular disorders
		Hematologic disorders
		  Polycythemia rubra vera
		Inflammatory disorders
		  Crohn's disease
		  Ulcerative colitis
		  Sarcoidosis
		Eclampsia

Sources: References 31, 32.

(e.g., endotoxins produced by Gram-negative bacteria) may disrupt the endothelium, resulting in platelet aggregation, activation of factor XII, and initiation of the intrinsic pathway. Activation of the extrinsic system may also occur when burns, trauma, obstetric accidents, or malignancies (especially leukemia) cause tissue injury or production of procoagulant material, resulting in the release of tissue thromboplastin.[31] Activation of the intrinsic or extrinsic pathway results in intravascular thrombin generation.

Intravascular Fibrin Clot Formation with End-Organ Damage

In the presence of thrombin, fibrinogen is cleaved into fibrinopeptides A and B and fibrin monomer (Fig. 15.3, left path). Fibrin monomer is then polymerized to form a fibrin clot. Polymerized fibrin is deposited in the microvascular circulation and entraps platelets, forming microthrombi. Platelet-rich microthrombi are subsequently replaced by fibrin-rich hyaline microthrombi.[32] Continued thrombin generation results in macrovascular thrombosis, ischemia, and eventual end-organ damage, which can be extensive.

Activation of the Fibrinolytic Systems

Fibrin clot activates the fibrinolytic system, beginning with plasminogen conversion to plasmin by t-PA (Fig. 15.4). Plasmin digests the fibrin clot by converting it to FDPs to exacerbate bleeding. FDPs also act independently as an anticoagulant by interfering with fibrin polymerization and forming soluble fibrin monomer, which will also worsen bleeding.

Depletion of Blood Coagulation Proteins and Platelets

The ongoing processes of fibrin formation and breakdown result in consumptive depletion of coagulation factors, natural anticoagulants, and platelets. The intensity and duration of the DIC determine the degree of depletion.

Pathophysiology Summary

The simultaneous presence of thrombin and plasmin in the systemic circulation generates a paradox of concurrent clotting and bleeding. Polymerized fibrin clot and microthrombi result in thrombosis and ischemia. At the same time, fibrinolysis, depletion of coagulation factors, natural

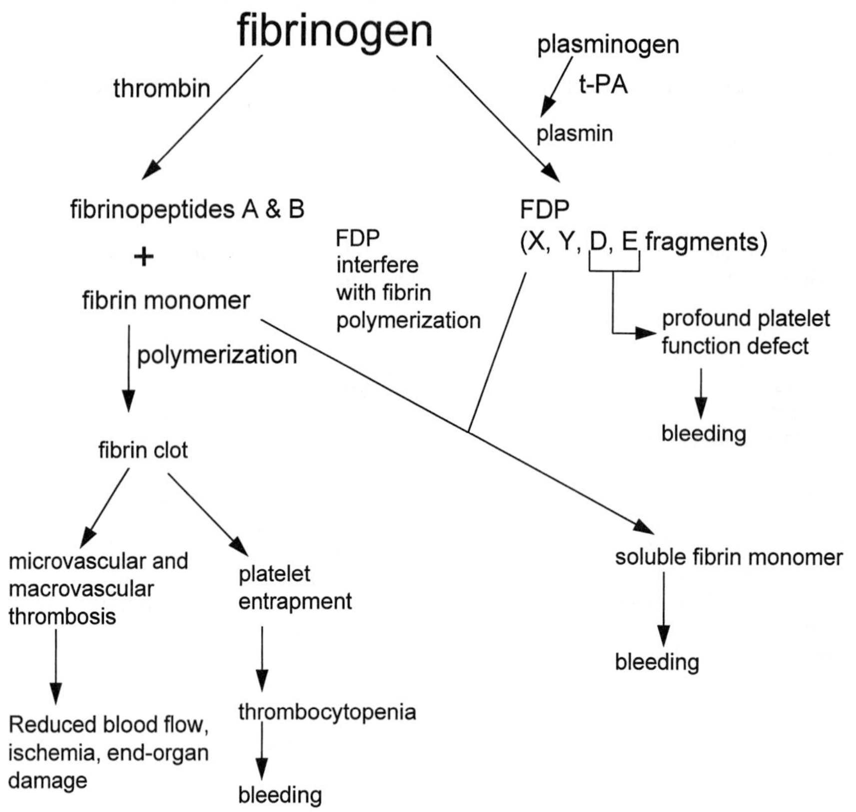

Figure 15.3. Pathogenesis of disseminated intravascular coagulation. *FDP,* fibrin degradation product; *t-PA,* tissue plasminogen activator.

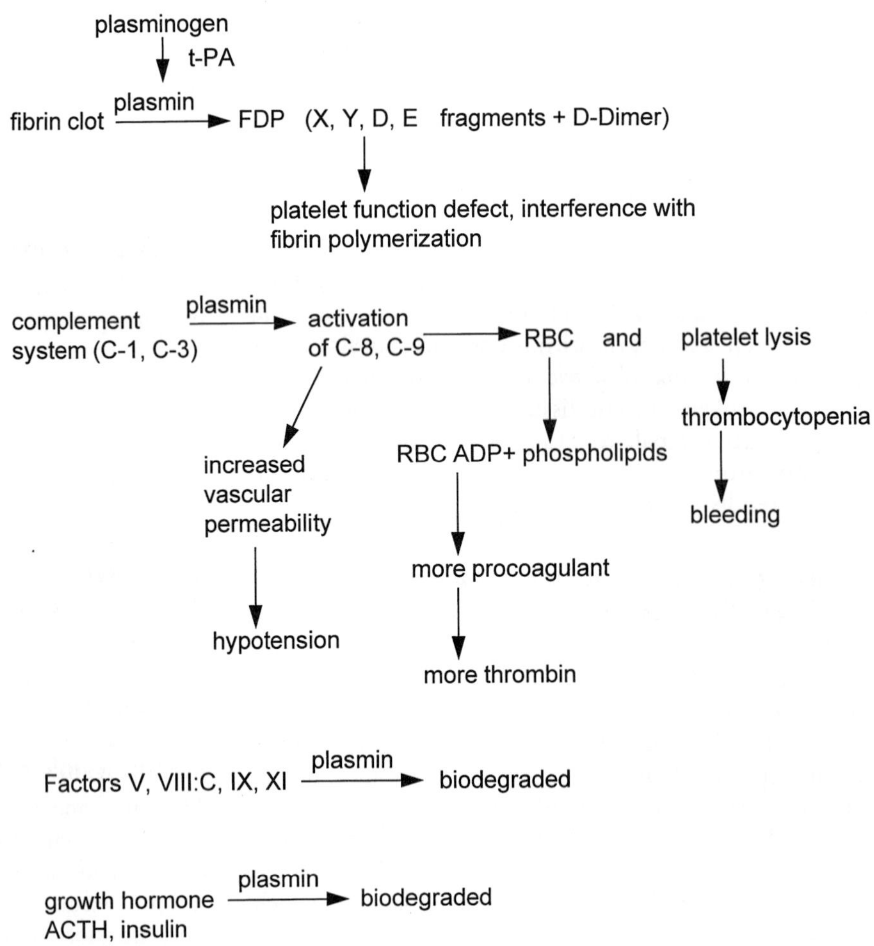

Figure 15.4. Additional actions of plasmin. *ACTH,* adrenocorticotropic hormone; *FDP,* fibrin degradation product; *RBC,* red blood cell; *t-PA,* tissue plasminogen activator.

anticoagulant proteins, and platelets, coupled with the platelet function disorder, cause hemorrhage. Depending on the balance between coagulation and fibrinolysis, both processes may be clinically evident in DIC, although sometimes one dominates over the other. In infection, thrombosis usually predominates. In acute leukemia, bleeding is the primary manifestation.[31]

CLINICAL PRESENTATION AND DIAGNOSIS

The diagnosis of DIC is established when all four processes above occur in a patient who also has a condition that is known to be a precipitating cause. Prompt diagnosis requires a high index of suspicion and aggressive laboratory testing. Signs and symptoms are variable and confusing because of the wide spectrum of manifestations contributed by the coagulopathy and the underlying disease. In some patients the diagnosis is obvious (e.g., gangrene of the extremities, bleeding, and multiorgan failure in a patient with meningococcemia). In others there may be mild or no bleeding at all, clinically silent microvascular thrombosis, and only subtle laboratory abnormalities. A single patient may manifest one or more of these findings alone, simultaneously, or serially at different times in the disease process.[33] The signs and symptoms of the underlying disorder further complicate the clinical presentation. The total picture for an individual patient therefore reflects both the DIC and the underlying disorder and depends on the tissues and organs that are involved and the severity of the DIC and disease processes. Vigilant correlation of physical examination and laboratory results is essential in the diagnosis, management, and evaluation of DIC.

In general, there are two modes of presentation of DIC: acute and chronic. Acute ("fulminant") DIC is more common than the chronic form. In acute DIC the clinical and laboratory features develop rapidly (over a few hours to days), often with catastrophic consequences. The patient is critically ill from the underlying disease as well as from the DIC. Acute DIC usually presents with both bleeding and thrombosis, bleeding being more clinically evident in most patients. Hemorrhage can range from low-grade oozing to massive bleeding. Bleeding from multiple sites is usually seen, because even small wounds lack normal hemostasis (Table 15.4). Areas of trauma, sites of surgical or other invasive procedures, or other area with pathologic manifestations are common sources of bleeding. In the skin, microvascular thrombosis of end-arterioles with concurrent bleeding results in symptoms ranging from petechiae to gangrene. End-organ dysfunction secondary to microvascular and macrovascular thrombosis is also common, although it should be recognized that organ failure may also be caused by the underlying disease. End-organ malfunction is often less evident clinically but requires early identification and treatment to avoid irreversible damage. The organ systems affected most often (respiratory, renal, central nervous, cardiovascular, and hepatic) will exhibit progressive organ failure (Table 15.4). Fluid and electrolyte disorders and fever are also commonly seen. Pallor and jaundice secondary to microangiopathic hemolytic anemia are less common. The intermingling of these findings with those of the underlying disease make the diagnosis of DIC impossible without coagulation studies.

Table 15.4 ▪ Signs and Symptoms of Acute Disseminated Intravascular Coagulation

Hemorrhage	Thrombosis
Surgical or trauma sites Wound bleeding Internal bleeding Skin and soft tissue Oozing at venipuncture, IV catheter insertion, and arterial-line sites Petechiae, purpura Ecchymoses Spreading hematomas Hemorrhagic bullae Ear, nose, throat Gingival or oral mucosal bleeding Epistaxis Respiratory Blood-tinged respiratory secretions Gastrointestinal Hematemesis Blood in nasogastric secretions (occult or gross) Fecal blood (occult or gross) Urinary Hematuria	Skin and soft tissue Cyanosis of hands, feet, nose, cheeks Acral cyanosis Cold, mottled fingers, toes, hands, feet Purpura Infarction, necrosis or gangrene of digits, hands, feet, nose, earlobes Venous thromboembolism End-organ dysfunction Lung (hypoxia, acidosis, respiratory failure, ARDS) Kidney (elevated BUN, creatinine, oliguria, proteinuria, hematuria, acute renal failure) Central nervous system (altered mental status, seizures, coma) Cardiovascular (hypotension, shock, hemodynamic instability or failure) Liver (elevated ALT, AST) Gastrointestinal (vomiting, diarrhea, abdominal distress, ileus)

Sources: References 31, 33.
ARDS, adult respiratory distress syndrome; *BUN,* blood urea nitrogen; *ALT,* alanine aminotransferase; *AST,* aspartate aminotransferase.

Coagulation test results associated with acute DIC encompass a wide spectrum. Unfortunately, there is no single test for DIC with acceptable specificity, sensitivity, and widespread availability. Specific criteria for the laboratory diagnosis of DIC have been published,[32] but they rely on assays of biochemical markers that are often available only in research institutions (e.g., prothrombin fragment 1 + 2, fibrinopeptides A and B, thrombin-antithrombin complex, plasmin-antiplasmin complex, α_2-antiplasmin). The most useful tests that are readily available include measurements of FDP (or D-dimer) level, platelet count, and fibrinogen level, the protamine sulfate test, and PT (Table 15.5).[32,33] FDP levels are elevated to greater than 40 mg/mL in almost all patients and are considered a sensitive but not specific test for DIC, because they do not distinguish between fibrin versus fibrinogen degradation. D-dimer is a specific biochemical

Table 15.5 ▪ Laboratory Findings in Acute Disseminated Intravascular Coagulation

	Reference Range	Findings in DIC
Fibrin degradation products	<10 μg/mL	Increased
D-dimer	<500 ng/mL	Increased
Platelet count	150,000–400,000/mm³	Decreased
Fibrinogen	200–400 mg/dL	Decreased
Protamine sulfate	Negative	Positive
Prothrombin time	0.88–1.12 INR	Increased

Sources: References 29, 59, 60.
INR, international normalized ratio.

marker for fibrin breakdown; assays are therefore more useful, although they are not always available.[31,32] Thrombocytopenia is a cardinal finding. The platelet count is less than 50,000 to 60,000/mm^3 in about 50% of patients (range 2,000 to 100,000/mm^3). Results of platelet function tests such as template bleeding time or platelet aggregation studies are abnormal in almost all patients as well.[31,32] The plasma fibrinogen level is less than 150 mg/dL in 70 to 80% of patients; levels less than 50 mg/dL are often associated with severe bleeding. A normal fibrinogen level may be observed in DIC associated with pregnancy, sepsis, or malignancy, because the baseline fibrinogen level may be elevated in these conditions.[33–35] Conversely, liver disease is associated with low baseline fibrinogen levels. The protamine sulfate test measures the presence of circulating soluble fibrin monomer. It is usually positive in patients with DIC, although it is not specific for this disease process. The PT is prolonged in 50 to 75% of patients with DIC, owing to factor consumption.[31] Unfortunately, the PT may be normal or even shorter than the control time in as many as 50% of patients; this test is therefore less useful for diagnosing DIC.

Other laboratory tests are commonly performed in the screening and evaluation of patients with suspected acute DIC but have limited value. These include the aPTT, thrombin clotting time (TT), euglobulin clot lysis time, coagulation factor assays, and peripheral blood smear examination. The aPTT is prolonged in 50 to 60% of patients with acute DIC, but it may also be normal or short[31,32] and is therefore unreliable for patient assessment. Likewise, the TT may be prolonged, the euglobulin clot lysis time may be shortened, and blood coagulation factor levels are often low, but these findings are not reliable and do not add meaningful information. Examination of a peripheral blood smear provides evidence of RBC fragmentation, mild reticulocytosis, mild leukocytosis with a mild to moderate shift to immature neutrophil forms ("left shift"), and thrombocytopenia with large young platelets. Unfortunately, these findings also lack specificity and sensitivity.

Chronic ("low-grade" or "compensated") DIC is characterized by abnormal low-grade coagulation and fibrinolysis accompanying an array of less acute conditions (Table 15.4). Chronic DIC is thought to be less common than the acute form. However, the subtle manifestations of this form may contribute to underdiagnosis. Many believe that acute and chronic DIC are simply different phases in the continuum of a single disease. Chronic DIC is not generally considered an emergency. Clinical findings are less florid, and laboratory abnormalities are more subtle. Enhanced turnover with increased production of platelets, fibrinogen, and coagulation proteins may yield normal or near-normal levels. If the rate of fibrinolysis is sufficient to balance the rate of fibrin formation, there may be no obvious clinical symptoms. Patients with chronic DIC uniformly have elevated D-dimer levels. Measurement of D-dimer (or FDP) levels is therefore very useful in establishing the diagnosis.

Over time these patients may develop overt problems, especially thrombotic complications such as thrombophlebitis, PE, or stroke.[33,35] Patients with metastatic malignancies often manifest DIC as a "hypercoagulable syndrome" with recurrent local or diffuse thrombotic events. Trousseau's syndrome, a recurrent migratory venous thrombosis, is a variant of this condition.[35] Subacute or "bothersome" bleeding may also be seen. It is important to recognize that patients with chronic DIC may develop the acute form with hemostatic stress, such as surgery or invasive procedures.

In summary, no single physical finding or laboratory test is diagnostic for acute or chronic DIC. Careful physical examination and laboratory assessment, combined with vigilance and good judgment, are essential in establishing the diagnosis. Normal D-dimer (or FDP) levels make DIC unlikely. A combination of elevated D-dimer (or FDP) level, thrombocytopenia, low or falling fibrinogen (in the absence of liver disease), a positive protamine sulfate test, and a prolonged PT in a patient with a disease known to cause DIC will establish the diagnosis in most patients with the degree of abnormality roughly correlating with disease acuity. These tests are also the most useful in monitoring the response to therapy.

MANAGEMENT

The cornerstone of DIC management is treatment of the underlying disease and supportive therapy for the signs and symptoms. This along with careful observation and follow-up may be the only measures required for some patients.

Acute DIC with life-threatening hemorrhage and thrombosis requires complex management and intensive monitoring. Prompt and aggressive treatment to control or correct the underlying disorder is imperative. Without this, the stimulus for DIC will continue, and additional corrective measures might not be successful. Patients also require vigorous supportive therapy. Acid-base, fluid and electrolyte, hemodynamic, respiratory, and renal disturbances must be effectively managed. Intramuscular medications and venipunctures should be minimized to avoid additional sites of bleeding and hematoma formation. Frequent clinical and laboratory monitoring is essential. If treatment of the underlying disease and supportive therapy are timely and successful and the laboratory parameters are improving, the need for additional treatment should be transient; in some cases, no further therapy will be required. Aggressive antibiotic therapy for sepsis or evacuation of the uterus for an obstetric accident are examples in which successful treatment of the underlying disorder alone may resolve the DIC. In other situations, efforts to treat the precipitating disease are unsuccessful or inadequate, and/or the manifestations fail to resolve. Patients with acute leukemia may even suffer an initial worsening of the DIC after administration of chemotherapy, owing to massive blast cell lysis with subsequent generation of large amounts of procoagulant.

Specific treatment modalities for acute DIC beyond supportive care and treatment of the underlying diseases are highly controversial, are poorly documented, and lack consensus. A general lack of prospective randomized clinical trials exists, largely because of the complex spectrum of underlying diseases and clinical manifestations. Published trials are difficult to compare because of differences in diagnostic and outcome criteria. Moreover, patient outcomes are often dependent more on the underlying disease than on the DIC. Individualization of therapy is essential. Treatment may involve measures to (1) interrupt the coagulation process, (2) replace depleted coagulation factors and platelets, and/or (3) interrupt fibrinolysis.

Measures to interrupt the coagulation process include administration of anticoagulants and replacement of natural anticoagulant proteins. Although bleeding is often more obvious and alarming, thrombosis is more dangerous and has more impact on morbidity and mortality because of its potential to cause irreversible ischemic end-organ damage.[31] Unfortunately, prospective, randomized studies of heparin use in DIC are lacking and impractical to perform because of variability in the clinical manifestations and precipitating disorders. Anecdotal evidence suggests that some patients benefit in terms of hemorrhage control and survival.[33,34] Heparin is clearly indicated for patients with thrombosis and has been associated with a reduction in mortality.[35] All patients should be carefully monitored for evidence of microvascular and macrovascular thrombosis, including progressive organ failure (Table 15.4). Immediate heparin therapy is required if necrosis, gangrene, and irreversible end-organ damage are to be prevented.

The use of heparin in the treatment of patients with DIC and hemorrhage but with no clear-cut evidence of fibrin deposition is controversial. Because bleeding in acute DIC is caused by massive coagulation cascade activation with subsequent depletion of clotting factors and platelets, it seems reasonable to interrupt this process with heparin. Heparin will also inhibit growth of existing thrombi, thereby stabilizing the coagulation system while the underlying disease is treated.[32,33,35] However, heparin is also a potent anticoagulant and carries its own risks, including further bleeding. Patients with acute DIC and bleeding therefore usually receive heparin in conjunction with blood component replacement.

The timing of heparin administration relative to blood component replacement in patients with hemorrhage but no clinical evidence of thrombosis is debatable. Many clinicians recommend anticoagulants before blood component replacement therapy. This is based on the theory that administration of more coagulation factors and platelets will only increase coagulation unless the thrombosis has been interrupted; moreover, the exogenous blood components will be rapidly depleted and therefore will not be effective for stopping the hemorrhage.[32,33] Others disagree on the premise that early administration of heparin may worsen bleeding. These clinicians base the initial treatment on the dominant abnormality (i.e., anticoagulants for thrombosis, replacement therapy for hemorrhage).[31]

Heparin dosing in patients with acute DIC is also controversial.[35] Many practitioners recommend a full therapeutic dose of heparin with a loading dose of 5,000 to 10,000 U followed by continuous infusion of 15 to 20 U/kg/hr (20,000 to 30,000 U/day). These doses are based on the theories that (1) the coagulation cascade has already been activated, (2) heparin-neutralizing components (e.g., platelet factor-4 and β-thromboglobulin) may be released from activated platelets, and (3) depletion of the natural anticoagulant antithrombin-III (AT-III) may limit heparin's effect.[33] Others recommend continuous administration of lower doses (5 to 10 U/kg/hr) without a loading dose. Another strategy is to give "low-dose" subcutaneous heparin (5,000 U every 12 hours), with the belief that these doses are at least as effective as higher intravenous doses, they have been associated with a reduction in mortality, and the risk of excessive bleeding is reduced.[32]

Specific aspects of the mechanism of action, pharmacokinetics, and adverse drug reaction profile of heparin are reviewed in Chapter 44, Thromboembolic Disease.

The potential for exacerbation of bleeding can be a significant deterrent to heparin use in treating acute DIC. Traditional heparin preparations are unfractionated mixtures containing several components. Purified LMWHs have been shown to be associated with a lower incidence of bleeding and may therefore be advantageous in treating patients with DIC. The anticoagulant effect of unfractionated heparin (UFH) occurs via complexation with AT-III, which inhibits activated coagulation factors, principally thrombin and factor Xa. LMWHs possess selective antifactor Xa properties and do not inhibit thrombin. They do not markedly prolong the aPTT and have less effect on platelet activation and aggregation than UFH does; these attributes have translated into a lower incidence of bleeding with LMWHs. This offers attractive possibilities in treating patients with DIC, because LMWHs may therefore abort thrombus formation without exacerbating bleeding. Several LMWH compounds have been identified, including enoxaparin (Lovenox or PK 10169), dalteparin (Fragmin, FR-860 or Kabi 2165), and fraxiparin (CY 216); enoxaparin and dalteparin are available in the United States. A double-blind randomized study of intravenous dalteparin versus UFH in 126 patients suggested a more favorable profile for dalteparin with respect to improvement of clinical symptoms and safety, although there was no difference in overall efficacy.[36] A dose-finding trial of dalteparin[37] and case studies using enoxaparin[38] have been reported with promising results. Large-scale randomized comparative trials should be performed to establish the role of LMWHs in acute DIC.

Contraindications to heparin in any form include CNS bleeding (e.g., intracranial or subarachnoid hemorrhage or subdural hematoma), bleeding into other closed spaces where vital functions might be compromised (e.g., intraspinal, pericardial, or peritracheal hemorrhage), and DIC associated with fulminant liver failure.[32,35] Caution should also be exercised in treating patients with a high risk of heparin-induced bleeding (e.g., those with intracranial metastases, severe hypertension, or a recent history of peptic ulcer disease).

Depletion of natural anticoagulant proteins (AT-III and proteins C and S) is another important contributor to clotting in patients with acute DIC. AT-III depletion may be particularly significant, because it is both an anticoagulant (Fig. 15.1) and required for the in vivo activity of heparin. Restoration and maintenance of adequate AT-III levels may therefore ameliorate the coagulopathy via both direct and indirect mechanisms. AT-III administration may be especially useful in treating patients with acute DIC with bleeding, because it does not exacerbate hemorrhage. Patients with apparent heparin resistance or those with severe bleeding may benefit from AT-III replacement via transfusion with FFP or AT-III concentrate. FFP has the advantages of containing multiple coagulation proteins and derivation from a single donor, but the large volumes that are required may be a limitation. AT-III concentrate (Thrombate-III, ATnativ) is a purified heat-treated concentrate made from human plasma. It has been studied alone and in combination with heparin in treating acute DIC. Randomized trials of AT-III concentrate versus placebo[39] or versus heparin alone or with AT-III[40] have demonstrated significantly shorter duration of DIC signs and symptoms in the AT-III groups. A significant effect on mortality was not observed.[39] An important finding in one study[40] was a significantly higher RBC transfusion requirement in the group receiving both AT-III and heparin, yielding the conclusion that AT-III alone was effective and had a more favorable safety profile. Clinical improvement has also been demonstrated in a cohort of children[41] and in a patient with recurrent multisite arterial thrombosis refractory to heparin.[42] Limited data also support efficacy in DIC associated with pregnancy or acute fatty liver of pregnancy. Adverse effects have been minimal. On the basis of these data, some clinicians therefore advocate early initiation of AT-III replacement in patients with fulminant DIC.[32] The Food and Drug Administration is currently conducting studies on whether DIC should be an approved use of AT-III.

Specific dosing and adverse effect information regarding AT-III concentrate are reviewed in the section of this chapter entitled "Hypercoagulable States." Two important considerations specific to its use in treating acute DIC are a shorter half-life, which necessitates twice-daily initial administration[40] and the interaction between AT-III and heparin. Some clinicians administer heparin only after AT-III functional levels greater than 70% have been established,[37,40] because the efficacy of heparin depends on the presence of AT-III. Patients who are already receiving heparin before AT-III may demonstrate a markedly enhanced heparin effect after AT-III is added. Careful monitoring of heparin dosing is therefore important in this scenario.

Protein C is another natural anticoagulant (Fig. 15.1) that is commonly depleted in acute DIC. Trials of protein C concentrate in limited numbers of patients with thrombosis have been favorable with respect to both efficacy and safety[43,44]; however, these are only preliminary results. Protein C concentrate is available in the United States on an investigational basis; details regarding its use are found in the section of this chapter entitled "Hypercoagulable States."

TREATMENT

Replacement of Depleted Coagulation Factors and Platelets

Blood component replacement therapy is indicated when the patient continues to have active bleeding after initial supportive measures or when an invasive procedure or surgery is required. If coagulation factor and platelet depletion is believed to be a major cause of bleeding, replenishment may slow hemorrhage. It is unnecessary in most patients with chronic DIC (factors not usually depleted) and may even be harmful for patients with gross thrombosis (may cause thrombus extension).

Replacement therapy includes platelets, FFP, and cryoprecipitate. If bleeding is severe, administration of packed RBCs will also be necessary. Factor VIII concentrates are not appropriate, because DIC depletes multiple coagulation factors. Prothrombin complex ("factor IX") concentrates may actually worsen or induce DIC. Platelet transfusions are indicated for marked thrombocytopenia (platelet count less than 20,000/mm^3) or for ongoing hemorrhage. At least 5 to 10 U of platelet concentrate (or 0.1 U/kg) should be given.[31] One or two units of FFP (or

10 to 15 mL/kg) or 15 U of cryoprecipitate (or 0.2 bag/kg) usually improve factor deficiencies.[31] Use of FFP requires administration of larger volumes but is advantageous because it contains clotting factors plus AT-III and proteins C and S. Cryoprecipitate contains 10 times more fibrinogen per unit than FFP. It is indicated for patients with very low fibrinogen levels (<50 mg/dL) or those with fibrinogen levels <100 mg/dL who are bleeding.

As was previously discussed, the timing of blood component administration in the management strategy of acute DIC is controversial. If given while clotting is still ongoing, exogenous coagulation factors will simply be integrated into the coagulation process; this will not elevate factor levels and may even worsen the thrombosis. Although this "fuel-the-fire" argument is theoretically possible and may rarely occur, it has not been well substantiated in clinical practice.[34,35] Nonetheless, many believe that factor replacement should be withheld until intravascular clotting has been suspended with heparin, especially when using components containing fibrinogen.[31,33] After intravascular clotting has been interrupted, any depleted component can be given and should raise factor levels and reduce bleeding. In situations in which heparin is contraindicated, products with high fibrinogen content (e.g., FFP and cryoprecipitate) should be avoided.

Vitamin K deficiency may occur in patients with acute DIC, depending on the degree and duration of DIC, whether factor replacement is given, the type of nutritional support given to the patient, and other issues such as administration of broad-spectrum antibiotics. In patients with vitamin K deficiency, supplementation will facilitate production of vitamin K-dependent clotting factors.

Interruption of Fibrinolysis

Fibrinolytic (or fibrinogenolytic) inhibitors such as ϵ-aminocaproic acid (Amicar) or tranexamic acid (Cyklokapron) are theoretically useful, because they will slow fibrinolysis of the microthrombi, thereby slowing bleeding. Successful use of intravenous tranexamic acid in acute DIC that is unresponsive to heparin, AT-III, and FFP has been reported.[45] However, use of antifibrinolytics may be dangerous. If intravascular clotting has not been suspended before use, they may cause catastrophic widespread fibrin deposition in the microcirculation, leading to irreversible ischemic multiorgan damage, which is sometimes fatal.[35] These agents should be used with extreme caution and always with concurrent heparin therapy. They should be restricted to last-recourse situations with life-threatening bleeding or evidence of extensive secondary fibrinolysis and after failure of other therapies.[31,35] An exception to this is the patient with acute promyelocytic leukemia, who may have primary activation of both the coagulation and fibrinolytic systems caused by the malignancy. When antifibrolytics are used in conjunction with other modalities, the benefits may outweigh the risks for these patients.

Other Therapies

Exchange transfusions are sometimes used in the treatment of DIC. Plasma exchange, plasmapheresis, leukopheresis, and whole blood exchange have been used. Their efficacy is thought to be related to removal of FDPs, activated clotting factors, and toxins from the patient's plasma, all of which aggravate bleeding.[34] Replacement of AT-III, proteins C and S, and other proteins in the exchanged plasma may also contribute to a successful outcome by reestablishing the normal balance of circulating coagulation factors and natural anticoagulants. Exchange transfusion is not considered part of the routine management of DIC because of its associated risks and the need for specialized equipment and trained personnel.

A number of drugs for the management of acute DIC are being clinically investigated. These include gabexate mesilate (FOY), a synthetic inhibitor of serine proteases in the coagulation, fibrinolysis, and other systems (complement, kinins, prostaglandins, superoxide). Gabexate has antithrombin and antiplasmin effects that are independent of AT-III and account for its efficacy in acute DIC.[46,47] Dermatan sulfate (MF-701) enhances the antithrombin effect of heparin cofactor II via a mechanism that is analogous to the effect of AT-III on thrombin.[48] Compounds that are undergoing preclinical trials include recombinant human soluble thrombomodulin (rhs-TM), recombinant hirudin (PEG hirudin), and an inhibitor of factor Xa (DX-9065).

MONITORING PARAMETERS FOR ACUTE DIC

All patients with acute DIC should have regular monitoring of fibrinogen levels, D-dimer (or FDP) levels, protamine sulfate test results, and platelet counts. Measurements of AT-III levels and other biochemical markers (prothrombin fragment 1 + 2, fibrinopeptides A and B) are also useful if available. Attainment and maintenance of adequate fibrinogen levels and platelet counts, with falling D-dimer (or FDP) levels, normal protamine sulfate test results, and stable hematocrit are indicators of successful interruption of the coagulopathy. Initial monitoring every 6 to 12 hours is appropriate, with once-daily assessment after the patient's condition is stable. Changes in the balance between fibrinogen synthesis and consumption can be seen within hours, whereas it may take 1 to 2 days for platelet and D-dimer (or FDP) levels to show meaningful trends.[34] In patients with some conditions, such as acute leukemia, D-dimer levels will increase initially, then fall. Clinical response begins shortly after improvement in laboratory parameters,[32] with stabilization of bleeding, thrombosis, and end-organ dysfunction. Blood pressure, cardiac output, systemic vascular resistance, the Glasgow coma score, and urine output may be measured, as well as arterial blood gases, serum BUN, creatinine, alanine aminotransferase, and aspartate aminotransferase. A reduction in the need for continued use of pressor agents, ventilators, dialysis, and transfusion of coagulation factors, platelets and packed RBCs also indicates improvement. It is essential to recognize that improvement or worsening of the underlying disease will also influence the patient's clinical status.

Patients who are receiving heparin require additional monitoring. aPTT, TT, PT, and hematocrit are measured 4 to 6 hours after initiation of heparin and every 12 to 24 hours thereafter. Although the aPTT is a primary tool for monitoring and adjusting heparin therapy in other situations, most patients with acute DIC have an abnormal baseline aPTT. The aPTT therefore provides limited guidance, as do plasma heparin levels. The inability to ameliorate the general manifestations of acute DIC as described earlier (D-dimer, fibrinogen, etc.) can indicate a need to increase the heparin dose. In general, heparin should be continued until fibrinogen levels are greater than 100 mg/dL and platelet counts are greater than 100,000/mm^3. The hematocrit should also be monitored frequently to assess both beneficial and adverse effects of heparin.

Patients who are receiving AT-III via FFP or AT-III concentrate should have plasma AT-III levels measured every 12 hours until their condition is stable and then daily. Clinical improvement should occur in 1 to 3 days.

Objective measures of successful management in patients who are receiving coagulation factor or platelet transfusions include an increase in platelet count and plasma fibrinogen concentration, as well as the criteria reviewed above for the general monitoring of acute DIC. Platelet and fibrinogen levels should be determined 30 to 60 minutes after a transfusion and every 6 to 12 hours thereafter until they are stable. With effective therapy the fibrinogen concentration and platelet count should stabilize and then increase. Similarly, clinical improvement, measured as a slowing and then cessation of bleeding, occurs over several days. A subsequent need for transfusion will depend on clinical response, treatment of the underlying disorder, and the half-life of the platelets and clotting factors. Once consumption is interrupted, the bone marrow and liver usually take several days to replenish endogenous platelet and fibrinogen levels.

Treatment of the precipitating disorder and supportive therapy for clinical manifestations should be the first steps for chronic DIC. For some patients, especially those who are asymptomatic and have a correctable underlying disease, these alone are adequate. Careful observation and follow-up are essential, because these patients can develop acute florid DIC when they are subjected to stressors such as surgery, invasive procedures, infection, or disease progression.[34,35]

Patients who have deep vein thrombosis (DVT) should be managed with intravenous heparin at standard therapeutic doses (20,000 to 30,000 U/day via constant intravenous infusion). Special care should be exercised when treating patients with intracranial metastases or other risk factors for bleeding. It is important to recognize that oral coagulants are only rarely successful in treating patients with thrombotic complications of chronic DIC. DIC associated with neoplastic disease is caused by direct activation of the extrinsic pathway via release of procoagulant material from the malignant cells. Warfarin and other coumarin derivatives are not effective in this situation because they simply reduce the amounts of activated vitamin K-dependent clotting factors but will not otherwise affect coagulation and fibrinolysis. Patients who require long-term secondary prophylaxis of thrombotic events in these situations should receive chronic subcutaneous heparin.[33] Patients with untreatable malignancies and other persistent symptoms of DIC should also be managed with subcutaneous heparin. The use of antiplatelet agents (e.g., aspirin and/or dipyridamole) and pentoxifylline is controversial. Some advocates believe that they may correct coagulation parameters and reduce bleeding or thrombosis[31]; others find no documented clinical benefit.[35] Replacement therapy with blood components or antifibrinolytic drugs is rarely necessary for patients with chronic DIC.

Monitoring parameters for chronic DIC include routine assessment of signs and symptoms. If treatment is given, D-dimer (or FDP) and fibrinogen levels, protamine sulfate test results, and platelet counts should be monitored. Patients receiving long-term heparin therapy should be monitored and counseled as described in Chapter 44.

PROGNOSIS

Much remains to be investigated to further clarify the pathophysiology and management of DIC. Randomized controlled large-scale trials have been difficult to perform because of the broad spectra of underlying diseases, diagnostic criteria, and outcome measurements. Most clinicians therefore base their treatment decisions on clinical judgment and prior experience.

Acute DIC may be an incidental preterminal event occurring in a variety of acute catastrophic illnesses. It may be brief and end promptly with effective treatment of the underlying disorder. Alternatively, patients may die from hemorrhage and progression of the underlying disorder. Mortality rates for patients with acute DIC are reported to be 50 to 85%. However, this may be more reflective of the mortality rates of the precipitating disorders rather than treatment of the DIC. Morbidity and mortality are reduced with early recognition and aggressive treatment of the DIC; however, the prognosis may not improve until better methods of prevention and treatment of the underlying disorders become available.

Some patients with chronic DIC may be asymptomatic with only laboratory evidence of the disorder. Others may have recurrent episodes of thromboembolism requiring long-term therapy with subcutaneous heparin for prophylaxis. In most cases the prognosis for chronic DIC is related to that of the precipitating disease rather than the treatment strategy.

Hypercoagulable States

Hypercoagulable states comprise a number of conditions that share the common endpoint of inappropriate thrombus formation. Patients with these disorders are at higher risk for both venous and arterial thromboembolic disease. Disruption of coagulation may occur on an inherited (primary) or acquired (secondary) basis. Inherited hypercoagulable disorders are abnormalities in the synthesis or function of various proteins in the coagulation and fibrinolytic systems. Exaggerated formation or impaired breakdown of fibrin results in clotting, which may occur in the microvasculature or in large vessels such as the iliac veins. Acquired disorders include a wide spectrum of conditions associated with an enhanced risk of thromboembolism. Acquired risk factors for venous thromboembolism (Table 15.6) are varied, including production of abnormal proteins, diseases, drugs, or clinical situations. This discussion will focus on the venous manifestations of hypercoagulable states. For a more detailed review of arterial diseases (myocardial infarction, cerebrovascular accident, peripheral vascular disease, etc.) the reader is referred to other chapters.

Table 15.6 ▪ Acquired Risk Factors for Venous Thromboembolism

Abnormal function of the coagulation cascade or fibrinolytic system
Surgery (especially orthopedic surgery of the lower limb)
Trauma
Pregnancy
Oral contraceptives
Infection (associated with DIC)
Nephrotic syndrome
Antiphospholipid syndrome
Hepatic insufficiency
Abnormal platelet number or function
Myeloproliferative disorder (such as essential thrombocytosis)
Paroxysmal nocturnal hemoglobinuria
Abnormal vessel endothelial cell function or blood rheology
Stasis (prolonged sitting or bed rest, acute hemiplegia or paraplegia, congestive heart failure, varicose veins)
Trauma
Abnormal blood rheology (previous venous thrombosis, extrinsic compression)
Hyperviscosity syndromes (including myeloproliferative syndromes such as polycythemia vera)
Artificial surfaces (heart valves, vascular patches)
Vasculitis
Miscellaneous
Malignancy
Obesity
Drugs (heparin-associated thrombocytopenia, warfarin skin necrosis, antineoplastic agents)

Sources: References 29, 59, 60.
DIC, disseminated intravascular coagulation.

Inherited Hypercoagulable States

As previously discussed, hemostasis is regulated by two major physiologic systems called the coagulation and fibrinolytic systems. Under normal conditions, both are intricately balanced to maintain the blood in a fluid state within the vessels while at the same time minimizing blood loss from the vasculature at sites of injury. Disruption of this intrinsic balance may result in either bleeding or thrombosis. Thrombosis occurs when large amounts of thrombin are produced via the coagulation cascade. Thrombin catalyzes the conversion of fibrinogen to fibrin, which then polymerizes to form an insoluble clot (Fig. 15.1). The fibrin clot is degraded by another endogenous cascade called the fibrinolytic system (Fig. 15.2). Physiologic inhibitors of coagulation act to either inhibit thrombin formation or enhance fibrinolysis. In this manner, almost every protein in the coagulation and fibrinolytic systems has a natural inhibitor or lytic mechanism.

A number of endogenous proteins act as major deterrents to thrombin formation and are sometimes called "natural" or "physiologic" anticoagulants. The best-understood include AT-III protein C, and protein S. Each has a critical role in preventing the formation of pathologic amounts of thrombin, depicted in Figure 15.1. Patterns of inheritance, prevalence, and site(s) of endogenous production are summarized in Table 15.7.

Table 15.7 ▪ Natural Inhibitors of Coagulation

			Prevalence		
	Half-Life	Inheritance	General Population	8 Reports of Unselected Patients with Thrombosis[a]	Site of Synthesis
Antithrombin III	2.5 days	Autosomal dominant	1/2,000 to 1/5,000	0.5–8%, mean 4%	Hepatocyte; vitamin K-independent
Protein C	6–8 hr	Autosomal dominant	1/15,000	1.5–11.5%, mean 5.4%	Hepatocyte; vitamin K-dependent
		Autosomal recessive	1/200 to 1/300		
Protein S	Unknown	Autosomal dominant	Unknown	1.5–13.2%, mean 5.9%	Hepatocyte; vitamin K-dependent α-Platelet granules Endothelial cells Megakaryocytes

Sources: References 29, 50, 57, 71.
[a]Data from reference 57.

Antithrombin-III Deficiency

AT-III is a serine protease inhibitor with a broad spectrum of activity in the coagulation cascade. AT-III irreversibly complexes with factors IXa, Xa, XIa, XIIa, thrombin, and plasmin (Fig. 15.1). Inactivation of factor Xa and thrombin is an especially important function. The entire process is markedly accelerated in the presence of heparin. AT-III is considered a crucial component in limiting ongoing activation of the coagulation cascade; it is sometimes called the primary physiologic inhibitor of in vivo coagulation. Assays for both the quantity (antigen) and function of AT-III are reported as a percentage compared to normal pooled plasma; normal values for both assays range from 70 to 120% of control. AT-III levels in 20-week fetuses and term babies are about 25 and 50% of control, respectively; adult levels are achieved at about 6 months of age. In utero or neonatal clotting is uncommon because of a concurrent physiologic reduction in procoagulant factor levels. AT-III plasma levels may be measured in patients taking warfarin but should be avoided during heparin therapy and during acute thromboembolic events.

AT-III deficiency is inherited in an autosomal dominant pattern. Homozygotes die in utero or during infancy. In the heterozygous AT-III-deficient population two subtypes are seen. Type I deficiency is more common and is characterized by decreased synthesis of a functionally normal AT-III molecule (i.e., a quantitative defect). In these persons, functional and antigenic assays yield similar values; most have approximately 40 to 70% of control levels.[29,49–51] Formation of a biologically dysfunctional form of AT-III (qualitative, or type II, deficiency) is less common. These persons have normal antigenic levels but abnormal AT-III activity as measured in functional assays. AT-III deficiency may be caused by more than one type of genetic abnormality; some investigators have suggested a relationship between specific aberrations and the prevalence and/or severity of thrombosis.[52]

The wide array of clinical manifestations reflect an inheritance pattern with variable expression. Only moderate reductions (50 to 70% of normal) of AT-III levels may induce thrombophilia. Some patients remain asymptomatic, although many clinically asymptomatic patients have laboratory evidence of a procoagulant state.[51] In evaluations of families with AT-III deficiency, the prevalence of venous thromboembolism in heterozygotes is about 50%.[53] The cumulative incidence of thrombosis increases with age with most patients having their first event in adolescence or young adulthood (10 to 35 years). By age 40 about 50% have had a thrombotic event, and by age 50 to 60 as many as 85 to 95% will have had at least one episode.[52–54] Recurrence is common (about 50 to 60%). Typically, the initial event is DVT of a lower extremity and/or PE. Thrombosis may also occur at unusual sites such as the upper extremity (axillary or brachial vein), viscera (mesenteric, renal, or retinal vein), cerebrum (the cerebral sinuses), or vena cava. Superficial thrombophlebitis and arterial thrombosis are relatively uncommon with AT-III deficiency. The initial event in AT-III deficiency usually occurs in the presence of a known thrombogenic risk factor (most commonly pregnancy or surgery/trauma but also during prolonged bed rest or exposure to other factors or drugs, as listed in Table 15.6). Apparent heparin resistance may occur rarely with AT-III deficiency and occasionally is a clue to its presence. For a discussion of the clinical manifestations and diagnosis of venous thromboembolism refer to Chapter 44.

AT-III deficiency is also associated with a high risk of maternal and fetal complications during pregnancy; 42 to 68% of pregnant women with untreated AT-III deficiency will develop venous thrombosis during pregnancy or in the immediate postpartum period.[50] Moreover, a significantly higher incidence of fetal morbidity and mortality is manifested as spontaneous abortions, intrauterine growth retardation, and preterm delivery. Widespread microvascular thrombosis with subsequent fibrosis of the placenta has been observed and is presumed to cause placental insufficiency.[52,55] It may occur at any stage of the pregnancy, and there is currently no way to prospectively identify patients who will develop these complications.

TREATMENT

The management of acute thromboembolism in AT-III-deficient patients is the same as that for the general population. UFH (porcine-derived) or LMWH should be administered, the dose being titrated according to the aPTT. Heparin resistance is uncommon at the AT-III levels that are typically seen in deficient patients; the dose of heparin that is required to attain a therapeutic aPTT is not related to the degree of AT-III deficiency. Warfarin therapy is initiated concomitant with the heparin, with a target prothrombin time international normalized ratio (INR) of 2.0 to 3.0. For further description of the management of acute DVT and PE, refer to Chapter 44.

AT-III concentrate (Thrombate-III, Miles Cutter Biological; ATnativ, KabiVitrum) is prepared as a purified (via heparin chromatography affinity) plasma concentrate that is then pasteurized to inactivate hepatitis B and HIV-1 viruses. One unit of AT-III concentrate is equal to the amount of AT-III present in 1 mL of normal plasma. AT-III concentrate is available in the United States as an orphan drug. Because of its considerable expense and short half-life, it is not indicated for long-term prophylaxis for AT-III-deficient patients. Approved indications are therefore limited to short-term prophylaxis and treatment of thromboembolism in patients with inherited AT-III deficiency, with or without concomitant heparin therapy.

Preventive indications include situations with a high risk of thrombosis, such as surgery, pregnancy and delivery, major trauma, and prolonged bed rest. After parturition and surgery, plasma AT-III levels are reduced for several days, concurrent with the high risk for thrombosis.[51,56] The plasma level reduction is accentuated in congenital deficiency, and AT-III concentrate is therefore given just before (when able) and for a period of 5 to 7 days after exposure, depending on the situation. The lack of bleeding risk associated with AT-III administration makes it a particularly attractive alternative to traditional anticoagulants for preventing venous thrombosis. Randomized controlled trials of efficacy are limited by the rarity of congenital deficiency and ethical considerations. Several small-scale trials have yielded very promising results in preventing thrombosis using AT-III concentrate either alone or with concurrent heparin.[50,51,53–55] AT-III-deficient patients with acute thrombosis may also benefit from the addition of AT-III concentrate to heparin therapy, especially those who experience thrombus extension while receiving heparin or those with apparent heparin resistance.[52,54] The use of AT-III concentrate in acquired AT-III deficiency states far exceeds that in inherited conditions, and there are many more reported trials, although these are technically not approved uses (see the discussion of acquired AT-III deficiency later in this chapter).

After intravenous administration, peak plasma AT-III levels are achieved in 15 to 30 minutes.[51] In vivo recovery is variable, ranging from 60 to 100% after administration to patients with stable congenital AT-III deficiency.[49,50] Plasma AT-III activity levels can be expected to increase 1 to 2% for each unit per kilogram administered. Another dosing strategy is to set a desired plasma AT-III level of 80 to 125% as the goal and a plasma volume of 40 mL/kg and then calculate the dose as follows:

$$\text{Dose (U)} = \frac{(\text{Desired [AT-III]\%}) - \text{pretreatment [AT-III]\%} \times 40\ \text{mL/kg} \times \text{weight (kg)}}{\text{Fraction recovered} \times 100}$$

If the pretreatment AT-III level is 50%, this corresponds to a loading dose of 30 to 50 U/kg.[50,51] Important dosing considerations include a lower goal concentration when used neonates and highly variable fraction-recovered values, both between and within patients, which are related to the disease being treated and its acuity. It is therefore important to measure AT-III levels in dosage calculation, rather than using fixed dosing methods. In asymptomatic patients with inherited AT-III deficiency, elimination of initial doses is biphasic through a decline in AT-III activity and antigen. This has been observed both immunologically and functionally. An initial half-life of AT-III activity of 22 hours has been reported,[51] with terminal half-lives ranging from 60 to 90 hours (AT-III activity) and 53 to 59 hours (AT-III antigen).[51,54] Prolonged administration yields single-phase second-order elimination. Once-daily administration is therefore usually sufficient, except in acute DIC, in which a 12-hour dosing interval is preferred because of a reduction in the half-life (4.5 hours) and fraction recovered (50%).[40,51]

Adverse drug reactions reported with AT-III concentrate have been minimal. Rarely chest tightness, dizziness, and fever have occurred.[51,54] An interesting finding in patients with DIC who received AT-III plus heparin was a greater need for RBC transfusion compared to that with either drug alone.[40] A higher incidence of wound hematoma and bleeding was also noted after joint replacement surgery, compared to dextran 40.[56] Conversion of hepatitis B antigen and antibody has been reported; however, these patients also received other blood products.[54] Hepatitis C and HIV-1 transmission have not been reported.

In administering AT-III concentrate and heparin concurrently, it is important to consider their interaction. Replenishment of AT-III to a deficient patient may result in a significantly lower dosage requirement for heparin. Empiric dosage reduction and/or frequent laboratory monitoring is appropriate when AT-III concentrate is added to heparin therapy.

Monitoring parameters for AT-III concentrate include plasma AT-III levels, hemoglobin, and hematocrit every 12 hours until stable, then every 24 hours. Care should be exercised during monitoring to ensure that AT-III functional rather than antigenic or immunologic levels are determined. Patients receiving heparin and warfarin should also have regular monitoring of aPTT, PT, and TT. Other laboratory indicators of ongoing thrombin formation such as fibrinopeptide A, prothrombin fragment 1 + 2, and thrombin-antithrombin complex levels should be assessed if available. The patient should be examined regularly for the signs and symptoms of thromboembolism such as lower extremity pain, swelling and warmth, shortness of breath, pleuritic chest pain, and hypoxemia. Occult blood monitoring of nasogastric aspirate, stools, and urine is appropriate.

LONG-TERM MANAGEMENT

Once a thrombotic event has occurred, the AT-III-deficient patient will have a significant lifelong risk of recurrence, which can happen spontaneously or in the presence of thrombosis risk factors. In a retrospective analysis of 238 patients from 73 families with inherited deficiency of either AT-III, protein C, or protein S, the incidence of an initial episode of venous thromboembolism was 1.3 per 100 patient-years; in contrast, the incidence of recurrent events was 4.8 per 100 patient-years.[53] This finding emphasizes the importance of long-term secondary prophylaxis. Lifelong replacement therapy with AT-III concentrate is neither indicated nor practical. Most investigators therefore advise lifelong therapy with oral anticoagulants after a single thrombotic event, adjusted to a target prothrombin time INR of

2.0 to 3.0.[29,50,57] Some take a more conservative approach, advising lifelong therapy only for patients with recurrent DVT, or a single episode if life-threatening, or a single episode if spontaneous.[53] The decision about long-term anticoagulant therapy should be made for each individual patient. Patients with dementia, peptic ulcer disease, or chronic bleeding or who have a history of frequent falls or trauma, poor or unreliable compliance with drug therapy, or alcohol abuse may not be suitable candidates for lifelong treatment.

The management of pregnant women (or those desiring pregnancy) merits special discussion. AT-III deficiency, whether inherited or acquired, is associated with both maternal and fetal complications. The incidence of maternal thrombosis during pregnancy is higher with AT-III deficiency than with protein C or S deficiency. Most investigators therefore recommend prophylaxis for all AT-III-deficient patients, regardless of the history of thrombosis.[29,53] Patients who are receiving warfarin should discontinue use in advance, if possible, because of its known teratogenic effects.[58] Subcutaneous heparin therapy should be initiated and maintained until the time of delivery. Patients with difficulty managing subcutaneous injections should receive heparin at least during the first trimester and the last 1 to 2 months of pregnancy and oral anticoagulants during the remainder of the pregnancy.[53,58] Twice-weekly AT-III concentrate infusions plus subcutaneous heparin have been successfully used in treating two women with congenital AT-III deficiency and heparin resistance.[51] For most patients, however, AT-III concentrate is withheld until the peripartum period, when it is given at the time of delivery and for several days thereafter.[54,55] Additionally, warfarin therapy (usually with a few days of concurrent heparin) should be promptly reinitiated postpartum. Warfarin is considered safe for an infant whose mother is breastfeeding[58]; however, it should be noted that this assessment of safety does not extend to other coumarin derivatives.

All AT-III-deficient patients who undergo surgery, incur trauma, or are exposed to other high-risk situations should receive prophylaxis with heparin, warfarin, and/or AT-III concentrate, whether or not they are receiving long-term oral anticoagulant therapy. Short-term prophylaxis should be given before, during, and for a few days after exposure to thrombosis risk factors.[53]

The use of long-term oral anticoagulant prophylaxis in patients with AT-III deficiency who have not experienced a thrombotic event (e.g., a person detected in family screening) is controversial. Short-term prophylaxis as described above during exposure to high-risk situations (including pregnancy) is appropriate. However, there are no studies demonstrating a definite benefit of long-term anticoagulant therapy for these patients.[57,59] The decision to initiate such treatment should therefore be individualized on the basis of the family history and after patient consultation regarding the risks and benefits of treatment. If the patient and clinician elect to treat with warfarin, it may be initiated on an outpatient basis without concomitant heparin.

The value of a management strategy that incorporated short-term prophylaxis for all patients and long-term anticoagulants for symptomatic patients with inherited deficiencies of AT-III, protein C, or protein S was evaluated in a retrospective study of 238 patients from 73 families.[53] At the time of diagnosis the incidence of recurrent venous thrombosis was 4.8 per 100 patient-years. This was reduced to 1.4 per 100 patient-years with the described treatment strategy; if those who complied poorly with the drug regimen were excluded, the incidence was further reduced to 0.3 per 100 patient-years. Specific analysis of AT-III-deficient patients yielded a reduction in the overall incidence (single event or recurrent, long-term prophylaxis or not) of major thrombotic events from 2.5 to 1.3 per 100 patient-years after implementation of the strategy (0.5 if those who complied poorly were excluded). Four AT-III-deficient women (two with and two without a prior history of thrombosis) became pregnant and were managed with heparin, with or without oral anticoagulants and AT-III concentrate; none had a thrombotic event. Six AT-III-deficient patients were given perioperative prophylaxis with heparin and/or AT-III concentrate, with no thrombotic events. During follow-up of 42 asymptomatic AT-III-deficient patients over a mean of 5.3 years, two developed major thrombotic manifestations. This last finding may argue for long-term prophylaxis for asymptomatic patients, although confirmation with larger patient populations is desirable.

IMPROVING OUTCOMES

Counseling for all patients with inherited AT-III deficiency should include a review of thrombosis risk settings and the importance of avoiding such situations. All patients should be informed of the symptoms of DVT and PE and the need for prompt medical evaluation should they occur. All patients should consider short-term prophylaxis with heparin, warfarin, and/or AT-III concentrate when risk factors are present. The following information should be given to patients who are receiving long-term warfarin therapy: rationale for treatment, symptoms of bleeding, necessity to avoid contact sports or activities, importance of consistent dietary intake of vitamin K, necessity to avoid aspirin in any form, abundance of drug interactions, and the need for regular coagulation studies and dosage adjustment (also refer to Chapter 44). Women of childbearing age who are receiving long-term anticoagulant therapy must be counseled regarding the teratogenic effects of coumarin derivatives and the need for effective contraception. Women who are not receiving long-term anticoagulant therapy should be informed of the maternal and fetal risks during pregnancy and the advisability of prophylaxis during pregnancy and shortly thereafter.

Acquired Antithrombin-III Deficiency

In addition to congenital aberrations of the physiologic anticoagulant and fibrinolytic proteins, certain diseases may alter their levels or function, resulting in acquired deficiencies. This may occur in patients with increased AT-III consumption (DIC, preeclampsia, major surgery, extensive acute DVT, or PE), decreased production (liver failure, fatty liver of pregnancy, malnutrition, or preterm infants), or increased plasma loss (nephrotic syndrome or inflammatory bowel disease).[52,60] Patients with malignancy may develop AT-III deficiency via an uncertain mechanism. Most patients with acquired AT-III deficiency do not develop thrombosis. Although nephrotic syndrome is associated with a high risk of thromboembolism, a causative relationship with AT-III deficiency remains unclear.[60] Prophylaxis for acquired AT-III deficiency is therefore not generally necessary. For patients with acute thromboembolism with known low plasma AT-III levels, DIC, fatty liver of pregnancy with DIC, or fulminant hepatic failure, the usefulness of AT-III concentrate has been demonstrated.[40,50,55] Patient counseling regarding avoidance of high-risk situations is appropriate.

Two randomized double-blind trials of AT-III concentrate, either alone or in combination with heparin, that involved patients with DIC have been reported. When compared to heparin[40] or placebo,[39] a significantly shorter duration of DIC in groups receiving AT-III was observed. One trial found a trend toward a reduction in mortality in patients receiving AT-III concentrate that was not statistically significant.[39] The need for RBC transfusion in patients receiving AT-III concentrate was higher in one study[40] than in the other.[39] Uncontrolled trials or case reports have been published on patients with fatty liver of pregnancy and DIC,[55] children with DIC,[41] and patients with DIC and arterial thrombosis that was unresponsive to heparin alone.[42] Whereas AT-III concentrate has been demonstrated to improve the clinical and laboratory markers for patients with DIC, the ultimate outcome as measured by mortality is primarily related to the underlying disease.

A third randomized trial of AT-III concentrate was performed in normals after total hip or knee replacement surgery.[56] Patients in the AT-III plus heparin group (treated for 5 days) had a significantly lower incidence of venous thrombosis compared to those who received dextran 40. An interesting finding was the occurrence of venous thrombosis in 100% of patients with AT-III plasma levels less than 65%, suggesting that this value may represent an important threshold.

Drug-induced AT-III deficiency has been reported with L-asparaginase, oral contraceptives, and heparin. L-Asparaginase is thought to cause thrombosis via reduced endogenous synthesis of the coagulation and fibrinolytic proteins and/or drug-induced endothelial damage. Thrombosis during or immediately after L-asparaginase administration is well documented, occurring in 3 to 5% of patients.[61] AT-III concentrate has been evaluated in a small cohort of patients undergoing induction therapy for acute lymphoblastic leukemia, yielding a reduction in laboratory test abnormalities and clinical thrombosis.[61]

Oral contraceptives are the triggering event for the initial episode of venous thrombosis in 5 to 10% of AT-III-deficient patients and are generally avoided in this population.[52,53] To assess the additional risk of oral contraceptives in 48 patients with hereditary thrombophilia, a retrospective study of AT-III-deficient women compared those who had taken oral contraceptives at least once with age-matched control subjects.[62] The AT-III-deficient patients who had taken oral contraceptives had a significantly higher probability for thrombosis (48 and 77% after 12 and 60 months, respectively), with a yearly incidence of 27.5% compared to 3.4% of control subjects. It was concluded that oral contraceptives were contraindicated for patients with AT-III deficiency and that relatives of those with known AT-III deficiencies should be screened before initiation of oral contraception. A limitation of this study was the very small sample size of 15 AT-III-deficient patients.

Protein C Deficiency

Protein C is a vitamin K-dependent proenzyme that circulates as an inactive zymogen. Activation occurs when thrombomodulin, a vascular endothelial cell receptor, binds to thrombin, thereby altering thrombin's substrate affinity in two important ways: (1) Thrombomodulin-bound thrombin does not catalyze the conversion of fibrinogen to fibrin, and (2) the thrombomodulin-thrombin complex is a powerful activator of protein C, forming protein Ca. Protein Ca inhibits thrombin formation by proteolytic inactivation of factors Va and VIIIa (Fig. 15.1). This effect is markedly enhanced in the presence of a cofactor called protein S. Protein Ca will also enhance fibrinolysis by inactivating tissue plasminogen activator inhibitor (PAI-1). In this capacity, protein Ca is a major physiologic modulator of blood fluidity and hemostasis.

Assays are available for determining both functional and immunologic (antigenic) protein C levels. The reference range of 65 to 130% that is used for both methods is expressed as a percentage of normal pooled plasma. Protein C levels are not affected by heparin. Assays in persons taking oral anticoagulants are difficult to interpret because protein C production is vitamin K-dependent and therefore altered by the warfarin. If discontinuation of the oral anticoagulant is deemed harmful, the magnitude of protein C reduction may be compared to that of another vitamin K-dependent protein such as factor X, but this has less precision in identifying deficient patients.

The inheritance pattern of protein C deficiency is intriguing. The commonly reported prevalence of 1:200 to 1:300 is not consistent with the pattern of clinical manifestations. This disparity may be due either to inheritance of a single congenital disorder with variable degrees of penetrance or to the existence of two separate phenotypes with different clinical manifestations. Recent research supports the latter hypothesis.[63–65] In the autosomal-recessive form, heterozygotes have protein C antigen levels of 30 to 60%, but most remain asymptomatic for life.[64,65] Homozygotes with this form have nonmeasurable plasma levels associated with neonatal purpura fulminans or severe thrombosis in infancy. This form has a prevalence in the general population of 1:200 to 1:300 (Table 15.7). Heterozygotes with the autosomal-dominant form have similar protein C levels of 30 to 60%[63,64,66] but have a high incidence of recurrent thrombosis beginning in early adulthood. Homozygotes have very low levels (5 to 20%) but often remain completely asymptomatic until adolescence or young adulthood, when they develop recurrent thrombosis in a pattern similar to that of heterozygotes with the same autosomal-dominant form; some may even remain asymptomatic for life.[66] The autosomal dominant form is found in about 60% of protein C-deficient patients, with a prevalence in the general population estimated at 1:15,000.[64] This hypothesis therefore yields "healthy" (autosomal-recessive) and "thrombosis-prone" (autosomal-dominant) families[63] and at least partially explains the discordance between the prevalence of deficiency and the incidence of thrombotic manifestations. Heterozygotes in either group may have either reduced levels of functionally normal protein C (type I, quantitative; more common) or "normal" levels of dysfunctional protein C (type II, qualitative; less common).

A new type of congenital protein C abnormality has recently been described. In this form, antigenic and functional protein C levels are normal, but factor Va is resistant to the proteolytic action of protein Ca. The procoagulant activity of factor Va is retained, which therefore favors thrombosis in affected patients. This disorder, called activated protein C resistance (APCR), is caused by a single point mutation of the gene for factor V and is inherited in an autosomal-dominant pattern. The prevalence of heterozygotes in the general population is very high (3 to 5%). Most are asymptomatic, which suggests that APCR alone is not a major risk factor for thrombosis. However, a high risk for thrombosis exists when APCR occurs concomitantly with a second abnormality such as AT-III, protein C or S deficiency, the lupus anticoagulant, or homozygous APCR. APCR may be found in as many as 50% of patients with hereditary thrombophilia, compared to 3 to 7% of healthy control subjects. APCR is therefore the most common hereditary abnormality identified to date. An attractive hypothesis suggests that APCR, protein C deficiency, or protein S deficiency, if present alone, results in a moderate increase in risk of thrombosis, whereas when two deficiencies coexist, the risk is markedly enhanced.[63]

CLINICAL PRESENTATION AND DIAGNOSIS

In neonatal purpura fulminans, homozygotes with the autosomal recessive form usually develop symptoms within hours after birth. Microvascular thrombosis with DIC is seen clinically as ecchymoses, purpura, and hemorrhagic bullae, followed by necrosis and gangrene, usually on the extremities, trunk, scalp, and pressure points (also occasionally in other organs). Laboratory findings resemble those of DIC, except for nondetectable protein C antigenic and functional levels. Skin biopsies reveal extensive thrombosis of the arterioles and venules. CNS and vitreous or retinal thrombosis with hemorrhage may occur in utero, resulting in mental retardation, developmental delay, and blindness, although fortunately these complications are attenuated by reduced hepatic synthesis of vitamin K-dependent coagulation factors. Neonatal extension of this protected state may suppress purpura fulminans, with affected babies instead developing massive thrombosis later in infancy.[64] Most reported infants with neonatal purpura fulminans have been the offspring of consanguineous parents.

In thromboembolic disease, both heterozygotes and homozygotes with the autosomal dominant (thrombosis-prone) form may develop a wide spectrum of thrombotic diseases. DVT and/or PE is the most frequent manifestation. Arterial events such as myocardial infarction, transient ischemic attacks, and ischemic stroke are uncommon overall, but the prevalence is higher with proteins C or S deficiency (8.4%) than with AT-III (1%) deficiency.[53] Superficial thrombophlebitis is also relatively more common with protein C deficiency. Events begin in adolescence or young adulthood with 80% of instances occurring before the age of 40 years.[53,60,66] About 50% of events occur during periods of thrombosis risk such as pregnancy or surgery. The risk is intensified in patients who are younger than 40 years old; the incidence of thromboembolism before age 40 is 120-fold and 14-fold higher in protein C-deficient males and females, respectively, than in the general population.[53] Thrombosis in unusual sites such as the upper extremities, viscera (renal, mesenteric veins), or brain (cerebral sinuses) occurs with a prevalence similar to that of other inherited deficiencies. Some patients may have only a single thrombotic episode, but about 50% have recurrent events.

The syndrome of warfarin-induced skin necrosis is characterized by the sudden onset of painful edematous erythema followed by hemorrhagic bullae, gangrene, and necrosis of the skin and subcutaneous tissues of the extremities, trunk, breasts, buttocks, or penis.[67,68] These symptoms typically occur 2 to 3 days after initiation and are more common with the older practice of large warfarin loading doses. Laboratory findings in severe cases resemble those of DIC. Histologic examination reveals microvascular thrombosis, a finding that was previously considered paradoxical, since the reaction was caused by an anticoagulant. It is now believed that warfarin-induced skin necrosis is caused by a transient hypercoagulable state that occurs because of the short half-life of protein C (6 to 8 hours) compared to that of the other vitamin K-dependent clotting factors, especially factors II, IX, and X (24 to 80 hours). When warfarin is begun, rapid depletion of protein C may be seen at a time when levels of factors II, IX, and X are almost normal.[60,67,68] This exaggerated imbalance causes the thrombosis and may also explain the association with large loading doses. At steady state, the reduction in protein C levels is comparable to that of the other factors, and the risk of thrombosis is therefore eliminated. Patients with inherited or acquired protein C deficiency are particularly susceptible to warfarin-induced skin necrosis because they have low baseline levels.

TREATMENT

For neonatal purpura fulminans, prompt recognition and treatment are essential for survival. Protein C may be replaced by infusion of FFP in doses of 8 to 12 mL/kg every 12 hours. This has been reported to halt the formation of new lesions and to induce regression of evolving lesions.[64] Alternative sources of protein C include prothrombin complex concentrate (factor IX concentrate) and protein C concentrate if available. Heparin, factor VIII concentrate, AT-III concentrate, vitamin K, and antiplatelet agents are not useful.[64] Supportive care for the dermatologic, neurologic, and ophthalmic manifestations should be provided. Replacement therapy should be continued until all lesions are healed. If the patient survives, healing occurs over 4 to 8 weeks, often with residual scarring and sometimes requiring plastic surgery or amputation.

Human protein C concentrate (Immuno-AG, Vienna, Austria) is available in the United States on an investigational basis. It is prepared as a monoclonal antibody-purified concentrate made from viral-inactivated prothrombin complex concentrate (factor IX concentrate). The product is then vapor heated for further virus inactivation. Protein C concentrate is undergoing trials in a number of conditions. In purpura fulminans, normalization of laboratory findings occurs over several days; actual resorption of retinal hemorrhage and healing of a necrotic leg lesion have also been reported.[69] One international unit of concentrate is equal to the protein C activity in 1 mL of normal pooled plasma. After intravenous administration the close correlation between antigenic and functional plasma levels suggests that the infused protein C retains its activity. Pharmacokinetic studies have demonstrated variability in the fraction recovered, depending on disease acuity. Biphasic elimination with initial and terminal half-lives of 6 and 11 hours, respectively, was observed in a neonate not receiving oral anticoagulants.[69] When concentrate was given at the time of oral anticoagulant initiation, the half-life of protein C activity was about 12 hours after the first dose and 18 hours with subsequent doses.[66] Short- (4 days), medium- (32 days), and long-term (8 months) maintenance therapy has been administered without adverse effects.[66,69,70]

Acute thromboembolism (acute DVT and PE) in protein C-deficient patients is managed with UFH or LMWH and warfarin in doses to produce the same target laboratory values as in the general population (refer to Chapter 44). An important precaution in protein C-deficient patients is to ensure that therapeutic doses of UFH or LMWH are being administered at the time of initial warfarin therapy and until a therapeutic prothrombin time INR is achieved. Warfarin must be started at low doses in conjunction with UFH or LMWH. This reduces the risk of warfarin-induced skin necrosis. Resistance to heparin may occur rarely in protein C-deficient patients. This was managed in a homozygous male with acute DVT by infusion of protein C concentrate during the warfarin titration period.[66]

For warfarin skin necrosis, prompt diagnosis and management are required to avoid ischemic necrosis of the subcutaneous tissues. It is managed with heparin (to stop the clotting process), FFP or cryoprecipitate (to replace protein C), and vitamin K (to facilitate endogenous protein C production). Protein C concentrate with intravenous heparin administration has also been reported to induce a rapid improvement in laboratory abnormalities and clinical manifestations over 24 hours, with complete healing over 15 days.[70] Appropriate supportive therapy to minimize complications such as infection is essential. Reconstructive surgery may be necessary in severe cases.

LONG-TERM MANAGEMENT

Until recently, neonatal purpura fulminans was considered a uniformly and rapidly fatal disorder. Advances in its diagnosis and management have improved short-term survival and allowed development of long-term treatment strategies. Protein C concentrate is not suitable for long-term maintenance use because of its short half-life and high cost. After complete resolution of the purpura fulminans, either FFP given daily or prothrombin complex concentrate (factor IX complex) given every other day may be used to sustain protein C levels that are adequate to halt ongoing coagulation.[64] Successful management for as long as 2 years has been reported.[71] Unfortunately, both products have significant disadvantages, including possible virus transmission and the need for venous access; hyperproteinemia, hypertension, or fluid overload and the need for daily infusions associated with FFP; and variable and unpredictable protein C content with the possibility of drug-induced thromboembolism with prothrombin complex concentrate. An alternative approach to long-term management is to reduce the levels of vitamin K-dependent coagulation factors (II, VII, IX, and X) to a degree sufficient to suppress clot formation. Oral warfarin carefully titrated to a prothrombin INR that is adequate to maintain an asymptomatic state is the most common long-term treatment.[64] Special considerations in the use of warfarin in protein C-deficient patients include delaying treatment until all lesions of purpura fulminans have healed and the need for 5 to 7 days of overlapping heparin or FFP when initiating therapy. The latter precaution is recommended to reduce the likelihood of warfarin skin necrosis. If the symptoms of purpura fulminans recur, prompt replacement of protein C with FFP or protein C concentrate is indicated (prothrombin complex concentrate may be harmful in this situation). Liver transplantation was reported to cure protein C deficiency in a single case.

Patients with protein C deficiency or APCR associated with recurrent thrombosis should be managed with lifelong warfarin therapy to a prothrombin INR goal of 2.0 to 3.0 (or sometimes higher). Symptomatic patients with APCR and a second inherited deficiency (AT-III, protein C, or protein S) should be similarly treated. LMWH (fraxiparin) has also been successfully used as long-term secondary prophylaxis in treating patients who have a history of warfarin skin necrosis.[65] Patients who refuse or are not suitable candidates for long-term anticoagulant therapy should be counseled regarding avoidance of thrombosis risk situations and the advisability of short-term prophylaxis.

Management of asymptomatic persons and those with a single thrombotic event is controversial because of variable and unpredictable clinical expression of the deficiency. The decision to maintain lifelong treatment is made only after individualized consultation regarding its potential risks and benefits. Many practitioners advise long-term prophylaxis after only one event if it is life-threatening or spontaneous. The value of this strategy was assessed in 141 protein C- or S-deficient patients who were followed for 598 patient-years.[53] The overall incidence (initial or recurrent events, with or without long-term prophylaxis) was reduced from 1.4 (protein C) to 2.0 (protein S) per 100 patient-years before the strategy was initiated to 0.8 (combined) per 100 patient-years after implementation. If oral anticoagulants were given and patients who complied poorly were excluded, this was further reduced to 0.5 per 100 patient-years. The reduction in recurrent thromboembolism was even more striking, from 4.8 per 100 patient-years (baseline incidence) to 1.4 after the strategy was initiated and 0.3 if patients who complied poorly were excluded. A disturbing finding in this report was the occurrence of major thrombosis in 2 of 51 protein C-deficient patients and 2 of 16 protein S-deficient patients who were asymptomatic at presentation and therefore did not receive long-term prophylaxis. Although this finding may support prophylaxis in all patients, it should be emphasized that the risk of treatment must also be considered for each patient. Patients who are unreliable, those who are subject to trauma, and those with a condition that has a risk of bleeding such as ulcer disease should be carefully evaluated before long-term anticoagulant therapy is given. An important therapeutic distinction in protein C-deficient patients is the need for either intravenous or subcutaneous heparin in doses to achieve a therapeutic aPTT before the first dose of warfarin and until a therapeutic prothrombin INR is achieved. Alternatively, FFP or protein C concentrate may be given during warfarin titration.[66]

Approximately 50% of major thrombotic events occur in association with a risk situation. Short-term prophylaxis should be given to all patients during exposure to high-risk situations such as surgery, trauma, or prolonged immobilization, regardless of the history of thrombosis. Heparin, warfarin, FFP, and/or protein C concentrate may be used. Limited evidence favors the use of replacement therapy, either alone or with heparin. Prophylaxis should be given before, during, and immediately after risk exposure and is especially important in patients younger than 40 years of age.[53]

The risk of maternal and fetal complications during pregnancy in protein C-deficient women is not as high as that seen with AT-III deficiency but is nonetheless higher than that of the general population. All patients should therefore receive prophylaxis, regardless of history of thrombosis. Pregnancy is managed as previously described in the discussion of AT-III deficiency, with the elimination of AT-III concentrate. FFP or protein C concentrate may be considered in the peripartum period. Warfarin should be initiated promptly after delivery, with overlapping heparin therapy.

MONITORING PARAMETERS

Frequent clinical assessment of the affected areas should be performed. Relevant laboratory studies in patients with purpura fulminans include markers of DIC (Table 15.5). If available, levels of fibrinopeptide A, prothrombin fragment 1 + 2, thrombin-antithrombin complex, and protein C are also useful in assessing response. Patients who receive FFP should be regularly assessed for fluid overload and hypertension, with periodic evaluation of cardiac, renal, and hepatic function. Indwelling intravenous catheters should be evaluated for function, patency, and infection. Patients who are receiving long-term warfarin therapy should have regular monitoring of prothrombin INR, hematocrit, and signs of bleeding. All patients should receive longitudinal assessment for recurrence of the thrombotic manifestations. Childhood growth and development should also be followed.

IMPROVING OUTCOMES

Counseling for patients with protein C deficiency is similar to that described in the discussion of AT-III deficiency. Patients should be apprised of both the potential for reduction in subsequent events with treatment and the lack of effect if compliance with treatment is poor. Family screening should be performed to identify other family members with this deficiency. Females who desire oral contraceptives should be advised of the potential for drug-induced thromboembolism. Although the incremental risk in protein C-deficient females who have taken oral contraceptives appears to be less than that for AT-III deficiency,[62] in one study oral contraceptives were the precipitating factor for five initial thrombotic events in 57 protein C-deficient patients.[53] Therefore, these patients should be advised to use other forms of contraception.

Acquired Protein C Deficiency

Protein C levels may be reduced in severe liver disease, DIC, acute respiratory distress syndrome, malignancy, and pregnancy and after surgery, but a causative relationship with risk of thrombosis is unclear. Patients with previously normal protein C levels may have reduced levels during extensive DVT or PE due to consumption. Drugs that may alter levels include oral anticoagulants and L-asparaginase. Open trials of protein C concentrate in cohorts of children[43] and adults[44] with DIC have identified improvement in both clinical and laboratory parameters. The lack of bleeding risk with protein C is appealing, and it was found to be very useful in treating one patient with severe gastrointestinal bleeding.

Protein S Deficiency

Protein S is a vitamin K-dependent entity synthesized in the liver. It differs from protein C in that it does not require activation and is not itself an anticoagulant but rather a cofactor for the actions of other proteins. Binding of protein Ca to protein S markedly augments the proteolytic activity of protein Ca on factors Va and VIIIa. Protein S may also be a cofactor for the profibrinolytic actions of protein C. Approximately 30 to 50% of body stores circulate in the free (active) form.[63] The remainder exists in an inactive membrane-bound complex with C4b binding protein, a regulator of the complement system. Protein S levels are altered by warfarin but not by heparin.

Protein S deficiency in the general population is now known to be common. The inheritance is autosomal dominant, and heterozygous patients have a strong tendency to develop DVT.[57,59,63] The prevalence in patients with venous thromboembolism is at least as high as that of AT-III and protein C deficiency.[63] Three types of deficiency have been described:

- Type I (quantitative) is the most common and is characterized by a reduction in both total and free protein S antigen. The protein S produced is of normal or moderately reduced activity. C4b binding protein levels are also reduced.
- Type II is a qualitative deficiency wherein normal amounts of protein S antigen are produced but it is functionally defective. This type is rare.
- In type III, total protein S antigen and C4b binding protein levels are normal, but the levels of free protein S are reduced.[63,72] In general, the functional protein S levels in type III patients are higher than in type I patients.[72]

CLINICAL PRESENTATION AND DIAGNOSIS

Like the other deficiency syndromes, protein S deficiency has variable clinical and biologic expression. Homozygous protein S deficiency manifests as death in utero or a syndrome similar to neonatal purpura fulminans as seen in protein C deficiency. Some heterozygotes are completely asymptomatic (even during exposure to risk factors). DVT and/or pulmonary thrombosis account for 64% of initial events,[72] which typically begin in young adulthood. Superficial thrombophlebitis (30% of events) occurs at a rate greater than that of AT-III deficiency and comparable to that of protein C deficiency. Venous thrombosis in unusual sites (axillary, cerebral sinuses, mesenteric, portal, jugular, etc.) is seen with a prevalence comparable to that of other deficiencies. Arterial thrombosis (primarily in the cerebrum or coronary arteries) occurs in 5 to 8% of patients.[54,72–74] Approximately one-half of initial events are spontaneous. Pregnancy is a common predisposing condition, especially for patients with combined protein S deficiency and APCR.[73,75] Recurrence is common with some patients reported to have as many as 15 thrombotic episodes. Warfarin-induced skin necrosis has also been reported in protein S deficiency.

Thrombotic events appear to be more common in isolated protein S deficiency than in protein C deficiency,[54] although some have suggested that the high incidence may be due to selection of severely affected families[73] or misdiagnosis in patients who actually have APCR.[63] At least 50 to 70% have their first episode before the age of 40.[53,72,73] Some investigators have suggested that with prolonged follow-up, all persons with heterozygous protein S deficiency will eventually develop thrombosis.[57,73] There is no relationship between the type of deficiency, the levels of antigenic or functional protein S, and the incidence of thrombosis,[72,73] a finding that suggests that factors other than the antigenic or functional concentration regulate the degree of clinical expression. Evidence suggests that patients with both protein S deficiency and APCR have a significantly greater incidence of thrombosis than do patients with either alone.[73,75]

TREATMENT

The acute and long-term management of patients with protein S deficiency is similar to that for protein C deficiency. UFH or LMWH is used for acute thrombosis, whereas maintenance therapy is long-term low-dose UFH, LMWH, or warfarin. Because of the higher incidence of thrombotic events, however, there is a greater tendency to give lifelong oral anticoagulants to patients with protein S deficiency after even one event. Some practitioners maintain a conservative approach, treating with long-term warfarin only patients with recurrent thrombosis.[60] When given in doses titrated to the standard desired prothrombin INR, warfarin has been found to be effective in preventing subsequent events[72,73]; detailed documentation of value is discussed in the section of this chapter titled "Protein C Deficiency."[53] Moreover, temporary discontinuation of warfarin resulted in recurrent thrombosis.[73] Asymptomatic patients are generally not treated with long-term warfarin. The occurrence of initial thrombotic events in 2 of 16 previously asymptomatic patients who were followed for a mean of 5.3 years, coupled with the severity of these events (stroke in a 23-year-old and myocardial infarction in a 42-year-old),[53] suggests that further studies should be performed to assess the value of long-term warfarin therapy in asymptomatic protein S-deficient patients. Replacement therapy with either FFP or prothrombin complex concentrate (factor IX concentrate) has been used both therapeutically and prophylactically.[57] The use of FFP requires larger volumes; however, it may otherwise be advantageous, since it exposes the patient to fewer infectious complications and does not have the potential to enhance thrombosis risk by providing other coagulant factors.

On the basis of available data, all protein S-deficient persons should receive short-term prophylaxis before, during, and immediately after exposure to risk situations such as surgery or trauma, regardless of the history of thrombosis. Pregnant females with isolated protein S deficiency have a lower risk of thrombosis than those with AT-III or protein C deficiency.[62] Most clinicians nonetheless prefer to give prophylaxis to pregnant patients in the same fashion as for patients with protein C deficiency.[53]

Liver disease, DIC, nephrotic syndrome, and pregnancy have all been associated with low protein S levels and are all seen in patients with acquired protein S deficiency. Drug-induced reductions in protein S levels may occur during treatment with oral anticoagulants, oral contraceptives,[74,75] estrogens, and L-asparaginase. The C4b binding protein that complexes with protein S is an acute phase reactant; therefore levels will increase in acute inflammatory processes (e.g., postoperative states or infection). This may reduce levels of free (active) protein S, thereby partially explaining the high risk of thrombosis associated with these conditions.[29,57]

As with other inherited thrombotic disorders, effective management includes familial studies to identify those at risk for thrombosis. Counseling for affected patients is important, so that risk factors, such as obesity, oral contraceptive use, and comorbidities, can be avoided, and prophylactic use of anticoagulants can be started in clinical situations such as pregnancy and delivery and after surgery.

Other Inherited Hypercoagulable States

The miscellaneous causes of hypercoagulable states may be broadly grouped into impaired fibrinolysis, abnormal fibrinogen, or heparin cofactor II deficiency. Fibrinolysis is a complex process that is regulated by numerous proteins (Fig. 15.2). Abnormalities in the fibrinolytic system are common in patients with acute thrombosis but in this context are probably due to the disease and are unlikely to be the cause of the thrombosis. Inherited deficiency, dysfunction, and impaired release of plasminogen, t-PA, PAI-1, or factor XII have been reported[29,57,60] and occur in an autosomal-dominant pattern. Acute ethanol ingestion, drugs (e.g., oral contraceptives), other conditions (e.g., acute myocardial infarction, malignancy, or infection), or surgery may also alter fibrinolysis. The clinical presentation of thrombosis is similar to that of AT-III or protein C or S deficiency.[29,60] However, abnormalities in fibrinolysis appear to be much less important, since associated thrombosis is rare. An important therapeutic consideration in these patients is that abnormal plasminogen function or activation may preclude the use of thrombolytic agents.

Abnormal inherited fibrinogen defects may result in inadequate quantity or function, the latter condition being more common. Congenital fibrinogen disorders are clinically asymptomatic in most patients and more commonly cause bleeding rather than thrombosis when symptoms are seen.[57,60] Thrombosis is rare; when present, it is caused by the production of abnormal fibrinogen that is resistant to lysis by plasmin. Acquired quantitative abnormalities are more common than the inherited form. A low fibrinogen level is one of the hallmark signs of DIC and contributes to its associated bleeding. Accelerated fibrinogen consumption by thrombolytic drugs and decreased production in liver disease are other causes of fibrinogenemia.

Heparin cofactor II has a specific antithrombin effect (Fig. 15.1) that is accelerated by heparin, dermatan sulfate, and dextran. Inherited deficiency may manifest clinically as arterial or venous thrombosis; however, the vast majority of heparin cofactor II-deficient patients are asymptomatic. Low levels are also seen in DIC but not in nephrotic syndrome or acute venous thrombosis.

Hemophilia

The hereditary deficiencies of factor VIII (antihemophilic factor, AHF) or factor IX (plasma thromboplastin component, PTC, Christmas factor) procoagulant activity are known as the hemophilias. They occur in an estimated 10 to 25 males per 100,000 and are the most common congenital plasma coagulation defects. Hemophilia results in spontaneous or posttraumatic bleeding into muscles, joints, and body cavities.

A defect or absence of the procoagulant portion of factor VIII or factor IX causes hemophilia A and B, respectively. Both are X-linked recessive disorders that are clinically indistinguishable. Lack of either functional factor decreases the conversion of factor X to factor Xa, diminishing the coagulation response to vascular injury. The abnormality causes an increase in the aPTT with no changes in PT, bleeding time, or platelet count. Hemophilia A accounts for 80% of hemophilias.

Factor deficiency is not absolute in hemophilia. Factor VIII and factor IX procoagulant levels remain relatively constant in a patient and correspond to hemorrhagic frequency and severity. Factor VIII or factor IX levels of 100% correspond to factor VIII or factor IX activity of 1.0 U/mL. Factor VIII and factor IX levels in a normal person range from 50 to 200% (0.5 to 2.0 U/mL).

Although hemostasis occurs at 25 to 30% of normal factor VIII activity, most symptomatic patients with hemophilia A have factor VIII levels less than 5%. Patients with factor VIII levels less than 1% (0.01 U/mL) are classified as having severe hemophilia. They average two to four hemorrhagic episodes monthly that often occur without discernible trauma. Patients with factor VIII levels greater than 5% are considered to have mild hemophilia. These patients usually hemorrhage only after trauma or surgery. Spontaneous bleeding may occur occasionally, especially in joints that have been damaged by previously undertreated posttraumatic hemorrhage. Patients with factor VIII levels between 1 and 5% are considered to have moderate hemophilia, with manifestations between the two extremes. Most patients with hemophilia A have factor VIII levels less than 5%.

CLINICAL PRESENTATION AND DIAGNOSIS

The clinical hallmarks of hemophilia A and B are (1) lack of excessive hemorrhage from minor cuts or abrasions, owing to the normalcy of platelet function; (2) joint and muscle hemorrhages leading to the most difficult to treat and disabling long-term sequelae; (3) easy bruising; (4) prolonged and potentially fatal postoperative hemorrhage; and (5) a panoply of social, psychological, vocational, and economic problems.[76]

Hemarthrosis is the most common and often the most disabling manifestation of hemophilia. The joints that are most often involved include the knees, elbows, ankles, shoulders, hips, and wrists. The spine and hands are rarely involved.

An aura consisting of joint warmth and tingling often signals the onset of hemorrhage. Mild discomfort gives way to pain, swelling, erythema, and decreased range of motion over the next several hours. Young children often display guarding, irritability, and decreased movement in an affected joint. Classic symptoms in a reliable patient are a sufficient basis for immediate treatment.

Joint hemorrhage should be treated when the earliest symptoms appear to limit acute and prevent long-term sequelae. Within 8 to 12 hours of treatment, symptoms of hemarthrosis begin to resolve. Initial treatment with factor VIII or factor IX concentrate requires that levels be increased to 30 to 50%.[77] Maintenance at a level of 15 to 25% may be required for several days. Once bleeding has stopped, blood is resorbed, and the joint returns to normal over several days to weeks. Use of nonsteroidal anti-inflammatory agents for joint pain should be avoided because of their disruptive effects on platelet function.

Many hemophiliac patients develop "target joints" that bleed more often. Frequent and undertreated hemarthrosis leads to synovitis, hemophilic arthropathy, joint capsule fibrosis, and chronic loss of joint mobility.

Microscopic and macroscopic hematuria is a common problem among hemophiliac patients. Treatment usually includes bed rest, increased fluid intake, and corticosteroids.[78] Treatment with factor concentrate to elevate levels to 40% for 2 to 4 days is necessary if conservative treatment is unsuccessful. The use of ϵ-aminocaproic acid should be avoided, since decreasing clot lysis may prevent removal of a clot occluding the ureter.[79]

Spontaneous and posttraumatic hematomas are frequent complications of hemophilia. Although most are small and resolve spontaneously, large soft-tissue bleeding episodes may cause anemia and compartment syndromes with ischemic and neurologic complications. Large hematomas require treatment with factor concentrates to increase levels to 50 to 60% or more. Maintenance therapy for several days may be required to reduce rebleeding. Aggressive therapy can reduce the incidence of long-term complications, including pseudocysts, calcifications, and fibrosis.[77]

Spontaneous or posttraumatic intracranial bleeding accounts for 25% of deaths of hemophiliac patients. Patients who survive are often left with mental retardation, seizure disorders, or motor impairment.[80] Treatment of intracranial bleeding should be immediate and aggressive. Any patient with a history of head trauma and signs of head injury, including abrasions, lacerations, or scalp hematoma, should be treated. Factor VIII or factor IX concentrates should be given to increase and maintain the level to 100%.[75,76]

Minor lacerations are usually managed with conservative treatment. Factor replacement to raise the factor level to 30 to 50% is usually limited to minor lacerations that are unresponsive to conservative therapy or serious lacerations.

Falls, with mucosal lacerations to the mouth, are common among toddlers. Application of ice and pressure may be helpful but difficult to accomplish. Factor replacement to a level of 40 to 50% is often indicated. Supplementation with ϵ-aminocaproic acid or tranexamic acid may be advantageous. Temporary restriction of oral intake and repeated treatment may be required if clot dislodgment is a problem.[77]

Gastrointestinal bleeding, gingival bleeding, epistaxis, and other forms of bleeding occur less commonly.

TREATMENT

Currently available modes of treatment for hemophilia center on increasing the concentration of deficient clotting factors or inhibiting fibrinolysis. Products that are used to increase clotting factor concentration include FFP, cryoprecipitate, factor concentrates, and desmopressin (DDAVP). Antifibrinolytic agents include α-aminocaproic acid and tranexamic acid.

Fresh Frozen Plasma

FFP is the fluid portion of 1 unit of whole blood, taken from a single donor. It contains about 1 U of factor VIII and 1 U of factor IX per mL of plasma. One unit of FFP contains 200 to 300 U of both factors, a sufficient quantity to increase factor concentrations by 5 to 10% in a 60-kg man.[77] Because of the large amount of fluid that would be required, FFP is not the optimal means of factor replacement. However, it is a readily available source of clotting factors that can be used until a more advantageous source is available.

Cryoprecipitate

Cryoprecipitate is prepared by thawing FFP and removing the cell-free fluid remaining after centrifugation. The residual precipitate contains 40 to 50% of the original factor VIII concentration. Cryoprecipitate contains no factor IX. Although less volume would be required to restore hemostasis than with FFP, cryoprecipitate is not a primary means of hemophilia A treatment.

Factor VIII Replacement

Purified factor VIII is isolated from pooled plasma generated from thousands of donors. To decrease the risk of viral transmission, early lyophilized products were usually heat-treated to 60°C for 10 to 30 hours. This method was abandoned because of the continued reports of hepatitis and HIV. Current virucidal techniques include treating the concentrate with solvent/detergent to disrupt viral lipid coats, heat treatment to higher temperatures for longer time periods, pasteurization, and vapor heating.

Immunosuppression due to alloantigens or viruses in factor concentrates has been combated with the advent of highly purified factor concentrates. Purity refers to the amount of non–factor VIII proteins in the final product. Isolation by affinity chromatography with monoclonal antibody techniques produces high-purity concentrates. Although extraneous proteins are removed, increasing purity does not decrease the risk of viral transmission.

More recently, human factor VIII cDNA has been introduced into mammalian cell lines to produce recombinant factor VIII products that appear to be equivalent to plasma-derived concentrates. The obvious advantage of recombinant factor concentrate is the decreased risk of viral transmission compared with plasma-derived factors. Currently, no recombinant factor IX is available. It is recommended that all patients with hemophilia, regardless of previous exposure to HIV or hepatitis, should receive treatment with high-purity concentrates or recombinant concentrates with the lowest possible risk of viral transmission (Table 15.8). Cost, however, remains a factor since high purity and recombinant concentrates are more expensive.

The goal of factor replacement therapy is to achieve hemostasis by maintaining adequate levels of deficient factor. The level of clotting factor to achieve this goal depends on the indication for treatment.

Factor volume of distribution, baseline concentration, half-life, and the presence of inhibitors are four pharmacokinetic factors that influence the dose of factor replacement required.

Factor VIII distributes to plasma volume and initially to extravascular space. The volume of distribution is approximately 50 mL/kg. A simple dose calculation based on volume of distribution is that each unit of factor VIII (equal to the amount found in 1 mL of plasma) infused per kilogram of body weight yields a 2% increase in plasma level (0.02 U/mL).

$$\text{Dose in U/kg} = \frac{(\text{Desired concentration} - \text{baseline patient concentration})}{2}$$

The half-life of factor VIII is biphasic. The early redistribution phase half-life is approximately 4 hours, and

Table 15.8 ▪ Factor VIII Concentrates

Product	Viral Inactivation	Manufacturer
Humate-P	Heat-treated, wet method; pasteurized	Armour
Melate	Solvent-detergent inactivation	Melville Biologics
Profilate OSD	Solvent-detergent inactivated	Alpha Therapeutics
Profilate SD	Heat-treated, wet method; solvent-detergent inactivated	Alpha Therapeutics
High-purity		
Monoclate-P	Heat-treated, wet method; pasteurized, monoclonal antibody purified	Armour
Hemofil M, Method M	Solvent-detergent inactivated, monoclonal antibody purified	Hyland
Koate-HP	Solvent-detergent inactivated, gel filtration purified	Miles
Antihemophilic factor (human)	Solvent-detergent inactivated, monoclonal antibody purified	American Red Cross
Recombinant		
Recombinant		
Kogenate		

Source: American Hospital Formulary Service Drug Information, American Society of Hospital Pharmacists, Inc., 1994.

the biologic half-life is approximately 12 hours. Therefore, 12 hours after an infusion, the plasma concentration of factor VIII will decrease to one-half of its postinfusion concentration. Infusions of one-half the original dose given every 12 hours should restore the factor concentration to the desired level.

Factor IX Replacement

Because cryoprecipitate does not contain factor IX and DDAVP does not increase endogenous concentrations of factor IX, elevations in factor IX concentration are accomplished through infusions of either FFP or purified factor IX concentrates.

Prothrombin complex concentrates have been the mainstay of treatment for patients with hemophilia B. These concentrates contain not only factor IX, but also significant quantities of the other vitamin K-dependent clotting factors II, VII, and X. Although these agents are effective, they increase the risk of thrombosis, especially when used at high doses.[81]

Highly purified factor IX concentrates are now available, containing only trace quantities of factors II, VII, and X. These concentrates should decrease the risk of thrombosis and myocardial infarction. Although more costly, they are the preferred source of factor IX in the treatment of hemophilia B (Table 15.9).

Because the molecular size of factor IX is one-fifth that of factor VIII, the volume of distribution of factor IX is twice that of factor VIII. A simple dose calculation based on volume of distribution is that each unit of factor IX (equal to the amount found in 1 mL of plasma) infused per kg of body weight yields a 1% increase in plasma level (0.01 U/mL). The minimum hemostatic level is 10 to 25%, a range that is significantly lower than the estimated 30% minimum for factor VIII.

$$\text{Factor IX dose in U/kg} = \frac{(\text{Desired concentration} - \text{baseline patient concentration})}{2}$$

The biologic half-life of factor IX is approximately 24 hours. Because of the long half-life compared to that of factor VIII, subsequent doses of factor IX can be administered at a 24-hour dosing interval. Factor IX levels should be monitored every few days to ensure adequate concentrations.

Treatment Complications

Approximately 10 to 15% of patients with severe hemophilia A develop factor VIII inhibitors after repeated doses of factor concentrate. These inhibitors are IgG antibodies that bind to and inactivate factor VIII. Anti-factor VIII development (titers expressed as Bethesda units [BU]) follow two patterns. Low responders (3 to 5 BU) have low inhibitor titers that do not rise after further exposure to factor VIII. High responders (65 to 75% of patients with inhibitors) have low inhibitor titers that rise markedly with further exposure to factor VIII (anamnestic response).[82] Inhibitor titers usually rise 2 to 3 days after

Table 15.9 ▪ Factor IX Concentrates

Product	Viral Inactivation	Manufacturer
Factor IX complex		
Bebulin VH Immuno	Heat-treated, wet method	Immuno-US
Konyne 80	Heat-treated, dry method	Miles
Profilnine heat-treated	Heat-treated, wet method; organic solvent	Alpha Therapeutics
ProPlex T	Heat-treated, dry method	Baxter
Human		
AlphaNine SD	Solvent-detergent inactivated	Alpha Therapeutics
Mononine	Monoclonal antibody purified	Armour

Source: American Hospital Formulary Service Drug Information, American Society of Hospital Pharmacists, Inc., 1994.

exposure, reach a maximum in 7 to 21 days, then decline slowly. Inhibitors may persist for 1 to 2 years after exposure to factor VIII.

Options for treatment of patients producing inhibitors are to (1) administer sufficient quantities of human or porcine factor concentrate to overwhelm antibodies that are present with an excess to produce hemostasis, (2) restore hemostasis with factors other than factor VIII, and (3) remove antibodies by plasmapheresis or extracorporeal adsorption.

Human factor VIII can be used to treat hemorrhages in patients with low or high responses with inhibitor levels less than 5 BU and in patients with inhibitor levels between 5 and 30 BU after inhibitor removal. To neutralize inhibitors and achieve therapeutic hemostatic concentrations of 30 to 50%, an adult patient can be given an initial factor VIII bolus of 70 to 140 U/kg followed by an infusion of 4 to 14 U/kg/hr.[83] Alternatively, factor VIII can be given every 1 to 4 hours (40 U/kg BU + 20 U/kg/BU).[84] Factor VIII levels should be monitored regularly to ensure that therapeutic concentrations are maintained.

Cross-reactivity to porcine factor VIII is approximately 25%. After treatment with porcine factor VIII, antiporcine and antihuman factor VIII antibody concentrations rise, but less than is seen after the infusion of human factor VIII. Many patients who are unresponsive to human factor VIII respond to porcine factor VIII.[85]

When factor VIII inhibitor levels are too high (>30 BU), an attempt to bypass factor VIII can be initiated with factor IX concentrate. Two types of factor IX concentrates are available: unactivated factor IX, as is used for the treatment of hemophilia B, and activated concentrate, with higher concentrations of "factor VIII-bypassing material." The activated concentrates, Autoplex and FEIBA, are designed specifically to treat hemorrhages in patients with high factor VIII inhibitor concentrations. The efficacy of both types of factor IX is unpredictable. Infusion-induced hypercoagulability with resultant thromboembolic events is a possible complication.[84]

Inhibitors to factor IX occur in approximately 12% of patients with severe hemophilia B. Like factor VIII inhibitors, factor IX inhibitors are IgG antibodies. Treatment of patients with factor IX inhibitors is usually accomplished with factor IX concentrates. The role of immunosuppressive therapy is under investigation.

Infectious complications from viruses that are transmitted by transfusion were first noted in hemophiliac patients in the late 1970s. Nearly all patients who were treated with concentrates before the use of current viral inactivation methods have developed antibodies to hepatitis C and/or hepatitis B. Patients who develop chronic carrier states are at increased risk for chronic liver disease and hepatocellular carcinoma. Despite current virucidal methods, sporadic cases of hepatitis have been reported. Therefore all patients with newly diagnosed hemophilia should receive the hepatitis B virus vaccination. Infants with newly diagnosed hemophilia should receive the series of three injections beginning soon after birth.

HIV was introduced into the U.S. blood supply in the 1970s. By 1982, 50% of hemophiliac patients were infected with the virus.[86] Since that time the virucidal treatment of concentrates has virtually eliminated the risk of HIV due to factor transfusion.

Allergic reactions to factor concentrate are mild and uncommon. Patients who have had allergic reactions to cryoprecipitate usually do not react to concentrates. Large doses of factor VIII may cause hemolytic anemia in recipients with type A or B erythrocytes, owing to the presence of anti-A or anti-B antibodies in the concentrate. If RBC transfusion is necessary, type O cells should be given.

Desmopressin

DDAVP is a synthetic analog of the hormone vasopressin. Although its mechanism is unknown, DDAVP produces a 2- to 4-fold increase in factor VIII concentrations in most mild hemophiliac patients.[87] DDAVP does not increase production of factor VIII but stimulates the release of stored factor VIII. DDAVP does not increase the concentration of factor IX. Therefore, patients with severe hemophilia A or with hemophilia B do not benefit from this therapy.

To determine whether patients are responsive to DDAVP, a plasma factor concentration is obtained after an infusion. Testing for responsiveness is often conducted while a patient is asymptomatic. This prevents the decision to use more aggressive forms of therapy from being delayed while DDAVP response is being assessed. Most patients with mild hemophilia A and factor VIII levels greater than 10% respond to DDAVP.

For patients who are known to respond and who do not have life-threatening bleeding, DDAVP is the treatment of choice.[77] The recommended intravenous dose is 0.3 to 0.4 mg/kg, diluted in 50 mL of normal saline (10 mL for children weighing ≤10 kg) and infused over 15 to 30 minutes. DDAVP may be administered daily for 2 to 3 days, after which tachyphylaxis may develop.[88] DDAVP can be infused 30 minutes before a planned minor surgical procedure for prophylaxis. Blood pressure, fluids, electrolytes, and heart rate should be monitored in patients receiving DDAVP, because it may cause a slight pressor response and fluid retention. Seizures secondary to hyponatremia have also been reported.[89]

Antifibrinolytic Agents

α-Aminocaproic acid and tranexamic acid are antifibrinolytic agents that are used to help stabilize clots. Their primary role is as a single-dose prophylactic agent after dental procedures. α-Aminocaproic acid is administered orally as a loading dose of 200 mg/kg (maximum 10 g) followed by maintenance doses of 100 mg/kg every 6 hours (maximum 30 g over 24 hours) for 5 to 7 days.

Tranexamic acid is administered orally at 25 mg/kg every 6 to 8 hours for 5 to 7 days. The two agents are generally well tolerated, gastrointestinal complaints being the most reported complication.

Prophylaxis

Prophylactic factor VIII or factor IX infusions can eliminate or minimize most bleeding complications if therapy is initiated before joint disease.[90] Once joint disease is present, prophylactic therapy in preventing progression is unproven.[77] The expense and inconvenience of prophylactic regimens are also limiting factors.

FUTURE THERAPIES

The only documented cure for hemophilia to date is liver transplantation. One report describes liver transplants in four hemophiliac patients with end-stage liver disease. Of the three surviving patients, all had return of normal factor VIII production and resolution of hemophilia.[91] The cloning of genes for factor VIII and factor IX ("gene therapy") may be the most practical cure currently under investigation. Transplanting human fibroblasts transfected with a human factor IX gene into mice has been successful in producing circulating human factor IX.[92] Additional experiments are in progress.

Antiphospholipid Syndrome

The antiphospholipid syndrome (APS), an acquired defect in most instances, consists of two closely related but distinct clinical syndromes: (1) the lupus anticoagulant syndrome (LAS) and (2) the anticardiolipin antibody syndrome (ACLAS).[92,93] Although the two are similar, there are distinct clinical, laboratory, and biochemical differences, especially regarding prevalence, cause, possible mechanisms, clinical presentation, laboratory diagnosis, and management. ACLAS is five times more common than LAS.[93–95] Both syndromes may be associated with arterial and venous thrombosis, fetal wastage, and thrombocytopenia in descending order of prevalence. However, ACLAS is commonly associated with both arterial and venous thrombosis, including typical DVT and PE, premature coronary and cerebrovascular disease, and retinal vascular disease. LAS, although sometimes associated with arterial disease, is more commonly associated with venous thrombosis. Also, patients with ACLAS develop more predictable types of thrombosis than do those with LAS, and management of thrombotic problems differs between the two syndromes. APS might be the most commonly acquired defect seen with thrombosis, with the lower leg being the most prevalent site.[96] Although both antiphospholipid syndromes can be seen in association with SLE, other connective tissue and autoimmune disorders, malignancy, HIV infection, drug ingestion, and other medical conditions, most persons who develop either ACLAS or LAS are otherwise healthy and harbor no other underlying medical condition. These patients are classified as having primary instead of secondary APS.[93–95]

CLINICAL PRESENTATION AND DIAGNOSIS

Anticardiolipin antibodies are associated with many types of venous thrombosis including DVT of the upper extremities, intracranial veins, inferior vena cava, hepatic veins (Budd-Chiari syndrome), portal vein, renal vein, and retinal veins and PE.[93,97,98] Arterial thrombotic sites associated with anticardiolipin antibodies include the coronary arteries, carotid arteries, cerebral arteries, retinal arteries, subclavian or axillary arteries, brachial arteries, mesenteric arteries, peripheral (extremity) arteries, and both the proximal and distal aorta.[93,97] Anticardiolipin antibodies have been associated with premature or precocious coronary artery disease, early angioplasty (percutaneous transluminal coronary angioplasty) failure, and early and late coronary artery bypass graft occlusion.[99]

The neurologic syndromes associated with anticardiolipin antibodies have included transient ischemic attacks, small stroke syndrome, arterial and venous retinal occlusive disease, cerebral arterial and venous thrombosis, migraine headache, Degos disease, Sneddon syndrome, Guillain-Barré syndrome, chorea, seizures, and optic neuritis.[100–103]

Anticardiolipin antibodies are associated with a high chance of fetal wastage; the characteristics of this syndrome are frequent abortion, particularly in the first trimester; recurrent fetal wastage in the second and third trimesters; placental vasculitis; and, less commonly, maternal thrombocytopenia. Women harboring anticardiolipin antibodies have about a 50 to 75% chance of fetal wastage, and successful anticoagulant therapy can increase the chances of normal term delivery to about 80%.[104]

When testing for the anticardiolipin antibody the laboratory test to be performed is the enzyme-linked immunosorbent assay. In this test, look for the levels of IgG, IgM, and IgA isotypes in the presence of β_2-glycoprotein. Interpret these values as mildly, moderately, or markedly elevated for each individual antibody isotype. Most commonly the IgM isotype will be low in titer and transient with the IgG and IgA isotypes being high in titer and persistent. Tests to order when looking for lupus anticoagulant are aPTT, kaolin clotting time, and dilute Russell's viper venom time.[96]

TREATMENT

Even though treatment for these patients is not yet clearly defined, some trials have implemented long-term anticoagulation therapy with warfarin to prevent recurrent thrombosis. In these patients, the INR was between 2.5 and 4.0. It was also found that lower-dose warfarin with an INR between 2.0 to 3.0 and aspirin therapy alone did not adequately prevent recurring thrombosis.[105]

The optimal therapy for fetal wastage syndrome has not yet been defined. Based upon available reports, the use of low-dose aspirin in combination with low-dose porcine mucosal heparin (5000 to 7500 IU subcutaneously twice a day with the dose depending on total body weight and heparin levels)[104] and steroids[105] appears to be the most effective therapy for term delivery at present.[104] If fetal loss continues to occur despite this treatment regimen, IVIG may be indicated during future pregnancies.[105]

Immediately after conception, low-dose porcine mucosal heparin is added to the aspirin, and both are used to term.[104] Anticardiolipin antibodies are also associated with a unique postpartum syndrome of spiking fevers, pleuritic chest pain, dyspnea and pleural effusion, patchy pulmonary infiltrates, cardiomyopathy, and ventricular arrhythmias. This syndrome characteristically occurs 2 to 10 days postpartum. Because most patients with postpartum syndrome recover spontaneously, usually no therapy other than symptomatic treatment is needed.[93,97,106]

ANTIPHOSPHOLIPID SYNDROMES AND THROMBOCYTOPENIA

Thrombocytopenia is associated with both types of APS. Moderate to severe thrombocytopenia is common and occurs in 50% of patients with secondary APS; however, it occurs in less than 10% of those with primary APS.[93,95,97]

Pathophysiology

The autoimmune pathophysiology is thought to be platelet sensitization by antibody attached to surface phospholipids. A high correlation between IgA anticardiolipin antibodies and thrombocytopenia exists, although thrombocytopenia may accompany IgG and IgM antibodies as well. Regardless of the severity of the thrombocytopenia, thrombosis, not bleeding, remains the major clinical consequence.

Treatment

IVIG or plasma exchange may be beneficial as additive therapy to the standard management of the antiphospholipid syndrome in patients with severe thrombocytopenia and thrombosis.[93,95,97]

Summary

This chapter stresses the common hereditary and acquired coagulation disorders associated with thrombosis and hypercoagulability. The most common of the hereditary defects appears to be APCR and antithrombin and proteins C and S deficiency, and the most common acquired defects are the presence of anticardiolipin antibodies and the lupus anticoagulant (antiphospholipid antibodies). Therefore, these are the defects that should first be looked for in an individual with unexplained thrombosis.

The importance of finding these defects has significant implications for therapy of the individual patient and for institution of familial studies to identify, inform, and possibly treat others at risk.

Finally, a diagnosis of thrombosis is only a generic and partial diagnosis; the cause must be clearly defined. Only in this manner can cost-effective and appropriate therapy for both primary treatment and secondary prevention be initiated. Treatment options are summarized in Table 15.10.

KEY POINTS

- Normal hemostasis requires three responses: the vascular response (vasoconstriction), formation of a platelet plug (primary hemostatic mechanism), and the formation of a fibrin clot (secondary hemostatic mechanism).
- Immediately after tissue injury, platelets clump together to form a primary hemostatic plug through a series of the following overlapping phases: adhesion, aggregation, secretion, and elaboration of procoagulant activity.
- The extrinsic, intrinsic, and common pathways are components of the coagulation cascade, which results in the formation of thrombin. Thrombin and platelets form a clot, which acts as a plug to minimize further blood loss.
- Naturally occurring anticoagulation proteins inhibit the action of clotting factors in an attempt to control thrombosis, fibrinolysis, and inflammation.

Table 15.10 ▪ Treatment Options for Coagulation Disorders

Coagulation Disorder	Treatment
Thrombocytopenia	Correct underlying conditions Discontinue drug therapies known to cause thrombocytopenia Administer coagulation factors and platelets if indicated Offer supportive care of associated signs and symptoms
Acute autoimmune thrombocytopenic purpura	Treatment is controversial: No treatment due to self-limiting nature and low incidence of side effects, or Treat when platelet count $<20{,}000/mm^3$ with: Prednisone High-dose IVIG Anti-Rh(D) (WinRho)
Chronic autoimmune thrombocytopenic purpura	Prednisone ± azathioprine Splenectomy If refractory to the above treatments: Azathioprine Cyclophosphamide Colchicine Vincristine Danazole Cyclosporine Vinblastine Anti-Rh(D) (WinRho) Interferon-α Anti-Fc receptor monoclonal antibodies High-dose ascorbic acid
HIV-associated thrombocytopenia	Control underlying virus If symptoms from thrombocytopenia: Corticosteroids IVIG Splenectomy Anti-Rh(D) (WinRho)
Thrombotic thrombocytopenic purpura	Give simultaneously: Plasma infusion or exchange Splenectomy Corticosteroids Antiplatelet agents (aspirin, dipyridamole) IVIG Other options: Cytotoxic agents (vincristine) Other antiplatelet agents (prostacycline, sulfinpyrazone, dextran)
Platelet function disorders	Avoid situations that are associated with a high risk of bleeding Avoid medications that alter platelet function or numbers Treat underlying disorder Decrease in platelets after bypass surgery: Platelet transfusion Uremia-associated decrease in platelets: Desmopressin, conjugated estrogens
Drug-induced immune thrombocytopenia	Type I heparin-induced thrombocytopenia: Monitor platelet counts every 2–3 days Type 2 heparin-induced thrombocytopenia: Discontinue heparin immediately Give alternative anticoagulants: Dextran Aspirin Warfarin Lepirudin Danaparoid Thrombolytics (if needed)
Acute disseminated intravascular coagulation	Treat underlying disease Give supportive therapy for signs and symptoms Interrupt the coagulation process: Heparin LMWH

(continued)

Table 15.10 *(continued)*

Coagulation Disorder	Treatment
Acute disseminated intravascular coagulation *(continued)*	Replacement of depleted coagulation factors and platelets: FFP Protein C concentrate AT-III concentrate Platelets Cryoprecipitate Interruption of fibrinolysis: Fibrinolytic inhibitors: ϵ-aminocaproic acid or tranexamic acid + heparin Other therapies: Exchange transfusions (plasma exchange, plasmapheresis, leukopheresis, whole blood exchange) Investigational drugs (see text)
Chronic disseminated intravascular coagulation	Treat underlying disease Give supportive therapy for clinical manifestations Treatment: heparin Prophylaxis: heparin, aspirin, dipyridamole, Pentoxifylline
Antithrombin-III deficiency	Acute thromboembolism, prevention of thromboembolism during high-risk situations, and long-term prophylaxis after first thrombotic event: Heparin or LMWH + warfarin AT-III concentrate Warfarin (long-term management only)
Protein C deficiency	Neonatal purpura fulminans treatment and long-term management: FFP Factor VIII concentrate Protein C concentrate Warfarin (long-term management only) Acute thromboembolism, prevention of thromboembolism during high-risk situations, and long-term prophylaxis after first thrombotic event: Heparin or LMWH + warfarin (must have therapy with heparin or LMWH before starting warfarin) FFP, Protein C concentrate (prevention in high-risk situations only) Warfarin skin necrosis: Stop warfarin Heparin FFP Cryoprecipitate Vitamin K Protein C concentrate + heparin
Protein S deficiency	Acute thromboembolism, prevention of thromboembolism during high-risk situations, and long-term prophylaxis after first thrombotic event: Heparin LMWH FFP Factor IX concentrate Factor VIII concentrate Warfarin (long-term prophylaxis only)
Hemophilia	Products that increase clotting factors: FFP Cryoprecipitate Desmopressin Factor VIII concentrate Factor IX concentrate Antifibrinolytic agents: ϵ-Aminocaproic acid Tranexamic acid
Antiphospholipid syndrome	Acute thromboembolism, prevention of thromboembolism during high-risk situations, and long-term prophylaxis after first thrombotic event: Heparin LMWH Warfarin (long-term prophylaxis only) Heparin + low-dose aspirin + corticosteroids (to prevent fetal wastage) IVIG or plasma exchange (treatment of associated thrombocytopenia)

IVIG, immune globulin; *LMWH*, low-molecular-weight heparin; *FFP*, fresh frozen plasma; *AT-III*, antithrombin III.

- The fibrinolytic system dissolves and removes excess fibrin deposits to preserve vascular patency and restore blood flow. Fibrinolysis is mediated by the enzyme plasmin.
- Platelets are formed in the bone marrow. They have an average life span of 7 to 10 days, and younger platelets are more physiologically active than older ones.
- Thrombocytopenia is defined as a decrease in the number of blood platelets and is one of the most common causes of abnormal bleeding. A decrease in platelets may occur from (1) a decrease in production, (2) altered distribution [sequestration], or (3) increased destruction of platelets.
- AITP causes shortened platelet survival due to immune-mediated platelet destruction by antiplatelet autoantibodies of the IgG or IgM subtypes. There are two forms of AITP: acute, affecting previously healthy children, and chronic, affecting mainly women from 20 to 40 years of age.
- HIV associated thrombocytopenia is best treated by controlling the virus with antiretroviral and protease inhibitor medications.
- TTP is an uncommon disorder that causes widespread occlusion by platelets and hyaline material in the capillaries and arterioles (but not the venules) of nearly all organs, resulting in high mortality. The treatment of choice is plasma infusion or exchange.
- Platelet function disorders may cause bleeding or thrombosis independent of the platelet count and are commonly associated with uremia, cardiac bypass, liver disease, dysproteinemias, and myeloproliferative disorders. The underlying disorder should be corrected or treated when possible.
- Drug-induced platelet disorders include those that alter platelet function and those that cause thrombocytopenia by decreased production or increased destruction of platelets.
- Drug-induced immune thrombocytopenia can be caused by the formation of an immunoglobulin-drug immune complex that attaches to and destroys the platelet or the binding of the drug to the platelet membrane, creating a hapten that ultimately results in the formation of antiplatelet antibodies.
- Heparin causes two types of drug-induced thrombocytopenia. Type I is a mild, gradual thrombocytopenia that develops over the first few days of treatment and usually resolves spontaneously even with continued heparin treatment. Type II generally appears 5 to 14 days after therapy or sooner if the patient has been previously exposed and is thought to be caused by the formation of a platelet-associated IgG that reacts with heparin.
- DIC is an intermediary syndrome caused by a second coexisting disease, which results in the simultaneous in vivo activation of the coagulation and fibrinolytic systems causing both thrombosis and hemorrhage. The cornerstone of DIC management is treatment of the underlying disease that is the stimulus for DIC and supportive care for the signs and symptoms associated with the syndrome. Other treatments include interruption of the coagulation process, replacement of depleted coagulation factors and platelets, and interruption of fibrinolysis.
- Hypercoagulable states comprise a number of conditions (AT-III deficiency, protein C deficiency, protein S deficiency, and antiphospholipid syndrome) that share the common endpoint of inappropriate thrombus formation. Patients with these disorders are at higher risk for both venous and arterial thromboembolic disease. Disruption of coagulation may occur on an inherited (primary) or acquired (secondary) basis.
- Treatments for acute thromboembolism for patients with AT-III deficiency, protein C deficiency, protein S deficiency, or antiphospholipid syndrome are heparin or LMWH with or without warfarin. Patients with protein C deficiency should be given heparin or LMWH before warfarin is initiated.
- All patients with AT-III deficiency, protein C deficiency, protein S deficiency, or antiphospholipid syndrome should receive short-term prophylaxis before, during, and immediately after exposure to situations with a high risk of thrombosis, such as surgery, pregnancy, delivery, major trauma, and prolonged bed rest with heparin or LMWH with or without warfarin regardless of thromboembolic history.
- Because of the high risk of recurrence after the first episode of thromboembolism, prophylaxis against future events should be considered in patients with inherited AT-III deficiency, protein C deficiency, protein S deficiency, or antiphospholipid syndrome especially after a life-threatening or spontaneous thrombotic event. Patients should be advised about the risks and benefits of treatment. Warfarin is generally the drug of choice.
- Pregnancy increases the risk of thromboembolism in patients with inherited AT-III deficiency, protein C deficiency, protein S deficiency, or antiphospholipid syndrome. Therefore, patients who become pregnant should receive anticoagulation prophylaxis therapy with heparin or LMWH, regardless of thrombotic history.
- Oral contraceptives can increase the risk of thrombosis in patients with AT-III deficiency, protein C deficiency, or protein S deficiency and should be avoided.
- Warfarin-induced skin necrosis can occur in patients who have inherited protein C deficiency when large warfarin loading doses are given. It is caused by a transient hypercoagulable state that occurs because of the short half-life of protein C compared to that of the other vitamin K-dependent clotting factors. Other acute complications of protein C deficiency include neonatal purpura fulminans and acute thromboembolism.

- Miscellaneous causes of hypercoagulable states may be broadly grouped into impaired fibrinolysis, abnormal fibrinogen, or heparin cofactor II deficiency.
- Hemophilia results in spontaneous or posttraumatic bleeding into muscles, joints, and body cavities. There is generally a lack of excessive hemorrhage from minor cuts or abrasions, owing to the normalcy of platelet function. A defect in or absence of the procoagulant portion of factor VIII or factor IX causes hemophilia A and B, respectively. Joint hemorrhage is the most common and often most disabling manifestation of hemophilia and should be treated at the earliest manifestation of symptoms to limit acute and prevent long-term sequelae.
- APS is an acquired defect in most instances and consists of two closely related but distinct clinical syndromes: LAS and ACLAS. Both syndromes may be associated with arterial and venous thrombosis, fetal wastage, and thrombocytopenia. However, LAS is more commonly associated with venous thrombosis.

REFERENCES

1. Saito H. Normal hemostatic mechanisms. In: Ratnoff OD, Forbes CD, eds. Disorders of hemostasis. Philadelphia: WB Saunders, 1991:18–47.
2. Goebel RA. Thrombocytopenia. Emerg Med Clin North Am 11:445–464, 1993.
3. Comp PC. Production of plasma coagulation factors. In: Williams WJ, Beutler E, Erslev AJ, et al., eds. Hematology. 4th ed. New York: McGraw-Hill, 1990:1285–1294.
4. Rutherford CJ, Frenkel EP. Thrombocytopenia: issues in diagnosis and therapy. Med Clin North Am 78:555–575, 1994.
5. Blanchette VS, Kirby MA, Turner C. Role of intravenous immunoglobulin G in autoimmune hematologic disorders. Semin Hematol 29(3 Suppl 2):72–82, 1992.
6. Waters AH. Autoimmune thrombocytopenia: clinical aspects. Semin Hematol 29:18–25, 1992.
7. Blanchette VS, Luke B, Andrew M, et al. A prospective, randomized trial of high-dose intravenous immune globulin G therapy, oral prednisone therapy, and no therapy in childhood acute immune thrombocytopenic purpura. J Pediatr 123:989–995, 1993.
8. Blanchette V, Imbach P, Andrew M, et al. Randomised trial of intravenous immunoglobulin G, intravenous anti-D, and oral prednisone in childhood acute immune thrombocytopenic purpura. Lancet 344:703–707, 1994.
9. Collins PW, Newland AC. Treatment modalities of autoimmune blood disorders. Semin Hematol 29:64–74, 1992.
10. Warkentin TE, Kelton JG. Current concepts in the treatment of immune thrombocytopenia. Drugs 40:531–542, 1990.
11. Albayrak D, Islek I, Kalayci G, et al. Acute immune thrombocytopenic purpura: a comparative study of very high oral doses of methylprednisolone and intravenously administered immune globulin. J Pediatr 125(6 Part 1):1004–1007, 1994.
12. Imbach P. Immune thrombocytopenic purpura and intravenous immunoglobulin. Cancer 68(Suppl):1422–1425, 1991.
13. Imbach P, Berchtold W, Hirt A, et al. Intravenous immunoglobulin versus oral corticosteroids in acute immune thrombocytopenic purpura in childhood. Lancet 2:464–468, 1985.
14. Nabi. The revolutionary advantages of WinRho SDF™. 1999.
15. Naouri A, Feghali B, Chabal J, et al. Results of splenectomy for idiopathic thrombocytopenic purpura. Acta Haematol 89:200–203, 1993.
16. Schattner E, Bussel J. Mortality in immune thrombocytopenic purpura: report of seven cases and consideration of prognostic indicators. Am J Hematol 46:120–126, 1994.
17. Oksenhandler E, Bierling P, Farcet JP, et al. Response to therapy in 37 patients with HIV-related thrombocytopenic purpura. Br J Haematol 66:491–495, 1987.
18. Tertian G, Risler W, Lebras P, et al. Intravenous gammaglobulin treatment for thrombocytopenic purpura in patients with HIV infection. Eur J Hematol 39:180–181, 1987.
19. Rose M, Rowe JM, Eldor A. The changing course of thrombotic thrombocytopenic purpura and modern therapy. Blood Rev 7:94–103, 1993.
20. Dabrow MB, Wilkins JC. Hematologic emergencies. Postgrad Med 93:193–194, 197–199, 202, 1993.
21. Bennett JS, Kolodziej MA. Disorders of platelet function. Dis Mon 38:579–631, 1992.
22. Bick RL. Platelet function defects associated with hemorrhage or thrombosis. Med Clin North Am 78:577–607, 1994.
23. Salama A, Mueller-Eckhardt C. Immune-mediated blood cell dyscrasias related to drugs. Semin Hematol 29:54–63, 1992.
24. Schmitt BP, Adelman B. Heparin-associated thrombocytopenia: a critical review and pooled analysis. Am J Med Sci 305:208–215, 1993.
25. Chong BH. Heparin-induced thrombocytopenia. Aust NZ J Med 22:145–152, 1992.
26. Kelton JG. The clinical management of heparin-induced thrombocytopenia. Semin Hematol 36(Suppl 1):17–21, 1999.
27. Warkentin TE, Chong BH, Greinacher A. Heparin-induced thrombocytopenia: towards consensus. Thromb Haemost 19:1–7, 1998.
28. Bodensteiner DC, Doolittle GC. Adverse haematological complications of anticancer drugs. Drug Saf 8:213–224, 1993.
29. Nachman RL, Silverstein R. Hypercoagulable states. Ann Intern Med 119:819–827, 1993.
30. Isaacs C, Robert NJ, Bailey FA, et al. Randomized placebo-controlled study of recombinant human interleukin-11 to prevent chemotherapy-induced thrombocytopenia in patients with breast cancer receiving dose-intensive cyclophosphamide and doxorubicin. J Clin Oncol 15:3368–3377, 1997.
31. Gilbert JA, Scalzi RP. Disseminated intravascular coagulation. Emerg Med Clin North Am 11:465–480, 1993.
32. Bick RL. Disseminated intravascular coagulation: objective criteria for diagnosis and management. Med Clin North Am 78:511–543, 1994.
33. Rubin RN, Coleman RW. Disseminated intravascular coagulation: approach to treatment. Drugs 44:963–971, 1992.
34. Colman RW, Rubin RN. Disseminated intravascular coagulation due to malignancy. Semin Oncol 17:172–186, 1990.
35. Feinstein DI. Treatment of disseminated intravascular coagulation. Semin Thromb Hemost 14:351–362, 1988.
36. Sakuragawa N, Hasegawa H, Maki M, et al. Clinical evaluation of low-molecular-weight heparin (FR-860) on disseminated intravascular coagulation (DIC): a multicenter co-operative double-blind trial in comparison with heparin. Thromb Res 72:475–500, 1993.
37. Oguma Y, Sakuragawa N, Maki M, et al. Treatment of disseminated intravascular coagulation with low molecular weight heparin. Semin Thromb Hemost 16(Suppl):34–40, 1990.
38. Gillis S, Dann EJ, Eldor A. Low molecular weight heparin in the prophylaxis and treatment of disseminated intravascular coagulation in acute promyelocytic leukemia. Eur J Haematol 54:59–60, 1995.
39. Fourrier F, Chopin C, Huart JJ, et al. Double-blind, placebo-controlled trial of antithrombin III concentrates in septic shock with disseminated intravascular coagulation. Chest 104:882–888, 1993.
40. Vinazzer H. Therapeutic use of antithrombin III in shock and disseminated intravascular coagulation. Semin Thromb Hemost 15:347–352, 1989.
41. Hanada T, Abe T, Takita H. Antithrombin III concentrates for treatment of disseminated intravascular coagulation in children. Am J Pediatr Hematol Oncol 7:3–8, 1985.
42. Wisecarver JL, Haire WD. Disseminated intravascular coagulation with multiple arterial thromboses responding to antithrombin-III concentrate infusion. Thromb Res 54:709–717, 1989.
43. Rivard GE, David M, Farrell C, et al. Treatment of purpura fulminans in meningococcemia with protein C concentrate. J Pediatr 126:646–652, 1995.
44. Okajima K, Imamura H, Koga S, et al. Treatment of patients with disseminated intravascular coagulation by protein C. Am J Hematol 33:277–278, 1990.
45. Takada A, Takada Y, Mori T, et al. Prevention of severe bleeding by tranexamic in a patient with disseminated intravascular coagulation. Thromb Res 58:101–108, 1990.
46. Tamaki S, Hiyoyama K, Minamikawa K, et al. Treatment of disseminated intravascular coagulation with gabexate mesilate. Clin Ther 15:1076–1084, 1993.
47. Okamura T, Niho Y, Itoga T, et al. Treatment of disseminated intravascular coagulation and its prodromal stage with gabaxate mesilate (FOY): a multi-center trial. Acta Haematol 90:120–124, 1993.
48. Cofrancesco E, Boschetti C, Leonardi P, et al. Dermatan sulphate for the treatment of disseminated intravascular coagulation (DIC) in acute leukaemia: a randomised, heparin-controlled pilot study. Thromb Res 74:65–75, 1994.

49. Hassouna HI. Laboratory evaluation of hemostatic disorders. Hematol Oncol Clin North Am 7:1161–1249, 1993.
50. Menache D. Antithrombin III concentrates. Hematol Oncol Clin North Am 6:1115–1120, 1992.
51. Schwartz RS, Bauer KA, Rosenberg RD, et al. Clinical experience with antithrombin III concentrate in treatment of congenital and acquired deficiency of antithrombin. Am J Med 87(Suppl 3B):53S–60S, 1989.
52. Hathaway WE. Clinical aspects of antithrombin III deficiency. Semin Hematol 28:19–23, 1991.
53. De Stefano V, Leone G, Mastrangelo S, et al. Clinical manifestations and management of inherited thrombophilia: retrospective analysis and follow-up after diagnosis of 238 patients with congenital deficiency of antithrombin III, protein C, protein S. Thromb Haemost 72:352–358, 1994.
54. Menache D, O'Malley JP, Schorr JB, et al. Evaluation of the safety, recovery, half-life, and clinical efficacy of antithrombin III (human) in patients with hereditary antithrombin III deficiency. Blood 75:33–39, 1990; Makris M. Safety of antithrombin III concentrate. Blood 76:649–650, 1990.
55. Owen J. Antithrombin III replacement therapy in pregnancy. Semin Hematol 28:46–52, 1991.
56. Francis CW, Pellegrini VD Jr, Harris CM, et al. Prophylaxis of venous thrombosis following total hip and total knee replacement using antithrombin III and heparin. Semin Hematol 28:39–45, 1991.
57. Bick RL. Hypercoagulability and thrombosis. Med Clin North Am 78:635–665, 1994.
58. Briggs GG, Freeman RK, Yaffe SJ. Drugs in pregnancy and lactation. Baltimore: Williams & Wilkins, 1994:223c–229c.
59. Alving BM. The hypercoagulable states. Hosp Pract 28:109–114, 119–121, 1993.
60. Eby CS. A review of the hypercoagulable state. Hematol Oncol Clin North Am 7:1121–1142, 1993.
61. Pogliani EM, Parma M, Baragetti I, et al. L-Asparaginase in acute lymphoblastic leukemia treatment: the role of human antithrombin III concentrates in regulating the prothrombotic state induced by therapy. Acta Haematol 93:5–8, 1995.
62. Pabinger I, Schneider B, GTH Study Group on Natural Inhibitors. Thrombotic risk of women with hereditary antithrombin III-, protein C- and protein S-deficiency taking oral contraceptive medication. Thromb Haemost 71:548–552, 1994.
63. Dahlback B. Molecular genetics of venous thromboembolism. Ann Med 27:187–192, 1995.
64. Marlar RA, Montgomery RR, Broekmans AW, Working Party. Diagnosis and treatment of homozygous protein C deficiency. J Pediatr 114(4 Part 1):528–534, 1989.
65. Pescatore P, Horellou HM, Conard J, et al. Problems of oral anticoagulation in an adult with homozygous protein C deficiency and late onset of thrombosis. Thromb Haemost 69:311–315, 1993.
66. De Stefano V, Mastrangelo S, Schwarz HP, et al. Replacement therapy with a purified protein C concentrate during initiation of oral anticoagulation in severe protein C congenital deficiency. Thromb Haemost 70:247–249, 1993.
67. Broekmans AW, Bertina RM, Loeliger EA, et al. Protein C and the development of skin necrosis during anticoagulant therapy [Letter]. Thromb Haemost 49:251, 1983.
68. McGehee WG, Klotz TA, Epstein DJ, et al. Coumarin necrosis associated with hereditary protein C deficiency. Ann Intern Med 101:59–60, 1984.
69. Dreyfus M, Magny JF, Bridey F, et al. Treatment of homozygous protein C deficiency and neonatal purpura fulminans with a purified protein C concentrate. N Engl J Med 325:1565–1568, 1991.
70. Schramm W, Spannagl M, Bauer KA, et al. Treatment of coumarin-induced skin necrosis with a monoclonal antibody purified protein C concentrate. Arch Dermatol 129:753–756, 1993.
71. Marlar RA, Sills RH, Groncy PK, et al. Protein C survival during replacement therapy in homozygous protein C deficiency. Am J Hematol 41:24–31, 1992.
72. Gouault-Heilmann M, Leroy-Matheron C, Levent M. Inherited protein S deficiency: clinical manifestations and laboratory findings in 63 patients. Thromb Res 76:269–279, 1994.
73. Zoller B, Berntsdotter A, Garcia de Frutos P, et al. Resistance to activated protein C as an additional genetic risk factor in hereditary deficiency of protein S. Blood 85:3518–3523, 1995.
74. Heistinger M, Rumpl E, Illiasch H, et al. Cerebral sinus thrombosis in a patient with hereditary protein S deficiency: case report and review of the literature. Ann Hematol 64:105–109.
75. Hellgren M, Svensson PJ, Dahlback B. Resistance to activated protein C as a basis for venous thromboembolism associated with pregnancy and oral contraceptives. Am J Obstet Gynecol 173:210–213, 1995.
76. Brettler DB, Levine PH. Clinical manifestations and therapy of inherited coagulation factor deficiencies. In: Coleman RW, Hirsch J, Marder VJ, et al., eds. Hemostasis and thrombosis. 3rd ed. Philadelphia: JB Lippincott, 1994:169.
77. Furie B, Limentani SA, Rosenfield CG. A practical guide to the evaluation and treatment of hemophilia. Blood 84:3–9, 1994.
78. Rizza CR, Kenoff PB, Matthews JM, et al. A comparison of coagulation factor replacement with and without prednisolone in the treatment of haematuria in haemophilia and Christmas disease. Thromb Haemost 37:86–90, 1977.
79. Hilgartner MW. Intrarenal obstruction in hemophilia. Lancet 2:486, 1966.
80. Eyster ME, Gill FM, Blatt PM, et al. Central nervous system bleeding in hemophiliacs. Blood 51:1179–1188, 1978.
81. Abildgaard CF. Hazards of prothrombin complex concentrates in the treatment of hemophilia. N Engl J Med 304:670–671, 1981.
82. Feinstein DI. Acquired disorders of hemostasis. In: Coleman RW, Hirsch J, Marder VJ, et al, eds. Hemostasis and thrombosis. 3rd ed. Philadelphia: JB Lippincott, 1994:881.
83. Blatt PM, White GC, McMillan CW, et al. Treatment of antifactor VIII antibodies. Thromb Haemost 38:514–523, 1977.
84. Kasper CK. The therapy of factor VIII inhibitors. Prog Hemost Thromb 9:57–86, 1989.
85. Brettler DB, Forsberg AD, Levine PH, et al. The use of porcine factor VIII concentrate (hyate:C) in the treatment of patients with inhibitor antibodies to factor VIII. Arch Intern Med 149:1381–1385, 1989.
86. Eyster EM, Goedert JJ, Sarngadhanan MG, et al. Development and natural history of HTLV-III antibodies in persons with hemophilia. JAMA 253:2219–2223, 1985.
87. Mannucci PM, Ruggeri ZM, Pareti FI, et al. 1-Deamino-8-*d*-arginine vasopressin: a new pharmacologic approach to the management of hemophilia and von Willebrand's disease. Lancet 8:869–872, 1977.
88. Mannucci PM, Bettega D, Cattaneo M. Patterns of development of tachyphylaxis in patients with haemophilia and von Willebrand's disease after repeated doses of desmopressin (DDAVP). Br J Heamatol 82:87–93, 1992.
89. Weinstein RE, Bona RD, Altman AJ, et al. Severe hyponatremia after repeated intravenous administration of desmopressin. Am J Hematol 32:258–261, 1989.
90. Nilsson IM. Experience with prophylaxis in Sweden. Semin Hematol 30(Suppl 2):16–19, 1993.
91. Bontempo FA, Lewis JH, Gorenc TJ, et al. Liver transplantation in hemophilia. Blood 69:1721–1724, 1987.
92. Palmer TD, Thompson AR, Miller AD. Production of human factor IX in animals by genetically modified skin fibroblasts. Blood 73:438–445, 1989.
93. Bick RL. The antiphospholipid thrombosis syndromes: lupus anticoagulants and anticardiolipin antibodies. Adv Pathol Lab Med 8:391, 1995.
94. Bick RL, Baker WF. Anticardiolipin antibodies and thrombosis. Hematol Oncol Clin North Am 6:1287–1299, 1992.
95. Bick RL, Baker WF. The antiphospholipid and thrombosis syndromes. Med Clin North Am 78:667–684, 1994.
96. Devine DV, Brigden ML. The anti-phospholipid syndrome. When does the presence of antiphospholipid antibodies require therapy? Postgrad Med 99:105–122, 1996.
97. Bick RL. Antiphospholipid thrombosis syndromes: etiology, pathophysiology, diagnosis and management. Int J Hematol 65:193–213, 1997.
98. Oppenheimer S, Hoffbrand B. Optic neuritis and myelopathy in systemic lupus erythematosus. Can J Neurol Sci 13:129–132, 1986.
99. Bick RL, Ismail Y, Baker WF. Coagulation abnormalities in patients with precocious coronary artery thrombosis and patients with failing coronary artery bypass grafting and percutaneous transcoronary angioplasty. Semin Thromb Hemost 19:412–417, 1993.
100. Englert H, Hawkes C, Boey M. Dagos' disease: association with anticardiolipin antibodies and the lupus anticoagulant. Br Med J 289:576, 1984.
101. Frampton G, Winer JB, Cameron JS. Severe Guillain-Barre syndrome: an association with IgA anti-cardiolipin antibody in a series of 92 patients. J Neuroimmunol 19:133,139 1988.
102. Hinton RC. Neurological syndromes associated antiphospholipid antibodies. Semin Thromb Hemost 20:46–54, 1994.
103. Levine SR, Welch K. The spectrum of neurologic disease associated anticardiolipin antibodies. Arch Neurol 44:876–883, 1987.
104. Khamashta MA, Cuadrado MJ, Mujic F, et al. The management of thrombosis in the antiphospholipid-antibody syndrome. N Engl J Med 332: 993–997, 1995.
105. Harris JM, Abramson N. Evaluation of recurrent thrombosis and hypercoagulability. Am Fam Physician 56:1591–1595, 1997.
106. Bick RL, Laughlin HR, Cohen B, et al. Fetal wastage syndrome due to blood protein/platelet defects: results of prevalence studies and treatment outcome with low-dose heparin and low-dose aspirin. Clin Appl Thromb Hemost 1:286, 1995.

CHAPTER 16

ADRENOCORTICAL DYSFUNCTION AND CLINICAL USE OF STEROIDS

Anne M. Hoffmeister and Karen J. Tietze

Overview of the Adrenal Glands

ANATOMY AND PHYSIOLOGY

There are two adrenal glands in the human body, each located posteromedially and occasionally attached to the superior pole of each kidney. The adult adrenal is a pyramidal structure, 2 to 3 cm wide, 4 to 6 cm long, and about 1 cm thick. The adrenals are supplied with blood by 11 or 12 small arteries from the abdominal aorta and renal and phrenic arteries. Drainage of the adrenal gland occurs via the renal vein on the left and the inferior vena cava on the right.

The adrenal gland is composed of two physiologically distinct organs: the adrenal cortex (90% of the total gland) and the adrenal medulla (10% of the total gland). Histologically, the adrenal cortex is differentiated into

Table 16.1 ▪ Glucocorticoid and Mineralocorticoid Equivalencies

	Equivalent Dosage	Glucocorticoid Potency	Mineralocorticoid Potency	Plasma $t_{1/2}$ (min)	Biologic $t_{1/2}$ (hr)
Glucocorticoids					
Short acting					
Cortisone	25	0.8	2	30	8–12
Hydrocortisone	20	1	2	80–118	8–12
Intermediate acting					
Prednisone	5	4	1	60	18–36
Prednisolone	5	4	1	115–212	18–36
Triamcinolone	4	5	0	200+	18–36
Methylprednisolone	4	5	0	78–188	18–36
Long acting					
Dexamethasone	0.75	20–30	0	110–210	36–54
Betamethasone	0.6–0.75	25–30	0	300+	36–54
Mineralocorticoids					
Aldosterone	—	0.3	300	15–20	8–12
Fludrocortisone	2	15	150	200	18–36
Deoxycorticosterone	—	0	20	70	—

Source: References 2, 3.

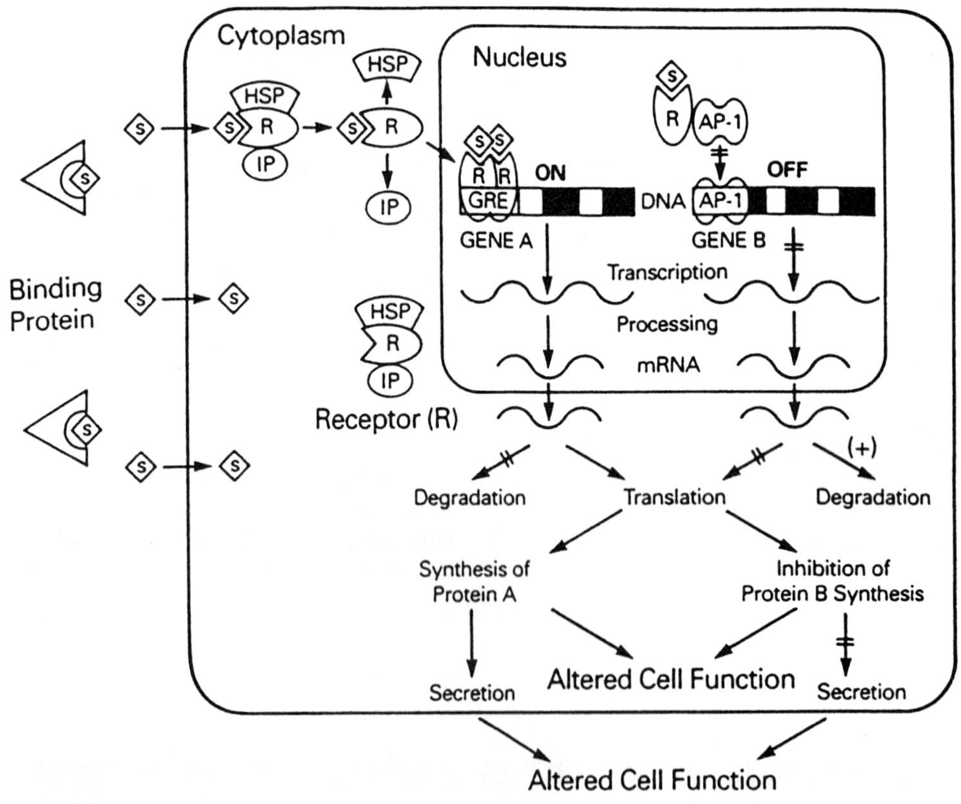

Figure 16.1. Mechanism of glucocorticoid action. Steroid hormone *(S)* circulates as a free molecule or as a complex with plasma-binding protein. After the steroid enters the cell, it binds to receptors *(R)* that reside in the cytosol complexed to heat-shock protein *(HSP)* and immunophilin *(IP)*. Binding of the ligand to the complex causes dissociation of HSP and IP. The receptor ligand is translocated into the nucleus, where it binds at or near the 5′-flanking DNA sequences of certain genes (glucocorticoid-responsive elements *[GRE]*). Receptor binding to the regulatory sequences of the responsive genes increases or decreases their expression. In the first instance *(ON)*, glucocorticoids increase the transcription or stability of messenger RNA, which is translated on ribosomes to the designated protein. In the second instance *(OFF)*, glucocorticoids repress *(cross-hatched arrows)* certain genes at the transcriptional level by interacting with and preventing the binding of nuclear factors required for activation of the gene (for example, activator protein *(AP)*-1 nuclear factor). In other instances, glucocorticoids exert their effects posttranscriptionally by either increasing the degradation of messenger RNA or inhibiting the synthesis or secretion of the protein. (Reprinted with permission from Chrousos GP. Mechanism of action. In: Boumpas DT, moderator. Glucocorticoid therapy for immune-mediated disease: basic and clinical correlates. Ann Intern Med 119:1198–1208, 1993.)

three separate zones: the zona glomerulosa, the zona fasciculata, and the zona reticularis. Functionally, the adrenal gland consists of two zones. The outer zone (glomerulosa) produces aldosterone. The inner zones (fasciculata/reticularis) produce androgens and cortisol. The principal glucocorticoid, cortisol, is secreted at a rate of 15 to 30 mg/day but can be as high as 200 to 500 mg/day when the patient is stressed.[1] The adrenal medulla is responsible for the secretion of catecholamines. Aldosterone is the principal mineralocorticoid; other adrenal steroids with some mineralocorticoid activity include cortisol, corticosterone, and deoxycorticosterone. Aldosterone normally is secreted at a rate of 40 to 160 μg/day. Sodium depletion or hyperreninism may cause the production rate to increase tenfold or more.

Although the name *glucocorticoid* is derived from the carbohydrate metabolic effects, glucocorticoids affect every system of the body. The physiologic actions of glucocorticoids include effects on glycogen metabolism, gluconeogenesis, peripheral glucose use, lipid metabolism, fluid and electrolyte homeostasis, and immunologic, bone, neuropsychiatric, gastrointestinal, and developmental processes.

Corticosteroids have mineralocorticoid and/or glucocorticoid activity (Table 16.1). Mineralocorticoids enhance the reabsorption of sodium and water from the distal tubule of the kidney and increase urinary potassium and hydrogen ion excretion. Glucocorticoids regulate cellular transcription, mitochondrial function, and membrane receptor activity.[4] Glucocorticoids affect nearly every inflammatory cell in the body and block the synthesis and release of multiple damaging mediators.[5]

Glucocorticoids inhibit or induce the secretion of end-effector proteins by regulating cellular transcription (Fig. 16.1).[3] Glucocorticoids circulate in the blood free or bound to cortisol-binding globulin (CBG). Free glucocorticoid diffuses through plasma membranes and binds with specific cytoplasmic receptors to form ligand–receptor complexes. The ligand–receptor complex undergoes a conformational change, translocates into the nucleus, and binds to specific elements within the DNA. The bound complex modulates the transcription of specific genes, resulting in either the production of end-effector proteins or the inhibition of specific proteins.

Glucocorticoids have a direct or indirect effect on circulating lymphocytes, eosinophils, neutrophils, macrophages, monocytes, mast cells, and basophils. Glucocorticoids interfere with arachidonic metabolism, reduce microvascular leakage, inhibit cytokine production and secretion, and increase the responsiveness of β-adrenergic receptors.[5] Low dosages inhibit lymphocyte movement and cellular immune responses; high dosages suppress leukocyte function and humoral immune response.

Hypothalamus–Pituitary–Adrenal Axis

The three major components of the axis function as an integrated feedback system (Fig. 16.2). Corticotropin-releasing hormone (CRH) is released from the hypothalamus in response to a variety of stimulants, including neurotransmitters, vasopressin, and catecholamines.[6] Adrenocorticotropic hormone (ACTH), the anterior pituitary hormone, is released into the systemic circulation in response to stimulation by CRH. ACTH simulates the adrenal cortex to produce cortisol. As serum cortisol levels increase, the biosynthesis and secretion of CRH and ACTH decrease in a classic negative feedback mechanism.

Circadian Rhythm

Circadian rhythms, synchronized to solar cycles and normally a reflection of sleep–wake patterns, influence the hypothalamus–pituitary–adrenal (HPA) axis.[7,8] ACTH, secreted in brief episodic bursts, cause sharp rises in the plasma concentrations of ACTH and cortisol (Fig. 16.3).[1] ACTH concentration peaks before and after awakening, declines throughout the morning, and is lowest in the evening.[9] Consequently, plasma cortisol concentrations peak at awakening (275 to 555 nmol/L, or 10 to 20 μg/dL), decline in the late afternoon and evening, and nadir an

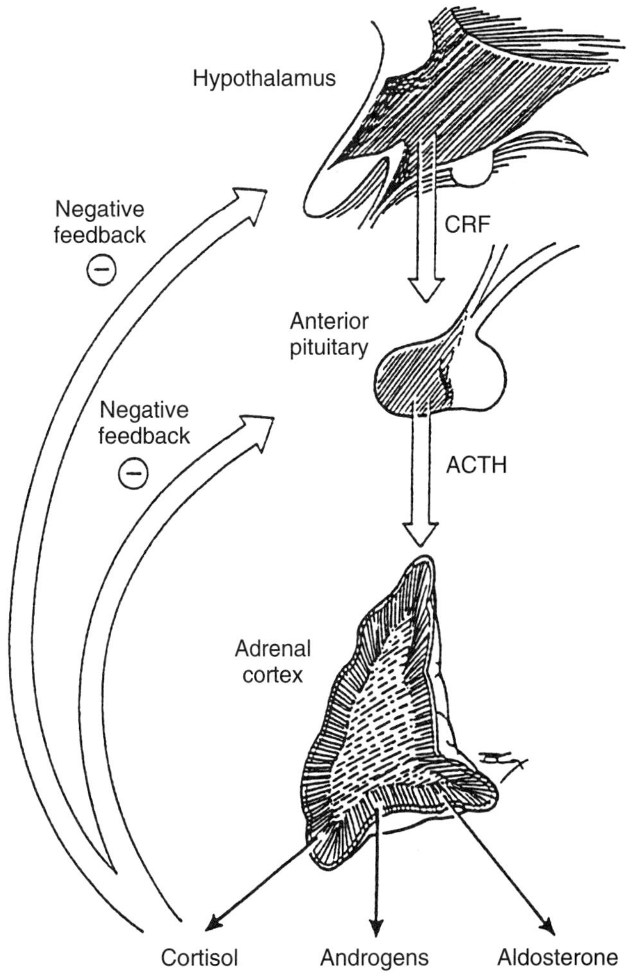

Figure 16.2. Normal function of the hypothalamus–pituitary–adrenal axis. Cortisol is synthesized in the adrenal cortex in response to adrenocorticotropic hormone *(ACTH)*, produced in the anterior pituitary. Pituitary release of ACTH is controlled by corticotropin-releasing hormone *(CRH)*, a hypothalamic peptide. (Reprinted with permission from Ackermann RJ. Adrenal disorders: know when to act and what tests to give. Geriatrics 49:32–37, 1994.)

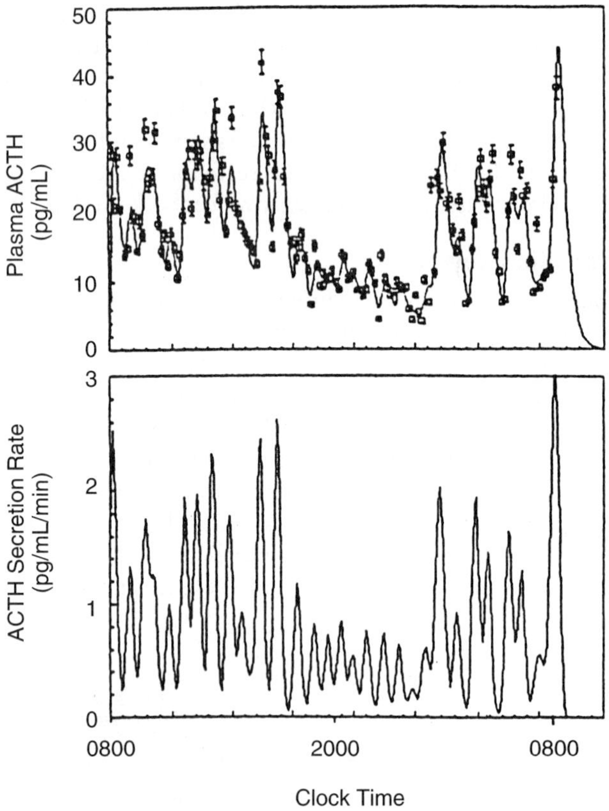

Figure 16.3. Pulse analysis of plasma ACTH sampled at 10-minute intervals for 24 hours. The upper panel shows the measured serial plasma ACTH concentrations *(boxes)*, the concentration-dependent standard deviation of the assay *(brackets)*, and the ACTH concentrations predicted by the deconvolution program *(solid line)*. The lower panel shows the computer-calculated ACTH secretion rate plotted as a function of time. (To convert pg/mL to pmol/L, multiply by 0.22.) Variation in the amplitude, not the frequency, of the pulses is responsible for the circadian rhythmicity of plasma ACTH concentration. (Reprinted with permission from Velduis JD, Iranmanesh A, Johnson ML, et al. Amplitude, but not frequency, modulation of adrenocorticotropin secretory bursts give rise to the nyctohemeral rhythm of the corticotropic axis in man. J Clin Endocrinol Metab 71:452–463, 1990. Copyright ©1990, by The Endocrine Society.)

hour or two after beginning sleep (less than 140 nmol/L, 5 μg/dL) (Fig. 16.4).[1,10]

Major factors controlling ACTH release include CRH, free cortisol plasma concentration, and the sleep–wake cycle. Additional secretory episodes of ACTH often occur during lunch and sometimes dinner, depending on the protein content.[11,12] Stress (pyrogens, surgery, hypoglycemia, exercise, severe emotional trauma) enhances ACTH

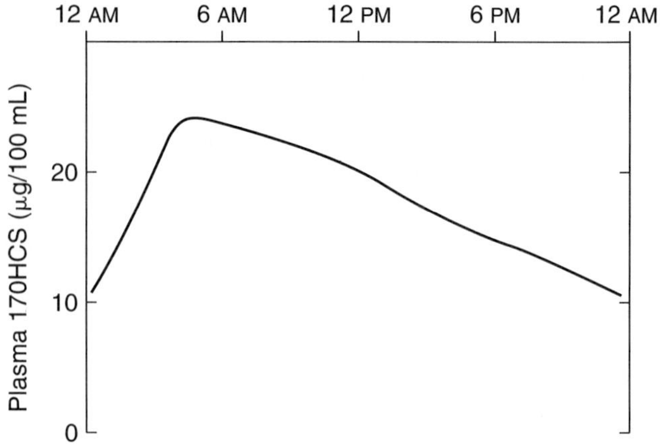

Figure 16.4. Diurnal variation in plasma cortisol. (Reprinted with permission from Pincus G, Nakao T, Tait JF, eds. Symposium on the dynamics of steroid hormones. New York: Academic Press, 1965:387.)

release and abolishes ACTH circadian rhythmicity. High-dose glucocorticoid administration suppresses stress-related ACTH release.

Cortisol Pharmacokinetics

Adrenocortical steroids are derived from endogenous and exogenous cholesterol (Fig. 16.5). Hepatic cytochrome P-450 enzymes are responsible for adrenal steroid conversion. Cortisol is produced via two cytochrome P-450–mediated hydroxylations at the 21-position, yielding 11-deoxycortisol, and at the 11-position, yielding cortisol. In physiologic concentration, 90 to 97% of circulating cortisol is protein bound. The major corticosteroid binding proteins include CBG (transcortin), testosterone-binding globulin, and albumin.[1] Cortisol and other steroids are also associated with erythrocytes; erythrocyte-associated cortisol exceeds albumin-bound or free cortisol.[13] Protein binding is not necessary for all steroid hormone transport. Protein-bound hormones act as reservoirs that prevent rapid fluctuations in free steroid concentration that occur with episodic cortisol secretions. Additionally, hormone-binding proteins may ensure uniform distribution to target tissues.[1] Cortisol undergoes extensive hepatic metabolism; cortisol metabolites are eliminated by glomerular filtration. The half-life of cortisol is 70 to 120 minutes, with less than 1% of unchanged cortisol excreted by the kidneys over 24 hours.

Cushing's Syndrome

DEFINITION

Cushing's syndrome, the constellation of clinical signs and symptoms resulting from chronic glucocorticoid excess, probably was first described by William Osler in 1899.[1] In 1912, Osler's colleague and friend, Harvey W. Cushing, reported on a 23-year-old woman with "painful obesity, hypertrichosis and amenorrhea" and postulated 20 years later that the "polyglandular syndrome" was caused by primary pituitary dysfunction.[14] The overall prevalence of Cushing's syndrome is difficult to estimate because of the widespread use of exogenous glucocorticoids.

TREATMENT GOALS: CUSHING'S SYNDROME

- Primarily, restore HPA function by eliminating glucocorticoid and mineralocorticoid excess.
- Reduce cortisol secretion to normal, eradicate tumors, and prevent dependency on medications.[15]
- With appropriate medical and/or surgical therapy, enable patients to live more normal lives.

EPIDEMIOLOGY

The overall incidence of spontaneous Cushing's syndrome is approximately two to four new cases per million per year.[16] ACTH-dependent Cushing's syndrome accounts for about 80% of endogenous cases. Primary pituitary ACTH hypersecretion, known as Cushing's disease, causes 70 to 80% of ACTH-dependent Cushing's syndrome cases; ectopic ACTH syndrome causes 10 to 20% of

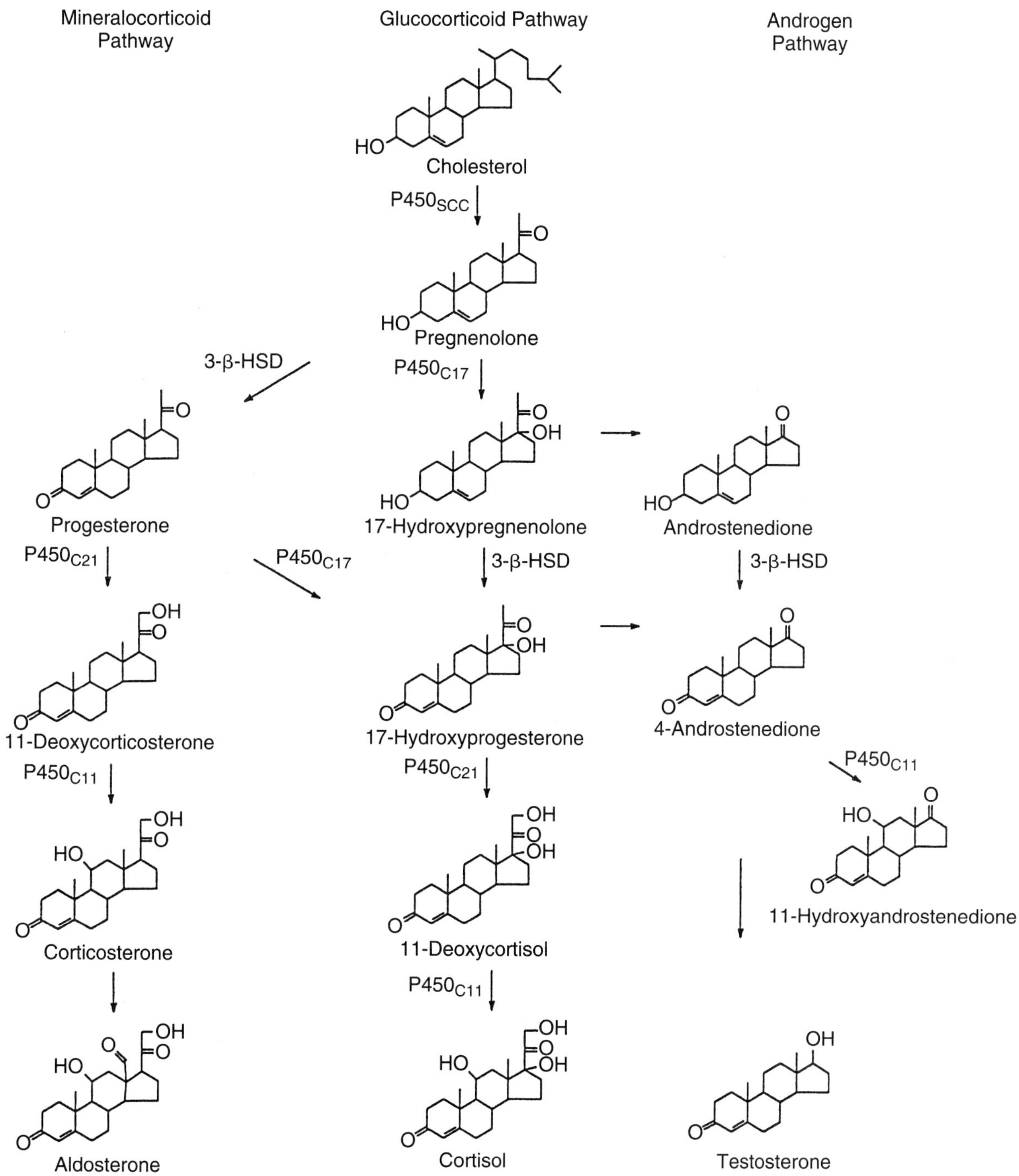

Figure 16.5. Biosynthetic pathways for adrenal steroid production; major pathways to mineralocorticoids, glucocorticoids, and androgens. *3-β-HSD,* 3-β-hydroxysteroid dehydrogenase; *$P450_{C11}$,* C11-hydroxylase; *$P450_{C17}$,* C17-hydroxylase; *$P450_{C21}$,* C21-hydroxylase; *$P450_{SCC}$,* cholesterol side chain cleavage enzyme.

cases.[17] Benign cortisol-secreting adenomas or adrenocortical carcinomas cause about 20% of endogenous cases. All other causes of Cushing's syndrome are rare. The incidence of exogenous Cushing's syndrome is increasing and far exceeds that of the endogenous forms.[18]

Gender distribution depends on the cause. Women are three to eight times more likely than men to develop Cushing's disease, approximately three times more likely to have either benign or malignant adrenal tumors, and four to five times more likely to have Cushing's syndrome associated with an adrenal tumor.[19] Ectopic ACTH secretion is more common in men, largely because of the higher incidence of lung cancer in men.[20]

PATHOPHYSIOLOGY

Cushing's syndrome is caused by prolonged exposure to excess glucocorticoids. Cushing's syndrome can be exogenous, resulting from chronic glucocorticoid or ACTH administration, or endogenous, resulting from increased cortisol or ACTH secretion. Endogenous Cushing's syndrome is caused by either excess ACTH secretion (ACTH-dependent) or autonomous cortisol hypersecretion (ACTH-independent).[1]

The three types of ACTH-independent Cushing's syndrome include primary adrenocortical adenomas and carcinomas, bilateral micronodular hyperplasia, and bilateral macronodular hyperplasia. The three types of ACTH-dependent Cushing's syndrome include primary pituitary ACTH hypersecretion (Cushing's disease), ectopic ACTH syndrome (nonpituitary secretion of ACTH), and ectopic CRH syndrome (ACTH hypersecretion caused by nonhypothalamic tumor CRH secretion). Pseudo-Cushing's syndrome, a nonendocrine disorder characterized by some of the clinical and biochemical manifestations of Cushing's syndrome, is associated with major depressive disorders and alcoholism.

CLINICAL PRESENTATION AND DIAGNOSIS

Signs and Symptoms

The clinical manifestations of Cushing's syndrome are insidious in onset and encompass multiple organ systems; none is pathognomonic (Table 16.2). Signs and symptoms depend on the degree and duration of hypercortisolism, the presence or absence of androgen excess, and additional tumor-related effects (adrenal carcinoma or ectopic ACTH syndrome).

Table 16.2 ▪ Clinical Signs and Symptoms of Cushing's Syndrome

General	Cardiovascular	Skin
Central obesity	Hypertension	Wide (>1 cm) striae
Facial plethora	Edema (ankle)	Spontaneous ecchymoses
Proximal muscle weakness	Congestive heart failure	Facial plethora
Headache		Hyperpigmentation
Abdominal pain		Acne
		Hirsutism
		Fungal skin infections
Endocrine and Metabolic		**Psychiatric**
Osteopenia, osteoporosis		Irritability, mild paranoia
Hypercalciuria and renal caliculi		Insomnia
Glucose intolerance, hyperinsulinemia, polyuria, polydipsia		
Menstrual disorders, decreased libido, impotence		
Elevated white blood cell count		

Source: References 1, 20.

General

Progressive obesity, the most common sign, usually is central, involving the face, neck, trunk, and abdomen, with the extremities spared. Facial fat accumulation produces moon facies, often accompanied by facial plethora. Fat pads that fill and bulge above the supraclavicular fossae are specific for Cushing's syndrome; an enlarged dorsocervical fat pad ("buffalo hump") accompanies major weight gain of any cause.[6] Weakness, usually associated with proximal muscle wasting, is caused by the catabolic effects of cortisol on muscle tissue; reduction in the arm muscle mass is most striking.[21] Those with severe disease may be unable to climb stairs, get up from a deep chair, or raise their arms long enough to comb their hair.

Cardiovascular

Moderate hypertension (diastolic blood pressure greater than 100 mm Hg) is common. Dependent edema is another sign of mineralocorticoid excess. Congestive heart failure has been reported in almost half of patients older than 40 years.[22]

Dermatologic

The skin is atrophic and fragile; there is loss of subcutaneous fat, allowing subcutaneous blood vessels to be seen. Loss of connective tissue results in easy bruisability. Striae, caused by stretched skin, appear purplish or reddish because the thin, transparent skin reveals the color of venous blood in the dermis. Striae, often more than 1 cm wide, appear most often on the breasts, hips, buttocks, upper abdomen, shoulders, and upper thighs and in the axillae. Androgen excess is manifested by oily facial skin, acne, and mild facial hirsutism. Thinning scalp hair is common. Oligomenorrhea in women, impotence in men, and decreased libido in both sexes are common.

Endocrine and Metabolic

Osteopenia and osteoporosis are caused by cortisol osteoblast inhibition[1]; back pain, vertebral compression fractures, pathologic rib fractures, and, less commonly, long bone fractures result. Hypercalcuria and renal caliculi may be present. Glucose intolerance and hyperinsulinemia are common. True diabetes mellitus occurs in less than 20% of patients, probably in those with a familial predisposition to this disorder; ketoacidosis is rare.

Psychological

More than half of patients with Cushing's syndrome experience psychological complications including emotional lability, agitated depression, loss of energy and libido, irritability, anxiety, panic attacks, and mild paranoia.[23–25] Most patients have increased appetite and weight gain. Insomnia is a common early symptom.

Other Signs and Symptoms

Phlebothrombosis and thromboembolic events may increase.[26] Glucocorticoids suppress immune function; infection occurs only with severe hypercortisolemia. Inflammatory and febrile responses are suppressed. Intraocular pressure is reversibly increased and aggravates preexisting glaucoma.

Laboratory Abnormalities

Packed red blood cell volume and hemoglobin concentration tend to be high normal. The total leukocyte count usually is normal but may be elevated. Half of all patients have a relative or absolute lymphopenia and one-third have eosinopenia. Hypercalcuria occurs in almost half of patients, but serum calcium and phosphorus are normal. Electrolyte levels are normal except in extreme hypercortisolism. Serum cholesterol and triglyceride concentrations often are elevated secondary to increased levels of very-low-density lipoprotein, low-density lipoprotein, and high-density lipoprotein. Clotting factors V and VIII and prothrombin may be elevated.[27]

Diagnosis

The diagnosis is based on recognition of multiple new signs and symptoms with documented endogenous hypercortisolism.[6] Further testing is required to determine the cause of the hypercortisolism. There is no current consensus on how best to confirm the diagnosis of Cushing's syndrome and define the cause; one typical scheme is shown in Figure 16.6.

Establishing Hypercortisolism

Urinary Free Cortisol

The 24-hour urinary free cortisol (UFC) excretion test is the best screening test for endogenous hypercortisolism.[18,28] At least two, preferably three consecutive 24-hour urine specimens are collected to minimize collection errors and hormonal secretion variability. Creatinine excretion is measured to assess adequacy of collection. Steroids, ACTH, CRH, adrenal enzyme inhibitors, and all other unnecessary medications should not be administered during collections. Basal UFC excretion more than three times the upper-normal limit (225 nmol, or 81 μg) indicates Cushing's syndrome.

Midnight Plasma or Salivary Cortisol

Midnight plasma samples are obtained on three consecutive evenings. The evening ACTH nadir is not preserved in patients with Cushing's syndrome. Consequently, a midnight plasma cortisol greater than 207 nmol/L (7.5 μg/dL) indicates Cushing's syndrome. Salivary cortisol concentration is a more accurate index of plasma free cortisol. Saliva is collected before brushing teeth twice daily (immediately after arising and just before retiring) for 3 days. Elevated evening salivary cortisol confirms the diagnosis of Cushing's syndrome.

Low-Dose Dexamethasone Suppression Test

Patients with Cushing's syndrome lack normal negative feedback cortisol regulation.[28] Dexamethasone does not cross-react in most radioimmunoassays for serum cortisol or UFC.[28,29] Suppression tests include the overnight (1 mg at 11 PM or 12 AM)[30] and the 2-day (0.5 mg every 6 hours for eight doses) low-dose dexamethasone suppression tests.[31] The overnight test is faster, but the 2-day test produces fewer false-positive results. In the overnight test, a single blood sample is drawn at 8 AM. Plasma cortisol greater than 138 nmol/L (5 μg/dL) indicates Cushing's syndrome. The 2-day test includes at least one 24-hour urine collection for cortisol metabolites and UFC. UFC greater than 28 μmol (10 μg)/24 hours or 17-hydroxycorticosteroid (OHCS) greater than 6.9 μmol (2.5 mg)/24 hours indicates Cushing's syndrome. Plasma ACTH is high normal or elevated in ectopic ACTH syndrome, normal in Cushing's disease, and undetectable in adrenal tumor.

Differential Diagnosis

Defining the precise cause of the Cushing's syndrome is essential to appropriate surgical management. Drug therapy is supportive and essentially the same regardless of the explicit diagnosis. Further diagnostic procedures are indicated when biochemical testing suggests the presence of specific lesions.

Basal Plasma Adrenocorticotropic Hormone Concentrations

Plasma ACTH concentrations are high in patients with ACTH-dependent Cushing's syndrome and low in patients with ACTH-independent Cushing's syndrome. At least two and preferably three plasma ACTH and cortisol concentrations are collected between midnight and 2 AM, but late afternoon samples are acceptable. Plasma cortisol greater than 415 nmol/L (15 μg/dL) and ACTH less than 1.1 pmol/L (5 pg/mL) indicate ACTH-independent cortisol secretion. Plasma cortisol greater than 415 nmol/L (15 μg/dL) and plasma ACTH greater than 3.3 pmol/L (15 pg/mL) indicate ACTH-dependent cortisol secretion.[1] Intermediate plasma ACTH values are less definitive but usually indicate that cortisol secretion is ACTH-dependent.

High-Dose Dexamethasone Suppression Test

Nonpituitary ACTH-independent Cushing's syndromes are not responsive to glucocorticoid negative feedback; pituitary ACTH-independent Cushing's syndrome is only slightly resistant.

Suppression tests include the standard (2 mg dexamethasone orally every 6 hours for 48 hours)[31] and the overnight (8 mg dexamethasone orally between 11 PM and

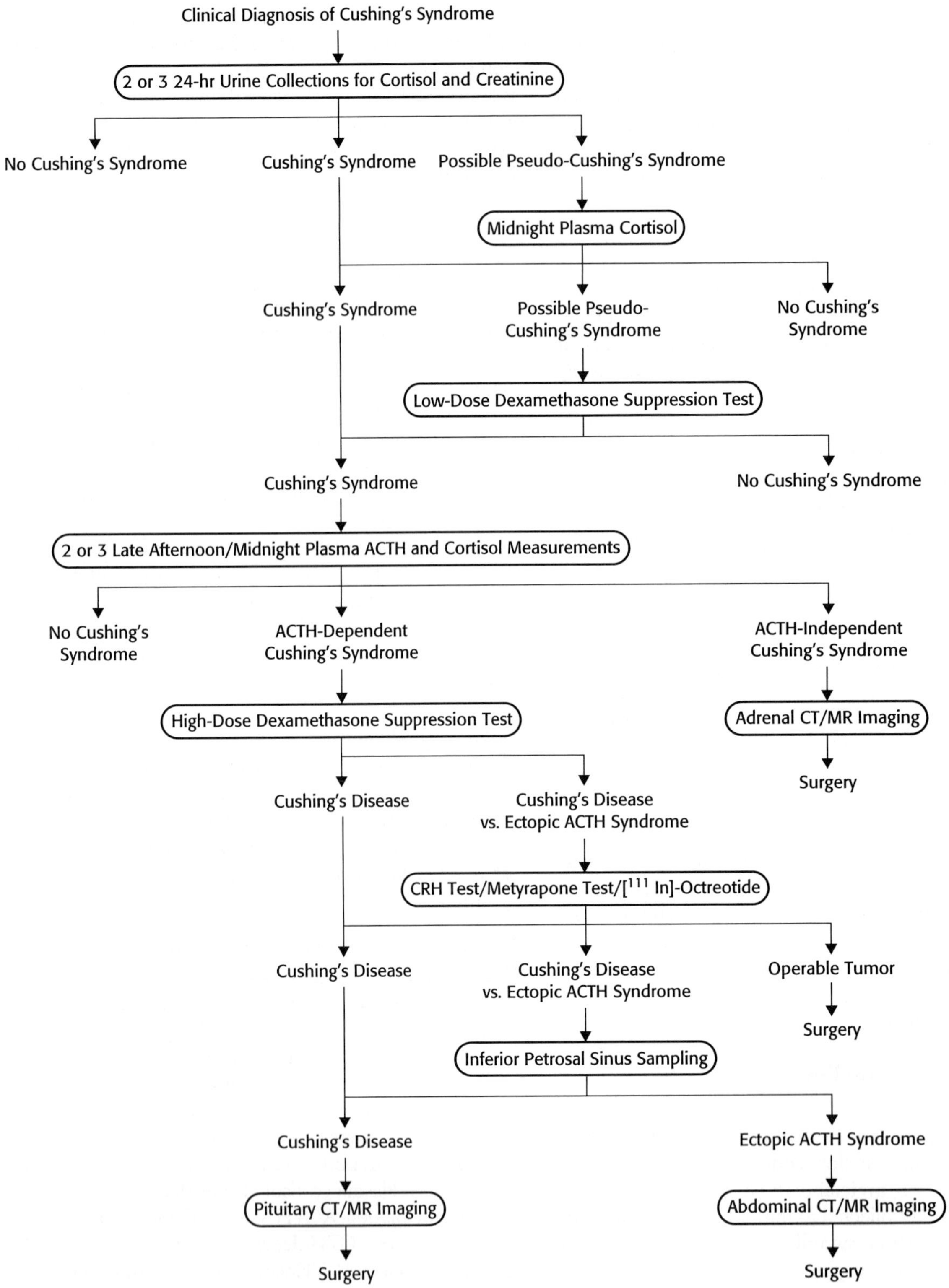

Figure 16.6. Algorithm for Cushing's syndrome. (Adapted with permission from Orth DN, Kovacs WJ. The adrenal cortex. In: Wilson JD, Foster DW, Kronenberg HM, et al. Williams textbook of endocrinology. 9th ed. Philadelphia: WB Saunders, 1998:517–664.)

12 AM)[32] high-dose dexamethasone suppression tests. In the standard test, at least one 24-hour urine specimen is collected throughout the duration of the test. Urinary 17-OHCS measurements less than 6.9 nmol (2.5 mg)/24 hours and UFC less than 14 nmol (5 mg)/24 hours suggest Cushing's disease. In the overnight test, a single blood sample is drawn at 8 AM the next morning. Plasma cortisol less than 140 nmol/L (5 μg/dL) suggests Cushing's disease.

Corticotropin-Releasing Hormone Stimulation Test

CRH stimulates ACTH secretion in patients with Cushing's disease but not ectopic ACTH-secreting tumors. An intravenous bolus dose (1 μg/kg body weight) of synthetic ovine CRH is injected. Blood samples for plasma ACTH and cortisol are obtained before and after CRH injection. Patients with Cushing's disease respond with an increase of 35% or more above basal plasma ACTH levels 10 to 15 minutes after CRH injection.[28] The plasma cortisol response is more variable.

The Metyrapone Test

Metyrapone blocks the synthesis of 11-deoxycortisol to cortisol at the level of the adrenal enzyme, 11β-hydroxylase, resulting in decreased circulating cortisol. Plasma 11-deoxycortisol increases in response to increased pituitary ACTH secretion; cortisol levels fall. Patients with Cushing's disease have a supranormal increase of plasma 11-deoxycortisol, whereas patients with ectopic ACTH-secreting tumors show little or no response and pituitary ACTH production is suppressed.[28]

^{111}In-Octreotide Scintigraphy

^{111}In-octreotide scintigraphy is a nonspecific test used to localize primary and metastatic neuroendocrine tumors. Tumors with neuroendocrine features (e.g., breast, brain, lymphoma) express receptors for somatostatin that are recognized by octreotide, a somatostatin analog. In patients with ACTH-dependent Cushing's syndrome, a single site of ^{111}In-octreotide uptake localizes the source of ectopic ACTH secretion. The exact location and size are determined by radiologic imaging.[1,20]

Radiologic Imaging

Adrenal adenomas (small, rounded, well-circumscribed unilateral masses) and carcinoma (larger than 5 cm, irregular, infiltrated masses) are distinguished by computed tomography (CT).[28] CT of the adrenals in patients with ACTH-dependent Cushing's syndrome shows bilaterally hyperplastic glands; 10 to 15% may also have nodular hyperplasia, and up to 30% of patients with proven Cushing's disease have normal adrenals.[28] CT of the chest and abdomen is indicated in patients with clinical and biochemical signs of ectopic ACTH production to identify the source.

Inferior Petrosal Sinus Catheterization

Inferior petrosal sinus catheterization (IPSC) determines the origin (pituitary versus ectopic) and lateralization (left versus right pituitary) of ACTH-secreting lesions. Catheters are placed into the left and right inferior petrosal venous system draining the pituitary gland. Blood is sampled simultaneously from both sides and in the periphery. The petrosal–peripheral gradient is greater than two or three in patients with a pituitary source. CRH administration during the procedure enhances the diagnostic accuracy.

PSYCHOSOCIAL ASPECTS

Cushing's syndrome is a potentially curable but life-threatening chronic disease. With appropriate medical or surgical therapy, patients with Cushing's syndrome can live nearly normal lives. Major depressive disorder is a severe and life-threatening complication of Cushing's syndrome. Psychiatric symptoms, ranging from anxiety to psychotic disturbances and cognitive impairment, may be present, though to a lesser degree than depression. A depressed mood has a profound influence on quality of life, how the patient experiences the disease process, and his or her interactions with others. Treatment to correct the hypercortisolism in Cushing's syndrome is more effective than antidepressant medication. The pharmacist must recognize and understand how these factors affect patients with Cushing's syndrome and work with patients to improve their quality of life.

TREATMENT

Pharmacotherapy

Pharmacotherapy of endogenous Cushing's syndrome is indicated to reduce cortisol production in preparing an extremely ill patient for surgery or maintain normal plasma cortisol levels while awaiting the full effects of surgical or radiation therapy or when severe physical or psychiatric consequences of hypercortisolism are present. Treatment of exogenous Cushing's syndrome consists of minimizing glucocorticoid or ACTH exposure.

Three types of drugs (steroidogenic inhibitors, neuromodulators of ACTH secretion, and glucocorticoid receptor antagonists) are used to treat Cushing's syndrome (Table 16.3).[33] Steroidogenic inhibitors, used almost exclusively to treat ACTH-dependent syndromes, are the most effective agents available for treating Cushing's syndrome. Results with neuromodulator agents have been disappointing.[34,35] Only one glucocorticoid receptor antagonist (mifepristone) is available.

Ketoconazole

Ketoconazole inhibits adrenocortical cytochrome P-450–dependent enzymes, thereby blocking the formation of pregnenolone and additional cortisol precursors. Ketoconazole is highly effective in lowering cortisol in patients with Cushing's syndrome.[33] Treatment is initiated with 200 mg orally every day and increased at 4- to 7-day intervals until UFC concentrations fall into the upper limits of normal (Table 16.3). Most studies report biochemical response with 600 to 800 mg/day. Antacids, histamine$_2$ antagonists, antisecretory agents, and sucralfate decrease the absorption of ketoconazole; coadministration should be separated by at least 2 hours. Isoniazid and rifampin decrease ketoconazole levels and should be avoided. Careful clinical monitoring, including serum drug levels when appropriate, is indicated when ketoconazole is coadministered with hepatically metabolized drugs including cyclosporine, warfarin, digoxin, and phenytoin.

Table 16.3 ▪ Cushing's Syndrome Medications

Medication	Dosage	Response Time	Hydrocortisone Replacement	Mechanism of Action	Major Adverse Effects
Ketoconazole	Initially: 800–1200 mg PO QD MD: 600–800 mg PO QD	4–6 wk	Not necessary	Inhibits cortisol synthesis	Nausea, vomiting, fatigue, pruritus, gynecomastia, hepatotoxicity
Metyrapone	Initially: 250 mg PO QD MD: Up to 1000 mg PO QID	Up to 4 mo	Necessary	Inhibits cortisol synthesis	Dizziness, sedation, rash, hirsutism, hypertension
Mitotane	Initially: 500 mg PO BID MD: 1000 mg PO QID	2 wk–6 mo	Necessary	Destruction of adrenocortical cells that secrete cortisol	Anorexia, nausea, vomiting, diarrhea, lethargy, impaired memory, hepatotoxicity
Aminoglutethimide	Initially: 250 mg PO QID MD: 500–2000 mg PO QD (divided QID)	Up to 4 mo	Necessary	Inhibits cortisol synthesis	Headache, sedation, dizziness, nausea, anorexia, rash, blood dyscrasias, tachycardia, hypotension
Bromocriptine	3.75–30 mg PO QD	4–6 wk	Not necessary	Inhibits ACTH secretion	Nausea, dry mouth, headaches, nasal congestion, postural hypotension
Cyproheptadine	Initially: 8 mg PO QD MD: Up to 24 mg PO QD	4–6 wk	Not necessary	Inhibits ACTH secretion	Somnolence, hyperphagia, weight gain, sedation

MD, maintenance dosage.

Metyrapone

Metyrapone is used to treat Cushing's syndrome when dose-limiting side effects occur with ketoconazole or as part of combination therapy with other steroidogenic inhibitors.[18,33,34] The initial dosage of metyrapone is 250 mg daily; dosages up to 2000 mg/day are well tolerated (Table 16.3). The incidence of side effects can be decreased with dosage reduction.[36] Metyrapone induces hepatic mixed-function oxidases; concurrent use of phenytoin or phenobarbital requires careful clinical monitoring.

Mitotane

Mitotane destroys adrenocortical-secreting cells and partially suppresses ACTH secretion.[37] Mitotane is most commonly used in conjunction with pituitary irradiation but may be used in combination with other steroidogenic inhibitors. Treatment is initiated with 500 mg twice daily and increased as required to normalize UFC concentrations (Table 16.3). Most patients (80 to 90%) respond to pituitary irradiation and do not require chronic mitotane therapy,[18] but mitotane accumulates in fatty tissues and persists in plasma for several months after discontinuation.[38] Glucocorticoid replacement therapy is initiated with mitotane after pituitary irradiation. Spironolactone may antagonize the effect of mitotane.[39]

Aminoglutethimide

Aminoglutethimide inhibits cortisol synthesis, but the effects are short-lived because of a compensatory rise in ACTH. The duration of effect is longer in patients with cortisol-secreting adenocarcinomas or when aminoglutethimide is used in combination with metyrapone or pituitary irradiation.[34,40] Treatment is initiated with 250 mg four times daily and increased as required to normalize UFC concentrations; dosages of less than 1 g/day usually are well tolerated (Table 16.3).[41] Requirements may increase with chronic therapy.[42]

Bromocriptine

Bromocriptine, a dopamine receptor agonist and prolactin inhibitor, has been used experimentally to induce a temporary remission of ACTH-dependent Cushing's syndrome.[43,44] Acute biochemical response to acute bromocriptine does not predict long-term efficacy.

Cyproheptadine

Cyproheptadine inhibits ACTH secretion by an antiserotonin effect on the hypothalamus. Data are limited. One study reported that treatment with 24 mg/day for at least 3 weeks was necessary to assess efficacy (Table 16.3).[45]

Other Pharmacotherapy

Valproic acid presumably enhances γ-aminobutyric acid (GABA) inhibition of hypothalamic CRH release by inhibiting GABA reuptake.[33] It is unclear whether valproic acid is useful in treating Cushing's syndrome. Several early reports documented valproic acid responsiveness, but subsequent placebo-controlled studies did not confirm the results.[33,46]

Octreotide is a long-acting somatostatin analog used primarily as an antisecretory agent. Octreotide has been reported to reduce ectopic ACTH secretion by some nonpituitary tumors.[47,48] Uptake of ^{111}In-octreotide predicts a positive response to the drug but has limited clinical value. Octreotide appears to have little role in treating Cushing's syndrome.

Mifepristone competitively binds to glucocorticoid receptors, blocking agonist-induced activation. Data about the use of mifepristone to treat Cushing's syndrome are limited.[49] In the largest study reported to date, dosages of mifepristone ranged from 5 to 22 mg/kg/day, and treatment durations varied from 4 weeks to 12 months.[50] Nausea was the most common side effect; two of three male patients developed gynecomastia and one male patient developed impotence. Additional studies are required to determine its place in therapy before routine use can be recommended.

Nonpharmacologic Therapy

Surgery

Transsphenoidal microadenomectomy is the surgery of choice for clearly circumscribed microdenomas.[6] With a cure rate of approximately 95%, this surgery preserves normal anterior pituitary function.[51] Most (85 to 90%) of the anterior pituitary is resected in the absence of a clearly identifiable microadenoma. Resection of nonpituitary ACTH- and CRH-secreting tumors is curative; however, most tumors are nonresectable[6] and the hypercortisolism is controlled with pharmacotherapy. Bilateral total surgical adrenalectomy is indicated for patients with bilateral micronodular or macronodular adrenal hyperplasia, with nonresectable ectopic tumors, when rapid hypercortisolism reduction is needed, or when all other therapies have failed. Unilateral adrenalectomy is indicated in patients with adrenal adenoma or carcinoma.[6]

Corticosteroid replacement therapy is indicated after successful transsphenoidal microadenomectomy, complete resection of an ACTH-secreting ectopic tumor, or unilateral or bilateral adrenalectomy. Corticosteroid replacement includes both glucocorticoids and mineralocorticoids.

Irradiation

Pituitary irradiation is indicated for treating Cushing's disease not cured by transsphenoidal surgery. Pituitary irradiation is curative in 15 to 65% of adults; another 25 to 30% sufficiently improve and require no additional therapy or only modest medical management.[1] Newer forms of radiotherapy, including computer-assisted linear accelerator (photon knife) or cobalt-60 (gamma knife) may be more effective, but experience is limited. Maximal benefits may not be observed until 12 to 18 months after pituitary irradiation. During this period, hypercortisolism is controlled with adrenal enzyme inhibitors. The combination of pituitary irradiation with drug therapy reduces serum cortisol concentrations rapidly and is more effective than pituitary irradiation alone.

Addison's Disease

DEFINITION

Addison's disease, also known as primary adrenal insufficiency, was first described in 1855 by Thomas Addison.[52] A rare disease primarily caused by autoimmune-mediated destruction of the adrenal cortex, the signs and symptoms of Addison's disease result from decreased production of glucocorticosteroids, mineralocorticoids, and sex hormones. The prevalence is estimated to be approximately 110 per million population, with an incidence of 5 to 6 per million per year.[53]

TREATMENT GOALS: ADDISON'S DISEASE

- Addison's disease is a potentially fatal disease for which there is no cure.
- The goal of therapy is to restore HPA hormonal balance by replacing glucocorticoids and mineralocorticoids.
- To accomplish this goal, patients must be taught how to manage chronic hormonal replacement therapy and intercurrent illnesses.

EPIDEMIOLOGY

Adrenal insufficiency is classified as primary, secondary, or tertiary. In Addison's disease the adrenal glands are destroyed by autoimmune, infectious, and other processes. Secondary and tertiary adrenal insufficiency are caused by other disorders that also lead to a decrease in adrenal hormonal secretion. Secondary adrenal insufficiency is caused by deficient pituitary ACTH secretion. Tertiary adrenal insufficiency is caused by deficient CRH or other ACTH secretagogues. Historically, tuberculosis was a common cause of Addison's disease. However, advances in preventing and treating tuberculosis have reduced the number of tuberculosis-associated Addison's disease cases. In 1995, Zelissen et al.[54] reported that 91.2% of patients had autoimmune-associated Addison's disease.

Addison's disease occurs as an isolated disorder or as one component of multiple coexisting endocrinopathies known as polyglandular autoimmune (PGA) syndromes.[55] As an isolated endocrine disorder, autoimmune adrenal insufficiency most commonly is first diagnosed in women in their third or fourth decade.

PATHOPHYSIOLOGY

All three zones of the adrenal glands are progressively destroyed and replaced by fibrotic tissue; the medulla is spared but may be atrophic. The onset of adrenal gland dysfunction may be gradual or sudden. Clinical signs and symptoms of adrenal insufficiency appear when 90% or more of the adrenal cortex is destroyed.[56] The zona glomerulosa is affected first, followed months to years later by zona fasciculata dysfunction. Acute adrenal gland hemorrhage or infection is associated with sudden and complete loss of adrenal function.

Autoantibodies are directed against adrenal cortex steroid-producing cells in autoimmune Addison's disease. Additional antibodies are found in PGA syndromes. Antibodies to at least three of the cytochrome P-450 enzymes involved in steroidogenesis, including 17α-hydroxylase, 21α-hydroxylase, and side-chain cleavage enzymes, have been identified.[57]

Several other mechanisms, including disseminated infection with *Mycobacterium tuberculosis*, histoplasmosis, and paracoccidioidomycosis; metastatic tumor; and acute hemorrhage associated with anticoagulation or meningococcemia, destroy the adrenal cortex. Adrenal metastases have been identified in 40 to 60% of patients with disseminated breast or lung cancer. Patients infected with the human immunodeficiency virus are at risk of Addison's disease on the basis of infection with cytomegalovirus, *Mycobacterium intracellulare avium* and cryptococcus, and metastatic Kaposi's sarcoma.[58] Drugs that interfere reversibly with steroidogenesis (aminoglutethimide, etomidate, ketoconazole, metyrapone, and mitotane)[59] or competitively inhibit glucocorticoid and progestogens (mifepristone) can cause Addison's disease. Rifampin, a potent inducer of hepatic enzymes, increases the metabolism of endogenous glucocorticoids and may precipitate an acute adrenal crisis.[60]

CLINICAL PRESENTATION AND DIAGNOSIS

Signs and Symptoms

Addison's disease has been called the "unforgiving master of non-specificity and disguise."[61] Addison's disease is considered when patients complain of persistent vague symptoms, especially in the presence of other autoimmune diseases, and when critically ill patients remain hypotensive despite maximal vasopressor therapy. The signs and symptoms range from vague, persistent feelings of unwellness to acute syncope and mental status changes (Table 16.4).[59,61] More than 90% of patients present with biochemical abnormalities including hyponatremia, hyperkalemia, hypoglycemia, azotemia, hypercalcemia, mild hyperchloremic metabolic acidosis, elevated blood urea nitrogen:creatinine, elevated aspartate transaminase, eosinophilia, lymphocytosis, neutropenia, anemia, and elevated erythrocyte sedimentation rate.[62] Serum cortisol and ACTH are unreliable markers of disease.

An adrenal crisis generally occurs in the setting of undiagnosed adrenal insufficiency and untreated stress. The signs and symptoms mimic septic shock and include profound anorexia with nausea and vomiting, severe dehydration, hypotension, shock unresponsive to pressors and inotropes, tachycardia, fever, hypoglycemia, progressively deteriorating mental status, and biochemical changes including hypoglycemia, hyponatremia, hyperkalemia, lymphocytosis, and eosinophilia.

Acute Addison's disease may occur in the setting of previously normal adrenal function or may be superimposed on chronic adrenal insufficiency. When acute Addison's disease occurs in isolation, patients are not hyperpigmented and serum sodium and potassium are normal. When an acute Addisonian crisis is superimposed on chronic adrenal insufficiency, dehydration, hyperpigmentation, hyponatremia, hyperkalemia, weight loss, and azotemia are present.

Diagnosis

Diagnosis begins with a high degree of clinical suspicion but depends on provocative testing of the HPA axis

Table 16.4 ▪ Clinical Signs and Symptoms of Addison's Disease

Glucocorticoid Deficiency	Mineralocorticoid Deficiency	Other
Fatigue	Dehydration	Hyperpigmentation
Lassitude, malaise	Hypotension	Salt craving
Weight loss	Orthostatic hypotension	Amenorrhea
Anorexia	↓ Cardiac output	↓ Libido
Nausea, vomiting, abdominal pain	↓ Catecholamine response	↓ Axillary and pubic hair
Diarrhea		Premature menopause
Steatorrhea		Multiple dental caries
Hypotension		Splenomegaly
Weakness, myalgias, arthralgias		Lymphoid hyperplasia
Depression		
Organic brain syndrome		
Psychosis		
Perceptual disturbances		
Electrocardiographic		
Changes secondary to hyperkalemia		
Radiologic		
Abdominal computed tomography: small, normal, enlarged adrenals (depending on the cause)		
Skull radiograph: enlarged sella turcica (chronic untreated or undertreated disease)		
Head computed tomography: enlarged pituitary		

Source: References 1, 59, 61.

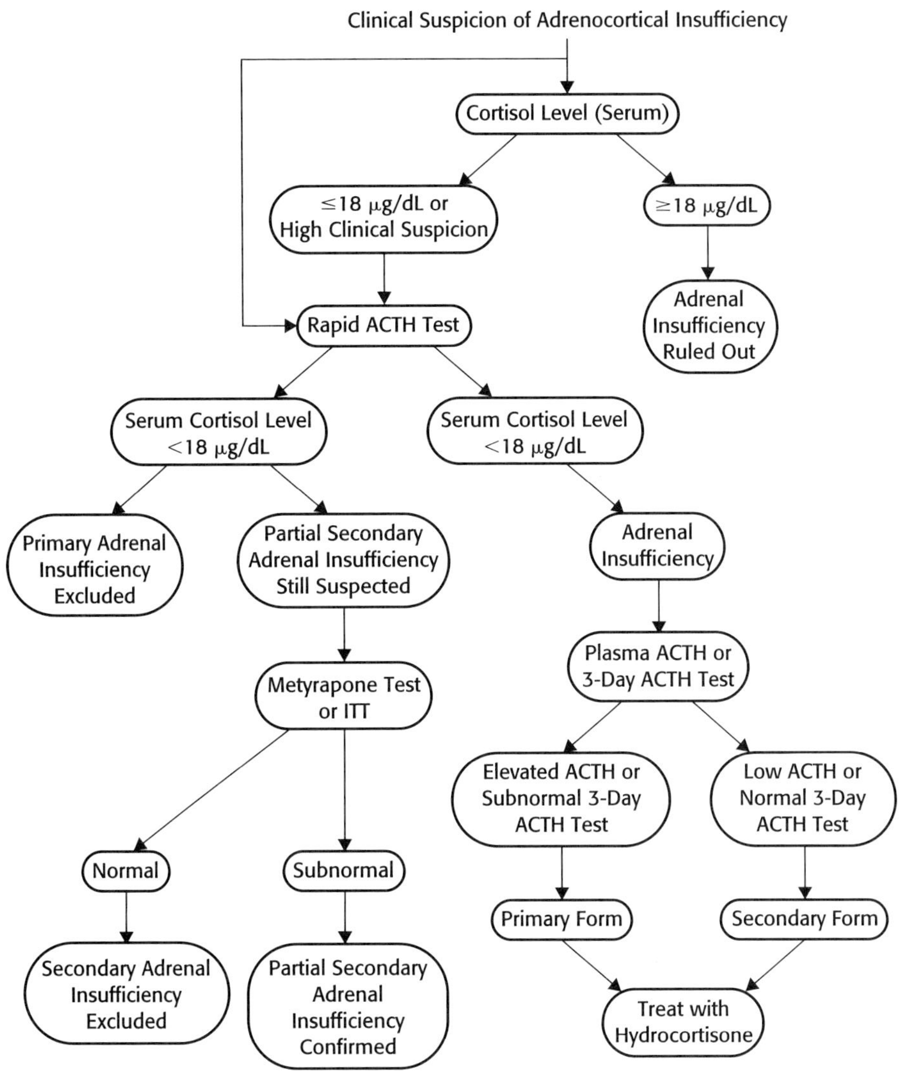

Figure 16.7. Algorithm for evaluating suspected adrenal insufficiency. (Adapted with permission from Chin R Jr, Zekan JM. Adrenal insufficiency. Probl Crit Care 4:312–324, 1990.)

(Figs. 16.2 and 16.7).[63] Initial screening tests for the cause of Addison's disease include complete blood count with differential, glucose, calcium, phosphorus, thyroid function tests, luteinizing hormone, and follicle-stimulating hormone. Tuberculosis and fungal disease are ruled out by chest radiograph, skin testing, and urinalysis. CT of the adrenals may reveal adrenal enlargement, atrophy, hemorrhage, or calcification.

Basal Serum Cortisol

Basal morning serum cortisol has some use but may be normal or nearly normal if partial adrenal function is preserved. Very low basal cortisol concentrations (less than 140 nmol/L, or 5 μg/dL) are consistent with adrenal dysfunction. Moderately low basal cortisol concentrations (less than 275 nmol/L, or 10 μg/dL) strongly suggest adrenal dysfunction. High basal cortisol serum concentrations (more than 550 nmol/L, or 20 μg/dL) rule out adrenal insufficiency. Twenty-four-hour UFC and cortisol metabolite assessment are more useful but inconvenient and susceptible to collection errors.

Short Adrenocorticotropic Hormone Test

Synthetic ACTH (cosyntropin; Cortrosyn) is used for the short ACTH and 3-day ACTH tests instead of human ACTH, which is allergenic. The short ACTH test can be conducted any time of the day and does not require fasting. Serum cortisol is measured before and 30 and 60 minutes after intramuscular or intravenous administration of 250 μg of cosyntropin; some clinicians prefer a single 45-minute cortisol sample. Addison's disease is ruled out if the 30-minute serum cortisol concentration is 500 nmol/L (18 μg/dL) or higher. The cosyntropin test does not distinguish between primary and secondary adrenal insufficiency and does not always predict the response to surgery, hypoglycemia, or other forms of stress.

Three-Day Adrenocorticotropic Hormone Test

The 3-day ACTH test distinguishes Addison's disease from secondary adrenal insufficiency and is more reliable than the short ACTH test. The adrenal glands require ACTH; prolonged deficiency causes a reversible inability to produce cortisol. ACTH 250 μg is infused over 8 hours on

3 consecutive days. Serum cortisol and 24-hour UFC are collected daily. In Addison's disease, serum cortisol is less than 553 nmol/L (20 μg/dL) and urinary 17-OHCS is low. In secondary adrenal insufficiency, serum cortisol is greater than 968 nmol/L (35 μg/dL) and urinary 17-OHCS is elevated by the end of the third day.

Metyrapone Test

Metyrapone blocks the synthesis of cortisol at the level of the adrenal enzyme 11β-hydroxylase, the final step in cortisol synthesis. The blockade causes a decrease in circulating cortisol and an increase in 11-deoxycortisol. The usual dosage is 300 mg/m^2 orally every 4 hours for 24 hours. A normal response is a decrease in serum cortisol to less than 277 nmol/L (10 μg/dL) and an increase in serum 11-deoxycortisol to more than 194 nmol/L (7 μg/dL). A subnormal response suggests primary or secondary adrenal insufficiency.

Insulin Tolerance Test

The insulin tolerance test (ITT), the most sensitive and accurate test of HPA axis function, is physiologically stressful and therefore contraindicated in patients with seizure disorders, cerebrovascular disease, and cardiovascular disease. Regular insulin is administered by continuous infusion until the patient has symptomatic hypoglycemia and a serum glucose less than 2.2 mmol/L (40 mg/dL). A normal response, defined as a plasma cortisol concentration greater than 497 mmol/L (18 mg/dL) at 60 to 90 minutes, rules out secondary adrenal insufficiency.

PSYCHOSOCIAL ASPECTS

Addison's disease is an incurable, potentially life-threatening disease. As with other serious chronic diseases, patients with Addison's disease must learn to live with the disease without letting it control their lives. With appropri-

Table 16.5 ▪ Treatment of Addison's Disease

Acute Adrenal Crisis
Establish intravenous access with a large-gauge needle.
Obtain blood for stat serum electrolytes, glucose, plasma cortisol, and ACTH.
Rapidly infuse 2–3 L 0.9% (154 mmol/L) sodium chloride or 5% (50 g/L) dextrose 0.9% (154 mmol/L) sodium chloride.
Inject 4 mg dexamethasone intravenously.
Chronic Replacement Therapy
Glucocorticoid: Dexamethasone 0.5 mg (0.25–0.75 mg) orally at bedtime; add hydrocortisone 5–10 mg orally midafternoon if indicated or hydrocortisone 15–20 mg orally on awakening and 5–10 mg orally midafternoon.
Mineralocorticoid: Fludrocortisone 0.1 mg (0.05–0.2 mg) orally daily.
Liberalize salt intake (unless concurrent essential hypertension).
Special Situations
Short-term minor stress or febrile illness
Double or triple the glucocorticoid dosage for 2–3 days; notify physician if illness persists.
Pregnancy
Maintain usual glucocorticoid and mineralocorticoid dosages; may need additional glucocorticoid during third trimester.
During labor, maintain saline hydration and give hydrocortisone 25 mg IV every 6 hr. Give hydrocortisone 100 mg every 6 hr if labor is prolonged.
Rapidly taper glucocorticoid to routine maintenance dosage over 3 days after delivery.
Emergency of severe stress or trauma
Give dexamethasone 4 mg IM immediately and get to emergency department as soon as possible.
Moderate stress
Increase hydrocortisone to 50 mg PO or IV twice daily; rapid taper to maintenance dosage when stress resolves.
Continue routine mineralocorticoid dosing.
Severe stress
Increase hydrocortisone to 100 mg IV every 8 hr; slowly taper to maintenance dosage when illness resolves.
Restart maintenance mineralocorticoid dosage when able to take oral medications.
Surgery
Give hydrocortisone 25 mg IM or IV at 6 PM and 12 AM the day before surgery.
Give hydrocortisone 100 mg IV during surgery.
Give hydrocortisone 100 mg IV every 8 hr the first postoperative day; rapidly taper to maintenance mineralocorticoid dosage.
Restart maintenance mineralocorticoid dosage when able to take oral medications.

Source: References 1, 59, 63, 68.

ate medical therapy, patients can live fairly normal lives. Patients with Addison's disease may present with or develop psychiatric symptoms, making it difficult to recognize secondary psychiatric complications such as reactive depression. Neuropsychiatric symptoms, including fatigue and depression, may occur if corticosteroid replacement therapy is tapered too quickly. The pharmacist must recognize and understand how these factors affect patients with Addison's disease and work with patients to improve their quality of life.

TREATMENT

Pharmacotherapy

Replacement glucocorticoid and mineralocorticoid drug therapy generally is continued indefinitely; some cases of subclinical autoimmune adrenal insufficiency may be self-limiting.[64] Supplemental glucocorticoid therapy is needed during periods of stress. Dexamethasone is the glucocorticoid of choice for patient-initiated rescue therapy, initial treatment of an adrenal crisis before the diagnosis is confirmed, and chronic replacement therapy. Dexamethasone does not interfere with serum cortisol measurements and has the advantage of prolonged ACTH suppression with minimal systemic glucocorticoid side effects.[65] Hydrocortisone, the intravenous drug of choice for the acute treatment of an Addison's crisis or for short-term parenteral use, has about 1% of the mineralocorticoid activity of aldosterone; large hydrocortisone dosages supply sufficient mineralocorticoid activity.[66]

Glucocorticoid dosage is titrated to relieve clinical signs and symptoms and normalize the morning plasma ACTH; hyperpigmentation may resolve with continued drug treatment. The mineralocorticoid dosage is titrated to relieve postural hypotension symptoms, normalize standing and sitting blood pressure, and normalize serum potassium and plasma renin activity. Atrial natriuretic peptide may be a useful adjunct to plasma renin activity when mineralocorticoid dosages are adjusted and may be a useful marker of excessive mineralocorticoid dosage.[67]

Acute Adrenal Crisis

Acute adrenal insufficiency is life-threatening. Empiric glucocorticoid replacement therapy and supportive therapy must be initiated before the diagnosis is confirmed or laboratory test results are available (Table 16.5). Mineralocorticoid deficiency is treated with saline and fluid loading; specific aldosterone replacement therapy is not necessary. Once the patient is stabilized, intravenous fluids are continued at a lower rate for 24 to 48 hours. Dexamethasone is replaced with hydrocortisone 100 mg every 8 hours once the diagnosis is confirmed; hydrocortisone is tapered to maintenance dosages after the precipitating illness resolves. Mineralocorticoid replacement therapy with fludrocortisone is started when the patient is stable and able to take oral medications.

Chronic Adrenal Insufficiency

Chronic replacement therapy consists of daily glucocorticoid and mineralocorticoid replacement therapy. Cortisol replacement (20 to 40 mg/day) is slightly higher than physiologic cortisol production. In the past, cortisone acetate was used for chronic replacement therapy twice daily to simulate normal circadian rhythms. However, this regimen causes fluctuating serum concentrations and transient adrenal insufficiency.[69] The current recommended regimen consists of dexamethasone 0.5 mg (0.25 to 0.75 mg) or prednisone 5 mg (2.5 to 7.5 mg) plus fludrocortisone 0.1 mg (0.05 to 0.2 mg) daily at bedtime. The dosages are based on clinical response. Patients who have drug-associated insomnia can take the drug upon arising. Supplemental hydrocortisone (5 to 10 mg) may be required.

Supplemental Stress-Dose Steroids

Patients physiologically stressed by acute medical illnesses or other trauma need supplemental steroids. Steroid supplementation is not needed for routine uncomplicated dental procedures, minor procedures performed with local anesthesia, or most radiologic procedures. If adrenal status is uncertain and time permits, adrenal cortical reserve can be assessed. For special situations, including short-term minor stress or febrile illnesses, pregnancy, emergency treatment of stress or trauma, and severe stress or febrile illness, refer to Table 16.5.

Nonpharmacologic Therapy

Nondrug therapy for normotensive patients consists of liberalizing the dietary salt intake. However, hypertensive patients should be maintained on salt-restricted diets; sodium-wasting diuretics and spironolactone must be avoided.

Clinical Use of Steroids

Corticosteroids, introduced into clinical practice in the late 1940s, are indicated for treating endocrine insufficiency diseases and virtually all immunologically mediated diseases. Marketed in numerous dosage forms, including oral, parenteral, topical, compartmental (i.e., intraarticular), and inhalational, corticosteroids have multiple effects on almost all cells involved in the inflammatory process. Mineralocorticoids are indicated as partial replacement for adrenocortical insufficiency in Addison's disease and for treatment of salt-losing adrenogenital syndromes.

PHARMACOKINETICS OF CORTICOSTEROIDS

Corticosteroid pharmacokinetics are complex and drug specific.[70] Oral bioavailability is high, ranging from nearly 100% with prednisone and methylprednisolone to about 70% with cortisol. The volume of distribution ranges from 0.5 L/kg with cortisol to 1.2 L/kg with dexamethasone and methylprednisolone. Corticosteroids are hepatically metabolized. Prednisone and cortisone are inactive until converted to prednisolone and cortisol, respectively. Prednisone, cortisol, methylprednisolone, and dexamethasone undergo extensive interconversion between active and inactive forms, reducing serum fluctuations and prolonging the half-life.

Corticosteroid receptor pharmacokinetics greatly influence the clinical response to corticosteroids.[71] Biologic activity depends on the corticosteroid–receptor interactions and activity of newly produced proteins. Corticosteroid–receptor interactions are influenced by receptor-binding affinity, corticosteroid–receptor association and disassociation rates, and corticosteroid–receptor complex half-life.[72] Limited corticosteroid–receptor pharmacokinetic data are available. Although lung receptor studies demonstrate clear differences among the corticosteroids, the clinical relevance is not known.

CORTICOSTEROID DOSING

Corticosteroid dosing depends on indication, route of administration, and acuity of disease. Physiologic or replacement dosages are indicated for deficiency diseases. Pharmacologic dosages are indicated for treating acute and chronic immune-mediated diseases such as acute organ transplant rejection. Corticosteroid dosages applied directly to a target tissues (skin, eyes, lungs, joints) are small compared to systemic dosages. To minimize toxicity, corticosteroids are used in the lowest effective dosage for the shortest period of time. Topical corticosteroids, usually associated with the least risk, may cause systemic side effects at high dosages. The benefit to risk ratio must be weighed when deciding whether to use corticosteroids during pregnancy. The fluorinated corticosteroids (fludrocortisone, triamcinolone, betamethasone, dexamethasone) readily cross the placenta and should be used with caution during pregnancy. Newborns exposed to high-dose fluorinated corticosteroids in utero must be evaluated for adrenal insufficiency.

Topical Corticosteroids

Cutaneous penetration depends on potency, concentration, formulation, application technique, skin condition, and site of application.[73] Systemic absorption is higher with potent drugs (betamethasone dipropionate, clobetasol dipropionate, diflorasone diacetate, and halobetasol propionate), higher drug concentrations, ointments, excipient use (urea or difluoromethylornithine), drug application to damaged or thin skin, increased skin hydration, occlusive dressing use, and continuous application. Creams are indicated for acute or weeping lesions, ointments for dry or chronic lesions, and lotions, creams, and gels for hairy areas.

Systemic Therapy

Initial systemic dosages are high to suppress immune-mediated processes and reduce subsequent tissue damage. Initial systemic dosages (0.6 to 1 mg/kg/day prednisone or equivalent) are given as single morning or twice-daily regimens; twice-daily regimens generally are preferred. Once the acute illness resolves, the dosage is changed to once daily and rapidly tapered off. Tapering is individualized according to the clinical response. Too rapid a taper may exacerbate the precipitating disease; too slow a taper increases the risk of corticosteroid side effects.

Pulse Therapy

Large daily intravenous dosages (methylprednisolone sodium succinate 1 gm/m^2) for short durations (less than 10 days) are indicated for the initial treatment of progressive immune-mediated diseases. Pulse therapy suppresses disease activity with minimal risk of HPA axis suppression.

Stress-Dose Therapy

Stress-dose therapy is indicated for patients who have received pharmacologic dosages of corticosteroids (more than 7.5 mg/day prednisone or equivalent) for more than 2 or 3 weeks and during the first 6 months after discontinuation of long-term corticosteroid therapy. Hydrocortisone 100 mg daily in two to three divided doses is indicated for minor stress or surgery; more severe stress requires 400 to 500 mg. Physiologic replacement dosages are continued for 4 weeks after resolution of the acute stress.

Tapering and Chronic Alternate Day Therapy

Corticosteroids can be rapidly tapered and discontinued abruptly if used for less than 2 to 3 weeks. Patients may experience corticosteroid withdrawal symptoms (anorexia, fatigue, nausea, vomiting, fever, orthostatic hypotension, dizziness, syncope, hypoglycemia, and exacerbation of immune-mediated disease) if the patient is adrenally suppressed and the corticosteroid is tapered too quickly. Chronic alternate day therapy reduces the risk of corticosteroid toxicity, allows recovery of HPA axis function, and minimizes the risk of infection and delayed growth in children.

There is no single rule for changing therapy from daily to an alternate day corticosteroid regimen except to slowly decrease the dosage while monitoring the patient closely. The goal is to place the patient on a regimen consisting of the lowest effective corticosteroid dosage on one day, alternating with no corticosteroid the next day. Each dose is given as a single morning dose. Some patients tolerate only very small dosage decreases (e.g., 1-mg decreases monthly). Underlying disease states masked by the corticosteroid therapy may be unmasked as the dosage is decreased. Patients should wear medical identification and have instructions on how to manage stress.

ADVERSE DRUG REACTIONS OF CORTICOSTEROIDS

Corticosteroids are associated with significant morbidity (Table 16.6).[74–76] Some side effects are apparent within days of initiation (e.g., euphoria, insomnia, leukocytosis) and some side effects are associated with long-term therapy (e.g., osteoporosis, cataracts, delayed growth). Strategies to limit systemic corticosteroid toxicity include alternate day regimens, use of lowest effective dosages for shortest period of time, exercise, low-fat diets, smoking cessation, single morning dose regimens, adequate dietary calcium (1000 mg/day), and limited alcohol intake.

Cardiovascular

Mineralocorticosteroids are associated with systemic hypertension and vascular disease. Retained sodium and water increase circulating volume and elevate systemic blood pressure. Multiple steroid-associated factors, including hypertension, obesity, hypercholesterolemia, hypertriglyceridemia, insulin resistance, hyperinsulinemia, electrolyte disturbances, endothelial cell damage, hypercoagulability, catecholamine potentiation, and altered monocyte and macrophage function, contribute to the development of thrombi and premature atherosclerosis.[79]

Gastrointestinal

Historically, corticosteroids were thought to increase the risk of peptic ulceration. However, the most recent data suggest that the combination of corticosteroids and nonsteroidal anti-inflammatory agents, especially in older adults, increases the risk of peptic ulceration.[80] Pancreatitis is a rare complication.

Growth

Corticosteroids delay linear bone growth and closure of bone epiphyses. Although the mechanism is unclear, corticosteroids decrease growth hormone secretion and competitively inhibit insulin and somatostatin receptors. Growth resumes and catches up if corticosteroids are discontinued before puberty.

Hypothalamus–Pituitary–Adrenal Axis Suppression

HPA axis suppression depends on the type of corticosteroid, dosage, dosage interval, time of administration, route of administration, and duration of corticosteroid therapy.[81,82] Recovery of function is slow and may take several months; patients should be considered adrenally suppressed for as long as 6 to 12 months after discontinuation of chronic corticosteroid therapy.[83]

Metabolic

Corticosteroids alter fat, glucose, and protein metabolism. Fat redistribution from the periphery to the trunk causes centripetal obesity, characterized by moon facies, buffalo hump, and protuberant abdomen. Easy bruisability occurs in 50% of patients and is the most common side effect associated with inhaled corticosteroids.[84] Hyperglycemia usually is mild but may persist for several months after the corticosteroid is discontinued. The risk of corticosteroid-induced hyperglycemia is dose related; the greater the dosage, the greater the risk. Corticosteroids are more likely

Table 16.6 ▪ Corticosteroid Side Effects

Cardiovascular and Renal
- Hypercalcuria[a]
- Hypertension[a]
- Hypokalemic metabolic alkalosis[a]
- Sodium and water retention[a]

Gastrointestinal
- Negative calcium balance[a]
- Pancreatitis[a]
- Fatty infiltration of liver

Immune System
- Immunosuppression
- Infections
- Impaired wound healing

Musculoskeletal
- Osteoporosis
- Aseptic necrosis
- Myopathy

Central Nervous System
- Insomnia[a]
- Mood disorders[a]
- Psychosis[a]
- Pseudotumor cerebri

Hematopoietic
- Leukocytosis
- Monocytopenia
- Lymphopenia
- Eosinopenia

Ophthalmic
- Cataracts
- ↑ Intraocular pressure
- Glaucoma
- Central serous choroidopathy

Endocrine and Metabolic
- Acne[a]
- Adrenal suppression
- Amenorrhea
- Delayed growth in children
- Carbohydrate intolerance
- Hyperinsulinemia
- Insulin resistance
- Diabetes mellitus
- Cushingoid features
- Impotence
- ↓ Thyroid-stimulating hormone and T_3
- Hypokalemia
- Hirsutism
- Hypercholesterolemia[a]
- Hyperosmolar nonketotic coma[a]
- Hypertriglyceridemia[a]
- Negative nitrogen balance[a]
- Impaired wound healing
- Subcutaneous tissue atrophy
- Increased appetite[a]

Source: References 76–78.

[a]May be evident within days of starting therapy.

to uncover latent diabetes mellitus and to increase the insulin requirement in known diabetics than to cause new cases of diabetes mellitus.

Muscle

Corticosteroid-associated myopathy usually presents as symmetric proximal muscle weakness that spreads from the pelvic girdle to the proximal shoulder muscles and may progress to generalized weakness. Myopathy is more commonly associated with prolonged courses of high-dose corticosteroids; a sedentary lifestyle increases the risk. The electromyogram is normal but muscle biopsy reveals atrophy of the type IIb muscle fibers. The myopathy usually is reversible upon discontinuation of the corticosteroid.

Ophthalmic

There is no consensus about the relative risks for corticosteroid-associated posterior subcapsular cataracts. Some of the factors that may be important include daily dosage, cumulative dosage, duration of corticosteroid use, age, and ethnicity. The cataracts develop slowly, are bilateral, and occur more often in children than in adults. Glaucoma, less predictable and not necessarily reversible, is more likely in patients with diabetes mellitus, myopia, or a family history of glaucoma.

Psychological

Corticosteroids cause numerous emotional disturbances, including euphoria, depression, mania, and psychotic reactions.[85] Corticosteroids generally make people feel well, although severe depression with suicidal ideation may occur. These effects usually are dose related, occur within a few days of initiation, and resolve spontaneously within a few weeks of discontinuation.[86] High-dose alternate day regimens may cause mood swings resembling manic–depressive states. A psychiatric history does not predispose patients to corticosteroid-associated psychological side effects. If an acute psychotic reaction occurs, taper the corticosteroid off over a period of several days to avoid rebound depression and increased anxiety.

Skeletal

Osteoporosis, one of the most serious corticosteroid-associated side effects, is caused by the combination of multiple factors including protein catabolism, osteoblast inhibition, growth hormone inhibition, decreased calcium absorption, decreased renal calcium reabsorption, and mild secondary hyperparathyroidism.[87] Skeletal decalcification occurs quickly; bone fractures are commonly reported during the first year of treatment. All bones are affected; however, lumbar spine compression and rib fractures are more common. Biochemical markers of bone turnover are not sensitive or specific predictors.

A combination of nondrug and drug therapy is recommended to preserve bone.[88] Lifestyle modification includes smoking cessation, avoidance of excessive alcohol intake, and adequate weight-bearing and resistive exercise (30 to 60 minutes per day). Drug therapy includes calcium (approximately 1500 mg/day unless contraindicated), vitamin D (800 IU/day or 50,000 U three times weekly), or calcitriol (0.5 mcg/day), hormonal replacement therapy in postmenopausal women, low-dose thiazide diuretic if hypercalcuria is detected, and bisphosphonates.

Table 16.7 ▪ Corticosteroid Drug Interactions

Drug	Effect
Aminophylline	Variable
Aminoglutethimide[a]	Decreased steroid effect
Antacids	Decreased steroid effect
Anticholinesterases	Refractory muscle depression
Anticoagulants	Variable
Barbiturates	Decreased steroid effect
Cholestyramine	Decreased steroid effect
Colestipol	Decreased steroid effect
Contraceptives, oral	Increased steroid effect
Cyclosporine	Increased steroid and cyclosporine effects
Ephedrine[a]	Increased steroid effect
Erythromycin	Increased steroid effect
Estrogens	Increased steroid effect
Interferon-α	Decreased interferon-α effect
Isoniazid	Decreased isoniazid effect
Ketoconazole	Increased steroid effect
Nondepolarizing muscle relaxants	Decreased nondepolarizing muscle relaxant effects
Phenytoin	Decreased steroid effect
Primidone	Decreased steroid effect
Rifabutin	Decreased steroid effect
Rifampin	Decreased steroid effect
Salicylates	Decreased salicylate effect
Theophylline	Variable
Troleandomycin	Increased steroid effect

Source: Reference 89.
[a]Dexamethasone only.

DRUG INTERACTIONS OF CORTICOSTEROIDS

Numerous drug interactions have been reported with corticosteroids (Table 16.7). Glycyrrhizin, the saponin of licorice root, increases the steroid effect. The effectiveness of glucocorticoids is greatly impaired by rifampin administration through induction of hepatic steroid-metabolizing enzymes. It is strongly recommended that in patients with compromised adrenal function, rifampin is accompanied by a doubling or tripling of the adrenal steroid dosage to maintain adequate replacement therapy.[90] In addition to these typical pharmacokinetic drug interactions, corticosteroids have numerous pharmacodynamic drug interactions. The hypokalemic effect of corticosteroids may exaggerate the hypokalemic effects of amphotericin B, potassium-depleting diuretics, and digitalis glycosides. Corticosteroids may inhibit the growth-promoting effect of growth hormone. The expected immune response to vaccines may be impaired in the presence of corticosteroids. The risk of duodenal ulcer is greatly increased when corticosteroids and nonsteroidal anti-inflammatory drugs are administered concomitantly.[80] Patients must be monitored closely and drug dosages adjusted to achieve the desired clinical effect.

KEY POINTS

Cushing's Syndrome

- The goal of therapy is to restore HPA hormonal balance by eliminating excess glucocorticoids and mineralocorticoids.
- Cushing's syndrome is a constellation of clinical signs and symptoms.
- Most cases of Cushing's syndrome are caused by iatrogenic administration of glucocorticoids.
- Other causes of Cushing's syndrome are rare, but are important because many are curable.
- Signs and symptoms of Cushing's syndrome are nonspecific and usually insidious in onset.
- Diagnosis depends on documenting hypercortisolism and identifying the precise cause.
- Treatment of exogenous Cushing's syndrome consists of minimizing glucocorticoid or ACTH exposure.
- Treatment of endogenous Cushing's syndrome consists of reducing cortisol production.
- Three types of drugs are used to treat Cushing's syndrome: steroidogenic inhibitors, neuromodulators of ACTH release, and glucocorticoid receptor antagonists.
- Nonpharmacologic therapy for Cushing's syndrome includes surgery for resectable tumors and pituitary irradiation for Cushing's disease not cured by surgery.

Addison's Disease

- The goal of therapy is to restore HPA hormonal balance by replacing glucocorticoids and mineralocorticoids.
- Addison's disease, also known as primary adrenal insufficiency, is a chronic, incurable disease.
- Most cases of Addison's disease are caused by autoantibodies directed against steroid-producing cells.
- Although the signs and symptoms of Addison's disease are nonspecific, nearly all patients present with biochemical abnormalities.
- The presenting signs and symptoms and biochemical findings depend on the acuity of presentation.
- Diagnosis depends on provocative tests of the HPA axis.
- An acute adrenal crisis is life-threatening; drug treatment cannot be delayed for diagnostic testing or blood chemistry results.
- The current recommended chronic replacement regimen consists of dexamethasone 0.5 mg plus fludrocortisone 0.1 mg daily at bedtime.
- Nondrug therapy for normotensive patients consists of liberalizing the dietary salt intake.

REFERENCES

1. Orth DN, Kovacs WJ. The adrenal cortex. In: Wilson JD, Foster DW, Kronenberg HM, et al. Williams textbook of endocrinology. 9th ed. Philadelphia: WB Saunders, 1998:517–664.
2. Hebel SK, ed. Drug facts and comparisons. St. Louis: Facts and Comparisons, 1998.
3. Chrousos GP. Mechanisms of action. In: Boumpas DT, moderator. Glucocorticoid therapy for immune-mediated diseases: basic and clinical correlates. Ann Intern Med 119:1198–1208, 1993.
4. Ramirez VD. How do steroids act? Lancet 347:630–631, 1996.
5. Bleecker E. Inhaled corticosteroids: current products and their role in patient care. J Allergy Clin Immunol 101:S400–S402, 1998.
6. Orth DN. Cushing's syndrome. N Engl J Med 332:791–803, 1995.
7. Moore-Ede MC, Czeisler CA, Richardson GS. Circadian timekeeping in health and disease. Part I. Basic properties of circadian pacemakers. N Engl J Med 309:469–476, 1983.
8. Czeisler CA, Chiasera AJ, Duffy JF. Research on sleep, circadian rhythms and aging: applications to manned spaceflight. Exp Gerontol 26:217–232, 1991.
9. Veldhuis JD, Iranmanesh A, Johnson ML, et al. Amplitude, but not frequency, modulation of adrenocorticotropin secretory bursts give rise to the cytohumoral rhythm of the corticotropic axis in man. J Clin Endocrinol Metab 71:452–463, 1990.
10. Pincus G, Nakao T, Tait JF, eds. Symposium on the dynamics of steroid hormones. New York: Academic Press, 1965:387.
11. Quigley ME, Yen SSC. A mid-day surge in cortisol levels. J Clin Endocrinol Metab 49:945–947, 1979.
12. Slag MF, Ahmed M, Gannon MC, et al. Meal stimulation of cortisol secretion: a protein induced effect. Metabolism 30:1104–1108, 1981.
13. Hiramatsu R, Nisula BC. Erythrocyte-associated cortisol: measurement, kinetics of dissociation, and potential physiological significance. J Clin Endocrinol Metab 64:1224–1232, 1987.
14. Cushing H. The basophil adenomas of the pituitary body and their clinical manifestations (pituitary basophilism). Bull Johns Hopkins Hosp 50:137–195, 1932.
15. Orth DN, Liddle GW. Results of treatment in 108 patients with Cushing's syndrome. N Engl J Med 285:243–247, 1971.
16. Ross NS. 1994 epidemiology of Cushing's syndrome and subclinical disease. Endocrinol Metab Clin North Am 23:539–546, 1994.
17. Becker M, Aron DC. 1994 Ectopic ACTH syndrome and CRH-mediated Cushing's syndrome. Endocrinol Metab Clin North Am 23:585–606, 1994.
18. Tsigos C. Differential diagnosis and management of Cushing's syndrome. Annu Rev Med 47:443–661, 1996.
19. Carpenter PC. Diagnostic evaluation of Cushing's syndrome. Endocrinol Metab Clin North Am 17:445–472, 1988.
20. Meier CA, Biller BMK. Clinical and biochemical evaluation of Cushing's syndrome. Endocrinol Metab Clin North Am 26:741–762, 1997.
21. Wajchenberg BL, Bosco A, Marone MM, et al. Estimation of body fat and lean tissue distribution of dual energy X-ray absorptiometry and abdominal body fat evaluation by computer tomography in Cushing's disease. J Clin Endocrinol Metab 80:2791–2794, 1995.
22. Ross EJ, Marshall-Jones P, Friedman M. Cushing's syndrome: diagnostic criteria. Q J Med 35:149–192, 1966.
23. Jeffcoate WJ, Silverstone JT, Edwards CRW, et al. Psychiatric manifestation of Cushing's syndrome: response to lowering of plasma cortisol. Q J Med 48:465–472, 1979.
24. Loosen PT, Chambliss B, DeBold CR, et al. Psychiatric phenomenology in Cushing's disease. Pharmacopsychiatry 25:192–198, 1992.
25. Dorn LD, Burgess ES, Dubbert B, et al. Psychopathology in patients with endogenous Cushing's syndrome: "atypical" or melancholic features. Clin Endocrinol 43:433–442, 1995.
26. Ross EJ, Linch DC. Cushing's syndrome–killing disease: discriminatory value of signs and symptoms aiding early diagnosis. Lancet 2:646–649, 1982.

27. Sjoberg HE, Blomback M, Granberg PO. Thromboembolic complications, heparin treatment and increase in coagulation factors in Cushing's syndrome. Acta Med Scand 199:95–98, 1976.
28. Perry LA, Grossman AB. The role of the laboratory in the diagnosis of Cushing's syndrome. Ann Clin Biochem 34:345–359, 1997.
29. Wood PJ, Barth JH, Freedman DB, et al. Evidence for the low dose dexamethasone suppression test to screen for Cushing's syndrome: recommendations for a protocol for biochemistry laboratories. Ann Clin Biochem 34:222–229, 1997.
30. Pavlatos FC, Smilo RP, Forsham PH. A rapid screening test for Cushing's syndrome. JAMA 193:720–723, 1965.
31. Liddle GW. Tests for pituitary adrenal suppressibility in the diagnosis of Cushing's syndrome. J Clin Endocrinol Metab 20:1539–1560, 1960.
32. Tyrrell JB, Findling JW, Aron DC, et al. An overnight high-dose dexamethasone suppression test for rapid deferential diagnosis of Cushing's syndrome. Ann Intern Med 104:180–186, 1986.
33. Miller JW, Crapo L. The medical treatment of Cushing's syndrome. Endocrinol Rev 14:443–458, 1993.
34. Atkinson AB. The treatment of Cushing's syndrome. Clin Endocrinol 34:507–513, 1991.
35. Koppeschaar HPF, Croughs RJM, Thijssen JHH, et al. Response to neurotransmitter modulating drugs in patients with Cushing's disease. Clin Endocrinol 25:661–667, 1986.
36. Child DF, Burke DM, Rees LH, et al. Drug control of Cushing's syndrome. Acta Endocrinol 82:330–341, 1976.
37. Schteingart DE, Tsao HS, Taylor CI, et al. Sustained remission of Cushing's disease with mitotane and pituitary irradiation. Ann Intern Med 92:613–619, 1980.
38. Hogan TF, Citrin DL, Johnson BM, et al. O,p′-DDD (mitotane) therapy of adrenal cortical carcinoma: observations on drug dosage, toxicity, and steroid replacement. Cancer 42:2177–2181, 1978.
39. Wortsman J, Goler NG. Mitotane. Spironolactone antagonism in Cushing's syndrome. JAMA 238:2527, 1977.
40. Thoren M, Adamson U, Sjoberg HE. Aminoglutethimide and metyrapone in the management of Cushing's syndrome. Acta Endocrinol 109:451–557, 1985.
41. Misbin RI, Canary J, Willard D. Aminoglutethimide in the treatment of Cushing's syndrome. J Clin Pharmacol 16:645–651, 1976.
42. Santen RJ, Misbin RI. Aminoglutethimide: review of pharmacology and clinical use. Pharmacotherapy 1:95–120, 1981.
43. McKenna MJ, Linares M, Mellinger RC. Prolonged remission of Cushing's disease following bromocriptine therapy. Henry Ford Hosp Med J 35:188–191, 1987.
44. Jeffcoate WJ. Treating Cushing's disease. BMJ 296:227–228, 1988.
45. Krieger DT. Cyproheptadine for pituitary disorders [letter]. N Engl J Med 295:394–395, 1976.
46. Calao A, Pivonello R, Tripodi FS, et al. Failure of long-term therapy with sodium valproate in Cushing's disease. J Endocrinol Invest 20:387–392, 1997.
47. Invitti C, de Martin M, Brunani A, et al. Treatment of Cushing's syndrome with the long-acting somatostatin analogue SMS 201-995 (Sandostatin). Clin Endocrinol 32:275–281, 1990.
48. Stalle GK, Brockmeier SJ, Renner U, et al. Octreotide exerts different effects in vivo and in vitro in Cushing's disease. Eur J Endocrinol 130:125–131, 1994.
49. Sartor O, Cutler G. Mifepristone: treatment of Cushing's syndrome. Clin Obstet Gynecol 39:506–510, 1996.
50. Chrousos GP, Laue L, Nieman LK, et al. Clinical applications of RU 486, a prototype glucocorticoid and progesterone antagonist. In: Baulieu EE, Segal SJ, eds. The antiprogestin steroid RU 486 and human fertility control. New York: Plenum, 1989:273–284.
51. Mampalan TJ, Tyrrell JB, Wilson CB. Transsphenoidal microsurgery for Cushing's disease. A report of 216 cases. Ann Intern Med 109:487–493, 1988.
52. Addison T. On the constitutional and local effects of disease of the supra-renal capsules. Med Classics 2:244–277, 1937.
53. Kong M-F, Jeffcoate W. Eighty-six cases of Addison's disease. Clin Endocrinol 41:757–761, 1994.
54. Zelissen PM, Bast EJ, Croughs RJ. Associated autoimmunity in Addison's disease. J Autoimmun 8:121–130, 1995.
55. Betterle C, Greggio NA, Volpato M. Autoimmune polyglandular syndrome type 1. J Clin Endocrinol Metab 83:1049–1055, 1998.
56. Barker NW. The pathologic anatomy in twenty-eight cases of Addison's disease. Arch Pathol 8:432–450, 1929.
57. Baker JR Jr. Autoimmune endocrine disease. JAMA 278:1931–1937, 1997.
58. Dluhy RG. The growing spectrum of HIV-related endocrine abnormalities. J Clin Endocrinol Metab 70:563–565, 1990.
59. Chin R Jr, Zekan JM. Adrenal insufficiency. Probl Crit Care 4:312–324, 1990.
60. Elansary EH, Earis JE. Rifampicin and adrenal crisis. BMJ 286:1861–1861, 1983.
61. Brosnan CM, Gowing NFC. Lesson of the week: Addison's disease. BMJ 312:1085–1087, 1996.
62. Nerup J. Addison's disease: clinical studies. A report of 108 cases. Acta Endocrinol 76:127–141, 1974.
63. Burke CW. Adrenocortical insufficiency. Clin Endocrinol Metab 14:947–976, 1985.
64. De Bellis A, Bizzarro A, Rossi R, et al. Remission of subclinical adrenocortical failure in subjects with adrenal autoantibodies. J Clin Endocrinol Metab 76:1002–1007, 1993.
65. Khalid BAK, Burke CW, Hurley DM, et al. Steroid replacement in Addison's disease and in subjects adrenalectomized for Cushing's disease: comparison of various glucocorticoids. J Clin Endocrinol Metab 55:551–559, 1982.
66. Ulick S. Cortisol as mineralocorticoid. J Clin Endocrinol Metab 81:1307–1308, 1996.
67. Cohen N, Gilbert R, Wirth D, et al. Atrial natriuretic peptide and plasma renin levels in assessment of mineralocorticoid replacement in Addison's disease. J Clin Endocrinol Metab 81:1411–1415, 1996.
68. Baylis RIS. Adrenal cortex. Clin Endocrinol Metab 9:477–486, 1980.
69. Scott RS, Donald RA, Espiner EA. Plasma ACTH and cortisol profiles in Addisonian patients receiving conventional substitution therapy. Clin Endocrinol 9:571–576, 1978.
70. Jusko WJ, Ludwig EA. Corticosteroids. In: Evans WE, Schentag JJ, Jusko WJ, eds. Applied pharmacokinetics: principles of therapeutic drug monitoring. 3rd ed. Vancouver, WA: Applied Therapeutics, Inc., 1992:1–34.
71. Derendorf H, Hochhaus G, Mollmann H, et al. Receptor-based pharmacokinetic-pharmacodynamic analysis of corticosteroids. J Clin Pharmacol 33:115–123, 1993.
72. Johnson M. Pharmacodynamics and pharmacokinetics of inhaled glucocorticoids. J Allergy Clin Immunol 97:169–176, 1996.
73. Giannotti B. Current treatment guidelines for topical corticosteroids. Drugs 36(suppl 5):9–14, 1988.
74. Balow JE. Complications of therapy. In: Boumpas DT, moderator. Glucocorticoid therapy for immune-mediated diseases: basic and clinical correlates. Ann Intern Med 119:1205–1206, 1993.
75. McEvoy CE, Niewoehner DE. Adverse effects of corticosteroid therapy for COPD. Chest 111:732–743, 1997.
76. Magiakou MA, Chrousos GP. Corticosteroid therapy, nonendocrine disease, and corticosteroid withdrawal. Curr Ther Endocrinol Metab 6:138–142, 1997.
77. Rossi SJ, Schroeder TJ, Hartharan S, et al. Prevention and management of the adverse effects associated with immunosuppressive therapy. Drug Saf 9:104–131, 1993.
78. Truhan AP, Ahmed AR. Corticosteroids: a review with emphasis on complications of prolonged systemic therapy. Ann Allergy 62:375–390, 1989.
79. Maxwell SRJ, Moots RJ, Kendall MJ. Corticosteroids: do they damage the cardiovascular system? Postgrad Med J 70:863–870, 1994.
80. Piper JM, Ray WA, Daugherty JR, et al. Corticosteroid use and peptic ulcer disease: role of nonsteroidal anti-inflammatory drugs. Ann Intern Med 114:735–740, 1991.
81. Helfer EL, Rose LI. Corticosteroids and adrenal suppression. Drugs 38:838–845, 1989.
82. Melby JC. Systemic corticosteroid therapy: pharmacology and endocrinologic considerations. Ann Intern Med 81:505–512, 1974.
83. Livanou T, Athens MD, Ferrimano D, et al. Recovery of hypothalamic–pituitary–adrenal function after corticosteroid therapy. Lancet 2:856–859, 1967.
84. Mak V, Melchor R, Spiro S. Easy bruising as a side-effect of inhaled corticosteroids. Eur Respir J 5:1068–1074, 1992.
85. Vincent FM. The neuropsychiatric complications of corticosteroid therapy. Compr Ther 21:524–528, 1995.
86. BCDSP. Acute adverse reactions to prednisone in relation to dosage. Clin Pharmacol Ther 13:694–698, 1972.
87. Picado C, Luengo M. Corticosteroid-induced bone loss. Drug Saf 15:347–359, 1996.
88. Anonymous. Recommendations for the prevention and treatment of glucocorticoid-induced osteoporosis. Arthritis Rheum 39:1791–1801, 1996.
89. Tatro DS, ed. Drug interaction facts. 5th ed. St. Louis: Facts and Comparisons, 1996.
90. Kyriazopoulou V, Parparousi O, Vagenakis AG. Rifampicin-induced adrenal crisis in Addisonian patients receiving corticosteroid replacement therapy. J Clin Endocrinol Metab 59:1204–1206, 1984.

CHAPTER 17

THYROID DISORDERS

Betty J. Dong

The thyroid disorders discussed in this chapter include hyperthyroidism, hypothyroidism, and thyroid nodules. Thyroid hormones are responsible for the optimal growth, development, and function of all metabolic processes and body systems. Therefore, a deficiency or excess in thyroid hormone secretion can affect multiple organ systems and result in a wide variety of complaints and physical findings. It is also important to recognize that the clinical presentation of thyroid disorders, especially in older adults, can masquerade as many different illnesses (e.g., atrial fibrillation), and it is essential to exclude an underlying thyroid disorder when considering the medical diagnosis. Thyroid disorders can also affect the treatment of concurrent illnesses (e.g., diabetes, depression, angina) and changes in thyroid function can alter the pharmacokinetics of drugs used in management of other illness.[1]

Overview of the Thyroid

ANATOMY AND PHYSIOLOGY

The gland synthesizes, stores, and releases two major metabolically active hormones: triiodothyronine (T_3) and thyroxine (T_4). T_3 is more active than T_4 because the thyroid receptor protein within the cell nucleus has about a tenfold higher affinity for T_3 than for T_4. Approximately 35 to 40% of the secreted T_4 is peripherally monodeiodinated to active T_3, which provides 80% of the total daily production of T_3 and 40% of reverse T_3 (rT_3), which has little or no thyroid activity. Many acute conditions, chronic disorders, and drugs can reduce peripheral conversion of T_4 to active T_3 and increase the conversion to inactive rT_3, which can cause diagnostic confusion if such laboratory findings are not properly recognized.[2]

The thyroid hormones circulate in both the active, free (unbound) form and the protein-bound or inactive form. T_4 is 99.89% bound; only 0.02% is free. This high affinity for the plasma proteins (thyroxine-binding globulin [TBG], 80%; thyroxine-binding prealbumin [TBPA], 10 to 15%; and albumin 4 to 5%) accounts for the high serum concentration and the slow metabolic degradation ($t_{1/2} = 7$ days) of T_4. In hyperthyroidism, the half-life of T_4 is shortened to 3 to 4 days, and in hypothyroidism the half-life is prolonged to 9 to 10 days. Similar changes in half-life are described for T_3.[1] T_3 is three times more potent metabolically than T_4, but its biologic activity is similar because the lower affinity of T_3 for the plasma proteins results in a lower serum concentration and greater clearance ($t_{1/2} = 1.5$ days). About 0.2% of T_3 is free and active.

Hormone synthesis and release is achieved by an intricate negative feedback mechanism involving the gland, the hypothalamic–pituitary axis (Fig. 17.1), and autoregulation of iodide uptake. Low circulating levels of thyroid hormone initiate the release of thyroid-stimulating hormone (TSH) or thyrotropin from the pituitary and secretion of thyrotropin-releasing factor (TRF) from the hypothalamus. Rising TSH levels increase iodide trapping by the gland, causing a subsequent increase in hormone synthesis and circulating hormone levels that shut off TRF and TSH secretion and prevent further hormone synthesis. As the hormone levels drop, the hypothalamic–pituitary centers once again become responsive to release of TSH and TRF. Physiologic factors (i.e., dopamine, stress) can also influence the hypothalamic–pituitary axis and hormone synthesis.

The gland can also regulate its own uptake of iodide to protect against excessive hormone production if a large iodide load is ingested (i.e., radiographic iodine dye). This autoregulation, known as the Wolff–Chaikoff block, is not overcome by TSH stimulation and occurs when a critical intrathyroidal iodide concentration effect is established within the gland. The normal gland escapes from the block within 7 to 14 days, which prevents subsequent development of hypothyroidism and goiter. Escape results from a decrease in iodide transport or an iodide leak, both of which tend to decrease the intrathyroidal iodide concentration and remove the block to further hormone synthesis. In certain thyroid disorders (e.g., Hashimoto's thyroiditis), the gland cannot escape from the Wolff–Chaikoff block, causing hypothyroidism. Conversely, hyperthyroidism results if this critical block does not occur (as in multinodular goiter).

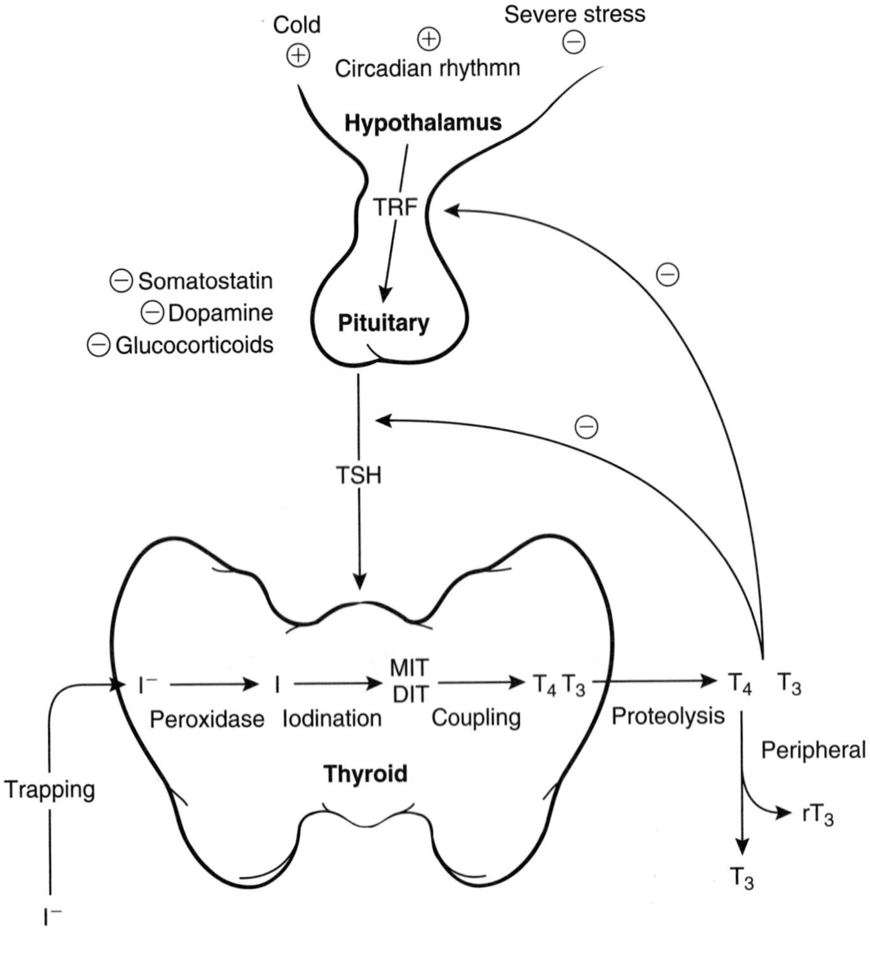

Figure 17.1. Hormone synthesis via negative feedback control on the hypothalamic–pituitary–thyroid axis. *DIT,* diiodotyrosine; *MIT,* monoiodotyrosine; *rT_3,* reverse triiodothyronine; *T_3,* triiodothyronine; *T_4,* thyroxine; *TRF,* thyrotropin-releasing factor; *TSH,* thyroid-stimulating factor. (Key: ⊖ = inhibitory influence; ⊕ = stimulatory influence.)

THYROID EVALUATION

The assessment of a patient with a suspected thyroid disorder should include the following:

- Symptoms of thyroid excess or deficiency
- Neck or thyroid symptoms (e.g., pain, tenderness, difficulty swallowing or breathing)
- A history of familial thyroid abnormalities
- A history of upper chest or neck irradiation during childhood
- Examination of the thyroid for enlargement, consistency, and nodularity
- Examination for thyroid hormone effects on target systems
- Medication history for ingestion of thyroid, antithyroid drugs, or drugs that can cause or be altered by thyroid disease
- Appropriate thyroid function tests

THYROID FUNCTION TESTS

Several laboratory tests are available to assess thyroid homeostasis and metabolic function.[2] These tests measure circulating T_4 and T_3 levels, iodine-trapping ability of the gland, hypothalamic–pituitary function, autoimmunity, and various nonspecific metabolic indices (Table 17.1). The normal range depends on the laboratory and the assay used. The most cost-effective screening test for thyroid disorders is a TSH or thyrotropin level. Routine TSH screening for thyroid illness is recommended, particularly in patients more than 50 years old.[3,4] A free thyroxine level (FT_4) or a free thyroxine index (FT_4I) can be obtained concurrently if the clinical suspicion for thyroid disease is high. A total triiodothyronine level (TT_3) is helpful only in evaluating hyperthyroidism and should not be obtained routinely. If the screening TSH level is abnormal, subsequent determinations of hormone levels are indicated. Thyroid antibodies confirm the presence of an autoimmune thyroid disorder only if an abnormal thyroid gland or clinical symptoms exist. A number of nonspecific indices, including the cholesterol, carotene, transaminase (e.g., serum glutamic-oxaloacetic transaminase [SGOT], serum glutamic-pyruvic transaminase [SGPT]), creatine phosphokinase (CPK), and lactic dehydrogenase (LDH) levels, can be abnormal in thyroid dysfunction because of impaired clearance in severe hypothyroidism or increased elimination in hyperthyroidism. It should be appreciated that several drugs and clinical conditions can alter laboratory values, interfere with proper interpretation of these tests, and make evaluation of thyroid status difficult (Table 17.2).[2,5] An algorithm for laboratory evaluation of thyroid disorders is presented in Figure 17.2.

Measurements of Circulating Hormone Levels

Tests of circulating hormone levels can measure either the free (active) or total (free and protein-bound) concentrations of T_4 and T_3 (Table 17.1). Measurements of FT_4 concentrations by equilibrium dialysis or by the analog tests are more accurate and should replace older measurements of the total thyroxine level (TT_4), which are affected by changes in protein binding. FT_4 levels also can be estimated by calculation of FT_4I.

The total T_3 (free and bound T_3) is most useful in evaluating hyperthyroidism because it can be elevated when T_4 levels are normal (e.g., in T_3 toxicosis and before the development of elevated T_4 levels). The TT_3 is not reliable in evaluating hypothyroidism or euthyroidism because it can be normal or low. Likewise, a low TT_3 does not prove hypothyroidism because multiple factors (e.g., age, acute or chronic disease) can cause a low TT_3 in the euthyroid patient by inhibiting the peripheral conversion of T_4 to T_3. Interference of the TT_3 by changes in protein binding can be corrected by calculation of the free T_3 index (FT_3I). Free T_3 (FT_3) can also be measured by equilibrium dialysis, but this test is not yet widely available.

The FT_4I and FT_3I are indirect, calculated estimates of the FT_4 and FT_3, as derived from TT_4 and TT_3 measurements. The FT_4I and FT_3I correct for fluctuations in TBG (Table 17.2), which do not accurately reflect the active or free hormone levels and are unchanged in a euthyroid state. An exception is in the euthyroid sick syndrome, where the FT_4I or FT_3I can be falsely low. Two methods can be used to calculate the index, and the method selected depends on the laboratory performing the assays (Table 17.1).

Thyrotropin or Thyroid-Stimulating Hormone

The sensitive TSH assay is the most accurate indicator of euthyroidism and thyroid dysfunction (Table 17.1). Serum TSH elevations often occur before overt clinical and laboratory manifestations of hypothyroidism are present. Therefore, the TSH can be elevated despite normal FT_4, TT_4, and FT_4I, findings that indicate early subclinical hypothyroidism or insufficient hormone replacement. Likewise, in subclinical hyperthyroidism or in overreplacement therapy, the TSH is suppressed into the subnormal range, even though circulating hormone levels are within the normal range. In overt hyperthyroidism, the TSH is often undetectable. The TSH also can be used to differentiate primary thyroid failure (elevated TSH) from secondary (central) pituitary deficiency (absent or low normal TSH). Finally, TSH is invaluable in excluding secondary thyroid failure in patients with the euthyroid sick syndrome. The sensitive TSH assays are not affected by the high levels of human chorionic gonadotropins (HCG) found in pregnancy. However, factors that affect dopamine, which physiologically controls TSH secretion, can alter the TSH level. Dopamine agonists (e.g., dopamine, levodopa, bromocriptine) and high-dose corticosteroids can suppress TSH secretion, and dopamine antagonists (e.g., metoclopramide) can increase TSH secretion.[2,5] These mild drug-induced alterations in TSH levels generally do not interfere with the diagnosis of thyroid dysfunction in patients with true thyroid disease.

Table 17.1 ▪ Thyroid Function Tests

Test	Normal Values	Measures	Hyperthyroidism	Hypothyroidism	Comments
TT_4	64–142 mmol/L (5–11 µg/dL)	Total T_4, both free and bound	↑	↓	Affected by changes in TBG
FT_4	9–24 pmol/L (0.7–1.9 ng/dL)	Direct measure of free T_4 by equilibrium dialysis or analog method	↑	↓	Levels reflect true thyroid status; not affected by changes in TBG
FT_4I	16–50 mmol/L (1.3–4.2) calculated index using product of RT_3U and TT_4 107–118 mmol/L (6.5–12.5) calculated index by dividing TT_4 by T_4 uptake	Indirect estimate of active free T_4 levels	↑	↓	Compensates for changes in TBG concentration; reflects true thyroid status except in euthyroid sick syndrome
RT_3U	0.25–0.37 (25–37%)	Indirect measure of degree of saturation of TBG sites by T_4	↑	↓	Affected by changes in TBG
T_4U	0.6–1.2	Available binding sites on TBG, prealbumin, and albumin	↑	↓	Affected by changes in TBG, prealbumin, and albumin
TT_3	1.1–2.0 nmol/L (70–132 ng/dL)	Total T_3 (free and bound)	↑	↓	Affected by changes in TBG; not useful in diagnosis of hypothyroidism
FT_3I	0.28–0.75 nmol/L (18–49 ng/dL)	Product of RT_3U and TT_3; calculated estimate of active free T_3 levels	↑	↓	See comments for FT_4I
^{131}I radioactive iodine uptake	5–15% at 5 hr 10–35% at 24 hr	Iodine-trapping ability of gland	↑	↓ or ↑ in subclinical hypothyroidism	Normals vary depending on degree of dietary iodide intake and geographic area; interfered by iodide intake (i.e., contrast dye)
TSH	0.5–4.7 mIU/L	Pituitary TSH	↓	↑	Most sensitive indicator of adequate circulating hormone levels
Thyroid antibodies					
ATgA	0–8%	Autoimmune process	Often positive (Graves' disease)	Often positive (Hashimoto's thyroiditis)	TPO more sensitive than ATgA, elevated even with remission
TPO	< 100 IU/L (< 100 IU/mL)	Autoimmune process	Often positive (Graves' disease)	Often positive (Hashimoto's thyroiditis)	
TrAb	Negative	Immunoglobulin G in Graves' disease	Often positive (Graves' disease)	Often negative	Indicates Graves' disease, predictive for neonatal Graves' disease during pregnancy
Thyroid scan	Isotopes scan with ^{123}I or $^{99}TcO_4$	Detects hypofunctioning (cold) and hyperfunctioning (hot) nodules and estimates size of gland	Diffusely enlarged; can have hot areas	Cold areas might occur with Hashimoto's disease	Not usually done unless discrete nodules are felt on physical examination

TT_4, total thyroxine; *T_4*, thyroxine; *TBG*, thyroxine-binding globulin; *FT_4*, free thyroxine; *FT_4I*, free thyroxine index; *RT_3U*, resin T_3 uptake; *T_4U*, T_4 uptake; *TT_3*, total T_3; *FT_3I*, free T_3 index; *T_3*, triiodothyronine; *TSH*, thyrotropin-stimulating hormone; *ATgA*, thyroglobulin antibody; *TPO*, thyroperoxidase antibody.

Thyroid Antibodies

The presence of thyroid antibodies, antithyroglobulin (ATgA) and thyroperoxidase (TPO), directed against the thyroglobulin and the peroxidase component of the thyroid gland usually indicates an underlying autoimmune process, such as Graves' disease or Hashimoto's thyroiditis. However, because positive antibodies can occur in patients without thyroid dysfunction or in patients with collagen vascular disorders, their presence is not diagnostic of thyroid illness in the absence of clinical findings. The levels of ATgA and TPO are consistently higher during the acute phases of autoimmune thyroid disease and decline during remission and after therapy. TPO is the more sensitive of the two antibodies because levels remain detectable after remission, whereas ATgA titers might revert to normal.

Thyroid receptor antibody (TRab*)* is an IgG immunoglobulin capable of stimulating the thyroid gland and found in approximately 90% of patients with Graves' disease. There is no need to run a TRab test on a patient with classic symptoms of Graves' disease because the test is expensive (approximately $100) and offers no additional therapeutic or diagnostic information. The TRab will help confirm the diagnosis of Graves' disease in clinically euthyroid patients with an atypical presentation (e.g., ophthalmopathy). The TRab should be monitored in all pregnant women with a history of Graves' disease because a high maternal TRab titer offers predictive information about the risk of neonatal Graves' disease. Finally, the presence or absence of TRab in patients with Graves' disease may act as a prognostic indicator of the potential for disease relapse and remission.

Radioactive Iodine Uptake and Scan

The radioactive iodine uptake (RAIU) measures only the iodine-trapping ability of the gland without regard to the iodine's ultimate fate. After a tracer dose of radioactive iodine (RAI), the percentage iodine uptake is measured at 5 and 24 hours. An elevated uptake (more than 35% at 24 hours) typically occurs in hyperthyroidism, whereas a depressed uptake (less than 30% in 24 hours) is seen in hypothyroidism. However, an elevated uptake can also occur in early hypothyroidism, indicating an attempt by the failing gland to increase iodine uptake and subsequent hormone synthesis. Fluctuations in the total iodide pool, through either dietary or therapeutic maneuvers, will falsely alter the true value of the RAIU (Table 17.2). A thyroid scan usually is obtained concurrently. An uptake and scan often is used to estimate a therapeutic dosage of RAI therapy for hyperthyroidism. The scan provides a

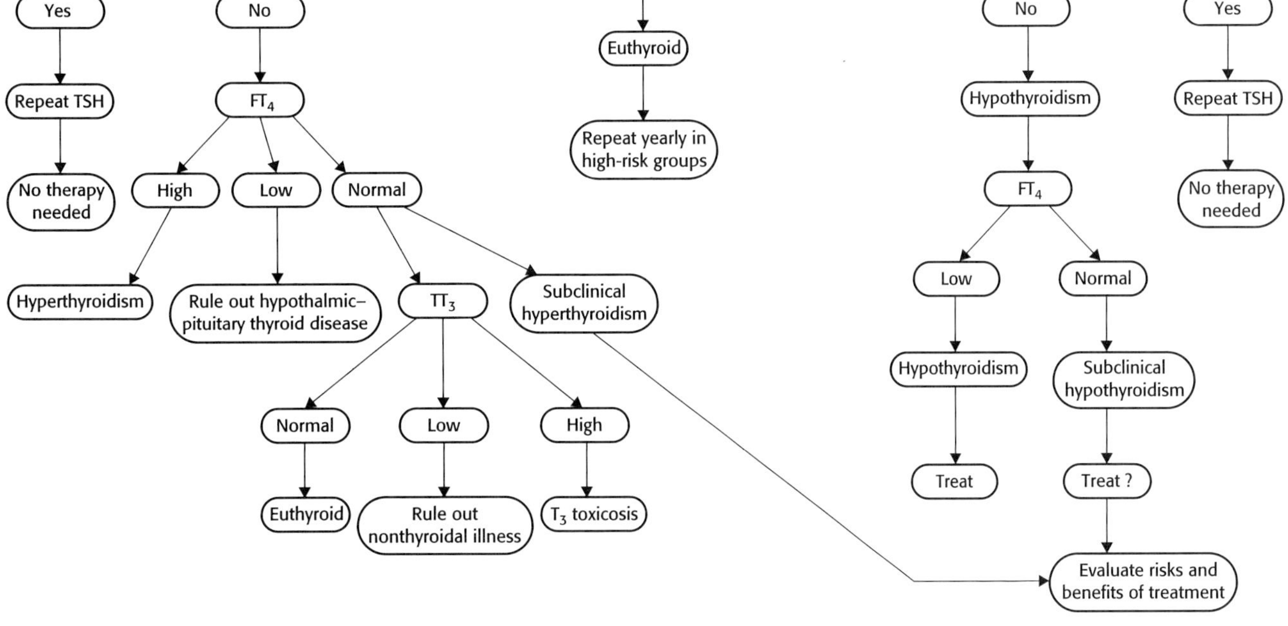

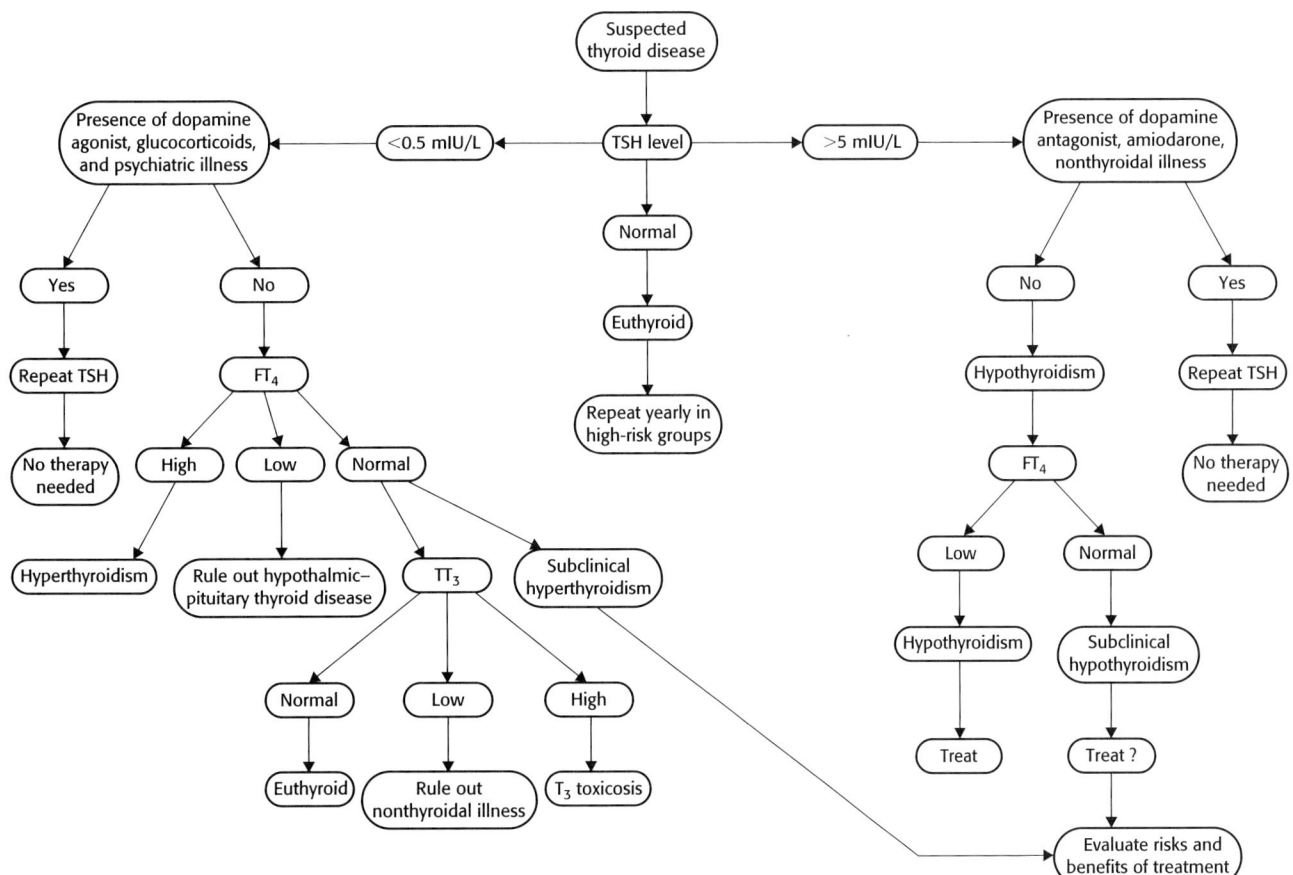

Figure 17.2. Algorithm for laboratory evaluation of thyroid disorders. *FT_4*, free thyroxine; *TSH*, thyroid-stimulating hormone; *T3*, triiodothyronine; *TT_3*, total triiodothyronine.

Table 17.2 ▪ Summary of Laboratory Alterations by Drug or Disease State[a]

Drug or Disease	Mechanism	TT_4	RT_3U	FT_4/FT_4I	TT_3	^{131}I Uptake	TSH	Comments
Estrogens, oral contraceptives, pregnancy, heroin, methadone, clofibrate, acute and chronic active hepatitis, familial ↑ TBG	↑ serum TBG concentrations	↑	↓	No change	↑	No change	No change	FT_4/FT_4I corrects for TBG alterations; TSH indicates true thyroid status
Glucocorticoids (stress dosages)	↓ serum TBG concentrations, ↓ TSH secretion, ↓ T_4 to T_3 conversion	↓	↑	↓	↓	Slight ↓	↓	Evaluate thyroid status after steroids are stopped
Androgens, anabolic steroids, danazol, L-asparaginase, nephrotic syndrome, cirrhosis, familial ↓ TBG	↓ serum TBG concentrations	↓	↑	No change	↓	No change	No change	FT_4/FT_4I corrects TBG alterations; TSH indicates true thyroid status
Phenytoin in vitro, high-dose heparin, furosemide, salicylates (level >15 mg/100 mL), phenylbutazone, fenclofenac, halofenate, mitotane, chloral hydrate, 5-fluorouracil	Displacement of T_4 and T_3 from TBG	↓	↑ or little to no change	No change	↓	No change	No change	FT_4/FT_4I corrects for TBG changes; TSH indicates true thyroid status
Serotonin reuptake inhibitors (e.g., sertraline)	↓ serum TBG concentrations; ? ↑ T_4 clearance	↓ or no change	↑ or ↓ or no change	↓ or no change	↓ or no change	↑ or no change	↑ or no change	Sertraline reported to cause hypothyroidism

Iodide-containing compounds, contrast media, providone–iodine, kelp, tincture of iodine, saturated solution potassium iodide, Lugol's solution, amiodarone	Dilution of total body iodide pools	No change if test not interfered by iodide (i.e., radioimmunoassay)	No change	No change	No change	↓	No change	No change in thyroid status
Strong diuresis by furosemide, ethacrynic acid; iodine deficiency	Decrease total body iodide pools	No change	No change	No change	No change	Might be ↑	No change	No change in thyroid status
Phenytoin, carbamazepine, rifampin, phenobarbital	Hepatic enzyme inducer of T_4 metabolism	↓ or normal	↑ or no change	↓ or normal	No change	No change	No change in euthyroid patients not on T_4 replacement	No change in euthyroid patients not on T_4 replacement
Propranolol, old age, fasting, malnutrition, acute and chronic systemic illness (e.g., euthyroid sick syndrome)	Impair peripheral conversion of T_4 to T_3; ↑ rT_3	Normal or ↓	No change	Normal or ↓	Usually low	No change	No change but in euthyroid sick syndrome, slight ↑ or ↓ in TSH might occur	Thyroid replacement not necessary
Dopamine, levodopa, high-dose glucocorticoids, bromocriptine	Dopamine suppresses TSH secretion	No change	No change	No change	No change	No change	↓ TSH secretion	Not enough to interfere with diagnosis of hyperthyroidism
Amiodarone, iopodate, iopanoate	Impair pituitary and peripheral conversion of T_4 to T_3	↑	No change	↑	↓	↓	Transient ↑	Thyroid abnormalities transient; should be normal within 3 mo; can cause thyroid dysfunction in predisposed patients

[a]See Table 17.1 for abbreviations.

camera picture of the gland, allowing visualization of hypofunctioning, non–iodine-concentrating cold areas, or hyperfunctioning, iodine-concentrating hot areas in the gland. A scan is particularly helpful if discrete thyroid nodules or irregularities are palpable. However, most clinicians prefer to use a fine-needle aspiration rather than an uptake and scan to evaluate a thyroid nodule.

EUTHYROID SICK SYNDROME

Many acute and chronic nonthyroid disorders (e.g., starvation, acute depression and other psychiatric disorders, acute infection, chronic cardiac, pulmonary, renal, hepatic, and neoplastic disorders, and acquired immunodeficiency syndrome) are associated with impaired peripheral conversion of T_4 to T_3, causing abnormal and confusing thyroid function tests in euthyroid patients.[2]

This euthyroid sick syndrome, most common in hospitalized patients, requires appropriate recognition to avoid dangerous and unnecessary hormone replacement. Abnormalities in thyroid function tests vary, but often include a low TT_4, TT_3, a low calculated free T_4 and T_3 index, normal or elevated FT_4, and usually a normal or slightly elevated TSH of less than 10 mIU/L. The slight elevations in TSH concentrations tend to be transient and indicate a recovery phase. Less often, hyperthyroxinemia (e.g., psychiatric illness) occurs. An abnormal binding inhibitor in the sera of sick patients probably accounts for some of the abnormal alterations. Reversal of the abnormal thyroid function tests is a good prognostic indicator of recovery and decreased mortality. Thyroid hormone supplementation is dangerous and unnecessary and might impair normal recovery of thyroid homeostasis.

Hyperthyroidism

DEFINITION

Hyperthyroidism or thyrotoxicosis is a syndrome caused by excessive production of both thyroid hormones and characterized by increased metabolism of all body systems. Thyroid storm, a medical emergency, is an exaggerated form of thyrotoxicosis. A suppressed TSH level with normal thyroid hormone levels is defined as subclinical hyperthyroidism; symptoms may not always be present.

TREATMENT GOALS: HYPERTHYROIDISM

- Reverse the signs and symptoms of hyperthyroidism, normalize thyroid hormone levels, minimize the deleterious effects of T_4 on organ systems, prevent thyroid storm, and improve overall functional capacity.
- Reverse hyperthyroid complaints.
- Reverse hyperthyroid physical findings.
- Normalize free T_4, T_3, and TSH levels.
- Reduce goiter size.
- Improve cardiac function and prevent systemic embolism.
- Preserve bone density and prevent osteoporosis.
- Improve emotional well-being and quality of life.
- Support placenta development and maintenance of pregnancy.
- Promote normal growth, and physical and mental development.

EPIDEMIOLOGY

Overview

Hyperthyroidism affects approximately 2% of women and 0.2% of men; the incidence of hyperthyroidism is reported to be 2.5 to 4.7 per 1000 women.[6,7] Hyperthyroidism in children is rare, accounting for about 1 to 5% of cases.[8] It is unusual in the first 5 years of life; the peak incidence occurs between the ages of 10 and 12 years. The frequency of subclinical hyperthyroidism has ranged from 2 to 16%; the percentage who progress to overt hyperthyroidism is low.[9] The causes of hyperthyroidism and subclinical hyperthyroidism are presented in Table 17.3.

The most common cause of hyperthyroidism is Graves' disease.[6,10] Graves' disease can occur at any age, although its peak onset is between ages 20 and 50. Like all other thyroid disorders, it is 8 to 10 times more common in women than in men; incidences of 80 per 100,000 women per year and 10 per 100,000 men have been reported.[10] There is a strong familial predisposition, but the mode of genetic transmission is unknown. The combination of pregnancy and Graves' thyrotoxicosis is rare, affecting 0.2

Table 17.3 ▪ Causes of Hyperthyroidism

Graves' disease	Autoimmune (see Table 17.6)
Toxic nodules	Single and multinodular
Subacute thyroiditis	Inflammatory thyroiditis, including postpartum thyroiditis, viral thyroiditis (e.g., de Quervain's, amiodarone)
Drug-induced	Iodides (Jod-Basedow), amiodarone, lithium, cytokines
Neonatal thyrotoxicosis	Transplacental passage of TRab
Hashitoxicosis	Hyperthyroid phase of Hashimoto's thyroiditis
T_3 toxicosis	Preferential secretion of T_3, often precedes T_4 toxicosis
Tumors	Secretion of thyroid-stimulating substances
Factitious	Self-administration of L-thyroxine

to 1.4% of the pregnant population. Usually the thyrotoxicosis and treatment antedate the pregnancy because most hyperthyroid patients have reduced fertility. Neonatal thyrotoxicosis develops in 1 to 1.4% of these pregnant women.

The incidence of hyperthyroidism from toxic multinodular goiters (TMG) ranges from 9 to 16%; incidences of 5 to 16 per 100,000 have been reported.[6,11] This is the most common cause of new-onset hyperthyroidism in adults in the fifth or sixth decade of life. Single toxic adenomas are less common; an incidence of 1.6% was noted in the United States, and a higher incidence, 9%, was noted in Europe.[11]

The incidence of hyperthyroidism from a subacute thyroiditis is variable. Postpartum thyroiditis (PPT) develops in 4 to 8% of women after delivery and in as many as 25% of women with insulin-dependent diabetes.[12,13] Cases of subacute thyroiditis (de Quervain's thyroiditis) tend to be seasonal and follow a viral infection.

The incidence of drug-induced thyroid dysfunction ranges from 6% for interferon-α, to 15 to 30% for lithium, to 2 to 24% for amiodarone.[13–16] Hyperthyroidism is less common than hypothyroidism. The incidence of amiodarone-induced hyperthyroidism is 10% in areas of endemic iodine deficiency but only 2 to 3% in iodine-sufficient areas such as the United States. Iodide-induced hyperthyroidism is known as Jod-Basedow.

Drug-Induced Thyrotoxicosis

Iodine-induced thyrotoxicosis (Jod-Basedow) was first described in the 1800s in residents of iodine-deficient areas who became symptomatic after adequate iodine supplementation. Most cases occurred in patients with multinodular goiters and autonomous functioning nodules that were activated by the increased iodine supplements. Iodides do not cause the underlying thyroid disease; they produce thyrotoxicosis in abnormal thyroid glands that have lost the protective Wolff–Chaikoff block. Hyperthyroidism has also been reported after injections of radiocontrast material or iodinated topical preparations.[17]

Lithium is associated with the development of hyperthyroidism, probably through an immune-modulating effect.[13,15,18] Paradoxically, because lithium acts like iodides in blocking hormone release, lithium has been suggested for treatment of hyperthyroidism if other options are not feasible.

Amiodarone, which contains 37.2% iodine by weight, has been implicated in causing two types of hyperthyroidism.[16,19,20] Hyperthyroidism can occur abruptly at any time during the course of amiodarone therapy. Excessive hormone production, caused by amiodarone's high iodine content and loss of the protective Wolff–Chaikoff effect in predisposed people (e.g., multinodular goiter with autonomous nodules, Graves' disease), is managed with the combination of thioamides, potassium perchlorate, and β-blockers. Corticosteroids for 2 to 3 months, in combination with thioamides, are recommended if there is an inflammatory thyroiditis associated with high interleukin-6 levels and hormone leakage into the circulation, causing the hyperthyroidism.[17,21] Because hyperthyroxinemia is a normal laboratory finding in euthyroid patients receiving amiodarone, true thyrotoxicosis should be documented by elevations in serum TT_3 levels, suppression of the TSH, and clinical symptoms. Worsening of cardiac symptoms requires investigation for amiodarone-induced hyperthyroidism. Typical laboratory findings in euthyroid patients on amiodarone include an elevated FT_4 or FT_4I, a subnormal T_3, and an initial transient elevated TSH level that returns to normal after the first 2 to 3 months of amiodarone therapy.

PATHOPHYSIOLOGY

Graves' disease is an autoimmune disorder caused by an abnormal thyroid receptor IgG-stimulating immunoglobulin (e.g., TRab) that binds to the TSH receptor to cause uncontrolled thyroid hormone production.[6,10] Lymphocytic infiltration of the thyroid gland, cytokines including interleukin 1, 4, 8, 10, and interferon-γ, and AtgA and TPO antibodies provide further evidence for an autoimmune process. A defect in suppressor T lymphocytes may be responsible for the formation of the TRab found in the blood of patients with active disease. Cure and spontaneous remission are unlikely as long as the TRab is present; however, how long the TRab persists is unknown. In pregnancy, spontaneous remission and improvement of hyperthyroid symptoms can result from falls in the concentrations of TRab and thyroid antibody titers. Transplacental passage of TRab from the maternal circulation can produce fetal and neonatal hyperthyroidism, which resolves 1 to 2 months after delivery as the antibody levels decline.[22,23] Graves' disease often occurs with other autoimmune processes, including Hashimoto's thyroiditis, type I diabetes mellitus, Addison's disease, vitiligo, and myasthenia gravis. Graves' disease and Hashimoto's thyroiditis have been postulated to be the same autoimmune process because Graves' disease can undergo spontaneous remission to hypothyroidism. Precipitation of Graves' disease has been reported after trauma, severe emotional stress, smoking, weight reduction involving diet restrictions, stimulants, thyroid hormone, and iodide administration (Jod-Basedow).[24]

Single or multiple nodules can produce hyperthyroidism because the nodules function independently of TSH control (autonomously).[11] Patients with autonomous nodules residing in an iodine-deficient area often experience toxemia when given an increased iodide substrate (e.g., iodinated contrast media, relocation to an iodine-sufficient area such as the United States).[17] Patients with a TMG often give a history of a large, firm, multinodular goiter and euthyroidism (normal thyroid status) before hyperthyroidism occurs. Similarly, a single adenoma can be quiescent for many years before becoming toxic. Multiple etiologic factors, including iodine deficiency, genetic abnormalities, and the immune system, have been implicated. Recent evidence suggests that the immune system may be involved, as in Graves' disease, because TPO and TRab antibodies have been detected in patients with TMG.[11]

Hyperthyroidism caused by a subacute thyroiditis results from dumping or leakage of thyroid hormones into the circulation from an inflamed gland.[12,13] de Quervain's thyroiditis is a spontaneous, remitting, inflammatory thyroid condition that is believed to have a viral origin; positive antibody titers to Coxsackievirus, mumps, and other viruses have been identified. PPT is most likely to occur in women with positive thyroid antibodies; 30 to 50% of women with positive thyroid antibodies during pregnancy or at the time of delivery developed PPT. Thyrotoxicosis should be differentiated from Graves' disease or other forms of hyperthyroidism. PPT may recur after subsequent pregnancies, and treatment does not prevent recurrences. Routine screening of women after pregnancy has been recommended. Amiodarone has also been associated with inflammatory thyroiditis.

T_3 thyrotoxicosis is characterized by normal levels of T_4 and elevated levels of T_3. T_3 toxicosis is seen in Graves' disease, toxic goiters, and carcinomas, and is reported in children. Preferential T_3 secretion, producing toxicity, is more prevalent in iodine-deficient areas. Elevated T_3 levels often precede the onset of frank T_4 toxicosis after withdrawal of antithyroid medications in patients with Graves' disease.

Subclinical hyperthyroidism is caused by the same disorders that cause overt hyperthyroidism.[4,9] A common cause of a suppressed TSH is partially treated Graves' disease after RAI therapy. Nonthyroidal illness, medications (Table 17.2), central hypothyroidism, and excessive L-thyroxine replacement therapy should be excluded as potential causes of subclinical hyperthyroidism. Treatment of subclinical hyperthyroidism is warranted. Among patients older than 60 years with untreated subclinical hyperthyroidism, a threefold greater risk of developing atrial fibrillation occurred during a 10-year period.[19] Other concerns include loss of bone density and an increased risk of osteoporosis, especially problematic in postmenopausal women.[20]

CLINICAL PRESENTATION AND DIAGNOSIS

Signs and Symptoms

The clinical symptoms of hyperthyroidism (Table 17.4) in adults reflect increased adrenergic activity, primarily cardiovascular and neurologic. Not all manifestations are present in the same patient. Exogenous ingestion of sympathomimetics or agents with sympathomimetic activity intensify the hyperthyroid symptoms and should be avoided during active disease. Concurrent medical conditions (e.g., diabetes, cardiac conditions) can be exacerbated, and drug action (e.g., digoxin, warfarin, theophylline, insulin) can be altered by the thyrotoxicosis (Tables 17.2 and 17.5).[1]

Thyrotoxicosis-induced increases in heart rate (HR), stroke volume (SV), and cardiac output can cause new or worsening angina, atrial fibrillation, extrasystoles, or congestive heart failure (CHF; high output) that usually are resistant to conventional treatment until euthyroidism occurs. Clinically, a rapid bounding pulse, an elevated systolic blood pressure, a wide pulse pressure, cardiomeg-

Table 17.4 ▪ Signs and Symptoms of Hyperthyroidism and Hypothyroidism

Body System	Hyperthyroidism	Hypothyroidism
General	Heat intolerance, weight loss, ↑ appetite, ↑ sweating, weight gain caused by ↑ appetite	Cold intolerance, weight gain despite ↓ appetite, hoarseness and lowering of voice pitch, ↓ sweating, easy fatigability
Head	Hair thinning and fine texture	Dry, brittle, sparse hair; thinning of the lateral aspects of the eyebrows; puffy facies, large tongue
Eyes	Prominence of the eyes, lid lag, lid retraction; can proceed to loss of visual acuity; Graves' ophthalmopathy	Edematous eyelids, ptosis
Neck	Soft, diffusely enlarged goiter or single or multiple nodules	Goiter in primary hypothyroidism, none found in pituitary disorders
Cardiac	Palpitations, high output failure, angina, edema, ↑ pulse and systolic pressure, wide pulse pressure, presence of systolic murmurs	Cardiac enlargement, poor heart sounds, pericardial pain, low output failure, dyspnea
Gastrointestinal	Diarrhea, loose bowels, or hyperdefecation	Constipation
Genitourinary	Amenorrhea or ↓ menstrual flow	Menorrhagia, dysmenorrhea
Extremities	Pretibial myxedema, Plummer's nails; hot, flushed, and moist skin; palmar erythema	Broad hands and feet, pretibial myxedema, cold and dry skin, brittle nails, yellowish skin
Neuromuscular	Fatigue, weakness, tremor, rapid deep tendon reflexes	Muscle pain and weakness, paresthesias, delayed deep tendon reflexes
Emotional	Nervousness, irritability, emotional lability, insomnia or shortened sleep cycles	Emotional instability, depression, lethargy, ↓ energy, ↑ sleep requirements, mental sluggishness

Table 17.5 ▪ Effect of Thyroid Status on Drug Action

Drug	Hyperthyroidism	Hypothyroidism	Comments
Sympathomimetics (e.g., asthma and cold preparations)	↑ sensitivity to catecholamines; exacerbation of thyrotoxic symptoms, especially cardiac	Blunted response to sympathomimetics (insignificant)	↑ hyperthyroid symptoms even if thyroid function tests normal
Digoxin and digitalis preparations	↑ volume of distribution and renal clearance of digoxin; might need ↑ dosages to achieve therapeutic effect	↑ sensitivity to digoxin therapeutic and toxic effect; ↓ digoxin needed to achieve therapeutic effect	Need to adjust dosages as thyroid function changes to maintain efficacy and avoid toxicity
Insulin	↑ insulin metabolism and clearance; exacerbation of diabetes	Prolonged insulin effect; ↑ risk of hypoglycemia and ↓ insulin to control type II diabetes	Need to adjust insulin dosages in patients with type II diabetes as thyroid status changes
Coumadin	↑ metabolism of clotting factors; ↓ half-life of clotting factors; ↓ coumadin needed for anticoagulation	↓ metabolism of clotting factors; ↑ half-life of clotting factors; ↑ coumadin needed for anticoagulation	Need to adjust dosages as thyroid function changes to maintain efficacy and avoid toxicity
β-Blockers (propranolol, metoprolol, atenolol)	↑ metabolic clearance	Not significant	Might require higher dosages for desired clinical response in hyperthyroidism
Respiratory depressants (e.g., barbiturates, phenothiazines, narcotics)	Not significant	Increased sensitivity to respiratory depressant effects of sedative–hypnotic agents	Increased CO_2 retention; might precipitate myxedema coma; use cautiously in hypothyroidism
Theophylline	Not significant	↓ metabolic clearance	Might need less drug for clinical response; monitor for toxicity
L-thyroxine	↓ serum half-life to 3–4 days	↑ half-life to 9–10 days	Changes in time to steady-state levels and monitoring of thyroid function tests
Cortisol	↓ serum half-life to 50 min	↑ half-life to 155 min	Might need ↑ steroids in management of hyperthyroidism

aly, and a systolic murmur are seen. Tachycardia, increased voltage, and a prolonged P-R interval are evident on electrocardiogram (ECG). It is important to eliminate thyrotoxicosis as causing or exacerbating the cardiac disease, particularly in older adults, in whom cardiac findings can predominate and systemic arterial embolism is of concern.

Thyroid storm is a medical emergency characterized by accentuation of the hyperthyroid symptoms and the acute onset of high fever. If untreated, cardiovascular collapse and shock can occur. Gastrointestinal symptoms can be profound, producing diarrhea, vomiting, abdominal pain, and liver enlargement. Central nervous system involvement can cause agitation and psychosis, leading to apathy, stupor, and coma.[25]

Occasionally, a patient with severe toxemia may exhibit none of the classic hyperthyroid symptoms. This "apathetic" or masked hyperthyroidism can be a typical finding in older adults. Presenting symptoms of anorexia, fatigue, apathy, listlessness, dull eyes, extreme weakness, CHF, delayed speech and mentation, and low-grade fever are confusing in such patients and obscure the diagnosis. Likewise, premature atrial contractions, atrial fibrillation with embolism, or tremor might be the only clue to occult hyperthyroidism in older adults. If the condition goes untreated, coma and death are certain. Therefore, the presence of any new or worsening cardiac, neurologic, or failure-to-thrive symptoms in older adults necessitate an evaluation for underlying thyroid disease. Occult thyrotoxicosis is confirmed easily by standard laboratory tests.

In children, the signs and symptoms are similar to those seen in the adult, with the notable exception of cardiovascular manifestation.[8] Excessive thirst, behavioral manifestations of restlessness, and inability to concentrate incur difficulties in school and family relationships and might be the initial presenting symptom.

Fetal hyperthyroidism usually appears during the second half of pregnancy and is characterized by tachycardia (HR greater than 160/minute), craniosynostosis, frontal bossing, mental retardation, intrauterine growth retardation, premature delivery, and a mortality rate of approximately 16%.[18]

The triad of hyperthyroidism, a diffusely enlarged and symmetric goiter, and infiltrative ophthalmopathy or dermopathy characterizes Graves' disease. A bruit, indicative of high blood flow, might be present in a severely toxic patient. Bruits usually are audible over the entire thyroid gland and disappear in euthyroidism. Not all of these clinical findings are present or necessary for the diagnosis.

The ocular findings are the most striking abnormalities of Graves' disease.[26] Graves' ophthalmopathy is not directly correlated with the thyroid status and can appear before, during, or even years after successful therapy of the hyperthyroidism. The ocular involvement can be unilateral or bilateral and might not reverse with euthyroidism. Progression and worsening of the eye signs can occur abruptly after RAI therapy, particularly in patients who have mild symptoms before RAI therapy, and prophylaxis with systemic corticosteroids is indicated.[26,27] It is not known why the eyes and the orbital muscles are involved whereas other organ systems are spared. Mild eye symptoms are found in 50% of patients; the most severe forms occur in less than 5%. The ophthalmopathy is more severe and progressive in smokers, who have higher levels of TRab than nonsmokers. The ocular manifestations include the noninfiltrative and the characteristic infiltrative ophthalmopathy of Graves' disease.

The noninfiltrative ocular abnormalities result from hyperactivity of the sympathetic system and can be found in any hyperthyroid condition. Increased sympathetic tone on Muller's superior palpebral muscle causes spasm and retraction of the upper lid, widening the palpebral fissure to give the characteristic stare or frightened expression. On physical examination, lid lag is present when the eyelid movement lags behind eye movement, and a narrow white rim of sclera becomes visible between the upper lid and the cornea. These ocular changes can cause symptoms of grittiness, dryness, tearing, itching, redness, and photophobia that improve with normalization of the hormone levels.

Exophthalmos or proptosis (protrusion of the cornea more than the normal 18 to 20 mm beyond the lateral margin of the orbit) is a characteristic feature of Graves' ophthalmopathy that results from an increase in the orbital contents. Histologic examination reveal lymphocytic infiltration and deposition of mucopolysaccharides, fat, and water in all retrobulbar tissue, causing the globes to be firmer and harder than normal. Proptosis can produce a wide-eyed stare, leading to increased tearing and irritation from the exposed conjunctiva. Soft tissue involvement can produce edema and swelling of the lids and periorbital tissue, causing chemosis, excessive tearing, photophobia, and conjunctivitis. Corneal scarring and ulceration result if the proptosis causes the lid to remain open, exposing and drying out the eye during sleep. Paralysis of extraocular muscles can limit eye movements, producing diplopia, loss of upward gaze, and loss of convergence. Blindness might result from venous congestion and hemorrhage of the retina and optic nerve.

The dermopathy of Graves' disease, also known as pretibial myxedema, can occur with the infiltrative ophthalmopathy. Mucopolysaccharide infiltration of the skin causes the cutaneous thickening and hyperpigmentation (i.e., orange-peel skin) usually seen over the tibial aspects of the leg. Similar lesions can appear on the dorsa of the feet and hands. Pretibial myxedema usually is asymptomatic but can be painful or pruritic. Like the infiltrative ocular symptoms, pretibial myxedema can occur at any time in the course of the disease. If necessary, the clinical diagnosis can be confirmed by tissue biopsy. Treatment with high-potency topical corticosteroids and plastic wrap often is effective.

Diagnosis

The American College of Physicians has established clinical guidelines for diagnosis and screening of hyperthyroidism.[3] The diagnosis of hyperthyroidism is confirmed by a finding of abnormally high levels of FT_4 or TT_3 and an undetectable TSH. The presence of positive antibodies (i.e., ATgA and TPO), ophthalmopathy, or dermopathy confirms the diagnosis of Graves' disease (Table 17.6). An elevated TT_3 and positive TRab can provide essential information in patients with atypical presentations. The RAIU is elevated but is not cost-effective or necessary for a diagnosis of Graves' in a patient with positive antibodies and the classic presentation. On scan, a diffusely enlarged, homogenous hot gland is found.

The presence of palpable nodules in a normal or enlarged goiter requires exclusion of a TMG or toxic adenoma. Diagnosis is confirmed by a finding of the typical hyperthyroid indices, a suppressed TSH in a mildly symptomatic or asymptomatic person, and an RAIU and scan revealing hot nodules. In some cases, the rest of the thyroid may not be visible on the thyroid scan if functioning thyroid tissue is suppressed by the hot nodule.

Conditions caused by subacute thyroiditis (e.g., PPT, amiodarone) can be confirmed by a finding of a low or undetectable RAIU, elevated thyroid hormone levels, and a suppressed or undetectable TSH level. de Quervain's subacute thyroiditis must be suspected if there is the acute onset of gland tenderness or pain with swallowing, a recent history of flulike symptoms, fever, malaise, and symptoms of either hyperthyroidism or hypothyroidism.[13] Other laboratory abnormalities include an elevated erythrocyte sedimentation rate (ESR), negative thyroid antibodies, and leukocytosis.

THERAPEUTIC PLAN

The American Thyroid Association and the American Association of Clinical Endocrinologists have published clinical guidelines for treatment of hyperthyroidism.[28,29]

Table 17.6 ▪ Characteristics of Graves' Disease

Hyperthyroidism, goiter, and ophthalmopathy or dermopathy
Positive family history
Female > male patients
Elevated FT_4 or FT_4I, TT_4, TT_3
Suppressed/Undetectable TSH level
Positive ATgA, TPO, TRab
Unknown duration of disease

FT_4, free thyroxine; *FT_4I*, free thyroxine index; *TT_4*, total thyroxine; *TT_3*, total triiodothyronine; *TSH*, thyroid-stimulating hormone; *ATgA*, thyroglobulin antibody; *TPO*, thyroperoxidase antibody; *TRab*, thyroid receptor antibody.

The major treatment modalities for the management of hyperthyroidism include thioamides, RAI, and surgery (Table 17.7).[6,7,30] Each has its own advantages and limitations, so treatment must be individualized. The cause of the hyperthyroidism, its severity, the patient's age, the size of the goiter, the presence of thyroid and nonthyroid complications, and social and economic issues are critical considerations for treatment selection. Depending on the cause of the hyperthyroidism, all three treatment options might be appropriate (e.g., Graves' disease); for another cause, one modality is preferred. In some cases, therapy might be transient because the disease is self-limiting (e.g., subacute thyroiditis, neonatal Graves' disease, PPT, drug-induced disease). Treatment algorithms such as the one in Figure 17.3 enable pharmacists to treat patients with hyperthyroidism effectively. Treatment adjuncts include iodides, iodinated contrast media, potassium perchlorate, adrenergic antagonists, corticosteroids, cholestyramine,[31] and rarely, lithium (Table 17.7).

Patients with uncomplicated Graves' disease, particularly children, might be treated medically with thioamides until remission occurs.[6–8] Theoretically, thioamides are preferred over RAI and surgery to treat the patient with uncomplicated Graves' because they do not destroy the gland and they control the disease. Therefore, chronic thyroid replacement, which is likely with RAI or surgery, might not be necessary if thioamides are used. This advantage of thioamides might be irrelevant because the natural history of Graves' disease appears to be eventual hypothyroidism even if no glandular destruction occurs. If RAI or surgery is selected, most older patients and all severely thyrotoxic patients should be pretreated with thioamides.[30] Pretreatment depletes the gland of stored hormones, reduces the hypermetabolic rate, and prevents leakage of hormone from the gland after RAI or during surgery, preventing thyroid storm.[25,30] However, the final decision in the patient with uncomplicated Graves' disease is often empiric, depending on available resources, the physician's experience, and the patient's personal preference. Treatment selection should be a joint patient–physician decision after a discussion of the benefits and risks of each method.

The preferred therapy of hyperthyroidism in patients with Graves' ophthalmopathy is unresolved.[6,7,26,27] Endocrinologists at the University of California at San Francisco prefer thyroid ablation with RAI or surgery (less desirable) to remove the antigen source (i.e., gland) and believe that these methods are more effective than thioamides to prevent progressive ophthalmopathy. However, worsening ocular symptoms have been reported after all types of treatment, particularly after RAI in patients with preexisting eye symptoms.[26,27] In such patients, prophylactic systemic corticosteroids (e.g., prednisone 30 to 40 mg daily starting within a few days of RAI and continuing for approximately 2 to 3 weeks) is indicated to prevent further progression of the ophthalmopathy. Hypothyroidism can also aggravate preexisting eye complaints. Regardless of the method of treatment selected, hyperthyroidism control and hypothyroidism prevention are essential to prevent deterioration of the ophthalmopathy.

A survey of practicing thyroidologists also showed considerable variation in the initial treatment selected for Graves' disease.[32,33] In the United States, RAI therapy is the preferred modality of choice, except in younger patients, for whom thioamides are chosen. In contrast, thioamides are selected as the treatment of choice by European and Japanese endocrinologists. All participants chose surgery as the last choice unless there were obstructive symptoms or concerns about malignancy. Concerns about ophthalmopathy were not addressed.

Although thioamides can normalize thyroid hormone levels, single or toxic multinodular disease is best managed with definitive treatment, such as RAI or surgery, because spontaneous remission is unlikely.[11]

The usual treatment choices in children are thioamides and subtotal thyroidectomy, although all three methods (surgery, RAI, and thioamides) have been used.[8,30,34] The risks of surgery must be weighed against the benefits of speedy correction of the thyrotoxicosis and the lack of need for the rigid dosing schedules of the thioamides. RAI usually is not recommended because of fear of genetic damage, leukemia, and carcinogenesis, although these risks are unsubstantiated.[30] Thyroid carcinoma and dysfunction have been reported in children exposed to external head and neck irradiation, although similar results have not been shown with internal RAI.

Hyperthyroidism can be difficult to manage during pregnancy. Pregnancy is best postponed until the hyperthyroidism is controlled permanently with either surgery or RAI to prevent disease flares and relapse during pregnancy and during and after delivery.[18,35] Spontaneous remission of the disease with improvement of symptoms can occur during pregnancy because of declines in TRab levels, and antithyroid medications often are not necessary.[13] Untreated maternal thyrotoxicosis can result in abortion, perinatal death, and prematurity, so proper treatment is crucial. Thioamides can be used if precautions are taken. RAI and iodides are absolutely contraindicated, and surgery in the second trimester is an option.

Infants with neonatal Graves' disease are extremely ill within hours of delivery. Supportive measures, including sedation, cooling, oxygen, fluid, and electrolyte replacement and short-term management of the hyperthyroidism by thioamides, iodides, or β-blockers, are required. Fortunately, the disease is self-limiting and symptoms disappear in 1 to 2 months as the level of TRab declines. Antithyroid drugs should be withdrawn at this time.

Subacute thyroiditis is self-limiting, and spontaneous recovery is common.[13] Treatment is symptomatic and consists of heat, rest, analgesics (e.g., nonsteroidal anti-inflammatory drugs), and β-blockers, if necessary, to control the symptoms of hyperthyroidism. Thioamides are not effective because hormone leakage from the gland rather than increased hormone synthesis causes the

Table 17.7 ▪ Management of Hyperthyroidism

Method	Drug	Dosage	Mechanism of Action	Toxicity	Comments
Thioamides	PTU 50-mg tablets; can be formulated for rectal administration	300–400 mg/day given every 6–8 hr initially; maintenance dosage of 50–150 mg daily	Blocks organification of hormone synthesis Inhibits peripheral conversion of T_4 to T_3 Immunosuppressive	Skin rashes, bitter taste, agranulocytosis, gastrointestinal symptoms, hepatocellular hepatitis	Remission rate of 20–30% Onset of action approximately 2–4 wk Used in pregnancy and during lactation
	Methimazole (Tapazole) 5- and 10-mg tablets; can be formulated for rectal administration	30–40 mg once daily initially, maintenance dosage of 5–15 mg daily	Blocks organification of hormone synthesis; immunosuppressive	See PTU Secreted in breast milk Might be teratogenic (e.g., scalp defects) Obstructive jaundice	DOC for once-daily dosing Remission rate of 20–30% Onset of action approximately 2–4 wk Appears to have little cross-sensitivity to PTU for maculopapular rashes
Iodides	Lugol's solution 8 mg iodide/drop; saturated solution of potassium iodide 50 mg/drop; intravenous potassium iodide available	6 mg iodide/day, although larger dosages are given	Block hormone release Decrease gland vascularity and increase gland firmness to facilitate surgical removal	Hypersensitivity reactions: rashes, rhinorrhea, parotid and submaxillary swelling Rarely anaphylactoid reactions Contraindicated in pregnancy	Provides symptomatic relief before onset of thioamides Use in thyroid storm and as a preoperative adjunct Do not use before RAI
Adrenergic antagonists	Propranolol (Inderal); Metoprolol (Lopressor); Atenolol (Tenormin) Various tablet strengths Intravenous propranolol 1 mg/mL Avoid β-blocker with intrinsic sympathomimetic activity	Propranolol 20–40 mg orally every 6 hr or equivalent β-blocker	Blocks the peripheral action of thyroid hormone No effect on disease state Blocks peripheral T_4 to T_3 conversion	Bradycardia, congestive heart failure, asthma Inhibits hyperglycemic response to hypoglycemia Avoid in pregnancy	Provides rapid symptomatic relief while awaiting activity of thioamides, RAI, or surgery
	Diltiazem (Cardizem) 30-, 60-, 90-, 120-mg tablets Sustained-release tablets might not be as effective	60 mg PO QID or 120 mg TID	Blocks the peripheral action of thyroid hormone No effect on disease state	Hypotension, bradycardia, pedal edema	Alternative for patients unable to tolerate β-blockers (e.g., asthma, insulin-dependent diabetes mellitus) Verapamil and dihydropyridine calcium channel blockers not as effective

RAI	^{131}I	80–150 μCi/g thyroid tissue Usual dosage 8–10 mCi	Destruction of the gland	Hypothyroidism, rarely radiation thyroiditis Fear of malignancy, leukemia, and genetic damage Contraindicated in pregnancy	Slow onset of action (approximately 2–4 wk) Full effects seen within 3–6 mo
Surgery	Iodides, thioamides, or β-blockers preoperatively to prevent storm and facilitate surgery	5–10 drops/day of iodides for 10–14 days before surgery	Removal of the gland Total thyroidectomy might be surgery of choice to prevent recurrent hyperthyroidism	Hypothyroidism, hypoparathyroidism, complications of surgery and anesthesia	Incidence of hypothyroidism indirectly proportional to gland remnant size
Iodinated contrast media	Ipodate, iopanoic acid 500-mg tablets	500 mg–1 g PO daily or 3 g PO every third day	Blocks T_4 to T_3 conversion, release of iodides	Similar to iodides: nausea, vomiting, abdominal cramps, diarrhea, dizziness, headache	Rapid onset of action Adjunct to thioamides Not for chronic use because effects are not sustained
Ionic exchange resin	Cholestyramine 4 g oral powder packets	4 g PO TID	Increases fecal excretion of T_4 by binding T_4 in the intestine	Gastrointestinal: bloating, flatulence, constipation Impairs absorption of concurrent medications	Adjunct to thioamides; useful when additional decline in hormone levels is desired
Monovalent anions	Potassium perchlorate 200-mg capsules	800–1000 mg/day PO in four divided doses for 2–6 wk	Competitive inhibitor of iodide binding Discharges nonorganified iodide from the gland	Gastric irritation, nausea, vomiting, fever, rashes Aplastic anemia, bone marrow suppression, and nephrotic syndrome when used chronically	Useful short-term adjunct to thioamides for amiodarone-induced hyperthyroidism
Lithium	Lithium carbonate, various dosage forms available	800–1200 mg/day in 2 to 3 divided doses	Acts similar to iodides to block hormone release	Nausea, vomiting, diarrhea, tremor, ataxia, dizziness, confusion, coma Maintain normal serum levels Avoid hyponatremia or sodium depletion	Reserved for special situations when other agents are contraindicated or ineffective

PTU, propylthiouracil; T_4, thyroxine; T_3, triiodothyronine; *DOC*, drug of choice; RAI, radioactive iodine.

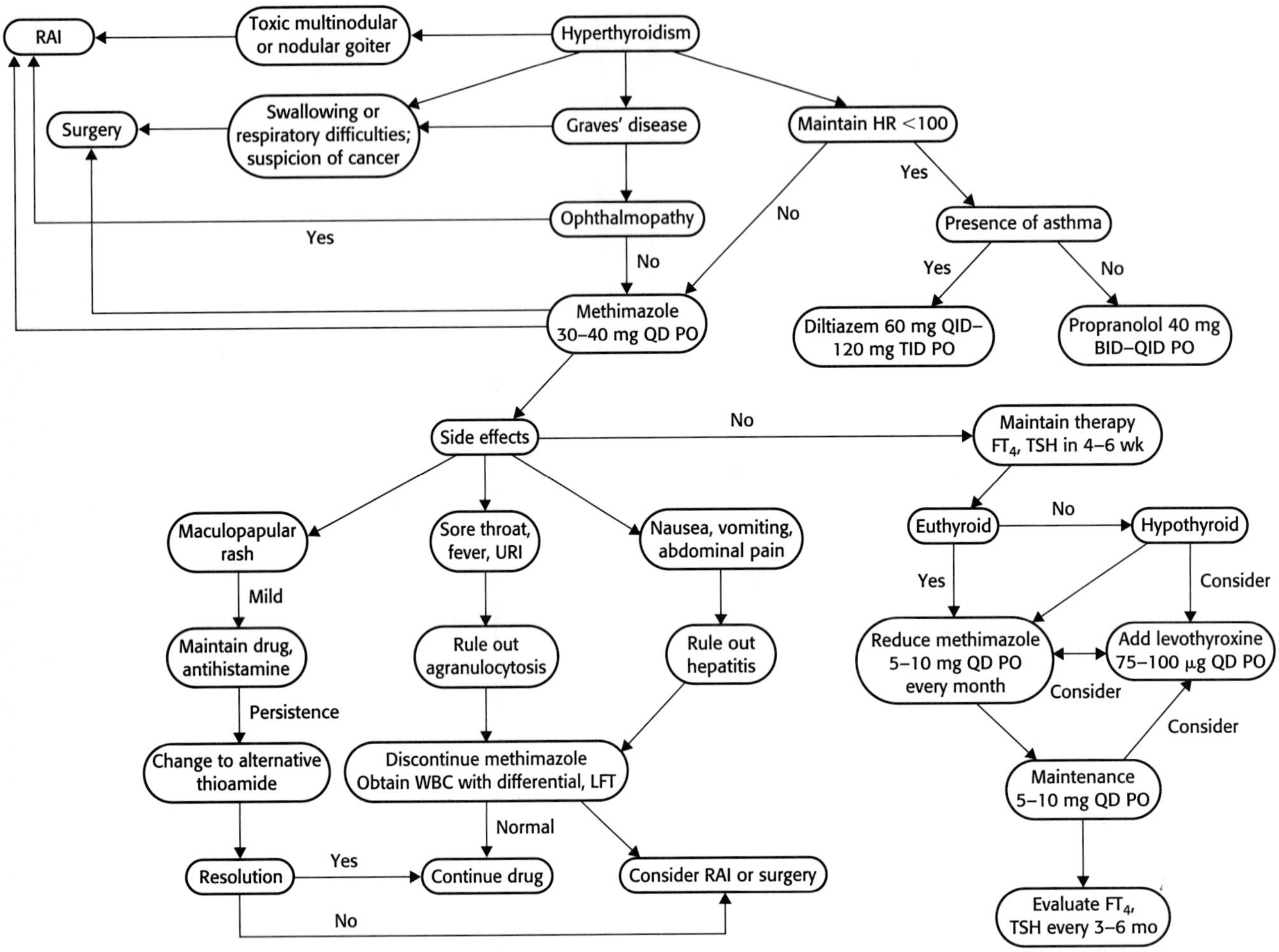

Figure 17.3. Treatment algorithm for management of hyperthyroidism from Graves' disease or autonomous nodules (single or multinodular). *FT_4*, free thyroxine; *HR*, heart rate; *LFT*, liver function test; *RAI*, radioactive iodine; *TSH*, thyroid-stimulating hormone; *URI*, upper respiratory tract symptoms.

elevated hormone levels. Corticosteroids are indicated for severe inflammation if analgesics are ineffective. In the hypothyroid phase, transient thyroid replacement might be necessary to suppress further TSH stimulation to the damaged gland and treat symptoms of hypothyroidism.

TREATMENT

Pharmacotherapy

Thioamides

Thioamides can be used as long-term primary therapy for Graves' hyperthyroidism, especially in adolescents and children, or given transiently to reduce thyroid hormone levels before definitive therapy with RAI or surgery.[6,7,36] Thioamides are the treatment of choice in patients with small goiters and mild disease, for whom a high remission rate is likely. The advantages of thioamides include the potential for remission without damage to the gland. Limitations include nonadherence, strict parental and physician supervision in children, low success rates, and the risks of adverse reaction.

The thioamides, propylthiouracil (PTU) and methimazole, prevent thyroid hormone synthesis by inhibiting the oxidation binding of iodide and its coupling to tyrosine residue. PTU (but not methimazole) inhibits the peripheral deiodination of T_4 to T_3, so serum T_3 levels decline 20 to 30% more rapidly in severely thyrotoxic patients. TSH receptor antibody levels also are suppressed by thioamides via an unknown immunosuppressive mechanism of action.[37]

Thioamide selection is based largely on the prescriber's personal preference, although certain pharmacologic differences should dictate the choice. Generally, PTU is preferred over methimazole in patients with thyroid storm or those with severe hyperthyroidism because it blocks the peripheral conversion of T_4 to T_3 and therefore might have a faster onset of action. PTU, and not methimazole, generally is considered the drug of choice in pregnancy because maternal use of methimazole is associated with congenital skin defects (i.e., aplasia cutis). However, some have concluded that the association between methimazole and congenital skin defects is not sufficiently supported to preclude the use of this drug during pregnancy, and methimazole has been used without deleterious effects.[38–40] PTU is preferred over methimazole in lactating women because insignificant amounts of PTU are excreted in the milk, whereas

7 to 16% of a methimazole dose is detected in breast milk.[35] Although PTU is more commonly prescribed, methimazole is preferred for several reasons. Methimazole can be given as a single daily dose, which improves patient compliance. It is more potent than PTU and requires fewer tablets. It is also less expensive, better tolerated, and at low dosages is less toxic than PTU.[36] Therefore, methimazole is the thioamide of choice except in patients unable to tolerate PTU and in the situations just identified, in which PTU might be preferable.

Methimazole is 10 times as potent as PTU (100 mg PTU = 10 mg methimazole), but they are equally effective if given in equipotent dosages. Both drugs are absorbed rapidly from the gastrointestinal tract, and peak plasma concentrations are reached within 30 minutes of ingestion. The serum half-lives of 4 to 6 hours for methimazole and 1 to 2 hours for PTU do not change as the thyroid status changes. However, the duration of action and frequency of dosing depend on the intrathyroidal half-life, not on the short plasma half-lives. The duration of action of methimazole is 24 to 36 hours, permitting once-daily administration. The intrathyroidal duration of PTU is much shorter, requiring initial dosing every 6 to 8 hours to be effective.

Initial therapy should begin with 30 to 40 mg/day orally of methimazole, given either as a single daily dose or in three divided doses, if needed to limit gastrointestinal intolerance. Alternatively, 300 to 400 mg/day of PTU can be given in three to four divided doses.[36] Dosage regimens for thioamides in children are similar to those used in adults. In neonates, PTU (5 to 10 mg/kg/day) or methimazole (0.5 to 1 mg/kg/day) is effective.[8] Initial single-dose regimens have been used successfully with PTU, but the best results are obtained by multiple daily dosing until euthyroidism is achieved, then changing to a single-dose maintenance regimen. Patients experiencing severe toxemia or thyroid storm may need dosages as high as 1200 mg/day of PTU or its equivalent, given in divided doses. There are no intravenous preparations, although both drugs can be formulated for rectal administration.[41,42] Tapering of the thioamide dosage should not begin until symptoms are reduced and T_4 levels are normal, usually 6 to 8 weeks (based on elimination of existing thyroid stores; $t_{1/2}$ = 7 days). The initial dosage can be reduced gradually, by one-third each month, until a daily maintenance dosage of 5 to 15 mg methimazole or 50 to 150 mg/day PTU is reached. If symptoms do not resolve within the specified time, nonadherence, incomplete blockage of synthesis by insufficient dosage, or an inadequate dosing interval should be considered as causes of failure. A change to methimazole is indicated if PTU was the initial drug because nonadherence is more likely to occur with PTU than with methimazole.

In pregnancy, the dangers of fetal goiter and hypothyroidism are reduced if initial dosages of PTU are maintained below 300 mg/day (given in divided doses) and maintenance dosages of 50 to 100 mg/day are used throughout pregnancy.[18] Equivalent dosages of methimazole appear to be as safe as PTU with respect to fetal hypothyroidism and could be used if necessary, although methimazole might pose a rare teratogenic risk of aplasia cutis.[38–40,43] Clinically, the mother should be maintained in a comfortable, mildly hyperthyroid state (FT_4I or FT_4 in the upper ranges of normal) to prevent fetal thyroid suppression. The appearance of an enlarged maternal goiter during therapy is alarming because it implies the development of maternal and fetal hypothyroidism. The concomitant use of thyroid hormone is not helpful because thyroid does not cross the placenta and might make maternal management more difficult. Fortunately, the intellectual development of offspring exposed to antithyroid drugs in utero appears to be no different from that of unexposed siblings.[44]

A baseline FT_4 or FT_4I, TSH, and white blood cell (WBC) count with differential should be obtained before thioamides are started. A baseline WBC with differential can help ascertain the development of thioamide-induced agranulocytosis because hyperthyroidism can be associated with a relative reduction in the neutrophil count. Thyroid hormone levels should normalize within 6 to 8 weeks after the start of therapy and parallel the clinical response. The FT_4 or FT_4I and TSH should be monitored routinely at 4 to 8 weeks after the start of therapy and after any change in the dosing regimen. Once a stable thioamide maintenance dosage is reached, thyroid function tests can be monitored routinely every 2 to 4 months.

The recommended duration of thioamide therapy for Graves' disease is empiric, generally 12 to 18 months. Courses of 3 to 6 months have been proposed, but lower remission rates of 20 to 40% result.[36] Several studies suggest that the remission rate might improve with a longer duration of therapy.[45,46] An 18-month treatment period yielded higher remission rates (61.8%) than 6-month therapy (41.7%). A study in children noted a 25% increase in the remission rate when the duration was increased by 1 year.[47] Therefore, 12 months is the minimum treatment duration recommended to maximize remission potential. Longer treatment durations can be used if there are no adverse effects and the patient is willing to continue antithyroid therapy.

Disappointing remission rates of 15% to 80% after stopping thioamides have led to progressive disenchantment with the antithyroid drugs as definitive therapy for Graves' disease. Permanent spontaneous remission is rare. It is unclear why some patients remain in remission while others relapse. No factors have been consistently predictive of successful long-term remission, and most studies have produced conflicting results. Factors associated with poor long-term remission rates include increased dietary intake of iodides, severe hyperthyroidism, a large goiter that does not regress with thioamide therapy, short duration of thioamide therapy, persistent high titers of TRab after stopping thioamides, recurrent hyperthyroidism, and presence of HLA antigen.[36,45–47]

An excellent indicator for remission is normalization of the goiter size during therapy. Patients with small goiters, mild and short duration of symptoms and illness, and disappearance of TRab during therapy might have a better chance of remission.[36,45–47] Analysis of HLA specificities (HLA-B8 and DW3) in conjunction with IgG levels may be highly predictive of remission or relapse after withdrawal of thioamides.

Factors associated with TRab titer reduction include therapy longer than 1 year, high blocking dosages of thioamides, and concomitant administration of levothyroxine (L-thyroxine) with thioamides. High thioamide blocking dosages (i.e., 600 to 800 mg PTU or 40 to 60 mg methimazole) given throughout therapy produced better remission rates (75.4%) than conventional therapy (41.6%) but produced greater toxicity and therefore cannot be recommended.[48] The initial enthusiasm and optimism generated by a study showing that adding L-thyroxine to antithyroid therapy could reduce relapse rates by suppressing TSH receptor antibody levels have quieted. Hashizume et al.[49] first reported a startling recurrence rate of 1.7% in Japanese patients who received methimazole for 6 months, followed by combined L-thyroxine and methimazole for a year, and then L-thyroxine alone for 3 years, compared with a relapse rate of 34.7% in those not receiving L-thyroxine. However, another study did not find that adding L-thyroxine resulted in greater TSH receptor antibody suppression than methimazole alone, suggesting that remission rates would not be different.[50] Unfortunately, several prospective studies, using similar designs, have been unable to duplicate Hashizume et al.'s favorable remission rates, and the benefits of using a more complicated and expensive combination regimen are questionable.[51,52] Some clinicians advocate the concomitant use of exogenous L-thyroxine during antithyroid therapy to prevent hypothyroidism and suppress goiter formation from excessive PTU or methimazole administration. Proper titration of the thioamide dosage should alleviate this problem, so concomitant L-thyroxine therapy is recommended only if proper titration is difficult.

Toxic reactions to PTU and methimazole occur in 1 to 5% of patients.[6,36] A pruritic maculopapular skin rash, without other systemic manifestations, is the most common adverse reaction. Therefore, all patients should be instructed to report symptoms of skin reactions. It is also important to distinguish a thioamide rash from a heat rash or hives caused by ectopic hyperthyroidism. In mild cases, the rash might disappear spontaneously despite continued therapy. Antihistamines can provide symptomatic relief of the pruritus. If the rash persists, the alternative thioamide can be substituted because little cross-sensitivity exists. However, if the rash is associated with systemic symptoms (i.e., fever, arthralgias) or if angioneurotic edema, hives, or other anaphylactoid reactions occur, substitution with another thioamide is not recommended because the risks of cross-sensitivity are high.

Hepatitis is more common than previously appreciated.[53,54] Hepatocellular and obstructive hepatitis have been reported with both agents; however, hepatocellular damage is more common with PTU, and obstructive jaundice occurs with methimazole, especially at dosages greater than 40 mg daily. The incidence of PTU-induced hepatotoxicity is estimated to be less than 0.5%, but the true incidence is unknown. Approximately 30% of patients on PTU can have asymptomatic hepatic transaminase elevations. Stopping PTU might not be necessary if the transaminases normalize within 3 months of a dosage reduction. In contrast, PTU should be stopped immediately to ensure complete recovery in patients with clinical evidence of hepatitis. PTU-induced hepatitis typically is associated with nonspecific hepatocellular necrosis on liver biopsy. The prognosis appears worse in those aged less than 11 years or more than 40 years, with duration of jaundice more than 7 days before onset of encephalopathy and with significant elevations in serum bilirubin (more than 300 μmol/L, or 17.5 mg/dL) and prothrombin time (more than 50 seconds). Circulating autoantibodies and in vitro peripheral lymphocyte sensitization to PTU indicate a possible autoimmune cause. These idiosyncratic reactions typically occur early in therapy, although delayed reactions have been noted. It is reversible if detected early, although fatalities have been reported. Because of the severity of the reaction and potential for cross-sensitivity, substitution with the alternative thioamide is not recommended. Routine monitoring of liver function tests should be considered in patients with a history of liver disease and risk factors for hepatitis (e.g., alcoholism). All patients should be educated about the symptoms of hepatitis and instructed to avoid alcohol and to immediately report any symptoms of hepatitis to their health care providers.

Rarely, hypoprothrombinemia (with PTU), serologic abnormalities (lupus erythematosus, antinuclear antibody), lupus, and lupuslike syndromes have also been reported. Recovery occurs after withdrawal of the drug or institution of steroids.

Agranulocytosis (fewer than 500 polymorphonuclear neutrophil leukocytes) is the most serious (but rare) adverse reaction to the thioamides. The incidence is between 0.5 and 6%.[6,36] The onset of fever higher than 101°F, malaise, gingivitis, and sore throat is so abrupt that routine WBC counts usually are not helpful. Although one study suggests that weekly monitoring of the WBC with differential during the first 3 months of therapy might identify early and asymptomatic agranulocytosis, routine monitoring is not indicated because it might hamper patient compliance and does not appear to be cost-effective.[55] All patients should be educated carefully about agranulocytosis and instructed to immediately report the onset of such symptoms to their pharmacists or physicians. Patients older than 40 years and those on high-dose methimazole (more than 40 mg/day) might be at greater risk of developing this toxic reaction, although it is not necessarily dose-related. Lower dosages (less than 30 mg/day) of methimazole might be safer than any dosage of PTU. Sex is not a predictive factor. This reaction is more likely to occur during the first 6 weeks of therapy, although it can occur at any time in the course of treatment. One study suggests that agranulocytosis might occur earlier with PTU therapy (i.e., 17.7 ± 9.7 days) than with methimazole therapy (36.9 ± 14.5 days).[55] Fortunately, complete resolution of symptoms and recovery of granulocytes are often seen within a few days to 3 weeks after the thioamides are stopped. Granulocyte colony-stimulating factor and corticosteroids might shorten the recovery period. If infection occurs, antibiotics, adrenal steroids, and possibly hospitalization (bacteria-free room) are indicated. Rechallenge with the same drug or an alternative thioamide is not recommended because the risk of recurrent agranulocytosis outweighs the benefits of therapy. The degree of cross-sensitivity is not known.

Potassium Perchlorate

Potassium perchlorate is a monovalent anion that interferes with iodide binding and causes the discharge of nonorganified iodide from the gland. Because perchlorate is a competitive inhibitor of iodide, it is particularly useful for the short-term management of amiodarone-induced hyperthyroidism, but its antithyroid effect can be overcome by iodine administration.[16,20] Short-term administration (e.g., 800 mg to 1 gm/day for 2 to 6 weeks) is well tolerated, but irreversible aplastic anemia and nephrotic syndrome have limited the usefulness of the monovalent anions for chronic therapy of hyperthyroidism.

Iodides

Although the iodides have been known to provide symptomatic relief of thyrotoxicosis since the 1920s, their clinical use has been largely superseded by the thioamides and β-blockers. Iodides act by several mechanisms of action: They inhibit organification (Wolff–Chaikoff effect) and hormone release and decrease gland vascularity.[17] The rapid relief of thyrotoxic symptoms after 2 to 7 days of iodide administration suggests that inhibition of hormone release is the predominant mechanism of action, rather than a block in organification, which would not be apparent for several weeks. This rapid effect is advantageous for patients in thyroid storm and for those awaiting the onset of thioamide therapy. However, iodides should not be used before RAI therapy (or if RAI is considered as subsequent treatment) because iodides can block effective RAI retention by the gland for several weeks after use.

Iodides are routinely given 10 to 14 days before surgery to facilitate surgical removal of the hyperplastic gland by decreasing its vascularity and increasing its firmness. Preoperatively, the combination of β-blockers and iodides can also be used, although the established regimen of thioamides and iodides is preferable.

Stable iodine is available as either Lugol's solution (5% iodine and 10% potassium iodide), containing 8 mg of iodide per drop, or as the more palatable saturated solution of potassium iodide (SSKI), containing 50 mg/drop. A parental preparation, potassium iodide, is also available (Table 17.7).

The major adverse effects of iodides are hypersensitivity reactions, including rashes, drug fever, sialadenitis, conjunctivitis, rhinitis, and collagen vascular disorders. In patients with underlying thyroid disorders, iodides can either produce hyperthyroidism (e.g., multinodular goiter) from failure of the Wolff–Chaikoff block, or cause goiter and hypothyroidism (e.g., Hashimoto's thyroiditis) in patients unable to escape from the Wolff–Chaikoff block.[17] Chronic iodide administration should be avoided throughout pregnancy because ingesting as little as 12 mg iodine has caused fetal goiter and asphyxiation. Vaginal povidone or topical iodine can produce high serum concentrations of iodine and should also be avoided.

Advantages of iodide therapy include simplicity, low cost, low toxicity, and no gland destruction. Limitations of treatment include escape, treatment relapse, allergic reactions, and interference with subsequent RAI therapy.

Adrenergic Antagonists

Because many of the signs and symptoms of thyrotoxicosis are mediated through the sympathetic nervous system, drugs that deplete or block the effects of thyroid hormones on tissue catecholamines can provide rapid symptomatic relief before thioamides, RAI, and surgery act. These agents do not affect the underlying disease process, so they should not be used as primary therapy.

Propranolol is the β-blocker most widely used and studied in the treatment of the hyperthyroidism and therefore the standard against which others are judged.[7,56] When propranolol is given orally in dosages of 20 to 40 mg three to four times a day as necessary, symptomatic relief of palpitations, tachycardia, anxiety, sweating, tremor, and diarrhea occurs. However, weight loss remains unaffected. Patients with severe toxemia might need as much as 480 mg/day to achieve symptomatic relief and maintain the HR below 100 bpm. Propranolol is also surprisingly effective in controlling the neuromuscular manifestations of hyperthyroidism, especially periodic paralysis. It can be used as an adjunct to thioamides and RAI during therapy of neonatal thyrotoxicosis, pregnancy, or thyroid storm and as a preoperative medication. Although β-blockers have been used successfully as sole agents preoperatively, they are not recommended in the patient with severe toxemia because inadequate control of severe thyrotoxicosis has resulted in storm. All the selective and nonselective β-blockers (e.g., nadolol, atenolol, metoprolol) appear to be equally effective in the symptomatic relief of hyperthyroidism. β-Blockers with intrinsic sympathomimetic activity (e.g., pindolol) are not recommended because they do not reduce the HR as much as β-blockers without intrinsic sympathomimetic activity. Chronic administration of β-blockers should be avoided during pregnancy, particularly in the last trimester, because of the risk of fetal respiratory depression, small placenta, intrauterine growth retardation, impaired responses to anoxic stress, and postnatal bradycardia and hypoglycemia. Propranolol is also excreted in breast milk and should be avoided during lactation. Such findings indicate that propranolol, like iodides, should be used only on a short-term basis in pregnancy.

The kinetics and blood levels of propranolol in patients with toxemia are subject to large interindividual variation.[56] This variation is attributed to a significant first-pass effect seen with oral administration, altered hepatic function in hyperthyroidism, and the presence of an active metabolite, 4-hydroxypropranolol. Propranolol clearance in thyrotoxicosis might increase as much as 50% because of enhanced liver blood flow and increased activity of drug-metabolizing enzymes. The volume of distribution increases and the elimination half-life is unchanged. Although the lower propranolol levels reported in hyperthyroidism might result from individual variations, data suggest that higher propranolol dosages are necessary in patients with toxemia because of the increased clearance rate. Similarly, larger dosages of metoprolol are needed because of hyperthyroidism-increased hepatic clearance. The converse is true in hypothyroidism. The clearance of β-blockers, such as atenolol and nadolol, which are excreted renally, is unaltered in hyperthyroidism and can be administered once daily to improve compliance.

The calcium-channel blockers, particularly diltiazem, might be a useful alternative when β-blockers are contraindicated (e.g., in patients with asthma, CHF, or insulin-dependent diabetes). Diltiazem (oral, 120 mg three times a day or 60 mg four times a day) is well tolerated and appears to be as effective as propranolol in suppressing thyrotoxicosis symptoms.[57] However, verapamil has produced detrimental effects in thyrotoxicosis. The potential synergistic benefits and toxicity of the calcium blockers and β-blockers in the management of thyrotoxicosis are unknown.

Radioactive Iodine

RAI therapy is indicated in postadolescent patients, those with Graves' ophthalmopathy or a history of thyroid surgery, those who are poor surgical candidates because of complicating nonthyroid illness, and those who fail or experience thioamide toxicity.[7,30] RAI is absolutely contraindicated in pregnancy because the RAI crosses the placenta and destroys the fetal thyroid, which begins functioning between the twelfth and fourteenth weeks of life. It is also the treatment of choice in older patients with cardiac disease and in those with TMGs.

^{131}I, which has a half-life of 8 days and delivers high-energy β-radiation to a maximal depth of 2 mm, is the isotope commonly used. ^{125}I, which has less tissue penetration and a half-life of 60 days, has not resulted in a lower incidence of hypothyroidism, as was initially anticipated. Because ^{125}I emits γ rays that penetrate only a few microns, larger therapeutic dosages are required, which increases considerably the total body radiation without reducing the incidence of hypothyroidism.

RAI dosage is calculated using a formula that incorporates an estimate of the gland size, the uptake of iodine at 24 hours, and the standard number of microcuries of iodine given per gram of thyroid tissue. At the University of California, patients receive approximately 80 to 150 μCi/g thyroid tissue. Despite this formula, the proper dosage (i.e., one that prevents both recurrent hyperthyroidism and subsequent hypothyroidism) is difficult to calculate or predict.

$$I^{131}\ (\text{mCi}) = [\text{Estimated gland weight (g)} \times 80\text{–}150\ \mu\text{Ci/g}] \div 100\%\ \text{24-hour RAI}$$

Pretreatment with thioamides for approximately 1 month to deplete the gland of stored hormones or with β-blockers before and after RAI therapy is necessary to prevent exacerbations of thyrotoxicosis within 10 to 14 days after RAI. Older adults, patients with heart disease, and those with large intraglandular stores of hormones are at greatest risk.[30] Iodides should not be used before RAI therapy because ^{131}I uptake and efficacy will be significantly impaired for several months. Thioamides should be discontinued 1 week before and after RAI therapy to facilitate optimal ^{131}I uptake and retention. Nevertheless, the RAI dosage might have to be increased by 25% in patients pretreated with thioamides.[30,36] β-Blockers and calcium-channel blockers can be used without compromising RAI therapy.

Resolution of the hyperthyroidism is slow after RAI treatment. Improvement of symptoms might be apparent by 3 to 6 weeks after RAI; however, maximum effects do not occur until 3 to 4 months after an ablative dose. Because of this delayed onset, iodides, ipodate, thioamides, or β-blockers might be necessary for symptomatic control after RAI is given. If a second dose is required, a larger dosage of RAI must be given to optimize gland uptake, exposing the body to more radiation.

The lowest appropriate age limit for RAI therapy is controversial. After more than 25 years of extensive clinical experience, RAI is generally accepted as safe for most adult patients under 35 years of age. Adolescents have also been safely treated with RAI, although its use is controversial.[8,30]

The major concerns about RAI therapy include carcinogenesis, leukemia, and genetic damage. So far, these hazards appear to be unfounded. Although a large retrospective cohort study found a small increase in cancer mortality, RAI did not result in a significant increase in total cancer mortality.[58] The radiation dosage to the gonads in patients treated with ^{131}I for hyperthyroidism is generally less than 3 rads, which is not significantly different from gonadal irradiation received from commonly used diagnostic tests such as barium enemas and pyelograms. The major complication of RAI is hypothyroidism, which is most common the first year after therapy and increases at a constant rate of 2.5%/year thereafter, accounting for a 20-year incidence of 30 to 70%. Immediate side effects of ^{131}I therapy are minimal and might include mild thyroid pain and tenderness, temporary hair thinning, and (rarely) dysphagia. Exacerbation of Graves' ophthalmopathy can occur after RAI therapy, and prophylactic systemic corticosteroids should be considered in patients with mild eye symptoms.[26,27] Generally, RAI therapy is effective, quick, easy, painless, and nontoxic.

Iodinated Contrast Media

An unlabeled use for iodinated contrast dye (e.g., ipodate, iopanoic acid) is the acute management of hyperthyroidism.[59] When ipodate is administered in a daily dosage of 500 mg to 1 g orally or 3 g every third day to thyrotoxic patients, dramatic improvement in both subjective and objective symptoms parallel the rapid fall in thyroid hormone levels. The changes in serum T_4, serum T_3, and rT_3 levels are consistent with inhibition of the peripheral deiodination of T_4 to T_3. Serum T_3 levels decline within 6 hours of ipodate administration, declining to 50% of baseline at 24 hours and 70% of baseline (nadir) at 48 hours. T_3 levels remain suppressed for 3 to 5 days after a single administration. Similarly, T_4 levels reach their nadir 3 days after administration and remain depressed for as long as 6 days after the last dose. When compared with PTU, ipodate produced earlier symptomatic and objective improvements and more rapid declines in T_3 hormone levels. Prolonged suppression of T_3 and T_4 levels suggests that hormone secretion inhibition, caused by the released iodine, might be an additional ipodate mechanism of action. Although similar inhibition of peripheral T_3 production is seen with most iodinated contrast media, such as iopanoic acid (Telepaque), ipodate (Oragrafin), which contains 61.4% iodine, is the most potent.

Because ipodate is nontoxic, it is a useful addition to the acute thyrotoxicosis treatment. Ipodate is recommended as an adjunct to thioamides in severe toxemia or thyroid storm and as an alternative in those allergic to thioamides. It may also be an effective preoperative preparation in lieu of iodides, but experience is very limited. Another potential use is patients who may eventually be treated with RAI therapy because ipodate does not appear to interfere with RAI retention as much as iodides do. These agents are not indicated for chronic therapy because the hormone level reductions seen within the first month of therapy are not sustained in most hyperthyroid patients.

Nonpharmacologic Therapy

Thyroidectomy is an effective therapy for patients in whom RAI or thioamides are contraindicated; those with large goiters, causing cosmetic disfigurement, respiratory embarrassment, or swallowing difficulties; those with suspected malignancies; and selected children and pregnant women.[60] Prior thyroid surgery should be considered a strong deterrent to further surgery because reoperation increases the hazard of vocal cord paralysis and hypoparathyroidism 10-fold and 30-fold, respectively. Other poor surgical candidates are patients with severe cardiac, respiratory, or debilitating diseases and women in the third trimester of pregnancy (because surgery can precipitate spontaneous labor). Surgery can be performed safely in the second trimester after suitable preparation with thioamides or short-term use of β-blockers.

The ideal surgical endpoint is a 3- to 8-g remnant of thyroid tissue that produces neither a recurrence of the thyrotoxicosis nor hypothyroidism.[60] The risk of recurrent thyrotoxicosis is directly proportional to the amount of thyroid remnant left. Increasing the remnant gland size by 1 g decreases the risk of postoperative hypothyroidism by 10%; conversely, increasing the remnant size above 10 g increases the risk of recurrent disease without changing the risk of hypothyroidism. Although euthyroidism might not always be feasible, one series reported a 94% euthyroid success rate using a modified subtotal thyroidectomy. A subtotal thyroidectomy is the most popular form of surgery for hyperthyroidism because it offers the best chance of euthyroidism. Others advocate a total thyroidectomy, despite the risk of hypothyroidism, to prevent recurrence of the hyperthyroidism. Surgery appears to be as safe as nonsurgical treatments for hyperthyroidism if it is performed by experienced surgeons on patients adequately prepared by the standard combination of thioamides, iodides, or β-blockers. In adequately prepared patients, operative mortality and risk of thyroid storm are low. Vocal cord paralysis and permanent hypoparathyroidism occur in fewer than 1% of patients after a subtotal thyroidectomy.

The major complication is hypothyroidism, which occurs in the first 6 months to 3 years postoperatively but can develop insidiously as late as 10 years postoperatively. Incidences of 5 to 75% are reported. The incidence of hypothyroidism is inversely proportional to the remnant of thyroid tissue left; remnants of 2 to 4 g result in an incidence of 70%.

The disadvantages of surgery include expense, need for hospitalization, risks of anesthesia, postoperative complications, and the patient's fear of surgery. These disadvantages may outweigh the advantages of rapid, definitive surgical intervention.

Special Treatment Issues

Subclinical Hyperthyroidism

Treatment of subclinical hyperthyroidism is controversial because no studies have been performed in patients before or following any antithyroid therapy.[3,9,61] Recommendations for antithyroid therapy must be individualized and may be considered for those at the greatest risk for morbidity (e.g., older adults with cardiac disease and patients with osteoporosis, especially postmenopausal women). In patients without risk factors, observation and routine TSH monitoring may be the optimal plan because progression to overt hyperthyroidism is uncommon.

Exophthalmos and Ophthalmologic Complications

Because the pathogenesis and progression of ophthalmopathy are not well understood, treatment of ocular complaints often is symptomatic until euthyroidism occurs.[26]

Periorbital edema and chemosis (inflammation of the conjunctiva) respond to elevation of the head of the bed to promote diuresis. Protective glasses, methylcellulose and hydrocortisone drops, and avoidance of smoke and dust might alleviate photophobia and external irritation. In patients whose eyes do not completely close during sleep, taping the eyelids shut at night is essential to prevent corneal scarring and drying.

Systemic corticosteroids are indicated for progressive inflammatory exophthalmos and decreasing visual acuity. Prednisone 60 to 120 mg/day, administered in divided doses for 1 to 3 weeks, often produces dramatic resolution of inflammatory eye symptoms. When symptoms resolve, the dosage can be tapered over 2 weeks and then gradually withdrawn. In addition to their anti-inflammatory action, corticosteroids suppress TRab levels and decrease T_3 levels by impairing the peripheral conversion of T_4 to T_3. Immunosuppressive agents, such as cyclophosphamide and azathioprine, have not been as effective as steroids. External orbital radiation therapy, which achieves similar results, can be used in patients with contraindications to steroids.

After euthyroidism is achieved and the eye symptoms are stable, lid or orbital surgery can provide cosmetic or visual corrections.

Atrial Fibrillation and Congestive Heart Failure

Hyperthyroidism or subclinical hyperthyroidism can cause new or worsening atrial fibrillation and CHF. Routine thyroid function tests should be obtained to exclude underlying thyroid disease.[3,9,20,61] The atrial fibrillation and heart failure often are difficult to control until euthyroidism occurs. A combination of medications, including β-blockers and calcium blockers, as well as larger dosages of digoxin (Table 17.5) might be needed to slow the HR and correct the heart failure. Hyperthyroid patients tend to be clinically resistant to the glycosides, whereas hypothyroid patients are very sensitive. A larger loading and maintenance dosage of digoxin are required in thyrotoxicosis because of a hyperthyroidism-induced increase in the digoxin volume of distribution and clearance.[1]

Anticoagulation with coumadin is recommended in patients with hyperthyroidism-related atrial fibrillation, valvular disease, and heart failure because of the high incidence of systemic emboli. Smaller dosages of coumadin (e.g. 2 to 3 mg) are needed for anticoagulation in hyperthyroidism (Table 17.5). An enhanced anticoagulant response occurs because the warfarin-induced decrease in clotting factor synthesis is combined with hyperthyroidism-induced increases in factor catabolism. The opposite occurs in hypothyroidism; the anticoagulant response decreases because of delayed catabolism of clotting factors. Therefore, thyrotoxic patients need less warfarin and myxedematous patients need more warfarin to achieve the same hypoprothrombinemic response.

The dosage of digoxin and warfarin must be adjusted as euthyroidism occurs to prevent toxicity and maintain therapeutic efficacy. Spontaneous conversion to normal sinus rhythm after euthyroidism is achieved is less likely if the patient has underlying heart disease or if the duration of the atrial fibrillation persists after 4 months of euthyroidism.

Thyroid Storm

The pathogenesis of storm is not well understood, but it appears to be an exaggerated form of thyrotoxicosis. Storm can be precipitated by childbirth, stress, infection, trauma, diabetic ketoacidosis, inadequate preparation before RAI or surgery, and nonadherence with antithyroid medication.[25]

Prompt recognition and immediate treatment can decrease the 100% mortality rate to 7% or better. Treatment is directed at five major areas:

- Supporting vital functions with sedation, oxygen, fluids, and antipyretics, treating infection, correcting electrolyte abnormalities, and using corticosteroids (hydrocortisone 100 to 200 mg intravenously every 6 hours) for unsuspected hypoadrenalism. Peripheral conversion to T_3 is also reduced by corticosteroids.
- Using thioamides and iodides to block synthesis and release of hormones. Preferably, large dosages of PTU (200 to 300 mg every 6 hours or 600 to 1200 mg/day) or methimazole (30 to 40 mg every 6 hours) should be given. Theoretically, iodides should be given 1 hour after thioamide administration so as not to interfere with the latter's effect and to prevent iodizing existing hormone stores, which will aggravate existing storm. Iodides (e.g., Lugol's solution 30 to 60 drops orally daily or potassium iodide 1 to 2 g intravenously daily) and the combination of thioamides often control symptoms within 1 day. Lithium can be given in dosages of 500 to 1500 mg/day if iodides are contraindicated, but it offers no advantages over iodides. Cholestyramine has also been recommended.[31]
- Blocking the metabolic effects by administering propranolol 20 to 80 mg orally every 6 hours or 0.5 to 2 mg intravenously every 4 hours or comparable β-blocker, or diltiazem 60 to 120 mg orally three to four times a day.
- Eliminating and correcting precipitating factors.
- Removing circulating hormone by plasmapheresis, exchange transfusion, and dialysis when routine measures fail.

Hypothyroidism

DEFINITION

Hypothyroidism is a clinical syndrome caused by thyroid hormone deficiency and characterized by a slowing of all body systems. An exaggeration of the signs and symptoms of severe and prolonged hypothyroidism, which can precede coma, is known as myxedema. Myxedema coma is the end stage of long-standing uncorrected hypothyroidism.[62] Cretinism or congenital hypothyroidism is hypothyroidism that develops in utero or in the neonate and leads to developmental impairment. Subclinical hypothyroidism exists when TSH levels are elevated and thyroid hormone levels are normal, usually in a patient without symptoms of hypothyroidism.

Primary hypothyroidism, or failure of the thyroid gland to secrete sufficient thyroid hormones, is the most common type of hypothyroidism. Central or secondary causes of hypothyroidism result from pituitary or hypothalamic injury.

TREATMENT GOALS: HYPOTHYROIDISM

- Reverse hypothyroid complaints.
- Reverse hypothyroid physical findings.
- Normalize the FT_4 level.
- Normalize the TSH level.
- Reduce goiter size, if applicable.
- Reduce diastolic blood pressure.
- Reduce serum cholesterol levels.
- Improve emotional well-being and quality of life.
- Prevent myxedema.
- Support placenta development and maintenance of pregnancy.
- In neonates and children, maintain normal growth and physical and mental development.

EPIDEMIOLOGY

Overview

Hypothyroidism affects approximately 8 million Americans. An incidence of 1.4% overt hypothyroidism in women and less than 0.1% in men has been reported.[63] Women are five to seven times more likely to develop hypothyroidism than men. Patients with a family history of thyroid or autoimmune disorders (e.g., diabetes, rheumatoid arthritis), older adults, particularly women, and those with a history of medically treated thyroid disease (e.g., radioactive therapy, thyroidectomy) are at greater risk of overt hypothyroidism.

Goitrous forms include Hashimoto's, thyroiditis, drug-induced thyroiditis, dyshormonogenesis, endemic thyroiditis, subacute thyroiditis, and multinodular goiters. Nongoitrous forms include cretinism (congenital hypothyroidism), idiopathic atrophy, or iatrogenic causes. Congenital hypothyroidism is reported in 1 in 4000 births.

Hashimoto's thyroiditis is the most common cause of goiter and hypothyroidism in the United States and is similar to Graves' disease in prevalence. Like other thyroid disorders, it is more common in women than men and has a strong familial predisposition. Its occurrence peaks in middle age, although any age group is at risk.

Iatrogenic hypothyroidism, caused by RAI or surgery, is the next most common cause of hypothyroidism, after Hashimoto's thyroiditis. Virtually all patients receiving RAI and about 50 to 75% of patients undergoing total thyroidectomies develop hypothyroidism.[30,60] Therefore, all patients with a history of RAI or surgery should be routinely monitored for development of hypothyroidism.

Postpartum thyroiditis, a type of subacute thyroiditis, can affect approximately 5% of women in the first year after delivery.[12,13] High-risk women include those with preexisting autoimmune disorders, including diabetes mellitus, autoimmune thyroiditis, collagen vascular disorders, and women with positive antibodies.

Pituitary causes (e.g., postpartum hemorrhage [Sheehan's], head injury, pituitary tumors, or idiopathic atrophy of the hypophysis) are uncommon. Concomitant disorders of the adrenals and gonads (Simmonds's disease or panhypopituitarism) may also occur. Hypothalamic hypothyroidism, caused by inadequate secretion of TRF, is rare.

Drug-Induced Hypothyroidism

Iodides and iodide-containing compounds (i.e., povidone iodine, amiodarone, iodinated contrast media) can produce hypothyroidism and goiter in patients with underlying thyroid abnormalities.[15,16,17] These patients (e.g., those with cystic fibrosis, and untreated Hashimoto's thyroiditis and those not receiving L-thyroxine with a history of RAI- or surgery-treated Graves' disease) are inordinately sensitive to iodides and unable to normally escape from the Wolff–Chaikoff block to resume hormone synthesis. Older adults and patients on long-term amiodarone also appear to be at greater risk of amiodarone-induced hypothyroidism. Unfortunately, the goiter or hypothyroidism may not always be reversible after the iodides or amiodarone are stopped. L-Thyroxine can be given concurrently, if necessary, to treat the hypothyroidism and goiter.

The prevalence of amiodarone-induced hypothyroidism ranges from 1.0 to 9.8%.[15,16] Each 200-mg tablet of amiodarone contains 75 mg organic iodide, of which 6 to 12 mg free iodine is released. An iodine load is produced that is 100 times greater than the normal daily intake of 0.5 mg. Patients at risk for hypothyroidism include those with a family history of thyroid disease, a multinodular goiter, or positive thyroid antibodies, indicating an autoimmune process (e.g., Hashimoto's). No relationship is identified between the development of thyroid dysfunction and the cumulative dosage or duration of therapy. Hypothyroidism usually develops within the first 2 years of therapy, or it may occur during the first year after therapy is stopped because of amiodarone's long half-life and accumulation in adipose tissue. Amiodarone-induced hypothyroidism may be difficult to recognize because symptoms of bradycardia and constipation can be attributed to either hypothyroidism or amiodarone. Suspected hypothyroidism should be confirmed by a TSH level higher than 10 mIU/L and a reduction in FT_4 levels. Routine monitoring of thyroid function tests is recommended at baseline and every 6 months thereafter in patients receiving amiodarone.

Lithium-induced hypothyroidism and goiter have been reported in 5 to 50% of patients on chronic therapy.[5,15] Risk factors include a family history of thyroid illness, presence of thyroid antibodies, abnormal thyroid glands, and underlying thyroid illness, although a few cases have occurred in patients without any risk factors. Lithium's antithyroid effect is similar to that of the iodides and was first identified in patients receiving treatment for bipolar disorder. The onset of a nontender, diffuse goiter with or without hypothyroidism is variable and may appear after 5 months to 2 years of therapy. Regression of the goiter and reversal of the hypothyroidism do not always occur after the lithium is stopped, but L-thyroxine can be added to permit continued lithium therapy.

The cytokines (e.g., interleukin-2 and interferon-α) have produced transient episodes of hypothyroidism.[14,15] Preexisting hypothyroidism can also worsen. Interleukin-2 has produced thyroid dysfunction in 10 to 41% of patients after two courses of therapy. Hypothyroidism can be permanent, requiring chronic thyroid therapy. Positive thyroid antibodies have been reported in 20% of patients receiving interferon-α.

Thiocyanate is a well-known inhibitor of iodide trapping, particularly if high blood concentrations are present. Thiocyanate-induced hypothyroidism can result from long-term use of nitroprusside in patients with renal insufficiency. Plants such as rutabagas, cabbage, and turnips contain thiocarbamides, which are metabolized in the body to thiocyanates. These dietary goitrogens do not produce a significant degree of hypothyroidism unless large amounts are ingested raw over a long time period.

Goiters can result from the use of certain drugs with antithyroid activity (Table 17.8). The thioamides and the monovalent anions can produce goiter if excessive dosages are used.

PATHOPHYSIOLOGY

Hashimoto's thyroiditis, an autoimmune process resulting from defects in suppressor T lymphocytes, is characterized by diffuse enlargement and lymphocytic infiltration of the thyroid gland, an immunologic disturbance, and hypothyroidism. AtgA and TPO antibodies usually are present. If the gland is able to maintain hormone synthesis in response to TSH stimulation, then euthyroidism is maintained. However, when the gland eventually fails to keep up with metabolic demands, goiter and hypothyroidism occur. Hashimoto's disease often coexists with other autoimmune disorders, including Graves' disease, pernicious anemia, rheumatoid arthritis, and other collagen vascular diseases. Some postulate that Graves' and Hashimoto's thyroiditis are actually the same disease because mild thyrotoxicosis can precede the onset of hypothyroidism. Findings of positive thyroid antibodies, similar histologic lymphocytic infiltration of the gland, and the presence of thyroid immunoglobulins that block rather than stimulate the TSH receptor strengthen the autoimmune association between Graves' and Hashimoto's

Table 17.8 ▪ Drug-Induced Thyroid Disease

Drug	Mechanism	Drug-Induced Thyroid Effect	Comments
Nitroprusside	Metabolized to thiocyanate, an anion inhibitor	Goiter, hypothyroidism	Increased risk with renal failure and duration of use
Lithium	Inhibits hormone release	Goiter, hypothyroidism, hyperthyroidism	Usually in patients with untreated thyroid disease (e.g., Hashimoto's thyroiditis)
Iodides and iodine-containing compounds (e.g., amiodarone, ipodate, iodinated contrast media)	Inability to escape from Wolff–Chaikoff block	Hypothyroidism, goiter	Usually in patients with untreated Hashimoto's thyroiditis or following treatment of Graves' disease with radioactive iodine or surgery and not receiving thyroid replacement
Iodides and iodine-containing compounds (e.g., amiodarone, ipodate, iodinated contrast media)	Provides substrate to iodide-deficient autonomous thyroid tissue; loss of Wolff–Chaikoff block	Hyperthyroidism	Usually in patients with multinodular goiters and autonomous nodules (Jod-Basedow disease)
Amiodarone	Destruction thyroiditis, with dumping of hormones into circulation	Hyperthyroidism	Associated with elevation of interleukin-6 levels
Sertraline	?? related to ↑ T_4 elimination	Hypothyroidism, thyroid-stimulating hormone elevation	Prevalence unknown; unknown whether disease occurs with other serotonin reuptake inhibitors
Sulfonylureas, sulfonamides, resorcinol, phenylbutazone	Inhibits organic binding and organification	Hypothyroidism, goiter	Rare cause of thyroid disease
Immunotherapy (e.g., interferon-α, interleukin-2)	Autoimmune process	Hypothyroidism, hyperthyroidism	Generally transient, resolves without treatment
Natural goitrogens (e.g., cabbage)	Contains thiocyanate and other goitrogens	Hypothyroidism, goiter	Rare; occurs only with consumption of large amounts of raw vegetables

thyroiditis. Likewise, hypothyroidism can be the result of long-standing Graves' disease.

Congenital, nongoitrous hypothyroidism, produced by a deficiency of thyroid hormone in utero or in the neonate, may result from defective hormone synthesis, pituitary or hypothalamic dysfunction, or incomplete growth of the gland (agenesis). Ectopic thyroid tissue, destruction of the gland by maternal autoantibodies, and destruction by RAI therapy are other possible causes of agenesis. Neonatal goitrous hypothyroidism has been reported after maternal ingestion of iodides and thioamide therapy.[35]

Endemic goiter is a descriptive term for a goiter caused by an iodine deficiency during the growth years. The amount of dietary iodine deficiency determines the degree of nodularity and gland enlargement. Patients may be euthyroid or hypothyroid.

Dyshormonogenesis is a group of familial thyroid disorders resulting from abnormalities in the synthesis, delivery, or peripheral action of thyroid hormones. Impaired hormone synthesis can result from defects in iodine accumulation or iodide organification, from a dehalogenase deficiency, and from a coupling abnormality.

Myxedema coma can be precipitated by cold weather (hypothermia), stress (surgery), infection, trauma, acid-base disturbances, and unrecognized concomitant illness (i.e., diabetes, arteriosclerotic cardiovascular disease). Respiratory depressants of any kind (i.e., anesthetics, narcotics, phenothiazines, and sedative–hypnotics), which are metabolized slowly in the hypothyroid patient, can precipitate coma by aggravating preexisting hypothermia and carbon dioxide retention. Immediate and aggressive therapy is required to prevent mortality, which occurs at a rate of 60 to 70%.[62]

Hypothyroidism from a subacute thyroiditis (e.g., PPT, de Quervain's thyroiditis) occurs if long-standing inflammation of the gland prevents further hormone synthesis after the initial hormone stores are depleted.[13] Patients often undergo a mild thyrotoxic phase before transient hypothyroidism develops. Transient L-thyroxine therapy may be necessary, although permanent hypothyroidism can occur (e.g., PPT).

CLINICAL PRESENTATION AND DIAGNOSIS

Signs and Symptoms

The classic symptoms of hypothyroidism include weakness, fatigue, lethargy, cold intolerance, constipation, and weight gain (Table 17.4). Normochromic, normocytic anemia or microcytic anemia caused by heavy menses in women may be present. In older adults, the diagnosis of hypothyroidism might be missed easily and is particularly difficult because symptoms may be absent, atypical, or wrongly attributed to normal aging. Hypothyroid symptoms from naturally occurring hypothyroidism (e.g., Hashimoto's thyroiditis) can be insidious, remain unnoticed by the patient, and occur with amazing placidity over several months to years before the appearance of a terminal myxedematous state. In contrast, symptoms resulting from iatrogenic causes (e.g., RAI therapy or surgery) occur rapidly and rarely go unrecognized by the patient. It should be appreciated that hypothyroid patients are inordinately sensitive to medications such as digoxin and the respiratory and central nervous system effects of respiratory depressants, including anesthetics, narcotics, phenothiazines, and sedative–hypnotics (Table 17.5). Likewise, medical treatment of concurrent medical conditions (e.g., diabetes, hyperlipidemia, cardiac conditions) can be influenced by hypothyroidism (Table 17.5).[64]

Marked physical findings, usually present in myxedema, include a puffy and masklike facies, edematous eyelids, thickened and doughy skin changes, especially over the pretibial aspects of the leg, hair loss from the lateral aspects of the eyebrows, a large tongue, cardiomegaly, and a yellowish tint to the skin. Myxedematous cachexia is characterized by intensifying hypothyroid signs and symptoms and often precedes the onset of myxedema coma. Significant clinical features of myxedema coma include hypothermia, hypoxia, carbon dioxide retention, hyponatremia, hypoglycemia, markedly delayed or absent deep tendon reflexes, altered sensorium ranging from stupor to coma, and shock. Paranoid psychosis has also been reported.[25,62]

The cardiovascular manifestations of hypothyroidism can mimic or exacerbate preexisting low-output CHF. Preexisting angina typically becomes quiescent; rarely, the severity and frequency of attacks can increase. Elevated cholesterol levels caused by impaired elimination might accelerate atherosclerotic changes, although this effect is speculative.[64] Clinical findings include cardiomegaly caused by loss of muscle tone and mucopolysaccharide deposition; dyspnea; edema; and pleural effusions caused by decreased cardiac output and SV and reduced myocardial contractibility. Characteristic ECG changes can resemble those of ischemia and include slow rate and low voltage, flattened or inverted T waves, and, occasionally, increased P-R interval and widened QRS complex. Although glomerular filtration rate (GFR) and renal plasma flow are reduced by decreased cardiac output and blood volume, overt evidence of renal failure does not occur. In severe myxedema, changes in GFR and inappropriate antidiuretic hormone secretion delay water excretion, producing edema and hyponatremia.

A goiter should always be considered an abnormal finding. Goiters are produced by prolonged TSH stimulation, usually in response to low levels of circulating hormone. However, some patients with a goiter can be euthyroid because the thyroid gland might transiently increase hormone secretion in response to the elevated TSH level. A very large goiter (e.g., multinodular goiter), producing pressure symptoms, a choking sensation, pain and difficulty swallowing, or regurgitation of food and liquids from compression of the trachea or the esophagus, is an indication for surgical removal. Clinically, patients can be euthyroid but often develop hyperthyroidism or hypothyroidism in later years.

Patients with Hashimoto's thyroiditis can present with thyrotoxicosis in the early stages (Hashitoxicosis), euthyroidism and goiter, hypothyroidism and goiter, or hypothyroidism without goiter in the later stages of the disease. Euthyroidism occurs if the gland is able to compensate for the inherent block in hormone synthesis by increasing hormone synthesis in response to TSH stimulation. Asymptomatic thyroiditis, characterized by euthyroidism, absence of goiter, normal levels of circulating hormones, and positive antithyroid antibodies, may precede the clinical manifestations of overt goiter and hypothyroidism. Idiopathic atrophy of the thyroid and destruction of the gland represent the end stages of Hashimoto's thyroiditis.

The clinical presentation of congenital hypothyroidism depends on the severity of the hypothyroidism, the age of onset, and the cause of the thyroid deficiency. Determining cord TSH levels at time of delivery is crucial because it permits early diagnosis of hypothyroidism. The clinical symptoms are so subtle that if the condition is not detected until the child is older, irreversible neurologic damage can occur. The earliest findings are a heavy expression, a piglike appearance of the eyes, hypothermia, prolonged jaundice, umbilical hernia, hoarseness, thick tongue, protuberant abdomen, constipation, and drooling. Delayed developmental characteristics, failure to thrive, poor appetite, and cretinoid facies might not be recognized until the infant is 3 to 6 months old and neurologic damage is irreversible.[65] Growth retardation, delayed physical development, and hypothyroid symptoms, similar to those seen in an adult, are of concern. Radiologic evidence of epiphyseal dysgenesis is pathognomonic of neonatal hypothyroidism.

Diagnosis

Clinical guidelines for screening and diagnosing hypothyroidism have been established by the American College of Physicians.[3] In adults, the diagnosis of hypothyroidism is confirmed by laboratory findings of a low FT_4I or FT_4 and an elevated TSH level (Table 17.1). Because T_3 levels can be normal in overt hypothyroidism, T_3 levels are not helpful or cost-effective and should not be obtained. In secondary hypothyroidism, FT_4 levels are low when the TSH level is low, and other features of pituitary or hypothalamic disease usually are apparent. The presence of positive antibodies indicates an underlying autoimmune process (e.g., Hashimoto's thyroiditis). An RAIU is not necessary for diagnosis of autoimmune hypothyroidism; it is usually decreased, but an elevated uptake may be present in the early stages of hypothyroidism. Serum SGOT, LDH, CPK, carotene, cholesterol, and triglyceride levels may be elevated from impaired elimination.

THERAPEUTIC PLAN

The American Thyroid Association and the American Association of Clinical Endocrinologists have published clinical guidelines for treating hypothyroidism.[28,29] Administering thyroid hormones provides adequate replacement therapy for hypothyroidism and prevents progression to myxedema coma. The average replacement dosage often is quoted as 100 to 200 μg L-thyroxine daily, which parallels the normal thyroid production. However, such a simplistic approach is inappropriate and dangerous. Dosing requirements depend on several factors, including patient age and weight, severity and cause of the illness, presence or absence of cardiac disease, and hormone absorption. Any existing goiter usually regresses in size because TSH production is suppressed (Fig. 17.1). Hypothyroid patients on L-thyroxine can be treated effectively by the pharmacist using a treatment algorithm (Fig. 17.4).

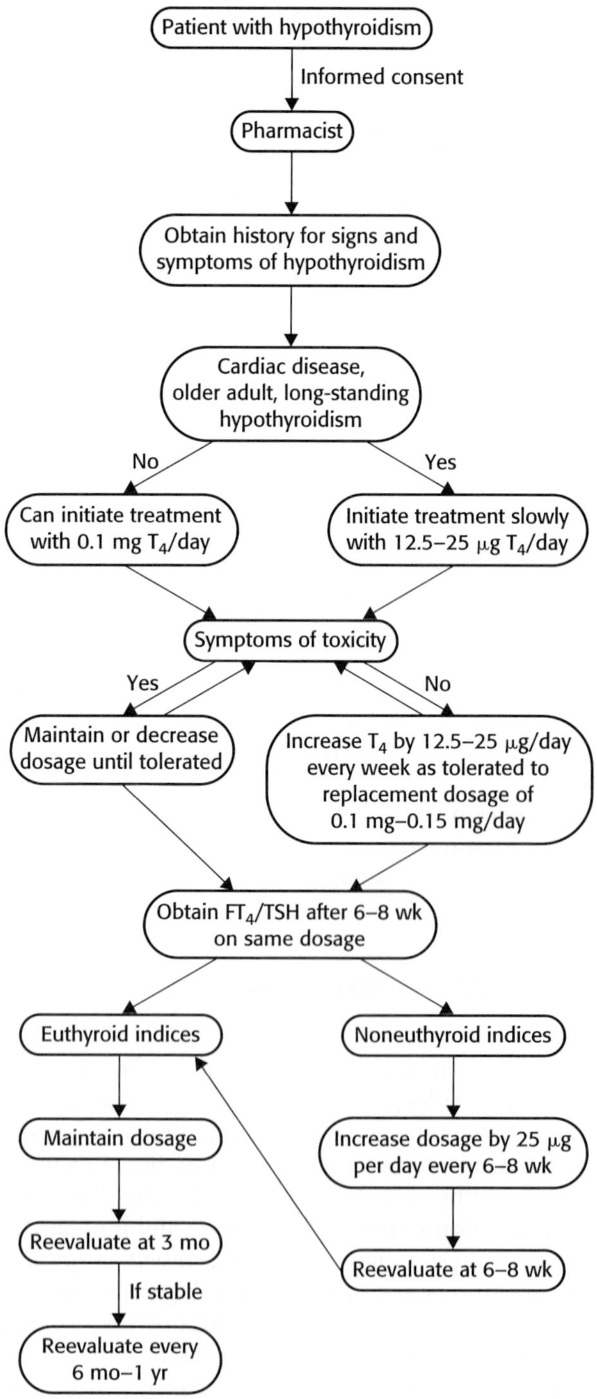

Figure 17.4. Treatment algorithm for management of hypothyroidism. *FT_4*, free thyroxine; *T_4*, thyroxine; *TSH*, thyroid-stimulating hormone.

Table 17.9 ▪ Thyroid Preparations in Treatment of Hypothyroidism

Preparation[a]	Content	Advantages	Disadvantages	Effect on Thyroid Tests	Comments
Desiccated thyroid, U.S. Pharmacopeia 0.25, 0.5, 1, 1.5, 2, 3, 4, or 5 grains	Defatted, dried pig thyroid powder containing 0.17–0.23% iodine	Inexpensive	Poor standardization, with variable hormonal content and T_4/T_3 ratio Deterioration with storage	Normal FT_4/FT_4I, TSH, normal or ↑ TT_3	Obsolete product Variable potency Problems inherent to all T_3-containing products
Sodium L-thyroxine,[a] (Levoxyl, Levothroid, Synthroid, various), 0.0125, 0.025, 0.05, 0.075, 0.088, 0.1, 0.112, 0.125, 0.137, 0.15, 0.175, 0.2, 0.3 mg; injectable 200, 500 μg	Synthetic, pure T_4	Stable, smooth action, inexpensive Long half-life (7 days) Generics and branded products bioequivalent	Slow onset of action, cumulative effects Various drugs can impair absorption	Normal thyroid function tests; TSH in normal range	Might be more potent than desiccated thyroid Should lower T_4 dosage by 0.5 grain to avoid toxicity when changing from >2 grains desiccated thyroid to L-thyroxine
Sodium L-thyronine (Cytomel), 5, 25, 50 μg; injectable 10 μg/mL (Triostat)	Synthetic, pure T_3	Uniform absorption, fast onset of action	Expensive; supraphysiologic T_3 levels can produce toxicity Requires twice-daily dosing	Low FT_4, normal or ↑ TT_3, normal TSH	Not DOC for hormone replacement Monitor T_3 and TSH levels
Liotrix 0.25, 0.5, 1, 2, 3 (Thyrolar)	Contains T_4 and T_3 in a ratio of 4:1 (mimics natural hormone secretion)	Both short- and long-acting effects	Expensive	Normal thyroid function values	No real need for Liotrix because T_4 is converted peripherally to T_3

[a]Approximate dosage equivalence: 1 grain desiccated thyroid = 0.1 mg L-thyroxine = 37.5 μg l-thyronine = Liotrix-1 (see Comments column).
T_4, thyroxine; *T_3*, triiodothyronine; *FT_4*, free thyroxine; *FT_4I*, free thyroxine index; *TT_3*, total triiodothyronine; *TSH*, thyroid-stimulating hormone; *DOC*, drug of choice.

TREATMENT

Pharmacotherapy

L-Thyroxine is the preparation of choice for hormone replacement, although other thyroid hormones preparations are available commercially (Table 17.9).[66]

The initial dosage of T_4 depends on the patient's age, the severity and duration of the hypothyroidism, and the presence or potential for underlying cardiac disease. In young, healthy patients with disease of short duration, L-thyroxine can be administered in nearly full replacement dosages (e.g., 100 to 150 μg daily) without fear of precipitating cardiac toxicity. This dosage can be adjusted as necessary, using the patient's symptoms and laboratory values obtained at steady state (i.e., after 6 to 8 weeks of therapy). However, in patients with long-standing and severe myxedema, in older adults, and in patients with cardiac disease (i.e., angina, CHF), who are likely to be extremely sensitive to the metabolic effects of thyroid hormone, minute dosages of L-thyroxine must be instituted cautiously to avoid cardiovascular complications of heart failure, angina, tachycardia, and myocardial infarction. Subtherapeutic L-thyroxine dosages can precipitate these complications, so careful monitoring is critical. Angina should be controlled before L-thyroxine therapy is attempted. If medically indicated, coronary bypass surgery can be performed safely in hypothyroid patients before L-thyroxine replacement. In the high-risk patient, initial dosages should not exceed 25 μg T_4 daily. The patient should be instructed to report any cardiac symptoms immediately. If after 1 week the initial dosage is well tolerated, the dosage can be increased by similar increments every 1 to 2 weeks until therapeutic levels are achieved. It is not necessary to monitor thyroid function tests at these subtherapeutic dosages. Complete euthyroidism might never be achieved in high-risk patients without further compromising the cardiac status.

The daily maintenance dosage of L-thyroxine for uncomplicated hypothyroidism is estimated to be 1.6 to 1.7 μg/kg, or about 0.7 to 0.8 μg/lb.[63,66,67] The average daily replacement dosage is 100 to 125 μg/day in women and 125 to 150 μg in men. In older adults, lower dosages of 50 to 100 μg daily (less than 1.6 μg/kg/day) might be sufficient to maintain euthyroidism. Lower replacement dosages are also appropriate in patients with hypothyroidism caused by RAI or surgery ablation than in those with spontaneous hypothyroidism.[68]

Approximately 75% of patients receiving adequate prepregnancy L-thyroxine replacement need a 20 to 30% increase from their replacement dosage during the first or second trimester to maintain a normal TSH level.[66] The fetal thyroid does not depend on the maternal thyroid hormones that do not cross the placenta. The greatest dangers to the fetus from inadequate maternal replacement therapy during the first trimester are poor placenta development and poor maintenance of the pregnancy. Although normal offspring have been reported in women who remained hypothyroid throughout pregnancy, congenital defects, abnormal fetal development, spontaneous abortions, stillbirths, and mental retardation have been associated with maternal myxedema. It is also important to remember that the use of iron supplements may impair L-thyroxine absorption. If hormone replacement therapy is adequate and maternal euthyroidism (normal TSH and FT_4I, or FT_4 level) is achieved, a normal pregnancy is expected. TT_4 levels will be elevated because of pregnancy-induced TBG levels. After delivery, the prepregnancy dosage of L-thyroxine can be reinstituted.

Malabsorption caused by short bowel or the concurrent administration of several drugs (Table 17.10) can affect the daily L-thyroxine replacement dosage.[69–72] Separating administration times of L-thyroxine and some medications (e.g., calcium, iron, cholesterol resin binders) can minimize impairment of L-thyroxine absorption. However, this strategy is not helpful with aluminum-containing antacids; if appropriate, these preparations should be avoided. An increase in the daily L-thyroxine dosage usually is necessary when enzyme inducers (e.g., phenytoin), aluminum-containing products, and sertraline are given concurrently.

Patients should notice improvement in typical hypothyroid symptoms after 3 to 4 weeks of daily medication adherence. Weight, skin, hair, and voice changes may not reverse for several months despite normalized thyroid function tests.

The TSH and FT_4 levels should be evaluated at steady state (e.g., after 2 to 3 months of daily dosing). Trough TSH levels, obtained either before the next dose or at least 10 hours after the last dose, are recommended to minimize transient high peak FT_4 levels and suppressed TSH levels and properly interpret laboratory results.[73] Once the dosage has been established, therapy should be evaluated

Table 17.10 ▪ Medications and Conditions Affecting L-Thyroxine Replacement Dosages

Condition or Medication	Mechanism	Recommendation	Comments
Resin binders (e.g., cholestyramine, colestipol)	Binds T_4 in gut, ↓ T_4 absorption	Separate administration times by 4–6 hr.	↑ dosage of T_4 might be needed.
Aluminum-containing preparations (e.g., sucralfate, aluminum hydroxide antacids)	Binds T_4 in gut, ↓ T_4 absorption	Separating administration times by 4–6 hr might not prevent this interaction.	Avoid aluminum-containing products; ↑ dosage of T_4 might be needed.
Iron sulfate	Binds T_4 in gut, ↓ T_4 absorption	Separating administration times by 4–6 hr might prevent this interaction.	Monitor and ↑ dosage of T_4 if necessary.
Calcium carbonate	? Binds T_4 in gut, ↓ T_4 absorption	Separating administration times by 4–6 hr appears effective.	Interaction does not seem to occur with all calcium preparations.
Sertraline	? unknown mechanism, ? ↑ T_4 elimination	Separating administration times by 4–6 hr might not prevent this interaction.	↑ T_4 dosage might be needed; ? similar effect with other serotonin reuptake inhibitors.
Lovastatin	? Binds T_4 in gut, ↓ T_4 absorption	Change to another lipid-lowering agent, monitor TFTs and ↑ dosage if needed.	Interaction not well documented; based on one case report.
Enzyme inducers (i.e., phenytoin, carbamazepine, rifampin, phenobarbital)	↑ metabolism and clearance of T_4	↑ T_4 dosage to normalize TSH level; free T_4 level might remain low.	Not significant in euthyroid patients.
Androgens	↓ TBG levels; possibly higher free T_4 and lower TSH levels	Might need to ↓ T_4 dosage by 25–50% to normalize TSH.	Not significant in euthyroid patients.
Pregnancy	↑ TBG levels and ↑ thyroxine demands	↑ T_4 dosage by 20–30% to achieve normal TSH level.	Not significant in euthyroid patients on birth control pills or postmenopausal hormone replacement.
Age	T_4 clearance ↓ with age	Lower dosages (<1.7 μ/kg/day) might be effective in those >60 yr.	Monitor TFTs yearly; reduce dosage with advancing age.
Malabsorption (i.e., diarrhea, short bowel syndrome)	↓ T_4 absorption	↑ T_4 dosage; monitor TSH to adjust dosage.	High-dose T_4 therapy might be necessary.

T_4, thyronine; *TFT*, thyroid function tests; *TSH*, thyroid-stimulating hormone; *TBG*, thyroxine-binding globulin.

at yearly intervals to ensure that the current L-thyroxine dosage is still appropriate. A dosage reduction might be necessary in patients whose dosage was determined before the availability of more potent products and the advent of the sensitive TSH assay, in adults as they age, and if there is significant weight loss. The FT_4 or FT_4I and TSH should be maintained within the normal range. Suppression of TSH to undetectable levels (less than 0.05 mIU/L) should be avoided in replacement therapy to minimize overreplacement and subclinical signs of hyperthyroidism.[9,61,63,66] Supraphysiologic dosages may predispose patients to an increased risk of bone loss, osteoporosis, and cardiac arrhythmia.[22,23,61] However, TSH levels on a stable dosage of L-thyroxine can be quite variable, and it is unknown whether toxicity is produced and a dosage adjustment is always necessary. Some clinicians arbitrarily accept TSH levels that vary from a suppressed TSH of 0.25 mIU/L to a high of 5.0 mIU/L.[74] In addition, retrospective studies show no difference in morbidity and mortality between patients with normal and variable TSH levels.[4,61,75]

L-Thyroxine is available in branded or generic preparations, with minor differences between formulations.[74,76,77] U.S. Food and Drug Administration (FDA) criteria for bioequivalence between a leading branded product and its competitor products have been demonstrated.[77] L-Thyroxine's potency, cost-effectiveness, lack of foreign protein antigenicity, and ease of dosing contribute to its popularity. L-Thyroxine is stable but loses about 6% of its potency per year.[78] Its long half-life of 7 days makes it amenable to once-a-day dosing, increasing patient compliance and allowing various convenient dosing schedules (e.g., daily except weekends). Once-weekly administration of L-thyroxine has been proposed for noncompliant patients but requires further study.[79] L-Thyroxine absorption is enhanced about 20% during fasting. The bioavailability of branded L-thyroxine preparations is 80%; the bioavailability of generic preparations appears to be similar. This similarity should be considered when changing from oral to intravenous or intramuscular dosing regimens. Previous problems with subpotent tablets have been improved considerably by the 1985 U.S. Pharmacopeia (USP) requirement that all L-thyroxine preparations be standardized by high-performance liquid chromatography assay for L-thyroxine tablet content. Additionally, the FDA requirement that all manufacturers that continue to market L-thyroxine submit a New Drug Application by the year 2000 should correct any existing potency concerns. L-Thyroxine replacement may produce TT_4 levels in the hyperthyroid ranges in about 20% of patients; however, no dosage adjustment is necessary if the TSH levels are normal and the patient is clinically euthyroid. T_3 levels often are within the normal range.[66]

T_3 is a chemically pure agent with predictable potency, excellent bioavailability, and a half-life of 1.5 days. Theoretically, T_3 rather than T_4 has been proposed as the drug of choice in patients with cardiovascular problems because its shorter half-life might permit any adverse effects on the heart to resolve more quickly (i.e., in 3 to 5 days) once T_3 is stopped (the half-life of T_4 is 7 to 10 days). However, because of T_3's rapid absorption, supraphysiologic T_3 levels occur after ingestion, producing symptoms of mild toxicity in susceptible patients.[66] The greater cardiotoxic potential of T_3 outweighs its advantage of rapid elimination, so its use cannot be recommended. It is also not recommended as routine thyroid replacement because of its high cost, the need for multiple daily dosing to ensure a uniform response, and greater difficulty in monitoring therapeutic and toxic responses. T_3 administration does not change pretreatment T_4 levels, which, if not properly recognized, can cause therapeutic confusion and potential overreplacement despite adequate hormone replacement. T_3 administration is best monitored by TSH and TT_3 levels. T_3 is used primarily as a diagnostic agent in the T_3 suppression test and when short-term hormone replacement therapy is indicated (e.g., in patients who need repeat scans and RAIU after total thyroidectomy for thyroid cancer). The thyroid hormones must be eliminated completely before the scan. Because T_3 has a short half-life, it is rapidly eliminated after discontinuation, producing a short duration of tolerable hypothyroidism before RAIU and scan. Because of its rapid onset of action (1 to 3 days), intravenous T_3 has been recommended as the drug of choice for myxedema coma. However, its routine use in this condition is limited by concerns about its potentially greater cardiotoxicity. Also, mortality has occurred despite the higher T_3 levels achieved after T_3 administration.[25,62] Approximately 25 to 37.5 μg T_3 is equivalent to 0.1 mg L-thyroxine. Patients should not receive T_3 as routine hormone replacement therapy.

Desiccated thyroid (USP) is obtained from animal thyroid glands (e.g., hog, cow, sheep). Because this preparation is standardized only by iodine content (0.17 to 0.23% iodine), the hormone ratio of T_4 to T_3 may vary from 2:1 (hog) to 3:1 (cow or sheep). Therefore, variability in potency might result from changes in the ratio of the two hormones or from the quantity of organic iodine present. Desiccated thyroid suffers from problems inherent to all T_3-containing preparations. Improper or prolonged tablet storage, causing a loss of potency, can also contribute to an unpredictable response. Desiccated thyroid tablets appear to be stable for 5 years or longer if they are kept dry. Inactive preparations, containing small amounts of T_4 and T_3 or iodinated casein, and tablets with excessive biological activity have been reported. Allergic reactions to the protein component might also occur. During therapy, the FT_4 levels (i.e., FT_4I or FT_4), TT_3, and TSH should remain within normal limits; however, thyroid function tests often are abnormal, especially if supraphysiologic levels of T_3 occur.[66] For these reasons, desiccated thyroid should be considered obsolete. However, desiccated thyroid remains on the market because this preparation is inexpensive and some patients prefer the high that results from the T_3 component. It is strongly recommended that all patients receiving desiccated thyroid be changed to L-thyroxine. Although 0.1 mg of L-thyroxine is theoretically equivalent to 1 grain or 60 mg of desiccated thyroid, such equivalents might not be valid if dosage titrations were initially based on inactive desiccated thyroid preparations. In one study, 60 μg L-thyroxine was equivalent to 1 grain desiccated thyroid.[80] This disparity in equivalence is especially important when patients needing more than 2 grains/day of desiccated thyroid are changed to L-thyroxine. A theoretically equivalent dosage of L-thyroxine might not be reasonable (e.g., 3 grains of desiccated thyroid equivalent to 300 μg of L-thyroxine) because of subpotent desiccated preparations, and dosage retitration is recommended.

Liotrix is a combination of synthetic T_4 and T_3 in a 4:1 ratio that mimics the natural secretion of hormones. It is available commercially as Thyrolar. Because this preparation approximates the normal thyroid production, it was once considered the agent of choice, before it was recognized that a significant amount of T_4 is converted peripherally to T_3. Liotrix is stable and chemically pure, is of predictable potency, and produces laboratory values similar to those seen after T_4 administration. In Thyrolar-1, 50 μg T_4 and 12.5 μg T_3 is equivalent to 1 grain thyroid. Because of its high cost, problems inherent to all T_3-containing preparations, and lack of therapeutic rationale, there is no advantage in using Liotrix.

Special Treatment Issues

Congenital Hypothyroidism

Normal growth and physical and mental development are determined by the age at which treatment is instituted and by how well euthyroidism is maintained.[65,81,82] The earlier treatment begins, the better the prognosis for normal mental and growth development. Mean IQ is higher in those who receive treatment before 3 months and achieve a serum T_4 level of 180 nmol/L (14 μg/dL) than in those who do not. If treatment is delayed until 6 months to 1 year, mental development is impaired despite subsequent treatment. Despite early therapy, neurologic deficits also occur if replacement is inadequate to increase the serum TT_4 above 103 mmol/L (8 μg/dL) and suppress the TSH into the normal range after 3 to 4 months of therapy. Dwarfism does not occur if therapy is delayed until age 5. Infants born athyreotic may have a poorer prognosis for normal mental development because of late detection compared with those born with an abnormal or ectopic thyroid gland.

The preparation of choice for hormone replacement is L-thyroxine. The appropriate T_4 replacement dosage depends on the infant's age and the presence of risk factors (Table 17.11).[65,82] Full replacement dosages can be started in the infant without cardiac disease or other complications. However, infants with long-standing and severe myxedema are extremely sensitive to minute dosages of thyroid, necessitating initiation with very small dosages of L-thyroxine to prevent toxicity (i.e., hyperactivity and irritability). In these infants, initial dosages of T_4 should not exceed 25% of the normal recommended dosage. If no toxicity occurs after 1 to 2 weeks, dosages can be increased gradually by similar increments every 1 to 2 weeks until full replacement dosages are achieved or until the dosage is limited by toxicity.

Table 17.11 ▪ T_4 Dosage for Infants and Children

Age	T_4 Dosage (μg/kg/day)
0–3 mo	10–15
3–6 mo	10–15
6–12 mo	5–7
1–10 yr	3–6
10–16 yr	2–4

Source: References 81, 82.

Normal physical and mental development and reversal of hypothyroid signs and symptoms indicate the optimal replacement dosage. Adequate replacement is achieved when the serum TT_4 level reaches 154 to 180 mmol/L (12 to 14 μg/dL).[81,82] TSH normalization should not be used as the sole criterion because the hypothalamic–pituitary system is not responsive to the negative feedback effect of thyroid hormone, causing TSH to remain elevated for months despite proper or excessive hormone replacement. TSH should normalize within 3 to 4 months after the start of therapy; attempts to normalize TSH earlier may result in overreplacement, producing symptoms of overmetabolism, irritability, brain dysfunction, and premature craniosynostosis.

Subclinical Hypothyroidism

It is controversial whether L-thyroxine therapy should be started in all patients with subclinical hypothyroidism or whether all patients will progress to overt hypothyroidism. Although many patients are older and asymptomatic, improvement in cardiac contractility, lipoprotein concentrations, and cognitive function have been reported.[4,61,64] The decision to start therapy should be based on several considerations, including the risks and benefits of treatment, the likelihood of overt hypothyroidism, the degree of TSH elevation, and history of thyroid disease. In patients receiving L-thyroxine therapy, the elevated TSH level indicates either nonadherence or inadequate replacement, and the dosage should be increased to normalize the TSH if nonadherence is not suspected. In patients with a history of partial thyroid ablation therapy (e.g., RAI, surgery), the likelihood of progression to overt hypothyroidism is high, and replacement therapy is strongly encouraged. In patients with a negative history for thyroid illness, a normal gland, negative thyroid antibodies, and TSH elevations less than 10 mIU/L, L-thyroxine therapy can be withheld if close monitoring of the TSH level every 3 to 4 months is feasible. In patients with an abnormal gland, positive thyroid antibodies, and TSH levels greater than 10 mIU/L, L-thyroxine replacement should be strongly considered if the potential benefits of improvement in cardiac contractility, lipoprotein concentrations, and cognitive function outweigh the risks and expense of therapy.

Myxedema Coma

Treatment includes hormone replacement and supportive measures.[62] There are no comparative trials between L-thyroxine and T_3 in myxedema coma. However, T_4 generally is recommended because of greater clinical experience with its administration than T_3. Fatalities have also been reported after T_3 administration even though higher T_3 levels were achieved. Replacement therapy with large dosages of L-thyroxine (400 μg intravenously) should be given to saturate the TBG. This dosage can be reduced if there are cardiac risk factors. Alternatively, T_3 20 to 50 μg intravenously every 8 hours can be administered. Maintenance dosages of 50 μg intravenous T_4 or 5 μg T_3 daily should be started as soon as possible. Hydrocortisone 50 to 100 mg intravenously every 6 hours must be given to prevent adrenal crisis in case undetected hypopituitarism exists.

Supportive measures include assisted ventilation, glucose infusions for hypoglycemia, fluid restriction because of hyponatremia, and use of plasma expanders for shock and circulatory collapse. Cooling blankets, which may further aggravate shock by vasodilatation, are not recommended. Finally, precipitating factors should be eliminated or corrected. If the proper treatment and support are provided, consciousness, restoration of normal vital functions, and normalization of TSH levels occur within 24 hours.

IMPROVING OUTCOMES

Patients must be aware that reversal of hypothyroid symptoms can be delayed for several weeks even if L-thyroxine adherence is excellent. Patients should be instructed about the proper timing of L-thyroxine in relation to meals and about drug interactions that can significantly impair L-thyroxine's efficacy. L-Thyroxine should be taken on an empty stomach to improve absorption.

PHARMACOECONOMICS

L-Thyroxine therapy is inexpensive, costing approximately \$50 to \$100 per year, depending on whether a brand name or generic preparation is prescribed. Approximately 8 to 12 million L-thyroxine prescriptions are filled annually. Yearly direct savings could amount to \$356 to \$534 million if a less costly brand or generic preparation is used instead of the top-selling brand name preparation. Costs for laboratory medical visits should also be included.

Thyroid Nodules

EPIDEMIOLOGY

The discovery of asymptomatic single or multiple nodules in a normal or enlarged thyroid gland is common, affects women more than men, and occurs in about 5 to 7% of all adults more than 30 years old.[83–85] Its incidence may be as high as 30 to 50%, based on ultrasonography in patients without evidence of clinical thyroid disease. Benign nodules may be present in 10 to 20 million people in the United States.

PATHOPHYSIOLOGY

The pathogenesis is not well understood, but may be related to iodide deficiency, irradiation, dietary goitrogens, and enzymatic defects. These nodules can be described as hypofunctioning ("cold") or autonomously functioning ("hot"). A significant increase in benign thyroid abnormalities (20 to 33%) and thyroid cancers (6 to 9%) has been observed in adults who received external irradiation to the thyroid, thymus, tonsils, adenoids, or upper head and neck region 20 to 25 years earlier.[84] Papillary, mixed papillary–follicular, and follicular malignancies and benign abnormalities, including focal hyperplasia, Hashimoto's thyroiditis, adenomas, Graves' disease, and colloid nodules have been reported. These malignant tumors are slow growing, and the prognosis is good if there are no metastases. Nonpalpable cancers have been found during surgery.

CLINICAL PRESENTATION AND DIAGNOSIS

Patients usually are asymptomatic and clinically euthyroid, although bothersome symptoms can occur. It is often difficult to determine clinically which nodule, if any, is cancerous. In general, 10 to 20% of "cold" nodules on thyroid scan are cancerous and "hot" nodules rarely are carcinogenic. The risk of malignancy is higher if a history of irradiation is present. Cold nodules in a multinodular goiter rarely are malignant; evidence of hypothyroidism or hyperthyroidism reduces but does not eliminate the risk of malignancy. A physician skilled in thyroid examinations should evaluate all patients with a history of childhood irradiation. A physical examination of the thyroid, base-

Table 17.12 ▪ Risk Factors for Thyroid Cancer

Evidence	Lower Index of Suspicion	Higher Index of Suspicion
History	Familial history of thyroid disease or endemic goiter	History of neck or head irradiation
Patient characteristics	Older women; multinodular goiter, soft nodule	Children, young adults, men; solitary firm, dominant nodule; vocal cord paralysis; enlarged lymph nodes; hoarseness
Laboratory characteristics	Negative thin-needle biopsy, positive thyroid antibodies, hot nodule on scan, cystic lesion on echo	Positive thin-needle biopsy, ↑ thyroglobulin after thyroid surgery, ↑ serum calcitonin levels, cold nodule on scan, solid lesion on echo
L-Thyroxine suppression therapy	Regression of nodule after 3–6 mo therapy	No regression, ↑ growth

line TSH, FT_4I or FT_4, and antibodies should be obtained even if the patient is clinically euthyroid and asymptomatic. If no abnormalities are found, routine yearly examinations are recommended. A fine-needle biopsy of the nodule, performed in the outpatient setting, can provide supporting information for or against surgery. Significant risk factors for malignancy are listed in Table 17.12.[84]

THERAPEUTIC PLAN

A high index of suspicion for thyroid carcinoma requires surgical intervention. In euthyroid patients with a nodule that is likely to be benign, no history of thyroid irradiation, and a low index of suspicion for cancer, a trial of TSH suppression therapy is warranted to prevent further growth and stimulation of the nodule. Higher dosages of L-thyroxine, 0.15 to 0.2 mg, may be required to achieve a suppressed TSH level of 0.1 to 0.5 mIU/L, raising concerns about L-thyroxine toxicity.[61,83,85] There is also the potential for overt hyperthyroidism, especially if exogenous L-thyroxine is added to endogenous thyroxine overproduction (e.g., hot nodule). If significant regression of the nodule occurs after 3 to 6 months of therapy, treatment may be continued indefinitely. However, therapy usually does not shrink the gland to normal size. Any growth of the nodule during thyroid suppression therapy is alarming and requires rebiopsy or surgical removal because of the risk of malignancy. A clinically euthyroid patient with a suppressed TSH level should be the goal of therapy. However, the use of TSH suppression in preventing nodule growth and potential symptoms has produced mixed results, leading some to criticize such use.[85]

KEY POINTS

- Hypothyroidism, hyperthyroidism, and nodular disease are common endocrine problems that affect 15% of women and 5% of men.
- Practitioners should be alert to drugs that cause thyroid illness, interfere with proper laboratory interpretation, or interact with effective medical management.
- Thyroid function tests are essential to detect, evaluate, and monitor thyroid disease in symptomatic patients and in older adults who have atypical symptoms.
- TSH is the most sensitive test for monitoring thyroid function.
- Many different treatment options are available for hyperthyroidism, hypothyroidism, and nodular disease.
- L-Thyroxine is the preparation of choice for managing hypothyroidism.
- Supraphysiologic T_4 dosages can cause osteoporosis and cardiac arrhythmias.
- Practitioners should integrate several patient and medication considerations in selecting the optimal treatment regimen for hyperthyroidism.
- The preferred thioamide for managing hyperthyroidism is methimazole.
- Rash, hepatotoxicity, and agranulocytosis can occur with thioamide therapy.
- An understanding of the detection, evaluation, medical management, and education of patients with thyroid disease is essential.

REFERENCES

1. O'Connor P, Feely J. Clinical pharmacokinetics and endocrine disorders. Therapeutic implications. Clin Pharmacokinet 13:345–364, 1987.
2. Surks MI, Chopra IJ, Mariash CN, et al. American Thyroid Association guidelines for use of laboratory tests in thyroid disorders. JAMA 263:1529–1532, 1990.
3. American College of Physicians. Screening for thyroid disease. Ann Intern Med 129:141–143, 1998.
4. Helfand M, Redfern CC. Screening for thyroid disease: an update. Ann Intern Med 129:144–158, 1998.
5. Surks MI, Sievert R. Drugs and thyroid function. N Engl J Med 333:1688–1694, 1995.
6. Lazarus JH. Hyperthyroidism. Lancet 349:339–343, 1997.
7. Gittoes NJL, Franklyn JA. Hyperthyroidism. Current treatment guidelines. Drugs 55:543–553, 1998.
8. Zimmerman D, Lteif AN. Thyrotoxicosis in children. Med Clin North Am 27:109–126, 1998.
9. Marqusee E, Haden ST, Utiger RD. Subclinical thyrotoxicosis. Med Clin North Am 27:37–49, 1998.
10. McIver B, Morris JC. The pathogenesis of Graves' disease. Med Clin North Am 27:73–89, 1998.
11. Siegel RD, Lee SL. Toxic nodular goiter: toxic adenoma and toxic multinodular goiter. Med Clin North Am 27:151–168, 1998.
12. Lazarus JH, Hall R, Othman S, et al. The clinical spectrum of postpartum thyroid disease. QJ M 89:429–435, 1996.
13. Ross DS. Syndromes of thyrotoxicosis with low radioactive iodine uptake. Med Clin North Am 27:169–185, 1998.
14. Koh LKH, Greenspan FS, Yeo PPB. Interferon-α induced thyroid dysfunction: three clinical presentations and a review of the literature. Thyroid 7:891–896, 1997.
15. Gittoes NJL, Franklyn JA. Drug-induced thyroid disorders. Drug Saf 13:46–55, 1996.

16. Harjai KJ, Licata AA. Effects of amiodarone on thyroid function. Ann Intern Med 126:63–73, 1997.
17. Bartalena L, Brogioni S, Grasso L, et al. Treatment of amiodarone-induced thyrotoxicosis, a difficult challenge: results of a prospective study. J Clin Endocrinol Metab 81:2930–2933, 1996.
18. Barclay MI, Brownlie BEW, Turner JG, et al. Lithium associated thyrotoxicosis: a report of 14 cases, with statistical analysis of incidence. Clin Endocrinol 40:759–764, 1994.
19. Sawin CT, Geller A, Wolf PA, et al. Low serum thyrotropin concentrations as a risk factor for atrial fibrillation in older persons. N Engl J Med 331:1249–1252, 1994.
20. Faber J, Galloe AM. Changes in bone mass during prolonged subclinical hyperthyroidism due to L-thyroxine treatment: a meta-analysis. Eur J Endocrinol 130:350–356, 1994.
21. Bartalena L, Grasso L, Brogloni S, et al. Serum interleukin-6 in amiodarone-induced thyrotoxicosis. J Clin Endocrinol Metab 78:423–427, 1994.
22. Mestman JH. Hyperthyroidism in pregnancy. Med Clin North Am 27:127–149, 1998.
23. Burrow GN. Thyroid function and hyperfunction during gestation. Endocr Rev 14:194–202, 1993.
24. Woeber KA. Iodine and thyroid disease. Med Clin North Am 75:169–178, 1991.
25. Gavin LA. Thyroid crises. Med Clin North Am 75:179–193, 1991.
26. Burch HB, Wartofsky LW. Graves' ophthalmopathy. Current concepts regarding pathogenesis and management. Endocr Rev 14:747–793, 1993.
27. Bartalena L, Marcocci C, Bogazzi F, et al. Relationship between therapy for hyperthyroidism and the course of Graves' ophthalmopathy. N Engl J Med 338:73–78, 1998.
28. Garcia M, Baskin HJ, Feld S, et al. AACE clinical practice guidelines for the evaluation and treatment of hypothyroidism and hyperthyroidism. Endocr Pract 1:54–62, 1995.
29. Singer PA, Cooper DS, Levy EG, et al. Treatment guidelines for patients with hyperthyroidism and hypothyroidism. JAMA 273:808–812, 1995.
30. Kaplan MM, Meier DA, Dworkin HJ. Treatment of hyperthyroidism with radioactive iodine. Med Clin North Am 27:205–223, 1998.
31. Mercado M, Mendoza-Zubieta V, Bautista-Osorio R, et al. Treatment of hyperthyroidism with a combination of methimazole and cholestyramine. J Clin Endocrinol Metab 81:3191–3193, 1996.
32. Wartofsky L, Glinoes D, Solomon B, et al. Differences and similarities in the diagnosis and treatment of Graves' disease in Europe, Japan, and the United States. Thyroid 1:129–135, 1991.
33. Solomon B, Glinoer D, Lagasse R, et al. Current trends in the management of Graves' disease. J Clin Endocrinol Metab 70:1518–1524, 1990.
34. Glaser NS, Styne DM. Predictors of early remission of hyperthyroidism in children. J Clin Endocrinol Metab 82:1719–1726, 1997.
35. Burrow GN. Thyroid function and hyperfunction during gestation. Endocr Rev 14:194–202, 1993.
36. Cooper DS. Antithyroid drugs for the treatment of hyperthyroidism caused by Graves' disease. Med Clin North Am 27:225–247, 1998.
37. Volpe R. Evidence that the immunosuppressive effects of antithyroid drugs are mediated through the action on the thyroid cell modulating thyrocyte-immunocyte signaling: a review. Thyroid 4:217–223, 1994.
38. Van Dijke CP, Heydendael RJ, De Kleine MJ. Methimazole, carbimazole, and congenital skin defects [letter]. Ann Intern Med 106:60–61, 1987.
39. Mandel SJ, Brent GA, Larsen PR. Review of antithyroid drug use during pregnancy and report of a case of aplasia cutis. Thyroid 4:129–133, 1994.
40. Momotani N, Ito K, Hamada N, et al. Maternal hyperthyroidism and congenital malformation in the offspring. Clin Endocrinol (Oxf) 20:695–700, 1984.
41. Walter RM, Bartle W. Rectal administration of propylthiouracil in the treatment of Graves' disease. Am J Med 88:69–70, 1990.
42. Nabil N, Miner DJ, Amatruda JM. Methimazole: an alternative route of administration. J Clin Endocrinol Metab 54:180–181, 1982.
43. Momotani N, Noh JY, Ishikawa N, et al. Effects of propylthiouracil and methimazole on fetal thyroid status in mothers with Graves' hyperthyroidism. J Clin Endocrinol Metab 82:3633–3636, 1997.
44. Eisenstein Z, Weiss M, Katz Y, et al. Intellectual capacity of subjects exposed to methimazole or propylthiouracil in utero. Eur J Pediatr 151:558–559, 1992.
45. Allannic H, Fauchet R, Orgiazzi J, et al. Antithyroid drugs and Graves' disease: a prospective randomized evaluation of the efficacy of treatment duration. J Clin Endocrinol Metab 70:675–679, 1990.
46. Feldt-Rasmussen U, Glinoer D, Orgiazzi J. Reassessment of antithyroid drug therapy of Graves' disease. Annu Rev Med 44:323–334, 1993.
47. Lippe BM, Landaw EM, Kaplan SA. Hyperthyroidism in children treated with long term medical therapy: twenty-five percent remission every two years. J Clin Endocrinol Metab 64:1241–1245, 1987.
48. Romaldini JH, Bromberg N, Werner RS, et al. Comparison of effects of high and low dosage regimens of antithyroid drugs in the management of Graves' hyperthyroidism. J Clin Endocrinol Metab 57:563–570, 1983.
49. Hashizume K, Ichikawa K, Sakurai A, et al. Administration of thyroxine in treated Graves' disease: effects on the level of antibodies to thyroid-stimulating hormone receptors and on the risk of recurrence of hyperthyroidism. N Engl J Med 324:947–953, 1991.
50. Rittmaster RS, Zwicker H, Abbott EC, et al. Effect of methimazole with or without exogenous L-thyroxine on serum concentrations of thyrotropin (TSH) receptor antibodies in patients with Graves' disease. J Clin Endocrinol Metab 81:3283–3288, 1996.
51. McIver B, Rae P, Beckett G, et al. Lack of effect of thyroxine in patients with Graves' hyperthyroidism who are treated with an antithyroid drug. N Engl J Med 334:220–224, 1996.
52. Tamai H, Hayaki I, Kawai K, et al. Lack of effect of thyroxine administration on elevated thyroid stimulating hormone receptor antibody levels in treated Graves' disease patients. J Clin Endocrinol Metab 80:1481–1484, 1995.
53. Liaw Y-F, Huang M-J, Fan K-D, et al. Hepatic injury during propylthiouracil therapy in patients with hyperthyroidism: a cohort study. Ann Intern Med 118:424–428, 1993.
54. Williams KV, Nayak S, Becker D, et al. Fifty years of experience with propylthiouracil-associated hepatotoxicity: what have we learned? J Clin Endocrinol Metab 82:1727–1733, 1997.
55. Tajiri J, Noguchi S, Murakami T, et al. Antithyroid drug-induced agranulocytosis: the usefulness of routine white blood cell count monitoring. Arch Intern Med 150:621–624, 1990.
56. Geffner DL, Hershman JM. Beta-adrenergic blockade for the treatment of hyperthyroidism. Am J Med 93:61–68, 1992.
57. Milner MR, Gelman KM, Phillips RA, et al. Double-blind crossover trial of diltiazem versus propranolol in the management of thyrotoxic symptoms. Pharmacotherapy 10:100–106, 1990.
58. Ron E, Doody MM, Becker DV, et al. Cancer mortality following treatment for adult hypothyroidism. JAMA 280:347–355, 1998.
59. Wang YS, Tsou CT, Lin WH, et al. Long term treatment of Graves' disease with iopanoic acid (Telepaque). J Clin Endocrinol Metab 65:679–682, 1987.
60. Weber CA, Clark OH. Surgery for thyroid disease. Med Clin North Am 69:1097–1115, 1985.
61. Cooper DS. Subclinical thyroid disease: a clinician's perspective. Ann Intern Med 129:135–138, 1998.
62. Nicoloff JT, LoPresti JS. Myxedema coma. A form of decompensated hypothyroidism. Endocrinol Metab Clin North Am 22:279–290, 1993.
63. Lindsay RS, Toft AD. Hypothyroidism. Lancet 349:413–417, 1997.
64. O'Brien T, Dinneen SF, O'Brien PC, et al. Hyperlipidemia in patients with primary and secondary hypothyroidism. Mayo Clin Proc 68:860–866, 1993.
65. LaFranchi S. Diagnosis and treatment of hypothyroidism in children. Compr Ther 13:20–30, 1987.
66. Toft AD. Thyroxine therapy. N Engl J Med 331:174–180, 1994.
67. Fish LH, Schwartz HL, Cavanaugh J, et al. Replacement dose, metabolism, and bioavailability of levothyroxine in the treatment of hypothyroidism. N Engl J Med 316:764–770, 1987.
68. Bearcroft CP, Toms GC, Willians SJ, et al. Thyroxine replacement in post-radioiodine hypothyroidism. Clin Endocrinol (Oxf) 34:115–118, 1991.
69. Schneyer CR. Calcium carbonate and reduction of levothyroxine efficacy [letter]. JAMA 279:750, 1998.
70. Mandel SJ, Brent GA, Larsen PR. Levothyroxine therapy in patients with thyroid disease. Ann Intern Med 119:492–502, 1993.
71. Sherman SI, Malecha SE. Absorption and malabsorption of levothyroxine. Am J Ther 2:814–818, 1995.
72. McCowen KC, Garger JR, Spark R. Elevated serum thyrotropin in thyroxine-treated patients with hypothyroidism given sertraline [letter]. N Engl J Med 337:1010–1011, 1997.
73. Ain KB, Pucino F, Shiver TM, et al. Thyroid hormone levels affected by time of blood sampling in thyroxine-treated patients. Thyroid 3:81–85, 1993.
74. Oppenheimer JH, Braverman LE, Toft A, et al. A therapeutic controversy. Thyroid hormone treatment: when and what? J Clin Endocrinol Metab 80:2873–2883, 1995.
75. Leese GP, Jung RT, Guthrie C, et al. Morbidity in patients on L-thyroxine: a comparison of those with a normal TSH level to those with suppressed TSH. Clin Endocrinol (Oxf) 37:500–503, 1992.
76. Escalante DA, Arem N, Arem R. Assessment of interchangeability of two brands of levothyroxine preparations with a third-generation TSH assay. Am J Med 98: 374–378, 1995.
77. Dong BJ, Hauck WW, Gambertoglio JG, et al. Bioequivalence of generic and brand-name levothyroxine products in the treatment of hypothyroidism. JAMA 277:1205–1213, 1997.
78. Stoffer SS, Szpunar WE. Levothyroxine loses potency with age [letter]. JAMA 255:1881–1882, 1986.

79. Grebe SKG, Cooke RR, Ford HC, et al. Treatment of hypothyroidism with once weekly thyroxine. J Clin Endocrinol Metab 82:870–875, 1997.
80. Sawin CT, Hershman JM, Fernandez-Garcia R, et al. A comparison of thyroxine and desiccated thyroid in patients with primary hypothyroidism. Metabolism 27:1518–1525, 1978.
81. Heyerdahl S, Kase BF, Lie SO. Intellectual development in children with congenital hypothyroidism in relation to recommended thyroxine treatment. J Pediatr 118:850–857, 1991.
82. Fisher DA, Foley BL. Early treatment of congenital hypothyroidism. Pediatrics 83:785–789, 1989.
83. Ridgway EC. Medical treatment of benign thyroid nodules: have we defined a benefit. Ann Intern Med 128:403–405, 1998.
84. Greenspan FS. The problem of the nodular goiter. Med Clin North Am 75:195–209, 1991.
85. Gharib H, Mazzaferri EF. Thyroxine suppressive therapy in patients with nodular thyroid disease. Ann Intern Med 128:386–394, 1998.

CHAPTER 18

PARATHYROID DISORDERS

Renu F. Singh and Betty J. Dong

To understand the treatment of common parathyroid disorders, one must first understand the effects of parathyroid hormone (PTH), the consequences of excessive secretion or lack of end-organ response, and its relationship to calcium metabolism.

There are four parathyroid glands, located posteriorly on the thyroid gland in the neck. PTH, the principal regulator of extracellular ionic calcium, is released from the parathyroid glands via a negative feedback system responsive to plasma calcium levels. Normal plasma ionic calcium is maintained through the action of PTH on kidney, bone, and intestine. Most of the total body calcium is in the form of hydroxyapatite in bone (99%), and only a small fraction of the calcium circulates in the bloodstream as the active (ionized) or inactive (bound) forms. Approximately 40% of the total serum calcium is bound, primarily to albumin, 15% is complexed with phosphate or other anions, and 45% is in the ionized active form. Therefore, reductions in serum albumin alter the concentration of protein-bound calcium and increase the free ionized fraction proportionally. The normal total serum calcium concentration is approximately 2.12 to 2.62 mmol/L (8.5 to 10.5 mg/dL), depending on the laboratory. In patients with hypoalbuminemia, the serum calcium can be adjusted by adding 0.2 mmol/L (0.8 mg/dL) for each 10 g/L of albumin below a normal level of 40 g/L to the measured serum calcium [$\text{Serum Ca}_{\text{corrected}}$ (mg/dL) $= \text{Serum Ca}_{\text{observed}} + 0.8\ (4 - \text{Serum albumin}_{\text{observed}})$]. This formula might not completely correct for albumin, and direct determination of ionized calcium levels might be useful.

PTH protects against hypocalcemia by the following mechanisms:

- Increasing calcium and phosphate release from osteoclastic bone resorption
- Increasing calcium and magnesium reabsorption from the renal tubule
- Increasing intestinal calcium absorption indirectly via vitamin D
- Increasing conversion of the metabolite 25-hydroxycholecalciferol to active vitamin D_3 (1,25-dihydroxycholecalciferol or 1,25-$[OH]_2D_3$ or calcitriol) by stimulating the activity of renal tubular 25-OH-1-α-hydroxylase
- Increasing renal bicarbonate excretion (bicarbonaturia), producing a metabolic acidosis that decreases the ability of circulating albumin to bind calcium, thus increasing calcium by physiochemical means
- Increasing renal phosphate excretion (hyperphosphaturia) and preventing elevations in plasma phosphate levels from increased bone resorption.

Thus, a reciprocal relationship between calcium and phosphate exists. In hyperparathyroidism, serum calcium is elevated and hypophosphatemia occurs. Conversely, in hypoparathyroidism, hypocalcemia and hyperphosphatemia are seen.

Hyperparathyroidism

DEFINITION

Primary hyperparathyroidism is an endocrine disorder characterized by excessive and incompletely regulated release of PTH from one or more parathyroid glands.

TREATMENT GOALS: HYPERPARATHYROIDISM

- Reverse symptoms resulting from severe hypercalcemia.
- Correct dehydration.
- Increase renal calcium excretion.
- Inhibit bone resorption.
- Prevent short-term and long-term complications resulting from hypercalcemia.

EPIDEMIOLOGY

Adenomatous parathyroid glands (single-gland involvement) account for 80% of hyperparathyroid cases, and hyperplastic (multiple-gland involvement) or malignant parathyroid glands account for 20% and less than 2% of cases, respectively. Hyperparathyroidism, associated with multiple endocrine neoplasia (MEN) syndromes, almost always involves multiple glands. The hallmark of hyperparathyroidism is hypercalcemia because the negative feedback cycle fails to suppress further PTH secretion. The cause of this disorder is unknown, although inheritance via an autosomal dominant trait is described. Hyperparathyroidism is more common than previously recognized. Earlier detection of asymptomatic disease has resulted from the widespread use of routine serum calcium measurements. Various studies before 1969 indicate an incidence of 10 to 20 cases per 100,000.[1] In a population-based study, an incidence of 7.8 cases/100,000 jumped to 42 cases/100,000 after routine calcium measurements were introduced.[2] This subsequently fell to 27.7 cases/100,000, a rate similar to those reported in England and Sweden.[3,4] The incidence of hyperparathyroidism increases with age, and it is two to four times more common in women than in men. Approximately 100,000 new cases develop each year in the United States.[5]

Patient Characteristic	Prevalence
Both sexes, 39 yr or younger	10:100,000
Both sexes, 40 yr or older	50:100,000
Women 60 yr or older	188:100,000
Men 60 yr or older	91:100,000

PATHOPHYSIOLOGY

Excessive PTH release causes hypercalcemia and hypophosphatemia via the mechanisms previously described. Mild to moderate hyperchloremic acidosis is caused by PTH-induced bicarbonaturia. Hypercalciuria results when the renal threshold for reabsorbing calcium is exceeded; serum calcium usually is less than 3.00 mmol/L (12 mg/dL). Complications of nephrolithiasis result from prolonged hypercalciuria in an alkaline medium (bicarbonaturia), resulting in calcium carbonate kidney stones. Other extraskeletal metastatic calcifications might produce rheumatologic complaints of calcific tendinitis and chondrocalcinosis.

CLINICAL PRESENTATION AND DIAGNOSIS

Signs and Symptoms

Most patients presenting with primary hyperparathyroidism in the United States today are asymptomatic. Earlier detection of the disease has changed the clinical presentation of hyperparathyroidism. With only mildly elevated serum calcium (more than 0.24 mmol/L, or 1 mg/dL of upper limits), most patients are asymptomatic or have nonspecific complaints of weakness and easy fatigue. High-risk older women might show confusion and dehydration. Before the routine use of serum calcium measurements, patients typically presented with symptoms resulting from severe hypercalcemia. Serum calcium levels greater than 3.00 mmol/L (12 mg/dL) commonly produce gastrointestinal symptoms (e.g., anorexia, nausea, and vomiting) and neurologic manifestations of proximal muscle weakness, delayed deep tendon reflexes, and altered mental status. Skeletal symptoms may include diffuse bone pain and arthralgias. Severe deforming disease, such as osteitis cystica, is rarely seen with primary hyperparathyroidism today but is still a problem with secondary hyperparathyroidism in patients with end-stage renal disease complicated by renal osteodystrophy. Hyperparathyroidism affects mainly cortical bone and spares cancellous bone such as the spine.

The clinical spectrum and complications of primary hyperparathyroidism are presented in Table 18.1. The severity of the clinical manifestations, especially the degree of hypercalcemia, generally is proportional to the degree of hyperfunctioning tissue and the level of PTH elevation.

Diagnosis

There are usually no abnormal physical findings on physical examination, so in 80 to 90% of cases the diagnosis of hyperparathyroidism is based on an elevated serum calcium level (usually more than 2.62 mmol/L, or 10.5 mg/dL) and an elevated PTH level. Immunoradiometric assay (IRMA) of the intact PTH level measured by is one of the most sensitive PTH assays and should be obtained to confirm the diagnosis of hyperparathyroidism. Total serum calcium levels should be elevated in three

Table 18.1 ▪ Signs and Symptoms of Hypercalcemia and Hyperparathyroidism

System	Symptoms	Complications	Laboratory Tests
General	Weakness, easy fatigability		
Gastrointestinal	Nausea, vomiting, anorexia, constipation, abdominal pain, weight loss	Peptic ulcer disease (10–15%), chronic pancreatitis, cholelithiasis, fecal impaction, intestinal obstruction	↑ Amylase, ↑ gastrin
Genitourinary	Polyuria, nocturia, polydipsia, dehydration, uremia symptoms, renal colic pain	Nephrolithiasis, nephrocalcinosis (20–30%), renal failure, pyelonephritis	Hematuria, inability to concentrate urine (low specific gravity), pyuria, ↓ Na, ↓ K, ↓ Mg
Skeletal	Vague aches and pains, arthralgias, localized swellings	Osteitis fibrosa cystica, chondrocalcinosis, pathologic fractures, bone cysts, calcium depositions leading to gout, pseudogout	Radiologic: subperiosteal bone resorption Dual energy absorptiometry: ↓ bone mineral density in regions of cortical bone
Neurologic	Emotional lability, slow mentation, poor memory, drowsiness, ataxia, coma	Depression, psychoses; headaches, myopathy (proximal), coma	Hyperactive deep tendon reflexes
Cardiovascular	Bradycardia	Hypertension (20–60%), cardiac arrest, bundle branch block, heart block, enhanced digitalis sensitivity	Electrocardiographic intervals: ↓ Q-T, ↑ P-R, ↑ QRS
Metabolic	Dehydration	Hyperchloremic acidosis, insulin hypersecretion, decreased insulin sensitivity	↓ HCO_3, ↑ Cl
Others	Pruritus caused by ectopic calcifications in skin; ectopic calcifications in lungs, kidneys, cornea; red eyes	Anemia, band keratopathy, thrombosis, malignancies in gastrointestinal tract, breast, thyroid	

separate measurements before hypercalcemia is established. Ionized serum calcium levels should be used in patients with low serum albumin. Drugs that can increase serum calcium concentrations, such as thiazide diuretics, should be withdrawn for several days. Chronic lithium therapy may produce hypercalcemia with an elevated serum PTH level. Lithium should be discontinued, if possible, to distinguish drug-induced hyperparathyroidism from other causes.

Other abnormal laboratory findings include hypophosphatemia, hyperphosphaturia, hypercalciuria, low serum bicarbonate concentration, elevated serum chloride levels, elevations in serum alkaline phosphatase and osteocalcin (markers of bone formation), and urinary hydroxyproline and collagen cross-link residues (markers of bone resorption). Serum urea nitrogen or creatinine levels can be helpful in evaluating renal function. Radiographic manifestations of osteitis fibrosa cystica, nephrolithiasis, or other extraskeletal calcifications can be present. Other causes of hypercalcemia should be eliminated (Table 18.2).

Table 18.2 ▪ Some Causes of Hypercalcemia

- Hyperparathyroidism
  - Primary: parathyroid adenomas, hyperplasia, or carcinoma
- Granulomatous disease (sarcoidosis, tuberculosis, histoplasmosis, coccidiomycosis, leprosy)
- Drugs
  - Vitamin A or D toxicity or calcium intoxification
  - Milk-alkali syndrome
  - Lithium
  - Thiazides and thiazidelike diuretics
  - Estrogens, antiestrogens, testosterone in breast cancer
- Malignancies
  - Nonhematologic (breast, bronchus)
  - Hematologic (myeloma, leukemia, lymphoma)
- Endocrine (adrenal insufficiency, thyrotoxicosis, acromegaly, pheochromocytoma)
- Immobilization
- Bone disorders (Paget's osteoporosis)
- Familial hypocalciuric hypercalcemia
- Parenteral nutrition
- Aluminum excess
- Acute and chronic renal disease

THERAPEUTIC PLAN

The National Institutes of Health Consensus Development Panel[5] concludes that the diagnosis of hyperparathyroidism in an asymptomatic patient does not always mandate surgery. In patients who are asymptomatic with only a mildly elevated serum calcium, no previous episodes of life-threatening hypercalcemia, and normal renal and bone status, the indications for surgery are less clear because the true progression of the disease is unknown.[5] There are no objective criteria to predict which patients will eventually need surgery and which patients can be treated medically. Generally, long-term follow-up studies indicate a benign course with stable hypercalcemia and, rarely, progressive loss of renal function. In a 10-year retrospective study of 248 patients with mild asymptomatic hyperparathyroidism, 51% ultimately needed surgical intervention because of complications of their disease and 49% had no deterioration in their clinical status.[6] In the latter group, 22% of patients died during this 10-year period (unrelated to the hyperparathyroidism) or were lost to follow-up. Patients who are unlikely to return for consistent follow-up or whose coexistent illness complicates management should be considered surgical candidates. Surgery is also recommended for young patients (less than 50 years of age) because the outcome of several decades of primary hyperparathyroidism is unknown. Many studies tend to favor early surgical intervention to normalize serum calcium levels, prevent further bone loss, and increase bone density even though surgery might be less effective in patients with mild disease and difficult-to-locate PTH abnormalities. If medical observation is selected, then patients should be monitored closely with serum calcium and phosphorus levels every 6 months and urinary calcium and creatinine determinations yearly. Annual abdominal radiography to detect renal stones also is recommended. Although bone density seems to remain stable in patients with mild hyperparathyroidism, bone density measurements should be obtained every 1 to 3 years to assess bone loss of both cortical (distal radius) and cancellous bone (lumbar spine). If the disease progresses, then surgical intervention is indicated.

TREATMENT

Surgical exploration of the neck and removal of adenomatous, hyperplastic, or malignant tissue is the definitive treatment of choice for symptomatic primary hyperparathyroidism.[7] Surgery is absolutely indicated in patients with sustained serum calcium levels >2.86 (>11.5 mg/dL); evidence of bony involvement (bone mineral density less than 2 SD below normal controls); evidence of renal involvement, including nephrolithiasis, nephrocalcinosis, hypercalciuria (more than 400 mg/day, or 9.98 mmol/L) or decreased creatinine clearance in the absence of any other cause; complications from hyperparathyroidism, including an episode of acute primary hyperparathyroidism; and coexisting disease states that might be exacerbated by elevations in serum calcium levels (e.g., hypertension).

Most critical to the surgical treatment of primary hyperparathyroidism is an experienced and skilled surgeon. In competent hands, the evidence of postoperative complications (i.e., vocal cord paralysis) is minimal, and the cure rate is greater than 90%.[8]

Neuromuscular symptoms often are reversed by successful parathyroidectomy, but somatic symptoms are not predictably improved by the operation. Postoperatively, serum calcium levels normalize or fall below normal within 24 to 48 hours. Hypocalcemia is usually mild and transient. Serum calcium levels should be monitored daily until levels stabilize, around the fifth to sixth postoperative day. Serum calcium should be maintained above 8 mg/dL. Hypocalcemic symptoms of tetany or pretetany should be treated intravenously with 10 to 20 mL 10% calcium gluconate, given slowly (not faster than 10 mL/minute) until symptoms are relieved. Modest degrees of postoperative hypocalcemia need not be treated except by ensuring an adequate calcium intake with dietary calcium or elemental calcium in oral dosages of 1 to 2 g/day. Most patients have a temporary hypocalcemia postsurgically that is normalized quickly as the parathyroid glands begin to regain function. A small percentage of patients develop permanent hypoparathyroidism, necessitating treatment with vitamin D. Parathyroid transplantation might be indicated for the patient with secondary hyperparathyroidism (renal osteodystrophy), primary parathyroid hyperplasia, persistent or recurrent hyperparathyroidism, or radical head and neck surgery including thyroidectomy.[9]

Pharmacotherapy

There is no pharmacologic substitute for the surgical management of hyperparathyroidism because surgery can correct the underlying disorder. However, medical management of hypercalcemia is indicated in symptomatic patients before surgery or in patients who refuse surgery, in those with life-threatening hypercalcemia, in those with resistant or recurrent hyperparathyroidism despite previous neck surgery, and in poor surgical candidates.

Several therapeutic options are available (Table 18.3). The goals are to correct dehydration, increase renal calcium excretion, and inhibit bone resorption. Many of these options are very effective and should lower serum calcium in virtually all patients. A single agent or a combination of agents might be needed, depending on the severity of the hypercalcemia, the extent of dehydration, and the duration and degree of effectiveness of the selected agent.

Hydration with intravenous saline is the initial treatment in the management of hypercalcemia (≥3 mmol/L; ≥12 mg/dL) from any cause.[10,11] Because hypercalcemia often causes vomiting and polyuria (resulting in dehydration, hypokalemia, and hypomagnesemia), adequate electrolyte replacement and volume expansion are critical. Typically, 2.5 to 4 L saline per day is administered, with the infusion rate adjusted to the degree of volume depletion and urine output. Increasing urine output should be observed in the initial hours of fluid repletion to guide adequacy of fluid load and the patient's ability to tolerate it (e.g., in congestive heart failure or renal failure). Adequate hydration should reverse mild hypercalcemic symptoms, restore the glomerular filtration rate, and increase calcium excretion. Serum calcium levels generally decrease by 0.25 to 0.5 mmol/L (1 to 2 mg/dL) within a few hours, but rarely does hydration alone lead to normalization of marked hypercalcemia.

In addition to hydration with saline, adjunctive diuretic

therapy with a loop diuretic, such as furosemide, may be effective. Loop diuretics inhibit calcium reabsorption in the thick ascending limb of the loop of Henle. Furosemide is given as 10 to 20 mg intravenously every 6 to 12 hours.[10] The use of diuretic therapy is well tolerated even in patients with moderate renal impairment and might reduce serum calcium levels by 0.75 mmol/L (3 mg/dL) within 24 hours. It is essential that patients be adequately hydrated throughout this diuresis and repletion of electrolytes such as magnesium and potassium be maintained. Thiazides and related diuretics, such as metolazone and indapamide, may reduce calcium excretion at distal tubular sites and should be discontinued in patients with primary hyperparathyroidism.

In emergent hypercalcemic crisis, the preceding methods might be used more aggressively. Forced diuresis with up to 6 L per day of normal saline and furosemide, 80 to 100 mg intravenously every 1 to 2 hours, to maintain urinary flow rates of above 200 mL/hour might be needed.[12] Such an approach reduces serum calcium levels by 0.5 to 1 mmol/L (2 to 4 mg/dL) within 24 hours but necessitates central venous pressure monitoring of fluid status and bladder catheterization in addition to continuous electrolyte repletion.

Because saline hydration rarely normalizes hypercalcemia, early initiation of an antiresorptive agent is prudent to avoid the potential complications of prolonged saline diuresis. In addition, saline does not affect calcium mobilization from bone, which is the major contributor of hypercalcemia. Bisphosphonates have become one of the primary treatment options for the management of hypercalcemia. Bisphosphonates are stable pyrophosphate analogs that bind to hydroxyapatite in bone and act as potent inhibitors of PTH-mediated osteoclastic bone resorption. The calcium-lowering effect varies among bisphosphonates, and the effect is significantly weaker in patients with primary hyperparathyroidism than in patients with tumor-induced hypercalcemia.

Etidronate, a first-generation bisphosphonate, is poorly absorbed and, like most bisphosphonates, is more effective when administered intravenously. Etidronate is approved for administration in a daily dosage of 7.5 mg/kg intravenously over 4 hours for 3 days. Serum calcium levels start to fall within 24 to 48 hours after administration, but maximal effect may take up to 7 days. Response rates are better in patients who are well hydrated with saline before etidronate administration and in those who continue to receive intravenous saline. Repeat dosing of etidronate is not recommended earlier than 7 days after the initial course. Etidronate may be discontinued after 3 days if serum calcium is reduced by more than 2 mg/dL or approaches the normal range. Oral etidronate can be given after a course of intravenous etidronate to maintain normocalcemia, although oral etidronate is less effective than intravenous etidronate in lowering serum calcium levels. The recommended oral dosage of etidronate is 20 mg/kg/day for 30 to 90 days. Etidronate therapy is generally well tolerated, with occasional transient elevations in serum creatinine and phosphate levels. Etidronate should be used cautiously in patients with renal dysfunction. Chronic administration of high-dose etidronate is associated with impaired bone mineralization, resulting in osteomalacia.

Pamidronate, a second-generation bisphosphonate, is a more potent agent than etidronate and less likely to inhibit bone mineralization or osteoblast activity.[13] Clinical studies comparing pamidronate to etidronate have demonstrated a greater reduction in serum calcium levels with pamidronate, although there was no difference in the duration of response or rate of hypercalcemic symptom resolution.[14,15] The time course of the fall in serum calcium is similar to that of etidronate. The higher the level of basal serum calcium, the greater the reduction in serum calcium level after treatment with pamidronate. Pamidronate is administered as a 60- or 90-mg intravenous infusion over 24 hours, depending on the severity of the hypercalcemia. In the United States, pamidronate is available only intravenously. However, in countries where oral pamidronate is available, the intravenous route would still be preferred because patients often experience gastrointestinal intolerance with oral pamidronate. Repeat pamidronate doses should not be given in less than 7 days. Intravenous pamidronate may cause a mild, transient fever, a small reduction in serum phosphate levels, and myalgias in 33% of patients. It should be used with caution in patients with renal dysfunction.

Calcitonin inhibits bone resorption and acutely reduces renal calcium excretion. Synthetic (salmon) and human calcitonin are available in the United States; most experience is with the more potent and longer-acting salmon calcitonin. Calcitonin has the most rapid onset of action among the available hypocalcemic agents but rarely produces normocalcemia. Calcium levels decrease rapidly within 2 to 4 hours after administration of 4 IU/kg subcutaneously or intramuscularly every 12 hours. Dosages can be increased to 8 IU/kg every 6 hours if the lower dosage is ineffective. The maximal calcium-lowering effect occurs within 12 to 24 hours of administration, but this effect often is followed by a return to the initial hypercalcemic level within 24 to 72 hours despite continued administration. Calcitonin is less potent than bisphosphonates and plicamycin, with serum calcium lowering rarely exceeding 2 mg /dL. Except in patients with mild hypercalcemia, normocalcemia rarely is achieved with calcitonin alone. Combination therapy of a bisphosphonate and calcitonin produces a more rapid fall in serum calcium levels than with a bisphosphonate alone, and this combination is especially useful in patients with severe hypercalcemia who need a rapid but sustained fall in serum calcium levels. Before this combination was developed, glucocorticoids were used with calcitonin but were not very effective in sustaining low serum calcium levels. Calcitonin is well tolerated; flushing and mild, transient nausea and abdominal cramps are the most common side effects. Because of its potential for anaphylactoid

Table 18.3 ▪ Treatment of Hypercalcemia

Method	Mechanism of Action	Dosage	Onset of Calcium-Lowering Effect	Maximal Effect	Adverse Effects	Comments
Hydration with saline, replacement of depleted electrolytes	Increases calcium excretion	100–150 mL/hr IV saline	Hours	Decreases serum calcium by 1–2 mg/dL	Volume overload	Cautious administration in patients with congestive heart failure, renal failure; careful fluid and electrolyte monitoring crucial
Hydration with saline and loop diuretic	Increases calcium excretion	Furosemide 10–20 mg IV q6–12hr	Within 4 hr	Decreases by 1–3 mg/dL	Volume depletion, serum calcium hypokalemia, hypomagnesemia	Avoid in dehydration; avoid thiazides, which decrease calcium excretion
Forced diuresis with saline	Increases calcium excretion	150–250 mL/hr IV saline plus furosemide 80–100 mg IV q1–2 hr	Hours	Decreases serum calcium by 2–4 mg/dL	Volume depletion hypokalemia, hypomagnesemia	Central venous pressure monitoring of fluid status and bladder catheterization needed; continuous electrolyte repletion crucial
Calcitonin	Inhibits bone resorption	4 IU/kg SC or IM q12hr; maximum of 8 IU/kg q6hr	2–4 hr	12–24 hr; decreases serum calcium by 1–2 mg/dL	Hypersensitivity reactions, nausea, abdominal cramps, flushing	Rapid rebound in hypercalcemia within 24–72 hr; combination with a bisphosphonate sustains calcium-lowering effect
Etidronate disodium	Inhibits bone resorption	7.5 mg/kg/day IV QD for 3 days	24–48 hr	7 days	Hyperphosphatemia, diarrhea, nausea, ↑ serum creatinine	Indicated for Paget's disease and hypercalcemia of malignancy; infuse over minimum of 2 hr; use with caution in renal dysfunction; do not repeat dose less than 7 days after initial course; for chronic maintenance therapy, may follow IV course with etidronate 20 mg/kg/day PO for 30–90 days

Pamidronate disodium	Inhibits bone resorption	60–90 mg IV over 24 hr	24–48 hr	7 days	Fever, myalgias, hypophosphatemia	Indicated for Paget's disease and hypercalcemia of malignancy; do not repeat dose earlier than 7 days after initial dose; use with caution in renal dysfunction
Plicamycin	Inhibits bone resorption	25 μg/kg IV every 2–4 days for 3 or 4 doses; 12.5 μg/kg if preexisting renal or hepatic dysfunction	24–48 hr	2–4 days	Nausea, vomiting, ↓ platelets, hemorrhage, hepatotoxicity, nephrotoxicity	Toxicity increases with dosages > 30 μg/kg or with consecutive doses; avoid in patients with coagulation disorders or bone marrow suppression; use lower dosage in patients with renal or hepatic disease; infuse in 1 L fluid over 4–6 hr to reduce gastrointestinal toxicity; observe extravasation precautions
Estrogens, progestins	Inhibits bone resorption	Ethinyl estradiol 30–50 μg PO QD	3 wk	2 mo; decreases serum calcium by 1 mg/dL Premarin 0.625–2.5 mg PO QD Norethindrone 5 mg PO QD	Risks of estrogen/progestin therapy	Effective in postmenopausal women with mild hyperparathyroidism
Dialysis	Removes calcium	Hemodialysis or peritoneal dialysis (using calcium-free dialysis fluid)	Immediately	24–48 hr; decreases serum calcium by 3–12 mg/dL	Complications of dialysis	Temporary hypocalcemic effect, with the calcium rebounding rapidly after cessation of dialysis; monitor and supplement serum phosphate levels if necessary

reactions, the manufacturer recommends initial skin testing with 1 IU/0.1 mL intracutaneously, especially in atopic patients or those with a history of hypersensitivity to calcitonin. However, true allergic reactions are rare and treatment should not be withheld while awaiting skin test results.

Gallium nitrate is a potent inhibitor of bone resorption and is approved for the treatment of hypercalcemia associated with malignancy. However, it is no longer manufactured in the United States. Gallium nitrate does not affect bone mineralization. Gallium nitrate 200 mg/m^2 as a continuous intravenous infusion daily for 5 days has been shown to be more effective than salmon calcitonin 8 IU/kg subcutaneously every 6 hours for 5 days[16] in achieving normocalcemia in patients with hypercalcemia of malignancy, and for longer duration (6 days versus 1 day). Gallium nitrate is administered as a 200-mg/m^2 24-hour infusion for 5 consecutive days. Patients with mild hypercalcemia may be given 100 mg/m^2 for 5 days. Onset of effect is in 24 to 48 hours after the first dose, with the maximum response observed within 7 to 10 days. The major adverse effect associated with gallium nitrate is nephrotoxicity. It should be avoided in patients with a serum creatinine above 221 μmol/L (2.5 mg/dL) or if concomitant nephrotoxic drugs such as aminoglycosides or amphotericin B are given. Patients should be well hydrated, and serum creatinine and blood urea nitrogen concentrations should be monitored. Other side effects include hypophosphatemia, hypocalcemia, and anemia (in high dosages).

Plicamycin (mithramycin), an antitumor antibiotic that inhibits bone resorption, is the oldest and least expensive agent for producing a prolonged antihypercalcemic effect. However, because of its high potential for toxicity and the current availability of effective, better-tolerated agents, plicamycin generally is reserved for patients who are intolerant to bisphosphonates or in whom they are ineffective. Serum calcium concentrations begin to fall 6 hours after a single intravenous dose of 25 μg/kg over 4 hours. Because maximum reductions in calcium levels might not occur for 2 to 4 days, it is advisable to wait at least 48 hours before administering additional doses to avoid hypocalcemia. Repeated doses (3 or 4) might be necessary. The duration of action is highly variable, ranging from 5 to 15 days. Reduced dosages of 12.5 μg/kg/day can be tried in patients with preexisting hepatic or renal dysfunction. Nausea is a common side effect and can be minimized by slow intravenous infusion. Care should be used to prevent local extravasation of plicamycin. Plicamycin can also cause hepatotoxicity, with serum aminotransferase elevation in 20% of patients, nephrotoxicity (increased serum creatinine and blood urea nitrogen concentration, and proteinuria), and thrombocytopenia. These adverse effects are more likely with repeated administration. Plicamycin is contraindicated in patients with hepatic or renal dysfunction, bone marrow suppression, or coagulation disorders.

Chronic oral administration of estrogens (e.g., conjugated estrogens 0.625 to 2.5 mg daily, ethinyl estradiol 30 to 50 μg daily) and progestins with androgenic properties (e.g., norethindrone 5 mg daily) have been shown in numerous studies to reduce serum calcium levels and calciuria and to decrease bone turnover in postmenopausal women with primary hyperparathyroidism.[17,18] Estrogens and progestins block PTH-mediated bone resorption without affecting circulating PTH levels. Normalization of serum calcium levels is more likely with estrogens than with progestins; therefore, estrogens are the agents of choice unless contraindications exist. Contraindications to estrogen therapy include a history of thromboembolic disorders, thrombophlebitis, liver disease, abnormal genital bleeding, and pregnancy. The serum calcium reductions are variable and modest; some women do not respond, and the decline in others might be less than 0.25 mmol/L (1 mg/dL). Nevertheless, estrogens can control hypercalcemia and hypercalciuria in more than half of postmenopausal women with hyperparathyroidism and have beneficial effects on osteoporosis and cardiovascular risk factors.

Intravenous or oral sodium and potassium phosphate are no longer used in the management of hypercalcemia.

Dialysis should be considered in hypercalcemia complicated by renal failure. Peritoneal dialysis and hemodialysis with calcium-free dialysis fluid are equally effective in rapidly removing large quantities of calcium from the blood. Serum calcium levels might be reduced by 0.7 to 3 mmol/L (3 to 12 mg/dL) over 24 to 48 hours. Because phosphate is also removed in dialysis, serum phosphate levels should be monitored after dialysis and supplemented if necessary.

Corticosteroids are not recommended for treating hypercalcemia from primary hyperparathyroidism because of the poor response,[19] although they may be effective in hypercalcemia of malignancy.

Nonpharmacologic Therapy

Supportive therapeutic measures for patients with hyperparathyroidism should include moderate restriction of dietary calcium intake. Severe calcium restriction may predispose the patient to bone loss over the long term. Prolonged bed rest should be avoided because immobilization can cause hypercalciuria and hypercalcemia through increased bone resorption and decreased bone formation.

FUTURE THERAPIES

There are no current alternatives to surgery in reducing both PTH secretion and serum calcium levels. However, new calcimimetic drugs are being investigated in clinical trials, prompted by the discovery of a calcium-sensing receptor on parathyroid cells that regulates PTH synthesis and secretion. When activated by increasing extracellular calcium, the calcium-sensing receptor signals the cell to raise the intracellular calcium concentration, thereby inhibiting PTH secretion. R-568 is a compound that mimics the effect of extracellular calcium on parathyroid tissue, and it reduces both PTH levels and serum calcium concentrations in postmenopausal women with primary hyperparathyroidism.[20] This agent may provide a medical alternative to parathyroid surgery.

IMPROVING OUTCOMES

In selecting an appropriate approach to managing hypercalcemia secondary to hyperparathyroidism, a patient's serum calcium level and clinical status must be assessed (Fig. 18.1). All patients with a serum calcium level 3 mmol/L (12 mg/dL) or higher should be hydrated immediately with intravenous saline. If both the clinical symptoms and hypercalcemia are mild (serum calcium 2.6 to 2.9 mmol/L [10.5 to 11.9 mg/dL), hydration alone often is sufficient, without the addition of drug therapy. In moderate hypercalcemia (serum calcium 3 to 3.5 mmol/L [12 to 14 mg/dL]), hydration with saline should be followed by a saline diuresis, with or without the addition of furosemide, depending on the patient's fluid status. If subsequent serum calcium levels remain above 3 mmol/L (12 mg/dL), pamidronate should be initiated. If the hypercalcemia is severe (serum calcium greater than 3.5 mmol/L, or 14 mg/dL) or the patient is severely symptomatic, a rapidly acting agent, calcitonin, should be administered along with hydration. Concurrently, pamidronate, a slower agent, should be initiated to provide a longer-lasting effect. If the patient does not respond or cannot tolerate pamidronate, plicamycin can be considered if there are no contraindications such as renal or hepatic dysfunction, thrombocytopenia, or coagulopathy. If the patient has marked hypercalcemia, but a less urgent reduction in serum calcium is appropriate (e.g., serum calcium is greater

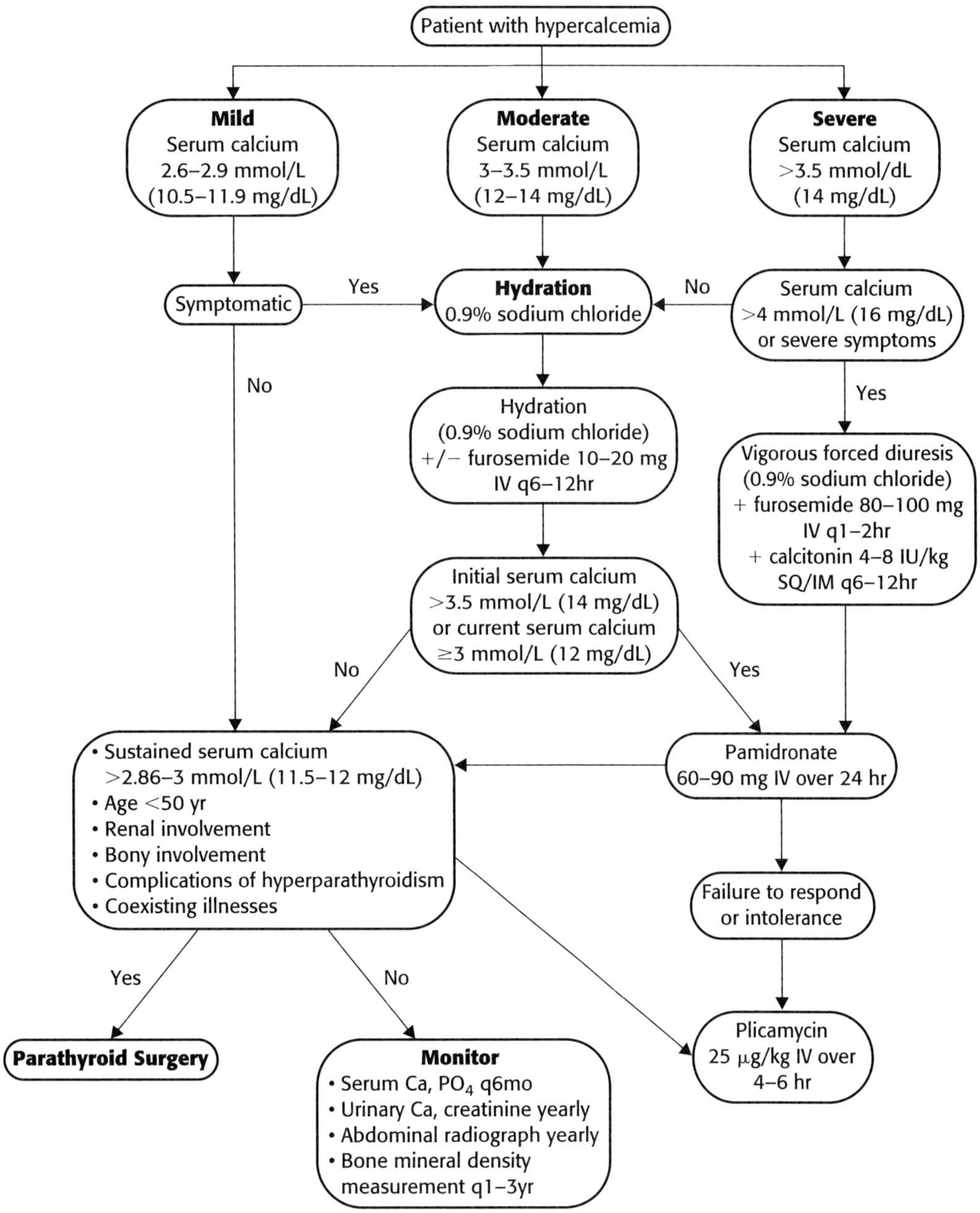

Figure 18.1. Algorithm for the management of hypercalcemia secondary to hyperparathyroidism.

than 3.5 mmol/L, or 14 mg/dL, with mild to moderate symptoms), pamidronate might be started with saline (with or without furosemide) rather than calcitonin. Postmenopausal women should be considered for chronic estrogen therapy if there are no contraindications. To minimize the risk of endometrial hyperplasia with unopposed estrogen therapy, women with an intact uterus should receive cyclic progestin therapy or start a daily low-dose progestin regimen. Parathyroid surgery is absolutely indicated in patients with sustained serum calcium levels below 3 mmol/L (12 mg/dL), renal or bony involvement, complications from hyperparathyroidism, or a coexisting illness that may be exacerbated by hypercalcemia. Surgery should also be considered in all patients under 50 years of age, regardless of symptoms, or in patients who are unlikely to return for regular follow-up monitoring.

Patient Education

Patients with asymptomatic, mild hyperparathyroidism under medical observation must be willing to follow up with a clinician at least every 6 months. Patients who do not follow up consistently should be considered for parathyroid surgery.

Methods to Improve Patient Adherence to Drug Therapy

Treatment for acute hypercalcemia caused by primary hyperparathyroidism usually necessitates hospitalization. However, a 24-hour intravenous infusion of pamidronate instead of a 3-day regimen with intravenous etidronate may enable the patient to be discharged earlier. In addition, any further courses of pamidronate may be administered as a home infusion, reducing patient anxiety about a prolonged hospital admission or treatment course.

PHARMACOECONOMICS

Saline hydration with or without a loop diuretic is an effective and inexpensive way to lower serum calcium. Calcitonin lowers serum calcium more rapidly but at a higher cost, and it should be reserved for symptomatic patients or patients with markedly elevated serum calcium levels who need a rapid reduction. In addition, calcitonin does not sustain calcium-lowering effects beyond 72 hours. A single dose of pamidronate 60 or 90 mg intravenously is considerably less expensive than a 3-day course of intravenous etidronate.[21] In addition, hospitalization and nursing time are reduced with pamidronate treatment. Pamidronate administered by a home infusion pharmacist or nurse may also prevent hospitalization. Because pamidronate is also slightly more effective in lowering serum calcium levels than etidronate and can be given as a single dose instead of over several days, it is the preferred bisphosphonate for treating hypercalcemia. Plicamycin is much less expensive than pamidronate, but its high potential for toxicity limits its use to patients who do not respond to or cannot tolerate bisphosphonates.

Hypoparathyroidism

DEFINITION

Hypoparathyroidism is an endocrine disorder characterized by decreased secretion or peripheral action of PTH, resulting in hypocalcemia and hyperphosphatemia.

TREATMENT GOALS: HYPOPARATHYROIDISM

- Increase serum calcium levels.
- Reverse signs and symptoms of hypocalcemia.
- Prevent complications resulting from hypocalcemia.
- Prevent vitamin D toxicity.

EPIDEMIOLOGY

The most common cause of hypoparathyroidism is surgical excision or exploration of the anterior neck. In experienced surgical hands, the risk of permanent hypoparathyroidism is less than 1% for all thyroid and parathyroid surgeries.[22,23] This risk increases significantly after subtotal parathyroidectomy for parathyroid hyperplasia (multiple-gland involvement) or after repeated neck surgery for recurrent disease.

Table 18.4 outlines other possible causes of hypocalcemia. Rare causes include idiopathic hypoparathyroidism, neonatal hypoparathyroidism, destruction of the parathyroid glands by radiation or metastatic disease, inactive PTH, and target organ resistance to PTH (pseudohypoparathyroidism). Nonparathyroid causes of hypocalcemia include functional hypoparathyroidism resulting from severe hypomagnesemia. Because magnesium is needed for normal release of PTH and for the action of PTH peripherally, hypocalcemia might persist until the hypomagnesemia is corrected. Some causes of hypomagnesemia include starvation, prolonged intravenous feeding, malabsorption, chronic alcoholism, diuretics, aminoglycosides, and *cis*-platinum therapy. Malabsorption and chronic pancreatitis can significantly reduce intestinal calcium and fat-soluble vitamin absorption, especially of vitamin D.

Table 18.4 • Causes of Hypocalcemia

Hypoparathyroidism
Surgical: thyroidectomy, parathyroidectomy, neck exploration
Idiopathic
Neonatal
Destruction of parathyroids (tumor, radiation)
Pseudohypoparathyroidism (end-organ resistance to parathyroid hormone)
Inactive parathyroid hormone
Magnesium deficiency (functional hypoparathyroidism)
Acute pancreatitis or malabsorption
Renal failure (secondary hypoparathyroidism)
Osteomalacia
Drugs: phenytoin, phenobarbital, cholestyramine; laxative abuse with phosphate enemas; aminoglycoside nephrotoxicity
Hyperphosphatemic states: rhabdomyolysis, chemotherapy (causing cell lysis), malignant hyperthermia
Vitamin D deficiency
Parenteral nutrition

The long-term use of anticonvulsants such as phenytoin, phenobarbital, and structurally related compounds increases the hepatic conversion of vitamin D_3 (cholecalciferol) and 25-OH-D_3 (25-hydroxycholecalciferol) to biologically inactive metabolites, causing decreased concentrations of 25-OH-D_3, malabsorption of calcium, hypocalcemia, and osteomalacia. This risk is greater in patients on long-term combination anticonvulsant therapy, with low dietary calcium intake, with little sunlight exposure, and with diseases predisposing to vitamin D malabsorption, and in blacks because of their greater resistance to the irradiating effects of sunlight. Changes in serum calcium, alkaline phosphatase and phosphate levels, and the bony changes of osteomalacia should be monitored closely in these patients.

Another iatrogenic cause of hypocalcemia and osteomalacia is long-term administration of cholestyramine, which binds the bile acids necessary for vitamin D absorption from the intestine. Therapy with higher dosages of vitamin D is necessary to overcome the gut inhibitory effects of cholestyramine on vitamin D absorption.

PATHOPHYSIOLOGY

Deficiency of PTH hormone decreases bone resorption, causes hyperphosphatemia and hypophosphaturia, decreases intestinal absorption of calcium, decreases levels of active 1,25-$(OH)_2$-vitamin D, causes hypocalcemia and hypercalciuria, and causes metabolic alkalosis resulting from decreased bicarbonate excretion.

CLINICAL PRESENTATION AND DIAGNOSIS

Signs and Symptoms

The clinical manifestations of hypoparathyroidism are related to the severity and chronicity of hypocalcemia. Abrupt declines in serum calcium level (e.g., within the first 48 hours after parathyroidectomy) are much more likely to produce hypocalcemic symptoms than gradual reductions of calcium levels. Changes in acid-base status also affect the symptoms. Metabolic alkalosis worsens the hypocalcemia by increasing the plasma protein binding of calcium and decreasing the free ionized fraction. Conversely, acidosis improves the hypocalcemia by increasing the free, active, ionized calcium levels. The signs and symptoms of hypocalcemia and hypoparathyroidism are presented in Table 18.5.

Diagnosis

Hypoparathyroidism should be suspected in the presence of hypocalcemia, hyperphosphatemia, low or undetectable levels of PTH, and a history of neck surgery. However, serum phosphate concentrations might not always be elevated because of dietary restrictions, use of aluminum-containing phosphate binders, or increased mineral uptake by bone. Normal or elevated PTH levels with hypocalcemia excludes the diagnosis of true hypoparathyroidism and strongly suggests end-organ resistance to PTH (pseudohypoparathyroidism) or secretion of inactive PTH hormone. Serum magnesium levels should be checked to exclude the diagnosis of functional hypoparathyroidism. Other causes of hypocalcemia, including drugs, should be excluded (Table 18.4).

THERAPEUTIC PLAN

Theoretically, the most appropriate therapy for hypoparathyroidism is PTH. However, no suitable oral preparation is available. An effective alternative to PTH therapy is high dosages of calcium supplements and vitamin D to increase intestinal calcium absorption.

TREATMENT

Pharmacotherapy

A daily intake of 1 to 2 g elemental calcium in three or four divided doses usually is sufficient to maintain calcium homeostasis in patients with mild hypoparathyroidism. Symptomatic patients with serum calcium levels below 1.87 mmol/L (7.5 mg/dL) often need concomitant therapy with vitamin D to maintain eucalcemia. Therapy directed at reducing serum phosphorus levels generally is not necessary because normalization of serum calcium levels reduces the renal threshold for phosphorus excretion and lowers serum phosphorus concentrations. However, if serum calcium levels remain low with high serum phosphorus concentrations after a few weeks of calcium supplementation, a phosphate binder such as aluminum hydroxide gel should be added to bind and prevent absorption of dietary phosphorus, and a moderately restricted phosphorus diet should be initiated to allow increased calcium absorption.

If dietary intake is inadequate, effective calcium supplementation can be provided through various calcium-

Table 18.5 ▪ Clinical Features of Hypocalcemia and Hypoparathyroidism

System	Signs and Symptoms	Complications	Comments
Musculoskeletal	Circumoral and distal numbness and tingling, muscle twitching, hyperreflexia, positive Chvostek's and Trousseau's signs	Tetany: carpopedal spasms, laryngeal stridor, convulsions	Emergency treatment with intravenous calcium needed
Neurologic	Papilledema, increased cerebrospinal fluid pressure, basal ganglia calcifications, extrapyramidal symptoms, abnormal electroencephalogram	Epilepsy, parkinsonism; complication in 20% of patients with hypoparathyroidism	Improves with eucalcemia, increased sensitivity to dystonic reactions with phenothiazines
Psychiatric	Irritability, paranoia	Depression, psychosis, mental retardation in 20% of children	May improve with eucalcemia
Integument	Dry, scaly skin, coarse, friable dry hair, longitudinal nail ridges	Exfoliative dermatitis, atopic eczema, psoriasis, candida infection	May improve with eucalcemia
Ocular	Visual impairment and lens opacities	Lenticular cataracts most common sequelae of hypoparathyroidism	Eucalcemia halts progression of cataracts
Cardiac	Symptoms of heart failure, irregular rhythm, ↑ Q-T interval, T-wave peaks, and inversions	Cardiac dilation	Improves with eucalcemia
Others	Impaired dental development, intestinal malabsorption with steatorrhea		Improves with eucalcemia
Laboratory results	Increased creatine phosphokinase, lactate dehydrogenase, ↓ calcium, ↑ phosphate, urinary phosphate low, urinary calcium low to absent, parathyroid hormone low		

containing salts. Calcium gluconate, containing small amounts of calcium, is not very palatable because a large number of tablets must be administered to attain a therapeutic dosage. Similarly, calcium chloride is most likely to cause gastric irritation. Calcium carbonate usually is preferred because it is well tolerated, fewer tablets are needed, and it is more effective than supplements containing small amounts of calcium (gluconate, lactate). Calcium must be in a soluble, ionized form in the intestine for absorption to occur. Ionization of calcium occurs in an acidic intestinal pH. Conversely, alkaline intestinal pH retards calcium absorption. Therefore, calcium carbonate is poorly absorbed in patients with achlorhydria, such as older adults, and should be administered with food in this population to facilitate absorption.[24] Calcium absorption is also poor in patients with renal osteodystrophy, steatorrhea, or uremia.

The following salts provide 1 g calcium:

Calcium carbonate	2.5 g (40% calcium)
Tricalcium phosphate	2.6 g (39% calcium)
Calcium chloride	3.7 g (27% calcium)
Calcium acetate	4.0 g (25% calcium)
Calcium citrate	4.75 g (21% calcium)
Calcium lactate	7.7 g (13% calcium)
Calcium gluconate	11.0 g (9% calcium)

Constipation is a potential problem with all calcium supplements and should be managed.

Vitamin D should be started for hypocalcemic symptoms as soon as possible. The general term *vitamin D* refers to any form of vitamin D. Vitamin D metabolism is depicted in Figure 18.2. Vitamin D_3 (cholecalciferol) is produced in the skin after ultraviolet sunlight exposure. Provitamin D_2 (ergosterol) is absorbed from the distal ileum from dietary sources and undergoes metabolism by ultraviolet sunlight exposure to ergocalciferol (vitamin D_2). The active form of vitamin D is 1,25-dihydroxyvitamin D, or 1,25-$(OH)_2$-D, which is activated in the kidney by the 1-α-hydroxylase enzyme after hepatic 25-hydroxylation; 1,25-$(OH)_2$-D_2 and 1,25-$(OH)_2$-D_3 are equally active. The selection of an appropriate vitamin D preparation depends on the cause of the hypocalcemia, onset of action, metabolism, duration of toxicity after discontinuation, and cost (Table 18.6).[25,26] The 1-hydroxylated forms of vitamin D are more potent and act more quickly because hepatic conversion to the active form is unnecessary. Serum calcium levels may increase from 1.5 mmol/L (6 mg/dL) up to 2.2 mmol/L (8.8 mg/dL) within a few days, rather than a few weeks for vitamin D_2 or vitamin D_3. In addition, serum calcium levels decrease more rapidly on discontinuation of 1-hydroxylated compounds, an advantage in the case of inadvertent overdose. However, the effects of vitamin D_2 or D_3 may take several weeks to months to disappear because they are stored in body fat and released slowly.

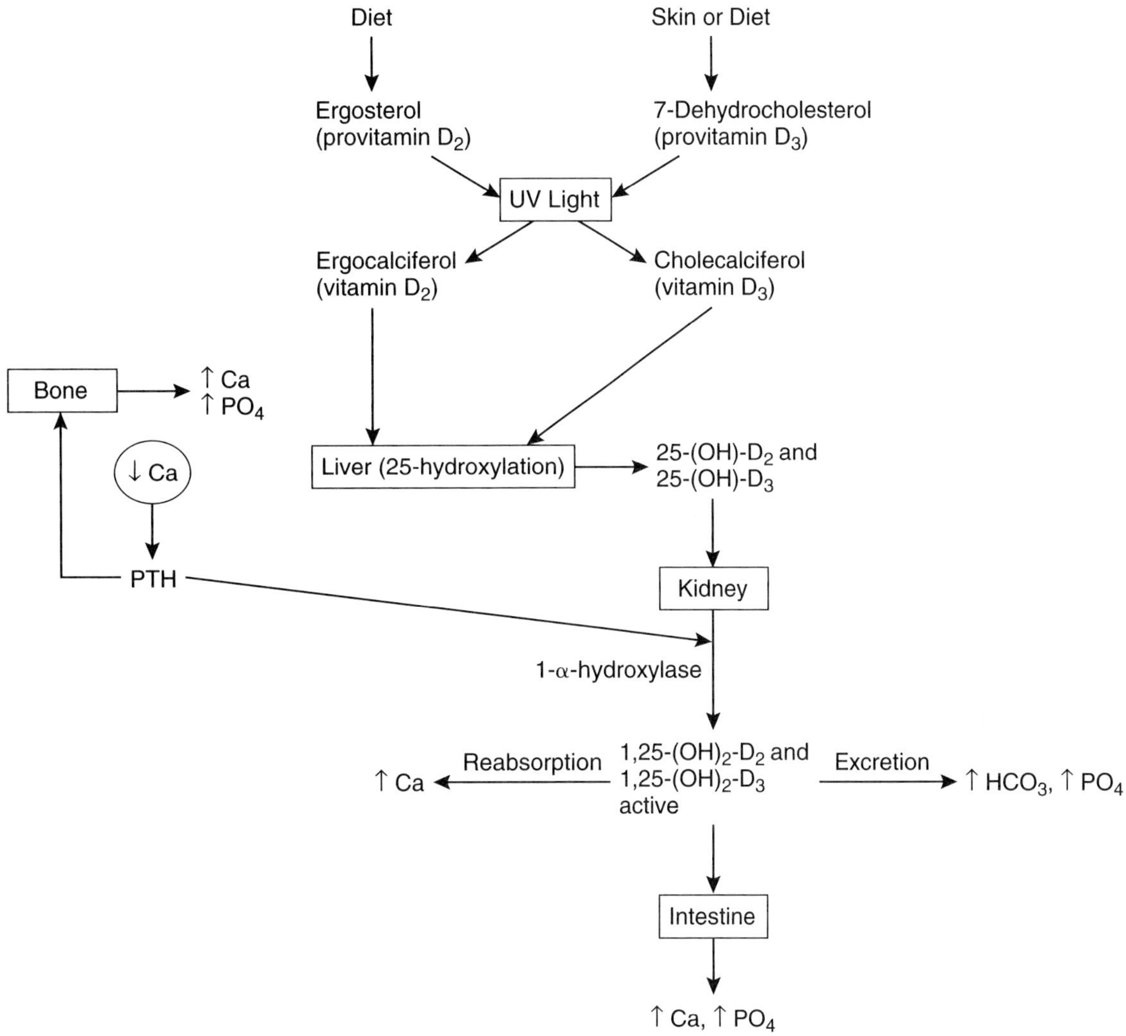

Figure 18.2. Relationship and metabolism of vitamin D to PTH and calcium.

Vitamin D products should not be interchanged without careful monitoring and consideration.[27] In addition, considerable confusion occurs about dosage equivalence because some preparations are dosed in international units, whereas others are dosed in weight (milligrams or micrograms); 1 mg vitamin D_2 (ergocalciferol) is equal to 40,000 IU.[25]

Vitamin D_2 is commonly used in patients with long-standing hypoparathyroidism because it is the least expensive of all the preparations. Vitamin D_2 therapy can be initiated with 50,000 IU/day and then gradually increased to maintenance dosages of 50,000 to 200,000 IU/day after steady-state serum calcium levels are achieved at each dosage level. Maximal effects on serum calcium usually are achieved in 4 to 6 weeks but can take up to 12 weeks. Because of its slow onset of effect, dosage titration must be gradual. Dihydrotachysterol (DHT) or calcitriol might be preferred in patients with newly diagnosed hypoparathyroidism. The initial dosage of DHT is 0.8 to 2.4 mg daily for several days, then a maintenance dosage of 0.2 to 1 mg daily. To shorten the time to maximal action, DHT is occasionally initiated with a loading dosage of four times the daily maintenance dosage for 2 days, followed by two times the daily maintenance dosage for 2 days. However, such an approach increases the risk of toxicity and must be monitored carefully. Calcitriol may be dosed initially at 0.25 to 0.5 μg once or twice daily. Serum calcium levels may be measured every 1 to 2 days if rapid stabilization is needed, with dosage adjustment every 2 to 3 days. Stabilization to a lower maintenance dosage is possible within 1 month. Calcitriol exerts its action more rapidly than vitamin D_2, DHT, or calcifediol (25-OH-D_3) because it bypasses renal as well as hepatic hydroxylation. Patients with widely fluctuating serum calcium levels because of medication noncompliance may be better treated with a longer-acting vitamin D_2 or D_3 product.

Because PTH and hypophosphatemia stimulate activity of renal 1-α-hydroxylase enzyme, a suitable vitamin D preparation in patients with hyperparathyroidism would already contain the 1-α-hydroxyl group (i.e., DHT or calcitriol). DHT still must undergo 25-hydroxylation by the liver, and therefore should be avoided in hepatic disease.

Table 18.6 ▪ Comparison of Vitamin D Preparations

Preparation	Abbreviation	Brand Name	Dosage	Characteristics	Activity	Comments
Calciferol Ergocalciferol Capsules 50,000 IU Tablets 50,000 IU Liquid 8,000 IU/mL Injection 500,000 IU/mL	Vitamin D_2	Calciferol, Drisdol, Deltalin	Initial: 50,000 IU/day Maintenance: 50,000–200,000 IU/day 1 mg = 40,000 IU 3 mg = 120,000 IU	Restores normocalcemia in 4–8 wk; maximal effects in 4–12 wk; long $t_{1/2}$; slow elimination; persists 6–18 wk after cessation	Biologically inactive; requires activation by hepatic 25-hydroxylation and renal 1-α-hydroxylase	Least expensive; bile salts needed for complete absorption in gut; short shelf-life
Dihydrotachysterol Tablets/capsules 125 µg Tablets 200 µg 400 µg Solution 0.2 mg/mL 0.25 mg/mL	DHT	Hytakerol	Initial: 0.8–2.4 mg/day Maintenance: 0.2–1 mg/day	Restores normocalcemia in 1–2 wk; maximal effect in 1–2 wk; persists 1–3 wk after cessation	Requires only hepatic 25-hydroxylation for activation; contains 1α-hydroxyl group so no kidney activation necessary	Three times more potent than vitamin D_2; main action is to increase intestinal calcium absorption; calcium supplementation recommended; more effective in chronic renal failure and hypoparathyroidism than vitamin D_2
Calcifediol (25-hydroxycholecalciferol) Capsules 20 µg 50 µg	25-(OH)-D_3	Calderol	Initial: 50 µg/day Maintenance: 50–100 µg/day	Restores normocalcemia in 2–4 wk; persists 4–12 wk after cessation	Requires kidney for bioactivation	1.5 times as potent as vitamin D_2; preparation of choice in intestinal malabsorption and hepatobiliary disease; also effective in renal osteodystrophy; therapeutic blood level monitoring available
Calcitriol (1,25-dihydroxyvitamin D_3) Capsules 0.25 µg 0.5 µg Injection 1 µg/mL 2 µg/mL	1,25-$(OH)_2$-D_3	Rocaltrol, Calcijex	Initial: 0.25 µg/day Maintenance: 0.5–2 µg/day	Restores normocalcemia in 3–7 days; $t_{1/2}$ 2–3 hr; persists 3–7 days after cessation	Active	Most potent and most expensive preparation available; requires calcium supplementation in hypoparathyroidism; major advantage is rapid onset and long duration of effect
Paricalcitol Injection 5 µg/mL	19-nor-1,25-$(OH)_2$-D_2	Zemplar	Initial: 0.04–0.1 µg/kg IV bolus 3 × /week (maximum 0.24µg/kg) during hemodialysis	$t_{1/2}$ 15 hr in chronic renal failure requiring hemodialysis; dosage may be increased q2–4wk	Active	Approved for prevention and treatment of secondary hypoparathyroidism associated with chronic renal failure; monitor serum calcium and phosphate levels monthly and parathyroid hormone levels q3mo

Conversely, patients with renal osteodystrophy or hypocalcemia secondary to chronic renal disease may have more predictable results with calcitriol or DHT. A new synthetic vitamin D analog, paricalcitol (19-nor-1-α-25-$[OH]_2$-D_2), contains both the 1-α-hydroxyl group and 25-hydroxyl group and has been approved for treating hyperparathyroidism secondary to chronic renal failure. Paricalcitol may be less likely to result in hypercalcemic and hyperphosphatemic complications than calcitriol in patients on chronic hemodialysis while effectively reducing PTH serum levels. It is available as an intravenous injection only and is administered on days of hemodialysis.

Antiseizure medications such as phenytoin and phenobarbital induce hepatic enzymes, resulting in decreased plasma concentrations of 25-hydroxylated ergocalciferol and cholecalciferol. If DHT or ergocalciferol is administered, higher dosages may be needed. However, any change in antiseizure medication may also necessitate a change in the vitamin D dosage. Calcifediol (25-$[OH]D_3$), which does not require hepatic hydroxylation, and calcitriol may be more stable choices.

To avoid hypercalcemia, dosages of all vitamin D preparations should be increased gradually and only after maximal effects are achieved. Serum calcium levels should be maintained between 2.12 and 2.25 mmol/L (8.5 and 9 mg/dL), leaving a margin for fluctuations. Serum calcium and phosphorus levels should be checked weekly at initiation of vitamin D therapy, then monthly during dosage adjustments and at least every 3 months thereafter. An abdominal radiograph or ultrasound should be considered before vitamin D therapy is started and should be repeated every few years to check for nephrocalcinosis or stone formation.[27] Patients should be monitored carefully for early signs of vitamin D intoxication, which include lassitude, anorexia, thirst, constipation, and bone pain. Frequent adjustments in vitamin D dosages might be necessary to prevent vitamin D intoxication. Higher dosages of vitamin D are needed for patients on anticonvulsants, oral contraceptives, and glucocorticoids. Estrogens decrease serum calcium by preventing bone resorption. Glucocorticoids reduce intestinal absorption of calcium by antagonizing vitamin D, decrease bone resorption by antagonizing PTH, and reduce renal tubular absorption of calcium. Patients needing massive blood transfusions might need more calcium because the citrate added to each unit of blood for anticoagulation purposes has a very high affinity for calcium.[28]

Toxicities of all vitamin D preparations include hypercalcemia, hypercalciuria, and nephrolithiasis, which can be prevented by close monthly monitoring of serum calcium, phosphorus, and alkaline phosphatase levels. Availability of 25-(OH)-D_3 and 1,25-$(OH)_2$-D_3 assays in more specialized centers might help prevent toxicity from hypercalcemia. Calcitriol has been associated with renal function deterioration in some patients with previously stable renal function. However, prospective, long-term studies have not confirmed these reports.[29]

Thiazide diuretics and sodium restriction have been shown to reduce urinary calcium excretion in patients with mild hypocalcemia, allowing calcium and vitamin D supplementation to be reduced. Serum calcium levels should be monitored carefully. This therapy might also protect against the development of kidney stones, a potential complication of the long-term management of hypoparathyroidism. Long-term studies are necessary to assess the role of this approach. Patients with hypoparathyroidism might be more sensitive to the calciuretic effects of loop diuretics such as furosemide, so they should be avoided.

Acute hypocalcemia complicated by tetany may occur after inadvertent parathyroidectomy during thyroid surgery. Such a situation necessitates emergency treatment with intravenous calcium. After the patient's airway is cleared, 1 mg/kg/hour elemental calcium is administered intravenously until symptoms are relieved or until the serum calcium level increases above 1.87 mmol/L (7.5 mg/dL). Serum calcium levels should be monitored every 6 hours. The plasma calcium level should increase by approximately 0.5 mg/dL/100 mg calcium load per 24 hours. Too vigorous treatment of the tetany can cause irreversible tissue calcifications. Hypomagnesemia should be corrected, and oral calcium and vitamin D supplements should be started immediately. Drugs that exacerbate hypocalcemia (i.e., loop diuretics) should be avoided. Phenothiazines should be used cautiously because dystonic reactions can occur. Also, inadvertent hypercalcemia can precipitate cardiac arrhythmias in patients receiving digoxin, and such patients need ECG monitoring while receiving intravenous calcium therapy.

Transient hypocalcemia commonly occurs after neck exploration, with normocalcemia reestablished within 1 week. Such patients should be given oral calcium supplements and reassessed in a few weeks. Vitamin D therapy may not be necessary at that point.

Nonpharmacologic Therapy

Parathyroid autografts or allografts have been transplanted successfully in a number of patients in whom accidental removal or devascularization of the parathyroid glands has occurred during thyroid or parathyroid surgery. Parathyroid tissue is transplanted into the forearm muscles or the sternomastoid muscles. Such patients need calcium supplementation for 4 weeks and then can be weaned off.[30]

IMPROVING OUTCOMES

Patients with long-standing hypothyroidism may start with the slow-acting vitamin D_2 (ergocalciferol). Patients with newly diagnosed hypoparathyroidism may need DHT or calcitriol for a more rapid response. Close monitoring of serum calcium and phosphate levels is important in ensuring adequate vitamin D dosages and preventing toxicity. The prognosis of hypoparathyroidism is excellent. Improvement of most symptoms can be expected with restoration of normal serum calcium levels. In surgery-associated hypoparathyroidism, vitamin D therapy usually is withdrawn after 6 to 8 weeks of treatment to assess whether the patient can maintain a normocalcemic state. Such an approach minimizes the risk of vitamin D intoxication.

Patient Education

Oral calcium absorption is most efficient with single doses of 500 mg or less, taken on an empty stomach.[27] However, calcium carbonate has reduced bioavailability in achlorhydric patients, such as older adults. Such patients should be instructed to take this preparation with meals. Calcium carbonate may reduce absorption of iron and certain drugs, such as tetracycline and norfloxacin, and should not be administered simultaneously with these products. Calcium citrate does not reduce iron absorption. Fiber does not significantly reduce absorption of calcium, although combination with wheat bran may.[31] Certain preparations of calcium (bone meal and dolomite) can be contaminated by lead and other heavy metals, although most commercial calcium products are tested to ensure that significant heavy metal contamination is not present. Dietary calcium may be an alternative to supplements (250 mL skim or whole milk provides approximately 300 mg elemental calcium). However, patients intolerant to dairy products should use calcium supplements.

Constipation is common in patients receiving calcium supplements. Patients should be instructed to increase their fiber and fluid intake; if necessary, a stool softener or bulk laxative may be added.

Methods to Improve Patient Adherence to Drug Therapy

Calcium carbonate has the highest amount of calcium per tablet. A tablet containing calcium carbonate 500 mg provides 40% elemental calcium, or 200 mg. Tablets containing the highest amounts of elemental calcium should be selected to reduce the number of calcium tablets needed per day. Calcium carbonate preparations generally are well tolerated and preferred over other calcium salts. Although preparations combining calcium with vitamin D are available commercially, the amount vitamin D contained in such supplements generally is too low for treatment of hypoparathyroidism.

PHARMACOECONOMICS

A large number of inexpensive calcium products are available over the counter. Vitamin D preparations are more costly than calcium preparations. Dihydrotachysterol is slightly more expensive than calcitriol or calcifediol. Ergocalciferol is available without a prescription in the United States, but its cost is comparable to calcifediol when administered in high dosages.[21]

In addition to cost, vitamin D selection depends on its onset of action and metabolism, the duration of toxicity after discontinuation, and the cause of the hypocalcemia (Table 18.6).

KEY POINTS

- Hyperparathyroidism results in hypercalcemia and hypophosphatemia.
- Patients often are asymptomatic.
- Parathyroid surgery is indicated for symptomatic hyperparathyroidism.
- Acute management of hypercalcemia is initiated with intravenous hydration.
- Calcitonin has the most rapid calcium-lowering effect, but effects are not sustained beyond 72 hours.
- Bisphosphonates have a slower onset of action but provide sustained decreases in serum calcium for at least 1 week.
- Hypoparathyroidism is caused by decreased secretion of PTH, resulting in hypocalcemia and hyperphosphatemia.
- A common cause of hypoparathyroidism is surgical excision or exploration of the neck.
- Treatment includes increased oral intake of calcium and vitamin D.
- Vitamin D selection depends on the preparation's onset of action, metabolism, duration of toxicity after discontinuation, and cost and the cause of the hypocalcemia.

REFERENCES

1. Melton LJ III. Epidemiology of primary hyperparathyroidism. J Bone Miner Res 6(2):S25–S29, 1991.
2. Heath H III, Hodgson SF, Kennedy MA. Primary hyperparathyroidism: incidence, morbidity and potential economic impact in community. N Engl J Med 302:189–193, 1980.
3. Mundy GR, Cove DH, Flaken R. Primary parathyroidism: changes in the pattern of clinical presentation. Lancet 1:1317–1320, 1980.
4. Stenstrom F, Heedman PA. Clinical findings in patients with hyperparathyroidism. Acta Med Scand 195:473–477, 1974.
5. Consensus Development Conference Panel. Diagnosis and management of asymptomatic primary hyperparathyroidism: Consensus Development Conference statement. Ann Intern Med 114:593–597, 1991.
6. Heath DA, Heath EM. Conservative management of primary hyperparathyroidism. J Bone Miner Res 6(Suppl 2):S117–S120, 1991.
7. Fischer JA. Asymptomatic and symptomatic primary hyperparathyroidism. Clin Invest 71:505–518, 1993.
8. Zahrani AA, Levine MA. Primary hyperparathyroidism. Lancet 349:1233–1238, 1997.
9. Baumann DS, Wells SA. Parathyroid autotransplantation. Surgery 113:130–133, 1993.
10. Bilezikian JP. Management of hypercalcemia. J Clin Endocrinol Metab 77:1445–1449, 1993.
11. Nussbaum SR. Pathophysiology and management of severe hypercalcemia. Endocrinol Metab Clin North Am 22:343–362, 1993.
12. Suki WN, Yium JJ, Von Minden M, et al. Acute treatment of hypercalcemia with furosemide. N Engl J Med 283:836–840, 1970.
13. Hall TG, Schaiff RA. Update on the medical management of hypercalcemia of malignancy. Clin Pharm 12:117–125, 1993.
14. Ralston SH, Gallacher SJ, Patel U, et al. Comparison of three intravenous bisphosphonates in cancer-associated hypercalcemia. Lancet 2:1180–1182, 1989.
15. Gucalp R, Ritch P, Wiernik PH, et al. Comparative study of pamidronate disodium in the treatment of cancer-related hypercalcemia. J Clin Oncol 10:134–142, 1992.

16. Warrell RP Jr, Israel R, Frisone M, et al. Gallium nitrate for acute treatment of cancer-related hypercalcemia: a randomized, double-blind comparison to calcitonin. Ann Intern Med 108:669–674, 1988.
17. Wishart J, Horowitz M, Need AG, et al. Treatment of postmenopausal hyperparathyroidism with norethindrone. Long term effects on forearm mineral content. Arch Intern Med 150:1951–1953, 1990.
18. Marcus R. Estrogens and progestins in the management of primary hyperparathyroidism. J Bone Miner Res 6(Suppl 2):S1–S165, 1991.
19. Schaiff RA, Hall TG, Bar RS. Medical treatment of hypercalcemia. Clin Pharm 8:108–121, 1989.
20. Silverberg SJ, Bone III HG, Marriott TB, et al. Short-term inhibition of parathyroid hormone secretion by a calcium-receptor agonist in patients with primary hyperparathyroidism. N Engl J Med 337:1506–1510, 1997.
21. Drug topics red book. Montvale, NJ: Medical Economics Company, 1998.
22. Weber CA, Clark OH. Surgery for thyroid disease. Med Clin North Am 69:1097–1115, 1985.
23. Clark OH, Duh QY. Primary hyperparathyroidism. A surgical perspective. Endocrinol Metab Clin North Am 18:701–713, 1989.
24. Recker RR. Calcium absorption and achlorhydria. N Engl J Med 313:70–73, 1985.
25. Kumar R, Riggs BL. Series on pharmacology in practice. 11. Vitamin D in the therapy of disorders of calcium and phosphorus metabolism. Mayo Clin Proc 56:327–333, 1981.
26. Haussler MR, Cordy PE. Metabolites and analogues of vitamin D. Which for what? JAMA 247:841–844, 1982.
27. O'Riordan JLH. Treatment of hypoparathyroidism. In: Bilezikian JP, et al. The parathyroids. Basic and clinical concepts. New York: Raven, 1994:801–804.
28. Netterville JL, Aly A, Ossoff RH. Evaluation and treatment of complications of thyroid and parathyroid surgery. Otolaryngol Clin North Am 23:529–552, 1990.
29. Halabe A, Arie R, Mimran D, et al. Hypoparathyroidism: a long term experience with 1α-vitamin D_3 therapy. Clin Endocrinol 40:303–307, 1994.
30. Shaha AR, Burnett C, Jaffe BM. Parathyroid autotransplantation during thyroid surgery. J Surg Oncol 46:21–24, 1991.
31. National Institutes of Health Conference Statement. Optimal calcium intake. JAMA 272:1942–1948, 1994.

CHAPTER 19

DIABETES

Stephen M. Setter, John R. White Jr., and R. Keith Campbell

Diabetes mellitus was recognized as early as 1500 B.C. by Egyptian physicians, who described a disease associated with "the passage of much urine." The term *diabetes* (the Greek word for siphon) was coined by Greek physician Aretaeus the Cappadocian around A.D. 2. Aretaeus noticed that patients with diabetes had a disease that caused the siphoning of the structural components of the body into the urine. Although it was known for centuries that the urine of patients with diabetes was sweet, it was not until 1674 that a physician named Willis coined the term *diabetes mellitus* (from the Greek word for honey).

Diabetes mellitus is a complex syndrome that affects multiple organ systems. There is still much to be learned about diabetes mellitus; however, recent pharmacologic and surgical advances have enhanced the understanding and treatment of this syndrome. The landmark Diabetes Control and Complications Trial (DCCT) demonstrated conclusively that the level of glycemic control is closely correlated with the appearance and progression of retinopathy, nephropathy, and neuropathy in patients with type 1 diabetes.[1] The results of the recently completed 20-year United Kingdom Prospective Diabetes Study (UKPDS) confirmed the benefit of strict glycemic control in patients with type 2 diabetes.[2–5] Strict glycemic control is within reach of many patients with diabetes, now that self-monitoring of blood glucose (SMBG) is commonly practiced and better education programs and new treatment protocols are available. The overall treatment goal for all patients with diabetes is to achieve glycemic control to prevent the long-term complications of diabetes. Individual management to achieve this goal varies between patients but generally involves SMBG, nutritional counseling, and training in self-management and problem solving.[6]

A thorough, positive, and empowering education program for the patient with diabetes that covers the disease, medication, monitoring, and hygiene is a major component of diabetes management. Studies have demonstrated that poor diabetes control is often the result of medication error, misinterpretation of test results, and ignorance of the disease.[7] Patient education is extremely important. Health care providers must explain the importance of diet control and the food exchange system. Patients need to develop a positive and proactive attitude, learn how to perform tests to monitor control, learn proper insulin injection technique, and keep records of factors that affect glycemic control. Health care providers need to answer patient questions about the disease, blood testing, drug therapy, diet products, and foot care and reinforce the information that other members of the team provide. The pharmacist is an invaluable asset to the health care team. Because patients with diabetes see pharmacists more often than any other health professional, the pharmacist is in a unique position to have a significant impact on their treatment and quality of life. Pharmacists must become competent in selecting, initiating, and individualizing drug therapy for the various types of diabetes. Thus, the pharmacist performs three significant functions: referral, monitoring, and education.

DEFINITION

Diabetes mellitus is spectrum of conditions that includes hyperglycemia as a common medical finding. Diabetes was once thought of as a single disease, but it is clearly a heterogeneous group of disorders that are secondary to various genetic predispositions and precipitating factors. Not only does type 1 diabetes (insulin-dependent diabetes, IDDM) differ from type 2 diabetes (non–insulin-dependent diabetes, NIDDM), but there appears to be heterogenicity within each of the two types.[8] Diabetes is a chronic disease characterized by disorders in carbohydrate, fat, and protein metabolism caused by an absolute or relative deficiency in the action of insulin and possibly abnormally high amounts of glucagon and other counter-regulatory hormones such as growth hormone, sympathomimetic amines, and corticosteroids. Insulin secretion in patients with type 1 diabetes is normally deficient to nonexistent, whereas those with type 2 disease may have normal, high, or low insulin secretion.

Table 19.1 ▪ Diabetes Mellitus: Etiologic Classification

- I. Type 1 diabetes (β-cell destruction, usually leading to absolute insulin deficiency)
  - A. Immune mediated
  - B. Idiopathic
- II. Type 2 diabetes (accompanied by insulin resistance)
- III. Other specific types
  - A. Genetic defects of β-cell function
    1. Chromosome 12, HNF-1α (formerly maturity-onset diabetes of youth 3)
    2. Others
  - B. Genetic defects in insulin action
    1. Type A insulin resistance
    2. Leprechaunism
    3. Others
  - C. Diseases of the exocrine pancreas
    1. Pancreatitis
    2. Neoplasia
    3. Cystic fibrosis
  - D. Endocrinopathies
    1. Acromegaly
    2. Cushing's syndrome
    3. Pheochromocytoma
    4. Others
  - E. Drug or chemical induced
    1. Nicotinic acid
    2. Glucocorticoids
    3. Thiazides
    4. Others
  - F. Infections
    1. Congenital rubella
    2. Cytomegalovirus
    3. Others
  - G. Uncommon forms of immune-mediated diabetes
    1. Stiff-man syndrome
    2. Anti-insulin receptor antibodies
    3. Others
  - H. Other genetic syndromes sometimes associated with diabetes
    1. Down's syndrome
    2. Klinefelter's syndrome
    3. Turner's syndrome
    4. Others
- IV. Gestational diabetes mellitus

Source: Expert committee on the diagnosis and classification of diabetes mellitus. Report of the expert committee on the diagnosis and classification of diabetes mellitus. Diabetes Care 20:1183–1197, 1997.

HNF, hepatocyte nuclear factor.

Table 19.2 ▪ Diabetes Mellitus: Diagnostic Criteria

Symptoms of diabetes plus casual plasma glucose concentration ≥200 mg/dL (11.1 mmol/L). *Casual* is defined as any time of day without regard to time since last meal. The classic symptoms of diabetes include polyuria, polydipsia, and unexplained weight loss.

or

Fasting plasma glucose ≥126 mg/dL (7.0 mmol/L). *Fasting* is defined as no caloric intake for at least 8 hr.

or

Two-hour plasma glucose ≥200 mg/dL during an oral glucose tolerance test. 75-g glucose load or equivalent is recommended when performing this test.

Source: Expert committee on the diagnosis and classification of diabetes mellitus. Report of the expert committee on the diagnosis and classification of diabetes mellitus. Diabetes Care 20:1183–1197, 1997.

Classifying the patient with diabetes into one of several categories in which hyperglycemia is a clinical finding is critical in developing a patient-specific treatment regimen. In the past many classification schemes were used that often resulted in confusion. Recently an expert panel revised the criteria for diagnosing and classifying diabetes mellitus. Table 19.1 summarizes the new etiologic classification system with the updated terminology, and the new diagnostic criteria for diabetes mellitus are outlined in Table 19.2.

Type 1 diabetes results from immune-mediated destruction of the β-cells of the pancreas, resulting in eventual absolute insulin deficiency. Roughly 5 to 10% of people with diabetes have type 1 disease.[9] Patients with type 1 disease are more likely to develop ketoacidosis than are patients with type 2. Patients with type 2 usually have some degree of insulin resistance with variable insulin secretion. Insulin secretion is said to be relatively deficient because many patients may have normal to elevated levels of insulin; however, their blood sugars remain elevated because of tissue resistance to the action of the insulin. Many patients with type 2 diabetes can survive without insulin; however, up to 40% use insulin sometime during the disease course. Table 19.3 compares the two major clinical types of diabetes.

TREATMENT GOALS: DIABETES

- Because diabetes is an incurable disease, focus on controlling blood sugars in the normal or near normal range and preventing the short- and long-term complications associated with this disease.
- Maintain normal growth and development in children.

- Promote SMBG at least three to four times a day in those with type 1 diabetes and a sufficient number of times daily or weekly to facilitate reaching glucose goals in patients with type 2 diabetes.
- Administer medical nutritional therapy that balances food intake with physical activity and pharmacologic therapies.
- Prevent symptoms of hyperglycemia such as polyuria, blurred vision, weight loss, recurrent infection, ketoacidosis, and hyperosmolar coma and prevent symptoms of hypoglycemia including mood changes, mental confusion, and coma.
- Prevent long-term complications (microvascular and macrovascular disease) by keeping blood glucose levels as close to normal as possible.
- Maintain appropriate blood pressure and lipid values.
- Treat other physiologic derangements when present.
- Provide comprehensive and ongoing education and reevaluate the patient's understanding and ability to control his or her disease.

EPIDEMIOLOGY

Diabetes mellitus is present in roughly 16 million U.S. citizens; however, only half of all people with this disease are diagnosed.[9] Close to 675,000 people have type 1 diabetes, and the majority of those remaining have type 2 disease. Girls experience a peak incidence of type 1 diabetes between 10 and 12 years of age, whereas boys have a higher incidence between 12 and 14 years. Diabetes in people older than 20 accounts for 90 to 95% of all cases.

Table 19.3 ▪ Distinguishing Features of Two Major Types of Diabetes Mellitus

	Type 1	Type 2
Age of onset	Usually but not always during childhood or puberty.	Often over 35.
Type of onset	Abrupt.	Usually gradual.
Prevalence	0.5%.	5–6%.
Incidence	<10–15%.	>75%.
Family history of diabetes	Rarely positive.	Commonly positive.
Primary cause	Pancreatic β-cell deficiency.	Insulin resistance.
Nutritional status at time of onset	Usually undernourished.	Usually obese.
Symptoms	Polydipsia, polyuria, polyphagia.	May be none.
Hepatomegaly	Common.	Uncommon.
Stability	Blood glucose fluctuates widely in response to small changes in insulin dosage, exercise, and infection.	Less marked blood glucose fluctuations.
Cause	Unknown.	Unknown.
Proneness to ketosis	Common, especially if treatment is insufficient.	Uncommon except in presence of unusual stress or sepsis.
Insulin defect	Defect in secretion; secretion is impaired early in disease; secretion may be totally absent late in disease.	*Insulin deficiency:* Most patients show failure of insulin secretion to keep pace with inordinate demands engendered by obesity; may appear initially as failure to respond to glucose alone, suggesting an impairment on the glucoreceptor of the pancreatic β-cell. *Insulin resistance:* Some patients have a defect in tissue responsiveness to insulin and evidence of hyperinsulinemia; in such patients insulin resistance may be mediated by receptor or postreceptor defects.
Plasma insulin (endogenous)	Negligible to zero.	Low, normal, or high.
Vascular complications of diabetes and degenerative changes	Uncommon until diabetes has been present for >5 yr.	Common.
Usual causes of death	Degenerative complications (e.g., renal failure caused by diabetic nephropathy).	Accelerated atherosclerosis (e.g., myocardial infarction); to a lesser extent, microangiopathic changes in target tissues (e.g., renal failure).
Diet	Mandatory in all patients.	If diet is used fully, antidiabetic drug therapy may not be needed.
Insulin	Necessary for all patients.	Necessary for 20–30% of patients.
Oral agents	Rarely efficacious.	Efficacious.

Half of all new cases of diabetes occur in adults over the age of 55, and approximately 11% of the older population (65 to 74 years) has diabetes. Certain ethnic groups have a higher incidence of diabetes than Caucasians, with African Americans having a 50 to 60% higher rate, Mexican Americans a 110 to 120% higher rate, and the Pima Indians of Arizona having the highest rate known in the world, with about half of this population afflicted with diabetes.[9,10]

Patients who are diagnosed with diabetes include 2.8% of the U.S. population, and they account for 5.8% of the total personal health care cost.[11] A new case of diabetes is diagnosed every 60 seconds, and 7 to 8% of hospital admissions are related to diabetes. The chance of developing diabetes doubles with every 20% increase above ideal body weight and every decade of life. Diabetes is the leading cause of new cases of blindness; diabetic patients are 25 times more prone to blindness than are nondiabetic patients. Patients with diabetes are 17 times more prone to kidney disease, with diabetic nephropathy being the primary cause of end-stage renal disease (ESRD) in adults.[12] Diabetic patients are twice as prone to heart disease and stroke as are nondiabetic people and 25 times more prone to developing gangrene. Also, diabetes is the leading cause of nontraumatic lower-limb amputations in the United States, and up to 50% of men with long-standing diabetes are sexually impotent.

The annual cost of diabetes in the United States is estimated at $100 billion per year, with the majority of these costs related to hospitalization and the treatment of long-term complications.[13] As an example of the cost of diabetic complications, approximately one-third of all cases of ESRD in the United States are the result of diabetes. The U.S. Renal Data System reported in 1993 that the cost of medical care for patients with ESRD was about $7.2 billion, with diabetes accounting for $2 to $3 billion of this cost per year.[14]

PATHOPHYSIOLOGY

The etiology of diabetes is incompletely understood, and numerous factors are associated with its development. Table 19.4 summarizes some of the factors linked with the development of diabetes. Patients with type 1 diabetes have a defect in pancreatic β-cell function related to faulty genetics or other external factors. These extrinsic factors affecting β-cell function include damage caused by viruses such as mumps or Coxsackie B4, by destructive cytotoxins and antibodies released by sensitized lymphocytes, or by autodigestion in the course of an inflammatory disorder involving the exocrine pancreas.

Genetic susceptibility to type 1 diabetes appears to be linked to two genes on chromosome 6. These genes control production of human lymphocyte antigens (HLAs) DR3 and DR4, and people with either or both of these antigens have a greater chance of developing diabetes than does a person lacking the antigens.[15] Ninety-five percent of patients with type 1 diabetes have one or both of these antigens; however, 40% of patients without diabetes have one or both of these antigens. Conversely, patients who carry HLA-DQA1* or HLA-DQB1*0602 are resistant to type 1 diabetes.[15]

Table 19.4 ▪ Etiologic Factors Associated with Diabetes Mellitus

Obesity
Increasing age
Heredity
Emotional stress
Autoimmune β-cell damage
Endocrine diseases (e.g., Cushing's disease)
Viral stress
Vasculitis in tissues highly perfused with capillaries (e.g., eye, kidney)
Insulin receptor or post–insulin receptor defects
Drugs (e.g., corticosteroids, thyroid, phenytoin, diazoxide, thiazide diuretics)

The reaction of predisposed patients to environmental stimuli (β-cell cytotoxic virus or chemicals) is abnormal and leads to destructive autoimmune-mediated mechanisms, or these patients experience lack of regeneration after β-cells are damaged. Intensive research is being done to test and identify the mechanisms involved. The majority of patients who develop type 1 diabetes have circulating antibodies, islet cell antibodies (ICAs), and insulin autoantibodies (IAAs) before overt type 1 disease develops.[16] The result is an absolute insulin deficiency.

On the other hand, many patients with type 2 diabetes have excess insulin secretion and are obese. In addition to hyperinsulinemia and obesity, many patients with type 2 disease have hypertension, dyslipidemia, and impaired fibrinolysis, a collection of conditions called syndrome X.[17] Patients with syndrome X are more likely to experience cardiovascular disease and develop long-term complications of diabetes. Hyperinsulinism and insulin resistance may be correlated with a decrease in insulin receptors, reduced insulin binding, or post–insulin-receptor signaling defects.

Insulin resistance is thought to be the primary underlying pathophysiologic defect in people with type 2 diabetes. Patients with type 2 diabetes and insulin resistance demonstrate the following two major metabolic defects: a decreased sensitivity of target tissues (primarily the liver and skeletal muscle) to the actions of insulin and a relative deficiency of endogenous insulin secretion.[18] Because the peripheral tissues (liver and muscle) are less able to respond to insulin, patients secrete higher levels of insulin in an attempt to compensate for the diminished activity of insulin, and plasma glucose levels rise. Impaired insulin secretion and increased glucagon contribute to continued hepatic glucose output, resulting in elevated fasting glucose levels.[19] Figure 19.1 schematically demonstrates the insulin resistance syndrome.

Blood glucose levels can be elevated by a variety of mechanisms. Some patients may have elevated blood glucose levels because of excessive glucagon or abnormal and excessive hepatic glucose production. Others may have a defect in somatostatin or an excess of growth hormone, cortisol, epinephrine, or other hormones that influence blood glucose regulation. Numerous drugs have also been implicated in increasing blood glucose levels, including corticosteroids, diazoxide, phenytoin, glucagon, caffeine, cyclophosphamide, lithium, epinephrine and other catecholamines, estrogens, furosemide, thiazide diuretics, thyroid preparations, and sugar-containing medications. Other drugs may cause lower-than-normal blood glucose levels, including anabolic steroids, sulfonylureas, disopyramide, ethanol, monoamine oxidase inhibitors, propranolol, and large dosages of salicylates.[20] Table 19.5 lists drugs associated with hyperglycemia or hypoglycemia and their clinical significance.

Numerous factors other than a relative or true lack of insulin may cause an increase in blood glucose. These include Cushing's disease, pheochromocytoma, aldosteronism, hyperthyroidism, pancreatitis, cirrhosis, pregnancy, emotional stress, and infections. Other factors can decrease blood glucose levels, such as an exogenous insulin excess, nonfasting reactive hypoglycemia, and fasting hypoglycemia.

Once hyperglycemia is established, elevated blood sugar values themselves can lead to glucotoxicity that causes an increase in insulin resistance and reduces insulin secretion. When hyperglycemia is reduced by pharmacotherapeutic means, glucotoxicity is lessened and insulin secretion is reduced, with a concomitant reduction in insulin resistance. Nonpharmacologic methods can also improve glycemic control. Modest weight loss has been shown to reduce hepatic glucose production, improve insulin secretion, and increase peripheral insulin action, all of which tend to lessen insulin resistance.[21] These measures, when combined with proper nutrition and exercise, are particularly useful in controlling blood sugars in patients with type 2 diabetes.

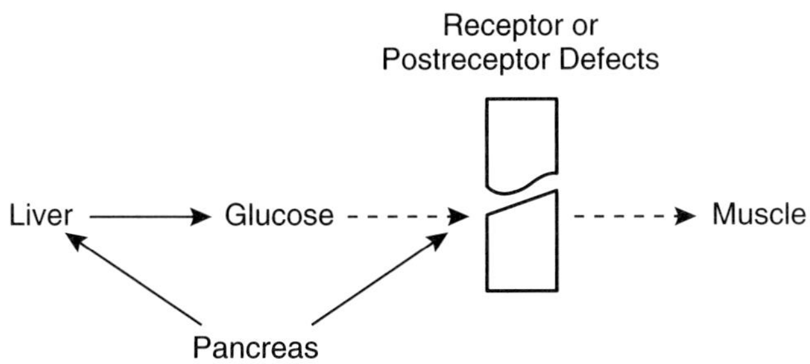

Figure 19.1. Characteristics of insulin resistance. Insulin resistance is defined by Polonsky et al. as "a diminished ability of insulin to exert its biologic action across a broad range of concentrations."[19]

We still have a great deal to learn about the specific cellular biochemical mechanisms involved in diabetes. The consequences of a lack of insulin or a lack of insulin effect are well known. The consequences of high blood glucose levels may be categorized into acute and chronic effects. The complex cellular effects of insulin provide numerous clues about the type of intervention that should be implemented to improve the prognosis of a patient with diabetes.

Normal Insulin Production and Effects

Insulin is a protein composed of 51 amino acids in two chains (A and B chains), connected by two disulfide bonds. Insulin is synthesized and stored in the β-cells of the islets of Langerhans, which are located in the pancreas. The pancreas produces a parent protein called preproinsulin. Preproinsulin is cleaved to form a smaller protein, proinsulin. Proinsulin is cleaved to form equimolar amounts of C-peptide and insulin.[22] The normal human pancreas contains approximately 200 U insulin, and a basal amount of insulin is secreted continuously at a rate of approximately 0.5 to 1.0 U/hour. Additional insulin is also released in response to blood glucose levels of 100 mg/dL or more. The average daily insulin secretory rate in the adult is 25 to 50 U/day. Insulin is cleared metabolically by the liver, peripheral tissues, and kidneys. Insulin follows first-order elimination kinetics, and the serum half-life is approximately 4 to 5 minutes.

The important metabolic sites that are sensitive to insulin include the liver, where glycogen is synthesized, stored, and broken down; skeletal muscle, where glucose oxidation produces energy; and adipose tissue, where glucose can be converted to fatty acids, glyceryl phosphate, and triglycerides. Insulin affects carbohydrate, protein, and lipid metabolism.

Carbohydrate Metabolism

In patients without diabetes, insulin acts in concert with glucagon, somatostatin, growth hormone, corticosteroids, epinephrine, and parasympathetic innervation to maintain blood glucose between 40 and 160 mg/dL at all times. Three cell types, α-cells, β-cells, and δ-cells, have been identified in the islets of Langerhans of the pancreas. The α-cells produce glucagon, a hormone that acts to increase blood glucose levels. The β-cells produce, store, and release insulin. The δ-cells produce somatostatin, which inhibits both insulin and glucagon secretion and suppresses growth hormone. The suppression of glucagon by somatostatin decreases blood glucose levels, and its effect persists for roughly 60 to 120 minutes.

Euglycemia is maintained by the three previously identified hormones working in concert. Ingestion of a carbohydrate load results in a prompt increase in the amount of insulin release and a concomitant decrease in plasma glucagon. Glucagon is released in response to low blood glucose levels and protein ingestion. Glucagon

Table 19.5 ▪ Drugs That May Alter Blood Glucose Levels

Drug	Mechanism of Action	Clinical Significance
Drugs That May Increase Blood Glucose Levels		
Acetazolamide	Unknown, but may enhance insulin or sulfonylurea elimination.	+
Alcohol (ethanol)	Glucose tolerance may worsen with chronic ingestion and may increase metabolism of tolbutamide. May result in chlorpropamide flush reaction or hypoglycemia.	+
Asparaginase	May inhibit insulin synthesis (diabetic ketoacidosis has been reported).	++
β-Adrenergic antagonists	Inhibit insulin secretion. Cardioselective agents less likely to produce this effect.	++
Caffeine	High dosages may stimulate gluconeogenesis.	+
Calcium channel antagonists	Inhibit insulin secretion.	+
Clonidine	May be related to release of growth hormone (transient and associated only with high dosages of clonidine).	+
Diazoxide	Inhibits insulin secretion. Decreases use of insulin.	+++
Diuretics	May be related to hypokalemia, leading to a decrease in insulin secretion. Thiazides show a greater increasing effect than loop diuretics, which show a greater effect than potassium-sparing diuretics.	++
Epinephrinelike agents (sympathomimetics, decongestants, anorexiants)	Increase glycogenolysis and gluconeogenesis.	++
Glucagon	Increases glycogenolysis.	+++
Glucocorticosteroids	Increase gluconeogenesis; depress insulin action.	+++
Glycerol	Unknown, probably volume depletion (hyperglycemic hyperosmolar nonketotic coma has been reported).	++
Immunosuppressives (cyclosporin and tacrolimus)	May induce insulin resistance.	++
Interferon (α and β)	Unknown.	+
Lithium salts	May decrease insulin secretion.	+
Niacin	Unknown, may worsen insulin resistance.	++
Nicotine	Vasoconstriction leading to a decreased absorption of injected insulin.	++
Oral contraceptives	Unknown. High-dose combination products can impair glucose tolerance (minimal effect with newer low-dose combination products).	++
Pentamidine	Toxic to pancreatic β-cells.	+++
Phenytoin	Inhibits insulin secretion.	++
Protease inhibitors	Unknown, possibly pancreatic toxicity.	+
Rifampin	Enhances tolbutamide metabolism.	+
Sugar-containing syrups	Increase sugar load.	++
Thyroid hormones	Increase metabolic clearance of insulin and hypoglycemic agents.	++

(continued)

release stimulates insulin secretion; insulin in turn inhibits glucagon release.

The presence of insulin favors the uptake and use of glucose by insulin-sensitive sites. In skeletal muscle, glucose uptake and subsequent energy production increase. In the liver, glucose uptake and the formation of glycogen increase in the presence of insulin.

A minimum blood glucose level of 40 mg/dL is needed to provide adequate fuel for the brain, which can use only glucose as fuel and does not depend on the presence of insulin for its use. Glucose spills into the urine, resulting in energy and water loss, when blood glucose levels exceed the renal threshold (180 mg/dL).

Protein Metabolism

The presence of insulin favors the production of structural proteins from constituent amino acids. When glucose is present intracellularly in sufficient quantities for needed energy production, most structural proteins retain their integrity. In the absence of insulin, structural protein

Table 19.5 *(continued)*

Drug	Mechanism of Action	Clinical Significance
Drugs That May Cause Hypoglycemia		
Alcohol (ethanol)	Impairs gluconeogenesis and increases insulin secretion.	+++
Anabolic steroids	Decrease glucose tolerance.	+
Angiotensin-converting enzyme inhibitors	May improve insulin sensitivity, particularly in skeletal muscle.	+
β-Adrenergic antagonists	Inhibit glycogenolysis; attenuate signs and symptoms of hypoglycemia.	++
Chloramphenicol	May inhibit metabolism of sulfonylureas.	++
Chloroquine	Unknown (hypoglycemia leading to death has been reported in overdose).	++
Clofibrate	Unknown.	+
Coumarins and dicumarol	Inhibit hepatic clearance of tolbutamide and chlorpropamide.	++
Disopyramide	Unknown; appears to result from endogenous insulin secretion.	++
Growth hormone	Unknown.	++
Monoamine oxidase inhibitors	May increase insulin release and decrease sympathetic response to hypoglycemia.	+
Pentamidine	Cytolytic response in pancreas accompanied by insulin release.	+++
Phenylbutazone	Reduces clearance of sulfonylureas.	++
Salicylates	Increase insulin secretion and sensitivity; may alter pharmacokinetic disposition of sulfonylureas.	++
Saquinavir	Unknown.	+
Sulfonamides	Alter clearance of sulfonylureas.	+
Triazole antifungals	Enhance the effect of sulfonylureas.	+++

Source: Reference 20.

+, low probability of occurrence or low level of glucose alteration expected in most patients; *++,* probability of occurrence in most patients is high, but degree of glucose alteration may or may not be clinically significant; *+++,* high probability of occurrence, clinically significant in many cases.

production is not favored, and intracellular glucose levels are insufficient to match energy demands. In an attempt to produce energy, skeletal muscle converts its structural proteins to constituent amino acids. The liberated amino acids are transported to the liver, where they are converted to glucose via gluconeogenesis. In patients with diabetes, glucose enters the blood but is not taken up by tissue because of a true or relative lack of insulin. Thus, hyperglycemia is escalated, and structural proteins are wasted.

Fat Metabolism

The presence of insulin favors the production of triglycerides from free fatty acids (FFAs). When insulin deficiency causes an energy deficit, FFAs are oxidized to β-hydroxybutyric acid, acetoacetic acid, and acetone. β-Hydroxybutyric acid can be used as an energy source, but in the absence of insulin the production of the keto acids eventually is greater than their metabolism and excretion. If insulin is not given to the patient, metabolic ketoacidosis ensues. The keto acids cause the blood pH to decline, and diuresis secondary to the elimination of ketones and glucose causes dehydration. The body's neutralizing factors eventually are depleted, and the patient continues to deteriorate to the point of coma and possibly death. Figure 19.2 shows the clinical manifestations of the untreated patient with type 1 diabetes who is insulinopenic (completely lacks insulin).

Patients with type 2 diabetes may have an elevated, normal, or low level of circulating insulin, depending on the chronicity of their disease, and have a relative lack of effective insulin. In patients with type 2 disease, insulin and glucose levels usually are adequate to prevent ketoacidosis development. However, glucose can accumulate in the blood and can reach extremely high levels (more than 400 mg/dL), resulting in nonketotic hyperosmolar syndrome (NKHS).

CLINICAL PRESENTATION AND DIAGNOSIS

Signs and Symptoms

Type 1 diabetes usually presents rapidly, typically with polydipsia, polyuria, polyphagia, weakness, weight loss, dry skin, and ketoacidosis (30% of all cases of diabetic ketoacidosis (DKA) occur in previously undiagnosed patients). On the other hand, type 2 diabetes typically is slow and insidious in onset and often unaccompanied by symptoms. Type 2 diabetes often is discovered when glucose is found in the urine or when elevated blood sugar is noticed during a routine examination. Patients with type 2 disease usually are over age 40 and often obese. Careful examination of these patients often reveals glucosuria, proteinuria, postprandial hyperglycemia, microaneurysms, and possibly retinal exudates.

Other symptoms of hyperglycemia that are associated with diabetes include blurred vision, tingling or numbness of the extremities, slow-healing skin infections, itching, drowsiness, and irritability. Patients with these symptoms and patients who have a family history of diabetes should be screened closely for hyperglycemia. Table 19.6 lists testing recommendations in previously undiagnosed patients. Monilial infections of the vagina and anus and a history of complications during pregnancy are also warning signs to test for diabetes. The earlier diabetes is diagnosed, the more easily it can be controlled and the better is the long-term prognosis.

Diagnosis

Type 1 diabetes usually is easy to diagnose because patients present with all of the classic symptoms of diabetes and high amounts of glucose in the urine and blood. Type 2 diabetes is more of a challenge to diagnose because patients often do not present with the classic symptoms. Table 19.6 reviews the screening criteria for diabetes mellitus and Table 19.2 summarizes the diagnostic criteria developed by the Expert Committee on the Diagnosis and Classification of Diabetes Mellitus in 1997.[6] Basically there are three ways in which diabetes can be diagnosed. Each method must be confirmed on another day by the same or a different method.

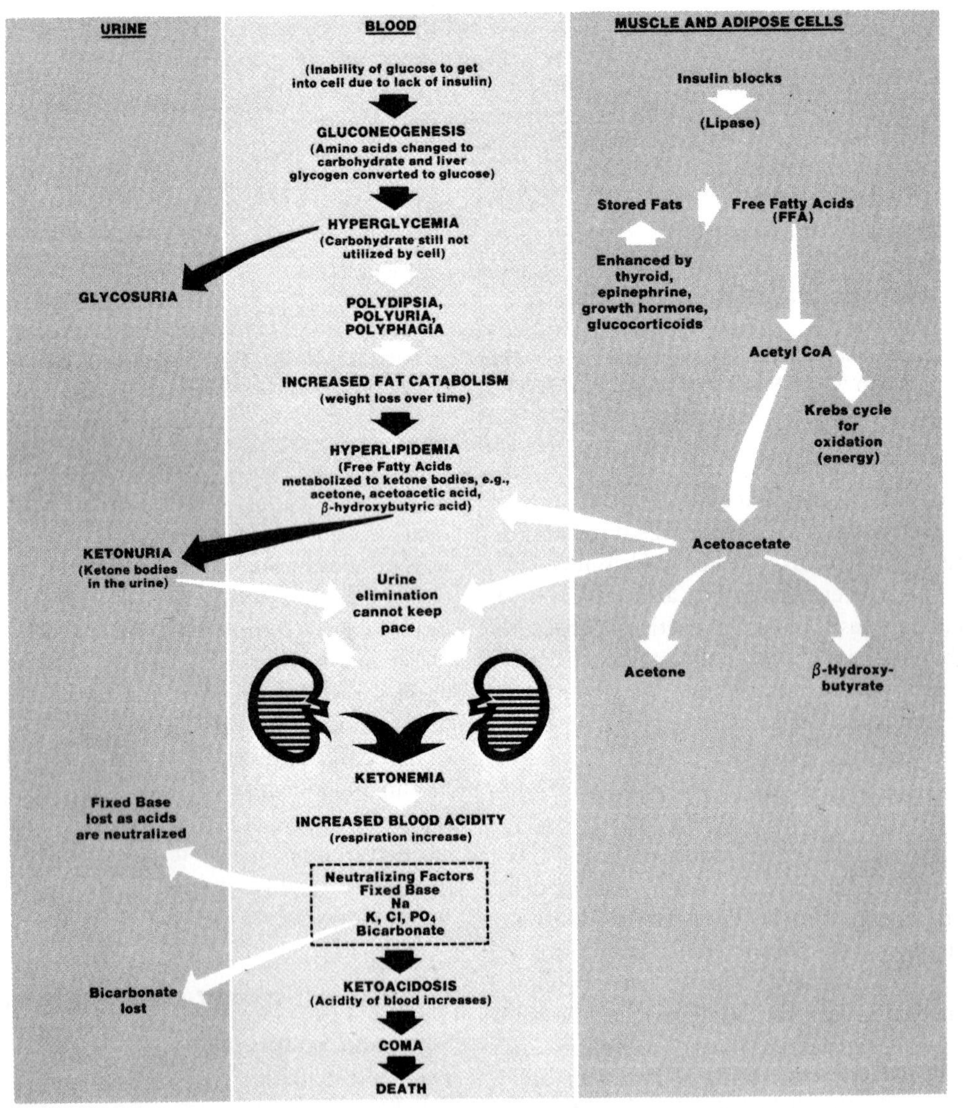

Figure 19.2. Clinical manifestations of a complete lack of insulin.

Table 19.6 • Screening Criteria for Diabetes

Testing should be considered in all patients age 45 yr and older. Repeat at 3-yr intervals.

Consider testing at younger age or test more often in patients who:
- Are obese (≥120% desirable body weight or body mass index ≥27 kg/m²)
- Have a first-degree relative with diabetes
- Are members of a high-risk ethnic group (e.g., African American, Hispanic, Native American)
- Have delivered a baby weighing >9 lb or have been diagnosed with gestational diabetes mellitus
- Are hypertensive (≥140/90)
- Have a high-density lipoprotein cholesterol level ≤35 mg/dL or a triglyceride level ≥250 mg/dL
- On previous testing had IGT or IFG

Source: Expert committee on the diagnosis and classification of diabetes mellitus. Report of the expert committee on the diagnosis and classification of diabetes mellitus. Diabetes Care 20:1183–1197, 1997.

IGT, impaired glucose tolerance; *IFG,* impaired fasting glucose.

Fasting plasma glucose is the preferred method for testing for diabetes. It is fast, economical, and commonly used. Blood is drawn from the patient after an overnight fast. Normal is in the range of 65 to 110 mg/dL, with minor variations between laboratories. The diagnosis of diabetes may be confirmed in patients with two or more fasting plasma glucose levels above 126 mg/dL (7 mmol/L; 1 mmol = 18 mg/dL glucose).

A less common and more cumbersome test is the oral glucose tolerance test (OGTT). This test measures the patient's ability to handle a glucose load over a period of time. After an overnight fast, a morning fasting blood sugar is drawn and the patient ingests a 75-g glucose load. Then blood samples are drawn at half-hour intervals for 2 hours and then at 3 hours.[23] In normal subjects, the blood glucose returns to normal in less than 2 hours. In patients with diabetes, the glucose peak is higher and occurs much later than in those without diabetes; levels also decline at a slower rate. A normal OGTT occurs when the fasting plasma glucose is less than 115 mg/dL, the 2-hour plasma glucose is less than 140 mg/dL, and the intervening glucose values are below 200 mg/dL. Because of criteria that accept random or fasting glucose levels as diagnostic, this test is not commonly performed. Infections, stress, pregnancy, metabolic abnormalities, and certain drugs can impair glucose tolerance and produce abnormal results, and these should be screened for when OGTT is used.

Diagnostic tests can be elevated by emotional stress, physical exertion, and stimulants such as tobacco, coffee, and tea. Therefore, caution should be exercised in using diagnostic tests for diabetes. A patient should not be diagnosed as having diabetes unless it is certain that the disease exists. To inappropriately label a patient with this diagnosis leads to personal frustration, including insurance riders, driver's license limitations in some states, and possible employment limitations. Health care providers who are monitoring older adults should be alert to the fact that as a person ages, tolerance to glucose decreases. This results in some older adults being labeled as diabetic and being placed on unnecessary medications.

MONITORING

Self-Monitoring of Blood Glucose

The objective of diabetes treatment is to achieve normal or near normal blood glucose levels through a program of education, diet, exercise, and medications. Achieving the objective entails active patient involvement to ensure that glycemic control is attained. One of the easiest and most practical methods of monitoring glycemic control is SMBG. SMBG is acceptable to many patients and it allows the patient to better understand the factors that affect blood glucose levels; gives an accurate reflection of the blood glucose after exercise, before and after meals, and when the patient is taking medications or is ill; helps the patient to better understand diabetes and the objectives of therapy; assists in detecting and therefore avoiding hypoglycemia; helps the patient understand the symptoms of hypoglycemia and hyperglycemia; improves the relationship between the health care professional and the patient; and helps the patient to become a more active, informed participant in diabetes management.

The disadvantages of SMBG, which include the increased expense and the annoyance of obtaining a drop of blood, are greatly outweighed by the many advantages. Several devices are now available to help the patient obtain a drop of blood easily and almost painlessly.[24] Several methods of determining blood glucose levels are available, and selection of a specific product can be made on the basis of cost, ability to perform the test accurately, and flexibility of the system. The manual dexterity needed and the ease of reading the result are additional factors to consider. Some systems have extended memories so that recordkeeping is easier, and newer products can download data to a computer, making trend analysis much easier and more convenient for health professionals to interpret.

Because blood sugar maintenance is impossible without measurement and because it is convenient and less costly for the patient to self-monitor, SMBG is highly recommended for all patients with diabetes. Pregnant patients, labile patients who have difficulty bringing their diabetes under control, and patients with frequent hypoglycemia are all excellent candidates for SMBG. Also, blood glucose monitoring is a necessity for patients who are using continuous subcutaneous insulin infusion.

Most of the tests available for use by patients involve the glucose oxidase and peroxidase reaction to detect glucose. Some of the tests use a reflective photometer to read the strip and give a digital readout of the blood glucose values. Other methods have a color reaction on the strip, which is compared to a chart on the side of the bottle that the patient reads visually. Although the visually read strips are less expensive and very portable, electronic blood glucose monitoring gives the patient a more accurate blood glucose determination. In general, the visually read strips are not recommended. Patients with type 1 diabetes generally should test their blood sugars three or four times daily.[25] The optimal monitoring frequency in patients with type 2 diabetes is not known, and testing frequency would be influenced by their dependence on oral or injectable therapy and their adherence to a diet and exercise program.

Urine Tests

Patient-performed urine tests are available for evaluating glucose, ketones, and protein values. Glucosuria is observed in many conditions and is not a persistent finding in diabetes. It occurs when the renal threshold is exceeded (blood glucose level of 180 mg/dL or higher); however, this value is not consistent for all patients. In particular, older patients with diabetes may not "spill" any glucose into the urine despite greatly elevated blood sugar values. Older patients may have overt diabetes that may not be detected by urinalysis. Therefore, urine testing in older adults would not reflect their level of glycemia accurately. Another problem for patients with diabetes, possibly more important, is the fact that residual urine in the bladder, even when the patient double-voids, can alter the level of glucose detected in the urine and may actually reflect blood glucose values from the previous 2 to 3 hours. Because of the problems inherent in urine glucose monitoring, this method is no longer recommended.

Available urine ketone tests include Acetest, Chemstrip K, and Ketostix. Urine ketone testing should be encouraged for the patient with diabetes during acute illness or stress or when blood glucose levels are not well controlled. Patients with type 1 disease should test for urine ketones when blood sugar readings are greater than 240 mg/dL and should report moderate or higher ketone readings to a health care professional.

Finally, urine tests are available for measuring urine proteins. Constant routine monitoring of urine protein usually is not warranted. Urine protein tests are used primarily as a screening tool for the presence of diabetic nephropathy. Patients who test negative with standard dipstick methods may be further evaluated with an in-office microalbumin test (Micro-Bumintest) or by 24-hour urine collections. These methods are much more sensitive than the standard dipstick method. Patients who have had type 1 diabetes for more than 5 years should be screened annually; patients with type 2 diabetes should be screened annually from the time of diagnosis.[26]

Glycosylated Hemoglobin

Hemoglobin glycosylation occurs when hemoglobin is exposed to ambient glucose concentrations in the blood. When higher concentrations of blood glucose are present, the percentage of HbA1c (glycosylated hemoglobin) increases because red blood cells are freely permeable to glucose. Because the average life span of the red blood cell is 120 days, the HbA1c reflects glycemic control for that time period and most precisely reflects the average blood sugar from the previous 60 to 90 days. HbA1c is an important measure of long-term glycemic control and is directly correlated with the long-term complications of diabetes. HbA1c is a subcategory of hemoglobin that can be glycosylated. Some laboratories measure all of the glycosylated hemoglobins (and not specifically the HbA1c portion), so it is important to know which test is being performed and that particular laboratory's normal ranges.

Typically the patient without diabetes has a HbA1c in the range of 4 to 6%, and those with diabetes may have values as high as 20%. In general, for each 1% rise in HbA1c value, the average serum blood sugar increases by 30 mg/dL. Therefore, a patient with an HbA1c value of 6% would correlate with an average blood sugar of 120 mg/dL, and a person with a 9% value would have an average blood glucose value corresponding to roughly 210 mg/dL.

Studies show that when a patient with uncontrolled diabetes brings his or her blood glucose under strict control, there is a dramatic improvement in glycosylated hemoglobin. The DCCT confirmed that there is a strong correlation between glycosylated hemoglobin concentrations and the progression of microvascular disease in patients with type 1 diabetes. This test is particularly useful for patients who have poor compliance in recordkeeping or who make an extra effort to achieve acceptable plasma glucose levels only at the time of the physician visit. The test can be performed at any time and is not affected by recent meals or physical activities. Glycohemoglobin testing should be performed in all patients with diabetes on a routine basis. The ideal frequency of testing is unknown, although it is generally recommended that two to four tests be performed per year. The number of tests to do per year depends on the degree of glycemic control, the number of therapeutic changes made, and the physician's clinical judgment. The therapeutic goal recommended by the American Diabetes Association for glycosylated hemoglobin is less than 7%, and treatment should be reevaluated for patients with multiple values higher than 8. Table 19.7 lists goals of therapy.

Table 19.7 ▪ Glycemic Control Parameters

Biochemical Index	Nondiabetic	Goal	Values That Warrant Corrective Action
Preprandial glucose (mg/dL)	<115	80–120	<80 or >140
Bedtime glucose (mg/dL)	<120	100–140	<100 or >160
Hemoglobin A1c (%)	<6	<7	>8

Source: American Diabetes Association. Standards of medical care for patients with diabetes mellitus. Diabetes Care 22(Suppl 1):S32–S41, 1999.

Glycated Serum Protein

Proteins in the bloodstream can become glycated, much like hemoglobin. The half-life of serum albumin ranges from 14 to 20 days and acts as a marker of glycemic control over a shorter time frame than HbA1c.[25] Serum fructosamine assay is a common method of measuring glycated albumin in the body and is highly correlated with HbA1c values. A serum fructosamine value gives information about the degree of glycemic control over the past 2 to 3 weeks and may be invaluable in monitoring patients whose glycemic status must be verified over a shorter period of time. Patients who may benefit from this include pregnant patients, those undergoing major changes in therapy, and older adults. Currently one product is available for home use that measures serum fructosamine with a fingerstick.

HYPERGLYCEMIA

Short-Term Effects

The short-term effects of hyperglycemia range from minor symptoms to life-threatening metabolic compromise. Short-term effects such as blurred vision, polydipsia, polyuria, increase in incidence of urinary tract infection, fatigue, or drowsiness may impair the quality of life of patients untreated or poorly treated for diabetes. Although these can lead to significant impairment (e.g., blurred vision), two life-threatening short-term complications necessitate prompt medical intervention: DKA and NKHS.

Diabetic Ketoacidosis

The physiologic events that lead to DKA are described in Figure 19.2. DKA is a life-threatening condition that occurs secondary to an insulin deficit. DKA may occur in patients with diabetes who have an active infection, those who have discontinued insulin therapy, or those subjected to other forms of stress (e.g., acute myocardial infarction, stroke). DKA necessitates prompt and proper treatment and has a 5 to 10% mortality rate.[27]

Signs and symptoms of DKA include polydipsia, polyuria, fruity breath, dry mucous membranes, tachycardia, and hypotension. Consciousness may be mildly to severely impaired. Common laboratory findings include elevated serum glucose, creatinine, blood urea nitrogen, hyponatremia, ketonuria, and glucosuria.

Insulin is usually administered initially with an intravenous bolus dose between 0.1 and 0.2 U/kg, followed by a continuous infusion of 0.1 U/kg/hour. Normal saline (0.9% NaCl) is administered at a rate of 0.5 to 1 L/hour until blood pressure and pulse are stabilized, at which point normal saline is substituted. When blood glucose approaches normal, D5 normal saline may be used. If potassium levels are elevated, supplemental potassium should not be administered. Once normokalemia has been achieved, 10 to 20 mEq/hour potassium is needed for maintenance. Hypokalemic patients need additional potassium supplementation beyond the maintenance rate, based on potassium serum levels (typically 20 to 40 mEq/L fluid). Phosphate administration is controversial because it can promote hypokalemia and hypomagnesemia; however, it can be provided to patients with low phosphorus levels at a rate of 5 to 10 mmol/hour. Bicarbonate should be administered only to patients whose arterial pH levels are less than 7.1 and in dosages of 44 mEq/hour.[28]

Nonketotic Hyperosmolar Syndrome

NKHS typically is characterized by blood glucose levels higher than 600 mg/dL and has a mortality rate up to 30%. Older adults with type 2 diabetes are at increased risk of NKHS and are much less likely to develop DKA. Certain diseases such as infections and renal or cardiac disease may precipitate the NKHS development, and prompt recognition and treatment are needed to prevent mortality. After a major insult (e.g., acute myocardial infarction, infection) the body releases cortisol and epinephrine, which has the effect of worsening hyperglycemia. With increased glycemia, dehydration and hyperosmolarity develop and increased amounts of glucose are lost in the urine. Ketone bodies are not formed because of the presence of insulin. Dehydration and hyperosmolarity occur that can result in altered consciousness and lethargy, with coma being less commonly recognized (an older term for this syndrome was *nonketotic hyperosmolar coma syndrome*).

Signs of dehydration in patients with NKHS include tachycardia, dry skin, and orthostatic hypotension. The primary treatment consists of rehydration, insulin, electrolyte replacement, and treatment of the underlying cause. Because older patients with diabetes are more prone to develop NKHS, health professionals must encourage regular serum glucose monitoring by older adults and advocate consistent recording and reporting of any upward trends in blood sugars.

Long-Term Effects

Although the short-term metabolic effects of hyperglycemia are life-threatening and necessitate prompt attention, the long-term effects are insidious and often unnoticed. However, the prolonged effects are serious, very often debilitating, and, if untreated, life-threatening over the long term. The chronic complications of diabetes include macrovascular disease (peripheral, cerebral, cardiovascular) microvascular disease (retinopathy and nephropathy), neuropathy (peripheral and autonomic), and foot problems. Although the molecular mechanisms leading to chronic complications have not been delineated conclusively, several abnormal biochemical pathways have been suggested. Most salient in this list of deleterious pathways is the production of high concentrations of advanced glycosylation end products (AGE) and sorbitol. There has been considerable debate about whether the lesions that develop within the diabetic patient's retina, kidneys, nerves, and vascular system result from a disorder in the structure and function of blood vessels or from prolonged hyperglycemia caused by inadequate metabolic control.

The bulk of the data suggests that microvascular disease and neuropathy are linked to hyperglycemia.[1–5]

The causes of macrovascular disease associated with diabetes are less well understood. Ischemic heart disease accounts for approximately 40% of the mortality in this population, with other cardiovascular disease and stroke accounting for an additional 25%.[29] Many patients with type 2 diabetes have hyperinsulinemia, are obese, and have hypertension along with high levels of triglycerides and low-density lipoprotein and low levels of high-density lipoprotein; all but hyperinsulinemia are known risk factors for cardiovascular disease. The role of hyperinsulinemia is not as clear, and definitive clinical trials assessing the role of hyperinsulinemia and exogenous insulin administration are critically needed to determine whether high insulin levels contribute to macrovascular disease.

Advanced Glycosylation End Products

Proteins throughout the body are nonenzymatically glycosylated at a rate that is proportional to the ambient glucose concentration. These glycosylated proteins are highly reactive, forming bonds with other glycosylated proteins, collagen, and other molecules, eventually forming AGEs (Fig. 19.3). Once formed, AGEs are very stable and are incorporated into the basement membrane matrix of capillaries. This process causes the thickening of basement membranes and a reduction of the production of active endothelium-derived relaxing factor, resulting in vasoconstriction.[30] The net result of this process is leakage across the basement membranes, which appears as hard exudates in the patient with diabetic retinopathy and as proteinuria in the patient with diabetic nephropathy. This process is thought to be one of the major pathways leading to the development of microvascular disease. To date there is no drug product available to alter the formation of AGEs; however, aminoguanidine, an AGE blocker, is under intense investigation.

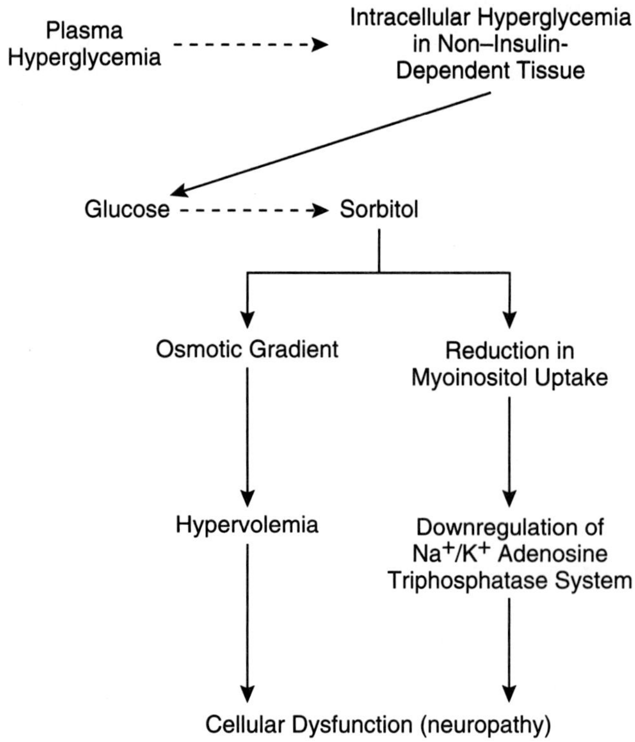

Figure 19.4. The sorbitol pathway.

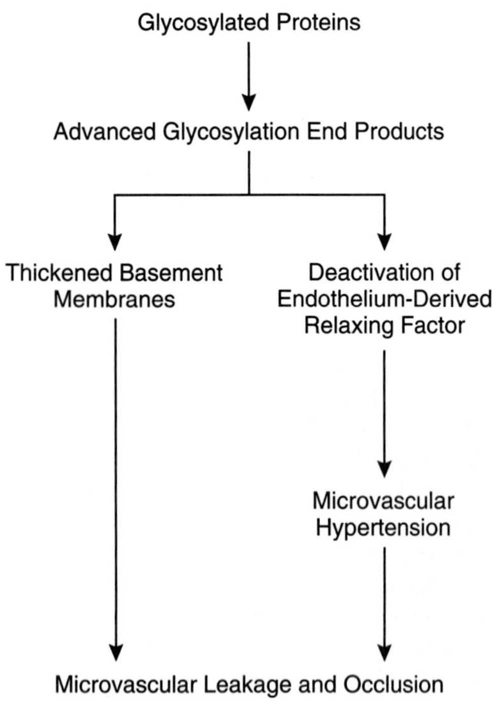

Figure 19.3. Advanced glycosylation end products and microvascular disease.

Sorbitol and Aldose Reductase Inhibition

The sorbitol pathway may be another clinically important biochemical mechanism by which chronic complications develop in patients with diabetes.[31] Many cell lines, such as the Schwann cell in the central nervous system, do not need insulin for glucose uptake. These cell types are subject to intracellular hyperglycemia during times of ambient hyperglycemia. Intracellular hyperglycemia causes an inordinately high fraction of glucose to be shunted into the sorbitol pathway (Fig. 19.4), leading to the production of high concentrations of sorbitol via the enzyme aldose reductase. High concentrations of sorbitol cause a reduction in myoinositol uptake, which in turn results in the downregulation of the Na^+/K^+ adenosine triphosphatase system, with a reduction in energy production. Additionally, sorbitol creates an intracellular osmotic gradient, resulting in hypervolemia of the cell, probably further compromising cellular function. This pathway may play a substantial role in neuropathy development in patients with diabetes. Aldose reductase inhibitors currently in clinical studies include zopolrestat, minalrestat, and zenarestat.

DIABETES STUDIES

Diabetes Control and Complications Trial

The landmark DCCT conclusively determined that glycemic control definitely affects the appearance and progression of chronic diabetic complications.[1] This study evaluated patients with type 1 disease, with patients randomized to receive either conventional therapy (one to two insulin injections per day and avoidance of acute symptoms of hyperglycemia) or intensive therapy (three or more injections per day or subcutaneous insulin infusion pump therapy and strict glycemic control). The interim analysis showed an overwhelming support for intensive therapy, and the study was stopped 1 year earlier than initially planned. Results were reported in terms of relative risk reduction or, simply stated, what level of risk reduction for the appearance or progression of a chronic complication is imparted by intensive therapy versus conventional therapy. The results are shown in Table 19.8. In addition to the significant chronic complication findings, the study also reported a threefold increase in hypoglycemic episodes and more weight gain in the patients who were treated with intensive insulin therapy. Despite these potential drawbacks to intensive therapy, there is a renewed emphasis on strict but reasonable glycemic control to prevent the severe and debilitating chronic complications of diabetes. Strict glycemic control is particularly important before and during pregnancy and has been shown to reduce the incidence of perinatal complications and mortality in mothers with diabetes.

United Kingdom Prospective Diabetes Study

The UKPDS was a 20-year study involving more than 4000 patients with type 2 diabetes.[2–5] Four separate trials were conducted and involved the following four components: effects of intensive blood glucose control with sulfonylureas or insulin, effects of intensive blood glucose control with metformin in overweight patients, effect of tight blood pressure control in hypertensive diabetic patients, and the effects of atenolol and captopril on blood pressure control. In the UKPDS study, intensive control was defined as achieving fasting plasma glucose of less than 6 mmol/L (108 mg/dL), and conventional treatment was treatment that resulted in fasting plasma glucose less than 15 mmol/L (270 mg/dL). Patients treated with conventional therapy were treated with diet and weight maintenance and with sulfonylureas, metformin, or insulin if severe or symptomatic hyperglycemia occurred. Blood sugars were controlled with chlorpropamide, glyburide, glipizide, or insulin in the intensively treated group. The following endpoints were evaluated: any diabetes-related endpoint (sudden death, death from hyperglycemia or hypoglycemia, fatal or nonfatal myocardial infarction), other cardiovascular events, amputation, or ophthalmic events; death related to diabetes including sudden death, stroke, peripheral vascular disease, renal disease, glycemic derangements, and death from myocardial infarction; or death from all causes. Single clinical endpoints examined included myocardial infarction, stroke, amputation, or death from peripheral vascular disease and microvascular complications.

HbA1c values over a 10-year period were 7.0% in the intensive group and 7.9% in the conventional group, with all agents having similar efficacy in the intensively treated patients. Patients in the intensively treated group had a 12% lower risk of any diabetes-related endpoint and a 25% lower risk of microvascular complications than those in the conventionally treated group. No significant differences in the risk of diabetes-related deaths, all-cause mortality, myocardial infarction, stroke, amputation, or death from peripheral vascular disease were noted. As in the DCCT, significant reductions in the risk of progression of retinopathy and microalbuminuria were noted. See Table 19.8 for the results of the DCCT and UKPDS studies.[2–5]

Table 19.8 ▪ Results of Two Landmark Studies

Diabetes Control and Complications Trial
60% reduction in clinical neuropathy development
35% reduction in microalbuminemia development
56% reduction in macroalbuminemia development
27% reduction in initial appearance of retinopathy
34–76% reduction in clinically significant retinopathy
45% reduction in progression to severe retinopathy
34% reduction in low-density lipoprotein concentration
41% reduction in risk of macrovascular disease
300% increase in incidence of severe hypoglycemia
United Kingdom Prospective Diabetes Study
Intensive blood glucose control with sulfonylureas or insulin
12% reduction of any diabetes-related endpoint
25% reduction in microvascular complications
29% reduction in photocoagulation
21% reduction in progression to retinopathy
34% reduction in progression to microalbinuria
Mean 3.1-kg weight gain in intensive group over 10 yr
Intensive blood glucose control with metformin in overweight patients
32% reduction in any diabetes-related endpoint
42% reduction in risk of diabetes-related death
36% reduction in mortality
39% reduction of myocardial infarction
Effect of tight blood pressure control (<150/85) in hypertensive patients
24% reduction in any diabetes-related endpoint
32% reduction in diabetes-related death
44% reduction in fatal and nonfatal stroke
37% reduction in microvascular disease
34% reduction in deterioration of retinopathy
Effect of atenolol and captopril in risk reduction of microvascular and macrovascular complications
Both agents equally effective in maintaining blood glucose control
No differences in risk of macrovascular or microvascular disease between the two groups

Table 19.9 • Treatment Objectives for Diabetes Mellitus

Normalize glucose metabolism
- Normalize glycosylated hemoglobin
- Urine glucose and ketones negative
- Fasting blood glucose: 3.9–6.6 mmol/L (70–120 mg/dL)
- 2-hr postprandial glucose level less than 8.8 mmol/L (160 mg/dL)

Avoid symptoms of diabetes mellitus.
Avoid hypoglycemia.
Normalize nutrition and maintain reasonable weight.
Achieve normal growth and development.
Minimize or prevent complications.
Accept diabetes with a realistic but positive attitude.
Enjoy normal and flexible lifestyle.
Promote emotional well-being; have patient take charge of condition.

THERAPEUTIC PLAN

The treatment objectives for diabetes are summarized in Table 19.9. In achieving the objectives, one must remember that diabetes is a heterogeneous condition and that there is tremendous variation among patients. The treatment protocol must be individualized and can be developed only after the type of diabetes has been categorized. In general, glucose metabolism is normalized in diabetic patients who achieve excellent control. The DCCT verified that strict glycemic control is associated with a reduction in the occurrence and progression of chronic complications in patients with type 1 diabetes. The results of the UKPDS confirm that intensive control of blood sugar results in a decrease in long-term complications and mortality in patients with type 2 disease. Excellent blood sugar control in patients with either type 1 or type 2 diabetes significantly improves the patient's quality of life.

The formula to achieve these objectives combines a program of weight control or loss with an individualized exercise program and the use of medications. Diet, exercise, and medications are greatly enhanced by a program of education and weight reduction.

TREATMENT

Although therapies exist for treating the chronic complications of diabetes, prevention should always be the goal. As demonstrated by the DCCT and UKPDS, good glycemic control can have dramatic effects on the development and progression of complications and should be attempted unless otherwise contraindicated.

Diabetes affects virtually every organ of the body, and complications often affect the eyes, nervous system, penile erectile function, kidneys, cardiovascular system, and extremities. Retinopathy can be treated successfully with laser photocoagulation. If retinal vitreous hemorrhage occurs, surgical vitrectomy can often restore the patient's vision. Diabetic cataracts may improve with strict glycemic control and may respond to treatment with aldose reductase inhibitors. Neuropathies may also respond to strict glycemic control, but other therapeutic modalities often are necessary. Table 19.10 lists neuropathies and their respective treatment options.

Many men with diabetes are sexually impotent. Self-injection or intrapenile insertion of prostaglandins, vacuum tumescence devices, and surgical prosthetic implants are viable options for the man with impotence. A class of drugs called phosphodiesterase type 5 inhibitors has recently revolutionized the treatment of erectile dysfunction.[32] These drugs selectively inhibit the phosphodiesterase type enzyme, thereby enhancing the activity of nitric oxide, which increases blood flow to the penis, resulting in enhanced penile pressure and erection maintenance. Sildenafil citrate is the first marketed drug in the class, and others are anticipated.

Patients with diabetes are more likely to develop nephropathy than those without diabetes; diabetic nephropathy is the most common cause of ESRD in the Western world.[14] Proteinuria is the first clinical manifestation, with progression to hypertension, azotemia, hypoalbuminemia, and edema. Treatment to control the complication of nephropathy and dialysis or transplantation may be necessary for patients who have progressive renal disease. Strict blood glucose control is necessary to reduce, or possibly prevent, pathologic changes caused by hyper-

Table 19.10 • Clinical Manifestations and Treatment of Neuropathies

Disturbance	Manifestation	Treatment
Cardiovascular abnormalities	Orthostatic hypotension	Fludrocortisone Midodrine
Motor disturbance of gastrointestinal tract	Gastroparesis	Metoclopramide Cisapride Erythromycin
	Constipation	Laxatives, stool softeners
	Diarrhea	Antidiarrheals
Genitourinary tract disturbances	Sexual dysfunction Male: impotence	Sildenafil Alprostadil (injection or penile suppository) Vacuum tumescent devices Testosterone
	Female: insufficient lubrication	Estrogen Vaginal lubricants
Peripheral neuropathy	Nerves of extremities	Amitriptyline Desipramine Imipramine Capsaicin Carbamazepine Phenytoin Mexiletine

glycemia. Although many antihypertensive drugs have been evaluated for preventing and treating diabetic nephropathy, angiotensin-converting enzyme inhibitors (ACEIs) have a greater effect on reducing diabetic proteinuria and slowing creatinine clearance reduction than other types of antihypertensive medications.[33] Additionally, ACEIs have an effect on proteinuria and creatinine that could not be explained by reductions in blood pressure alone, and an ACEI-mediated nephroprotective effect was hypothesized. Currently, many practitioners are treating patients who have diabetic proteinuria, with or without hypertension, with ACEIs in an attempt to slow the progression of nephropathy.

Training the patient with diabetes to monitor foot care and vigorously treat any foot problems can reduce the incidence of infection and gangrene that often necessitates amputation. Patients with diabetes are 15 to 40 times more likely to need lower limb amputation than those without the disease.[34] Ulceration of the foot with subsequent infection often is the initiating lesion. Peripheral vascular disease caused by atherosclerosis, deceased pain sensation caused by nephropathy, and poor immune function may all contribute to the development of foot lesions. Patients with diabetes should thus be instructed to monitor foot care daily, never go barefoot, strictly control blood glucose, and avoid trauma to the feet by properly cutting toenails and selecting shoes that fit properly. The hemorheologic agent pentoxifylline may improve impaired circulation, slow neuropathy development, improve healing, and correct blood flow defects common to patients with diabetes.[35] Becaplermin gel, a topical agent that is genetically engineered platelet-derived growth factor, may promote wound healing and decrease the time to complete ulcer closure in patients with neuropathic lower extremity ulcers.[36] Despite effective treatment modalities, prevention of foot ulcers is always preferred because 20% of people with foot ulcers need amputation.[37]

Nonpharmacologic Therapy

Education

The patient with diabetes spends 365 days a year caring for the condition and monitoring the results of his or her efforts. Each patient with diabetes must understand the disease and be able to follow specific steps to treat the condition and evaluate whether the treatment protocol is achieving its objectives.

Patient education entails a health team approach that includes a physician, nurse, dietitian, pharmacist, and possibly a social worker, psychologist, and exercise physiologist. It is also important that the patient be educated continually and interact with other patients who have diabetes. This can be achieved by active involvement in the Juvenile Diabetes Foundation or the local affiliate of the American Diabetes Association. The educational effort must be well organized and assess each individual's patient's needs. It is also important that patients be evaluated periodically for their competence in performing blood tests, mixing and injecting insulin, rotating injection sites, using the diet exchange system, and following a prescribed exercise program. Education should be broken down into at least three areas:

- Initial management of the diabetes, which provides necessary information to bring the condition under control and gives the patient time to adjust to the condition. This level of education is based on the limitations of the patient and family to accept or assimilate all there is to know about diabetes at the time of diagnosis and the limitations of some settings to provide additional education. During this time the patient is taught the initial skills needed for basic self-care (insulin injection technique, recognition of signs and symptoms of hypoglycemia).
- Home management of diabetes places emphasis on increasing knowledge and flexibility as some experience is gained in adapting and living with diabetes. This level is essential for every patient but must be tailored to each person's needs and capacity. This type of educational experience is preferably offered in a nonhospital environment that is as close to home as possible.
- Lifestyle improvement is the third area in which educational guidelines should be developed. This form of education deals with advanced learning and is viewed as enriching the patient's life with flexibility, insight, and self-determination. This level also provides education on how to respond to special situations such as adjusting insulin dosages when traveling across time zones or using devices designed to assist vision-impaired patients. Unfortunately, many patients with diabetes are left to discover this information by trial and error.

Physical Activity (Exercise)

Physical activity, or exercise, has many positive physical and psychological benefits and should be practiced in some form by most patients with diabetes. Although physicians nearly always recommend exercise as part of diabetes treatment, it is seldom prescribed or followed. Recently, more health care professionals have begun to understand how exercise improves the control of diabetes, and programs are available specifically for patients with diabetes. Exercise improves insulin sensitivity or the ability to drive glucose into the cell. This is particularly important in patients with type 2 diabetes. Exercise also lowers blood glucose by allowing glucose to penetrate the muscle cell and be metabolized without the assistance of insulin. Glucose can be used to varying degrees without insulin in all types of cells. Additionally, exercise improves circulatory function, helps maintain normal body weight, and aids in breathing, digestion, and metabolism. An exercise log may help the patient maintain a regular daily schedule, and patients who monitor their own blood glucose become motivated to exercise because they easily see the beneficial effects of exercise on blood sugar control.

An exercise program should be prescribed and followed by patients with type 1 and type 2 diabetes. Patients should be evaluated before the exercise prescription is determined. The patient's health, interests, preferences, and motivation to exercise should be taken into consideration in developing a specific method of exercising. If blood glucose is greater than 300 mg/dL, exercise can result in an excessive rise in counterregulatory hormones that in the presence of inadequate insulin availability can decrease muscle glucose uptake and increase liver glucose production, causing more pronounced hyperglycemia. Therefore, patients with type 1 diabetes should know their blood glucose level before beginning exercise. If the blood glucose is less than 300 mg/dL, injected insulin that has been absorbed subcutaneously can be absorbed more rapidly, resulting in excessive insulin, which, in combination with the exercise, can cause a serious drop in blood glucose. Patients over the age of 40 and those who have had diabetes for more than 25 years should have an exercise stress test and an individualized graded exercise program should be prescribed. Patients with peripheral sensory neuropathy or vascular insufficiency should avoid exercise that may cause trauma to the feet. Patients with proliferative retinopathy should avoid strenuous exercise, which may induce hemorrhage and resultant blindness.

Exercise-induced hypoglycemia is another concern in patients who exercise. Additional carbohydrate consumed 30 minutes before exercise can help prevent hypoglycemia. Patients should also inject insulin at a nonexercise site (e.g., in the abdomen if the patient intends to run). The patient should log the exercise and monitor what effect it has on his or her blood glucose control. By doing this, a patient will be encouraged to exercise regularly. If hypoglycemia is a recurrent problem, a decrease in the insulin dosage may be warranted. Patients should also be warned to wear an identification bracelet or necklace when exercising in case of an emergency. All patients should carry a quick source of sugar with them when exercising in case hypoglycemia develops. General guidelines for all people with diabetes who exercise include the following: use proper footwear and other protective clothing, avoid exercising in extreme temperatures, inspect feet daily and after each exercise session, and avoid exercise when glycemic control is erratic.[38]

Diet

Nutritional therapy, or diet, is one of the most challenging and difficult aspects of therapy to maintain consistently. For this reason, the American Diabetes Association in recent years has begun to focus on developing nutrition goals that can be achieved with a wide range of diets. Therefore, there is no one "diabetic diet" or "American Diabetes Association diet." Rather, nutritional and therapy goals are established for each patient, taking into consideration the patient's lifestyle, food preferences, cultural background, and other factors that may influence the foods consumed. Table 19.11 provides an overview of diabetes diet therapy and outlines the goals of medical nutrition therapy. It should be stressed that the overall goal of nutrition therapy is to "assist people with diabetes in making changes in nutrition and exercise habits leading to improved metabolic control."[39]

Table 19.11 ▪ Diabetes Diet Therapy and Goals of Medical Nutritional Therapy

Maintain near-normal blood glucose levels by balancing food intake with insulin or oral glucose-lowering medications and activity levels.
Achieve optimal serum lipid levels.
Maintain reasonable weight for adults and growth and development rates in children and adolescents, and meet increased metabolic needs during pregnancy and lactation or recovery from catabolic illnesses. (Reasonable weight is the weight a patient and health care provider acknowledge as achievable and maintainable; it need not be the same as the traditionally defined ideal body weight.)
Prevent and treat acute complications (hypoglycemia, short-term illness, exercise-related problems) and chronic complications such as renal disease, neuropathy, hypertension, and cardiovascular disease.
Improve health by optimizing nutrition.

Source: American Diabetes Association. Nutrition recommendations and principles for people with diabetes mellitus. Diabetes Care 22(Suppl 1):S42–S45, 1999.

Patients should be taught to read labels carefully because many sugarless and dietetic products actually contain a high number of calories and are not effective in helping those with diabetes achieve or maintain ideal body weight. Ingestion of animal (saturated) fats should be minimized because of the increased incidence of atherosclerotic disease in diabetic patients. Some excellent studies have been done that show the importance of increasing fiber in the diet of patients with diabetes. However, each patient needs to see how he or she responds to the various types of fiber. Some fibers that have a high degree of pectin can cause constipation; other fiber products, because of their bulk nature, can cause flatulence and diarrhea. Fiber may have a role in the prevention of colon cancer and can have a beneficial effect on lipid profile. Dietary fiber intake of 20 to 35 g generally is recommended.

To achieve the objectives of diet therapy, the patient must spend time with a dietitian to specifically determine individual goals and outline a method to achieve those goals. Blood glucose monitoring, HbA1c, lipids blood pressure, and renal function are all critical factors in assessing nutrition therapy. In general, protein should be restricted to 10 to 20% of total calories, and in those with renal dysfunction, lower protein intakes may be advised. Protein should be derived from both animal and plant sources.

If 10 to 20% of total calories is derived from protein, then the remaining 80 to 90% will be derived from carbohydrates and fats. In contrast to older dietary recommendations, there are no guidelines on how many calories should come from these latter sources. Simple sugars are no longer shunned, and complex carbohydrates are no longer the only type of carbohydrate recommended. It has been demonstrated that fruits and milk have a lower glycemic index than most starches, and the glycemic response to bread, rice, and potatoes may be similar to that to sucrose. Adjustment of type and proportion of carbohydrate intake is dictated by the goals for that individual patient and should take into account the patient's glucose and lipid profile. Nonnutritive sweeteners approved by the U.S. Food and Drug Administration (FDA), such as saccharin and aspartame, are safe for all patients with diabetes.

Of all the calories consumed, less than 10% should consist of saturated fats and up to 10% from polyunsaturated fats. The desired glucose, lipid, and body weight goals influence the amount of fat to consume. Patients with normal lipid levels and a reasonable weight should receive 30% or less of total calories from total fat and less than 10% of calories as saturated fat. On the other hand, if obesity and weight loss are concerns, a further reduction in fat intake is warranted.

Patients with diabetes need to learn the simple diabetic exchange system, which allows patients to have a large variety of foods. Diet therapy with type 2 diabetes has a high degree of failure and often creates feelings of frustration, pessimism, and anger, which in turn result in poorly informed and inadequately motivated patients. Successful diet programs entail behavior modification. Patients should be encouraged to join groups such as Weight Watchers and to keep a diet log. For a period of 4 to 10 days, each time he or she eats, the patient should write down how much he or she eats and why (whether because of social pressure, loneliness, depression, or nervousness or because nourishment is truly needed). By using smaller plates, taking only one helping of food at a time, and being conscious of why they eat, patients can change their dietary behavior.

One reason diet therapy may fail is that changes in the patient's diet are not accompanied by an appropriate change in the dosage of insulin or other medication. The first steps in diet therapy should be to prescribe an exercise program, lower the medication dosage, and put the patient on a diet containing fewer calories. Insulin overtreatment probably is one of the most common causes of inadequate diabetes control and weight gain. In one group of diabetic patients, 75% needed a reduction in insulin dosage of at least 10%; 35% of the overtreated patients had large appetites, and 30% had hepatomegaly and headaches.[40] Patients taking too much insulin tend to eat up to that level of insulin and therefore gain weight. Also, many patients with type 2 diabetes already have excess serum insulin levels and they still feel hungry after eating a large meal, presumably because of their excess insulin levels.

Alcohol Use

If a patient's diabetes is well controlled, modest amounts of alcohol will significantly alter blood glucose levels. In general, the same guidelines of alcohol use applicable to the general public apply to patients with diabetes. Two government agencies recommend that no more than two drinks per day for men and one drink a day for women are considered safe and reasonable.[41] Pregnant women and patients with a history of alcoholism or alcohol abuse should avoid alcohol. Likewise, if other medical conditions exist that could be exacerbated by alcohol (e.g., pancreatitis, neuropathy), then abstention from alcohol would be prudent. Alcohol should always be ingested along with a meal, and patients on insulin or sulfonylureas may be more susceptible to altered blood glucose levels when consuming alcohol. Two first-generation sulfonylureas, tolbutamide and chlorpropamide, have been reported to interact with alcohol, resulting in a disulfiramlike reaction. The second-generation agents do not appear to cause such a reaction.

Patients who consume alcoholic beverages must consider the caloric content of the beverage and should be encouraged to choose low-calorie drinks. The sugar content of wines and mixed drinks also must be considered.

Blood Pressure and Lipid Control

The presence of hypertension or dyslipidemias in patients with diabetes contributes to the chronic complications that include nephropathy, retinopathy, cerebrovascular disease, and cardiovascular disease. In general, diabetes places patients at risk for atherosclerotic vascular disease, and this risk increases when hypertension or dyslipidemias are present. Additionally, obesity and smoking can further contribute to the development of vascular complications. Table 19.12 lists current guidelines for blood pressure and lipid control in patients with diabetes.

Pharmacotherapy

The therapeutic options available in the United States for managing diabetes mellitus have expanded greatly in the past few years. Currently, six categories of FDA-approved medications for treating diabetes are available: insulin,

Table 19.12 ▪ Treatment Goals for Blood Pressure and Lipids

Blood Pressure	
Adults	<130/85 mm Hg
Isolated systemic hypertension of ≥180 mm Hg	<160 mm Hg
Systolic 160–179	Reduce by 20 mm Hg
Lipids	
LDL	≤100 mg/d
Triglycerides	<200 mg/dL
HDL (men)	>35 mg/dL
HDL (women)	>45 mg/dL

Source: American Diabetes Association. Standards of medical care for patients with diabetes mellitus. Diabetes Care 22(Suppl 1):S32–S41, 1999.

LDL, low-density lipoprotein; *HDL,* high-density lipoprotein.

Table 19.13 ▪ Factors Considered in Comparing Insulins

Kinetic formulation and time activity profile
Species source (human, pork, beef)
Strength (U-100, U-500)
Methods of achieving long action (e.g., protein such as protamine)
Purity
Mixability
Cost
Manufacturer dependability and availability

sulfonylureas, biguanides, α-glucosidase inhibitors, thiazolidinediones, and meglitinides. All six categories of medicines can treat patients with type 2 diabetes effectively, but insulin is the only diabetic medication needed for those with type 1 disease.

Because the recent expansion in the number of antidiabetic drugs available, choosing the optimal medication or combinations for the management of hyperglycemia in patients with diabetes is not easily reduced to a single treatment algorithm. Treating the patient with diabetes remains an art and entails constant reevaluation and assessment of the patient's response to proven therapies. Although some situations clearly warrant the use of one product over another, the choice of medications usually is not clear-cut, and cost considerations, amount of glycemic lowering needed, compliance issues, and the patient's age, weight, and lipid profile all factor into the decision-making process.

Insulin

Insulin has been used since 1922 as monotherapy in patients with type 1 disease and since the late 1950s in combination or monotherapy in patients with type 2 disease. Typically, patients who have type 1 diabetes and need insulin initially tend to be younger than 30 years old, lean, markedly hyperglycemic, and prone to developing ketoacidosis.

Children with diabetes should begin giving their own injections around age 8 or 9, although parents should periodically administer insulin to stay in practice and should inject in areas that are difficult for the child to reach. All patients on insulin therapy should be strongly encouraged to self-monitor blood glucose levels. Insulin regimens should be tailored to each patient's individual needs, desired metabolic control, and age. Tighter glycemic control is best achieved with three or four insulin injections per day or with an infusion pump, although not all patient populations are best served by regimens offering strict glycemic control (e.g., the very old, the very young).

Choice of Insulins

The time action profile, effects of mixing, species, strength, and cost of insulin all must be considered in choosing insulin. Factors to consider when choosing insulin are outlined in Table 19.13, and Table 19.14 summarizes the currently available insulins.

Time Activity Profile. Insulins may be categorized in the following groups on the basis of their time activity profiles: ultra-short-acting, short-acting, intermediate-acting, and long-acting. Figure 19.5 shows the kinetic parameters of the four categories of insulin. Each patient may experience variations in clinical response to any particular class of insulin, and the characteristics of each insulin (time of onset, time to peak, duration of action) can vary from patient to patient. Table 19.15 describes some of the factors that may alter the time activity profiles of insulin.

The only ultra–short-acting insulin available is the insulin analog insulin lispro. Human insulin analogs have a similar structure and function to human insulin but are developed with DNA recombinant technology. By altering the amino acid sequence in human insulin, manufacturers

Table 19.14 ▪ Insulins Available in the United States

Product	Manufacturer	Strength
Ultra–short-acting		
Humalog (Insulin lispro)	Lilly	U-100
Short-acting		
Pork		
Iletin II Regular	Lilly	U-100, U-500
Purified Pork Regular	Novo-Nordisk	U-100
Beef and pork		
Iletin I Regular	Lilly	U-100
Human		
Humulin Regular	Lilly	U-100
Novolin R	Novo-Nordisk	U-100
Velosulin Human R	Novo-Nordisk	U-100
Intermediate-acting		
Pork		
Iletin II Lente	Lilly	U-100
Iletin II NPH	Lilly	U-100
Purified Pork Lente	Novo-Nordisk	U-100
Purified Pork NPH	Novo-Nordisk	U-100
Beef and pork		
Iletin I NPH	Lilly	U-100
Iletin I Lente	Lilly	U-100
Human		
Humulin L (Lente)	Lilly	U-100
Humulin N (NPH)	Lilly	U-100
Novolin L (Lente)	Lilly	U-100
Novolin N (NPH)	Lilly	U-100
Long-acting		
Human		
Humulin U (Ultralente)	Lilly	U-100
Fixed combinations (all are U-100 insulins)		
Human		NPH/Regular
Humulin 70/30	Lilly	70/30
Novolin 70/30	Novo-Nordisk	70/30
Humulin 50/50	Lilly	50/50

NPH, neutral protamine Hagedorn.

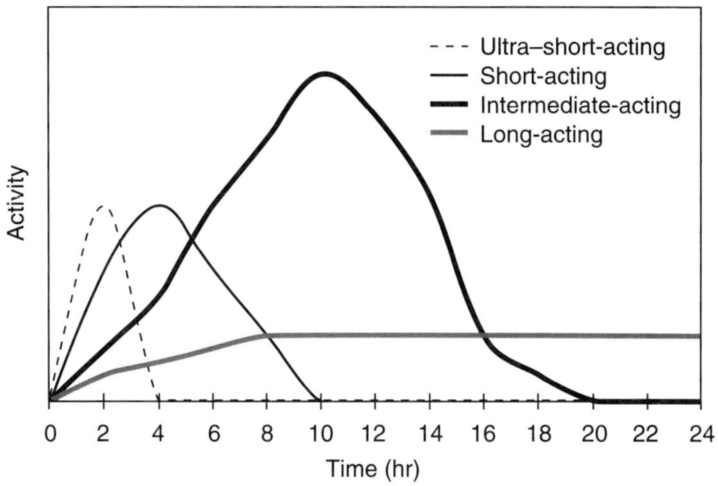

Insulin Type	Onset	Peak	Duration
Ultra–short-acting	0–0.25 hr	1–2 hr	2–4 hr
Short-acting	0.5–1 hr	2–4 hr	6–8 hr
Intermediate-acting	1–4 hr	6–10 hr	16–24 hr
Long-acting	4–6 hr	18 hr	24–36 hr

Figure 19.5. Time activity profiles for insulin.

Table 19.15 ▪ Factors Affecting Serum Insulin Concentrations

Injection site (abdomen, arm, thigh)
Exercise (enhances absorption)
Depth of injection
Concentration of insulin
Increase in ambient temperature (increases absorption)
Massage of site (increases absorption)
Insulin antibodies (attract and hold insulin)
Variance in degrading enzymes at site (yields day-to-day variation)
Insulin interaction with receptors

can create various alterations in the actions of insulin. Insulin lispro has the normal sequence of proline (Pro) and lysine (Lys) reversed at the twenty-eighth and twenty-ninth positions. The change in amino acid sequence results in rapid absorption from the subcutaneous tissues, resulting in a faster physiologic action than human regular insulin.[42] Insulin lispro can be administered immediately before a meal and provides added flexibility, particularly for young patients and those with erratic meal schedules. Because of its unique rapidity of action, it may be safer and more predictable in regard to the development of hypoglycemia. Insulin aspart is another ultra–short-acting insulin that is expected to gain FDA approval in the near future.

The short-acting insulins include semilente, regular, and regular buffered insulins. Regular and buffered insulin formulations are clear and contain solubilized crystalline insulin. Regular insulin and insulin lispro are the only two insulins that can be given intravenously, but regular is the only insulin used in this fashion because intravenous use of insulin lispro would be more expensive and would not provide any advantage over regular insulin. The only FDA-approved insulin for use in insulin pumps is Velosulin BR (buffered regular human insulin); however, human regular insulin has been safely used for many years, and insulin lispro is commonly used with this mode of delivery with excellent results. Velosulin BR may soon be available as a genetically engineered product. Semilente is an amorphous precipitate of insulin and zinc in the form of a suspension, with a slightly delayed onset and peak and a greater duration of action than regular insulin.

Intermediate-acting insulins include neutral protamine Hagedorn (NPH) and lente insulins. NPH insulin preparations contain a suspension of zinc–insulin crystals and protamine, which is a protein derived from fish sperm. A small number of patients are or can become allergic to protamine. Lente insulin is composed of a 30:70 mixture of semilente and ultralente. The lente insulins are produced form various forms of the zinc–insulin complex and were particularly useful in patients sensitive to protamine. The only available long-acting insulin is ultralente.

Currently, two strengths of insulin are available in the United States: U-100 and U-500. U-500 can be obtained only by prescription and must be special ordered from Eli Lilly. In Europe insulin is available only by prescription and in one strength, U-40.

Species Source and Purity. Species source is becoming less of a concern as more and more patients are switched to or are started on human forms of insulin. The following sources of insulin are available: beef, pork, beef and pork mixtures, biosynthetic human, semisynthetic human, and analogs of human insulin. Pork insulin is less antigenic than beef insulin, and roughly 80% of patients with persistent local allergy to mixed beef–pork insulin improve when treated with pure pork insulin or human insulin.[43] Purified pork insulin has no clear advantages over human insulin, and its availability may cease in the near future.

Human insulin is the least antigenic of the available insulins and tends to be more soluble than animal insulins. This results in more rapid absorption and shorter duration of action, so a patient being switched from one source of insulin to another should be monitored closely. Close monitoring is also needed for patients switching from a short-acting insulin to ultra–short-acting insulin lispro.

Biosynthetic insulin and semisynthetic insulin are all therapeutically equivalent. Biosynthetic insulins include an insulin formed by recombinant DNA using *Escherichia coli* (Eli Lilly), insulin formed by biosynthetic recombinant DNA using baker's yeast (Novo-Nordisk), and semisynthetic insulin (Novo-Nordisk). Insulin is produced through recombinant processes by the insertion of the human gene for proinsulin into the *E. coli* or baker's yeast genome. These genetically altered organisms are fermented in an appropriate medium that is conducive to the production of proinsulin (or a miniproinsulin). The proinsulin is harvested, enzymatically altered to form insulin, and purified. Human insulin is also produced via a semisynthetic method by the enzymatic transpeptidation of pork insulin at position 30 of the B chain with the substitution of threonine for alanine.

The recommendations for dosing insulin when changing from beef to human insulin or from conventional to purified insulin are summarized in Table 19.16. Human insulin is indicated for the patient types listed in Table 19.17. All patients with insulin allergy should be placed on human insulin.

Another factor that may affect insulin choice is purity. Most forms of insulin available today are highly purified and are unlikely to contain substances that affect the action of the insulin. All of the insulins listed in Table 19.14 are classified as highly purified because they have fewer than 10 parts per million of proinsulin. Highly purified insulins are less likely to produce lipoatrophy or cause insulin antibody formation.

Insulin Dosing

A number of dosing regimens are used in administering insulin to patients with type 1 diabetes (Fig. 19.6). Commonly used methods include the following:

1. Single daily injection of intermediate-acting insulin.
2. Two daily injections of intermediate-acting insulin.
3. Two daily injections of 70:30 intermediate:short-acting premixed insulin.
4. Two daily injections of split and mixed intermediate and short-acting insulin.
5. Three daily injections of short-acting (or ultra–short-acting) insulin in combination with a single injection of long-acting insulin.
6. Continuous subcutaneous insulin infusion (insulin infusion pump).
7. Sliding scale (multiple daily injections of short-acting or ultra–short-acting insulin).

Table 19.16 ▪ Recommendations for Dosing Insulin When Changing from Beef to Human or Conventional to Purified Insulin

Highly variable from patient to patient; monitor patient closely (decreases of 9–20% reported).
Recommend 10% decrease of normal dosages.
Recommend 20% decrease if patient receiving more than 50 U/day.

Table 19.17 ▪ Patients Who Should Use Human Insulin

Patients with insulin resistance (using more than 100–200 U/day)
Patients with insulin allergy (e.g., local cutaneous reactions, rashes)
Patients with lipoatrophy or lipohypertrophy
All patients with type 2 diabetes using insulin for a short period of time (e.g., during surgery, infections)
Any patient using insulin intermittently (e.g., patients with gestational diabetes, those on total parenteral nutrition)
All newly diagnosed patients with type 1 diabetes
Pregnant patients (antibodies are passed to the fetus)

The level of practitioner motivation, patient ability to monitor glucose control and adjust dosages, and level of control desired affect the choice of regimen. The daily insulin need of the typical patient with type 1 diabetes is 0.5 to 1.0 U/kg/day. This total daily dosage may be given as one injection (method 1) or may be divided into several doses to more closely mimic physiologic insulin secretion. Premeal doses of insulin are adjusted; approximately 1 to 2 U insulin is given for each 50 mg/dL of desired decrease in blood glucose levels.

Insulin can be delivered through different devices, the most common being the syringe. Insulin pumps, jet injectors, and insulin pens are additional methods of delivery. When syringes are used properly, the injections are not painful because of finer needles and the use of special coatings that allow easy insertion. Insulin pumps are small, computerized, externally worn devices that deliver a steady dose of insulin through a small plastic tube and a small needle that is inserted and taped into place in the abdominal region. A bolus dose of insulin can be given upon command before meals. Jet injectors force a pressurized stream of insulin through the skin, thereby avoiding puncturing of the skin. This mode of injecting may cause some skin bruising. Insulin pen devices are small and convenient and look much like old-fashioned cartridge pens. The insulin is stored in prefilled cartridges that can be replaced. Additionally, insulin pens can be adjusted easily to deliver a precise amount of insulin, and some devices are disposable. The insulin pen device is well suited for patients with limited coordination (e.g., older adults) and for people leading active lives.

Method Comparison

Method 1. A single injection of intermediate-acting insulin is not sufficient to control blood glucose levels for a 24-hour period. This regimen usually results in hyperglycemia before the next dose and may cause hypoglycemia that coincides with peak levels about 8 hours after the

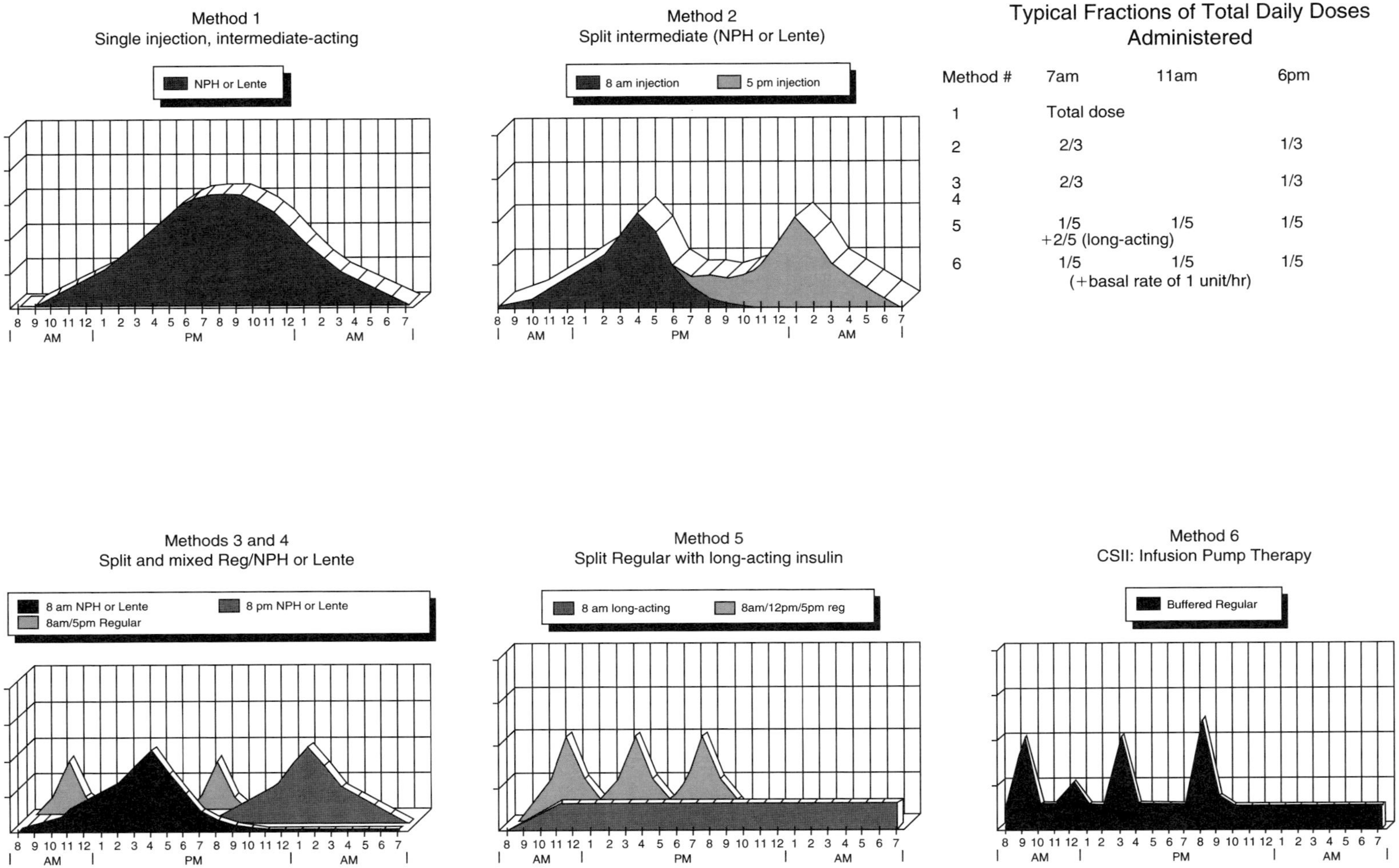

Typical Fractions of Total Daily Doses Administered

Method #	7am	11am	6pm
1	Total dose		
2	2/3		1/3
3 4	2/3		1/3
5	1/5 +2/5 (long-acting)	1/5	1/5
6	1/5 (+basal rate of 1 unit/hr)	1/5	1/5

Figure 19.6. Commonly used insulin regimens.

dose. A dose that is high enough to cover the patient for 24 hours usually will also cause hypoglycemia at the peak. Ketoacidosis may be avoided, but erratic blood glucose swings are common. HbA1c levels attained with this regimen typically fall in the range of 11 to 13%, which is unacceptable blood glucose control.

METHOD 2. Glycemic control is slightly greater than that with method 1. With method 2, two-thirds of the total daily insulin requirement is injected before breakfast and one-third is injected just before dinner. Intermediate-acting insulin is used. The chance of developing hypoglycemia is less with this method than with method 1, but the glycemic control attained is only slightly better than that of method 1.

METHODS 3 AND 4. These two methods provide average to above-average control with two injections per day. The only difference between the two methods is that with method 3 the patient can only increase or decrease the individual doses but not alter the ratio of short-acting to intermediate-acting insulin. The patient usually takes two-thirds of the total daily dose before breakfast and one-third before dinner. The split and mixed regimen is initiated with a 70:30 mixture of intermediate:short-acting insulin, but this ratio may be altered according to insulin needs. Blood sugar must be monitored before meals and at bedtime and the insulin dosage adjusted accordingly. Method 4 is the preferred over method 3. A common variation of method 3 is to administer a mixed (intermediate and short-acting) dose before breakfast, a dose of short-acting insulin before dinner, and a dose of intermediate-acting insulin at bedtime. Glycemic control expected with these methods may provide HbA1c values in the range of 7 to 9%, with few symptoms.

METHOD 5. This multidose method uses doses of short-acting or ultra–short-acting insulin before each meal in combination with one or two daily doses of a longer-acting insulin. Variations of this method include administering regular or insulin lispro before each meal with a dose of intermediate-acting insulin at bedtime. This regimen entails a great deal of patient motivation but provides excellent glycemic coverage and allows the patient a great deal of latitude with regard to meals.

METHOD 6. Continuous subcutaneous insulin infusion is an excellent method. Initially, this method requires intensive patient training, but the increased flexibility and freedom are unparalleled by other dosage regimens. This method provides the patient with a continuous basal amount of insulin (0.5 to 1 U/hour) in combination with pulsatile doses to cover meals. Currently available pumps are about the size of a deck of cards and weigh only a few ounces. Insulin reaches the patient via a small plastic catheter and through a subcutaneous needle. Table 19.18 summarizes the criteria that are used for selecting patients to use.[44] Factors to be considered for insulin pump selection include availability of safety and clinical features (low-battery alarm, programmable basal rates), durability, service level of manufacturer, ease of use, and cosmetic appeal. HbA1c values commonly achieved with methods 5 and 6 fall in the range of 6 to 7%.

Table 19.18 ▪ Criteria for Prescribing Insulin Pumps

Selecting patients
- Pregnant patients
- Patients with early complications
- Renal transplant recipients
- Patients with difficult-to-control diabetes
- Motivated patients with type 1 diabetes
- Not suitable for children and patients with type 2 diabetes
- All patients must be
  - Willing and highly motivated
  - Capable of learning to use pump correctly
  - Responsible for keeping records and following specific procedures
  - Willing to perform and log blood tests daily
  - Willing to be hospitalized for 2–4 days if necessary

Pump selection
- Safety features (e.g., low-battery alarm)
- Durability
- Service level by manufacturer
- Degree of training provided by manufacturer
- Ease of use
- Clinical features (e.g., programmable basal rates)
- Cosmetic appeal

METHOD 7. The sliding scale method is reserved for hospitalized patients who undergo frequent blood glucose monitoring. Insulin dosage adjustments in patients who are acutely ill require more insulin than normal, and the scales used in these patients vary from institution to institution. The following is an example of a sliding scale that uses regular insulin for an adult:

Blood Glucose	Subcutaneous Insulin Dosage
<140 mg/dL	0 U
140–200 mg/dL	2 U
201–300 mg/dL	5 U
301–400 mg/dL	10 U
>400 mg/dL	12 U

The scale is adjusted on the basis of patient response to various dosages of insulin.

Interpretation of Blood Glucose Levels

Several problems may be encountered in SMBG. Proper patient technique and understanding of a patient's particular method should always be ascertained before insulin dosage is adjusted. Patients who are being treated with methods 3 through 6 should routinely check blood glucose levels four times daily, before meals and at bedtime. Additionally, early morning (3:00 to 4:00 AM) and postprandial levels may be checked on a nonroutine basis as needed. Patients who use method 1 should also be instructed to check blood glucose levels. However, it is difficult to target particular out-of-range levels because only one dose is administered daily.

Generally, an increase in insulin dosage of 1 U can be expected to decrease the blood glucose level by approximately 50 mg/dL. Some patients adjust dosages daily on the basis of the previous day's response. This approach may be reasonable for some; however, it is probably more prudent to alter dosages only after a trend has been identified.

Two potential problems observed with the interpretation of morning fasting blood glucose levels include the dawn effect and the Somogyi phenomenon. The dawn effect results from a rise in blood glucose levels that increases insulin need starting at about 5:00 AM and continuing until about 9:00 AM. The early morning glucose rise can be caused by insufficient treatment, but in studies involving patients with continuous subcutaneous insulin infusion, the dawn phenomenon can still occur. Food ingestion is another factor that could influence early morning rise. Yet studies of fasting patients show that blood glucose levels can increase in the early morning. Although the phenomenon and its prevalence are not totally understood, it is a cause for concern for patients who are trying to achieve strict control. The most logical mechanism for the dawn phenomenon is an increased glucose production or decreased glucose use caused by the morning rise of cortisol levels or other circadian influences.

The Somogyi phenomenon is a condition in which there is early morning hyperglycemia secondary to hypoglycemia. The diabetic patient suffers an episode of hypoglycemia during sleep that results in the release of hormones that increase blood glucose levels such as cortisol, glucagon, and adrenaline. These hormones cause blood glucose levels to increase, and when the patient arises in the morning and tests his or her blood glucose, it is elevated. Because hypoglycemia is the precipitating cause of this phenomenon, the necessary step in treatment is to decrease the insulin dosage.

The assessment of morning hyperglycemia must include an early morning (3:00 AM to 4:00 AM) blood glucose determination. If hypoglycemia is observed, then the bedtime or evening insulin dosage should be decreased. If the level is within normal limits or high, then a slight increase in the evening insulin dosage is warranted.

Mixing and Storing Insulin

Insulin can be stored at room temperature for up to 1 month and should be injected at room temperature for patient comfort. Unused vials of insulin may be stored in the refrigerator, but they should not be exposed to extreme temperatures. Patients should be cautioned to store insulin properly when traveling in very hot or very cold climates.

Regular and NPH insulin are stable when mixed together in any ratio, and they are the mixture of choice when short- and intermediate-acting insulin is needed.[45] Patients should adhere to the following sequence when mixing NPH and regular insulin:

1. Inject the appropriate quantity of air into the NPH insulin vial.
2. Inject the appropriate quantity of air into the regular insulin vial.
3. Withdraw the dose of regular insulin.
4. Withdraw the dose of NPH insulin.

Insulin lispro can also be mixed in the same syringe with NPH insulin or insulin zinc suspension insulins. As with regular insulin, always draw the insulin lispro into the syringe first, then introduce the other insulin into the syringe. Regular and lente (also ultralente) insulin interact when mixed, the result being a blunting of the short-acting insulin. Patients should be instructed to either inject immediately after mixing or consistently inject after a measured period of time. The reaction between lente and regular insulin continues for 24 hours, so the response from an injections that is taken immediately after mixing may be significantly different from the response from an injection taken 24 hours after mixing. Velosulin regular insulins should not be mixed with lente insulins. The phosphate buffers precipitate the zinc from these formulations, resulting in an increased activity of short-acting insulin. Lente insulins may be mixed with each other in any ratio without affecting the time activity profile of the components, and mixtures of this nature remain stable for up to 18 months.

Adverse Reactions to Insulin

The most common and serious reaction to insulin therapy is hypoglycemia. Previously, when less pure sources of insulin were used, lipoatrophy, insulin allergy, and insulin antibody formation were more common, but they are now uncommon.

HYPOGLYCEMIA. All patients with diabetes should know the signs and symptoms of hypoglycemia, particularly patients on insulin therapy (oral hypoglycemic therapy, discussed shortly). Factors that predispose the patient to hypoglycemia include insufficient food intake (skipping meals, vomiting, or diarrhea), poor timing of injections in relation to food intake, excessive exercise, inaccurate measurement of insulin, concomitant intake of hypoglycemic drugs, termination of diabetogenic conditions or drugs, and strict glycemic control. Symptoms of hypoglycemia include a parasympathetic response (nausea, hunger, or flatulence), diminished cerebral function (confusion, agitation, lethargy, or personality changes), sympathetic responses (tachycardia, sweating, or tremor), coma, and convulsions. Ataxia and blurred vision also are common. In older adults with decreased nerve function, patients with advanced neuropathy, patients with diabetes of 10 years or more duration, or patients receiving β-blockers, the symptoms of hypoglycemia sometimes are blunted or absent and the condition may go undetected and untreated. All manifestations of hypoglycemia are relieved rapidly by glucose administration. In unconscious patients, injections of glucagon or intravenous glucose or dextrose may be needed.

Because of the potential danger of insulin reactions, the diabetic patient should always carry packets of table sugar or candy for use at the onset of hypoglycemic symptoms. Note also that if a hypoglycemic person is mistakenly thought to be hyperglycemic and is given insulin, severe hypoglycemia and subsequent brain damage may result. Thus, when there is doubt as to whether a diabetic person is hypoglycemic or hyperglycemic, sugar should be given initially until the condition can be evaluated accurately. Spouses or caregivers of patients with diabetes should be trained to administer glucagon in the event of hypoglycemic-induced unconsciousness. Glucagon (1 mg) should be administered subcutaneously or intramuscularly. Glucagon may cause nausea and vomiting; therefore, the unconscious patient should be positioned lying on his or her side or on his or her stomach to avoid aspiration.

Virtually every patient treated with insulin experiences hypoglycemia at some time. Ten percent of insulin-treated patients need assistance for at least one episode of severe hypoglycemia per year. Mortality secondary to hypoglycemia in insulin-treated patients may be as high as 3%.[45] Patients in the DCCT who were treated with intensive insulin therapy had an incidence of hypoglycemia three times higher than that of patients treated with conventional therapy.[1]

LIPOHYPERTROPHY. Lipohypertrophy is a problem encountered by patients who do not rotate injection sites. With repeated use of a single injection site, the area becomes anesthetized. Fatty tumors occur and usually resolve after the patient begins to rotate sites. Because this problem probably is not immunologic in nature, switching to a more highly purified product is not warranted.

LIPOATROPHY. Atrophy of the fatty tissue appears to be an immunologic process, and lipoatrophy may occur at the injection site or at a distant location. Female patients are affected more than male patients. The treatment of choice is to switch to human insulin. Human insulin should be injected directly into the atrophied area until the site has filled in. After resolution, the patient should be instructed to continue to inject the area every 2 to 3 weeks to prevent recurrence.[46]

Oral Medications for Treating Type 2 Diabetes

Oral therapy is very efficacious in treating patients with type 2 diabetes, but all patients should first be tried on course of diet and exercise for 3 months before oral therapy is used. Certain situations dictate the use of intravenous therapy over oral agents in patients with type 2 diabetes (e.g., development of NKHS, presence of severely elevated blood glucose values), but the importance of diet and exercise can not be overstated. Some patients with type 2 diabetes can totally manage their disease by losing weight and following a strict exercise program. Even if oral medication is needed, patients who exercise regularly and are on a proper diet can manage their condition on less medicine than those not on a suitable diet or exercise program.

Sulfonylureas

Sulfonylureas have been the mainstay of therapy for patients with type 2 diabetes since the late 1970s. This class of agents will continue to be widely used for treating diabetes, but as more is learned about the pathophysiology of insulin resistance and type 2 diabetes, agents with other mechanisms of action than the sulfonylureas (insulin secretagogues) will play an important role in diabetes treatment.

Sulfonylureas have demonstrated both pancreatic and extrapancreatic effects but are useful only in patients with intact and functioning β-cells.[47] Sulfonylureas increase insulin secretion directly and decrease glucagon release. Additionally, sulfonylureas may affect glucose levels by increasing insulin receptor binding affinity, increasing insulin effect by postreceptor action, and decreasing hepatic insulin extraction. The clinical effects of these extrapancreatic effects continue to be a subject of research and debate.

The following patient characteristics sometimes predict a positive clinical response to sulfonylureas: The patient is not diagnosed with diabetes until after age 40, the duration of diabetes is less than 5 years, the patient is near or above his or her ideal body weight, there has been no prior insulin treatment or the disease has been controlled with less than 40 U insulin per day, and the fasting blood glucose is less than 180 mg/dL.

The available sulfonylureas are summarized in Table 19.19. Chlorpropamide has the longest half-life of the first-generation agents and is associated in the highest incidence of adverse events. Chlorpropamide generally is not recommended for newly diagnosed patients. The second-generation agents tend be less potent, so higher dosages are needed. They also tend to displace drugs from protein-binding sites and are more likely to have drug interactions. Drug interactions with the first-generation agents include alcohol, anabolic steroids, β-blockers, dicoumarol, monoamine oxidase inhibitors, salicylates, and sulfonamides. Second-generation sulfonylureas are more potent and tend to have fewer drug interactions because they bind nonionically and are present at much lower concentrations than the first-generation agents. Tolbutamide, tolazamide, and glipizide are metabolized to inactive or weakly active metabolites and are favored in patients with renal failure. The newest sulfonylurea, glimepiride, has similar effects as the other sulfonylureas and can be given once daily. Additionally, glimepiride is reported to have a lower incidence of hypoglycemia than other sulfonylureas, perhaps making it an attractive choice in older adults.[48]

The primary side effects of sulfonylureas include hypoglycemia and weight gain. The incidence of hypoglycemia is variable and depends on the agent and patient characteristics. One study reported a 20% chance of developing hypoglycemia in every 6 months of continuous sulfonylurea therapy.[47] Weight gain in the range of 1.8 to 2.8 kg has been documented in clinical studies. Conditions in which the sulfonylureas usually are contraindicated include acidosis, severe infections, major surgery, sulfa sensitivity, and pregnancy. Approximately 40% of patients with type 2 diabetes do not achieve satisfactory control with the sulfonylureas.[49] Ten percent of all patients do not respond initially and are considered to be primary failures. Secondary failure occurs with long-term use and approaches 30%.

In general, therapy should be started with a low dosage and gradually titrated until desired effect is achieved. Low dosages are given once daily before breakfast; higher dosages are split and given two or more times per day, depending on the half-life and formulation of the drug. Table 19.20 lists counseling points for each category of oral agents.

Biguanides

Metformin is a biguanide that lowers blood glucose by reducing hepatic glucose production and glycogen metabolism in the liver and enhancing insulin-mediated glucose uptake by skeletal muscle. Phenformin, a cousin of metformin, was removed from the market because of a high incidence of lactic acidosis (64 cases per 100,000 patient years). Roughly 5 to 9 patients per 100,000 patients treated with metformin develop lactic acidosis, mainly those with contraindications to its use.[50] Metformin has a much lower incidence of lactic acidosis, and when recommended prescribing guidelines are followed, it is extremely rare.

Abdominal bloating, nausea, intestinal cramping, and diarrhea are common adverse effects of metformin, particularly when therapy is initiated. With continued use many of these side effects dissipate, and side effects can be lessened by always taking with food and starting with a low dosage and slowly titrating to a maximum of 2550 mg. In one dose–response trial, the greatest glycemic effect was observed at a dosage of 2000 mg per day, and dosages greater than that have less of an effect.[51] Metformin typically is started at 500 mg twice daily and then titrated every 1 to 2 weeks by 500 mg. If the patient is started on 850 mg, this is usually given once daily and then titrated as needed. This drug should always be taken with food.

Metformin is not metabolized and is secreted primarily by the renal tubules, so it is contraindicated in patients with renal dysfunction (serum creatinine greater than 1.5 mg/dL in male patients or greater than 1.4 in female patients), clinical laboratory evidence of hepatic dysfunction, acute or chronic lactic acidosis, or a history of alcoholism or binge drinking, or in patients who need pharmacologic management of congestive heart failure (CHF). Metformin should be withheld temporarily in patients experiencing conditions that may predispose them to acute renal failure or acidosis, such as cardiovascular collapse, acute myocardial infarction, or acute exacerbation of CHF, or undergoing a major surgical procedure. Lastly, metformin should be discontinued before intravenous iodinated contrast media are administered and not restarted until 48 hours after the procedure and upon documentation of normal renal function.

Monotherapy with metformin reduces fasting plasma glucose levels an average of 58 mg/dL and HbA1c an average of 1.8%. Additionally, metformin is associated with a reduction in triglyceride concentrations (16%), low-density lipoprotein (LDL) cholesterol (8%), and total cholesterol (5%) and is associated with a slight increase in high-density lipoprotein (HDL) cholesterol (2%).[52] Many patients lose a small amount of weight when metformin is used, which is useful for the many overweight patients with type 2 diabetes.[51] Metformin can also be used in combination with insulin or sulfonylureas for patients with type 2 diabetes. As with oral antidiabetic agents, the risk of hypoglycemia increases when it is used with insulin secretagogues (sulfonylureas) or insulin.

α-Glucosidase Inhibitors

α-Glucosidase enzymes in the brush border of the small intestines, along with pancreatic α-amylase, are responsible for the hydrolysis of complex starches, oligosaccharides, trisaccharides, and disaccharides. Acarbose, an α-glucosidase and α-amylase inhibitor, works by reducing the rate of complex carbohydrate digestion and subsequent absorption of glucose, thereby lowering postprandial glucose excursions in patients with diabetes.[53] Acarbose is particularly effective for patients who experience postprandial hyperglycemia. Miglitol is another α-glucosidase inhibitor that works similarly to acarbose and likewise is effective in controlling postprandial hyperglycemia.

Dose-related side effects of the α-glucosidase inhibitors are mainly gastrointestinal in nature and include flatulence, diarrhea, and abdominal pain. Slow titration of these agents may lessen the severity of side effects, and patients who can continue to take the medicine may develop tolerance to the side effects. Although the α-glucosidase inhibitors by themselves are not considered hypoglycemic agents, when they are used in combination with insulin or a sulfonylurea, hypoglycemia can occur. Hypoglycemic episodes in patients taking α-glucosidase inhibitors must be treated with oral glucose tablets or gel because oral complex carbohydrates cannot be digested and absorbed.

Patients with inflammatory bowel disease, colonic ulceration, obstructive bowel disorders, or any gastrointestinal condition in which excess intestinal gas would be detrimental should not receive these agents. Patients with serum creatinine levels higher than 2.0 mg/dL should not receive α-glucosidase inhibitors. The α-glucosidase inhibitors can interact with intestinal adsorbents such as charcoal, and supplemental pancreatic or intestinal enzyme replacements containing amylase, pancrelipase, or

Table 19.19 ▪ Oral Antidiabetic Agents

Generic	Brand	Mechanism of Action	Dosing	Side Effects
First-Generation Sulfonylureas				
Acetohexamide	Dymelor	Stimulates the release of insulin from pancreatic β-cells	250 mg QD; titrate to a maximum dosage of 1.5 g/day (divided)	GI, blood dyscrasias, SIADH, disulfiram reaction, and hypoglycemia
Chlorpropamide (not recommended)	Diabinese		250 mg QD; titrate to a maximum dosage of 750 mg/day (divided) Older adults, 100–125 mg QD	GI, blood dyscrasias, disulfiram reaction, dilutional hyponatremia, and prolonged hypoglycemia
Tolazamide	Tolinase		100–250 mg QD; titrate to a maximum of 500 mg BID Adults over 65, 50–125 mg QD; titrate	GI, blood dyscrasias, disulfiram reaction, and hypoglycemia
Tolbutamide	Orinase		1–2 g QD; titrate to a maximum dosage of 3 g (divided)	GI, blood dyscrasias, disulfiram reaction, dilutional hyponatremia, and hypoglycemia
Second-Generation Sulfonylureas				
Glimepiride	Amaryl	Stimulates the release of insulin from pancreatic β-cells	1–2 mg QD; titrate to a maximum dosage of 8 mg/day	GI, blood dyscrasias, cholestatic jaundice, and hypoglycemia
Glipizide	Glucotrol and Glucotrol XL		5 mg QD; titrate to a maximum dosage of 40 mg/day (divided)	GI, blood dyscrasias, cholestatic jaundice, disulfiram reaction, and hypoglycemia
Glyburide	Diabeta, Micronase, and Glynase (micronized)		2.5–5 mg QD; titrate to a maximum dosage of 20 mg/day Micronized: 1.5–3 mg QD; titrate to a maximum dosage of 12 mg/day	GI, visual changes, blood dyscrasias, cholestatic jaundice, hepatitis, increased LFT values, and hypoglycemia
α-Glucosidase Inhibitor				
Acarbose	Precose	Competitive and reversible inhibition of intestinal α-glucoside hydrolase and pancreatic α-amylase, resulting in delayed carbohydrate metabolism and absorption	25 mg TID with first bite of food of each main meal; titrate every 4–8 wk to a maximum dosage of 50–100 mg TID ≤60 kg: 50 mg TID; ≥60 kg: 100 mg TID	GI and increase in LFT values
Miglitol	Glyset		25 mg TID with first bite of food of each main meal; titrate over 4–8 wk up to 50 mg TID; if not at HgAlc goal in 3 mo, titrate up to 100 mg TID	GI

		Biguanide		
Metformin	Glucophage	Decreases hepatic glucose production and increases peripheral insulin sensitivity	500 mg BID or 850 mg QD; titrate 500 mg weekly to a maximum dosage of 2500 mg/day or 850 mg every 2 wk to a maximum dosage of 2550 mg/day (maximum of 2000 mg/day just as effective as higher dosage)	GI, megaloblastic anemia, lactic acidosis, and alterations in taste
		Thiazolidinediones		
Troglitazone	Rezulin	Increases skeletal muscle cell sensitivity to insulin and decreases hepatic glucose production	Combination therapy: 200 mg QD; titrate every 2–4 wk to a maximum dosage of 600 mg/day	Liver failure, risk of pregnancy in anovulatory women, and hypoglycemia when used in combination with insulin or sulfonylureas
Rosiglitazone	Avandia		Monotherapy or combination with Metformin; 4 mg QD or BID or 8 mg QD	Mild to moderate edema, anemia, increase in blood cholesterol
Pioglitazone	Actos			
		Meglitinides		
Repaglinide	Prandin	Increases insulin secretion by the pancreas Sulfonylurea like	Monotherapy: 0.5 to 0.4 mg before each meal Combination therapy: with metformin or insulin	Hypoglycemia, weight gain

GI, gastrointestinal; *SIADH,* syndrome of inappropriate antidiuretic hormone; *LFT,* liver function tests.

Table 19.20 ▪ Counseling Points for Oral Antidiabetic Agents

Sulfonylureas
- Review signs and symptoms of hypoglycemia.

α-Glucosidase inhibitors
- Take with first bite of each meal.
- If a meal is missed, do not take dose.
- May cause diarrhea, flatulence, abdominal pain, especially at initiation of therapy.
- Report any persistent or severe signs or symptoms of gastrointestinal discomfort.

Biguanides
- Take with food.
- Mild gastrointestinal symptoms may be noted early in therapy.
- Signs and symptoms of hypoglycemia should be reviewed if taking with sulfonylureas or insulin.
- Report any unusual signs or symptoms to a health care professional (diarrhea, severe muscle pain or cramping, shallow and fast breathing, unusual tiredness and weakness, and unusual sleepiness may be signs of lactic acidosis).

Thiazolidinediones
- Take with food.
- Review signs and symptoms of hypoglycemia if taking with sulfonylurea or insulin.
- Report the following symptoms of hepatic dysfunction to a health care professional: nausea, vomiting, abdominal pain, fatigue, anorexia, or dark urine.

Meglitinides
- Review signs and symptoms of hypoglycemia.
- Take 30 min to immediately before a meal.
- If a meal is missed, do not take.

other related enzymes can decrease the effectiveness of α-glucosidase inhibitors.

Reductions in fasting plasma glucose of 5.4 to 20 mg/dL and 38 to 50 mg/dL have been reported with acarbose. Reductions in HbA1c of roughly 0.5% could be expected with the α-glucosidase class of medicines.

Thiazolidinediones

Troglitazone, a thiazolidinedione agent, is an insulin sensitizer that lowers blood glucose by enhancing the action of insulin and reducing insulin resistance. Its main action is on muscle tissue, where it increases glucose disposal, and to a lesser degree in the liver, where it decreases hepatic glucose production. Two other thiazolidinediones, rosiglitazone and pioglitazone, act similarly to troglitazone, and each has been approved recently in the United States.

Troglitazone is well tolerated; however, it is associated with rare idiosyncratic hepatocellular injury that has resulted in liver transplant or death. Routine liver function testing is recommended for all patients taking troglitazone, and the most recent recommendations are outlined in Table 19.21. If signs or symptoms of liver impairment (e.g., nausea, jaundice) occur during therapy, troglitazone should be discontinued and the origin of the problem identified. Troglitazone is hepatically metabolized and is an inducer of the cytochrome P-450 (CYP) 3A4 and therefore can interact with other drugs metabolized by this enzyme system (e.g., cyclosporine, tacrolimus). Cholestyramine decreases the absorption of troglitazone and has been shown to reduce plasma concentrations of some estrogen-containing drugs (e.g., ethinyl estradiol) and therefore could compromise the contraceptive efficacy of the estrogens.

Troglitazone is approved for combination use in patients on insulin or a sulfonylurea and as triple therapy for those on metformin and a sulfonylurea. When it is used in combination with other agents, often the dosage of the other agent can be decreased. In clinical trials, roughly 15% of patients taking insulin and troglitazone were able to discontinue the use of insulin. Of those unable to completely stop insulin, many were able to decrease their total daily dosage or frequency of insulin use.

Troglitazone may result in increases of LDL (up to 13%), HDL (up to 16%), and total cholesterol levels (as much as 5%), but the ratios of these are not altered. Postprandial and fasting triglyceride levels may be reduced by up to 26%.[49] Reductions in HbA1c of roughly 0.5% are seen when troglitazone is used as monotherapy, with drops of 1.4 and 1.8% reported when it is used in combination with insulin or sulfonylureas, respectively. Modest weight gain is reported when troglitazone is used in combination with other oral agents or insulin.

Rosiglitazone is indicated as monotherapy or in combination with metformin. Pioglitazone is FDA approved to be used as a monotherapy or in combination with a sulfonylurea, metformin, or insulin.

Meglitinides

The meglitinides are unrelated to the sulfonylureas, although they have a similar clinical effect, with both classes causing an increase in insulin secretion from the pancreas and therefore needing functioning β-cells for their action. Repaglinide is the first agent of this class to be made available in the United States.

Repaglinide is rapidly absorbed and eliminated ($t_{1/2}$ less than 1 hour) and is most effective when given within 30 minutes preprandially. Adverse events common with repaglinide therapy include weight gain and hypoglyce-

Table 19.21 ▪ Troglitazone: Recommendations for Liver Enzyme Monitoring

Check ALT levels
- At the start of therapy
- Every month during the first 12 mo
- Every 3 mo thereafter

Perform liver function tests at the first symptoms of hepatic dysfunction (e.g., nausea, vomiting, abdominal pain, fatigue, anorexia, dark urine).

If ALT levels are moderately elevated (>1.5 times normal limits) repeat liver function testing within 1 wk, then weekly until levels return to normal or rise to >3 times normal. If more than 3 times normal, troglitazone should be discontinued.

ALT, alanine aminotransferase.

mia, which is not surprising considering its mechanism of action. Modest weight gain has been reported (3.3%). Hypoglycemia appears to be more likely in sulfonylurea-naive patients with HbA1c values less than 8%, whereas those who have received sulfonylureas and have HbA1c values of 8% or more have no increased incidence in hypoglycemia. Antifungal agents such as ketoconazole and miconazole and the antibiotic erythromycin may inhibit the metabolism of repaglinide. Also, hepatic inducers of the CYP 3A4 isoenzyme (e.g., carbamazepine, barbiturates) can increase the metabolism of repaglinide.

Because repaglinide is hepatically metabolized and excreted via the feces, cautious use is advised in patients with hepatic impairment. In patients with renal compromise, lower starting dosages and longer intervals between dosage increases also are recommended. Currently, repaglinide is approved for monotherapeutic use or in combination with insulin or metformin. Its clinical effect is most pronounced in the first couple weeks of therapy, and HbA1c reductions of 1.7 to 2.1% are reported.[54]

Combination Therapy

Combination therapies are becoming much more common in the treatment of patients with type 2 diabetes. A second agent may be given to a patient who is poorly controlled on a single agent, and sometimes a third drug may be needed to achieve the desired clinical goal. In general, oral agents should not be substituted for one another, but rather a second or third drug should be added to the regimen. Clinical studies demonstrate that if antidiabetic drugs are simply substituted, no increase in therapeutic effect is seen, and in many cases glycemic control is compromised. Insulin may be used in combination with sulfonylureas, acarbose, metformin, troglitazone, or repaglinide. Keep in mind that insulin needs may decrease when oral agents are added to the regimen.

Role of Aspirin

Aspirin has been shown to reduce the risk of myocardial infarction and other vascular adverse events (stroke, transient ischemic attack) through its inhibition of thromboxane A_2. Thromboxane A_2 is a potent platelet aggregator and vasoconstrictor. The use of enteric coated aspirin (81 to 325 mg) is recommended in patients with diabetes who have evidence of large vessel disease (e.g., history of myocardial infarction, stroke, angina) and in those with a family history of coronary heart disease, cigarette smoking, hypertension, hyperlipidemia, obesity, or albuminuria. Contraindications to aspirin therapy include aspirin allergy, bleeding disorder, history of gastrointestinal bleeding, and active hepatic disease.

CONCLUSION

Diabetes mellitus is a complex, heterogeneous endocrine disorder that necessitates a health team effort to achieve treatment objectives. Through a combination of diet, exercise, medications, and most importantly education that results in the patient's taking charge of the condition, the outlook for the patient with diabetes is improving continually. Because of the rapid expansion of available therapeutic agents to treat this disease, the pharmacist's role in caring for patients with diabetes has expanded. Pharmacists can educate their patients about the proper use of medications, screen for drug interactions, explain monitoring devices, and make recommendations for ancillary products and services.

Health care providers, including pharmacists, must make a concerted effort to educate diabetic patients about treatment and monitoring. Members of the health care team must communicate and reinforce the information they provide to the patient with diabetes. These health care providers should participate actively in diabetes associations, keep up on the various educational methods and programs relating to diabetes, and become active in the American Association of Diabetes Educators. Health care providers should familiarize themselves with all available diabetes care products. The opportunity for specialists in the care of diabetes is great, and those who participate will find that the rewards are even greater.

KEY POINTS

- Diabetes is an incurable disease, so the overall goals of treatment include maintaining blood sugars in the normal or near normal range and preventing the short- and long-term complications associated with this disease.
- Type 1 diabetes is seen primarily in children and adolescents, whereas type 2 diabetes most commonly affects those over age 45.
- Measuring glycosylated hemoglobin (HbA1c) is the gold standard for monitoring patients with diabetes, and all patients with diabetes should have this test performed one to four times yearly.
- SMBG should be performed by most patients with diabetes, and the results of this activity should be reviewed regularly with a health care professional.
- Uncontrolled diabetes results in kidney, eye, and nerve disease that greatly compromise the quality of life of patients with diabetes, so normalization or near normalization of blood glucose is a primary treatment goal.
- Educating the patient with diabetes is critical to the successful management of this chronic disease.
- In addition to insulin, the therapeutic options to control diabetes include an array of agents that have various effects on the pancreas, muscle, and liver.
- The successful treatment of diabetes requires a team approach that incorporates the expertise of physicians, nurses, pharmacists, and dieticians.

REFERENCES

1. Diabetes Control and Complications Trial Research Group. The effect of intensive treatment on the development and the progression of long-term complications in insulin-dependent diabetes mellitus. N Engl J Med 329:977–986, 1993.

2. UK Prospective Diabetes Study (UKPDS) Group. Intensive blood-glucose with sulfonylureas or insulin compared with conventional treatment and risks of complications in patients with type 2 diabetes (UKPDS 33). Lancet 353:837–853, 1998.
3. UK Prospective Diabetes Study (UKPDS) Group. Effect of intensive blood-glucose with metformin on complications in overweight patients with type 2 diabetes (UKPDS 34). Lancet 352:854–865, 1998.
4. UK Prospective Diabetes Study (UKPDS) Group. Tight blood pressure control and risk of macrovascular and microvascular complications in type 2 diabetes (UKPDS 38). BMJ 317:703–713, 1998.
5. UK Prospective Diabetes Study (UKPDS) Group. Efficacy of atenolol and captopril in reducing risk of macrovascular and microvascular complications in type 2 diabetes (UKPDS 39). BMJ 317:13–20, 1998.
6. American Diabetes Association. Standards of medical care for patients with diabetes mellitus. Diabetes Care 20(Suppl 1):S5–S13, 1997.
7. Watkins JD, Robers DE, Williams TF, et al. Observation of medication errors made by diabetic patients at home. Diabetes 16:883, 1967.
8. Salans LB. Diabetes mellitus, a disease that is coming into focus. JAMA 247:590, 1982.
9. Diabetes 1996 vital statistics. Alexandria, VA: American Diabetes Association, 1996:1–102.
10. Epidemiological correlates of NIDDM in Hispanics, whites, and blacks in the U.S. population. Diabetes Care 14(Suppl 1):639–648, 1991.
11. Anonymous. Direct and indirect costs of diabetes in the United States in 1992. Alexandria, VA: American Diabetes Association, 1993.
12. Fioretto P, Steffes MW, Sutherland DER, et al. Reversal of lesions of diabetic nephropathy after pancreas transplantation. N Engl J Med 339:69–75, 1998.
13. Eastman RC, Javitt JC, Herman WH, et al. Model of complications of NIDDM. Diabetes Care 20:735–744, 1997.
14. United States Renal Data System. USRDS 1993 annual report. Bethesda, MD: 1993.
15. Atkinson MA, Maclaren NK. The pathogenesis of insulin-dependent diabetes mellitus. N Engl J Med 331:1428–1436, 1994.
16. Skyler JS, Marks JB. Immune intervention in type 1 diabetes mellitus. Diabetes Rev 1:15–42, 1993.
17. Reaven GM. Banting lecture 1988. Role of insulin resistance in human disease. Diabetes 37:1595–1607, 1988.
18. DeFronzo RA, Bonadonna RC, Ferrannini E. Pathogenesis of NIDDM. A balanced overview. Diabetes Care 15:318–368, 1992.
19. Polonsky KS, Sturis J, Bell GI. Non-insulin-dependent diabetes mellitus: a genetically programmed failure of the beta cell to compensate for insulin resistance. N Engl J Med 334:777–783, 1996.
20. White JR, Campbell RK. Drug/drug and drug/disease interactions and diabetes. Diabetes Educator 21:283–289, 1995.
21. Henry RR, Wallace P, Olefsky JM. Effects of weight loss on mechanisms of hyperglycemia in obese non-insulin-dependent diabetes mellitus. Diabetes 35:990–998, 1986.
22. Galloway JA, Potvin JH, Shuman CR, eds. Diabetes mellitus. 9th ed. Indianapolis: Lilly Research Laboratories, 1988.
23. Anonymous. The physician's guide to type II diabetes (NIDDM): diagnosis and treatment. Alexandria, VA: American Diabetes Association, 1992.
24. Anonymous. Buyer's guide to diabetes products, 1998. Alexandria, VA: American Diabetes Association, 1998.
25. Anonymous. Tests of glycemia in diabetes. Diabetes Care 20(Suppl 1):S18–S20, 1997
26. Anonymous. Diabetic nephropathy. Diabetes Care 20(Suppl 1):S24–S27, 1997.
27. Lipsky M. Management of diabetic ketoacidosis. Am Fam Physician 49:1607–1612, 1994.
28. Fish LH. Diabetic ketoacidosis. Postgrad Med 93:75–96, 1995.
29. Stern MP. The effect of glycemic control on the incidence of macrovascular complications of type 2 diabetes. Arch Fam Med 7:155–162, 1998.
30. Brownlee M. Glycation products and the pathogenesis of diabetic complications. Diabetes Care 15:1838, 1992.
31. Frank R. The aldose reductase controversy. Diabetes 43:169–172, 1994.
32. Goldstein I, Lue TF, Padma-Nathan H, et al. Oral sildenafil in the treatment of erectile dysfunction. N Engl J Med 338:1397–1404, 1998.
33. Kasiske BL, Kalil RSN, Ma JZ, et al. Effect of antihypertensive therapy on the kidney in patients with diabetes: a meta-regression analysis. Ann Int Med 118:129–138, 1993.
34. Pecoraro RE, Reiber GE, Burgess EM. Pathways to diabetic limb amputation: basis for prevention. Diabetes Care 13:513–521, 1990.
35. Campbell RK. Clinical update on pentoxifylline therapy for diabetes-induced peripheral vascular disease. Ann Pharmacother 27:1099–1105, 1993.
36. Steed DL and the Diabetic Ulcer Study Group. Clinical evaluation of recombinant human platelet-derived growth factor for the treatment of lower extremity diabetic ulcers. J Vasc Surg 21:71–81, 1995.
37. Bureau of Primary Health Care. LEAP Into Primary Care conference proceedings. Washington, DC: Health Resources and Services Administration, 1995.
38. Anonymous. Diabetes mellitus and exercise. American Diabetes Association. Diabetes Care 20(Suppl 1):S51, 1997.
39. American Diabetes Association. Nutrition recommendations and principles for people with diabetes mellitus. Diabetes Care 20(Suppl 1):S14–S17, 1997.
40. Richter EA, Ruderman NB, Schneider SH. Diabetes and exercise. Am J Med 70:201, 1981.
41. US Department of Agriculture, US Department of Health and Human Services. Nutrition and your health: dietary guidelines for Americans. 4th ed. Hyattsville, MD: USDA Human Nutrition Information Service, 1995.
42. Campbell RK, Campbell LK, White JR. Insulin lispro: its role in the treatment of diabetes mellitus. Ann Pharmacother 30:1263–1271, 1996.
43. Galloway JA, Potvin JH, Shuman CR, eds. Diabetes mellitus. 9th ed. Indianapolis: Lilly Research Laboratories, 1988.
44. Anonymous. Continuous subcutaneous insulin infusion. American Diabetes Association. Diabetes Care 20(Suppl 1):50, 1997.
45. White J, Campbell RK. The guide to mixing insulins. Hosp Pharm 26:1046–1050, 1991.
46. Valenta LJ, Elias AN. Insulin-induced lipodystrophy in diabetic patients resolved by treatment with human insulin. Ann Intern Med 102:790–791, 1985.
47. Gerich JE. Oral hypoglycemic agents. N Engl J Med 321:1232–1245, 1989.
48. Campbell RK. Glimepiride: role of a new sulfonylurea in the treatment of type 2 diabetes mellitus. Ann Pharmacol 32:1044–1052, 1998.
49. Maggs DG, Buchanan TA, Burant CF, et al. Metabolic effects of troglitazone monotherapy in type 2 diabetes mellitus. Ann Intern Med 338:176–185, 1998.
50. Misbin RI, Green L, Stadel BV, et al. Lactic acidosis in patients with diabetes treated with metformin [letter]. N Engl J Med 338:265–266, 1997.
51. Garber AJ, Duncan TG, Goodman AM, et al. Efficacy of metformin in type II diabetes: results of a double-blind, placebo-controlled, dose-response trial. Am J Med 102:491–497, 1997.
52. DeFronzo RA, Goodman AM, and the Multicenter Metformin Study Group. Efficacy of metformin in patients with NIDDM. N Engl J Med 333:541–549, 1995.
53. Santeusanio F, Compagnucci P. A risk-benefit appraisal of acarbose in the management of non-insulin-dependent diabetes mellitus. Drug Saf 11:432–444, 1994.
54. Cheatham WW. Repaglinide: a new oral blood glucose lowering agent. Clin Diabetes 16:70–72, 1998.

CHAPTER 20

HYPERLIPIDEMIA

Camille W. Thornton and James M. Holt

Cardiovascular disease is one of the leading causes of morbidity and mortality in the United States. Heart disease causes an estimated 500,000 deaths yearly, and the total annual cost of managing cardiovascular disease is $20 to $40 billion per year.[1] Risk factors associated with the development of cardiovascular disease include gender, age, cigarette smoking, diabetes, hypertension, and hyperlipidemia.[2,3] Hyperlipidemia, hypertension, and cigarette smoking are considered treatable risk factors. Cholesterol and blood pressure reduction and smoking cessation have been proven to reduce the risk of cardiovascular disease.[4] The past decade has seen an increase in media coverage and public awareness of medical issues. Hyperlipidemia and the medications used to lower cholesterol have received generous exposure. As a result, the public is aware that high cholesterol is a risk factor for cardiovascular disease.

DEFINITION

Hyperlipidemia is defined as the presence in the blood of an abnormally high concentration of fats such as cholesterol, cholesterol esters, triglycerides, and phospholipids. The clinical importance of these abnormal elevations depends on which components are affected and to what extent. For instance, studies have demonstrated that elevated low-density lipoprotein (LDL) levels are an independent and proven risk factor for cardiovascular disease.[3,5] Hypertriglyceridemia has been associated with certain lipoprotein disorders and with pancreatitis and uncontrolled diabetes mellitus, but has not been identified as an independent risk factor for cardiovascular disease.[5–8]

The association between elevated cholesterol levels and cardiovascular disease is proven, but there is controversy over the proper methods used to lower cholesterol and the benefits of those interventions. Clinical studies have been criticized for using biased reporting methods and applying the results of cholesterol reduction in certain study subgroups to the general population. Several groups have developed certain definitions and various treatment guidelines for hypercholesterolemia. Of these, the National Cholesterol Education Program Adult Treatment Panel II (NCEP-ATPII) guidelines are the most widely accepted.[2,5,9–11] Most clinicians agree that lowering cholesterol is important in reducing the risk of cardiovascular disease. A low-fat diet should be the foundation of all cholesterol reduction interventions. Only in patients with significantly elevated cholesterol levels with or without the presence of other cardiovascular risk factors, or if diet therapy fails to lower cholesterol to desired levels, should drug therapy be considered. Even when drug therapy is instituted, patients should maintain a healthful diet.[12]

TREATMENT GOALS: HYPERLIPIDEMIA

- Reduce morbidity and mortality from coronary heart disease (CHD) and decrease mortality from all causes in patients with established CHD.[5]
- Reduce new CHD events and CHD mortality in patients without established CHD.[5]
- Decrease the risk of myocardial infarction (MI), unstable angina, stroke (in patients with established CHD), and transient ischemic attack (in patients with established CHD) and the need for coronary artery bypass grafts and angioplasty.[3,4,11]

EPIDEMIOLOGY

Etiology

Hyperlipidemia can be caused by primary (genetic predisposition) or secondary causes (diet, medications, or underlying disease). Primary hyperlipidemia is associated

Table 20.1 ▪ Secondary Causes of Hyperlipidemia

Conditions Causing Hypertriglyceridemia	Conditions Causing Hypercholesterolemia
Acromegaly	Anorexia nervosa
Alcoholism	Cholestasis
Burns	Cushing's syndrome
Chronic renal failure	Growth hormone deficiency
Diabetes mellitus	Hypothyroidism
Glycogen storage disease	Myelomatosis (immunoglobulins A and G)
Hyperandrogenism in women	Nephrotic syndrome
Lipodystrophy	Obstructive liver disease
Pancreatitis	
Systemic lupus and polyclonal gammopathy	
Weight gain	

Source: References 14, 20.

with high morbidity and mortality. A defect often occurs in lipid metabolism or transport in primary hyperlipidemia, resulting in reduced LDL receptor activity and accumulation of LDL cholesterol in the plasma, leading to atherogenesis. Patients usually need medication and diet and exercise education.

Two types of genetic lipid receptor alterations can occur. A heterozygous receptor abnormality can occur when there is a mutant gene for the LDL receptor such that only half the LDL receptors are functional. Patients usually have cholesterol levels that are twice normal, causing increased risk of premature heart disease, angina, or MI (generally by age 30 or 40). A homozygous receptor alteration occurs when two mutant genes for the LDL receptor are present, leaving patients with essentially no functional LDL receptors. Cholesterol levels can be as high as 1000 mg/dL and CHD may develop in the first or second decade of life.[13]

All patients should be evaluated for secondary causes of hyperlipidemia. After dietary reasons, hypothyroidism is the most common cause of secondary hyperlipidemia. The mechanism by which this happens is not fully understood but it is thought that hypothyroidism increases triglycerides, possibly by reducing the clearance of very low-density lipoprotein (VLDL) secondary to a reduction in lipoprotein lipase activity or through increasing production of VLDL remnants. Thyroid hormone replacement used to correct thyroid levels lowers lipid levels in these patients. However, this effect is not seen in people with normal thyroid function, and levothyroxine should not be used for lipid lowering in euthyroid patients. Diseases such as diabetes mellitus, Cushing's syndrome, obstructive liver disease, nephrotic syndrome, and alcoholism are also common causes of high cholesterol.[14] Tables 20.1 and 20.2 list conditions and drugs that are common causes of secondary hyperlipidemia.

Special Concerns

Screening for hyperlipidemia is recommended for children older than 2 years whose parents or grandparents had documented CHD at or before age 55 years or whose parents have serum cholesterol levels above 6.2 mmol/L (240 mg/dL). Obese children or those who smoke are judged to be at higher risk for CHD and should also be screened for hyperlipidemia. If a family history is not available, children can be screened for hyperlipidemia at the discretion of the health care provider. Medical treatment should be reserved for children over 10 years of age with LDL levels above 4.9 mmol/L (190 mg/dL) or LDL levels above 4.1 mmol/L (160 mg/dL) with multiple risk factors. The desired LDL level for children is less than 2.8 mmol/L (110 mg/dL). These values are lower than those for adults because during the first two decades of life, overall lipid values are lower.

Treating hyperlipidemia in older adults may not necessarily prolong life significantly. However, therapy can extend the active life expectancy and improve the quality of life of these patients. In addition, it may reduce the need for expensive long-term care and help contain health care costs. Decisions about diagnostic or therapeutic interventions should not be based on the patient's chronologic age, but rather on the patient's physiologic age, presence and severity of concomitant diseases, mental status, cognitive ability, and expectations for medical care.[15] Although no clinical trials have been done exclusively in older adults, the Scandinavian Simvastatin Survival Study (4S) and the Cholesterol and Coronary Events (CARE) trial demon-

Table 20.2 ▪ Medications That Can Induce Hyperlipidemia

Medication	Total Cholesterol	LDL	HDL	TG	VLDL
Amiodarone	↑	–	–	–	–
Anabolic steroids	↑	↑	↓	–	–
Anticonvulsants	–	–	↑	–	–
β-Blockers (non-ISA)	–	–	↓	↑	↑
Chlorinated hydrocarbon insecticides	↑	–	–	–	–
Corticosteroids	↑	↑	↑	↑	↑
Cyclosporine	↑	↑	–	–	–
Estrogen therapy	↓	↓	↑	↑	↑
Isotretinoin	↑	–	↓	↑	–
Phenothiazines	↑	–	↓	–	–
Progestins	↑	↑	↓	–	–
Retinoids	↑	↑	↓	↑	↑
Thiazide diuretics	↑	↑	–	↑	↑

Source: References 14, 20, and Henkin Y, Como J, Oberman A. Secondary dyslipidemia: inadvertent effects of drugs in clinical practice. JAMA 267: 961–968, 1992.

LDL, low-density lipoprotein; *HDL,* high-density lipoprotein; *TG,* triglycerides; *VLDL,* very low density lipoprotein; *ISA,* intrinsic sympathomimetic activity.

strated a statistically significant decrease in both morbidity and mortality in older adults with established coronary artery disease.[16]

Hyperlipidemia is common after cardiac transplantation and affects about 70% of transplant recipients. Accelerated coronary artery disease remains a major cause of morbidity and mortality in patients who are alive more than 1 year after transplantation. Niacin is of benefit if the patient does not have impaired glucose tolerance. Resins interfere with cyclosporine absorption and raise triglyceride levels. Fibrates are well tolerated and reduce triglycerides but may increase LDL levels, limiting their effectiveness as a lipid-lowering agent. Statins have been shown to lower total cholesterol and LDL levels in transplant recipients but are not without risk. The incidence of rhabdomyolysis in heart transplant recipients treated with a statin and cyclosporine is about 1%. Pravastatin may be less likely to cause this adverse effect and should be considered first in this patient population.[17]

Homocysteine levels above 15 μmol/L are an important risk factor for MI, stroke, peripheral vascular disease, and thrombosis. There is a genetic link in patients with hyperhomocysteinemia; therefore, relatives of patients with this condition should be screened for increased risk of atherosclerosis. Plasma levels of homocysteine are increased by inadequate intake of folic acid and vitamins B_6 and B_{12} as well as by drugs, concomitant illnesses, age, and gender. Treatment with folic acid 1 to 2 mg/day alone or in combination with pyridoxine (vitamin B_6) 10 to 25 mg/day and vitamin B_{12} 400 mμg/day is an effective way to reduce elevated levels of homocysteine, although the clinical benefit of this intervention has not been tested fully.

PATHOPHYSIOLOGY

Cholesterol, a lipid, is one of the primary components of cell membranes and a precursor in steroid hormone and bile acid metabolism. Cholesterol is obtained through diet and endogenous manufacture: 40 to 60% of measured cholesterol in the blood is endogenous, with the remainder coming from diet.[12]

Lipoproteins transport cholesterol, triglycerides, and other lipid particles throughout the body. The components of the spherically shaped lipoproteins divide them into five categories: LDL, composed primarily of cholesterol; high-density lipoproteins (HDLs), composed of cholesterol; VLDLs, composed primarily of triglycerides; intermediate-density lipoproteins (IDLs), composed of triglycerides and cholesterol esters, also known as VLDL remnants; and chylomicrons, composed of triglycerides, cholesterol, and apolipoproteins obtained exogenously (diet) or assembled in the gut.

LDL accounts for 60 to 70% of total serum cholesterol. When LDL particles are transferred from the plasma to the subendothelial tissue, they become oxidized. This oxidation causes LDL to become cytotoxic and contributes to the development of atherosclerosis. HDL accounts for 20 to 30% of the total serum cholesterol. It reverses cholesterol transport by retrieving free cholesterol from cells and tissues and transferring it to the liver and kidney to be metabolized. VLDL, which is composed mainly of triglycerides, is about 10 to 15% of total serum cholesterol. Triglycerides are constructed of free fatty acids and are used as an energy substrate. They are obtained through fats in the diet and through the conversion of excess carbohydrates in the liver. IDLs, or VLDL remnants, are intermediate products between VLDL and the formation of LDL particles and have a short life span. Cholesterol and triglycerides contained in them do not contribute significantly to total serum cholesterol.[1,18–20]

There are two lipoprotein transport systems in the body (Fig. 20.1). The exogenous system involves the metabolism and transportation of chylomicron particles and remnants. Cholesterol and triglycerides obtained from diet form the triglyceride-rich chylomicrons in the intestinal endothelium, which then enters the lymphatic system, where they are transported throughout the bloodstream. Once in the general circulation, chylomicrons can be hydrolyzed through an enzymatic process with lipoprotein lipase on the vascular endothelium into a chylomicron remnant. Through this process, the triglycerides in the chylomicron are hydrolyzed into free fatty acids and monoglycerides, which are absorbed by muscle and adipose tissue and used as an energy substrate. Therefore, the remnant is smaller, contains less triglyceride, and is more concentrated with cholesterol. These cholesterol-rich chylomicron remnants also retain apolipoproteins B-48 and E. They are taken up by the liver and metabolized by LDL-related receptor proteins. These receptor proteins metabolize the cholesterol in chylomicron remnants into bile salts, which are excreted into the intestine. Bile salts solubilize dietary fats in the intestine to increase their absorption.[18,19]

Lipids and triglycerides produced by the body are transported through the endogenous pathway by VLDL, LDL, and HDL. The liver secretes triglycerides into the bloodstream as VLDL. VLDL particles contain about five times as much triglycerides as cholesterol. They also contain apolipoproteins B-100, E, and C-II. The B and E apolipoproteins interact with B/E LDL receptors on cell surfaces. Apolipoprotein C-II is a cofactor for the enzyme lipoprotein lipase. Once secreted into the bloodstream, triglycerides contained in the VLDL particles are hydrolyzed by lipoprotein lipase in the vascular endothelium. These IDL particles, or VLDL remnants, are smaller and have a lower triglyceride content but retain practically all of the cholesterol initially carried by the VLDL particle.

VLDL remnants undergo delipidation through lipoprotein lipase and hepatic lipase to form much smaller, cholesterol-rich LDL particles. By the time LDL particles are formed, the apolipoproteins E and C have been shed, leaving only apolipoprotein B-100. About half of VLDL remnants are cleared from the bloodstream by the LDL receptor, and the other half is converted to LDL particles.

LDL particles transport cholesterol to various body

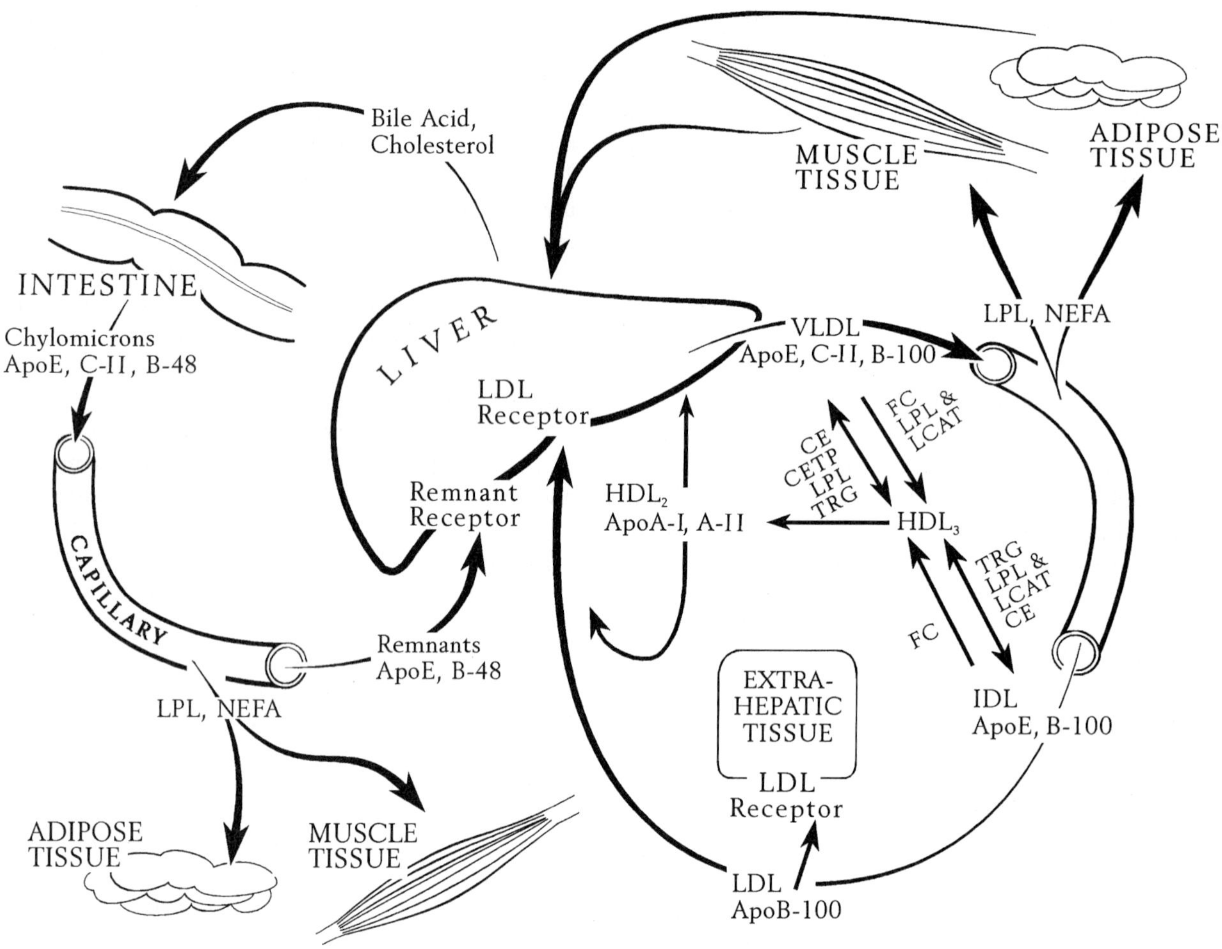

Figure 20.1. Schematic of lipoprotein transport systems in the body. *ApoA-I,* apolipoprotein A-I; *ApoA-II,* apolipoprotein A-II; *ApoB-48,* apolipoprotein B-48; *ApoB-100,* apolipoprotein B-100; *ApoC-II,* apolipoprotein C-II; *ApoE,* apolipoprotein E; *CE,* cholesterol ester; *CETP,* cholesteryl ester transfer protein; *FC, HDL,* high-density lipoprotein; *LCAT,* lecithin:cholesterol acyl transferase; *LDL,* low-density lipoprotein; *LPL,* lipoprotein lipase; *NEFA, TRG,* triglyceride. (Reprinted with permission from Israel M, Sisson E. Hyperlipidemias. In: Carter B, Lake K, Raebel M, et al., eds. Pharmacotherapy Self-Assessment Program. 3rd ed. Kansas City, MO: American College of Clinical Pharmacy, 1998:174.)

tissues, where they interact with LDL receptors on cell membranes. LDL particles taken up by cells are used for steroid synthesis or as part of the cell membrane. Excessive circulating LDL cholesterol causes cholesterol to be deposited outside the cell, causing atherogenic plaques to form in the vascular endothelium. Qualitative differences in particle size exist within the LDL population. Among the LDL population, very small, dense LDL particles have a greater ability to penetrate into subendothelial tissue and contribute to the development of atherosclerosis. LDL particles surrounded by a plasminogenlike glycoprotein apolipoprotein (a), called lipoprotein Lp(a), appear to be associated strongly with CHD risk.[18,19,21]

HDL particles are cholesterol rich and are involved in the process of reverse cholesterol transport. HDL acts as a receptacle for circulating free cholesterol in the tissues by returning it to the liver and kidney to be catabolized. HDL particles have been subclassified into HDL_3 and HDL_2 particles. The smaller HDL_3 particles are converted to larger HDL_2 particles through the acquisition of triglycerides and cholesterol from peripheral cells. HDL particles contain apolipoproteins A-I, A-II, and C. Apolipoprotein A-I is more strongly correlated with reduced CHD risk than apolipoprotein A-II.

Apolipoprotein A-I activates the transport of cholesterol from the periphery to the liver by causing the enzyme lecithin:cholesterol acyl transferase (LCAT) to convert cholesterol in HDL particles to insoluble cholesterol esters. Cholesteryl ester transfer protein (CETP) activates the exchange of cholesterol esters from HDL particles for triglycerides in VLDL particles and remnants. Once the cholesterol esters are transferred to the VLDL particles and remnants, they travel to the liver, where they are eliminated.

The VLDL-LDL and LDL pathway is responsible for carrying cholesterol and triglycerides from the liver to the cells for use and back to the liver for elimination. VLDL-LDL delivers triglycerides and LDL carries cholesterol. Cells upregulate the synthesis of B/E LDL receptors if cellular concentrations of cholesterol and triglycerides become low. New B/E LDL receptors travel to an area on the cell surface known as the coated pits. Circulating VLDL particles and remnants have a higher binding affinity for these LDL receptors than LDL particles do because they contain the apolipoproteins B and E. Once binding occurs, the lipoproteins are engulfed by the cell and broken down into elemental substances for use by the cell. The receptor then returns to the cell surface to bind with other circulating apolipoproteins B or E containing lipoproteins.[8,21]

CLINICAL PRESENTATION AND DIAGNOSIS

Signs and Symptoms

LDL cholesterol is the lipid component most closely associated with the risk of CHD. Increased serum cholesterol levels are also directly linked to the risk of CHD. Clinical trials have demonstrated that lowering serum cholesterol levels is associated with reduced morbidity and mortality. For every 1% reduction in total serum cholesterol, there is a 2 to 3% decrease in the risk of CHD. Conversely, increased HDL reduces the risk of CHD.[5]

Hypertriglyceridemia has not been associated directly with increased risk of CHD but is generally indicative of an underlying lipid abnormality. High triglycerides usually result in low HDL, which is a known risk factor for CHD. Triglycerides below 2.3 mmol/L (200 mg/dL) are considered normal according to NCEP-ATP II; above 4.5 mmol/L (400 mg/dL) is defined as high. There is disagreement on whether triglyceride levels below 11.3 mmol/L (1000 mg/dL) warrant treatment for increased CHD risk. Reducing triglyceride levels with an associated increase in HDL cholesterol may be beneficial for the patient. Triglyceride levels above 11.3 mmol/L (1000 mg/dL) do warrant intervention because of the risk of acute pancreatitis, lipemia, retinalis, and eruptive skin xanthomas.[5,14,20]

LDL cholesterol levels can be calculated from measured total cholesterol, HDL, and triglycerides by the Friedewald formula:

$$\text{LDL} = \text{Total cholesterol} - \text{Triglycerides}/5 - \text{HDL}$$

Triglycerides above 4.5 mmol/L (400 mg/dL) result in a falsely low LDL value and the formula becomes invalid. The cause of the hypertriglyceridemia should be identified and treated. If after treatment or adequate trials of exercise, diet, and drug therapy the triglyceride level remains elevated, a direct measurement of LDL can be done. This may be especially important in the patient with established CHD, who is at the greatest risk.

Table 20.3 lists a number of clinical trials that have studied the effect of dietary or pharmacologic interventions for cholesterol reduction in patient populations with no existing CHD (primary prevention) and with established CHD (secondary prevention). The line between primary and secondary prevention has become less distinct in recent years because of ongoing emphasis on risk of disease progression in patients with hypercholesterolemia, which has been promoted by the NCEP-ATP II guidelines and newer clinical trials.

Some of the older studies (Lipid Research Clinic Coronary Primary Prevention Trial, Helsinki Heart Study, Coronary Drug Project Niacin Study, Oslo Study Diet and Antismoking Trial) conducted in the 1970s and early 1980s using interventions such as gemfibrozil, clofibrate, niacin, and cholestyramine were attacked for stating the benefit of cholesterol reduction on outcomes as a reduction in relative risk instead of absolute risk.[22–27] Challengers maintained that reporting results in terms of relative risk led professionals to believe that there are greater benefits to cholesterol reduction than actually exist.[28,29] Also, a majority of these trials were conducted in a study population of middle-aged men with elevated cholesterol levels. The question of whether the results could be applied to the population as a whole was raised. Also, some of the older trials showed an increase in total mortality in treatment groups, which clouded the issue of when to treat and whether lipid-lowering agents were safe.

Newer trials using 3-hydroxy-3-methylglutaryl coenzyme A (HMG CoA) reductase inhibitors (West of Scotland Coronary Prevention Study, CARE, 4S, Air Force/Texas Coronary Atherosclerosis Prevention Study [AFCAPS/TexCAPS], and Long-Term Intervention with Pravastatin in Ischemic Disease [LIPID] study) were conducted on a broader range of patients, including women, older adults, and subjects with average cholesterol levels. This permitted interpretation of cholesterol reduction in these populations, which was found to be just as beneficial.[16,30–33] The 4S trial demonstrated that patients with CHD showed a 30% reduction in total mortality and no increase in noncardiovascular mortality, which alleviated concerns about lipid-lowering death and non–CHD mortality.[16] These newer trials support the guidelines put forth by the NCEP-ATPII.

Most experts agree that the apparent benefit of cholesterol reduction in study patients at risk for CHD warrants interventions in the general population for those at increased risk with or without evidence of preexisting CHD.[5] This position is strengthened by studies in patients with CHD or previous MI, where lipid-lowering interventions reduced the incidence of cardiac events and resulted in the regression of measurable coronary lesions.[34,35]

Diagnosis

Table 20.4 lists NCEP-ATPII appropriate levels for lipids and triglycerides. Treatment decisions are based on a patient's LDL level, risk factor status, and presence of known CHD or atherosclerotic disease. Patient risk factors are listed in Table 20.5. Patients are placed in one of three risk categories to determine the most appropriate intervention and the goals of that intervention. Patients with known CHD or other atherosclerotic disease have the highest risk for a future event and are considered to be in the secondary prevention group. Experts are debating whether patients

Table 20.3 ▪ Events and Death Rates in Primary and Secondary Prevention Trials

Study	Intervention	Nonfatal Cardiac Events (%)	Death Rate (%)					
			CAD	OVD	Cancer	A&V	Other	Total
Primary								
LRC-CPPT	Resin	N/C	1.7	0.3	0.8	0.6	0.2	3.6
	D/P	N/C	2.3	0.2	0.8	0.2	0.3	3.7
HHS	Fibric	2.2	0.7	0.4	0.5	0.5	0.1	2.2
	D/P	3.5	0.9	0.2	0.5	0.2	0.2	2.1
OSDAT	Diet	2.2	1.2	0.3	1.0	0.7	0.0	3.1
	N/I	3.5	2.7	0.2	1.6	0.3	0.2	4.9
WOSCOPS	Pravastatin	5.8	1.3	0.3	1.3	0.2	0.2	3.2
	D/P	7.8	1.9	0.4	1.5	0.2	0.2	4.1
AFCAPS/TexCAPS	Lovastatin	N/A	0.5	N/A	7.6	0.03	N/A	2.4
	D/P	N/A	0.8	N/A	7.8	0.09	N/A	2.3
Secondary								
CDP-NS	Niacin	10.4	38.8	3.6	4.0	1.1	4.6	52.0
	D/P	14.7	43.7	4.0	4.4	0.9	5.2	58.2
POSCH	PIB	10.0	7.6	0.7	1.9	0.7	0.7	11.6
	Diet	14.8	10.6	1.2	1.9	0.7	0.5	14.9
4S	Simvastatin	15.9	5.0	1.1	1.5	0.3	0.3	8.2
	D/P	22.6	8.5	0.8	1.6	0.3	0.3	11.5
CARE	Pravastatin	8.3	4.6	2.6	8.3	0.4	0.5	8.6
	D/P	11.1	5.7	3.8	7.7	0.2	0.7	9.4
LIPID	Pravastatin	N/A	6.4	7.3	2.8	0.1	0.9	11.0
	D/P	N/A	8.3	9.6	3.1	0.2	1.3	14.1

Source: Reference 21.

CAD, coronary artery disease; *OVD,* other vascular disease; *A&V,* accidents and violence; *LRC-CPPT,* Lipid Research Clinic Coronary Primary Prevention Trial; *Resin,* bile acid resin; *N/C,* not collected; *D/P,* diet and placebo; *HHS,* Helsinki Heart Study; *fibric,* fibric acid derivative; *OSDAT,* Oslo Study Diet and Antismoking Trial; *N/I,* no intervention; *WOSCOPS,* West of Scotland Coronary Prevention Study; *AFCAPS/TexCAPS,* Air Force/Texas Coronary Atherosclerosis Prevention Study; *N/A,* not available; *CDP-NS,* Coronary Drug Project Niacin Study; *POSCH,* Program on the Surgical Control of the Hyperlipidemias; *PIB,* partial ileal bypass; *4S,* Scandinavian Simvastatin Survival Study; *CARE,* Cholesterol and Coronary Events trial; *LIPID,* Long-Term Intervention with Pravastatin in Ischemic Disease study group.

Table 20.4 ▪ Classification of Cholesterol and Triglyceride Levels Based on NCEP-ATPII Guidelines

	Desirable	Borderline	High Risk
Cholesterol	<5.2 mmol/L (200 mg/dL)	5.2–6.2 mmol/L (200–239 mg/dL)	>6.2 mmol/L (240 mg/dL)
Low-density lipoprotein	<3.4 mmol/L (130 mg/dL)	3.4–4.1 mmol/L (130–159 mg/dL)	>160
High-density lipoprotein	>1.5 mmol/L (60 mg/dL)	–	<0.9 mmol/L (35 mg/dL)
Triglycerides	<2.3 mmol/L (200 mg/dL)	2.3–4.5 mmol/L (200–400 mg/dL)	4.5–11.3 mmol/L (400–1000 mg/dL)

Source: References 5, 20.

without known CHD and diabetes should be included in the high-risk group. Diabetic patients are two to four times more likely to develop CHD than nondiabetics. Patients with a strong family history of CHD may also be moved into this group. Patients with elevated cholesterol levels and multiple risk factors but no known CHD are at intermediate risk. Finally, patients with no risk factors or known CHD but elevated cholesterol levels have a modestly increased risk. Patients with no known CHD are considered to be in the primary prevention group.

Positive risk factors are those that, if present, increase the risk of developing CHD. Factors such as age, sex, and family history cannot be modified. Hypertension and diabetes are risk factors that respond to medical intervention but remain positive risk factors for CHD even when controlled. Smoking is also a modifiable risk factor, but history of smoking is not counted as a positive risk factor, which is one reason why cessation is vital for patients who smoke.

Negative risk factors are those that decrease the risk of developing CHD. HDL greater than 60 mg/dL is considered a negative risk factor and, if it is present, one positive risk factor can be subtracted.[5,21]

Intervention goals of dietary and drug therapy for patients with high LDL levels are listed in Table 20.6. LDL cholesterol levels should be determined on two separate occasions and the results averaged to determine the patient's risk category. If the two levels differ by more than 0.7 mmol/L (30 mg/dL), a third level should be taken and all three averaged to make an assessment. These levels can be drawn on consecutive days if the patient is metabolically stable. Acute ischemic events such as an MI or surgical revascularization may reduce serum cholesterol levels below the true baseline. Levels should return to normal within 6 weeks. When making treatment decisions based on laboratory values, it is important to be working with a reliable laboratory. The laboratory measuring these values should adhere to established standards for cholesterol measurement.[5]

The NCEP-ATPII guidelines recommend screening all adults 20 years or older for elevated cholesterol levels by obtaining a total cholesterol and HDL reading every 5 years for primary prevention. Total cholesterol levels of 5.2 mmol/L (200 mg/dL) or less are classified as desirable, between 5.2 and 6.2 mmol/L (200 to 239 mg/dL) as borderline high cholesterol, and 6.2 mmol/L (240 mg/dL) or more as a high cholesterol level. As mentioned earlier, HDL less than 0.9 mmol/L (35 mg/dL) is also a CHD risk factor. Figure 20.2 outlines screening guidelines for primary and secondary prevention. Monitoring and treatment decisions are based on total cholesterol, HDL, and LDL. Patients in the primary prevention category should be evaluated for secondary causes of hyperlipidemia. Information including the patient's past medical history and current medication profile is important in making this determination. All patients should receive proper dietary and physical activity counseling, regardless of classification.

Table 20.5 ▪ Risk Factors for Coronary Heart Disease

Positive Risk Factors	Comments
Sex and age	Men age ≥45; women age ≥55 or premature menopause without estrogen replacement
Family history of heart disease	MI or sudden death before age 55 in father or other male first-degree relative or before age 65 in mother or other female first-degree relative[a]
Atherosclerotic disease	History of peripheral vascular disease, MI, or cerebrovascular accident
Current cigarette smoking	
Hypertension	Blood pressure ≥140/90 mm Hg or use of antihypertensive medications
Low HDL	≤35 mg/dL
Diabetes	

Negative Risk Factors	Comments
High HDL	≥60 mg/dL (if present, subtract a positive risk factor)

Source: References 5, 20.

[a]First-degree relative: sister or brother.

MI, myocardial infarction; *HDL*, high-density lipoprotein.

Table 20.6 ▪ NCEP-ATPII Recommended Interventions Based on LDL Cholesterol Levels

	LDL Level at Start of Therapy, mmol/L (mg/dL)	Goal LDL Level, mmol/L (mg/dL)
Dietary therapy		
Without CHD		
<2 risk factors	≥4.1 (160)	<4.1 (160)
>2 risk factors	≥3.4 (130)	<3.4 (130)
With CHD[a]	>2.6 (100)	≤2.6 (100)
Drug therapy[b]		
Without CHD		
<2 risk factors	≥4.9 (190)	<4.1 (160)
>2 risk factors	≥4.1 (160)	<3.4 (130)
With CHD	≥3.4 (130)	≤2.6 (100)

Source: References 5, 20.

LDL, low-density lipoprotein; *CHD*, coronary heart disease.

[a]Should begin step 2 diet immediately.

[b]In young men (age <35) and premenopausal women, drug therapy should be reserved for those with very high LDL levels (>220 mg/dL) unless the patient has multiple risk factors, particularly diabetes mellitus or a positive family history of CHD.

TREATMENT

Once a patient has been diagnosed with hyperlipidemia and classified according to the presence of risk factors, treatment options are the next area of consideration. No matter what the lipid disorder, diet therapy is a necessary part of any treatment plan. Secondary causes of hyperlipidemia such as hypothyroidism, diabetes, diet, and drugs should be treated and the impact of treatment on the lipid profile measured before hyperlipidemia treatment is started.

The 27th Bethesda Conference developed four evidence-based risk factor categories to help prioritize intervention approaches (Table 20.7). Category I risk factors, such as cigarette smoking and hypertension, have interventions that have been proven to lower CHD risk

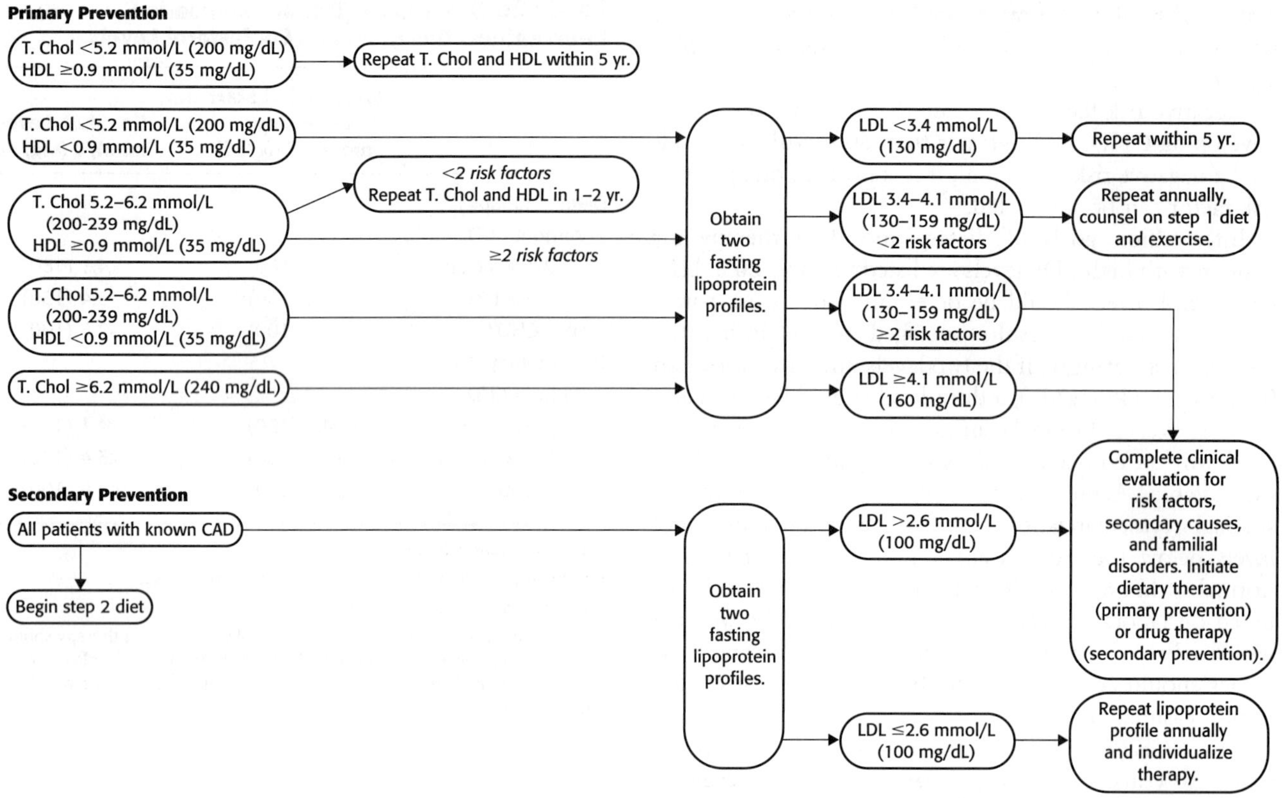

Figure 20.2. Screening algorithm. *CAD,* coronary artery disease; *HDL,* high-density lipoprotein; *LDL,* low-density lipoprotein; *T. Chol.,* total cholesterol. (Adapted from reference 21.)

and therefore should be addressed early in the patient's therapy. Cigarette smoking is associated with decreased levels of HDL cholesterol. Smoking cessation can increase HDL levels by 10 to 30% within several weeks of quitting. Controlling hypertension also decreases the risk of CHD. Categories II and III list risk factors that have interventions that are likely to lower CHD risk, but the evidence is not as strong as that for category I. Physical inactivity is in category II. Aerobic exercise stimulates lipoprotein lipase activity, thereby decreasing the number of triglyceride particles and increasing levels of HDL cholesterol. Excess body weight is positively correlated with LDL cholesterol and negatively associated with HDL cholesterol. Weight loss stimulates lipoprotein lipase activity, decreasing triglyceride and increasing HDL levels. Another added benefit of weight reduction and increased physical activity is a decrease in blood pressure and the risk of developing diabetes mellitus.[36] Modifiable risk factors in categories I, II, and III should be part of any treatment plan. Category IV lists risk factors that are not modifiable and are associated with increased risk of CHD.[37]

Diet

Diet is the cornerstone of treatment for hyperlipidemia. Efforts to reduce the dietary intake of total fat, saturated fat and cholesterol, and caloric intake beyond daily needs are the goals of diet therapy. Several dietary protocols have been developed, and most follow the recommendations of the NCEP-ATPII and the American Heart Association.[5,38] These diets recommend reducing total fat intake to less than 30% of calories and reducing saturated fat intake while increasing polyunsaturated and monounsaturated fats. Cholesterol consumption should be reduced and daily total caloric intake should be decreased to help patients reach and maintain an ideal weight. Proteins and carbohydrates should be consumed in appropriate ratios for a balanced diet.

NCEP-ATPII has developed two diets: the step 1 diet, which is generally used first, and the step 2 diet, which is implemented if the patient does not achieve his or her dietary goals on the step 1 diet or if the patient has CHD. The recommendations for step 1 and step 2 diets are listed in Table 20.8. Diet therapy alone can reduce cholesterol levels by 10% or more in compliant patients. Diet interventions should be given a 6-month trial to determine their effectiveness in lowering cholesterol levels (Fig. 20.3). Patients should receive dietary advice from trained professionals. Complying with dietary guidelines is difficult; therefore, patients should receive encouragement and reinforcement at every visit to help them reach their goals. Involving family members in the process is helpful because they can offer support to the patient.[5,20]

Table 20.7 ▪ Risk Factor Stratification and the Impact of Intervention on CHD Risk

Category I (risk factors for which interventions have been proven to lower CHD risk)
Cigarette smoking
LDL cholesterol
High-fat or high-cholesterol diet
Hypertension
Left ventricular hypertrophy
Thrombogenic factors
Category II (risk factors for which interventions are likely to lower CHD risk)
Diabetes mellitus
Physical inactivity
HDL cholesterol
Triglycerides; small, dense LDL
Obesity
Postmenopausal status in women
Category III (risk factors associated with increased risk of CHD that, if modified, might lower risk)
Psychosocial factors
Lipoprotein (a)
Homocysteine
Oxidative stress
No alcohol consumption
Category IV (risk factors associated with increased risk of CHD that cannot be modified)
Age
Male gender
Low socioeconomic status
Family history of early-onset CHD

Source: Reference 4.

CHD, coronary heart disease; *LDL,* low-density lipoprotein; *HDL,* high-density lipoprotein.

Patients should be instructed on which foods to choose or avoid (Tables 20.9 and 20.10). Increased intake of fruits and vegetables should be encouraged. In general, highly processed foods and most snack products are high in calories and fat and should be avoided. Remind patients that a product that is low in fat or cholesterol is not necessarily low in calories. Oils, meat, dairy products, and condiments can also be a significant source of fat in the diet. Patients should read labels and check for total calories, fat, and cholesterol content of a serving of the product. A conversion of fat content in grams to calories (9 kcal/g) reveals whether it represents more than 30% of calories.[38,39]

Bran, fish oil, antioxidant vitamins, red wine, and other foods may lower serum cholesterol or reduce CHD risk. Confusion over health claims for these and other products led to the development of the U.S. Nutrition Labeling and Education Act of 1990. This act resulted in the Food and Drug Administration's final rule regarding seven accepted health claims, two of which address CHD risk reduction. First, fruits, vegetables, and grain products that contain fiber, particularly soluble fiber, are associated with a reduction in CHD risk. The second claim states that diets low in saturated fats and cholesterol may reduce the risk of CHD.[40] No other products may be promoted as reducing the risk of CHD at this time.

Pharmacotherapy

Patients in whom treatment with lifestyle modifications fails should be started on lipid-lowering agents. Patients with multiple risk factors and very high cholesterol levels may need early intervention with drug therapy because diet therapy may not reduce LDL cholesterol to the goal range. Drug therapy may be delayed in men under 35 years old, premenopausal women, or older adults for whom the benefit-to-risk ratio of intervention is uncertain. Figure 20.4 describes when to begin drug therapy.

The following considerations determine which drug should be tried first: the type of hyperlipidemia, past medical history, the adverse effect profile of the drug, the effectiveness of the drug, the patient's adherence history, and cost. Diet therapy should be continued when drug therapy is instituted. Dosages should be increased until goals are achieved, the maximum dosage is reached, or the patient experiences intolerable adverse effects. If goals are not achieved after an adequate trial, a more effective agent should be considered, or a second drug that has a different mechanism of action can be added to the regimen.

Bile Acid Resins

Bile acid resins exchange an anion, usually sodium, for bile acids in the intestinal tract. This interrupts the recycling of bile acids through enterohepatic circulation, causing hepatic cells to be stimulated to convert more cholesterol into bile acids. This process upregulates the LDL receptors

Table 20.8 ▪ Dietary Recommendations of NCEP-ATPII for Treating Hypercholesterolemia

Nutrient	Step 1 Diet	Step 2 Diet
Total fat[a]	30%	30%
Saturated fat[a]	<10%	<7%
Polyunsaturated fat[a]	<10%	<10%
Monounsaturated fat[a]	5–15%	5–15%
Carbohydrate[a]	50–70%	50–70%
Protein[a]	10–20%	10–20%
Cholesterol	<300 mg	<200 mg
Calories	To maintain optimal weight	To maintain optimal weight

Source: Schaefer EJ. New recommendation for the diagnosis and treatment of plasma lipid abnormalities. Nutr Rev 51:246–252, 1993.

[a]Percentage of total daily calories.

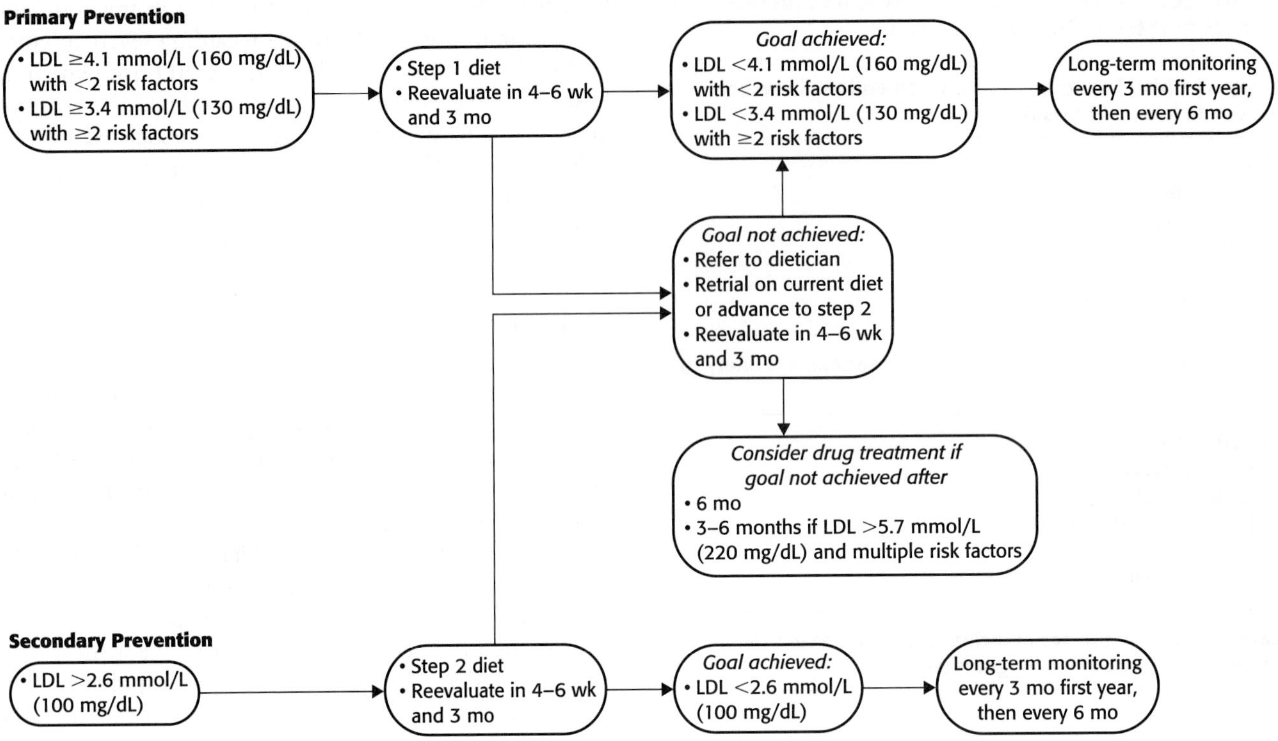

Figure 20.3. Diet therapy algorithm. *LDL,* low-density lipoprotein. (Adapted from reference 5.)

Table 20.9 ▪ Recommended Diet Modifications to Lower Blood Cholesterol

Products	Increase	Decrease
Fruits and vegetables	Fresh, frozen, canned, or dried fruits and vegetables	Vegetables prepared in butter, creams, or other sauces
Meat, poultry, and fish	Fish, poultry without skin, lean cuts of beef, lamb, pork, or veal, shellfish	Fatty cuts of beef, lamb, pork, spare ribs, organ meats, regular cold cuts, sausage, hot dogs, bacon, sardines
Bread, cereals, and grains	Rice, pasta	Egg noodles
	Whole-grain breads and cereals (oatmeal, whole wheat, rye, bran, multigrain)	Breads in which eggs are a major ingredient
	Homemade baked goods using unsaturated oils sparingly, angel food cake, low-fat crackers, low-fat cookies	Commercial baked goods: pies, cakes, doughnuts, croissants, pastries, muffins, biscuits, high-fat crackers, high-fat cookies
Eggs	Egg whites (two egg whites equal one egg in recipes), cholesterol-free egg substitutes	Egg yolks
Dairy products	Skim or 1% fat milk (liquid, powdered, evaporated), buttermilk	Whole milk, regular, evaporated, condensed milk; cream, half-and-half, 2% milk, imitation milk products, most nondairy creamers, whipped toppings
	Nonfat or low-fat yogurt	Whole-milk yogurt
	Low-fat cottage cheese (1–2%)	Whole-milk cottage cheese (4% fat)
	Low-fat cheeses, farmer or pot cheeses (all should be labeled no more than 2–6 g fat per ounce)	All natural cheeses (e.g., bleu, roquefort, camembert, cheddar, swiss), cream cheese, sour cream
	Sherbet, sorbet	Ice cream
Fats and oils	Baking cocoa	Chocolate
	Unsaturated vegetable oils; corn, olive, canola, safflower, sesame, soybean, sunflower oil; margarine or shortenings made from unsaturated oils, diet margarine	Butter, coconut oil, palm oil, lard, bacon fat
	Mayonnaise, salad dressings made with unsaturated oils, low-fat dressings	Dressings made with egg yolk
	Seeds and nuts	Coconut

Source: The Expert Panel. Report of the National Cholesterol Education Program Expert Panel on Detection, Evaluation, and Treatment of High Blood Cholesterol in Adults. Arch Intern Med 148:36–69, 1988.

Table 20.10 ▪ Fatty Acid Composition of Vegetable Oils and Animal Fats

High in saturated fats	
	Coconut oil
	Cocoa butter
	Palm kernel oil
	Palm oil
	Butterfat
	Beef tallow
High in monounsaturated fats, low in saturated fats	
	Olive oil
	Peanut oil
	Canola (rapeseed) oil
High in polyunsaturated fats, low in saturated fats	
	Soybean oil
	Corn oil
	Sunflower oil
	Safflower oil

Source: American Medical Association Council on Scientific Affairs. Saturated fatty acids in vegetable oils. JAMA 263:693–695, 1990.

and enhances LDL clearance from the plasma. Therefore, bile acid resins exert their primary effect on LDL cholesterol. Colestipol and cholestyramine lower total cholesterol and LDL by 15 to 30%. HDL may be increased moderately, by 3 to 5%. Triglycerides can be increased by about 7% acutely and 2 to 3% after prolonged therapy in patients with normal triglyceride levels. Clinicians should use resins with caution in patients with mild to moderate triglyceride elevations because the increase in triglycerides may be pronounced in these patients and may precipitate pancreatitis. Bile acid resins can decrease the risk of CHD, are safe, and have no long-term risks.[5,23,24]

Because resins are not absorbed from the gastrointestinal (GI) tract, they have no systemic side effects. These agents are ideal for younger patients, including women considering pregnancy. The most common side effects involve the GI tract and include constipation, abdominal pain, belching, bloating, gas, heartburn, and nausea. Constipation occurs in about 20% of patients and can be reduced with stool softeners and increased intake of soluble fiber. Psyllium can be used to increase dietary soluble fiber and has the added benefit of further reducing LDL levels. Resin dosages should be titrated slowly to allow patients to develop tolerance to the GI complaints. Side effects may become more tolerable with prolonged therapy.

Resins are also known to interfere with the absorption of medications taken concurrently. Patients should take other medications at least 1 hour before or 4 hours after the resin. Interactions with digoxin, warfarin, thyroid hormones, thiazide diuretics, antibiotics, β-blockers, HMG CoA reductase inhibitors, iron salts, and phenobarbital have been documented.

Dosing is usually initiated at 4 g for cholestyramine and 5 g for colestipol, with maximum amounts of 24 g and 30 g, respectively, generally given in two to four divided doses. A common regimen is to divide the total daily dosage by the number of meals the patient has each day. Resins should be given in at least 4 oz of a beverage or soup or sprinkled on a pulpy fruit. The dose should be sprinkled on top of the desired liquid to allow hydration before mixing. The drug should not be taken dry because of the risk of esophageal irritation or blockage. Colestipol beads are odorless and tasteless and may be preferable to some patients; 1-g tablets of colestipol are also available. They should be taken whole, not crushed.

The taste and side effects of resins make them difficult to tolerate as a lifelong regimen. This should be considered if the patient has a history of noncompliance. For this reason, bile acid resins typically are used as second-line agents. The addition of low-dose resin therapy to other cholesterol-lowering agents can produce an additional 9 to 16% reduction in total cholesterol and LDL.

Niacin

Niacin (nicotinic acid) is a water-soluble B vitamin that exerts its lipid-lowering effect by inhibiting the production of VLDL particles in the liver. This results in a decrease in triglycerides and LDL. Niacin may also increase HDL levels by reducing its catabolism. Niacin lowers LDL by 10 to 25%, decreases triglycerides by 20 to 50%, and increases HDL by 15 to 35%.[5] These cholesterol-lowering effects are dose-related, and more than 1500 mg/day niacin usually is needed. Niacin is an ideal agent for patients who have elevated LDL and triglycerides and a normal or low HDL level. The Coronary Drug Project trial showed a decrease in the risk of recurrent MI in patients taking niacin. In the 15-year follow-up group, total mortality decreased by 11% in the niacin arm of the trial.[26]

Despite the favorable effects of niacin on the lipid profile, many patients cannot tolerate the medication's side effects. The most common symptoms include flushing, tingling, itching, rash, and headaches, which are thought to be produced by prostaglandin-mediated vasodilation. These side effects are seen mainly at the beginning of therapy, with subsequent dosing changes, and when therapy is resumed after missed doses. Tolerance to these side effects quickly develops with continued dosing. Patients are instructed to take niacin with food to reduce GI side effects and with aspirin 30 minutes before administration to reduce the prostaglandin-mediated vasodilation. These side effects can also be minimized by slowly titrating to the recommended dosage of 1500 to 3000 mg/day (Table 20.11).

Niacin can cause abdominal pain and discomfort, and some clinicians avoid niacin in patients with a history of peptic ulcer disease (PUD) because of concern that it may aggravate PUD or interfere with the clinical presentation.

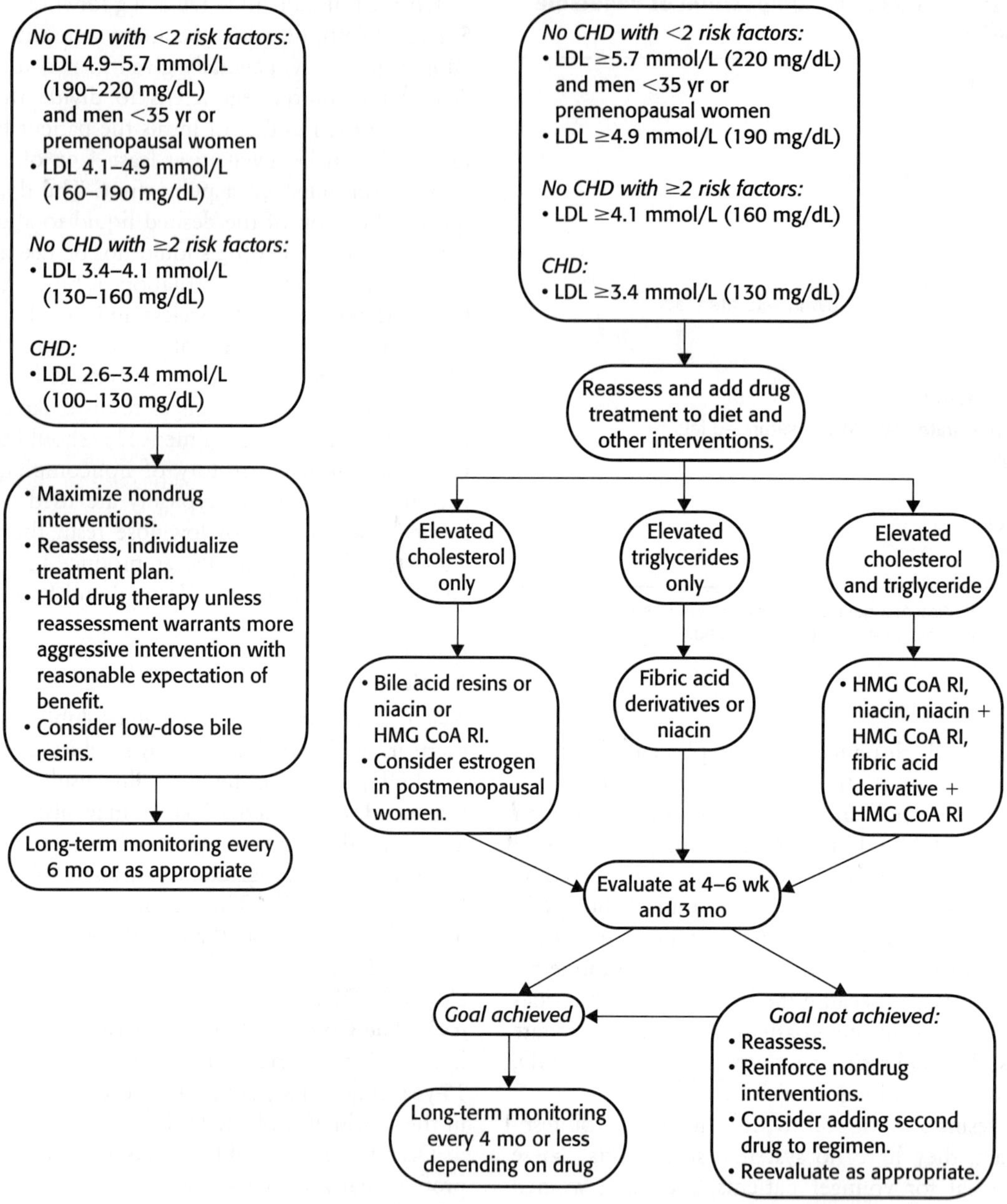

Figure 20.4. Drug therapy algorithm. *CHD,* coronary heart disease; *HMG CoA RI,* 3-hydroxy-3-methylglutaryl coenzyme A (HMG CoA) reductase inhibitor; *LDL,* low-density lipoprotein. (Adapted from reference 5.)

Niacin is contraindicated in patients with chronic liver disease and active PUD. Sustained-released preparations are available that may decrease the prostaglandin-mediated side effects and the GI discomfort, but they are generally less effective cholesterol-lowering agents and have been associated with an increase in the risk of hepatotoxicity.[41] The difference in toxicity may be the result of differences in the metabolism of the immediate-release and sustained-release formulations. In clinical trials of a new extended-release niacin tablet, fewer than 1% of patients with normal liver function tests (LFTs) at baseline had elevations to more than three times the upper limit of normal. This product also demonstrated effects on the lipid profile similar to that of immediate-release niacin. Starting dosages of this extended-release product are 375 mg once daily at bedtime, titrating up to a maximum dosage of 2000 mg/day.

Other side effects include elevations in LFTs, uric acid levels, and blood glucose levels. For these reasons, niacin should be used with caution in patients with gout or diabetes. Elevation in liver enzymes can occur at any time but usually occurs if the niacin dosage is increased too quickly. Patients should undergo baseline LFTs when niacin is started and regular monitoring thereafter. NCEP-ATPII guidelines recommend a maximum dosage of immediate-release niacin of 3000 mg/day, which is usually given in three divided doses, but niacin can be dosed up to 6000 mg/day with appropriate monitoring.

3-Hydroxyl-3-Methylglutaryl-Coenzyme A Reductase Inhibitors

Atorvastatin, cerivastatin, fluvastatin, lovastatin, pravastatin, and simvastatin, or the statin drugs, competitively inhibit the enzyme HMG CoA reductase, which is responsible for the conversion of HMG CoA to mevalonic acid. Mevalonic acid is a precursor to cholesterol in its synthesis. When this process is inhibited, cholesterol production is reduced, which results in an upregulation of LDL receptors and further reduction of circulating free cholesterol.

HMG CoA reductase inhibitors are the most potent LDL-lowering drugs available and generally are preferred in patients with elevated LDL because they are more effective and better tolerated than other cholesterol-lowering agents. Statins reduce LDL by 20 to 60%, decrease triglycerides by 10 to 40%, and increase HDL by 5 to 15%.[5] Table 20.12 lists the pharmacokinetic properties of the available statins.

Primary and secondary prevention trials have shown that these agents reduce the risk of CHD and total mortality. The 4S study was the first trial to show a benefit in total mortality, with a 30% risk reduction.[16] Investigators for this trial also reported 42% lower coronary mortality among patients with CHD and a mean baseline LDL of 188 mg/dL who were treated with simvastatin than in those receiving placebo. The CARE trial looked at survivors of MI and mean baseline LDL of 139 mg/dL who were treated with pravastatin 40 mg/day.[31] At the end of 5 years, these study patients had a 24% lower incidence of coronary events than those given placebo. LIPID, also a secondary prevention trial, demonstrated a 24% risk reduction of death from CHD in patients included in the pravastatin treatment arm of this study.[33] AFCAPS/TexCAPS reported a 37% reduction in the risk for first acute major coronary events, defined as fatal or nonfatal MI, unstable angina, or sudden cardiac death in a primary prevention population treated with lovastatin.[32]

Dose-ranging studies show that statins are most effective when the dosage is divided into a twice-daily regimen. There is a loss of about 3 to 6% in total cholesterol and 2 to 4% in LDL reduction when the total dose is given in the evening. If the same dosage is administered in the morning, there is a loss of 6 to 12% total cholesterol and 4 to 9% LDL. The exception is atorvastatin, which has a sufficiently long half-life of to allow once-daily administration without loss of effect. Nevertheless, evening administration of statins has become the preferred administration time because of improved compliance with once-daily administration, which may overcome the slight loss of efficacy with long-term use. In addition, evening administration of statins allows the peak concentration of statin to occur during peak cholesterol synthesis, between midnight and 3 am. Lovastatin should be dosed with meals to enhance its bioavailability. The bioavailability of pravastatin is slightly lower when it is given with meals; however, this does not seem to affect its LDL-lowering effect. Therefore, pravastatin can be given without regard to meals.

The statins generally are well tolerated, but safety beyond 5 years has not been established. The most common side effects are GI effects, including abdominal pain, flatulence, and constipation, which occur in approximately 3% of patients. Headaches, liver enzyme elevations, and skin rashes are seen in approximately 0.6 to 1.3% of

Table 20.11 ▪ Schedule for Titrating Niacin

Week 1	125 mg BID
Week 2	250 mg BID
Week 3	500 mg BID
Week 4	500 mg BID
Week 5	1000 mg BID
Week 6	1500 mg BID

Source: Reference 20.

Table 20.12 ▪ Pharmacokinetics of HMG CoA Reductase Inhibitors

	Atorvastatin	Cerivastatin	Fluvastatin	Lovastatin	Pravastatin	Simvastatin
Dosage	10–80 mg	0.2–0.3 mg	20–80 mg	20–80 mg	10–40 mg	5–80 mg
Relative potency	3	0.5	0.5	1	1	2
Average low-density lipoprotein reduction	39–60%	25–28%	22–24%	20–40%	20–40%	28–45%
Average triglyceride reduction	26–45%	5–15%	7–12%	10–19%	9–15%	4–19%
Average high-density lipoprotein increase	5–15%	5–10%	2–4%	7–10%	12–16%	5–12%
Effect of food	No effect	No effect	No effect	Bioavailability ↑ by 50%	No effect	No effect
Active metabolites	Yes	Yes	No	Yes	Yes	Yes
Protein binding	≥98%	>99%	98%	95%	50%	95%
Crosses blood-brain barrier	N/A	N/A	No	Yes	No	Yes
T_{max} [14]	1–2 hr	2–5 hr	0.5 hr	2–4 hr	1–2 hr	1–2 hr
Elimination	Hepatic	Hepatic/renal	Hepatic	Hepatic	Hepatic	Hepatic/renal

Source: References 21, 41.

patients. LFTs for most of the statins should be performed at the start of therapy, 6 and 12 weeks after initiation of therapy or when the dosage is increased, and periodically thereafter. Fluvastatin, pravastatin, and simvastatin have fewer LFT monitoring requirements than the other statins. In patients on fluvastatin or pravastatin, LFTs should be checked at baseline and 12 weeks after initiation of therapy or dosage increase. For simvastatin, LFTs should be checked at initiation of therapy and semiannually for the first year or until 1 year after the last dosage increase. In patients who are titrated to the 80 mg/day dosage, LFTs should be evaluated 3 months after that dosage is established. If aspartate aminotransferase (AST) and alanine aminotransferase (ALT) levels increase to more than three times the upper limit of normal, the drug should be discontinued. The likelihood of drug-induced hepatotoxicity increases if AST and ALT elevation is accompanied by a substantial reduction in cholesterol levels. Elevations in liver enzymes generally are reversible upon discontinuation of the drug.

Myopathy with elevated creatine kinase, possibly resulting in rhabdomyolysis and acute renal failure, occurs rarely (in 0.8% of patients) but can be a serious, life-threatening event. Patients should be warned of this potential side effect and advised to report promptly any unexplained muscle weakness or pain. Creatine kinase levels typically are not useful in routine monitoring of asymptomatic patients because they can increase as the result of exercise or minor muscle trauma. The incidence of myopathy and rhabdomyolysis increases when statins are given concomitantly with cyclosporine, niacin, gemfibrozil, erythromycin, protease inhibitors, and possibly other HMG CoA reductase inhibitors, but it would be unusual to give two statins simultaneously. Statins have been used safely with cyclosporine and gemfibrozil in studies, but side effects and LFTs must be monitored more often. Some evidence suggests that pravastatin may be the HMG CoA reductase inhibitor of choice in this setting because of its hydrophilicity and lack of metabolism via the cytochrome P-450-3A4 system. Active liver disease, unexplained elevation of the liver enzymes, pregnancy, and hypersensitivity are the recommended contraindications for these agents.[17,42,43]

Fibric Acid Derivatives

Fibrates principally lower triglycerides by increasing the activity of lipoprotein lipase, the enzyme responsible for the hydrolysis of triglycerides from VLDL and IDL particles. By increasing the catabolism of VLDL, a precursor to LDL, fibrates also slightly decrease LDL levels. Fibric acid derivatives effectively reduce triglycerides by 20 to 30%, decrease LDL by approximately 15%, and increase HDL by 10 to 20%.[5] In the Helsinki Heart Study,[25] a primary prevention trial, a significant reduction in the rates of both fatal and nonfatal CHD events was seen among patients taking gemfibrozil. The greatest benefit occurred among those with high LDL, low HDL, and high triglyceride levels. There was no benefit in patients with high LDL levels alone. In a 3.5-year follow-up of the trial, there was a suggestion of increased total mortality secondary to an increase in noncoronary deaths in patients treated with gemfibrozil. This finding was inconclusive, and gemfibrozil use has not been associated with fatal side effects.

Fibric acid derivatives are considered first-line therapy in patients with isolated hypertriglyceridemia. Gemfibrozil is indicated for patients with high triglycerides and for primary CHD prevention in patients with elevated LDL and triglycerides. It is not recommended as single-drug therapy in patients with established CHD. The usual dosage is 600 mg twice daily. Clofibrate, another fibric acid agent, is not commonly used because of a significantly higher rate of total mortality in clinical trials, malignant GI disease, and a higher rate of cholecystectomy for gallstones.[22] The usual dosage for clofibrate is 1 g twice daily. Fenofibrate has been available outside the United States for many years. The new micronized form, which is now available in the United States, is more rapidly and completely absorbed. The starting dosage is 67 mg daily, with a maximum dosage of 201 mg/day.

Gemfibrozil and fenofibrate generally are well tolerated but may cause GI disturbances in some patients. Nausea, abdominal pain, and diarrhea occur in 4 to 5% of patients. Other reported adverse effects include altered LFTs, muscle pain, and skin rash. Caution is indicated when fibric acid derivatives and HMG CoA reductase inhibitors are used concomitantly because of the risk of rhabdomyolysis. In addition, use of warfarin in combination with gemfibrozil or fenofibrate can increase the anticoagulant effects of warfarin. For patients taking this type of drug regimen, the international normalized ratio (INR) should be monitored closely after the fibric acid derivative is added or discontinued. Absolute contraindications to fibric acid use include severe renal or hepatic dysfunction, pregnancy, and gallbladder disease.

Other Agents

Men are at greater risk for heart disease than premenopausal women. CHD typically occurs 10 years later in women than in men. In addition, CHD develops later in women who take conjugated estrogens after menopause than in those who do not take estrogen. Therefore, hormone replacement therapy is considered first-line treatment for lipid management in postmenopausal women. Estrogen, with or without progestin, decreases LDL by 15%, increases HDL by 15%, and slightly increases triglycerides.[44,45] Caution is warranted when estrogen is used in patients with significantly elevated triglycerides and in those in whom estrogen may exacerbate a medical condition, such as estrogen-receptor–positive breast cancer. Lipid profiles should be repeated within 6 months after hormone replacement therapy is started, and the decision about further drug treatment should be based on this measurement.

In a 20-year observational study conducted in the Netherlands,[46] middle-aged men who consumed 30 g fish daily had 50% lower cardiovascular mortality than those who did not eat fish. In another study,[47] more than 2000 MI survivors were randomly assigned to three different groups. Patients assigned to the fish group had a 29% reduction in all-cause mortality, but the rate of reinfarction was not affected. The beneficial effects of fish oil result from the reduction in the production of VLDL and plasma homocysteine levels. Fish oil also impairs the scavenger receptor pathway that leads to the synthesis of lipid-rich foam cells. Fish oil is indicated only for patients with severe hypertriglyceridemia or chylomicronemia and for those at risk for pancreatitis who are refractory to niacin or fibric acid derivatives. Fish oil is available in capsules containing 600 mg of Ω-3 fatty acids. The starting dosage is three capsules twice daily with meals. If therapeutic goals are not met at the 6- to 8-week follow-up, the dosage should be increased to four to five capsules twice a day, which is the maximum dosage.

Fish oil should be used cautiously in patients with increased bleeding tendencies and thrombocytopenia. The dosage should be decreased or the drug discontinued if easy bruising or evidence of bleeding tendency develops. Patients may gain weight while taking fish oil capsules because of the fat content. Patients with type 2 diabetes should not take fish oil because it impairs glucose tolerance by increasing hepatic glucose production and inhibiting insulin secretion.[36]

There is a dose-related relationship between alcohol and HDL cholesterol. On average, people who consume 1 oz alcohol daily (i.e., 24 oz beer, 8 oz table wine, or two shots of proof spirit) have HDL levels 6 to 7 mg/dL higher than those of people who do not drink alcohol. However, people who consume more than this are at risk for cardiovascular and other health problems. Patients with hypertriglyceridemia should use alcohol sparingly because it can increase triglyceride levels.[48]

Probucol can cause a 10 to 21% reduction in total cholesterol, LDL, and HDL. Its effect on triglycerides varies. Because this drug reduces HDL, it is rarely used in treating hyperlipidemia. Adverse effects tend to be minor and transient. They include diarrhea in about 10% of patients, abdominal pain, flatulence, nausea, and vomiting. Headache, dizziness, and paresthesias have also been reported in a small number of patients. The usual adult dosage is 500 mg twice daily, given with the morning and evening meals. Daily dosages should not exceed 1 g.

Several studies have documented the cholesterol-lowering ability of the aminoglycoside neomycin.[49,50] The drug may reduce the absorption of cholesterol from the gut, but the exact mechanism of action is not known. Neomycin has no role as a lipid-lowering agent because of potential nephrotoxicity and ototoxicity, the possibility of selecting resistant pathogens, decreasing the effective use of aminoglycosides, and the availability of safer agents.

Recent evidence indicates that the antioxidant vitamins C, E, and β-carotene may be effective in the treatment and prevention of CHD. The Cambridge Heart Antioxidant Study (CHAOS)[51] trial looked at the effect of vitamin E in the secondary prevention of CHD. The investigators found total mortality to be slightly but not significantly lower in the vitamin E group than in the placebo group. Unfortunately, the study was too small to examine mortality. Interpretation and extrapolation of these results are difficult because of the baseline differences in the two study groups and variations in vitamin E dosage during the trial. Nevertheless, it raised interesting questions about the use of vitamin E in this patient population. It is thought that vitamin E works by reducing lipid peroxidation and macrophage recruitment, resulting in plaque stabilization. Further study is needed to elicit the true benefit, if any, of vitamin E and other antioxidants.

Garlic is thought to lower cholesterol levels by decreasing hepatocyte cholesterol synthesis. A review of clinical trials assessing the lipid-lowering effects of garlic showed that garlic decreased total cholesterol by 10% on average.[52] Most of these trials were done with small numbers of study patients for short lengths of time and with different garlic preparations. These different preparations of garlic have not been equated to a specific dosage. Also, there are several constituents in garlic products, and it is not know which are responsible for the lipid-lowering effect. More clinical trials involving larger numbers of study subjects using standard dosing of garlic are needed to assess its true benefit as a hyperlipidemic agent.

PHARMACOECONOMICS

Most cost analyses show that cholesterol-lowering drug therapy is clearly cost-effective for secondary prevention in all patients regardless of age or sex. The 4S trial conducted an economic evaluation of the impact of simvastatin on hospital resources.[53] The evaluation was reported in U.S. dollars and based on the significantly lower rates of hospitalization for revascularizations (26% lower), hospitalizations for coronary artery disease events (32% lower), and average length of stay (7.1 versus 7.9 days) in the simvastatin group compared to the placebo group. The investigators concluded that the cost of using lipid-lowering medications is offset by the decrease in the numbers of procedures, hospitalizations, and other medical interventions.

Cost-effectiveness of cholesterol-lowering drugs in primary prevention is highly dependent on age and coronary risk factors. Because of the low incidence of coronary events in otherwise healthy young men and women, drug therapy appears to be much less cost-effective than other forms of intervention. Dietary therapy and other lifestyle modifications appear to be most cost-effective in this patient population.

CONCLUSION

Early diagnosis and treatment of hyperlipidemia are very important in decreasing the incidence of cardiovascular disease. Drug therapy should be started in patients who do not achieve adequate LDL reductions with lifestyle modifications. By lowering lipid levels, we should see decreases in morbidity and mortality from cardiovascular disease and realize significant cost savings.

The NCEP-ATPII recommendations were last revised in 1993. New guidelines should be developed in the next few years and should address areas such as triglycerides as a risk factor for CHD and treatment of hyperlipidemia in older adults. They may also move patients with diabetes and a strong family history into the most aggressive treatment group, which is now reserved for patients with preexisting CHD.

KEY POINTS

- Cardiovascular disease is one of the leading causes of morbidity and mortality in the United States.
- One of the major risk factors for the development of CHD is hyperlipidemia.
- A low-fat diet should be the foundation of all cholesterol reduction interventions and should be tried before any other interventions are used.
- Hyperlipidemia can be caused by primary (genetic predisposition) or secondary causes (diet, medications, or underlying diseases).
- LDL cholesterol is the lipid component most closely associated with CHD risk and elevated serum cholesterol.
- Low HDL levels are a risk factor for CHD.
- Treatment decisions are based on a patient's LDL level, risk factor status, and presence of CHD or atherosclerotic disease.
- Fruits, vegetables, and grain products that contain fiber, particularly soluble fiber, and a diet low in saturated fat and cholesterol are associated with a reduction in the risk of CHD.
- The choice of which drug to begin should be based on the type of hyperlipidemia, past medical history, adverse effect profile of the drug, effectiveness of the drug, patient's adherence history, and cost.
- Bile acid resins lower total cholesterol and LDL by 15 to 30%, increase HDL by 3 to 5%, and increase triglycerides 2 to 3% after prolonged therapy. These drugs are effective treatment for hypercholesterolemia.
- Niacin decreases LDL by 10 to 25%, decreases triglycerides by 20 to 50%, and increases HDL by 15 to 35% but should be used with caution in patients with a history of PUD, chronic liver disease, gout, and diabetes. Niacin is effective in treating hypercholesterolemia and hypertriglyceridemia.
- HMG CoA reductase inhibitors reduce LDL by 20 to 60%, reduce triglycerides 10 to 40%, and increase HDL by 5 to 15%. Statins are effective for treating hypercholesterolemia and hypertriglyceridemia.
- Fibric acid derivatives reduce LDL by 15%, reduce triglycerides 20 to 30%, and increase HDL by 10 to 20%. They are useful for treating hypertriglyceridemia.

REFERENCES

1. National Cholesterol Education Program. Second report of the Expert Panel on Detection, Evaluation and Treatment of High Blood Cholesterol in Adults (Adult Treatment Panel II). Circulation 89:1329–1345, 1994.
2. Working Group on Management of Patients with Hypertension and High Blood Cholesterol. National Education Programs Working Group report on the management of patients with hypertension and high blood cholesterol. Ann Intern Med 114:224–237, 1991.
3. Pekkanen J, Linn S, Heiss G, et al. Ten-year mortality from cardiovascular disease in relation to cholesterol level among men with and without preexisting cardiovascular disease. N Engl J Med 322:1700–1707, 1990.
4. Fuster V, Pearson T. 27th Bethesda Conference. Matching the intensity of risk factor management with the hazard for coronary disease events. J Am Coll Cardiol 27:957–1047, 1996.
5. The Expert Panel on Detection, Evaluation and Treatment of High Blood Cholesterol in Adults. Summary of the second report of the National Cholesterol Education Program (NCEP) Expert Panel On Detection, Evaluation and Treatment of High Blood Cholesterol in Adults (Adult Treatment Panel II). JAMA 269:3015–3023, 1993.
6. National Institute of Health Office of Medical Applications of Research. Treatment of hypertriglyceridemia. JAMA 251:1196–1200, 1994.
7. Austin M, Hokanson J. Epidemiology of triglycerides, small dense low density lipoprotein, and lipoprotein (a) as risk factors for coronary heart disease. Med Clin North Am 78:99–115, 1994.
8. NIH Consensus Conference. Triglycerides, high density lipoprotein, and coronary heart disease. JAMA 269:505, 1993.
9. Gotto A, Bierman E, Connor W, et al. Recommendations for treatment of hyperlipidemia in adults. Circulation 69:1065A–1090A, 1994.
10. National Institutes of Health Office of Medical Research. Lowering blood cholesterol to prevent heart disease. JAMA 253:2080–2086, 1985.
11. American College of Physicians. Guidelines for using serum cholesterol, high density lipoproteins cholesterol, and triglyceride levels as screening tests for preventing coronary heart disease in adults. Ann Intern Med 124:515–517, 1996.
12. McKenney J. Lovastatin: a new cholesterol lowering agent. Clin Pharmacol Ther 7:21–36. 1988.
13. Havel R, Rapaport E. Management of primary hyperlipidemia. N Engl J Med 332:1491–1498, 1995.
14. Stone N. Secondary causes of hyperlipidemia. Med Clin North Am 78:117–141, 1993.
15. Welch G, Loscalzo J. Homocysteine and atherothrombosis. N Engl J Med 338:1042–1050, 1998.
16. Scandinavian Simvastatin Survival Study Group. Randomized trial of cholesterol lowering in 4,444 patients with coronary heart disease: the Scandinavian Simvastatin Survival Study (4S). Lancet 334:1383–1389, 1994.
17. Schectman G, Hiatt J. Dose-response characteristics of cholesterol-lowering drug therapies: implications for treatment. Ann Intern Med 125:990–1000, 1996.
18. Schaefer E, Levy R. Pathogenesis and management of lipoprotein disorders. N Engl J Med 312:1300–1310, 1985.
19. Ginsberg H. Lipoprotein metabolism and its relationship to atherosclerosis. Med Clin North Am 78:1–20, 1994.
20. Clark A, Holt J. Identifying and managing patients with hyperlipidemia. Am J Man Care 3:1211–1219, 1997.
21. Israel M, Sisson E. Hyperlipidemias. In: Carter B, Lake K, Raebel M, et al., eds. Cardiology module 1. Pharmacotherapy self-assessment program (PSAP). 3rd ed. Kansas City, MO: American College of Clinical Pharmacy, 1998:173–201.
22. Oliver M, Heady J, Morris J, et al. A cooperative trial in the primary prevention of ischemic heart disease using clofibrate. Br Heart J 40:1069–1118, 1978.
23. Lipid Research Clinics Program. The lipid research clinics coronary primary prevention trial results I. Reductions in incidence of coronary heart disease. JAMA 251:357–364, 1984.
24. Lipid Research Clinics Program. The lipid research clinics coronary primary prevention trial results II. The relationship of reduction in incidence of coronary heart disease to cholesterol lowering. JAMA 251:365–374, 1984.
25. Frick M, Elo O, Haapa K, et al. Helsinki heart study; primary prevention trial with gemfibrozil in middle aged men with dyslipidemia. N Engl J Med 317:1237–1245, 1987.

26. Coronary Drug Project Research Group. Clofibrate and niacin in coronary heart disease. JAMA 231:360–381, 1975.
27. Hjermann I, Holme I, Velve Byrne K, et al. Effect of diet and smoking intervention on the incidence of coronary heart disease. Report from the Oslo Study Group of a randomized trial in healthy men. Lancet 11:1303–1310, 1981.
28. Grumbach K. How effective is drug treatment of hypercholesterolemia? A guided tour of the major clinical trials for the primary care physician. J Am Board Fam Pract 4:437–445, 1991.
29. Labreche D. Reassessment of the value of lowering serum cholesterol: how should physicians interpret the published data for patients. Clin Pharmacol Ther 7:592–603, 1988.
30. Shepherd J, Cobbe S, Ford I, et al. Prevention of coronary heart disease with pravastatin in men with hypercholesterolemia. N Engl J Med 333:1301–1307, 1995.
31. Sacks F, Pfeffer M, Moye L, et al. The effects of pravastatin on coronary events after myocardial infarction in patients with average cholesterol levels. N Engl J Med 335:1001–1009, 1996.
32. Buchwald H, Matts J, Fitch L, et al. Changes in sequential coronary arteriograms and subsequent coronary events. Surgical control of the hyperlipidemias (POSCH) group. JAMA 268:1429–1433, 1992.
33. The Post Coronary Artery Bypass Graft Trial Investigators. The effect of aggressive lowering of low density lipoprotein cholesterol levels and low dose anticoagulation on obstructive changes in saphenous-vein coronary artery bypass grafts. N Engl J Med 336:153–162, 1997.
34. Miller M, Vogel R. The practice of coronary disease prevention. Baltimore: Williams & Wilkins, 1996:76–78.
35. Fuster V, Pearson T. 27th Bethesda Conference: matching the intensity of risk factor management with the hazard for coronary disease events. J Am Coll Cardiol 27:957–1047, 1996.
36. American Heart Association Nutrition Committee. Dietary guidelines for healthy American adults. Circulation 77:721A–724A, 1988.
37. Anonymous. Mandatory nutrition labeling: FDA's final rule. Nutr Rev 51:101–105, 1993.
38. Anonymous. The FDA's final regulations on health claims for foods. Nutr Rev 51:90–93, 1993.
39. McKenney J, Proctor J, Harris S, et al. A comparison of the efficacy and toxic effects of sustained versus immediate-release niacin in hypercholesterolemic patients. JAMA 271:672–676, 1994.
40. Morgan J, Capuzzi D, Guyton J, et al. Treatment effect of Niaspan, a controlled-release niacin, in patients with hypercholesterolemia: a placebo-controlled trial. J Cardiovasc Pharmacol Ther 1:195–202, 1996.
41. Blum C. Comparisons of properties of four inhibitors of 3-hydroxy-3-methylglutaryl-coenzyme A reductase. Am J Cardiol 73:3D–11D, 1994.
42. Stampfer M, Colditz G, Willett W, et al. Postmenopausal estrogen therapy and cardiovascular disease: ten-year follow-up from the nurses' health study. N Engl J Med 325:756–762, 1991.
43. Writing Group for PEPI Trial. Effects of estrogen or estrogen/progestin regimens on heart disease in postmenopausal women: The postmenopausal estrogen/progestin trial. JAMA 273:199–208, 1995.
44. Keli S, Feskens, Kromhount D. Fish consumption and risk of stroke. The Zutphen study. Stroke 25:328–332, 1994.
45. Burr M, Gilbert J, Holliday R, et al. Effects of changes in fat, fish and fibre intakes on death and myocardial reinfarction: diet and reinfarction trial (DART). Lancet 2:757–761, 1989.
46. Gazian J, Buring J, Breslow J, et al. Moderate alcohol intake, increased levels of high-density lipoprotein and its subfractions, and decreased risk of myocardial infarction. N Engl J Med 329:1829–1834, 1993.
47. Hoeg J, Schaefer E, Romano C, et al. Neomycin and plasma lipoproteins in type II hyperlipoproteinemia. Clin Pharmacol Ther 36:555–565, 1984.
48. Miettenen T. Effects of neomycin alone and in combination with cholestyramine on serum cholesterol and fecal steroids in hypercholesterolemic subjects. J Clin Invest 301:595–597, 1979.
49. Stephens N, Parsons A, Schofield P, et al. Randomized controlled trial of vitamin E patients with coronary disease: Cambridge Heart Antioxidant Study (CHAOS). Lancet 347:781–786, 1996.
50. Warshafsky S, Damer RS, Sivak S. Effect of garlic on total serum cholesterol. Ann Intern Med 119:599–605, 1993.
51. Pederson T, Kjekshus J, Berg K, et al. Cholesterol lowering and the use of healthcare resources: results of the Scandinavian Simvastatin Survival Study. Circulation 93:1796–1802, 1996.
52. Frost P, Davis B, Burlando A, et al. Serum lipids and incidence of coronary heart disease: findings from the Systolic Hypertension in the Elderly Program (SHEP). Circulation 94:2381–2388, 1996.
53. Lewis S, Moye L, Sacks F, et al. Effect of pravastatin on cardiovascular events in older patients with myocardial infarction and cholesterol levels in the average range. Ann Intern Med 129:681–689, 1998.

CHAPTER 21

ACUTE RENAL DISEASE

Jay F. Mouser

The literature defines acute renal failure (ARF) in a variety of ways. Broadly categorized, ARF is abrupt deterioration in renal function that results in the inability of the kidney to regulate water and solute balance.[1] Clinicians also rely on acute increases in serum creatinine (Scr) concentration of 44 μmol/L (0.5 mg/dL) when the baseline Scr is less than 265 μmol/L (3 mg/dL) or an increase of 88 μmol/L (1 mg/dL) when the baseline Scr is more than 265 μmol/L (3 mg/dL) to define ARF.[2] Mild ARF has been defined as a rise in Scr concentration to 177 to 265 μmol/L (2.0 to 3.0 mg/dL). Severe cases are associated with rises of Scr above 442 μmol/L (5 mg/dL).[2] However, the rate of creatinine rise varies depending on the extent of renal injury, dietary intake, and muscle mass of the patient.

ARF is classified according to the amount of urine produced per day as anuric ARF (less than 50 mL/day), oliguric ARF (50 to 400 mL/day), and nonoliguric ARF (more than 400 mL/day).[1] Although ARF is often thought of as a decrease in urine output, nonoliguric ARF accounts for up to 60% of cases of ARF.[3] Patients with nonoliguric ARF do not concentrate the urine that is produced and continue to retain urea, creatinine, and other waste products of metabolism.

Approximately 5% of hospitalized patients and up to 20% of all patients in an intensive care unit (ICU) develop ARF.[4,5] The course of the illness is highly variable, ranging from transient disease lasting less than 1 week and associated with full recovery of renal function to a disease persisting for longer than 6 weeks and necessitating dialysis and intensive care management.[6] Several important causes and pathophysiologic mechanisms that underlie renal dysfunction and improved supportive care have become better understood recently.[5,7] This has led to the increased use of continuous hemofiltration and various modifications of continuous renal replacement therapy (CRRT). Despite these advances, survival in critically ill patients with ARF has not significantly improved, and optimal treatments and the preferred form of renal replacement therapy (RRT) remain controversial.[4,6,8–10] In the critically ill patient, ARF carries a dismal prognosis, with mortality recently reported to be 58%.[8] Possible explanations for the lack of substantial improvement in survival may be that older patients, often with multiorgan failure and septicemia, are being hospitalized.[10] Also, more surgical procedures are being performed in older adults, thus contributing to the mortality statistics.[1] When factored by illness acuity or injury severity, this may imply that ARF outcomes actually are improving.

Patients with ARF often have other major medical problems necessitating aggressive drug therapy and often resulting in a high incidence of adverse drug reactions. In treating these patients, the clinician must be able to assess the degree of renal insufficiency, recognize pharmacologic agents that can worsen renal function, and perform adjustments of drug dosages. Treating these patients entails an understanding of the underlying pathophysiology and consists of preventive measures, supportive care, and efforts to preserve renal function. This chapter examines the causes, clinical course, and treatment of ARF. Because there are many causes of ARF, only the major causes are discussed.

DEFINITION

ARF has been defined as an increase in Scr of more than 44 μmol/L (0.5 mg/dL) over the baseline value, an increase of more than 50% in Scr, a reduction in calculated creatinine clearance (Ccr) of 50%, or a decrease in renal function that results in the need for dialysis.[7] In addition to changes in Scr, a sudden, sustained decline in glomerular filtration rate (GFR), usually associated with azotemia and a fall in urine output, has also been used to define ARF.[11]

TREATMENT GOALS: ACUTE RENAL DISEASE

- Recognize ARF early and anticipate and prevent potential problems and further renal injury.
- Reverse the underlying cause (if possible).
- Correct or maintain euvolemia and restore electrolyte and acid-base balance.
- Provide support until the patient recovers.
- Maintain the patient's nutritional status.
- Prevent and treat infectious complications.
- Enhance urine flow rates.
- Reverse azotemia.

EPIDEMIOLOGY

ARF is most often a hospital-acquired illness. Risk factors for development of ARF in the ICU include sepsis, hypotension, volume depletion, hemorrhage, mechanical ventilation, and surgery.[12] Numerous surgical and medical insults are associated with ARF. The highest incidence is associated with abdominal aneurysm resection, severe trauma, and open heart surgery.[12] The exact incidence of ARF is difficult to distinguish partly because of the lack of standardized definitions of ARF. In hospitalized patients, the incidence of ARF ranges from less than 1% to about 5%, depending on whether the institution is a primary care facility or a tertiary care referral center.[4,13] Mortality rates in ARF range from approximately 7% among patients admitted to a hospital with prerenal azotemia[14] to more than 80% among patients with postoperative ARF or those with multiple organ failure.[7]

Classification

ARF usually is classified into three categories: prerenal or hypoperfusion states, intrarenal or intrinsic renal parenchymal injury, and postrenal ARF or urinary obstructive disorders.[15]

Prerenal Azotemia

Prerenal azotemia is the most common cause of ARF.[16] It occurs when renal blood flow (RBF) decreases to a level adequate to sustain cells but inadequate to maintain normal GFR. Therefore, cellular injury does not occur and the GFR can be normalized rapidly once the pathophysiologic state is corrected.[17] Reduced RBF may be secondary to any event that results in decreased renal perfusion or intense compensatory afferent arteriolar vasoconstriction. Various causes of prerenal azotemia are listed in Table 21.1.[17–19] Vascular diseases (e.g., renal artery emboli, atheroembolic renal disease) may reduce RBF and cause prerenal ARF. Thrombocytopenic purpura and hemolytic uremic syndrome may also lead to prerenal ARF, but more commonly, they also cause significant glomerular injury.

Mild hypoperfusion, caused by volume depletion, leads to prerenal azotemia with a mild decrease in GFR. The kidneys attempt to increase intravascular volume by conserving salt and water through increased proximal and distal reabsorption as well as increased antidiuretic hor-

Table 21.1 ▪ Causes of Prerenal Acute Renal Failure

Decreased cardiac output
Congestive heart failure
Pericardial tamponade
Pulmonary embolism
Cardiomyopathy
Myocardial infarction
Hypovolemia
Major trauma
Burns
Hemorrhage (surgical, postpartum)
Volume depletion (renal losses, skin, vomiting, diarrhea)
Sequestration (hypoalbuminemia, pancreatitis, peritonitis)
Increased renal vascular resistance
Renal vasoconstriction (norepinephrine, dopamine)
Systemic vasodilation (sepsis, vasodilatory agents)
Anesthesia
Surgery
Systemic vasodilation
Bacterial sepsis
Antihypertensives
Afterload reduction
Renovascular obstruction[a]
Renal artery (atherosclerosis, thrombosis, embolism)
Renal vein (thrombosis)

Source: Reference 18.

[a]In bilateral renal disease or single functioning kidney.

Table 21.2 ▪ Urinary Indices to Differentiate Causes of Acute Renal Failure

	Prerenal	Acute Tubular Necrosis	Postrenal Obstruction
Protein	–	2–4+	–
WBC	–	2–4+	1+
RBC	–	2–4+	Variable
Casts	±	RTE, WBC	–
Osmolality (m Osm/kg)	>400	<350	<350
Specific gravity	>1.013	<1.013	–
U_{Na} (mmol/L)	<20	>40	Variable
FE_{Na} (%)	<1	>2	>1
BUN:Scr ratio	>20:1	<20:1	–
Ucr:Scr ratio	>40	<20	<20
RFI	<1	>4	>1.5

WBC, white blood cell count; *RBC,* red blood cell count; U_{Na}, urine sodium concentration; FE_{Na}, fractional excretion of sodium; *BUN,* blood urea nitrogen; *Ucr,* urine creatinine concentration; *Scr,* serum creatinine concentration; *RFI,* renal failure index.

Table 21.3 ▪ Causes of Postrenal Acute Renal Failure

- Bilateral ureteral obstruction
  - Intraureteral (emboli, stones, crystals)
  - Extraureteral (tumor, retroperitoneal fibrosis)
  - Papillary necrosis (acute pyelonephritis)
- Bladder obstruction
  - Mechanical (prostate hypertrophy, malignancy, infection)
  - Functional (anticholinergics, ganglionic blockers, neuropathy)
- Urethral obstruction

mone (ADH) release. GFR is maintained initially, but only small amounts of concentrated urine are produced. This urine is low in sodium and has a high urine creatinine: plasma creatinine ratio and a low (less than 1) fractional excretion of sodium (FE_{Na}). Because urea reabsorption is also increased, a disproportionate increase in blood urea nitrogen (BUN) relative to Scr occurs; therefore, the BUN:Scr ratio often is more than 20:1. Other factors that may help to differentiate prerenal ARF from intrinsic or postrenal ARF are shown in Table 21.2. Rapid correction of prerenal azotemia can prevent ischemic injury and the associated morbidity and mortality.

Postrenal Acute Renal Failure

Obstruction of the collecting system generally must involve both kidneys (or a solitary kidney) to cause significant renal failure. Obstruction of the urinary tract may result from bladder outlet obstruction caused by prostate enlargement, tumor, or urethral stricture; urethral obstruction from tumor, stone, or fibrosis; or even crystal (uric acid, calcium oxalate, sulfonamide, acyclovir, methotrexate) deposition in the tubules.[7] Obstruction should be considered in patients with acute anuria, particularly in those with a recent history of alternating polyuria and oliguria. Postrenal azotemia is simply an accumulation of nitrogenous wastes secondary to obstruction of urine flow. This disorder accounts for approximately 15% of cases of ARF.[19] Causes of postrenal azotemia are listed in Table 21.3. These causes should be ruled out initially because they are often easily corrected, preventing the progression to intrinsic renal damage.

Intrinsic Acute Renal Failure

Intrinsic ARF is a decrease in renal function resulting from more severe or prolonged ischemic, toxic, or immunologic mechanisms (Table 21.4) and is associated with structural damage to glomeruli, tubules, vascular supply, or interstitial tissue.[19] Such damage to the renal parenchyma often follows prerenal or postrenal azotemia, and if the degree of insult or duration of hypoperfusion or obstruction is sufficient, it is not immediately reversible. Recovery from intrarenal disease commonly takes 10 to 14 days but may take 6 weeks to more than a year.[6] *Intrinsic ARF* is commonly used interchangeably with *acute tubular necrosis* (ATN), which denotes a histologic finding signifying necrotic damage to the renal tubules.

Acute Renal Failure from Therapeutic Agents

The kidneys are uniquely vulnerable to toxic injury because relative to their weight, they have the largest endothelial surface area and highest blood flow of any organ. Concentration of potential nephrotoxins occurs within the renal tubules through secretion and reabsorption, thus exposing the tubular lumen and peritubular cells to high concentrations of potential toxins. Renal medullary and

Table 21.4 ▪ Intrinsic Causes of Acute Renal Failure

- Sequelae of prolonged prerenal azotemia
- Nephrotoxic agents (drugs and radiocontrast)
- Ischemic events
  - Massive hemorrhage
  - Pregnancy (preeclampsia, postpartum renal failure)
  - Crush injury
  - Septic shock
  - Transfusion reaction
  - Venous occlusion
  - Arterial thrombosis
- Glomerular
  - Systemic lupus erythematosus
  - Poststreptococcal glomerulonephritis
  - Drug-induced vasculitis
  - Malignant hypertension
- Tubulointerstitial
  - Acute tubular necrosis
  - Acute interstitial nephritis
  - Acute pyelonephritis
  - Hyperuricemia
  - Hypercalcemia

papillary tissues are vulnerable to toxic damage because of a combination of low blood flow and extremely high solute concentration. Also, the kidneys are highly active metabolic organs capable of transforming innocuous substances, such as acetaminophen, into highly reactive metabolites.[20,21] The lesions associated with drug-induced nephropathy can be divided into three major categories: ATN, acute tubulointerstitial disease (ATID), and glomerulonephritis. A list of drugs and chemicals associated with each of these lesions is provided in Table 21.5.

ATN is a nonspecific response to ischemia or direct toxic insult. ARF may result from cellular debris of tubular necrosis obstructing the proximal tubule. As intratubular pressure increases and glomerular filtration decreases, filtered wastes regain access to the circulation by leaking across transtubular membranes.[22–24] The type of cellular injury associated with ATN varies with the type of renal insult. In a study of 121 patients who developed ATN, hypotension (27%) and dehydration (27%) were the sole causes of ARF. More than one acute insult was identified in 62% of these patients.[25]

ATID, also known as acute interstitial nephritis, is characterized by interstitial edema and renal cellular infiltrates made up of monocytes, large and small lymphocytes, and plasma cells. Eosinophils may or may not be present. Tubular damage is suggested by the presence of cellular infiltrates located along the tubular basement membrane or between tubular epithelial cells.[26] Drug-induced ATID appears to be a hypersensitivity reaction and often is associated with systemic signs of an allergic reaction such as fever, skin rash, eosinophilia, and arthralgia. Hypersensitivity is further suggested by the small number of patients developing the reaction, the lack of dose-related effect, and a sudden recurrence with reinstitution of therapy.[27,28] Other less common causes of ATID include autoimmune diseases (e.g., lupus), infiltrative disease (e.g., sarcoidosis), and infectious agents (e.g., *Legionella pneumophila*).[7] ARF caused by ATID often is reversible after the underlying disease is treated or the offending medication is discontinued. In cases of ATID in which infection can be excluded, corticosteroids may accelerate renal function recovery.

Glomerulonephritis may be caused by several different mechanisms. In some cases there is a direct dose-dependent effect on glomerular structures; in the majority, however, the glomerulus is involved through immunologic reactions. Drugs may act as haptens or antigens that either produce circulating antigen–antibody complexes or cause complex formation within the glomerulus. Damage to or alteration of the glomerular basement membrane produces proteinuria, a hallmark of this disease. The most common drug-induced lesion is membranous glomerulonephritis with proteinuria and nephrotic syndrome. Prompt treatment of glomerulonephritis using immunosuppressive agents or plasma exchange may reduce the risk of end-stage renal disease.[7]

Table 21.5 ▪ Agents Associated with Nephrotoxicity

- Acute tubular necrosis
  - Antibiotics
    - Aminoglycosides
    - Amphotericin B
    - Bacitracin and polymyxins
    - Cephalosporins
    - Sulfonamides
  - Metals
    - Bismuth
    - Mercurials
    - Platinum
  - Radiocontrast media
  - Miscellaneous agents
    - Acetaminophen
    - Cisplatin
    - Cyclosporine
    - Methotrexate
    - Tacrolimus
- Glomerulonephritis
  - Allopurinol
  - Ampicillin
  - Captopril
  - Cocaine
  - Cyclophosphamide
  - Daunorubicin
  - Gold
  - Hydralazine
  - Methicillin
  - Penicillamine
  - Penicillin
  - Rifampin
  - Thiazides
- Acute tubulointerstitial disease
  - Penicillins
    - Ampicillin, amoxicillin
    - Methicillin
    - Nafcillin
    - Oxacillin
    - Penicillin
  - Other antibiotics
    - Cephalosporins
    - Erythromycin
    - Rifampin
    - Sulfonamides
  - Metals
    - Bismuth
    - Gold
  - Miscellaneous agents
    - Captopril
    - Furosemide
    - Nonsteroidal anti-inflammatory drugs
    - Phenytoin
    - Thiazides

Aminoglycosides

Aminoglycosides are avidly concentrated within the renal cortex. After initial binding to tubular brush border membranes, they are vacuolized and taken up by the proximal tubular cells. Once within the cell, they are transported to the lysosomes. Continued uptake results in lysosomal dysfunction and eventual degeneration, allowing lysosomal enzymes to act on other cell organelles. Tubular cell necrosis may result from continued exposure. The initial manifestations of nephrotoxicity include release of brush border and lysosomal enzymes, glycosuria, aminoaciduria, and tubular proteinuria. Defects in proximal tubular transport may be indicated by the presence of β_2-microglobulin. Hypokalemia, hypomagnesemia, and loss of concentrating ability may also be seen. Patients who develop aminoglycoside nephrotoxicity are most often nonoliguric. The occurrence of toxicity is most closely related to treatment duration and usually is seen after 7 to 10 days of therapy. Additional risk factors for the development of nephrotoxicity include age, dosage, high trough serum concentrations, and low urine flow rates. Selecting patients correctly, based on culture and sensitivity data, withdrawing unnecessary therapy early, adjusting dosages to ensure therapeutic levels, and maintaining good urine output during therapy help to minimize toxicity.[29–35]

Amphotericin B

Interaction of amphotericin B with membrane sterols disrupts cell membranes. The possibility of direct vasoconstriction of the renal vasculature has also been suggested. Toxicity is dose related and is seen in up to 80% of patients treated with a cumulative dosage of 2 to 3 g. Early manifestations of amphotericin B nephrotoxicity include renal concentrating defects, distal renal tubular acidosis with potassium wasting, and modest proteinuria. The occurrence of renal failure usually is associated with proximal tubular necrosis. Because nephrotoxicity often limits a full course of therapy, many attempts to limit toxicity have been tried. To date, no regimen or manipulation in therapy has been found to attenuate the toxicity consistently, although encouraging results have been seen with sodium supplementation of 150 mEq/day. Alternate-day therapy may be used when toxicity is recognized, and discontinuation is recommended when the BUN exceeds 50 mg/dL.[29,36,37] In addition, new amphotericin products have been formulated to reduce nephrotoxicity. Liposomal amphotericin B has a lower nephrotoxicity profile, although it is 20 to 50 times more expensive than conventional therapy.

Cyclosporine

Cyclosporine has a major role in the prevention of allograft rejection. The most common side effect is a dose-dependent decline in GFR, with reversible increases in Scr and BUN concentrations. This toxicity can complicate treatment of renal transplant recipients because distinguishing between graft rejection and cyclosporine toxicity is difficult, even with the use of decision algorithms.[38,39] Enhanced toxicity may occur with the simultaneous use of acyclovir, ketoconazole, amphotericin B, aminoglycosides, and cotrimoxazole. Reduction in toxicity has been attempted by prolonging the infusion time to up to 24 hours and administering transdermal clonidine and thromboxane synthetase inhibitors.[40,41] Attempts have been made to monitor plasma levels of cyclosporine and to maintain trough concentrations of 100 to 250 ng/mL. In vitro data suggest that there is little immunosuppression in mixed lymphocyte cultures at concentrations below 100 ng/mL. The search for a therapeutic window using pharmacokinetic monitoring continues to be an important function at transplantation centers.[42–44] (See Chapter 104, Transplantation.)

Radiographic Contrast Media

The increased use of contrast media associated with intravenous pyelography, angiography, and computed tomography has led to greater recognition of this class of agents as an important cause of ARF. The diagnosis must be considered when one of these agents is used in a high-risk patient who subsequently develops any degree of renal failure. Mild nonoliguric renal failure may be transient, with Scr reaching a peak in 3 to 5 days and returning to baseline within 10 to 14 days. Severe oliguric renal failure may occur within 24 hours of the contrast administration, with a return to baseline within 3 weeks, residual renal impairment, or renal failure necessitating dialysis. High-risk patients include those with diabetes mellitus, preexisting renal disease, multiple myeloma, advanced age, coexisting liver disease, peripheral vascular disease, hypertension, dehydration, and prior exposure to contrast media. However, the overall risk of developing ARF from contrast media is less than 0.01% for all patients undergoing these procedures.[45] The precise mechanism of nephrotoxicity is unknown but may include impaired renal perfusion, glomerular injury, tubular injury, and tubular obstruction. Prevention is aimed at avoiding unnecessary procedures, providing vigorous hydration (particularly in high-risk patients), avoiding nonsteroidal anti-inflammatory drugs (NSAIDs), using low dosages of contrast media, and avoiding multiple procedures that involve the use of contrast. The use of hyperosmolar (1500 mOsm/kg) or less hyperosmolar (750 mOsm/kg) nonionic contrast agents does not significantly influence the risk of nephrotoxicity in patients with normal renal function.[46] Extracellular volume expansion with 800 mL/hour normal saline during the procedure and liberal oral or parenteral fluids both before and after the procedure have reduced toxicity significantly, even in high-risk patients.[29,47] Clinical trials performed in patients with moderate renal insufficiency (Scr 1.4 to 2.4 mg/dL) have demonstrated a lower incidence of renal dysfunction in patients receiving newer nonionic, low-osmolality agents than in those receiving ionic agents. However, because they are much more expensive, the use of nonionic contrast agents should be restricted to high-risk patients, such as those with Scr above 2 mg/dL, particularly if they are diabetic.[47,48]

Angiotensin-Converting Enzyme Inhibitors

Acute reversible nonoliguric renal failure may occur after initiation of angiotensin-converting enzyme (ACE) inhibitor therapy in patients with bilateral renal artery stenosis or renal artery stenosis in a solitary kidney. Low renal perfusion stimulates the renin–angiotensin system. Angiotensin II causes renal vasoconstriction and increases efferent arteriolar tone, which acts to maintain glomerular filtration pressure. ACE inhibition leads to dilation of efferent arterioles, which causes an abrupt decline in renal function in those dependent on efferent tone to maintain GFR.[49,50]

Nonsteroidal Anti-Inflammatory Drugs

Local prostaglandin (PG) production promotes dilation of medullary blood vessels and maintains local blood flow. Although RBF is not dependent on these PGs in normal patients, in certain clinical situations (e.g., systemic hypotension, severe hemorrhage, pancreatitis, liver disease, third-space losses from burns, cardiogenic shock), RBF becomes dependent on intrarenal PG production and these patients are susceptible to NSAID-induced renal failure.[46,51] The association between NSAID-induced ARF with diuretic use may be related to the edematous state (and decreased effective blood volume) or stimulation of vasodilator PGs. Cyclosporine increases urinary excretion of vasodilator PGs, probably because of its renal vasoconstrictive effect, and increases the risk of NSAID-induced ARF.

Cisplatin

Cisplatin is highly concentrated in the proximal tubular cells. Intracellular transformation of the chloride ligands on the molecule into a highly reactive aquated compound is thought to occur because of the low intracellular chloride concentration. This transformed molecule is then able to alkylate purine and pyrimidine bases of DNA. ATN occurs because cellular degeneration results in a proximal tubular obstruction from cellular debris. The incidence and severity of renal toxicity is both dose and duration dependent. A rise in Scr and BUN levels may be preceded by proteinuria, tubular casts, enzymuria, and the presence of β_2-microglobulin in the urine. Cisplatin nephrotoxicity has been reduced with prehydration with saline. One such approach is administering 5% dextrose in 0.45 to 0.9% sodium chloride at a rate of 250 mL/hour beginning 2 hours before cisplatin. The cisplatin dose is administered in 250 mL 3% sodium chloride solution. Mannitol 12.5 g is given immediately before cisplatin and then infused at the rate of 10 g/hour for 3 hours. This technique provides enough chloride to prevent the aquation reaction within the cisplatin container and provides an osmotic diuresis to minimize exposure of proximal tubular cells.[29,52,53]

PATHOPHYSIOLOGY

Normal Renal Function

A basic understanding of normal kidney function facilitates a clinical appreciation of ARF. The primary function of the kidney is to maintain the body's internal environment by regulating body fluid volume, electrolyte composition, and acid-base balance. The kidneys are also responsible for producing and secreting various hormones and enzymes. Erythropoietin is produced by the renal cortical cells and stimulates erythrocyte maturation in the bone marrow. Also, 1,25-dihydroxycholecalciferol (the active form of vitamin D) is formed in the proximal tubule cells and plays an important role in regulating body calcium and phosphate balance. Therefore, complications of renal disease reflect impairment of the normal physiologic functions of the kidney, primarily regulation of water and electrolyte balance, arterial blood pressure, erythrocyte production, and vitamin D activity and excretion of metabolic waste products. A logical approach to understanding abnormal renal function is to divide the kidney into basic components of renal circulation, glomerular hemodynamics, and nephron function.

Renal Circulation

The renal arteries carry approximately one-fifth of cardiac output to the kidneys. After reaching the kidney, the renal artery bifurcates into smaller artery branches, eventually leading to afferent arterioles, which supply the glomeruli. As blood leaves the glomeruli, the capillaries coalesce into the efferent arteriole, which then bifurcates to form the peritubular capillary network. Thus, RBF passes through two extensive capillary networks, the glomerular bed and peritubular capillary bed, and the latter nourishes the tubular cells and brings substances to the tubules for secretion. The afferent arterioles supply blood to the glomerulus, and the efferent arterioles carry blood from the glomerulus (Fig. 21.1).

Glomerular Hemodynamics

The glomerulus is located at the proximal end of the renal tubule and is the area where the afferent and efferent arterioles connect. The transcapillary hydrostatic pressure produced by glomerular surface area and vascular resistance across the arterioles is responsible for glomerular ultrafiltrate production. Afferent arteriolar tone is determined predominantly by the vasoconstrictor effects of angiotensin II and the vasodilator effects of PGs. Efferent arteriolar tone is determined by local concentrations of angiotensin II. Glomerular ultrafiltrate production is decreased by pathophysiologic processes and medications that alter afferent or efferent arteriolar tone and reduce

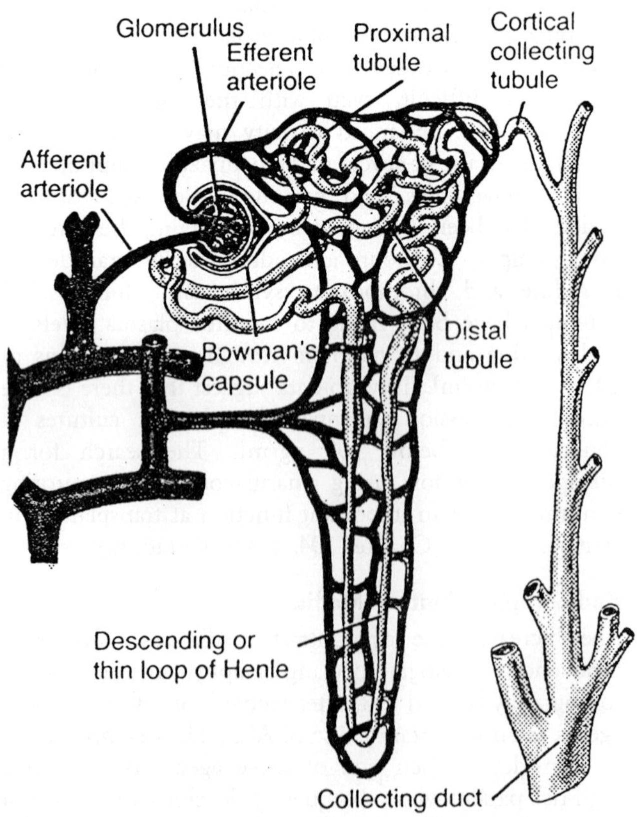

Figure 21.1. The nephron. (Reprinted with permission from Smith HW. The kidney: structure and functions in health and disease. New York: Oxford University Press, 1951.)

glomerular hydrostatic pressure (i.e., hypercalcemia, ACE inhibitors, and NSAIDs).

Nephron Function

Each nephron consists of a glomerular capillary network surrounded by Bowman's capsule, a proximal tubule, a loop of Henle, a distal tubule, and a collecting duct (Fig. 21.1). There are about a million nephrons in each kidney. A plasma ultrafiltrate is formed in the glomerular capillary with collection of the filtered fluid in Bowman's capsule. The filtrate then enters the proximal tubule, where approximately two-thirds of the filtered sodium and water is reabsorbed. More than 90% of filtered bicarbonate and nearly all of filtered glucose and amino acids are also reabsorbed in the proximal tubule. The loop of Henle consists of the terminal portion of the proximal tubule, the thin descending and ascending limbs, and the thick ascending limb. The loop of Henle is responsible for urine dilution and is also the site of magnesium reabsorption. The distal tubule and collecting duct make the final adjustments in urine composition. Here, ADH regulates water reabsorption and aldosterone regulates sodium reabsorption and potassium excretion.

Abnormal Renal Function

Although considerable experimental work using animal models has resulted in several theories, the pathogenesis of ARF remains unclear. Several mechanisms are thought to be involved in the development of renal dysfunction. Again, these theories can be categorized as circulatory, glomerular, and tubular events.

Circulatory Disturbances

RBF reduction, if severe enough, can lead to ischemia and is the most common mechanism of ARF.[1,7,11] In response to reduced RBF, vasodilating PGs (e.g., PGI_2 and PGE_2) reduce afferent arteriolar tone and increase blood flow to the kidney.[7] NSAIDs inhibit PG synthesis and limit the kidney's production of these vasodilatory substances. This appears to be particularly detrimental in patients with congestive heart failure (CHF) who have low effective arterial blood volume and in those with actual volume depletion.[54] Other clinical situations in which diminished RBF may lead to ischemic ARF include severe extracellular fluid volume depletion, systemic hypotension, severe hemorrhage, gastrointestinal losses, pancreatitis, liver disease, third-space losses from burns, cardiogenic shock, or surgical procedures in which repair of renal artery lesions entails aortic cross-clamping proximal to the renal arteries. RBF may also become structurally impaired by renal artery lesions or atheromatous disease. In these situations, GFR becomes dependent on angiotensin II for maintaining efferent arteriolar tone. Treatment with ACE inhibitors reduces the glomerular capillary filtration pressure by decreasing efferent arteriolar tone, and GFR falls. When the ACE inhibitor is discontinued, GFR increases rapidly.

α-Adrenergic receptor-mediated systemic vasoconstriction associated with norepinephrine or high-dose dopamine can also result in marked RBF reductions. Severe renal hypoperfusion also is associated with eclamptic complications of pregnancy.[55] Nephrotoxic agents, especially aminoglycosides, amphotericin B, and radiocontrast media, are commonly associated with the development of ARF. Finally, endotoxin-mediated renal vasoconstriction may occur in sepsis.[56]

In response to diminished RBF, the kidney attempts to maintain intravascular volume by conserving sodium and water through increased reabsorption in the proximal and distal tubules and by increasing ADH release. Despite these compensatory mechanisms, ischemia may occur if RBF diminishes to the extent that nutrient and oxygen supplies cannot meet metabolic demands of the renal tubular cells. During the ischemic insult, the lack of oxygen causes mitochondrial oxidative phosphorylation to stop, leading to depletion of adenosine triphosphate (ATP) stores.[57] Thus, cells with the greatest dependence on mitochondrial ATP production may be most susceptible to oxygen deprivation-induced ATP depletion.[58] In experimental models, renal epithelial cell ATP concentrations decrease shortly after ischemic insult, and exogenous administration of ATP results in accelerated recovery of ATP levels and a shortened duration of ARF.[59]

Severe ATP depletion may be expected to disable many energy-dependent processes, including active transport and the maintenance of intracellular homeostasis and cell structure.[1] Cellular volume regulation depends on Na–K adenosine triphosphatase (ATPase) pump activity, which is limited by decreased ATP during ischemia, such that accumulation of intracellular sodium and water leads to cell swelling and disruption of cell membranes.[60]

Calcium homeostasis is disrupted by low calcium ATPase concentrations. This may increase intracellular calcium concentrations, leading to further mitochondrial injury and exacerbating ATP depletion.[61] A high intracellular calcium concentration may activate phospholipases and proteases, which then alter membrane lipid composition, further contributing to cellular damage.[58]

During reperfusion, injury may worsen as oxygen free radicals are produced. This occurs when xanthine oxidase converts hypoxanthine to xanthine while donating an electron to generate superoxide radicals from the products of purine metabolism (e.g., adenosine monophosphate degradation).[58] Experimentally, oxygen free radicals increase membrane permeability via lipid peroxidation and may also cause oxidation of important sulfhydryl groups on proteins, including important renal transporter proteins.[62]

Tubular and Glomerular Events

Besides intrarenal vasoconstriction, various other explanations for diminished renal function have been postulated.[1,11,18] These include backleak of glomerular filtrate into peritubular fluid through damaged tubular epithelia, tubular obstruction from cellular debris, and decreased glomerular capillary permeability. Urine flow and tubular capacity to reabsorb can be diminished by sloughing of the brush border membranes and cast formation within the tubular lumen. The sloughing of tubular membranes disrupts tubular integrity and allows backleak of glomerular ultrafiltrate via disrupted tubular epithelium into the peritubular circulation. This increased permeability results in the return of urea, creatinine, and other waste products into the systemic circulation. Tubular obstruction also increases intratubular hydraulic pressure, which opposes glomerular filtration pressure, leading to an unfavorable glomerular filtration pressure gradient and reducing GFR.[18]

Another theory suggests that GFR declines because of an altered glomerular capillary ultrafiltration coefficient (K_f). Substantial reductions in the effective surface area for filtration cause a decrease in GFR. Experimental data indicate that the reduction in K_f may result from angiotensin II production.[19] Damage to the glomeruli can also result from immunologic reactions, and vascular occlusive diseases (e.g., hemolytic–uremic syndrome, renal artery thrombosis, or embolic diseases) are thought to cause glomerular damage by a mechanism similar to mechanisms described earlier for ischemic events of the kidney.[18,19]

COMPLICATIONS

Complications of ARF are shown in Table 21.6. Before dialytic therapies were developed, the most common causes of death in patients with ARF were progressive uremia, hyperkalemia, and complications of volume overload. With the advent of dialysis, the most common causes of death are sepsis, cardiovascular and pulmonary dysfunction, and withdrawal of life support measures.

CLINICAL PRESENTATION AND DIAGNOSIS

Signs and Symptoms

The clinical course of ARF often is divided into four sequential phases: initiation or injury, maintenance, diuresis, and recovery. Characteristic of the initiation phase is a significant change in hemodynamics and markedly decreased in renal function. The maintenance phase of ARF usually lasts from several days to weeks and is commonly associated with oliguria. Treatment is focused on minimizing fluids and maintaining electrolyte balance until renal function returns. Impaired renal function may coexist with cellular repair processes. Surviving tubular cells appear to regenerate new tubular cells necessary to restore functional capacity. This process probably is influenced by a variety of peptide growth factors.[63,64] Renal cells release growth factors, including epidermal growth factor (EGF) and insulin-like growth factor (IGF-1), which may mediate repair of injured cells and recovery of renal function. Also, there appears to be some role for purine nucleotides in stimulating renal epithelial cell growth.[65]

Once kidney repair begins, it is typical to see a diuretic phase, which begins before measurable reductions in Scr and urea nitrogen. This diuresis is thought to result from the return of glomerular filtration function before complete correction of tubular reabsorption capacity. An osmotic diuretic effect may also result from accumulated uremic toxins and fluid during the oliguric phase. It is important to provide patients with adequate volume and electrolyte repletion during the diuretic phase of ARF.

Table 21.6 ▪ Complications in Acute Renal Failure

Sodium and water imbalance	Carbohydrate intolerance
Acid-base imbalance	Hypertension
Potassium imbalance	Gastrointestinal disturbances
Anemia	Neuromuscular disturbances
Hemostatic defects	Renal osteodystrophy
Calcium and phosphate abnormalities	Dermatologic disorders
Hyperuricemia	Psychological disorders

Diagnosis

Patient History and Physical Examination

Evaluation of the patient's history and physical examination often reveal the cause of ARF. For example, the findings of volume depletion or a recent history of exposure to a nephrotoxic medication or a radiocontrast agent could provide important diagnostic information necessary for prompt intervention. Additional diagnostic clues may include sudden anuria, suggesting postrenal ARF, or a rash in the case of allergic interstitial nephritis.

Urinalysis

Further important diagnostic information is obtained from a urinalysis and evaluation of various urine indices. A urinalysis usually is performed on a random sample of urine and consists of the following major components:

- Physical and chemical properties
- pH
- Concentrating ability
- Protein content
- Cells and casts
- Sodium excretion

Physical and Chemical Properties

The urine should be clear but usually has a faint yellow tinge from the presence of urochromes. Erythrocytes and white blood cells cause turbid urine. Agents that may cause urine to change color are shown in Table 21.7. Concentrated urine has a deepened color. Increasing amounts of bilirubin produce colors ranging from yellow-brown to deep olive green. Urine containing old blood, hemosiderin, or myoglobin is brown to black. Small amounts of red blood cells produce a characteristic smoky appearance. Patients with porphyria may void a normal-colored urine,

Table 21.7 ▪ Agents Causing Changes in Urine Color Not Related to Disease

Color	Drug
Darkening on standing	Cascara Chloroquine Levodopa Methocarbamol Methyldopa Metronidazole Nitrofurantoin Phenytoin
Red	Anthraquinone Daunorubicin Deferoxamine Doxorubicin Ibuprofen Phenolsulfonphthalein
Orange-brown	Cascara Chloroquine Chlorzoxazone Furazolidone Ibuprofen Iron sorbitex Phenazopyridine Phenytoin Primaquine Quinine Senna Sulfamethoxazole Sulfasalazine
Blue-green	Amitriptyline Doan's Pills Indigo blue Methylene blue Resorcinol Triamterene
Deep yellow	Cascara Fluorescein Quinacrine Riboflavin

but the sample may develop a deep purple or brownish color on standing. Food pigments, such as the pigment in beets, can color the urine red.[66,67]

pH

Urine pH varies between 4.5 and 8 in patients with healthy kidneys. The pooled daily urine specimen usually is acidic (pH 6). Decreased pulmonary ventilation during sleep causes respiratory acidosis and the development of a highly acidic urine. After meals, the urine becomes alkaline for a few hours. Thus, pH varies widely depending on the time of collection. Highly concentrated urine usually is strongly acidic and may be irritating. When urine stands it becomes alkaline as urea breaks down to ammonia. Therefore, a pH test should always be done on freshly voided urine. Urine that is persistently acid or alkaline may suggest the presence of systemic or urinary tract disease. Conditions associated with persistently acid or alkaline urine are listed in Table 21.8.[67] Some agents known to alter urine pH are listed in Table 21.9.[66]

Concentrating Ability

Specific gravity is the most convenient way to measure the amount of dissolved solids in the urine (e.g., urea, sodium, and chloride) and provides an accurate assessment of renal concentrating ability. By definition, the specific gravity of urine is the ratio of urine weight to the weight of an equal volume of distilled water. In health, the specific gravity may range from 1.003 to 1.030. Concentrated and dilute urine have specific gravities greater than or less than 1.010, respectively. Specific gravity is a useful tool in differentiating between prerenal azotemia and ATN. Usually in prerenal azotemia, the kidney should conserve sodium and water, leading to a specific gravity greater than 1.030. Conversely, during ATN, the kidney loses its ability to concentrate, leading to a lower urine specific gravity.

Osmolality measurement is more accurate and less influenced by large, dense molecules such as protein and radiographic contrast media. To test concentrating ability, the patient is either deprived of water for a number of

Table 21.8 ▪ Conditions Associated with Persistent Changes in Urine pH

Persistently Acid (pH <7.0)
Metabolic acidosis
Respiratory acidosis
Pyrexia
Phenylketonuria
Alkaptonuria
Persistently Alkaline (pH >7.0)
Urinary tract infection with urea-splitting organisms
Metabolic alkalosis
Carbonic anhydrase inhibitors
Hyperaldosteronism
Cystinosis

Table 21.9 ▪ Agents Causing a Change in Urine pH

Increased pH	Decreased pH
Acetohexamide	Ammonium chloride
Amiloride	Ascorbic acid
Amphotericin B	Corticotropin
Citrates (potassium or sodium)	Diazoxide
Epinephrine	Glucose
Niacinamide	Methenamine mandelate
Sodium bicarbonate	Metolazone
Triamterene	Niacin
	Sucrose

hours or given vasopressin 10 units subcutaneously. Failure to concentrate urine to more than 800 mOsm/kg or 1.020 specific gravity demonstrates decreased concentrating ability. When renal function approaches 20% of normal, the specific gravity and osmolality become fixed and stabilize at 1.010 and 300 mOsm/kg, respectively. The term *isosthenuria* is used to describe urine that is consistently at 1.010 or 300 mOsm/kg.

Protein Content

Normally, nearly all filtered protein is reabsorbed or catabolized by the proximal tubular cells, and less than 150 mg protein is excreted in the urine per day. Proteinuria is an important indicator of renal disease. Its evaluation entails a knowledge of factors that cause proteinuria without renal disease. Nonpathologic or functional proteinuria is transient and usually occurs in young adults. Proteinuria can occur with excessive exercise, exposure to cold, postural changes (such as standing from a recumbent position), and pregnancy. Proteinuria associated with renal disease results from numerous disorders (Table 21.10).[68] Proteinuria is a common characteristic of nearly every form of glomerular disease and contributes to several nephrotic syndrome complications.

Protein in the urine is measured by sulfosalicylic acid, heat and acetic acid, or dipstick methods. Because of its simplicity, the dipstick method often is used as a screening test for proteinuria. Various urine dipstick products are commercially available to detect and quantitate urine protein. In general, if protein losses are greater than 3 g/day, a glomerular origin is suspected. Protein losses of less than 3 g/day are nondiagnostic, and the source is often unclear. The source of protein loss is also evaluated using electrophoresis, which differentiates prerenal, glomerular, or tubular origin.

Table 21.10 ▪ Diseases Associated with Proteinuria

Infectious disease
Poststreptococcal glomerulonephritis
Infective endocarditis
Syphilis
Neoplastic disease
Lymphoma
Leukemia
Carcinoma (colon, lung, breast, stomach, kidney)
Multisystem and connective tissue diseases
Systemic lupus erythematosus
Polyarteritis
Sarcoidosis
Sjögren's syndrome
Amyloidosis
Diabetes mellitus
Miscellaneous conditions
Allergic reactions (bee stings, serum sickness)
Chronic allograft rejection
Preeclampsia

Source: Reference 68.

Cells and Casts

Normal urine contains a small number of red blood cells, white blood cells, and hyaline casts. Casts are cylindrical elements with parallel sides that derive their shape and size from the tubular segment in which they were formed. Factors favoring cast formation are an acid pH, highly concentrated urine, proteinuria, and stasis within the tubules. The transparent hyaline casts are composed entirely of protein. Cellular casts represent red blood cells, white blood cells, or renal epithelial cells trapped within the protein matrix. Granular casts represent degraded cellular casts and usually indicate renal parenchymal damage.

Sodium Excretion

Renal tubular sodium reabsorption (i.e., the difference between the amount of sodium filtered and the amount excreted) is the predominant mechanism that regulates sodium excretion. Tubule reabsorption accounts for more than 99% of filtered sodium under normal conditions. For example, when the GFR is 2 mL/second (120 mL/minute) and the plasma sodium concentration is 145 mmol/L, approximately 17 mmol of sodium is filtered per minute. Over the course of a day this is equivalent to about 25,000 mmol (or 575 g) of filtered sodium. However, only 100 to 250 mmol of sodium is excreted per day (less than 1%).

FE_{Na} is the fraction of filtered sodium excreted in urine using creatinine as an estimate for GFR. Thus, FE_{Na} (%) is calculated as follows:

$$FE_{Na} = U_{Na} \times Pcr/Ucr \times P_{Na} \times 100 \qquad (21.1)$$

where U_{Na} is urine sodium concentration (mmol/L), Pcr is plasma creatinine concentration (μmol/L), Ucr is urine creatinine concentration (μmol/L), and P_{Na} is plasma sodium concentration (mmol/L).

FE_{Na} is a useful guide to distinguish whether an abrupt rise in BUN is the result of impaired renal perfusion (i.e., prerenal azotemia) or ATN. During ATN, tubular sodium transport is impaired and FE_{Na} values usually exceed 2%. FE_{Na} values less than 1% suggest prerenal azotemia. However, values between 1 and 2% may have little predictive value. FE_{Na} may be elevated in patients receiving diuretics. The renal failure index (RFI) has also been proposed to help differentiate prerenal ARF from ATN. The RFI is determined by dividing the urine sodium concentration by the urine:plasma creatinine ratio. RFI values less than 1 suggest prerenal failure and values greater than 4 may indicate ATN.[69]

Laboratory Data

Determination of Glomerular Filtration Rate or Inulin Clearance

GFR is approximated by measuring the urinary excretion rate of a marker substance known to be filtered and excreted in equal amounts. Properties of the ideal marker substance are that it is neither absorbed nor secreted by the renal tubules and is filtered freely across glomerular membranes, not metabolized in renal tubules or produced by the kidneys, and not eliminated by nonrenal routes. These critical properties are satisfied ideally by inulin. To measure inulin clearance, a continuous intravenous infusion of inulin is given, several samples of blood and urine are collected at specified times, and these samples are assayed for inulin concentrations. Because the filtered amount of inulin is equal to the amount of inulin excreted, the following equation applies:

$$GFR = U_{in} \times \dot{V}/P_{in} \qquad (21.2)$$

where GFR is glomerular filtration rate (mL/second), U_{in} is urine inulin concentration (μmol/L), P_{in} is plasma inulin concentration (μmol/L), measured at the midpoint of the collection period, and $\dot{V}$ is volume per unit time (i.e., the total urine volume collected divided by the total time of collection, in mL/second). Because GFR varies according to body size, values typically are expressed by standardizing them to body surface area. The average GFR in young men is approximately 2 mL/second/1.73 m^2 (120 mL/minute/1.73 m^2). This value usually is 10 to 15% lower in women.

Creatinine Clearance

In clinical practice Ccr is the index of GFR most often used. Determination of Ccr is convenient, inexpensive, and easily calculated from a timed urine collection assayed for creatinine and a single Scr measurement. Measurement is most accurate if the urine collection interval is 24 hours and a blood sample is obtained at the midpoint of this timed collection. The calculation of Ccr is similar to that of GFR, except that urine and Scr concentrations are substituted for inulin concentrations.

Creatinine production results from the nonenzymatic hydrolysis of muscle stores of creatine and creatine phosphate. Creatinine is produced at a fairly constant daily rate: Approximately 1 mg creatinine is produced daily from about 20 g muscle.[70] Therefore, creatinine production depends on muscle mass and is influenced by age and gender. After age 20, creatinine production decreases by approximately 2 mg/kg/24 hours per decade of life in both men and women.[71] Because creatinine is filtered by the glomerulus and is also secreted in the proximal tubule, its clearance approximates but is always greater than GFR.[72] If GFR is greater than 0.4 mL/second (25 mL/minute), then Ccr approximates GFR reasonably well. However, creatinine secretion is enhanced in patients with lower GFR, and especially in disease states affecting primarily the glomeruli (i.e., acute glomerulonephritis), leading to overestimation of GFR.

Often it is difficult to obtain accurate 24-hour urine collections. Therefore, Ccr may be estimated using the following formula, derived by Cockroft and Gault:[73]

$$Ccr(men) = (140 - Age) \times Weight/72 \times Scr \qquad (21.3)$$

where Ccr is creatinine clearance (mL/minute), age is in years, weight is in kilograms, and Scr is the serum creatinine concentration (mg/dL). In women, Equation 21.3 is multiplied by 0.85. Factors other than a decreased GFR can alter the Scr level and must be considered in assessing renal function. Patients with decreased muscle mass as a result of old age or cachexia have a decreased creatinine production and therefore a low or normal Scr level, even though their renal function may be impaired.[74,75]

Creatine is the amino acid precursor of creatinine. Synthesis of creatine from glycine, arginine, and methionine occurs in the liver. Thus, patients with advanced liver disease have decreased creatine production and decreased body pools of creatine. This results in decreased creatinine production and Scr concentrations below expected values for any given level of renal function. In patients with liver disease, formulas that estimate renal function based on a Scr level should not be used because they will greatly overestimate renal function.[76] Creatine is also contained in meat. Cooking converts creatine to creatinine, which is absorbed and contributes to the total body creatinine pool. Patients who do not eat meat will have a lower intake of creatine and creatinine, which results in a smaller body pool of these substances. This accounts for a lower than usual Scr, even though these patients may have normal renal function.

Laboratory determination of Scr is based on the alkaline picrate method of Jaffe, modified for increased specificity and to accommodate automation.[71] Because this is a colorimetric test, other noncreatinine chromogens can result in overestimation of Scr. Some of these agents are listed in Table 21.11.[77] Large elevations in Scr levels without appreciable changes in the BUN should alert the clinician to possible laboratory interference. Some drugs (e.g., cimetidine) compete with creatinine for tubular secretion and thus result in elevated Scr concentrations.

Table 21.11 ▪ Agents That Cause a False Elevation in Serum Creatinine as Measured by the Jaffe Method

Acebutolol	Fluorescein
Acetoacetate	Fructose
Acetohexamide	Glucose
Acetone	Levodopa
Aminohippuric acid	Methyldopa
Ascorbic acid	Moxalactam
Cefamandole	Nitrofurantoin
Cefoperazone	Phenolsulfonphthalein
Cefoxitin	Pyruvate
Cephalothin	Sulfobromophthalein

Source: References 66, 77, 78.

Blood Urea Nitrogen

Urea nitrogen is derived from hepatic deamination of amino acids, causing liberation of ammonia, which combines with available carbon dioxide. Urea is eliminated primarily by the kidney through glomerular filtration and undergoes reabsorption in the proximal tubule. The extent of reabsorption depends on the urine flow rate, such that 40% of the filtered urea is reabsorbed with diuresis and 60% is reabsorbed with antidiuresis. Normal BUN concentrations are 3.6 to 5.4 mmol/L (10 to 15 mg/dL) but may increase to more than 54 mmol/L (150 mg/dL) with severe renal failure. In general, BUN concentrations greater than 36 mmol/L (100 mg/dL) are associated with higher risks of complication during renal failure and the need for dialysis. BUN is less accurate than Scr or Ccr levels in assessing renal function. The major limitations are related to a number of factors that can alter urea generation and urea clearance in the absence of changes in renal function. Urea generation depends on protein catabolism and therefore is altered by changes in dietary intake, liver disease, blood in the gastrointestinal tract, steroid-induced catabolism, and the antianabolic effect of most tetracyclines. Because the amount of urea reabsorbed is inversely proportional to the urine flow rate, low-flow states elevate BUN disproportionately to changes in Scr concentration. Any factors that lower the absolute or effective blood volume (and hence RBF) increase BUN. Table 21.12 lists factors responsible for BUN elevation in the absence of renal impairment.[67,77]

Renal Imaging and Renal Biopsy

In patients who present with severe oliguria or anuria, a renal ultrasound is a useful examination to quickly rule out a urinary tract obstruction. The ultrasound may be followed by contrast studies to establish the precise location of an obstruction. Renal biopsy usually is not necessary in evaluating the patient with ARF. However, when prerenal and postrenal causes have been excluded by other measures (e.g., history, laboratory and imaging studies), histologic analysis may establish an intrarenal diagnosis and guide management.

THERAPEUTIC PLAN

Managing ARF consists of preventive measures, removal of underlying causes or complications, supportive care, and pharmacotherapeutic agents. In the majority of cases, ARF is reversible, but it has multiple causes, occurs in a variety of clinical settings, and presents in various forms (i.e., oliguric versus nonoliguric). Preventive therapy may be designed to avoid nephrotoxic drugs or maintain a euvolemic state and adequate renal perfusion pressure. Supportive care during the ARF episode is directed at treating infectious complications, maintaining adequate fluid, electrolyte, and acid-base balance, and providing optimal nutritional support. Specific treatment of ARF is aimed at increasing urine output and RBF, restoring normal fluid and electrolyte balance, removing metabolic wastes, and minimizing further nephrotoxic injury.

Table 21.12 ▪ Factors Elevating Blood Urea Nitrogen Without Renal Impairment

High-protein diet	Hypovolemia
Febrile illness with catabolism	Decreased cardiac output
Gastrointestinal bleeding	Steroids
Hyperthyroidism	Tetracyclines

PREVENTION

In the patient who suddenly develops oliguria with rising BUN and Scr concentrations, it is important to distinguish whether the underlying disease process is prerenal or postrenal because rapid correction of these conditions can prevent progression to ischemic injury and development of ARF. Adequate correction of volume deficits can lead to prompt restoration of renal perfusion. Therapeutic agents known to further reduce blood flow must be withdrawn and potential nephrotoxins, such as aminoglycosides, radiocontrast dye, NSAIDs, and ACE inhibitors should be administered cautiously, if at all. Initial efforts should also be directed at ruling out urinary tract obstruction. Factors suggesting obstruction include a normal urinalysis, rapid changes in urine output, and residual urine on postvoiding catheterization. If renal calculi are present, a radiograph of the abdomen will detect the 90% that are radiopaque. In the absence of obstruction, urinary indices provide the most reliable method of distinguishing prerenal azotemia from ATN.

Table 21.2 will help in distinguishing reversible prerenal failure from ATN, but its usefulness is limited after diuretics are administered or in patients with underlying chronic renal failure (CRF). It is important to differentiate between prerenal and intrinsic ARF on the basis of these clinical laboratory measurements. If prerenal azotemia is suspected, aggressive fluid resuscitation should result in an increased urine output. If urine flow does not increase, additional fluids should be given cautiously, if at all, because fluid overload is likely to ensue if ARF is already established. Also, a fluid challenge can be detrimental to the patient with intrinsic renal damage (ATN). Thus, the patient who presents with a high urinary sodium (in the absence of diuretic use) and FE_{Na} greater than 2% probably has ATN and should not receive fluid resuscitation.

Preventing associated complications, such as infection and gastrointestinal bleeding, is very important. Careful maintenance of intravenous lines, minimal use of indwelling urinary bladder catheters, and early recognition and treatment of wound and other infections are necessary. Monitoring for signs of blood loss (e.g., testing stools for occult blood, monitoring the hematocrit, and controlling gastric pH with H_2 antagonists or antacids) minimizes the morbidity associated with bleeding.

In clinical situations, when exposure to potential nephrotoxic insults is likely to occur, specific preventive measures, such as hydration and volume repletion before and during nephrotoxin exposure, are recommended. For example, when using amphotericin B or aminoglycosides, ensuring that patients are well hydrated may eliminate or reduce the severity of renal damage. Normal saline or mannitol infusion 1 hour before amphotericin B administration may reduce the degree of renal injury (possibly by maintaining urinary output with increased solute excretion and preventing tubular obstruction).[79] Other preventive measures to consider are therapeutic drug monitoring of aminoglycoside concentrations, fluid hydration before cisplatin therapy, and the use of allopurinol and urine alkalinization during high-dose chemotherapy to avoid uric acid nephropathy. Combination therapy with more than one nephrotoxic agent carries additional risk and should be avoided if possible. Substitution of less nephrotoxic agents should be considered in older adults and others at risk for renal dysfunction (Table 21.13). For example, in high-risk patients, it may be possible to avoid radiocontrast agents and use less invasive diagnostic techniques such as ultrasonography. Nephrotoxins should be avoided or discontinued, and dosages of medications whose pharmacokinetics or pharmacodynamics are affected by renal dysfunction should be adjusted. Several common medications whose dosage must be adjusted during renal insufficiency are listed in Table 21.14. Dosage adjustments must be based on the patient's degree of renal dysfunction and the characteristics of the medication. The goal is to maintain efficacious drug therapy while avoiding toxicity (see also Drug Dosing Issues later in this chapter).

SUPPORTIVE CARE

ARF often persists for several days or weeks, necessitating prolonged supportive care. The minimum daily fluid needs include replacement of measurable losses (i.e., urine output, nasogastric suction, vomiting, chest tube drainage, and fistula output) and insensible losses through the skin and lungs (approximately 600 to 900 mL/day). The choice of fluid intake should be determined by the need for colloid or crystalloid, electrolytes, and calories.

Table 21.13 ▪ Preventing Acute Renal Failure

Identify patients at risk
- Older adults
- Patients with abnormal renal function or diabetes
- Volume-depleted patients

Avoid nephrotoxic agents
- Nonsteroidal anti-inflammatory drugs
- Aminoglycosides
- Amphotericin B
- Angiotensin-converting enzyme inhibitors in volume-depleted patients

Use prevention strategies
- Contrast media (extracellular fluid volume expansion)
- Rhabdomyolysis (correct intravascular volume, urinary alkalinization, mannitol infusion)
- Tumor lysis syndrome (allopurinol, diuresis, urinary alkalinization)
- Surgical procedures (optimize volume status, avoid multiple insults and hypotension)

Table 21.14 ▪ Selected Medications for Which Dosage Adjustment is Needed in Renal Insufficiency

Antimicrobial
- Aminoglycosides (amikacin, gentamicin, tobramycin)
- Antifungal agents (fluconazole, flucytosine, itraconazole)
- Antitubercular agents (ethambutol, pyrazinamide)
- Antiviral agents (acyclovir, cidofovir, didanosine, famciclovir, foscarnet, ganciclovir, lamivudine, stavudine, zalactabine, zidovudine)
- Cephalosporins (cefamandole, cefazolin, cefmetazole, cefonicid, cefotaxime, cefotetan, cefoxitin, ceftazidime, ceftizoxime, cefuroxime, cephalothin)
- Fluoroquinolones (ciprofloxacin, levofloxacin, ofloxacin)
- Macrolides (clarithromycin, erythromycin)
- Penicillins (ampicillin, methicillin, mezlocillin, penicillin, piperacillin, ticarcillin)
- Tetracyclines (minocycline, tetracycline)
- Others (aztreonam, chloramphenicol, imipenem, meropenem, trimethoprim–sulfamethoxazole,vancomycin)

Cardiovascular
- Angiotensin-converting enzyme inhibitors (benazepril, captopril, enalapril, lisinopril, quinapril, ramipril)
- Antiarrhythmic agents (bretylium, flecainide, procainamide, quinidine, sotalol) β-Blockers (acebutolol, atenolol, carteolol, nadolol, pindolol)
- Others (digoxin, milrinone, nitroprusside)

Other
- Analgesics (codeine, ketorolac, meperidine, morphine)
- Barbiturates (phenobarbital, thiopental)
- Gastrointestinal agents (cimetidine, famotidine, metoclopramide, ranitidine)
- Hypoglycemic agents (acetohexamide, chlorpropamide, glyburide, insulin)
- Neuromuscular blocking agents (neostigmine, pancuronium, pyridostigmine, tubocurarine, vecuronium)
- Others (allopurinol, lithium carbonate, paroxetine, phenytoin)

Fluid Management

The normal kidney is critical to the maintenance of volume homeostasis, which permits constant circulatory and extracellular fluid volumes despite varying water and salt consumption and varying loss. The presence of pedal or sacral edema or pulmonary edema in the setting of ARF implies that water or salt intake has exceeded the injured kidney's ability to excrete the water and salt load. This situation can be anticipated in the oliguric or anuric patient but often complicates nonoliguric ARF as well. Most patients with ARF lose the ability to concentrate or dilute the urine and as a consequence excrete a constant volume of urine regardless of fluid intake. For example, a patient with ATN whose urine output is fixed at 500 mL/day but receives 1000 mL/day of parenteral nutrition (PN) along with various intravenous antibiotics will gradually develop volume overload and edema unless the volume administered is adjusted. Volume status management is based on careful physical examination, and the patient must be examined daily to measure supine and standing blood pressure and pulse, skin turgor, and mucous membrane hydration; auscultate the lungs for evidence of pulmonary congestion; perform a general examination for sacral or pedal edema; review daily intake and output; and measure daily (serial) weight changes accurately.

The prescription for fluid and sodium intake should be specified. In general, a patient who is euvolemic should be given an additional 300 to 500 mL/day of electrolyte-free water to replace insensible water losses. A sodium intake of less than 2 g/day should be prescribed. Patients with increased insensible fluid loss, such as those with burns or severe diarrhea, have much larger fluid needs. However, because insensible fluid losses can not be measured accurately, it is imperative that a patient's volume status be assessed accurately on a daily basis and the fluid prescription modified as necessary. The patient with clinical evidence of fluid overload should be restricted to a fluid intake less than the daily urine output. Patients with clinical evidence of volume depletion should be given additional volume to achieve a euvolemic state. Sustained hypovolemia may worsen renal injury or delay recovery from renal failure. Increased fluid needs should be anticipated during the polyuric recovery phase of ARF.

In the ICU, clinical assessment of volume status can be confounded by surgical wound loss, severe pneumonia, or edema caused by altered capillary permeability. Here, measurements of central venous pressure and capillary wedge pressure are important adjuncts to volume status monitoring. These patients often are receiving multiple parenteral medications that constitute a large obligatory volume load. Often these medications can be given slowly in a concentrated solution to minimize the volume administered. Likewise, the volume of PN should be adjusted to optimize calories and protein in a minimum volume. The clinician must keep in mind the solutions in which various medications are delivered.

Electrolyte Homeostasis

Electrolyte abnormalities that occur in ARF include disorders of sodium, potassium, phosphate, magnesium, and calcium homeostasis. Hypernatremia and hyponatremia often are observed in patients with ARF. Because abnormal serum sodium concentrations are caused by disorders of water metabolism, sodium homeostasis is linked to volume management. Hyponatremia usually results from an excess of free water relative to solute, whereas hypernatremia results when free water intake is inadequate. It is important to keep track of the amount of free water delivered in intravenous solutions and to limit this free water whenever necessary. For example, administering 500 mL 0.45% saline is equivalent to giving 250 mL 0.9% (normal) saline and 250 mL electrolyte-free water. Other sources of free water excess include parenteral and enteral feedings.

Hyperkalemia can be a serious consequence of ARF; potassium intake can exceed the injured kidney's reduced potassium excretory capacity. In addition, there can be shifts between intracellular and extracellular compartments secondary to acid-base balance. Hyperkalemia usually is prevented by restricting potassium intake to less than 50 mEq/day. Certain food types, such as fruits, chocolates, and nuts, must be eliminated from the diet. Often, potassium is omitted from parenteral fluids, and it is important to not overlook nondietary exogenous sources of potassium. These include drugs such as potassium penicillin G and salt substitutes. Finally, drugs that impair renal potassium excretion, such as potassium-sparing diuretics, NSAIDs, and ACE inhibitors, should be avoided if possible.

If potassium restriction is inadequate to prevent hyperkalemia, sodium polystyrene sulfonate can be used to exchange sodium for potassium in the bowel and increase intestinal excretion of potassium. Although usually administered orally (15 to 30 g in 20% sorbitol), in the presence of an ileus, potassium binding resins are effective as enemas. Because these compounds exchange sodium for potassium, large sodium loads can worsen volume overloads or cause hypernatremia. Repeated administration can lead to diarrhea as a result of sorbitol intake, and this may complicate acidosis by increasing intestinal bicarbonate loss. Persistent hyperkalemia despite potassium intake restriction and sodium polystyrene administration is an indication for dialysis. However, other endogenous causes of hyperkalemia (e.g., severe acidosis, insulinopenia, hemolysis, rhabdomyolysis, and ischemic tissue injury) should also be investigated.

Hypocalcemia may occur secondary to the hypomagnesemia associated with cisplatin, amphotericin B, or aminoglycoside administration. Hypomagnesemia also inhibits synthesis and release of parathyroid hormone, which may cause hypocalcemia. Decreased synthesis of 1,25-dihydroxyvitamin D by the injured kidney reduces intestinal calcium absorption and can contribute to hypocalcemia. Additionally, hypocalcemia can result from frequently administered blood products preserved in citrate. Hypocalcemia is prevented and treated with generous calcium supplementation either orally in dosages of 3 to 4 g/day in divided doses or, for symptomatic hypocalcemia, as calcium acetate, calcium gluconate, or calcium chloride. Magnesium should be repleted (cautiously) orally or parenterally. Avoiding magnesium-containing antacids decreases the potential for hypermagnesemia.

Phosphorus accumulates during renal failure and may result in hyperphosphatemia. Although hyperphosphatemia is much more problematic in patients with CRF, high serum phosphorus levels can contribute to hypocalcemia. Restricting dietary phosphate and administering phosphate-binding antacids (e.g., calcium-containing antacids) usually maintains serum phosphate within normal ranges.

TREATMENT

Three basic therapeutic interventions are currently used in ARF: pharmacologic, dialytic, and nutritional therapies.

Despite considerable recent research, none of these has been found to improve mortality rates or hasten renal function recovery significantly. Thus, the initial care of a patient with ARF should focus on reversing the underlying cause, correcting fluid and electrolyte imbalances, and preventing further renal injury by providing supportive measures (Fig. 21.2).

Pharmacotherapy

Therapeutic modalities for treating ARF are designed to increase RBF, increase urine output, maintain fluid and electrolyte balance, remove metabolic wastes, and slow or reverse kidney damage.

Diuretics

Although diuretic therapy (e.g., mannitol and furosemide) helps to protect the kidney from injury in experimental ischemia, most clinical trials have failed to demonstrate effectiveness of these agents in treating or preventing ischemic ARF. If administered early in the course of ARF, both furosemide and mannitol can convert oliguric ARF to a nonoliguric state. Because evidence suggests that nonoliguric ARF is associated with less morbidity and mortality, clinicians have often tried to convert oliguric ARF to nonoliguric ARF. However, no prospective controlled clinical trials confirm that pharmacologic conversion from oliguria to nonoliguria reduces mortality

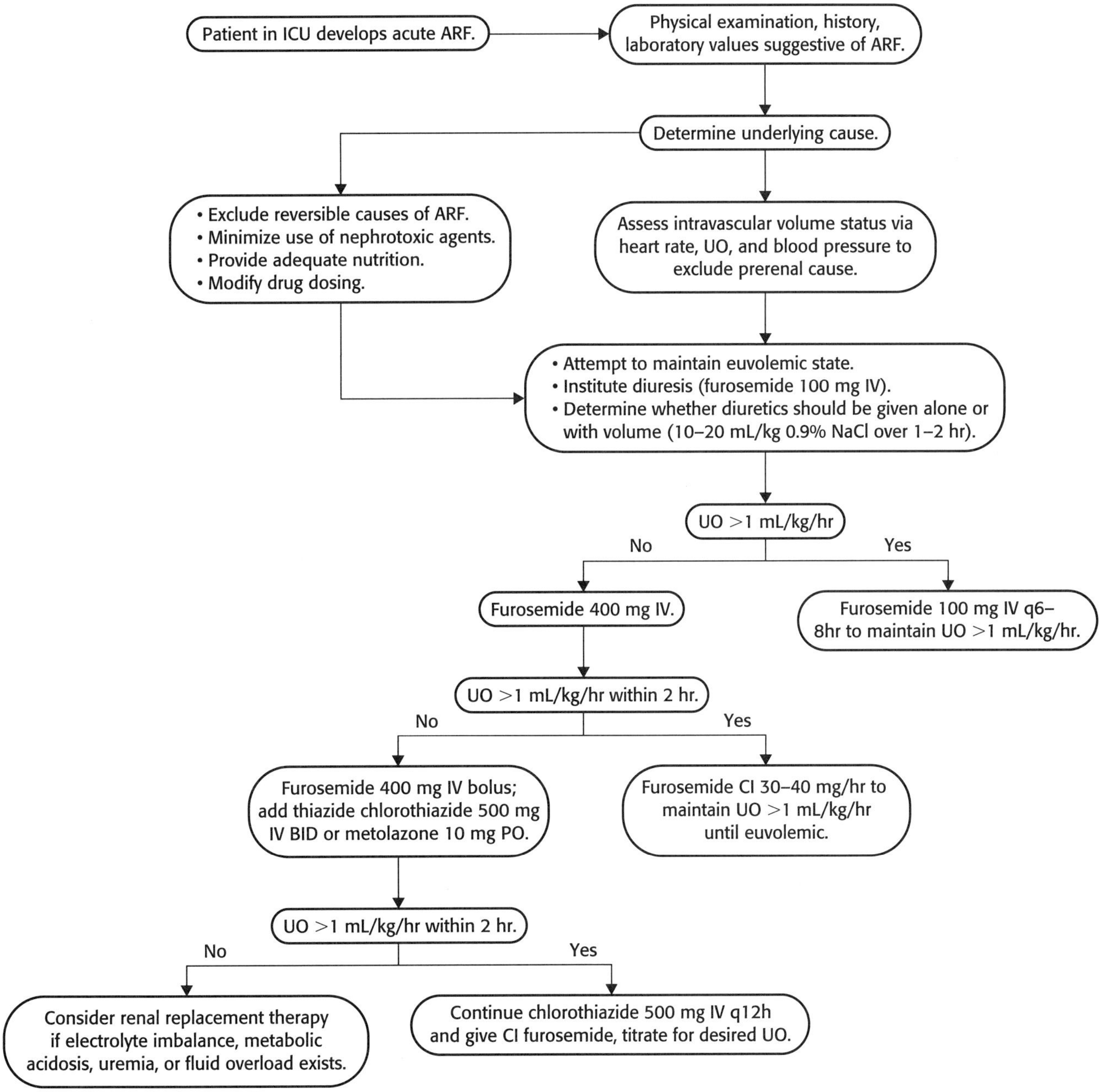

Figure 21.2. Treatment algorithm for patients with suspected ARF. *ARF,* acute renal failure; *CI,* continuous infusion; *ICU,* intensive care unit; *UO,* urine output.

or time to recovery in established ARF. However, most clinicians would agree that nonoliguric patients are easier to treat than oliguric patients and have fewer complications, less need for dialysis, and shorter hospital courses than those with oliguric renal failure.[6] Maintaining a high urine output may prevent volume overload and allow increased nutritional support.

At present, loop diuretics or mannitol should be used to optimize fluid management in newly apparent intrinsic ARF. Diuretics should be avoided in the setting of contrast nephropathy and as routine prophylaxis of ARF because resultant hypovolemia could accelerate the progression from prerenal azotemia. Instead, urine flow rates and intravascular volume are greater after saline administration than after diuretic use.[80] It is also clear that high-dose diuretics are of no value when administered after intrinsic ARF is firmly established.[81,82]

Mannitol

This was the first pharmacologic substance used in ARF, and many nephrologists continue to use mannitol to treat ARF. Proposed mechanisms of benefit include increased filtration pressure, improved urine flow rates, reduced tubular cell inflammation, and improved RBF caused by a decrease in renal vascular resistance.[6,81] Mannitol is also a free radical scavenger. Despite these theoretical benefits, there are several reports of mannitol-induced ARF, and consistent benefit in patients with ARF has not been demonstrated.

As soon as possible after a decrease in urine output is noted, a short course of mannitol might be tried. In adults, a wide range of mannitol dosages sufficient to expand intravascular volume and increase renal perfusion pressure have been tried.[69] In general, 20% mannitol solution dosed at 0.5 g/kg can be infused over 30 to 60 minutes, then repeated in an hour if there is no response. If urine output follows, additional doses are titrated to maintain urine output. If a diuresis does not occur and additional doses are given, intravascular volume overload and CHF may occur. Mannitol is recommended for prevention and early treatment of myoglobinuric ARF[83] and is used with adequate hydration to prevent cisplatin-associated nephrotoxicity.

Loop Diuretics

Loop diuretics usually are considered the diuretics of choice in patients with renal insufficiency.[84] The beneficial effects of loop diuretics in early ARF are thought to result from decreased tubule obstruction, reduction of active transport processes and oxygen demand in the tubular cells, or renal vasodilation resulting in increased RBF.[18,85] All loop diuretics (i.e., furosemide, torsemide, ethacrynic acid, and bumetanide) affect the ascending limb of the loop of Henle to increase solute diuresis. However, ethacrynic acid is not used in patients with renal failure because of accumulation and ototoxicity. Bumetanide is an effective and potent loop diuretic and can be used in patients with ARF; however, its use in these patients has not been studied extensively. Torsemide is the newest loop diuretic available in the Unites States. Compared to furosemide, torsemide's advantages include a high oral bioavailability (80 to 100%) and a long duration of activity (12 to 24 hours).

The use of furosemide has been evaluated in both animals and humans. Although the majority of experimental studies are not in models of well-established experimental ATN, the effects of loop diuretics in animal models are consistently positive. In various clinical trials, furosemide use in patients with oliguric ARF has been associated with a response rate of 40 to 100% for conversion to a nonoliguric state.[81,86] Levinsky and Bernard[81] performed a meta-analysis of 19 studies and found significantly greater survival in patients with early oliguric ATN who responded to diuretic therapy. However, these authors proposed that a diuretic may simply predict better outcome on the basis of less severe injury rather than decreasing morbidity and mortality.[81] Studies clearly suggest that if any benefits are to be gained, therapy with diuretics or mannitol should begin during the first 24 hours after an insult.[84,85] Two reports indicate possible deleterious effects when furosemide is used as prophylaxis to prevent contrast nephropathy.[80,87]

Although the use of loop diuretics remains controversial, they should be considered after an inadequate response to a fluid challenge. Because the window of opportunity may be narrow, an initial intravenous furosemide dose 1.5 to 3 mg/kg (100 to 200 mg) should be infused over 15 to 30 minutes.[85,88] If urine output does not increase within an hour, the dosage should be doubled and a thiazide added. If there is no response, therapy should be discontinued. Dosages greater than 500 mg are unlikely to be of benefit. If urine output increases, additional doses can be given to maintain urine flow. Patients who have a poor response to intermittent doses of a loop diuretic may benefit from a continuous furosemide infusion in a dosage of 10 to 40 mg per hour, titrated according to the patient's urine output.[84,85] It is thought that maintaining effective amounts of diuretic within the luminal tubule will enhance the diuretic response.[84] Before a continuous infusion of a loop diuretic is started, a loading dose should be given to decrease the time necessary to achieve therapeutic drug concentrations.

Vasoactive Agents

Dopamine (Efficacy Studies)

Dopamine appears to be helpful in converting oliguric ARF to nonoliguric ARF. Whether this conversion affects the outcome of patients with ARF is not known. Dopamine infusions are used to increase cardiac output and cause renal artery vasodilation, increasing RBF and GFR. The mechanisms by which dopamine modulates RBF differ depending on the rate of infusion. Dopaminergic effects (i.e., intrarenal vasodilation and increased RBF) occur at dosages of 1 to 3 μg/kg/minute, and adrenergic effects (i.e., vasoconstriction) predominate at dosages of

5 to 20 μg/kg/minute. Dopamine may also decrease renal oxygen demand by inhibiting Na–K ATPase and tubular sodium reabsorption. Because of its different mechanism of action (i.e., increasing RBF through renal artery vasodilation), the combination of low-dose dopamine administered with furosemide may increase urine output in early oliguric ARF unresponsive to diuretics alone. If urinary output does not increase within 6 hours, dopamine should be discontinued.[89]

Results of clinical studies assessing the use of renal dose dopamine are controversial. Weisberg et al.[90] found no protective effect of dopamine (2 μg/kg/minute) against radiocontrast nephrotoxicity in patients with underlying renal disease compared to those treated with saline. More recently, Flancbaum et al.[89] showed that low-dose dopamine infusions can significantly increase urine output in ICU patients with oliguric renal failure. It is widely assumed that dobutamine in combination with dopamine could improve cardiac index, cause arterial vasodilation, and maximize RBF and natriuresis in oliguric patients with left ventricular dysfunction. However, although urine output may be enhanced, it has not been established whether dopamine prevents ARF or improves outcome in this setting.[91] Another recent trial[92] questioned the routine administration of dopamine. The placebo group in the anaritide ARF study received either low-dose (less than 3 μg/kg/minute), high-dose (more than 3 μg/kg/minute), or no dopamine. In these 256 patients, there was no significant difference in relative risk of mortality or the need for dialysis, regardless of whether dopamine was administered.[92] Additional placebo-controlled trials are needed to delineate the safety and efficacy of low-dose dopamine in the patients with ARF.

Calcium Channel Blockers

After ischemic ARF, calcium channel blockers may protect against ARF by inhibiting vasoconstrictive responses of the afferent arterioles and increasing GFR. In addition, calcium antagonists may prevent damage from elevated intracellular calcium after hypoxic injury. These agents have been examined extensively in experimental ARF models, yet few clinical studies confirm their beneficial effects. In 12 patients with ARF, Lumlertgul et al.[93] compared verapamil (100 μg/minute intrarenally for 3 hours) and furosemide (0.8 mg/kg/hour intravenously for 24 hours) with control subjects receiving only furosemide. These investigators reported a more rapid recovery of GFR in the verapamil-treated group. Also, in the setting of renal transplantation, verapamil improves early graft function when administered to donors before kidney harvest. Furthermore, calcium channel blockers may reduce the vasoconstrictive effects associated with cyclosporin and radiocontrast agents.[7]

Atrial Natriuretic Peptide

Atrial natriuretic peptide (ANP) is a hormone synthesized by the cardiac atria that increases GFR by dilating afferent arterioles while constricting efferent arterioles. The hormone also inhibits tubular reabsorption of sodium and chloride, redistributes renal medullary blood flow, and disrupts tubuloglomerular feedback. Anaritide is a 25–amino acid synthetic form of ANP. In a multicenter, randomized, double-blind, placebo-controlled clinical trial of 504 patients with ATN, Allgren et al.[92] showed that anaritide may improve dialysis-free survival in patients with oliguria. Conversely, in patients without oliguria, anaritide may actually worsen dialysis-free survival, possibly by causing drug-induced hypotension. More clinical studies are needed to further evaluate this agent in the setting of ARF.

Growth Factors

Renal regeneration to restore structural injury and renal function starts immediately after an acute renal insult. Several mitogenic growth factors, including EGF, transforming growth factor-α, IGF-1, and hepatocyte growth factor (HGF) have been shown to promote regeneration of tubular cells.[64] When administered to animals subjected to ischemic renal injury, EGF, IGF-1, and HGF reduce the extent of kidney damage and accelerate renal function recovery. On the basis of these animal data, two clinical trials evaluating the efficacy of IGF-1 in ARF have been performed with differing results.[94,95] IGF-1 may increase Ccr in patients with less severe renal injury who do not need RRT,[94] whereas there is no benefit for patients with severe renal damage.[95]

Drug Dosing Issues

In patients with renal failure, a number of factors can affect drug absorption: uremic gastroparesis, changes in gastric pH, gut wall edema, and alterations in first-pass metabolism. It is also important to appreciate some pharmacodynamic changes likely to occur in renal failure. For example, because the sensitivity of β-receptors decreases in renal failure, it may be necessary to increase the propranolol dosage despite an increased bioavailability. In renal failure, the volume of distribution may change because of changes in body composition and decreased plasma protein binding (PPB). PPB reduction is clinically significant for agents highly bound to albumin. This may occur secondary to hypoalbuminemia, drug displacement from binding sites on albumin by accumulated organic acids, and diminished drug affinity by albumin. With reduced PPB, a therapeutic free (active) serum concentration occurs at a lower total serum concentration. Additionally, renal failure may increase or decrease nonrenal (hepatic) drug clearance and decrease renal drug metabolism and excretion. Finally, the degree to which a drug is removed via dialysis determines whether a supplemental dose is necessary.

Changes in renal function make it necessary to alter the dosage or dosing interval for drugs excreted by the kidney. Renal insufficiency influences drug disposition through changes in drug bioavailability, reduced protein binding, altered apparent volume of distribution, and altered renal metabolism. Tailoring regimens to targeted drug concentrations and monitoring free or unbound concentrations may minimize risks of drug toxicity associated with renal failure.[96] For more extensive reviews, see Chapter 1 and the comprehensive tables published by Benet.[97,98]

Dosing guidelines have also been established for use in patients receiving intermittent hemodialysis (IHD) or CRRT.[99–101] However, many of these recommendations were determined in patients with CRF, and for drugs with significant nonrenal clearance (which may be preserved in ARF) it may be necessary to distinguish between ARF and CRF. Drug clearance in conventional IHD therapies is substantially different from that in CRRT (hemofiltration). Dosing becomes even more complicated when newer RRT techniques are used that combine diffusive and convective drug loss. A more complete discussion of estimating clearance by dialysis appears in Chapter 23, Dialytic and Pharmacotherapy for End-Stage Renal Disease.

Nutritional Support

With renal failure, the kidney can no longer regenerate bicarbonate, and metabolic acidosis ensues. This acidosis accelerates proteolysis and branched-chain amino acid oxidation and can be corrected with sodium bicarbonate.[102] ARF in the setting of multiple organ failure is associated with lean body mass catabolism, malnutrition, and a high rate of mortality.[103] Attempting to enhance patient outcomes through nutritional support remains controversial. An early clinical study showed greater survival rates and enhanced recovery of renal function in patients receiving small dosages of essential amino acids plus glucose than in patients receiving glucose alone.[104] Subsequent studies suggested that such supplementation might improve renal function and patient outcomes, but these results are not conclusive.

Unfortunately, the dietary restrictions needed to manage ARF may offset efforts to optimize nutritional support, and the possible benefits of avoiding short-term dialysis must be weighed against the potential increase in morbidity and mortality caused by impaired nutrition. The need for nutrition support varies according to the patient's nutritional status, degree of hypercatabolism, GFR, clinical condition, and plans for dialysis or ultrafiltration therapy. For example, very low protein diets (0.3 to 0.5 g essential amino acids/day) have been advocated to prevent uremia and avoid dialysis in nonhypercatabolic patients with ARF and little or no protein depletion.[105] However, this essential amino acid regimen remains controversial and this level of protein restriction is not recommended for more than 2 weeks. In the nonhypercatabolic patient with better residual renal function (i.e., GFR greater than 10 mL/minute), a mixture of essential and nonessential amino acids or protein may be provided at 0.6 to 0.8 g/kg/day. Amino acid or protein needs may be considerably higher in very ill or severely wasted hypercatabolic patients with ARF who are expected to need dialysis. Generally about 1.2 g amino acids/kg/day is prescribed for patients receiving IHD, and protein needs may even be higher in patients receiving CRRT. PN often is necessary in patients with ARF, but the composition of the PN solution must be modified in accordance with the loss of renal function. In general, most clinicians agree that patients who are severely ill do better if they are given sufficient caloric intake (25 to 35 kcal/kg/day) to attenuate gluconeogenesis and minimize negative nitrogen balance. For further discussion of nutrition needs in ARF, see Chapter 10, General Nutrition.

Renal Replacement Therapy

The early use of dialysis to treat ARF has been associated with increased survival. A small prospective study of casualties during the Vietnam War demonstrated that patients whose BUN was maintained below 18 mmol/L (50 mg/dL) and whose Scr concentration was maintained below 442 (5 mg/dL) had a mortality rate of 37%, whereas those given dialysis for a BUN above 43 mmol/L (120 mg/dL) and Scr concentration above 884 μmol/L (10 mg/dL) had a mortality rate of 80%.[106] It is postulated that early dialysis provides a better biochemical environment for fighting infections and for wound healing. IHD, peritoneal dialysis (PD), or CRRT may be indicated in patients with neurologic signs and symptoms of uremia, severe hyperkalemia, volume overload, or severe acidosis.

For the past several decades, IHD has been the conventional RRT for severe ARF. Recently, continuously administered (e.g., venovenous and arteriovenous) RRTs have emerged. The advantages of CRRT over IHD include more precise fluid and metabolic control, less hemodynamic instability, better removal of harmful cytokines, and the ability to deliver unlimited nutritional support. The drawbacks to CRRT include the need for prolonged anticoagulation, and the procedure entails constant sophisticated surveillance. Currently the choice of one therapy over another often is based on personal preference, hemodynamic stability of the patient, or availability of a particular method.

In ARF, the role of RRT is to prevent morbidity associated with complications of ARF and to provide temporary support until the renal insufficiency resolves. The decision to initiate dialysis and the frequency of dialysis should be based on the patient's clinical condition rather than a particular BUN or Scr concentration. Unfortunately, there is no consensus on the timing with dialysis intervention in ARF. Absolute indications for dialysis are pericarditis and uremic symptoms because these can be resolved only by dialysis. Relative indications include volume overload, hyperkalemia, and acidosis. In these cases, dialysis should be instituted when other conservative approaches have failed or are impractical. These indications for dialytic intervention are summarized in Table 21.15.[107] In general, a reasonable goal is to maintain predialysis BUN less than 29 mmol/L (80 mg/dL). Further details of the dialysis prescription are beyond the scope of this discussion and are covered in Chapter 23.

Table 21.15 ▪ Indications for Renal Replacement Therapy

Electrolyte imbalance (hyperphosphatemia, hyperkalemia, hypermagnesemia)
Acid-base abnormalities (metabolic acidosis)
Fluid overload
Uremia (maintenance of blood urea nitrogen <100 mg/dL)
Drug toxicities (lithium, methanol, theophylline)

FUTURE THERAPIES

Calpain and Nitric Oxide Synthase Inhibitors

During ischemic injury, depletion of cellular ATP increases cytosolic calcium concentrations. In addition to its vasoconstrictive effects, calcium can activate proteases and phospholipases and interfere with mitochondrial energy metabolism. Intracellular calcium chelation protects against hypoxic tubular injury in experimental models. Two potential calcium-dependent enzymes (calpain and nitric oxide synthase) are thought to mediate hypoxic proximal tubular injury.[108] Inhibiting these enzymes using the newly developed calpain inhibitors and nitric oxide synthase inhibitors may have important clinical application in treating ischemic and reperfusion injury.[108]

Intercellular Adhesion Molecules

Intercellular adhesion molecule-1 (ICAM-1) mediates ischemic ARF by potentiating the adhesion of neutrophils to endothelial cells, resulting in tissue damage. Increased systemic levels of tumor necrosis factor and interleukin-1 may upregulate ICAM-1 after ischemia and reperfusion injury.[109] Administering a monoclonal antibody against ICAM-1 protects animals from ischemic ARF, even when it is given 2 hours after the ischemic event.[110] These agents may have clinical implications for treating ischemic ARF and preventing renal injury in allograft recipients.

Other Agents

Other therapeutic approaches to counteract the vasoconstrictive component of ARF include adenosine receptor antagonists, endothelin receptor antagonists, and phosphodiesterase inhibitors. These agents have shown promise in experimental models and may lead to improved outcomes in patients with ARF. In addition, lazaroids and antioxidants decrease the formation or action of free radicals. Despite some positive animal data that show that antioxidants or scavengers of reactive oxygen species may prevent functional tissue damage, there is no compelling evidence to support their use in patients with ARF. Arg-Gly-Asp peptides, which ameliorate adhesion between cells in the tubular lumen and may prevent tubular obstruction, are also being considered for use in ARF.[111] Finally, the selective dopamine (DA-1) agonists (e.g., fenoldopam) activate dopamine receptors without stimulating α- or β-adrenoreceptors. Thus, DA-1 agonists increase RBF and GFR with fewer unwanted side effects.[112] Several studies in normal and hypertensive patients support controlled clinical testing of these agents in preventing or treating ARF.

IMPROVING OUTCOMES

Despite major advances in dialysis and intensive care, the mortality associated with ARF continues to be high, probably because the age of these patients continues to rise and coexisting illnesses are increasingly common. Therefore, clinicians' efforts should focus on preventing ARF. Identifying risk factors for developing ARF is the first step (Table 21.13). Preventing postsurgical ARF begins with preoperative risk assessment and optimal volume status. Avoiding intraoperative volume depletion, hypotension, and nephrotoxic agents is also an important preventive measure. Aggressive intravascular volume restoration reduces the incidence of ATN after trauma. Adequate hydration and high urinary flow rates protect against toxicity from chemotherapeutic agents.

In 1996, the French Study Group on ARF[8] identified the following seven variables that predicted ARF death in 20 French ICUs: advanced age, poor health before admission, hospitalization before ICU admission, development of ARF later in the ICU admission (as compared to early on), sepsis, oliguria, and elevated initial disease severity score. These same factors have been identified in almost every trial of this type and suggest that extra vigilance is needed when treating patients with these characteristics.[16,25]

Biocompatible Membranes

The choice of dialysis membrane in ARF may effect morbidity and mortality. Cuprophane membranes lead to activation of the alternative pathway of complement.[113] This can upregulate leukocyte adhesion molecules and aggravate tissue damage in ischemic kidneys. Synthetic membranes, (e.g., polyacrylonitrile, polymethylmethacrylate, and polysulfone) activate complement to a lesser extent than cuprophane membranes. In a prospective study involving 72 patients with ARF, Hakim et al.[114] compared the biocompatible membrane (polymethylmethacrylate) with cuprophane. Improved patient survival and more rapid recovery of renal function occurred when dialysis was performed using the biocompatible membranes. These results have recently been confirmed in two additional randomized, prospective clinical trials.[115,116] In a multicenter study of 153 patients with ARF, dialysis with biocompatible membranes resulted in significantly better rates of survival (57 versus 46%) and renal function recovery (64 versus 43%).[116]

Intermittent Hemodialysis Versus Continuous Renal Replacement Therapy

IHD is the most widely used RRT method for ARF. However, various modifications of CRRT have gained popularity in the ICU setting. Few prospective randomized clinical studies have compared CRRT with IHD in treating ARF. Randomized studies are being conducted to determine whether CRRT improves renal function recovery and offers a survival advantage over intermittent therapies. Nevertheless, some indirect evidence suggests that CRRT may be superior to conventional IHD in certain settings.

It has been suggested that decreased urine output, hypotensive episodes, and complement activation may perpetuate renal injury and delay renal function recovery in patients with ARF occurring during treatment with IHD.[88] Removal of excess volume and urea may decrease urine output and increase the work load of the remaining functional nephrons (fractional reabsorption) and predispose to worsening of tubular obstruction. In addition, hypotension further compromises RBF, which may cause further ischemic insults in the kidney. Furthermore, bioincompatible (cellulose) membranes used for conventional IHD may activate the complement system and lead to mobilization of neutrophils, which infiltrate the kidney and prolong ATN.

Patients who are hemodynamically unstable, such as those with sepsis, are not suitable candidates for IHD. Therefore, CRRT may be preferred in patients whose major complication is fluid overload, those who need ongoing administration of large volumes of fluids, or those whose blood pressure is unstable. However, CRRT entails meticulous monitoring and is associated with complications related to access, anticoagulation, lack of portability, and higher costs.[107] The need for anticoagulation and the resultant hemorrhagic risk are significant disadvantages of either method of dialysis. PD, an effective modality for fluid removal and solute clearance for children and adolescents with ARF, obviates vascular access and therefore anticoagulation. Dialysis techniques are discussed extensively in Chapter 23. It is often pointed out that mortality from ARF remains high despite recent improvements in therapy. It may therefore be questioned whether CRRT using hemofiltration has real benefit, despite its advantages.

CONCLUSION

The normal kidney is a remarkable organ that maintains the internal environment of the body by regulating body fluid volume, electrolyte composition, acid-base balance, and hormone and enzyme production. Although it is highly vulnerable to a variety of toxins, the kidney has the unique ability to regenerate new tubular cells and often recover from iatrogenic misadventures. Many therapeutic approaches have been undertaken to prevent ischemic or nephrotoxic renal injury and, once ARF has developed, to enhance renal function recovery and reduce mortality. Unfortunately, data supporting the efficacy of many of these interventions are inadequate, probably because ARF has a wide spectrum of causes and often occurs along with other comorbid factors, it occurs with varying severity and in a variety of clinical settings, and controlled studies are difficult to perform when the mortality rate of a disorder approaches 50%. The goals of successful management are to remove underlying causes, prevent associated complications, provide symptomatic care, and normalize the internal environment through dietary restriction, drugs, and dialysis.

KEY POINTS

- Prevention is the best treatment for ARF. To date, conventional therapy offers little benefit to patients with established ARF (i.e., mortality remains high and renal function recovery cannot be improved).
- Use alternative agents whenever possible and avoid nephrotoxic drugs (i.e., substitute a third-generation cephalosporin for an aminoglycoside).
- When nephrotoxins must be administered, consider aggressive hydration to improve renal perfusion and reduce tubular work load.
- Maintaining euvolemia is essential in treating established ARF.
- In nearly every epidemiologic study of ARF, patients with nonoliguric ARF have a significantly lower mortality rate than anuric or oliguric patients.
- When necessary, use RRT to support the patient awaiting renal function recovery.

REFERENCES

1. Brady HR, Brenner BM, Lieberthal W. Acute renal failure. In: Brenner BM, ed. The kidney. 5th ed. Philadelphia: WB Saunders, 1996:1200–1252.
2. Rose BD. Acute renal failure: prerenal disease versus acute tubular necrosis. In: Rose BD. Pathophysiology of renal disease. 2nd ed. New York: McGraw-Hill, 1987:63–117.
3. Anderson RJ, Linas SL, Barns AS, et al. Nonoliguric acute renal failure. N Engl J Med 296:1134–1138, 1977.
4. Hou SH, Bushinsky DA, Wish JB, et al. Hospital-acquired renal insufficiency: a prospective study. Am J Med 74:243–248, 1983.
5. Alkhunaizi AM, Schrier RW. Management of acute renal failure: new perspectives. Am J Kidney Dis 28:315–328, 1996.
6. Finn WF. Recovery from acute renal failure. In: Lazarus JM, Brenner BM. Acute renal failure. 3rd ed. New York: Churchill Livingstone, 1993:553–596.
7. Thadhani R, Pascual M, Bonventre JV. Acute renal failure. N Engl J Med 334:1448–1460, 1996.
8. Brivet FG, Kleinknecht DJ, Loirat P, et al. Acute renal failure in intensive care units: causes, outcome, and prognostic factors of hospital mortality; a prospective, multicenter study. French Study Group on Acute Renal Failure. Crit Care Med 24:192–198, 1996.
9. van Bommel EF, Leunissen KM, Weimar W. Continuous renal replacement therapy for the critically ill: an update. J Intensive Care Med 9:265–280, 1994.
10. Elasy TA, Anderson RJ. Changing demography of acute renal failure. Semin Dial 9:438–443, 1996.
11. Nissenson AR. Acute renal failure: definition and pathogenesis. Kidney Int 53(Suppl 66):S7–S10, 1998.
12. Jochimsen F, Schafer JH, Maurer A, et al. Impairment of renal function in medical intensive care: predictability of acute renal failure. Crit Care Med 18:480–485, 1990.
13. Kjellstrand CM, Solez K. Treatment of acute renal failure. In: Schrier RW, Gottschalk CW. Diseases of the kidney. 5th ed. Boston: Little, Brown, 1992:1371–1404.
14. Kaufman J, Dhakal M, Patel B, et al. Community acquired renal failure. Am J Kidney Dis 17:191–198, 1991.

15. Harter HR, Martin KJ. Acute renal failure: classification, evaluation, and clinical consequences. Postgrad Med 72:243–248, 1982.
16. Bullock ML, Umen AJ, Finkelstein M, et al. The assessment of risk factors in 462 patients with acute renal failure. Am J Kidney Dis 5:97–103, 1985.
17. Conger JD, Schrier RW. Renal hemodynamics in acute renal failure. Annu Rev Physiol 42:603–614, 1980.
18. Conger JD, Brinner VA, Schrier RW. Acute renal failure: pathogenesis, diagnosis, and management. In: Schrier RW. Renal and electrolyte disorders. 4th ed. Boston: Little, Brown, 1992:495–537.
19. Conger JD, Anderson RJ, Schrier RW, et al. Acute renal failure. In: Schrier RW, ed. Renal and electrolyte disorders. 6th ed. Boston: Little, Brown, 1996:1069–1113.
20. Matzke GR, Millikin SP. Influence of renal function and dialysis on drug disposition. In: Evans WE, Schentag JJ, Jusko WJ, eds. Applied pharmacokinetics: principles of therapeutic drug monitoring. 3rd ed. Vancouver, WA: Applied Therapeutics, 1992:8-1–8-49.
21. Duggin GG. Mechanisms in the development of analgesic nephropathy. Kidney Int 18:553–561, 1980.
22. Myers BD, Moran SM. Hemodynamically mediated acute renal failure. N Engl J Med 314:97–105, 1986.
23. Stein JH, Fried TA. Experimental models of nephrotoxic acute renal failure. Transplant Proc 17:72–80, 1985.
24. Solez K, Racusen LC, Olsen S. The pathology of drug nephrotoxicity. J Clin Pharmacol 23:484–490, 1983.
25. Rasmussen HH, Ibels LS. Acute renal failure: multivariate analysis of causes and risk factors. Am J Med 73:211–218, 1982.
26. Antonovych TT. Drug-induced nephropathies. In Sommers SC, Rosen PP. Pathol Annu 19(2):165–196, 1984.
27. Laberke HG. Drug-associated nephropathy part II: tubulointerstitial lesions. In: Berry CL et al, eds. Current topics in pathology. New York: Springer-Verlag, 1980:183–215.
28. Revert L, Montoliu J. Acute interstitial nephritis. Semin Nephrol 8:82–88, 1988.
29. Bennett WM, Elzinga LW, Porter GA. Tubulointerstitial disease and toxic nephropathy. In: Brenner BM, ed. The kidney. 5th ed. Philadelphia: WB Saunders, 1996:1430–1496.
30. Matzke GR, Lucarotti RL, Shapiro HS. Controlled comparison of gentamicin and tobramycin nephrotoxicity. Am J Nephrol 3:11–17, 1983.
31. Sawyers CL, Moore RD, Lerner SA, et al. A model for predicting nephrotoxicity in patients treated with aminoglycosides. J Infect Dis 153:1062–1068, 1986.
32. Williams PJ, Hull JH, Sarubbi FA, et al. Factors associated with nephrotoxicity and clinical outcome in patients receiving amikacin. J Clin Pharmacol 26:79–86, 1986.
33. Johnson MW, Mitch WE, Heller AH, et al. The impact of an educational program on gentamicin use in a teaching hospital. Am J Med 73:9–14, 1982.
34. Garrison MW, Rotschafer JC. Clinical assessment of a published model to predict aminoglycoside-induced nephrotoxicity. Ther Drug Monit 11:171–175, 1989.
35. Contreras AM, Gamba G, Cortes J, et al. Serial trough and peak amikacin levels in plasma as predictors of nephrotoxicity. Antimicrob Agents Chemother 33:973–976, 1989.
36. Heidemann HT, Gerkens JF, Spickard WA, et al. Amphotericin B nephrotoxicity in humans decreased by salt repletion. Am J Med 75:476–481, 1983.
37. Sacks P, Fellner SK. Recurrent reversible acute renal failure from amphotericin. Arch Intern Med 147:593–595, 1987.
38. Kahan BD. Clinical summation. An algorithm for the management of patients with cyclosporine-induced renal dysfunction. Transplant Proc 17:303–308, 1985.
39. Neild GH, Taube HE, Hartley RB, et al. Morphological differentiation between rejection and cyclosporin nephrotoxicity in renal allografts. J Clin Pathol 39:152–159, 1986.
40. Luke J, Luke DR, Williams LA, et al. Prevention of cyclosporine-induced nephrotoxicity with transdermal clonidine. Clin Pharm 9:49–53, 1990.
41. Smeesters C, Chaland P, Giroux L, et al. Prevention of acute cyclosporine A nephrotoxicity by a thromboxane synthetase inhibitor. Transplant Proc 20(Suppl 2):663–669, 1988.
42. Luke RG, Greifer I. Posttransplant risks of cyclosporine: nephrotoxicity. Am J Kidney Dis 5:342–343, 1985.
43. Whiting PH, Simpson JG. The enhancement of cyclosporine A included nephrotoxicity by gentamicin. Biochem Pharmacol 32:2025–2028, 1983.
44. Burckart GJ, Canafax DM, Yee GC. Cyclosporine monitoring. Drug Intell Clin Pharm 20:649–652, 1986.
45. Conlon PJ, Schwab SJ. Time to abandon nonionic contrast? J Am Soc Nephrol 5:123–124, 1994.
46. Coffman TM. Renal failure caused by therapeutic agents. In: Greenberg A. Primer on kidney diseases. 2nd ed. San Diego: Academic Press, 1998:260.
47. Rudnick MR, Goldfarb S, Wexler L, et al. Nephrotoxicity of ionic and nonionic contrast media in 1196 patients: a randomized trial. Kidney Int 47:254–261, 1995.
48. Steinberg EP, Moore RD, Powe N, et al. Safety and cost effectiveness of high-osmolality compared to low-osmolality contrast material in patients undergoing cardiac angiography. N Engl J Med 326:425–430, 1992.
49. Textor SC, Gephardt GN, Bravo EL, et al. Membranous glomerulopathy associated with captopril therapy. Am J Med 74:705–711, 1983.
50. Packer M. Identification of risk factors predisposing to the development of functional renal insufficiency during treatment with converting-enzyme inhibitors in chronic heart failure. Cardiology 76(Suppl 1):50–55, 1989.
51. Perneger TV, Whelton PK, Klag MJ. Risk of kidney failure associated with the use of acetaminophen, aspirin, and nonsteroidal antiinflammatory drugs. N Engl J Med 331:1675–1679, 1994.
52. Litterst CL. Alterations in the toxicity of cis-dichlorodiamine-platinum-II and in tissue localization of platinum as a function of NaCl concentration in the vehicle of administration. Toxicol Appl Pharmacol 61:99–108, 1981.
53. Finley RS, Fortner CL, Grove WR. Cisplatin nephrotoxicity: a summary of preventative interventions. Drug Intell Clin Pharm 19:362–367, 1985.
54. Galler M, Folkert VW, Schlondorff D. Reversible acute renal insufficiency and hyperkalemia following indomethacin therapy. JAMA 246:154–155, 1981.
55. Grunfeld JP, Ganeval D, Bournerias F. Acute renal failure in pregnancy. Kidney Int 18:179–191, 1980.
56. Auguste LJ, Stone AM, Wise L. The effects of *Escherichia coli* bacteremia on in vitro perfused kidneys. Ann Surg 192:65–68, 1980.
57. Trifillis AL, Kahng MW, Trump BF. Metabolic studies of glycerol-induced acute renal failure in the rat. Exp Mol Pathol 35:1–13, 1981.
58. Weinberg JM. The cell biology of ischemic renal injury. Kidney Int 39:476–500, 1991.
59. Siegel N, Avison MJ, Reilly HF, et al. Enhanced recovery of renal ATP with postischemic infusion of ATP-$MgCl_2$ determined by ^{31}P. Am J Physiol 245:F530–F534, 1983.
60. Shanley PF, Brezis M, Spokes K, et al. Transport-dependent cell injury in the S3 segment of the proximal tubule. Kidney Int 29:1033–1037, 1986.
61. Brezis M, Shina A, Kidroni G, et al. Calcium and hypoxic injury in the renal medulla of the perfused rat kidney. Kidney Int 34:186–194, 1988.
62. Paller MS, Hoidal JR, Ferris TF. Oxygen free radicals in ischemic acute renal failure in the rat. J Clin Invest 74:1156–1164, 1984.
63. Humes HD, Cieslinski DA, Coimbra TM, et al. Epidermal growth factor enhances renal tubule cell regeneration and repair and accelerates the recovery of renal function in postischemic acute renal failure. J Clin Invest 84:1757–1761, 1989.
64. Schena FP. Role of growth factors in acute renal failure. Kidney Int 53:S11–S15, 1998.
65. Lake EW, Humes HD. Acute renal failure: directed therapy to enhance renal tubular regeneration. Semin Nephrol 14:83–97, 1989.
66. Young DS. Effects of drugs on clinical laboratory tests. 3rd ed. Washington, DC: American Association of Clinical Chemistry, 1990.
67. Friedman RB, Young DS. Effects of disease on clinical laboratory tests. 2nd ed. Washington, DC: American Association of Clinical Chemistry, 1990.
68. Kaysen GA. Proteinuria and the nephrotic syndrome. In: Schrier RW, ed. Renal and electrolyte disorders. 4th ed. Boston: Little, Brown, 1992:681–726.
69. Mann HJ, Fuhs DW, Hemstrom CA. Acute renal failure. Drug Intell Clin Pharm 20:421–438, 1986.
70. Alleyne GA, Millward DJ, Scullard GH. Total body potassium, muscle electrolytes, and glycogen in malnourished children. J Pediatr 76:75–781, 1970.
71. Bjornsson TD. Use of serum creatinine concentrations to determine renal function. In: Gibaldi M, Prescott L, eds. Handbook of clinical pharmacokinetics. New York: ADIS Press, 1983:277–300.
72. Walser M, Drew HH, LaFrance ND. Creatinine measurements often yield false estimates of progression in chronic renal failure. Kidney Int 34:412–418, 1988.
73. Cockroft DW, Gault MH. Prediction of creatinine clearance from serum creatinine. Nephron 16:31–41, 1976.
74. Goldberg TH, Finklestein MS. Difficulties in estimating glomerular filtration rate in the elderly. Arch Intern Med 147:461–463, 1987.
75. Hatton J, Parr MD, Blouin RA. Estimation of creatinine clearance in patients with Cushing syndrome. Ann Pharmacother 23:974–947, 1989.
76. Hull JH, Hak LJ, Koch GG, et al. Influence of range of renal function and liver disease on predictability of creatinine clearance. Clin Pharmacol Ther 29:516–521, 1981.
77. Siest G, Galteau MM. Drug effects on laboratory test results. Analytical interferences and pharmacological effects. St Louis: Year Book, 1988.

78. Ross DL, Neely AE. Textbook of urinalysis and body fluids. Norwalk, CT: Appleton-Century-Crofts, 1983:68–122.
79. Valdes ME, Landau SE, Shah DM, et al. Increased glomerular filtration rate following mannitol administration in man. J Surg Res 26:473–477, 1979.
80. Solomon R, Werner C, Mann D, et al. Effects of saline, mannitol, and furosemide on acute decreases in renal function induced by radiocontrast agents. N Engl J Med 331:1416–1420, 1994.
81. Levinsky NG, Bernard DB. Mannitol and loop diuretics in acute renal failure. In: Brenner BM, Lazarus JM, eds. Acute renal failure. 2nd ed. New York: Churchill Livingstone, 1988:841–856.
82. Conger JD. Interventions in clinical acute renal failure: what are the data? Am J Kidney Dis 26:565–576, 1995.
83. Better OS, Stein JH. Early management of shock and prophylaxis of acute renal failure in traumatic rhabdomyolysis. N Engl J Med 322:825, 1990.
84. Brater DC. Diuretic Therapy. N Engl J Med 339:387–395, 1998.
85. Majumdar S, Kjellstrand CM. Why do we use diuretics in acute renal failure? Semin Dial 9:454–459, 1996.
86. Shilliday IR, Quinn KJ, Allison MEM. Loop diuretics in the management of acute renal failure: a prospective, double blind, placebo-controlled, randomized study. Nephrol Dial Transplant 12:2592–2596, 1997.
87. Weinstein JM, Heyman S, Brezis M. Potential deleterious effect of furosemide in radiocontrast nephropathy. Nephron 62:413–415, 1992.
88. Klahr S, Miller SB. Acute oliguria. N Engl J Med 338:671–675, 1998.
89. Flancbaum L, Choban PS, Dasta JF. Quantitative effects of low-dose dopamine on urine output in oliguric surgical intensive care unit patients. Crit Care Med 22:61–68, 1994.
90. Weisberg LS, Kurnik PS, Kurnick BR. Dopamine and renal blood flow in radiocontrast induced nephropathy in humans. Ren Fail 15:61–68, 1993.
91. Denton MD, Brady HR. Renal-dose dopamine for the treatment of acute renal failure: scientific rationale, experimental studies and clinical trials. Kidney Int 49:4–14, 1996.
92. Allgren RL, Marbury TC, Rahman SN, et al. Anaritide in acute tubular necrosis. N Engl J Med 336:828–834, 1997.
93. Lumlertgul D, Hutdagoon P, Sirivanichai C. Beneficial effect of intrarenal verapamil in human acute renal failure. Ren Fail 11:201–208, 1990.
94. Franklin SC, Moulton M, Sicard GA, et al. Insulin-like growth factor I preserves renal function postoperatively. Am J Physiol 272:F257–F259, 1997.
95. Kopple JD, Hirschberg R, Guler HP, et al. Lack of effect of recombinant human insulin-like growth factor-1 (IGF-1) in patients with acute renal failure (ARF) [abstract]. J Am Soc Nephrol 7:1375, 1996.
96. Toto RD. Approach to the patient with acute renal failure. In: Greenberg A, ed. Primer on kidney diseases. 2nd ed. San Diego: Academic Press, 1998:253.
97. Benet LZ, Williams RL. Design and optimization of dosage regimens: pharmacokinetic data. In: Gilman AG, Rall TW, Nies AS, et al. The pharmacologic basis of therapeutics. 8th ed. New York: Pergamon, 1990: 1650–1735.
98. Benet LZ, Massoud N. Pharmacokinetics. In: Benet LZ, Massoud N, Gambertoglio JG, eds. Pharmacokinetic basis for drug treatment. New York: Raven, 1984:1–28.
99. Bickley SK. Drug dosing during continuous arteriovenous hemofiltration. Clin Pharm 7:198–206, 1988.
100. Bressolle F, Kinowski JM, de la Coussaye JE, et al. Clinical pharmacokinetics during continuous hemofiltration. Clin Pharmacokinet 26:451–471, 1994.
101. Reetze-Bonorden P, Bohler J, Keller E. Drug dosage in patients during continuous renal replacement therapy. Clin Pharmacokinet 24:362–379, 1993.
102. Hara Y, May RC, Kelly RA, et al. Acidosis, not azotemia, stimulates branched-chain amino acid catabolism in uremic rats. Kidney Int 32:808–814, 1987.
103. Hak LJ. Nutrition in renal failure. In: Torosian MH, ed. Nutrition for the hospitalized patient: basic science and principles of practice. New York: Marcel Dekker, 1995:499–503.
104. Abel RM, Beck CH, Abbott WM, et al. Improved survival from acute renal failure after treatment with intravenous L-amino acids and glucose. N Engl J Med 288:695–699, 1973.
105. Kopple JD. The nutrition management of the patient with acute renal failure. JPEN 20:3–12, 1996.
106. Lordon RE, Burton JR. Posttraumatic renal failure in military personnel in southeast Asia. Am J Med 53:137–142, 1972.
107. Mehta RL. Continuous renal replacement therapies in the acute renal failure setting: Current concepts. Adv Ren Replace Ther 4(Suppl 1):81–92, 1997.
108. Edelstein CL, Ling H, Wangsiripaisan A, et al. Emerging therapies for acute renal failure. Am J Kidney Dis 30(Suppl 4):S89–S95, 1997.
109. Kelly KJ, Williams WWJ, Colvin RB, et al. Intercellular adhesion molecule-1 deficient mice are protected against ischemic renal injury. J Clin Invest 97:1056–1063, 1996.
110. Kelly KJ, Williams WWJ, Colvin RB, et al. Antibody to intercellular molecule-1 protects the kidney against ischemic renal injury. Proc Natl Acad Sci USA 91:812–816, 1994.
111. Goligorsky MS, Dibona GF. Pathogenic role of Arg-Gly-Asp recognizing integrins in acute renal failure. Proc Natl Acad Sci USA 90:5700–5704, 1993.
112. Singer I, Epstein M. Potential of dopamine A-1 agonists in the management of acute renal failure. Am J Kidney Dis 31(5):743–755, 1998.
113. Hakim RM, Fearon DT, Lazarus JM. Biocompatibility of dialysis membranes: effects of chronic complement activation. Kidney Int 26:194–200, 1984.
114. Hakim RM, Wingard RL, Parker RA. Effect of dialysis membrane in the treatment of patients with acute renal failure. N Engl J Med 331:1338–1342, 1994.
115. Schiffl H, Lang SM, Konig A, et al. Biocompatible membranes in acute renal failure: prospective case-controlled study. Lancet 344:570–572, 1994.
116. Himmelfarb J, Tolkoff-Rubin N, Chandran P, et al. A multicenter comparison of dialysis membranes in the treatment of acute renal failure requiring dialysis. J Am Soc Nephrol 9:257–266, 1998.

CHAPTER 22

CHRONIC RENAL DISEASE

Amy Galpin Krauss and Lawrence J. Hak

DEFINITION

Chronic renal disease (CRD) can be defined as a persistent or progressive deterioration in renal function. Left untreated, many forms of chronic renal disease will progress over several years to a complete loss of renal function. As the kidney increasingly fails to regulate volume, electrolyte, acid-base, metabolic, and endocrine homeostasis, a multisystem syndrome called uremia emerges (Table 22.1). Soon thereafter, initiation of a renal replacement therapy becomes necessary to control uremic symptoms and to sustain life, at which point an individual is said to have entered into end-stage renal disease (ESRD). Currently available options for chronic renal replacement therapy include kidney transplantation and dialysis. Chronic dialysis modalities (hemodialysis and peritoneal dialysis) are discussed in Chapter 23, and kidney transplantation is discussed in Chapter 104.

TREATMENT GOALS: CHRONIC RENAL DISEASE

- Preserve remaining renal function; maintain acceptable metabolic, nutritional and volume status; reduce uremic complications to other organ systems; prevent or control patient symptoms; and adjust drug and other therapies as indicated by disease progression.
- Achievement of these goals requires a multidisciplinary effort that usually includes referral to a specialty clinician or center.
- Several key principles can help foster success in approaching these goals:
  - Recognize risk factors for the development of renal disease at an *early* timepoint.
  - Minimize progression of renal disease through *early* intervention: drug, diet, and lifestyle measures.
  - Monitor the progression of renal disease at regular intervals.
  - Identify and remove factors exacerbating renal decline (e.g., drugs, volume depletion).
  - Include dietary measures as a cornerstone of disease, metabolic, and symptom control.
  - Institute appropriate drug therapy to manage volume, acid-base, electrolyte, cardiovascular, hematologic, musculoskeletal, gastrointestinal, and endocrine abnormalities.
  - Be aware of polypharmacy and polyprescribing in the CRD population.
  - Consider pharmacokinetic alterations as CRD progresses and adjust drug regimens accordingly.
  - Educate patients *in advance* of reaching ESRD about options for renal replacement therapy and the drug, diet, financial, and psychosocial issues commonly encountered in ESRD.

Table 22.1 ▪ Uremic Complications of Chronic Renal Disease

Fluid-electrolyte
- Volume control: hypervolemia, impaired sodium-water regulation
- Electrolytes: hyperkalemia, hypermagnesemia, hyperphosphatemia, hypocalcemia, hypercalcemia

Metabolic-nutritional
- Acid-base status: chronic metabolic acidosis, elevated anion-gap acidosis
- Protein: azotemia, hypoalbuminemia, protein malnutrition
- Carbohydrate: prolonged insulin action, peripheral insulin resistance, glucose intolerance
- Lipid: dyslipidemia, hyperlipidemia

Endocrine: hyperparathyroidism; deficiency in erythropoietin, calcitriol, and gonadal hormones

Hematologic: anemia, thrombocytopenia, impaired hemostasis, uremic bleeding

Cardiovascular: hypertension, left-ventricular hypertrophy, congestive heart failure, pericarditis, arrythmias

Musculoskeletal: osteodystrophy, hyperuricemia, amyloidosis, extraskeletal calcification

Gastrointestinal: dyspepsia, peptic ulcer disease, anorexia, nausea and vomiting, uremic fetor, constipation

Neurologic: peripheral neuropathy, altered mentation, uremic seizures, restless legs syndrome, poor sleep

Dermatologic: pruritis, discoloration, dryness/scaliness of skin

Infectious: impaired immune response, increased susceptibility to infections

Psychosocial: loss of autonomy, depression, loss of employment, financial hardships

Source: References 12, 49, 79, 80.

EPIDEMIOLOGY

Incidence and U.S. Renal Data Systems Statistics

Chronic renal disease is a major cause of morbidity and mortality in the United States and has been steadily on the rise. In the United States, extensive data describing the demographics, treatment, and outcomes of ESRD patients are collected and reported through a government-sponsored network referred to as the U.S. Renal Data Systems (USRDS). According to 1998 network statistics, the ESRD population had more than doubled in the prior decade to over 300,000 patients and was estimated to be growing by approximately 5% per year.[1] Data characterizing the pre-ESRD population are less complete; however, the number of individuals suffering from chronic renal disease in the United States is estimated at over 1.6 million.[2] The ESRD figures portray only a final endpoint in the continuum of chronic renal disease, but nevertheless are assumed to indirectly reflect overall trends in renal disease, as well as a fraction of its impact on health care today.

The incidence and prevalence of ESRD vary according to sex, age, race, and underlying disease.[1] Approximately 80,000 new individuals enter into ESRD yearly, the majority having followed a predictable course of CRD progression. The crude prevalence of ESRD is greater than 1000 per million of population, is slightly higher in males than females, and increases with age. The 65 and older age-group has been the most rapidly growing segment of the ESRD population, which exhibits an overall age distribution as follows: 20 to 44 years, 25%; 45 to 64 years, 39%; and 65 years and older, 34%. Compared with Caucasians, the prevalence of ESRD is higher within African American, Asian American, and Native American populations by 4.5-fold, twofold, and threefold, respectively. The primary disorders most commonly leading to ESRD are diabetes, hypertension, and glomerulonephritis.[1]

Chronic renal disease carries a poor prognosis. Historically, most individuals who have developed mild to moderate renal insufficiency have continued a relentless deterioration to ESRD. Before the availability of dialysis and renal transplant, ESRD became uniformly fatal within days to weeks. Despite the use of these therapies, unfortunately, the remaining life expectancy of an ESRD patient is still only one-half to one-fifth as long as that of an age-matched population free from renal disease.[1] The mortality rate in the U.S. ESRD population averages 22% yearly but appears to be influenced by additional factors, such as patient age, sex, race, concurrent disease, and renal replacement modality. More than half of the deaths in ESRD patients are attributed to cardiovascular causes (e.g., myocardial infarction, congestive heart failure, arrhythmias), followed by infection and voluntary withdrawal from renal replacement therapy.[1]

Chronic renal disease is costly. In the United States, medical care to ESRD patients incurred over $11 billion in direct expenditures in 1997 and is projected to now approach $16 billion annually. These treatment costs are borne largely by the federal government through its present Medicare End-Stage Renal Disease program. In 1997, annual Medicare payments averaged $43,000 per ESRD patient and ranged from $17,000 to more than $100,000 per patient year, depending on the treatment modality and complicating factors.[1] When costs for the management of chronic renal disease and acute renal failure are considered in conjunction with ESRD, a sizeable amount of health care resources is spent treating renal disease.

Etiology

Chronic renal disease can result from a primary intrinsic renal disease, from anatomic or obstructive abnormalities, as a secondary complication of another systemic disease, or from acute renal failure that never fully resolves. The major diseases leading to chronic renal failure and new cases of ESRD are diabetes (33 to 40%), hypertension (25%), and glomerulonephritis (18%). Less common causes of ESRD are detailed in Table 22.2.[1] Notably, diabetes mellitus (DM) now accounts for nearly 40% of new ESRD cases. Only 5 to 10% of patients with type II diabetes develop end-stage nephropathy, but they account for nearly two thirds of diabetes-related ESRD, in part due to the 20-fold higher prevalence of type II in comparison with type I diabetes. In contrast, nearly 25 to 40% of patients with type

I diabetes are estimated to enter into ESRD as a result of diabetic nephropathy. Those who have received kidney transplants comprise an expanding fraction of the CRD population. Although the kidney transplant cures their ESRD, the transplanted kidney may eventually fail for a number of reasons, including recurrent damage from the original systemic disorder, acute or chronic rejection, or drug-related nephrotoxicity associated with the use of certain immunosuppressants (e.g., cyclosporine, tacrolimus). Renal transplant recipients (RTRs) are a highly specialized subset of patients; however, many of the issues managed in CRD remain pertinent to the RTR population.

Progressive Nature

Aggressive treatment or elimination of the primary disease, such as diabetes or hypertension, can potentially retard or interrupt the progression of renal disease.[3,4] Toward this end, *early* intervention appears to be crucial in maximizing the success of preventive efforts. Intensive control of blood glucose has been shown to reduce or slow the onset of diabetic nephropathy in insulin-dependent diabetics,[5,6] pancreas transplant recipients,[7] and patients with type II diabetes.[8,9] Although interventions to reduce the U.S. prevalence of hypertension have led to significant reductions in secondary stroke and myocardial infarction, only a minor impact on the incidence of hypertensive renal disease has thus far been realized. The discrepancy in target organ outcomes suggests that more aggressive measures are needed to improve renal outcomes in the hypertensive population, and this appears to be especially true for male African Americans.

Table 22.2 ▪ Etiologies of Chronic Renal Failure

Primary Disease	New Cases (%)
Systemic disorders	
Diabetes (type 1, type 2, unspecified)	40
Hypertension (e.g., essential hypertension, renal artery stenosis)	27
Vasculitis/secondary glomerulonephritis (e.g., lupus erythematosus, scleroderma, polyarteritis, Wegener's granulomatosis, hemolytic-uremic syndrome)	2.4
Primary renal disorders	
Glomerulonephritis (e.g., acute, chronic, or rapidly progressive; postinfectious; focal glomerulosclerosis; Goodpasture's syndrome; IgA nephropathy)	11
Congenital anomalies/diseases (e.g., polycystic kidney disease, hypoplastic kidneys)	3.4
Neoplasms/tumors (e.g., renal/urologic, Wilms' tumor, multiple myeloma)	1.7
Drug-induced (e.g., analgesic abuse, other nephrotoxins)	0.7
Miscellaneous	6.3
Uncertain/data missing	7.5

Source: Reference 1.

A number of pathophysiologic processes are believed to perpetuate renal damage through a common pathway, regardless of the initiating insult or disease.[10,11] Understanding how these factors contribute to the progression of renal failure could lead to improved strategies for preserving renal function in individuals at risk of proceeding to ESRD.

PATHOPHYSIOLOGY

Several aspects of renal anatomy and physiology are reviewed in Chapter 21. The reader is referred to this material as background for the following discussion on the pathogenesis and pathophysiology of chronic renal disease.

Glomerular Hyperfiltration and Intraglomerular Hypertension

When the number of functioning nephrons is reduced because of renal insult or disease, the remaining nephrons compensate by enlarging (hypertrophy) and by increasing their individual glomerular filtration rates (GFRs). By escalating glomerular blood flow and intraglomerular capillary pressure, a state of increased glomerular perfusion can be attained, but at the expense of simultaneously inducing a degree of intraglomerular hyperfiltration and hypertension.[10–12] Referred to as renal reserve capacity, these glomerular adaptations accomplish the short-term goal of improving or restoring total renal GFR. Paradoxically, sustained elevations of blood flow and pressure within the glomeruli cause damage to remaining nephrons, ultimately proving *maladaptive* toward the long-term preservation of renal function.[10,11] Glomerular injury is also believed to result from increased capillary permeability (reduced permselectivity), which allows proteins and other macromolecules to leak through capillaries into the renal tubules. Microalbuminuria is one of the earliest clinical manifestations that indicates such glomerular damage is occurring. The abnormal urine solute load caused by these processes may, in turn, promote the secretion of proinflammatory mediators[11] and induce renal mesangial cells to deposit an extracellular glycoprotein matrix,[13] leading to a type of renal fibrosis and scarring termed *sclerosis.* Sclerosis can involve the entire nephron (nephrosclerosis), extending from the glomerulus (glomerulosclerosis) to the tubules and renal interstitium.

Hyperglycemia, systemic hypertension, and excessive dietary protein are able to initiate or exacerbate glomerular hyperfiltration. Intervention strategies targeting glycemic control, systemic hypertension, and protein intake are believed to retard progression of renal disease, in part, by attenuating glomerular hyperperfusion and its subsequent complications.

Although therapeutic interventions that reduce intraglomerular hyperperfusion might offer some protection against the progression of CRD, they can also interfere with the recruitment of renal reserve. When such measures are instituted clinically, it is not uncommon to observe an acute drop in GFR, accompanied by mild elevation of serum creatinine (SCr) that is reversible on cessation of therapy. Ironically, the hemodynamic effects resulting in this short-term loss of renal reserve (i.e., reversal of intraglomerular hypertension and hyperfiltration) also appear to be a chief mechanism of conferring long-term protection against CRD. In most instances, the initial sacrifice in GFR is offset by continued therapy because of the subsequently slower rate of renal decline.[14] Provided the acute drop in GFR is clinically tolerated, it may be the "price" paid to retard renal disease via nephroprotective maneuvers that reduce glomerular hyperfiltration.

Protein Intake and Therapeutic Implications

A high-protein diet has been found to increase renal blood flow (RBF) and GFR by several potential mechanisms. One could therefore theorize that excessive protein intake would heighten glomerular hyperfiltration, and hence long-term risk of renal disease. Conversely, protein restriction might help limit hyperfiltration and renal disease in certain individuals. Over the past decade, the effect of dietary protein restriction on the progression of renal disease has been the subject of several clinical investigations, which have yielded conflicting findings.

Early animal and pilot clinical studies in humans with moderate to severe diabetic nephropathy had demonstrated that moderate to strict protein restriction could significantly reduce the rate and number of patients progressing toward ESRD.[15,16] However, two larger trials subsequently failed to show a similar benefit from moderate to marked degrees of protein restriction, over a 3-year study period.[17,18] These landmark studies, one of which is known as the Modification of Diet in Renal Disease (MDRD) study,[17] were conducted in populations with largely nondiabetic forms of advanced renal disease. Because of the divergent findings between trials, considerable controversy exists over the value of dietary protein restriction in slowing CRD progression. Disagreement between the MDRD and earlier findings has been partially attributed to differences in the study populations and study designs, including the use of additional interventions in later trials, which helped lower the rate of disease progression in control groups (e.g., aggressive blood pressure control, the use of angiotensin converting enzyme inhibitors (ACEIs), and levels of protein intake within "control" groups that were well below usual dietary practice in the United States and Europe).

Reanalysis of the original MDRD findings now favors the argument that protein restriction was indeed beneficial to retarding CRD progression, particularly in individuals with moderate disease (GFR 25 to 55 mL/min) or a rapidly declining GFR at enrollment.[19] Similar to the pattern of response described earlier with interventions that reduce hyperfiltration, small drops in GFR were noted after the initiation of protein restriction, which were later followed by slower rates of GFR decline when compared with controls. Unfortunately, the primary 3-year endpoint may have proven too early to demonstrate differences in absolute outcome between groups, owing to initial losses in GFR experienced by treatment groups. With extended follow-up, the renal-sparing benefits of protein restriction might have become fully apparent, as the reduced rate of GFR decline in restricted groups began to compensate for early drops in GFR. Two meta-analyses examining the effect of dietary protein restriction on CRD progression also support the notion that dietary protein restriction is beneficial for some patients, especially diabetics and nondiabetics with moderate to severe disease.[20–22] In contrast, others maintain that the benefit is modest, relative to other interventions such as control of hypertension.[21]

Thus, despite the considerable attention this question has received, controversy persists about the benefit of protein restriction in retarding GFR decline, the optimal level of protein intake, which types or stages of renal disease are most likely to benefit, and whether other interventions are of greater importance. In practice, most nephrologists advise CRD patients to avoid *excessive* protein intake, and many advocate dietary protein restrictions to 0.6 to 0.8 g/kg/day for the purpose of slowing renal decline.[22,23]

Proteinuria

The appearance of protein (e.g., albumin) in the urine is usually interpreted as a harbinger of incipient nephropathy. In this sense, proteinuria is thought to indicate the presence of intraglomerular hypertension and abnormal glomerular permeability, as detailed in preceding sections. However, because tubular protein deposits can elicit proteolytic inflammatory responses, proteinuria itself is suspected to contribute independently to renal damage. The appearance or worsening of proteinuria is believed to predict the likelihood for progression of diabetic and other types of nephropathies.[24] Moreover, therapies that reduce proteinuria (such as ACEIs) have in many studies been associated with a salutary effect on renal disease progression. For these reasons, proteinuria has been emphasized as a clinical monitoring parameter in those recognized to be at risk of renal disease.

The nephroprotective benefit of antiproteinuric therapies has mostly been ascribed to reductions in glomerular hypertension.[10,25] However, nonhemodynamic effects may also contribute, such as the modification of glomerular permeability or reduced inflammatory stimulus from urine protein content. The degree of reduction in proteinuria is sometimes assessed as a surrogate endpoint for adjusting therapies that are prescribed to reduce intraglomerular hypertension. In general, a 30 to 50% reduction from baseline urinary albumin excretion (UAE) rate has been targeted clinically. More experience is needed to determine how consistently antiproteinuric responses will predict long-term renal outcomes for various interventions and types of renal disease.

Hypertension

Moderate to severe hypertension is strongly correlated with the risk of developing ESRD, consistent with observations that systemic hypertension can both cause and result from renal disease. Assuming that an elevated systemic blood pressure is transmitted to the glomerulus, systemic hypertension could be anticipated to exacerbate CRD progression, by contributing to intraglomerular hypertension and hyperfiltration. Arteriosclerosis, another hypertensive complication, can also contribute to nephron loss through ischemic mechanisms. Antihypertensive therapies have been postulated to protect against glomerulopathy by several mechanisms, including the reduction of blood pressure or blood flow reaching the glomerulus; the attenuation of intraglomerular hypertension via reductions in afferent or efferent arteriolar tone; the alteration of nonhemodynamic factors such as membrane permselectivity, inflammation, and oxidative stress; or possibly some combination of these mechanisms.[4,12]

Antihypertensive Differences

In theory, correction of hypertension by any agent *should* help reduce the risk of nephropathy.[4,17,26,27] However, all antihypertensives do not appear to provide equal protection against the progression of renal disease. Different antihypertensives alter glomerular hemodynamics to differing extents, depending on the interplay of their effect on systemic hemodynamics and afferent versus efferent renal arteriolar tone. Accumulating data suggest that for any given level of systemic blood pressure reduction, ACEIs and nondihydropyridine calcium channel blockers (diltiazem and verapamil) produce superior antiproteinuric and renoprotective effects, especially in diabetics[25,28–30] and individuals with established proteinuria.[31–33] Beyond effective blood pressure control, the advantage of ACEIs is believed to result from preferential dilation of the efferent renal artery, which should lower intraglomerular hypertension more consistently than other agents dilating the afferent arteriole. ACEIs and nondihydropyridine calcium channel blockers (non-DHP CCBs) are also proposed to influence the local renal environment in a manner that contributes to protective effects through nonhemodynamic mechanisms.[34–36] The use of antihypertensives in CRD is discussed in greater detail later in this chapter.

Hyperlipidemia

In patients with diabetes or hypertension, the presence of proteinuria is recognized as an independent risk factor for cardiovascular morbidity and mortality.[37] A common finding in these patients is elevation in the low-density lipoprotein (LDL) cholesterol and lipoprotein A lipid fractions, accompanied by reduced levels of high-density lipoprotein (HDL) cholesterol.[38] The observed lipid profile alterations presumably result from impaired breakdown of lipoprotein fractions or from increased hepatic lipoprotein production.[39,40]

Experimental and clinical data suggest a probable relationship between lipid abnormalities and the progression of renal disease.[41–44] In humans with renal disease, glomerular lipoprotein deposits, atheromatous lesions, and foam cells have been noted on renal biopsy. These may develop in parallel with systemic atherosclerotic disease as a consequence of the oxidative modification of LDL. Interestingly, renal mesangial cells possess LDL receptors and are capable of LDL uptake and oxidation. Moreover, in model systems, oxidized LDL can act as a direct toxin to mesangial cells that induces the production and release of inflammatory cytokines, vasoactive substances, and macrophage chemotactic factors. Macrophages subsequently recruited into the area can also oxidize LDL, transforming into foam cells that augment local inflammatory mediator release and glomerular scarring.

In theory, lipid-lowering therapies could prove clinically useful in reducing forms of renal damage linked to such processes, and are presently under investigation for this purpose. Results from a preliminary trial of simvastatin in normotensive diabetics with hypercholesterolemia and microalbuminuria have demonstrated a 25% reduction in albumin excretion rates after 1 year of lipid-lowering therapy.[45] Other small trials have suggested a reduction in renal disease progression attributable to antihyperlipidemic interventions.[44,46] Alternatively, control of proteinuria is proposed to indirectly limit excessive lipoprotein production and its associated cardiovascular risks. Ongoing clinical studies should offer insights regarding the role of lipid-lowering interventions to reduce both renal and cardiovascular disease in at-risk populations, such as diabetics and nephrotics.

Diabetes-Associated Chronic Renal Disease and Therapeutic Implications

Diabetes is the single most important disease leading to ESRD in the Western hemisphere. The incidence of diabetic nephropathy peaks after 10 to 15 years of diabetes; however, functional renal abnormalities are often present within 2 years of the onset of type I DM. Because the diagnosis of type II DM is often delayed from actual onset, renal changes are usually present at diagnosis in this population. Aside from hyperglycemia, comorbidities such as hypertension and hyperlipidemia are common in diabetics and are believed to contribute to progression of nephropathy in most cases.[3,47,48] As alluded to earlier, less than half of all diabetics progress completely to ESRD. This fraction is disproportionately high in certain racial groups such as Pima Indians, Native Americans, Hispanics, and Asian/Pacific Islanders. Therefore, racial or hereditary factors are believed to influence the likelihood of developing end-stage diabetic nephropathy. Improved characterization of the natural history of diabetic nephropathy has led to a new classification scheme for type I diabetic nephropathy. Table 22.3 summarizes this scheme, relevant clinical findings, and strategies for intervention.[49] Nephropathy in type II DM appears to be of a complex nature, involving heterogeneous mechanisms in addition to those typical of type I DM.[3,49]

Drug Exacerbation of Chronic Renal Disease and Other Reversible Factors

Residual renal function, as measured by GFR, is usually assumed to decline at a constant rate within a given individual, although the rate of loss varies considerably

Table 22.3 ▪ Stages of Diabetic Nephropathy in Type 1 (Insulin-Dependent) Diabetes

Stage*	Functional Alterations	Onset from Diagnosis of Diabetes Mellitus	Suggested Strategies for Intervention
I	Early hyperfunction Glomerular hyperfiltration and hypertrophy	0–2 years	Glycemic control Systemic blood pressure control
II	"Silent stage" Glomerular lesions developing (thickened basement membrane, mesangial expansion) Microalbuminuria not persistently present	2–5 years; may stabilize for several decades	Glycemic control Systemic blood pressure control† Avoid excessive dietary protein
III	"Incipient nephropathy" Persisent microalbuminuria (>20 μg/min or >30–300 mg/24 hr) GFR normal or elevated Intraglomerular hypertension present Systemic hypertension commonly arises Progression to overt nephropathy may still be preventable with appropriate intervention	7–15 years	Glycemic control ACEI: antiproteinuric Systemic blood pressure control† Avoid excessive dietary protein; consider dietary protein restriction
IV*	"Overt nephropathy" Clinical proteinuria (>0.5 g/24 hr) Systemic hypertension usually present GFR begins to fall by approximately 1 mL/min per month; may be slowed but not completely prevented Nephrotic syndrome may develop in patients with large urinary protein losses (>3 g/day)	15–25 years	Glycemic control‡ Systemic blood pressure control† ACEI: antiproteinuric Dietary protein restriction Reduce hyperlipidemia‡ Phosphate control Smoking cessation‡ See text—specialized approach
V*	Advanced renal insufficiency → azotemia → end-stage renal disease and uremia	Usually >20 years (or within 10–20 years after onset of stage IV)	Similar to stage IV, plus conventional measures for CRD complications Relaxation of glycemic control may be required

Source: Reference 49.

ACEI, angiotensin converting enzyme inhibitor; *CRD,* chronic renal disease; *GFR,* glomerular filtration rate.

*Stages IV and V are zones of irreversible nephropathy; interventions may slow but generally do not reverse progression to end-stage renal disease.

†Systemic blood pressure goals: less than 130/85 in absence of clinical proteinuria (urinary albumin excretion less than 1 g/day) or less than 125/75 if proteinuria is present (greater than 1 g/day); ACEIs are the preferred front-line antihypertensive.

‡Benefit in retarding late nephropathy is unclear; favored also to reduce cardiovascular risks.

between individuals. Patient features that have been identified to predict more rapid progression of renal disease include race (African American), hypertension, low serum HDL cholesterol, overt proteinuria, and diabetic microalbuminuria.[50] Exceptions to this generalization are noted, particularly when treatment to forestall GFR decline has been successful. As an example, if a patient exhibits a stable decline in GFR of 4 mL/min per year, one would predict that in the absence of successful intervention, his GFR would drop from a present value of 40 mL/min to 10 mL/min, over the next 7 to 8 years. After this point, dialysis would become necessary within 1 year. However, if institution of ACEI therapy were to slow the rate of decline by 50% (i.e., 2 mL/min per year), the need for dialysis could be delayed for 15 rather than 8 years.

Abrupt worsening or acceleration of the GFR decline can be a signal that new factors have begun to hasten renal deterioration. This situation is sometimes termed *acute renal failure (ARF) superimposed on chronic renal failure (CRF).* Because the responsible factors are often reversible or correctable, potential causes should be sought and eliminated when renal function acutely worsens over a previously established rate of decline. Examples of acute drug and nondrug exacerbators of renal dysfunction are described in Table 22.4. Several of these are included among the causes of ARF, as described in Chapter 21. In the setting of decreased renal reserve, drugs capable of inducing tubular necrosis and of reducing renal perfusion or volume status require particularly cautious use. Agents such as ACEIs and some other antihypertensives can be viewed as either nephroprotective or nephrotoxic, depending on the clinical context of their use.

Histologic Features

Nephron dropout is seen in several forms of CRD and refers to the loss of functional nephron units, which can occur in a scattered or regional pattern throughout the kidney. Hypertrophy in remaining (remnant) nephrons usually accompanies this finding, reflecting the adaptive (or maladaptive) pathophysiologic changes discussed in preceding sections. Most renal biopsies are described, in part, by which aspects of renal architecture are disrupted (e.g., glomerulus, tubule, interstitium).

Hallmark lesions of type I diabetic nephropathy include glomerular basement membrane thickening, glomerular hypertrophy, mesangial matrix expansion, and hyalinization or sclerosis of glomerular capillaries. Histologic findings in type II DM often include these lesions, as well as a mixture of others. Hypertensive kidney disease is typified by arteriolar thickening and vascular luminal narrowing, which promote ischemic damage in glomeruli and tubules. Deposition of hyaline, a proteinaceous material, is often observed throughout the nephron and leads to nephrosclerosis. In some forms of glomerulonephritis and immune-mediated renal disease, glomerular deposition of immune complexes or antibodies occurs in patterns that can be characterized only by special staining or electron microscopy techniques. A variety of histologic findings are associated with other types of intrinsic renal diseases; a full discussion of these is beyond the scope of this chapter.

Metabolic and Systemic Consequences of Chronic Renal Disease

The extent to which renal dysfunction reduces urinary solute excretion has been found to vary for different substances. For example, rises in urea and creatinine are observed early in CRD and inversely correlate with GFR, whereas the renal excretion of potassium, urate (uric acid), phosphorus, and hydrogen ion is generally preserved until GFR falls to below 25% of normal. Excretion of these solutes can be enhanced by increased tubular secretion or reduced reabsorption until GFR is 25 to 30 mL/min or less, at which point accumulation becomes unavoidable and plasma levels of these solutes also begin to rise. Finally, the renal handling of other solutes (e.g., Na^+, Cl^-) may be well preserved late into CRD but is noted to differ substantially among types of renal disease.

Table 22.4 ▪ Correctable Factors That Can Precipitate Renal Decline in Chronic Renal Disease

Reduction in renal perfusion Diuretics—overzealous diuresis leading to volume or sodium deficits ACEIs/ARBs—modest decline in GFR common; monitor for marked declines NSAIDs—in states of prostaglandin-dependent renal blood flow Antihypertensives—if excessive lowering of cardiac output or systemic blood pressure occurs Sudden reductions in sodium or fluid intake Excessive volume losses—diarrhea, vomiting, sweating, etc.	Direct nephrotoxins Antimicrobials—amphotericin, aminoglycosides, foscarnet, cidofovir, indinavir, high-dose acyclovir Radiocontrast dyes (especially high-osmolality) Anticancer agents—cisplatin, carboplatin, ifosfamide, high-dose methotrexate Immunosuppressants—cyclosporine, tacrolimus
Urologic abnormalities Urinary tract infection Urinary obstruction (stones, anatomic, prostatic hypertrophy)	Other factors High-protein diets (e.g., rapid weight loss) Excessive calcium or phosphorus intake (dietary or pharmaceutical)

ACEIs, angiotensin converting enzyme inhibitors; *ARBs,* angiotensin receptor blockers; *GFR,* glomerular filtration rate; *NSAIDs,* nonsteroidal anti-inflammatory drugs.

Azotemia refers to the systemic accumulation of nitrogenous wastes, such as blood urea nitrogen (BUN) and creatinine. "Uremia" is a clinical syndrome that encompasses not only a symptomatic degree of azotemia, but also a constellation of signs and symptoms referable to the other organ systems secondarily affected by ESRD. Although the concentration of urea can be correlated with the degree of renal impairment and overall severity of symptoms, no specific uremic toxins have been identified as being responsible for all the complications of the uremic syndrome. Aside from urea, additional toxins have been identified to accumulate in uremia, including ammonia, guanidine, guanidinosuccinic acid, methyl guanidine, phenols, myoinositol, and others.[12,49]

Of the numerous complications of CRD listed in Table 22.1, the pathophysiology of only the most common and clinically relevant features is discussed here. The therapeutic management of each of these complications is discussed in the next section of this chapter. In general, many of the metabolic derangements and symptoms of CRD relate directly to an imbalance between dietary intake and urinary excretion.

Volume, Sodium, and Water Balance

Because daily sodium intake usually exceeds requirements, the kidneys are able to maintain sodium balance by simply reducing urinary Na^+ reabsorption (i.e., increasing the fractional excretion of sodium or FE_{Na}). Conversely, if sodium intake is below output, the kidney is usually able to increase its conservation of sodium, except in certain salt-wasting nephropathies. At creatinine clearances below 25 mL/min, however, renal adaptation to wide fluctuations in sodium or water intake is sluggish and incomplete. The kidney becomes unable to concentrate or dilute urine efficiently, and urinary excretion of water and salt tends to become fixed at nearly iso-osmotic concentrations, in volumes of about 2 L/day. Because iso-osmotic fluid reabsorption is preserved until late in CRD, serum sodium concentrations are maintained within normal limits. In contrast, regulation of volume status becomes significantly impaired. As ESRD is neared, daily urine volumes decrease further in most patients. When salt and water intake are below output, volume depletion can develop rapidly. More commonly intake exceeds output, leading to volume retention, which exacerbates hypertension. As volume overload worsens, weight gain, edema, and finally pulmonary congestion or other cardiovascular complications can arise.

Electrolyte Balance: Potassium and Magnesium

Even though potassium is excreted almost exclusively in the urine, hyperkalemia is not common in patients having a GFR above 10 mL/min, unless acute changes in potassium intake have occurred. As GFR declines, potassium balance is maintained through increased secretion in the distal renal tubule and increased intestinal potassium secretion. Factors that jeopardize potassium homeostasis include increased potassium intake, the administration of potassium-sparing diuretics, ACEIs or angiotensin receptor blockers (ARBs), β-blockers, and several other drugs. In addition, acidosis commonly arises in advanced CRD and promotes shifting of potassium from the intracellular to the extracellular compartment. As renal reserve diminishes over time, the likelihood escalates for hyperkalemic complications from any of these factors. Chronic hyperkalemia of a mild to moderate degree is generally well tolerated by ESRD patients, when compared with patients who develop acute elevations in serum K^+ of similar magnitude. However, cardinal electrocardiograph changes (i.e., peaked T waves and a widened QRS complex) are usually observed once serum K^+ exceeds 7 to 7.5 mEq/L and represent the most common electrolyte emergency in the ESRD population. Hyperkalemic patients are usually asymptomatic, but occasionally they exhibit confusion or complain of muscle weakness, flaccidity, or paresthesias. Additional risk factors and complications from hyperkalemia are discussed in Chapter 9.

The primary route of magnesium excretion is renal. Mild, asymptomatic elevations in serum magnesium can occur in patients with advanced CRD. Provided that dietary intake is not unusually excessive, life-threatening hypermagnesemia is uncommon. However, pharmaceutical sources of magnesium such as antacids and magnesium-based cathartics can markedly elevate serum magnesium if used chronically or in large quantities. Many of these products are available over the counter; hence thorough medication histories and patient education are paramount to judicious use of such products. Potassium-sparing diuretics also tend to promote magnesium retention, particularly if magnesium supplements are in concurrent use.

Acid-Base Regulation

A normal adult consuming a mixed diet generates approximately 1 mEq/kg of metabolic acid daily. This hydrogen is rapidly buffered by circulating bicarbonate and is excreted by the lungs as respiratory acid (CO_2). Bicarbonate lost during this process is regenerated by the kidney through the excretion of acid (H^+), which must be buffered by ammonia (forming NH_4^+) or other urinary buffers. In kidney disease, renal ammonia formation (ammoniagenesis) is generally impaired as a consequence of reduced nephron mass. Because urinary acid secretion and renal regeneration of bicarbonate are coupled to the availability of ammonia, these associated processes become impaired in CRD. Bicarbonate is also filtered into the urine and must be reclaimed by reabsorption; however, this tends to remain intact until CRD is far advanced. The metabolic acidosis of CRD typically begins as a normal anion gap acidosis, characterized by low serum bicarbonate and mild hyperchloremia. As GFR falls below 10 mL/min, various organic acids accumulate, and the picture evolves toward that of an "elevated anion-gap" acidosis, with bicarbonate levels near or above 12 to 15 mEq/L. The metabolic acidosis appears to be clinically tolerated, but it is thought to promote bone resorption and to contribute to a chronic catabolic state, by stimulating branched-chain amino acid breakdown.[12,51] In addition, patients with renal disease may not withstand acute acid-base challenges well (such as sepsis or ketoacidosis) because their overall buffer reserve is diminished.

Calcium, Phosphorus, and Bone Homeostasis

In CRD, calcium, phosphorus, and bone metabolism can assume a variety of disturbances, but is most often characterized by a combination of hyperphosphatemia, hypocalcemia, hyperparathyroidism, and abnormal bone turnover. The normal regulation of calcium-phosphate homeostasis through the actions of parathyroid hormone and vitamin D on the gut, kidney, and bone are briefly summarized in Table 22.5. A more detailed review can be found in Chapters 23 and 35.

The normal kidney is able to maintain serum calcium and phosphate homeostasis by balancing tubular reabsorption of these minerals against dietary intake and their deposition into bone (as calcium phosphate). Parathyroid hormone (PTH) promotes bone turnover and mobilization of bone calcium phosphate stores to the serum while enhancing renal phosphate wasting but calcium reabsorption. PTH secretion is stimulated by low ionized calcium levels or elevated serum phosphate (directly or indirectly) and is inhibited by calcitriol (1,25-dihydroxyvitamin D_3).

Table 22.5 ▪ Major Changes in Calcium and Phosphorus Homeostasis Related to End-Stage Renal Disease

Regulatory Hormone	Stimulatory Signals	Effect at Major Target Organs	Outcome on Serum Ca, PO_4	Alterations in End-Stage Renal Disease
Parathyroid hormone (PTH)	Increased by ↓Ca, ↑PO_4 Decreased by calcitriol	Bone: ↑turnover, ↑Ca, PO_4 release Kidney: ↓PO_4, ↑Ca reabsorption, ↑calcitriol formation Gut: ↑PO_4 absorption (?)	↑Serum Ca ↓→Serum PO_4	↑PTH half-life Impaired renal PO_4 excretion ↓Calcitriol negative feedback regulation of PTH
Calcitriol (1,25-dihydroxyvitamin D3)	Increased by ↑PTH, ↓PO_4 Decreased by ↑PO_4	Bone: ↑mineralization, ↑turnover Kidney: ↑PO_4, ↑Ca reabsorption Gut: ↑Ca, ↑PO_4 absorption Parathyroid: ↓PTH secretion	↑Serum Ca ↑Serum PO_4	↓Calcitriol formation

Under normal conditions, the net effect of PTH secretion is to increase serum calcium and bone turnover while maintaining or decreasing serum phosphate levels. Calcitriol is the most physiologically active form of vitamin D and is produced by the renal hydroxylation of 25-hydroxycholecalciferol to 1,25-dihydroxycholecalciferol. Calcitriol facilitates PTH-mediated bone turnover, enhances gut calcium absorption, and increases the renal tubular reabsorption of both calcium and phosphate. Calcitriol production is stimulated by low ionized calcium or elevated PTH levels, but it can be blunted by the presence of hyperphosphatemia. Normally, the net effect of calcitriol is to elevate both serum calcium and phosphate, facilitating the mineralization of newly forming bone. PTH is thought to promote renal calcitriol production, whereas calcitriol inhibits PTH secretion, providing a form of negative feedback regulation. Finally, ionized serum calcium and phosphate share a reciprocal relationship, in that the elevation of one tends to reduce the serum level of the other, by either complexation, precipitation as calcium phosphate, or other poorly understood hormonal mechanisms. Precipitation of calcium phosphate is thought to occur when elevations in the serum calcium or phosphate result in a calcium phosphate product that exceeds their solubility value, approximately 65 to 75 or greater at blood pH. The calcium phosphate product can be computed by multiplying the total serum calcium (mg/dL) by serum phosphorus (mg/dL), using total serum calcium levels that are corrected for hypoalbuminemia. Extraskeletal calcium phosphate precipitation, also called ectopic or metastatic calcification, can occur in vessels, soft tissues, joints and tendons, and other vital organs, leading to numerous complications.[12,49]

The primary disturbance in CRD is nephron loss, which limits renal capacity for phosphate excretion and calcitriol production, especially once the GFR falls below 25 to 30 mL/min. These changes invoke secondary responses (such as increased PTH secretion) that ultimately perpetuate a cycle of dysregulation.[52–54] The following sequence of events is characteristic of early homeostatic responses in renal disease: as renal function initially diminishes, urinary phosphorus excretion also declines, inducing a modest elevation in serum phosphorus. Ionized serum calcium levels fall as phosphorus rises, both of which are thought to stimulate PTH secretion. Elevation in PTH then promotes bone resorption, releasing bone calcium and phosphate stores into serum while enhancing renal tubular excretion of phosphorus and reabsorption of calcium. Overall, this response serves to normalize serum phosphorus downward and calcium levels upward, but it is maintained at the expense of increased circulating PTH levels. Later, as renal mass progressively declines, the kidney becomes unable to excrete phosphorus even in the face of rising PTH. Sustained elevations in serum phosphate provide a continued stimulus for PTH secretion, which continues to accelerate bone turnover but is ineffective in promoting renal phosphate excretion. Unless reductions in dietary phosphorus intake can offset the accelerated turnover of bone phosphate into the serum and renal phosphate retention, a relentless cycle of hyperphosphatemia and hyperparathyroidism becomes established.

The renal conversion of 25-hydroxycholecalciferol to calcitriol is inhibited by elevations in serum phosphorus, which is partially offset by the concomitant elevations in PTH that promote calcitriol formation. However, as renal disease progresses, the kidneys become unable to produce sufficient quantities of calcitriol, regardless of stimulatory signals. A state of relative calcitriol deficiency ensues, which impairs not only inhibition of PTH release, but also intestinal calcium absorption and bone response to PTH. In conjunction with persistent hyperphosphatemia, calcitriol deficiency is thought to contribute to hypocalcemic tendencies in ESRD. Blunted calcitriol levels and alterations in bone metabolism are thought to begin at mild to moderate stages of renal failure (e.g., CrCl less than 65 mL/min).[55]

Renal degradation of PTH is impaired in advanced renal disease, as is clearance of inactive PTH metabolites. In these patients, measure of the active N-terminus moiety, called iPTH (intact parathyroid hormone), provides a more accurate reflection of parathyroid status than nonspecific assays. Secondary hyperparathyroidism is noted in a majority of untreated CRD patients, as a result of both prolonged iPTH half-life and increased PTH release driven by sustained hyperphosphatemia, hypocalcemia, and low calcitriol activity. Hyperparathyroidism is a concern not only because it abnormally accelerates bone turnover, but also because PTH is suspected to mediate other aspects of the uremic syndrome. Subclinical hyperparathyroidism is now recognized to emerge at GFRs above 50 mL/min, preceding overt hyperphosphatemia in many patients with CRD.

Renal osteodystrophy is a term that collectively refers to the diverse skeletal abnormalities observed in individuals with renal disease. Osteitis fibrotica, the most common manifestation, is associated with secondary hyperparathyroidism, elevated rates of bone turnover, and "brittle" fibrous bone. Osteomalacia and adynamic (low-turnover) subtypes of bone disease are observed in a smaller fraction of patients, in association with low PTH levels (usually as the iatrogenic result of overzealous suppressive treatment), variable elevations in body aluminum stores, and poor mineralization of bone. Osteoporosis, osteosclerosis, and mixed forms of bone disease can also plague ESRD patients. These disturbances in bone and calcium phosphate metabolism progress insidiously, but eventually lead to increased fracture rates (especially hip), bone pain, muscle weakness, musculoskeletal discomfort, and pathologic calcification of soft tissue, organs, nerves, and blood vessels. Although these complications are well recognized in long-term ESRD patients, there is a growing appreciation that they begin at earlier stages in chronic renal disease and should be amenable to intervention before the point of ESRD.[55]

Anemia of Chronic Renal Disease

Anemia is observed in virtually all patients with chronic renal failure and tends to become clinically manifest at serum creatinine values near 3 mg/dL.[12,49] Early signs and symptoms of anemia include pallor, reduced energy, decreased exercise tolerance, exertional dyspnea, altered cognition, and fatigue. At GFRs exceeding 10 mL/min, hematocrit values tend to remain above 30%, but then drift downward to 20 to 25% as GFR falls further. In the absence of severe cardiopulmonary disease, acute clinical deteriorations are uncommon because most patients are able to physiologically "adapt" as the anemia gradually develops. Clearly, however, untreated anemia compromises quality of life and functional status in patients with CRD.[56,57] Moreover, even moderate degrees of anemia are suspected to contribute to the early development of cardiac enlargement and other cardiovascular abnormalities, which are notably prevalent in the ESRD population.[58,59]

Anemia of CRD is caused by a number of factors that are listed in Table 22.6. The primary causes are a decrease in renal erythropoietin (EPO) production that parallels the decline in functional nephrons and a reduction in red blood cell (RBC) life span. Natural EPO is produced and secreted by the kidney in response to hypoxia and enhances erythropoiesis by stimulating the bone marrow to produce erythroid cells. In nonanemic states, normal EPO plasma levels range from 15 to 25 mU/mL. When nonuremic patients develop anemia, serum EPO levels rise to 10 to 100 times the normal level, in order to generate a compensatory increase in RBC production and hematocrit. In contrast, patients with CRD are unable to mount proportionate increases in EPO production, resulting in a blunted marrow response to anemic conditions. For some patients, increased hepatic production of EPO, normally accounting for 10% of endogenous EPO, may help sustain hematocrits.

In advanced CRD or uremia, RBC life span is also reduced from the normal value of 90 to 120 days to only 60 to 90 days on average, thereby raising the basal RBC production rate needed to maintain hematocrit. Increased RBC turnover has been attributed to the "toxic" uremic environment; however, the specific factors responsible for shortening RBC life span have not been clearly identified. Anemia that is due purely to renal disease should be normocytic and normochromic. In practice, a mixed picture is often observed because of the presence of additional factors contributing to anemia in this population, such as iron deficiency, aluminum toxicity, and folate or vitamin B_{12} deficiency. Other causes of normocytic, normochromic anemia in the CRD population include inflammatory or infectious processes, acute or chronic blood loss (iatrogenic, gastrointestinal, or pathologic), hypersplenism, and severe osteitis fibrotica.

Table 22.6 ▪ Causes of Anemia of Chronic Renal Failure

Decreased erythropoietin activity
Shortened red blood cell lifespan
Gastrointestinal blood loss
Dialysis
Iron deficiency from dialyzer blood loss
Folic acid deficiency from dialysis removal
Red cell destruction from hemolysis
Splenic sequestration

Cardiovascular Disease: Hypertension and Heart Disease

Hypertension is present in 65 to 90% or more of the CRD population, showing a higher prevalence in Blacks and in those with more severe renal dysfunction.[60] If not the preexisting cause of renal failure, hypertension invariably develops along the course of renal disease and can accelerate its progression.[12,27,49,61,62] The kidney plays a major role in the control of blood pressure by regulating sodium retention, extracellular fluid volume, and the renin-angiotensin system. Expanded extracellular fluid (ECF) volume is presumed to be a major factor contributing to hypertension in most CRD patients, followed by elevated renin-angiotensin activity.[12,49,63] Imbalances between endogenous vasoconstrictive (e.g., endothelin) and vasodilatory substances (e.g., nitric oxide) have also been recognized as a probable factor underlying hypertension in CRD.[12,64,65] Increased pulse pressure and isolated systolic hypertension are also more common in the CRD population, consistent with the concept of expanded ECF volume and reduced vascular compliance.

Hypertension significantly increases the risk for cardiac disease and stroke in the general population. This holds true for the ESRD population as well, in which cardiovascular mortality is 10 to 20 times higher.[66] In ESRD, the prevalence of left ventricular hypertrophy (LVH), coronary artery disease, and congestive heart failure (CHF) is epidemic, approaching 40%, 75%, and 40%, respectively. Although data describing cardiovascular disease in pre-ESRD patients are scant, LVH has been observed in 25 to 50% of individuals with moderate to severe degrees of chronic renal insufficiency. It seems reasonable to suspect that cardiovascular risk actually begins to increase *before* entering ESRD, in parallel with or as a consequence of chronic renal disease. Risk factors common to the progression of both cardiovascular and renal disease are present in the majority of those with CRD and often include hypertension, hyperlipidemia, diabetes, and altered neurohumors (e.g., renin-angiotensin, endothelin, and nitric oxide).[67] Elevated homocysteine levels and possibly oxidative stress are implicated in promoting cardiovascular disease in several populations and are suspected to rise progressively during the course of CRD.[68] The potential importance of homocysteine in the ESRD population is discussed in Chapter 23.

Hypertension is an important risk factor for the progression of renal disease. As discussed in earlier sections, renal damage is thought to result from exaggerated intraglomerular hypertension and hyperfiltration, perhaps in conjunction with ischemic damage due to arteriosclerotic changes in renal vasculature. As renal disease advances, achieving good control of hypertension can become challenging, but it is still important in minimizing or slowing end-organ damage.

Dyslipidemias

In chronic renal disease, the prevalence of dyslipidemia is higher than in the general population, ranging from 30 to 90% or more.[38] The pattern of abnormality varies by lipid fraction among types and stages of renal disease and is also affected by concurrent metabolic conditions, such as diabetes. Reduced HDL, increased triglycerides, and elevated lipoprotein A are common in nearly all forms of renal disease, whereas increased very low density lipoprotein (VLDL), LDL, and total cholesterol are most common in patients with nephrotic syndrome, renal transplants, or in ESRD receiving dialysis. The mechanisms underlying the different patterns of lipoprotein abnormality are not clear, in that evidence exists for both increased production and altered catabolism of lipoproteins.

In patients with heavy urinary protein losses (greater than 3 g/day; i.e., nephrotic syndrome), the degree of hyperlipidemia and cardiovascular risk is thought to correlate directly with urine protein excretion and inversely with serum albumin levels.[38,39] In these individuals, most of whom are extremely hypoalbuminemic, increased hepatic lipoprotein production is hypothesized to compensate for low serum oncotic pressure.[12,39,49] However, evidence suggests that impaired lipid catabolism may also contribute to hyperlipidemia.[40] In at least one pilot study, measures to reduce urine protein excretion were associated with secondary reductions in hyperlipidemia.[69]

As in the general population, increased LDL and total cholesterol fractions in the CRD population are associated with elevated cardiovascular risk. At present, the cardiovascular risks associated with other observed lipoprotein abnormalities–increased triglycerides, decreased HDL, and increased Lp(a) lipoprotein–are not well defined in the general or the CRD population. Dyslipidemia may contribute to renal disease progression through atherogenic and other mechanisms, as discussed in earlier sections of this chapter.

Bleeding and Other Hematologic Abnormalities

An increased tendency toward bleeding is common in uremia and may be manifested by bruising, purpura, epistaxis, and bleeding from venipuncture and gastrointestinal sites. Less common but potentially fatal complications can include hemorrhage from trauma sites, intracranial bleeding, and pericardial bleeding. No single mechanism has been identified that fully explains the various hemostatic defects noted in uremics. However, abnormalities in platelet number and function are thought to play a more predominant role than clotting factor deficits.[12,49] Consistent with this, the clinical risk of bleeding is thought to correlate roughly with the degree of prolongation in bleeding time, whereas tests of coagulation (e.g., prothrombin time) are generally found to be normal.[70]

Impairment of platelet adhesion, aggregation, and activation, processes critical to primary hemostasis, is thought to be an important aspect of uremic platelet dysfunction. Thrombocytopenia, possibly due to increased peripheral platelet destruction, is noted to a moderate degree in more than half of patients, although platelet counts below 50,000/mL are rare. Reduced von Willebrand factor (vWF) levels or ineffective interactions among vWF, platelet GPIIb-IIIa receptors, and fibrinogen are suspected to contribute to faulty platelet aggregation or adhesion to vascular wall collagen.[71] The ability of dialysis to improve hemostatic deficits implies a role for accumulated uremic toxins, although the mechanism or mechanisms by which these substances interfere with hemostasis are not well understood.[12,49] The activity of at least one procoagulant, platelet factor III, has been correlated inversely with levels of guanidinosuccinic acid, a uremic toxin that is dialyzable. Production of nitric oxide, a powerful inhibitor of platelet aggregation, is also generally elevated in CRD. Finally, anemia of CRD reduces the enhancing influence of RBC mass on platelet-vessel interactions and the intravascular dispersion of platelets. Coupled with the aforementioned abnormalities, the use of heparin or other drugs with antiplatelet or anticoagulant effects can further heighten bleeding risk.

Carbohydrate, Protein, and Nitrogen Metabolism

A hallmark of chronic renal disease is the progressive accumulation of nitrogenous waste products, which are the byproducts of protein catabolism from both dietary and endogenous protein sources. The most commonly measured substances, urea and creatinine, generally correlate with severity of symptoms, especially as GFR falls below 25 to 30 mL/min; however, other unmeasured amino acids and nitrogenous wastes almost certainly contribute.[12,49]

Catabolism of protein is thought to become accelerated by chronic metabolic acidosis, insulin resistance, or excessive protein intake.[12,49] Inadequate protein intake (e.g., due to anorexia or dietary restriction) can also induce a shift from an anabolic to a catabolic state. Protein malnutrition and loss of lean muscle mass is becoming increasingly recognized in the pre-ESRD population and is not uncommon in individuals with ESRD receiving dialysis (discussed extensively in Chapter 23). Although serum albumin is used clinically as a nonspecific index of visceral protein stores, its utility is reduced in individuals with large urinary protein (i.e., albumin) losses and volume overload, such as those with nephrotic syndrome.

The kidneys are normally responsible for clearing approximately 40% of circulating insulin, through glomerular filtration and intrarenal metabolism. As renal failure progresses, renal insulin clearance is reduced and the half-life and activity of insulin are prolonged, resulting in lower exogenous insulin requirements in diabetics with advancing CRD. In patients receiving oral agents, hypoglycemic episodes may occur as a result of the accumulation of renally eliminated hypoglycemics or their active metabolites (e.g., chlorpropamide, glyburide). Changes in insulin disposition are paralleled, however, by increasing degrees of peripheral insulin resistance in both nondiabetic[72] and diabetic forms of kidney disease. Despite the fact that endogenous insulin secretion is blunted in proportion to blood glucose, hyperinsulinemia may develop. As a result, the majority of nondiabetic CRD patients develop glucose intolerance of varying severity, evidenced by elevated postprandial blood glucose levels in the face of normal fasting blood glucose values.[73] The clinical relevance of glucose intolerance, hyperinsulinemia, and insulin resistance in nondiabetic CRD is not entirely clear. However, recent data support earlier suspicions that hyperinsulinemia may accelerate atherosclerotic processes and cardiovascular disease.[74] In addition, peripheral insulin resistance is likely to interfere with the anabolic actions of insulin, which normally promote nitrogen retention and inhibit protein catabolism.

Endocrine and Hormonal Abnormalities

Abnormalities in female and male gonadal hormones are common in ESRD and result in a high incidence of infertility and sexual dysfunction.[75] Hyperprolactinemia is common, and gonadotropin, follicle-stimulating hormone (FSH), and luteinizing hormone (LH) levels may be low in both men and women. Women may cease to ovulate or menstruate, or only do so irregularly. Although pregnancy is still possible, these are considered high-risk cases and only 40% result in successful deliveries. Decreased libido and erectile dysfunction are common in men with ESRD, which may be related not only to reduced testosterone levels, but also concurrent malaise, anemia, vascular, and neurologic abnormalities.

The regulation and function of other hormonal systems that are affected by ESRD have been discussed separately, including parathyroid hormone, calcitriol, erythropoietin, and insulin disposition and action. Many ESRD patients also exhibit a form of secondary hypothyroidism called sick euthyroid syndrome, characterized by low T3 and total T4 levels but normal free T4 index and thyroid-stimulating hormone (TSH) levels.[76] Evaluation of thyroid abnormalities in ESRD is complicated by alterations in hormone protein binding and the frequent presence of concurrent diseases with overlapping symptoms.

Gastrointestinal Disease

Patients with advanced renal failure commonly have gastrointestinal complications such as anorexia, nausea, and vomiting.[12] These symptoms become pronounced as ESRD advances, to a degree that often prompts initiation of dialysis. They may complain of a metallic or salty taste, and their breath may smell of ammonia, referred to as uremic fetor. Uremic patients have high concentrations of urea in their saliva, which undergoes conversion to ammonia in the presence of bacterial ureases. As a consequence of the irritative effects of ammonia and probably other factors, mucosal and submucosal ulcerations often develop along the alimentary tract; these may take the form of stomatitis, parotitis, esophagitis, erosive gastritis, and colitis. Peptic ulcer disease is common in uremic patients; however, the relative importance of ammonia versus gastric acidity, *Helicobacter pylori*, and other pathogenic factors has not been clearly defined.[77] Coupled with defects in hemostasis, blood loss from gastrointestinal sites is thought to contribute significantly to anemia in advanced CRD. In diabetic uremics, it is not uncommon for gastroparesis to be superimposed on the aforementioned abnormalities, compounding nausea, vomiting, and gastroesophageal reflux. Constipation is a nearly universal complaint in ESRD, which partly stems from the use of constipating medications, along with fluid and dietary restrictions.

Pruritis and Dermatologic Changes

Generalized pruritus is common in CRD and may be one of the most recalcitrant and frustrating symptoms that patients experience. Causative factors are thought to include dry skin, accumulation of uremic wastes, elevations in serum calcium phosphate product (leading to integumentary calcification), hyperparathyroidism, altered neurologic sensory input, hypervitaminosis A, and increased levels of histamine and serotonin.[12,49] A sallow yellowish or bronze pigmentation of the skin is common, as is pallor in extremely anemic patients. Bruises and hematomas reflect the heightened bleeding tendency and become even more evident as patients begin to undergo frequent venipunctures and invasive procedures.

Musculoskeletal and Neurologic Abnormalities

Uric acid is the end product of purine metabolism. It circulates primarily as urate, is filtered at the glomerulus, and is almost completely reabsorbed in the proximal tubules. Renal excretion of uric acid is impaired when the GFR falls below 25 to 30 mL/min, resulting in elevated serum uric acid levels. Potential complications from hyperuricemia include gouty attacks, uric acid kidney stones, and urate nephropathy.[12,49] For unknown reasons, chronic renal failure patients rarely develop gout unless there is a previous history of underlying gout. Chronic hyperuricemia may also contribute to the progression of renal disease; however, the true nature of this association is unclear. In more than one-third of long-standing ESRD patients, arthropathies, tendinitis, or carpal tunnel syndrome results from the accumulation and widespread deposition of an amyloid protein called β_2-microglobulin.[12,78]

More than 60% of uremic patients exhibit some evidence of peripheral neuropathy once GFR falls below 5 mL/min.[78] Early symptoms may include tingling or numbness, paresthesias, painful cramps, and restless legs syndrome (an intense, irresistible urge to move the legs). In severe cases, reduced or absent tendon reflexes, proximal muscle wasting, weakness, and ataxia may develop. Uremic polyneuropathy is presumed to involve axonal degeneration of motor and sensory nerve fibers, but generally improves or stabilizes with institution of renal replacement therapies. Diabetic neuropathy is commonly superimposed on uremic polyneuropathy.

CLINICAL PRESENTATION AND DIAGNOSIS

Signs and Symptoms

Table 22.7 summarizes terminology that has been used to describe progressive stages of renal disease and the usual associated clinical findings. It should be remembered that these terms are not rigorous definitions and that several of these descriptors are applied variably in clinical practice. Most patients experience few symptoms of CRD until less than 25% of normal renal function remains. CRD can therefore progress insidiously over months to years, evident only through abnormal biochemical parameters, such as gradually rising levels of BUN and SCr or falling creatinine clearance values. Nonspecific complaints such as malaise, fatigue, and nocturia may be present. Urine output may be diminished or nearly normal. Hypertension may develop and, if discovered, presents a critical opportunity to investigate renal implications. Unless patients are recognized to be at risk of and are monitored for renal disease, they usually do not seek medical attention until the onset of uremic symptoms. At this point, interventions to forestall progression to ESRD are largely unfruitful.

Diagnosis

When a patient is newly discovered to have renal dysfunction, an effort should be made to discern whether this is the result of a long-standing chronic process, an acute reversible form of renal failure, or a combination of both.[79,80] Several other systemic diseases can manifest initially with renal dysfunction. Diagnostic tests to rule out other causes such as autoimmune, malignant, and thrombotic disorders may be necessary. An extensive history should be conducted to uncover exposure to nephrotoxins (especially drugs), previously unrecognized urinary tract symptoms, or risk factors for renal disease. A renal biopsy can provide information that is helpful in confirming the etiology of renal disease, its extent, and the overall prognosis, especially when causes other than diabetes or hypertension are suspected. In general, biopsies are performed only if a treatable form of systemic disease is suspected, and the information will alter or guide therapeutic decisions.[12,49] Renal ultrasound (sonography) can be helpful in assessing kidney size and in ruling out obstructive processes, often associated with hydronephrosis. Small kidney size generally implies a long-standing, irreversible or advanced form of disease. Renal arteriography may be considered in order to rule out the presence of renal artery stenosis or other vascular or perfusion abnormalities. Although serum creatinine values can provide a rough estimate of remaining GFR, measured urinary creatinine clearance studies will more accurately assess residual renal function (see Chapter 21). Urinalysis is usually performed, but it is generally less informative in differentiating chronic renal disease subtypes as compared with its utility in ARF. Nonetheless, quantifying the amount of proteinuria can be helpful as a prognostic feature or in establishing a baseline for antiproteinuric interventions. Metabolic and hematologic panels

Table 22.7 ▪ Continuum of Progression: Pre-ESRD to End-Stage Renal Disease

Stage	Diminished Renal Reserve	Renal Insufficiency	Chronic Renal Failure	Uremia	End-Stage Renal Disease
Percent of function	50–75%	20–50%	10–25%	<10%	<5–10%
Usual SCr* (mg/dL)	1.4–2	1.8–4.5	4–10	8–12+	>8 (variable)
Creatinine clearance (mL/min)	60–90	30–60	10–30	<10	<5–10
Clinical signs, laboratory findings, and symptoms	↑BUN, ↑SCr Asymptomatic	Nocturia Hypertension ↓Hematocrit (mild) ↑iPTH (mild) Proteinuria	Urine volume ↓ or → Mild hypervolemia ↑Hypertension ↓Hematocrit ↑↑iPTH ↑PO_4^{2-}, ↓Ca^{2+} ↑K^+ (mild) Acidosis (mild) ↓Calcitriol Anorexia, dysguesia Fatigue, malaise	↓Urine volume Hypervolemia Hypertension ↓↓Hematocrit ↑↑iPTH ↑↑PO_4^{2-}, ↓↓Ca^{2+} ↑↑K^+ ↑Acidosis ↓↓Calcitriol Severe nausea or vomiting ↑↑Malaise Pruritis ↓Mental status Neuropathy	Dialysis needed to control signs and symptoms of uremia Emergent indications for dialysis: seizures, pericarditis, hypervolemia acidosis or hyperkalemia (severe) Uremic signs and symptoms, to left, generally present

Source: References 79–81.

BUN, blood urea nitrogen; *iPTH,* intact parathyroid hormone; *SCr,* serum creatinine.

*Conversion to International System of Units: SCr in μmol/L = 88.4 × (SCr in mg/dL).

aid in assessing the degree of multiorgan involvement present as part of the uremic syndrome.

Identification of factors that could potentially aggravate progression of renal disease is crucial. Correction of reversible factors may help partially restore renal function toward baseline and preserve remaining function. Destabilizing variables might include the initiators of ARF superimposed on CRF (Table 22.4), as well as uncontrolled hypertension or excessive protein intake. Depending on how advanced the renal failure is, efforts to reduce proteinuria, correct dyslipidemia, and optimize glycemic control (in diabetics) may still prove helpful with respect to retarding progression to ESRD.

Nephrotic Syndrome

Nephrotic syndrome is the metabolic and clinical consequence of continued heavy proteinuria, usually greater than 3.5 g of protein per day. In addition to proteinuria, this syndrome is characterized by hypoalbuminemia, edema, hyperlipidemia, and hypercoagulability. A variety of glomerulonephropathies have been associated with nephrotic syndrome, including those caused by systemic, metabolic, and endocrine diseases; allergens; microorganisms; drugs; and toxins.[12,49]

Increased glomerular permeability to plasma protein leads to each of the clinical and metabolic derangements associated with nephrotic syndrome.[81] Hypoalbuminemia is the direct result of albumin loss in the urine, which accounts for 60 to 90% of urinary protein. Loss of larger molecular weight proteins, including immunoglobulins, is associated with abnormalities in immune response and increased susceptibility to serious infections. Enhanced hepatic synthesis of lipoproteins is thought to result from hypoalbuminemia and a reduction in colloid oncotic pressure, inducing a hyperlipidemic state that is suspected to increase risk of ischemic heart disease.[82] Edema is due to sodium retention by the kidney and a reduction in intravascular colloid oncotic pressure. Edema seen with nephrotic syndrome is marked by a distribution pattern that includes the face and periorbital region, particularly in the morning. Edema of the lower extremities can be seen as the day progresses. Numerous defects in clotting factors, the fibrinolytic system, and platelet function are responsible for the hypercoagulable state. Low levels of antithrombin III are thought to correlate with the clotting defects.

PSYCHOSOCIAL ASPECTS

Numerous studies have shown that the development of ESRD is often accompanied by significant losses in quality of life, functional status, and autonomy.[83,84] In turn, at least one study in this population has found that impairments in mental status, performance status, and quality of life are independently correlated with risk of mortality.[85] Many of the challenges to maintaining quality of life are rooted in medical causes, but they are compounded by constraints within the health care delivery system, the type of renal replacement therapy (RRT) administered, financial difficulties, and societal misunderstanding of renal disease. Several barriers, both practical and artificial, exist against employing ESRD patients. Although these are not insurmountable, fewer than 10% of ESRD patients below 60 years of age are able to maintain gainful employment.

THERAPEUTIC PLAN

Retarding Progression of Chronic Renal Disease

It is unlikely that the primary diseases leading to CRD (diabetes, hypertension, and glomerulonephritis) will be eradicated in the near future. In the meantime, a more reasonable clinical goal is to minimize the number of individuals progressing into ESRD, or to at least forestall this event by several years. The interrelationship that chronic renal disease shares with diabetes, hypertension, and hyperlipidemia is becoming increasingly recognized. Through recently developed clinical practice guidelines, groundwork for an integrated approach to management of these disease states has been laid. These guidelines represent a collaborative effort and consensus between the National Heart, Lung and Blood Institute (through JNC-VI),[86] the National Cholesterol Education Program (through NCEP II),[87] the National Kidney Foundation (NKF), and the American Diabetes Association (ADA);[88,89] excerpts pertaining to renal disease are summarized in Table 22.8.

Strategies for slowing renal disease progression are often divided into measures for diabetic versus nondiabetic individuals. In practice, however, these groupings differ primarily in the threshold for their implementation and in the amount of clinical evidence supporting their beneficial role. Obviously, measures targeting glycemic control pertain to the diabetic population.[48,49]

Recognizing Risk Factors of Chronic Renal Disease

Early recognition of nephropathy or of risk factors for CRD remains one of the greatest challenges to the timely institution of nephroprotective measures. Diabetics are the most obvious target population on which to focus preventive efforts and screening for early evidence of nephropathy. Current World Health Organization (WHO) and ADA recommendations are to screen yearly for microalbuminuria, beginning at the time of diagnosis in type II diabetics and within 5 years of onset in type I diabetics (or at puberty in juvenile-onset DM).[88] In diabetics who develop hypertension or elevations in serum creatinine, more frequent screening for microalbuminuria is advised (e.g., every 3 to 6 months).[90] Because other factors can transiently elevate urinary albumin excretion (UAE), positive screens should be confirmed within 3 to 6 months, and antiproteinuric treatment should be instituted only if two separate evaluations show evidence of microalbuminuria.

In contrast, most nondiabetics with hypertension do

Table 22.8 ▪ Proposed Strategies for Retarding Chronic Renal Disease Progression

Strategy for Intervention	Diabetic Individual	Nondiabetic Individual
Screening for microalbuminuria	Type 1: yearly starting at fifth year after onset Type 2: yearly from onset of diagnosis If hypertension develops: increase to every 3–6 months until detected and confirmed	NR
Screening for proteinuria	Yearly—may follow from above	Should be considered in presence of hypertension or elevated SCr
Antiproteinuric therapy (ACEI preferred; if intolerant, ARB is an acceptable alternative)	Type 1: all with mAU (even normotensives) Type 2: all with mAU and hypertension; assess and treat normotensives individually	If UAE >1 g/day in presence of hypertension, nephrotic syndrome, or hyperlipidemia Not yet routine for normotensives or in lesser degrees of proteinuria
Blood pressure goals and preferred antihypertensives (diabetics = JNC-VI group C; non-DM = variable group; non-DM with CRI identified = JNC-VI group C)	Lifestyle modifications; consider Na^+ restriction at early time If no microalbuminuria: ▪ Goal <130/85 (any agent*) ▪ ACEI† *suggested,* or CCB ▪ Diuretic, α-adrenergic antagonist If UAE 30 mg–1 g/day: ▪ Goal <130/85 ▪ ACEI† front-line (+ diuretic, CCB, others) If proteinuria ≥1 g/day: ▪ Goal <125/75 ▪ ACEI† front-line (+ CCB, diuretic, others)	Lifestyle modifications; Na^+ restriction in established CRD No known renal insufficiency/TOD: ▪ Goal <140/90 (any agent*) ▪ African American: consider more aggressive control Renal insufficiency established: If proteinuria <1 g/day: ▪ Goal <130/85 ▪ Any agent, but ACEI *suggested* in presence of CRI (+ diuretic, others) If proteinuria ≥1 g/day: ▪ Goal <125/75 ▪ ACEI† front-line (+ diuretic, CCB, others)
Dietary protein restriction	Institute at overt DN (UAE >0.3–0.5 g/day) ▪ Intake: 0.8 g/kg/day ▪ If GFR falling and nutrition permits, consider decrease to 0.6 g/kg/day	Institute at GFR <55 mL/min, if falling ▪ Intake: 0.8 g/kg/day ▪ At GFR <25 mL/min, consider further decrease to 0.6 g/kg/day
Hyperlipidemic control	Highly recommended at any stage, especially if microalbuminuria present (CVD risks) May help retard nephropathy	If CRI/proteinuria present, treat as highest risk category for CVD May help retard nephropathy
Glycemic control	Type 1: definitely beneficial before stage IV Type 2: presumably beneficial Benefit at or beyond stage IV DN: unclear	NR

Source: References 49, 86–90.

ACEI, angiotensin converting enzyme inhibitor; *ARB,* angiotensin receptor blocker; *CCB,* calcium channel blocker; *CRD,* chronic renal disease; *CRI,* chronic renal insufficiency; *CVD,* cardiovascular disease; *DN,* diabetic nephropathy; *GFR,* glomerular filtration rate; *mAU,* microalbuminuria (UAE >30–300 mg/day); *NR,* not routinely recommended; *SCr,* serum creatinine; *TOD,* target organ damage; *UAE,* urinary albumin excretion.

*Base selection on standard criteria (additional comorbidities, side effect profile, etc.).

†If intolerant to ACEI, preferred alternative is ARB; both are contraindicated in pregnant patients.

not appear to be routinely screened for evidence of nephropathy despite JNC recommendations, nor is the most cost-effective means of doing so clear at this time. Past National Institutes of Health (NIH) recommendations had been that women or men exhibiting a serum creatinine of greater than 1.5 or 2 mg/dL (132 or 177 µmol/L), respectively, should be referred to a renal specialty team as "pre-ESRD" candidates. More recently, a task force has condoned a definition of renal insufficiency that includes all renal transplant recipients and anyone manifesting a serum creatinine value of greater than 1.2 mg/dL (106 µmol/L) or greater than 1.4 mg/dL (124 µmol/L) in females and males, respectively.[91] Within the general medical community, however, the importance of early renal assessment and intervention may be underrecognized, comprising a significant barrier against timely initiation of nephroprotective measures.[92] In this regard, pharmacists can provide crucial input when making recommendations for diabetic care, antihypertensive therapies and goals, lipid management, and the prevention of drug-induced exacerbations of CRD.

Monitoring Progression of Chronic Renal Disease

When a patient is identified to have renal disease, regular periodic assessments should be performed to determine the rate of GFR decline and to confirm the efficacy of interventions intended to slow renal demise. Regular monitoring also facilitates the detection of sudden deteriorations in GFR due to reversible factors. Early detection and management of complications that begin to develop before ESRD (e.g., anemia, bone disease, malnutrition, hypertension, and heart disease) may help minimize morbidity and mortality. Maintaining an accurate gauge of renal status should help prompt the adjustment of dose or regimen for renally eliminated drugs, preventing toxicity or dangerous drug accumulation.

The reciprocal of SCr (1/SCr) has been stated to decline in a linear fashion and is sometimes used clinically to predict when the point of ESRD will be reached and dialysis will become necessary. However, the accuracy of this approach has been debated, because the relationship between SCr and GFR is subject to several nonrenal influences (lean body mass, liver disease, etc.). As GFR declines, even measured creatinine clearance values tend to overestimate GFR because of the increasing contribution of tubular secretion to overall creatinine excretion. Although no surrogate marker of renal function is failproof, GFR estimation and assessment of metabolic status are advocated at 3-month intervals, if not more often. Serial measures of proteinuria appear to be less precise than GFR in monitoring progression of renal disease, but are valuable in establishing the presence and gross extent of nephropathy and in assessing antiproteinuric interventions.

TREATMENT

Pharmacotherapy

Diuretics—Volume Management

Until patients become dialysis dependent, diuretic therapy is a mainstay of fluid and volume management. When used as single agents, thiazides lose much of their diuretic efficacy once GFR falls below 20 to 30 mL/min; however, their vasodilatory actions can still modestly contribute to blood pressure reduction. At this point, loop diuretics such as furosemide, bumetanide, and torsemide become drugs of choice in maintaining volume balance. These agents enter the urine through tubular secretion, producing dose-dependent diuretic responses that require a "threshold" urinary concentration to be present. In patients with CRD, drug entry into urine is impaired, and administration of doses 2 to 10 times higher than those in normal renal function may be required to produce a comparable diuretic response.

Clinical resistance to loop diuretics can occur and may result from impaired drug entry into the urine (due to diminished tubular secretion or renal perfusion), rebound sodium retention at distal tubular sites, altered protein binding, concurrent use of nonsteroidal anti-inflammatory drugs (NSAIDs), or other factors.[12,93,94] One of the first steps in overcoming diuretic resistance has traditionally been to escalate the dose until an effective diuresis is achieved, thereby establishing a "threshold" diuretic dose. In this circumstance, administration of a single larger dose of loop diuretic will more reliably elicit a diuresis than if the same total amount were divided into smaller intermittent doses that are below the threshold. The use of longer-acting agents (e.g., torsemide) or repeated doses of shorter-acting agents (furosemide, bumetanide) may further improve diuretic responsiveness by maintaining urinary drug levels and by reducing compensatory postdiuresis sodium retention. Repeat doses that are administered later in the day should be no smaller than the threshold effective dose. Although no loop diuretic is clearly superior, some differences exist between the agents. The bioavailability of torsemide and bumetanide is nearly complete, whereas that of oral furosemide averages only 50% (range 20 to 80%). Conversion from parenteral to oral furosemide dosing should account for this difference and generally requires a doubling of dose. In addition, severe gastrointestinal edema may reduce the bioavailability and efficacy of these agents, necessitating initial intravenous therapy, especially in the case of furosemide. In severe renal impairment, nonrenal clearance is more significant for bumetanide than furosemide, and the usual milligram equivalency ratio of bumetanide to furosemide is reduced from 1:40 mg to 1:20 mg. Furosemide is highly protein bound and as such becomes bound to urinary albumin, reducing active urinary levels. In patients with high urine protein content (e.g., nephrotic syndrome), dose escalation becomes necessary to overcome protein binding in the tubular fluid and to achieve desired diuretic responses. Although ototoxicity is possible with any of these agents, there may be a slightly greater incidence with furosemide, partly because of the higher doses and systemic accumulation noted in CRD. The risk of ototoxicity is generally greatest with high-dose intravenous bolus/infusion regimens and when additional ototoxins are used concurrently, such as aminoglycosides or cisplatin. Because of its even greater ototoxic potential, ethacrynic acid is generally reserved for patients with an established hypersensitivity to sulfa-based thiazides and other loop diuretics.[12]

The addition of metolazone (or another thiazide) to a loop diuretic can greatly enhance diuretic response, presumably by blunting distal tubular sodium reabsorption. Many clinicians prefer to institute combination therapy before escalating to extremely high doses of loop diuretic. These synergistic combinations occasionally result in an exaggerated diuretic response associated with large urinary sodium, potassium, and magnesium losses. Volume status, blood pressure, and electrolytes should therefore be closely monitored in robust responders. If thiazides and loop diuretics are used in combination, their administration should be timed to ensure that both drugs are simultaneously present in the tubule. When both agents are being given by the same route (oral or intravenous), simultaneous administration is appropriate. However, an oral agent (usually the thiazide or metolazone) should be given at least 30 to 60 minutes before an intravenous loop diuretic, to allow adequate time for its absorption. At present, chlorothiazide is the only thiazide diuretic available in the United States in an intravenous formulation.

Finally, if a patient fails to respond to escalation of a loop diuretic and to combination therapy, inpatient therapy with escalating IV bolus or continuous infusion loop diuretic may become necessary. Following administration of an effective loading bolus, continuous infusions of loop diuretic are thought to maintain urine drug concentrations and diuretic response more effectively than intermittent boluses.[93] The use of continuous loop diuretic infusions is also discussed in Chapter 21. In most instances of severe diuretic resistance, it is advisable to discontinue any agents capable of interfering with diuretic response, particularly NSAIDs (including selective cyclooxygenase-2 [COX-2] inhibitors).

Bed rest is beneficial in mobilizing interstitial fluid to the intravascular compartment. By expanding the central blood volume, renal perfusion improves and enhances delivery of sodium and diuretic to the tubule. For this reason, diuretics are best given immediately after arising from the daily sleep (or even before bedtime, if patients are able to withstand arising to urinate). Patients with edema or diminishing diuretic responsiveness should be placed on a salt-restricted diet to assist in reducing positive sodium balance or rebound sodium retention (2 g/day of sodium). On a practical basis, this means no added salt to the home-cooked diet, as well as restricting intake of processed foods, especially meals from fast food restaurants. Significant reductions in dietary sodium intake are best instituted gradually in CRD, because renal adaptation to abrupt changes in volume status is inefficient. As urinary volume diminishes, restriction of daily fluid intake becomes necessary to prevent volume overload. Fluid intake is generally allowed to match the daily urine output plus insensible losses (which average 500 mL/day under usual conditions).

Potassium-Lowering Agents

The acute management of life-threatening hyperkalemia is discussed in Chapter 9. Acute management does not differ significantly for CRD patients, with the exception that sodium bicarbonate may not be as efficacious in shifting K^+ intracellularly, when compared with its use in patients who have developed an acute acidosis.[12] If glucose and insulin are given, it is appropriate to monitor for delayed-onset hypoglycemia because of the prolonged duration of insulin action in CRD. For ESRD patients already receiving hemodialysis, initiation of a hemodialysis treatment to reduce serum potassium levels can be more readily performed than in patients without suitable vascular access already established.

Because CRD patients generally tolerate a mild degree of chronic hyperkalemia, goal serum potassium levels of 4.5 to 5.5 mEq/L (mmol/L) are usually accepted. Chronic hyperkalemia is managed through dietary potassium restriction to approximately 1 mEq/kg per day, as well as curtailing the use of medications that can interfere with potassium excretion (e.g., ACEIs, angiotensin receptor blockers, potassium-sparing diuretics, β-blockers, trimethoprim). The addition of a potassium-binding resin such as sodium polystyrene sulfonate (Kayexalate, SPS Suspension) may become necessary when semi-urgent lowering is needed or control cannot be maintained by dietary measures and the elimination of offending medications. When dosed orally, SPS Suspension is typically administered as a commercially available suspension in sorbitol, which serves not only as a vehicle but also as a cathartic to hasten resin removal. Maintenance doses usually range from 10 to 30 g/day (dosed by SPS content) in divided doses after meals or at bedtime. Constipation itself can interfere with gut potassium secretion and should therefore be prevented, while taking care to avoid bulk laxatives that contain a significant potassium content. For ESRD patients receiving hemodialysis, an additional management option is to modify the hemodialysis bath to promote greater potassium removal.

Acid-Base Management: Systemic Alkalinizers

Metabolic acidosis can be corrected by the administration of sodium bicarbonate or sodium citrate. The required amount of buffer varies among individual patients and whether additional forms of renal tubular acidosis (RTA) are present, but it is generally titrated to achieve serum bicarbonate levels near 20 mEq/L (mmol/L). Bicarbonate doses typically range from 20 to 40 mEq/day (0.5 to 2.0 mEq/kg per day); however, much higher doses may be needed when proximal (type II) RTA is present.[12] Sodium bicarbonate is available in oral tablet and powder forms; each 325 mg tablet provides 4 mEq of bicarbonate. After oral administration, the bicarbonate reacts with gastric hydrochloric acid, generating carbon dioxide, which must be eliminated through belching. For patients in whom the elimination of stomach gas is difficult or painful, the use of Shohl's solution (a combination of sodium citrate and citric acid) provides an alternative buffer source. The sodium citrate in this formulation combines with hydrochloric acid to form citric acid, which is then absorbed and metabolized to carbon dioxide and water, without the generation of stomach gas. Per milliliter, Shohl's solution contains 1 mEq of sodium and 1 mEq of basic buffer. The use of potassium citrate solutions in CRD patients should be avoided because of their potential to precipitate hyperkalemia. Citrate can also enhance the absorption of aluminum salts. Thus, for patients receiving both sodium citrate and aluminum-based antacids or phosphate binders, the administration of each should be separated by 2 to 3 hours in order to reduce the risk of chronic aluminum intoxication. In hemodialysis patients, the inclusion of bicarbonate in the dialysis bath provides an additional source of alkaline buffer.

Renal Osteodystrophy

The goals of therapy include maintaining serum phosphorus and calcium levels near normal, inimizing secondary elevations in PTH, and preventing or correcting relative calcitriol deficiency. Although these are only intermediate endpoints, it is hoped that control of these parameters will ultimately serve to minimize long-term abnormalities in bone turnover, structure, and mineralization. Figure 22.1 outlines an algorithm for the management of phosphorus, calcium, and PTH in progressive renal disease. In addition, correction of the chronic metabolic acidosis through measures discussed in the preceding section may help curtail bone demineralization.[12,51]

Early conservative management consists of dietary phosphorus restriction through reducing the intake of foods high in phosphorus such as meat, milk, legumes, beer, and colas. Because dietary protein sources tend to be rich in phosphate, institution of a low-protein diet also helps reduce phosphorus intake and may be sufficient to maintain serum phosphate within the normal range of 2.5 to 4.5 mg/dL (0.84 to 1.45 mmol/L).

As renal failure progresses and GFR falls below 30 mL/min, dietary restriction alone becomes inadequate to prevent hyperphosphatemia. The use of phosphate-binding gels that decrease dietary phosphorus absorption and promote removal of phosphate through the gut generally becomes necessary, as does acceptance of slightly higher serum phosphorus goals (4.5 to 6.0 mg/dL; 1.45 to 1.94 mmol/L). The divalent and trivalent cations Mg^{2+}, Ca^{2+}, and Al^{3+} can all work effectively as phosphate binders when given during or immediately preceding mealtime. Because systemic absorption of each of these cations occurs to some extent, calcium salts have emerged as preferred agents and often serve a dual purpose as a calcium supplement. Before the 1990s, aluminum salts were a mainstay of phosphate-binding regimens; however, accumulation syndromes, associated with encephalopathy, osteomalacia, myopathy, and microcytic anemia, were common. Aluminum-based binders are now reserved for short-term use in severely hyperphosphatemic patients (e.g., serum phosphate greater than 6.5 mg/dL [greater than 2.1 mmol/L]) or in hypercalcemic patients, in whom the initiation or escalation of calcium salts could present the danger of driving the calcium phosphate product beyond 70. Of the presently available calcium salts, calcium carbonate and calcium ace-

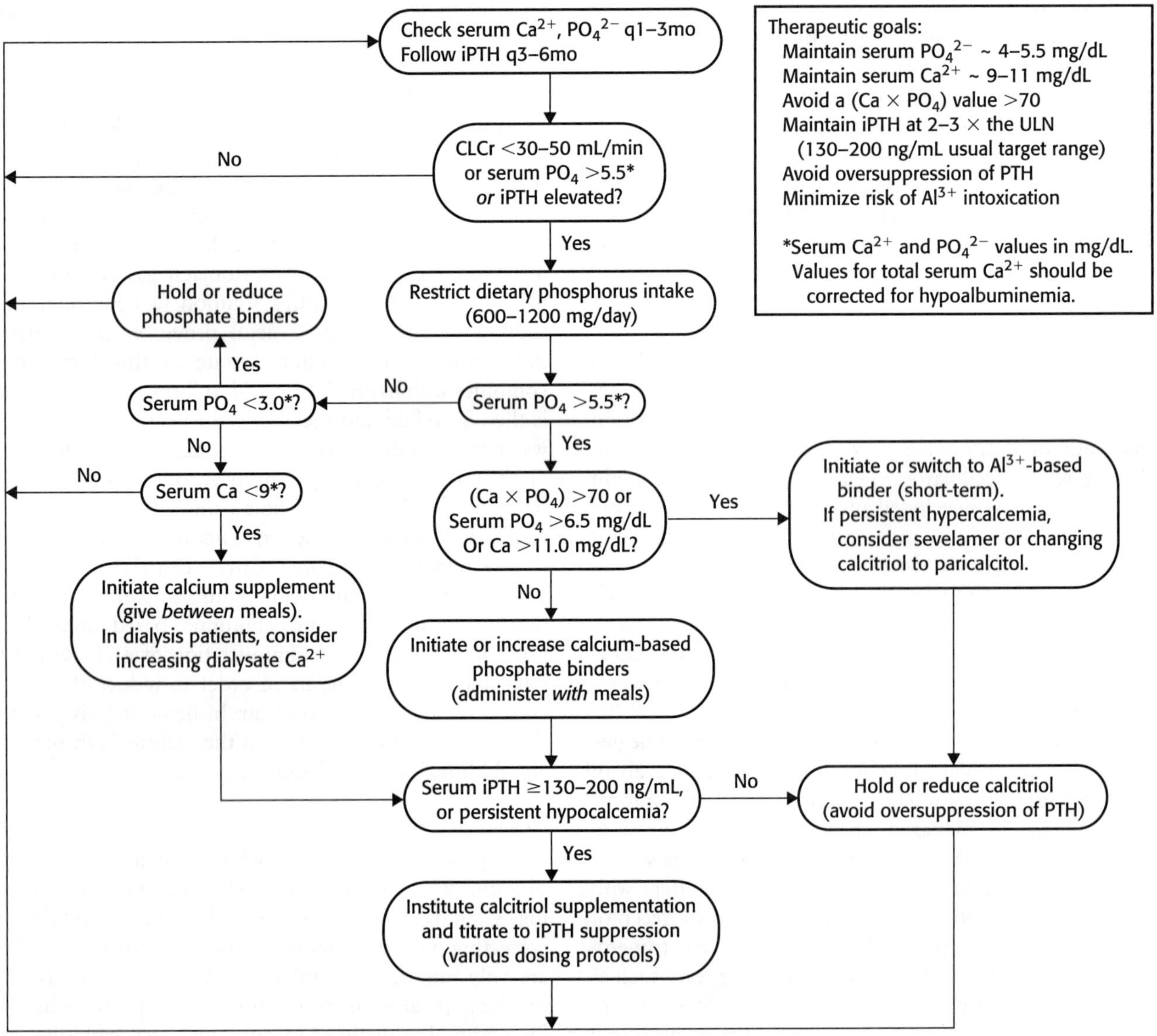

Figure 22.1. Algorithm for the management of renal osteodystrophy in CRD.

Table 22.9 • Commonly Used Dietary Phosphorus-Binding Agents

Agent, Trade Name, and Dosage Form	Elemental Mineral Content/Unit	Usual Dosing and Instructions
Calcium-based products		
Calcium carbonate (40% Ca)	Ca content:	Initial, then titrate: Elemental Ca^{2+} 500 mg–1 g with each meal plus 200–500 mg with high-PO_4 snacks
Tums 500 mg, 750 mg, 1000 mg	200 mg, 300 mg, 400 mg	Chewing encouraged if chewable product (and dentition intact)
Oscal-500	500 mg	
$CaCO_3$ (various) 1250 mg	500 mg	
Caltrate-600	600 mg	
$CaCO_3$ 1250 mg/5 mL	500 mg/5 mL	Sorbitol content may cause diarrhea
CalCarb HD 6.5 g packets	2400 mg/packet	Can be mixed into food
Calcium acetate (25% Ca)		
Phoslo 667 mg	167 mg	Initial: 2 tablets TID with meals. Large tablet–chew if possible
Phos-Ex 62.5 167, 125, 250 mg	62.5, 167, 125, and 250 mg	Tablets chewable and flavored
Calcium citrate (21% Ca)		
Citracal 950 mg, 2376 mg liquitab	200 mg; 500 mg	Not commonly used Separate from Al^{3+}-containing products by at least 2 hr
Aluminum-based products		*All products*
Aluminum hydroxide		Initial, then titrate: 300–900 mg $Al(OH)_3$ with meals and 300–400 mg with high-PO_4^{2-} snacks
Amphojel 600 mg tablets	Dosed by $Al(OH)_3$ content as labeled	Separate from citrate-containing products (Shohl's, Ca citrate)
Amphojel 320 mg/5 mL liquid		Reserved for temporary use in patients with serum PO_4^{2-} >6.5, ↑serum Ca^{2+} (>11.0), or ($Ca^{2+} \times PO_4^{2-}$) product >65–70
AlternaGEL 600 mg/5 mL liquid		
Alu-Cap 400 mg		Tend to be constipating
Alu-Tab 500 mg		Caution: may interfere with absorption of other medicines
Dialume 500 mg capsules		
Aluminum carbonate gel, basic		
Basaljel 608 mg tablets, capsules	500 mg $Al(OH)_3$ equivalent	
Basaljel liquid	400 mg $Al(OH)_3$/5 mL equivalent	
Sucralfate		Not indicated as phosphate binder, but may decrease serum PO_4^{2-} in use as antiulcer agent
Carafate 1 g tablet		Significant Al^{3+} absorption possible with chronic use
Carafate 1 g/10 mL suspension		
Aluminum and Calcium Free		
Sevelamer		Initial: three times daily with meals according to serum PO_4^{2-}: 6–7.5 mg/dL: 2 capsules/dose 7.5–9 mg/dL: 3 capsules/dose ≥9 mg/dL: 4 capsules/dose
Renagel 403 mg capsules		May cause bloating and diarrhea Use cautiously in conditions of impaired gastric motility Caution: may interfere with absorption of other medicines

tate are the most commonly used as phosphate binders in patients with CRD (Table 22.9). Both also provide calcium supplementation and systemic alkalinizing effects. Because the efficiency of phosphate binding depends on solubilization of the calcium salt, the use of products not meeting United States Pharmacopeia (USP) dissolution standards (such as those marketed as dietary supplements) may compromise therapeutic efficacy. Concomitant therapy with agents that markedly suppress gastric acid secretion, such as H_2-antagonists[95] and proton pump inhibitors,[96] may also interfere with calcium solubilization and therefore phosphate control; however, the clinical significance of this has been questioned.[96] The selection of dietary phosphorus binding agents is discussed more fully in Chapter 23. Patients should be counseled about the importance of taking these agents immediately before or with meals and snacks and about separating their administration from other drugs for which absorption could be impaired by simultaneous ingestion. Some patients learn to successfully "titrate" their phosphate-binder dose according to dietary variations in phosphate intake, but others require more stringent dosing instructions. The initiation of dialytic therapies affords the additional removal of about 500 mg (16 mmol) phosphate per hemodialysis session and helps compensate for the liberalization of protein intake usually implemented after beginning dialysis.

Sevelamer, an oral phosphorus-binding gel that is devoid of calcium, aluminum, and magnesium, has recently become available. It is intended for use in situations where hypercalcemia precludes or limits the use of calcium-based phosphate binders. Published clinical experience is thus far limited to use in hemodialysis patients, and data concerning chronic use in the pre-ESRD population are not yet available.[97,98] Sevelamer also modestly lowers lipid levels, but it has the significant potential to interfere with the absorption of other drugs.

In the past, vitamin D therapy was reserved for individuals in whom serum calcium and PTH could not be normalized with the aforementioned measures, and barring contraindications, it became needed by most patients with advanced CRD. Current trends are toward initiating therapy at earlier stages of renal disease, although the optimal time at which to begin vitamin D (calcitriol) therapy is still under debate.[55] Calcitriol (1,25-dihydroxyvitamin D_3) offers some advantages over other forms of vitamin D, such as ergocalciferol (vitamin D_2) and cholecalciferol (vitamin D_3). Not only is calcitriol the most potent and specific congener that becomes deficient in renal disease, but it directly suppresses PTH suppression and has a shorter onset and duration of action than the others. The potential for vitamin D intoxication is a major hazard associated with pharmacologic doses of vitamins D_2 and D_3, and it can induce sustained hypercalcemia and hyperphosphatemia that may require weeks to resolve. In contrast, calcitriol-associated hypervitaminosis reverses much more readily after cessation of therapy. Calcitriol is usually withheld, interrupted, or reduced if hypercalcemia or hyperphosphatemia develops or if there is evidence that PTH secretion has become overly suppressed (less than two to three times the upper limit of normal), because overcorrection of hyperparathyroidism in CRD is thought to lead to low-turnover forms of osteodystrophy. Calcitriol is usually given orally to the pre-ESRD and peritoneal dialysis population, but it is generally administered intravenously to patients undergoing hemodialysis. When compared with daily dosing, larger intermittent "pulse" doses of calcitriol (e.g., three times weekly) may produce superior PTH suppression with less risk of inducing hypercalcemia or hyperphosphatemia.[99] The rationale for selection between dosing schedules is discussed in greater detail in Chapter 23. A new vitamin D analog, paricalcitol, has recently been approved and is being marketed for patients in whom hypercalcemia limits the utility of calcitriol. At this time, clinical experience with paricalcitol has been limited to an intravenous dosage form used in hemodialysis populations.[100,101] Clinical trials directly comparing paricalcitol to calcitriol are needed to help define the role of paricalcitol in the general CRD population.

Anemia of Chronic Renal Disease: Erythropoietin, Iron, and Other Supplements

Before the introduction of recombinant human erythropoietin (epoetin alfa [EPO]) in the late 1980s, anabolic steroids and red cell transfusions were the primary modalities by which anemia was treated in the CRD population. Anabolic steroids (e.g., Deca-Durabolin) were only marginally effective, RBC transfusions were (and are still) costly, and each of these approaches was associated with significant safety concerns. The availability of EPO revolutionized anemia management in the ESRD population, but despite more than a decade of clinical use, opinions are still evolving regarding the most appropriate manner of EPO use, optimal therapeutic hemoglobin (or hematocrit) goals, and their associated risk-benefit ratios. Two recombinant DNA human EPO products, Epogen and Procrit, are available. Although considered to be similar in pharmacologic effect and interchangeable by most practitioners, only Epogen carries a Food and Drug Administration (FDA) indication for use in hemodialysis patients. A third human erythropoietin product, produced by a novel gene-activated technology, is also under development for use and is anticipated to be clinically available by 2001.

In 1997, the Dialysis Outcomes Quality Initiative (DOQI) workgroup, a multidisciplinary expert task force, reviewed the dearth of published clinical data examining the relationship between hematocrit (hemoglobin) level and physiologic outcomes or quality of life in the CRD population. From these efforts, new clinical practice guidelines were formulated that encourage an earlier and more aggressive approach to anemia management.[102] Their recommendations, in part, included the following: (1) a target hematocrit (hemoglobin) range for EPO therapy of 33 to 36% (11 to 12 g/dL); (2) initiation of anemia workup and therapy once hematocrit (hemoglobin) falls below 33% (11 g/dL) in premenopausal females or below 37% (12 g/dL) in males and postmenopausal females; (3) inclusion of the pre-ESRD population meeting these criteria as candidates for EPO therapy (in addition to the ESRD and dialysis populations); and (4) the use of hemoglobin (in lieu of hematocrit) as a more reliable and reproducible laboratory index of RBC mass. Several trials have demonstrated that elevation of hematocrit (hemoglobin) to even higher ranges (36 to 42% [12 to 14 g/dL]) may further benefit cardiopulmonary status, quality of life, and symptoms.[56–59,103,104] However, because a small number of studies have suggested that the use of aggressive EPO or iron therapy to achieve normal hematocrit values may be associated with other risks, higher hematocrit target ranges have not yet been adopted as a routine therapeutic goal.[105,106] Data specific to anemia management in the pre-ESRD population are limited, hence whether the therapeutic approach for this subgroup should distinctly differ from that for ESRD patients is the subject of ongoing exploration.[103,107] In support of attaining goal hematocrits and optimizing EPO response, additional therapeutic goals should include (1) the maintenance of adequate iron, folate, and vitamin B_{12} stores; (2) the correction of any coexisting nonrenal forms of anemia; and (3) consideration of EPO administration route as a determinant of dosing requirements; in this sense, the subcutaneous route often provides a dose-sparing effect relative to intravenous administration of EPO.[102,108]

EPO can be administered either subcutaneously (SQ) or intravenously (IV). Predialysis and peritoneal dialysis patients typically receive EPO SQ divided into 1 or 2 doses per week, whereas most hemodialysis patient are given EPO by the intravenous route, in a schedule that coincides with their hemodialysis sessions (i.e., three times weekly). The DOQI-recommended initial adult EPO dosing range in terms of weekly total is 80 to 120 U/kg per week (SQ) divided into 2 or 3 doses or 120 to 180 U/kg per week (IV) divided into 3 doses. Younger pediatric patients (less than 5 years) may require 2 to 3 times these doses. The time to reach new steady-state hematocrit values after an EPO dose adjustment ranges from 1 to 4 months and is influenced not only by the EPO dose and iron stores, but also by the turnover rate of the existing RBC mass. At the aforementioned doses, the average rate at which hematocrit rises in usual responders is 1% per week (range 0.5 to 1.5%). A variety of dosing strategies are acceptable; however, most algorithms make EPO dose adjustments as a fractional increment of the previous EPO dose, based on the actual hematocrit value along with the rate of hematocrit rise (Fig. 22.2). Hematocrit monitoring is recommended at 1- to 2-week intervals, accompanied by EPO dosage titration at approximately 2- to 4-week intervals until a stable

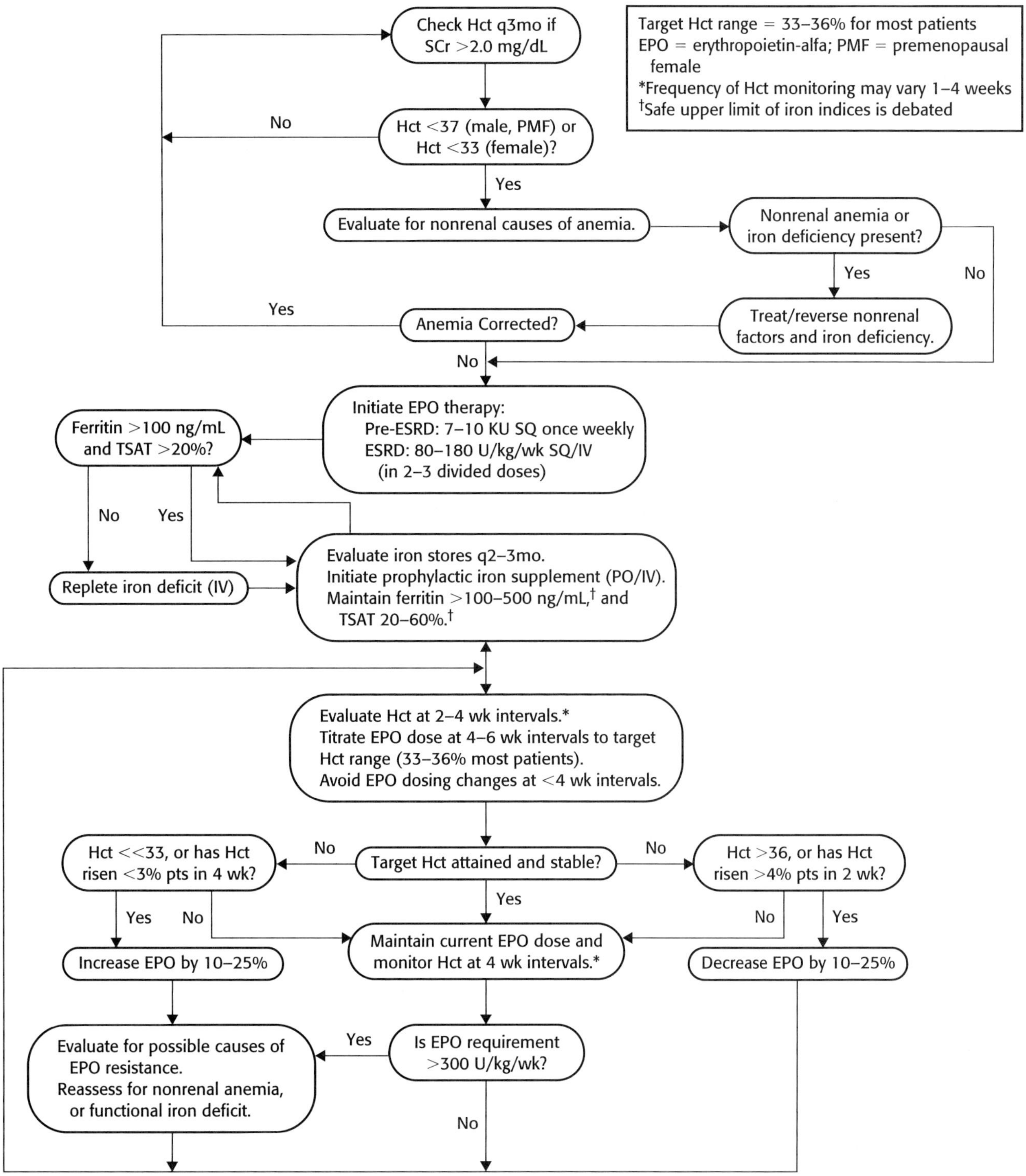

Figure 22.2. Algorithm for the management of anemia in CRD.

hematocrit and EPO dose have been achieved. For patients exhibiting an exaggerated or unusually rapid hematocrit rise (e.g., greater than 4% in a 2-week period or 8% in a 4-week period), EPO dosage reduction is suggested, whereas suboptimal responders may benefit from early EPO dosage increases to minimize the time to reach target hematocrit values (ideally within 2 to 4 months).[102] Following stabilization of response, less frequent monitoring of hematocrit (every 2 to 4 weeks) and EPO dose adjustments (every 4 weeks) generally suffice and tend to be more cost-efficient in centers managing large numbers of patients. Reticulocyte response is not routinely monitored in EPO recipients demonstrating an adequate response. In the United States, reimbursement constraints have influenced EPO dosing practices–an unfortunate but nonetheless germane factor.[109]

EPO therapy is generally well tolerated. Hypertension occurs or is exacerbated in approximately 25% of patients receiving EPO for reasons that may relate to expansion of blood volume, elevation of endothelin levels, or other poorly understood mechanisms. Regular blood pressure monitoring and measures to adequately control hypertension are therefore standards of care in EPO recipients. Although rare, seizures have occurred and have been postulated to result from overly rapid rises in hematocrit. For these reasons, it is considered prudent to reduce EPO dose when hematocrit increases by more than 4% in a 2-week period (or 8% in 1 month). In dialysis patients, hematocrit elevations pursuant to EPO therapy have been suspected to increase thrombosis of vascular access devices, reduce dialytic efficiency, and promote hyperkalemia. However, these complications have not proven clearly attributable to EPO therapy, are readily managed, and would not outweigh the benefits of EPO.[102] For patients receiving EPO subcutaneously, use of the benzyl-preserved multidose product may help reduce injection site stinging and increase patient acceptance.[102]

Several factors can blunt or inhibit response to EPO therapy (Table 22.10), especially iron deficiency. Adequate iron stores should be established before initiating therapy, and most patients require ongoing iron supplementation during EPO therapy. Although neither of the following indices of iron status is entirely physiologically accurate, DOQI guidelines suggest maintaining transferrin saturation (TSAT) at 20% or greater and ferritin concentrations of at least 100 ng/mL (μg/L). Even at values above these ranges, a functional iron deficiency may be manifested by poor EPO response, which improves after additional iron supplementation. Unfortunately, aggressive iron supplementation may also present unforeseen risks, and the safe upper limit for iron therapy is under debate. At TSAT values greater than 50% or ferritin greater than 500 to 800 ng/mL (μg/L), many experts advise reduction or interruption of iron supplementation; however, opinions vary widely on this matter.[102,110] To predialysis and peritoneal dialysis patients, iron supplementation is usually given orally in doses of 150 to 200 mg of elemental iron daily (i.e., oral ferrous sulfate, 300 mg three times daily). Iron is more efficiently absorbed on an empty stomach, and phosphate-binding agents (given at mealtime) tend to further reduce iron absorption. Therefore, oral iron would optimally be taken between meals–a schedule that most patients find difficult to comply with on a chronic basis, due to gastrointestinal intolerance or impracticality. Because oral iron supplementation is ineffective in maintaining adequate iron stores for a large fraction of patients, parenteral iron supplementation has become increasingly popular, especially for the hemodialysis population, in whom venous access is convenient and chronic blood loss escalates iron deficits.[102,111] The intraperitoneal route of iron and EPO administration has also been explored for use in the peritoneal dialysis population. Folic acid deficiency can result from elevated rates of erythropoiesis or from its removal by hemodialysis, necessitating daily supplementation of folate (0.8 to 1 mg/day) in order to optimize EPO response. Specialized aspects of managing anemia in the dialysis population are discussed in Chapter 23.

Table 22.10 ▪ Potential Causes of Poor Response to Erythropoietin Therapy for Anemia of Chronic Renal Disease

Iron deficiency (relative or absolute)
Folate or vitamin B_{12} deficiency
Malnutrition
Inflammatory, infectious, or malignant process
Unrecognized hemoglobinopathy (e.g., thalassemias)
Severe osteitis fibrosa
Aluminum intoxication or elevated Al^{3+} stores
Severe uremia or inadequate dialysis
Unrecognized blood loss or hemolysis (nondialysis related)
Excessive known blood loss (dialysis related, vascular surgery)
Pharmacokinetic variability–consider switch of administration route (SQ ↔ IV)
Concurrent medications: marrow-suppressive agents; angiotensin converting enzyme inhibitors or possibly angiotensin receptor blockers

Cardiovascular Disease: Antihypertensives

Goals of Therapy

According to JNC-VI criteria, the presence of renal disease signifies target organ damage and places an individual in the highest risk group for cardiovascular and renal complications of hypertension (group C). The JNC guidelines do not clearly define nephropathy, but do recommend evaluations of SLR and urinalysis as a routine part of the initial hypertensive workup. Proteinuria greater than 1 g/day implies significant renal disease, and should be detectable by UA, whereas more sensitive tests for CrCl or microalbuminuria are suggested as optimal. From the Hypertension Detection and Follow-up Program (HDFP) conducted in the 1980s, an SCr value greater than 1.7 mg/dL (greater than 150 μmol) had been identified as a predictor of increased risk for cardiovascular mortality.[112] More recently, an NIH consensus statement has advocated that all renal transplant recipients be considered renally insufficient, as well as anyone manifesting a serum creatinine value greater than 1.2 mg/dL (106 μmol/L) in females or greater than 1.4 mg/dL (124 μmol/L) in males.[91] Toward reducing the incidence of hypertensive nephropathy, JNC-VI adopted target blood pressure goals below the usual normotensive range (less than 140/90) as potentially beneficial in populations at risk of developing ESRD. If early renal disease or renal insufficiency is present, an "optimal" blood pressure is considered to be 130/80 or less. Drug therapy is recommended when blood pressure persists above 135/85, despite standard dietary and lifestyle measures (discussed in Chapter 39). Table 22.8 summarizes additional blood pressure goals for the major CRD subsets, as defined by diabetic and proteinuric status.[60,66,86,89]

In the pre-ESRD population, some question remains regarding which antihypertensives are the most likely to maximize antiproteinuric and nephroprotective benefits (refer also to earlier section on progression of CRD). As in the general population, selection of an antihypertensive regimen requires consideration of other comorbidities, such as reactive airway disease, coronary artery disease, cardiac conduction deficits, prostatic hypertrophy, and other conditions. At present, ACEIs are favored as first-line antihypertensives in the setting of CRD. This recommendation is primarily based on the tendency of ACEIs to reduce proteinuria, and presumably intraglomerular pressure, to a greater extent than other agents exerting equivalent levels of blood pressure control. Despite inconsistencies noted in earlier trials, the preponderance of available data supports the efficacy and utility of ACEIs as renoprotective agents in diabetic and nondiabetic forms of renal disease.[17,25,29–32] Thus in the JNC-VI guidelines, front-line inclusion of an ACEI is recommended in the presence of diabetes, proteinuria, or established nephropathy. For ACEI-intolerant individuals, nondihydropyridine CCBs or ARBs are perceived as useful, and potentially advantageous as renoprotectants, relative to other antihypertensive classes.[36,113,114] Because hypertension in CRD is usually volume sensitive, salt restriction and diuretics are also included as a mainstay of blood pressure control. Unfortunately, regardless of how well blood pressure is controlled, approximately 10 to 20% of patients experience relentless deterioration in renal function. Achieving control of blood pressure has been especially challenging in the African American population, for reasons that are not entirely elucidated. Moreover, in this population suboptimal hypertensive control appears to be a key factor allowing progression to ESRD.[115]

In diabetics, the presence of microalbuminuria (greater than 30 to 300 mg/24 hr) portends a high risk for progression to overt nephropathy (proteinuria greater than 300 to 500 mg/24 hr). At present, blood pressure goals for diabetics exhibiting albuminuria of less than 1 g/day are not distinctly different from those of nondiabetics; however, this is an area of controversy and research. For normotensive type I diabetics with microalbuminuria, institution of ACEI therapy is recommended as an antiproteinuric measure. In these patients, therapy has generally been titrated to minimize UAE rates *as tolerated*, rather than targeting systemic blood pressure reductions. In normotensive type II diabetics, the role of antiproteinuric ACEI therapy is not clearly defined; however, consideration of these measures is suggested in the face of worsening proteinuria or renal dysfunction.[89,90]

For individuals who have entered ESRD and are dialysis dependent, blood pressure goals do not differ significantly from the general population (i.e., <140/90).[60] If clinically achievable and tolerated, lower blood pressure goals may be appropriate in patients with additional nonrenal target organ damage. Blood pressure tends to parallel volume status, rising and peaking before intermittent hemodialysis treatments and then falling during and shortly after sessions; thus, the optimal time point at which to assess blood pressure in hemodialysis patients is under debate. In addition, maintaining predialysis pressures greater than 140/90 may be necessary to avoid hypotensive episodes from fluid removal during hemodialysis. The management of hypertension in the ESRD dialysis population is discussed fully in Chapter 23.

Specific Antihypertensive Classes

Although thiazide diuretics lose their saluretic efficacy at CrCl below 25 to 30 mL/min, they possess vasodilatory actions that contribute to antihypertensive activity more significantly than for loop diuretics. Diuretic therapy (see preceding section) is clearly indicated when volume excess or fluid retention is a component of hypertension, as is presumably true in most CRD patients. Concern exists that when used alone, diuretics may stimulate the renin-angiotensin system, exacerbating intraglomerular hypertension. Thus in CRD, diuretics are usually combined with agents that offset renin-angiotensin aldosterone (RAA) axis stimulation, such as ACEIs or β-adrenergic blockers. Because of the tendency toward hyperkalemia in CRD, potassium-sparing agents and combination products should be avoided or used with extreme caution, especially if combined with ACEIs, ARBs, or β-blocking agents. In addition, excessive diuresis may induce intravascular volume depletion, which can precipitate ARF in those with decreased renal reserve or receiving ACEIs, ARBs, NSAIDs, or nephrotoxins such as cyclosporine, tacrolimus, aminoglycosides, and others (see Chapter 21). Once a patient becomes dialysis dependent, diuretics are usually supplanted by the dialytic therapy as the mainstay of volume and blood pressure control. A small fraction of dialysis-dependent individuals maintain sufficient urine output to assist in managing blood pressure and volume status.

Angiotensin Converting Enzyme Inhibitors and Angiotensin Receptor Blocking Agents

ACEIs have emerged as front-line antihypertensives in CRD, in part because of their presumed nephroprotective benefits. This class seems a logical choice because elevated systemic or intrarenal RAA activity is thought to contribute

Table 22.11 ▪ Initial Dosage Recommendations of Angiotensin-Converting Enzyme Inhibitors in Renal Insufficiency

Drug	C_{cr} (30–60 mL/min)	C_{cr} (10–30 mL/min)	C_{cr} (<10 mL/min)
Captopril	12.5 mg twice daily	6.25–12.5 mg twice daily	6.25–12.5 mg once daily
Benazepril	5–10 mg once daily	5 mg once daily	?
Enalapril	5 mg once daily	2.5 mg once daily	1.25 mg once daily
Fosinopril	10 mg once daily	10 mg once daily	10 mg once daily
Lisinopril	10 mg once daily	5 mg once daily	2.5 mg once daily
Quinapril	5 mg once daily	2.5 mg once daily	?
Ramipril	1.25–2.5 mg once daily	1.25 mg once daily	?

Source: Carter BL. Dosing of antihypertensive medications in patients with renal insufficiency. J Clin Pharmacol 35:81–6, 1995; Hoelscher DD, Weir MR, Bakris GL. Hypertension in diabetic patients: an update of interventional studies to preserve renal function. J Clin Pharmacol 35:73–80, 1995; and Olin B. Cardiovascular agents. In: Drug Facts and Comparisons. St. Louis, MO: Facts and Comparisons, Inc., 1995: 135d–166.

C_{cr}, creatinine clearance.

to hypertension in most cases of CRD. In combination with diuretics, ACEIs blunt diuretic-induced RAA activation and act synergistically to control volume status. As in the non-CRD population, ACEIs as single agents in African American CRD patients may not be as effective as CCBs, but they are still a desired component of the antihypertensive regimen because of their nephroprotective benefit. When used for essential hypertension, ACEIs do not markedly reduce RBF or GFR. However, in situations where GFR and renal perfusion pressure are dependent on RAA activation and efferent arteriolar vasoconstriction, ACEIs can induce a mild to significant fall in GFR, owing to their preferential dilation of efferent arterioles. Clinical circumstances presenting this likelihood include CRD with intrarenal vascular disease, nephrosclerosis, renovascular hypertension (i.e., bilateral or unilateral renal artery stenosis), intravascular volume depletion, and CHF. Patients with RAA-driven renovascular hypertension may have exaggerated hypotensive responses to ACEI initiation. Close monitoring of clinical status, serum creatinine, and potassium in the first week after ACEI initiation is suggested in the aforementioned populations. Sodium and volume status may not restabilize for 2 to 4 weeks after ACEI initiation or dose escalation, and eventual volume depletion may necessitate a reduction in diuretic dose or ACEI. In the setting of CHF, short-acting ACEIs (e.g., captopril) have been characterized as less likely than longer-acting agents (e.g., enalapril) to reduce GFR after initiation of therapy.[116] However, cautious titration using low initial doses of longer-acting agents may be equally as safe.[117] Given their lower relative potency and available dosage strengths, captopril and enalapril may allow more precise titration at the lowest end of the ACEI dosing range. Mild elevations in SCr of 1 mg/dL or less need not preclude ACEI continuation and may be offset by chronic renoprotective or cardiovascular benefits, as discussed in earlier sections.

With the exception of fosinopril, all of the presently available ACEIs are renally eliminated or have active metabolites that are renally eliminated; fosinopril, moexipril, ramipril, trandolapril, and quinapril undergo fecal elimination, which may partially compensate for situations of reduced renal clearance. Dosage modification and cautious titration are therefore required in renal impairment; Table 22.11 provides initial ACEI dosage suggestions in renal insufficiency. Fosinopril, quinapril, and possibly benazepril do not appear to be removed significantly by hemodialysis. Of these three, fosinopril may afford the most straightforward dosage titration in hemodialysis-dependent individuals.[118] In azotemic patients, careful monitoring of serum potassium is necessary to prevent life-threatening hyperkalemia associated with ACEIs. Hyperkalemic tendencies are increased by concurrent use of potassium-sparing diuretics, NSAIDs, trimethoprim, cyclosporine, tacrolimus, β-blockers, and ARBs.

In the CRD population, ARBs are thought to have similar antihypertensive efficacy as ACEIs. In contrast to ACEIs, the ARBs do not inhibit the breakdown of bradykinin, nor do they reduce angiotensin II type-2 receptor-mediated activity. ARBs may also provide blockade against the receptor effects of angiotensin II formed through non-ACE mediated pathways. At this time, the significance of these two class differences in relation to the treatment of hypertension and prevention of CRD is not clear. Because ACEI-mediated reductions in efferent arteriolar tone are believed to be partially kinin dependent, ARBs have been theorized to alter intraglomerular hemodynamics less profoundly than ACEIs, a potential advantage for populations in whom short-term reductions of GFR are not desirable (e.g., severe CHF).[119] On the other hand, in the absence of enhanced kinin activity, the long-term renal effects of ARBs should not be assumed to replicate those of ACEIs, despite the fact that they have demonstrated comparable antiproteinuric effects. At present, ARBs are generally accepted as reasonable substitutes in patients intolerant of ACEIs (e.g., due to cough or angioedema). Combination therapy with ACEI and ARB has been reported as advantageous in certain animal models of hypertension and CHF, but clinical experience is too limited to surmise what the role of this approach should be in the CRD population.[120] Compared with ACEIs, the ARBs are thought to have similar or slightly less potential to induce short-term elevations in serum creatinine and promote hyperkalemia.

Of the clinically available ARBs, losartan, irbesartan, telmisartan, and valsartan are eliminated primarily by hepatic mechanisms, but experience in severe renal insufficiency is limited. Losartan possesses a potent active metabolite that undergoes significant renal elimination, and both moieties appear to accumulate at creatinine clearances below 30 mL/min. Eprosartan and candesartan possess dual hepatic and renal elimination pathways, each of which partially compensates for impairment of the other. In the presence of significant renal (CrCl less than 30 mL/min) or hepatic dysfunction, systemic exposure to both of these agents exceeds that observed in normal subjects. Whereas routine dosage adjustment for renal dysfunction has not yet been recommended for eprosartan, initial maintenance doses of candesartan should be reduced by approximately one-third in the elderly and by one-half in those with severe renal insufficiency. Hemodialysis does not appear to appreciably alter the kinetics or dosage requirement of most of the ARBs except for eprosartan, for which removal has been reported as variable, but occasionally significant.[121]

Calcium Channel Blockers

Calcium channel antagonists are generally useful in the treatment of hypertension associated with CRD and are believed to maintain their efficacy in volume-expanded states, which prevail in CRD. CCBs exert vasodilatory actions on both afferent and efferent renal arterioles, resulting in decreased intraglomerular pressure but variable effects on GFR. The dihydropyridine CCBs are believed to dilate afferent arterioles significantly, raising concern that glomerular blood flow and glomerular hyperfiltration could be accentuated rather than reduced. Data from animal and clinical studies are in conflict regarding the nephroprotective benefits of dihydropyridine CCBs.[36] In renal transplant recipients, for example, such vasodilatory effects may be advantageous in offsetting cyclosporine-induced vasospasm and its associated nephrotoxicity. Of the entire CCB class, the nondihydropyridine CCBs, diltiazem and verapamil, have most consistently demonstrated antiproteinuric and nephroprotective efficacy beyond that attributable to systemic blood pressure control.[34–36] These benefits are postulated to result from nonhemodynamic mechanisms and are thought to be additive when combined with ACEIs. The negative inotropic and chronotropic effects of diltiazem and verapamil should be considered before their use in a given patient. Such actions may be advantageous in patients with angina or coronary artery disease, but they could be deleterious to those with systolic dysfunction, CHF, or cardiac conduction defects. Diltiazem and verapamil are relatively potent inhibitors of the cytochrome P450 3A4 drug metabolic pathway and can therefore result in clinically significant drug interactions; elevation of cyclosporine and tacrolimus blood levels is one example pertinent to the RTR population.

After oral administration, most CCBs undergo extensive hepatic first-pass metabolism. Some metabolites, such as norverapamil, are mildly active and renal impairment may reduce their elimination. Therefore, although initial dosage adjustment for renal failure may not be necessary for the CCBs, the possibility of long-term metabolite accumulation and slow titration of maintenance doses should be considered. Advanced renal failure can also alter the hepatic metabolism of several CCBs; non-renal clearance is generally reduced for verapamil, nicardipine, and nimodipine, whereas increased clearance has been noted for nifedipine.[122]

β-Adrenergic Blocking Agents

β-Blockers lower blood pressure primarily by reducing cardiac output. They also inhibit renin release and thus may be especially useful in the setting of renovascular hypertension or renal failure or in combination with renin-activating agents (such as diuretics). Although β-blockers reduce renal blood flow, renal autoregulatory mechanisms generally prevent clinically significant reductions in GFR from occurring.[12] β-Blocking agents may be appropriate as first- or second-line antihypertensives in CRD patients with ischemic heart disease (although in the CRD population, nondihydropyridine CCBs could be a rational alternative). The nonselective β-blockers are suspected to promote hyperkalemia by inhibiting β_2-mediated K^+ translocation across cell membranes, which traps K^+ extracellularly; reduced renin secretion may compound the hyperkalemic tendency. In practice, β-blocker–associated elevations in serum K^+ are usually observed only when other risk factors for hyperkalemia are also present. Acebutolol and pindolol are agents with partial agonist activity and are thought to suppress renin release, myocardial workload, and K^+ translocation to a lesser extent than other agents of this class. Labetolol and carvedilol combine α-blockade with nonselective β-blocking effects, do not directly produce significant alterations in GFR, and are thought to be tolerated comparably between the CRD and non-CRD population.

The more highly lipophilic β-blockers are extensively metabolized by the liver to inactive metabolites and are not thought to require dosage modifications in renal dysfunction (propranolol, metoprolol, labetalol, pindolol, and timolol). In contrast, the less lipophilic agents are excreted primarily by the kidneys and may require dosage adjustment when creatinine clearance falls below 50 mL/min (atenolol, acebutolol, nadolol, betaxolol, bisoprolol, and carteolol). Although carvedilol is almost completely metabolized, elevated plasma AUCs of the α-blocking R-enantiomer have been noted in the presence of moderate to severe renal impairment.[123] Carvedilol dosage reduction for renal dysfunction is not routinely recommended, but conservative titration of carvedilol dose may be prudent in those with advanced CRD.

Other Adrenergic Blocking Agents

The centrally acting α_2-adrenergic agonists (methyldopa, clonidine, guanabenz, and guanfacine) are useful in reducing blood pressure in patients with chronic renal failure. Because methyldopa and its active metabolite accumulate with decreased renal function, dosing adjustments and cautious titration are necessary. At creatinine clearances below 50 mL/min, reduction of clonidine dosage should also be considered, along with extended observation for symptoms of prolonged accumulation (excessive hypotension, bradycardia, somnolence, etc.). Neither guanabenz nor guanfacine is thought to require routine dosage adjustment in renal insufficiency, despite the observation that moderate accumulation of guanfacine may occur.[12] These agents tend to produce sedation and xerostomia (dry mouth), making adherence to fluid restrictions difficult for some patients.

The α_1-adrenergic blockers (prazosin, terazosin, doxazosin) reduce blood pressure by producing arterial and venous vasodilation. They can be useful adjunctive or second-line agents in patients with renal failure, particularly in the presence of other conditions that could benefit from α_1-blockade, such as benign prostatic hypertrophy or hyperlipidemia. These agents do not generally require dosage reduction in the presence of renal dysfunction.

Other Antihypertensives

The direct-acting vasodilators, hydralazine and minoxidil, decrease peripheral vascular resistance primarily in arterial but also in venous beds. Blood pressure reduction is usually accompanied by compensatory activation of the sympathetic nervous system and renin release, leading to reflex tachycardia, increased cardiac output, and fluid retention. Because of these secondary effects, hydralazine and minoxidil are generally used in combination with agents that counteract fluid retention (e.g., diuretics) and tachycardia (e.g., β-blockers, which also blunt renin release). The long-term influence of these agents on progression of renal disease is controversial; in fact, some data suggest that they may actually exacerbate glomerular hyperfiltration.[12,124] Although both of these agents are extensively metabolized, minoxidil disposition may be prolonged in renal insufficiency. Despite its rapid and powerful onset, hypotensive effects may not plateau for an additional 5 to 10 days, necessitating cautious minoxidil titration. As discussed in Chapter 6, hydralazine demonstrates polymorphic differences in metabolism according to acetylator phenotypes. Slow acetylators may be predisposed to drug accumulation in CRD and thus require dosage titration and close monitoring.

Dyslipidemia: Lipid-lowering Agents

For the classification, initiation of treatment, and target cholesterol levels, NCEP II guidelines are generally followed in the CRD population, with the following caveats: (1) it has been suggested that the CRD population should be considered part of the highest risk group; (2) drug therapy is usually needed in addition to step I dietary modifications; and (3) the step II diet may prove too restrictive in ESRD patients, who are already under several dietary constraints.[38] Target total and LDL cholesterols levels, respectively, are 200 mg/dL or less and 100 mg/dL or less (5.2 mmol/L or less and 2.6 mmol/L or less); corresponding LDL thresholds for the initiation of diet and drug therapy are 100 mg/dL or greater and 130 mg/dL or greater (2.6 mmol/L or greater and 3.4 mmol/L or greater). Although the primary goal of lipid-lowering therapy is to reduce cardiovascular disease, the benefit of treatment may extend to slowing of renal disease progression in some individuals, as discussed in earlier sections. Some clinicians also base their treatment approach to hyperlipidemia according to whether nephrotic syndrome (greater than 3 g/day urinary protein excretion) is present, in which case control of the primary disease and antiproteinuric interventions (e.g., ACEIs, NSAIDs, and possibly ARBs) may enhance lipid control.

For all CRD subgroups exhibiting elevated total and LDL cholesterol, the HMG-CoA reductase inhibitors are probably the most effective agents, with reasonable safety and tolerability.[38] Myositis and rhabdomyolysis can occur at high doses, particularly if used in combination with fibrates or in transplant recipients receiving cyclosporine or (presumably) tacrolimus. Bile acid sequestrants are reasonable alternatives, but they may elevate triglycerides, interfere with fluid restrictions, and further complicate complex drug administration schedules because of their potential to reduce the absorption of concurrent medications. When lipid elevation is primarily in the triglyceride fraction, fibric acid derivatives are effective, but the more potent HMG-CoA reductase inhibitors (atorvastatin, cerivastatin) may also lower triglyceride levels to a moderate extent. Clofibrate and fenofibrate are generally avoided in advanced CRD because of their tendency to accumulate in renal dysfunction and thus precipitate myopathies. Of the fibrates, gemfibrozil is thought to undergo the least pharmacokinetic alteration in ESRD and is the preferred agent of this class. For the other patterns of lipid alteration commonly described in CRD, the role of corrective therapy remains to be defined. Measures to control diabetes and optimize insulin sensitivity may also improve dyslipidemia in diabetics with CRD.

Bleeding and Hemostatic Defects

In the absence of clinical bleeding or situations of increased risk for bleeding (e.g., invasive or surgical procedures), no specific therapy is required. In general, bleeding diathesis can be reduced by adequate treatment of the uremic state through hemodialysis or peritoneal dialysis and by avoiding unnecessary use of agents having antiplatelet effects.[12] Through EPO therapy (or transfusions), correction of the hematocrit to levels above 30%

may help enhance platelet–endothelial interactions. Although the benefit has largely been attributed to improved intravascular dispersion of platelets by RBC mass, EPO has been proposed to increase the expression of platelet membrane GPIIb-IIIa receptors.[125]

Acute treatment for severe bleeding necessitates red cell transfusion and, in life-threatening circumstances, administration of cryoprecipitate. The role of platelet transfusion is more controversial, given that repeated platelet transfusions are likely to promote the development of antiplatelet antibodies. Moreover, platelets transfused into the uremic environment are thought to become deficient in function, in the manner described in earlier sections for native platelets. Relatively rapid improvements in bleeding time can be produced in most uremic patients through the administration of desmopressin (DDAVP) 3 to 4 μg/kg by IV infusion. Desmopressin is thought to increase the release of von Willebrand factor (vWF), a glycoprotein that complexes with factor VIII, from endothelial storage sites. Desmopressin has proven clinically useful and well tolerated in the prophylaxis and acute management of uremic bleeding episodes. Unfortunately, its effects are short-lived (4 to 24 hours), and repeated short-term administration of desmopressin eventually leads to tachyphylaxis, presumably due to depletion of vWF stores.[126] Conjugated estrogens may be useful in reducing bleeding time, particularly when a more prolonged effect is desired. The mechanisms by which estrogens serve to shorten bleeding time are not completely understood but are believed to involve reductions in nitric oxide or precursor synthesis, possibly through estrogen-receptor–mediated control of nuclear transcription pathways.[125] The hemostatic benefit of estrogens is dose dependent; however, the optimal dose of conjugated estrogens for control of uremic bleeding is unclear, in that reportedly effective doses have ranged widely (10 to 60 mg/day; 0.1 to 0.6 mg/kg/day).[127] With repeated dosing, hemostatic effects generally begin within 24 hours, peak at 5 to 7 days, and can persist for more than 1 week after discontinuation. Because high doses are usually needed, estrogen-related side effects may limit their long-term utility in uremic bleeding.

Gastrointestinal Complications

Antacids were once used heavily in CRD patients for relief of dyspepsia or gastrointestinal irritation. In the setting of renal insufficiency, many of these agents present potential problems. Bicarbonate-based products can result in the inadvertent administration of large sodium loads, but they may be useful in controlling metabolic acidosis. When magnesium-containing antacids or cathartics are given chronically in renal failure, accumulation of magnesium becomes a concern as creatinine clearance falls below 30 mL/min. Serum magnesium levels may rise above 6 mEq/L (3 mmol/L), leading to central nervous system depression, lethargy, somnolence, and loss of deep tendon reflexes. Dialysis removes magnesium effectively and may be indicated in cases of severe toxicity. As discussed in earlier sections, chronic use of aluminum-based antacids or phosphate binders may lead to aluminum intoxication syndromes.

H_2-receptor antagonists have largely replaced chronic antacid use for dyspepsia in the CRD and other populations. Most of these agents are eliminated renally, hence dosage reduction has traditionally been recommended at CrCl less than 30 to 50 mL/min; however, their elimination by active tubular secretion helps preserve renal drug clearance at reduced GFRs. The majority of accumulation-related adverse experiences have been reported in association with cimetidine and ranitidine, consisting primarily of encephalopathy and mental status alterations. When evaluating H_2-antagonist dose, it is appropriate to remember that these agents have a wide dosing range depending on their therapeutic purpose; therefore, renal dose reductions may not be called for in situations where aggressive acid suppression is needed. Proton-pump inhibitors do not undergo significant pharmacokinetic alterations in CRD. Their use could be anticipated to reduce the efficacy of calcium carbonate–based phosphate binders, which are dependent on gastric acidity for solubilization;[95] however, available data do not consistently support a significant degree of interference.[96]

Constipation is a common complaint in advanced CRD and is likely to be exacerbated by diet and fluid restrictions, Al^{3+}- or Ca^{2+}-based phosphate-binding agents, iron supplements, calcium channel blockers, and other medications. Bulk-forming laxatives are not front line agents, as they are in the general population, because concomitant fluid restrictions reduce their efficacy and safety; some products also contain a significant potassium content. The use of cathartics that are magnesium or phosphate based (e.g., Phospho-Soda) should be minimized because of their potential for systemic accumulation. Chronic use of stimulant laxatives is permitted to a greater extent in patients with CRD than in the general population. Lactulose and the osmotic cathartic sorbitol are also prescribed, but they may generate patient disfavor because of the flatulence and bloating that often accompany their use.

Pruritis

A variety of topical and systemic therapies have been reported as beneficial in reducing or relieving uremic pruritus (Table 22.12).[128–130] Unfortunately, none of these has proven uniformly effective, often necessitating a trial-and-error approach. Topical therapies that moisten dry, scaly skin or produce a counterirritant effect are generally safe and are an appropriate initial measure that may provide partial relief. Ensuring optimal control of serum phosphate and calcium levels along with minimizing secondary hyperparathyroidism may help reduce the overall tendency toward severe itching episodes but usually does not lead to immediate symptomatic improvement. The use of large quantities of antihistamine and antiserotonergic agents (systemically or topically) is common, but patients should

Table 22.12 ▪ Management of Uremic Pruritis: Empiric and Anecdotal Approaches

Rule out drug, diet, and environmentally induced causes
Topical therapies
- Emollients and moisturizers: lanolin based, hypoallergenic lotion, superfatted soaps, oatmeal baths
- Counterirritants: camphorated or mentholated lotions
- Antipruritics: topical antihistamines, doxepin, anesthetics* (caution if widespread application)
- Capsaicin (0.025% strength)
- Phototherapy (ultraviolet B exposure; not commonly used)*

Systemic therapies
- Antihistamines (H_1 and H_2), serotonin-blocking antihistamines (cyproheptadine)
- Opiate antagonists (oral naloxone)*
- Toxin adsorption/removal*: oral cholestyramine, activated charcoal
- Optimize intensity of dialysis
- Optimize control of hyperparathyroidism, serum phosphate, and calcium levels
- Erythropoietin therapy, hematocrit optimization, or both

Source: References 128–130.
*Anecdotal approaches.

be monitored for intoxication syndromes and the inability to adhere to fluid restrictions because of the xerostomia that these drugs tend to produce.

Musculoskeletal Complaints

Control of acute gouty attacks is often achieved through cautious use of traditional agents such as NSAIDs (e.g., indomethacin) and colchicine. On NSAID initiation, patients should be monitored closely for bleeding, worsened renal function, and loss of diuretic efficacy. When used chronically in renal impairment, colchicine accumulation can induce a peripheral neuropathy that may be mistakenly attributed to other factors. For chronic prevention of gouty attacks, uricosurics lose much of their efficacy in advanced CRD. Allopurinol, which decreases uric acid production, is the preferred prophylactic agent; because it possesses an active metabolite (oxypurinol) that is renally eliminated, doses are usually reduced to 100 to 200 mg daily in advanced CRD.

Pharmacokinetic Considerations and Drug Dosing

The presence of renal failure can alter the disposition and patient response to many drugs. For renally eliminated agents, a major clinical concern is the potential for drug accumulation and heightened risk of related systemic toxicities, especially if normal doses are used. In addition, some drugs damage the kidney, hence their use may further compromise renal function. Because several nephrotoxins also happen to be eliminated renally, both of these aspects may dictate the need for cautious use in the setting of CRD. A complete discussion of CRD-associated pharmacokinetic and pharmacodynamic alterations is beyond the scope of this chapter, but fundamental principles and classic examples are briefly summarized. Issues specific to drug removal and dosing requirements in hemodialysis and peritoneal dialysis recipients are discussed in Chapter 23.

Pharmacokinetic Changes

Absorption. CRD is thought to alter the absorption of several agents, but most of the described changes are believed to be of minor clinical significance.[131] Drug absorption may be reduced in the presence of severe gastrointestinal edema, as could occur in nephrotic syndrome (furosemide, digoxin). However, a more clinically significant cause of impaired drug absorption may result from concurrent administration of phosphorus-binding and acid-suppressive agents (fluoroquinolones, iron, itraconazole). Gastroparesis is common among diabetic CRD patients and may retard drug absorption or necessitate greater temporal separation of doses, when attempting to circumvent such interactions.

Distribution. The volume of distribution of several drugs may be increased or decreased as a result of changes in plasma protein and tissue-binding characteristics.[12,131] Drug-binding alterations have been characterized most consistently in long-standing uremia, whereas changes in moderate CRD or acute renal failure have proven less predictable. The plasma protein binding of acidic drugs (phenytoin, warfarin, mycophenolic acid) is generally decreased in uremia, leading to an increased V_d or elevated free fraction of drug. Depending on the drug, reduced binding has been attributed to binding competition with uremic toxins, hypoalbuminemia, systemic acidosis, and the accumulation of renally eliminated metabolites. For these agents, appropriate interpretation of serum drug levels reported as total (bound plus unbound) values may require adjustment of the target range to account for elevated free (active) fractions, or "correction" to values that would correspond to situations of normal protein binding. Formulas such as the following have been developed to aid in the interpretation of phenytoin levels when uremia or hypoalbuminemia is present:[131]

$$C_{normal} = C_{observed}\,[1/(\alpha \cdot \text{Alb} + 0.1)]$$

where

$\alpha = 0.1$ in uremic subjects or 0.2 in nonuremic subjects

Alb = the patient's measured serum albumin (g/dL)

This equation "corrects" the reported total phenytoin value in uremic and hypoalbuminemic subjects to a value that would have been observed were drug protein binding normal. In uremic patients with normal albumin levels (4 to 4.4 g/dL), uncorrected total phenytoin levels of 4 to 10 μg/mL would correspond to a corrected therapeutic range of approximately 10 to 20 μg/mL.

For some drugs (e.g., digoxin), decreased tissue binding or uptake results in a reduced V_d and an elevated ratio of plasma to tissue levels. In such cases, an elevated plasma drug level may not necessarily be associated with symptoms of excess target tissue activity.[131]

METABOLISM. Uremia has been associated with both decreases and increases in the hepatic metabolism of drugs. Thus, even if a drug is eliminated primarily by hepatic means, its disposition may be altered indirectly by CRD. The accumulation of renally eliminated metabolites may become a concern when they contribute to the therapeutic or toxic effects of the parent drug (e.g., procainamide, morphine, meperidine, codeine, cefotaxime, zidovudine, clofibrate, verapamil, allopurinol). For these drugs, initial dosage requirements may be similar to those in nonuremic subjects, whereas maintenance regimens may require dose reduction or close observation for signs and symptoms of excessive accumulation. Although the kidney has become increasingly recognized as a site of drug metabolism and detoxification, much less information is available to characterize the clinical relevance of these pathways in normal versus reduced renal function.[12,131]

EXCRETION. The processes of glomerular filtration, tubular secretion, and renal metabolism may contribute by differing extents to the renal elimination of a drug. Apart from issues discussed previously, the presence of renal disease has the greatest implications for drug dosing when a significant fraction (greater than 30%) of parent drug or active metabolite elimination is renal and compensatory elimination pathways are impaired or absent. The most commonly used gauge for approximating renal drug elimination capacity is the measured or estimated creatinine clearance. Pitfalls associated with interpretation of SCr and calculated creatinine clearance values are discussed in Chapter 21. Despite the fact that creatinine clearance is an imperfect surrogate marker of renal drug clearance, in most medical centers it remains the most practical approach through which to guide dosing adjustments. Most drug dosing guidelines are based on either (1) specific ranges of creatinine clearance, (2) individualized approximations of drug clearance based on pharmacokinetic formulas that correlate creatinine clearance with drug clearance, or (3) pharmacokinetic individualization based on measured in vivo drug concentrations. Maintenance dosing adjustments may be accomplished through alteration of dose, reduction of frequency, or a combination of both, depending on the significance of peak-to-trough serum level fluctuations and other factors, such as convenience and available dosage increments.

PHARMACODYNAMIC. Drug response has been noted to be both increased (morphine, codeine, alprazolam) and decreased (digoxin, propranolol) in uremics. Although many of these apparent alterations in drug response can be accounted for by closely examining changes in disposition, it appears that sensitivity to the action of some drugs is affected by the uremic state.

Practical Clinical Approach

With a few important exceptions, the majority of drugs in clinical use do not routinely require dosage adjustment until creatinine clearance values fall below 50 to 60 mL/min. However, several renally eliminated agents of narrow therapeutic index merit dosage individualization at even milder degrees of renal impairment. These include, but are not limited to, aminoglycosides, digoxin, metformin, procainamide, foscarnet, ganciclovir, cidofovir, flucytosine, carboplatin, lepirudin, and vancomycin. References should be routinely consulted to ascertain the need for dosage adjustment (Table 22.13), especially at creatinine clearance values below 60 mL/min. Knowing the fraction of drug or active metabolite that is renally eliminated under normal circumstances can help to more efficiently identify drugs requiring renal dosage adjustment. Drug interactions and impairment of alternate elimination pathways may increase the significance of renal impairment.

One should be aware that dosage recommendations are sometimes based on creatinine clearance values that have

Table 22.13 ▪ Useful Resources in Determination of Renal Dosing Requirements

Compendia

- Manufacturer's product literature; consider specific inquiry to medical information department
- American Hospital Formulary Service (AHFS): *Drug Information*
- *Drug Facts and Comparisons*
- CD-ROM and drug information databases: Micromedex (Drugdex), Excerpta Medica CD, Clinical Pharmacology, AHFS: Drug Information Fulltext
- Martindale's: *The Extra Pharmacopoeia*

Tertiary References

- Textbook treatise: pharmacology, pharmacotherapeutic textbooks
- Specialty related: nephrology or specialty related to drug indication
- Pharmacokinetic: Applied Pharmacokinetics—Principles of Therapeutic Drug Monitoring
- Pharmacotherapy Self-Assessment Program (PSAP)—Nephrology module(s)

Pocket Guides

- Bennett WM et al eds. Drug prescribing in renal failure. 4th ed. American College of Physicians, 1999.
- Gilbert DN, Moellering RC, Sande MA, eds. The Sanford guide to antimicrobial therapy. Vienna, VA: Antimicrobial Therapy, Inc. (published yearly; antimicrobials only).
- Dosing charts provided by manufacturers of ESRD care–related products (Amgen, Fresenius, Gambro, Baxter, etc.).

Literature Search

- Review articles (e.g., Talbert RL. Drug dosing in renal insufficiency. J Clin Pharmacol 34:99–110, 1994; St Peter WL, Redic-Kill KA, Halstenson CE. Clinical pharmacokinetics of antibiotics in patients with impaired renal function. Clin Pharmacokinet 22:169–210, 1992)
- Primary literature search

Source: Carter BL, Angaran DM, Lake KD, et al., eds. Pharmacotherapy Self Assessment Program. 2nd ed. St Louis, MO: ACCP, 1996: Module 6, 123–160.

been normalized to weight or body surface area and adjust calculations accordingly. Values for creatinine clearance (and therefore drug clearance) that have been calculated from SCr carry an inherent margin of error averaging 10 to 25%. Clinical judgment as to the risks of underestimation versus overestimation of dosage requirements must be exercised in each individual case, especially when calculated drug clearance values fall near cutoff values for dose adjustment or when renal function appears to be changing. Finally, it is not uncommon to find conflicting recommendations for dosage adjustment from different resources. Clinical judgment and scrutiny of the conditions and patient characteristics from which dosage guidelines were derived may help in selecting the most appropriate strategy. If therapeutic drug level monitoring is not feasible, monitoring parameters for both therapeutic failure and accumulation-related toxicities should be identified and closely followed.

Aminoglycoside Pulse Dosing

Dosing strategy is thought to influence the nephrotoxic potential of certain agents, such as aminoglycosides. The traditional approach to dosing gentamicin and tobramycin has been to administer doses of 1 to 3 mg/kg at 8- to 24-hour intervals (adjusted according to renal drug clearance), in order to achieve target peak (4 to 10 μg/mL) and trough (less than 2 μg/mL) concentrations that were presumed to be associated with therapeutic efficacy, as well as an accepted incidence of nephrotoxicity or ototoxicity. However, newer pharmacodynamic models of the antimicrobial activity and nephrotoxic potential of aminoglycosides have provided a rationale for alternative dosing practices using larger "pulse" doses (e.g., 4 to 7 mg/kg for gentamicin or tobramycin) at extended time intervals (24 to 48 hours).[132] These approaches are based on the assumptions that (1) the duration and extent of gram-negative antimicrobial activity is proportional to peak aminoglycoside concentration and (2) renal uptake of aminoglycoside, a major determinant of nephrotoxicity, occurs to a lower extent during pulse drug exposure than during traditional regimens that result in constant renal tubular drug exposure. With once-daily consolidated pulses, the extended dosing interval is thought to permit less renal drug accumulation (and therefore nephrotoxic risk), while the high peak level achieved (12 to 25 μg/mL for gentamicin) is postulated to enhance concentration-dependent microbe killing, enhance tissue penetration, and sustain a postantibiotic effect throughout periods of "subtherapeutic" serum drug levels.

Continued clinical experience with pulse aminoglycoside strategies in select populations suggests that antimicrobial efficacy is preserved, while nephrotoxicity is less than[133] or similar to[134] that observed with conventional dosing. Various methods of applying the pulse dosing approach have been developed; at present, clinical data are insufficient to advocate one protocol over another.[135] Because many protocols use fewer serum drug levels to guide dose adjustment than traditional aminoglycoside dosing, they may also prove to be more cost-effective. It is important to note that pulse dosing of aminoglycosides has generally *not* been advocated as monotherapy for systemic infections; in gram-positive infections; or in patients with highly altered kinetic profiles, such those with ARF or advanced renal disease (e.g., creatinine clearance values less than 20 to 30 mL/min or requiring a dosing interval longer than 48 hours for drug washout), pregnancy, extensive burns, or significant ascites.

Nonpharmacologic Therapy

Diet

To a great extent, many of the symptoms and complications of CRD are explainable by imbalances between the dietary intake and urinary excretion of several solutes. Dietary interventions have been mentioned previously and are generally regarded to be of equal importance to pharmacologic therapies for disease and symptom control. Dietitians are integral members of most specialized renal care teams and can complement the pharmacist's efforts to educate patients on appropriate use of their phosphorus binders and calcium, iron, and calcitriol supplements.

In the face of mild to moderate renal disease (e.g., GFR less than 60 mL/min), restriction of dietary intake to 0.6 to 0.8 g/kg/day of high-biologic-value protein is now presumed to retard the progression of renal disease. Protein restriction also helps limit phosphorus intake and the symptoms attributed to accumulation of nitrogenous waste products. Thorough dietary instruction is crucial, and continued supervision may help ensure that protein malnutrition does not occur, especially in those with excessive urinary protein losses (e.g., nephrotic syndrome). After initiation of dialysis, protein intake is generally liberalized to prevent or correct protein malnutrition, as discussed in Chapter 23. Once GFR falls below 25 to 30 mL/min, reduction of dietary phosphorus intake becomes necessary in order to curtail hyperphosphatemia, secondary hyperparathyroidism, and the subsequent progression of renal bone disease. For a 70 kg individual, a 42 g low-protein diet (0.6 mg/kg/day) provides approximately 26 mmol (approximately 800 mg) of phosphorus per day, which is within the suggested range (10 mg/kg/day or less [0.32 mmol/kg/day or less]) of early phosphorus restriction.[12] As GFR declines to less than 10 to 15 mL/min, limitation of dietary sodium and fluid intake often becomes essential to maintaining control of blood pressure and blood volume status. Changes in both of these should be instituted gradually because renal adaptation mechanisms are often sluggish. Restriction of dietary potassium generally is required once GFR is less than 10 mL/min, in order to avoid life-threatening hyperkalemic episodes. Patients should be advised to use caution in selecting sodium substitutes, because many of these contain high amounts of potassium. For CRD patients who also suffer from diabetes or hyperlipidemia, adherence to dietary measures to control these diseases is generally advocated to improve outcomes. However, if unrealistic restrictions are imposed on protein, carbohydrate, *and* fat intake, it may become an impossible task to maintain adequate caloric intake (30 to 35 kcal/kg/day or more).

Supplementation with moderate quantities of B-complex vitamins, folic acid, and other water-soluble vitamins is usually recommended in predialysis and dialysis patients, because dietary intake of these nutrients is generally inadequate on restricted diets, and removal is enhanced by dialysis.[12] Daily doses of vitamin C (ascorbic acid) exceeding 250 mg have been implicated in precipitating oxalosis and therefore require caution in advanced CRD. Interest has recently emerged in using ascorbic acid to enhance iron mobilization from reticuloendothelial storage sites, but experience with this approach is limited.[136] Administration of vitamin D analogs is typically individualized according to osteodystrophy status. Serum levels of vitamins A and E have been noted to be elevated in uremic patients. Although the clinical significance of this is not clear, routine supplementation of vitamins A, E, and K is not generally advised in advanced CRD. Recently, high-dose tocopherol (vitamin E) has been advocated for numerous maladies (restless legs syndrome, antioxidant protection, etc.); however, the long-term safety of pharmacologic doses of tocopherol has not yet been rigorously assessed in the ESRD setting. Variable derangements of trace mineral balance have been observed in uremic and dialysis patients and may be influenced by the trace mineral content of dialysate water sources. Supplementation of trace minerals has not been routine in CRD; if undertaken, the potential for prolonged accumulation and associated toxicities should be considered.

FUTURE THERAPIES

Receptor antagonists of endothelin, an endogenous vasoconstrictor derived from the vascular endothelium, are under clinical development. These "-entans" (e.g., bosentan) are thought to be promising in the setting of both renal and cardiovascular disease, conditions in which endothelin levels are noted to be elevated and are suspected of perpetuating vascular and target organ damage. Although they are not yet clinically available, their anticipated utility in managing hypertension, cardiovascular disease, and the progression of CRD is likely to generate a significant amount of clinical study.[137,138] Ongoing and future studies of other presently available therapies should help clarify the optimal strategies for retarding the progression of CRD and its related comorbidities. Patients with limited renal reserve, who are likely to be further compromised by exposure to nephrotoxins, may benefit from renal-sparing alternatives that have recently become available for several therapeutic classes of drugs (Table 22.14); use of these therapies may help reduce the number of patients whose entry in ESRD has been hastened iatrogenically.

Table 22.14 ▪ Renal-Sparing Alternatives to Nephrotoxic Therapies: Potential Approaches

Nephrotoxin	Possible Alternative or Renal-Sparing Approach*
Aminoglycoside	Fluoroquinolones, aztreonam, imipenem, meropenem, ceftazidime, cefepime Once-daily "pulse" dosing strategies
Cyclosporine, tacrolimus	Sirolimus (rapamycin)
Amphotericin B	Liposomal or lipid complex formulations Itraconazole, fluconazole
Cisplatin	Carboplatin Nephroprotection with amifostine
Radiocontrast media	Low-osmolality or nonionic contrast agents Nephroprotection protocols; fenoldopam†

*Appropriateness of these alternatives depends on the specific patient, indication, and situation.

†Animal studies–human clinical data preliminary (Bakris GL, Lass NA, Glock D. Renal hemodynamics in radiocontrast medium–induced renal dysfunction: a role for dopamine-1 receptors. Kidney Int 56:206–210, 1999).

IMPROVING OUTCOMES

Patient Education

Individuals with advanced renal disease are expected to understand and follow complex dietary, medication, and physical care regimens. Data indicate that intense educational effort in ESRD is associated with increased patient autonomy, improved quality of life, increased compliance with therapies, and the medical ability to delay initiation of dialysis.[83] The need for renal replacement therapy (RRT) can often be predicted more than 1 year in advance, providing ample opportunity for early education of patients facing ESRD (and their caregivers). Patient referral to a renal care specialty team may help ensure that the patient gains an adequate understanding of kidney disease and participates in decisions regarding options for renal replacement modality. Educational programs generally emphasize patient comprehension of: the most common complications of kidney disease (anemia, bone disease, hypertension), measures to slow progression of renal disease (if still feasible), dietary management (protein, phosphorus, potassium, sodium, and fluid restrictions), medication management (reason for use, manner of use, and precautions), choice of RRT modality and physical preparation for this (catheter or fistula placement, transplantation referral, etc.), options for medical care and prescription coverage, and possibilities for vocational support. Individuals with renal disease could be considered fortunate, in that the renal community offers numerous organizations from which to draw educational information, psychosocial support, and financial guidance. A partial list of organizations and programs that offer patient-focused

Table 22.15 ▪ Chronic Renal Disease: Patient-Oriented Organizations and Resources Providing Education, Advocacy, and Support Services (Partial Listing)

Kidney Disease (General)	
Organizations and programs	
American Association of Kidney Patients	www.aakp.org
The Life Options Rehabilitation Council	www.lifeoptions.org
National Kidney Foundation	www.kidney.org
The Renal Association	www.renal.org
Kidney Dialysis Foundation	www.kdf.org
American Diabetes Association	www.diabetes.org
National Kidney and Urologic Diseases Information Clearinghouse/NIDDK	www.niddk.nih.gov
IgA Nephropathy Foundation American Kidney Fund	www.igan.org
Web-based link site and search engines	
Kidney Information Clearing House	www.renalnet.org
The Nephron Information Center	www.nephron.com
Transplantation	
Organizations and programs	
Organ Transplant Fund	
National Transplant Assistance Fund	
Transplant Recipients International Organization (TRIO)	
United Network for Organ Sharing	www.unos.org
Web-based link sites and search engines	
The National Institute of Transplantation	www.transplantation.com
Transplantation Resources on the Internet	www.transweb.org
The Kidney Transplant Patient Partnering Program	www.ktppp.com

Many of these organizations and resources are primarily informational. Financial assistance, grants, and other support services are available through some of these organizations, in addition to government, private, and nonprofit agencies.

resources for those suffering from renal disease is provided in Table 22.15. Numerous resources oriented toward renal health professionals exist, some of which are also accessible through these sites.

Pharmacists can address several facets of medication use to foster patient acceptance, compliance, and safety. For those receiving nephroprotective medications as part of an effort to forestall ESRD, continued reinforcement and encouragement regarding the rationale for therapy may be necessary. Patients should understand that the safety and elimination of medication might change as their renal disease progresses, necessitating dosage adjustments or a change to alternative medications; anyone prescribing or dispensing medication to CRD patients should be made aware of their *present* renal status. Patients should be encouraged to seek advice before using over-the-counter products, because even over-the-counter products can worsen renal function (e.g., NSAIDs), prove dangerous (e.g., certain antacids, laxatives, NSAIDs), or require dosing precautions (e.g., H_2 antagonists used in excessive quantity).

Methods to Improve Patient Adherence to Drug Therapy

The median number of maintenance medications prescribed in ESRD exceeds 8 per patient,[1] and medications are often prescribed by multiple practitioners who are not fully aware of the patient's entire medication regimen. Given that the likelihood of drug interactions and drug-related misadventures increases with regimen complexity, a role for regular review of medication profiles becomes evident. Patients should be encouraged to communicate and verify information about their *actual* medication routine on a regular basis, because dosing changes are often communicated verbally from prescriber to patient, and medical records or dispensing profiles may not reflect actual practice.

Examples of instructions specific to medications commonly used in the CRD population are included in Table 22.16. Cognitive deficits and patient misunderstanding of the medication regimen are common barriers to compli-

Table 22.16 ▪ Medication Counseling in Chronic Renal Disease: Some General Points

General Information

- Ensure that all prescribers are aware of your kidney disease.
- Continue to inquire about special dosing for kidney disease (new prescriptions and as kidney function changes).
- Seek advice before self-medication with over-the-counter agents, especially laxatives, antacids, and nonsteroidal anti-inflammatory drugs.
- Vaccination yearly against influenza and every 5 years against pneumococcus is recommended.
- Ingestion of medications with soft, juicy foods may facilitate adherence to fluid restrictions.

Specific Medications

- Phosphate binders: take with or immediately after meal; $CaCO_3$-based binders are best taken immediately before the meal.
- Phosphate binders may interfere with the absorption of other medications; inquire specifically.
- Oral iron supplements are best taken between meals, if tolerated, on an empty stomach and separate from phosphate binders.

Hemodialysis Patients

- Check to see if medication should be specifically taken before or after dialysis (because some drugs are removed by dialysis); avoid changes in this "routine" unless approved by physician.
- Long-acting antihypertensives: ask physician if you should take before dialysis on hemodialysis days.
- Hepatitis B vaccination series and boosters are recommended (often performed at hemodialysis center).
- Epoetin administered subcutaneously: patients may require instructions on self-administration and appropriate storage.

ance. Reviewing the rationale for a medication's use, along with discussing the results of examinations, laboratory tests, and diagnostic tests, may help reinforce to the patient the value of compliance with diet, medication, and other treatments. Some patients are motivated by trade-offs between dietary restriction and medication regimen complexity. For example, learning to estimate dietary phosphorus intake and accordingly titrate phosphate binder dose may afford flexibility and autonomy to patients who are capable of managing such alternatives. On the other hand, dietary indiscretion leading to episodes of hyperphosphatemia, hyperkalemia, or volume overload could necessitate therapies associated with undesirable effects, such as aluminum-based phosphate binders (worsened constipation), SPS Suspension (flatulence and bloating), or additional dialysis sessions (inconvenience). Symptomatic improvements can often be attributed at least partly to compliance with specific interventions, and this may help tangibly illustrate to the patient the benefits of adhering to therapy.

Disease Management Strategies to Improve Patient Outcomes

Over the past decade, our understanding of the factors that influence morbidity and mortality in the ESRD population has grown considerably. In addition to research efforts, much information has been gained through the establishment of registries that support the collection and analysis of data relating patient variables and trends in ESRD care to measurable outcomes. Strategies to further develop and apply this knowledge toward improving future pre-ESRD and ESRD outcomes have been identified and summarized.[139] However, concerns regarding the quality of care delivered to the pre-ESRD subgroup are equally significant, as well as the need to better track this poorly characterized segment of the CRD population. Standards for care of the pre-ESRD population have not been well defined.[139] However, it is becoming evident that the general level of care delivered to pre-ESRD candidates is widely suboptimal, and that as a probable consequence, outcomes in the ESRD population have suffered.[92,140,141] In the coming decade, a concerted effort to measure and define standards for pre-ESRD care will be undertaken. Initiatives for improvement in care are likely to target earlier detection and tracking of renal disease; increased utilization of interventions to retard CRD; earlier management of uremic complications (anemia, bone disease, acidosis, malnutrition); more aggressive management of comorbid conditions (such as diabetes, hyperlipidemia, and cardiovascular disease); earlier initiation of RRT; and preparation of patients, both medically and psychosocially, farther in advance for this event.[142] The most efficient and cost-effective approach for identifying those at risk of CRD, particularly nondiabetics, must be established; hypertensives may be the most logical population on which to focus. It is encouraging to note that although the ESRD population continues to grow, the *rate* of increase in new ESRD cases during the 1990s declined from 10% to 5% yearly.

Recent advances in transplantation and supportive care have improved both patient and graft survival in renal transplant recipients. Because transplant patient outcomes (in terms of survival rates, quality of life, and rehabilitation) are superior and the average overall cost per patient year of therapy is actually less than dialysis, transplantation has become the preferred renal replacement modality for otherwise appropriate candidates. When feasible, a kidney from a living related donor (LRD) is used over a cadaveric organ source. Not only do LRD transplants provide longer patient and graft survival rates, they allow cadaveric kidneys to be allocated to those who lack a suitable living donor. Unfortunately, advanced age or certain comorbidities may preclude undergoing a transplant. Moreover, limited availability of donor organs has resulted in lengthy periods (1 to 3 years) on dialysis for many individuals in ESRD awaiting transplantation. Before reaching ESRD, patients are now encouraged to consider and prepare for transplantation from an LRD; such a preemptive approach may help avoid the demise in overall patient status associated with prolonged dialytic therapies. A combined kidney-pancreas transplant may also be an option for younger type 1 diabetics in end-stage nephropathy who are free of significant cardiovascular disease and meet additional criteria (see Chapter 104).

PHARMACOECONOMICS

By the year 2000, it is estimated that 85,000 individuals will enter into ESRD annually, incurring yearly medical expenditures of approximately $50,000 per individual. ESRD patients are estimated to consume more than 10 times the health care resources of the average U.S. citizen.[143] Given the outlay of resources for even 1 year of renal replacement therapy, one might anticipate that interventions that are successful in delaying ESRD could easily prove cost-effective. To date, surprisingly few published studies have addressed such pharmacoeconomic issues in detail. However, Rodby and colleagues recently exemplified the potential benefits of reducing ESRD in the diabetic population, in a cost-effectiveness analysis of captopril for prevention of diabetic nephropathy.[143] In their model, the initiation of captopril in type 1 or 2 diabetics with proteinuria was projected to result in a cumulative health care cost savings of $2.4 billion over a 10-year period (1995–2005), primarily through a reduction in ESRD-related care costs. Significant indirect savings, in terms of lost productivity and functional status, were also modeled. This analysis provides impetus to prospectively confirm the cost-effectiveness of nephroprotective strategies in the diabetic population and to explore these approaches in nondiabetic forms of renal disease.

Several studies have documented the effectiveness of EPO therapy in ameliorating the anemia of renal disease, improving quality of life, reducing transfusion requirements, and reversing left ventricular hypertrophy. However, additional pharmacoeconomic studies are needed to delineate the most cost-effective approach to anemia management in ESRD and pre-ESRD. Analysis strategies would ideally incorporate additional variables, such as manner of iron supplementation,[144,145] route of EPO administration,[146] differing hematocrit goals, reimbursement policies,[109] and other factors affecting EPO response, including adequacy of dialysis and concurrent illness.

KEY POINTS

- Chronic renal disease is a significant and growing source of morbidity, mortality, and health care expenditure in the United States and worldwide.
- Much has been learned about the pathophysiology of CRD in the past decade; however, prevention and treatment strategies based on this new knowledge are still at early stages of clinical evaluation.
- Advanced CRD and uremia affect several organ systems, leading to secondary metabolic, hematologic, cardiovascular, skeletal, neuromuscular, gastrointestinal, endocrine, and other complications.
- A critical area for improvement in renal care is the earlier recognition of renal disease or those at risk of CRD, followed by aggressive intervention to forestall progression to ESRD.
- Improvement in the management of the pre-ESRD population is needed and may be paramount to improving outcomes in the later continuum of renal disease.
- Pharmacologic therapies are a mainstay of managing the complications of uremia, but they should be coupled with dietary interventions for optimal results.
- Medication regimen complexity and altered drug disposition in the CRD population provide a significant opportunity for pharmacists to improve patient outcomes, at an individual and a population level.

REFERENCES

1. The United States Renal Data System (USRDS). 1998 annual data report. Bethesda, MD: National Institute of Diabetes, Digestive and Kidney Diseases, 1998.
2. Obrador GT, Arora P, Kausz AT, et al. Pre-end-stage renal disease care in the United States: a state of disrepair. J Am Soc Nephrol 9:S44–S54, 1998.
3. DeFronzo RA. Diabetic nephropathy: etiologic and therapeutic considerations. Diabetes Rev 3:510–564, 1995.
4. Brown TE, Carter BL. Hypertension and endstage renal disease. Ann Pharmacother 28:359–366, 1994.
5. Diabetes Control and Complications Trial Research Group. The effect of intensive treatment of diabetes on the development and progression of long-term complications in insulin-dependent diabetes mellitus. N Engl J Med 329:977–986, 1993.
6. Bangstad HJ, Ostersby R, Dahl-Jorgensen K, et al. Improvement of blood glucose control in IDDM patients retards the progression of morphological changes in early diabetic nephropathy. Diabetologia 37:483–490, 1994.
7. Fioretto P, Steffes MW, Sutherland DE, et al. Reversal of lesions of diabetic nephropathy after pancreas transplantation. N Engl J Med 339:69–75, 1998.
8. UK Prospective Diabetes Study (UKPDS) Group. Intensive blood-glucose control with sulphonylureas or insulin compared to conventional treatment and risk of complications in patients with type 2 diabetes (UKPDS 33). Lancet 352:837–853, 1998.
9. Ohkubo Y, Kishikawa H, Araki E, et al. Intensive insulin therapy prevents the progression of diabetic microvascular complications in Japanese patients with non-insulin-dependent diabetes mellitus: a randomized prospective 6-year study. Diabetes Res Clin Pract 28:103–117, 1995.
10. Mackenzie HS, Brenner BM. Current strategies for retarding progression of renal disease. Am J Kidney Dis 31:161–170, 1998.
11. Remuzzi G, Ruggenenti P, Benigni A. Understanding the nature of renal disease progression. Kidney Int 51:2–15, 1997.
12. Brenner BM. The kidney. 5th ed. Philadelphia: Saunders, 1996.
13. Peten EP, Striker LJ. Progression of glomerular disease. J Intern Med 236:241–249, 1994.
14. Apperloo AJ, de Zeeuw D, de Jong PE. A short-term antihypertensive treatment-induced fall in glomerular filtration rate predicts long-term stability of renal function. Kidney Int 51:793–797, 1997.
15. Zeller KR. Low-protein diets in renal disease. Diabetes Care 14:856–866, 1991.
16. Zeller K, Whittaker E, Sullivan L. Effect of restricting dietary protein on the progression of renal failure in patients with insulin-dependent diabetes mellitus. N Engl J Med 324:78–84, 1991.
17. Klahr S, Levey AS, Beck GJ, et al, for the Modification of Diet in Renal Disease (MDRD) Study Group. The effects of dietary protein restriction and blood-pressure control on the progression of chronic renal disease. N Engl J Med 330:877–884, 1994.
18. Locatelli F, Alberti D, Graziani G, et al. Prospective, randomized multicentre trial of effect of protein restriction on progression of chronic renal insufficiency. Lancet 337:1299–1304, 1991.
19. Levey AS, Adler S, Greene T, et al. Effects of dietary protein restriction on the progression of moderate renal disease in the Modification of Diet in Renal Disease Study. Am J Kidney Dis 27:652–653, 1996.
20. Pedrini MT, Levey AS, Lau J, et al. The effect of dietary protein restriction on the progression of diabetic and nondiabetic renal diseases: a meta-analysis. Ann Intern Med 124:627–632, 1996.
21. Kasiske BL, Lakatua JD, Ma JZ, et al. A meta-analysis of the effects of dietary protein restriction on the rate of decline in renal function. Am J Kidney Dis 31:954–961, 1998.
22. Levey AS, Greene T, Beck GJ, et al. Dietary protein restriction and the progression of chronic renal disease: what have all of the results of the MDRD study shown? J Am Soc Nephrol 10:2426–2439, 1999.
23. Maroni BJ. Protein restriction in the pre-end-stage renal disease (ESRD) patient: who, when, how, and the effect on subsequent ESRD outcome. J Am Soc Nephrol 9:S100–S106, 1998.
24. Bennett PH, Haffner S, Kasiske BL, et al. Screening and management of microalbuminuria in patients with diabetes mellitus: recommendations to the Scientific Advisory Board of the National Kidney Foundation from an ad hoc committee of the Council on Diabetes Mellitus of the National Kidney Foundation. Am J Kidney Dis 25:107–112, 1995.
25. Mogensen CE, Keane WF, Bennett PH, et al. Prevention of diabetic nephropathy with special reference to microalbuminuria. Lancet 346:1080–1084, 1995.
26. Hannedouche T, Pandais P, Goldfarb B, et al. Randomised controlled trial of enalapril and B blocker in non-diabetic chronic renal failure. BMJ 309:833–837, 1994.
27. Peterson JC, Adler S, Burkart JM, et al., for the MDRD Study Group. Blood pressure control, proteinuria, and the progression of renal disease. Ann Intern Med 123:754–762, 1995.
28. Erley CM, Haefele U, Heyne N, et al. Microalbuminuria in essential hypertension. Hypertension 21:810–815, 1993.
29. Lewis EJ, Hunsicker LG, Bain RP, et al, for the Collaborative Study Group. The effect of angiotensin-converting-enzyme inhibition on diabetic nephropathy. N Engl J Med 329:1456–1462, 1993.
30. Kasiske BL, Kalil RSN, Ma JZ, et al. Effect of antihypertensive therapy on the kidney in patients with diabetes: a meta-regression analysis. Ann Intern Med 118:129–138, 1993.
31. Machio G, Alberti D, Janin G, et al, for the Angiotensin-Converting-Enzyme Inhibition in Progressive Renal Insufficiency Study Group. Effect of the angiotensin-converting-enzyme inhibitor benazepril on the progression of chronic renal insufficiency. N Engl J Med 330:877–884, 1996.
32. Giatras I, Lau J, Levey AS, for the Angiotensin Converting Enzyme and Progressive Renal Disease Study Group. Effect of angiotensin-converting-enzyme inhibitors on the progression of nondiabetic renal disease: a meta-analysis of randomized trials. Ann Intern Med 127:337–345, 1997.
33. The GISEN Group. Randomized placebo-controlled trial of effect of ramipril on decline in glomerular filtration rate and risk of terminal renal failure in proteinuric, non-diabetic nephropathy. Lancet 349:1857–1863, 1997.
34. Hoelscher D, Bakris G. Antihypertensive therapy and progression of diabetic renal disease. J Cardiovasc Pharmacol 23:S34–S38, 1994.

35. Maki DD, Ma JZ, Louis TA, et al. Long-term effects of antihypertensive agents on proteinuria and renal function. Arch Intern Med 155:1073–1080, 1995.
36. Reams GP. Do calcium channel blockers have renal protective effects? Drugs Aging 5:263–287, 1994.
37. Ljungman S, Wikstrand J, Hartford M, et al. Urinary albumin excretion–a predictor of risk of cardiovascular disease. A prospective 10-year follow-up of middle-aged nondiabetic normal and hypertensive men. Am J Hypertens 9:770–778, 1996.
38. Kasiske BL. Hyperlipidemia in patients with chronic renal disease. Am J Kidney Dis 32:S142–S156, 1998.
39. Wheeler DC, Bernard DB. Lipid abnormalities in the nephrotic syndrome: causes, consequences and treatment. Am J Kidney Dis 23:331–346, 1994.
40. Demant T, Mathes C, Gutlich K, et al. A simultaneous study of the metabolism of apolipoprotein B and albumin in nephrotic patients. Kidney Int 54:2064–2080, 1998.
41. Walker WG. Relation of lipid abnormalities to progression of renal damage in essential hypertension, insulin-dependent and non insulin-dependent diabetes mellitus. Miner Electrolyte Metab 19:137–143, 1993.
42. Keane WF, Mulcahy WS, Kasiske BL, et al. Hyperlipidemia and progression of renal disease. Kidney Int 39:S41–S48, 1991.
43. Scanferla F, Landini S, Fracasso A. Risk factors for the progression of diabetic nephropathy: role of hyperlipidemia and its correction. Diabetologia 29:268–272, 1992.
44. Cappelli P, Di Liberato L, Albertazzi A. Role of dyslipidemia in the progression of chronic renal disease. Renal Failure 20:391–397, 1998.
45. Tonolo G, Ciccarese M, Brizzi P, et al. Reduction of albumin excretion rate in normotensive microalbuminuric type 2 diabetic patients during long-term simvastatin treatment. Diabetes Care 20:1891–1895, 1997.
46. Lam KSL, Cheng IKP, Januse ED, et al. Cholesterol-lowering therapy may retard the progression of diabetic nephropathy. Diabetologia 38:604–609, 1995.
47. Hostetter TH. Mechanisms of diabetic nephropathy. Am J Kidney Dis 23:188–192, 1994.
48. Marks JB, Raskin P. Nephropathy and hypertension in diabetes. Med Clin North Am 82:877–907, 1998.
49. Schrier RW, Gottschalk CW, eds. Diseases of the kidney. Boston: Little, Brown, 1997.
50. Hunsicker LG, Adler S, Caggiula A, et al, for the MDRD Study Group. Predictors of the progression of renal disease in the modification of diet in renal disease study. Kidney Int 51:1908–1919, 1997.
51. Franch HA, Mitch WE. Catabolism in uremia: the impact of metabolic acidosis. J Am Soc Nephrol 9:S78–S81, 1998.
52. Coen G, Mazzaferro S. Bone metabolism and its assessment in renal failure. Nephron 67:383–401, 1994.
53. Slotopolsky E, Delmez AJ. Pathogenesis of secondary hyperparathyroidism. Am J Kidney Dis 23:229–236, 1994.
54. Fesenfeld AJ, Lach F. Parathyroid gland function in chronic renal failure. Kidney Int 43:771–789, 1993.
55. Coburn JW, Elangovan L. Prevention of metabolic bone disease in the pre-end-stage renal disease setting. J Am Soc Nephrol 9:S71–S77, 1998.
56. Beusterien KM, Nissenson AR, Port FK, et al. The effects of recombinant human erythropoietin on functional health and well-being in chronic dialysis patients. J Am Soc Nephrol 7:763–773, 1996.
57. Revicki DA, Brown RE, Feeny DH, et al. Health-related quality of life associated with recombinant human erythropoietin therapy for predialysis chronic renal disease patients. Am J Kidney Dis 25:548–554, 1995.
58. Mann JF. What are the short-term and long-term consequences of anaemia in CRF patients? Nephrol Dial Transplant 14:S29–S36, 1999.
59. Eckhardt KU. Cardiovascular consequences of renal anaemia and erythropoietin therapy. Nephrol Dial Transplant 14:1317–1323, 1999.
60. Mailloux LU, Levey AS. Hypertension in patients with chronic renal disease. Am J Kidney Dis 32:S120–S141, 1998.
61. Whelton PK, Perneger TV, He J, et al. The role of blood pressure as a risk factor for renal disease: a review of the epidemiologic evidence. J Hum Hypertens 10:683–689, 1996.
62. Klag MJ, Whelton PK, Randall BL, et al. Blood pressure and end-stage renal disease in men. N Engl J Med 334:13–18, 1996.
63. Henrich WL. Approach to volume control, cardiac preservation, and blood pressure control in the pre-end-stage renal disease patient. J Am Soc Nephrol 9:S63–S65, 1998.
64. Kohan DE. Endothelins in the normal and diseased kidney. Am J Kidney Dis 29:2–26, 1997.
65. Kone BC. Nitric oxide in renal health and disease. Am J Kidney Dis 30:311–333, 1997.
66. Meyer KB, Levey AS. Controlling the epidemic of cardiovascular disease in chronic renal disease: report from the National Kidney Foundation Task Force on Cardiovascular Disease. J Am Soc Nephrol 9:S31–S42, 1998.
67. Coresh J, Longenecker JC, Miller ER, et al. Epidemiology of cardiovascular risk factors in chronic renal disease. J Am Soc Nephrol 9:S24–S30, 1998.
68. Hasselwander O, Young IS. Oxidative stress in chronic renal failure. Free Radic Res 29:1–11, 1998.
69. Keilani T, Schleuter WA, Levin ML, et al. Improvement of lipid abnormalities associated with proteinuria using fosinopril, an angiotensin-converting enzyme inhibitor. Ann Intern Med 188:246–254, 1993.
70. Eberst ME, Berkowitz LR. Hemostasis in renal disease: pathophysiology and management. Am J Med 96:168–179, 1994.
71. Gawaz MP, Dobos G, Spath M, et al. Impaired function of platelet membrane glycoprotein IIb-IIIa in end-stage renal disease. J Am Soc Nephrol 5:36–46, 1994.
72. Fliser D, Pacini G, Engelleiter R, et al. Insulin resistance and hyperinsulinemia are already present in patients with incipient renal disease. Kidney Int 53:1343–1347, 1998.
73. Mak RH. Renal disease, insulin resistance and glucose intolerance. Diabetes Rev 2:19–28, 1994.
74. Pyorala M, Miettinen H, Laakso M, et al. Hyperinsulinemia predicts coronary heart disease risk in healthy middle-aged men: the 22-year follow-up results of the Helsinki Policeman Study. Circulation 98:398–404, 1998.
75. Hou S. What are the clinically important consequences of ESRD-associated endocrine dysfunction? Semin Dialysis 10:11–13 (related comments 18–21), 1997.
76. Amorosa LF. Thyroid function in end-stage renal disease. Semin Dialysis 10:13–16, 1997.
77. Mandelbrot DA. Gastrointestinal bleeding in patients on dialysis. Semin Dialysis 11:161–166, 1998.
78. Young GB, Bolton CF. Peripheral nervous system complications in hemodialysis patients. Semin Dialysis 10:46–51, 1997.
79. Fauci AS, Braunwald E, Isselbacher KJ, et al, eds. Harrison's principles of internal medicine. 14th ed. New York: McGraw-Hill, 1997.
80. Bennett CJ, Plum F, eds. Cecil textbook of medicine. 20th ed. Philadelphia: Saunders, 1996.
81. Orth SR, Ritz E. The nephrotic syndrome. N Engl J Med 338:1202–1211, 1998.
82. Ordonez JD, Hiatt RA, Killebrew EJ, et al. The increased risk of coronary artery disease associated with nephrotic syndrome. Kidney Int 44:638–642, 1993.
83. Latham CE. Is there data to support the concept that educated, empowered patients have better outcomes? J Am Soc Nephrol 9:S141–S144, 1998.
84. Ifudo O, Paul H, Mayers JD, et al. Pervasive failed rehabilitation in center-based maintenance hemodialysis patients. Am J Kidney Dis 23:394–400, 1994.
85. DeOreo PB. Hemodialysis patient-assessed functional health status predicts continued survival, hospitalization, and dialysis-attendance compliance. Am J Kidney Dis 30:204–212, 1997.
86. The Sixth Report of the Joint National Committee on Prevention, Detection, Evaluation, and Treatment of High Blood Pressure. Arch Intern Med 157:2413–2446, 1997.
87. Expert Panel on Detection, Evaluation, and Treatment of High Blood Cholesterol in Adults. Summary of the Second Report of the National Cholesterol Education Program (NCEP) (Adult Treatment Panel II). JAMA 269:3015–3023, 1993.
88. American Diabetes Association. Diabetic nephropathy (position statement). Diabetes Care 21:S50–S53, 1998.
89. American Diabetes Association. Standards of medical care for patients with diabetes mellitus (position statement). Diabetes Care 21:S23–S31, 1998.
90. American Diabetes Association. Consensus development on the diagnosis and management of nephropathy in patients with diabetes mellitus (consensus statement). Diabetes Care 17:1357–1361, 1994.
91. NIH consensus statement. Morbidity and mortality of dialysis. Ann Intern Med 121:62–70, 1994.
92. Arora P, Obrador GT, Ruthazer R, et al. Prevalence, predictors, and consequences of late nephrology referral at a tertiary care center. J Am Soc Nephrol 10:1281–1286, 1999.
93. Brater DC. Diuretic therapy. N Engl J Med 339:387–395, 1998.
94. Andreucci M, Russo D, Fuiano G, et al. Diuretics in renal failure. Miner Electrolyte Metab 25:32–38, 1999.
95. Tan CC, Harden PN, Rodger RSC, et al. Ranitidine reduces phosphate binding in dialysis patients receiving calcium carbonate. Nephrol Dial Transplant 11:851–853, 1996.

96. Hardy P, Sechet A, Hottelait C, et al. Inhibition of gastric acid secretion by omeprazole and efficiency of calcium carbonate in the control of hyperphosphatemia in patients on chronic hemodialysis. Artif Organs 22:569–573, 1998.
97. Bleyer AJ, Burke SK, Dillon M, et al. A comparison of the calcium-free phosphate binder sevelamer hycrochloride with calcium acetate in the treatment of hyperphosphatemia in hemodialysis patients. Am J Kidney Dis 33:694–701, 1999.
98. Chertow GM, Burke SK, Dillon MA, et al. Long-term effects of sevelamer hydrochloride on the calcium × phosphate product and lipid profile of hemodialysis patients. Nephrol Dial Transplant 12:2907–2914, 1999.
99. Daisley-Kydd RE, Mason NA. Calcitriol in the management of secondary hyperparathyroidism of renal failure. Pharmacotherapy 16:619–630, 1996.
100. Martin KJ, Gonzalez EA, Gellens M, et al. 19-nor-1-alpha-25-dihydroxyvitamin D2 (paricalcitol) safely and effectively reduces the levels of intact parathyroid hormone in patients on hemodialysis. J Am Soc Nephrol 9:1427–1432, 1998.
101. Goldenberg MM. Paricalcitol, a new agent for the management of secondary hyperparathyroidism in patients undergoing chronic renal dialysis. Clin Ther 21:432–441, 1999.
102. NKF-DOQI Anemia Workgroup. NKF-DOQI clinical practice guidelines for the treatment of anemia of chronic renal failure. New York: National Kidney Foundation, 1997.
103. Portoles J, Torralbo A, Martin P, et al. Cardiovascular effects of recombinant human erythropoietin in predialysis patients. Am J Kidney Dis 29:541–548, 1997.
104. Macdougall IC. Quality of life and anemia: the nephrology experience. Semin Oncol 25:S39–S42, 1998.
105. Besarab A, Kline Bolton W, Browne JK, et al. The effects of normal as compared with low hematocrit values in patients with cardiovascular disease who are receiving hemodialysis and epoetin. N Engl J Med 339:584–590, 1998.
106. Besarab A. Iron and cardiac disease in the end-stage renal disease setting. Am J Kidney Dis 24:S18–S24, 1999.
107. Foley RN, Parfrey PS. Anemia in predialysis chronic renal failure: what are we treating? J Am Soc Nephrol 9:S82–S84, 1998.
108. Kaufman JS, Reda DJ, Fye CL, et al. Subcutaneous compared with intravenous epoetin in patients receiving hemodialysis. N Engl J Med 339:578–583, 1998.
109. Greer JW, Milam RA, Eggers PW. Trends in use, cost, and outcomes of human recombinant erythropoietin, 1989–98. Health Care Financ Rev 20:55–62, 1999.
110. Fishbane S. Iron treatment: impact of safety issues. Am J Kidney Dis 32:S5152–S5156, 1998.
111. Macdougall IC. Strategies for iron supplementation: oral versus intravenous. Kidney Int 69:S61–S66, 1999.
112. Shulman NB, Ford CE, Hall D, et al. Prognostic value of serum creatinine and effect of treatment of hypertension on renal function: results from the Hypertension Detection and Follow-up Program. Hypertension 13:S80–S93, 1989.
113. Russo D, Pisani A, Balletta MM, et al. Additive antiproteinuric effect of converting enzyme inhibitor and losartan in normotensive patients with IgA nephropathy. Am J Kidney Dis 33:851–856, 1999.
114. Ruilope LM, Lahera V, Alcazar JM, et al. Randomly allocated study of the effects of standard therapy versus ACE inhibition on micro-albuminuria in essential hypertension. J Hypertension 12:559–563, 1994.
115. Hebert LA, Kusek JW, Greene T, et al, for the MDRD Study Group. Effects of blood pressure control on progressive renal disease in blacks and whites. Hypertension 30(3 pt 1):428–435, 1997.
116. Packer M, Lee WH, Yushak M, et al. Comparison of captopril and enalapril in patients with severe chronic heart failure. N Engl J Med 315:847–853, 1986.
117. Oster JR, Materson BJ. Renal and electrolyte complications of CHF and effects of therapy with angiotensin-converting enzyme inhibitors. Arch Intern Med 152:704–710, 1992.
118. White CM. Pharmacologic, pharmacokinetic and therapeutic differences among ACE inhibitors. Pharmacotherapy 18:588–599, 1998.
119. Sica DA, Deedwania PC. Cardiorenal implications of angiotensin-receptor antagonist therapy. Congest Heart Fail 4:35–40, 1998.
120. Menard J, Campbell DJ, Aziz M, et al. Synergistic effects of ACE inhibition and ANGII antagonism on blood pressure, cardiac weight, and renin in spontaneously hypertensive rates. Circulation 96:3072–3078, 1997.
121. Kovacs SJ, Tenero DM, Martin DE, et al. The pharmacokinetics and protein binding of eprosartan in hemodialysis patients with end-stage renal disease. Pharmacotherapy 19:612–619, 1999.
122. DePiro JT, Talbert RL, Yee GC, et al, eds. Pharmacotherapy: a pathophysiologic approach. 3rd ed. Stamford, CT: Appleton & Lange, 1997.
123. Gehr TW, Tenero DM, Boyle DA, et al. The pharmacokinetics of carvedilol and its metabolites after single and multiple dose oral administration in patients with hypertension and renal insufficiency. Eur J Clin Pharmacol 55:269–277, 1999.
124. Anderson S, Rennke HG, Garcia DL, et al. Short and long term effects of antihypertensive therapy in the diabetic rat. Kidney Int 36:526–536, 1989.
125. Rose, B. Platelet dysfunction in uremia. UpToDate. Wellesley: UpToDate, Inc., Vol 7.1, 1999.
126. Lethagen S. Desmopressin (DDAVP) and hemostasis. Ann Hematol 69:173–180, 1994.
127. Heunisch C, Resnick DJ, Vitello JM, et al. Conjugated estrogens for the management of gastrointestinal bleeding secondary to uremia of acute renal failure. Pharmacotherapy 18:210–217, 1998.
128. Cho YL, Liu HN, Huang TP, et al. Uremic pruritis: roles of parathyroid hormone and substance P. J Am Acad Dermatol 36:538–543, 1997.
129. De Marchi S, Cecchin E, Villalta D, et al. Relief of pruritis and decreases in plasma histamine concentrations during erythropoietin therapy in patients with uremia. N Engl J Med 326:969–974, 1992.
130. Henrich WL. Uremic Pruritis. UpToDate. Wellesley: UpToDate, Inc., Vol 7.1, 1999.
131. Evans WE, Schentag JJ, Jusko WJ, eds. Applied pharmacokinetics: principles of therapeutic drug monitoring. Vancouver: Applied Therapeutics, 1992.
132. Periti P. Preclinical and clinical evaluation of once-daily aminoglycoside chemotherapy. J Chemother 7:311–337, 1995.
133. Rybak MJ, Abate BJ, Kang SL, et al. Prospective evaluation of the effect of aminoglycoside dosing regimen on rates of observed nephrotoxicity and ototoxicity. Antimicrob Agents Chemother 43:1549–1555, 1999.
134. Morris RG, Sallustio BC, Vinks AA, et al. Some international approaches to aminoglycoside monitoring in the extended dosing interval era. Ther Drug Monit 21:379–388, 1999.
135. Nicolau DP, Wu AH, Finocchiaro S, et al. Once-daily aminoglycoside dosing: impact on requests and costs for therapeutic drug monitoring. Ther Drug Monit 18:263–266, 1996.
136. Tarng DC, Wei YH, Huang TP, et al. Intravenous ascorbic acid as an adjuvant therapy for recombinant erythropoietin in hemodialysis patients with hyperferritinemia. Kidney Int 55:2477–2486, 1999.
137. Benigni A, Remuzzi G. Endothelin antagonists. Lancet 353:133–138, 1999.
138. Wolf SC, Brehm BR, Gaschler F, et al. Protective effects of endothelin antagonists in chronic renal failure. Nephrol Dial Transplant 14:S29–S30, 1999.
139. Pereira BJ, Burkart JM, Parker TM. Strategies for influencing outcomes in pre-ESRD and ESRD patients: summary and recommendations. Am J Kidney Dis 32(6 Suppl 4):S2–S4, 1998.
140. Obrador GT, Ruthazer R, Arora P, et al. Prevalence of and factors associated with suboptimal care before the initiation of dialysis in the United States. J Am Soc Nephrol 10:1793–1800, 1999.
141. Ritz E, Koch M, Fliser D, et al. How can we improve prognosis in diabetic patients with end-stage renal disease? Diabetes Care (Suppl 2):B80–83, 1999.
142. Obrador GT, Pereira BJ. Early referral to the nephrologist and timely initation of renal replacement therapy: a paradigm shift in the management of patients with chronic renal disease. Am J Kidney Dis 31:398–417, 1998.
143. Rodby RA, Firth LM, Lewis EJ. An economic analysis of captopril in the treatment of diabetic nephropathy. Diabetes Care 19:1051–1061, 1996.
144. Driver PS. Cost-effectiveness impact of iron dextran on hemodialysis patients' use of epoetin alfa and blood. Am J Health Syst Pharm 55:S12–S16, 1998.
145. Macdougall IC, Chandler G, Elston O, et al. Beneficial effects of adopting an aggressive intravenous iron policy in a hemodialysis unit. Am J Kidney Dis 34:S40–S46, 1999.
146. Kaufman JS. Subcutaneous erythropoietin therapy: efficacy and economic implications. Am J Kidney Dis 32:S147–S151, 1998.

CHAPTER 23

DIALYTIC AND PHARMACOTHERAPY FOR END-STAGE RENAL DISEASE

Gary R. Matzke and Winnie M. Yu

End-stage renal disease (ESRD) may result from primary injury to the nephron or develop secondary to systemic diseases such as diabetes mellitus, hypertension, and certain autoimmune disorders (e.g., systemic lupus erythematosus). Intrarenal diseases (e.g., polycystic kidney disease, primary glomerulonephritis), or postrenal factors (e.g., ureteral obstruction and neoplasm) account for approximately 20% of cases. Exposure to toxic substances (e.g., amphotericin B, aminoglycosides, compound analgesics) is a rare cause of ESRD. As renal function declines to less than 10 to 15% of normal, accumulation of nitrogenous wastes and other toxins leads to uremia, which is clinically defined as symptomatic renal failure.[1] These uremic signs and symptoms encompass myriad complications affecting most major organ systems, including the cardiovascular, pulmonary, neuromuscular, and central nervous systems.[1,2] If the patient does not receive a kidney transplant, dialysis becomes necessary to sustain life.

TREATMENT GOALS: END-STAGE RENAL DISEASE

- Extend the patient's remaining life span to age-normalized values observed in the general population and enhance his or her quality of life.
- Treat co-existing medical conditions such as diabetes mellitus and coronary artery disease.
- Treat conditions associated with ESRD, including anemia, hypertension, hyperlipidemia, metabolic acidosis, malnutrition, and renal osteodystrophy.
- Reverse the symptoms of uremia.
- Maintain adequate nutritional status.

- Minimize patient inconvenience.
- Optimize compliance with the complicated pharmacotherapeutic regimens.
- Facilitate physical and economic rehabilitation (i.e., return to work).

EPIDEMIOLOGY

In the last decade, the number of patients with ESRD has increased at an annual rate of 6 to 7%.[3] Despite advances in treating chronic renal failure, ESRD remains a major cause of morbidity and mortality in the United States. The life expectancy of people 45 to 49 years old is 28 to 36 years in the general U.S. population and 5 to 7 years in those with ESRD. The United States Renal Data System (USRDS), a national database of all Medicare-treated patients with ESRD, has facilitated the characterization of the ESRD population and provides a means to monitor trends in treatment outcomes in this population.[4] In 1996, more than 283,000 patients were treated for ESRD under the Medicare program and 73,901 new patients began ESRD treatment. The prevalence and incidence rates increase with age and reach a peak at age 65 to 69 and age 70 to 74 years, respectively. The incidence of ESRD is three times higher in blacks than in whites in the United States.[5] Cardiac events are the most common cause of death in patients with ESRD, accounting for 50% of the reported cases. Infection is the second most common cause and is more prevalent in younger, female, and black patients than in older, male, and white patients.[6] The economic burden of ESRD in the United States is estimated to exceed $14.5 billion per year, or about $43,500 for each patient with ESRD per year. With the increasing incidence and health care expenditures on ESRD, improving the outcomes and quality of care of patients with ESRD is a major national priority.[7] Because patients on hemodialysis used a median of 8 different medications in 1996 and more than 34% of the patients were prescribed 10 or more medications, the potential role of pharmacists in the care of this growing population is significant.[8] This chapter discusses the causes of ESRD and available therapeutic options, the principles of various dialysis modalities, pharmacotherapeutic issues in treating patients with ESRD, and drug dosing considerations.

ESRD can be caused by an acute irreversible insult to the kidney, a primary kidney disease, or a systemic illness. In the last few years, the number of new ESRD cases caused by diabetes mellitus has increased significantly; diabetes mellitus is the most common cause of ESRD, accounting for 39.2% of all new cases.[5] Hypertension accounts for about 28% of all cases, and it is a predominant cause of ESRD in African Americans. Other causes include glomerulonephritis, interstitial nephritis, and cystic kidney disease (Fig. 23.1).

THERAPEUTIC ALTERNATIVES

The kidneys are involved not only in water and electrolyte homeostasis, but also in the production and metabolism of many peptide hormones, including insulin, erythropoietin, parathyroid hormone (PTH), and 1,25-dihydroxyvitamin D_3 (calcitriol). Therefore, dialysis can never completely replace normal renal function or return the patient to a normal state of health. At best, dialysis provides waste removal that is equivalent to a glomerular filtration rate (GFR) of 10 to 20 mL/minute without compensating for the endocrine and metabolic activities of the kidney.[9] Dialysis is used to remove toxic metabolites, electrolytes, and large quantities of accumulated fluid in order to avoid volume overload, correct acid-base balance, and prevent congestive heart failure and pulmonary edema. The ultimate goals of dialysis are to improve quality of life and decrease morbidity and mortality.[9] Although dialysis therapy prolongs patient survival, morbidity and mortality rates remain high, partly because of the number of complications associated with available modalities.

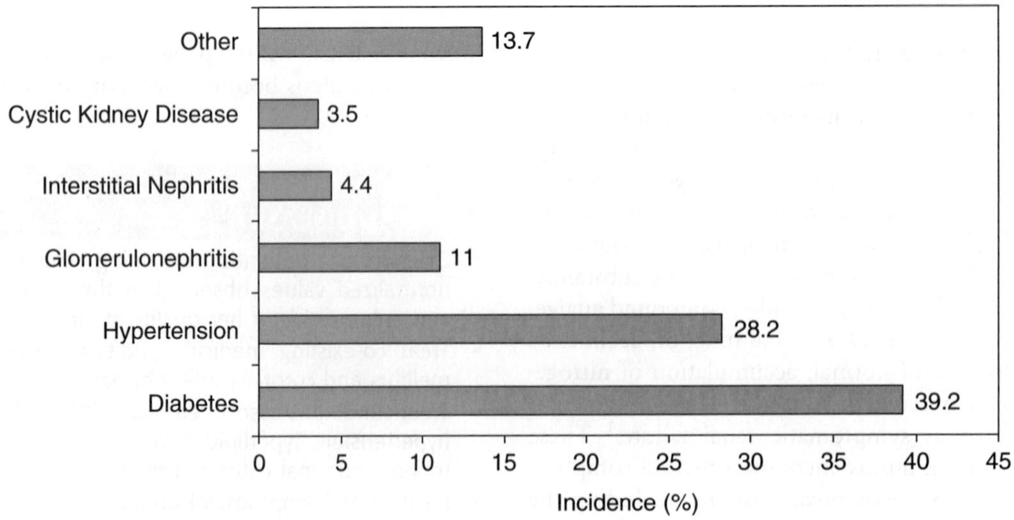

Figure 23.1. Primary diagnoses of end-stage renal disease. (Data from The United States Renal Data System, Reference 3.)

The three forms of renal replacement therapy available to patients with ESRD are renal transplantation, hemodialysis, and peritoneal dialysis. Despite its high initial cost, transplantation is the treatment of choice because of its favorable cost and outcomes.[10,11] However, the long waiting time for cadaveric organs, the presence of medically disqualifying comorbid conditions, and an overall low transplantation rate indicate that dialysis will remain the primary mode of renal replacement therapy for the near future.[12] According to the USRDS, 62.6% of all patients with ESRD received in-center hemodialysis, 28.2% had a functioning renal transplant, and 8.7% received peritoneal dialysis in 1997.[13] Dialysis therapy is by no means standardized. Choices of vascular access, peritoneal catheters, heparin dosing, dialyzers, dialysis machines, dialysate composition, and base buffers vary among centers. The choice of renal replacement modality also varies greatly between countries.[14]

The use of home hemodialysis and peritoneal dialysis, which some prefer over in-center hemodialysis, has decreased during the 1990s in most countries.[14] The percentage of patients with ESRD receiving home hemodialysis ranges from 1.0% in the United States and Japan to 18% in New Zealand; for peritoneal dialysis the range is from 5% in Japan, Uruguay, and Chile to 79% in Hong Kong. Transplantation offers patients the greatest likelihood of a return to their pre-ESRD lifestyle. The percentage of patients with a functioning transplant, which ranges from 20% or less in Chile and Uruguay to 73% in Ireland, is influenced by cultural, legal, and socioeconomic factors.

UREMIC TOXINS

The constellation of signs and symptoms associated with uremia has been attributed in part to the accumulation of compounds that are collectively labeled uremic toxins. These toxins include well-known molecules such as hydrogen ion, inorganic phosphorus, potassium, and several small (300 to 500 Da) and middle-molecular-weight (1500 to 5000 Da) substances.[15] Nearly all potential uremic toxins are products of protein metabolism.[15] However, a cause-and-effect relationship between these compounds and the clinical manifestations of uremia has not been established clearly. Nonetheless, throughout the history of renal replacement therapy, the dialysis prescription has been based on the removal of these "uremic toxins."

The ideal marker of uremia has the following characteristics: It accumulates in renal failure, it is removable by dialysis, it has proven toxicity, its production and elimination are representative of other potential toxins, it demonstrates a concentration-dependent clinical outcome, and it is easily measured in blood, urine, and dialysate.[15] Not surprisingly, no marker meets all these criteria. Given the lack of an ideal uremic marker, a combination of several markers together with clinical signs and symptoms is used to monitor patients on dialysis.[16]

Urea or blood urea nitrogen (BUN) is the prototypic marker of protein intake and small solute uremic toxins.[17] It is easy to measure and is the only solute for which the concentration has been correlated with outcome.[18] Because a patient with low BUN concentration may be severely undernourished or underdialyzed (i.e., receiving inadequate hemodialysis), one cannot predict patients' uremic status by BUN levels alone.

Middle molecules, such as vitamin B_{12}, have been used as a marker of middle molecular solute clearance. Although perhaps not as important as small solutes, middle molecules are important in the development of dialysis-related complications such as arthropathy and malnutrition.[19] Other potential uremic toxins include PTH and β_2 microglobulin.

Transplantation

INDICATIONS AND PATIENT EVALUATION

Numerous factors must be considered before it can be determined that transplantation is the optimal ESRD treatment for a given patient.[20,21] The initial assessment focuses on the overall health status of the patient and his or her physiologic and chronologic age. Patients with severe pulmonary disease, diabetes mellitus, or obesity often are poor surgical candidates.[22] Although immunosuppression may increase the risk of cancer recurrence or life-threatening infections, a history of either of these entities should not preclude renal transplantation. The only exceptions to this are dialysis-related peritonitis in the month preceding transplantation and documented human immunodeficiency virus infection. The risk of cardiovascular and cerebrovascular events such as ischemic heart disease and transient ischemic attacks increases after transplantation. Therefore, pharmacologic or surgical therapy may be initiated before transplant to minimize subsequent risk. Psychosocial, urologic, and gastrointestinal (GI) assessments, as well as blood and tissue typing, are considered important parts of the evaluation of renal transplant candidates.[21]

Once it is determined that a patient has ESRD and does not have any contraindications to transplantation, living donors, related and unrelated, should be screened.[23] Living donor (LD) transplantation provides superior patient and graft survival and can dramatically reduce the waiting time, which exceeds 2 years for a cadaveric kidney.[24]

ACCESS TO TRANSPLANTATION

In addition to the limited supply of cadaveric organs, a number of factors reduce the likelihood that a patient will receive a transplant. Medical suitability is a limiting factor for many older patients. Patients with historically lower medical use rates (e.g., racial and ethnic minorities, those with lower educational levels, and the poor) are less likely to be evaluated prospectively and listed for transplant before they are in imminent need of dialysis.[25]

Pediatric patients (0 to 19 years of age) are most likely to receive a kidney transplant,[24] but as a group they receive only 6.0% of the total number of primary transplants. Patients between 51 and 65 years old are the least likely to receive an LD or cadaveric donor transplant. According to the latest USRDS data, the primary transplantation rate in all three recipient age groups has declined dramatically.[24] Rates fell by 38.5% in 0- to 19-year-olds, 29.6% in 20- to 24-year-olds, and 15.5% in 45- to 64-year-olds. However, repeat cadaveric transplantation rates have remained consistent for all but the youngest patients.

Male patients are more likely than female patients to receive a primary cadaveric transplant, and they have a higher percentage of functioning transplants (30.8 versus 24.8%).[24] Blacks of either gender had markedly lower transplantation rates during 1994–97 than non-Blacks among those more than 20 years old. Although graft survival rates in Blacks were significantly lower in the late 1980s, these differences have diminished, and as of 1996 the LD and cadaveric 1-year survival rates are similar: 93.5 versus 94.1% (Blacks versus Caucasians) and 86.6 versus 88.9%, respectively. The lower transplantation rate and poor graft survival earlier in the decade contributed to the finding that in 1997 only 15.6% of black patients with ESRD had a functioning transplant, compared with 28% of non-Blacks.[13]

Primary ESRD diagnosis seems to have a dramatic effect on renal transplantation outcome. Only a small percentage of patients with diabetes and hypertension had functioning transplants in 1997 (17.9 and 16.3%, respectively). In stark contrast, 44.6 and 50.6% of patients with glomerulonephritis and cystic kidney disease had functioning transplants.[13] Physicians must consider these findings as they evaluate patients as potential transplant recipients. Because of the growing disparity between the number of patients on the waiting list and the number of transplants performed annually between 1988 and 1997, the waiting period for transplantation has increased. This finding has serious implications for patient morbidity, mortality, and quality of life and increases the cost of ESRD care.

ECONOMICS

Annual costs for ESRD treatment are lowest in the young ($23,000 per person per year for ages 0 to 19) and steadily rise to $57,000 per person per year for those 75 years of age and older.[11] Medicare payments for transplant recipients in all age groups were markedly less ($14,000 to 23,000 per person per year). These costs exclude the one-time donor acquisition payment of $25,000, which is paid by Medicare. Even when this additional cost is factored in, transplantation becomes the most cost-effective ESRD therapy for patients of all ages within 1 year. Although these data suggest that transplantation is the most cost-effective therapy, the complications of chronic immunosuppression (e.g., hypertension, hyperlipidemia, fluid retention, gout, and increased risk of infection) may markedly reduce a patient's quality of life and dramatically increase total Medicare expenditures.[26]

Dialysis

PRINCIPLES

Despite continuous modifications in the biotechnology of dialysis, the basic principles of hemodialysis and peritoneal dialysis have remained unchanged since they were introduced more than 50 years ago. The three basic components of a hemodialysis system are a blood compartment, a dialysate compartment, and a semipermeable membrane that separates the blood and dialysate compartments. Fundamentally, hemodialysis consists of the perfusion of heparinized blood and physiologic salt solution (i.e., dialysate) on opposite sides of a semipermeable membrane. The waste products of protein metabolism and other toxins move from the blood compartment into the dialysate by passive diffusion along concentration gradients (Fig. 23.2).[27] Conversely, if a substance is present in the dialysate in a higher concentration than in the blood (e.g., bicarbonate), this solute will diffuse from the dialysate into the systemic circulation.

The second process that occurs during dialysis is ultrafiltration, which is the movement of water and nonprotein plasma component down the hydrostatic pressure gradient from the blood into the dialysate. This is the primary mode for removal of excess body fluids. Ultrafiltration (expressed in mL/hr/mm Hg) can be maximized by increasing the hydrostatic pressure gradient (mm Hg) across the dialysis membrane. The amount of fluid removed during a dialysis session depends on the ultrafiltration coefficient of the dialysis filter (Table 23.1). Through trial and error, a post-dialysis target weight is determined for every patient, such that 0 to 5 kg typically is removed during each dialysis session. If a patient needs a large amount of fluid removal during each dialysis session, a dialyzer with a larger ultrafiltration coefficient is most appropriate.

Diffusion and ultrafiltration usually occur simultaneously during standard hemodialysis procedures. However, for selected patients these two processes may be performed in sequence. This form of sequential hemodialysis therapy is particularly beneficial for patients who have extensive fluid gains between dialysis periods, as well as for patients with poor cardiac function who are unable to tolerate simultaneous, extensive ultrafiltration.[28] With sequential dialysis, some patients may tolerate removal of as much as 4 L fluid per hour. The primary problem of long-term sequential dialysis treatment is that the reduced diffusion time may not allow adequate removal of uremic waste products.

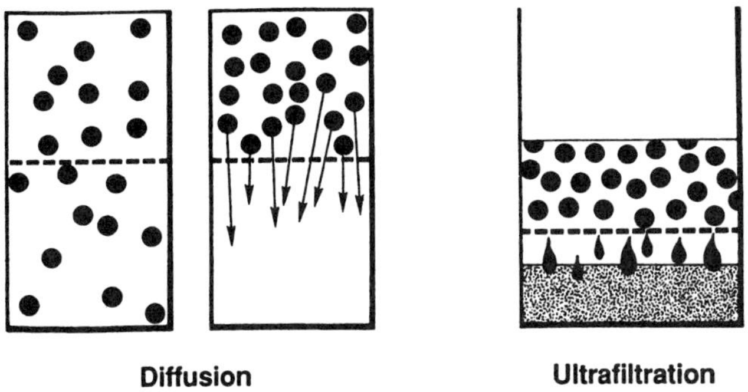

Figure 23.2. Diffusion and ultrafiltration. Diffusion of endogenous solutes from the blood to the dialysate *(left panel)* is limited by the pore size of the membrane *(dashed line)*, the molecular size of the solute, and the time that the dialysate fluid is in contact with the blood. Ultrafiltration *(right panel)* is the removal of plasma water with or without the accompaniment of solute. The limiting processes for water removal are the amount of pressure the membrane can tolerate without rupturing and the pressure difference across the membrane.

The three principles of dialysis also apply to peritoneal dialysis. Like hemodialysis, dialysis across the peritoneal membrane consists of diffusion and ultrafiltration.[29] Diffusion occurs from the blood to the dialysate or from the dialysate to the blood, depending on the concentration gradient for the particular substance (Fig. 23.2). The degree of diffusion is critically influenced by the thickness of the peritoneal membrane, the effective surface area of the membrane that is exposed to the dialysate, the peritoneal capillary blood flow, the dialysate flow rate, the volume of instilled dialysate, and the temperature of the dialysate.[29,30]

With hemodialysis, the membrane that separates the blood from the dialysate compartment can be selected to attain the optimal diffusion and ultrafiltration goals. In contrast with peritoneal dialysis, only one membrane is available per patient. Ultrafiltration during peritoneal dialysis can be enhanced by changing the dextrose concentration in the dialysate. An increase in dextrose concentration increases the osmolality of the peritoneal compartment, resulting in an increase in fluid removal.

INDICATIONS FOR DIALYSIS

The indications for dialysis are different in patients with acute or chronic renal failure. When a patient presents with severe metabolic acidosis, life-threatening electrolyte abnormalities, refractory volume overload, or symptoms of uremia, initiation of dialysis therapy is warranted to sustain life and prevent worsening of the condition (Table 23.2). The criteria for initiation of dialysis in patients with chronic renal failure are less well defined. Although chronic dialysis therapy is expensive and is associated with

Table 23.1 ▪ Characteristics of Frequently Used Dialyzers

Manufacturer and Model	Membrane	Surface Area (m^2)	Ultrafiltration Coefficient (mL/hr/mm Hg)	Clearance (Q_b = 200 mL/min) Urea	Clearance (Q_b = 200 mL/min) Vitamin B_{12}
Hollow fiber					
Baxter					
CT 110G	CTA	1.1	22	185	109
CT 190G	CTA	1.9	36	192	137
Fresenius					
Hemoflow F 40	PS	0.7	20	165	75
Hemoflow F 60	PS	1.25	40	185	115
Toray					
B3-2.0A	PMMA	2.0	11	190	100
BK-2.1U	PMMA	2.1	19	194	125
Parallel-plate (flat plate)					
Gambro					
Lundia IC-3H	CU	0.8	5.2	159	43
Lundia IC-6N	CU	1.6	9	182	63
Hospal					
1800-S	AN69	0.7	30	145	55
3000-S	AN69	1.2	50	180	80

CTA, cellulose triacetate; *PS*, polysulfone; *PMMA*, polymethylmethacrylate; *CU*, cuprophane; *AN69*, polyacrylonitrile.

Table 23.2 ▪ Indications for Dialysis

Absolute Indications	Conditions
Acidosis	Metabolic acidosis
Electrolyte abnormalities	Hyperkalemia
Overload	Refractory hypertension, congestive heart failure
Uremia	Uremic encephalopathy Blood urea nitrogen >100 mg/dL Serum creatinine >12 mg/dL in a nonedematous patient >70 kg
Miscellaneous	Bleeding diathesis Pericarditis

Relative Indications	Conditions
Nutritional	Anorexia, nausea and vomiting, unexplained weight loss, altered biochemical indices (e.g., falling albumin, prealbumin, transferrin), decreased fat-free edema-free body mass, falling caloric or protein intake by history
Neurologic	Lethargy, decreased mentation, peripheral neuropathy, change in sleep–wake cycle, restless leg syndrome
Dermatologic	Pruritus

numerous complications, late initiation of dialysis therapy is associated with high rates of mortality and hospitalization.[31] Therefore, appropriate timing for initiation of dialysis therapy should be based on a global assessment of the subjective and objective signs of renal failure. The goal of therapy should be improvement of the patient's well-being and quality of life.[32] Elevated serum creatinine alone is an unreliable indicator for dialysis because creatinine concentrations may be only moderately elevated in some patients because of a loss of somatic mass secondary to a reduction in physical activity and dietary intake.[33] Therefore, it should be used only as supportive evidence in conjunction with other indices of uremia. Because progression of renal disease is associated with spontaneous reduction in dietary protein intake, malnutrition should be used as an early sign of uremia.[32] Patients with anorexia, unexplained weight loss, or falling nutritional indices such as albumin, prealbumin, or transferrin should receive dietary counseling, and initiation of dialysis should be planned. In particular, early dialysis and aggressive nutritional support may be indicated in patients with diabetic nephropathy and gastroparesis because they may experience a more rapid decline in the renal function and are more susceptible to malnutrition. Abnormal neurologic findings and persistent pruritus also suggest worsening uremia. According to the National Kidney Foundation's Dialysis Outcomes Qualitative Initiative (NKF-DOQI) guidelines, hemodialysis should be started in nondiabetic patients who have one or more of the signs and symptoms just described when their creatinine clearance is 9 mL/minute/1.73 m^2. In patients with diabetes mellitus, dialysis should be initiated earlier (i.e., when creatinine clearance is between 9 and 14 mL/min/1.73 m^2).[34]

Preparations for initiation of dialysis should begin before the patient's GFR drops below 25 mL/minute. Treatment options should be discussed with the patient. It may be beneficial for the patient to visit a hemodialysis unit and talk with other patients who are undergoing hemodialysis or those who have undergone renal transplantation. Videotapes and reading materials are available to inform patients about their disease, its progress, and the various treatment options.

CHOICE OF DIALYTIC MODALITY

The choice of one dialysis method over another depends on several personal, medical, economic, and psychosocial factors. However, in certain situations the patient may not have a choice in selecting a mode of renal replacement therapy. For example, if a patient has lost all viable vascular sites for an arteriovenous fistula, continuous ambulatory peritoneal dialysis (CAPD) is the only choice. Similarly, hemodialysis may be the only remaining choice for a patient on CAPD who has lost ultrafiltration capacity because of extensive peritoneal fibrosis.

Which Method in Which Condition?

The answer to this question depends on the effect of hemodialysis and CAPD on several aspects of morbidity and mortality. In many clinical situations the use of peritoneal dialysis is preferred to hemodialysis (Table 23.3).[35,36] Because the hemodialysis procedure routinely entails the use of heparin to prevent fistula clotting, CAPD is more suitable for a patient with bleeding diathesis. Similarly, the rapid removal of fluid and electrolytes during hemodialysis stresses the heart to an extent that a patient with coronary artery disease may not be able to tolerate. Therefore, such patients may benefit from the slow and continuous nature of CAPD.[29]

Ease of Blood Pressure Control

Treating hypertension in patients with ESRD is difficult and often involves multiple drugs. Because of its slow correction and more stable control of sodium and water balance, hypertension management is easier in CAPD than in hemodialysis. In fact, a significant number of patients on CAPD may not need antihypertensive drugs.[35,36]

Slow and Sustained Ultrafiltration

Rapid fluid removal during a typical thrice-weekly hemodialysis session causes intravascular fluid volume depletion and can lead to hypotension. In predisposed patients, sustained hypotension may lead to complications of ischemic vascular disease, such as stroke and myocardial infarction.[35] Because of its slower rate of ultrafiltration and minimal risk of hypotension, patients with severe cardiovascular disease (e.g., diabetics) may benefit from CAPD.[35,37,38]

Preservation of Residual Renal Function

Residual renal function, even at low levels,has significant clinical importance, including a substantial contribution to the removal of small solutes and middle molecules.[39,40] In addition, the increased removal of sodium, potassium, phosphate, and hydrogen ions allows a less restrictive fluid and dietary intake.[35,40] Patients on CAPD tend to preserve their residual renal function for a longer period than patients on hemodialysis do.[40] This may be because of better removal of toxins involved in residual nephron damage, preservation or enhancement of growth factors that are beneficial to the maintenance of GFR and renal blood flow, less ischemic injury to the kidneys because of a more stable hemodynamic status,[16] and lack of membrane-induced inflammatory changes (e.g., production of tumor necrosis factor and interleukin-1), which may cause vascular or immunologic renal injury.[35]

Because residual renal function is preserved longer, CAPD is recommended for patients who have uncontrolled hypertension, heart failure, severe nephrotic syndrome, rapidly progressive renal failure, analgesic nephropathy, chronic urinary obstruction, and cholesterol emboli.[40]

Table 23.3 ▪ Potential Advantages and Disadvantages of Continuous Ambulatory Peritoneal Dialysis Compared to Standard Hemodialysis

Advantages	Disadvantages
Steady-state biochemical parameters	Excessive glucose load
Hemodynamic stability (slow and sustained ultrafiltration)	Continued need for sterile exchange
Better removal of larger molecules (e.g., β_2-microglobulin	Requires patient motivation for compliance
Better preservation of residual renal function	Higher protein loss
No need for heparin	Peritonitis
Lesser degree of anemia	Increased intraabdominal pressure
Lower serum parathyroid hormone concentration	Higher mortality among older (>40 yr) diabetic patients
Lower incidence of high-turnover bone disease	
Higher aluminum clearance	
Lower mortality among younger (≤40 yr) diabetic patients	
Possibly better among older nondiabetic patients	
Easier access for dialysis	
No machine dependence	
Allows long-distance travel	
Allows uninterrupted employment and social activities	
Better glycemic control with intraperitoneal insulin	

Effect on Anemia

Virtually all patients with ESRD develop a normocytic, normochromic anemia. Without treatment, the hematocrit (Hct) stabilizes between 20 and 25%. Causes include reduced erythropoietin (EPO) synthesis by the kidneys, decreased red blood cell survival, GI bleeding, presence of inhibitors of erythropoiesis (e.g., aluminum, PTH), and blood loss caused by hemodialysis.[41] Historically, patients on hemodialysis were more anemic and had a higher blood transfusion requirement than patients on CAPD.[41] Patients on CAPD have higher EPO concentrations because of higher clearance of uremic toxins, which may inhibit EPO production; EPO production by stimulated peritoneal macrophages (caused by infusion of dialysate); and better preservation of residual renal function.[40,41] Thus, EPO dosage needs are lower and the maintenance of target Hct values generally is easier in patients on CAPD.

Effect on Mineral Metabolism and Renal Bone Disease

Hyperphosphatemia, hyperparathyroidism, hypocalcemia, and vitamin D resistance are common in chronic renal failure and can lead to secondary complications such as renal osteodystrophy (i.e., defective bone formation), myocardial calcification, and myocardial fibrosis. Chronic renal failure is associated with two predominant types of bone disease: high-turnover disease, characterized by fibrous tissues in the bone marrow, and low-turnover disease, characterized by reduced osteoblastic activity.[42,43] Hyperparathyroidism, also known as osteitis fibrosa cystica, is the main cause of high-turnover bone disease, although metabolic acidosis may cause or worsen the condition. The major cause of low-turnover bone disease is excessive suppression of PTH as the result of aggressive vitamin D therapy.[42]

Compared to patients on hemodialysis, patients on CAPD have a lower incidence of high-turnover bone disease. This may be because CAPD has a higher clearance of PTH and because, with CAPD, the serum ionized calcium increases because of absorption of calcium from the peritoneal dialysate; therefore, the risk of hypocalcemia-induced stimulation of PTH secretion is reduced with CAPD. Given the potential cardiotoxicity of PTH,[44] the lower serum PTH concentration associated with CAPD provides a theoretical advantage over hemodialysis.

Choice for Patients with Diabetes

Diabetic patients who are on dialysis often have a worse prognosis than nondiabetic patients, so kidney transplantation is clearly the preferred mode of renal replacement therapy.[35] These patients often start on dialysis with advanced comorbid conditions (e.g., coronary artery disease), which often progress during the course of dialysis. Furthermore, because younger diabetic patients with minimal comorbid conditions often are selected for transplantation, the remaining patients on dialysis have advanced coexisting conditions that increase the incidence of mortality.[35] Therefore, it is not surprising that diabetic patients need a higher dosage of dialysis than do nondiabetic patients.[45]

Among the benefits of CAPD for diabetic patients is the ability to administer insulin intraperitoneally. The bioavailability of intraperitoneal insulin is approximately 50% after an 8-hour dwell time. Intraperitoneal insulin diffuses across the visceral peritoneum into the portal venous circulation. Within the liver, insulin inhibits glycogenolysis, gluconeogenesis, and ketogenesis and stimulates glycogen and fatty acid synthesis.[35,46] This absorption profile allows better glycemic control and a lower risk of hypoglycemia, possibly because of the presence of a basal insulin concentration.[35] For a given insulin dosage, intraperitoneal administration produces lower serum insulin concentrations than subcutaneous insulin does; however, intraperitoneal administration allows more rapid, consistent, and physiologic absorption of insulin. The lower serum concentrations resulting from intraperitoneal insulin administration may be important in view of the increasing evidence implicating hyperinsulinemia as an atherogenic risk factor.[35]

Technique Failure

Peritonitis is the most common cause of technique failure with CAPD, accounting for 40 to 47% of cases. Loss of peritoneal function (15 to 19%) and access-related problems (9 to 15%) are other common causes of dropouts. The most common causes of technique failure with hemodialysis are cardiovascular instability and loss of vascular access. The method failure rate is higher with CAPD; however, if peritonitis is removed as a cause, the failure rates are similar.[46]

Mortality

In general, mortality rates with CAPD and hemodialysis are similar.[47–51] Older diabetic patients treated with CAPD appear to have a higher mortality rate than patients treated with hemodialysis.[51] Because the use of biocompatible hemodialysis membranes may result in lower mortality rates, their recent popularity may translate in a few years to a lowered hemodialysis mortality rate.

HEMODIALYSIS

Principles

Effective dialysis entails convective bulk fluid removal, ultrafiltration, and diffusion of toxic materials down a concentration gradient from blood to dialysate. Convection is the process by which solutes are lost during ultrafiltration. Ultrafiltration depends on the difference in blood and dialysate transmembrane colloid osmotic pressure, membrane permeability, and blood dilution.[16] The use of high dialysate and blood flow rates with high-flux (larger-pore) and high-efficiency (larger surface area) dialyzers has necessitated precise ultrafiltration control systems to avoid excessive fluid loss, dehydration, and hypotension.[52,53]

Vascular Access

Dialysis access can be achieved at the bedside by insertion of a catheter into the internal jugular, femoral, or subclavian vein. Significant complications can occur with these initial temporary access devices, including venous thrombosis, emboli, and infection.[54] Permanent vascular access for hemodialysis may be accomplished by several techniques.[55] The simple arteriovenous fistula has the longest survival of all blood access devices and the lowest complication rate. An arteriovenous fistula is formed by surgical anastomosis of an artery and a vein that allows access to the circulation by skin puncture. Polytetrafluoroethylene (PTFE) grafts are extensively used for chronic dialysis access, especially when fistula placement is unsuccessful or not feasible. The choice of a blood access device depends primarily on how soon the patient needs dialysis and the adequacy of the patient's vascular system.[56] An arteriovenous fistula must be placed 1 to 2 months before hemodialysis is initiated to allow proper healing and maturation of the fistula. In contrast, a PTFE graft may be used within 2 weeks of surgery.

Dialyzers

In recent years, numerous hemodialyzers have become available.[27,57] Two basic forms of dialyzers, the hollow fiber dialyzer and the flat plate dialyzer, now predominate (Table 23.1). Most dialysis centers use several types of dialyzers and select the optimal dialysis filter for the individual patient. For stable young patients without cardiac or bleeding problems, the dialyzer that has the highest clearance of urea and creatinine, the two primary uremic waste products, should be selected. For older patients, very small patients, and those with multiple medical complications, greater attention to individualization is needed.

The interaction of blood with the extracorporeal circuit has been viewed as a significant cause of morbidity and possibly mortality. This has led to the unofficial categorization of dialyzers as biocompatible or bioincompatible. Biocompatible membranes have a smaller effect on blood constituents (e.g., monocytes, macrophages, lymphocytes, and neutrophils) and do not cause some of the systemic reactions that arise from acute and chronic exposure to biocompatible dialyzers. Polysulfone, polyacrylonitrile, polymethylmethacrylate, polycarbonate, and polyamide membranes are examples of synthetic biocompatible membranes. Although most biocompatible membranes are also high-flux, such membranes may also have low to moderate ultrafiltration coefficients.[58]

A bioincompatible membrane (e.g., cuprophan and cellulose acetate) activates the complement system, suppresses the immune system, induces cytokine release, enhances production of β_2 microglobulin, and increases the risk of morbidity and possibly mortality.[58] As a result, such membranes may increase the risk of infection and malignancy, cause intradialytic cardiovascular instability, increase protein catabolism, and potentiate musculoskeletal effects of long-term hemodialysis.[58]

Technique

Hemodialysis consists of pumping the patient's heparinized blood through the blood compartment of the dialysis filter at a rate of 300 to 600 mL/minute (Fig. 23.3).[27,59] Generally, anticoagulation is achieved by infusing heparin continuously or intermittently into the blood line of the dialyzer. The dialysate is prepared from a commercially available concentrated liquid or dried salts and treated water. This fluid is warmed to body temperature and then perfused through the dialysate compartment of the dialysis filter. Although several types of hemodialysis machines are available, most of the current generation of dialysis machines provide precise volumetric fluid removal.

The duration of dialysis therapy has decreased steadily since the 1970s, from approximately 12 hours three times a week to 3 hours three times a week.[60] Recent advances in dialysis technology, including precise volumetric control systems and dialyzers with larger pores (high flux) and larger surface areas (high efficiency), have allowed the removal of the same amount of small solutes over a shorter period than is possible with cellulosic membranes.[52] However, inappropriately short dialysis sessions with low-flux biocompatible or incompatible dialyzers are associated with multiple complications.[61,62]

Adequacy of Hemodialysis

In the early years of hemodialysis, the dialysis prescription was not individualized and usually consisted of 4- to 5-hour sessions, thrice weekly, using blood flow rates of 200 to 300 mL/minute and a dialysate flow rate of 500 mL/minute. In the late 1980s and early 1990s, it became evident that inadequate dialysis was associated with an increase in the frequency of adverse clinical outcomes and high mortality rates.[52,63–65] In response to the widespread concern about underdialysis, a number of investigators attempted to quantitatively define adequate dialysis. Idealistically, adequate dialysis can be defined as the dosage of dialysis that returns the patient's lifestyle and life expectancy to what it would have been if he or she never had renal disease.[66] Clinically, it is the lowest dosage of dialysis needed to ensure good short-term (less than 5 years) outcomes (e.g., survival similar to that of transplant recipients), good quality of life, and reversal of signs and symptoms of uremia. Identification of underdialysis using clinical parameters is difficult because many of the signs and symptoms of morbid events are the same in adequately dialyzed patients as in underdialyzed patients.

In 1974, the National Institutes of Health (NIH) initiated the multicenter National Cooperative Dialysis Study (NCDS) to evaluate quantitative methods for prescribing hemodialysis therapy on an individualized

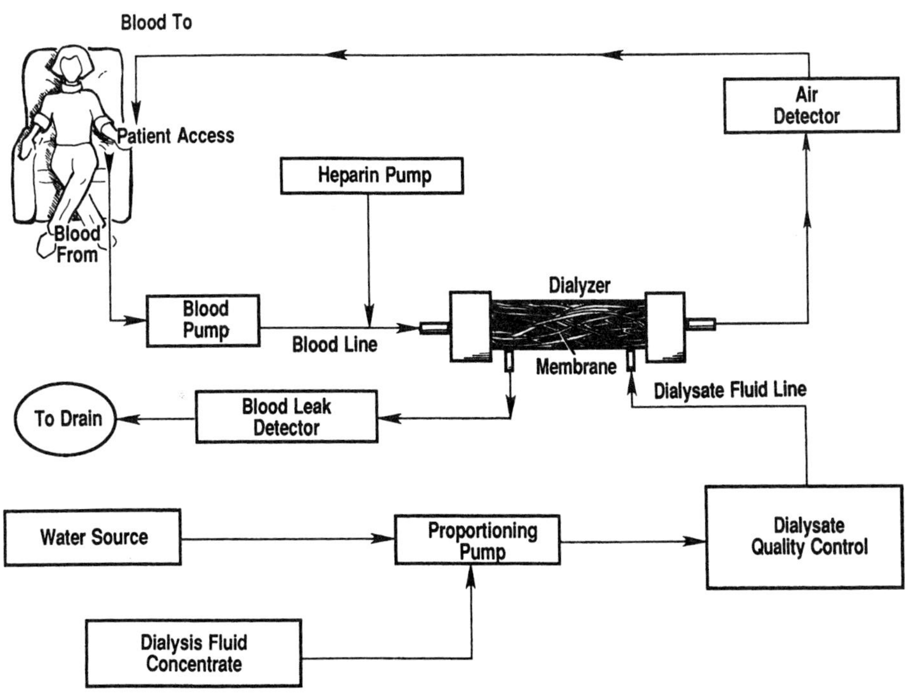

Figure 23.3. Outline of the blood flow and dialysate flow pathways during hemodialysis. Blood flows from the patient via the blood pump at rate of 200 to 500 mL/minute through the dialyzer and back to the patient. Heparin is administered into the blood line to prevent clotting in the dialyzer. The dialysate is a combination of dialysis fluid concentrate and water that is pumped at a rate of 500 to 800 mL/minute through the dialysate side of the dialyzer.

basis.[17] In this study of 151 patients, four treatment groups were divided according to two parameters: dialysis treatment time (2.5 to 3.5 hours versus 4.5 to 5.0 hours) and time-averaged BUN concentration or the area under the BUN curve divided by time (TAC, 20 to 50 mg/dL versus 50 to 100 mg/dL). BUN concentration was considered a surrogate marker for small molecules, and treatment time was considered a marker for middle molecules. However, because removal of middle molecules is also a function of membrane surface area and because different dialyzers were used in the study, treatment time was not an appropriate marker for dialysis of middle molecules.[67]

Patients in the low dialysis dosage group (TAC of 50 to 100 mg/dL) withdrew from the study for medical reasons at a significantly higher rate than did those in the high dialysis dosage group (TAC of 20 to 50 mg/dL). Hospitalization was also greater in the low dialysis dosage group. Although it was originally believed that dialysis treatment time would have no significant effect, a post hoc analysis of the NCDS's findings indicated that reducing the dialysis time increased the hospitalization rate by 181%, especially for patients who had received the low dosage of dialysis.[68] Indeed, the short-time (2.5 to 3.5 hours), low-dose group was discontinued early because a preliminary analysis indicated excessive hospitalization and medical withdrawal in this group. The results of this study revealed that four factors can affect outcome independently: BUN concentration (a higher TAC urea was associated with greater morbidity), protein catabolic rate (a lower PCR or dietary protein intake is associated with greater morbidity), the presence of comorbid conditions (which was associated with greater morbidity), and dialysis time (a shorter dialysis time is associated with greater morbidity).

In 1985, Gotch and Sargent,[69] in their reanalysis of the NCDS data, developed a means by which to quantify dialysis. Kt/V is a dimensionless parameter that takes into account dialyzer urea clearance (K), the duration of the dialysis procedure (t), and the patient's urea volume of distribution (V). This yields the prescribed fractional clearance of urea from total body water. The amount of delivered dialysis may be quantified by direct measurement of K, t, and V or approximated by using predialysis and postdialysis blood urea concentrations along with the change in the patient's weight: $Kt/V = -\ln(R - 0.008t) + [(4 - 3.5R)(UF/Weight_{post})]$, where R is the ratio of postdialysis BUN to predialysis BUN, t is the duration of dialysis in hours, and UF is the predialysis weight minus the postdialysis weight.[70] This equation takes into consideration the efficiency of the treatment as a function of the treatment time and the convective removal of urea in the ultrafiltrate (UF/Weight). Alternatively, urea kinetic modeling can be used to calculate Kt/V using a two-compartment model.

The fractional urea clearance during a single dialysis session may be approximated by calculating the urea reduction ratio: $URR = (BUN_{predialysis} - BUN_{postdialysis})$ divided by $BUN_{predialysis}$ multiplied by 100.[71] Therefore, URR is the percentage reduction in blood urea concentration during the course of one dialysis session. It offers the advantage of determining dialysis dosage independent of patient size, dialysis time, blood and dialysis flow rates, and dialyzer urea clearance. The relationship between Kt/V and URR is curvilinear,[72] such that to achieve a Kt/V of 1.0, 1.2, or 1.4, a URR of 58, 65, and 70%, respectively, would be needed.

Quantification of Delivered Dialysis Dosage

Ideally, the delivered dosage should be consistent with the prescribed dosage; however, calculation of the Kt/V parameters is associated with a multitude of errors because its individual components, K, t, and V, are all subject to inaccuracies that often lead to overestimation of the actual delivered dosage of dialysis. The delivered dosage of dialysis when accurately measured generally is 20 to 30% lower than the prescribed dosage.[73] Therefore, the actual amount of dialysis delivered must be measured and compared with the prescribed dosage.

Shortening dialysis times without monitoring adequacy closely by subjective and objective means may have deleterious consequences.[16] The reduction in dialysis times during the 1980s was correlated with an increased mortality rate among the U.S. hemodialysis population.[52,59] This increase probably was caused by the associated reduction in delivered dialysis dosage.[74] Indeed, patients dialyzed less than 3.5 hours had a higher mortality rate than do those who are dialyzed for longer periods.[61] Some investigators believe that dialysis time may be a predictor of mortality, independent of Kt/V.[63] In long-term, uncontrolled studies of patients who undergo dialysis for more than 10 years, survivors have consistently had longer dialysis times than did nonsurvivors.[52] The lower rates of ESRD morbidity and mortality in Europe and Japan may be related to longer dialysis times. Whereas the average weekly dialysis time in the United States is 9 hours, those in Europe and Japan are 12 hours and 15 hours, respectively.[59]

Dialyzer Reuse

Over the past 20 years, the number of centers in the United States reusing dialyzers increased from 18% to more than 70%.[75] With repeated dialyzer use, the effective clearance (K) is reduced. It is currently recommended that dialyzers be discarded once the volume of the dialyzer drops below 80% of the initial value. With reuse, there is also a small potential risk of death from sepsis caused by inadequate sterilization of the dialyzer.[62] However, dialysis reuse may be performed safely under the established sterilization guidelines of the Association for the Advancement of Medical Instrumentation. Therefore, the National Kidney Foundation Ad Hoc Committee on Reduction of Morbidity and Mortality in U.S. Maintenance Dialysis Patients concludes that when appropriately performed, dialyzer reuse is safe and decreases the cost of treatment, thus allowing the delivery of a larger dialysis dosage.[76] Furthermore, because protein film coats the membrane,[58] the reuse of cellulosic membranes has been associated with decreased intradialytic complement activation, which may reduce the incidence of certain intradialytic symptoms.[77]

The evaluation of dialysis adequacy must include all three parameters: BUN, PCR, and Kt/V (or URR). It is strongly emphasized that the goal of adequate dialysis is not only high urea removal, but also adequate dietary protein (i.e., at least 1.2 g/kg/day) and caloric intake (i.e., at least 35 kcal/kg/day). The adequacy of dialysis must be based on the dosage delivered rather than the dosage prescribed. The patient's residual renal function must be included in such an assessment to allow a more valid estimation of clearance values, and the dialysis dosage should be increased as residual renal function deadlines. A hemodialysis session should provide a minimum Kt/V of 1.2 (or URR of 60%); however, a Kt/V of 1.3 to 1.4 is recommended because further reductions in morbidity and mortality may be obtained past this threshold. Diabetic patients may respond better to even higher dosages.[78] According to one estimate, for every Kt/V increase of 0.1, there is a 7% reduction in mortality.[59]

Long-term prospective data about dialysis adequacy or optimization should be available shortly. The results of the NIH-sponsored hemodialysis (HEMO) study, which was initiated in 1995 and is due to be completed in 2001, should address this critical issue. This prospective randomized multicenter clinical trial was designed to compare the benefits of a high (Kt/V = 1.6) and conventional (Kt/V = 1.2) dialysis dosage in patients receiving hemodialysis with low- and high-flux dialyzers.[79] Until these data are available, patients should be monitored monthly for dialysis adequacy and protein calorie malnutrition (PCM). The monitoring should include edema-free postdialysis body weight and the serum concentrations of albumin and BUN. In addition, dietary intake should be monitored at least every 6 months. If the patient is underdialyzed, the dialysis time may be increased or the effective dialyzer clearance of urea may be increased by using a different dialyzer or higher blood or dialysate flow rates.

Complications

Cardiovascular Complications

Cardiovascular disease is the most common cause of mortality among the dialysis population, accounting for 50% of deaths.[80,81] Myocardial infarction, coronary artery disease, moderate to severe congestive heart failure, vascular stroke, and peripheral vascular disease are present in one-third or more of hemodialysis patients.[81] The presence of cardiovascular disease at the initiation of dialysis is an independent predictor of mortality.[44] The hemodialysis procedure per se is associated with both acute (e.g., hypotension, sudden death) and chronic (e.g., left ventricular hypertrophy, heart failure, coronary artery disease) cardiovascular complications.

Predisposing factors to chronic cardiovascular complications include predialytic hypertension, chronic anemia, hyperparathyroidism, volume overload, high-output cardiac failure, and dyslipoproteinemias.[81,82] Treatment strategies such as smoking cessation, correction of hypertension, and regular aerobic exercise may reduce the cardiovascular morbidity and mortality during chronic dialysis.[83] It is unclear, however, whether modifications of the common dyslipoproteinemias (e.g., hypertriglyceridemia) in patients with chronic renal failure and ESRD positively affect mortality rates.[84] Because myocardial calcification and fibrosis contribute to one-half of heart failure cases (especially diastolic dysfunction), control of calcium, phosphorus, vitamin D, and PTH abnormalities may help to prevent both cardiovascular and bone diseases.[80]

Left Ventricular Hypertrophy

The majority of patients on hemodialysis have left ventricular hypertrophy, which is the most important pathogenic factor in the development of diastolic dysfunction.[83] Because left ventricular hypertrophy often is associated with left atrial dilation, patients are at risk for development of atrial fibrillation. Indeed, left ventricular hypertrophy may be a risk factor for sudden death of patients on hemodialysis.[38,44] In contrast, the systolic function usually is normal or high. Patients on hemodialysis are often in a state of volume overload. Because of a decreased left ventricular distensibility, the left ventricular pressure is unusually high, predisposing the patient to pulmonary congestion and edema. During rapid intradialytic fluid removal, the left ventricular pressure is reduced rapidly, resulting in intradialytic hypotension; therefore, dialysis hypotension may signal the presence of left ventricular hypertrophy and a patient who is at risk for sudden death.[38,82] In patients with significant vascular disease (e.g., coronary, carotid, or peripheral artery diseases), prolonged hypotension leads to ischemic symptoms and possibly myocardial infarction and stroke.[35] In the absence of atrial fibrillation, positive inotropic drugs rarely are of value. Large and rapid changes in intravascular volume should be avoided during dialysis.[38] Ideally, hypertension and anemia should be treated aggressively before dialysis to reduce the degree of left ventricular hypertrophy.

Coronary Artery Disease

Coronary artery disease, which is common among patients on ESRD, can be exacerbated by intradialytic hypotension, which increases oxygen demand, and anemia of chronic renal failure, which increases myocardial oxygen demand and decreases supply. The balance of oxygen supply and demand also may be affected by the presence of an arteriovenous fistula. Arteriovenous fistulas with high flow rates may precipitate heart failure, even in the absence of coronary artery disease.[38] Treating anemia with EPO can reduce the left ventricular hypertrophy[85] and reduce myocardial ischemia.[86] For patients with significant coronary artery disease, CAPD may be preferred because of the absence of an arteriovenous fistula, adequately maintained left ventricular end-diastolic pressure (an important factor for myocardial perfusion), and absence of rapid volume shifts.[38]

Vascular Access Complications

Complications related to the vascular access (clotting and stenosis) are the leading cause of morbidity among patients on hemodialysis[54] and perhaps the major factor limiting continued use of hemodialysis.[87] Clotting of the arteriovenous fistula or graft may be amenable to pharmacotherapy[88] or surgical revision.[89]

Before the age of renal replacement therapy, infections were a major cause of death of patients with chronic renal failure.[90] In this era, infection is a major cause of morbidity and the second most common cause of mortality, accounting for 15 to 30% of all deaths among patients on dialysis. The costs associated with access infections have been estimated to exceed $1 billion annually.[91] Patients on dialysis are at an increased risk of infection for three main reasons: malnutrition, decreased immune function, and invasion of the skin and other integuments for the purpose of placing dialysis catheters and performing hemodialysis. Hemodialysis with a bioincompatible membrane can adversely affect the patient's immune system and serve as an additional risk factor for infection.[92] The use of biocompatible membranes is associated with as much as a 50% reduction in the incidence of infection.[91]

Staphylococcus aureus and *S. epidermidis* are the pathogens most often responsible for infection at the vascular access site, with or without associated bacteremia.[93] Patients are also at risk for developing pneumonia and urinary tract infection, in addition to infections caused by *Mycobacterium tuberculosis,* hepatitis A, hepatitis B, and hepatitis C.[90] Cefazolin, a first-generation cephalosporin, is the drug of choice for antibiotic prophylaxis before access placement. With the outbreak of vancomycin-resistant enterococcus (VRE) in hospitals and nursing homes and the increasing reports of VRE colonization in patients on dialysis, use of vancomycin for antibiotic prophylaxis is not recommended.[94] The optimal approach to manage an access infection depends on the type of access involved and the extent of the infection. Guidelines for optimum treatment have been recommended by the NKF-DOQI working group and are outlined in Figure 23.4.[95]

The nasal carriage of *S. aureus* has been identified as a risk factor for the development of infections (e.g., bacteremia) by this microorganism in patients on hemodialysis. At the time of initiation of hemodialysis, more than 40% of patients on hemodialysis are nasal carriers of *S. aureus*. Administering mupirocin 2% ointment (a topical

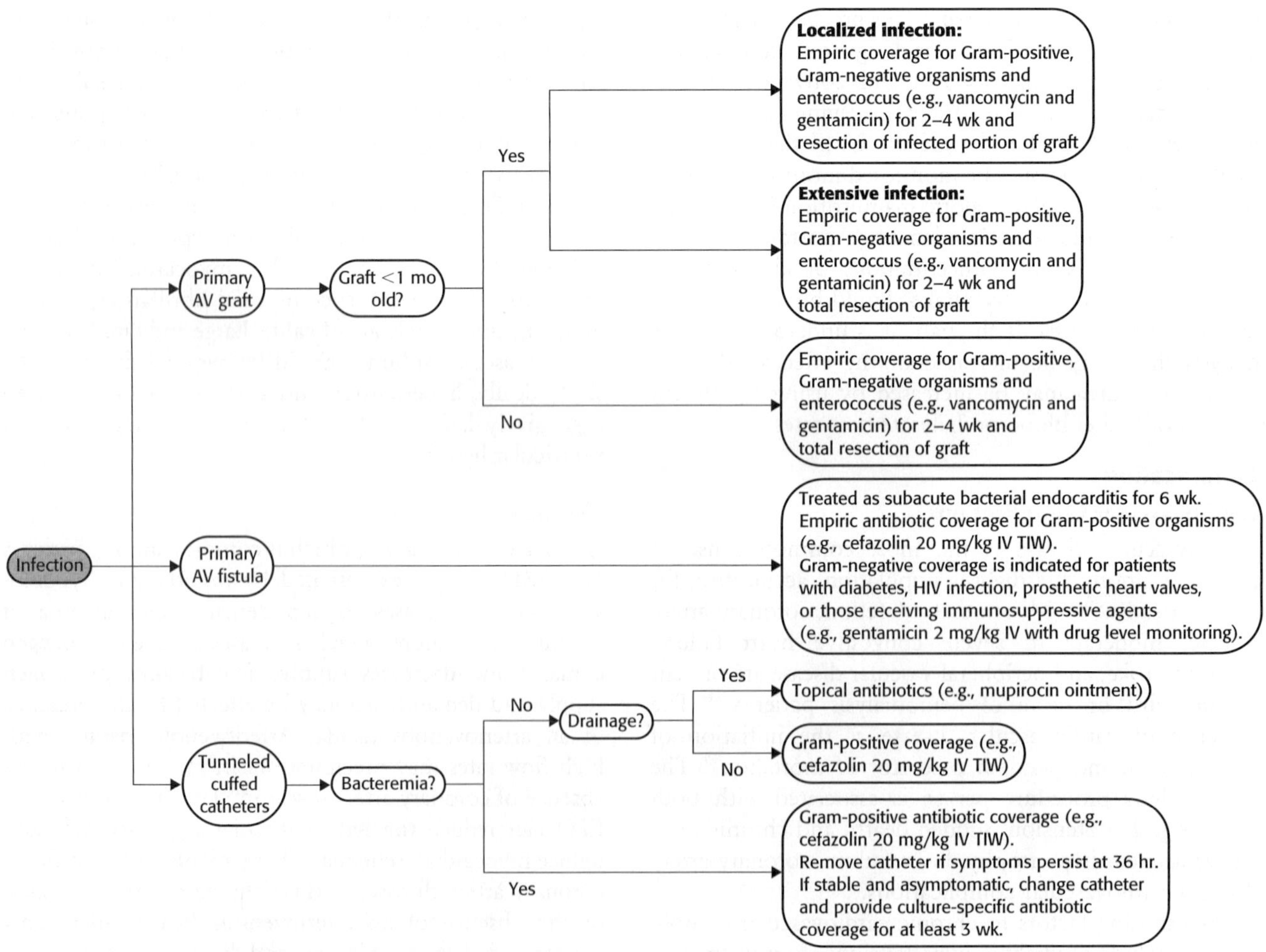

Figure 23.4. Algorithm for treatment of access infections.

antistaphylococcal agent) intranasally once per week has been shown to be effective in reducing the incidence of *S. aureus* infections and is only rarely associated with the emergence of mupirocin resistance.[96]

Immune System Dysfunction

Patients with ESRD manifest a number of immune function abnormalities, some of which are worsened by hemodialysis. These abnormalities are part of a multifactorial process that predisposes patients to infection.[1] Although neutrophil counts may be normal or modestly elevated, patients on hemodialysis have multiple neutrophil functional defects, including decreased chemotaxis, phagocytosis, and in vitro killing of bacteria.[97] This is caused by iron deficiency or iron overload, PCM, hyperparathyroidism, and the presence in some patients of a specific granulocyte inhibitory protein.[98]

Lymphocytes, natural killer cells, monocytes, and macrophages constitute the cell-mediated arm of the immune system. Evidence of defects in cell-mediated immunity in patients on ESRD comes from the following observations: prolonged survival of skin allografts, impairment of cutaneous delayed-type hypersensitivity to common antigens (e.g., *Candida*), remission of systemic lupus erythematosus when renal function reaches end stage, increased incidence of tuberculosis, and an abnormally high incidence of malignant tumors.[97,99] Humoral immunity appears for the most part to be unaffected.

Intradialytic Symptoms

The exposure during dialysis of large volumes of blood to a foreign surface (i.e., dialyzer), extracorporeal circuit, and substances introduced during manufacture and sterilization is associated with a number of intradialytic symptoms, including muscle cramps, chest or back pain, hypoxemia, fever, nausea, vomiting, seizures, and cardiac arrhythmias. During rapid fluid removal, patients may experience hypotension and muscle cramps. With the advent of newer, more precise ultrafiltration systems and sodium modeling, ultrafiltration is now more precise and gradual. This change has resulted in a reduction in many of the nonspecific intradialytic symptoms. The replacement of acetate with bicarbonate as the dialysate base buffer has led to a reduction in the incidence of nausea, vomiting, and hypotension. In addition, the use of bicarbonate dialysate is associated with improved survival.

Muscle Cramps

The pathogenesis of muscle cramps during dialysis is not well understood. Plasma volume contraction appears to be the initiating event, and sympathetic activation may also play a role.[100] Dialysis-associated muscle cramps may be acutely relieved by boluses of hypertonic saline, hypertonic glucose, or mannitol.[100,101] Low-dose prazosin (0.25 to 1.0 mg) given at the start of dialysis may reduce the frequency of cramps, although an increased incidence of hypotension may also be observed during and after hemodialysis.[102] Low-dose l-carnitine (500 mg/day) is also effective in improving muscular symptoms by restoring carnitine tissue levels.[103]

Table 23.4 ▪ Dialyzer Reactions

Type A Reaction	Type B Reactions
Immediate onset	Onset within 40 min
Manifestations:	Manifestations
Abdominal cramps	Back pain
Angioedema	Chest pain
Skin flushing	Dyspnea (if severe)
Hypotension	Fever (low grade)
Laryngeal edema	Mild hypoxemia
Nausea and vomiting	Postdialytic fatigue
Pruritus	Role for complement activation
Sensation of heat	
Urticaria	
Role for ethylene oxide and formaldehyde	
Predisposing factors:	
Angiotensin-converting-enzyme inhibitors	
Atopy	
Atopy inverted total serum immunoglobulin E	
Eosinophilia	

Intradialytic Hypotension

Intradialytic hypotension is a common complication of hemodialysis, and enhanced nitric oxide production may be involved in its development.[104] Strategies that have been used to manage hypotensive episodes include cooling dialysate to 35°C, infusing hypertonic saline, and administering medications such as vasopressin, caffeine, carnitine, ephedrine sulfate, adenosine, and midodrine.[105–111] These strategies have been used with various degrees of success, and no universal recommendations can be made for all patients on hemodialysis.

Dialyzer Reactions

There are two types of dialyzer reactions (Table 23.4). Type A is an anaphylactoid or allergic reaction to some component of the hemodialysis circuit that develops within the first 20 minutes of a dialysis session, often immediately after blood flow is initiated. Signs and symptoms are similar to those of a drug-induced anaphylactic reaction and may result from sensitization to a component of the extracorporeal circuit. Atopic patients and those receiving angiotensin-converting enzyme (ACE) inhibitor therapy are at an increased risk of developing type A dialyzer reactions. Polyacrylonitrile membranes should be used with extreme caution for patients who are taking ACE inhibitors.[58] Treatment involves immediate discontinuation of dialysis and the institution of standard therapy for anaphylactic reactions, such as epinephrine, antihistamines, corticosteroids, and, if necessary, ventilatory support.[112]

Type B reactions occur within 20 to 40 minutes of initiating dialysis and involve primarily chest and back pain. Usually, symptoms subside with continued dialysis. However, in severe cases, dyspnea may develop, necessitating discontinuation of dialysis. Type B reactions may be caused by intradialytic complement activation.[112]

Postdialytic Symptoms

Often, the patient feels weak and fatigued after a dialysis session. This is probably caused by intradialytic cytokine and complement activation. Biocompatible polymer membranes (e.g., polysulfone, polyacrylonitrile, polymethylmethacrylate) have permeability and blood interactive characteristics that are different from those of cellulosic membranes. Therefore, complement and cytokine stimulation may not be as amplified with these dialyzers, and the postdialysis symptoms, if any, may be less intense.[112]

Dialysis Disequilibrium Syndrome

Dialysis disequilibrium syndrome is one of a number of central nervous system abnormalities seen in patients with ESRD.[28] It occurs predominantly in patients who are undergoing rapid dialysis or patients who have recently started hemodialysis. Although the exact mechanism is unclear, the signs and symptoms of dialysis disequilibrium syndrome are caused by the increased intracranial pressure that results from dialysis-induced cerebral edema.[28] Younger patients, especially pediatric patients, and those with a previous neurologic disorder (e.g., head trauma, stroke, malignant hypertension) appear to be at a higher risk for this syndrome. The minor disequilibrium symptoms include headache, restlessness, dizziness, nausea, vomiting, and muscular twitching. Major signs and symptoms include disorientation, hypertension, tremors, and seizures.[28,113]

β_2 Microglobulin Amyloidosis

Patients who receive long-term hemodialysis (typically for 10 or more years) commonly suffer from a syndrome of pain and osteoarthropathy called dialysis-related amyloidosis.[19,114] Amyloid fibrils may be made primarily of immunoglobulins, β_2 microglobulin, or other proteins. The tissue deposition of these fibrils leads to organ damage. Dialysis-related amyloidosis may lead to the development of carpal tunnel syndrome, destructive arthropathy of the medium-sized joints (e.g., knees, wrists, shoulders, pelvis, vertebral column), and periarticular cystic bone lesions.[114] The signs and symptoms of carpal tunnel syndrome include diminished sensitivity to stimulation (hypesthesia); abnormally low sensitivity to pain (hypalgesia); tenderness, weakness, and wasting of the lateral (radial) side of the palms; and decreased motor nerve conduction velocity.[19] The signs and symptoms of the arthropathy include pain, noninflammatory swelling, joint dysfunction, and pathologic fractures. With progressive amyloidosis the hips become affected, resulting in pathologic fractures of the femoral neck. Symptomatic spinal damage may also occur with progressive disease.[114] The risk of carpal tunnel syndrome is related to the duration of dialysis. The incidence in patients who are hemodialyzed for less than 8 years is low; it increases to 30 to 50% after 15 years and approaches 100% after 20 years of hemodialysis with biocompatible dialyzers.[19,114] Dialysis-related amyloidosis is less common in patients who are dialyzed with biocompatible synthetic membranes (e.g., polyacrylonitrile).[115]

Patients on hemodialysis have serum β_2 microglobulin concentrations that may reach 60 times the normal values of 1 to 3 mg/L.[19] The retention of β_2 microglobulin in ESRD appears to be a necessary but not sufficient factor in the development of dialysis-related amyloidosis. Dialysis-related amyloidosis can also occur in patients on long-term CAPD.[114] The incidence of carpal tunnel syndrome in patients on CAPD is only slightly less than that in patients on hemodialysis.[52] However, patients on CAPD typically have lower serum β_2 microglobulin concentrations than do patients on hemodialysis. This may be because of better preservation of residual renal function (a major determinant of serum β_2 microglobulin clearance) in the CAPD population or the greater permeability to middle molecules of the peritoneal membrane compared to bioincompatible membranes.[16]

Although carpal tunnel syndrome can be treated surgically, there is no established treatment for amyloidosis. Attempts should be made to remove as much β_2 microglobulin as possible because the maintenance of low concentrations may slow the progression of amyloidosis.[114] The high-flux biocompatible membranes (e.g., polysulfone, polyacrylonitrile, cellulose triacetate, and polymethylmethacrylate) are preferred for preventing and slowing the progression of dialysis-related amyloidosis,[115,116] especially for patients older than 50.

PERITONEAL DIALYSIS

Peritoneal dialysis has undergone several modifications over the last 20 years. CAPD was a dramatic innovation that increased the proportion of patients receiving peritoneal dialysis. However, it was still associated with multiple adverse events; peritonitis is the predominant factor that forces patients to switch to hemodialysis. During the 1990s several variants on CAPD were introduced in an attempt to enhance patient acceptance and improve the delivered dosage of dialysis.[117] The popularity of these automated methods has increased dramatically during the last 5 years.[118] Irrespective of the mode and time frame in which dialysate resides in the peritoneal cavity, the principles of peritoneal dialysis solute, fluid, and drug removal are similar.

Peritoneal Membrane

The peritoneal cavity comprises a single-layered membrane that lines the abdomen and the visceral organs. The side of the peritoneal cavity that covers the abdominal wall is called the parietal surface, and the visceral surface covers the visceral organs. The peritoneal surface area of adults approximates the body surface area, and ranges from 1 to 2 m^2. The adult peritoneal cavity contains approximately 100 mL of lipid-rich fluid that acts as a lubricating agent. The peritoneal space can accommodate several liters of fluid in the presence of ascites or by instillation of dialysate solution.[29,30]

The peritoneal membrane has pores that are large enough to allow the passage of middle- to high-molecular-weight compounds. Therefore, CAPD clears larger substances more effectively than conventional cellulosic hemodialysis membranes. The routes of absorption from the peritoneal cavity differ for small solutes and macromolecules (molecular weights greater than 20,000 Da), such as albumin and dextrans). Whereas small solutes diffuse down their concentration gradient into the systemic circulation, macromolecules are absorbed primarily via the subdiaphragmatic lymphatic system.[119] With chronic peritoneal dialysis, the character of the mesothelial layer may change, mostly because of the hyperosmolarity of the dialysate solutions.[29] These alterations may lead in some patients to peritoneal fibrosis (thickening), decreased permeability, and diminished ultrafiltration.[30,120]

Mechanics of Peritoneal Dialysis

Like hemodialysis, peritoneal dialysis has three basic components: a blood compartment (systemic circulation), a dialysate compartment (peritoneal cavity), and a semipermeable membrane that separates the blood and dialysate compartments (peritoneal membrane). Peritoneal dialysis is a procedure by which the dialysis solution is instilled into the peritoneal cavity via an indwelling catheter. In the presence of dialysate, solute transfer occurs via diffusion and convection bidirectionally across the peritoneal membrane to and from the blood compartment.[29] Because the dialysis fluid contains glucose (dextrose) as an osmotic agent, fluid is pulled from the intravascular space into the peritoneal cavity by ultrafiltration. This osmotic effect is lost as the dialysate glucose is absorbed, especially if the duration of dialysate residence, called dwell time, is prolonged.

Peritoneal Access Devices and Placement Techniques

Permanent access to the peritoneal cavity for peritoneal dialysis may be accomplished by several techniques. The first catheter developed for long-term peritoneal dialysis was described by Tenckhoff in 1968. Several other catheters for long-term peritoneal dialysis have been introduced in the last few years.[121] The multiple types of indwelling catheters and administration sets were designed to prevent contamination and to reduce infectious complications of peritoneal dialysis. The chronic (permanent) indwelling catheters are made of silicone rubber, polyurethane, and other soft materials. The Tenckhoff catheter, which is the most commonly used peritoneal catheter, has two sections, intraperitoneal and extraperitoneal. The intraperitoneal portion is placed via a surgical procedure in the left or right lower peritoneum, preferably in one of the pelvic gutters just above the hips.[29] The extraperitoneal end is passed through subcutaneous layers and placed approximately halfway between the umbilicus and the pubis in the caudal direction. The indwelling catheter is then immobilized to allow healing, prevent leaks, and act as a barrier for migration of skin microorganisms. For this purpose, one or preferably two Dacron cuffs are placed above or below the abdominal muscle layers, and the patient is allowed to heal before peritoneal dialysis is begun.[121] During this healing period, the patient undergoes training for self-administration of dialysis and care of the catheter using sterile technique. The waiting period between catheter placement and dialysis initiation varies among patients. The healing period is usually 4 to 6 weeks for patients with potentially impaired wound healing, such as diabetic patients and those receiving high-dose steroids. A young and otherwise healthy patient can often start dialysis 2 weeks after catheter placement. Patients who are about to undergo continuous cycling peritoneal dialysis (CCPD) may start even sooner because they can use lower initial volumes with no daytime dwell.

Dialysate Solutions

The peritoneal dialysis solution is hypertonic because it contains dextrose, which is necessary to create a diffusive gradient between the peritoneal and blood compartments and to augment ultrafiltration. The dialysate contains electrolytes such as sodium, potassium, chloride, magnesium, and calcium in addition to hydrous dextrose.[30] Although other osmotic agents have been used experimentally, including glycerol, icodextrin, and amino acids, none are available commercially.[122] A variety of additives, including potassium, calcium, and lactate, may be added to the dialysate to control the balance of electrolytes and to correct the metabolic acidosis associated with ESRD.

Continuous Ambulatory Peritoneal Dialysis

In CAPD, as the name implies, patients are dialyzed continuously, 24 hours a day, 7 days a week. Given its demanding and time-consuming nature, the patient must be reliable and highly motivated. Omission of only a few exchanges per week reduces the urea clearance, with the potential of increasing morbidity and mortality. A typical CAPD regimen involves four daily exchanges: three with a dialysate dwell time of about 4 to 6 hours and one with an overnight dwell time of about 10 to 12 hours.[29,117] Commercial CAPD solutions are available in volumes of 1 to 3 L in flexible polyvinyl chloride plastic bags similar to those of large-volume parenterals. The bags have a port for connecting an administration set and a port for administering excipients (e.g., insulin, antibiotics).

The fresh dialysate bag is connected to the permanent indwelling catheter via an administration set. A volume of dialysate (commonly 2 L) is warmed to body temperature and infused by gravity into the peritoneal cavity over 10 to

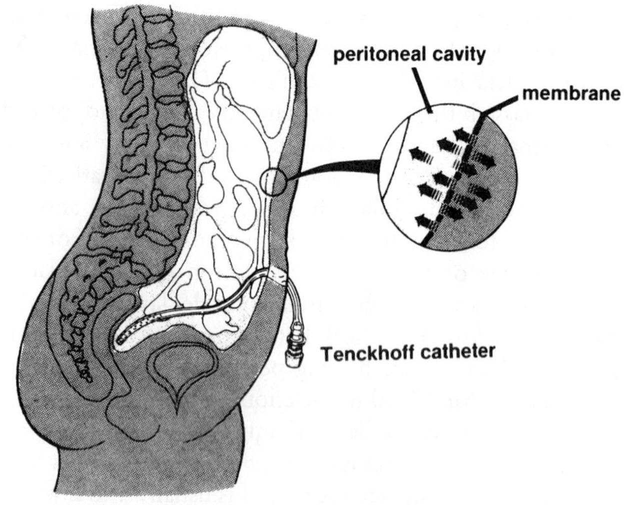

Figure 23.5. Diffusion and ultrafiltration occur across the peritoneal membrane. These processes are bidirectional; that is, solutes and water can be absorbed from the peritoneal cavity or drawn into the cavity. The rate-limiting process is the concentration of a particular solute and dextrose in the dialysis fluid.

20 minutes (Fig. 23.5). The dialysate is warmed to prevent pain and cramping during the initial minutes of an exchange. Depending on the catheter and administration set, the empty bag is either removed and tucked inside the patient's clothing or carried inside a separate belt underneath the clothing while still connected to the catheter.[29,30] After the prescribed dwell time, the same bag is connected to the administration set and placed at a level that is lower than the peritoneal cavity to allow drainage by gravity, which also takes 10 to 20 minutes. When the drainage has ceased, the tubing is again clamped, and using sterile technique (mask and gloves), the patient disconnects the bag of drained fluid. Then a fresh bag of sterile dialysate fluid is connected to the tubing and allowed to infuse into the peritoneal cavity. Fresh, unused dialysate is clear and colorless; spent or used dialysate is clear and straw-colored. During bouts of peritonitis, the spent dialysate becomes cloudy; this is considered a diagnostic sign of infection.

Automated Peritoneal Dialysis

The four main forms of automated peritoneal dialysis are CCPD, daily ambulatory peritoneal dialysis (DAPD), nightly intermittent peritoneal dialysis (NIPD), and nightly tidal peritoneal dialysis (NTPD).[117] These procedures involve the use of a dialysate cycling machine, which automatically instills and drains peritoneal dialysate solutions. In CCPD, the most common variation of CAPD, four 2-L exchanges are performed at night while the patient is sleeping. In the daytime, the patient may carry 0 to 2 L of dialysate in the peritoneal cavity. Patients on NIPD perform no exchanges during their waking hours. However, while they sleep, six to eight 2.5-L exchanges of dialysate are delivered by the cycler. With NTPD, a minimal dwell volume (often 1 L) remains in the peritoneal cavity during the night. The cycler instills fresh dialysate at regular intervals to minimize the amount of drain and fill times during which no effective dialysis takes place, maintain an optimum transmembrane solute gradient to enhance solute removal, and minimize the stagnant fluid layer that is in contact with the peritoneal membrane.[123]

Adequacy of Peritoneal Dialysis: Dialysis Quantification

During the early years of this therapy, patients on CAPD routinely received a standard daily therapy consisting of four 2-L exchanges. For the purpose of quantifying dialysis dosage, creatinine rather than BUN was proposed as a marker for quantification of CAPD.[124] On the basis of clinical experience, a normalized weekly creatinine clearance of about 60 L/1.73 m^2 of body surface area has been suggested as minimally adequate.[34] The weekly Kt/V for the standard CAPD regimen of four daily 2-L exchanges is approximately 1.7 (1.5 to 1.8) per week, compared to a weekly Kt/V of 3.0 to 3.6 for hemodialysis.[104,124] The low CAPD Kt/V is similar to that of the low-dose hemodialysis regimen used in the NCDS study (i.e., high-failure) groups; however, the mortality rates are equal to or lower than those of the hemodialysis population.[125] There are two possible explanations for this incongruity. First, because of its continuous nature, the concentrations of blood urea (or other uremic toxins) with CAPD are at a fairly constant steady state, whereas a sawtooth profile is observed with hemodialysis (i.e., peak predialysis concentrations followed by trough postdialysis concentrations).[67]

The second possible reason for the discrepant minimum dialysis dosage needs is that residual renal function is better preserved during CAPD than during hemodialysis.[16,40] To illustrate, in calculating Kt/V for urea, K should include both dialyzer and renal clearances. For example, CAPD and hemodialysis may both provide a dialysis dosage that is equivalent to a GFR of 10 mL/minute. However, if the patient on CAPD has a native GFR of 5 mL/minute and the patient on hemodialysis has lost all residual renal function, the patient on CAPD will have a much higher total urea clearance (K) of 15 versus 10 mL/minute.

Although both urea and creatinine kinetics are associated with clinical outcome in CAPD patients, creatinine appears to be a more sensitive predictor of outcome.[67,126] The Kt/V method of assessing dialysis adequacy offers two additional advantages: It allows the assessment of dietary protein intake, and it allows prospective prescription of a dialysis dosage.[34,123] The use of urea modeling (Kt/V) together with weekly creatinine clearance values provides a comprehensive method of assessing the adequacy of dialysis. Although few well-controlled studies have assessed the adequacy of peritoneal dialysis, a minimum weekly Kt/V of 2.0 has been recommended.[34]

Peritoneal dialysis adequacy should be determined every 3 months and include parameters such as BUN, PCR, Kt/V, and creatinine clearance. Assessment of urea and creatinine clearances must include the contribution from residual renal function. In the presence of adequate nutrition (dietary protein intake 1.2 g/kg/day, caloric intake 35 kcal/kg/day) the delivered weekly Kt/V should be at least 2.0.[34] Alternatively, a weekly creatinine clearance (CAPD plus renal clearance) of 60 L/1.73 m^2 of body surface area may be used as the target. Patients should be monitored monthly for PCM; the monitoring should include body weight (measured with an empty peritoneum) and serum concentrations of albumin and transferrin. In addition, dietary intake should be monitored at least every 6 months.[34]

Complications

Exit Site and Tunnel Infections

Exit site infections and tunnel infections occur at a rate of about one episode every 1 to 2.5 patient-years.[127] An infected exit site is characterized by redness, induration, or purulent discharge. Other symptoms include heat, drainage, odor, tenderness, and pain. Crust formation around the exit site and positive cultures from the exit site in the absence of inflammation do not indicate infection.[128] If the infection infiltrates the deeper subcutaneous tissues, the patient is said to have a tunnel infection. Edema, redness, and tenderness over the subcutaneous path of the catheter indicate the presence of a tunnel infection. However, it may be difficult to differentiate between exit site and tunnel infections.[29,37] Tunnel infections often precede the development of peritonitis.

Treatment of exit site infections has included systemic and intraperitoneal antibiotics, topical antibiotics and disinfectants, debridement of the infected subcutaneous cuff, and catheter removal.[29,129] The presence of erythema alone may be an early sign of infection, and topical therapy with chlorhexidine, mupirocin, or hydrogen peroxide may be considered. When an exit site infection is suspected, the patient should be instructed to cleanse the site frequently with hydrogen peroxide and povidone iodine. When purulent discharge is present, a Gram stain and culture should be obtained.[129]

Empiric oral antibiotics are used against the common causative organisms (*S. aureus* and *S. epidermidis*), starting with a first-generation cephalosporin (e.g., cephalexin, cephradine), dicloxacillin, or trimethoprim–sulfamethoxazole.[129] Vancomycin should be reserved for persistent infections. Once the culture results are known, they should be used to guide antibiotic treatment. The optimal duration of therapy has not been established; however, 2 to 3 weeks often is sufficient. Prolonged antibiotic use is a predisposing factor for the development of fungal peritonitis.[130] If within 1 week of starting treatment for *S. aureus* infection there is no sign of improvement, rifampin 600 mg daily may be added.[129] For Gram-negative infections, oral ciprofloxacin 500 mg twice daily is recommended.[129] To avoid decreased absorption, ciprofloxacin must be dosed several hours before or after phosphate binders. If no improvement is observed within 2 to 3 weeks, catheter removal may be indicated.

Peritonitis

Peritonitis is the most prevalent infectious complication of CAPD, occurring at a rate of 1 to 2 episodes per patient-year.[30,131] CAPD peritonitis is responsible for the death of 1.3 to 1.9% of all patients on CAPD.[46] Breakdown in aseptic technique during dialysis exchanges is one of the major risk factors for the development of peritonitis. The peritonitis-causing organism may enter directly through the catheter lumen or migrate along the catheter through a tunnel. The development of catheter biofilms or exit site infections may also contribute to peritonitis.[132] Rarely, peritonitis is caused by intestinal or genitourinary sources or from hematogenous seeding.

Patients on peritoneal dialysis have many immune deficiencies. In addition, the presence of a low-pH, hyperosmolar dialysate solution inhibits phagocytosis, chemotaxis, bactericidal killing, free oxygen radical generation, and leukotriene synthesis of peripheral neutrophils and peritoneal macrophages.[77,133] This diminished intraperitoneal immune capacity may contribute to the development of peritonitis. Bacterial colonization of the nares with *S. aureus* is a risk factor for both exit site infection and peritonitis.[132] Recurrent peritonitis occurs in up to one-third of the patients and is a major cause of technique failure (i.e., discontinuation of this dialysis modality).[29]

Peritonitis associated with CAPD is typically less serious than that caused by GI perforation. Most of the cases are of bacterial origin, although other forms, such as chemical, viral, mycobacterial, and fungal, also are observed. Up to 60% of peritonitis episodes are caused by *Staphylococcus* species, mostly *S. epidermidis*.[134] Gram-negative organisms, mostly Enterobacteriaceae, *Pseudomonas* species, and *Acinetobacter* species, cause up to 35% of cases. Polymicrobial peritonitis accounts for 5% of cases and may be indicative of intraabdominal viscus perforation. Sterile peritonitis may be caused by a transient allergic reaction to some component of the CAPD catheter or poor laboratory culture techniques.[129,134]

Initial Assessment

Peritonitis diagnosis is based on the presence of two of the following three symptoms: abdominal pain with or without rebound tenderness, the presence of more than 100 white blood cells per cubic millimeter of peritoneal fluid (with more than 50% neutrophils), and a positive dialysate culture.[129] A cloudy effluent is the most common presenting sign of peritonitis; however, the effluent may be clear or may remain cloudy after microbiologic cure.[129] When peritonitis is suspected, a Gram stain of the dialysate should be obtained. The Gram stain is positive in up to 40% of cases. Culture of the spent dialysate must also be obtained, but therapy should not await the results. Although intravenous antibiotics can produce effective drug concentrations within the peritoneal cavity, usually within 2 to 4 hours after dosing,[135] intraperitoneal administration of antibiotics rapidly produces high local concentrations because of the large difference in the volumes of the peritoneal and systemic compartments.[135,136]

Initial Management

Because CAPD peritonitis is less severe than other forms of peritonitis, it usually is treated on an outpatient basis. However, the following circumstances may necessitate patient hospitalization: inability or unwillingness to self-administer antibiotics, noncompliance with therapy or follow-up, and presence of significant systemic symptoms, such as fever, vomiting, abdominal pain, or hypotension.[120] Once CAPD peritonitis has been diagnosed, two or three rapid dialysis exchanges of 20 minutes each may provide symptomatic benefit.[120] Also, the addition of heparin (1000 U/L) to the fresh dialysate may help to reduce the number of subsequent peritoneal adhesions and reduce postinfectious complications.[134]

Before the causative organism is determined, empiric broad-spectrum antibiotic therapy must be initiated against common Gram-positive or Gram-negative bacteria, which cause approximately 90% of all CAPD peritonitis cases.[129] Intraperitoneal administration is favored over the intravenous route, and combinations of a first-generation cephalosporin with an aminoglycoside are recommended. Current dosing recommendations include the choice between intermittent (i.e., one large dose in one exchange per day) and continuous (i.e., a smaller dose in each exchange per day) therapy. Cefazolin, the prototypical cephalosporin, can be given as 500 mg/L in the first bag, with 125 mg/L in each subsequent bag, or as 1000 mg in one bag each day. The dosage recommendations for gentamicin (the prototypic aminoglycoside) are 8 mg/L into the first bag, with 4 mg/L in each subsequent bag, or 0.6 mg/kg in one bag each day. The intermittent dosage (once a day) of both agents should be increased if the patient has significant urine output (more than 500 mL/day).

Gram-Positive Organisms on Culture

If a Gram-positive organism is identified on culture, the choice of therapy should be guided by the sensitivity pattern of the organism. *S. aureus* infections usually can be managed with continuation of the first-generation cephalosporin and the addition of oral rifampin 600 mg per day. Aminoglycoside therapy should be discontinued in this case, as well as with the isolation of any other Gram-positive organism except enterococci. The isolation of enterococci mandates discontinuation of the cephalosporin and the addition of ampicillin at a dosage of 125 mg/L. The usual duration of therapy is 3 weeks for *S. aureus* infections and 2 weeks for all other Gram-positive species.[129]

Gram-Negative Organisms on Culture

The presence of a Gram-negative organism indicates the possibility of an intraabdominal disorder (e.g., bowel perforation). In such a circumstance, surgical exploration should be considered, especially if a polymicrobial infection is present. If multiple organisms or anaerobes are cultured, metronidazole 500 mg orally or intravenously every 8 hours should be added.[129] The presence of a single nonpseudomonal Gram-negative organism (e.g., *Escherichia coli*) usually can be treated for 14 days with an aminoglycoside, cephalosporin (e.g., ceftazidime), or extended-spectrum penicillin (e.g., piperacillin). The agent should be chosen on the basis of sensitivity patterns. With the presence of *Pseudomonas* or *Stenotrophomonas* species, dual therapy is needed (e.g., ceftazidime plus an aminoglycoside, ciprofloxacin, or aztreonam).[129] If an extended-spectrum penicillin is to be used with an aminoglycoside, it is best to administer the penicillin intravenously to avoid intraperitoneal inactivation of the aminoglycoside. Peritonitis caused by *Pseudomonas* or *Stenotrophomonas* often necessitates removal of the peritoneal catheter and 3 to 4 weeks of antibiotic therapy.[129]

Fungal Organisms on Culture

Previously, catheter removal was recommended uniformly as part of the treatment of fungal peritonitis.[137] However, current guidelines suggest that treatment may commence with the catheter in place, especially for treating nonfilamentous (yeast) peritonitis. Treatment consists of oral or intraperitoneal fluconazole 100 to 200 mg every day plus oral flucytosine 1 g/day for 4 to 6 weeks. If clinical improvement is not observed within 4 to 7 days, the catheter should be removed. Antifungal treatment should be continued with oral fluconazole 100 mg and flucytosine 1 g daily for 10 days after the catheter is removed.[129]

Infection Prevention

Infection prevention strategies have been designed to reduce CAPD-related morbidity, method failure, and possibly mortality. Because CAPD entails frequent manipulation of the dialysis catheter through repeated connections and disconnections of the administration set, the patient or caregiver must be trained to use aseptic techniques. Recent advances in the disconnect systems using the flush-before-fill technique (e.g., Y-connector set) have limited the manipulations needed during exchanges, thus reducing the incidence of peritonitis and exit site and tunnel infections caused by touch contamination,[128,138] mainly by reducing *S. epidermidis*, polymicrobial, and other Gram-positive infections.[138] Unfortunately, the rates of *S. aureus* and Gram-negative infections have not changed.[132,138]

The nasal carriage of *S. aureus* is an established predisposing factor for peritonitis and tunnel and exit site infections.[139] Up to 60% of patients on dialysis are nasal carriers of this organism, compared to 10 to 30% of the general population; the carriage rate is even higher among diabetic patients.[12] Eradicating nasal *S. aureus* can reduce catheter loss after peritonitis or exit site infection.[140] Eradicating nasal *S. aureus* with intranasal mupirocin 2% ointment, administered twice daily for 5 days of every month, can reduce the incidence of peritonitis and exit site infection by *S. aureus*;[141] however, the incidence of infections by other Gram-positive and Gram-negative bacteria may simultaneously increase. Rifampin 300 mg twice daily for 5 consecutive days every 12 weeks can prevent peritonitis and exit site infections without a significant effect on nasal carriage of *S. aureus*.[142] Thus, patients with recurrent CAPD infections may benefit from one of these intermittent treatment regimens.

Cardiovascular Complications

Many of the cardiovascular complications of ESRD that are associated with hemodialysis are less prevalent in CAPD patients.[38] The continuous nature of CAPD prevents the large, rapid volume shifts of hemodialysis, thus minimizing the risk of rapid reduction in left ventricular pressure and hypotension. However, aggressive fluid removal with the use of hypertonic (4.25% hydrous dextrose) solutions can occasionally result in hypotension (usually orthostatic).[46] Compared with undialyzed patients, patients on CAPD have lower left ventricular end-diastolic and end-systolic volumes, a lower stroke index and cardiac index, and a faster myocardial contraction speed.[38] Therefore, CAPD is the preferred mode of dialysis for patients with significant cardiovascular disease (e.g., preexisting left ventricular hypertrophy and coronary artery disease).

Increased Intraabdominal Pressure

The infusion of peritoneal dialysate increases the intraabdominal pressure up to five times without a significant increase in pressure inside the stomach or at the lower esophageal sphincter.[143] This increased intraabdominal pressure can increase the stress on structures of the abdomen and lead to a number of complications, including a sensation of bloating and symptoms of esophageal reflux.[120] The dialysate-induced increase in intraabdominal pressure can push against the diaphragm in a manner similar to that observed during pregnancy or obesity. The resulting upward displacement of the diaphragm decreases the functional residual capacity of the lungs. If severe enough, it may lead to small airway collapse, ventilation–perfusion mismatch, and arterial hypoxemia. Paradoxically, a less severe displacement may actually improve the efficiency of diaphragmatic contraction and improve ventilation.[143] A serious complication of peritoneal dialysis is the leakage of dialysate across the diaphragm, resulting in hydrothorax (i.e., fluid in the pleural cavity).[29] Although mild hydrothorax may be asymptomatic, life-threatening respiratory compromise may occur in severe cases.[143] The most common clinical manifestations include dyspnea, chest pain, hypotension, and, in rare instances, atrial fibrillation.[144]

The goal of treatment is to resolve the pleural effusion and prevent its recurrence. CAPD should be discontinued temporarily until the effusion regresses spontaneously.[143] For severe dyspnea or cardiovascular instability, a chest tube may be placed to allow draining of fluid.[144] If hydrothorax recurs, surgical repair may be necessary. Alternatively, the pleural space can be closed off with talcum powder, iodized talc, triamcinolone acetonide, fibrin adhesive, or autologous blood instillation.

The increased intraabdominal pressure places excess stress on the lumbar vertebrae. In the presence of poor abdominal muscle tone, the spinal stress increases, leading to back pain or sciatica. Treatment involves the use of smaller dialysate volumes, although this may compromise dialysis adequacy. The optimal solution may be to start the patient on NIPD.[143]

Hernias

Up to one-quarter of patients on CAPD may develop a hernia, most commonly at the site of incision for catheter insertion, the inguinal canal, or the umbilicus.[143] If the hernia is left untreated, bowel incarceration and strangulation may ensue, necessitating emergency surgery. Hernia treatment usually involves surgical correction.[145]

Loss of Ultrafiltration

Although rare, a loss of ultrafiltration is troublesome because it may necessitate discontinuation of CAPD. There are two types of ultrafiltration failure. Most cases are type I failure, in which the permeability of the peritoneal membrane to glucose is increased, resulting in rapid absorption of intraperitoneal glucose and loss of transmembrane osmotic gradient. Although the ability to remove fluid is lost, the clearance of other solutes, such as creatinine or urea, is maintained or even increased because their removal depends on diffusion. Type I ultrafiltration failure usually occurs in patients who are on long-term CAPD but can also occur during bouts of peritonitis when peritoneal permeability and intraperitoneal glucose absorption increase. Treating type I ultrafiltration failure involves the use of hypertonic dialysate (4.25%) and more frequent dialysis exchanges.[133]

Type II ultrafiltration failure is caused by a reduction in effective peritoneal surface area that results from extensive scar tissue formation (fibrosis) and peritoneal adhesions. Permeability to glucose remains normal or is decreased. Type II failure most commonly results from severe and prolonged peritonitis, usually caused by *S. aureus* or a fungus and often necessitates discontinuation of CAPD.[133]

PHARMACOTHERAPEUTIC CONSIDERATIONS FOR PATIENTS ON DIALYSIS

Anemia

The primary cause of anemia in patients with ESRD is a relative EPO deficiency, for which therapy with recombinant human EPO alfa (epoetin) has been available since the late 1980s. The kidneys synthesize about 90% of circulating EPO, and secretion increases in response to hypoxia.[146,147] Although the Hct, an index of the red blood cell count, begins to decline when the serum creatinine is more than 2 mg/dL, it usually is maintained above 30% until GFR declines to 30 mL/minute or less.

Other factors such as blood loss; iron, folic acid, or vitamin B_{12} deficiency; severe renal bone disease; systemic infection or inflammatory illness; and aluminum toxicity may also contribute to the development of anemia in patients on dialysis. Although renal anemia typically is associated with normochromic and normocytic cells, iron deficiency can result in a microcytic, hypochromic pattern, whereas vitamin B_{12} or folate deficiency can lead to a macrocytic anemia. Because the cause of anemia in patients on dialysis often is multifactorial, multiple hematologic and iron studies should be assessed before the patient begins epoetin.

Fatigue, exertional dyspnea, dizziness, headache, angina, congestive heart failure, and decreased cognition are common in patients with ESRD. Reversal of the signs and symptoms of tissue oxygen deprivation and left ventricular hypertrophy, improvement in exercise capacity, and ultimately an improvement in the quality of life are the primary therapeutic goals of anemia management. Because the signs and symptoms of anemia tend to resolve in patients who have achieved and maintained Hct between 30 and 38%, the DOQI working group recommended a target Hct range of 33 to 36%.[148]

Currently, epoetin is the therapy of choice for maintaining Hct levels in patients on dialysis. It is reasonable to begin epoetin therapy when the patient's Hct drops below 33%. Before epoetin therapy is initiated, iron status (serum ferritin and transferrin saturation [TSAT]) should be assessed. Serum ferritin values tend to correlate with body stores of iron. Unfortunately, ferritin is an acute phase reactant and its values can rise independently of body iron stores in response to inflammation, liver disease, malignancy, or infection. The TSAT is a measure of the transferrin-bound iron that is readily available to the bone marrow for erythropoiesis. To optimize hematopoiesis in patients on dialysis receiving epoetin, ferritin and TSAT values of at least 100 ng/mL and 20%, respectively, should be maintained.[148]

Ideally, iron deficiency should be corrected before epoetin therapy is initiated. Although oral iron generally is not sufficient to maintain adequate iron stores in patients on hemodialysis, in part because of their ongoing blood losses, it is a reasonable option for patients on peritoneal dialysis. Initially, ferrous salts (sulfate, gluconate, and fumarate) should be used to provide approximately 200 mg elemental iron per day for adults. If nausea, vomiting, constipation, or diarrhea are noted, oral iron can be taken with a snack or another dosage form or product can be tried. Unfortunately, absorption is reduced when iron is ingested with food and phosphate binders. Some clinicians suggest giving vitamin C concomitantly with oral iron to enhance absorption.

Epoetin can be administered intravenously or subcutaneously at a dosage of 90 to 180 U/kg/week. Subcutaneous administration is recommended for all patients with ESRD.[148] Although the bioavailability of subcutaneous epoetin is low, the half-life is prolonged[149] and Hct response is at least as good as or better than with intravenous administration. The preponderance of data indicates that the target Hct may be maintained with weekly subcutaneous epoetin dosages that are about 30% lower than the intravenous dosages.[150]

The initiation of epoetin therapy may lead to functional or absolute iron deficiency because of the elevated degree of erythropoiesis, even if oral iron intake is started. Thus, maintenance dosages of intravenous iron are recommended for patients on hemodialysis to prevent iron deficiency and sustain erythropoiesis.[148] Parenteral iron has been shown to improve responsiveness to epoetin and reduce the amount of epoetin needed to achieve and maintain the desired Hct.[148] One-time large (500- to 2000-mg) infusions and intermittent 100-mg doses given during hemodialysis for 10 consecutive sessions have been used to treat iron deficiency. Although these dosage regimens usually replete iron stores acutely, they do not sustain erythropoiesis indefinitely. To maintain iron stores in adults on hemodialysis, the DOQI anemia working group recommended that 50 mg iron dextran be given each week for 10 weeks, with measurement of TSAT and ferritin 2 weeks after the tenth dose. Earlier measurement may yield erroneous results because of the presence of circulating iron dextran. The iron dosage can be individualized (25 to 100 mg per week) to maintain adequate ferritin and TSAT values. The intravenous iron products available in the United States are the dextrans INFeD (165,000 Da) and DexFerrum (267,000 Da), or the sodium ferric gluconate complex, Ferrelicit.[151] Iron dextran is not immediately available to the bone marrow for heme synthesis; it must be processed by the reticuloendothelial system before being released to transferrin. Iron dextran infusions have been associated with acute anaphylactic reactions in fewer than 1% of patients and with delayed side effects such as arthralgias, myalgias, and serum sickness–like symptoms. Although the need for a test dose is controversial, DOQI guidelines recommend that a one-time dose of 25 mg should be administered intravenously before iron therapy is initiated.

Hypertension

Hypertension is a major modifiable cardiovascular risk factor in patients with ESRD and it is found in 60% and 24% of the hemodialysis and general U.S. populations, respectively.[152,153] Inadequate hypertension control can accelerate atherosclerosis and increase cardiovascular morbidity secondary to heart disease and stroke.[154,155] Predialysis mean arterial blood pressure (MAP) greater than 115 mm Hg has been associated with a significant increase in morbidity and mortality in patients on hemodialysis.[156] A 10-mm Hg increase in MAP also is associated with a sevenfold increase in the risk of left ventricular hypertrophy and a twofold increase in the risk of heart failure.[157] In patients with preexisting ischemic heart disease, mortality from myocardial infarction is the lowest when the treated diastolic blood pressure is reduced to 85 to 90 mm Hg.[158] Recent results from the Hypertension Optimal Treatment (HOT) study indicate that the incidence of cardiovascular events is the lowest when diastolic blood pressure is reduced to 83 mm Hg or less. Moreover, subgroup analysis of patients with diabetes mellitus revealed a 51% lower incidence of major cardiovascular events in the target group (diastolic blood pressure 80 mm Hg or less) than in those who had a diastolic blood pressure of 80 to 90 mm Hg.[159]

Despite the high prevalence of hypertension in the ESRD population, the mechanism of high blood pressure in these patients is not well understood. Sodium retention is believed to be one of the mechanisms responsible for the development of ESRD hypertension. However, extracellular volume expansion alone does not produce hypertension. In fact, patients on dialysis seldom have profound edema, and increased peripheral vascular resistance is found in almost all patients.[160] In a survey conducted in 649 patients on hemodialysis, visible edema was observed in less than 10% of patients, yet 70% of these patients were receiving antihypertensive medications or had predialysis blood pressure higher than 150/90 mm Hg.[161] Studies examining the relationship between changes in vascular volume and blood pressure suggest that short- and intermediate-term physiologic mechanisms buffer the direct effects of fluid overload on MAP. These mechanisms include significant reductions in plasma arginine vasopressin and angiotensin II and an increase in atrial natriuretic peptide.[162] Impairment of these compensatory mechanisms can lead to increased systemic vascular resistance and sympathetic tone and hence susceptibility to volume-induced hypertension.[163]

Hypertension in patients on dialysis can be treated by dialytic removal of sodium and water or the use of antihypertensive medications. Blood pressure patterns in these patients lack diurnal variation, and interdialytic blood pressure may be estimated by the predialysis and postdialysis blood pressure.[164] In general, volume control by adequate dialysis is a more effective way to lower blood pressure than pharmacologic therapy.[165,166] In patients who have high blood pressure despite adequate fluid removal, use of antihypertensive medications is indicated. According to the recommendations from the sixth report of the Joint National Committee on the Prevention and Treatment of Hypertension (JNC-6), lifestyle modifications (e.g., reduced intake of dietary salt to less than 2 g/day, reduced saturated fat and cholesterol intake, smoking cessation, weight loss) are recommended as adjunctive therapy for all patients before pharmacologic therapy is initiated.[167] Therapy selection should take into consideration other comorbid conditions such as diabetes mellitus, coronary heart disease, myocardial infarction, and depression. Lower starting dosages are necessary in older adults and when agents that are predominantly renally eliminated are being used. Higher dosages may be needed on nondialysis days than on dialysis days. Agents that are removable by dialysis may be given after dialysis on dialysis days. In general, ACE inhibitors, long-acting calcium channel blockers, β-blockers, and angiotensin receptor antagonists are effective for management of hypertension in patients with ESRD. The use of short-acting calcium channel blockers, especially in patients with diabetes mellitus, is controversial because of the potentially increased risk of cardiac events such as myocardial infarction and stroke.

Hyperlipidemia and Atherosclerosis

Hyperlipidemia, especially hypertriglyceridemia, is a common cardiovascular risk factor that occurs in 30 to 70% of patients undergoing maintenance hemodialysis.[168] Although hypercholesterolemia is less common in patients on hemodialysis, it is often seen in patients undergoing CAPD.[169] Measuring total cholesterol (TC) and triglyceride (TG) levels may underestimate the magnitude and scope of the problem because there may be an accumulation of very low density lipoproteins and intermediate-density lipoproteins despite normal TC and TG levels. High-density lipoprotein levels may be reduced despite normal low-density lipoprotein (LDL) levels. Impaired function of key enzymes such as lipoprotein and hepatic TG lipases appears to be important in the pathogenesis of lipid metabolism in these patients.[168]

The role of homocysteine in the pathogenesis of atherosclerotic diseases in patients on dialysis has been an area of intense research. Hyperhomocysteinemia has been identified as an independent risk factor for atherosclerotic vascular diseases in the general population.[170] Homocysteine, a metabolite of methionine, is highly protein bound, and approximately 20% of plasma homocysteine is present in the form of cysteine–homocysteine conjugates, homocysteine–homocysteine dimers, and free homocysteine.[171] Several studies have demonstrated elevated homocysteine levels in patients on hemodialysis and peritoneal dialysis, ranging from two to four times those of patients with normal renal function, despite folic acid supplementation with 1 mg daily.[172,173] The cause of hyperhomocysteinemia in patients on dialysis is unclear because less than 1% of total homocysteine produced is excreted unchanged in urine.[171] Recent data suggest that the kidney may play a role in homocysteine remethylation, and the loss of renal mass may impair this function.[174] Pharmacologic dosages of folic acid (i.e., 5 to 15 mg/day) reduce homocysteine levels in one-third of patients on dialysis, although elevated levels persist in the rest of the patients.[175] To date, no studies have demonstrated that lowering homocysteine levels leads to improved cardiovascular outcomes in the general population or the dialysis population. Further research efforts should focus on identifying better methods to treat homocysteinemia and evaluate the effects of treatment on patient outcomes and survival.

Hypertriglyceridemia of more than 500 mg/dL should be treated with dietary modification and, if necessary, lipid-lowering therapy.[176] An isocaloric, low-saturated-fat, low-cholesterol diet is recommended by the Adult Treatment Panel of the National Cholesterol Education Program (NCEP).[177,178] Clofibrate and fenofibrate are eliminated predominantly by the kidney and therefore are not recommended for use in patients on dialysis. Gemfibrozil, on the other hand, is not metabolized appreciably by the kidney, so dosage adjustment is unnecessary in patients with renal impairment. Therefore, it is the drug of choice in patients on dialysis who have severe hypertriglyceridemia, and the starting dosage is 600 mg twice daily.[179] Hypercholesterolemia (LDL more than 130 mg/dL), although less commonly observed in patients on dialysis, should be treated aggressively in patients at high risk for cardiovascular disease. To date, no randomized, controlled clinical trials have demonstrated that treating hypercholesterolemia in patients receiving renal replacement therapy prevents cardiovascular diseases and improves survival. However, the West of Scotland Coronary Prevention Study, Scandinavian Simvastatin Survival study, Cholesterol and Recurrent Events study, Air Force/Texas Coronary Atherosclerosis Prevention Study, Long-Term Intervention with Pravastatin in Ischaemic Disease Study, and Atorvastatin Versus Revascularization Treatments trial provide overwhelming evidence to support the use of β-hydroxy-β-methylglutaryl-conezyme A (HMG-CoA) inhibitors, also known as statins, for primary and secondary prevention of cardiovascular diseases in the nondialysis high-risk population.[180–185] Because cardiovascular diseases such as myocardial infarction, cardiac failure, and stroke account for more than 50% of all deaths in patients on dialysis, hypercholesterolemia should be treated aggressively with statin therapy, despite the lack of outcome data to support the benefits of treatment in this patient population. Statins can be given safely to patients on dialysis because they are metabolized predominantly by the liver. Nicotinic acid such as niacin should be used with caution in patients on dialysis; if started, initial dosages should be reduced (e.g., to 100 mg three times daily) to prevent flushing, hypotension, GI distress, and impaired glucose tolerance.

Metabolic Acidosis

Acid-base homeostasis in patients on hemodialysis is accomplished by bicarbonate transfer across the dialysis membrane, and this rate of transfer depends on the transmembrane bicarbonate gradient (Fig. 23.6).[186] The interdialytic acid production rate in patients on dialysis is approximately 28 mEq/day, much lower than that of the normal population (60 mEq/day). Predialysis bicarbonate levels are determined by factors such as the rate of endogenous acid production, characteristics of the dialysis prescription, organic anion loss during dialysis, and loss or gain from the gastrointestinal tract (Table 23.5).[186] Uncorrected chronic metabolic acidosis has significant clinical effects on bone, electrolyte balance, and protein metabolism.[187] A predialysis bicarbonate level of 17 mEq/L or less is deleterious for bone metabolism and can result in bone demineralization, increased bone resorption, and decreased bone formation.[188] Reduced plasma bicarbonate also stimulates PTH secretion and suppresses vitamin D synthesis. Acidosis also stimulates protein catabolism and amino acid oxidation and worsens uremia.[188] Associated

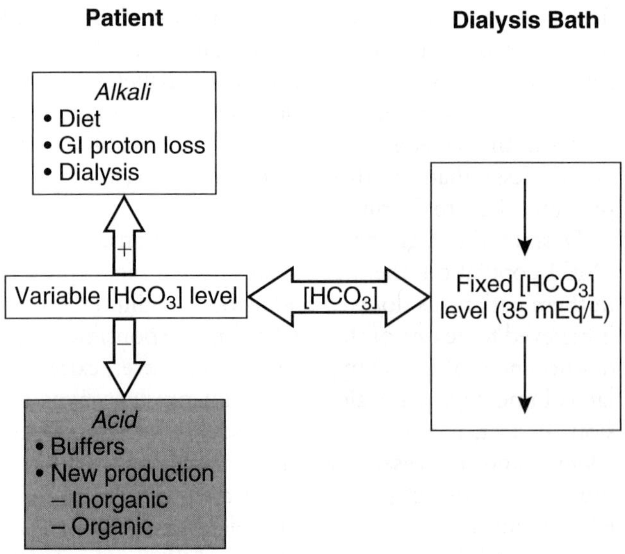

Figure 23.6. Diagrammatic representation of the events governing bicarbonate transfer during hemodialysis.

Table 23.5 ▪ Determinants of Predialysis Bicarbonate Level

Dialysis prescription
Bath alkali concentration
Duration of treatment
Blood flow rate
Organic anion loss during dialysis
Endogenous acid production
Weight gain
Gastrointestinal acid and alkali losses

electrolyte derangements such as hyperkalemia may result in fatigue, decreased exercise tolerance, and reduced cardiac contractility.

Metabolic acidosis in these patients should not be managed by simple addition of more alkali in the dialysate.[186] Instead, the best approach is predicated on the cause of the low predialysis bicarbonate level in each individual patient. Dietary modifications can reduce interdialytic acid production. Treating concurrent diarrhea can reduce bicarbonate loss from the GI tract. Oral alkali supplementation is indicated when other nondrug attempts fail to correct the serum bicarbonate level. Low starting dosages of alkali (e.g., sodium bicarbonate or Shols solution) such as 0.5 mEq/kg/day divided in two or three doses may be initiated to minimize GI distress. Dosage titration is recommended to maintain a target predialysis bicarbonate level of more than 20 mEq/L. Interdialytic weight gain secondary to the sodium content in the alkali supplement should be monitored during dosage titration.

Malnutrition

Healthy adults need a minimum of 0.75 g/kg/day of high-quality protein and a calorie intake of 30 to 35 kcal/kg/day to maintain a neutral or positive nitrogen balance.[189] By contrast, patients on hemodialysis need 1.2 g/kg/day of primarily high-quality protein and a caloric intake of at least 35 kcal/kg/day.[63,190] This higher protein requirement is due to a higher protein catabolism as a result of metabolic acidosis, infections, the blood–dialyzer interaction (especially with bioincompatible membranes), and losses of protein and amino acid in the dialysate that range from 10 to 13 g per session.[63] Unfortunately, most patients have nutritional intakes below the recommended level; this explains the high prevalence of PCM among patients on hemodialysis.[190] There are numerous causes of anorexia and decreased dietary intake in the ESRD population, including inadequate dialysis.[191,192]

PCM is an important risk factor for morbidity and mortality in the ESRD population.[190] Signs of PCM include reduced energy stores (subcutaneous fat stores); reduced muscle mass as indicated by lower serum creatinine concentrations or as measured by anthropometric methods; low total body nitrogen; low serum concentrations of albumin, transferrin, and other visceral proteins; and abnormalities in the plasma and intracellular amino acids profiles.[190] The risk of death is inversely related to the predialysis serum concentrations of creatinine (marker of muscle mass), BUN (marker of dietary protein intake), albumin (marker of visceral proteins), and cholesterol (marker of dietary intake).[123,193] The serum albumin concentration is by far the most useful laboratory predictor of mortality in patients on hemodialysis and CAPD. The risk of death increases exponentially with decreasing serum albumin values. With a reference value of 4 g/dL, a serum albumin value of 3.5 to 4.0 g/dL, which is still within the normal reference range for most laboratories, is associated with a twofold increase in mortality rate.[192] The mortality risk increases nearly 7-fold when the albumin concentration is 3.0 to 3.5 g/dL and 15-fold when it is 2.5 to 3.0 g/dL.

The bioincompatible dialysis membranes (e.g., cuprophan) can adversely affect protein intake and catabolism, thus influencing a patient's overall nutritional status. The high-flux, biocompatible membranes (e.g., polyacrylonitrile, polysulfone) have a clear advantage in that they have little or no effect on protein catabolism. This is probably because the high-flux membranes have a higher clearance for middle molecules for the same amount of urea removal.[63] Thus, the adequacy of dialysis should ideally be based on removal of both small (e.g., urea) and larger (e.g., β-microglobulin) solutes. Another explanation for this membrane effect may be that the biocompatible membranes do not stimulate production of activated complement components, interleukin-1, and tumor necrosis factor, which may suppress appetite and increase muscle catabolism.[63]

The therapeutic options for preventing PCM include dietary counseling and prescribing adequate protein and calorie intake. Optimizing the hemodialysis dosage and avoiding metabolic acidosis and catabolic diseases such as infections may minimize the likelihood of PCM in a given patient.[194–197] Nutritional intervention for the management of PCM in nondialysis patients as described in Chapter 12, Enteral and Parenteral Nutrition, can also be used in patients on hemodialysis and peritoneal dialysis. Unfortunately, there are few data on the efficacy of enteral nutrition in adults on hemodialysis.[197] Total parenteral nutrition support for hemodialysis or peritoneal dialysis is associated with many complications ranging from the lack of vascular access, fluid overload, and electrolyte abnormalities to economic and logistical consequences. Its use is therefore limited to patients with severe GI tract abnormalities that preclude enteral nourishment. Although intradialytic parenteral nutrition (IDPN) was described more than 25 years ago, the clinical scientific data do not clearly indicate a broad role for its use. Foulks evidence-based evaluation suggests that this means of intermittent nutrition administration is associated with marked reductions in hospitalizations (67%), mortality (48%), and odds ratio for death and an increase in life span of about 1 year.[196] The associations between IDPN and outcomes are weak, and stringent reimbursement policies have restricted its use.[194] Currently, IDPN should be used only for patients who meet the NKF guidelines for the use of IDPN.[196]

Patients on CAPD lose approximately 6 g/day of albumin and 9 g/day of total protein into the dialysate. This amount increases to 15 g/day during bouts of peritonitis. As in hemodialysis, a low serum albumin concentration (3.5 g/dL) is a strong predictor of morbidity and mortality in the CAPD population.[123] The dietary protein intake of patients on CAPD depends on the dialysis dosage, such that for a malnourished and underdialyzed patient an increase in the dialysis dosage results in increased dietary protein intake within a few weeks.[63,198] For a given dialysis dosage (Kt/V), patients on CAPD tend to have a higher dietary protein intake than those on hemodialysis, possibly because of improved appetite and well-being associated with CAPD's enhanced removal of middle molecules.[124] In addition to standard nutrition support options, investigators recently have shown that daily losses of amino acids and proteins can be offset by the administration of a 1.1% amino acid peritoneal dialysis solution during one exchange per day.[199] Although the results of previous studies were controversial, these results are encouraging. Long-term comparative clinical trials are needed to establish the safety, efficacy, and economic outcomes associated with this novel therapeutic approach.

Renal Osteodystrophy and Secondary Hyperparathyroidism

Bone disease is a major cause of morbidity in patients undergoing chronic dialysis treatment. Although several types of bone lesions have been identified from bone biopsies of patients on dialysis, a high-turnover bone disease called osteitis fibrosa cystica, which results from high circulating concentrations of PTH, is the classic lesion.[200,201] Osteomalacia and an adynamic lesion have also been characterized. Histologically, the adynamic lesion shows low amounts of fibrosis or osteoid tissue and is associated with low bone formation rates. The incidence of adynamic lesions has increased dramatically over the last 10 years, and they may be seen in up to 50% of patients on dialysis.[201] This is predominantly because of aggressive management of osteitis fibrosa cystica with vitamin D therapy.[200,202]

Phosphate retention is one of the primary derangements that leads to secondary hyperparathyroidism (i.e., high-turnover bone disease). Phosphorus retention decreases ionized calcium, and the resultant hypocalcemia is a major stimulus for PTH secretion. High phosphorus concentrations may also directly increase PTH secretion.[203] The increase in PTH results in a compensatory decrease in proximal tubular phosphate reabsorption that maintains phosphate balance until the GFR falls below 30 mL/minute. The second primary derangement is a decrease in the production of 1,25 dihydroxyvitamin D_3 (calcitriol). The serum levels of this hormone are reduced by about 50% in patients with GFRs of approximately 65 mL/minute and progressively decline with further decreases in GFR. This results in impaired intestinal absorption of calcium and stimulates PTH release and thus may contribute to defective bone mineralization. Common signs and symptoms of secondary hyperparathyroidism include fatigue and musculoskeletal and GI complaints. Metastatic calcification of joints, vessels, and soft tissue can also be seen especially when the serum calcium–phosphorus product exceeds 70.[204,205] Clinical bone symptoms are rare in patients with mild to moderate renal insufficiency. Renal osteodystrophy often progresses insidiously for several years before patients become symptomatic. When bone pain and skeletal fractures occur, the disease is not easily amenable to treatment. Bone marrow fibrosis and decreased hematopoiesis may also be evident in cases of severe secondary hyperparathyroidism.

Serum calcium, phosphorus, PTH, and alkaline phosphatase are the principal biochemical markers used to diagnose and monitor the status of renal osteodystrophy. Transiliac bone biopsy, although rarely used, is the only method that clearly differentiates between the different causes and thus is the gold standard for evaluation of renal osteodystrophy. Tetracycline administration before bone biopsy provides information about bone turnover rate.[206] Bone mineral densitometry studies are also useful in monitoring the outcome of therapeutic interventions.

The goals of therapy are to control serum phosphorus and PTH concentrations and normalize serum calcium concentration. Dietary phosphorus should be restricted to 800 to 1200 mg/day (10 to 17 mg/kg/day) once dialysis is initiated.[204] This usually entails a major dietary adjustment because many foods or beverages such as meats, dairy products, dried beans, nuts, peanut butter, colas, and beer are high in phosphorus. In addition, most patients on dialysis need a combination of a phosphate-binding medication and calcium supplement or vitamin D therapy to alter the progressive effects of secondary hyperparathyroidism.

Calcium-, aluminum-, and magnesium-containing phosphate-binding agents retard phosphorus absorption from the gut if they are ingested just before or with meals. The dosage should be titrated to achieve serum phosphorus concentrations in the range of 4.5 to 6.0 mg/dL for patients on hemodialysis and peritoneal dialysis. Medication counseling is essential to enhance compliance because many phosphate binders are marketed primarily as antacids or calcium supplements, so many patients on dialysis do not take them correctly for this off-label use.[207] Aluminum salts once were widely used, but their use should be reserved for patients with severe hyperphosphatemia and high serum calcium concentrations. Sucralfate is an effective phosphate binder. However, because the aluminum contained in sucralfate appears to be better absorbed than that from aluminum hydroxide,[208] its use should be avoided. Calcium carbonate and calcium acetate may partially correct the metabolic acidosis, increase ionized calcium concentrations, and thereby decrease PTH secretion and reduce GI phosphorus absorption. Thus, oral calcium compounds have emerged as first-line agents for controlling serum phosphorus and calcium concentrations.

Multiple studies have shown that calcium carbonate alone can achieve the desired phosphate concentrations in most patients on dialysis; however, large dosages (6 to 14 g/day calcium carbonate) may be needed.[209,210] The relationship between ingested dietary phosphorus and the amount of calcium carbonate needed to achieve the phosphorus concentration goal in patients with ESRD, derived from the work of Delmez and Slatopolsky,[205] can be used to guide initial dosage recommendations. Calcium carbonate is marketed in a variety of dosage forms and is inexpensive. Unfortunately, many calcium carbonate products are marketed as food supplements and are not subject to U.S. Pharmacopeia standards. Calcium carbonate is more soluble in an acidic medium and therefore should be administered before meals. Furthermore, concomitant use with ranitidine and other H_2 antagonists can reduce the phosphate-binding activity of calcium carbonate by increasing gastric pH.[211]

Calcium acetate binds approximately twice as much phosphorus as calcium carbonate when comparable dosages of elemental calcium are ingested.[212,213] Furthermore, calcium acetate is more soluble and therefore better absorbed than calcium carbonate in an alkaline pH. Thus, the incidence of hypercalcemia is similar to that of calcium carbonate when equivalent phosphorus concentrations are achieved.[212,213] Although the chloride and citrate salts of calcium can be used as phosphate binders, these agents exhibit several disadvantages.[214] Citrate-containing compounds should not be combined with aluminum-containing compounds since they increase the absorption of aluminum.

Magnesium-containing antacids also bind phosphorus, although serum potassium and magnesium concentrations may rise and diarrhea is a problem. Magnesium carbonate is less well absorbed and better tolerated than the other magnesium salts. However, magnesium and potassium serum concentrations must be monitored closely with all agents. Finally, a nonabsorbable hydrogel phosphate-binding agent that does not contain any aluminum, calcium, or magnesium appears to effectively lower phosphorus, PTH, and total and LDL cholesterol concentrations.[215] This agent (RenaGel) has recently been approved for use in the United States, and its role in the management of hyperphosphatemia is unclear.

Once the desired serum phosphorus level has been achieved, changes in the phosphate-binding regimen may be needed to achieve normocalcemia. Although dietary calcium intake often is subnormal in patients on dialysis because of the reduced intake of phosphate-containing dairy products, calcium-containing phosphate binders usually achieve positive calcium balance. Therefore, calcium supplementation is no longer necessary in the majority of patients.

Vitamin D therapy should be added in patients who do not achieve normocalcemia or those with an elevated PTH concentration despite the use of calcium-containing binders. Calcitriol is the predominant vitamin D preparation used for the management of renal osteodystrophy in the United States because it inhibits PTH secretion directly and stimulates intestinal calcium absorption. The most effective route of administration (oral versus intravenous) and the optimal dosage or dosage interval (daily or intermittent) are controversial.[216,217] Low-dose oral daily therapy with 0.25 to 0.5 μg is a reasonable strategy for the persistently hypocalcemic patient. Calcitriol enhances phosphorus and calcium absorption from the gut and can thus aggravate the patient's hyperphosphatemia.[218,219] Daily oral doses of calcitriol are more commonly associated with hypercalcemia and hyperphosphatemia than intravenous calcitriol. Strategies to maximize PTH suppression with minimal impact on phosphate and calcium levels have included intermittent dosing and administration at bedtime or between meals when gut calcium and phosphorus content is lowest.[216] If the predominant problem is markedly elevated PTH levels, higher dosages (1 to 4 μg three times a week) probably are needed. The dosage for each patient should be guided by his or her degree of PTH elevation.

19-Nor-1-α-25-dihydroxyvitamin D_2 (paricalcitol) was approved in 1998 for use in the United States. Data from three human trials showed that intravenous paricalcitol significantly reduced PTH levels with a mean ending dosage of 0.12 μg/kg, whereas serum calcium and phosphorus values rose only slightly during the study.[220,221] The value of this new therapeutic addition remains to be determined. In patients on hemodialysis with moderate hyperparathyroidism, oral 1-α-hydroxyvitamin D_2 (doxercalciferol) has also been shown to effectively suppress PTH with mean dosages of about 5 μg after each dialysis. Calcium and phosphorus concentrations increased slightly in these patients as well.[222] This oral product was approved in 1999. Although the efficacy and safety profiles of these two new agents look promising, comparative trials with calcitriol are needed to establish their role in therapy.

Parathyroidectomy should be undertaken as a therapeutic option for patients with secondary hyperparathyroidism who have persistent hypercalcemia, a calcium–phosphorus product above 70, progressive radiographic lesions, and intractable pruritus. Subtotal parathyroidectomy or total parathyroidectomy with transplantation of some parathyroid tissue to an accessible site (e.g., the forearm) is the most common surgical procedure. Postoperative hypocalcemia, hypophosphatemia, and hypomagnesemia may be severe and necessitate treatment with supplemental calcium and calcitriol for weeks or months. After surgery, continual efforts to prevent hyperphosphatemia and the recurrence of secondary hyperparathyroidism may be necessary.

DRUG DOSING CONSIDERATIONS FOR PATIENTS ON DIALYSIS

Patients who receive chronic dialysis therapy need dosage modification for most commonly used drugs.[223,224] The disposition of drugs that depend largely on the kidney for elimination (i.e., the fraction that is excreted unchanged by the kidney exceeds 60%) may be influenced greatly by changes in renal function. Furthermore, the pharmacokinetics of many drugs that are eliminated predominantly by hepatic routes may also be markedly affected by changes in nonrenal clearance and alterations in protein binding and volume of distribution.[225] Thus, during development, all new drugs should be evaluated for use by patients with renal insufficiency. This information can be used to individualize drug therapy regimens for patients on dialysis.

The effects of the hemodialysis or peritoneal dialysis procedure itself on the pharmacokinetics of a drug and its serum concentration–time profile are complex. Because multiple dialyzers are available and several techniques are in use for hemodialysis therapy, use of yes-or-no information in terms of dialyzability is inappropriate. Rather, references that provide quantitative estimates of the effect of hemodialysis or peritoneal dialysis on the elimination half-life or total body clearance of a drug should be used.[135,223,226] A compilation of data for many commonly used antibiotics is given in Table 23.6. This clearance information, together with the estimated patient-specific pharmacokinetic parameters, can be used to design a dosing regimen for a given patient.

For the patient on dialysis, the clearance of the drug from the plasma (CL_d) can be defined as the sum of the patient's residual renal clearance (CL_{pt}), the nonrenal clearance (CL_{nr}), and the dialysis clearance (CL_{hd} or CL_{pd}):

$$CL_d = CL_{pt} + CL_{nr} + (CL_{hd} \text{ or } CL_{pd})$$

The characteristics of a drug that has the greatest degree of dialyzability include a low molecular weight, low

Table 23.6 ▪ Effect of Hemodialysis and Intermittent Peritoneal Dialysis on Clearance and Half-Life of Selected Antimicrobial Agents

	Half-Life (hr)		Effect of Dialysis			
Drug	**Normal**	**ESRD**	**CL_{hd} (mL/min)**	**$t_{½,hd}$ (hr)**	**CL_{pd}**	**$t_{½,pd}$**
Amikacin	1.6	39	70.6	3.5	6.7	18–26
Ampicillin	1.3	10–20	30–154	2.9–5.0	2.7	9.5
Aztreonam	2.0	7.0	43	2.7	2.1	7.0
Cefazolin	2.2	28.0	NR	2.6–5.0	NR	32
Cefotaxime	0.9	2.5	91.2	2.1	6.7	2.3
Ceftazidime	1.8	26.0	50–155	1.2–3.2	8.5	8.7
Cefuroxime	1.3	15–22	103	1.6–3.5	2.9	15
Ciprofloxacin	4.4	8.4–12	48.6	5.3	ND	ND
Gentamicin	2.2	53	24–116	3.0–11.3	12.5	8.5
Imipenem	0.9	2.9	73.5	1.6	ND	ND
Penicillin G	0.7	4.1	37.5	2.3	3.9	17.6
Piperacillin	1.2	3.9	92.4	1.3	3.6	2.2
Ticarcillin	1.2	14.8	46.6	2.7	7.2	10.6
Tobramycin	2.5	58	31–120	4.3–6.7	4.7	25
Trimethoprim	14	26–40	29–66	5–9.4	5.1	17–24
Vancomycin	6.9	161	16.1–150	4.5–24	2.3–14.2	30–43

ESRD, end-stage renal disease; CL_{hd}, hemodialysis clearance; $t_{½,hd}$, hemodialysis half-life; CL_{pd}, peritoneal dialysis clearance; $t_{½,pd}$, peritoneal dialysis half-life; *NR*, not reported; *ND*, not done.

protein binding, a small volume of distribution, a rapid rate of equilibration between tissue binding sites and blood, and a limited amount of nonrenal metabolism and excretion. The additional effect of dialysis clearance usually is not considered important unless the procedure increases overall plasma clearance by at least 30% or the fractional drug removal by dialysis exceeds 0.30.[223]

Drug Dosing in Hemodialysis

The actual amount of drug that is removed by hemodialysis is the product of the concentration of the drug in the recovered dialysate and the dialysate volume. This value divided by the total body stores of the drug before dialysis (product of predialysis concentration and volume of distribution) yields the actual fraction of drug removed by dialysis (F_{hd}). Often it is not clinically feasible or analytically practical to measure dialysate drug concentrations. Several methods to predict F_{hd} have been proposed.[227] It is important before using these formulas to differentiate clearance by dialysis (CL_{hd}) from the clearance during dialysis (CL_d); the latter is the sum of the patient's residual renal and nonrenal clearance ($CL_{pt} + CL_{nr}$) and CL_{hd}. The fractional drug removal by dialysis is calculated as follows:

$$F_{hd} = (CL_{hd}/CL_d) \times (1 - e^{-t \times CLd/Vd})$$

where V_d is the volume of distribution of the drug and t is the duration of dialysis.

Alternatively, F_{hd} may be estimated by using the off-dialysis and during-dialysis elimination rate constants. Again, the overall elimination rate constant, K_d, must be differentiated from the dialysis elimination rate constant, K_{hd}, and the patient's residual elimination rate constant, K_{pt}. The off-dialysis half-life divided into 0.693 yields K_{pt}, and 0.693 divided by the half-life during dialysis yields K_d. The dialysis elimination rate constant (K_{hd}) can be approximated as $K_d - K_{pt}$. Therefore, F_{hd} may also be calculated as follows:

$$F_{hd} = (K_{hd}/K_d) \times (1 - e^{-Kd \times t})$$

F_{hd} assessment may help to optimize individualized drug therapy for patients on hemodialysis. For several drugs, the clearance and half-life on and off dialysis have been determined. For example, if a patient on dialysis received 140 mg of gentamicin intravenously just before 4 hours of dialysis, the F_{hd} could be calculated as follows by using a literature value for clearance of 116 ml/mm [228] and steady-state volume of distribution (23.1 L or 0.33 L/kg):

Gentamicin clearance off dialysis, CL_{pt}, is 0.30 L/hour. Gentamicin clearance by dialysis, CL_{hd}, is 6.96 L/hour.

$$CL_d = CL_{hd} + CL_{pt} = 6.96\ L/hr + 0.30\ L/hr = 7.26\ L/hr$$

$$F_{hd} = (6.96\ L/hr/7.26\ L/hr) \times (1 - e^{-4hr \times (7.26L/hr/23.1L)}) = 0.69$$

Endogenous clearance of a drug during the period between dialyses may also affect the drug regimen design. Knowledge of the amount of drug that is removed both during and between dialysis treatments often is needed to design an optimal therapeutic regimen. Patients may need postdialytic or interdialytic dosing when serum concentrations must be maintained within a narrow range to maximize efficacy or minimize toxicity. Unfortunately, accurate information on the dialysis kinetics of many drugs is not readily available. However, if one assumes that drug removal by dialysis and during the interdialytic period follows first-order kinetics–that is, that the drug concentration declines monoexponentially depending on the clearance, volume of distribution, and time between observations–then the serum concentration–time profile and dosing regimen for an individual patient can be predicted, as demonstrated in the following case study.

Case Study

A.Y. is a 70-kg man who was admitted to the hospital with fever. He has been maintained on hemodialysis for 2 years. On admission, gentamicin 140 mg intravenously was given once over 0.5 hour and cefazolin 1.5 g was administered to treat a possible access infection. He was scheduled to receive conventional hemodialysis for 4 hours three times weekly. The gentamicin dose was given right after the dialysis session.

- What is the predicted gentamicin level right after the infusion (C_{max}), right before the next hemodialysis session (C_{bhd}), and right after the hemodialysis session (C_{ahd})?

The first step is to calculate the patient's volume of distribution (V_d):

$$V_d = V_d^* \times \text{Total body weight} = 0.33 \times 70 \text{ kg} = 23.1 \text{ L}$$

where V_d^* is the average value for patients on dialysis, derived from the literature, expressed in liters per kilogram.

$$CL_{pt} \times C_{max} = (140/0.5) \times (1 - e^{-kpt \times tin})$$
$$\text{Therefore, } C_{max} = 6.05 \text{ mg/L}$$

where $CL_{pt} = 0.3$ L/hr (as calculated in the previous example), $k_{pt} = 0.013$ hr – 1, $t_{in} = 0.5$ hr.

$$C_{bhd} = C_{max} \times e^{-kpt \times 43.5hr}$$
$$= 6.05 \times e^{-0.013 \times 43.5}$$
$$= 3.44 \text{ mg/L}$$
$$C_{ahd} = C_{bhd} \times e - (CL_d/V_d) \times 4 \text{ hr}$$
$$= 3.44 \times e - (3.12/23.1) \times 4 \text{ hr}$$
$$= 2.0 \text{ mg/L}$$

where $CL_d = 3.12$ L/hr and $V_d = 23.1$ L

- What postdialysis dosage should be given to achieve a desired peak concentration of 10 mg/L?

Because the half-life of gentamicin in A.Y. is prolonged in comparison to the infusion time, the bolus model may be used to estimate the dosage needed.

$$\text{Dosage} = V_d \times (C_{peak} - C_{min})$$
$$\text{Dosage} = 23.1 \text{ L} \times (10 - 2) \text{ mg/L} = 184.8 \text{ mg}$$

Therefore, to achieve a desired peak concentration of 10 mg/L, the postdialysis dosage that should be given to A.Y. is 184.8 mg, or approximately 180 mg.

Drug Dosing in Continuous Ambulatory Peritoneal Dialysis

Factors that increase drug removal by peritoneal dialysis include a low molecular weight, low protein binding, a small volume of distribution, a rapid rate of equilibration between tissue binding sites and blood, and a limited amount of nonrenal metabolism and excretion. Keller and colleagues described several factors that may limit drug removal by CAPD: a low dialysate outflow rate, a low ratio of dialysate to body volume of distribution, a low peritoneal-to-body clearance ratio, and drug protein binding.[229] As a general rule, if the amount of drug removed by peritoneal dialysis is more than 20% of the administered dosage, supplemental doses are needed.[230] Lower values are less significant because of the large intersubject variability in the pharmacokinetics of many drugs. Aminoglycosides, most cephalosporins, and vancomycin meet this rule and nearly always require higher dosages for patients on CAPD than for nondialyzed patients.[229–231] However, many other commonly used drugs do not require a dosing regimen different from those for an anuric patient because of their low clearance by CAPD.[229] Many of these agents are not cleared adequately by CAPD because of their pharmacokinetic properties. Drugs with volumes of distribution well above 0.05 L/kg body weight (e.g., digoxin), high nonrenal clearances (e.g., cimetidine), or high protein binding (e.g., tricyclic antidepressants) are not cleared to any significant extent by CAPD.

Pharmacokinetics of Systemically Administered Drugs

Because pharmacokinetic data on the effect of CAPD are not available for many drugs, consideration of certain general principles allows the physician to predict whether dosing adjustment is needed. This estimation requires knowledge of several factors that influence drug movement across the peritoneal membrane.[231]

To assess the amount of drug that is removed by CAPD, both the peritoneal clearance (CL_{pd}) and the volume of distribution (V_d) of the drug must be known. CL_{pd} is calculated by dividing the total amount of drug recovered in the spent dialysate from one or more dwell periods (A_{0-t}) by the area under the plasma concentration–time curve during the same period (AUC_{0-t}).[229] Alternatively, if at the end of the each dwell period equilibrium is reached between the drug concentrations in blood and the peritoneal cavity and if there is no significant plasma protein binding, the CL_{pd} is roughly equivalent to the dialysate flow rate. Given the continuous nature of CAPD, the dialysate flow rate rarely exceeds 5 to 7 mL/minute, which limits the amount of drug that is removed by CAPD.[229,230] In estimating the supplemental dosage of a drug, the amount of drug or the fraction of the dosage (f_{pd})

removed by CAPD may be determined from the following formula:

$$f_{pd} = CL_{pd}/CL_d$$

where CL_d is the systemic clearance, which includes the CL_{pd} and CL_{pt} of the drug. The CL_{pt} and CL_{pd} may be estimated from the literature values for patients with ESRD (Table 23.6). Because plasma protein binding is the main limiting factor for diffusion of a drug into the peritoneal cavity, the unbound drug fraction (f_u) should be included in the preceding equation:

$$f_{pd} = (CL_{pd}/CL_d) \times f_u$$

The equation indicates that the higher the clearance ratio of CL_{pd} to CL_d, the higher the fraction of the drug removed by CAPD.[229,231] This method provides a reasonable estimation of the fraction of a dose that is removed by CAPD.

Pharmacokinetics of Intraperitoneally Administered Drugs

Intraperitoneal administration is the preferred route in at least three clinical situations: administering deferoxamine to treat aluminum overload, administering antibiotics to patients with CAPD peritonitis, and administering insulin.[230] Intraperitoneal administration of a low-molecular-weight drug, such as most antibiotics, rapidly achieves high local drug concentrations. This concentration gradient leads to rapid movement (diffusion) of the drug from the peritoneal cavity into the systemic circulation. The reverse movement from the systemic circulation into the peritoneal cavity is much slower and restricted.[229,230] As a result, intraperitoneal antibiotics used to treat peritonitis (e.g., cephalosporins, aminoglycosides) are 50 to 80% bioavailable during a 6-hour dwell period. Despite this rapid peritoneal absorption, there is insignificant loss of antibacterial activity with penicillins, cephalosporins, aminoglycosides, and vancomycin during a normal dwell period.[230] During bouts of peritonitis, because of the higher permeability of the peritoneal membrane, both the rate and the extent of intraperitoneal absorption for certain drugs (e.g., vancomycin, gentamicin, and various β-lactam antibiotics) increase and remain high for days after the episode.[229,230] One concern about the intraperitoneal administration of drugs is the potential for irritation of the peritoneal membrane. Imipenem plus cilastatin, vancomycin, and amphotericin B have all been reported to cause chemical peritonitis in some patients.[230]

CONCLUSION

The advent of dialysis has led to a substantial reduction in morbidity and mortality for patients with chronic renal failure. However, despite their benefits, hemodialysis and CAPD are associated with a number of medical and mechanical complications that can affect morbidity and mortality. In recent years, attention has been focused on the adequacy of dialysis. It is now clear that dialysis therapy is not very successful if the patient is malnourished. Therefore, at times the dialysis dosage must be increased to affect the patient's nutritional state. Treating patients with ESRD is facilitated by a multidisciplinary approach involving physicians, pharmacists, nurses, and social workers.

Although there is some general consensus about what constitutes adequate dialysis, the optimum level of dialysis is unclear. Given the high rate of mortality from ESRD, this issue is of utmost importance. Future research will address the effect of aggressive nutritional support on malnourished patients before dialysis; the effect of higher dialysis dosages on morbidity and mortality; clinical effects of biocompatible, high-flux membranes; modification of cardiovascular risk factors; and immunomodulation. Meanwhile, as new drugs and new dialysis membranes are introduced, clinical pharmacokinetics research must continue to provide drug dosing information to aid in ascertaining the best possible outcome for patients on dialysis.

KEY POINTS

- ESRD may result from primary injury to the nephron, systemic diseases, or exposure to toxic substances.
- Renal transplantation can improve quality of life and is the most cost-effective therapy for patients with ESRD. The low availability of organs limits its wider use.
- Dialysis may be necessary to manage fluid and electrolyte balance and prevent uremia in patients with renal failure.
- Dialysis has led to a substantial reduction in morbidity and mortality in patients with chronic renal failure.
- Hemodialysis and peritoneal dialysis are associated with medical and mechanical complications, which can affect morbidity and mortality.
- Although there is a consensus about what constitutes adequate dialysis, the optimum level of dialysis is unclear.
- Dosage modifications for drugs may be necessary in patients on dialysis.
- The effects of hemodialysis and peritoneal dialysis on the pharmacokinetics of a drug are complex. Drug dosing should be individualized for each patient.

REFERENCES

1. May RC. Pathophysiology of uremia. In: Brenner BM, Rector FCJ, eds. The kidney. 4th ed. Philadelphia: WB Saunders, 1991:1997–2018.
2. Alfrey AC, Chan L. Chronic renal failure: manifestations and pathogenesis. In: Schrier RW, ed. Renal and electrolyte disorders. 4th ed. Boston: Little, Brown, 1992:539–579.
3. The United States Renal Data System. 1998 annual data report. Chapter V. Patient mortality and survival. Am J Kidney Dis 32(2, Suppl 1):S69–S80, 1998.
4. United States Renal Data System. USRDS 1998 annual data report. Bethesda, MD: National Institutes of Health, the National Institute of Diabetes and Digestive Kidney Diseases, 1998.

5. The United States Renal Data System. 1998 annual data report. Chapter II. Incidence and prevalence of ESRD. Am J Kidney Dis 32(2, Suppl 1):S38–S49, 1998.
6. The United States Renal Data System. 1998 annual data report. Chapter VI. Causes of death. Am J Kidney Dis 32(2, Suppl 1):S81–S88, 1998.
7. The United States Renal Data System. 1998 annual data report. Chapter X. The economic cost of ESRD and medicare spending for alternative modalities of treatment. Am J Kidney Dis 32(2, Suppl 1):S118–S131, 1998.
8. The United States Renal Data System. 1998 annual data report. Chapter IV. Medication use among dialysis patients in the DMMS. Am J Kidney Dis 32(2, Suppl 1):S60–S68, 1998.
9. Hakim RM. Initiation of dialysis. Adv Nephrol Necker Hosp 23:295–309, 1994.
10. Eggers P. Comparison of treatment costs between dialysis and transplantation. Semin Nephrol 12:284-9, 1992.
11. United States Renal Data System. USRDS 1999 annual data report. Chapter X. The economic cost of ESRD and Medicare spending for alternative modalities of treatment. Bethesda, MD: National Institutes of Health, the National Institute of Diabetes and Digestive Kidney Diseases, 1999:145–161.
12. Consensus Development Conference Panel. Morbidity and mortality of renal dialysis: NIH consensus conference statement. Ann Intern Med 121:62–70, 1994.
13. The United States Renal Data System. 1999 annual data report. Chapter III. Treatment modalities for ESRD patients. Bethesda, MD: National Institutes of Health, the National Institute of Diabetes and Digestive Kidney Diseases, 1999:39–56.
14. The United States Renal Data System. 1999 annual data report. Chapter XII. International comparisons of ESRD therapy. Bethesda, MD: National Institutes of Health, the National Institute of Diabetes and Digestive Kidney Diseases, 1999:173–184.
15. Ringoir S. An update on uremic toxins. Kidney Int 62:S2–S4, 1997.
16. Vanholder RC, Ringoir SM. Adequacy of dialysis: a critical analysis. Kidney Int 42:540–558, 1992.
17. Gotch FA, Sargent JA. A mechanistic analysis of the National Cooperative Dialysis Study. Kidney Int 28:526–534, 1985.
18. Lowrie EG, Laird NM, Parker TF III, et al. Effect of hemodialysis on patient morbidity: report from the National Cooperative Dialysis Study. N Engl J Med 305:1176–1181, 1981.
19. Gejyo F, Homma N, Arakawa M. Long-term complications of dialysis: pathogenic factors with special reference to amyloidosis. Kidney Int 43(Suppl 41):S78–S82, 1993.
20. Nissenson AR, Prichard SS, Chen IKP, et al. Non-medical factors that impact on ESRD modality selection. Kidney Int 43(Suppl 40):S1–S8, 1993.
21. Kaisike BL, Ramos EL, Gaston RS, et al. The evaluation of renal transplant candidates: clinical practice guidelines. J Am Soc Nephrol 6:1–34, 1995.
22. Bertram LK. The evaluation of prospective renal transplant recipients. In: Greenberg A, Cheung AK, Coffman TM, et al., eds. Primer on kidney diseases 2nd ed. San Diego: Academic Press, 1998:477–481.
23. Kasiske BL, Ravenscraft M, Ramos EL, et al. The evaluation of living renal transplant donors: clinical practice guidelines. J Am Soc Nephrol 7:2288–2313, 1996.
24. United States Renal Data System. USRDS 1999 annual data report. Chapter VI. Renal transplantation: access and outcomes. Bethesda, MD: National Institutes of Health, the National Institute of Diabetes and Digestive Kidney Diseases, 1999:101–112.
25. Kasiske BL, London W, Ellison WD. Race and socioeconomic factors influencing early placement on the kidney transplant waiting list. J Am Soc Nephrol 9(11):2142–2147, 1998.
26. Lundin AP. The doctor who is a patient: conflicting or complementary roles? Nephrol Dial Transplant 14:1082–1084, 1999.
27. Cheung AK. Hemodialysis and hemofiltration. In: Greenberg A, Cheung AK, Coffman TM, et al., eds. Primer on kidney diseases. San Diego: Academic Press, 1994:258–265.
28. Arieff AI. Dialysis disequilibrium syndrome: current concepts on pathogenesis and prevention. Kidney Int 45:629–635, 1994.
29. Bailie GR, Eisele G. Continuous ambulatory peritoneal dialysis: a review of its mechanics, advantages, complications, and areas of controversy. Ann Pharmacother 26:1409–1420, 1992.
30. Piraino B. Peritoneal dialysis. In: Greenberg A, Cheung AK, Coffman TM, et al., eds. Primer on kidney diseases. San Diego: Academic Press, 1998: 416–421.
31. Jungers P, Zingraff J, Albouze G, et al. Late referral to maintenance dialysis: detrimental consequences. Nephrol Dial Transplant 8:1089–1093, 1993.
32. Hakim RM, Lazarus JM. Initiation of dialysis. J Am Soc Nephrol 6(5):1319–1328, 1995.
33. Lucas PA, Meadows JH, Roberts DE, et al. The risks and benefits of a low protein-essential amino acid keto acid diet. Kidney Int 29:995–1003, 1986.
34. NKF-DOQI. Clinical practice guidelines for dialysis adequacy. Am J Kidney Dis 30(Suppl 2):S1–S136, 1997.
35. Khanna R. Dialysis considerations for diabetic patients. Kidney Int 43(Suppl 40):S58–S64, 1993.
36. Diax-Buxo JA. Modality selection. J Am Soc Nephrol 9(12, Suppl):S112–S117, 1998.
37. Khanna R, Oreopoulos DG. Peritoneal dialysis. In: Schrier RW, Gottschalk CW, eds. Diseases of the kidney. 5th ed. Boston: Little, Brown, 1993:2969–3030.
38. Wizemann V, Timio M, Alpert MA, et al. Options in dialysis therapy: significance of cardiovascular findings. Kidney Int 43(Suppl 40):S85–S91, 1993.
39. Burkart JM. Clinical experience: how much earlier should patients really start renal replacement therapy? J Am Soc Nephrol 9:S118–S123, 1998.
40. Rottembourg J. Residual renal function and recovery of renal function in patients treated by CAPD. Kidney Int 43(Suppl 40):S106–S110, 1993.
41. Himmeltarb J. Hematological manifestations of renal failure. In: Greenberg A, Cheung AK, Coffman TM, et al., eds. Primer on kidney diseases. San Diego: Academic Press, 1998:465.
42. Sheperd DJ. Aplastic bone: a nondisease of medical progress. Adv Ren Replace Ther 2:20–23, 1995.
43. Sherrard DJ, Hercz G, Pei Y, et al. The spectrum of bone disease in end stage renal disease: an evolving disorder. Kidney Int 43:436–442, 1993.
44. Parfrey PS, Harnett JD. Long-term cardiac morbidity and mortality during dialysis therapy. Adv Nephrol Necker Hosp 23:311–330, 1994.
45. Collins AJ. High flux, high efficiency procedures. In: Henrich WE, ed. Principles and practice of dialysis. Baltimore: Williams & Wilkins, 1994:22–37.
46. Maiorca R, Cancarini GC, Brunori G, et al. Morbidity and mortality of CAPD and hemodialysis. Kidney Int 43(Suppl 40):S4–S15, 1993.
47. Bloembergen WE, Port FK, Mauger EA, et al. A comparison of mortality between patients treated with hemodialysis and peritoneal dialysis. J Am Soc Nephrol 6:177–183, 1995.
48. Bloembergen WE, Port FK, Mauger EA, et al. A comparison of cause of death between patients treated with hemodialysis and peritoneal dialysis. J Am Soc Nephrol 6:184–191, 1995.
49. Fenton SSA, Schaubel DE, Desmeules M, et al. Hemodialysis versus peritoneal dialysis: a comparison of adjustment mortality rates. Am J Kidney Dis 30:334–342, 1997.
50. Foley RN, Parfrey PS, Harnett JD, et al. Mode of dialysis therapy and mortality in end-stage renal disease. J Am Soc Nephrol 9:267–276, 1998.
51. Vonesh EF, Moran J. Mortality in end-stage renal disease: a reassessment of differences between patients treated with hemodialysis and peritoneal dialysis. J Am Soc Nephrol 10:354–365, 1999.
52. Hakim RM. Assessing the adequacy of dialysis. Kidney Int 37:822–832, 1990.
53. Parker TF III. Trends and concepts in the prescription and delivery of dialysis in the United States. Semin Nephrol 12:267–75, 1992.
54. Uldall PR. Temporary vascular access for hemodialysis. In: Nissenson AR, Fine RN, eds. Dialysis therapy. 2nd ed. Philadelphia: Hanley & Belfus, 1993:5–10.
55. Tomasula JR, Delaney V, Butt KMH. Vascular access for chronic hemodialysis. In Nissenson AR, Fine RN, eds. Dialysis therapy. 2nd ed. Philadelphia: Hanley & Belfus, 1993:10–14.
56. NKF-DOQI. Patient evaluation prior to access placement. Am J Kidney Dis 30(Suppl 3):S154–S161, 1997.
57. Cheung AK. Dialyzer biocompatibility: practical considerations. In: Nissenson AR, Fine RN, eds. Dialysis therapy. 2nd ed. Philadelphia: Hanley & Belfus, 1993:75–77.
58. Lazarus JM, Owen WF. Role of biocompatibility in dialysis morbidity and mortality. Am J Kidney Dis 24:1019–1032, 1994.
59. Held PJ, Carroll CE, Liska DW, et al. Hemodialysis therapy in the United States: what is the dose and does it matter? Am J Kidney Dis 24:974–980, 1994.
60. Lazarus JM, Hakim RM. Medical aspects of hemodialysis. In: Brenner BM, Rector FC, eds. The kidney. 4th ed. Philadelphia: WB Saunders, 1991:2223–2299.
61. Held PJ, Levin NW, Boubjerg RR, et al. Mortality and duration of hemodialysis treatment. JAMA 265:871–875, 1991.
62. Shaldon S. Unanswered questions pertaining to dialysis adequacy in 1992. Kidney Int 43(Suppl 41):S274–S277, 1993.
63. Bergstrom J. Nutrition and adequacy of dialysis in hemodialysis patients. Kidney Int 43(Suppl 41):S261–S267, 1993.
64. Held PJ, Port FK, Wolfe RA, et al. The dose of hemodialysis and patient mortality. Kidney Int 50:550–556, 1996.
65. Bloembergen WE, Stannard DC, Port FK, et al. Relationship of dose of hemodialysis and cause-specific mortality. Kidney Int 50:557–565, 1996.
66. Burkart JM. Adequacy of peritoneal dialysis. In: Henrich WL, ed. Principles of practice of dialysis. Baltimore: Williams & Wilkins, 1994:111–129.

67. Keshaviah P. Urea kinetic and middle molecule approaches to assessing the adequacy of hemodialysis and CAPD. Kidney Int 43(Suppl 40):S28–S38, 1993.
68. Harter HR. Review of significant findings from the National Cooperative Dialysis Study and recommendations. Kidney Int 23(Suppl 13):S107–S112, 1983.
69. Gotch FA, Sargent JA. A mechanistic analysis of the National Cooperative Dialysis Study (NCDS). Kidney Int 28:526–534, 1985.
70. Daugirdas JT, Depner TA. A nomogram approach to hemodialysis urea modeling. Am J Kidney Dis 23:33–40, 1994.
71. Lowrie EG, Lew NL. Death risk in hemodialysis patients: the predictive value of commonly measured variables and an evaluation of death rate differences between facilities. Am J Kidney Dis 15:458–482, 1990.
72. Daugirdas JT. Chronic hemodialysis prescription: a urea kinetic approach. In: Daugirdas JT, Ing TS, eds. Handbook of hemodialysis. 2nd ed. Boston: Little, Brown, 1994:92–120.
73. Sargent J. Short falls in the delivery of dialysis. Am J Kidney Dis 15:500–510, 1990.
74. Hakim RM, Breyer J, Ismail N, et al. Effects of dose of dialysis on morbidity and mortality. Am J Kidney Dis 23:661–669, 1994.
75. National Kidney Foundation report on dialyzer reuse. Task force on reuse of dialyzer, Council on Dialysis, National Kidney Foundation. Am J Kidney Dis 30(6):859–871, 1997.
76. Kopple JD, Hakim RM, Held PJ, et al. Recommendations for reducing the high morbidity and mortality of United States maintenance dialysis patients. Am J Kidney Dis 24:968–973, 1994.
77. Parker TF III. Role of dialysis dose on morbidity and mortality in maintenance hemodialysis patients. Am J Kidney Dis 24:981–989, 1994.
78. Collins AJ, Ma JZ, Umen A, et al. Urea index and other predictors of hemodialysis patient survival. Am J Kidney Dis 23:272–282, 1994.
79. Depner T, Beck G, Daugirdas J, et al. Lessons from the hemodialysis study: an improved measure of the actual hemodialysis dose. Am J Kidney Dis 33(1):142–149, 1999.
80. Consensus Development Conference Panel. Morbidity and mortality or renal dialysis: NIH Consensus Conference statement. Ann Intern Med 121:62–70, 1994.
81. Foley RN, Parfrey PS, Sarnak MJ. Epidemiology of cardiovascular disease in chronic renal disease. J Am Soc Nephrol 9:S16–S23, 1998.
82. Ritz E, Deppisch R, Stier E, et al. Atherogenesis and cardiac death: are they related to dialysis procedure and biocompatibility? Nephrol Dial Transplant 9(Suppl 2):165–172, 1994.
83. Meyer KB, Levey AS. Controlling the epidemic of cardiovascular disease in chronic renal disease: report from the National Kidney Foundation Task Force on Cardiovascular Disease. J Am Soc Nephrol 9:S31–S42, 1998.
84. Cheung AK, Wu LL, Kablitz C, et al. Atherogenic lipids and lipoproteins in hemodialysis patients. Am J Kidney Dis 22:271–276, 1993.
85. Silberberg J, Racine N, Barre P, et al. Regression of left ventricular hypertrophy in dialysis patients following correction of anemia with recombinant human erythropoietin. Can J Cardiol 6:1–4, 1990.
86. Nissenson AR. Optimal hematocrit in patients on dialysis therapy. Am J Kidney Dis 32(6, Suppl 4):S142–S146, 1998.
87. NKF-DOQI. Management of complications: when to intervene? Am J Kidney Dis 30(4, Suppl 3):S170–S172, 1997.
88. Crain M. Management of fibrin sheaths I: percutaneous fibrin sheath stripping. Semin Dial 11(6):336–341, 1998.
89. Lund GB. Management of fibrin sheaths II: thrombolytic therapy. Semin Dial 11(6):342–346, 1998.
90. Khan IH, Catto GR. Long-term complications of dialysis: infection. Kidney Int 43(Suppl 41):S143–S148, 1993.
91. Feldman Hi, Kobrin S, Wasserstein A. Hemodialysis vascular access morbidity. J Am Soc Nephrol 7:523–535, 1996.
92. Himmelfarb J, Hakin RM. Biocompatibility and risk of infection of hemodialysis patients. Nephrol Dial Transplant 9(Suppl 2):138–144, 1994.
93. Marr KA, Kong L, Fowler VG, et al. Incidence and outcome of Staphylococcus aureus bacteremia in hemodialysis patients. Kidney Int 54:1684–1689, 1998.
94. Roghmann MC, Fink JC, Polish L, et al. Colonization with vancomycin-resistant enterococci in chronic hemodialysis patients. Am J Kidney Dis 32(2):254–257, 1998.
95. NKF-DOQI. Management of complications: optimal approaches for treating complications. Am J Kidney Dis 30(4, Suppl 3):S173–S178, 1997.
96. Boelaert JR. *Staphylococcus aureus* infection in haemodialysis patients. Mupirocin as a topical strategy against nasal carriage: a review. J Chemother 2:19–24, 1994.
97. Descamps-Latscha B, Herbelin A. Long-term dialysis and cellular immunity: a critical survey. Kidney Int 43(Suppl 41):S135–S142, 1993.
98. Rhinehart A, Collins AJ, Keane WF. Host defenses and infectious complications in maintenance hemodialysis patients. In: Replacement of renal function by dialysis. In: Jacobs C, Kjellstrand CM, Koch KM, et al., eds. 4th ed. Boston, MA: Kluwer Academic Publishers, 1996:1103–1122.
99. Moran J, Blumenstein M, Gurland HJ. Immunodeficiencies in chronic renal failure. Contrib Nephrol 86:91–110, 1990.
100. Sherman RA, Goodling KA, Eisinger RP. Acute therapy of hemodialysis-related muscle cramps. Am J Kidney Dis 2:287–288, 1982.
101. Hagstam KE, Lingergard B, Tibbling G. Mannitol infusion in regular hemodialysis treatment for chronic renal insufficiency. Scand J Urol Nephrol 3:257–263, 1969.
102. Sidhom OA, Odeh YK, Krumlovsky FA, et al. Low dose prazosin in patients with muscle cramps during hemodialysis. Clin Pharmacol Ther 56:445–451, 1994.
103. Sakurauchi Y, Matsumoto Y, Shinzato T, et al. Effects of L-carnitine supplementation on muscular symptoms in hemodialyzed patients. Am J Kidney Dis 32(2):258–264, 1998.
104. Nishimura M, Takahashi H, Maruyama K, et al. Enhanced production of nitric oxide may be involved in acute hypotension during maintenance dialysis. Am J Kidney Dis 31(5):809–817, 1998.
105. Shinzato T, Miwa M, Naka S, et al. Role of adenosine in dialysis induced hypotension. J Am Soc Nephrol 4:1987–1994, 1994.
106. Jost CMT, Agarwal R, Khair-El-Din T, et al. Effects of cooler temperature dialysate on hemodynamic stability in problem dialysis patients. Kidney Int 44:605–612, 1993.
107. Sadowski RH, Allred EN, Jabs K. Sodium modeling ameliorates intradialytic and interdialytic symptoms in young hemodialysis patients. J Am Soc Nephrol 4:1192–1198, 1993.
108. Lindberg JS, Copley JB, Melton K, et al. Lysine vasopressin in the treatment of refractory hemodialysis induced hypotension. Am J Nephrol 10:269–275, 1990.
109. Ahmad S, Robertson MT, Golper TA, et al. Multicenter trial of L-carnitine in maintenance hemodialysis patients. II. Clinical and biochemical effects. Kidney Int 38:912–918, 1990.
110. Hirszel IP, Martin RH, Mizell MW, et al. Uremic autonomic neuropathy: evaluation of ephedrine sulfate therapy for hemodialysis-induced hypotension. Int Urol Nephrol 8:313–321, 1976.
111. Blowey DL, Balfe W, Gupta I, et al. Midodrine efficacy and pharmacokinetics in a patient with recurrent intradialytic hypotension. Am J Kidney Dis 28(1):132–136, 1996.
112. Salem M, Ivanovich PT, Ing TS, et al. Adverse effects of dialyzers manifesting during the dialysis session. Nephrol Dial Transplant 9(Suppl 2):127–137, 1994.
113. Swartz RD. Hemodialysis-associated seizure activity. In: Nissenson AR, Fine RN, eds. Dialysis therapy. 2nd ed. Philadelphia: Hanley & Belfus, 1993:113–116.
114. Drueke TB. Dialysis related amyloidosis. Nephrol Dial Transplant 13(Suppl 1):58–64, 1998.
115. Hakim RM, Wingard RL, Husni L, et al. The effect of membrane biocompatibility on plasma β_2 microglobulin levels in chronic hemodialysis patients. J Am Soc Nephrol 7:472–478, 1996.
116. Koda Y, Nishi SI, Miyazaki S, et al. Switch from conventional to high-flux membrane reduces the risk of carpal tunnel syndrome and mortality of hemodialysis patients. Kidney Int 52:1096–1101, 1997.
117. Brophy DF, Mueller BA. Automated peritoneal dialysis: new implications for pharmacists. Ann Pharmacother 31:756–764, 1997.
118. USRDS 1998 data on PD methods. NIH Publication No. 99-4578. Bethesda, MD, 1999.
119. Mactier RA. Peritoneal cavity lymphatics. In: Nolph KD, ed. Peritoneal dialysis. 3rd ed. Boston: Kluwer, 1989:28–47.
120. Niezgoda JA, Wolfson AB. Continuous ambulatory peritoneal dialysis. Emerg Med Clin North Am 12:759–769, 1994.
121. Ash SR. Peritoneal access devices and placement techniques. In: Nissenson AR, Fine RN, eds. Dialysis therapy. 2nd ed. Philadelphia: Hanley & Belfus, 1993:23–28.
122. La Greca, Feriani M, Ronco C, et al. Proceedings of the 6th International Course on PD. Perit Dial Int 17 (Suppl 2):S47–S83, 1997.
123. Teehan BP, Schleifer CR, Brown J. Adequacy of continuous ambulatory peritoneal dialysis: morbidity and mortality in chronic peritoneal dialysis. Am J Kidney Dis 24:990–1001, 1994.
124. Gotch FA. Adequacy of peritoneal dialysis. Am J Kidney Dis 21:96–98, 1993.
125. Coles GA, Williams JD. What is the place of peritoneal dialysis in the integrated treatment of renal failure? Kidney Int 54:2234–2240, 1998.
126. Brandes JC, Piering WF, Beres JA, et al. Clinical outcome of continuous ambulatory peritoneal dialysis predicted by urea and creatinine kinetics. J Am Soc Nephrol 2:1430–1435, 1992.
127. Flanagan MJ, Hochstetler LA, Langholdt D, et al. CAPD catheter infections: diagnosis and management. Perit Dial Int 15:248–254, 1995.

128. Twardowski ZJ. Peritoneal catheter exit-site and tunnel infections. In Nissenson AR, Fine RN, eds. Dialysis therapy. 2nd ed. Philadelphia: Hanley & Belfus, 1993:165–168.
129. Keane WF, Alexander SR, Bailie GR, et al. Peritoneal dialysis-related peritonitis treatment recommendations: 1996 update. Perit Dial Int 16:557–573, 1996.
130. Michel C, Courdavault L, al Khayat R, et al. Fungal peritonitis in patients on peritoneal dialysis. Am J Nephrol 14:113–120, 1994.
131. Holley JL, Bernardini J, Perlmutter JA, et al. A comparison of infection rates among older and younger patients on continuous peritoneal dialysis. Perit Dial Int 14:66–69, 1994.
132. Nolph KD. Access problems plague both peritoneal dialysis and hemodialysis. Kidney Int 43(Suppl 40):S81–S84, 1993.
133. Chaimovitz C. Peritoneal dialysis. Kidney Int 45:1226–1240, 1994.
134. Vas SI. Treatment of peritonitis. Perit Dial Int 14(Suppl 3):S49–S55, 1994.
135. Taylor C, Abel-Rahman E, Zimmerman SW, et al. Clinical pharmacokinetics during continuous ambulatory peritoneal dialysis. Clin Pharmacokinet 31(4):293–308, 1996.
136. Bailie GR, Eisele G. Pharmacokinetic issues in the treatment of CAPD-associated peritonitis. J Antimicrob Chemother 35:563–567, 1995.
137. The Ad Hoc Advisory Committee on Peritonitis Management. Continuous ambulatory peritoneal dialysis (CAPD) peritonitis treatment recommendations: 1989 update. Perit Dial Int 9:247–256, 1989.
138. Holley JL, Bernardini J, Piraino B. Infecting organisms in continuous ambulatory peritoneal dialysis patients on the Y-set. Am J Kidney Dis 23:569–573, 1994.
139. Luzar MA. Exit-site infection in continuous ambulatory peritoneal dialysis: a review. Perit Dial Int 11:333–340, 1991.
140. Perez-Fontan M, Garcia-Falcon T, Roasales M, et al. Treatment of *Staphylococcus aureus* nasal carriers in CAPD with mupirocin: long-term results. Am J Kidney Dis 22:708–712, 1993.
141. Piraino B, Lu VL. Nasal mupirocin: its role in dialysis patients. Semin Dial 10:145–147, 1997.
142. Zimmerman SW, Ahrens E, Johnson CA, et al. Randomized controlled trial of prophylactic rifampin for peritoneal dialysis-related infections. Am J Kidney Dis 18:225–231, 1991.
143. Bargman JM. Complications of peritoneal dialysis related to increased intraabdominal pressure. Kidney Int 43(Suppl 40):S75–S80, 1993.
144. Spinowitz BS, Charytan C, Gupta B. Hydrothorax and peritoneal dialysis. In: Nissenson AR, Fine RN, eds. Dialysis therapy. 2nd ed. Philadelphia: Hanley & Belfus, 1993:189–191.
145. Spinowitz BS, Charytan C. Abdominal hernias in CAPD. In: Nissenson AR, Fine RN, eds. Dialysis therapy. 2nd ed. Philadelphia: Hanley & Belfus, 1993:187–188.
146. Jelkmann W. Erythropoietin: structure, control of production, and function. Physiol Rev 72:449–489, 1992.
147. Koury ST, Koury MJ. Erythropoietin production by the kidney. Semin Nephrol 13:78–86, 1993.
148. NKF-DOQI. Clinical practice guidelines for the treatment of anemia of chronic renal failure. Am J Kidney Dis 30(4, Suppl 3):S192–S224, 1997.
149. Jensen JD, Madsen JK, Jensen LW, et al. Reduced production, absorption, and elimination of erythropoietin in uremia compared with healthy volunteers. J Am Soc Nephrol 5:177–185, 1994.
150. Kaufman JS. Subcutaneous erythropoietin therapy: efficacy and economic implications. Am J Kidney Dis 326(6, Suppl 4):S147–151, 1998.
151. Matzke GR. Intravenous iron supplementation in ESRD patients. Am J Kidney Dis 33(3):595–597, 1999.
152. Burt VL, Whelton P, Roccella EJ, et al. Prevalence of hypertension in the U.S. adult population: results from the National Health and Nutrition Examination Survey, 1988–91. Hypertension 25:305–313, 1995.
153. ESRD Networks. 1995 Core Indicators Project: initial results. Opportunities to improve care for adult in-center hemodialysis patients. Baltimore: Department of Health and Human Services, Health Care Financing Administration, Health Standards and Quality Bureau, 1996.
154. Linder A, Charra B, Sherrand DJ, et al. Accelerated atherosclerosis in prolonged maintenance hemodialysis. N Engl J Med 290:697–701, 1974.
155. Vincenti F, Amend W, Abele J, et al. The role of hypertension in hemodialysis-associated atherosclerosis. Am J Med 68:363–369, 1980.
156. Fernandez JM, Carbonell ME, Mazzuchi N, et al. Simultaneous analysis of morbidity and mortality factors in chronic hemodialysis patients. Kidney Int 41:1029–1034, 1992.
157. Foley RN, Parfrey PS, Harnett JD, et al. Impact of hypertension on cardiomyopathy, morbidity and mortality in end-stage renal disease. Kidney Int 49:1379–1385, 1996.
158. Cruickshank J, Thorp J, Zacharias F. Benefits and potential harm of lowering high blood pressure. Lancet 1(8533):581–584, 1987.
159. Hansson L, Zanchetti A, Carruthers SG, et al. Effects of intensive blood-pressure lowering and low-dose aspirin in patients with hypertension: principal results of the Hypertension Optimal Treatment (HOT) randomised trial. Lancet 351(9118):1755–1762, 1998.
160. Shemin D, Dworkin LD. Sodium balance in renal failure. Curr Opin Nephrol Hypertens 6:128–132, 1997.
161. Salem MM. Hypertension in the hemodialysis population: a survey of 649 patients. Am J Kidney Dis 26:461–468, 1995.
162. Luik AJ, van Kuijk WM, Spek J, et al. The effects of hypervolemia on interdialytic hemodynamics and blood pressure control in hemodialysis patients. Am J Kidney Dis 30:466–474, 1997.
163. Flanigan MJ. Dialysis and hypertension: worthy of investigation? Semin Dial 11(2):109–112, 1998.
164. Coomer RW, Schulman G, Breyer JA, et al. Ambulatory blood pressure monitoring in dialysis patients and estimation of mean interdialytic blood pressure. Am J Kidney Dis 29(5):678–684, 1997.
165. Salem MM. Hypertension in the hemodialysis population: any relationship to 2-years survival? Nephrol Dial Transplant 14:125–128, 1999.
166. Dorhout Mees EJ. Hypertension in hemodialysis patients: who cares? Nephrol Dial Transplant 14:28–30, 1999.
167. Joint National Committee. The sixth report of the Joint National Committee on Detection, Evaluation, and Treatment of High Blood Pressure. Arch Intern Med 57:2413–2446, 1998.
168. Attman PO, Samuelsson O, Alaupovic P. Lipoprotein metabolism and renal failure. Am J Kidney Dis 21:573–592, 1993.
169. Wheeler DC. Abnormalities of lipoprotein metabolism in CAPD patients. Kidney Int 50(Suppl 56):S41–S46, 1996.
170. Boushey CJ, Beresford SA, Omenn GS, et al. A quantitative assessment of plasma homocysteine as a risk factor for vascular disease. Probable benefits of increasing folic acid intakes. JAMA 274:1049–1057, 1995.
171. Yuen JY. The role of homocysteine in end-stage renal disease. Semin Dial 11(2):95–101, 1998.
172. Bostom AG, Shemin D, Nadeau MR, et al. Short term betaine therapy fails to lower elevated fasting total plasma homocysteine concentrations in hemodialysis patients maintained on chronic folic acid supplementation. Atherosclerosis 113:129–132, 1995.
173. Tamura T, Johnston KE, Bergman SM. Homocysteine and folate concentrations in blood from patients treated with hemodialysis. J Am Soc Nephrol 7:2414–2418, 1996.
174. Bostom AG, Lathrop L. Hyperhomocystinemia in end-stage renal disease: prevalence, etiology and potential relationship to atherosclerotic outcomes. Kidney Int 52:10–20, 1997.
175. Bostom AG, Shermin D, Lapane KL, et al. High dose vitamin B treatment of hyperhomocystinemia in dialysis patients. Kidney Int 49:147–152, 1996.
176. Kasiske BL. Management of lipid abnormalities in the patient with renal disease. In: Mitch WE, Klahr S, eds. Handbook of nutrition and the kidney. 3rd ed. Boston: Little, Brown, 1998:123–143.
177. Wheeler DC. Should hyperlipidemia in dialysis patients be treated? Nephrol Dial Transplant 12:19–21, 1997.
178. Expert Panel on Detection, Evaluation, and Treatment of High Blood Cholesterol in Adults. Summary of the second report of the National Cholesterol Education Program (NCEP) Expert Panel on Detection, Evaluation, and Treatment of High Blood Cholesterol in adults. JAMA 269(23): 3015–3023, 1993.
179. Kasiske BL. Hyperlipidemia in patients with chronic renal disease. Am J Kidney Dis 32(5, Suppl 3): S142–S156, 1998.
180. Shepherd J, Cobbe SM, Ford I, et al. Prevention of coronary heart disease with pravastatin in men with hypercholesterolemia. N Engl Med 333:1301–1307, 1995.
181. Scandinavian Simvastatin Survival Study Group. Randomized trial of cholesterol lowering in 4444 patients with coronary heart disease: the Scandinavian Simvastatin Survival Study. Lancet 344:1383–1389, 1994.
182. Sacks FM, Pfeffer MA, Moye LA, et al. The effect of pravastatin on coronary events after myocardial infarction in patients with average cholesterol levels. N Engl J Med 335:1001–1009, 1996.
183. Downs J, Clearfield M, Weis S, et al. Primary prevention of acute coronary events with lovastatin in men and women with average cholesterol levels: results of AFCAPS/TexCAPS. JAMA 279(20):1615–1622, 1998.
184. The Long-Term Intervention with Pravastatin in Ischaemic Disease (LIPID) Study Group. Prevention of cardiovascular events and death with pravastatin in patients with coronary heart disease and a broad range of initial cholesterol levels. N Engl J Med 339:1349–1357, 1998.
185. McCormick LS, Black DM, Waters D, et al. Rationale, design, and baseline characteristics of a trial comparing aggressive lipid lowering with atorvastatin versus revascularization treatments (AVERT). Am J Cardiol 80(9):1130–1133, 1997.

186. Gennari FJ. Acid-base homeostasis in end-stage renal disease. Semin Dial 9(5):404–411, 1996.
187. Graham KA, Goodship TH. Does metabolic acidosis have clinically important consequences in dialysis patients? Semin Dial 11(1):14–15, 1998.
188. Lefebvre A, DeVernejoul MC, Gueris J, et L. Optimal correction of acidosis changes progression of dialysis osteodystrophy. Kidney Int 36:1112–1118, 1989.
189. Young VR. Nutritional requirements of normal adults. In: Mitch WE, Klahr S, eds. Handbook of nutrition and the kidney. 3rd ed. Boston: Little, Brown, 1998:1–24.
190. Ikizler TA, Hakim RM. Nutritional requirements of hemodialysis adults. In: Mitch WE, Klahr S, eds. Handbook of nutrition and the kidney. 3rd ed. Boston: Little, Brown, 1998:253–268.
191. Mamoun AH. Anorexia in patients with chronic renal failure: progress towards understanding the molecular basis. Nephrol Dial Transplant 13:2460–2463, 1998.
192. Mitch WE, Maroni BJ. Factors causing malnutrition in patients with chronic uremia. Am J Kidney Dis 33(1):176–179, 1999.
193. Lowrie EG, Lew NL. Death risk in hemodialysis patients: the predictive value of commonly measured variables and an evaluation of death rate differences between facilities. Am J Kidney Dis 15:458–482, 1990.
194. Lazarus JM. Recommended criteria for initiating and discontinuing intradialytic parenteral nutrition therapy. Am J Kidney Dis 33(1):211–216, 1999.
195. Hakim RM. Proposed clinical trials in the evaluation of intradialytic parenteral nutrition. Am J Kidney Dis 33(1):217–220, 1999.
196. Foulks CJ. An evidence-based evaluation of intradialytic parenteral nutrition. Am J Kidney Dis 33(1):186–192, 1999.
197. Kopple JD. Therapeutic approaches to malnutrition in chronic dialysis patients: the different modalities of nutritional support. Am J Kidney Dis 33(1):180–185, 1999.
198. Gokal R, Harty J. Nutrition and peritoneal dialysis. In: Mitch WE, Klahr S, eds. Handbook of nutrition and the kidney. 3rd ed. Boston: Little, Brown, 1998:269–293.
199. Jones MR, Gehr TW, Burkart JM, et al. Replacement of amino acid and protein losses with 1.1% amino acid peritoneal dialysis solution. Perit Dial Int 18:210–216, 1998.
200. Sherrard DJ. Aplastic bone: a nondisease of medical progress. Adv Ren Replace Ther 2:20–23, 1995.
201. Sherrard DJ, Hercz G, Pei Y, et al. The spectrum of bone disease in end-stage renal failure: an evolving disorder. Kidney Int 43:436–442, 1993.
202. Malberti F, Corradi B, Imbasciati E. Effect of CAPD and hemodialysis on parathyroid function. Adv Perit Dial 12:239–244, 1996.
203. Kates DM, Sherrard DJ, Andress DL. Evidence that serum phosphate is independently associated with serum PTH in patients with chronic renal failure. Am J Kidney Dis 30:809–813, 1997.
204. Brookhyser J, Pahre SN. Dietary and pharmacotherapeutic considerations in the management of renal osteodystrophy. Adv Ren Replace Ther 2:5–13, 1995.
205. Delmez JA, Slatopolsky E. Hyperphosphatemia: its consequences and treatment in patients with chronic renal disease. Am J Kidney Dis 19:303–317, 1992.
206. Coen G, Mazzaferro S. Bone metabolism and its assessment in renal failure. Nephron 67:383–401, 1994.
207. Cleary DJ, Matzke GM, Alexander AM, et al. Medication knowledge and compliance among patients receiving long-term dialysis. Am J Health Syst Pharm 52:1895–1900, 1995.
208. Roxe DM, Mistovich M, Barch DH. Phosphate-binding effects of sucralfate in patients with chronic renal failure. Am J Kidney Dis 13:194–199, 1989.
209. Fournier A, Drüeke T, Morinière P, et al. The new treatments of hyperparathyroidism secondary to renal insufficiency. Adv Nephrol 21:237–306, 1992.
210. Fournier A, Morinière P, Hamida FB, et al. Use of alkaline calcium salts as phosphate binder in uremic patients. Kidney Int 42(Suppl 38):S50–S61, 1992.
211. Tan CC, Harden PN, Rodger RSC, et al. Ranitidine reduces phosphate binding in dialysis patients receiving calcium carbonate. Nephrol Dial Transplant 11:851–853, 1996.
212. Schaefer K, Scheer J, Asmus G, et al. The treatment of uraemic hyperphosphataemia with calcium acetate and calcium carbonate: a comparative study. Nephrol Dial Transplant 6:170–175, 1991.
213. Morinière P, Djerad M, Boudailliez B, et al. Control of predialytic hyperphosphatemia by oral calcium acetate and calcium carbonate. Nephron 60:6–11, 1992.
214. Nolan CR, Califano JR, Butzin CA. Influence of calcium acetate or calcium citrate on intestinal aluminum absorption. Kidney Int 38:937–941, 1990.
215. Chertow GM, Burke SK, Lazarus JM, et al. Poly[allylamine hydrochloride] (Renagel): a noncalcemic phosphate binder for the treatment of hyperphosphatemia in chronic renal failure. Am J Kidney Dis 29:66–71, 1997.
216. Daisley-Kydd RE, Mason NA. Calcitriol in the management of secondary hyperparathyroidism of renal failure. Pharmacotherapy 16:619–630, 1996.
217. Fernandez E, Llach F. Guidelines for dosing of intravenous calcitriol in dialysis patients with hyperparathyroidism. Nephrol Dial Transplant 11(Suppl 3):96–101, 1996.
218. Fischer ER, Harris DCH. Comparison of intermittent oral and intravenous calcitriol in hemodialysis patients with secondary hyperparathyroidism. Clin Nephrol 40:216–220, 1993.
219. Malberti F, Surian M, Cosci P. Effect of chronic intravenous calcitriol on parathyroid function and set point of calcium in dialysis patients with refractory secondary hyperparathyroidism. Nephrol Dial Transplant 7:822–828, 1992.
220. Llach F, Keshav G, Goldblat MV, et al. Suppression of parathyroid hormone secretion in hemodialysis patients by a novel vitamin D analogue: 19-nor-1,25-dihydroxyvitamin D_2. Am J Kidney Dis 32(4, Suppl 2):S48–S54, 1998.
221. Martin KJ, Gonzalez EA, Gellens ME, et al. Therapy of secondary hyperparathyroidism with 19-nor-1-alpha, 25-dihydroxyvitamin D_2. Am J Kidney Dis 32(4, Suppl 2):S61–S66, 1998.
222. Tan AU Jr, Levine BS, Mazess RB, et al. Effective suppression of parathyroid hormone by 1a-hydroxy-vitamin D_2 in hemodialysis patients with moderate to severe secondary hyperparathyroidism. Kidney Int 51:317–323, 1997.
223. Matzke GR, Millikin SP. Influence of renal disease and dialysis on pharmacokinetics. In: Evans WE, Schentag JJ, Jusko WJ, eds. Applied pharmacokinetics: principles of therapeutic drug monitoring. 3rd ed. Spokane, WA: Applied Therapeutics, 1992.
224. Aronoff GR, Berns JS, Brier ME, et al., eds. Drug Prescribing in renal failure. 4th ed. Boston: Little, Brown, 1998:123–143.
225. Elston AC, Bayliss MK, Park GR. Effect of renal failure on drug metabolism by the liver. Br J Anaesth 71:282–290, 1993.
226. St Peter W, Redic-Kill KA, Halstenson CE. Clinical pharmacokinetics of antibiotics in patients with impaired renal function. Clin Pharmacokinet 22(3):169–210, 1992.
227. Lee CC. The assessment of fractional drug removal by extracorporeal dialysis. Biopharm Drug Dispos 3:163–173, 1982.
228. Amin NB, Padhi D, Touchette MA, et al. Gentamicin removal by the F-80 membrane in patients with end stage renal disease. Am J Kidney Dis 34:222–227, 1999.
229. Keller E. Peritoneal kinetics of different drugs. Clin Nephrol 30(Suppl 1): S24–S28, 1988.
230. Keller E, Reetze P, Schollmeyer P. Drug therapy in patients undergoing continuous ambulatory peritoneal dialysis: clinical pharmacokinetic considerations. Clin Pharmacokinet 18:104–117, 1990.
231. Paton TW, Cornish WR, Manuel MA, et al. Drug therapy in patients undergoing peritoneal dialysis: clinical pharmacokinetic considerations. Clin Pharmacokinet 10:404–125, 1985.

CHAPTER 24

PEPTIC ULCER DISEASE

Robert P. Henderson and Roger D. Lander

Peptic ulcer disease (PUD) is a chronic inflammatory condition involving a group of disorders characterized by ulceration in regions of the upper gastrointestinal (GI) tract where parietal cells secrete pepsin and hydrochloric acid. The most common sites are the duodenum and stomach, where the major forms are duodenal and gastric ulceration. Additionally, Barrett ulcer of the esophagus, postbulbar ulcer, some cases of Meckel's diverticulum, and stomal or jejunal ulcers after surgery for peptic ulceration also are classified as PUD. Early in the twentieth century, PUD was believed to be related to stress and dietary factors. Later, the concept arose that PUD was caused by the injurious effects of digestive secretions such as gastric acid. PUD results from an imbalance between aggressive factors (acid secretion) and protective factors (mucosal defense; Table 24.1).

TREATMENT GOALS: PEPTIC ULCER DISEASE

- Relieve pain, enhance ulcer healing, prevent complications such as GI bleeding or perforation, and prevent ulcer recurrence.
- Apply drug therapy for PUD to neutralize stomach acid (antacids), protect the stomach mucosa (sucralfate, misoprostol), prevent acid secretion (H_2 antagonists, proton pump inhibitors [PPIs]), and detect and eradicate *Helicobacter pylori* as a cause of PUD.
- Avoid use of ulcerogenic drugs.
- Encourage patients to stop smoking, avoid alcohol intake, avoid caffeine intake, refrain from eating after dinner so as not to stimulate acid secretion during the night.
- Promote stress management.

Overview of Peptic Ulcer Disease

EPIDEMIOLOGY

The lifetime prevalence of PUD is 5 to 10% in the general population.[1,2] There are approximately 3.9 million patients with PUD in the United States, with 200,000 to 400,000 new cases reported each year. The peak incidence is between 50 and 70 years of age. Peptic ulcer typically is a recurrent disease, with 50 to 90% of patients with duodenal ulcer (DU) having a recurrence within 1 year of diagnosis; the relapse rate is lower for gastric ulcer (GU). Recent findings suggest that PUD may have an infectious

Table 24.1 ▪ Factors That Influence Peptic Ulcer Disease Development

Aggressive Factors	Protective Factors
Hydrochloric acid, pepsin	Mucus secretion
Alcohol, nicotine	Rapid gastric epithelial cell turnover
Gastric mucosal ischemia	Gastric and duodenal mucosal blood flow
Helicobacter pylori	Normal pyloric function (motility)
Ulcerogenic drugs	Bicarbonate secretion
Aspirin	
Nonsteroidal anti-inflammatory drugs	
Corticosteroids	
Iron salts	
Potassium chloride	
Erythromycin	
Chemotherapeutic agents	
Alendronate	
Zidovudine	

component (*H. pylori*), and this may largely account for the recurrent nature of the disease.

DUs are approximately four times more common than GUs. DUs rarely are cancerous, but approximately 5% of GUs are malignant; therefore, careful evaluation and close follow-up are extremely important in patients with GU disease.

PUD is a dynamic condition, and the incidence varies with age, gender, ulcer type, and geographic location, with DU being more common than GU in the United States. Peptic ulcer and its complications tend to occur and recur during autumn and winter rather than summer.[1] DU was previously thought to be more common in men; however, recent trends indicate that the incidence among women may be similar to that in men. DU tends to occur between ages 25 and 55 years and peaks at 40 years. GU usually does not occur before age 40, peaks between 55 and 65 years of age, and probably is influenced by use of ulcerogenic medications.

The number of PUD-related hospitalizations has declined over the last several decades, with a shift of care to the outpatient setting seen with the introduction of H_2-receptor antagonists and other new therapeutic agents. The incidence of PUD-related surgery has decreased in all age groups except older adults. Mortality from PUD has decreased among people of all ages and both sexes.[2] Despite these observations, PUD remains one of the most common GI diseases, resulting in substantial human suffering and high costs.[3,4]

PATHOPHYSIOLOGY

Regulation of Gastric Acid Secretion

Gastric hydrochloric acid secretion is intimately related to PUD. A peptic ulcer does not develop when there is no acid secretion. In fact, with few exceptions, therapeutic approaches follow Schwarz's dictum: No acid, no ulcer.

There are three anatomically and functionally distinct regions in the stomach: the cardia (superior region); the body, which accounts for 80 to 90% of the stomach mass; and the antrum (lower prepyloric region). The cardia contains mucus-secreting cells. The body, which includes the fundus, contains parietal cells, responsible for hydrochloric acid and intrinsic factor secretion, and chief cells, responsible for pepsinogen secretion. The antrum contains G cells, responsible for gastrin secretion.

Parietal cells are located in the walls of the oxyntic glands, the secretory units of the gastric mucosa. Hydrochloric acid secretion by parietal cells is the result of the activation of a unique proton pump, hydrogen–potassium ion adenosine triphosphatase (H^+/K^+-ATPase). This magnesium-dependent enzyme is found only on the membranes of parietal cells and exchanges one potassium ion from the canalicular fluid for one hydrogen ion from the cytoplasm. The normal stomach contains approximately 1 billion parietal cells that can secrete hydrogen ions into the gastric lumen against a 3 million : 1 concentration gradient, producing concentrations as high as 160 mEq/L. Gastric mucosal integrity normally is maintained by resisting attack from these very high acid concentrations.

Three pathways stimulate gastric acid secretion: the neurocrine pathway, which causes acetylcholine release from postganglionic vagal neurons in the stomach; the endocrine pathway, which causes gastrin release from antral G cells; and the paracrine pathway, which releases histamine from the mast cells in the lamina propria.[5] The neurocrine pathway involves acetylcholine release at parietal and G cells by central mediation of local cholinergic nerves, stimulation of postganglionic branches of the vagus nerve, and distension of the stomach that is mediated through receptors in the gastric wall. These actions result in acid secretion by acting on muscarinic M_3 cholinergic receptors. Acetylcholine also causes G cells to release gastrin, further increasing acid secretion.[6] These cholinergic actions can be blocked by atropine.

Gastrin is a key factor in acid secretion and is secreted by antral G cells in two principal forms: G-34 (big gastrin), a 34–amino acid peptide, is the predominant form in serum; G-17 (little gastrin), a 17–amino acid peptide, is identical to the C-terminal half of G-34 and is the principal form in gastric antral mucosa.[6,7] Both forms of gastrin are equally potent in stimulating gastric acid secretion. Gastrin has several physiologic actions, including stimulation of gastric acid and pepsinogen secretion, hepatic bile flow, insulin release from the pancreas, and pancreatic secretions. In addition, gastrin stimulates gastric and intestinal motility and increases lower esophageal sphincter (LES) pressure, which promotes closure of the sphincter.

Gastrin may be measured accurately in the blood by radioimmunoassay; the normal level is less than 200 pg/mL. Gastrin levels are not elevated in chronic PUD; however, these patients may be more sensitive to the effects of gastrin. A gastrin assay is necessary for the diagnosis of the gastrin-producing pancreatic adenoma (Zollinger–Ellison [ZE] syndrome), in which fasting blood gastrin levels are extremely high, typically between 200 pg/mL and 1000 pg/mL.

Histamine is present in many body tissues, including the gastric mucosa. In 1971, Sir James Black discovered the H_2 receptor and identified the important physiologic role of histamine in gastric acid secretion. Histamine is contained throughout the stomach in enterochromaffin-like cells in the lamina propria. These cells are found in proximity to parietal cells and receive cholinergic innervation. Histamine plays an important role in gastric acid secretion, but the role of enterochromaffin-like cells in the pathophysiology of PUD is not well understood.

Gastric acid secretion occurs continuously, and is called interdigestive, or basal, when no stimuli are present. Basal acid output usually ranges from 0 to 5 mEq/hour but can rise to 20 mEq/hour or higher with appropriate stimulation. Acid output is highest between 2:00 PM and 1:00 AM and lowest between 5:00 AM and 11:00 AM. Gastric secretion can be divided into three phases based on origin: cephalic, gastric, and intestinal.

The cephalic phase represents gastric acid secretion in response to the thought, sight, taste, smell, or chewing of food. Vagal stimulation causes acetylcholine release, which causes the parietal cell to secrete hydrochloric acid and antral G cells to release gastrin. The gastric phase begins when food causes stomach distension and is mediated by both gastrin and cholinergic nerves, leading vagus nerve stimulation. Amino acids and peptides from protein cause further secretion of acid through gastrin release. Gastrin causes histamine release, which stimulates acid and pepsinogen secretion. Pepsinogen causes pepsin formation, at pH less than 4. Pepsins are proteolytic enzymes that exhibit maximal activity at pH 2 to 3.3 and lose their activity above pH 5. The role of pepsin in the pathogenesis of PUD involves its ability to disrupt the mucus–bicarbonate barrier, which normally protects the gastric epithelial surface and mucosa from acid. As the gastric pH decreases, gastrin output in response to amino acids decreases. The intestinal phase begins when food enters the proximal portion of the small intestine. Gastric secretion can be decreased through negative feedback when the pH in the small intestine becomes too low. A number of other substances are secreted by the stomach, including vasoactive intestinal peptide, cholecystokinin–pancreozymin, serotonin, somatostatin, platelet-activating factor, growth factors, and prostaglandins (PGs).

The normal gastric mucosa is protected from ulceration by several mechanisms. Gastric epithelial cells secrete mucus and bicarbonate, which helps to protect the mucosa from damage. Mucus and bicarbonate act as a barrier to hydrogen ion back-diffusion across the gastric mucosa, normally keeping the pH almost neutral at the surface of the mucosa, even when the luminal pH is around 2.0. If ultimately damaged, these mucosal epithelial cells regenerate rapidly and allow the gastric mucosa to heal itself. Rapid gastric mucosal blood flow allows removal of hydrogen ions that cross the gastric mucosa, and if this blood flow is compromised, the risk of mucosal damage increases. PGs (e.g., PGE) stimulate mucus and bicarbonate secretion and maintain gastric mucosal blood flow. Normal pyloric function allows stomach emptying and negative feedback mechanisms to reduce acid secretion when acid is excessive. Normally these protective mechanisms counteract aggressive forces on the gastric mucosa. Ulceration typically develops when there is a deficiency in protective factors or an excess in aggressive factors.

Duodenal Ulcer

A DU is an ulcer in the wall of the duodenum, rarely malignant, extending into the muscularis mucosa. Practically all DUs occur in the duodenal bulb. Ulcers that occur beyond the bulb are uncommon and are called postbulbar ulcers. About 10% of patients have multiple DUs.[8] DUs usually are round or oval and less than 1 cm in diameter but may be larger and irregular in shape. The true cause of DU is unknown, although it has been assumed for years that they are related to excessive parietal cell hydrochloric acid secretion. This could result from increased parietal cell mass, increased vagal or hormonal drive to secrete acid, increased gastric emptying rate, or defective inhibition of acid secretion. Only one-third to one-half of patients with DUs have excessive acid secretory rates, as evidenced by basal gastric hypersecretion and increased peak acid secretion.

DU disease is both chronic and recurrent. Approximately 60% of healed DUs recur within 1 year and 80 to 90% within 2 years.[7] DUs probably represent a stage in a dynamic disease process that begins with acute inflammation of the duodenal mucosa and progresses through more severe stages of duodenitis until an ulcer develops. The ulcer usually persists for 4 to 6 weeks but may on occasion heal rapidly. The whole process may repeat itself. A recurrent ulcer may or may not develop in the same location as the previous one. Certain risk factors such as cigarette smoking, chronic use of aspirin and other nonsteroidal anti-inflammatory drugs (NSAIDs), or alcohol contribute to increased risk of ulcer development. Genetic factors appear to be important, with first-degree relatives of patients with DUs developing ulcers three times as often as the general population. Smokers have earlier and more frequent recurrence, with increased mortality. Psychosomatic factors probably do not play an important role in ulcer development. A variety of stress situations appear to be weakly associated with new ulcer development. The role of *H. pylori* as an infectious cause of PUD and recurrence is under investigation and is discussed later in this chapter.

Gastric Ulcer

In the United States, GU occurs about one-fourth as often as DU. Like DU, it is more common in men than in women. The incidence increases after 50 years of age, peaks in the sixth decade, and is unusual in younger people. Benign GU can occur anywhere in the stomach but is most commonly found at the junction between the antrum and the fundus of the stomach, on the lesser curvature, the so-called saddle ulcer. They are rarely found in the fundus and usually are accompanied by antral gastritis. Benign GUs are similar to DUs histologically but are deep and usually exhibit more extensive gastritis surrounding the ulcer crater.

Unlike DUs, GUs tend to be associated with lower rates of acid secretion. However, 10 to 20% of patients with GUs also have DUs, with acid secretory rates paralleling those of DU. GUs may be caused primarily by the breakdown of the mucosal barrier and subsequent back-diffusion of acid across the gastric mucosa. Normally, less than one-tenth of the gastric HCl secreted by the parietal cells is reabsorbed through the gastric mucosa by back-diffusion. In patients with GUs, the figure tends to be much higher. GU healing does not result in normalization of the gastric mucosal barrier to back-diffusion. Back-diffusion remains high, even if the ulcer has disappeared. The mucosal barrier defect appears to be generalized, rather than localized, because the ulcer does not necessarily recur at the previous ulcer site. Pyloric sphincter dysfunction and reflux of bile salts also appear to be involved in GU genesis.

The plasma membrane and mucus of surface epithelial cells constitutes the mucosal barrier. The barrier is rendered impermeable to ionized substances because of the high phospholipid content and the tight junctions between these cells. A number of agents can damage the mucosal barrier, allowing rapid back-diffusion of hydrogen ion from the lumen into the mucosa, causing cellular destruction and increasing capillary permeability within the damaged mucosa. This results in extravasation of plasma proteins, producing mucosal edema. The rapid cell turnover of the gastric mucosa is also disrupted, leading to desquamation and loss of gastric epithelial cells in the area. NSAIDs are responsible for a significant number of GUs, presumably due in part to reduced synthesis of cytoprotective PGs.

Helicobacter pylori

Insight into an important pathogenic factor in PUD was provided when a spiral shaped, Gram-negative, flagellated, urease-producing organism was found in the narrow interface between the gastric epithelial cell surface and the overlying mucus gel layer (mucosal barrier). The organism was originally named *Campylobacter pyloridis* and subsequently *Campylobacter pylori* because of its similarity to other *Campylobacter* species. The name *Helicobacter pylori* was given in 1989 based on functional and enzymatic properties. Early studies found that the presence of this organism was associated with antral gastritis, DUs, and GUs. *H. pylori* is a common gastric infection affecting more than 50% of the world's population and is a major cause of gastritis and PUD.[1] Most patients with DU have *H. pylori* gastritis; thus, infection with *H. pylori* may be a prerequisite for the majority of DUs in the absence of other precipitating factors (such as NSAID use or ZE syndrome).[1,9] It is important to note the role of *H. pylori* in patients with ulcer disease; however, the majority of *H. pylori*–infected patients do not develop DUs or GUs.

H. pylori is found below the mucous layer next to the gastric epithelium in the stomach, esophagus, duodenum, and Meckel's diverticulum. It is able to burrow through the mucous layer because of its motility and spiral shape. *H. pylori* produces a urease enzyme that catalyzes urea, forming ammonium and bicarbonate, allowing it to withstand the harsh gastric environment. Current methods of detection rely on this reaction for positive results. The organism is very sensitive to gastric acid and the ammonium forms a protective alkaline microenvironment. Transmission appears to occur via human-to-human spread, most likely through the fecal–oral route.[9]

Prevalence depends on socioeconomic class, race, and country of residence. In Western countries, the incidence is low before 20 years of age and increases to 40 to 60% at age 60. In the United States, Hispanics and blacks appear to have markedly higher rates than whites. Lower socioeconomic class and crowding tend to result in higher rates, up to 80% in family members of infected patients.

CLINICAL PRESENTATION AND DIAGNOSIS

Signs and Symptoms

The clinical findings of PUD are nonspecific and variable. Patients can be asymptomatic or experience anorexia, nausea, vomiting, belching and bloating, and heartburn or epigastric pain. Patients with DU usually describe epigastric pain or tenderness as burning, gnawing, and aching between the xiphoid and umbilicus, often relieved with food intake. GU typically involves diffuse pain over the midepigastrium and may be worsened by food.[7] Pain occurring when the stomach is empty, such as between meals and at night, is typical of DU. Pain occurring within an hour or two of eating is typical of GU. The differences can be slight, making differentiation difficult based on symptoms alone. Patients may occasionally describe pain that radiates to other areas, such as the back or lower abdomen. Some patients may perceive abdominal pressure or a hunger sensation. Changes in the character of pain may herald the development of complications, such as penetration, perforation, gastric outlet obstruction, or hemorrhage. It should be emphasized that some patients have a silent ulcer and do not experience symptoms with active ulcer disease, especially with recurrences. Many NSAID-induced ulcers and ulcers in older adults bleed without any prior symptoms. Therefore, the presence or absence of pain is not reliable in diagnosing or assessing healing with therapy in PUD.

Diagnosis

Radiology and Endoscopy

The diagnosis of PUD depends on radiologic or endoscopic visualization (esophagogastroduodenoscopy) of the ulcer. Radiologic study with barium contrast (upper GI series) is still a common initial method of diagnosis for PUD. At best, single-contrast barium studies with radiographs can detect 70 to 80% of ulcers found with endoscopy; detection rises to approximately 90% with double-contrast barium. Endoscopy generally is not needed when an ulcer is found with barium radiographic study. However, endoscopy is useful for detecting suspected ulcers not found radiographically, visualizing and performing biopsies of GUs, collecting gastric biopsies for detection of *H. pylori,* and identifying sources of active GI bleeding. Because up to 10% of GUs are malignant, it is important to have follow-up endoscopy in these patients. Endoscopy permits direct examination of the esophagus, stomach, and duodenum. Thus, most areas in which upper GI disease occurs are readily accessible to direct visualization and biopsy. Equivocal lesions can be biopsied easily, and superficial erosions can be visualized that were not detected radiographically. Endoscopy is the preferred diagnostic procedure in evaluation of upper GI disorders in pregnant women, in whom radiation is to be avoided. The diagnostic accuracy rate of endoscopy in ulcer disease is about 95%.

Diagnosis of *H. pylori*

Bicarbonate produced by the urease reaction is largely excreted as carbon dioxide by the lungs and forms the basis of measuring urease activity. Diagnostic tests can be divided into invasive and noninvasive measures and are summarized in Table 24.2. Invasive measures include endoscopy with gastric biopsy and histologic demonstration of organisms, biopsy with direct detection of urease activity in the tissue specimen, and biopsy with culture of the *H. pylori* organism. Noninvasive measures include serologic tests for immunoglobulin G antibodies to *H. pylori* and breath tests of urease activity using orally administered urea labeled with carbon 14 or carbon 13. It is important to note that with the exception of serologic assays, all tests may be falsely negative in patients who have recently taken antibiotics, bismuth compounds, or acid pump inhibitors in the recent past. Also, antibody levels decrease slowly after successful eradication of *H. pylori* infection. Currently, there is no readily available, inexpensive, and accurate noninvasive method to monitor eradication of *H. pylori*. Even if there were, it is not necessary to test all patients in view of the high efficacy of treatment and the low reinfection rate.

THERAPEUTIC PLAN

The goals of treatment for PUD are to relieve pain, enhance ulcer healing, prevent complications such as GI bleeding or perforation, and prevent ulcer recurrence. Although sophisticated drug therapy is available for PUD, other measures involving lifestyle modifications and avoidance of ulcerogenic drugs are important to optimize therapy. Patients should be advised to stop smoking and avoid alcohol intake because both can impair ulcer healing. Ulcerogenic drugs, such as aspirin and other NSAIDs, should be avoided. Caffeine is a gastric acid stimulant and should be avoided. Foods and beverages that aggravate their symptoms should be avoided. Patients should refrain from eating after dinner so as not to stimulate acid secretion during the night. Stress management may help in reducing ulcer symptoms. Drug therapy for PUD is oriented primarily toward neutralizing (antacids) or reducing the amount of acid secreted (H_2 receptor antagonists, PPIs) or protecting the gastric mucosa from the effects of acid (sucralfate, PGs). As the role of *H. pylori* is becoming better understood, treatment with antibiotics is becoming an important part of PUD therapy and recurrence prevention.

TREATMENT

Pharmacotherapy

Antacids

Antacids can provide symptomatic relief and heal peptic ulcers. Although intensive antacid therapy has been shown to be less expensive than and as effective as the H_2 receptor antagonists and sucralfate, it is no longer common to find antacids used as sole therapy because of the inconvenience of the regimens used, palatability, and adverse effects. However, antacids are still widely used on an as-needed basis for symptom control. Common antacid preparations include sodium bicarbonate, calcium carbonate, and salts

Table 24.2 ▪ Diagnostic Tests for *Helicobacter pylori*

Test	Sensitivity (%)	Comments
Urease testing: breath testing (nonradioactive C_{13}, radioactive C_{14})	90–95	Noninvasive; rapid (60 min); represents the entire mucosa; may be used to monitor therapy. Entails ingestion of radiolabeled carbon 13 or 14.
Biopsy	90–98	Invasive; endoscopy needed to obtain sample for testing (culture, histology, urease); rapid *Campylobacter*-like organism test can provide results within 30 min with specificity and sensitivity of 80–90%.
Histology	70–95	Invasive; endoscopy needed with 2 or more biopsies (1 or more from the antrum); special stains (Giemsa, Warthin–Starry silver) may be needed.
Culture	60–95	Invasive; entails endoscopy; may take 1 wk to grow; poor predictive value without histology; may become necessary if antibiotic resistance develops.
Serology	90–95	Noninvasive; does not differentiate active and past infection; possible cross-reactivity with similar bacteria, so reliability is questionable; epidemiologic tool; titers decrease with eradication.

of aluminum and magnesium. Magnesium and aluminum hydroxide are the most commonly used antacids for PUD.

Antacids heal DUs by neutralizing gastric acid, which also inhibits the action of pepsin when the gastric pH increases above 4. The acid-neutralizing capacity (ANC) is a primary consideration in selecting an antacid. The ANC varies for commercial preparations and is expressed in milliequivalents per milliliter (the amount of acid needed to keep an antacid suspension at pH 3 for 2 hours in vitro; Table 24.3). Antacids with a high ANC usually are more effective in vivo, and less volume is needed for a given ability to neutralize acid. However, the most potent antacids are not necessarily the most useful for chronic therapy. Sodium bicarbonate and calcium carbonate have the greatest ANC but produce unacceptable side effects when administered chronically. Antacids may provide additional benefit by suppressing *H. pylori* growth.[10]

Frequent administration of antacid is necessary to buffer the constant secretion of acid produced by the stomach. The stomach in a fasting state empties its contents into the duodenum as often as every 30 minutes to 1 hour, limiting the amount of antacid in the stomach. Acid secretion is greatest in response to a meal and at night. A regimen that administers antacids several times between meals and at bedtime maximizes the buffering ability of the antacid at the times of greatest acid output. The regimen most commonly used is 30 mL of a high-potency antacid 1 hour and 3 hours after a meal and at bedtime. Lower dosages of antacids (15 mL six times daily) have proven to be effective and may be more conducive to patient compliance.[11–13] Because antacid must be present in the stomach to work, the patient may be awakened at night with pain caused by nocturnal acid secretion. A treatment period of 4 to 6 weeks is necessary to heal 70 to 80% of DUs. Treatment for longer than 6 weeks does not offer any additional advantage, except possibly in smokers.

Antacid adverse effects are problematic and contribute to noncompliance. Sodium bicarbonate and calcium carbonate are potent antacids, but have side effects that preclude their use in PUD. Sodium bicarbonate produces gas from CO_2 formation in the stomach, has a tendency to induce systemic alkalosis, and delivers a high sodium load when used chronically. Calcium that is absorbed from calcium carbonate stimulates gastrin release to produce acid rebound. Chronic administration of large dosages of calcium carbonate can be associated with the milk-alkali syndrome, producing hypercalcemia, hyperphosphatemia, increased blood urea nitrogen (BUN), and systemic alkalosis. This can cause renal insufficiency and renal calcinosis. Magnesium-containing antacids can cause diarrhea, the main dose-limiting adverse effect, and are rarely used alone for PUD therapy. Aluminum hydroxide is a weaker antacid than magnesium hydroxide and can cause constipation. Magnesium–aluminum combination products were developed in an attempt to minimize diarrhea. Occasionally, if diarrhea persists, a combination magnesium–aluminum product can be alternated with doses of aluminum hydroxide. Other adverse effects include hypermagnesemia and hyperalbuminemia in the presence of renal failure. Phosphorus depletion can occur in patients taking chronic doses of aluminum salts because of phosphate binding in

Table 24.3 ▪ Comparison of Selected Liquid Antacid Products

Product Name	Ingredients per 5 mL	Acid-Neutralizing Capacity (per 5 mL)	Sodium (mg)
Maalox suspension	225 mg aluminum hydroxide 200 mg magnesium hydroxide	9	1.4
Maalox TC suspension	500 mg aluminum hydroxide 300 mg magnesium hydroxide	27.2	0.8
Mylanta liquid	200 mg aluminum hydroxide 200 mg magnesium hydroxide 20 mg simethicone	12.7	0.68
Mylanta II liquid	400 mg aluminum hydroxide 400 mg magnesium hydroxide 40 mg simethicone	25.4	1.14
Riopan suspension	540 mg magaldrate (hydroxymagnesium aluminate)	15	<0.1
Riopan extra strength	1080 mg magaldrate	30	<0.3
Camalox suspension	225 mg aluminum hydroxide 200 mg magnesium hydroxide 250 mg calcium carbonate	18.5	1.2
Titralac Plus liquid	500 mg calcium carbonate	11	0.0005
Amphojel suspension	320 mg aluminum hydroxide	10	<2.3
ALternaGEL Liquid	600 mg aluminum hydroxide with simethicone	16	<2.5
Basaljel suspension	Aluminum carbonate equivalent to 400 mg aluminum hydroxide	12	2.9

Consult a comprehensive product reference guide for a complete list of available products.

the intestinal tract. Long-term complications may include osteoporosis.

Antacids can cause drug interactions, usually by interfering with absorption or chelation of the drug (e.g., tetracycline). Antacids have been reported to significantly reduce the serum concentrations of digoxin, ketoconazole, tetracycline, ferrous sulfate, isoniazid, and fluoroquinolones (e.g., ciprofloxacin) when administered concomitantly. Antacids can increase quinidine serum concentrations by enhancing renal tubular reabsorption of quinidine through an increase in urine pH.

H_2 Receptor Antagonists

The development and use of H_2 receptor antagonists significantly enhanced the management of PUD when cimetidine was introduced in 1976. Currently, four H_2 receptor antagonists are marketed in the United States (cimetidine, ranitidine, famotidine, and nizatidine), and they are used often to treat PUD.[14,15] This use has decreased significantly with the approval of the PPIs, but the most significant change has resulted from the growing recognition of *H. pylori* infection in PUD. All of these agents are available without prescription and are useful in the acute and chronic treatment of DU, benign GU, hypersecretory conditions, and gastroesophageal reflux and in preventing upper GI bleeding caused by stress ulceration.

H_2 receptor antagonists competitively and reversibly bind to the H_2 receptor of the parietal cells, causing a dose-dependent inhibition of gastric acid secretion. They differ in potency, chemical structure, adverse effects, and ability to cause drug interactions. Famotidine is the most potent, followed by nizatidine, ranitidine, and cimetidine.

H_2 receptor antagonists are more effective than placebo in healing DUs and GUs, with 80% of DUs healed after 4 weeks and more than 90% healed after 8 weeks. GUs usually take longer to heal; often at least 8 weeks of treatment are needed.

H_2 receptor antagonists can be given in divided daily doses or daily as a single dose for acute initial therapy for duodenal and GUs, with similar efficacy rates.[17] The dosage regimens are equivalent and may be administered for up to 8 weeks (Table 24.4). Maintenance therapy for DU should be given as a single daily dose.

DU recurrence is reported to be approximately 60 to 80% within 12 months after cessation of therapy.[7] Risk factors associated with recurrence of peptic ulcers include cigarette smoking, gastric hypersecretion, male sex, presence of *H. pylori* in the original ulcer, low-fiber diet, NSAIDs (including acetylsalicylic acid), and poor compliance. Full-dose H_2 antagonist therapy (Table 24.4) may be given intermittently to patients at low risk if there is evidence of ulcer recurrence. It may be prudent to screen these patients for *H. pylori* and treat if necessary. Patients with risk factors for recurrence should receive daily maintenance H_2 antagonist therapy after the ulcer is initially healed. Treatment may be needed indefinitely in some cases.

Table 24.4 ▪ Dosing Schedule for Drugs Used to Treat Peptic Ulcer Disease

Drug	Acceptable Regimens for Initial Therapy	Maintenance Therapy
Cimetidine	300 mg QID 400 mg BID 800 mg HS	400 mg HS
Ranitidine	150 mg BID 300 mg HS	150 mg HS
Famotidine	20 mg BID 40 mg HS	20 mg HS
Nizatidine	150 mg BID 300 mg HS	150 mg HS
Sucralfate	1 g QID 2 g BID	1 g BID
Omeprazole	20 mg QD	10 mg QD
Lansoprazole	15 mg QD 30 mg QD	15 mg QD

Cimetidine

Cimetidine is approved for acute and chronic treatment of DU, active benign GU, hypersecretory conditions, and gastroesophageal reflux disease (GERD).[17] Cimetidine has an oral bioavailability of 60 to 70%, with peak levels produced within 1 hour of administration. Cimetidine is metabolized in the liver and has an elimination half-life of about 2 hours in patients with normal renal function. The half-life increases as the renal function diminishes, extending to approximately 5 hours in anephric patients.

Cimetidine, like the other H_2 receptor antagonists, has very few major side effects. Diarrhea, usually mild and transient, dizziness, and headache have been reported in 1 to 7% of patients.[14,18] Mental status alteration (confusion, agitation, anxiety, disorientation) may occur, especially in severely ill patients (with renal or hepatic impairment) and in older adults if the dosage is not adjusted appropriately. Gynecomastia has been reported in about 4% of patients receiving high-dose cimetidine for long-term treatment of ZE syndrome. Mild and transient increases in several laboratory test results (aspartate aminotransferase, alanine aminotransferase, alkaline phosphatase, and serum creatinine levels) have occurred but usually are not clinically important. Cimetidine inhibits hepatic CYP1A2, CYP2C8-10, CYP2D6, and CYP3A3-5 enzymes in the liver, resulting in several important drug interactions (Table 24.5).[18] The oral dosing regimens for cimetidine may be found in Table 24.4. Cimetidine may also be administered intramuscularly or intravenously in dosages of 300 mg every 6 to 8 hours. In patients with a creatinine clearance less than 30 mL/minute, it is recommended that the dosage be decreased by 50%.

Ranitidine

Ranitidine is available in oral and parenteral dosage forms. It is well absorbed after oral administration, with peak serum levels occurring in 2 to 3 hours. Ranitidine undergoes significant first-pass metabolism, with a bioavailability of approximately 50%. The elimination half-life of ranitidine averages 1.7 to 3.2 hours in patients with normal renal function but is prolonged to 6 to 10 hours in patients with creatinine clearances less than 30 mL/minutes and in older adults. Ranitidine is metabolized in the liver and excreted in the urine and by the biliary system.[19]

Adverse effects of ranitidine are similar to those of cimetidine. Ranitidine appears to have less effect on endocrine and gonadal function than does cimetidine, but gynecomastia and impotence have occurred rarely.

Ranitidine inhibits hepatic CYP2D6 and CYP3A3-5 enzymes, but to a lesser extent than cimetidine, and thus appears to produce fewer clinically significant drug interactions (Table 24.5).[18] It only minimally inhibits hepatic metabolism of drugs such as warfarin, theophylline, diazepam, and propranolol.

Dosing information for ranitidine may be found in Table 24.4. Ranitidine may also be administered intermittently via the intramuscular or intravenous route in dosages of 50 mg every 6 to 8 hours, or it may be given by continuous intravenous infusion at a starting dosage of 6.25 mg/hour. The dosage should be reduced to one-third to one-half the usual dosage in patients with creatinine clearances less than 50 mL/minute.[17]

Famotidine

Famotidine is absorbed incompletely from the GI tract after oral administration, with an oral bioavailability of 40 to 50%. Famotidine has the longest elimination half-life of the currently available H_2 receptor antagonists, an average of 2.5 to 4 hours. The half-life is approximately 12 hours in patients with creatinine clearances less than 30 mL/minute. Famotidine is metabolized in the liver and excreted in the urine via glomerular filtration and tubular secretion. Side effects of famotidine are similar to those of the other H_2 receptor antagonists, except that it does not appear to exhibit antiandrogenic activity or affect the hepatic clearance of other drugs to the extent that cimetidine does.[17,20]

Oral dosing information for famotidine is given in Table 24.4. Famotidine may also be given by slow intravenous injection in dosages of 20 mg every 12 hours or by continuous intravenous infusion at a rate of 3.2 to 4.0 mg/hour. Dosage should be reduced to 20 mg/day in patients with creatinine clearances less than 10 mL/minute.

Nizatidine

Nizatidine was the fourth H_2 antagonist to be marketed in the United States and is currently available only in an oral dosage form. Nizatidine is well absorbed orally from the GI tract, with a bioavailability of approximately 70%. Peak plasma concentrations occur within about 1 hour after administration. Nizatidine is approximately one-third metabolized in the liver and two-thirds excreted unchanged in urine. The elimination half-life ranges from 1 to 2 hours in normal patients and is increased in patients with renal impairment.[20]

The adverse effects seen with nizatidine are similar to those of other H_2 receptor antagonists. There is no evidence of antiandrogen effects, and no serious effects on the central nervous system have been reported. There is no effect on the cytochrome P-450 enzyme system, making nizatidine a favorable choice when other drugs that might interact with other H_2 receptor antagonists are being administered.

Dosing information for nizatidine is presented in Table 24.4. In patients with creatinine clearances between 20 and 50 mL/minute, a 50% reduction in dosage is recommended.[17]

Table 24.5 ▪ Drug Interactions with Antiulcer Medications

Interacting Drug	Cimetidine	Ranitidine	Famotidine	Nizatidine	Omeprazole	Lansoprazole	Sucralfate
Fluoroquinolone antibiotics							Decreased absorption
Ketoconazole	Decreased absorption	Decreased absorption	Decreased absorption	Decreased absorption	Decreased absorption	Decreased absorption	Decreased absorption
Theophylline	Decreased clearance	Minimally decreased clearance	Negligible	Negligible	Negligible	Minimally increased clearance	Decreased absorption
Phenytoin	Decreased clearance	Minimally decreased clearance	Negligible	Negligible	Decreased clearance	Decreased clearance	Decreased absorption
Warfarin	Decreased clearance	Minimally decreased clearance	Negligible	Negligible	Decreased clearance	Decreased clearance	Decreased absorption
Diazepam	Decreased clearance	Minimally decreased clearance	Negligible	Negligible	Decreased clearance	Decreased clearance	Negligible
Procainamide	Decreased clearance	Minimally decreased clearance	No effect	No effect	No effect	No effect	No effect
Metronidazole	Decreased clearance	Minimally decreased clearance	No effect	No effect			No effect
Lidocaine	Decreased clearance	Decreased clearance	No effect	No effect	No effect	No effect	No effect
Clarithromycin	Decreased clearance	Decreased clearance	No effect	No effect	Decreased clearance	Decreased clearance	No effect

Sucralfate

Sucralfate is a unique therapeutic agent used for the acute and chronic treatment of DUs, treatment of GUs, and prevention of stress ulceration. It is an aluminum salt of a sulfated disaccharide that exerts its action locally on the GI mucosa. Sucralfate binds to positively charged molecules to form a gelatinous layer at the ulcer site, which protects the ulcer or involved mucosa from the aggressive action of acid, pepsin, and bile salts. It has also been shown to adsorb pepsin and bile salts and may stimulate the secretion of endogenous cytoprotective PGs.[21] Sucralfate undergoes very limited absorption form the GI tract (3 to 5%), although the aluminum ions released by its interaction with gastric acid may be absorbed significantly.[22,23]

Because of its lack of significant systemic bioavailability, sucralfate generally is well tolerated. Its most common adverse effects are constipation (2%), diarrhea, nausea, vomiting, bloating, flatulence, dry mouth or metallic taste, and indigestion (each less than 1% incidence). The small amount of aluminum absorbed from sucralfate is readily excreted by the kidney in patients with normal renal function. However, patients with chronic renal failure and patients who need dialysis may accumulate the aluminum systemically, leading to aluminum toxicity. The resulting complications include osteomalacia, osteodystrophy, and encephalopathy or seizures. Therefore, it is recommended that sucralfate be given cautiously to patients with renal impairment.[17]

The development of gastric bezoars has also been reported.[19] Drug interactions with sucralfate have been investigated in recent years, and significant interactions are shown in Table 24.5. The most significant of these are with the fluoroquinolones; it may be best to place the patient receiving fluoroquinolones on alternative antiulcer medications until the antibiotic course is completed.[17] Sucralfate dosing information is given in Table 24.4. No adjustments in renal or hepatic impairment are necessary.

Proton Pump Inhibitors

Omeprazole and lansoprazole are both benzimidazole derivatives that irreversibly bind to and inhibit the H^+/K^+-ATPase (acid pump) on the apical membrane of parietal cells, the final phase in acid secretion.[24,25] The maximum effect occurs within 2 hours of administration, reducing peak acid output by 80% or more. At 24 hours there is 50% of maximum inhibition, and effects may persist for up to 72 hours after a dose, until new H^+/K^+-ATPase can be synthesized. The antisecretory activity of omeprazole or lansoprazole is greater than that of the H_2 receptor antagonists. Other PPIs under investigation include rabeprazole and pantoprazole.[24]

Because these agents are acid unstable, they have been formulated using an enteric coating, which delays release, allowing them to pass through the stomach before release. Bioavailability of omeprazole varies between 30 and 70%, whereas that of lansoprazole is between 80 and 90%.[26] Both drugs undergo hepatic metabolism, but the parent drug in both cases must be metabolized in the parietal cells of the stomach to the active metabolites, which in turn inhibit H^+/K^+-ATPase production. This metabolism in the acid space of the parietal cell is acid dependent, so administering these agents before food intake is preferred. This potent effect on acid secretion can cause gastrin concentrations to increase twofold to fourfold. Serum gastrin returns to pretreatment concentrations within 2 weeks of discontinuation.[24]

The PPIs are recommended as part of the initial treatment of PUD related to *H. pylori* infection because they play a primary role in eradicating *H. pylori*. In DUs, disease healing occurs with 2 to 4 weeks of single daily doses of PPIs, compared to 4 to 8 weeks with H_2 receptor antagonists.[24,25] The PPIs also are rapidly effective in treating GUs and GERD and are used extensively in the long-term treatment of GI hypersecretory conditions such as ZE syndrome.

The initial omeprazole dosage is 20 mg daily, given approximately 30 minutes before a meal, for 4 to 8 weeks. Increasing the dosage to 40 mg daily should be considered in patients with an unhealed ulcer after 8 weeks of treatment with 20 mg daily. The initial lansoprazole dosage is 15 mg daily for DU and 30 mg daily for GU and GERD. Lansoprazole should also be given approximately 30 minutes before a meal. Higher dosages of both agents may be necessary, with as much as 180 mg daily of lansoprazole and 360 mg daily of omeprazole in refractory patients or those with ZE syndrome.[20]

Adverse effects of PPIs include headache, diarrhea, abdominal pain, and nausea in less than 5% of patients. Hyperplasia of enterochromaffin-like cells and gastric carcinoid tumors have been observed in rats given PPIs, presumably because of marked hypergastrinemia. However, no cases of enterochromaffin-like cell hyperplasia or gastric tumors have been reported in humans. Forty patients with ZE syndrome were given omeprazole 82 ± 31 mg per day with no evidence of gastric tumors for up to 4 years (6 to 51 months).[27]

PPIs inhibit cytochrome P-450 enzymes and may interact with drugs metabolized by this pathway.[28] Significant interactions are shown in Table 24.5.

Anticholinergics

Anticholinergics are of little importance in DU treatment. They can reduce acid secretion by 30 to 35%, as compared to 85 to 90% with H_2 receptor antagonists. Anticholinergics have been used with antacids in patients with DU to help reduce stomach emptying and prolong the buffering activity of antacids. Anticholinergics have no place in the treatment of patients with GUs. The minor antisecretory activity of this class of drugs is offset by the ability to reduce the motility of the GI tract. This causes retention of acid and pepsin in the stomach.

Treatment of *H. pylori*

Despite the initial efficacy of available therapeutic agents for PUD, the recurrence rate after complete healing remains high. DUs treated by acid suppression therapy alone, without maintenance, recur in about 80% of patients within 12 months.[29,30] The major role of therapy directed toward eradicating *H. pylori* is to reduce ulcer recurrence to less than 10% or eliminate recurrence in some cases.[31–36] Reinfection in some cases may be caused by different strains of *H. pylori,* obtained from sources such as family members, environmental reservoirs, and endoscopic equipment.[36]

The combination of an antisecretory agent, such as omeprazole or lansoprazole, with an antibiotic generally is necessary for ulcer healing and *H. pylori* eradication.[37,38] Success rates are poor with antibiotics alone for DU,[39] but some evidence suggests that antibiotics alone may heal GUs as effectively as omeprazole.[40]

H. pylori resides under the mucus gel layer in the highly acidic milieu of the stomach. Data suggest that *H. pylori* eradication therapy depends on topical, local mucosal delivery of antibiotics. The oral route of antibiotic administration is preferred and produces high, transient drug concentrations in the gastric mucosa.[41–43] In addition, H_2 receptor antagonists have been shown to be effective in increasing antibiotic concentrations in the gastric mucosa, which may explain, in part, the greater efficacy seen when antisecretory agents are combined with antibiotics than when antibiotics are used alone.[44]

There is no suitable animal model to study therapy, so most available information about drug selection is based on small trials in humans. A variety of antibiotics have activity against *H. pylori,* including tetracycline, metronidazole, amoxicillin, clarithromycin, and azithromycin. The best combination of agents is a continuing subject of debate, but eradication rates of 80 to 90% can be achieved with appropriate therapy. Eradication rates of 90% or higher have been documented with three- and four-drug regimens. Various combinations of agents and durations of therapy are being studied in the attempt to optimize eradication within the shortest time frame. Table 24.6 provides a summary of effective regimens. Three- and four-drug regimens generally produce higher eradication rates.

Single-antibiotic therapy should be avoided because of high rates of resistance.[38] Eradication rates of 80 to 90% have been documented with the combination of omeprazole 20 mg twice daily and amoxicillin 1.5 to 2.0 g/day.[36,39,45–47] Omeprazole should be given with the antibiotic rather than before because evidence suggests that pretreatment with omeprazole may reduce the regimen's effectiveness. However, this combination generally is not considered first-line therapy.

Triple therapy includes several bismuth-based and PPI-based regimens (Table 24.6).[37,38] An example is bismuth subsalicylate two tablets four times daily, tetracycline 500 mg four times daily, and metronidazole, 250 mg three times daily, given for 14 days.[38,39,48–50] Other triple regimens include lansoprazole, clarithromycin, and metronidazole or amoxicillin given for 7 to 14 days. Tetracycline is said to have in vitro synergism with metronidazole against 30 to 40% of metronidazole-resistant strains.[51] Substitution of oxytetracycline[52] or doxycycline[53] for tetracycline has been shown to reduce eradication to 83% and 65%, respectively. Similar eradication rates have been demonstrated with the combination of ranitidine 150 mg twice daily, metronidazole 500 mg three times daily, and amoxicillin 750 mg three times daily.[54,55]

Quadruple therapy involves use of bismuth subsalicylate two tablets four times daily, omeprazole 20 mg twice daily, tetracycline 500 mg four times daily, and metronidazole 500 mg three times daily for 7 to 12 days.[37,38] Eradication rates greater than 95% have been reported.

Table 24.6 ▪ Regimens for Eradicating *Helicobacter pylori*

Regimen	Eradication Rate (%)
Dual therapy[a]	
Lansoprazole 30 mg BID + clarithromycin 400 mg BID for 14 days	73
Omeprazole 40 mg QD for 28 days + clarithromycin 500 mg TID for 14 days	64–83
Triple therapy	
Ranitidine bismuth citrate (Tritec) 400 mg BID for 28 days + clarithromycin 500 mg TID for 14 days	82–94
Bismuth subsalicylate 2 tablets QID + metronidazole 250 mg QID + amoxicillin 500 mg QID for 14 days	80–86
Bismuth subsalicylate 2 tablets QID + metronidazole 500 mg TID + amoxicillin 500 mg TID for 14 days	84
Bismuth subsalicylate 2 tablets QID + clarithromycin 500 mg TID + tetracycline 500 mg QID for 14 days	93
Bismuth subsalicylate 2 tablets QID + metronidazole 250 mg QID + tetracycline 500 mg QID for 14 days	88–90
Bismuth subsalicylate 2 tablets QID + metronidazole 250 mg QID + tetracycline 500 mg QID for 7 days	85–90
Bismuth subsalicylate 2 tablets QID + metronidazole 250 mg QID + amoxicillin 500 mg QID for 7 days	75–80
Omeprazole 20 mg BID + metronidazole 500 mg BID + clarithromycin 500 BID for 7 days	87–91
Omeprazole 20 mg BID + metronidazole 250 mg BID + amoxicillin 1 g QD for 7–14 days	77–83
Omeprazole 20 mg BID + clarithromycin 500 mg BID + amoxicillin 1 g QD for 7 days	86–91
Lansoprazole 30 mg BID + clarithromycin 500 mg BID + amoxicillin 1 g QD for 14 days	86–91
Quadruple therapy	
Bismuth subsalicylate 2 tablets QID + metronidazole (250 mg QID or 500 mg TID) + tetracycline 500 mg QID + omeprazole 20 mg BID for 7 days	94–98
Bismuth subsalicylate 2 tablets QID + metronidazole 250 mg QID + tetracycline 250 mg QID + omeprazole 20 mg BID for 12 days	98

[a]Triple and quadruple therapy generally are preferred because they offer better eradication rates.

Two- or three-drug regimens typically should be 2 weeks long, although 1-week regimens have been reported to be successful in some patients.[56–59] Resistance has been documented, particularly with nitroimidazoles such as metronidazole, but does not appear to be a widespread problem with other agents. Single-antibiotic regimens without antisecretory drugs do not appear to be effective and have led to enhanced antimicrobial resistance and are thus discouraged. Generally, antisecretory therapy should continue for a total of 6 weeks if the patient has an active ulcer. If an H_2 antagonist was started, then it can be continued; if a PPI was used, after 2 weeks the dosage can be reduced or the patient may be switched to a less expensive H_2 antagonist.

Treatment Summary

The H_2 receptor antagonists appear to be equal in effect in their treatment of DUs and GUs. Use of these products should be determined by potential for adverse effects, drug interactions, and cost. Sucralfate can be used as an alternative to H_2 receptor antagonists, but there is no convincing evidence that the combination of sucralfate with an H_2 receptor antagonist is any more beneficial than either agent alone. Omeprazole has demonstrated better healing of DUs than conventional therapy. *H. pylori* eradication can reduce peptic ulcer recurrence and has become an important consideration in therapy.

PHARMACOECONOMICS

Several factors should be considered in PUD management. It is important to assess therapeutic efficacy, safety, tolerance, and recurrence reduction when choosing therapy for PUD. A less effective regimen probably will result in more PUD recurrence and thus be more costly in the long run.[60] Patient tolerance and compliance also affect the success or failure of a regimen. A more expensive regimen that is more effective may be associated with less recurrence and greater cost savings in the long term.

Treatment of Specific Diseases

Zollinger-Ellison (Gastrinoma Syndrome)

ZE syndrome is an ulcerogenic neoplasm that occurs in less than 1% of patients with PUD and is one of several hypersecretory syndromes. It is caused by a gastrin-producing adenoma, usually in the pancreas and duodenal wall. The basal gastrin concentration in patients with DU disease without gastrinoma usually is less than 200 pg/mL. A serum gastrin concentration of 200 to 1000 pg/mL with compatible clinical findings supports the diagnosis of ZE syndrome. Serum gastrin concentrations can exceed 1000 pg/mL.[6,7] In more than 70% of patients, the basal gastric acid output exceeds 15 mEq/hour.[6]

ZE syndrome characteristically produces numerous severe, often unremitting recurrences of peptic ulcers. These may either be single or multiple DUs or GUs occurring in unusual locations such as the distal portion of the duodenum or even the jejunum. These patients typically have persistent ulcer pain and diarrhea. ZE syndrome occurs in adults with equal frequency in both sexes and rarely in children.

TREATMENT

Proton Pump Inhibitors

Until omeprazole was introduced, many cases of ZE syndrome were treated with combination therapy with H_2 receptor antagonists and sucralfate. Omeprazole and lansoprazole usually control acid output with a single daily dose and, other than curative surgery, are considered to be the best treatment for this disorder. The omeprazole or lansoprazole dosage should be adjusted for each patient to produce a basal gastric acid secretion rate of less than 5 mEq/hour before the next dose.[6,20,25] The usual omeprazole dosage for patients with ZE syndrome is 60 or 70 mg daily (20 to 360 mg) and 60 mg daily for lansoprazole (15 mg every other day to 180 mg daily).

H_2 Receptor Antagonists

Before the availability of PPIs, H_2 receptor antagonists were the mainstay of therapy for ZE syndrome. To achieve the degree of acid suppression needed, they usually must be given in higher dosages or with greater frequency than is recommended for GUs or DUs. However, at this time they offer no advantage over PPIs.

Octreotide

Octreotide may suppress gastrin levels and provide symptomatic relief in carefully selected patients with ZE syndrome.[61] It inhibits both gastric acid and gastrin production and secondary peptides released by gastrinomas. However, octreotide is expensive, is administered intravenously, and may be impractical in many cases.

CONCLUSION

PPIs are considered the drugs of choice in treating this disorder. Patients have been safely treated for several years with no major adverse effects, but further evaluation of long-term safety is needed. A cure rate of 20 to 30% may be possible if the gastrinoma is resectable.

Gastroesophageal Reflux Disease

GERD is the syndrome consisting of esophageal mucosal damage produced by retrograde flow of gastric contents into the esophagus. Heartburn, an epigastric burning sensation, is the most common clinical manifestation of this illness, brought about primarily by an ineffective or incompetent LES.[7,62] The LES normally remains closed except during swallowing. It is kept in this closed position by its inherent muscular tone and through vagal stimulation. As a result of decreased LES tone, gastric contents are refluxed into the esophagus, where the acidity of this material may irritate and damage the mucosa. Increases in intragastric pressure or volume make reflux more likely, but decreased LES tone is necessary for reflux to occur. Other symptoms (in addition to heartburn) include dysphagia, odynophagia, hypersalivation, and regurgitation of liquid into the mouth, which may even produce morning hoarseness or result in pulmonary aspiration, with resultant pneumonitis or chronic asthma. Although many people experience heartburn occasionally, severe or recurrent symptoms warrant investigation.

Between 10 and 15% of patients with erosive esophagitis develop Barrett's esophagus, which is associated with midesophageal strictures, esophageal ulcers, and histologic changes in the lower esophageal mucosa.[62] These changes become cancerous in 5 to 10% of patients, usually by the time of diagnosis, and approximately one-third of all esophageal cancers are linked with Barrett's esophagitis. The incidence of esophageal cancer, especially adenocarcinoma, has risen rapidly over the last few decades.[63] There is evidence of a strong association between gastroesophageal reflux and the risk of esophageal cancer, regardless of the presence of Barrett's esophagus.[64]

Diagnosis of GERD is based on clinical history. Esophagitis may be demonstrated by barium swallow, esophagoscopy with or without esophageal mucosal biopsy, and esophageal motility and clearance studies. Many substances can worsen reflux by altering LES pressure or intragastric pressure (Table 24.7).

TREATMENT

The goals of treatment for GERD include reducing or eliminating symptoms, decreasing reflux, neutralizing the refluxate, improving esophageal clearance, and protecting and inducing esophageal mucosa healing.[7]

Lifestyle changes may be sufficient to reduce the intensity or frequency of GERD in mild cases and include dietary avoidance of offensive foods, especially during the evening or at bedtime, weight reduction, and elevation, or "blocking," of the head of the bed. This should be accomplished by placing the bed legs on 6- to 8-inch blocks or placing a wedge under the mattress to achieve a straight incline from foot to head. In addition, the patient should stop smoking and reduce his or her ethanol intake, if applicable. Each of these measures should be tried in all patients where applicable but should be continued only if they improve symptoms. In addition, the patient should be instructed to avoid certain offending medications when possible (Table 24.7).

Acid suppression is the mainstay of therapy for GERD. Mild, uncomplicated cases of occasional heartburn can be treated effectively with antacids or nonprescription H_2 receptor antagonists.[65] If necessary, antacids in a dosage that provides 40 to 80 mEq of ANC or use of over-the-counter H_2 receptor antagonists may be added to these nonpharmacologic measures.

Although most cases can be managed with lifestyle modifications and antacids, some patients with moderate to severe disease with esophagitis may need additional intervention with prescription medications, including the H_2 receptor antagonists, PPIs, or prokinetic agents such as bethanechol, metoclopramide, or cisapride.

If standard-dose H_2 receptor antagonists are not fully effective in patients with moderate to severe GERD, then these agents can be given in higher dosages to, usually 1.5 to 2 times the standard dosage. One study compared oral ranitidine 150 mg twice a day with ranitidine 300 mg four

Table 24.7 • Factors That Decrease Lower Esophageal Sphincter Pressure and May Worsen Gastroesophageal Reflux Disease Symptoms

Smoking (nicotine)
Food
Chocolates
Fatty foods
Garlic
Onions
Spearmint
Peppermint
Drugs and other substances
α-Adrenergic antagonists
Anticholinergic agents
Barbiturates
β_2-Agonists
Calcium channel antagonists
Cholecystokinin
Diazepam
Dopamine
Ethanol
Estrogen
Gastric acid
Glucagon
Meperidine
Morphine
Nitrates
Progesterone
Prostaglandins (E_1, E_2, A_2)
Secretin
Somatostatin
Serotonin
Theophylline
Tricyclic antidepressants
Vasoactive intestinal peptide

times a day. At the end of 8 weeks of therapy, the healing rate was significantly better in the high-dose than the low dose-group (response rate of 75% versus 54%).[66] Sometimes it is necessary to give dosages such as this for long treatment periods (8 weeks) for initial therapy, and 3 to 6 months of high-dose therapy may be needed if the patient has a recurrence.

Omeprazole 20 to 40 mg/day or lansoprazole 30 to 60 mg/day can be used to treat GERD and esophagitis. Ambulatory esophageal pH recordings have shown almost total control of reflux episodes in patients given these regimens.[67] Omeprazole and lansoprazole have been evaluated in patients who have failed to respond to various H_2 receptor antagonists. In a dosage of 40 mg/day, omeprazole treatment for 12 weeks successfully healed almost 90% of such cases.[68] Another study compared lansoprazole 30 mg/day with ranitidine 150 mg twice a day and found a significant difference in healing rates at 8 weeks (89% versus 38%, respectively).[69] However, after discontinuation of therapy, many patients have clinical recurrences of esophagitis. Therefore, patients whose esophagitis recurs usually are placed on long-term maintenance therapy. At this point, PPIs may be considered the most efficacious maintenance therapy. Further experience with the long-term use of these agents will be helpful in determining their safety.

Prokinetic agents such as metoclopramide and cisapride are sometimes used to treat GERD. These agents increase LES pressure, thereby reducing the number of reflux episodes. Metoclopramide and cisapride hasten gastric emptying.[70] Metoclopramide usually is administered in a regimen of 10 mg four times daily, before meals and at bedtime. It is often combined with an H_2 antagonist or PPI. Side effects of metoclopramide include blurred vision, dry mouth, depression, and pseudoparkinsonism.

Cisapride has some indirect cholinomimetic effects and also appears to cause serotonergic stimulation. After oral administration, cisapride is very well absorbed but appears to have a bioavailability of approximately 40 to 50%. Peak serum concentrations are reached within 2 hours of administration, and food increases bioavailability. It is extensively metabolized by the liver and has an elimination half-life of 7 to 10 hours. Cisapride is given in an oral dose of 10 mg three to four times daily, 15 minutes before meals and at bedtime, with an increase to 20 mg/dose if necessary. The efficacy of cisapride in treating GERD must be studied further, but it appears to be more effective than placebo when given in sufficient dosages.[70]

Cisapride generally is well tolerated, with GI adverse effects such as diarrhea and cramping being the most commonly reported. It appears to cause fewer extrapyramidal effects than metoclopramide.

CONCLUSION

GERD often can be managed effectively through lifestyle changes. When they do not alleviate symptoms completely, drug therapy may be instituted, with first-line therapy being antacids on an as-needed basis. For moderate to severe esophagitis, H_2 receptor antagonists, PPIs, and prokinetic agents, used individually or in combination where appropriate, provide healing in the majority of cases. Recurrence rates are high, necessitating long-term maintenance therapy in some patients. These chronic therapies do not appear to present long-term risks to this patient population.

Stress-Related Ulceration

Stress ulceration is defined as superficial erosions of the gastric mucosa that develop when severe physiologic demands are placed on a critically ill patient.[7] This type of ulceration differs from traditional PUD in a number of ways. Stress ulcerations often are small and numerous. The lesions are superficial rather than deep or penetrating and are most commonly located in the acid-secreting portion of the stomach but may also occur in the duodenum or gastric antrum. Stress ulceration also tends to be painless, with the major clinical manifestation being bleeding. Approximately 80% of untreated seriously ill patients develop stress ulcers, with serious hemorrhage occurring in 5 to 20%. The associated mortality with hemorrhage ranges from 50 to 80%. The incidence of stress-related ulceration has declined with the increased use of prophylactic drug therapy and better nutritional and ventilatory support of critically ill patients. However, stress-related ulceration remains a significant and potentially life-threatening complication in the critically ill patient.

EPIDEMIOLOGY

All seriously ill patients are at risk for stress-related ulceration. Patients with severe burns (more than 35% of body surface), sepsis, hemodynamic shock from a variety of causes, and other severe illnesses are at increased risk. The Canadian Critical Care Trials Group study showed that two strong independent risk factors for the development of GI bleeding among critically ill patients were respiratory failure, defined as a need for mechanical ventilation for more than 48 hours, and the presence of coagulopathy.[71]

PATHOPHYSIOLOGY

The pathogenic mechanisms involved in stress ulcer formation include reduced mucosal blood flow, presence of gastric acid, and disruption of mucosal barriers. The gastric mucosal epithelium normally has a very high oxygen requirement, making it particularly susceptible to reductions in mucosal blood flow. Gastric acid output is sometimes but not always high in patients who develop stress ulcerations. However, it appears that the presence of acid is necessary for the development of these superficial erosions. The presence of gastric acid, in concert with the breakdown in natural mucosal barriers, leads to hydrogen ion back-diffusion into the mucosal cells, causing mucosal damage, which then develops into superficial ulceration. The mucosal damage also leads to a decrease in mucus production and bicarbonate secretion and inhibits mucosal PG synthesis. During long periods of stress or a lack of adequate nutrition and oxygenation, regeneration of gastric epithelium is also impaired. Eventually, these ulcers predispose the patient to hemorrhage, which may occur in small amounts as quickly as 24 to 48 hours after the onset of injury or severe stress. Larger amounts of blood loss, often leading to hemodynamic compromise and mortality, usually occur 3 or more days after the initial injury or stress event.[7,72]

CLINICAL PRESENTATION AND DIAGNOSIS

Blood loss, as represented by gross examination of gastric contents or positive guaiac of nasogastric aspirate, usually is the first sign of ulceration. Although not all patients with minor blood loss progress to clinically important bleeding, upper GI endoscopic examination is the most reliable method for confirming ulceration. Radiographic examination is less reliable than endoscopic examination for detecting acute stress-induced mucosal erosion.[7]

TREATMENT

The need for routine prophylactic therapy for all patients in intensive care units remains controversial. High-risk patients are targeted by many institutions and receive prophylactic therapy. Therapeutic goals in these patients include maintaining gastric pH above 4.0, protecting gastric mucosa, and enhancing mucosal barriers. Antacids, H_2 receptor antagonists, and sucralfate all have been used as prophylactic therapy against stress ulceration.

Antacids originally were used heavily in the prophylaxis of stress ulceration. However, large dosages often are needed to maintain intragastric pH above 4. Monitoring pH from gastric aspirates is also essential in adjusting the antacid dosage to achieve this pH goal.

H_2 receptor antagonists also are effective in raising the intragastric pH above 4 and are given either as intermittent bolus therapy or by continuous infusion. Continuous infusion of H_2 receptor antagonists generally has been shown to produce a more consistent elevation of intragastric pH, with dosages ranging from cimetidine 37.5 to 100 mg/hour, ranitidine 6.25 to 12.5 mg/hour, and famotidine 3.2 to 4.0 mg/hour.[73] Continuous-infusion cimetidine was shown to be more effective than placebo in preventing GI hemorrhage in critically ill patients.[74]

Sucralfate has also been used effectively to prevent stress ulceration.[72] A recent study compared sucralfate 1 g every 4 hours to a continuous ranitidine infusion of 6.25 mg/hour and to an antacid suspension with a buffering capacity of 1.2 mEq/mL, given in a starting dosage of 20 mL every 2 hours and titrated to maintain intragastric pH above 4.[75] No difference in the occurrence of macroscopic bleeding was found between the groups. Sucralfate can be administered every 4 hours as a suspension either orally or via nasogastric tube.

Currently, it is suspected that stress ulcer prophylaxis may play a role in the development of bacterial pneumonia in these critically ill patients. The proposed mechanism involves gastric pH changes produced by H_2 receptor antagonists and antacids: A pH above 4 may promote growth of Gram-negative bacteria because low intragastric pH normally functions as a deterrent to bacterial growth. This increased colonization of the stomach may increase the risk of aspiration of these bacteria into the respiratory tract.[76] Because sucralfate does not raise intragastric pH significantly, some clinicians believe that it may offer an advantage in this regard.[75] Further investigation may better delineate any differences between sucralfate, H_2 receptor antagonists, antacids, and other therapies with regard to resultant pneumonia.

Drug-Induced Ulceration

Drug-induced GI adverse effects are common and can result in significant morbidity. Drugs such as erythromycin, iron salts, corticosteroids, and potassium chloride can cause gastroduodenal damage; however, the drugs most often associated with acute and chronic gastroduodenal injury, including ulceration, are NSAIDs. NSAID-induced adverse GI effects may be seen in 2 to 30% of patients.[77–79] The incidence of ulcers is approximately 15 to 20% in patients taking NSAIDs for osteoarthritis or rheumatoid arthritis.[80] Prolonged ingestion of NSAIDs is a significant cause of GU, and more than 10% of patients receiving NSAIDs have endoscopically verified peptic ulcers. The risk of developing NSAID-induced ulcers and complications increases with advancing age, previous history of peptic ulcer or GI bleeding, higher NSAID dosages, concomitant cardiovascular disease, and concomitant use of corticosteroids or anticoagulants.[80] In one retrospective study, NSAID users were found to be four times more likely to die of PUD or upper GI bleeding than nonusers.[81]

Cigarette smoking can increase the risk of ulceration and its complications in patients taking NSAIDs. Patients who smoke have impaired healing and greater recurrence of ulcers, as well as an increased likelihood that surgery will be needed for ulcer repair.

PATHOPHYSIOLOGY

NSAIDs are thought to induce damage of the gastric mucosa via two mechanisms: direct effects of the acidic agent on the gastric mucosa and decreased production of protective PGs. Gastric mucus provides a barrier that protects the stomach epithelium from gastric contents through several mechanisms: The mucosa secretes bicarbonate, via receptor-mediated active transport, which buffers acidic contents; the mucus layer thickens in response to epithelial injury, allowing rapid epithelialization to take place after insults from agents such as aspirin and ethanol; and gastric mucosal blood flow helps to protect the mucosa from injury. If the mucous barrier is disrupted, a compensatory increase in mucosal blood flow helps to remove the H^+ ions that can damage the mucosa. When the blood flow does not increase, cell death follows.[7]

PGs are stimulated by stress or trauma to the cell membranes. These protective substances have an antisecretory effect on gastric acid production and defend the stomach against acid and other noxious substances. PGs have a variety of GI effects but are thought to aid the gastric mucosal defense primarily by stimulating bicarbonate secretion and mucus synthesis.

NSAIDs inhibit PG synthesis, allowing disruption of PG-mediated mucosal defenses. NSAIDs act as weak organic acids that can increase basal levels of gastric acid secretion and can also alter and disrupt cell membranes, allowing back-diffusion of H^+ ions to occur. Once these weak acids disrupt cell membranes, they become trapped within the mucosal cells, inducing alterations in the morphology of exposed mucosal cells.

TREATMENT

Discontinuing NSAID use is not always feasible, particularly in patients with rheumatoid arthritis and osteoarthritis. Consequently, availability of effective therapies to prevent and treat NSAID-induced ulceration is important.

Misoprostol and other PGE_1 analogs have been studied for efficacy in protecting the gastric mucosa against ulcerogenic agents.[80,82–84] Other analogs include enprostil, arbaprostil, trimoprostil, rioprostil, enisprostil, and ornoprostil. PGs appear to facilitate regeneration of the mucosa after injury by NSAIDs and should be effective in healing and preventing mucosal damage. Misoprostol aids in mucosal defense by enhancing mucus secretion and increasing bicarbonate production and mucosal blood flow. Misoprostol has some antisecretory effects, but they probably provide little protective effect because the more potent antisecretory H_2 receptor antagonists do not appear to be effective in preventing NSAID-induced ulceration.

Prophylactic use of misoprostol has been shown to reduce NSAID-induced GU by 75% and 95% in dosages of 100 μg or 200 μg four times daily, respectively. Misoprostol and other PG analogs have been shown to be comparable to conventional therapy in healing peptic ulcers, but their propensity to cause diarrhea precludes their routine use for therapy.

Currently, misoprostol is the only agent indicated for preventing NSAID-induced gastric ulceration. Patients who should receive misoprostol prophylaxis include those at high risk of developing ulcers, such as older adults, patients with concomitant diseases, and patients with a history of peptic ulceration.[85–87] This agent is rapidly and extensively absorbed and exhibits plasma protein binding of 80 to 90%. Plasma concentrations of misoprostol decrease when the dose is administered with food, and concomitant use of antacids decreases total bioavailability. The recommended misoprostol dosage is 200 μg four times daily with meals. A dosage of 100 μg four times daily with food is suggested for patients who do not tolerate the higher dosage. Dosage adjustment is not necessary in the presence of renal or hepatic insufficiency.[20]

Misoprostol produces minor adverse effects including nausea, abdominal discomfort, headache, dizziness, and diarrhea. Diarrhea is the most troublesome adverse effect and has occurred in 14 to 40% of patients. These adverse effects are similar to the symptoms seen with GUs. The diarrhea may be dose related, tends to occur early in the course of therapy, and may be self-limited or may necessitate discontinuation of the drug in some patients. In women, menstrual disturbances, spotting, and abdominal cramping may occur. Misoprostol can induce abortions and is contraindicated during pregnancy (U.S. Food and Drug Administration pregnancy category X). Women in their childbearing years must not be pregnant when therapy is initiated and should use effective contraception while on misoprostol therapy. If pregnancy occurs during misoprostol therapy, the patient should discontinue therapy and contact her physician immediately. Patients should be counseled accordingly.

H_2 antagonist prophylaxis with ranitidine has been shown to reduce the incidence of NSAID-induced DU, but no consistent effect on GU has been observed.[85,88,89] Once an ulcer has formed after NSAID therapy, other commonly used therapeutic agents should be used in preference to misoprostol. Any of the commonly used drugs already discussed appear to heal ulcers once NSAID treatment is stopped. A PPI is the agent of choice when NSAIDs must be continued in the presence of ulcer disease.[80,83]

KEY POINTS

- The goals of treatment for PUD are to relieve pain, enhance ulcer healing, prevent complications such as GI bleeding or perforation, and prevent recurrence of the ulcer.
- Depending on the cause of PUD these goals can be achieved through drug therapy for PUD to neutralize stomach acid with antacids or prevent acid secretion with an H_2 antagonist or a proton pump inhibitor; possibly protect the stomach mucosa (sucralfate, misoprostol), and detect and eradicate *H. pylori* as a cause of PUD in many cases of ulcer not associated with drug-induced causes or ZE syndrome.

- It is important for patients with PUD to avoid ulcerogenic drugs and to stop smoking, avoid alcohol and caffeine, refrain from eating after dinner so as not to stimulate acid secretion during the night, and reduce stress.
- GERD is a syndrome in which an ineffective or incompetent LES allows the reflux of gastric contents into the esophagus, producing an epigastric burning sensation known as heartburn.
- Several different medications and lifestyle practices may decrease LES competence and predispose a patient to GERD. Lifestyle modification should be initiated and continued throughout the GERD treatment course.
- Antacids and over-the-counter H_2 receptor antagonists are appropriate initial therapy for GERD.
- Acid suppression is the mainstay of therapy for GERD. Higher dosages of H_2 receptor antagonists or use of PPIs may be necessary in the treatment of moderate to severe GERD. Long-term, continuous use of these agents may be warranted because of the chronic nature of GERD.
- Great strides have been made in PUD treatment over the last two decades. New therapies continue to be developed. The emergence of *H. pylori* as a cause of peptic ulcers and gastritis adds yet another dimension to the complexity of these disorders. Effective antiulcer and antibiotic therapy can reduce the recurrence of DUs and GUs.
- The pathophysiology of PUD is complex, with considerable etiologic diversity. Each patient should be evaluated carefully and therapy individualized to maximize therapeutic and pharmacoeconomic outcomes. Emphasis should be placed not just on healing the initial ulcer but also on preventing recurrence.

REFERENCES

1. Del Valle J, Cohen H, Laine L, et al. Acid-peptic disorders. In: Yamada T, Alpers DH, Owyang C, eds. Textbook of gastroenterology. 3rd ed. Philadelphia: Lippincott, 1999:1370–1444.
2. Drea EJ. Evaluation of outcomes achieved through peptic ulcer disease state management. Am J Man Care 4:S272-S279, 1998.
3. Kurata JH. Ulcer epidemiology: an overview and proposed research framework. Gastroenterology 96:569–580, 1989.
4. Bloom BS. Cross national changes in the effects of peptic ulcer disease. Ann Intern Med 114:558–562, 1991.
5. Wolfe MM, Soll AH. The physiology of gastric acid secretion. N Engl J Med 319:1707–1715, 1988.
6. Feldman M. Peptic ulcer diseases. In: Dale DC, Federman DD, eds. Scientific American medicine. New York: Scientific American, 1997:Section 4-II, 1–15.
7. Friedman LS, Peterson WL. Peptic ulcer and related disorders. In: Fauci AS, Braunwald E, Isselbacher KJ, et al., eds. Harrison's principles of internal medicine. 14th ed. New York: McGraw-Hill, 1998:1596–1616.
8. Hui WM, Lam SK. Multiple duodenal ulcer. Gut 28:1134–1141, 1987.
9. Fennerty MB. *Helicobacter pylori.* Arch Intern Med 154:721–727, 1994.
10. Berstad A, Alexander B, Weberg R, et al. Antacids reduce *Campylobacter pylori* colonization without healing the gastritis in patients with nonulcer dyspepsia and erosive prepyloric changes. Gastroenterology 95:619–624, 1988.
11. Weberg R, Aubert E, Dahlberg O, et al. Low dose antacids for duodenal ulcer. Gastroenterology 95:1465–1469, 1988.
12. Berstad A, Rydning A, Aadland E, et al. Antacid therapy of duodenal ulcer: effects of smaller doses. Scand J Gastroenterol 17:953, 1982.
13. Nauert C, Caspary WF. Duodenal ulcer therapy with low-dose antacids: a multicenter trial. J Clin Gastroenterol 13(Suppl 1):S149–S154, 1991.
14. Feldman M, Burton ME. Histamine$_2$-receptor antagonists (part one). N Engl J Med 323:1672–1680, 1990.
15. Feldman M, Burton ME. Histamine$_2$-receptor antagonists (part two). N Engl J Med 323:1749–1755, 1990.
16. Brooks WS. Short- and long-term management of peptic ulcer disease: current role of H_2-antagonists. Hepatogastroenterology 39:47–52, 1992.
17. Anonymous. Drugs used in disorders of the upper gastrointestinal tract, section 9: gastrointestinal drugs. In: Bennet DR, ed. Drug evaluations. Chicago: American Medical Association, 1994:1:1–1:31.
18. Smallwood RA. Safety of acid-suppressing drugs. Dig Dis Sci 40(Suppl):63S–80S, 1995.
19. Reddy AN. Sucralfate gastric bezoar. Am J Gastroenterol 81:149–150, 1986.
20. Anonymous. Miscellaneous GI drugs. In: McEvoy GK, ed. AHFS 98 drug information. Bethesda, MD: American Society of Health-Systems Pharmacists, 1998:2417–2469.
21. Szabo S. Pathways of gastrointestinal protection and repair: mechanisms of action of sucralfate. Am J Med 86(Suppl 6A):23–31, 1989.
22. Lauritsen K, Laursen LS, Rask-Madsen J. Clinical pharmacokinetics of drugs used in the treatment of gastrointestinal diseases. Part I. Clin Pharmacokinet 19:11–31, 1990.
23. Lauritsen K, Laursen LS, Rask-Madsen J. Clinical pharmacokinetics of drugs used in the treatment of gastrointestinal diseases. Part II. Clin Pharmacokinet 19:94–125, 1990.
24. Sachs G. Proton pump inhibitors and acid-related diseases. Pharmacotherapy 17(1):22–37, 1997.
25. Langtry HD, Wilde MI. Lansoprazole: an update of its pharmacological properties and clinical efficacy in the management of acid-related disorders. Drugs 54(3):473–500, 1997.
26. Gerloff J, Mignot A, Barth H, et al. Pharmacokinetics and absolute bioavailability of lansoprazole. Eur J Clin Pharmacol 50:293–297, 1996.
27. Maton PN, Vinayer R, Furcht H, et al. Long-term efficacy and safety of omeprazole in patients with Zollinger–Ellison syndrome: a prospective study. Gastroenterology 97:827–836, 1989.
28. Welage LS, Berardi RR. Drug interactions with antiulcer agents: considerations in the treatment of peptic ulcer disease. J Pharm Pract 7:177–195, 1994.
29. Gudmand-Hoyer E, Jensen KB, Krag E, et al. Prophylactic effect of cimetidine in duodenal ulcer disease. BMJ 1:1095–1097, 1978.
30. Boyd EJS, Penston JG, Johnston DA, et al. Does maintenance therapy keep duodenal ulcer healed? Lancet 1:1324–1327, 1988.
31. Marshall BJ, Goodwin CS, Warren JR, et al. Prospective double blind trial of duodenal ulcer relapse after eradication of *Campylobacter pylori.* Lancet 2:1437–1441, 1988.
32. Borody T, Cole P, Noonan S, et al. Long-term *Campylobacter* recurrence post-eradication. Gastroenterology 94:A43, 1988.
33. Graham DY, Lew GM, Klein PD, et al. Effect of treatment of *Helicobacter pylori* infection on the long-term recurrence of gastric or duodenal ulcer: a randomized, controlled study. Ann Intern Med 116:705–708, 1992.
34. Coghlan JG, Gilligan D, Humphries H, et al. *Campylobacter pylori* and recurrence of duodenal ulcers: a 12-month follow-up study. Lancet 2:1109–1111, 1987.
35. Adamek RJ, Wegener M, Labenz J, et al. Medium-term results of oral and intravenous omeprazole/amoxicillin *Helicobacter pylori* eradication therapy. Am J Gastroenterol 89:39–42, 1994.
36. Abu-Mahfouz MZ, Prasad VM, Sautograde P, et al. *Helicobacter pylori* recurrence after successful eradication: 5 year follow-up in the United States. Am J Gastroenterol 92:2025–2027, 1997.
37. Howden CW, Hunt RH. Guidelines for the management of *Helicobacter pylori* infection. Am J Gastroenterol 93:2330–2338, 1998.
38. Salcedo JA, Al-Kawas F. Treatment of *Helicobacter pylori* infection. Arch Intern Med 158:842–851, 1998.
39. Chiba N, Babu VR, Rademaker JW, et al. Meta-analysis of the efficacy of antibiotic therapy in eradication of *Helicobacter pylori.* Am J Gastroenterol 87:1716–1727, 1992.
40. Sung JJY, Chung SCS, Ling TKW, et al. Antibacterial treatment of gastric ulcers associated with *Helicobacter pylori.* N Engl J Med 332:139–142, 1995.
41. Scembri M, Lambert J, Loncar B, et al. Amoxicillin concentrations in the gastric mucosa are determined by luminal levels. Microb Ecol Health Dis 4:S182, 1991.
42. Lambert HR, Loncar B, Schembri MA, et al. Luminal amoxicillin determines gastric mucosal concentrations. Gastroenterology 100:A104, 1991.
43. Lamouliatte H, Cayla R, Meyer M, et al. Pharmacokinetics of oral and intravenous amoxicillin in human gastric mucosa. Ital J Gastroenterol 23(Suppl 2):109, 1990.
44. Westblom TU, Duriex DE. Enhancement of antibiotic concentrations in gastric mucosa by H_2-receptor antagonists: implications for treatment of *Helicobacter pylori* infection. Dig Dis Sci 36:25–28, 1991.

45. Bayerdorffer E, Mannes GA, Sommer A, et al. High dose omeprazole treatment combined with amoxicillin eradicates *Helicobacter pylori*. Gastroenterology 102:A38, 1992.
46. Labenz J, Gyenes E, Ruhl GH, et al. Amoxicillin plus omeprazole versus triple therapy for eradication of *Helicobacter pylori* in duodenal ulcer disease. Gut 34:1167–1170, 1993.
47. Labenz J, Ruhl GH, Bertrams J, et al. Medium- or high-dose omeprazole plus amoxicillin eradicates *Helicobacter pylori* in gastric ulcer disease. Am J Gastroenterol 89:726–730, 1994.
48. Borody TJ, Brandl S, Andrews P, et al. Use of high efficacy, lower dose triple therapy to reduce side effects of eradicating *Helicobacter pylori*. Am J Gastroenterol 89:33–38, 1994.
49. Axon ATR. *Helicobacter pylori* therapy: effect on peptic ulcer disease. J Gastroenterol Hepatol 6:131–137, 1991.
50. Graham DY, Lew GM, Evans DG, et al. Effect of triple therapy (antibiotics plus bismuth) on duodenal ulcer healing. Ann Intern Med 115:266–269, 1991.
51. Xia HX, Daw MA, Sant S, et al. Clinical efficacy of triple therapy in *Helicobacter pylori*-associated duodenal ulcer. Eur J Gastroenterol Hepatol 5:141–144, 1993.
52. Lynch D, Sobala GM, Gallacher B, et al. Effectiveness of a five times daily triple therapy regime for eradicating *Helicobacter pylori*. Irish J Med Sci 161(Suppl 10):92, 1992.
53. Borody TJ, George LL, Brandl S, et al. *Helicobacter pylori* eradication with doxycycline-metronidazole-bismuth subcitrate triple therapy. Scand J Gastroenterol 305:502–504, 1992.
54. Hentschel E, Brandstatter G, Dragosics B, et al. Effect of ranitidine and amoxicillin plus metronidazole on the eradication of *Helicobacter pylori* and the recurrence of duodenal ulcer. N Engl J Med 328:308–312, 1993.
55. Goh KL, Peh SC, Parasakthi N, et al. Omeprazole 40 mg o.m. combined with amoxicillin alone or with amoxicillin and metronidazole in the eradication of *Helicobacter pylori*. Am J Gastroenterol 89:1789–1792, 1994.
56. Logan RPH, Gummett PA, Misiewicz JJ, et al. One week eradication regimen for *Helicobacter pylori*. Lancet 2:1249–1252, 1991.
57. Hosking SW, Ling TKW, Yung MY, et al. Randomized controlled trial of short term treatment to eradicate *Helicobacter pylori* in patients with duodenal ulcers. BMJ 305:502–504, 1992.
58. Sung JJY, SC Chung S, Ling TKW, et al. One-year follow-up of duodenal ulcers after 1-week triple therapy for *Helicobacter pylori*. Am J Gastroenterol 89:199–202, 1994.
59. Hunt RH. Eradication of *Helicobacter pylori* infection. Am J Med 100:42S–51S, 1996.
60. Fennerty MB. Clinical issues and cost effectiveness of treating *H. pylori*. Am J Managed Care 4:S253–S258, 1998.
61. Mozell EJ, Cramer AJ, O'Dorsio TM, et al. Long term efficacy of octreotide in the treatment of Zollinger–Ellison syndrome. Arch Surg 127:1019–1026, 1992.
62. Kahrilas PJ. Gastroesophageal reflux disease and its complications. In: Feldman M, Scharschmidt BF, Sleisinger MH, eds. Sleisinger and Fordtran's gastrointestinal and liver disease: pathophysiology/diagnosis/management. 6th ed. Philadelphia: Saunders, 1998:498–517.
63. Cohen S, Parkman HP. Heartburn: a serious symptom. N Engl J Med 340:878–879, 1999.
64. Lagergren J, Bergstrom R, Lindgren A, et al. Symptomatic gastroesophageal reflux as a risk factor for esophageal adenocarcinoma. N Engl J Med 11:825–831, 1999.
65. DeVault KR, Castell DO. Updated guidelines for the diagnosis and treatment of gastroesophageal reflux disease. Am J Gastroenterol 94:1434–1442, 1999.
66. Johnson NJ, Boyd EFS, Mills JG, et al. Acute treatment of reflux esophagitis: a multicentre trial to compare 150 mg ranitidine b.d. with 300 mg. q.d.s. Aliment Pharmacol Ther 3:259–266, 1989.
67. Pasqual JC, Henery P, Bruley S, et al. Comparison of the effects of two doses of omeprazole on 24-hour esophageal pH in gastroesophageal reflux disease [abstract]. Gastroenterology 92:1567, 1987.
68. Sontag SJ. The medical management of reflux esophagitis: role of antacids and acid inhibition. Gastroenterol Clin North Am 19:683–712, 1990.
69. Feldman M, Harfore WV, Fisher RS, et al. Treatment of reflux esophagitis resistant to H_2 receptor antagonists with lansoprazole, a new H^+/K^+-ATPase inhibitor: a controlled, double blind study. Am J Gastroenterol 88:1212–1217, 1993.
70. Barone JA, Jessen LM, Colaizzi JL, et al. Cisapride: a gastrointestinal prokinetic drug. Ann Pharmacother 28:488–500, 1994.
71. Cook DJ, Fuller HD, Guyatt GH, et al. Risk factors for gastrointestinal bleeding in critically ill patients. N Engl J Med 330:377–381, 1994.
72. Kleiman RL, Adair CG, Ephgrave KS. Stress ulcers: current understanding of pathogenesis and prophylaxis. Ann Pharmacother 22:452–460, 1988.
73. Smythe MA, Zarowitz BJ. Changing perspectives of stress gastritis prophylaxis. Ann Pharmacother 28:1073–1085, 1994.
74. Ben-Menachem T, Fogel R, Patel RV, et al. Prophylaxis for stress related gastric hemorrhage in the medical intensive care unit. Ann Intern Med 121:568–575, 1994.
75. Prod'hom G, Leuenberger P, Koerfer J, et al. Nosocomial pneumonia in mechanically ventilated patients receiving antacid, ranitidine or sucralfate as prophylaxis for stress ulcer. A randomized clinical trial. Ann Intern Med 120:653–662, 1994.
76. Tryba M. The gastropulmonary route of infection: fact or fiction? Am J Med 91(Suppl 2A):135S–146S, 1991.
77. Lewis JH. Gastrointestinal injury due to medicinal agents. Am J Gastroenterol 81:819–834, 1986.
78. Agrawal NM. Anti-inflammatories and gastroduodenal damage: therapeutic options. Eur J Rheumatol Inflamm 13:17–24, 1993.
79. Bianchi PG, Lazzaroni M. Prevention and treatment of non-steroidal gastroduodenal lesions. Eur J Gastroenterol Hepatol 5:420–432, 1993.
80. Lanza FL. A guideline for the treatment and prevention of NSAID-induced ulcers. Am J Gastroenterol 93:2037–2045, 1998.
81. Griffin MR, Ray WA, Schaffner W. Nonsteroidal antiinflammatory drug use and death from peptic ulcer in elderly persons. Ann Intern Med 109:359–363, 1988.
82. Graham DY, Agrawal NM, Roth SH. Prevention of NSAID-induced gastric ulcer with misoprostol: multicentre, double-blind, placebo controlled trial. Lancet 2:1277–1280, 1988.
83. Walt RP. Misoprostol for the treatment of peptic ulcer and antiinflammatory-drug-induced gastroduodenal ulceration. N Engl J Med 327:1575–1580, 1992.
84. Roth SH. Misoprostol in the prevention of NSAID-induced gastric ulcer: a multicenter, double-blind, placebo-controlled trial. J Rheumatol 17(Suppl 20):20–24, 1990.
85. Graham DY. Prevention of gastroduodenal injury induced by chronic nonsteroidal antiinflammatory drug therapy. Gastroenterology 96:675–681, 1989.
86. Jones MP, Schubert ML. What do you recommend for prophylaxis in an elderly woman with arthritis requiring NSAIDs for control? Controversies, dilemmas, and dialogues. Am J Gastroenterol 86:264–265, 1991.
87. Smith JL. What do you recommend for prophylaxis in an elderly woman with arthritis requiring NSAIDs for control? Am J Gastroenterol 86:266–267, 1991.
88. Ehsanullah RSB, Page MC, Tildesley G, et al. Prevention of gastroduodenal damage induced by nonsteroidal anti-inflammatory drugs: controlled trial of ranitidine. BMJ 297:1017–1021, 1988.
89. Robinson MG, Griffin JW, Bowers J, et al. Effect of ranitidine on gastroduodenal mucosal damage induced by nonsteroidal anti-inflammatory drugs. Dig Dis Sci 34:424–428, 1989.

CHAPTER 25

INFLAMMATORY BOWEL DISEASE

Rosemary R. Berardi

DEFINITION

Inflammatory bowel disease (IBD) describes two major chronic, nonspecific inflammatory disorders of the gastrointestinal (GI) tract, ulcerative colitis (UC) and Crohn's disease (CD), the causes of which remain unknown. UC usually is limited to the colon and rectum (Fig. 25.1). It may affect the rectum alone (proctitis), only the descending and sigmoid colon and rectum (proctosigmoiditis), or the entire colon (pancolitis). In contrast, CD may affect any part of the GI tract from mouth to anus; it may involve only the terminal ileum (TI; ileitis), regions of the small intestine (regional enteritis), only the colon (colitis), or both the small intestine and colon (Fig. 25.1). The anatomic location is important because the response to drug therapy may vary, depending on the site of involvement. Both UC and CD are characterized by recurrent acute inflammatory episodes and periods of remission.

TREATMENT GOALS: INFLAMMATORY BOWEL DISEASE

- Tailor treatment to severity of symptoms; extent, location, and severity of inflammatory process; and response to previous medications. Acute exacerbations, quiescent symptom-free periods, and chronic symptomatic periods warrant individualized treatment.
- Terminate the acute attack and induce remission.
- Maintain remission during quiescent symptom-free periods.
- Control symptoms during chronic symptomatic periods.
- Prevent or control complications.
- Maintain or improve quality of life.
- Use the most cost-effective drug regimen.

EPIDEMIOLOGY

IBD afflicts approximately 2 million Americans, usually before age 40. In the United States, complications of these diseases are believed to claim 1000 lives a year. The epidemiologies of UC and CD share many features (Table 25.1) but differ with geographic location.[1–3] Both diseases are more common in Western populations and in urban rather than rural areas. There is a higher rate of IBD among Jewish people born in the United States and Europe than in Israeli Jews. In the United States, UC and CD are more prevalent in Caucasians and in women. UC and CD have been reported in different members of the same family.[1–3] Although IBD can occur at any age, the peak age of incidence is in the teens or early twenties. A second but controversial peak may occur later in life. The incidence of smoking in UC and CD differs from that of the general population.

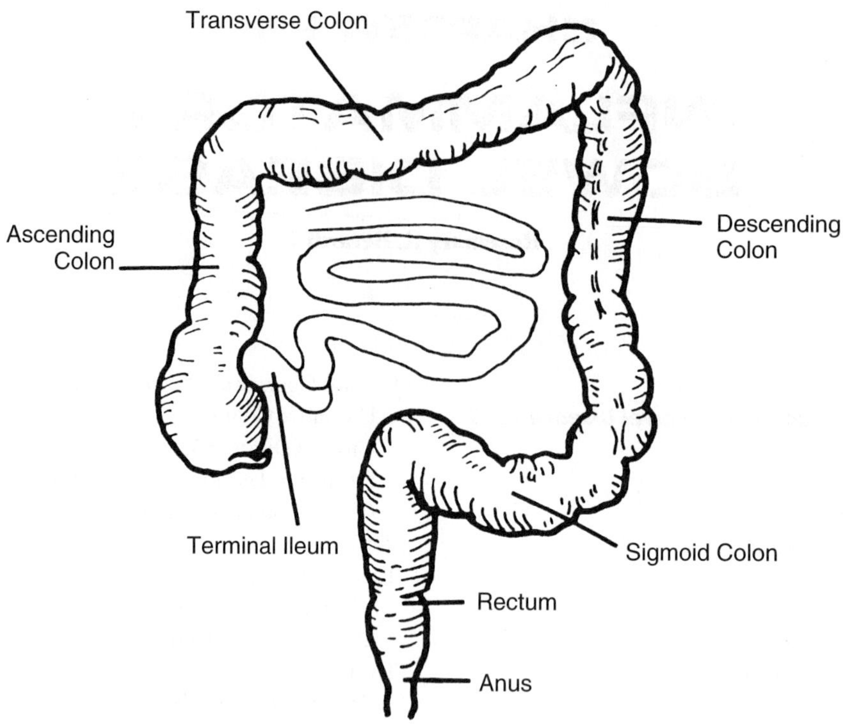

Figure 25.1. Anatomic location of various segments of the bowel.

Table 25.1 ▪ Epidemiology of Ulcerative Colitis and Crohn's Disease

Factor	Ulcerative Colitis	Crohn's Disease
Incidence (per 100,000)	2–10	1–6
Prevalence (per 100,000)	35–100	10–100
Location	More common in urban than rural areas	More common in urban than rural areas
Ethnicity	More common in Jewish than non-Jewish people	More common in Jewish than non-Jewish people
Race	More common in Caucasians than African Americans, Asians, Hispanics, or Native Americans	More common in Caucasians than African Americans, Asians, Hispanics, or Native Americans
Sex	Slightly more common in women than men	Slightly more common in women than men
Age of onset	15–25, ?50–80	15–25, ?50–80
Cigarette smoking	Less common in smokers than nonsmokers	More common in smokers than nonsmokers
Socioeconomic status	More common in higher socioeconomic level	More common in higher socioeconomic level

Source: References 1–3.

Genetic Influences

There appears to be a higher incidence of IBD among relatives of patients with IBD. The incidence of IBD among first-degree relatives is 30 to 100 times that of the general population.[1-3] Studies with monozygotic twins also support the presence of a genetic influence. No specific genetic marker has been identified for either UC or CD.

Cigarette Smoking

Cigarette smoking is an established risk factor for CD.[4,5] Ex-smokers also seem to be at higher risk, but the risk is less than that for current smokers. In contrast, smoking reduces the risk of UC.[4,5] However, former smokers are at greater risk than those who have never smoked. How smoking protects patients with UC is unknown, but it probably involves nicotine. Patients with IBD should stop smoking because of its health hazards and the uncertainty of its protective effect in UC.

Nonsteroidal Antiinflammatory Drugs

Nonsteroidal antiinflammatory drugs (NSAIDs) can cause a variety of effects in patients with IBD, ranging from asymptomatic mucosal inflammation to strictures, obstruction, perforation, and hemorrhage.[6] NSAIDs have also been linked to colitis in patients without previous IBD and may activate quiescent IBD.[4,6,7] Because NSAIDs often are used to treat the arthropathy that accompanies IBD, patients taking NSAIDs should be monitored closely for signs of obstruction, perforation, or bleeding.

Psychological Factors

Emotional and psychological factors have been implicated in the etiology of IBD, but there is no evidence that stress is causative and that psychotherapy is effective.[1–3] However, psychological factors may influence the clinical course of the disease and the patient's response to therapy because acute flares of activity often occur in association with stressful events.[8,9] Thus, it is possible that the nervous system has a regulatory effect on the immune system. IBD management should include the realization that the symptoms of IBD, such as diarrhea, pain, and rectal bleeding, are in themselves likely to cause various psychological responses.

PATHOPHYSIOLOGY

The cause and pathogenesis of IBD remain unknown. Both UC and CD appear to be immunologically mediated and influenced by genetic and environmental factors.[7,10–15] Current etiologic theories are listed in Table 25.2. Abnormal immunologic findings often appear with the active inflammatory process and subside with quiescence. Inflammation and tissue damage usually are confined to the GI tract. Various pathogens, dietary antigens, and the patient's own intestinal epithelial cells (autoimmune) have been implicated as proinflammatory triggers (Table 25.2). Similarities between UC and CD suggest that they may be heterogeneous disorders with different antigenic triggers. Factors that may lead to IBD relapse include activation of eosinophils by environmental stimuli, systemic and enteric infections, use of NSAIDs, mesalamine sensitivity, changes in smoking status, and treatment noncompliance.[4]

Proinflammatory Triggers

Microbial antigens are likely proinflammatory triggers. Clinical and experimental evidence suggests that normal luminal microbial flora (especially anaerobic bacteria) can induce and perpetuate chronic intestinal inflammation.[7,10] It is hypothesized that the normal host develops tolerance to these bacteria and maintains homeostasis through a number of host protective factors (Table 25.2). This balance can be disrupted by genetic defects in immunoregulation or mucosal barrier function and by various environmental factors. Once mucosal inflammation is triggered in a susceptible host, chronic inflammation and mucosal permeability ensue. No conclusive evidence has linked a specific pathogen to UC or CD. However, *Mycobacterium paratuberculosis* and the measles virus may play a pathogenic role in CD.[2,7]

Dietary antigens represent most of the nonpathogenic antigens presented to the intestinal mucosa.[7,10] Chronic exposure to dietary luminal antigens produces a low-grade chronic inflammation of the lamina propria in healthy patients. Failure to suppress the inflammatory response to normal dietary antigens could result in the immune activation observed in IBD. Chemical food additives, cow's milk, high consumption of refined sugars, and low intake of dietary fiber have been linked to IBD, but evidence supporting a primary etiologic role is not compelling. It is possible that dietary antigens play a secondary role, which is mediated by genetic factors. Other potential proinflammatory triggers are identified in Table 25.2.

Altered Immune Response

Alterations in the mucosal immune system are central to the pathogenesis of IBD. However, no consistent immunologic abnormality has been established as the primary defect in UC or CD. Proinflammatory triggers (Table 25.2) in the intestinal lumen appear to activate macrophages and T-lymphocytes to release numerous endogenous mediators (e.g., cytokines, arachidonic acid metabolites, and growth factors) of inflammation in IBD. Many of the mediators of tissue damage also amplify the immune response and pro-

Table 25.2 ▪ Pathogenic Factors and Etiologic Theories of Inflammatory Bowel Disease

Proinflammatory triggers	Host protective factors	Modifying factors
Normal luminal microflora	Impermeable mucosal barrier	*Genetic*
Dietary antigens	Protective prostaglandins	Immunoregulation
Bacterial antigens	Corticosteroids (e.g., cortisol)	Mucosal barrier
Digestive enzymes	Interleukin-1ra	*Environmental*
Bile acids	Interleukin-4	Diet
Cell wall polymers	Interleukin-10	Stress
Chemotactic peptides	Transforming growth factor-β	Smoking
Lipopolysaccharide	Inhibitory neuropeptides	Nonsteroidal antiinflammatory drugs
Etiologic theories	T_2 lymphocytes	Infections
Specific infectious pathogen	Short-chain fatty acids	Antiinflammatory mediators
Permeable mucosal barrier	Proinflammatory mediators	T-Suppressor lymphocytes
Defective epithelial healing	Cytotoxic T-lymphocytes	Interleukin-1ra
Abnormal immune response	Leukotrienes	Interleukin-4
	Interleukin-1	Interleukin-10
	Interleukin-12	s-Tumor necrosis factor-R
	Tumor necrosis factor	Non–complement-fixing immunoglobulin A
	Platelet activating factor	
	Complement-fixing immunoglobulin G	
	Reactive oxygen radicals or nitrous oxide	

Source: References 7, 10–15.

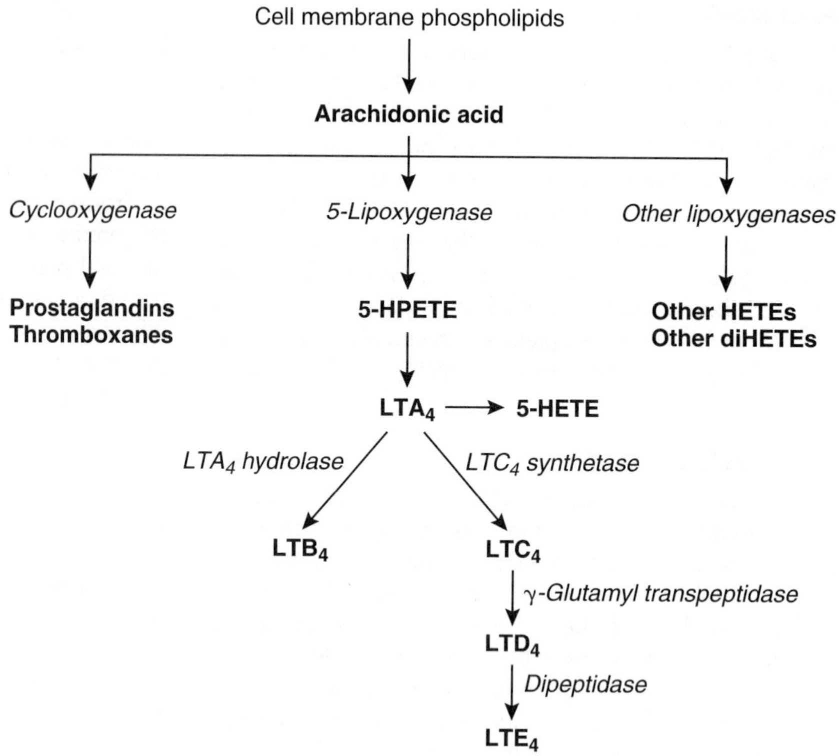

Figure 25.2. Arachidonic acid metabolism and leukotriene formation. *LTA$_4$–LTE$_4$*, leukotrienes A$_4$–E$_4$; *5-HETE*, 5-hydroxyeicosatetraenoic acid; *5-HPETE*, 5-hydroxyperoxyeicosatetraenoic acid; *HETE*, hydroxyeicosatetraenoic acid; *diHETE*, dihydroxyeicosatetraenoic acid.

mote further inflammation. Cytokines, prostaglandins, neuropeptides, and metabolites of arachidonic acid, including leukotrienes (Fig. 25.2), often correlate with disease activity and provide a rationale for drug therapy.[11–15] Increased production of potent proinflammatory cytokines, including interleukin-1 (IL-1), IL-12, tumor necrosis factor (TNF), platelet-activating factor (PAF), and interferon-γ (IFN-γ) stimulate epithelial, endothelial, and mesenchymal cells and activate immune cells (Table 25.2). The chemotactic cytokines, IL-8, macrophage chemotactic and activating factor (MCAF), and other chemotactic substances such as leukotriene B$_4$ (LTB$_4$) increase macrophage and neutrophil migration from the circulation into the inflamed mucosa. This process may be related to ischemic injury involving the release of superoxide and other reactive oxygen species. Mucosal and serum prostaglandin concentrations are elevated in IBD, but there is evidence against their role as mediators of inflammation because NSAIDs have failed to provide clinical improvement.

COMPLICATIONS

Local Complications

Local complications arise from the intestinal component of IBD and include pseudopolyps, perianal fissures, abscesses, fistulas, intestinal obstruction, colonic perforation, massive hemorrhage, toxic megacolon, and colon cancer.[1,2] The incidence of abscesses and fistula formation is higher in CD than in UC and may be the initial presentation of the disease. Fistulas occur most often in the perianal and perirectal areas, with enterocutaneous, enterovaginal, and enteroenteric fistulas occurring less often. Small bowel obstruction is a common complication of CD and may result from inflammation and edema of the involved intestine or the narrowing of the bowel secondary to scar formation. Colonic perforation is uncommon in CD but may complicate toxic megacolon in UC. The risk of perforation and peritonitis is greatest during an initial severe attack and is associated with a high mortality.

Toxic Megacolon

Toxic megacolon may occur in CD of the colon but is more likely to complicate severe attacks of UC.[1,2] This serious complication is preceded by a rapidly deteriorating clinical course and is associated with a high morality. It is characterized by acute dilation of the transverse colon to a diameter greater than 6 cm with accompanying systemic toxicity. The pathogenesis of the acute dilation is related to the deep inflammatory process, which involves all layers of the colon and results in the inability of the colon to contract. Toxic megacolon may be triggered by anticholinergics, opiates, and other antimotility agents used to treat diarrhea or by severe electrolyte abnormalities such as hypokalemia. Medications that decrease intestinal motility should be withdrawn.

Colon Cancer

The risk of colon cancer is greater in patients with IBD than in the general population, with a higher incidence observed in UC than in CD.[1,2] The risk of developing cancer in UC increases when the duration of the disease is more than 8 years and when the disease involves the entire colon.[1] Because colonic cancer in UC is virulent, algorithms for surveillance recommend performing colonoscopy with biopsy every 1 to 2 years in most patients with pancolitis of 8 to 10 years' duration.[1] A prophylactic total colectomy will cure UC and prevent colonic cancer.

Table 25.3 ▪ Important Anatomic, Pathologic, and Clinical Features of Ulcerative Colitis and Crohn's Disease

Feature	Ulcerative Colitis	Crohn's Disease
Anatomic		
Small bowel only	+	+++
Small bowel and colon	+	++++
Colon only	++	+++
Anorectal only	++++	+
Diffuse, continuous involvement	++++	++
Cobblestoning	+	++++
Pathologic		
Transmural	+	++++
Fissures and fistulas	++	+++
Crypt abscesses	++++	++
Strictures	+	+++
Shortening of the colon	+++	+
Pseudopolyps	+++	+
Clinical		
Rectal bleeding	++++	++
Diarrhea	++++	++++
Abdominal pain	++	++++
Malaise, fever	++	++++
Weight loss	+++	++++
Extraintestinal manifestations	++	++
Perianal disease	++	+++
Intestinal obstruction	+	+++
Toxic megacolon	+++	++
Risk of malignancy	+++	++

Frequencies are estimates, categorized as consistent (++++), frequent (+++), infrequent (++), or rare (+). None of the features are always present or always absent.

CLINICAL PRESENTATION AND DIAGNOSIS

Signs and Symptoms

Ulcerative Colitis

UC affects primarily the mucosa and submucosa of the rectum and the left colon, with the rectum involved histologically in more than 90% of the cases.[1] Distal UC may be described as proctitis or proctosigmoiditis, depending on the location of mucosal inflammation. Lesions usually develop in the rectum and spread proximally; however, initial disease may involve the entire colon (Fig. 25.1). The disease extends to the total colon (universal or pancolitis) in 5 to 10% of patients and may involve a minimal portion of the TI (backwash ileitis). In severe forms of UC, such as toxic megacolon, deeper layers of the colon may be involved.

The inflammatory process in UC is continuous with no intervening areas of normal mucosa; deeper layers of the bowel usually are not involved (Table 25.3). Chronic recurrent mucosal inflammation with concomitant tissue repair may lead to characteristic findings such as the formation of crypt abscesses, pseudopolyps, shortening of the colon (foreshortening), and a "lead pipe" appearance. Dysplasia in colonic biopsies may represent a premalignant change and a risk of carcinoma.

The clinical features of UC vary with disease severity (Table 25.4). Determining whether the disease is mild, moderate, or severe is important because treatment and prognosis are related to disease severity.[1] Clinically mild disease usually involves only the sigmoid and rectum. Diarrhea and rectal bleeding are mild, and systemic symptoms usually are absent. Diarrhea, with varying degrees of rectal bleeding, usually is the major presenting symptom in moderate disease. Abdominal cramping is more prominent but is often relieved by defecation. Severe UC is characterized by a sudden onset of profuse diarrhea, rectal bleeding, and severe abdominal cramps. The patient usually is febrile, dehydrated, and profoundly weak. Blood loss can

Table 25.4 ▪ Clinical Features of Ulcerative Colitis Based on Disease Severity

	Mild	Moderate	Severe
Frequency	60%	20–25%	10–15%
Location	Rectum and distal colon	Rectum and ⅓–½ of colon	Rectum and entire colon
Weight loss	Uncommon	<10 lb	>10 lb
Fever	Uncommon	Intermittent	Persistent
Abdominal pain	Uncommon	Common	Severe
Bowel sounds	Normal	Normal	Absent
Diarrhea	3–5 stools/day	>5 stools/day	Hourly
Rectal bleeding	Intermittent	Common	Severe
Tachycardia	Uncommon	Frequently	Common
Anemia	Uncommon	Hematocrit >30%	Hematocrit <30%
Leukocytosis	Uncommon	Common	Common
Albumin	Normal	Normal	Low
Extraintestinal manifestations	Uncommon	Common	Severe
Risk of malignancy	Not increased	Increased after 10 yr	Increased after 10 yr
Mortality (acute attack)	<0.5%	2%	10–25%

Table 25.5 ▪ Clinical Features of Crohn's Disease Based on Disease Location

	Small Bowel	Ileocolitis	Colitis
Diarrhea	>90%	>90%	>90%
Abdominal pain	Common	Common	Very common
Malnutrition	Common	Common	Less common
Fistula	10–20%	30–50%	10–30%
Obstruction	30–40%	40–50%	10–20%
Perianal disease	Uncommon	Common	Very common

result in a rapid pulse, low blood pressure, and anemia. Death may occur during the acute attack.

Crohn's Disease

The distal ileum and right colon (ileocolitis) are the most common sites of involvement in CD (Table 25.3). Although the TI usually is involved, other areas of the small bowel may be affected. The small bowel and colon are involved in about two-thirds of patients, with about 15 to 20% having only colonic involvement. In the majority of patients with CD of the colon, the rectum is spared. Sections of bowel that appear normal by radiography or colonoscopy can have histologic features of CD.

In contrast to UC, CD is characterized by chronic inflammation extending through all layers of the bowel wall as well as the mesentery and regional lymph nodes.[2] The transmural process can lead to fissure and fistula formation and a thickened, edematous bowel, which can result in obstruction (Table 25.3). The disease often involves segments of the bowel separated by normal-appearing bowel called skip lesions. In advanced cases, the mucosa has a nodular or cobblestone appearance. Although certain anatomic and pathologic features enable CD of the colon to be distinguished from UC, this distinction is not possible in about 20% of cases.

The clinical features of CD vary but usually reflect the anatomic location of the disease (Table 25.5). A low-grade fever occurs in more than 50% of patients in the absence of any complications. Malabsorption and nutritional deficiencies result in weight loss in more than 80% of patients. Abdominal pain tends to be steady and localized to the right lower quadrant. A colicky or cramping pain, usually associated with bowel movements, may be superimposed on the steady pain. When CD is confined to the small bowel, diarrhea often occurs without bleeding. With colonic involvement, diarrhea is accompanied by rectal bleeding in about 50% of patients. Most patients have recurrent episodes of diarrhea, abdominal pain, and fever lasting from a few days to several months. Perianal fissures, fistulas, and abscesses may be the presenting feature. Acute CD may be mild, moderate, or severe depending on the extent of involvement.

Nutritional Disorders

Nutritional disorders are more common and complex in CD because of food avoidance and the potential for malabsorption and malnutrition. Mechanisms include inadequate food intake; inflammatory involvement of the small bowel resulting in decreased absorption of nutrients, lactase deficiency, and protein-losing enteropathy; small bowel bacterial overgrowth with associated malabsorption of cobalamin and altered bile salt metabolism; intestinal surgery; and the catabolic effects of chronic inflammation.[2] Prolonged periods of poor nutrition and disease can result in dehydration, acid-base and electrolyte disturbances, protein calorie malnutrition, and deficiencies of vitamins A, D, K, B_{12}, and folic acid. Consequences of these disorders can be especially serious in children with CD and may lead to growth retardation and delayed sexual maturation.

Extraintestinal Manifestations

Many extraintestinal manifestations are associated with IBD and may precede or accompany the underlying intestinal disorder (Table 25.6). These manifestations may be related to the clinical activity of the inflammatory process, its anatomic location, or to the disordered physiology of the small intestine.[1,2,16] The arthritic, skin, and eye manifestations occur more often in patients with UC and Crohn's colitis than in patients with CD of the small intestine. The arthritis usually is asymmetric and affects the joints of the knees, hips, ankles, wrists, and elbows. In most patients, it tends to parallel the activity and severity of the bowel disease, often subsiding with therapy, colectomy, or spontaneous remission. In contrast, ankylosing spondylitis may appear years before bowel symptoms and runs a course independent of the intestinal disease.

Minor abnormalities in hepatic transaminases commonly occur in patients with IBD. but clinically important

Table 25.6 ▪ Extraintestinal Manifestations of Inflammatory Bowel Disease

Manifestation	Incidence (%)	Related to Intestinal Disease Activity
Arthritis and arthralgias	25–30	Yes
Aphthous mouth ulcers	5–10	Yes
Episcleritis or uveitis (iritis)	5–10	Yes
Erythema nodosum	1–5	Yes
Pyoderma gangrenosum	1–5	Usually
Sacroiliitis	10–15	No
Ankylosing spondylitis	1–2	No
Abnormal liver transaminases	30–50	No
Liver disease	1–3	No
Sclerosing cholangitis	1–4	No
Cholelithiasis[a]	20–30	No
Nephrolithiasis[a]	25–35	No
Renal disease[a]	1–3	No

In general, the extraintestinal manifestations in ulcerative colitis and Crohn's colitis are similar in type and prevalence.

[a]This manifestation is seen primarily in Crohn's disease of the small intestine.

liver disease is uncommon. Cirrhosis, chronic hepatitis, and sclerosing cholangitis, although rare, tend to occur more often in UC.[1] Cholelithiasis may occur in CD with ileal involvement or resection and results from diminished bile salt reabsorption. Nephrolithiasis also occurs in ileal CD and results from increased oxalate absorption secondary to malabsorption of fatty acids. Renal amyloid may cause nephrotic syndrome and renal failure in CD.[2]

The most common hematologic complication is iron deficiency anemia secondary to blood loss.[1,2] Chronic anorexia and malabsorption can lead to other complex anemias. Some patients may develop an idiopathic hemolytic anemia or a hemolytic anemia associated with sulfasalazine. Thromboembolic events resulting from abnormalities of clotting factors during active episodes may complicate the course of both diseases. Treatment involves the risk of colonic bleeding during anticoagulation.

Diagnosis

A diagnosis of IBD should be considered in all patients who present with persistent abdominal pain and diarrhea or bloody diarrhea. Occasionally, fever, weight loss, or extraintestinal manifestations may overshadow the intestinal symptoms. Because UC and CD are nonspecific diseases, the diagnosis usually is made by exclusion and relies on the clinical picture, stool findings, sigmoidoscopic or colonoscopic appearances, and histologic assessment.[1,2] Once the diagnosis of IBD is established, the distinction between UC and CD of the colon often is possible.

Laboratory tests usually are nonspecific and do not establish the diagnosis. Leukocytosis and an elevated erythrocyte sedimentation rate may reflect the inflammatory process. Electrolyte abnormalities, particularly hypokalemia, exist when there is severe diarrhea. Hypoalbuminemia may reflect the patient's poor nutritional status and overall clinical condition. Anemia often accompanies chronic blood loss.

Sigmoidoscopic or colonoscopic examination of the bowel is most important in establishing mucosal inflammation in both UC and CD. A rectal or colonic biopsy usually confirms the presence of an abnormal and inflamed mucosa. Radiography (with or without contrast) also provides essential information and complements endoscopy. Barium contrast studies are used in CD when involvement of the small bowel or fistula is suspected. A plain film of the abdomen may be indicated in patients in whom a barium enema and endoscopy are contraindicated. Computed axial tomography and ultrasonography are useful in diagnosing abscess and fluid collections.

CLINICAL COURSE AND PROGNOSIS

Ulcerative Colitis

The initial attack of UC often is abrupt, with symptoms ranging from nonbloody diarrhea to fulminant diarrhea and colonic hemorrhage. In 50% of patients, the first attack is mild, 30% are of moderate severity, and 20% have severe disease.[1] The majority of patients have highly variable intermittent attacks with varying intervals of asymptomatic remissions. A smaller number are troubled by continuous symptoms with intermittent flares of disease activity. More than 90% of patients with active UC respond to drug therapy. Patients with mild UC have a prognosis similar to that of the general population. Morbidity is greatest when the onset of symptoms is severe, colonic involvement is extensive, or toxic megacolon develops. About 50% of patients with severe initial disease need a colectomy within 2 years; the same percentage of patients with pancolitis need a colectomy in 5 years.[1] Disease-related complications and the risk of colon cancer contribute to the clinical course and prognosis.

Crohn's Disease

CD, like UC, follows a clinical course of acute exacerbations and remissions. The disease is characterized by recurrent attacks of diarrhea, abdominal pain, and low-grade fever, resulting in gradual deterioration over a period of years. Blood loss and poor nutrition lead to anemia, weight loss, malnutrition, and fatigue. Approximately 60% of patients with CD need surgery within 10 years of the initial diagnosis; of these, about half eventually need another operation.[2] Partial or complete obstruction is the most common indication for surgery and occurs more rapidly in patients with ileocolitis. Perianal or perirectal disease develops in about one-half of patients with colonic involvement. Patients with sclerosing cholangitis or ankylosing spondylitis may be more troubled by extraintestinal manifestations than by the underlying intestinal disease. The prognosis for CD is not as favorable as for UC because of the variable nature of the disease, the less-than-optimum response to drug therapy, the need for surgery, and postoperative disease recurrence. Morbidity and mortality, often associated with peritonitis and sepsis, increase with disease duration.

Pregnancy, Lactation, and Fertility

In the majority of IBD patients, pregnancy does not alter the course of disease, nor does the disease adversely affect the outcome of pregnancy or fertility. However, men should be informed that salicylazosulfapyridine (SASP) reversibly inhibits spermatogenesis. Folic acid supplementation may be necessary in pregnant mothers taking SASP. Pregnant or nursing mothers with active IBD usually are unable to discontinue their medications. This may be of concern because many of these drugs (or their metabolites) cross the placental barrier and are secreted in breast milk.[17] SASP, mesalamine, and glucocorticosteroids (GCSs) are safe in pregnancy and during lactation.[17–20] Alternatively, metronidazole (MTZ), azathioprine (AZA), 6-mercaptopurine (6-MP), cyclosporine, methotrexate (MTX), and infliximab should be avoided in pregnancy because of the risk of fetal growth retardation, prematurity, or congenital malformation.[17,18] Breastfeeding is not recommended in mothers treated with these medications.

Children and Adolescents

When IBD begins in childhood, the clinical course is similar to that observed when the onset occurs later in life. However, growth retardation is more common in children with CD than those with UC. Because malnutrition contributes to growth failure, nutritional supplementation must be pursued aggressively. Medications used to treat IBD in children are similar to those used to treat adults. However, prolonged use of high-dose GCS may suppress growth and cause other steroid-related adverse effects. Although MTZ and the immunomodulators have been used in children, they should be used with caution because of their potentially serious complications.[21–25]

PSYCHOSOCIAL ASPECTS

Psychosocial factors are an important component of treatment in patients with IBD.[8,9,26] Many of the symptoms (e.g., diarrhea, bloating, abdominal cramps) are exacerbated by stressful life events. The patient's psychological state (especially depression) appears to correlate with disease severity.[8,9] Patients with IBD often express concerns about abdominal pain, fatigue, body image, surgery, and cancer potential.[8,9] Thus, it is important to incorporate psychosocial information into the daily care plan. A number of IBD-related quality-of-life questionnaires have been developed to assess the patient's perception of his or her well-being, daily functioning, psychological state, job satisfaction, and interpersonal relationships.[8,9] Once this information is obtained, health care practitioners should work with the patient to develop a psychosocial plan that includes patient education, coping strategies, stress reduction techniques, social and family support, self-help groups, or psychological referral when appropriate. These efforts are likely to improve the outcome of drug treatment and the overall health of the patient.

THERAPEUTIC PLAN

The therapeutic plan for UC or CD is based on an assessment of disease location and severity. Disease severity is determined by evaluating the local inflammatory, obstructive, or fistulizing processes, the presence of systemic and extraintestinal manifestations, and the global impact of IBD on the patient's quality of life.[27,28] Recommendations for remission induction and maintenance are presented for UC and CD and discussed according to disease type, severity and location.

Ulcerative Colitis

Severe Colitis

Patients with severe active UC (Fig. 25.3) should be treated with an intravenous GCS (e.g., methylprednisolone 40 to 80 mg/day).[1,27] If the patient improves during the next 7 to 10 days, an oral GCS should replace the intravenous drug. Failure to demonstrate significant improvement after 10 days is an indication for surgery or investigational therapy with intravenous cyclosporine. Once remission is induced, the oral GCS should be withdrawn and oral sulfasalazine (SASP) maintenance therapy instituted. If the patient is intolerant of SASP, a 5-aminosalicylic acid (5-ASA, mesalamine) preparation such Asacol or Pentasa should be used. Patients with toxic megacolon should be treated with fluid and electrolyte replacement, blood transfusions if indicated, and intravenous GCS.[1,27] Intravenous therapy with broad-spectrum antibiotics directed at enteric Gram-negative, enterococcal, and anaerobic pathogens should be instituted. The initial 24 to 48 hours is crucial and determines future treatment.

Mild to Moderate Extensive Colitis

Patients with mild to moderate active UC (Fig. 25.3) should be treated with oral SASP, Asacol, or Pentasa.[1,27,29–31] Most patients respond to oral dosages of 3 to 4 g/day of SASP, but up to 6 g/day can be given. Lower SASP dosages may be attempted initially and then gradually increased as tolerance to the drug's adverse effects develops. Treatment with Asacol (800 to 1600 mg three times/day) or Pentasa (1 g four times/day) may be useful in patients who do not tolerate SASP. Symptomatic improvement with SASP, Asacol, or Pentasa takes 2 to 4 weeks. The addition of a GCS or 5-ASA enema may provide additional benefit.

If an immediate response is needed, or if the response to SASP or 5-ASA is inadequate, these drugs should be discontinued and an oral GCS (e.g., prednisone) instituted in a dosage of 20 to 60 mg/day. When clinical improvement occurs, the prednisone dosage should be tapered (usually 5 to 10 mg/week until 20 mg is reached, then 2.5 mg/week until discontinued) and maintenance therapy initiated with low-dose SASP, Asacol, Pentasa, or olsalazine. If the patient remains steroid-dependent, the addition of AZA or 6-MP may permit withdrawal of the GCS in those wanting to avoid a colectomy. However, 3 to 6 months of treatment usually is needed to obtain the optimal effect of AZA or 6-MP. Antidiarrheals (e.g., diphenoxylate or loperamide) may be used to control diarrhea in patients with mild to moderate chronic UC.

Mild to Moderate Distal Colitis

Patients with mild to moderate active distal UC (e.g., proctitis, proctosigmoiditis, left-sided colitis) usually respond to oral SASP, oral mesalamine (Asacol or Pentasa), topical mesalamine, or topical GCS.[1,27,29–31] The therapeutic plan often depends on the patient's preference for either oral or topical therapy because both are effective (Fig. 25.3). Although mesalamine enemas (1 to 4 g/day) are effective in inducing and maintaining remission in distal colitis, the cost of a course of therapy is many times that of oral SASP or steroid enemas. Thus, their use often is reserved for patients with mild to moderate active disease of the distal colon who do not respond to topical GCSs or SASP. Topical GCSs (e.g., 100 mg hydrocortisone enema or 10% hydrocortisone foam) are effective in inducing remission but are ineffective in maintaining remission in

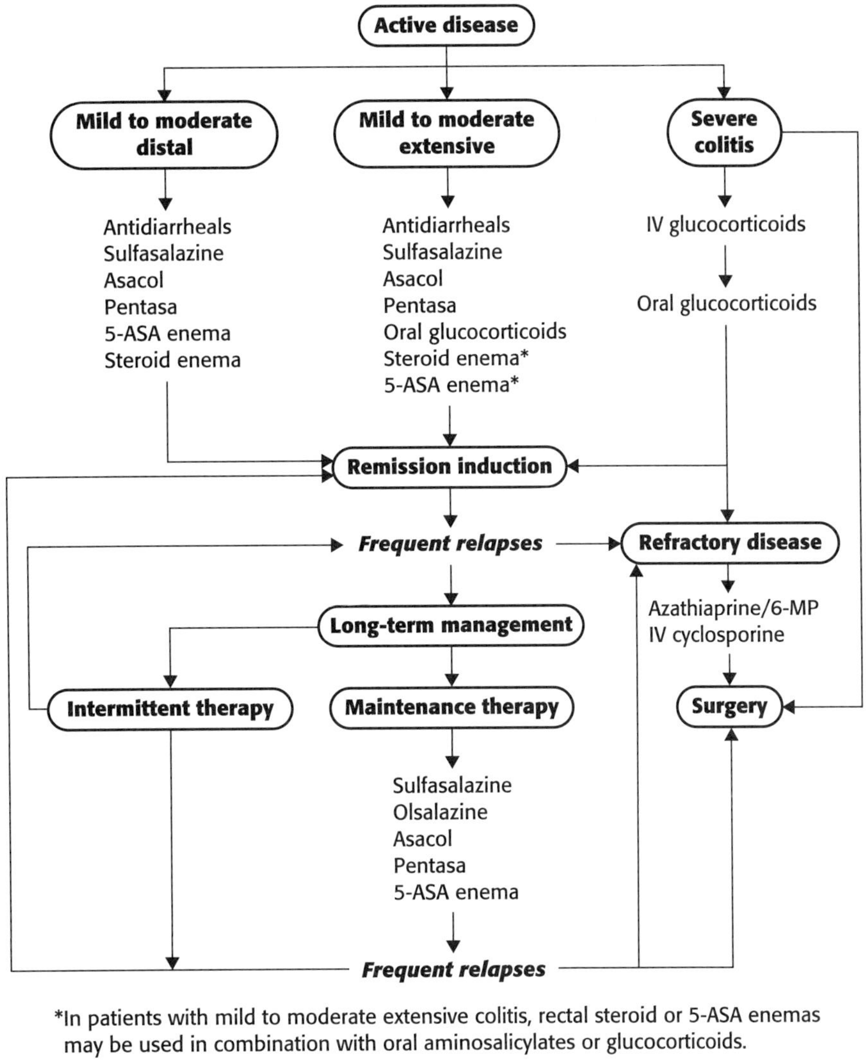

Figure 25.3. Algorithm for managing ulcerative colitis. *5-ASA,* 5-aminosalicylic acid; *6-MP,* 6-mercaptopurine.

distal colitis. Frequent relapses may warrant maintenance therapy with low-dose SASP. Pentasa, Asacol, or olsalazine should be reserved for patients intolerant to SASP. Mesalamine suppositories (500 mg twice daily) may be used to maintain remission in patients with proctitis.

Crohn's Disease

Severe Fulminant Disease

Once infection or an abscess has been excluded, intravenous GCS is indicated for patients with severe fulminant CD (Fig. 25.4) in dosages similar to those used in severe UC.[2,28,31,32] Patients who do not improve within 10 days should be considered surgical candidates. Patients who respond to parenteral therapy should be transferred gradually to an oral GCS until symptomatic relief is obtained. In patients whose symptoms worsen when GCSs are withdrawn, adding AZA or 6-MP in an attempt to withdraw or reduce the GCS dosage should be considered. There appears to be no specific role for parenteral nutrition in addition to GCSs, but nutritional support (either total parenteral nutrition or elemental tube feedings) is indicated for patients unable to tolerate an oral diet for more than 5 to 7 days. Broad-spectrum antibiotics should be instituted when an inflammatory mass is present.

Moderate to Severe Disease

Therapy for patients with moderate to severe active CD (Fig. 25.4) should be initiated with 40 to 60 mg/day of oral prednisone after infection or abscess is excluded.[2,28,31,32] Oral GCSs typically are administered until symptoms resolve and weight gain resumes (usually 1 to 4 weeks). Approximately 50% of patients treated with GCSs become steroid-dependent or resistant after the acute course. Although there is no advantage to using 5-ASA in patients with active colonic CD, Asacol or Pentasa may be useful in patients with ileal involvement and in maintaining remission in nonsurgical patients and after surgical resection once GCSs are withdrawn. In patients unable to discontinue GCSs, AZA or 6-MP should be added to the regimen in an attempt to lower the steroid dosage. Investiga-

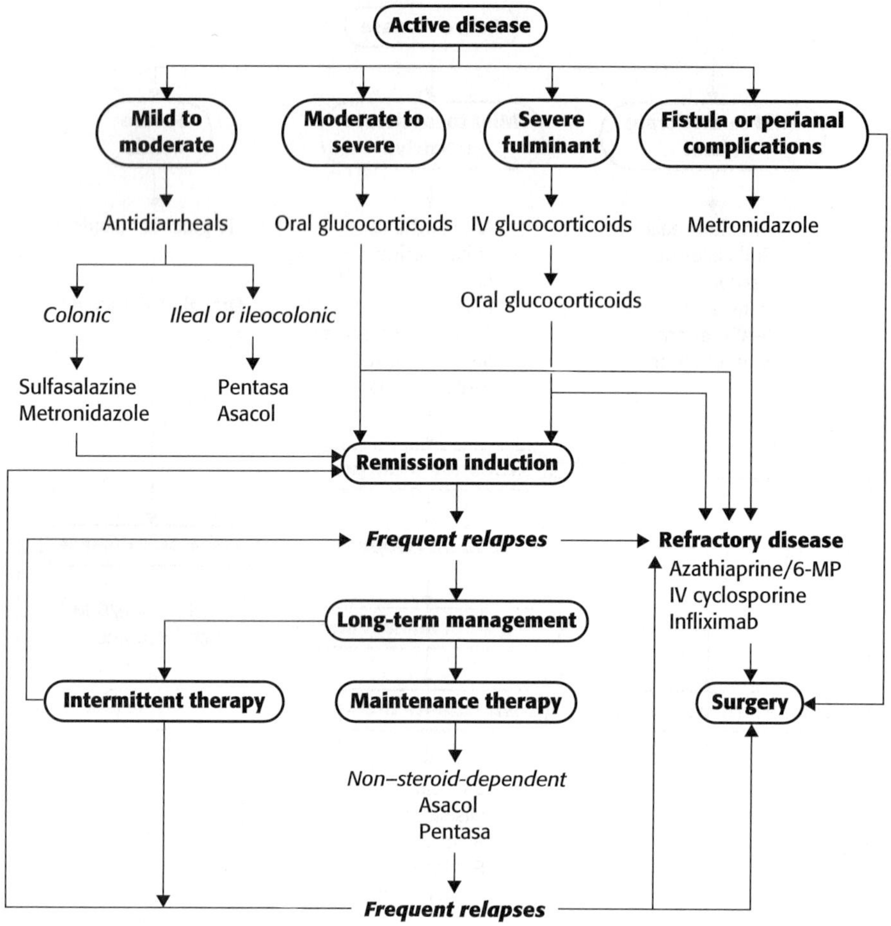

Figure 25.4. Algorithm for managing Crohn's disease. *6-MP,* 6-mercaptopurine.

tional intravenous cyclosporine or infliximab may be helpful in patients with severe CD who cannot discontinue steroids.[28] GCSs should not be used as long-term maintenance therapy.

Mild to Moderate Disease

Patients with mild to moderate active ileal or ileocolonic disease (Fig. 25.4) should be treated with oral Pentasa or Asacol because SASP has not been consistently effective in patients with CD involving the small bowel.[2,28,31,32] SASP or MTZ may be used in patients with mild to moderate active Crohn's colitis. Topical mesalamine or GCSs may be of value when the rectum is involved. Antibiotics (other than MTZ) have not been evaluated adequately despite their widespread use. The response to initial therapy should be evaluated after several weeks and continued until symptomatic remission or failure to improve. If the response to SASP, Asacol, Pentasa, or MTZ is inadequate, an oral GCS should be instituted. If symptomatic remission is achieved, maintenance therapy should be initiated with Asacol or Pentasa.

Perianal or Fistulizing Disease

Perianal or fistulizing disease warrants treatment if the patient is symptomatic. Drugs that reduce inflammation and diarrhea are likely to reduce perianal discharge.[32,33] Nonsuppurative perianal complications (Fig. 25.4) often respond to MTZ alone or in combination with ciprofloxacin, although symptoms usually recur when the antibiotic is discontinued.[14,32,33] GCSs may reduce diarrhea but are ineffective in treating fistulas. AZA or 6-MP may be helpful in healing perianal or fistulizing complications, but there is concern about their long-term safety. Refractory fistulas may respond to intravenous cyclosporine followed by AZA or 6-MP.[14,32] A trial of infliximab may be warranted.[14,15] Perianal or fistulizing disease warrants surgical drainage if suppuration is present.[2,33]

TREATMENT

Pharmacotherapy

Antidiarrheals, Antispasmodics, Analgesics

Antidiarrheals, antispasmodics, and analgesics provide symptomatic relief without affecting IBD activity. Antidiarrheals, such as diphenoxylate and loperamide, are useful in patients with mild chronic IBD and in those who have diarrhea resulting from small bowel resection. Symptomatic treatment of diarrhea may permit a reduction in the dosage of other medications, thereby reducing adverse effects. Antidiarrheals are contraindicated in severe IBD because they may precipitate toxic megacolon. In addition, they are ineffective in severe disease because the diarrhea results from a loss of colonic absorptive capacity caused by widespread destruction of the colonic mucosa.

Cholestyramine is used to treat bile salt diarrhea resulting from resection of the terminal ileum.[34] The formation of oxalate kidney stones and steatorrhea may also be prevented with cholestyramine. Clonidine or octreotide may be used to enhance fluid and electrolyte absorption in refractory diarrhea, but their utility is limited because of the numerous adverse effects associated with their use.[34]

Antispasmodics, including tincture of belladonna or opium and other anticholinergics, may be effective in reducing cramps and rectal urgency. They should be given before meals to decrease peristalsis associated with eating. Antispasmodics should be avoided if obstruction is suspected and are contraindicated in severe IBD.

Pain management should be aimed at controlling disease activity. Analgesics may be used to supplement treatment but should not become the mainstay of chronic pain control. Narcotics, when used to relieve severe pain, should be scheduled around the clock.[35] Iatrogenic drug addiction is a common problem among patients with CD but is minimized by having only one clinician prescribe and manage pain medications.

Sulfasalazine

Sulfasalazine (salicylazosulfapyridine, SASP) is a conjugate of 5-ASA and sulfapyridine (SP) linked by a diazo bond (Fig. 25.5). About 20% of the oral SASP dosage is absorbed, some of which is excreted in the bile.[1,31,32] The remainder of the parent drug passes unchanged into the colon, where colonic bacteria cleave the diazo bond to form 5-ASA and SP (Table 25.7). Most of the liberated 5-ASA remains in the colon and is excreted in the feces. SP is absorbed, metabolized (in part by acetylation in the liver), and excreted in the urine. Because 5-ASA and SP are absorbed when given orally, the diazo linkage provides a delivery system by which higher concentrations of 5-ASA can reach the diseased intestine.[31,32,36] SASP 1 g releases about 400 mg 5-ASA. Increased intestinal transit (diarrhea) or concomitant antibiotics may reduce SASP breakdown. Bacterial overgrowth may permit SASP metabolism in the small bowel. The exact mechanism by which SASP acts in IBD is uncertain. However, SASP and 5-ASA, the primary active moiety, interfere with arachidonic acid metabolism.[1,31,32] Both inhibit the lipoxygenase pathway and decrease the synthesis of chemotactically active leukotrienes in peripheral blood neutrophils and within the intestinal mucosa. SASP and 5-ASA also inhibit the cyclooxygenase pathway and lower intestinal prostaglandin concentrations. 5-ASA also may act as a free radical scavenger or an inhibitor of immunoglobulin secretion.[32]

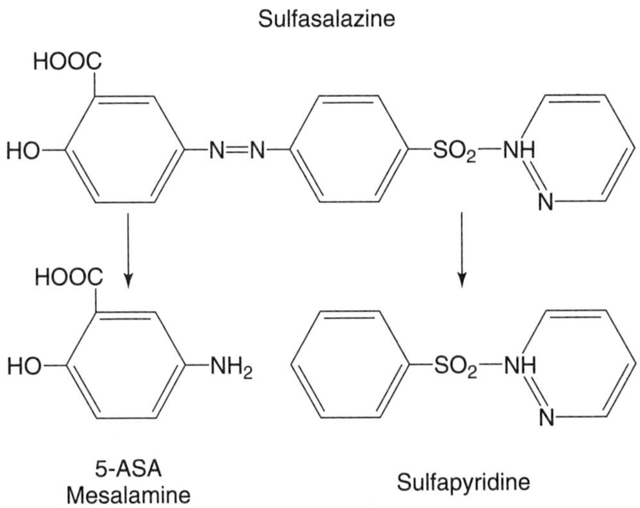

Figure 25.5. Structures of sulfasalazine, 5-aminosalicylic acid *(5-ASA)*, and sulfapyridine.

Table 25.7 ▪ Comparison of Aminosalicylate Preparations

Product	Formulation	Delivery Site	Urinary Recovery of 5-ASA (%)
Sulfasalazine	5-ASA linked to sulfapyridine carrier by azo-bond	Colon	17–37
Olsalazine	Two 5-ASA linked by azo-bond	Colon	14–27
Balsalazide	5-ASA linked to aminobenzoyl–alanine carrier by azo-bond	Colon	15–25
Mesalamine (Asacol)	5-ASA coated with Eudragit-S; delayed release (pH >7)	Distal ileum and colon	20–35
Mesalamine (Pentasa)	5-ASA encapsulated in ethylcellulose microgranules; sustained release	Pylorus throughout small and large bowel	30–55
Mesalamine (Salofalk, Claversal)	5-ASA coated with Eudragit-L; delayed release (pH >6)	Ileum and colon	23–54
Mesalamine (Rowasa)	Enema; 60-mL suspension	Left colon	
Mesalamine (Rowasa)	Suppository	Rectum	

Source: References 30–32.
5-ASA, 5-aminosalicylic acid.

SASP is effective in treating mild to moderate active UC (Tables 25.8, 25.9). Higher SASP dosages (6 to 8 g/day) sometimes are tried, but they are often intolerable. Adverse effects can be minimized by initiating treatment at a lower dosage (500 mg twice a day) and gradually increasing the dosage by 500 mg every 2 to 3 days, administering SASP with meals, or using enteric-coated tablets. Clinical response to SASP usually occurs within 2 to 4 weeks. SASP is effective in maintaining remission, but the relapse rate varies inversely with the daily dosage.[1,27,37] In most patients, the optimal maintenance dosage is 2 g/day.[36] Although the duration of maintenance therapy remains unresolved, most clinicians favor prolonged or indefinite treatment. SASP is effective in treating mild to moderate active CD (Tables 25.8, 25.9). However, patients with ileal disease respond less favorably to SASP than those with colonic involvement.[2,32] Release of 5-ASA in the colon probably accounts for the difference in efficacy. Combining SASP with oral GCS offers no increase in efficacy or steroid-sparing effect. Controlled clinical trials do not support the efficacy of SASP maintenance therapy in nonsurgical or postoperative patients with CD.[2,32,37]

Table 25.8 ▪ Drug Regimens Used to Treat Inflammatory Bowel Disease

	Route	Active Therapy	Maintenance Therapy
Aminosalicylates			
Sulfasalazine	Oral	3–6 g/day	2–4 g/day
Olsalazine	Oral	Not indicated	1.5–3 g/day
Balsalazide	Oral	2–6 g/day (?)	2–6 g/day (?)
Asacol	Oral	2.4–4.8 g/day	800 mg–4.8 g/day
Salofalk/Claversal	Oral	1.5–3 g/day	750 mg–1.5 g/day
Pentasa	Oral	2–4 g/day	1.5–3 g/day
Mesalamine enema	Rectal	1–4 g/bedtime	1–2 g/bedtime
Mesalamine suppository	Rectal	1–1.5 g/day	500 mg/bedtime
Corticosteroids			
Methylprednisolone	IV	40–80 mg/24 hr	Not indicated
Prednisone	Oral	20–60 mg/day	Not indicated
Hydrocortisone enema	Rectal	100–200 mg/day	Not indicated
Immunomodulators			
Azathioprine	Oral	2.0–3.0 mg/kg/day	2.0–3.0 mg/kg/day
6-Mercaptopurine	Oral	1.0–1.5 mg/kg/day	1.0–1.5 mg/kg/day
Cyclosporine A	IV	4 mg/kg/day	Not indicated
	Oral	10 mg/kg/day	Not indicated
Methotrexate	IM	25 mg/week	Not indicated
	Oral	12.5–25 mg/week	Not indicated
Infliximab	IV	5 mg/kg	Not indicated
Antibiotics			
Metronidazole	Oral	10–20 mg/kg/day	Not indicated

Dosage ranges based on data reported in references 1, 2, 27–33.

Table 25.9 ▪ Efficacy of Drug Therapy Used to Treat Ulcerative Colitis and Crohn's Disease

	Ulcerative Colitis		Crohn's Disease		
Drug	**TX**	**MTN**	**TX**	**MTN**	**Fistula**
Sulfasalazine	++	++	++	–	–
Olsalazine	++	++	++	–	–
Asacol	++	++	++	+	–
Pentasa	++	++	++	+	–
Corticosteroids	++	–	++	–	–
Metronidazole	–	–	++	–	+
Ciprofloxacin	–	–	+	–	+
Azathioprine/6-mercaptopurine[a]	+	+	+	+	+
Cyclosporine A[a]	+	–	+	–	+
Methotrexate[a]	–	–	+	–	–
Infliximab[a]	–	–	+	–	+

TX, active disease; *MTN*, remission maintenance; ++, effective; +, likely to be effective; –, documented efficacy lacking.
[a]Refractory disease.

Table 25.10 ▪ Adverse Effects of Medications Used to Treat Inflammatory Bowel Disease

Sulfasalazine	**Mesalamine (5-aminosalicylic acid)**	**Metronidazole**	**Cyclosporine A**
Dose-dependent	Fever	Dyspepsia	Tremor
Nausea	Skin rash	Metallic taste	Paresthesias
Vomiting	Nausea	Skin rash	Headache
Dyspepsia	Diarrhea	Dark urine	Nausea
Diarrhea	Pancreatitis	Glossitis	Anorexia
Anorexia	Hepatitis	Disulfiramlike reaction	Hypertrichosis
Headache	Nephrotoxicity	Peripheral neuropathy	Gingival hyperplasia
Malaise	Headache	Neutropenia	Nephrotoxicity
Male infertility	Alopecia	Pancreatitis	Hypertension
Dose-independent	**Glucocorticosteroids**	**Azathioprine or 6-mercaptopurine**	**Methotrexate**
Fever	Major	Bone marrow depression	Anorexia
Skin rash	Infection	Nausea	Nausea
Hemolytic anemia	Hypertension	Diarrhea	Vomiting
Agranulocytosis	Psychosis	Fever	Diarrhea
Pulmonary complications	Hypokalemia	Skin rash	Stomatitis
Hepatitis	Hyperglycemia	Infection	Fever
Pancreatitis	Osteoporosis	Arthralgias	Headache
Neurologic toxicity	Cataracts	Pancreatitis	Alopecia
	Glaucoma	Hepatitis	Leukopenia
	Minor	**Infliximab**	Pneumonitis
	Moon face	Upper respiratory tract and other infections	Nephrotoxicity
	Acne	Acute or delayed hypersensitivity reactions	Hepatic fibrosis and cirrhosis
	Hirsutism	Lupus-like reaction	
	Insomnia	Lymphoma?	
	Striae		
	Weight gain		
	Vascular fragility		

The frequency of adverse effects associated with SASP ranges from 20 to 45%.[36] Dose-dependent effects (Table 25.10) tend to correlate with SP concentrations in the blood and may be more common in slow acetylators.[1,32,36] Hemolysis and leukopenia are thought to be related to SP blood concentrations and slow acetylator status. SASP alters sperm morphology, motility, and counts, leading to male infertility. This effect is thought to be highest in slow acetylators but is reversible within several months of discontinuing SASP. Dose-independent adverse effects (Table 25.10) include hypersensitivity reactions typical of the sulfonamides.[1,32,36] Skin rashes occur commonly, and in 2 to 3% of patients the drug must be withdrawn. Hematologic effects include hemolytic anemia and bone marrow suppression. Fever, pulmonary infiltrates, hepatitis, pancreatitis, polyneuritis, agranulocytosis, thrombocytopenia, and a lupuslike syndrome with polyarthritis and vasculitis have been reported.[1,32,36] A desensitization program can be undertaken in which low, incremental, dosages of SASP are increased over a prolonged period of time.

SASP inhibits folic acid absorption and interferes with folate metabolism in the jejunal brush border.[1,32] Some clinicians recommend folic acid supplementation of 1 mg/day with long-term SASP therapy. The interaction between SASP and other highly protein-bound drugs (e.g., warfarin) may lead to displacement of these drugs from their protein binding sites. Concomitant administration of SASP and digoxin may decrease digoxin bioavailability and reduce digoxin serum concentrations. Administering iron and SASP may result in chelation and possibly decreased blood levels of both drugs. The clinical importance of many of these interactions is uncertain.

Newer Oral Aminosalicylates

Several strategies have been used to create SP-free oral dosage forms that deliver higher concentrations of 5-ASA to the distal small bowel and colon, which may be better tolerated.[31,32,36,38–41] Second-generation preparations include azo-bond coupling of 5-ASA with agents other than SP, delayed-release pH-dependent enteric-coated tablets, and sustained-release products (Table 25.7). Oral mesalamine preparations under investigation include balsalazide, Salofalk, and Claversal. A hypersensitivity reaction to 5-ASA occurs in about 10 to 20% of patients (Table 25.10). Therefore, patients allergic to aspirin should not take mesalamine. The potential for nephrotoxicity exists in patients receiving high daily dosages or concomitant 5-ASA-liberating medications and those with preexisting renal disease.

Olsalazine consists of two salicylate molecules linked by a diazo bond (Table 25.7). On a molar basis, olsalazine delivers twice as much 5-ASA to the colon as SASP. Its efficacy in treating active UC and in maintaining remission is similar to that of SASP when equivalent 5-ASA dosages are used.[1,40] However, the higher dosages (1.5 to 3 g/day) are not used because of the greater potential for a dose-dependent secretory diarrhea.[1,31,40] Thus, olsalazine is used primarily for remission maintenance in UC when patients are intolerant of SASP (Tables 25.8, 25.9). Diarrhea also occurs in up to 17% of patients receiving 1 g/day; however, the incidence of diarrhea may be less than previously reported.[40] Patients should be counseled to report any change in stool frequency or volume after initiating therapy with olsalazine.

Asacol, a delayed-release tablet (Table 25.7), contains 400 mg 5-ASA coated with an acrylic resin (Eudragit-S). Upon oral administration, 5-ASA is released in the ileum or colon when the intestinal pH is sufficient (pH greater than 7) to dissolve the enteric coating.[32,36,38,39] Because intestinal pH and motility may vary, Asacol may not provide reliable site-specific release of 5-ASA. In 2 to 3% of patients, intact or partially intact tablets have been found in the stool. Patients should be instructed to observe for intact tablets in the stool. Therapy in UC or CD (Tables 25.8, 25.9) usually is initiated with 2.4 g/day in three divided doses and may be increased to 4.8 g/day, if necessary.[32,36,38,39] Studies in UC demonstrate similar efficacy to SASP when used to treat mild to moderate active disease and in remission maintenance.[36,38,39] Remission maintenance in CD appears to be of most benefit in the postsurgical patient and in patients with ileal involvement.[42] In maintenance therapy, there appears to be greater absorption of 5-ASA from Asacol than from SASP or olsalazine.[43]

Pentasa, a sustained-release dosage form (Table 25.7), contains 250 mg 5-ASA microgranules, which slowly and continuously dissolve in the small intestine and colon. Approximately 20 to 50% of the 5-ASA is released in the small bowel, with the remainder released in the colon.[39,44] In contrast to Asacol, Pentasa's release characteristics are primarily time dependent rather than pH dependent.[39] Patients should be advised that small beads may be left in the stool after the 5-ASA is released. The efficacy of Pentasa (4 g/day in four divided doses) in treating mild to moderate active UC and maintaining remission (2 g/day in two divided doses) has been established.[36,38,39] Clinical trials indicate that Pentasa is also effective in inducing and maintaining remission in mild to moderate CD, regardless of disease location, and after curative surgery for CD.[32,36,38,39,42]

Topical Aminosalicylates

Topical 5-ASA exerts a local antiinflammatory effect and is useful in treating active distal UC.[27,29–31] The 5-ASA rectal enema (4 g/60 mL) is indicated for treating ulcerative proctitis and proctosigmoiditis (Table 25.8). The enema should be administered at bedtime and retained for 8 hours. Improvement usually occurs within a week, but the usual course of therapy is 3 to 6 weeks depending on symptoms and sigmoidoscopic findings. In patients with mild to moderate active UC, the 5-ASA enema is as effective as oral SASP or GCS enema.[29,30,45] Additionally, patients refractory to oral SASP and oral or rectal GCS may respond to rectal 5-ASA alone or combined with oral therapy.[29,30] Rectal suppositories (500 mg twice/day), indicated for distal ulcerative proctitis, should be retained at least 1 to achieve maximum benefit. Lower daily dosages of the enema and the suppository (Table 25.8), as well as alternate-day dosing, are effective in maintaining remission, but the optimal regimen has not been determined.[29,30] Remission maintenance may also be achieved by combining oral 5-ASA and intermittent 5-ASA enemas.[46] Topical 5-ASA should be used only in patients with distal CD.

Topical 5-ASA is associated with fewer adverse effects than oral mesalamine and SASP, presumably because systemic availability is lower.[29,30,45] Less than 15% of the rectally administered 5-ASA dosage is absorbed. Adverse effects occur in 1 to 10% of patients and include headache, flatulence, abdominal pain, diarrhea, dizziness, and fatigue, many of which are indistinguishable from the underlying disease. Anal irritation or a hypersensitivity reaction to 5-ASA or the sulfite contained in the topical suspension may occur. Most patients intolerant of SASP tolerate the 5-ASA enema or suppository. The monthly cost of 5-ASA enemas, as well as patient acceptance and compliance, should be considered when less costly and more convenient treatment alternatives are available.

Glucocorticosteroids

The efficacy of systemic GCSs in treating moderate to severe active UC and CD (Table 25.10) is well established.[1,2,27,28,32] Topical GCSs are effective in treating mild to moderate distal UC.[1,27,29,30] The exact mechanism by which GCSs suppress intestinal inflammation is unknown, but theories include interaction with the immune system, prostaglandin inhibition, lysosomal membrane stabilization, and kinin release blocking.[47] The dosage regimen and route of administration (parenteral, oral, or topical) vary with disease severity and activity (Table 25.8). The potential adverse effects of systemic GCSs limit their long-term use in IBD (Table 25.10).

Continuous or intermittent intravenous GCS (prednisolone-equivalent 60 mg/24 hours in divided doses) induces remission in most patients with moderate to severe active UC.[1,27] Although few studies have assessed the relative value of the available GCS and specific dosing regimens, methylprednisolone 40 to 80 mg/24 hours often is preferred in the very ill patient. Higher GCS dosages or pulsed intravenous methylprednisolone therapy (1 g/24 hours) appears to be no more effective than conventional intravenous regimens.[1,48] Intravenous GCS treatment is superior to adrenocorticotropic hormone (ACTH) because it does not depend on adrenal responsiveness. However, parenteral ACTH (120 U/24 hours) may be used in patients with new-onset UC or those who have not received recent GCS therapy. ACTH is rarely used in the United States to treat severe IBD.[1,27]

Most patients with mild to moderate active UC respond favorably to oral GCSs, with improvement or remission occurring in several weeks.[1,27] In an attempt to mimic the natural diurnal rhythm of GCS secretion and to minimize adverse effects, a single morning dose or alternate-day dosing often is advocated. For most patients, a single morning GCS dose is as effective as a divided daily dosage.

However, some patients may respond best when the dosage is divided. The GCS should be taken as a single morning dose or the largest portion of the dosage should be taken in the morning. Because a decrease in adverse effects often parallels a diminution in therapeutic effect, alternate-day therapy is not recommend for patients with IBD. Alternatively, growth-stunted children who need maintenance GCS may benefit from this regimen.

Patients with mild active distal UC often respond to rectal instillation of GCS.[1,27,29,30] Although topical administration results in up to 50% of the GCS being absorbed, the degrees of adrenal suppression and adverse effects are less than that observed with the equivalent oral dosage of the same drug. The volume and composition of the fluid vehicle, the GCS dosage, and the dwell time contribute to variations in systemic absorption. Whether acute intestinal inflammation alters drug absorption is unclear. Retention enemas should be administered at bedtime to permit overnight contact with the inflamed mucosa. An additional dose may be given in the morning after the first bowel movement. Once remission occurs, usually within 2 to 3 weeks, an alternate-night schedule may be used for an additional 2 weeks. Patients should be instructed to instill the enema in the supine position and then change to the left, right, and prone positions for at least 20 minutes each to facilitate maximal topical coverage. An enema may spread as far proximally as the hepatic flexure, but their use should be limited to left-sided colitis or proctosigmoiditis. Rectal foams are useful in patients unable to retain an enema because of local inflammation, tenesmus, or diarrhea. However, foams usually do not spread beyond the sigmoid colon. Although convenient, they should be used only in patients with disease confined to the sigmoid or rectum.

The use of GCS to treat CD is similar to that described for UC, although the results are not always as dramatic and remission is more difficult to achieve.[2,28,32] Patients with ileal or ileocolonic disease respond more favorably to GCS than those with colonic CD. GCS enemas may be effective in patients with left-sided colitis. Although this treatment is not supported in the literature, some clinicians maintain patients with CD on a minimum GCS dosage for about 1 to 2 months before beginning the steroid taper. Continuing GCS therapy after remission induction usually does not alter the frequency of recurrence or the frequency of relapse after surgery.[2,28,32] Older patients with CD receiving GCS are at increased risk of developing hypertension, hypokalemia, and mental status changes.[49] GCS should be used with caution in patients with fistula, abscess, or malnutrition because of the increased risk of infection and the potential for fluid and electrolyte disturbances.

Immunomodulators

Azathioprine and 6-Mercaptopurine

AZA or 6-MP is effective (Table 25.9) in treating refractory UC and CD, fistulizing CD, and steroid-dependent UC and CD and maintaining UC and CD remission.[14,27,28,31–33,50–54] AZA is metabolized to 6-MP and subsequently converted to inactive 6-thiouric acid by xanthine oxidase. The specific mechanism by which AZA and 6-MP act in IBD is uncertain but probably is related to their ability to inhibit nucleotide biosynthesis and purine nucleotide interconversion.[50–52] The effect of 6-MP on T-cells and its antiinflammatory effect may contribute to its efficacy in IBD. AZA and 6-MP have similar therapeutic and toxic effects.

Controlled trials of AZA (1.0 to 3.0 mg/kg/day) or 6-MP (1.5 mg/kg/day) support their efficacy (Tables 25.8, 25.9) as single agents and in conjunction with GCS to reduce the steroid dosage.[50–53] The typical AZA or 6-MP starting dosage is 0.5 to 1.5 mg/kg/day. A lower dosage (50 mg/day) of 6-MP may be associated with minimal hematologic toxicity.[54] The daily dosage should be reduced by at least 50% in patients receiving allopurinol. The response to AZA or 6-MP takes 3 to 6 months or longer.[50–53] It is possible that an intravenous loading dose of AZA (20 to 44 mg/kg over 36 hours) decreases the time to response.[52] When either drug is continued after the GCS is withdrawn, remission usually is sustained. Unfortunately, there is a high relapse rate when these agents are tapered or withdrawn.[50–53] AZA and 6-MP also are effective in relieving some extraintestinal manifestations and in healing fistulas.[14,52]

The long-term use of AZA and 6-MP has been associated with toxic effects (Table 25.10). However, a lower incidence of adverse effects has been observed with lower daily dosages.[52–54] Because of the potential for bone marrow suppression, blood counts must be monitored regularly, especially when therapy is initiated. Drug fever and arthralgias often occur within weeks of treatment initiation. Despite an improved safety profile, patients on long-term AZA or 6-MP should be monitored closely for signs of infection, pancreatitis, and hepatitis. A theoretical risk of developing neoplasia, particularly non-Hodgkin's lymphoma, exists after long-term treatment with AZA or 6-MP, but this increased risk has not been confirmed in patients with IBD.[55]

Cyclosporine A

Cyclosporine A (CYA), a potent inhibitor of cell-mediated immunity, may be effective (Table 25.9) in severe UC or CD refractory to GCS therapy and fistulizing CD.[14,32,50,51,56–58] CYA exerts its immunosuppressant activity by inhibiting T-cell production of cytokines including IL-2, IL-3, IL-4, and IFN-γ.[50,56] A number of trials have been conducted in patients with UC and CD using intravenous, oral, or topical dosage forms.[50,51,56–58] Results indicate that in CD, low-dose CYA (5 mg/kg/day orally or less) is not effective for treating active disease or maintaining remission. Higher dosages (4 mg/kg/day intravenous or 10 mg/kg/day oral) may be effective for severe active UC, CD, and fistulizing CD (Table 25.8). CYA enemas (5 mg/kg/day or less) for left-sided colitis are not effective. When CYA is used to treat active disease, improvement usually is observed within several weeks, but relapse occurs when the drug is withdrawn.

The use of CYA must be weighed against the risk of irreversible nephropathy and other serious adverse effects (Table 25.10). In most cases, the adverse effects are dose dependent. Paresthesias, hypertension, and renal insufficiency occur in 26%, 11%, and 6% of patients, respectively.[50] Severe infections may complicate CYA therapy, especially if the patient is on concomitant GCS. The usual starting dosage is 2 to 4 mg/kg/day intravenously or 8 mg/kg/day orally.[50,56] Maintaining an adequate blood level with oral CYA in patients with CD often is difficult because of inflammation or resection of the small bowel. There is a strong correlation between clinical response and whole blood concentrations in IBD when comparing high-dose (whole blood CYA concentration greater than 400 ng/mL) with low-dose (whole blood CYA concentration less than 200 ng/mL) therapy.[56] It is unclear whether the relationship between clinical response and whole blood CYA concentration between 200 and 400 ng/mL is linear or whether there is a threshold for clinical response. Patients receiving CYA should be monitored for drug interactions with other medications that interact with hepatic cytochrome P-4503A4.

Methotrexate

MTX, a folic acid antagonist, is under investigation for treating severe refractory IBD.[14,32,50,59] MTX exerts its effect on proliferating cells while sparing resting cells. Among its numerous effects, MTX inhibits purine synthesis and decreases LTB4 and IL-1 production.[50] When given weekly as an oral or intramuscular injection (Tables 25.8, 25.9), MTX improves symptoms and reduces the GCS needs in patients with severe active CD and UC.[59] However, relapses occur when the drug is withdrawn. Of major concern are the teratogenic and toxic effects, which limit its usefulness (Table 25.10).

Infliximab

Infliximab, a chimeric monoclonal antibody to TNF-α (anti–TNF-α), is a new treatment option for patients with moderate to severe or fistulizing CD resistant to other treatments.[14,15,60,61] Its exact mechanism of action is unknown, but it appears to confirm the central role of TNF-α in the inflammatory process. A single intravenous infusion (Table 25.8) achieves remission within 4 weeks (in about two-thirds of patients with CD), lasts for about 4 to 6 months, and is well tolerated.[61] In patients with fistula, the infusion can be repeated at 2 and 6 weeks. Because TNF is a mediator of inflammation and the cellular immune response, the potential for infections and malignancies remains a concern. Maintenance regimens are under investigation.

Antibiotics

Antibiotic or antibiotic combinations do not alter the long-term course of IBD.[14,27,32,62,63] Preliminary reports of benefit in UC have not been confirmed.[14,63] Although MTZ and ciprofloxacin are effective in CD,[14,62] limited data support the use of other antibiotics.

Metronidazole

MTZ is beneficial in treating mild to moderate active colonic or fistulizing CD (Table 25.9) but is less effective in patients with CD and ileal disease or active UC.[2,14,28,32] The mode by which MTZ acts in IBD is unclear but is probably related to its immunosuppressive and antibacterial properties. Effective dosages range from 10 to 20 mg/kg/day (Table 25.8), and response to treatment usually takes several months. Higher dosages may be needed in patients with fistula or perineal disease. Most patients with mild to moderate Crohn's colitis or ileocolitis usually respond to 250 mg MTZ four times daily. Dosage reduction or discontinuation often is associated with worsening disease. The use of MTZ to maintain remission of CD is not well studied, but it may be effective in preventing recurrence after ileal resection.[2,32,37] Numerous adverse effects have been reported with short-term use of MTZ (Table 25.10). Peripheral neuropathy occurs in up to 50% of patients and appears to be dose dependent.[2,32] Although MTZ has not been proven to be mutagenic, teratogenic, or carcinogenic in humans, its long-term safety remains in question. MTZ should be discontinued after several months if it is ineffective or tapered after 3 to 4 months.

Nonpharmacologic Therapy

Nutrition

Replacement of vitamins, minerals, and other nutrients is indicated whenever there is clinical or laboratory evidence of deficiency.[64,65] Iron, folic acid, and B_{12} deficiencies should be identified and treated appropriately. Because oral iron may aggravate IBD, it may be preferable to give the iron parenterally or as a blood transfusion. Fat malabsorption in patients with CD may contribute to malabsorption of vitamins A, D, and K; replacing these vitamins may be necessary. Patients with CD involving the small intestine may present with deficiencies of calcium, magnesium, B complex vitamins, and vitamin C. Lactose-intolerant patients should avoid dairy products or use lactase-containing preparations. Patients should be instructed to limit *only* the foods that consistently and reliably produce symptoms.

The use of enteral or parenteral nutrition as adjunct therapy in IBD to restore a balanced nutritional state is well established.[64,65] Indications for supplemental parenteral nutrition in IBD include short bowel syndrome, high output stomas or fistulas, and perioperative support of the severely malnourished patient. The efficacy of nutritional support as primary therapy in IBD patients is not well established. Although parenteral nutrition is considered a valuable adjunct to therapy in both severe UC and CD, there is little evidence that the overall course of either of these diseases is altered by bowel rest and nutrition. Thus, parenteral nutrition should be used to improve the nutritional status of severely ill patients with IBD who cannot be fed enterally and in selected patients with CD in whom bowel rest may be of value.

Surgery

Surgery is indicated after medical management fails or for actual or impending complications. The decision to operate must be weighed against the disabilities of the disease and the adverse effects of long-term drug therapy. A colectomy is curative in UC and may rid the patient of systemic complications. Indications for surgery in UC include medical therapy failure, toxic megacolon, colonic perforation or hemorrhage, anal complications, and the risk of developing colon cancer.[1] Although a prophylactic colectomy has been recommended for children and adults with long-standing pancolitis, the most reasonable approach is periodic colonoscopy and histologic examination of biopsies for precancerous changes. Total proctocolectomy with a permanent ileostomy is the procedure of choice. Postoperative mortality is 3% in elective colectomy, 10 to 15% in patients undergoing emergency surgery for severe active disease, and 50% in those who have had colonic perforation.

Surgery in CD is influenced by the site of involvement and the fact that it is not curative. Indications include medical management failure, intestinal obstruction, strictures, fistulas, abscess formation, perforation, and hemorrhage.[2] Approximately 60% of patients need surgery within 10 years of initial symptoms, with the rate of recurrence after intestinal resection reported to be as high as 75% after 15 years.[3] Because of the high recurrence rate after resection, conservative intestinal resection of diseased bowel with primary bowel anastomosis usually is the procedure of choice. Increasing losses of the small bowel through resection and disease may eventually limit its absorptive surface and result in malabsorption and malnutrition.

FUTURE THERAPIES

A better understanding of the immune and inflammatory cascades in the pathogenesis of IBD has led to the development of novel treatment modalities.[14,47,66–72] Studies with agents that inhibit 5-lipoxygenase and prevent leukotriene synthesis (e.g., Zileuton) and members of the ω3 fatty acid family may be effective in treating UC.[66] Adding transdermal nicotine to conventional therapy appears to improve symptoms in patients with active UC, but does not appear to be effective in maintaining remission.[38,68,69] A limited number of studies have been conducted using clonidine, sucralfate, lidocaine, sodium cromoglycate, short-chain fatty acids (butyrate), heparin, and bismuth salts.[66,67] The efficacy and safety of these agents have not been established and their role in treating IBD is unknown.

The GCS are unsurpassed in treating IBD, but their beneficial effects often are offset by troublesome adverse effects. New approaches to this problem include using prodrug conjugates in which conventional GCSs are linked to inert molecules such as dextran and then detached by bacterial enzymes in the distal bowel, using delayed- or sustained-release enteric coatings, and identifying GCSs that have high tissue uptake and affinity for GCS receptors as well as rapid and extensive biotransformation in the liver. Among the new GCSs, tixocortol pivalate, fluticasone propionate, and budesonide are the principal contenders for use in IBD.[70–72] Of these, budesonide has emerged as the most promising. An oral dosage form appears to be efficacious in active ileocolonic CD, causing less suppression of endogenous plasma cortisol levels and fewer adverse effects than oral prednisolone.[70,71] The efficacy of budesonide enema is similar to that of conventional GCSs when used to treat active UC but does not appear to have appreciable effects on adrenal gland function.[70,72]

A number of novel biologicals and newer immunomodulators are emerging for treatment of CD.[14,15,67] Biological agents–including humanized IGg4 anti-TNF–α, anti–α4 integrin antibody, recombinant human IL-10, IL-11, and antisense oligonucleotide–are currently under investigation. Early reports with tacrolimus, mycophenolate mofetil, and thalidomide suggest that they may be of benefit. Reactive oxygen species, neuropeptide modulators, and proinflammatory cytokine antagonists offer intriguing approaches to treatment.

IMPROVING OUTCOMES

Patients with IBD should be educated about their disease and drug therapy. In addition, patients should be counseled to stop smoking and to avoid the use of NSAIDs. Adequate nutrition and psychosocial information should be incorporated into the patient's daily care plan. Adherence to drug therapy and, in some cases, surgery should improve the patient's overall health. Quality-of-life parameters, including social activities, work, recreation, ability to sleep, sexual relationships, and indoor and outdoor activities should also be evaluated in order to ensure improvement in patient outcomes.[9,73,74]

PHARMACOECONOMICS

The economic impact of IBD and issues that affect the cost-effectiveness of medical management are reviewed elsewhere.[74] The efficacy and safety of the newer oral 5-ASA formulations has been compared to SASP for treating UC.[75] Although this meta-analysis suggests that the newer oral 5-ASA products may be slightly better than SASP for inducing remission, the 5-ASA preparations were not superior to SASP for remission maintenance. There were significantly more patients with adverse effects to SASP than 5-ASA in patients with active disease, but this difference was not found in the patients receiving maintenance therapy. Because the newer 5-ASA formulations are three or four times more expensive than SASP, the 5-ASA products should be reserved for SASP-intolerant patients and men concerned about fertility. Alternatively, the newer 5-ASA formulations may be more cost-effective in treating ileal CD and maintaining remission.

KEY POINTS

- The goal of medical therapy in IBD is to induce and maintain remission, control symptoms, and prevent or control complications.
- Drug selection, dosage, and route of administration are determined by the location, extent, and severity of intestinal involvement.
- Maintaining adequate nutrition is an important goal in patients with IBD, especially when there is extensive intestinal involvement or bowel resection.
- Psychosocial factors are an important component of IBD treatment and should be included in the daily care plan.
- Antidiarrheals are contraindicated in severe IBD because they may precipitate toxic megacolon.
- Because the newer oral 5-ASA formulations are more expensive than SASP, they should be reserved for SASP-intolerant patients with UC and men concerned about fertility.
- The newer oral 5-ASA formulations are more effective than SASP for treating CD patients with ileal involvement and in maintaining remission.
- Patients with severe IBD should be treated with intravenous GCSs. Failure to improve after 10 days signals the need for surgery or intravenous immunomodulator therapy.
- MTZ is most beneficial in treating patients with mild to moderate active colonic or fistulizing CD.
- The use of AZA or 6-MP should be limited to treating refractory UC and CD, fistulizing CD, and steroid-dependent UC and CD.
- CYA should be used only as rescue therapy as a bridge to other agents (e.g., AZA or 6-MP), which take longer to act.
- Parenteral nutrition should be used to improve the nutritional status of severely ill patients with IBD who cannot be fed enterally and in selected patients with CD in whom bowel rest may be of value.
- A colectomy is curative in UC and may rid the patient of systemic complications.
- Surgery in CD is not curative and is influenced by response to drug therapy and impending complications.
- Educating patients and improving quality-of-life parameters contribute to improvement in IBD patient outcomes.

REFERENCES

1. Jewell DP. Ulcerative colitis. In: Feldman M, Scharschmidt BF, Sleisenger MH, eds. Sleisenger & Fordtran's gastrointestinal and liver disease: pathophysiology/diagnosis/management. 6th ed. Philadelphia: WB Saunders, 1998:1735.
2. Kornbluth A, Sachar DB, Saloman P. Crohn's disease. In: Feldman M, Scharschmidt BF, Sleisenger MH, eds. Sleisenger & Fordtran's gastrointestinal and liver disease: pathophysiology/diagnosis/management. 6th ed. Philadelphia: WB Saunders, 1998:1708.
3. Andres PG, Friedman LS. Epidemiology and the natural course of inflammatory bowel disease. Gastroenterol Clin North Am 28:225–281, 1999.
4. Miner PB. Factors influencing the relapse of patients with inflammatory bowel disease. Am J Gastroenterol 92(Suppl):1S–4S, 1997.
5. Thomas GAO, Rhodes J, Green JT. Inflammatory bowel disease and smoking: a review. Am J Gastroenterol 93:144–149, 1998.
6. Faucheron JL. Toxicity of non-steroidal anti-inflammatory drugs in the large bowel. Eur J Gastroenterol Hepatology 11:389–392, 1999.
7. Sartor RB. Pathogenesis and immune mechanisms of chronic inflammatory bowel disease. 92(Suppl):3S–11S, 1997.
8. Ferry GD. Quality of life in inflammatory bowel disease: background and definitions. J Ped Gastroenterol Nutrition 28(Suppl):S15–S18, 1999.
9. Irvine EF. Quality of life issues in patients with inflammatory bowel disease. Am J Gastroenterol 92(Suppl):18S–24S, 1997.
10. Sartor RB. Review article: role of the enteric microflora in the pathogenesis of intestinal inflammation and arthritis. Aliment Pharmacol Ther 11(Suppl 3):17–23, 1997.
11. Van Dullemen H, Meenan J, Stronkhorst, et al. Mediators of mucosal inflammation: implications for therapy. Scand J Gastroenterol 32(Suppl 223):92–98, 1997.
12. Rogler G, Andus T. Cytokines in inflammatory bowel disease. World J Surg 22:382–389, 1998.
13. Papadakis KA, Targan SR. Current theories on the causes of inflammatory bowel disease. Gastroenterol Clin North Am 28:283–296, 1999.
14. Sands BE. Therapy of inflammatory bowel disease. Gastroenterology 119(Suppl):S68–S82, 2000.
15. Sandborn WJ, Hanauer SB. Antitumor necrosis factor therapy for inflammatory bowel disease: a review of agents, pharmacology, clinical results, and safety. Inflamm Bowel Dis 5:119–133, 1999.
16. Das KM. Relationship of extraintestinal involvements in inflammatory bowel disease: new insights into autoimmune pathogenesis. Dig Dis Sci 44:1–13, 1999.
17. Connell WR. Safety of drug therapy for inflammatory bowel disease in pregnant and nursing women. Inflamm Bowel Dis 2:33–47, 1996.
18. Connell W, Miller A. Treating inflammatory bowel disease during pregnancy: risks and safety of drug therapy. Drug Safety 21:311–323, 1999.
19. Diav-Citrin O, Park YH, Veerasuntharam G, et al. The safety of mesalamine in human pregnancy: a prospective controlled cohort study. Gastroenterology 114:23–28, 1998.
20. Bell CM, Habal FM. Safety of topical 5-aminosalicylic acid in pregnancy. Am J Gastroenterol 92:2201–2202, 1997.
21. Winter HS, Ng S. Consensus conference on the evaluation of drugs to treat children with inflammatory bowel disease. Inflamm Bowel Dis 4:101–131, 1998.
22. Winter HS, Grand RJ. Medical therapy for children with inflammatory bowel disease. Inflamm Bowel Dis 2:269–275, 1996.
23. Kam L. Ulcerative colitis in young adults: complexities of diagnosis and management. Postgrad Med 103:45–59, 1998.
24. Baldassano RN, Piccoli DA. Inflammatory bowel disease in pediatric and adolescent patients. Gastroenterol Clin North Am 28:445–458, 1999.
25. D'Agata ID, Vanounou T, Seidman E. Mesalamine in pediatric inflammatory bowel disease: a 10 year experience. Inflamm Bowel Dis 2:229–235, 1996.
26. Drossman DA. Psychosocial factors in gastrointestinal disorders. In: Feldman M, Scharschmidt BF, Sleisenger MH, eds. Sleisenger & Fordtran's gastrointestinal and liver disease: pathophysiology/diagnosis/management. 6th ed. Philadelphia: WB Saunders, 1998:69.
27. Kornbluth A, Sachar DB. Ulcerative colitis practice guidelines in adults. Am J Gastroenterol 92:204–211, 1997.
28. Hanauer SB, Meyers S. Practice guidelines: management of Crohn's disease in adults. Am J Gastroenterol 92:559–566, 1997.
29. Michetti P, Peppercorn MA. Medical therapy of specific clinical presentations. Gastroenterol Clin North Am 28:371–390, 1999.
30. Ardizzone S, Bianchi Porro G. A practical guide to the management of distal ulcerative colitis. Drugs 55:519–542, 1998.
31. Stein RB, Hanauer SB. Medical therapy for inflammatory bowel diseases. Gastroenterol Clin North Am 28:297–321, 1999.

32. Elton E, Hanauer SB. Review article: the medical management of Crohn's disease. Aliment Pharmacol Ther 10:1–22, 1996.
33. Steinhart AH, McLeod RS. Medical and surgical management of perianal Crohn's disease. Inflamm Bowel Dis 2:200–210, 1996.
34. Barrett KE, Dharmsathaphorn K. Pharmacological aspects of therapy in inflammatory bowel diseases: antidiarrheal agents. J Clin Gastroenterol 10:57–63, 1988.
35. Kaplan MA, Korelitz BI. Narcotic dependence in inflammatory bowel disease. J Clin Gastroenterol 10:275–278, 1988.
36. Goldenberg MM. Critical drug appraisal: mesalamine in the treatment of inflammatory bowel disease. P & T (October):498–512, 1997.
37. Tremaine WJ. Maintenance therapy in inflammatory bowel disease. Inflamm Bowel Dis 4:292–301, 1998.
38. Bonapace CR, Mays DA. The effect of mesalamine and nicotine in the treatment of inflammatory bowel disease. Ann Pharmacother 31:907–913, 1997.
39. Small RE, Schraa CC. Chemistry, pharmacology, pharmacokinetics, and clinical applications of mesalamine for the treatment of inflammatory bowel disease. Pharmacotherapy 14:385–398, 1994.
40. Wadworth AN, Fitton A. Olsalazine: a review of its pharmacodynamic and pharmacokinetic properties, and therapeutic potential in inflammatory bowel disease. Drugs 41:647–664, 1991.
41. Prakash A, Spencer CM. Balsalazide. Drugs 56:83–89, 1998.
42. Camma C, Giunta M, Rosselli M, et al. Mesalamine in the maintenance treatment of Crohn's disease: a meta-analysis adjusted for confounding variables. Gastroenterology 113:1465–1473, 1997.
43. Stretch GL, Campbell BJ, Dwarakanath AD, et al. 5-Aminosalicylic acid absorption and metabolism in ulcerative colitis patients receiving maintenance sulphasalazine, olsalazine, or mesalazine. Aliment Pharmacol Ther 10:941–947, 1996.
44. Layer PH, Goebell H, Keller J, et al. Delivery and fate of oral mesalamine microgranules within the human small intestine. Gastroenterology 108:1427–1433, 1995.
45. Kam L, Cohen H, Dooley C, et al. A comparison of mesalamine suspension enema and oral sulfasalazine for treatment of active distal ulcerative colitis in adults. Am J Gastroenterol 91:1338–1342, 1996.
46. d'Albasio G, Pacini F, Camarri E, et al. Combined therapy with 5-aminosalicylic acid tablets and enemas for maintaining remission in ulcerative colitis: a randomized double-blind study. Am J Gastroenterol 92:1143–1147, 1997.
47. Thiesen A, Thomson ABR. Review article: older systemic and newer topical glucocorticosteroids and the gastrointestinal tract. Aliment Pharmacol Ther 10:487–496, 1996.
48. Rosenberg W, Ireland A, Jewell DP. High-dose methylprednisolone in the treatment of acute ulcerative colitis. J Clin Gastroenterol 12:40–41, 1990.
49. Akerkar GA, Peppercorn MA, Hamel MB, et al. Corticosteroid-associated complications in elderly Crohn's disease patients. Am J Gastroenterol 92:461–464, 1997.
50. Sandborn WJ. A review of immune modifier therapy for inflammatory bowel disease: azathioprine, 6-mercaptopurine, cyclosporine, and methotrexate. Am J Gastroenterol 91:423–433,1996.
51. Scholmerich J. Immunosuppressive therapy for chronic inflammatory bowel disease. Digestion 58(Suppl 1):94–97, 1997.
52. Sandborn WJ. Azathioprine: state of the art in inflammatory bowel disease. Scand J Gastroenterol 33(Suppl 225):92–99, 1998.
53. Pearson DC, May GR, Fick GH, et al. Azathioprine and 6-mercaptopurine in Crohn's disease: a meta-analysis. Ann Intern Med 122:132–142, 1995.
54. Bernstein CN, Artinian L, Anton PA, et al. Low-dose 6-mercaptopurine inflammatory bowel disease is associated with minimal hematologic toxicity. Dig Dis Sci 39:1638–1641, 1994.
55. Connell WR, Kamm MA, Dickson M, et al. Long-term neoplasia risk after azathioprine treatment in inflammatory bowel disease. Lancet 343:1249–1252, 1994.
56. Sandborn WJ. A critical review of cyclosporine therapy in inflammatory bowel disease. Inflamm Bowel Dis 1:48–63, 1995.
57. Lichtiger S, Present DH, Dornbluth A, et al. Cyclosporine in severe ulcerative colitis refractory to steroid therapy. N Engl J Med 330:1841–1845, 1994.
58. Santos J, Baudet S, Casellas F, et al. Efficacy of intravenous cyclosporine for steroid refractory attacks of ulcerative colitis. J Clin Gastroenterol 20:285–289, 1995.
59. Feagan BD. Methotrexate treatment of Crohn's disease. Inflamm Bowel Dis 4:120–121, 1998.
60. Wall GC, Heyneman C, Pfanner TP. Medical options for treating Crohn's disease in adults: focus on antitumor necrosis factor–α-chimeric monoclonal antibody. Pharmacotherapy 19:1138–1152, 1999.
61. Targan SR, Hanauer SR, van Deventer SJH, et al. A short-term study of chimeric monoclonal antibody cA2 tumor necrosis factor-α for Crohn's disease. N Engl J Med 337:1029–1035, 1997.
62. Colombel JF, Lemann M, Cassagnou M et al. A controlled trial comparing ciprofloxacin with mesalazine for the treatment of active Crohn's disease. Am J Gastroenterol 94:674–678, 1999.
63. Mantzaris GJ, Archavilis E, Christoforidis P, et al. A prospective randomized controlled trial of oral ciprofloxacin in acute ulcerative colitis. Am J Gastroenterol 92:454–460, 1997.
64. O'Sullivan MA, O'Morain CA. Nutritional therapy in Crohn's disease. Inflamm Bowel Dis 4:45–53, 1998.
65. Han PD, Burke A. Baldassano RN, et al. Nutrition and inflammatory bowel disease. Gastroenterol Clin North Am 28:423–443, 1999.
66. Rhodes J, Thomas G, Evans BK. Inflammatory bowel disease: some thoughts on future drug developments. Drugs 53:189–194, 1997.
67. Sands BE. Novel therapies for inflammatory bowel disease. Gastroenterol Clin North Am 28:323–351, 1999.
68. Pullan RD, Rhodes J, Ganesh S, et al. Transdermal nicotine for active ulcerative colitis. N Engl J Med 330:811–815, 1995.
69. Thomas GAO, Rhodes J, Mani V, et al. Transdermal nicotine as maintenance therapy for ulcerative colitis. N Engl J Med 332:988–992, 1995.
70. Spencer CM, McTavish D. Budesonide: a review of its pharmacological properties and therapeutic efficacy in inflammatory bowed disease. Drugs 50:854–872, 1995.
71. Thomsen O, Cortot A, Jewell D, et al. A comparison of budesonide and mesalamine for active Crohn's disease. N Engl J Med 339:370–374, 1998.
72. Lofberg R. New steroids for inflammatory bowel disease. Inflamm Bowel Dis 1:135–141, 1995.
73. Feagan BG. Review article: economic issues in Crohn's disease–assessing the effects of new treatments on health-related quality of life. Aliment Pharmacol Ther 13(Suppl 4):29–37, 1999.
74. Ward FM, Bodger K, Daly MJ, et al. Clinical economics review: medical management of inflammatory bowel disease. Aliment Pharmacol Ther 13:15–25, 1999.
75. Sutherland LR, Roth DE, Beck PL. Alternatives to sulfasalazine: a meta-analysis of 5-ASA in the treatment of ulcerative colitis. Inflamm Bowel Dis 3:65–78, 1997.

CHAPTER 26

NAUSEA AND VOMITING

Bruce D. Clayton and Carla B. Frye

DEFINITION

Nausea is the unpleasant sensation of the awareness of the urge to vomit. It is often preceded or accompanied by a variety of autonomic signs such as pallor, sweating, tachycardia, salivation, and increased respiratory rate.

Vomiting is the reflex expulsion of the stomach contents via the esophagus and mouth, usually associated with nausea and retching. Nausea and retching can occur without expulsion, and occasionally expulsion occurs without prior nausea and retching. This is known as projectile vomiting.

Retching is the involuntary but unsuccessful effort to vomit. It involves mainly the respiratory muscles of the abdomen, diaphragm, and chest and often is accompanied by bradycardia.

TREATMENT GOALS: NAUSEA AND VOMITING

- Review the cost-effectiveness of medications used regularly in a particular practice setting or diagnosis.
- Analyze the usage patterns, efficacy, and pharmacoeconomics of medications used.
- Develop treatment protocols for the practice setting based on outcomes and cost-effectiveness.
- Treat the cause of nausea and vomiting, if this can be identified.
- Assess the contribution of concurrent diseases to the occurrence of nausea and vomiting.
- Assess for fluid and electrolyte loss.
- Individualize appropriate symptomatic drug treatment after considering contraindications and adverse drug effects.
- For patients undergoing clinical events in which nausea and vomiting are likely to occur (i.e., chemotherapy, surgery, motion sickness), maintain adequate hydration; recommend that the patient eat small, light meals, avoiding sweet, greasy, or spicy foods; premedicate with an antiemetic regimen specific for the patient and the chemotherapy to be administered; ensure that the patient has adequate knowledge of nonpharmacologic preventive measures; and educate the patient about the risks and benefits of the medications that will be used.

PATHOPHYSIOLOGY

The vomiting reflex is found in many species and probably evolved as a protective mechanism to limit the effects of ingested toxic materials.[1] In humans, the tendency to experience nausea and vomiting varies greatly. Causes of nausea and vomiting are listed in Table 26.1.

The principal anatomic elements involved in vomiting are shown diagrammatically in Figure 26.1. Coordination of the vomiting reflex occurs in the vomiting center (VC), located in the lateral reticular formation of the medulla. Afferent fibers from sensory receptors in the pharynx, stomach, intestines, and other viscera connect directly with the VC through the vagus and splanchnic nerves and produce vomiting when stimulated. The center also responds to stimuli originating in other tissues, such as the cerebral cortex, vestibular apparatus of the inner ear, and blood. These so-called central stimuli are believed to travel first to the chemoreceptor trigger zone (CTZ), which then activates the VC to induce vomiting. The CTZ is located in the medullary region known as the area postrema, located on the caudal margin of the fourth ventricle. An important function of the CTZ is to sample blood and spinal fluid for potentially toxic substances and, when detected, to initiate the vomiting reflex. It is therefore appropriate that the CTZ is located in the area postrema, a region of the brain that is not protected by the blood–brain barrier. The CTZ cannot initiate emesis independently but only by stimulating the VC.[2] Both the VC and the CTZ are bilateral and are much smaller than shown in Figure 26.1.

Table 26.1 ▪ Causes of Vomiting

Ingestion of certain substances present in food and the environment	Renal diseases such as renal failure, pyelonephritis, uremia, and uremic colic
Ingestion of certain drugs, particularly opiates, general anesthetics, and antineoplastic drugs	Metabolic and endocrine disorders and conditions such as diabetic ketoacidosis, hyperparathyroidism, adrenal insufficiency, and pregnancy
Motion or other effects on the vestibular apparatus	Gynecologic disorders such as pelvic inflammation and complications or pregnancy
Infection (part of the prodrome of many infections)	Normal pregnancy
Respiratory problems such as violent coughing	Neurologic disorders such as increased cranial pressure, hemorrhage, epilepsy, meningitis, migraine, vertigo, Ménière's syndrome, and brain metastases
Cardiovascular disease such as infarction	Psychiatric disorders including bulimia, rumination, and anorexia nervosa
Disorders of the gastrointestinal tract:	Drug withdrawal syndromes
Gastrointestinal tract obstruction	Radiation therapy
Mucosal lesions such as ulcers, inflammation, and atrophy	
Liver disease	
Pancreatic and small intestinal diseases	
Diseases of the components of the gut wall (collagen, smooth muscle, nerve)	
Peritonitis	

The higher centers of the brain can be a source of stimulus or inhibition of the VC (Fig. 26.1). Vomiting can occur as a conditioned response (e.g., the pretreatment nausea that occurs in some patients about to receive a course of anticancer chemotherapy) or as a reaction to unpleasant sights and smells. The cerebrum can greatly modify the vomiting response to stimuli from other sources such as visceral or vestibular nerve pathways, enhancing or repressing vomiting. The large placebo response seen in many trials of antiemetics can be explained in these terms, as can repression of motion sickness by the patient's concentration on some mental activity. Psychological factors can thus play an important role in nausea and vomiting, although they are usually outweighed by physical factors.

Anatomically, the VC is well placed to coordinate the various efferent functions associated with vomiting (Fig. 26.1). When the VC is stimulated, efferent impulses are sent to the salivary, vasomotor, and respiratory centers and to cranial nerves VIII and X. The vomiting reflex begins with a sudden deep inspiration that increases abdominal pressure (Fig. 26.2), which is further increased by contraction of the abdominal muscles. The soft palate rises and the epiglottis closes, thus preventing the aspiration of vomitus into the lungs. The pyloric sphincter contracts and the cardiac sphincter and esophagus relax, allowing stomach contents to be expelled. The flow of saliva increases to aid the expulsion.[3]

Drugs that exert an emetic effect by acting on the CTZ include apomorphine, cardiac glycosides, morphine, the ergot alkaloids, anesthetics, and many antineoplastic agents. There is considerable interspecies difference in the sensitivity of the CTZ to emetic drugs as well as great variation in the extent to which emesis is stimulated by other routes, such as stimulation of the sensory receptors of the viscera. Apomorphine is the only drug that produces vomiting solely by direct action on the CTZ in all species. The complexity of the pharmacology of emetic drugs is illustrated by morphine, which can act on the CTZ directly or indirectly via the vestibular afferent system. It can also antagonize the emetic action of other drugs by direct depression of the VC.

The neurochemical control of vomiting is not completely understood, but four neurotransmitter systems appear to play significant roles in mediating the emetic response: dopaminergic, histaminic, cholinergic, and 5-hydroxytryptamine$_3$ (5-HT$_3$). Dopamine receptors are found in both the CTZ and the gastrointestinal (GI) tract. Dopamine agonists, such as apomorphine and levodopa, produce emesis by acting on the CTZ and peripheral dopamine receptors that stimulate the CTZ, whereas dopamine antagonists, such as the phenothiazines and metoclopramide, block emesis. Histamine (H_1 and H_2) receptors also are found in the CTZ, but histamine receptor blockade results in antiemetic activity limited to vestibular causes. The neurotransmitters involved in motion sickness are better understood. The sensory disorientation that occurs in motion sickness results in an imbalance in cholinergic and adrenergic activity in the region of the medulla near the VC and CTZ. The result is excess acetylcholine that affects the VC either directly or, more likely, through an effect on the CTZ.[1] Studies indicate that serotonergic receptors (subtypes 5-HT$_3$ and 5-HT$_4$) appear to be principal mediators in the emetic reflex. High concentrations of the 5-HT$_3$ receptors have recently been identified in the area postrema–nucleus tractus solitarii region of the medulla.[4] About 90% of the 5-HT$_3$ in the adult human body is located in the enterochromaffin cells of the GI tract, and the remainder is present in the central nervous system and the platelets. It is thought that chemotherapeutic agents (e.g., cisplatin) produce nausea and vomiting by releasing serotonin from the enterochromaffin cells and that the released serotonin then activates 5-HT$_3$ receptors located on afferent vagal

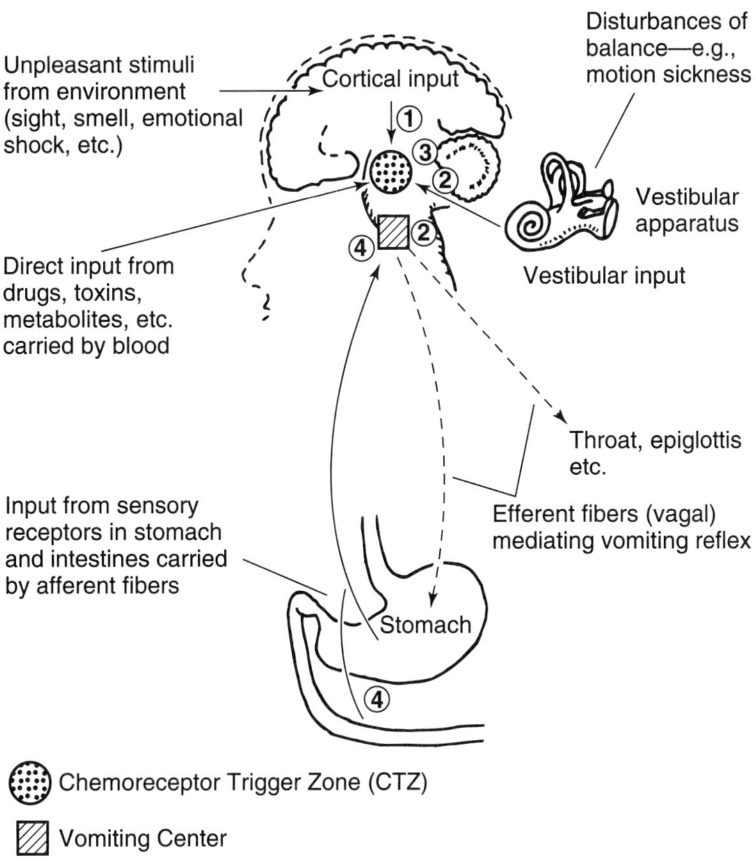

Figure 26.1. Anatomic structures involved in the vomiting reflex. Sites of action of common antiemetic drugs are labeled as follows: 1, site of action of sedative; 2, site of action of antihistamines and anticholinergics; 3, site of action of dopamine antagonists; and 4, proposed sites of action of serotonin antagonists. The vomiting reflex is mediated through the vomiting center. This center receives impulses from afferent fibers from the stomach and intestines and from fibers in the chemoreceptor trigger zone. It sends out impulses via afferent fibers to the muscles of the throat, epiglottis, and stomach, as shown in Figure 26.2.

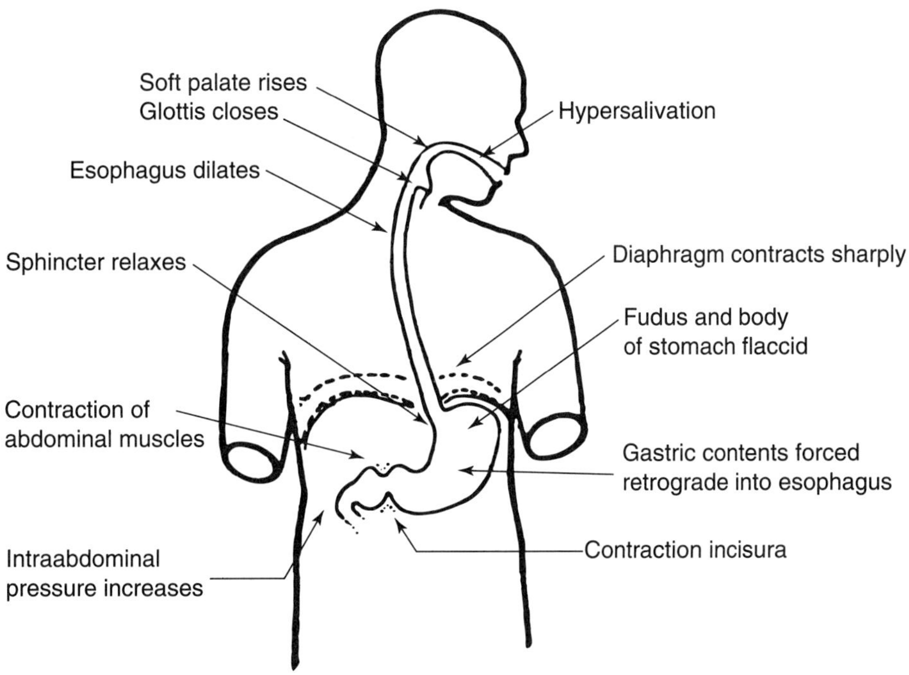

Figure 26.2. The mechanism of the complex act of vomiting. (Reprinted with permission from Whelan G. Targeting therapy: the patient with nausea, retching and vomiting. Curr Ther 26[12]:26, 1985.)

nerve terminals to initiate the vomiting reflex.[5] The serotonin antagonists act as antiemetics by selectively inhibiting 5-HT_3 receptors.

Other receptors may initiate emesis for drugs such as the cardiac glycosides, copper sulfate, and the opiates. Other neurotransmitters and peptides, including enkephalin, arginine vasopressin, substance P, peptide YY, and catecholamines stimulate the CTZ and may play a role in triggering emesis.[3] Emesis is thus mediated through a variety of receptor types and it is probable that more pathways will be discovered, leading to more effective and more disease-specific antiemetic therapy.

CLINICAL PRESENTATION AND DIAGNOSIS

Signs and Symptoms

The signs and symptoms of vomiting-induced metabolic disturbances include the following:

- Dehydration, suggested by oliguria, weight loss, mental confusion, and reduced tissue turgor
- Sodium depletion, suggested by thirst and hypotension
- Potassium depletion, suggested by muscle weakness or cardiac rhythm disturbances
- Alkalosis, which can result from loss of hydrogen ions in the vomitus, and the concentration of extracellular fluid secondary to fluid loss

Sodium, potassium, and chloride depletion result mainly from loss in the vomitus but also from other metabolic disturbances.

Diagnosis

An accurate diagnosis is essential before treatment for nausea and vomiting begins because symptomatic therapy may be contraindicated (e.g., in GI obstruction, acute appendicitis, or cerebral edema), or assessment of the underlying disease could be complicated by the sedative properties of most antiemetic therapy. The causes of vomiting should be kept in mind (Table 26.1) in developing the treatment plan.

The appearance, frequency, and timing of nausea and vomiting, together with associated specific and nonspecific symptoms such as jaundice, dehydration, diarrhea, weight loss, pain, and fever are important in making a diagnosis. Blood in the vomitus, an important sign, can be fresh and bright red (as from an esophageal tear) or altered, having the appearance of coffee grounds (indicating a GI bleed). Bile in the vomitus gives it a green or yellow color and suggests that the pyloric sphincter is open, allowing reflux of duodenal contents into the stomach.

The cause of vomiting usually is obvious (e.g., pregnancy, motion, or the use of certain drugs), but in some cases diagnosis can be difficult, especially if psychogenic factors are involved. With unexplained vomiting, the first step in assessment is eliminating the possibility of upper GI tract lesions or systemic conditions such as meningitis or uremia. The need to treat the sequelae of prolonged vomiting, such as fluid and electrolyte depletion, should also be assessed.

Chronic vomiting, with or without weight loss, can be psychogenic. This is suggested when the vomiting has been occurring for some time (especially if the patient has delayed seeking help), there is a family history of vomiting, the patient is able to suppress vomiting, or vomiting rarely occurs in a public place.

THERAPEUTIC PLAN

The patient experiencing nausea or vomiting is in acute need of pharmaceutical care. The pharmacist's primary goals are to recognize patients and circumstances that have a higher incidence of nausea and vomiting and prevent or minimize the frequency of nausea and vomiting. The pharmacist must use the accumulated knowledge about the causes and impact of nausea and vomiting to design an individualized pharmaceutical care plan that addresses drug efficacy, disease remission, and patient well-being to effectively treat this disorder with minimal patient morbidity. In preparation for individualized patient therapy, pharmacists should do the following:

- Treat the cause if it can be identified.
- Assess for fluid and electrolyte loss. In most cases this entails giving adequate fluids orally, particularly those containing glucose. If fluid loss leads to metabolic disturbances, the patient should be hospitalized and given appropriate intravenous fluids.
- Give appropriate symptomatic drug treatment after considering contraindications and adverse drug reactions. The choice of drug and dosage must be individualized.
- For unexplained vomiting, continue with diagnostic examinations.[6]

TREATMENT

Pharmacotherapy

Antiemetic Drugs

Considerable effort has been spent in developing antinausea drugs. In the past, most research focused on treating motion sickness and nausea of pregnancy (hyperemesis gravidarum), but more recently it has focused on treating nausea and vomiting caused by antineoplastic agents. Nausea and vomiting are common complications of chemotherapeutic regimens, often so severe as to cause the patient not to return for further treatment.

When selecting drugs to treat nausea and vomiting, it is important to remember that therapy must be individualized. This disorder can be caused by a variety of stimuli, and correlations between serum levels and efficacy have not been established for most antiemetics. For these reasons, treatment regimens should be regarded only as guidelines.

Dopamine Antagonists

The dopamine D_2 receptor antagonists include the phenothiazines, butyrophenones, and substituted benzamides (e.g., metoclopramide). The antiemetic action of the compounds is thought to result, at least in part, from inhibition of dopamine receptors in the CTZ. Unfortunately, the antiemetics that act as dopamine antagonists may also produce symptoms of dystonia, parkinsonism, akathisia, and tardive dyskinesia because the extrapyramidal nigrostriatal system is highly innervated by dopaminergic fibers.[7]

PHENOTHIAZINES. The phenothiazines have been the most widely used antiemetics since the 1950s. Two key modifications of the phenothiazine heterocyclic structure improve antiemetic activity. Halogenation (prochlorperazine, perphenazine) or thiethylation (thiethylperazine) of position 2 (R1), in combination with the attachment of a piperazine side chain at the 10 position (R2), enhances antiemetic (as well as extrapyramidal) activity. The phenothiazines also have varying amounts of anticholinergic and antihistaminic activity that may inhibit the vestibular pathway and the VC of the brain.[8]

Adverse effects of the phenothiazines include orthostatic hypotension and excessive sedation, which may limit use in ambulatory patients. Extrapyramidal effects occur most often with perphenazine but are readily controlled with diphenhydramine or benztropine. The phenothiazines can be given orally, parenterally, and rectally. The latter routes are useful when vomiting precludes oral administration.

Phenothiazines are used primarily to treat mild to moderate nausea and vomiting associated with anesthesia and surgery, radiation therapy, and anticancer chemotherapy.

Prochlorperazine has been the phenothiazine most widely used and studied as an antiemetic. Onset of action is 10 to 20 minutes for intramuscular administration, 30 to 40 minutes for oral tablet administration, and 60 minutes for rectal suppository administration. The duration of action is 3 to 4 hours, regardless of the route. Prochlorperazine has routinely been administered in a dosage of 10 mg every 4 to 6 hours, orally or intramuscularly, or 25 mg every 6 hours rectally to provide optimal antiemetic efficacy. At these dosages, comparative studies of cancer chemotherapy indicate that it is more effective than placebo, equivalent in potency to low-dose metoclopramide (0.1 to 0.3 mg/kg/dose) and droperidol, and less effective than tetrahydrocannabinol (THC), high-dose metoclopramide (1 to 3 mg/kg/dose), and nabilone.[7] Studies have demonstrated significantly greater antiemetic activity when dosages of 30 to 40 mg of prochlorperazine were administered by slow intravenous infusion. There was no substantial increase in adverse effects if diphenhydramine was administered prophylactically to prevent extrapyramidal reactions.[8–10]

BUTYROPHENONES. The butyrophenones, like the phenothiazines, are dopamine D_2 receptor antagonists and are effective antiemetic agents with similar uses and side effects. The main side effect is sedation, although extrapyramidal side effects do occur. The butyrophenones are less likely to produce hypotension than the phenothiazines. Droperidol is an effective antiemetic for use in cytotoxic therapy and in combination with fentanyl for postoperative nausea and vomiting (PONV), but it is for parenteral administration only. The onset of pharmacologic action of droperidol occurs within 3 to 10 minutes, but peak pharmacologic effects may not be apparent until 30 minutes after injection. Duration of antiemetic action is 2 to 4 hours, but sedating and tranquilizing effects may persist for up to 12 hours after a single dose.

Haloperidol is used occasionally as an antiemetic. It is usually given in dosages of 1 to 3 mg orally or intramuscularly every 3 hours. Oral bioavailability is 60%. Peak plasma concentrations occur within 2 to 6 hours. Haloperidol appears to undergo first-pass metabolism and enterohepatic recirculation. After intramuscular administration, peak plasma concentrations occur with 10 to 20 minutes, with peak pharmacologic action within 30 to 45 minutes.

METOCLOPRAMIDE. Metoclopramide has dual action as an antagonist of both dopamine D_2 and 5-HT_3 receptors, protecting against the emetic effects of dopamine and serotonin agonists. The action of metoclopramide is more selective than that of the phenothiazines in that it shows neuroleptic activity only at very high dosages. Through a peripheral action, possibly as a partial agonist of enteric postsynaptic neurons,[11] metoclopramide also increases the motility of the stomach and small intestine and relaxes the pyloric sphincter, increasing the activity of the upper regions on the GI tract. The antidopaminergic and antiserotonergic effects of metoclopramide on the gut complement the central antiemetic effect and are particularly useful in treating nausea and vomiting associated with GI cancer, gastritis, peptic ulcer, radiation sickness, and migraine. Metoclopramide is contraindicated in patients with intestinal obstruction who are at high risk for colonic rupture. It appears to be of little value in treating motion sickness, although it has been widely used for this purpose in Europe.

Early clinical trials of metoclopramide at dosages of 0.1 to 0.3 mg/kg showed only minimal antiemetic effect for a variety of antineoplastic agents, but high-dose (1 to 3 mg/kg) metoclopramide therapy was much more effective as an antiemetic.[12]

There are no major differences in the pharmacokinetics of conventional- and high-dose metoclopramide.[13] Oral doses are rapidly absorbed, but variable first-pass metabolism provides an oral bioavailability of 32 to 100%.[14] Peak levels occur in about 1 hour. High lipophilicity results in a large volume of distribution (2.8 to 4.5 L/kg). Approximately 85% of an orally administered dose appears in the urine within 72 hours. Of the 85% eliminated in the urine, about half is present as free or conjugated metoclopramide. The terminal half-life is 4.5 to 8.8 hours. One study to date indicates that there is substantial pharmacokinetic variability between patients with various cancers. The authors attribute this variability primarily to differences in body weight and serum alkaline phosphatase levels.[15] Although an early study indicated that serum levels greater than 800 ng/mL were necessary to achieve maximum protection against cisplatin-induced emesis, more recent trials have failed to show that serum metoclopramide concentrations predict antiemetic response or adverse effects.

Several controlled and uncontrolled studies have investigated routes of administration for optimal antiemetic therapy, ease and expense of administration, and frequency of adverse effects. Although optimal dosages and time schedules have not been delineated completely, the studies indicate that oral, continuous intravenous, and intermittent intravenous administration provide comparable antiemetic activity against a variety of chemotherapeutic agents. Oral therapy tends to be associated with a greater frequency of loose stools than intravenous administration, and scheduled dosing may be difficult if vomiting occurs. Rectal administration shows significant variation in the bioavailability of extemporaneously compounded suppositories (30 to 86%) but is successful in reducing the frequency of emesis as described in a case report of one patient.[16] Other points such as legal aspects of compounding, formulation stability, and cost must also be considered.[17]

Adverse effects associated with metoclopramide therapy include diarrhea, sedation, dizziness, and extrapyramidal symptoms. Diarrhea occurs in about 50% of patients receiving high-dose metoclopramide and cisplatin, but this may be related to cisplatin therapy. Mild sedation is observed in most patients who receive higher dosages. The extrapyramidal symptoms include akathisia, restlessness, and dystonic reactions (including torticollis, oculogyric crisis, and Parkinson-like symptoms). The overall frequency is 3 to 5%, but as many as 30% of men under the age of 30 years may suffer from extrapyramidal effects. Extrapyramidal symptoms subside within 5 minutes of intravenous diphenhydramine administration. When high-dose metoclopramide is used as an antiemetic, many cancer chemotherapy protocols now include routine doses of diphenhydramine to minimize extrapyramidal symptoms (see Chemotherapy-Induced Emesis).

Serotonin Receptor Antagonists

The serotonin ($5\text{-}HT_3$) receptor antagonists have made a major impact in the treatment of emesis associated with cancer chemotherapy, radiation therapy, and PONV. Three serotonin ($5\text{-}HT_3$) receptor antagonists, ondansetron, granisetron, and dolasetron, are now available. Table 26.2 compares the pharmacokinetic properties of these agents. Serum concentrations do not correlate with antiemetic efficacy, and there does not appear to be accumulation after multiple dosing. Ondansetron is extensively metabolized, with only 5% recovered in the urine as unchanged drug. The primary metabolic pathway is hydroxylation of the indole ring followed by glucuronide or sulfate conjugation.[18] Granisetron is metabolized by *N*-demethylation and aromatic ring oxidation followed by

Table 26.2 ▪ Pharmacokinetics of Serotonin Antagonists

Variable	Ondansetron		Granisetron		Dolasetron	
	PO (8 mg)	IV (0.15 mg/kg)	PO (1 mg)	IV (40 μg/kg)	PO (hydrodolasetron)	IV (hydrodolasetron)
Bioavailability	56%		NA		75%	
Half-life (hr)						
Patients with cancer		4.0		9	7.9[a]	7.5[b]
Volunteers						
20–40 yr	3.3	3.5	6.2[c]	4.9	8.1[d]	7.3[e]
60–75 yr[f]	4.5	4.7		7.7	7.2[g]	6.9[h]
>75 yr[f]	5.5	5.5				
Liver impairment						
Moderate		9.2	NA	NA	NA	NA
Severe		20.6	NA	NA	11	11.7
Protein binding	70–76%	70–76%	65%	65%	69–77%	
Volume of distribution (L/kg)			3.97		5.8	

Source: References 18, 19, 22.
[a]25–200 mg PO.
[b]1.8 mg/kg IV.
[c]No age differentiation with 39 normal volunteers.
[d]200 mg PO.
[e]100 mg IV.
[f]No dosage adjustment needed in older adults.
[g]2.4 mg/kg PO.
[h]2.4 mg/kg IV.

conjugation. Animal studies suggest that some of the metabolites may also have 5-HT_3 receptor antagonist activity. In normal volunteers, approximately 12% is eliminated unchanged in the urine in 48 hours. The remainder is excreted as metabolites, 49% in the urine and 34% in the feces. Dolasetron is rapidly ($t_{1/2}$ less than 10 minutes) reduced to hydrodolasetron, the primary active agent, by carbonyl reductase. Hydrodolasetron is further metabolized by oxidation of the indole ring; *N*-oxidation also occurs before it is excreted as glucuronide, sulfate conjugates, and *N*-oxide.[19,20] Two-thirds of the administered dose is eliminated in the urine and one-third in the feces.

Ondansetron, granisetron, and dolasetron are metabolized by the cytochrome P 2D6 isoenzyme of the hepatic cytochrome P-450 enzyme system[21]; inducers or inhibitors of these enzymes may change the clearance and the half-life of these serotonin antagonists. Blood levels of hydrodolasetron increased 24% when dolasetron was coadministered with cimetidine for 7 days and decreased 28% with coadministration of rifampin for 7 days.[19] At this time, no dosage adjustments are recommended, only close monitoring for adverse effects. Ondansetron, granisetron, and dolasetron do not induce or inhibit the cytochrome P-450 enzyme system.[18,19,22] A particular advantage of this group of antiemetics is minimal dopaminergic blockade, demonstrated by few reports of extrapyramidal adverse effects.[18,19,23,24]

Tables 26.3 and 26.4 compare the frequency of adverse effects of the serotonin antagonists. Note that the clinical studies cited for frequency of adverse effects of granisetron used a dosage of 40 μg/kg. Because no statistical difference in antiemetic efficacy has been demonstrated between 10 μg/kg and 40 μg/kg, the recommended dosage in the United States is now 10 μg/kg.[22] Studies indicate that dolasetron may induce electrocardiographic interval changes (PR, QTc, JT prolongation, and QRS widening). These changes are dose related; some patients have interval prolongations for 24 hours or more. There have been rare reports of interval prolongation leading to heart block and cardiac arrhythmias. Dolasetron should be administered with caution in patients who have or may develop prolonged conduction intervals. This side effect is more common in patients with hypokalemia or hypomagnesemia and those taking diuretics, antiarrhythmic drugs, or other drugs that lead to QT prolongation and in patients on a cumulative high-dose anthracycline therapy.[19]

Cisplatin, a potent serotonin agonist, is well recognized for its almost 100% emetic potential when administered to patients without emesis prophylaxis. It is therefore the primary agent against which the efficacy of antiemetics is measured. The serotonin antagonists have been shown to actively control nausea and vomiting associated with cisplatin and several other emetogenic chemotherapeutic agents in both animals and humans. Comparative studies between ondansetron and metoclopramide conclude that ondansetron is more effective than metoclopramide in the control of high-dose cisplatin-induced nausea and vomiting.[23,25–28] Several single-center and multicenter, double-blind, randomized studies comparing the efficacy and safety of ondansetron, granisetron, and dolasetron in controlling cisplatin-induced acute emesis conclude that there are no significant differences between any of the treatment groups with respect to emetic control, nausea, or adverse reactions. These studies also bear out the impact of the dosage of highly emetogenic agents (cisplatin) and

Table 26.3 ▪ Frequency of Adverse Effects Reported in Clinical Trials After Oral Administration

	Ondansetron (8 mg BID)	Granisetron (2 md QD)	Dolasetron[a] (100 mg QD)
CIE[b]			
Headache	24%	20%	22.9%
Fatigue	13	NA	5.7
Constipation	9	14	NA
Diarrhea	6	9	5.3
Dizziness	5	NA	3.1
Asthenia	NA	18	NA
Dyspepsia	NA	6	2.2
PONV			
Headache	9	NA[c]	7
Fever	8		3.5
Dizziness	7		4.4

Adverse effects listed are those that had a reported incidence higher than the incidence reported with placebo.

Source: References 18, 19, 22.

CIE, chemotherapy-induced emesis; PONV, postoperative nausea and vomiting.

[a]Dolasetron not compared with placebo in CIE studies.

[b]Ondansetron and cyclophosphamide regimen, granisetron and cyclophosphamide or cisplatin regimen, dolasetron and cyclophosphamide or doxorubicin regimen.

[c]Granisetron not tested in PONV.

Table 26.4 ▪ Frequency of Adverse Effects Reported in Clinical Trials After Intravenous Administration

	Ondansetron	Granisetron	Dolasetron
CIE[a,b]			
Headache	25%	14%	24.3%
Diarrhea	8	4	12.4
Fever	7	NA	4.3
Fatigue	NA	NA	3.6
PONV[c]			
Headache	17	NA[d]	9.4
Dizziness	12		5.5
Drowsiness	8		2.4

Adverse effects listed are those that had a reported incidence higher than the incidence reported with placebo.

Source: References 18, 19, 22.

CIE, chemotherapy-induced emesis; PONV, postoperative nausea and vomiting.

[a]Chemotherapy received was predominantly cisplatin.

[b]Dosage (single dose): Ondansetron = 32 mg; Granisetron = 40 mg/kg; Dolasetron = 1.8 mg/kg.

[c]Dosages (single dose): Ondansetron = 4 mg; Dolasetron = 12.5 mg.

[d]Granisetron not tested in PONV.

moderately emetogenic agents (cyclophosphamide, doxorubicin) in comparing studies with different rates of control of emesis and nausea. For higher-dose cisplatin, 35 to 50% of patients receiving serotonin antagonists have no episodes of emesis, and 50 to 70% have two or fewer episodes of emesis. Emesis is controlled in 50 to 70% of patients receiving moderately emetogenic chemotherapy. Headache is the most frequently reported drug related adverse effect, occurring in 9 to 24% of all patients.[29–38] More recently, the serotonin antagonists have been shown to be more effective against chemotherapy-induced nausea and vomiting when combined with dexamethasone (see Corticosteroids) than when administered as monotherapy.

The serotonin antagonists have become a common choice for preventing and treating PONV. The FDA approved ondansetron for this use in 1993, and dolasetron followed in 1997. When used properly, these drugs have very few adverse effects. Alexander and Fennelly[39] compared ondansetron with metoclopramide and placebo for reducing nausea and vomiting after major surgery and found that oral premedication with ondansetron 8 mg was more effective than metoclopramide 10 mg and placebo. Tang et al.[40] studied the timing of ondansetron administration for PONV in the ambulatory setting and found that giving 4 mg ondansetron immediately before the end of surgery was the most efficacious in patients undergoing outpatient laparoscopy. The expense of the serotonin antagonists limits their cost-effectiveness for preventing and treating PONV, but their therapeutic efficacy must be considered in evaluating potential drug therapy.

Anticholinergic Drugs

Anticholinergic drugs include muscarinic antagonists such as scopolamine and H_1 receptor antagonist antihistamines. These drugs are used to treat motion sickness and, in the case of the antihistamines, for treating nausea and vomiting associated with pregnancy. The antiemetic effects of the antihistamines result primarily from their anticholinergic activity, not the blocking of histamine receptors.[41]

The most commonly used anticholinergic antiemetic drugs include scopolamine (hyoscine) and the antihistamines promethazine, diphenhydramine, cyclizine, and meclizine. The choice of drug depends on the period for which antinausea protection is needed and the side effects. Clinical studies indicate that oral scopolamine (0.2 to 0.6 mg) is the drug of choice for brief periods of motion and an antihistamine is the drug of choice for longer periods.[1] Of the antihistamines, promethazine (25 mg) is the drug of choice.[41] Although higher dosages have a longer duration of action, sedation usually is a problem. Cyclizine (50 mg) has fewer side effects than promethazine but has a shorter duration of action and is less effective for severe conditions. Meclizine (50 mg) is similar to cyclizine, and both drugs are used when nausea is mild and protection is needed for short periods. Diphenhydramine has a long duration, but excessive sedation usually is a problem. For very severe conditions, sympathomimetic drugs such as ephedrine are used in combination with scopolamine or antihistamines.

The transdermal (patch) delivery system for administering scopolamine has produced good results.[42] The 2-mm-thick patch with a surface area of 2.5 cm^2 contains 1.5 mg of scopolamine. Part of the dosage is contained in the hypoallergenic contact adhesive and is released immediately to saturate skin binding sites and initiate absorption. The remainder of the dosage is contained in a reservoir separated from the contact surface by a membrane that releases the drug at a constant rate of about 5 μg/hour for a period of approximately 66 hours. The patch is backed by a water-resistant layer. The manufacturers recommend that the patch be applied to the postauricular skin (a highly permeable skin site of the body) 4 to 6 hours before the user expects to be in motion.

About 67% of people using transdermal scopolamine complain of dryness of the mouth, although this is not a contraindication. Drowsiness occurs in about 17% of patients, and blurred vision is experienced by about 12% of users and probably results in some cases from transfer of drug to the eyes by the fingers. Potential users should be advised to try the patches before using them in a travel situation and to wash their hands after applying the patch. The patches should not be used in children and adolescents, during pregnancy, in patients with glaucoma or a family history of glaucoma, and in those with psychosis.

A gel form of scopolamine for topical use has been compounded by many pharmacists and used at a time when production problems caused the patch to be withdrawn from the market. This dosage form has similar effects as the marketed patch.[43]

Corticosteroids

A variety of studies have shown that dexamethasone and, to a lesser extent, methylprednisolone, can be effective antiemetics as single agents or in combination with other antiemetics. The antiemetic mechanism of action is unknown, but it has been suggested that the drugs act by inhibiting prostaglandin synthesis in the hypothalamus. Other actions of the corticosteroids, such as mood elevation, increased appetite, and a sense of well-being, may be responsible for patient acceptance and positive outcomes.[44]

The antiemetic effects of dexamethasone are comparable to those of high-dose metoclopramide (1 to 3 mg/kg) in controlling nausea and vomiting associated with low-dose cisplatin (less than 60 mg/m^2) therapy and standard dosages of chemotherapeutic agents with moderately emetogenic activity. However, metoclopramide appears to be more effective than dexamethasone against high-dose cisplatin (120 mg/m^2) and other highly emetogenic cancer chemotherapy agents. Dexamethasone also appears to be more effective against emesis induced by moderately emetogenic agents than standard dosages of oral prochlorperazine (10 mg).[44] Kris et al.[45] also demonstrated that the overall antiemetic activity can be improved when dexamethasone is added to metoclopramide and prochlorperazine therapy. A randomized, double-blind, parallel-group study comparing ondansetron plus dexamethasone with metoclopramide plus dexamethasone demonstrated that ondansetron plus dexamethasone is highly effective and is significantly superior to metoclopramide plus dexamethasone preventing carboplatin-induced emesis. In the ondansetron plus dexamethasone group, 97% reported complete or major control of emesis (0 to 2 emetic episodes) on the first day of carboplatin therapy, compared with 74% of the metoclopramide plus dexamethasone group. Furthermore, 87% of the ondansetron plus dexamethasone group reported 0 to 2 emetic episodes on the worst day of the study, whereas 66% of the metoclopramide plus dexamethasone group reported only 0 to 2 episodes.[46] Recent studies demonstrated significantly less nausea and vomiting with the combination of dexamethasone plus a serotonin antagonist for both moderately emetogenic chemotherapy[47–49] and highly emetogenic chemotherapy.[50,51] The dexamethasone dosage used in these studies ranged from 8 to 20 mg. Kris et al.[50] demonstrated that oral dolasetron and dexamethasone is as effective in preventing emesis as intravenously administered antiemetics.

Although few studies have been completed, methylprednisolone may be useful as a single antiemetic agent during chemotherapy with mildly to moderately emetogenic agents, but it is not recommended as a single agent with the use of highly emetogenic agents such as cisplatin.[44] Further trials are needed to establish the optimum dosing regimens for use with the various antineoplastic agents and the advantages of combining corticosteroids with other antiemetics.

The advantage of the steroids, apart from their efficacy, is their relative lack of side effects with short-term use. Lethargy, weakness, euphoria, a sense of well-being, insomnia, increased appetite, and generalized swelling are the more common side effects of corticosteroids. Other rare effects reported include headache, metallic taste, abdominal discomfort, itchy throat, and a swollen feeling in the mouth. Adverse effects associated with the long-term use of corticosteroids are not applicable in this setting. Dexamethasone is also reported to significantly decrease the incidence of diarrhea and sedation associated with metoclopramide therapy.[45]

Cannabinoids

In light of numerous reports that smoking marijuana reduces nausea, the antiemetic properties of the active ingredients Δ-8- and 9-THC and synthetic analogs such as nabilone and levonantradol have been studied extensively. Proposed mechanisms of action are that the cannabinoids act in the cerebral cortex to inhibit pathways to the VC, exert an anticholinergic effect on cholinergic terminals in Auerbach's plexus, and possibly mediate the prostaglandin cyclic nucleotide system.[52] Other studies indicate that there is no dopaminergic antagonist activity.[53]

Pharmacokinetic studies of THC show that absorption from the GI tract is slow and erratic, with bioavailability less than 10%, although this may depend on the formulation. THC is highly protein bound (97%). Peak plasma concentrations are attained in about 1 hour after oral administration, with serum levels in the 5 to 10 ng/mL range producing antiemetic activity. Higher serum levels are associated with greater antiemetic effect but with substantially more adverse effects. The terminal half-life of THC is 20 to 30 hours, but other active metabolites take 1 to 2 days for elimination. Patients report a correlation with the peak serum concentrations and a euphoric high. The high following oral administration usually begins 30 to 60 minutes after ingestion, peaks in 1 to 3 hours, and lasts for 4 to 6 hours. Smoking THC cigarettes raises bioavailability (to about 20%), with onset of action in 6 to 12 minutes. Peak levels are attained in 30 to 120 minutes, with a duration lasting 3 to 4 hours. Normal behavior is observed 24 hours after administration.[52,53]

THC has been shown to be more effective than placebo and as effective as prochlorperazine in patients receiving moderately emetogenic chemotherapy. It is less effective than metoclopramide and associated with more side effects when used to prevent emesis secondary to cisplatin therapy. Most common adverse effects associated with THC therapy include dry mouth, sedation, orthostatic hypotension, dizziness, and confusion. Dysphoric effects such as depressed mood, dreaming or fantasizing, perception distortion, and elated mood are more common with dosages greater than 5 mg/m^2. Younger patients appear to tolerate these side effects better than older patients or patients who have not previously used marijuana.[54] Voth and Schwartz[55] evaluated research published between 1975 and 1996 on the medical uses, complications, and legal precedents for the use of THC and crude marijuana. They conclude that pure THC is beneficial in treating nausea associated with cancer chemotherapy, but with the availability of other effective antiemetic agents and pure THC (dronabinol) as a prescription, crude marijuana need not be made available for medicinal purposes.

Nabilone is rapidly and well absorbed orally (96%), with an elimination half-life of about 2 hours. Studies indicate that nabilone is more effective than placebo and prochlorperazine against moderately emetogenic chemotherapeutic agents. However, it is not as effective as metoclopramide with vomiting associated with cisplatin therapy. Nabilone has been reported to have fewer euphoric effects than THC.[56]

Because of the mind-altering effects of the cannabinoids and the potential for abuse, these agents have been used as antiemetics only in patients receiving chemotherapy. The cannabinoids have more utility in younger patients who are refractory to other antiemetic regimens and in whom combination therapy may be more effective.

Benzodiazepines

The benzodiazepines, diazepam, lorazepam, and midazolam, are effective in reducing not only the frequency of nausea and vomiting, but also the anxiety often associated with chemotherapy.[57,58] This action probably results from a combination of effects, including sedation, reduction in anxiety, possible depression of the VC, and an amnesic effect. Of these, the amnesic effect appears to be the most important in treating patients with cancer, and in this respect lorazepam and midazolam are superior to diazepam. The sedative and amnesic effects are dose-related, with higher dosages (4 mg or more) of lorazepam inducing amnesic effects that persist for a longer period of time and occur in a larger percentage of patients. Amnesia does not correlate well with sedation because sedation may remain high while the amnesic effects decline.

After intravenous administration of lorazepam or midazolam, the onset of sedative, anxiolytic, and amnesic action usually occurs within 1 to 5 minutes. The duration of action after intravenous administration of midazolam usually is less than 2 hours; however, dose-dependent actions may persist for up to 6 hours in some patients. After intramuscular administration, the onset of action of lorazepam is 15 to 30 minutes, and the duration of action is 12 to 24 hours. After intramuscular administration of midazolam, onset of action occurs within 5 to 15 minutes but may not be maximal for 20 to 60 minutes; the duration of action is about 2 hours, although the range is 1 to 6 hours. The onset of action of orally administered lorazepam is about 30 minutes, with peak activity occurring within 2 hours. Duration of action is 4 to 6 hours. The elimination half-life of lorazepam is 10 to 20 hours, with no active metabolites, whereas that of midazolam is 1 to 12 hours, with active metabolites.

Clinically, midazolam and lorazepam are most useful in combination with other antiemetics such as metoclopramide and dexamethasone. The anxiolytic and amnesic effects result in marked subjective support from patients.[59] The greatest benefit from benzodiazepine therapy is derived by patients who have not received prior chemotherapy and who have not developed negative conditioning by episodes of nausea and vomiting (see Anticipatory Nausea and Vomiting). Side effects associated with benzodiazepine therapy are drowsiness and dizziness. Patients should not be left unattended in the sedated, amnesic state because vomiting may still occur and could lead to aspiration. Because of its short half-life and short duration of action, midazolam may be the more appropriate adjunctive antiemetic for outpatient use.

Treatment of Selected Causes of Nausea and Vomiting

Chemotherapy-Induced Emesis

Chemotherapy-induced emesis (CIE) is the most unpleasant adverse effect associated with the use of antineoplastic agents. Many patients regard it as the most stressful aspect of their disease, more so even than the prospect of dying. Because the object of therapy in many cases is to prolong life for a short period, the effect of CIE on the quality of life must be considered. Also, many patients whose prognosis is good find it difficult to adhere with chemotherapy regimens and may request that they be discontinued because of CIE. Before contemporary treatment regimens for CIE were tested, one multicenter survey found that as many as 10% of patients refused to continue with chemotherapy because of nausea and vomiting.[60]

Three types of emesis have been identified in patients receiving chemotherapy:

- Anticipatory nausea and vomiting
- Acute CIE
- Delayed emesis

Patients may also have emesis for reasons other than chemotherapy, perhaps induced by medications such as analgesics, or tumor-related complications such as intestinal obstruction. Addressing these matters usually is more important than selecting antiemetic therapy.[61] Apart from distressing the patient, severe vomiting complicates the patient's medical condition, causing dehydration, metabolic alkalosis, electrolyte deficiencies, nutritional impairment including cachexia, and physical injury, including esophageal tears and bone fractures.

Anticipatory Nausea and Vomiting

The patient's fear of CIE may lead to anticipatory nausea or vomiting (ANV). Anticipatory nausea alone has been reported in up to 78% of patients[62] and anticipatory vomiting in up to 38%.[63] Patients who develop ANV are more likely to have increased pretreatment anxiety, greater posttreatment dizziness and vomiting, and a delayed onset of postchemotherapy nausea and vomiting.[62] Patients who experience ANV are more likely to be younger and to have received twice as many courses of chemotherapy with more drugs for about three times longer than patients who do not experience ANV.[63,64] ANV correlates with the emetic potential of chemotherapy regimens and with the severity of nausea and vomiting after chemotherapy. Although considerable interpatient variability is observed, the onset of ANV usually starts 2 to 4 hours before treatment and is most severe at the time of drug administration.[65] It is believed that ANV is a conditioned response triggered by the sight or smell of the clinic or hospital or by the knowledge that treatment is imminent. ANV tends to become more severe as treatments progress unless behavior therapy modifies the conditioned response.[66] Such treatments include progressive muscle relaxation, mind diversion, hypnosis, self-hypnosis, and systematic desensitization. People with a negative attitude toward therapy, such as the belief that it will be of no benefit, are more likely to develop ANV than those with a positive attitude. A positive relationship between the patient and health care professionals is important in the success of behavioral treatment of CIE. The patient must be able to communicate freely with the staff about real and imagined fears about therapy and thereby develop positive attitudes toward his or her treatment. In this age of managed care, health maintenance organizations, and rotating medical staff in teaching hospitals and clinics, the patient may not always see the same health care provider.[66]

Complications associated with ANV underscore the need to accompany the initial course of emesis-producing chemotherapy with the most effective antiemetic regimen and continue vigorous therapy with each subsequent cycle of chemotherapy.[48,61] Adding lorazepam to antiemetic regimens induces an amnesic effect about chemotherapy and emesis in some patients[67] and has received subjective support from patients.[68] If delayed emesis is associated with any of the agents in the chemotherapeutic regimen, effective antiemetic therapy should be continued long enough to reduce the frequency of nausea and emesis, thus minimizing the risk of preconditioning the patient against further chemotherapy and ANV.

Acute Chemotherapy-Induced Emesis

The choice of antiemetic therapy for patients receiving antineoplastic therapy should take into account both patient and drug factors.

Patient Factors. The incidence and severity of CIE generally are greater among people of advanced age, those in poor general health (especially if cachetic), and those with metabolic disturbances, (i.e., dehydration, uremia, GI tract obstruction, or infection). Patient age can also influence the response to antiemetic drugs. For example, patients under age 30 are more sensitive to the extrapyramidal effects of dopaminergic blockade from phenothiazines or high-dose metoclopramide than older patients. On the other hand, younger patients tolerate cannabinoids better than older people. Patients who have a history of chronic heavy alcohol usage (more than 5 mixed drinks per day) tolerate chemotherapy with fewer bouts of emesis than those without this history.[61] Patients who are prone to motion sickness seem to be more sensitive to the emetic effects of cytotoxic agents. Because these two types of emesis are mediated by different mechanisms, this correlation probably reflects a psychogenic component. Finally, the patient's mental outlook and attitude toward therapy can influence the frequency and severity of emetic reactions considerably.

Drug Factors. The emetogenic potential of antineoplastic drugs varies greatly, ranging from more than 90% in the case of cisplatin to 10% or less with chlorambucil. Table 26.5 classifies chemotherapeutic agents in terms of emetogenicity, although emetogenicity is also influenced by the dosage, duration, and frequency of courses. The effects of combinations of chemotherapeutic agents on vomiting are poorly understood.

The extensive literature on testing antiemetics for use with antineoplastic agents often is difficult to interpret. Comparisons between trials are difficult because of differences in protocol, cytotoxic drugs, and patient characteristics.[57,69] Most prospective clinical trials that test efficacy of antiemetics use patients who have not had prior exposure to chemotherapy (chemotherapy-naive patients). Success rates of antiemetic regimens are substantially more variable after multiple courses of chemotherapy. Some studies rely entirely on objective data alone (i.e., the frequency of vomiting and the volume of vomitus) without investigating patient attitudes, performance capabilities, or quality of life issues. A patient who vomits only occasionally but experiences nausea continually may have a poorer quality of life than someone who vomits more frequently but has little intervening nausea. Hesketh et al.[70] have proposed a new classification of emetogenicity of chemotherapeutic agents that may serve as a framework to allow more accurate comparisons of the antiemetic effects of medicines with subsequent development of treatment guidelines.

It is clear that major progress has occurred in treating CIE,[71] and the following general recommendations can be made:

- Antiemetics are most effective when administered prophylactically against nausea and vomiting. Because most nausea and vomiting starts 1 to 4 hours after chemotherapy is initiated, in general, antiemetics should be administered 30 to 60 minutes before chemotherapy is administered. Dosages, efficacies, and severity of adverse effects of primary antiemetic drugs are

Table 26.5 ▪ Relative Emetic Activity of Chemotherapeutic Agents

Very high emetic incidence (>90%)	Low emetic incidence (10–30%)
Carmustine >250 mg/m^2	Docetaxel
Cisplatin >50 mg/m^2	Etoposide
Cyclophosphamide >1500 mg/m^2	5-Fluorouracil <1000 mg/m^2
Dacarbazine >500 mg	Gemcitabine
Dactinomycin	Methotrexate 50–250 mg/m^2
Lomustine >60 mg	Mitomycin
Mechlorethamine	Paclitaxel
Streptozocin	Very low emetic incidence (<10%)
High emetic incidence (60–90%)	Bleomycin
Carboplatin	Busulfan
Carmustine <250 mg/m^2	Chlorambucil (oral)
Cisplatin <50 mg/m^2	2-Chlorodeoxyadenosine
Cyclophosphamide 750–1500 mg/m^2	Fludarabine
Cytarabine >1g/m^2	Hydroxyurea
Dacarbazine <500 mg	Methotrexate <50 mg/m^2
Doxorubicin >60 mg/m^2	L-Phenylalanine mustard (oral)
Ifosfamide >1.5 g	Thioguanine (oral)
Lomustine <60 mg	Vinblastine
Methotrexate >1000 mg/m^2	Vincristine
Procarbazine (oral)	Vinorelbine
Moderate emetic incidence (30–60%)	
Cyclophosphamide <750 mg/m^2	
Cyclophosphamide (oral)	
Doxorubicin 20–60 mg/m^2	
Epirubicin <90 mg/m^2	
Hexamethylmelamine (oral)	
Idarubicin	
Ifosfamide	
Methotrexate 250–1000 mg/m^2	
Mitoxantrone <15 mg/m^2	

Source: References 70, 87.

given in Table 26.6. Therapy must be individualized, and the dosages and treatment schedules given are meant as guidelines only. All antiemetics except antimuscarinics (anticholinergics andantihistamines) have been found useful in treating CIE.

- All patients being treated with moderate to very high emetogenic chemotherapeutic agents (Table 26.5) should receive prophylactic antiemetic therapy before antineoplastic therapy is initiated. Combinations of ondansetron, granisetron, or dolasetron plus dexamethasone, plus lorazepam, plus prochlorperazine are the drugs of choice in treating cisplatin-induced emesis.[72] An alternative for the patient who cannot tolerate serotonin receptor antagonists is high-dose metoclopramide, dexamethasone, and diphenhydramine.[61,73–76] Antiemetic therapy should be continued for 4 to 7 days to prevent or minimize delayed vomiting (see Delayed Emesis).
- Emesis induced by moderately emetogenic agents such as methotrexate and 5-fluorouracil can be treated prophylactically with metoclopramide and dexamethasone, and therapy should be continued for 24 hours.[77]
- A phenothiazine (prochlorperazine) or dexamethasone alone is recommended if the chemotherapy is of low emetic potential. An alternative for this group may be a cannabinoid plus a phenothiazine to ameliorate central nervous system side effects.[77]

Table 26.6 ▪ Efficacy, Dosage, and Toxicity of Antiemetics Used to Treat Cytotoxic-Induced Emesis

Drug	Antiemetic Activity[a]	Dosage Range (dosages must be individualized)[b]	Adverse Effects[c]
Phenothiazines			
Prochlorperazine	++	5–10 mg q2–4h PO. 5–10 mg q3–6h IM/IV[d], 25 mg PR q6h.	+/++
Chlorpromazine	++	25–50mg q3–6h PO. 25 mg q4–6h PO/IM/IV[d]/PR.	+/++
Thiethylperazine	++	10 mg q8h PO/IM/PR.	+/++
Butyrophenones			
Droperidol	++	1–3 mg q4–6h IV or 5 mg IV 30 min before chemotherapy, then continuous infusion of 1–1.5 mg/hr for 9–12 hr.	+/++
Haloperidol	++	1–3 mg q4–6h PO/IM/IV.[d]	+/++
Metoclopramide			
High dose	+++	1–3 mg/kg IVPB over 15 min 0.5 hr before and q2h × 3–4 doses after chemotherapy.	++
Low dose	0/+	0.1–0.3 mg/kg q4h PO/IM/IV.	+
Corticosteroids			
Dexamethasone	+++	4–25 mg PO/IV before chemotherapy and q4–6h × 1–2 days.	0/+
Methylprednisolone	+++	125–500 mg PO/IV 2 hr before chemotherapy and 2 hr after or as infusion.	0/+
Benzodiazepines			
Lorazepam	++/+++	1–4 mg q4–6h PO/IV; can begin when patient arrives for chemotherapy.	+/++
Cannabinoids			
Δ-9-tetrahydrocanabinol (Dronabinol)	++[e]	5–15 mg/m² q4h PO; begin night before chemotherapy.	++/+++
Serotonin antagonists			
Granisetron	+++	1 mg PO within 60 min before starting chemotherapy. Repeat once at 12 hr	
		10 μg/kg IVPB over 5 min within 30 min before starting chemotherapy.	++
Ondansetron	+++	8 mg PO q4h × 3 doses beginning 30 min before start of emetogenic chemotherapy. Follow chemotherapy with 8 mg q8hr for 1–2 days.	++
		32 mg IVPB as a single dose or 0.15 mg/kg IVPB q4h × 3 doses. Infuse dose over 15 min beginning 30 min before start of emetogenic chemotherapy.	++
Dolsetron	+++	100 mg PO within 60 min before chemotherapy. 1.8 mg/kg or 100 mg IVPB over up to 15 min within 30 min before starting chemotherapy.[f]	++

PR, per rectum; IVPB, intravenous piggyback.

[a]Antiemetic activity against cisplatin; 0, little or none, to +++, high.

[b]Dosages are examples only and represent the ranges given in the references cited in the text. Best results usually are obtained with a combination of antiemetics. Dosing often is begun before chemotherapy.

[c]0, little or none, to +++, high incidence.

[d]Can be administered by slow (15–20 min) IV administration.

[e]May have marked efficacy in young patients.

[f]May also be given undiluted IV as 100 mg/30 sec.

The rationale for using combinations of antiemetic agents is based on the assumption that cytotoxic agents produce emesis by multiple mechanisms. Antiemetics also act by multiple mechanisms, and a combination could have a synergistic action. Side effects also are a factor in the choice of an antiemetic, and combinations of drugs acting by different mechanisms are less likely to produce adverse reactions than the highest dosage of a single drug. In some cases a second antiemetic agent may reduce the side effects of the first drug (e.g., dexamethasone, diphenhydramine, or lorazepam is added to high-dose metoclopramide).

The availability of the 5-HT_3 antagonists has made significant impact in reducing the frequency of nausea and vomiting episodes in patients receiving moderately and highly emetogenic chemotherapy. Unfortunately, the cost of the wide use of serotonin receptor antagonists for most cases of CIE, regardless of emetogenicity, has become prohibitive. These high costs have necessitated the development of guidelines for using the antiemetic agents.[78–80] Multidisciplinary teams of physicians, nurses, and pharmacists have developed highly successful guidelines for use of antiemetics based on the emetic potential of the chemotherapy, lower effective ondansetron dosages,[80,81] higher effective dosages of non–5-HT_3 antagonist antiemetics,[81] use of oral rather than parenteral dosage forms,[50,82] and avoidance of treatment of delayed-onset nausea and vomiting with 5-HT_3 antagonists.[72,83]

There has been a general perception among health care providers that the 5-HT_3 receptor antagonists improve the patient's quality of life because the frequency of nausea and vomiting is reduced by these agents. Assessment tools are now being used to measure the impact of chemotherapy and antiemetics on patients' quality of life.[84,85] Comparison with pre–serotonin antagonist studies is difficult because of differing patient populations, use of much more aggressive chemotherapy, newer antineoplastic agents, and the availability of the new antiemetics. The serotonin antagonists have also brought the concept of delayed emesis much more clearly into focus as a separate entity (see Delayed Emesis), and preventing delayed emesis is much less successful than preventing acute emesis. de Boer-Dennert et al.[86] repeated a study published in 1983 that cited nausea and vomiting as the two most distressing side effects associated with chemotherapy. The new study, following the use of serotonin antagonists, reported that nausea, hair loss, and vomiting were the three most distressing side effects of chemotherapy, even though the incidence and severity of acute nausea and vomiting were reduced significantly.

The Functional Living Index–Emesis (FLIE) provides an assessment of the impact of CIE on a patient's daily functioning.[85] Farley et al.[87] designed a multicenter study to measure the impact of serotonin antagonists on quality of life and to determine whether there was a difference in scores between those treated with ondansetron or granisetron. The study demonstrated significantly lower FLIE scores in patients who had nausea and vomiting after chemotherapy but no difference in scores of patients receiving granisetron or ondansetron.

The European Organization for Research and Treatment of Cancer (EORTC) Core Quality of Life Questionnaire (QLQ-C30) is another quality of life assessment tool consisting of 30 questions that measure five functional domains, a global quality of life domain, three symptom domains, five additional symptoms, and an item on financial status.[88] Osoba et al.[89] reported that patients who received either moderately or highly emetogenic chemotherapy who developed CIE had significantly lower physical, role, and social function scores as well as lower global quality of life scores than did those who were emesis-free. This study suggested that pretreatment quality scores could predict which patients are at greater risk for CIE, so that additional measures may be taken to minimize the severity of CIE. The discussion section of this paper is particularly comprehensive in comparing literature in this area describing shortfalls of studies that should be considered in designing new investigations.

Delayed Emesis

Delayed emesis is a distinct syndrome that occurs 24 or more hours after chemotherapy is administered. It has been reported in as many as 93% of patients receiving high-dose cisplatin. It is particularly severe in patients receiving dosages greater than 100 mg/m^2. Symptoms may occur 24 to 120 hours after cisplatin administration but are most severe at 48 to 72 hours. Patients who have incomplete control of acute emesis often experience delayed emesis. Delayed nausea and vomiting usually are less severe than those that may occur acutely but can still be important in developing ANV and reducing activity, nutritional state, and hydration. The causes of delayed nausea and vomiting are not known, but different mechanisms appear to play a role in acute and delayed emesis.[90] Symptoms may be caused directly by the action of chemotherapeutic agents or their metabolites on the nervous system or GI tract.[91] In addition to delayed emesis caused by chemotherapy or its metabolites, episodes of delayed vomiting often are associated with provocative events such as brushing teeth, using mouthwash, manipulating dentures, seeing food, and, in the morning, standing up after getting out of bed. A combination of prochlorperazine 10 mg, lorazepam 0.5 mg, and diphenhydramine 50 mg all given orally 1 hour before breakfast, lunch, and dinner has been reported to be successful in controlling delayed emesis secondary to cisplatin therapy.[92] In a randomized, double-blind trial, the combination of oral dexamethasone and metoclopramide decreased the frequency of delayed vomiting.[93] The Italian Group for Antiemetic Research found similar protection in treating cisplatin-induced delayed emesis when ondansetron plus dexamethasone or high-dose metoclopramide plus dexamethasone was used. Their study also reinforced the observation that patients who had complete control of acute emesis had a much lower incidence of delayed-onset emesis.[94] The 5-HT_3 receptor antagonists have been no more effective than placebo in controlling delayed emesis secondary to cisplatin therapy when given alone.[95–97]

It has been noted recently that if complete 24-hour control after cisplatin administration is not achieved, emesis usually begins at 17 to 22 hours. This raises the question of whether this is the start of delayed emesis, even though, by definition, 24 hours had not passed.[50,98] Gralla et al.[98] devised a study that demonstrated that ondansetron plus dexamethasone started 16 hours after cisplatin administration was more successful (62% versus 52%) than metoclopramide plus dexamethasone[93] in controlling delayed vomiting.

Postoperative Nausea and Vomiting

PONV is a complication of many surgical procedures. Its incidence is multifactorial, and it is often associated with concurrent illnesses, analgesic use, preoperative level of anxiety, age (children have a higher incidence than adults), length of surgical procedure, type of procedure, anesthetics or type of anesthesia, history of motion sickness, and sex (women have a higher incidence than men). Over the last few years, this disorder has received greater attention because of the increase in outpatient surgical procedures. PONV can lengthen the patient's recovery time and significantly delay release from an ambulatory surgical center, even to the point of necessitating hospital admission.[99] Serious complications of PONV are uncommon, but the patient can become dehydrated or experience electrolyte abnormalities that can delay wound healing or lead to other complications. Because the incidence of PONV varies widely and results from a variety of causes, the clinician must look carefully at many factors (including cost-effectiveness) when choosing prophylactic or therapeutic drug therapy for this disorder.

Scopolamine has long been used to prevent and treat PONV because it decreases the volume of gastric secretions and reduces GI motility. Several investigators have looked at the use of transdermal scopolamine to manage PONV. In outpatient ear surgery, the drug reduced but did not eliminate PONV and vertigo.[100] In patients undergoing outpatient laparoscopic procedures, transdermal scopolamine proved to be slightly better than placebo and allowed patients to be discharged from the outpatient center earlier.[101] The drug can cause hallucinations, delirium, and coma in the high dosing ranges as well as the more common anticholinergic effects of constipation, urinary retention, blurred vision, and dry mouth.

The antihistamines (promethazine and cyclizine) and the phenothiazines (perphenazine and prochlorperazine) have been long used to prevent and treat PONV. They are inexpensive and have been proven in many studies over many years. Promethazine and cyclizine should be used only with caution in children because they may be at greater risk of experiencing the central nervous system stimulant effects often associated with antihistamines. Perphenazine and prochlorperazine also have limited usefulness in both children and adults because they may cause extrapyramidal symptoms.

Droperidol is another effective agent for PONV, and at one time it was available as a combination product with fentanyl (Innovar) for neuroleptic anesthesia. This agent has been studied extensively for preventing and treating PONV. Droperidol has been studied in combination with propofol[102] and also added to patient-controlled analgesia[103] with varying degrees of effectiveness for PONV.

Metoclopramide has also been used extensively for PONV. Like droperidol and the phenothiazines, metoclopramide can cause extrapyramidal reactions. Metoclopramide and droperidol have been compared often in studies of PONV and have been found to have similar efficacy rates.

As one might expect, serotonin antagonists have proven to work in preventing and treating PONV. Ondansetron and dolasetron have been studied and found to have very few adverse effects. Tramer et al. completed a systematic review of randomized placebo-controlled trials using ondansetron to prevent PONV and found that if the risk of PONV was very high, for every 100 patients receiving an adequate dosage of ondansetron, 20 patients would not vomit who would have vomited had they received placebo.[104]

Many other therapies for PONV have been tried with varying success. Maintaining good hydration and adequate blood pressure and avoiding excess movement of the patient limits the incidence of PONV. The anesthetic induction and maintenance agent propofol,[105] nitrous oxide anesthesia,[106] ephedrine,[107] ginger,[108] and various combinations of antiemetics have all been studied and found to be effective for PONV. Unfortunately, no one medication or combination has been found to be the therapy of choice for this disorder. The serotonin antagonists may have the best efficacy, but because there is no good way to predict which patients will develop PONV, it is not cost-effective to use these drugs in all patients undergoing operative procedures. When determining which antiemetic to use, the clinician should consider the patient's preoperative level of anxiety, previous history of nausea and vomiting with surgery or opioids, experience with motion sickness, and response to particular antiemetics in the past. Careful evaluation of the individual patient should direct the choice of therapy in this disorder.

Motion Sickness

Motion sickness is not a true sickness but rather a normal response to an abnormal situation. Any healthy person can experience this response given the right type and degree of stimulation. The susceptibility to motion sickness varies greatly, with approximately one-third of people being very sensitive, one-third reacting only to rough conditions, and one-third reacting only to extreme conditions. Although there is no question about the physical basis of motion sickness, it is also very clear that psychological factors play an important part in both suppressing and enhancing the tendency to be sick.

The stimuli that produce motion sickness arise in the labyrinth of the inner ear. They are carried by afferent fibers that synapse in the vestibular region of the medulla, where they are thought to stimulate the release of an excessive amount of acetylcholine that acts on the CTZ, which then stimulates the VC.[1,109] A proposed theory suggests that motion sickness arises when there is conflict between the sensory information being transmitted by the eyes, vestibular system, and nonvestibular proprioceptors, particularly as it relates to previous experience. As a result of this conflict, an imbalance of cholinergic and sympathetic transmitters occurs in the medulla, which can be corrected by giving anticholinergic drugs or sympathomimetics. The vestibular system plays the central role. True immunity to motion sickness is possible only in a person who lacks a normally functioning peripheral vestibular system.

Nausea is the most common symptom of motion sickness, but most patients experience several other symptoms including pallor, yawning, restlessness, and cold sweats. Vomiting does not inevitably result from nausea because elimination of the offending stimulus can prevent it. The importance of conflicting sensory stimuli as a cause of motion sickness is illustrated in a practical way by the relief obtained when the person can establish a satisfactory stable visual reference. For example, looking out of a car window (particularly from the front seat) can give marked relief, whereas reading in a car (particularly in the rear seat) can provoke motion sickness.

Despite the very extensive literature on anti–motion sickness drug testing, there is a distinct lack of basic clinical pharmacology such as dose-response relationships and pharmacokinetic parameters. In accordance with the sensory conflict theory of motion sickness, drugs used to treat motion sickness would need to block acetylcholine or enhance norepinephrine activity in the central nervous system. Drugs that have proven effective include sympathomimetics and anticholinergics (Table 26.7). The choice of drug or drug combination depends on the expected duration and severity of the reaction. For very severe conditions, as might be experienced by an astronaut adapting to weightlessness, combinations of scopolamine and dexamphetamine or amphetamine have shown the greatest efficacy.[110] Such combinations have the advantage that the stimulatory effects of the amphetamine offset the drowsiness caused by the scopolamine. Unfortunately, the tendency for amphetamines to be abused limits their usefulness in this disorder. Combinations of ephedrine and promethazine also are very effective and have been ranked just below the amphetamine–scopolamine combination.[41] Dosages are given in Table 26.7.

Of the single drugs, oral scopolamine (0.2 to 0.6 mg) is the most effective for short periods of exposure (less than 6 hours). Unfortunately, the commercially prepared oral dosage form is not available in the United States. For longer periods or for moderate to mild conditions, the antihistamines are the drugs of choice. Of these, promethazine 25 mg and dimenhydrinate 50 to 100 mg appears to be the most effective.[41] Transdermal scopolamine has been used successfully to treat motion sickness of several days' duration. It can be applied before entering situations in which motion sickness is likely to occur. All anti–motion sickness drugs are more effective if used prophylactically rather than after sickness has developed.

For patients with severe motion sickness, the oral route may be unavailable and therapy can be given by the intramuscular route. Scopolamine (0.2 mg) or promethazine (50 mg) (adult dosages) may be given. Promethazine probably is the preferred injectable medication for acute motion sickness, and transdermal scopolamine could be used if a rapid onset is not necessary.

In therapeutic dosages, all drugs used to treat motion sickness cause side effects. Anticholinergic drugs produce dry mouth, sedation, and blurred vision. The sympathomimetics produce tachycardia. In the case of scopolamine, the total dosage should not exceed 1 mg in 24 hours because of effects on the central nervous system.

Nonpharmacologic therapy has also proven very suc-

Table 26.7 ▪ Dosages and Duration of Action of Anti–Motion Sickness Drugs

Severity of Sickness	Drug	Oral Dosage[a]	Duration of Action (hr)
Severe	Scopolamine and dexamphetamine	0.2–0.6 mg scopolamine and 5–10 mg dexamphetamine[b]	6
Severe	Promethazine and ephedrine	25 mg promethazine and 25 mg TID ephedrine	12
Severe	Scopolamine	0.2–0.6 mg q6h[c]	4
Severe	Promethazine	25 mg TID	12
Moderate	Dimenhydrinate	50 mg 2–3 × daily	6
Mild	Cyclizine	50 mg 2–3 × daily	4
Mild	Meclizine	50 mg 2–3 × daily	6

[a]Antimotion drugs are most effective if therapy is initiated before exposure to motion. Therapy usually should be initiated about 30 min before departure and repeated if necessary.

[b]Used only under special circumstances (e.g., by service personnel).

[c]No more than four doses should be taken in 24 hr.

cessful in preventing and treating motion sickness. Behavioral modification can be effective for people whose employment involves frequent exposure to motion (e.g., pilots, sailors). Powdered ginger root was used in a double-blind, placebo-controlled study in passengers on an ocean cruise and found to significantly reduce the tendency to vomit and have cold sweats.[111] Acupuncture and acupressure have also been studied extensively. In acupressure techniques, a wrist band with a pressure button located over the Neiguan (P6) acupoint is worn by the patient. This technique has been found quite effective in preventing motion sickness and treating PONV.[112]

Psychogenic Vomiting

Psychogenic vomiting can be self-induced or it can occur involuntarily in response to situations that the person considers threatening or distasteful (e.g., eating food whose origin is considered repulsive).

When a person presents with chronic or recurrent vomiting, a diagnosis of psychogenic vomiting is made after all other possible causes are eliminated (Table 26.1). The person with psychogenic vomiting usually does not lose weight and can control vomiting in certain situations (e.g., in public). It may not be possible to identify the causes of psychogenic vomiting and resolve the problem. A short course of an antiemetic drug such as metoclopramide or antianxiety drugs may be prescribed, along with counseling to treat psychogenic vomiting.

CONCLUSION

Nausea and vomiting ranges from a minor inconvenience of a transient GI infection to a severe and limiting adverse reaction to drug therapy. The consequences of vomiting can be severe. The cause of the nausea and vomiting should be determined before treatment is begun, and specific therapy should be chosen for each cause. Drug regimens specifically designed for the patient and the cause of nausea and vomiting, based on valid clinical studies, have a high success rate in treating this disorder. However, care should be taken to minimize any side effects from the antiemetic drugs.

KEY POINTS

Nausea and Vomiting

- An accurate diagnosis is essential before treatment of nausea and vomiting begins.
- Treat the cause if it can be identified.
- Assess for fluid and electrolyte loss.

Chemotherapy-Induced Emesis

- There are three types of CIE: ANV, acute CIE, and delayed emesis.
- The emetogenic potential of antineoplastic drugs varies significantly (Table 26.6).
- Antiemetics are most effective when administered 30 to 60 minutes before chemotherapy is administered.
- All patients being treated with moderate to very high emetogenic chemotherapeutic agents should receive prophylactic antiemetic therapy. Combinations of a serotonin antagonist plus dexamethasone, plus lorazepam, plus prochlorperazine are the drugs of choice.
- Emesis induced by moderately emetogenic agents may be treated prophylactically with metoclopramide and dexamethasone.
- Prochlorperazine or dexamethasone alone is recommended if the chemotherapy is of low emetic potential.

Postoperative Nausea and Vomiting

- The causes of PONV are multifactorial.
- A review of the patient's previous history can help determine who would benefit from prophylactic antiemetic therapy.
- Maintaining good hydration and adequate blood pressure and avoiding excess movement of the patient limit the incidence of PONV.
- No one medication or combination has been found to be the therapy of choice for PONV. Scopolamine, phenothiazines, metoclopramide, droperidol, and the serotonin antagonists often are used to prevent PONV.
- The serotonin antagonists have good success rates and the fewest side effects but are the most expensive.

Motion Sickness

- Antiemetics are most effective when administered 30 to 60 minutes before activities that may induce motion sickness.
- Anticholinergic drugs have been studied the most extensively and are most frequently recommended (e.g., scopolamine, promethazine, diphenhydramine).
- Patients who experience motion sickness routinely because of their occupation might best be treated with behavioral therapy rather than drugs.

REFERENCES

1. Barnes JH. The physiology and pharmacology of emesis. Mol Aspects Med 7:397–508, 1984.
2. Grunberg SM. Control of chemotherapy-induced emesis. N Engl J Med 329:1790–1796, 1993.
3. Mitchelson F. Pharmacological agents affecting emesis. Drugs 43:295–315, 1992.
4. Cubeddu LX, Hoffmann IS, Fuenmayor NT, et al, Efficacy of ondansetron (GR38032F) and the role of serotonin in cisplatin-induced nausea and vomiting. N Engl J Med 322:810–816, 1990.
5. Bermudez J, Boyle EA, Miner WD, et al. The antiemetic potential of the 5-hydroxytryptamine$_3$ receptor antagonist BRL 43694. Br J Cancer 58:644–650, 1988.
6. Malagelada JR, Camilleri M. Unexplained vomiting: a diagnostic challenge. Ann Intern Med 101:211–218, 1984.
7. Wampler G. Pharmacology and clinical effectiveness of phenothiazines and related drugs for managing chemotherapy-induced emesis. Drugs 25(Suppl 1):35–51, 1983.
8. Carr B, Doroshow J, Blayney D, et al. Toxicity and dose-response studies of prochlorperazine for cisplatin-induced emesis [abstract]. Proc Am Soc Clin Oncol 5:252, 1986.

9. Olver IN, Bishop JF, Hollcoat BL, et al. A phase-I dose finding study for intravenous prochlorperazine as an antiemetic for chemotherapy induced emesis [abstract]. Proc Am Soc Clin Oncol 7:287, 1988.
10. Carr BI, Somlo G, McDevitt J, et al. Pharmacokinetic profiles of high- and low-dose prochlorperazine [abstract]. Proc Am Soc Clin Oncol 7:294, 1988.
11. Fozard JR. Neuronal 5-HT receptors in the periphery. Neuropharmacol 23:1473–1486, 1984.
12. Gralla RJ. Metoclopramide: a review of antiemetic trials. Drugs 25:63–73, 1983.
13. McGovern EM, Grevel J, Bryson SM. Pharmacokinetics of high-dose metoclopramide in cancer patients. Clin Pharmacokinet 11:415–424, 1986.
14. Bateman DN. Clinical pharmacokinetics of metoclopramide. Clin Pharmacokinet 8:523–529, 1983.
15. Grevel J, Whiting B, Kelman AW, et al. Population analysis of the pharmacokinetic variability of high-dose metoclopramide in cancer patients. Clin Pharmacokinet 14:52–63, 1983.
16. Parrish RH, Bonzo SM. Use of metoclopramide suppositories. Clin Pharm 2:395–396, 1983.
17. Tami JA, Waite WW. Metoclopramide suppository considerations. Drug Intell Clin Pharm 22:268–269, 1988.
18. Product information for Zofran. Research Triangle Park, NC: GlaxoWellcome, December 1996.
19. Product information for Anzemet. Kansas City, MO: Hoechst Marion Roussel, October 1997.
20. Balfour JA, Goa KL. Dolasetron. Drugs 54:273–298, 1997.
21. Sanwald P, David M, Jow J. Characterization of the cytochrome P-450 enzymes involved in the in vitro metabolism of dolasetron. Drug Metab Dispos 24:602–609, 1996.
22. Product information for Kytril. Philadelphia: SmithKline Beecham, October 1997.
23. Marty M, Pouillart P, Scholl S. Comparison of the 5-hydroxytryptamine$_3$ (serotonin) antagonist ondansetron (GR38032F) with high-dose metoclopramide in the control of cisplatin-induced emesis. N Engl J Med 322:816–821, 1990.
24. Mathews H. Extrapyramidal reaction caused by ondansetron. Ann Pharmacother 30:196, 1996.
25. De Mulder PHM, Selynaeve C, Vermorken JB, et al. Ondansetron compared with high-dose metoclopramide in prophylaxis of acute and delayed cisplatin-induced nausea and vomiting. Ann Intern Med 113:834–840, 1990.
26. Hesketh PJ. Comparative trials of ondansetron vs. metoclopramide in the prevention of acute cisplatin-induced emesis. Semin Oncol 19(Suppl 10):33–40, 1992.
27. Sledge G Jr, Einhorn L, Nagy C. Phase III double-blind comparison of intravenous ondansetron and metoclopramide as antiemetic therapy for patients receiving multiple-day cisplatin-based chemotherapy. Cancer 70: 2524–2528, 1992.
28. Tsavaris N, Charalambidis G, Ganas N, et al. Ondansetron versus metoclopramide as antiemetic treatment during cisplatin-based chemotherapy. Acta Oncol 34:243–246, 1995.
29. Ruff P, Paska W, Goedhals L, et al. Ondansetron compared with granisetron in the prophylaxis of cisplatin-induced acute emesis: a multicenter double-blind, randomized, parallel-group study. Oncology 51:113–118, 1994.
30. Jantunen I, Muhonen T, Kataja V, et al. 5-HT$_3$ receptor antagonists in the prophylaxis of acute vomiting induced by moderately emetogenic chemotherapy: a randomized study. Eur J Cancer 29A:1669–1672, 1993.
31. Noble A, Bremer K, Goedhals L, et al. A double-blind, randomized, crossover comparison of granisetron and ondansetron in 5-day fractionated chemotherapy: assessment of efficacy, safety and patient preference. Eur J Cancer 30A:1083–1088, 1994.
32. Gebbia V, Cannata G, Testa A, et al. Ondansetron versus granisetron in the prevention of chemotherapy induced nausea and vomiting: results of a prospective, randomized trial. Cancer 74:1945–1952, 1994.
33. Navari R, Gandara D, Hesketh S, et al. Comparative clinical trial of granisetron and ondansetron in the prophylaxis of cisplatin-induced emesis. J Clin Oncol 13:1242–1248, 1995.
34. Park J, Rha S, Yoo N, et al. A comparative study of intravenous granisetron versus intravenous and oral ondansetron in the prevention of nausea and vomiting associated with moderately emetogenic chemotherapy. Am J Clin Oncol 20:569–572, 1997.
35. Hesketh P, Navari R, Grote T, et al. Double-blind, randomized comparison of the antiemetic efficacy of intravenous dolasetron mesylate and intravenous ondansetron in the prevention of acute cisplatin-induced emesis in patients with cancer. J Clin Oncol 14:2242–2249, 1996.
36. Fauser AA, Duclos B, Chemaissani A, et al. Therapeutic equivalence of single oral doses of dolasetron mesylate and multiple doses of ondansetron for the prevention of emesis after moderately emetogenic chemotherapy. Eur J Cancer 32A:1523–1529, 1996.
37. Pater J, Lofters W, Zee B, et al. The role of the 5-HT$_3$ antagonists ondansetron and dolasetron in the control of delayed onset nausea and vomiting in patients receiving moderately emetogenic chemotherapy. Ann Oncol 8:181–185, 1997.
38. Audhuy B, Cappelaere P, Martin M, et al. A double-blind, randomized comparison of the anti-emetic efficacy of two intravenous doses of dolasetron mesylate and granisetron in patients receiving high dose cisplatin chemotherapy. Eur J Cancer 32A:807–813, 1996.
39. Alexander R, Fennelly M. Comparison of ondansetron, metoclopramide and placebo as premedicants to reduce nausea and vomiting after major surgery. Anaesthesia 52:695–703, 1997.
40. Tang J, Wang B, White PF, et al. Effect of timing on ondansetron administration on its efficacy, cost-effectiveness, and cost-benefit as a prophylactic antiemetic in the ambulatory setting. Anesth Analg 86:274–282, 1998.
41. Wood CD. Antimotion sickness and antiemetic drugs. Drugs 17:471–479, 1985.
42. Clissold SP, Heel RC. Transdermal hyoscine (scopolamine): a preliminary review of its pharmacodynamic properties and therapeutic efficacy. Drugs 29:189–207, 1985.
43. Allen LV. Scopolamine topical gel for travelers. US Pharmacist March:22–23, 1995.
44. Cersosimo RJ, Karp DD. Adrenal corticosteroids as antiemetics during cancer chemotherapy. Pharmacotherapy 6:118–127, 1986.
45. Kris MG, Gralla RJ, Tyson LB, et al. Improved control of cisplatin-induced emesis with high-dose metoclopramide and with combinations of metoclopramide, dexamethasone and diphenhydramine. Cancer 55:527–534, 1985.
46. du Bois A, McKenna C, Andersson H, et al. A randomised, double-blind, parallel-group study to compare the efficacy and safety of ondansetron (GR38032F) plus dexamethasone with metoclopramide plus dexamethasone in the prophylaxis of nausea and emesis induced by carboplatin chemotherapy. Oncology 54:7–14, 1997.
47. Italian Group for Antiemetic Research. Dexamethasone, granisetron, or both for the prevention of nausea and vomiting during chemotherapy for cancer. N Engl J Med 332:1–5, 1995.
48. Italian Group for Antiemetic Research. Persistence of efficacy of three antiemetic regimens and prognostic factors in patients undergoing moderately emetogenic chemotherapy. J Clin Oncol 13:2417–2426, 1995.
49. Kirchner V, Aapro M, Terrey J-P, et al. A double-blind crossover study comparing prophylactic intravenous granisetron alone or in combination with dexamethasone as antiemetic treatment in controlling nausea and vomiting associated with chemotherapy. Eur J Cancer 33:1605–1610, 1997.
50. Kris M, Pendergrass K, Navari R, et al. Prevention of acute emesis in cancer patients following high-dose cisplatin with the combination of oral dolasetron and dexamethasone. J Clin Oncol 15:2135–2138, 1997.
51. Pectasides D, Mylonakis A, Varthalitis J, et al. Comparison of two different doses of ondansetron plus dexamethasone in the prophylaxis of cisplatin-induced emesis. Oncology 54:1–6, 1997.
52. Vincent BJ, McQuiston DJ, Einhorn LH, et al. Review of cannabinoids and their antiemetic effectiveness. Drugs 25(Suppl 1):52–62, 1983.
53. Anderson PO, McGuire GG. Delta-9-tetrahydrocannabinol as an antiemetic. Am J Hosp Pharm 38:639–646, 1981.
54. Devine ML, Dow GJ, Greenberg BR, et al. Adverse reactions to delta-9-tetrahydrocannabinol given as an antiemetic in a multicenter study. Clin Pharm 6:319–322, 1987.
55. Voth E, Schwartz R. Medicinal applications of delta-9-tetrahydrocannabinol and marijuana. Ann Intern Med 126:791–798, 1997.
56. Ward A, Holmes B. Nabilone: a preliminary review of its pharmacological properties and therapeutic use. Drugs 30:127–144, 1985.
57. Kearsley JH, Tattersall MHN. Recent advances in the prevention and reduction of cytotoxic-induced emesis. Med J Aust 143:341–346, 1985.
58. Bishop JF, Oliver IN, Wolf MM, et al. Lorazepam: a randomized double-blind crossover study of a new antiemetic in patients receiving cytotoxic chemotherapy and prochlorperazine. J Clin Oncol 2:691–695, 1984.
59. Kris MG, Gralla RJ, Clark RA, et al. Consecutive dose-finding trials adding lorazepam to the combination of metoclopramide plus dexamethasone: improved subjective effectiveness over the combination of diphenhydramine plus metoclopramide plus dexamethasone. Cancer Treat Rep 69:1257–1262, 1985.
60. Penta JS, Poster DS, Bruna S, et al. Cancer chemotherapy induced nausea and vomiting in adult and pediatric patients. Am Soc Clin Oncol 4:396, 1981.
61. Gralla RJ, Tyson LB, Kris MG, et al. The management of chemotherapy-induced nausea and vomiting. Med Clin North Am 70:289–301, 1987.
62. Chin S, Kucuk O, Peterson R, et al. Variables contributing to anticipatory nausea and vomiting in cancer chemotherapy. Am J Clin Oncol 15:262–267, 1992.

63. Moher D, Arthur AZ, Pater JL. Anticipatory nausea and/or vomiting. Cancer Treat Rev 11:257–264, 1984.
64. Alba E, Roma B, de Andres L, et al. Anticipatory nausea and vomiting: prevalence and predictors in chemotherapy patients. Oncology 46:26–30, 1989.
65. Dolgin MJ, Katz ER, McGinty K, et al. Anticipatory nausea and vomiting in pediatric cancer patients. Pediatrics 75:547–552, 1985.
66. Stoudemire A, Cotanch P, Laszlo J. Recent advances in the pharmacologic and behavioral management of chemotherapy-induced emesis. Arch Intern Med 144:1029–1033, 1984.
67. Laszlo J, Clark RA, Hanson DC, et al. Lorazepam in cancer patients treated with cisplatin: a drug having antiemetic, amnesic and anxiolytic effects. J Clin Oncol 3:864–869, 1985.
68. Kris MG, Gralla RJ, Clark RA, et al. Consecutive dose-finding trails adding lorazepam to the combination of metoclopramide plus dexamethasone: improved subjective effectiveness over the combination of diphenhydramine plus metoclopramide plus dexamethasone. Cancer Treat Rep 69:1257–1262, 1985.
69. Pater JL, Willian AR. Methodologic issues in trials of antiemetics. J Clin Oncol 2:484–497, 1984.
70. Hesketh P, Kris M, Grunberg S, et al. Proposal for classifying the acute emetogenicity of cancer chemotherapy. J Clin Oncol 15:103–109, 1997.
71. O'Brien MER, Cullen MH. Are we making progress in the management of cytotoxic drug-induced nausea and vomiting? J Clin Pharmacol Ther 13:19–31, 1988.
72. Berard C, Mahoney C. Cost-reducing treatment algorithms for antineoplastic drug-induced nausea and vomiting. Am J Health Syst Pharm 52:1879–1885, 1995.
73. Smith DB, Newlands ES, Spruyt OW, et al. Ondansetron (GR380032F) plus dexamethasone: effective antiemetic prophylaxis for patients receiving cytotoxic chemotherapy. Br J Cancer 61:323–324, 1990.
74. Cunningham D, Turner A, Hawthorn J, et al. Ondansetron with and without dexamethasone to treat chemotherapy-induced emesis. Lancet 1:1323, 1989.
75. Italian Group for Antiemetic Research. Ondansetron + dexamethasone vs metoclopramide + dexamethasone + diphenhydramine in prevention of cisplatin-induced emesis. Lancet 340:96–99, 1992.
76. Chevallier B. The control of acute cisplatin-induced emesis: a comparative study of granisetron and a combination regimen of high-dose metoclopramide and dexamethasone. Br J Cancer 68:176–180, 1993.
77. Craig JB, Powell BL. Review: the management of nausea and vomiting in clinical oncology. Am J Med Sci 293:34–44, 1987.
78. Browman GP, Levine MN, Mohide EA, et al. The practice guidelines development cycle: a conceptual tool for practice guidelines development and implementation. J Clin Oncol 13:502–512, 1995.
79. Mahoney CD, Berard CM, Simas EA, et al. Implementing a chemotherapy practice standard in an integrated health care system. Hosp Pharm 33:954–960, 1998.
80. Osoba D, Warr DG, Fitch MI, et al. Guidelines for the optimal management of chemotherapy-induced nausea and vomiting: a consensus. Can J Oncol 5:381–399, 1995.
81. Trovato J, Stull D, Finley R. Outcomes of antiemetic therapy after the administration of high-dose antineoplastic agents. Am J Health Syst Pharm 55:1269–1274, 1998.
82. Perez E, Hesketh P, Sandbach J, et al. Comparison of single-dose oral granisetron versus intravenous ondansetron in the prevention of nausea and vomiting induced by moderately emetogenic chemotherapy: a multicenter, double-blind, randomized parallel study. J Clin Oncol 16:754–760, 1998.
83. Nolte M, Berkery R, Pizzo B. Assuring the optimal use of serotonin antagonist antiemetics: the process for development and implementation of institutional antiemetic guidelines at Memorial Sloan-Kettering cancer center. J Clin Oncol 16:771–778, 1998.
84. Schipper H, Clinch J, McMurray A, et al. Measuring the quality of life of cancer patients. The functional living index, cancer: development and validation. J Clin Oncol 2:472–483, 1984.
85. Lindley CM, Hirsch JD, O'Neill CV, et al. Quality of life consequences of chemotherapy-induced emesis. Qual Life Res 1:331–340, 1992.
86. de Boer-Dennert M, de Wit R, Schmitz P, et al. Patient perceptions of the side effects of chemotherapy: the influence of $5HT_3$ antagonists. Br J Cancer 76:1055–1061, 1997.
87. Farley P, Dempsey C, Shillington A, et al. Patients' self-reported functional status after granisetron or ondansetron therapy to prevent chemotherapy-induced nausea and vomiting at six cancer centers. Am J Health Syst Pharm 54:2478–2482, 1997.
88. Osoba D, Zee B, Pater J, et al. Psychometric properties and responsiveness of the EORTC Quality of Life Questionnaire (QLQ-C30) in patients with breast, ovarian and lung cancer. Qual Life Res 3:353–364, 1994.
89. Osoba D, Zee B, Warr D, et al. Quality of life studies in chemotherapy-induced emesis. Oncology 53(Suppl 1):92–95, 1996.
90. Morrow G, Hickok J, Burish T, et al. Frequency and clinical implications of delayed nausea and delayed emesis. Am J Clin Oncol 19:199–203, 1996.
91. Kris MG, Gralla RJ, Clark RA, et al. Incidence, course, and severity of delayed nausea and vomiting following the administration of high dose cisplatin. J Clin Oncol 3:1379–1384, 1985.
92. Sridhar KS, Donnelly E. Combination antiemetics for cisplatin chemotherapy. Cancer 61:1508–1517, 1988.
93. Kris MG, Gralla RJ, Tyson LB, et al. Controlling delayed vomiting: double blind, randomized trial comparing placebo, dexamethasone alone and metoclopramide plus dexamethasone in patients receiving cisplatin. J Clin Oncol 7:108–114, 1989.
94. Italian Group for Antiemetic Research. Ondansetron versus metoclopramide, both combined with dexamethasone, in the prevention of cisplatin-induced delayed emesis. J Clin Oncol 15:124–130, 1997.
95. Kris MG, Tyson LB, Clark RA, et al. Oral Ondansetron for the control of delayed emesis after cisplatin. Cancer 70(Suppl):1012–1016, 1992.
96. Pater J, Lofters W, Zee B, et al. The role of the 5-HT_3 antagonists ondansetron and dolasetron in the control of delayed onset nausea and vomiting in patients receiving moderately emetogenic chemotherapy. Ann Oncol 8:181–185, 1997.
97. Hesketh P. Management of cisplatin-induced delayed emesis. Oncology 53(Suppl 1):73–77, 1996.
98. Gralla R, Rittenberg C, Peralta M, et al. Cisplatin and emesis: aspects of treatment and a new trial for delayed emesis using oral dexamethasone plus ondansetron beginning at 16 hours after cisplatin. Oncology 53(Suppl 1):86–91, 1996.
99. Gold BS, Kitz DS, Lecky JH, et al. Unanticipated admission to the hospital following ambulatory surgery. JAMA 262:3008–3010, 1989.
100. Reinhart DJ, Klein KW, Schroff E. Transdermal scopolamine for the reduction of postoperative nausea in outpatient ear surgery: a double-blind, randomized study. Anesth Analg 79:281–284, 1994.
101. Bailey PL, Streisand JB, Pace NL, et al. Transdermal scopolamine reduces nausea and vomiting after outpatient laparoscopy. Anesthesiology 72:977–980, 1990.
102. Wagner BKJ, Berman SL, Devitt PA, et al. Retrospective analysis of postoperative nausea and vomiting to determine antiemetic activity of droperidol added to propofol: a possible drug interaction. Pharmacotherapy 14:586–591, 1994.
103. Woodhouse A, Mather LE. Nausea and vomiting in the postoperative patient-controlled analgesia environment. Anaesthesia 52:770–775, 1997.
104. Tramèr MR, Reynolds JM, Moore RA, et al. Efficacy, dose-response, and safety of ondansetron in prevention of postoperative nausea and vomiting. Anesthesiology 87:1277–1289, 1997.
105. Montgomery JE, Sutherland CJ, Kestin IG, et al. Infusions of subhypnotic doses of propofol for the prevention of postoperative nausea and vomiting. Anaesthesia 51:554–557, 1996.
106. Hovorka J, Korttila K. Nitrous oxide does not increase nausea and vomiting following gynaecological laparoscopy. Can J Anaesth 36:145–148, 1989.
107. Liu YC, Kang HM, Liou CM, et al. Comparison of antiemetic effect among ephedrine, droperidol and metoclopramide in pediatric inguinal hernioplasty. Acta Anaesthesiol Sin 30:37–42, 1992.
108. Philips S, Ruggier R, Hutchinson SE. *Zingiber officinale* (ginger): an antiemetic for day case surgery. Anaesthesia 48:111–120, 1993.
109. Reason JT, Brand JJ. Motion sickness. New York: Academic Press, 1975.
110. Wood CD, Manno JE, Wood MJ, et al. Mechanisms of antimotion sickness drugs. Aviat Space Environ Med 58(Suppl):A262–265, 1987.
111. Grontved A, Brask T, Kambskard J, et al. Ginger root against seasickness. A controlled trial on the open sea. Acta Otolaryngol 105:45–49, 1988.
112. Stein DJ, Birnback DJ, Danzer BI, et al. Acupressure versus intravenous metoclopramide to prevent nausea and vomiting during spinal anesthesia for cesarean section. Anesth Analg 84:821–825, 1997.

CHAPTER 27

CONSTIPATION AND DIARRHEA

Valerie W. Hogue

Constipation and diarrhea are common disorders of the gastrointestinal system that most people experience at some time in their lives. Generally, these symptoms are self-limiting and may not necessitate intervention. However, patients may consider intervention necessary because of their beliefs and attitudes toward normal bowel function. Constipation and diarrhea can affect the ability to carry out work or school responsibilities, and loss of productivity usually necessitates prompt and effective intervention.

Symptoms of diarrhea and constipation may result from various disease states, medications, dietary changes, food or water contamination, and even psychological distress. Many over-the-counter (OTC) products are available in the United States for resolving the symptoms. The pharmacist's consultation is important for proper use of these products during self-treatment. The pharmacist must ascertain the possible cause of these symptoms to prevent masking a serious medical problem and to deter laxative and antidiarrheal abuse.

Constipation and Diarrhea

DEFINITION

The definitions of diarrhea and constipation have been debated for several years, primarily because of variations in the definition of normal bowel habits. Most clinicians agree that no single definition describes either medical problem effectively.

Clinicians generally incorporate two primary aspects in the definition of constipation: difficulty passing stools and infrequent stools. However, patients may describe constipation as less frequent defecation than is normally observed, lower stool volume, difficulty passing stool, hard or firm stool, straining upon defecation, a sensation of

Table 27.1 ▪ General, Systemic, and Psychological Causes of Constipation

Lifestyle factors	
	Inadequate fluid intake
	Decreased food intake
	Ignored defecation urge
	Immobility
External factors	
	Medications
Endocrine and metabolic	
	Hypothyroidism
	Hypercalcemia
	Porphyria
Neurologic	
	Parkinson's disease
	Multiple sclerosis
	Spinal lesions
	Damage to sacral parasympathetic nerves
	Autonomic neuropathy
	Autonomic failure
Psychological	
	Depression
	Eating disorders (e.g., anorexia nervosa)
	Misconceptions about "inner cleanliness"
	Denied bowel activity

Source: Adapted with permission. Lennard-Jones JE. Constipation. In: Feldman M, Scharschmidt BF, Sleisenger MH. Gastrointestinal and liver disease: pathophysiology/diagnosis/management. 6th ed. Philadelphia: WB Saunders, 1998:176.

incomplete evacuation of bowel, or the lack of an urge to stool. A study of young adults not seeking health care asked 568 subjects to define constipation. They emphasized function (straining) and consistency (hard stools) rather than the number of stools in their definition.[1] Therefore, determining the patient's definition is essential.

Diarrhea has been described more consistently than constipation. Generally, it is defined as three or more loose or unformed bowel movements per day, accompanied by symptoms of fever, abdominal cramps, or vomiting. It has been further described as a condition of abnormal increases in stool weight and liquidity. An increase in stool water excretion above 150 mL every 24 hours is an objective parameter for acute diarrhea.[2]

TREATMENT GOALS: CONSTIPATION AND DIARRHEA

- For diarrhea, alleviate the loose stools and accompanying symptoms.
- For constipation, relieve the difficulty in passing stools and the irregularity of bowel movements.
- Prevent complications associated with diarrhea, including dehydration and electrolyte losses.
- Prevent complications associated with constipation, including hemorrhoids and anal fissures.
- Restore normal bowel habits by increasing or decreasing frequency of defecation based on presenting problem.
- Restore normal bowel consistency.

Table 27.2 ▪ Gastrointestinal Causes of Constipation and Related Symptoms

Gastrointestinal tract	
	Obstruction
	Aganglionosis (Hirschsprung's disease, Chagas' disease)
	Myopathy
	Neuropathy
	Systemic sclerosis
	Megarectum or megacolon
Anorectum	
	Anal atresia or malformation
	Hereditary internal anal sphincter myopathy
	Anal stenosis
	Weak pelvic floor
	Large rectocele
	Internal intussusception
	Anterior mucosal prolapse
	Prolapse
	Solitary rectal ulcer

Source: Reprinted with permission. Lennard-Jones JE. Constipation. In: Feldman M, Scharschmidt BF, Sleisenger MH. Gastrointestinal and liver disease: pathophysiology/diagnosis/management. 6th ed. Philadelphia: WB Saunders, 1998:177.

Table 27.3 ▪ Medication-Induced Constipation

Antacids (e.g., calcium- and aluminum-containing)
Anticholinergics
Barium sulfate
Bismuth
Calcium channel blockers (e.g., verapamil, diltiazem)
Central α-adrenergic agonists (e.g., clonidine, guanabenz, guanfacine)
Clozapine
Diuretics
Ganglionic blocking agents
Iron
Laxatives (overuse)
Monoamine oxidase inhibitors
Opiates
Phenothiazines
Resins (e.g., cholestyramine, colestipol, polystyrene sulfonate)
Sucralfate
Tricyclic antidepressants
Vincristine

Source: Adapted with permission. Tedesco FJ, DiPiro JT. Laxative use in constipation. Am J Gastroenterol 80(4):303–309, 1985.

EPIDEMIOLOGY

Etiology

Constipation

Constipation may result from underlying systemic disorders or general lifestyle factors (Table 27.1). Diseases producing constipation may be localized to the gastrointestinal tract or anorectum (Table 27.2). Drugs, including the chronic use of laxatives, may induce constipation (Table 27.3). In addition, psychological factors may cause changes in bowel habits, leading to constipation.[3]

Diarrhea

Diarrhea may be caused primarily by inhibition of ion absorption, stimulation of ion secretion, retention of fluid in the intestinal lumen, and disorders of intestinal motility. Retention of fluid in the bowel lumen may be precipitated by carbohydrate malabsorption, disaccharidase deficiencies, lactulose therapy, poorly absorbable salts (magnesium sulfate, sodium phosphate, sodium citrate, antacids), and ingestion of mannitol and sorbitol. Secretagogues from tumors such as vasoactive intestinal polypeptide (VIP), serotonin, and calcitonin may be mediators of secretory diarrhea. Certain medications may act as mediators also (Table 27.4). Disorders of motility may lead to symptoms of diarrhea in irritable bowel syndrome (IBS), diabetic neuropathy, or thyrotoxicosis. Bacterial and viral infections often cause diarrhea (e.g., travelers' diarrhea [TD]). Food intolerance associated with disaccharidase (lactose) deficiency also may result in diarrhea.[4]

Prevalence

Constipation

Although constipation is a common disorder, its prevalence is difficult to define because it lacks a standard definition. However, several studies have assessed its prevalence based on patients' self-report. The incidence of self-reported constipation, diarrhea, and defecation frequency in the United States was estimated from the results of a national, population-based survey.[5] Respondents ranged in age from 25 to 74 years. The majority of the respondents reported daily defecation (73.3% of European Americans, 63.7% of African Americans). The frequency of defecation differed significantly with regard to race and gender but not age. Regardless of gender or race, self-reported constipation was positively correlated with age.

Table 27.4 ▪ Medication-Induced Diarrhea

Acarbose
Antacids (magnesium-containing)
Antineoplastic agents
Auranofin
Cisapride
Colchicine
Guanethidine
Laxatives
Metformin
Metoclopramide
Misoprostol
Quinidine
Reserpine
Serotonin reuptake inhibitors
Tacrine
Tacrolimus

Source: Hogue VW. The management of constipation and diarrhea. Drug Store News for the Pharmacist 6(3):56–64, 1996. Adapted by permission–Copyright Drug Store News for the Pharmacist, March 1996.

This difference may reflect a difference in the perception of constipation by older adults because the frequency of defecation did not change as age progressed.

In a study of 15,014 men and women aged 12 to 74 years, the overall incidence of self-reported constipation was 12.8% in the U.S. population.[6] It was observed most often in African Americans (17.3%), women (18.2%), and people over 60 years (23%).

Diarrhea

It has been estimated that the incidence of diarrhea in the United States and other industrialized nations is, on average, one episode per person annually.[7] It is of special concern in older adults because the majority of deaths associated with diarrheal illnesses in the United States occur in this population. In addition, adults who care for infants in day care facilities, international travelers, homosexual men, immunosuppressed patients, and those exposed to contaminated food and water are at greater risk.[8]

PATHOPHYSIOLOGY

An understanding of the normal physiologic flow rate of fluid and electrolytes and the process of defecation is the basis for discussing the development of constipation and diarrhea. Three major aspects of bowel function exist: colonic absorption, colonic motility, and defecation reflexes.

The daily volume of fluid traversing the duodenum is 9 L for people consuming three meals daily. Approximately 8 L fluid per day are absorbed by the small bowel. However, the colon absorbs 0.9 to 1.4 L per day, which is 90% of the fluid presented initially. The absorptive capacity of the colon exceeds that of the small intestine, which absorbs only 75% of the fluid presented initially. Daily fecal output is less than 200 mL, which contains approximately 5 mEq sodium and 8 mEq potassium.

Colonic motility involves three patterns of muscle contractions controlled by the autonomic nervous system: nonpropulsive segmental contractions, which churn the contents of the lumen; short-segment propulsive contractions, which move contents forward and backward, promoting absorption; and long-segment propulsive contractions, which move contents forward over long distances. The urge to defecate occurs when gastric filling and increased physical activity trigger the gastroenteric reflex to produce massive peristalsis. The feces move from the sigmoid colon to the rectum, producing an urge to defecate. This occurs most often after breakfast.[9]

Defecation is initiated by the distension of the rectum by feces. Normally, the rectum can differentiate distension produced by fluids, flatus, and feces through defecation reflexes. Evacuation occurs after the internal and external anal sphincters relax in conjunction with the contraction of the rectosigmoid segment and increased intraabdominal pressure. Voluntary relaxation of the external anal sphincter allows evacuation of the bowel. Conversely, voluntary contraction of the sphincter inhibits defecation.[9]

Constipation

An intact nervous system is vital for normal defecation. Many patients develop constipation secondary to colonic motility disorders caused by congenital or acquired abnormalities of the nervous system. Outlet obstruction, a mechanism of constipation, may be secondary to a hyperactive rectosigmoid junction, increased storage capacity of the rectum, rectal spasticity, and hypertonicity of the anal canal.[3]

Diarrhea

Four physiologic mechanisms may contribute to the development of diarrhea: increased osmolality, intestinal ion secretion, impaired absorption, and inflammatory and ulcerative processes. An understanding of the mechanisms of fluid loss aids in comprehending the mechanism of action of antidiarrheals.[4]

Increased Osmolality (Osmotic Diarrhea)

In general, osmotic diarrhea is caused by the retention of fluid by nonabsorbable solutes in the bowel lumen. Peristalsis is stimulated by the increased fluid volume in the lumen, resulting in increased transit of the fecal matter by the colon. Because the colon is very efficient in the reabsorption of sodium chloride and water, increased transit through the colon promotes diarrhea.

Osmotic diarrhea also is evident when enzymes such as lactase are deficient. Lactase deficiency is common among certain racial groups, such as those of African and Asian descent. Lactase is responsible for the degradation of lactose to glucose and galactose, which are absorbed by the mucosa. In the absence of this enzyme, lactose retains fluid, thereby increasing the volume of water in the stool.

Intestinal Ion Secretion (Secretory Diarrhea)

Two factors contribute to secretory diarrhea: inhibition of ion absorption and intestinal ion secretion. As a result, the stool contains an excess of monovalent ions and water. Enterotoxins produced by certain bacteria stimulate intestinal fluid secretion. Laxatives such as senna and dioctyl sodium sulfosuccinate may also cause this type of diarrhea. Certain hormones such as serotonin, calcitonin, prostaglandin E_1, and VIP have been implicated as mediators of secretory diarrhea.[2]

Altered Intestinal Motility

Changes in intestinal motility may affect fluid and electrolyte absorption within the gut lumen. Increased activity may reduce the surface area and limit the contact time for nutrient absorption.

Inflammatory and Ulcerative Processes

Inflammation and ulceration of the intestinal mucosa often result in the release of mucus, serum proteins, and blood into the lumen. The absorption of water and electrolytes is impaired. This malabsorption is the presumed cause of diarrhea in patients with ulcerative colitis.

Consequences of Diarrhea

Although diarrhea may be uncomplicated and self-limiting, persistent diarrhea may cause serious consequences. Sodium and water deficits secondary to fluid loss are common in persistent diarrhea. Potassium losses of approximately 6 to 7 mEq/kg may be observed in untreated patients, which places the patient at risk of developing paralytic ileus and cardiac arrhythmias if potassium is not replaced appropriately. Fecal loss of bicarbonate and impaired renal excretion of acids may cause metabolic acidosis.

CLINICAL PRESENTATION AND DIAGNOSIS

Constipation

The clinician must obtain a complete history to diagnose constipation. During the interview, the patient's definition of normal bowel function must be ascertained to determine the impact of the change in bowel habit. The onset and duration of constipation, a description of the stool, and the presence of symptoms are necessary information. Medication use should be determined, especially that of OTC laxatives. The physical examination should include an abdominal examination, a digital examination of the rectum, and a proctosigmoidoscopy. A barium enema should be initiated in chronically constipated patients and patients with a recent history of constipation to determine whether obstruction is present.

Diarrhea

A careful history and physical examination are essential for the diagnosis of diarrhea. Ascertaining the duration of diarrhea, the description of the stool (consistency, color, odor, presence or absence of melanic stool), the frequency of bowel movements, associated symptoms, and any underlying disorders is essential to obtaining a thorough history. Distinguishing between large-stool and small-stool diarrhea helps determine whether the underlying disorder originates from the small bowel or proximal colon or the left colon and rectum, respectively.

Several signs and symptoms of diarrhea suggest underlying disease states. Generally, the passage of blood may indicate inflammatory, infectious, or neoplastic disease. Pus or exudate in the stool may indicate inflammation or infection. Infection caused by *Shigella* has a characteristic blood-tinged mucus without an odor. *Salmonella* infections and *Escherichia coli* infections in infants usually are characterized by green, soupy stools. Passage of nonbloody mucus often suggests IBS, particularly when it is associated with intermittent diarrhea and constipation. Fecal incontinence and nocturnal diarrhea are associated with rectal sphincter dysfunction secondary to neurologic problems. Less specific signs of diarrhea associated with a patient's desire to lose weight may suggest laxative abuse.

PSYCHOSOCIAL ASPECTS

The decision to self-medicate for constipation or diarrhea depends largely on the patient's perception of abnormal bowel habits. In a survey of public perceptions of digestive health and disease, researchers found that 62% of American respondents believed that a bowel movement each day is necessary for good digestive health.[10] This idea may have been influenced by the notion of autointoxication, which stated that noxious substances in the colon increase cellular degeneration and promote aging.[9] Although this notion is obsolete, the belief appears to be common among older adults, whose concern for regularity of bowel movements is shown by their frequent use of laxatives.

Normal bowel habits may range between 3 and 21 stools per week.[11] This demonstrates a wide variation of bowel habits among healthy people and may suggest an equivalent variation in laxative use.

THERAPEUTIC PLAN

Because constipation and acute, nonspecific diarrhea often are self-limiting and self-managed, there are no national guidelines for treatment. However, the American Gastroenterological Association is developing guidelines for treating all forms of constipation. Specific disorders such as acute infectious diarrhea (including TD) and IBS have recommendations for their management that are described later in this chapter.

TREATMENT OF CONSTIPATION

Pharmacotherapy

The classification of laxatives is controversial. They have been categorized primarily by their mechanism of action, although the exact mechanisms are unclear. Most laxatives alter intestinal fluid and electrolyte transport mechanisms, thereby causing defecation.[12] The therapeutic options are many. Agents available for use are varied and include bulk-forming agents, hyperosmotic agents, stool softeners, lubricants, saline, and stimulant laxatives (Table 27.5). Several dosage forms are available for laxatives. Some agents such as psyllium and senna are formulated in wafers and tea bags, respectively.

In general, there are no differences in efficacy between laxatives, but there are differences in their uses. However, one study suggests that the stool-softening and laxative effect of psyllium (a bulk-forming agent) compared with that of docusate sodium (a stool softener) was significantly better in patients with chronic idiopathic constipation.[15] More study is needed to verify whether there is a significant clinical difference between these and other laxatives.

Bulk-Forming Laxatives

Bulk-forming agents include nonabsorbable polysaccharide and cellulose derivatives. These agents swell in water, forming an emollient gel that increases bulk in the intestines. Peristalsis is stimulated by the increased fecal mass, which decreases the transit time. It is proposed that microflora metabolize polysaccharides to osmotically active metabolites. The metabolites may alter intestinal motility and electrolyte transport.

Bulk-forming agents generally produce a laxative effect within 12 to 24 hours, but they may take 2 to 3 days to exert their full effect. They are generally safe, and minimal side effects are associated with their use. Flatulence may occur if dosages are increased rapidly. Intestinal and esophageal obstruction may occur if insufficient liquid is administered with the dose. Therefore, patients should be cautioned to take each dose with at least one 240-mL glass of liquid. Bulk-forming laxatives should not be recommended for patients with intestinal stenosis, ulceration, or adhesions. Rare reports of allergic reactions to karaya have been noted, characterized by urticaria, rhinitis, dermatitis, and bronchospasm.[12]

Hyperosmotic Agents

Glycerin and lactulose are hyperosmotic laxatives. They increase osmotic pressure within the intestinal lumen, which results in luminal retention of water, softening the stool. Lactulose is an unabsorbed disaccharide metabolized by colonic bacteria primarily to lactic, formic, and acetic acids. It has been proposed that these organic acids may contribute to the osmotic effect.[12]

Glycerin is available only for rectal administration (suppository or enema) for treating acute constipation. Its laxative effect occurs within 15 to 30 minutes. Lactulose may take effect in 24 to 48 hours. It should be reserved for acute constipation because it is as effective as other less costly medications.

Side effects of glycerin include rectal irritation and burning; hyperemia of the rectal mucosa may occur. Lactulose is associated with flatulence, abdominal cramps, and diarrhea. Caution should be exercised when this agent is administered because it may also cause significant electrolyte imbalances and dehydration.[14]

Stool Softeners

Stool softeners are also called emollient laxatives. They include calcium, potassium, and sodium salts of dioctyl sulfosuccinate. Stool softeners are anionic surfactants that lower the fecal surface tension in vitro, allowing water and lipid penetration. It has been proposed that in vivo these agents stimulate water and electrolyte secretion into the colon.[12]

Softening of the feces generally occurs after 1 to 3 days. Some products (e.g., docusate sodium with casanthrol) combine a stool softener with a laxative. Adverse effects are rare with docusates. Mild gastrointestinal cramping may occasionally develop. Throat irritation has occurred following use of the docusate sodium solution. Docusate has been associated with hepatotoxicity when used in combination with oxyphenisatin or dantrol.[15]

Lubricants

The primary lubricant laxative is mineral oil. Its mechanism of action involves lubrication of the feces and hindrance of water reabsorption in the colon. Mineral oil is indigestible and its absorption is limited considerably in the nonemulsified formulation. Greater absorption from

Table 27.5 ▪ Laxatives for the Management of Constipation

Laxative Category	Dosage Per Day: Adult	Dosage Per Day: Pediatric	Dosage Form	Onset of Action	Patient Information
Bulk-forming					
Bran	>12 yr: up to 14 g	6–11 yr: up to 7 g 2–5 yr: up to 3.5 g	O	12–72 hr	Should be administered with 240 mL liquid/dose; additional fluid intake encouraged; recommended in pregnancy.
Karaya	>12 yr: up to 14 g	–	O		
Malt soup extract	>12 yr: up to 64 g	6–11 yr: up to 32 g 2–5 yr: up to 16 g	O		
Methylcellulose and sodium carboxymethylcellulose	>12 yr: up to 6 g	6–11 yr: up to 3 g	O		
Polycarbophil	>12 yr: up to 6 g	6–11 yr: up to 3 g 3–5 yr: up to 1.5 g	O		
Psyllium hydrophilic mucilloid	>12 yr: up to 30 g	6–11 yr: up to 15 g	O		
Stimulants					
Bisacodyl[a]	>12 yr: 5–15 mg >12 yr: 10 mg	>3 yr: 0.3 mg/kg 2–11 yr: 5–10 mg <2 yr: 5 mg	O RS	6–12 hr 15 min–2 hr	May cause a pink or red discoloration of the urine. May cause skin rash; discontinue medication and contact pharmacist or physician. Tablets should not be chewed.
Casanthranol[a]	>12 yr: 30–90 mg	2–12 yr: 15–45 mg <2 yr: 7.5–22.5 mg	O		
Dehydrocholic acid	>12 yr: 750–1500 mg	–	O		
Phenolphthalein[b]	>12 yr: 30–270 mg	6–11 yr: 30–60 mg 2–5 yr: 15–30 mg	O		
Sennosides[a]	>12 yr: 12–75 mg	6–11 yr: 6–33 mg 2–6 yr: 3–12.5 mg	O		
	>12 yr: 30–60 mg		RS		
Saline agents					
Magnesium citrate	>12 hr: 11–25 g	6–11 yr: 5.5–12.5 g 2.5 yr: 2.7–6.25 g	O	30 min–6 hr	
Magnesium hydroxide	>12 yr: 2.4–4.8 g	6–11 yr: 1.2–2.4 g 2.5 yr: 0.4–1.2 g	O		
Magnesium sulfate	>12 yr: 10–30 g	6–11 yr: 5–10 g 2–5 yr: 2.5–5 g	O		
Sodium phosphate, monobasic	>12 yr: 9.1–20.2 g	10–11 yr: 4.5–10.1 g 5–9 yr: 2.2–5.05 g	O		
	>12 yr: 18.24–20.16 g	2–11 yr: 9.12–10.08 g	RE	2–15 min	
Sodium phosphate dibasic	>12 yr: 3.42–7.5 g	10–11 yr: 1.71–3.78 g 5–9 yr: 0.86–1.89 g	O		
	>12 yr: 6.84–7.56 g	2–11 yr: 3.42–2.78 g	RE	2–15 min	

(continued)

the emulsion formulation has been reported, but the clinical significance is unsubstantiated.

The onset of action of orally administered mineral oil is 6 to 8 hours. Although adverse effects occur rarely with mineral oil, potentially significant effects may occur. Chronic use of mineral oil has been reported to cause impaired absorption of fat-soluble vitamins (A, D, E, and K). Aspiration of the product may cause a lipoid pneumonia, so its oral use should be avoided in young children (less than 6 years), older adults, and debilitated patients. Administration at bedtime should be avoided to prevent aspiration. Foreign-body reactions in the lymphoid tissue of the intestinal tract have resulted from its limited amount of absorption. Seepage of the product from the rectum following high-dose oral or rectal administration may cause pruritus ani, increased infection, and decreased healing of anorectal lesions.[12,14]

Saline Laxatives

Magnesium, sulfate, phosphate, and citrate salts are used when rapid bowel evacuation is needed. The mechanism of action of these poorly absorbed ions is unclear, but it is believed that they produce an osmotic effect that increases intraluminal volume and stimulates peristalsis. Magnesium

Table 27.5 *(continued)*

Laxative Category	Dosage Per Day: Adult	Dosage Per Day: Pediatric	Dosage Form	Onset of Action	Patient Information
Hyperosmotic agents					
Glycerin	>12 yr: 3 g	>6 yr: 2–3 g 5–15 mL <6 yr: 1–1.7 g 2–5 mL	RS RE RS RE	15–30 min	May cause rectal burning or irritation.
Lactulose	>12 yr: 10–20 g, then up to 40 g	<12 yr: 5 g[c]	O, RE		May be mixed in fruit juice to increase palatability. May cause belching, flatulence, or abdominal cramps. Pediatric dose should be given after breakfast.
Lubricants					
Mineral oil	>12 yr: 15–45 mL >12 yr: 120 mL	6–11 yr: 5–15 mL 6–11 yr: 30–60 mL	O R	6–8 hr	Should not be administered to children <6 yr, pregnant women, or debilitated patients. Bedtime doses should be avoided. May cause pruritus ani, especially when administered rectally.
Surfactants					
Dioctyl sulfosuccinate (calcium, potassium, sodium)	No official recommendation		O, RE		Oral solutions may be diluted with 120 mL milk, fruit juice, or infant formula; solutions may cause throat irritation.

O, oral; *RS*, rectal suppository; *RE*, rectal enema.

[a]The U.S. Food and Drug Administration (FDA) has proposed the reclassification of these agents from category I (generally recognized as safe and effective and not misbranded) to category III (further testing needed; reference 21).

[b]The FDA has proposed a ban on over-the-counter sale and reclassification of agent to category II (not generally recognized as safe and effective; reference 21).

[c]Use currently is not included in the FDA-approved labeling.

may cause cholecystokinin release from the duodenal mucosa, promoting increased fluid secretion and motility of the small intestine and colon.[16]

The laxative effect of the orally administered magnesium and sodium phosphate salts occurs within 0.5 to 6 hours. Phosphate-containing rectal enemas evacuate the bowel within 2 to 15 minutes.

Saline laxatives are safe for short-term management of constipation. They are useful in preparing for endoscopic examinations, eliminating parasites and toxic anthelmintics before or after therapy, removing poisons, and treating fecal impaction. They may cause significant fluid and electrolyte imbalances when used for prolonged periods or in certain patients. Dehydration may result from repeated administration without appropriate fluid replacement. The risk of hypermagnesemia in patients with renal dysfunction should be considered when magnesium salts are initiated because 10 to 20% of the dose may be absorbed systemically. Caution should be exercised when administering the sodium phosphate salts to patients with congestive heart failure when sodium restriction is necessary. These agents are not recommended for children under 2 years of age because of the potential for hypocalcemia in this population.

Stimulant Laxatives

Anthraquinone (casanthrol, cascara sagrada, danthron, sennosides, and aloe) and diphenylmethane (bisacodyl, phenolphthalein) derivatives, castor oil, and dehydrocholic acid are stimulant laxatives. They are called stimulants because they stimulate peristalsis via mucosal irritation or intramural nerve plexus activity, which results in increased motility. Although this has been long regarded as the mechanism of action for these agents, their activity actually may be related to their effect on the colonic mucosal cells. It is proposed that stimulant laxatives modify the permeability of these cells, resulting in intraluminal fluid and electrolyte secretion.

Defecation occurs 6 to 12 hours after oral administration of these agents. Therefore, a single bedtime dose promotes a morning bowel movement. The laxative effects of phenolphthalein may persist for several days because up to 15% of the oral dose is absorbed and undergoes enterohepatic recirculation. Unlike the other stimulant laxatives, dehydrocholic acid is administered at least three times daily. Rectal administration of bisacodyl and senna produces catharsis within 15 minutes to 2 hours.

Adverse effects of these medications include abdominal cramps, nausea, electrolyte disturbances (e.g., hypokalemia, hypocalcemia, metabolic acidosis, or alkalosis), and rectal burning and irritation with suppository use. Anthraquinone derivatives have been noted to cause melanosis coli (discoloring of colonic mucosa), which is harmless and reversible. Hypersensitivity reactions may occur (rarely) with phenolphthalein and dehydrocholic acid, causing dermatologic manifestations (e.g., skin eruptions, rashes, pigmentation, pruritus). These agents may also cause a pink or red discoloration of the urine.

Currently, the U.S. Food and Drug Administration (FDA) is proposing to ban the OTC sale of phenolphthalein because of its potential to cause cancer in humans.[17] The proposal to reclassify this agent as "not generally recognized as safe and effective" results from a review of animal carcinogenicity studies. Studies revealed that rats and mice administered phenolphthalein developed tumors at dosages 50 to 100 times the dosage recommended for humans. These results have caused some manufacturers to reformulate their products to contain other laxatives (e.g., docusate sodium) instead of phenolphthalein.

Chronic use of stimulant laxatives should be discouraged and use beyond 1 week should be avoided. These agents may produce a "cathartic colon" if used for several years (15 to 40). The colon develops abnormal motor function, and the condition resembles ulcerative colitis on roentgenogram. Usually, discontinuation of laxative use restores normal bowel function.

Danthron-containing laxatives were removed from the market in 1987 because of their potential for causing intestinal and hepatic tumors in humans. Chronic administration of danthron at high dosages produced tumors in rats.[18] Although only insignificant amounts distribute into the milk of nursing mothers, stimulant laxatives should be avoided during lactation.

Other Agents

Data suggest a role for other agents in treating constipation. Cisapride and naloxone have been used to treat chronic idiopathic constipation.

Cisapride is a piperidinyl benzamide that is chemically related to metoclopramide. It is a prokinetic agent that enhances gastrointestinal motility throughout the entire length of the gastrointestinal tract. The mechanisms by which cisapride facilitates gastrointestinal motility have not been elucidated. However, a proposed mechanism involves its enhancement of acetylcholine release in the myenteric plexus of the gut.[19] Cisapride has no antidopaminergic effects.

Cisapride, in oral dosages of 5 to 20 mg, is absorbed rapidly and almost completely from the gastrointestinal tract. The oral bioavailability is approximately 40 to 50% and is enhanced by food. Its tissue distribution in humans is not known; however, it is metabolized extensively to metabolites with minimal pharmacologic activity. Its elimination half-life after oral administration is approximately 7 to 10 hours. Some evidence suggests that the half-life of cisapride may increase in older adults and those with hepatic impairment.[19]

Cisapride at a dosage of 20 mg twice daily was investigated in patients with chronic idiopathic constipation or chronic laxative use. Cisapride increased stool frequency by 50% and reduced mean laxative intake by half.[20] In another study, cisapride was used to treat constipation at dosages of 5 mg and 10 mg three times daily for 12 weeks. Stool frequency was increased by approximately 70% with both dosages, compared to 43% with placebo.[21]

The side effect profile of cisapride is moderate, based on current experience. Common side effects include abdominal cramping, borborygmi (intestinal rumbling), and diarrhea. Central nervous system (CNS) side effects, such as somnolence and fatigue, have been reported less often.

Concomitant administration of cisapride with specific agents has caused drug interactions. Cimetidine coadministration may cause a 45% increase in the bioavailability of cisapride.[19] Cisapride may enhance acenocoumarol absorption; therefore, monitoring coagulation times is advisable with anticoagulants.[19] Because cisapride can accelerate gastric emptying, patients should be monitored during concomitant use of agents with narrow therapeutic windows (e.g., digoxin and phenytoin).

It has been postulated that endogenous opiates regulate colonic propulsive activity.[22] Consequently, the role of opiate receptor antagonists in treating constipation has been investigated. Naloxone (an opiate receptor antagonist) has reversed chronic idiopathic constipation at intravenous and oral dosages of 20 to 30 mg/day.[23] In addition, naloxone causes acceleration of colonic transit, although it has not been shown to affect the number of bowel movements per 48 hours.[24] Further studies are needed to define the role of this agent in treating chronic constipation.

Nonpharmacologic Therapy

Some of the primary causes of constipation may necessitate nonpharmacologic intervention for symptom relief. Deficient fluid and fiber intake have been suggested as causative factors. However, two large-scale studies have not demonstrated an association between fiber consumption and self-reported constipation.[5,6] Fiber may be useful in preventing constipation. Fiber increases stool bulk, based on the ability of the polysaccharides to absorb and retain water and the extent of bacterial fermentation of these polysaccharides in the gut. A dietary bulk-forming agent such as bran may be useful in preventing constipation because it is only partially fermented by bacteria, resulting in increased stool bulk, accelerated transit time, and promotion of normal defecation.

Fiber intake may have other health benefits. The FDA recently ruled that labels on certain foods (i.e., breakfast cereals) containing soluble fiber from psyllium seed husk (PSH) may claim that, as part of a diet low in saturated fat and cholesterol, they can reduce the risk of coronary heart disease.[25] The ruling is based on evidence that consumption of approximately 7 g/day soluble fiber from PSH showed significant lowering of total and low-density lipoprotein cholesterol.

Increased fiber intake should be recommended cautiously. Rapid increases in dietary roughage may cause abdominal bloating and flatulence. Adequate fluid intake is also necessary to prevent fecal impaction. Generally, 240 to 360 mL fluid with each tablespoon of bran is sufficient.

Immobility and inactivity, common among debilitated patients and older adults, are risk factors for the development of constipation.[26] Regular exercise such as walking or jogging may improve constipation associated with a sedentary lifestyle. Pharmacologic intervention (e.g., laxatives) may be necessary if lifestyle modifications are unsuccessful.

TREATMENT OF ACUTE, NONSPECIFIC DIARRHEA

For most people, diarrhea is a transient, self-limiting complaint. This form of diarrhea is often called acute, nonspecific diarrhea that is not caused by underlying diseases or etiologic agents. However, the symptoms may often interfere with activities and contribute to loss of productivity. The management of acute, nonspecific diarrhea consists of adequate oral rehydration and symptom relief. Several nonprescription agents are effective in managing the associated symptoms of diarrhea (Table 27.6).

Pharmacotherapy

Various medications, both prescription and OTC, are available for the symptomatic relief of diarrhea. Recently, the FDA reevaluated the safety and efficacy of OTC products for diarrhea. The Advisory Review Panel on OTC Laxative, Antidiarrheal, Emetic, and Antiemetic Drug Products reviewed several products in 1975 for their safety and efficacy. The FDA evaluated the panel's recommendations and published tentative rulings in 1986.[27] Currently, the only OTC products considered safe and effective treatments of diarrhea are attapulgite, kaolin (without pectin), polycarbophil, and loperamide.

Table 27.6 ▪ Recommended Over-the-Counter Antidiarrheals

Medication	Dosage	Maximum Dosage per Day
Attapulgite	>12 yr: 1.2 g at onset, then repeat after each loose stool	8.4 g
	6–11 yr: 0.6 g at onset, then repeat after each loose stool	4.2 g
	3–5 yr: 0.3 g at onset, then repeat after each loose stool	2.1 g
Kaolin	>12 yr: 26.2 g after each stool	262.0 g
	<12 yr: consult physician	
Polycarbophil and calcium polycarbophil	>12 yr:1.2 g TID–QID	4–6 g
	6–11 yr: 0.5–1 g TID	3 g
	3–5 yr: 0.33–0.5 g TID	1.5 g
Loperamide[a]	>12 yr: 4 mg at onset, then 2 mg after each loose stool	8 mg;[b] 16 mg
	9–11 yr: 2 mg at onset, then 1 mg after each loose stool	6 mg
	6–8 yr: 1 mg at onset, then 1 mg after each loose stool	4 mg
	<6 yr:[c] 1 mg at onset, then 1 mg after each loose stool	3 mg

Source: Minutes of the Nonprescription Drugs Advisory Committee and the Gastrointestinal Drugs Advisory Committee Meeting of the FDA, April 9, 1993. Facts and Comparisons, 1998.

[a]Therapy should not exceed 2 days.

[b]Travelers' diarrhea.

[c]Use only under medical supervision.

Attapulgite is a naturally occurring hydrous magnesium aluminum silicate that adsorbs approximately eight times its weight in water because of its large surface area. This adsorbent property reduces the liquidity of the stool. Side effects are minimal with attapulgite because it is not absorbed systemically. It is administered at the onset of symptoms, followed by smaller dosages after each loose stool (Table 27.6).

Kaolin is a naturally occurring hydrated aluminum silicate with adsorbent properties. It is effective in treating acute nonspecific diarrhea, based on its ability to improve stool consistency within 24 to 48 hours. Kaolin is no longer approved for OTC use in combination with pectin for treating diarrhea. Studies have not demonstrated that the fixed combination (kaolin and pectin) is more effective than kaolin alone. Like attapulgite, kaolin has minimal side effects. Recommended dosages for adults and children older than 12 years are listed in Table 27.6.

Polycarbophil has been used to treat diarrhea and constipation. It is a hydrophilic polyacrylic resin that, like attapulgite, has adsorbent properties. It is not absorbed systemically, with no systemic side effects. Epigastric pain and bloating are common sequelae. Administering smaller dosages spaced more evenly throughout the day may provide relief from bloating. Minimal fluid intake is encouraged for patients with diarrhea.

Loperamide is a synthetic congener of meperidine, which decreases gastrointestinal motility through its effect on the circular and longitudinal muscles of the intestines. CNS penetration of the drug is low. It does not elicit the CNS side effects associated with opiate use and lacks potential for abuse.

Loperamide relieves symptoms of acute nonspecific diarrhea, and it is effective in treating nondysenteric TD.[28–30] It has been compared with attapulgite in acute diarrhea.[29] The dosage of loperamide was 4 mg initially, then 2 mg after every unformed stool, not exceeding 8 mg in 24 hours. Attapulgite was administered initially as 3 g, followed by up to 6 g after each unformed stool, to a maximum dosage of 9 g in 24 hours. The mean number of unformed stools was significantly lower in the loperamide group in the first and second 12-hour intervals. However, no significant difference was observed in duration of relief from diarrhea after the initial dose.

Although generally well tolerated, loperamide can cause abdominal pain, constipation, drowsiness, fatigue, dry mouth, nausea, and vomiting. Dosages for adults should not exceed 8 mg/day for OTC use; however, maximum daily dosages of 16 mg are permitted under medical supervision. Children under 6 years of age should not receive loperamide unless medically supervised. The medication should be discontinued after 48 hours if clinical improvement is not evident.

Opiates (opium powder, tincture, and paregoric) have been used extensively to treat acute, nonspecific diarrhea. Opiates contain morphine, which promotes increased smooth muscle tone of the gastrointestinal tract, inhibits gastrointestinal motility and propulsion, and reduces digestive secretions. Paregoric is commonly used at dosages of 5 to 10 mL one to four times daily for adults and 0.25 to 0.5 mL/kg one to four times daily for children.[31] Opium tincture contains 25% more morphine than paregoric; therefore, the dosage is 0.3 to 1 mL four times daily, with a maximum daily dosage of 6 mL. Although these agents are considered safe and effective antidiarrheals, they are not recommended in nonprescription combination products.[32]

Other derivatives of morphine, such as codeine and the meperidine congener diphenoxylate can be used for diarrhea. At dosages of 15 to 30 mg orally every 6 hours, codeine reduces the frequency of loose stools. However, its use has been limited in favor of the various nonnarcotic alternatives for diarrhea currently available. Diphenoxylate, which has activity similar to that of morphine on intestinal smooth muscle, is used in combination with atropine sulfate at dosages of 2.5 to 5 mg orally four times daily. Unlike loperamide, diphenoxylate can produce euphoria and suppress opiate withdrawal symptoms at high dosages. Consequently, abuse potential exists with diphenoxylate alone. Atropine sulfate has been added to discourage abuse.

Nonpharmacologic Therapy

Fluid losses in acute, nonspecific diarrhea in adults generally are not severe and necessitate only simple replacement of fluid and electrolytes lost in the stool. However, special consideration should be given to older and immunocompromised adults. Patients should be advised to ingest 2 to 3 L clear liquids (e.g., flat ginger ale and decaffeinated cola, tea, broth, or gelatin) within the first 24 hours. For 24 hours, the diet should consist of bland foods including rice, soup, bread, salted crackers, cooked cereals, baked potatoes, eggs, and applesauce.[33] A regular diet may be resumed after 2 to 3 days.

Untreated diarrhea in the pediatric population is a major cause of morbidity and mortality, especially in developing countries. Infants and young children are more susceptible to the acute losses of fluid caused by diarrhea because the intestinal surface area of infants and children is greater in relation to their body size. Consequently, oral rehydration solutions (ORSs) are recommended for acute diarrhea. Infants and children with a 5 to 7.5% weight loss should receive an ORS at a dosage of 40 to 50 mL/kg administered in the first 4 to 6 hours. Oral maintenance can be administered at a rate of 150 mL/kg/day once rehydration is achieved.[34] The World Health Organization (WHO) provides the standard ORS, which contains glucose (20 g/L), sodium (90 mEq/L), potassium (20 mEq/L), chloride (80 mEq/L), and citrate (10 mEq/L) as a base. It is prepared by mixing one packet with 1 L boiled or treated water. The solution should be discarded within 12 hours if kept at room temperature and within 24 hours if refrigerated. Packets are available in stores or pharmacies in all developing countries. Other ORSs are available commercially in the United States as ready-to-use preparations.

TREATMENT OF INFECTIOUS DIARRHEA

The role of antiperistaltic agents in infectious diarrhea has been questioned. The body normally defends itself from invading bacteria by eliminating these organisms during diarrhea. Antiperistaltic agents such as diphenoxylate and loperamide inhibit this process by increasing gastrointestinal transit time. Therefore, these agents are not recommended for treating diarrhea induced by invasive organisms such as enterotoxigenic *E. coli* (ETEC), *Salmonella,* or *Shigella.*[35,36] They should also be avoided in patients with fecal leukocytes, fever, or blood in the stools. The risk of toxic megacolon exists when these agents are given to patients with pseudomembranous colitis or ulcerative colitis.[36]

Although infectious diarrhea can be treated with antimicrobial therapy, the use of these agents is controversial. However, antimicrobial therapy is indicated when diarrhea persists for more than 48 hours, when the patient passes six or more loose stools in 24 hours, or when diarrhea is associated with fever, blood, or pus in the stools. Table 27.7 describes the common organisms and their therapy.

TREATMENT OF DIARRHEA IN IMMUNOCOMPROMISED PATIENTS

Diarrhea in immunocompromised patients (e.g., those having acquired immunodeficiency syndrome [AIDS], organ transplant, or chemotherapy) poses a challenge. Often, these patients (particularly those with AIDS) experience symptoms that are refractory to conventional therapy. Some patients may respond to opium tincture when loperamide is not successful.[8] Octreotide, a synthetic analog of somatostatin, may be effective. It should be recommended only after other therapies have failed because it is given subcutaneously and is expensive.

Infectious diarrhea in these patients also warrants special consideration because it is often difficult to identify a pathogen or control symptoms once a pathogen is known. Specific antimicrobial therapy for infectious diarrhea in immunocompromised patients is described in Table 27.8.

ALTERNATIVE THERAPIES

Several OTC products are marketed as herbal remedies for constipation, diarrhea, and other common ailments of the gastrointestinal tract. Although products for constipation contain roots and bark of various plants and trees, their main ingredients often include aloe, psyllium seed, senna, or cascara sagrada. Some products also contain prune concentrate. Prunes are high in fiber and well regarded as

Table 27.7 ▪ Antimicrobial Therapy for Common Causes of Infectious Diarrhea

Organism	Suggested Antimicrobial Therapy	Duration
Salmonella		
Uncomplicated	None	
Hyperpyrexia and systemic toxicity	TMP/SMX 160/800 mg PO BID	5–7 days
	Fluoroquinolones[a]	
Shigella	TMP/SMX 160/800 mg PO BID (if acquired in U.S.)	3 days
	Fluoroquinolones[a] (if acquired internationally)	3–5 days
Enteropathogenic *E. coli*	Fluoroquinolones[a]	3–5 days
Enterotoxigenic *E. coli*	Fluoroquinolones[a]	1–5 days
Enteroinvasive *E. coli*	TMP/SMX 160/800 mg BID (if acquired in U.S.)	3 days
	Fluoroquinolones[a] (if acquired internationally)	3–5 days
Enterohemor-rhagic *E. coli*	Antimicrobials usually withheld except in particularly severe cases	
Campylobacter spp.	Erythromycin stearate 500 mg PO BID	5 days
	Fluoroquinolones,[a] if susceptible	
	Azithromycin (for quinolone-resistant cases)	
Yersinia spp.	Fluoroquinolones[a]	3–5 days
	Ceftriaxone 1 g IV QD (severe cases)	5 days
Noncholera *Vibrio*	Fluoroquinolones[a]	3–5 days
Clostridium difficile	Vancomycin 125–500 mg PO QID	10 days
Giardia lamblia	Metronidazole 250 mg PO QID	7 days
	Quinacrine 100 mg PO TID (where available)	7 days
	Tinidazole 2 g single dose-(where available)	
Cryptosporidium		
Uncomplicated	None	
Severe	Paromomycin 500 mg PO TID	7 days
Isospora	TMP/SMX 160/800 mg PO BID	7 days
Cyclospora	TMP/SMX 160/800 mg PO BID	days

Source: Adapted with permission. DuPont HL. Guidelines on acute infectious diarrhea in adults. Am J Gastroenterol 92(11):1962–1975, 1997.

TMP/SMX, trimethoprim–sulfamethoxazole.

[a]Oral fluoroquinolones include norfloxacin 400 mg, ciprofloxacin 500 mg, and ofloxacin 300 mg at BID dosing.

a dietary intervention for constipation. Rhubarb root often is included in many herbal products for constipation because of its natural laxative effect.[37,38]

Many herbal remedies for diarrhea include substances known as tannins. They have astringent properties, thereby reducing intestinal inflammation and restricting secretions. Edible berry plants (i.e., blackberry, blueberry, and raspberry) are commonly used. Dried blueberries are recommended over fresh because the latter are high in fiber and may produce a laxative effect. Table 27.9 describes herbs commonly used for constipation and diarrhea and their therapeutic ingredients.[37,38]

Disorders leading to chronic constipation may be aided by other alternative therapies for relief of symptoms. Patients who experience pelvic floor dyssynergia (an inability to relax the pelvic floor muscles during defecation) may benefit from biofeedback training. Patients with diarrhea or abdominal pain associated with IBS may also respond to biofeedback, in addition to hypnosis, cognitive and behavioral treatment, relaxation and stress management, or psychotherapy.[39]

Table 27.8 ▪ Indications for Specific Antimicrobial Therapy in Infectious Diarrhea in Immunocompromised[a] Patients

Indication for Antimicrobial Therapy	Suggested Antimicrobial Therapy
Shigellosis	If acquired in the U.S., give TMP/SMX 160/800 mg PO BID for 7–10 days. If acquired during international travel, treat as febrile dysentery; check for susceptibility of drug used.
Intestinal salmonellosis	TMP/SMX 160/800 mg PO BID or quinolone[b] NF 400 mg, CF 500 mg, OF 300–400 mg PO BID for 14 days; repeat stool cultures 1 wk after treatment.
Cryptosporidium diarrhea	Paromomycin 500 mg PO QID with food for 14–28 days, then 500 mg BID indefinitely; with treatment failures, may try azithromycin 2.4 g PO day 1, then 1.2 g/day for 27 days, then 600 mg/day for maintenance treatment given indefinitely.
Isospora diarrhea	320 mg TMP/1600 mg SMX po BID for 2–4 wk, then 160–320 mg TMP/800–1600 mg SMX PO QD.
Cyclospora diarrhea	TMP/SMX 160/800 mg PO QID for 10 days, then 160/800 mg three times a week indefinitely.
Microsporidiosis	Albendazole 400 mg PO BID ≥4 wk or metronidazole 500 mg PO TID or atovaquone 750 mg PO TID continued indefinitely.
Cytomegalovirus diarrhea	Ganciclovir 5 mg/kg IV q12hr or q8hr 14–21 days and foscarnet 60 mg/kg IV q8hr or 90 mg/kg IV q12hr for 14–21 days.
Mycobacterium avium–intracellulare complex	Clarithromycin 500 mg PO BID, ethambutol PO 15 mg/kg/day, plus one of the following: CF 500–750 mg PO BID, clofazimine PO 100 mg/day, rifampin 600 mg PO QD, or rifabutin 300 mg/day PO indefinitely.

Source: Reprinted with permission. DuPont HL. Guidelines on acute infectious diarrhea in adults. The Practice Parameters Committee of the American College of Gastroenterology. Am J Gastroenterol 92(11):1962–1975, 1997.

TMP/SMX, trimethoprim–sulfamethoxazole.

[a]Patients with AIDS, after organ transplantation, and during cancer chemotherapy.

[b]Fluoroquinolones include norfloxacin (*NF*), ciprofloxacin (*CF*), and ofloxacin (*OF*).

Table 27.9 ▪ Common Herbal Remedies for Constipation and Diarrhea

Herb	Active Therapeutic Ingredient	Effect	Dosage	Comments
Constipation				
Aloe	Anthraquinone glycosides: aloin A and B	Stimulant (potent)	None described	Little use in U.S.; use dried bitter yellow latex or juice of plant only, not gel.
Buckthorn bark	Anthraquinone derivatives: glucofrangulin A and B, frangulin A and B	Stimulant (gentle)	1 g	Bark must be aged 1 yr before use.
Cascara sagrada	Cascarosides A, B, C, and D	Stimulant (gentle)	1 g (1/2 tsp)	Bark must be aged 1 yr before use.
Plantago seed (psyllium seed)	*Plantago psyllium L* or *Plantago indica L*	Bulk-producing (gentle)	7.5 g (2 rounded tsp)	Stir husks into glass of water, juice, or milk; drink before mixture thickens. Patients should drink plenty of fluids. May have positive effects on cholesterol.
Senna	Dianthrone glycosides: sennosides A, A_1, B, C, D, G	Stimulant	0.5–2 g to prepare a bitter tea	A more palatable beverage can be prepared by soaking leaflets in cold water for 10–12 hr.
Rhubarb	Dried rhizome and root of *Rheum officinale*	Stimulant (potent)	None described	Differs from common garden rhubarb. Causes intestinal griping or colic and is rarely used.
Diarrhea				
Blackberry leaves	Tannin (8–14%)	Astringent	Boiling water over 1–2 tsp of leaves	Drink up to 6 times/day.
Blueberry leaves	Tannin (up to 10%)	Astringent	Same	
Raspberry leaves	Tannin	Astringent	Same	
Dried blueberries	Tannin	Astringent	Chew and swallow 3 tbsp	
	Pectin	Adsorbent		

Source: Adapted with permission. Tyler VE. Herbs of choice: the therapeutic use of phytomedicinals. New York: Pharmaceutical Products Press, 1994:46–54.

IMPROVING OUTCOMES

Patient Education and Improving Adherence to Drug Therapy

To provide patient medication counseling for constipation, the pharmacist must determine the patient's perception of normal bowel habits. Only then can the pharmacist determine whether nonpharmacologic or pharmacologic treatment is appropriate. A discussion of bowel habits should emphasize that although constipation often is self-limiting, it may be a symptom of a more serious disease. Consequently, counseling should include questions about the onset and duration of constipation and a history of medical illnesses. The patient's medication profile should be reviewed for possible drug-induced constipation and for a history of the patient's laxative use. Diet and lifestyle activities are ascertained because the lack of exercise and fiber is associated with the development of constipation. Finally, educating patients (especially children) to respond to the urge to defecate is essential.

Several patient education materials are available, in print and online, for constipation and diarrhea. The National Digestive Diseases Information Clearinghouse has several publications for order via facsimile or electronic mail. Flow charts for self-diagnosis and care of problems such as diarrhea and constipation are available online from the American Academy of Family Physicians. In addition, the International Foundation for Functional Gastrointestinal Disorders provides support and educational information for people affected by gastrointestinal disorders such as constipation, diarrhea, and IBS.

Disease Management Strategies to Improve Patient Outcomes

If a recommendation for a laxative is appropriate, the pharmacist should consider the following guidelines:

- Laxative use should not exceed 1 week of self-medication.
- Laxatives are inappropriate in the presence of abdominal pain or cramping, nausea, vomiting, or bloating.
- Daily administration of bulk-forming agents should be the first choice in uncomplicated chronic constipation.
- Pharmacists may recommend one of the following for 1 week or less: a low-dose saline laxative, stimulant laxative at bedtime, or glycerin suppository.
- Institutionalized or bedridden patients may need laxatives in addition to daily bulk-forming agents to prevent fecal impaction (e.g., weekly intermittent doses of stimulant laxatives, lactulose 30 mL/day, and milk of magnesia).
- Mineral oil should be avoided in older adults, young children (less than 6 years), and debilitated patients because of the risk of aspiration.
- Patients with histories of myocardial infarction, anal fissures, hernias, and colorectal surgery are candidates for prophylactic laxative therapy to prevent straining. Acceptable agents

include docusate, milk of magnesia, glycerin suppository, and bulk-forming products.
- Pregnant patients should use only bulk-forming agents and stool softeners if a laxative is needed.

Patient education for acute diarrhea should include information about the prevention of subsequent episodes (especially for pediatric diarrhea and TD). Pharmacists should inform the parents of children to do the following:

- Keep ORSs in the home at all times.
- Check the expiration dates of all ORSs regularly.
- Recommend use of newer dosage forms (e.g., freezer pops) and more palatable flavors to enhance compliance.
- Pack a diarrhea prevention kit when traveling that includes oral rehydration packets, water purification tablets, antidiarrheal medications, and a thermometer.
- Monitor children for signs and symptoms of diarrhea upon the initiation of any antibiotic medication.
- Recognize the importance of early intervention of acute diarrhea to prevent complications of dehydration and electrolyte losses.

PHARMACOECONOMICS

The financial impact of constipation and diarrhea in the United States is significant. Currently, an estimated $2 billion is spent on antacids and digestive aids, primarily antidiarrheals and laxatives.[40] One factor contributing to the increased usage is the rise in patient self-treatment with OTC products. A survey of consumer OTC usage trends revealed that of 1356 household respondents, 26% used products for constipation and 28% used products for diarrhea over a 6-month period.[41] Women and people over the age of 60 years used nonprescription laxatives more often. No correlation was observed in these two populations with the use of antidiarrheals.

In a study of 1059 rural older adults taking OTC medications, 9.7% of those interviewed used laxatives. Results indicated that the use of laxatives was significantly associated with a higher number of physician visits, hospitalizations, emergency room visits, and number of prescriptions 6 months before the interview. The use of home health services was also significantly associated with laxative use.[42]

Related Disorders

Two disorders related to uncomplicated constipation and diarrhea warrant special discussion: TD and IBS. Although treating these disorders often incorporates several of the therapeutic interventions mentioned previously, they are unique and specific disorders that warrant additional discussion.

Traveler's Diarrhea

DEFINITION AND EPIDEMIOLOGY

Each year, 10% of the American population travels to other countries. Specifically, more than 8 million travel to developing countries.[43] Often their excursions are interrupted by TD, an infectious disease of the gastrointestinal tract in people traveling outside their home country that results in a twofold or greater increase in the frequency of unformed bowel movements, with associated symptoms. The risk of TD depends on the traveler's destination. Approximately 20 to 50% of travelers develop TD.[44] The disease affects primarily people traveling from industrialized nations to developing countries. People traveling from the United States, Canada, or northern Europe would be at risk of developing TD when traveling to Latin America, Africa, the Middle East, or Asia. The incidence is slightly greater in young adults than in older adults.

CLINICAL PRESENTATION AND DIAGNOSIS

The abrupt onset of diarrhea generally is self-limiting, with a median duration of 3 to 5 days. Although persistent diarrhea is uncommon in TD, 10% of the cases may continue for more than 1 week. Travelers should be aware that TD may occur more than once during a trip, so appropriate precautions should be taken throughout the travel period. TD develops from food or water that is contaminated with fecal material containing bacteria, viruses, parasites, or combinations of microbes. The most common offending organism is enterotoxigenic *E. coli,* which accounts for more than 40% of cases. *Salmonella* and *Shigella* species as well as *Campylobacter jejuni* also cause TD. Other potential bacterial pathogens include *Aeromonas hydrophila, Yersinia enterocolitica, Plesiomonas shigelloides, Vibrio parahaemolyticus,* and other *Vibrio* species. Viruses such as rotavirus and Norwalk virus often contaminate water, but they are not common causes of TD in adults. Parasitic enteric pathogens including *Giardia lamblia, Entamoeba histolytica,* and *Cryptosporidium* cause fewer cases of TD.

PREVENTION

Pharmacotherapy

Although there is a consensus in the health community about food and water precautions for TD prevention, chemoprophylaxis for TD prevention is controversial. Several studies have provided data that demonstrate efficacy for both antimicrobial and nonantimicrobial agents in decreasing the incidence of diarrhea. The nonantimicrobial agent bismuth subsalicylate has been shown to prevent diarrhea in up to 65% of subjects receiving two tablets (524 mg) four times daily for 21 days beginning on the first day of travel. Lower protection rates (40%) were observed in subjects receiving one tablet (262 mg) four times daily.[45] In a previous trial of the liquid preparation, 60 mL four times daily for 3 weeks resulted in a 62% reduction in illness.[46] Bismuth subsalicylate has side effects, including darkening of the tongue and stool and mild tinnitus. Patients taking aspirin concurrently for arthritis may be at increased risk for developing tinnitus secondary to the salicylate component in bismuth subsalicylate. This agent is contraindicated in patients with renal insufficiency, gout, or allergies to aspirin. Caution should be exercised when administering this medication to adolescents and children with chicken pox or flu because of the risk of Reye's syndrome. This agent is not indicated for children less than 3 years old. Patients with AIDS may be at greater risk of developing encephalopathy from consuming excessive dosages of bismuth subsalicylate.[47] Concurrent use of anticoagulants, probenecid, or methotrexate is contraindicated with this agent. Bismuth subsalicylate appears to be effective for TD prophylaxis and is recommended by the Centers for Disease Control for use not longer than 3 weeks.

Several antibiotics have been investigated for TD chemoprophylaxis. One of the earliest agents studied was doxycycline. Dosages of 100 mg/day for 21 days are effective in areas where enterotoxigenic *E. coli* were sensitive to the drug.[48,49] However, the protection rate decreased in geographic areas with resistant strains.[48] In addition, side effects including photosensitivity and diarrhea and contraindications in pregnancy and lactation and in children (less than 8 years of age) increase its risk:benefit ratio for prophylactic use.

Trimethoprim–sulfamethoxazole (TMP/SMX) in regimens of 160 mg/800 mg twice daily for 21 days and daily for 14 days has demonstrated efficacy in preventing TD.[50,51] TMP alone at dosages of 200 mg daily for 14 days is effective for diarrhea prevention.[51] Although significant compared with placebo, the protection rate of TMP alone was less than that of the combination (95% versus 52%). Side effects noted in the studies were primarily dermatologic, including rashes and skin eruptions. Because TMP/SMX can cause serious skin eruptions such as Stevens–Johnson syndrome, the risk of taking these agents for TD prophylaxis is of concern.

Quinolone carboxylic acid derivatives are useful for TD chemoprophylaxis. Norfloxacin and ciprofloxacin have been studied widely. Norfloxacin 400 mg orally once daily for 14 days is effective.[52] Fewer patients developed diarrhea on norfloxacin than on placebo (7% versus 61%). Norfloxacin provided an 88% protection rate. Resistance was not evident among aerobic Gram-negative bacilli. Adverse reactions were limited to one case of a generalized rash 11 days after therapy with norfloxacin, which resolved upon discontinuation. In another study, ciprofloxacin 500 mg daily was compared with placebo in people traveling to Tunisia.[53] Ciprofloxacin provided a 94% protection rate and was well tolerated. One case of serious sunburn was observed that may have been drug related. Ciprofloxacin did not appear to affect aerobic bacterial flora 5 weeks after travel.

Although prophylactic management of TD with antimicrobial agents has demonstrated benefits, the uncertainty of the risk of widespread use must be evaluated. These agents have the potential for side effects such as skin rashes, photosensitivity reactions, blood disorders, Stevens–Johnson syndrome, and staining of the teeth in children. In addition, infections secondary to antimicrobial therapy (e.g., *Candida* vaginitis, antibiotic-associated colitis, and *Salmonella* enteritis) are a risk. Therefore, prophylactic antimicrobial agents are not recommended for travelers. Alternatively, instructing travelers about proper food and water precautions and early treatment of TD provide better outcomes without the risks associated with widespread prophylaxis.

Nonpharmacologic Therapy

Instructing travelers about safe food and water precautions is the mainstay of TD prevention. Travelers should be advised to avoid drinking or brushing their teeth with tap water. Ice cubes should be avoided because they may have been made with contaminated water. Boiled water (as in hot tea or coffee), carbonated beverages, beer, and wine generally are safe to consume. Two reliable methods of purification are vigorous boiling of water and chemical disinfection with iodine. Chemical disinfection can be accomplished by using tincture of iodine or tetraglycine hydroperiodide tablets. These tablets are available in pharmacies. However, disinfection with iodine often leaves an unpleasant taste. Foods that should be avoided are undercooked or raw foods, salads, and unpasteurized milk and milk products. Foods safe for consumption include bread or crackers, peeled fruit or vegetables, and well-cooked foods.[44]

TREATMENT

Approaches to treating TD include many of the remedies for treating acute nonspecific diarrhea: fluid replacement and symptomatic relief with adsorbents, antimotility agents, and short-term antimicrobial therapy. The self-limiting nature of TD generally allows successful management with nonspecific agents. However, antimicrobial agents may be useful in persistent diarrhea.

Bismuth subsalicylate is effective for relieving symptoms of mild to moderate TD. Dosages of 30 mL every 30 minutes for 8 doses generally are effective in relieving abdominal pain and cramping and reducing unformed stools.[54,55] Bismuth subsalicylate has not been shown to improve the nausea and vomiting of TD.

Loperamide, an antimotility agent, is approved for the symptomatic relief of TD at dosages up to 8 mg/day.

Loperamide was compared with bismuth subsalicylate for treating TD.[55] Dosages of loperamide were administered at 4 mg initially, then 2 mg after each unformed stool, and bismuth subsalicylate was administered at recommended dosages. Loperamide demonstrated significantly more relief (disappearance) of diarrhea and abdominal pains and a greater decrease in severity of symptoms than bismuth subsalicylate. There was no significant difference in the duration of diarrhea. Loperamide-treated patients with shigellosis did not experience prolongation of diarrhea.[55] This is consistent with the results of a study involving 43 patients; two patients infected with *Shigella* species were treated with loperamide without prolongation of diarrhea.[56]

Although using antimicrobial agents to treat TD is controversial, they may be appropriate in patients who develop persistent diarrhea. Travelers with diarrhea unresponsive to conventional therapy, three or more loose stools in an 8-hour period, and associated symptoms of nausea, vomiting, abdominal cramps, fever, or blood in the stools may benefit from a short course of therapy. Selection of an appropriate agent may depend on the traveler's symptoms, the location of travel, the climate, and the type of chemoprophylaxis received before treatment.[57] The recommended duration of treatment is 3 days.[44]

TMP/SMX (160 mg/800 mg) twice daily or TMP 200 mg alone twice daily for 3 to 5 days is effective in reducing the number of unformed stools and decreasing symptoms, including abdominal cramps, pain, and nausea.[58] The efficacy of ciprofloxacin 500 mg twice daily and TMP/SMX (160 mg/800 mg) twice daily, each for 5 days, was compared with that of placebo.[59] Both agents were equally effective. Ciprofloxacin may offer an alternative for patients with hypersensitivity to TMP/SMX. As resistance to TMP/SMX increases, fluoroquinolones may have greater benefit.

In general, fluoroquinolones are the drugs of choice for adults traveling to high-risk areas (e.g., Latin America, Africa, the Middle East, and Asia).[57] Data suggest the use of combination therapy with antimotility agents (loperamide) and antibiotics (TMP/SMX) initially in patients with moderate to severe diarrhea.[60] However, further study on the efficacy and safety is warranted.

FUTURE THERAPIES

Future developments in TD prophylaxis and treatment may include the use of poorly absorbed antimicrobial agents such as bicozamycin and oral aztreonam.[61,62] These agents should be safe in pregnant women and children. Zaldaride maleate, an intestinal calmodulin inhibitor, is another agent under investigation for TD because of its antisecretory properties.[63] However, more data about the safety and efficacy of these agents are needed.

Irritable Bowel Syndrome

DEFINITION

IBS is one of the most common disorders of the gastrointestinal tract among young to middle-aged adults. It is defined as a combination of chronic or recurrent gastrointestinal symptoms not explained by structural or biochemical abnormalities, attributed to the intestines, and associated with symptoms of pain and disturbed defecation or symptoms of bloating and distension.[64]

EPIDEMIOLOGY AND PATHOPHYSIOLOGY

The impact of IBS on health care is significant. It is estimated that IBS accounts for 2.4 to 3.5 million physician visits annually in the United States.[65,66] In a recent study, health care costs attributed to IBS in 1 year were $742 dollars, compared with $429 for patients without IBS.[67] Loss of work days is three times greater in people with IBS than in those without bowel symptoms.[68]

Although this syndrome comprises 41% of all functional gastrointestinal disorders, little is known about the pathogenesis of IBS. It is believed that IBS results from disordered intestinal motility and increased visceral sensitivity, with psychological stress contributing to its recurrence and exacerbation.[64,69]

CLINICAL PRESENTATION AND DIAGNOSIS

Clinical manifestations of IBS may vary. The diagnosis is made by identifying symptom-based criteria, known as the Rome criteria (Table 27.10), and excluding symptoms of diseases that may mimic IBS. A physical examination is warranted to exclude other diagnoses. Additional diagnostic tests can be initiated based on the patient's symptomatic subgroup (Table 27.11).

THERAPEUTIC PLAN

Treatment should be initiated to alleviate the predominant symptom (i.e., constipation, diarrhea, or pain, gas, or bloating). Therapy generally should be reassessed after 3 to 6 weeks.

TREATMENT

Pharmacotherapy

Several pharmacologic agents have been investigated for treating IBS. Bulk-forming laxatives generally are recommended for patients with constipation. Cisapride has been used in these patients; however, it may be less effective in patients with severe or refractory constipation.[39,70]

Table 27.10 ▪ Rome Diagnostic Criteria for Irritable Bowel Syndrome

At least 3 mo of continuous or recurrent symptoms of the following:
- Abdominal pain or discomfort
  - Relieved with defecation or
  - Associated with change in frequency of stool or
  - Associated with a change in consistency of stool
- Two or more of the following, at least one-fourth of occasions or days:
  - Altered stool frequency (for research purposes *altered* may be defined as more than three bowel movements each day or fewer than three bowel movements each week)
  - Altered stool form (lumpy/hard or loose/watery stool)
  - Altered stool passage (straining, urgency, or feeling of incomplete evacuation)
  - Passage of mucus
  - Bloating or feeling of abdominal distension

Source: Reprinted with permission. American Gastroenterological Association Patient Care Committee. American Gastroenterological Association medical position statement: irritable bowel syndrome. Gastroenterology 112: 2118–2119, 1997.

Table 27.11 ▪ Initial Treatment of Irritable Bowel Syndrome

	Symptomatic Subgroup		
	Constipation	Diarrhea	Pain, Gas, or Bloating
Review diet history	Yes	Yes	Yes
Additional tests	No	Lactose-H_2 breath test	Plain abdominal radiograph
Therapeutic trial	Increase roughage Osmotic laxative	Loperamide	Antispasmodic

Source: Adapted with permission. American Gastroenterological Association Patient Care Committee. Irritable bowel syndrome: a technical review for practice guideline development. Gastroenterology 112:2120–2137, 1997.

In treating diarrhea, data suggest that the opiate agonist loperamide is safe and effective. Studies demonstrate that patients with IBS taking loperamide experience improvement in diarrhea associated with decreases in stool frequency, passage of unformed stools, and incidence of urgency.[71,72] In patients with IBS and constipation, loperamide may worsen the symptoms.[72] An appropriate dosage for loperamide in IBS has not been determined. However, dosages ranging from 2 mg twice daily to 4 mg four times daily have been used for relief of symptoms. Cholestyramine, a bile acid sequestrant, may be beneficial in patients with IBS and diarrhea and a history of cholecystectomy or idiopathic bile acid malabsorption.[39]

Antispasmodics (anticholinergic agents) are commonly used in the United States for treating symptoms of abdominal pain associated with IBS. These agents suppress the postprandial contractile response of the gastrointestinal tract, thereby reducing its tone and motility. Examples of these agents are belladonna alkaloids, dicyclomine hydrochloride, and hyoscyamine sulfate. Before therapy with these agents is initiated, patients should be informed of their anticholinergic side effects. Antispasmodic medications may be contraindicated in patients with a history of cardiac arrhythmia, glaucoma, and urinary retention.

Psychotropic medications, such as tricyclic antidepressants, are indicated for patients who experience severe or refractory symptoms with associated depression or panic attacks. These patients have generally failed psychological treatment methods (e.g., cognitive and behavioral treatment, hypnosis, relaxation and stress management, or psychotherapy). Dosages used for IBS are often lower than those used for depression. Although selective serotonin reuptake inhibitors have been used clinically because of their favorable side effect profile, no published controlled studies are available for review. Anxiolytics have been used but generally are not recommended because of their potential for physical dependence and drug interactions.[64]

Nonpharmacologic Therapy

Treating IBS incorporates lifestyle modifications and pharmacologic management based on the patient's predominant symptoms. Although its use is controversial, it is recommended that patients with IBS and constipation increase their dietary fiber intake to 25 g per day. Patients with symptoms of diarrhea should avoid foods that may aggravate diarrhea such as dairy products, caffeine, alcoholic beverages, sorbitol-containing foods, and fatty foods. If symptoms of bloating and gas persist, avoiding gas-producing foods (e.g., beans, cabbage, certain fruits) may be helpful. Certain medications may aggravate gastrointestinal symptoms and should be avoided (e.g., stimulant laxatives and antacids).

KEY POINTS

- Constipation and diarrhea are common disorders of the gastrointestinal tract that are more often self-reported by older adults.
- The pharmacist is essential in counseling patients on the self-management of constipation and diarrhea.
- The primary goals in the management of constipation and diarrhea should be to relieve symptoms, prevent complications, and restore normal bowel habits. Because these disorders often are self-limiting, intervention may be of short duration.
- Definitions of constipation vary but most often incorporate straining, hard or firm stool, less frequent defecation, and a feeling of incomplete evacuation.
- Diarrhea generally is defined as three or more loose or unformed bowel movements per day with symptoms of fever, abdominal cramps, or vomiting.

- Agents available for treating constipation include bulk-forming agents, hyperosmotic agents, stool softeners, lubricants, saline, and stimulant laxatives.
- Laxatives should not be used for more than 1 week without medical supervision, nor should they be used in the presence of abdominal pain or cramping, nausea, or vomiting.
- Patients should be instructed to increase fluid intake and participate in regular exercise to prevent constipation.
- Infants and young children are more susceptible to acute losses of fluid through diarrhea and may need ORSs.
- Attapulgite, kaolin, and polycarbophil are agents with adsorbent properties used to treat acute nonspecific diarrhea.
- Loperamide should be discontinued after 48 hours if clinical improvement of diarrhea is not observed.
- People from industrialized nations traveling to developing countries often experience TD.
- Safe food and water precautions are the mainstay of TD prevention. Prophylactic antimicrobial agents are not recommended for travelers.
- TD can be managed successfully with bismuth subsalicylate and loperamide. Persistent TD may necessitate 3 days of antimicrobial therapy.
- The diagnosis of IBS can be made using the Rome criteria. Treatment is based on predominant symptoms.
- Constipation-predominant IBS can be managed with bulk-forming agents or cisapride. Diarrhea-predominant IBS is managed primarily with loperamide. Abdominal pain is relieved by antispasmodics. Psychotropic medications are reserved for patients who are refractory to other medications and have certain psychiatric disorders.

REFERENCES

1. Sandler RS, Drossman DA. Bowel habits in young adults not seeking health care. Dig Dis Sci 32:841–845, 1987.
2. Binder HJ. Pathophysiology of acute diarrhea. Am J Med 88(Suppl 6A):2S–4S, 1990.
3. Lennard-Jones JE. Constipation. In: Sleisinger MH, Fordtran JS. Gastrointestinal and liver disease: pathophysiology, diagnosis, and management. 6th ed. Philadelphia: WB Saunders, 1998:174–197.
4. Fine KD. Diarrhea. In: Sleisinger MH, Fordtran JS. Gastrointestinal and liver disease: pathophysiology, diagnosis, and management. 6th ed. Philadelphia: WB Saunders, 1998:128–152.
5. Everhart JE, Liang V, Johannes RS, et al. A longitudinal survey of self-reported bowel habits in the United States. Dig Dis Sci 34:1153–1162, 1989.
6. Sandler RS, Jordan MC, Shelton BJ. Demographic and dietary determinants of constipation in the US population. Am J Public Health 80:185–189, 1990.
7. Garthwright W, Archer D, Kvenberg J. Estimates of incidence and cost of intestinal infectious diseases in the United States. Public Health Rep 103:107–15, 1988.
8. DuPont HL. Guidelines on acute infectious diarrhea in adults. The Practice Parameters Committee of the American College of Gastroenterology. Am J Gastroenterol 92(11):1962–1975, 1997.
9. Koch TR. Constipation. In: Haubrich WS, Schaffner F, Berk JE. Bockus gastroenterology. 5th ed. Philadelphia: WB Saunders, 1995:103–104.
10. Ruben BD. Public perceptions of digestive health and disease. Pract Gastroenterol 10:35–40, 1986.
11. Cohnell AM, Hilton C, Irvin G, et al. Variation of bowel habit in two population samples. BMJ 2:1095–1102, 1965.
12. Brunton LL. Agents affecting gastrointestinal water flux and motility: emesis and antiemetics; bile acids and pancreatic enzymes. In: Hardman JG, Limbird LE, Molinoff PB, et al. Goodman & Gilman's the pharmacological basis of therapeutics. 9th ed. New York: McGraw-Hill, 1996:917–928.
13. McRorie JW, Daggy BP, Morel JG, et al. A clinical study comparing stool softening and laxative efficacy of psyllium vs. docusate sodium. Gastroenterology 112(Suppl):A787, 1997.
14. Tedesco FJ, Dipiro JT. Laxative use in constipation. Am J Gastroenterol 80:303–309, 1985.
15. Anonymous. Safety of stool softeners. Med Lett 19:45–46, 1977.
16. Donowitz M. Current concepts of laxative action: mechanisms by which laxatives increase stool water. Clin Gastroenterol 1:777–784, 1979.
17. Anonymous. Laxative drug products for over-the-counter human use: proposed amendment to the tentative final monograph. Federal Register 62 FR 46223, September 2, 1997.
18. Anonymous. Laxatives. Replacing danthron. Drug Ther Bull 26:53–56, 1988.
19. Baron JA, Jessen LM, Colaizzi JL, et al. Cisapride: a gastrointestinal prokinetic drug. Ann Pharmacother 28:488–500, 1994.
20. Muller-Lissner SA. Treatment of chronic constipation with cisapride and placebo. Gut 28:1033–1038, 1987.
21. Verheyen K, Vervaeke M, Demyttenaere P, et al. Double-blind comparison of two cisapride dosage regimens with placebo in the treatment of functional constipation. Curr Ter Res 41:978–985, 1987.
22. Hedner T, Cassieto J. Opioids and opioid receptors in peripheral tissues. Scand J Gastroenterol Suppl 130:36–40, 1987.
23. Kreek MJ, Schaefer RA, Hahn EF, et al. Naloxone, a specific opioid antagonist, reverses chronic idiopathic constipation. Lancet 1:261–262, 1983.
24. Kaufman PN, Krevsky B, Malmud LS, et al. Role of opiate receptors in the regulation of colonic transit. Gastroenterology 94:1351–1356, 1988.
25. Anonymous. Final rule: psyllium health claims. Federal Register 63 FR 8103, February 18, 1998.
26. Kinnunen O. Study of constipation in a geriatric hospital, day hospital, old people's home and at home. Aging 3:161–170, 1991.
27. Anonymous. Antidiarrheal drug products for over-the-counter human use: tentative final monograph. Federal Register 51:16138–16149, 1986.
28. DuPont HL, Sanchez JF, Ericsson CD, et al. Comparative efficacy of loperamide hydrochloride and bismuth subsalicylate in the management of acute diarrhea. Am J Med 88(Suppl 6A):15S–19S, 1990.
29. Dupont HL, Ericsson CD, DuPont MW, et al. A randomized open-label comparison of non-prescription loperamide and attapulgite in the symptomatic treatment of acute diarrhea. Am J Med 88(Suppl 6A):20S–23S, 1990.
30. Johnson PC, Ericsson CD, DuPont HL, et al. Comparison of loperamide with bismuth subsalicylate for the treatment of acute travelers' diarrhea. JAMA 225:757–760, 1986.
31. Anonymous. Opium preparations. American Hospital Formulatory Service drug information 1998. Bethesda, MD: American Society of Health-Systems Pharmacists, 1998: 2385–2386, Section 56.08.
32. Anonymous. Status of certain over-the-counter drug category II and III ingredients. Federal Register 55:20434–20438, 1990.
33. Brownlee HJ. Family practitioner's guide to patient self-treatment of acute diarrhea. Am J Med 88(Suppl 6A):27S–29S, 1990.
34. Anonymous. Oral fluids for dehydration. Med Lett 29:63–64, 1987.
35. DuPont HL, Hornick RB. Adverse effect of Lomotil therapy in shigellosis. JAMA 226:1525–1528, 1973.
36. Brown JW. Toxic megacolon association with loperamide therapy. JAMA 241:501–502, 1979.
37. Tyler VE. Herbs of choice: the therapeutic use of phytomedicinals. New York: Pharmaceutical Products Press, 1994:1.
38. Tyler VE. The honest herbal: a sensible guide to the use of herbs and related remedies. 3rd ed. 1993:336–351.
39. American Gastroenterological Association Patient Care Committee. Medical position statement: irritable bowel syndrome. Gastroenterology 112:2118–2119, 1997.
40. Gannon K. The next five years: the hot and not so hot OTC drugs. Drug Top (May 7):28–32, 1990.
41. Gannon K. Who's buying what in OTCs. Drug Top (Jan. 8):32–48, 1990.
42. Stoehr GP, Ganguli M, Seaberg EC, et al. Over-the-counter medication use in an older rural community: the Movies Project. J Am Geriatr Soc 45:158–165, 1997.

43. Salata RA, Olds GR. Infectious diseases in travelers and immigrants. In: Warren KS, Mahmoud AF. Tropical and geographic medicine. 2nd ed. New York: McGraw-Hill, 1990:228.
44. U.S. Department of Health and Human Services. Health information for international travel. Atlanta: HHS Publication No. (CDC) 96-8280, 1996–97.
45. DuPont HL, Ericsson CD, Johnson PC. Prevention of travelers' diarrhea by the tablet formulation of bismuth subsalicylate. JAMA 257:1347–1350, 1987.
46. DuPont HL, Sullivan P, Evans DG, et al. Prevention of travelers' diarrhea (emporiatric enteritis): prophylactic administration of bismuth subsalicylate. JAMA 243:237–241, 1980.
47. Mendelowitz PC, Hoffman RS, Weber S. Bismuth absorption and myoclonic encephalopathy during bismuth subsalicylate therapy. Ann Intern Med 112:140–141, 1990.
48. Sack DA, Kaminsky DC, Sack RB, et al. Prophylactic doxycycline for travelers' diarrhea: results of a prospective double-blind study of Peace Corps volunteers in Kenya. N Engl J Med 298:758–763, 1978.
49. Sack RB, Frochlich JL, Zulich AW, et al. Prophylactic doxycycline for travelers' diarrheas: results of a prospective double-blind study of Peace Corps volunteers in Morocco. Gastroenterology 76:1368–1373, 1979.
50. DuPont HL, Evans DG, Rios N, et al. Prevention of travelers' diarrhea with trimethoprim–sulfamethoxazole alone. Gastroenterology 84:75–80, 1983.
51. DuPont HL, Galindo E, Evans DG, et al. Prevention of travelers' diarrhea with trimethoprim–sulfamethoxazole and trimethoprim alone. Gastroenterology 84:75–80, 1983.
52. Johnson PC, Ericsson CD, Morgan DR, et al. Lack of emergency of resistant fecal flora during successful prophylaxis of travelers' diarrhea with norfloxacin. Antimicrob Agents Chemother 30:671–674, 1986.
53. Rademaker CM, Hoepelam IM, Wolfhagen MJ. Results of a double-blind placebo-controlled study using ciprofloxacin for prevention of traveler's diarrhea. Eur J Clin Microbiol Infect Dis 8:690–694, 1989.
54. DuPont HL, Sullivan P, Pickering LK, et al. Symptomatic treatment of diarrhea with bismuth subsalicylate among students attending a Mexican university. Gastroenterology 73:715–718, 1997.
55. Johnson PC, Ericsson CD, DuPont HL. Comparison of loperamide with bismuth subsalicylate for the treatment of acute travelers' diarrhea. JAMA 255:757–760, 1986.
56. Van Loon FP, Bennish ML, Butler C. Double-blind trial of loperamide for treating acute watery diarrhea in expatriates in Bangladesh. Gut 30:492–495, 1989.
57. DuPont HL, Ericsson CD. Prevention and treatment of travelers' diarrhea. N Engl J Med 328:1821–1827, 1993.
58. DuPont HL, Reves RR, Galindo E, et al. Treatment of travelers' diarrhea with trimethoprim/sulfamethoxazole and with trimethoprim alone. N Engl J Med 307:841–844, 1982.
59. Ericsson CD, Johnson PC, DuPont HL, et al. Ciprofloxacin or trimethoprim–sulfamethoxazole as initial therapy for travelers' diarrhea. Ann Intern Med 106:216–220, 1987.
60. Ericsson CD, DuPont HL, Mathewson JJ, et al. Treatment of travelers' diarrhea with sulfamethoxazole and trimethoprim and loperamide. JAMA 263:257–261, 1990.
61. Ericksson CD, DuPont HL, Sullivan P, et al. Bicozamycin, a poorly absorbable antibiotic, effectively treats travelers' diarrhea. Ann Intern Med 98:20–25, 1983.
62. DuPont HL, Ericsson CD, Mathewson JJ, et al. Oral aztreonam, a poorly absorbed yet effective therapy for bacterial diarrhea in U.S. travelers to Mexico. JAMA 267:1932–1935, 1992.
63. DuPont HL, Ericsson CD, Mathewson JJ, et al. Zaldaride maleate: an intestinal calmodulin inhibitor in the therapy of traveler's diarrhea. Gastroenterology 104(3):709–715, 1993.
64. American Gastroenterological Association Patient Care Committee. Irritable bowel syndrome: a technical review for practice guideline development. Gastroenterology 113:2120–2137, 1997.
65. Everhart JE, Renault PF. Irritable bowel syndrome in office-based practice in the United States. Gastroenterology 100:998–1005, 1991.
66. Sandler RS. Epidemiology of irritable bowel syndrome in the United States. Gastroenterology 99:409–415, 1990.
67. Talley NJ, Gabriel SE, Harmsen WS, et al. Medical costs in community subjects with irritable bowel syndrome. Gastroenterology 109:1736–1741, 1995.
68. Drossman DA, Li Z, Andruzzi E, et al. U.S. household survey of functional gastrointestinal disorders: prevalence, sociodemography and health impact. Dig Dis Sci 38:1569–1580, 1993.
69. McGill B. Functional diarrhea. Evaluation and management. Pract Gastroenterol 4:16–20, 1980.
70. Van Outryve M, Milon R, Toussaint J, et al. "Prokinetic" treatment of constipation-predominant irritable bowel syndrome. A placebo-controlled study of cisapride. Clin Gastroenterol 13:49–57, 1991.
71. Cann PA, Read NW, Holdsworth CD, et al. Role of loperamide and placebo in the management of irritable bowel syndrome. Dig Dis Sci 29:239–247, 1984.
72. Hovdenak N. Loperamide treatment of the irritable bowel syndrome. Scand J Gastroenterol 130(Suppl):81–84, 1987.

CHAPTER 28

HEPATITIS, VIRAL AND DRUG-INDUCED

Mary F. Hebert

DEFINITION

Hepatitis is inflammation of the liver that can be caused by viruses (e.g., hepatitis B or hepatitis C), medications (e.g., methyldopa or isoniazid), or immunologic abnormalities (e.g., autoimmune hepatitis). Hepatitis can occur as acute or chronic disease. Chronic disease generally is defined as that persisting for 6 months or longer.

Viral Hepatitis

Because of the great deal of overlap between the symptoms and incubation periods for the various hepatitis viruses, symptoms and time course alone cannot be used for differentiating between the virus types. Therefore, viral serologies are needed to distinguish between infections caused by each of the viruses. There are many hepatitis viruses, including all the letters of the alphabet from A to G. Although each of the viruses from A to G is mentioned briefly (Table 28.1), this chapter focuses on hepatitis A, B, and C viruses.

Drug-Induced Hepatitis

Drug-induced liver injury is highly variable in the type of reactions seen and individual patient susceptibility. Drug-induced liver injury is most often asymptomatic until extensive damage is done. For some agents, elevations in serum aminotransferases can be transient despite continuation of therapy. For others, continuation of the offending agent can result in extensive hepatocellular necrosis and death. Although other types of drug-induced liver injury occur, this chapter addresses only drug-induced hepatitis. (For further discussion on other types of drug-induced liver injury, such as hepatocellular necrosis and cholestasis, see Chapter 2.)

TREATMENT GOALS: VIRAL HEPATITIS

- Prevent hepatitis viral infection by avoiding exposure (e.g., avoiding contaminated food and water, practicing good personal hygiene, avoiding reuse of intravenous needles, practicing safer sex, avoiding recapping needles after blood drawing, and using sterile technique with acupuncture and tattooing).
- Prevent hepatitis viral infection by following prophylaxis regimens when exposure is expected.
- When prevention fails, clear the virus as measured by polymerase chain reaction.
- Improve or normalize serum aminotransferases.
- Improve or normalize histologic changes associated with hepatitis.
- Prevent progression of hepatic disease.
- Maintain compliance with therapy.
- Minimize and manage adverse effects associated with therapy.
- Manage the complications of end-stage liver disease.

Table 28.1 ▪ Hepatitis Viruses

Virus	Other Names	Family	Type	Usual Route of Transmission
Hepatitis A	Infectious hepatitis	Picornavirus	RNA	Oral–fecal
Hepatitis B	Serum hepatitis	Hepadnaviridae	DNA	Blood or sexual
Hepatitis C	Non-A, non-B	Flaviviridae	RNA	Blood
Hepatitis D	Delta hepatitis	Delta viridae	RNA	Blood or sexual
Hepatitis E		Caliciviridae	RNA	Fecal–oral
Hepatitis F				Fecal–oral
Hepatitis G		Flaviviridae		Blood

TREATMENT GOALS: DRUG-INDUCED HEPATITIS

- Avoid, if possible, giving agents known to cause hepatitis to patients with liver disease (risks and benefits should be weighed before therapy is started).
- Detect drug-induced hepatitis early and discontinue the offending agent.
- Avoid significant liver damage.
- Treat drug-induced liver disease as clinically appropriate.

EPIDEMIOLOGY

Viral Hepatitis

Hepatitis A

Approximately 125,000 to 200,000 patients are infected with hepatitis A in the United States each year.[1] It takes approximately 2 to 7 weeks (average 4 weeks) from the time of infection to the development of hepatitis symptoms such as jaundice, malaise, and right upper quadrant pain.[2–4] The contagious period for hepatitis A appears to start 1 to 2 weeks before the onset of symptoms and end shortly (10 to 15 days) thereafter.[5–7] Because high concentrations of hepatitis A are found in the stool of infected patients, the usual mode of transmission is by direct fecal–oral contact or fecal contamination of food or water. There is no carrier state for hepatitis A. Therefore transmission of hepatitis A through a blood transfusion is very rare.[8–13]

Hepatitis B

It is estimated that more than 1 million people in the United States are chronically infected with hepatitis B virus.[14] Approximately 140,000 to 320,000 people per year become acutely infected with the hepatitis B virus in the United States. Of those infected, 70,000 to 160,000 become symptomatic, 8400 to 19,000 are hospitalized, 8000 to 32,000 develop chronic infections, and 140 to 320 die of fulminant disease each year.[14] Chronic infections are most likely to occur in very young patients infected with hepatitis B (90% of infections in infants, 25 to 50% in children less than 5 years and 6 to 10% in adults). Approximately one-fourth of the patients with chronic hepatitis B infections develop chronic active hepatitis, which often progresses to cirrhosis. These patients also are at a much greater risk for developing liver cancer (12 to 300 times normal risk). In addition, 5000 to 6000 patients die each year from liver disease related to hepatitis B.[14,15] In 1995, 6.8% of the liver transplants performed in the United States were in patients infected with hepatitis B virus.[16]

Hepatitis B can be transmitted by blood or sexual exposure.[17,18] Hepatitis B transmission through infected blood exposures can occur when contaminated fluid splashes into an eye or when sterile techniques are not used with intravenous needles, tattooing, body piercing, or acupuncture.[19–23] The virus remains in the blood approximately 6 weeks with an acute infection. In addition, a carrier state exists for hepatitis B.[24] A carrier is a person who is persistently (more than 6 months) hepatitis B surface antigen (HB_sAg) positive. Patients who test positive for HB_sAg are potentially infectious, but those testing positive for hepatitis B e antigen (HB_eAg) have the highest degree of infectivity.[15] The incubation period from the time of infection to the onset of symptoms is 4 months on average but ranges from 1.5 to 5 months.[15]

Hepatitis C

Almost 4 million patients in the United States are thought to be infected with hepatitis C virus.[25] An estimated 36,000 hepatitis C infections occur in the United States each year; 85% of these infections go on to become chronic infections.[26,27] Approximately 1 to 5% of patients with chronic hepatitis C develop hepatocellular carcinoma after 20 years of infection. Once cirrhotic, 1 to 4% of the patients per year develop hepatocellular carcinoma.[25] Non-A, non-B, or hepatitis C alone, or in combination with hepatitis B or alcoholic liver disease, accounted for 32.6% of the liver transplants performed in the United States in 1995.[16] Hepatitis C appears to be transmitted primarily through infected blood exposures such as blood transfusions, needlesticks, or tattooing.[28–30] Although the incidence is not as clear, perinatal (mother to infant) transmission and transmission through sexual contact probably also occur.[31,32]

Drug-Induced Hepatitis

Drug-induced liver disease is rare, although as many as 1000 agents have been associated with the various types of hepatic disease. Some agents or their metabolites have been found to be directly hepatotoxic, whereas others appear to produce an allergic reaction that results in hepatic injury. Between 1 in 600 and 1 in 3500 hospital admissions and 2 to 3% of all admissions for drug-induced adverse reactions are related to drug-induced hepatic injury. In addition, approximately 5% of hospital admissions for jaundice, 20 to 50% of nonviral chronic hepatitis, and 15–30% of fulminant hepatic failure cases appear to be drug induced.[33,34] Many factors affect drug-induced hepatotoxicity. Some of the factors associated with an increased susceptibility to drug-induced liver injury are listed in Table 28.2.

PATHOPHYSIOLOGY

Viral Hepatitis

Hepatitis A

Hepatitis A infections are asymptomatic in approximately one-third of the patients. Another third develop mild nonspecific symptoms, and the last third develop more severe symptoms including jaundice. A month after infection, patients typically experience the acute onset of symptoms, which last about 4 weeks. Patients with more severe symptoms have an increase in their serum aspartate aminotransferase (AST), alanine aminotransferase (ALT), and bilirubin, which resolve over 4 to 6 months.

Hepatitis B and C

Hepatitis B infections are asymptomatic in approximately two-thirds of patients. Acute hepatitis occurs in another third, with progression to fulminant hepatitis in less than 1%. Of the adults infected, 5 to 10% develop chronic hepatitis B infection. Some of those chronically infected are asymptomatic, and others go on to develop hepatic cirrhosis or hepatocellular carcinoma. About 30% of those chronically infected with hepatitis B go on to develop cirrhosis. Similarly, two-thirds of patients with hepatitis C acute infection are asymptomatic. Unfortunately, more than 85% of the infections become chronic, and approximately 70% of patients develop chronic liver disease. Between 8000 and 10,000 deaths per year result from chronic liver disease related to hepatitis C.[14,27] The 5-year chronic hepatitis C survival for patients with compensated cirrhosis is 91%. In contrast, those with decompensated cirrhosis (concomitant liver failure, ascites, variceal hemorrhage, or encephalopathy) have a 5-year survival of 50%.[25]

Acute hepatitis B typically is associated with high elevations in AST and ALT (more than a 100-fold increase over normal) and bilirubin (20-fold increase over normal). Serum AST, ALT, and bilirubin increase in acute hepatitis C infection, but the increases tend not to be as high as in hepatitis B. Jaundice is a common finding in acute hepatitis but is rare with chronic hepatitis unless the liver disease becomes quite severe. Chronic hepatitis, on the other hand, is associated with mild elevations in AST and ALT (up to 20 times normal) and generally normal alkaline phosphatase and γ-glutamyl transpeptidase. Platelet and white blood cell counts also remain normal until the liver disease becomes severe and splenomegaly develops. Liver biopsies, although not always performed, can be helpful in determining the severity of disease, establishing the cause, and predicting the outcome of therapy, particularly with hepatitis C. Chronic hepatitis is associated with an inflammatory infiltrate with mononuclear cells in the liver. There may also be hepatocyte necrosis.

Drug-Induced Hepatitis

Several different types of hepatitis have been reported as adverse drug reactions (Table 28.2). Nonspecific hepatitis is characterized by focal hepatocellular necrosis with a mononuclear infiltrate and variable amounts of portal inflammation. Viral-like hepatitis is characterized by an inflammatory infiltrate, variable amounts of hepatocyte necrosis, bile stasis, and lobular disarray. Severe cases can exhibit bridging submassive or massive necrosis. Granulomatous hepatitis is characterized by aggregates of epithelioid histiocytes with variable types and amounts of inflammatory cells. Autoimmunelike hepatitis is characterized by a hepatitis picture with positive antinuclear antibodies. Inflammation may be severe, and an elevated number of plasma cells may be seen in the liver biopsy. Cholestatic hepatitis is characterized by prominent cholestasis, variable amounts of hepatocellular necrosis, and portal and lobular mononuclear, neutrophilic, or eosinophilic inflammation. Some medications have been reported to cause more than one type of liver injury.

CLINICAL PRESENTATION AND DIAGNOSIS

Signs and Symptoms

Viral Hepatitis

Hepatitis A

Hepatitis A is associated with the abrupt onset of symptoms, including fever in about 50% of patients, nausea, anorexia, malaise, abdominal discomfort, dark urine, and jaundice. The severity of illness appears to be age dependent. In most cases children are asymptomatic, whereas adults usually become symptomatic and jaundiced. Hepatitis A viral infection generally is considered the most benign of the three viruses presented here. The fatality rate for hepatitis A infection is less than 1%.[15]

Hepatitis B and C

Acute Hepatitis. After the incubation period, patients who become symptomatic characteristically develop nonspecific, flulike symptoms such as malaise, weakness, anorexia, nausea, vomiting, and right upper quadrant

Table 28.2 ▪ Drug-Induced Hepatitis

Agent	Type of Hepatitis Reaction	Time to Onset (frequency of hepatitis or jaundice)	Host Factors That Increase Susceptibility to Liver Damage	Expected Outcome	Comments
Allopurinol	Viral-like or granulomatous hepatitis	<5 wk	Diuretic use Renal disease	Rarely fatal.	
Amiodarone	Alcoholiclike, cholestatic, and granulomatous hepatitis	1 mo to several years (1%)		Insidious onset; hepatotoxicity may persist several months after discontinuation; death from liver failure has been reported.	
Angiotensin-converting enzyme inhibitors	Cholestatic hepatitis	1 wk–20 mo (<1%)		Slow recovery after discontinuation; submassive necrosis and fulminant liver failure have occurred with continued therapy.	
Aspirin	Nonspecific or viral-like hepatitis	Several days to weeks (0.1–0.5%)	Chronic rheumatic disease Children with acute rheumatic fever Low albumin Defect in mitochondrial β-oxidation	Reversible with discontinuation.	Dose-dependent reaction, most common with concentrations >25 mg/dL (3–5 g/day for adults); can occur with concentrations <10 mg/dL in 2% of the reactions.
Carbamazepine	Granulomatous or cholestatic hepatitis	(5–10%)[a]		Mild asymptomatic increases in liver function values are common; more severe cases can take months to resolve.	
Dantrolene	Viral-like acute or chronic hepatitis	>1 mo (1–2%)	Age >30 yr	22–28% fatal.	Monitor liver function tests in all patients on dantrolene.
Diclofenac	Nonspecific acute or autoimmunelike chronic hepatitis	1 wk–14 mo (<1%)		Most resolve with discontinuation; fatalities from massive necrosis have occurred.	Monitor liver function tests every 3–6 mo; discontinue if more than threefold increase.
Disulfiram	Acute viral-like hepatitis	<2 mo (<1%)	Women	Fulminant hepatic failure has occurred.	
Erythromycin estolate	Cholestatic hepatitis	1–4 wk (0.1–0.5%)		Usually rapid and complete resolution after discontinuation; fulminant hepatic failure has been reported.	Less common with other erythromycin salts.
Etretinate	Chronic hepatitis	1 mo (1.5%)		Most commonly causes transient increases in liver function values, more serious reactions have occurred.	
Halothane	Viral-like acute hepatitis	Several days to 3 wk after exposure, shortened to a few days after repeat exposure (<0.001%)	Repeat exposures Female patients Obesity Older adults	Usually mild, subclinical increase in liver function values, acute hepatitis is rare but fatal in 80% of cases.	If repeat anesthetic exposure is necessary, avoid halothane.

Isoniazid	Viral-like hepatitis	Most cases <3 mo; can be delayed as long as 1 yr (<1%)	Age >50 yr Women	Reactions range from mild acute reactions to liver failure and death; case fatality rate approximately 10%.	
Methyldopa	Acute and chronic viral-like, cholestatic, or autoimmunelike hepatitis	<3 mo (0.1–0.5%)		Usually transient, asymptomatic increases in liver function values, recovery can take months, fatal massive necrosis is not uncommon.	Rechallenge has been fatal in some cases.
Monoamine oxidase inhibitors	Acute viral-like hepatitis	(<1%)		Often fatal.	
Niacin	Hepatitis	<3 mo, sometimes within days (50%)[a]		Fulminant failure has been reported in some patients.	
Nitrofurantoin	Autoimmunelike or granulomatous hepatitis	Usually <1 mo; delayed cases have been reported (<1%)	Women (although this may reflect usage pattern)	Usually complete recovery after discontinuation; fatalities have been reported particularly if continued despite evidence of liver injury.	
Oxacillin	Nonspecific focal hepatitis	>1 wk		Resolution within several weeks after discontinuation.	Associated with high-dose intravenous therapy.
Phenytoin	Viral-like acute or chronic and granulomatous hepatitis	Usually 4–6 wk; may occur as early as 1–2 wk (0.5–1%)		Usually resolves with discontinuation; advanced cases may be slow to resolve or progress and be fatal over weeks to months.	Often associated with fever, malaise, rash, and eosinophilia.
Procainamide	Granulomatous hepatitis			Usually resolves with discontinuation of agent.	
Quinidine	Granulomatous or hepatocellular–cholestatic hepatitis	1–2 wk		Usually reversible with discontinuation.	
Rifampin	Viral-like acute hepatitis	(<1%)	Concomitant administration of isoniazid Slow acetylators		
Sulfonamides	Nonspecific, autoimmune-like or granulomatous chronic hepatitis	Usually <2 wk; may be delayed (0.5–1%)	Human immunodeficiency virus infection	Usually complete recovery within weeks to a few months after discontinuation; a few deaths have been reported.	
Tetracycline	Viral-like hepatitis			Reaction often is progressive.	
Trazodone	Chronic hepatitis			Reversible with discontinuation.	

Source: References 33–59.

[a]Hepatitis incidence not found; percentage reported for patients with elevated liver function values.

abdominal pain (over the liver). These symptoms start about a week before jaundice develops. The onset of clinical symptoms is insidious and usually continues for a few weeks after the development of dark urine, jaundice, and serum bilirubin values of 2.5 mg/dL or more. The appearance of jaundice or dark urine often prompts a visit to the doctor. Before that, patients often feel as if they have had a very bad flu. A small percentage of patients develop fulminant viral hepatitis, with symptoms of liver failure and encephalopathy. The fatality rate from fulminant viral liver failure is approximately 1 to 1.5% of those infected.[15]

Chronic Hepatitis. For many patients, chronic hepatitis is asymptomatic. Other patients experience mild symptoms intermittently. Sometimes the diagnosis of chronic hepatitis is not made until the patient develops cirrhosis.[60,61] The most common symptoms of chronic hepatitis are fatigue, weakness, and malaise. In a small subset of these patients, the fatigue is so severe that it impairs their ability to perform daily activities. Although less common than fatigue, some patients experience tenderness in the right upper quadrant of the abdomen, nausea, anorexia, and muscle or joint pain. Once cirrhosis develops, the fatigue, anorexia, weight loss, and weakness become more severe. In addition, patients may develop ascites, jaundice, muscle wasting, hepatic encephalopathy, and esophageal varices (see Chapter 29 for further discussion). A small group of patients can develop extrahepatic symptoms of chronic viral hepatitis such as arthritis, polyuria, and urticaria.

Drug-Induced Hepatitis

The signs and symptoms of drug-induced hepatitis are highly variable and can present as acute or chronic disease. Some patients may have only asymptomatic transient elevations in their serum aminotransferases, and others progress to fulminant hepatic failure. Patients may develop fever, rash, arthralgias, nausea, jaundice, abdominal complaints, lymphadenopathy, hepatomegaly, and eosinophilia. All patients have elevations in at least some liver enzymes (AST, ALT, alkaline phosphatase, and bilirubin). The magnitude of the elevations and the enzymes involved depend on the offending agent and the severity and stage of the liver damage. Patients with very severe liver injury can develop encephalopathy and symptoms of portal hypertension such as ascites and esophageal varices (see Chapter 29 for further discussion). The case fatality rate for drug-induced hepatic injury is approximately 5% overall. Unfortunately, the fatality rate for some agents is much higher.

Diagnosis

Viral Hepatitis

Hepatitis A

The diagnosis of acute hepatitis A cannot be made on clinical symptoms alone. Diagnosis is based on measurement of immunoglobulin M (IgM) antibodies to hepatitis A in the serum. Later, IgG antibodies to hepatitis A appear in the serum and protect against reinfection.

Hepatitis B

Several markers can be measured for diagnosis of hepatitis B. HB_sAg can be measured in the serum 30 to 60 days after exposure to hepatitis B virus. Antibodies against HB_sAg develop in response to an infection with hepatitis B and provide long-term immunity. IgM antibodies against the hepatitis B core antigen also develop in response to an acute hepatitis B infection and persist for about 6 months. The IgM antibodies against the core antigen can be used as markers for acute hepatitis B infection. HB_eAg is a marker of rapid viral replication. The development of antibodies to HB_eAg correlates with loss of replicating virus and decreased infectivity of the virus.

Hepatitis C

Hepatitis C virus infections can be diagnosed by detection of antibodies against the hepatitis C virus or hepatitis C viral RNA in the patient's serum. Antibodies against hepatitis C can be measured 6 to 9 weeks after infection depending on the assay.[28] Hepatitis C RNA can be measured within 1 week of infection.[26] About 15% of patients test positive for antibodies against hepatitis C and negative for hepatitis C viral RNA. These patients have resolved infection.

Drug-Induced Hepatitis

Because the symptoms of drug-induced hepatitis can be quite similar to those of hepatitis from other origins, the diagnosis of drug-induced liver injury requires exclusion of other causes. Ultimately, the diagnosis depends on the history of exposure, time course, consistent clinical and laboratory findings, exclusion of other causes, and resolution of the injury after discontinuation of the offending agent. Although rechallenge with the suspected etiologic agent can confirm drug-induced injury, this usually is not done and should not be recommended because of the risk of further injury and the availability of alternative agents in most cases.

Often the pharmacist is asked to evaluate whether the patient's medications could be contributing to liver disease. Although this is difficult to determine with any level of certainty, the first step in the evaluation is to determine for each medication (prescription and over-the-counter) the scope of liver injury that has been reported in the literature. A comparison between the time course, frequency, and type of injury the patient is exhibiting and those that have been reported in the literature is helpful in determining the likelihood that a particular reaction is drug induced.

PSYCHOSOCIAL ASPECTS

Three main psychosocial issues should be addressed in patients with chronic hepatitis B or C. The first is related to the disease process itself. Many patients become depressed following their diagnosis. Because hepatitis B and C are potentially life-threatening diseases with limited cure rates, even if patients are given information about the options, they often walk away with the perception that they are terminally ill and about to die. Patients may need to be told more than once that chronic hepatitis is a slowly progressive disease, that most patients live for many years after diagnosis, that treatments are available that provide clinical improvement or cure in some patients, that lifestyle changes such as discontinuation of ethanol consumption and illegal drug use may be helpful in prolonging life, and that for patients who do not respond to therapy, liver transplantation may be an option.

The second psychosocial issue is related to compliance with drug therapy. Although most patients are compliant with their treatment regimens, for some the adverse effects are prohibitive. It is helpful to educate patients about the severity and types of expected adverse effects before starting treatment. Patients should be encouraged to continue therapy as clinically appropriate and taught which symptoms are expected to decline with continued treatment. Finally, because patients with chronic viral hepatitis (particularly B) can transmit the virus to their partners through sexual contact, education about safer sex practices is important. Changes in sexual practices for people with chronic hepatitis C in monogamous relationships are controversial because the sexual transmission rate is low.

TREATMENT

Pharmacotherapy

Viral Hepatitis

Hepatitis A: Preexposure Prophylaxis

The Centers for Disease Control currently recommend hepatitis A vaccination of children (over 2 years), adolescents, and adults planning to live in or make multiple visits to intermediate- or high-risk areas for hepatitis A. This includes areas of the world endemic with hepatitis A, particularly rural areas of developing countries with poor sanitation. There are two inactivated hepatitis A vaccines that should be administered into the deltoid muscle. The vaccine takes about 4 weeks to induce a protective immune response, which lasts at least 20 years. The most common side effects of the hepatitis A vaccine are soreness at the injection site, headache, fatigue, and anorexia, which usually are mild and resolve within 2 days. Although rare, anaphylactic reactions have been reported. Children less than 2 years of age making multiple visits or planning to live in hepatitis A endemic areas for long periods of time and those 2 years of age and older needing only short-term protection, should receive intramuscular immune globulin. A single 0.02-mL/kg dose generally is adequate for short trips (less than 3 months), but 0.06 mL/kg every 5 months is necessary for longer visits.[62] Guidelines for travel prophylaxis are summarized in Table 28.3. Intramuscular injection of immune globulin can result in pain, swelling, and muscle stiffness at the injection site. Less commonly, urticaria, angioedema, headache, malaise, fever, and nephrotic syndrome have been reported. Severe reactions including anaphylactic shock have been reported rarely. Patients who will need repeat doses of immune globulin in a developing country should make sure that the product they receive meets licensing requirements for the United States. Immune globulin products produced in developing countries may not meet U.S. standards for purity.

Hepatitis A: Postexposure Prophylaxis

The need for immune globulin postexposure prophylaxis for hepatitis A virus depends on the nature of the exposure. Immune globulin prophylaxis for hepatitis A is recommended for patients with household or sexual contact with people infected with hepatitis A, employees or attendees of a day care center if other children or employees are diagnosed as having a hepatitis A infection, those in close contact with people infected with hepatitis A in prisons or other group facilities, coworkers of a food handler infected with hepatitis A, or patrons of a restaurant in which a food handler infected with hepatitis A (with poor hygienic practices or diarrhea) has been preparing food, without wearing gloves, that will not be cooked before eaten. In addition, patients must be identified and treated within 2 weeks of exposure.[15] Immune globulin (0.02

Table 28.3 ▪ Hepatitis Travel Prophylaxis

Hepatitis Type	When to Give Prophylaxis	Comments	Age	Recommendation
Hepatitis A	Travelers to hepatitis A endemic areas	Visit >3 mo or repeat visits	≥2 yr	Hepatitis A vaccine
		Visit <3 mo	All	Immune globulin 0.02 mL/kg IM single dose
		Visit >3 mo or repeat visits	<2 yr (or ≥2 yr and not vaccinated)	Immune globulin 0.06 mL/kg IM every 5 mo
Hepatitis B	Travelers to hepatitis B endemic areas	Visit >6 mo or short visits with high-risk of blood or sexual exposure to hepatitis B	All	Hepatitis B vaccine

mL/kg intramuscularly) has been found to be 80 to 90% effective in preventing hepatitis A infections after exposure if it is given early in the incubation period.[63,64] Giving immune globulin more than 2 weeks after exposure is not recommended.

Hepatitis B: Preexposure Prophylaxis

Hepatitis B vaccine is routinely given to infants and children in the United States. Patients who have not received the hepatitis B vaccine series and plan to live in an area with high levels of endemic hepatitis B virus for longer than 6 months, or short-term travelers with a high likelihood of exposure to hepatitis B through blood or sexual contact with natives of a hepatitis B endemic area, should receive the hepatitis B vaccine series. Guidelines for travel prophylaxis are summarized in Table 28.3. In addition, people at high risk for exposure to hepatitis B (e.g., intravenous drug users, sexually active heterosexuals with multiple partners, homosexual men, sexual and household contacts of infected patients, health care workers, and patients on hemodialysis) should also receive the hepatitis B vaccine series.

Hepatitis B: Postexposure Prophylaxis

Hepatitis B immune globulin (HBIG) is produced from plasma that contains high titers of antibody against HB_sAg. It is used to provide passive immunity against hepatitis B infection. The Immunization Practices Advisory Committee (ACIP) recommends HBIG for unvaccinated patients or those with an inadequate response to the hepatitis B vaccine who are exposed to HB_sAg-positive individuals through a needlestick or human bite, direct mucous membrane contact (oral or ophthalmic), birth (neonates), sexual or intimate contact, and household exposure for infants less than 12 months old. Prophylaxis of other household contacts is not routinely necessary unless there is an identifiable exposure to blood such as sharing razors or toothbrushes.[15] HBIG is 75% effective in preventing transmission of acute hepatitis B infection through sexual contact.[65] Because HBIG provides only short-term protection against hepatitis B, the hepatitis B vaccine series or booster doses should also be given to these patients as appropriate. HBIG (0.06 mL/kg for adults and 0.5 mL for infants) should be administered by intramuscular injection, preferably into the deltoid muscle or the anterolateral aspect of the thigh as soon after exposure to the hepatitis B virus as possible. The value of HBIG when given more than 7 days after the exposure is unclear. The most common adverse reactions of HBIG are local pain, swelling, and erythema at the injection site. Allergic reactions, body and joint pain, muscle cramps, malaise, and fever have also been reported.

The hepatitis B vaccine is a recombinant product in which common baker's yeast is used to produce HB_sAg. The series of three intramuscular injections (second and third doses are given 1 and 6 months after the first dose) produces an adequate antibody response in 90% of adults and 95% of children. Clinical trials have demonstrated that the hepatitis B vaccine is 80 to 95% effective in preventing hepatitis B infection in high-risk groups.[66,67] Infants with perinatal exposures should receive the hepatitis B vaccine in combination with HBIG, which has been shown to be 85 to 95% effective in preventing the hepatitis B carrier state.[67–70] The deltoid muscle is the recommended location for injection for adults and children because injections into the buttocks produce a lower response rate.[71] The anterolateral thigh muscle should be used for infants and neonates. Table 28.4 describes the available hepatitis B vaccine products and dosing information. Larger dosages (two to four times the normal dosage) or one additional dose (total four doses) are needed to produce an adequate immune response in many immunocompromised patients or those on hemodialysis.[72,73] Some immunocompromised patients do not respond to the vaccine even when higher dosages are given. Local reactions, such as soreness, pain, ecchymosis, and swelling are the most common side effects of the hepatitis B vaccine. Mild systemic symptoms such as fever, malaise, headache, and fatigue have also been reported. Allergic reactions such as rash, anaphylaxis, and serum sickness, although uncommon, have been reported. The hepatitis B vaccine is contraindicated in patients allergic to yeast or any of the other ingredients contained in the vaccine.

Table 28.4 ▪ Hepatitis B Vaccine

Trade Name	Patients	Product Concentration	Dosage
Recombivax HB	≤10 yr	2.5 μg/0.5 mL	2.5 μg
	11–19 yr or infants born to HB_sAg+ mothers	5 μg/0.5 mL	5 μg
	≥20 yr	10 μg/mL	10 μg
	Dialysis or immunocompromised	40 μg/mL	40 μg
Engerix-B	≤10 yr	10 μg/0.5 mL	10 μg
	11–19 yr	10 μg/0.5 mL or 20 μg/mL	10–20 μg
	≥20 yr	20 μg/mL	20 μg
	Dialysis or immunocompromised	20 μg/mL	40 μg (divided between two sites)

Chronic Hepatitis B

Interferon was the first approved agent used to treat chronic hepatitis B. Several types of interferons are commercially available (interferon α-2A and α-2B, interferon α-n3, interferon alfacon-1, interferon β-1A and β-1B, and interferon γ-1B). Interferon has both antiviral and immune stimulatory properties that may be beneficial in treating viral hepatitis. Interferon α-2B (5 million IU subcutaneously daily or 10 million IU three times weekly for 16 weeks) has been used to treat chronic hepatitis B infection with some success. Virologic response (loss of HB_eAg and hepatitis B DNA) occurred in 36 to 37% of the patients and 7% of controls. In addition, 43 to 44% had a biochemical response (normalization of serum ALT), as compared to 19% of controls. Sustained virologic response after discontinuation of therapy was 34 to 37%.[74] Interferon treatment often is associated with flulike symptoms (fever, fatigue, headache, and myalgia). Dosing the interferon at bedtime can improve the tolerability of this agent. Acetaminophen should be used for fever and headache management. However, patients with liver disease should limit the amount of acetaminophen to 2 g per day for adults. Gastrointestinal symptoms (nausea, diarrhea, and anorexia), arthralgias, weakness, alopecia, and rigors also are common. Anemia, leukopenia, and thrombocytopenia are significant problems that can be dose limiting. Although less common, depression can be a very serious problem in these patients. Suicides have been reported with interferon therapy. Interferon can also induce various autoimmune diseases. Some patients also have photosensitivity reactions while on interferon and should be counseled on the use of sunscreen and protective clothing. Interferon therapy should be reduced or discontinued if the patient develops anemia, leukopenia, thrombocytopenia, depression, or autoimmune disease. Interferon can be quite difficult to tolerate: 10 to 40% of patients need dose reduction and 5 to 10% need discontinuation of therapy.[25]

Another class of agents has recently come on the scene for treating hepatitis B. Lamivudine, (–) 2′, 3′-dideoxy, 3′thiacytidine (3TC), is an irreversible inhibitor of reverse transcriptase that inhibits hepatitis B viral replication. Lamivudine has been effective in lowering hepatitis B DNA by more than 90%.[75,76] When treatment durations were extended to 12 to 18 months, 9 of 24 patients became HB_eAg negative in one study.[77] In another study, it was found that lamivudine 100 mg daily for 1 year was more effective than 25 mg daily of lamivudine or placebo in improving liver histology in patients with chronic hepatitis B. Virologic response (loss of HB_eAg, development of antibodies against HB_eAg, and undetectable hepatitis B viral DNA) and biochemical response (sustained normalization of ALT) were found in 16% and 72% of the patients receiving lamivudine 100 mg daily, respectively.[76] One of the greatest concerns with lamivudine is the high incidence of hepatitis B viral mutation and drug resistance. Lamivudine is not effective for the RNA viruses. The most common adverse effects are headache, malaise, fatigue, nausea, vomiting, diarrhea, neuropathy, cough, congestion, and musculoskeletal pain. Less common but serious adverse events include neutropenia, anemia, thrombocytopenia, pancreatitis, and increased liver function tests. One study found that 100 mg lamivudine daily had comparable adverse reaction rates to placebo.[76] Dosage adjustments must be made for patients with renal insufficiency.

Hepatitis C

The majority of clinical trials for treating chronic hepatitis C have studied interferon α-2B, although interferon α-2A and interferon alfacon-1 also are approved for treating chronic hepatitis C. Initially, interferon α-2B was approved for treating chronic hepatitis C at a dosage of 3 million IU subcutaneously three times weekly for 6 months. This resulted in an end-of-treatment biochemical response (ALT normalization) rate of 40 to 50% and virologic response (loss of serum hepatitis C RNA) of 30 to 40%. Unfortunately, relapse was common, and 6 months after treatment was completed, the biochemical response rate declined to 15 to 20% and virologic response to 10 to 20%. Prolonging interferon α-2B treatment to 12 months did not increase the end-of-treatment response rates but did decrease the biochemical relapse rates, such that 20 to 30% of patients had a sustained biochemical response. In addition to the biochemical and virologic improvements, patients also had histologic improvements based on liver biopsies.[78,79] Interferon treatment durations of 18 to 24 months have been associated with similar results. To date, no published studies have compared 12 months to 18 or 24 months of interferon therapy. Although it is clear that at least 12 months of therapy should be given, additional studies are needed to determine the optimum duration of treatment. A few factors appear to predict a good therapeutic outcome. Patients with hepatitis C virus genotype 2 or 3, hepatitis C virus RNA levels less than 1,000,000 copies/mL, and no cirrhosis on liver biopsy tend to do better with interferon than those not having these characteristics. Interestingly, patients who do not respond (persistent elevations in ALT and hepatitis C RNA) in the first 3 months of interferon treatment probably will not respond at all. These patients seem to have resistant hepatitis C virus. However, patients who have an initial biochemical response to interferon but relapse during the 6 months after treatment have a 75 to 85% end-of-treatment biochemical response and 30 to 40% sustained biochemical response when re-treated with interferon for an additional 12 months.[80]

Ribavirin, a nucleoside analog with antiviral properties, initially was approved in combination with interferon for treating chronic hepatitis C in compensated liver disease following relapse after interferon therapy. Although ribavirin monotherapy is associated with a significant biochemical response (decreased ALT), no effect is seen on hepatitis C viral RNA levels.[81] Therefore, ribavirin monotherapy is not recommended for treating chronic hepatitis

C. However, 6 months of combination therapy with oral ribavirin, in combination with interferon α-2B in patients with hepatitis C who had relapsed following interferon therapy alone, resulted in a 21 to 60% sustained virologic response and 49% sustained histologic response as compared with less than 20% sustained virologic response and 36% sustained histologic response with interferon alone.[78,79,82,83] One disturbing side effect of ribavirin is hemolytic anemia within the first 2 to 4 weeks of therapy. The anemia can be associated with a significant number of cardiac and pulmonary events. Central nervous system side effects such as insomnia, depression, and irritability also are common. Allergic reactions such as rash and pruritus may also occur. Ribavirin is also known to be teratogenic. The ribavirin dosage is based on the patient's body weight. Adult patients with normal renal function, weighing 75 kg or less should receive 400 mg every morning and 600 mg every evening orally. Patients weighing more than 75 kg should receive 600 mg orally twice daily. Ribavirin is eliminated by the kidney and not removed by dialysis. Dosage reduction or discontinuation should be instituted for patients who develop anemia, leukopenia, thrombocytopenia, or depression. Recently, ribavirin in combination with interferon received FDA approval for primary treatment of chronic hepatitis C. This combination has quickly become the treatment of choice. In previously untreated patients with chronic hepatitis C, ribavirin in combination with interferon α-2B resulted in an end-of-treatment virologic response of 52 to 90% and sustained response of 43 to 47%, compared with an end-of-treatment response of 42 to 53% and sustained response of 6 to 23% for interferon alone.[83,84]

Drug-Induced Hepatitis

The most important step that can be taken in a suspected clinically significant drug-induced liver injury is discontinuation of the offending agent. Management of the liver injury should be supportive (see Chapter 29 for management of severe disease).

Nonpharmacologic Therapy

The development of end-stage liver disease and cirrhosis can be hastened in some patients by ethanol consumption.[25] In addition, many liver transplant programs and insurance carriers require very long periods of ethanol abstinence before transplantation regardless of the cause of liver disease. Therefore, it is very important for patients to be counseled on the need to discontinue all alcohol consumption.

ALTERNATIVE THERAPIES

Interest in herbal remedies for treating liver disease and other medical problems appears to be growing. Several herbal remedies have been reported to cause liver dysfunction, such as germander (*Teucrium chamaedrys*), chaparral (*Larrea divaricata*), skullcap (*Scutellaria laterifolia*), and valerian (*Valeriana officinalis*).[85–88] Milk thistle (*Silybum marianum*), on the other hand, has been used to treat liver disease.[89] Several clinical studies have reported positive results with silymarin (derived from the milk thistle plant), suggesting that it decreases complications and hastens recovery from hepatitis. Most clinical studies have been with small numbers of patients, a wide range of causes and severity of illness studied within each study, and in most cases the lack of control or evaluation of ethanol consumption.[89] Other products such as ji gu cao pill (*Fructus abri* 40%, *Agkistrodan* 15%, *Margarita* 3%, *Calculus Bovis* 10%, *Radix Angelicae Sinensis* 10%, *Fructus Lycii Chinensis* 7%, and *Radix Salviae Miltiorrhizae* 15%), li gan pian liver strengthening tablets (*Herba Jinqiancao* 70% and *Fellis Bovis* 30%), yin chen hao tang (*Herba Artemisiae Scopariae* 43%, *Fructus Gardeniae* 28.5%, *Radix Rhizoma Rhei* 28.5%), ta chai hu tang (*Bupleurum falcatum*), and jujube (*Zizyphus jujuba*) are herbal remedies with claims of beneficial effects for the liver. Controlled clinical trials are needed to determine their efficacy and safety.

FUTURE THERAPIES

Several new antiviral agents appear to have efficacy against the hepatitis B virus. One of the promising new agents for treating chronic hepatitis B and possibly preventing hepatitis B recurrence after liver transplantation is famciclovir, a prodrug of penciclovir. Famciclovir has been shown to dramatically reduce hepatitis B viral DNA levels.[90] Adefovir and lobucavir also are being evaluated for hepatitis B. Additional controlled trials are necessary to determine the place in therapy for the new agents. It is likely that combination therapy with interferon and an antiviral agent will become the mainstay for chronic hepatitis B treatment.

IMPROVING OUTCOMES

Patient education for hepatitis should address several points. First, the ways to avoid exposure to and transmission of hepatitis should be addressed for travelers as well as patients with hepatitis. Avoiding food or beverages that may be contaminated with hepatitis A is important. In particular, water (or ice), uncooked shellfish, and uncooked fruits or vegetables that patients did not peel themselves may be contaminated with the hepatitis A virus and result in transmission. Second, educating patients about prescribed medication regimens, expected side effects, and side effect management is essential. For some medications, such as interferon, detailed education on administration technique and product handling is necessary. In addition to safer sex counseling, patients receiving ribavirin, a known teratogen, need to be informed about the risk to the fetus in the event of pregnancy. Because of the long half-life of ribavirin, the risk of teratogenicity extends 6 months after discontinuation of treatment. Compliance is another important area for patient education, particularly for patients receiving the hepatitis B vaccine series, which includes three doses over 6 months, and for those receiving antiviral therapy because efficacy is diminished with noncompliance.

PHARMACOECONOMICS

For hepatitis A, the only pharmacoeconomic evaluation that has been reported is related to travelers' prophylaxis. Intramuscular immunoglobulin is less expensive than hepatitis A vaccination for travelers visiting endemic areas fewer than five times in a 10-year period.[91]

Pharmacoeconomic analysis for hepatitis B affects how we monitor before and after vaccination. Routine testing of patients for antibodies to hepatitis B core antigen or antibodies to HB_sAg before vaccination is a cost-effectiveness issue that must be resolved at each center. It may be reasonable to screen high-risk patients before vaccination but not low-risk patients. This decision depends on the cost of the vaccine, the cost of testing, and the expected prevalence of immunity. Postvaccination testing for immune response to the hepatitis B vaccine is not recommended for healthy people because of the very high expected response rate (90%). However, people who would be expected to have a suboptimal response (e.g., immunocompromised patients and those on hemodialysis) would be advised to have postvaccination testing for antibody response to the vaccine 1 to 6 months after completion of the series. Revaccination of those who did not have an adequate response to the initial series with one additional dose results in 15 to 25% of the patients having an adequate antibody response. Repeating the entire series (three additional doses) results in 30 to 50% having an adequate antibody response.[92]

A meta-analysis evaluating the cost-effectiveness of interferon α-2B found that it prolonged life at a reasonable marginal cost per year of life saved in patients with chronic hepatitis B (HB_eAg positive),[93] but the ultimate role of interferon alone for chronic hepatitis B is not clear. Early studies with several antiviral agents for treating chronic hepatitis B suggest that interferon alone may not be the mainstay of treatment. Instead, chronic hepatitis B probably will be managed with a combination of agents, for which the pharmacoeconomic impact has not yet been evaluated.

As is the case for hepatitis B, therapy for hepatitis C is changing rapidly. This has limited the usefulness of cost-effectiveness analysis performed with interferon alone. Nonetheless, the cost-effectiveness of interferon α-2B has been studied using meta-analysis and a mathematical model of the natural history of chronic hepatitis C.[94] It was found that interferon α-2B alone prolonged life expectancy at a reasonable cost per year of life gained for patients with chronic mild hepatitis C, particularly for young patients. The relative cost-effectiveness of the combination of interferon and ribavirin versus interferon alone has not been determined.

KEY POINTS

- If possible, viral hepatitis should be prevented through precautions such as avoiding contaminated food and water, practicing good personal hygiene, not reusing intravenous needles, practicing safer sex, avoiding recapping needles after blood drawing, and using sterile technique with acupuncture, tattooing, or body piercing.
- When traveling to hepatitis A and B endemic areas of the world, follow prophylaxis regimens to avoid hepatitis transmission.
- Treating chronic hepatitis B and C with interferon and/or antiviral therapy can promote clearance of the virus, improve liver function tests, improve liver histology, and prolong life.
- Maintaining compliance with therapy is essential to efficacy, particularly for completion of the hepatitis B vaccine series and antiviral therapy.
- Many patients have difficulty tolerating interferon therapy. Evening dosing and judicious use of acetaminophen (less than 2 g per day) for fevers and headaches may improve tolerability.
- The teratogenicity during and 6 months after ribavirin therapy must be discussed with patients.
- The risks and benefits should be weighed before agents with hepatotoxic potential are initiated in patients with preexisting liver disease.
- Early detection and discontinuation of agents causing hepatitis may minimize liver injury.
- When a patient presents with possible drug-induced hepatitis, assessing all agents the patient has been taking for hepatotoxic potential (focusing on duration of exposure, type of injury, and clinical and laboratory findings) is helpful in determining the most likely culprit. However, exclusion of other causes and resolution of symptoms after discontinuation of the offending agent ultimately are necessary to confirm the cause.
- Treatment of end-stage liver disease caused by hepatitis should be supportive.

REFERENCES

1. CDC hepatitis A fact sheet. Available at: http://www.cdc.gov/ncidod/diseases/hepatitis/a/fact.htm. Accessed October 29, 1999.
2. Havens WP Jr. Period of infectivity of patients with experimentally induced infectious hepatitis. J Exp Med 83:2521, 1946.
3. Giles JP, Liebharber H, Krugman S, et al. Early viremia and viruria in infectious hepatitis. Virology 24:107, 1964.
4. Havens WP Jr, Ward R, Drill LA, et al. Experimental production of hepatitis by feeding icterogenic materials. Proc Soc Exp Biol Med 57:206, 1944.
5. Dienstag JL, Feinstone SM, Kapikian AZ, et al. Fecal shedding of hepatitis-A antigen. Lancet 1:765, 1975.
6. Rakela J, Mosley JW. Fecal excretion of hepatitis A virus. J Infect Dis 135:933, 1977.
7. Hollinger FB, Bradley DW, Maynard JE, et al. Detection of hepatitis A viral antigen by radioimmunoassay. J Immunol 115:1464, 1975.
8. Krugmean S, Giles JP, Hammond J. Infectious hepatitis: evidence for two distinctive clinical epidemiological and immunological types of infection. JAMA 200:365, 1967.

9. Barbara JAJ, Howell DR, Briggs M, et al. Post-transfusion hepatitis A. Lancet 1:738, 1982.
10. Hollinger FB, Khan NC, Oefinger PE, et al. Posttransfusion hepatitis type A. JAMA 250:2313, 1983.
11. Corey L, Holmes KK. Sexual transmission of hepatitis A in homosexual men: incidence and mechanism. N Engl J Med 302:435, 1980.
12. Neefe JR, Stokes J Jr. An epidemic of infectious hepatitis apparently due to a waterborne agent. JAMA 128:1063, 1945.
13. Denes AE, Smith JC, Hindman SH, et al. Foodborne hepatitis A infection: a report of two urban restaurant-associated outbreaks. Am J Epidemiol 105:156, 1977.
14. CDC hepatitis B fact sheet. Available at: http://www.cdc.gov/ncidod/diseases/hepatitis/b/fact.htm. Accessed January 7, 2000.
15. Protection against viral hepatitis recommendations of the immunization practices advisory committee (ACIP). MMWR Morb Mortal Wkly Rep 39:1, 1990.
16. Belle SH, Beringer KC, Detre KM. Recent findings concerning liver transplantation in the United States. Clin Transpl 15, 1996:15.
17. Beeson PB. Jaundice occurring one to four months after transfusion of blood or plasma. Report of 7 cases. JAMA 121:1332, 1943.
18. Alter MJ, Margolis HS. The emergence of hepatitis B as a sexually transmitted disease. Med Clin North Am 74:1529, 1990.
19. Kew MC. Possible transmission of serum (Australia-antigen–positive) hepatitis via the conjunctiva. Infect Immun 7:823, 1973.
20. Seeff LB, Zimmerman HJ, Wright EC, et al. Hepatic disease in asymptomatic parenteral narcotic drug abusers: a Veterans Administration collaborative study. Am J Med Sci 270:41, 1975.
21. Roberts RH, Stul H. Homologous serum jaundice transmitted by a tattooing needle. Can Med Assoc J 62:75, 1950.
22. Johnson CJ, Anderson H, Spearman J, et al. Ear piercing and hepatitis: nonsterile instruments for ear piercing and the subsequent onset of viral hepatitis. JAMA 227:1165, 1974.
23. Carron H, Epstein BH, Grand B. Complication of acupuncture. JAMA 228:1552, 1974.
24. Tiku ML, Bentner KR, Ramirez RI, et al. Distribution and characteristics of hepatitis B surface antigen in body fluids of institutionalized children and adults. J Infect Dis 134:342, 1976.
25. National Institutes of Health. Consensus development statement. Management of hepatitis C, 1997. odp.od.nih.gov/consensus/statements/cdc/105/105_stmt.html.
26. Kato N, Yokosuka O, Hosoda K, et al. Detection of hepatitis C virus RNA in acute non-A, non-B hepatitis as an early digestive tool. Biochem Biophys Res Commun 192:800, 1993.
27. CDC hepatitis C fact sheet. Available at: http://www.cdc.gov/ncidod/diseases/hepatitis/c/fact.htm. Accessed October 29, 1999.
28. Alter HJ, Purcell RH, Shih JW, et al. Detection of antibody to hepatitis C virus in prospectively followed transfusion recipients with acute and chronic non-A, non-B hepatitis. N Engl J Med 321:1494, 1989.
29. Seeff LB. Hepatitis C from a needlestick injury. Ann Intern Med 115:411, 1991.
30. Ko YC, Ho MS, Chiang TA, et al. Tattooing as a risk of hepatitis C infection. J Med Virol 38:288, 1992.
31. Everhart JE, Di Bisceglie AM, Murray LM, et al. Risk for non-A, non-B (type C) hepatitis through sexual or household contact with chronic carriers. Ann Intern Med 112:544, 1990.
32. Thaler MM, Park CK, Landers DV, et al. Vertical transmission of hepatitis C virus. Lancet 338:17, 1991.
33. Lewis JH, Zimmerman HJ. Drug-induced liver disease. Med Clin North Am 73:775, 1989.
34. Bass NM, Ockner RK. Drug-induced liver disease. In: Zakim D, Boyer TD. Hepatology. A textbook of liver disease. 3rd ed. Philadelphia: WB Saunders, 1996:962.
35. Lee WM. Drug-induced hepatotoxicity. N Engl J Med 333:1118, 1995.
36. Hagley MT, Hulisz DT, Burns CM. Hepatotoxicity associated with angiotensin-converting enzyme inhibitors. Ann Pharmacother 27:228, 1993.
37. Swank LA, Chejfec G, Nemchausky BA. Allopurinol-induced granulomatous hepatitis with cholangitis and a sarcoid-like reaction. Arch Intern Med 138:997, 1978.
38. Kalantzis N, Gabriel P, Mouzas J, et al. Acute amiodarone hepatitis. Hepatogastroenterology 38:71, 1991.
39. Wolfe JD, Metzger AL, Holdstein RC. Aspirin hepatitis. Ann Intern Med 80:74, 1974.
40. Horowitz S, Patwardhan R, Marcus E. Hepatotoxic reactions associated with carbamazepine therapy. Epilepsia 29:149, 1988.
41. Utili R, Boitnott JK, Zimmerman HJ. Dantrolene-associated hepatic injury. Gastroenterology 72:610, 1977.
42. Iveson TJ, Ryley NG, Kelly PM, et al. Diclofenac-associated hepatitis. J Hepatol 10:85, 1990.
43. Schade RR, Gray JA, Dekker A, et al. Fulminant hepatitis associated with disulfiram. Report of a case. Arch Intern Med 143:1271, 1983.
44. Carson JL, Strom BL, Duff A, et al. Acute liver disease associated with erythromycins, sulfonamides and tetracyclines. Ann Intern Med 119:576, 1993.
45. Sanchez MR, Ross B, Rotterdam H, et al. Retinoids hepatitis. J Am Acad Dermatol 28:853, 1993.
46. Neuberger JM. Halothane and hepatitis: a model of immune mediated drug hepatotoxicity. Clin Sci 72:263, 1987.
47. Black M, Mitchell JR, Zimmerman HJ, et al. Isoniazid-associated hepatitis in 144 patients. Gastroenterology 69:289, 1975.
48. DaPrada M, Kettler R, Keller HH, et al. Preclinical profiles of the novel reversible MAO-A inhibitors, moclobemide and brofaromine, in comparison with irreversible MAO inhibitors. J Neural Transm 28:5, 1989.
49. Rodman JS, Deutsch DJ, Gutman SI. Methyldopa hepatitis. A report of six cases and review of the literature. Am J Med 60:941, 1976.
50. Mullin GE, Greenson JK, Mitchell MC. Fulminant hepatic failure after ingestion of sustained release nicotinic acid. Ann Intern Med 111:253, 1989.
51. Sharp JR, Ishak KG, Zimmerman HJ. Chronic active hepatitis and severe hepatic necrosis associated with nitrofurantoin. Ann Intern Med 92:14, 1980.
52. Onorato IM, Axelrod JL. Hepatitis from intravenous high-dose oxacillin therapy. Findings in an adult population. Ann Intern Med 89:497, 1978.
53. Roy AK, Mahoney HC, Levine RA. Phenytoin-induced chronic hepatitis. Dig Dis Sci 38:740, 1993.
54. Rotrensch HH, Yust I, Siegman-Igra Y, et al. Granulomatous hepatitis: a hypersensitivity response to procainamide. Ann Intern Med 89:646, 1978.
55. Knobler H, Levij IS, Gavish D, et al. Quinidine-induced hepatitis: a common and reversible hypersensitivity reaction. Arch Intern Med 146:526, 1986.
56. Scheuer PJ, Summerfield JA, Lal S, et al. Rifampicin hepatitis. Clinical and histological study. Lancet 1:422, 1974.
57. Ivarson I, Lundlin P. Multiple attacks of jaundice associated with repeated sulfonamide treatment. Acta Med Scand 206:219, 1979.
58. Peters RL, Edmondson HA, Mikkelsen WP, et al. Tetracycline-induced fatty liver in nonpregnant patients. A report of six cases. Am J Surg 113:622, 1967.
59. Beck PL, Bridges RJ, Demetrick DJ, et al. Chronic active hepatitis associated with trazodone therapy. Ann Intern Med 118:791, 1993.
60. Redeker AG. Viral hepatitis: clinical aspects. Am J Med Sci 270:9, 1975.
61. Merican I, Sherlock S, McIntyre N, et al. Clinical, biochemical and histological features in 102 patients with chronic hepatitis C virus infection. Q J Med 86:119, 1993.
62. Centers for Disease Control, Department of Health and Human Services. Vaccine recommendations for travelers health-care provider information, 1996. www/cdc/gov/travel/hcwvax.htm.
63. Drake ME, Ming C. Gamma globulin in epidemic hepatitis: comparative value of two dosage levels approximately near the minimal effective level. JAMA 155:1302, 1954.
64. Mosley JW, Reisler DM, Brachott D, et al. Comparison of two lots of immune serum globulin for prophylaxis of infectious hepatitis. Am J Epidemiol 87:539, 1968.
65. Redeker AG, Mosley JW, Gocke DJ, et al. Hepatitis B immune globulin as a prophylactic measure for spouses exposed to acute type B hepatitis. N Engl J Med 293:1055, 1975.
66. Szmuness W, Stevens CE, Harley EJ, et al. Hepatitis B vaccine: demonstration of efficacy in a controlled clinical trial in a high-risk population in the United States. N Engl J Med 303:833, 1980.
67. Stevens CE, Taylor PE, Tong MJ, et al. Yeast-recombinant hepatitis B vaccine: efficacy with hepatitis B immune globulin in prevention of perinatal hepatitis B virus transmission. JAMA 257:2612, 1987.
68. Beasley RP, Hwang L-Y, Lee GC, et al. Prevention of perinatally transmitted hepatitis B virus infections with hepatitis B immune globulin and hepatitis B vaccine. Lancet 2:1099, 1983.
69. Wong VCW, Ip HMH, Reesink HW, et al. Prevention of the HB_sAg carrier state in newborn infants of mothers who are chronic carriers of HB_sAg and HB_eAg by administration of hepatitis-B vaccine and hepatitis-B immunoglobulin: double-blind randomised placebo-controlled study. Lancet 1:921, 1984.
70. Stevens CE, Toy PT, Tong MJ, et al. Perinatal hepatitis B virus transmission in the United States: prevention by passive-active immunization. JAMA 253:1740, 1985.
71. CDC. Suboptimal response to hepatitis B vaccine given by injection into the buttock. MMWR Morb Mortal Wkly Rep 34:105, 1985.
72. Stevens CE, Alter HJ, Taylor PE, et al. Hepatitis B vaccine in patients receiving hemodialysis. Immunogenicity and efficacy. N Engl J Med 311:496, 1984.
73. Collier AC, Croey L, Murphy VL, et al. Antibody to human immunodeficiency virus and suboptimal response to hepatitis B vaccination. Ann Intern Med 109:101, 1988.

74. Perrillo RP, Schiff ER, Davis GL, et al. A randomized, controlled trial of interferon alfa-2B alone and after prednisone withdrawal for treatment of chronic hepatitis B. N Engl J Med 323:295, 1990.
75. Dienstag JL, Perrillo RP, Schiff ER, et al. A preliminary trial of lamivudine for chronic hepatitis B infection. N Engl J Med 333:1657, 1995.
76. Lai C-L, Chien R-N, Leung NWY, et al. A one-year trial of lamivudine for chronic hepatitis B. N Engl J Med 339:61, 1998.
77. Dienstag JL, Schiff ER, Mitchell M, et al. Extended lamivudine retreatment for chronic hepatitis B. Hepatology 24:188A, 1996.
78. Carithers RL, Emerson S. Therapy of hepatitis C: meta-analysis of interferon alfa-2B trials. Hepatology 26:83S, 1997.
79. Poynard T, Leroy V, Cohard M, et al. Meta-analysis of interferon randomized trials in the treatment of viral hepatitis C: effects of dose and duration. Hepatology 24:778, 1996.
80. Alberti A, Chemello L, Noventa F, et al. Therapy of hepatitis C: re-treatment with alpha interferon. Hepatology 26:137S, 1997.
81. DiBisceglie A, Conjeevaram H, Fried M, et al. Ribavirin as therapy for chronic hepatitis C: a randomized, double-blind, placebo-controlled trial. Ann Intern Med 123:897, 1995.
82. Reichard O, Norkrans G, Fryd'en A, et al. Randomised, double-blind, placebo-controlled trial of interferon alpha-2B with and without ribavirin for chronic hepatitis C. The Swedish Study Group. Lancet 351:78, 1998.
83. Schalm SW, Brouwer JT, Chemello L, et al. Interferon–ribavirin combination therapy for chronic hepatitis C. Dig Dis Sci 41:131S, 1996.
84. Reichard O, Schvarcz R, Weiland O. Therapy of hepatitis C: alpha interferon and ribavirin. Hepatology 26:108S, 1997.
85. Dunbabin DW, Tallis GA, Popplewell PY, et al. Lead poisoning from Indian herbal medicine (Ayurveda). Med J Aust 157:835, 1992.
86. Pauwels A, Thierman-Duffaud D, Azanowsky JM, et al. Acute hepatitis caused by wild germander. Hepatotoxicity of herbal remedies. Two cases. Gastroenterol Clin Biol 16:92, 1992.
87. Gordon DW, Rosenthal G, Hart J, et al. Chaparral ingestion. The broadening spectrum of liver injury caused by herbal medications. JAMA 273:489, 1995.
88. MacGregor FB, Abernethy VE, Dahabra S, et al. Hepatotoxicity of herbal remedies. BMJ 299:1156, 1989.
89. Flora K, Hahn M, Rosen H, et al. Milk thistle (*Silybum marianum*) for the therapy of liver disease. Am J Gastroenterol 93:139, 1998.
90. Main J, Brown JL, Howells C, et al. A double blind, placebo-controlled study to assess the effect of famciclovir on virus replication in patients with chronic hepatitis B virus infection. J Viral Hepat 3:211, 1996.
91. Fenn P, McGuire A, Gray A. An economic evaluation of vaccination against hepatitis A for frequent travelers. J Infect 36:17, 1998.
92. Hadler SC, Francis DP, Maynard JE, et al. Long term immunogenicity and efficacy of hepatitis B vaccine in homosexual men. N Engl J Med 315:209, 1986.
93. Wong JB, Koff RS, Tine F, Pauker SG. Cost-effectiveness of interferon-α2B treatment for hepatitis B e antigen–positive chronic hepatitis B. Ann Intern Med 122:664, 1995.
94. Bennett WG, Inoue Y, Beck JR, et al. Estimates of the cost-effectiveness of a single course of interferon-α2B in patients with histologically mild chronic hepatitis C. Ann Intern Med 127:855, 1997.

CHAPTER 29

CIRRHOSIS

Richard Brown

DEFINITION

Cirrhosis is characterized by a diffuse increase in the fibrous connective tissue of the liver, with areas of necrosis and regeneration of parenchymal cells, imparting a nodular or glandular texture histologically. In its later stages, cirrhosis leads to such deformity of the liver that it interferes with hepatobiliary function and the circulation of blood both to and from the liver.

TREATMENT GOALS: CIRRHOSIS

- Currently, no specific medical therapy exists for cirrhosis except prevention. However, several drugs are used to treat the complications of this disorder.
- Primary goal of therapy is to prevent symptoms and maintain a reasonable quality of life.
- Specific complications of the disease are treated to reduce morbidity and the need for frequent hospitalizations.
- Once the diagnosis of cirrhosis is established, it is of utmost importance therapeutically that patient discontinue consumption of all alcohol.

EPIDEMIOLOGY

It is difficult to cite an incidence of cirrhosis because patients often do not exhibit signs or symptoms. Postmortem data from various hospitals show an incidence of 3 to 15%. Cirrhosis is the ninth leading cause of death in the United States.[1] Worldwide, the annual death rate from cirrhosis of all causes is as high as 15 to 40 per 100,000 population.[2] However, death and hospitalization rates of patients with chronic liver disease and cirrhosis are on the decline in the United States. In 1989, chronic liver disease was the underlying cause of death for 26,720 people and a contributing cause of death for an additional 14,101 people. From 1980 through 1989 the age-adjusted death rate for chronic liver disease decreased 23%, from 13.5 to 10.4 per 100,000 people. Chronic liver disease appeared as the first diagnosis in an estimated 72,232 hospitalizations in 1989 and as a secondary diagnosis in an additional 218,156 hospitalizations. From 1980 through 1989 the hospitalization rate attributed to chronic liver disease and cirrhosis declined 44%, from 50.6 to 28.2 per 100,000 people.[3] Table 29.1 lists the relative frequencies of the various types of cirrhosis that are encountered clinically. The largest percentage is Laennec's cirrhosis, which occurs principally in patients between 40 and 60 years of age and is found most often in men. In the United States, 50 to 90% of these patients have a history of chronic alcoholism. The quantity of ethanol needed to cause cirrhosis is 80 g/day for 5 years. With approximately 11 to 12 g per average drink, six or seven drinks per day over this period could be considered an etiologic factor in cirrhosis. In developing countries, children often are affected by maternally acquired hepatitis B.[1,2,4]

PATHOPHYSIOLOGY

Several major types of cirrhosis have been described (Table 29.1), but cirrhosis associated with alcohol abuse, or Laennec's cirrhosis, is by far the most commonly encountered form in the United States.[4] Alcoholic liver disease usually begins with severe fatty changes in the liver. In the early stages this fatty infiltration is not associated with fibrosis and scarring. Later stages are marked by a prominent inflammation, an increase in fibrous tissue, and a progressive shrinkage, nodularity, and hardening of the liver.

In experimental animals, dietary derangements can induce significant fatty changes in the liver, with subsequent development of cirrhosis. Therefore, it is often claimed

Table 29.1 ▪ Cirrhosis: Incidence and Causes

Type	Frequency (%)	Causes
Alcohol-associated (Laennec's)	60–70	Alcohol abuse and protein deficiency inducing fatty changes, inflammation, and scarring liver
Biliary (primary and secondary)	10–15	Obstruction to bile flow (e.g., immune complexes, stones, and carcinoma); often secondary to long-standing bacterial infection
Postnecrotic	10–15	Scarring following massive hepatic necrosis such as that seen in chronic viral hepatitis, after exposure to hepatotoxic drugs, or in immune-mediated hepatitis
Metabolic	5–10	Excessive iron (hemochromatosis) or copper (Wilson's disease) deposition, α_1-antitrypsin deficiency, other inborn errors of metabolism

that dietary indiscretion in alcoholics may be an important underlying associated cause of cirrhosis. This concept is supported by the observation that when a chronic alcoholic is hospitalized and placed on an adequate diet, excess fat can be mobilized and the liver structure and function may return to normal. This reversibility is less clear if fibrosis has already occurred. Other evidence implicates alcohol as a direct hepatotoxin. One group of investigators was able to demonstrate development of cirrhosis in baboons that were maintained on a balanced diet but given large daily dosages of alcohol.[5]

Biliary cirrhosis is cirrhosis caused by chronic obstruction of bile flow (cholestasis). Primary biliary cirrhosis (PBC) follows long-standing cholestasis that is generally of unknown origin, but it may have an underlying immunologic basis with elevated immunoglobulin M (IgM), autoantibodies, and circulating complement-fixing immune complexes. Secondary biliary cirrhosis may be caused by stones or a tumor obstructing bile flow, leading to an inflammatory reaction and scarring.

Less common causes of cirrhosis are related to chronic viral hepatitis, immune-mediated chronic hepatitis, and various metabolic disorders (Table 29.1).

CLINICAL PRESENTATION AND DIAGNOSIS

Signs and Symptoms

Cirrhosis is insidious in its development and often produces no clinical manifestations. Up to 50% of all cases are discovered only at the time of postmortem examination. Many patients seek medical help, complaining of vague, nonspecific symptoms such as weight loss, loss of appetite, nausea, vomiting, and ill-defined digestive disturbances. Others enter the hospital acutely ill with the full syndrome of acute alcoholic hepatitis (a precursor to cirrhosis). These patients have jaundice (bilirubin levels range from 2 mg/dL to more than 40 mg/dL), mildly elevated serum alanine and aspartate aminotransferase (ALT and AST) and alkaline phosphatase levels, a low serum albumin level, evidence of impaired coagulation (prolonged prothrombin time and INR), and right upper quadrant pain. In the later stages of cirrhosis, patients may have the complications of cirrhosis: ascites, gastrointestinal (GI) bleeding, and mental deterioration. The clinical manifestations include visible collateral venous engorgement on the abdominal wall or caput medusa, testicular atrophy, parotid glandular enlargement, nail clubbing, skin hyperpigmentation, amenorrhea, jaundice, edema, palmar erythema, fetor hepaticus, loss of body hair, spider angiomas, gynecomastia, ascites, splenomegaly, and muscle wasting. Hepatocellular carcinoma develops in as many as 10% of subjects with long-standing cirrhosis.

Diagnosis

The complications of cirrhosis generally relate to abnormalities in the portal venous system. The portal vein receives blood draining from the arterial and capillary system of the entire GI tract. This system is unique in that although it is a venous system, it has a second set of microvasculature (or sinusoids) that runs throughout the liver and then rejoins to empty into the hepatic veins and eventually the inferior vena cava. The main function of the portal venous network is to act as a pathway for detoxification and metabolism by the liver of substances absorbed from the GI tract. The portal venous system does not provide oxygenated blood to the liver (this is done by the hepatic artery). The anatomy of the portal system allows first-pass (presystemic) metabolism of orally administered drugs such as propranolol, verapamil, and morphine. As scarring and nodularity increase in the liver during cirrhosis, the blood flow through the portal system becomes obstructed, leading to a dramatic rise in the pressure of the portal vein and its tributaries in the GI tract (i.e., portal hypertension). Blood also may be shunted around the liver to empty directly into the systemic circulation (inferior vena cava). The clinical problems that arise secondary to portal hypertension include ascites, GI bleeding (varices), and encephalopathy.

Ascites

Ascites, characterized by the accumulation of protein-rich fluid in the peritoneal cavity, is one of the most striking features of cirrhosis. Complaints associated with ascites include a rapidly developing inability to fit into one's clothes, abdominal and back pain, gastroesophageal reflux, and shortness of breath secondary to impaired diaphragm movement or pleural effusions. The amount of fluid in the abdomen can vary from a few liters to 20 or more, leading to a large protuberant abdomen and an umbilical hernia.

Ascitic fluid is a good culture medium for bacterial growth, and infections can occur spontaneously (spontaneous bacterial peritonitis, SBP). An unexplained high fever or elevated white blood cell count is an indication for obtaining an aspirate culture from the ascitic fluid or initiating appropriate antibiotic therapy.

Several mechanisms have been postulated to explain the formation of ascites (Fig. 29.1), none of which is fully accepted as the definitive answer.[6,7] Most of the postulates agree that disruption of hepatic architecture and blood flow caused by inflammation, cell necrosis, fibrosis, or obstruction leads to hemodynamic alterations, causing an elevated lymphatic pressure within hepatic sinusoids, which eventually causes excessive transudation (weeping) of protein-rich fluid from the surface of the liver into the peritoneal cavity. According to the underfill theory, both the lymphatic leakage and high prehepatic venous pressure (portal hypertension) cause a net flow of volume from the vascular spaces to the third space of the peritoneal cavity via hydrostatic forces. The high protein content of the ascitic fluid may also help to draw volume out of the vasculature. As a result, effective vascular volume throughout the body decreases, causing secondary sodium and water retention by the kidney. The renin–angiotensin system is a major mediator of the sodium and water retention, ultimately causing release of aldosterone by the adrenal gland. Antidiuretic hormone (ADH) release may also increase. Serum levels of aldosterone and ADH remain elevated because of impaired metabolism secondary to liver failure. These processes are accentuated by the reduced oncotic pressure within the intravascular space.

A major inconsistency with the underfill theory is that some patients have an increased, not decreased, total blood volume and not all patients have demonstrable hyperaldosteronism. According to the overfill theory, the primary defect in ascites formation is excessive renal reabsorption of sodium and water. As plasma volume expands, ascites results from overflow of fluid out of the splanchnic circulation and increased pressure in the portal system. This implies that an unknown primary renal stimulus initiates the volume expansion. Increased sympathetic activity and a variety of hormonal substances have been proposed as factors affecting renal function in cirrhotic patients.[8]

Schrier et al.[6] propose an integration of these two theories, citing a possible systemic intravascular vasodilation that causes a relative decrease in effective plasma volume or pressure, followed by excessive renal retention of sodium and water. Central blood volume has a primary influence on renal circulation. In cirrhotic patients, measurement of this vascular space reveals a reduced circulating volume even in patients who had not yet developed ascites. This volume reduction results from a vasodilated peripheral vascular system. The kidneys and arterial baroreceptors sense a peripheral vascular shift from the central circulation, activate vasoconstrictive systems, and enhance sodium reabsorption. The renin–angiotensin–aldosterone system and the release of vasopressin act to increase central vascular filling.[9] Rocco and Ware[7] believe that both intrahepatic hypertension and a primary renal defect are responsible for the early stages of ascites.

Hypoalbuminemia, secondary to decreased hepatic synthesis and lymphatic leakage into the peritoneum, may contribute to further accumulation of ascites. A low serum albumin concentration causes a reduced serum osmotic (oncotic) pressure that again favors flow of fluid from the vasculature into the extravascular third space. Not all patients with cirrhosis have hypoalbuminemia, but those who do may have both ascites and extensive peripheral edema with a relative systemic hypovolemia. Portal hypertension resulting in ascites can be distinguished from other causes (hepatoma, pancreatic ascites, biliary ascites) by evaluation of a serum albumin–ascites gradient. If the value of the gradient (serum albumin – ascites albumin) exceeds 1.1 g/dL, with 97% certainty, portal hypertension is present.[10] Patients often have hyponatremia from retention of free water, induced by elevated ADH levels. Hypokalemia may develop secondary to hyperaldosteronism and excessive vomiting.

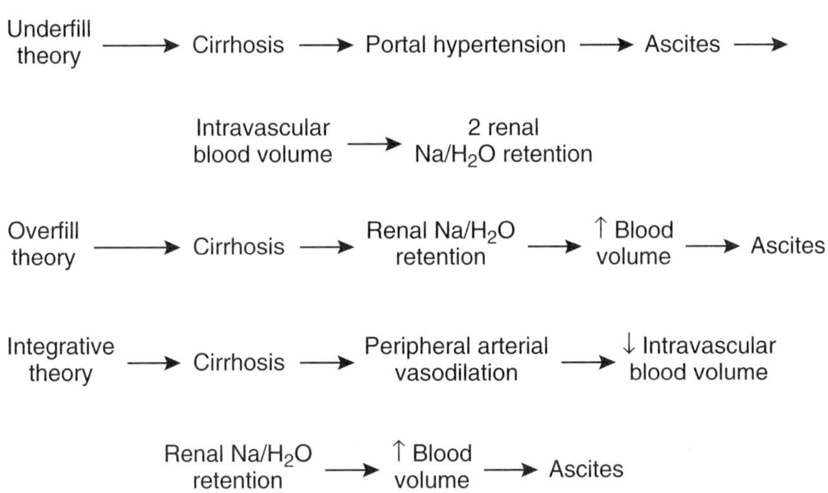

Figure 29.1. Mechanisms of ascites development.

Gastrointestinal Bleeding

GI hemorrhage occurs in about one-fourth to one-third of patients. About one-third of these patients die from the initial hemorrhage. Even nonfatal GI hemorrhages tend to be massive. The major cause of GI bleeding associated with cirrhosis is shunting of blood away from the high-pressure portal system to low-pressure systemic collaterals in the esophagus (esophageal varices), rectum (hemorrhoids), and other parts of the GI tract. These veins become enlarged and tortuous and can rupture easily. Bleeding may be increased by deficiencies in the vitamin K–dependent clotting factors. Esophageal varices account for about 50 to 60% of the GI bleeding observed in cirrhosis, and peptic ulcer disease accounts for another 25%. Presence of varices in the cirrhotic patient accounts for a 20% higher 2-year mortality and a 30% higher 5-year mortality rate.

Hepatic Encephalopathy

The ultimate result of advanced cirrhosis or severe hepatitis is liver failure and hepatic coma (hepatic encephalopathy). This is characterized by increasing drowsiness, personality changes, and mental confusion, with a characteristic flapping tremor of the fingers and hands when the wrists are hyperextended (liver flap or asterixis). Eventually, a deepening coma and death follow. Neurologic complications include incoordination, tremor, nystagmus, and incontinence. As the disease progresses, a characteristic sweet, pungent odor (fetor hepaticus) may be present in the patient's breath. The cause of the odor is unclear but may be related to exhalation of mercaptans.

The diagnosis of hepatic encephalopathy may be complicated by other neurologic disorders including alcohol withdrawal–induced tremors, Wernicke's disease (mental disturbances, ataxia, and nystagmus from acute thiamine deficiency), Korsakoff's syndrome (psychosis and confabulation from chronic thiamine deficiency), and cerebellar damage from chronic alcohol ingestion. The presence of asterixis is a major differentiating factor.

The pathogenesis of hepatic encephalopathy is not well understood, but it may be related in part to increased arterial and central nervous system (CNS) ammonium levels. Although no direct cause-and-effect relationship has been shown between encephalopathy and blood ammonium concentration, when factors that influence ammonium production are decreased, the patient's sensorium often clears. Ingestion of food or bleeding into the GI tract (e.g., esophageal bleeding) introduces a rich source of protein into the intestinal tract. Ammonia is produced in the lower GI tract when these proteins and urea are metabolized by bacterial enzymatic action. The ammonia is then absorbed into the bloodstream and converted to ammonium ion. Normally, the liver converts the ammonium into urea for excretion by the kidney, but when the liver is malfunctioning or the blood is being shunted away from it, as in advanced cirrhosis, serum ammonium levels increase, and encephalopathy ensues. It is theorized that the cerebrotoxicity of ammonia results from inhibition of oxidative metabolism by the citric acid cycle in the brain. α-Ketoglutarate combines with ammonia to produce high CNS levels of glutamine (a byproduct of ammonium metabolism) while robbing the citric acid cycle of the α-ketoglutarate needed for production of high-energy adenosine triphosphate (ATP). Serum ammonium levels and cerebrospinal fluid (CSF) glutamine sometimes are measured to confirm hepatic encephalopathy.

An alternative explanation for the pathogenesis of hepatic encephalopathy concerns derangements in plasma and brain amino acid patterns.[11–13] Characteristically, there is a relative elevation in methionine and aromatic amino acid (AAA) levels (e.g., phenylalanine, tyrosine, and tryptophan) and a corresponding relative deficiency in branched-chain amino acids (BCAA; e.g., valine, leucine, and isoleucine). These derangements lead to an imbalance of brain neurotransmitters, causing elevated levels of serotonin, octopamine, and phenylethanolamine and a decrease in dopamine and possibly norepinephrine. Serotonin is an end product of tryptophan metabolism, whereas phenylethanolamine and octopamine are byproducts of phenylalanine and tyrosine metabolism.

Although the exact reason for these derangements in plasma and brain amino acids is unknown, a number of observations have been made.[7–9] The normal ratio of BCAAs to AAAs is 4:1 to 6:1. In both sepsis and liver failure, catabolic states lead to a negative nitrogen balance and preferential use of BCAAs as a source of energy. As ammonia levels rise, glucagon secretion is stimulated, which in turn stimulates hepatic gluconeogenesis to convert amino acids into glucose for energy. In response to gluconeogenesis, insulin is secreted, which leads to increased uptake and metabolism of BCAAs by skeletal muscle. As liver failure progresses, the liver can no longer store or release glucose in adequate amounts, so greater quantities of BCAAs must be metabolized by skeletal muscle for energy.

Simultaneously, the plasma clearance of AAAs and methionine, which depends on hepatic metabolism, is diminished. The net result is an alteration of the BCAA:AAA ratio. In acute liver failure the AAAs rise dramatically while BCAAs remain normal. In chronic hepatic disease the AAAs remain abnormally high while BCAA concentrations drop to low levels, further lowering the BCAA:AAA ratio. In addition to alterations in amino acid metabolism, there appears to be a derangement of the blood-brain barrier during chronic liver disease. In people with hepatic encephalopathy, there is a selective increase in transport of AAAs across the blood-brain barrier, possibly via an exchange of CSF glutamine (from ammonia metabolism) for AAAs in the plasma. The arterial concentration of ammonium and other amines may be accentuated by excessive dietary protein consumption, GI hemorrhage (source of protein), overdiuresis leading to dehydration, or other conditions that lead to severe electrolyte imbalance and metabolic alkalosis.

An entirely different avenue of research suggests that

the γ-aminobutyric acid (GABA) benzodiazepine receptor complex is involved in the pathogenesis of hepatic encephalopathy.[14] GABA is the primary inhibitory neurotransmitter in the CNS. According to this theory, an increase in CNS GABA-ergic neurotransmission may partially account for the behavioral and electrophysiologic manifestations of encephalopathy. This hypothesis is based on the observation that an accentuation of CNS inhibitory neurotransmitter tone can cause ataxia, sedation, and coma. Although GABA levels do not seem to be elevated in patients with encephalopathy, it is speculated that other endogenous or exogenous GABA-like ligands may be involved. Not surprisingly, these patients also demonstrate unusual sensitivity to benzodiazepinelike drugs that elicit GABA-ergic–like activity.

Other Associated Disorders

Anemia and other hematologic disorders commonly accompany cirrhosis. Chronic alcohol abusers tend to malabsorb folic acid and iron. In addition, their diets may be deficient in both iron and folate. Iron deficiency may be further aggravated by a blocking of iron uptake into the bone marrow induced by chronic alcoholism and by slow GI bleeding caused by gastritis. Thrombocytopenia and leukopenia may occur because of folic acid deficiency and hypersplenism secondary to portal hypertension.

Endocrine disorders are seen in advanced cirrhosis because of the liver's inability to metabolize the steroid hormones of the adrenals and gonads. In men, increased circulating estrogen levels cause gynecomastia, testicular atrophy, loss of body hair, impotence, spider angiomas, and palmar erythema.

The concurrent impairment of renal function with hepatic failure is called hepatorenal syndrome (HRS). HRS develops in about 4% of patients with decompensated cirrhosis and is associated with a poor prognosis. More than 95% of these patients die within a few weeks after onset of azotemia. HRS is characterized by increased renal vascular resistance and decreased systemic vascular resistance. The complex hemodynamic changes occur in response to vasoactive agents that produce different effects on the systemic and renal circulation. The vasoactive agents and systems involved in HRS are the renin–angiotensin–aldosterone system, the sympathetic nervous system, ADH, and the renal prostaglandin and kinin systems. HRS may occur acutely or progressively. The acute onset generally occurs in patients with end-stage cirrhosis or with other complications such as encephalopathy, bacterial infections, and bleeding. Clinical symptoms include oliguria that develops within a few days, along with a rapid increase in plasma urea and creatinine levels, tense ascites, dilutional hyponatremia, hypotension, and jaundice. A slower progressive type involving other chronic types of renal conditions associated with liver disease exhibits a gradual decrease in glomerular filtration rate that may last for several weeks or months. These patients may also demonstrate ascites that is poorly responsive to diuretics.[15]

PSYCHOSOCIAL ASPECTS

It is generally accepted that more than 90% of Americans drink alcohol at some time. This social drug clearly is the most widely abused substance in our society. Problems associated with the chronic use of alcohol are impressive in pathologic magnitude and costs incurred by society. Additionally, the physical and socioeconomic harm from its use is not limited to the patient. The alcoholic patient's life often is characterized by decreased productivity, an increase in vehicular accidents, criminal behavior, physical problems, mental illness, and disruption of the family. This sociologic disruption may extend into the community and workplace. The question of why some patients may drink alcohol excessively and others do not remains unanswered. This behavior is seen even in those who are well educated about the complications associated with chronic alcohol use. For the alcoholic patient with cirrhosis, psychological consultation with consideration for structured rehabilitation should be a component of the overall care plan.

THERAPEUTIC PLAN

Management of cirrhosis is largely symptomatic (Table 29.2). In Laennec's cirrhosis the primary treatment is to encourage the patient to abstain from alcohol. Fluid and electrolyte balance should be maintained by parenteral administration or oral therapy. If the patient is vomiting, antiemetics may be used. However, the phenothiazine-type antiemetics (e.g., prochlorperazine) have been associated with cholestasis and should be used with caution. Analgesics may be administered cautiously for abdominal pain. Aspirin-containing products and nonsteroidal anti-inflammatory drugs may worsen gastritis or GI bleeding. Also, acetaminophen hepatotoxicity may be more prevalent in alcoholic patients. Narcotics may lead to profound CNS and respiratory depression if the patient's liver status is severely compromised or if the patient is already obtunded. Sedatives and hypnotics should be avoided if there is any danger of hepatic coma. If there are no signs of impending hepatic coma, the patient should be maintained on a 2000- to 3000-calorie diet with 1 g protein per kilogram of body weight. If encephalopathy is present, dietary supplements that are rich in BCAAs and low in AAAs (e.g., Hepatic-Aid) have been used in an attempt to prevent negative nitrogen balance in patients who are intolerant to standard proteins.

TREATMENT

Pharmacotherapy

Hypoprothrombinemia

Vitamin replacement is essential in most cirrhotic patients, especially those with a recent alcoholic history. Replacement of thiamine at 50 to 100 mg/day along with a good diet may improve mentation, decrease symptoms of nutritional polyneuropathy, and improve gait disorders.

Table 29.2 ▪ Drugs Used in Cirrhotic Patients

Thiamine
- Reason: reverse mental confusion secondary to thiamine deficiency (Wernicke's syndrome) and decrease peripheral neuropathies
- Dosage: 100–200 mg/day, occasionally higher
- Monitoring parameters
  - Mental status
  - Decrease in nystagmus, peripheral neuropathies; more than 10 days of therapy is unwarranted

Vitamin K (phytonadione) (AquaMethyton preferred)
- Reason: prevent bleeding secondary to decreased production of factors II, VII, IX, and X (vitamin K–dependent factors)
- Dosage: 10–15 mg/day, not to exceed 3 doses
- Monitoring parameters
  - Hypersensitivity (fever, chills, anaphylaxis, flushing, sweating)
  - Prothrombin time

Spironolactone
- Reason: diuresis in ascites; specific for antagonism of preexisting hyperaldosteronism
- Dosage: 200–400 mg/day, occasionally higher; may be given as a single daily dose
- Monitoring parameters
  - Weight (avoid more than 1-kg weight loss per day)
  - Mental status
  - Serum K^+
  - Urine Na^+ and K^+ (Na^+ should not exceed K^+ at therapeutic dosages)
  - Abdominal girth
  - Blood urea nitrogen (increased in dehydration)
  - Gynecomastia (prolonged use)
  - Blood pressure

Loop diuretics
- Reason: diuresis in ascites after failure of high-dose spironolactone
- Dosage: start at 40 mg, titrate to 1-kg weight loss per day; occasionally very high dosages (200–600 mg/day) needed
- Monitoring parameters
  - Same as spironolactone except urine electrolytes of no value
  - Possible hearing loss with rapid IV bolus

Vasopressin
- Reason: vasoconstrictor for esophageal bleeding
- Dosage: 0.2–0.4 IU/min IV infusion
- Monitoring parameters
  - Rate of GI bleeding
  - Signs of ischemia (chest pain, elevated blood pressure, bradycardia)
  - GI cramping
  - Serum Na^+

Sodium tetradecyl sulfate, ethanolamine oleate, or sodium morrhuate
- Reason: sclerosing agent for esophageal bleeding
- Dosage: 0.5–2 mL of 1–1.5% tetradecyl, 5% ethanolamine, or 5% sodium morrhuate solution in each varix about 2 cm apart
- Monitoring parameters
  - Signs of GI bleeding
  - Chest pain, fever, local ulceration

Propranolol
- Reason: prevent GI bleeding
- Dosage: 40–320 mg/day titrated to 25% reduction in resting pulse rate if tolerated

Propranolol *(continued)*
- Monitoring parameters
  - Signs of GI bleeding
  - Mental changes
  - Vital signs: pulse >60, blood pressure >100/70
  - Signs of congestive heart failure, bradycardia
  - Signs of bronchospasm
  - Renal function

Lactulose
- Reason: hepatic encephalopathy; converted to lactic acid to lower bowel pH and prevent absorption of NH_3
- Dosage: 20–30 g QID or 300 mL 50% lactulose QS to 700–1000 mL as rectal enema titrated to 3–4 soft stools per day
- Monitoring parameters
  - Mental status, liver flap
  - Diarrhea

Neomycin
- Reason: hepatic encephalopathy; sterilizes gut to prevent bacterial breakdown of protein and thus decreases serum NH_3 levels
- Dosage: 2–6 g/day, orally or rectally
- Monitoring parameters
  - Mental status, liver flap
  - Diarrhea, bacterial overgrowth
  - Renal function
  - Signs of ototoxicity

Hepatamine and Hepatic-Aid[a]
- Reason: hepatic encephalopathy; replace branched-chain amino acids
- Dosage: Titrate to caloric and nitrogen needs
- Monitoring parameters
  - Mental status
  - Serum ammonia, cerebrospinal fluid glutamine
  - Serum amino acid levels (branched-chain: aromatic amino acid ratio)
  - Electrolyte balance

Dopamine[a]
- Reason: hepatorenal syndrome
- Dosage: 1–4 μg kg/min
- Monitoring parameters
  - Mental status, liver flap
  - Urine output
  - Blood pressure

Cochicine[a]
- Investigational use only; efficacy unclear
- Reason: antiinflammatory and antifibrotic effects
- Dosage: 0.6 mg PO BID or 1 mg PO QD 5 days/wk
- Monitoring parameters
  - Nausea, abdominal pain, diarrhea

Norfloxacin[a] (ciprofloxacin, sulfamethoxazole–trimethoprim)
- Reason: prevention of spontaneous bacterial peritonitis
- Dosage: 400 mg daily or 400 mg BID (ciprofloxacin 750 mg weekly, SMX/TMP 1 DS QD M–F)
- Monitoring parameters
  - Reduction in incidence of spontaneous bacterial peritonitis

Flumazenil[a]
- Investigational use only; efficacy unclear
- Reason: reversal of hepatic encephalopathy
- Dosage: 0.2–0.4 mg titrated to response
- Monitoring parameters
  - Reversal of mental obtundation

GI, gastrointestinal.

[a]Not recommended for all patients.

Continuation of thiamine therapy beyond 1 or 2 weeks is of questionable value because it is a water-soluble vitamin whose stores are rapidly replaced. Up to 1 g per day occasionally may be needed if the patient displays severe nystagmus, Wernicke's encephalopathy, or oculogyric crisis. Iron replacement or folic acid supplements are needed if the patient is anemic. Iron deficiency is confirmed by measurement of serum iron, total iron-binding capacity, and ferritin concentrations (see Chapter 13, Iron Deficiency and Megaloblastic Anemias).

Vitamin K 10 mg subcutaneously daily for 3 or more days is given if the prothrombin time is elevated. If the prothrombin time is not reversed after three to five doses, further doses should be avoided because an occasional patient demonstrates a paradoxical lengthening of the prothrombin time from excessive vitamin K. This paradoxical effect is theorized to be a result of consumptive processes induced by overstimulation of the production of clotting factors, leading to an eventual depletion of the body stores. Vitamin K_1, or phytonadione (AquaMephyton), gives a more rapid response when given parenterally than does either vitamin K_3 (menadione) or vitamin K_4 (menadiol). In giving vitamin K parenterally, the subcutaneous route is preferred, but it may also be given by very slow intravenous infusion in 50 mL of 5% dextrose in water (D_5W) over 15 to 20 minutes. Intramuscular injections are contraindicated if the patient has a prolonged prothrombin time or thrombocytopenia because of the possibility of hematoma and further complications. Because phytonadione is a colloidal suspension, there is a small risk of development of fever, chills, and even anaphylactic reactions with rapid intravenous injection. If the patient is malabsorbing fats, menadiol is the vitamin K of choice for oral administration because it is water soluble and is absorbed independently of bile acids.

Ascites

Ascites reversal is a time-consuming process that entails weeks or months of conservative management including bed rest to decrease plasma renin release, salt restriction (500 mg to 2 g/day), and, in some cases, fluid restriction. Approximately 5% of patients have a spontaneous diuresis with bed rest alone, and another 10 to 25% respond to salt restriction.[7] Fluid restriction is warranted only in cases of hyponatremia because excessive fluid restriction may lead to decreased renal blood flow and azotemia. Hospitalization usually is recommended for these patients for three reasons: intensive education on medications and diet; close monitoring of serum and urine electrolytes, urea nitrogen, and creatinine; and investigation of the cause of the liver disease.

Diuresis is the cornerstone of drug therapy of ascites, but the diuresis must be slow. If urinary losses exceed the volume of fluid reabsorbed from ascites or peripheral edema, volume depletion with hypotension and renal insufficiency can ensue. In patients treated with sodium restriction alone, no more than 300 mL of ascites can be reabsorbed per day. Even with the use of a diuretic, the maximum rate of reabsorption is 1440 mL per 24 hours.[16,17] Diuresis should be limited to 0.2 to 0.3 kg weight loss per day in those without edema and 0.5 to 1 kg per day in patients with edema.[7] Others allow a slightly more liberal diuresis of 0.75- to 2-kg weight loss per day.[17] These recommendations assume that each liter of volume lost is equivalent to a 1-kg weight loss. In patients with concurrent peripheral edema, a greater diuresis may be acceptable for the first 1 to 2 days because peripheral edema equilibrates more readily with the vasculature than does ascitic fluid. Other monitoring parameters include volume of urine output, changes in abdominal girth, postural blood pressures, blood urea nitrogen (avoiding prerenal azotemia), increase in urine potassium:sodium ratio from pretreatment baseline, and mental status changes.

Although slow diuresis with any diuretic is acceptable for treating ascites, the first diuretic given usually is spironolactone (Aldactone). It is a gentle, slow-acting diuretic specific for antagonizing the effects of the hyperaldosteronism that exists in many of these patients. In contrast to the small dosages of spironolactone that are used as an adjunct in hypertension, the dosage in ascites is begun at 50 to 100 mg per day. A 3- to 5-day lag period exists for the onset and maximum response from spironolactone, so frequent dosage adjustments should be avoided. Dosages are titrated upward in 50- to 100-mg intervals every 3 to 5 days, 400 mg per day being needed eventually in 75% of patients. Even greater dosages, up to 1 g per day, have been used, but this is expensive, and other diuretics such as furosemide usually are added before dosages of this magnitude are tried. The delayed onset and long duration of spironolactone result from the long half-life (approximately 17 hour) of its active metabolite, canrenone. For patient convenience, once-daily dosing should be recommended. Multiple daily doses are not necessary unless the patient cannot swallow the necessary number of tablets without gastric distress. Triamterene (Dyrenium) or amiloride (Midamor) can be slightly more rapid in onset, but they are not specific aldosterone inhibitors. Clinically, they probably are equal in effect to spironolactone, although the response of ascites to these drugs in comparison with spironolactone has not been studied extensively.

Besides the general monitoring parameters cited for diuretic therapy, serum and urine electrolyte levels, especially potassium, must be monitored. If hyperaldosteronism is present, it is not uncommon to see very little or no urinary sodium excretion and exceedingly large urinary potassium losses. One measure of having achieved the desired spironolactone dosage is a reversal of the urine electrolyte pattern to normal (i.e., sodium loss greater than potassium loss). Patients with urine sodium:potassium ratios greater than 1 tend to respond to lower dosages of spironolactone (100 to 150 mg/day); those with ratios less than 1 often need larger dosages, averaging 400 mg/day.[7]

Hyperaldosteronism, if present, may also cause a reduction in serum potassium concentration. Although the use of spironolactone with potassium supplements is nearly always contraindicated in treatment of other diseases because of a high risk of inducing hyperkalemia, this combination may be necessary early in the treatment of ascites, especially if the patient has GI losses of potassium secondary to vomiting or diarrhea. Serum potassium must be monitored daily to avoid hypokalemia or hyperkalemia. Because these patients often are placed on low-sodium diets, salt substitute use should be discouraged to further limit the complexity of potassium supplementation in this setting. Long-term use of spironolactone can lead to gynecomastia, a problem that is common in cirrhosis independent of diuretic use.

High spironolactone dosages may not produce the desired diuresis in some patients or may cause hyperkalemia. In these situations the addition of more potent diuretics such as thiazides and loop diuretics may be warranted. The dosage should be started low, 50 mg/day of hydrochlorothiazide or 20 to 40 mg/day of furosemide, and gradually increased. Some patients are especially refractory, needing several hundred milligrams per day of furosemide to obtain the desired 0.5- to 1-kg/day weight loss. One drawback to the use of thiazides and loop diuretics is that they cause a significant natriuresis, which negates the value of monitoring urine electrolytes. Intravenous furosemide should be avoided if possible because it can decrease glomerular filtration rates.[18] Nonsteroidal anti-inflammatory drug use should also be discouraged to avoid possible blunting of diuretic action and the renal blood flow reduction often associated with their use.

Paracentesis (aspiration of peritoneal fluid with a needle), except for removal of small volumes (250 to 1500 mL) to decrease pain and respiratory distress from abdominal stretching, has traditionally been discouraged because of the risk of abdominal perforation and introduction of infection. If large volumes are removed, 15 to 100% (mean 58%) of the fluid reaccumulates over the next 24 to 48 hours, leading to transient hypovolemia and the possibility of shock, encephalopathy, or acute renal failure.[16]

Recently, however, the combination of therapeutic paracentesis with intravenous albumin infusions (to hold volume in the vascular space) has become an accepted mode of therapy.[19–22] A typical regimen is removal of 4 to 6 L/day via paracentesis, with replacement of 40 to 50 g albumin after each tap. Paracentesis with albumin replacement is superior to diuretic therapy; it decreases ascites faster and shortens hospital stay without significant worsening of hepatic, renal, or cardiovascular function. Single large-volume (5-L) paracentesis without albumin replacement also appears to be safe in patients with painful, tense ascites,[23] but repeated large-volume paracentesis without albumin replacement may result in hyponatremia or renal impairment in some patients.[20] Another possible concern is an increased risk of SBP secondary to reduced ascitic fluid opsonic activity.[24] Arguments about the high cost of albumin are counterbalanced by decreased hospitalization time. The use of dextran as a volume expander after paracentesis has been looked at as an alternative to albumin.[25] It has been shown to help prevent the asymptomatic abnormalities in lab values at a lower cost.[18] Although its use remains controversial,[26] albumin has also been used without paracentesis in an attempt to increase intravascular volume and induce diuresis. The drawbacks to this treatment are a short duration of response, the risk of inducing variceal hemorrhage, and high cost. Generally, treatment with albumin without paracentesis is to be avoided unless all other therapies have failed. In Europe, ascites recirculation with removal, concentration, and reinfusion of peritoneal fluid has been found to be safe and effective.[27] The possibility of reaccumulation of ascites after paracentesis necessitates continuation of a low-sodium diet and diuretics.

A peritoneovenous shunt (LeVeen shunt), in use extensively for the last 18 to 20 years, was devised for use in refractory ascites.[28,29] The shunt consists of a surgically implanted one-way valve in the abdominal wall, an intraabdominal cannula, and an outflow tube tunneled subcutaneously from the valve to a vein that empties directly into the inferior vena cava. As the diaphragm descends, the pressure in the intrathoracic veins drops and intraperitoneal pressure rises. This pressure differential pumps the ascitic fluid into the venous system. The results may be dramatic, with urine output as high as 15 L occurring during the first 24 hours. Supplemental diuresis with furosemide may be needed to prevent vascular overload. However, use of this procedure is limited by such complications as fever, shunt occlusions, hypokalemia, infection, shunt leaks, disseminated intravascular coagulopathy, and (less often) variceal hemorrhage, bowel obstruction, pulmonary edema, and pneumothorax.[28] A Veterans Administration Cooperative study involving 3860 patients demonstrated no improvement in survival and significant morbidity rates in patients treated with peritoneovenous shunt compared with those treated with diuretic therapy.[29] However, shunting alleviated disabling ascites more rapidly than medical management did.

Spontaneous Bacterial Peritonitis

By definition, SBP is the spontaneous infection of ascitic fluid without any evidence of an intraabdominal or extraabdominal source of infection. SBP occurs in approximately 30 to 40% of all cirrhotic patients.[30] Although some patients may be asymptomatic, commonly observed signs and symptoms include fever, chills, vomiting, abdominal pain or tenderness, decreased bowel sounds, and encephalopathy. Diagnosis is made through paracentesis. Positive cultures or polymorphonuclear cell counts greater than 250/mm^3 indicate SBP.[31,32]

The exact pathophysiology of SBP is unclear, but several potential mechanisms have been proposed. One of the most likely routes is through hematogenous spread. Portal blood flow in cirrhotic patients may bypass the liver, permitting circulating bacteria to avoid removal by the hepatic reticuloendothelial filtering system. Second, portal hypertension causes congestion in the lymphatic and splanchnic veins, resulting in inflammation and edema in the bowel wall. A decrease in local resistance to bacterial invasion via bowel translocation may occur in these patients.[31]

The organisms of primary concern in SBP are the enteric Gram-negative bacilli and some *Streptococcus* strains. Anaerobes are only rarely reported as causative organisms in SBP, and pseudomonal and staphylococcal species are not a concern. Empiric therapy has traditionally been ampicillin or a first-generation cephalosporin in combination with an aminoglycoside. More recently, clinical use of less toxic alternative agents such as cefotaxime, ampicillin–sulbactam, ticarcillin–clavulanate, or second-generation cephalosporins such as cefotetan or cefoxitin have also provided acceptable outcomes. Caution is advised with cefotetan because the presence of the methylthiotetrazole side chain may further complicate an existing hypoprothrombinemic state. Cefotaxime generally is accepted as the current drug of choice for SBP.[33,34] Either drug can be used until final culture and sensitivity information is available. Duration of therapy may be shortened to 5 days because of the low inoculum of organisms in the ascitic fluid.[35]

Some patients are at greater risk for development of SBP and its complications. These include cirrhotic patients with ascites who have GI hemorrhage, encephalopathy, or a history of previous episodes of SBP; patients with decreased protein levels in their ascitic fluid; and those awaiting liver transplant. Prevention of SBP in these patients has been attempted. Norfloxacin 400 mg once daily has been used successfully as prophylactic treatment for high-risk patients. This fluoroquinolone causes a selective intestinal decontamination that eliminates the Gram-negative bacilli but preserves the remaining normal flora. Norfloxacin was shown to markedly reduce the incidence of SBP in patients with previous SBP episodes and is considered a safe and effective long-term treatment for SBP prophylaxis.[36] Twice-daily dosing of the drug may be needed in patients experiencing GI hemorrhage.[37] Singh et al.[38] have also shown trimethoprim–sulfamethoxazole to be of value in SBP prevention. Recently, a single dose of 750 mg ciprofloxacin administered weekly was shown to be effective in preventing SBP.[39] The simplicity of a single weekly dosage has popularized this approach in many medical centers. Because the quinolone is given only once weekly, it is especially important that concomitant administration of divalent and trivalent cations be avoided and that doses be spaced adequately (see Chapter 3, Drug Interactions).

Gastrointestinal Bleeding

Bleeding from esophageal varices is a grave sign and may be difficult to stop. Multiple transfusions often are needed. Even if the bleeding is stopped, the chances of the patient hemorrhaging again are high. One way to control a simple bleed is by direct pressure. Placing a lumened, inflatable balloon tube (Linton, Minnesota, or Sengstaken–Blakemore tube) to slow the bleeding by compression has been tried, with varied results. The balloon inflates, and the varix is compressed between the balloon and esophageal wall, leading to a clotting of the laceration. This procedure is complicated by vomiting and a high rate of aspiration or recurrence of bleeding as soon as the balloon is deflated. Bleeding is stopped in 40 to 80% of patients, but use of this procedure, by current standards, is only a temporary measure.

Injecting sclerosing agents into esophageal varices is receiving increased interest.[40–45] This approach is considered by many to be the therapy of choice. Although not a new technique, sclerotherapy remained impractical until the widespread availability of the flexible fiberoptic esophagoscope in the 1970s. Percutaneous transhepatic sclerotherapy or embolization is a major operative procedure involving insertion of a catheter into the gastric and coronary veins via initial entry into the portal vein. Hypertonic glucose or Gel Foam is then injected into the vessels to obliterate them and prevent flow to the esophageal vessels. A less invasive procedure involves direct injection of bleeding varices with a sclerosing agent via an endoscope. The most commonly used sclerosants in the United States are sodium tetradecyl sulfate (Sotradecol), ethanolamine oleate (Ethamolin), and sodium morrhuate (Scleromate). Injection of these agents into a bleeding varix leads to intense inflammatory response, thrombus formation, and cessation of bleeding within 2 to 5 minutes. A more permanent fibrotic obliteration of the vessel develops over several days.

Sclerotherapy controls acute variceal bleeding in 90 to 95% of patients, nearly twice the rate of benefit achieved with balloon tamponade or vasopressin.[40] A single treatment controls bleeding in 90% of subjects; the remainder need one or more repeated treatments over several weeks. Success rates are lower for treating actively bleeding patients than for controlling bleeding initially by more conservative methods. Failure of therapy is defined as continuation of bleeding after two injections of a sclerosing agent during a single admission.[46] Compared with portacaval and splenorenal shunt procedures, sclerotherapy is almost equally effective in stopping bleeding, there is no difference in survival, and there is much lower morbidity.[42,43] Prophylactic sclerotherapy in patients with endoscopic evidence of varices but no history of past or current bleeding is of no apparent clinical benefit.[44,45]

A 0.5 to 3% solution of tetradecyl, a premixed solution of ethanolamine 5% or morrhuate 5% for injection, is used. After the endoscope is passed, approximately 0.5 to 2 mL of sclerosing solution is injected into each varix at points about 2 to 4 cm apart. If bleeding recurs, therapy can be repeated. Although it appears that sclerotherapy is effective in stopping acute bleeding and preventing rebleeding, more than 50% of patients rebleed, and long-term mortality is not lower than with conventional therapy. Side effects associated with sclerotherapy include pericarditis, chest pain, dysphagia, pyrexia, cardiac tamponade, formation of esophagobronchial fistulae, and local ulcerations.

After sclerotherapy, prophylaxis with antacids, histamine-2 (H_2) antagonists, proton pump inhibitors, or sucralfate may be initiated. Dosing of these drugs is the same as that recommended for treating peptic ulcer disease or reflux esophagitis (see Chapter 24, Peptic Ulcer Disease). Careful monitoring of mental status in patients who are treated with cimetidine is a must because cirrhosis may predispose them to the mental confusion associated with this agent.[47] The pharmacokinetics of ranitidine may also be altered in cirrhosis, resulting in its accumulation.[48] Sucralfate suspension has been used to prevent ulcers at the sclerosis site. Investigators using endoscopy have shown that the drug complex coats the varices and decreases ulcer formation.[49] The aluminum component of sucralfate may complex with coadministered norfloxacin or ciprofloxacin, resulting in poor absorption. The importance of divalent and trivalent cations complexing with quinolones could be questioned in SBP prophylaxis because of local intestinal rather than systemic action. However, because the complex does not enter bacteria as well,[50] it is prudent to adequately space doses of these agents even in SBP prophylaxis.

A newer endoscopic technique for control of variceal bleeds is endoscopic variceal banding therapy (EBT). The success rate of this procedure may be as high as 90%.[51] The procedure involves endoscopic placement of a small rubber band over a distal varix. A large varix is drawn by suction aspiration of into the end portion of the sleeve, and the band is triggered over the base of the varix. A specially modified endoscope that carries a triggering device and rubber band on a small sleeve over the objective end of the scope is needed. Though not widely used, EBT has a control rate of 86% for acute bleed. It has also been associated with a lower complication rate, although the risk of rebleeding may be slightly higher than that of sclerotherapy.[52,53]

The natural hormone vasopressin (ADH) often was used to treat bleeding varices before the advent of sclerotherapy. Vasopressin significantly decreases portal blood flow and pressure by constricting portal and other splanchnic arterioles. This slows or stops bleeding long enough to allow thrombus formation at the site of bleeding. The use of this drug is declining and remains controversial because the benefits in morbidity and mortality have never been clearly proven.[54] Sclerotherapy has been shown consistently to be more effective than vasopressin, but vasopressin may be given first to slow bleeding and make visualizing bleeding varices by endoscope easier.

The major limitation to vasopressin therapy is side effects. The intense vasoconstrictor action decreases cardiac output and may cause coronary ischemia. This is especially a problem in patients who have coronary artery disease or hypertension, but ischemic changes also have been reported in patients with no prior evidence of ischemic disease.[54] Bradycardia caused by stimulation of the vagus nerve is the most widely observed side effect of vasopressin.[54] It also may produce skin blanching, GI cramping, and even bowel necrosis by stimulating smooth muscle contraction. Women may experience uterine pain similar to menstrual cramps. Finally, vasopressin may lead to excess water retention and a dilutional hyponatremia.[54]

In an attempt to reduce toxicity, continuous intravenous infusions starting at 0.2 to 0.4 U/minute or direct intraarterial infusion via a catheter into the superior mesenteric artery at 0.05 to 0.4 IU/minute have been tried.[54] The maximum recommended intravenous infusion rate is 0.9 IU/minute. Infusions may be continued for up to 72 hours with a slow tapering of the dosage over time. The results have been varied, with some authors claiming up to 50 to 70% effectiveness.[54] Others claim poor response and a high incidence of complications, including bleeding from the site of catheter insertion and septicemia.[55]

A combination of vasopressin infusion and intravenous nitroglycerin (40 μg/minute titrated according to blood pressure to a maximum of 400 μg/minute)[56] or sublingual nitroglycerin (0.6 mg every 30 minutes for 6 hours)[57] may cause an additional decrease in portal pressure. In the study using intravenous nitroglycerin, there was less bleeding in the combination therapy group; in the trial with sublingual nitroglycerin, the rate of bleeding cessation was equal to that with vasopressin alone. In both studies, combination therapy led to a marked reduction in cardiac complications.

The use of somatostatin has also been evaluated in controlling variceal bleed. Somatostatin reduces portal pressure and blood flow with continuous intravenous administration. It offers efficacy equal to that of vasopressin with considerably fewer side effects. Its use is limited by its significantly higher cost; therefore, it is not considered as a first-line therapy.[42,58]

Bleeding from other GI sites, especially bleeding caused by gastritis and peptic ulcer, usually is treated with nasogastric suction, tap water lavage, H_2 antagonists, proton pump inhibitors, or hourly antacids.[59] Occasionally, 20 IU vasopressin, 1 to 2 ampules of norepinephrine, or ice is used in a gastric lavage to cause localized vasoconstriction in an attempt to slow bleeding. No evidence documents these latter maneuvers to be any more effective than tap water lavage or H_2 antagonists alone; therefore, their use generally is discouraged.

It has been suggested that because propranolol and possibly other β-adrenergic blockers decrease portal venous pressure, they may prevent GI bleeding associated with portal hypertension.[60–65] Primary therapy is defined as treatment of patients with known varices but without a history of active bleeding. Secondary intervention involves administering the drug after resolution of an acute bleeding episode. Although data are limited, overall analysis of the benefit of primary therapy is positive.[60–62] For example, in the European Cooperative study group, a median dosage of 160 mg/day (range 40 to 320 mg) led to a cumulative 74% of patients in the propranolol group who were free of bleeding after 2 years, compared with 39% in the placebo group. Two-year survival was 72% in the treated patients and 37% in the untreated subjects.[62] Propranolol also appears to be a cost-effective approach, with savings between $450 and $14,600 over 5 years in 1997 dollars.[63]

The results for secondary prophylaxis are also encouraging but somewhat more complex. Lebrec et al.[64] showed that oral propranolol in dosages that reduced the heart rate by 25% led to a significantly lower frequency of rebleeding than did placebo, during a 2-year study in chronic alcoholic patients with a history of esophageal bleeding. Only 21% of patients in the propranolol group had recurrence of bleeding, compared with 68% in the placebo group. Cumulative survival was 90% in the propranolol group and 57% in the placebo group. None of the patients showed deterioration of hepatic or renal function while taking propranolol, but because propranolol may decrease cardiac output and liver blood flow, patients should be monitored closely.

A similar study by Burroughs et al.[65] failed to confirm the findings of Lebrec. However, the patients in Burroughs et al.'s study had more severe liver disease and included some with cirrhosis from causes other than chronic alcoholism. Selective β-blockade with atenolol or metoprolol is less effective than sclerotherapy in arresting acute variceal bleeding.[60,61]

A follow-up study by Poynard et al.[66] confirms the benefits of propranolol, with 71% of subjects free of bleeding at 1 year and 57% at 2 years. In this study, five factors were identified that increased the risk of rebleeding: hepatocellular carcinoma, continued alcohol abuse, lack of suppression of pulse rate by propranolol, a history of rebleeding, and noncompliance with drug therapy. Of particular concern, 12 of 14 (86%) patients who discontinued β-blocker therapy rebled abruptly. The time of greatest risk for rebleeding is within the first 3 to 4 days of stopping therapy, but it may occur up to 150 days later.[60,61,66–68] It is not possible to be certain that drug discontinuation is responsible for rebleeding in the cases in which the occurrence is delayed.

A recent randomized controlled study by Teres et al.[69] in Barcelona compared sclerotherapy with propranolol in prevention of rebleeding for varices. Although rebleeding was less with sclerotherapy (26 of 58 subjects) than with propranolol (37 of 58 subjects) titrated to reduce resting heart rate by 25%, complications were significantly more common and of greater severity with sclerotherapy. The authors could not recommend either approach on the basis of the study findings. Another published trial compared isosorbide-5-mononitrate with propranolol in long-term follow-up (128 patients followed over 7 years). Isosorbide-5-mononitrate was as effective as propranolol in reducing mortality.[70] Additional perspective on this approach is offered in the accompanying editorial.[71]

Surgical treatment may be needed for patients who have repeated GI bleeding (especially esophageal varices) or those who have bleeding that cannot be stopped by the more conservative measures already described.[40] A portacaval shunt involves anastomosis of the portal vein directly to the inferior vena cava, thus bypassing the cirrhotic liver. This decreases portal hypertension and lowers backpressure on the abdominal venous system. Unfortunately, these patients have a poor prognosis because the only way to carry toxins to the liver for detoxification is now the hepatic artery. If they survive the initial surgery, patients may die of sepsis or develop hepatic failure and encephalopathy. The Warren shunt decompresses varices by shunting splenic blood flow to the renal vein (splenorenal shunt) and may decrease hepatic perfusion less.

Hepatic Encephalopathy

Clinical manifestations of hepatic encephalopathy should be recognized and addressed promptly because most are reversible with appropriate therapy.[72] If the patient develops signs of an impending hepatic coma (e.g., confusion, drowsiness, asterixis), lactulose is indicated, and dietary protein should be decreased to 20 to 30 g/day. Use of CNS depressants should be minimized. Except for cautious use of spironolactone, diuretics usually should be withheld at this stage because hypovolemia, hypokalemia, and metabolic alkalosis tend to aggravate encephalopathy.

Lactulose is a synthetic disaccharide of galactose and fructose that is neither absorbed nor hydrolyzed in the small bowel. It is degraded by colonic bacteria to lactic, acetic, and formic acids, thus decreasing the pH of the colonic contents to an endpoint of approximately 5.5. The effect of lactulose was originally attributed to replacement of proteolytic bacteria such as *Escherichia coli, Proteus,* and *Bacteroides* with organisms such as *Lactobacillus* that thrive in a more acidic medium and lack urease and other enzymes that are used in the production of ammonia. However, most investigators cannot demonstrate a marked change in the colonic flora and attribute the effects of lactulose solely to the pH changes that occur. As the colon becomes more acidic, the ratio of ammonium ion to ammonia increases, and less absorption of the ammonia occurs. There may also be back-diffusion of ammonia from the blood to the intestinal lumen under acidic pH conditions. In any event, lactulose therapy results in a decrease in arterial ammonium levels.[73]

Each 15 mL lactulose oral liquid contains 10 g lactulose, and it is usually given in a dosage of 30 to 40 mL three to four times daily. Use of retention enemas of 300 mL of 50% lactulose diluted to 700 to 1000 mL with tap water has also been reported.[74] Onset of effect by either route is 12 to 48 hours. Once improved mental state has been achieved, the dosage can be tapered slowly to identify the smallest effective dosage. Patient tolerance can be improved by diluting the drug in fruit juice or carbonated beverages. In most patients, lactulose can be discontinued after several days to a few weeks if the patient's mental status improves. In a few patients, prolonged therapy for months or years may be needed if discontinuation of the drug causes a recurrence of symptoms.

The most common complaints of patients treated with lactulose are nausea (because of the sweet taste of the drug), gaseous distension, bloating, belching, or diarrhea caused by osmotic effects in the bowel. Diarrhea may account for part of the therapeutic effects of lactulose,[75] but compared with sorbitol, lactulose is more effective in overcoming the encephalopathy, indicating that other mechanisms are working. The dosage usually is adjusted so that the patient has two to three soft, semiformed stools daily. Watery diarrhea should be avoided. Of course, if the patient's mental state improves at a dosage that produces fewer than two to three stools per day, it is not logical to give a larger dosage.

The success rate with lactulose has been reported to be around 85%. Unfortunately, a few patients become resistant after prolonged therapy, and others die from complications of the disease, even though their encephalopathy has cleared. Fluid losses secondary to diarrhea should be considered in monitoring lactulose therapy. Serum sodium should be monitored to detect hyponatremia associated with loss of free water from osmotic diarrhea.

An alternative to lactulose is neomycin in dosages of 1 to 2 g four times daily. Neomycin destroys colonic bacteria, slowing the degradation of protein to ammonia. If the patient does not respond, the dosage of the neomycin should be increased to 8 to 12 g/day and the protein restriction should be lowered to 0 to 20 g/day. For patients who cannot take medications orally, a retention enema of 2 to 4 g neomycin in 200 mL of saline thickened with methylcellulose may be used morning and night. When the patient improves, the maintenance dosage of neomycin may be lowered to 2 to 4 g/day.

The duration of therapy varies with lactulose and neomycin and may last for less than 1 week in most cases or up to months and even years in poorly controlled patients. Some degree of protein restriction may be indicated because an intolerance to protein intake may be observed in certain patients. Many patients who look well compensated can deteriorate rapidly after eating a single high-protein meal.

One well-controlled study[76] failed to show a clear superiority of neomycin (83% effective) or lactulose (90% effective) in treating acute encephalopathy. For long-term use, lactulose has the potential advantage of less toxicity, but it is considerably more expensive. The possibility that sterilization of the gut by neomycin might decrease the effectiveness of lactulose appears to be of minimal consequence;[77] in fact, the two drugs are more effective when used together.[78]

Neomycin is considered a nonabsorbable antibiotic. However, 1 to 3% of a dose is absorbed,[79] and there are several reported cases of ototoxicity in patients on chronic oral neomycin therapy.[80] Most of these patients had been taking neomycin for at least 8 months and had coexisting renal dysfunction. Annual auditory testing should be performed, and the patient should be observed for subjective changes in hearing status if the drug is to be used for prolonged periods.

Neomycin has also been implicated in development of HRS. Although neomycin is renal toxic when given parenterally, it is difficult to determine whether the renal changes with oral dosing are drug-induced or a progression of the disease process itself. The consensus is that the latter mechanism prevails.

Another consequence of neomycin therapy is diarrhea from changes in the bowel flora. This may not be a serious problem because patients often are given cathartics to cleanse the bowel and eliminate excess ammonia. However, cathartics alone are not effective in moderating encephalopathy, and they should always be accompanied by lactulose or neomycin and protein restriction. Because cathartics can cause fluid and electrolyte imbalance, they may worsen encephalopathy. Adequate intravenous infusions of dextrose or saline with potassium supplements should be maintained. Daily metronidazole or rifaximin, a derivative of rifamycin, has also been used with some success.[72]

Therapeutic Value of Corticosteroids

Cirrhotic patients with biopsy-proven alcoholic hepatitis may benefit from the anti-inflammatory and antifibrotic effects of corticosteroid therapy. The beneficial effect may be related to the corticosteroid's inhibition of cytokine production.

The efficacy of steroids in treating liver disease remains controversial. Clinical trials have shown conflicting results in regard to mortality. A meta-analysis of the randomized trials was completed to determine the efficacy of steroids on short-term mortality in patients with alcoholic hepatitis. The combined data indicate that steroids provide a protective efficacy of 27% in patients with hepatic encephalopathy. This figure increased in patients without active GI bleeding. Among subjects without hepatic encephalopathy, steroids had no protective efficacy. These data suggest that only patients with severe disease would benefit from steroid therapy. Patients with severe disease are defined as those with hepatic encephalopathy or a discriminant function higher than 32 (Discriminant function = 4.6 [Patient's prothrombin time − Control time] + Bilirubin). Patients with severe disease who have active GI bleeding or need treatment for active infection should be excluded from steroid therapy.[81]

Prednisolone is the most studied and appears to be the preferred steroid. The dosing regimen is 40 mg/day for 4 weeks and is then tapered over 2 to 4 weeks.[82]

Therapeutic Value of γ-Aminobutyric Acid Antagonists

As was introduced in the section on clinical findings and diagnosis, some investigators believe that endogenous or exogenous GABA-ergic–like compounds that stimulate the GABA–benzodiazepine receptor complex in the brain may be responsible for symptoms of encephalopathy.[14,83]

Preliminary data suggest that the benzodiazepine antagonist flumazenil may be valuable in both short-term and long-term management of encephalopathy.

In a series of 14 subjects, 71% of patients had short-term improvement in symptoms after intravenous administration of flumazenil.[84] Arousal was greatest in patients with deeper coma (stage III to IV encephalopathy). Although response was rapid, the duration of effect was only 1 to 2 hours with parenteral therapy. The usual dosage was 0.2 to 0.4 mg, and some subjects receiving up to 10 doses.

A single case report describes long-term use of oral therapy.[85] A patient given 25 mg twice daily experienced complete reversal of symptoms for 14 months. Previously, this patient had experienced 12 attacks of coma over a 2-year period. Discontinuation of the drug led to a recurrence of symptoms within 48 hours.

A randomized double-blind placebo-controlled crossover trial from Canada shows a significant clinical improvement in 5 of 11 (45%) hepatic coma patients receiving flumazenil in the initial treatment phase and 1 of 2 (50%) in the crossover phase of the study. The authors conclude that the agent is efficacious and safe for relieving neurologic symptoms in cirrhotic patients with hepatic coma.[86] This trial has been criticized.[87] The use of benzodiazepine receptor antagonist therapy in these patients remains investigational and controversial.

Therapeutic Value of Dopamine

Dopamine and norepinephrine are important mediators of normal sympathetic activity in both the CNS and the periphery, especially in the kidney. Some of the neurologic manifestations of hepatic failure, as well as HRS, may be caused by accumulation of other β-hydroxylated phenylethylamines such as octopamine and serotonin. These compounds may replace normal transmitters and act as false neurotransmitters in sympathetic nerve terminals and granules. Precursors of false neurotransmitters, such as phenylalanine and tyrosine (Fig. 29.2), are produced from protein in the gut by bacterial amino acid decarboxylases. Normally, these precursors are metabolized rapidly in the liver by monoamine oxidase (MAO), allowing norepinephrine that is formed elsewhere in the body to predominate. When hepatic function is impaired or when blood is shunted away from the liver, these false neurotransmitters may replace normal transmitters. Systemically, this may lead to lowered peripheral vascular resistance and shunting of blood away from the kidney. Similarly, asterixis and other signs of hepatic encephalopathy might result from displacement of transmitters such as dopamine and norepinephrine in the basal ganglia and other areas in the brain.

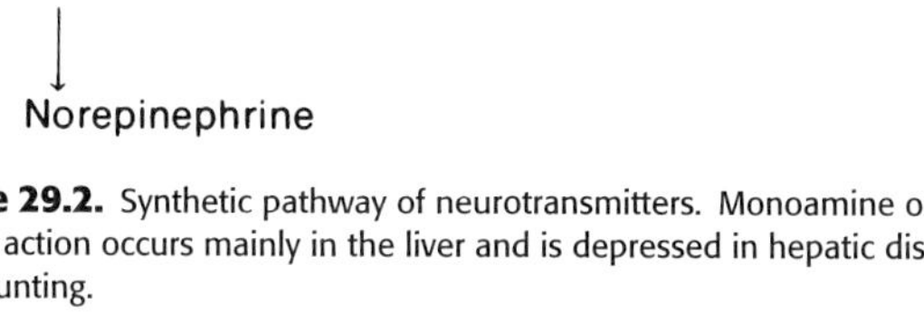

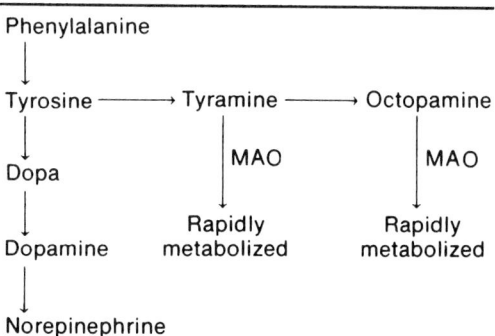

Figure 29.2. Synthetic pathway of neurotransmitters. Monoamine oxidase (*MAO*) action occurs mainly in the liver and is depressed in hepatic disease and shunting.

If the displacement of normal central and peripheral transmitters by less active amines can account for hepatic coma and its cardiovascular complications, then the restoration of normal transmitter stores might restore normal function. For hospitalized patients this is accomplished with low-dose infusions of dopamine at 1.3 to 5 μg/kg/minute.[88] This may increase renal blood flow and help to reverse HRS. Unfortunately, the mortality rate of patients with HRS approaches 100%, even in those who receive dopamine. Failure to improve urine output or increase blood pressure within the first 24 hours of dopamine treatment is a poor prognostic sign. Because dopamine does not cross the blood-brain barrier, encephalopathy may not be helped. However, as shown in Figure 29.2, dopamine is also a precursor to norepinephrine, which may help to restore natural neurotransmitter balance in a second way.

Pharmacotherapy of Primary Biliary Cirrhosis

Colchicine, a drug with both anti-inflammatory and antifibrotic properties, has been evaluated as a potential disease-modifying agent for several years. In one study, 57 patients with biopsy-proven PBC were treated with 0.6 mg colchicine twice daily or placebo.[89] The colchicine-treated patients had significant improvement in biochemical parameters (serum bilirubin and transferase levels) but no difference (compared with placebo) in histologic progression. A second group of investigators conducted a randomized, double-blind, placebo-controlled trial of colchicine, 1 mg/day, 5 days per week, in 100 patients with cirrhosis caused by alcohol abuse or a history of hepatitis.[90] Median survival was 3.5 years in the placebo group and 11 years in the colchicine-treated patients, and deaths from liver failure were 24% in the placebo group and 15% in the treatment group. Side effects in both trials were mild, consisting primarily of nausea, abdominal pain, and diarrhea. Although these results are encouraging, flaws in the study design and the small number of subjects treated prevent widespread endorsement of colchicine therapy at this time.

Numerous other drugs have been tried in treating PBC, including penicillamine, chlorambucil, azathioprine, cyclosporine, corticosteroids, and methotrexate.[91] Each of these therapies is based on the hope that anti-inflammatory or immunomodulating effects may alter the disease process. Cyclosporine showed modest improvement in symptoms, enzyme levels, and histologic findings in a controlled trial for treating PBC. However, toxicity with this drug is a limiting factor in therapy. A controlled, multicenter trial with ursodeoxycholic acid also showed improvement in symptoms, enzyme levels, and histologic findings in some patients but showed little effect in patients with advanced disease.[92] In addition, sequestration of copper by penicillamine may have a therapeutic effect. Unfortunately, most of the trials with these drugs have been limited by a small sample size without adequate controls, and the improvement obtained has been only marginal. At this time, none of these drugs can be recommended. Ursodiol may be effective in slowing the progression of PBC and may decrease the need for transplantation.[93]

Nonpharmacolgic Therapy

One of the goals of progressive liver disease management is to provide adequate nutritional support, including protein and calories. Positive nitrogen balance must be established without exacerbating hepatic encephalopathy caused by inappropriate combinations of amino acids. In experimental animals and to a lesser extent in humans, diets that are high in BCAAs and low in AAAs and methionine may help to restore normal amino acid balance and reduce encephalopathy.[11–13,94] An 8% amino acid solution (Hepatamine) is marketed that contains more BCAAs than standard parenteral nutrition solutions. The ratio of BCAAs to AAAs in Hepatamine is 37:1, compared with 5:1 in conventional crystalline amino acid solutions. Mixing 500 mL Hepatamine with 500 mL 50% dextrose in water yields 40 g/L of amino acids. Indications for use of this therapy and its efficacy are debated. The high cost and questionable efficacy of Hepatamine have led most institutions to limit the use of BCAA solutions to patients with life-threatening encephalopathy refractory to conventional therapy and those with documented elevated serum ammonia levels. In most cases an amino acid screen is used to assess the ratio of BCAA:AAA in the patient. The cost of an amino acid screen is approximately equal to 1 day's therapy with Hepatamine.

For the alert patient without central venous access, enteral therapy has been proposed. One such dietary supplement is Hepatic-Aid, a complex of carbohydrate, protein, and fat in a readily digestible form. One package of Hepatic-Aid mixed in a blender with 250 mL water yields 340 mL suspension for oral or nasogastric administration that contains 2.2 g nitrogen (15 g protein), 98 g carbohydrate, 12 g fat, and 560 calories (500 nonprotein calories). One to four packages can be given per day, but the administration rate should be slow at first to prevent glucose overload. Use of oral BCAAs is discouraged because of questionable efficacy, high cost, and disagreeable taste. American Society of Parenteral and Enteral Nutrition (ASPEN) Medical Practice Guidelines for nutritional supplementation in patients with liver disease, with specific recommendations, are available.[95] Severe growth hormone resistance is also been associated with the protein catabolic state seen in cirrhosis. From the limited data available, it appears that treatment with growth hormone can possibly improve nitrogen use.[96] Additionally, because *Helicobacter pylori* has strong urease activity, some evidence supports treatment, if present. *H. pylori* eradication can lead to reduced hyperammonemia.[97]

ALTERNATIVE THERAPY

The naturally occurring whole extract of the milk thistle (*Silybum marianum*) is known as silymarin. This flavonoid complex has been shown to have a liver protective effect in experimental models of liver intoxication, including acetaminophen, ethanol, carbon tetrachloride, and phenylhydrazine intoxication. Use of silymarin has been popularized by lay press, Internet sources, and some scientific efficacy validation. Silymarin has been found to prevent lipid peroxidation, changes in phospholipid composition of membranes, and hepatic glutathione depletion. It also appears to normalize hepatic function markers in patients with alcoholic liver disease. This positive effect may be attributed to the selective inhibition of leukotriene formation by Kupffer cells achieved with an isomer of the silymarin complex known as silibinin.[98]

IMPROVING OUTCOMES

The therapeutic outcome for patients with cirrhosis depends entirely on the stage of the disease and the presence of complications. If the cause of the cirrhosis is alcoholism and the patient continues to drink, the prognosis is poor. Conversely, discontinuation of drinking increases survival. Patient education with a goal of total abstinence from alcohol is a primary issue in dealing with this population of patients. Use of alcohol in any amount is strictly forbidden. Rigid compliance with diet and drug therapy is critical. Generally, adherence to a diet of at least 1 g protein per kilogram of body weight, with an intake of 2000 to 3000 calories per day, is acceptable. Patients must be weighed daily to adjust diuretic dosage.

PROGNOSIS

In one series of 1155 patients with cirrhosis from a variety of causes, the overall 5-year survival was about 40%.[99] The causes of death were liver failure in 49%, hepatocellular carcinoma in 22%, bleeding in 14%, HRS in 8%, and other causes in the remainder. Patients who entered the study with compensated cirrhosis (mild or absent symptoms) became symptomatic at the rate of 10% per year. Survival was higher in this group of patients (54% at 6 years). People who entered the study with symptoms already present (ascites, history of bleeding, or encephalopathy) had a survival rate of only 21% at 6 years and a much higher incidence of hepatocellular carcinoma.

PHARMACOECONOMICS

The management of cirrhosis can have a major economic impact, primarily because of the chronicity and progressive nature of the disease. Patients who do not abstain from alcohol and comply with a low-protein diet and drug therapy can be expected to have multiple hospital admissions as the disease progresses. End-stage cirrhosis management is expensive. The preventive approaches discussed in this chapter that minimize morbidity, such as SBP prophylaxis, diuretics, encephalopathy prevention, vitamin supplementations, and dietary modification, are cost-effective and must be implemented early in a care plan. It is important to develop rapport with family members or other caregivers to ensure their support of the treatment plan and thereby lessen the risk of noncompliance and recidivism. Family and caregiver support is an especially important component of a successful alcohol rehabilitation effort.

KEY POINTS

- In the United States, cirrhosis is one of the five most common causes of death in people over age 40.[1]
- Despite extensive investigation of liver function and pathologies, there is no effective therapy for many liver diseases.
- Discontinuation of alcohol intake in patients with proven cirrhosis is of primary importance. Use of naltrexone in an effort to decrease craving may prove valuable in this setting.[100]
- Although therapy for cirrhosis focuses mainly on symptomatic management, other forms of chronic liver disease such as hepatitis B and autoimmune hepatitis can be treated specifically with modern antiviral therapy (see Chapter 28, Hepatitis: Viral and Drug-Induced).
- Although the lesions of advanced cirrhosis are irreversible, it is estimated that 70% or more of liver tissue must be destroyed before the body is unable to eliminate drugs and toxins via the liver.[101] Unfortunately, it is difficult to tell which patients have reached this stage of involvement, so practitioners should always be aware of the potential inability of patients with advanced liver disease to metabolize various hepatically cleared drugs and adjust dosages accordingly.
- Limited pharmacokinetic dosing research and guidance are available for the aging liver[102] and the diseased liver.[103] However, dosage reductions continue to be done empirically because data specifically quantifying the degree of adjustment necessary in liver disease generally are unavailable.

REFERENCES

1. Anonymous. Trends in mortality from cirrhosis and alcoholism: United States. MMWR Morb Mortal Wkly Rep 35:703–705, 1983.
2. World health statistics annual. Geneva: World Health Organization, 1985.
3. Anonymous. Deaths and hospitalizations from chronic liver disease: United States. MMWR Morb Mortal Wkly Rep 41:969–973, 1993.
4. Cotran R, Kumar V, Robbins S. Pathological basis of disease. 4th ed. Philadelphia: WB Saunders, 1989:941–957.
5. Rubin E, Lieber C. Fatty liver, alcoholic hepatitis, and cirrhosis produced by alcohol in primates. N Engl J Med 290:128, 1974.
6. Schrier R, Arroyo V, Bernardi M, et al. Peripheral arterial vasodilation hypothesis: a proposal for the initiation of renal sodium and water retention in cirrhosis. Hepatology 8:1151–1157, 1988.
7. Rocco V, Ware A. Cirrhotic ascites: pathophysiology, diagnosis, and management. Ann Intern Med 105:573–585, 1986.
8. Porayko M, Wiesner R. Management of ascites in patients with cirrhosis. Postgrad Med 92(8):156, 1992.
9. Wood LJ, Massie D, McLean AJ, et al. Renal sodium retention in cirrhosis: tubular site and relation to hepatic dysfunction. Hepatology 8(4):831, 1988.
10. Runyon B, Montano A, Akriviadis E, et al. The serum–ascites albumin gradient in the differential diagnosis of ascites is superior to the exudate/transudate concept. Ann Intern Med 117:215, 1992.
11. Fraser C, Arieff A. Hepatic encephalopathy. N Engl J Med 313:869–873, 1985.
12. Bode J, Shafer K. Pathophysiology of chronic hepatic encephalopathy. Hepatogastroenterology 32:259–265, 1985.
13. Sax H, Talamini M, Fischer J. Clinical use of branched-chain amino acids in liver disease, sepsis, trauma and burns. Arch Surg 121:358–366, 1986.
14. Basile A, Gammal S. Evidence for the involvement of benzodiazepine receptor complex in hepatic encephalopathy; implications for treatment with benzodiazepine receptor antagonists. Clin Neuropharmacol 11:401–422, 1988.
15. Badalamenti S, Graziani G, Salerno F, et al. Hepatorenal syndrome: new perspectives in pathogenesis and treatment. Arch Intern Med 153:1957–1967, 1993.
16. Shear L, Ching S, Gabuzda G. Compartmentalization of ascites and edema in patients with hepatic cirrhosis. N Engl J Med 282:1391–1396, 1970.
17. Pockros P, Reynolds T. Rapid diuresis in patients with ascites from chronic liver disease: the importance of peripheral edema. Gastroenterology 90:1827–1833, 1986.
18. Daskalopoulos G, Laffi G, Morgan T, et al. Immediate effects of furosemide on renal hemodynamics in chronic liver disease with ascites. Gastroenterology 92:1859, 1987.
19. Gines P, Arroyo V, Quintero E, et al. Comparison of paracentesis and diuretics in the treatment of cirrhotics with tense ascites; results of a randomized study. Gastroenterology 93:234–241, 1987.
20. Gines P, Tito L, Arroyo V, et al. Randomized comparative study of therapeutic paracentesis with and without intravenous albumin in cirrhosis. Gastroenterology 94:1493–1502, 1988.
21. Panos MZ, Moore K, Vlavianos P, et al. Single, total paracentesis for tense ascites: sequential hemodynamic changes and right atrial size. Hepatology 11:662, 1990.
22. Tito LI, Gines P, Arroyo V, et al. Total paracentesis associated with intravenous albumin in the management of patients with cirrhosis and ascites. Gastroenterology 98:146, 1990.
23. Pinto P, Amerian J, Reynolds T. Large-volume paracentesis in nonedematous patients with tense ascites: its effect on intravascular volume. Hepatology 8:207–210, 1988.
24. Runyon B, Antillon M, Montano A. Effect of diuresis versus therapeutic paracentesis on ascitic fluid opsonic activity and serum complement. Gastroenterology 97:158–162, 1989.
25. Runyon B. Care of patients with ascites. N Engl J Med 330(5):340, 1994.
26. Vermelulen LC, Ratko TA, Erstad BL, et al for the UHC Consensus Exercise on the Use of Albumin, Nonprotein Colloid and Crystalloid Solutions. A paradigm for consensus: the University Hospital Consortium guidelines for the use of albumin, nonprotein colloid and crystalloid solutions. Arch Intern Med 155:373–379, 1995.
27. Smart H, Triger D. A randomised prospective trial comparing daily paracentesis and intravenous albumin with recirculation in diuretic refractory ascites. J Hepatol 10:191–197, 1990.
28. Epstein M. Peritoneovenous shunt in the management of ascites and the hepatorenal syndrome. Gastroenterology 82:790–799, 1980.
29. Stanley M, Ochi S, Lee K, et al. Peritoneovenous shunting as compared with medical treatment in patients with alcoholic cirrhosis and massive ascites. N Engl J Med 321:1632–1638, 1989.
30. Gines P, Arrovo V, Rodes J. Pharmacotherapy of ascites associated with cirrhosis. Drugs 43(3):325, 1992.
31. Conn H, Fessell JM. Spontaneous bacterial peritonitis in cirrhosis: variations on a theme. Medicine 50:161, 1991.
32. Friedman SL. Cirrhosis of the liver and its major sequelae. In: Cecil textbook of medicine. 20th ed. Philadelphia: WB Saunders, 1996:795.
33. Ariza J, Xiol X, Esteve M, et al. Aztreonam versus cefotaxime in the treatment of Gram-negative spontaneous bacterial peritonitis in cirrhotic patients. Hepatology 14:91–98, 1991.

34. Felisart J, Rimola A, Arroyo V, et al. Cefotaxime is more effective than is ampicillin-tobramycin in cirrhotics with severe infections. Hepatology 5:457–462, 1985.
35. Fong TL, Akriviadis EA, Runyon BA, et al. Polymorphonuclear cell count response and duration of antibiotic therapy in spontaneous bacterial peritonitis. Hepatology 9:423–426, 1989.
36. Gines P, Rimola A, Planas R, et al. Norfloxacin prevents spontaneous bacterial peritonitis recurrence in cirrhosis: results of a double-blind, placebo-controlled trial. Hepatology 12:716–724, 1990.
37. Soriano G, Guarner C, Tomas A, et al. Norfloxacin prevents bacterial infection in cirrhotics with gastrointestinal hemorrhage. Gastroenterology 103:477, 1991.
38. Singh N, Gayowski T, Yu VL, et al. Trimethoprim–sulfamethoxazole for the prevention of spontaneous bacterial peritonitis in cirrhosis: a randomized trial. Ann Intern Med 122:595–598, 1995.
39. Rolachon A, Cordier L, Bacq Y, et al. Ciprofloxacin and long term prevention of spontaneous bacterial peritonitis: results of a prospective controlled trial. Hepatology 22:1171–1174, 1995.
40. Terblanche J, Burroughs A, Hobbs K. Controversies in the management of bleeding esophageal varices. N Engl J Med (part 1) 320:1393–1397, 1989; (part 2) 320:1469–1475, 1989.
41. Cello J, Crass R, Grendell J, et al. Management of the patient with hemorrhaging esophageal varices. JAMA 256:1480–1484, 1986.
42. Rice T. Treatment of esophageal varices. Clin Pharm 8:122–131, 1989.
43. Henderson J, Kutner M, Millikan W, et al. Endoscopic variceal sclerosis compared with distal splenorenal shunt to prevent recurrent variceal bleeding in cirrhosis. Ann Intern Med 112:262–269, 1990.
44. Santangelo W, Dueno M, Estes B, et al. Prophylactic sclerotherapy of large esophageal varices. N Engl J Med 318:814–216, 1988.
45. Sauerbruch T, Wotzka R, Kopcke W, et al. Prophylactic sclerotherapy before the first episode of variceal hemorrhage in patients with cirrhosis. N Engl J Med 319:8–15, 1988.
46. Goff J. Gastroesophageal varices: pathogenesis and therapy of acute bleeding. Gastroenterol Clin North Am 22(4):779, 1993.
47. Ziemniak J, Bernhard H, Schentag J. Hepatic encephalopathy and altered cimetidine kinetics. Clin Pharmacol Ther 34(3):375, 1983.
48. Gonzalez-Martin G, Paulos C, Veloso B, et al. Ranitidine disposition in severe hepatic cirrhosis. Int J Clin Pharmacol Toxicol 25:139–142, 1987.
49. Roark G. Treatment of postsclerotherapy esophageal ulcers with sucralfate. Gastrointest Endosc 30:9–10, 1984.
50. Lecomte S, Baron MH, Chenon MT, et al. Effect of magnesium complexation by fluoroquinolones on their antibacterial properties. Antimicrob Agents Chemother 38:2810–2816, 1994.
51. Stiegmann GV, Goff JS, Sun JH, et al. Endoscopic ligation of esophageal varices. Am J Surg 159:21–26, 1990.
52. Van Stiegmann G, Cambre T, Sun JH. A new endoscopic elastic band ligating device. Gastrointest Endosc 32:230–233, 1986.
53. Stiegmann GV, Goff JS, Michaletz-Onody PA, et al. Endoscopic sclerotherapy as compared with endoscopic ligation for bleeding esophageal varices. N Engl J Med 326:1527–1532, 1992.
54. Stump D, Hardin T. The use of vasopressin in the treatment of upper gastrointestinal haemorrhage. Drugs 39:38–53, 1990.
55. Fogel M, Knaver C, Andres L, et al. Continuous intravenous vasopressin in active upper gastrointestinal bleeding: a placebo controlled trial. Ann Intern Med 96:565–569, 1982.
56. Gimson A, Westaby D, Hegarty J, et al. A randomized trial of vasopressin plus nitroglycerin in the control of acute variceal hemorrhage. Hepatology 6:410–413, 1986.
57. Tsai Y, Lay C, Lai K, et al. Controlled trial of vasopressin plus nitroglycerin versus vasopressin alone in bleeding esophageal varices. Hepatology 6:406–409, 1982.
58. Lamberts SWJ, Von der Lely A, Herder WW, et al. Octreotide. N Engl J Med 334:246–254, 1996.
59. Laine L, Peterson W. Bleeding peptic ulcer. N Engl J Med 331(11):717–727, 1994.
60. Lewis J, Davis J, Allsopp D, et al. Beta-blockers in protal hypertension: an overview. Drugs 37:62–69, 1989.
61. Hayes P, Davis J, Lewis J, et al. Meta-analysis of value of propranolol in prevention of variceal hemorrhage. Lancet 336:153–156, 1990.
62. Pascal J, Cales P, et al. Propranolol in the prevention of first upper gastrointestinal tract hemorrhage in patients with cirrhosis of the liver and esophageal varices. N Engl J Med 317:856–861, 1987.
63. Teran JC, Imperiale TF, Mullen KD, et al. Primary prophylaxis of variceal bleeding in cirrhosis: a cost effectiveness analysis. Gastroenterology 112:473–482, 1997.
64. Lebrec O, Poynard T, Bernuau J, et al. A randomized controlled study of propranolol for prevention of recurrent gastrointestinal bleeding in patients with cirrhosis. Hepatology 4:355–384, 1984.
65. Burroughs A, Jenkins W, Sherlock S, et al. Controlled trial of propranolol for the prevention of recurrent gastrointestinal bleeding in patients with cirrhosis. N Engl J Med 309:1539–1542, 1983.
66. Poynard T, Lebrec D, Hillon P, et al. Propranolol for prevention of recurrent gastrointestinal bleeding in patients with cirrhosis: a prospective study of factors associated with rebleeding. Hepatology 7:447–451, 1987.
67. Lebrec D, Bemuau J, Rueff B, et al. Gastrointestinal bleeding after abrupt cessation of propranolol administration in cirrhosis. N Engl J Med 307:560, 1982.
68. Alabaster S, Gogel H, McCarthy D. Propranolol withdrawal and variceal hemorrhage. JAMA 250:3047, 1983.
69. Teres J, Bosch J, Bordas J, et al. Propranolol versus sclerotherapy in preventing variceal rebleeding: a randomized controlled trial. Gastroenterology 105: 1508–1514, 1993.
70. Angelico A, Carli L, Piat C, et al. Effects of isosorbide-5-mononitrate compared with propranolol on first bleeding and long term survival in cirrhosis. Gastroenterology 113:1632–1639, 1997.
71. Groszmann RJ. Beta adrenergic blockers and nitrovasodilators for the treatment of portal hypertension: the good, the bad, the ugly [editorial]. Gastroenterology 113:1794–1797, 1997.
72. Riordan SM, Williams R. Treatment of hepatic encephalopathy. N Engl J Med 337:473–479, 1997.
73. Avery GS, Davies EF, Brogden RN. Lactulose: a review. Drugs 4:7–48, 1972.
74. Kersh ES, Rifkin H. Lactulose enemas. Ann Intern Med 78:81–84, 1973.
75. Rodgers JB Jr, Kiley JE, Balint JA. Comparison of results of long term treatment of chronic hepatic encephalopathy with lactulose and sorbitol. Am J Gastroenterol 60:459–465, 1973.
76. Conn HO, Leevy CM, Vlahcevic J, et al. Comparison of lactulose and neomycin in the treatment of chronic portal systemic encephalopathy. Gastroenterology 72:573, 1977.
77. Conn HO. Interactions of lactulose and neomycin. Drugs 4:4–6, 1972.
78. Weber F, Fresard K, Lally B. Effects of lactulose and neomycin on urea metabolism in cirrhotic subjects. Gastroenterology 82:213–217, 1982.
79. Breen K, Bryant R, Levinson J, et al. Neomycin absorption in man. Ann Intern Med 76:211–218, 1972.
80. Berk D, Chalmer T. Deafness complicating antibiotic therapy of hepatic encephalopathy. Ann Intern Med 73:393–396, 1970.
81. Imperiale T, McCullough A. Do corticosteroids reduce mortality from alcoholic hepatitis? Ann Intern Med 113:299–307, 1990.
82. Ramond M, Poynard T, Rueff B, et al. A randomized trial of prednisolone in patients with severe alcoholic hepatitis. N Engl J Med 326:507–512, 1992.
83. Basile AS, Hughes RD, Harrison PM, et al. Elevated brain concentrations of 1,4-benzodiazepines in fulminant hepatic failure. N Engl J Med 325(7):473–478, 1991.
84. Bansky G, Meier P, Riederer E, et al. Effects of the benzodiazepine receptor antagonist flumazenil in hepatic encephalopathy in humans. Gastroenterology 97:744–750, 1989.
85. Ferenci P, Grimm G, Meryn S, et al. Successful long-term treatment of portal-systemic encephalopathy by benzodiazepine antagonist flumazenil. Gastroenterology 96:240–243, 1989.
86. Pomier LG, Giguere JF, Lavoie J, et al. Flumazenil in cirrhotic patients in hepatic coma. Hepatology 19:32–37, 1994.
87. Sterling R, Shiffman M, Schubert M. Flumazenil for hepatic coma: the elusive wake-up call? Gastroenterology 107:1204–1205, 1994.
88. Chan TYK. Beneficial effects of low dose dopamine in cirrhosis and renal insufficiency. Ann Pharmacother 29:433, 1995.
89. Bodenheimer H, Schaffner F, Pezzullo J. Evaluation of colchicine therapy in primary biliary cirrhosis. Gastroenterology 95:124–129, 1988.
90. Kershenobich D, Vargas F, Barcia-Tsao G, et al. Colchicine in the treatment of cirrhosis of the liver. N Engl J Med 318:1709–1713, 1988.
91. Stavinoha M, Soloway R. Current therapy of chronic liver disease. Drugs 39:814–840, 1990.
92. Fennerty MB. Primary sclerosing cholangitis and primary biliary cirrhosis. Postgrad Med 94(6):81, 1993.
93. Poupon R, Poupon R, Balkau B, et al. Ursodiol for the long-term treatment of primary biliary cirrhosis. N Engl J Med 333(19):1342–1347, 1994.
94. Horst D, Grace N, Conn H, et al. Comparison of dietary protein with an oral, branched chain-enriched amino acid supplement in chronic portal–systemic encephalopathy: a randomized controlled trial. Hepatology 4:279–287, 1984.
95. Anonymous. Guidelines for the use of parenteral and enteral nutrition in adult and pediatric patients. JPEN J Parenter Enteral Nutr 17(Suppl 4):14–15SA, 1993.

96. Donaghy A, Ross R, Wicks C, et al. Growth hormone therapy in patients with cirrhosis: a pilot study of efficacy and safety. Gastroenterology 113:1617–1622, 1997.
97. Miyaji H, Ito S, Auuma T. Effects of *Helicobacter pylori* eradication therapy on hyperammonaemia in patients with liver cirrhosis. Gut 40(6):726–730, 1997.
98. Dehmlow C, Erhard J, De Groot H. Inhibition of Kupffer cell function as an explanation for hepatoprotective properties of silibinin. Hepatology 23:749–754, 1996.
99. D'Amico G, Morabito A, Pagliaro L, et al. Survival and prognostic indicators in compensated and decompensated cirrhosis. Dig Dis Sci 31:468–475, 1986.
100. Anonymous. Approval of naltrexone for use in chronic alcoholism. Washington, DC: Food and Drug Administration, Jan. 1995.
101. Bass N, Williams R. Guide to drug dosage in hepatic disease. Clin Pharmacokinet 15:396–420, 1988.
102. LeCouteur DG, Mclean AJ. The aging liver: drug clearance and an oxygen diffusion barrier hypothesis. Clin Pharmacokinet 34:359–373, 1998.
103. Morgan DJ, McLean AJ. Clinical pharmacokinetic and pharmacodynamic considerations in patients with liver disease. Clin Pharmacokinet 29:370–391, 1995.

CHAPTER 30

PANCREATITIS

Katherine C. Herndon and Paula A. Thompson

Pancreatic inflammatory disease can be classified as acute or chronic, based on the reversibility of the functional and structural changes that arise within the gland. After clinical resolution of an acute attack of pancreatitis, the pancreas recovers normal exocrine and endocrine function and morphology. Most attacks have a mild, self-limited course, but severe disease complicated by multiple organ system failure and life-threatening infection may develop. Although pancreatic necrosis can result in transient or, occasionally, permanent derangement of gland function and structure, acute pancreatitis rarely progresses to chronic disease.[1,2]

In contrast, the persistent inflammation of chronic pancreatitis is associated with a permanent and often progressive loss of pancreatic exocrine and endocrine function and irreversible structural damage. Recurrent exacerbations of pancreatitis, which often complicate chronic disease, are virtually impossible to distinguish clinically from discrete attacks of acute pancreatitis.[2,3]

Reliable incidence and prevalence data are difficult to obtain. The incidence of both acute and chronic forms varies considerably among geographic areas as a consequence of differences in regional environmental and genetic factors.[3,4] However, the incidence of pancreatic inflammatory disease appears to have increased 10-fold over the past 20 years. This may be because of an increase in alcohol abuse or may only reflect improved diagnostic techniques.[5]

Both acute and chronic pancreatitis are discussed after a brief review of pancreatic anatomy and physiology. An understanding of normal structure and function is a necessary background for this discussion.

ANATOMY AND PHYSIOLOGY OF THE PANCREAS

Anatomy

The adult pancreas is a flattened and elongated gland, usually ranging from 12 to 20 cm in length and weighing 70 to 110 g. It lacks a fibrous capsule and is soft and lobular, rather like the salivary glands. The pancreas lies retroperitoneally, the head nestled within the curve of the duodenum as it exits the stomach and the tail extending obliquely to the left (Fig. 30.1).[6,7]

Blood is supplied to the pancreas by the celiac and superior mesenteric arteries, and the blood ultimately drains into the hepatic portal vein. The lymphatic vessels draining the pancreas terminate primarily in the pancreaticosplenic and pancreaticoduodenal lymph nodes. Sympathetic innervation is predominantly through splanchnic neurons synapsing in the celiac plexus, and parasympathetic innervation is derived from the vagus nerve.[6,7]

The pancreas contains both exocrine (about 80%) and endocrine (about 2%) tissue. The remaining 18% is ductular. The secretory unit of the exocrine pancreas is the acinus, from the Latin word for "berries in a cluster." Each acinus consists of 20 to 50 pyramid-shaped cells surrounding a central lumen. The acini are connected to the main pancreatic duct through a network of interconnecting ductules.

The islets of Langerhans (pancreatic islets) make up the endocrine pancreas and are composed of four major cell types, each apparently secreting a single hormone. Approximately 75 to 80% of the islet cell mass is made up of β-cells, which secrete insulin. Glucagon, somatostatin, and pancreatic polypeptide are secreted by α-cells, δ-cells, and PP cells, respectively. Insulin and glucagon are critical in the regulation of carbohydrate metabolism (see Chapter 19, Diabetes). In addition to their systemic effects, these hormones also play a role in the regulation of pancreatic exocrine secretion. Insulin may potentiate the actions of stimulatory factors, whereas glucagon, somatostatin, and pancreatic polypeptide exert inhibitory effects.[6–8]

Physiology

Overview of Exocrine Function

Pancreatic exocrine function is complex and incompletely understood. During the course of a day, the pancreas can secrete 1 to 2.5 L of isosmotic alkaline fluid containing more than 20 enzymes and proenzymes (zymogens). This fluid, commonly called pancreatic juice, is produced by acinar and ductular cells. The acinar cells synthesize and secrete the digestive enzymes (Fig. 30.1). Proximal ductular cells, called centroacinar cells, extend into the lumen of the acinus and are primarily responsible for secretion of water and electrolytes. The intralobular ductules draining the acini coalesce with interlobular ductules, ultimately emptying into the main pancreatic duct. This duct and the common bile duct enter the duodenum at the ampulla of Vater (hepatopancreatic ampulla). The sphincter of Oddi (sphincter of the hepatopancreatic ampulla) regulates flow from both ducts.[8–10]

Secretion of Water and Electrolytes

The principal cations of pancreatic juice are sodium and potassium, which are secreted at fixed concentrations similar to their plasma concentrations. The principal anions are bicarbonate and chloride, which vary reciprocally in concentration, maintaining a fairly constant sum of approximately 150 mEq/L (Fig. 30.2). Bicarbonate is secreted by centroacinar cells, whereas secretions from the acinar cells are rich in chloride. The relative concentration of each reaching the duodenum depends on the amount secreted and the exchange of bicarbonate for chloride in the ductules. The concentration of bicarbonate, physiologically the most important electrolyte, increases with increasing flow rates. Flow rates range from a basal level of 0.2 to 0.3 mL/minute to 4 mL/minute during stimulation. At

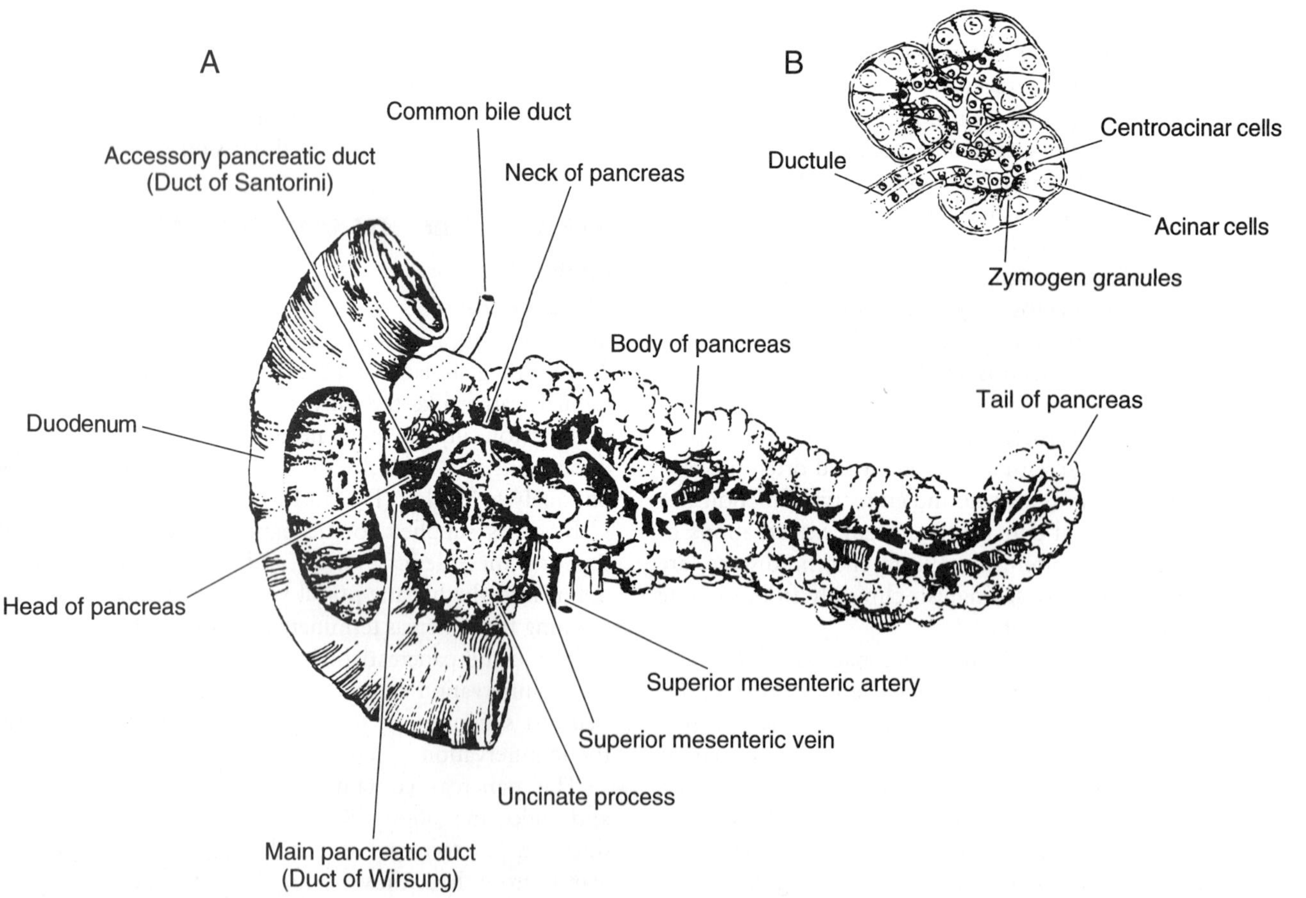

Figure 30.1. Structure of the pancreas. **A,** Dissected to show ductal system. **B,** Enlargement of a representative acinus.

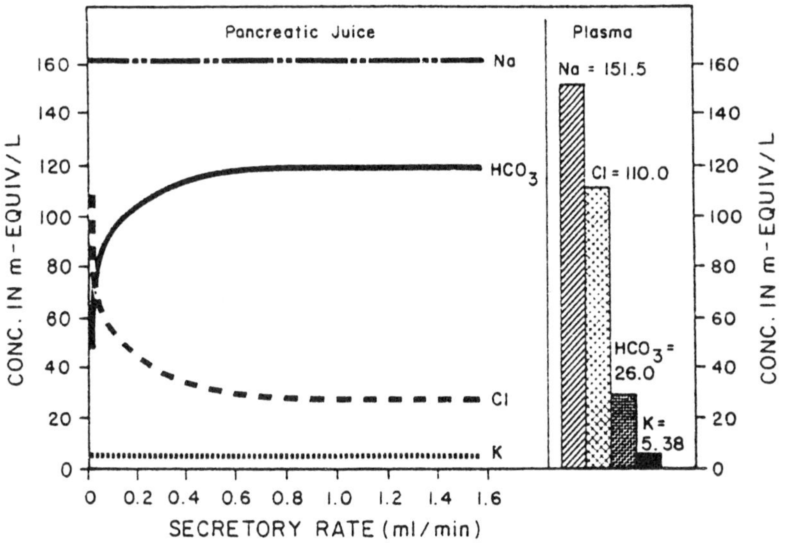

Figure 30.2. Relationship between ion concentration in pancreatic juice and secretory flow rate. (Reprinted with permission from Pandol S. Pancreatic physiology. In: Sleisenger MH, Fordtran JS. Gastrointestinal disease: pathophysiology/diagnosis/management. 5th ed. Philadelphia: WB Saunders, 1993:1586.)

maximal rates of secretion, bicarbonate concentration approaches 120 mEq/L, and the pH of the resulting pancreatic juice is approximately 8.3. This alkalinity buffers the acidic chyme delivered to the duodenum from the stomach and maintains a pH that is optimal for the functioning of pancreatic enzymes. Other ions present in pancreatic juice include calcium and trace amounts of magnesium, zinc, phosphate, and sulfate. Water enters the ductules passively down the concentration gradient established by the active transport of solute, maintaining isosmolality.[8–10]

Enzymes

Protein constitutes up to 10% of pancreatic juice, and more than 90% of this protein consists of digestive enzymes and proenzymes.[9,10] These enzymes are synthesized in the rough endoplasmic reticulum of the acinar cells and are stored in secretory vesicles (zymogen granules) before their release by exocytosis. There are four major categories of enzymes corresponding to the four classes of organic compounds found in food: proteins, carbohydrates, lipids, and nucleic acids (Table 30.1). The proteases and phospholipases are secreted as inactive zymogens, which become active in the intestinal lumen through the action of enterokinase produced by the duodenal mucosa. Enterokinase cleaves a small fragment of trypsinogen to form active trypsin, which can then activate other zymogens, including additional trypsinogen molecules.

The pancreas is protected from autolysis not only by secretion of proteolytic enzymes in zymogen form, but also by the presence of trypsin inhibitor, which binds to trypsin in a 1:1 ratio, rendering it inactive. This protein is present in sufficient quantity to protect against small amounts of trypsin that may become active in the ductules, but its activity is insignificant in the duodenal lumen.[8,9,11]

Regulation of Exocrine Function

A discussion of all the putative regulatory factors of pancreatic exocrine function, both neural and hormonal, is beyond the scope of this text. The roles of secretin, cholecystokinin (CCK), and cholinergic neurons in pancreatic secretions are well established and are reviewed briefly here. Inhibition of secretion also is addressed.

Table 30.1 ▪ Major Digestive Enzymes Secreted by the Pancreas

Proteolytic
Trypsinogen (3)[a] $\xrightarrow{\text{Enterokinase, Trypsin}}$ Trypsin
Chymotrypsinogen (2)[a] $\xrightarrow{\text{Trypsin}}$ Chymotrypsin
Proelastase (2)[a] $\xrightarrow{\text{Trypsin}}$ Elastase
Procarboxypeptidase A (2)[a] $\xrightarrow{\text{Trypsin}}$ Carboxypeptidase A
Procarboxypeptidase B (2)[a] $\xrightarrow{\text{Trypsin}}$ Carboxypeptidase B
Amylolytic
α-Amylase
Lipolytic
Lipase
Procolipase $\xrightarrow{\text{Trypsin}}$ Colipase (cofactor essential for optimum lipase activity)
Prophospholipase A_2 $\xrightarrow{\text{Trypsin}}$ Phospholipase A_2
Carboxylesterase lipase
Nucleolytic
Deoxyribonuclease
Ribonuclease

[a]Number of molecular forms described.[10]

Stimulation

Secretin, a peptide hormone released from the mucosa of the duodenum and jejunum, stimulates bicarbonate and water secretion, primarily in response to the presence of acid in the small intestine. The pH threshold for secretin release is 4.5. The presence of bile salts and some fatty acids within the intestinal lumen can also trigger secretin release. In addition to its effect on bicarbonate, secretin may cause a weak stimulation of pancreatic enzyme release.

CCK, also a peptide hormone secreted by the mucosa of the small bowel, causes the release of an enzyme-rich juice from the pancreas. CCK production occurs when amino acids or fatty acids enter the duodenum. Intravenous CCK also stimulates enzyme release, and pancreatic response is reduced substantially by the CCK antagonists. The combined release of secretin and CCK potentiates the pancreatic response, increasing bicarbonate and volume secretion.

Secretin and CCK exert their effects, at least in part, through the binding to specific receptor sites on the pancreatic cell membranes. Vasoactive intestinal peptide (VIP), structurally similar to secretin, increases bicarbonate release by binding to the secretin receptor. Gastrin shares the C-terminal structure of CCK, and its binding triggers a weak release of enzymes. A muscarinic receptor mediates cholinergic stimulation of bicarbonate and enzyme release, and other receptor sites have also been identified. Possibly the most intriguing is a site for bombesin, a tetradecapeptide isolated from amphibian skin (gastrin-releasing peptide is the mammalian analog). It is postulated that bombesin stimulates enzyme-rich secretion through a direct effect on the acinar cell and indirectly by stimulating CCK release. Finally, substance P receptors can bind substance P–like neurotransmitters released from intrapancreatic neurons, resulting in increased pancreatic secretion. The physiologic importance of the latter two mediators has not been established.

The response of pancreatic cells to the binding of these ligands appears to be mediated by two intracellular transducer systems. The formation of an agonist–receptor complex stimulates adenosine 3′,5′-cyclic monophosphate synthesis through the activation of adenylate cyclase (secretin and VIP) or formation of other intracellular messengers (including calcium released from intracellular stores) via phosphoinositide-specific phospholipase C (CCK, gastrin, bombesin, substance P, and acetylcholine).[8,9,12]

Inhibition

Inhibitory mechanisms are less well understood than stimulatory ones. Intravenous infusions of amino acids or glucose inhibit pancreatic function, probably at least in part because of the release of glucagon and somatostatin from islet cells. Pancreatic polypeptide may also decrease exocrine function by modulating cholinergic pathways, although the physiologic significance of this effect has not been delineated. Lipid in the colon inhibits CCK-stimulated pancreatic output, possibly acting through a mediator called peptide YY.[8–10,12] A negative feedback loop also has been demonstrated whereby trypsin in the intestinal lumen inactivates a CCK-releasing peptide, decreasing CCK release and pancreatic enzyme secretion.[8,9,11,13] Increasing our understanding of these inhibitory mechanisms may help to guide the development of effective therapeutic modalities.

Phases of Pancreatic Secretion

Pancreatic function can best be described in terms of interdigestive (fasting) and digestive (postprandial) periods. Digestive secretion can be further subdivided into cephalic, gastric, and intestinal phases. The pancreas is not quiescent between meals, but rather displays a cyclic basal secretion. Although overall secretion is low, there are fluctuations that parallel changes in gastrointestinal motility.

Vagal nerves mediate the cephalic phase, in which pancreatic secretion can be stimulated by the sight, smell, or taste of food. In sham feeding experiments (patients chew food without swallowing it), pancreatic enzyme secretion increased to approximately 50% of the maximal secretion elicited by intravenous CCK. Gastric acid production also is stimulated during this phase, triggering secretin release, which increases bicarbonate and enzyme secretion.

The gastric phase begins when food enters the stomach. Gastric distension causes increased pancreatic secretion mediated through a gastropancreatic vagovagal reflex, but the relative contribution of this gastric phase has not been determined in humans.

The most important phase is triggered when chyme enters the small intestine. This intestinal phase is regulated by the hormones secretin and CCK and by enteropancreatic vagovagal reflexes triggered by volume or hyperosmolality in the gut. During all phases of pancreatic secretion, the interplay of neural and hormonal factors results in the coordinated response of the pancreas to feeding.[8–11]

Acute Pancreatitis

DEFINITION

Acute pancreatitis is an acute inflammatory process of the pancreas that is initiated by intrapancreatic activation of proteolytic and lipolytic digestive enzymes. The inflammation may remain localized in the pancreas or involve peripancreatic tissues and even remote organ systems.[14] Approximately 80% of patients have interstitial pancreatitis, which is characterized by interstitial edema with or without mild peripancreatic fat necrosis.[15–17] The remaining patients develop necrotizing pancreatitis with diffuse or focal areas of nonviable pancreatic parenchyma and large areas of peripancreatic fat necrosis.[14,16] Acute pancreatitis is also classified clinically as mild or severe.[14] Although interstitial pancreatitis may be associated with serious systemic toxicity, its clinical course is usually mild, with minimal organ dysfunction and a resultant mortality of less than 2%. In contrast, the mortality of severe acute pancreatitis, involving organ failure or local complications such as abscess or pseudocyst, remains in the range of 10 to 30%.[15,16] Severe pancreatitis is most often the clinical expression of pancreatic necrosis.

TREATMENT GOALS: ACUTE PANCREATITIS

- Correct intravascular volume and electrolyte loss with aggressive fluid resuscitation.
- Relieve pain with parenteral analgesia.
- Minimize pancreatic exocrine secretion by eliminating oral intake.
- Provide nutritional support when oral intake is suspended for an extended period.
- Recognize systemic complications early and provide immediate intensive supportive care.
- Manage infected pancreatic necrosis with appropriate antibiotic therapy and surgical debridement.
- Identify and correct factors that may have precipitated the acute attack.

EPIDEMIOLOGY

The incidence of acute pancreatitis varies widely and depends on the incidence of precipitating factors among populations.[4] The incidence of acute pancreatitis in the United States is thought to range from 54 to 238 episodes per 1 million per year.[18] Disease incidence has been extensively studied in the United Kingdom and appears to have increased 10-fold from the 1960s to the 1980s.[5] This may reflect an increase in alcohol abuse as well as diagnostic advances.

Acute pancreatitis is associated with many other disease processes and events (Table 30.2). Biliary tract stone disease and ethanol abuse account for 60 to 80% of acute bouts of pancreatitis, with the incidence of each depending on the patient population being evaluated.[4,15] Female patients and those living in suburban areas tend to have pancreatitis as a result of biliary tract stone disease, whereas ethanol abuse is more often associated with pancreatitis in men and inner-city dwellers.[4,15] A number of miscellaneous causes account for 10 to 15% of pancreatitis attacks, with another 10 to 15% of cases classified as idiopathic.[5,15] However, recent studies suggest that up to two-thirds of idiopathic cases may be caused by biliary microlithiasis.[4]

Cholelithiasis increases a patient's relative risk of developing acute pancreatitis; however, the condition develops in only a small percentage of these patients.[19] Biliary pancreatitis may be associated with recurrent episodes of acute disease, but chronic pancreatitis is rare. In contrast, many patients with alcoholic pancreatitis have consumed large amounts of alcohol for many years before the initial onset of symptoms. Because these patients often have functional and morphologic pancreatic damage before their first attack, it appears that many cases of acute alcoholic pancreatitis actually represent acute inflammation of chronic pancreatitis.[4,5,15] However, alcoholic pancreatitis is not invariably associated with chronic pancreatic damage.[4,5] Because clinical pancreatitis develops in only 5% of alcoholics, unidentified factors must affect susceptibility to pancreatic injury.[5]

Gallstones are the most common obstructive cause of acute pancreatitis, but inflammation may also result from other lesions that interfere with the flow of pancreatic juice through the ductal system. Thus, pancreatitis may result from ductal strictures, sphincter of Oddi dysfunction, or tumors of the pancreas, ampulla, or duodenum.[1,5] Blunt trauma to the abdomen may also cause pancreatitis by disrupting the pancreatic ductal system. Similarly, pancreatitis can occur as a postoperative complication of procedures that involve manipulation of the pancreas or during endoscopic retrograde cholangiopancreatography (ERCP), in which a side-viewing endoscope is passed into the duodenum and a catheter introduces a radiopaque contrast medium into the pancreatic duct. Certain viral, parasitic, and bacterial infections may also precipitate acute attacks. Other causes of acute pancreatitis include penetrating duodenal ulcer, vascular compromise, hypertriglyceridemia, and various toxins.[1,4,5] Debate continues about the association of acute pancreatitis with pancreas divisum, a congenital abnormality in which the dorsal and ventral pancreatic ducts fail to fuse. Because pancreas divisum is a common

Table 30.2 ▪ Causes of Acute Pancreatitis

Obstruction
Gallstones
Sphincter of Oddi spasm or stenosis
Periampullary or pancreatic tumors
Periampullary duodenal diverticula
Pancreas divisum with accessory duct obstruction
Infection
Parasitic: ascariasis, clonorchiasis
Viral: Coxsackie B virus, mumps, rubella, Epstein–Barr virus, cytomegalovirus, varicella, hepatitis A, hepatitis B
Bacterial: mycoplasma, *Legionella* species, *Salmonella* species, *Shigella* species, *Mycobacterium tuberculosis, Campylobacter* species
Toxins
Alcohol
Drugs (Table 30.3)
Scorpion venom
Organophosphate insecticides
Trauma
Postoperative trauma
Endoscopic retrograde cholangiopancreatography
Endoscopic sphincterotomy
Coronary artery bypass
Blunt abdominal trauma
Metabolic
Hypertriglyceridemia
Hypercalcemia
Vascular
Vasculitis
Atherosclerotic emboli
Hypoperfusion
Miscellaneous
Idiopathic
Hereditary pancreatitis
Cystic fibrosis
Penetrating duodenal ulcer
Inflammatory bowel disease
Hypothermia

Source: References 1, 4, 5.

anatomic abnormality with an overall incidence of about 7%, it may be an incidental finding in many patients with idiopathic pancreatitis.[4,5]

More than 85 drugs have been associated with acute pancreatitis, although the frequency of drug-induced disease generally is low.[20–32] Because scattered case reports make up the bulk of the literature on drug-induced pancreatic disease, it usually is difficult to link drugs with pancreatic inflammation conclusively. Mallory and Kern[21] classified drugs into three categories based on the clinical evidence implicating them in the development of acute pancreatitis: definite, probable, and questionable. The association is considered definite when drug therapy results in abdominal pain combined with hyperamylasemia that resolves when therapy is discontinued or recurs when the drug is reintroduced (Table 30.3). Because drug-induced acute pancreatitis cannot be distinguished clinically from that induced by other causes, it should be considered when other causes of disease have been ruled out.

Table 30.3 ▪ Agents Associated with Acute Pancreatitis

Definite association	Questionable association
Amiodarone	Acetaminophen
Angiotensin-converting enzyme inhibitors	Ampicillin
Asparaginase	Carbamazepine
Azathioprine	Cholestyramine
Codeine	Cisplatin
Cytarabine	Clonidine
Didanosine	Colchicine
Estrogens	Cyclosporine
Furosemide	Cyproheptadine
Isoniazid	Diazoxide
Losartan	Diphenoxylate
Mercaptopurine	Ergotamine
Mesalamine	Erythromycin
Metronidazole	Gold compounds
Pentamidine	Indomethacin
Sulfonamides	Interleukin-2
Sulindac	Isotretinoin
Tetracycline	Ketoprofen
Thiazides	Mefenamic acid
Valproic acid	Metolazone
Probable association	Naproxen
Bumetanide	Nitrofurantoin
Chlorthalidone	Opiates
Cimetidine	Oxyphenbutazone
Clarithromycin	Phenolphthalein
Clozapine	Piroxicam
Corticosteroids	Propoxyphene
Ethacrynic acid	Ranitidine
Ifosfamide	Tryptophan
Ketorolac	
Methyldopa	
Phenformin	
Procainamide	
Salicylates	
Sulfasalazine	
Zalcitabine	

Source: References 20–32.

PATHOPHYSIOLOGY

The inflammation and necrosis of acute pancreatitis begin as an autodigestive process initiated by the inappropriate activation and release of proteolytic and lipolytic enzymes into the interstitium of the organ. The activation of trypsinogen to trypsin within the acinar cells is the initial step in the pathogenesis of acute pancreatitis.[1] Trypsin can then activate other pancreatic proteases, including elastase, chymotrypsin, and carboxypeptidase, as well as phospholipase A_2, which then contribute to acinar cell inflammation. Elastase causes vascular damage by dissolving the elastic fibers of blood vessels. Chymotrypsin augments this vascular damage and the resulting edema, and phospholipase A_2 destroys acinar cell membranes. These pancreatic enzymes leak from the damaged acinar cells into the interstitium, causing local inflammation. Lipase is also liberated from peripheral acinar cells, resulting in peripancreatic fat necrosis. The kinin and complement systems are activated by trypsin, leading to the release of vasoactive peptides, which cause vasodilation, increased vascular permeability, and accumulation of leukocytes.[15] In severe disease, pancreatic enzymes, vasoactive peptides, and other toxic factors extravasate from the pancreas into peripancreatic spaces and the peritoneal cavity, causing a widespread chemical irritation.[16] These materials may also reach the systemic circulation through retroperitoneal lymphatic and venous circulation to contribute to systemic complications, including shock, respiratory failure, and renal failure.[16]

Factors that contribute to the transformation of acute pancreatitis from a local inflammatory process into a multiorgan illness are not entirely understood. Recently, the contribution of leukocytes and their products in amplifying pancreatic inflammation into a generalized systemic inflammatory response has been recognized.[1,33] Neutrophils, macrophages, and monocytes invade the inflamed pancreas and release destructive mediators such as elastase, phospholipase A_2, platelet activating factor, nitric oxide, oxygen free radicals, and cytokines.[1] The inflammatory cytokines, particularly interleukin-1, interleukin-6, and tumor necrosis factor, appear to be the most important systemic mediators of acute pancreatitis.[33] Cytokines are produced not only locally, but also systemically in sites such as the spleen, liver, and lung, where they have been linked to organ dysfunction. Circulating levels of cytokines are higher in patients with severe acute pancreatitis, and these levels can be predictive of disease severity, end-organ failure, and mortality.[34,35] Consequently, cytokine antagonism may prove beneficial in treating patients with acute pancreatitis. Furthermore, impairment of the pancreatic microcirculation by the deleterious effects of leukocyte products on the vascular endothelium appears to be an important mechanism in pancreatic necrosis.[36]

The mechanism by which pancreatic enzymes become prematurely activated within the gland to initiate the cascade of events that causes acute pancreatitis is unknown. Proposed mechanisms focus on biliary tract stone disease, postulating that reflux of hepatic bile or duodenal contents into the pancreatic ductal system may activate enzymes within the pancreatic parenchyma.[1,4] More recently, investigators have proposed that activation of trypsin may occur within the pancreatic acinar cell rather than in the ductal or intercellular space.[1,5] Obstruction in the pancreatic duct could disturb the normal events that maintain segregation of lysosomal enzymes, including cathepsin B, from digestive enzymes, thus allowing them to mix intracellularly. Cathepsin B can convert trypsinogen to trypsin, which could then activate the remaining digestive zymogens. The mechanism of ethanol-induced pancreatitis is not understood but may include relaxation or spasm of the sphincter of Oddi, obstruction of small pancreatic ductules by proteinaceous plugs, or direct toxic effects of ethanol or one of its metabolites.[1,4]

The pathogenesis of drug-induced pancreatic injury is unknown, but it does not appear to differ substantially from that of acute pancreatitis induced by other causes. Possible mechanisms include pancreatic ductal constriction, immune suppression, arteriolar thromboses, direct cellular toxicity, hepatic production of free radicals, and osmotic or metabolic effects.[22]

CLINICAL PRESENTATION AND DIAGNOSIS

Signs and Symptoms

The classic presentation of acute pancreatitis consists of abdominal pain, nausea, and vomiting. The abdominal pain is usually located in the epigastrium or diffusely throughout the upper abdomen.[1] Pain is usually sudden in onset and increases to maximal intensity within 10 to 30 minutes.[37] Pain may be severe, and it is most commonly described as a steady, dull, or boring pain that often radiates to the back. Patients may move about continually in search of a comfortable position and may find partial relief by sitting and leaning forward or lying on their side in the fetal position.[4] Pain resolves over 1 to 3 days in mild cases but may last many days to weeks during severe attacks. Painless pancreatitis has been reported infrequently. Nausea and vomiting are almost invariably present and usually are preceded by the onset of pain. Epigastric tenderness is a consistent finding on abdominal examination, as is mild abdominal distension. Bowel sounds often are diminished but not absent. Fever in the range of 100°F to 102°F is seen in most patients as the pyrogenic products of pancreatic injury enter the circulation. Tachycardia and hypotension progressing to circulatory shock can occur in severe cases as a result of hypovolemia caused by vomiting, hemorrhage, and fluid sequestration within the retroperitoneal space. Circulating kinins and cytokines contribute to this circulatory instability through vasodilatory effects and increased vascular permeability.[15] Disorientation, delirium, or hallucinations are sometimes observed, although most patients present without changes in mental status.[1]

Diagnosis

The diagnosis of acute pancreatitis is based on careful clinical evaluation of the patient, laboratory tests, and radiographic imaging. Mild cases of acute pancreatitis often represent a diagnostic dilemma because symptoms may be nonspecific and pancreatic enzyme levels and imaging studies are often virtually normal.[15] Occasionally, acute pancreatitis must be distinguished from other processes that present with abdominal pain and hyperamylasemia, such as acute cholecystitis or appendicitis, intestinal ischemia or infarction, perforated gastric or duodenal ulcer, intestinal obstruction, ectopic pregnancy, and common bile duct obstruction.[37]

Laboratory Tests

Leukocytosis, ranging from 10,000 to 25,000 cells/mm^3, is a common finding during routine laboratory evaluation of patients with acute pancreatitis.[1,15] Hyperglycemia, transient hypertriglyceridemia, and hypoalbuminemia also are common. Liver function tests often reveal mild hyperbilirubinemia and elevations in serum alkaline phosphatase and transaminase levels, which tend to be more pronounced with biliary pancreatitis. Hypovolemia may result in hemoconcentration, as evidenced by elevated hematocrit, blood urea nitrogen, and serum creatinine levels.

Pancreatic Enzymes

Elevation of serum amylase has remained central to the diagnosis of acute pancreatitis since its first association with the disease in 1929.[5,15] The pancreas and salivary glands account for most of the serum amylase activity in healthy people. The serum amylase level typically rises rapidly (from the normal range of 35 to 118 IU/L) during the initial hours of an attack and then declines over the following 3 to 10 days.[1,4] The sensitivity of the test may be compromised if patients do not present early in the course of the disease. Furthermore, the test lacks specificity because hyperamylasemia is associated with a variety of nonpancreatic conditions, including diseases of the biliary tract, intestines, female genitourinary tract, lungs, prostate, and salivary glands.[38] Generally, patients with biliary pancreatitis present with a more marked hyperamylasemia than do patients with alcohol-related disease.[15,38] The measurement of serum amylase isoenzymes has been largely abandoned because most nonpancreatic abdominal diseases that simulate pancreatitis are associated with increased pancreatic rather than nonpancreatic amylase levels.[38] In contrast, serum lipase is derived almost exclusively from the pancreas (normal range 2.3 to 20 IU/dL). Thus, it is more specific for acute pancreatitis and remains normal in a variety of conditions associated with elevations of serum amylase, including salivary gland disease, gynecologic disorders, and macroamylasemia associated with renal insufficiency.[1] However, hyperlipasemia may also occur in nonpancreatic acute abdominal conditions.[4,38] Although serum lipase typically parallels amylase in onset of elevation, lipase elevation persists longer, thus enhanc-

Table 30.4 ▪ Ranson's Prognostic Criteria

	Nonbiliary Pancreatitis	Biliary Pancreatitis
On admission		
Age (yr)	>55	>70
WBC/mL	>16,000	>18,000
Glucose (mg/dL)	>200	>220
LDH (IU/L)	>350	>400
AST (IU/L)	>250	>250
Within 48 hr of admission		
Decrease in Hct (points)	>10	>10
Increase in BUN (mg/dL)	>5	>2
Calcium (mg/dL)	<8	<8
Pao_2 (mm Hg)	<60	–
Base deficit (mEq/L)	>4	>5
Fluid deficit (L)[a]	>6	>4

Source: Reference 39.

WBC, white blood cells; *LDH,* lactate dehydrogenase; *AST,* aspartate transaminase; *Hct,* hematocrit; *BUN,* blood urea nitrogen; *Pao_2,* partial pressure of oxygen.

[a]Input minus output.

ing its utility in patients who present several days after the onset of symptoms.

In summary, elevations in serum amylase and lipase activity support the diagnosis of acute pancreatitis. The assays are widely available and can be performed rapidly and reliably at low cost.[38] Values of serum amylase and lipase greater than three times the upper limit of normal are characteristic of acute pancreatitis and rarely occur in nonpancreatic conditions.[1] The magnitude of increase in serum amylase and lipase activity has no prognostic value and does not correlate with the severity of the acute attack.[37] Furthermore, daily measurement of pancreatic enzymes has little value in assessing a patient's progress or prognosis.[1] The use of other pancreatic enzymes such as immunoreactive trypsinogen, chymotrypsin, elastase, and phospholipase A_2 as markers for acute pancreatitis does not appear to provide any diagnostic advantage over the determination of serum amylase and lipase activity. Additionally, measuring the urinary amylase level and the amylase:creatinine clearance ratio offers little benefit in improving diagnostic accuracy.[15,38]

Imaging

Radiographic studies play an important role in confirming the diagnosis of pancreatitis and provide important etiologic and prognostic information. Although the abdominal radiograph is not considered diagnostic, it has several uses in this setting.[38] Most importantly, it may help to exclude nonpancreatic diseases that may simulate pancreatitis, including bowel obstruction and perforated viscus. The primary role of ultrasonography is in evaluating the biliary tract for stones, dilation, or obstruction.[38] Recent guidelines from the American College of Gastroenterology recommend performing an abdominal ultrasound within 24 to 48 hours of hospitalization for the initial episode of acute pancreatitis.[37] Computed tomography (CT) is useful for excluding other serious intraabdominal conditions, but its importance early in the course of an acute attack is controversial.[37] Dynamic contrast-enhanced CT scan, the best test for identifying pancreatic necrosis, should be performed after the first 3 days in patients with severe acute pancreatitis to distinguish interstitial from necrotizing disease.[37]

Assessing Severity

Multiple clinical criteria systems have been developed to assess the severity and prognosis of pancreatitis. Predictors of severity allow early identification of patients with the greatest likelihood of developing severe pancreatitis.[14,15,37] Ranson and colleagues developed 11 prognostic criteria that can be measured 48 hours after hospital admission to assess the severity of an acute attack (Table 30.4).[37,39] Although more complex than Ranson's criteria, the Acute Physiology and Chronic Health Evaluation II (APACHE-II) is another list of clinical and laboratory values used to assess patients with acute pancreatitis that can be calculated within hours of admission and at daily intervals thereafter.[4,5,40] Table 30.5 lists the variables evaluated under the APACHE-II system.[40] Severe acute pancreatitis is characterized by three or more Ranson criteria or at least eight APACHE-II points.[14] According to recent guidelines, the APACHE-II score should be generated on the day of admission.[37] After 48 hours, the APACHE-II or Ranson's score may be used to follow the course of the patient with pancreatitis.[37]

Complications

The clinical course of acute pancreatitis is uncomplicated in approximately 80% of attacks. Thus, the majority of patients with acute pancreatitis have mild disease that resolves promptly with conservative therapy.[14–16] The remaining patients develop severe disease that is usually the clinical expression of pancreatic necrosis.[14] Although the mortality of interstitial pancreatitis remains low (less than 2%), necrotizing pancreatitis has an associated mortality ranging from 10% (sterile necrosis) to 30% (infected necrosis).[16]

Acute pancreatitis may be complicated by either local or systemic events (Table 30.6). Local events include the development of acute fluid collections located in or near the pancreas, occurring early in the course of 30 to 50% of

Table 30.5 ▪ APACHE II Variables

Temperature	Serum sodium
Heart rate	Serum potassium
Mean arterial pressure	Serum creatinine
Respiratory rate	Hematocrit
Oxygenation	White blood count
Arterial pH	Glasgow coma score
Age points	Chronic health assessment points

Source: Reference 40.

Table 30.6 • Complications of Acute Pancreatitis

Local	
	Necrosis (sterile or infected)
	Pancreatic fluid collection (sterile or infected)
	Pseudocyst
	Abscess
	Pancreatic ascites
	Blood vessel rupture or thrombosis
	Bowel necrosis, obstruction, perforation
	Ileus
	Fistula
Systemic	
	Shock
	Renal failure
	Pulmonary insufficiency (including adult respiratory distress syndrome)
	Coagulopathy
	Gastrointestinal hemorrhage
	Encephalopathy
	Retinopathy
	Hypocalcemia
	Hyperglycemia

Source: References 4, 5.

attacks.[41] Acute fluid collections lack a well-defined wall and regress spontaneously in 50% of cases.[41] Fluid collections may also progress to become pseudocysts or abscesses. A pseudocyst is a collection of pancreatic juice enclosed by a well-defined wall of fibrous tissue forming 4 or more weeks after the onset of an acute attack.[41] Approximately 40% of these acute pseudocysts resolve within 6 weeks.[41] Pseudocysts may be clinically silent or they may cause severe abdominal pain and elevation of pancreatic enzymes. Pancreatic abscess, another late-developing complication, is a circumscribed intraabdominal collection of pus containing little or no pancreatic necrosis.[41] The term *pancreatic abscess* is also used to describe infection within a pseudocyst. In contrast, the development of pancreatic necrosis is an early event appearing within the first 4 days of an acute attack. Necrosis can be found in approximately 20% of acute pancreatitis cases and is necessary for the subsequent development of infection. Pancreatic infection, which occurs in 30 to 50% of patients, usually develops in the second to third week of illness.[37] Infectious complications account for 80% of deaths from acute pancreatitis.[4,14,15]

Severe acute pancreatitis may be complicated by multiple organ system failure, which most commonly involves the cardiovascular, renal, and pulmonary systems.[4,5] Organ failure is the most important indicator of severity of acute pancreatitis.[14,16] Cardiovascular decompensation, the result of hypovolemia and vasodilation caused by circulating vasoactive peptides and cytokines, has the highest associated mortality. Acute renal failure is a consequence of hypovolemia and decreased renal perfusion. Pulmonary complications vary from mild arterial hypoxemia, usually detected during the first 2 days of an attack, to adult respiratory distress syndrome, the result of pulmonary parenchymal injury caused by circulating inflammatory mediators.[1] Systemic complications related to organ failure are responsible for death early in the course of acute pancreatitis.

THERAPEUTIC PLAN

In the absence of effective specific therapy for the underlying disease process, the treatment of acute pancreatitis remains largely supportive. In patients with mild disease, principles of management include eliminating oral intake, maintaining adequate hydration with intravenous fluid, and providing parenteral analgesia to relieve pain.[5,37] With standard conservative therapy, the majority of cases of acute pancreatitis subside within 3 to 10 days.[15] In contrast, severe acute pancreatitis almost invariably warrants treatment in an intensive care unit. Quantification of attack severity with the APACHE-II system or Ranson's criteria is an important early step.[18,37] A dynamic contrast-enhanced CT scan should be performed in patients with severe acute pancreatitis, as evidenced by the development of organ failure, to detect necrotizing pancreatitis (Fig. 30.3).[37] In the absence of clinical improvement, a CT-guided percutaneous aspiration should be performed to detect infected necrosis that necessitates surgical debridement.[37] Patients must be reassessed and monitored throughout the attack for the development of complications, particularly organ failure and infection. In addition, eliminating factors that precipitated the acute attack may improve the patient's course and prevent recurrence of disease.[5,15]

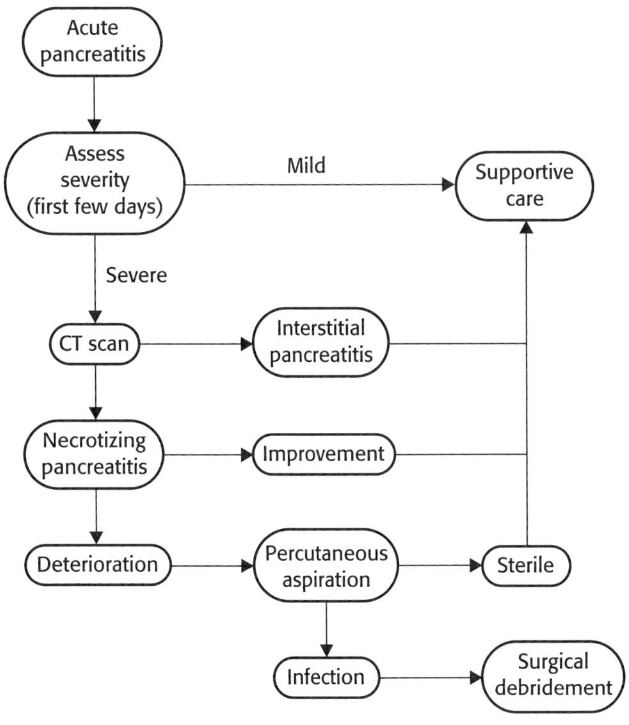

Figure 30.3. Algorithm for the management of acute pancreatitis. (Adapted with permission from Banks PA. Practice guidelines in acute pancreatitis. Am J Gastroenterol 92[3]:384, 1997.)

TREATMENT

Acute pancreatitis may be associated with severe intravascular volume contraction and hypovolemia that results from exudation of protein-rich fluid into the inflamed peripancreatic retroperitoneum and peritoneal cavity, as well as sequestration of fluid within the bowel affected by ileus. In addition, volume losses are incurred through vomiting, hemorrhage, and nasogastric suction. The primary goal of therapy early in the course of acute pancreatitis is to replace intravascular volume and electrolytes to avoid cardiovascular compromise and renal failure. Aggressive fluid resuscitation may also support the pancreatic microcirculation, limiting the development of necrosis. Volume replacement with crystalloid solutions is adequate for most patients, but intravenous colloids may be needed if protein-rich fluid losses are massive. Potassium, calcium, and magnesium losses may also necessitate intravenous replacement. Hyperglycemia should be managed with insulin as needed. Clinical status, vital signs, and appropriate laboratory and radiographic studies should be reassessed frequently. Severe acute pancreatitis for which aggressive fluid resuscitation and maximal supportive care are needed should be managed in the intensive care setting. The complicated course of severe disease often necessitates continuous hemodynamic and arterial blood gas monitoring, as well as intensive management of cardiovascular, pulmonary, renal, and septic complications.

It is standard practice to eliminate oral intake of food and liquids early in the course of an acute attack to minimize pancreatic exocrine secretion and halt the autodigestive process. There are no precise guidelines for refeeding. After abdominal pain and tenderness resolve and bowel sounds and appetite return, feeding may be reintroduced with liquids and the diet advanced as tolerated.[4,37] Although it is reasonable to restrict fat and protein intake to limit pancreatic stimulation, there is little evidence to support the benefit of a low-fat, low-protein diet.[1] Total parenteral nutrition (TPN) is an important adjunct to therapy for patients with severe or protracted disease, when oral intake may be suspended for an extended period during a time of increased caloric need.[42] TPN should be used in patients when oral nutrition will be withheld for at least 7 days.[37] Lipids may be included in the formulation as long as serum triglyceride levels are less than 500 mg/dL.[37,42] Nasogastric suction has not been shown to improve the clinical course of mild to moderate pancreatitis.[43,44] However, it is appropriate therapy for patients with severe nausea and vomiting or significant abdominal distension and ileus.[4,5,15,17]

Analgesia

Narcotic analgesics are usually needed to control the severe abdominal pain that often accompanies acute pancreatitis. Transient elevations in serum amylase and lipase that often follow administration of opiates should not preclude their use because these effects do not appear to be detrimental to the disease course. Therapy is commonly initiated with meperidine administered parenterally at regular intervals in dosages of 50 to 100 mg because it reportedly causes less spasm of the sphincter of Oddi than morphine and its derivatives.[15] However, because there is little evidence to suggest a clinically significant difference in the degree of sphincter spasm produced by any particular opiate, efficacy should be the primary guide for analgesic treatment of these patients.[1]

Unproven Medical Therapies

Medical therapies designed to decrease pancreatic enzyme secretion, inhibit activity of proteolytic enzymes, or modulate the pancreatic inflammatory response generally have not been successful in preventing complications or improving the course of acute pancreatitis (Table 30.7).[1,4,5,45] Attempts to treat acute pancreatitis by pharmacologically reducing pancreatic exocrine secretion with glucagon, calcitonin, atropine, 5-fluorouracil, histamine-2 (H_2) receptor antagonists, somatostatin, and the long-acting somatostatin analog octreotide have been disappointing.[4,5,15,45] A meta-analysis of six controlled studies evaluating the use of somatostatin in acute pancreatitis suggested a reduction in mortality, but subsequent randomized studies have not supported these results.[46–48] However, octreotide may decrease complication rates in patients with severe disease.[48] Inhibiting pancreatic secretion may not prove to be a rational therapeutic approach to managing acute pancreatitis because exocrine pancreatic secretion is strongly inhibited in animal models of the disease.[45]

Inhibiting pancreatic enzymes that are responsible for parenchymal damage and systemic complications has also proven ineffective. Protease inhibitors, including aprotinin, gabexate, and camostate, as well as the phospholipase A_2 inhibitor $CaNa_2$ ethylenediaminetetraacetic acid have failed to generate significant reductions in complications or mortality in patients with severe disease.[5,15,45] Similarly, administering fresh frozen plasma to replenish circulating antiprotease activity has met with little success.[5,45] Clinical trials evaluating peritoneal lavage as a method of washing out inflammatory mediators have been

Table 30.7 • Unproven Medical Therapies for Acute Pancreatitis

Glucagon	$CaNa_2$ ethylenediaminetetraacetic acid
Calcitonin	Indomethacin
Somatostatin	Prostaglandin E_2
Antacids	Corticosteroids
Cimetidine	Fluorouracil
Atropine	Propylthiouracil
Aprotinin	Dextran
Gabexate mesilate	Heparin
Camostate	Vasopressin
Fresh frozen plasma	(ϵ-Aminocaproic acid)

Source: References 1, 4, 5, 45.

ineffective in reducing morbidity or mortality.[45] Modulating local and systemic inflammation with nonsteroidal anti-inflammatory drugs or prostaglandin E_2 has yielded mixed results in animal studies and has not been evaluated in humans.[45]

Antibiotics

Even though infection has emerged as an important cause of death in acute pancreatitis, the role of prophylactically administered antibiotics remains to be established. Early studies evaluating the use of antibiotics in patients with mild disease failed to show any clinical benefit.[49] Secondary pancreatic infection is limited to patients with necrotizing disease, so the applicability of these studies in clinical practice is unclear. A recent study suggested that imipenem reduced the incidence of pancreatic infections, but the incidence of organ failure and the mortality rate were not affected.[50] Sainio et al.[51] demonstrated reduced mortality but no decrease in infections after prophylaxis with cefuroxime. Similarly, a study of selective digestive decontamination with topical and intravenous antimicrobial therapy yielded a slight survival benefit.[52] However, these data are insufficient to mandate prophylactic antibiotic therapy in the management of acute pancreatitis because of weaknesses in study design and methods.[1,49] It is certainly appropriate to initiate empiric antibiotic therapy in patients with pancreatic necrosis confirmed by dynamic contrast-enhanced CT scan and clinical evidence of infection or a deteriorating clinical condition. The presence of infected necrosis should be confirmed with CT scan–guided percutaneous needle aspiration of fluid from necrotic areas for Gram stain and culture (Fig. 30.3).[16,37] Pathogens most often isolated from infected necrosis include *Escherichia coli, Klebsiella pneumoniae, Enterococcus* species, *Staphylococcus aureus, Pseudomonas aeruginosa, Proteus mirabilis, Enterobacter aerogenes,* and *Bacteroides fragilis,* presumably originating in the colon.[53] Antibiotics that can achieve bactericidal concentrations in pancreatic tissue, such as the fluoroquinolones, metronidazole, and imipenem, should be used.[16,49,53] Once infection develops in the necrotic pancreas, surgical debridement is mandatory.[37]

Correcting Biliary Tract Disease

Virtually all clinicians agree that removing residual biliary tract stones is necessary to prevent recurrent attacks of biliary pancreatitis. However, the optimal timing of stone removal and the choice between endoscopic and surgical treatment are subjects of continuing debate. Early ERCP (within 72 hours of admission) is recommended for patients with gallstone pancreatitis who have evidence of biliary sepsis or organ failure.[1,37] Stones in the common bile duct should be removed and a sphincterotomy performed.[37] Otherwise, it appears that either surgical or endoscopic procedures for biliary duct clearance should be performed before discharge from the hospital once pancreatic inflammation has resolved.[4,15]

FUTURE THERAPIES

Although medical treatment of acute pancreatitis is currently supportive, major goals in the future should include limiting systemic complications and preventing pancreatic necrosis.[37] Attempts at inflammatory mediator antagonism have focused on activated pancreatic enzymes; however, the destructive products of leukocytes, including elastase, phospholipase A_2, platelet activating factor, nitric oxide, and cytokines, have not been addressed in prospective, randomized trials. Preliminary studies with the platelet activating factor antagonist lexipafant have demonstrated that a therapeutic window exists for cytokine antagonism.[54,55] Animal studies have also demonstrated that colloidal hemodilution may improve the pancreatic microcirculation and minimize necrosis.[1] Well-designed, controlled, prospective studies are warranted to establish the value of these medical therapies. Additional studies are also needed to determine the optimal use of prophylactic antibiotics for improving mortality in patients with pancreatic necrosis.

IMPROVING OUTCOMES

Early identification of severe acute pancreatitis is an important management principle that may enhance patient outcome.[37] Formalized scoring systems and clinical evidence of organ failure can assist the clinician in this regard. Severe disease almost invariably warrants management in an intensive care unit for aggressive cardiovascular and pulmonary support. Patients must be reassessed and monitored throughout the attack for complications, particularly organ failure and infection. When infection is suspected, pharmacists should assist in selecting and monitoring appropriate antibiotic therapy. Invasive procedures such as surgical debridement of infected necrosis and endoscopic or surgical removal of gallstones also are important for optimizing patient outcome.[37] Cytokine antagonism may eventually have a role in reducing the morbidity and mortality of severe acute pancreatitis.[33] In addition, eliminating factors that precipitated the acute attack may improve the patient's course and prevent recurrence of disease.[5,15] Pharmacists can assist in identifying drug-induced pancreatitis and recommend therapeutic alternatives for the offending agent. Because alcoholic pancreatitis is associated with chronic pancreatic damage, substance abuse counseling should be offered to support patient efforts to abstain.[4,5]

PHARMACOECONOMICS

Although data about the economic impact of acute pancreatitis are sparse, experts have recognized the resource demands of intensive care management in severe disease.[56] Because survivors of severe acute pancreatitis report excellent quality of life, these substantial costs may be justified.[56] As disease-specific therapies, such as cytokine antagonists, become available, their contribution to cost containment must be analyzed.

Chronic Pancreatitis

DEFINITION

Chronic pancreatitis is an inflammatory disease process leading to irreversible damage to pancreatic structure and function. All patients experience loss of exocrine tissue and fibrosis, and many lose endocrine function as well. The clinical course may consist of recurrent acute attacks, which are difficult to distinguish from acute pancreatitis, or chronic symptoms, which usually progress.

Further subclassification of chronic pancreatitis based on etiologic, pathologic, radiologic, or other criteria has proved difficult. One classification system is the Marseilles–Rome system, which distinguishes three types:[57]

- Chronic calcifying pancreatitis is the most common, accounting for more than 95% of cases.[58] It usually results from alcohol abuse and is characterized by intraductal protein plugs and, often, calcified stones.
- Chronic obstructive pancreatitis is uncommon and results from obstruction of the main pancreatic duct by tumor, stricture, or congenital abnormalities. This type is notable in that protein plugs and stones are absent, and damage may be reversible in part when obstruction is alleviated.
- Chronic inflammatory pancreatitis is characterized by fibrosis, infiltration by monocytes, and atrophy of exocrine tissue. This form has been associated with autoimmune disease.

Students of medical history are referred to Pitchumoni's review of chronic pancreatitis from the first description of the pancreas in 300 B.C. to the present.[59]

TREATMENT GOALS: CHRONIC PANCREATITIS

- Control pain through the use of analgesics, enzyme replacement, or endoscopic and surgical treatment.
- Manage exocrine insufficiency, usually manifested as malabsorption, through enzyme replacement.
- Manage diabetes resulting from endocrine insufficiency. This is covered in detail in Chapter 19. One key difference between type 1 diabetes mellitus and pancreatic diabetes should be mentioned, however. In chronic pancreatitis, there is loss of glucagon as well as insulin secretion, leading to very hard to control, or "brittle," diabetes.

EPIDEMIOLOGY

As mentioned in the introduction to this chapter, incidence and prevalence data are meager and specific to geographic area. Prevalence estimates range from 0.03 to 5%, and incidence is approximately 3.5 to 8.2 per 100,000 inhabitants per year. Men are significantly more likely to be affected than women.[1–3,59]

Ethanol abuse is by far the most common cause of chronic pancreatitis, particularly in Western countries, accounting for 70 to 80% of reported cases. As many as 45% of alcoholics show evidence of the disease at autopsy (approximately 50 times the incidence in nondrinkers).[1,3] A hereditary form of chronic pancreatitis, transmitted by an autosomal dominant gene with incomplete penetrance, has been described, and trauma can precipitate this disease. A tropical form also exists in some African and Asian countries in which malnutrition and perhaps dietary toxins are presumed to play a role. Other etiologic factors that have been proposed include hyperparathyroidism, hyperlipidemia, autoimmune disease, and pancreas divisum, although a definitive role in disease initiation and progression has not been delineated for any of these. Up to 40% of cases are classified as idiopathic, and this form appears to have two subsets: juvenile, or early onset, and senile, or late onset. Although gallstone disease may coexist with chronic pancreatitis, cholelithiasis does not appear to predispose a patient to this disease (Table 30.8).[1–3,59–62]

PATHOPHYSIOLOGY

Although many questions remain about the mechanisms involved in the initiation and progression of chronic pancreatitis, it appears that alcohol changes the nature of pancreatic secretions. The absolute amount of protein in secretions increases, facilitating the formation of protein plugs, particularly in the smaller ductules. GP2, a 97-kDa protein that is analogous to the renal cast protein uromodulin, has been isolated from ductal plugs and may play a role in their formation.[63] The resulting obstruction can lead to inflammation and fibrosis, and protein plugs act as a nidus for the formation of calcium carbonate stones.[1–3]

At least one protein appears to be secreted in lower concentrations in the presence of alcohol. Lithostatine, formerly known as pancreatic stone protein, normally inhibits the formation of insoluble calcium salts in the ductules. Therefore, a deficiency of this protein may allow increased precipitation of calcium salts, exacerbating obstruction, inflammation, and fibrosis.[1,2,64]

CLINICAL PRESENTATION AND DIAGNOSIS

Signs and Symptoms

Pain and malabsorption are the hallmarks of chronic pancreatitis, although a significant number of patients also develop diabetes mellitus, pseudocysts, or jaundice.[1,3,60,65]

Table 30.8 ▪ Causes of Chronic Pancreatitis (approximate percentage in the United States)

Alcohol (70%)	Other *(continued)*
Idiopathic (20%)	Heredity
Juvenile (early onset)	Hyperparathyroidism
Senile (late onset)	Hypertriglyceridemia
Other (10%)	Autoimmunity
Trauma	Malnutrition (tropical pancreatitis)
Obstruction	Pancreas divisum

The causes of pain have not been delineated, but increased intraductal and parenchymal pressure, ischemia, pseudocyst, obstruction of the bile duct, or inflammation, especially in and around the pancreatic nerves, may be involved.[1,66–68] This pain, sometimes accompanied by nausea and vomiting, is similar to that of acute pancreatitis. It is epigastric and often described as deep and penetrating, with a characteristic radiation to the back in 65% of cases. Relief may be obtained by leaning forward from a sitting position, and pain usually is aggravated by eating. Pain with eating, in addition to malabsorption, contributes to the weight loss often observed in these patients.[1,3] Up to 20% of patients may be pain-free, but this is more commonly the case with idiopathic rather than alcoholic pancreatitis.[2,59,69]

Loss of exocrine function occurs in all cases of chronic pancreatitis, but it may remain subclinical until fairly late in the course of the disease. Malabsorption does not manifest itself until less than 10% of pancreatic secretory function remains. Lipase activity decreases more than protease activity, so steatorrhea presents earlier and usually is more severe than azotorrhea.[1,3,70] Although some decrease in absorption of carbohydrates and fat-soluble vitamins does occur, symptoms rarely develop.[3,71] Bicarbonate secretion also declines with disease progression.[58,72]

The following scenario summarizes the clinical course of a representative patient. He is an alcoholic man who began to drink heavily at age 25 and started to experience attacks of pain by age 35. Within 5 years, abdominal radiographs showed calcification of the pancreas, and he developed symptoms of diabetes. At 45 years of age, pancreatic insufficiency had progressed to the point that steatorrhea was troublesome. He was dead at 50, probably from complications of alcoholism rather than pancreatitis per se.[2,73] Major predictors of mortality appear to be age at diagnosis (the older the patient, the worse the prognosis), smoking, and drinking.[74] Chronic pancreatitis also is associated with an increased risk of pancreatic cancer.[75]

Diagnosis

A diagnosis of chronic pancreatitis generally is straightforward in an alcoholic patient with recurrent bouts of epigastric pain and evidence of calcification of the pancreas by radiography. Diagnosis is more difficult if the patient is without pain or if a distinction is sought between chronic pancreatitis and recurring acute pancreatitis or pancreatic cancer. Physical examination and routine laboratory tests are of limited utility because they usually are within normal limits. Even serum amylase and lipase levels generally are normal, although they may be elevated during acute exacerbations or decreased late in the course of the disease. Imaging techniques and pancreatic function tests provide the most useful diagnostic tools.[1–3] They are presented here in approximately the order in which they should be considered, based on effectiveness, invasiveness, and expense.

Imaging Studies

Radiography can reveal calcifications (usually diagnostic) and displacement of the stomach or duodenum, indicating the presence of a pseudocyst. Ultrasonography usually demonstrates calcifications, pancreatic enlargement, and pseudocysts, although CT is superior in detecting pseudocysts and can reveal dilated pancreatic ducts as well as pancreatic enlargement and calcifications. ERCP is the most sensitive procedure for viewing changes in the ductal system and is currently considered the gold standard of imaging.[1,3,76] Two newer techniques, endoscopic ultrasonography and magnetic resonance cholangiopancreatography (MR-CP), show promise but must be studied further.[1,76]

Table 30.9 ▪ Selected Diagnostic Tests for Chronic Pancreatitis

Imaging techniques
Plain abdominal radiography
Ultrasonography
Abdominal
Endoscopic
Computed tomography
Magnetic resonance cholangiopancreatography
Endoscopic retrograde cholangiopancreatography[a]
Pancreatic function tests
Direct tests: measurement of pancreatic exocrine secretions
Secretin–pancreozymin test[a]
Lundh test
Indirect tests: measurement of enzyme action
Bentiromide (NBT-PABA) test
Fecal chymotrypsin concentration
Fecal fat analysis

[a]Currently considered gold standards.[1,3,69]

Pancreatic Function Tests

These tests, which can be classified as direct or indirect, have been reviewed extensively elsewhere.[1,3,77,78] Direct tests, including the secretin–pancreozymin and Lundt tests, are invasive, necessitating intubation of the duodenum. In the secretin–pancreozymin test, the gold standard for measuring pancreatic secretory function, a patient is given intravenous secretin and CCK, and the subsequent increase in secretion is measured. The Lundh test is similar, with pancreatic secretion measured after the ingestion of a test meal.

Indirect tests measure markers of pancreatic function in the blood, urine, breath, or stool. Indirect tests are of limited usefulness because of their relative lack of sensitivity early in the course of chronic pancreatitis. Examples of indirect tests include measuring fat or chymotrypsin in stool samples and measuring urinary excretion of paraaminobenzoic acid (PABA) after hydrolytic cleaving of PABA from NBT-PABA (N-benzoyl-L-tyrosyl-p-aminobenzoic acid) by chymotrypsin in the intestine (bentiromide test). A combination of imaging studies and pancreatic function tests may be necessary for a definitive diagnosis of chronic pancreatitis, particularly early in the course of the disease (Table 30.9).

PSYCHOSOCIAL ASPECTS

Many patients develop chronic pancreatitis as a result of alcoholism, and this patient population can be very difficult to manage. If the patient is still drinking actively, every effort should be made to convince him or her to abstain. Unfortunately, however, this may not slow the course of the disease.[2] Alcoholics may also be at increased risk for addiction to opioid analgesic agents, complicating pain management. Treatment regimens and follow-up must be tailored to individual patient profiles.

THERAPEUTIC PLAN

Chronic pancreatitis usually is progressive and, with the possible exception of the obstructive form, irreversible. Therefore, treatment is directed at managing the pain, malabsorption, and other complications that arise from this disease.

TREATMENT

Pain

The pain of chronic pancreatitis, which may be episodic or persistent, is a poorly understood phenomenon, complicating decisions about therapy. Furthermore, few clinical trials have compared treatment regimens rigorously. As a result, there is no universally accepted standard of care for these patients. Warshaw et al.[79] sought to address this problem in their excellent 1998 review of pain management, and they proposed an algorithm for treating pain in chronic pancreatitis (Fig. 30.4).[80]

Treatable causes of pain such as pseudocyst, biliary stricture, duodenal stenosis, peptic ulcer disease, and pancreatic cancer should be identified and addressed as the first

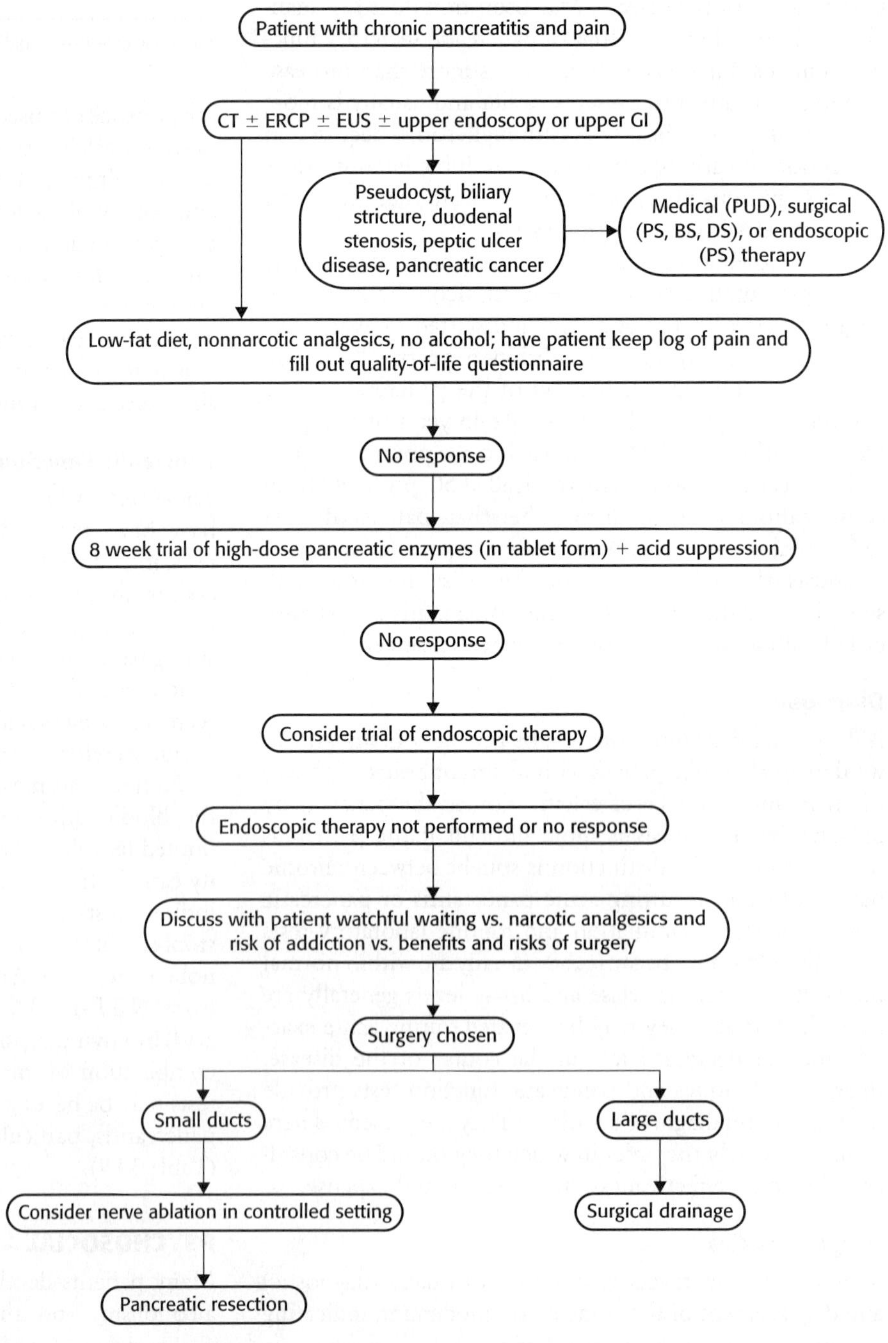

Figure 30.4. Algorithm for treatment of pain in chronic pancreatitis. *BS,* biliary stricture; *CT,* computed tomography; *DS,* duodenal stenosis; *ERCP,* endoscopic retrograde cholangiopancreatography; *EUS,* endoscopic ultrasonography; *GI,* gastrointestinal; *PS,* pseudocyst; *PUD,* peptic ulcer disease. (Reprinted with permission from Warshaw AL, Banks PA, Fernandez-del Castillo C. AGA technical review on treatment of pain in chronic pancreatitis. Gastroenterology 115[3]:763–764, 1998.)

step in managing chronic pancreatic pain. Abstinence from alcohol may reduce pain in up to 50% of patients, but the majority need some form of analgesia.[67,69,71] Warshaw et al. recommend that patients keep a log of their pain to aid in assessment. Salicylates, nonsteroidal anti-inflammatory drugs, or acetaminophen should be tried initially, perhaps in conjunction with a low-fat diet. Adjunctive antidepressant therapy may prove beneficial in some patients, although evidence of efficacy is merely anecdotal.[69,79]

Enzyme replacement therapy may help to alleviate pain, especially in patients with nonalcoholic chronic pancreatitis.[1,62,79,81] Clinical trial data have not always shown effectiveness, however.[1,79,82] It is presumed that the presence of exogenous proteases in the duodenum suppresses pancreatic function through a negative feedback mechanism. This mechanism involves degradation of a CCK-releasing peptide by trypsin in the duodenum, inhibiting the release of CCK.[1,13,79,83] Enzymes contained in non–enteric-coated preparations may be delivered to the duodenum more reliably than enzymes from enteric-coated dosage forms because the latter sometimes are released in more distal portions of the small intestine. This is because of the low duodenal pH caused by decreased bicarbonate secretion in chronic pancreatitis.[58,72] As a result, nonenteric preparations may be more effective at suppressing CCK release and reducing pain.[62,79] In theory, the addition of an H_2-receptor antagonist or a proton pump inhibitor could decrease acid-stimulated pancreatic secretion and diminish pain, but this has not been demonstrated. However, these agents often are tried because of their ease of use and relative safety.[79]

Other agents may also be used to control pain. Octreotide, a somatostatin analogue, has not consistently demonstrated efficacy in chronic disease,[79] but it may have a role in managing pancreatic pseudocysts[81,84] and decreasing complications after pancreatic surgery.[85] Antioxidant therapy may also prove beneficial because patients with chronic pancreatitis seem to be deficient in endogenous antioxidants.[1,79] Further study is needed before specific recommendations can be made, however.

For patients still experiencing pain, the choices remaining are opioid analgesics and interventional therapy. Unfortunately, there are no well-defined criteria for making this decision. Opioid analgesics may prove very effective, although there is a very real risk of addiction, particularly in this patient population.[79,86] Refer to Chapter 54, Pain Management, for a discussion of these agents.

Despite maximum medical management, up to 30% of patients still experience pain.[73] This pain may diminish, or "burn out," over time as the pancreas becomes progressively more fibrotic, but this phenomenon may not occur in as many patients as was once thought.[1,79] Some patients need endoscopic or surgical intervention to control pain.

Endoscopic treatment may be effective for stenosis, strictures, or stones. Stent placement relieves intraductal pressure and pain in many patients, although there is a risk of ductal injury. Patients may also experience pain relief with the elimination of intraductal pancreatic stones by lithotripsy or pancreatic duct sphincterotomy. Improvement is reported in 50 to 85% of patients undergoing endoscopic therapy, but many questions remain.[1,79,87]

Surgery usually is reserved for the patients with intractable pain. The procedure of choice for patients with dilated ducts (more than 6 mm) is surgical drainage with a procedure called lateral pancreaticojejunostomy. For patients with small duct disease, surgical denervation or pancreatic resection are options. These procedures are reviewed extensively elsewhere.[1,62,79,88]

Steatorrhea

Patients with documented weight loss and steatorrhea should receive treatment for malabsorption. Two types of pancreatic enzyme replacement preparations are currently available. Pancreatin is derived from freeze-dried porcine or bovine pancreases and contains at least 2 U.S. Pharmacopeia (USP) units of lipase and 25 USP units each of protease and amylase per milligram. Pancrelipase, extracted from porcine pancreases, is more potent, containing at least 24, 100, and 100 USP units of lipase, protease, and amylase per milligram, respectively (Table 30.10).[89]

Rapid-release and enteric-coated dosage forms are available. Although rapid-release forms more reliably deliver proteases to the upper duodenum, where they may exert a negative feedback inhibitory effect, they expose lipase to the acid environment of the stomach. Lipase is pH-labile, maximally active at pH 8 and irreversibly inactivated at pH less than 4. Enteric coatings that dissolve at approximately pH 5.6 to 6.0 better protect lipase from gastric acidity, but enzyme release may be delayed. Although rapid-release forms are preferable for pain control, enteric-coated products are more effective in treating steatorrhea.[62]

Because lipid malabsorption and steatorrhea are the primary clinical problems associated with pancreatic insufficiency, the lipase dosage to be delivered to the duodenum is a paramount concern. Maximal postprandial delivery of lipase from a normal pancreas is 140,000 U/hour for 4 hours. Supplying 5 to 10% of this dosage significantly decreases steatorrhea; therefore, the enzyme supplement usually should provide at least 28,000 U over a 4-hour period, although regimens should be individualized for each patient.[1,60]

Efficacy of therapy can be assessed by monitoring the fat content of stools. If steatorrhea persists, another agent can be added to increase gastric pH in an attempt to increase the delivery of active lipase to the duodenum. Agents that may be useful include H_2-receptor antagonists and omeprazole.[11,89,90] Sodium bicarbonate and aluminum-containing antacids may also increase the efficacy of supplements, but calcium- and magnesium-containing antacids worsen steatorrhea.[62] Even with careful management of supplements, however, eliminating steatorrhea is very difficult.[11] Figure 30.5 presents one possible approach to enzyme replacement therapy for steatorrhea.

Patients should be counseled to take supplements just before or with meals. The microspheres or microtablets contained in capsules should not be crushed, but they may be mixed with soft food such as applesauce, if necessary.

The pH of the food should be less than 5 to avoid premature dissolution of the enteric coating. Brands should not be changed without consulting a physician or pharmacist.

Problems that may be encountered with enzyme-replacement therapy, especially at high dosages, include abdominal pain, oral and perianal irritation, nausea, vomiting, diarrhea, and rare hypersensitivity. There have also been reports of hyperuricosuria, although this appears to be more common in patients with cystic fibrosis receiving very high dosages of pancreatic enzymes. Finally, patient compliance often is less than optimal because of the large numbers of capsules needed, gastrointestinal distress, and the expense of the regimen,[12,60] although the overall safety and tolerability of pancreatic extracts appears to be good.[91]

Two approaches currently under study may improve control of steatorrhea. Microbial lipases, which are more acid-resistant than mammalian lipases, seem to be effective. Decreasing levels of proteases in pancreatic preparations may also be an option, slowing proteolytic degradation of lipase in the gastrointestinal tract,[1] although this may render these preparations less effective in treating pain.

FUTURE THERAPIES

Chronic pancreatitis is a very heterogeneous condition, and it is likely that response to a therapeutic modality depends, at least in part, on the cause or clinical course of the disease in a particular patient. This has not been addressed to date in clinical trials, however, because the study populations generally reflect the heterogeneity of the population at large. Defining which patient subgroup may benefit from a particular therapy will help to guide treatment.

IMPROVING OUTCOMES

This patient population presents challenges, particularly if there is continuing alcohol consumption. Substance abuse programs may help to establish and maintain abstinence. Referral to a pain clinic may also be warranted, and one physician should manage narcotic analgesics. Although few studies have attempted to assess quality of life in patients with chronic pancreatitis, this is beginning to be better addressed.[69]

Table 30.10 ▪ Some Commercial Pancreatic Enzyme Preparations

			Enzyme Content (USP units)		
Product[a]	Formulation	Dosage Form	Lipase	Protease	Amylase
Rapid release					
Cotazym	PL	C	8,000	30,000	30,000
Donnazyme	PC	T	1,000	12,500	12,500
Ilozyme	PL	T	11,000	30,000	30,000
Ku-Zyme HP	PL	C	8,000	30,000	30,000
Pancreatin 4 × USP	PC	T	12,000	60,000	60,000
8 × USP	PC	T	22,500	180,000	180,000
Panokase	PL	T	8,000	30,000	30,000
Viokase	PL	T	8,000	30,000	30,000
Viokase	PL	P	16,800	70,000	70,000
Delayed-release capsules					
Cotazym-S	PL	MS	5,000	20,000	20,000
Creon 5 minimicrospheres	PL	MS	5,000	18,750	16,600
Creon 10 minimicrospheres	PL	MS	10,000	37,500	33,200
Creon 20 minimicrospheres	PL	MS	20,000	75,000	66,400
Encron 10	PL	MS	10,000	37,500	33,200
Pancrease	PL	MS	4,000	25,000	20,000
Pancrease MT-4	PL	MT	4,000	12,000	12,000
Pancrease MT-10	PL	MT	10,000	30,000	30,000
Pancrease MT-16	PL	MT	16,000	48,000	48,000
Pancrease MT-20	PL	MT	20,000	44,000	56,600
Pancron 10	PL	MS	10,000	37,500	33,200
Protilase	PL	MT	4,000	25,000	20,000
Protilase MT-16	PL	MT	16,000	48,000	48,000
Ultrase	PL	MS	6,000	25,000	20,000
Ultrase MT6	PL	MT	6,000	19,500	19,500
Ultrase MT12	PL	MT	12,000	39,000	39,000
Ultrase MT18	PL	MT	18,000	58,500	58,500
Ultrase MT20	PL	MT	20,000	65,000	65,000
Zymase	PL	MS	12,000	24,000	24,000

[a] These products, available before passage of the 1938 Food, Drug, and Cosmetic Act, are not approved by the FDA and cannot be considered pharmaceutically or therapeutically equivalent.[11]

USP, U.S. Pharmacopeia; *PL*, pancrelipase; *C*, capsule; *PC*, pancreatin; *T*, tablet; *P*, powder; *MS*, enteric-coated microspheres; *MT*, enteric-coated microtablets.

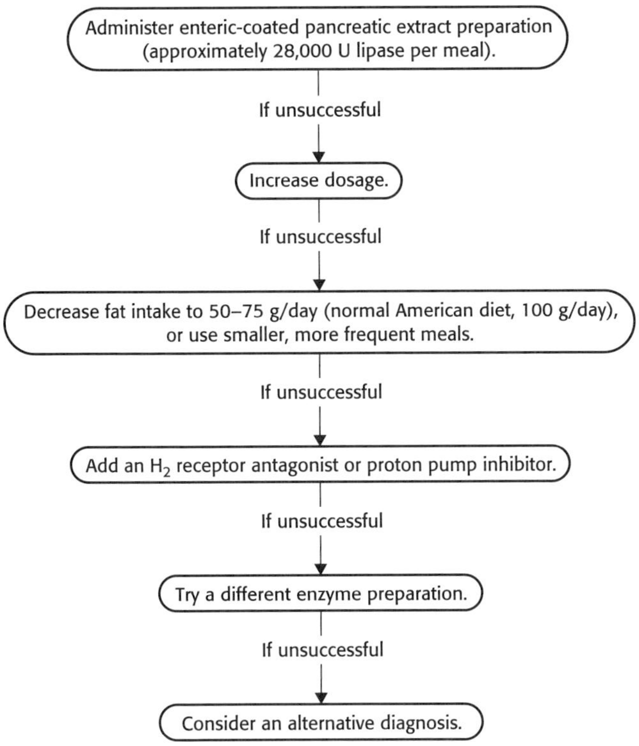

Figure 30.5. Algorithm for treatment of steatorrhea. (Adapted from reference 1.)

PHARMACOECONOMICS

To date, no studies have been published evaluating the economic impact of chronic pancreatitis or its therapy. This information will be needed to refine emerging therapeutic algorithms.

KEY POINTS

- Acute and chronic pancreatitis appear to be distinct clinical entities that are often, although not always, alcohol related. Acute pancreatitis is an autodigestive process characterized by inflammation, edema, and necrosis, whereas chronic pancreatitis is associated with intraductal protein plugs and calculi leading to irreversible loss of functional tissue. An acute process may evolve into chronic disease, but this is uncommon and cannot be predicted.
- Controlled clinical trials are needed to assess the role of medical therapy directed at the underlying pathogenesis of acute and chronic pancreatic disease.

Acute Pancreatitis

- The mortality associated with acute pancreatitis ranges from 5 to 10%.
- The most common causes of acute pancreatitis are alcohol and gallstones.
- Severe acute pancreatitis should be identified early in the course of the disease.
- Therapy for acute pancreatitis is supportive. Future therapies will be directed at curtailing inflammation.
- Patients should be assessed throughout the course of an acute attack for complications such as organ failure and infection.

Chronic Pancreatitis

- Most cases are alcohol related and usually progressive and irreversible.
- Clinical course varies widely, complicating diagnosis and therapy.
- Treatment is directed at managing pain, steatorrhea, diabetes, and other complications.
- Future trials should stratify cases by cause or clinical course, compare treatment regimens, determine cost-effectiveness of therapy, and assess patient quality of life.

REFERENCES

1. Banks PA, Acute and chronic pancreatitis. In: Feldman M, Sleisenger MH, Scharschmidt BF. Gastrointestinal and liver disease: pathophysiology/diagnosis/management. 6th ed. Philadelphia: WB Saunders, 1998:809.
2. Steer ML, Waxman I, Freedman S. Chronic pancreatitis. N Engl J Med 332:1482–1490, 1995.
3. Owyang C, Levitt MD. Chronic pancreatitis. In: Yamada T. Textbook of gastroenterology. 2nd ed. Philadelphia: Lippincott, 1995:1874.
4. Gorelick FS. Acute pancreatitis. In: Yamada T. Textbook of gastroenterology. 2nd ed. Philadelphia: Lippincott, 1995:2064.
5. Steinberg W, Tenner S. Acute pancreatitis. N Engl J Med 330(17):1198–2010, 1994.
6. Grendell JG, Ermak TH. Anatomy, histology, embryology, and developmental anomalies of the pancreas. In: Feldman M, Sleisenger MH, Scharschmidt BF. Gastrointestinal and liver disease: pathophysiology/diagnosis/management. 6th ed. Philadelphia: WB Saunders, 1998:761.
7. Mulholland MW, Moossa AR, Liddle RA. Pancreas: anatomy and structural anomalies. In: Yamada T. Textbook of gastroenterology. 2nd ed. Philadelphia: Lippincott, 1995:2051.
8. Pandol SJ. Pancreatic physiology and secretory testing. In: Feldman M, Sleisenger MH, Scharschmidt BF. Gastrointestinal and liver disease: pathophysiology/diagnosis/management. 6th ed. Philadelphia: WB Saunders, 1998:771.
9. Owyang C, Williams JA. Pancreatic secretion. In: Yamada T. Textbook of gastroenterology. 2nd ed. Philadelphia: Lippincott, 1995:361.
10. Valenzuela JE. Pancreatic physiology. In: Valenzuela JE, Reber HA, Ribet A. Medical and surgical diseases of the pancreas. New York: Igaku-Shoin, 1991:1.
11. Lebenthal E, Rolston DDK, Holsclaw DS. Enzyme therapy for pancreatic insufficiency: present status and future needs. Pancreas 9(1):1–12, 1994.
12. Chey WY. Regulation of pancreatic exocrine secretion. Int J Pancreatol 9:7–20, 1991.
13. Owyang C, Louie DS, Tatum D. Feedback regulation of pancreatic enzyme secretion: suppression of cholecystokinin release by trypsin. J Clin Invest 77:2042–2047, 1986.
14. Bradley EL. A clinically based classification system for acute pancreatitis. Arch Surg 128(5):586–590, 1993.
15. Marshall JB. Acute pancreatitis: a review with an emphasis on new developments. Arch Intern Med 153(10):1185–1198, 1993.
16. Banks PA. Acute pancreatitis: medical and surgical management. Am J Gastroenterol 89(8 Suppl):S78–S85, 1994.
17. DiMagno EP. Treatment of mild acute pancreatitis. In: Bradley EL. Acute pancreatitis: diagnosis and therapy. New York: Raven, 1994:261–263.
18. Gupta PK, Al-Kawas FH. Acute pancreatitis: diagnosis and management. Am Fam Physician 52(2):435–443, 1995.
19. Moreau JA, Zinsmeister AR, Melton LJ, et al. Gallstone pancreatitis and the effect of cholecystectomy: a population-based cohort study. Mayo Clin Proc 63:466, 1988.
20. Underwood TW, Frye CB. Drug-induced pancreatitis. Clin Pharmacy 12:440–448, 1993.

21. Mallory A, Kern F. Drug-induced pancreatitis: a critical review. Gastroenterol 78:813–820, 1980.
22. Runzi M, Layer P. Drug-associated pancreatitis: facts and fiction. Pancreas 13(1):100–109, 1996.
23. Goyal SB, Goyal RS. Ketorolac tromethamine-induced acute pancreatitis. Arch Intern Med 158:411, 1998.
24. Bosch X. Losartan induced acute pancreatitis. Ann Intern Med 127:1043–1044, 1997.
25. Gerson R, Serrano A, Villalobos A, et al. Acute pancreatitis secondary to ifosfamide. J Emerg Med 15(5):645–647, 1997.
26. Bosch X, Bernadich O. Acute pancreatitis during treatment with amiodarone. Lancet 350:1300, 1997.
27. Liviu L, Yair L, Yehuda S. Pancreatitis induced by clarithromycin. Ann Intern Med 125:701, 1996.
28. Hastier P, Longo F, Buckley M, et al. Pancreatitis induced by codeine: a case report with positive rechallenge. Gut 41(5):705–706, 1997.
29. Fernandez J, Sala M, Panes J, et al. Acute pancreatitis after long-term 5-aminosalicylic acid therapy. Am J Gastroenterol 92(12):2302–2303, 1997.
30. McBride CE, Yavorski RT, Moses FM, et al. Acute pancreatitis associated with continuous infusion cytarabine therapy: a case report. Cancer 77(12):2588–2591, 1996.
31. Madsen JS, Jacobsen IA. Angiotensin converting enzyme inhibitor therapy and acute pancreatitis. Blood Press 4(6):369–371, 1995.
32. Castiella A, Lopez P, Bujanda L, et al. Possible association of acute pancreatitis with naproxen. J Clin Gastroenterol 21(3):258, 1995.
33. Norman J. The role of cytokines in the pathogenesis of acute pancreatitis. Am J Surg 175:76–83, 1998.
34. Leser HG, Gross V, Scheibenbogen B. Elevations of serum interleukin-6 concentration precedes acute-phase response and reflects severity in acute pancreatitis. Gastroenterology 101:782–785, 1991.
35. Exley AR, Leese T, Holliday MP. Endotoxemia and serum tumor necrosis factor as prognostic markers in severe acute pancreatitis. Gut 33:1126–1128, 1992.
36. Bassi D, Kollias M, Fermamdez-del C. Impairment of pancreatic microcirculation correlates with the severity of acute experimental pancreatitis. J Am Coll Surg 179:257, 1994.
37. Banks PA. Practice guidelines in acute pancreatitis. Am J Gastroenterol 92(3):377–386, 1997.
38. Agarwal N, Pitchumoni CS, Sivaprasad AV. Evaluating tests for acute pancreatitis. Am J Gastroenterol 85(4):356–365, 1990.
39. Ranson JHC. Etiological and prognostic factors in human acute pancreatitis: a review. Am J Gastroenterol 77:633–638, 1982.
40. Agarwal N, Pitchumoni CS. Assessment of severity in acute pancreatitis. Am J Gastroenterol 86(10):1385–1391, 1991.
41. Baron TH, Morgan DE. The diagnosis and management of fluid collections associated with pancreatitis. Am J Med 102:555–563, 1997.
42. McClave SA, Snider H, Owens N, et al. Clinical nutrition in pancreatitis. Dig Dis Sci 42(10):2035–2044, 1997.
43. Sarr MG, Sanfey H, Cameron JL. Prospective, randomized trial of nasogastric suction in patients with acute pancreatitis. Surgery 100(3):500–504, 1986.
44. Levant JA, Secrist DM, Resin H, et al. Nasogastric suction in the treatment of alcoholic pancreatitis. JAMA 229(1):51–52, 1974.
45. Niederau C, Schulz HU. Current conservative treatment of acute pancreatitis: evidence from animal and human studies. Hepatogastroenterology 40:538–549, 1993.
46. Carballo F, Dominguez E, Fernandez-Calvet L, et al. Is somatostatin useful in the treatment of acute pancreatitis? A meta-analysis. Digestion 49:12–13, 1991.
47. McKay C, Baxter J, Imrie C. A randomized, controlled trial of octreotide in the management of patients with acute pancreatitis. Int J Pancreatol 21(1):13–19, 1997.
48. Paran H, Neufeld, Mayo A, et al. Preliminary report of a prospective randomized study of octreotide in the treatment of severe acute pancreatitis. J Am Coll Surg 181:121–124, 1995.
49. Barie PS. A critical review of antibiotic prophylaxis in severe acute pancreatitis. Am J Surg 172(Suppl 6A):38S–43S, 1996.
50. Pederzoli P, Bassi C, Vesentini S, et al. A randomized multicenter clinical trial of antibiotic prophylaxis of septic complications in acute necrotizing pancreatitis with imipenem. Surg Gynecol Obstet 176:480–483, 1993.
51. Sainio V, Kemppainen E, Puolakkainen, et al. Early antibiotic treatment in acute necrotising pancreatitis. Lancet 346:663–667, 1995.
52. Luiten EJ, Hop WC, Lange JF, et al. Controlled clinical trial of selective decontamination for the treatment of severe acute pancreatitis. Ann Surg 222:57–65, 1995.
53. Buchler M, Malfertheiner P, Frie H, et al. Human pancreatic tissue concentration of bactericidal antibiotics. Gastroenterology 103:1902–1908, 1992.
54. McKay CJ, Curran F, Sharples C, et al. Prospective placebo-controlled randomized trial of lexipafant in predicted severe acute pancreatitis. Br J Surg 84:1239–1243, 1997.
55. Kingsnorth AN. Early treatment with lexipafant, a platelet activating factor antagonist reduces mortality in acute pancreatitis: a double blind, randomized, placebo controlled study. Gastroenterology 112:A453, 1997.
56. Neoptolemos JP, Raraty M, Finch M, et al. Acute pancreatitis: the substantial human and financial costs. Gut 42(6):886–890, 1998.
57. Sarles H, Adler G, Dani R, et al. The pancreatitis classification of Marseilles–Rome 1988. Scand J Gastroenterol 24:641–642, 1989.
58. Sarles H, Bernard JP, Johnson C. Pathogenesis and epidemiology of chronic pancreatitis. Annu Rev Med 40:453–468, 1989.
59. Pitchumoni CS. Chronic pancreatitis: a historical and clinical sketch of the pancreas and pancreatitis. Gastroenterologist 6(1):24–33, 1998.
60. Mergener K, Baillie J. Chronic pancreatitis. Lancet 350:1379, 1997.
61. Ito T, Nakano I, Koyanagi S. Autoimmune pancreatitis as a new clinical entity: three cases of autoimmune pancreatitis with effective steroid therapy. Dig Dis Sci 42(7):1458–1468, 1997.
62. Toskes PP. Medical management of chronic pancreatitis. Scand J Gastroenterol 30(208):74–80, 1995.
63. Freedman SD, Sakamoto K, Venu RP. GP2, the homologue to the renal cast protein uromodulin, is a major component of intraductal plugs in chronic pancreatitis. J Clin Invest 29:83–90, 1993.
64. Yamadera K, Moriyama T, Makino I. Identification of immunoreactive pancreatic stone protein in pancreatic stone, pancreatic tissue, and pancreatic juice. Pancreas 5(3):255–260, 1990.
65. Larsen S. Diabetes mellitus secondary to chronic pancreatitis. Dan Med Bull 40(2):153–162, 1993.
66. Ebbehoj N. Pancreatic tissue fluid pressure and pain in chronic pancreatitis. Dan Med Bull 39(2):128–133, 1992.
67. Karanjia ND, Rever HA. The cause and management of the pain of chronic pancreatitis. Gastroenterol Clin North Am 19(4):895–904, 1990.
68. Tenner S, Levine RS, Steinberg WM. Drug treatment of acute and chronic pancreatitis. In: Lewis JH. A pharmacologic approach to gastrointestinal disorders. Baltimore: Williams & Wilkins, 1994:311.
69. Glasbrenner B, Adler G. Evaluating pain and the quality of life in chronic pancreatitis. Int J Pancreatol 22(3):163–170, 1997.
70. Layer P, Holtmann G. Pancreatic enzymes in chronic pancreatitis. Int J Pancreatol 15(1):1–11, 1994.
71. Ladas SD, Giorgiotis K, Raptis SA. Complex carbohydrate malabsorption in exocrine pancreatic insufficiency. Gut 34:984–987, 1993.
72. Beglinger C. Relevant aspects of physiology in chronic pancreatitis. Dig Dis 10:326–329, 1992.
73. Young HS. Diseases of the pancreas. Sci Am 4:1–17, 1994.
74. Lowenfels AB, Maisonneuve P, Cavallini G, et al. Prognosis of chronic pancreatitis: an international multicenter study. Am J Gastroenterol 89(9): 1467–1471, 1994.
75. Lowenfels AB, Maisonneuve P, Cavallini G, et al. Pancreatitis and the risk of pancreatic cancer. N Engl J Med 328(20):1433–1437, 1993.
76. Outwater EK, Siegelman ES. MR imaging of pancreatic disorders. Top Magn Reson Imaging 8(5):265–289, 1996.
77. Goldberg DM, Durie PR. Biochemical tests in the diagnosis of chronic pancreatitis and in the evaluation of pancreatic insufficiency. Clin Biochem 26:253–275, 1993.
78. Ribet A, Moreau J, Valenzuela JE. Diagnosis of chronic pancreatitis. In: Valenzuela JE, Reber HA, Ribet A. Medical and surgical diseases of the pancreas. New York: Igaku-Shoin, 1991:113.
79. Warshaw AL, Banks PA, Fernandez-Del Castillo C. AGA technical review: treatment of pain in chronic pancreatitis. Gastroenterology 115:765–776, 1998.
80. Warshaw AL, Banks PA, Fernandez-del Castillo C. AGA technical review on treatment of pain in chronic pancreatitis. Gastroenterology 115(3):763–764, 1998.
81. Malfertheiner P, Dominguez-Munoz JE, Buchler MW. Chronic pancreatitis: management of pain. Digestion 55(Suppl 1):29–34, 1994.
82. Brown A, Hughes M, Tenner S. Does pancreatic enzyme supplementation reduce pain in patients with chronic pancreatitis: a meta-analysis. Am J Gastroenterol 92(11):2032, 1997.
83. Garces MC, Gomez-Cerozo J, Condoceo R. Postprandial cholecystokinin response in patients with chronic pancreatitis in treatment with oral substitutive pancreatic enzymes. Dig Dis Sci 43(3):562–566, 1998.
84. Buchler MW, Binder M, Friess H. Role of somatostatin and its analogues in the treatment of acute and chronic pancreatitis. Gut (Suppl 3):S15–S19, 1994.
85. Friess H, Klempa I, Hermanek P, et al. Prophylaxis of complications after pancreatic surgery: results of a multicenter trial in Germany. Digestion 55(Suppl 1):35–50, 1994.

86. Isenhower HL, Mueller BA. Selection of narcotic analgesics for pain associated with pancreatitis. Am J Health Syst Pharm 55:480, 1998.
87. Waxman I, Freedman SD, Zeroogian JM. Endoscopic therapy of chronic and recurrent pancreatitis. Dig Dis 16(3):134–143, 1998.
88. Ho HS, Frey CF. Current approach to the surgical management of chronic pancreatitis. Gastroenterologist 5(2):128–136, 1997.
89. Kraisinger M, Hochhaus G, Stecenko A, et al. Clinical pharmacology of pancreatic enzymes in patients with cystic fibrosis and in vitro performance of microencapsulated formulations. J Clin Pharmacol 34:158–166, 1994.
90. Bruno MJ, Rauws EAJ, Hoek FJ, et al. Comparative effects of adjuvant cimetidine and omeprazole during pancreatic enzyme replacement therapy. Dig Dis Sci 39(5):988, 1994.
91. Gullo L, Pezzilli R, Gaiani S. Tolerability and safety of the long-term administration of pancreatic extracts [letter]. Pancreas 14(2):210–212, 1997.

CHAPTER 31

RHEUMATOID ARTHRITIS

Eric G. Boyce

DEFINITION

Rheumatoid arthritis (RA) is a highly variable, chronic inflammatory condition of unknown cause affecting mostly diarthrodial (hingelike) joints but often with periarticular and systemic involvement. The word *rheuma* was defined by ancient Greek physicians to mean "flowing," which fit well with their humoral theory of disease. The term *rheumatism* was used in the 1600s by a French physician as an inexact label for a systemic condition with joint ailments. *Rheumatoid arthritis* was coined in 1858 as a label for cases reported in 1800 by a French medical student.[1]

TREATMENT GOALS: RHEUMATOID ARTHRITIS

- Provide safe, effective, and inexpensive treatment that diminishes pain, improves well-being, prevents or slows disease progression in those predisposed, and reduces the need for health care and disability services. The pathogenesis of the disease remains unknown and the vast majority of current therapies are nonspecific and rarely curative, despite continuous advances in knowledge.
- Use basic nondrug treatment modalities (proper diet, exercise, rest, education, psychosocial support) in an effort to diminish the signs, symptoms, and associated features of RA and to enhance the patient's overall health and well-being.
- Use the least toxic and least expensive method of suppressing the patient's chronic inflammation in a manner that is individualized to the patient's disease course, general health, and socioeconomic status, generally starting with nonsteroidal anti-inflammatory drugs (NSAIDs).
- Initiate effective, safe therapy with second-line therapies to prevent or diminish the progressive nature of RA as soon as possible in patients determined to have an aggressive, destructive, or unrelenting course of disease.
- Provide methods to correct deformities and enhance ability to function when needed.
- Provide effective and safe therapy to manage RA flares and treat extraarticular manifestations of the disease as needed.
- Continue monitoring for beneficial and adverse effects of therapy, both acutely and chronically.

EPIDEMIOLOGY

The cause of RA is unknown, but ongoing research continues to develop and test theories that implicate genetic, infectious, endocrinologic, gastrointestinal, atmospheric, environmental, and other etiologic factors. Single or multiple factors may be involved. The autoimmune nature of RA is documented by the presence of immune cell reactivity and production of antibodies to endogenous elements such as immunoglobulins, collagen, and cellular components.

A genetic predisposition appears to play a major role in RA. A greater prevalence of RA is found in patients with select major histocompatability complex (MHC) antigens, which are genetically determined components that appear on cell surfaces and assist in cell recognition and immune reactions. MHC class I antigens (human lymphocyte antigens HLA-A, HLA-B, and HLA-C) are expressed on the surface of all nucleated cells and red blood cells and are markers for cytotoxic T cell ($CD8^+$) and natural killer (NK) cell activation for removal of abnormal cells. MHC class II antigens (HLA-DR, HLA-DP, HLA-DQ) are expressed on the surface of macrophages and helper T-lymphocytes ($CD4^+$) and interact to assist in activating and regulating the immune response to an antigen. RA and the development of more severe RA are associated with HLA-DR4 and HLA-DR1 in many populations (odds ratios of 2 to 4), HLA-A2 and HLA-B40 in Asian Indians, HLA-A23 and HLA-Aw33 in African Americans, and subtypes of these HLA antigens. Shared epitopes of specific amino acid chain sequences in the antigen-recognizing hypervariable region of the HLA-DRB1 unit and possibly on HLA-DP and HLA-DQ also predispose patients to RA and to more severe RA. Many endogenous elements (e.g., collagen, cartilage glycoprotein, rheumatoid factor (RF), bacterial products) have affinity for the shared epitope and may activate an immune response in RA. Conversely, select HLA types, subtypes, and epitopes appear to be less commonly associated with or protective against RA. Other genetically determined factors associated with RA include the homozygous C-κ genotype (constant region of immunoglobulin G [IgG]), T-cell receptor chains, defects in T-cell proliferation, and complement C4 allotypes. These associations provide strong evidence that immunogenetics play an important role in RA. However, bone marrow transplantation from a patient with RA did not lead to development of RA in the recipient, who was also the donor's sibling.[2] This case raises many questions and illustrates the complexity and limits of current knowledge in RA pathogenesis.

Infectious causes of RA are supported by a number of findings, many of which overlap with genetic and autoimmune causes. Patients with RA demonstrate hyperreactivity or increased antibody titers to Epstein–Barr virus, human T-cell lymphoma I/II virus, *Mycobacterium tuberculosis, Proteus mirabilis,* possibly *Escherichia coli* and *Klebsiella pneumonia,* normal human gut flora antigen, and the superantigen staphylococcal enterotoxin B. The shared epitope amino acid sequence in the hypervariable region of HLA-DRB1 that predisposes patients to RA is similar to the amino acid sequence of proteins produced by *E. coli, Brucella ovis, Lactobacillus lactis,* and Epstein–Barr virus. Single or chronic exposure to one of these organisms could trigger the expression of HLA antigens and subsequent activation of the immune system, resulting in a chronic immunologic and inflammatory reaction to an endogenous antigen. However, only a few antimicrobial agents have demonstrated efficacy against RA, and those agents have immune system actions that may explain their effects in RA.[3–7]

Endocrinologic etiologic links to RA are supported by the greater risk of RA in female patients and after breastfeeding, lower risk associated with a history of pregnancy or possibly oral contraceptive use, and lower severity in patients who used oral contraceptives before the onset of RA. In pregnant women with RA, approximately 75% have decreases in the activity of RA, but increases and no change can also be seen. Decreases in RA activity during pregnancy may result from decreased production of certain inflammatory cytokines or abnormal immunoglobulins. Both prolactin, which has proinflammatory effects, and arginine vasopressin are elevated in patients with RA. Patients with RA have a suppressed cortisol response to inflammation.[8] Additionally, there appears to be a weak association between thyroid disorders and RA. Neuroendocrinologic causes are supported by a decrease in RA in a limb affected by a stroke but not in unaffected limbs.

Gastrointestinal factors may play a role through the presence of hyperreactivity or antibodies to enteric organisms and to gluten. In general, however, food antigens are unlikely to be responsible for T-cell activation in RA. Changes in the atmosphere, particularly changes in barometric pressure, are associated with acute worsening of the disease.

The causes of RA remain a mystery. The differences among various populations with respect to association with HLA allele, clinical presentation, and severity complicate efforts to determine causation. However, it appears that genetic, other endogenous, and exogenous factors are important in the development of RA.

RA affects 0.3 to 1.5% of the population and is two to three times more common in women than in men. Genetic predisposition is suggested by the greater incidence of RA in certain families, monozygote twins, and people with specific HLA genetic markers, as noted earlier. It can be seen in any culture or race. RA occurs at any age, with the peak incidence in women occurring between 30 and 60 years of age. Children with chronic arthritis who meet certain diagnostic criteria are given a diagnosis of juvenile RA, which is a different diagnosis than RA. Age of onset of RA may also be associated with HLA typing. RA onset in older Japanese adults was more strongly associated with a different shared epitope amino acid sequence than in younger patients with RA or in control subjects.

PATHOPHYSIOLOGY

A normal diarthrodial joint is a functional interface that supports and limits the relative movement of two or more bones over defined ranges. The joint capsule surrounds the joint space and connects to the surrounding bones (Fig. 31.1). The synovium, or synovial tissue, is the internal structure of the joint capsule that secretes synovial fluid and contains many blood vessels and immunologically active cells. Connective tissue surrounds the synovial tissue and provides stability to the joint capsule and the synovial lining membrane. Tendons, ligaments, and muscles also stabilize the joint. Cartilage, which is composed of a proteoglycan matrix and 70% water, is bathed in synovial fluid and cushions the forces between the opposing bones during movement and compression. Synovial fluid provides nutrients, removes wastes from the cartilage, and helps maintain the structure of the cartilage

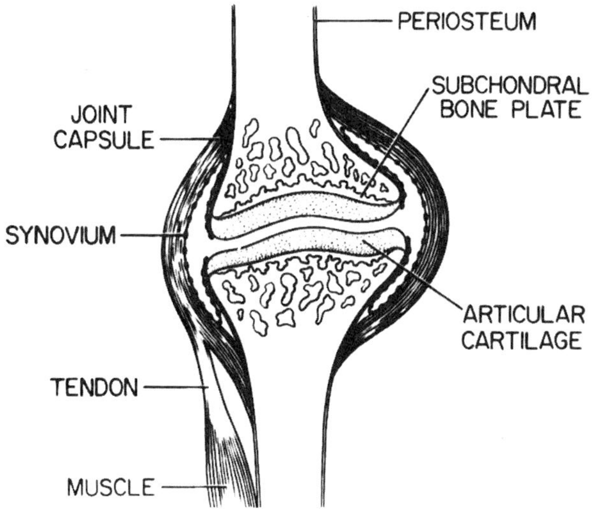

Figure 31.1. Normal diarthrodial joint. The typical diarthrodial joint, such as the knee, is freely movable. The articulating surfaces are covered by a smooth layer of hyaline cartilage and are enclosed in a fibrous capsule. The fibrous capsule merges externally with periosteum, tendons, ligaments, and fascia and internally with the synovial membrane that lines the joint cavity. Articular cartilage is not covered by synovial membrane. A small amount of synovial fluid normally is present within the joint cavity.

through hydration. Normal anatomy and physiology are altered in RA by immunologically and inflammatory mediated changes in bone, cartilage, supporting tissues, and synovial tissue and fluid.

A normal immune reaction to an antigen begins with nonspecific phagocytosis, followed by the development and activation of specific, adaptive processes, and results in antigen removal and memory immune cell formation. Macrophages initially engulf and process the antigen, present the antigen to helper T-lymphocytes (T_H-cells, $CD4^+$) and B-lymphocytes (B cells), and secrete interleukin-1 (IL-1) to activate T_H cells. MHC class II antigens and cellular adhesion molecules are expressed on the surface of macrophages and other antigen-processing cells in association with processed antigen and regulate the interaction with activated helper T cells. Once activated, T_H cells secrete IL-2, which in turn activates and enhances proliferation of T_H cells, cytotoxic T cells (T_C cells, $CD8^+$), suppressor T cells (T_S cells, $CD8^+$), B cells, NK cells, memory T and B cells, macrophages, and other phagocytes. Activated T_H cells also secrete interferon-γ (IFN-γ), which enhances the expression of MHC-II antigens and the function of macrophages. Through genetic rearrangement, clones of B cells and T cells develop variable reactive regions that become much more specific for the antigen, resulting in secretion of specific immunoglobulins by B cells and enhanced binding by T cells. Immunoglobulins (or antibodies) bind to the antigen and facilitate its removal by macrophages and other phagocytes. The stimulation of numerous cells and development of antigen-specific binding sites greatly enhance the rate and specificity of the reaction to the antigen. As the antigen is removed and through action of suppressor T cells, the immune reaction to the antigen diminishes. Specific memory B- and T-lymphocytes remain dormant until a subsequent exposure to that antigen, at which time they initiate a rapid, specific response to the antigen. The normal immune reaction is much more complicated than indicated in this overview, involving numerous other cytokines. Little or no tissue destruction is expected in a normal immune response, but abnormalities in the immune response associated with RA result in inflammation and damage both within and outside the joint.

The pathophysiology of the joint changes seen in RA involves changes at tissue, cellular, biochemical, and molecular levels.[1,9–14] The chronic inflammation, synovial proliferation, and bone and cartilage destruction seen in RA appear to be associated with abnormalities in immune, inflammatory, and repair responses that result from secretions and other activity by macrophages, fibroblasts (which may be specialized macrophages), lymphocytes, neutrophils, mast cells, and other immune cells.

The antigen responsible for initiating the immunologic events in RA is unknown. Potential candidates include the Fc (constant) portion of IgG, collagen (from cartilage, synovium, and blood vessels), cartilage components, numerous infectious agents or their products, and superantigens. Synovial macrophages appear to be in a hyperactive state in patients with RA, possibly activated by immune complexes, complement, IFN-γ, and the antigens listed earlier (Table 31.1).[9–11] Hyperreactivity to the antigens may be linked to the MHC class II antigens, adhesion molecules, or chronic exposure to the antigen. The expression of MHC class I antigens, which is associated with cytotoxicity, and the increased expression of adhesion molecules on the surface of rheumatoid synovial fibroblasts are enhanced by IL-1, tumor necrosis factor-α (TNF-α), and IFN-γ.[9–11]

Macrophages release a number of factors that are important in the pathophysiology of RA, including IL-1, TNF, destructive enzymes (collagenase, proteases), inflammatory prostaglandins (PGE_2) and leukotrienes (LTB_4), and other factors (granulocyte–macrophage colony-stimulating factor [GM-CSF]). IL-1 stimulates the activation and proliferation of helper T cells ($CD4^+$) and secretion of tissue growth factor. IL-1 and TNF are chemotactic, enhance the expression of adhesion and MHC class antigens, and stimulate the secretion of PGE_2, destructive enzymes (collagenase, proteases), substance P (a pain mediator), and other cytokines (e.g., GM-CSF, IL-6).[9–11] TNF-α is secreted with IL-1 and correlates with rheumatoid cachexia.[12] Levels of IL-1, TNF-α, GM-CSF, and soluble IL-2 receptors are elevated in the blood, synovial fluid, and synovial tissue in patients with RA and may correlate with disease activity. IL-1 and TNF secretion is inhibited by IFN-γ, IL-4, IL-10, and IL-13. Inhibitors of the action of IL-1 and TNF include receptor antagonists (IL-1Ra), soluble receptors (soluble TNF receptors), and IL-10. IL-10 also inhibits GM-CSF secretion and synovial monocyte proliferation.

T-lymphocytes are activated by IL-1, IL-2, enhanced HLA-DR antigen expression, other interleukins (IL-12, IL-15), and numerous antigens including chondrocyte

Table 31.1 ▪ Actions of Immunologic Mediators in Rheumatoid Arthritis

Substance	Source	Stimulates (Inhibits)
IL-1, TNF	Macrophages	MHC-I expression, chemotaxis Release of PGE_2, IL-6, GM-CSF, collagenase, metalloprotease, substance P
IL-1	Macrophages	Lymphocyte proliferation and activation Growth factor release
IL-6	Fibroblasts T-Lymphocytes	T-cell and B-cell function GM-CSF release
IL-10	Synovial cells B cells Memory $CD4^+$ T cells	IgM and Ig G release (Inhibits TNF-α action) (Inhibits activation of antigen-processing cells and T cells)
IL-13	Synovial macrophages	(Inhibits production of IL-1β, TNF-α) HLA-DR expression
IL-15	Synovial endothelial cells	T-cell migration and activation TNF production by T cells and macrophages
IFN-γ	T-Lymphocytes	MHC-I and MHC-II expression (Inhibits collagenase and PGE_2 release)
GM-CSF	Macrophages Lymphocytes	Bone marrow cell formation, IL-1 production PMN activation, monocyte attraction
PGE_2	Fibroblasts	Growth factor release, cartilage degradation, inflammation, pain
Collagenase	Fibroblasts	Cartilage degradation
Growth factors		Synovial tissue proliferation
Transforming growth factor		Synovial tissue proliferation, IL-1 production, monocyte chemotaxis (Inhibits lymphokine and protease secretion, synoviocyte growth, and HLA-DR expression)

IL, interleukin; *TNF*, tumor necrosis factor; *MHC*, major histocompatibility complex; *PG*, prostaglandin; *GM-CSF*, granulocyte–macrophage colony-stimulating factor; *Ig*, immunoglobulin; *HLA-DR*, human lymphocyte antigen type DR; *IFN*, interferon; *PMN*, neutrophils.

membrane, synovial cell antigen, superantigen, human collagen (types I, II, IV, V), cartilage proteoglycans and metalloproteases, *Mycobacterium tuberculosis, M. bovus* heat shock protein, tetanus toxoid, and a synovial protein similar to the Fc portion of IgG. IL-15 and soluble adhesion molecules from synovial endothelial cells mediate T-cell migration into the synovial capsule. In RA synovium, T cells appear to accumulate, be autoreactive, and display atypical proliferation and differentiation. Few antigens appear to be primarily responsible for T-cell activation, and those antigens appear to change over time. T cells from patients with RA demonstrate markers for activated ($CD3^+$) and suppressor/cytotoxic ($CD8^+$) T cells, increased activation of surface adhesion and signaling lymphocytic activation molecules, and mature and hyperreactive memory T cells.[11] Synovial T cells and peripheral $CD8^+$ T cells have fewer β-adrenergic receptors, which may decrease the inhibitor effect of catecholamines on T-cell activity.[13] Patients with RA have gone into remission when infected with the human immunodeficiency virus,[14] implicating a key role of helper T cells in RA.

T cells are responsible for secreting IL-2, IL-6, IL-8, IL-10, IFN-γ, and GM-CSF. IL-6 is elevated in inflammatory synovial fluid and increases production of GM-CSF, immunoglobulins, and acute phase reactants after secretion from monocytes, T cells, and fibroblasts (Table 31.1).[11] IL-6 production is stimulated by IL-1-β, GM-CSF, IFN-γ, and TNF-α but inhibited by IL-10, IL-4, IL-13, IL-1Ra, and anti-CD14 monoclonal antibody. GM-CSF, secreted from numerous sources, promotes the growth of certain bone marrow cell lines, increases MHC class II expression on synovial macrophages, stimulates IL-1 production, activates neutrophils, and attracts monocytes (Table 31.1).[11] IL-8 is secreted by T-cell–stimulated synoviocytes in RA and appears to be a chemoattractant for neutrophils. IFN-γ increases MHC class I and II antigen expression and macrophage activation.

Despite the role of T cells in RA and the accumulation of T cells in RA synovium, T-cell function in RA synovium is actually suppressed. This suppression has been documented by low numbers of activated T_H cells, hyporesponsive T cells, diminished expression of activation receptors,[11] and T_H-cell defects in proliferation and production of IL-2, IL-4, TNF-α, IFN-γ, and IL-6. T-cell activation appears to be suppressed by suppressor T cells, IL-4, IL-10, soluble vascular cell adhesion molecule, selective antigen MHC class II activation, site-specific alterations in activation, and TNF-α. The suppressed T-cell state may explain the T cell accumulation and continued inflammatory activity in synovial tissue resulting from direct activation by antigens.

B cells (B-lymphocytes) become activated plasma cells and then produce and secrete specific antibody and IL-10. The stimuli for this activation are IL-2, IL-10, and select synovial antigens including mitochondria from destruction of synovial cells or cartilage. Plasma cells are the most prevalent, highly active monocyte in synovial tissue and blood vessels in RA. Normal and mutated clonal rearrangement patterns for the hypervariable region of the secreted immunoglobulins have been found. Memory B cells appear to accumulate and reside for long periods of time in synovial membrane in RA.

Antibodies and the consequences of antibody release (immune complexes and complement activation) also increase in patients with RA. RF is an autoantibody directed against the Fc portion of IgG that is positive in 80% of patients with RA. RF from patients with RA has a higher affinity for antigens and is a potent activator of complement compared to RF from people without RA. Hyaluronic acid, a normal component of synovial fluid, appears to facilitate the formation of immune complexes of RF and IgG. RF may also bind native and inactivate C1q, part of the complement cascade, because of the similarity in antigenicity of C1q and type II collagen. IgG antibodies to collagen chains are seen early in the course of erosive RA but decrease over the first year of the disease. Immune complexes containing *N*-acetylglucosamine, a cartilage glycoprotein, are higher in RA than in other inflammatory disorders. IgG lacking galactose in the Fc portion is increased in patients with RA and in those with more active disease and decreased during pregnancy. Other autoantibodies are also seen in RA. The increased secretion of antibody and formation of immune complexes in RA appear to sustain the immune reaction and may be responsible for joint and extraarticular manifestations of the disease.

Phagocytic and immune cells found in synovial fluid and tissue include macrophages, NK cells (found in early rheumatoid synovial tissue), neutrophils (activated by IFN-γ), and mast cells. Macrophages may also be the target of destruction by activated T-cytotoxic cells. Neutrophils may be in a primed, semiactivated state in RA. Mast cells are found in invasive synovial tissue and may be important in cartilage destruction and inflammatory edema because of their association with increases in IL-1, TNF, stromelysin-1, and collagenase, in addition to enhancing production of PGE_2 and proteases. Phagocytic cells are responsible for removing damaged cells and debris and initiating repair. However, the immune dysregulation in RA leads to damage by these cells.

Synovial tissue proliferates in RA, becomes hypervascular, and develops into an invasive tissue known as the pannus. Growth factors (platelet-derived, epidermal, transforming, basic fibroblast) and receptors for these growth factors in synovial fluid and tissue may lead an autocrine, tumorlike growth of synovial tissue and synovial blood vessels in RA. IL-1 and PGE_2 (Table 31.1) regulate platelet-derived growth factor. Transforming growth factor decreases lymphokine and protease secretion, synoviocyte growth, and HLA-DR expression but enhances collagen and fibronectin gene transcription, protease inhibitor and IL-1 production, monocyte chemotaxis, and immunosuppression. Migrating circulatory macrophages may also help maintain the hyperplastic, invasive synovium.

The bone resorption and cartilage destruction of RA generally are progressive over time and are caused by cellular activities and secretions. Collagenase, PGE_2, plasminogen activator, and stromelysin are able to degrade cartilage or collagen and are produced by synovial fibroblasts or chondrocytes after stimulation by IL-1 or TNF. The effect of IL-1 and TNF on collagenase and PGE_2 production is diminished by IFN-γ (Table 31.1). Decreased secretion of IFN-γ may be associated with increased joint destruction. Erosive disease also is associated with increased secretion of IgG to collagen early in the course of the disease, induction of osteoclastogenesis by IL-6 and soluble IL-6 receptors, stimulation of osteoclast differentiation by IL-11, hyperreactivity of T-cells to chondrocyte membrane, and phagocytosis of cartilage and type II collagen. Cartilage repair may be reduced by a decrease in the formation of cartilage precursors by synovial cells. Plasma parathyroid hormone and calcitriol levels may also correlate with periarticular bone loss in patients with RA. This destruction of bone and cartilage is an endpoint of the pathologic process of RA, but fortunately it occurs in less than 30% of patients with RA.

The inflammation, synovial proliferation, and collagen destruction of RA lead to changes in synovial fluid, synovial tissue, cartilage, and bone. The pressure within the joint increases from vacuum or subatmospheric pressures in the normal joint to supraatmospheric pressures when inflamed. Rheumatoid synovial fluid is similar to that seen in other inflammatory joint diseases with respect to leukocytosis (mostly polymorphonuclear cells) and decreased viscosity. The synovial tissue becomes hypervascular and blood flow increases with vasodilation, but this may not be enough to meet the metabolic demands resulting from the inflammation. Lactate levels are high in inflamed synovial fluid. Increased synovial fluid, synovial tissue proliferation, and cartilage destruction lead to discomfort and limit movement. Cartilage and bone destruction and the disruption of positioning and functioning of tendons and ligaments further destabilize the joint.

CLINICAL PRESENTATION AND DIAGNOSIS

Signs and Symptoms

The onset of RA varies from slow and insidious to rapidly progressive. The course of the disease is also highly variable: 10 to 20% of patients have a short course with subsequent remission, 70 to 80% have mild to moderate disease with cyclic exacerbation, and 10 to 20% develop progressive, destructive disease. More severe disease at onset and follow-up can be seen in patients from poor socioeconomic settings.[15] Restricted activity is noted in 70% of patients with RA and 89% of patients with RA and comorbid disorders.[16] Proper assessment of the patient's abilities is needed to adequately assess their disease. Functional classification enables the physician to follow a patient's global ability to perform daily living activities (Table 31.2). More specific activities of daily living questionnaires and quality of life surveys are also useful but are not widely used clinically.

Table 31.2 ▪ Functional Classes

Class	Description
I	Able to perform daily living activities without restriction
II	Moderate restrictions but still able to do normal activities
III	Major restriction in performing work or self-care activities
IV	Unable to perform self-care or confined to bed or wheelchair

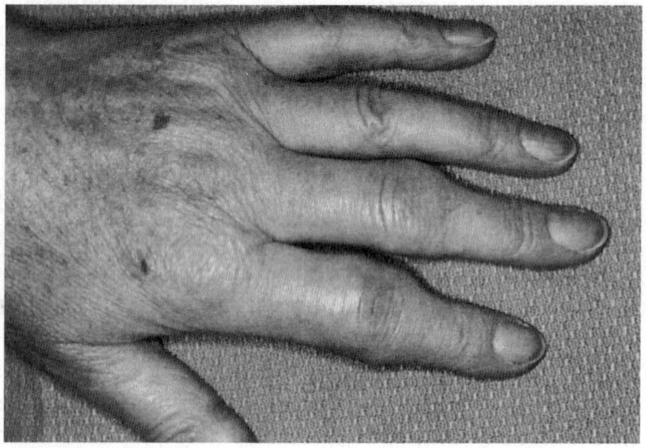

Figure 31.2. Rheumatoid arthritis: hand, fusiform swelling. Soft tissue swelling occurs as an early finding in rheumatoid arthritis and usually appears as typical fusiform or spindle-shaped enlargement of proximal interphalangeal joints. The second and third fingers of this patient are most involved. These proximal interphalangeal joints are tender and have a limited range of motion. (Reprinted from the Clinical Slide Collection on the Rheumatic Diseases, copyright 1991, 1995, 1997. Used by permission of the American College of Rheumatology.)

Joints are the primary areas of involvement in RA, ranging from quiescent or mild synovitis to severe synovitis, considerable synovial thickening or proliferation, detectable synovial fluid, and obvious bone deformity. RA usually affects diarthrodial joints including the joints of the hands (Fig. 31.2) and feet such as the proximal interphalangeal (PIP) joints, metacarpal–phalangeal (MCP) joints, metatarsal–phalangeal (MTP) joints, wrists, and ankles. Elbows, shoulders, sternoclavicular joints, temporomandibular joints, knees, and hips are commonly involved. Cervical spine involvement may lead to severe pain and subluxation.

Stiffness is a gellike sensation experienced in the joints or more generally in patients with RA when they attempt to move after waking in the morning or after a period of inactivity. Patients are likely to describe it as pain or discomfort. The degree of stiffness diminishes with movement, usually over the first few hours after awakening in the morning or after moving about after a period of inactivity. Plasma levels of keratan sulfate, a large cartilage proteoglycan degradation product, are inversely proportional to the duration of morning stiffness.

Erosive joint disease, mostly in the hands, is seen within the first 2 years of RA in 67 to 73% of patients with progressive destructive RA, progresses most rapidly over the first 5 years, and continues to progress over at least 20 years.[17,18] Joint destruction in RA has been correlated or associated with RF titers (total, IgA, IgM), rheumatoid nodules, HLA-DR4, specific shared epitopes of HLA-DRB1, IgG lacking galactose, memory T cells, erythrocyte sedimentation rate (ESR), C-reactive protein (CRP), and antikeratin antibody titers. Conversely, select epitopes of HLA-DP and HLA-DR are associated with nonerosive disease. These bone erosions and joint deformities are caused by destruction of periarticular bone by inflammatory mediators, enzymes, phagocytosis, and physical stress. Common deformities seen in RA include ulnar deviation, swan neck deformities, boutonnière deformities, hammer or cock-up toe formation, and ankylosis (Figs. 31.3 to 31.6). Opposing or compensating forces lead to a zigzag pattern of deformity. In the late stages of progressive disease, bony deformities may predominate and acute inflammation may be absent or minimal. Joints are destabilized by bone, muscle, tendon, ligament, or joint capsule changes. The amount of joint destruction can be quantified by three techniques (Steinbrocker stage, Larsen score, modified Sharp score), but these measures have only fair correlation with patient function. Prevention of these deformities is likely to progress considerably if the use of HLA typing and other clinical variables are found to have reasonable sensitivity, specificity, availability, and affordability for assessing patient risk.

General constitutional symptoms are common in RA. Fatigue, which occurs in many patients, particularly during active RA, may be related to abnormal sleep patterns, anemia, depression, muscle weakness, and neuropeptides. Depression, anxiety, and social problems also are common in patients with RA. The cachexia and muscle weakness that occur in RA are associated with inactivity, catabolic effects of inflammatory mediators (TNF), use of corticosteroids, and other factors.[12] The generalized osteopenia

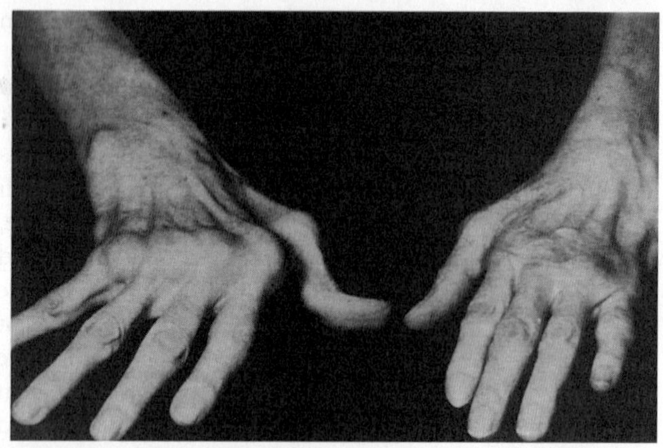

Figure 31.3. Rheumatoid arthritis: hands, ulnar deviation, and muscle atrophy. Ulnar deviation and subluxation of metacarpophalangeal joints have occurred in the patient's right hand. These joints also appear swollen. Muscle atrophy has developed in the dorsal musculature of both hands. (Reprinted from the Clinical Slide Collection on the Rheumatic Diseases, copyright 1991, 1995, 1997. Used by permission of the American College of Rheumatology.)

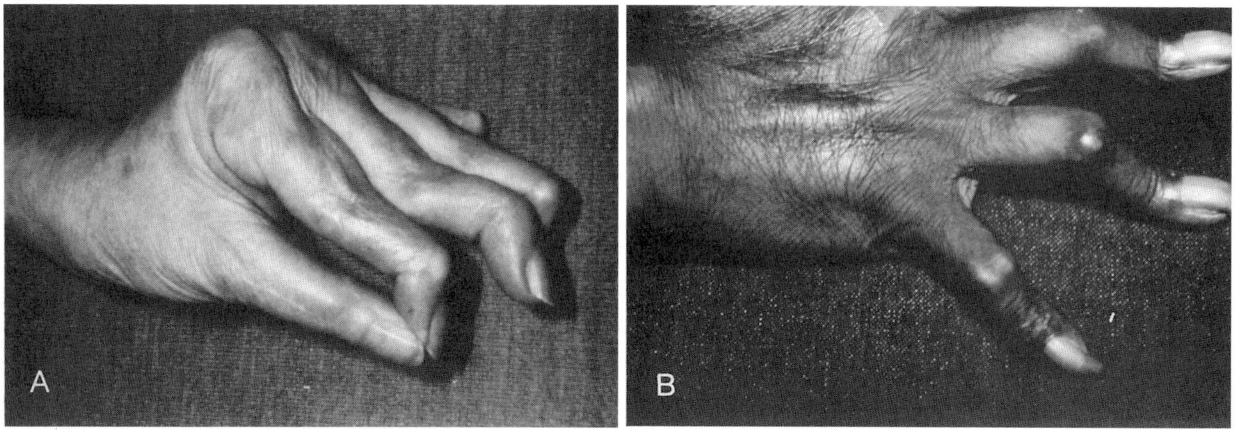

Figure 31.4. Rheumatoid arthritis. **A,** Swan neck deformities are present in the second and third fingers of this patient with rheumatoid arthritis. This deformity results from contracture of the interosseous and flexor muscles and tendons, resulting in a flexion contracture of the metacarpophalangeal joint, hyperextension of the proximal interphalangeal joint, and flexion of the distal interphalangeal joint. There is no rupture of the extensor apparatus, and the metacarpophalangeal joints are not dislocated. When a swan neck deformity is present, the patient may be unable to flex the proximal interphalangeal joint if the metacarpophalangeal joint of the involved finger is held in extension. **B,** Boutonnière deformities, present in the third, fourth, and fifth fingers, are characterized by persistent flexion of the proximal interphalangeal joint and hyperextension of the distal interphalangeal joint. This deformity is caused by weakening of the central slip of the extrinsic extensor tendon and a palmar displacement of the lateral bands to the flexor side of the joint fulcrum. Because the mechanism of this deformity resembles a knuckle being pushed through a buttonhole, it has become known as the boutonnière deformity. (Reprinted from the Clinical Slide Collection on the Rheumatic Diseases, copyright 1991, 1995, 1997. Used by permission of the American College of Rheumatology.)

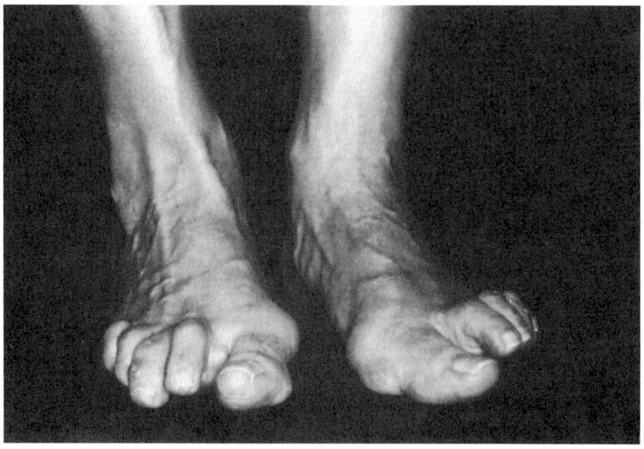

Figure 31.5. Rheumatoid arthritis: foot deformities. The most common foot deformities in rheumatoid arthritis are hallux valgus and hammer toes. The cock-up toe deformities in this patient are associated with subluxation of the metatarsophalangeal joints. Superimposed painful corns and bunions result from irritation caused by faulty shoes. (Reprinted from the Clinical Slide Collection on the Rheumatic Diseases, copyright 1991, 1995, 1997. Used by permission of the American College of Rheumatology.)

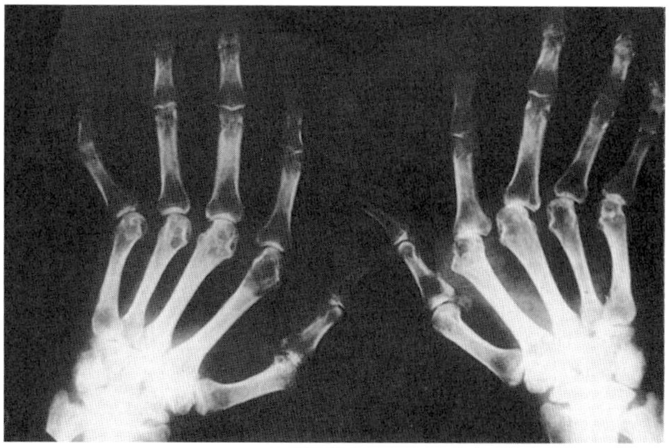

Figure 31.6. Rheumatoid arthritis: hands, advanced deformity (radiograph). The metacarpophalangeal joints demonstrate marked narrowing with subluxation and ulnar deviation. Erosions are seen in the metacarpal heads. The proximal interphalangeal joints are narrowed, but there is no reactive bone change. Demineralization is present in bones adjacent to the metacarpophalangeal and proximal interphalangeal joints. The carpal spaces are narrowed and the carpal bones and ulnar styloid processes also reveal erosions. (Reprinted from the Clinical Slide Collection on the Rheumatic Diseases, copyright 1991, 1995, 1997. Used by permission of the American College of Rheumatology.)

seen in patients with RA is related to or worsened by inflammatory mediators, immobility, corticosteroids, and age-related effects in postmenopausal women and older adults.

Extraarticular involvement in RA is more common in patients who have a positive RF, IgA RF, HLA-DR4, HLA-DR1, HLA-DR3, select shared epitopes for HLA-DRB1 chain sequences, higher proportions of a specific helper T cell, circulating immune complexes, male sex, and more severe arthritis. Extraarticular features include rheumatoid nodules, vasculitis, vital organ effects, anemia, thrombocytopenia, Felty's syndrome, Sjögren's syndrome, and ocular inflammation in addition to the generalized constitutional symptoms. Extraarticular manifestations demonstrate the systemic immune effects associated with RA.

Rheumatoid nodules (Fig. 31.7), which contain monocytes and macrophages surrounding a necrotic area, occur in 25% of patients with RA, almost all of whom are RF positive. Other risk factors for developing rheumatoid nodules include longer duration of RA, more severe RA,

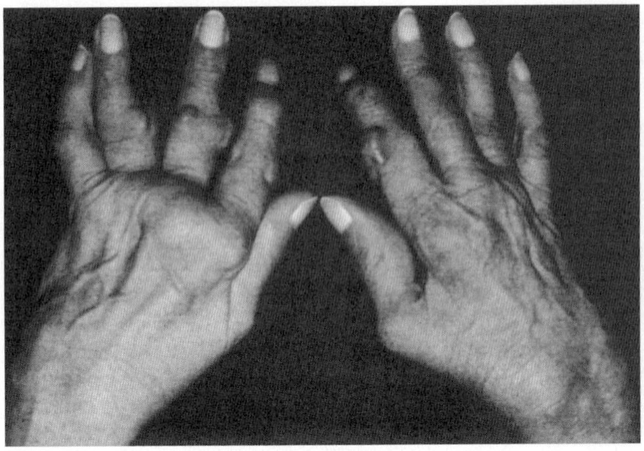

Figure 31.7. Rheumatoid arthritis: subcutaneous nodules, fingers. Multiple subcutaneous nodules can be seen in the fingers of this patient with rheumatoid arthritis. Subcutaneous nodules are most common on the dorsal forearm surface distal to the olecranon process but also may appear in the fingers, over the Achilles tendon, on the occiput, and at other pressure points such as the ischial tuberosity and sacrum. They are most common in rheumatoid arthritis and rheumatic fever but also may occur in other rheumatic diseases such as systemic lupus erythematosus and mixed connective tissue disease. This patient also displays marked synovial proliferation with subluxation of metacarpophalangeal joints of the left hand. (Reprinted from the Clinical Slide Collection on the Rheumatic Diseases, copyright 1991, 1995, 1997. Used by permission of the American College of Rheumatology.)

other extraarticular manifestations, and a specific shared epitope of the HLA-DRB1 chain sequence. Methotrexate (MTX) may increase the number of rheumatoid nodules in some patients.[19] Rheumatoid nodules generally occur subcutaneously over bone in pressure point areas but may be found in other tissues and organs.

Vasculitis is most common in patients with severe, nodular, seropositive RA and those with a specific shared epitope of the HLA-DRB1 chain sequence, perinuclear antineutrophilic cytoplasmic antibody (pANCA), or a high ESR. Male patients may be at higher risk for vasculitis. The vasculitis varies from minor skin lesions to major organ vascular involvement. Clues to the presence of vascular inflammation include the presence of the spectrum of skin manifestations from palpable purpura to digital infarcts, ischemic ulcers, and progression to gangrene and necrosis (Fig. 31.8). Larger-vessel involvement with major organ compromise is seen on rare occasions.

Anemia of chronic inflammatory disease is seen in patients with RA, and it worsens as the arthritis worsens. This anemia is related to the inability to use iron stores and responds poorly to iron therapy. Anemia of chronic disease may occur in conjunction with iron deficiency. Hemolytic anemia and autoimmune thrombocytopenia are rare features of RA. Anemia may also be caused by the drugs used to treat RA, gastrointestinal ulcers with bleeding (caused by NSAIDs, systemic corticosteroids), bone marrow suppression (caused by MTX, azathioprine, gold salts, cyclophosphamide), hemolytic or immune anemia (caused by sulfasalazine, antimalarials, gold salts, penicillamine, sulfasalazine), and numerous other nonrelated causes. Drug-associated thrombocytopenia is also seen.

The combination of RA, splenomegaly, and leukopenia (sometimes in association with thrombocytopenia, lymphadenopathy, leg ulcers, and infections) defines Felty's syndrome. Felty's syndrome is also more common in patients with severe, seropositive, nodular RA. Joint infections may occur more commonly in patients with RA, particularly in those with prosthetic joints. Amyloidosis may be more common in RA because of inflammatory mediator-induced production of amyloid protein by the liver. Leukopenia and immunosuppression are seen with many drugs used to treat RA.

Vital organs are also affected in RA. Rheumatoid lung disease occurs in up to 20% of patients with RA and is characterized by pulmonary effusions, pleuritis, and possibly fibrosis. Rheumatoid lung may be associated with pANCA. Other causes of lung disorders include the therapy for RA (e.g., MTX, gold salts, penicillamine, cyclophosphamide), rheumatoid nodules, and genetic and environmental factors. Renal disease secondary to RA is presumed to be rare, but a study in 143 Japanese patients with RA revealed that 21 (15%) had mesangial proliferation glomerulonephritis (12 of whom had IgA-related nephritis), 7 had membranous nephropathy, 7 had amyloid nephropathy, and 6 had minor abnormalities.[20] Rarely, renal disease in patients with RA has been associated with pANCA. However, subclinical renal dysfunction is found, particularly in patients with progressive RA. Renal abnormalities in RA may be caused more commonly by medications (NSAIDs, cyclosporine, gold salts, penicillamine) or amyloidosis secondary to long-standing inflammation. The most common cardiac manifestation in RA is asymptomatic pericarditis with or without effusions. Heart valve dysfunction, embolic phenomena, conduction defects, aortitis, and myocardiopathy are less common. Serositis (pericarditis and pleuritis) may be more common in male patients.

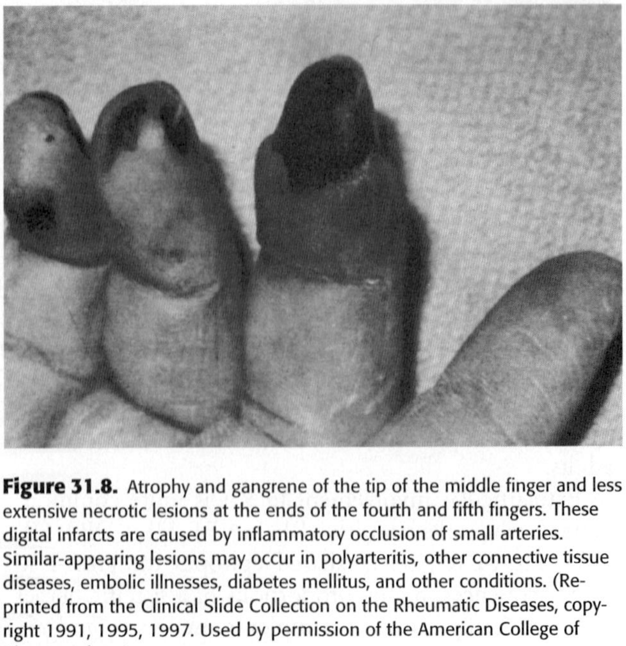

Figure 31.8. Atrophy and gangrene of the tip of the middle finger and less extensive necrotic lesions at the ends of the fourth and fifth fingers. These digital infarcts are caused by inflammatory occlusion of small arteries. Similar-appearing lesions may occur in polyarteritis, other connective tissue diseases, embolic illnesses, diabetes mellitus, and other conditions. (Reprinted from the Clinical Slide Collection on the Rheumatic Diseases, copyright 1991, 1995, 1997. Used by permission of the American College of Rheumatology.)

Keratoconjunctivitis sicca with complaints of dry eyes (xerophthalmia) and dry mouth (xerostomia) indicates the presence of secondary Sjögren's syndrome. Keratoconjunctivitis sicca is associated with a higher proportion of a specific B cell and IgA RF. Other ocular abnormalities in patients with RA include episcleritis, scleritis, and scleromalacia perforans.

Neurologic complications are common in RA. Their pathogenesis usually is related to myelopathies associated with cervical spine instability, entrapment of peripheral nerves through confined compartments (such as carpal tunnel syndrome), or ischemic neuropathies related to vasculitis often presenting as a mononeuritis multiplex. A peripheral neuropathy commonly associated with ganglioside antibodies is seen in patients with severe RA. Cyclosporine, gold salts, and penicillamine may also cause neurologic disorders.

Rheumatoid factors (RFs) are autoantibodies (IgM, IgG, and IgA) directed against the Fc portion of IgG and found in blood and synovial fluid. Plasma titers of RF are positive in approximately 80% of patients with RA but also in up to 5% of the population at large and in patients with a variety of inflammatory or infectious disorders such as endocarditis, tuberculosis, and systemic lupus erythematosus. RF is measured in both titers and units. The titers that define a positive RF may vary, but in general are 1:32 or greater. In patients with RA and a positive rheumatoid factor (RF+), higher plasma titers of RF usually are associated with more active RA. IgM RF and IgA RF are associated with more severe disease. Numerous factors are associated with the presence or absence of RF in patients with RA, as noted earlier, but HLA-DR4 is associated with RF+ RA and HLA-DR1 with RF– RA. Does seronegative (RF–) RA exist? The answer is unclear. It is more likely that secretion of RF is on a continuum in which all patients have B cells that can secrete RF but only 80% of those patients secrete a sufficiently large amount of RF. Additionally, fractionation has revealed hidden IgM RF in seronegative patients with RA.

Other antibodies found in patients with RA include antinuclear antibodies (ANAs), antifilaggrin antibodies (antikeratin antibodies and antiperinuclear antibodies), anti-RA 33 antibodies, and antithyroid antibodies. ANAs, which are autoantibodies against nuclear proteins in patients with systemic lupus erythematosus and other autoimmune disorders, are found in low titers in patients with RA. Antifilaggrin antibodies, such as antiperinuclear antibodies and antikeratin antibodies, may be more specific for the diagnosis of RA than RF, but they are not yet used clinically. Antiperinuclear antibodies are found in 45 to 60% of patients with RA. Antikeratin antibodies are found in 16% of Greeks with RA and may be associated with positive RF, HLA-DR1, male sex, and radiographic progression of RA. ANCA is seen in 5 to 20% of patients with RA but globally is unrelated to serology and severity, except for some clinical features as noted earlier. Also as noted earlier, IgG lacking galactose on the Fc component is found in RA, more often with active disease.

ESR is a nonspecific but clinically useful indicator of inflammation that correlates with synovial tissue inflammation and vasculitis. ESR is measured by placing anticoagulated whole blood in a small tube for 1 hour, allowing red blood cells to settle to the bottom of the tube, and then measuring the number of millimeters that the red blood cells have vacated. Normal ESRs are generally 0 to 15 mm/hour but vary depending on method and sex. CRP concentrations and platelet counts are nonspecific acute phase reactants that are elevated in patients with active RA and may also assist in clinical assessment. Plasma hyaluronic acid levels correlate with the number of tender or swollen joints but are not used clinically.

Joint radiographs are helpful in assessing and following up on patients with RA. Early radiographic findings include soft tissue swelling. Periarticular bone loss may occur within 3 to 4 months of RA onset. Bone erosions, bone cysts, and deformities may become evident as the disease progresses (Fig. 31.6). Radiographic classification is useful in following patients over time. Joint scintigraphy may be useful in detecting soft tissue swelling in early RA but adds nothing to the clinical examination. Magnetic resonance imaging (MRI) scans are well suited for evaluating soft tissue (such as synovial tissue), cartilage, ligaments, and changes in bone marrow but are not used as commonly as joint radiographs. The evaluation of synovial proliferation by MRI scans is more sensitive and correlates better with clinical deterioration or improvement than to an evaluation using joint radiographs.

The prognosis in most patients with RA is expected to be good, but depends on the course of the disease. Approximately 10 to 20% of patients with RA have a mild single cycle of the disease that remits spontaneously, 70 to 80% have multiple cycles of mild to moderate arthritis, and 10 to 15% have multiple cycles of progressive, severe disease. Patients with RA may experience temporary or permanent disability, considerable morbidity from medications or the systemic features of the disease, and some decrease in survival, particularly in those with more severe disease. Patients with extraarticular manifestations of RA have mortality rates two to three times higher than those of patients with no extraarticular manifestations. A common cause of death among patients with RA appears to be heart disease. Quality of life, which can be assessed by a number of questionnaires, is affected in many patients at some time during the course of the disease. A very small number of patients with RA are confined to a wheelchair or bed.

Diagnosis

The American College of Rheumatology revised the criteria for classifying RA in 1988.[21] These criteria (Table 31.3) are intended to serve as the standard in research and to aid in the clinical setting but are not intended to supersede a diagnosis of RA based on clinical findings and impressions. These classification criteria emphasize the chronic, symmetric, and small peripheral joint involvement in RA in conjunction with signs of its underlying pathophysiology. Despite these revised criteria and extensive educational

Table 31.3 ▪ Classification of Rheumatoid Arthritis Based on the 1987 Revised "Traditional" Method

The patient must meet four of the following seven criteria to be classified to have rheumatoid arthritis:
- Morning stiffness of or near joints lasting 1 hr before maximum benefit.[a]
- Arthritis, as demonstrated by soft tissue swelling or fluid, in three or more joint areas including right or left PIP, MCP, wrist, elbow, MTP, ankle, or knee joints.[a,b]
- Arthritis, as demonstrated by soft tissue swelling or fluid, in the hand joints (PIP, MCP, or wrist).[a,b]
- Symmetric arthritis in the areas noted in second criterion. PIP, MCP, and MTP joint area symmetry need not be absolute to meet this criterion.[a,b]
- Rheumatoid nodules as noted by subcutaneous nodules near bones or joints or on extensor surfaces.[b]
- Positive rheumatoid factor determined by a test positive in less than 5% of normal subjects.
- Radiologic changes of the hands or wrists including erosions or bone decalcification in or next to involved joints.

Source: Reference 17.

PIP, proximal interphalangeal joint(s); *MCP,* metacarpophalangeal joint(s); *MTP,* metatarsophalangeal joint(s).

[a] Present for at least 6 wk.

[b] Must be observed by physician.

efforts, the diagnosis of RA may be delayed 36 weeks (median; range 4 weeks to 10 years) after onset of symptoms and 18 weeks after first medical encounter.[22]

PSYCHOSOCIAL ASPECTS

The psychosocial impact of RA can be dramatic. Initially, the diagnosis may or may not be readily apparent. The patient has little control over the process and may not have a diagnosis. Once diagnosed, the disease provides a chronic pattern of inflammation along with the prospect of deformity. Many patients do not accept the diagnosis or are overly frustrated by the inability to dramatically alter the course of progressive disease. This may lead them to try numerous other modalities for treatment. There is also the hope that this is just a temporary condition.

The patient's family and friends may not be able to recognize when the patient is in pain or not feeling well. A hearty handshake from a well-intentioned friend can cause considerable acute pain and discomfort in a patient with active RA of the hands. A change in the patient's ability to perform daily functions can affect all aspects of his or her life, including self-worth, family life, occupation, recreation and hobbies, and responsibilities. Depression is common in patients with RA and may affect their perceptions of disease activity. The association between depression and disease activity is unclear except that depression is associated with loss of valued activities.[23] Fortunately, the vast majority of patients effectively deal with RA once the patient and his or her family gain a better understanding of the disease and appropriate care is instituted.

THERAPEUTIC PLAN

The goals of RA therapy are to improve or maintain current function in the patient's daily living activities, diminish progression of the patient's joint and extraarticular disease, and minimize adverse drug effects using beneficial, safe, and cost-effective means.[24] Therapy should be individualized for each patient based on the course of RA, degree of articular and extraarticular disease, concurrent diseases and therapies, age, need for relief, and a host of other factors. Nonspecific drug and nondrug therapies are used to control the acute inflammation and attempt to control the progression of the disease, but very few patients achieve a cure. Specific measures, such as surgery, are useful in correcting deformities and enhancing the ability to perform certain tasks.

Therapeutic algorithms are useful in clinical decision making. Many treatment approaches and algorithms have been used in RA, but the pyramid approach and its modifications continue to be the standard. The pyramid approach includes a series of levels of therapy, depending on the patient's disease. The first level of therapy includes the fundamental, first-line therapies needed for almost all patients and includes proper amounts of rest and exercise, appropriate diet and education, and chronic use of NSAIDs. Patients with progressive or continued active disease may progress to chronic use of second-line drugs, which are added to the first line of therapy. Patients may sequentially proceed through the list of second line drugs because of inefficacy or adverse effects and may then become candidates for more toxic or experimental therapies. Physical and occupational devices to assist with ambulation and daily living activities, intraarticular injections of anti-inflammatory agents, surgery, and treatment of extraarticular manifestations of RA are added when needed at any level.

Early in the course of disease it may be difficult to predict whether a patient's RA will follow a rapidly progressive, slowly progressive, nonprogressive, or remitting course. Therapeutic decisions are thus complicated and restricted by the currently available options. Many investigators promote approaches other than this traditional pyramid, particularly the use of second-line agents earlier in a patient's course. Others recommend a stepdown approach in early RA that begins with a combination of second-line drugs and high dosages of systemic corticosteroids but eventually decreases the corticoid dosage and discontinues one of the second-line agents.[25] This stepdown approach was associated with earlier control of arthritis and slower radiographic progression than the use of a single drug (sulfasalazine).

TREATMENT

Pharmacotherapy

Nonsteroidal Anti-Inflammatory Drugs

NSAIDs are considered an integral part of RA treatment. However, recent data indicate that NSAID use has diminished so that only 76% of patients with RA are taking an NSAID.[26] NSAIDs are used to treat acute synovitis in all stages of RA because they inhibit prostaglandin synthesis, membrane-related enzyme activities, membrane anion transport, arachidonate precursor uptake and insertion into monocyte membranes, collagenase release, and neutrophil function.[27] The D-isomer (S(+) isomer) of the propionate derivatives (Table 31.4) has anti-inflammatory activity. Subtherapeutic levels of NSAIDs may enhance prostaglandin secretion in vitro, but PGE levels in synovial fluid continue to be suppressed even after synovial levels of the NSAID drop to very low levels. NSAIDs also enhance cytotoxic and suppressor T-cell activity, which may inhibit B-cell activity. Certain NSAIDs, such as ibuprofen and naproxen, decrease T-cell responses to IL-2 by blocking IL-2 binding. Most currently available NSAIDs increase or do not alter leukotriene levels, but ketoprofen and investigational agents inhibit leukotriene synthesis and bradykinin activity. Glycosaminoglycan synthesis in joint cartilage is inhibited by sodium salicylate, but other NSAIDs are noted to inhibit cartilage destruction. The clinical significance of many of these differences is unclear.

NSAID-induced inhibition of cyclooxygenase-mediated prostaglandin synthesis appears to be responsible for many of the beneficial and harmful effects of NSAIDs. Prostaglandins are locally active components derived from phospholipids that have two major activities: regulation of organ function and reaction to damage. Cyclooxygenase-1 (COX-1) is involved in the synthesis of prostaglandins that regulate organ function (e.g., vasodilation, vasoconstriction, bronchoconstriction, bronchodilation, gastric secretion, insulin secretion).[26] Cyclooxygenase-2 (COX-2) is involved in the synthesis of prostaglandins that react to damage and result in inflammation and pain.[28] Most currently available NSAIDs are nonspecific COX inhibitors and inhibit both COX-1 and COX-2 to similar degrees.[28] Meloxicam, which is approved for use in Europe but not yet in the United States, is intermediate in COX-2 selectivity. Celecoxib and rofecoxib (which is not yet indicated for RA) are highly selective for COX-2 and do not inhibit COX-1 at therapeutic dosages. NSAIDs with increased COX-2 selectivity are more effective than placebo and as effective as other NSAIDs[29] and are expected to cause fewer effects than nonspecific COX-inhibiting NSAIDs. Selective COX-2 inhibiting NSAIDs may be preferred in select patients with high risk for adverse effects, but it is unclear whether they will be preferred over nonspecific COX inhibitors for use in all patients. The potential decrease in adverse effects of gastrointestinal ulceration and bleeding, renal dysfunction, and inhibition of platelet aggregation by COX-2–specific NSAIDs may be offset by an increase in cardiovascular events and acquisition costs of the medications.

Table 31.4 ▪ Nonsteroidal Anti-Inflammatory Drugs Used in Rheumatoid Arthritis

Class	Drug (active metabolite)	Normal Half-Life (hr)	Half-Life in ESRD (hr)	Daily Dosage (mg/day)	Doses per day
Acetic acids	Diclofenac	1–2	1–2	150–200	3–4
	Etodolac	7	NC	800–1200	3–4
	Indomethacin	1–16	NC	100–200	3–4
	Indomethacin SR	1–16	NC	150	1–2
	Nabumetone			1000–2000	1–2
	(acetic acid)	22–30[a]	39		
	Sulindac	8	NC	300–400	2
	(sulfide)	16–18			
	Tolmetin	1–5		1600–2000	3–4
Fenamates	Meclofenamate	1–3		300–400	3–4
Oxicams	Piroxicam	30–86	44	10–20	1
Propionates	Fenoprofen	1.5–4		1600–3200	3–4
	Flurbiprofen	3–6		200–300	2–4
	Ibuprofen	1–2.5	2.5	1600–3200	3–4
	Ketoprofen	1–4	3.2	150–300	3–4
	Ketoprofen SR	1–4	3.2	200	1
	Naproxen	9–17	15	500–1500	2–3
	Oxaprozin	42–50		1200–1800	1
Salicylates	Aspirin	0.2–0.3	NC	2400–6500	3–5
	(salicylate)	2–30	NC		
	Diflunisal	5–20	15–138	500–1500	2–3
	Salsalate	2–30	NC	2000–3000	3–4
	Other	2–30	NC	2400–6500	3–5
COX-2 selective	Celecoxib	11		200–400	1–2
	Rofecoxib	17		12.5–25	1[b]

ESRD, end-stage renal disease; *NC*, no change; *SR*, sustained release.

[a]Longer half-life in older adults.

[b]Rofecoxib is not indicated for use in rheumatoid arthritis but is indicated for use in osteoarthritis.

All NSAIDs are equally effective in treating RA, although some patients appear to be helped more by certain NSAIDs than others. The impression that nonacetylated salicylates are less effective is not documented by clinical studies.[27] The onset of anti-inflammatory effect of NSAIDs in RA occurs within a few days to a week (longer for agents with longer half-lives), with maximum effects seen in 1 to 4 weeks. Analgesic and antipyretic effects of NSAIDs are seen within hours. NSAIDs decrease ESR, CRP, RF, and the number of circulating activated T cells in patients with RA. Hemoglobin and hematocrit, if decreased by an anemia of the chronic inflammatory process of RA, may not increase even if the patient has had a good response to the NSAID. This minimal response of the anemia is caused by increased bleeding or limited effects on the underlying disease process.

NSAIDs are traditionally considered to be part of the background therapy for mild to late and early to advanced RA, but long-term toxicity limits their use, so many patients decrease the dosage or stop the NSAID when the response to second-line drugs is evident. Adverse effects, cost, and ease of administration are major factors in choosing an NSAID. If a patient does not tolerate or respond to maximum anti-inflammatory dosages after 2 weeks or loses response, subsequent selections can be taken from a different or the same chemical class. Less than 50% of those starting an NSAID are on that agent after 12 months.[30] Aspirin is inexpensive and may be safer than previously thought,[31] but it is still reserved for use in those not responding to other NSAIDs. Because ibuprofen is inexpensive and is available in a variety of dosage forms, it may be the preferred NSAID in the low-risk patient. The high NSAID dosages needed to treat RA increase the likelihood of toxicity.

NSAIDs generally are well absorbed after oral administration and highly bound to albumin. Plasma protein binding of salicylates is more than 95% at low levels but diminishes as the salicylate level increases as binding sites become saturated. The half-lives and dosing of NSAIDs vary considerably (Table 31.4).[27] Synovial fluid levels of NSAIDs rise and fall at rates slower than their serum levels, with synovial fluid levels becoming greater than serum levels at times proportional to their half-life. This may explain in part why ibuprofen, which has a half-life of 2.1 hours, is effective when given two to four times daily.[27] Synovial fluid levels of NSAIDs with longer half-lives generally do not exceed serum levels during the dosing interval. Most NSAIDs undergo hepatic metabolism, but appreciable amounts are excreted unchanged in urine. Glucuronidation of ketoprofen and possibly other NSAIDs may be reversed in patients with renal failure.[27] Aspirin is rapidly deacetylated in plasma to salicylic acid, which then displays nonlinear pharmacokinetics at anti-inflammatory plasma levels of 150 to 250 mg/L. Sulindac is metabolized to an inactive, renally excreted metabolite and its active metabolite. Nabumetone is metabolized to its active component. At high dosages, naproxen is unusual in that its excretion is increased and serum levels are lower than expected from the dosage increase. End-stage renal disease prolongs the half-life of diflunisal (Table 31.4). Dosage adjustments may be needed in patients with end-stage renal or hepatic disease, depending on the specific drug.

Adverse Effects

Adverse effects from NSAIDs involve many organ systems, demonstrate considerable interpatient variability, and warrant careful monitoring.[32] Indomethacin and meclofenamate are more commonly associated with severe adverse effects. Older studies demonstrated that aspirin was associated with more adverse effects than other NSAIDs, but recent studies have demonstrated a safer profile for aspirin than for nonaspirin products. This safer profile for aspirin may result from the current use of lower dosages of aspirin (2665 mg/day on average), compared with previous higher dosages (2600 to 5000 mg/day), or patient selection.[31] Nonacetylated salicylates appear to be associated with fewer effects on certain organ systems than other NSAIDs.

Gastrointestinal effects are the most common problem with NSAIDs and include discomfort, distress, nausea, vomiting, diarrhea, bleeding, and ulceration.[33] Meclofenamate has a high incidence of diarrhea. Microbleeding is greater from aspirin than from other NSAIDs. Gastric ulceration or bleeding occurs in 0.5 to 3% of patients on NSAIDs, but mucosal damage is found in up to 75% of patients on chronic NSAIDs.[33] The ulcerogenic effects of NSAIDs result in part from an increase in gastric acidity found after 1 month of NSAID therapy.[34] Celecoxib, etodolac, nabumetone, and rofecoxib appear to cause less gastric or duodenal ulceration than other NSAIDs.[33] Patients at high risk for peptic ulceration or bleeding include older adults and those with a history of peptic ulcer disease, gastrointestinal bleeding, or liver or renal disease, those on high dosages of NSAIDs, and those receiving corticosteroids chronically. There is no apparent association between NSAID-induced ulceration and *Helicobacter pylori* infection, but patients with an NSAID-associated ulcer and *H. pylori* infection should be treated for the ulcer and the infection. Misoprostol, a PGE_1 analog, protects against both gastric and duodenal ulceration associated with chronic NSAID use but is also associated with considerable diarrhea and gastrointestinal cramping. Misoprostol is contraindicated in pregnancy because it can induce abortions. Misoprostol is cost-effective in high-risk patients if the initial estimates on the rates of ulceration and bleeding are accurate. A misoprostol–diclofenac combination product (Arthrotec, 50 and 75 mg of diclofenac) provides a convenient and possibly less expensive method of drug administration in patients at risk for ulceration. Proton pump inhibitors are effective in protecting against gastrointestinal ulceration.[35] Histamine-2 receptor antagonists are less effective in preventing NSAID-associated gastric ulceration or bleeding but are useful in preventing duodenal ulceration or bleeding in high-risk patients.[33] Sucralfate has little protective effect against NSAID-induced ulceration. Histamine-2 antagonists and sucralfate diminish the dyspepsia associated with NSAIDs. Treatment of NSAID-induced gastric or duodenal ulcers includes histamine-2 antagonists and proton pump inhibitors. Proton pump inhibitors or increased duration of histamine-2 antagonists leads to higher ulcer healing rates than does a standard course of histamine-2 antagonist therapy in patients who remain on an NSAID or who smoke cigarettes.

Commonly occurring NSAID-induced central nervous effects are also common and include dizziness, fussiness, and headache. These are particularly common in older adults. The use of indomethacin is limited by the high percentage of central nervous system effects including hallucinations, dizziness, headaches, confusion, disorientation, and nightmares. Aseptic meningitis occurs rarely, mostly in patients with systemic lupus erythematosus taking ibuprofen, but has occurred with other NSAIDs and in patients with RA or other disorders.

The most common NSAID-induced renal disorder is a decrease in renal blood flow caused by prostaglandin inhibition, but interstitial nephritis, tubular necrosis, and papillary necrosis also are seen. Patients with cardiovascular conditions or cirrhosis, older adults, those on loop diuretics or high-dose NSAIDs, or those with renal insufficiency are at higher risk of NSAID-induced renal disease. These patients need increased levels of vasodilating renal prostaglandins to maintain sufficient renal blood flow and glomerular filtration. Nabumetone, sulindac, celecoxib, rofecoxib, and possibly etodolac and nonacetylated salicylates have less effect on renal prostaglandins than other NSAIDs and may be preferred in high-risk patients. NSAID-induced prostaglandin-mediated renal dysfunction generally is reversible, but chronic renal failure has been reported. Much less often, NSAIDs cause renal dysfunction as a result of papillary necrosis, interstitial nephritis, and rhabdomyolysis.

NSAIDs inhibit platelet aggregation through concentration-dependent inhibition of platelet thromboxane production. Production of vascular prostacyclin, an antithrombosis prostaglandin, may also be inhibited. Celecoxib, rofecoxib, nabumetone, etodolac, and nonacetylated salicylates have minimal effects on thromboxane or prostacyclin production. Aspirin causes irreversible inhibition of platelet aggregation that persists for 3 to 7 days, but the effect is reversible with other NSAIDs. In patients about to undergo surgery, it would be preferable to use an NSAID that does not affect platelet function. A second option would be to use an NSAID with a short half-life because its antiplatelet effect generally disappears within 24 hours after the drug is stopped. Severe aspirin toxicity is associated with hypoprothrombinemia. Agranulocytosis and aplastic anemia are rarely associated with NSAIDs. Infertility is a rare complication of NSAID use.[36]

NSAIDs also are associated with cholestatic or cellular hepatotoxicity. Aspirin, diclofenac, sulindac, and possibly other salicylates may increase the risk of liver toxicity.[27] Aspirin-induced hepatotoxicity has been associated with more active arthritis. NSAID-associated hepatotoxicity generally is reversible but may lead to chronic liver failure, need for a liver transplant, or death.

Hypersensitivity reactions to NSAIDs include bronchoconstriction, nasal polyps, urticaria, rhinitis, angioedema, and anaphylaxis. Bronchospasm and nasal polyps may be caused by prostaglandin synthesis inhibition, which is consistent with the cross-sensitivity among these drugs.[37] Nonacetylated salicylates have been suggested as safe alternatives in sensitive patients, but cross-sensitivity with nonacetylated salicylates has occurred.[38] Photosensitivity may also be associated with NSAIDs.

Drug Interactions

Drug interactions associated with NSAIDs generally are mediated by pharmacodynamic or pharmacokinetic effects. NSAIDs may diminish the effectiveness of antihypertensives (β-blockers, angiotensin-converting enzyme inhibitors) and loop diuretics because of their effects on renal prostaglandins, but the effect varies from serious to unimportant. Renal function inhibition may alter the pharmacokinetics of renally excreted drugs. Lithium levels increase after many NSAIDs other than aspirin and sulindac. Salicylates inhibit the action of uricosurics. Aspirin interacts with warfarin through antiplatelet effects and protein binding, but all NSAIDs that exhibit antiplatelet effects increase the bleeding potential in patients on warfarin. Warfarin metabolism is inhibited by celecoxib, which inhibits isoenzyme CYP2D6, and rofecoxib, which mildly inhibits isoenzyme CYP3A4. Rofecoxib also enhances midazolam metabolism, probably through induction of gastric mucosal CYP3A4. High-dose MTX may be much more toxic when used with NSAIDs, but the low dosages of MTX used to treat RA usually are administered safely with most NSAIDs. Aspirin plus MTX leads to a higher incidence of increases in liver enzymes than other NSAIDs plus MTX.[39] Acetazolamide levels are increased by aspirin, which displaces the protein binding and decreases the renal clearance of acetazolamide. NSAIDs may increase the renal toxicity of nephrotoxic drugs such as cyclosporine and tacrolimus and the ulcerogenic potential of corticosteroids.

NSAIDs may be the target of pharmacokinetic or pharmacodynamic interactions. Salicylate levels are decreased by magnesium–aluminum hydroxide combination antacids, which increase urine pH and enhance salicylate renal excretion, and corticosteroids, which increase liver metabolism and renal clearance. Cyclosporine markedly increases the serum concentrations of diclofenac, leading to the need to decrease the diclofenac dosage when the two drugs are used concomitantly. Rifampin dramatically enhances rofecoxib clearance by inducing cytochrome P-450 enzymes, and fluconazole inhibits celecoxib metabolism by inhibiting isoenzyme CYP2C9. Drugs causing gastrointestinal or renal toxicity may increase NSAID toxicity. NSAIDs interact with each other pharmacokinetically and pharmacodynamically, but only the additive toxicity is of clinical relevance.

Leukotriene Inhibitors

Inhibitors of the synthesis or action of leukotrienes have been approved for treating asthma and may be of benefit in RA. Zileuton (Zyflo), an inhibitor of 5-lipoxygenase and leukotriene B4 synthesis, at dosages of 2400 mg/day was found to be superior to placebo and ibuprofen 2400 mg/day in patients with RA.[40] Montelukast (Singulair) and zafirlukast (Accolate) are leukotriene receptor antagonists that may also be of benefit.

Second-Line Antirheumatic Drugs

Second-line agents, also called disease-modifying, disease-controlling, or slow-acting antirheumatic drugs, include antimalarials (chloroquine and hydroxychloroquine), MTX, azathioprine, sulfasalazine, injectable gold salts, auranofin (an oral gold salt), cyclosporine, tetracyclines minocycline and doxycycline, cyclophosphamide, penicillamine, and more recently leflunomide, etanercept, and infliximab. These drugs have varied activities on the immune system, but the mechanisms of action in RA remain unclear for most of these agents.

The traditional use of second-line agents has been in patients with potentially reversible progressive disease. The use of these agents in RA is increasing, with approximately 50% of patients with RA now receiving these drugs.[26] Rheumatologists are more likely than general practitioners to use second-line drugs and to use those drugs earlier in the disease in an attempt to reduce long-term joint destruction. Beneficial anti-inflammatory effects of second-line agents are seen over 1 to 6 months and may lead to remission or decreased progression of the disease in up to 5% of patients.[41,42] Second-line drugs probably diminish the progression of joint disease, but studies are conflicting. This research has been somewhat hampered by the lack of consistent drug effects and disease progression, definitive measures, and knowledge of the usual course of progression. A small case control study revealed that patients not using second-line drugs had 57% more damaged joints and 122% higher overall radiographic score than those who received such drugs did.[43] However, many studies have found decreases in progression of bony erosions with various agents over periods of 5 years or longer.[44]

In patients with recently diagnosed, early RA without progressive disease, the use of second-line agents is somewhat controversial because of the difficulty in predicting which patients will go on to progressive, erosive disease and determining whether the toxicity and cost will be offset by the potential benefits. Factors that predict which patients are at high risk for progressive joint destruction include specific HLA-DRB1 chain sequences, higher baseline ESR, first-year progression, female sex, and a combination of RF+, involvement of at least two large joints, and disease lasting more than 3 months.[45,46] High-risk patients appear to have less progressive disease with earlier, aggressive treatment with select second-line drugs or a stepdown combination regimen.[25] Large, long-term studies evaluating the use of early second-line agents have not yet been performed.

Choosing among second-line agents has become somewhat difficult because of the growing number of agents available and the complexity of evaluating relative efficacy, safety, and costs.[32] The second-line drug of choice to initiate in patients with RA depends on the patient's current and previous disease activity and therapy, duration of RA, prescriber experience, clinical pathway guidelines (if available), associated costs, efficacy, and adverse effects. In general, a patient with severely progressive or unrelenting RA despite adequate NSAID and other first-line therapy who is naive to second-line agents should be given at least one of the following: MTX, leflunomide, possibly low-dose corticosteroid, or any of these in combination with other second-line agents. However, MTX is considered the initial second-line drug of choice in severe RA by many clinicians. Although not indicated as initial second-line therapy in patients with RA, etanercept, infliximab plus MTX, and cyclosporine may eventually be found to be very useful as initial drugs in patients with severe RA. In moderately active RA, the following agents should be considered as the first agents: MTX, leflunomide, azathioprine, sulfasalazine, auranofin, and possibly minocycline or doxycycline. Mycophenolate and tacrolimus may also prove more useful as initial therapy depending on the results of future studies and use in RA. Hydroxychloroquine is useful in combinations but is effective only in suppressing mild RA. Injectable gold, cyclophosphamide, and penicillamine probably should be used only for refractory cases. MTX, azathioprine, cyclophosphamide, and cyclosporine are also useful in treating extraarticular manifestations such as steroid-resistant rheumatoid lung or vasculitis. These recommendations are based on data from individual clinical studies and collections of pooled data.

MTX, gold sodium thiomalate, and cyclophosphamide appear to be among the most efficacious second-line drugs; MTX was among the least toxic and injectable gold salts were among the most toxic.[41,42] Hydroxychloroquine and auranofin were ranked as least effective, with hydroxychloroquine among the least toxic and auranofin with intermediate toxicity. Sulfasalazine ranking varies from least effective to mostly effective, and it is intermediately toxic. Azathioprine was of intermediate efficacy and among the least toxic.[41] Penicillamine was ranked as intermediately to mostly efficacious but was among the most toxic. In other studies, leflunomide has proven to be as effective as MTX. Comparative studies on newer agents have not been carried out.

Additionally, patients generally cannot stay on these agents very long despite the chronic nature of RA. MTX is an exception. Only 50% of those starting the drug will be on oral gold (auranofin) after 10 months; on hydroxychloroquine, penicillamine, injectable gold, or azathioprine after 20 to 27 months; and on MTX after 60 months.[30] Other reports have found that 70% of patients are able to continue MTX for 5 years or more. Many agents were not included in these analyses, particularly newer agents.

Second-line agents are combined with or added to current second-line drug therapy to increase efficacy because they have different mechanisms of action without increases in adverse effects. Numerous combinations of two to four drugs such as antimalarials, MTX, azathioprine, oral and injectable gold, sulfasalazine, penicillamine, cyclophosphamide, chlorambucil, and pulse methylprednisolone have been studied.[25,47–53] However, only select regimens of multiple second-line drugs appear to be more effective than single second-line drug regimens.[47] Other regimens demonstrated greater toxicity or no additional benefit.[47] Cyclosporine, etanercept, infliximab, hydroxychloroquine, sulfasalazine, or gold salts combined with MTX appears to be superior to MTX alone.[48–50] The combination of MTX, sulfasalazine, and hydroxychloroquine also appears to be superior to those agents used alone,[51] particularly in patients with the shared HLA-DR1 epitope. A stepdown approach used in early RA involves starting with the combination of sulfasalazine, MTX, and prednisolone (60 mg/day) and then slowly decreasing the dosages of MTX and the corticoid and stopping them at 28 and 40 weeks, respectively.[25] This approach was associated with earlier control of arthritis and slower radiographic progression than the use of sulfasalazine alone. Regimens containing MTX may have better efficacy:toxicity ratios than other currently used MTX-free combinations. Auranofin, azathioprine, or sulfasalazine plus MTX may not be better than MTX alone, except when combined in patients who have lost their initial response to MTX. Another method of using combination second-line drugs includes initiating therapy with two drugs, such as MTX and hydroxychloroquine, then stopping one of them (MTX) when a response has stabilized.[52] The use of cyclophosphamide in combinations is limited by concerns of secondary tumor development and has been replaced by either azathioprine or MTX. A few regimens have been associated with reversal of bony erosions. Combinations of second-line drugs should be considered in refractory patients.

Numerous experimental second-line treatments are continually being explored in RA treatment as a result of advances in the understanding of RA pathophysiology and drug action. Plasminogen activation inhibitors, for example, may decrease the bony destruction seen in RA. Herbal remedies, such as Chinese thunder god wine, and antioxidants, such as *N*-acetylcysteine, have immunologic actions that may prove useful in RA.

Antiproliferative Agents

The antiproliferative drugs used in RA inhibit the proliferation of lymphocytes and other white blood cells in the bone marrow as a major part of their action in RA, but they have other effects on the immune system and the proliferation of other cells, perhaps including the proliferating synovium of RA. These agents are mostly anticancer drugs with antimetabolite or alkylator activity, and they inhibit DNA replication. The most widely used antimetabolites in RA include MTX and azathioprine, but mycophenolate mofetil (MMF) and leflunomide probably will see increased use in the future. Cyclophosphamide is the most common alkylator reported to have been used in RA, but mechlorethamine (nitrogen mustard) and chlorambucil (Leukeran) have been effective in treating RA according to case reports. Nitrogen mustard appears to have a rapid onset of 1 to 2 weeks. Paclitaxel (Taxol), an antimitotic alkaloid, has diminished synovial inflammation and neovascularization in animal models and has been effective in RA.

Methothexate

MTX (Rheumatrex) is effective in RA at dosages ranging from 7.5 to 20 mg orally, intramuscularly, or subcutaneously administered weekly in one dose or in three equal doses every 12 hours. An oral solution using 10 mg injectable MTX mixed in 8 ounces of water can be substituted for oral tablets,[53] to reduce costs. High-dose MTX (500 mg/m^2) followed by leucovorin rescue every 2 weeks has been of some use in patients with refractory RA.[54] The mechanisms of action of MTX include leukotriene synthesis inhibition and dihydrofolate reduction inhibition–associated decreases in proliferation of T- and B-lymphocytes and rapidly dividing (but not slowly dividing) synoviocytes. MTX differs from other second-line agents in its rapid response (as early as 4 to 6 weeks), a flare in the arthritis flare seen soon after MTX withdrawal,[55] and an increase in rheumatoid nodules during its use.[19] MTX was most effective in decreasing tender joint counts in a meta-analysis of older second-line agents[42] and appears to slow the progress of erosive RA. Patients who initially respond to MTX and then have a worsening in RA are likely to respond to an increase in the MTX dosage. MTX is contraindicated in pregnant women.

MTX oral absorption averages 70% but is highly variable, diminishes after cholecystectomy, and reportedly decreases by 13.5% over time in patients with RA.[56] Oral tablets and oral use of diluted intravenous MTX appear to have equal bioavailability.[53] MTX is found in high levels in synovial membrane and bone even after serum levels have diminished. Approximately 10% of MTX is metabolized to an active metabolite, 7-hydroxy-MTX. Biliary excretion may account for 9 to 26% of MTX elimination and 2 to 5% of 7-hydroxy metabolite elimination after low dosages of MTX. MTX clearance is lower in older adults or patients who have impaired renal function, is increased by hemodialysis, and is not altered by peritoneal dialysis.

Patients are monitored every 2 weeks initially, then eventually every 6 weeks, for adverse effects from MTX. Pooled clinical studies have revealed that withdrawals from MTX are caused by hepatic effects (10.3%), mucous membrane effects (2.6%), nausea or vomiting (2.1%), gastrointestinal effects (2.1%), leukopenia (1%), blood effects (1.5%), and diarrhea (0.5%).[42] The majority of the liver effects were elevations of liver enzymes rather than abnormalities on liver biopsy. Liver biopsies are the definitive method of detecting hepatotoxicity but are not routinely recommended in patients with RA receiving MTX because of the low incidence of hepatotoxicity and the morbidity, mortality, and costs associated with liver biopsy. An increased incidence of abnormalities in liver enzymes has been found in patients on MTX plus aspirin[39] (but not in all studies) or those with alcoholism, diabetes, or obesity. Although usually irreversible, severe liver toxicity is occasionally reversible. Sustained elevation of mean corpuscular volume in a patient treated with MTX may indicate folate deficiency and may predict MTX hematologic toxicity. Severe neutropenia, thrombocytopenia, anemia, and pancytopenia may develop with low MTX dosages, especially in older adults and patients with renal disease, hypoalbuminemia, and concomitant antiproliferative agents. MTX-induced pancytopenia may respond to pulse methylprednisolone and granulocyte colony-stimulating factor.[57] MTX causes immunosuppression and possibly an increase in postsurgical infections, but there is no consensus on whether it should be stopped before major surgery. MTX induces or reactivates infections, such as herpes zoster or Epstein–Barr viral infections, which may be followed by complications such as shingles or Epstein–Barr virus–associated lymphoma, respectively. Patients with RA have a higher incidence of MTX-induced pulmonary toxicity, particularly older adults and patients with a history of smoking, preexisting interstitial pulmonary disorders, rheumatoid lung, diabetes, hypoalbuminemia, and previous adverse effects from disease-modifying drugs.[58–60] The influence of previous pulmonary disorders in general may or may not predispose patients to this effect. MTX-induced lung toxicity begins as a pneumonitis with symptoms of cough, shortness of breath, and fever and then may progress to pulmonary fibrosis and possibly death.[61] The pulmonary problems recur upon rechallenge with MTX, with an increased risk of mortality.[61] The incidence is reportedly low but has been as high as 2%. Hypersensitivity, rashes, and vasculitis are rarely associated with MTX.

Concurrent folic acid and leucovorin administration may diminish MTX-induced stomatitis and macrocytic anemia, but leucovorin use can diminish MTX efficacy.[62] Folic acid usually is administered at dosages of 1 mg/day for 4 days per week by omitting the day before, day of, and day after MTX administration. Folic acid dosages up to 27.5 mg/week have been used. Folic acid also diminishes the risk of hyperhomocystinemia and therefore may decrease the risk of cardiovascular disease.[63] Severe MTX toxicity is reversed by leucovorin. Allopurinol mouthwashes (5 mg/mL suspension in water) have been useful in treating MTX-induced stomatitis, but patients should be discouraged from swallowing the suspension. Severe, refractory MTX-induced vomiting may respond to ondansetron.

Drug interactions involving MTX may have serious consequences. As noted earlier, aspirin is associated with increases in MTX hepatotoxicity. Salicylate and probenecid inhibit MTX excretion. However, a recent study found no clinically relevant effects of NSAIDs (aspirin, diclofenac, ibuprofen, indomethacin, and naproxen) on MTX pharmacokinetics.[64] Cholestyramine binds to MTX and enhances its excretion. Trimethoprim and antiproliferative drugs increase the toxicity of MTX. Folinic acid may reverse the efficacy of MTX,[62] depending on the dosage and timing of administration.

Leflunomide

Leflunomide (Arava) was approved for treating RA in 1998 at dosages of 10 to 25 mg/day efficacy was demonstrated in placebo- and active-control studies.[65] It appears to be as effective as MTX and has also been studied in the prevention of solid organ transplant rejection. Leflunomide is rapidly metabolized to an active metabolite (A77 1726), a malononitrilamide with a half-life of 11 to 16 days that is more than 99% plasma protein bound.[65] This metabolite inhibits B- and T-cell proliferation, antibody secretion, and cellular adhesion. Leflunomide's active metabolite inhibits nucleotide (pyrimidine) synthesis by inhibiting dihydroorotate dehydrogenase. Animal studies have revealed that a combination of low-dose leflunomide and cyclosporine suppresses chronic antigen-induced arthritis. The major adverse effects of leflunomide include gastrointestinal disturbances, weight loss, allergic reactions, transient elevations of liver transaminases, and reversible alopecia. Decreases in hematocrit, hemoglobin, and platelets are seen less often but usually do not necessitate drug discontinuation. Both efficacy and adverse effects are more common with higher leflunomide dosages. Cholestyramine and activated charcoal decrease plasma levels of the active metabolite by 40 to 50%.

Azathioprine

Azathioprine (Imuran) has demonstrated efficacy in treating RA at dosages of 1.0 to 2.5 mg/kg/day or 50 to 200 mg per day. Azathioprine has a half-life of 0.2 to 1 hour, is removed by hemodialysis, and is converted to 6-mercaptopurine, its active form. Purine inhibition by 6-mercaptopurine inhibits proliferation of lymphocytes and other white blood cells. Allopurinol inhibits azathioprine metabolism, so the azathioprine dosage must be decreased by 67 to 75%.

Azathioprine and MTX have common adverse effects. The risk of adverse effects from azathioprine has been of concern, but a postmarketing surveillance study has revealed a safe adverse effect profile in RA. Monitoring complete blood cell counts and liver function tests and examining mucous membranes every 2 to 6 weeks is still necessary to evaluate azathioprine-induced gastrointestinal distress, leukopenia, anemia, stomatitis, pancreatitis, pneumonitis, and liver toxicity. Infections and pulmonary toxicity have also been reported. Severe bone-marrow suppression is rarely seen and may be associated with deficiencies in purine metabolic enzymes.

Mycophenolate Mofetil

MMF (CellCept) has been used and approved for use in preventing transplant rejection but has also been used to treat RA at dosages of 2000 mg/day.[1,66] MMF is a prodrug for mycophenolic acid, which is a noncompetitive, reversible inhibitor of inosine monophosphate dehydrogenase and disrupts the synthesis of guanine nucleotides. MMF appears to inhibit the proliferation of lymphocytes more than other cells. In patients with RA, MMF decreased RF, swelling, and pain in patients with RA. However, only 8 of 28 patients responded in one study.[1] The drug is well tolerated in patients with RA; reversible gastrointestinal effects including nausea, vomiting, abdominal pain, and diarrhea are the most common adverse effects. However, bone marrow suppression and liver toxicity have been seen in transplant recipients.

Cyclophosphamide

Cyclophosphamide (Cytoxan) is effective in RA at dosages of 75 to 150 mg (0.68 to 3.4 mg/kg) per day but has considerable short- and long-term toxicity even at lower dosages. Dosages generally are adjusted to keep the white blood cell count within the normal or low normal range. Low dosages (50 mg/day) of oral cyclophosphamide are better tolerated and result in fewer secondary tumors than usual dosages of 75 to 150 mg/day, but efficacy is poor. Intravenous cyclophosphamide at high dosages (500 mg/m^2) every 4 to 6 weeks for six cycles may be useful in treating rheumatoid vasculitis but it is poorly tolerated, minimally to somewhat effective, and associated with arthritis reactivation soon after completion of the course in patients with refractory RA.[67]

Cyclophosphamide is inactive and converted in the liver to active metabolites, which are 56% plasma protein bound. The half-life of cyclophosphamide increases from 5 to 7 hours in normal renal function to 4 to 12 hours in end-stage renal disease. Renal dysfunction decreases cyclophosphamide metabolite excretion, leading to increased toxicity and necessitating a dosage decrease. Cyclophosphamide is removed by hemodialysis.

Cyclophosphamide is associated with short- and long-term toxicity. Leukopenia, hemorrhagic cystitis, hair loss, gastrointestinal disturbance, infertility, inappropriate secretion of antidiuretic hormone, and immunosuppression are serious effects. Hemorrhagic cystitis, a mild to severe effect caused by the direct effects of a toxic metabolite of cyclophosphamide on the urinary bladder lining, is more common with chronic oral therapy than with pulse intravenous therapy and with inadequate hydration. Immunosuppression leads to a higher incidence of parasitic, fungal, viral, and bacterial infections. Cyclophosphamide causes pneumonitis and pulmonary fibrosis. The occurrence of malignancies was four times greater in a group of patients with RA who had received cyclophosphamide than in those who had not. Other than physical findings, complete blood cell counts and urinalyses are used to monitor cyclophosphamide therapy. Cyclophosphamide interacts with other agents that affect bone marrow function.

Biologic Immunotherapy

Biologic immunotherapy is defined in this chapter as normally occurring or modified immune system components, including soluble receptors, immunoglobulins, and antigens. Corticosteroids are covered elsewhere in this chapter. These agents modify the immunologic and inflammatory response of RA in a specific manner. This section of biologic immunotherapy is expected to expand considerably and should provide more targeted and selective therapeutic options that are effective without the serious adverse effects seen with other therapies. TNF inhibitors, which include soluble TNF receptors and anti-TNF antibodies, are the first of the specific biologic immunotherapies that have been approved as treatment for progressive RA.[49,50,68,69]

Etanercept

Etanercept (TNFR:Fc, Enbrel), a recombinant human TNF receptor (p75)-Fc fusion protein preparation, was approved in 1998 for RA treatment. This preparation contains a soluble TNF-α receptor attached to the Fc portion of human IgG_1. The receptor binds TNF-α. The complex is then removed by phagocytic cells, leading to a decrease in TNF-α concentrations. Etanercept has proven beneficial in RA without significant adverse reactions or the development of antibodies against the product.[68] Subcutaneous etanercept at dosages of 16 mg twice weekly for 3 months was associated with more than 50% response in patients with refractory RA.[68] Adverse effects include discomfort at the injection site and minor upper respiratory tract symptoms. Inhibition of the action of TNF can lead to immunosuppression with subsequent development of infections or tumors, particularly with chronic therapy. Tumor has not been a problem to date, but patients on etanercept appear to have a higher incidence of respiratory tract infections. Therefore, etanercept currently is reserved for patients with refractory arthritis. Etanercept has also been effective when added to MTX therapy.[49]

Infliximab

Infliximab (Remicade), a TNF monoclonal antibody, is also approved for use in patients with RA but only in combination with MTX.[1,50,69] If it is not combined with MTX, patients receiving infliximab develop neutralizing antibodies that inactivate infliximab. Infliximab decreases in circulating TNF and decreases in IL-1, IL-6, and IL-8 secretion.

Lymphocyte Removal or Replacement

Removal or replacement of lymphocytes may also be of benefit in patients with RA. Stem cell (bone marrow) transplantation has been found to induce a sustained remission in some patients with RA and an initial remission followed by an attenuated relapse in others.[2] Total lymphoid irradiation and thoracic duct drainage have been of benefit in patients with RA.

Immunosuppressive Agents (Cyclosporine, Tacrolimus)

Cyclosporine

Cyclosporine (CyA, cyclosporin A, Neoral, Sandimmune), which inhibits helper T-cell secretion of IL-2, has been effective in RA. Initial dosages of 2.5 mg/kg/day are given in two doses, then increased to a recommended maximum of 4 mg/kg/day, but dosages up to 10 mg/kg/day have been used. It is indicated for use after MTX has failed. Cyclosporine is more effective than placebo and at least as effective as chloroquine[70,71] and is effective in combination with MTX.[48] Cyclosporine plus an oral corticosteroid may also be beneficial in treating rheumatoid lung.

Cyclosporine has complicated, variable pharmacokinetics including variable absorption, binding to lipoproteins and red blood cells, and extensive hepatic metabolism via the cytochrome P-450 system. A microencapsulated formulation (Neoral) is preferred because it provides enhanced, more rapid, and more consistent bioavailability than the older preparation (Sandimmune). However, it is not necessary to decrease the cyclosporine dosage when initially switching from Sandimmune to Neoral despite the expected increase in bioavailability. A small dosage adjustment (a 15% decrease on average), eventually may be needed after a switch to the microencapsulated product. Cyclosporine concentrations usually are not measured to monitor patients with RA because low dosages are used compared to those used to prevent transplant rejection. To interpret the measured value, the clinician must know the type of sample (blood versus plasma or serum) and assay (immunoassay versus HPLC) in addition to the timing relative to the dosage.

The use of cyclosporine is somewhat limited by adverse effects and the needed monitoring every 2 to 6 weeks. Nephrotoxicity, hypertension, infection, gingival hyperplasia, hypertrichosis, fatigue, and gastrointestinal and neurologic complaints (paresthesias) are common in transplant recipients but less common with the lower dosages used in patients with RA. The decrease in renal function in patients on cyclosporine for RA rarely leads to irreversible structural damage. Infections associated with cyclosporine include *Pneumocystis carinii,* fungal, viral, and bacterial infections.

Drug interactions with cyclosporine are numerous and involve both pharmacokinetic and pharmacodynamic mechanisms. Drugs that enhance (e.g., rifampin, phenytoin) or inhibit (e.g., cimetidine, ketoconazole, ciprofloxacin) CYP3A4 alter the clearance of cyclosporine. Drugs with renal toxicity may also enhance the renal toxicity of cyclosporine. The use of NSAIDs with cyclosporine to treat RA usually does not lead to renal toxicity, probably in part because lower dosages of cyclosporine are used in treating RA than in preventing transplant rejection. Cyclosporine increases the serum concentrations of diclofenac and serum creatinine.

Tacrolimus

Tacrolimus (Prograf, FK-506) is similar to cyclosporine in many respects. Tacrolimus also inhibits secretion of IL-2 by helper T cells, results in immunosuppression and prophylaxis against rejection of transplants, and inhibits IL-6 release. Additionally, the pharmacokinetic and adverse effect profiles of tacrolimus are very similar to those of cyclosporine. It has been studied in animal models of RA and can be expected to have effects in RA that are similar to those of cyclosporine.

Nonspecific Immunotherapy and Antirheumatic Therapy

The group of miscellaneous immunotherapies includes modalities that do not fall into the other groups because of their nonspecific or other effects on the immune system. This group includes commonly used drugs such as antimalarials, gold salts, sulfasalazine, tetracyclines, and penicillamine.

Antimalarials

Antimalarials have been used to treat RA since publication of a 1951 report of a patient whose RA improved after mepacrine was used to treat the patient's discoid lupus.[72] Chloroquine (Aralen) became widely used but has been widely replaced by hydroxychloroquine in RA treatment, although chloroquine may be more effective.[42] Hydroxychloroquine diminishes the functions of macrophages but also increases pain thresholds. Hydroxychloroquine is used at dosages of 2 to 4 mg/kg or 200 to 400 mg/day orally. Chloroquine oral dosages range from 200 to 300 mg of the base per day, but some clinicians recommend no more than 3.5 mg/kg/day. Antimalarials are used in milder disease or in combination with other second-line drugs.

Hydroxychloroquine (Plaquenil) is readily absorbed after oral administration, with peak levels in 1 to 3 hours. Hydroxychloroquine is 45% bound to serum albumin, distributes into red blood cells and other tissues, and has a half-life of approximately 40 days. Dosage adjustments are not needed in renal dysfunction because only 22 to 34% of hydroxychloroquine is excreted unchanged in urine. Chloroquine's pharmacokinetics are similar, with a half-life of 6 to 50 days and lack of appreciable removal by hemodialysis.

Pooled data from clinical studies reveal that chloroquine and hydroxychloroquine are among the least toxic of the second-line drugs. Adverse effects include gastrointestinal tract (4.6%), rash (2.3%), ocular (0.7%), and, less commonly, mucous membrane, leukopenia, central nervous system, neuromuscular, and cardiac effects.[42] Corneal deposits occur in at least 20% and symptomatic retinopathy in 2 to 17% of those receiving chloroquine, with higher frequencies seen in older adults and patients on higher dosages. Hydroxychloroquine appears to be rarely discontinued because of retinopathy at the dosage ranges listed in this section, which has led experts to question the need for complete ophthalmic exams by an ophthalmologist every 6 to 12 months during therapy. However, hydroxychloroquine may also exacerbate psoriasis and cause allergic rashes, hemolytic anemia, and gastrointestinal and neurologic effects. Chloroquine has decreased the normal response to intradermal rabies vaccine in normal subjects and may induce heart block.

Sulfasalazine

Sulfasalazine (Azulfidine) was designed in the 1940s to treat RA but only recently has been used widely to treat RA after promising studies were conducted.[42] Sulfasalazine is broken down to sulfapyridine and aminosalicylate in the gut. Both sulfasalazine and its sulfapyridine metabolite have effects against RA. Sulfasalazine decreases secretion of IL-6, immunoglobulins, and RFs in RA. It is often used in patients with mild RA but is also effective in patients with moderate to severe disease.

The adverse effect withdrawal rate from sulfasalazine is less than for gold but similar to that of penicillamine,[42] but the occurrence of serious adverse effects of sulfasalazine is lower. Sulfasalazine was withdrawn for nausea or vomiting (12.5%), skin rash (3.8%), liver effects (1.6), leukopenia (1.1%), mucous membrane effects (1.1%), fever (1.1%), anemia (0.5%), and lung effects (0.5%).[42] Folate deficiency may be common in patients on sulfasalazine and may be associated with chronic hemolytic anemia in some patients. Toxic epidermal necrolysis and drug-induced lupus are rarely seen with sulfasalazine. Monitoring for toxicity involves an examination and questioning for signs and symptoms of gastrointestinal intolerance, allergic reactions (e.g., skin rashes), and other problems.

Gold Salts

Gold salts have been used intramuscularly to treat RA since the 1920s and orally since the early 1980s. The intramuscular dosages used at first were 100 to 200 mg/week and were associated with unacceptable toxicity. The currently used lower dosages are much more tolerable. Currently two test doses, one of 10 mg then one of 25 mg, are used for the first two weekly intramuscular injections of the injectable gold salt and are followed by 25 to 50 mg/week if no problems arise. If the patient maintains a sustained response for a few months on the weekly maintenance dose, then the dosage interval may be widened to every 2 weeks, then every 3 weeks, and so on. An oral form of gold, auranofin, is effective at dosages of 3 to 9 mg daily. Auranofin appears to be less effective but also less toxic than injectable gold.[42] Auranofin is of little benefit in patients previously treated with injectable gold salts.

Injectable gold salts and auranofin (Ridaura) are 50% and 28% elemental gold, respectively. Two injectable gold salt forms are available. Aurothiomalate (gold sodium thiomalate, Myochrysine) is a water-soluble solution and aurothioglucose (Solganal) is a less water soluble suspension. Auranofin is 20 to 25% absorbed orally, but the injectable forms are poorly absorbed orally. Gold is extensively bound to serum albumin and widely distributes to kidneys, liver, reticuloendothelial system, spleen, synovial membrane, skin, hair, and nails. Skin acts as a large storage site after chronic injectable gold administration. A higher percentage of injectable gold than of auranofin is retained in body tissues. The half-lives of both forms of gold are at least 1 week. Most of the absorbed gold salt is excreted in urine, but 85% of auranofin is recovered in feces. Gold is removed by peritoneal dialysis but not by hemodialysis.

Injectable gold was discontinued because of adverse effects more than other second-line agents.[42] The reasons for withdrawal included skin rash (13%), proteinuria (3.7%), mucous membrane effects (1.8%), leukopenia (1.5%), thrombocytopenia (1.1%), gastrointestinal effects (1.3%), hepatic (0.9%) and blood effects (0.9%), and, less commonly, diarrhea, fever, alopecia, and renal, lung, and ocular effects.[42] Nitritoid reactions, characterized by flushing and syncope, may occur up to 30 minutes after an injection of gold salts, particularly with aurothiomalate. If the nitritoid reaction occurs, the patient should be asked to sit or lie down for 20 to 30 minutes after each injection or the patient may be switched to aurothioglucose, which is a suspension and is less rapidly absorbed. Gold storage in skin can lead to chrysiasis, a bronze-like appearance. Injectable gold-induced proteinuria is associated with HLA-DRw3 or HLA-B8. In some patients, gold-induced skin toxicity is associated with the presence of anti-Ro (SSA) autoantibody or with nickel contamination in patients allergic to nickel. Safe monitoring of injectable gold salts entails an evaluation of complete blood and platelet count, urinalysis, skin, and mucous membranes just before each injection. Auranofin adverse reaction withdrawal rates were lower than those of other second-line agents and included diarrhea (3.9%), skin rash (3.2%), gastrointestinal effects (1.1%), proteinuria (0.9%), and, less commonly, thrombocytopenia, leukopenia, anemia, taste alteration, nausea, vomiting, and mucous membrane, hepatic, lung, and central nervous system effects.[42] Auranofin-induced diarrhea is not altered by concurrent use of bulk-forming laxatives, except in some patients soon after auranofin initiation. Auranofin monitoring includes an evaluation of complete blood and platelet count, urinalysis, skin, mucous membranes, and the gastrointestinal tract every 2 to 4 weeks. Other organ toxicity, such as lung and liver, also warrants monitoring for either type of gold. Rarely, gold salts induce a decrease in immunoglobulin production that varies from a mild to severe immunocompromised state. Severe diarrhea, bloody gastroenteritis, proteinuria, mucositis, rash, hematologic or pulmonary toxicity, or other serious abnormalities usually indicate discontinuation of gold. Gold-induced pulmonary toxicity may respond to gold discontinuation or to systemic corticosteroids.

Tetracyclines

Tetracyclines, minocycline (Minocin) and doxycycline (Doryx, Vibramycin, Vibra-Tabs), may be of benefit in treating RA in a pattern similar to other second-line agents, with a slow onset of effect and no loss of effect shortly after discontinuation of the drug.[3–6] Tetracyclines decrease IL-6 and RF and are postulated to decrease collagenase production and therefore decrease the inflammation and destruction caused by those enzymes.[5] Minocycline 100 mg twice daily was effective as early as after 1 month of therapy in open-label and placebo controlled studies.[4,6] The major adverse effects from tetracyclines include gastrointestinal effects, dizziness, and photosensitivity.

Penicillamine

Penicillamine (Cuprimine, Depen) is effective in treating severe, progressive RA by starting at low dosages of 125 to 250 mg/day and increasing every 2 to 4 weeks to a maximum of 500 or 750 mg/day, although dosages up to 1500 mg/day have been used. Studies of penicillamine in early RA have been disappointing. Efficacy and toxicity do not correlate with serum levels. Bucillamine, a similar agent, is as effective and appears to be safer than penicillamine.

Peak plasma levels of penicillamine are seen 1 to 3 hours after administration, but only 30 to 70% is absorbed in fasting patients and less in patients recently fed or given iron tablets or antacids containing aluminum or magnesium hydroxides. Penicillamine is 70 to 80% bound to serum albumin. Approximately 2 to 8% of penicillamine is hepatically metabolized to its methyl metabolite, but the major route of elimination is urinary excretion. The half-life of penicillamine is 1.5 to 3 hours. Penicillamine is removed by hemodialysis. In patients with end-stage renal disease on hemodialysis three times weekly and RA, penicillamine dosages of 250 mg three times weekly yielded serum drug and metabolite levels that were similar to those seen after higher daily dosages in patients with normal renal function.

The use of penicillamine is limited by adverse effects, many of which increase as the dosage increases. Withdrawals from penicillamine were caused by skin rash (7.1%), proteinuria (5%), thrombocytopenia (2.5%), taste alterations (2.5%), nausea or vomiting (2%), leukopenia (1%), and less commonly fever, diarrhea, and hepatic, renal, lung, breast, and mucous membrane effects.[42] Patients who undergo poor sulfoxidation are almost times more likely to experience toxicity to penicillamine at comparable dosages than those who undergo ample sulfoxidation are, but without a difference in efficacy. Penicillamine-induced proteinuria is associated with HLA-DRw3 or HLA-B8. Penicillamine induces autoimmune disorders such as myasthenia gravis, systemic lupus erythematosus, Goodpasture's syndrome, polymyositis, hemolytic anemia, and pemphigus. Penicillamine-induced peripheral neuropathy may respond to pyridoxine. Because penicillamine is a minor metabolite of penicillin, caution should be used when administering penicillamine to penicillin-allergic patients, although it is generally considered safe. Fetal abnormalities, including connective tissue defects, may occur when penicillamine is given during pregnancy. At the initiation of therapy, patients should be monitored every 2 to 4 weeks for adverse effects by urinalysis, complete blood cell count, and examination of skin and mucous membranes. Once the patient's condition is stable, monitoring every 4 to 6 weeks may suffice. Penicillamine may chelate iron salts and lead to malabsorption of both agents from the gastrointestinal tract.

Corticosteroids

Corticosteroids have been used to treat RA by low oral daily dosages in 30 to 40% of patients, intraarticular injections in less than 10% of patients, and intravenous pulses of high dosages rarely.[26] Iontophoresis has also been used to administer corticosteroids.[73] Corticosteroids inhibit the activity of T and B cells, chemotaxis and migration of leukocytes, numbers of mast cells in rheumatoid synovium, and release of collagenase and lysosomal enzymes.

Low-Dose Oral Corticosteroids

Low-dose oral corticosteroids, at prednisone-equivalent dosages of 2.5 to 15 mg/day, can dramatically decrease the swelling and tenderness and improve the sense of well-being in patients treated with NSAIDs, just started on slow-acting antirheumatic drugs, or not responding to a second-line agent.[74] Low-dose oral corticosteroids may decrease bone turnover but not cartilage turnover. Chronic systemic corticosteroid use probably is not associated with an increase in bony erosions. However, the risk of cumulative toxic effects on the skeleton, metabolism, and other organ systems limits the chronic use and dosage of corticosteroids. MTX may enhance corticoid-induced demineralization in the lumbar spine but not in the femoral neck. A minority of patients taking systemic corticosteroids also take calcium, estrogens, or other prophylactic therapy. Calcitonin, alendronate, and supplementation with calcium and vitamin D are helpful in preventing or treating corticosteroid-induced osteoporosis.[75–77] Corticosteroids may increase the incidence of peptic ulcer and gastrointestinal hemorrhage, particularly in patients receiving NSAIDs. Hypothalamic–pituitary–adrenal suppression can be seen even with the use of low-dose corticosteroids. Low-dose oral corticosteroids are superior in efficacy to placebo and to NSAIDs in RA and appear to be acceptable if used intermittently.[78] The use of low-dose corticosteroids early in the course of progressive RA can diminish inflammation without long-term consequences if the drugs are used for a limited time.[51] An unconventional use of corticosteroids in RA includes an approach similar to patient-controlled analgesia and may result in lower average daily dosages. High-dose corticosteroids are the initial drug of choice for severe extraarticular features of RA, such as vasculitis and rheumatoid lung.

Corticosteroid Intraarticular Injections

Intraarticular injections of corticosteroids should be used judiciously, preferably into only a few joints that are inflamed to the point of considerably limiting the patient's ability to function or rehabilitate. Intraarticular injections of corticosteroids involve compounds that are insoluble salts of active corticosteroids. A needle with attached syringe is inserted into a joint space under aseptic conditions. Synovial fluid is removed and should be analyzed further for white blood cells and differential, bacteria, crystals, and other features. With the needle still in place, the syringe is changed and the corticosteroid is injected. A dosage of 2.5

to 10 mg prednisolone tebutate equivalents would be used in a small joint such as a PIP, MCP, or MTP joint of a hand or foot; 10 to 25 mg in a wrist, ankle, or elbow; and 20 to 50 mg in a shoulder, ankle, knee, or hip. These insoluble corticosteroid salts may also benefit tenosynovitis, bursitis, and carpal tunnel syndrome. After injection of the joint or other structure, brief passive range of motion or activity can be used to enhance spread of the drug, followed by a period of joint rest lasting 24 to 48 hours. Intra-articular corticosteroids may cause a crystal synovitis because they are insoluble. Joint infections are rare, but multiple injections to the same joint may result in breakdown of articular cartilage. However, joint replacement was not more common in joints receiving the highest number of corticoid injections.[79] The effects of this modality can be dramatic and may last for months to years.

Iontophoresis

Iontophoresis techniques of administering corticosteroids involve the use of electrically charged ions to assist in the transport of drug through the skin. The active, soluble corticosteroids are applied on the skin near the joint over a series of treatments three times weekly. A 1-week series of iontophoresis treatments to a knee using dexamethasone (4 mg in 1:1 water solution per treatment) led to improvements in pain and range of motion.[73] However, long-term efficacy and toxicity have not been well studied.

Pulse, High-Dose Methylprednisolone

Pulse, high-dose methylprednisolone (1 g daily intravenously for 1 to 3 days) may produce short-term benefits in treating refractory RA or in patients with severe extraarticular disease. It does not appear to have long-term effects or retard disease progression. Pulse methylprednisolone can decrease synovial fluid polymorphonuclear cells, lymphocytes, immune complexes, and CRP. Severe adverse effects to high-dose, pulse corticosteroids include short-term dose-related effects of corticosteroids (e.g., hyperglycemia, immunosuppression, sodium and fluid retention), dysgeusia in more than 50% of patients, hypotension, and the rare occurrence of seizures, cardiac arrhythmias, sudden death, and gastrointestinal ulceration or perforation.[80]

Systemic and Topical Analgesics

Systemic and topical analgesics may benefit selected patients with RA. Systemic analgesics, such as acetaminophen and opioid analgesics, generally are considered to be of limited benefit because of the inflammatory nature of this disease but may help occasionally as adjuncts to anti-inflammatory medications. Topical ointments, creams, and liniments provide some local relief. Although they are designated as topical, systemic absorption is possible and may lead to toxicity or drug interactions such as increased effect of warfarin in patients using topical salicylates. Capsaicin cream inhibits substance P and relieves the pain associated with joint inflammation, but its effects are not anti-inflammatory.

Other Adjunctive Therapy

Adjunctive therapy is needed to treat general and extra-articular manifestations of RA. Antidepressant, antianxiety, and sedative–hypnotic agents should be used when needed. The bedtime use of benzodiazepines results in improved sleep, diminished morning stiffness, and less sleepiness during the daytime. Sjögren's syndrome is treated with methylcellulose eye drops and glycerol oral solutions to lubricate the eyes and mouth, respectively. Rheumatoid nodules can be removed surgically if needed. The anemia of chronic inflammatory disease responds to decreases in the inflammation of RA or to erythropoietin administration, as long as iron stores are adequate.[81] RA-associated hemolytic anemia, autoimmune thrombocytopenia, pulmonary disease, and vasculitis generally respond to moderate to high dosages of systemic corticosteroids (0.5 to 2.0 mg/kg/day of prednisone or equivalent). Added cyclophosphamide (oral or pulse intravenous), MTX, azathioprine, cyclosporine, or pulse methylprednisolone (0.25 to 1 g/day for 3 days) may be needed in refractory cases. Refractory thrombocytopenia may also respond to the addition of danazol.

Nonpharmacologic Therapy

Rest and Exercise

Rest and exercise must be balanced. Rest spares joints and decreases inflammation, and ideally leads to repair of damaged tissues. Patients with RA and fatigue should not diminish activity completely but should be encouraged to rest on a routine basis each day. Prolonged immobility may lead to increased stiffness and diminished mobility of joints and strength. For selected patients, hospitalization with rest and possibly minor revisions in drug therapy may have dramatic results. Intensive hospitalization for 14 days resulted in a threefold improvement in RA at a 2.5-fold higher cost than no hospitalization, with the effects of hospitalization lasting for at least 2 years in some patients. Treating patients with RA in a day care treatment center appears to be as effective as hospitalization but much less expensive.

Physical Therapy

Physical therapists assist patients by developing appropriate exercise programs that decrease joint inflammation, maintain range of motion, and increase overall well-being through range of motion, cardiovascular fitness, or strength-building programs that do not overstress joints and muscles. Such exercise programs may also diminish the development of osteoporosis in patients on corticosteroids or those otherwise at risk. Exercise has been shown to improve physical function in patients with RA but does not change the number or activity of immune cells or mediators except a possible decrease in peripheral $CD4^+$ T-cell count. Physical therapists also help patients develop methods to remain more mobile and perform daily living activities.

Occupational Therapy

Occupational therapists assist in the design and use of special eating utensils, grooming aids, working aids, and other self-help aids that are useful in maintaining patients' self-reliance. Splints may be useful in stabilizing a weak joint, resting an active joint, or possibly diminishing the rate of joint destruction. Walking aids or wheelchairs may dramatically improve a patient's mobility and stability. Cold packs, hot packs, and hot paraffin wax treatments may decrease inflammation and discomfort.

Surgery

Surgery is very useful in RA to repair or replace damaged joints, fuse joints for stability, correct tendon or ligament instability, release carpal tunnel syndrome, or remove invasive synovium. Radical surgical synovectomy may be beneficial in refractory patients, particularly in those who are HLA-DRB1*0405 negative. Initial studies show that photodynamic laser therapy, which includes photosensitizing agents followed by laser ablation of synovial tissue, has been beneficial in RA.

Nutrition

Nutrition is important to help patients lose weight if overweight, but patients must have sufficient protein intake to maintain or enhance muscle mass and sufficient calcium intake to diminish periarticular osteopenia. Sodium fluoride can diminish spinal bone loss associated with RA. Calcium supplementation may also be beneficial in diminishing bone loss, particularly in patients on chronic, systemic corticosteroids. After finding that patients with RA on second-line agents had lower levels of selenium than normal subjects, selenium supplementation in patients with RA led to the use of lower dosages of NSAIDs and systemic corticosteroids.[82] Vitamin E supplementation (α-tocopherol 1200 mg/day) provides a small amount of pain relief in addition to the effects of anti-inflammatory drugs in patients with RA.[83]

ALTERNATIVE THERAPIES

Altering the fatty acid precursors of prostanoids and leukotrienes through the use of γ-linolenic acid (GLA),[84,85] eicosapentaenoic acid (EPA) and docosahexaenoic acid (DHA),[86,87] and vegetarian and elemental diets has also shown some benefit.[88,89] GLA (n-9 or ω9 fatty acids found in borage seed oil, evening primrose oil, and black currant seed oil) and EPA and DHA (n-3 or ω3 fatty acids found in fish oil) lead to the formation of anti-inflammatory or less inflammatory prostaglandins and leukotrienes than PGE_2 or LTB_4, which are derived from arachidonic acid (n-6 or ω6 fatty acid). Fish oil supplementation also decreases IL-1 concentrations and may provide sufficient relief for patients to be able to stop taking NSAIDs. However, α-linolenic acid, a precursor of n-3 fatty acids found in flaxseed oil, was of no benefit in RA. Vegetarian diets lead to decreases in RF and other inflammatory measures.[88] An uncooked vegetarian diet rich in *lactobacilli* alters gut bacteria, may also be of benefit in RA, but is difficult to tolerate. An elemental diet is a hypoallergenic diet composed of amino acids, glucose, trace elements, and vitamins. Use of an elemental diet followed by careful reintroduction of regular foods may decrease the activity of RA but is difficult to tolerate.[89] The effects of supplementation or special diets generally lead to modest benefits. Supplementation with fatty acid precursors may lead to some gastrointestinal intolerance (e.g., nausea, diarrhea). Vegetarian and elemental diets may be difficult for some patients to tolerate and may lead to deficiencies of vitamins or minerals. For patients not willing or able to take supplements or dramatically change their diet, increasing the amount of vegetables and deep sea fish and decreasing the amount of other animal fats in their diets may provide some benefit for their arthritis and their health in general.

Other nontraditional therapies abound. Patients must be cautioned about using anecdotal or unproven therapies including copper bracelets, herbal remedies, megadose vitamins, bee venom, and snake venom. Such remedies may provide relief in anecdotal reports, but few stand up to the rigor of controlled clinical study.

FUTURE THERAPIES

Advances in understanding and assessing RA, immunology, molecular biology, and the effects of currently used and investigational therapies should lead to advances in RA therapy. The goals appear to be designing therapies that specifically act against possible defects in the HLA-DR4 antigen, macrophages, lymphocytes, mast cells, or other components of the immune system in patients with RA.

Oral type II collagen (derived from chicks) in low dosages has been found to be of some benefit in treating patients with RA,[90] particularly in patients with higher concentrations of antibody to collagen. A low dosage of 20 μg/day proved to be superior to higher dosages and to placebo.[90] Other formulations of type II collagen have been effective in RA. This follows the hypothesis that low oral dosages of an autoantigen (type II collagen in this case) can desensitize patients to that autoantigen, lead to a decrease in antibodies to the autoantigen, and result in manifestations of the autoimmune disease. Adverse effects to the oral collagen were rare or not seen.

Miscellaneous other biologic agents have provided somewhat disappointing effects in RA despite initial promising tissue and animal studies. Monoclonal antibodies targeted against lymphocytes have been tested. Anti-CD4 monoclonal antibody has been somewhat disappointing in RA despite a decrease in circulating $CD4^+$ T cells (T_H cells) that is sustained until the therapy is stopped. Selective depletion of $CD4^+$ lymphocytes, except for activated/memory cells, and production of antimonoclonal antibodies may have diminished the effect of the monoclonal antibody. Campath-1H, a humanized rat anti–human CD52 monoclonal antibody that lyses helper T cells, given subcutaneously twice weekly was associated with an initial modest improvement in RA, but the effect diminished as a result of the production of antibodies to the product. Anti-CD5 antibodies and anti-CD7 antibodies have also proven to be ineffective in RA. Lymphocytes are also the target of total lymphoid irradiation, thoracic duct drainage, antilymphocyte globulin, antithymocyte globulin, and a monoclonal antibody to intercellular adhesion molecule 1. Interferon-γ and interferon-β have demonstrated some efficacy in RA in open-label studies or case reports. However, a placebo-controlled, double-blind study found that the beneficial effects of IFN-γ were equal to those of placebo, but the interferon was associated with more adverse effects.[91] The search continues for specific biologic agents that are safe and effective.

A number of other miscellaneous therapies have been tested or tried in patients with RA but can be considered to be of little use or are not approved at this time. Dapsone is used in a variety of autoimmune disorders but should be reserved for highly refractory RA because of its adverse effects. Metronidazole (Flagyl) was effective in patients with RA who could tolerate it, but the level of toxicity was unacceptable.[7] Pentoxifylline (Trental), which has some anti-inflammatory activity related to TNF-α inhibition, was associated with remission in a patient with RA but provided only pain relief when given for 1 month to patients with refractory RA. Pentoxifylline plus thalidomide was associated with some benefit but also considerable toxicity in patients with RA. Bromocriptine, an inhibitor of prolactin secretion, was somewhat effective in two small, open-label studies. Acupuncture, which provides pain relief, has been shown to decrease serum concentrations of IgG, IgM, and IgA, but not IgE. Tenidap is an experimental agent that inhibits synovial fibroblasts, T cells, and release of IL-1, IFN-γ, and TNF-α. Tenidap was more effective than placebo in patients with RA withdrawn from NSAIDs. Ciamexon and amiprilose have shown initial promise in treating RA.

IMPROVING OUTCOMES

Enhancing patient outcomes continues to be the major focus of therapy in patients with RA because of the chronic inflammation and progressive nature of the disease. Methods for improving outcomes include the proper selection of initial and subsequent therapy, particularly the use of second-line, potentially disease-modifying antirheumatic drugs early in patients with aggressive disease. However, patient education and adherence also play an important role.

Patient Education

Education and other nondrug therapies are widely used in all stages of RA. Patients should be well informed of the nature and possible progression of their disease to promote self-awareness, self-determination, and self-reliance as well as the knowledge of when to seek help from others. Family support is essential, with negative attitudes toward the patient's disease leading to less coping and adaptation and more stress. Education programs can lead to improved exercise, rest, and joint protection.

Methods to Improve Patient Adherence to Drug Therapy

Adherence is a problem in some patients with RA, but most patients are compliant because of the chronic inflammatory nature of the disease. However, the second-line agents are somewhat slow acting and patients must be routinely reminded of that fact because many may not appropriately adhere to the regimen if they do not see immediate benefits. Also, once stabilized on a therapeutic regimen, patients may not adhere to the regimen and experience an increase in inflammation acutely or over the long run. A thorough discussion, complete with explanations and realistic expectations, followed by a final agreement on the treatment course between the patient and the clinicians involved, is very important in ensuring adherence. Routine visits with a physical therapist, for example, also promote adherence with an exercise program. Alternatively, many patients have very active disease and disability but do little to seek help. They do not want to be a bother or complain too much. These patients need reassurance that it is important to try to diminish these inflammatory episodes and the potential joint destruction, discomfort, and lack of function seen with flares of disease activity.

Disease Management Strategies to Improve Patient Outcomes

As noted earlier, the most effective disease management strategies include using the basic nonpharmacologic therapies (rest, exercise, assist devices, education, and support) continually, selecting the appropriate NSAID and protective agents given the patient's other disorders, using NSAIDs at high enough dosages, using systemic corticosteroids at low dosages and only when needed, and initiating therapy with second-line agents in patients who have RA that is progressive, persistent, or highly likely to become progressive. Early aggressive therapy with second-line, potentially disease-modifying agents is currently the best way to diminish the short- and long-term destruction, discomfort, and disability associated with RA.

PHARMACOECONOMICS

Patients with RA are extensive users of health care services, with usage rates and costs that are two to three times greater than those of the general population.[16] The costs of drug therapy and the associated costs of monitoring and treating adverse effects account for up to 80% of this expenditure. Additional considerations in any pharmacoeconomic assessment include the costs of workup, diagnosis, and monitoring of the disease plus the gains in quality of life and productivity.

Each specific drug class is associated with costs associated with drug acquisition and administration and the prevention, monitoring, and treating of adverse events. The acquisition costs for NSAIDs vary considerably, with ibuprofen and aspirin being the least expensive and many new products being more than five times more expensive. However, select newer NSAIDs may also be less toxic. Although it is unlikely that the less toxic, more expensive NSAIDs will be less costly overall, they are most likely to decrease patient morbidity and possibly mortality.[92] In high-risk patients, however, adding a protective agent may prove cost-effective. Patients prescribed NSAIDs may be twice as likely to be prescribed an ulcer-protecting agent.[93] Those who develop NSAID-associated adverse effects are expected to have a 45% increase in the cost of the NSAID-based therapy.[94] A single NSAID-induced gastrointestinal adverse effect that is treated on an outpatient basis costs approximately $500 for the workup and treatment.[95]

The costs associated with chronic, low-dose corticosteroids and second-line drugs have been less well studied. The cost of drug acquisition and monitoring is low for chronic corticosteroids but high for most second-line agents. Second-line drug therapy costs (drug, monitoring, and toxicity, in 1995 U.S. dollars) differed among agents, with per patient per month estimates of $155 for auranofin and hydroxychloroquine; $185 to $225 for penicillamine, MTX, and azathioprine; and $295 for injectable gold.[96] One extreme example is that of etanercept, which has an acquisition cost of more than $10,000 per year, but monitoring costs are very low. It is unclear whether this high cost will prove worthwhile in the long term. However, this apparently high cost for more specific biologic immunotherapy may prove cost-effective if the efficacy rates and extent of response are high and toxicity remains low.

KEY POINTS

- RA is a chronic autoimmune disease of unknown cause that affects joints and other tissues and organs.
- Alterations in the immune, inflammatory, and related systems result in the tumorlike proliferation of synovial tissue and destruction of bone and cartilage.
- The variable course of RA may or may not be altered by the drug and nondrug therapies used.
- Nondrug therapies are used to help the patient cope and to maintain or correct the problems associated with RA.
- NSAIDs are used as a baseline measure to treat acute inflammation but may also have effects on the immune system and on cartilage formation and destruction. Safer NSAIDs are on the horizon.
- In patients with progressive or probable progressive disease, second-line agents are used despite a poor therapeutic ratio, inability to sustain therapy with any one agent, questionable effects on the progression of the disease, and lack of consensus on which agent or agents to use and how early to initiate this type of therapy. The current second-line drugs of choice appear to be MTX, leflunomide, or combination therapy for severe disease and those agents or others for mild to moderate RA. Etanercept and the combination of infliximab and MTX may prove to be drugs of choice in the future. Combinations and more toxic agents may be used in refractory disease.
- The release of a specific biologic agent against TNF may lead to improved therapy and development of other specific therapies.
- Extraarticular manifestations warrant aggressive treatment, particularly in patients with more severe RA.
- It is hoped that research will lead to effective, more specific, and less toxic therapies.
- Early intervention in patients with unresponsive inflammation, rapidly progressive disease, or high RF titers should diminish the relentless progression of the disease in the 10 to 15% of those who develop severe RA.

REFERENCES

1. Schiff M. Emerging treatments for rheumatoid arthritis. Am J Med 102(Suppl 1):11S–15S, 1997.
2. Snowden JA, Kearney P, Kearney A, et al. Long-term outcome of autoimmune disease following allogeneic bone marrow transplantation. Arthritis Rheum 41:453–459, 1998.
3. Tilley BC, Alarcon GS, Heyse SP, et al. Minocycline in rheumatoid arthritis: a 48-week, double-blind, placebo-controlled trial. Ann Intern Med 122:81–89, 1995.
4. O'Dell JR, Haire CE, Palmer W, et al. Treatment of early rheumatoid arthritis with minocycline or placebo: results of a randomized, double-blind, placebo-controlled trial. Arthritis Rheum 40:842–848, 1997.
5. Nordstrom D, Lindy O, Lauhio A, et al. Anti-collagenolytic mechanism of action of doxycycline treatment in rheumatoid arthritis. Rheumatol Int 17:175–180, 1998.
6. Lai NS, Lan JL. Treatment of DMARDs-resistant rheumatoid arthritis with minocycline: a local experience among the Chinese. Rheumatol Int 17:245–247, 1998.
7. Marshall DA, Hunter JA, Capell HA. Double blind, placebo controlled study of metronidazole as a disease modifying agent in the treatment of rheumatoid arthritis. Ann Rheum Dis 51:758–760, 1992.
8. Gudbjornsson B, Skogseid B, Oberg K, et al. Intact adrenocorticotropic hormone secretion but impaired cortisol response in patients with active rheumatoid arthritis. Effect of glucocorticoids. J Rheumatol 23:596–602, 1996.
9. Feldman M, Brennan FM, Maini RN. Role of cytokines in rheumatoid arthritis. Annu Rev Immunol 14:397–440, 1996.
10. Williams RC Jr. Autoimmune mechanisms involved in the pathogenesis of rheumatoid arthritis. Adv Dental Res 10:47–51, 1996.
11. Goronzy JJ, Weyand CM. T cells in rheumatoid arthritis. Paradigms and facts. Rheum Dis Clin North Am 21:655–674, 1995.
12. Boubenoff R, Roubenoff RA, Selhub J, et al. Abnormal vitamin B_6 status in rheumatoid cachexia: association with spontaneous tumor necrosis factor α production and markers of inflammation. Arthritis Rheum 38:105–109, 1995.
13. Baerwald CG, Laufenberg M, Specht T, et al. Impaired sympathetic influence on the immune response in patients with rheumatoid arthritis due to lymphocyte subset-specific modulation of beta 2-adrenergic receptors. Br J Rheumatol 36:1262–1269, 1997.
14. Calabrese LH, Wilke WS, Perkins AD, et al. Rheumatoid arthritis complicated by infection with the human immunodeficiency virus and the development of Sjögren's syndrome. Arthritis Rheum 32:1453–1457, 1989.
15. McEntegart A, Morrison E, Capell HA, et al. Effect of social deprivation on disease severity and outcome in patients with rheumatoid arthritis. Ann Rheum Dis 56:410–413, 1997.
16. Yelin EH, Felts WR. A summary of the impact of musculoskeletal conditions in the United States. Arthritis Rheum 33:750–755, 1990.
17. Pincus T, Fuchs HA, Callahan LF, et al. Early radiographic joint space narrowing and erosion and later malalignment in rheumatoid arthritis: a longitudinal analysis. J Rheumatol 25:636–640, 1998.

18. Kaarela K, Kautiainen H. Continuous progression of radiological destruction in seropositive rheumatoid arthritis. J Rheumatol 24:1285–1287, 1997.
19. Bautista BB, Boyce E, Koronkowski M, et al. Effects of second line drugs on progression or regression of rheumatoid nodules. J Clin Rheum 1(4):213–218, 1995.
20. Nakano M, Ueno M, Nishi S, et al. Determination of IgA- and IgM-rheumatoid factors in patients with rheumatoid arthritis with and without nephropathy. Ann Rheum Dis 55:520–524, 1996.
21. Arnett FC, Edworthy SM, Bloch DA, et al. The American Rheumatism Association 1987 revised criteria for the classification of rheumatoid arthritis. Arthritis Rheum 31:315–324, 1988.
22. Chan KA, Felson DT, Yood RA, et al. The lag time between onset of symptoms and diagnosis of rheumatoid arthritis. Arthritis Rheum 37:814–820, 1994.
23. Katz PP, Yelin EH. The development of depressive symptoms among women with rheumatoid arthritis. Arthritis Rheum 38:49–56, 1995.
24. Anonymous. Guidelines for the management of rheumatoid arthritis. Arthritis Rheum 39:713–722, 1996.
25. Boers M, Verhoeven AC, Markusse HM, et al. Randomised comparison of combined stepdown prednisolone, methotrexate and sulphasalazine with sulphasalazine alone in early rheumatoid arthritis. Lancet 350:309–318, 1997.
26. Ward MM, Fries JF. Trends in antirheumatic medication use among patients with rheumatoid arthritis, 1981–1996. J Rheumatol 25:408–416, 1998.
27. Furst DE. Review: are there differences among nonsteroidal antiinflammatory drugs? Comparing acetylated salicylates, nonacetylated salicylates, and non-acetylated nonsteroidal antiinflammatory drugs. Arthritis Rheum 37:1–9, 1994.
28. Jouzeau JY, Terlain B, Abid A, et al. Cyclo-oxygenase isoenzymes: how recent findings affect thinking about nonsteroidal anti-inflammatory drugs. Drugs 53(4):563–582, 1997.
29. Simon LS, Lanza FL, Pipsky PE, et al. Preliminary study of the safety and efficacy of SC-58635, a novel cyclooxygenase 2 inhibitor: efficacy and safety in two placebo-controlled trials in osteoarthritis and rheumatoid arthritis, and studies of gastrointestinal and platelet effects. Arthritis Rheum 41:1591–1602, 1998.
30. Pincus T, Callahan LF. Variability in individual responses of 532 patients with rheumatoid arthritis to first-line and second-line drugs. Agents Actions 44(Suppl):67–75, 1993.
31. Fries JF, Ramey DR, Singh G, et al. A reevaluation of aspirin therapy in rheumatoid arthritis. Arch Intern Med 153:2465–2471, 1993.
32. Anonymous. Guideline for monitoring drug therapy in rheumatoid arthritis. Arthritis Rheum 39:723–731, 1996.
33. Lichtenstein DR, Syngal S, Wolfe MM. Nonsteroidal antiinflammatory drugs and the gastrointestinal tract: a double edged sword. Arthritis Rheum 38:5–18, 1995.
34. Savarino V, Mela GS, Zentilin P, et al. Effect of one-month treatment with nonsteroidal antiinflammatory drugs (NSAIDs) on gastric pH of rheumatoid arthritis patients. Dig Dis Sci 43:459–463, 1998.
35. Hawkey CJ, Karrasch JA, Szczepanski L, et al. Omeprazole compared with misoprostol for ulcers associated with nonsteroidal antiinflammatory drugs. Omeprazole versus Misoprostol for NSAID-Induced Ulcer Management (OMNIUM) Study Group. N Engl J Med 338:727–734, 1998.
36. Akil M, Amos RS, Stewart P. Infertility may sometimes be associated with NSAID consumption. Br J Rheumatol 35:76–78, 1996.
37. Szczeklik A, Gryglewski RJ, Czerniawska-Mysik G. Relationship of inhibition of prostaglandin biosynthesis by analgesics to asthma attacks in aspirin-sensitive patients. BMJ 1:67–69, 1975.
38. Chudwin DS, Strub M, Golden HE, et al. Sensitivity to non-acetylated salicylates in a patient with asthma, nasal polyps, and rheumatoid arthritis. Ann Allergy 57:133–134, 1986.
39. Fries JF, Singh F, Lenert L, et al. Aspirin, hydroxychloroquine, and hepatic enzyme abnormalities with methotrexate in rheumatoid arthritis. Arthritis Rheum 33:1611–1619, 1990.
40. Weinblatt ME, Kremer JM, Coblyn JS, et al. Zileutin, a 5-lipoxygenase inhibitor, in rheumatoid arthritis. J Rheumatol 19:1537–1541, 1992.
41. Furst DE. Rational use of disease-modifying antirheumatic drugs. Drugs 39:19–37, 1990.
42. Felson DT, Anderson JJ, Meenan RF. The comparative efficacy and toxicity of second-line drugs in rheumatoid arthritis: results of two metaanalyses. Arthritis Rheum 33:1449–1461, 1990.
43. Abu-Shakra M, Toker R, Flusser D, et al. Clinical and radiographic outcomes of rheumatoid arthritis patients not treated with disease-modifying drugs. Arthritis Rheum 41:1190–1195, 1998.
44. Ferraccioli GF, Della Casa-Alberighi O, Marubini E, et al. Is the control of disease progression within our grasp? Review of the GRISAR study. Br J Rheumatol 35(Suppl 2):8–13, 1996.
45. Fex E, Jonsson K, Johnson U, et al. Development of radiographic damage during the first 5–6 yr of rheumatoid arthritis. A prospective follow-up study of a Swedish cohort. Br J Rheumatol 35:1106–1115, 1996.
46. Brennan P, Harrison B, Barrett E, et al. A simple algorithm to predict the development of radiological erosions in patients with early rheumatoid arthritis: prospective cohort study. BMJ 313:471–476, 1996.
47. Felson DT, Anderson JJ, Meenan RF. The efficacy and toxicity of combination therapy in rheumatoid arthritis: a meta-analysis. Arthritis Rheum 37:1487–1491, 1994.
48. Stein CM, Pincus T, Yocum D, et al. Combination treatment of severe rheumatoid arthritis with cyclosporine and methotrexate for forty-eight weeks: an open-label extension study. The Methotrexate–Cyclosporine Combination Study Group. Arthritis Rheum 40:1843–1851, 1997.
49. Weinblatt ME, Kremer JM, Bankhurst AD, et al. A trial of etanercept, a recombinant tumor necrosis factor receptor:Fc fusion protein, in patients with rheumatoid arthritis receiving methotrexate. N Engl J Med 340:253–259, 1999.
50. Maini RN, Breedveld FC, Kalden JR, et al. Therapeutic efficacy of multiple infusions of anti-tumor necrosis factor alpha monoclonal antibody combined with low-dose methotrexate in rheumatoid arthritis. Arthritis Rheum 41(9): 1552–1563, 1998.
51. Verhoeven AC, Boers M, Tugwell P. Combination therapy in rheumatoid arthritis: updated systematic review. Br J Rheumatol 37(6):612–619, 1998.
52. Clegg DO, Dietz F, Duffy J, et al. Safety and efficacy of hydroxychloroquine as maintenance therapy for rheumatoid arthritis after combination therapy with methotrexate and hydroxychloroquine. J Rheumatol 24:1896–1902, 1997.
53. Marshall PS, Gertner E. Oral administration of an easily prepared solution of injectable methotrexate diluted in water: a comparison of serum concentrations vs methotrexate tablets and clinical utility. J Rheumatol 23:455–458, 1996.
54. Shiroky JB, Neville C, Skelton JD. High dose intravenous methotrexate for refractory rheumatoid arthritis. J Rheumatol 19:247–251, 1992.
55. Kremer JM, Rynes RI, Bartholomew LE. Severe flare of rheumatoid arthritis after discontinuation of long-term methotrexate therapy: double-blind study. Am J Med 82:781–786, 1987.
56. Hamilton RA, Kremer JM. Why intramuscular methotrexate may be more efficacious than oral dosing in patients with rheumatoid arthritis. Br J Rheumatol 36:86–90, 1997.
57. Kondo H, Date Y. Benefit of simultaneous rhG-CSF and methylprednisolone "pulse" therapy for methotrexate-induced bone marrow failure in rheumatoid arthritis. Int J Hematol 65:159–163, 1997.
58. Ohosone Y, Okano Y, Kameda H, et al. Clinical characteristics of patients with rheumatoid arthritis and methotrexate induced pneumonitis. J Rheumatol 24:2299–2303, 1997.
59. Alarcon GS, Kremer JM, Macaluso M, et al. Risk factors for methotrexate-induced lung injury in patients with rheumatoid arthritis. A multicenter, case-control study. Methotrexate–Lung Study Group. Ann Intern Med 127(5):356–364, 1997.
60. Saag KG, Kolluri S, Koehnke RK, et al. Rheumatoid arthritis lung disease. Determinants of radiographic and physiologic abnormalities. Arthritis Rheum 39:1711–1719, 1996.
61. Kremer JM, Alarcon GS, Weinblatt ME, et al. Clinical, laboratory, radiographic, and histopathologic features of methotrexate-associated lung injury in patients with rheumatoid arthritis: a multicenter study with literature review. Arthritis Rheum 40:1829–1837, 1997.
62. Ortiz Z, Shea B, Suarez-Almazor ME, et al. The efficacy of folic acid and folinic acid in reducing methotrexate gastrointestinal toxicity in rheumatoid arthritis. A metaanalysis of randomized controlled trials. J Rheumatol 25:36–43, 1998.
63. Morgan SL, Baggott JE, Lee JY, et al. Folic acid supplementation prevents deficient blood folate levels and hyperhomocystinemia during longterm, low dose methotrexate therapy for rheumatoid arthritis: implications for cardiovascular disease prevention. J Rheumatol 25:441–446, 1998.
64. Iqbal MP, Baig JA, Ali AA, et al. The effects of non-steroidal anti-inflammatory drugs on the disposition of methotrexate in patients with rheumatoid arthritis. Biopharm Drug Disp 19:163–167, 1998.
65. Mladenovic V, Domljan Z, Rozman B, et al. Safety and effectiveness of leflunomide in the treatment of patients with active rheumatoid arthritis. Results of a randomized, placebo-controlled, phase II study. Arthritis Rheum 38:1595–1603, 1995.
66. Goldblum R. Therapy of rheumatoid arthritis with mycophenolate mofetil. Clin Exp Rheumatol 11(Suppl 8):S117–S119,1993.
67. Lacki JK, Leszczynski P, Mackiewicz SH. Intravenous cyclophosphamide combined with methylprednisolone in the treatment of severe refractory rheumatoid arthritis: the effect on lymphocytes. J Invest Allergol Clin Immunol 6:232–236, 1996.
68. Moreland LW, Baumgartner SW, Schiff MH, et al. Treatment of rheumatoid arthritis with a recombinant human tumor necrosis factor receptor (p75)-Fc fusion protein. N Engl J Med 337:141–147, 1997.

69. Kalden-Nemeth D, Grebmeier J, Antoni C, et al. NMR monitoring of rheumatoid arthritis patients receiving anti-TNF-alpha monoclonal antibody therapy. Rheumatol Int 16:249–255, 1997.
70. Landewé RBM, Goei Thé HS, van Rijthoven AWAM, et al. A randomized, double-blind, 24-week controlled study of low-dose cyclosporine versus chloroquine for early rheumatoid arthritis. Arthritis Rheum 37:637–643, 1994.
71. van den Borne BE, Landewe RB, The HS, et al. Low dose cyclosporine in early rheumatoid arthritis: effective and safe after two years of therapy when compared with chloroquine. Scand J Rheumatol 25:307–316, 1996.
72. Page F. Treatment of lupus erythematosus with mepacrine. Lancet 2:755–758, 1951.
73. Li LC, Scudds RA, Heck CS, et al. The efficacy of dexamethasone iontophoresis for the treatment of rheumatoid arthritic knees: a pilot study. Arthritis Care Res 9:126–132, 1996.
74. Saag KG, Criswell LA, Sems KM, et al. Low-dose corticosteroids in rheumatoid arthritis. A meta-analysis of their moderate-term effectiveness. Arthritis Rheum 39:1818–1825, 1996.
75. Buckley LM, Leib ES, Cartularo KS, et al. Calcium and vitamin D_3 supplementation prevents bone loss in the spine secondary to low-dose corticosteroids in patients with rheumatoid arthritis. A randomized, double-blind, placebo-controlled trial. Ann Intern Med 125:961–968, 1996.
76. Kotaniemi A, Piirainen H, Paimela L, et al. Is continuous intranasal salmon calcitonin effective in treating axial bone loss in patients with active rheumatoid arthritis receiving low dose glucocorticoid therapy? J Rheumatol 23:1875–1879, 1996.
77. Saag KG, Emkey R, Schnitzer TJ, et al. Alendronate for the prevention and treatment of glucocorticoid-induced osteoporosis. Glucocorticoid-Induced Osteoporosis Intervention Study Group. N Engl J Med 339:292–299, 1998.
78. Gotzsche PC, Johansen HK. Meta-analysis of short-term low dose prednisolone versus placebo and non-steroidal anti-inflammatory drugs in rheumatoid arthritis. BMJ 316:811–818, 1998.
79. Roberts WN, Babcock EA, Breitbach SA, et al. Corticosteroid injection in rheumatoid arthritis does not increase rate of total joint arthroplasty. J Rheumatol 23:1001–1004, 1996.
80. Baethge BA, Lidsky MD, Goldberg JW. A study of adverse effects of high-dose intravenous (pulse) methylprednisolone therapy in patients with rheumatic disease. Ann Pharmacother 26:316–320, 1992.
81. Pincus T, Olsen NJ, Russell IJ, et al. Multicenter study of recombinant human erythropoietin in correction of anemia in rheumatoid arthritis. Am J Med 89:161–168, 1990.
82. Heinle K, Adam A, Gradl M, et al. [Selenium concentration in erythrocytes of patients with rheumatoid arthritis. Clinical and laboratory chemistry infection markers during administration of selenium]. [German] Med Klinik 92(Suppl 3):29–31, 1997.
83. Edmonds SE, Winyard PG, Guo R, et al. Putative analgesic activity of repeated oral doses of vitamin E in the treatment of rheumatoid arthritis. Results of a prospective placebo controlled double blind trial. Ann Rheum Dis 56:649–655, 1997.
84. Leventhal LJ, Boyce EG, Zurier RB. Treatment of rheumatoid arthritis with gamma-linolenic acid. Ann Intern Med 119:867–873, 1993.
85. Leventhal LJ, Boyce EG, Zurier RB. Treatment of rheumatoid arthritis with blackcurrant seed oil. Br J Rheumatol 33:847–852, 1994.
86. Fortin PR, Lew RA, Liang MH, et al. Validation of a meta-analysis: the effects of fish oil in rheumatoid arthritis. J Clin Epidemiol 48:1379–1390, 1995.
87. Ariza-Ariza R, Mestanza-Peralta M, Cardiel MH. Omega-3 fatty acids in rheumatoid arthritis: an overview. Semin Arthritis Rheum 27:366–370, 1998.
88. Kjeldsen-Kragh J, Mellbye OJ, Haugen M, et al. Changes in laboratory variables in rheumatoid arthritis patients during a trial of fasting and one-year vegetarian diet. Scand J Rheumatol 24:85–93, 1995.
89. Kavanaghi R, Workman E, Nash P, et al. The effects of elemental diet and subsequent food reintroduction on rheumatoid arthritis. Br J Rheumatol 34:270–273, 1995.
90. Barnett ML, Kremer JM, St Clair EW, et al. Treatment of rheumatoid arthritis with oral type II collagen. Results of a multicenter, double-blind, placebo-controlled trial. Arthritis Rheum 41:290–297, 1998.
91. Veys EM, Menkes CJ, Emery P. A randomized, double-blind study comparing twenty-four-week treatment with recombinant interferon-gamma versus placebo in the treatment of rheumatoid arthritis. Arthritis Rheum 40:62–68, 1997.
92. McCabe CJ, Akehurst RL, Kirsch J, et al. Choice of NSAID and management strategy in rheumatoid arthritis and osteoarthritis. Pharmacoeconomics 14(2): 191–199, 1998.
93. Smalley WE, Griffin MR. The risks and costs of upper gastrointestinal disease attributable to NSAIDs. Gastroenterol Clin North Am 25(2):373–396, 1996.
94. Bloom BS. Direct medical costs of disease and gastrointestinal side effects during treatment for arthritis. Am J Med 84(Suppl 2A):20–24, 1988.
95. Burke TA, Triadafilopoulos G, Kaye BR. Costs of NSAID-induced nonhospitalized gastrointestinal discomfort among arthritis patients: a retrospective claims analysis coupled with expert opinion. Pharmacotherapy 19(4):497, 1999.
96. Prashker MJ, Meenan RF. The total costs of drug therapy for rheumatoid arthritis: a model based on costs of drug, monitoring, and toxicity. Arthritis Rheum 38:318–325, 1995.

CHAPTER 32

OSTEOARTHRITIS

Amy L. Whitaker and Ralph E. Small

DEFINITION

Osteoarthritis (OA) is the most common form of arthritis and is a major cause of morbidity and disability, especially among the older population.[1] OA creates more dependency in walking, climbing stairs, and other activities involving the lower extremities than any other disease which affects older adults.[2] The management of OA is an economic burden on the health care system. The cost of managing OA in the United States is estimated to be $15.5 billion dollars, three times the cost of managing rheumatoid arthritis.[3] More than half of these costs are indirect; they are due to time lost from work.

OA is a disease that affects mainly the weight-bearing joints of the peripheral and axial skeleton. This leads to pain, decreased range of motion, deformities, and progressive disability. Other terms are often used to describe OA such as degenerative joint disease, hypertrophic arthritis, or osteoarthrosis. These terms focus on a single aspect of the disease rather than on the entire disease process; therefore, it is difficult to state a single definition. A group of health care professionals specializing in OA defined OA as a group of overlapping distinct diseases, which may have different etiologies but have similar biologic, morphologic, and clinical outcomes. The disease processes affect not only the articular cartilage, but involve the entire joint, including the subchondral bone, ligaments, capsule, synovial membrane, and periarticular muscles. Ultimately the articular cartilage deteriorates with fibrillation, fissures, ulceration, and full-thickness loss of the joint surface.[4]

TREATMENT GOALS: OSTEOARTHRITIS

- Monitoring and goals of treatment for patients with OA are individualized. It is important to consider patient age, concurrent disease states, and the extent of joint involvement when establishing the patient's goals.
- Goals of therapy for patients with OA could include[5,6]:
  - control of pain
  - minimization of disability
  - decrease in joint stiffness
  - maintenance of mobility and functioning
  - maintenance or improvement of quality of life
  - education of patients and family members about OA and its therapies

EPIDEMIOLOGY

The etiology of OA remains unknown; however, several theories have been developed to explain the pathogenesis of OA. Systemic and local factors have been identified that may contribute to the likelihood of a joint developing OA.[7,8] Systemic factors include age, sex, and genetic predisposition. It is believed that these systemic factors make the cartilage more susceptible to daily injury and less efficient with respect to repair. Systemic factors may alter the effects of growth factor and cytokines that contribute to the development of cartilage matrix. An example of such a change would be the decreased responsiveness of chondrocytes to growth factor that stimulates repair as a person ages. Other factors may increase deterioration of cartilage through increased activity of matrix metalloproteinases and collagenolytic enzymes. With the systemic component in place, local factors such as repetitive joint injury, obesity, muscle weakness, and joint deformity begin to cause joint breakdown.

Approximately 60 to 80% of people older than age 55 have radiographic evidence of OA.[9] Many of these patients will experience significant pain and disability.[9] The prevalence and incidence of OA increase with advancing age. Men have a higher prevalence and incidence of OA than women before the age of 50; however, after age 50, women have a higher prevalence and incidence.[10] It is believed that the increased incidence of OA in older women is a result of postmenopausal estrogen deficiency. The incidence and prevalence of OA do plateau after age 80 for both men and women.[11]

The development of OA in one joint is associated strongly with the development of OA in other joints throughout the body.[12] In patients who have OA of the hand, involvement within various hand joints (distal interphalangeal, carpometacarpal, and wrist joints) is more likely than co-occurrence in the hands and knees or in the hands and hips.

Children of parents who developed OA are at increased risk of developing OA themselves, especially if the onset of OA in the parent was in middle age or earlier, or the disease was polyarticular in nature.[10] A mutation involving type II procollagen has been discovered in families in which there is an extensive history of early-onset severe OA. The application of this genetic finding and the development of OA in the general population are still being examined.[13] Inheritance plays an important role in the development of OA of the hand with a greater than 50% occurrence associated with a family history. In OA of the knee the percentage is smaller, partially because OA develops more as a function of repeated mechanical injury to the joint.[14,15]

Suggestions that subchondral bone deformations protect articular cartilage from damage during impact loading of the joint[16] and findings that osteoporosis and OA were inversely related in more than 80% of the cross-sectional studies reviewed[17] reveal a lower than expected rate of OA in patients with osteoporosis.[18] Additionally, patients with OA have a higher bone density than age-matched control subjects.[19] Increased bone density and OA are both linked to obesity; however, the association of OA with high bone density is independent of body mass index.[20] This increase in bone density is believed to be linked to the presence of circulating bone growth factor and the formation of osteophytes.

Increased body weight has been closely associated with the development of OA of the knee and less strongly for OA of the hip.[10] Weight is believed to act via two mechanisms to cause OA. First, increased weight on the body increases the amount of force across the weight-bearing joints, which may cause cartilage breakdown.[21] Second, excess adipose tissue may increase the presence of metabolic components such as hormones and growth factor, which affect cartilage or bone in such a way to predispose to the development of OA.[10] Weight change also impacts the risk of developing OA. In women who were considered obese, a weight loss of 11 pounds was shown to decrease the risk of developing symptomatic OA of the knee by 50%.[22]

Major injury to the joint or surrounding tissue is a common cause of OA. Injury increases the stress on a joint and the surrounding cartilage and leads to the progressive changes associated with OA.[10] In the Framingham study, men with a history of major knee injury (cruciate ligament damage or meniscal tears) had a five to six times greater risk of developing OA of the knee than those without knee injury. For women, the risk was greater than 3-fold.[23] Development of OA has also been associated with repetitive joint use. Occupations such as farming, mill working, moving, and mining place repeated stress on the hips, hands, and knees. Several studies have indicated a high correlation and increased risk of developing OA in persons working in these professions.[10] Athletic activities have also been examined for the risk of developing OA. The effect of sports is difficult to assess because major injury may occur to athletes during sporting events. The effects of endurance, high-intensity, and high-impact activity on the development of OA is difficult to establish; however, studies have indicated that athletes are at increased risk of developing OA, especially in weight-bearing joints.[24,25] Soccer players and weight lifters have been identified as having an increased risk of developing premature OA of the knee. [26] This risk may be due to knee injuries associated with soccer or an increase in body mass seen in weight lifters. Participants in sports that involve repetitive nontraumatic loading (e.g. running, jogging, or shooting) have a small risk of developing premature OA.[26]

PATHOPHYSIOLOGY

OA is no longer considered a disease of aging and wear and tear on the joint, but rather a condition that is dynamic in nature. It involves not only biomechanical forces, but also inflammatory, biochemical, and immunologic components. Changes seen in OA are visible not only in the articular cartilage and associated joint, but also in subchondral bone.[1] Pathologic changes within the joint may be reparative, rather than destructive, because normal function of the joint is trying to be maintained.[1]

Normal cartilage dissipates the force and stress caused by weight bearing, owing to the unique elasticity and compressibility of its molecular components.[27] Within the diarthrodial joint, cartilage provides a low friction surface that covers both the concave and convex ends of the bone. Two essential roles of joint cartilage include the ability to promote joint stability during use and to distribute load across the joint, thereby preventing concentrations of stress within the joint. Upon weight bearing at the joint, cartilage is compressed (up to 40%), providing a large contact area that disperses the force uniformly to the underlying bone. Because of the relative thinness of the cartilage layer (1 to 4 mm), other shock-absorbing mechanisms must be in place to protect the joint.

Efficient functioning of the diarthrodial joint and its components is greatly impaired in OA. Changes that occur within the cartilage matrix include increased water and proteoglycan content. Although an exact mechanism is not known, this is related to a breakdown within the collagen fibers and release of proteoglycans. The cartilage then increases its hydration and thickens. Owing to disruption of the cartilage matrix, metalloproteinases are released, which degrade proteoglycans and initiate the repair process within the joint. The increase in degradation stimulates chondrocyte activity; however, the capacity of chondrocyte proliferation is limited and proteoglycan degradation continues while water content increases. The resulting cartilage is thin and shows signs of softening, fibrillation, and ulceration on the surface.

Significant changes also occur within the subchondral bone as OA progresses. The destruction of protective cartilage leads to exposure of underlying bone and abrasion within the joint. As the cartilage layer is completely eroded away, dense, smooth bone is exposed. This grinding motion stimulates osteoclast/osteoblast activity, and bone resorption and vascular changes begin to occur. Without cartilage, dispersion of weight across the joint no longer occurs, thereby leading to microfractures and cysts in the subchondral plate. New bone is formed to help repair the fracture at the joint margin, thus leading to the formation of osteophytes. Formation of these bony projections may be an attempt by the body to repair and stabilize the joint; however, this leads to further disfiguration and friction within the joint.

Joint capsule and synovium changes occur secondary to OA. The release of matrix components, as well as bony formations, leads to inflammation within the synovium. This may be a prostaglandin-mediated process or an immune response to cartilage antigens. The degree of inflammation within the joint is significantly less than that seen in rheumatoid arthritis.

CLINICAL PRESENTATION AND DIAGNOSIS

Signs and Symptoms

The clinical presentation of OA depends upon the duration of disease, joints affected, and the severity of joint involvement. Pain is a common finding among patients with OA and occurs early in the disease process. Initially, patients experience pain only upon use of the joint and describe it as dull and aching. Relief is achieved when the joint is at rest or when weight is removed. However, as OA progresses, the pain becomes constant and increases in severity. The pain may vary for patients as changes in weather or barometric pressure occur. Because articular cartilage is aneural, pain arises from other structures such as microfractures in subchondral bone, synovitis, stretching of the joint capsule due to muscle spasm or joint instability, hypertension within the bone marrow related to thickening of subchondral bone, and stretched nerve endings around osteophytes.[28] Other factors such as anxiety, depression, muscle weakness, and physical demands (either occupational or physiologic) also contribute to pain in OA.[29]

Joint stiffness is another complaint that is often expressed by patients with OA. This stiffness, unlike that in patients with rheumatoid arthritis, is relatively short in duration.[29] Stiffness is related to periods of inactivity and resolves upon movement of the joint. In the morning, a patient with OA may awaken with joint stiffness, which resolves within 30 minutes, whereas a patient with rheumatoid arthritis may have stiffness that persists for several hours after awakening. As OA progresses, quick recovery from joint stiffness is slowed. Stiffness may also worsen with changes in weather or barometric pressure.

Crepitus, or joint "cracking" and "popping," is related to irregularities that develop on the joint surface and loss of cartilage within the joint. This is experienced when the joint is moved and most commonly occurs in OA of the knee.[29] Crepitus may not only be felt by the patient but may also be heard at times. Development of bony proliferations leads to the development of joint enlargement. Synovitis and swelling of the joint capsule may also lead to the appearance of an enlarged joint. Any warmth, redness, or tenderness associated with enlargement of a joint should be evaluated for the presence of inflammation.

Joint deformity is another common finding in OA, especially as the disease advances. Physical examination of a patient with OA provides more information regarding the physical presentation of disease and the extent of deformity. OA involvement with the hand typically affects the distal and proximal interphalangeal (DIP and PIP) and first carpometacarpal joints. Heberden's (most common) and Bouchard's nodes, osteophytes on the DIP and PIP, respectively, are commonly seen joint deformities. Isolation of knee pain and symptoms is important, because it allows the practitioner to identify the specific area of the knee that is involved. Bowlegged deformities are associated with the medial region whereas knock-knee deformities correspond to lateral involvement. In patients with OA of the hip, as well as the knee, the development of a limp is a source of concern. This may be caused by either changes within the joint or compensation of surrounding muscle due to instability or muscle atrophy.

There are few laboratory changes that occur in patients with OA. Erythrocyte sedimentation rate, electrolyte and hematologic markers, and urinalysis are generally found to be within normal limits. Patients will not have a positive test result for rheumatoid factor, and analysis of synovial fluid may indicate the presence of mild leukocytosis (<2000 white blood cells/mm^3). This contrasts to the laboratory findings for patients with rheumatoid arthritis.

Diagnosis

When diagnosing OA, many factors must be considered including a careful evaluation of the patient's history, physical examination of any affected joint(s), and radiographic findings. A complete evaluation of a patient with OA would include classification of the disease, identification of the joint(s) involved, radiologic and clinical staging, notation of any physical deformities (contracture or atrophy), and assessment of the functional capacity of the patient.[27]

Classification of OA clinically is beneficial for understanding the underlying pathogenesis of the disease. OA

Table 32.1 ▪ American College of Rheumatology Classification Criteria for Osteoarthritis of the Hip

Traditional format
Hip pain **and** at least 2 of the following 3 items:
Erythrocyte sedimentation rate <20 mm/hr
Radiographic femoral or acetabular osteophytes
Radiographic joint space narrowing
Classification tree
Hip pain **and** radiographic femoral or acetabular osteophytes
Or
Hip pain **and** radiographic joint space narrowing **and** erythrocyte sedimentation rate <20 mm/hr

Source: Reference 5.

Table 32.2 ▪ American College of Rheumatology Classification Criteria for Osteoarthritis of the Knee

Traditional format
Knee pain **and** radiographic osteophytes **and** at least 1 of the following 3 items:
Age >50 yr
Morning stiffness ≤ 30 min in duration
Crepitus on motion
Classification tree
Knee pain **and** radiographic osteophytes
Or
Knee pain **and** age ≥ 40 yr **and** morning stiffness ≤ 30 min in duration **and** crepitus on motion

Source: Reference 41.

can be divided into either primary or secondary forms.[30] The cause of primary OA is not clearly understood. Development may be linked to either thickening of the cartilage and sclerosis of the subchondral bone, which damages the shock-absorbing capabilities of the joint, or imbalance of hormonal and metabolic control in cartilage formation/degradation, leading initially to cartilage hyperplasia and later to increased breakdown of cartilage.[31] Secondary OA may be caused by overuse/repetitive use of the joint, trauma, inflammatory joint disease, metabolic processes that may weaken cartilage, or congenital/acquired anatomical deformities.[32] To further aid in the classification of OA, the American College of Rheumatology (ACR) has developed criteria, which review clinical, laboratory, and radiographic findings seen in OA, as well as location of joint involvement[33–35] (Tables 32.1 and 32.2).

Radiographic evaluation is a necessity for diagnosing OA; however, the need for comparative x-rays, as well as reference standards, imposes limitations on the interpretation of radiographs.[36] With disease progression, joint space narrowing due to cartilage degeneration, fractures in subchondral bone, and osteophytes and cysts along the joint margin are visible. Arthroscopic evaluation of the joint may determine the extent of joint involvement in OA. This procedure is generally more prognostic than diagnostic in function.

PSYCHOSOCIAL ASPECTS

Psychosocial factors play an important role in OA. Depression, anxiety, avoidance and decreased quality of life are several factors that may influence the way patients perceive pain and disability associated with their disease.[37] It is important to identify and address these factors to optimize patient therapy.

The degree of seriousness with which OA is initially viewed by patients is critical to their ability to cope with the disease.[38] Those who saw the disease as threatening were more likely to be depressed than those who accepted the diagnosis and strategies for treatment. Anxiety and avoidance are two factors that are closely related. Patients with increased pain often focused on activities and stressors in their lives, which led to avoidance of physical activity and anticipation regarding performance of activities of daily living (ADL).[39] Perceived quality of life (QOL) also is important in managing patients with OA. Using QOL instruments, patients with OA were found to have lower life satisfaction than those patients receiving dialysis, and the more severe the symptoms of OA that were present, the lower the QOL rating.[40]

THERAPEUTIC PLAN

Current treatment of patients with OA focuses on symptom control because there are no disease-modifying osteoarthritic agents available.[1] Effectiveness of therapy can be measured subjectively by lessening of pain and decreasing joint stiffness, or objectively by evaluation of joint range-of-motion and radiographic changes. Treatment guidelines have been published by the ACR for the management of OA of both the hip and knee[5,41] (Tables 32.3 and 32.4). A therapeutic plan should be developed for each patient individually based upon the extent and distribution of joint involvement, as well as other concurrent diseases that may be present.[1]

Table 32.3 ▪ Medical Management of Patients with Osteoarthritis of the Hip

Nonpharmacologic therapy
Patient education
Self-management programs
Health professional social support via telephone contact
Weight loss (if overweight)
Physical therapy
Range-of-motion exercises
Strengthening exercises
Assistive devices for ambulation
Occupational therapy
Joint protection and energy conservation
Assistive devices for activities of daily living
Aerobic aquatic exercise programs
Pharmacologic therapy
Nonopioid analgesics (acetaminophen)
Nonsteroidal anti-inflammatory drugs
Opioid analgesics (propoxyphene, codeine, oxycodone)

Source: Reference 5.

Table 32.4 ▪ Medical Management of Patients with Osteoarthritis of the Knee

- Nonpharmacologic therapy
  - Patient education
    - Self-management programs
  - Health professional social support via telephone contact
  - Weight loss (if overweight)
  - Physical therapy
    - Range-of-motion exercises
    - Quadriceps strengthening exercises
    - Assistive devices for ambulation
  - Occupational therapy
    - Joint protection and energy conservation
    - Assistive devices for activities of daily living
  - Aerobic exercise programs
- Pharmacologic therapy
  - Intra-articular steroid injections
  - Nonopioid analgesics (acetaminophen)
  - Topical analgesics (capsaicin, methylsalicylate creams)
  - Nonsteroidal anti-inflammatory drugs
  - Opioid analgesics (propoxyphene, codeine, oxycodone)

Source: Reference 41.

TREATMENT

Pharmacotherapy

Pain relief is the primary indication for initiating drug therapy in patients with OA (Figures 32.1 and 32.2).[5] Because there are no medications currently available that reverse or alter the structural and biochemical changes associated with OA, drug therapy is targeted at symptom control. Individualization of patient therapy is important when dealing with medications. Many patients with OA are older and may have concurrent diseases. Careful selection and evaluation of agents is important to minimize adverse effects and maximize efficacy.

Analgesics

Acetaminophen is the recommended initial drug of choice for treating symptomatic OA.[5] Doses up to 4 g/day may be used with minimal occurrence of side effects.[42] Comparative studies between acetaminophen and nonsteroidal anti-inflammatory drugs (NSAIDs) have shown no difference in efficacy, even in the presence of inflammatory symptoms such as synovitis and joint swelling.[43,44] Other studies have confirmed that anti-inflammatory doses of NSAIDs are no more beneficial than acetaminophen for the treatment of OA symptoms.[45,46] Although equivalency has been shown, patients who are not responding to acetaminophen therapy should be given an NSAID for pain relief.[5]

Use of acetaminophen has been linked to the development of liver toxicity.[5] The occurrence of this side effect is rare; it is generally seen in patients with underlying liver conditions, in patients who consume alcohol on a chronic basis, or in situations when the maximum daily dosage exceeds recommended quantities.[47–49] Long-term consumption of acetaminophen has also been linked to the development of renal failure.[50] Data collected to support this finding are confounded because the sequence of drug administration and development of renal failure was not established.[51] It is important to remember that the development of renal failure has also been associated with long-term use of NSAIDs.[51]

Other analgesics such as tramadol and opioid derivatives are beneficial for the management of pain associated with OA.[5] Use of these agents should be short term and for the management of acute exacerbations of pain. Long-term use should be avoided, if possible, because there is potential for the development of dependence. However, use of these agents should not be restricted based upon the fear of developing dependence. Appropriate patient education and dosing of these agents can provide significant improvement in a patient's quality of life.

Nonsteroidal Anti-Inflammatory Drugs

Principles of appropriate NSAID (Table 32.5) use for patients with OA include use of the minimum effective dose, use of no more than one NSAID simultaneously, assessment of benefit after a period of 1 month (change or discontinue therapy if no benefit seen), and patient education regarding intelligent nonadherence so that the patient is not taking the medication if no pain is felt.[1]

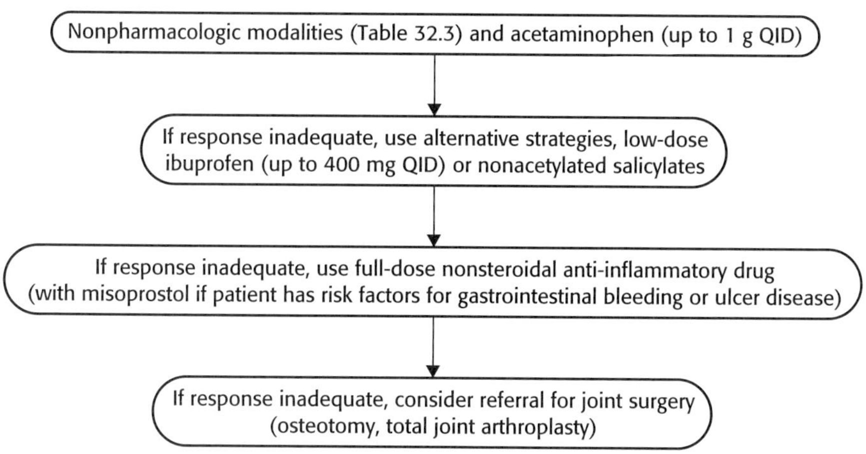

Figure 32.1. Treatment algorithm for osteoarthritis of the hip.

Short-term benefit with NSAIDs has been demonstrated; however, data regarding chronic administration indicated an increased incidence of side effects and no additional improvement in efficacy.[49,52]

Development of toxicity is a significant reason not to recommend the use of NSAIDs as first-line agents.[5] Among people age 65 and older, as many as 30% of all hospitalizations and deaths related to peptic ulcer disease (PUD) can be attributed to NSAID use.[53] In addition to age, other risk factors associated with NSAID-induced PUD include a history of PUD or upper gastrointestinal (GI) bleeding, concomitant use of corticosteroids or oral anticoagulants, high NSAID dose, and possibly smoking and alcohol consumption.[54,55] NSAIDs may also increase the risk of developing chronic renal disease in patients who are over the age of 65 and have hypertension or congestive heart failure.[5] Monitoring of serum creatinine should be performed to detect changes in renal function.

Pharmacokinetic profiles of individual NSAIDs are generally similar with the major difference being half-life.[56] Absorption of NSAIDs is extensive and all are highly protein bound. Elimination is via hepatic metabolism to inactive metabolites, except for sulindac and nabumetone, which are converted to active metabolites. Analgesic effects are generally seen within 1 to 2 hours after taking the NSAID, while maximum anti-inflammatory effects are obtained after 2 to 3 weeks of continuous administration.

Selection of a NSAID should be based upon frequency of dosing, cost, efficacy, and toxicities. There are dozens of NSAIDs available on the U.S. market, both prescription and nonprescription (over the counter [OTC]). All have equivalent efficacy and comparable toxicity. Aspirin, ibuprofen, naproxen, and ketoprofen are all available OTC and may be available at a lower cost than prescription NSAIDs. The ACR suggests the use of low-dose ibuprofen (<1600 mg/day) on an as-needed basis initially because of its lesser cost, similar efficacy, and fewer GI toxicities.[5,41] Because there is a great deal of variation in symptoms experienced by patients with OA, both during the day and from one day to the next, the use of short half-life NSAIDs on an as-needed basis is preferred if adequate pain relief is achieved.[5]

The variation in GI side effect profiles of NSAIDs may be a result of the cyclo-oxygenase (COX) selectivity of individual drugs.[57] COX serves as the rate-limiting enzyme in prostaglandin production. Inhibition of this enzyme decreases prostaglandin-induced initiation and maintenance of inflammatory responses.[58] COX has been identified to have two isoforms (COX-1 and COX-2).[58] COX-1 is beneficial in helping to maintain normal cellular physiologic processes in the GI tract, kidneys, and blood. In the gut, COX-1 stimulates the secretion of bicarbonate and mucus and reduces stomach acid secretion.[59] All of these actions are protective for the lining of the stomach

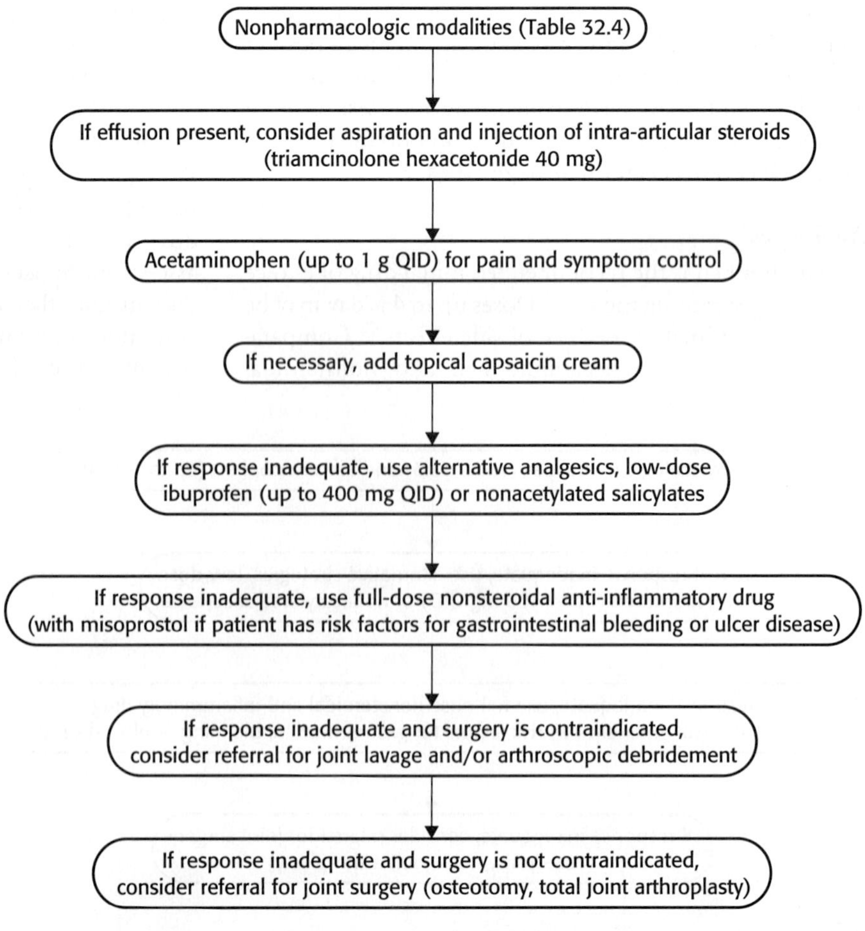

Figure 32.2. Treatment algorithm for osteoarthritis of the knee.

Table 32.5 ▪ Appropriate Use of Nonsteroidal Anti-Inflammatory Drugs

Class/Drug	Half-Life (hr)	Maximum Recommended Daily Dose (mg)
Nonprescription		
Propionic acids		
Ibuprofen	1.8–2.5	1200
Ketoprofen	2–4	75
Naproxen sodium	12–15	660
Prescription		
Propionic acids		
Fenoprofen	2–3	3200
Flurbiprofen	5.7	300
Ibuprofen	1.8–2.5	3200
Ketoprofen	2–4	300
Naproxen	12–15	1500
Naproxen sodium	12–13	1375
Oxaprozin	42–50	1800
Acetic acids		
Diclocfenac sodium	1–2	200
Etodolac	7.3	1200
Indomethacin	4.5 (SR 4.5–6)	200 (SR150)
Nabumetone	22.5–30	2000
Sulindac	7.8/(16.4)	400
Tolmetin	1–1.5	2000
Fenamates/anthranilic acids		
Meclofenamate sodium	2–3.3	400
Mefenamic acid	2–4	1000
Oxicams		
Piroxicam	30–86	20
Nonacetylated salicylates		
Choline magnesium trisalicylate	2–19	3000
Magnesium salicylate	2–19	4800
Salsalate	2–19	3000
Diflunisal	2–19	1500
Cyclo-oxygenase inhibitors		
Celecoxib	11.2	400
Rofecoxib	17	25

SR, sustained release.

against irritants. COX-2 is involved in selectively activating proinflammatory cytokines and does not have a gastroprotective effect.[59] Therefore, the ideal NSAID would selectively inhibit COX-2 to reduce the inflammatory response, but also maintain the GI and renal protective nature of COX-1. Several agents have been developed that are COX-2 selective, including meloxicam, celecoxib, and rofecoxib. Although the clinical relevance of COX-2-selective NSAIDs is unclear, they may prove beneficial for patients requiring long-term NSAID therapy who have a predisposition for developing adverse GI effects.

Topical Agents

For patients who do not respond to oral analgesics or those who refuse to take systemic therapy, the use of topical lineaments, gels, and creams is appropriate.[41] Local application of agents avoids systemic side effects and allows the use of more potent agents.[60] Capsaicin is a topical rubefacient derived from the pepper plant. The primary effects of capsaicin are related to its activity in the peripheral portion of the sensory nervous system. It works to excite nociceptive C-afferent neurons causing the release of substance P.[61] Substance P is an essential chemical mediator in the transmission of pain from the peripheral to central nervous system. Upon repeated application of capsaicin substance P is depleted, thus, leading to inhibition of pain sensation.[61]

Capsaicin should be applied to the affected joint(s) four times a day.[41] After several weeks of continual application, maximal pain relief is noted and the frequency of application may be reduced.[61] Capsaicin may be used either as monotherapy or in combination with oral agents.[41] Associated side effects include a mild stinging or burning sensation, but patients rarely discontinue therapy because of this reaction. Because capsaicin is safe and effective and does not have systemic side effects, it should be considered for the management of pain associated with OA.

Corticosteroids

The role of corticosteroids in the management of OA remains controversial. Systemic corticosteroids should be avoided, because prolonged use leads to the development of side effects that outweigh any benefits of therapy.[62] On the other hand, intra-articular injections of corticosteroids may be beneficial. For OA of the hip, the efficacy of such injections has not been determined, and they are not recommended as a part of routine medical management.[5] For patients with OA of the knee, the use of intra-articular injections of corticosteroids may be appropriate.[63] Triamcinolone acetonide or hexacetonide at a dose of 40 mg is beneficial in reducing pain, especially when signs of effusion or local inflammation are present.[41] It is recommended that injections not be performed more than three to four times per year, because there is concern that repeated injections into the joint may lead to progressive cartilage damage.[5,41] Patients may experience synovitis after an injection, which is due to a local reaction to the suspended steroid crystals.[41] This reaction is mild and lasts for a short period of time.

Hyaluronic Acid Derivatives

Hyaluronan and hylan G-F 20 are two glycosaminoglycan polysaccharide compounds, which have been approved by the Food and Drug Administration for the treatment of pain associated with OA of the knee.[64] These agents, also known as hyaluronic acid, are indicated for patients who have not responded adequately to nonpharmacologic therapy and treatment with analgesics.[65,66] In patients with OA, both elasticity and viscosity within the synovial fluid are reduced.[6] Vicosupplementation, administration of hyaluronic acid and its derivatives, is believed to restore the composition of synovial fluid such that normal tissue regeneration and function may occur.

Data from clinical trials have shown that both agents are safe and effective in the treatment of OA of the knee. The most common side effect reported with both agents is pain at injection site.[65,66] Other side effects such as swelling, effusion, warmth, and redness at the injection site have also been reported. It is not recommended that either agent be administered with anesthetics or other medications concurrently, because they may become diluted such that safety and efficacy may be compromised. However, subcutaneous local anesthetics may be administered. Dosing for hyaluronan is 2 ml injected intra-articularly on a weekly basis for 5 weeks. It has not been established how often this cycle may be repeated. Some studies examined readministration every 3 to-4 months while others waited for symptoms to reappear. Hylan G-F 20 is injected intra-articularly on a weekly basis for 3 weeks at a dose of 2 ml. As with hyaluronan, frequency of readministration has not been established. Practitioners are recommending that no more than six injections be given within 6 months and a minimum of 4 weeks should pass between cycles. Hyaluronan and hylan G-F 20 should be considered for patients not responding to other therapies and before joint replacement. Because comparative data are lacking, the exact place in therapy for these agents in the management of OA is to be determined but should be reserved for patients in whom conventional treatment has failed or for those who were unable to tolerate NSAIDs or analgesics.[67]

Nonpharmacologic Therapy

Physical and occupational therapies play a crucial role in the management of patients with OA who have functional limitations.[5] Physical therapists assess muscle strength, range of motion, mobility, and ambulation. Instruction can then be provided about appropriate exercises, and the use of modalities such as heat and cold to aid range of motion and mobility. Application of warm compresses or warm water soaks may be beneficial before exercise to help relieve joint pain and stiffness.[5] Occupational therapists assess ADL and recommend devices such as splints, canes, wall bars, and raised toilet seats, which improve patient independence and accommodate functional disability. Appropriate assessment and intervention in ADL, mobility, and ambulation have a significant impact on the quality of life of the patient.

The goals of exercise for patients with OA should include reduction of joint impairment, improvement in joint function, protection of the joint from further damage, and prevention of disability.[68] Before a patient begins an exercise program, complete cardiac assessment should be performed to identify any underlying disease and to establish a target heart rate.[69] An exercise program should consist of both aerobic and range-of-motion and strengthening exercises.[44] Aquatic aerobics programs target these areas and should be recommended to patients with OA.[5] To sustain benefit, exercise programs require a long-term commitment of both time and effort on the part of the patient.[5]

For patients who may be overweight, weight reduction may reduce the symptoms of OA, especially in the weight-bearing joints.[1] Comprehensive weight management should include counseling on appropriate diet choices and involvement in aerobic exercise activities.[5] Specific changes to the diet (restricted meats, no preservatives, fish oil, alfalfa, and zinc) have not been shown to be beneficial for patients with OA and are not recommended.[70]

Surgical intervention is indicated for patients who are experiencing severe pain that has failed to respond to medical therapy and has progressively decreased their ADL.[5] Arthroscopic debridement and lavage of the joint space are beneficial for patients who refuse surgery or those for whom surgery is not recommended. The removal of matrix debris and inflammatory mediators have been suggested as possible reasons for benefit from lavage. Osteotomy, the surgical cutting and repositioning of bone, may provide relief to patients because restructuring and repositioning of the bone places the joint back into normal alignment. This procedure may help to prevent disease progression in patients who are not candidates for arthroplasty, also known as joint replacement.[5] Complete joint arthroplasty is responsible for a dramatic improvement in quality of life in patients with OA. Careful consideration needs to be given to the patient's health status, the surgeon performing the procedure, the hospital where it will be performed, and postoperative management and rehabilitation before arthroplasty is performed.[71,72]

ALTERNATIVE THERAPIES

The combination of glucosamine sulfate and chondroitin sulfate has been touted as the "miracle cure" for patients suffering from OA. Both compounds are found naturally in the body and are essential to formation of cartilage.[73] Glucosamine is a basic component of articular cartilage glycosaminoglycans and acts as a substrate in the synthesis of proteoglycans.[74] With aging, the body decreases the synthesis of glucosamine, and the synovial fluid becomes thin and is no longer effective in lubricating the joint.[75] The rationale for the use of glucosamine sulfate in OA is to provide the building blocks for cartilage regeneration.[76] Chondroitin is another constituent in the cartilage matrix.[77] Because of its chemical nature, is has a strong ability to retain water and gives cartilage its shock-absorbing characteristics.[78] The primary function of chondroitin is to prevent premature breakdown of existing cartilage by partially inhibiting the proteolytic enzyme elastase.[79] Chondroitin also serves to stimulate RNA synthesis of chondrocytes.[80] Whereas chondroitin may be used alone in the management of OA, the combination of glucosamine sulfate and chondroitin sulfate is believed to have a synergistic effect by stimulating cartilage production and inhibiting its destruction.[76]

In clinical trials, doses of both glucosamine and chondroitin varied based upon route of administration and study design. Side effects associated with the use of these agents include mild gastric discomfort, dyspepsia, nausea, and euphoria.[81] Chondroitin sulfate does have potential anticoagulant activity; however, laboratory evaluation of patients before and after treatment suggested no significant hematologic changes with chondroitin use for 6 months.[82] Many of the studies involving glucosamine and chondroitin are flawed by poor study design, bias, and inadequate sample size. The results that demonstrate relief of symptoms are questionable. There are no long-term studies demonstrating relief of symptoms or slowing of the disease process. The Arthritis Foundation does not recognize either agent as treatment for OA and continues to support the ACR guidelines for appropriate management of OA.

FUTURE THERAPIES

Until recently, OA was considered an inevitable and irreversible part of aging. However, research has led to a better understanding of the disease and new ways to manage it. New therapies are being developed, which one day may prevent, stop, reverse, or even cure OA. Development of safer NSAIDs, evaluation of gene therapy, application of currently available medications for new indications, and exploration into the role of cytokines in OA are just some of the areas of research and development.

COX-2 inhibitors have advanced NSAID therapy; however, more selective agents are being developed to minimize or eliminate the GI and renal side effects seen with currently available agents. Because OA may develop from genetic defects in collagen, researchers are targeting therapies to specifically block defective genes. Transfer of genes directly into the joint that stimulate cartilage formation or inhibit cartilage breakdown are being evaluated for therapeutic use.[83] Control of tissue inhibitors of metalloproteinases and metalloproteinase genes would provide an opportunity to control a patient's disease.[84] Doxycycline, in canine models, has been shown to inhibit collagenase activity in articular cartilage.[85] This activity prevented proteoglycan loss, cell death, and deposition of weak collagen matrix in vitro. Therapies that interact with cytokines are also in development. Administration of tumor growth factor-β via liposomes may induce repair of articular cartilage lesions.[86] While structure or disease-modifying agents for OA have not yet been developed, research is underway to determine if such agents are realistic.

IMPROVING OUTCOMES

The ultimate outcome for treating patients with OA is to have patients reach their therapeutic goals. Many interventions can help patients to reach these goals and have been proven to be beneficial for the management of patients with OA.

Patient Education

Patient education provides the cornerstone of nonpharmacologic management of OA. Education of family members, friends, and caregivers is integral, because they provide a support structure for the patient.[5] Patients should be encouraged to become involved in self-help programs or support groups offered at local community centers, hospitals, or through local or national chapters of the Arthritis Foundation.[5] The Arthritis Foundation is available to provide educational materials for patients and families, information regarding providers, identification of other agencies offering both physical and economic support to patients, and information on various drugs used to treat OA.[87] The Arthritis Foundation may be reached at 1-800-283-7800.

Providing patients with social support emphasizes the importance not only of personal patient contact, but also the significant impact for interventions in improving patient care and outcomes.[5] Trained lay personnel can review items such as joint pain, medication and treatment adherence, drug toxicities, appointments with providers, and overall patient quality of life.[5] This provides another source of information regarding treatment effectiveness and reinforces the collaborative effort needed for optimal patient care. Self-management and support groups for patients have led to decreased pain, decreased number of physician visits, and improved overall quality of life for participants.[88] Use of social support networks has been shown to improve the patient's pain and functional status, while not significantly increasing costs.[89]

The benefits of aerobic exercise and weight reduction have also been demonstrated by a decrease in symptoms and improvement in ambulation.[90] Development and execution of an appropriate therapeutic plan allow patients to receive maximal benefit and reach therapeutic goals.

Providing education has a positive impact on both the health and psychosocial status of patients dealing with OA.[91] Education should not only be offered to the patient, but also to family, friends, and caregivers.[5,41] Topics that should be discussed include understanding the development and progression of OA, pain control, appropriate use of medications, side effects or adverse events from medications, appropriate techniques for exercise and rest, weight reduction (if appropriate), modifications/adaptations for ADLs, and support services. It is also important for patients to understand the waxing/waning nature of their disease and the necessity to adjust their care plans accordingly. Encouraging patients to become involved in self-management programs empowers them and allows them to be active participants in their own care. Benefits of such programs include decreased pain, less frequent physician visits, and overall improvement in quality of life.[5,41] Educational materials such as videos, pamphlets, and newsletters, as well as information regarding support services available, may be obtained from either local chapters or the national office of the Arthritis Foundation, 1330 W. Peachtree St., Atlanta, GA 30309; phone (404) 872-7100 or 1-800-283-7800; web site: *http://www.arthritis.org.*

Methods to Improve Patient Adherence to Drug Therapy

Adherence with both pharmacologic treatment regimens is essential to ensure optimal patient outcomes. Many factors may contribute to nonadherence such as: failure to understand the importance of therapy, failure to understand instructions, multiple drug therapy, frequency of administration, adverse events, fear of becoming drug dependent, symptoms disappear, comorbid conditions, and the cost of treatment.[92] Recognizing and identifying these factors can aid in developing appropriate treatment plans.

Use of patient education and support groups greatly increases patients' understanding of the disease process and the role of therapy in improving their condition.[87–89] With this understanding comes improved outcomes and increased adherence. Evaluation of patients with OA has shown significant improvement in medication and therapy (physical and occupational) adherence in patients involved with self-management programs.[93] The frequency of medication administration also has an impact on adherence to therapy. Data show that as the frequency of administration increases, adherence decreases dramatically. By choosing extended-release formulations or medications with longer half-lives, administration once or twice a day may be possible, leading to improved adherence and outcomes. Adherence may also be improved by the use of special packaging. Nonsafety tops on prescription bottles may ease opening of containers for patients with OA who may also have involvement in their hands or wrists. For patients with complicated medication regimens or those who may cognitively or visually impaired, the use of blister packaging may assist in appropriate medication usage.

To improve patient adherence it is important to identify factors that may lead to nonadherence, develop a treatment plan which correlates with the patients' normal activities, educate the patient and family members, and monitor therapy on a regular basis. These steps allow both patient and practitioner to meet therapeutic goals and optimize care.

Disease Management Strategies to Improve Patient Outcomes

An appropriately designed therapeutic plan focuses on both pain relief and minimization of disability because as of yet there are no disease-modifying drugs for OA. Combination therapy with both pharmacologic and nonpharmacologic modalities has proven to be beneficial in improving patient outcomes. Data suggest that exercise programs should be routines recommended along with standard pharmacologic therapy and occupational therapy may be beneficial to patients in helping them adapt to functional limitations imposed by OA.[94,95]

Principles of pharmacologic therapy include selection of an appropriate agent, optimal therapeutic dosing, usage of the minimal effective dose of NSAIDs to minimize side effects, and appropriate duration of therapy with selected agents.[1] Assessment of benefit should be performed after 1 month of therapy at which point either dosage adjustments or selection of another agent may be necessary if optimal results are not being achieved. Analgesia is the cornerstone of pharmacologic therapy and appropriate therapeutic agents should be chosen to meet this goal.

Other important components of disease management are monitoring and evaluation of therapy. Both subjective and objective parameters should be used to assess disease progression and patient outcomes. Quality of life indicators, walking distance, ACR criteria, pain ratings, and WOMAC scores are beneficial in completely assessing the patient with OA.[96,97]

Because OA is a chronic disease with multiple etiologies and risk factors, it may be possible to look at prevention as a disease management strategy.[10] Primary prevention measures include reduction of known risk factors such as obesity and preventing major joint injury. Secondary prevention has not been established but may include screenings for persons who may have early, asymptomatic disease. Tertiary prevention involves prevention of disability for those who already have active disease. Ongoing research in this area will provide practitioners with strategies to both prevent and more effectively treat OA in the future.

PHARMACOECONOMICS

The World Development Report estimates that there are 11.2 million disability-adjusted life-years lost each year as a result of OA.[98] Pain, the predominant symptom of OA, accounts for much of the disability and impaired quality of life associated with OA, as well as the increased use of health care resources by patients with OA.[50] Evaluating the pharmacoeconomics of OA provides not only a means to compare costs, but also examines the benefits and effectiveness associated with different therapies.

Research supports the use of pure analgesics instead of NSAIDs in the management of mild-to-moderate OA for proof of clinical effectiveness, safety, and pharmacoeconomics.[49,50] In an economic analysis comparing acetaminophen to NSAIDs either with or without misoprostol prophylaxis, the costs associated with treating patients with NSAIDs were significantly higher than costs of treatment with acetaminophen.[99] This study examined not only drug costs, but also the associated costs of treating adverse events and the costs of prophylaxis for patients receiving NSAIDs in a managed care organization. Using retrospective medical and prescription claims data, the investigators determined that the average expected treatment costs for NSAIDs were $61 per treatment month compared to acetaminophen at $19 per treatment month. The costs associated with treating adverse events in NSAID users were $106 in patients not receiving prophylaxis and $55 in patients who received prophylaxis compared to $12 in patients receiving acetaminophen. Acetaminophen was determined to be the most cost-effective choice of therapy for patients with mild-to-moderate OA, due to decreased cost, and decreased incidence and cost of side effects. When acetaminophen was compared to low-cost NSAIDs (ibuprofen) at $18 per treatment month in drug costs, the costs of treating adverse effects associated with NSAID use still made acetaminophen the least costly treatment alternative.

KEY POINTS

- Control pain.
- Minimize disability.
- Decrease joint stiffness.
- Maintain mobility and functioning.
- Maintain or improve quality of life.
- Educate patients and family members about OA and its therapies.
- Use nonpharmacologic modalities in conjunction with pharmacologic modalities in the management of patients with OA.
- Acetaminophen is considered first-line therapy and is a cost-effective treatment for OA.
- Psychosocial factors may influence patient perception of pain and disability associated with OA.
- Future therapies in OA may include agents produced to target specific cytokines or drugs disease-modifying drugs for OA.
- Resources are available for patients and health care practitioners from the Arthritis Foundation.

REFERENCES

1. Creamer P, Hochberg M. Osteoarthritis. Lancet 350(9076):503–509, 1997.
2. Guccione A, Felson D, Anderson J, et al. The effects of specific medical conditions on functional limitations of elders in the Framingham Study. Am J Public Health 84:351–358, 1994.
3. Yelin E. The economics of osteoarthritis. In: Brandt K, Doherty M, Lohmander L, eds. Osteoarthritis. New York: Oxford University Press, 1998:23–30.
4. Kuettner K, Goldberg V. Introduction. In: Kuettner K, Goldberg V, eds. Osteoarthritic disorders. Rosemont, IL: American Academy of Orthopedic Surgeons, 1995:xxi–xxv.
5. Hochberg M, Altman R, Brandt K, et al. Guidelines for the medical management of osteoarthritis: part I. Osteoarthritis of the hip. Arthritis Rheum 38:1535–1540, 1995.
6. Blackburn W. Management of osteoarthritis and rheumatoid arthritis: prospects and possibilities. Am J Med 100(Suppl 2A):24S–30S, 1996.
7. Dieppe P. The classification and diagnosis of osteoarthritis. In: Kuettner K, Goldberg V, eds. Osteoarthritic disorders. Rosemont, IL: American Academy of Orthopedic Surgeons, 1995:5–12.
8. Dieppe P, Cushnaghan J, Shepstone L. The Bristol "OA500" Study: progression of osteoarthritis (OA) over 3 years and the relationship between clinical and radiographic changes at the knee joint. Osteoarthritis Cartilage 5:57–97, 1997.
9. Oddis C. New perspectives on osteoarthritis. Am J Med 100(Suppl 2A):10S–15S, 1996.
10. Felson D, Zhang Y. An update on the epidemiology of knee and hip osteoarthritis with a view to prevention. Arthritis Rheum 41:1343–1355, 1998.
11. Oliveria S, Felson D, Reed J, et al. Incidence of symptomatic hand, hip, and knee osteoarthritis among patients in a health maintenance organization. Arthritis Rheum 38:1134–1141, 1995.
12. Hirsch R, Lethbridge-Cejku M, Scott W Jr, et al. Association of hand and knee osteoarthritis: evidence for a polyarticular disease subset. Ann Rheum Dis 55:25–29, 1996.
13. Ritvaniemi P, Korkko J, Bonaventure J, et al. Identification of COL2A1 gene mutations in patients with chondrodysplasias and familial osteoarthritis. Arthritis Rheum 38:999–1004, 1995.
14. Spector T, Cicuttini F, Baker J, et al. Genetic influences on osteoarthritis in women: a twin study. Br Med J 312:940–944, 1996.
15. Felson D, Couropmitree N, Chaisson C, et al. Evidence for a Mendelian gene in a segregation analysis of generalized radiographic osteoarthritis; the Framingham Study. Arthritis Rheum 41:1064–1071, 1998.
16. Radin E. Mechanical aspects of osteoarthritis. Bull Rheum Dis 26:862–865, 1976.
17. Dequeker J, Boonen S, Aerssens J, et al. Inverse relationship between osteoarthritis-osteoporosis: what is the evidence? What are the consequences? Br J Rheumatol 35:813–820, 1996.
18. Hart D, Mootoosamy I, Doyle D, et al. The relationship between osteoarthritis and osteoporosis in the general population: the Chingford Study. Ann Rheum Dis 53:158–162, 1994.
19. Dequeker J, Goris P, Utterhoven R. Osteoporosis and osteoarthritis (osteoarthrosis): anthropometric distinctions. JAMA 249:1448–1451, 1983.
20. Hannan M, Anderson J, Zhang Y, et al. Bone mineral density and knee osteoarthritis in elderly men and women: the Framingham Study. Arthritis Rheum 36:1671–1680, 1993.
21. Schipplein O, Andriacchi T. Interaction between active and passive knee stabilizers during level walking. J Orthop Res 9:113–119, 1991.
22. Felson D, Zhang Y, Anthony J, et al. Weight loss reduces the risk for symptomatic knee osteoarthritis in women. Ann Intern Med 116:535–539, 1992.
23. Zhang Y, Glynn R, Felson D. Musculoskeletal disease research: should we analyze the joint or the person? J Rheumatol 23:1130–1134, 1996.
24. Spector T, Harris P, Hart D, et al. Risk of osteoarthritis associated with long term weight-bearing sports: a radiologic survey of the hips and knees in female ex-athletes and population controls. Arthritis Rheum 39:988–995, 1996.
25. Vingard E, Alfredsson L, Goldie I, et al. Sports and osteoarthrosis of the hip: an epidemiologic study. Am J Sports Med 21:195–200, 1993.
26. Kujala U, Kettunen J, Paananen H, et al. Knee osteoarthritis in former runners, soccer players, weight lifters, and shooters. Arthritis Rheum 38:539–546, 1995.
27. Pinals R. Mechanisms of joint destruction, pain and disability in osteoarthritis. Drugs 52(Suppl 3):14–20, 1996.
28. Schaible H, Neugebauer V, Schmidt R. Osteoarthritis and pain. Semin Arthritis Rheum 18:30–34, 1989.
29. Hochberg M, Lawrence R, Everett D, et al. Epidemiologic association of pain in osteoarthritis of the knee; data from the National Health and Nutrition Examination Survey and the National Health and Nutrition Examination–I. Epidemiologic follow-up survey. Semin Arthritis Rheum 18:4–9, 1989.
30. Balint G, Szebenyi B. Diagnosis of osteoarthritis: guidelines and current pitfalls. Drugs 52(Suppl 3):1–13, 1996.
31. Buckwalter J. Osteoarthritis and articular cartilage use, disuse and abuse: Experimental studies. J Rheumatol 22(Suppl 43):13–15, 1995.
32. Schumacher R Jr. Secondary osteoarthritis. In: Moskowitz R, Howell D, Goldberg V, et al, eds. Osteoarthritis. Diagnosis and medical/surgical management. 2nd ed. Philadelphia: WB Saunders, 1992:367–398.
33. Altman R, Asch E, Bloch D, et al. Development of criteria for the classification and reporting of osteoarthritis. Classification of osteoarthritis of the knee. Arthritis Rheum 29:1039–1049, 1986.
34. Altman R, Alarcon G, Appelrouth D, et al. The ACR criteria for the classification and reporting of osteoarthritis of the hand. Arthritis Rheum 33:1601–1610, 1990.
35. Altman R, Alarcon G, Appelrouth D, et al. The ACR criteria for the classification and reporting of osteoarthritis of the hip. Arthritis Rheum 34:505–514, 1991.
36. Hart D, Spector T. Radiographic criteria for epidemiologic studies of osteoarthritis. J Rheumatol 22(Suppl 43):46–48, 1995.
37. Creamer P, Hochberg M. The relationship between psychosocial variables and pain reporting in osteoarthritis of the knee. Arthritis Care Res 11:60–65, 1998.
38. Hampson S, Glasgow R, Zeiss A. Coping with osteoarthritis by older adults. Arthritis Care Res 9:133–141, 1996.
39. Dekker J, Boot B, van der Woude LH, et al. Pain and disability in osteoarthritis: a review of behavioral mechanisms. J Behav Med 15:189–214, 1992.
40. Kee C, Harris S, Booth L, et al. Perspectives on the nursing management of osteoarthritis. Geriatr Nurs 19:19–27, 1998.
41. Hochberg M, Altman R, Brandt K, et al. Guidelines for the medical management of osteoarthritis: Part II. Osteoarthritis of the knee. Arthritis Rheum 38:1541–1546, 1995.
42. Batchlor E, Paulus H. Principles of drug therapy. In: Moskowitz R, Howell D, Goldberg V, et al., eds. Osteoarthritis: diagnosis and medical/surgical management. 2nd ed. Philadelphia: WB Saunders, 1992.
43. Bradley J, Brandt K, Katz B, et al. Comparison of an anti-inflammatory dose of ibuprofen, an analgesic dose of ibuprofen, and acetaminophen in the treatment of patients with osteoarthritis of the knee. N Engl J Med 325:87–91, 1991.
44. Bradley J, Brandt K, Katz B, et al. Treatment of knee osteoarthritis: relationship of clinical features of joint inflammation to the response to a nonsteroidal anti-inflammatory drug or pure analgesic. J Rheumatol 19:1950–1954, 1992.
45. Dieppe P, Cushnaghan J, Jasani M, et al. A 2-year, placebo controlled trial of nonsteroidal anti-inflammatory therapy in osteoarthritis of the knee joint. Br J Rheumatol 32:595–600, 1993.

46. Doyle D, Dieppe P, Scott J, et al. An articular index for the assessment of osteoarthritis. Ann Rheum Dis 40:75–78, 1981.
47. Farrell G. The hepatic side effects of drugs. Med J Aust 145:600–604, 1986.
48. Acetaminophen, NSAIDs and alcohol. Med Lett Drugs Ther 1996 Jun 21; 38(977):55–56.
49. Benison H, Kaczynski J, Wallerstedt S. Paracetamol medication and alcohol abuse: a dangerous combination for the liver and kidney. Scand J Gastroenterol 22:701–704, 1987.
50. Perneger T, Whelton P, Klag M. Risk of kidney failure associated with the use of acetaminophen, aspirin, and nonsteroidal anti-inflammatory drugs. N Engl J Med 331:1671–1679, 1994.
51. Ronco P, Flahaut A. Drug induced end stage renal disease [Editorial]. N Engl J Med 331:1711–1712, 1994.
52. Scholes D, Stergachis A, Penna P, et al. Nonsteroidal anti-inflammatory drug discontinuation in patients with osteoarthritis. J Rheumatol 22:708–712, 1995.
53. Griffin M, Piper J, Daughtery J, et al. Nonsteroidal anti-inflammatory drug use and increased risk for peptic ulcer disease in elderly persons. Ann Intern Med 114:257–263, 1991.
54. Lichtenstein D, Syngal S, Wolfe M. Nonsteroidal anti-inflammatory drugs and the gastrointestinal tract: the double edged sword. Arthritis Rheum 35:5–18, 1995.
55. Henry D, Dobson A, Turner C. Variability in the risk of major gastrointestinal complications from nonaspirin nonsteroidal anti-inflammatory drugs. Gastroenterology 105:1078–1088, 1993.
56. Furst D. Are there differences among nonsteroidal anti-inflammatory drugs? Arthritis Rheum 1:1–9, 1994.
57. Brater DC, Cummings DM, Lofholm PW, et al. Advances in nonsteroidal anti-inflammatory drug therapy: practical considerations for optimizing product selection. Philadelphia: PCPS, 1997.
58. Siebert K, Masferrer JL. Role of inducible cyclo-oxygenase (COX-2) inflammation. Receptor 4:17–23, 1994.
59. Simon LS. Nonsteroidal anti-inflammatory drugs and their effects: the importance of COX "selectivity." J Clin Rheumatol 2:135–140, 1996.
60. Wollheim F. Current pharmacological treatment of osteoarthritis. Drugs 52(Suppl 3):27–38, 1996.
61. Fusco B, Giacovazzo M. Peppers and pain. The promise of capsaicin. Drugs 53:909–914, 1997.
62. Moskowitz R, Goldberg V. Osteoarthritis: clinical features and treatment. In: Schumacher H, ed. Primer on the rheumatic diseases. 10th ed. Atlanta: Arthritis Foundation, 1993.
63. Neustadt D. Intraarticular steroid therapy. In: Moskowitz R, Howell D, Goldberg V, et al., ed. Osteoarthritis. Diagnosis and medical/surgical management. 2nd ed. Philadelphia: WB Saunders, 1992.
64. Levien T, Baker D. Hyaluronic acid. Hospital Pharm 33:698–713, 1998.
65. Package insert. Hyalgan. New York: Sanofi-Synthelabo, June 1997.
66. Package insert. Synvisc. Philadelphia: Wyeth-Ayerst, August 1997.
67. Simon L. Vicosupplementation therapy with intra-articular hyaluronic acid. Fact or fantasy? Rheum Dis Clin North Am 25:345–357, 1999.
68. Minor M. Exercise in the management of osteoarthritis of the knee and hip. Arthritis Care Res 7:198–204, 1994.
69. Semble E, Loeser R, Wise C. Therapeutic exercise for rheumatoid arthritis and osteoarthritis. Semin Arthritis Rheum 20:32–40, 1990.
70. Panush R. Is there a role for diet or other questionable therapies in managing rheumatic diseases? Bull Rheum Dis 42:1–4, 1993.
71. Peterson M, Hollenberg J, Szatrowski T, et al. Geographic variations in the rates of elective total hip and knee arthroplasties among Medicare beneficiaries in the United States. J Bone Jt Surg Am 74:1530–1539, 1992.
72. Lavernia C, Guzman J. Relationship of surgical volume to short-term mortality, morbidity, and hospital charges in arthroplasty. J Arthroplasty 10:133–140, 1995.
73. Horstman J. Glucosamine and chondroitin. Arthritis Today Sept/Oct:46–51, 1998.
74. Reichelt A, Forster K, Fischer M, et al. Efficacy and safety of intramuscular glucosamine sulfate in osteoarthritis of the knee: a randomized, placebo-controlled, double-blind study. Arzneimittelforschung 44:75–80, 1994.
75. Rosenfeld I. Dr. Rosenfeld's guide to alternative medicine: what works, what doesn't and what's right for you. New York: Random House, 1996.
76. Glucosamine. In: The Lawrence review of natural products. St Louis: Facts and Comparisons, 1996.
77. Morreale P, Maupulo R, Galati M, et al. Comparison of the antiinflammatory efficacy of chondroitin sulfate and diclofenac sodium in patients with knee osteoarthritis. J Rheumatol 23:1385–1391, 1996.
78. Tripple S. Articular cartilage research. Curr. Opin. Rheumatol 2:777–782, 1990.
79. Pipitone V. Chondroprotection with chondroitin sulfate. Drugs Exp Clin Res 17:3–7, 1991.
80. Soldani G, Romagroli J. Experimental and clinical pharmacology of glycosaminoglycans (GAGs).Drugs Exp Clin Res 17:81–85, 1991.
81. Chavez M. Glucosamine sulfate and chondroitin sulfates. Hosp Pharm 32:1275–1285, 1997.
82. Olivero U, Sorrentino G, DePaola P, et al. Effects of the treatment with Matrix on elderly people with chronic articular degeneration. Drugs Exp Clin Res 17:45–51, 1991.
83. Evans CH, Robbins PD. Potential treatment of osteoarthritis by gene therapy. Rheum Dis Clin North Am 25:333–344, 1999.
84. Lozasa C, Altman R. Chondroprotection in osteoarthritis. Bull Rheum Dis 46:5–7, 1997.
85. Cole A, Chubinskaya S, Luchene L, et al. Doxycycline disrupts chondrocyte differentiation and inhibits cartilage matrix degradation. Arthritis Rheum 32:1727–1734, 1994.
86. Hunziker E, Rosenburg L. Induction of repair in partial thickness articular cartilage lesions by timed release of TGF-beta. In: Transactions of the 40th Annual Meeting of the Orthopedic Research Society. 19(Sect 1):236, 1994.
87. Arthritis Foundation, Atlanta.
88. Lorig K, Lubeck D, Kraines T, et al. Outcomes of self-help education for patients with arthritis. Arthritis Rheum 28:680–685, 1985.
89. Weinberger M, Tierney W, Booher P, et al. Can the provision of information to patients with osteoarthritis improve functional status? A randomized, controlled trial. Arthritis Rheum 32:1577–1583, 1989.
90. Minor M, Hewitt, Webel R, et al. Efficacy of physical conditioning exercise in patients with rheumatoid arthritis and osteoarthritis. Arthritis Rheum 32:1396–1405, 1989.
91. Lorig K, Konkol L, Gonzalez V. Arthritis patient education: a review of the literature. Patient Educ Couns 10:207–252, 1987.
92. Gourley DR, Ueda CT. Patient factors that influence dosage form selection. In Banker GS, Chalmer RK, eds. Pharmaceutics and Pharmacy Practice. Philadelphia, PA: Lippincott, 1982.
93. Barlow JH, Turner AP, Wright CC. Long-term outcomes of an arthritis self-management programme. Br J Rheumatol 37:1315–1319, 1998.
94. Puett DW, Griffin MR. Published trials of nonmedicinal and noninvasive therapies for hip and knee osteoarthritis. Ann Intern Med 121:133–140, 1994.
95. Ettinger WH, Burns R. Messier SP, et al. A randomized trial comparing aerobic exercise and resistance exercise with a health education program in older adults with osteoarthritis. JAMA 277:25–31, 1997.
96. Wolfe F. Determinants of WOMAC function, pain and stiffness scores: evidence for the role of low back pain, symptom counts, fatigue and depression in osteoarthritis, rheumatoid arthritis and fibromyalgia. Rheumatology (Oxford) 38:355–361, 1999.
97. La Montagna G, Tirri F, Cacace E, et al. Quality of life assessment during six months of NSAID treatment. Clin Exp Rheumatol 16:49–54, 1998.
98. Tugwell P. Economic evaluation of the management of pain in osteoarthritis. Drugs 52(Suppl 3):48–58, 1996.
99. Holzer S, Cuerdon T. Development of an economic model comparing acetaminophen to NSAIDs in the treatment of mild-to-moderate osteoarthritis. Am J Manag Care 2(Suppl): s15–s26, 1996.

CHAPTER 33

GOUT AND HYPERURICEMIA

Pierre A. Maloley and Gina R. Westfall

DEFINITION

Gout is a chronic metabolic disease, most commonly afflicting men over 30 years old. It was recognized as a human malady and treated before the ancient Greeks ruled the Mediterranean world. Gout was associated with wealthy intellectuals who were known to overindulge in food and drink. Despite this long history, no specific cause was identified until 1848, when Sir Alfred Garrod identified uric acid as the cause of gout. One of the major therapeutic advances of the nineteenth century was the use of colchicine to treat the symptoms of the disease. As the role of purines in the disease process was discovered, specific dietary recommendations were also made for patients with gout. Treatment improved in the twentieth century with the development of new drugs. Acute attacks were treated with colchicine and later with indomethacin or phenylbutazone. The use of uricosuric agents closely followed these advances, and since 1965 allopurinol has also been used for the long-term management of gout.

Uric acid is an end product of protein catabolism. In humans it is the final product resulting from the breakdown of purines. DNA and RNA are degraded, yielding the nucleosides adenosine and guanosine. The enzyme xanthine oxidase (XO) converts guanosine directly to xanthine and converts adenosine first to hypoxanthine then to xanthine; finally, xanthine is converted into uric acid. At a physiologic pH of 7.4 the monovalent form of uric acid is the predominant form.[1]

Total body content of uric acid ranges from 1.0 to 1.2 g in a normal man, with a daily turnover rate of 600 to 800 mg. These values are slightly lower for women. In a normal person this turnover constitutes 50 to 60% of the urate pool each day. Almost 70% of the uric acid is excreted in the urine; the remainder is secreted into the gastrointestinal (GI) tract by a passive process and is degraded by intestinal microorganisms to ammonia and carbon dioxide.[2,3]

A four-component hypothesis for urate handling by the kidney best explains the actions of drugs to increase or decrease uric acid levels. These four components are filtration, reabsorption, secretion, and postsecretory reabsorption in the later part of the proximal tubule or in the distal tubule. Approximately 95% of the serum uric acid is filtered freely across the glomerulus. The other 5% of plasma urate is protein bound. Of the filtered urate, 98 to 100% is reabsorbed in the early part of the proximal tubule. A variable percentage of the filtered load is secreted back into the tubular lumen in a more distal part of the proximal tubule. The fourth component may occur in the distal part of the proximal tubule or in the distal tubule.[2]

Hyperuricemia is defined as a urate level greater than 480 μmol/L (8.0 mg/dL) in men and 420 μmol/L (7.0 mg/dL) in women. These values are more than two standard deviations above the mean population values. The lower value for women results from an estrogen-dependent sex difference. This difference, which manifests at puberty and is related to greater urate clearance, diminishes or disappears after menopause.[4]

Two laboratory methods are used to measure serum urate concentrations. The colorimetric method is used by most autoanalyzers. It is nonspecific, and false elevations can result from amino acids in the test sample, uremia, high dosages of vitamin C, and other xanthines such as caffeine, theobromine, and theophylline, as well as levodopa.

The uricase method is more specific and yields levels that are lower by 24 to 60 μmol/L (0.4 to 1.0 mg/dL) than the colorimetric values. The clinician must know which method is used to analyze uric acid serum levels. The definitions of hyperuricemia given here are based on colorimetric determinations.[1]

TREATMENT GOALS: GOUT AND HYPERURICEMIA

- Terminate the acute attack and resolve the pain.
- Gradually reduce the serum uric acid concentration.
- Prevent recurrent gout attacks.

EPIDEMIOLOGY

Hyperuricemia and gout traditionally are classified as either primary or secondary. *Primary gout* refers to cases in which the basic metabolic defect is unknown or, if it is known, the main manifestation is that of hyperuricemia and gout. *Secondary gout* refers to cases in which hyperuricemia is part of some other acquired disorder or in which the basic metabolic defect underlying the hyperuricemia is known but the main clinical characteristics are not those of gout. The distinctions may not always be clear.[2]

Patients with primary hyperuricemia and gout have elevated serum uric acid levels that are caused by increased production or impaired clearance of uric acid. Between 10 and 20% of patients with primary gout and hyperuricemia are overproducers of uric acid. Overproducers of uric acid can be identified with a 24-hour urinary uric acid excretion test. Patients who overproduce uric acid generally have a miscible urate pool that is more than two to three times normal. On a diet that is essentially free of purine-containing foods for more than 5 days, normal men excrete 975 to 3497 mmol (164 to 588 mg) of uric acid per day.[5] Patients who excrete more than 3569 mmol (600 mg) of uric acid in 24 hours on a purine-restricted diet or more than 4758 to 5948 mmol (800 mg to 1 g) of uric acid on a normal diet can be classified as overproducers.[3] Another method for quantitative analysis of uric acid production involves the use of a spot urine specimen. This method expresses uric acid in terms of excretion per deciliter of glomerular filtrate. With this method, a urinary uric acid value of 0.4 mg/dL (20 μmol/L) of glomerular filtrate is considered normal. Patients who are overproducers have values above 0.7 mg/dL (42 μmol/L).[6]

Primary hyperuricemia and gout may also (rarely) result from one of two identified enzymatic defects. Patients who lack hypoxanthine guanine phosphoribosyltransferase (HGPRT) activity show one of two phenotypes. Complete HGPRT deficiencies present as the Lesch–Nyhan syndrome. This syndrome is associated with hyperuricemia, hyperuricaciduria, renal calculi, and a neurologic disorder characterized by self-mutilation, mental retardation, choreoathetosis, and spasticity. Patients with partial deficiency may have only gouty arthritis, hyperuricemia, hyperuricosuria, and renal calculi in the second or third decade of life. Patients with phosphoribosyl-1-pyrophosphate (PRPP) synthetase variants have increased de novo purine production. These patients may have gouty arthritis in their teens or early twenties.[7]

Secondary hyperuricemia is associated with increased nucleic acid turnover, decreased renal function, increased purine production, or drug-induced decreased elimination of uric acid. A deficiency of glucose-6-phosphatase can also lead to hyperuricemia from infancy. This results from increased purine biosynthesis and decreased uric acid clearance from hyperlactacidemia.[7]

Drug-induced hyperuricemia is the most common of the secondary hyperuricemias. Of the responsible drugs, diuretics are the most commonly implicated. The mechanism of diuretic-induced hyperuricemia is not clear, but it may relate to an increased reabsorption of uric acid in the proximal tubule. Another possible explanation is a decreased tubular secretion or an increased postsecretory reabsorption of uric acid. Spironolactone is the only diuretic that does not cause hyperuricemia.

Aspirin can increase serum urate concentrations when it is ingested in dosages of less than 2 g/day. Dosages of more than 2 g cause a uricosuric effect. Low dosages preferentially inhibit tubular secretion, and high dosages inhibit reabsorption of uric acid.

Pyrazinamide inhibits urate secretion. It markedly decreases urinary excretion of urate even when there are high levels of filtered urate. Another antitubercular drug, ethambutol, is also associated with decreased renal clearance of uric acid. Other drugs that are known to increase serum levels of uric acid include nicotinic acid, ethanol, cyclosporine, methoxyflurane, levodopa, and epinephrine.[2,8]

Hyperuricemia may be associated with any disorder that causes an increase in the cell proliferation rate. This leads to an increase in purine production and an elevation of the urate pool. Hyperuricemia occurs with lymphoid and myeloid proliferative disorders and may also occur with diseases such as psoriasis and dissemination of solid tumors. Hyperuricemia occurs in up to half of patients with chronic myelogenous leukemia. Patients with chronic lymphocytic leukemia rarely present with hyperuricemia. Hyperuricemia often occurs in myeloid metaplasia and polycythemia vera. Patients with sickle cell anemia, hemolytic anemia with secondary erythrocytosis, and thalassemia may have hyperuricemia, even though it is uncommon in primary red blood cell disorders.[2]

Chronic lead ingestion leading to nephropathy is associated with gout and hyperuricemia. Lead presumably causes a defect in the tubular secretion of urate and inhibits guanase, the enzyme that deaminates guanine to xanthine. In these cases of saturnine gout, uric acid clearance is reduced markedly, even though creatinine clearance may be only slightly decreased.[2]

Patients who fast for 1 or 2 days have elevated levels of serum urate. In most cases these elevations result from a decreased urinary output of uric acid because urate excretion is inhibited by elevated ketone levels. Alcohol (112 to 135 g) given with food is associated with an important increase in blood lactate concentration, decreased urinary uric acid output, and overproduction of uric acid. The combination of fasting and ethyl alcohol may have an additive effect on uric acid retention.[9]

Hyperuricemia may also result from other causes of increased ketoacids and lactic acid, such as exercise and uncontrolled diabetes. Additionally, hypothyroidism, hyperparathyroidism, and hypoparathyroidism have all been associated with hyperuricemia, presumably because they reduce the renal urate excretion.[3]

Many studies have related gout to racial, geographic, dietary, and other socioeconomic factors. The one consistent marker is the relationship between elevated uric acid levels and gout. The epidemiology of gout was studied as a part of the Heart Disease Epidemiology Study at Framingham, Massachusetts. This study involved 5127 subjects aged 30 to 59 on initial evaluation. Thirteen subjects, 0.2% of the total population, had experienced a gouty attack before entry in the study. The mean age of the population at the beginning of the study was 44 years. Fourteen years later, when the mean age of the population was 58, 1.5% of the population (76 subjects) had experienced an attack of gout. Gout had occurred in 2.8% of the men and 0.4% of the women. The prevalence of gouty arthritis was found to increase with increasing uric acid levels. The frequency of gout was 0.6% in men with uric acid levels under 360 μmol/L (6 mg/dL). The rate was 1.9% with levels of 360 to 410 μmol/L (6 to 6.9 mg/dL) and 20% with uric acid levels above 420 μmol/L (7 mg/dL).[10] Ninety percent of men had gout when levels exceeded 530 μmol/L (9 mg/dL).

PATHOPHYSIOLOGY

A combination of factors probably is responsible for urate crystal formation in patients with gout. The degree of hyperuricemia, joint location, abrupt changes (increases or decreases) in serum uric acid levels, physical state of the joint, resolution of joint effusions, the presence of certain protein polysaccharides, and joint temperature all are involved in urate crystal formation.

Acute attacks of gout develop when monosodium urate (MSU) crystals deposit in the synovium of joints. These crystals are derived from either preformed synovial deposits or de novo synthesis. Characteristically, acute attacks affect the peripheral joints; the most distal joints are more likely to be affected early in the course of a patient's gouty arthritis. A possible explanation for this involves joint temperature because MSU solubility varies directly with temperature. The solubility of urate in physiologic saline is 400 μmol/L (6.8 mg/dL) at 37°C but only 270 μmol/L (4.5 mg/dL) at 30°C. Joint temperatures decrease distally. The average temperature of the knee is 33°C, and that of the ankle is 29°C. However, this factor alone cannot explain why gout develops in some people and not in others who have similar uric acid levels. Also involved may be the increased solubility of urate in proteoglycans, chondroitin sulfate, and hyaluronic acid, which are abundant in the synovial fluid and cartilage. Urate solubility may be affected by genetic or environmental alterations in these substances that predispose the patient to, or even initiate, attacks of gout.[2]

Another explanation was proposed by Simkin, who was concerned with the predisposition of gout in the first metatarsophalangeal joint. Gout in this joint is called podagra, and more than 50% of first attacks of gout occur in this joint. Ultimately, most patients with gout experience podagra. The base of the big toe is subjected to extreme forces in the normal process of walking. Shoes compound the problem by forcing the joint to endure these forces in an unnatural position. The joint that has experienced degenerative changes or recent trauma, including trauma that may have been unnoticed, is likely to be the site of a synovial effusion. At night while the patient sleeps, the effusion resolves. Water leaves the joint faster than urate does; the result is a transiently high intraarticular urate concentration that favors crystal formation. This explains the common nocturnal onset of gout in the big toe and may help to explain the occasional attack of gout that develops in a person with a normal urate serum concentration.[11]

Urate crystals in the synovial fluid or surrounding tissues and the reaction of the body's defense mechanisms to these crystals cause the typical gouty attack. This reaction begins within 4 to 8 hours of the presence of these crystals in the synovial fluid. Many factors are involved in this acute inflammatory response. MSU crystals have sharp, irregular crystal facets with multiple outward projections. These surface irregularities favor the absorption of immunoglobulin G and other polypeptides. Adsorption of these polypeptides increases crystal phagocytosis by polymorphonuclear leukocytes (PMNs). In addition, MSU crystals are electronegative and therefore bind, denature, and cleave Hageman factor (clotting factor XII). This activates the clotting, kininogen, plasminogen, and complement cascades. Prostaglandins play a role in the inflammatory response of gout, causing vasodilation, increased vascular permeability, and release of chemotactic substances that attract PMNs. Although the extent of involvement of these other factors is unclear, the role of PMNs is well established.[2]

Synovial fluid from patients with gout has an average leukocyte count of 19.5×10^9/L (19,500 cells/mm^3), 90% or more of which are neutrophils. PMNs, monocytes, and synovial cells phagocytize MSU crystals that are coated with protein. This causes a fusion of lysosomes with a phagosome, producing a phagolysosome that contains enzymes. The protein coat on the crystal is digested by the enzymes, allowing hydrogen bond–mediated membranolysis to occur. Cellular autolysis results when the phagolysosome is lysed and hydrolytic enzymes are released into the cytoplasm. This also leads to increased permeability of the outer membrane of the cell and a subsequent release of enzymes into the extracellular medium. Urate crystals are digested by peroxidases in phagocytic cells, which can also adsorb leukocyte-derived proteins that may terminate the stimulus for further phagocytosis. This series of events causes the clinical findings that mark the beginning and the resolution of an acute attack of gout.[12]

CLINICAL PRESENTATION AND DIAGNOSIS

Signs and Symptoms

Acute attacks of gout are most often characterized by the sudden onset of unbearable pain in one joint of the lower extremities. The first attack is not associated with other symptoms and usually is monoarticular, although polyarticular involvement in a first attack occurs in about 10% of cases. The attack lasts a variable but limited period of time and is followed by a completely asymptomatic period.

These periods between attacks are called intercritical periods. Although a rare patient may never experience a reoccurrence, most patients experience a second attack within 6 months to 2 years. As the disease progresses, the intercritical periods become shorter and the attacks become polyarticular, more severe, and longer lasting. Eventually, patients enter a phase of chronic gout without pain-free intercritical periods.

Over time the periods between attacks become shorter, and the symptoms of the attack do not resolve completely. This leads to chronic crippling arthritis. The peak age of onset of gout is between 30 and 50 years in men. When women develop gout, it is almost always after menopause. Gout in patients of either sex before age 30 should lead to an investigation for possible enzyme defects, purine overproduction, or renal disease. Gout rarely affects patients this young.

Other commonly affected joints, in order of frequency of involvement, are the instep, ankle, heel, knee, wrist, finger, and elbow. Although acute gout initially is predominantly a disease of the joints of the lower extremities, later in the course any joint may be involved. Rare sites of involvement are the shoulder, hip, spine, sacroiliac, sternoclavicular, and temporomandibular joints.[11,13]

Patients may report several trivial episodes of pain in the big toe or ankle before the first attack of gout. Most patients have their initial attack during periods of good health. Attacks commonly occur while the patient is sleeping; many patients are awakened by excruciating pain. Occasionally, patients first detect the symptoms as their feet touch the cold floor when they get up in the morning. Three or 4 hours after the onset of an attack, the skin over the affected joint becomes red, hot, swollen, and exquisitely painful and tender. Inflammation is slight at first but progresses and can resemble a bacterial cellulitis. The systemic signs of the attack include fever, leukocytosis, and elevation of the erythrocyte sedimentation rate.[4,7] Systemic signs are more common in patients with polyarticular involvement. Temperatures may reach values as high as 39.4°C. In one study, neither fever nor leukocytosis correlated with the number of joints involved.[13] Untreated attacks of gout may last for hours to several weeks. As the patient recovers, the skin over the affected joint often desquamates. Even though an attack may be severe, with marked swelling and incapacitation, recovery from the first attack generally is complete. Patients return to their preattack state of health until the next attack.[7]

Modern treatment of gout with allopurinol and uricosurics has all but eliminated the occurrence of chronic tophaceous gout. Before these agents became available, 50 to 70% of patients with gout developed the chronic tophaceous form. It now affects approximately 3% of patients. Tophaceous gout is a consequence of consistently levated levels of uric acid, and it correlates directly with the levels of urate. In one series the mean serum urate concentration was 540 μmol/L (9.1 mg/dL) (uricase method) in 722 nontophaceous patients, 590 to 650 μmol/L (10 to 11 mg/dL) in 456 patients with minimal to moderate tophaceous deposits, and above 650 μmol/L (11 mg/dL) in 111 patients with extensive tophaceous deposits. Tophi usually are firm and movable, with thin and reddened overlying skin. They are commonly found on the helix or antihelix of the ear; the finger, hand, knee, foot, or toe; the ulnar surface of the forearm; the olecranon bursa; or the Achilles tendon. The thin skin overlying the tophi may break down and extrude a milky white substance composed mainly of urate crystals. Infection by skin flora may develop in these areas and heals slowly. Eventually, these deposits destroy the articular cartilage and portions of the subchondral bone.[7,14,15]

Renal involvement in gout is the most serious and second most common clinical manifestation. Two forms of renal disease are possible: urate nephropathy or uric acid nephropathy. Urate nephropathy results from the deposition of MSU salt crystals in the renal interstitium and the accompanying inflammation. This progresses slowly but is not thought to decrease life expectancy. It is not known whether the urate deposits cause a deterioration in renal function. Uric acid nephropathy results from the deposition of uric acid crystals in the collecting tubules. Acute renal failure occurs in patients who overproduce and overexcrete uric acid as a result of aggressive chemotherapy, lymphoma, leukemia, or enzymatic defects. This renal failure correlates not with the serum urate concentration but with the amount of uric acid excreted. Before the advent of hemodialysis, renal failure accounted for 17 to 25% of deaths in the gouty population. Kidney damage in gout usually occurs when there is diabetes, hypertension, renal vascular disease, glomerulonephritis, pyelonephritis, renal calculi with urinary tract infection, congenital nephropathy, or some other cause of primary nephropathy that is not directed from gout. It is currently accepted that asymptomatic hyperuricemia does not result in renal destruction until uric acid levels exceed 650 μmol/L (11 mg/dL) for prolonged periods.[16–18]

Diagnosis

Many criteria have been developed for establishing the diagnosis of gout. A diagnosis of gout must be firmly established before expensive and potentially toxic therapy is instituted. Gout should be considered in a patient with an acute onset of monoarticular or asymmetric polyarticular arthritis of the distal extremities. The diagnosis of acute gouty arthritis may be established by the demonstration of MSU crystals in white cells of synovial fluid or a tophus. The synovial fluid in gouty patients is cloudy and less viscous than normal. Leukocyte counts average 13.5×10^9/L (13,500 cells/mm^3, range 1.0 to 70.0×10^9/L, or 1000 to 70,000 cells/mm^3), with a predominance of PMNs. Total protein is normal, as is the glucose concentration. The Gram stain and culture of the aspirate should be negative. Needle-shaped crystals 2 to 10 μm long are present. When viewed with a polarized light microscope with a first-order red decompensator, the crystals are negatively birefringent. Urate crystals may not be found in patients with gout because of the difficulty in aspirating fluid from

Table 33.1 ▪ American Rheumatism Association Criteria for Diagnosis of Acute Gout

Definite	
	Demonstration of sodium urate crystals in affected joint
Suggestive[a]	
	More than one attack of arthritis
	Development of maximum inflammation within 1 day
	Oligoarthritis attack
	Redness over joint
	Painful or swollen first metatarsophalangeal joint
	Unilateral attack on first metatarsophalangeal joint
	Unilateral attack on tarsal joint
	Tophus
	Hyperuricemia
	Asymptomatic swelling within a joint

[a]A minimum of six criteria should be present.

involved joints. Acutely inflamed joints have intracellular urate crystals in 85% of patients with gout. A probable diagnosis of gout may be established by using criteria established by the American Rheumatism Association (Table 33.1). In addition to these criteria, complete resolution of synovitis with colchicine treatment may suggest the diagnosis. The clinical findings of pseudogout, acute sarcoidosis, psoriatic arthritis, and acute calcific tendonitis may mimic those of gout. Pseudogout and sarcoidosis may even respond to a trial of colchicine therapy, especially if it is given intravenously. If uric acid levels are normalized in a patient for a prolonged period without resolution of joint symptoms, another diagnosis should be sought.[4,7,19]

Assessment of the gouty patient should begin with a detailed history and physical examination. A family history may demonstrate a predisposition for gout, and all medications should be checked for their potential to induce hyperuricemia. It is also important to classify the hyperuricemia as a problem with overproduction or underexcretion. A 24-hour urine collection should be obtained to measure urine uric acid and creatinine. At the same time, samples for serum creatinine and blood urea nitrogen levels should be obtained to assess kidney function. Uric acid excretion above 3569 mmol (600 mg) in 24 hours in a patient on a low-purine diet for 4 to 5 days should be considered abnormal. In the absence of a purine-free diet, excretion of more than 5948 mmol (1000 mg) per 24 hours is diagnostic of overproduction. Hyperuricemia with a normal 24-hour excretion indicates underexcretion.[19]

THERAPEUTIC PLAN

Gout and hyperuricemia are treated using a two-step approach. The first step is to terminate the acute attack and resolve the pain. Once the acute attack is resolved, the goal is to gradually reduce the serum uric acid concentration. Anti-inflammatory agents that are useful for acute attacks include colchicine (Table 33.2) and nonsteroidal anti-inflammatory drugs (NSAIDs) (Table 33.3). Serum uric acid levels should not be reduced until the acute attack has been terminated. Uric acid levels should be lowered slowly and cautiously because rapid lowering of uric acid levels may precipitate another acute attack. In some mild cases, patients may be able to control the hyperuricemia by diet modifications and weight reduction. Agents that decrease uric acid levels include the XO inhibitor allopurinol and the uricosuric drugs probenecid and sulfinpyrazone (Table 33.2). Hypouricemic therapy is used to decrease the body stores of urate in an attempt to prevent or reverse the complications of urate deposition.

TREATMENT

Acute Gouty Arthritis

The treatment of acute gout is directed at alleviating the pain rapidly and attempting to restore joint mobility. It is often beneficial to immobilize the affected joint and,

Table 33.2 ▪ Drugs for Acute and Chronic Gout and Hyperuricemia

Drug (trade name)	Dosage Form (mg)	Initial Dosage (average maintenance)	Comments
Probenecid (Benemid)	Tablets (500)	250 mg BID (500 mg BID)	Hydrate well; avoid salicylates; use with caution in peptic ulcer disease and renal impairment; take with meals.
Sulfinpyrazone (Anturane)	Tablets (100) Capsules (200)	50 mg BID (100–200 mg BID)	Same as for probenecid.
Allopurinol (Zyloprim, Lopurin)	Tablets (100, 300)	100 mg QD (300 mg QD)	Hydrate well; adjust dosage in renal impairment; report any rash; take with meals.
Colchicine	Tablets (0.5, 0.6)	0.5–1.2 mg PO followed by 0.5–1.2 mg q1–2 hr	Use with caution in gastrointestinal, renal, and hepatic disorders; bone marrow depression occurs with long-term use.
	Injection (1 mg/2 mL)	Refer to text	
Probenecid and colchicine (ColBenemid)	Tablets (500 probenecid, 0.5 colchicine)	1 tablet QD (1 tablet BID)	

Table 33.3 ▪ Nonsteroidal Anti-Inflammatory Drugs for Gout

Drug (trade name)	Dosage[a] (mg)	Dosing Interval	Dosage Form (mg)
Piroxicam (Feldene)	40	QD	Capsules (10, 20)
Sulindac (Clinoril)	200	BID	Tablets (150, 200)
Naproxen (Naprosyn)	750 load, then 250	TID	Tablets (250, 375, 500)
(Anaprox, naproxen sodium)[b,c]			Tablets (275, 550)
Ketoprofen (Orudis)	100	TID	Capsules (25, 50, 75)
Ibuprofen (Motrin, Rufen)[c]	800	TID	Tablets (200, 300, 400, 600, 800)
Indomethacin (Indocin)	50	TID–QID	Capsules (10, 25, 50, 75) Suspension (25/5 mL) Suppositories (50)
Tolmetin (Tolectin)	400	TID–QID	Tablets (200, 600) Capsules (400)
Fenoprofen (Nalfon)	600–800	QID	Capsules (200, 300) Tablets (600)
Flurbiprofen (Ansaid)	400 load, then 50–100	BID–QID	Tablets (50, 100)
Etodolac (Lodine)	200–400	BID–QID	Capsules (200, 300)

[a]Recommended dosages for treating acute gouty attacks.
[b]275 mg naproxen sodium is equivalent to 250 mg naproxen.
[c]Also available over the counter under various trade names.

in severe cases, to use analgesics in addition to anti-inflammatory therapy. Anti-inflammatory medications should be started as soon after the onset of pain as possible.

Colchicine

Extracts of colchicum have been used to treat acute episodes of gout for more than 1200 years. Colchicine, an alkaloid of colchicum, was isolated in 1820, and although it is one of the oldest treatments for gout, it remains useful in certain cases. It is effective in alleviating acute attacks of gout and preventing future attacks. Colchicine is also effective in treating pseudogout, sarcoid arthritis, and calcific tendonitis. Colchicine may be used to establish a probable diagnosis of gout because the anti-inflammatory action is limited to these conditions.[20] This action is particularly useful in cases in which small joints are involved; aspirating synovial fluid and isolating uric acid crystals from these joints often are difficult. Response to colchicine is between 75 and 90%. Response rates depend on how quickly therapy is initiated after the onset of an attack. Colchicine is most effective when given within the first 12 to 36 hours of an attack. Signs and symptoms of inflammation abate within 12 to 24 hours; in 90% of patients the pain is gone within 24 to 48 hours. Most patients should be treated first with indomethacin or another of the NSAIDs that tend to be less toxic than colchicine when used in the short term.[3,7,21–23]

Colchicine has anti-inflammatory activity but no analgesic activity. It has no effect on serum levels of urinary excretion of uric acid. The mechanism of action of colchicine is not yet fully understood. Possible mechanisms include diminished PMN chemotaxis, metabolism, and lysosomal enzyme release. The mechanism of decreased chemotaxis is related to colchicine's ability to impair chemotactic factor. Colchicine also interferes with sodium urate deposition by decreasing lactic acid production by PMNs.[24]

After oral administration, colchicine is rapidly absorbed from the GI tract and partially metabolized in the liver. Unchanged drug may be reabsorbed from the intestine after biliary secretion. Concentrations of colchicine and metabolites decrease after 1 to 2 hours and then increase as a result of reabsorption of unchanged drug. The acute GI toxicity related to colchicine may be related to this drug recycling. Colchicine is concentrated in leukocytes but also appears in other tissues, including the kidneys, liver, and intestinal tract. The plasma half-life after intravenous dosing is approximately 20 minutes. The half-life in leukocytes averages 60 hours. Colchicine and its metabolites are excreted primarily in the feces; smaller amounts are excreted in the urine. Colchicine may have a prolonged half-life in patients with severe renal disease as a result of large decreases in renal excretion, and measurable quantities of drug have been found in urine for up to 10 days after therapy has been discontinued in patients with normal renal function.[22,25]

Colchicine has a very narrow therapeutic index. Acute gout attacks are treated with an initial oral dose of 0.5 to 1.2 mg colchicine. This is followed by 0.5 to 0.6 mg every hour or 1.0 to 1.2 mg every 2 hours. Therapy is continued until the patient improves, adverse GI effects (nausea, vomiting, or diarrhea) develop, or a maximum of 8 to 10 mg has been administered. The effective dosage usually is between 4 and 8 mg.[3,7,22] Death has occurred after administration of as little as 7 mg.[26] As many as 80% of patients experience some adverse GI effects, including vomiting, diarrhea, abdominal pain, and nausea, that necessitate dosage modification. Patients with preexisting Crohn's disease, diverticulitis, peptic ulcer disease, or a history of GI bleeding should not be given oral colchicine. If colchicine is deemed necessary for these patients, it may be given intravenously. Colchicine for intravenous use should be mixed with 0.9% sodium chloride or sterile water for injection because dextrose 5% in water or bacteriostatic saline may cause precipitation. A 1- to 2-mg dose should be mixed with 10 to 20 mL of the appropriate diluent and injected slowly over a period of 2 to 5 minutes or into the line of a flowing intravenous solution. Care should be taken to ensure that the intravenous injection site is patent and not infiltrating. Colchicine causes severe local irritation to the skin and tissues and should never be given subcutaneously or intramuscularly. After an initial intravenous dose of 2 mg, 0.5 mg may be given every 6 hours until a response occurs. Alternative dosing methods include a one-time dose of 3 mg or 1 mg initially, followed by 0.5 mg once or twice daily if needed. The total daily recommended intravenous dosage is 4 mg. No more than 5 mg total intravenous dosage should be given during any one treatment period. Additional courses of therapy should not be given for at least 3 days because of risk of GI toxicity.[3,25,26]

Colchicine may cause bone marrow depression with agranulocytosis, thrombocytopenia, leukopenia, and aplastic anemia. These adverse effects are rare and usually occur only in patients who have received excessive dosages or those who have decreased renal or hepatic function. Other rare adverse effects that may occur with prolonged administration include loss of body and scalp hair, rashes, peripheral neuropathy, myopathy, vesicular dermatitis, anuria, renal damage, or hematuria. Increased serum concentrations of alkaline phosphatase may also occur with colchicine administration.[27]

Colchicine may still be considered as primary therapy in patients who have used it successfully in the past. These patients generally know the total dosage of colchicine that worked for them previously and should be given half the total dosage at one time and the rest in 0.5- to 0.6-mg increments every hour until the total dosage is given. Patients who have hypersensitivity reactions to aspirin and the NSAIDs may also be candidates for colchicine therapy. Some patients who are taking warfarin should not take NSAIDs and should use colchicine. Other patients with a relative contraindication to NSAIDs include those with renal failure, congestive heart failure, and hypertension. NSAIDs in these patients can cause decreased renal function and sodium and water retention. If these patients cannot tolerate colchicine, sulindac, which may have a safer renal profile, should be tried cautiously.[28]

Gouty patients with alcoholic cirrhosis also should be treated with colchicine. Because these patients may have preexisting GI distress, renal insufficiency, and ascites, the intravenous colchicine dosage should be reduced by one-half.[29]

The frequency of recurrent attacks of gout may be reduced by prophylactic treatment with colchicine. Patients who experience fewer than one attack per year may be given 0.5 to 0.6 mg colchicine one to four times each week. If attacks are more frequent, the dosage usually is 0.5 to 0.6 mg each day. Some patients may need as much as three times this dosage each day to control the disease. Patients with a history of gout who are undergoing surgical procedures should receive 0.5 to 0.6 mg colchicine three times daily for 3 days before and 3 days after surgery.[30]

Indomethacin

Indomethacin is a potent anti-inflammatory drug that also has antipyretic and analgesic properties. It is considered by many to be the agent of choice for treating acute gouty attacks. Indomethacin should be started as soon as possible after the onset of an acute gouty attack. Unlike colchicine, it usually is effective even when treatment is delayed by several days. The probable mechanism of action of indomethacin is potent inhibition of prostaglandin synthesis. In addition, indomethacin may exert an inhibitory effect on the mobility of PMNs.[3,7,21,29]

Indomethacin given orally is rapidly and completely absorbed. Peak plasma concentrations are attained within 30 to 120 minutes. Absorption of indomethacin that is administered with food is delayed, but the serum concentration–time profile is similar to that observed in fasting subjects. Indomethacin suppositories are available for patients who are unable to take oral doses. Peak concentrations from rectal administration generally are more rapid but lower than those achieved with similar oral dosages. Bioavailability from suppositories is approximately 80%. The half-life of indomethacin ranges from 1 to 16 hours. Possibly, this large range results from extensive enterohepatic recycling and unpredictable biliary discharge. Indomethacin is metabolized primarily by the hepatic microsomal enzyme system and extramicrosomal deacylation. All metabolites are inactive.[30]

An initial dose of 50 to 75 mg of indomethacin should be given, followed by 50 mg every 6 hours. This dosage is continued for 24 to 48 hours, and then it is tapered gradually. Treatment after an acute gouty attack generally is continued for at least 2 weeks. Common adverse effects include headache, dizziness, nausea, and vomiting. These adverse effects generally are better tolerated than those seen with colchicine. Additionally, sodium and water retention, hyperkalemia, and renal dysfunction may occur in some patients.[2,3,29] Because it irritates the gastric mucosa, indomethacin should be given with food, milk, or an antacid.[29] Indomethacin should be used with caution by older adults, patients with congestive heart failure,[21] and patients with a history of peptic ulcer disease.

When indomethacin is given concurrently with probenecid, indomethacin serum levels increase, probably because of a decrease in biliary secretion.[30]

Other Anti-Inflammatory Agents

There are many other NSAIDs, and most are useful in treating gout. Agents such as sulindac, Tolectin, ibuprofen, piroxicam, naproxen, and ketoprofen are just a few of the many available drugs. These compounds also inhibit prostaglandin synthesis. Many of the newer agents may have a lower overall rate of adverse effects than indomethacin, particularly in older adults. Dosages of the drugs used to treat gout usually are the same as or higher than the dosages used to treat rheumatoid arthritis. These drugs should not be used by patients who are allergic to aspirin or by asthmatic patients with nasal polyps. The most common adverse effect with these agents is GI disturbance, and they should all be taken with food or milk. These drugs should be used with caution by patients who have a history of GI bleeding. GI hemorrhage can be life-threatening and has occurred with all of these drugs.[31–34]

Asymptomatic Hyperuricemia

Hyperuricemia exists when the serum concentration of urate exceeds the solubility limits. This level generally is considered to be 420 μmol/L (7 mg/dL) with the uricase method or 480 μmol/L (8 mg/dL) with the less specific colorimetric method.[4] Once hyperuricemia is diagnosed, the decision to treat must be based on careful evaluation of the patient's clinical condition. Treatment entails lifelong therapy and therefore includes the risk of adverse reactions and a substantial cost. Treatment of asymptomatic hyperuricemia is controversial. It is impractical and perhaps imprudent to treat every person who has mild hyperuricemia because the risks of gout and its sequelae are small.[16,35] Some clinicians believe that drug therapy is not warranted unless uric acid levels exceed 720 μmol/L (12 mg/dL) in the truly asymptomatic patient. These concentrations may be associated with joint changes and renal complications. Patients who have developed hyperuricemia as a result of other medications may need treatment if the causative agent must be continued. Hypouricemic agents also should be used for patients with recurrent episodes of gout. Patients who have developed tophi or other complications of gout should be treated with urate-lowering drugs, even in the absence of clinical disease.

Once the decision to treat has been made, two options are available: XO inhibitors and uricosurics (Fig. 33.1). Two uricosuric agents, probenecid and sulfinpyrazone, are available to increase renal elimination of uric acid. Allopurinol is the XO inhibitor. Therapy is generally based on the cause of the hyperuricemia and the patient's overall physical condition. Uricosuric agents are considered the logical choice for patients who are underexcreters of uric acid. Overproducers should be started on therapy with allopurinol. Allopurinol is also a rational choice for patients with tophi, renal stones, or moderate to severe renal dysfunction. All forms of hyperuricemia may be treated with allopurinol, but the toxicity profiles of the agents must be taken into consideration.

Probenecid

Probenecid competitively inhibits the active reabsorption of uric acid at the proximal convoluted tubule. This tubular blocking action promotes the urinary excretion of uric acid, thereby decreasing serum urate concentrations.[36]

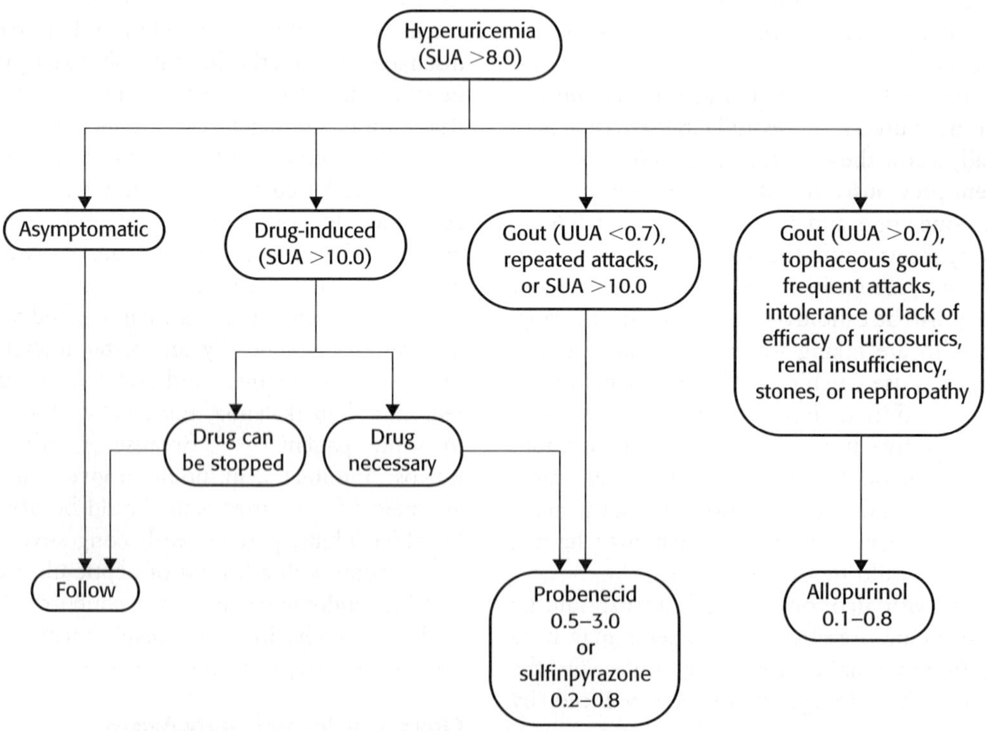

Figure 33.1. Algorithm for managing hyperuricemia. Serum urate *(SUA)* is expressed in milligrams per deciliter, measured by the colorimetric method. Urinary uric acid *(UUA)* excretion is expressed in milligrams per deciliter of glomerular filtrate. Dosages of hypouricemic drugs (probenecid, sulfinpyrazone, and allopurinol) are in grams, with the starting dosage on the left and the maximum dosage on the right. Most patients' hyperuricemia is well controlled by intermediate dosages. (*Source:* Reference 29.)

Probenecid absorption is rapid and complete; peak levels are achieved in 1 to 5 hours. The peak action of the drug occurs at about 2 hours and lasts for about 8 hours. Probenecid is highly protein bound, primarily to albumin. The drug accumulates in the kidney but not in other organs. Probenecid is metabolized by oxidation of the alkyl side chains and glucuronide conjugation. These processes account for about 90% of the metabolism. The elimination half-life is dose-dependent, approximately 2 to 6 hours with 0.5- to 1-g doses and 4 to 12 hours with a 2-g dose. Renal elimination is dose-independent but also depends on the pH and rate of urine formation. Urine alkalinization increases probenecid elimination.[37]

Dosages of 1 to 2 g of probenecid can cause a fourfold to sixfold increase uric acid elimination.[21] Active metabolites of probenecid contribute little to uric acid elimination.[37] Probenecid therapy should not be started during an acute attack of gout because it may exacerbate and prolong the inflammatory phase. Therapy should begin with 250 mg twice a day during the first week of therapy and then increase gradually in increments of 250 to 500 mg/week. A dosage of 1 g/day results in adequate urate lowering in approximately 60% of patients.[3] Dosages should be adjusted to maintain serum uric acid levels below 420 µmol/L (7 mg/dL). The dosage may also be increased if the 24-hour urine uric acid excretion is not above 4160 mmol (700 mg).[7] The drug may increase the frequency of acute attacks during the first year of therapy, even if urate concentrations are maintained at or below normal.

Patients should be advised to drink large quantities of fluid, at least 2 L/day, while taking probenecid. This decreases the risk of uric acid stone formation.[3] Urine alkalinization to a pH greater than 6 greatly increases the solubility of uric acid; the resulting increase in probenecid elimination is not therapeutically important.[37] Probenecid may not be effective in and should not be used by patients with renal impairment who have a creatinine clearance of less than 50 mL/minute.[22]

Probenecid usually is well tolerated; the adverse effects most commonly associated with probenecid are GI discomfort in 8 to 18% of patients, hypersensitivity reactions in 5%, precipitation of uric acid stones in 10%, and precipitation of acute gouty attacks in 10%. GI complaints may be decreased by taking each dose with food.[3,36]

Probenecid should be used cautiously by patients with a history of peptic ulcer disease, and it should not be used by patients with a blood dyscrasia or uric acid kidney stones. The drug should never be used to treat hyperuricemia caused by cancer chemotherapy, myeloproliferative neoplastic diseases, or radiation because of greatly increased risks of uric acid nephropathy.

Because probenecid inhibits renal tubular secretion of many weak organic acids, it causes many interesting drug interactions. Probenecid inhibits the secretion of the penicillins, cephalosporins, nalidixic acid, rifampicin, and nitrofurantoin. This leads to higher levels of antibiotics for prolonged periods. This drug interaction has been used therapeutically to increase the duration and plasma concentrations of the penicillins and cephalosporins. The efficacy of nitrofurantoin is decreased by this interaction, and the toxicity is increased. The renal elimination of naproxen, indomethacin, and sulfinpyrazone is also decreased. The naproxen and indomethacin dosages must be decreased, but the concomitant use of probenecid and sulfinpyrazone does not increase adverse reactions. In contrast, allopurinol clearance increases in the presence of probenecid, but the effects of the two drugs are additive, and the combination may be used to therapeutic advantage.

The diuresis produced by furosemide and the thiazides increases because their renal elimination decreases when they are given with probenecid. Concomitant administration with heparin has been reported to increase clotting time. In patients receiving chlorpropamide, blood sugar levels should be monitored closely at the start of probenecid therapy because the half-life of chlorpropamide may increase and may result in hypoglycemia. Interactions with other sulfonylureas may occur. Low-dose aspirin is an absolute contraindication with probenecid or sulfinpyrazone therapy because aspirin blocks uric acid excretion, reducing the therapeutic effect of these uricosuric agents.

Sulfinpyrazone

Like probenecid, sulfinpyrazone competitively inhibits active reabsorption of uric acid at the proximal convoluted tubule, thereby promoting the urinary excretion of uric acid and reducing serum urate concentrations. Sulfinpyrazone is a potent uricosuric agent that is chemically related to phenylbutazone. In addition, it reduces platelet adhesiveness and can result in prolonged platelet survival.[22]

Oral administration of sulfinpyrazone results in rapid and complete absorption. Peak plasma levels usually are obtained within 1 hour. The half-life is short, ranging from 1 to 3 hours. Approximately 98% of plasma sulfinpyrazone is bound to proteins, and 25 to 45% of a dose is excreted unchanged in the urine, with most of the excretion occurring within 6 hours. The uricosuric action of the drug results from inhibition of the tubular reabsorption of uric acid in the nephron.[36]

On a weight-for-weight basis, sulfinpyrazone is three to six times as potent as probenecid as a uricosuric. Therapy should be started with a daily dosage of 100 mg, given as 50 mg twice a day, for about the first week. The dosage is then increased by 100-mg increments each week until an effective dosage is reached. A typical regimen might be 50 mg twice a day for 1 week, 100 mg twice a day for 1 week, 150 mg twice a day for 1 week, and so on, until a maintenance dosage of 200 to 400 mg/day is achieved. The drug may increase the frequency of acute attacks during the first year of therapy, even if urate concentrations are maintained at or below normal. There is evidence that administering prophylactic dosages of colchicine, 1 mg/day or less, during the first 6 months decreases the frequency of subsequent attacks. Most clinicians agree with the prophylactic use of colchicine or NSAIDs for patients taking uricosuric agents during this phase.[7,21,22]

Like probenecid, this drug should not be used when creatinine clearance is less than 50 mL/minute. Periodic blood counts should be performed during sulfinpyrazone therapy because of the rare occurrence of anemia, leukopenia, thrombocytopenia, and agranulocytosis. No uricosuric should be used by patients who are overproducers of uric acid.

When used in recommended dosages, sulfinpyrazone usually is well tolerated, with a low rate of adverse effects. The most common adverse effects are those affecting the GI tract (nausea or peptic ulcer reactivation). These may occur in as many as 15% of patients. As with probenecid, there is the risk of inducing uric acid crystalluria; therefore, patients who are on this therapy should consume large quantities of fluid.[36] Bronchoconstriction may occur in some patients who are aspirin sensitive. In addition to these adverse effects, sulfinpyrazone has been noted to cause an immunoallergic acute interstitial nephritis. These changes are for the most part reversible.

Although sulfinpyrazone inhibits the renal tubular secretion of many weak organic acids, the elevation in plasma concentrations of penicillins and cephalosporins is not clinically useful. Sulfinpyrazone decreases the antiinfective action of nitrofurantoin and increases its toxicity. Salicylates should not be used with sulfinpyrazone because they block the uricosuric action.

Allopurinol

Allopurinol is the most commonly used agent for the long-term control of chronic gout. Allopurinol inhibits XO, the enzyme that catalyzes the conversion of xanthine to uric acid and hypoxanthine to xanthine. Allopurinol itself is metabolized by XO to oxypurinol, which also inhibits XO (Fig. 33.2). The inhibition of XO by allopurinol and oxypurinol decreases the concentrations of serum and urinary uric acid. The decrease in uric acid concentrations is accompanied by an increase in urinary concentrations of xanthine and hypoxanthine. The solubilities of uric acid, xanthine, and hypoxanthine are independent, thus greatly reducing the chances of crystalluria.[38–40]

These actions result not only from XO inhibition but also from a decrease in de novo purine biosynthesis. Allopurinol is converted to a ribonucleotide by HGPRT. The critical rate-limiting enzyme in purine biosynthesis, PRPP amidotransferase, is inhibited by the allopurinol ribonucleotide. Patients who are deficient in HGPRT activity, such as those with Lesch–Nyhan syndrome, do not demonstrate this decrease in purine biosynthesis.[2,41]

Allopurinol is well absorbed from the intestinal tract and has a half-life of only 2 to 3 hours. The half-life of oxypurinol is much longer than that of allopurinol (18 to 30 hours). The long half-life of the active metabolite allows once-daily dosing in chronic therapy.[25]

Allopurinol is the drug of choice for overproducers of uric acid, but it is also efficacious for patients who are underexcreters. Many clinicians prescribe allopurinol because of the decreased risk of nephrolithiasis. However, because of uncommon but potentially dangerous adverse effects associated with allopurinol, it should be recommended only in the following cases: tophaceous gout, major uric acid overproduction (urinary excretion of more than 5350 mmol, or 900 mg, uric acid per 24 hours on a diet with rigid purine restriction), frequent gouty attacks that are unresponsive to prophylactic colchicine, intolerance or lack of efficacy of uricosuric agents, recurrent uric acid calculi, renal insufficiency, recurrent calcium oxalate, renal calculi associated with hyperuricosuria, and prevention of acute urate nephropathy in patients receiving cytotoxic therapy for malignancies. Asymptomatic hyperuricemia, uncomplicated gout, and acute gouty attacks are not considered proper indications for the use of allopurinol.[42]

Allopurinol is effective in dosages of 100 to 300 mg/day. The average dosage for an adult with gout and normal renal function is 300 mg once a day. For cases of moderately severe tophaceous gout, dosages of 400 to 600 mg/day in divided doses may be needed. A single daily dose is possible for normal patients because of the prolonged half-life of the active allopurinol metabolite oxypurinol. In patients with impaired renal function, allopurinol and oxypurinol may accumulate, and the dosage should be reduced. The usual dosage of 300 mg/day should be reduced to 200 mg when the creatinine clearance is 0.17 to 0.33 mL/second (10 to 20 mL/minute) and to 100 mg when the creatinine clearance is less than 0.17 mL/second (10 mL/minute). For patients with a creatinine clearance less than 0.05 mL/second (3 mL/minute), a 300-mg dose twice a week should

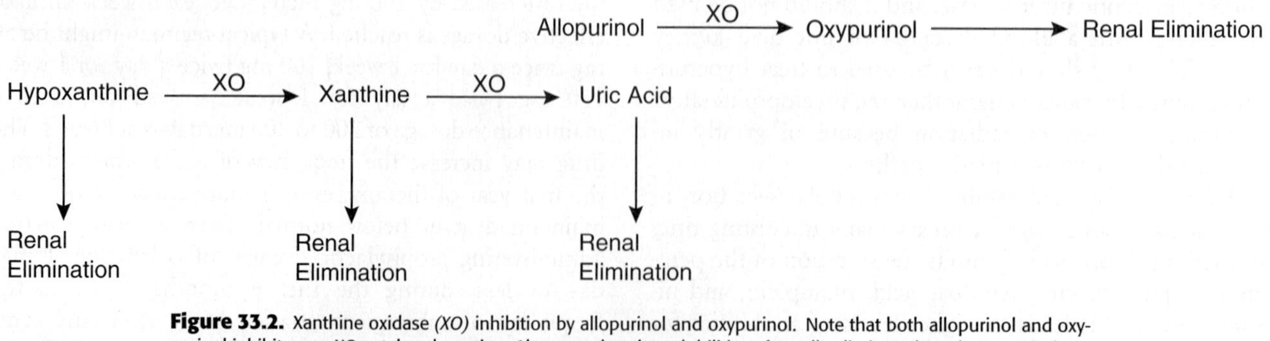

Figure 33.2. Xanthine oxidase *(XO)* inhibition by allopurinol and oxypurinol. Note that both allopurinol and oxypurinol inhibit every XO-catalyzed reaction. Also note that the solubilities of renally eliminated products are independent of one another, increasing the body's ability to eliminate products of purine metabolism.

be adequate to reduce serum urate concentrations. To reduce the risk of an acute gouty attack when initiating therapy, the dosage should begin at 100 mg/day and be increased by 100 mg weekly until serum urate levels fall below 360 μmol/L (6 mg/dL) or the maximum recommended dosage of 800 mg/day is reached. When begun after an acute gouty attack, prophylactic NSAIDs or colchicine 0.5 to 1.2 mg/day may be administered with allopurinol to decrease the risk of another acute attack. When at all possible, let the acute gouty attack resolve before initiating therapy to lower uric acid. If the acute attacks occur after therapy has been started, dosages should not be adjusted. Allopurinol therapy should be continued indefinitely; intermittent therapy is of little benefit and may place the patient at risk of an acute attack.[7,21,22]

Allopurinol is also used to treat or prevent hyperuricemia associated with tissue breakdown resulting from cancer chemotherapy or radiation. It also reduces the chances of the patient developing secondary uric acid nephropathy from myeloproliferative neoplastic diseases.

Allopurinol generally is well tolerated, with an overall adverse effect rate less than 1%. The frequency of adverse effects increases in the presence of renal insufficiency. The most common adverse effect is a pruritic maculopapular rash. Exfoliative, urticarial, erythematosus, hemorrhagic, and purpuric skin eruptions also occur. Stevens–Johnson syndrome has rarely been reported. Skin reactions may be delayed and have occurred as long as 2 years after therapy is started. These reactions sometimes are severe and associated with a hypersensitivity reaction that can be fatal. Symptoms include a variety of skin eruptions, fever, lymphadenopathy, eosinophilia, and generalized vasculitis. Renal and hepatic damage may occur if the reaction is severe and generalized. Less common adverse effects include alopecia, exfoliative dermatitis, leukopenia and neutropenia, hepatitis as part of a generalized hypersensitivity reaction, and nephrolithiases.[41–46]

Drug Interactions

Allopurinol and oxypurinol inhibit the metabolism of azathioprine and 6-mercaptopurine, increasing their potential toxicity. When administered concomitantly, the dosages of these drugs should be reduced by 25 to 33%. Patients who are receiving allopurinol with ampicillin or amoxicillin have an increased frequency of rash. In addition, patients who are receiving uricosuric therapy with allopurinol have an increased excretion of oxypurinol. This effect can reduce XO inhibition. Even though this occurs, the effect of combined allopurinol and a uricosuric generally is additive, and no dosage adjustments are necessary.[21,22]

KEY POINTS

- Gout is characterized by hyperuricemia that results from an overproduction or underexcretion of uric acid. It is an acute inflammatory joint disease in which uric acid crystals are deposited in the affected joints.
- Disease progression is variable and patient dependent. The risk of progression to a debilitating chronic disease is lower today because effective treatments have been developed.
- Treatment with hypouricemic agents for long-term control should be based on careful patient assessment. When this therapy is deemed necessary, treatment is lifelong.
- Occasional gout or asymptomatic hyperuricemia may not warrant drug treatment. In these cases, alterations in diet and lifestyle may be enough to keep a patient symptom-free.

REFERENCES

1. Bell JE. Uric acid. Hosp Pharm 7:356–357, 1972.
2. Boss GR, Seegmiller JE. Hyperuricemia and gout: classification, complications and management. N Engl J Med 300:1459–1468, 1979.
3. Mangini RJ. Drug therapy reviews: pathogenesis and clinical management of hyperuricemia and gout. Am J Hosp Pharm 36:497–504, 1979.
4. Lo B. Hyperuricemia and gout. West J Med 142:104–107, 1985.
5. Seegmiller JE, Grayzel AI, Laster L, et al. Uric acid production in gout. J Clin Invest 40:1094–2098, 1962.
6. Simkin PA, Hoover PL, Paxson CS, et al. Uric acid excretion: quantitative assessment from spot, midmorning serum and urine samples. Ann Intern Med 91:44–47, 1979.
7. German DC, Holmes EW. Hyperuricemia and gout. Med Clin North Am 70:419–436, 1986.
8. Demartine FE. Hyperuricemia induced by drugs. Arthritis Rheum 8:823–829, 1965.
9. Maclachlan MJ, Rodnan GP. Effects of food, fast and alcohol on serum uric acid and acute attacks of gout. Am J Med 42:38–57, 1967.
10. Hall AP, Barry PE, Dawber TR, et al. Epidemiology of gout and hyperuricemia: a long term population study. N Engl J Med 42:27–37, 1967.
11. Simkin PA. The pathogenesis of podagra. Ann Intern Med 86:230–233, 1977.
12. McCarty DJ. Pathogenesis and treatment of crystal-induced inflammation. In: McCarty DJ, ed. Arthritis and allied conditions. 10th ed. Philadelphia: Lea & Febiger, 1985:1494–1514.
13. Hadler NM, Franck WA, Bress NM, et al. Acute polyarticular gout. Am J Med 56:715–719, 1974.
14. Krane SM. Crystal-induced joint disease. In: Rubenstein E, Federman DD, eds. Medicine. New York: Scientific American, 1982;2:1–15.
15. Holmes EW. Clinical gout and the pathogenesis of hyperuricemia. In: McCarty DJ, ed. Arthritis and allied conditions. 10th ed. Philadelphia: Lea & Febiger, 1985:1445–1480.
16. Liang MH, Fries JF. Asymptomatic hyperuricemia: the case for conservative management. Ann Intern Med 88:666–670, 1978.
17. Yu TF, Berger L. Impaired renal function in gout, its association with hypertensive vascular disease and intrinsic renal disease. Am J Med 72:95–100, 1982.
18. Palella TD, Kelley WN. An approach to hyperuricemia and gout. Geriatrics 39:89–102, 1984.
19. Yu TF, Berger L. Renal function in gout. IV: an analysis of 524 gouty subjects including long-term follow-up studies. Am J Med 59:605–613, 1975.
20. Wallace SL, Bernstein D, Diamond H. Diagnostic value of the colchicine therapeutic trial. JAMA 199:525–528, 1967.
21. Bergman HD. Drug therapy in gout. US Pharm 2:58–64, 1977.
22. Emmerson BT. Drug control of gout and hyperuricemia. Drugs 16:158–166, 1978.
23. Lomen PL. Flurbiprofen in the treatment of acute gout. Am J Med 80(3A):134, 1986.
24. Spilberg I, Mandell B, Mehta J, et al. Mechanism of action of colchicine in acute urate crystal-induced arthritis. J Clin Invest 64:775–780, 1979.
25. Flower RJ, Moncada S, Vane JR. Analgesic-antipyretics and anti-inflammatory agents: drugs employed in the treatment of gout. In: Gilman GA, Goodman LS, Rall TW, et al., eds. The pharmacological basis of therapeutics. 7th ed. New York: Macmillan, 1985:674–715.
26. Freeman DL. Frequent doses of intravenous colchicine can be lethal [letter]. N Engl J Med 309:310, 1983.

27. Naidus RM, Rodvien R, Mielke CH. Colchicine toxicity: a multi-system disease. Arch Intern Med 137:394–396, 1977.
28. Ciabattoni G, Cinotti GA, Pierucci A, et al. Effects of sulindac and ibuprofen in patients with chronic glomerular disease. N Engl J Med 310:279–283, 1984.
29. Nashel DJ, Chandra M. Acute gouty arthritis, special management considerations in alcoholic patients. JAMA 247:58–59, 1982.
30. Simkin PA. Management of gout. Ann Intern Med 90:812–816, 1979.
31. Helleberg L. Clinical pharmacokinetics of indomethacin. Clin Pharmacokinet 6:245–258, 1981.
32. Brogden RN, Heel RC, Speight TM, et al. Piroxicam: a reappraisal of its pharmacology and therapeutic efficacy. Drugs 28:292–323, 1984.
33. Widmark PH. Piroxicam: its safety and efficacy in the treatment of acute gout. Am J Med 72(2A):63–65, 1982.
34. Schweitz MC, Nashel DJ, Alpea P. Ibuprofen in the treatment of acute gouty arthritis. JAMA 239:34–35, 1978.
35. Warnock DG. Treatment of hyperuricemia and gout [letter]. N Engl J Med 301:1240, 1979.
36. Kantor T. Ketoprofen: a review of its pharmacologic and clinical properties. Pharmacotherapy 6(3):93–103, 1986.
37. Gutman AB. Uricosuric drugs, with special reference to probenecid and sulfinpyrazone. Adv Pharmacol 4:91–136, 1966.
38. Cunningham RF, Israili ZH, Dayton PG. Clinical pharmacokinetics of probenecid. Clin Pharmacokinet 6:135–151, 1981.
39. Yu TF. The effect of allopurinol in primary and secondary gout. Arthritis Rheum 8:905–906, 1965.
40. Houpt JB. The effect of allopurinol (HPP) in the treatment of gout. Arthritis Rheum 8:899–904, 1965.
41. Klineberg JR. The effectiveness of allopurinol in the treatment of gout. Arthritis Rheum 8:891–895, 1965.
42. Rundles RW. The development of allopurinol. Arch Intern Med 145:1492–1502, 1985.
43. Singer JZ, Wallace SL. The allopurinol hypersensitivity syndrome: unnecessary morbidity and mortality. Arthritis Rheum 29:82–87, 1986.
44. Vincent PC. Drug-induced aplastic anemia and agranulocytosis: incidence and mechanisms. Drugs 31:52–63, 1986.
45. Ohsawa T, Ohtsubo M. Hepatitis associated with allopurinol. Drug Intell Clin Pharm 19:431–433, 1985.
46. Worth CT, Hussein SM. Peripheral neuropathy due to long term ingestion of allopurinol. BMJ 291:1688, 1985.

CHAPTER 34

SYSTEMIC LUPUS ERYTHEMATOSUS

Stephen H. Fuller and Carlos da Camara

Systemic Lupus Erythematosus

DEFINITION

Systemic lupus erythematosus (SLE) is a complex autoimmune disorder affecting many organ systems, with clinical manifestations varying significantly between patients. Although significant advances of recent years have refined our understanding of the immunologic mechanisms of the disease, many uncertainties about the main causes remain. Advances in diagnosis and management have substantially improved the prognosis, mortality, and overall quality of life of patients with SLE. Because of these improvements, other areas such as disease comorbidities and drug therapy complications are receiving greater attention.

Most of the disease manifestations of SLE are related to the key immunologic response: inflammation.[1] Dermatologic and joint manifestations are the most prominent features of SLE. Organ systems commonly affected include the kidneys, central and peripheral nervous systems, heart, lungs, and circulatory system.[2,3] Although many of these organs can be affected by the disease, the name *lupus erythematosus* arose from early recognition of the characteristic cutaneous manifestations in the mid-nineteenth century.[3]

Clinically distressing symptoms such as heat, swelling, pain, tenderness, and local tissue destruction all relate to the inflammatory process. However, no single theory can completely explain the pathologic process, so researchers suspect multiple causes and triggering mechanisms (e.g., one defect triggers the immune response and another perpetuates a significant antibody reaction). Other etiologic factors include a genetic predisposition, drugs, viral infections, ultraviolet (UV) rays, hormones, environmental agents, and emotional stress. Therefore, SLE may not be a single disease entity but rather a complex immunologic phenomenon resulting in signs and symptoms produced by different causes.[4]

TREATMENT GOALS: SYSTEMIC LUPUS ERYTHEMATOSUS

- Relieve symptoms of the disease.
- Slow or prevent the inflammatory response and subsequent tissue destruction.
- Improve the patient's overall quality of life.
- Prolong survival.
- Closely monitor for disease manifestations.
- Avoid precipitating factors.
- Educate the patient about the manifestations of the disease and side effects of drug therapy.[5]

EPIDEMIOLOGY

SLE has recently been estimated to affect 14.6 to 50.8 people per 100,000 in the United States, compared to 12 to 30 cases per 100,000 in other countries. SLE has an annual incidence rate of almost 8 new cases per 100,000, an increase from the 2 cases per 100,000 observed 30 years ago. SLE can occur in all races but is two to four times more common in blacks, Hispanics, and Asians than in Caucasians. In younger age groups (less than 40 years), SLE is seen primarily in women (9:1 female:male ratio), but this predominance fades in patients who are diagnosed after 65 years of age (2:1 female:male ratio). More than 60% of patients are diagnosed between ages 15 and 55; 20% or less are diagnosed before 15 years or after 65 years of age. A hereditary component also appears to be involved, with multiple genes being emphasized as affecting regulation of the immune system and sex hormones. First-degree family members of patients with SLE have SLE rates of 5 to 12%, several hundred times higher than in the general population. Although SLE occurs primarily in women of childbearing age, many etiologic factors still are not understood.[1,6–9]

PATHOPHYSIOLOGY

Although the causes of SLE remain largely unknown, it is evident that much of the pathogenic process results from a loss of self-tolerance.[10] Genetic, viral, endocrine, and other environmental factors are thought to play an important role in the pathogenesis of the disease, but the exact mechanism remains to be determined.[4] The most important feature of this disorder is the production of autoantibodies directed against proteins found in the nucleus and cytoplasm and on cellular surfaces.[4,10] Specific factors triggering development of these pathogenic proteins are being investigated. These abnormal autoimmune-mediated responses result in the characteristic clinical manifestations of SLE.[4] The important autoantibodies expressed in patients with SLE include those directed against the cell nucleus (antinuclear antibodies, ANAs).[11] The presence of these autoantibodies is characteristic of SLE; they can be found in more than 95% of cases.[12]

Although they are capable of binding to DNA, RNA, nuclear proteins, and other protein nucleic acid complexes, two are highly specific for patients with SLE.[1] Double-stranded (ds) DNA antibodies and those directed against components of a small RNA protein (called anti-Smith [anti-Sm]) are found exclusively in patients with SLE. Although both are used as markers for SLE, they have different patterns of expression, associated clinical events, and target antigens. For example, these ANAs have been shown to be involved in immune complex–mediated organ inflammation and damage (e.g., glomerulonephritis), autoimmune-mediated cellular dysfunction (e.g., autoimmune cytopenias), and immune interference with cell surface phospholipid molecules (e.g., antiphospholipid syndrome).[2,3] In the case of glomerulonephritis, a clear correlation has been shown between anti-DNA antibody serum levels and disease activity.[11,13] Although assays have been developed to detect anti-DNA antibodies, their application is mostly for diagnosis rather than monitoring.[1]

In addition to excessive autoantibody production, patients with SLE have hyperactivation of B cells and T cells, monocyte function abnormalities, and disturbances in deposition and disposal of the complement system.[1,4] This abnormal activation produces hyperglobulinemia (immunoglobulin M [IgM], IgG, IgA), an increase in the number of cells that produce antibodies, and an increase in the response to many antigens (self and foreign). There is also strong evidence of a general failure of the immunoregulatory system to downregulate the excessive activation of these cells.[4]

Patients with SLE clearly have enhanced activity of B cells at stages of cell maturation. Activation of B cells in patients with SLE occurs in a nonspecific manner that results in a generalized or polyclonal production of antibody-forming B-lymphocytes.[14] Why so many different pathogenic antibodies form in patients with SLE is unclear. Besides hyperactivated B cells, recent evidence shows that other factors, such as interleukin-6 (IL-6) and IL-10 may play a role in activating, perpetuating, and increasing the stimulation of specific autoantigens.[4] Although it is unclear which of these specific autoantibodies contribute to the disease process, there appears to be a strong correlation between the number of pathogenic antibodies and the level of disease activity in patients with SLE.[14,15]

T-cell abnormalities also figure prominently in the disease process.[4] The total number of suppressor T cells is reduced in many patients with SLE (probably because of the effects of antilymphocyte antibodies), but the remaining T cells may stimulate B cells to increase production of pathogenic anti-DNA antibodies.[4] Therefore, it appears that the enhanced level of autoantibody production by B cells is a T cell–dependent immune response. In fact, several studies show a good correlation between T-cell lymphopenia and disease severity.[14] T-cell subsets that may promote autoantibody production in patients with SLE include $CD4^+/CD8^-$, $CD4^-/CD8^+$, and the phenotypes $CD4^-/CD8^-$ α/β and γ/δ.[14] In addition to the increased production of immune complexes, it has been postulated that impaired immune complex clearance in patients with SLE may play a role.[1,4] Factors that may impair immune complex handling and clearance include primary complement deficiency, defective complement function, and abnormal distribution of IgG fragment constant (Fc) receptors.[15] The degree of hypocomplementemia also correlates directly with the severity of disease activity, with extreme hypocomplementemia occurring in patients with renal and central nervous system (CNS) disease. During immune complex formation, chemotactic factors are released, attracting phagocytic cells, which results in the production of lysosomal enzymes, causing immune complex–mediated inflammation and tissue destruction. The characteristic SLE pathologic changes include three histologic lesions: hematoxylin bodies (bluish, globular masses suspected of being the inclusion bodies of lupus cells), onionskin lesions (characteristic concentric perivascular fibrosis found in central and penicillary arteries of the spleen), and Libman–Sacks verrucous endocarditis (characteristic lesions consisting of nonbacterial vegetations on heart valves (especially the mitral valve), chordae tendineae, and endocardium of the papillary muscle. Pathologic involvement in most other organs relates to vasculitis or mononuclear cell infiltrates.[1]

Many factors can contribute to SLE disease susceptibility. Genetic factors play a significant role in the disease development, with immunologic abnormalities being found more often in family members of patients with SLE than in the general population. There is a 14 to 57% incidence of the trait in monozygotic twins, compared to approximately 5 to 9% frequency in dizygotic twins and other first-degree relatives of patients with SLE. In addition, certain ethnic groups have a high prevalence of SLE. For example, SLE is three times more common in black people than in the general population.[1,16] Numerous other genetic relationships point to causality. The best-defined genes that have been linked to SLE in humans can be found on chromosome 6, which encodes for human leukocyte antigen (HLA) genes, especially those in classes II (DR, DQ, DP) and III (C2, C4).[4]

Viruses and other transmissible infectious agents have received a lot of attention because electron microscopic observations in SLE tissues reveal tubuloreticular structures and the nucleoprotein core of paramyxoviruses. Serologic levels of antiviral antibodies in patients with SLE often are elevated; however, they are usually directed toward several unrelated viruses, which suggests a nonspecific B-cell lymphocyte activation rather than a unique antigenic exposure. Although direct viral isolation from tissue of patients with SLE has been attempted, conventional or cocultivation techniques have not been successful in identifying specific viruses.[4] Therefore, it remains to be determined whether virus expression is the result or cause of SLE.

The high incidence of SLE in women of reproductive age suggests that hormonal factors may play an important role in the this disorder. Selected animal models of SLE show that female mice have earlier appearances of dsDNA antibodies, more severe complications (e.g., nephritis), and shorter life spans.[4] Administering androgens appears to improve survival and reduce nephritic complications in these animals. Furthermore, estrogen hormones enhance and androgen hormones suppress immune reactivity.[4] Although the effects of these mechanisms are not known, it is thought that estrogens depress T cell–mediated immunity (the natural killer cell function) and allow B-cell antibody proliferation. By contrast, androgens inhibit both B-cell and T-cell maturation and depress the reactivity of passively transferred lymphocytes, thereby depressing immune reactivity.[17]

Environmental factors also may contribute to the development of SLE. UV light (especially UVB), thermal burns, and other physical stresses (e.g., infection, pregnancy, or surgery) have been implicated in modifying the disease process. Other factors such as drug-induced SLE, the presence of antibodies in laboratory workers exposed to SLE sera, household contacts of patients with SLE, hair dyes, and specific diets may also support the development of SLE in genetically susceptible people.[4,10]

CLINICAL PRESENTATION AND DIAGNOSIS

Signs and Symptoms

The diagnosis of SLE is based on the presence of clinical features, as outlined in the Revised Criteria for the Classification of SLE (Table 34.1); the presence of at least four criteria is considered mandatory for a diagnosis of SLE to be considered.[12] The most problematic symptoms of SLE are fatigue, fever, and weight loss, which occur in 80 to 100% of patients and often can lead to misdiagnosis. Fatigue usually is a patient's initial and most common complaint because it is very debilitating, and it often responds to exercise or medication. However, fatigue may be present when no other clinical symptoms are obvious, and it worsens with acute exacerbations of the disease. Episodic fevers (up to 101°F) occur in 80% of patients with SLE; however, infectious disease processes must be ruled out if fevers are persistently higher than 101°F. Weight loss (more than 5 pounds) often occurs before the actual diagnosis of SLE and is thought to be related to the loss of appetite from SLE-induced gastrointestinal inflammation. This results in dyspepsia, difficulty swallowing, and gastroesophageal reflux disease. However, these gastrointestinal symptoms and peptic ulcer disease also can result from the medications patients receive to treat SLE (nonsteroidal anti-inflammatory drugs [NSAIDs], steroids, immunosuppressants).[9,18]

Musculoskeletal manifestations are found in 80 to 95% of patients with SLE and often precede the diagnosis by several months. Joint involvement is symmetric and involves primarily the wrists, small joints of the hand, knees, and less often ankles, elbows, hips, and shoulders.

Radiologic findings show soft tissue swelling and periarticular demineralization.[9] In contrast to rheumatoid arthritis, morning stiffness and joint involvement tend to be nonerosive and nondeforming. Other common sources of musculoskeletal pain in SLE include avascular necrosis, septic arthritis, and myositis. Some patients may experience swan neck deformities, subcutaneous nodules, and sacroiliac joint involvement, but these are not common and usually suggest other disease processes such as mixed connective tissue disease or rheumatoid arthritis.[3,12] Patients receiving high-dose steroids on a chronic basis may be predisposed to avascular necrosis (osteonecrosis) or steroid-induced osteoporosis, which can result in demineralization of trabecular bone, causing fractures of the hip or spine. In addition, steroids may cause joint pain and swelling due to fluid retention or muscle tenderness (steroid myopathy) in addition to the symptoms already present.[3,18]

Skin lesions are present in 90% of patients with SLE and occur with systemic flares of lupus or upon exposure to sunlight (usually UVB rays) or other sources of UV light

Table 34.1 ▪ 1982 Revised Criteria for Classification of Systemic Lupus Erythematosus

Criterion	Definition
Malar rash	Fixed erythema, flat or raised, over the malar eminences, tending to spare the nasolabial folds.
Discoid rash	Erythematous raised plaques with adherent keratotic scaling and follicular plugging; atrophic scarring may occur in older lesions.
Photosensitivity	Skin rash as a result of unusual reaction to sunlight, as determined through history taking or physician observation.
Oral ulcers	Oral or nasopharyngeal ulceration, usually painless, observed by a physician.
Arthritis	Nonerosive arthritis involving two or more peripheral joints, characterized by swelling, tenderness, or effusion.
Serositis	Pleuritis (convincing history of pleuritic pain or rub heard by physician or evidence of pleural effusion) or pericarditis (documented by electrocardiogram, rub, or evidence of pericardial effusion).
Renal disorder	Persistent proteinuria (>0.5 g/day or >3 if quantitation is not performed) or cellular casts (red cell, hemoglobin, granular, mixed).
Neurologic disorder	Seizures or psychosis in the absence of offending drugs or known metabolic problems (uremia, ketoacidosis, or electrolyte imbalance).
Hematologic disorder	Hemolytic anemia (with reticulocytosis), leukopenia (<4000/mm^3 total on two or more occasions), lymphopenia (<1500/mm^3 on two or more occasions), or thrombocytopenia (<100,000/mm^3 in the absence of offending drugs).
Immunologic disorder	Positive lupus cell preparation, anti-DNA antibodies, anti-Sm antibodies, false-positive serologic test for syphilis known to be positive for at least 6 mo and confirmed by *Treponema pallidum* immobilization or fluorescent treponemal antibody absorption test.
Antinuclear antibody	An abnormal titer of antinuclear antibody by immunofluorescence or an equivalent assay at any time and in the absence of drugs known to cause drug-induced lupus syndrome.

Source: Reference 6.

The proposed classification is based on 11 criteria. For the purpose of clinical studies, a patient shall be said to have systemic erythematous lupus if any 4 or more of the 11 criteria are present, serially or simultaneously, during any interval of observation.

(fluorescent light). Dermatologic manifestations are labeled as acute cutaneous lupus erythematosus (ACLE), subacute cutaneous lupus erythematosus (SCLE), and discoid lupus erythematosus (DLE); ACLE and SCLE involve sensitivity to sunlight, especially in Caucasian patients. ACLE is responsible for more than half of the skin disease in patients with SLE and usually appears as the classic butterfly or malar rash (40% of patients), which derives its name from the butterfly-shaped erythema covering the cheeks and bridge of the nose.[19] The malar rash is acute in onset and may last for hours to days and may be worsened upon exposure to sunlight. Other ACLE rashes include morbilliform eruptions and bullous lesions.

SCLE occurs in 15 to 20% of patients with SLE, and the lesions are small, superficial, papulosquamous, annular, nonscarring lesions typically located on the shoulders, neck, forearms, and upper torso. Most patients (70%) are photosensitive, and have anti-Ro antibodies, high ANA titers, possible decreases in complement, and very mild or no systemic involvement.

DLE lesions occur in 10 to 20% of patients with lupus and present as round, well-defined, red-purple, scaly plaques that occur primarily on the head, neck, and upper torso. The severity of the rash often depends on the intensity of the UV exposure, but DLE lesions can occur in areas not exposed to the sun. DLE lesions are deeper than SLCE lesions and may result in depigmentation and scarring. In addition, DLE lesions may be chronic and not associated with other symptoms of SLE; however, approximately 10% of patients with DLE are at risk of developing SLE. Vascular lesions can occur in up to 50% of patients and are believed to form from leukocyte infiltration, resulting in vascular damage. These lesions affect different vessel locations and can result in urticaria, purpura, and petechiae on the hands or feet. Mucous membranes are involved in more than 25% of patients and often appear as discoid lesions on the lips or mouth.[3,9,19]

Almost all SLE patients demonstrate renal abnormalities, including clinical nephropathy, within 36 months of diagnosis. Although serum creatinine estimates renal function, it usually underestimates the severity of renal disease in lupus patients. Other markers of clinical renal disease include proteinuria (more than 500 mg/24 hours), the presence of casts (red blood cell [RBC], hemoglobin, tubular, granular, or mixed), pyuria (more than 5 white blood cells per high-power field [WBC/HPF]), and hematuria (more than 5 RBC/HPF). Sudden increases in proteinuria (more than 500 mg/24 hour change) or urinary sediments may necessitate a renal biopsy to determine the type of lesion and possibly the prognosis (see the World Health Organization classification of lupus nephritis in Table 34.2). In general, mesangial nephropathy (class II), membranous nephropathy (class V), and focal proliferative nephropathy (class III) involve fewer lesions and have better prognoses. Active lesions represent acute inflammatory changes, which are more responsive to aggressive therapy with steroids or immunosuppressive therapies than are fibrotic chronic lesions.[1,2,9,20–23]

Pulmonary manifestations occur in more than 50% of patients with lupus; symptoms of pleurisy, coughing, and dyspnea are the most common patient complaints and usually the first clue of lung involvement. Pleurisy, or chest wall pain, often is the only patient complaint and occurs upon movement and often disturbs the patient's sleep. Because many patients experience benign chest wall pain caused by muscle inflammation, patients should be evaluated by listening (via stethoscope) to inspirations for pleural friction rubs. The rough sound of the pleural membranes rubbing together, along with the radiographic presence of a pleural effusion, usually indicates pleuritis as a sign of lupus lung involvement. Because chest pain with pleuritis can be severe, patients must be evaluated for a pulmonary embolus or infectious pneumonia.[2,9]

Atelectasis (progressive shrinking of lungs with decreased lung volumes) is seen in many patients with SLE and causes basal infiltration and diaphragmatic elevation, leading to dyspnea. Acute lupus pneumonitis and pulmonary hemorrhage are less common but have high short-term mortality rates (50 to 90%); patients experience high fever, dyspnea, tachycardia, pulmonary infiltration, and possibly cyanosis. The mechanism of this fatal pulmonary manifestation is thought to be acute alveolar damage by immune complexes. In general, corticosteroids with or without immunosuppressants are considered first-line therapy for these conditions. Other pulmonary manifestations include chronic lupus pneumonitis and pulmonary hypertension. Most pulmonary manifestations of SLE show restrictive lung disease patterns on pulmonary function tests, with reduction in carbon monoxide diffusion capacity and fibrosis of the lungs.[1,2,9]

Many patients (up to 66%) with SLE experience neuropsychiatric symptoms during the course of their disease. Neurologic disorders include headaches, seizures, stroke, movement disorders, and neuropathies. Headaches can be muscular or migrainous in origin, and virtually all patients with lupus complain of headaches as the disease progresses. Seizures occur in 15 to 20% of patients and usually are generalized tonic–clonic seizures, but patients have been reported to experience petit mal and temporal seizures. Seizures may be secondary to other organic disorders (metabolic abnormalities, uremia) and should be considered a part of CNS lupus only if other symptoms of organic brain disease or lupus develop concomitantly. Other neurologic manifestations, such as cranial or peripheral neuropathies and stroke, occur in 10 to 15% of patients. These disorders can result in diplopia, nystagmus, visual field deficits, hallucinations, weakness of the lower extremities, and loss of bowel and bladder continence.[1,2,9,24]

The psychiatric manifestations include depression, anxiety, mania, psychoses, and organic brain syndrome. Depression is found in a majority of patients and is thought to be caused by autoantibody induction of cerebral dysfunction. Many patients recover through the support of family and SLE support groups and with the use of medications; however, some patients continue to experience psychosomatic insomnia, constipation, and fatigue. Psychoses are thought to be caused by functional or organic abnormalities as well as medications (steroids, NSAIDs, sedatives, and narcotics). Ironically, high dosages of steroids often improve psychotic manifestations. Organic brain syndrome (dementia), which occurs in up to 20% of patients with SLE, results in memory impairment, apathy, agitation, and loss of orientation and judgment.[1,2,9]

Cardiovascular involvement occurs in 30 to 50% of patients with SLE; the most prominent cardiac manifestations are pericarditis, myocarditis, valvular abnormalities, and accelerated atherosclerosis. Pericardial SLE is seen in up to 50% of patients and can be suspected if a patient suffers from substernal chest pain or an audible pericardial rub with electrocardiographic (ECG) abnormalities or detection of fluid. Many of these patients can be treated with NSAIDs and low-dose steroids, but these medications

Table 34.2 ▪ Clinical, Laboratory, and Pathologic Findings in Patients with Lupus Nephritis

Parameter	Normal Glomeruli (class I)	Mesangial GN (class II)	Focal Proliferative GN (class III)	Diffuse Proliferative GN (class IV)	Membranous GN (class V)	Sclerosing GN (class VI)
Incidence	Rare	40%	15%	30%	10%	3%
Hypertension	None	None	Occasional	Common	Late onset	Common
Proteinuria (g/day)	None	<1	<2	1–20	3.5–20	Severe
Hematuria (RBC/HPF)	None	5–15	5–15	Many	None	Many
Pyuria (WBC/HPF)	None	5–15	5–15	Many	None	Many
Casts	None	Occasional	Many	Many	None	Many
Glomerular filtration rate (mL/min)	Normal	Normal	60–80	<60	Normal	Severe
Total complement activity	Normal	Normal to low	Low	Largely low	Normal	Low
Anti-DNA	Normal	Normal to high	High	Largely high	Normal	High
Immune complexes	Normal	Normal to high	High	Largely high	Normal	High
Renal prognosis	Excellent	Good	Moderate	Poor	Moderate	Poor

Source: References 4, 13.

GN, glomerulonephritis; *RBC,* red blood cells; *HPF,* high-power field; *WBC,* white blood cells.

can exacerbate existing hypertension and coronary heart disease, making manifestations of myocarditis worse. Myocarditis, which is seen in 10% of patients, results in congestive heart failure (CHF) and is suspected when patients present with resting tachycardia, unexplained cardiomegaly, and ECG abnormalities. Patients with SLE also have a high incidence (20 to 70%) of valvular heart disease, which can be caused by antiphospholipid antibodies resulting in valvular leaflet thickening, nonbacterial endocarditis (Libman–Sacks), and regurgitation. Patients often become symptomatic (systolic murmurs, tachycardia, anemia) and may need valve replacement. In addition, the valvular lesions may place them at risk for infectious endocarditis, and many experts recommend that patients with valvular abnormalities routinely receive antibiotic prophylaxis before surgical and dental procedures. Atherosclerosis occurs at a much higher rate (up to nine times higher) in patients with SLE than in the general population, and it is believed to be multifactorial because patients with SLE also have a higher incidence of hypertension, obesity, renal disease, and hyperlipidemia.[1,2,9]

Anemia occurs in up to 80% of patients with SLE and is thought to result from a combination of the chronic inflammatory process of lupus, the decrease of erythropoiesis from renal insufficiency, and the adverse effects of medications (i.e., intestinal blood loss and bone marrow suppression). Therefore, most patients present with a normochromic, normocytic anemia with a decrease in the number of reticulocytes. In addition, 30 to 50% of patients with lupus suffer from leukopenia (WBC count less than 4000/mm^3) or thrombocytopenia (less than 150,000/mm^3). Leukopenia is caused by antilymphocyte antibodies and is a marker of overall SLE disease activity; however, WBC counts usually do not fall below 1500/mm^3 unless additional factors are involved. Thrombocytopenia usually is caused by antiplatelet or antiphospholipid antibodies, with platelet counts often falling below 50,000/mm^3. In one subset of patients, the thrombocytopenia that corresponds with acute flares of SLE probably is caused by antiphospholipid antibodies and responds to immunosuppressive therapies. Other patients experience a decreased platelet count (around 20,000/mm^3) without any other symptoms of SLE activity and usually need no intervention.[2,25]

Up to 25% of patients with SLE may have the antiphospholipid antibody syndrome, which places them at risk for thromboembolic events caused by the presence of antibodies to clotting factors. The presence of lupus anticoagulant results in a prolonged partial thromboplastin time, whereas the presence of anticardiolipin antibodies (which inhibit clotting factors) places the patient at risk for thrombosis. Many of these patients are treated successfully, primarily with heparin or warfarin, aspirin, and, if necessary, immunosuppressive therapies.[1,2,3,9,25]

Diagnosis

Because many of the symptoms described are present with other connective tissue conditions, SLE initially can be misdiagnosed as rheumatoid arthritis, scleroderma, Sjögren's syndrome, fibromyalgias, or other connective tissue diseases. In addition, patients may have a false-positive syphilis test result, leukopenia, thrombocytopenia, or an elevated prothrombin time, which can cause clinicians to consider other diagnoses before SLE. Therefore, clinicians should use the 1982 American Rheumatoid Association (ARA) criteria (Table 34.1) to make the diagnosis of SLE. These clinical symptoms combined with laboratory findings will confirm the diagnosis of SLE in most patients. The most widely accepted lab screening test for SLE is the fluorescent ANA test, which should be used when SLE is suspected. Most patients with SLE exhibit a positive ANA and have very high titers (antibody concentrations much greater than a dilution of 1:320). The ANA test is positive in approximately 99% of patients with SLE; very few patients with clinical lupus are ANA negative. Therefore, patients with negative ANAs usually do not undergo further antibody tests unless their symptoms strongly suggest a connective tissue disorder. However, the ANA test is not specific to SLE. Some studies show that up to 30% of healthy older adults have a false-positive ANA test with low titers (less than 1:320) that exhibit a homogeneous pattern of fluorescence. In addition, the ANA test is positive in up to 50% of patients with rheumatoid arthritis, scleroderma, and Sjögren's syndrome.

Traditionally, the pattern of the fluorescence of the ANA test is observed to increase the specificity of the diagnosis. The ANA fluorescence patterns observed in-

Table 34.3 • Percentage of Patients with Antinuclear Antibodies in Several Conditions

Antibodies	ANA (% positive)	dsDNA	Sm	ssDNA	Histone	U_1RNP	Ro	La	RiboP
Normal	<5	0	0	0	0	0	0	0	0
Systemic lupus erythematosus	99	75	25	>75	25	30–40	35–40	10–15	10–20
Rheumatoid arthritis	25–50	70	Rare	50–60	—	47	—	—	—
Scleroderma	75	0	Rare	—	—	20	95	—	—
Sjögren's syndrome	68	Rare	Rare	14	—	5–60	—	15–85	—
Drug-related lupus	95	Rare	Rare	60	90	20	—	—	—

Source: References 1, 12, 24.

ANA, antinuclear antibody; *dsDNA,* double stranded DNA; *Sm,* anti-Smith; *ssDNA,* single-stranded DNA; *U_1RNP,* U_1 ribonucleoprotein; *Ro,* anti-Ro; *La,* anti-La; *RiboP,* ribosomal P.

clude homogeneous, nuclear rim, speckled, and nucleolar. In general, the homogeneous and rim patterns are more specific for SLE, but most clinicians use additional laboratory tests to detect more specific antibodies and increase the accuracy of the diagnosis (Table 34.3).

There are several different antibody tests, which are characterized according to whether the antibodies bind nucleic acids (DNA), nucleic acid binding proteins (histones, ribonucleoproteins [RNPs]), or cell membrane antigens (antiphospholipids). Some DNA tests include the dsDNA and single-stranded DNA (ssDNA) tests. RNA tests include the U_1 ribonucleoprotein (U_1RNP), Sm, Ro, and La antibody tests. The presence of dsDNA and Sm antibodies and decreasing levels of total complement (CH_{50}) are considered highly specific for SLE. However, 73 to 80% of patients produce anti-dsDNA antibodies, with only 20 to 30% of patients producing antibodies to Sm. Studies have shown that anti-dsDNA antibodies correlate strongly with disease activity and lupus nephritis, whereas anti-Sm antibodies correlate with milder renal and CNS disease and overall disease activity.[11] Other antibodies that are less specific for SLE include antibodies to ssDNA, ribonucleoproteins (U_1RNP, Ro, and La), and ribosomal P. Anti-ssDNA antibodies occur in up to 90% of patients with SLE and predict less severe renal disease, but they are not specific and occur in several other rheumatologic disorders. U_1RNP antibodies are found in 30 to 40% of patients with SLE but also are found in patients with scleroderma. They are often associated with myositis, Raynaud's disease, and a good renal prognosis. Ro and La antibodies occur in 35 to 40% and 10 to 15% of SLE patients, respectively, and are strongly linked to Sjögren's syndrome. Ro is correlated with photosensitive skin, rash, pulmonary disease, and lymphopenia, and La is associated with the neonatal lupus syndrome and late-onset SLE.[11] Ribosomal P antibodies occur in 10 to 20% of patients with SLE and are related to psychiatric symptoms of lupus. The presence of histone antibodies (antibodies that form drug–nuclear protein complexes) are found in 90% of patients with drug-induced lupus. All antibodies tend to decrease within normal limits when patients are treated successfully and in remission.[1,9,11]

TREATMENT

SLE is an inflammatory disease that results in acute and chronic complications; therefore, treatment is aimed at relieving acute symptoms and preventing chronic complications. Specific goals of therapy must be tailored to the clinical manifestations of each patient; they include minimizing the signs and symptoms of active disease and normalizing laboratory values used to monitor SLE disease activity. These goals are achieved through nonpharmacologic and pharmacologic treatment and the discriminate use of laboratory tests (Table 34.4).

Table 34.4 ▪ Specific Goals of Therapy in Treating Systemic Lupus Erythematosus

Minimize Signs and Symptoms	Treatment: Nonpharmacologic	Treatment: Pharmacologic
Fatigue	Rest, minimize exercise	
Arthralgias and myalgias	Rest	NSAIDs, steroids (if severe)
Fever	Watch for infection	Acetaminophen, antibiotics
Rash	Avoid sun, use sunscreen	Antimalarials, steroids
Pulmonary signs	Avoid smoking	NSAIDs, steroids, antimalarials, antibiotics
Nephritis		Steroids, immunosuppressants
Central nervous system signs	Psychotherapy	Antidepressants, antipsychotics, steroids
Hematologic		Steroids, therapy for anemia type
Normalize Laboratory Values		
Antibody	Decrease levels	
Complement	Increase levels	
Immune complexes	Decrease levels	
Glomerular filtration rate	Increase	
Proteinuria	Decrease	
Hematuria	Decrease	

NSAIDs, nonsteroidal anti-inflammatory drugs.

Pharmacotherapy

Pharmacologic treatment varies with disease severity. Nonmajor organ involvement usually necessitates only short-term symptomatic treatment because clinical features are not life-threatening. Arthritis and arthralgias, rashes, pleurisy, pericarditis, myositis, and constitutional symptoms such as fever and fatigue and often can be managed with NSAIDs, antimalarial drugs (hydroxychloroquine 400 mg/day), or low-dose glucocorticoids (15 to 30 mg/day oral prednisone). In some cases of myositis and fatigue, larger glucocorticoid dosages (more than 40 mg prednisone daily) may be useful to decrease fatigue and muscle weakness and reverse enzyme abnormalities.[26,27] Rashes are common in photosensitive patients, so patients should use sunscreens and topical steroid therapy. Mild- to moderate-potency topical steroids should be used (especially in the facial area) for 2 or more weeks with antimalarials, and systemic glucocorticoids (prednisone) should be reserved for more difficult cases (e.g., discoid lupus). A rash that develops during tapering of oral steroid therapy usually will resolve if the steroid dosage is increased.[26,27]

More aggressive therapy should be initiated when life-threatening flares involving renal, CNS, pulmonary, vascular, and hematologic manifestations occur. Major organ manifestations that respond to steroid therapy include vasculitis, severe serositis (pleuritis, pericarditis, peritonitis), myocarditis, immune-mediated hematologic abnormalities (e.g., hemolytic anemia or thrombocytopenia), glomerulonephritis, severe CNS disease, and other severe constitutional symptoms. Some manifestations such as vascular occlusions (e.g., strokes), pure membranous glomerulonephritis, and resistant thrombocytopenia or hemolytic anemia may not respond to steroid therapy.[9]

Patients not responding to steroids or experiencing steroid-related adverse effects often receive cytotoxic agents such as cyclophosphamide or azathioprine. Cyclophosphamide administered intravenously once a month for several months has been shown to be more effective than steroids or azathioprine at decreasing disease flares and preserving renal function. Unfortunately, one-third of patients relapse after therapy, and the adverse effects can be very serious. In patients with refractory nephritis, some clinicians use a combination of high-dose steroids, azathioprine, and cyclophosphamide, and some clinicians try plasmapheresis.[9,26,27]

Plasmapheresis (plasma exchange to reduce the concentration of circulating antibodies and immune complexes in the bloodstream) is performed two to four times a week for 4 weeks in combination with immunosuppressive drugs to treat acute, severe glomerulonephritis. However, a comparison of plasmapheresis combined with cyclophosphamide and glucocorticoids versus cyclophosphamide and glucocorticoids alone for 2 to 3 years suggests that plasmapheresis is not very useful for treating lupus nephritis.[28] If all these therapeutic modalities fail, the patient will progress to end-stage renal disease and need dialysis or renal transplantation.[21,26]

Diagnosing CNS involvement is difficult because the clinical presentation can be caused by other factors. There are no laboratory tests specific for CNS involvement in patients with lupus (although the presence of anti-Sm or ribosomal P antibodies suggests CNS activity), and high dsDNA antibodies and low serum complement do not necessarily correlate with CNS manifestations. Therefore, CNS involvement in lupus is a diagnosis of exclusion, and therapy consists of medications to treat each manifestation. Patients experiencing stroke may have a hypercoagulable state that can be confirmed by the presence of antiphospholipid antibodies. For these patients, long-term anticoagulation therapy with warfarin should be considered. Patients with depressive or psychotic disorders should receive antidepressants and antipsychotics, respectively. Patients with seizure disorders secondary to CNS lupus are treated with anticonvulsant therapy. Patients with mild cognitive disorders (organic brain syndrome) usually are not treated; however, data suggest that patients with more extensive impairment may respond to prednisone at a dosage of at least 30 mg/day for several weeks.[18,19,26]

Many of the pulmonary manifestations of lupus (such as pulmonary edema) may be secondary to other underlying problems associated with lupus (renal failure or CHF), and treatment entails controlling the primary problems. Serious pulmonary complications seen in patients with SLE include diffuse pneumonitis and bacterial pneumonia. Antibiotics and steroid therapy should be used to treat the pneumonia and pneumonitis, respectively.[2,26,27] A small percentage of patients experience clotting abnormalities (lupus anticoagulant or anticardiolipin antibodies) as the primary manifestation of SLE. These patients should receive warfarin (INR treatment goal 2.0 to 3.0) but usually are not treated with steroids or other immunosuppressive therapies because lupus anticoagulant and anticardiolipin antibodies respond poorly to these agents.[26]

Patients with active SLE often develop severe anemia of chronic disease that reverses occasionally with NSAID therapy but most often with low-dose steroid therapy. Some patients experience a mild, transient thrombocytopenia that usually does not necessitate therapy. If platelet levels are less than 100,000/mm^3, patients often respond to oral prednisone (60 to 100 mg/day) until the platelet count rises to within normal limits.[25,26] If this is unsuccessful, other therapies include intravenous γ-globulin (6 to 15 mg/kg/day or 400 to 1000 mg/day for 4 to 7 days) or danazol (400 to 800 mg/day). Patients usually begin to respond in a few weeks.

Nonsteroidal Anti-Inflammatory Drugs

The first-line therapy for mild manifestations of SLE includes aspirin (salicylates) or other NSAIDs (Table 34.5). Salicylates and NSAIDs have antipyretic, analgesic, and anti-inflammatory effects, making them good treatment choices for lupus. These agents work primarily by inhibiting the cyclo-oxygenase enzyme, which is responsible for converting arachidonic acid to prostaglandins, which mediate inflammation. Other postulated mechanisms include inhibition of lipoxygenase and leukotriene formation, decreasing chemotaxis, T- and B-cell proliferation, and inhibition of free radical formation. Most clinical trials show that there are few differences in efficacy between aspirin and the NSAIDs, with slight differences in their adverse effect profiles. Therefore, selection of an NSAID for SLE often is based on factors such as physician or patient preference, patient's tolerance to side effects, frequency of administration, and cost of therapy.[29,30] However, the recent discovery of two isoenzymes of cyclooxygenase (COX-1 and COX-2) may help scientists to develop NSAIDs that have fewer side effects. COX-2 appears to be responsible for the formation of prostaglandins, causing inflammation and disease manifestations, whereas COX-1 is responsible for the formation of prostaglandins, which protect the stomach and kidneys. An NSAID that can selectively inhibit COX-2 with little effect on COX-1 should be as effective as current therapies with less gastrointestinal and renal adverse effects. Although data suggest that the new COX-2 inhibitor celecoxib is as effective as other NSAIDs, with a lower incidence of gastrointestinal adverse effects, long-term clinical trials comparing the efficacy and adverse effects of COX-2 inhibitors must be completed. Until then, we should regard most NSAIDs as having similar adverse effect profiles. Unfortunately, many NSAID-induced adverse effects are similar to symptoms seen with flares of SLE and include renal, psychiatric, and hepatic manifesta-

Table 34.5 ▪ Nonsteroidal Anti-Inflammatory Drugs

Drug	Trade Name	Half-Life (hr)	Daily Dosage (mg)	Dosing Schedule
Diclofenac	Voltaren, Cataflam	2–3	100–200	BID–QID
Diflunisal	Dolobid	7–15	500–1000	BID
Etodolac	Lodine	7–8	400–900	BID–QID
Fenoprofen	Nalfon	2–3	1200–3200	TID–QID
Flurbiprofen	Ansaid	5–6	200–300	BID–TID
Ibuprofen	Motrin, Rufen	1–3	1200–3200	TID–QID
Indomethacin	Indocin	3–4	50–200	BID–QID
Ketoprofen	Orudis, Oruvail	2–4	150–300	TID–QID
Ketorolac	Toradol	4–9	20–40	TID–QID
Meclofenamate	Meclomen	2–3	200–400	QID
Nabumetone	Relafen	22–30	500–2000	QD–BID
Naproxen	Naprosyn, Anaprox	12–15	500–1100	BID
Oxaprozin	Daypro	50–60	600–1800	QD
Piroxicam	Feldene	30–86	10–20	QD
Sulindac	Clinoril	16–18	200–400	BID
Tolmetin	Tolectin	2–7	600–2000	QID
Celecoxib[a]	Celebrex	11–12	200–400	QD–BID
Rofecoxib[a]	Vioxx	12–16	125–50	QD

[a]Celecoxib and Rofecoxib are COX-2 inhibitors (see text).

tions. NSAIDs cause decreased renal perfusion and interstitial nephritis; psychiatric manifestations such as headache, psychoses, depression, and dizziness; and hepatitis characterized by increases in liver transaminases. Fortunately, these NSAID-induced adverse effects are reversible upon discontinuation of the medication.[26,27,29]

Information about the pharmacokinetics, dosage and administration, adverse effects, and drug interactions of NSAIDs is outlined in Chapter 31. Upon selection of NSAID therapy to treat lupus, patients should receive therapy for 1 to 2 weeks to evaluate the efficacy of the NSAID. If a particular NSAID is found to be ineffective or causes adverse effects, another NSAID should be selected and used for another 1- to 2-week trial period. Using more than one NSAID at a time will not result in greater efficacy but may result in increased side effects and therefore is not recommended.[26,29,30] If NSAID therapy fails, immunosuppressive agents such as glucocorticoids or antimalarials often are tried, depending on the lupus manifestation.

Antimalarials

Patients presenting with lupus-induced rashes (SLE, discoid lupus, or subacute lupus) are candidates for antimalarial treatment. The efficacy of antimalarial treatment has been well documented in patients with dermatologic manifestations (DLE, SCLE), with 60 to 90% of patients responding to treatment.[26,31] Although antimalarials are not considered effective for the major organ manifestations of SLE, they have been shown to be beneficial for treating and preventing mild or nonmajor organ involvement (arthritis, fever, myositis, fatigue, serositis). In addition, antimalarial therapy has allowed clinicians to reduce steroid dosages in some patients when treating mild to moderate SLE conditions.[31,32] Several mechanisms of action have been proposed for antimalarial medications. These include stabilization of lysosomal membranes inhibiting lysosomal enzyme release; binding to DNA substrates, thus interfering with DNA antibody attacks; decreasing prostaglandin and leukotriene production; and decreasing T-cell activation and releasing IL-1 and tumor necrosis factor α (TNF-α).[26,31,32] The antimalarials most often used to treat SLE manifestations are chloroquine and hydroxychloroquine. Patients initially receive chloroquine (250 mg/day) or hydroxychloroquine (400 to 600 mg/day) for the first 1 to 2 weeks of therapy, with most patients showing some regression of erythematous skin lesions during the first 2 weeks. However, a maximal response may not be seen for 4 to 6 weeks. Once the patient has a good response, the dosage should be reduced by 50% (chloroquine 125 mg/day or hydroxychloroquine 200 mg/day) for several months until the SLE manifestations have resolved completely. The optimal duration of therapy is not well established, but the incidence of lupus flares is lower in patients on antimalarial maintenance therapy than in patients who discontinue medication. If the medication is to be discontinued, attempts should be made to taper antimalarial therapy by administering very low dosages two or three times a week before discontinuation. Unfortunately, 90% of patients relapse within 3 years of discontinuation.[31,32]

The antimalarials are rapidly and almost completely absorbed from the gastrointestinal tract upon oral administration. When they are taken with food, absorption is enhanced. These drugs are widely distributed throughout the body, which explains adverse effects such as mild

Table 34.6 ▪ Corticosteroids and Immunosuppressive Agents

Drug	Trade Name	Dosing Schedule	Indications
Hydroxychloroquine	Plaquenil	200–600 mg PO divided BID	Mild disease
Chloroquine	Aralen	125–500 mg PO divided BID	Rashes, arthritis
Prednisone	Various	0.5–1.0 mg/kg PO daily 1.0–2.0 mg/kg PO daily	Mild disease Moderate to severe disease Renal, central nervous system, refractory symptoms
Methylprednisolone	Various	10–30 mg/kg daily or 0.5–1 g IV daily for 3–6 days	Severe disease
Azathioprine	Imuran	1–3 mg/kg PO daily	Severe disease
Cyclophosphamide	Cytoxan	2–4 mg/kg PO daily 0.75–1.0 g/m² every 1–3 mo	Severe disease
Methotrexate	Rheumatrex	7.5–20 mg each wk	Moderate to severe disease
Cyclosporin	Sandimmune	5 mg/kg daily	Severe disease
Azathioprine with cyclophosphamide		Azathioprine 1.5–2.5 mg/kg/day PO and cyclophosphamide 1.5–2.5 mg/kg/day PO	Severe disease

neurotoxicity, retinal deposits, and drug-induced rashes. Antimalarials are eliminated primarily by renal excretion (70 to 75%), with the remainder being metabolized. Little information about adjusting antimalarial drug dosages in hepatic or renal impairment is available.[31,32]

Antimalarial medications generally are considered safe. Hydroxychloroquine is reported to have half the side effects of chloroquine. The most common adverse effects are gastrointestinal (epigastric burning, abdominal bloating, nausea, vomiting), which usually begin shortly after initiation of therapy. These and other adverse effects appear to be dose related and can be minimized by splitting the total daily dosage (200 mg twice a day instead of 400 mg each morning), administering antimalarials with food, and using small maintenance dosages after the initial treatment period.[26,31]

Because antimalarial medications are well distributed into the skin, patients may experience cutaneous lesions or pigmentary changes. Rashes tend to be morbilliform, maculopapular, or urticarial. Pigmentation changes include graying of the hair or blue-black discoloration of the skin. Neurologic side effects include headache, insomnia, and nervousness, which usually are mild and can be minimized by using lower dosages. A neuromuscular syndrome can occur that includes muscle weakness in the proximal lower extremities, abnormal creatine kinase levels, and abnormal muscle biopsy results. Although uncommon, it has been reported after patients have received several months of antimalarial therapy and often is confused with glucocorticoid-induced muscle weakness.[26,31]

Antimalarials can cause three types of ocular toxicity; two of these (accommodation changes causing blurred or double vision and corneal deposits associated with halos around lights) are benign and reversible. The most serious and publicized adverse effect of antimalarials is retinal toxicity, which can lead to permanent loss of vision. The two types of retinal lesions are described as premaculopathy and pigmentary changes. Premaculopathy results in changes in color vision, with a loss of ability to see red due to destruction of rods and cones caused by deposition of these medications in the pigment layers of the retina. These patients usually have mild pigmentary changes, and the visual changes are reversible if the medication is discontinued. Patients with extensive pigmentary changes develop a bull's-eye retinal lesion that leads to permanent visual field defects.[31,32] Hydroxychloroquine has caused fewer documented cases of retinal damage than chloroquine, and the risk of retinal toxicity is related to the total daily dosage, not the duration of therapy or cumulative dosage. Patients at risk for retinal toxicity usually are more than 65 years old and have received daily dosages greater than 6.5 mg/kg (400 mg) hydroxychloroquine or 3 to 4 mg/kg (150 mg) chloroquine. If patients are discovered to have retinal lesions (even if asymptomatic), therapy should be discontinued. If these dosages are not exceeded, retinal toxicity is not common. Although many of the retinal lesions reverse upon discontinuation of antimalarial therapy, ophthalmic examinations (funduscopy, visual acuity, color tests) should be performed before initiation of therapy and every 6 months during antimalarial therapy.[31,32]

Corticosteroids

Corticosteroid therapy is considered a mainstay in the treatment of SLE and can be used for various manifestations of the disease (Table 34.6). They should be used whenever patients present with serious and life-threatening forms of lupus, especially when they do not respond to NSAIDs or antimalarial therapy. The beneficial therapeutic effects are thought to result from the anti-inflammatory and immunosuppressive activity of these agents.[33] Because of the potential risks for serious toxicities and anticipated long-term use in patients with SLE, steroids should not be used as first-line therapy for mild SLE.

The goals of treatment with corticosteroids are to relieve symptoms, improve abnormal laboratory parameters, and sustain improvement of clinical manifestations (Table 34.7). Patients with severe manifestations of SLE such as nephritis, serositis, and vasculitis often receive high-dose corticosteroids for 3 to 6 days (pulse therapy) in an effort to accelerate the patient's response to treatment and decrease potential long-term adverse events. Methylprednisolone is the most common intravenous corticosteroid form (10 to 30 mg/kg over 30 minutes).[27,34] It commonly results in prompt relief of fulminant disease and can be lifesaving in many cases. Data from uncontrolled trials of intravenously administered steroids show that most patients (75%) experience significant disease improvements within a few days, with markers of renal disease (serum creatinine, blood urea nitrogen) worsening at first, then improving. Proteinuria usually improves after 4 to 10 weeks of glucocorticoid therapy. In addition, complement serum levels and DNA antibodies increase and decrease, respectively, in 1 to 3 weeks. Less severe manifestations (vasculitis, serositis, hematologic abnormalities, CNS abnormalities) usually respond in 5 to 19 days. Pulse therapy with methylprednisolone is followed by oral prednisone given for several weeks.[9,26,27]

Oral prednisone is used more often than dexamethasone because of its shorter biologic half-life and subsequent ease in switching to alternate-day therapy. Prednisone dosages range from 0.5 to 1 mg/kg/day in mild SLE to 1 to 2 mg/kg/day in acute, severe SLE. Once the therapeutic goals are achieved, further treatment decisions are based on controlling signs and symptoms and minimizing drug toxicity. After the disease has been controlled for at least 2 weeks, the steroid regimen should be changed to once-daily dosing. After the patient has been asymptomatic for another 2 weeks, the dosage should be tapered with the ultimate goal of alternate-day dosing and possibly discontinuation. Special precautions are warranted when tapering prednisone dosages of 20 mg per day or less and switching to alternate-day dosing because adrenal insufficiency caused by hypothalamic–pituitary–2adrenal (HPA) suppression from steroid use can occur.

An example of a tapering schedule is shown in Table 34.8. This schedule may take 6 months to a year or even longer if disease exacerbations occur. A patient with non-major organ involvement may benefit from a faster tapering schedule, and patients with severe disease may need slower tapering schedules. Flares without major organ involvement (e.g., fatigue, fever, arthralgias, or serositis) may simply respond to a return to the previous dosage until the symptoms resolve or the addition of NSAIDs or hydroxychloroquine. Major organ involvement during a flare (e.g., nephritis) may not always be controlled by a return to the previous dosage; in these cases, it may be necessary to use very high dosages to control these signs and symptoms; a new, slower tapering schedule will be needed. Recent studies suggest that high-dose oral prednisone, low-dose oral cyclophosphamide, or pulse intravenous cyclophosphamide may reduce lupus nephritis morbidity, maintain renal function, and stabilize serologic markers.[21,22,28]

High-dose corticosteroids should be used with caution in patients with SLE who have comorbid conditions that can predispose them to increased risks. These include the previously described HPA suppression, fluid and electrolyte disturbances, hypertension, peptic ulceration, osteoporosis, osteonecrosis, myopathy, increased susceptibility to infections including tuberculosis, cataracts, growth arrest, hyperglycemia, and Cushing's habitus.[33] All of these adverse events and their management are discussed in more detail in Chapter 31, which covers systemic corticosteroid therapy.

Table 34.7 ▪ Systemic Lupus Erythematosus Manifestations Usually Responsive to Glucocorticoids

Severe dermatitis	Vasculitis
Polyarthritis	Polyserositis
Lupus pneumonitis	Myocarditis
Glomerulonephritis	Hemolytic anemia
Myelopathies	Thrombocytopenia
Peripheral neuropathies	Organic brain syndrome
Serious central nervous system defects	Lupus crisis

Source: References 2, 3, 15.

Table 34.8 ▪ Example of a Prednisone Tapering Schedule

Dosage (mg)	Duration (wk)
20	2
17.5	3
15	4
15 alternating with 12.5	2–4
15 alternating with 10	2–4
15 alternating with 7.5	2–4
15 alternating with 5	2–4
15 alternating with 2.5	2–4
20 alternating with 0	4
17.5 alternating with 0	4
15 alternating with 0	4

Cyclophosphamide

Other medications that often are used to treat moderate to severe SLE include the alkylating agents. These cytotoxic agents work by disturbing cell growth, mitotic activity, and cell differentiation and function.[35] They inhibit DNA formation (unrelated to cell cycle), resulting in the death of T and B cells and neutrophils that contribute to the inflammatory response. Suppression of B-lymphocytes results in a direct suppression of antibody (IgG) formation, which additionally reduces the inflammatory response. Unfortunately, high-dose therapy with these medications can cause immunosuppression, which may increase the risk of neutropenia and infection in these patients.[36] Therefore, regular monitoring of WBC, hematocrit, and platelet counts is mandatory. Because of the high risk of teratogenicity, pregnancy testing and birth control measures should be used whenever female patients of childbearing age are exposed to these agents.

Cyclophosphamide is the most widely used and studied alkylating agent used to treat SLE. Usually it is reserved for patients with severe lupus nephritis who are resistant to less toxic therapies. In patients with renal disease, monthly infusions of intravenous cyclophosphamide have been shown to be more effective than prednisone alone in controlling signs and symptoms of nephritis, slowing the progression of renal scarring, and decreasing the risk of end-stage renal failure.[2] It is also effective in treating patients with SLE and diffuse CNS disease, thrombocytopenia, and interstitial pulmonary infiltrates.[1]

Although cyclophosphamide appears to be effective in treating severe SLE, its use is controversial.[9] There are conflicting reports about its efficacy in severe SLE, and there are concerns that it may not change long-term outcome, especially in the face of the large number of undesirable side effects. Additional questions remain, especially with regard to optimal dosage, route of administration, treatment interval, duration of cyclophosphamide pulse therapy, rate of relapse, and duration of disease remission.

Cyclophosphamide is well absorbed and can be administered either orally or intravenously. Approximately 70% of the drug is metabolized and 30% remains unchanged and is excreted by the kidney; therefore, dosages must be adjusted in renally impaired patients.[37] Although cyclophosphamide is metabolized by the cytochrome oxidase pathway, medications known to affect microsomal enzymes (e.g., cimetidine and barbiturates) usually do not cause clinically significant drug interactions.[36]

Both low oral dosages and high pulse intravenous dosages of cyclophosphamide have been used in patients with SLE. Orally administered dosages of cyclophosphamide range from 1 to 4 mg/kg/day for 4 to 8 weeks and intravenous dosages range from 8 to 20 mg/kg every 1 to 3 months, as determined by patient response.[36–38] Clinical effects usually are seen within 2 to 3 weeks of therapy, with WBC counts (primarily neutrophils) also reaching nadirs at this point. Immunosuppressive effects are thought to be worse with daily oral cyclophosphamide than with intermittent monthly intravenous boluses. However, the patient's granulocyte count must be monitored frequently to maintain cell counts not less than $300/mm^3$. If granulocyte levels fall below $300/mm^3$, dosages should be adjusted appropriately.[36,37]

Cyclophosphamide has been shown to decrease proteinuria, DNA antibodies, and serum creatinine (slightly) and to increase complement (C3) levels when the lupus nephritis is resolving. Studies show that adding cyclophosphamide to the drug therapy of patients with lupus nephritis refractory to high-dose steroid therapy decreases the progression to end-stage renal disease and lowers the daily glucocorticoid needs.[36,39–43] Because recent studies have evaluated the long-term efficacy and safety of low-dose or intermittent boluses of cyclophosphamide with oral steroids, future studies must concentrate on comparing therapies to determine the most effective approach to treating and preventing renal deterioration.

Although many consider cyclophosphamide to be the most effective agent available for treating severe lupus, its toxicities can be substantial. In addition to immunosuppression and the increased risk of infection (especially herpes zoster), other common adverse effects include dose-related nausea and vomiting, diarrhea, and alopecia. Most patients experience nausea and vomiting with intravenous administration, and this side effect can be treated easily with antiemetics. Alopecia may be severe in some patients, and they must be reassured that their hair will regrow even when therapy is continued. Chronic administration of cyclophosphamide can result in ovarian failure and decreased sperm production. Ovarian failure is nearly universal in women over age 30, and recovery is unpredictable.[44]

Azathioprine

Azathioprine is a second-line cytotoxic agent that can be used to treat severe SLE. It is used as an alternative in patients who are intolerant to cyclophosphamide, but it is considered less effective and far less toxic. It can be used alone or in combination to treat SLE; however, in short-term studies (i.e., 1 to 2 years' duration) it has been shown to be less effective than corticosteroids in treating symptomatic, multisystemic SLE when used alone.[9] It is most effective in patients with resistant discoid lupus and in those with minimal renal involvement.[36,38] Azathioprine augments glucocorticoid therapy in patients with SLE and renal disease and during acute, severe episodes of SLE not fully controlled with prednisone alone or prednisone and cyclophosphamide. Austin et al.[39] demonstrated that patients had better outcomes when treated with low-dose azathioprine or cyclophosphamide combined with low-dose prednisone than when given prednisone alone. Felson and Anderson pooled results from several studies and showed that azathioprine reduced proteinuria, improved or stabilized renal function, and reduced mortality.[45]

Azathioprine is given orally in dosages starting at 0.5 mg/kg/day and titrated upward to dosages of 3 mg/kg/day. In general, clinicians should expect a 6- to 12-month delay before the full benefits of azathioprine can be appreciated. After the disease has been well controlled with a combination of steroids and azathioprine, the steroid dosages should be tapered to the lowest possible levels. After this, azathioprine should be tapered, with the ultimate goal of discontinuing the therapy if the disease is well controlled. Patients on azathioprine should be monitored for hematopoietic or lymphoreticular toxicity every 2 weeks during the first 3 months of therapy while dosages are being adjusted, then monthly with chronic therapy. Baseline liver function tests should be performed and liver function should be monitored every 6 months while the patient is being treated.[4,36]

Azathioprine generally is well tolerated by patients with SLE and is less toxic than cyclophosphamide. The most common toxicities of azathioprine include gastrointestinal complaints and bone marrow suppression (especially leukopenia). Blood counts should be monitored regularly during azathioprine therapy, and the drug should be discontinued or the dosage decreased if there is evidence of marrow suppression. Patients with SLE on chronic azathioprine therapy are at greater risk of developing hematopoietic and lymphoreticular malignancies (e.g., non-Hodgkin's lymphoma and leukemia).[16] Other potentially serious adverse effects include herpes zoster, sterility, and hepatic toxicity.[27,38,39,46]

Experimental Pharmacotherapy

Cyclosporine

Cyclosporine, a potent inhibitor of T-lymphocyte activation, is effective in inhibiting nephritis in animal models of SLE.[47] In humans with SLE, cyclosporine is considered an experimental or investigational agent, and experience with this agent has been very limited.[4,27,48] Some investigators have shown that combining low dosages of cyclosporine (e.g., 3 to 5 mg/kg/day) and glucocorticoids may improve the renal and extrarenal manifestations of SLE.[48,49] Obviously, the major concern about the use of cyclosporine in patients with SLE is its toxicity. Most patients treated with cyclosporine develop elevations in blood pressure or increases in serum creatinine, which can be particularly harmful in patients with SLE.[4] To minimize cyclosporine-induced renal toxicities in patients with autoimmune diseases, some recommend that the drug not be administered in dosages higher than 5 mg/kg/day and that elevations in serum creatinine not be permitted to rise above 30% of the patient's baseline level.[50] Other cyclosporine adverse effects include transient hirsutism, tremor, and gingival hyperplasia. Hussein et al.[51] has recently recommended that cyclosporine be used to treat lupus nephritis in pregnant women because of its established safety with regard to teratogenicity in renal transplant recipients. Further study in this area is highly recommended because the majority of the patients in this study developed hypertension. Cyclosporine should be considered only in patients with severe steroid-resistant SLE who are not candidates for cytotoxic agents.

Methotrexate

Limited studies have been performed using methotrexate to treat SLE and its manifestations.[4,27] Rothenberg et al.[45] suggest that methotrexate is a rational therapeutic alternative to antimalarials or low-dose corticosteroids and may be particularly useful in the management of SLE in the presence of arthritis, skin rashes, serositis, or fever. Case reports and uncontrolled studies show that methotrexate may control joint symptoms and spare corticosteroids in 50 to 60% of patients.[5] The usual recommended methotrexate dosage for treating SLE is 7.5 to 15 mg orally once a week, which is comparable to the dosage regimens used in rheumatoid arthritis. Adverse effects of methotrexate include leukopenia, thrombocytopenia, hepatotoxicity, gastrointestinal disturbances and oral mucositis, teratogenicity, and renal impairment.[5] Therefore, patients receiving methotrexate for SLE should be monitored in a similar manner as patients receiving methotrexate for rheumatoid arthritis (Chapter 31). Methotrexate should be used with caution and dosages must be adjusted in patients with renal impairment.

Nonpharmacologic Therapy

Nonpharmacologic therapy includes educating the patient and his or her family; developing proper exercise, diet, and rest habits; and providing psychological and supportive therapies. Patients should be educated about the severity of their SLE, acute symptoms, the need for compliance with medications, and the adverse effects of medications.[9,26] Patients should be instructed to minimize their exposure to direct sunlight (and fluorescent light in some patients) especially if they have a history of photosensitivity upon exposure to UV light. These patients should apply sunscreens that block both UVA and UVB radiation (sunlight protection factor 15) liberally to exposed body parts and should wear long-sleeved shirts and broad-brimmed hats to minimize sun exposure. Patients should also be warned that unexplained fever may be a sign of infection, which is particularly common if they have received cytotoxic therapy or high-dose steroids. To further minimize infections, patients should receive the influenza vaccine annually and prophylactic antibiotics if they have valvular disease.[26,27] To deal with the psychological and psychosocial aspects of SLE, patients should be aware of SLE educational programs and support groups. These can be reached through the Lupus Foundation of America (800-558-0121).

Pregnancy, Estrogen, and Systemic Lupus Erythematosus Treatment

Several important issues characterize the relationship between pregnancy (estrogen) and SLE. These issues include the effect of estrogen therapies and pregnancy on lupus activity (flares), the impact of SLE on fetal outcome and premature delivery, and the use of medications for SLE in pregnant patients. The association of oral contraceptive or estrogen replacement therapy with increased lupus activity is very controversial. Much of the information about a possible twofold increase in SLE activity with estrogen therapies was not statistically significant. In addition, many studies involved case-control, retrospective reports of many patients who did not meet the four diagnostic criteria of SLE. Although some sources say that these medications should not be used, there are data to indicate that patients should avoid these therapies, which have other proven benefits.

Many studies report that 50 to 60% of pregnant patients experience a flare of their lupus, usually during the third trimester of pregnancy. However, controlled clinical trials report that lupus flare rates for pregnant women are no different from those in nonpregnant patients, with many complications, such as renal impairment, hypertension, and proteinuria, occurring in women with lupus and pregnancy-induced toxemia. Maternal complications other than flare and toxemia are rare, and flares usually are mild to moderate (85%); little or no increase in dosage (prednisone) or additional medication is needed, and few flares result in renal failure. Laboratory values consistent with an increase in lupus activity usually reveal a decrease in complement levels, rising anti-DNA antibodies, and worsening renal values. Although many pregnant patients with SLE carry their pregnancies to full term, SLE activity during pregnancy can cause 12 to 30% more fetal loss (miscarriage, stillbirth) and 20 to 50% more premature deliveries than in pregnant patients without lupus. Fetal loss and premature delivery are directly related to the following exacerbations during pregnancy: worsening renal disease and hypertension, elevations of anti-dsDNA and antiphospholipid antibodies (e.g., lupus anticoagulant and cardiolipin antibodies), and possibly decreased levels of serum complement. The neonatal lupus syndrome is associated with anti-Ro and anti-La antibodies and occurs in 5 to 8% of SLE pregnancies and results in transient rash and rarely congenital heart block (less than 3% of patients). However, the heart block usually is permanent and may be responsible for deaths during the neonatal period. Therefore, clinicians should consider monitoring pregnant patients (especially as they enter the second trimester) for changes in blood pressure, serum creatinine, complete blood cell count, and urine protein.[3,52,53]

Most women need to maintain lupus medication treatment during their pregnancy to prevent maternal and fetal adverse outcomes. Corticosteroids are considered the drugs of choice in pregnant patients because of their efficacy and because they have fewer adverse effects than other medications. Although corticosteroids cross the placenta, much is metabolized by placental hydroxygenase before it reaches the fetus. Few problems are noted in the mother or fetus when patients have received prednisone or other steroids to treat SLE. In addition, steroids may actually promote fetal lung maturation. NSAIDs and aspirin are fairly safe (pregnancy category B) during the first and second trimesters but are considered harmful (pregnancy category D) during the third trimester because of their effects on premature closure of the ductus arteriosus. Low-dose aspirin (81 mg/day) with or without heparin can be used during lupus pregnancies complicated by antiphospholipid antibodies (lupus anticoagulant, anticardiolipin antibodies) to decrease fetal complications; however, steroid therapy does not improve fetal outcome in patients with antiphospholipid antibodies. If NSAIDs or aspirin are used during pregnancy, use should be restricted to the first trimester and to the lowest possible dosage.

Although data on the use of antimalarial drugs in pregnancy are sparse, the information available does not indicate that these medications are teratogenic (pregnancy category C). Although dosages used for malaria prophylaxis do not seem to predispose the fetus to risk of teratogenic abnormalities, dosages of antimalarials used for SLE have been associated with congenital abnormalities in a few case reports, with chloroquine appearing to be more teratogenic than hydroxychloroquine. Despite the possible risk of antimalarials, most experts agree that a patient with uncontrolled (active) lupus has a greater chance of experiencing spontaneous abortion or neonatal death than teratogenic effects. Therefore, if a patient is on antimalarial medications when she becomes pregnant, she should remain on these medications throughout the pregnancy. Immunosuppressant medications (azathioprine, cyclophosphamide) have been associated with teratogenicity (pregnancy category D) and should be avoided if possible.[3,53]

PROGNOSIS

The prognosis for patients with SLE has improved over the last 30 years, with 5- and 10-year survival rates improving from 65 and 55%, respectively, in the 1960s to more than 90% for both in the 1990s. This is believed to be a result of earlier detection with widespread use of the ANA test, improved treatment modalities, and the availability of renal dialysis and transplantation.

Several prognostic indicators related to a poor outcome in patients with SLE are used along with clinical signs and symptoms to monitor disease progression. Non-SLE factors thought to be related to a poorer prognosis include early age at onset (15 to 30 years), female gender, black race, and low socioeconomic status. However, recent data show that the significance of these risk factors is very controversial. Some studies have shown that women are at greater risk, and others suggest that men are at greater risk.

Although most data indicate that severe disease (nephritis) at an early age suggests a worse prognosis, other studies report that diagnosis at a later age is a risk factor for death. When evaluating the effects of race (primarily for black patients) and socioeconomic status on prognosis, it is often difficult to separate these two factors; however, it appears that socioeconomic status plays a more important role than racial influences.[7,9,22,23,54–56]

Lupus-specific factors that predict a poor prognosis include overall disease activity at the time of presentation, the extent of major organ damage, and infection. Most studies show that patients who present with severe renal and CNS manifestations within the first 5 years of diagnosis have a poorer prognosis. Specifically, patients with diffuse proliferative nephritis, a high acute activity index, chronic sclerotic lesions on biopsy, elevated serum creatinine, increased proteinuria, and onset of nephritis at a younger age are at greater risk for renal failure, renal transplantation, and death.

In patients with evidence of neurologic involvement (psychoses, seizures, stroke, cognitive impairment), permanent CNS damage that increases the risk of morbidity and mortality can occur.

Laboratory values associated with a poor prognosis and active disease include azotemia, elevated serum creatinine, increased urinary protein excretion, high levels of dsDNA antibodies, low complement levels, the presence of complement fixation by the dsDNA antibodies, and prolonged and severe anemia and possibly thrombocytopenia or hemolytic anemia. Because many of these laboratory values change with acute and active disease, they are used along with clinical symptoms to monitor the progression of SLE. High levels of dsDNA antibodies and low levels of CH_{50} are associated with active renal disease, and these laboratory values normalize as the disease is treated successfully. Death during the first 5 to 10 years of SLE usually results from an acute exacerbation of the disease, whereas death after 10 years of the disease usually is caused by infection, atherosclerosis, or other complications of the disease or the medications used to treat lupus.[7,9,22,23,54–56]

Drug-Related Lupus

The first drug-related lupus (DRL) syndromes involved sulfonamides and penicillins in the late 1940s and early 1950s, with anticonvulsants and cardiovascular medications implicated in the late 1950s and early 1960s. Since that time more than 50 drugs have been implicated as causing a positive ANA and at least five associated with DRL syndrome; procainamide and hydralazine are the most common culprits (Table 34.9).

EPIDEMIOLOGY

Etiology

Although several theories have been proposed to explain DRL, the exact cause cannot be explained. Some medications (e.g., hormone therapies) are thought to exacerbate symptoms in patients with existing lupus conditions, whereas other medications (hydralazine, procainamide) produce lupuslike symptoms in patients not previously diagnosed with idiopathic SLE. DRL is more common in patients who are genetically slow acetylators (linked to HLA-DR4), which results in a slow rate of drug acetylation by the *N*-acetyltransferase enzyme. This causes an accumulation of drug, which forms a complex with nuclear proteins (DNA, histones). ANAs are then formed against the complexes, resulting in T- and B-cell stimulation, antibody formation, and an inflammatory response. Further evidence shows that a slow acetylation phenotype may predispose a patient to becoming ANA positive and developing lupus symptoms sooner than a fast acetylator. However, patients with a fast acetylator phenotype can develop a positive ANA and DRL symptoms. DRL is related to the medication dosage, duration of therapy, and probably other unidentifiable factors.[9,57–59]

Table 34.9 ▪ Drug-Related Lupus: Implicated Medications

Definite	Possible		Unlikely
Hydralazine	Anticonvulsants	Propylthiouracil	Griseofulvin
Procainamide	Phenytoin	Methimazole	Penicillin
Isoniazid	Carbamazepine	Penicillamine	Gold salts
Chlorpromazine	Valproic acid	Sulfasalazine	
Methyldopa	Ethosuximide	Sulfonamides	
	β-Blockers	Nitrofurantoin	
	Propranolol	Levodopa	
	Metoprolol	Lithium	
	Labetalol	Cimetidine	
	Acebutolol	Tacrolimus	
		Captopril	
		Lisinopril	
		Enalapril	
		Oral contraceptives	

Source: References 35–37.

Procainamide

Procainamide-induced SLE is the most common drug-induced lupus, with 80 to 100% of patients having positive ANA titers within 1 year of starting therapy. Approximately 25% of these patients develop clinical signs of lupus within 3 months to 2 years.[57–59] There appears to be a total dosage relationship to procainamide-induced lupus, with most patients having received more than 1600 mg daily. The most common signs and symptoms of procainamide-induced lupus are arthritis, pleuritis, and pleural effusions.[57–59]

Hydralazine

The number of patients reported to have a positive ANA on hydralazine varies from 4 to 14%, with 4% of patients developing symptoms of DRL. The incidence of hydralazine-induced lupus is directly related to the dosage, with no cases reported in patients receiving less than 50 mg/day. Incidence rates increase from 4 to 12% as patients receive 100 mg/day and 200 mg/day, respectively. Hydralazine-induced symptoms are characterized as early and late onset. Patients with early-onset hydralazine-induced lupus complain primarily of fever and malaise that usually occur within the first 30 days of hydralazine therapy. Patients complaining of late-onset hydralazine-induced lupus have signs and symptoms that usually start 2 years after therapy is initiated and include arthritis, myalgias, and rash. A few patients have reported renal manifestations.[58,59]

Other Medications

Other medications that can cause positive ANA tests include isoniazid, chlorpromazine, β-blockers, methyldopa, and quinidine; however, few patients develop clinical features.[58,59]

Table 34.10 ▪ Comparison of Drug-Related and Idiopathic Lupus

	Idiopathic	Drug-Related
Clinical features		
Age	20–50 yr	60–70 yr
Sex (F:M)	9:1	6:4
Race	Blacks > whites	Whites > blacks
Acetylation type	Slow–fast	Slow
Onset of symptoms	Slow	Abrupt
Fever and malaise	>75%	25–50%
Arthralgia and arthritis	90%	>75%
Renal disease	50–75%	5%
Pleuropericarditis	50%	50%
Skin rash	75%	10–10%
Central nervous system disease	25–50%	0%
Hematologic disease	50–75%	Unusual
Hepatomegaly	25–50%	25%
Immune abnormalities		
Antinuclear antibodies	>95%	>95%
Lupus erythematosus cells	90%	90%
Anti–double-stranded DNA	80%	Rare
Antihistone	25%	95%
Anti-U_1 ribonucleoprotein	30–40%	20%
Anti-Smith	25%	Rare
Complement	Reduced	Normal
Immune complexes	Elevated	Normal

Source: References 35–37.

Patient Profile

Patients with DRL differ greatly from patients with idiopathic SLE (Table 34.10). DRL occurs most often in older patients (50 to 70 years), whereas the average age of onset for idiopathic SLE is 20 to 50 years. This difference probably reflects the use of procainamide and hydralazine by older patients. Women make up approximately 90% of patients with idiopathic SLE and 40% of patients with DRL. Caucasian patients represent almost all DRL cases but less than half of idiopathic SLE cases. Although there are differences in the populations that acquire DRL and SLE, many of the clinical presentations are similar.[57–59]

CLINICAL PRESENTATION AND DIAGNOSIS

Signs and Symptoms

In differentiating between idiopathic SLE and DRL, evaluating the clinical presentation and laboratory values can be helpful (Table 34.10). Patients with DRL typically have a milder clinical presentation with lesser organ involvement. Predominant clinical features include arthralgias, myalgias, fever, weight loss, malaise, and cardiopulmonary involvement. Joint involvement tends to be nondeforming, migratory, and less severe than in idiopathic SLE and involves the smaller joints of the hands, elbows, knees, shoulders, and feet. Cardiopulmonary lesions can result in dyspnea, hemoptysis, pleuritis, pleural effusion, and pericarditis in 30 to 50% of patients. Renal and CNS findings are not common (less than 5%) in DRL, with dermatologic manifestations (urticaria, purpura, malar rash) being less common in DRL (10 to 20%) than in idiopathic SLE. Hematologic abnormalities (leukopenia, thrombocytopenia) can occur, but they are much less severe than in idiopathic SLE. Signs and symptoms of drug-induced lupus usually occur within 3 months to 2 years after drug therapy is initiated; however, a few cases of DRL have occurred as early as 2 weeks and as late as 4 years after initiation of drug therapy.

Diagnosis

The laboratory tests commonly used to help clinicians diagnose DRL include the ANA, dsDNA, and histone antibody tests. The commonly used ANA test is positive in 95% of patients with DRL and idiopathic SLE, so a positive ANA may not differentiate between DRL and idiopathic SLE. However, the ANA staining usually is homogeneous in DRL, indicative of antibodies to nuclear histones. A positive antihistone test is very common (90%) with DRL and less common (25%) with idiopathic SLE, whereas a positive dsDNA antibody test is indicative of idiopathic SLE (but not DRL). If the ANA test is negative, DRL can be ruled out. Because many patients develop a positive ANA test before having signs and symptoms of DRL, the combination of an ANA and clinical features is necessary for a patient to be considered to have DRL (Table 34.10).[57–59]

TREATMENT

Treatment of DRL consists of discontinuing the medication if symptoms of DRL are present and watching for resolution of signs and symptoms. Medications often are used to treat the signs and symptoms of DRL based on the severity of the clinical features. Aspirin and other NSAIDs are used for patients complaining of arthralgias and myalgias. Patients with more severe signs and symptoms may receive glucocorticoids (prednisone 0.5 to 1.0 mg/kg) for several weeks to resolve the drug-induced lupus more quickly.[57,59]

PROGNOSIS

DRL also is different from idiopathic SLE in that it is reversible, and signs and symptoms fade within 4 to 6 weeks after discontinuation of the medication; however, serologic markers of disease may remain elevated for more than a year.[9,57–59]

KEY POINTS

- SLE is a multisystem disease consisting primarily of abnormal autoantibody production.
- Today, health care providers have greater opportunities in disease identification, prognosis indicators, refined therapies, and improved guidelines for drug therapy use.

- SLE is a chronic inflammatory disease (similar to rheumatoid arthritis) that involves many organ systems and occurs primarily (80%) in black or Hispanic women less than 40 years old.
- The symptoms and prognosis for each patient are determined by the organs affected, with early involvement (younger than 30 years) of the renal system and CNS being poor prognosticators. Common symptoms include joint and muscle pain, fatigue, fevers, and weight loss. The disease course and prognosis are highly variable among patients, but marked improvement in survival and quality of life provide hope.
- Anti-inflammatory medications (NSAIDs, low-dose corticosteroids) and hydroxychloroquine are used to treat mild disease flareups such as joint and muscle pain, fatigue, and rashes.
- High-dose corticosteroids, azathioprine, and cyclophosphamide are used to treat severe exacerbations involving the renal, cardiac, and central nervous systems. If patients are unresponsive or cannot tolerate these medications, cyclosporine and methotrexate can be used to suppress the inflammation associated with SLE.
- In terms of monitoring, laboratory values are used to assess disease activity or monitor drug toxicity. Common laboratory values monitored in patients with SLE include the ANA test (increases with disease activity), dsDNA antibodies (increases with disease activity), serum complement (CH_{50}, decreases with disease activity), serum creatinine (increases with disease activity and drug toxicity), and the complete blood cell count (RBC, hemoglobin, hematocrit, elevated with disease activity and drug toxicity).

REFERENCES

1. Pisetsky DS, Gladman DD, Urowitz MB. Systemic lupus erythematosus: epidemiology, pathology, pathogenesis, and clinical and laboratory features. In: Schumacher HR. Primer on rheumatic diseases. 11th ed. Atlanta: Arthritis Foundation, 1997:246–257.
2. Boumpas DT, Austin HA, Fessler BJ, et al. Systemic lupus erythematosus: emerging concepts. Part 1: renal, neuropsychiatric, cardiovascular, pulmonary, and hematologic disease. Ann Intern Med 122:940–950, 1995.
3. Boumpas DT, Fessler BJ, Austin HA, et al. Systemic lupus erythematosus: emerging concepts. Part 2: dermatologic and joint disease, the antiphospholipid antibody syndrome, pregnancy and hormonal therapy, morbidity and mortality, and pathogenesis. Ann Intern Med 123:42–53, 1995.
4. Hahn BH. Pathogenesis of systemic lupus erythematosus. In: Kelley WN, Harris ED, Ruddy S, et al., eds. Textbook of rheumatology. 5th ed. Philadelphia: WB Saunders, 1997:1015–1027.
5. Schroeder JO, Euler HH. Recognition and management of systemic lupus erythematosus. Drugs 554:422–434, 1997.
6. Hochberg MC. Epidemiology of systemic lupus erythematosus. In: Lahita RG, ed. Systemic lupus erythematosus. 2nd ed. New York: Churchill-Livingstone, 1992:103–116.
7. Klippel JH. Systemic lupus erythematosus: demographics, prognosis, and outcome. J Rheumatol 24(Suppl 48):67–71, 1997.
8. Johnson AE, Gordon C, Hobbs FDR, et al. Undiagnosed systemic lupus erythematosus in the community. Lancet 347:367–369, 1996.
9. Lahita RG. Clinical presentation of systemic lupus erythematosus. In: Kelley WN, Harris ED, Ruddy S, et al., eds. Textbook of rheumatology. 5th ed. Philadelphia: WB Saunders, 1997:1028–1039.
10. Steinberg AD, Gourley MF, Klinmann DM, et al. NIH conference. Systemic lupus erythematosus. Ann Intern Med 115:548–559, 1991.
11. Peng SL, Hardin JA, Craft J. Antinuclear antibodies. In: Kelley WN, Harris ED, Ruddy S, et al., eds. Textbook of rheumatology. 5th ed. Philadelphia: WB Saunders, 1997:250–266.
12. Tan EM. Antinuclear antibodies: diagnostic markers for autoimmune diseases and probes for cell biology. Adv Immunol 44:93–151, 1989.
13. Pisetsky DS. Anti-DNA antibodies in systemic lupus erythematosus. Rheum Dis Clin North Am 18:437–454, 1992.
14. Blaese RM, Grayson J, Steinberg AD. Elevated immunoglobulin secreting cells in the blood of patients with active systemic lupus erythematosus: correlation of laboratory and clinical assessment of disease activity. Am J Med 69:345–350, 1980.
15. Davies KA. Complement, immune complexes and systemic lupus erythematosus. Br J Rheumatol 35:5–23, 1996.
16. Hopkinson N. Epidemiology of systemic lupus erythematosus. Ann Rheum Dis 51:1292–1294, 1992.
17. McCruden AB, Stimson WH. Sex hormones and immune function. In: Ader R, Felton DL, Cohen N, eds. Psychoneuroimmunology. San Diego: Academic Press, 1991:475–493.
18. Venables PJ. Diagnosis and treatment of systemic lupus erythematosus. BMJ 307:663–667, 1993.
19. Sontheimer RD, Gilliam JN. Systemic lupus erythematosus and the skin. In: Lahita RG. Systemic lupus erythematosus. 2nd ed. New York: Churchill-Livingstone, 1992:657–681.
20. Gladman DD. Indicators of disease activity, prognosis, and treatment of systemic lupus erythematosus. Curr Opin Rheumatol 5:587–595, 1993.
21. Ponticelli C. Current treatment recommendations for lupus nephritis. Drugs 40:19–30, 1990.
22. Appel GB, Cohen DJ, Pirani CL, et al. Long-term follow-up of patients with lupus nephritis: a study based on the classification of the World Health Organization. Am J Med 83:877–885, 1987.
23. Pollack VE, Kant KS. Systemic lupus erythematosus and the kidney. In: Lahita RG, ed. Systemic lupus erythematosus. 2nd ed. New York: Churchill-Livingstone, 1992:683–706.
24. West SG. Neuropsychiatric lupus. Rheum Dis Clin North Am 20(1):129–158, 1994.
25. Laurence J, Wing JL, Nachman R. The cellular hematology of systemic lupus erythematosus. In: Lahita RG, ed. Systemic lupus erythematosus. 2nd ed. New York: Churchill-Livingstone, 1992:771–805.
26. Hahn BH. Management of systemic lupus erythematosus. In: Kelley WN, Harris ED, Ruddy S, et al., eds. Textbook of rheumatology. 5th ed. Philadelphia: WB Saunders, 1997:1040–1056.
27. Klippel JH. Systemic lupus erythematosus: treatment. In: Schumacher HR. Primer on rheumatic diseases. 11th ed. Atlanta: Arthritis Foundation, 1997:258–262.
28. Lewis EJ, Hunsicker LG, Lan S-P, et al. The lupus nephritis collaborative study group: a controlled trial of plasmapheresis therapy in severe lupus nephritis. N Engl J Med 326:1373–1379, 1992.
29. Clements PJ, Paulus HE. Nonsteroidal anti-inflammatory drugs (NSAIDs). In: Kelley WN, Harris ED, Ruddy S, et al., eds. Textbook of rheumatology. 5th ed. Philadelphia: WB Saunders, 1997:707–740.
30. Furst DE. Are there differences among nonsteroidal antiinflammatory drugs? Arthritis Rheum 37(1):1–9, 1994.
31. Rynes RI. Antimalarial drugs. In: Kelley WN, Harris ED, Ruddy S, et al., eds. Textbook of rheumatology. 5th ed. Philadelphia: WB Saunders, 1997:747–757.
32. Nayak V, Esdaile JM. The efficacy of antimalarials in systemic lupus erythematosus. Lupus 5(Suppl 1):23–27, 1996.
33. Boumpas DT, Chrousos GP, Wilder RL, et al. NIH conference. Glucocorticoid therapy for immune-mediated diseases: basic and clinical correlates. Ann Intern Med 119:1198–1208, 1993.
34. Schimmer BP, Parjer KL. Adrenocorticotropic hormone. Adrenocortical steroids and their synthetic analogs: inhibitors of the synthesis and actions of adrenocortical hormones. In: Hardman JG, Limbird LE, Molinoff PB, et al., eds. Goodman & Gilman's the pharmacological basis of therapeutics. 9th ed. New York: McGraw-Hill, 1996:14359–14385.
35. Donadio JV, Glassock RJ. Immunosuppressive drug therapy in lupus nephritis. Am J Kidney Dis 21:239–250, 1993.
36. Fauci AS, Young KR Jr. Immunoregulatory agents. In: Kelley WN, Harris ED, Ruddy S, et al., eds. Textbook of rheumatology. 5th ed. Philadelphia: WB Saunders, 1997:805–827.
37. Allegra CJ, Curt GA, Calabresi P, et al. Antineoplastic agents. In: Hardman JG, Limbird LE, Molinoff PB, et al., eds. Goodman & Gilman's The pharmacological basis of therapeutics. 9th ed. New York: McGraw-Hill, 1996:1233–1287.

38. Dinant HT, Decker JL, Klippel JH, et al. Alternate modes of cyclophosphamide and azathioprine therapy in lupus nephritis. Ann Intern Med 96:728–736, 1982.
39. Austin HA, Klippel JH, Balow JE, et al. Therapy of lupus nephritis: controlled trial of prednisone and cytotoxic drugs. N Engl J Med 314:614–619, 1986.
40. Levey AS, Lan S-P, Corwin HL, et al. The Lupus Nephritis Collaborative Study Group: progression and remission of renal disease in the lupus nephritis collaborative study. Ann Intern Med 116:114–123, 1992.
41. McCune WJ, Golbus J, Zeldes W, et al. Clinical and immunologic effects of monthly administration of intravenous cyclophosphamide in severe systemic lupus erythematosus. N Engl J Med 318:1423–1431, 1988.
42. Boumpas DT, Austin HA, Balow JE, et al. Therapy of lupus nephritis: controlled trial of pulse methylprednisolone versus two different regimens of pulse cyclophosphamide. Lancet 340:741–744, 1992.
43. Moroni G, Banfi G, Ponticelli C. Clinical status of patients after 10 years of lupus nephritis. Q J Med 84:681–689, 1992.
44. Wang CL, Wang F, Bosco JJ. Ovarian failure in oral cyclophosphamide treatment for systemic lupus erythematosus. Lupus 4:11–14, 1995.
45. Rothenberg RJ, Graziano FM, Grandone JT, et al. The use of methotrexate in steroid-resistant systemic lupus erythematosus. Arthritis Rheum 31:612–615, 1988.
46. Balow JE. Lupus nephritis: natural history, prognosis and treatment. Clin Immunol Allergy 6:353–366, 1986.
47. Mountz JD, Smith HR, Wilder RL, et al. CS-A therapy in MRL-lpr/lpr mice: amelioration of immunopathology despite autoantibody production. J Immunol 138:157–163, 1987.
48. Favre H, Miescher PA, Huang YP, et al. Cyclosporine in the treatment of lupus nephritis. Am J Nephrol 9(Suppl 1):57–60, 1989.
49. Tokuda M, Kurata N, Mizoguchi A, et al. Effect of cyclosporin A on systemic lupus erythematosus disease activity. Arthritis Rheum 37:551–558, 1994.
50. Feutren G, Mihatsch MJ. Risk factors for cyclosporine-induced nephropathy in patients with autoimmune diseases. International kidney biopsy registry of cyclosporine in autoimmune diseases. N Engl J Med 326:1654–1660, 1992.
51. Hussein MM, Mooij JM, Roujouleh H. Cyclosporine in the treatment of lupus nephritis including two patients treated during pregnancy. Clin Nephrol 40:160–163, 1993.
52. Kreidstein S, Urowitz MB, Gladman DD, et al. Hormone replacement therapy in systemic lupus erythematosus. J Rheumatol 24:49–52, 1997.
53. Petri M. Systemic Lupus erythematosus and pregnancy. Rheum Dis Clin North Am 20(1):87–118, 1994.
54. Urowitz MB, Gladman DD, Abu-Shakra M, et al. Mortality studies in systemic lupus erythematosus. Results from a single center. III. Improved survival over 24 years. J Rheumatol 24:1061–1065, 1997.
55. Gladman DD. Prognosis and treatment of systemic lupus erythematosus. Curr Opin Rheumatol 8:430–437, 1996.
56. Ward MM, Pyun E, Studenski S. Mortality risks associated with specific clinical manifestations of systemic lupus erythematosus. Arch Intern Med 156:1337–1344, 1996.
57. Hess EV, Mongey AB. Drug-related lupus: the same or different from idiopathic disease? In: Lahita RG, ed. Systemic lupus erythematosus. New York: Churchill-Livingstone, 1992:893–904.
58. Stratton MA. Drug-induced systemic lupus erythematosus. Clin Pharm 4:657–663, 1985.
59. Rich MW. Drug-induced lupus. Postgrad Med 100(3):299–308, 1996.

CHAPTER 35

OSTEOPOROSIS AND OSTEOMALACIA

Louise Parent-Stevens

Osteoporosis and osteomalacia are two diseases of the calcified connective tissue (bone). They differ from each other etiologically, but the primary pathologic difference is that although both cause deficient mineralization of bone, osteoporosis also results in bone matrix loss. These disorders may be silent for an extended period, resulting in a delay of diagnosis. Patients can have both disorders concomitantly. Typically, osteomalacia is diagnosed visually in children by the bending of long bones. Osteoporosis is confirmed after a fracture or multiple fractures have occurred, which leads to significant morbidity and loss of independence for many, particularly older adults. As the population ages, these bone diseases, especially osteoporosis, become increasingly prevalent. More than $10 billion is spent annually on treatment of these potentially preventable disorders.[1] Therefore, prevention must become the cornerstone of therapy. This chapter addresses the pathophysiology and etiology of osteoporosis and osteomalacia, then focuses on the various diagnostic, therapeutic, and preventive modalities currently in use.

Osteoporosis

DEFINITION

Osteoporosis has been defined as "low bone mass [and] microarchitectural deterioration of bone tissue, leading to enhanced bone fragility and a consequent increase in fracture risk."[1] The World Health Organization (WHO) has established general diagnostic categories of bone loss based on the degree of deviation from the mean bone mineral density in normal young adults (T score; Table 35.1).[2]

TREATMENT GOALS: OSTEOPOROSIS

- Prevent disease by maximizing and maintaining bone mass.
- Prevent further bone loss in patients with disease.
- Decrease the risk of fractures by maximizing bone mineral density.

Table 35.1 ▪ World Health Organization Diagnostic Criteria for Osteoporosis and Osteopenia

	Bone Mineral Density (T Score[a])
Normal	<1 SD below normal
Osteopenia	1–2.5 SD below normal
Osteoporosis	≥2.5 SD below normal, no history of fractures
Severe (established) osteoporosis	≥2.5 SD below normal, history of non-violent fractures

Source: Reference 2.

[a]SD from mean of young adult bone mineral density.

EPIDEMIOLOGY

Osteoporosis can be divided into several types. Type I (postmenopausal osteoporosis) is associated with accelerated bone loss (2 to 3% of total bone per year) beginning with the onset of menopause and lasting approximately 10 years if no intervention is implemented. Loss is greater in trabecular bone than cortical bone. This results in an increased risk of vertebral compression and distal forearm fractures in the 10 to 20 years after onset. Type II (senile osteoporosis) is more insidious, causing progressive bone loss in both cortical and trabecular bone (approximately 0.5 to 1% per year) over many years, resulting in hip and vertebral fractures in both men and women over age 70.[3] Therefore, osteoporosis is primarily a disease of older adults. The Third National Health and Nutrition Examination Survey (NHANES III), which measured bone mineral density of the proximal femur in a random population of U.S. residents, documented an osteoporosis rate of 13 to 18% in women over age 50 and a 37 to 50% rate of osteopenia in this population. Based on this prevalence, an estimated 4 to 6 million women over 50 years of age in the United States have osteoporosis and an additional 13 to 17 million have osteopenia.[4] As the proportion of older adults in the United States increases, greater numbers of patients will be at risk for complications of low bone density.

Type III (secondary osteoporosis) may be caused by disease or medications (Table 35.2). Bone loss can also result from immobilization caused by accidents or serious illness. Secondary osteoporosis can occur at any age.

Postmenopausal Osteoporosis

Menopause is defined as the loss of ovarian function. The ovaries no longer respond to the hypothalamic secretion of gonadotropin-releasing hormone (GnRH) or the anterior pituitary secretion of follicle-stimulating hormone (FSH) and luteinizing hormone (LH). Endogenous estrogen production from the ovaries is therefore lost. Women still have some endogenous estrogen production that results from conversion of androstenedione to estrone in peripheral fat tissue. As a general rule, obese women have a greater rate of estrone production than thin women. This loss of ovarian estrogen is accompanied by bone loss. Several theories describe this relationship. Estrogen may be involved in the stimulation of calcitonin secretion, thus inhibiting bone resorption. Additionally, activation of the estrogen receptors present on osteoblasts suppresses the activation of cytokines, including interleukins 1 and 6 and tumor necrosis factor (TNF). These agents are involved in the stimulation of bone resorption.[5] In type I or postmenopausal osteoporosis, osteoclast activity is enhanced in the presence of normal osteoblast function, leading to accelerated bone loss. This bone loss is greater from trabecular sites than cortical sites.

Senile Osteoporosis

Although the precise cause of senile osteoporosis is not known, it is probably the result of several changes that occur during the aging process. These include an age-related decrease in gastrointestinal (GI) calcium absorption, a gradual increase in serum parathyroid hormone (PTH) concentration, and a decreased rate of vitamin D activation.[6]

Drug-Induced Osteoporosis

Glucocorticoids

Corticosteroid-induced bone loss has been recognized since Cushing first described hypercortisolism in the 1930s, but the incidence of osteoporosis in patients receiving steroids is not known. One study reported an 11% incidence of vertebral and rib fractures in asthmatic patients on corticosteroids for at least 1 year.[7] Proposed mechanisms for this drug-induced side effect include an alteration in calcium absorption and elimination leading to secondary hyperparathyroidism, an inhibitory effect on sex hormone production, and direct inhibition of osteoblast function.[8] The effect of glucocorticoids on bone appears to be dose and duration dependent, with the greatest loss

Table 35.2 ▪ Causes of Type III (Secondary) Osteoporosis

Diseases	Drugs
Hyperadrenalism	Corticosteroids
Hyperthyroidism	Excessive thyroid hormone
Hyperparathyroidism	Heparin (>6 mo)
Inflammatory arthritis	Anticonvulsants
Hypogonadism	Furosemide
Chronic renal failure	Aluminum-containing antacids
Chronic liver disease	Methotrexate
Malabsorption syndromes	Medroxyprogesterone acetate
Alcoholism	Gonadotropin-releasing hormone agonists
Calcium deficiency	Etretinate
Multiple myeloma	Cyclosporine A

Table 35.3 ▪ American College of Rheumatology Guidelines for the Prevention and Treatment of Glucocorticoid-Induced Osteoporosis

For all patients
- Choose the corticosteroid regimen with the lowest risk
  - Inhaled or topical
  - Lowest possible dosage
  - Alternate-day therapy not protective
- Encourage appropriate lifestyle modifications
  - Cessation of tobacco use
  - Limited alcohol intake
  - Regular exercise regimen
- Prescribe dietary modifications and nutritional supplements
  - Calcium 1500 mg/day
  - Vitamin D 50,000 units 3 times/wk or 800 IU/day or calcitriol 0.5 μg/day

For patients on long-term therapy
- Evaluate
  - Bone mineral density
  - Gonadal function
  - Calcium balance
- Consider thiazide diuretic if otherwise indicated (e.g., patient is hypertensive)
- Correct hypogonadal state if present
  - Premenopausal women: oral contraception
  - Postmenopausal women: hormone replacement therapy (estrogen with or without progesterone)
  - Men: testosterone
- Consider alternative or additional therapy in patients unable to take hormonal therapy or those who have established osteoporosis
  - Bisphosphonates (alendronate, etidronate)
  - Calcitonin

Source: Reference 8.

occurring during the first 6 months of therapy. Prednisone at a dosage of 7.5 mg or more per day is associated with significant bone loss, with trabecular bone loss being greater than cortical bone loss. It is unclear whether physiologic dosages have deleterious effects on bone, but alternate-day dosing does not appear to be safer than daily dosing.[8] Inhaled corticosteroids do not decrease bone density at low to moderate dosages but may have some effect at higher dosages.[9] Men are equally affected, and no protection appears to be offered by race. Some bone mass restoration may occur upon withdrawal of glucocorticoid therapy.[8] The recommendations developed by the American College of Rheumatology Task Force on Osteoporosis Guidelines for minimizing bone loss associated with corticosteroid therapy are summarized in Table 35.3.

Heparin

Heparin was first reported to cause osteoporosis in 1965.[10,11] Although the number of identified cases is small, one study estimated the incidence of symptomatic osteoporosis after long-term heparin to be as high as 2%. Some studies suggest that the risk of developing osteoporosis with heparin is dose and duration dependent (e.g., more than 15,000 U/day for more than 4 months).[12] Potential mechanisms include increased osteoclast activity and decreased osteoblast activity, a hypocalcemia-induced increase in PTH activity, heparin-induced increase in collagenase activity, and a decrease in the production of 1,25-hydroxyvitamin D (1,25-$(OH)_2$-D) caused by decreased renal conversion enzyme activity. This bone loss has been shown to reverse after heparin is discontinued. One group particularly at risk is pregnant women needing anticoagulation, in whom warfarin therapy is contraindicated. Whether calcium and vitamin D supplementation during heparin therapy is beneficial is not known, but it is considered prudent. Initial studies suggest that the risk of osteoporosis also exists with low-molecular-weight heparin but to a lesser degree than with heparin.[12]

Gonadotropin-Releasing Hormone Agonists

The GnRH agonists leuprolide, goserelin, and nafarelin are associated with bone loss in women[13] and men.[14] Initial stimulation of the hypothalamic–pituitary–ovarian or hypothalamic–pituitary–testicular axis is followed by shutdown of these axes because of downregulation of receptors. The net result is a hypoestrogenic or hypotestosterone state. Trabecular bone loss can be rapid, varying from 2 to 6% over 1 year. It is recommended that the use of these agents be limited to 6 months.[15] Therapy with estrogen and progesterone (called add-back therapy) or progesterone alone may minimize the osteoporotic effects of GnRH agonists, allowing longer use in women. However, hormone replacement therapy (HRT) may limit the therapeutic effects of the GnRH agonist in conditions such as endometriosis, leiomyomata, or premenstrual syndrome.[16,17] Alternatively, the bisphosphonate etidronate has been shown to prevent the bone density changes associated with GnRH agonist therapy.[18]

Other Substances

Furosemide and other loop diuretics are known to cause calciuria, as are caffeine and phosphorus-containing sodas. Conversely, thiazide diuretics, which decrease urinary calcium excretion and may inhibit bone resorption, appear to be protective of bone mass.[19] High phosphorus content in the GI tract inhibits calcium absorption, as does alcohol. Cigarette smoking appears to have an antiestrogenic effect.[20] Although these compounds are not known to result in overt bone loss, they are often prescribed or ingested by those at risk for osteoporosis. Minimizing ingestion of these compounds is prudent.

Other Causes of Osteoporosis

Anorexia nervosa can decrease bone density by two mechanisms: dietary calcium and vitamin D deficiency and pseudomenopause induction. Many anorexic women have estrogen deficiency and cease to have menstrual cycles. The bone loss associated with anorexia resembles that of menopause. Likewise, premature ovarian failure and premenopausal surgical castration (oophorectomy) result in estrogen deficiency that will accelerate bone loss unless HRT is initiated.

Patients with quadriplegia or paraplegia, as well as posttraumatic immobilization resulting in traction or prolonged bed rest, are at risk for bone loss. Daily weight-bearing activity improves bone density and is essential to good skeletal health.[21]

Men may be protected from osteoporosis by several factors, including a higher peak bone mass than women and no distinct cessation of sex hormone production equivalent to female menopause. However, based on results of the NHANES III study, the incidence of osteoporosis in men over age 50 is estimated at 3 to 6% (1 to 2 million) and that for osteopenia is 28 to 47% (8 to 13 million).[4] Approximately 14% of all vertebral compression fractures and almost 25% of all hip fractures occur in men. Secondary causes assume a much greater role, but hypogonadism resulting in low testosterone is a primary cause. Because low serum testosterone may not impair sexual function, patients may be unaware of their increased risk. Other causes of osteoporosis in men are diseases such as Cushing syndrome, hyperthyroidism, cancer, glucocorticoid therapy, chronic alcohol ingestion and other dietary factors, smoking, and prolonged immobilization. Treatment options are the same as those for women except that exogenous testosterone instead of estrogen is used if a deficiency is identified.[22]

PATHOPHYSIOLOGY

Skeletal formation begins during the sixth week of embryologic development, when mesenchymal cells differentiate into chondrocytes, which form a cartilaginous skeleton. Shortly thereafter, calcification begins and growth plates are formed on the ends of bone.[23] The skeletal mass of infants doubles in the first year of life, and 37% of the total skeletal mass is accumulated during adolescence. Skeletal growth continues until genetic height is attained, but bone mineralization continues until the third decade.[24,25] Infants, children, and adolescents have a greater ability to retain ingested calcium than adults, which aids in attaining desired peak bone mass. Adequate calcium intake during the years of skeletal growth and mineralization obviously is vital. Exercise to produce dense bone is also very important. Multiple factors, including growth hormone, are involved in optimal bone production, but their full roles have not been elucidated.

Bone loss (resorption) and formation is a dynamic process that occurs throughout life. These two opposing processes are usually coupled in bone-remodeling units (BRUs); there are more than 1 million active BRUs, involving 15 to 20% of the bone surface, at any given time.[26] This is shown schematically in Figure 35.1.[27] BRUs serve two important functions: to provide the serum with

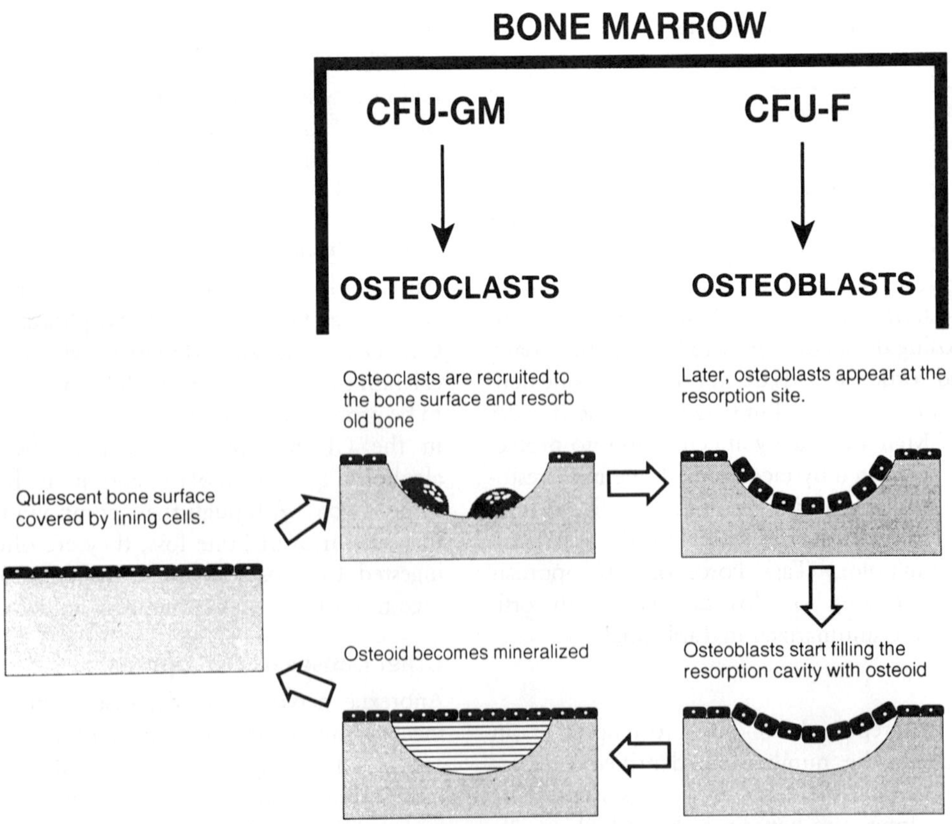

Figure 35.1. Relationship between bone marrow and the bone-remodeling process. Replenishment of osteoclasts and osteoblasts from their respective hematopoietic progenitors (granulocyte–macrophage colony-forming units *[CFU-GM]*) and mesenchymal progenitors (fibroblast colony-forming units *[CFU-F]*) in the bone marrow is critical for remodeling, which is accomplished by cycles involving the resorption of old bone by osteoclasts and the subsequent formation of new bone by osteoblasts. (Reprinted with permission from Manolagas SC, Jilka RL. Bone marrow, cytokines, and bone remodeling. Emerging insights into the pathophysiology of osteoporosis. N Engl J Med 332:305–311, 1995.)

a readily available source of calcium for maintaining physiologic processes such as muscle contraction and nerve conduction and to strengthen, revitalize, and rehydrate the bone matrix.

One of the first signals to bone matrix to initiate bone resorption is a decrease in serum calcium below the normal values of 9 to 11 mg/dL. Hypocalcemia causes secretion of PTH from the four parathyroid glands located in the neck adjacent to the thyroid gland. PTH not only initiates bone resorption but also causes three additional actions aimed at increasing serum calcium: inhibition of renal phosphorus resorption, increased renal calcium resorption, and increased renal production of 1,25-$(OH)_2$-D, which increases dietary calcium absorption from the GI tract. Gut absorption of calcium is by active transport in the distal duodenum and proximal jejunum. 1,25-$(OH)_2$-D induces calcium-binding proteins to carry calcium through the gut cell wall. If GI concentrations of phosphorus, dietary phytates or oxalates, or free fatty acids are high, this process is impaired. In an acidic medium, calcium can also undergo passive absorption if GI concentrations are high enough.

When bone resorption begins, evidence suggests that surface osteocytes (inactive osteoblasts) contract to allow osteoclast exposure to mineralized bone matrix (Fig. 35.1). Osteoclasts secrete collagenases and proteinases that solubilize the bone matrix to a depth of approximately 1 mm^3. The goal of calcium release is therefore accomplished. This is followed in several days by the influx of osteoblasts, which begin new bone synthesis. Osteoblasts promote collagen synthesis into new bone matrix, also known as osteoid, over about 10 days. Next, the new bone must become mineralized with hydroxyapatite, a compound consisting primarily of calcium and phosphorus, having the chemical structure $Ca_{10}(PO_4)_6(OH)_2$. The bone matrix also contains sodium, potassium, magnesium, and carbonate. The complete mineralization and hardening process takes several months. The now inactive osteoblasts become sequestered in bone tissue as flattened lining cells (surface osteocytes) on the new bone.

Bone resorption occurs on the bone surface, and the type of bone with the greatest surface area is trabecular, or cancellous, bone. Trabecular bone is found primarily in the vertebrae and the metaphyses of long bones. The long bone shafts are primarily cortical (compact) in structure. Approximately 25% of trabecular bone is remodeled each year, compared to approximately 2 to 3% of cortical bone.[28]

Table 35.4 ▪ Factors That Increase or Decrease Risk of Developing Osteoporosis

Risk Factors	Protective Factors
General	High normal body mass
Slender build (thin, small frame)	African or Mediterranean race
Caucasian or Asian race	Weight-bearing exercise
Female sex	Estrogen replacement therapy
Menopause	Adequate lifetime calcium intake
Oophorectomy during reproductive years	Avoidance of risk factors
Positive family history	Thiazide diuretic use
Medical therapy	Oral contraceptive use
Glucocorticoids	
Loop diuretic	
Gonadotropin-releasing hormone agonists	
Heparin	
Diet	
Chronic low calcium intake	
Chronic high phosphorus intake	
Personal habits	
Smoking	
Heavy caffeine consumption	
Heavy alcohol consumption	
Inactivity	
Falls	

CLINICAL PRESENTATION AND DIAGNOSIS

Signs and Symptoms

An early symptom of osteoporosis is back pain in the lumbar or thoracic spinal region; however, many patients may not identify this as early disease. The pain is precipitated by usual activity that in the patient's past would not have been considered stressful. Spinal movement may be restricted. The patient may notice a loss in height of several inches, or this may be identified during yearly physical examinations. Progressive kyphosis, or curvature of the spine, may develop as compression fractures worsen. This may result in the classic dowager's hump. The ribs eventually rest on the iliac crest of the pelvis, causing abdominal protrusion due to the loss of truncal space.

Wrist fractures, primarily of the distal radius, may occur if the patient falls and lands on an instinctively outstretched hand. Falls also are associated with fractures of the proximal femur, proximal humerus, and pelvis. Fractures of this type are associated with significant morbidity, particularly as the patient ages. Fractures resulting in surgery or prolonged hospitalization place the patient at risk for thromboembolic sequelae, pneumonia, and worsening of disease caused by immobilization. Many people who sustain hip fractures lose their ability to live independently. Some, fearful of additional fractures, restrict their activities, leading to isolation and depression.

Diagnosis

As noted, many cases of osteoporosis are not identified until a fracture occurs. However, patients can be screened for osteoporotic risk factors and the condition may be diagnosed early enough for intervention to produce a beneficial effect. Risk factors are listed in Table 35.4. Although Caucasian or Asian race has long been considered a risk factor, recent evidence shows that black women with a slender body habitus and other risk factors listed in Table 35.4 are also at risk for osteoporosis.[29]

Routine serum or urine chemistries generally are not helpful in osteoporosis diagnosis. Serum calcium, phosphorus, total alkaline phosphatase, PTH, 25-hydroxyvitamin D (25-OH-D), and 1,25-$(OH)_2$-D usually are within normal limits. Byproducts of collagen catabolism, such as pyridinoline and deoxypyridinoline, and the collagen telopeptides, N-telopeptide-to-helix and c-telopeptide-to-helix, are markers of bone resorption; urinary levels of these compounds may be useful for distinguishing patients with rapid rates of bone resorption. Bone-specific alkaline phosphatase and serum osteocalcin (bone Gla-protein) reflect osteoblast activity and therefore may be useful as markers of bone formation, especially in evaluating response to antiresorptive drug therapy, such as estrogen or calcitonin.[30] These tests are not a replacement for bone mineral density measurements.

Several radiographic techniques may be considered for diagnosing osteoporosis, but authorities differ in their recommendations for widespread use of these techniques (Table 35.5). A routine spinal radiograph, often performed in symptomatic patients, will not detect osteoporosis until 20 to 50% of spinal bone has been lost.[32] This technique is not useful to follow progression of bone loss or assess efficacy of medical intervention. Single-photon absorptiometry (SPA) is an inexpensive measure of cortical bone mineral density at one discrete site. The site (usually the distal forearm) is exposed to a beam of photons, and the transmitted fraction is measured in grams per square centimeter. The greater the bone density, the lower the transmitted fraction. Unfortunately, SPA information is not applicable to the entire skeleton. Dual-photon absorptiometry, dual-energy x-ray absorptiometry, and quantitative computed tomography (QCT) are better indicators of density of trabecular bone, such as the vertebrae. QCT is the most expensive and exposes the patient to the greatest amount of radiation. The newest technique, ultrasonography, uses sound waves to evaluate bone density. This method is less expensive than those involving radiation but is not as well validated as the radiologic tests.[31] Clinical use of these measurements is evolving, but acceptable uses with regard to osteoporosis include early screening, diagnosis, and assessing response to dietary and pharmacologic therapy.[33]

PREVENTION AND TREATMENT

The goals of osteoporosis management include prevention and treatment. Preventive therapy includes maximizing bone mass during the formative years and then maintaining bone mass once peak bone mass has been achieved. For patients with established osteoporosis, the optimal treatment goal is to replenish bone mass. Unfortunately, currently available therapies have not been shown to replace significant amounts of lost bone. Therefore, osteoporosis treatment focuses on preventing further bone loss and decreasing the risk of fractures. Figure 35.2 is a decision algorithm for osteoporosis prevention and treatment in postmenopausal women.

Calcium

Calcium is an important adjunct therapy for osteoporosis. Alone, it does not completely retard the rapid bone loss occurring at menopause. However, adequate calcium intake is vital for adequate response to other antiosteoporotic agents. Based on currently available information, the National Institutes of Health[34] recommends higher calcium intakes for some age groups than the currently established recommended daily intakes (Table 35.6). Adequate calcium intake throughout life is essential for attaining peak bone mass and may affect the rate at which bone is lost later in life. Calcium is a threshold nutrient. The daily calcium intake below which the body must obtain calcium from bone is approximately 400 mg. Women with optimal calcium intake are not likely to receive additional benefit from calcium supplements, whereas women with very low intake receive significant

Table 35.5 ▪ Bone Mineral Density Measurement Methods

Method	Evaluable Sites	Radiation Dosage	Comments
Single-energy photon absorptiometry	Forearm Calcaneus (heel)	Very low	10- to 15-min scan time Accurate and precise Limited to peripheral bone
Dual-energy x-ray absorptiometry	Spine Lateral lumbar spine Proximal femur Total body	Low	Scan time <5 min Correlated with fracture risk Accurate and precise High cost
Quantitative computed tomography	Spine Radius	High Low	High cost Not well correlated with fracture risk
Broadband ultrasound attenuation	Calcaneus Patella	None	Inexpensive Portable Correlated with fracture risk

Source: Reference 31.

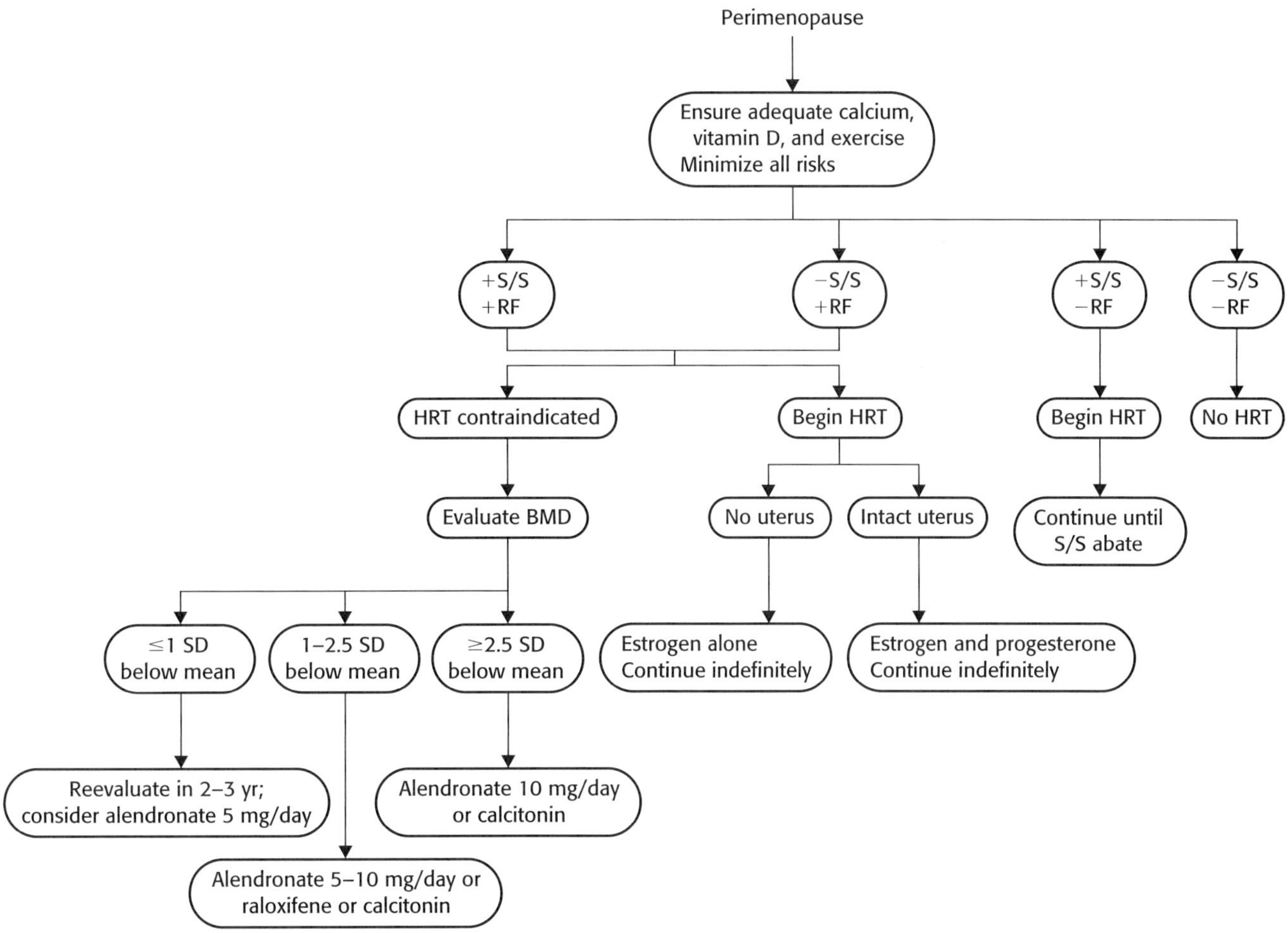

Figure 35.2. Decision algorithm for osteoporosis treatment and prevention in perimenopausal women. *BMD,* bone mineral density; *HRT,* hormone replacement therapy; *RF,* risk factors; *S/S,* signs/symptoms (vasomotor, urogenital).

benefit.[35] Dietary calcium and supplements are equally efficacious if ingestion (in milligrams of elemental calcium) is equal. Calcium carbonate and tribasic calcium phosphate have the greatest percentage of elemental calcium, 40% and 39%, respectively. Table 35.7 lists the variety of calcium supplements available. As a general rule, when calculating calcium intake, one can estimate 250 mg from each full serving of a dietary source known to be high in calcium. These include dairy products, fortified juices, canned fish including bones, and some green vegetables, such as collard greens, broccoli, and rhubarb. Calcium absorption is rate-limited; divided doses are better absorbed than a large single daily dose.

Older adults may have decreased calcium absorption caused by lower vitamin D concentrations, resulting in less active transport of calcium, or by achlorhydria. Taking supplements with meals enhances passive absorption. Although it contains less elemental calcium than calcium carbonate, calcium citrate is not dependent on gastric pH for absorption and may be a good choice for older adults.

Zealous support for calcium therapy may lead some patients to overmedicate themselves. However, homeostatic mechanisms decrease intestinal fractional absorption

Table 35.6 ▪ Recommended Calcium Intakes

	Elemental Calcium (mg/day)	
Group	**Current RDA**	**NIH Consensus**
Infant		
Birth–6 mo	400	400
6–12 mo	600	600
Children		
1–5 yr	800	800
6–10 yr	800	800–1200
Adolescents		
11–18 yr	1200	1200–1500
Men		
19–24 yr	1200	1200–1500
25–65 yr	800	1000
>65 yr	800	1500
Women		
19–24 yr	1200	1200–1500
25–50 yr	800	1000
>50 yr on estrogen	800	1000
>50 yr not on estrogen	800	1500
>65 yr	800	1500
Pregnant or lactating	1200	1200–1500

Source: Reference 34.

Table 35.7 ▪ Selected Calcium Supplements

Salt	Elemental Calcium (%)	Solubility	Selected Products	Calcium/Tablet (mg)	Relative Cost/1000 mg
Calcium carbonate	40	Insoluble	Generic	600	$
			OsCal	500	$–$$
			Caltrate	600	$
			Tums	200, 300, 400	$–$$
Tribasic calcium phosphate	39	Insoluble	Posture	600	$$
Calcium citrate	21	Soluble	Generic	200	$
			Citracal	200	$$
Calcium lactate	18	Soluble	Generic	84	$$$
Calcium gluconate	9	Soluble	Generic	45, 58	$$–$$$$

Table 35.8 ▪ Estrogen Equivalencies for Osteoporosis Therapy

Component	Route	Antiosteoporotic Dosage (mg)	Available strengths (mg)
Conjugated estrogens	Oral	0.625	0.3, 0.625, 0.9, 1.25, 2.5
Esterified estrogens	Oral	0.3	0.3, 0.625, 1.25, 2.5
17β-Estradiol, micronized	Oral	0.5	0.5, 1, 2
Piperazine estrone sulfate (estropipate)	Oral	1.25	0.625, 1.25, 2.5
17β-estradiol	Transdermal	0.05	0.0375, 0.05, 0.075, 0.1

when intake is great. In the absence of excessive vitamin D, the use of calcium supplements is rarely associated with hypercalciuria or renal calcium stones. The primary side effects from calcium supplements are gastrointestinal, including nausea and constipation. Fiber impairs absorption, as does iron therapy. Patients should take tetracycline compounds and calcium at least 2 hours apart to avoid intestinal chelation.

Estrogen

The data in support of estrogen replacement therapy (ERT) at menopause onset are unequivocal. The bone loss rate is lower in those prescribed estrogen than in those not taking estrogen, resulting in a 50% lower fracture rate.[36,37] There is increasing evidence that estrogen is beneficial more than 10 years after menopause for minimizing further bone loss.[38] However, not all women entering menopause develop osteoporosis, so screening for osteoporotic risk factors (Table 35.2) and contraindications to estrogen therapy are vital. Contraindications to estrogen therapy have traditionally included history of endometrial or breast cancer, but there may be exceptions to this rule.[39] Other contraindications include liver disease, undiagnosed genital bleeding, active thromboembolic disorder, history of thromboembolic disorder caused by hormonal therapy, and known or suspected pregnancy.

Estrogens are available as several different compounds and by various routes of administration. The two routes proven to provide osteoporosis prevention are oral and transdermal. The daily estrogen dosage shown to preserve bone mineral density is equivalent to 0.625 mg of conjugated estrogens, although some studies suggest that 0.3 mg may provide adequate antiosteoporotic activity.[40] The 0.3-mg dosage of esterified estrogens was recently approved by the U.S. Food and Drug Administration (FDA) for preventing osteoporosis.[41] Larger dosages may be needed to control menopausal symptoms in some women. See Table 35.8 for marketed estrogens and equivalent osteoporotic therapeutic dosages. Although prices vary between products, therapy can be achieved at a cost of approximately 30 to 80 cents per day, or about $100 to $300 per year, making preventive therapy very cost-effective. Combination products of estrogen and progestin simplify regimens and may enhance compliance.

Benefits Other Than Osteoporosis Prevention

Estrogen also brings relief from other conditions associated with menopause, such as vasomotor symptoms (hot flashes) and urogenital atrophy manifesting as vaginal itching and dryness. Although not FDA approved for prevention of heart disease, estrogens are known to favorably affect the lipid profile by increasing high-density lipoprotein (HDL) and decreasing low-density lipoprotein (LDL) level. This effect is greater with oral products than transdermal, but transdermal estrogens do provide some benefit and decrease triglyceride levels.[42] Other potential cardioprotective mechanisms include endothelial function improvement and effects on fibrinogen and the fibrinolytic system.[43] Based on retrospective studies, it is estimated that estrogen therapy can reduce a woman's risk of cardiovascular mortality by 50%.[44] However, role of estrogen therapy in treating heart disease is unclear. The Heart and Estrogen/Progestin Replacement Study (HERS), a prospective trial of HRT use in women with preexisting heart disease, did not show any overall benefit in relation to cardiovascular mortality, although there was a trend to improved outcomes after 4 years of treatment. Of concern in this study was the higher incidence of coronary events in the treatment group during the first year of the study.[45] Other long-term clinical trials, such as the Women's Health Initiative, which is scheduled to be completed in 2007, should help clarify the effect of estrogen therapy on cardiovascular disease. Adding a progestin reduces but does not eliminate the beneficial effects of estrogen on the lipid profile.[46] The limited number of studies available suggests that the cardiovascular benefits of estrogen are maintained with combination therapy.[47]

Recent evidence suggests that estrogen therapy may reduce the risk of dementia and colorectal cancer.[48,49] However, additional studies are needed before HRT can be recommended specifically for these diseases.

Risks

Prolonged exposure to estrogen at high dosages is associated with endometrial hyperplasia and endometrial cancer in women with an intact uterus. Concomitant cyclic or continuous progestin therapy can prevent endometrial tissue hyperplasia.[50] Many regimens have been used, and the most commonly advocated are described in Table 35.9. After hysterectomy, women do not need concomitant progestin.

The risk of thromboembolism secondary to ERT increases during the first year of therapy with oral or transdermal estrogen but falls off significantly thereafter.[51] In the 3-year Postmenopausal Estrogen/Progestin Interventions (PEPI) trial, women receiving estrogen therapy did not demonstrate any significant changes in blood pressure.[46] However, some patients taking oral estrogen may exhibit increases in blood pressure; these women may do better on a transdermal product. The incidence of cholecystitis appears to be two to three times higher[52] and might be prevented by use of transdermal estrogen. All underlying risk factors should be addressed before ERT is initiated.

Multiple studies have examined the effect of estrogens on breast cancer, but the results remain equivocal. Several meta-analyses do not support an increased risk from all use of estrogen therapy but suggest that long-term use (more than 5 years) is associated with a higher risk of breast cancer.[53] Adding progestin to estrogen does not appear to decrease the risk of breast cancer, but whether combination therapy increases breast cancer risk remains to be determined. Self-breast examination, yearly physical examination, and mammograms are recommended for women on estrogen replacement, as they are for all women more than 50 years old.

The most common side effects of estrogen therapy include breast tenderness, peripheral edema, and headaches. Cyclic administration may be effective in relieving these side effects. Women receiving combination therapy experience withdrawal vaginal bleeding, although with the continuous regimens this should abate over time. Transdermal products may irritate the skin. Rotating patch placement and placement on the buttocks may reduce skin reactions. Enzyme inducers such as rifampin and phenobarbital may increase hepatic metabolism of estrogen; therefore, response to estrogen should be monitored and estrogen dosage increased if indicated. Estrogens may increase the effects of both corticosteroids and tricyclic antidepressants; therefore, patients prescribed these combinations should be monitored closely.

Biphosphonates

The bisphosphonates are compounds that adsorb onto hydroxyapatite crystals at sites of active bone resorption and inhibit osteoclastic activity without a subsequent effect on osteoblastic activity.

Alendronate is FDA approved for preventing and treating osteoporosis. In women with osteoporosis, with or without preexisting fractures, alendronate has been shown

Table 35.9 ▪ Estrogen and Progestin Regimens for Osteoporosis

Estrogen	Progestin	Dosing	Bleeding Pattern
Patient with intact uterus			
Oral estrogen[a] or estradiol transdermal patch (0.05 mg)	Progestin (equivalent to 5–10 mg medroxyprogesterone)	Estrogen: days 1–25 of each month Progestin: days 1–12 or 16–25 of each month (at least 10 days/mo)	Monthly withdrawal bleeding 1–2 wk after progestin dose
Oral estrogen or estradiol transdermal patch (0.05 mg)	Progestin (equivalent to 2.5 mg medroxyprogesterone)	Estrogen: daily Progestin: daily	Irregular for first 6–12 mo; many patients cease bleeding after 1 yr of continuous therapy
After hysterectomy			
Oral estrogen or estradiol transdermal patch (0.05 mg)	None	Daily	None

[a]See Table 35.8 for estrogen dosages.

to progressively increase bone mass and prevent vertebral, hip, and wrist fractures.[54,55] In postmenopausal women without osteoporosis, alendronate preserves bone mass to almost the same degree as estrogen therapy.[56,57] The drug has also been shown to increase bone density in patients receiving glucocorticoids.[58] The combination of estrogen therapy and alendronate in women with osteoporosis is more effective than estrogen alone.[59]

The alendronate dosage depends on the indication (10 mg daily for treatment, 5 mg daily for prevention). Oral bioavailability is approximately 0.78% in women. To optimize absorption, alendronate should be taken upon arising in the morning. Patients should be instructed to ingest the tablet with 6 to 8 oz water at least 30 minutes before ingesting other foods, beverages, or other medications. The patient should not lie down for 30 minutes after ingesting the medication. Esophagitis has been reported and in many cases was felt to be caused by inappropriate drug administration; proper drug use should be reinforced at each visit. Adequate calcium and vitamin D through dietary sources or supplements is also necessary to ensure optimal increases in bone mineral density.

Alendronate is not metabolized; drug not adsorbed onto bone is excreted unchanged in urine and feces. It is contraindicated in patients with creatinine clearances less than 35 mL/minute. The side effect profile of alendronate is limited primarily to GI complaints such as abdominal pain or distension, nausea, dyspepsia, constipation, flatulence, and dysphagia. Alendronate should be used cautiously in patients with a history of preexisting GI problems.

Alendronate should be considered in patients with or at risk for osteoporosis in whom estrogen is contraindicated or refused. Alendronate therapy is estimated to cost the patient approximately $750 per year.

Etidronate, a bisphosphonate currently marketed for Paget's disease and hypercalcemia, has been evaluated in patients with osteoporosis. Regimens with etidronate administered 400 mg orally daily for 2 weeks followed by 10 to 14 weeks of calcium were designed to mimic the bone remodeling cycle. Improved bone mineral density and decreased fracture rates were observed in women with osteoporosis.[60,61] A combination of estrogen and etidronate has also been shown to be more effective than either agent alone.[62] Etidronate is well tolerated, the most common side effects being gastrointestinal.

Three other bisphosphonates, risedronate, pamidronate, and tiludronate, are marketed in the United States. These agents are not approved for treating osteoporosis; however, clinical trials are in progress. Investigational bisphosphonates include ibandronate and zoledronate.

Selective Estrogen Receptor Modulators

Selective estrogen receptor modulators (SERMs) are synthetic compounds that exhibit estrogenic properties in some tissues while exerting antiestrogenic activities in other tissues. Tamoxifen, the first commercially available SERM, has antiestrogenic effects in breast tissue but has estrogenic properties in bone, the lipoprotein system, and the uterus. Currently, tamoxifen is approved only for treating and preventing breast cancer. Raloxifene, a SERM that is an estrogen agonist in bone and lipids but an estrogen antagonist in breast and endometrial tissue, is approved for prevention and treatment of postmenopausal osteoporosis. Additional SERMs under investigation for managing osteoporosis include droloxifene, idoxifene, and levormeloxifene.

Raloxifene, like estrogen, inhibits bone resorption. In postmenopausal women, 60 mg daily raloxifene has been shown to promote significantly greater bone mineral density than placebo, but its effects on bone may not be as great as those seen with ERT.[63] Currently, no data are available on fracture rates in women taking raloxifene. Raloxifene decreases total cholesterol and LDL levels in a fashion similar to ERT, but it has less marked effects on HDL and HDL_2 cholesterol and triglycerides.[64] These changes suggest that raloxifene may exert some degree of the cardioprotective effects attributed to estrogen, but clinical trials are needed to define such a benefit. Postmenopausal women taking raloxifene do not demonstrate endometrial tissue proliferation, indicating a minimal risk of endometrial cancer.[65] Raloxifene's antiestrogenic effects on breast tissue suggest a possible use for treating or preventing breast cancer; however, clinical trials are needed to fully elucidate its role.[66]

Dosing of raloxifene is 60 mg daily without regard to meals, and 60% of the dose is absorbed. The drug has a high first-pass metabolism, and the major route of elimination is in the feces. Use of raloxifene in patients with significant liver impairment has not been studied. Adverse effects include hot flashes and leg cramps. The risk of thromboembolism increases with raloxifene, especially during the first 4 months of therapy. Patients who will be immobilized for a prolonged period of time should have therapy discontinued 72 hours before the start of immobilization or as soon as possible thereafter.

Based on currently available information, raloxifene should be reserved for postmenopausal women at risk for osteoporosis who cannot take ERT or bisphosphonates. Annual cost for raloxifene is approximately $700.

Calcitonin

Calcitonin is an endogenous hormone secreted by the thyroid gland in response to dietary or elevated serum calcium. Women have been shown to have less endogenous calcitonin secretion in response to dietary calcium than men, which suggests a basis for lower bone density in women. Calcitonin prevents bone resorption by inhibiting osteoclast activity. The drug has been shown to significantly increase bone mineral density and decrease fracture rates in women with established osteoporosis.[67] The drug has its greatest effect on the spine and is most effective in patients with high bone turnover rates. Calcitonin also has an analgesic effect; women with osteoporotic vertebral fractures report symptomatic pain improvement after therapy with intranasal or injectable salmon calcitonin.[68]

Current administration routes include subcutaneous or intramuscular and intranasal. Calcitonin's effect is dose related. The recommended injectable dosage is 100 IU (subcutaneous or intramuscular) and the intranasal dosage is 200 IU(one spray)/day. Patients should ingest adequate calcium and vitamin D during calcitonin treatment. Studies 1 to 3 years long show evidence of continued benefit, but long-term use has been associated with a waning of effect, possibly caused by receptor downregulation.[69] Some studies suggest that intermittent or discontinuous dosing (1 year on drug, 1 year off) may prevent resistance.[70]

Side effects with injectable calcitonin include nausea and GI discomfort in approximately 8 to 10% of patients; this may be minimized by bedtime administration. Initially, facial flushing and dermatitis may occur in 2 to 5% of patients, but these effects usually abate with continued therapy. Pruritus at the injection site is also problematic. To minimize these side effects, patients should be instructed to administer calcitonin subcutaneously rather than intramuscularly. The intranasal formulation appears to be better tolerated; rhinitis is the most commonly reported side effect. Although antibodies have been reported in patients receiving salmon calcitonin, they do not appear to affect clinical response.

Calcitonin is a viable therapeutic option for patients who cannot tolerate other antiosteoporotic agents. It may also be considered in patients with back pain caused by vertebral fractures, glucocorticoid-induced osteoporosis, bone loss caused by immobilization, or hypoestrogenic states resulting from therapy with GnRH agonists. It has an excellent safety profile and few additional metabolic effects. The nasal spray has better patient acceptance than the injectable formulation. The annual cost of intranasal calcitonin is approximately $550.

Vitamin D

Vitamin D is a fat-soluble vitamin that might be more appropriately considered a hormone because of its physiologic function. The two exogenous sources of vitamin D are ergosterol (vitamin D_2) from plant sources and cholecalciferol (vitamin D_3) from animal sources, such as fish liver oils. Endogenous production of vitamin D_3 in the skin requires ultraviolet light exposure. These compounds first undergo hydroxylation in the liver to 25-OH-D, then are further hydroxylated in the kidney to result in the physiologically active compound 1,25-$(OH)_2$-D. The production of 1,25-$(OH)_2$-D is influenced by PTH, calcium, and phosphorus. Its presence enhances GI absorption of calcium. Therefore, a confounding factor in impaired calcium absorption may be inadequate vitamin D status. Optimal serum 25-OH-D serum concentrations range from 20 to 30 ng/mL. Many older adults have low dietary intake of vitamin D, and their exposure to sunlight may be minimal, especially if they are homebound or institutionalized. Production of 1,25-$(OH)_2$-D usually is within normal limits until serum 25-OH-D concentrations decrease below 7 ng/mL. Several studies have demonstrated that osteoporotic patients have deficient 25-OH-D serum concentrations. The combination of vitamin D_3 and calcium has been shown to decrease the incidence of nonvertebral fractures in older adults.[71,72] In patients with preexisting vertebral compression fractures, calcitriol (1,25$(OH)_2$-D) proved to be more effective than calcium alone in preventing further vertebral fractures.[73]

Patients at risk for vitamin D deficiency, such as older adults or patients on corticosteroids or anticonvulsant therapy, should be given vitamin D_2 or vitamin D_3 at dosages of 800 IU/day. In those receiving glucocorticoids, vitamin D_2 up to 50,000 IU three times weekly has been recommended. Calcitriol 0.5 μg/day is used for patients with established osteoporosis. This product is available by prescription only. When calcium and vitamin D are used concomitantly, the amount of calcium needed may be lower because intestinal calcium absorption should be enhanced. For patients receiving calcitriol, the calcium dosage should not exceed 800 mg/day. After calcitriol therapy is initiated, serum calcium and 24-hour urine calcium excretion should be assessed to ensure efficacy and the absence of hypercalcemia.[74] Concomitant use of thiazide diuretics and calcitriol may increase the risk of adverse effects. Patients exhibiting symptoms of anorexia, nausea, and weakness should be evaluated for possible hypercalcemia. For a comparison of vitamin D supplements, see Table 35.10.

ALTERNATIVE THERAPY

Phytoestrogens, plant-based compounds with weak estrogenic activity, have been credited as a protective factor contributing to interracial differences in the incidence of hormone-related disease. Some of these compounds, including lignins, which are found in a wide range of plant foods, and isoflavones, which are found primarily in soybeans, have demonstrated weak estrogenic and antiestrogenic activity in humans.[75] Epidemiologic studies indicate that diets rich in phytoestrogens have a protective effect against hot flashes and hormone-dependent cancers, such as breast cancer. A prospective study comparing soy protein supplementation with placebo has shown a beneficial effect on the frequency of hot flashes.[76] Additional studies are needed to confirm these benefits and determine their effects on osteoporosis, heart disease, and breast cancer. Diets rich in phytoestrogens appear to be well tolerated and could be recommended as adjunctive therapy to other risk-reducing behaviors.

FUTURE THERAPIES

Fluoride

It has long been recognized that people living in areas with high-fluoride water have very dense bone, but those with fluoride toxicity (fluorosis) have brittle bone. Dental programs including fluoridated water, rinses, and toothpastes are known to prevent caries development. Sodium fluoride is not FDA approved for osteoporosis treat-

Table 35.10 ▪ Vitamin D Preparations[a]

Product	Component	Strength	Availability
Ergocalciferol	D_2	8000 IU/mL (drops) 50,000 IU (tablets, capsules)	OTC Rx
Cholecalciferol	D_3	400 IU (tablets) 1000 IU (tablets)	OTC
Calcifediol	25-OH-D_3	20 μg, 50 μg (capsules)	Rx
Calcitriol	1,25-$(OH)_2$-D_3	0.25 μg, 0.5 μg (capsules), 1 mcg/mL (solution)	Rx
Dihydrotachysterol	Synthetic D_2	0.125 mg (tablets, capsules) 0.2 mg, 0.4 mg (tablets) 0.2 mg/mL (solution)	Rx

OTC, over-the-counter; *Rx*, prescription.
[a] 1 IU vitamin D activity = 0.025 μg vitamin D_3; 40,000 IU vitamin D activity = 1 mg vitamin D_3.

ment in the United States but is approved in many European countries.

Fluoride increases bone mineral density in several ways.[77] In the presence of therapeutic amounts of fluoride, fluoride substitutes for the hydroxyl ion in the crystal lattice, resulting in fluoroapatite instead of the physiologic compound hydroxyapatite. The newly synthesized bone appears to be more resistant to remodeling than bone containing hydroxyapatite.[78] Second, an increased number of osteoblasts appear on bone surfaces, thus uncoupling the BRU in favor of anabolism. At low dosages (sodium fluoride less than 30 mg/day) this new bone is lamellar, or normal in appearance, but at high dosages (80 mg/day or more) this bone may be abnormal. Fluoride also stimulates collagen synthesis and calcium deposition. Fluoride exerts most of its effect on trabecular bone, which has a higher turnover rate than cortical. For appropriate mineralization to occur, it is vital that therapeutic amounts of calcium be administered during fluoride therapy. If adequate calcium is not provided, clinical osteomalacia may result.

Studies have consistently shown that fluoride increases spinal bone mass up to 5% per year for a period of up to 4 years without significant effects on appendicular bone. However, studies evaluating fracture rates have yielded conflicting results.[79–81] The variation in the outcomes of these studies may be related to differences in the fluoride dosage and the degree of severity of osteoporosis being studied. One study found that patients with severe osteoporosis had no change in vertebral fracture incidence after fluoride therapy, whereas patients with milder osteoporosis experienced a significant decrease in vertebral fracture rates.[79] An early study of fluoride found a higher incidence of proximal femur fractures. Although this has not been confirmed by subsequent studies, concern about a possible cortical stealing effect of fluoride must be resolved before the drug can be widely used. Approximately 70% of patients respond to fluoride therapy, but currently no tool is available to predict who will have a positive response. Twelve to 24 months of therapy are necessary before response can be assessed.[78]

The optimal fluoride dosage has not been established. However, the minimum effective sodium fluoride dosage appears to be 30 mg/day. Based on limited data, a therapeutic range of fasting serum fluoride of 5 to 10 μmol (95 to 190 ng/mL) has been proposed; this must be confirmed. Dosage modification may be needed for patients with renal impairment. Plain sodium fluoride tablets have greater bioavailability and more rapid absorption than slow-release tablets.[78] Bioavailability is impaired when sodium fluoride is ingested concomitantly with antacids, milk or dairy products, calcium, iron, or magnesium. Ingestion of these substances and fluoride should be spaced by at least 2 hours. Sodium monofluorophosphate bioavailability, which is similar to that of sodium fluoride, is not affected by meals or calcium salts.

The most common side effect of fluoride therapy is gastrointestinal; the drug may induce chemical gastritis. Adverse effects, including pain, nausea, diarrhea, or constipation, have been reported in up to 50% of patients taking uncoated tablets. Use of a sustained-release product or sodium monofluorophosphate is associated with improved GI tolerance. Up to 20% of patients may experience painful lower extremity syndrome. This acute-onset leg pain may be caused by cortical bone stress fractures.[80] Tooth mottling may occur in children. Case reports of rheumatoid arthritis exacerbations limit sodium fluoride's use in this population.[82]

At this time, fluoride therapy cannot be recommended for routine use, but moderate dosages in combination with calcium may produce optimal bone density. It should be used with caution in patients with rheumatoid arthritis, renal impairment, or GI bleeding.

Parathyroid Hormone

PTH, the primary regulator of calcium homeostasis, has a dual effect on bone. A continuous infusion of PTH stimulates bone resorption. However, once-daily injections of PTH have been shown to increase trabecular bone formation, with a potentially detrimental effect on cortical bone.[83] Clinical trials of human PTH in women who were estrogen deficient secondary to treatment with GnRH agonists demonstrated a greater bone-saving effect of the combination than that of a GnRH agonist alone.[84] In osteoporotic women receiving estrogen, adding PTH resulted in further increases in bone mineral density and fewer new vertebral fractures. The effect was greatest in the spine, but no detrimental effects were seen in the peripheral skeleton, perhaps because of the antiresorptive effects of estrogen.[85] The most common adverse effects of PTH are administration related (pain and erythema at the injection site). Nausea and arthralgias have also been reported. Research on alternative delivery systems is under way. Additional studies are needed to determine the optimal application of PTH in osteoporosis.

Ipriflavone

Ipriflavone is a synthetic derivative of naturally occurring phytoestrogens. Although it has no apparent estrogenic activity in humans, it has been shown to have an inhibitory effect on osteoclasts while stimulating osteoblasts.[86] Several studies in postmenopausal women have shown the drug to have a protective effect against bone loss. The drug appears to be well tolerated; GI side effects are most common. The results of ongoing studies will further define the usefulness of this agent in treating osteoporosis.

IMPROVING OUTCOMES

Many women are unaware of the risks for osteoporosis and how they can protect themselves.[87] The pharmacist is in a key position to provide the counseling and education needed for successful preventive therapy. Adolescents and premenopausal women should be advised to increase their calcium intake and exercise so that they meet menopausal years with optimal bone mass. Perimenopausal and postmenopausal women likewise should be encouraged to ingest adequate calcium, participate in weight-bearing exercise, have adequate exposure to sunlight for vitamin D production, and minimize the risk factors listed in Table 35.4. Although HRT has benefits beyond relieving menopausal symptoms, many women avoid or prematurely discontinue therapy because of concern about adverse effects.[88] Patients must be thoroughly educated about the benefits and risks of HRT. Bone density in patients at risk for osteoporosis should be evaluated to assist in decision making. HRT regimens used vary widely; instructions should be reinforced during counseling sessions. Women should have annual physical exams, including annual mammography after the age of 50, and they should be competent in self-breast examination. For women who cannot or will not take HRT, alendronate, raloxifene, and calcitonin are alternative therapies. Thorough counseling on proper use of these agents is important to ensure optimal response.

CONCLUSION

Maximizing bone mineral density before the onset of menopause or the initiation of drugs that induce osteoporosis may decrease the risk of fractures. Minimizing alcohol and caffeine, avoiding high phosphorus intake, and ceasing smoking may also decrease risks. Adequate calcium and vitamin D intake should be strongly encouraged. For women with a propensity for osteoporotic fracture, adding estrogen with or without progesterone protects bone. Fortunately, women can adhere to this regimen at a total cost of less than $1 per day, making prevention truly cost-effective. For women who are not candidates for estrogen therapy, alendronate, raloxifene, and calcitonin are alternative agents. The best course for patients at risk for osteoporotic fractures is prevention through early intervention. A decision algorithm such as the one in Figure 35.2 can be used for therapeutic decision making. Therapy for osteoporosis is still in evolution, and it will take several generations to define the optimal protocol.

Osteomalacia

DEFINITION

Osteomalacia is an osteopenia manifested by inadequate bone mineralization that usually results in bone deformities. Rickets, which occurs in childhood, is osteomalacia involving the growth plate as well as formed bone. Osteomalacia does not involve the epiphyses and occurs in adults. Osteomalacia was first described in 1645 in northern Europe during the industrial revolution, when many children and adults worked long hours with very little exposure to sunlight. However, it was not until the 1800s that an association with lack of sunlight was suggested. The identification of vitamin D and its sources has prevented most cases of vitamin-D–deficient rickets, but several circumstances may put patients at risk for osteomalacia today.

TREATMENT GOALS: OSTEOMALACIA

- Base treatment on underlying disorder.
- Large dosages of vitamin D may be needed to treat vitamin D deficiency.

EPIDEMIOLOGY

When phosphorus and calcium are not available for production of hydroxyapatite, the mineralized compound of bone matrix, osteomalacia may develop. The causes may vary and include inadequate dietary intake of calcium, phosphorus, or vitamin D; genetic or acquired deficiencies of enzymes; and neoplasia.[89,90] A unique group at risk are premature infants being fed by total parenteral nutrition

(TPN). These infants miss the greatest opportunity for in utero accretion of calcium and phosphorus during the third trimester of pregnancy. It is difficult to solubilize adequate calcium and phosphorus in TPN, but the development of pediatric amino acid solutions has allowed an increased capability.[91] Table 35.11 lists types of osteomalacia, causes, and general treatment guidelines.

CLINICAL PRESENTATION AND DIAGNOSIS

Although there are varied and multiple pathogenic causes, patient manifestations are similar with all causes. Infants and young children may have marked stunting of growth, and they may be apathetic, irritable, and hypotonic. Often, they have an enlarged abdomen, called rachitic potbelly. They may have impaired dentition, resulting in extensive caries. Joint enlargement at the ankles, knees, and elbows may be present. Kyphosis and bowing of long bones is evident. The child may present with fractures.

Adult osteomalacia manifests similarly; the most common complaint is diffuse bone pain. Pressing on long bones elicits pain. Depending on the length of time the disease has been present, adults may also present with bone deformities.

In children, radiographic observation reveals abnormalities of the epiphyseal plate because bone growth is abnormal. In both children and adults, cortical and trabecular mineralized bone are covered by a large osteoid seam, an area of unmineralized bone. Looser's lines, also known as pseudofractures, are a prominent finding, especially on bone scan. These may result in clinical fractures after minimal trauma.

On serum chemistry analysis, PTH and alkaline phosphatase are elevated. Serum calcium, phosphorus, and 25-OH-D usually are depressed. Urinary calcium typically is low unless the patient has phosphorus deficiency. These findings can differentiate osteoporosis and osteomalacia because these values are within normal limits in osteoporosis.

Another diagnostic test used in adults is an assessment of tetracycline uptake in bone. Typically, tetracycline is administered for 2 to 3 days; 10 to 11 days later, another 2- or 3-day course of tetracycline is given. Bone biopsy of the iliac crest is performed 3 to 5 days after the second course. This site is used because it contains both cortical and trabecular bone. The distance between the two tetracycline bands is observed and measured via fluorescent microscopy. It can be used as an assessment of the rate of bone

Table 35.11 ▪ Osteomalacia Causes and Treatments

Type	Cause	Treatment
VDDR	Inadequate sunlight Inadequate dietary intake Unsupplemented breastfeeding	Ultraviolet lamp or increased sun exposure Vitamin D
Inadequate calcium absorption	Chelators in diet: phytates, oxalates, excess phosphate	Dietary changes Calcium supplements
Inadequate calcium intake	Lack of dietary calcium	Dietary changes Calcium supplements
Phosphorus deficiency	Aluminum ingestion Prematurity with prolonged feeding of low-phosphorus formula or TPN	Avoidance of aluminum antacids, contaminated sources Increased phosphorus intake
Gastric rickets	Gastrectomy Achlorhydria	Calcium citrate or other highly soluble calcium salt
Biliary rickets	Abnormal fat metabolism	Injectable vitamin D
Enteric rickets	Injury to small bowel by diseases such as Crohn's, coeliac sprue, short bowel syndrome	Injectable vitamin D
Hypophosphatemic rickets (Albright's syndrome)	Genetic or acquired fault of phosphorus reabsorption in proximal tubule	Phosphate, 1,25-$(OH)_2$-D
Type I VDDR	Genetic or acquired deficiency of 25-hydroxyvitamin D-1-hydroxylase	1,25-$(OH)_2$-D
Type II VDDR	Intracellular 1,25-$(OH)_2$-D receptor defect	1,25-$(OH)_2$-D and calcium
Renal tubular acidosis	Varied, results in calcium wasting	Alkalinization with sodium bicarbonate
Oncogenic or tumor-induced osteomalacia	Bone and soft tissue neoplasia	Tumor resection Bisphosphonates, vitamin D, phosphorus
Anticonvulsant-induced osteomalacia (phenytoin, phenobarbital)	Stimulation of cytochrome P-450 enzyme pathway resulting in accelerated metabolism and deficient 25-OH-D	1,25-$(OH)_2$-D
TPN-induced rickets in premature infants	Inadequate calcium and phosphorus in TPN solution	Increase calcium and phosphorus to maximum solubility

1,25-$(OH)_2$-D, 1,25-hydroxyvitamin D; *TPN,* total parenteral nutrition; *VDDR,* vitamin D–deficient rickets.

mineralization and can also differentiate osteoporosis from osteomalacia.[92]

TREATMENT

The treatment of osteomalacia depends on the underlying disorder identified, as seen in Table 35.11. If the cause is vitamin D deficiency, large dosages may be needed for 4 to 6 weeks but can be reduced as healing ensues. Therapy with vitamin D can be monitored with serum alkaline phosphatase, which decreases as body stores of vitamin D are repleted and therapeutic action occurs. Table 35.10 lists the vitamin D preparations and typical dosages available. The success of treatment depends on the underlying disorder.

CONCLUSION

The best prognosis for osteomalacia is obtained by preventive measures. Early identification and treatment can prevent bone deformities; therefore, patients at risk, such as premature infants on TPN, patients on phenytoin therapy, patients who have undergone gastrectomy, and others listed in Table 35.11 should be monitored closely. After acute disease resolves, dietary therapy may be adequate to prevent relapse, depending on the underlying cause.

KEY POINTS

- Osteoporosis is a disease characterized by loss of bone mass and is clinically silent until a fracture occurs.
- As the population ages, there will be a significant increase in the number of people at risk for osteoporotic fractures.
- Preventive measures, such as exercise and risk avoidance, are key to maximizing bone mass and reducing risk of fractures.
- Adequate calcium, through diet or supplementation, should be recommended for all patients.
- Screening for patients at risk, through risk assessment and bone mineral density measurements, can lead to early intervention and decreased risk of fractures.
- Patients on medications that may cause bone loss, such as glucocorticoids, should institute preventive measures and be monitored closely for the development of osteoporosis.
- Estrogen therapy, with or without progestin supplementation, prevents postmenopausal bone loss and may provide cardiovascular benefits, but risk of cancer may increase in some patients.
- Alendronate, a bisphosphonate, decreases the risk of fractures in women with established osteoporosis and prevents bone loss in nonosteoporotic postmenopausal women.
- Raloxifene, a selective estrogen receptor modulator, maintains the bone and possibly the cardiovascular benefits of estrogen while minimizing its adverse effects on uterine and breast tissue.
- In addition to decreasing bone resorption, calcitonin provides significant analgesic benefit for patients who have back pain caused by vertebral compression fractures.
- Osteomalacia and rickets, two disorders of bone mineralization, often are caused by diet, drug, or disease-induced deficiencies in vitamin D, calcium, or phosphorus.

REFERENCES

1. Consensus Development Conference. Prophylaxis and treatment of osteoporosis. Am J Med 90:107–110, 1991.
2. Kanis JA, Melton J III, Christiansen C, et al. The diagnosis of osteoporosis. J Bone Miner Res 9:1137–1141, 1994.
3. Riggs BL, Melton LJ III. Involutional osteoporosis. N Engl J Med 314:1676–1686, 1986.
4. Looker AC, Orwoll ES, Johnston CC Jr, et al. Prevalence of low femoral bone density in older U.S. adults from NHANES III. J Bone Miner Res 12:1761–1768, 1997.
5. Rosen CJ, Kessenich CR. The pathophysiology and treatment of postmenopausal osteoporosis: an evidence-based approach to estrogen replacement therapy. Endocrinol Metab Clin North Am 26:295–311, 1997.
6. Resnick NM, Greenspan SL. "Senile" osteoporosis reconsidered. JAMA 261:1025–1029, 1989.
7. Adinoff AD, Hollister JR. Steroid-induced fractures and bone loss in patients with asthma. N Engl J Med 309:265–268, 1983.
8. American College of Rheumatology Task Force on Osteoporosis Guidelines. Recommendations for the prevention and treatment of glucocorticoid-induced osteoporosis. Arthritis Rheum 39:1791–1801, 1996.
9. Ip M, Lam K, Yam L, et al. Decreased bone mineral density in premenopausal asthma patients receiving long-term inhaled steroids. Chest 105:1722–1727, 1994.
10. Griffith GC, Nichols G, Asher JD, et al. Heparin osteoporosis. JAMA 193:91–94, 1965.
11. Jaffe MD, Willis PW. Multiple fractures associated with long-term sodium heparin therapy. JAMA 193:152–154, 1965.
12. Nelson-Piercy C. Heparin-induced osteoporosis. Scand J Rheumatol 27:S68–S71, 1998.
13. Uemura T, Mohri J, Osada H, et al. Effect of gonadotropin-releasing hormone agonist on the bone mineral density of patients with endometriosis. Fertil Steril 62:246–250, 1994.
14. Goldray D, Weisman Y, Jaccard N, et al. Decreased bone density in elderly men treated with the gonadotropin-releasing hormone agonist decapeptyl (D-Trp_6-GnRH). J Clin Endocrinol Metab 76:288–290, 1993.
15. Comite F. GnRH analogs and safety. Obstet Gynecol Surv 44:319–325, 1989.
16. Mezrow G, Shoupe D, Spicer D, et al. Depot leuprolide acetate with estrogen and progestin add-back for long-term treatment of premenstrual syndrome. Fertil Steril 62:932–937, 1994.
17. Hornstein MD, Surrey ES, Weisberg GW, et al. Leuprolide acetate depot and hormonal add-back in endometriosis: a 12-month study. Obstet Gynecol 91:16–24, 1998.
18. Mukherjee T, Barad D, Turk R, et al. A randomized, placebo-controlled study on the effect of cyclic intermittent etidronate therapy on the bone mineral density changes associated with six months of gonadotropin-releasing hormone agonist treatment. Am J Obstet Gynecol 175:105–109, 1996.
19. Feskanich D, Willett WC, Stampfer MJ, et al. A prospective study of thiazide use and fractures in women. Osteoporos Int 7:79–84, 1997.
20. Kiel DP, Baron JA, Anderson JJ, et al. Smoking eliminates the protective effect of oral estrogens on the risk for hip fracture among women. Ann Intern Med 116:716–721, 1992.
21. Eisman JA, Sambrook PH, Kelly PJ, et al. Exercise and its interaction with genetic influences in the determination of bone mineral density. Am J Med 91(Suppl 5B):5S–9S, 1991.
22. Jackson JA, Kleerekoper M. Osteoporosis in men: diagnosis, pathophysiology, and prevention. Medicine 69:137–152, 1990.
23. Iannotti JP. Growth plate physiology and pathology. Orthoped Clin North Am 21:1–17, 1990.

24. Matkovic V. Calcium intake and peak bone mass. N Engl J Med 327:119–120, 1992.
25. Ettinger B. Role of calcium in preserving the skeletal health of aging women. South Med J 85(Suppl 2):22S–30S, 1992.
26. Kanis JA. The restoration of skeletal mass: a theoretic overview. Am J Med 91(Suppl 5B):29S–36S, 1991.
27. Manolagas SC, Jilka RL. Bone marrow, cytokines, and bone remodeling. Emerging insights into the pathophysiology of osteoporosis. N Engl J Med 332:305–311, 1995.
28. Silverberg SJ, Lindsay R. Postmenopausal osteoporosis. Med Clin North Am 71:41–57, 1987.
29. Grisso JA, Kelsey JL, Strom BL. Risk factors for hip fracture in black women. N Engl J Med 330:1555–1559, 1994.
30. Eyre DR. Bone biomarkers as tools in osteoporosis management. Spine 22:17S–24S, 1997.
31. Hodgson SF, Johnston CC. AACE clinical practice guidelines for the prevention and treatment of postmenopausal osteoporosis. Jacksonville, FL: American Association of Clinical Endocrinologists, 1996.
32. Hall FM, Davis MA, Baran DT. Bone mineral screening for osteoporosis. N Engl J Med 316:212–214, 1986.
33. Miller PD, Bonnick SL, Rosen LJ, et al. Clinical utility of bone mass measurements in adults: consensus of an international panel. Semin Arthritis Rheum 25:361–372, 1996.
34. NIH Consensus Development Panel on Optimal Calcium Intake. Optimal calcium intake. JAMA 272:1942–1947, 1994.
35. Dawson-Hughes B, Dallal GE, Krall EA, et al. A controlled trial of the effect of calcium supplementation on bone density in postmenopausal women. N Engl J Med 323:878–883, 1990.
36. Kiel DP, Felson DT, Anderson JJ, et al. Hip fracture and the use of estrogens in postmenopausal women. The Framingham study. N Engl J Med 317:1169–1174, 1987.
37. Ettinger B, Genant HK, Conn CE. Long-term estrogen replacement therapy prevents bone loss and fractures. Ann Intern Med 102:319–324, 1985.
38. Felson DT, Zhang Y, Hannan MT, et al. The effect of postmenopausal estrogen therapy on bone density in elderly women. N Engl J Med 329:1141–1146, 1993.
39. ACOG Committee Opinion. Estrogen replacement therapy in women with previously treated breast cancer. Washington, DC: American College of Obstetricians and Gynecologists (ACOG) Technical Bulletin no. 135, 1994.
40. Lindsay R, Hart DM, Clark DM. The minimum effective dose of estrogen for prevention of postmenopausal bone loss. Obstet Gynecol 63:759–763, 1984.
41. Genant HK, Lucas J, Weiss S, et al. Low-dose esterified estrogen therapy: effects on bone, plasma estradiol concentrations, endometrium, and lipid levels. Arch Intern Med 157:2609–2615, 1997.
42. Jewelewicz R. New developments in topical estrogen therapy. Fertil Steril 67:1–12, 1997.
43. Bush DE, Jones CE, Bass KM, et al. Estrogen replacement reverses endothelial dysfunction in postmenopausal women. Am J Med 104:552–558, 1998.
44. Stampfer MJ, Colditz GA. Estrogen replacement therapy and coronary heart disease: a quantitative assessment of the epidemiologic evidence. Prev Med 20:47–63, 1991.
45. Hulley S, Grady D, Bush T, et al. Randomized trial of estrogen plus progestin for secondary prevention of coronary heart disease in postmenopausal women. JAMA 280:605–613, 1998.
46. The Writing Group for the PEPI Trial. Effects of estrogens or estrogen/progestin regimens on heart disease risk factors in postmenopausal women: the Postmenopausal Estrogen/Progestin Interventions (PEPI) trial. JAMA 273:199–208, 1995.
47. Sotelo MM, Johnson SR. The effects of hormone replacement therapy on coronary heart disease. Endocrinol Metab Clin North Am 26:313–328, 1997.
48. Yaffe K, Sawaya G, Lieberburg I, et al. Estrogen therapy in postmenopausal women: effects on cognitive function and dementia. JAMA 279:688–695, 1998.
49. Grodstein FA, Martinez E, Platz EA, et al. Postmenopausal hormone use and risk for colorectal cancer and adenoma. Ann Intern Med 128:705–712, 1998.
50. PEPI Trial Writing Group. Effects of hormone replacement therapy on endometrial histology in postmenopausal women: the Postmenopausal Estrogen/Progestin Interventions (PEPI) trial. JAMA 275:370–375, 1996.
51. Gutthann SP, Rodriguez LAG, Castellsague J, et al. Hormone replacement therapy and risk of venous thromboembolism: population based case-control study. BMJ 314:796–800, 1997.
52. Boston Collaborative Drug Surveillance Program. Surgically confirmed gall bladder disease, venous thromboembolism, and breast tumors in relation to postmenopausal estrogen therapy. N Engl J Med 290:15–19, 1974.
53. Brinton LA. Hormone replacement therapy and risk for breast cancer. Endocrinol Metab Clin North Am 26:361–378, 1997.
54. Liberman UA, Weiss SR, Broll J, et al. Effect of oral alendronate on bone mineral density and the incidence of fractures in postmenopausal osteoporosis. N Engl J Med 333:1437–1443, 1995.
55. Black DM, Cummings SR, Karpf DB, et al. Randomised trial of effect of alendronate on risk of fracture in women with existing vertebral fractures. Lancet 348:1535–1541, 1996.
56. Hosking D, Chilvers CED, Christiansen C, et al. Prevention of bone loss with alendronate in postmenopausal women under 60 years of age. N Engl J Med 338:485–492, 1998.
57. McClung M, Clemmesen B, Daifotis A, et al. Alendronate prevents postmenopausal bone loss in women without osteoporosis: a double-blind, randomized, controlled trial. Ann Intern Med 128:253–261, 1998.
58. Saag KG, Emkey R, Schnitzer TJ, et al. Alendronate for the prevention and treatment of glucocorticoid-induced osteoporosis. N Engl J Med 339:292–299, 1998.
59. Lindsay R, Cosman F, Cary DJ, et al. Effect of alendronate added to ongoing hormone replacement therapy in the treatment of postmenopausal osteoporosis [abstract]. Osteoporos Int 8(Suppl 3):12, 1998.
60. Storm T, Thamsborg G, Steiniche T, et al. Effect of intermittent cyclical etidronate therapy on bone mass and fracture rate in postmenopausal women with osteoporosis. N Engl J Med 322:1265–1271, 1990.
61. Miller PD, Watts NB, Licata AA, et al. Cyclical etidronate in the treatment of postmenopausal osteoporosis: efficacy and safety after seven years of treatment. Am J Med 103:468–476, 1997.
62. Wimalawansa SJ. A four-year randomized controlled trial of hormone replacement and bisphosphonate, alone or in combination, in women with postmenopausal osteoporosis. Am J Med 104:219–226, 1998.
63. Balfour JA, Goa KL. Raloxifene. Drugs Aging 12:335–341, 1998.
64. Walsh BW, Kuller LH, Wild RA, et al. Effects of raloxifene on serum lipids and coagulation factors in healthy postmenopausal women. JAMA 279:1445–1451, 1998.
65. Delmas PD, Bjarnason NH, Mitlak BH, et al. Effects of raloxifene on bone mineral density, serum cholesterol concentrations, and uterine endometrium in postmenopausal women. N Engl J Med 337:1641–1647, 1997.
66. Jordan VC. Antiestrogenic action of raloxifene and tamoxifen: today and tomorrow. J Natl Cancer Inst 90:967–971, 1998.
67. Overgaard K, Hansen MA, Jensen SB, et al. Effect of salcatonin given intranasally on bone mass and fracture rates in established osteoporosis: a dose–response study. BMJ 305:556–561, 1992.
68. Pun KK, Chan LWL. Analgesic effect of intranasal salmon calcitonin in the treatment of osteoporotic vertebral fractures. Clin Ther 11:205–209, 1989.
69. Gennari C, Camporeale A. Calcitonin in the treatment of osteoporosis. Osteoporos Int 7(Suppl 3)S159–S162, 1997.
70. Overgaard K, Hansen MA, Nielsen V, et al. Discontinuous calcitonin treatment of established osteoporosis: effects of withdrawal of treatment. Am J Med 89:1–6, 1990.
71. Chapuy MC, Arlot ME, Duboef F, et al. Vitamin D_3 and calcium to prevent hip fractures in elderly women. N Engl J Med 327:1637–1642, 1992.
72. Dawson-Hughes B, Harris SS, Krall EA, et al. Effect of calcium and vitamin D supplementation on bone density in men and women 65 years of age or older. N Engl J Med 337:670–676, 1997.
73. Tilyard MW, Spears GF, Thomson J, et al. Treatment of postmenopausal osteoporosis with calcitriol or calcium. N Engl J Med 326:357–362, 1992.
74. Gallagher JC. Vitamin D metabolism and therapy in elderly subjects. South Med J 85(Suppl 2):S43–S47, 1992.
75. Knight DC, Eden JA. A review of the clinical effects of phytoestrogens. Obstet Gynecol 87:897–904, 1996.
76. Albertazzi P, Pansini F, Bonaccorsi G, et al. The effects of dietary soy supplementation on hot flashes. Obstet Gynecol 91:6–11, 1998.
77. Riggs BL, Hodgson SF, O'Fallon WM, et al. Effect of fluoride treatment on the fracture rate in postmenopausal women with osteoporosis. N Engl J Med 322:802–809, 1990.
78. Kleerekoper M. The role of fluoride in the prevention of osteoporosis. Endocrinol Metab Clin North Am 27:441–442, 1998.
79. Pak CY, Sakhaee K, Adams-Huet B, et al. Treatment of postmenopausal osteoporosis with slow-release sodium fluoride: final report of a randomized controlled trial. Ann Intern Med 123:401–408, 1995.
80. Meunier PJ, Sebert JL, Reginster JY, et al. Fluoride salts are no better at preventing new vertebral fractures than calcium–vitamin D in postmenopausal osteoporosis: the FAVO Study. Osteoporos Int 8:4–12, 1998.
81. Reginster JY, Meurmans L, Zegels B, et al. The effect of sodium monofluorophosphate plus calcium on vertebral fracture rate in postmenopausal women with moderate osteoporosis: a randomized, controlled trial. Ann Intern Med 129:1–8, 1998.
82. Duell B, Chesnut CH. Exacerbation of rheumatoid arthritis by sodium fluoride treatment of osteoporosis. Arch Intern Med 151:783–784, 1991.

83. Cosman F, Lindsay R. Is parathyroid hormone a therapeutic option for osteoporosis?: a review of the clinical evidence. Calcif Tissue Int 62:476–480, 1998.
84. Finkelstein JS, Klibanski A, Arnold AL, et al. Prevention of estrogen deficiency-related bone loss with human parathyroid hormone-(1-34): a randomized controlled trial. JAMA 280:1067–1073, 1998.
85. Lindsay R, Nieves J, Formica C, et al. Randomised controlled study of effect of parathyroid hormone on vertebral-bone mass and fracture incidence among postmenopausal women on oestrogen with osteoporosis. Lancet 350:550–555, 1997.
86. Reginster JY, Taquet AN, Gosset C. Therapy for osteoporosis: miscellaneous and experimental agents. Endocrinol Metab Clin North Am 27:453–463, 1998.
87. Ailinger RL, Emerson J. Women's knowledge of osteoporosis. Appl Nurs Res 11:111–114, 1998.
88. Mattsson LA, Milsom I, Stadberg E. What do women want? Br J Obstet Gynecol 103(Suppl 13):104–107, 1996.
89. Mankin HJ. Rickets, osteomalacia, and renal osteodystrophy. An update. Orthoped Clin North Am 21:81–96, 1990.
90. Econs MJ, Drezner MK. Tumor-induced osteomalacia: unveiling a new hormone. N Engl J Med 330:1679–1681, 1994.
91. Koo WW, Tsang RC. Calcium, magnesium, phosphorus, and vitamin D. In: Tsang RC, Lucas A, Uauy R, et al., eds. Nutritional needs of the preterm infant. Baltimore: Williams & Wilkins, 1993:135–155.
92. Recker RR. Bone biopsy and histomorphometry in clinical practice. In: Favus MJ, ed. Primer on the metabolic bone diseases and disorders of mineral metabolism. 3rd ed. Philadelphia: Lippincott-Raven, 1996:164–167.

CHAPTER 36

ASTHMA

Kathryn Blake

DEFINITION

The National Asthma Education and Prevention Program (NAEPP) of the Heart, Lung, and Blood Institute updated the *Guidelines for the Diagnosis and Management of Asthma* in 1997.[1] These guidelines can be downloaded from the Internet at http://www.nhlbi.nih.gov/nhlbi/lung/asthma/prof/asthgdln.pdf. According to these guidelines, the current definition of asthma is "a chronic inflammatory disorder of the airways in which many cells and cellular elements play a role, in particular, mast cells, eosinophils, T lymphocytes, macrophages, neutrophils, and epithelial cells." This definition emphasizes that asthma is an inflammatory disease of the airways and not simply a disease of smooth muscle bronchoconstriction, as was once thought.

There is also increasing evidence that a fixed or irreversible component may be present with advanced disease. Based on these features, asthma research focuses on its immunologic aspects. Treatment recommendations have also changed and now emphasize earlier institution of anti-inflammatory therapy to reflect the inflammatory processes present in the disease.

TREATMENT GOALS: ASTHMA

- Prevent chronic and troublesome symptoms (e.g., coughing or breathlessness at night, in the early morning, or after exertion).[1]
- Maintain near-normal pulmonary function.[1]
- Maintain normal activity levels (including exercise and other physical activity).[1]
- Prevent recurrent exacerbation of asthma and minimize the need for emergency department (ED) visits or hospitalizations.[1]
- Provide optimal pharmacotherapy with the fewest adverse effects.[1]
- Meet patients' and families' expectations for asthma care.[1]
- Develop simple drug regimens (to facilitate adherence with therapy) at a reasonable cost according the patient's insurance or payment method.

EPIDEMIOLOGY

An estimated 13.7 million people (5.4% of the population) in the United States had self-reported asthma as of 1994. This is an increase from 6.8 million in 1980. Thirty percent of asthmatic patients are under 14 years and another 30% are between 14 and 34 years of age. Children under age 14 account for 35% of hospital admissions, with girls having 20% more admissions than boys. African Americans accounted for 25% of all hospitalizations for asthma in 1994 and are 2.5 times more likely to die from asthma than Caucasians. There were 5400 deaths from asthma in 1994, an increase from 2745 deaths in 1980.[2] The risk factors for death from asthma are shown in Table 36.1.[1]

PATHOPHYSIOLOGY

Asthma is a complex disease. Airway obstruction is responsible for its clinical manifestations, but underlying airway inflammation and bronchial hyperresponsiveness also are characteristic features.

Histologic and Morphologic Changes

Histologic and morphologic changes occur in the airways and lungs of patients with asthma (Fig. 36.1).[3] Airway inflammation and epithelial damage have been observed in all degrees of asthma, including newly diagnosed cases.[4] These changes lead to airflow obstruction and are characterized by acute bronchoconstriction, which may be induced by allergens, aspirin or nonsteroidal anti-inflammatory drugs (NSAIDs), exercise, cold air, irritants, and perhaps stress; airway edema caused by increased microvascular permeability and leakage, resulting in a stiffer and more narrow airway; chronic mucus plug formation, which is always present in severe asthma; and airway remodeling, which results from subepithelial fibrosis or collagen deposition in the basement membrane, which may or may not be a reversible process.[1]

Table 36.1 ▪ Risk Factors for Death from Asthma

History of sudden, severe exacerbations
Prior intubation for asthma
Prior admission for asthma to an intensive care unit
Two or more hospitalizations for asthma in the past year
Three or more emergency care visits for asthma in the past year
Hospitalization or an emergency care visit for asthma within the past month
Use of >2 canisters per month of inhaled short-acting β_2-agonist
Current use of systemic corticosteroids or recent withdrawal from systemic corticosteroids
Difficulty perceiving airflow obstruction or its severity
Comorbidity, as from cardiovascular disease or chronic obstructive pulmonary disease
Serious psychiatric disease or psychosocial problems
Low socioeconomic status and urban residence
Illicit drug use
Sensitivity to *Alternaria*

Source: Reference 1.

Bronchial Hyperresponsiveness

Bronchial hyperresponsiveness is an exaggerated bronchoconstrictive response to stimuli such as cold air, exercise, allergens, viral infection, and certain chemicals. The degree of hyperresponsiveness can be measured by inhalation challenge testing with histamine or methacholine and is thought to correlate with disease severity and medication needs. Bronchial hyperresponsiveness is caused by an interaction between an asthmatic patient's baseline bronchial responsiveness and airway changes caused by inflammation[5] and appears to be one manifestation of airway inflammation in asthma.[6] There is evidence that a greater number of inflammatory cells in the airways corresponds to a greater degree of airway hyperresponsiveness; however, the mechanisms by which inflammatory cells and their mediators promote airway hyperresponsiveness are not clear.[6]

Airway Inflammation

Airway inflammation is a complex interaction of various cells and mediators that results in bronchial hyperresponsiveness and airway obstruction as well as ongoing inflammation (Fig. 36.2).[7] Our understanding of these

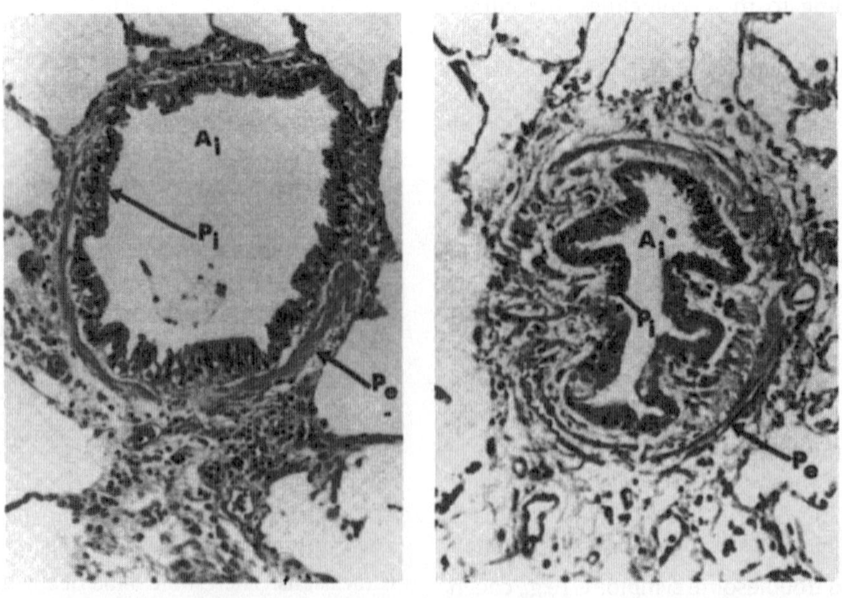

(a) (b)

Figure 36.1. Diagram of the changes present in a fully contracted small airway *(right)* compared with a fully relaxed small airway *(left)*. (Reprinted from Hogg JC. Post-mortem pathology in asthma. In: Kay AB. Allergy and allergic diseases. Oxford, UK: Blackwell, 1997:1360–1365, with permission.)

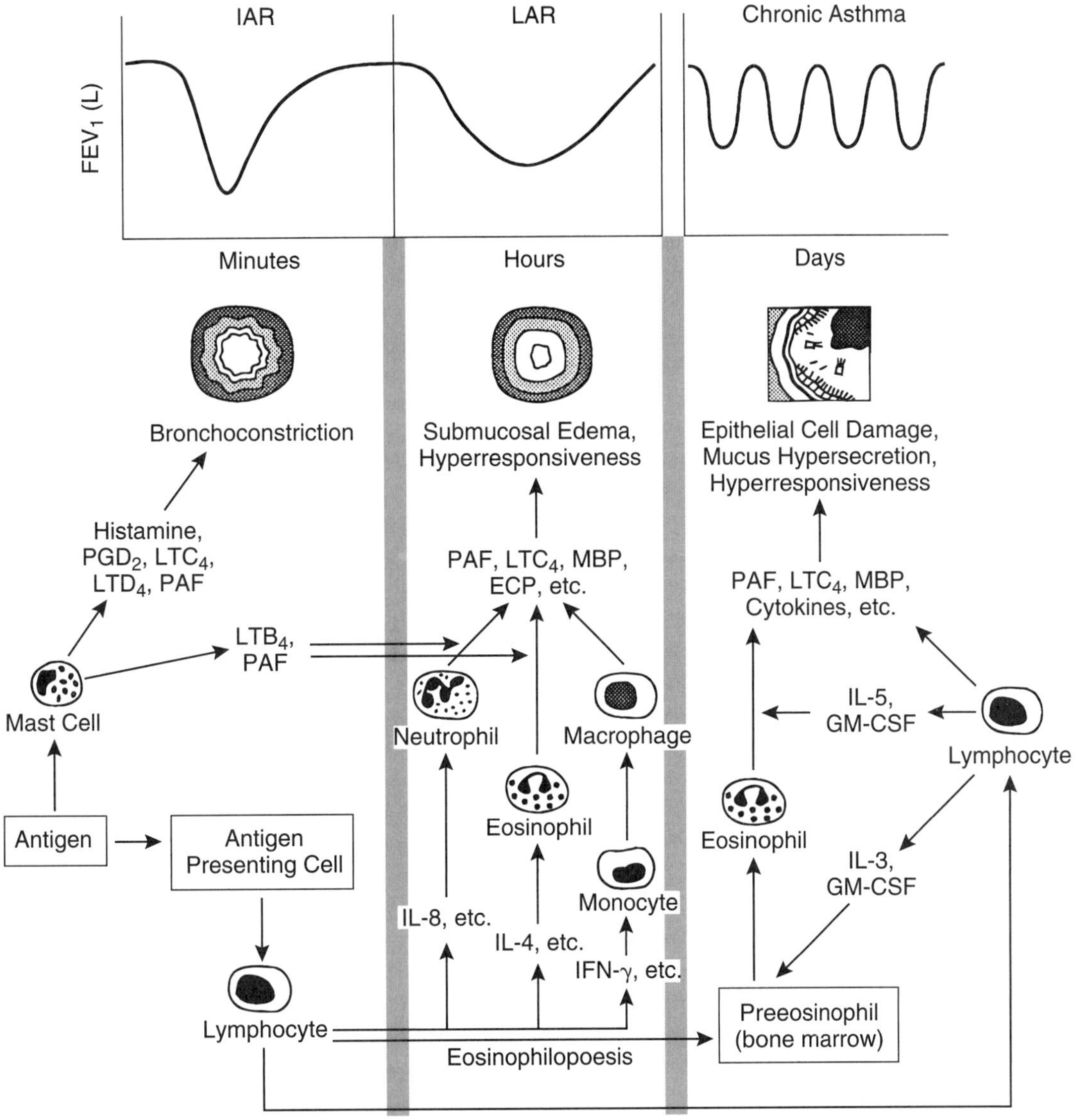

Figure 36.2. Greatly simplified diagram illustrating the relationships between immediate asthmatic response *(IAR)*, late asthmatic response *(LAR)*, and chronic asthma, and inflammatory cells, cytokines, and mediators. *ECP*, eosinophil cationic protein; *FEV_1*, forced expiratory volume in 1 sec; *GM-CSF*, granulocyte–macrophage colony-stimulating factor; *IFN-γ*, interferon-γ; *IL*, interleukin; *LTB_4*, leukotriene B_4; *LTC_4*, leukotriene C_4; *LTD_4*, leukotriene D_4; *MBP*, major basic protein; *PAF*, platelet-activating factor; *PGD_2*, prostaglandin D_2. (Reprinted from Kay AB. Asthma and inflammation. J Allergy Clin Immunol 87:893–910, 1991, with permission.)

interactions, though vastly increased in recent years, is still not complete.

Inflammatory Cells

A variety of cells are important in the inflammatory response because they produce and liberate mediators, which in turn recruit other cells or have direct toxic effects, perpetuating this vicious cycle.

Mast cells, known as acute response cells,[8] are important in initiating inflammatory responses after exposure to allergens and the resulting immediate bronchoconstriction. After the allergen binds to immunoglobulin E (IgE)-bound high-affinity receptors on the surfaces of mast cells, various immediate-acting mediators such as histamine, leukotrienes, prostaglandins, and platelet-activating factor (PAF) are released that cause immediate bronchoconstriction.[9,10] In addition, several longer-acting mediators are released such as eosinophil and neutrophil chemotactic factors, tumor necrosis factor-α (TNF-α), and cytokines such as interleukin-4 (IL-4), IL-8, and IL-13, which promote an airway inflammatory response.[8,9] However, it appears that other cells such as macrophages, eosinophils, and T lymphocytes are more important than mast cells in maintaining the chronic airway inflammatory processes.[8] Further evidence of the importance of the mast cell is the finding of greater numbers of degranulated mast cells in the airways of asthmatic patients who died from fatal attacks.[11]

The importance of eosinophils in the pathogenesis of asthma has been known for many years, primarily because of the association between asthma and peripheral blood eosinophilia. Eosinophils are present in the peripheral blood, bronchial mucosa, and bronchoalveolar lavage fluid of patients with asthma, and the number of cells has been correlated with the degree of bronchial hyperresponsiveness.[8] Eosinophils are a source of lipid-derived mediators (leukotrienes), and eosinophil granules contain major basic protein (MBP), eosinophil cationic protein (ECP), eosinophil-derived neurotoxin, and eosinophil peroxidase. Cytokines also are generated by eosinophils and appear to regulate the function of eosinophils rather than having broader inflammatory effects. MBP and ECP are detectable in the sputum of asthmatic patients and may be responsible for much of the damage to airway epithelium, which may in turn contribute to bronchial hyperresponsiveness.[4,7] The importance of adhesion molecules in drawing eosinophils to the site of inflammation is discussed later in this chapter.

Alveolar macrophages, normally present in the lumen of large and small airways, produce and release a number of mediators thought to be involved in the initiation and amplification of the inflammatory process. These include leukotrienes, PAF, and eosinophil and neutrophil chemotactic factors. Additionally, macrophages may be activated by IgE-dependent mechanisms. Macrophages may act as antigen-presenting cells by preparing antigen for presentation to T lymphocytes.[8,12] Interestingly, macrophages may also have some anti-inflammatory effects, depending on the stimulus for activation, but the mechanisms have not been defined.[8]

Neutrophils are a source of proteases and oxygen radicals, which can cause tissue damage, and lipid mediators, such as leukotriene B_4 (LTB_4) and PAF, which act as chemoattractants for recruiting additional neutrophils into the area of inflammation.[13] Because neutrophils can be produced rapidly in large amounts by the bone marrow and have a very short half-life, it is thought that these cells have a greater role in acute asthma episodes than in chronic asthma symptoms.[8,14] In support of this concept, high numbers of neutrophils have been found in the airways of patients who died from sudden-onset asthma, suggesting a role for this cell type in sudden-onset fatal asthma.[15]

T lymphocytes play an important role in the pathogenesis of asthma by coordinating the inflammatory response. Whereas B lymphocytes are involved in IgE production, T lymphocytes produce cytokines, which promote inflammation. The T lymphocytes include the subsets Th0, Th1, and Th2; each subset secretes specific cytokines, although the distinction between Th1 and Th2 cells is less clear than was once thought. Because Th0 cells secrete cytokines also secreted by Th1 and Th2 cells, it is thought that the Th0 subset may actually be a precursor for the Th1 and Th2 subsets.[8] Cytokines produced by T lymphocytes include IL-2, IL-3, IL-4, IL-5, IL-6, IL-10, granulocyte–macrophage colony-stimulating factor (GM-CSF), interferon-γ (IFN-γ), and TNF-β. Several of these cytokines are important in the recruitment and survival of eosinophils and the maintenance of mast cells in the airways.

Mediators

The cells involved in inflammatory processes present in asthma produce and release numerous mediators responsible for many of the pathophysiologic changes. It has been proposed that for a substance to be defined as a mediator, three criteria must be fulfilled:

- It must be capable of producing the pathologic changes observed in asthma or physiologic changes that define asthma.
- It must be produced in the lung during an asthmatic episode and measurable in body fluids.
- Removal by specific inhibition or antagonism results in amelioration or attenuation of the asthmatic response.[16]

A number of substances have been implicated as mediators of asthma. These may be preformed or may be rapidly produced by cells after activation or stimulation. Those thought to be important in the pathogenesis of asthma include histamine and the many products of arachidonic acid metabolism such as leukotrienes, prostaglandins, thromboxanes, and PAF. Actions of mediators that are pertinent to the pathophysiology of asthma include epithelial damage, smooth muscle contraction, mucosal edema and inflammation, and mucus secretion (Table 36.2).[10] Specific antagonists of mediators and inhibitors of enzymes involved in their production have shed light on the importance of the various mediators in the pathophysiology of asthma, and the leukotriene modifiers represent the first class of antimediator drugs to be used in treating asthma.

Table 36.2 ▪ Mediators, Their Sources, and Their Actions Relevant to Asthma

Mediator	Source	Action
Major basic protein	Eosinophils	Epithelial damage
Histamine	Mast cells	Smooth muscle constriction, mucosal edema, mucus secretion
Leukotrienes (LTB_4, LTC_4, LTD_4, LTE_4)	Mast cells, basophils, eosinophils, neutrophils, macrophages, monocytes	Smooth muscle constriction, mucosal edema and inflammation
Prostaglandins (PGD_2, PGE_2, $PGF_2\alpha$, PGI_2)	Mast cells, endothelial cells	Smooth muscle constriction, mucosal edema, mucus secretion
Thromboxanes (TXA_2)	Macrophages, monocytes, platelets	Smooth muscle constriction, mucus secretion
Platelet-activating factor	Mast cells, basophils, eosinophils, neutrophils, macrophages, monocytes, platelets, endothelial cells	Smooth muscle constriction, mucosal edema and inflammation, mucus secretion, bronchial hyperresponsiveness

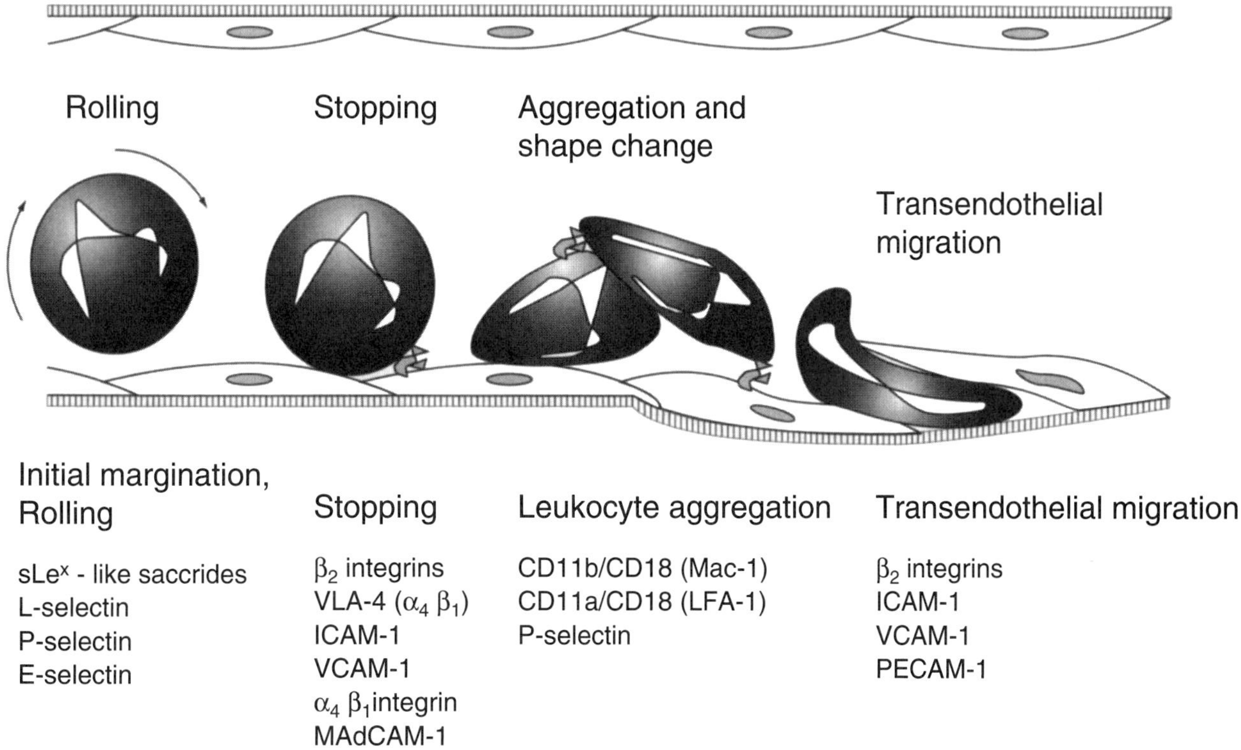

Figure 36.3. Leukocyte emigration during inflammation. The sequence of intravascular events for leukocyte emigration is depicted with the relevant adhesion molecules for each step. *ICAM-1,* intracellular adhesion molecule 1; *LFA-1,* leukocyte function-associated antigen 1; *Mac-1,* membrane attack complex 1; *MAdCAM-1,* mucosal adressin cell adhesion molecule 1; *PECAM-1,* platelet endothelial cell adhesion molecule 1; *sLe^x^,* sialyl Lewis X; *VCAM-1,* vascular cell adhesion molecule 1; *VLA-4,* very late antigen 4. (Modified from Smith C. Cellular adhesion and interactions. In: Rich RR, Fleisher TA, Schwartz BD, et al. Clinical immunology principles and practice. St Louis: Mosby, 1996:176–191, with permission.)

Adhesion Molecules

Adhesion of inflammatory cells to surfaces of the vasculature is an important early step in the inflammatory response because it allows relevant cells to infiltrate and migrate to sites of inflammation. To facilitate this process, glycoproteins or adhesion molecules are expressed by cell membranes of basophils, granulocytes, lymphocytes, neutrophils, monocytes, platelets, and endothelial and epithelial cells after their activation by mediators or other cells and permit cell-to-cell and cell-to-substratum attachment. Adhesion molecules have other functions, such as promoting cell activation, cell–cell communication, and cell migration and infiltration. Complex interactions whereby mediators affect the expression of adhesion molecules, which in turn result in production of mediators, also exist.[17,18] More than 35 adhesion molecules have been identified.

Adhesion molecules are divided into families based on their chemical structures, and those thought to be of particular importance in inflammation include the integrins, immunoglobulin supergene family, selectins, and carbohydrate ligands. A major role of adhesion molecules in inflammation is the recruitment of leukocytes from the vascular lumen to tissue sites. To facilitate this process, transient and reversible binding of the adhesion molecules to specific ligands on endothelial cells occurs, resulting in slowing or rolling of the circulating leukocyte along the surfaces of the vasculature (Fig. 36.3).[19] In response to the initial adhesion event or mediators, activation of the leukocyte or endothelial cell follows. Finally, firm adhesion occurs, anchoring the leukocyte to the endothelial cell surface and allowing diapedesis between endothelial cells and migration into the extracellular matrix and site of inflammation.[17,18]

Characterizing the precise role of adhesion molecules is an area of active study. Adhesion molecule knockout mice (mice specifically bred to lack the genes encoding for adhesion molecule production) have been developed to study the role of adhesion molecules in the inflammatory response. Peptide antagonists and monoclonal antibodies to the functional epitopes of adhesion molecules are entering clinical trials and will facilitate a better understanding of the cells and their interactions and ultimately the roles of adhesion molecules in the pathophysiology of asthma and other inflammatory diseases. These immunomodulators may become a novel therapeutic approach or a complement to existing anti-inflammatory asthma therapy.

Transcription Factors

Production of inflammatory proteins such as cytokines, adhesion molecules, and enzymes can be augmented by an

Table 36.3 ▪ Classification of Asthma Severity

	Clinical Features Before Treatment[a]		
	Symptoms[b]	Nighttime Symptoms	Lung Function
Step 4: severe persistent	Continual symptoms Limited physical activity Frequent exacerbations	Frequent	FEV_1 or PEF ≤60% predicted PEF variability >30%
Step 3: moderate persistent	Daily symptoms Daily use of inhaled short-acting β_2-agonist Exacerbations affect activity Exacerbations ≥2 times/wk; may last days	>1 time/wk	FEV_1 or PEF 60–80% predicted PEF variability >30%
Step 2: mild persistent	Symptoms >2 times/wk but <1 time/day Exacerbations may affect activity	>2 times/mo	FEV_1 or PEF ≥80% predicted PEF variability 20–30%
Step 1: mild intermittent	Symptoms ≤2 times/wk Asymptomatic and normal PEF between exacerbations Exacerbations brief (from a few hours to a few days); intensity may vary	≤2 times/mo	FEV_1 or PEF ≥80% predicted PEF variability <20%

FEV_1, forced expiratory volume at 1 sec; *PEF*, peak expiratory flow.

[a]The presence of one of the features of severity is sufficient to place a patient in a category. A patient should be assigned to the most severe grade in which any feature occurs. The characteristics noted in this table are general and may overlap because asthma is highly variable. Furthermore, a patient's classification may change over time.

[b]Patients at any level of severity can have mild, moderate, or severe exacerbations. Some patients with intermittent asthma experience severe and life-threatening exacerbations separated by long periods of normal lung function and no symptoms.

increase in the transcription of selected target genes. Nuclear factor-κB (NF-κB) is one transcription factor that can be activated by cytokines and oxidants already present to further increase production of inflammatory cytokines, chemokines, and adhesion molecules. Corticosteroids are potent inhibitors of the activity of NF-κB, thus supporting the role of NF-κB in airway inflammation.[20]

Nitric Oxide

Nitric oxide is produced constitutively by endothelial and neuronal nitric oxide synthase, which regulates vascular tone, platelet activation, and neurotransmission. Production of nitric oxide from inducible nitric oxide synthase is induced by certain cytokines and lipopolysaccharides from many cells, including endothelial cells, when exposed to inflammatory processes. The amount of nitric oxide induced during inflammation is much greater than that produced constitutively and appears to have protective effects such as relaxation of the bronchi.[21] Pulmonary nitric oxide levels increase in asthma, and there is interest in monitoring exhaled nitric oxide levels in response to disease changes and treatment effects.[21]

Neural Mechanisms

Neural regulation of the airways is complex and involves the parasympathetic, sympathetic, and sensory systems. These systems affect airway functioning by regulating epithelial, vascular, glandular, and smooth muscle activity through release of neurotransmitters and neuropeptides. These effects are classified as cholinergic (bronchoconstrictor), adrenergic (bronchodilator), inhibitory nonadrenergic noncholinergic bronchodilator, and excitatory nonadrenergic noncholinergic bronchoconstrictor effects and result from the specific combinations of neurotransmitters and neuropeptides within the sensory, parasympathetic, and sympathetic systems. No longer is the nonadrenergic noncholinergic system considered to be a separate system of nerves. Because of the complex interrelationships of nerve type and peptides and transmitters, one cannot impute the functions of nerve populations to specific neurotransmitters.

The parasympathetic nerves contain acetylcholine and vasoactive intestinal peptide, which causes bronchoconstriction and glandular exudation. Asthmatic patients show an increased responsiveness to cholinergic stimuli. Changes in the muscarinic receptor or increases in cholinergic sensitivity might increase parasympathetic tone and cause reflex bronchoconstriction in asthmatic patients, but these mechanisms appear only partially responsible for the bronchospasm that follows inhalation of relevant agents.

The sympathetic system has little direct innervation into the airway smooth muscle, and effects are mediated through circulating catecholamines principally by acting on the β_2-receptor. Epinephrine has bronchodilator effects in asthma, but its activity on the β_2-receptor may be diminished by coexisting airway inflammation.

The sensory nervous system present in the human airway contains neuropeptides, such as substance P and neurokinin A (collectively called tachykinins), which are bronchoconstrictive to asthmatic patients and, perhaps more importantly, cause increased vascular permeability, mucus secretion, and leukocyte infiltration.[22] Neutral endopeptidase (NEP), the enzyme that degrades neuropeptides, has been shown to be present in all cells that have neuropeptide receptors, and induction or suppression of NEP affects the activity of neuropeptides, such as tachykinins. Tachykinins are potent inducers of airway inflammation, so NEP can have an important role in regulating airway inflammation. NEP activity is reduced by external factors such as cigarette smoke, viral infections, and pollution, and the presence of these aggravators augments tachykinin-induced airway inflammation. Research is ongoing to evaluate ways of regulating NEP activity.[23,24]

CLINICAL PRESENTATION AND DIAGNOSIS

Signs and Symptoms

Symptoms of asthma include shortness of breath or dyspnea, wheezing, cough, and sputum production. Chest tightness is a common complaint among asthmatic patients. Objective signs of the disease are reduced airflow, increased airway resistance and reduced conductance, hyperinflation of the lungs, and bronchial hyperresponsiveness. In acutely obstructed patients, tachypnea, tachycardia, retractions, cyanosis, and hypoxemia may also be present. The NAEPP guidelines base treatment recommendations on the classification of asthma as mild intermittent, mild persistent, moderate persistent, or severe persistent (Table 36.3).[1]

Airflow is measured easily, and although reduced airflow is a characteristic feature of asthma, other diseases may present with similar obstruction. Airflow typically is measured by spirometry or peak expiratory flow (PEF; Fig. 36.4*A* and *B*), and normal (predicted) values based on height, age, gender, and race are established. Forced expiratory volume in 1 second (FEV_1) is the most commonly used spirometric evaluation of pulmonary function and consists of the volume of air expelled within the first second of forced expiration after maximal inhalation. It is normally more than 70% of the total volume of expired air or the forced vital capacity (FVC), but in obstructive processes such as asthma, FEV_1 is decreases, as does FVC (though to a lesser extent); therefore, the FEV_1/FVC ratio decreases. PEF is the maximal rate at which air is exhaled from the lungs with a forced expiratory maneuver, and it correlates fairly well with FEV_1 (although for some patients it does not correlate well with symptoms). Peak flow meters

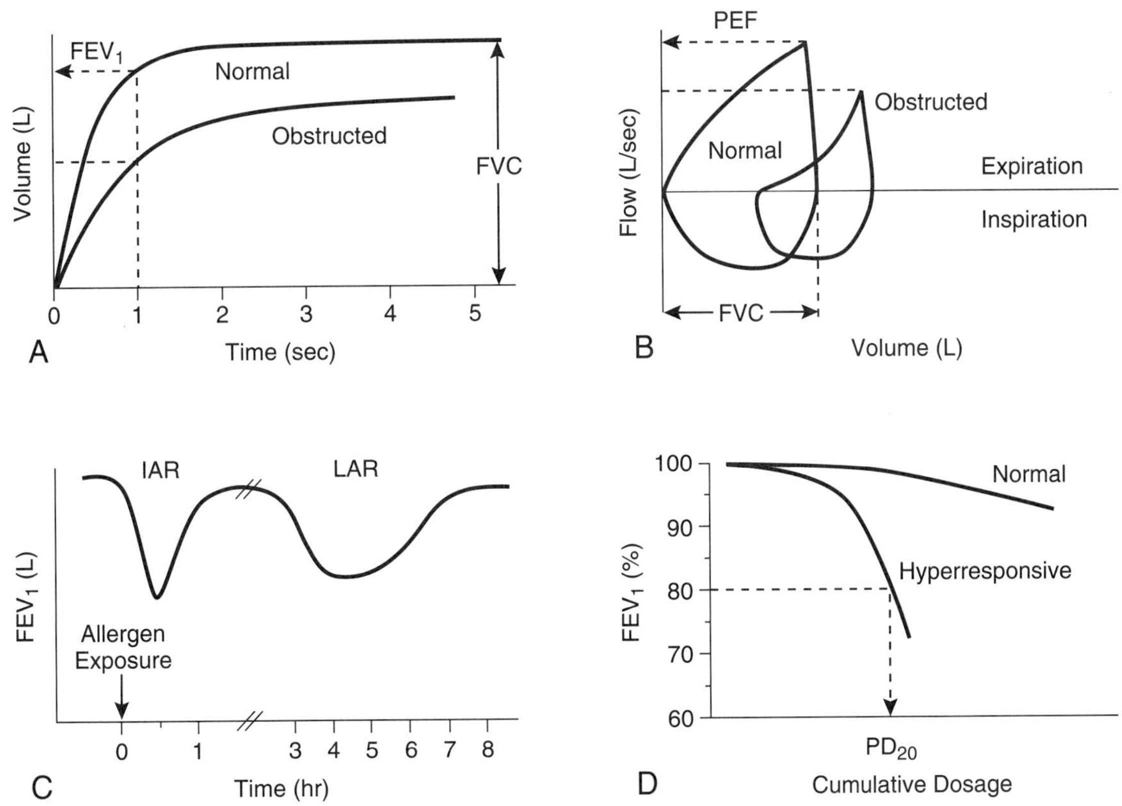

Figure 36.4. **A,** Typical spirometry of normal and obstructed patients. Note the lower forced expiratory volume at 1 sec *(FEV_1)*, forced vital capacity *(FVC)*, and FEV_1/FVC ratio in the obstructed patient. **B,** Typical flow–volume loops of a normal and obstructed patient. Note the lower peak expiratory flow *(PEF)*, greater lung volume, and typical "scooped out" expiratory curve in the obstructed patient. **C,** Typical immediate asthmatic response *(IAR)* and late asthmatic response *(LAR)* seen after exposure to relevant allergen. IAR occurs within minutes, whereas LAR occurs several hours after exposure. Patients may demonstrate an isolated IAR, isolated LAR, or dual responses. **D,** Typical pulmonary function seen with histamine or methacholine challenge testing in normal and hyperresponsive patients. Concentration or dosage of histamine or methacholine needed to elicit a drop of FEV_1 of 20% *(PC_{20} or PD_{20})* is inversely proportional to bronchial hyperresponsiveness.

are simple, portable, and inexpensive devices that facilitate accurate and objective self-monitoring of pulmonary function. Patients should be encouraged to use the same brand of peak flow device during monitoring because different brands can give clinically significant different measurements. A disadvantage of both FEV_1 and PEF is their dependence on patient effort.[1]

Asthma often occurs with a predominance of nocturnal symptoms, and this is reflected in a typical pattern of lower pulmonary function in the early morning. Allergies, atopic dermatitis, rhinitis, and sinusitis are commonly associated with asthma. Because asthma is a chronic disease with the potential for acute exacerbations, symptoms may be episodic, continuous, or continuous with episodic exacerbations. Symptoms can occur seasonally, perennially, or perennially with seasonal exacerbations. Exacerbations may be slowly progressing or have rapid onset. Even patients with mild intermittent or mild persistent asthma can have severe and rapidly progressive exacerbations. A number of factors may trigger asthma symptoms or exacerbations, such as allergens (pollens, molds, mites, animal danders), viral respiratory tract infections, environmental irritants (smoke, strong odors, cold dry air), exercise, food additives (sulfites, tartrazine), and medications (aspirin, NSAIDs, β-blockers). Although the psychological effects of emotions do not induce asthma, the physiologic response to certain emotions (hard laughter, crying) may precipitate asthma symptoms. After exposure to a relevant allergen, an immediate asthmatic response (IAR), a drop in pulmonary function occurring within minutes, and a late asthmatic response (LAR), a second drop in pulmonary function may occur after several hours of exposure (Fig. 36.4*C*). The LAR is characterized by a progressive inflammatory response in the lungs. It is believed that many of the symptoms of persistent asthma are caused by the unrelenting inflammatory responses triggered by continued exposure to allergens or other provocateurs. Although isolated IAR or LAR may occur, a dual response after exposure is also common.

As described previously, bronchial hyperresponsiveness is the exaggerated bronchoconstrictor response to exposure to physical and chemical stimuli and may persist for weeks or months after exposure to stimuli such as viral respiratory infections. Bronchial hyperresponsiveness can be measured by inhalation challenge testing, with patients inhaling increasing dosages of histamine or methacholine, with the endpoint being the dosage needed to elicit a 20% or greater fall in pulmonary function, typically FEV_1. The provocative concentration or dosage needed for a 20% fall in FEV_1 (PC_{20} or PD_{20}) is inversely proportional to bronchial hyperresponsiveness, so a lower PD_{20} is indicative of more reactivity (Fig. 36.4*D*). Not only can measures of bronchial hyperresponsiveness be used for diagnosing asthma, but changes in PD_{20} over time can be useful for gauging response to treatment.

Diagnosis

The diagnosis of asthma usually is based on clinical history and objective measures of pulmonary function. It can be elusive because a number of other diagnoses, including foreign body aspiration, laryngotracheomalacia, bronchiolitis, and cystic fibrosis, may also present with wheezing (Table 36.4).[1] Recurrent exacerbations; provoking factors such as allergens, irritants, exercise, or viral respiratory infections; and a history of nocturnal symptoms are particularly characteristic of asthma. Although the history is of great importance in narrowing the diagnosis of the disease, it is not diagnostic. The physical examination may be normal when no symptoms are present. Chest radiographs (posterior–anterior) may be normal in mild disease, but signs of air trapping (hyperinflation) are more often present with severe, chronic asthma. Rhinitis, sinusitis, eczema, blood eosinophilia, and nasal secretion and sputum eosinophilia may also be present.[1,25]

Table 36.4 ▪ Differential Diagnosis of Asthma

Infants and Children	Adults
Allergic rhinitis and sinusitis	Chronic obstructive pulmonary disease (chronic bronchitis or emphysema)
Foreign body in trachea or bronchus	Congestive heart failure
Vocal cord dysfunction	Pulmonary embolism
Vascular rings or laryngeal webs	Laryngeal dysfunction
Laryngotracheomalacia, tracheal stenosis, or bronchostenosis	Mechanical obstruction of the airways (tumors)
Enlarged lymph nodes or tumor	Pulmonary infiltration with eosinophilia
Viral bronchiolitis or obliterative bronchiolitis	Cough secondary to drugs
Cystic fibrosis	Vocal cord dysfunction
Bronchopulmonary dysplasia	
Heart disease	
Aspiration from dysfunctions of swallowing	
Recurrent cough not caused by asthma	
Mechanism dysfunction or gastroesophageal reflux	

Source: Reference 1.

Objective measures of pulmonary function showing reversible airflow obstruction (either spontaneously or with treatment) are critical in establishing the diagnosis of asthma. Demonstrating bronchial hyperresponsiveness by inhalation challenge testing with histamine, methacholine, or exercise can also be helpful in making the diagnosis, but these tests can pose some danger, and sufficient precautions are needed. For safety reasons, provocation with specific allergens is rarely recommended.[25] A number of other techniques have been implemented in the diagnosis of asthma, such as IgE antibody testing, allergen skin testing, examination of spontaneously produced or induced sputum, and direct investigative methods (bronchoalveolar brushings, lavage, and biopsy), but the latter are limited by low specificity, their experimental nature, and potential safety risks.[1,25]

PSYCHOSOCIAL ASPECTS

Patients with asthma may also suffer from psychosocial problems that affect their ability to care for themselves and thus adversely affect their overall health and quality of life. Patients with brittle asthma (asthma characterized by frequent and significant fluctuations in daily peak flow readings or sudden, severe exacerbations in otherwise stable disease) or those who have had near death from asthma or ultimately died from asthma often have had psychosocial problems (Table 36.5).[26] Psychiatric illnesses (primarily depression) may exist in up to 40% of these patients and denial in nearly 60% of patients. In patients with near-fatal asthma, most are women, exacerbations are common on Sundays, asthma is characterized as severe persistent and has an adverse effect on work or school, visits to the ED or intensive care unit are frequent, and routine asthma care is considered suboptimal. In addition to these characteristics, patients who have died from asthma also are from lower socioeconomic groups. In patients with near-fatal asthma or fatal asthma, psychosocial issues are believed to have contributed to the event in more than 80% of cases.[26]

Factors that have been identified as being associated with asthma deaths include an underestimation of the severity of the disease caused by lack of objective measures of lung function (such as PEF) in evaluating the patient's disease, failure of the patient and his or her family to appreciate the severity of episodes because the patient is used to having a suboptimal level of health, and underuse of oral and inhaled corticosteroids for chronic treatment.[26] It is interesting to note that with the introduction of more effective treatment for asthma such as inhaled corticosteroid therapy in the 1970s, there has been diminished interest in the psychological and psychosocial aspects of the disease.[26] In fact, two extensive textbooks on asthma published since 1997 do not include chapters on these issues.

Table 36.5 ▪ Adverse Psychosocial Factors on Near Fatal and Fatal Asthma

	Near-Fatal Asthma	Fatal Asthma
Depression or other psychiatric illness	+	+
Denial	+	+
Personality disorder		+
Psychiatric caseness	+	+
Current or recent use of major tranquilizers or sedatives	+	+
Deliberate self-harm		+
Learning disability or mental retardation	+	+
Psychiatric disorder in a first-degree relative	+	+
Alcohol or drug abuse	+	+
Recent bereavement		+
Severe domestic stress	+	+
Social isolation, living alone, homelessness	+	+
Unemployment, self-employment, threatened unemployment	+	+
Marital problems		+
Separated or single parenthood	+	+
Extreme poverty		+
Childhood abuse		+
Smoking or passive smoking	+	+
Legal problems		+

Many patients had more than one adverse factor.

Source: Reprinted with permission from Harrison BD. Psychosocial aspects of asthma in adults. Thorax 53:519–525, 1998.

Poor adherence with prescribed medications is associated with increased mortality from asthma. Patients who are nonadherent with their medications tend to be younger, have higher scores for depression on certain scales, feel ashamed, embarrassed, or angry about their disease, and be concerned about side effects of corticosteroids and becoming addicted to their medications.[26] Adolescents, in particular, are poorly adherent with their medications because of denial, peer pressure, lack of perception of disease, reluctance to seek medical advice, ignorance, and desire for a simpler medication regimen.[27] However, once adolescents realize that asthma does not have to be disabling and that participation in sports is encouraged, medication adherence improves because of their desire to be normal.[27] Interestingly, patients are no more adherent with a quick-relief β-agonist regimen than with a long-term control inhaled corticosteroid regimen.[26]

The NAEPP guidelines include *Education for a Partnership in Asthma Care* as one of the four components of asthma management.[1] Although this component does not directly address the psychosocial issues surrounding asthma, it does emphasize the need for patient and family involvement with all members of the health care team. This partnership encourages joint development of treatment goals, regular review of these goals and outcomes, open communication, and teaching and reinforcement of self-management techniques. These processes can be expected to improve the patient's psychosocial well-being.

THERAPEUTIC PLAN

Treatment Guidelines

Interest in asthma management has increased dramatically in the last decade and has led to the development and update of a number of asthma treatment guidelines and consensus statements. The first formal treatment guidelines were published in 1989 to provide uniformity in asthma management for children.[28] These were followed by published guidelines from many countries, including the United States (NAEPP),[29] and several international and global guidelines were developed in an attempt to consolidate these regionally specific guidelines. The following discussion of chronic and acute asthma management reviews the treatments outlined in the most recent update of the NAEPP *Guidelines for the Diagnosis and Prevention of Asthma,* Expert Panel Report 2, from the National Heart, Lung, and Blood Institute of the National Institutes of Health.[1] These treatment guidelines will be revised continually as new information on the pathophysiology of the

Treatment | **Preferred treatments are in bold print**

	Long-Term control	**Quick Relief**	**Education**
Step 4: Severe Persistent	Daily Medications • **Anti-inflammatory: inhaled corticosteroid (high dosage)** AND • Long-acting bronchodilator: either **long-acting inhaled β_2-agonist,** sustained-release theophylline, or long-acting β_2-agonist tablets AND • Corticosteroid tablets or syrup long term (2 mg/kg/day, generally do not exceed 60 mg per day).	• Short-acting bronchodilator: **inhaled β_2-agonists** as needed for symptoms. • Intensity of treatment depends on severity of exacerbation. • Use of short-acting inhaled β_2-agonists on a daily basis, or increasing use, indicates the need for additional long-term control therapy.	Steps 2 and 3 actions plus: • Refer to individual education and counseling.
Step 3: Moderate Persistent	Daily Medication • Either **Anti-inflammatory: inhaled corticosteroid (medium dosage)** OR **Inhaled corticosteroid (low–medium dosage)** and add a long-acting bronchodilator, especially for nighttime symptoms: either **long-acting inhaled β_2-agonist,** sustained-release theophylline, or long-acting β_2-agonist tablets. • If needed Anti-inflammatory: **inhaled corticosteroids (medium–high dosage)** AND **Long-acting bronchodilator,** especially for nighttime symptoms; either **long-acting inhaled β_2-agonist,** sustained-release theophylline, or long-acting inhaled β_2-agonist tablets.	• Short-acting bronchodilator: **inhaled β_2-agonists** as needed for symptoms. • Intensity of treatment depends on severity of exacerbation. • Use of short-acting inhaled β_2-agonists on a daily basis, or increasing use, indicates the need for additional long-term control therapy.	Step 1 actions plus: • Teach self-monitoring. • Refer to group education if available. • Review and update self-management plan.
Step 2: Mild Persistent	One Daily Medication • **Anti-inflammatory:** either **inhaled corticosteroid** (low dosages) or **cromolyn or nedocromil** (children usually begin with a trial of cromolyn or nedocromil). • Sustained-release theophylline to serum concentrations of 5–15 μg/mL is an alternative but not preferred therapy. Zafirlukast, zileuton or montelukast may also be considered, although their position in therapy is not fully established.[a]	• Short-acting bronchodilator: **inhaled β_2-agonists** as needed for symptoms. • Intensity of treatment depends on severity of exacerbation. • Use of short-acting inhaled β_2-agonists on a daily basis, or increasing use, indicates the need for additional long-term control therapy.	Step 1 actions plus: • Teach self-monitoring. • Refer to group education if available. • Review and update self-management plan.
Step 1: Mild Intermittent	No daily medication is needed.	• Short-acting bronchodilator: **inhaled β_2-agonists** as needed for symptoms. • Intensity of treatment depends on severity of exacerbation. • Use of short-acting inhaled β_2-agonists on a daily basis, or increasing use, indicates the need for additional long-term control therapy.	• Teach basic facts about asthma. • Teach inhaler, spacer, or holding chamber technique. • Discuss roles of medications. • Develop self-management plan. • Develop action plan for when and how to take rescue actions, especially for patients with a history of severe exacerbations. • Discuss appropriate environmental control measures to avoid exposure to known allergens and irritants.

↓ **Step Down**
Review treatment every 1 to 6 mo; a gradual stepwise reduction in treatment may be possible.

↑ **Step Up**
If control is not maintained, consider step up. First, review patient medication technique, adherence, and environmental control (avoidance of allergens or other factors that contribute to asthma severity).

Note:

- **The stepwise approach presents general guidelines to assist clinical decision making; it is not intended to be a specific prescription. Asthma is highly variable; clinicians should tailor specific medication plans to the needs and circumstances of individual patients.**
- Gain control as quickly as possible, then decrease treatment to the least medication necessary to maintain control. Gaining control may be accomplished by either starting treatment at the step most appropriate to the initial severity of the condition or starting at a higher level of therapy (e.g., a course of systemic corticosteroids or higher dosage of inhaled corticosteroids).
- A rescue course of systemic corticosteroids may be needed at any time and at any step.
- Some patients with intermittent asthma experience severe and life-threatening exacerbations separated by long periods of normal lung function and no symptoms. This may be especially common with exacerbations provoked by respiratory infections. A short course of systemic corticosteroids is recommended.
- At each step, patient should control his or her environment to avoid or control factors that make asthma worse (e.g., allergens, irritants); this requires specific diagnosis and education.

Referral to an asthma specialist for consultation or comanagement is recommended if there are difficulties achieving or maintaining control of asthma or if the patient needs step 4 care. Referral may be considered if the patient needs step 3 care.

[a]Montelukast can be used in children as young as 6 yr; zafirlukast can be used in children as young as 7 yr; zileuton can be used in patients $\geq$12 yr.

Figure 36.5. Stepwise approach for managing asthma in adults and children older than 5 years. (Modified from National Asthma Education and Prevention Program. Expert panel report 2: guidelines for the diagnosis and management of asthma. Bethesda, MD: US Department of Health and Human Services, Public Health Service, National Institutes of Health, National Heart, Lung, and Blood Institute, pub. no. 97-4051, April 1997.)

disease is discovered and new classes of drugs enter the market.

The NAEPP recommends establishing a four-part program for effective asthma management:[1]

- Measures of assessment and monitoring
- Control of factors contributing to asthma severity
- Pharmacologic therapy
- Education for a partnership in asthma care

Selected algorithms for the management of chronic and acute asthma are presented in Figures 36.5–36.7.[1]

Chronic Asthma

Because inflammation in asthma is believed to cause most of the chronic symptoms and pathologic changes observed, much of the current treatment emphasizes the use of anti-inflammatory drugs. However, before any therapy is initiated, the severity of asthma symptoms must be assessed because all guidelines base treatment on whether asthma is mild, moderate, or severe.

Classification of Asthma Severity

The NAEPP guidelines classify asthma severity into four categories: mild intermittent, mild persistent, moderate persistent, and severe persistent (Table 36.3).[1] The distinction between mild intermittent and mild persistent is made to distinguish patients whose symptoms are mild but occur infrequently (e.g., reappearing in intervals of weeks or months) from those whose symptoms are mild but occur frequently (e.g., several days a week). An example of someone with mild intermittent asthma would be a patient who has symptoms only upon exercising.

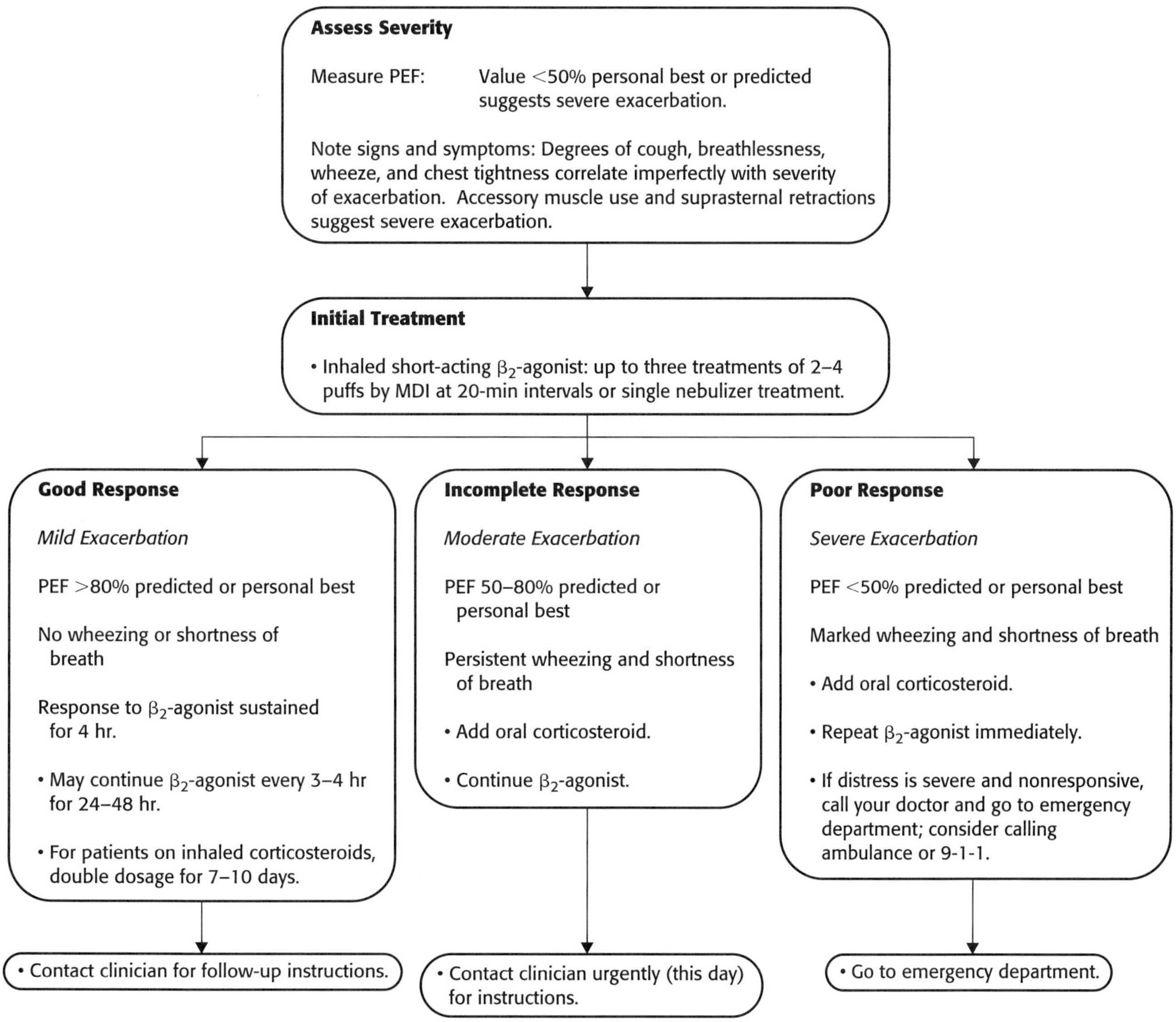

Figure 36.6. Management of asthma exacerbations: home treatment. Patients at high risk of asthma-related death should receive immediate clinical attention after initial treatment. *MDI,* metered-dose inhaler; *PEF,* peak expiratory flow. (Modified from National Asthma Education and Prevention Program. Expert panel report 2: guidelines for the diagnosis and management of asthma. Bethesda, MD: US Department of Health and Human Services, Public Health Service, National Institutes of Health, National Heart, Lung, and Blood Institute, pub. no. 97-4051, April 1997.)

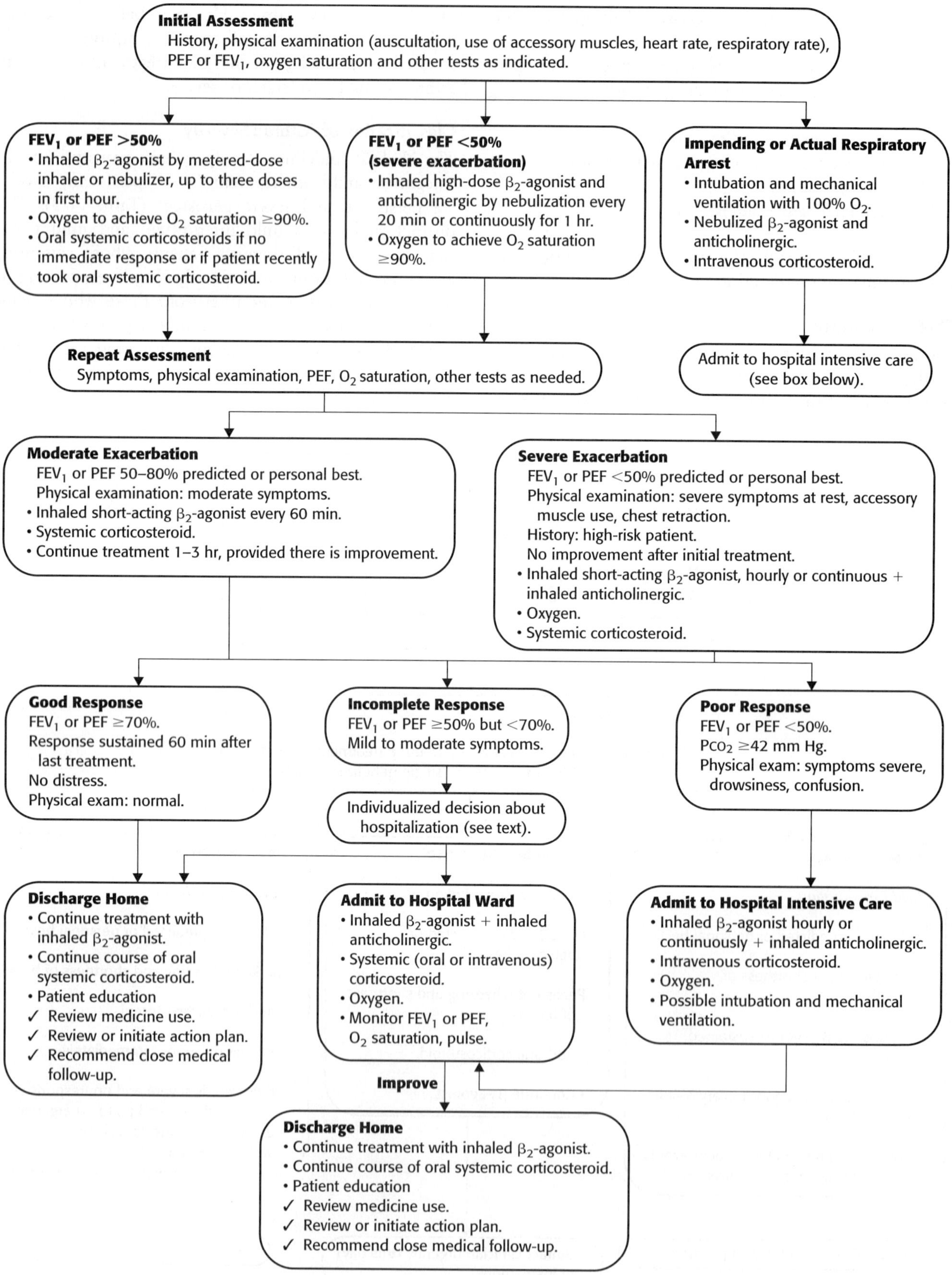

Initial Assessment
History, physical examination (auscultation, use of accessory muscles, heart rate, respiratory rate), PEF or FEV_1, oxygen saturation and other tests as indicated.
FEV_1 or PEF >50%
• Inhaled β_2-agonist by metered-dose inhaler or nebulizer, up to three doses in first hour.
• Oxygen to achieve O_2 saturation ≥90%.
• Oral systemic corticosteroids if no immediate response or if patient recently took oral systemic corticosteroid.
FEV_1 or PEF <50% (severe exacerbation)
• Inhaled high-dose β_2-agonist and anticholinergic by nebulization every 20 min or continuously for 1 hr.
• Oxygen to achieve O_2 saturation ≥90%.
Impending or Actual Respiratory Arrest
• Intubation and mechanical ventilation with 100% O_2.
• Nebulized β_2-agonist and anticholinergic.
• Intravenous corticosteroid.
Repeat Assessment
Symptoms, physical examination, PEF, O_2 saturation, other tests as needed.
Admit to hospital intensive care (see box below).
Moderate Exacerbation
FEV_1 or PEF 50–80% predicted or personal best.
Physical examination: moderate symptoms.
• Inhaled short-acting β_2-agonist every 60 min.
• Systemic corticosteroid.
• Continue treatment 1–3 hr, provided there is improvement.
Severe Exacerbation
FEV_1 or PEF <50% predicted or personal best.
Physical examination: severe symptoms at rest, accessory muscle use, chest retraction.
History: high-risk patient.
No improvement after initial treatment.
• Inhaled short-acting β_2-agonist, hourly or continuous + inhaled anticholinergic.
• Oxygen.
• Systemic corticosteroid.
Good Response
FEV_1 or PEF ≥70%.
Response sustained 60 min after last treatment.
No distress.
Physical exam: normal.
Incomplete Response
FEV_1 or PEF ≥50% but <70%.
Mild to moderate symptoms.
Individualized decision about hospitalization (see text).
Poor Response
FEV_1 or PEF <50%.
P_{CO_2} ≥42 mm Hg.
Physical exam: symptoms severe, drowsiness, confusion.
Discharge Home
• Continue treatment with inhaled β_2-agonist.
• Continue course of oral systemic corticosteroid.
• Patient education
✓ Review medicine use.
✓ Review or initiate action plan.
✓ Recommend close medical follow-up.
Admit to Hospital Ward
• Inhaled β_2-agonist + inhaled anticholinergic.
• Systemic (oral or intravenous) corticosteroid.
• Oxygen.
• Monitor FEV_1 or PEF, O_2 saturation, pulse.
Admit to Hospital Intensive Care
• Inhaled β_2-agonist hourly or continuously + inhaled anticholinergic.
• Intravenous corticosteroid.
• Oxygen.
• Possible intubation and mechanical ventilation.
Improve
Discharge Home
• Continue treatment with inhaled β_2-agonist.
• Continue course of oral systemic corticosteroid.
• Patient education
✓ Review medicine use.
✓ Review or initiate action plan.
✓ Recommend close medical follow-up.

Figure 36.7. Management of asthma exacerbations: emergency department and hospital care. *FEV_1*, forced expiratory volume in 1 sec; *P_{CO_2}*, partial pressure of carbon dioxide; *PEF*, peak expiratory flow. (Modified from National Asthma Education and Prevention Program. Expert panel report 2: guidelines for the diagnosis and management of asthma. Bethesda, MD: US Department of Health and Human Services, Public Health Service, National Institutes of Health, National Heart, Lung, and Blood Institute, pub. no. 97-4051, April 1997.)

Patients with mild intermittent asthma have daytime symptoms no more often than twice a week and nighttime symptoms no more often than twice a month. Pulmonary function tests (the FEV_1 and PEF) indicate normal lung function (80% or more of predicted value), and peak flow measurements performed in the morning and afternoon over several weeks during a stable period of the disease fluctuate no more than 20%. Severe but brief exacerbations (periods of increased symptoms beyond the usual) necessitating oral corticosteroids may occur, and the frequency and characteristics of these episodes are highly individualistic.

The symptoms of patients with mild persistent asthma occur more often than twice a week but not daily. Nocturnal symptoms occur at least twice a month. When symptoms are stable, pulmonary function appears normal (80% or more of predicted values), but peak flow measurements show a 20 to 30% variability between morning and afternoon measurements when measured over 1 to 2 weeks.

In patients with moderate persistent asthma, symptoms occur daily and necessitate the use of an inhaled short-acting bronchodilator (e.g., albuterol) daily. Nocturnal awakenings occur at least once a week. Pulmonary function is abnormal, ranging from more than 60% to less than 80% predicted. Peak flow measurements show more than 30% variability between morning and afternoon measurements when measured over 1 to 2 weeks. Exacerbations, generally reflected in the increased need to use a short-acting β_2-agonist inhaler or nebulizer solution for several days, occur more often than twice a week and can last for several days.

Patients with severe persistent asthma have continuous symptoms with frequent exacerbations. Their activity level is severely limited and they have frequent nighttime symptoms. Pulmonary function is less than 60% predicted, and peak flow measurements show more than 30% variability between morning and afternoon measurements when measured over 1 to 2 weeks.

A patient's symptoms rarely fall into a discrete category; symptoms often overlap between levels. Therefore, patients are placed in the category that corresponds to their most severe symptoms. For example, a patient with symptoms 3 days/week (mild persistent) and nocturnal awakenings once a week (moderate persistent) should be classified in the moderate persistent asthma category. The same principle applies when classifying patients already taking medications: The most severe category according to the current medication needs and level of symptom control should be chosen. Because the medication selected to treat a patient's asthma is based on his or her severity classification, it is necessary to know the severity classification in order to make recommendations for stepping up or stepping down a patient's current medication level.

Step Care Approach to Asthma Management

The medications used in treating asthma are shown in Figure 36.5.[1] Drugs are categorized as long-term control medications, used to achieve and maintain control in patients with persistent asthma, and quick-relief medications, used to treat acute symptoms and exacerbations in patients with intermittent and persistent asthma. Higher levels of therapy (i.e., a short course of systemic corticosteroids or a higher dosage of inhaled corticosteroids) should be initiated to achieve control in persistent asthma, and once control is achieved, therapy should be stepped down to the lowest level needed to control symptoms.

Quick-relief medications (i.e., inhaled β_2-agonists) are to be used only as needed for symptom control in all patients with asthma. They should be used prophylactically 15 to 30 minutes before exercise or cold air exposure. Cromolyn and nedocromil can prevent asthma symptoms when used before exercise or cold air exposure, but they are not nearly as effective as inhaled β_2-agonists and thus are not recommended for this purpose. Increased use of inhaled β_2-agonist therapy may indicate the need for additional long-term control medications or may signal the onset of an acute exacerbation.

Patients with mild intermittent asthma are treated with short-acting inhaled β_2-agonists as needed, but daily use signals the need for additional therapy to control symptoms. Symptoms usually are triggered by exercise or exposure to irritants, allergens, or respiratory infections.

Mild persistent asthma is poorly controlled by episodic administration of short-acting inhaled β_2-agonists. These patients are treated with daily medication that provides long-term control of symptoms, with either low-dose inhaled corticosteroids or cromolyn or nedocromil as the recommended therapies. Sustained-release theophylline may be considered as an alternative therapy, and montelukast and zafirlukast may be used in patients as young as 6 and 7 years old, respectively. Zileuton may be considered for patients at least 12 years old.

Patients with moderate persistent asthma are treated with a medium dosage of inhaled corticosteroids or a low dosage of inhaled corticosteroids plus a long-acting bronchodilator, such as a long-acting β_2-agonist or sustained-release theophylline. The dosages of inhaled corticosteroids are increased as necessary to provide symptom control. In patients with moderate persistent asthma who have increasingly frequent symptoms, a short-term oral corticosteroid burst followed by maintenance inhaled corticosteroid therapy is recommended, with the goal of relieving symptoms and preventing the need for emergency medical care.

Patients who have severe persistent asthma need inhaled corticosteroids plus a long-acting bronchodilator to treat their continual symptoms. Because these patients have limited physical activity and frequent exacerbations of symptoms, they may need frequent oral corticosteroid bursts or continuous maintenance therapy with oral corticosteroids at as low a dosage as possible in combination with high-dose inhaled corticosteroids and other antiasthma long-term control medications.

Children are treated similarly, based on disease severity, although the measurement of peak flow may be less reliable, especially in children less than 5 years old. Symptoms such as cough, wheeze, disruption of activity, and nocturnal awakenings are useful in defining disease severity. These last two symptoms reflect significant airway obstruction typical of moderate persistent asthma, but even disruption of activity and nocturnal awakenings can be the result of other diseases. Young children often cannot use a metered-dose inhaler (MDI) successfully and therefore must use a nebulizer, an MDI with a spacer (with or without a face mask), or possibly a dry powder inhaler (DPI). Children with mild intermittent asthma are treated with short-acting inhaled β-agonists, whereas children with mild persistent disease are given a trial of inhaled cromolyn sodium and, if it is ineffective, switched to inhaled corticosteroids. Sustained-release theophylline is an alternative therapy in children under 5 years who have moderate persistent asthma; however, there is concern about the narrow therapeutic index of the drug. With regular use of these drugs to control disease symptoms, β-agonists should be used infrequently to relieve any additional symptoms.

A reduction or "stepdown" in therapy can be considered if there is less than 10 to 20% variability in PEF or if the PEF is consistently higher than 80% of the patient's personal best (determination of personal best is described later in this chapter). Symptoms must be minimal and there must be little need for short-acting inhaled β_2-agonists, an absence of nighttime awakenings, and no activity limitations over at least a 3-month period. The pharmacologic therapy should be reduced gradually because asthma can deteriorate at a highly variable rate and intensity. The NAEPP guidelines generally recommend that the last medication that was added to the patient's regimen be the first medication to be reduced. However, the rate of reduction and interval for evaluation have not been established with certainty. The guidelines recommend that the dosage of inhaled corticosteroids can be reduced approximately 25% every 2 to 3 months to the lowest dosage possible that maintains control of asthma. Patients with persistent asthma need daily anti-inflammatory medications to suppress airway inflammation. Asthma may worsen if inhaled corticosteroids are discontinued completely.

To assess asthma control, physicians should schedule follow-up examinations at 1- to 6-month intervals. They also should determine whether the appropriate stepdown in therapy was instituted. Pharmacists can also provide care at this point by ensuring that the medications have been taken as prescribed and helping the patient to monitor peak flow readings.

In treating asthma, consideration must be given to the management of other diseases or stimuli that may precipitate asthma symptoms, especially when asthma symptoms persist despite optimal pharmacotherapy and compliance.[30] Allergic rhinitis and asthma are closely related pathophysiologically, and treating allergic rhinitis may improve symptoms of asthma. Similarly, acute or chronic sinusitis may aggravate asthma symptoms even in the absence of a bacterial infection. Gastroesophageal reflux may cause nocturnal coughing in some infants and may be mistaken for asthma symptoms. Also in adults, gastroesophageal reflux disease may precipitate asthma symptoms, and in some women asthma symptoms worsen just before and during menstruation.

A key to the outpatient management of asthma is self-monitoring of asthma signs and symptoms by the patient. Home PEF monitoring is an objective way to assess symptom severity and response to therapy, and daily monitoring is recommended for patients with moderate or severe persistent asthma.[1] However, all patients may need peak flow monitoring during an exacerbation to monitor response to therapy. Airway obstruction can be detected and treated even before wheezing is audible or the patient experiences symptoms. Patients should be instructed to determine their personal best value from which green, yellow, and red zones are calculated. To obtain a reliable PEF measurement, the patient must place the mouthpiece between the teeth, ensuring that the tongue is not obstructing the mouthpiece, and exhale rapidly with maximal force. The personal best PEF is determined by having the patient record the best of three PEF measurements taken between noon and 2 PM each day for 2 to 3 weeks and after each use of his or her inhaled β_2-agonist. The highest number recorded over this time period is considered the patient's personal best and is used for comparison with all subsequent PEF measurements. The green zone indicates "all clear": Symptoms are not present and medications are to be taken as usual. The green zone is usually 80 to 100% of predicted PEF or personal best. The yellow zone, 50 to 80% of predicted PEF or personal best, indicates "caution," and the usual medication regimen may need to be modified. The red zone, below 50% predicted PEF or personal best, indicates "medical alert," and patients are to use inhaled β_2-adrenergic agonist medication immediately and follow up with medical personnel. Additional information on peak flow monitoring and examples of peak flow diaries that can be distributed to patients are available in the NAEPP guidelines.[1]

Consideration of the cost of therapy is essential in the management plan for any chronic illness. If patients cannot afford the medications prescribed, adherence will be poor and symptom recurrence will be common. Medication adherence is especially important in treating asthma, a life-threatening disease in which death can occur within minutes of an acute severe exacerbation. In addition, many asthmatic patients are atopic and may need costly therapy to treat allergic rhinitis, allergic conjunctivitis, or eczema. Before recommending treatment, health care providers should obtain detailed information about payment methods.

Acute Exacerbations

Self-Management of Acute Exacerbations

The NAEPP guidelines recommend that all patients have a written action plan to guide self-management.[1] However, patients with risk factors for death from asthma should always seek medical care early during an exacerbation and be taught how to obtain emergency transportation to an ED. Similarly, the parents or guardians of infants should always seek medical care because of the risk of respiratory failure.[1] Patients with symptoms of severe asthma such as the inability to speak in complete sentences or walk 100 feet without stopping, use of accessory muscles or suprasternal retractions, severe wheezing or breathlessness, or PEF less than 50% predicted need medical intervention.

Self-management of asthma exacerbations by patients outside a health care facility is shown in Figure 36.6.[1] However, any individualized written action plan for a patient supersedes the steps shown in Figure 36.6. Patients who show an incomplete or poor response after initial treatment should be treated with oral corticosteroids, and patients with a good response who are currently treated with an inhaled corticosteroid should increase their dosage of the inhaled corticosteroid for the next 7 to 10 days. Children whose asthma is precipitated by an upper respiratory tract infection may begin a short course of oral corticosteroids at the first symptom of an upper respiratory tract infection even in the absence of wheezing. This can reduce the number of days with wheezing, ED visits, and hospitalizations.[31] Children should be seen by a medical professional, but adults may continue with self-observation and seek medical care if symptoms do not improve.

Emergency Department Management of Acute Exacerbations

ED management of asthma exacerbations is shown in Figure 36.7.[1] Patients with mild or moderate exacerbations (pulmonary function more than 50% of predicted value on presentation to the ED) can be treated with an MDI or nebulized β_2-adrenergic agonists administered three times during the first hour, but patients with severe exacerbations (pulmonary function less than 50% of predicted value) should be treated with nebulized β_2-agonists rather than from an MDI. Numerous studies have demonstrated that high dosages of β_2-adrenergic agonists from an MDI attached to a spacer in the ED are efficacious, but nebulized treatment is more effective in patients who are unable to coordinate proper use of an MDI because of their age, agitation during the event, or severity of the event. Laboratory assessments may include arterial blood gas measurement, complete blood count, theophylline, and serum electrolyte measurement. A chest radiograph is indicated only in patients with a complicating cardiopulmonary process such as pneumothorax or atelectasis. Supplemental oxygen is indicated for all patients who are hypoxemic. In patients with mild or moderate exacerbations whose symptoms persist after initial treatment, frequent or continuous nebulized β_2-adrenergics are begun and systemic corticosteroids are indicated. Systemic corticosteroids are started concurrently with nebulized β_2-adrenergic treatment plus anticholinergic therapy if symptoms are severe. Patients with severe exacerbations should be assessed after the initial dose of nebulized β_2-adrenergic treatment plus anticholinergic therapy because the response to the initial treatment in the ED is a better predictor of the need for hospitalization than the severity of the exacerbation on presentation. Patients with mild or moderate exacerbations are assessed after the initial three doses of nebulized β_2-adrenergic treatment. Intravenous aminophylline is no longer indicated for treating asthma in the ED except in patients who take theophylline to treat chronic symptoms. All patients who are discharged from the ED should receive a course of oral corticosteroids.[1]

Patients who are admitted to the hospital continue treatment with frequent inhaled β_2-agonists plus inhaled anticholinergics and systemic corticosteroids. Most studies of intravenous aminophylline in hospitalized patients have failed to show an improved benefit over optimal dosages of inhaled β_2-adrenergic agonists and systemic corticosteroids. However, patients who do not improve and those admitted to the intensive care unit should received intravenous aminophylline. Patients in the intensive care unit may benefit from subcutaneous, intramuscular, or intravenous β-adrenergic agonists, intravenous magnesium, or heliox (a mixture of helium and oxygen) therapy.[1] In general, patients may be discharged when pulmonary function returns to 70% or more of the predicted value or personal best.

Patient education about discharge medications, PEF monitoring, and the importance of a follow-up visit is an essential component of discharge procedures. Inhaled corticosteroids are initiated at discharge while the patient continues treatment with oral corticosteroids. Initiating inhaled corticosteroid therapy at this time with patient education reinforces to the patient the importance of this therapy in achieving long-term control. Patients who received theophylline treatment in the hospital may need to continue using oral theophylline. All patients should be taught correct techniques for inhaled β_2-adrenergic therapy, whether administered by nebulizer, MDI with or without a spacer, or a DPI because this therapy is essential for maintaining optimal lung function.

TREATMENT

Pharmacotherapy

As outlined in the NAEPP guidelines,[1] treatment includes providing optimal pharmacotherapy with minimal or no adverse effects. Maintaining affordable care with reasonable medication regimens (facilitating better adherence) could also be included in this list of treatment goals. Because asthma is a chronic condition with periodic exacerbations, therapy entails continuous attention with efforts to prevent or minimize acute symptoms.

The medications used to treat asthma can be divided into the general categories of bronchodilators and anti-inflammatory agents. The NAEPP guidelines categorize medications into quick-relief medications, which include short-acting inhaled β_2-agonists, anticholinergics, and short-term use of systemic corticosteroids, and long-term control medications, which include inhaled and systemic corticosteroids, cromolyn and nedocromil, long-acting β_2-agonists, methylxanthines, and leukotriene modifiers. Not only must the symptoms of bronchoconstriction be treated, but the underlying inflammation must be addressed as well.

Bronchodilators

β-Adrenergic Agonists

β-Adrenergic agonists are potent bronchodilators. Two classes of β-adrenergic agonists exist: short-acting (albuterol, bitolterol, metaproterenol, pirbuterol, terbutaline) and long-acting (salmeterol and formoterol, which is investigational). These two types have very different roles in treating asthma. Currently available β-adrenergic agonists stimulate the α, β_1, and β_2 receptors, but it is the action on the β_2 receptors that produces the therapeutic response in asthma. Drugs with modifications of the catecholamine ring and side chains have been developed to prolong the duration of effect, enhance β_2 receptor selectivity, and confer oral bioavailability over the catecholamines. A different modification exists for bitolterol mesylate, which is a prodrug slowly hydrolyzed in the lung to colterol; colterol has a similar duration of action to isoproterenol.

Adrenergic receptors belong to the G-protein–linked rhodopsin-related receptor superfamilies. When a β_2-adrenergic agonist binds to the receptor on the cell membrane, guanosine diphosphate is released from G protein, which is a membrane-associated heterotrimer. This enables guanosine triphosphate to bind to the β-receptor, which activates adenylyl cyclase, catalyzing formation of cyclic 3′,5′ adenosine monophosphate (cAMP). Cytosolic calcium ion concentration decreases and smooth muscle relaxation ensues.[32] Other mechanisms of smooth muscle relaxation include shifting of myosin light-chain kinase to a less active form, cAMP inhibition of phospholipase C and reduction of 1,4,5-triphosphate formation (reducing intracellular calcium), stimulation of a calcium-activated potassium channel, and inhibition of acetylcholine release from cholinergic neurons.[32] The long duration of effect for salmeterol is believed to result from the binding of the lipophilic side chain to an exocite, which is adjacent to the active portion of the β-receptor. The exocite anchors the agonist and permits nearly continuous stimulation of the β-receptor. The mechanism for the long duration of activity of formoterol is less clear but is believed to result from its extreme lipophilicity and high affinity for the β-receptor.[33] Although β-adrenergic agonists have certain anti-inflammatory effects, including inhibition of preformed and newly generated mediators released from mast cells, reduction of microvascular leakage, and enhancement of mucociliary clearance, the clinical significance has not been determined. However, neither short-acting nor long-acting drugs affect inflammation when evaluated by lung biopsy.[34,35]

Nine polymorphisms of the β_2-receptor have been identified;[36] four are nondegenerate (coded for a change in the protein sequence). Two of these nondegenerate polymorphisms encode an amino acid change at position 16 from arginine (Arg16) to glycine (Gly16) and at position 27 from glutamine (Gln27) to glutamate (Glu27). These changes have clinical significance for asthma phenotypes and treatment. Patients with the Gly16 genotype may have more severe asthma, more frequent nocturnal symptoms, and greater airway hyperresponsiveness, and patients with the Glu27 genotype have less airway hyperresponsiveness.[36] In addition, patients with the Arg16 genotype have a greater response to β_2-agonists (defined as at least a 15% improvement in FEV_1) and are less susceptible to β-receptor desensitization than patients with the Gly16 genotype.[37] Patients with the Glu27 genotype also show less susceptibility to β-receptor desensitization.[36] Characterizing β-receptor genotype may allow for better individualization of drug therapy and predictability of response to medications.

β_2-Adrenergic agonists may be given orally, subcutaneously, or by inhalation. When given orally, much larger dosages must be used than with the inhaled route because of high first-pass metabolism. The subcutaneous route is less often used because highly potent β_2-selective drugs are available that may be given via inhalation. In addition, inhalation provides a more rapid onset of action and fewer systemic adverse effects. Inhaled β_2-adrenergic agonists may be administered via a number of ancillary devices, described in detail later in this chapter. β_2-Adrenergic agonists also can be administered intravenously in patients with impending respiratory failure, but potentially life-threatening adverse effects greatly limit the safety of this route of administration.[38] It is believed that the intravenous route allows drug to reach airways poorly accessed by the inhaled route when diminished tidal volumes and small airway obstruction with mucous plugs and edema are present in patients with severe bronchoconstriction. Interestingly, the intravenous route has been advocated for rapid reduction of serum potassium in patients with severe hyperkalemia with other causes.[39]

β_2-Adrenergic agonists have both bronchodilator and bronchoprotective effects, and differences in these effects can distinguish between the drugs and dosages. All are functional antagonists and can reverse smooth muscle constriction from any stimulus. Irrespective of device or drug administered, equipotent dosages at the β_2-receptor produce equivalent response, but the duration of effect and magnitude of adverse effects vary between drugs. Inhaled short-acting agents have an onset of effect within minutes and peak effect in 30 to 90 minutes. In contrast, salmeterol, the only long-acting agent available in the United States, has a much slower onset of effect (10 to 20 minutes) and a longer time to peak effect (2 to 4 hours). Formoterol has a more rapid onset (3 minutes) than salmeterol. Short-acting β_2-adrenergic agonists provide bronchodilation for about 4 to 6 hours and protection from provocateurs for about 2 to 4 hours. In contrast, long-acting agents provide bronchodilation and bronchoprotection up to 12 hours and possibly 24 hours after a single dose.

Clear dose–response relationships for peak effect and duration of effect are apparent for inhaled β_2-adrenergic agonists. This is particularly important in severe acute asthma, when repeated dosing with as much as a fivefold to tenfold increase in dosage is needed to reverse bronchoconstriction. This dose–response relationship is not relevant to the long-acting β_2-adrenergic agonists because use of these agents is confined to the management of chronic asthma. Both short- and long-acting agents protect against exercise-induced asthma, but the latter sustain this effect for at least 12 hours after a dose. Both short- and long-acting agents protect against the early fall in pulmonary function after exposure to allergen, but only the long-acting agents inhibit bronchoconstriction during the LAR.[40] This effect on the LAR is believed to result from a combination of functional antagonism and anti-inflammatory effects.

Adverse effects may occur after acute use (minutes to hours) or chronic regular use (weeks to years). Acute adverse effects are seen after oral and inhaled administration and are caused principally by β_2-receptor stimulation in skeletal muscle and vascular smooth muscle, producing tremors, reflex tachycardia, and headache, and β_1- and β_2-stimulation in the heart, resulting in tachycardia and palpitations. Other acute effects include activation of Na^+, K^+ adenosine triphosphatase in skeletal muscle (which may result in hypokalemia), gluconeogenesis, and increased insulin secretion (possibly enhancing hypokalemia). Tachyphylaxis to systemic effects usually occurs within 2 weeks with continued therapy.[41]

There has been concern in recent years about the potential for β_2-adrenergic agonists to worsen asthma with regular or excessive use. The package insert for these drugs states the maximum daily dosage as two inhalations four to six times daily. In one study, patients treated with fenoterol, two inhalations four times daily for 6 months, had worse asthma symptoms than patients on as-needed therapy,[42] and a follow-up study with this same drug has supported this finding.[42] In another study, patients who used excessive amounts of albuterol or fenoterol were found to have an increased risk of death or near death from asthma.[42] It is believed that the increased need for β-adrenergic therapy over days or months is an indication of worsening asthma rather than of toxicity from the drugs themselves. In addition, long-term, regular administration of β_2-adrenergic agonists can increase bronchial hyperreactivity,[42] diminish the duration of bronchoprotective effects,[43] and decrease the bronchodilator duration but not peak effect.[42] However, other studies have not shown tolerance or tachyphylaxis to the bronchoprotective or bronchodilator effects with regular use.[42] Because few studies report data on individual subjects, it is not known whether contributing factors are present that protect against or predispose certain asthmatic patients to this effect. These data indicate that short-acting β_2-adrenergic agonists should be used on demand rather than regularly scheduled in the chronic treatment of asthma symptoms. This will avoid the worsening of asthma symptoms described in several studies and provides a means of evaluating asthma control and the need for additional therapy.

It has been suggested that the deleterious effects from β_2-agonists (with a focus on albuterol) may result from the activity of the S-isomer of the drug. Albuterol exists as a racemic mixture of R-albuterol and S-albuterol. The biologically active form of albuterol, R-albuterol, is responsible for the therapeutic effects and the commonly seen adverse effects of albuterol, such as tremor and tachycardia. Studies in animals with S-isoproterenol, S-terbutaline, and S-albuterol have demonstrated an increase in airway hyperresponsiveness induced by histamine, PAF, leukotrienes, and antigen. These effects do not appear to be mediated by the β_2-receptor.[44] Several clinical trials have been completed and others are ongoing to evaluate the effect of R-albuterol in comparison with the albuterol racemate.[44] Long-term studies will be needed to determine whether use of R-albuterol provides a greater safety margin than racemic albuterol. It is expected that the first R-albuterol product will be approved by the U.S. Food and Drug Administration (FDA) in 1999.

In contrast to the short-acting agents, long-acting β_2-adrenergic agonists are not to be used on demand but rather are prescribed on a twice-daily basis and are described as a long-term control medication (rather than quick relief) by the NAEPP guidelines. In addition, salmeterol has a slower onset of action (10 minutes or more) than other short-acting inhaled β_2-agonists. The misconception that salmeterol has a rapid onset of action may have contributed to the approximately 20 deaths that occurred within 8 months after the release of salmeterol in the Unites States. Formoterol, but not salmeterol, appears to cause desensitization with prolonged (at least 4 weeks) use.[45] The clinical significance of this finding is not known because desensitization is not associated with a worsening of asthma control.[45] The long-acting agents may be used prophylactically for exercise-induced asthma or as a replacement for other oral bronchodilators (theophylline or oral β_2-adrenergic agonists). The NAEPP guidelines state that they should be used only in patients who are already taking an inhaled corticosteroid and continue to be symptomatic. Several studies with salmeterol and formoterol have confirmed that adding a long-acting β_2-agonist to low-dose inhaled corticosteroid therapy provides better control of symptoms than doubling the dosage of the inhaled corticosteroid.[45] Long-acting β_2-adrenergic drugs probably will replace other oral bronchodilators in most asthma treatment plans. However, syrup formulations of β_2-adrenergic agonists will continue to have a place in treating asthma in young children who cannot effectively use these drugs by the inhaled route.

Theophylline

Methylxanthines have been used to treat acute and chronic asthma for more than 50 years; theophylline is the primary drug. Dyphylline, caffeine, and theobromine (found in chocolate) are methylxanthines with much weaker bronchodilator properties than theophylline, and enprofylline, though more potent, has unacceptable cardiovascular effects. Salts of theophylline have been developed to improve solubility and absorption. Because theophylline absorption is related to lipophilic characteristics rather than water solubility, only the ethylenediamine salt (aminophylline), used for intravenous administration, is of clinical importance. Oral salt formulations (choline, calcium salicylate, sodium glycinate) simply contain less anhydrous theophylline by weight, and it is the fraction of theophylline in these dosage forms that determines the prescribed dosage.

Although theophylline has long been used to treat asthma, its complete mechanism of action is still largely unknown. Theophylline has well-known concentration-dependent bronchodilator effects, but the mechanism by which they occur has only recently become clear. Because adenosine is a potent bronchoconstrictor in asthmatic airways, it was previously thought that theophylline antagonism of adenosine-induced bronchoconstriction was the mechanism for the bronchodilator effects. This theory has been discarded because enprofylline, which does not antagonize adenosine, has similar bronchodilator effects to theophylline at approximately 1/4 to 1/6 the serum concentrations.[46]

Evidence is mounting that theophylline exerts its bronchodilator effects via inhibition of phosphodiesterase (PDE). PDE III, IV, and V catalyze the breakdown of intracellular cAMP and cyclic 3′,5′ guanosine monophosphate (cGMP), respectively. PDE isoenzymes may have differential expression depending on the cell type studied; PDE III, IV, and possibly V are present in smooth airway muscle, whereas PDE IV is the predominant isoenzyme in inflammatory cells. PDE III and IV inhibition increase cAMP, which opens maxi-K^+ channels. These channels assist in recovery and stability of excitable cells following activation; opening these channels contributes to smooth muscle relaxation. Because theophylline, a nonselective PDE inhibitor, minimally inhibits PDE at therapeutic concentrations and relaxes airways without modifying cyclic nucleotide levels, this potential mechanism, a popular theory several decades ago, has received little attention until recently. It has been suggested that PDE expression may be activated in asthmatic airways, thus enhancing the effect of theophylline. The fact that theophylline has bronchodilator activity in asthmatic but not nonasthmatic subjects provides foundation for this hypothesis. In addition, recent observations suggest that theophylline inhibits isoenzymes of PDE at clinically relevant therapeutic concentrations.[46]

Theophylline is now believed to have modest anti-inflammatory or immunomodulatory effects as well. Theophylline inhibits adenosine-stimulated release of mediators from mast cells at therapeutic serum concentrations. At low therapeutic serum concentrations, theophylline inhibits eosinophil activation and degranulation, decreases the total number of eosinophils beneath the basement membrane, and attenuates eosinophil cationic protein release from eosinophils after allergen challenge.[46]

The anti-inflammatory effects of theophylline at the cellular level may result largely from its actions on T lymphocytes. Studies in the last several years have focused on the effect of theophylline on $CD4^+$ and $CD8^+$ T cell activation and numbers. Theophylline withdrawal resulted in a fall in peripheral blood monocytes and activated $CD8^+$ T cells and a simultaneous increase in airway $CD4^+$ and $CD8^+$ T cells in one study. This effect was seen in patients with theophylline levels above 27.5 μmol/L (5 μg/mL) but not in patients with lower levels. In patients in whom theophylline was added, there was a decrease in epithelial $CD8^+$ T cells, although no change was noted in airway $CD4^+$ or $CD8^+$ T cells. In addition, after allergen challenge, theophylline decreases the number of peripheral $CD4^+$ and increases peripheral $CD8^+$ T cells and reduces activated eosinophils. These studies illustrate that theophylline modulates T-cell activity, possibly by altering the movement of T cells between the periphery and the airways, but the precise molecular mechanisms are not fully understood. The contribution to clinical efficacy is likewise unknown.[46]

Other related pharmacologic actions of theophylline include increased right and left ventricular ejection fraction, reduced fatigue of the diaphragmatic muscles (which may decrease work of breathing), decreased vascular permeability, and enhanced mucociliary clearance, although some of these effects have not been observed consistently in all studies.[47]

Theophylline is a weaker bronchodilator than are inhaled β_2-adrenergic agonists. However, like the β_2-adrenergic agonists, theophylline is a functional antagonist and can inhibit bronchospasm induced by various stimuli, including histamine, methacholine, exercise, and distilled water, in a serum concentration–related manner.[47] Protection has been noted at serum concentrations less than 55 μmol/L (10 μg/mL) for exercise- and methacholine-induced bronchoconstriction. However, results of studies examining the long-term effects of theophylline in reducing bronchial hyperresponsiveness measured by bronchoprovocation with histamine or methacholine have conflicted.[47] It appears that theophylline is effective in preventing the fall in airway function during both IAR and LAR after inhaled allergen and inhibiting the subsequent increase in airway responsiveness to histamine.[48] The effect seen with theophylline is similar to that after inhaled cromolyn from an MDI.[48]

Theophylline is administered orally, intravenously, and rectally, although the latter is rarely used because of unpredictable absorption. Theophylline has no antiasthma effects when inhaled. Familiarity with the pharmacokinetics of theophylline is essential to safe and effective use of this drug. In addition, recognizing that differences in the formulations of slow-release products can result in significant differences in the rate and extent of absorption is also important. Clinicians who use this drug must stay abreast of new information about therapeutic efficacy and toxicity (pharmacokinetics of slow-release formulations, drug interactions, combination therapy with other antiasthma therapy). Inappropriate use leading to toxicity can have dire consequences for the patient.

The therapeutic range was previously defined as 55 to 110 μmol/L (10 to 20 μg/mL); currently, a lower range of

Table 36.6 ▪ Clinically Significant Drug Interactions with Theophylline

Drug	Type of Interaction	Effect[a]
Adenosine	Theophylline blocks adenosine receptors.	Higher dosages of adenosine may be needed to achieve desired effect.
Alcohol	A single large dose of alcohol (3 mL/kg whiskey) decreases theophylline clearance for up to 24 hr.	30% increase.
Allopurinol	Decreases theophylline clearance at allopurinol dosages ≤600 mg/day.	25% increase.
Aminoglutethimide	Increases theophylline clearance by inducing microsomal enzyme activity.	25% decrease.
Carbamazepine	Similar to aminoglutethimide.	30% decrease.
Cimetidine	Decreases theophylline clearance by inhibiting cytochrome P-450 1A2.	70% increase.
Ciprofloxacin	Similar to cimetidine.	40% increase.
Clarithromycin	Similar to erythromycin.	25% increase.
Diazepam	Benzodiazepines increase CNS concentrations of adenosine, a potent CNS depressant, whereas theophylline blocks adenosine receptors.	Larger benzodiazepine dosages may be needed to produce desired level of sedation. Discontinuing theophylline without reducing diazepam dosage may result in respiratory depression.
Disulfiram	Decreases theophylline clearance by inhibiting hydroxylation and demethylation.	50% increase.
Enoxacin	Similar to cimetidine.	300% increase.
Ephedrine	Synergistic CNS effects.	Increased frequency of nausea, nervousness, and insomnia.
Erythromycin	Erythromycin metabolite decreases theophylline clearance by inhibiting cytochrome P-450 3A3.	35% increase. Erythromycin steady-state serum concentrations decrease by a similar amount.
Estrogen	Estrogen-containing oral contraceptives decrease theophylline clearance in a dose-dependent fashion. The effect of progesterone on theophylline clearance is unknown.	30% increase.
Flurazepam	Similar to diazepam.	Similar to diazepam.
Fluvoxamine	Similar to cimetidine.	Similar to cimetidine.
Halothane	Halothane sensitizes the myocardium to endogenous catecholamines; theophylline increases endogenous catecholamine release.	Increased risk of ventricular arrhythmias.
Interferon, human recombinant α-A	Decreases theophylline clearance.	100% increase.
Isoproterenol (IV)	Increases theophylline clearance.	20% decrease.
Ketamine	Pharmacologic.	May lower theophylline seizure threshold.

(continued)

27.5 to 82.5 μmol/L (5 to 15 μg/mL) is standard.[1] However, whereas some studies have documented increased asthma symptoms when the serum theophylline concentration (STC) drops below 55 μmol/L (10 μg/mL), others have noted a flattening of the serum concentration–response curve in patients at STCs above approximately 82.5 μmol/L (15 μg/mL). It seems reasonable to conclude that the majority of patients will have the greatest improvement in pulmonary function when STCs are 55 to 82.5 μmol/L (10 to 15 μg/mL) but some will have adequate response at lower concentrations and others will need higher concentrations for maximum effect.[46]

Theophylline pharmacokinetics depend largely on factors influencing hepatic metabolism after 1 year of age, when approximately 90% of a dose is metabolized in the liver. Below 1 year of age, nearly half a dose is excreted as unchanged theophylline in the urine. *N*-Demethylation and hydroxylation are the major metabolic pathways and are regulated by several P-450 enzymes including 1A2, 2E1, and 3A3. Both pathways are saturable within the therapeutic range, and patients with high initial clearance rates may be at greatest risk. Factors influencing hepatic metabolism of theophylline include age, concurrent diseases, and drug interactions. Hyperthyroidism, cystic fibrosis, smoking, and ingestion of a high-protein, low-carbohydrate diet are common conditions known to increase theophylline clearance, whereas age less than 1 year or over 60 years, congestive heart failure, prolonged fever (higher than 102°F), hypothyroidism, and liver disease are some conditions known to decrease theophylline clearance. Ninety drugs have been evaluated for their effect on theophylline clearance, and approximately half have clinically important interactions (Tables 36.6 and 36.7).[49] Theophylline rarely affects the pharmacokinetics of other drugs.

Table 36.6 *(continued)*

Drug	Type of Interaction	Effect[a]
Lithium	Theophylline increases lithium renal clearance.	Lithium dosage needed to achieve a therapeutic serum concentration increased an average of 60%.
Lorazepam	Similar to diazepam.	Similar to diazepam.
Methotrexate	Decreases theophylline clearance.	20% increase after low-dose MTX; higher-dose MTX may have a greater effect.
Mexiletine	Similar to disulfiram.	80% increase.
Midazolam	Similar to diazepam.	Similar to diazepam.
Moricizine	Increases theophylline clearance.	25% decrease.
Pancuronium	Theophylline may antagonize nondepolarizing neuromuscular blocking effects, possibly because of phosphodiesterase inhibition.	Larger pancuronium dosage may be needed to achieve neuromuscular blockade.
Pentoxifylline	Decreases theophylline clearance.	30% increase.
Phenobarbital	Similar to aminoglutethimide.	25% decrease after 2 wk of concurrent phenobarbital.
Phenytoin	Phenytoin increases theophylline clearance by increasing microsomal enzyme activity. Theophylline decreases phenytoin absorption.	Serum theophylline and phenytoin concentrations decrease about 40%.
Propafenone	Decreases theophylline clearance; pharmacologic interaction.	40% increase. β_2-blocking effect may decrease the efficacy of theophylline.
Propranolol	Similar to cimetidine; pharmacologic interaction.	100% increase. β_2-blocking effect may decrease efficacy of theophylline.
Rifampin	Increases theophylline clearance by increasing cytochrome P-450 1A2 and 3A3 activity.	20–40% decrease.
Sulfinpyrazone	Increases theophylline clearance by increasing demethylation and hydroxylation. Decreases renal theophylline clearance.	20% decrease.
Tacrine	Similar to cimetidine; also increases renal theophylline clearance.	90% increase.
Thiabendazole	Decreases theophylline clearance.	190% increase.
Ticlopidine	Decreases theophylline clearance.	60% increase.
Troleandomycin	Similar to erythromycin.	33–100% increase depending on troleandomycin dosage.
Verapamil	Similar to disulfiram.	20% increase.
Zafirlukast	Decreases theophylline clearance.	120% increase.
Zileuton	Decreases theophylline clearance.	73% increase.

Source: Updated with permission from Hendeles L, Jenkins J, Temple R. Revised FDA labeling guidelines for theophylline oral dosage forms. Pharmacotherapy 15:409–427, 1995.

CNS, central nervous system; *MTX,* methotrexate.

[a]Average effect on steady-state theophylline concentration or other clinical effect for pharmacologic interactions. Individual patients may experience larger changes in serum theophylline concentration than the value listed.

Dosing schemes and monitoring guidelines for theophylline administration in acute and chronic asthma are presented in Table 36.8 and Figure 36.8, respectively.[46,50] However, the dosages listed are merely guidelines for attaining serum concentrations within the therapeutic range and should be confirmed with serum concentration measurement.

Adverse effects to theophylline generally are mild and temporary when serum concentrations are less than 110 μmol/L (20 μg/mL) and include caffeinelike effects such as nausea and vomiting, headache, and insomnia. The severity of adverse effects worsens as the serum concentration exceeds 110 μmol/L (20 μg/mL).[51] However, minor symptoms of toxicity such as nausea and vomiting may not precede more severe toxicity and cannot be relied on as a dosing endpoint. Only serum concentration measurement can reliably predict the potential for severe or life-threatening toxicity. Effects not related to serum concentration are uncommon. Controlled studies and meta-analyses have failed to show an adverse effect of theophylline on behavior and school performance.[46]

Theophylline toxicity is not as clearly related to serum concentrations as was once thought. It is now evident that the method of intoxication (acute, chronic, acute on chronic) is extremely relevant to the morbidity from theophylline toxicity. Acute intoxication is defined as a single large (greater than 10 mg/kg) ingestion or multiple ingestions within 24 hours, chronic intoxication is defined as excessive doses taken over a period of more than 24 hours, and acute on chronic intoxication is defined as large ingestions in addition to therapeutic chronic dosing. Acute on chronic intoxication presents similarly to chronic intoxication with regard to life-threatening events.[46] Dosing errors by parent or physician are the most common reason for intoxication, particularly chronic intoxication. The majority of dosing errors involve theophylline tablets or capsules that result in dosages above age and weight recommendations or calculation errors in converting aminophylline dosing to theophylline equivalents.[46]

Patients with acute single overdosage have higher serum concentrations and may exhibit hypotension, hypokalemia, or low serum bicarbonate and are less likely to suffer seizures or death than those with chronic or acute on chronic overdosing. Generalized seizures and arrhythmias often develop in patients with chronic overdosing at serum concentrations of 165 to 385 μmol/L (30 to 70 μg/mL);[52] patients over 60 years and children less than 2 years of age are at greatest risk.[46,53] In contrast, life-threatening events usually do not occur in cases of acute overdose unless the serum concentration exceeds 550 μmol/L (100 μg/mL).[46] Treatments for toxicity include oral activated charcoal, phenobarbital or diazepam for seizures, antiarrhythmics for life-threatening arrhythmias, and charcoal hemoperfusion.

Table 36.7 ▪ Drugs That Have Been Documented Not to Interact with Theophylline or That Produce No Clinically Significant Interaction with Theophylline

Albuterol (systemic and inhaled)	Medroxyprogesterone
Amoxicillin	Methylprednisolone
Ampicillin (with or without sulbactam)	Metoprolol
Atenolol	Metronidazole
Azithromycin	Montelukast
Caffeine (dietary ingestion)	Nadolol
Cefaclor	Nifedipine
Co-trimoxazole (trimethoprim and sulfamethoxazole)	Nizatidine
Diltiazem	Norfloxacin
Dirithromycin	Ofloxacin
Donepezil	Omeprazole
Enflurane	Pantoprazole
Famotidine	Prednisone, prednisolone
Felodipine	Ranitidine
Finasteride	Rifabutin
Hydrocortisone	Roxithromycin
Influenza vaccine	Sorbitol (purgative doses do not inhibit theophylline absorption)
Isoflurane	Sucralfate
Isoniazid	Terbinafine
Isradipine	Terbutaline (systemic)
Ketoconazole	Terfenadine
Lansoprazole	Tetracycline
Levofloxacin	Tocainide
Lomefloxacin	Trovafloxacin
Mebendazole	

Source: Updated with permission from Hendeles L, Jenkins J, Temple R. Revised FDA labeling guidelines for theophylline oral dosage forms. Pharmacotherapy 15:409–427, 1995.

Until inhaled β_2-adrengeric agonists were introduced in the early 1970s and 1980s, theophylline had a well-established role in treating acute asthma. Many well-designed studies have been published demonstrating that adding theophylline to optimal inhaled β_2-adrenergic agonists plus systemic corticosteroids in both the ED and in hospitalized patients provides no added benefit over optimal treatment with inhaled β_2-adrenergic agonists plus systemic corticosteroids alone in acute severe asthma.[46] Therefore, intravenous theophylline should be reserved for patients who do not respond to high-dose inhaled β_2-adrenergic agonists and systemic corticosteroids.[46]

Similarly, theophylline's role in treating chronic asthma has also lessened with the introduction of potent inhaled corticosteroids, long-acting inhaled β_2 agonists, and leukotriene modifiers. Despite the regular use of inhaled corticosteroids, some patients have fewer symptoms, less inhaled β-adrenergic agonist use, and fewer exacerbations necessitating systemic corticosteroids with the addition of theophylline.[47] The NAEPP guidelines reserve theophylline as second-line therapy in mild persistent asthma and as a second-line choice after long-acting inhaled β_2-agonist therapy in patients already treated with inhaled corticosteroids.[1]

Anticholinergics

Anticholinergic drugs have been used to treat asthmalike symptoms for more than 400 years. Until the introduction of quaternary ammonium derivatives such as ipratropium, glycopyrrolate, atropine methonitrate, and oxitropium, central nervous systemic adverse effects limited their use. Recent information suggests that acetylcholine stimulation of the muscarinic receptor may activate an inhibitory G protein and decrease the activity of adenylate cyclase, resulting in decreased cAMP, causing smooth muscle contraction. Two other mechanisms include activation of phospholipase C via a different G protein, which releases stores of intracellular calcium, producing smooth muscle contraction, and formation of a second messenger, diacylglycerol, which activates protein kinase C and causes a slow and prolonged contraction.[54]

The parasympathetic nervous system is largely responsible for the control of baseline airway caliber. Therefore, anticholinergic drugs, which are competitive antagonists rather than functional antagonists, are most useful in patients whose symptoms are caused by excessive cholinergic stimulation. Unfortunately, it is not possible to predict whose asthma symptoms may be caused by excessive cholinergic stimulation. Because most mediators, such as histamine, allergens, and exercise, cause bronchoconstriction only partially through cholinergic stimulation, anticholinergics are less effective than β_2-adrenergic agonists and theophylline, which are functional antagonists.

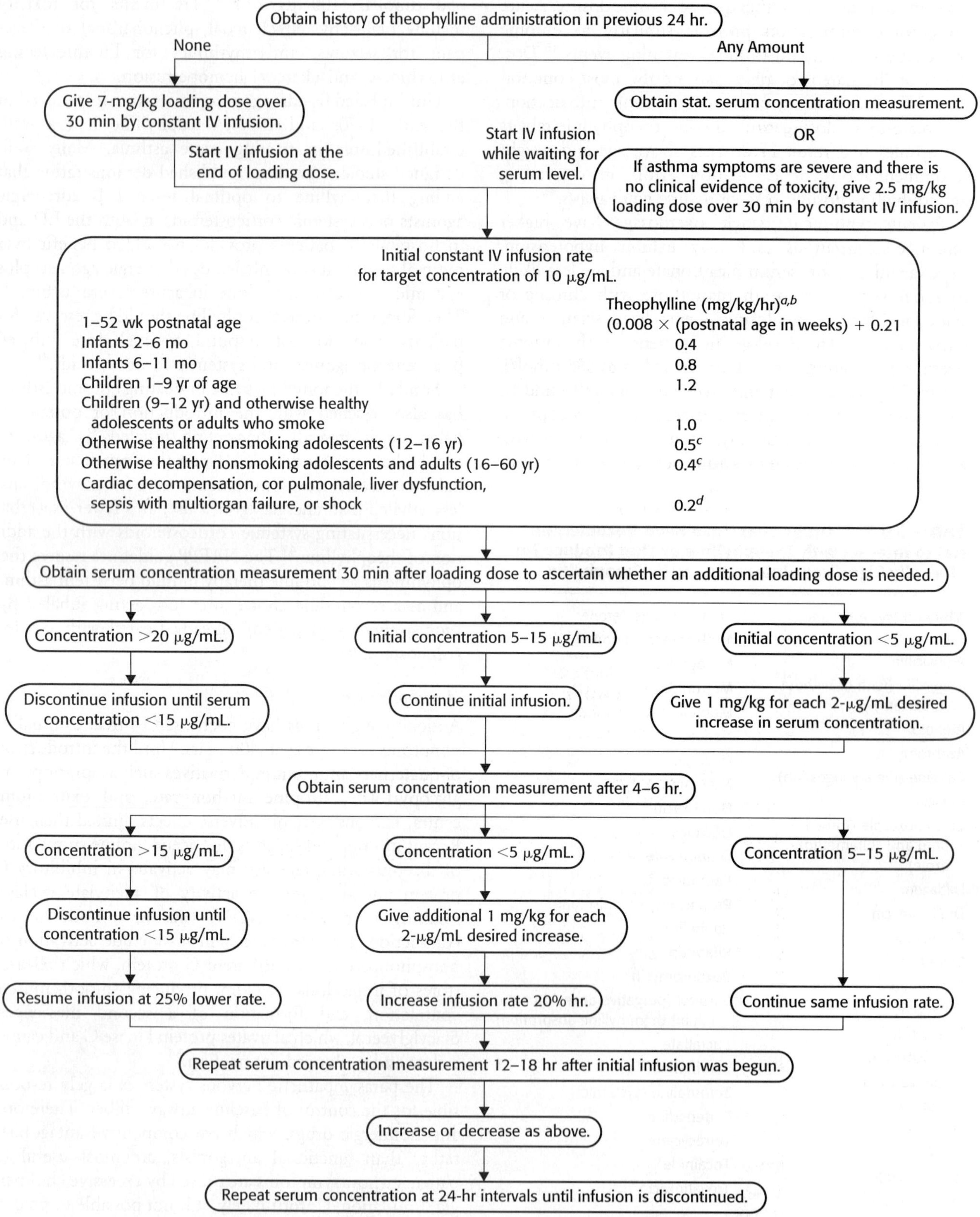

[a]Aminophylline = Theophylline dosage ÷ 0.8.
[b]Use ideal body weight for obese patients; lower initial dosage may be needed for patients receiving other drugs that alter theophylline clearance.
[c]Not to exceed 900 mg/day unless serum concentration levels indicate the need for a larger dosage.
[d]Not to exceed 400 mg/day unless serum concentration levels indicate the need for a larger dosage.

Figure 36.8. Algorithm for intravenous theophylline use in acute asthma. (Adapted from Blake K. Theophylline. In: Murphy S, Kelly HW. Pediatric asthma. New York: Marcel Dekker, 1999:363–431, with permission.)

Currently available anticholinergics are nonselective competitive antagonists at the muscarinic receptor. Recently, five muscarinic receptor subtypes have been discovered; three receptors have been characterized pharmacologically (Fig. 36.9).[54,55] Stimulation of M_1 receptors on the terminal of parasympathetic preganglionic neurons facilitates cholinergic transmission. M_2 receptors, located on the postganglionic terminal, inhibit acetylcholine release when stimulated and thus function as inhibitory feedback receptors. It is believed that abnormal functioning or absence of the M_2 receptors is responsible for asthma induced by β-blocker drugs[54] because blockade of the β_2-adrenergic receptor on cholinergic nerves stimulates release of acetylcholine, which is normally turned off by

Table 36.8 ▪ Dosage Guidelines for Theophylline in Children Older Than 6 Months and Adults Who Have No Risk Factors for Decreased Theophylline Clearance[a]

Variable	Weight-Adjusted and Maximal Dosage	Comments	Dosage Adjustment
Initial dosage	~10 mg/kg body weight/day; maximum 300 mg/day	If initial dosage is tolerated, increase the dosage no sooner than 3 days later to the first increment.	
First increment	~13 mg/kg/day; maximum 450 mg/day	If the first incremental increase is tolerated, increase the dosage no sooner than 3 days later to the second increment.	
Second increment	~16 mg/kg/day; maximum 600 mg/day	Measure the peak serum concentration after at least 3 days at the highest tolerated dosage.[b]	
Serum theophylline concentration (μg/mL)			
<10			Increase approximately 25%.
10–15			Maintain dosage if tolerated.
15.1–19.9			Consider a reduction of approximately 10%.[c]
20–25			Withhold next dose, then resume treatment with next lower dosage increment.
>25			Withhold next 2 doses, then resume treatment with initial dosage or lower dosage.

Source: Reprinted with permission from Weinberger M, Hendeles L. Theophylline in asthma. N Engl J Med 334:1380–1388, 1996.

[a]For infants 6 wk to 6 mo of age, the initial daily dosage is calculated according to the following regression equation: Dosage (mg/kg/day) = (0.2)(Age in weeks) + 5.0. Subsequent dosage increases in this age group should be based on peak serum concentrations measured no sooner than 3 days after the start of therapy. The guidelines listed use dosages that are lower than in previous guidelines to account for the most recent assessment of population dosage needs and to minimize the risk of even minor adverse effects. With the use of these guidelines, one to two measurements of serum theophylline usually are sufficient to determine the dosage needed, with annual checks thereafter unless clinical indications suggest the need for more frequent assessment.

[b]The length of time to the peak serum concentration depends on the rate of absorption, rate of elimination, and dosing interval.

[c]This decreases the likelihood of side effects caused by fluctuations in the absorption or elimination rate that may result in serum concentrations above 20 μg/mL and is especially important for patients who need dosages higher than those used in the second increment.

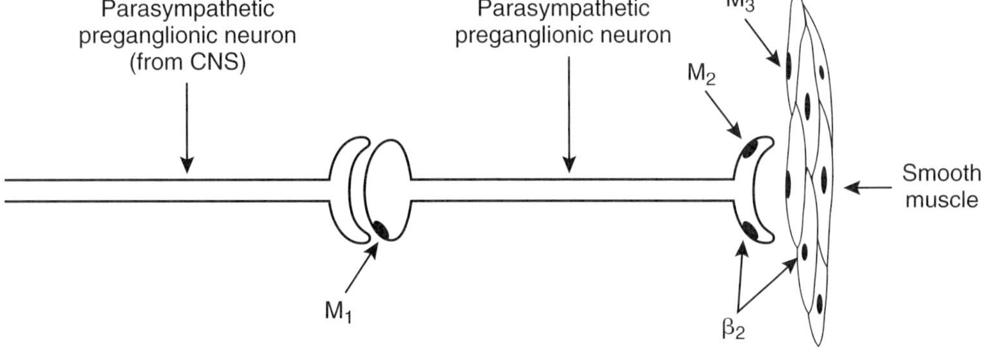

Figure 36.9. Diagram of parasympathetic nervous system illustrating location of M_1, M_2, M_3, and β_2 receptors. *CNS,* central nervous system.

the M_2 receptor. Dysfunction of the M_2 receptor allows continued release of acetylcholine, resulting in exaggerated bronchoconstriction. M_3 receptors located on airway smooth muscle also facilitate cholinergic transmission. Therefore, selective blockers at the M_1 and M_3 receptors probably would have greater benefit than nonselective muscarinic receptor blockers. Antagonism of M_3 receptors, also located on mucus glands, will cause drying of secretions, so drugs must be developed for inhalation use to avoid unwanted systemic adverse effects.[55]

With the availability of ipratropium bromide, a quaternary amine, for nebulization, there is no longer any reason to use nebulized atropine sulfate. Atropine sulfate is rapidly absorbed when inhaled, resulting in dose-related adverse effects including tachycardia, meiosis causing blurred vision, difficulty swallowing, and flushing. Ipratropium is remarkably free of unwanted adverse effects because of its minimal systemic absorption. Adverse effects may include dry mouth, irritated throat, or bitter taste.

Anticholinergics do not produce maximal bronchodilation when compared with β_2-adrenergic agonists in asthmatics but do have a longer duration of effect. Maximum bronchodilation occurs in 1.5 to 2 hours, but 50% of the eventual maximum occurs within 3 to 5 minutes and 80% within 30 minutes,[56] which is comparable clinically to the time of peak effect (30 minutes) with inhaled β_2-adrenergic agonists. Several inhaled anticholinergic compounds are under development that have a duration of effect of approximately 12 hours. The NAEPP guidelines recommend the use of nebulized anticholinergic therapy in combination with β_2-agonist therapy to treat acute severe asthma.[1] Adding several doses (versus a single dose) of an anticholinergic decreases the risk of hospital admissions by approximately 30%.[57] In patients who are hospitalized, the combination of anticholinergic and β_2-agonist therapy should be continued for at least 36 hours to reduce the length of hospitalization.[58] The NAEPP guidelines do not include therapy with anticholinergics to manage chronic asthma because more effective drugs are available.[1] Limited data indicate that anticholinergics may be effective in psychogenic asthma.

Anti-Inflammatory Agents

Cromolyn and Nedocromil

Cromolyn sodium has been available for treating asthma for nearly three decades, and nedocromil sodium has been available in the last decade. Though structurally distinct and possibly pharmacologically distinct, these two drugs often are discussed together. Neither drug has acute bronchodilator effects. The exact mechanisms of action for each are largely unknown, but both can inhibit the IgE-mediated release of mediators from mast cells. However, this effect seems to vary depending on the species and the cell type tested, and other drugs with greater mast cell stabilizing activity do not have therapeutic efficacy.[54] Cromolyn also is effective in preventing mast cell degranulation induced by nonimmunologic stimuli such as phospholipase A, dextran, and polymyxin B. The mechanism by which cromolyn and nedocromil inhibit mediator release at the cellular level is unclear but probably involves regulation of intracellular calcium by phosphorylation of a specific membrane protein that inhibits calcium influx into the cell. Cromolyn and nedocromil also inhibit the release of mediators from eosinophils, alveolar macrophages, neutrophils, and monocytes.[59] Other effects regulated by cromolyn include inhibition of PDE, modification of the vagal reflex, and inhibition of irritant receptors. Cromolyn and nedocromil also inhibit chemotaxis of inflammatory mediators and may inhibit release of inflammatory neuropeptides, which induce bronchoconstriction through efferent cholinergic pathways.[54,59]

Neither cromolyn nor nedocromil is effective orally or intravenously. Cromolyn and nedocromil, which are systemically absorbed, are largely excreted unchanged in the urine or the bile. The half-life for clinical effectiveness is short (less than 4 hours), so these drugs must be administered three to four times daily.[59] In some patients, particularly children, twice-daily dosing may also be effective. Symptoms should be brought under control with three- or four-times-daily dosing before further dosage reductions are tried. Adverse effects of cromolyn and nedocromil are rare and most often include transient bronchospasm, cough, and dry throat. Bronchospasm is relieved quickly by an inhaled β_2-adrenergic agonist. Infrequent adverse effects include anaphylaxis, generalized or facial dermatitis, myositis, gastroenteritis, and immunologic reactions in the lung. Because of the lack of systemic effects, cromolyn is often regarded as the safest anti-inflammatory therapy for asthma for use in children and during pregnancy.

Both cromolyn and nedocromil inhibit the IAR and LAR to inhaled allergen after a single dose, in contrast to inhaled corticosteroids, which inhibit only the LAR after a single dose. They also prevent exercise-induced asthma (though to a much lesser extent than inhaled β_2-adrenergic agonists), and inhaled β_2-agonists are the drugs of choice for exercise prophylaxis. Despite the variety of effects, cromolyn and nedocromil are most valued for their ability to decrease airway hyperresponsiveness, measured by histamine- or methacholine-induced bronchoconstriction, when given for at least 12 weeks. Cromolyn and nedocromil have effects similar in magnitude to that of low-dose inhaled corticosteroids (less than 400 μg/day beclomethasone equivalent) on airway reactivity, although their effects have not been found to be uniformly consistent. This variability may indicate that patients may be responders or nonresponders to these drugs. There appears to be no benefit to adding cromolyn or nedocromil to high-dose inhaled corticosteroids (more than 1000 μg/day beclomethasone equivalent) or oral corticosteroids or theophylline. However, some patients on moderate dosages of inhaled corticosteroids may achieve a reduction in corticosteroid dosage with added cromolyn or nedocromil.[41,59]

Cromolyn and nedocromil are not indicated for relieving acute symptoms of asthma because neither has bronchodilator effects. Although clinical effects may be noted within 1 week of starting therapy, 4 weeks generally is needed to determine whether a patient is responding to therapy. The NAEPP guidelines[1] recommend cromolyn or nedocromil only in mild persistent asthma, and they may be the preferred initial anti-inflammatory therapy in children.

Leukotriene Modifiers

The leukotriene modifiers (zileuton, zafirlukast, and montelukast) are the first new pharmacologic class of drugs for treating asthma in more than 20 years. The leukotrienes are released from inflammatory cells in the airway and interact with specific receptors to cause bronchoconstriction, airway hyperresponsiveness, increased microvascular permeability leading to edema, leukocyte activation, eosinophilia, and enhanced mucus secretion. Leukotrienes are formed when the enzyme 5-lipoxygenase, in conjunction with the co-factor 5-lipoxygenase–activating protein, metabolizes arachidonic acid. An unstable intermediate product (LTA_4) is formed initially. Further conversion occurs to form the cysteinyl leukotrienes (CysLTs) LTC_4, LTD_4, and LTE_4 or, via a separate pathway, to form LTB_4. The bronchoconstriction produced by LTD_4 has been estimated to be 1000 to 10,000 times greater than the activity of histamine and methacholine. LTC_4, LTD_4, and LTE_4 are highly potent inducers of airway smooth muscle contraction and bronchoconstriction, with an approximate equal potency between LTC_4 and LTD_4; however, LTE_4 is only about 10% as potent.[60] LTC_4 is rapidly (minutes) converted to LTD_4, which is then converted to LTE_4 over approximately 30 minutes.[61] LTC_4, LTD_4, and LTE_4 act by binding to a common receptor, $CysLT_1$, but because LTD_4 is extremely potent and has the longest half-life of the leukotrienes, it has been the focus of antimediator drug development. Leukotriene modifiers block leukotriene-mediated effects, either by preventing the enzymatic conversion of arachidonic acid to LTA_4, as with zileuton, or by blocking the binding of leukotrienes to the $CysLT_1$ receptor site, in the case of zafirlukast and montelukast.

The leukotriene modifiers are administered orally and do not have clinically significant effects when inhaled. The pharmacokinetics and adverse effects differ significantly between zileuton, zafirlukast, and montelukast. Zileuton is dosed four times daily, zafirlukast twice daily, and montelukast once daily. Montelukast should be dosed at bedtime to provide the highest serum concentrations of montelukast during the night and early morning hours, when asthma symptoms tend to be worst. Montelukast and zafirlukast are approved for use in children as young as 6 or 7 years old, respectively. Zafirlukast bioavailability is significantly reduced by concomitant food ingestion, so it must be dosed 1 hour before or 2 hours after a meal. Drug interactions occur with zileuton and zafirlukast but to date have not been found with montelukast. Zileuton decreases warfarin and theophylline clearance, and zafirlukast decreases the clearance of warfarin, corticosteroids, theophylline (rare cases reported), and possibly other drugs metabolized by the cytochrome P-450 2C9 isoenzyme, such as, tolbutamide, phenytoin, and carbamazepine.[62]

Zileuton can cause liver dysfunction, and liver function monitoring is recommended before therapy begins, every month for the first 3 months, and every 3 months for the next 9 months. Reports of Churg–Strauss syndrome, characterized by eosinophilia, pulmonary infiltrates, and myocardial dysfunction, have occurred in patients treated with zafirlukast and montelukast who were being weaned from oral corticosteroid therapy. It is believed that this syndrome is being unmasked by the withdrawal of oral corticosteroid therapy rather than being caused by zafirlukast and montelukast because the syndrome also has been observed after treatment with inhaled corticosteroids during oral corticosteroid withdrawal.[62] Given the convenience of once-daily dosing, the lack of food and drug interactions, and approval for use in children, montelukast is the preferred leukotriene modifier for use in patients with persistent asthma.

The leukotriene modifiers are effective in attenuating induced asthma and all have similar clinical efficacy in asthma treatment. After allergen inhalation, these drugs attenuate the IAR and LAR by approximately 50% after a single dose but are not effective in inhibiting the increased airway hyperresponsiveness that occurs 24 hours later. Similarly, these drugs attenuate the fall in pulmonary function after exercise after a single dose by 50 to 80%, but significant bronchospasm can still occur at the end of the dosing interval.[60] In asthmatic patients with aspirin sensitivity, leukotriene modifiers are extremely effective in preventing bronchoconstriction, which can occur after ingestion of aspirin or NSAIDs.[60] Clinical trials indicate that therapy with leukotriene modifiers can improve pulmonary function by approximately 10 to 12%, reduce inhaled β_2-agonist use by 30%, and decrease nocturnal awakenings caused by asthma by 30%.[60] However, in these studies, significant asthma symptoms remained when leukotriene modifiers were used as monotherapy. Most published clinical trials evaluated these drugs in patients with moderate to severe persistent asthma, however, so it is not surprising that these drugs did not provide complete control of asthma symptoms. These drugs are less effective than low-dose inhaled corticosteroid therapy (beclomethasone 400 μg/day), but it appears that certain patients achieve significant improvement in pulmonary function comparable to that obtained with inhaled corticosteroids.[63]

These drugs currently have no role in treating acute asthma, and it is not clear where these drugs should be used in the management of chronic asthma. The NAEPP guidelines currently recommend using leukotriene modifiers as single-drug therapy to treat mild persistent asthma as an alternative after considering therapy with inhaled corticosteroids, cromolyn, or nedocromil. There is evidence that leukotriene modifiers may provide additive effects to inhaled corticosteroid therapy, and the combination of a leukotriene modifier with low-dose inhaled

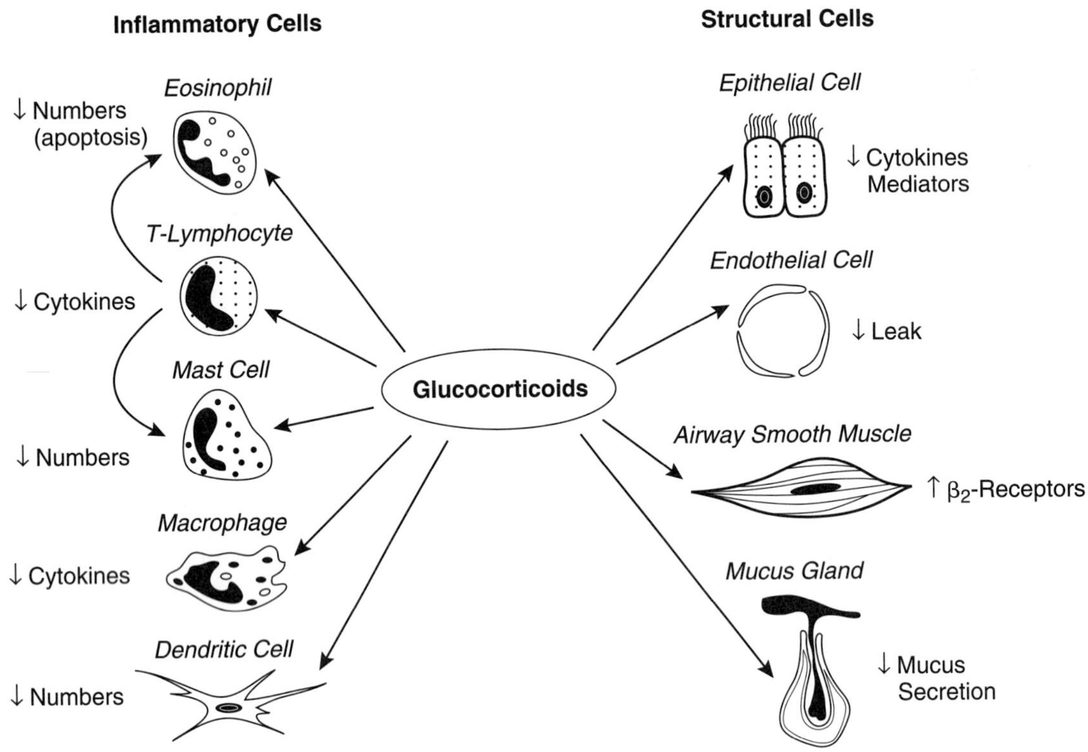

Figure 36.10. Effects of corticosteroids on inflammatory and structural cells involved in asthmatic inflammation. (Reprinted from Barnes PJ. Efficacy of inhaled corticosteroids in asthma. J Allergy Clin Immunol 102:531–538, 1998, with permission.)

corticosteroid may be preferable in some patients to increasing the inhaled corticosteroid dosage.[64] In addition, these drugs may be used to decrease the dosage of inhaled corticosteroids while maintaining control of asthma symptoms. Probably the greatest advantage of leukotriene modifiers is that they are available in oral dosage forms. Studies indicate that patients prefer and are more adherent with oral than inhaled asthma therapy.[65,66]

Corticosteroids

With the new emphasis on anti-inflammatory therapy, corticosteroids, particularly inhaled, are now a cornerstone in asthma treatment. Inhaled anti-inflammatory agents are recommended in all asthmatic patients who need regular inhaled bronchodilator treatments. Systemic corticosteroids are reserved for severe persistent asthma and acute exacerbations.

SYSTEMIC. Corticosteroids have been used to treat asthma for more than 40 years. Structural changes to cortisone have resulted in synthetic corticosteroids with enhanced potencies and prolonged duration of action. Cortisone itself is inactive and must be interconverted at the 11-ketone group to a hydroxy molecule via metabolic pathways to its active form, cortisol or hydrocortisone, just as prednisone must be converted to prednisolone. The specific mechanism of action of corticosteroids is not well established despite their long history in asthma treatment, but many of their biochemical actions are known.

Corticosteroids have many actions that may contribute to their effectiveness in controlling inflammation (Fig. 36.10).[67] After the drug penetrates the cell wall, a number of complex steps involving activation and binding of the corticosteroid receptor and its subunits are necessary. Ultimately, binding to a specific sequence of DNA within the nucleus, called the glucocorticoid responsive element (GRE), occurs, resulting in increased transcription of genes coding for anti-inflammatory proteins.[68] Other effects independent of the GRE include inhibiting the expression of multiple genes coding for inflammatory proteins through action on transcription factors such as nuclear factor-κB, activator protein-1, and the transcription coactivator cAMP response element binding protein. The result is conformational changes in DNA structure that can prevent gene expression of inflammatory proteins.[68]

Corticosteroids are known to prevent and reverse downregulation of β_2-receptors and induce increases of receptor density. Lymphocyte, eosinophil, monocyte, and basophil circulating cell counts are reduced, cytokine-mediated eosinophil survival is inhibited, and eosinophil and neutrophil chemotaxis are reduced. Physiologic effects of corticosteroids include inhibition of microvascular leakage and, of particular relevance to asthma, reduction of bronchial hyperresponsiveness.[69]

Because of their structural modifications, the various corticosteroids differ in their potencies and durations of action (Table 36.9). These effects in turn influence their recommended dosages and the risk of adverse effects, as do their pharmacokinetic parameters. Corticosteroids are generally well absorbed after oral administration.

A slow onset of action and slow dissipation of effects, consistent with clinical responses by patients with asthma, is a characteristic feature of corticosteroid pharmacodynamics. Effects after a single oral dose may not occur for 3 hours, with maximal effects not reached for 9 to 12 hours.[41] Certain drug and disease interactions can affect corticosteroid effects (Table 36.10).[70]

Prolonged use of systemically administered corticosteroids is limited by adverse effects (Table 36.11). These can be severe and debilitating and necessitate use of the lowest possible dosages. However, limited short courses may be necessary for treating acute exacerbations. Typically, 30 to 80 mg/day of prednisolone (or equivalent) is administered for 3 to 10 days depending on response, with tapering of the dosage needed only after approximately 2 weeks or more of therapy. There is no difference in efficacy between oral and intravenous corticosteroid administration, and oral therapy is preferred because it is less invasive.[1]

Table 36.9 ▪ Relative Potencies and Equivalent Dosages of Corticosteroids Commonly Used to Treat Asthma

Corticosteroid	Relative Anti-Inflammatory Potency	Equivalent Dosage (mg)
Hydrocortisone	1	20
Prednisolone	4	5
Methylprednisolone	5	4
Dexamethasone	25	0.75

Table 36.10 ▪ Potential Drug Interactions with Corticosteroids

Interacting Medication, Disease State, or Factor	Effect on Corticosteroid
Antacids	Decreased bioavailability
Ketoconazole	Impaired elimination
Erythromycin, troleandomycin	Impaired methylprednisolone elimination
Oral contraceptives	Impaired elimination
Hypothyroidism	Possibly impaired elimination
Aminoglutethimide	Enhanced elimination
Carbamazepine	Enhanced elimination
Ephedrine	Enhanced elimination
Phenobarbital	Enhanced elimination
Phenytoin	Enhanced elimination
Rifampin	Enhanced elimination
Hyperthyroidism	Possibly enhanced elimination

Source: Reprinted with permission from Szefler SJ. Glucocorticoid therapy for asthma: clinical pharmacology. J Allergy Clin Immunol 88:147–165, 1991.

Table 36.11 ▪ Adverse Effects of Systemic Corticosteroid Therapy

Acne
Adrenal suppression and insufficiency
Avascular necrosis of the femoral head
Behavioral disturbances
Cushingoid habitus (moon facies, buffalo hump, central obesity)
Ecchymosis
Fluid and electrolyte imbalances
Growth suppression
Hirsutism
Hyperglycemia
Hypertension
Increased susceptibility to infection
Myopathy
Osteoporosis
Peptic ulcers
Posterior subcapsular cataracts
Striae

If maintenance oral corticosteroids are needed to control chronic symptoms, it is important that the lowest effective dosages be given and that therapy be reevaluated periodically to minimize the patient's risk of severe adverse effects. Alternate-day regimens, as compared to daily doses, pose a somewhat lower risk of corticosteroid adverse effects.[70]

INHALED. Inhaled corticosteroids, created by a further modification of the basic glucocorticoid molecule, are a potent therapy for asthma. Those available in the United States are administered by inhalation via MDIs or DPIs and include beclomethasone dipropionate, budesonide, flunisolide, fluticasone propionate, and triamcinolone acetonide. These anti-inflammatory agents have also been shown to improve the inflammation and bronchial hyperresponsiveness characteristic of asthma, but with a much lower potential for systemic toxicities than systemic administration. Anti-inflammatory therapy is recommended for all patients with persistent asthma, and dosages are based on the level of asthma severity (Fig. 36.5).[1] Corticosteroids for nebulized administration have been evaluated in controlled clinical trials, and a budesonide nebulizing product should be available in 2000.

Local adverse effects with inhaled corticosteroid therapy include oropharyngeal candidiasis (thrush), coughing, dysphonia, and hoarseness. Myopathy of the vocal cords may be the mechanism for dysphonia development. These effects appear to be dose-dependent, so treatment should consist of the lowest possible dosage that allows control of asthma symptoms. Auxiliary spacer devices used with MDIs reduce oropharyngeal deposition of the corticosteroid and reduce the incidence and severity of these effects, and are therefore recommended. Mouth rinsing with water or mouthwash after treatments can also reduce the risk of topical adverse effects.[1]

The risk of systemic adverse effects with inhaled corticosteroids has received increasing attention in recent years because of the use of these agents as first-line anti-inflammatory therapy. Although this remains an area of controversy, most agree that the risk of such effects increases with higher dosages, especially 1000 μg/day or more (beclomethasone equivalent). Adrenal suppression, the development of cataracts or glaucoma, growth suppression in children, and osteoporosis are of greatest concern.

The concern about growth-suppressive effects in children from inhaled corticosteroids has received increasing attention in the past few years.[71] In general, it appears that low dosages (<400 μg/day beclomethasone equivalent) do not impair growth in the majority of children but that moderate and high dosages (400 μg/day or more beclomethasone equivalent) can suppress growth in some children by approximately 1 to 2 cm/yr.[71] The majority of this information comes from studies with beclomethasone and budesonide, and newer inhaled corticosteroids that have high activity in the lung and rapid systemic inactivation must be evaluated independently for effects on growth. In November 1998, the FDA issued a requirement for labeling changes on all inhaled and intranasal corticosteroids to include a statement in the *Precautions, Pediatric Use* about the possibility of growth suppression in children. Further confounding this issue is the number of new delivery forms for inhaled corticosteroids. Hydrofluoroalkane-propelled MDIs, nebulizers, spacers attached to MDIs, and powder devices deliver different dosages to the lung than standard CFC-propelled MDI formulations. Therefore, not only must each new drug be evaluated for effects on growth, but each delivery method must be evaluated. The potential for these effects appears to have considerable interpatient variability but can be reduced by using spacers with MDIs and rinsing the mouth after inhalation treatments. Monitoring for these adverse effects, particularly with high-dose treatment, is appropriate.[72]

A number of clinical trials have been compared the efficacy of inhaled corticosteroids.[73] Available information from clinical trials and topical skin blanching tests suggests the following relative order of potency: flunisolide = triamcinolone acetonide < beclomethasone dipropionate = budesonide < fluticasone propionate in a ratio of 0.25: 0.5:1, with 1 being the most potent (fluticasone propionate).[73] However, potency should not be confused with efficacy because many clinical trials have demonstrated similar efficacy between inhaled corticosteroid regimens.[73] Rather, more potent inhaled corticosteroids or larger dosages delivered to the lungs are likely to permit once- or twice-daily dosing with fewer inhalations, which promotes adherence and thus effectiveness. Table 36.12 presents comparative dosages for available inhaled corticosteroids.[1]

Recent evidence suggests that there is a diurnal responsiveness for efficacy with inhaled corticosteroids. It has long been recommended that oral corticosteroids be administered in the morning to minimize adrenal suppressive effects. Two studies now indicate that dosing an inhaled corticosteroid once daily between 3:00 PM and 5:30 PM is as effective in controlling asthma symptoms as giving the same total daily dose divided four times daily.[74,75] Such a strategy could improve adherence and effectiveness of inhaled corticosteroid therapy. Several ongoing clinical trials of investigational inhaled corticosteroids include treatment arms that compare once-daily dosing in the evening with twice-daily dosing. Two of the newer, more potent inhaled corticosteroids, budesonide and fluticasone propionate, have been used more successfully than previous agents in weaning patients from long-term oral corticosteroid use. However, as stated earlier, efficacy depends on potency and the delivery method used for the inhaled corticosteroid.

Inhaled Drug Delivery

Administering medications by inhalation allows delivery directly to the site of action. Inherent to this is a lower dosage need, less risk of systemic adverse effects, and potential for improved efficacy and a faster onset of action than with oral administration. Unfortunately, inhaled drug delivery can be affected immensely by a number of factors, such as the aerosol particle size, inhalation technique, propellants, and delivery device used.

Inhaled aerosol particles are deposited primarily by inertial impaction, sedimentation, and diffusion. Inertial impaction is the means by which larger particles, those unable to flow in the airstream with changes in direction, are deposited. This typically occurs with particles more than 5 μm in aerodynamic diameter and results in oropharyngeal deposition as well as deposition into the bifurcations of the larger airways. Smaller particles, those that flow in the slower airstream in conducting airways, are deposited by gravitational sedimentation, especially with breath-holding maneuvers. Finally, particles less than 0.5 μm in diameter deposit by random Brownian diffusion, but because they contain an extremely small proportion of the total aerosol and drug mass, they are less important for inhaled drug delivery. Thus, the ideal or respirable range of aerosol particles for deposition in the lower respiratory tract is 0.5 to 5 μm aerodynamic diameter.[54,76]

Therapeutic aerosols are created by nebulizers, MDIs, and DPI devices. Product factors that can affect aerosol deposition include the aerosol particle size, density and shape, dispersion (monodisperse versus heterodisperse), hygroscopic nature of the drug, and effects of electrical charges. Patient factors include inspiratory flow, inspiratory volume, breath-holding, breathing frequency, lung volume at which inhalation commences, anatomic variations of the airways, and airway narrowing. The use of auxiliary devices such as spacers with MDIs can also affect inhaled drug delivery.[54,76] Each type of delivery device–nebulizers, MDIs, and DPIs–has distinct advantages and disadvantages (Table 36.13).

Nebulizers

Two nebulizer types are available: compressed air (jet) and ultrasonic. Aerosols from ultrasonic nebulizers are produced by a piezoelectric transducer vibrating at a

Table 36.12 ▪ Estimated Comparative Daily Dosages for Inhaled Corticosteroids

Drug	Low Dosage	Medium Dosage	High Dosage
Adults			
Beclomethasone dipropionate 42 µg/puff 84 µg/puff	168–504 µg (4–12 puffs, 42 µg) (2–6 puffs, 84 µg)	504–840 µg (12–20 puffs, 42 µg) (6–10 puffs, 84 µg)	>840 µg (>20 puffs, 42 µg) (>10 puffs, 84 µg)
Budesonide Turbuhaler 200 µg/dose	200–400 µg (1–2 inhalations)	400–600 µg (2–3 inhalations)	>600 µg (>3 inhalations)
Flunisolide 250 µg/puff	500–1000 µg (2–4 puffs)	1000–2000 µg (4–8 puffs)	>2000 µg (>8 puffs)
Fluticasone MDI: 44, 110, 220 µg/puff	88–264 µg (2-6 puffs, 44 µg) or (2 puffs, 100 µg)	264–660 µg (2–6 puffs, 110 µg)	>660 µg (>6 puffs, 110 µg) or (>3 puffs, 200 µg)
DPI: 50, 100, 250 µg/dose	(2–6 inhalations, 50 µg)	(3–6 inhalations, 100 µg)	(>6 inhalations, 100 µg) or (>2 inhalations, 250 µg)
Triamcinolone acetonide 100 µg/puff	400–1000 µg (4–10 puffs)	1000–2000 µg (10–20 puffs)	>2000 µg (>20 puffs)
Children			
Beclomethasone dipropionate 42 µg/puff 84 µg/puff	84–336 µg (2–8 puffs, 42 µg) (1–4 puffs, 84 µg)	336–672 µg (8–16 puffs, 42 µg) (4–8 puffs, 84 µg)	>672 µg (>16 puffs, 42 µg) >8 puffs, 84 µg)
Budesonide Turbuhaler 200 µg/dose	100–200 µg	200–400 µg (1–2 inhalations, 200 µg)	>400 µg (>2 inhalations, 200 µg)
Flunisolide 250 µg/puff	500–750 µg (2–3 puffs)	1000–1250 µg (4–5 puffs)	>1250 µg (>5 puffs)
Fluticasone MDI: 44, 110, 220 µg/puff	88–176 µg (2–4 puffs, 44 µg)	176–440 µg (4–10 puffs, 44 µg) or (2–4 puffs, 110 µg)	>440 µg (>4 puffs, 110 µg) or (>2 puffs, 220 µg)
DPI: 50, 100, 250 µg/dose	(2–4 inhalations, 50 µg)	(2–4 inhalations, 100 µg)	(>4 inhalations, 100 µg) or (>2 inhalations, 250 µg)
Triamcinolone acetonide 100 µg/puff	400–800 µg (4–8 puffs)	800–1200 µg (8–12 puffs)	>1200 µg (>12 puffs)

The most important determinant of appropriate dosing is the clinician's judgment of the patient's response to therapy. The clinician must monitor the patient's response on several clinical parameters and adjust the dosage accordingly. The stepwise approach to therapy emphasizes that once control of asthma is achieved, the medication dosage should be titrated carefully to the minimum dosage needed to maintain control, thus reducing the potential for adverse effect.

The reference point for the dosage range for children is data on the safety of inhaled corticosteroids in children, which suggest that the dosage ranges are equivalent to beclomethasone dipropionate 200–400 µg/day (low dosage), 400–800 µg/day (medium dosage), and >800 µg/day (high dosage).

Some dosages may be outside package labeling.

MDI dosages are expressed as the actuator dose (the amount of drug leaving the actuator and delivered to the patient), which is the labeling required in the United States. This is different from the dosage expressed as the valve dose (the amount of drug leaving the valve, not all of which is available to the patient), which is used in many European countries and in some of the scientific literature. DPI dosages are expressed as the amount of drug in the inhaler after activation.

Source: Reference 1.

MDI, metered-dose inhaler; *DPI,* dry powder inhaler.

high frequency (1 to 3 MHz). Most nebulizers have a "dead" or residual volume, the amount of liquid that is not aerosolized, and up to 75% of the aerosol output is not available to the patient. Therefore, nebulizers are inefficient methods for delivering medications, and more medication is needed than with other inhaled delivery methods. Aerosol generation and drug delivery via nebulizers depend on the choice of nebulizer (considerable brand-to-brand and lot-to-lot differences exist), use of vents and triggers, driving gas flow rate, humidity, temperature, volume fill, and characteristics of the solution to be nebulized. Advantages of nebulizers are that little coordination is needed and they can be used by infants and young children and in ventilator circuits. The major disadvantages of nebulizers are their inefficiency and inconvenience. Nebulizers are expensive, use an electrical power source (some battery-powered compressors are available), are time-consuming to use, and must be cleaned after treatments to avoid contamination and possible infection. Also, the medication must be water soluble, and there is potential for mechanical difficulties and chemical breakdown of the drug (because of the heat and vibrations produced by ultrasonic nebulizers).[54,76]

Table 36.13 ▪ Advantages and Disadvantages of the Various Inhalation Delivery Systems

Device	Advantages	Disadvantages
Nebulizer	Simple to use (minimal coordination needed) Can use in mechanically ventilated patients	Water-soluble drug needed. Inefficient delivery. Significant drug waste (residual volume). Numerous factors can affect delivery. Device variability (brand to brand, lot to lot). Inconvenient, bulky, and time-consuming. Electrical power source needed. Nebulizer must be cleaned (potential for infection). Potential for breakdown of drug (ultrasonic). Costly.
MDI	Minimal time needed for treatments Small, portable Can use in mechanically ventilated patients	Significant coordination needed. Chlorofluorocarbon propellants to be phased out. Difficulty in determining number of doses remaining. Numerous excipients.
MDI with spacer	Significantly less coordination needed Better pulmonary drug deposition Less risk of adverse effects	Bulky, costly. Overall cost of drug treatment may decrease with increased delivery of drug to the lung (greater efficacy) and less oropharyngeal deposition (fewer systemic effects).
Breath-actuated MDI	Minimal coordination needed Potential for better pulmonary drug deposition	No additional benefit if good inhaler technique used. Cannot use with spacer (potential for adverse effects). Difficulty in determining number of doses remaining. Cannot use in mechanically ventilated patients. Chlorofluorocarbon propellants to be phased out.
Dry powder inhaler	Breath-actuated, minimal coordination needed Better pulmonary drug deposition Lactose excipients Some are single-dose units that must be assembled	Young children and acutely obstructed patients may not generate adequate inspiratory flow to actuate. Change in inhalation technique needed. Greater oropharyngeal drug deposition and systemic absorption increases risk of systemic adverse effects. Potential for drug to aggregate. Potential to provoke cough (not widely reported). Cannot use in mechanically ventilated patients.

MDI, metered-dose inhaler.

Table 36.14 ▪ Recommended Technique for the Proper Use of a Metered-Dose Inhaler

1. Remove cap.
2. Shake canister.
3. Exhale (to functional residual capacity or fully if slow exhalation).
4. Hold inhaler upright and
   a. Place lips around mouthpiece or
   b. Place mouthpiece ~2 in. or 2 fingerwidths from mouth or
   c. Place lips around spacer mouthpiece (if using a spacer device).
5. Start to inhale slowly (≥30 L/min) immediately before actuation.
6. Actuate inhaler while continuing to inhale.
7. Inhale completely and hold breath for 10 sec (or at least 4 sec).
8. Wait 1 min.
9. Repeat treatment (steps 2–7) if more than one inhalation prescribed.
10. For inhaled steroids, rinse mouth with water or mouthwash and expel contents.

Metered-Dose Inhalers

MDIs are the standard method of delivery, but because the chlorofluorocarbons (CFCs) used as propellants are being phased out of production, hydrofluoroalkane propellant alternatives (non-CFC) and powder delivery devices have become available. The hydrofluoroalkane propellant in MDIs increases the amount of drug delivered to the lungs. Therefore, dosage reduction may be needed when converting from a CFC-containing MDI to a hydrofluoroalkane-propelled MDI. This is not true for Proventil HFA, which was formulated to deliver the same dosage to the lungs as the CFC-containing albuterol MDIs. Patients should be counseled that the hydrofluoroalkane-propelled MDIs deliver a less forceful and warmer spray than CFC-containing MDIs but that the drug is still reaching the lungs. MDIs have simplified delivery of inhaled medications because they are more convenient and portable and little time is needed for treatments. Unfortunately, significant hand–lung coordination is needed for the proper use of MDIs (Table 36.14). Spacers (Fig. 36.11)[77] reduce the amount of coordination needed to use MDIs properly, allowing younger children to use them. Use can also result in improved pulmonary drug deposition and reduce the risks of topical and systemic adverse effects from medications. Thus, the use of spacer devices often is worth the extra cost and bulkiness.[54,76] Breath-actuated devices have further simplified use of MDIs by significantly lessening the degree of coordination needed, but they provide no advantage in patients with good inhaler technique and cannot be used with spacer devices, which have many advantages of their own.

Dry Powder Inhalers

Development of DPIs such as the Rotahaler, Rotadisk, Diskus, and Turbuhaler has been facilitated in part by the phaseout of CFC propellants for MDIs. DPIs are breath-actuated devices that allow medication to be inhaled in the form of a dry, micronized powder. Because they are breath actuated, minimal coordination is needed, but a different inhalation technique from that used with MDIs is needed. With DPIs, deep and forceful inspiration of more than 60 L/minute (30 L/minute or less for MDIs) is needed for optimal pulmonary drug delivery.[54,76] However, breath-actuated DPIs are under development that disperse drug at inspiratory flows as low as 15 L/minute. The greater inspiratory flow needed with DPIs and their inability to be used with spacers probably increases oropharyngeal drug deposition. This along with increased pulmonary drug deposition and absorption may increase the risks of topical and systemic adverse effects from medications, particularly corticosteroids, if the dosage is not adjusted. Drug aggregation caused by high humidity has largely been overcome by use of lactose fillers, and the potential for provoking cough has not been widely reported. A continuing concern is whether young children or acutely obstructed asthmatic patients can generate enough inspiratory flow to actuate DPIs.[72]

Nonpharmacologic Therapy

Environmental control measures are an integral component of successful asthma therapy. Environmental controls include allergen and trigger avoidance measures (Table 36.15). Patients must be counseled that environmental controls must be adhered to consistently to achieve any beneficial effect.

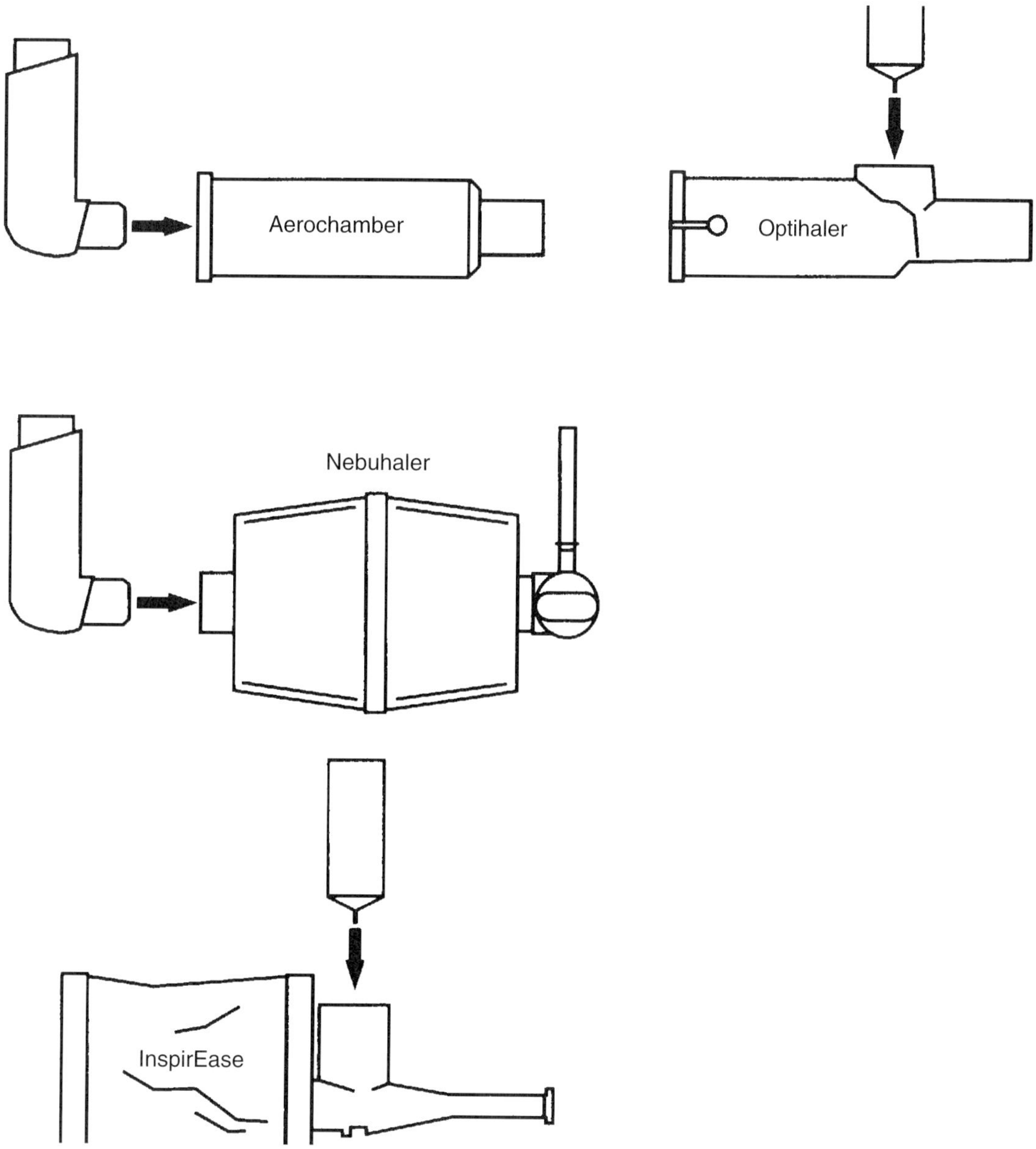

Figure 36.11. Diagram of the various spacer devices. (*Source:* Reference 77.)

Immuntherapy by subcutaneous administration of standardized allergen extracts generally is reserved for patients who have incomplete symptom control with drug therapy despite adherence with the regimen, have intolerable adverse effects from drug therapy, or cannot avoid exposure to the allergen. A single subcutaneous injection often contains multiple allergens to which the patient is sensitive. Physician visits are frequent (once or twice a week, initially), and it may take as much as 6 months to obtain symptom relief. Because treatment can continue up to 5 years or more, it is imperative to assess a patient's commitment before beginning treatment. Approximately 80 to 85% of patients have significant relief if they continue therapy.[78] If no improvement is noted after 1 year, clinical allergen sensitivities or the method of immunotherapy should be reassessed. For example, if too many allergens are included in each injection, none may be at a sufficient concentration to stimulate an immune response. After 1 to 2 years of being symptom free or having good control, the patient may discontinue therapy. Patients with coronary artery disease, severe hypertension, severe asthma, or severe atopic dermatitis should not receive immunotherapy because anaphylaxis to the allergen injection would increase the risk of life-threatening consequences. Immunotherapy may be continued in women who become pregnant but should not be initiated in pregnant patients. In addition, patients who need β-blockers or monoamine oxidase inhibitors should not receive immunotherapy because the presence of these drugs hampers treatment of anaphylaxis with adrenergic agonist drugs. Immunotherapy has been proven effective for grass, ragweed, birch, and mountain cedar pollens, dust mite, and cat allergen; efficacy of mold immunotherapy is still being evaluated.

The efficacy of immunotherapy may involve several mechanisms, including generating a rise in serum IgG antibodies that bind but do not cross-link allergens, suppressing IgE antibody levels, and reducing basophil and lymphocyte responsiveness to allergens. Only allergens to which the patient has demonstrated IgE-mediated sensitivity and positive clinical history should be included in an immunotherapy plan. No improvement in symptoms will be noted for about 6 months, and immunotherapy should be continued for at least 3 years because relapse is common when therapy is discontinued sooner. Patients should be much improved or symptom free for at least 1 year before discontinuation.

Table 36.15 ▪ Strategies to Reduce Allergen Exposure

Indoor allergen control	
Dust mite	Encase mattresses and pillows in mite-proof coverings. Remove carpeting entirely from home, if possible, or at least from bedrooms. Replace upholstered furniture with vinyl or leather. Wipe down surfaces of dressers, windowsills, and blinds weekly. Wash bedding (sheets, mattress covers, blankets) weekly in water at least 130°F. Remove stuffed animals and toys from the bedroom. Place stuffed animals and toys in dryer at 140°F for 1 hr or place in freezer overnight. Vacuum wearing a face mask or use HEPA filter on vacuum to avoid inhaling mite fecal balls. Apply acaricides[a] to carpet and upholstered furniture. Keep relative humidity in home below 45% and temperature below 70°F by using refrigerated air conditioning. Vacuum baseboard and wall heaters weekly.
Cats[b]	Remove cat from household or at least from bedroom; keep outdoors if possible. Wash and wipe walls weekly. Use HEPA filters or electrostatic filters on forced air central heating and cooling units to remove cat allergen from air.[c] For room air filtration, use HEPA filters; do not use electrostatic room air filters, which release ozone. Encourage children to play in homes that are cat free. Keep clothing in closet with door closed.
Molds	Use 5% bleach solution to clean bathrooms and kitchens to kill mold. Remove stacks of old newspapers and books. Use a dehumidifier. Change air filters monthly. If building a home, create airspace between cement floor and carpeting or use vinyl tile. Keep plants outdoors.
Cockroaches	Use professional extermination services.
Outdoor allergen control	
Pollens	Keep windows in car and home closed during pollen season and use air conditioning. Shower and wash hair nightly to remove pollen.
Molds	Avoid mowing grass, which releases mold spores into the air.

[a]Benzyl benzoate products are acaricidal; tannic acid–containing products denature the allergenic protein but are not acaricidal and thus are not recommended. Do not use if there is a toddler in the household. May need to apply products more frequently than stated in instructions.

[b]Products applied directly to the cat's fur are not effective in reducing cat allergen load.

[c]Filters can also remove dust mite fecal balls when they are airborne (i.e., after vacuuming).

Table 36.16 ▪ Properties of Alternative Asthma Treatments

Treatment	Bronchodilator	Steroid-Sparing	Hyperresponsiveness	Major Adverse Effects and Limitations
Methotrexate	–	+	–	Liver toxicity, GI upset
Troleandomycin	–	+	±	Potential for increased steroid adverse effects, increased liver enzymes, GI upset, reduces theophylline clearance
Gold	–	+	±	Renal toxicity, rash, GI upset
Intravenous immunoglobulin	–	+	–	Intravenous administration, costly
Cyclosporine	–	+	?	Renal toxicity, hypertension, paresthesias, potential for immunosuppression

–, no benefit reported; +, benefit reported; *GI,* gastrointestinal; ±, variable effects reported; *?,* effects unknown.

ALTERNATIVE THERAPIES

Because of the many toxicities and adverse effects associated with chronic oral corticosteroid use, a number of other therapies have been investigated for patients with severe persistent asthma. These include methotrexate, troleandomycin, gold, intravenous γ-globulin, and cyclosporine. Alternative treatments are reserved for patients with severe, steroid-dependent asthma. Not all patients respond to treatment, and each carries a risk of adverse effects (Table 36.16). Although the goal of therapy usually is to reduce systemic corticosteroid dosages, some studies have demonstrated improvements in pulmonary function (although none are bronchodilators in the traditional sense) and bronchial hyperresponsiveness.[79] For alternative treatments it is particularly important to define the goal of therapy because improving pulmonary function may not be realistic in the severely asthmatic patient with concomitant corticosteroid dosage reductions.

Patients with asthma also are increasingly using alternative and complementary therapies such as herbs, vitamins, massage, acupuncture, prayer, healing touch, and homeopathy (Table 36.17).[80–82] In a survey conducted in the United Kingdom, of the 41% of survey respondents who had used complementary therapies for asthma, the most commonly used treatments were breathing techniques (30%), homeopathy (12%), and herbalism (11%).[81] Practitioners (both MDs and non-MDs) tend to recommend primarily dietary and nutritional measures followed by herbs, meditation, and homeopathy.[83]

Pharmacists are most likely to be questioned about herbal and dietary therapies. Many herbs used for asthma have a pharmacologic basis for effect, but most are less potent than traditional medications used for asthma. Few herbal and dietary therapies have been studied in controlled clinical trials, and because formulations of products and possibly potencies vary between manufacturers, results of a trial with one specific product may not be applicable to another product of the same herb. A thorough review of herbal therapies in asthma is presented in reference 80. Intravenous and oral magnesium has been evaluated in controlled clinical trials. However, interest in this treatment was greatest in the early 1990s, with few studies published in recent years. Most studies had significant flaws, which precludes making a recommendation for its use in asthma treatment. The NAEPP guidelines do not include magnesium as an alternative for the usual management of acute or chronic asthma. Because asthma can result in death in a matter of minutes, it is important to

Table 36.17 ▪ Herbal Remedies Used in Asthma

Herb	Side Effects and Drug Interactions	Purported Mechanism
Coffee and tea	Tachycardia, insomnia, jitters, decreased appetite, potential interaction with β-agonist	Methylxanthines Increased intracellular cAMP Bronchodilator
Shinpi-to	Unknown; potential increase in steroid side effects	Inhibits 11 β-hydroxylase Blocks 5-lipoxygenase Inhibits PAF
Ma huang *(Ephedra sinica)*	Cardiovascular and CNS toxicity Deaths reported Potential interaction with β-agonists	β-Agonist Bronchodilator
Licorice root *(Glycyrrhiza glabra radix)*	Unknown	Inhibits 11 β-hydroxylase and cortisol breakdown
Coleus forskohlii	Unknown	Decreases cAMP metabolism Bronchodilator
Tylophora indica	Unknown	Unknown
Gingko biloba	Unknown	PAF antagonist Antioxidant
Onions *(Allium cepa)*	Hypersensitivity (rarely)	Blocks leukotriene synthesis
Bee pollen	Anaphylaxis	Unknown

Source: Adapted with permission from Kemper KJ, Lester MR. Alternative asthma therapies: an evidence-based review. Contemp Pediatr 16:162–195, 1999.

cAMP, cyclic adenosine monophosphate; *PAF,* platelet-activating factor; *CNS,* central nervous system.

counsel patients not to use alternative treatments in place of prescribed therapies as treatment delays could have grievous consequences.[84]

FUTURE THERAPIES

With increased research and knowledge of the pathophysiology of asthma, many novel treatment modalities are on the horizon. Inhibitors of PDE isoenzymes, which may have both bronchodilator and anti-inflammatory action, are being investigated for their use in treating asthma.[55] PDE isoenzymes regulate the breakdown of cAMP and cGMP within cells. Data from animal models and in vitro studies show the ability of isoenzymes III, IV, and V to relax precontracted smooth muscle and inhibit contraction. Inhibitors of PDE IV (and possibly III) are thought to suppress the infiltration and activation of inflammatory cells and their release of cytokines. A number of agents, both selective isoenzyme and dual PDE III/IV inhibitors, are undergoing development, but the presence of adverse effects (nausea and vomiting) has limited clinical trial progress. There is evidence of bronchodilator (antibronchoconstrictor) activity with PDE III inhibitors, but these agents cannot be considered potential replacements for β_2-agonists. The proposed anti-inflammatory effects of dual PDE III/IV inhibitors, along with bronchodilator activity, make for an intriguing potential new asthma therapy.[85]

Therapies directed at reducing concentrations of IgE with monoclonal antibodies have been evaluated in allergen challenge and short-term studies.[86] Anti-IgE monoclonal antibodies bind to IgE antibodies in the serum. Therefore, the effectiveness of these agents depends in part on how rapidly IgE bound to mast cells turns over because it is the IgE bound to mast cells that initiates the bronchospastic and inflammatory responses in most asthmatic patients. These agents have been effective in preventing the IAR and LAR to allergen when administered intravenously for several weeks before the challenge.[86] A study published in 1999 indicates that intravenous treatment improves asthma symptoms.[87]

A number of other agents are in early stages of development or clinical trials. Those being studied as potential anti-inflammatory agents include "soft" inhaled corticosteroids, which are designed to exert their pharmacologic effect locally and then be metabolized rapidly to inactive metabolites; phospholipase A_2 and cyclooxygenase inhibitors; antagonists of cytokines, thromboxane, bradykinin, and PAF; cell adhesion blockers; inhibitors of neurogenic inflammation; immunomodulators, and IgE suppressors. Potassium channel activators, calcium antagonists, and selective anticholinergics may represent novel bronchodilators.[55]

IMPROVING OUTCOMES

Outcome studies comparing the effects of different interventions (including improving medication adherence, teaching self-management strategies, and providing intensive follow-up) on the morbidity, mortality, and quality of life of patients with asthma have recently received increased interest. Such studies have become more important for guiding treatment of patients covered by health maintenance organizations and other health insurers and as part of the FDA drug approval process. Many insurers are developing asthma management programs for their enrollees in an attempt to better control expensive asthma outcomes such as ED visits and hospitalizations. The NAEPP guidelines provide extensive information on how to educate patients about asthma self-management.[1]

Patient Education

Patient education strategies are well described in the NAEPP guidelines.[1] The emphasis in these guidelines is on developing a partnership between the patient (and family) and caregivers. This partnership gives the patient and family members the education and skills needed for appropriate self-management with regular feedback and reinforcement from the caregivers. Areas that should be covered in patient education sessions include the following:

- Basic facts about asthma
- Roles of medications (especially the distinction between quick-relief and long-term control medications)
- Skills for proper inhaler use with or without a spacer, peak flow meter monitoring, and self-assessment
- Environmental control measures
- Appropriate use of rescue plans and medications

Educational materials and forms for self-monitoring are available for photocopy in these guidelines or can be downloaded from the Internet at http://www.nhlbi.nih.gov/nhlbi/lung/asthma/prof/asthgdln.pdf. Strategies written directly for pharmacists have also been published by the National Heart, Lung, and Blood Institute and can be implemented in both institutional and community pharmacy settings.[88]

Methods to Improve Patient Adherence to Drug Therapy

Patients with asthma, like others with chronic diseases, are poorly adherent with drug therapy. Rates of medication nonadherence among asthmatic patients range from 30% to 70%.[89] Adherence seems to improve as the disease severity worsens from mild to moderate asthma but then declines in patients with severe asthma; as expected, adherence declines with an increase in the number of times per day a medication is prescribed.[89] Patients with severe asthma whose treatment is unsuccessful probably will need intensive and individualized intervention. This is difficult to achieve in a typical clinical practice unless a dedicated member of the health care team is devoted to the care of these patients. Unfortunately, there appear to be no common patient characteristics that are predictive of medication nonadherence except that nonadherence is closely linked with the presence of psychopathologic problems.

Psychological disorders can lead to denial and predictably poor outcomes, and dysfunctional family interactions can lead to frequent changes in health care providers, conflicts between parent and child, erratic asthma management, and loss of faith in the value of therapy, all of which affect treatment adherence.[89]

The NAEPP guidelines stress a partnership between the patient and caregivers, including the pharmacist. A satisfying relationship with caregivers is the most important factor for changing health care behavior, including medication adherence.[89] Skills that the pharmacist should use include the following:

- Make direct eye contact.
- Express genuine interest.
- Explain all recommendations thoroughly and in language the patient can understand.
- Praise good medication adherence.
- Express a willingness to modify the treatment plan in accord with the patient's concerns (the pharmacist may need to communicate the patient's desires to the physician).[89]

Once a positive relationship is established, other changes that can be negotiated, which may lead to improved adherence, include the following:

- Prescribe less costly medications.
- Prescribe medications with fewer adverse effects that are of concern to the patient.
- Work with the patient to determine appropriate reminders to help with taking medications on schedule.
- Change dosing schedules to accommodate work or school.
- Reduce the number of medications.[89]

Adolescents are predictably nonadherent with medication regimens. Suggestions given by adolescents for improving communication with the health care provider include the following:

- Provide practical information on how to prevent symptoms.
- Explain how medications work and the purpose of each medication (especially important when there are multiple medications).
- Provide information in person, not as written material.
- Use language understood by adolescents.
- Use drawings, pictures, or videos to illustrate information (this could include demonstrations on using MDIs, DPIs, or peak flow meters).
- Keep drawings simple to facilitate remembering.[90]

Although many of these recommendations are generalized for any health care provider, the pharmacist could easily tailor these strategies for instruction on medication use and follow-up of medication use.

Disease Management Strategies to Improve Patient Outcomes

The NAEPP guidelines explain the methods needed to establish a comprehensive asthma management program.[1] These guidelines, initially published in 1991,[91] have been implemented community-wide in several metropolitan areas and have been found to reduce ED visits and hospitalizations.[92,93]

Pharmacists have implemented several programs that have improved asthma outcomes. These programs have been implemented in the ED,[94,95] clinics,[96,97] and community pharmacies.[98,99] The improved asthma outcomes include fewer hospitalizations, fewer ED visits, fewer physician visits (all reducing direct costs of care), and greater satisfaction with care and quality of life. Suggestions on how to develop and implement pharmacy-based services have also been published.[100]

PHARMACOECONOMICS

Direct and indirect costs associated with asthma continue to escalate. The annual cost of asthma in the United States is estimated to range from $5.8[101] to 7.8 billion.[102] Based on an estimate of 14 to 15 million patients with asthma, this figure represents annual costs exceeding $400 per patient.

Direct costs related to asthma include inpatient hospitalization, outpatient hospital services, physician services, emergency room services, and medications. The ability of drug therapy to reduce disease symptoms and minimize asthmatic exacerbations probably translates into cost savings.

Indirect costs are more difficult to quantify but reflect lost school days, which represent decreased earnings by the child's primary caretaker, loss of outside employment or housekeeping because of restricted activity or days spent in bed, and mortality costs, calculated from a person's normal life expectancy, which reflect lower employment or housekeeping productivity resulting from premature death. In addition, the psychosocial impact, such as unrealized patient potential, is impossible to estimate. In a recent publication, Barnes and Kharitonov[103] concluded that indirect costs account for 50% of total costs. Children accounted for almost 40% of these indirect costs, largely because of caregiver costs and the high prevalence of pediatric asthma.

The cost-effectiveness, quality of care, and financing of asthma management programs have been reviewed extensively by the NAEPP Task Force.[104] This group reviewed the published literature on the cost-effectiveness of asthma care based on studies conducted around the world. Medications reviewed for cost-effectiveness include inhaled corticosteroids, long-acting β_2-agonists, inhaled cromolyn, and a few other less commonly used medications. Comparisons included inhaled corticosteroids versus placebo, high versus low dosages of inhaled corticosteroids, inhaled corticosteroids versus fixed dosages of short-acting β_2-agonists, long-acting β_2-agonists versus placebo, and cromolyn versus placebo. The task force also included information on how to conduct and evaluate an intervention study and obtain cost savings information. Finally, the task force provided recommendations on improving asthma care financing. Although more recent studies have been conducted, the task force report provides a framework for evaluating newly available publications.

KEY POINTS

- Asthma is now recognized as much more than bronchoconstriction and may well represent a number of defects with similar clinical presentations.
- Therapy must target not only the symptoms resulting from bronchospasm but also the underlying inflammation and characteristic bronchial hyperresponsiveness.
- As new therapies and delivery systems are developed, choices between potentially equally efficacious regimens will become more complex. It is extremely important that treatment goals be developed through collaboration between the health care providers and the patient.
- The NAEPP goals of asthma management are to prevent chronic and troublesome symptoms (e.g., coughing or breathlessness in the night, in the early morning, or after exertion), maintain nearly normal pulmonary function, maintain normal activity levels (including exercise and other physical activity), prevent recurrent exacerbation of asthma and minimize the need for ED visits or hospitalizations, provide optimal pharmacotherapy with fewest adverse effects, and meet patients' and families' expectations of asthma care.[1]
- With implementation of an individualized asthma management plan, which includes use of appropriate medications and appropriate asthma education, both of which can be provided by pharmacists, patients with asthma should have a realistic chance of reaching these goals.

REFERENCES

1. National Asthma Education and Prevention Program. Expert panel report 2: guidelines for the diagnosis and management of asthma. Bethesda, MD: U.S. Department of Health and Human Services, Public Health Service, National Institutes of Health, National Heart, Lung, and Blood Institute, pub. no. 97-4051, April 1997.
2. Mannino DM, Homa DM, Pertowski CA, et al. Surveillance for asthma: United States, 1960–1995. MMWR CDC Surveill Summ 47:1-27, 1998.
3. Hogg JC. Post-mortem pathology in asthma. In: Kay AB. Allergy and allergic diseases. Oxford, UK: Blackwell, 1997:1360–1365.
4. Holgate ST. Asthma: past, present and future. Eur Respir J 6:1507–1520, 1993.
5. Pauwels R. Physiological aspects of airway, pulmonary and respiratory muscle function in asthma. In: Kay AB. Allergy and allergic diseases. Oxford, UK: Blackwell, 1997:682–691.
6. O'Byrne PM. Airway hyperresponsiveness. In: Middleton E Jr, Reed C, Ellis E, et al., eds. Allergy principles & practice. 5th ed. St Louis: Mosby, 1998;1: 859-866.
7. Kay AB. Asthma and inflammation. J Allergy Clin Immunol 87:893–910, 1991.
8. Barnes PJ. Pathophysiology of allergic inflammation. In: Middleton E Jr, Reed C, Ellis E, et al., eds. Allergy principles & practice. 5th ed. St Louis: Mosby, 1998:356–365.
9. Church MK, Bradding P, Walls AF, et al. Human mast cells and basophils. In: Kay AB. Allergy and allergic diseases. Oxford, UK: Blackwell, 1997;1: 149–170.
10. Barnes PJ, Chung KF, Page CP. Inflammatory mediators of asthma: an update. Pharmacol Rev 50:515–596, 1998.
11. Carroll N, Carello S, Cooke C, et al. Airway structure and inflammatory cells in fatal attacks of asthma. Eur Respir J 9:709–715, 1996.
12. Holt PG. Macrophages and dendritic cells in allergic reactions. In: Kay AB. Allergy and allergic diseases. Oxford, UK: Blackwell, 1997:228–243.
13. O'Byrne PM. Biology of neutrophils. In: Middleton E Jr, Reed CE, Ellis EF, et al., eds. Allergy principles & practice. 5th ed. St Louis: Mosby, 1998:237–241.
14. Haslett C, Chilvers ER. The neutrophil. In: Kay AB. Allergy and allergic diseases. Oxford, UK: Blackwell, 1997:198–213.
15. Sur S, Crotty TB, Kephart GM, et al. Sudden onset fatal asthma. A distinct entity with few eosinophils and relatively more neutrophils in the airway submucosa? Am Rev Respir Dis 148:713–719, 1993.
16. Smith HR, Henson PM. Mediators of asthma. Semin Respir Med 8:287–301, 1987.
17. Wardlaw AJ. Leukocyte adhesion in allergic inflammation. In: Kay AB. Allergy and allergic diseases. Oxford, UK: Blackwell, 1997:244–262.
18. Bochner BS. Cellular adhesion in inflammation. In: Middleton E Jr, Reed CE, Ellis EF, et al., eds. Allergy principles & practice. 5th ed. St Louis: Mosby, 1998:94–107.
19. Smith C. Cellular adhesion and interactions. In: Rich RR, Fleisher TA, Schwartz BD, et al., eds. Clinical immunology principles and practice. St Louis: Mosby, 1996:176–191.
20. Barnes PJ, Adcock IM. Transcription factors and asthma. Eur Respir J 12:221–234, 1998.
21. Gustafsson LE. Exhaled nitric oxide as a marker in asthma. Eur Respir J 26(Suppl):49S–52S, 1998.
22. Casale TB, Baraniuk JN. Neurogenic control of inflammation and airway function. In: Middleton E Jr, Reed C, Ellis E, et al., eds. Allergy principles & practice. 5th ed. St Louis: Mosby, 1998:183–203.
23. Barnes PJ. Neural mechanisms in asthma: new developments. Pediatr Pulmonol 16(Suppl):82–83, 1997.
24. Di Maria GU, Bellofiore S, Geppetti P. Regulation of airway neurogenic inflammation by neutral endopeptidase. Eur Respir J 12:1454–1462, 1998.
25. Fabbri LM, Caramori G, Maestrelli P. Definition, clinical features, investigations and differential diagnosis of asthma. In: Kay AB. Allergy and allergic diseases. Oxford, UK: Blackwell, 1997:1347–1359.
26. Harrison BD. Psychosocial aspects of asthma in adults. Thorax 53:519–525, 1998.
27. Randolph C, Fraser B. Stressors and concerns in teen asthma. Curr Probl Pediatr 29:82–93, 1999.
28. Warner GO, Gotz M, Landau LI, et al. Management of asthma: a consensus statement. Arch Dis Child 64:1065–1079, 1989.
29. International Consensus Report on Diagnosis and Management of Asthma. Bethesda, MD: US Department of Health and Human Services, Public Health Service, National Institutes of Health, National Heart, Lung, and Blood Institute, pub. no. 92-3091, March 1992.
30. Woolcock AJ. Steroid resistant asthma: what is the clinical definition? Eur Respir J 6:743–747, 1993.
31. Brunette MG, Lands L, Thibodeau LP. Childhood asthma: prevention of attacks with short-term corticosteroid treatment of upper respiratory tract infection. Pediatrics 81:624–629, 1988.
32. Bai TR. Adrenergic agonists and antagonists. In: Kay AB. Allergy and Allergic Diseases. Oxford, UK: Blackwell, 1997:568–583.
33. Lofdahl CG, Chung KF. Long acting β_2 adrenoceptor agonists: a new perspective in the treatment of asthma. Eur Respir J 4:218–226, 1991.
34. Laitinen LA, Laitinen A, Haahtela T. A comparative study of the effects of an inhaled corticosteroid, budesonide, and of a β_2-agonist, terbutaline, on airway inflammation in newly diagnosed asthma. J Allergy Clin Immunol 90:32–42, 1992.
35. Roberts JA, Bradding P, Walls AF, et al. The influence of salmeterol xinafoate on mucosal inflammation in asthma. Am Rev Respir Dis 145:A418, 1992.
36. Liggett SB. Polymorphisms of the beta$_2$-adrenergic receptor and asthma. Am J Respir Crit Care Med 156:S156–S162, 1997.
37. Martinez FD, Graves PE, Baldini M, et al. Association between genetic polymorphisms of the beta$_2$-adrenoceptor and response to albuterol in children with and without a history of wheezing. J Clin Invest 100:3184–3188, 1997.
38. Cheong B, Reynolds SR, Rajan G, et al. Intravenous β agonist in severe acute asthma. BMJ 297:448–450, 1988.
39. Murdock IA, Anjos RD, Haycock GB. Treatment of hyperkalemia with intravenous salbutamol. Arch Dis Child 66:527–528, 1991.
40. Twentyman OP, Finnerty JP, Harris A, et al. Protection against allergen-induced asthma by salmeterol. Lancet 336:1338–1342, 1990.

41. Jenne JS, Murphy SA. Drug Therapy for asthma: research and clinical practice. New York: Marcel Dekker, 1987.
42. Boulet LP. Long- versus short-acting beta 2-agonists. Implications for drug therapy [published erratum appears in Drugs 48(2):326, 1994]. Drugs 47:207–222, 1994.
43. Ramage L, Lipworth BJ, Ingram CG, et al. Reduced protection against exercise induced bronchoconstriction after chronic dosing with salmeterol. Respir Med 88:363–368, 1994.
44. Ind PW. Salbutamol enantiomers: early clinical evidence in humans [editorial; comment]. Thorax 52:839–840, 1997.
45. Moore RH, Khan A, Dickey BF. Long-acting inhaled beta$_2$-agonists in asthma therapy. Chest 113:1095–1108, 1998.
46. Blake K. Theophylline. In: Murphy S, Kelly HW. Pediatric asthma. New York: Marcel Dekker, 1999:363–431.
47. Barnes PJ, Pauwels RA. Theophylline in the management of asthma: time for reappraisal? Eur Respir J 7:579–591, 1994.
48. Hendeles L, Harman E, Huang D, et al. Theophylline attenuation of airway responses to allergen: comparison with cromolyn metered-dose inhaler. J Allergy Clin Immunol 95:505–514, 1995.
49. Hendeles L, Jenkins J, Temple R. Revised FDA labeling guideline for theophylline oral dosage forms. Pharmacotherapy 15:409–427, 1995.
50. Weinberger M, Hendeles L. Theophylline in asthma. N Engl J Med 334:1380–1388, 1996.
51. Hendeles L, Bighley L, Richardson RH, et al. Frequent toxicity from IV aminophylline infusions in critically ill patients. Drug Intell Clin Pharm 11:12–17, 1977.
52. Olson KR, Benowitz NL, Woo OF, et al. Theophylline overdose: acute single ingestion versus chronic repeated overmedication. Am J Emerg Med 3:386–394, 1985.
53. Shannon M. Predictors of major toxicity after theophylline overdose. Ann Intern Med 119:1161–1167, 1993.
54. Anonymous. In: Witek TJ, Schachter EN, eds. Pharmacology and therapeutics in respiratory care. Philadelphia: WB Saunders, 1994.
55. Barnes PJ. New drugs for asthma. Eur Respir J 5:1126–1136, 1992.
56. Pakes GE, Brogden RN, Heel RC, et al. Ipratropium bromide: a review of its pharmacological properties and therapeutic efficacy in asthma and chronic bronchitis. Drugs 20:237–266, 1980.
57. Plotnick LH, Ducharme FM. Should inhaled anticholinergics be added to beta$_2$ agonists for treating acute childhood and adolescent asthma? A systematic review. BMJ 317:971–977, 1998.
58. Brophy C, Ahmed B, Bayston S, et al. How long should Atrovent be given in acute asthma? Thorax 53:363–367, 1998.
59. Brogden RN, Sorkin EM. Nedocromil sodium: an updated review of its pharmacological properties and therapeutic efficacy in asthma. Drugs 45:693–715, 1993.
60. Drazen JM, Israel E, O'Byrne PM. Treatment of asthma with drugs modifying the leukotriene pathway. N Engl J Med 340:197–206, 1999.
61. Dahlen SE, Kumlin M, Bjorck T, et al. Airway smooth muscle and disease workshop: leukotrienes and related eicosanoids. Am Rev Respir Dis 136:S24–S28, 1987.
62. Deykin A, Israel E. Newer therapeutic agents for asthma. Dis Mon 45:117–144, 1999.
63. Malmstrom K, Rodriguez-Gomez G, Guerra J, et al. Oral montelukast, inhaled beclomethasone, and placebo for chronic asthma. A randomized, controlled trial. Montelukast/Beclomethasone Study Group. Ann Intern Med 130:487–495, 1999.
64. Blake KV. Montelukast: data from clinical trials in the management of asthma. In review with Ann Pharmacother 33:1299–1314, 1999.
65. Kelloway JS, Wyatt RA, Adlis SA. Comparison of patients' compliance with prescribed oral and inhaled asthma medications. Arch Intern Med 154:1349–1352, 1994.
66. Ringdal N, Whitney JG, Summerton L. Problems with inhaler technique and patient preference for oral therapy: tablet zafirlukast vs inhaled beclomethasone [abstract]. Am J Respir Crit Care Med 157:A416, 1998.
67. Barnes PJ. Efficacy of inhaled corticosteroids in asthma. J Allergy Clin Immunol 102:531–538, 1998.
68. Barnes PJ. Anti-inflammatory actions of glucocorticoids: molecular mechanisms [editorial]. Clin Sci (Colch) 94:557–572, 1998.
69. Taylor IK, Shaw RJ. The mechanism of action of corticosteroids in asthma. Respir Med 87:261–277, 1993.
70. Szefler SJ. Glucocorticoid therapy for asthma: clinical pharmacology. J Allergy Clin Immunol 88:147–165, 1991.
71. Allen DB. Influence of inhaled corticosteroids on growth: a pediatric endocrinologist's perspective. Acta Paediatr 87:123–129, 1998.
72. Kamada AK. Therapeutic controversies in the treatment of asthma. Ann Pharmacother 28:904–914, 1994.
73. Kelly HW. Comparison of inhaled corticosteroids. Ann Pharmacother 32:220–232, 1998.
74. Pincus DJ, Szefler SJ, Ackerson LM, et al. Chronotherapy of asthma with inhaled steroids: the effect of dosage timing on drug efficacy. J Allergy Clin Immunol 95:1172–1178, 1995.
75. Pincus DJ, Humeston TR, Martin RJ. Further studies on the chronotherapy of asthma with inhaled steroids: the effect of dosage timing on drug efficacy. J Allergy Clin Immunol 100:771–774, 1997.
76. Newman SP. Delivery of drugs from the respiratory tract. In: Chung KF, Barnes PJ. Pharmacology of the respiratory tract. New York: Marcel Dekker, 1993:701–728.
77. National Asthma Education and Prevention Program. Practical guide for the diagnosis and management of asthma. Based on the Expert Panel Report 2: guidelines for the diagnosis and management of asthma. Bethesda, MD: US Department of Health and Human Services, Public Health Service, National Institutes of Health, National Heart, Lung, and Blood Institute, pub. no. 97-4053, October 1997.
78. Druce HM. Allergic and nonallergic rhinitis. In: Middleton E Jr, Reed CE, Ellis EF, et al., eds. Allergy principles and practice. St Louis: Mosby, 1993:1433–1453.
79. Szefler SJ. Alternative therapy in severe asthma: rationale and guidelines for applications. In: Middleton E Jr, Reed CE, Ellis EF, et al., eds. Principles and practice. 3rd ed. St Louis: Mosby, 1991:1–14.
80. Bielory L, Lupoli K. Herbal interventions in asthma and allergy. J Asthma 36:1–65, 1999.
81. Ernst E. Complementary therapies for asthma: what patients use. J Asthma 35:667–671, 1998.
82. Kemper KJ, Lester MR. Alternative asthma therapies: an evidence-based review. Contemp Pediatr 16:162–195, 1999.
83. Davis PA, Gold EB, Hackman RM, et al. The use of complementary/alternative medicine for the treatment of asthma in the United States. J Investig Allergol Clin Immunol 8:73–77, 1998.
84. Blanc PD, Kuschner WG, Katz PP, et al. Use of herbal products, coffee or black tea, and over-the-counter medications as self-treatments among adults with asthma. J Allergy Clin Immunol 100:789–791, 1997.
85. Torphy TJ. Phosphodiesterase isozymes: molecular targets for novel anti-asthma agents. Am J Respir Crit Care Med 157:351–370, 1998.
86. Demoly P, Bousquet J. Anti-IgE therapy for asthma [editorial; comment; published erratum appears in Am J Respir Crit Care Med 156(5):1707, 1997]. Am J Respir Crit Care Med 155:1825–1827, 1997.
87. Milgrom H, Fick RB Jr, Su JQ, et al. Treatment of allergic asthma with monoclonal anti-IgE antibody. rhuMAb-E25 Study Group. N Engl J Med 341(26):1966–1973, 1999.
88. The role of the pharmacist in improving asthma care. Bethesda, MD: US Department of Health and Human Services, Public Health Service, National Institutes of Health, National Heart, Lung, and Blood Institute, July 1995.
89. Bender B, Milgrom H, Rand C. Nonadherence in asthmatic patients: is there a solution to the problem? Ann Allergy Asthma Immunol 79:177–185, 1997.
90. van Es SM, le Coq EM, Brouwer AI, et al. Adherence-related behavior in adolescents with asthma: results from focus group interviews. J Asthma 35:637–646, 1998.
91. National Asthma Education and Prevention Program. Expert panel report: guidelines for the diagnosis and management of asthma. Bethesda, MD: US Department of Health and Human Services, Public Health Service, National Institutes of Health, National Heart, Lung, and Blood Institute, pub. no. 91-3042, August 1991.
92. Wilson SR, Scamagas P, Grado J, et al. The Fresno Asthma Project: a model intervention to control asthma in multiethnic, low-income, inner-city communities. Health Educ Behav 25:79–98, 1998.
93. Greineder DK, Loane KC, Parks P. A randomized controlled trial of a pediatric asthma outreach program. J Allergy Clin Immunol 103:436–440, 1999.
94. Kelso TM, Self TH, Rumbak MJ, et al. Educational and long-term therapeutic intervention in the ED: effect on outcomes in adult indigent minority asthmatics. Am J Emerg Med 13:632–637, 1995.
95. Pauley TR, Magee MJ, Cury JD. Pharmacist-managed, physician-directed asthma management program reduces emergency department visits. Ann Pharmacother 29:5–9, 1995.
96. Kelso TM, Abou-Shala N, Heilker GM, et al. Comprehensive long-term management program for asthma: effect on outcomes in adult African-Americans. Am J Med Sci 311:272–280, 1996.

97. Im J. Evaluation of the effectiveness of an asthma clinic managed by an ambulatory care pharmacist. Calif J Hosp Pharm 5:5–6, 1993.
98. Knoell DL, Pierson JF, Marsh CB, et al. Measurement of outcomes in adults receiving pharmaceutical care in a comprehensive asthma outpatient clinic. Pharmacotherapy 18:1365–1374, 1998.
99. Rupp MT, McCallian DJ, Sheth KK. Developing and marketing a community pharmacy-based asthma management program. J Am Pharm Assoc (Wash) NS37:694–699, 1997.
100. Ferro LA, Im J, Iverson P, et al. Developing and implementing pharmacy-based asthma services. J Am Pharm Assoc (Wash) 38:551–565, 1998.
101. Smith DH, Malone DC, Lawson KA, et al. A national estimate of the economic costs of asthma. Am J Respir Crit Care Med 156:787–793, 1997.
102. Weiss KB, Gergen PJ, Hodgson TA. An economic evaluation of asthma in the United States. N Engl J Med 326:862–868, 1992.
103. Barnes PJ, Jonsson B, Klim JB. The costs of asthma. Eur Respir J 9(4):636–642, 1996.
104. Anonymous. National asthma education and prevention program task force report on the cost effectiveness, quality of care, and financing of asthma care. Am J Respir Crit Care Med 154:(3)S81–S130, 1996.

CHAPTER 37

CHRONIC OBSTRUCTIVE PULMONARY DISEASE

Tracey L. Goldsmith and Jeffrey J. Weber

DEFINITION

The term *obstructive pulmonary disease* encompasses several separate and distinct sets of pathologic changes, including asthma, chronic bronchitis, and emphysema. Interference with ventilation from an obstruction to airflow is the common element, in contrast to restrictive lung disease, in which the defect is reduced lung expansion capability. Asthma (discussed in detail in Chapter 36) is characterized by narrowing of the airways as a result of bronchial hyperreactivity, excessive bronchial secretions, and airway inflammatory changes. The resulting airflow obstruction is usually reversible.

In contrast, chronic obstructive pulmonary disease (COPD) describes the presentation of chronic cough, expectoration, varying degrees of exertional dyspnea, and a significant and progressive reduction in expiratory airflow.[1] This airflow obstruction may respond to varying therapeutic options, but it is largely irreversible. Chronic bronchitis and emphysema, potentially with a component of airway hyperreactivity, usually cause COPD. Chronic bronchitis is defined by chronic or recurrent excess mucus secretion into the bronchial tree that occurs on most days during a period of at least 3 months of the year for at least 2 consecutive years.[1] Emphysema is characterized by abnormal permanent enlargement of the airspaces distal to the terminal bronchioles, accompanied by destruction of their walls, and without obvious fibrosis.[1] Chronic bronchitis and emphysema are often indistinguishable on clinical examination, and many patients have components of both diseases. Of the two diagnoses, emphysema is the more disabling presentation.

TREATMENT GOALS: COPD

- Individualize approach to treatment as appropriate.
- Alter environmental influences.
- Correct airflow obstruction.
- Improve patient's functional status.
- Initiate pulmonary rehabilitation.
- Prevent acute disease exacerbations.
- Optimize drug-therapy regimens.
- Maintain adequate nutrition.

EPIDEMIOLOGY

Chronic obstructive pulmonary disease is the fourth leading cause of death in the United States.[2] More than 100,000 deaths per year are attributable to the disease. Cigarette smoking plays a major role in the occurrence of COPD, with current estimates suggesting that 80 to 90% of cases are attributable to smoking. The COPD mortality rate remains higher in Whites than Blacks and in males than females. This latter trend is changing, however, with predictions that within 10 to 20 years there will be an equal number of deaths between men and women related to cigarette consumption.[3] The mortality rate from COPD is increasing, particularly among older patients.[4] This rising mortality rate occurs at a time when deaths from heart disease and strokes are decreasing. Various estimates of the number of people in the United States affected by COPD range as high as 30 million,[5] but these numbers are likely underestimates of the prevalence due to the number of as yet undiagnosed patients with early or mild disease.

COPD is strongly associated with cigarette smoking, although only 10 to 26% of smokers go on to develop obstruction.[6] Passive smoking has been identified as a possible factor in COPD development, and other environmental factors such as pollution and occupational exposures have also been implicated. Cigarette smoking, in particular, causes increased bronchial reactivity and inflammation. Ciliary function is depressed, resulting in decreased clearance of mucus and particles. Macrophage function is similarly inhibited. Release of lysosomal enzymes destroys the connective tissue in the lung. Other factors such as increasing age, male sex, and existing impairment of lung function are also associated risks for COPD.

Inborn errors resulting in enzyme deficiencies are rare causes of emphysema (less than 1%). An imbalance between elastase (an enzyme that degrades elastin in the lung parenchyma) and elastase inhibitors results in alveolar destruction. A deficiency of α_1-antitrypsin (or α_1-proteinase inhibitor), an elastase inhibitor, is the genetic basis for alveolar wall destruction in these rare cases.

PATHOPHYSIOLOGY

The normal function of the respiratory system is to exchange oxygen (O_2) and carbon dioxide (CO_2) so that oxygen is delivered to and carbon dioxide is removed from the blood. CO_2 is the major stimulus for the respiratory center, located in the medulla of the brain. When $Paco_2$ levels increase, ventilation is stimulated, resulting in increased removal of CO_2. These gases move through the upper airway (nose, pharynx, larynx, trachea, and bronchi) and the lower respiratory tract (bronchioles, alveolar ducts, alveolar sacs, and alveoli). Exchange of O_2 and CO_2 occurs between the alveoli and the vascular supply (capillaries). Normal airway integrity is maintained through the relationship of pressures in and around the airway and the elasticity of the airway.

With obstructive pulmonary disease, air exchange is impaired in several ways. Airway integrity is compromised through smooth muscle contraction, inflammation, edema, and peribronchiolar fibrosis. Changes in pulmonary vasculature result from hypoxia. Pulmonary hypertension, with elevated mean pulmonary artery pressures and pulmonary vascular resistance, may develop. Cor pulmonale, or hypertrophy of the right ventricle due to primary lung disease, may then develop and progress to heart failure.

Contributing further to the abnormalities, respiratory drive becomes less responsive to changes in arterial pH and $Paco_2$ in COPD patients. Hypoxic drive begins to play a larger role. A patient with respiratory failure who receives oxygen administration will have an increase in $Paco_2$. This increase may be due to an effect on hypoxic drive, but it may also be due to changes in ventilation/perfusion caused by alleviation of hypoxia-induced vasoconstriction. Stable COPD patients rarely experience significant $Paco_2$ increases during oxygen therapy, but during acute exacerbations leading to respiratory failure, larger increases (10 to 13 mm Hg) in $Paco_2$ can occur, leading to further alterations in mental status and acidosis. However, concerns about oxygen supplementation causing narcosis should not prohibit its administration.[7]

High $Paco_2$ levels are not as ominous as once thought. Adaptive changes in chronic COPD allow patients to tolerate high $Paco_2$ levels. In mechanically ventilated patients, the concept of permissive hypercapnia (allow the $Paco_2$ to climb) is thought to be less harmful than mechanical ventilation that is required to keep values "normal." The patient compensates by retaining bicarbonate, and a pH as low as 7.25 may be fairly well tolerated. Occasionally, additional bicarbonate can be administered if needed.

Physical obstruction of the airways due to chronic or recurrent excessive mucus secretion, accompanied with inflammation, also interferes with normal mechanisms to maintain airway integrity in chronic bronchitis. This excessive mucus production is the result of irritation of the airway by smoke or other irritants. With chronic irritation, the mucous glands increase in number and size and their ducts dilate within the bronchial mucosa. The resulting excess mucus produces plugs or consolidations primarily in the small peripheral airways. Destruction of alveoli and further functional air exchange area reduction occurs. Airway obstruction is not necessarily always present in chronic bronchitis and may occur only during acute exacerbations. Each of the observed changes is thought to occur from repeated exposure to irritants, particularly cigarette smoke.

Finally, the primary culprit in emphysema contributing to loss of airway integrity is destruction of distal airspaces, including the bronchioles, alveolar ducts, and alveolar sacs. Loss of elastic recoil results. Elastic recoil contributes to the force of expiration; if decreased, distal airways collapse during expiration and trap air. A hereditary form of emphysema due to α_1-antitrypsin deficiency is characterized by destruction of all areas of the pulmonary lobule.[1]

CLINICAL PRESENTATION AND DIAGNOSIS

Signs and Symptoms

By the time they seek medical attention, patients are usually far advanced in their disease, with symptoms of airway obstruction. This delay in medical intervention occurs because the pathologic changes have been progressing for years, but overt clinical symptoms occur later. Screening programs to identify patients at risk for COPD, or in the earliest stages of the disease, are not prevalent compared with programs for detection of heart disease or cancer. A new national health care initiative, the National Lung Health Education Program (NLHEP),[5] is directed at primary care providers to assist in the early identification and intervention in COPD and related disorders. This initiative aims at preventing or forestalling premature morbidity and mortality from COPD and related disorders.[5]

Significant overlap between the clinical presentation of chronic bronchitis and emphysema exists. The usual presentation of chronic bronchitis begins with morning cough productive of sputum. Cough and increased sputum production are not generally present in emphysema. The patient may report a decline in exercise tolerance, although he or she may not have appreciated this decline until questioned. Fatigue also correlates with worsening pulmonary function.[8] Weight loss (sometimes profound) may be reported by the patient with primary emphysema; however, the patient with chronic bronchitis is typically obese. Dyspnea occurs later in the course of COPD and may be worsened by exposure to cold, dampness, pollution, or acute infection. Considerable interpatient variation exists in the subjective perception of dyspnea, but there is a close intrapatient correlation between dyspnea and worsening degree of airway obstruction in patients with advancing COPD.[9]

On physical examination, a prolonged expiratory effort may be seen as a sign of airway obstruction in primary emphysema. These patients may also exhale through pursed lips in an attempt to control the rate of expiration. Grunting may be heard on inspiration. Patients with predominant emphysema may prefer an upright, forward-leaning posture. The patient may be using the accessory respiratory muscles to aid in breathing. An overall increase in respiratory rate is common. Wheezes may be heard during bouts of airway obstruction in both chronic bronchitis and emphysema. An increase in the anteroposterior diameter of the chest and the classic "barrel chest" may occur in both diseases. These signs and symptoms do not correlate well with severity of illness. The chest x-ray may demonstrate emphysematous bullae or marked vascular changes.

As COPD progresses, other acute and chronic complications may develop. Patients in whom chronic bronchitis predominates may undergo repeated episodes of acute respiratory failure. These patients may develop cor pulmonale and right-sided congestive heart failure. The term *blue bloater* has been associated with this type of COPD patient. Hypoxemia and respiratory acidosis are common findings. Acute respiratory failure is rare until the end stages of emphysema. These patients are termed *pink puffers* because alveolar ventilation is maintained until the terminal stages of the disease. Table 37.1 summarizes the pertinent clinical features distinguishing chronic bronchitis and emphysema.

Respiratory infections of bacterial, viral, and mycoplasmal etiology can trigger an acute COPD exacerbation, especially in the patient with chronic bronchitis.[10] Alternatively, bacteria can be secondary invaders following viral or mycoplasmal infections.[10] *Haemophilus influenzae, Streptococcus pneumoniae,* and *Moraxella catarrhalis,* common colonizers of the upper airway, cause most of the bacterial respiratory infections.[10] Mucus hypersecretion predisposes to repeated infections. Decreased removal of bronchial secretions physically impairs the defenses of the lungs against infection, and the mucus provides a good growth medium for bacteria. The bacteria, together with the host's immune responses, contribute to further lung tissue damage.[10,11] It is unclear whether colonization or recurrent infection contributes to the progression of COPD by accentuating the rate of decline of pulmonary function.

Table 37.1 ▪ Clinical Presentation of Chronic Obstructive Pulmonary Disease

	Chronic Bronchitis (Blue Bloater)	Emphysema (Pink Puffer)
Symptoms	Chronic cough, heavy sputum production	Dyspnea, minimal cough, minimal sputum production
Weight	Obesity common	Marked weight loss
Smoking history	Common	Common
Blood gases	Low Pa_{O_2}	Normal or slightly low Pa_{O_2}
	Elevated Pa_{CO_2}	Normal or slightly high Pa_{CO_2}
	Respiratory acidosis	Normal pH or mild respiratory acidosis
Cor pulmonale	Early development	Late development
Respiratory failure	Repeated episodes	Rare until end stage
Pulmonary function tests	Decreased FEV_1 Decreased FVC Increased residual volume	Decreased FEV_1 Decreased FVC Greatly increased residual volume

Diagnosis

No specific laboratory information is useful in differentiating the various forms of COPD, with the exception of emphysema due to α_1-antitrypsin deficiency. This diagnosis is made by a serum protein electrophoretic study. Sputum and blood eosinophilia, usually associated with asthma, may be present if the COPD patient also has an asthma component. This information could be useful in determining the role of bronchodilator therapy and possibly the use of corticosteroids.

Pulmonary function tests (spirometry) provide the best information on the degree of airway obstruction and also help assess the efficacy of drug therapy. However, before discussing their utility, a brief review of the parameters forced expiratory volume (FEV_1), forced vital capacity (FVC), and FEV_1/FVC ratio is necessary. FEV_1 is the volume of air exhaled during forced exhalation in the first second. This parameter is decreased in the patient with an obstruction to outflow, such as COPD. FEV_1 above 2 L is usually not associated with dyspnea with normal activity. With a 50% decrease in FEV_1, dyspnea on exertion is present. A 75% decrease is associated with dyspnea at rest. There can be considerable day-to-day variability in FEV_1, with most stable COPD patients showing up to 20% fluctuation.[12] Up to 30% of patients have an increase of 15% or more in FEV_1 after inhalation of a β-agonist. The absence of a significant increase after a single dose does not justify withholding bronchodilator therapy.[1] FVC denotes the volume of gas expelled from the lungs during rapid and complete exhalation and is also reduced in COPD. In a patient without lung disease, the FEV_1/FVC ratio is normally 0.8 or greater. Therefore, a patient with chronic or acute airway obstruction would have an FEV_1/FVC ratio less than 0.8. These parameters are measured through spirometry testing, which is performed with the patient exhaling as rapidly and forcefully as possible for a minimum of 6 seconds through a device that measures airflow.

Appropriately performed and interpreted, spirometry testing serves as an early screening tool for identifying patients at risk for COPD, identifies patients with COPD and other disorders, provides positive reinforcement to patients attempting smoking cessation, and assesses response to drug therapy. It also allows staging of COPD. The American Thoracic Society has published the following staging criteria based on FEV_1:[13]

Stage I: $FEV_1 \geq 50\%$ predicted–no significant effect on health-related quality of life

Stage II: FEV_1 35 to 49% predicted–significant impact on health-related quality of life

Stage III: $FEV_1 < 35\%$ predicted–profound impact on health-related quality of life

These and other criteria are useful for initially assessing the severity of disease of the COPD patient and for following progression of disease over time.

ETHICAL DIMENSIONS

Discussion of end-of-life decisions is difficult for patients, families, and health care providers; COPD is no exception. Therapy of COPD is not currently curative, and progression of disease is inevitable. However, COPD patients are no more likely than other patients to have expressed their wishes about end-of-life decisions to their physicians or families.[14] The crucial decision usually centers around mechanical ventilation: Does the patient want to be placed on mechanical ventilation for respiratory failure? If mechanical ventilation is initiated, and the patient does not improve, does the patient wish to be removed from mechanical support? Physicians may be reluctant to remove a patient from mechanical ventilation, particularly in light of family objections. However, the patient's right for self-determination in these cases should outweigh concerns for legal liability or personal beliefs. Open discussion, before the point of medical crisis, should occur between caregivers, patient, and family. Decisions to not implement mechanical support or to withdraw mechanical support once begun are both ethically appropriate, but are only made harder when the patient has not expressed his or her wishes.

THERAPEUTIC PLAN

The therapy of COPD is discussed, with areas of particular benefit in primary chronic bronchitis or primary emphysema highlighted. There are no clearly agreed on standards of therapy in COPD. Until definitive standards are established and more is known about the pathogenesis of COPD, therapy should be minimally aimed at halting or slowing the progression of the pathologic changes, improving the patient's quality of life, and preventing acute exacerbations of the disease. An individualized approach to therapy is necessary, but general recommendations follow.

Alter Environmental Influences

A normal decline in FEV_1 occurs with aging; however, environmental influences can accelerate that decline. Smoking is the primary environmental risk factor for COPD, yet smoking cessation can be extremely challenging. This is made more difficult by the fact that only 10 to 26% of smokers develop clinical manifestations of COPD. Although the explanation for this is elusive, it has been emphasized in a recent publication from the National Lung Health Education Program[5] that those patients who will develop severe COPD can be identified early on in their smoking history through the documentation of an early and dramatic decline in airflow. In the Lung Health Study, patients in the early stages of COPD were randomized to three groups: usual care with no specific smoking intervention; smoking intervention and the use of ipratropium bromide; or smoking intervention and a placebo inhalation.[15] Rates of decline in FEV_1 were followed over 5 years. This study provided strong evidence that smoking cessation results in substantial benefit to lung function, with FEV_1 improving over the first year. During the second year after smoking cessation, FEV_1 continued unchanged and thereafter exhibited a similar rate of decline as nonsmokers. Smoking cessation is therefore the most important and beneficial intervention and is associated with immediate and sustained health benefits. See Chapter 63 for a more extensive review of smoking cessation therapies. Because smoking cessation is extremely difficult to achieve, prevention may be the key. The prevalence of smoking has declined dramatically since the 1960s; however, there has been little change in the prevalence since 1990. This is due primarily to the steady pace of young teenagers who are taking up smoking.

Exposure to other pollutants such as environmental or industrial pollutants should also be limited as much as possible. Humidification of inspired gases may be beneficial during use of artificial airways (either endotracheal tubes or tracheostomies), even in the patient not on mechanical ventilation.[1]

Correct Airflow Obstruction

Several therapeutic modalities have been studied, including inhaled and oral bronchodilators, corticosteroids, and mucolytics. Individual agents or combinations of agents have met with varying rates of success.

Improve Patient's Functional Status

Many attempts to demonstrate objective improvement in pulmonary function tests with drug therapy have resulted in varying degrees of improvement. Significant subjective improvement noted by the patient has varied between studies. However, if the patient's outlook improves, subjective improvement should not be taken lightly. A perception of increasing dyspnea and decreasing exercise tolerance can be detrimental to the patient's outlook and therefore detrimental to the treatment program.

Initiate Pulmonary Rehabilitation

Rehabilitation for patients with chronic lung diseases is well established as a means of improving the quality of life and preventing or forestalling morbidity and mortality. Rehabilitation programs include a variety of interventions that include education, exercise, and psychosocial counseling. An expert panel recently reviewed the literature and published evidence-based guidelines for pulmonary rehabilitation. Despite this support, pulmonary rehabilitation programs are still seldom used.[16]

Exercise training of both the lower and upper extremities can be helpful. Improved lower extremity muscle training improves ambulation and therefore the ability to do routine daily tasks. Upper extremity training can be important because arm activities can produce shortness of breath due to competition with accessory respiratory muscles. Even though these exercises may not improve pulmonary function, they improve motivation and quality of life by enhancing the patient's ability to carry out daily activities. Most randomized controlled trials do not support the use of ventilatory muscle training as an essential component of pulmonary rehabilitation. Many of these trials may not have used the necessary training intensity, and it is possible that individual patients may achieve benefit.[16]

Depression and anxiety are common in patients with COPD. Studies are lacking, but psychosocial interventions are believed by patients and physicians to be an important part of a pulmonary rehabilitation program. This may include smoking cessation efforts for those patients who have not already quit smoking. Quitting can be very difficult for patients who are feeling anxious or depressed. Adherence to other treatment interventions can also be improved.

Randomized clinical trials have shown that dyspnea improves with rehabilitation. The development of several instruments that measure dyspnea has led to increased emphasis on this parameter when discussing quality-of-life issues. The recent development of instruments that measure quality of life has also supported the benefit of pulmonary rehabilitation programs. COPD patients are heavy users of the health care system, and studies have demonstrated that rehabilitation can decrease the length of hospital stays.

Prevent Acute Disease Exacerbations

Because acute respiratory decompensations are commonly associated with respiratory infections, vaccination against common sources of infection is warranted. The long-term use of prophylactic antibiotics is controversial and not without risk of adverse effects; therefore, this practice is not usually recommended in the United States. The patient should be protected from rapid environmental changes, including cold, dampness, or heavy pollution, because they can trigger acute deterioration.

Optimize Drug Therapy Regimens

Although no specific drug or combination of drugs will reverse the damage already done to the respiratory tract, drug therapy is important in controlling symptoms and managing progression of the disease. The patient may be exposed to any number of drugs with additive adverse effect profiles, and close monitoring is essential to ensure compliance and limit adverse effects. Concomitant drug therapy that could reduce ventilatory drive or increase the work of breathing should be avoided whenever possible. Drugs that aggravate sequelae of COPD (such as arrhythmias) should also be used with caution.

Maintain Adequate Nutrition

COPD is often associated with significant loss of weight and muscle mass. Decreased caloric intake, increased energy expenditure due to the increased work of breathing, and declining pulmonary function measures are possible explanations.[17] The suggestion that weight loss may be the result of the same destructive processes responsible for emphysema is worthy of additional study.[17] Many patients have a body weight less than 90% of ideal. The degree of weight loss affects time of survival–patients with less than 90% of ideal body weight have a survival rate of less than 70% at 3 years.[17] There is some suggestion that COPD patients who develop acute respiratory failure may have a poorer nutritional status than those with stable COPD.[18] Substantial weight loss has been noted in both hospitalized and nonhospitalized[19] COPD patients. Malnutrition can result in decreased respiratory muscle function and depressed immune function, which may predispose the patient to infection. Hypophosphatemia also contributes to poor respiratory muscle function, so supplementation should provide adequate phosphates to avoid this complication.

TREATMENT

A summary of the drug therapy of COPD can be found in Table 37.2. An algorithm for the management of COPD is shown in Figure 37.1.

Pharmacotherapy

Anticholinergics

Anticholinergic therapy is now first-line therapy in stable COPD.[20] Data regarding its role during acute exacerbations is inconclusive, and β-agonists play a primary role. Cholinergic stimulation increases the activity of guanyl cyclase, the enzyme responsible for catalyzing the formation of cyclic guanosine 3′,5′-monophosphate (GMP). Cyclic GMP stimulates bronchoconstriction; therefore, administration of an anticholinergic agent prevents the formation of cyclic GMP. The result is inhibition of bronchoconstriction.

Table 37.2 ▪ Drug Therapy of Stable Chronic Obstructive Pulmonary Disease

Step 1	**Ipratropium** metered-dose inhaler (MDI) (with spacer*) or nebulizer for those patients who cannot master the proper technique; instruct patient on proper administration technique; 2–6† inhalations 4 times a day; instruct patient about importance of regular use; side effects of dry mouth and bitter taste. If drug trial results in <20% improvement in FEV_1, go to step 2.
Step 2	Add a **β_2-agonist** MDI (with spacer*) or nebulizer for those patients who cannot master the proper technique; instruct patient on proper administration technique; dose based on product selected; instruct patient about importance of regular use; side effects of tachycardia and tremor. If follow-up spirometry fails to demonstrate improvement, discontinue the β_2-agonist. If improvement is noted but overall outcome is still suboptimal, go to step 3.
Step 3	Add **theophylline** beginning with up to 400 mg/day as a long-acting dosage form; adjust dose at 3-day intervals by 25% to maintain serum level between 10–15 μg/mL; monitor for side effects of tachycardia, tremor, nervousness, gastrointestinal side effects. If no objective or subjective improvement noted and outcome is still suboptimal, discontinue theophylline and go to step 4.
Step 4	Trial of **corticosteroids: prednisone** 30–40 mg/day for 2–4 weeks; assess objective response with spirometry (i.e., improvement in FEV_1 of at least 20%); titrate dose to the lowest effective dose (<10 mg/day); consider trial of inhaled corticosteroids; patients unable to maintain a similar response with inhaled corticosteroids can be placed back on the oral dosage form.

*Spacers are preferred for most patients who use MDIs.

†There are few controlled studies showing benefits of doses greater than 2 puffs every 6 hours.

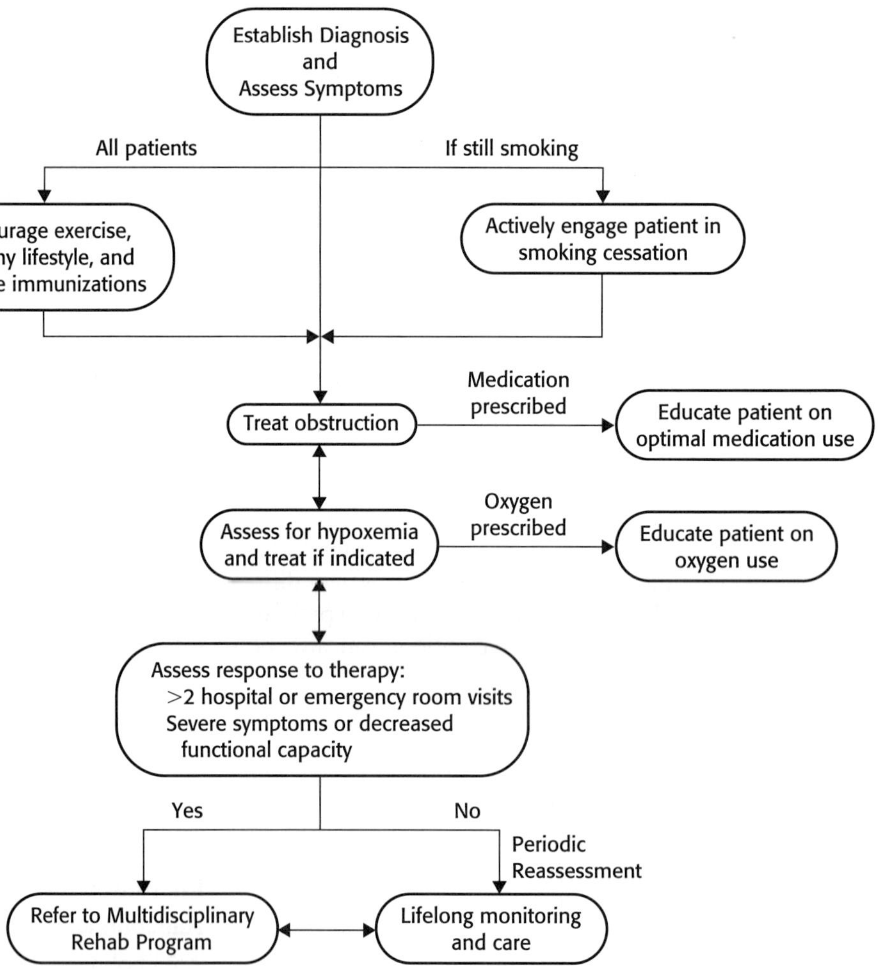

Figure 37.1. Management of COPD. (Reproduced with permission from the American Lung Association. In: Standards for the diagnosis and care of patients with chronic obstructive pulmonary disease [COPD] and asthma. Am J Respir Crit Care Med 152[5, part 2] Supplement, p. S84, 1995.)

The anticholinergic drugs atropine and ipratropium have been used in COPD. Atropine by nebulization is effective and is associated with a decreased incidence of systemic adverse effects compared with parenteral atropine. Some systemic absorption does occur, so the patient should be closely monitored for signs of systemic adverse effects, such as dry mouth, blurred vision, or tachycardia. Because of potentially additive adverse cardiovascular effects, care should be taken when using combinations of atropine and β-agonists or theophylline. The dose of atropine by nebulization is 0.025 mg/kg three to four times a day, with a range of 1 to 2.5 mg per dose. Because of safer alternatives with quaternary compounds, many experts prefer to avoid atropine sulfate.

Ipratropium bromide is an analog of atropine. It acts as a bronchodilator by the same mechanism as atropine; however, because it is a quaternary compound, little systemic absorption occurs. Studies comparing ipratropium to β-agonists in stable COPD patients show that ipratropium bromide produces equal or greater bronchodilation at usual doses.[21,22] At maximal doses, the bronchodilation produced by β-agonists probably equals that of ipratropium in COPD,[23] but adverse effects are more common. Ipratropium bromide produces a response within 15 minutes when inhaled, with effects seen for 4 to 6 hours.[21] Because of its slower onset compared with β-agonists, patients may prefer β-agonists for acute bronchospasm, with ipratropium being used on a scheduled basis. Ipratropium bromide is administered as 2 inhalations 4 times a day, increasing to 6 inhalations if needed. Adverse effects are uncommon and consist of dryness of the mouth and throat, bitter taste, cough, and nausea.

When prescribed therapy with ipratropium or other inhaled aerosol, the patient should be instructed on the proper use of metered-dose inhalers (MDIs). Metered-dose inhalers are a convenient way to deliver aerosolized drugs. However, many patients find it difficult to actuate the inhaler properly and synchronize inhalation and exhalation for maximum drug deposition. In one study of MDI use, 89% of adults were unable to perform all steps correctly.[24] Aerosol deposition within the airways is decreased in these cases. Patients have also been known to exhale during actuation of the inhaler, preventing any airway deposition of drug. Pharmacologic activity occurs only when sufficient drug is deposited at bronchial receptors. Many authorities have made recommendations on the optimal use of MDIs. One group recommends inhalation of the aerosol during a slow, deep inhalation with breath holding for 10 seconds.[25] Actuation of the MDI between tightly closed lips and actuation up to 2 inches in front of widely opened lips are both recommended, and study results disagree on the optimal technique. However, properly performed closed-mouth technique is as efficacious as using an add-on auxiliary device (spacer).[26] Therefore, either open- or closed-mouth technique is acceptable.

Thorough, repeated instructions, involving observation of the patient's technique whenever possible, should be given with each patient visit. Instructions to the patient for appropriate use of MDIs should include the following:

1. Use the inhaler only in the frequency and dose prescribed. If symptoms worsen, seek medical attention before routinely increasing the dose.
2. Shake the MDI canister thoroughly immediately before use.
3. Exhale slowly and completely.
4. Inhale slowly and deeply while depressing the MDI canister.
5. Hold breath for 10 seconds (or as long as possible if not able to do so for 10 seconds).
6. Wait at least 1 minute between multiple doses.
7. Clean MDI case and cap thoroughly with water once per day.

Many experts prefer to use spacers routinely. Spacers decrease particle size, resulting in decreased particle deposition in the upper airway and greater delivery of drug to the more distal airways. In doing so, these devices protect against deposition of aerosols in the oral mucosa and systemic absorption. These auxiliary systems may be useful in patients who fail to properly use MDIs despite education, although many patients may benefit equally from proper explanation and reinforcement of correct MDI use. Because the incidence of inappropriate technique is so high,[23] spacers should be routinely offered to patients.

Ipratropium may also be administered by nebulizer. For nebulization, a dose of 0.5 mg every 4 to 6 hours as needed is used. Because of their expense, size, and lack of increased efficacy, a nebulizer may be useful for patients unable to use MDIs with spacers, seriously ill patients who are not fully alert, and patients who psychologically would benefit from the use of a nebulizer.[27] Considerable debate exists about the role of nebulizers in inhalational therapy.

Sympathomimetics

Sympathomimetics, or β-agonists, are frequently used in COPD to control dyspnea and improve exercise tolerance. These drugs work by activating adenyl cyclase and increasing levels of cyclic adenosine monophosphate (cAMP), resulting in airway smooth muscle relaxation. There is also some evidence that these drugs may increase diaphragmatic contractility[28] and improve cor pulmonale.[29] β-Agonists were considered by many to be first-line therapy in COPD patients. This is currently controversial, because anticholinergic inhalers are equally or more efficacious.

The earliest β-agonists included drugs such as epinephrine, ephedrine, and isoproterenol. Although inhaled β-agonists are more efficacious, epinephrine remains useful in acute reversal of bronchospasm for some patients. However, its short duration of action, nonselectivity, development of refractoriness, and lack of an oral dosage form obviously limit chronic use. Ephedrine and isoproterenol use has been replaced by newer, safer β-agonists.

The most commonly used β-agonists are inhaled β_2-agonists administered via inhalation, although oral and parenteral products are also used. Systemic therapy is associated with more frequent adverse effects and lower efficacy. Rapid airway response is seen with inhaled β-agonists, whereas the onset of action with oral therapy in acute airway obstruction is delayed. Therefore, inhaled β-agonists are preferred in patients capable of using the devices. Standard dosing recommendations are usually applied to the COPD patient, but they have not been well studied for optimum response in these patients.

β-Agonists should be compared on the basis of selectivity for β_2-receptors, available dosage forms, onset and duration of action, and cost. Terbutaline, albuterol, bitolterol, salmeterol, and pirbuterol are all relatively β_2-specific agents. β_2-Receptor selectivity results in a decreased rate of systemic adverse effects, particularly adverse cardiovascular effects, compared with the nonselective agents. Because of this specificity, these drugs are commonly prescribed. Terbutaline, albuterol, bitolterol, salmeterol, and pirbuterol are all available for inhalation. They vary in onset and duration of action, with salmeterol having the longest onset and duration of action at up to 20 minutes and 12 hours, respectively. Because of the prolonged onset of action, salmeterol is not appropriate for treatment of acute bronchospasm or acute exacerbations of COPD. Patient education is important to ensure that this difference between salmeterol and other quick-onset β-agonists is understood. Another concern is the potential for therapeutic duplication when Combivent, a combination product of albuterol and ipratropium, is prescribed with salmeterol. In this instance, albuterol should be prescribed separately on an as needed basis. Salmeterol has been studied extensively in COPD and offers a valuable alternative for patients who have difficulty with adherance to more frequent administrations of short-acting agents.[30–32] The side effect profiles are similar in nature but vary in frequency. Minimal cardiovascular adverse effects are seen with the β_2-selective agents. Tremor is common to all the agents and is the primary adverse effect of albuterol and bitolterol. Transient hypokalemia may be induced by high doses of these agents. Combined therapy with inhaled and oral β-agonists may be seen, but additive adverse effects are likely to occur.

Appropriate instruction for MDI use should accompany β-agonist inhaler therapy, just as with ipratropium. β-Agonists may also be delivered via nebulization, but this practice is subject to the same concerns as with ipratropium. The relative doses of β-agonists for nebulization are similar to doses used in asthma and are higher than those for MDI inhalation because of the reduced efficiency of nebulizers in delivering the drug. However, patients who are severely dyspneic may benefit from nebulizer therapy if the MDI has not proven effective. Part of this improved response may relate to delivery of the drug as a wet aerosol.

Aerosol Bronchodilators (Ventilated Patients)

Aerosols are routinely used in the treatment of critically ill intubated patients. Little information exists regarding the most effective method of delivery, proper dose, and optimum ventilator settings to ensure delivery. Recommendations based on current knowledge include the following:

1. When using MDIs in the ventilated patient, the clinician should be aware that adequate amounts of medication may not reach the patient's airways. Physiologic parameters such as airway mechanics and close observation for systemic effects should be used to titrate and determine optimal dosing. MDIs administered through an in-line spacing device have been shown to have greater efficiency of aerosol deposition to lung tissue when compared with jet nebulization.[33]
2. For jet nebulizers, it is recommended to use the largest possible volume of fill.
3. Ventilators should be set at reduced inspiratory flows (40 to 50 mL/min) to prolong inspiratory time, although caution is advised for those patients with excessive amounts of intrinsic peak end-expiratory pressure (PEEP).[34]

Recently, continuous β-agonist nebulization has been tried in many intensive care units. Tachycardia and hypokalemia have been observed, so careful titration according to physiologic effect is necessary.[35] Further research must be done on this mode of delivery.

Combination β-Agonist/Anticholinergic

Data regarding the effects of using an anticholinergic medication with a β-agonist have been conflicting. The overall weight of the evidence favors an additive effect with chronic use but not acute use. Additive effects during chronic use have been recently supported by a large multicenter trial called Combivent.[36] The study found an additional bronchodilation of 20 to 40% for the combination over single agents. Despite this finding, clinical COPD symptom scores were not significantly different. A stepwise approach to the selection of a bronchodilator based on objective measurements such as peak flow or spirometry is thought to be more useful than using only symptomatic endpoints. Patients can be started on a single bronchodilator initially, and the combination can be tried if objective tests indicate a suboptimal response. On the other hand, if pulmonary function studies improve without subjective relief of dyspnea, it will have little relevance to the patient. The increased effectiveness of the combination is not surprising because the two classes of drugs have different mechanisms and sites of action. Anticholinergic drugs are believed to act primarily in the central airways where cholinergic receptors are abundant; the β-agonists' site of action includes peripheral as well as central airways.[37]

Several studies conducted in emergency rooms examined the effect of combination therapy during acute exacerbations. Results demonstrated significant benefit with either ipratropium or sympathomimetics as the initial agent, but were unable to demonstrate significant improvement with the combination.[38–40] If the combination is used during the acute treatment of COPD, an attempt should be made to determine whether a single agent would be sufficient once the patient is stable. The following step-care approach has been suggested: (1) obtain baseline spirometry; (2) administer ipratropium; (3) repeat spirometry 30 minutes later; (4) administer inhaled β-agonist; and (5) repeat spirometry.[41]

Methylxanthines

At one time, theophylline was the mainstay of bronchodilator therapy in the COPD patient. With more effective bronchodilators now available, theophylline's role in COPD has declined. However, theophylline may still be beneficial in the management of chronic COPD, especially if a bronchoconstrictive component can be identified. Theophylline, when added to regimens of inhaled anticholinergics or β-agonists, produces additive bronchodilation.[42–44] Once therapy is maximized with inhaled bronchodilators with suboptimal response, patients may be given a trial of theophylline followed by pulmonary function testing to assess response to therapy. Significant improvement can be demonstrated through pulmonary function testing,[44–46] as well as through decreased dyspnea[44,46] and quality-of-life measures.[44] Theophylline may also reduce overnight declines in FEV_1 and resultant morning respiratory symptoms when administered as an evening dose, and it may still have an important role in this setting.[47]

Theophylline, as intravenous aminophylline, has been evaluated in acute exacerbations of COPD.[48] In addition to a regimen consisting of β-agonists, corticosteroids, antibiotics, and oxygen (when needed), patients received either intravenous aminophylline or placebo. The results were not promising, with no significant improvement seen with the addition of theophylline. Because study numbers were small, questions remain about the role of theophylline in acute COPD exacerbations. Until further study shows benefit when added to standard therapies in acute exacerbations of COPD, this drug cannot be recommended for routine initial use.

In addition to questions regarding the overall efficacy of theophylline in COPD, the mechanisms by which it may produce beneficial effects are unclear. Proposed effects on the cardiac and respiratory systems include bronchodilation, improved respiratory muscle contractility and reserve, stimulation of central ventilatory drive, increased mucociliary clearance, decreased mean pulmonary artery pressure and pulmonary vascular resistance, increased collateral ventilation, and improved biventricular cardiac performance.[46,49] Although demonstrated in several small trials, the significance of these effects has not been fully examined in COPD patients on a large scale. Indeed it is likely that a combination of these effects is responsible for any positive benefit seen. Theophylline does not possess the bronchodilatory potency of β-agonists. Improved respiratory muscle reserve appears to account for improvement in dyspnea in patients with stable, severe COPD.[46] The ability to lower mean pulmonary artery pressure and decrease pulmonary vascular resistance has been demonstrated in both acute and long-term studies of theophylline, although study populations have been small.[50] Infusion of intravenous theophylline results in a significant decrease in these parameters, as well as a direct inotropic action; both are advantageous in the patient who has progressed to cor pulmonale and heart failure. Ventricular afterload is reduced and biventricular cardiac function is improved as a result.

Theophylline probably produces these effects through a number of actions, including inhibition of phosphodiesterase, alteration in calcium movement, blockade of adenosine receptors, prostaglandin antagonism, and alteration of cAMP binding to the binding protein.[49] Phosphodiesterase inhibition has traditionally been accepted as the mechanism of action of theophylline, but it is questionable whether this accounts for its effects at clinically used doses. The other effects have been noted at clinically useful levels and thus may be responsible for the efficacy of the drug.[51]

When initiating therapy, the clinician must address several issues related to theophylline. A multitude of dosage forms and salts of theophylline are available. The acuity of the situation dictates choice of dosage form (e.g., the patient in acute respiratory failure who cannot take oral medication is best managed by parenteral therapy). However, chronic therapy decisions must include an assessment of patient compliance, dosage form preference, factors that influence the clearance of theophylline, and cost. See Chapter 36 for a detailed discussion of theophylline, including dosage form comparisons, detailed pharmacokinetics, and drug interactions.

Recommendations for dosing of theophylline in COPD are similar to those for asthma. Continuous infusions for acute therapy are generally in the range of 0.2 to 0.7 mg/kg/hr, whereas oral dosages for chronic therapy start at up to 400 mg/day and increase by 25% at 3-day intervals until the desired dose is achieved.[52] Serum concentrations up to 20 μg/mL show a linear correlation with improvement in FEV_1 in the COPD patient.[52] However, as serum concentration exceeds 15 μg/mL, benefits may be outweighed by risk of toxicity. The general goal is to achieve serum concentrations of 8 to 12 μg/mL.[1] When used in COPD, theophylline therapy should be monitored closely to assess the degree of benefit the patient is receiving (primarily symptomatic control). Careful monitoring is also warranted to prevent or limit adverse effects that may be more common in these patients (e.g., they may be particularly sensitive to the arrhythmogenic effects of theophylline).[53] Many COPD patients continue to smoke, thereby increasing theophylline clearance. The clearance of theophylline may be reduced in advanced stages of COPD or in the presence of cor pulmonale with or without heart failure, and careful monitoring of serum concentrations is essential.

Given the adverse effect profile of theophylline, evidence of significant benefit should be obtained before subjecting the patient to long-term therapy. Preferably, pulmonary function testing should be used before and after theophylline, as well as dyspnea scoring. The clinician must be able to monitor the patient for side effects and toxicity such as nausea, vomiting, tremors, headaches, confusion, arrhythmias, and seizures. Further evidence of objective benefits on diaphragmatic contractility, stimulation of hypoxic drive, and improved cardiac performance may define the role of theophylline in COPD more clearly.

Corticosteroids

The role of corticosteroids, both systemic and inhaled, in COPD has been the subject of much debate. Studies have been contradictory, with positive studies tending to include patients who have a high level of reversibility following the use of a bronchodilator, suggesting the inclusion of more patients with an asthma component. Both asthma and COPD are characterized by the presence of airway inflammation. In asthma, this is manifested by an increase in the number of eosinophils and mast cells that stimulate cytokines and further the inflammatory process. COPD is characterized by a predominance of neutrophilic and lymphocytic infiltrates that result in a differing pattern of cytokine stimulation.[54] In a recent trial of severe COPD patients, inhaled budesonide (800 μg BID) was administered, and response was measured through lung function tests, symptom scores, and inflammatory indices.[54] Sputum assays for a variety of inflammatory markers were conducted. Because of the possibility of poor drug delivery to the lower airways in patients with severe COPD, a similar group of patients received oral prednisolone therapy. Known asthma patients were included as a control group. There was no clinical benefit in either lung function or symptom scores, and no significant change in the anti-inflammatory indices in either the oral or inhaled corticosteroid groups, while the asthmatic group exhibited marked decreases in inflammatory indices. This study supports the clinical impression that COPD is largely resistant to the anti-inflammatory effect of corticosteroids.

Yet evidence exists supporting a benefit from oral corticosteroids. A meta-analysis summarized studies performed in more stable COPD patients and concluded that oral corticosteroids improve baseline FEV_1 by 20% or greater approximately 10% more often than patients receiving placebo.[55] Subjective improvements in exercise tolerance and dyspnea have been reported.[56] Subjective improvement can occur without actual improvement in pulmonary function tests, exercise tolerance, or arterial oxygen saturation.[56,57] Oral corticosteroids can result in euphoria, especially in higher doses, and reports of subjective improvement may reflect a side effect of oral corticosteroid therapy. Improvement in quality-of-life measures during treatment with oral corticosteroids in COPD patients has been suggested.[58] Longer-term studies are needed to fully measure the extent of improvement. Only with longer periods of observation would measures such as exercise tolerance be evaluable, due to the lag time in muscle recovery following renewed or increased use.

Because bronchodilator therapy alone has been associated with increasing mortality and an accelerated rate of decline in FEV_1 in patients with asthma and COPD,[59] interest has been growing regarding the addition of oral corticosteroids to reverse this trend. Studies[60,61] designed to examine the spectrum of obstructive airways disease have shown improvement in morbidity, hyperresponsiveness, and rate of decline in FEV_1 with the combination of corticosteroids and bronchodilators. Subgroup analysis demonstrates that the greatest benefit is seen in patients with an asthmatic clinical presentation, but suggests that some benefit may also be achieved in some patients with COPD and some hyperresponsivity. This subgroup of patients may be those COPD patients with features of asthma such as reticular basement membrane thickening and eosinophilic inflammation. It has been demonstrated that patients with increased eosinophils in peripheral blood, bronchoalveolar lavage fluid, sputum, and bronchial biopsies are more like to respond to corticosteroids.[62,63] This may be difficult to apply clinically, but it strongly suggests the presence of this intermediate group between asthma and those with irreversible COPD.

In COPD exacerbations, intravenous steroids are usually added to bronchodilator therapy, but the number of clinical trials supporting this intervention is small. Systemic corticosteroids have resulted in a demonstrable increase in FEV_1 in both outpatients and hospitalized patients experiencing exacerbations of COPD given corticosteroids, even in patients who have not responded during stable periods of their disease.[64,65] High corticosteroid doses are usually recommended, although the effects of lower doses have not been adequately studied. A small clinical trial of parenteral methylprednisolone versus placebo in patients with COPD undergoing abdominal surgery indicated that methylprednisolone hastened recovery of pulmonary function following surgery.[66]

A trial of corticosteroids can be tried in patients suboptionally responding to bronchodilators. The duration of the trial is unclear and should take into accout the route of drug delivery chosen. Hudson and Monti[67] recommend a trial of oral corticosteroids for 1 to 2 weeks in patients with significant airflow obstruction. Weir and colleagues[68] demonstrated that some responders do not show maximum response for at least 2 weeks and recommended a longer corticosteroid trial. Several different corticosteroid regimens can be selected. When oral therapy is selected, methylprednisolone 20 to 40 mg daily or prednisone equivalent may be initiated. Improvements in FEV_1 of 20% are traditionally used to indicate a positive response; however, this criterion may be overly stringent, demanding an all-or-nothing response, because an increase of greater than 20% can be difficult to achieve even with the use of bronchodilators in moderate to severe asthma. Subjective improvements in dyspnea and exercise tolerance should also be noted. If the patient responds, the dose of corticosteroid should be tapered to the lowest effective dose due to the well-known systemic side effects with corticosteroids.

Evidence demonstrates that clinically used corticosteroid doses can produce muscle weakness.[69] Regimens that averaged 1.4 to 21.3 mg/day methylprednisolone equivalent, either as continuous therapy or in repeated short-course regimens over a 6-month period, produced this effect.[69] Both respiratory and peripheral muscles are affected. Respiratory muscle involvement may enhance dyspnea, thereby appearing as though COPD is worsening. The mechanism behind this finding has not been elucidated, and the overall significance of steroid-induced muscle weakness to the use of corticosteroids in COPD remains unclear.

The role of inhaled corticosteroids in COPD is even more controversial. A review of this topic points out that since 1972, more than 100 studies have attempted to answer this question.[70] Twelve of these were randomized, placebo-controlled studies, with two of them suggesting a benefit.[71,72] Paggiaro and colleagues[72] studied the efficacy of high-dose inhaled corticosteroids in COPD patients who demonstrated less than a 15% reversibility with bronchodilators. There was a small but clinically significant improvement in peak expiratory flow. Although there was no difference in the number of exacerbations, there were significantly fewer moderate to severe exacerbations in the fluticasone group than the placebo group. Studies evaluating oral versus inhaled corticosteroids have demonstrated efficacy differences, with fewer patients responding to inhaled corticosteroids than to an oral regimen.[73] However, in a study in which a spacer device was used to deliver inhaled beclomethasone, this mode of therapy was as effective as oral prednisolone.[58]

Despite their frequent use, available data suggest a limited role for inhaled corticosteroids in the treatment of COPD. Several large trials of anti-inflammatory treatment for COPD are currently underway, including the EUROSCOP, Lung Health II, ISOLDE, and Copenhagen Lung Study.[74,74a,74b] In the meantime, patients who exhibit a poor response to bronchodilator therapy should be given a trial of corticosteroids, either orally or with high-dose inhaled agents. If patients are thought to be responders, inhaled corticosteroids can be continued. Over a period of several months, if peak flow has been improved by at least 15 L/min and the severity and number of exacerbations is believed to be less, the patient can continue therapy. Inhaled corticosteroids offer the advantage of significantly less systemic side effects, although at high doses they also have the potential for systemic effects.

Several inhaled corticosteroid products are available, although fluticasone and budesonide offer potency and dosage forms that allow for the convenience of fewer puffs per day when compared with other agents. Budesonide is available as a dry powder inhaler that may offer an easier administration technique for many patients. For long-term use, budesonide also offers the most cost-effective choice. High-dose budesonide is generally 600 to 1000 μg/day (3 to 5 inhalations), and low-dose maintenance therapy can be 200 to 400 μg/day (1 to 2 puffs). The highest strength of fluticasone (220 μg/puff) can be used in the high-dose range of 660 to 1540 μg/day (3 to 7 puffs/day). The maintenance dose of fluticasone is generally in the range of 220 to 440 μg/day. Systemic side effects do not usually occur until daily dosing exceeds 1000 μg/day over a long period. More detailed information on inhaled corticosteroid products can be found in Chapter 36.

Antibiotics and Vaccines

Frequent isolation of *Streptococcus pneumoniae, Haemophilus influenzae,* and *Moraxella catarrhalis,* both in stable and exacerbated COPD patients, presents a dilemma to the clinician. This finding may represent colonization of the airway, not infection. Even if infection is present, but remains confined to the bronchial mucosa, spontaneous resolution without antibiotic treatment may occur.[75] The presence of two of three findings (increased dyspnea, increased sputum volume, and sputum purulence) has been recommended as an indicator for antibiotic treatment.[76] Improved clinical outcomes, fewer therapeutic failures, and more rapid recovery of lung function were noted in antibiotic-treated patients.[76] This finding is reinforced by a meta-analysis of antibiotic trials in COPD patients that also identified a statistical improvement in patients treated with antibiotics versus placebo.[77]

Despite the lack of consensus on the value of antibiotic use and the prevalence of viral infections in these patients, the fact remains that antibiotics are commonly prescribed in COPD patients. This practice results in increased drug therapy expense and almost certainly contributes to the widespread problem of antibiotic resistance. Common antibiotics prescribed include doxycycline, ampicillin or amoxicillin, cephalosporins, and cotrimoxazole. However, newer and broader-spectrum antibiotics continue to be introduced to the market and are commonly prescribed as well. Quinolones, clarithromycin or azithromycin, and β-lactamase inhibitor combination drugs are also commonly used. Oral therapy is indicated unless pneumonia complicating acute respiratory failure is present. In this latter case, the patient may be best managed with parenteral therapy, although oral options should be considered early. Local susceptibility patterns, previous patient exposure to antibiotics, and cost should govern the final selection of the antibiotic regimen. Duration of antibiotic therapy is usually 7 to 10 days.

Vaccination with pneumococcal and influenzae virus vaccines is recommended in high-risk patient groups. Pneumococcal vaccine is formulated to provide prophylaxis against the most common strains of *S. pneumoniae.* Clear evidence that COPD patients are at an increased risk of infection by *S. pneumoniae* and thus increased risk of death has not been presented.[78] Antibody titers to the organisms may be elevated in COPD, probably as a result of chronic upper airway colonization. When given the vaccine, these patients respond by further increasing their antibody titers. Therefore, many clinicians recommend giving the vaccine to individuals with COPD. The most current dosing recommendation for adults is 0.5 mL by subcutaneous or intramuscular injection. Because antibody titers decline with time, the question of revaccination has been posed. Revaccination of COPD patients every 5 to 10 years has been suggested.[79]

Influenza virus vaccine provides active immunity to the virus. As opposed to pneumococcal vaccine, influenza virus vaccine should be given annually to patients with COPD. The vaccine is reformulated periodically to cover the most common strains. The usual adult dose is 0.5 mL intramuscularly. Amantadine 100 mg twice daily for 14 days may be given during outbreaks of influenza A to high-risk patients who have not been immunized or during acute influenza if started within the first 48 hours.[80]

Oxygen Therapy

Oxygen therapy is an option for patients with severe chronic hypoxemia, cor pulmonale, and nocturnal or exercise-induced hypoxemia. In the setting of severe COPD, long-term oxygen therapy improves the survival rate in these patients.[81–83] It is usually considered when the baseline Pa_{O_2} drops below 55 mm Hg or below 60 mm Hg with concomitant right-sided heart failure, polycythemia, or impaired mentation. Oxygen can be administered by devices that allow for ambulation or by fixed devices. Devices that allow the patient to ambulate are preferable. It can be administered continuously, during exercise, or nocturnally. The number of hours per day the patient uses oxygen continuously seems to relate to the effectiveness of this therapy, with those patients who use oxygen for at least 15 hours per day showing the greatest benefit.[81] Patients may be reluctant to use continuous oxygen therapy, so nocturnal use may be more attractive. Oxygen use in combination with a structured exercise program may improve exercise tolerance. From 1 to 4 L of oxygen by nasal cannulae is usually required. The goal of therapy is to maintain oxygen saturation at or above 90%.

Mucolytic/Expectorant Agents

No clinical benefit of mucolytic or expectorant agents has been established in COPD patients. Acetylcysteine thins secretions in chronic bronchitics[84] but does not improve airflow in COPD patients.[85] Acetylcysteine can induce airway irritation and bronchospasm, requiring bronchodilator use. Because of the lack of demonstrated value, attention should be focused instead on decreased mucus production by limiting exposure to cigarette smoking and other airway irritants.[5]

Respiratory Stimulants

Chronic hypercapnia in the COPD patient is usually well tolerated and may be compensatory to reduce respiratory muscle fatigue.[86] It is best managed by proper muscle conditioning and bronchodilators. Although respiratory stimulants such as doxapram, medroxyprogesterone, and acetazolamide are available and used, any beneficial effect is short-lived. The potential risks of therapy are also significant concerns. Further respiratory fatigue from overstimulation of respiratory muscles may worsen respiratory failure.[5] At this time, their use cannot be recommended.

α_1-Proteinase Inhibitors

Approximately 1 to 13% of patients with emphysema have a deficiency of α_1-antitrypsin (AAT).[87] This deficiency leads to progressive destruction of elastin tissues and alveolar destruction caused by unopposed neutrophil elastase activity. A replacement product (Prolastin) is obtained from pooled human plasma. Maintenance of AAT serum concentrations above 70 mg/dL should slow the rate of lung destruction. This treatment is not indicated for patients who have not developed signs and symptoms of emphysema, those patients with other forms of emphysema, or those patients with FEV_1 less than 20% of predicted.

Treatment with α_1-proteinase inhibitor requires weekly therapy. The regimen is costly, averaging $500 to 1500 per week depending on patient weight. A dose of 60 mg/kg/wk intravenously appears to maintain the inhibitor at an appropriate level within the lungs.[88] The drug is well tolerated without adverse cardiovascular, respiratory, or hematologic effects. Although AAT from pooled human plasma is found to be nonreactive for the human immunodeficiency virus (HIV) antibody and hepatitis B surface antigen, hepatitis B immunization is still recommended with hepatitis B vaccine. Hepatitis B immune globulin, 0.06 mL/kg intramuscularly, may be given with the first dose of vaccine if therapy with α_1-proteinase inhibitor is indicated before the vaccination regimen can be administered.

Nonpharmacologic Therapy

Surgery

Lung volume resection surgery is a technique used to resect large emphysematous bullae or diffusely emphysematous lung. By reducing lung volume, postoperative lung elastic recoil is probably enhanced. This reduces the effort needed to maintain the same ventilatory pressure.[89] One series reports a 1-year increase in FEV_1 of 45% and improved exercise tolerance.[90] Identification of appropriate candidates and timing of surgical intervention are unresolved questions.

Lung transplantation for COPD has been a viable surgical treatment for COPD since the 1980s. Initially, double-lung and heart-lung transplantations were considered preferable to single-lung transplantations because of perceived ventilation/perfusion mismatches between the emphysematous lung and the transplanted lung. Subsequent work demonstrated that single-lung transplantation is effective, although FEV_1 returns to only 50 to 60% of predicted within the first 2 years.[91] Although this is less than the improvement noted with double-lung or heart-lung transplantation, acceptable return of functional capability of the patient is noted. Survival rates are 67% at the end of 2 years with single-lung transplantation.[91] Single-lung transplantation allows a greater number of patients to benefit from lung transplantation than double-lung or heart-lung transplantation, but each of these techniques is currently performed. Bronchiolitis obliterans syndrome, related to chronic rejection, remains a major reason for progressive loss of graft function. COPD is the most common diagnosis for lung transplantation. As with all solid organ transplants, access to donor organs is a common barrier to more widespread application of this treatment option.

Management of Other Complications

Breathlessness

The discomfort of breathlessness is one of the major factors affecting quality of life for many patients with COPD. It may significantly restrict the patient's ability for any level of exercise. Breathlessness worsens as pulmonary function declines, but there is a great deal of interpatient variability in the relationship between this symptom and commonly measured physiologic lung parameters. Factors contributing to breathlessness include mechanical, sensory, and behavioral components.[92]

Because the primary mechanical abnormality involves expiratory flow limitation, the onset of inspiration occurs before expiratory flow is complete. With each breath, inspiratory muscles must overcome the elastic recoil associated with expiration, placing more demand on already compromised respiratory muscles, including the diaphragm. The resultant lung hyperinflation is thought to cause negtive mechanical and sensory stimuli that contribute to the feeling of breathlessness. Anxiety also accompanies the feeling of breathlessness and may itself contribute to the symptom.[92]

Bronchodilators can relieve feelings of breathlessness even with the achievement of only small changes in FEV_1.[46] Anticholinergic medications may also reduce breathlessness. The mechanism for both medications is probably a reduction in gas trapping and lung hyperinflation, which results in a reduction in motor and sensory stimulation of breathlessness.

Supplemental oxygen has been shown to relieve breathlessness. This is probably related to decreased ventilatory demand due to altered peripheral chemoreceptor sensitivity. It is also possible that oxygen has central effects on the perceived discomfort of breathlessness. Beneficial effects of supplemental oxygen have been observed in patients who do not meet current American Thoracic Society criteria for long-term oxygen therapy.[93]

Opiates have been reported to substantially increase the exercise capacity of patients with COPD.[94,95] Probable mechanisms include a reduction in ventilatory drive in response to carbon dioxide, hypoxia, and exercise, as well as an altered central perception of inspiratory effort with the relief of anxiety. Improvements in workload and duration of exercise during opiate therapy have been suggested to be greater than those seen with anticholinergics and β-adrenergic stimulants. A recently reported study contradicts these findings, however. Poole and colleagues[96] conducted a randomized, double-blind, placebo-controlled crossover trial in which sustained-release morphine was given to 16 COPD patients with breathlessness caused by COPD. The primary endpoint was a quality-of-life assessment, and secondary endpoints included a 6-minute walk, distance, and breathlessness scores. There was no difference between treatments, and side effects (primarily nausea and vomiting) were common. One patient was described as having spectacular success with the therapy, suggesting a possible small subset of patients that may respond. Special precautions are necessary because of the possible excess respiratory depression that may occur. Current use is primarily restricted to palliative care patients due to adverse effects such as sedation and the problem of physical tolerance.

Benzodiazepines have not been shown to provide consistent beneficial effects when compared with placebo. They may be used in patients whose breathlessness has a significant anxiety component.[92]

Pulmonary Hypertension and Cor Pulmonale

Pulmonary hypertension develops in response to chronic hypoxemia. Cor pulmonale, or hypertrophy of the right ventricle, is a subsequent result. Right ventricular or biventricular failure may develop. Because sustained hypoxemia is postulated to be the major stimulus behind increased pulmonary vascular resistance and pulmonary hypertension, oxygen therapy is one of the primary therapies used in cor pulmonale. Diuretics have been used to manage dyspnea and edema. Digoxin may be beneficial in the patient with biventricular failure resulting from cor pulmonale, but its usefulness in isolated right ventricular failure is limited. Vasodilators reduce right ventricular afterload and may be used in patients with resistant pulmonary hypertension or right ventricular failure. Aggressive management of the underlying pulmonary disease, prevention of sustained hypoxemia, and patient education are the best means to reduce the incidence of this complication.

Acute Respiratory Failure

Acute respiratory failure may be precipitated by infection, use of central nervous system depressant drugs, bronchospasm, mucous plugging, or changes in environmental pollutants. Other stresses (e.g., surgery) may precipitate acute respiratory failure. The patient may have signs of diaphragmatic fatigue noted as asynchronous breathing. The PaO_2 is usually below 50 mm Hg, the $PaCO_2$ above 45 mm Hg, and the pH acidotic. Oxygen therapy and possibly mechanical ventilation are required. Mechanical ventilation is reserved until absolutely necessary, because it is difficult and slow to wean the COPD patient from ventilatory support. Supportive drug therapy, including β-agonists, corticosteroids, anticholinergics, and theophylline, may be instituted based on clinical symptoms (Table 37.3). Antibiotic therapy should be initiated in the patient with signs of infection. Cardiac failure or arrhythmias should be treated by appropriate measures. Invasive cardiopulmonary monitoring should be instituted at this time. Nutritional support should be instituted early to prevent further loss of muscle mass.

PROGNOSIS

The best indicators of prognosis are degree of obstruction and age.[97] Complications such as cor pulmonale and hypoxia are negative indicators for survival. FEV_1 obtained after bronchodilators is a good predictor of survival.[97] Once FEV_1 decreases below 0.75 L, severe airway obstruction is present and is associated with increased 5-year mortality rates. When patients have dyspnea, the mortality rate increases; up to 50% of patients die within 5 years. Multiple exacerbations, hospitalizations, and multiple-drug therapies to treat symptoms or prevent progression will probably characterize their course. Poor nutrition and exercise intolerance commonly develop, and patients undergo important alterations in lifestyle in severe disease.

Table 37.3 ▪ Drug Therapy of Acute Respiratory Failure

Oxygenation	Relief of hypoxemia with nasal cannula at 2–4 L/min or Venturi mask of 24–28%. Goal is to achieve 90% saturation of a normal hemoglobin level. If oxygenation is adequate and mental status deteriorates (secondary to increased $Paco_2$), oxygen can be decreased.
Bronchodilators	β_2-agonists are preferred in the emergency department due to faster onset of action and peak effect. Evidence of a significant clinical benefit is lacking for the combined use with ipratropium in the acute setting.* Monitor for common side effects such as tremor, tachycardia, hypokalemia. Less frequent adverse effects include exacerbation of arrhythmias such as atrial fibrillation/flutter, multifocal atrial tachycardia, and premature ventricular contractions.
	Ipratropium 4–6 inhalations (or 0.5 mg by nebulizatiom, which is preferred for acute respiratory failure) 4–6 times per day. May be the preferred agent over β_2-agonists in COPD for cardiac patients due to fewer systemic adverse effects.
Corticosteroids	Methylprednisolone 0.5 mg/kg IV every 6 hours or hydrocortisone 100–250 mg IV every 6 hours. Begin to taper by the third day. The rate of tapering of the corticosteroid dose is based on severity of disease and clinical response.
Antibiotics	Assess likelihood of infection. Institute appropriate antibiotics, if necessary.
Theophylline	Although there are no data supporting use, in a life-threatening situation it is warranted until benefits are disproven. Benefit/risk ratio must be carefully assessed due to adverse effects of nervousness, tremor, tachycardia, worsening arrhythmias, and gastrointestinal side effects. A loading dose of 5 mg/kg IV should be given if the patient was not previously on theophylline; maintenance infusion rates should range from 0.2–0.7 mg/kg/hr individualized based on patient history, concomitant drugs, and target blood levels of 8–12 μg/mL.
Fluids and electrolytes	Ensure adequate fluid intake with appropriate electrolyte replacement, including phosphates.
Nutrition	Initiate nutrition as soon as possible. Overfeeding should be avoided due to increased CO_2 production associated with excess caloric intake.
Mucolytics	Acetylcysteine may be used, especially for patients on mechanical ventilation with excessive secretions resulting in mucous plugging. They are not recommended for routine use because they are bronchial irritants and may promote bronchospasm.
Respiratory stimulants	Use is controversial and cannot be routinely recommended.
Physiotherapy	Although commonly employed, the value of physiotherapy in acute respiratory failure is not determined.

*Although many clinicians use anticholinergics concurrently, there is no evidence of additive effect in COPD (as there is in asthma).

KEY POINTS

- Chronic obstructive pulmonary disease is a potentially preventable disease. Recognition that smoking contributes to the majority of COPD cases logically leads to the conclusion that cessation of smoking would dramatically decrease its incidence. Public education about the hazards of smoking should continue. Obviously, health care professionals should model wellness by not smoking, and they should make concerted efforts to have patients stop smoking.
- Once COPD develops, those affected with moderate-to-severe disease are faced with a multitude of drug therapies with clearly debatable efficacy.
- The progressive nature of the disease means the cost to the patient, both personally and financially, and the cost to society is high.
- Ongoing evaluation of the benefits of screening for early diagnosis and intervention in patients at risk for COPD holds future promise.

REFERENCES

1. American Thoracic Society. Standards for the diagnosis and care of patients with chronic obstructive pulmonary disease (COPD) and asthma. Am J Respir Crit Care Med 152(5, pt 2):S77–S121, 1995.
2. National Center for Health Statistics. Monthly Vital Statistics Report 42(12):19, 1994.
3. Peto R, Lopez AD, Boreham J, et al. Mortality from tobacco in developed countries: indirect estimation from national vital statistics. Lancet 339:1269–1278, 1992.
4. Thom TJ. International comparisons in COPD mortality. Am Rev Respir Dis 140:S27–S34, 1989.
5. National Lung Health Education Program (NLHEP) Committee. Strategies in preserving lung health and preventing COPD and associated diseases–The National Lung Health Education Program (NLHEP). Chest 113:2 (Feb Suppl):123–163, 1998.
6. Fletcher C, Peto R, Tinker C, Speizer FE. The natural history of chronic bronchitis and emphysema. New York: Oxford University Press, 1976:82–84.
7. Carroll GC, Rothenberg DM. Carbon dioxide narcosis. Chest 102:986, 1992.
8. Breslin E, van der Schens C, Breukink S, Meek P. Perception of fatigue and quality of life in patients with COPD. Chest 114(4):958–964, 1998.
9. Altose MD. Assessment and management of breathlessness. Chest 88(2 Suppl):77S–83S, 1985.
10. Murphy TF, Sethi S. Bacterial infection in chronic obstructive pulmonary disease. Am Rev Respir Dis 146:1067–1083, 1992.
11. Wilson R, Dowling R, Jackson A. The biology of bacterial colonization and invasion of the respiratory mucosa. Eur Respir J 9:1523–1530, 1996.
12. Mendella LA, Manfreda J, Warren CPW, Anthonisen NR. Steroid response in stable chronic obstructive pulmonary disease. Ann Intern Med 96:17–21, 1982.
13. American Thoracic Society. Lung function testing: selection of reference values and interpretative strategies (Comments). Am Rev Respir Dis 144:1201–1218, 1991.
14. Pfeifer MP. End-of-life decision-making: special considerations in the COPD patient. Medscape Respiratory Care 2(5) (on-line publication). Available at http://www.medscape.com. Accessed March 20, 2000.
15. Anthonisen NR, Connett JE, Kiley JP, et al. Effects of smoking intervention and the use of an inhaled anticholinergic bronchodilator on the rate of decline of FEV_1: the Lung Health Study. JAMA 272:1497–1505, 1994.

16. ACCP/AACVPR Pulmonary Rehabilitation Guidelines Panel. Special report: pulmonary rehabilitation: joint ACCP/AACVPR evidence-based guidelines. Chest 112:1363–1396, 1997.
17. Wilson DO, Rogers RM, Wright EC, Anthonisen NR. Body weight in chronic obstructive pulmonary disease–the National Institutes of Health intermittent positive-pressure breathing trial. Am Rev Respir Dis 139:1435–1438, 1989.
18. Driver AG, McAlvey MT, Smith VL. Nutritional assessment of patients with COPD and acute respiratory failure. Chest 82:568–571, 1982.
19. Braun SR, Keim NL, Dixon RM, et al. The prevalence and determinants of nutritional changes in chronic obstructive pulmonary disease. Chest 86(4):558–563, 1984.
20. Braun SR, Levy SF. Comparison of ipratropium bromide and albuterol in chronic obstructive pulmonary disease: A three-center study. Am J Med 91(4A):28S–32S, 1991.
21. Tashkin DP, Ashutosh K, Bleecker ER, et al. Comparison of the anticholinergic bronchodilator ipratropium bromide with metaproterenol in chronic obstructive pulmonary disease. Am J Med 81(5A):81–90, 1986.
22. Ashutosh K, Lang H. Comparison between long-term treatment of chronic bronchitic airway obstruction with ipratropium bromide and metaproterenol. Ann Allergy 53(5):401–406, 1984.
23. Easton PA, Jadue C, Dhingra S, Anthonisen NR. A comparison of the bronchodilating effects of a beta-2 adrenergic agent (albuterol) and an anticholinergic agent (ipratropium bromide), given by aerosol alone or in sequence. N Engl J Med 315:735–739, 1986.
24. Epstein SW, Manning CP, Ashley MJ, et al. Survey of the clinical use of pressurized aerosol inhalers. Can Med Assoc 120(7):813–816, 1979.
25. Newman SP, Clark SN. Inhalation technique with aerosol bronchodilators: does it matter? Pract Cardiol 9:157–164, 1983.
26. Rachelefsky GS, Rohr AS, Wo J, et al. Use of a tube spacer to improve the efficacy of a metered-dose inhaler in asthmatic children. Am J Dis Child 140(11):1191–1193, 1986.
27. Self TH, Rumbak MJ, Kelso TM. Correct use of metered-dose inhalers and spacer devices. Postgrad Med 92(3):95–106, 1992.
28. Aubier M, Vires N, Murciano D, et al. Effects and mechanism of action of terbutaline on diaphragmatic contractility and fatigue. J Appl Physiol 56:922–929, 1984.
29. Brent BN, Mahler D, Bueger HJ, et al. Augmentation of right ventricular performance in chronic obstructive pulmonary disease by terbutaline: a combined radionuclide and hemodynamic study. Am J Cardiol 50:313–319, 1982.
30. Boyd G, Morice AH, Poundsford JC, et al. An evaluation of salmeterol in the treatment of COPD. Eur Respir J 10:815–821, 1997.
31. Ramirez-Venegas A, Ward J, Lentine T, et al. Salmeterol reduces dyspnea and improves lung function in patients with COPD. Chest 112:336–340, 1997.
32. Grove A, Lipworth BJ, Reid P, et al. Effects of regular salmeterol on lung function and exercise capacity in patients with COPD. Thorax 51:689–693, 1996.
33. Fuller HD, Dolovich MB, Posmituck G, et al. Pressurized aerosol versus jet aerosol delivery to mechanically ventilated patients: comparison of dose to the lungs. Am Rev Respir Dis 141:440–444, 1990.
34. Manthous CA, Hall JB. Administration of therapeutic aerosols to mechanically ventilated patients. Chest 106:560–571, 1994.
35. Lin RY, Smith AJ, Hergenroeder P. High serum albuterol levels and tachycardia in adult asthmatics treated with high-dose continuously aerosolized albuterol. Chest 103:221–225, 1993.
36. Combivent Inhalation Aerosol Study Group. In chronic obstructive pulmonary disease, a combination of ipratropium and albuterol is more effective than either agent alone: an 85-day multicenter trial. Chest 105:1411–1419, 1994.
37. Ohrui T, Yanai M, Sekizawa K, et al. Effective site of bronchodilation by beta-adrenergic and anti-cholinergic agents in patients with chronic obstructive pulmonary disease: direct measurement of intrabronchial pressure with a new catheter. Am Rev Respir Dis 146:88–91, 1992.
38. O'Driscoll BR, Taylor RJ, Horsley MG, et al. Nebulised salbutamol with and without ipratropium bromide in acute airflow obstruction. Lancet 1418–1420, 1989.
39. Patrick DM, Dales RE, Stark RM, et al. Severe exacerbations of COPD and asthma: incremental benefit of adding ipratropium to usual therapy. Chest 98(2):295–297, 1990.
40. Rebuck AS, Chapman KR, Abboud R, et al. Nebulized anticholinergic and sympathomimetic treatment of asthma and chronic obstructive airways disease in the emergency room. Am J Med 82:59–64, 1987.
41. LeDoux EJ, Morris JF, Temple WP, et al. Standard and double dose ipratropium bromide and combined ipratropium bromide and inhaled metaproterenol in COPD. Chest 95:1013–1016, 1989.
42. Bleecker ER. Acute bronchodilating effects of ipratropium bromide and theophylline in chronic obstructive pulmonary disease. Am J Med 91(4A):24S–27S, 1991.
43. Filuk RB, Easton PA, Anthonisen NR. Responses to large doses of salbutamol and theophylline in patients with chronic obstructive pulmonary disease. Am Rev Respir Dis 132:871–874, 1985.
44. Guyatt GH, Townsend M, Pugsley SO, et al. Bronchodilators in chronic air-flow limitation: Effects on airway function, exercise capacity, and quality of life. Am Rev Respir Dis 135:1069–1074, 1987.
45. Eaton ML, MacDonald FM, Church TR, Niewoehner DE. Effects of theophylline on breathlessness and exercise tolerance in patients with chronic airflow obstruction. Chest 82:538–542, 1982.
46. Murciano D, Auclair MH, Pariente R, et al. A randomized, controlled trial of theophylline in patients with severe chronic obstructive pulmonary disease. N Engl J Med 320(23):1521–1525, 1989.
47. Martin RJ, Park J. Overnight theophylline concentrations and effects on sleep and lung function in chronic obstructive pulmonary disease. Am Rev Respir Dis 145:540–544, 1992.
48. Rice KL, Leatherman JW, Duane PG, et al. Aminophylline for acute exacerbations of chronic obstructive pulmonary disease–a controlled trial. Ann Intern Med 107:305–309, 1987.
49. Aubier M, Roussos C. Effect of theophylline on respiratory muscle function. Chest 88(2 Suppl):91S–97S, 1985.
50. Matthay RA. Effects of theophylline on cardiovascular performance in chronic obstructive pulmonary disease. Chest 88(2 Suppl):112S–117S, 1985.
51. Lakshminarayan S, Sahn SA, Weil JV. Effect of aminophylline on ventilatory responses in normal man. Am Rev Respir Dis 117:33–38, 1978.
52. Whiting B, Kelman AW, Barclay J, Addis GJ. Modelling theophylline response in individual patients with chronic bronchitis. Br J Clin Pharmacol 12:481–487, 1981.
53. Levine JH, Michael JR, Guarnieri T. Multifocal atrial tachycardia: a toxic effect of theophylline. Lancet 12–14, 1985.
54. Keatings VM, Jatakanon A, Worsdell M. Effects of inhaled and oral glucocorticoids on inflammatory indices in asthma and COPD. Am J Respir Crit Care Med 155:542–548, 1997.
55. Callahan CM, Dittus RS, Katz BP. Oral corticosteroid therapy for patients with stable chronic obstructive pulmonary disease: a meta-analysis. Ann Intern Med 114:216–223, 1991.
56. Strain DS, Kinasewitz GT, Franco DS, George RB. Effect of steroid therapy on exercise performance in patients with irreversible chronic obstructive pulmonary disease. Chest 88(5):718–721, 1985.
57. Evans JA, Morrison IM, Saunders KB. A controlled trial of prednisone, in low dosage, in patients with chronic airflow obstruction. Thorax 29:401–406, 1974.
58. Weir DC, Burge PS. Effects of high dose inhaled beclomethasone dipropionate, 750 mcg and 1500 mcg twice daily, and 40 mg per day oral prednisolone on lung function, symptoms, and bronchial hyperresponsiveness in patients with non-asthmatic chronic airflow obstruction. Thorax 48:309–316, 1993.
59. Van Schayck CP, Dompeling E, Van Herwaarden CL, et al. Bronchodilator treatment in moderate asthma or chronic bronchitis: continuous or on demand? A randomized controlled study. BMJ 303:1426–1431, 1991.
60. Dompeling E, van Schayck CP, van Grunsven PM, et al. Slowing the deterioration of asthma and chronic obstructive pulmonary disease observed during bronchodilator therapy by adding inhaled corticosteroids. Ann Intern Med 118:770–778, 1993.
61. Kerstjens HAM, Brand PLP, Hughes MD, et al. A comparison of bronchodilator therapy with or without inhaled corticosteroid therapy for obstructive airways disease. N Engl J Med 327(20):1413–1410, 1992.
62. Chanez P, Vignola AM, O'Shaugnessy T, et al. Corticosteroid reversibility in COPD is related to features of asthma. Am J Respir Crit Care Med 155:1529–1534, 1997.
63. Pizzichini E, Pizzichini MM, Gibson P, et al. Sputum eosinophilia predicts benefit from prednisone in smokers with chronic obstructive bronchitis. Am J Respir Crit Care Med 158:1511–1517, 1998.
64. Albert RK, Martin TR, Lewis SW. Controlled clinical trial of methylprednisolone in patients with chronic bronchitis and acute respiratory insufficiency. Ann Intern Med 92:753–758, 1980.
65. Thompson WH, Nielson CP, Carvalho P, et al. Controlled trial of oral prednisone in outpatients with acute COPD exacerbation. Am J Respir Crit Care Med 154:2:407–412, 1996.
66. Fraser IM, Hyland RH, Hutcheon MA, et al. Preliminary study of the effects of postoperative methylprednisolone therapy on lung function recovery in patients with chronic obstructive pulmonary disease. Clin Pharm 8:214–219, 1989.
67. Hudson LD, Monti CM. Rationale and use of corticosteroids in chronic obstructive pulmonary disease. Med Clin North Am 74(3):661–690, 1990.
68. Weir DC, Robertson AS, Gove RI, et al. Time course of response to oral and inhaled corticosteroids in non-asthmatic chronic airflow obstruction. Thorax 45:118–121, 1990.

69. Decramer M, Lacquet LM, Fagard R, et al. Corticosteroids contribute to muscle weakness in chronic airflow obstruction. Am J Respir Crit Care Med 150:11–16, 1994.
70. Barnes PJ, Pederson S, Busse WW. Efficacy and safety of inhaled corticosteroids. Am J Respir Crit Care Med 157:S1–S46, 1998.
71. Thompson AB, Mueller MB, Heires AJ, et al. Aerosolized beclomethasone in chronic bronchitis: improved pulmonary function and diminished airway inflammation. Am Rev Respir Dis 146:389–395, 1992.
72. Paggiaro PL, Dahle R, Bakran I, et al. Multicentre randomised placebo-controlled trial of inhaled fluticasone propionate in patients with chronic obstructive pulmonary disease. Lancet 351:773–780, 1998.
73. Weir DC, Gove RI, Robertson AS, et al. Corticosteroid trials in non-asthmatic chronic airflow obstruction: a comparison of oral prednisolone and inhaled beclomethasone dipropionate. Thorax 45:112–117, 1990.
74. Lofdahl CG, Postma DS, Laitinen LA, et al. The European Respiratory Society study on chronic obstructive disease (EUROSCOP): recruitment methods and strategies. Respir Med 92(3):467–472, 1998.
74a. Vestbo JT, Sorensen P, Lange A, et al. Long-term effect of inhaled budesonide in mild and moderate chronic obstructive pulmonary disease: a randomized controlled trial. Lancet 353:1819–1823, 1999.
74b. Pauwels RA, Lofdahl CG, Laitinen LA, et al. Long-term treatment with inhaled budesonide in persons with mild chronic obstructive pulmonary disease who continue smoking. N Engl J Med 340:1948–1953, 1999.
75. Murphy TF, Seithi S. State of the art: bacterial infection in chronic obstructive lung disease. Am Rev Respir Dis 146:1067–1083, 1992.
76. Anthonisen NR, Manfreda J, Warren CPW, et al. Antibiotic therapy in exacerbations of chronic obstructive pulmonary disease. Ann Intern Med 106:196–204, 1987.
77. Saint S, Bent S, Vittinghoff E, et al. Antibiotics in chronic obstructive pulmonary disease exacerbations: a meta-analysis. JAMA 273:957–960, 1995.
78. Williams JH, Moser KM. Pneumococcal vaccine and patients with chronic lung disease. Ann Intern Med 104:106–109, 1986.
79. Butler JC, Breinan RF, Campbell JF, et al. Pneumococcal polysaccharide vaccine efficacy: an evaluation of current recommendations. JAMA 270:1826–1831, 1993.
80. Recommendations of the Immunization Practices Advisory Committee, Center for Disease Control. Ann Intern Med 107:521–525, 1987.
81. Nocturnal Oxygen Therapy Trial Group. Continuous or nocturnal oxygen therapy in hypoxemic chronic obstructive lung disease. Ann Intern Med 93:391–398, 1980.
82. Report of the Medical Research Council Working Party: long-term oxygen therapy in chronic hypoxic cor pulmonale complicating chronic bronchitis and emphysema. Lancet 1:681–686, 1981.
83. Cooper CB, Waterhouse J, Howard P. Twelve-year clinical study of patients with hypoxic cor pulmonale given long-term domiciliary oxygen therapy. Thorax 42:105–110, 1987.
84. Bowman G, Backer U, Larsson S, et al. Oral acetylcysteine reduces exacerbation rate in chronic bronchitis: report of a trial organized by the Swedish Society for Pulmonary Diseases. Eur J Respir Dis 64:405–415, 1983.
85. British Thoracic Society Research Committee. Oral *N*-acetylcysteine and exacerbation rates in patients with chronic bronchitis and severe airways obstruction. Thorax 40:832–835, 1985.
86. Begin P, Grassino A. Inspiratory muscle dysfunction and chronic hypercapnia in chronic obstructive pulmonary disease. Am Rev Respir Dis 143:905–912, 1991.
87. Hutchison DCS, Barter CE, Cook PJL, et al. Severe pulmonary emphysema: a comparison of patients with and without alpha-1-antitrypsin deficiency. Q J Med 41:301–315, 1972.
88. $Alpha_1$-proteinase inhibitor. Facts and comparisons. St. Louis: Lippincott, 1998:187c–187d.
89. Celli BR. Standards for the optimal management of COPD: a summary. Chest 113:283S–287S, 1998.
90. Cooper JD. The history of surgical procedures for emphysema. Ann Thorac Surg 63:312–319, 1997.
91. Levine SM, Anzueto A, Peters JI, et al. Medium term functional results of single-lung transplantation for endstage obstructive lung disease. Am J Respir Crit Care Med 150:398–402, 1994.
92. O'Donnell DE. Breathlessness in patients with chronic airflow limitation: mechanisms and management. Chest 106:904–912, 1994.
93. Dean NC, Brown KJ, Himelman RB, et al. Oxygen may improve dyspnea and endurance in patients with chronic obstructive pulmonary disease and only mild hypoxia. Am Rev Respir Dis 146:941–945, 1992.
94. Light RW, Muro JR, Sato RI, et al. Effects of oral morphine on breathlessness and exercise tolerance in patients with chronic obstructive pulmonary disease. Am Rev Respir Dis 139:126–133, 1989.
95. Johnson MA, Woodcock AA, Geddes DM. Dihydrocodeine for breathlessness in pink puffers. BMJ 286:675–677, 1993.
96. Poole PJ, Veale A, Black PN. The effect of sustained-release morphine on breathlessness and quality of life in severe chronic obstructive pulmonary disease. Am J Respir Crit Care Med 157:1877–1880, 1998.
97. Anthonisen NR, Wright EC, Hodgkin JE, and the IPPB Trial Group. Prognosis in chronic obstructive pulmonary disease. Am Rev Respir Dis 133:14–20, 1986.

CHAPTER 38

CYSTIC FIBROSIS

Paul Beringer

Cystic fibrosis (CF) is the most common lethal genetic disease in the United States today, affecting nearly 30,000 children and young adults.[1] It is caused by a single gene mutation on the long arm of chromosome 7, whose protein product is the cystic fibrosis transmembrane regulator (CFTR). According to current theory, CFTR regulates sodium and chloride transport across the apical membrane of epithelial cells. CFTR is present in many organs throughout the body, including sweat glands, respiratory tract, pancreas, gastrointestinal, hepatobiliary, and reproductive organs. The primary clinical characteristics of CF are malabsorption caused by pancreatic insufficiency (PI, 80 to 90%), chronic sinopulmonary infections, and male infertility. The major causes of morbidity and mortality are bronchiectasis and obstructive pulmonary disease, accounting for more than 90% of deaths.

Improvements in airway clearance techniques, pancreatic enzyme replacement, and treatment of pulmonary infections provided at CF care centers have greatly improved longevity, increasing median survival from 14 years in 1969 to 31 years in 1996 (Fig. 38.1). The percentage of adult patients has also increased: Adults represented 29.5% of the population with CF in 1988 and this increased to 37% in 1998. The rapid pace of research into the pathophysiology of the disease promises to bring new treatment strategies that will contribute to even greater improvements.

TREATMENT GOALS: CYSTIC FIBROSIS

- Slow the progressive deterioration in pulmonary function and maintain normal growth and maturation.
- Treat infection and inflammation and reduce airway obstruction to improve or maintain pulmonary function.
- Replace pancreatic enzymes and ensure adequate caloric intake to achieve normal growth.

EPIDEMIOLOGY

CF is an autosomal recessive trait that affects 1 of every 3300 live births.[1] To inherit CF, an individual must receive a defective copy of the CF gene from each parent. If both parents are carriers, there is a 25% chance of inheriting CF, a 50% chance of becoming a carrier, and a 25% chance of being unaffected. Currently 1 in 29 Americans (nearly 10 million) is an asymptomatic carrier of this disease.

Because of the great degree of variability in the clinical course of CF, much work is being conducted to identify specific mutations. Since the discovery of the gene responsible for CF, more than 800 different mutations have been identified. A classification scheme for mutations on the basis of CFTR protein alterations has been proposed.[2] The four classes include defects in protein production, processing, regulation, and conduction. The most common mutation (accounting for 70% among Caucasians) is a processing defect (class II mutation) arising from a 3-bp deletion resulting in the loss of the amino acid phenylalanine at position 508 in the CFTR protein (ΔF508). Patients who are homozygous for ΔF508 (both genes carry the mutant allele) are pancreatic insufficient. Patients who are pancreatic sufficient tend to have a better overall prognosis than their pancreatic-insufficient counterparts. In some cases, therefore, knowing a patient's genotype provides information about the phenotype. This type of classification scheme may serve as a prognostic indicator and provide a framework for specific treatments based on the class of mutation involved.

PATHOPHYSIOLOGY

The present theory holds that the basic defect in CF is decreased chloride transport. A reduction in chloride transport is accompanied by alterations in sodium and water transport, leading to dehydrated, thickened secretions. These thickened secretions are associated with obstruction and eventual destruction of exocrine glands involved. The primary systems affected include sweat, respiratory, pancreas, gastrointestinal, hepatobiliary, and reproductive organs.

Sweat Gland

In the sweat duct, CFTR reabsorbs chloride from sweat. Dysfunctional CFTR therefore causes impermeability to chloride, resulting in a nearly fivefold elevation in sweat chloride concentrations. This aberration is the principal laboratory criterion for diagnosis. This defect predisposes patients with CF to heat prostration. Adequate attention to dietary salt and fluid intake, especially during the summer, is necessary.

Reproductive System

Male and female infertility is common. More than 95% of men with CF have congenital bilateral absence of the vas deferens (CBAVD) and are therefore sterile. In women with CF, cervical mucus is dehydrated and fails to increase during midcycle, which can reduce fertility.[3] Pregnancy is of concern because it is thought to result in increased health risk to the mother. However, results of a recent study of 258 women with CF indicate that pregnancy does not alter the rate of deterioration in pulmonary function.[4]

Gastrointestinal Tract

Pancreas

One of the primary functions of the pancreas is secretion of lipase and colipase, which are responsible for hydrolyzing a large proportion of dietary triglycerides. PI results in malabsorption principally of fat through incomplete digestion. In addition, secretion of bicarbonate by the pancreas is reduced in both pancreatic sufficient and insufficient patients. This impairs digestion because an alkaline environment is necessary for optimal activity of both endogenous and exogenous pancreatic enzymes. Although the exact function of CFTR in the pancreatic duct cells has not been identified, it is presumed that its dysfunction results in reduced chloride and water secretion, leading to protein precipitation and ductule plugging.[5] Progression of pancreatic disease is associated with the onset of cystic fibrosis–related diabetes mellitus (CFRDM). Recent evidence suggests that CFRDM results from insulin resistance and decreased insulin secretion and is associated with worsened clinical status.[6]

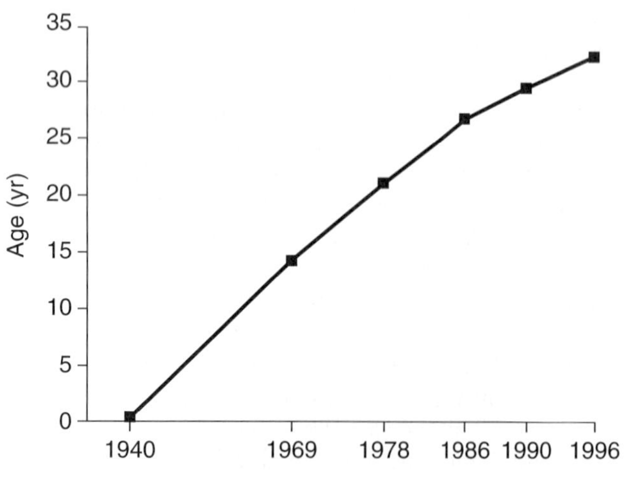

Figure 38.1. Median survival age for patients with cystic fibrosis in the United States.

Stomach and Esophagus

Gastroesophageal reflux results from an increased number of inappropriate transient relaxations of the lower esophageal sphincter (LES).[7] Cough, forced expirations during chest physiotherapy, and hyperinflation of the lung increase the abdominothoracic pressure gradient and thereby contribute to reflux.[8]

Liver and Gallbladder

The pathogenesis of liver disease in CF is currently unclear; however, the presence of CFTR in epithelial cells lining the biliary ductules suggests a deficiency in biliary electrolyte and fluid secretion, leading to obstruction and biliary cirrhosis if severe.[9,10] The development of cholelithiasis (gallstones) increases with age, occurring in 15% of young adults, and is also associated with PI.[11] Fecal loss of bile acids, resulting in diminished reserves, is thought to be the predisposing factor in the formation of gallstones in patients with CF.[12]

Lung

Respiratory disease is of major importance in patients with CF because it is the primary factor responsible for repeated hospitalizations, pulmonary function decline, and more than 90% of the mortality. Chronic bronchitis that progresses to bronchiectasis and eventual respiratory failure characterizes this process. Although the exact pathophysiologic mechanism linking defective CFTR to lung disease has not been established clearly, ineffective local host defense mechanisms resulting in chronic infection, inflammation, and tissue damage are probable mechanisms (Fig. 38.2). Three proposed defects responsible for initiation of infection include the following: Impaired mucociliary clearance caused by abnormally thickened mucus results in persistence of bacteria within the lungs,[13] host defense proteins (β-defensins) are inactivated by elevated salt concentrations in the airway surface fluid,[14] and CFTR acts as a receptor for ingestion of bacteria (e.g., *Pseudomonas aeruginosa*).[15]

Neutrophil elastase plays a central role in perpetuating the chronic cycle of infection, inflammation, and tissue damage (Fig. 38.3). In the normal host, proteases (e.g., neutrophil elastase) are released in response to an infectious insult and digest the bacteria, while lung tissue is

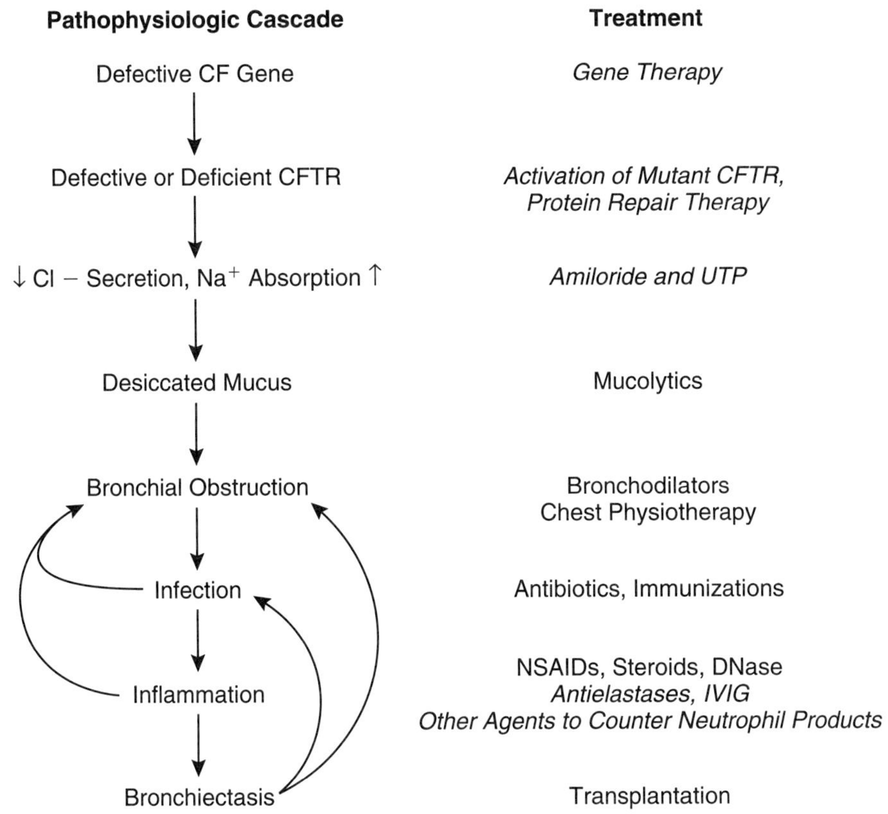

Figure 38.2. Proposed pathophysiologic cascade for cystic fibrosis *(CF)* lung disease and the therapeutic interventions targeted at each step. Although all the items in the right cascade occur in CF lung disease, their causal relations have not been established clearly. Treatments that are still in clinical testing are shown in italic print. *CFTR,* cystic fibrosis transmembrane regulator; *IVIG,* intravenous immunoglobulin; *NSAIDs,* nonsteroidal anti-inflammatory drugs; *UTP,* uridine triphosphates. (Reprinted with permission from Davis PB, Drumm M, Konstan MW. Cystic Fibrosis. Am J Respir Crit Care Med 1154:1239.)

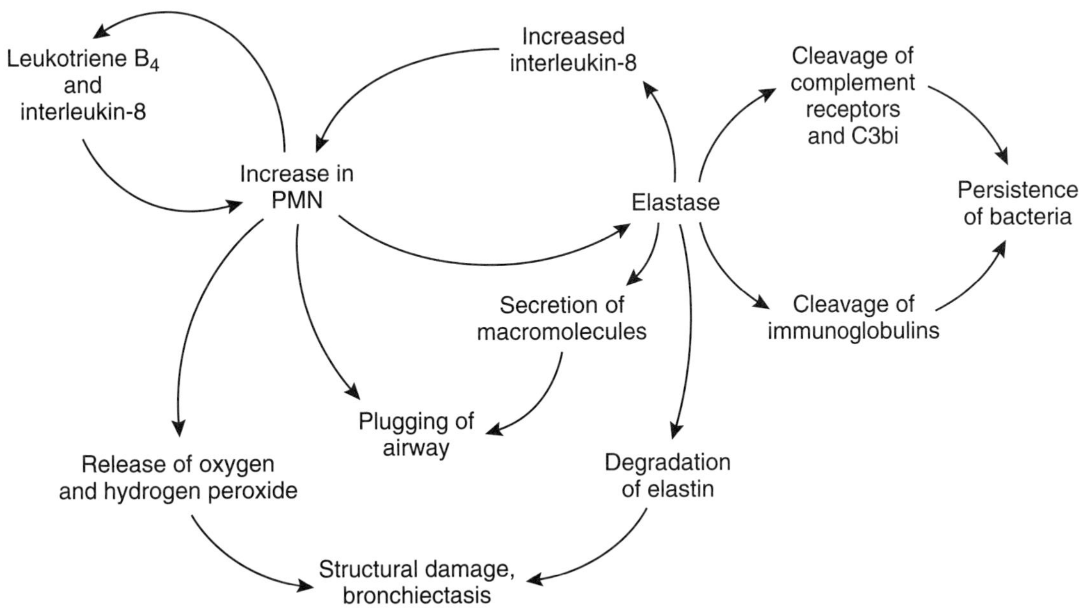

Figure 38.3. Products derived from polymorphonuclear leukocytes and their secondary effects on inflammation in the airways of patients with lung disease caused by cystic fibrosis. Leukotriene B_4 and interleukin-8 are chemoattractant substances that elicit an influx of more polymorphonuclear leukocytes *(PMN),* which release large quantities of elastase and other proteolytic enzymes as they die. These enzymes degrade structural proteins such as elastin and stimulate the hypersecretion of mucus. Elastase can inhibit phagocytosis of bacteria by cleaving immunoglobulins, complement receptors, and proteins of the complement cascade (C3bi). (Reprinted with permission from Ramsey BW. Drug therapy: management of pulmonary disease in patients with cystic fibrosis. N Engl J Med 335:179–188, 1996. Copyright © 1996 Massachusetts Medical Society. All rights reserved.)

protected by the presence of antiproteases. However, there is an exaggerated response in patients with CF because the persistence of bacteria in the lungs overwhelms the antiproteases. Free elastase impairs phagocytosis, causes direct and indirect (through release of free radicals) tissue damage, contributes to airway plugging, and increases neutrophil migration, resulting in further increases in elastase. Various pharmacologic interventions designed to disrupt this cycle are being evaluated. Direct inhibition of neutrophil elastase is being attempted through exogenous administration of antiproteases (α_1-protease inhibitor, recombinant secretory leukoprotease inhibitor, DMP-777). Mucolytic agents have been developed to improve airway plugging and are currently in use (recombinant DNase). Also, agents that inhibit neutrophil migration (pentoxifylline) are being evaluated.

The microbiology of lung infection changes with age (Fig. 38.4). In the typical patient, *Staphylococcus aureus* and *Haemophilus influenzae* are present in the airway at a very young age. However, *Pseudomonas aeruginosa* becomes the predominant pathogen in late childhood. Chronic infection with *P. aeruginosa* typically is preceded by a period of colonization followed by an acute infection. Infection is endobronchial, involving first the smaller airways and moving more proximally to involve the larger airways as the disease progresses. Once established, *P. aeruginosa* begins to produce the characteristic mucoid exopolysaccharide (MEP) capsule and the microcolony (biofilm) mode of growth. MEP provides protection against host defenses (impaired complement- and antibody-mediated phagocytosis) and a barrier to antibiotic penetration. The slow-growing nature of the microcolonies confers a survival advantage by reducing susceptibility to antimicrobial agents. The alterations in host and microbial factors combine to result in persistence of *P. aeruginosa* within the airway of patients with CF. Conversion to the mucoid *P. aeruginosa* phenotype is of concern because it has been associated with progression of pulmonary disease (Fig. 38.4) and can become multi-drug resistant.

Occasionally infections involve atypical organisms, including *Stenotrophomonas maltophilia* (3.9%) or *Burkholderia cepacia* (3.6%). Infections involving *B. cepacia* are of particular concern because it is typically multi-drug resistant, can be transmitted from patient to patient, and can result in deterioration in pulmonary function.[16,17] *Aspergillus* species present a unique challenge in patients with CF. The presence of these organisms ignites an immunologic response in some patients called allergic bronchopulmonary aspergillosis (ABPA).[18] The disease is not invasive; however, damage to the airways as a result of eosinophilic infiltration occurs.[19] The drug of choice for treating ABPA is corticosteroids. Antifungals have also been used as adjunctive therapy, but their effectiveness is not established.

Pulmonary function tests are useful tools in assessing respiratory status. They are typically used periodically to assess disease progression or the effect of a therapeutic intervention (e.g., bronchodilators, a course of antibiotics). The benefit of such interventions is determined by comparison of pulmonary function tests after the intervention with a baseline measurement. The two most commonly used measures are the forced expiratory volume in 1 second (FEV_1) and the forced vital capacity (FVC), the latter representing the total volume of air expelled through the mouth during forced maximal expiration after maximal inspiration. A classification scheme for stratifying patients based on severity of pulmonary disease has been developed. Mild disease is defined as an FEV_1 greater than 70%, moderate as FEV_1 40 to 69%, and severe as FEV_1 less than 40% of predicted value for a person of same age and

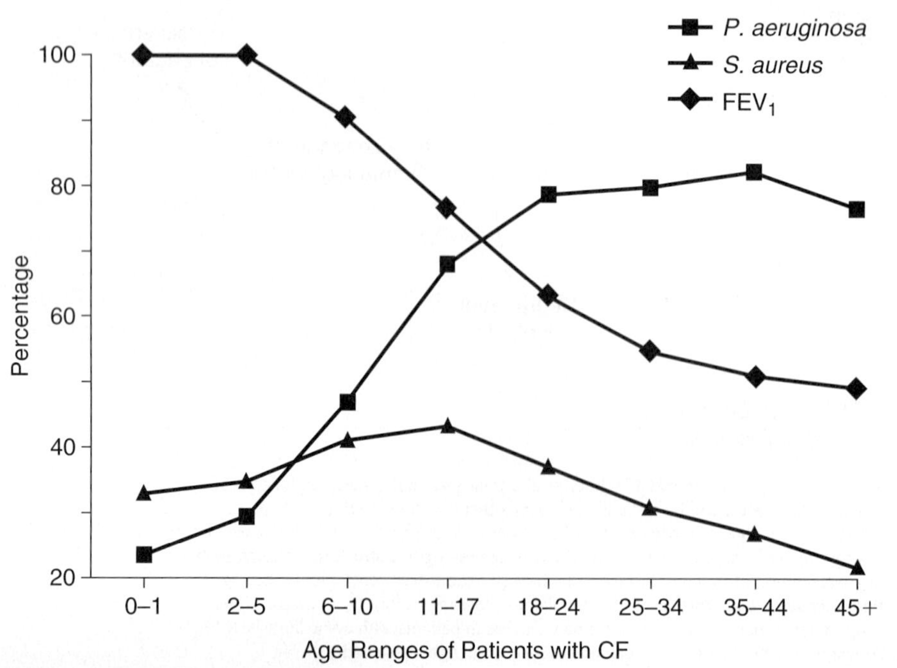

Figure 38.4. Age-related changes in microbiology and pulmonary function in patients with cystic fibrosis.

weight with normal lung function.[20] Pulmonary function as measured by FEV_1 declines steadily throughout childhood, adolescence, and early adulthood (Fig. 38.4).

CLINICAL PRESENTATION AND DIAGNOSIS

Signs and Symptoms

Pancreatic Insufficiency

Pancreatic dysfunction is one of the principal abnormalities in patients with CF. According to the Cystic Fibrosis Foundation (CFF), more than 90% of patients with CF in the United States currently receive pancreatic supplements. In a majority of patients, PI manifests at birth or shortly thereafter as failure to grow or gain weight despite adequate oral intake. Additional symptoms include crampy abdominal pain after high-fat meals and frequent, bulky, foul-smelling stools. Fifteen percent of patients with CF are pancreatic sufficient.[21] However, PI eventually develops in 10 to 20% of these patients.[22] Pancreatitis is a potential complication that occurs in both pancreatic sufficient and insufficient patients. A number of different direct and indirect methods of diagnosing PI have been described. The most widely used is the 72-hour fecal fat analysis, which provides a quantitative measurement of fecal fat losses caused by malabsorption. This tool can also be used to determine adequacy of the pancreatic enzyme replacement regimen.

Diabetes Mellitus

A period of glucose intolerance usually precedes CFRDM onset. The association of the occurrence of CFRDM with advancing age suggests that this problem will become more prevalent as further improvements in survival are made. The cumulative incidence identified in a recent prospective evaluation was 3%, 24%, and 76% at ages 10, 20, and 30, respectively. Periodic monitoring of the oral glucose tolerance test has recently been recommended as a screening tool for CFRDM.[23] The incidence of diabetic complications including retinopathy, nephropathy, and neuropathy is similar in diabetic patients with and without CF.[24] In addition, the presence of CFRDM may increase mortality.[25] Pharmacologic management is similar to that of type I diabetes. However, dietary considerations differ significantly. A low-fat, low-carbohydrate diet typically is recommended for diabetic patients. Because patients with CF typically are malnourished, this approach is not recommended.

Gastroesophogeal Reflux

Gastroesophogeal reflux is a common symptom of CF. Heartburn and regurgitation are reported in 20% of patients.[26] Progression to esophagitis as evidenced by endoscopy is present in more than 50% of patients with prominent respiratory symptoms.[27] Treatment is similar to that of patients without CF and includes both nonpharmacologic and pharmacologic approaches. Special attention is necessary to avoid possible drug interactions (antacid–quinolones, cimetidine–theophylline) and medications that can decrease LES pressure (theophylline, α-adrenergic agents).

Meconium Ileus and Distal Intestinal Obstruction Syndrome

In the neonate, reduced chloride and water secretion in the intestine are responsible for the presence of meconium ileus (intestinal obstruction) in 10 to 15% of patients.[28] With rare exception, meconium ileus occurs in patients with PI. Pancreatic replacement therapy therefore should be considered in affected patients. Treatment typically involves a therapeutic enema or surgical removal as a last resort. Distal intestinal obstruction syndrome (DIOS) is an analogous complication present in 15% of adolescents and adults.[26] This syndrome typically presents with abdominal pain, nausea and vomiting, and a palpable mass in the right lower quadrant. The use of oral polyethylene glycol electrolyte solution is the preferred treatment. Because of its recurrent nature, maintenance therapy with a high-fiber diet and laxatives is recommended. Prokinetic agents (e.g., cisapride) or stimulant laxatives can be used in patients with persistent symptoms.[21]

Cirrhosis and Cholelithiasis

Liver disease is the second leading cause of death among patients with CF (2% annual mortality).[1] The prevalence increases with age, so the overall incidence is expected to increase as further improvements in lung disease treatment are made. Liver disease is more common in patients with PI.[21] Most patients with mild disease are asymptomatic, with the only clinical sign being the presence of a firm, enlarged, or tender liver. Further progression in some patients is evidenced by the clinical manifestations of portal hypertension, variceal bleeding, and liver failure. Laboratory data typically are unremarkable. Elevations in γ-glutamyltranspeptidase are the only significant evidence of cirrhosis.[11] The primary determinants of morbidity and mortality are the presence of portal hypertension and variceal hemorrhaging.[21]

The clinical presentation of cholelithiasis is similar to that of other disorders, with intermittent right upper quadrant pain, nausea, vomiting, jaundice, and dietary fat intolerance. Cholecystectomy is the treatment of choice and is considered in patients who are symptomatic.

Malnutrition

Nutritional deficits can significantly affect the growth and survival of patients with CF.[29] The causes of malnutrition are multifactorial, influenced by energy intake, losses, and use. Recurrent vomiting caused by coughing or gastroesophageal reflux, chronic respiratory infections, and psychosocial stresses have been implicated in reduced energy intake. PI and reduced bile acid secretion result in malabsorption and loss of fat, protein, and carbohydrates. Increased resting energy expenditure correlates with severity of pulmonary disease.[30]

Deficiencies of fat-soluble vitamins (A, D, E, and K) can occur in patients with CF as a result of PI. Clinical symptoms as a result of deficiencies are uncommon but have been reported.[21] Vitamin D deficiency is found predominantly in patients with inadequate sunlight exposure or cholestatic liver disease. Rickets is extremely rare among patients with CF; however, bone demineralization has been reported.[31] Vitamin K production by intestinal flora is reduced during antibiotic use and therefore warrants replacement, particularly in patients with frequent pulmonary exacerbations. Hemorrhagic diathesis resulting from inadequate vitamin K levels is a serious complication that can be prevented by giving supplements to patients at greatest risk.

The CFF recommends routine nutritional status assessment, including quarterly anthropometric measurements (e.g., height, weight, triceps skinfold thickness), annual dietary intake and 3-day fat balance, and laboratory studies (e.g., complete blood count, vitamins A and E) to facilitate early intervention. Pancreatic replacement therapy, a high-fat and high-calorie diet, and aggressive pulmonary therapy are essential to improving nutritional status.

Respiratory Disease

The presentation of pulmonary disease is unique, accounting for its importance in establishing the diagnosis of CF. Chronic cough and sputum production are almost universally present. The frequency of cough and the quantity and appearance of sputum are useful in monitoring for acute exacerbations. Patients also commonly experience wheezing, shortness of breath, and chest tightness as a result of airway obstruction. Hemoptysis is seen occasionally, particularly during exacerbations. Episodes of hemoptysis typically resolve spontaneously after a few days, but medications that may exacerbate bleeding (e.g., nonsteroidal anti-inflammatory drugs [NSAIDs]) should be avoided. Pneumothorax occurs in 5 to 8% of patients and presents with simultaneous onset of dyspnea and unilateral chest pain.[19] Impaired gas exchange, leading to respiratory failure, is observed in patients with severe lung disease or during a severe pulmonary exacerbation in patients with moderate pulmonary disease. In severe cases, respiratory failure can result in pulmonary hypertension and cor pulmonale. Aggressive therapy to treat infection and inflammation is necessary to improve gas exchange. Supplemental oxygen and mechanical ventilation may also be necessary.

CF also affects the upper respiratory tract, manifesting as chronic sinusitis. In addition to the pain, pressure, and congestion it causes, infection can be transmitted to the lower respiratory tract. Sinus surgery is needed in 10 to 20% of patients with recurrent disease and is beneficial in reducing pulmonary exacerbations. Chronic antibiotic lavage has been recommended in patients who need repeated surgical treatments.[32]

Acute pulmonary exacerbations of chronic infection are an inevitable consequence of pulmonary disease in most patients with CF. Pulmonary exacerbations are characterized by increased cough and sputum production, decreased exercise tolerance, weight loss, new findings on chest exam, and fever.[26] Thirty-six percent of patients registered with the Cystic Fibrosis Foundation in 1996 experienced at least one pulmonary exacerbation. Although the exact inciting event is not known, improvement in the signs and symptoms is highly correlated with a reduction in sputum bacterial density.[33] *S. aureus, H. influenzae,* and particularly *P. aeruginosa* are commonly cultured pathogens. The goals of therapy in acute pulmonary exacerbations are to reduce bacterial density and improve pulmonary function and nutritional status.

Diagnosis

CF is most commonly diagnosed based on the presence of typical signs and symptoms (Table 38.1) and confirmed by laboratory evidence of CFTR dysfunction. Because of its sensitivity, an abnormal sweat chloride concentration (more than 60 mEq/L) is the recommended method of identifying CFTR dysfunction. Additional diagnostic methods include abnormal nasal potential differences and genetic mutational analysis, which may be useful in patients with atypical presentations.

Identification of the genetic defect responsible for CF has opened the door for genetic testing. Potential benefits of genetic testing are the identification of carriers of a single gene with a mutation and early diagnosis of CF. However, because there are more than 800 known mutations, many of which are currently not tested for, a negative result on genetic analysis does not exclude the

Table 38.1 ▪ Clinical Features Consistent with a Diagnosis of Cystic Fibrosis

Chronic sinopulmonary disease manifested by
- Persistent colonization with typical cystic fibrosis pathogens including *S. aureus,* nontypable *H. influenzae,* mucoid and nonmucoid *P. aeruginosa,* and *B. cepacia*
- Chronic cough and sputum production
- Persistent chest radiograph abnormalities (e.g., bronchiectasis, atelectasis, infiltrates, hyperinflation)
- Airway obstruction manifested by wheezing and air trapping
- Nasal polyps, radiographic or computed tomographic abnormalities of the paranasal sinuses
- Digital clubbing

Gastrointestinal and nutritional abnormalities, including
- Intestinal: meconium ileus, distal intestinal obstruction syndrome, rectal prolapse
- Pancreatic: pancreatic insufficiency, recurrent pancreatitis
- Hepatic: chronic hepatic disease manifested by clinical or histologic evidence of focal biliary cirrhosis or multilobular cirrhosis
- Nutritional: failure to thrive (protein/calorie malnutrition), hypoproteinemia and edema, complications secondary to fat-soluble vitamin deficiency

Salt loss syndromes: acute salt depletion, chronic metabolic alkalosis

Male urogenital abnormalities resulting in obstructive azoospermia

Source: Reprinted with permission from Clinical Practice Guidelines for Cystic Fibrosis, Cystic Fibrosis Foundation, 1997.

possibility that the patient has CF or is a carrier of the defective gene. For this reason, a 1997 consensus panel of experts did not recommend routine genetic screening for the entire population.[34]

TREATMENT

Reproductive Dysfunction

Treatment for infertility in both men and women is available. In men, sperm can be removed from the testes and used for artificial insemination of the partner. In women, infertility has been overcome by artificial insemination beyond the obstructing cervical mucus. However, this raises a number of psychosocial issues, including increased risk of CF in the fetus, perpetuation of an abnormal gene, and increased risk of early parental loss.

Liver Disease

The beneficial effects of ursodeoxycholic acid (UDCA) for treating liver disease in patients with CF have been demonstrated in a number of recent studies. UDCA improves liver function by reducing bile viscosity and preventing obstruction. UDCA is thought to increase clearance and inhibit intestinal absorption of toxic bile acids.[21] Treatment for a 1-year period was associated with significant improvement in clinical score (Shwachman) and liver function tests when compared with placebo in the largest controlled trial conducted to date.[35] However, the biochemical parameters have been shown to reverse to pretreatment values upon discontinuation of UDCA.[21] A prospective study using liver biopsies demonstrated a significant improvement in liver morphology (based on a subjective scoring system reflecting inflammation, bile duct proliferation, and fibrosis) over a 2-year treatment period with UDCA. In addition, UDCA has been shown to improve lipoprotein metabolism, resulting in improvement in essential fatty acid deficiency and correction of vitamin A levels.[36] The long-term benefit in terms of slower progression to portal hypertension is unknown. Guidelines for use of UDCA in CF liver disease currently do not exist; however, patients enrolled in the studies cited here had biochemical evidence of liver disease and abnormal morphology on liver biopsy or ultrasound. The dosages used were 15 to 20 mg/kg day and were well tolerated.

Pancreatic Disease

PI is treated with supplementation of exogenous pancreatic enzymes derived from bovine or porcine sources. The available products contain varying quantities of pancreatin or pancrelipase, protease, and amylase contained in powders, tablets, enteric-coated tablets, and enteric-coated microencapsulated tablets or spheres. The microencapsulated formulations are the most widely used because they provide the greatest protection against inactivation of enzymes by the acidic gastric environment. However, reduced bicarbonate secretion within the CF pancreas fails to provide the optimal pH for dissolution in the intestine. In addition, lipase is inactivated at pH values below 4, which may further reduce the activity of pancreatic enzyme supplements.[37] Therefore, normal absorption characteristics typically are not achieved in patients with CF; however, treatment usually is sufficient to control symptoms and promote adequate nutrition for most patients. In patients in whom enzyme supplementation is inadequate (symptomatic at dosages of 1000 to 2000 units lipase/kg/meal), the use of histamine (H_2) receptor blockers has been shown to increase body weight and reduce stool fat and nitrogen.[37] In addition, alternative factors contributing to an inadequate response including poor adherence, alterations in diet, and outdated prescriptions should be considered.

Dosing of pancreatic enzymes is based on lipase content. Ideally, dosing should be based on the amount of fat grams ingested to mimic the normal physiologic response. It has been estimated that patients will need on average 1800 lipase units per gram of fat per day.[26] A more practical method is to base the dosage on weight. Recommended initial dosages for children under age 4 is 1000 lipase units/kg/meal, and 500 units/kg/meal for patients older than 4 to account for the reduced fat intake per kilogram of body weight.[26] Dosages can be increased after several days if symptoms persist; however, dosages should not exceed 2500 lipase units/kg/meal unless they are determined to be effective based on 72-hour fecal fat measurements. Colonic strictures have been associated with dosages exceeding 6000 units/kg/meal and should be avoided.[38,39]

Nutrition

In addition to pancreatic supplements, an adequate caloric intake is necessary to achieve normal nutritional status. A high-fat diet in combination with pancreatic enzymes is recommended because fat is a dense source of energy. A study in children (mean age 12 years) with CF found that a target of 100 fat grams per day provided more than 110% of the recommended daily intake for energy.[40] A common method for assessing nutritional status is to determine the patient's weight for height ratio. In patients who are unable to maintain adequate nutrition (weight:height ratio less than 90% of ideal) despite appropriate pancreatic supplementation and dietary modifications, oral nutritional supplements are indicated. More aggressive nutritional management (enteral or parenteral support) is necessary for patients in whom significant improvements have not been made within 3 months or whose weight:height ratio declines to less than 85% of ideal. Nutritional status of patients with CF is closely related to pulmonary status, so aggressive pulmonary therapy also improves nutritional status.

Fat-soluble vitamins (A, D, E, and K) are replaced by administration of one or two multivitamins daily. In addition, supplementation with water-miscible forms of vitamin A (5000 IU) and vitamin E (100 to 400 IU) is needed to normalize the vitamin levels. Alternatively, a higher dosage of the fat-soluble form of vitamin E (200 to 800 IU) may be more cost-efficient. Additional vitamin D supplementation typically is not necessary unless the patient has little sunlight exposure. Similarly, vitamin K supplementation above that provided by the standard multivitamin preparation is not necessary unless the patient receives frequent antibiotic exposures or has liver disease. Supplemental dosages are individualized based on measured levels (vitamins A and E) or clinical response (prothrombin time, vitamin K). Multivitamin preparations containing water-miscible preparations of vitamins A, D, E, and K are available and may be helpful in improving patient adherence.

Lung Disease

Reducing Airway Obstruction

The primary method of mobilizing thickened pulmonary secretions is through chest physiotherapy. The basic components of chest physiotherapy have been chest percussion and vibration to loosen the mucus, combined with postural drainage to facilitate mobilization and removal via cough. Although effective, this method is time-consuming and a partner is needed. More recently, newer techniques such as airway oscillation (Flutter device) and high-frequency chest oscillation (ThAIRapy Vest) have been shown to provide similar or greater improvement in pulmonary function and sputum production with greater independence.[41] The choice of method is determined on an individual basis after effectiveness and compliance have been considered.

Bronchodilators

Response to bronchodilators in patients with CF is variable; patients may demonstrate improvement, no change, or even deterioration in pulmonary function. One method of determining whether a patient may exhibit a positive response to bronchodilators is by bronchoprovocation studies using methacholine and histamine to evaluate patients for airway hyperreactivity. The degree of hyperresponsiveness correlates with airflow limitation severity.[42] However, more commonly in the clinical setting bronchodilator therapy is considered in patients who demonstrate an increase of 10% or more in FEV_1 after use of an inhaled bronchodilator. However, response within an individual patient may vary over time.[43] Inhaled adrenergic agonists (e.g., albuterol) and parasympatholytic agents (e.g., ipratropium) used alone and in combination have been shown to improve pulmonary function in clinical trials. In addition, β_2-agonists may assist in airway clearance and are often used before chest physiotherapy.[44] The recommended dosages of agents used are similar to those recommended for asthma treatment. Preliminary evidence suggests that the long acting β_2-agonist salmeterol provides greater improvement in pulmonary function and symptoms than short acting β_2-agonists.[45]

Mucolytics

Accumulation of DNA from dead neutrophils contributes significantly to the viscoelasticity of airway secretions. Recombinant human DNase digests extracellular DNA and has been shown to reduce the viscoelasticity of sputum in vitro.[46] Treatment with recombinant human DNase has been associated with significant improvement in pulmonary function and a reduction in the risk of pulmonary exacerbations necessitating intravenous antibiotics.[47] Recombinant human DNase has been recommended for use in patients with chronic endobronchial infection with mucopurulent secretions and an obstructive pattern on pulmonary function testing. However, because of its high cost, some have questioned the value of its routine use in this population. Recombinant human DNase has been shown to form a precipitate when combined with tobramycin solution,[48] and its activity is inhibited when it is combined with macrolides.[49]

Managing Infection

Treatment of pulmonary infections has been integral in the management of CF and has significantly improved survival of this population. Several approaches to the use of antibiotics in CF have been proposed. Intermittent courses of intravenous antibiotics during acute exacerbations have been the primary mode of administration at CF care centers for a number of years. More recently, maintenance therapy with oral or inhaled antibiotics has been instituted to control the bacterial burden with the intention of extending the time period between pulmonary exacerbations. In addition, in a few preliminary reports, prophylactic antibiotic therapy has been instituted to prevent chronic infection.

Pulmonary Exacerbations

The value of antibiotic therapy in treating pulmonary exacerbations has been demonstrated in a placebo-controlled study that compared the addition of antibiotic therapy with a regimen of chest physiotherapy and bronchodilators alone. A moderate improvement in pulmonary function as measured by FEV_1 (6.6%) was demonstrated in patients treated with chest physiotherapy and bronchodilators alone. The addition of intravenous antibiotics resulted in further improvement in FEV_1 (16%). The improvement was highly correlated with a decline in the density of *P. aeruginosa* in sputum.

Selection of Antibiotic

Antibiotic selection is based on sputum culture and susceptibility data. In the absence of these data, empiric therapy directed at the most commonly occurring organisms (*P. aeruginosa, S. aureus,* and *H. influenzae*) is recommended. Two antibiotics with different mechanisms of action often are used when *P. aeruginosa* is suspected or known to be involved to prevent the development of resistance and provide potential synergistic activity. For these reasons, the combination of an antipseudomonal β-lactam and an aminoglycoside is the recommended treatment regimen.

Multi-drug-resistant *P. aeruginosa* isolates (defined as resistance to all agents in two of the following classes of antibiotics: β-lactams, aminoglycosides, or the quinolones) are to be expected among patients who have received frequent courses of antibiotic treatment. Synergy testing may be useful under these conditions to identify combinations of antibiotics with activity that would not be identifiable using standard susceptibility testing of individual compounds. The combinations of a β-lactam (e.g., ticarcillin, piperacillin, or aztreonam) with tobramycin and ciprofloxacin with piperacillin have been shown to consistently provide synergistic activity against multi-drug resistant *P. aeruginosa* isolates.[50]

Dosage

The antibiotics most commonly used to treat acute pulmonary exacerbations and their dosage ranges are listed in Table 38.2. Typical dosage regimens used in other populations may be inadequate in patients with CF because of altered pharmacokinetics, reduced lung penetration, decreased activity in sputum, presence of biofilm with *Pseudomonas* isolates, heavy bacterial inocula, and more resistant isolates. Oral antibiotics are used to treat patients with mild to moderate exacerbations, and parenteral administration is reserved for patients with severe exacerbations or those who do not respond to oral therapy.

Antimicrobial Pharmacokinetics and Pharmacodynamics

The pharmacokinetics of a number of compounds appears to be altered in patients with CF. Currently no unifying mechanism linking the altered pharmacokinetics to a specific alteration in patients with CF exists.[51,52] Therefore, the appropriate dosage should be determined on the basis of data derived from controlled pharmacokinetic studies or by individualization using measured serum concentrations if possible. In general, higher dosages or more frequent dosing is needed in patients with CF in order to achieve similar peak and trough serum antibiotic concentrations. This approach maximizes lung penetration and antibiotic concentrations at the site of infection.

AMINOGLYCOSIDES. Results of controlled trials of aminoglycoside (amikacin, gentamycin, and tobramycin) pharmacokinetics indicate that the total body clearance and volume of distribution are greater for patients with CF than for age-matched controls.[53–55] The increased clearance of tobramycin has been attributed to increased nonrenal clearance (e.g., biliary),[55] whereas an increased renal clearance was identified with amikacin.[52] The

Table 38.2 ▪ Intravenous Antibiotic Dosage Recommendations for Treating Pulmonary Exacerbations in Patients with Cystic Fibrosis

Antibiotic	Dosage (mg/kg/day)	Doses per Day	Maximum Daily Dosage (g) or Desired Serum Concentration
Amikacin	30	2 or 3	Peak 25–30
		1[a]	Trough <5
Ampicillin-sulbactam	100–150	4	9
Aztreonam	150–200	3 or 4	8
	100	CI	8
Cefepime	150–200	3 or 4	8
Ceftazidime	150–200	3 or 4	8
	100	CI	8
Cefuroxime	100–150	3	4.5
Ciprofloxacin	20–30	2 or 3	1.2
Ciprofloxacin (PO)	40	2 or 3	2.25
Colistin	2.5–5	3	0.2
Gentamicin	10	2 or 3	Peak 8–12
		1[a]	Trough <2
Imipenem–cilastatin	50–100	4	4
Nafcillin	100–200	4	12
Piperacillin, ± tazobactam	400[b]	4	18
Ticarcillin, ± clavulanate	400[b]	4	18
Tobramycin	10	2 or 3	Peak 8–12
		1[a]	Trough <2
Trimethoprim–sulfamethoxazole	10–20	2	20 mg/kg/day (trimethoprim)

Source: References 85–87.

CI, continuous infusion.

[a]Efficacy data with once-daily aminoglycoside administration are limited; a large, randomized, multicenter clinical trial is ongoing.

[b]Refers to dosing of piperacillin and ticarcillin components.

increased volume of distribution may result from reduced adipose tissue in patients with CF. Because aminoglycosides distribute poorly into adipose tissue, the volume of distribution when expressed per kilogram of body weight therefore appears elevated.[56]

The aminoglycoside antibiotics exhibit concentration-dependent bactericidal activity and demonstrate postantibiotic effects (PAEs) against Gram-negative organisms, including *P. aeruginosa*. The goal of therapy with these agents is to maximize the peak concentrations relative to the minimal inhibitory concentration (MIC) of the infecting organism, preferably to a ratio of 8 or more.[57] Because the median MIC for *P. aeruginosa* isolates obtained from patients with CF is 1 μg/mL, peak concentrations in the range of 8 to 12 mg/L are desirable. However, because of the risk of potential nephrotoxicity and ototoxicity with excessive tissue accumulation, serum trough concentrations greater than 2 mg/L for gentamicin or tobramycin should be avoided.[58] More recently, studies evaluating once-daily aminoglycoside dosing have been performed.[59] The goal of these dosage regimens is to administer higher dosages of aminoglycosides at prolonged intervals to maximize the peak concentration (and bactericidal activity) while minimizing accumulation (and risk of toxicity). In theory, the presence of the PAE provides some protection against bacterial regrowth between doses. Currently, data on efficacy with this dosing modality in treating pulmonary exacerbations in patients with CF are limited.[60,61] A large, randomized, multicenter clinical trial sponsored by the CFF is being conducted to compare the efficacy and safety of this dosing regimen with those of the traditional multiple daily dosing regimens.

Routine monitoring of serum aminoglycoside concentrations is recommended to maximize efficacy and minimize the risk of toxicity. An initial gentamicin or tobramycin dosage of 10 mg/kg/day divided into two or three doses results in the desired serum concentrations in many patients. Because many patients with CF receive multiple courses of aminoglycosides (average 1 pulmonary exacerbation per year) sometimes for extended durations (more than 2 weeks), they are particularly predisposed to developing nephrotoxicity and ototoxicity. Despite this concern, the incidence of renal failure among patients with CF is low (0.2%). However, considering the potential for concurrent use of a nephrotoxic agent (e.g., cyclosporine, ibuprofen, colistin) vigilant monitoring is an appropriate measure. Auditory toxicity affects high-frequency hearing; appropriate audiometric testing is needed for early detection. Thus, audiometric testing may be appropriate in patients with frequent exacerbations and in those who receive prolonged course of treatment (more than 21 days).

β-LACTAMS. Results of controlled pharmacokinetic studies indicate that the clearances of several commonly prescribed intravenous β-lactams are higher (ticarcillin,[62] ceftazidime,[63,64]) or unchanged (cefepime)[65,66] compared to those in matched controls. Similarly, the volume of distribution is shown to be greater (ceftazidime)[63,64] or unchanged (ticarcillin, cefepime) compared to that in matched controls.

In contrast to the aminoglycosides, β-lactams do not demonstrate any appreciable PAE against Gram-negative organisms. In addition, they do not exhibit concentration-dependent bactericidal activity if serum concentrations at least 4 times the MIC are achieved. The goal of therapy with this class of antibiotics is therefore to maintain concentrations above this threshold for the entire dosing interval. Because there is no advantage to higher concentrations (those exceeding 4 times the MIC), some have suggested administering β-lactams as a continuous infusion.[67] Studies with continuous-infusion ceftazidime have demonstrated that this method of administration more consistently maintains concentrations above the MIC of *P. aeruginosa* in patients with CF than does intermittent dosing. In addition, continuous infusion appears to be more efficient: One-third less drug per day is needed to maintain therapeutic concentrations (100 mg/kg/day compared with 150 mg/kg/day for continuous and intermittent dosing, respectively).[68] Although a few open-label studies have demonstrated positive clinical and microbiological results with this dosing strategy, these study findings must be confirmed in comparative trials evaluating larger numbers of patients.[69]

FLUOROQUINOLONES. The pharmacokinetics of the fluoroquinolones, particularly ciprofloxacin, have been extensively evaluated in patients with CF. Conflicting results have been demonstrated with respect to differences in pharmacokinetics when compared with age-matched controls.[70–73]

The pharmacodynamic characteristics of the fluoroquinolones are similar to those of the aminoglycosides, demonstrating concentration-dependent bactericidal activity and PAEs against Gram-negative organisms, including *P. aeruginosa*. Data about ciprofloxacin pharmacodynamics in CF are limited.

Monitoring Antibiotic Therapy

The typical treatment duration of an acute exacerbation is 10 to 14 days but can extend to 21 days or more if the signs and symptoms have not improved significantly. Research studies evaluating new antibiotics have often used improvements in sputum bacterial density or formal measures of pulmonary function (e.g., FEV_1) to assess treatment outcomes. In the clinical setting, improvement in subjective signs and symptoms (decreased cough and sputum production) and a return to baseline peak flow measurements may be all that is necessary. Although slight elevations in temperature and white blood cell counts occur with acute exacerbations, they do not correlate closely with the clinical status of the exacerbation. Elevations in erythrocyte sedimentation rate (ESR) can also occur during exacerbations, reflecting an increase in inflammation. However, ESR is a nonspecific marker of inflammation and therefore may be elevated secondary to other processes (e.g., arthritis).

The availability of home infusion services has enabled patients to be treated for pulmonary exacerbations at home. The advantages of home intravenous antibiotic therapy are that it is less disruptive to normal daily activities and it is substantially less expensive than hospitalization. Home therapy should be considered for patients with mild to moderate exacerbations in whom the home environment supports this therapy.

Chronic Maintenance Therapy

Recognition of the progressive decline in pulmonary function despite aggressive treatment of acute exacerbations and the availability of oral and inhaled therapies with activity against typical CF pathogens has led to increased use of chronic maintenance antibiotic therapy. The goal is to suppress the bacterial infection with the hope of reducing the frequency and severity of pulmonary exacerbations and to slow the progressive deterioration in lung function. Results of recent trials have established the benefit of chronic inhaled tobramycin in improving these outcomes. Currently the fluoroquinolones are the only oral antibiotics with significant activity against *P. aeruginosa;* however, because of rapid emergence of resistance during therapy, some clinicians suggest that these agents be reserved for acute exacerbations. Antibiotics and dosage recommendations are listed in Table 38.3. Other approaches such as prophylactic administration of oral or inhaled antibiotics to prevent or delay the onset of chronic infection are being evaluated. Of concern with this approach is the potential for development of resistance or superinfections with intrinsically resistant organisms.

Administering antibiotics via inhalation has the advantage of achieving high concentrations at the site of infection while minimizing systemic exposure and resultant toxicity. A number of different trials evaluating various antibiotics (aminoglycosides, β-lactams, and polymyxins) have demonstrated clinical benefit in chronic maintenance with this route of administration. The most widely studied drug is tobramycin, which has recently been approved by the U.S. Food and Drug Administration for use in patients with CF who are colonized with *P. aeruginosa.* Therapy with inhaled tobramycin significantly improves pulmonary function (improvement in FEV_1 of 9 to 14%), reduces the risk of hospitalization, and reduces the need for intravenous antipseudomonal antibiotics.[74] These benefits must be weighed against the high cost of aerosolized tobramycin solution (average wholesale price $12,000/year).

Managing Inflammation

Recognition of the potent inflammatory response to chronic infection in the airways and its destruction of the lung has led to investigations of various anti-inflammatory agents. The goal of such therapies is to interrupt the infection–inflammation cycle with the intent of slowing the deterioration in pulmonary function. As previously mentioned, the course of the lung disease progresses rapidly throughout childhood and adolescence, so early therapy is desirable to slow the deterioration (Fig. 38.4). Therapeutic agents that have been evaluated include oral and inhaled corticosteroids and oral nonsteroidals. Because of an increased incidence of growth retardation, cataracts, and glucose intolerance in children, prolonged therapy (more than 2 years) is not recommended.[75]

Inhaled corticosteroids are an attractive treatment option because in theory they could provide efficacy similar to that of oral corticosteroids without the systemic toxicities. Several short-term trials of inhaled corticosteroids have been reported, demonstrating marginal benefit

Table 38.3 ▪ Oral and Inhaled Antibiotic Dosage Recommendations for Chronic Suppressive Therapy in Patients with Cystic Fibrosis

Antibiotic	Dosage (mg/kg/day)	Doses per Day	Maximum Daily Dosage (g)
Oral			
Amoxicillin, ± clavulanate	50[a]	4	2
Cephalexin	100	4	4
Cefuroxime	50	2	2
Chloramphenicol	75	4	
Ciprofloxacin	40	2 or 3	2.25
Doxycycline	4	2	
Trimethoprim–sulfamethoxazole	10[b]	2	0.32 (trimethoprim)
Inhaled			
Colistin	150 mg/day	2 or 3	–
Tobramycin	600 mg/day	2	–

Source: References 85–87.

[a]Based on amoxicillin component.

[b]Based on trimethoprim component.

in pulmonary function. Larger trials evaluating longer-term use are necessary to determine the role of inhaled corticosteroids in managing chronic inflammation.

NSAIDs are also beneficial in controlling airway inflammation. High-dose ibuprofen can inhibit neutrophil migration and activation. It has been shown to be beneficial in children aged 5 to 13 with mild lung disease.[76] Dosage individualization is recommended because of the high dosages needed to achieve therapeutic concentrations (50 to 100 μg/mL) and the large interpatient variability in the pharmacokinetic parameters. Although results of this trial indicate that ibuprofen therapy is well tolerated, concern about adverse effects (e.g., bleeding, renal failure) has limited the widespread use of this agent. The concern about renal failure is relevant because concurrent aminoglycoside therapy for pulmonary exacerbations may increase the nephrotoxic potential of these agents.[77]

Lung Transplantation

Lung transplantation has been a potential treatment option for patients with end-stage lung disease since the mid-1980s. To date more than 350 lung transplants have been performed in patients with CF in the United States according to the CFF. Bilateral lung transplantation is the most common operative procedure; however, living-donor lobar transplantation is an alternative that is becoming more common because of a shortage of available organs. The current 5-year survival rate for patients with CF is 48% and appears comparable between the two transplant procedures (bilateral lung versus living-donor lobar). A patient should be considered for transplantation if his or her survival is expected to just exceed the expected waiting period for donor lung availability (currently 6 to 24 months). Specific criteria for lung transplantation include progressive pulmonary function impairment (i.e., FEV_1 less than 30% predicted, severe hypoxemia and hypercarbia), increased frequency and duration of hospitalization for pulmonary exacerbations, the presence of life-threatening pulmonary complications (e.g., massive hemoptysis), and increasing antibiotic resistance of bacteria infecting the lungs.[78] Contraindications to lung transplantation include inability to adhere to the complex treatment plan, major complications affecting other organ systems (e.g., hepatic or renal insufficiency, diabetes with end organ damage, malignancy), and active infection (human immunodeficiency virus, hepatitis B, *Mycobacterium tuberculosis*). Currently the lack of sufficient organ donors limits the availability of this treatment for many patients who meet these criteria.

FUTURE THERAPIES

Advances in the understanding of the pathophysiology of lung disease have led to investigations of new therapies that act against infection and inflammation and correct the basic defect (impaired chloride conductance). Agents in clinical trials include $rBPI_{21}$ and antipseudomonal vaccines for infection, exogenous antiproteases (α_1-antiprotease, SLPI, DMP-777) for inflammation and phenylbutyrate, CPX, UTP, amiloride, and gene therapy for correcting the basic defect.

Infection

The emergence of multi–drug resistant isolates of *P. aeruginosa, S. maltophilia,* and *B. cepacia* poses a difficult challenge in infection managements in patients with CF. Current research efforts are directed at enhancing the activity of current antibiotic therapy and preventing or delaying the onset of chronic infection.

$rBPI_{21}$ is a recombinant product based on a host defense protein, bactericidal permeability increasing protein (BPI), which has intrinsic bactericidal activity against many Gram-negative organisms including multi–drug resistant isolates. In addition, $rBPI_{21}$ binds to Gram-negative endotoxin (lipopolysaccharide, LPS) and may therefore reduce inflammation also. In vitro experiments demonstrated a fourfold reduction in MICs of commonly prescribed antibiotics against *P. aeruginosa*.[79] A phase I trial is being conducted to evaluate pharmacokinetics and safety in patients with CF and acute pulmonary exacerbations.

An additional strategy currently being investigated is early treatment of airway colonization with current antibiotics to determine whether the onset of chronic infection can be delayed. Active immunization directed against *P. aeruginosa* endotoxin (LPS) using vaccines has also been evaluated extensively as a means of preventing initial infection; however, early attempts have been unsuccessful. Despite these disappointing results, research continues in this area.[80]

Inflammation

Recognition of the significant contribution of chronic inflammation to lung destruction has led to investigations of a number of agents. As mentioned previously, neutrophil elastase plays a central role in sustaining airway inflammation. Exogenous antiproteases have been administered in an attempt to inhibit the activity of neutrophil elastase. α_1-Antitrypsin (α_1-AT) and secretory leukoprotease inhibitor are naturally occurring antiproteases found in the airways. Exogenous administration of both compounds is associated with a reduction in neutrophil elastase activity.[81] DMP-777 is a third antiprotease agent that is undergoing phase I evaluation. The effect of these agents on reducing inflammation and the associated decline in pulmonary function awaits longer-term evaluation in larger numbers of patients.

Correcting the Basic Defect

Three strategies directed at correcting the basic defect include activation of mutant CFTR, modulation of electrolyte (sodium and chloride) transport, and gene therapy. The advantage of these approaches is that they are directed at the primary defect of CF and therefore are potentially curative. Phenylbutyrate and CPX increase the activity of mutant CFTR by enhancing CFTR delivery to the cell surface. A pilot trial of phenylbutyrate in ΔF508 homozygous patients with CF demonstrated partial restoration of CFTR chloride channel function.[82] Phase I trials of CPX are under way. The discovery of alternative chloride channels provides another avenue for potential drug development. One such agent, UTP, activates chloride conductance by raising intracellular calcium concentration. A controlled trial of UTP in combination with amiloride (a sodium channel blocker) significantly improved mucociliary clearance in adults with CF.[83] The most promising area of research is gene replacement therapy. A number of clinical trials are evaluating the safety and effectiveness of gene therapies mediated by viral and liposomal vectors. The current obstacle is a lack of an efficient delivery system to provide sufficient expression of the gene.[84] With the development of an effective gene transfer strategy, there is hope that this therapy could be curative.

KEY POINTS

- CF is a genetic disorder resulting from impairment of chloride transport across epithelial cells, causing obstruction of exocrine glands, including sweat glands, respiratory tract, pancreas, gastrointestinal, hepatobiliary, and reproductive organs.
- Respiratory disease characterized by chronic endobronchial infection and inflammation resulting in tissue damage is the primary cause of morbidity and mortality, accounting for more than 90% of deaths.
- Nonpharmacologic therapies (chest physiotherapy) and pharmacologic therapies (bronchodilators, mucolytics) are used to reduce airway obstruction.
- Intermittent courses of antibiotics are used to treat acute pulmonary exacerbations to decrease bacterial burden.
- Patients with CF exhibit altered pharmacokinetics of many antibiotics and other drugs, necessitating the use of CF-specific dosage guidelines or individualization based on measured concentrations.
- Chronic administration of inhaled antibiotics is used to suppress infection and disrupt the cycle of infection and inflammation leading to tissue destruction.
- Pancreatic enzyme replacement and a high-fat, high-calorie diet are needed to ensure adequate absorption of food and nutrients necessary to achieve and maintain normal growth.
- As lung disease treatment improves, the incidence of complications involving other organs (e.g., cirrhosis, diabetes mellitus) is likely to increase.
- The most promising area of clinical research is gene replacement therapy. There is hope that this treatment may be curative. However, until it is developed, conventional therapies directed at maintaining pulmonary function and nutritional status remain the best treatment strategies.

REFERENCES

1. Cystic Fibrosis Foundation. Patient registry 1996 annual data report. Bethesda, MD: August 1997.
2. Welsh MJ, Smith AE. Molecular mechanisms of CFTR chloride channel dysfunction in cystic fibrosis. Cell 73:1251–1254, 1993.
3. Kotloff RM. Reproductive issues in patients with cystic fibrosis. Semin Respir Crit Care Med 15:402–413, 1994.
4. Fiel SB. Pulmonary function during pregnancy in cystic fibrosis: implications for counseling. Curr Opin Pulm Med 2:462–465, 1996.
5. Kopelman H, Durie P, Gaskin K, et al. Pancreatic fluid secretion and protein hyperconcentration in cystic fibrosis. N Engl J Med 312:329–334, 1985.
6. Hardin DS, LeBlanc A, Lukenbaugh S, et al. Insulin resistance is associated with decreased clinical status in cystic fibrosis. J Pediatr 130:948–956, 1997.
7. Cucchiara S, Santamaria F, Andreotti MR, et al. Mechanisms of gastroesophageal reflux in cystic fibrosis. Arch Dis Child 66:617–622, 1991.
8. Stern RC. Cystic fibrosis and the gastrointestinal tract. In: Davis PB, ed. Cystic fibrosis. Lung biology in health and disease. New York: Marcel Dekker, 1993;64:401–434.
9. Cohn JA, Strong TV, Picciotto MR, et al. Localization of the cystic fibrosis transmembrane conductance regulator in human bile duct epithelial cells. Gastroenterology 105:1857–1864, 1993.
10. Columbo C, Battezzati PM, Podda M. Hepatobiliary disease in cystic fibrosis. Semin Liver Dis 14:259–269, 1994.
11. Roy CC, Weber AM, Morin CL, et al. Hepatobiliary disease in cystic fibrosis: a survey of current issues and concepts. J Pediatr Gastroenterol Nutr 1:469–478, 1982.
12. Watkins JB, Tercyak AM, Szczepanik P, et al. Bile salt kinetics in cystic fibrosis: influence of pancreatic enzyme replacement. Gastroenterology 72:1023–1028, 1977.
13. Smith A. Pathogenesis of bacterial bronchitis in cystic fibrosis. Pediatr Infect Dis J 16:91–96, 1997.
14. Goldman MJ, Anderson GM, Stolzenberg ED, et al. Human beta-defensin-1 is a salt sensitive antibiotic in lung that is inactivated in cystic fibrosis. Cell 88:553–560, 1997.
15. Pier GB, Grout M, Zaidi TS. Cystic fibrosis transmembrane conductance regulator is an epithelial cell receptor for clearance of *Pseudomonas aeruginosa* from the lung. Proc Natl Acad Sci USA 94:12088–12093, 1997.
16. Muhdi K, Edenborough FP, Gumery L, et al. Outcome for patients colonised with *Burkholderia cepacia* in a Birmingham adult cystic fibrosis clinic and the end of an epidemic. Thorax 51:374–377, 1996.
17. Smith DL, Gumery LB, Smith EG, et al. Epidemic of *Pseudomonas cepacia* in an adult cystic fibrosis unit: evidence of person-to-person transmission. J Clin Microbiol 31:3017–3022, 1993.
18. Greenberger PA. Immunologic aspects of lung diseases and cystic fibrosis. JAMA 278:1924–1930, 1997.
19. Stern RC. Pulmonary complications. In: Davis PB, ed. Cystic fibrosis. Lung biology in health and disease. New York: Marcel Dekker, 1993;64:345–373.
20. Fiel SB, FitzSimmons S, Schidlow D. Evolving demographics of cystic fibrosis. Semin Respir Care 15:349–355, 1994.
21. Shalon LB, Adelson JW. Cystic fibrosis: gastrointestinal complications and gene therapy. Pediatr Clin North Am 43:157–196, 1996.
22. Waters DL, Dorney SA, Gaskin KJ, et al. Pancreatic function in infants identified as having cystic fibrosis in a neonatal screening program. N Engl J Med 322:303–308, 1990.
23. Lanng S, Hansen A, Thorsteinsson B, et al. Glucose tolerance in patients with cystic fibrosis: five year prospective study. BMJ 311:655–659, 1995.
24. Lanng S, Thorsteinsson B, Lund-Andersen C, et al. Diabetes mellitus in Danish cystic fibrosis patients: prevalence and late diabetic complications. Acta Paediatr 83:72–77, 1994.
25. Finkelstein SM, Wielinski CL, Elliott GR, et al. Diabetes mellitus associated with cystic fibrosis. J Pediatr 112:373–377, 1988.
26. Cystic Fibrosis Foundation. Clinical practice guidelines for cystic fibrosis. Bethesda, MD: Author, 1997.
27. Feigelson J, Girault F, Pecau Y. Gastroesophageal reflux and esophagitis in cystic fibrosis. Acta Paediatr Scand 76:989–990, 1987.
28. Kerem E, Cory M, Kerem B, et al. Clinical and genetic comparisons of patients with cystic fibrosis, with or without meconium ileus. J Pediatr 114:767–773, 1989.
29. Corey M, McLaughlin FJ, Williams M, et al. A comparison of survival, growth, and pulmonary function in patients with cystic fibrosis in Boston and Toronto. J Clin Epidemiol 41:583–563, 1988.

30. Vaisman N, Pencharz PB, Corey M, et al. Energy expenditure of patients with cystic fibrosis. J Pediatr 111:496–500, 1987.
31. Reiter EO, Brugman SM, Pike JW, et al. Vitamin D metabolites in adolescents and young adults with cystic fibrosis: effects of sun and season. J Pediatr 106:21–26, 1985.
32. Moss RB, King VV. Management of sinusitis in cystic fibrosis by endoscopic surgery and serial antimicrobial lavage: reduction in recurrence requiring surgery. Arch Otolaryngol Head Neck Surg 121:566–572, 1995.
33. Regelmann WE, Elliott GR, Warwick WJ, et al. Reduction of sputum *Pseudomonas aeruginosa* density by antibiotics improves lung function in cystic fibrosis more than do bronchodilators and chest physiotherapy alone. Am Rev Respir Dis 141:914–921, 1990.
34. Centers for Disease Control and Prevention. Newborn screening for cystic fibrosis: a paradigm for public health genetics policy development. Proceedings of a 1997 workshop. MMWR 46(RR-16):1–24, 1997.
35. Colombo C, Battezzati PM, Podda M, et al. Ursodeoxycholic acid for liver disease associated with cystic fibrosis: a double-blind multicenter trial. Hepatology 23:1484–1490, 1996.
36. Lepage G, Paradis K, Lacaille F, et al. Ursodeoxycholic acid improves the hepatic metabolism of essential fatty acids and retinol in children with cystic fibrosis. J Pediatr 130:52–58, 1997.
37. Cotton CU, Davis PB. The pancreas in cystic fibrosis. In: Davis PB, ed. Cystic fibrosis. New York: Marcel Dekker, 1993:161–192.
38. Fitzsimmons SC, Burkhart GA, Borowitz D, et al. High-dose pancreatic-enzyme supplements and fibrosing colonopathy in children with cystic fibrosis. N Engl J Med 336:1283–1289, 1997.
39. Stevens JC, Maguiness KM, Hollingsworth J, et al. Pancreatic enzyme supplementation in cystic fibrosis patients before and after fibrosing colonopathy. J Pediatr Gastroenterol Nutr 26:80–84, 1998.
40. Collins CE, O'Loughlin EV, Henry RL. Fat gram target to achieve high energy intake in cystic fibrosis. J Paediatr Child Health 33:142–147, 1997.
41. Hardy KA. A review of airway clearance: new techniques, indications, and recommendations. Respir Care 39:440–445, 1994.
42. Mitchell I, Corey M, Woenne R, et al. Bronchial hyperreactivity in cystic fibrosis and asthma. J Pediatr 93:744–748, 1978.
43. Pattishall EN. Longitudinal response of pulmonary function to bronchodilators in cystic fibrosis. Pediatr Pulmonol 9:80–85, 1990.
44. Cropp GJ. Effectiveness of bronchodilators in cystic fibrosis. Am J Med 100(Suppl 1A):19S–29S, 1996.
45. Bargon J, Viel K, Dauletbaev N, et al. Short-term effects of regular salmeterol treatment on adult cystic fibrosis patients. Eur Respir J 10:2307–2311, 1997.
46. Shak S, Capon DJ, Hellmiss R, et al. Recombinant human DNase I reduces the viscosity of cystic fibrosis sputum. Proc Natl Acad Sci USA 87:9188–9192, 1990.
47. Fuchs HJ, Borowitz DS, Christiansen DH, et al. Effect of aerosolized recombinant human DNase on exacerbations of respiratory symptoms and on pulmonary function in patients with cystic fibrosis. N Engl J Med 331:637–642, 1994.
48. Cipolla D, Clark A, Pearlman R, et al. Pulmozyme rhDNase should not be mixed with other nebulizer medications [abstract 236]. North American Cystic Fibrosis Conference, 1994.
49. Ripoll L, Reinert P, Pepin LF, et al. Interaction of macrolides with alpha dornase during DNA hydrolysis. J Antimicrob Chemother 37:987–991, 1996.
50. Saiman L, Mehar F, Niu WW, et al. Antibiotic susceptibility of multiply resistant *Pseudomonas aeruginosa* isolated from patients with cystic fibrosis, including candidates for transplantation. Clin Infect Dis 23:532–537, 1996.
51. De Groot R, Smith AL. Antibiotic pharmacokinetics in cystic fibrosis: differences and clinical significance. Clin Pharmacokinet 13:228–253, 1987.
52. Spino M. Pharmacokinetics of drugs in cystic fibrosis. Clin Rev Allergy 9:169–210, 1991.
53. Vogelstein B, Kowarski AA, Lietman PS. The pharmacokinetics of amikacin in children. J Pediatr 91:333–339, 1977.
54. Kearns GL, Hilman BC, Wilson JT. Dosing implications of altered gentamicin disposition in patients with cystic fibrosis. J Pediatr 100:312–318, 1982.
55. Levy J, Smith AL, Koup JR, et al. Disposition of tobramycin in patients with cystic fibrosis: a prospective controlled study. J Pediatr 105:117–124, 1984.
56. Kavanagh RE, Unadkat JD, Smith AL. Drug disposition in cystic fibrosis. In: Davis PB, ed. Cystic fibrosis. New York: Marcel Dekker, 1993:91–136.
57. Moore RD, Lietman PS, Smith CR. Clinical response to aminoglycoside therapy: importance of the ratio of peak concentration to minimal inhibitory concentration. J Infect Dis 155:93–99, 1987.
58. Dahlgren JG, Anderson ET, Hewitt WL, et al. Gentamicin blood levels: a guide to nephrotoxicity. Antimicrob Agents Chemother 8:58–62, 1975.
59. Bates RD, Nahata MC, Jones JW, et al. Pharmacokinetics and safety of tobramycin after once-daily administration in patients with cystic fibrosis. Chest 112:1208–1213, 1997.
60. Vic P, Ategbo S, Turck D, et al. Efficacy, tolerance, and pharmacokinetics of once daily tobramycin for pseudomonas exacerbations in cystic fibrosis. Arch Dis Child 78:536–539, 1998.
61. Powell SH, Thompson WL, Luthe MA, et al. One-daily vs. continuous aminoglycoside dosing: efficacy and toxicity in animal and clinical studies of gentamicin, netilmicin and tobramycin. J Infect Dis 147:918–932, 1983.
62. de Groot R, Hack BD, Weber A, et al. Pharmacokinetics of ticarcillin in patients with cystic fibrosis: a controlled prospective study. Clin Pharmacol Ther 47:73–78, 1990.
63. Leeder JS, Spino M, Isles AF, et al. Ceftazidime disposition in acute and stable cystic fibrosis. Clin Pharmacol Ther 36:355–362, 1984.
64. Hedman A, Adan-Abdi Y, Alvan G, et al. Influence of the glomerular filtration rate on renal clearance of ceftazidime in cystic fibrosis. Clin Pharmacokinet 15:57–65, 1988.
65. Huls CE, Prince RA, Seilheimer DK, et al. Pharmacokinetics of cefepime in cystic fibrosis patients. Antimicrob Agents Chemother 37:1414–1416, 1993.
66. Hamelin BA, Moore N, Knupp CA, et al. Cefepime pharmacokinetics in cystic fibrosis. Pharmacotherapy 13:465–470, 1993.
67. Mouton JW, Vinks AATMM. Is continuous infusion of β-lactam antibiotics worthwhile? Efficacy and pharmacokinetic considerations. J Antimicrob Chemother 38:5–15, 1996.
68. Vinks AATMM, Touw DJ, Heijerman GH, et al. Pharmacokinetics of ceftazidime in adult cystic fibrosis patients during continuous infusion and ambulatory treatment at home. Ther Drug Monitor 16:341–348, 1994.
69. Vinks AATMM, Brimicombe RW, Heijerman HG, et al. Continuous infusion of ceftazidime in patients with cystic fibrosis during home treatment: clinical outcome, microbiology and pharmacokinetics. J Antimicrob Chemother 40:125–133, 1997.
70. Lebel M, Bergeron MG, Vallee F, et al. Pharmacokinetics and pharmacodynamics of ciprofloxacin in cystic fibrosis patients. Antimicrob Agents Chemother 30:260–266, 1986.
71. Davis RL, Koup JR, Williams-Warren J, et al. Pharmacokinetics of ciprofloxacin in cystic fibrosis. Antimicrob Agents Chemother 31:915–919, 1987.
72. Reed MD, Stern RC, Myers CM, et al. Lack of unique ciprofloxacin pharmacokinetic characteristics in patients with cystic fibrosis. J Clin Pharmacol 28:691–699, 1988.
73. Christensson BA, Nilsson-Ehle I, Ljungberg B, et al. Increased oral bioavailability of ciprofloxacin in cystic fibrosis patients. Antimicrob Agents Chemother 36:2512–2517, 1992.
74. Ramsey B, Burns JL, Smith AL. Safety and efficacy of tobramycin solution for inhalation in patients with cystic fibrosis: the results of two phase III placebo controlled clinical trials. Abstract S10.4, Eleventh Annual North American Cystic Fibrosis Conference, Nashville, TN, 1997.
75. Rosenstein BJ, Eigen H. Risks of alternate-day prednisone in patients with cystic fibrosis. Pediatrics 87:245–246, 1991.
76. Konstan MW, Byard PJ, Hoppel CL, et al. Effect of high-dose ibuprofen in patients with cystic fibrosis. N Engl J Med 332:848–854, 1995.
77. Kovesi TA, Swartz R, MacDonald N. Transient renal failure due to simultaneous ibuprofen and aminoglycoside therapy in children with cystic fibrosis [letter]. N Engl J Med 338:65–66, 1998.
78. Yankaskas JR, Mallory GB. Lung transplantation in cystic fibrosis: consensus conference statement. Chest 113:217–226, 1998.
79. Lambert L, Mitchell C, Scannon P. Recombinant bactericidal/permeability-increasing protein (rBPI21) is bactericidal in vitro against *Pseudomonas aeruginosa* strains isolated from cystic fibrosis patients [abstract E-149:140]. Proceedings of the 37th Conference on Antimicrobial Agents and Chemotherapy, Toronto, September 28–October 1, 1997.
80. Pier GB. *Pseudomonas aeruginosa:* a key problem in cystic fibrosis. ASM News 64:339–347, 1998.
81. Allen ED. Opportunities for the use of aerosolized α_1-antitrypsin for the treatment of cystic fibrosis. Chest 110:256S–260S, 1996.
82. Rubenstein RC, Zeitlin PL. A pilot clinical trial of oral sodium 4-phenylbutyrate (Buphenyl) in ΔF508-homozygous cystic fibrosis patients. Am J Respir Crit Care Med 157:484–490, 1998.
83. Bennett WD, Olivier KN, Aeman KL, et al. Effect of uridine 5′-triphosphate plus amiloride on mucociliary clearance in adult cystic fibrosis. Am J Respir Crit Care Med 153:1796–1801, 1996.
84. Wagner JA, Gardner P. Toward cystic fibrosis gene therapy. Annu Rev Med 48:203–216, 1997.
85. Mouton JW, Kerrebyn KF. Antibacterial therapy in cystic fibrosis. Med Clin North Am 74:837–850, 1990.
86. Ramsey BW. Management of pulmonary disease in patients with cystic fibrosis. N Engl J Med 335:179–188, 1996.
87. Turpin SU, Knowles MR. Treatment of pulmonary disease in patients with cystic fibrosis. In: Davis PB, ed. Cystic fibrosis. Lung biology in health and disease. New York: Marcel Dekker, 1993;64:277–344.

CHAPTER 39

HYPERTENSION

Robert T. Weibert

Blood pressure control continues to be important in reducing cardiovascular risk, along with the modification of other cardiovascular risk factors, especially cholesterol levels. Lifestyle modification to reduce blood pressure may control stage 1 hypertension and is important adjunctive therapy in treating all hypertension. Drug treatment should be based on evidence of improved outcomes and individualized to account for patient age, race, and other disease states, effect on quality of life, drug costs, and patient compliance. The adverse consequences of antihypertensive drugs should be minimized, and stepdown drug therapy can be attempted after a sustained period of controlled blood pressure.

The majority of hypertensive patients need long-term antihypertensive drug treatment, and more pharmacologic agents are available for treating hypertension than for any other condition. Clinicians can provide information about the pharmacology, pharmacokinetics, drug interactions, and adverse effects of these agents. In addition, maintaining patients on long-term drug treatment allows pharmacists to participate in providing follow-up care. Although the number of cardiovascular deaths has decreased over the past 25 years, achieving long-term control of hypertension in millions of patients remains an important objective.

DEFINITION

Blood pressure varies from minute to minute and is influenced by measurement technique, time of day, emotion, pain, discomfort, hydration, temperature, exercise, posture, and drugs. The dividing line between normal blood pressure and hypertension is arbitrary.[1,2] Early insurance industry actuarial data showed a continuum; the higher the blood pressure, the greater the risk of complications. The 1997 Report of the Joint National Committee on Detection, Evaluation and Treatment of High Blood Pressure (JNC VI) criteria for establishing a diagnosis of hypertension are as follows: After screening, the diagnosis of hypertension is confirmed when the average of two or more diastolic blood pressure (DBP) measurements is 90 mm Hg or higher or the average of two or more systolic blood pressure (SBP) measurements is consistently greater than 140 mm Hg. JNC VI classifies blood pressures as shown in Table 39.1. Single, casual measurements of blood pressure may inaccurately classify patients as having hypertension and cause unnecessary emotional, social, and financial problems.[1]

Table 39.1 ▪ Classification of Blood Pressure

Classification	Systolic Pressure (mm Hg)		Diastolic Pressure (mm Hg)
Optimal blood pressure	<120	and	<80
Normal blood pressure	<130	and	<85
High normal blood pressure	130–139	or	85–89
Stage 1	140–159	or	90–99
Stage 2	160–179	or	100–109
Stage 3	180	or	110

TREATMENT GOALS: HYPERTENSION

- Educate patients about consequences of untreated hypertension
- Control blood pressure by nonpharmacologic interventions when possible
- Initiate drug therapy when nonpharmacologic interventions are unsuccessful

EPIDEMIOLOGY

Etiology

Essential Hypertension

More than 90% of patients with sustained elevation of arterial blood pressure have essential hypertension with no identifiable cause. The term *essential hypertension* evolved from the mistaken belief that high blood pressure was essential for adequate tissue perfusion.

Remediable Hypertension

A small percentage of patients may have potentially curable hypertension caused by renal disease, adrenal disease, coarctation of the aorta, or another rare condition.[1] Renovascular hypertension, which is considered the most prevalent remediable cause of hypertension, is estimated to cause hypertension in less than 0.5% of the hypertensive population.[3]

Drug-Induced Hypertension

Hypertension may occur in up to 5% of patients who take oral contraceptives. However, most women show small but measurable increases (9/5 mm Hg) in blood pressure during the first 2 years on the pill.[4] Factors that may increase the likelihood of oral contraceptive hypertension include age greater than 35 years, smoking, obesity, and a family history of hypertension. Although the estrogen is the most important component, the amount and type of progestin may further influence the effect on blood pressure. Proposed mechanisms for contraceptive-induced hypertension include stimulation of the renin–angiotensin–aldosterone system and sodium and fluid retention. Oral contraceptive–induced hypertension may develop gradually over 1 to 2 years and is usually reversible within 1 to 8 months after therapy is stopped. However, if blood pressure does not normalize within 3 months, further evaluation and therapy are appropriate. Oral contraceptive–induced hypertension is best prevented by checking blood pressure every 6 months and using the agent that has the lowest effective estrogen dosage (less than 30 μg) and a progestin content of 1 mg or less.[4] Women who are at higher risk or who actually develop hypertension may need alternative forms of contraception (see Section 18).

Other drugs may also significantly increase blood pressure. A double dose of the sympathomimetic diet drug phenylpropanolamine (PPA) causes a significant increase in blood pressure to a peak of 173/103 mm Hg.[5] There are reports of intracranial hemorrhage after PPA use. A meta-analysis of the effect of nonsteroidal anti-inflammatory drugs (NSAIDs) on blood pressure demonstrated that NSAIDs elevate supine mean blood pressure by 5.0 mm Hg.[6] NSAIDs antagonized the antihypertensive effects of β-blockers (6.2-mm Hg increase) to a greater extent than they antagonized vasodilators or diuretics.[5] Cyclosporine causes vasoconstriction and sodium retention, inducing hypertension in a high percentage of patients. Recombinant human erythropoietin (rHuEPO) causes hypertension that is not responsive to antihypertensive therapy and must be managed by a dosage reduction or discontinuation of rHuEPO.[1] Also, corticosteroids, monoamine oxidase inhibitors, and products that contain large quantities of sodium, such as effervescent solutions, may increase blood pressure.

Prevalence

The National Health and Nutrition Examinetics survey found that more than 50 million Americans have blood pressure higher than 140/90 mm Hg or are taking antihypertensive medications.[1] The majority have stage 1 or 2 hypertension, with DBPs ranging from 90 to 104 mm Hg. The prevalence of hypertension increases with age and is greater among African Americans than Caucasians and is greater in people with less education. Men and women of the same race are affected approximately equally. Massive public health efforts have increased patient and practitioner awareness of the need to identify and treat hypertension.[1] Although 68% of adults in the United States are now aware that they have hypertension, only 53% are on treatment and only 27% have achieved control of their blood pressure. From 1950 to 1989 the increased use of antihypertensive medications has reduced the prevalence of hypertension from 18.5% to 9.2% among men and from 28.0% to 7.7% among women. Thus, the major challenge for health care providers continues to be long-term hypertension control.[1]

PATHOPHYSIOLOGY

Blood pressure is maintained within a fairly constant range, despite changes in posture and wide variations in the demand for blood supply. Although much is known about the complex system that regulates blood pressure, the pathogenesis of essential hypertension remains unknown. Early theories suggested that renal sodium retention expanded vascular volume, increasing cardiac output. The increased cardiac output was believed to have led to increased vascular resistance. Further investigations suggest that natriuretic hormones may initiate sodium retention. Another theory suggests that inherited cellular defects cause increased intracellular sodium, leading to increases in ionic calcium and increased vascular tone and reactivity. A possible primary role of the sympathetic nervous system has also been suggested. It is likely that several interrelated mechanisms, rather than a single causative defect, control blood pressure in essential hypertension. A relationship between hypertension and obesity, insulin resistance, hyperinsulinemia, glucose intolerance, and hypertriglyceridemia has been reported. This relationship has been called "the deadly quartet" or "syndrome X." This has led to the theory that hyperinsulinemia is a cause of hypertension.[7] However, even with continued insights into the regulation of blood pressure, essential hypertension remains a process that must be controlled rather than a curable disorder.

Table 39.2 ▪ Risk Stratification for Treatment

Risk Group	Risk Factors	Blood Pressure to Begin Drug Therapy
A	No TOD or CCD No risk factors	Stages 2 and 3 (160/100 mm Hg) Stage 1 (140–159/90–99 mm Hg) after 12 mo of lifestyle modification
B	No TOD or CCD 1 risk factor except diabetes mellitus	Stages 2 and 3 (160/100 mm Hg) Stage 1 (140–159/90–99 mm Hg) after 6 mo of lifestyle modification
C	TOD, CCD, or diabetes with or without other risks	High-normal (130–139/85–89 mm Hg) Stage 1 (140–159/90–99 mm Hg) Stages 2 and 3 (160/100 mm Hg)

TOD, target organ damage; *CCD,* clinical cardiovascular disease.

COMPLICATIONS

Target organ disease (TOD) from arterial hypertension can be cardiac, cerebrovascular, peripheral vascular, renal, and ocular. The risk of complications and premature death is related to the degree of blood pressure elevation. Hypertension is additive with other risk factors in the development of coronary heart disease (CHD) and stroke. JNC VI recommends risk stratification to determine when drug therapy is indicated (Table 39.2).[1] Risk stratification is based on presence of TOD, clinical cardiovascular disease (CCD), and other cardiovascular risk factors including diabetes, dyslipidemia, and smoking.

Data from the Multiple Risk Factor Intervention Trial (MRFIT) study describe the combined effects of cardiovascular risk factors.[8] In men less than 46 years of age, a DBP greater than 90 mm Hg increased deaths to a rate 1.6 times the rate for men without risks, having two risk factors increased the rate 3 to 4 times, and having all three major risk factors increased the death rate six times (Table 39.3). The major correctable and noncorrectable risk factors are shown in Table 39.4.

Left ventricular hypertrophy (LVH) and left ventricular dysfunction are important complications related to hypertension.[9] Echocardiography demonstrates that left ventricular muscle mass is increased in 15 to 20% of patients with hypertension. Cardiovascular events occur more than twice as often in hypertensive patients with LVH (26%) than in patients without LVH (12%). Patients with LVH have a five to six times higher risk of sudden death or other cardiovascular mortality than do those without LVH.

The major complications associated with hypertension are stroke and CHD. A meta-analysis of nine prospective observational studies of 420,000 patients with a mean 10-year follow-up assessed these risks.[10] The combined data demonstrated a positive, continuous increase in risk

Table 39.3 ▪ Effect of Combined Risk Factors in Total Deaths per 1000 in the Multiple Risk Factor Intervention Trial

	Men Age 35–45 yr		Men Age 46–57 yr	
Risk Factor	Deaths/1000	Increase[a]	Deaths/1000	Increase[a]
None	5.4		19.3	
DBP >90	8.4	1.6	25.8	1.3
Cholesterol >250 mg/dL	10.0	1.9	25.4	1.3
Smoking	12.8	2.4	38.8	2.0
DBP + cholesterol	15.8	2.9	37.9	2.0
DBP + smoking	23.2	4.3	56.4	2.9
DBP/cholesterol/smoking	33.2	6.1	70.7	3.7

[a]Increased risk = deaths for men with risk factor/deaths for men with no risks.

within the range of DBP 70 to 110 mm Hg. There was no evidence of a threshold DBP, and lower blood pressures always were associated with less risk. Higher blood pressures even within the range that is considered normotensive are associated with increasing cardiovascular risks. A prolonged difference in DBP of 10 mm Hg was associated with 56% less stroke and 37% less CHD.[10]

CLINICAL PRESENTATION AND DIAGNOSIS

Hypertension usually is an asymptomatic disease and is most often detected by screening. Because hypertension is easily detected and effective therapy is available, screening is recommended for all adults.[1] Although headache, epistaxis, and tinnitus were once thought to be symptoms of high blood pressure, no relationship has been demonstrated between these symptoms and either SBP or DBP.[11] Work-site screening programs produce minimal psychosocial consequences.[12] Increased absenteeism after a diagnosis of hypertension is associated with higher baseline anxiety levels, and reassurance may be beneficial for these patients.[12]

The initial evaluation of patients with possible hypertension is an important process with several objectives:[1]

- *Establish a diagnosis of hypertension.*[1] The average of two or more measurements of blood pressure after an elevated blood pressure at screening confirms the diagnosis of hypertension. JNC VI classifications are shown in Table 39.1.
  - Correct measurement techniques are crucial in determining whether a casual screening or office blood pressure reflects a true increase in blood pressure. The SBP is the first sound (phase 1) and the DBP is the disappearance of sound (phase 5). Accurate blood pressure measurement involves correct cuff width (two-thirds of the length between the shoulder and elbow), correct arm position, a bared arm, and the lightest possible pressure on the stethoscope head. Patients should be comfortably seated and relaxed with the arm held passively at the level of the heart. They should not have smoked or ingested caffeine in the preceding 30 minutes. Twenty-one percent of patients with untreated borderline hypertension were shown to have "white-coat hypertension," based on ambulatory blood pressure monitoring.[13] This exaggerated pressor response is more pronounced when blood pressure is measured by a physician than by a technician and may be specific to the physician's office. White-coat or office hypertension occurs more often in female patients, younger patients, and patients who were recently diagnosed as hypertensive.[13] The health consequences of white-coat hypertension are benign compared to those of sustained hypertension.[14]
  - Ambulatory blood pressure monitoring (ABPM) for 24 hours or longer is possible by using portable monitoring devices.[1,15] ABPM is not cost-effective for all patients but may be useful in evaluating patients with high normal blood pressure who have target organ damage, drug-resistant hypertension, episodic hypertension, transient hypotension, office hypertension, or syncope. Damage to target organs appears to correlate best with data from ABPM.
- *Avoiding early dropout.* The problem of early dropout from hypertension treatment programs is well documented. The rate of dropout from care during the first year of treatment often approaches 50%.[16] The most important part of the initial visit is to ensure that the patient will return for further follow-up.
- *Evaluation for the presence of cardiovascular risk factors and quantitation of hypertensive vascular disease.* The medical history, physical examination, and laboratory testing are directed toward identifying risk factors, the extent of any existing vascular damage, and the presence of concurrent diseases. The JNC has provided guidelines for evaluating patients (Table 39.5).[1]
- *Screening for secondary causes of hypertension.* Most patients with elevated blood pressure have essential hypertension. Any patient whose medical history or physical examination suggests a possible cause of secondary hypertension warrants additional diagnostic evaluation (Table 39.6).[1]
- *Explanation of findings.* To avoid early dropout and to work toward long-term control of hypertension, patients need to become active participants in their own care. Patients must understand the following:
  - The potential benefits and risks of therapy
  - That their blood pressure exceeds normal limits
  - The possible consequences of uncontrolled hypertension
  - That hypertension usually is asymptomatic and that symptoms do not indicate the blood pressure level reliably
  - That prolonged follow-up and therapy are needed
  - That treatment will control but not cure high blood pressure
  - Their target goal blood pressure
  - The presence of any other cardiovascular risk factors and how these affect the patient's probability of developing cardiovascular disease

Table 39.4 ▪ Cardiovascular Risk Factors and Target Organ Damage

Major Risk Factors	Target Organ Damage
Smoking	Heart disease
Dyslipidemia	Left ventricular hypertrophy
Diabetes mellitus	Angina or prior myocardial infarction
Age >60 yr	Prior coronary revascularization
Sex: men and postmenopausal women	Heart failure
Family history of cardiovascular disease: women <65 yr or men <55 yr	Stroke or transient ischemic attack
	Nephropathy
	Retinopathy

The initial evaluation documents the presence of hypertension, begins to establish long-term compliance, and establishes the extent of target organ damage and the existence of other risk factors.[15,16] This allows a rational basis for planning treatment.

ANTIHYPERTENSIVE THERAPY TRIALS

Information from observational studies has clearly demonstrated that a lower DBP is associated with a lower risk of stroke and CHD. However, the effects of differences in blood pressure may develop over decades. Whether maintaining blood pressure reductions over a few years will

Table 39.5 ▪ Evaluation of Hypertensive Patients

A. Medical history
  1. Family history of hypertension and hypertensive complications
  2. History of cardiovascular, cerebrovascular, or renal disease or diabetes mellitus
  3. Duration and level of elevated blood pressure
  4. Effectiveness and side effects of previous drug treatment
  5. Medication history for drugs that elevate blood pressure
  6. Lifestyle and health habits:
     a. Smoking
     b. Ethanol excess
     c. Sodium intake
     d. Caffeine
     e. Exercise
     f. Emotional stress

B. Physical examination
  1. Two or more blood pressure measurements with patient supine or seated and standing
  2. Verification of blood pressure in the contralateral arm
  3. Height and weight
  4. Fundoscopic examination for arteriolar narrowing, arteriovenous compression, hemorrhages, exudates, and papilledema
  5. Neck examination for carotid bruits, distended veins, and enlarged thyroid
  6. Cardiac examination for increased rate, size, precordial heave, murmurs, arrhythmias, and S3 and S4 heart sounds
  7. Abdominal examination for bruits, enlarged kidneys, and aortic dilation
  8. Extremity examination for edema and decreased or absent pulses
  9. Neurologic assessment

C. Laboratory tests
  1. Hemoglobin and hematocrit
  2. Urinalysis
  3. Serum potassium
  4. Serum creatinine
  5. Fasting plasma glucose
  6. Total and high-density lipoprotein cholesterol
  7. Serum uric acid

Source: Reference 1.

decrease these cardiovascular risks is a question that randomized trials have attempted to answer. A detailed epidemiologic analysis has recently summarized the findings from 14 unconfounded randomized trials of antihypertensive drugs that were reported between 1965 and 1986.[17] There were a total of 37,000 patients, 30,000 of whom were treated for mild hypertension.[17] Most trials used a stepped-care (SC) approach, starting with a diuretic. Two trials started with a β-blocker. The usual goal of treatment was to reduce DPB to 90 mm Hg or less, and the mean time of follow-up was 5 years. The average difference in blood pressure between the treatment and control groups was 6 mm Hg. This reduction in blood pressure produced a highly significant reduction in stroke, a decrease of 42%. This benefit of stroke reduction appears soon after blood pressure decreases. The effect of blood pressure reduction on CHD was much smaller (14%), and the reduction in fatal CHD (11%) was not significant. The reduction in the rate of stroke was 33 to 50% in the clinical trials, which corresponds to the 35 to 40% predicted from observational studies. The reduction in the CHD rate was 4 to 22% in the clinical trials, which was less than the 20 to 25% predicted from observational studies. The shortfall in CHD reduction could have resulted from chance, the influence of chronic atherosclerotic processes that were not reversed by blood pressure reduction, or cardiotoxic adverse effects of the treatments that limited CHD reduction. An analysis that included the Systolic Hypertension in the Elderly Program (SHEP), Swedish Trial in Old Patients with Hypertension (STOP-Hypertension), and Medical Research Council (MRC) trials found that the benefit of drug therapy on CHD rises to 16% and stroke reduction was similar (45%).[18]

In summary, a 5- to 6-mm Hg reduction of DBP with diuretic-based regimens produced risk reductions of 45% for stroke and 16% for CHD. The World Health Organization (WHO) 1999 guidelines confirm that a prolonged 5-mm Hg reduction in DBP is associated with a 35 to 40% reduction in stroke and a 25% reduction in CHD.[2]

Improved compliance with antihypertensive therapy and an 8- to 10-mm Hg reduction in DBP should reduce stroke by 50% and CHD by 20%. Because CHD is more common, the absolute benefit of a 20% decrease in CHD could exceed the benefit of a 50% decrease in stroke. But other therapies for CHD (smoking cessation, cholesterol reduction, aspirin, and β-blockers) show stronger evidence of cardiac benefit and should be emphasized for high-risk patients. A high risk of stroke is a clearer indication for antihypertensive therapy than is an increased risk of CHD. Older adults have a 2% annual incidence of stroke, and patients with a prior transient ischemic attack have a 5% incidence.

Veterans Administration Cooperative Study

The Veterans Administration (VA) Cooperative Study clearly demonstrated that reducing blood pressure to normal or near-normal levels decreases the occurrence of complications and provided early evidence of the benefits of drug treatment.[1,19,19a] Complications developed three times as often in untreated patients. Treating moderate hypertension (DBP greater than 104 mm Hg) abolished hypertensive complications (congestive heart failure, accelerated hypertension, renal failure) and reduced cerebrovas-

Table 39.6 ▪ Clinical Findings Suggestive of Secondary Hypertension

Finding	Secondary Cause
Abdominal bruit	Renovascular disease
Abdominal or flank mass	Polycystic kidney disease
Hypokalemia	Hyperaldosteronism
Headache, palpitations, sweating, "spells"	Pheochromocytoma
Delayed or absent femoral pulse	Aortic coarctation
Truncal obesity	Cushing's syndrome

cular accidents by 75%. However, treatment did not decrease the incidence of myocardial infarction. Finally, the VA study has shown that even partial reduction of blood pressure (DBP 90 to 104 mm Hg) decreases cardiovascular complications.[20]

Hypertension Detection and Follow-Up Program Cooperative Study

The Hypertension Detection and Follow-Up Program (HDFP) randomized almost 11,000 patients to referred-care (RC) or stepped-care (SC) groups.[21–23] Seventy percent of the patients had mild hypertension (DBP 90 to 104 mm Hg). The treatment goal for HDFP patients was the lesser of a 10 mm Hg decrease from entry blood pressure or a DBP less than 90 mm Hg. The 5-year DBP averaged 84 mm Hg for the SC group and 89 mm Hg for the RC group, a difference of only 5 mm Hg. The rate of strokes was 45% lower, and the rate of death from myocardial infarction was 26% lower. The 5-year mortality was 16.9% lower for the SC group than for the RC group. Mortality was 20.3% lower for the SC subgroup with entry DBP of 90 to 104 mm Hg (5.9 versus 7.4 per 100). The subgroup with DBP 90 to 140 mm Hg and no evidence of end-organ damage at entry had 28.6% fewer deaths at 5 years. The HDFP did not demonstrate a significant reduction in mortality for white women or for patients younger than 50 years because the death rate was low in both groups. A post-trial surveillance study followed HDFP participants for an additional 2 years, providing 6.7-year mortality data. Mortality differences increased further, to 95.1 per 1000 SC patients compared to 116.3 per 1000 RC patients.[24]

Multiple Risk Factor Intervention Trial

The MRFIT followed 12,800 men over 7 years.[25] A special intervention (SI) group, which received SC treatment for hypertension, counseling for cigarette smoking, and dietary advice to lower cholesterol, was compared with a usual-care (UC) group. Risk factors in the SI group decreased in comparison to those in the UC group. However, the SI group showed only a nonsignificant 7% lower rate of CHD mortality. The possibility that antihypertensive drug therapy had an adverse effect on some patients has been raised as a potential explanation for the similar mortality despite the reduction of risk factors. Follow-up analysis described a 3.34% higher risk of CHD death in men with baseline electrocardiogram (ECG) abnormalities who were given diuretic drugs than in men who were not treated with diuretics.[26] Men without ECG abnormalities had a risk of 0.95%. However, no relationship was demonstrated between CHD mortality and hypokalemia or diuretic dosage.

European Working Party on High Blood Pressure in the Elderly Trial

The European Working Party on High Blood Pressure in the Elderly (EWPHE) trial assessed the effects of antihypertensive drug therapy on patients over 60 years of age.[27] In this trial, 840 patients with entry DBP of 90 to 119 mm Hg were randomized to treatment or placebo and followed over 12 years. Treatment reduced total mortality (9%) and cardiovascular mortality (27%). Therapy with combined hydrochlorothiazide (HCTZ) and triamterene adversely affected glucose tolerance, serum uric acid, and creatinine. Subanalysis showed little or no benefit from treating patients over 80 years of age, most of whom were women.[28]

Systolic Hypertension in the Elderly Program

The SHEP trial assessed the effects of antihypertensive drug therapy on the risk of nonfatal and fatal stroke in patients over 60 years of age with isolated systolic hypertension (ISH).[29] In this trial, 4736 patients with entry SBP of 160 to 219 mm Hg and DBP less than 90 mm Hg were randomized to treatment with chlorthalidone or placebo over an average 4.5-year follow-up. The 5-year incidence of total stroke was 5.2 per 100 treated patients and 8.2 per 100 placebo patients. Treating ISH reduced stroke by 37% and reduced all cardiovascular events by 32%. The number needed to treat (NNT) to prevent one stroke was 43 in the SHEP trial.

Swedish Trial in Old Patients with Hypertension

STOP-Hypertension assessed the effects of antihypertensive drug therapy on the risk of nonfatal and fatal stroke, myocardial infarction, and other cardiovascular complications in patients over 70 years of age with diastolic hypertension.[30] In this trial, 1627 patients with entry SBP of 180 to 230 mm Hg and DBP greater than 90 mm Hg were randomized to treatment with β-blockers, a diuretic, or placebo over an average 2-year follow-up. Treatment reduced primary endpoints (94 versus 58 events) and total stroke (53 versus 29 events), and benefits were discernible up to age 84. The NNT to prevent one stroke was 34 in the STOP trial. There was a significant reduction in total mortality of 43%.

Medical Research Council Trial in Older Adults

The MRC trial assessed the effects of diuretics or a β-blocker on the risk of stroke, CHD, and death in 4396 adults aged 65 to 74 years over a mean 5.8-year period.[31] Treated patients had a 25% lower rate of stroke and a 19% lower rate of coronary events than patients given a placebo. The β-blocker group showed no significant reduction in endpoints. The reduction in stroke was greatest in nonsmokers taking diuretics. The NNT to prevent one stroke was 70 in the MRC trial.

Treatment of Mild Hypertension Study

The Treatment of Mild Hypertension Study (TOMHS) assessed the effects of five antihypertensive drug therapies and a sustained lifestyle modification program on the risk of developing LVH, the effect on quality of life, and the risk of clinical cardiovascular events over a 4-year period.[32] In this trial, 902 patients with an entry DBP of 90 to 99 mm Hg were randomized to placebo or one of five antihypertensive agents in addition to nutritional and hygienic intervention. Greater reduction in blood pressure was achieved with drug treatment (–15.9/–9.1 mm Hg) than with nutritional invention plus placebo (–12.2/–8.6 mm Hg). Drug treatment resulted in lower rates of nonfatal cardiovascular events and progression to LVH by ECG than did nutritional intervention. Drug treatment also improved quality of life, although differences between the treatment groups were modest and inconsistent. In these mild hypertensive patients without a history of cardiovascular disease, no evidence of a *J*-shaped curve relationship was found. Nutritional intervention resulted in substantial reductions in blood pressure. However, if a target blood pressure of less than 140/90 mm Hg is not reached after 3 to 6 months, an antihypertensive drug should be added.

Hypertension Optimal Treatment Trial

The Hypertension Optimal Treatment (HOT) study is the largest hypertension treatment trial ever completed, with 19,000 hypertensive patients treated with drug combinations to target DBP of 85 to 90 mm Hg, 80 to 85 mm Hg, or less than 80 mm Hg.[33] Although the difference between adjacent groups was only 2 mm Hg, the conclusion of this study was that the optimal blood pressure was 138/83 mm Hg and further reduction in blood pressure had no beneficial effect. The HOT study did not support the *J*-curve hypothesis.

Summary of Treatment Studies

Early studies clearly demonstrated the benefit of treating hypertension with lifestyle modification and drug therapy. The JNC recommends that patients without target organ damage or CCD (risk groups A and B) with stage 1 hypertension first attempt to lower blood pressure by nonpharmacologic methods for 6 to 12 months (Table 39.2).[1] If this fails to lower blood pressure, then drug treatment should be started. Drug therapy is recommended for all patients with stage 2 or 3 hypertension and for all patients with TOD, CCD, or diabetes.[1] Trials of antihypertensive drugs in mild hypertension have shown a reduction in stroke, LVH, congestive heart failure, and accelerated hypertension. The goal of therapy is a SBP less than 140 mm Hg and a DBP less than 90 mm Hg, and treatment to lower blood pressure levels appears beneficial.[1]

TREATMENT

Pharmacotherapy

Drug therapy should be initiated for stages 2 and 3 hypertension, for all patients with TOD or CCD, and for hypertensive patients with coexisting diabetes.[1] Other hypertensive patients should attempt lifestyle modification for 6 to 12 months, based on risk stratification. In initiating drug therapy it is important to remember that hypertension is a disease of decades. Unless hypertension is severe, it is important to start a simple drug regimen that minimizes side effects and encourages long-term compliance. A continuing principle is that clinical drug therapy should be based on well-tested drugs that have been shown to prevent cardiovascular disease and reduce mortality rather than extrapolation of intermediate indicators.[34,35]

Understanding the site and mechanism of action of the various antihypertensive drugs is important in planning therapy. All current drugs impair normal homeostatic mechanisms, and most reduce peripheral vascular resistance. Pharmacologic classification and dosage information are presented in Table 39.7. Common adverse effects and special precautions for antihypertensive drugs are given in Table 39.8. The hemodynamic and hormonal effects are shown in Table 39.9. Drug interactions are listed in Table 39.10.

Diuretics

Thiazide and related diuretics were the mainstay of therapy in most randomized antihypertensive drug trials and have been proven to reduce cardiovascular events.[1,2,35] Thiazide diuretics are preferred when hypertensive patients have heart failure or ISH. Thiazide diuretics also have a favorable effect on osteoporosis. Thiazide-type diuretics are effective in small dosages, equivalent to 12.5 to 25 mg HCTZ. Using these lower dosages may reduce the incidence and severity of the metabolic abnormalities of hypokalemia, hyperglycemia, and hyperuricemia. Reducing HCTZ from 50 mg/day to 25 mg/day resulted in a 5-mm Hg increase in SBP with no change in DBP.[36] This dosage reduction led to a decrease in uric acid and an increase in serum potassium, but fasting and postprandial glucose, hemoglobin A_1C, and serum lipids were unchanged.[37] Serum lipids and hemoglobin A_1C decreased significantly after diuretics were discontinued. Diuretics add to the effectiveness of most other antihypertensive drugs and can reverse the fluid retention associated with some antihypertensive drugs. HCTZ has proven efficacy, can be administered once daily, is inexpensive, and is available in a variety of combination products.

Hypokalemia is dose related, and moderate hypokalemia (3.0 to 3.5 mEq/L) occurs in 2% of patients who are treated with HCTZ 25 mg/day, compared to 11% of patients treated with HCTZ 50 mg/day.[37] Hypokalemia is worsened by high-sodium diets and can be minimized by sodium restriction. The risk of ventricular arrhythmias and sudden death may be increased by hypokalemia in patients with baseline ECG abnormalities.[26] The risk of primary cardiac arrest is increased by high-dose thiazide diuretic therapy.[36] Hypokalemia should be minimized by using low-dose thiazide therapy, restricting sodium intake, using potassium supplements, and adding potassium-sparing drugs. Correcting diuretic-induced hypokalemia, a 0.5 mmol/L increase, can further reduce blood pressure by 6/5 mm Hg.[38] In trials using thiazide diuretics alone (MRFIT and the Oslo Study), patients with baseline ECG abnormalities had worse outcomes. In the EWPHE trial, which used a potassium-sparing combination agent, there was a reduction in total cardiac mortality.

Table 39.7 ▪ Antihypertensive Drug Products

Drug	Brand Name	Drug Class	Dosage Range	Extended Release
Benazepril	Lotensin	ACE inhibitor	10–40 mg	
Captopril	Capoten	ACE inhibitor	12.5–150 mg	
Enalapril	Vasotec	ACE inhibitor	2.5–40 mg	
Fosinopril	Monopril	ACE inhibitor	10–40 mg	
Lisinopril	Prinivil or Zestril	ACE inhibitor	5–40 mg	
Moexipril	Univasc	ACE inhibitor	7.5–30 mg	
Quinapril	Accupril	ACE inhibitor	5–80 mg	
Ramipril	Altace	ACE inhibitor	1.25–20 mg	
Trandolapril	Mavik	ACE inhibitor	1–4 mg	
Candesartan	Atacand	AII antagonist	8–32 mg	
Irbesartan	Avapro	AII antagonist	150–300 mg	
Losartan	Cozar	AII antagonist	25–100 mg	
Telmisartan	Micardis	AII antagonist	40–80 mg	
Valsartan	Diovan	AII antagonist	80–320 mg	
Atenolol	Tenormin	β-Blocker	25–100 mg	
Betaxolol	Kerlone	β-Blocker	5–40 mg	
Bisoprolol	Zebeta	β-Blocker	5–40 mg	
Metoprolol	Lopressor	β-Blocker	50–200 mg	Toprolol-XL
Nadolol	Corgard	β-Blocker	20–240 mg	
Propranolol	Inderal	β-Blocker	40–240 mg	Inderal-LA
Timolol	Blocadren	β-Blocker	10–40 mg	
Acebutolol	Sectral	ISA β-blocker	200–1200 mg	
Cartelol	Cartrol	ISA β-blocker	2.5–10 mg	
Penbutolol	Levatol	ISA β-blocker	20–80 mg	
Pindolol	Visken	ISA β-blocker	10–60 mg	
Carvedilol	Coreg	α–β-Blocker	12.5–50 mg	
Labetalol	Normodyne or Trandate	α–β-Blocker	200–1200 mg	
Amlodipine	Norvasc	Dihydropyridine calcium blocker	2.5–10 mg	
Felodipine	Plendil	Dihydropyridine calcium blocker	2.5–10 mg	
Isradipine	DynaCirc	Dihydropyridine calcium blocker	5–10 mg	DynaCirc-CR
Nicardipine	Cardene	Dihydropyridine calcium blocker	60–120 mg	Cardene-SR
Nifedipine	Procardia	Dihydropyridine calcium blocker	30–90 mg	Adalat CC, Procardia XL
Nisoldipine	Sular	Dihydropyridine calcium blocker	10–60 mg	
Diltiazem	Cardizem	Calcium channel blocker Calcium channel blocker Calcium channel blocker	120–360 mg	Cardizem CD and SR Dilacor XR, Diltia XT Tiamate, Tiazac
Verapamil	Calan	Calcium channel blocker Calcium channel blocker	120–480 mg	Calan SR, Isoptin SR Covera-HS, Verelan
Prazosin	Minipress	α-Adrenergic blocker	1–20 mg	
Terazosin	Hytrin	α-Adrenergic blocker	1–20 mg	
Doxazosin	Cardura	α-Adrenergic blocker		
Clonidine	Catapres	Central α-adrenergic agonist	250–2000 mg	Catapares TTS (transdermal)
Guanabenz	Wytensin	Central α-adrenergic agonist	4–64 mg	
Guanfacine	Tenex	Central α-adrenergic agonist	1–3 mg	
Methyldopa	Aldomet	Central α-adrenergic agonist	250–2000 mg	
Guanethidine	Ismelin	Peripheral adrenergic antagonist	10–50 mg	
Guanadrel	Hylorel	Peripheral adrenergic antagonist	10–75 mg	
Reserpine		Peripheral adrenergic antagonist	0.05–0.1 mg	

(continued)

Table 39.7 *(continued)*

Combination	Drug	Drug	Dosage	Brand
Hydralazine	Apresoline	Vasodilator	10–50 mg	
Minoxidil	Loniten	Vasodilator	2.5–40 mg	
Diuretic Combination	HCTZ	Spironolactone	25/25 mg or 50/50 mg	Aldactazide
		Triamterene	25 mg/37.5 mg	Dyazide, Maxzide
		Amiloride	50 mg/5 mg	Moduretic
β-Blocker and diuretic	Atenolol	Chlorthalidone	50, 100 mg/25 mg	Tenoretic
	Bisoprolol	HCTZ	2.5, 5, 10 mg/6.25 mg	Ziac
	Metoprolol	HCTZ	50, 100 mg/25 or 50 mg	Lopressor HCT
	Propranolol	HCTZ	40, 80 mg/25 mg	Inderide
	Propranolol extended release	HCTZ	80, 120, 160 mg/50 mg	Inderide LA
	Timolol	HCTZ	10 mg/25 mg	Timolide
ACE inhibitor and diuretic	Benazepril	HCTZ	5, 10, 20 mg/6.25, 12.5, 25 mg	Lotensin HCT
	Captopril	HCTZ	25, 50 mg/15, 25 mg	Capozide
	Enalapril	HCTZ	5, 10 mg/12.5, 25 mg	Vasretic
	Lisinopril	HCTZ	10, 20 mg/12.5, 25 mg	Prinzide
	Moexipril	HCTZ	7.5, 15 mg/12.5, 25 mg	Uniretic
AII blocker and diuretic	Losartan	HCTZ	50, 100 mg/12.5, 25 mg	Hyzaar
	Valsartan	HCTZ	80, 160 mg/12.5 mg	Diovan HCT
Calcium blocker and ACE inhibitor	Amlodipine	Benazepril	2.5, 5 mg/10, 20 mg	Lotrel
	Diltiazem	Enalapril	180 mg/10 mg	Teczem
	Felodipine	Enalapril	2.5, 5 mg/5 mg	Lexxel
	Verapamil extended release	Trandopril	180, 240 mg/1, 2, 4 mg	Tarka
Vasodilator and diuretic	Hydralazine	HCTZ	25, 50 mg/25, 50 mg	Apresazide
Central adrenergic agonist and diuretic	Methyldopa	HCTZ	250, 500 mg/15, 25, 30, 50 mg	Aldoril
	Clonidine	Chlorthalidone	0.1, 0.2, 0.3 mg/15 mg	Combipres

ACE, angiotensin-converting enzyme; *AII,* angiotensin II; *ISA,* intrinsic sympathomimetic activity; *HCTZ,* hydrochlorothiazide.

Thiazide diuretics may produce other metabolic abnormalities, including an increase in total cholesterol, LDL cholesterol, and triglycerides. A low-fat diet decreases the thiazide-induced changes. Thiazide-induced glucose intolerance is related to the degree of hypokalemia and is minimized by preventing potassium depletion. In the VA Cooperative studies, an average increase in fasting glucose was 6 mg/dL, and 3% of patients developed a fasting glucose greater than 140 mg/dL. Thiazides increase serum uric acid by approximately 1 mg/dL, which is not associated with adverse effects on renal function and does not warrant uric acid-lowering drugs unless the patient has symptomatic gout.[39]

Diuretics were associated with impotence at a frequency of 19.6 per 1000 patient-years in the MRC trial. Male patients taking thiazide diuretics reported significantly greater sexual dysfunction than did control subjects; diuretic therapy did not adversely affect other aspects of quality of life.[40]

Thiazide diuretics are particularly effective for patients with low-renin hypertension, which is often seen in older adults and African Americans. Thiazide diuretics may slow the rate of bone loss in older adults and reduce the incidence of hip fractures.[41]

The declining use of diuretics is not supported by the evidence.[42] Diuretic-induced metabolic effects and hypokalemia are minor with the smaller dosages of diuretics currently recommended, and cardiovascular mortality has been reduced even in patients with dyslipidemia and diabetes.[42] Blood pressure control in hypertensive patients will be improved with increased use of diuretic therapy.[42]

Loop Diuretics

Furosemide has a shorter duration of action than do the thiazide diuretics and causes less blood pressure reduction. Newer loop diuretics, torsemide and bumetanide, have longer durations of action. Loop diuretics often are used for patients with fluid retention who are unresponsive to thiazide diuretics or patients with decreased renal function.[43] Thiazide diuretics are ineffective for patients with impaired renal function (creatinine clearance less than 30 mL/minute). These patients can be treated with the loop diuretics metolazone or indapamide. Furosemide (40 mg/day) has also been shown to produce less hypokalemia than does HCTZ (50 mg/day) in hypertensive patients.[37] Furosemide and bumetanide appear to have a less marked effect on serum lipids than do thiazide diuretics.[44]

Table 39.8 ▪ Adverse Effects of Antihypertensive Drugs

Drug	Adverse Effects	Special Precautions
Thiazide diuretics	Hypokalemia, hyperuricemia, glucose intolerance, dyslipidemia, sexual dysfunction, dehydration, hyponatremia, hypomagnesemia, skin rash, photosensitivity	LVH, CHD, diabetes mellitus, gout, renal failure, digitalis, lithium
Loop diuretics	Similar to thiazide diuretics	Effective in patients with renal insufficiency
β-Blockers	Fatigue, insomnia, nightmares, depression, sexual dysfunction, dyslipidemia, rash, GI upset, worsening of psoriasis, withdrawal rebound CHD, bradycardia, decreased exercise tolerance, bronchospasm, Raynaud's phenomenon, masked symptoms of hypoglycemia	Asthma, COPD, CHF, heart block, diabetes mellitus, peripheral vascular disease
ISA β-blockers	Less bradycardia and dyslipidemia, drug-induced lupus erythematosus	
α–β-Blockers	Orthostatic hypotension, hepatotoxicity	No dyslipidemia
ACE inhibitors	Hyperkalemia, cough, hypotension, angioedema, rash, loss of taste, proteinuria, renal failure, neutropenia, cholestasis, rash, blood dyscrasias, increased fetal mortality	Renal failure, pregnancy, renal artery stenosis
Angiotensin receptor antagonists	Similar to ACE inhibitors but do not cause cough	
Calcium channel blockers	Headache, flushing, hypotension, dizziness, palpitations, nausea	CHF, heart block
Dihydropyridines	Edema, tachycardia	
Diltiazem	Lupuslike rash	
Verapamil	Constipation, atrioventricular block, bradycardia	Digitalis
Central antiadrenergics	Sedation, dry mouth, fatigue, sexual dysfunction, postural hypotension, impaired mental concentration, withdrawal rebound hypertension, contact dermatitis from patch	Depression; taper dosage when discontinuing to avoid rebound
Methyldopa	Hepatitis, Coombs'-positive hemolytic anemia, colitis, drug-induced lupus erythematosus	
Peripheral antiadrenergics	Sexual dysfunction, nasal congestion, orthostatic hypotension, dizziness, Na and fluid retention	Asthma, CHF, advanced age
α-Adrenergic blockers	Syncope after first dose or dosage increase, orthostatic hypotension, headache, dizziness, drowsiness, tachycardia, Na and fluid retention, priapism	Advanced age, first dose
Vasodilators	Headache, tachycardia, dizziness, Na and fluid retention	Angina, CHF
Hydralazine	Positive ANA, lupuslike syndrome, hepatitis, nasal congestion, GI disturbances	
Minoxidil	Hypertrichosis, facial coarsening, pleural or pericardial effusion	

LVH, left ventricular hypertrophy; *CHD,* coronary heart disease; *GI,* gastrointestinal; *COPD,* chronic obstructive pulmonary disease; *CHF,* congestive heart failure; *ISA,* intrinsic sympathomimetic activity; *ACE,* angiotensin-converting enzyme; *ANA,* antinuclear antibody.

Table 39.9 ▪ Hemodynamic and Hormonal Effects of Antihypertensive Agents

Drug	PVR	CO	HR	PRA	GFR
ACE/ARB	–	0/+	0	+	+/0/–
α_2-Agonists	–	–/0	–	–	0
β-Blockers	0/–	–	–	–	0/–
Calcium blockers	0/–	–/0	–/0/+	0/+	0
Labetalol	–	0	–	–	0/+
Loop diuretics	–	–	0	+	+
Peripheral antiadrenergics	–	–/0	–	–	0/–
α-Adrenergic blockers	–	0	0/+	–	0
Thiazide diuretics	–	–	0	+	–
Vasodilators	–	+	+	+	+

+ = increase, – = decrease, 0 = no change.

PVR, peripheral vascular resistance; *CO,* cardiac output; *HR,* heart rate; *PRA,* plasma renin activity; *GFR,* glomerular filtration rate.

Table 39.10 ▪ Antihypertensive Drug Interactions

Drug Class	Increased Antihypertensive Effect	Decreased Antihypertensive Effects	Other Drug Interaction Effects
Loop diuretics	ACE, antipsychotics, β-blockers, calcium channel blockers, ethanol, antiadrenergic agents	ASA/NSAIDs, anticonvulsants, bile acid resins, sympathomimetics	ACE ↑ renal insufficiency Carbenoxolone ↓ K Corticosteroids ↓ K Digoxin ↑ toxicity from hypokalemia Fibric acids ↓ albumin binding ↑ Lithium toxicity SSRIs: severe hyponatremia
Thiazide diuretics	ACE, antipsychotics, β-blockers, calcium channel blockers, ethanol, antiadrenergic agents	ASA/NSAIDs, bile acid resins, sympathomimetics	Calcium: milk alkali syndrome Carbenoxolone ↓ K ↑ Digoxin toxicity from hypokalemia ↑ Lithium toxicity ↓ Hypoglycemic agent effects from antagonism
β-Blockers	α-blockers, antipsychotics, calcium channel blockers, ethanol, antiadrenergic agents, H_2 blockers, SSRIs, antiarrhythmics, quinolones (↑ β-blocker)	ASA/NSAIDs, antacids, sympathomimetics ↓β-blocker levels: Barbiturate Carbamazepine Rifampin and rifabutin Sulfasalazine	α_1-Blockers and α_2-agonists ↑ rebound hypertension Amiodarone: bradycardia, cardiac arrest Contrast media (IV): ↑ anaphylaxis ↓ Diazepam metabolism Digoxin: bradycardia, ↑ digoxin levels with carvedilol Ergot alkaloids: ↑ vasoconstriction Hypoglycemic agents: mask hypoglycemic symptoms ↓ Quinidine effect with hepatic metabolized β-blockers Sympathomimetics: ↑ blood pressure, ↑ terbutaline levels, ↑ theophylline levels
Calcium blockers	Antipsychotics, β-blockers, diuretics, ethanol (postural hypotension) ↑ Calcium blocker levels: α_1-Blockers Cimetidine Erythromycin Grapefruit juice (↑ DHP) Proton pump inhibitors Quinidine Valproic acid	ASA/NSAIDs, sympathomimetics ↓ Calcium blocker levels: Carbamazepine Barbiturates Rifampin and rifabutin	↑ ASA antiplatelet activity β-Blockers: ↑ cardiac depression ↑ Carbamazepine levels with diltiazem or verapamil ↑ Cyclosporine levels ↑ Digoxin levels except DHP ↑ Ethanol ↑ Lithium neurotoxicity ↑ Phenytoin levels with nifedipine ↑ Quinidine levels with nifedipine ↑ Quinidine bradycardia and hypotension with verapamil ↑ TCA levels ↑ Theophylline levels with verapamil
ACE inhibitors and angiotensin receptor blockers	Antipsychotics, β-blockers, diuretics, ergot alkaloids	ASA/NSAIDs, sympathomimetics, antacids (captopril)	Azathioprine/6MP toxicity ↑ Lithium levels, hyperkalemia with K-sparing diuretics
α_1-Blockers	ACE inhibitors, antipsychotics, β-blockers, calcium blockers, diuretics, ethanol	ASA/NSAIDs, sympathomimetics	↑ Orthostatic hypotension with diuretics
α_2-Agonists	Antipsychotics, diuretics, ethanol, nitrates	ASA/NSAIDs, MAOIs, TCAs, trazodone, phenothiazines, sympathomimetics	↑ Cyclosporine levels with clonidine TTS ↓ Symptoms of hypoglycemia with clonidine ↑ Rebound hypertension with β-blockers ↑ Bradycardia with β-blockers ↑ CNS depression with all CNS depressants ↑ Lithium levels with methyldopa

(continued)

Table 39.10 *(continued)*

Drug Class	Increased Antihypertensive Effect	Decreased Antihypertensive Effects	Other Drug Interaction Effects
Potassium-sparing diuretics	Antipsychotics, ethanol, nitrates	ASA/NSAIDs, sympathomimetics	↑ Amantadine levels with triamterene ↑ Digoxin levels with spironolactone Acute renal failure with indomethacin and triamterene ↑ Hyperkalemia with ACE/ARB ↑ Quinidine toxicity with amiloride
Vasodilators	Antipsychotics, β-blockers, diuretics, ethanol	ASA/NSAIDs, sympathomimetics	
Peripheral adrenergic blockers	Diuretics, ethanol	ASA/NSAIDs, antipsychotics, MAOIs, sympathomimetics	

ACE, angiotensin-converting enzyme; *NSAIDs,* nonsteroidal anti-inflammatory drugs; *SSRIs,* selective serotonin reuptake inhibitors; *TCAs,* tricyclic antidepressants; *6MP,* 6-mercaptopurine; *MAOIs,* monoamine oxidase inhibitors; *TTS,* transdermal therapeutic system; *CNS,* central nervous system.

Thiazidelike Diuretics

Chlorthalidone is a long-acting diuretic similar to thiazides that produces greater hypokalemia and was the primary therapy in the SHEP trial. Metolazone is a thiazidelike diuretic that is effective for patients with renal impairment and is markedly effective in producing diuresis when combined with furosemide. Indapamide is a sulfonamide diuretic with antihypertensive effects that does not appear to elevate serum lipids.

Potassium-Sparing Diuretics

The potassium-sparing diuretics amiloride, spironolactone, and triamterene are used mainly to prevent or correct hypokalemia from other diuretics. Neither amiloride or triamterene has a significant antihypertensive effect. There is a potential risk of hyperkalemia with these agents in patients with renal dysfunction or diabetes or those who also take angiotensin-converting enzyme (ACE) inhibitors. Combination products with thiazide diuretics may provide less hypokalemia and improved blood pressure with reasonable costs.

Amiloride

Amiloride is a potassium-sparing diuretic that acts in the distal tubule. Amiloride is excreted in the urine as unchanged drug and has natriuretic and antikaliuretic effects for approximately 24 hours. The primary adverse effect is hyperkalemia. The presence of diabetes, cirrhosis, renal insufficiency, concomitant ACE inhibitor therapy, or potassium supplements increases the risk of hyperkalemia.

Spironolactone

Spironolactone is a competitive aldosterone antagonist used in combination with thiazide diuretics to prevent or correct hypokalemia or as an alternative diuretic for patients with gout or diabetes.[45] Food enhances the absorption of spironolactone, which is rapidly metabolized to pharmacologically active metabolites, including canrenone. Spironolactone may be superior to potassium supplements in correcting diuretic-induced hypokalemia and also corrects coexisting magnesium deficiency. Hyperkalemia occurs in 3% of spironolactone-treated patients who have normal renal function and are not taking potassium supplements.[45] In contrast, 25% of patients with renal insufficiency who are taking potassium supplements can develop hyperkalemia. Gynecomastia is related to dosage and duration of treatment and has occurred in more than 50% of male patients.[45] Impotence, hirsutism, menstrual irregularities, and gastrointestinal (GI) symptoms are adverse effects that can limit therapy. Limiting spironolactone dosage to less than 100 mg/day appears to reduce the incidence of adverse effects.

Triamterene

Triamterene is used principally in combination products to reduce the potassium loss with thiazide diuretics. Triamterene–HCTZ combinations can produce hypokalemia or hyperkalemia. The risk of hyperkalemia is increased by the presence of other risks, including renal impairment, potassium supplementation, ACE inhibitors, and diabetes mellitus. A triamterene urinary sediment (triamterene crystals) has developed in more than 50% of patients. This has caused nephrolithiasis and may be a risk factor for interstitial nephritis.[46] Triamterene–HCTZ decreases production of the renoprotective prostaglandin PGE_2, and amiloride–HCTZ increases renal PGE_2 production.[47] Finally, the combination of indomethacin and triamterene may cause reversible acute renal failure.[48] In high-risk patients or when hypokalemia develops, potassium-sparing agents are effective in preventing or reversing hypokalemia.

β-Blockers

β-Blockers are effective antihypertensive agents, particularly for young Caucasian patients, and have been proven to reduce mortality in randomized clinical trials. β-Blockers have additional favorable effects in patients with coexisting angina pectoris, atrial fibrillation or atrial tachycardia, essential tremor, hyperthyroidism, migraine headaches, or myocardial infarction. β-Blockers should be avoided or used with caution in patients with bronchospastic disease, depression, diabetes, dyslipidemia, second- or third-degree heart block, heart failure (recent evidence demonstrates benefits when β-blockers are added when heart failure is well controlled), and peripheral vascular disease (PVD).

Pharmacology

β-Blockers competitively inhibit catecholamine neurotransmitters at both cardiac receptors (β_1) and noncardiac receptors (β_2).[49] Cardiac effects include reductions in heart rate, venous return, cardiac output, and cardiac work. In addition, β-blockers reduce plasma renin activity, reduce norepinephrine release, and prevent the pressor response to exercise or stress catecholamine release.

Effectiveness

In the VA Cooperative Study Group, β-blockers were equivalent to HCTZ in Caucasian patients, but HCTZ was more effective in African Americans and older adults.[19] β-Blockers may provide primary protection from CHD, and they reduce the secondary risk after myocardial infarction.[49] β-Blockers are effective in producing LVH regression.

Comparison of β-Blockers

Although the available β-blockers are similar in efficacy and safety, there are two important differences in pharmacology. Cardioselective (β_1-selective) agents produce fewer negative effects on the heart in patients with congestive heart failure or conduction system disease. Cardioselective β-blockers may be better tolerated by patients with chronic obstructive pulmonary disease and PVD. Cardioselective (β_1-selective) agents produce less impairment in response to hypoglycemia in diabetic patients. Unfortunately, cardioselectivity is reduced or lost at higher dosages. Drugs with β-agonist activity or intrinsic sympathomimetic activity (ISA) may avoid the decrease in cardiac output and heart rate. ISA β-blockers are preferred for patients who experience bradycardia with other β-blockers. ISA β-blockers may also produce fewer problems for patients with PVD, lipid disorders, or diabetes mellitus. However, ISA β-blockers are not cardioprotective.

β-Blockers can also be classified into two groups on the basis of their pharmacokinetic properties. The β-blockers that are eliminated by hepatic metabolism are highly lipophilic, absorbed in the small intestine, undergo extensive first-pass metabolism, have variable bioavailability, have short plasma half-lives, and more readily penetrate the blood–brain barrier. β-Blockers that are eliminated unchanged by the kidney are hydrophilic, are incompletely absorbed throughout the gut, have longer plasma half-lives, and are less able to penetrate the central nervous system (CNS). Because the antihypertensive effect of β-blockers appears to outlast the presence of the drug in plasma, all agents can be used on a twice-daily schedule, and the longer-acting drugs can be given once daily. The bioavailability of propranolol and metoprolol increases approximately 60% when the drugs are taken with food. Propranolol has a wide dosage range, and plasma concentrations from a fixed dosage may vary 20-fold between patients. The hydrophilic agents (atenolol and nadolol) have flat dose–response curves but accumulate in renal failure.

Several disease states contraindicate the use of β-blockers or influence the selection of a β-blocker, and the choice of agents should be individualized. Although pregnancy was once considered a contraindication, studies indicate that β-blockers improve fetal outcome when they are used to treat hypertension in pregnancy.

Adverse Effects

Many adverse effects are related to β-adrenergic blockade in predisposed patients. Adverse effects from β_1-blockade include bradycardia, conduction abnormalities, and left ventricular failure.[49] Adverse effects of β_2-blockade include bronchospasm, cold extremities, and worsening claudication. A meta-analysis concluded that β-blocker therapy did not worsen claudication in patients with mild to moderate PVD.[50] These adverse effects tend to occur early in therapy even at low dosages. CNS effects may be most common with propranolol, and frank depression or vivid visual hallucinations can occur. However a large case control analysis did not demonstrate that β-blockers were causally related to depression.[51] Some patients have a pressor response to propranolol with worsening hypertension. Dermatologic reactions have included marked exacerbation of psoriasis. Adding propranolol doubled the HCTZ-induced increase in fasting glucose and glycosylated hemoglobin levels.[52] β-Blockers decrease HDL cholesterol, increase triglycerides, and blunt the effectiveness of dietary modification to lower cholesterol. Lipid changes are not associated with ISA β-blockers. Treatment with glucose tolerance factor chromium reversed the adverse effects of β-blockers on HDL cholesterol.[53]

Withdrawing β-blockers may produce β-adrenergic supersensitivity. Both abrupt cessation and gradual withdrawal over 4 to 8 days have caused overshoot hypertension and cardiovascular complications within 48 to 72 hours after the last β-blocker dose.[54] Symptoms of the withdrawal syndrome are nervousness, restlessness, anxiety, malaise, fatigue, headaches, insomnia, vivid dreams, tachycardia, palpitations, tremors, diaphoresis, excessive salivation, abdominal cramps and pain, anorexia, nausea, and vomiting. Cardiovascular morbidity has included encephalopathy, cerebrovascular accidents, unstable angina, myocardial infarction, and sudden death. β-Blocker withdrawal syndrome can be reversed by readministration of small dosages of the β-blocker. To prevent β-adrenergic supersensitivity, the β-blocker dosage should be reduced over 7 to 10 days to the equivalent of 30 mg/day of propranolol and then maintained at this low dosage for 2 additional weeks. The risk of β-blocker withdrawal is not only for patients with known ischemic heart disease. Withdrawing β-blockers in patients who are free of CHD resulted in a fourfold increase in new onset of CHD.[54] ISA β-blockers do not cause a withdrawal syndrome and are not cardioprotective.[54]

α-β-Blocker

Labetalol is a nonselective β-blocker and an α-blocker that reduces the β_2-blockade increase in peripheral vascular resistance and sustains blood flow to the extremities and kidney. Labetalol does not reduce HDL cholesterol but may cause orthostatic hypotension and sexual dysfunction. Labetalol may be more effective than other β-blockers for older adults or black patients and has been used by patients with pulmonary disease.

Angiotensin-Converting Enzyme Inhibitors

ACE inhibitors block the generation of angiotensin II (AII), a potent vasoconstrictor and a stimulator of aldosterone secretion. The antihypertensive efficacy of ACE inhibitors is comparable to that of diuretics and β-blockers as monotherapy for hypertension. ACE inhibitors are more effective in younger and white patients and somewhat less effective in black patients unless higher dosages are used or they are combined with diuretics.[55] The combination of low-dose diuretic therapy and ACE inhibitors may control blood pressure in up to 85% of patients.[55] ACE inhibitors are also synergistic with calcium entry blockers and additive with β-blockers. ACE inhibitors prolong the survival of patients with severe congestive heart failure and produce regression of LVH. ACE inhibitors also improve insulin sensitivity. They are also used to treat renovascular hypertension. Another unique benefit of ACE inhibitors is the reduction of AII-mediated intraglomerular capillary pressure. This effect appears to retard the progression of diabetic renal disease, stabilize renal function, and decrease proteinuria.[55] Finally, the CAPP trial found captopril to be equal to diuretics and β-blockers in preventing cardiovascular morbidity and mortality.[55a,56] ACE inhibitors avoid many of the adverse effects that were common to earlier antihypertensive drugs. They do not alter plasma lipids, glucose, or uric acid, nor do they aggravate bronchospastic disease or PVD. ACE inhibitors also do not cause CNS depression or sexual dysfunction. They may increase alertness and produce mood elevation, which may have contributed to the positive effect on the quality of life seen with captopril.[55]

Initial ACE inhibitor therapy is an indirect means of classification of renin status and controls blood pressure in about 50% of patients. Patients with a poor decrease in blood pressure from ACE inhibitors are likely to have low-renin hypertension. For patients who do not respond to initial ACE inhibitor therapy, adding low dosages of a thiazide diuretic controls blood pressure in up to 85% of patients by working synergistically with ACE inhibitor treatment.

Comparison of ACE Inhibitors

The available ACE inhibitors differ in pharmacokinetics. Captopril binds to ACE by a sulfhydryl, and the other ACE inhibitors do not.[55] Benazepril, enalapril, fosinopril, perindopril, quinapril, and ramipril are administered as prodrugs; this delays their onset of action and prolongs the effect. Captopril should be taken without food and should be taken twice daily. Some clinicians use captopril three times a day, but twice a day is preferable for most patients. Other agents are given once daily. The primary route of elimination is the kidney, and dosage should be reduced in renal insufficiency. Benazepril, trandolapril, and fosinopril are eliminated by both renal excretion and hepatic metabolism, and dosage reductions are not needed for patients with renal dysfunction.

Adverse Effects

Adverse effects that are common to all ACE inhibitors are hypotension, hyperkalemia, cough, angioedema, and renal insufficiency.[55] Hypotension occurs when patients are sodium depleted or have high renin and is more common with captopril because of its rapid onset of action. To reduce this risk, diuretics should be discontinued for 3 days before the initial ACE inhibitor dose. The risk of hyperkalemia is greater for patients with diabetes or renal insufficiency, if sodium intake is restricted, and if potassium-sparing diuretics, potassium supplements, or NSAIDs are given. Intractable, dry cough, warranting discontinuation of ACE inhibitor therapy, may develop in more than 20% of patients. Inhaled sodium cromoglycate may be effective in treating ACE inhibitor–induced cough.[57] Cough develops more often with enalapril than with captopril and is believed to be caused by an effect of ACE inhibitor on vagal C fibers.[55] Adverse effects of captopril also include neutropenia, skin rash, proteinuria, and taste disturbances.[55] Using lower captopril dosages has dramatically reduced the incidence of these complications. ACE inhibitors may also increase the risk of hypoglycemia.[58]

Angiotensin II Antagonists

The newest pharmacologic class of drugs is the AII type 1 receptor (AT_1) antagonists. The AT_1 antagonists displace AII from the type 1 receptor subtype, antagonizing smooth muscle contraction, sympathetic pressor response, and aldosterone release.[59] AT_1 antagonists lower blood pressure and have cardiac and renal protective effects. However, AT_1 antagonists are not yet approved by the U.S. Food and Drug Administration for heart failure, left ventricular dysfunction, myocardial infarction, or diabetic nephropathy. The first five marketed drugs are candesartan, irbesartan, losartan, telmisartan, and valsartan. The drugs differ in their metabolism, with twice-daily dosing needed for losartan and possibly candesartan. AT_1 antagonists are contraindicated in pregnancy. The AT_1 antagonists have few adverse effects and are indicated for patients unable to tolerate ACE inhibitors (usually because of cough).

Calcium Antagonists

Calcium antagonists may be the most controversial class of drugs that are considered to be effective monotherapy for initial hypertension treatment. Calcium antagonists impair the transport of calcium through the voltage-sensitive calcium channels in vascular smooth muscle cells; this decreases contractile force, vascular smooth muscle tone, and peripheral resistance. The calcium antagonists are particularly effective for patients with low-renin hypertension (i.e., hypertensive older adults and African Americans) and have greater antihypertensive efficacy with higher pretreatment blood pressures. Calcium antagonists now appear to be effective in treating ISH.[60] Verapamil is equally effective for black or white hypertensive patients.[61] Calcium antagonists are also used to treat angina, variant angina, certain arrhythmias, and migraine headaches; this makes them attractive antihypertensive agents for patients with those conditions. Calcium antagonists also do not adversely affect asthma, gout, peripheral vascular disease (PVD), lipids, and diabetes mellitus.

Comparison of Calcium Entry Blockers

There are three chemical classes of calcium antagonist. Verapamil is a phenylalkylamine, diltiazem is a benzothiazepine, and amlodipine, felodipine, isradipine, nicardipine, and nifedipine are dihydropyridines. All calcium antagonists that are used for hypertension have comparable efficacy but differ in their adverse effect profiles. The calcium antagonists have limited oral bioavailability because of first-pass hepatic metabolism. Only diltiazem (35%) has significant renal elimination. Because of short plasma half-lives, extended-release products are available for verapamil, diltiazem, and nifedipine, allowing once- or twice-daily administration. Extended-release products may also decrease dose-related adverse effects. However, postinfarction trials of calcium antagonists have not demonstrated cardioprotection. Adding a diuretic to a calcium entry blocker usually has only minimal additive effect; this may be due in part to the natriuretic effect of the calcium entry blockers.

Adverse Effects

The adverse effects of the calcium antagonists are primarily extensions of their pharmacologic actions and can be categorized as vasodilation, negative inotropic effects, conduction disturbances, GI effects, and metabolic effects. Vasodilatory side effects include headaches, flushing, palpitations, hypotension, and peripheral edema. Vasodilation is more common with dihydropyridine calcium antagonists. Negative inotropic effects are least with the dihydropyridines and greatest with verapamil. Although diltiazem has an intermediate negative inotropic effect, it can produce or worsen congestive heart failure in patients with preexisting left ventricular dysfunction. Conduction disturbances are greatest with verapamil, intermediate with diltiazem, and uncommon with dihydropyridines. Calcium antagonists do not increase the risk of GI bleeding, but β-blockers may prevent GI bleeding.[62] Verapamil often causes constipation, which may be relieved with stool softeners. Verapamil decreases digoxin elimination and can increase serum digoxin levels by 50 to 75%. Other calcium antagonists may also interact with digoxin but usually to a lesser degree. If a calcium antagonists is used in combination with a β-blocker, a dihydropyridine agent is preferred to reduce the additive cardioinhibitory and cardiodepressive effects.

Controversy has arisen about the possible increased risk of myocardial infarction associated with the use of calcium channel blockers.[63] The Appropriate Blood Pressure Control in Diabetes (ABCD) trial[64] and the Fosinopril versus Amlodipine Cardiovascular Events Randomized Trial (FACET)[65] raised the concern that dihydropyridine calcium antagonists may be dangerous in diabetic patients with hypertension, increasing the risk of myocardial infarction. The Systolic Hypertension in Europe (Syst-Eur) trial found that nitrendipine reduced cardiovascular complications in older adults with ISH.[60] Also, in the HOT study, 1500 diabetic patients with hypertension treated with felodipine had a significant reduction in cardiovascular mortality.[33] Data from the Framingham Heart Study found no difference in mortality among subjects using a calcium antagonist compared with those who were not.[66] Current recommendations are to avoid short-acting dihydropyridine calcium antagonists in patients with CHD; data from the large Antihypertensive Lipid-Lowering Treatment to Avoid Heart Attack (ALLHAT) trial are awaited for further clarification of the risks of ischemic heart disease associated with calcium blockers.[67]

Sympathetic Inhibitors

Many antihypertensive drugs interfere with the sympathetic nervous system. These agents may act in the CNS or peripheral nervous system.

α_1-Adrenergic Blocking Agents

These drugs produce a selective postsynaptic α_1-adrenoceptor inhibition, causing decreased peripheral resistance and vasodilation without reducing cardiac output or inducing a reflex tachycardia. These agents produce a slightly greater decrease in standing blood pressure than in supine blood pressure. They have additive effects with β-blockers and diuretics. α-Adrenergic blockers are considered for initial treatment of hypertension for patients with dyslipidemia and prostatism.[1] Their advantages include a favorable lipid profile effect, equal efficacy in all age and race groups, and a favorable effect on plasma glucose.[1] Doxazosin, in contrast to enalapril, reduced total cholesterol and triglycerides and increased HDL cholesterol while resulting in a similar reduction in blood pressure.[68] This resulted in a greater reduction in calculated CHD risk than does enalapril treatment.[68] α_1-Adrenergic inhibitors may also reduce preload and afterload in severe chronic congestive heart failure. Another group that may benefit from

α_1-adrenergic inhibitors is patients with benign prostatic hypertrophy (BPH). α_1-Adrenergic inhibitors increase urine flow and decrease urinary frequency in patients with BPH by inhibiting norepinephrine-induced contraction of prostate smooth muscle.

COMPARISON OF α_1-ADRENERGIC BLOCKERS. The three α_1-adrenergic inhibitors appear to have similar antihypertensive effects and adverse effects. The α_1-adrenergic inhibitors undergo substantial hepatic first-pass metabolism. The newer agents, doxazosin and terazosin, have a longer duration of action than does prazosin and can be dosed once daily.

ADVERSE EFFECTS. The most striking adverse effect of the α_1-adrenergic inhibitors is the first-dose syncope. Profound orthostatic hypotension with syncope can occur 1 to 3 hours after the first dose in patients with a low plasma volume from diuretic therapy or patients who are taking other antihypertensive drugs that blunt their response to the acute decrease in blood pressure. To avoid this problem, the initial dose should be limited to the equivalent of 1 mg prazosin and should be taken at bedtime or when the patient can be observed.

Central α_2-Agonists

Central α_2-adrenergic agonists stimulate α_2-adrenergic receptors in the lower brainstem, which decreases sympathetic outflow to the cardiovascular system. Some agents also block peripheral α_2-adrenergic receptors. The combined sympatholytic effects cause a decrease in peripheral vascular resistance.[69] The central α_2-adrenergic agonists are equally effective in all age and race subgroups and can be used for patients with renal insufficiency, diabetes mellitus, bronchospastic disease, and ischemic heart disease. The efficacy of these drugs is similar to that of other antihypertensives when used as monotherapy for initial hypertension treatment. Unlike peripheral sympatholytics, the central α_2-adrenergic agonists do not cause significant sodium and fluid retention. The central α_2-adrenergic agonists do not adversely effect glucose metabolism and have neutral or favorable effects on plasma lipids.[69] These agents also produce a regression in LVH. In addition to its use in hypertension, clonidine has increased the success of smoking cessation, particularly for women, and decreasing craving as well as withdrawal symptoms.

COMPARISON OF α_2-ADRENERGIC AGONISTS. Newer formulations of the central α_2-adrenergic agonists provide sustained antihypertensive efficacy with less frequent dosing and have reduced the occurrence of symptomatic side effects. Clonidine can be given twice daily; often a daily bedtime dose is effective and lessens sedation. A clonidine suppression test has been used to assess the contribution of increased sympathetic outflow in patients with essential hypertension. Clonidine is also available as a transdermal therapeutic system (TTS) that is applied once weekly. Transdermal clonidine controls blood pressure in 60 to 80% of patients with mild hypertension.[70] Severe withdrawal rebound hypertension is less likely to occur with transdermal therapy than with oral clonidine.[70] The transdermal system is a convenient form of treatment with equal efficacy and fewer adverse effects than oral clonidine; the main adverse effect is a contact dermatitis that develops in 10 to 15% of patients.

Guanfacine is a long-acting central α_2-adrenergic agonist that is metabolized by the liver (70%) and excreted unchanged by the kidneys (30%), with a prolonged elimination half-life of 16 to 23 hours. The long duration of action allows once-daily dosing and reduces adverse effects. Guanfacine also has a flat dose–response curve, with little increase in antihypertensive effect from dosages greater than 1 mg.

Guanabenz is a guanidine derivative that blocks central sympathetic vasomotor impulses and produces a guanethidinelike postganglionic blockage. Guanabenz decreases cholesterol and triglycerides without changing HDL cholesterol. Guanabenz is used on a twice-daily dosing schedule.

Methyldopa, the first central α_2-adrenergic agonist, has largely been replaced by the newer agents. A methyldopa metabolite, α-methyl norepinephrine, is the active agonist that reduces CNS sympathetic outflow. Methyldopa has an orthostatic effect greater than that of clonidine, but both cardiac output and renal function usually are preserved. Because sodium and water retention can produce a pseudotolerance, methyldopa normally is combined with a diuretic. Methyldopa can be used on a twice-daily dosing schedule and has a long history of use in treating hypertension in pregnancy.

ADVERSE EFFECTS. Sedation and dry mouth are the most common adverse effects of central α_2-adrenergic agonists. These symptoms often disappear after the first few weeks. Saliva substitutes or sugarless gum or candy can provide relief from dry mouth. Sedation is additive to the effects of other sedating drugs including alcohol; patients should be cautioned about these combinations and driving. Serious hypersensitivity reactions have occurred with methyldopa, including drug fever, colitis, hepatotoxicity, a positive Coombs' test, and hemolytic anemia. The risk of serious toxicity and impaired mental function makes alternative antihypertensive drugs preferable to methyldopa.

Abrupt discontinuation of clonidine has caused an acute withdrawal syndrome (AWS) characterized by a rapid increase in blood pressure, headaches, palpitations, tremor, restlessness, diaphoresis, and nausea. AWS appears to be rare with transdermal clonidine and guanfacine. The risk of AWS is higher in younger patients with severe hypertension who are treated with high dosages and multiple antihypertensive agents. Combination with β-blockers increases the risk of a hypertensive episode on discontinuation of clonidine.[71] This combination should be avoided; if it is used, the β-blocker should be tapered and stopped before the clonidine is tapered. Avoiding excessive dosages, encouraging patient compliance, and tapering clonidine slowly may help to prevent AWS. However, patients should be warned to seek immediate medical help if they develop signs and symptoms of AWS. Treatment by restarting medications usually is effective in reversing AWS, and labetalol has been effective for combined central agonist–β-blocker AWS.[72]

Peripheral Sympatholytics

Guanethidine is actively transported into the peripheral adrenergic neuron, where it depletes norepinephrine and produces a postural hypotension. Guanethidine decreases venous return to the heart, decreases cardiac output, and interferes with the sympathetic reflexes that control the resistance (arteriolar) and capacitance (venous) vessels. Because guanethidine depletes myocardial catecholamines, it can worsen congestive heart failure. Guanethidine is slowly and variably absorbed, undergoing partial first-pass hepatic metabolism. With chronic administration the half-life of guanethidine is 5 days, with 50% of the drug excreted unchanged in the urine. Because of the long half-life, guanethidine can be taken once daily, and dosage adjustments should be made only after 2 to 3 weeks. Prolonged standing, exercise, and heat increase postural hypotension. The guanethidine dosage should be adjusted on the basis of standing blood pressure, and blocks can be used to elevate the head of the bed to sustain a nighttime postural effect. Guanadrel is an adrenergic blocking agent that also depletes norepinephrine from peripheral neurons. Guanadrel has a more rapid onset and shorter duration of action than guanethidine. Because of the postural effect, standing blood pressure must always be measured. These agents are reserved for treating resistant hypertension.

Adverse Effects. The major problem with both guanethidine and guanadrel is postural and exercise hypotension. Patients should be warned to rise slowly from supine or sitting positions, to flex their arms and legs before arising, and to avoid additive vasodilating factors such as prolonged standing, hot showers, and alcohol. Postural effects are most pronounced in the morning on arising. Other dose-related problems include sexual dysfunction and diarrhea, which may necessitate discontinuation of therapy. A pseudotolerance caused by fluid retention may develop unless diuretic therapy is adequate. Because guanethidine diffuses poorly into the CNS, sedation and depression are infrequent problems. Several drugs can interfere with the uptake of the sympatholytics into the adrenergic neuron and rapidly block the antihypertensive effects. Guanadrel may cause less sexual dysfunction and orthostasis than does guanethidine. However, patients should be given similar precautions to minimize the risks of postural hypotension. Diuretics are needed to reduce sodium and water retention and weight gain.

Reserpine. Reserpine acts in both the central and peripheral sympathetic nervous systems, depleting norepinephrine and serotonin stores in the brain and peripheral adrenergic nerve endings. Reserpine also increases vagal tone; this contributes to the reduced heart rate and increased gastric acid secretions. The onset of action of reserpine may take several days; maximal hypotensive effects may take weeks. Adverse effects are common with high dosages and include nasal congestion from cholinergic stimulation. CNS changes include drowsiness, sedation, dizziness, sleep disturbances, impaired concentration, poor memory, and depression. Other antihypertensive agents are preferred because of greater efficacy and fewer adverse effects.

Vasodilators

Vasodilators directly relax arteriolar smooth muscle and decrease peripheral vascular resistance. They do not interfere with autonomic reflexes or produce postural hypotension. This stimulates carotid sinus baroreceptors, producing reflex increases in heart rate, renin release, and sodium and water retention. These drugs usually have been used in combination with a diuretic and a β-blocker or sympatholytic agent to prevent the reflex increases in cardiac output and fluid retention that blunt the effect of vasodilators when they are used alone. Older adults develop less reflex tachycardia.

Comparison of Vasodilators

Hydralazine is metabolized by hepatic acetylation with substantial first-pass elimination. Hydralazine is effective when taken twice daily; food increases bioavailability. The acetylation rate is genetically determined; slow acetylators experience greater hypotensive effects and usually should not receive more than 200 mg hydralazine daily.

Minoxidil is a potent vasodilator that markedly reduces peripheral vascular resistance and is reserved for severe hypertension. It can produce blood pressure reductions of 30 to 40 mm Hg when combined with diuretics and β-blockers. Minoxidil is well absorbed and undergoes hepatic metabolism. Despite a short half-life, the antihypertensive effect persists for 12 to 24 hours, and minoxidil is dosed twice daily. Minoxidil produces marked sodium and water retention, and large dosages of loop diuretics often are needed to control the edema. Reflex tachycardia and increased cardiac output are prevented by adequate β-blocker therapy.

Diazoxide is a nondiuretic thiazide that dilates peripheral arterioles and is used to treat hypertensive emergencies. Intravenous injection produces a profound decrease in both SBP and DBP that does not warrant continuous infusion and rarely causes hypotension. Diazoxide is metabolized in the liver and excreted in urine, with a duration of action of 2 to 24 hours. Diazoxide is administered as a minibolus (1 to 3 mg/kg) every 10 minutes, with a maximum of 150 mg, or as a 15-mg/minute infusion. Diazoxide produces sodium and water retention, and diuretic therapy is needed to maintain blood pressure control. Hyperglycemia is a problem with prolonged use. Patients with renal failure or myocardial ischemia are predisposed to the adverse effects of diazoxide.

Nitroprusside is an instant-acting vasodilator that is useful in virtually all hypertensive emergencies. Nitroprusside relaxes both arteriolar and venous smooth muscles. Nitroprusside reacts with cysteine, forming nitrocysteine, which activates guanylate cyclase, leading to increased cyclic guanylic acid, which relaxes vascular smooth muscle. Controlled intravenous nitroprusside infusions are highly effective in treating hypertensive emergencies. The onset and cessation of the hypotensive action are immediate. Nitroprusside is unstable and must be protected from light. The nitroprusside metabolite thiocyanate may rapidly accumulate with impaired renal function, and plasma thiocyanate concentrations greater than 10 mg/dL are toxic. Nitroprusside decreases peripheral resistance and can improve left ventricular function in patients with congestive heart failure or with impaired cardiac output after a myocardial infarction.

Adverse Effects

Adverse effects from reflex sympathetic stimulation or direct vasodilation include headache, dizziness, postural hypotension, tachycardia, and palpitations.[73] The reflex tachycardia can precipitate or aggravate angina pectoris. Hydralazine commonly causes throbbing headaches and also causes a pyridoxine deficiency–induced peripheral neuropathy. A positive antinuclear antibody (ANA) develops in 15 to 20% of hydralazine-treated patients, which can lead to a lupuslike syndrome, particularly if dosages greater than 200 mg/day are used. Symptoms can include arthralgia, arthritis, fever, malaise, rash, and weight loss. Symptoms can resolve rapidly and often disappear within 6 months; however, rheumatoid symptoms and a positive ANA can persist for years.

Minoxidil causes marked sodium and water retention, leading to weight gain, peripheral edema, cardiac enlargement, pulmonary hypertension, and pericardial effusion.[73] Minoxidil causes hypertrichosis in nearly all patients. This can be partly controlled with depilatories but limits its use by women. Coarsening of facial features can also occur.

Clinical Use of Antihypertensive Drugs

JNC VI recommends a diuretic or a β-blocker as initial therapy unless there are "compelling or specific indications for another drug."[1] The German HANE study comparing HCTZ, atenolol, nitrendipine, and enalapril did not find better control of blood pressure or fewer adverse effects with the newer agents.[74] Although newer trials attempt to establish whether newer classes of drugs are superior, most hypertensive patients who need drug therapy should receive diuretics or β-blockers.[56]

Other general JNC VI drug therapy guidelines include the following:

- Start with a low dosage and titrate upward based on age, need, and response.
- An optimal formulation should provide 24-hour efficacy with a once-daily dose, with at least 50% of the peak effect remaining at the end of the 24 hours.
- The advantages of 24-hour efficacy are better adherence, lower cost by using fewer tablets, persistent and smooth control of blood pressure, and protection against cardiovascular events caused by the abrupt increase in blood pressure after arising from overnight sleep.
- Combining low dosages of two agents from different classes increases efficacy and reduces dose-dependent adverse effects.

One of the most significant changes in JNC VI is the support of combination therapy.[1] JNC VI indicates that low dosages of two agents from different classes increase antihypertensive efficacy and reduce does-dependent adverse effects. The combination of a thiazide diuretic with other agents usually potentiates blood pressure lowering.[75] Combining ACE inhibitors and calcium antagonists can further reduce proteinuria and cause less pedal edema. Many of the major antihypertensive trials combined agents. Combination therapy results in blood pressure reductions approximately twice those of monotherapy.[2] Effective drug combinations include the following:

- Diuretics and β-blockers, ACE inhibitors, or AII antagonists
- Calcium antagonists and β-blockers or ACE inhibitors
- α-Blockers plus β-blockers

Low-dose combination products appear to be an important tool to reduce the continuing undertreatment of hypertension and often are less expensive than high-dose monotherapy.[76]

A limited number of trials have compared drug therapy using agents from several classes of antihypertensive drugs. An early VA Cooperative study used a goal DBP less than 90 mm Hg.[77] Diltiazem was the most effective therapy, with a 59% success rate. Diltiazem also ranked first for black patients (64%). Captopril and prazosin were least successful (42%). HCTZ (46%), clonidine (50%), and atenolol (51%) had intermediate success rates. Drug intolerance was most common with clonidine (14%) and prazosin (12%). The fewest dropouts occurred with diuretics (3%).

The TOMHS study found that all drug classes except ACE inhibitors were equally effective in reducing blood pressure.[32,78] All drugs were well tolerated, and 72% of patients continued their initial treatment, most not needing any dosage increase. An unexpected finding was that the greatest improvement in the quality of life was for patients taking a diuretic or β-blocker. Chlorthalidone was most effective in reducing LVH.

A real-world study of antihypertensive efficacy in VA hypertension clinics found that regimens of a diuretic or diuretic plus β-blocker were associated with the lowest blood pressures.[79] Calcium antagonists were associated with the highest blood pressures. ACE inhibitors were associated with higher DBP but with SBP similar to that achieved with diuretics.

If the initial drug therapy is not tolerated, another drug from a different class should be substituted. If blood pressure response is inadequate with alternative monotherapy but the initial drug is well tolerated, a second agent from a different class should be added, usually a diuretic, and low-dose combination therapy considered.

For hypertension that is not controlled by two drugs, the JNC VI recommendations are to continue adding agents from different classes. Additional drugs should be added or substituted in gradually increasing dosages until blood pressure is controlled, side effects are intolerable, or maximal recommended dosages are reached. Usually, an interval of 1 to 2 months allows maximal antihypertensive action before changes are made. In many instances, using smaller dosages of drugs with different sites of action is preferred to maximal dosages of a single drug. This method exploits the additive effects of drugs while minimizing side effects. More aggressive drug therapy is important to control hypertension. A VA trial found that 40% of antihypertensive men had a blood pressure ≥160/90 mm Hg despite an average of six hypertension-related visits per year and that therapy was increased at only 6.7% of visits.[80]

Refractory Hypertension

Patients with blood pressure that is not controlled (160/100 mm Hg or higher) by a triple-drug regimen are considered resistant. Several potential causes should be evaluated, including the following:

- Patient noncompliance
- Inadequate drug dosages
- Drug combinations that act at the same site
- Volume overload (excess sodium intake, inadequate diuretic therapy, renal insufficiency)
- Obesity
- Renovascular hypertension
- Excess alcohol intake
- Drug interactions
- Drug-induced hypertension

Step-Down Therapy

For patients who have maintained control of their blood pressure (DBP less than 85 mm Hg) for at least 1 year, a stepwise reduction in antihypertensive medications may be attempted.[1] Short-term studies described a high success rate (40 to 50%) of discontinuation of drug treatment, but a long-term evaluation found that only 8% of previously treated patients remained normotensive off medications.[81] Virtually all hypertensive patients who are off medication can be expected to relapse unless effective lifestyle modifications are implemented. A reasonable approach is to step down to one medication after blood pressure is controlled for 1 year on multiple drugs. Drug therapy cessation should be reserved for patients with no medical complications and mild hypertension who have demonstrated weight loss, sodium reduction, or increased exercise. Drug withdrawal is more likely to be successful in patients who adhere to weight loss and sodium reduction.[82] Patients who are off drugs should have their blood pressure measured every 3 to 6 months. They should be informed that permanent remission is rare and that eventual reinstitution of drug treatment is likely.

Hypertensive Emergencies and Urgencies

A hypertensive emergency is a clinical presentation in which blood pressure must be lowered immediately to limit target organ damage, including hypertensive encephalopathy, intracranial bleeding, myocardial infarction, acute heart failure, dissecting aortic aneurysm, or ecalampsia.[1,72] If end-organ damage is absent, it is a hypertensive urgency. Hypertensive crises may involve an abrupt increase in vascular resistance secondary to increased circulating vasoconstrictor substances, leading to ischemia, which triggers the further release of vasoconstrictors.[1,71] Therapy should interrupt this cycle and decrease blood pressure to lower levels while avoiding an abrupt decrease to normotensive or hypotensive blood pressures, which may cause ischemia or infarction. For a hypertensive emergency the target usually is to lower blood pressure 25% and then to 160/100 mm Hg within 2 to 6 hours. Excessive falls in blood pressure may precipitate renal, cerebral, or coronary ischemia and must be avoided.[1] Treatment options include sodium nitroprusside infusion, intravenous nicardipine, intravenous labetalol, enalaprilat, and hydralazine.[1,72] Sublingual or buccal fast-acting nifedipine has caused significant adverse effects and should not be used.[1]

Complicated Hypertension

The presence of hypertensive complications or coexisting disease states can influence the selection of antihypertensive drugs (Table 39.11).

Congestive Heart Failure and Left Ventricular Hypertrophy

The presence of LVH is an independent risk factor for cardiac dysrhythmias and sudden death. Premature ventricular contractions are 40 to 50 times more prevalent in hypertensive patients, and the risk of sudden death is increased five to six times by their presence.[9] Most of the antihypertensive drugs reduce LVH, including β-blockers, calcium entry blockers, ACE inhibitors, and central adrenergic agonists.[1] Diuretics may be less effective in reversing LVH and can increase cardiac risk by causing electrolyte disturbances. Vasodilators can increase left ventricular mass and should not be used as monotherapy. For patients with overt congestive heart failure, blood pressure control improves cardiac function and reduces clinical heart failure and cardiovascular mortality.[1] Substantial evidence demonstrates that ACE inhibitors reduce mortality in patients with heart failure (see Chapter 40, Congestive Heart Failure).[1] The α–β-blocker carvedilol also is beneficial in treating heart failure.

Renal Insufficiency

Treating hypertension can slow the progression of renal disease.[1,6,83] JNC VI guidelines suggest lowering blood pressure to 130/85 mm Hg (or to 125/75 mm Hg in

Table 39.11 ▪ Antihypertensive Drugs: Indications and Contraindications

Drug Class	Compelling Indications	Possible Indication	Contraindications
Diuretics	Heart failure Older adults Systolic hypertension	Diabetes	Gout
β-Blockers	Ischemic heart disease Acute myocardial infarction Tachyarrhythmias	Heart failure Pregnancy Diabetes	Asthma and chronic obstructive pulmonary disease Heart block
ACE inhibitors	Heart failure Left ventricular dysfunction Acute myocardial infarction Diabetic nephropathy		Pregnancy Hyperkalemia
Calcium antagonists	Angina Older adults Systolic hypertension	Peripheral vascular disease	Heart block
α-Blockers	Prostatic hypertrophy	Glucose intolerance Dyslipidemia	
Angiotensin II antagonists	ACE inhibitor cough	Heart failure	Pregnancy Bilateral renal artery stenosis Hyperkalemia

ACE, angiotensin-converting enzyme.

patients with proteinuria).[1] If the serum creatinine is greater than 2.5 mg/dL, a loop diuretic, furosemide, bumetanide, or metolazone is needed because thiazide diuretics are ineffective.[1,6] Sodium retention becomes a major factor in treating patients with renal insufficiency; larger dosages of loop diuretics may be added to most regimens. Other drugs that are effective for patients with renal disease and do not adversely affect renal blood flow or glomerular filtration are ACE inhibitors, calcium entry blockers, central antiadrenergics, and vasodilators.[84,85] ACE inhibitors and calcium entry blockers appear to have unique benefits for patients with renal disease. These agents increase renal blood flow and glomerular filtration rate, prevent tubular sodium reabsorption, and may limit the progression of renal disease.[84–86] ACE inhibitors' renoprotective effects include reduction of systemic and glomerular hypertension and renal fibrosis.[83] The risk of hyperkalemia from ACE inhibitors or AII blockers increases substantially if the serum creatinine is greater than 3 mg/dL. For hypertensive patients with renal insufficiency, blood pressure should be reduced to 130/85 mm Hg, and further reduction to 120/75 mm Hg in African Americans with renal disease may be beneficial.[86]

Dosage reductions are needed for antihypertensive drugs that are excreted by the kidney, and patients with chronic renal failure may exhibit an increased sensitivity to some drugs, including α-blockers and ACE inhibitors.

Coronary Artery Disease

The benefits of antihypertensive treatment in preventing the complications of coronary artery disease have been less than were predicted. To prevent coronary artery disease complications, emphasis should be given to correcting other cardiovascular risk factors, especially smoking, hyperlipidemia, and diabetes mellitus.[1] Calculating an individual coronary risk profile can aid in treatment.[87] Patients with angina pectoris or a previous myocardial infarction can be treated with β-blockers or calcium blockers, which reduce angina. β-Blockers are also shown to reduce mortality after myocardial infarction, at least in men. ACE inhibitors also reduce mortality after myocardial infarction, particularly in patients with left ventricular dysfunction. However, despite the documented benefits of β-blockers for secondary prevention of myocardial infarction, they continue to be underused[88] (see Chapter 41). Because of the increase of arrhythmias, caution must be exercised to avoid diuretic-induced hypokalemia and hypomagnesemia. Drugs that cause reflex tachycardia, such as hydralazine, should be avoided.

Cerebrovascular Disease

Antihypertensive therapy can reduce the overall risk of recurrent stroke by 42% and is an important component of therapy for patients with cerebrovascular disease.[89] Hypertension is also a risk factor for intracerebral hemorrhage (ICH). The risk of ICH is highest in younger patients, current smokers, and those who discontinue antihypertensive therapy.[90] It is important to avoid orthostatic hypotension, and antihypertensive drug therapy should be started cautiously because older adults with cerebrovascular disease are more likely to develop hypotension from these drugs.

Diabetes Mellitus

Hypertension is twice as common in diabetic patients than in nondiabetics, with 50% of diabetic patients becoming hypertensive.[91] Insulin resistance and hyperinsulinemia may contribute to the pathogenesis of hypertension in these patients.[7,91] Diabetic vascular disease and associated serum lipid abnormalities compound the cardiovascular risks. Nephropathy develops in up to 50% of patients with insulin-dependent diabetes mellitus (IDDM) and 40% of patients with non–insulin-dependent diabetes mellitus (NIDDM).[91]

Recent trials show that treating hypertension produces a greater reduction in cardiovascular mortality and events in diabetic patients than in nondiabetic patients.[92] The United Kingdom Prospective Diabetes Study (UKPDS) trial of tight control of blood pressure achieved blood pressures of 144/82 mm Hg versus 154/87 mm Hg in the loose control group.[93] The improved blood pressure control reduced both diabetic microvascular and cardiovascular complications. The reduction in complications was also found to be cost-effective.[93a] Thus the blood pressure goal for diabetic patients is now below 130/85 mm Hg.[1] The ABCD trial demonstrated a lower rate of myocardial infarction with enalapril than with nisoldipine.[64] This result was contrasted by the Syst-Eur trial, in which a nitrendipine-based therapy lowered cardiovascular mortality.[18,60,93b] In the FACET study, diabetic patients treated with an ACE inhibitor, fosinopril, had fewer cardiovascular events than patients treated with a calcium antagonist, amlodipine, which produced lower SBP.[65] The importance of diabetes as a combined risk factor is emphasized in the JNC VI recommendation to initiate drug therapy in at high-normal blood pressure in diabetic patients who also have TOD or CCD.[1]

Hypertension treatment should lower blood pressure without worsening diabetic control, serum lipids, or diabetic complications. Thiazide diuretics worsen glucose control and increase cholesterol, and these effects may not reverse with dosage reduction.[91,94] The adverse effects of thiazide diuretics on insulin release are abolished with adequate potassium supplementation.[95] In diabetic patients treated with thiazide diuretics, dosages of HCTZ in combination with other antihypertensive agents usually should be limited to 25 mg/day.[92] Discontinuation of HCTZ reduced mean fasting glucose from 130 mg/dL to 101 mg/dL.[96] Loop diuretics may produce less impairment of glucose control.[94] The mechanism of diuretic glucose elevation probably is hypokalemia, which suppresses insulin secretion and increases insulin resistance.[91] Patients with IDDM whose glycemic control is from exogenous insulin do not have this complication. β-Blockers adversely affect glucose by blocking insulin release and glycogenolysis.[52,91] β-Blockers also abolish catecholamine-mediated symptoms of hypoglycemia, such as tremor and tachycardia, and should be avoided in diabetic patients who have frequent episodes of hypoglycemia.[91,92] These agents can worsen PVD, which is 30 times more common in diabetic patients. Cardioselective β-blockers have less effect on glycemic control, and β-blockers that are cardioselective and not lipophilic are preferred for patients with type 2 diabetes.[85,91,95] β-Blockers are indicated for diabetic patients who have ischemic heart disease.[95] The risk of serious hypoglycemia was not increased by the use of nonselective β-blockers except for a statistically insignificant higher risk in patients using insulin.[97] β-Blockers that are cardioselective and not lipophilic are preferred for patients with NIDDM.[94] ACE inhibitors do not adversely effect glycemic control or lipid metabolism and can decrease proteinuria and slow the progression of diabetic renal disease.[21,98] Because of their renoprotective effects, ACE inhibitors are preferred for patients with diabetic nephropathy.[1] Close monitoring of renal function is needed because of the risk of ACE inhibitors accelerating renal insufficiency in patient with renal artery stenosis. Information about the effect of calcium entry blockers on glycemic control is conflicting. Nifedipine has increased serum glucose; verapamil has improved glycemic control.[99] Diltiazem can decrease proteinuria in diabetic patients as effectively as lisinopril, and calcium antagonists are considered to be renoprotective.[1,100,101] Amlodipine was associated with a higher rate of cardiovascular events,[65] and nisoldipine had a higher incidence of myocardial infarction.[64] Guanfacine may improve glycemic control, and α-blockers can blunt the deterioration in glucose tolerance caused by β-blockers.[100] Autonomic neuropathy and orthostatic hypotension are 30 times more common in diabetic patients than in nondiabetics, and drugs that produce postural hypotension should be used cautiously. Finally, sexual dysfunction is a common problem in diabetic men; drugs that cause sexual dysfunction should be avoided.

Older Adults

Nearly two-thirds of the 29 million people in the United States who are 65 years of age or older have some blood pressure elevation.[1] The HDFP and EWPHE trials have demonstrated benefit for older adults (up to age 80) who are treated for diastolic hypertension (DBP 90 mm Hg or higher).[102] ISH, defined as SBP greater than 160 mm Hg and DBP less than 90 mm Hg, is more prevalent above age 60.[103] ISH is associated with an increased risk of stroke and cardiovascular disease that is independent of other risk factors.[102] The SHEP trial demonstrated a 36% reduction in stroke for 4.5 years in patients age 60 years and older who were treated for ISH.[103] Drug treatment in SHEP was low-dose chlorthalidone (12.5 to 25 mg) and atenolol 25 mg, with potassium supplements if needed.[104] An important further analysis found that this drug treatment of ISH did not cause deterioration in measures of cognition, emotional state, physical function, or leisure activities.[105] A meta-analysis of antihypertensive trials involving older adults concluded that treatment reduced both stroke and CHD mortality without evidence of a *J*-curve phenomenon.[103] The Syst-Eur trial recently showed a 42% reduction in stroke using a nitrendipine-based SC treatment for older adults with ISH.[59] More than 50% were treated with calcium antagonist monotherapy and had a reduction in cardiovascular mortality.[106]

The selection of drug therapy for older adults may be

complicated by physiologic changes. Hypertensive older adults usually have a reduced cardiac output, intravascular volume, and heart rate and an increased peripheral vascular resistance.[107] Older adults often have LVH, which impairs coronary reserve and is associated with a possible increased risk of ventricular ectopy and sudden death.[107] Diminished baroreflexes increase the risk of postural hypotension, and renal function may be impaired. α_1-Blockers, labetalol, guanethidine, and guanadrel can increase orthostatic hypotension; this limits their use by older adults. Calcium entry blockers are effective, are physiologically appropriate, and do not adversely affect renal function. Their adverse effects are similar to those seen in younger patients. Although plasma renin activity decreases with age, the ACE inhibitors are effective in older adults. The ACE inhibitors do not have adverse metabolic effects and reduce the incidence of arrhythmias in cardiac failure.[107] Diuretic-based therapy in the SHEP trial was effective in patients with renal dysfunction and had mild effects on other cardiovascular risk factors.[108,109] Older adults should be treated with an individualized approach to drug therapy, and initial treatment should be guided by the axiom "start low and go slow."

Pregnancy

Hypertension complicates 10% of pregnancies and is more common in nulliparous women and women who have had multiple pregnancies.[110] Hypertension during pregnancy can be caused by chronic hypertension and preeclampsia (increased blood pressure with proteinuria and edema).[1] Chronic hypertension usually is well tolerated during pregnancy if DBP remains below 100 mm Hg. Preeclampsia can be life-threatening to both the fetus and the mother and usually develops near term with a pathophysiology of a marked increase in peripheral resistance.[111] Signs of preeclampsia include proteinuria, edema, hemoconcentration, hypoalbuminemia, increased urate, and hepatic or coagulation abnormalities.[111] Life-threatening complications are hemolytic anemia and marked hepatic dysfunction. Progression to seizures is called eclampsia, which is a major cause of maternal death.

Methyldopa has a long history of safe use in pregnancy, with normal follow-up evaluations in children up to 10 years after treatment.[111] β-Blockers, labetalol, thiazide diuretics, and hydralazine have also been used to treat hypertension during pregnancy with apparent success. β-Blockers are also considered to be safe when used later in pregnancy.[1] Limited information is available about the use of calcium entry blockers in pregnancy. ACE inhibitors and atenolol are avoided because they reduce uterine blood flow.[110,111] Intravenous hydralazine is commonly used to treat severe hypertension during pregnancy.[112] Diazoxide is used for refractory hypertension. Parenteral labetalol may become the second-choice agent. Calcium entry blockers are also effective, but concurrent magnesium sulfate may potentiate their effect and cause a precipitous fall in blood pressure. Calcium entry blockers also reduce uterine blood flow.[110]

Racial Differences

The prevalence of hypertension among African Americans is substantially higher than among Caucasians (38% versus 29%), and hypertension-related morbidity and mortality are three to five times higher than in Caucasians.[104,113,114] There is a higher prevalence of stage 3 hypertension in African Americans, and hypertension is often poorly controlled in African American patients. Environmental factors, including dietary excess, high sodium consumption, and low dietary potassium, calcium, and magnesium, may contribute to these differences.[104,114] The development of obesity and insulin resistance may be an important mechanism in hypertensive African Americans. Approximately 50% of hypertensive African Americans show salt sensitivity, and hypertension often is associated with low plasma renin and volume dependence.[114] Thiazide diuretics are effective therapy for hypertensive African Americans. In addition, thiazides offer cost-effective treatment. However, approximately 50% of hypertensive African Americans need two or more drugs.[104] African Americans have a lower response rate to β-blockers and ACE inhibitors than do hypertensive Caucasians. This difference may be smaller if higher drug dosages are used or β-blockers and ACE inhibitors are used in combination with diuretics. A comparison of different antihypertensive drugs in hypertensive African Americans demonstrated blood pressure control of 60% with atenolol, 57% with captopril, and 73% with verapamil.[115] Long-acting dihydropyridine calcium blockers effectively lower blood pressure in African Americans with hypertension.[116]

The use of age–race subgroups to predict response to initial antihypertensive therapy has also been shown to be a useful approach in VA patients.[117] The best response rates for treating stage 1 hypertension were 90% for prazosin in younger black men, 97% for diltiazem in older black men, 92% for atenolol in younger white men, and 95% for diltiazem in older white men.[117]

The prevalence of hypertension in the Hispanic population appears to be equal to or higher than that in Caucasians but lower than in African Americans.[1,112] Mexican Americans are likely to be obese and to have diabetes mellitus. Hypertension in Hispanics often is unrecognized or poorly controlled.[112]

Asians and Pacific Islanders also have a lower incidence of hypertension than Whites, but this appears to be modified by socioeconomic factors. Racial differences in drug response may be particularly important in the Asian population. Men of Chinese descent have a twofold greater sensitivity to the β-blocking effects of propranolol[118] than Caucasians. Men of Chinese descent had a greater decrease in both heart rate and blood pressure, despite a significantly higher metabolic clearance of propranolol than white subjects.[118] Asian patients also have a lower metabolism of nifedipine and often develop palpitations.[119] Because of possible racial differences in drug response and metabolism, antihypertensive drugs should be started at low dosages in treating Asian patients.

Adverse Drug Effects

Because of the long-term nature of hypertension, it is extremely important that drug therapy have minimal adverse effects. Adverse drug effects are listed in Table 39.8.

Quality of Life and Cost of Care

The cost of treatment and the adverse effects of antihypertensive drugs on the quality of life are important concerns. Drug therapy may produce subtle changes in emotion, behavior, and physical and cognitive function.[1] In an early study, physicians thought that all patients had improved, but only 48% of the patients agreed.[120] However, 99% of relatives thought that the patient had gotten worse since starting antihypertensive treatment. Problems included decreased memory, irritability, depression, hypochondria, and decreased sexual interest.[120] Captopril improved general well-being, caused fewer side effects, and had higher quality-of-life scores than methyldopa or propranolol.[121] Adding a diuretic worsened outcome for all drug treatment groups. For hypertensive African Americans there was no difference in quality of life with atenolol, captopril, or verapamil.[122] However, verapamil produced a significantly greater decrease in blood pressure. The Trial of Antihypertensive Interventions and Management (TAIM) evaluated the effects of a low-sodium and high-potassium diet, a weight loss diet, and a placebo, chlorthalidone, or atenolol on sexual function and quality of life.[123] Few drug-related side effects were found. Chlorthalidone produced erection problems in 28% of men on a usual diet, but a weight loss diet removed this effect. The weight loss diet reduced physical complaints and increased health satisfaction. The TAIM findings emphasize the importance of weight reduction in addition to drug regimens for overweight hypertensive patients.[124] A comparison of captopril and enalapril found higher quality-of-life scores with captopril, with similar blood pressure control and adverse effects.[124] Treatment with active drugs (chlorthalidone, acebutolol, doxazosin, amlodipine, or enalapril) produced lower blood pressure and better quality-of-life indexes than lifestyle intervention alone.[125]

Cost–benefit issues must be assessed to reduce medical costs while providing high-quality patient care. The costs of antihypertensive medications are widely variable. Combination diuretic products cost three or more times as much as HCTZ. β-Blockers and calcium entry blockers also show a wide cost variation.[126] ACE inhibitors and calcium entry blockers are 4 to 20 times more expensive than generic diuretics or generic β-blockers.[79] With the increasing cost of antihypertensive medications, some patients are not compliant because they cannot afford expensive drugs. Earlier estimates of the long-term cost-effectiveness projected that the cost per year of life saved was $10,900 for propranolol, $16,400 for HCTZ, $31,600 for nifedipine, $61,900 for prazosin, and $72,100 for captopril.[127] Lowering DBP by 1 mm Hg was estimated to be equivalent to lowering cholesterol by 6%.[127] However, these cost estimates have been severely criticized because of the multiple assumptions and the wide differences in the patient populations between the many studies that were compared.[128] A cost minimization analysis attempted to compare the total costs of antihypertensive therapy including drug acquisition cost, laboratory monitoring, supplemental drug acquisition costs, clinic visits, and treatment of side effects.[129] Mean total costs for antihypertensive drug classes were $895 for β-blockers, $1043 for diuretics, $1165 for central α-agonists, $1243 for ACE inhibitors, $1288 for α_1-blockers, and $1425 for calcium channel blockers. The use of calcium antagonists and ACE inhibitors has substantial cost implications. A VA systemwide study concluded that each 1% conversion from calcium antagonists to β-blockers or diuretics would result in annual cost savings of more than $700,000.[129a]

Managed care organizations often view hypertension as a long-term payoff disease.[96] However, evidence shows that the short-term costs of a disease management approach to successfully control blood pressure are lower than those of treating uncontrolled patients who need continued modification of their antihypertensive regimen.[96]

The choice of antihypertensive agent should be based on patient characteristics, concomitant diseases, and the cost of drug therapy.

Sexual Dysfunction

Antihypertensive drugs can cause erectile dysfunction (ED), ejaculation difficulties, and decreased libido.[130] Sexual dysfunction is reported by 4 to 7% of normotensive controls. The incidence of antihypertensive-induced sexual dysfunction is difficult to quantitate. Reports often range from 9 to 25% or higher, with increased frequency when multiple-drug therapy is used and with advancing age.[130] The MRC trial reported an increased frequency of erectile dysfunction with both bendrofluazide and propranolol. Sexual symptom distress scores were worsened by methyldopa and propranolol but not by captopril either alone or combined with a diuretic.[131] The risk of sexual dysfunction is greatest with peripheral adrenergic inhibitors and less with central α-agonists and diuretics. Lower incidences of sexual problems are also described with β-blockers.[130] The drugs that are least likely to cause sexual problems are the ACE inhibitors, calcium blockers, α_1-blockers, and direct vasodilators.[130] Analysis of sexual dysfunction from TOMHS found a threefold greater risk of ED in men treated with chlorthalidone, but the overall incidence was low.[131a] However, it must be recognized that ED has multiple causes; a study of Danish men with ED found a higher incidence associated with more severe hypertension, ischemic heart disease, and claudication, but not with antihypertensive drug use.[132]

Depression

Depletion of biogenic amines may be pathogenic in depression. Antihypertensive medications that interfere with the sympathetic nervous system and neurotransmitter concentrations may induce depression.[133] There is substantial evidence that reserpine and methyldopa can induce or worsen depression. β-Blockers may produce CNS effects, and an increased use of antidepressant drugs has been seen in patients treated with β-blockers.[133] Diuretics, calcium blockers, and ACE inhibitors have the lowest association with depression and are the preferred agents for patients at risk for depression.[133]

J-Curve

There is controversy about a *J*-shaped curve relationship between treated DBP and cardiac mortality in which lowering blood pressure below a critical point leads to an increase in mortality. Mortality appeared to increase in patients with preexisting ischemic heart disease whose DBP was lowered to less than 85 mm Hg.[134] In the EWPHE trial a *U*-shaped relationship was described in which total mortality increased in patients with the lowest treated SBP and DBP.[135] A review of 13 studies with a combined total of 48,000 patients found a consistent *J*-shaped relationship between cardiac events and treated DBP.[136] There was no increase in stroke at lower treated blood pressures. A proposed mechanism is increased myocardial ischemia in hypertensive patients with LVH when DBP is lowered below 85 mm Hg. A suggested compromise is to "be cautious in lowering blood pressure levels below 85 mm Hg in patients with known ischemic heart disease."[136] The risk of myocardial infarction was higher among treated hypertensive patients who achieved DBPs of less than 80 mm Hg.[137] JNC VI states that the *J*-curve may be of some concern only in patients with hypertension and preexisting coronary disease[1] and that lowering DBP to less than 90 mm Hg and SBP to less than 140 mm Hg is appropriate.

Serum Lipids

The combination of elevated blood pressure and dyslipidemia creates a synergistic increased risk of cardiovascular disease.[138] Lifestyle modifications (diet, exercise, weight reduction, and smoking cessation) are the foundation of the management of both hypertension and dyslipidemia. The potential effects of antihypertensive drugs on serum lipids must be considered in treated patients who are both hypertensive and dyslipidemic.[138,139] Thiazide-type diuretics produce a modest (5- to 10-mg/dL) increase in total cholesterol, LDL cholesterol, and triglycerides. Diuretic increases in cholesterol are greater with higher dosages and worse in blacks than in nonblacks.[139] However, the dyslipidemic effects of thiazide and loop diuretics are unlikely to occur with low-dose thiazide therapy and can be reduced or eliminated with diet modification.[1]

β-Blockers, except those with ISA or α-blocking properties, reduce HDL cholesterol and increase serum triglycerides.[1] Drugs that have minimal effects on serum lipids include calcium entry blockers, ACE inhibitors, ISA β-blockers, labetalol, hydralazine, minoxidil, and possibly indapamide. The α_1-adrenergic blockers and the central α_2-adrenergic agonists may slightly decrease total and LDL cholesterol. In the Coronary Primary Prevention Trial, the thiazide diuretics reduced the effect of lipid-lowering drugs on LDL cholesterol.[138] However, not all patients who are taking diuretics experience adverse lipid alterations, and a low-fat, low-cholesterol diet may minimize lipid changes. Some studies suggest that the hyperlipemic effects of diuretics may not persist more than 1 year.[138,139] Patients with CHD and hypertension need aggressive cholesterol-lowering therapy and careful lowering of blood pressure. β-Blockers may be needed for patients with CHD for antianginal effects and secondary prevention of myocardial infarction despite their adverse effects on serum triglycerides and HDL cholesterol. Antihyperlipidemic treatment may slow the progression of atherosclerosis and possibly induce plaque regression. The Primary Prevention Trial demonstrated that a reduction of both blood pressure and cholesterol is needed to reduce cardiovascular morbidity.[140]

A VA-based trial of the effects of six different antihypertensive drugs found no major adverse effects on lipids or lipoproteins after 1 year of therapy with HCTZ, atenolol, captopril, clonidine, diltiazem, or prazosin.[83] The study did find a reduction in HDL_2 cholesterol, but the evidence of reduced mortality from antihypertensive therapy with thiazide diuretics and β-blockers supports current guidelines.[141]

Drug Interactions

The effect of many antihypertensive drugs can be increased or decreased by the concurrent use of other drugs.[142,143] In addition, antihypertensive drugs can interact with other drugs. Often, potentially interacting drugs can be used successfully in combination if the possibility of the interaction is recognized, the effects are monitored, and drug dosages are adjusted if needed. Common interactions are listed in Table 39.10.

Nonpharmacologic Therapy

Lifestyle modification to reduce blood pressure should be the initial approach for young patients with mild hypertension and no other cardiovascular risk factors. Lifestyle modification is also continued to augment drug therapy.

Sodium Restriction

Restriction of sodium to less than 100 mmol daily (6 g sodium chloride or 2.4 g sodium) is achievable and may control hypertension in some patients with stage 1 hypertension with an average decrease of 6.3/2.2 mm Hg.[33] The Trials of Hypertension Prevention I (TOHP I) study demonstrated only a modest (1.7/0.9 mm Hg) reduction in blood pressure with sodium reduction.[144] This degree of sodium restriction can be achieved by refraining from adding salt at the table and avoiding highly salted processed foods.[145]

Weight Reduction

The prevalence of hypertension is 50% greater in overweight adults than in normal-weight adults.[146] The TOHP I study also found that a weight loss of 3.9 kg led to a reduction in blood pressure of 2.9/2.3 mm Hg.[144] Weight reduction is the most effective nonpharmacologic intervention to lower blood pressure. The JNC recommends that all overweight hypertensive patients (body mass index of 27 or greater) should lose weight. Reductions in blood pressure can occur with a weight loss as small as 4.5 kg (10 pounds). The TOHP II study documented reductions in blood pressure with weight loss (–3.7/–2.7 mm Hg), sodium restriction (–2.9/–1.6 mm Hg), and both interventions (–4.0/–2.8 mm Hg).[147] It is well recognized that weight reduction is difficult to achieve and sustain, and weight reduction programs should involve caloric restriction and increased physical activity.

Combination Diet

The most important advance in lifestyle modification was shown in the Dietary Approaches to Stop Hypertension (DASH) study.[148] The DASH study found that a combination diet rich in fruits and vegetables, high in calcium from low-fat dairy foods, and low in total saturated fat produced a greater reduction in blood pressure than traditional approaches of sodium restriction and weight reduction. The DASH diet resembled the Mediterranean diet and emphasized low-fat dairy foods. The DASH diet is also high in potassium. The greatest reductions in blood pressure were seen in patients with the highest levels of hypertension. The DASH combination was particularly effective in African Americans with hypertension.[149]

Exercise

Regular aerobic physical activity achieving a moderate level of physical fitness is also beneficial.[1] Exercise training decreases blood pressure in hypertensive patients an average of 11/8 mm Hg.[150] Exercise training is also beneficial in weight reduction, lowers plasma triglycerides, and improves insulin sensitivity.[150] Aerobic exercise was particularly effective in reducing stage 1 or 2 blood pressure in older, sedentary men.[151] A regular physical activity program should be started gradually, with 30 to 45 minutes of brisk walking on most days of the week. This level of exercise may control blood pressure without drug therapy.

Dynamic endurance exercises (walking, running, cycling, and swimming) are recommended; isometric exercises (rowing and competitive sports) are not suitable.[152] Because hypertensive patients may show exaggerated blood pressures during exercise, intensive training should not be started until DBPs are below 105 mm Hg.[152] Drugs that are effective in treating superelevated blood pressures (SBP greater than 200 mm Hg) during exercise include cardioselective β_1-blockers, verapamil, clonidine, and ACE inhibitors.[152]

Tobacco Avoidance

The coexistence of hypertension and smoking dramatically increases the risk of cardiovascular disease.[1,99] Cigarette smoking acutely raises blood pressure by 3/5 to 12/10 mm Hg.[153] Although office blood pressures do not differ for smokers, 24-hour ABPM has shown higher daytime blood pressures in smokers, particularly in Caucasians above age 50.[153] However, the most accepted view is that smokers have lower blood pressure than nonsmokers.[99] Smoking was also shown to interfere with the reduction of blood pressure by propranolol in black patients, and nonselective β-blockers should be avoided in hypertensive patients who smoke.[99,154] Finally, the reduction of cardiovascular risk by antihypertensive treatment is not as great in smokers as in nonsmokers.[1,99] The JNC recommends that a smoking cessation program is a key component of hypertension treatment.

Alcohol

Moderate to heavy alcohol intake increases the incidence of hypertension.[1,155] The JNC recommendations are to limit alcohol consumption to 30 mL ethanol daily (2 oz whiskey, 8 oz wine, or 24 oz beer).[1] Alcohol also interferes with antihypertensive drug treatment independently of noncompliance, and alcohol use should be evaluated in patients with resistant hypertension.[156] The Prevention and Treatment of Hypertension Study (PATHS) evaluation of 641 moderate to heavy drinkers did not find a significant reduction in blood pressure with a cognitive–behavioral alcohol reduction intervention program that produced an average decrease of 1.3 drinks per day.[157] But a U.K. study did not find evidence that light to moderate alcohol intake reduced mortality from CHD; rather, there is an increase in overall mortality with increasing alcohol consumption.[158]

Caffeine

Caffeine increases blood pressure in people who do not regularly consume methylxanthines, but habitual consumption of caffeine is believed to be associated with the development of complete tolerance to its pressor effect.[159] However, ABPM of habitual coffee drinkers demonstrated a consistent 4/4-mm Hg work-site increase in blood pressure and a 12/9–mm Hg increase during formal stress testing.[160] Men who drank three or more cups of coffee per day had twice the risk of thromboembolic stroke as nondrinkers of coffee.[161] Because of the possibility of increase blood pressure and stroke risk, hypertensive patients should be advised to limit coffee to two cups daily and to avoid coffee consumption before blood pressure measurement. JNC VI places no limitations on consumption of caffeine-containing beverages.

Potassium and Cation Supplementation

A low dietary potassium intake may increase blood pressure, and high dietary potassium may protect against hypertension. JNC VI recommends adequate dietary potassium (90 mmol/day), and the DASH diet is high in potassium.[1,149]

Although low calcium intake is associated with a higher prevalence of hypertension, there is no evidence to recommend calcium supplements for lowering blood pressure.[1] Meta-analysis of calcium supplementation shows only average reductions of 1–2/1 mm Hg.[162] Similarly, lower dietary magnesium is associated with higher blood pressure, but the effects of a high-magnesium intake are small (–2.4/–1.4 mm Hg).[163] However, a high dietary calcium intake is believed to be an important component of the DASH diet.

Stress Reduction: Relaxation and Biofeedback

The use of relaxation and biofeedback therapy to reduce behavioral stress and lower reduce blood pressure was ineffective in the TOHP I study and produced conflicting results in other studies.[1] JNC VI does not recommend relaxation therapies for definitive therapy of hypertension.[1]

Summary of Lifestyle Modifications

The JNC concluded that weight control and sodium restriction have been shown to independently reduce blood pressure, and their effects are additive with those of pharmacologic agents.[1] The Trial of Nonpharmacologic Interventions in the Elderly (TONE) found that modest salt restriction and weight loss enabled a large number of older adults to discontinue antihypertensive medications.[164] A nutritional program to lose weight and restrict sodium and alcohol achieved a 39% success in normalizing blood pressure without drug therapy.[89] The DASH diet, which did not restrict sodium or focus on weight loss, appears to be the most effective approach to lifestyle modification.[149] Alcohol restriction also is recommended. Smoking cessation and exercise programs are recommended for all hypertensive patients. Lifestyle modification alone should be tried for all patients with stage 1 hypertension if they are without target organ damage, CCD, or diabetes.[1,87] Patients who do not normalize blood pressure after 6 to 12 months of lifestyle modification should start drug treatment.

IMPROVING OUTCOMES

The single most important factor in successful hypertension treatment is patient compliance. Untreated and uncontrolled hypertension in aware hypertensive patients remains an important problem.[165,166] Public awareness programs have identified the majority of people with hypertension, but the problems of patient dropout and noncompliance with treatment still result in fewer than 50% of hypertensive patients having controlled blood pressure. Continuous effort is needed to prevent patient dropout, encourage lifestyle changes, and improve medication compliance.

Noncompliance is a complex problem, and prediction of compliance by clinicians is poor. Factors associated with poor compliance include younger age, urban dwelling, and smoking.[167] A systematic procedure to screen for medication noncompliance can help to identify patients who need extra attention to achieve blood pressure control. A patient-tracking system and a missed-appointment follow-up program are needed to achieve long-term attendance and blood pressure control. Failure to achieve blood pressure control is twice as great in nonattenders (no appointment in 6 months) as in attenders (67% versus 30%).[166]

Several important areas must be considered in attempting to overcome noncompliance. Combinations of techniques usually are needed.

Patient Education

Education about the consequences of untreated hypertension and the role of drug and nondrug treatments serves as a foundation for compliance. The patient must understand and believe that hypertension is a serious condition that needs treatment.

Methods to Improve Patient Adherence to Drug Therapy

- Simplifying the drug regimen can improve compliance.
- Avoid side effects by starting with low dosages and individually selected drugs.
- Schedule drug doses once or twice daily.
- Label prescriptions with clear, explicit directions, and indicate the purpose of the drug.
- Tailor medication times to coincide with existing daily habits.
- Provide written schedules or pillbox organizers for patients who are taking multiple drugs.
- Encourage the use of prompting cues such as stickers or calendars to remind patients to take medications.
- Discuss potential problems such as drug costs, confusion with other drugs, and previous problems with drug therapy.

Disease Management Strategies to Improve Patient Outcomes

- Involve the patient by providing feedback of blood pressure response or self-monitoring of blood pressure.
- Encourage or reward patients for keeping appointments, taking medications, and reducing blood pressure.
- Screen for noncompliance by monitoring attendance, patient self-reports, blood pressure response, and changes in biochemical or physical parameters (e.g., pulse or serum potassium).
- Provide close professional supervision, and establish a positive relationship with patients.

Pharmacists and Hypertension

The major opportunity for pharmacists is to assist in achieving long-term control of blood pressure. Pharmacists can provide patient education, monitor prescription drug use for noncompliance, implement medication refill reminder systems, screen for drug interactions and adverse drug reactions, and monitor blood pressure response.[165–171] In specialized settings, clinical pharmacists have treated hypertensive patients with improved compliance and blood pressure control.[170,171] Despite the tremendous increase in knowledge about hypertension and the explosion of drug therapy options, there remains a large gap in professional following of JNC guidelines and, more importantly, the consistent control of blood pressure in patients. Hypertension remains a largely untapped area for pharmacist participation in collaborative drug therapy management to optimize control of blood pressure in a vast patient population.

KEY POINTS

- Hypertension continues to be a national health problem. However, hypertension must be viewed as one of several major cardiovascular risk factors.
- Treatment must address all cardiovascular risks.
- The greatest patient benefit may be from controlling blood pressure by nonpharmacologic interventions.
- For patients who are unable to control blood pressure, drug therapy can effectively reduce risks if long-term control of hypertension is achieved.

RESOURCES

American College of Cardiology	http://www.acc.org
American Heart Association	http://www.americanheart.org
American Society of Hypertension	http://www.ash-us.org
Hypertension Network	http://www.bloodpressure.com
National Guideline Clearinghouse	http://www.guidelines.gov

Nutritional strategies efficacious in the prevention or treatment of hypertension.

Automated ambulatory blood pressure and self-measured blood pressure monitoring devices: their role in the diagnosis and management of hypertension.

National Heart, Lung, and Blood Institute	http://www.nhlbi.nih.gov/nhlbi/nhlbi.htm

The Sixth Report of the Joint National Committee (JNC VI) on High Blood Pressure

JNC VI Quick Reference Card

Working Group reports:

Ambulatory Blood Pressure Monitoring

High Blood Pressure in Pregnancy

Hypertension in Diabetes

REFERENCES

1. The sixth report of the Joint National Committee on Detection, Evaluation and Treatment of High Blood Pressure (JNC VI). Arch Intern Med 157:2413–2446, 1997.
2. Guidelines Sub-Committee. 1999 World Health Organization–International Society of Hypertension guidelines for the management of hypertension. J Hypertens 17:151–185, 1999.
3. Working Group on Renovascular Hypertension. Detection, evaluation and treatment of renovascular hypertension. Arch Intern Med 147:820–824, 1987.
4. Woods JW. Oral contraceptives and hypertension. Hypertension 11(Suppl I):11–14, 1988.
5. Lake CR, Zaloga G, Bray J, et al. Transient hypertension after two phenylpropanolamine diet aids and the effects of caffeine: a placebo-controlled follow-up study. Am J Med 86:427–432, 1989.
6. Johnson AG, Nguyen TV, Day RD. Do nonsteroidal anti-inflammatory drugs affect blood pressure? A meta-analysis. Ann Intern Med 121:289–300, 1994.
7. Reaven GM. Insulin resistance, hyperinsulinemia, and hypertriglyceridemia in the etiology and clinical course of hypertension. Am J Med 90(Suppl 2A):7S–11S, 1991.
8. Kannel WB, Wentworth D, et al. Overall and coronary heart disease mortality rates in relation to major risk factors in 325,348 men screened for MRFIT. Am Heart J 112:825–836, 1986.
9. Lavie CJ, Venture HO, Messerli FH. Regression on increased left ventricular mass by antihypertensives. Drugs 42:945–961, 1991.
10. MacMahon S, Peto R, Cutler J, et al. Blood pressure, stroke, and coronary heart disease. 1: prolonged differences in blood pressure: prospective observational studies corrected for regression dilution bias. Lancet 335:765–774, 1990.
11. Weiss NS. Relation of high blood pressure to headache, epistaxis and selected other symptoms. N Engl J Med 287:631–633, 1972.
12. Rudd P, Price MG, Graham LE, et al. Consequences of worksite hypertension screening: differential changes in psychosocial function. Am J Med 80:853–860, 1986.
13. Pickering TG, James GD, Boddie C, et al. How common is white coat hypertension? JAMA 259:225–228, 1988.
14. Khattar RS, Senior R, Lahiri A. Cardiovascular outcome in white-coat versus sustained mild hypertension. A 10-year follow-up study. Circulation 98:1892–1897, 1998.
15. National High Blood Pressure Education Program Coordinating Committee. National High Blood Pressure Education Program Working Group report on ambulatory blood pressure monitoring. Arch Intern Med 150:2270–2280, 1990.
16. Klein LE. Compliance and blood pressure control. Hypertension 11(Suppl II):61–64, 1988.
17. Collins R, Peto R, MacMahon S, et al. Blood pressure, stroke, and coronary heart disease. 2: short-term reductions in blood pressure: overview of the randomized drug trials in their epidemiological context. Lancet 335:827–838, 1990.
18. Herbert PR, Moser M, Mayer J, et al. Recent evidence on drug therapy of mild to moderate hypertension and decreased risk of coronary heart disease. Arch Intern Med 153:578–581, 1993.
19. Veterans Administration Cooperative Study Group on Antihypertensive Agents. Effects of treatment on morbidity in hypertension: results in patients with diastolic blood pressure averaging 90 through 104 mm Hg. JAMA 213:1143–1152, 1970.
19a. Veterans Administration Cooperative Study Group on Antihypertensive Agents. Effects of treatment on morbidity in hypertension: results in patients with diastolic blood pressure averaging 115 through 129 mm Hg. JAMA 202:1028–1034, 1967.
20. Taguchi J, Freis ED. Partial reduction of blood pressure and prevention of complications in hypertension. N Engl J Med 291:329–331, 1974.
21. Hypertension Detection and Follow-up Program Cooperative Group. Five year findings of the hypertension detection and follow-up program. I: reduction in mortality of persons with high blood pressure, including mild hypertension. JAMA 242:2562–2571, 1979.
22. Hypertension Detection and Follow-up Program Cooperative Group. Five year findings of the hypertension detection and follow-up program. II: mortality by race, sex and age. JAMA 242:2572–2577, 1979.
23. Hypertension Detection and Follow-up Program Cooperative Group. The effect of treatment on mortality in mild hypertension. N Engl J Med 307:976–980, 1982.
24. Hypertension Detection and Follow-up Program Cooperative Group. Persistence of reduction in blood pressure and mortality of participants in the Hypertension Detection and Follow-up Program. JAMA 259:2113–2122, 1988.
25. Multiple Risk Factor Intervention Trial Group. Risk factors changes and mortality results. JAMA 248:1465–1477, 1982.
26. Multiple Risk Factor Intervention Trial Group. Baseline rest electrocardiographic abnormalities, antihypertensive treatment, and mortality in the Multiple Risk Factor Intervention Trial. Am J Cardiol 55:1–14, 1985.
27. European Working Party on High Blood Pressure in the Elderly Trial (EWPHE). Mortality and morbidity results from the European Working Party on High Blood Pressure in the Elderly Trial. Lancet 1:1349–54, 1985.
28. European Working Party on High Blood Pressure in the Elderly Trial (EWPHE). Efficacy of antihypertensive drug treatment according to age, sex, blood pressure, and previous cardiovascular disease in patients over the age of 60. Lancet 2:589–592, 1986.
29. SHEP Cooperative Research Group. Prevention of stroke by antihypertensive

drug treatment in older persons with isolated systolic hypertension: final results of the Systolic Hypertension in the Elderly Program (SHEP). JAMA 265:3255–3264, 1991.
30. Dahlof B, Lindholm LH, Hannson L, et al. Morbidity and mortality in the Swedish Trial in Old Patients with Hypertension (STOP-Hypertension). Lancet 338:1281–1285, 1991.
31. MRC Working Party. Medical Research Council trial of treatment of hypertension in older adults: principal results. BMJ 304:405–411, 1992.
32. Neaton JD, Grimm RH Jr, Prineas RJ, et al. Treatment of mild hypertension study: final results. JAMA 270:713–724, 1993.
33. Hansson L, Zanchetti A, Carruthers SG, et al. Effects of intensive blood-pressure lowering and low-dose aspirin in patients with hypertension; principal results of the Hypertension Optimal Treatment (HOT) randomized trial: HOT Study Group. Lancet 351:1755–1762, 1998.
34. Alderman MH. Which antihypertensive drugs first–and why? JAMA 267: 2786–2887, 1992.
35. Psaty BM, Smith NL, Siscovick DS, et al. Health outcomes associated with antihypertensive therapies used as first-line agents: a systematic review and meta-analysis. JAMA 277:739–745, 1998.
36. Siscovick DS, Psaty BM, Koepsell TD, et al. Diuretic therapy for hypertension and the risk of primary cardiac arrest. N Engl J Med 330:1852–1857, 1994.
37. Licht JH, Haley RJ, Pugh B, et al. Diuretic regimens in essential hypertension: a comparison of hypokalemic effects, BP control, and cost. Arch Intern Med 143:1694–1699, 1983.
38. Kaplan NM, Carnegie A, Raskin P, et al. Potassium supplementation in hypertensive patients with diuretic-induced hypokalemia. N Engl J Med 312:746–749, 1985.
39. Langford HG, Blaufox D, Borhani NO, et al. Is thiazide-produced uric acid elevation harmful? Analysis of data from the Hypertension Detection and Follow-up Program. Arch Intern Med 147:645–649, 1987.
40. Chang SW, Fine R, Siegel D, et al. The impact of diuretic therapy on reported sexual function. Arch Intern Med 151:2402–2408, 1991.
41. Wasnich R, Davis J, Ross P, et al. Effect of thiazide on rates of bone mineral loss: a longitudinal study. BMJ 301:303–305, 1990.
42. Moser M. Why are physicians not prescribing diuretics more frequently in the management of hypertension. JAMA 279:1813–1816, 1998.
43. Kramer BK, Schweda F, Riegger GAJ. Diuretic treatment and diuretic resistance in heart failure. Am J Med 106:90–96, 1999.
44. van der Heijden, Donders SH, Cleophas TJ, et al. A randomized, placebo-controlled study of loop diuretics in patients with essential hypertension: the bumetanide and furosemide on lipid profile (BUFUL) clinical report study. J Clin Pharmacol 38:630–635, 1998.
45. Skluth HA, Gums JG. Spironolactone: a re-examination. Drug Intell Clin Pharm 24:52–59, 1990.
46. Spence JD, Wong DG, Lindsay RM. Effects of triamterene and amiloride on urinary sediment in hypertensive patients taking hydrochlorothiazide. Lancet 2:73–75, 1985.
47. Zawada ET. Antihypertensive therapy with triamterene-hydrochlorothiazide vs amiloride-hydrochlorothiazide: comparison of effects on urinary prostaglandin E2 excretion. Arch Intern Med 146:1312–1314, 1986.
48. Favre L, Glasson P, Valloton MB. Reversible acute renal failure from combined triamterene and indomethacin: a study in healthy subjects. Ann Intern Med 96:317–318, 1982.
49. Hampton JR. Choosing the right β-blocker: a guide to selection. Drugs 48:549–568, 1994.
50. Radack K, Deck C. β-adrenergic blocker therapy does not worsen intermittent claudication in subjects with peripheral arterial disease: a meta-analysis of randomized controlled trials. Arch Intern Med 151:1769–1776, 1991.
51. Bright RA, Everitt DE. β-blockers and depression: evidence against an association. JAMA 267:1783–1787, 1992.
52. Dornhorst A, Powell SH, Pensky J. Aggravation by propranolol of hyperglycaemic effect of hydrochlorothiazide in type II diabetics without alteration of insulin secretion. Lancet 1:123–126, 1985.
53. Roeback JR Jr, Hla KM, Chambless LE, et al. Effects of chromium supplementation on serum high-density lipoprotein cholesterol levels in men taking beta-blockers. Ann Intern Med 115:917–924, 1991.
54. Psaty BM, Koepsell TD, Wagner EH, et al. The relative risk of incident coronary heart disease associated with recently stopping the use of β-blockers. JAMA 263:1653–1657, 1990.
55. Leonetti G, Cuspidi C. Choosing the right ACE inhibitor: a guide to selection. Drugs 49:516–535, 1995.
55a. Hansson L, Lindholm LH, Niskaen A, et al. Effect of angiotensin-converting-enzyme inhibition compared with conventional therapy on cardiovascular morbidity and mortality in hypertension: the Captopril Prevention Project (CAPP) randomized trial. Lancet 353:611–616, 1999.
56. Culter JA. Commentary. Which drug for the treatment of hypertension? Lancet 353:604–605, 1999.
57. Hargreaves MR, Benson MK. Inhaled sodium cromoglycate in angiotensin-converting enzyme inhibitor cough. Lancet 345:13–16, 1995.
58. Herings RMC, de Boer A, Stricker BHC, et al. Hypoglycaemia associated with use of inhibitors of angiotensin converting enzyme. Lancet 345:1195–1198, 1995.
59. Baauer JH, Reams GP. The angiotensin II type 1 receptor antagonists: a new class of antihypertensive drugs. Arch Intern Med 155:1361, 1995.
60. Staesen JA, Fagard R, Thijs L, et al. Randomized double-blind comparison of placebo and active treatment for older patients with isolated systolic hypertension: the Systolic Hypertension in Europe (Syst-Eur) trial. Lancet 352:1347–1351, 1998.
61. Cubeddu LX, Aramda K, Somgj B, et al. A comparison of verapamil and propranolol for the initial treatment of hypertension: racial differences in response. JAMA 256:2214–2221, 1986.
62. Suissa S, Bourgault C, Barkun A, et al. Antihypertensive drugs and the risk of gastrointestinal bleeding. Am J Med 105:230–235, 1998.
63. Phillips BG, MacFarlane LL, Carson DS. Calcium-channel blockers and risk of myocardial infarction: more hype than harm. Circulation 92:1074, 1079, 1326, 1995.
64. Estacio RO, Jeffers BW, Hiatt WR, et al. The effect of nisoldipine as compared with enalapril on cardiovascular outcomes in patients with non-insulin dependent diabetes and hypertension. N Engl J Med 338:645–652, 1998.
65. Tatti, P, Pahor M, Byington RP, et al. Outcome results of the Fosinopril versus Amlodipine Cardiovascular Events Randomized Trial (FACET) in patients with hypertension and NIDDM. Diabetes Care 21:597–603, 1998.
66. Absascal VM, Larson MG, Evans JC, et al. Calcium antagonists and mortality risks in men and women with hypertension in the Framingham Heart Study. Arch Intern Med 158:1882–1886, 1999.
67. Cuter JA. Calcium-channel blockers for hypertension: uncertainty continues. Editorial. N Engl J Med 338:679–681, 1998.
68. Khoury AF, Kaplan NM. Alpha-blocker therapy of hypertension: an unfulfilled promise. JAMA 266:394–398, 1991.
69. Weber MA. Clinical pharmacology of centrally acting antihypertensive agents. J Clin Pharmacol 29:598–602, 1989.
70. Langley MS, Heel RC. Transdermal clonidine: a preliminary review of its pharmacodynamic properties and therapeutic efficacy. Drugs 35:123–142, 1988.
71. Mehta JL, Lopez LM. Rebound hypertension following abrupt cessation of clonidine and metoprolol: treatment with labetalol. Arch Intern Med 147:389–390, 1987.
72. Kaplan NM. Management of hypertensive emergencies. Lancet 344:1335–1338, 1994.
73. Pettinger WA, Mitchell HC. Side effects of vasodilator therapy. Hypertension 11(Suppl II):II34–36, 1988.
74. Philipp T, Anlauf M, Distler A, et al. Randomized double blind, multicenter comparison of hydrochlorothiazide, atenolol, nitrendipine and enalapril in antihypertensive treatment: results of the HANE study. BMJ 315:154–159, 1997.
75. Frishman WH, Bryzinski BS, Coulson LR, et al. A multifactorial trial design to assess combination therapy in hypertension. Arch Intern Med 154:1461–1468, 1994.
76. Frishman WH, Bryzinski BS, Coulson LR, et al. A multifactorial trial design to assess combination therapy in hypertension. Arch Intern Med 154:1461–1468, 1994.
77. Matterson BJ, Reda DJ, Cushman WC, et al. Single-drug therapy for hypertension in men: a comparison of six antihypertensive agents with placebo. N Engl J Med 328:914–921, 1993.
78. Black HR. Treatment of mild hypertension study: the more things change . . . [editorial]. JAMA 270:757–759, 1993.
79. Perry MH Jr, Binham S, Horney A, et al. Antihypertensive efficacy of treatment regimens used in Veterans Administration hypertension clinics. Hypertension 31:771–779, 1998.
80. Berlowitz DR, Ash AS, Hickey EC, et al. Inadequate management of blood pressure in a hypertensive population. N Engl J Med 23:1957–1963, 1998.
81. Dannenberg AL, Kannel WB. Remission of hypertension: the "natural" history of blood pressure treatment in the Framingham study. JAMA 257:1477–1483, 1987.
82. Espeland MA. Lifestyle interventions improve success rate of antihypertensive withdrawal in the elderly. Arch Fam Med 8:228–236, 1999.
83. Lakshman MR, Reda DJ, Materson BJ, et al. Diuretics and beta-blockers do not have adverse effects at 1 year on plasma lipid and lipoprotein profiles in men with hypertension. Arch Intern Med 159:551–558, 1999.
84. Schlueter WA, Batle DC. Renal effects of antihypertensive drugs. Drugs 37:900–925, 1989.
85. Inman SR, Stowe NT, Vidt DG. Role of the renal microcirculation in antihypertensive therapy. Cleve Clin J Med 61:356–361, 1994.

86. Moore MA, Epstein M, Agoddoa L, et al. Current strategies for management of hypertensive renal disease. Arch Intern Med 159:23–28, 1999.
87. Anderson KM, Wilson WF, Odell PM, et al. An updated coronary risk profile: a statement for health professionals. Circulation 83:356–361, 1991.
88. McCormick D, Gurwitz HJ, Lessard D, et al. Use of aspirin, beta-blockers and lipid-lowering medications before recurrent myocardial infarction. Missed opportunities for prevention? Arch Intern Med 159:561–567, 1999.
89. Stamler R, Stamler J, Grimm R, et al. Nutritional therapy for high blood pressure. Final report of a four-year randomized controlled trial: the hypertension control program. JAMA 257:1484–2491, 1987.
90. Thrift AG, McNeil, Forbes A, et al. Three important subgroups of hypertensive persons at greater risk of intracerebral hemorrhage. Hypertension 31:1223–1229, 1998.
91. Christlieb AR. Treatment selection considerations for the hypertensive diabetic patient. Arch Intern Med 150:1167–1174, 1990.
92. Peters AL, Hsueh W. Antihypertensive agents in diabetic patients: great benefits, special risks. Arch Intern Med 159:541–542, 1999.
93. UK Prospective Diabetes Study Group. Tight blood pressure control reduces the risk of macrovascular and microvascular complications in Type 2 diabetes (UKPDS 38). BMJ 317:703–713, 1998.
93a. UK Prospective Diabetes Study Group. Cost effectiveness analysis of improved blood pressure control in hypertensive patients with type 2 diabetes (UKPDS 40). BMJ 317:720–726, 1998.
93b. Tuomilehto J, Rastenyte D, Birkenhager WH, et al. Effects of calcium-channel blockade in older patients with diabetes and systolic hypertension. N Engl J Med 340:677–684, 1999.
94. O'Bryne S, Feely J. Effects of drugs on glucose tolerance in non-insulin dependent diabetics (part I). Drugs 40:6–18, 1990.
95. MacLeod MJ, McLay J. Drug treatment of hypertension complicating diabetes mellitus. Drugs 56:189–202, 1998.
96. Elliot WJ. Glucose and cholesterol elevations during thiazide therapy: intention-to-treat versus actual on-therapy experience. Am J Med 99:261–269, 1995.
97. Shorr RI, Ray WA, Daugherty JR, et al. Antihypertensives and the risk of serious hypoglycemia in older persons using insulin or sulfonylureas. JAMA 278:40–43, 1997.
98. Kasiske BL, Kalil RSN, Ma JZ, et al. Effect of antihypertensive therapy on the kidney in patients with diabetes: a meta-regression analysis. Ann Intern Med 118:129–138, 1993.
99. Pardell H, Tresserras R, Salto E, et al. Management of the hypertensive patient who smokes. Drugs 56:177–187, 1998.
100. O'Bryne S, Feely J. Effects of drugs on glucose tolerance in non-insulin dependent diabetics (part II). Drugs 40:203–219, 1990.
101. Slataper R, Vicknair N, Sadler R, et al. Comparative effects of different antihypertensive treatments on the progression of diabetic renal disease. Arch Intern Med 153:973–980, 1993.
102. Bennet NE. Hypertension in the elderly. Lancet 344:447–449, 1994.
103. Applegate WB, Pressel S, Wittes J, et al. Impact of the treatment of isolated systemic hypertension on behavioral variables: results from the Systolic Hypertension in the Elderly Program. Arch Intern Med 154:2154–2160, 1994.
104. Cooper ES, Kuller LH, Saunders E, et al. Cardiovascular diseases and stroke in African-Americans and other racial minorities in the United States: a statement for health professionals. Circulation 83:1462–1480, 1991.
105. Insua JT, Sacks HS, Lau TS, et al. Drug treatment of hypertension in the elderly: a meta-analysis. Ann Intern Med 121:355–362, 1994.
106. Staessen JA, Thijs L, Fagard R, et al. Calcium channel blockade and cardiovascular prognosis in the European trial on isolated systolic hypertension. Hypertension 32:410–416, 1998.
107. O'Malley K, Cox JP, O'Brien E. Choice of drug treatment for elderly hypertensive patients. Am J Med 90(Suppl 3A):27S–33S, 1991.
108. Pahor M, Shorr RI, Somes GW, et al. Diuretic-based treatment and cardiovascular events in patients with mild renal dysfunction enrolled in the systolic hypertension in the elderly program. Arch Intern Med 158:1340–1345, 1998.
109. Savage PJ, Pressel SL, Curb D, et al. Influence of long-tern, low-dose, diuretic-based, antihypertensive therapy on glucose, lipid, uric acid, and potassium levels in older men and women with isolated systolic hypertension. Arch Intern Med 158:741–751, 1998.
110. National High Blood Pressure Education Program Working Group report on high blood pressure in pregnancy. Am J Obstet Gynecol 163:1691–1712, 1990.
111. Galley EDM. Hypertension in pregnancy: practical management recommendations. Drugs 49:555–562, 1995.
112. Cangiano JL. Hypertension in Hispanic Americans. Cleve Clin J Med 61:345–350, 1994.
113. Eisner GM. Hypertension: racial differences. Am J Kidney Dis 16(Suppl 1):35–40, 1990.
114. Rutledge DR. Race and hypertension: what is clinically relevant. Drugs 47:914–932, 1994.
115. Saunders E, Weir MR, Kong W, et al. A comparison of the efficacy and safety of a β-blocker, a calcium channel blocker, and a converting enzyme inhibitor in hypertensive blacks. Arch Intern Med 150:1707–1713, 1990.
116. Hall WD, Reed JW, Flack JM, et al. Comparison of the efficacy of dihydropyridine calcium channel blockers in African American patients with hypertension. Arch Intern Med 158:2029–2034, 1998.
117. Preston RA, Materson BJ, Reda DJ, et al. Age-race subgroup compared with renin profile as predictors of blood pressure response to antihypertensive therapy. JAMA 280:1168–1172, 1998.
118. Zhou HH, Koshakji RP, Silbertein DJ, et al. Racial differences in drug response: altered sensitivity to and clearance of propranolol in men of Chinese decent as compared to American whites. N Engl J Med 320:565–570, 1989.
119. Ahsan CH, Macklin RB, Challenor VF, et al. Ethnic differences in the pharmacokinetics of oral nifedipine. Br J Clin Pharmacol 31:399–403, 1991.
120. Perez-Stable EJ. Management of mild hypertension: selecting an antihypertensive regimen. West J Med 154:78–87, 1991.
121. Croog SH, Levine S, Testa MA, et al. The effects of antihypertensive therapy on the quality of life. N Engl J Med 314:1657–1664, 1986.
122. Croog SH, Kong W, Levine S, et al. Hypertensive black men and women: quality of life and effects of antihypertensive medications. Arch Intern Med 150:1733–1741, 1990.
123. Wassertheil-Smoller S, Blaufox D, Oberman A, et al. Effect of antihypertensives on sexual function and quality of life: the TAIM study. Ann Intern Med 114:613–620, 1991.
124. Testa MA, Anderson RB, Nackley JF, et al. Quality of life and antihypertension therapy in men: a comparison of captopril and enalapril. N Engl J Med 328:907–913, 1993.
125. Lewis CE, Grandits GA, Flack J, et al. Efficacy and tolerance of antihypertensive treatment in men and women with stage 1 diastolic hypertension: results of the Treatment of Mild Hypertension Study. Arch Intern Med 156:377–385, 1996.
126. Friedman RB, Katt JA. Cost-benefit issues in the practice of internal medicine. Arch Intern Med 151:1165–1168, 1991.
127. Edelson JT, Weinstein MC, Tosteson ANA, et al. Long-term cost-effectiveness of various initial monotherapies for mild to moderate hypertension. JAMA 263:407–413, 1990.
128. Kaplan NM. Cost-effectiveness of antihypertensive drugs: fact or fancy? Am J Hypertens 4:478–480, 1991.
129. Hilleman DE, Mohiuddin SM, Lucas D Jr, et al. Cost-minimization analysis of initial antihypertensive therapy in patients with mild-to-moderate essential diastolic hypertension. Clin Ther 16:88–102, 1994.
129a. Siegel D, Lopez J, Meier J. Pharmacologic treatment of hypertension in the department of Veterans Affairs during 1995 and 1996. Am J Hypertens 11:1271–1278, 1998.
130. Materson BJ. Sexual dysfunction during antihypertensive treatment. Prog Pharmacol 6:117–124, 1985.
131. Croog SH, Levine S, Sudilovsky A, et al. Sexual symptoms in hypertensive patients. Arch Intern Med 148:788–794, 1988.
131a. Grimm RH, Grandits GA, Prineas RJ, et al. Long term effects on sexual function of five antihypertensive drugs and nutritional hygienic treatment in hypertensive men and women. Treatment of Mild Hypertension Study (TOMHS). Hypertension 29:8–14, 1997.
132. Jensen J, Lendorf A, Stimpel H, et al. The prevalence and etiology of impotence in 101 male hypertensive outpatients. Am J Hypertens 12:271–275, 1999.
133. Beers MH, Passman LJ. Antihypertensive medications and depression. Drugs 40:792–799, 1990.
134. Cruickshank JM, Thorp JM, Zacharias FJ. Benefits and potential harm of lowering high blood pressure. Lancet 1:581–583, 1987.
135. Staessen J, Bulpitt C, Clement D, et al. Relation between mortality and treated blood pressure in elderly patients with hypertension: report of the European Working Party on High Blood Pressure in the Elderly. BMJ 298:1552–1556, 1989.
136. Farnett L, Mulrow CD, Linn WD, et al. The *J*-curve phenomenon and the treatment of hypertension: is there a point beyond which pressure reduction is dangerous? JAMA 265:489–495, 1991.
137. McCloskey LW, Psaty BM, Koepsell TD, et al. Level of blood pressure and risk of myocardial infarction among treated hypertensive patients. Arch Intern Med 152:513–520, 1992.
138. Working Group on Management of Patients with Hypertension and High Blood Cholesterol. National education programs working group report on the management of patients with hypertension and high blood cholesterol. Ann Intern Med 114:224–237, 1991.
139. Kasiske BL, Ma JZ, Kalil RSN, et al. Effects of antihypertensive therapy on serum lipids. Ann Intern Med 122:133–141, 1995.

140. Samuelsson O, Wilhelmsen L, Andersson OK, et al. Cardiovascular morbidity in relation to change in blood pressure and serum cholesterol levels in treated hypertension: results from the Primary Prevention Trial in Goteborg, Sweden. JAMA 258:1768–1776, 1987.
141. Golomb BA, Criqui MH. Antihypertensive: much ado about lipids [editorial]. Arch Intern Med 159:535–537, 1999.
142. Francis Lam YW, Shepherd MM. Drug interactions in hypertensive patients: pharmacokinetic, pharmacodynamic and genetic considerations. Clin Pharmacokinet 18:295–317, 1990.
143. Brown J, Dollery C, Valdes G. Interaction of nonsteroidal anti-inflammatory drugs with antihypertensive and diuretic agents: control of vascular reactivity by endogenous prostanoids. Am J Med 81(Suppl 2B):43–57, 1986.
144. MacGregor GA, Sagnella GA, Markandu ND, et al. Double-blind study of three sodium intakes and long-term effects of sodium restriction in essential hypertension. Lancet 2:1244–1247, 1989.
145. Midgley JP, Matthew AG, Greenwood CMT, et al. Effect of reduced dietary sodium on blood pressure: a meta-analysis of randomized controlled trials. JAMA 275:1590–1597, 1996.
146. Schotte D, Stunkard AJ. The effect of weight reduction on blood pressure in 301 obese patients. Arch Intern Med 150:1701–1704, 1990.
147. The Trials of Hypertension Prevention Collaborative Research Group. Effects of weight loss and sodium reduction intervention on blood pressure and hypertension incidence in overweight people with high-normal blood pressure. The Trials of Hypertension Prevention II (TOHP II). Arch Intern Med 157:657–667, 1997.
148. Appel LJ, Moore TJ, Obarzanek E, et al. A clinical trial of the effects of dietary patterns on blood pressure. DASH (Dietary Approaches to Stop Hypertension) Collaborative Research Group. N Engl J Med 336:117–1124, 1997.
149. Svetkey LP, Simons-Morton D, Vollmer WM, et al. Effect of dietary patterns on blood pressure: subgroup analysis of Dietary Approaches to Stop Hypertension (DASH) randomized clinical trial. Arch Intern Med 159:285–293, 1999.
150. Hagberg JM, Seals DR. Exercise training and hypertension. Acta Med Scand 711(Suppl):131–136, 1990.
151. Dengel DR, Galecki AT, Hagberg JM, et al. The independent and combined effects of weight loss and aerobic exercise on blood pressure and oral glucose tolerance in older men. Am J Hypertens 11:1405–1412, 1998.
152. Klaus D. Management of hypertension in actively exercising patients: implications of drug selection. Drugs 37:212–218, 1989.
153. Mann SJ, James GD, Wang RS, et al. Elevation of ambulatory systolic blood pressure in hypertensive smokers: a case control study. JAMA 265:2226–2228, 1991.
154. Materson BJ, Reda D, Freis ED, et al. Cigarette smoking interferes with treatment of hypertension. Arch Intern Med 148:2116–2119, 1988.
155. Beevers DG, Maheswaran R, Potter JF. Alcohol, blood pressure and antihypertensive drugs. J Clin Pharmacol Ther 15:395–397, 1990.
156. Puddy JB, Beilin LJ, Vandongen R. Regular alcohol use raises blood pressure in treated hypertensive subjects: a randomized controlled trial. Lancet 1:647–651, 1987.
157. Cushman WC, Cutler JA, Hanna E, et al. Prevention and Treatment of Hypertension Study (PATHS): effects of an alcohol treatment program on blood pressure. Arch Intern Med 158:1197–1207, 1998.
158. Hart CL, Smith GD, Hole DJ, et al. Alcohol consumption and mortality from all causes, coronary heart disease and stroke: results from a prospective cohort study of Scottish men with 21 years of follow up. BMJ 318:1725–1729, 1999.
159. Sharp DS, Bentowitz NL. Pharmacoepidemiology of the effect of caffeine on blood pressure. Clin Pharmacol Ther 47:57–60, 1990.
160. Jeong DU, Dimsdale JE. The effects of caffeine on blood pressure in the work environment. Am J Hypertens 3:749–753, 1990.
161. Hakim AA, Ross GW, Curb D, et al. Coffee consumption in hypertensive men in older middle-age and the risk of stroke. The Honolulu Heart Program. J Clin Epidemiol 51:487–494, 1998.
162. Griffith LE, Guyatt GH, Cook RJ, et al. The influence of dietary and nondietary calcium supplementation on blood pressure. An updated meta-analysis of randomized controlled trials. Am J Hypertens 12:84–92, 1999.
163. Kawano Y, Matsuoka H, Takishita S, et al. Effects of magnesium supplementation in hypertensive patients. Hypertension 32:260–265, 1998.
164. Whelton PK, Appel LJ, Espland M, et al. Trial of Nonpharmacologic Interventions in the Elderly (TONE). JAMA 279:839–846, 1998.
165. Winickoff RN, Murphy PK. The persistent problem of poor blood pressure control. Arch Intern Med 147:1393–1396, 1987.
166. McClellan WM, Hall W, Brogan D, et al. Continuity of care in hypertension: an important correlate of blood pressure control among aware hypertensives. Arch Intern Med 148:525–528, 1988.
167. Vaur L, Vaisse B, Genes N, et al. Use of electronic pill boxes to assess risks of poor treatment compliance. Results of a large-scale trial. Am J Hypertens 12:374–380, 1999.
168. Lachman BE. Increasing patient compliance through tracking systems. California Pharmacist 34:54–58, 1987.
169. Oto-Kent DS. Controlling hypertension: pharmacists can make a difference. Calif Pharm 36:42–43, 1989.
170. McKenney JM, Slining JM, Henderson HR, et al. The effect of clinical pharmacy services on patients with essential hypertension. Circulation 48:1104–1111, 1973.
171. Hawkins DW, Fiedler FP, Douglas HL, et al. Evaluation of a clinical pharmacist in caring for hypertensive and diabetic patients. Am J Hosp Pharm 36:1321–1326, 1979.

CHAPTER 40

CONGESTIVE HEART FAILURE

Paul E. Nolan Jr. and Dawn G. Zarembski

Although there is no precise definition of congestive heart failure (CHF), CHF can be defined as a progressive, complex clinical syndrome characterized by dyspnea, fatigue, and fluid retention.[1,2] These symptoms may arise from any cardiac disorder that causes left ventricular (LV) dysfunction and diminished cardiac output (CO). These disorders activate a number of cardiac and peripheral neurohormonal compensatory adaptive responses, which with continued stimulation become maladaptive and ultimately affect fluid retention, disease progression, and mortality. However, a subgroup of patients with LV dysfunction are asymptomatic.[2] This subgroup is considered to have heart failure (HF) but without symptoms. The primary cardiac mechanisms that underlie the clinical syndrome of CHF and asymptomatic HF are systolic (i.e., contracting) and diastolic (i.e., filling) dysfunction, usually in combination.

TREATMENT GOALS: CONGESTIVE HEART FAILURE

- Relieve symptoms of central and peripheral circulatory congestion.
- Improve quality of life.
- Reduce neurohormonal activation.
- Prevent occurrence of CHF.
- Minimize or prevent acute CHF exacerbations.
- Slow progression of CHF.
- Increase survival.
- New therapies should neither worsen symptoms nor shorten life.

Overview

EPIDEMIOLOGY

Etiology

Some disparity exists in the reported frequencies of hypertension (HTN) and coronary artery disease (CAD) as causes of CHF. The Framingham Study, a community-based, longitudinal cohort investigation, reported an antecedent diagnosis of HTN, either alone or in conjunction with other causes in 74% of the patients diagnosed with CHF.[3] In contrast, a summary of 13 multicenter CHF drug trials published over the past 10 years and involving more than 20,000 patients listed CAD as the primary cause for CHF in almost 70% of the patients.[4] One possible explanation for the discrepant findings is that in the Framingham Study, diastolic dysfunction was not distinguished from systolic dysfunction, whereas in the summary of the drug trials, CHF was caused principally by systolic dysfunction. Nonetheless, in the Framingham Study a majority of patients (54%) had CAD as an attributable cause of CHF, and CAD was found with accompanying HTN 31% of the time.[3] Additional causes of CHF include idiopathic dilated cardiomyopathy, valvular heart disease, viruses, genetic abnormalities that promote familial hypertrophic or dilated cardiomyopathies, congenital heart disease, thyrotoxicosis, and atrial fibrillation. Any of these causes ultimately can engender decreases in the contractile performance of the heart (i.e., systolic dysfunction) or the ability of the heart to fill adequately during diastole (i.e., diastolic dysfunction; Table 40.1).

Drug-Induced Disease

Drugs are an uncommon cause of CHF (Table 40.1).[5] Antineoplastic agents such as the anthracycline antineoplastic agents, daunorubicin, and doxorubicin are well-described causes of CHF. Other antineoplastic agents, some immunomodulating drugs, ethanol, and cocaine also may produce CHF.

Prevalence

Largely because of an aging population and the enhanced survival after acute myocardial infarction (AMI), CHF is becoming an increasingly prevalent health care problem with notable socioeconomic consequences.[6] An estimated 4.6 million Americans, with nearly equal numbers of men and women, have CHF and are alive today.[7] For Caucasian, African American, and Mexican American men and women age 20 and older, the percentages of people with CHF are 2.8% and 2.2%, 3.2% and 2.8%, and 2.1% and 3.1%, respectively.[7] The prevalence of CHF increases considerably with age. For the age ranges of 45 to 54, 55 to 64, 65 to 74, and 75 and older, CHF is present in less than 2%, almost 5%, roughly 7%, and nearly 10%, respectively.[7] There are about 400,000 new cases of CHF per year.[7] The incidence of CHF, which also increases markedly with age, approaches 10 per 1000 population after age 65.[7] Patients with CHF accounted for 870,000 hospital discharges in 1996, which is more than twice the estimated number for 1979.[7] For people 65 years and older, CHF is the most common cause of hospitalization.[7]

Table 40.1 ▪ Causes of Heart Failure

A. Systolic dysfunction
  1. Echocardiographic and hemodynamic characteristics: ↓ LVEF, ↑ LVEDV, ↑ LVEDP
  2. Hypertension
  3. Coronary artery disease
  4. Idiopathic
  5. Valvular disease (e.g., mitral or aortic regurgitation)
  6. Viral
  7. Genetic abnormalities
  8. Drug-induced
     a. Anticancer drugs
        i. Anthracyclines
        ii. Cyclophosphamide
        iii. ?Paclitaxel
        iv. Mitoxantrone
        v. 5-Fluorouracil
        vi. ?Herceptin
     b. Ethanol
     c. Immunomodulating drugs
        i. Interferon-α
        ii. ?Interferons-β and -γ
        iii. Interleukin-2
     d. Cocaine

B. Diastolic dysfunction
  1. Echocardiographic and hemodynamic characteristics: normal or ↑ LVEF, ↑ LVEDP, normal or ↓ LVEDV
  2. Hypertension
  3. Advanced age
  4. Coronary artery disease
  5. Restrictive cardiomyopathies (e.g., amyloidosis)
  6. Valvular heart disease (e.g., aortic stenosis)
  7. Hypertrophic cardiomyopathy (e.g., idiopathic hypertrophic subaortic stenosis)
  8. Genetic abnormalities

LVEF, left ventricular ejection fraction; *LVEDV,* left ventricular end-diastolic volume; *LVEDP,* left ventricular end-diastolic pressure.

PATHOPHYSIOLOGY

Several generalized pathophysiologic conditions can lead to HF. These include pressure overload of the heart (e.g., HTN or aortic stenosis), volume overload (e.g., mitral or aortic valve regurgitation), loss of functional myocardial tissue (e.g., AMI), a generalized decrease in myocardial contractility (e.g., several types of dilated cardiomyopathies), and restricted filling (e.g., constrictive pericarditis or amyloidosis). Clinically, these conditions manifest as a reduction in systolic emptying (i.e., systolic dysfunction) or diastolic relaxation and filling (i.e., diastolic dysfunction). Either systolic or diastolic dysfunction can lead to a decrease in stroke volume (SV) and CO. The decrease in CO is sensed as a decrease in end-organ perfusion pressure principally by arterial baroreceptors.

In response to decreased CO, a number of compensatory (i.e., adaptive) responses, many of which are neurohormonally mediated, become activated (Fig. 40.1). Within the heart, ventricular dilation and hypertrophy (i.e., ventricular remodeling) occur. Ventricular dilation develops in response to an elevated end-diastolic pressure, a consequence of either systolic or diastolic dysfunction. An elevated end-diastolic pressure produces mechanical stretch, which stimulates myocyte lengthening through replication of sarcomeres in series (i.e., ventricular dilation or eccentric hypertrophy).[8] Ventricular dilation is an attempt to increase end-diastolic volume or preload to increase CO. As the ventricular chamber increases in size, it can fill to a greater extent during diastole, so SV increases during systole. This response often is depicted by the Frank–Starling relationship between systolic performance and diastolic filling. Preload is determined largely by the extracellular fluid volume and venous return. However, an increase in preload may raise systolic wall tension or stress. According to the LaPlace relationship, systolic wall tension equals the product of aortic pressure (P) and the internal radius of the ventricle (R) divided by the two times the wall thickness ($2h$): $T = (P \times R)/2h$. Preload is a component of

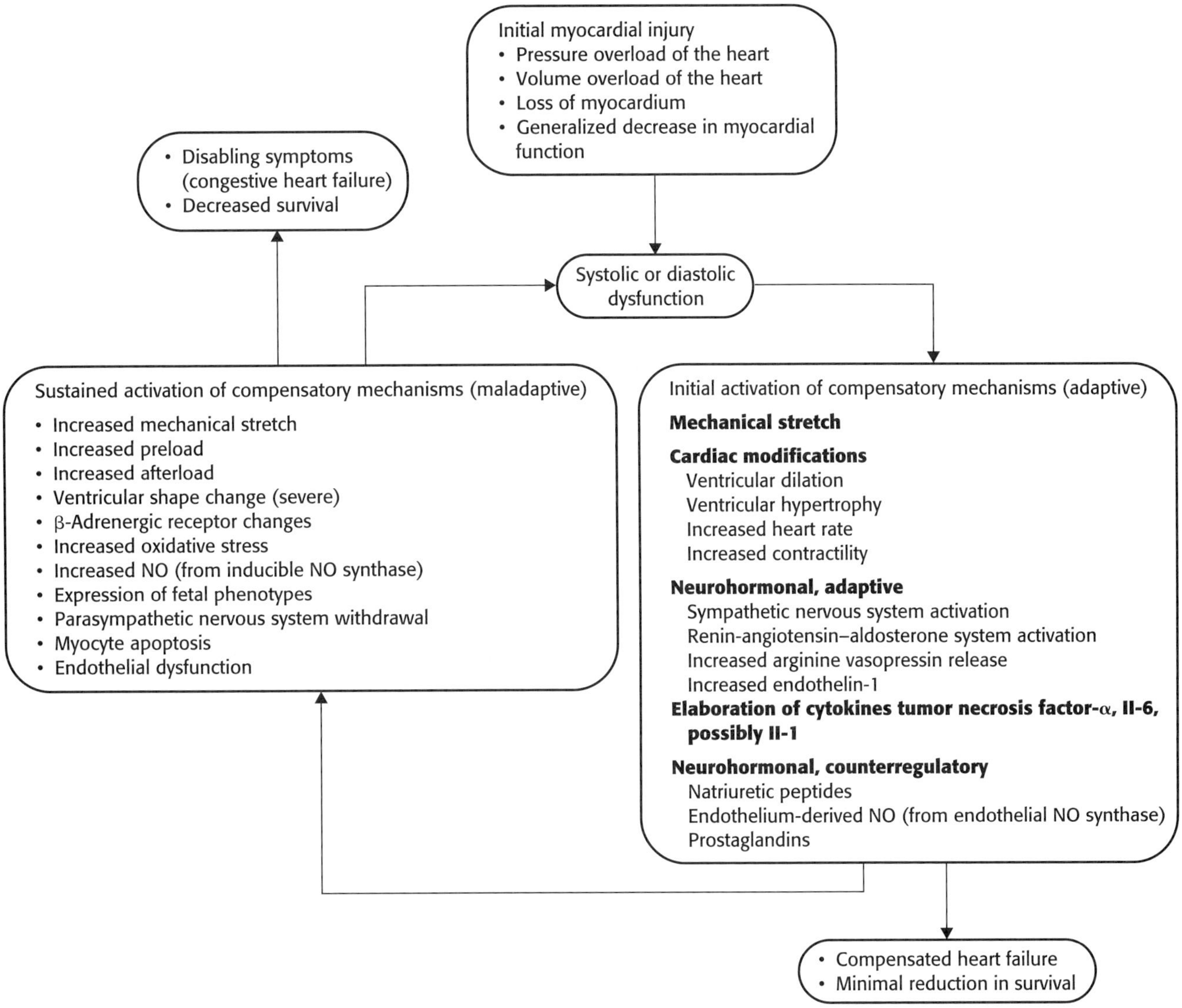

Figure 40.1. Pathogenesis of congestive heart failure. *IL*, interleukin.

wall tension in that it corresponds to the internal radius of the ventricular chamber. Therefore, increases in preload increase wall tension.

Cardiac myocyte hypertrophy or an increase in wall thickness also occurs, especially in response to the pressure overload of HTN or aortic stenosis, and is the result of an increase in the diameter of myocytes through the parallel addition of new sarcomeres (i.e., concentric hypertrophy).[8] This response is analogous to a weightlifter's increase in skeletal muscle size in response to lifting heavier weights. According to the LaPlace equation, the increase in wall thickness should result in a reduction in wall tension (or afterload) imposed on individual myocytes. Afterload is the hemodynamic load against which the ventricle must contract to deliver its SV. Afterload corresponds to the systolic wall tension defined previously. A major peripheral component of afterload is the systemic arteriolar tone or systemic vascular resistance, which also is a component of blood pressure (i.e., *P* in the LaPlace equation). In CHF it is common to see both parallel and series addition of sarcomeres.[8]

In addition to mechanical stretch, ventricular remodeling is mediated predominantly by initial activation of the sympathetic nervous system (SNS) and secondary activation of the renin–angiotensin–aldosterone (RAA) system (Fig. 40.1).[9,10] Norepinephrine (NE) and decreased renal perfusion pressure stimulate the release of renin by the kidney. Renin, both systemically and locally in the myocardium, first acts on angiotensinogen to convert it to angiotensin I (AI). AI is then converted to angiotensin II (AII) by angiotensin-converting enzyme (ACE). AII also can be synthesized locally via chymase, an ACE-independent pathway.[10] NE and AII act as mitogens for cardiac myocytes to increase the number of sarcomeres (i.e., cardiac hypertrophy).[8] AII enhances SNS activity by facilitating presynaptic NE release.[10] AII also stimulates the release of aldosterone from the adrenals and facilitates secretion of arginine vasopressin (AVP). In turn, aldosterone and AVP trigger renal sodium and water retention, respectively.[10] Blood volume is expanded, so preload is augmented. AII also enhances the formation of preproendothelin by endothelial cells. Preproendothelin is cleaved by endothelin-converting enzyme (ECE) to form endothelin-1 (ET-1), which stimulates further release of renin and aldosterone as well as further conversion of AI to AII in endothelial cells.[11] Therefore, ET-1 also promotes sodium retention. Furthermore, myocardial contractility is enhanced because NE, AII, and ET-1 are positive inotropic agents, the former via stimulation of β_1 receptors.[9–11] NE also increases heart rate (HR) via β-receptor stimulation.[9] In addition, cytokines such as tumor necrosis factor-α (TNF-α) and interleukin-6 (IL-6), the former being secreted by cardiomyocytes, become elaborated and probably play a role in facilitating early ventricular dilation by stimulating increased activity of matrix metalloproteinases (MMPs).[12,13] MMPs are enzymes that degrade extracellular matrix, thereby augmenting LV remodeling. Thus, neurohormonally mediated increases in contractility, HR, preload, and myocardial hypertrophy along with cytokine-mediated ventricular remodeling maintain CO after initial myocardial injury.

In the peripheral circulation NE, AII, and ET-1 promote systemic vasoconstriction via stimulation of vascular α-receptors, AII type 1 receptor (AT_1), and ET-1 type A (ET_A) receptors, respectively, to maintain perfusion pressure.[9–11] However, systemic vasoconstriction causes an increase in afterload. Sustained increases in afterload can lead to a decreased SV and CO, especially in advanced CHF. Nonetheless, the increase in afterload initially is compensated by release of atrial and brain natriuretic peptides (ANP and BNP) in response to atrial and ventricular stretch, respectively, which result from increased ventricular dilation.[14] ANP, and presumably BNP, decrease renin secretion, attenuate the stimulatory effects of AII on aldosterone release, inhibit the release of NE through stimulation of vagal afferents, inhibit growth of vascular smooth muscle and endothelial cells, and produce vasodilatory and natriuretic effects to reduce the hemodynamic load on the heart.[14] Recently a fourth natriuretic peptide, dendroaspis natriuretic peptide (DNP), has been identified in human atria and in the circulation of patients with CHF.[15] However, the role of DNP in the neurohormonal activation characteristic of CHF has not been determined. In addition to ANP and BNP, vasodilation is also promoted by nitric oxide (NO) synthesized by endothelium-derived nitric oxide synthase (eNOS or NOS_3), which is expressed in cardiomyocytes and endothelial cells and upregulated by mechanical stress.[16] Prostaglandins, prostacyclin (PGI_2) and prostaglandin E_2, also contribute to vasodilation. The increase in nitric oxide and prostaglandin synthesis may result from ET-1 stimulation of endothelial ET_B receptors.[11]

Thus, after the initial myocardial damage there appears to be a balance between vasoconstrictive and vasodilatory systems as well as sodium and fluid-retaining and excreting systems. However, over time, the initial neurohormonal adaptive responses overshoot (i.e., become maladaptive), producing a progressive, vicious cycle in the disease process, leading to the signs and symptoms of CHF and ultimately death (Fig. 40.1). Within the heart there is NE-, AII-, and ET-1–mediated deposition of collagen and other components of the extracellular matrix among cardiomyocytes.[8] This increases chamber stiffness, decreases compliance, reduces delivery of nutrients to cardiomyocytes, and further elevates end-diastolic pressure and therefore mechanical stress. Conversely, continued eccentric ventricular remodeling may result from the dissolution of collagen and other extracellular matrix tethers by MMP, causing side-to-side slippage of myocytes, further ventricular dilation, and increased preload and wall stress.[8,13] Continued cardiomyocyte hypertrophy and extracellular matrix production also may result in cardiomyocyte energy starvation.[17] This can result from reductions in oxygen supply caused by a decreased capillary density; oxygen diffusion impairment caused by myocyte hypertrophy and adjacent fibrosis, both of which increase the distance between perfusing capillaries and the adenosine triphosphate (ATP)-consuming myofibrils; or impairments in mitochondrial ATP production. Each of these in turn may contribute to the development of cardiomyocyte apoptosis.

Continued activation of neurohormonal responses, although intended to maintain an effective CO, becomes deleterious. Diminished contractile response actually results from sustained, increased concentrations of NE caused by downregulation of principally myocardial β_1 receptors and uncoupling of β1 and β_2 receptors. β-Receptor uncoupling is caused by phosphorylation of the β-receptor, which, in effect, inactivates the receptor; upregulation of inhibitory G-proteins; or sequestration of the receptors.[18] Impaired contractility may also result from alterations in other cardiac gene expressions such as the downregulation of sarcoplasmic reticulum ATPase, a protein important in excitation–contraction coupling in the heart, and upregulation of β-myosin heavy chain (MyHC), a fetal form of MyHC that produces less energy for muscle contraction than adult α-MyHC.[9,18] In addition, elevated, persistent activation of the SNS promotes myocardial apoptosis[8] and impairs parasympathetic influence on the heart,[19] which diminishes the normal arterial baroreceptor response and increases the risk of proarrhythmia. AII and ET-1 also promote myocyte apoptosis.[8] Peripheral vasoconstriction is further augmented and vasodilatory capacity impaired by NE, AII, and ET-1 along with increased sodium content of peripheral blood vessels. In addition, persistently increased levels of TNF-α and IL-6 diminish endothelium-mediated vasorelaxation and produce negative inotropic effects, largely by stimulating inducible nitric oxide synthase (iNOS or NOS_2) in cardiomyocytes.[16,20,21] This greatly increases myocardial concentrations of NO, which attenuate responsiveness to β-adrenergic stimulation and enhances myocyte apoptosis, perhaps by generating oxygen free radicals.[16,20,21] The counterregulatory vasodilator responses mediated by ANP, BNP, NO (produced by eNOS), and prostaglandins become overwhelmed. In addition, unrelenting stimuli that trigger sodium and water retention override counterbalancing salt-excreting systems (natriuretic peptides and prostaglandins) and further expand intravascular volume and pressure, resulting in circulatory congestion and edema. Altered skeletal muscle structure and function combined with decreased perfusion produce fatigue and exercise intolerance.

In summary, HF begins when myocardial and peripheral adaptive responses are activated to maintain an effective perfusion pressure after initial myocardial damage. HF progresses when these compensatory, chiefly neurohormonally and cytokine-mediated responses persist. This leads to a series of deleterious effects on the heart, circulation, and end organs such as the kidney and liver, resulting in CHF, that are manifest by classic physical and laboratory signs, disabling symptoms, and ultimately death.

CLINICAL PRESENTATION AND DIAGNOSIS

Knowledge of the pathophysiology of CHF easily predicts the expected signs, symptoms, and associated laboratory findings (Table 40.2).[22] However, many patients with impaired LV systolic function (i.e., left ventricular ejection fraction [LVEF] less than 40%) may exhibit no signs or

Table 40.2 ▪ Pathophysiologic Mechanisms Responsible for the Signs and Symptoms of Heart Failure

Left-Sided Sign or Symptom	Pathophysiologic Mechanism
Orthopnea Paroxysmal nocturnal dyspnea	Reintroduction of pooled blood from lower extremities after the patient assumes a supine position produces an abrupt increase in preload. The failing heart is unable to accommodate such abrupt increases in LVEDP, leading to pulmonary congestion and edema.
Pulmonary edema Bibasilar crackles	The failing heart is unable to accommodate increases in LVEDP, leading to pulmonary congestion, increased pulmonary vein hydrostatic pressure, and pulmonary edema.
Cough	Pulmonary congestion. Bradykinin accumulation secondary to the use of angiotensin-converting enzyme inhibitors.
Right-Sided Sign or Symptom	**Pathophysiologic Mechanism**
Peripheral edema Increased body weight	Sodium and water retention produces an increase in blood volume and venous hydrostatic pressure. Transudation of fluid into the subcutaneous tissue ensues. Albumin usually is decreased because of reduced hepatic synthesis and altered nutrition. Oncotic pressure is altered by the reduction in serum albumin.
Hepatomegaly Increased INR	Chronic venous congestion produces congestion of the liver. Synthesis of clotting factors can be reduced.
Jugular venous distension	Central blood volume is increased, leading to an increase in central venous pressure upon compression of the liver.
Nonspecific Sign or Symptom	**Pathophysiologic Mechanism**
Resting tachycardia Atrial fibrillation Ventricular arrhythmias	The reduction in cardiac output produces a compensatory increase in sympathetic nervous system activity, leading to an increase in heart rate and intracellular influx of calcium. The increase in norepinephrine along with parasympathetic withdrawal, myocardial architectural changes, and electrolyte disturbances predispose patients to arrhythmias.
Ventricular dilation and remodeling Enlarged heart (cardiac heave) Increased cardiothoracic ratio on chest roentgenograph	The ventricle dilates to accommodate increases in preload. Consequently, the natural elliptical shape of the ventricle is lost and the ventricle becomes spherical and baggy. Thus, the ratio of the size of the heart to thoracic cavity increases.
Fatigue and diminished exercise tolerance	Cardiac output is diminished, limiting oxygen delivery to brain and skeletal muscle. In addition, the ability to increase cardiac output in the face of exercise is reduced. Consequently, the skeletal muscles quickly become hypoxic. There are also defects in skeletal and respiratory musculature that contribute to fatigue and exercise limitations.
Altered mental status, confusion	Reduced cardiac output and oxygen delivery to central nervous system.
Hypotension	Blood pressure decreases secondary to a reduction in cardiac output ($MAP \approx CO \times SVR$).
Nocturia	Reintroduction of pooled blood from lower extremities after the patient assumes a supine position produces an increase in venous return. An increase in blood flow to the kidney occurs.
Oliguria Increased blood urea nitrogen and serum creatinine Increased urine specific gravity Hyponatremia	Reductions in cardiac output and secondary increases in norepinephrine, angiotensin II, and other neurohormones reduce blood flow to the kidney, leading to a reduction in urine output. Urea and creatinine are not filtered normally. Effects of increased arginine vasopressin result in dilutional hyponatremia, a concentrated urine, and inability to excrete free water.

LVEDP, left ventricular end-diastolic pressure; *MAP*, mean arterial pressure; *CO*, cardiac output; *SVR*, systemic vascular resistance.

symptoms of CHF. Up to 20% of patients with LVEF less than 40% may not meet clinical criteria diagnostic for CHF.[23] Nonetheless, most patients with LVEF less than 40% exhibit signs and symptoms of CHF. An understanding of the essential elements of the cardiovascular physical examination is key to appropriate monitoring of HF therapy.

The underlying reduction in CO that occurs in CHF stimulates compensatory mechanisms, leading to sodium and water retention and increased sympathetic activity. Sodium and water retention produces an increase in preload, which the failing heart is unable to manage. As is characteristic in most patients with CHF, systemic and pulmonary congestion ensues. Signs and symptoms of congestion relate to the failing ventricle. Pulmonary congestion develops secondary to failure of the left ventricle, whereas systemic congestion occurs secondary to failure of the right ventricle. LV failure is more common, however, because the ventricles share a common wall, and given considerable interventricular dependence, most patients eventually develop biventricular failure and consequently exhibit both systemic and pulmonary congestion.

Pulmonary pressures are increased in CHF by the diminished ability of the left ventricle to accept or eject the excess blood volume. Pulmonary congestion is manifest by varying degrees of breathlessness: dyspnea on exertion (DOE); orthopnea (dyspnea that occurs in the supine position); paroxysmal nocturnal dyspnea (PND), an exaggerated form of orthopnea that occurs when the patient is awakened abruptly at night with a feeling of suffocation; dyspnea at rest; and pulmonary edema (fluid accumulation in the alveoli). Some patients complain of cough or asthma symptoms.

Typically, DOE is the first symptom of CHF.[24] As the disease progresses, the degree of physical activity that produces dyspnea decreases. The level of activity that produces dyspnea can be used to monitor disease severity. Patients with severe CHF complain of dyspnea at rest and may demonstrate Cheyne–Stokes breathing (alternating hyperventilation and apnea). Orthopnea occurs within minutes after the patient assumes a supine position. A supine position places the lower extremities on the same vertical plane as the heart. Venous pooling, which occurs while the patient is standing, is reduced and the fluid is reintroduced into the central circulatory system, leading to pulmonary congestion. Sitting upright relieves orthopnea once it occurs. Increasing the number of pillows the patient uses to sleep often circumvents orthopnea, and changes in the number of pillows used while sleeping can be used to monitor the patient's condition. PND awakens the patient after 2 to 4 hours of sleep with the feeling of suffocation. Relief is obtained by maintaining an upright position and may take up to 30 minutes to occur. Severe pulmonary congestion, with accumulation of fluid in the alveoli, can occur, producing pulmonary edema. Patients may experience severe shortness of breath and anxiety as a result. Often patients with pulmonary edema expectorate a pink, frothy sputum. On physical examination, bibasilar rales (a crackling sound) may be heard upon lung auscultation. Rales are consistent with fluid accumulation in the alveoli. Pulmonary congestion may also be observed in a chest roentgenogram. Findings consistent with pulmonary congestion include pleural effusions and Kerley lines. Careful interpretation of the physical examination is warranted in patients with CHF. For instance, because of a compensatory increase in lymphatic drainage, patients with chronic CHF can have very high LV filling pressures but no detectable rales. Therefore, the absence of rales does not preclude the existence of elevated pulmonary pressures.

Systemic venous congestion may manifest as weight gain, dependent peripheral edema, jugular venous distension (JVD), and congestive hepatomegaly. Hepatic edema may cause right upper quadrant pain. Generalized visceral edema may also occur and cause abdominal distension, anorexia, nausea, and constipation. Patient weight should be assessed frequently because an increase in fluid retention is observed before the onset of peripheral edema. Short-term weight changes can be used to assess short-term fluctuations in fluid status. A gain of approximately 10 lb of extracellular fluid volume must occur before peripheral edema is noted. This edema usually develops in the gravity-dependent areas of the body such as the ankles and feet, or above the shinbone (i.e., pretibial) in ambulatory patients and in the sacral area when the patient is supine. Peripheral edema may be physically uncomfortable as well as cosmetically unattractive. Peripheral edema is specific for CHF in less than 30% of patients.[25] Additional populations at risk for peripheral edema include older adults, obese patients, and patients with peripheral vascular disease. In addition, the presence or absence of peripheral edema can be affected by the use of diuretics and vasodilators.

Central venous pressure (CVP) is estimated by elevating the patient's head to a 45° angle and observing the peak of the maximal venous pulsation in the internal jugular vein. In this position, the CVP normally does not exceed 2 cm of vertical distance above the sternal angle. Because the sternal angle usually lies about 5 cm above the right atrium, the CVP can be estimated by noting the vertical distance and adding 5 cm to the value. The liver is also characteristically congested in CHF and is generally palpable several centimeters below the right costal margin. Pressure on the abdomen further increases the jugular venous pressure (because the right ventricle cannot accept the increased blood returned to the heart) and produce a positive hepatojugular reflex. Visual examination of the jugular veins remains a reliable way to noninvasively assess the overall fluid status of the patients, provided the assessment is performed appropriately.[26] In addition, a quick assessment of the jugular veins may be useful in determining which patients warrant further attention by a physician.[27] Again, it is important to remember that signs of systemic congestion may be affected by the use of diuretics and vasodilators. In addition, systemic signs of fluid overload reflect elevated right-sided pressures and can occur secondary to conditions other than CHF, such as mitral stenosis and pulmonary HTN.

Systemically, inadequate perfusion of the skeletal muscles often leads to easy fatigability and weakness. Exercise tolerance is diminished, and patients adjust their lifestyles accordingly, such as no longer walking up a flight of steps. Nocturia (increased urine formation at night), which results from redistribution of blood flow to the kidney during recumbency, often occurs early in the course of CHF. Oliguria may become manifest later as the patient's HF worsens. A host of cerebral symptoms may also be observed and can include memory impairment, confusion, and insomnia.

A number of cardiac and systemic physical findings are observed with varying frequencies. An early diastolic third heart sound, S_3 (i.e., "Ken-tuc-KY," where "Ken," "tuc," and "ky" represent S_1, S_2, and S_3 respectively) is believed to be related to impaired diastolic relaxation of the ventricle and suggests an elevated end-diastolic pressure. An S_3 is a hallmark of moderate to severe HF.[28] A resting sinus tachycardia is often present. Objective cardiac findings often include an enlarged heart (palpable as a cardiac heave) and an increased cardiothoracic ratio (more than 0.50) as determined by chest roentgenogram. LV ejection fraction (LVEF) is most commonly assessed via a two-dimensional echocardiogram.[1] Patients with an LVEF less than 40% are considered to have systolic dysfunction. In addition, echocardiography can be used to assess LV chamber size, geometry, wall thickness, and valve function. Segmental wall motion abnormalities, suggesting an ischemic cardiomyopathy, can be observed on echocardiography, but coronary angiography is needed to assess the presence and severity of atherosclerotic heart disease. Furthermore, an assessment of viability may be needed before revascularization is attempted. Coronary angiography and radionuclide ventriculography are alternatives to echocardiography that can be used to assess LVEF. LV function measurement may be indicated every 12 to 24 months in unstable patients.

Numerous laboratory abnormalities are observed in patients with CHF. Simple laboratory tests (i.e., body weight, serum electrolytes, serum creatinine [Scr] and blood urea nitrogen [BUN], and serum digoxin concentration [SDC]), body weight, and chest roentgenogram are used most often in monitoring ambulatory patients with CHF.[29] At home, patients should monitor their weight daily. Serum electrolytes and markers of renal function can be checked every 1 to 3 months depending on the patient's clinical status and provided there are no changes in therapy. Total body sodium (Na^+) often is increased. However, a dilutional hyponatremia is commonly seen because of a diminished ability to excrete free water. Hyponatremia may worsen with diuretic treatment. Patients with CHF generally have deficits of both total body and intracellular potassium (K^+) and magnesium (Mg^{+2}), which may or may not be reflected in the serum concentrations of these cations.[30] These electrolyte deficiencies coupled with increased neurohormones may predispose patients to the development of potentially lethal ventricular arrhythmias. Impaired hepatic function may occur secondary to venous congestion and may be characterized by elevations in plasma concentrations of hepatic enzymes. Reductions in renal blood flow and glomerular filtration rate (GFR) are reflected by increases in both Scr and BUN levels. The urine usually is concentrated, with a high urine specific gravity, and there may be associated proteinuria.

A LVEF less than 40% indicates LV systolic dysfunction. CHF is a clinical diagnosis that can be observed in patients with either systolic or diastolic dysfunction. No one symptom can be considered the diagnostic gold standard of CHF. Rather, the presence of any single symptom warrants echocardiographic assessment of LV function with consideration of CHF as a possible cause. It is important to remember that symptoms alone are not indicative of CHF, and proper evaluation includes consideration of the clinical presentation and potential underlying causes. Past medical history is important to elicit the presence of prior myocardial infarction, HTN, and valvular disease and may aid in the diagnosis of CHF. In the future, measurement of circulating BNP may be a useful screening tool for LV systolic dysfunction.[31,32]

To evaluate both the severity of HF and the responses to therapy, two classification systems have been developed: the New York Heart Association (NYHA) Functional Classification[33] and a classification based on maximal exercise tolerance[34] (Table 40.3). Unfortunately, these classification systems do not correlate well. The NYHA classification, despite its reliance on subjective findings during exertion, is commonly used to classify the severity of CHF.[33] Initially, patients may present with severe symptoms (NYHA class IV) despite well-preserved LV function. In addition, patients often downgrade their expectations for exercise tolerance as CHF progresses. Consequently, the NYHA classification system may not correlate accurately with disease severity. The NYHA classification probably will remain popular among practitioners because of its simplicity and convenience. In addition to NYHA classification, quality of life can be assessed via a variety of methods, including the Minnesota Living with Heart Failure Questionnaire, the Chronic Heart Failure Questionnaire, the Specific Activity Scale, the Yale Scale, and the Quality of Life Questionnaire in Severe Heart Failure.[35]

The exercise tolerance classification system uses an incremental treadmill exercise protocol and noninvasive monitoring of respiratory gas exchange, HR, and blood pressure to grade the severity of chronic CHF.[34] Maximal oxygen uptake (Vo_{2max}, expressed in mL/minute/kg) is determined by maximal CO and by the maximal extraction of oxygen by the exercising muscles. Despite its relative objectivity and prognostic utility, it is a more complex, costly, and time-consuming method for evaluating CHF severity and responses to therapy. Furthermore, it

Table 40.3 ▪ Classification Systems for Congestive Heart Failure

Functional Capacity	Objective Assessment
New York Heart Association functional classification	
Class I. Patients with cardiac disease but without resulting limitation of physical activity. Ordinary physical activity does not cause undue fatigue, palpitation, dyspnea, or anginal pain.	A. No objective evidence of cardiovascular disease
Class II. Patients with cardiac disease resulting in slight limitation of physical activity. They are comfortable at rest. Ordinary physical activity results in fatigue, palpitation, dyspnea, or anginal pain.	B. Objective evidence of minimal cardiovascular disease
Class III. Patients with cardiac disease resulting in marked limitation of physical activity. They are comfortable at rest. Less than ordinary activity causes fatigue, palpitation, dyspnea, or anginal pain.	C. Objective evidence of moderately severe cardiovascular disease
Class IV. Patients with cardiac disease resulting in inability to carry out any physical activity without discomfort. Symptoms of heart failure or the anginal syndrome may be present even at rest. If any physical activity is undertaken, discomfort is increased.	D. Objective evidence of severe cardiovascular disease
Classification of heart failure based on maximal exercise tolerance	
Class A: No impairment: Vo_{2max} ≥20 mL/min/kg	
Class B: Mild to moderate impairment: Vo_{2max} = 16–20 mL/min/kg	
Class C: Moderate to severe impairment: Vo_{2max} = 10–15 mL/min/kg	
Class D: Severe impairment: Vo_{2max} <10 mL/min/kg	

Vo_{2max}, maximal oxygen (O_2) uptake. It is a function of the maximum cardiac output that the heart can generate and the maximum amount of oxygen that the exercising tissues can extract.

is effort dependent and may not be representative of the usual degree of physical activity for the typical patient. Its most appropriate uses may be to identify the patient's suitability for employment, rehabilitation programs, and cardiac transplantation.[1] An alternative measure of quantifying exercise capacity and its response to treatment is the 6-minute walk, which may better represent the patient's usual degree of physical activity.[36]

THERAPEUTIC PLAN

Therapeutic goals are achieved using a combination of patient and family education and support, nonpharmacologic, and pharmacologic, therapies, and surgical and related interventions (Table 40.4).[37,38] Nonpharmacologic treatment incorporates salt restriction, initial reduction of the heart's work load with abbreviated rest followed by exercise training upon recovery, lifestyle changes, and identification, treatment, and removal of precipitating causes.[37,38] Current pharmacologic therapy for CHF caused by systolic dysfunction consists of vasodilators (usually ACE inhibitors [ACEIs]), β-adrenergic receptor blockers, diuretics, and mild inotropic enhancement with digoxin (Fig. 40.2).[38] Surgical and related interventions include coronary artery bypass graft (CABG) surgery, orthotopic heart transplantation (OHT), and the use of artificial ventricles as bridges to transplantation.[39]

The majority of this chapter is devoted to the treatment of symptomatic HF (i.e., CHF) caused by systolic dysfunction (Fig. 40.2). HF secondary to diastolic dysfunction is treated very differently and is therefore discussed in a separate section (Fig. 40.3). A treatment algorithm also is included for asymptomatic systolic dysfunction (Fig. 40.4).

Table 40.4 ▪ General Nonpharmacologic and Pharmacologic Components in Treating the Patient with Heart Failure

- Patient and family education
  - Discussions and pamphlets on signs and symptoms of heart failure
  - Discussions and pamphlets on medications
  - Emphasis on compliance with complete treatment agenda
  - Instructions on when to contact health care providers (see Table 40.5)
- Diet
  - Daily weight chart
  - Individualized diet according to needs, preferences, and lifestyle
  - Sodium restriction, mild (<3 g/day) or moderate (<2 g/day)
  - Information about sodium content in foods
  - Information about potassium content in foods
  - Weight loss when appropriate
  - Alcohol restriction
  - Fluid restriction: ~2 L/day
  - Nutritional supplements (e.g., vitamins)
  - Emphasize importance of compliance
- Other
  - Smoking cessation
  - Pharmacologic treatment of hyperlipidemia
  - Pharmacologic treatment of diabetes
  - Pharmacologic treatment of hypertension
- Exercise
  - Consultation and prescription
- Psychosocial services
  - Evaluate emotional needs and presence of depression
  - Use individualized counseling or antidepressants
  - Evaluate financial needs
  - Support groups
  - End-of-life issues
- Intensive follow-up
  - Telephone calls
  - Home visits
  - Outpatient clinic visits

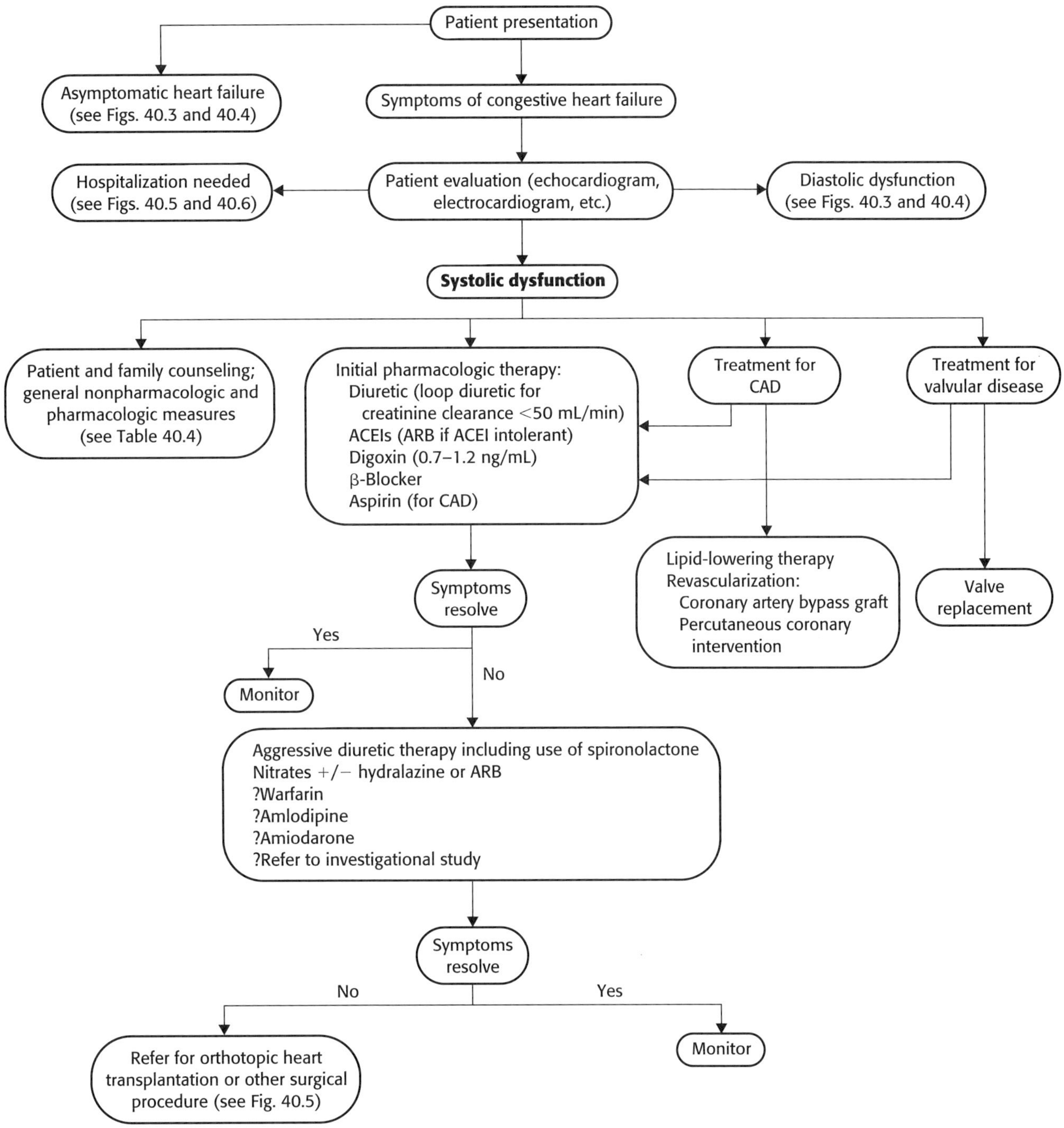

Figure 40.2. Treatment algorithm for symptomatic systolic dysfunction. *ACEI,* angiotensin-converting enzyme inhibitor; *ARB,* angiotensin II type 1 receptor blocker; *CAD,* coronary artery disease.

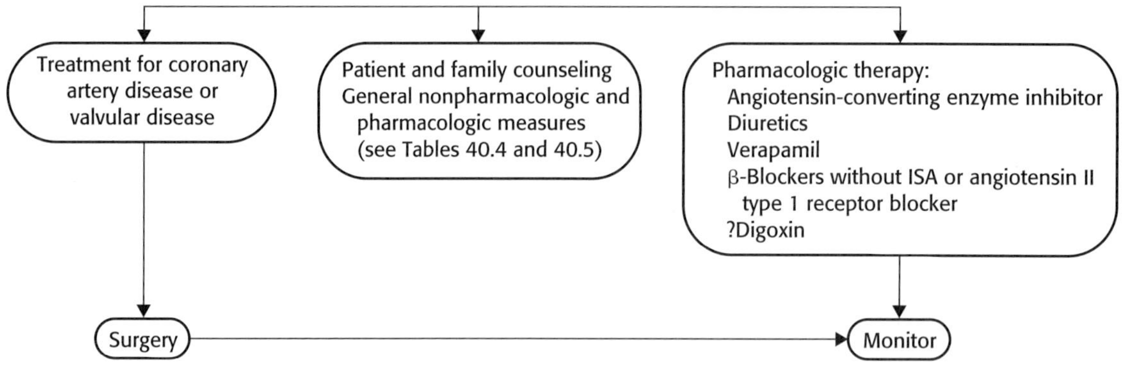

Figure 40.3. Treatment algorithm for symptomatic diastolic dysfunction.

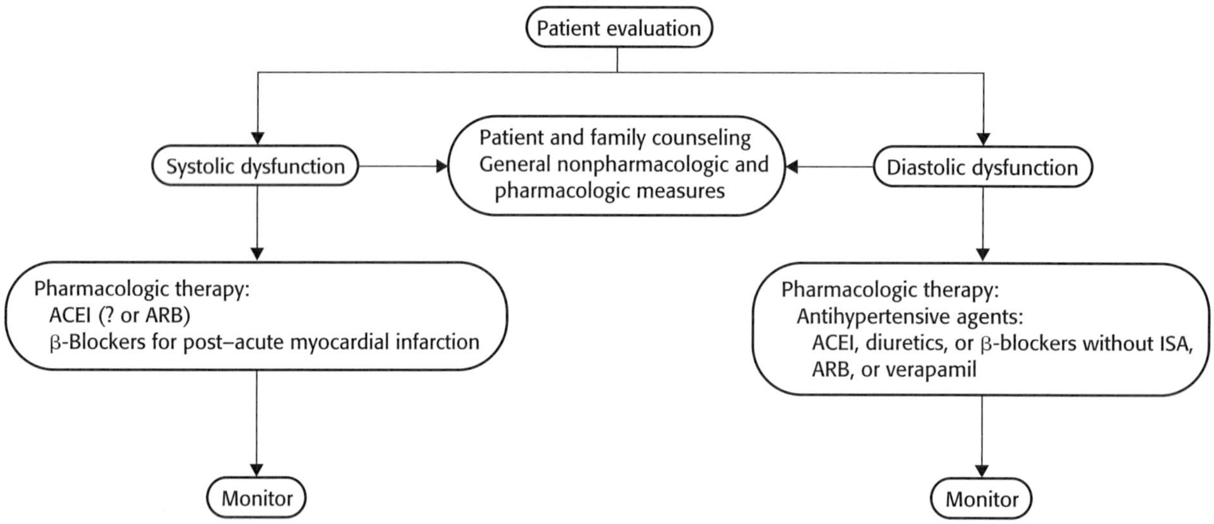

Figure 40.4. Treatment algorithm for asymptomatic heart failure. *ACEI,* angiotensin-converting enzyme inhibitor; *ARB,* angiotensin II type 1 receptor blocker.

Chronic Congestive Heart Failure Secondary to Systolic Dysfunction

TREATMENT

General Nonpharmacologic and Pharmacologic Measures

Initial measures in CHF management (Table 40.4) should focus on preventing the disease.[40] For example, alteration of correctable risk factors for CAD, a major etiologic factor for CHF, should be attempted. Proper prevention should include attempts to normalize serum lipids, blood pressure, and body weight. Patient education should also emphasize the importance of smoking cessation and moderate exercise.

Proper CHF management includes attempts to modify or correct systemic diseases causing or precipitating CHF exacerbations.[40] CAD, if present, may impair ventricular function through ongoing myocardial ischemia. Attempts at revascularization in appropriate patients may enhance ventricular function and survival. Patients with valvular disease may benefit from attempts to surgically repair or replace defective myocardial valves. In patients with symptomatic bradycardia, optimal CO can be ensured through the maintenance of sinus rhythm with pacemaker placement. Additional precipitating factors include systemic infection, pulmonary embolism, hypocalcemia, anemia, and endocrine disorders (e.g., hyperthyroidism). Acute CHF exacerbations may be prevented through judicious administration of pneumococcal and influenza vaccines.[40]

Initial restriction of physical activity to some degree is used to treat virtually any patient with CHF.[40] However, severe restrictions on physical activity may worsen a patient's exercise tolerance and lead to additional psychological problems. Many patients with CHF benefit from a carefully prescribed cardiac rehabilitation program. However, the actual minimum level of physical exertion needed to achieve improvements has not been defined. The actual type of physical activity that affords the greatest benefit to patients with CHF also is unknown. However, some form of regular aerobic exercise can enhance the cardiovascular system and improve exercise tolerance.[41,42] General improvement in physical condition can be accompanied by hemodynamic benefits, including reduction of the resting HR, reduction of exercise-associated peak systolic blood pressure (SBP), and an improvement in the tissue oxygen extraction. Long-term participation in exercise training may reduce mortality and improve quality of life for patients with CHF.[43]

Exercise capacity varies widely. Patients with severe CHF may be unable to tolerate low-intensity exercise, and more strenuous physical activity may not be tolerated even in patients with compensated CHF. Therefore, each patient should receive individualized instruction. It is not possible to predict exercise tolerance from either LVEF or other clinical parameters. However, patients who cannot increase their CO with exercise probably will do poorly. These patients often experience a drop in SBP while exercising, a finding that suggests that no cardiac reserve remains. Such patients may not tolerate any exercise program. Similarly, patients who have recently experienced a myocardial infarction should begin exercising only under the direction of a health care practitioner. Patients with HF should "begin low and go slow," thereby avoiding overexertion. Most cardiac rehabilitation programs include a combination of aerobic training and very light resistive exercises.[44] Many patients prefer walking programs. Such programs may improve mental health and combat some of the psychological problems typically seen in patients with CHF.

Patient education (Tables 40.4 and 40.5) should also focus on proper nutrition, with special attention to the potential harm of excess sodium intake,[37] because sodium overload is a leading cause of acute decompensation.[46] Limiting a patient's salt intake helps counteract the exaggerated renal retention of sodium. Higher or more frequent diuretic doses are needed to attenuate the effect of high sodium intake. However, increasing diuretic dosages are not desirable given their ability to further activate the RAA system. Instead, dietary sodium restriction should be encouraged. Initial guidelines typically encourage dietary intake be restricted to 3 g of sodium or less per day. Eliminating added salt and removing high-sodium foods (e.g., salted nuts, pretzels, salt-cured meats, potato chips, pickles, olives, processed meats, some canned vegetables and soups) will decrease daily sodium intake to about 1.5 to 3.0 g (3.75 to 7.5 g sodium chloride; 1.0 g Na = 2.5 g NaCl). The typical American diet usually contains twice this amount of sodium. Patients should be instructed to read the nutritional labels of packaged foods and to use the Internet for additional information about the sodium (www.ianr.unl.edu/pubs/FOODS/g916.htm) and potassium (www.consumermedhelp.com/HHPoCHrt.htm) content of foods. Excluding all salt from cooking further reduces the patient's sodium intake to 1.2 to 1.5 g. However, excessive sodium restriction may reduce the palatability of food and secondarily compromise adequate nutrition. Using spices to flavor various foods should be encouraged and may enhance patient compliance with a low-sodium diet. Any family members involved in food preparation also should receive dietary education. In addition, over-the-counter medications may be a hidden source of sodium intake, and the patient can consult his or her pharmacist about appropriate selection.

Fluid restriction may also be recommended, particularly for patients with severe CHF. Fluid intake, when limited to 2 L/day or less, may reduce overall diuretic use.[47] Patients adhering to a fluid restriction should be reminded to consider foods high in water, such as fruits and soup, in their total fluid intake. In addition, patients should be encouraged to abstain from alcohol. Ethanol and its metabolite acetaldehyde produce dose-related

Table 40.5 ▪ Instructions on When to Contact a Health Care Provider

UNIVERSITY MEDICAL CENTER
1501 N. Campbell Avenue
Tucson, Arizona 85724

Heart Failure Program

Signs and Symptoms of Heart Failure

Call your health care provider if you experience any of the following:

- Shortness of breath, especially if it does not go away with rest
- Difficulty breathing when lying down or waking up at night with shortness of breath
- Persistent cough or wheezing
- Fatigue or weakness with little or no energy for routine activities
- Weight gain of 2–3 lb in 2 days or 4–5 lb over 5–7 days, or if you do not achieve your desired weight after changing your diuretic dosage in response to the weight gain if you have been instructed to do so
- Swelling in your ankles, feet, legs, or abdomen
- Nausea or feeling full early with meals
- Abdominal pain or tenderness
- Confusion or difficulty with concentration

Also call your health care provider if you have

- Unusually prolonged or severe chest pain or angina
- Changes in the regularity of your heartbeat
- Dizziness or feeling faint when you stand up from a sitting position
- Any side effect from any of your medications

IN CASE OF A MEDICAL EMERGENCY, CALL 911 IMMEDIATELY.

Emergencies may include

- Chest pain or pressure not relieved with rest or after taking three nitroglycerin tablets 5 min apart
- Extreme shortness of breath
- Coughing up pink, frothy sputum
- Fainting spell, severe sweating, or passing out

Note: This is a sample list intended to serve as a guideline. It is not intended to include all potential medical problems for which a person with heart failure should seek urgent medical advice.

Source: Reference 190.

reductions in contractility via inhibition of actin and myosin coupling.[48] In addition, short-term alcohol intake can produce histologic alterations in the myocardium and is arrhythmogenic.[48] Chronic alcohol intake has been associated with the development of asymptomatic and symptomatic LV dysfunction, and abstinence has been associated with improvements in LV function and should therefore be encouraged.[49]

Patients should be informed about the use of herbal licorice, which is often advocated for gastrointestinal complaints but has mineralocorticoid properties that may antagonize the effects of the diuretic spironolactone.[50] The active component of licorice, glycyrrhizic acid, reduces 11-β-hydroxysteroid dehydrogenase activity, leading to excess mineralocorticoid effects. Consequently, sodium retention can occur, leading to an acute CHF exacerbation. In addition, hypokalemia may develop, increasing the patient's risk of arrhythmic complications. Patients with CHF should be advised to avoid using herbal licorice.

Patient noncompliance with prescribed medical and pharmacologic regimens often precipitates worsening of CHF. In a study of patients admitted to a Chicago hospital for HF treatment, 64% were noncompliant with their medical regimens.[51] Almost one-half of the patients in this study had uncontrolled HTN as a precipitating factor for HF. Hospital admissions may be reduced through proper attention to patient education.[37] Patient compliance improved in older adults with CHF enrolled in a 3-month patient education program provided by a pharmacist.[52] In addition, multidisciplinary interventions involving intensive patient education with detailed information about diet, medications, and instructions for calling health providers (Table 40.5); increased patient monitoring through visits by pharmacists and nurses; and improved access to health care providers have been demonstrated in randomized trials to reduce hospital readmissions, reduce length of stay, improve quality of life, enhance patient knowledge and medication compliance, improve functional capacity, and increase patient satisfaction.[53–56]

Some prescription medications may exacerbate CHF.[5] β-Adrenergic blocking therapy initiated at the usual antihypertensive dosages and first-generation calcium channel blocking agents (e.g., verapamil, diltiazem and nifedipine) are representative examples. Furthermore, adding antiarrhythmic agents with negative inotropic properties can worsen preexisting HF. Nonsteroidal anti-inflammatory drugs (NSAIDs) inhibit cyclooxygenase activity, leading to a reduction in vasodilatory prostaglandins, which oppose the renal and systemic effects of AII in patients with CHF.[5] Administering NSAIDs to patients with CHF produces a reduction in GFR and renal blood flow and an increase in sodium and water retention. Chronic use of NSAIDs in older adults with CHF is associated with increased hospitalization rates secondary to acute CHF decompensation.[57] NSAIDs are widely available and can be obtained without the knowledge or advice of a health care professional. Improved education about the possible detrimental effects of chronic NSAID use in patients with CHF is warranted. The impact of selective cyclooxygenase-2 (COX-2) inhibitors in patients with CHF is unknown. However, COX-2 is constitutively expressed in the kidney and is partially responsible for synthesis of some renal prostaglandins.[58]

Pharmacist-conducted "brown bag" reviews may be of particular importance in patients with CHF because they can help identify drugs that may contribute to CHF exacerbations.[37] Stricter attention to these precipitating factors could significantly reduce the number of hospitalizations and ease the clinical and economic burden of CHF for patients and society.

Pharmacotherapy

Vasodilators

Vasodilator therapy shows new promise in CHF treatment.[59] These agents through varied mechanisms have been shown to alter the capacitance (preload) and resistance (afterload) of vessels, either directly or indirectly. The net result is that vasodilators enhance physiologic performance of the diseased left ventricle, they relieve symptoms of dyspnea, and they improve exercise tolerance. Since investigations of the early 1970s, vasodilator therapy has become an integral component of chronic CHF treatment. Most importantly, vasodilator therapy reduces mortality in patients with CHF.[60,61] In general, the selection and dosing of a vasodilating agent for chronic CHF management should be based on studies that have evaluated the long-term beneficial and adverse effects of an agent (Table 40.6). The following section describes several classes of vasodilators used in to treat CHF.

Angiotensin-Converting Enzyme Inhibitors

The ACEIs, such as captopril, enalapril, fosinopril, lisinopril, quinapril, and ramipril, competitively block the conversion of AI to AII. AII is a potent peripheral arteriolar vasoconstrictor. AII also stimulates the release of aldosterone and AVP and facilitates both central and peripheral activity of the SNS. In addition, the enzyme that converts AI to AII is identical to kinase II, the enzyme that degrades bradykinin, an endogenous vasodilator and smooth muscle relaxant.[62] Therefore, the vasorelaxant effects of these substances may be accentuated in the presence of ACEIs. Thus, the reductions both in preload and afterload seen after an ACEI is administered may result from a number of different but interrelated mechanisms. Individual ACEIs vary with respect to a number of different pharmacologic characteristics. Captopril contains a sulfhydryl group that binds directly to the zinc moiety of the enzyme. The remaining ACEIs do not contain sulfhydryl groups and most, with the exception of fosinopril, bind via carboxyl groups. Fosinopril binds to ACE via a phosphoryl group. Captopril and lisinopril are active upon administration, and the remaining ACEIs are prodrugs that must be activated.

Table 40.6 ▪ Dosing Considerations for Vasodilators

Drugs	Starting Dosage	Target Dosage (survival)	Maximum Dosage	Adverse Effects	Altered Kinetics	Monitoring Parameters
Angiotensin-converting enzyme inhibitors						
Captopril	3.125–6.25 mg TID	50 mg TID	100 mg TID	Hypotension	Renal dysfunction	Blood pressure
Enalapril	1.25–2.5 mg BID	10 mg BID	20 mg BID	Renal dysfunction	(dosage adjustments needed)	Renal function
Lisinopril	2.5–5 mg QD	10 mg QD	40 mg QD	Angioedema		Potassium
Ramipril	2.5 mg BID	5 mg BID	10 mg BID	Cough		Cough
Quinapril	2.5–5 mg BID	20 mg BID	20 mg BID			Angioedema
Fosinopril	5–10 mg QD	20 mg QD	40 mg QD			Volume status CHF SS
Angiotensin II type I receptor blockers[a]						
Losartan	25–50 mg QD	?50 mg QD	?100 mg QD	Hypotension Renal dysfunction	Hepatic dysfunction	Blood pressure Renal function Hepatic function CHF SS
Isosorbide dinitrate	10–20 mg TID	120 mg QD in 3 divided doses while ensuring a 12-hr nitrate-free interval		Hypotension Headache		Blood pressure CHF SS
Hydralazine	25 mg TID	300 mg QD in 2 or 3 divided doses		Hypotension Headache Tachycardia Systemic lupus erythematosus	Renal dysfunction (dosage adjustments probably needed)	Blood pressure Heart rate CHF SS

CHF SS, signs and symptoms of congestive heart failure.
[a]Not approved by the U.S. Food and Drug Administration for treating heart failure.

ACEIs have emerged as the cornerstone in the medical management of CHF.[59] Currently captopril, enalapril, fosinopril, lisinopril, quinapril, and ramipril are approved by the U.S. Food and Drug Administration (FDA) for this indication.

Reductions in mortality and hospitalization rates have been demonstrated in patients with CHF receiving ACEI therapy regardless of the patient's NYHA functional class before treatment (Table 40.3).[60,61] Interestingly, in the patients with severe CHF (NYHA class IV), the reduction in total mortality was primarily a result of a reduction in progression of HF, whereas in the patients with mild to moderate CHF (NYHA class II to III) the mortality reduction was caused primarily by a reduction in sudden cardiac death. These findings have important implications for the mechanism through which ACEIs exert their beneficial effects. AII antagonism, reductions in sympathetic nerve activity and circulating NE,[63] and a direct protective effects on the myocardium or coronary vasculature have been postulated as potential mechanisms through which ACEIs affect mortality. In addition, the majority of health care costs attributed to CHF are direct costs of hospitalization. A 25% reduction in the hospitalization rate would lead to a $2-billion reduction in direct health care costs, or a net savings of more than $1 billion per year through the use of ACEIs alone.[64]

ACEIs also have important CHF-preventive effects when administered soon after AMI in patients with asymptomatic LV dysfunction (EF less than 40%; Fig. 40.4).[65] These trials were based on the ability of ACEIs to diminish the progressive ventricular remodeling observed soon after large myocardial infarctions. A meta-analysis of the trials in which ACEI therapy was initiated within 36 hours of MI and continued for 4 to 6 weeks showed a 7% reduction in mortality.[65] On average, approximately 5 lives would be saved per 1000 patients treated with ACEI therapy. Approximately 85% of the mortality benefit occurs early, within the first week of therapy. Patients with large anterior infarcts and patients at high risk for post-AMI complications (Killip class 2 to 3, HR greater than 100 bpm) derived the greatest benefit. A reduction in the frequency of CHF exacerbations also was observed. ACEI therapy was not associated with excess adverse effects in any subgroup, but hypotensive patients and patients in cardiogenic shock generally were excluded from analysis. In addition, a higher incidence of renal dysfunction and hypotension was observed in patients more than 75 years old.

ACEIs appear to consistently improve the clinical status and longevity of patients with CHF. ACEI therapy should be initiated early when signs and symptoms of CHF are absent or mild (i.e., NYHA class I and II). Current guidelines recommend the use of ACEIs as first-line therapy before digoxin or diuretics in the absence of troubling symptoms and in combination with these agents and β-blockers (Fig. 40.2).[40] In addition, ACEIs should be initiated early (post-AMI days 1 and 2) for patients presenting with AMI if there is no evidence of cardiogenic shock or hypotension (SBP less than 100 mm Hg). Despite this extensive evidence of its beneficial effects, ACEI therapy remains underused in patients with CHF. Analysis of prescribing patterns at an academic medical center in 1986 and 1994 indicated a significant but unsatisfactory increase in ACEI prescriptions among patients hospitalized for CHF (43% and 71%, respectively).[66] Additional analyses indicate that only 30 to 50% of patients with CHF receive ACEIs.[67,68] Similar evaluations in older adults with CHF have indicated underuse of ACEI therapy with an associated increase in adverse cardiovascular events in this population.[69,70]

ACEI dosages vary, but therapy generally should be initiated at low dosages (Table 40.6). ACEI therapy initiation typically involves captopril dosages of 12.5 mg every 8 hours, enalapril maleate dosages of 5 mg twice daily, lisinopril 5 mg daily, or equivalent dosages of alternative ACEIs. However, the actual ACEI dosage used depends on the patient's clinical status and his or her risk of hypotension.[60] Risk factors associated with hypotension secondary to ACEI therapy include hyponatremia (serum sodium concentration less than 130 mEq/L), volume depletion after increased diuretic therapy or concurrent use of a potassium-sparing diuretic, and an elevated Scr concentration (more than 1.7 mg/dL).[71] The lowest possible starting dosage (e.g., captopril 3.125, enalapril, 1.25, and lisinopril 2.5 mg) should be used in the aforementioned patients.

After therapy is initiated, current recommendations involve titrating the ACEI dosage upward, at 3- to 7-day intervals, to achieve the target dosages studied in the clinical trials.[60] Longer titration intervals may be indicated in patients at risk for adverse effects. Therefore, clinical observations, such as SBP, renal function, and the appearance of other adverse effects should be used to guide dosage adjustments until the target dosage is achieved. The beneficial effects of ACEI therapy appear to be dose related and every effort should be made to achieve the target dosage.[72,73] In support of this recommendation, results from the recent Assessment of Treatment with Lisinopril and Survival (ATLAS) trial indicated a trend toward lower mortality rates in patients receiving the higher lisinopril dosages (mean dosage difference 19 mg).[74] In addition, the higher-dose group was associated with greater improvements in the combined endpoint of mortality and progressive CHF. In contrast to the ATLAS study, the NETWORK trial did not demonstrate a significant dose-related reduction in mortality and morbidity for patients receiving 2.5 mg, 5 mg, and 10 mg twice daily.[75] However, the NETWORK trial was small, with relatively wide 95% confidence intervals. Despite data from the NETWORK trial, current recommendations suggest that ACEI dosages should be maximized to those used in clinical trials. Examples of target regimens used in clinical trials include captopril 50 mg every 8 hours, enalapril 10 mg twice daily, and lisinopril 10 mg daily (Table 40.6).[60] Patients unable to achieve target dosages should be maintained at the maximally tolerated dosage. Daily maintenance dosages probably can be reduced and the dosing interval extended (i.e., every 12 hours for captopril, every 24 hours for enalapril and quinapril, and every other day for lisinopril and ramipril) for patients with diminished renal function (i.e., estimated creatinine clearance [CL_{Cr}] less than 30 to 40 mL/minute; Table 40.6).

The most common adverse effect of ACEIs is hypotension. Peak hypotensive effects vary depending on the ACEI used. The peak hypotensive response to captopril generally occurs within 30 to 90 minutes of dosing, whereas this effect often occurs within 2 to 4 hours after enalapril and 7 hours after lisinopril. A single study showed that hypotension often was more severe and prolonged after enalapril than after captopril.[76] However, this investigation used large, fixed dosages of both drugs rather than optimizing the dosage of each agent to either hemodynamic or clinical effects. It is best to administer the first ACEI dose under the watchful eye of a clinician so that first-dose syncope or presyncope can be treated appropriately. Blood pressure should be assessed before an ACEI is administered and closely monitored during the time period of expected maximal hypotensive effects.[60] An absolute blood pressure under which ACEI administration is contraindicated has not been identified.[60] Administration of an ACEI in patients with SBPs below 90 mm Hg is left to the clinical judgment of the health care professional. Patients who are dehydrated or hyponatremic or have low intravascular fluid volume are particularly susceptible to ACEI-induced orthostasis and syncope. Therefore, if possible, diuretic dosages should be held the day of first dose administration or perhaps for 24 hours before the first ACEI test dose is administered.

Renal dysfunction is a worrisome adverse effect associated with ACEI therapy. Compensatory stimulation of AII production preserves renal blood flow in patients with CHF.[76] Therefore, after ACEI therapy is initiated, GFR is reduced and acute increases in BUN and Scr can occur, particularly during the first 6 weeks of therapy.[60] BUN and Scr normalization may occur with continued therapy or after decreases in the diuretic dosage in hypovolemic patients. Nonetheless, renal function may not improve and some degree of renal insufficiency may persist in some patients. Use of an ACEI is not contraindicated in patients with underlying renal insufficiency because baseline renal function does not predict the development of subsequent renal dysfunction.[77] Interestingly, there is a strong association between long-term preservation of renal function and acute increases in Scr of less than 30% above baseline that stabilize within the first 2 months of ACEI therapy.[78] The relationship persists for patients with baseline Scr greater than 1.4 mg/dL. ACEI withdrawal should be considered only when Scr increases more than 30% above baseline within the first 2 months of ACEI therapy.[78] However, special attention is needed to detect patients who may have both CHF and bilateral renal artery stenosis (or single renal artery stenosis in patients with only one kidney). Because many patients with CHF have severe CAD, atherosclerosis of other arteries is expected. In a study of 89 patients referred to a HF unit, 6 (7%) had renal artery stenosis.[79] The suspicion of renal artery stenosis is raised when the Scr abruptly increases after ACEI therapy is initiated. Another clue to renal artery stenosis is late-onset (more than 50 years) HTN. Once renal artery stenosis is confirmed (usually with digital subtraction angiography), angioplasty or surgery can correct the stenosis. The patient can then safely receive ACEI therapy for CHF. The ACEI must be discontinued if surgical or mechanical correction of the renal artery stenosis proves impossible.

ACEI-induced cough often contributes to the discontinuation of therapy.[60] The mechanism through which an ACEI produces cough is believed to involve the accumulation of bradykinin, a known mediator of bronchoconstriction.[80,81] The consequence is the development of a dry, nonproductive cough. However, cough in patients with CHF may also result from pulmonary edema. Consequently, the actual incidence of ACEI-induced cough is difficult to ascertain. The clinician should try to determine the cause of cough before ACEI therapy is discontinued. The ACEI should be discontinued or the dosage reduced only if the cough is believed to be related to the ACEI and is intolerable to the patient. Switching to an alternative ACEI[60] or to an AII type 1 receptor blocker (ARB)[82] may be helpful.

Urinary K^+ excretion is reduced and serum K^+ increased in patients receiving ACEI therapy. All diuretic and electrolyte therapy should be assessed before ACEI therapy is initiated. Discontinuation or dosage reductions of potassium supplements may be necessary and should be considered in patients with high serum K^+ concentrations.

One week after ACEI therapy begins and after any dosage adjustments, BUN, Scr, and K^+ concentrations should be assessed.[60] Routine laboratory assessments should be obtained every 3 months. Maculopapular rashes, taste disturbances, leukopenia, and proteinuria have been observed during ACEI administration. Therefore, it is prudent to check a baseline complete blood cell count with differential and repeat it in 2 weeks and again every 6 months after ACEI therapy begins.

Pharmacodynamic drug interactions involving excessive hypotension can occur in patients receiving ACEI concurrently with other vasodilators. In addition, hyperkalemia can develop in patients receiving potassium supplements or potassium-sparing diuretics in combination with ACEI therapy.[60] NSAIDs, including aspirin, can attenuate the vasodilatory effects of ACEIs in patients with CHF.[60] Chronic use of NSAIDs should be avoided, as previously discussed. The interaction between aspirin and ACEIs has been evaluated in a limited number of clinical trials involving small numbers of patients. Single-dose aspirin administration has been associated with variable hemodynamic effects. Retrospective reviews indicate that the concurrent use of aspirin may reduce the mortality benefit produced by ACEIs. However, a recent analysis of data from the Benzabrate Infarction Prevention (BIP) trial contradicts these findings.[83] In the BIP trial, mortality among patients with CAD and CHF was lower for patients receiving aspirin and ACEIs than for those not taking aspirin (24% versus 34%, respectively, $p = 0.001$). Consequently, concurrent use of ACEIs and aspirin depends on the presence of additional indications for aspirin therapy and is warranted in patients with CAD. Although pharmacokinetic interactions with ACEIs are rare, captopril has been shown to decrease digoxin clearance.

Angiotensin II Type 1 Receptor Blockers

Despite reductions in mortality, use of ACEIs in patients with CHF does not completely suppress AII formation. In addition, AII formation can occur independently of ACE-mediated pathways.[10,84] Vasoconstriction, myocardial remodeling, and sodium and water retention result from binding of AII to the AII type 1 (AT_1) receptors. Recently, agents have been developed that bind to the AT_1 receptor, thereby blocking the deleterious effects of AII. Consequently, the ARBs may provide more complete suppression of AII activity than that achieved during ACEI therapy. However, ARBs, unlike ACEIs, do not facilitate bradykinin accumulation. Given their different mechanisms of action, different clinical effects can be expected between the two classes.

ARBs produce dose-dependent inhibition of AII activity.[84] The individual ARBs vary in their pharmacokinetic profiles (Table 40.6). Losartan is metabolized to an active metabolite (E3174). Losartan and E3174 both antagonize the AT_1 receptor, but the metabolite is 10 times more potent and demonstrates noncompetitive receptor inhibition. Candesartan also is a prodrug, that is converted in the gastrointestinal tract to the active compound (CV-11974). Valsartan, telmisartan, and irbesartan do not need activation after administration. All of the currently available agents selectively inhibit AII binding to the AT_1 receptor. Significant differences in clinical response to the agents remain to be determined.

The efficacy of AT_1 receptor blockade via administration of ARBs including losartan, irbesartan, valsartan, and candesartan has recently been evaluated in a number of small clinical trials. The Evaluation of Losartan in the Elderly (ELITE) trial randomized 722 patients with symptomatic HF (NYHA class II and III) greater than 65 years of age to losartan (50 mg/day) or captopril (50 mg three times a day).[82] The trial was undertaken primarily to compare the safety of the two agents in patients with CHF. Patients enrolled were not previously receiving ACEI therapy. Duration of the trial was 48 weeks. Losartan administration was associated with a 32% lower mortality rate than that of the captopril group (4.8% versus 8.7%, $P = 0.035$). The difference in mortality resulted primarily from a difference in the rate of sudden death. Significant differences in renal function were not observed between the two agents. No difference in the incidence of hospital admission rates was observed between the two agents, and NYHA functional class improved equally in both treatment groups.

The results in the ELITE trial were not substantiated by the Randomized Evaluation of Strategies for Left Ventricular Dysfunction (RESOLVD) study, a dose-ranging trial comparing three different dosages of candesartan with enalapril alone or in combination with candesartan.[85] Data obtained from the RESOLVD trial indicate a 60% higher mortality associated with the use of candesartan than with enalapril. It is possible that the use of different ARBs in ELITE and RESOLVD may have contributed to the contrasting survival results. Currently, the role of ARBs in patients with CHF awaits further clarification. Until data from larger clinical trials comparing the ARBs with ACEI therapy are available, ARBs should be considered as second-line therapy in patients unable to tolerate ACEIs (Fig. 40.2).

Alternatively, limited data suggest that the combination of an ARB and maximal ACEI therapy may provide additional benefit. Combination ARB and ACEI therapy would inhibit AII production via ACE-independent pathways while maintaining bradykinin concentrations and antagonize the effects of AII produced by non-ACE pathways. In the RESOLVD trial, aldosterone production was reduced with combination candesartan and enalapril therapy.[85] Similar reductions in plasma aldosterone and NE were observed after valsartan was added to ACEI therapy.[86] In addition, improvements in NYHA functional class, LVEF, exercise tolerance, and peak exercise capacity have been observed with the combination of losartan and ACEI therapy.[87,88] However, the benefit of combined ARB and ACEIs on morbidity and mortality compared with ACEI therapy alone remains to be determined.

Adverse effects associated with the ARBs are similar to those observed during ACEI therapy. The incidence of hypotension and renal dysfunction observed with ARB therapy appears equal to that observed during ACEI therapy. However, the incidence of cough is lower during ARB therapy, as would be expected given the absence of bradykinin accumulation.[82]

Nitrates

Nitrates were one of the initial groups of vasodilating agents used to manage CHF.[89] The beneficial effects of nitrates are believed to be mediated by nitric oxide formation. Nitric oxide, through cyclic guanosine monophosphate (cGMP) formation, reduces intracellular calcium concentrations, leading to vasodilation. Nitrates decrease preload predominantly through vasodilation of venous capacitance vessels. Nitrates may also decrease afterload via dilation of large arteries and arterioles when administered in high dosages. LV filling pressures, mean pulmonary artery pressure, systemic vascular resistance, severity of mitral regurgitation, and SBP decrease while cardiac index (CI) increases during exercise after nitrates are administered in patients with chronic CHF.[89] Improvements in treadmill exercise times, systolic function, CHF symptoms, and hospitalization rates have been observed after nitrates were added to ACEI therapy. Therefore, nitrates may be added to ACEIs, but their impact on mortality is not known.[89]

Nitrate tolerance has been demonstrated consistently when the vascular endothelium is constantly exposed to nitroglycerin.[89] Investigation into this issue has revealed that tolerance appears to be mediated by excessive free radical formation caused by continuous exposure of the vascular tissue to organic nitrates. Free radicals impair nitric oxide release, thereby preventing cGMP-mediated vasodilation. Inhibition of nitrate tolerance via antioxidant administration is under investigation. Currently, the most frequently used method of avoiding nitrate tolerance involves intermittent administration, which provides a daily washout period. Of the available nitrate formulations used to treat chronic CHF, isosorbide dinitrate (ISDN) is the most frequently prescribed and well-studied agent (Table 40.6). Although many large clinical trials have used a four-times-daily dosing strategy, 10 to 80 mg three rimes daily, administered at 7 AM, 12 noon, and 5 PM, for example, would retain a 12-hour nitrate-free dosing interval. Similarly, if nitroglycerin patches are prescribed, they should be applied for 12 hours and then removed for 12 hours. Isosorbide mononitrates, although not well studied, also are used in CHF. Because most patients experience DOE during the waking hours, the nitrate-free interval usually is at night. These intermittent dosing regimens do not preclude using short-acting sublingual tablets or lingual spray nitroglycerin for episodes of acute dyspnea or angina.

The most common adverse nitrate effect is headache that often responds to mild analgesics such as acetaminophen (Table 40.6). Headaches usually disappear after several days of nitrate administration. Some patients continue to experience severe headaches with nitrates and may not tolerate any nitrate administration. Dizziness, flushing, postural hypotension, weakness, and occasionally skin rash have also been reported. In summary, nitrates are safe and effective vasodilators useful as adjunctive therapy to ACEIs or in combination with hydralazine in CHF treatment.

Hydralazine

Hydralazine is a direct-acting arteriolar dilator that principally reduces afterload. Reductions in afterload by hydralazine may also result in moderate reductions in preload because of the dependence of LV filling pressure on the resistance to ventricular emptying during systole. Hydralazine can markedly reduce LV filling pressure in patients with mitral or aortic valve regurgitation. Clinically, hydralazine is most commonly used in combination with other vasodilators with greater preload-reducing properties, such as nitrates.[90,91]

Studies using hydralazine monotherapy in patients with CHF (in dosages up to 225 mg per day) indicate that hydralazine, although improving quality of life, does not improve survival.[92,93] However, the combination of oral ISDN with hydralazine was the first pharmacologic therapy found to reduce mortality from CHF.[90] The Veterans Administrative Cooperative Study on Vasodilator Therapy of Heart Failure I (VHeFT-I) showed that the ISDN–hydralazine combination improved systolic function and reduced 2-year CHF mortality by 34%.[90] However, in VHeFT-II, enalapril conferred a greater survival benefit than the ISDN–hydralazine combination.[91] Consequently, combination ISDN–hydralazine therapy should be reserved for patients unable to tolerate ACEI therapy.

Hydralazine dosages for treating patients with chronic CHF vary greatly even though the placebo-controlled trials used fixed dosage regimens.[93] Baseline estimates of a patient's SBP, resting HR, and renal function should be determined before therapy is initiated. Hydralazine and ISDN dosages for patients receiving both agents in the VHeFT trials were 270 and 136 mg per day, respectively.[90,91] The total daily dosage can be divided into equal doses administered every 6, 8, or 12 hours, although the every-8-hours or three-times-daily schedule works best with current recommendations for prescribing ISDN (Table 40.6). Current data suggest that the dosage should be titrated to approximately 300 mg/day while SBP (not less than 95 mm Hg), HR (avoidance of a resting tachycardia), improvements in pulmonary and systemic symptoms, and the development of adverse effects are monitored. Patients with the highest elevations in CVP have required dosages as high as 2400 mg per day, and those with CL_{Cr} less than 35 mL/minute may exhibit the longest duration of action (at least 12 hours). Unfortunately, side effects increase with increasing daily dosages (Table 40.6). Side effects forced discontinuation of therapy in 19% of patients receiving ISDN–hydralazine in the VHeFT-I trial.[90] The most common adverse effects include headache, palpitations, postural hypotension, nausea, vomiting, and systemic lupus erythematosus (seen particularly in dosages higher than 200 mg per day). Salt and water retention may occur during long-term therapy with hydralazine. Mild to moderate increases in resting HR and myocardial ischemic events in patients with CHF also have been reported after hydralazine administration.

Prazosin

Prazosin is a specific, competitive antagonist of postsynaptic α_1-receptors located in the walls of precapillary arteriolar resistance vessels and postcapillary venous capacitance vessels. Therefore, prazosin is considered a balanced vasodilator in that it reduces both preload and afterload to approximately the same degrees. Prazosin therapy was one of the treatment arms in the VHeFT-I trial.[90] However, prazosin therapy did not result in lower mortality rates than did placebo. Therefore, little enthusiasm remains for using prazosin as a primary vasodilator to treat CHF.

Calcium Channel Blockers

Several theoretical reasons exist for considering calcium channel blockers in CHF treatment: These agents are powerful arteriolar dilators and thus reduce LV afterload; they produce hemodynamic effects similar to those of hydralazine, which has improved survival in patients with mild to moderate CHF; they have anti-ischemic effects, which make them an attractive therapeutic option for treating CHF caused by CAD; and these drugs improve diastolic dysfunction, a significant cause of HF symptoms, through their beneficial effects on LV relaxation.[94] However, the first-generation calcium channel antagonists, verapamil, diltiazem, and nifedipine, have universally produced hemodynamic and clinical deterioration in patients with HF caused by systolic dysfunction. Possible explanations for these detrimental effects include direct negative inotropic properties, further activation of deleterious neurohormonal responses, and an increase in blood volume, which may increase afterload. Nonetheless, in patients with severe asymptomatic aortic regurgitation and normal LV systolic function, nifedipine significantly reduces and delays the need for aortic valve replacement.[95] In addition, nifedipine may have a role in treating CHF caused by chronic severe mitral regurgitation.[96]

Two recent placebo-controlled trials evaluated the effects of second-generation dihydropyridines, amlodipine and felodipine, when added to ACEIs, digoxin, and diuretics.[97–99]

In the Prospective Randomized Amlodipine Survival Evaluation (PRAISE) trial, amlodipine significantly reduced combined morbidity and mortality by 31% and all-cause mortality by 45% in patients with nonischemic CHF.[97] Reductions in both sudden cardiac death and death secondary to progressive HF were observed.[98] No beneficial effect was observed in patients with CHF secondary to ischemic cardiomyopathy. PRAISE II is investigating the role of amlodipine in patients with nonischemic cardiomyopathy. VHeFT-III compared the addition of felodipine (5 mg twice daily) with placebo in 450 male patients (NYHA class II and III) already receiving enalapril and a diuretic.[99] Felodipine did not significantly reduce mortality (13.8% versus 12.8%) or hospitalization rates (43% versus 42%) during an average follow-up period of 18 months. In summary, the role of second-generation calcium channel blockers in CHF management awaits further clarification.

β-Adrenergic Blocking Agents

Despite the often assumed risk of precipitating an acute HF episode when using β-adrenergic blocking agents in patients with CHF, clinical evidence now indicates that patients with HF can benefit significantly from carefully up-titrated β-blocker therapy.[100] Chronic activation of the SNS in patients with CHF is associated with alterations in the structure and function of the myocardium, particularly in β-receptor density and sensitivity. Interruption of SNS activity by β-adrenergic blockers counteracts the deleterious effects previously discussed. β-Adrenergic receptor blockers antagonize the adverse effects of excessive activation of the SNS, leading to a reduction in plasma NE and upregulation of myocardial β_1-receptors.

Three generations of β-blockers are available.[100] First-generation β-blockers nonspecifically block both β_1- and β_2-adrenergic receptors. Second-generation β-blockers include the β_1-specific antagonists, metoprolol and bisoprolol, and the third-generation β-blockers, bucindolol and carvedilol, produce nonspecific β-blockade but have additional vasodilatory properties. Carvedilol produces vasodilation via α_1-blockade, inhibits vascular smooth muscle proliferation, and is an antioxidant. On the other hand, bucindolol produces vasodilation independent of α_1-blocking mechanisms. The efficacy of the different β-blockers has been examined in several large randomized trials.

Two different formulations of metoprolol have been studied in prospective, randomized, placebo-controlled trials.[101,102] The Metoprolol in Dilated Cardiomyopathy (MDC) trial evaluated the use of conventional-release metoprolol in 383 patients with dilated cardiomyopathy.[101] Metoprolol therapy was associated with improvements in exercise tolerance, quality of life, NYHA functional class, and the number of CHF exacerbations necessitating hospitalization. A significant difference in mortality (19 deaths in the metoprolol group and 23 in the placebo group, $P = 0.69$) was not observed. However, in a more recent study of nearly 4000 patients with predominantly NYHA class II or III CHF, controlled release/extended release (CR/XL) metoprolol conferred a 34% reduction in mortality.[102] Both sudden deaths and deaths caused by worsening CHF were significantly decreased.

The Cardiac Insufficiency Bisoprolol Study II (CIBIS-II) randomized 2647 patients (NYHA class III and IV) to receive bisoprolol (maximum dosage 10 mg) or placebo.[103] The trial was stopped early (mean follow-up, 1.3 years) upon observation of a 34% reduction in mortality, a 44% reduction in sudden death, and a 20% reduction in hospitalization rates in the group receiving bisoprolol.

The efficacy of carvedilol has been assessed in the U.S. Carvedilol trial involving 1094 patients with predominantly NYHA class II and III CHF.[104] The relative reductions in mortality and hospitalization for patients randomized to carvedilol were 65% and 36%, respectively. Reductions in mortality caused by progressive pump failure and sudden cardiac death were observed. Based on data extrapolated from the U.S. study, the cost per life-year saved for carvedilol ranges between $12,799 and $29,477, indicating that carvedilol therapy compares favorably with commonly used medical interventions.[105]

Given the reduction in mortality and hospitalization observed in these trials, β-blockers are currently advocated in patients with stable CHF who lack contraindications to β-blockade. Patients should be euvolemic and optimized on adequate vasodilator therapy before a β-blocker is added.[100] However, despite these favorable effects, several questions remain with respect to β-blocker therapy. For instance, debate continues as to which generation of β-blockers affords the greatest clinical benefit. A meta-analysis that combined the results of 18 trials indicated a 49% reduction in mortality for patients receiving nonselective β-blockers (carvedilol, bucindolol), with a more modest 18% reduction in the group receiving β_1-selective agents (metoprolol, bisoprolol).[106] However, a small, prospective, randomized, open-label trial involving patients with predominantly mild to moderate HF (NYHA class II to III) directly compared the effects of carvedilol ($n = 37$) and metoprolol ($n = 30$).[107] After 6 months of therapy, no significantly different effects on mortality, quality of life, ejection fraction (EF), exercise capacity, and incidence of adverse effects were observed between the two agents. Both drugs were well tolerated during initiation and up-titration of therapy, and no difference in the ability to achieve the target dosage was observed between the two groups. Data from large, ongoing, randomized trials directly comparing metoprolol and carvedilol are needed to conclusively determine the superiority of one agent. Carvedilol is available in very low dosages (3.125 mg, 6.25 mg, and 12.5 mg), suggesting that carvedilol may be a more attractive option than metoprolol because its higher-dose tablets must be crushed or compounded before administration.

The benefit of β-blockers in patients with severe CHF is unknown. Preliminary data indicate a greater risk of adverse effects associated with β-blocker therapy in patients with NYHA class IV CHF.[108] Finally, the ideal time to initiate β-blocker therapy in patients with LV dysfunction is also unknown. Although most studies of β-blockers for CHF have enrolled NYHA class II or III CHF patients,[106] retrospective analyses of the Survival and Ventricular Enlargement (SAVE) and Study of Left Ventricular Dysfunction (SOLVD) prevention trials reveal that the combination of β-blockers and ACEIs significantly reduces mortality in patients with asymptomatic LV dysfunction but without CHF (Fig. 40.4).[109,110] Data from ongoing trials are needed to assess the impact of β-blockade in patients with regard to these issues. Additional data are needed about the use of β-blockers in older adults because the majority of trials enrolled patients less than 80 years old.

As with ACEIs, initiation of β-blocker therapy begins with low dosages that are increased slowly and carefully (Table 40.7). The carvedilol dosage begins at 3.125 mg twice daily and is doubled every 2 weeks to a maximum of 25 mg twice a day (weight less than 85 kg) or 50 mg twice a day (weight more than 85 kg). In the CIBIS trial, bisoprolol was initiated at a dosage of 1.25 mg a day.[103] The dosage was increased gradually at weekly intervals to 10 mg according to patient tolerance. For immediate-release metoprolol, the starting dosage was 5 mg twice daily for 2 to 7 days, increased slowly to 50 to 75 mg twice

Table 40.7 ▪ Dosing Considerations for β-Blockers

Drugs	Starting Dosage	Target Dosage	Adverse Effect	Altered Kinetics	Monitoring Parameters
Carvedilol	3.125–6.25 mg BID	25 mg BID (wt <85 kg) 50 mg BID (wt >85 kg)	Hypotension Bradycardia CHF exacerbation	Hepatic dysfunction Concomitant administration of CYP2D6 inhibitors or substrates Poor metabolizers of CYP2D6	Blood pressure Heart rate CHF signs and symptoms Hepatic function Initiation of agents that inhibit CYP2D6
Metoprolol[a] (immediate release)	6.25–12.5 mg BID	50–100 mg BID	As for carvedilol	As for carvedilol	As for carvedilol
Metoprolol CR/XL[a]	12.5–2.5 mg QD	200 QD	As for carvedilol	As for carvedilol	As for carvedilol

CHF, congestive heart failure; *CR/XL,* controlled release/extended release; *CYP,* cytochrome P-450.
[a]Not approved by the U.S. Food and Drug Administration for treating CHF.

each day.[101] The starting dosage for metoprolol CR/XL was 12.5 mg and 25 mg once daily for 2 weeks for NYHA class III to IV and II, respectively.[102] Thereafter, the dosage was increased to 50 mg once daily for 2 weeks, then 100 mg daily for 2 weeks, and finally to the target dosage of 200 mg per day.

Close patient monitoring is needed when initiating and titrating β-blocker therapy (Table 40.7). Blood pressure and HR should be assessed before initiation of therapy or dosage adjustment and after the first dose of the new dosing regimen is administered. Commonly observed adverse effects associated with β-blocker therapy include symptomatic and asymptomatic hypotension and bradycardia. Clinical decompensation of CHF can occur, and initiating β-blocker therapy in patients with CHF entails extensive patient education to ensure compliance with the medication regimen. Expected benefits are achieved after several months of continued drug use. Before therapy begins, patients should understand that although acutely their symptoms may worsen, long-term improvements in their CHF may be obtained with the use of β-blocker therapy. In addition, dosage adjustments of their other medications, especially diuretics and ACEI, may be needed to alleviate symptoms during the initial titration period. It may be necessary to reduce the β-blocker dosage or withdraw therapy during severe CHF exacerbations.

Diuretics

Diuretics continue to be an integral component of symptomatic CHF management; most patients are maintained on some diuretic regimen (Figs. 40.2 to 40.6). Principally through the excretion of excess sodium and water, the major beneficial effect of chronically administered diuretics is the relief of pulmonary and systemic congestive signs and symptoms.[111,112] Diuretics also may indirectly provide favorable hemodynamic effects by decreasing intraventricular wall tension. This occurs principally through a reduction in preload and secondary to venodilation. Thus, preload reduction may slightly improve systolic function. In addition to improving signs and symptoms, a home-based flexible diuretic regimen, adjusted by the patient according to changing dietary factors and weight, may enhance other quality-of-life aspects such as patient's control over this frustrating chronic condition and a decreased need for office visits or hospitalization. Diuretics as monotherapy do not prolong life. However, adding spironolactone (25 to 50 mg/day) to a regimen of an ACEI, loop diuretic, and digoxin in NYHA class III and IV patients resulted in a 30% reduction in the risk of mortality and a 35% decrease in the risk of hospitalization for worsening HF. There was also a 32% reduction in risk of death from cardiac causes. Spironolactone was well tolerated, with 10% of patients developing gynecomastia. The incidence of serious hyperkalemia was minimal.[113,114]

ACEIs do not completely suppress aldosterone production. Spironolactone antagonizes aldosterone, which mediates sodium retention, potassium loss, myocardial NE uptake, and myocardial fibrosis.[114,115] In addition, diuretics play an important preventive role by decreasing the occurrence of CHF in patients with HTN.[116] Further enhancement of neurohormonal activation is a negative aspect of the use of thiazides or loop diuretics in CHF.

Principles of Diuretic Use

Before diuretic therapy is initiated for a patient with symptomatic CHF, a number of general principles of diuretic usage should be considered:[117,118]

- Therapy to rid patients of all traces of peripheral edema often is unnecessary and may be harmful.
- Begin therapy with the smallest effective dosage and titrate upward to minimize electrolyte imbalances and a patient's weight loss to 0.5 to 1.0 kg/day, except in extreme cases of pulmonary edema.
- The more proximally a diuretic acts within the nephron, the greater is the loss of fluid and electrolytes.
- Diuretics, which act proximally to the terminal distal tubule, where sodium is exchanged for both potassium and hydrogen, probably will produce both hypokalemia and metabolic alkalosis.
- Diuretics that induce hypokalemia often cause hypomagnesemia.

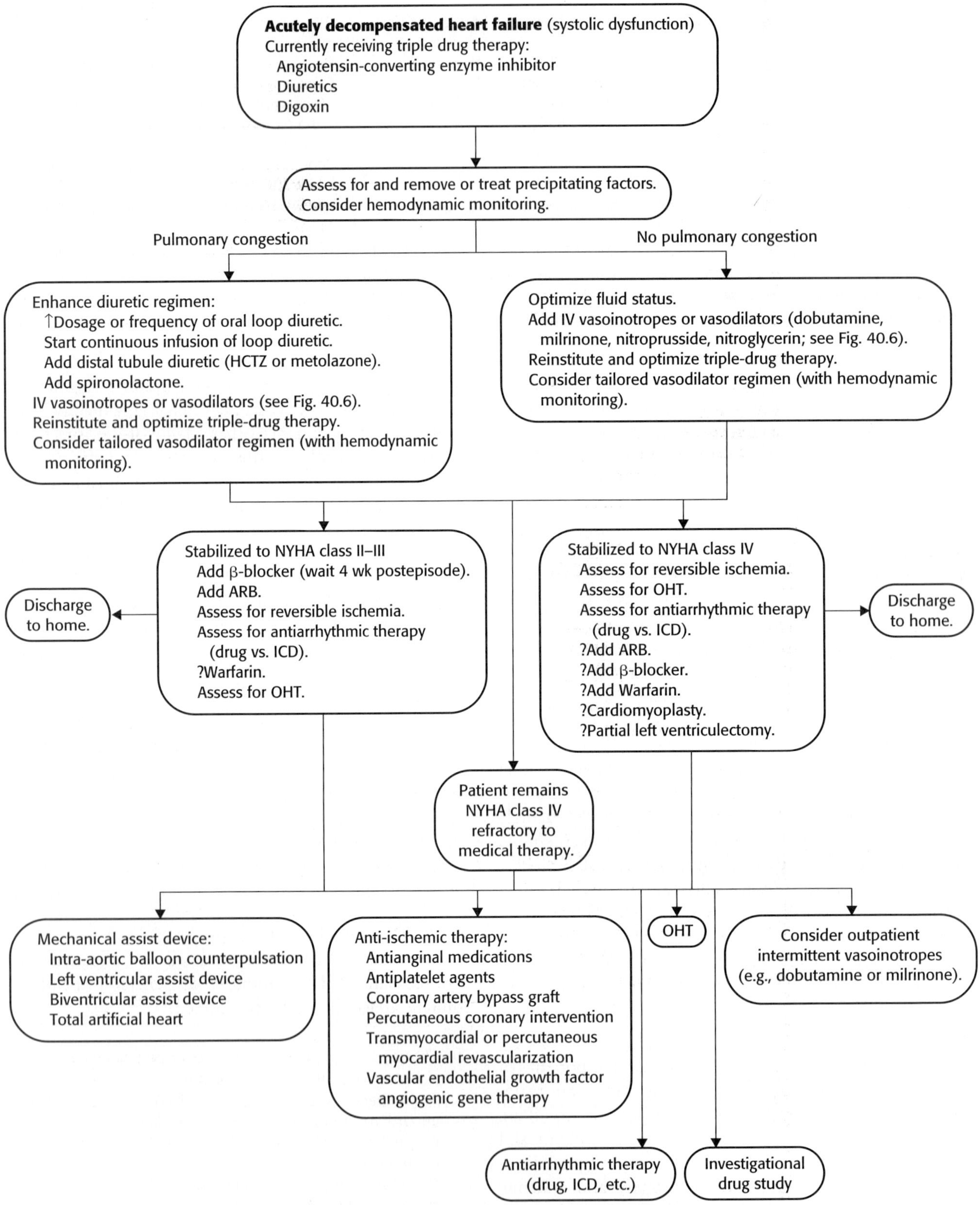

Figure 40.5. Algorithm for management of patient with acutely decompensated heart failure. *ARB,* angiotensin II type 1 receptor blocker; *HCTZ,* hydrochlorothiazide; *ICD,* implantable cardioverter–defibrillator; *NYHA,* New York Heart Association; *OHT,* orthotopic heart transplantation;

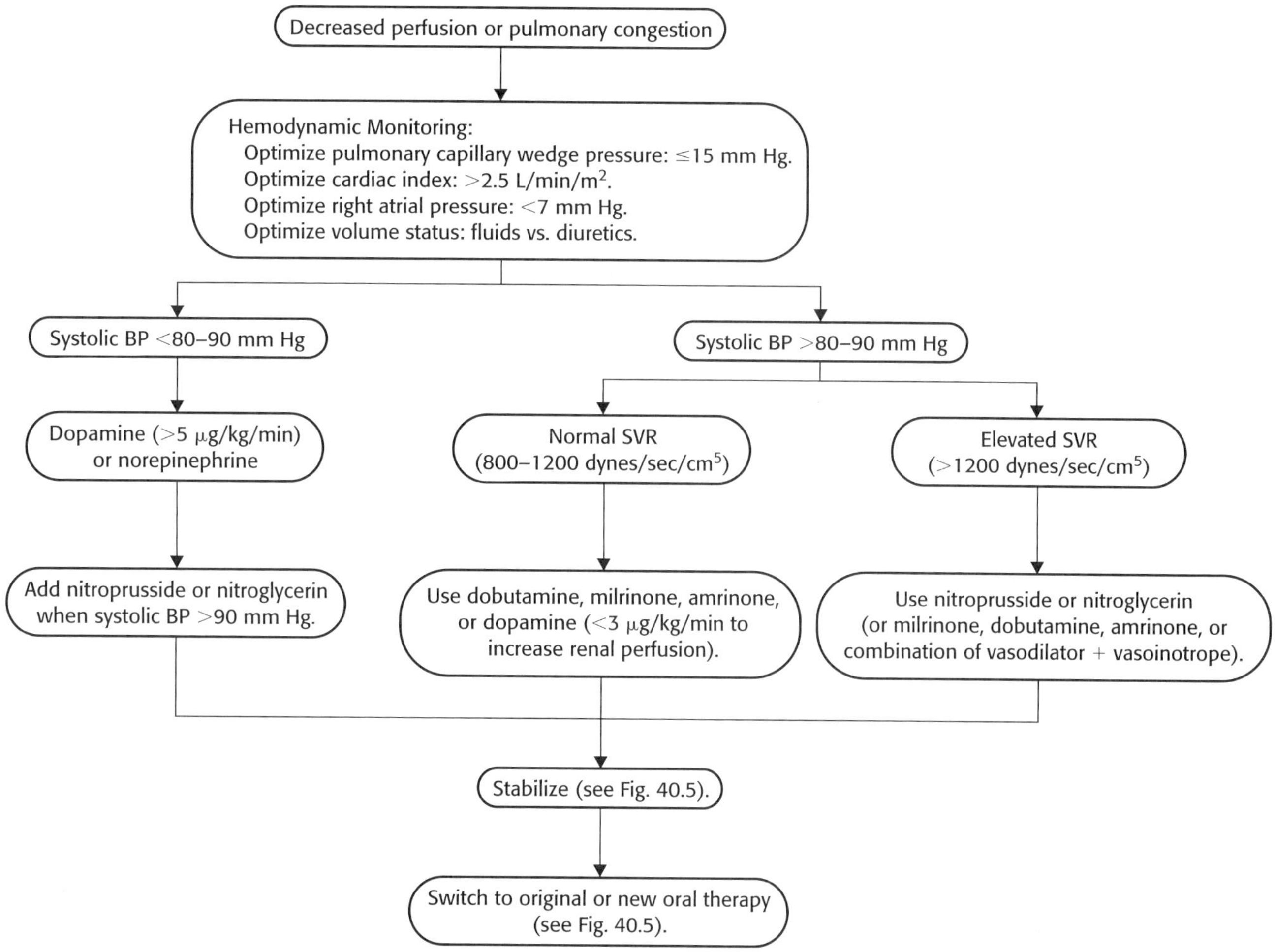

Figure 40.6. Algorithm for using vasoinotropes and vasodilators for patients hospitalized for congestive heart failure with acute decompensation. *BP,* blood pressure; *SVR,* systemic vascular resistance.

- Diuretics should be administered as frequently (or infrequently) as necessary.
- Combination diuretic therapy may be needed as a patient's CHF worsens.
- Osmotic diuretics generally are not useful in CHF management.
- Mild (less than 3 g/day) to moderate (less than 2 g/day) dietary Na^+ restriction is important for maintaining diuretic effectiveness.
- With the exception of spironolactone, all diuretics act at ionic luminal transport sites via access to renal tubular fluid.
- Potassium supplementation or a potassium-sparing diuretic generally is needed when large dosages of loop diuretics are prescribed, especially in combination with thiazide diuretics.

Classification of Diuretics

THIAZIDES. The major site of diuretic action of the thiazides is the early to mid-distal convoluted tubule, where they block the electroneutral sodium chloride transporter (Table 40.8).[117,118] This results in a maximal fractional excretion of sodium approximately 3 to 6%.[117] Thus, these compounds are considered moderately potent diuretics. The effectiveness of thiazide diuretics depends on the proximal tubule organic acid secretory pathway and GFR for delivery to the site of action.[118] Because individual thiazide agents are essentially interchangeable in terms of diuretic effectiveness, hydrochlorothiazide (HCTZ) generally is prescribed because of its low cost. Unless the patient has impaired renal function (i.e., CL_{Cr} less than 50 mL/minute) or moderate to severe congestive symptoms, conditions when a loop diuretic is indicated, a thiazide is a rational initial diuretic choice.[118] Mild HF with preserved renal function (i.e., CL_{Cr} greater than 50 mL/minute) may respond to daily dosages of HCTZ of 25 to 50 mg given once or twice daily (Table 40.8).[118] HCTZ dosages greater than 50 mg/day, generally in combination with a loop diuretic, are needed in instances of reduced renal function or worsening HF, at the risk of causing more severe electrolyte imbalances (Table 40.8).[118] Thiazide diuretic absorption may be delayed in CHF.[111] Adverse effects that may occur secondary to thiazide administration include hypokalemia, hyponatremia, hypomagnesemia, hyperuricemia, hyperlipoproteinemia (i.e., increases in total cholesterol, low-density lipoproteins, and triglycerides and decreases in high-density lipoproteins), and impaired carbohydrate tolerance (Table 40.8). NSAIDs and organic acids such as

Table 40.8 ▪ Diuretics Used to Treat CHF

Class	Pharmacokinetics	Pharmacodynamics	Dosing Guidelines	Adverse Effects	Drug Interactions	Monitoring Parameters
Thiazides SOA: early to mid DCT						
HCTZ[a]	F: 65–75% $t_{1/2}$: RI: >2.5 hr CHF: ND	Onset: 2 hr Peak: 4–6 hr Duration: 6–12 hr	PO 25–50 mg/day (CL_{Cr} >50 mL/min) 50–100 mg/day (CL_{Cr} 20–50 mL/min) 100-200 mg/day (CL_{Cr} <20 mL/min)	Hypokalemia Hyponatremia Hypomagnesemia Azotemia Hyperlipoproteinemia Hyperglycemia Rash Pancreatitis Cholestatic jaundice	Loop diuretics (excessive hypokalemia) NSAIDs (antagonize diuretic effects) Probenecid (competes for secretion)	Body weight Serum electrolytes: K^+, Mg^{+2}, Na^+ Signs and symptoms of CHF Blood pressure BUN, Scr Drug interactions
Chlorothiazide[a]	F: 30–50% $t_{1/2}$: 1.5 hr (N) RI: ND CHF: ND	Onset: (IV): 15 min Peak (IV): 30 min Duration (IV): 2 hr	IV 250 mg q12hr (CL_{Cr} >50 mL/min) 500 mg q12 hr (CL_{Cr} 20–50 mL/min) 1 g q12 hr (CL_{Cr} <20 mL/min)	As above	As above	As above
Metolazone SOA: early to mid-DCT and possibly PCT	F: 40–65% $t_{1/2}$: 14 hr (N) RI: ND CHF: ND	Onset: 1 hr Peak: 2–8 hr Duration: 12–24 hr	PO: 2.5–20 mg/day or every other day	As for thiazides	As for thiazides	As for thiazides
Loop diuretics SOA: TAL						
Furosemide	F: 10–100% $t_{1/2}$: RI: ~3 hr CHF: ~3 hr	Onset PO: 30 min IV: 5 min Peak PO: 1–2 hr IV: 30 min Duration PO: 6–8 hr IV: 2 hr	PO: 40–80 mg × Scr IV infusion 40 mg LD, then 10 mg/hr (CL_{Cr} >75 mL/min) 40 mg LD, then 10–20 mg/hr (CL_{Cr} 25–75 mL/min) 40 mg LD, then 20–40 mg/hr (CL_{Cr} <25 mL/min)	As for thiazides except for hypocalcemia, transient tinnitus, or deafness	As for thiazides Thiazides or metolazone (excessive hypokalemia)	As for thiazides

Bumetanide	F: 80–100% $t_{1/2}$: RI: 1.6 hr CHF: 1.3 hr	Onset PO: 0.5–1 hr IV: 5 min Peak PO: 1–2 hr IV: 30–45 min Duration PO: 4–6 hr IV: 2 hr	PO: 1 mg × Scr IV infusion 1 mg LD, then 0.5 mg/hr (CL_{Cr} >75 mL/min) 1 mg LD, then 0.5–1 mg/hr (CL_{Cr} 25–75 mL/min) 1 mg LD, then 1–2 mg/hr (CL_{Cr} <25 mL/min)	As above	As above	As above
Torsemide	F: 80–100% $t_{1/2}$: RI: 4–5 hr CHF: 6 hr	Onset PO: 1 hr IV : 10 min Peak PO: 1–2 hr IV : 1 hr Duration PO: 8–12 hr IV: 6–8 hr	PO: 10 mg × Scr IV infusion 20 mg LD, then 5 mg/hr (CL_{Cr} >75 mL/min) 20 mg LD, then 5–10 mg/hr (CL_{Cr} 25–75 mL/min) 20 mg LD, then 10–20 mg/hr (CL_{Cr} <25 mL/min)	As above	As above	As above
Potassium-sparing						
Spironolactone SOA: terminal DCT, aldosterone-dependent Na^+/K^+ exchange site	F: conflicting data $t_{1/2}$: >15 hr (N) (active metabolites) RI: ND CHF:ND	Onset: 3 days (active metabolites)	12.5–25 mg/day up to 200 mg/day	Hyperkalemia Gynecomastia	ACEIs, NSAIDs, or K^+ supplements (↑ risk of hyperkalemia) Digoxin (↑ SDC)	As for thiazides
Triamterene SOA: $Na^+/K^+/H^+$ exchange site, aldosterone-independent	F: >80% $t_{1/2}$: RI: >5 hr CHF: ND	Onset: 2–4 hr Peak: 2–4 hr Duration: 7–9 hr	100 mg BID	Hyperkalemia Azotemia Renal stones	ACEIs, NSAIDs, or K^+ supplements (↑ risk of hyperkalemia) H_2-Antagonists and trimethoprim (compete for renal tubular secretion)	As for thiazides
Amiloride SOA: same as triamterene	F: Conflicting data $t_{1/2}$: RI: 100 hr CHF: ND	Onset: 2 hr Peak: 3–4 hr Duration: 24 hr	5–10 mg/day up to 40 mg/day	Hyperkalemia Azotemia	As for triamterene	As for thiazides

Source: References 111, 118.

F, bioavailability; *N,* normals; *ND,* no data; *RI,* renal insufficiency; *CL_{Cr},* creatinine clearance; *Scr,* serum creatinine; *ACEI,* angiotensin-converting enzyme inhibitor; *LD,* loading dose; *BUN,* blood urea nitrogen; *SDC,* serum digoxin concentration; *SOA,* site of action within nephron; *DCT,* distal convoluted tubule; *PCT,* proximal convoluted tubules; *TAL,* thick ascending limb of the loop of Henle; *HCTZ,* hydrochlorothiazide.

[a]Not effective as a single agent if CL_{Cr} < 50 mL/min.

probenecid can diminish the response to thiazides (Table 40.8).[118] The former enhance sodium reabsorption in the thick ascending limb of the loop of Henle, and the latter impair proximal tubular secretion of the thiazide diuretic.

METOLAZONE. Metolazone is a thiazide-type drug that acts principally at the distal convoluted tubule (Table 40.8).[117] Metolazone also may have proximal tubular effects that further reduce sodium reabsorption. Major differences between metolazone and the thiazides are that metolazone retains its effectiveness even when renal function is markedly reduced and has a duration of action (elimination half-life of about 2 days) longer than that of most thiazides.[118] Metolazone and the thiazides produce similar adverse effects (Table 40.8). As a single diuretic, metolazone can be used in dosages starting at 2.5 mg daily. However, it is often used in combination with loop diuretics (i.e., sequential diuresis) and therefore may be prescribed as 2.5 mg every 1 to 4 days.[111–113,117–119] When metolazone is administered in conjunction with loop diuretics, it is advisable to administer metolazone (or any thiazide diuretic) about 1 hour before the loop diuretic to achieve maximal diuresis.[119]

LOOP DIURETICS. These drugs act principally at the thick ascending limb of the loop of Henle, where they block the sodium–potassium–chloride transporter and may increase the fractional excretion of sodium up to 25% (Table 40.8).[117] Like thiazides, loop diuretics depend on secretion into the proximal tubule via the organic acid pathway.[117,118] Loop diuretics also can increase renal blood flow by enhancing production of the renal vasodilatory prostaglandin. This effect contributes to the natriuretic effects of the loop diuretics. Loop diuretics remain effective despite reductions in GFR, although larger than usual dosages are needed in the setting of renal dysfunction (Table 40.8).

Furosemide, bumetanide, and torsemide are loop diuretics currently available in the United States. Furosemide is the most commonly prescribed agent in this subgroup because of cost. These agents differ predominantly with respect to milligram-to-milligram potency and pharmacokinetics (Table 40.8). Torsemide has a significantly longer $t_{1/2}$ than the other two agents.[118] In addition, in CHF furosemide absorption is delayed and erratic, bumetanide absorption is delayed; and torsemide absorption is unaffected.[118] Adverse effects of loop diuretics are similar to those of the thiazide diuretics (Table 40.8).[118] However, loop diuretics may produce hypocalcemia and transient ototoxicity, which are not shared with the thiazide compounds or metolazone. Initial dosages of furosemide (40 mg daily), bumetanide (1.0 mg daily), or torsemide (10 mg daily) can promote a prompt diuresis. However, as HF and secondary renal dysfunction progress, increasingly larger and more frequent doses are needed. Although dosages vary widely, patients with end-stage HF may need two or three oral daily doses of a loop diuretic (e.g., furosemide 160 to 400 mg).[118] A good rule for estimating the initial dosage of furosemide is 40 mg multiplied by the patient's Scr.[112]

POTASSIUM-SPARING DIURETICS. Spironolactone, triamterene, and amiloride exert their diuretic effects at the terminal portion of the distal convoluted tubule (Table 40.8).[117] Spironolactone, which is converted to the active metabolite canrenone, acts at an aldosterone-sensitive site, whereas triamterene and amiloride, which are secreted into the proximal tubule via the organic base pathway, block aldosterone-independent apical sodium channels. Potassium-sparing agents are considered weak diuretics because they induce a fractional excretion of sodium of only 1 to 2%.[117] Potassium-sparing diuretics are useful mainly as adjuncts with thiazides, metolazone, and loop diuretics to counteract the hypokalemia and hypomagnesemia often induced or exacerbated by these other drugs. Hypokalemia and hypomagnesemia are directly arrhythmogenic and may potentiate arrhythmias secondary to either digoxin or circulating catecholamines.[118] These combined electrolyte disturbances appear to be best prevented by potassium-sparing diuretics. However, therapy with potassium-sparing agents should be individualized.

In selecting a potassium-sparing diuretic, it should be noted that spironolactone is effective only in relative hyperaldosteronemic states such as CHF (Table 40.8).[117,118] Triamterene and amiloride are effective even when aldosterone levels are not elevated. Both triamterene and amiloride attain steady-state effects in about 1 to 1.5 days. Spironolactone's effects do not peak for several days because it takes 3 to 4 days for active metabolites to attain steady-state concentrations. Likewise, the effects of spironolactone persist for several days after cessation of therapy because of the presence of the active metabolite. Adding single daily doses of spironolactone ranging from 12.5 to 75 mg to a regimen of digoxin, loop diuretic, and an ACEI significantly increases urinary excretion of aldosterone and serum potassium levels and decreases atrial natiuretic factor (ANF) plasma concentrations.[120] As noted previously, spironolactone administration also is associated with almost a one-third reduction in 2-year mortality and hospitalization for HF.[113,114]

A potential consequence of prescribing any potassium-sparing diuretic is hyperkalemia. However, hyperkalemia appears to be dose related[120] and is more likely to occur in patients with severe renal dysfunction or in patients receiving concomitant potassium supplements, salt substitutes (which contain potassium), NSAIDs, ACEIs, or ARB (Table 40.8). On the other hand, trimethoprim and H_2-receptor blockers, both of which are organic bases, may compete for the secretion of amiloride and triamterene.[118] Spironolactone can induce gynecomastia. Triamterene-containing renal stones have been reported.

DIURETIC RESISTANCE. To optimize diuretic therapy in patients with CHF, the clinician must be familiar with the physiologic and pharmacologic factors that mediate a diminished clinical response to diuretics (i.e., diuretic resistance).[111–113,118,119] Patient noncompliance with the prescribed diuretic regimen minimizes the effectiveness of the drug. Noncompliance can be minimized through patient education.[52] Also, an increased Na^+ intake can offset the natriuretic effects of the diuretic. Therefore, a reduction in Na^+ consumption usually must accompany diuretic therapy (Table 40.4).[37]

Uremia may diminish the response to loop diuretics, which chemically are highly protein bound organic acids.[118] To reach their site of action within the nephron, loop diuretics depend largely on the proximal tubule organic acid secretory pump, which can be blocked by increased circulating concentrations of endogenous organic acids seen in uremia and renal dysfunction. This example of diuretic resistance may be overcome either by using more frequent and much higher dosages of the loop diuretic or by combining the loop diuretic with another diuretic that has a different site of action within the nephron, such as a thiazide or metolazone.[112–113,118,119] A continuous infusion of a loop diuretic also may be useful in this clinical setting.[118]

NSAIDs significantly diminish the natriuretic effect of loop diuretics. NSAIDs block the renal hemodynamic effects of these agents by inhibiting prostaglandin synthesis.[57] The effect was initially reported with indomethacin and has subsequently been shown to occur with ibuprofen, sulindac, naproxen, and aspirin. The use of NSAIDs in patients with CHF taking diuretics is associated with a twofold higher need for hospitalization for CHF.[57] NSAID-induced diuretic resistance can be counteracted by discontinuing the offending agent, if possible, by using larger or more frequent doses of loop diuretics, or by combining the loop diuretic with a thiazide or metolazone.[111–113,118,119]

CHF also can partially attenuate the response to loop diuretics by a number of mechanisms.[111–113,118,119] In CHF, the natriuretic response is reduced secondary to neurohormonally mediated enhanced sodium reabsorption. In addition, in CHF the rate of gastrointestinal absorption of orally administered thiazide and some loop diuretics may decrease, slowing delivery of the diuretic to its site of action and thereby delaying or diminishing response.[118] A more effective diuresis can be achieved by administering more frequent doses of the oral loop diuretic, adding a thiazide diuretic or metolazone, or administering the loop diuretic intravenously, either as a single dose or via continuous infusion.[111–113,118,119] The coexistence of renal dysfunction also warrants higher dosages of the loop or thiazide diuretic.[118]

Patient-Adjusted Diuretic Therapy

After appropriate patient education, some patients may be able to assume responsibility for making minor adjustments in their diuretic regimen based on changes in weight, salt and fluid intake, symptoms of dyspnea, and increasing peripheral edema. A simple but useful monitoring tool is a daily log of the patient's weight.[37] Careful attention to clinical parameters at home with concomitant adjustments in the diuretic regimen may lead to reductions in the frequency of HF exacerbations and resultant hospital admissions.

Digoxin

Digitalis glycosides classically have been used as inotropic drugs to treat CHF. However, only recently have clinical studies better defined the actual value and role of these agents in CHF management.[121] In the discussion that follows, digoxin is the only cardiac glycoside extensively reviewed because of its predominant use in clinical medicine.

Mechanism of Action

The inotropic effects of digoxin are produced indirectly, through inhibition of the sarcolemmal transport enzyme sodium–potassium adenosine triphosphatase (Na^+–K^+ ATPase).[122] This enzyme complex catalyzes Na^+ efflux from the myocardial cell in exchange for K^+. When Na^+ efflux is inhibited by digoxin, high intracellular concentrations of Na^+ result. Sodium is subsequently exchanged for calcium (Ca^{+2}) via an Na^+–Ca^{+2} exchange carrier. The increased intracellular concentrations of Ca^{+2} ultimately enhance myocardial contractility through a complex series of intracellular Ca^{+2} movements. In the failing human myocardium there appears to be an increased sensitivity to the inotropic effects of digoxin, which is caused in part by decreased expression of Na^+K^+ ATPase.[122]

Digoxin also has several neurohormonal effects. Digoxin increases parasympathomimetic activity, which slows both HR and atrioventricular (AV) conduction.[123] These effects may increase diastolic filling time and decrease myocardial oxygen consumption. Digoxin also decreases sympathetic activity, plasma renin, and aldosterone.[124] The combination of inotropic and neurohormonal-modulating effects may account for the recently observed beneficial outcomes in patients with CHF.[121]

Pharmacokinetics

A vast amount of literature describes the absorption, distribution, metabolism, and elimination of digoxin.[125] Digoxin is available parenterally and as a tablet, elixir, and capsule. For the oral preparations, the systemic availability is independent of the dosage administered and averages 70 to 80%, 75 to 85%, and 90 to 100%, respectively.

Digoxin is widely distributed into various tissues.[125] The highest concentrations of digoxin are found in the kidneys, heart, liver, adrenal glands, diaphragm, and intestinal tract. However, approximately 50% of the apparent total body stores of digoxin are found in the skeletal muscles. As a result of this extensive distribution to lean tissue, digoxin generally should be dosed using an estimate of the patient's ideal body weight (IBW). The plasma protein binding of digoxin is independent of concentration and averages 20 to 30%. Albumin is the principal binding protein. In patients with normal renal function, the volume of distribution at steady state (V_{ss}) averages 6 to 7 L/kg.

Digoxin undergoes metabolism primarily by two different pathways.[125] One of these pathways involves sequential hydrolysis of digitoxose sugar moieties, and the other route results in the formation of reduced metabolites. The reduced (i.e., dihydro) metabolites are inactive. In contrast, the hydrolysis products, digoxigenin bis- and mono-digitoxosides, have potencies that approach that of the parent compound. However, the contribution of these two metabolites to overall digoxin activity in humans is unknown. In adults with normal renal and hepatic function, the systemic clearance (CL_S) of digoxin averages approximately 180 mL/minute/1.73 m^2. Renal digoxin clearance (CL_R), which exceeds creatinine and inulin clearances, generally accounts for about 70% of the CL_S. The nonrenal clearance (CL_{NR}) of digoxin includes metabolism, biliary excretion, and possibly intestinal secretion and resultant fecal elimination. The CL_S of digoxin is linearly correlated, but the elimination half-life ($t_{1/2}$) is inversely correlated with creatinine clearance (CL_{Cr}). The $t_{1/2}$ of digoxin averages 36 hours in young adults with normal renal and hepatic function.

Numerous clinical conditions can alter digoxin pharmacokinetics (Table 40.9).[125–128] The bioavailability of digoxin tablets can be reduced by abdominal radiation, by various malabsorption syndromes such as hypermotility, diarrhea, and subtotal villus atrophy, and by several drugs.[125,126] In contrast, digoxin absorption may be enhanced by hypochlorhydria,[128] propantheline (and perhaps other anticholinergic drugs),[126] and oral antibiotics such as tetracycline and macrolides.[126,127] These anti-

Table 40.9 ▪ Conditions of Altered Digoxin Pharmacokinetics or Pharmacodynamics

Condition	Clinical Management
A. Reduced bioavailability	
1. Abdominal radiation	1. Consider administering digoxin as elixir or capsule.
2. Malabsorption syndromes	2. Same as above.
a. Hypermotility	
b. Diarrhea	
c. Subtotal villus atrophy	
3. Drugs	3. Consider administering digoxin 1–2 hr before or 2–3 hr after a, b, c, e, f, and g; consider administering digoxin as capsule or elixir for d.
a. Cholesterol-binding resins	
b. Kaolin–pectin	
c. Large dosages (e.g., 30 mL) of antacid	
d. Metoclopramide (oral)	
e. Sulfasalazine	
f. Neomycin (oral)	
g. Sucralfate	
B. Enhanced bioavailability	
1. Propantheline (and perhaps other anticholinergics)	1. Be alert for possible digoxin toxicity.
2. Oral antibiotics	2. Thought to be a problem in 10% of population who extensively metabolize digoxin to inactive reduction products by colonic bacteria; avoid antibiotics if possible. If antibiotics must be administered, be alert for possible occurrence of digoxin toxicity.
a. Erythromycin, clarithromycin, roxithromycin	
b. Tetracycline	
3. Hypochlorhydria, achlorhydria	3. Be alert for possible occurrence of digoxin toxicity.
C. Reduced systemic clearance	
1. Renal dysfunction	1. Adjust digoxin dosages to the reductions in creatinine clearance.
2. Aging	2. As for C1: also monitor SDCs every few months.
3. Drugs	
a. Quinidine	a. Reduce digoxin dosage by 50% upon start of quinidine; monitor SDCs.
b. Verapamil	b. Consider reducing digoxin dosage by about 50% on initiation of verapamil, monitor SDCs, and look for additive effects on SA and AV nodes.
c. Diltiazem	c. Monitor SDCs; be alert for additive effects on SA and AV nodes.
d. Spironolactone	d. Consider reducing digoxin dosage by about 50%, monitor SDCs, and be alert for signs and symptoms of toxicity.
e. Amiodarone	e. Consider reducing digoxin dosage by about 50%, monitor SDCs, and look for additive effects on SA and AV nodes.
f. Captopril	f. Routine reduction of digoxin appears to be unnecessary; monitor SDCs and be alert for signs and symptoms of toxicity.
g. Propafenone	g. Consider reducing digoxin dosage by about 25%, monitor SDCs, and be alert for signs and symptoms of toxicity.
D. Altered pharmacodynamics	
1. β-Blockers	1. Be alert for additive effects on SA and AV nodes.
2. Other inotropic drugs	2. Try to avoid because they may increase risk of digoxin-induced arrhythmias.
3. Diuretics	3. May produce hypokalemia or hypomagnesemia, which increase risk of digoxin-induced arrhythmias; replace depleted electrolytes.

SDCs, serum digoxin concentrations; *SA*, sinoatrial; *AV*, atrioventricular.

biotics decrease the number of colonic bacteria that metabolize digoxin to inactive reduced metabolites. The V_{SS} of digoxin is reduced by chronic renal failure but increased by physical activity.[125] Chronic renal failure also increases the $t_{1/2}$ of digoxin. Drugs that consistently reduce the CL_S of digoxin include quinidine, verapamil, spironolactone, amiodarone, and propafenone.[126] Inhibition of the active drug transporter *P*-glycoprotein, for which digoxin acts as a substrate, is the likely mechanism for the reduced CL_S.[129] Captopril, hypothyroidism, and advanced CHF also decrease the CL_S of digoxin.[126] Hyperthyroidism, rifampin, and orally administered cholesterol-binding resins and activated charcoal increase the CL_S of digoxin.[125,126] Pharmacodynamic interactions may occur with β-adrenergic blocking drugs, amiodarone, verapamil, and diltiazem, all of which enhance the effects of digoxin on decreasing AV nodal conduction and sinoatrial (SA) nodal rate (Table 40.9).

Serum Digoxin Concentration–Response Relationships

Although many clinical laboratories and reference texts list the therapeutic range for digoxin as 0.5 or 0.8 to 2.0 ng/mL, relationships between the SDC and the intensity of its inotropic response, autonomic and neurohormonal effects, and the development of digoxin toxicity are not clearly defined. This lack of a definitive therapeutic range reflects digoxin's rather modest inotropic effects, the apparently flat dose–response curve with respect to digoxin's autonomic and neurohormonal modulating effects, and the overlap between therapeutic and toxic SDCs. In addition, many assay techniques used to quantify SDCs are nonspecific, failing to distinguish digoxin from active and inactive metabolites as well as endogenous digoxinlike immunoreactive substances. However, recent findings may lead to a better definition of the therapeutic range of digoxin.[130–132] For example, in patients with CHF caused by systolic dysfunction, SDCs ranging from 0.9 to 1.2 ng/mL were associated with significantly higher maximal treadmill exercise time than that of placebo.[130] This improvement was of the same magnitude as that observed at SDCs greater than 1.2 ng/mL but superior to that of SDCs ranging from 0.5 to 0.9 ng/mL. In another study, a near doubling of the SDC from 0.7 to 1.2 ng/mL resulted in a small increase in EF, a trend toward increased exercise time, but no further decrease in circulating neurohormones.[131] Other investigators reported no additional reductions in HR or sympathetic activity or improvements in ventricular performance after a near doubling of SDCs from 0.8 to 1.5 ng/mL.[132] Furthermore, at mean SDCs less than 1.0 ng/mL (and within a targeted range 0.5 to 2.0 ng/mL) the combined endpoint of death or hospitalization due to HF was significantly decreased by digoxin in the Digitalis Investigation Groug (DIG) trial.[121] Last, despite considerable overlap between therapeutic and toxic SDCs, a review of data from more than 1000 patients reported a mean SDC of 1.4 ng/mL in patients without toxicity, whereas SDCs two to three times greater were noted in patients with overt toxicity.[133] Collectively these observations suggest that SDCs between 0.7 to 1.2 ng/mL should maximize the hemodynamic, clinical, and neurohormonal benefits of digoxin and minimize the risk of digoxin toxicity.

Dosing Guidelines

Several pharmacokinetic equations provide prospective dosing guidelines for digoxin. However, most equations show a poor correlation between predicted and measured SDCs.[134] Nonetheless, because the equations generally overestimate the measured SDC, they provide safe initial approximations of a patient's digoxin dosage. However, the method of Koup et al.,[135] using a CL_{NR} of 20 mL/minute/1.73 m^2, best correlates the predicted and measured steady-state SDC.[134]

To use this method, first estimate the patient's IBW:

$$IBW_{male} = 50 \text{ kg} + 2.3 \times \text{Height in inches above 5 ft}$$

$$IBW_{female} = 45 \text{ kg} + 2.3 \times \text{Height in inches above 5 ft}$$

If the patient's actual weight is less than the estimated IBW, use the actual weight. Next estimate the patient's body surface area (BSA) in square meters:

$$BSA \text{ m}^2 = IBW \text{ (kg)}^{0.425} \times \text{Height (cm)}^{0.725} \times 0.007184$$

Thereafter, estimate the patient's CL_{Cr} using the Cockgroft and Gault equation:[136]

$$CL_{Cr} = \frac{(140 - Age) \times ABW}{72 \times Scr} \times \frac{1.73\text{m}^2}{BSA}$$

where Age is the patient's age (in years), ABW is the patient's actual body weight (in kg), and Scr is the patient's Scr (in mg/dL). If the patient is female, multiply the result by 0.85.

Then estimate the CL_S for digoxin:

$$CL_S = (1.303 \times CL_{Cr}) + 20 \text{ mL/minute/1.73 m}^2$$

The initial estimate of the patient's daily digoxin dosage is computed using the steady-state equation and a target SDC (i.e., 1.0 ng/mL):

$$C_{SS} = \frac{F \times D}{CL_S \times \tau}$$

where

D = dosage (ng)
C_{SS} = steady-state digoxin level (ng/mL)
CL_S = systemic clearance (mL/minute/1.73 m^2)
τ = dosing interval (1440 minutes/day)
F = fraction absorbed (0.75 for tablets)

These digoxin dosing guidelines for patients with CHF should result in a low probability of achieving a potentially toxic SDC. A trough SDC can be obtained either after a few days, to verify that a serious overprediction or underprediction of the measured SDC has not occurred, or at the attainment of steady state (usually 7 to 10 days for most adults). General indications for measuring SDCs include establishing initial dose–SDC relationship, assessing known or suspected pharmacokinetic digoxin–drug interactions, evaluating the effect of a change in physiologic function known or suspected to alter the disposition of digoxin (e.g., renal dysfunction), monitoring after a change in the dosage form of digoxin, confirming suspected digoxin toxicity, evaluating a poor response to initial therapy or a decline in response after early therapeutic success, and assessing patient compliance. In addition, older adults may benefit from routine measurement of SDCs because of the difficulty of predicting digoxin dosages in this subgroup. Again it must be emphasized that SDCs do not predict efficacy or toxicity and should therefore be used only to complement good clinical judgement. Strict attention should be given to the timing of blood collection and its relationship to the time of last dose. Collecting blood during the distribution phase (lasting up to 12 hours after an oral dose) may cause the SDC to be falsely elevated and potentially useless in evaluating possible risk of toxicity.

Table 40.10 ▪ Signs and Symptoms of Digoxin Intoxication

Noncardiac	Common cardiac arrhythmias[a]
Gastrointestinal: anorexia, nausea, vomiting	VPDs, including multifocal VPDs and bigeminy or trigeminy
Neurologic: fatigue, malaise, delirium, acute psychosis, neuralgic pain	First-degree AV block
Ocular: halo vision, green (chloropsia) or yellow (xanthopsia) vision	Mobitz type I AV block
Miscellaneous: gynecomastia and sexual dysfunction (men)	Nonparoxysmal junctional tachycardia
	Supraventricular tachycardia with block
	Ventricular tachycardia (including bidirectional ventricular tachycardia)

VPDs, ventricular premature depolarizations; *AV*, atrioventricular.
[a]Virtually every known cardiac arrhythmia has occurred secondary to digitalis intoxication.

Table 40.11 ▪ Factors That May Predispose Patients to Developing Digoxin Intoxication

Electrolyte abnormalities	Hypoxia
Hypokalemia	Renal dysfunction
Hypomagnesemia	Hypothyroidism
Hypercalcemia	Drug interactions (see Table 40.9)
Advanced age	
Acid-base disturbances	
Alkalosis	

Digoxin Toxicity

Despite the objective means used to develop rational dosing guidelines for digoxin, digoxin toxicity remains a worrisome clinical problem. Previous estimates of the frequency of digitalis toxicity in hospitalized patients taking digoxin ranged from 4 to 35% and were accompanied by a high mortality rate of up to 41%.[133] However, today the incidence of definite or possible digoxin toxicity consistently approaches about 4%,[137,138] with hospitalization for digoxin toxicity needed for 1.5[138] to 2%[121] of patients receiving digoxin.

The diagnosis of digoxin intoxication is challenging. It can be acute or chronic, and it generally results from excessive ingestion, a change in disposition, or an increased sensitivity to digoxin. Digoxin intoxication can manifest as a number of noncardiac symptoms (Table 40.10), the most common of which are anorexia, nausea, and vomiting.[139,140] In addition, virtually any cardiac arrhythmia or conduction disturbance can be associated with digoxin toxicity. These rhythm disturbances are common manifestations and may be the first sign of digoxin toxicity. Digoxin-induced arrhythmias are generally classified as decreases in impulse conduction, enhancement of automaticity, or a combination of both. In a recent study, the most commonly observed arrhythmias for patients with definite or probable digoxin toxicity were AV block and sinus bradycardia.[137] However, in the DIG trial, the most common arrhythmias for suspected digoxin toxicity were ventricular fibrillation or tachycardia, supraventricular arrhythmia, and second- or third-degree AV block.[121]

Digoxin toxicity is largely preventable[141] given the number of known, usually modifiable and monitorable risk factors that predispose patients to digoxin toxicity, with the most common being older adults with impaired renal function (Table 40.11).[139] Older adults also may exhibit an increased sensitivity to the Na^+–K^+–ATPase inhibitory effects of digoxin. Renal dysfunction alone predisposes patients to digoxin toxicity because of decreases in the volume of distribution and elimination of digoxin. Hypokalemia and hypomagnesemia are associated with an increased incidence of digitalis-induced arrhythmias. Hypokalemia appears to increase myocardial uptake of digoxin. Magnesium (Mg^{+2}) acts as a cofactor for the enzyme Na^+–K^+ ATPase, so hypomagnesemia may decrease intracellular potassium. Alkalosis also decreases serum concentration and total body stores of K^+ and thereby increases the sensitivity to digitalis. Diuretic-induced alkalosis, even in the setting of normal serum K^+, increases the frequency of digoxin-associated arrhythmias. Hypothyroidism and hypoxia, through unidentified mechanisms, increase a patient's sensitivity to digoxin. Finally, the development of digoxin toxicity may be enhanced by other inotropic drugs, drugs that produce electrolyte disturbances (e.g., diuretics), agents that slow AV nodal conduction or sinus rate (i.e., β-blockers), or drugs that decrease the CL_S of digoxin or increase its absorption (Table 40.9).

Treating Digoxin Toxicity

The severity of digoxin toxicity should be assessed before a treatment plan is initiated. In general, blood should be obtained for determination of serum K^+, Mg^{+2}, and digoxin levels. Efforts should be made to identify and remove predisposing factors. Discontinuation of digoxin and supportive treatment may be sufficient to manage most noncardiac symptoms as well as asymptomatic cardiac manifestations such as first-degree AV block or Mobitz type I second-degree AV block.[140]

In the setting of an accidental or suicidal ingestion of large amounts of digoxin, syrup of ipecac can decrease absorption if administered within an hour of ingestion. Gastric lavage can be attempted if the patient presents within 2 hours of ingestion.[140] However, gastric lavage may provoke fatal arrhythmias. Orally administered activated charcoal, cholestyramine, or colestipol can also minimize absorption but may induce vomiting.

Altered potassium homeostasis often is observed in the setting of digoxin toxicity and can exacerbate digoxin-induced bradyarrhythmias or tachyarrhythmias.[139,140] Potassium should be administered if the potassium level is low or normal unless serum K^+ is 5.0 mEq/mL or higher, the patient is ingesting K^+-conserving drugs, severe renal insufficiency is present, markedly delayed AV conduction is observed (i.e., greater than first-degree AV block), or the patient has ingested a massive overdose of digoxin. Normal saline may be a better choice than 5% dextrose solution for diluting the potassium, avoiding the occasional paradoxical worsening of the hypokalemia sometimes observed in the severely K^+-depleted patient. Hyperkalemia, which generally reflects extracellular distribution of K^+ secondary to inhibition of Na^+–K^+ ATPase, is best managed by administering digoxin-specific antibodies (Fab fragments, Digibind). Fab antibodies bind to tissue-bound, intravascular, and interstitial digoxin.[139,140]

Select digoxin-induced arrhythmias such as nonparoxysmal AV junctional tachycardia, atrial tachycardia with block, ventricular premature depolarizations (VPDs), and ventricular tachycardia may be suppressed by potassium.[139] Magnesium also can suppress digitalis-induced ventricular arrhythmias even in the setting of mildly elevated Mg^{+2} levels.[140] The use of magnesium should be avoided in patients with severe renal insufficiency, a greater than first-degree AV block, or severe hypermagnesemia. The class IB antiarrhythmic drugs, lidocaine, and rarely phenytoin also may be useful in treating digitalis-induced ventricular arrhythmias. Other antiarrhythmics may be proarrhythmic in the setting of digoxin toxicity or may pharmacokinetically or pharmacodynamically interact with digoxin.[139,140] Cardioversion may produce severe arrhythmias or asystole in digoxin-intoxicated patients.[140]

Fab therapy is the most effective antiarrhythmic treatment for life-threatening ventricular arrhythmias secondary to digoxin toxicity.[139,140] An initial response, consisting of a 10- to 20-fold increase in total serum digoxin, a decrease in serum potassium, and a reversal of the adverse electrophysiologic effects of digoxin, often is observed less than 20 minutes after the Fab infusion. These digoxin-specific antibodies often completely reverse the toxic effects of digoxin within a few hours. A treatment response is expected in at least 90% of patients with definitive life-threatening digoxin toxicity. Caution must be exercised in administering Fab fragments to patients with digoxin toxicity and concomitant severe renal impairment. However, plasmapheresis appears to be effective in removing the digoxin–antidigoxin antibody complexes in this setting.[142]

To reverse symptomatic digoxin-induced bradycardia or mild SA or AV conduction delays, atropine administered in intravenous dosages of 0.5 to 2.0 mg is indicated.[140] If the bradycardia or conduction delays are hemodynamically significant and refractory to atropine, Fab therapy should be administered.[139,140] Temporary pacing is associated with a high complication rate in digoxin-intoxicated patients.[140]

Use of Digoxin in Congestive Heart Failure

Digoxin offers several benefits for patients in normal sinus rhythm with CHF secondary to systolic dysfunction who are receiving concurrent treatment with diuretics and ACEIs. Digoxin decreases symptoms, increases exercise performance, improves sympathetic/parasympathetic imbalances, reduces levels of harmful circulating neurohormones, and decreases hospital admissions secondary to HF. The latter effects especially may contribute to an estimated annual savings of $100 million.[143] Furthermore, in patients with coexistent atrial fibrillation, digoxin can offer the additional benefit of decreasing the ventricular rate response. The DIG trial also suggests that patients with CHF secondary to diastolic dysfunction may benefit from digoxin through a reduction in the need for hospitalization.[121] However, the currently limited information on the use of digoxin in these patients does not justify its routine use in this setting. The use of digoxin can result in digoxin toxicity, some of which is life-threatening. However, it should be emphasized that the incidence of digoxin toxicity is declining. Also, the majority of cases of digoxin toxicity today are benign and can be prevented by targeting initial dosing to a lower SDC, monitoring SDC, and monitoring for risk factors for digoxin toxicity and adjusting the dosage accordingly (Tables 40.9 to 40.11). Furthermore, all drugs used to treat CHF produce intolerable and difficult to manage adverse effects. In summary, for patients with CHF secondary to systolic dysfunction, digoxin can be recommended as initial therapy in combination with diuretics, ACEIs, and, if possible, β-blockers (Fig. 40.2).[40] However, future post hoc analyses of β-blocker trials may suggest that little incremental benefit is associated with the use of digoxin with respect to hospitalization, sudden death, or HR response rates in patients with CHF treated with a β-blocker, ACEI, and diuretic.[124]

Additional Inotropic Drugs

A number of inotropic drugs have been investigated in chronic CHF management.[144] Each of these agents raises intracellular concentrations of calcium within myocardial cells, resulting in increases in contractility. Unfortunately, enthusiasm about positive inotropic agents has waned because of their tendency to increase mortality in patients with CHF. Recently, many clinicians have begun to advocate the use of intermittent intravenous milrinone and dobutamine in patients with CHF in an effort to improve quality of life, reduce hospitalization rates, and reduce health care costs. The use of these agents has been based on anecdotal data and small, nonrandomized trials. Typical regimens involve administering intermittent 4- to 6-hour infusions several days a week, 24-hour infusions several times a month, or continuous infusion of the drug. Unfortunately, chronic use of intermittent intravenous inotropes has not been demonstrated to reduce mortality and may actually reduce survival.[145] Inotropic agents may precipitate ischemia and arrhythmias in patients with CHF. Consequently, intravenous inotropes should be reserved for temporary use in patients with acute CHF exacerbation or for hemodynamic support during diagnostic or surgical procedures.[146] Chronic, intermittent administration of intravenous inotropes either in a CHF clinic or at home are not routinely recommended by many cardiovascular specialists because of the lack of data demonstrating their efficacy.[40] Rather, every effort should be made to maximize the patient's CHF medications. Intermittent or continuous inotropic infusions with dobutamine or milrinone or perhaps the combination of milrinone plus a β-blocker[147] should be reserved for patients with end-stage CHF who are awaiting cardiac transplantation or in whom alternatives do not exist.[146]

Preventing Thromboembolic Complications

In the setting of LV dysfunction, abnormal, sometimes static flow through dilated cardiac chambers along with increases in platelet aggregability, coagulation activity, and neuroendocrine activation may predispose the patient to form an intraventricular thrombus and consequent emboli.[148] The incidence of arterial thromboembolism or stroke is approximately 1.9 per 100 patient-years.[148] Analysis of data from the SOLVD trial demonstrated that the risk of embolic events was directly related to the severity of LV dysfunction.[149] Consequently, the use of oral anticoagulants has been proposed in an effort to reduce thromboembolic complications of LV dysfunction. Based on a number of small trials, the efficacy of oral anticoagulation in the prevention of thromboembolic events may be related to the cause of CHF. Early trials indicating a benefit secondary to oral anticoagulant therapy included primarily patients with idiopathic dilated cardiomyopathies.[148] However, recent studies, which included patients with ischemic heart disease, have not shown a beneficial reduction in thromboembolic events in anticoagulated patients.[148]

Any beneficial reduction in thromboembolic events must be weighed against the risk of anticoagulant therapy. The annual risk of a major bleed for patients receiving oral anticoagulant therapy has been estimated at 2%, and the estimated risk of a fatal bleed is 0.8%.[148] Consequently, the risk of experiencing an adverse thromboembolic event is equivalent to and perhaps greater than the risk of experiencing a significant hemorrhagic adverse effect of anticoagulation. Anticoagulation management in patients with CHF is difficult because of a predilection to hepatic congestion and dysfunction, which can decrease warfarin metabolism. Results from CHF trials in which there was uncontrolled use of antiplatelet therapy also are contradictory with respect to favorable outcomes.[148] Thus, large randomized controlled trials that assess warfarin anticoagulation and antiplatelet therapy in patients with CHF and in normal sinus rhythm are needed before these treatments can be recommended routinely. However, for patients with coexisting atrial fibrillation, a history of thromboembolic events, or other known predisposing conditions, warfarin anticoagulation targeted to an international normalized ratio of 2.0 to 3.0 generally is indicated. Antiplatelet therapy probably is indicated for patients with CHF and concurrent CAD.

Arrhythmias in Congestive Heart Failure

Patients with LV dysfunction are at high risk of ventricular arrhythmia and subsequent sudden cardiac death. The risks predisposing patients with HF to sudden death are multifactorial. Structural changes in the myocardium, such as enhanced protein deposition leading to fibrosis and stretching of tissues, may enhance arrhythmogenesis.[150] Also, neurohormonal activation with elevated circulating catecholamines[9] coupled with parasympathetic withdrawal[19] may stimulate arrhythmia development, as can hemodynamic derangements. Electrolyte disturbances, such as hypokalemia and hypomagnesemia, can occur secondary to diuretic therapy and further predispose patients to arrhythmias.[118] In addition, inotropic agents[145] and antiarrhythmic agents[151] can be proarrhythmic.

The use of antiarrhythmic agents to reduce sudden cardiac death has been evaluated in a number of clinical trials. Class Ic agents, such as flecainide, have negative inotropic, proarrhythmic effects and, as demonstrated in the Coronary Arrhythmia Suppression Trial, are associated with an increased mortality in patients with diminished LV function (LVEF less than 30%).[151] Surprisingly, mortality was increased despite suppression of ventricular premature complexes, thus demonstrating the proarrhythmic potential of antiarrhythmic agents. Consequently, the use of class Ic antiarrhythmic agents for extended durations is contraindicated in patients with LV dysfunction. Conversely, class III antiarrhythmic agents, such as amiodarone and dofetilide, may have therapeutic benefit in patients with LV dysfunction.

Currently, amiodarone is the most commonly used antiarrhythmic agent in patients with LV dysfunction. The efficacy of prophylactic amiodarone administration in patients with LV dysfunction and asymptomatic, non–life-threatening ventricular arrhythmias has been evaluated in two clinical trials. In the Grupo de Estudia de la Sobrevida en la Insuficienca Cardiaca en Argentina trial, treatment with amiodarone (300 mg per day) was associated with a 30% reduction in mortality.[152] Reduction in both sudden cardiac death and progressive cardiac failure was observed. However, in the Congestive Heart Failure Survival Trial of Antiarrhythmic Therapy (CHF-

STAT), amiodarone (300 mg per day) was associated with a trend of improved survival only in patients with CHF secondary to nonischemic causes.[153] Thus, amiodarone may be considered if antiarrhythmic therapy is used in patients with LV dysfunction and asymptomatic, non–life-threatening ventricular arrhythmias.

Dofetilide, a class III antiarrhythmic agent, was recently evaluated in patients with LV dysfunction in the Danish Investigations of Arrhythmia and Mortality on Dofetilide trial.[154] A 25% reduction in HF hospitalizations was observed. The role of dofetilide in patients with LV dysfunction must be elucidated, however.

A history of life-threatening ventricular arrhythmias warrants placement of an implantable cardioverter defibrillator (ICD).[155] Since their development in the 1980s, ICDs have revolutionized the management of life-threatening ventricular arrhythmias in the setting of LV dysfunction. Technological improvements in the ICD now permit surgical insertion in a manner similar to pacemaker implantation. Current ICDs are capable of delivering high-energy shock to patients with ventricular fibrillation and rapid ventricular tachycardia or providing antitachycardia pacing to patients with monomorphic ventricular tachycardia. Several trials have been conducted to compare the efficacy of antiarrhythmic therapy and ICD placement.[155] Based on the results of these trials, mild to moderate LV dysfunction and documented sustained or nonsustained ventricular tachycardia warrant placement of an ICD. In patients with severe CHF, the ICD may be used as a bridge to transplantation. In the absence of sustained, nonsustained, or inducible ventricular arrhythmias, sufficient data are currently lacking for empiric placement of an ICD in patients with LV dysfunction. Results from large, ongoing trials such as the Sudden Cardiac Death in Heart Failure trial are being awaited.

In addition to ventricular arrhythmias, atrial fibrillation occurs in 10% to 50% of patients with CHF, and its incidence increases with worsening CHF severity.[156] Elevated atrial pressures lead to hypertrophy and interstitial fibrosis, both of which in conjunction with increased concentrations of circulating NE and other neurohormones can alter the normal electrophysiologic properties of the atria, leading to multiple reentry circuits and atrial fibrillation. In CHF, atrial fibrillation can lead to systemic embolization, adverse hemodynamic effects, worsening symptoms, decreased exercise tolerance, and increased mortality.[156] Retrospective analyses of the SOLVD trials also describe an association between atrial fibrillation and an increased risk of mortality and CHF progression.[157] If ventricular rate control is the goal of therapy, then digoxin, a β-blocker, or amiodarone can be tried.[156] If pharmacologic maintenance of normal sinus rhythm is the goal of therapy, then amiodarone is the drug of choice, and class I antiarrhythmics should be avoided.[156] Dofetilide may offer an alternative to amiodarone in the future. Warfarin anticoagulation, unless there are contraindications, is also indicated for patients with CHF and concomitant atrial fibrillation.[156]

Surgery and Related Therapies

Orthotopic Heart Transplantation

During the last three decades, OHT has emerged as the standard definitive therapy for patients with severe CHF refractory to medical therapy.[39] In the United States, the 1- and 5-year post-OHT survival rates are approximately 85% and 69%, respectively,[158] both of which far exceed corresponding survival rates for patients with severe CHF.[39] However, the number of patients needing OHT far outstrips the limited availability of donor hearts, thereby restricting the annual number of OHTs to 2300, with nearly 4100 patients currently or soon to be listed for OHT.[39] These figures do not begin to address the potential 40,000 patients in the United States who might benefit from OHT.[158]

Given the shortage of available donor hearts, patients referred for cardiac transplantation undergo a specific evaluation to prioritize those most likely to benefit from OHT. Most patients referred for OHT are adults 50 to 64 years old with severe ventricular dysfunction (a resting LVEF under 25%) secondary to advanced CAD or nonischemic cardiomyopathy.[39,158] The cause of CHF is determined for each patient; potentially reversible and precipitating factors are corrected; medical therapy, if possible, should be maximally tailored to delay the need for transplantation and to preserve end-organ function; and patients are evaluated with a measurement of exercise performance, $V_{O_{2max}}$.[39] Other comorbid conditions that may affect post-OHT morbidity or mortality (i.e., malignancy or a life-threatening infectious disease) should be identified.[39,158] These diagnostic and therapeutic efforts are used to stratify potential recipients as United Network for Organ Sharing (UNOS) status I or II patients. The former is the highest-priority status and specifies that potential recipients should be receiving inpatient parenteral pharmacologic (e.g., dobutamine or milrinone) or mechanical (e.g., intra-aortic balloon pump or ventricular support device) support to maintain effective CO. All other patients are listed as UNOS status II patients.[39]

Proper selection and management of donor hearts and donor–recipient matching are essential to transplant success. Ideally, donors are under 40 years old and without cancer, cardiac disease, or active infection.[158] Potential donors also must meet both medical and legal criteria for brain death.[158] Donor hearts are allocated according to ABO blood type compatibility, accrued waiting time on the transplant list, body weight, and geographic region.[39,158] Recent data suggest that minimizing human lymphocyte antigen mismatches improves graft survival after transplantation.[39] Recipients are screened for preformed immunoglobulin G circulating antibodies against a panel of donor antigens (i.e., panel reactive antibodies) that are likely to trigger hyperacute rejection during the immediate post-OHT period.[39]

The impressive survival after OHT can be traced largely to improved immunosuppression and perhaps most specifically to the introduction of cyclosporine. Cyclosporine is most commonly coprescribed with corticosteroids (usually prednisone) and mycophenolate mofetil (MMF) or azathioprine (i.e., triple-drug therapy) after OHT.[39] A recent study comparing triple-drug therapy using MMF or azathioprine as the antiproliferative agent showed that MMF significantly reduced 1-year mortality and the need for antirejection treatment.[39] In addition, tacrolimus is replacing cyclosporine at some institutions. Immunosuppressive therapy must be tailored for each patient, with careful monitoring for potential adverse effects, cyclosporine or tacrolimus whole blood concentrations, drug interactions, signs and symptoms of rejection, and infectious complications. Induction therapy with antilymphocyte antibodies, usually rabbit or equine polyclonal antithymocyte globulin, may be used to facilitate earlier corticosteroid tapering or withdrawal and to hasten the development of immune tolerance, which should delay the mean time to initial allograft rejection. In addition, antilymphocyte antibodies are used to treat corticosteroid-resistant or hemodynamically severe allograft rejection.

Posttransplant complications may include a variety of bacterial, viral, fungal, or protozoal infections.[39] Perhaps the most worrisome is cytomegalovirus (CMV) infection because of its association with the development of coronary allograft vasculopathy (CAV).[39] CAV is a rapidly progressive, obliterative vasculopathy that leads to concentric myointimal hyperplasia in the coronary arteries of the donor heart and is the principal cause of death in long-term OHT survivors.[39] Preemptive treatment with intravenous ganciclovir may reduce the incidence of post-OHT CMV disease.[159] In addition, prophylactic intravenous ganciclovir administration may reduce CAV.[160] Posttransplant HTN and renal dysfunction remain common post-OHT complications, and the incidence of skin cancers and lymphoproliferative disorders increases after OHT.[39]

Newer medical therapies are emerging for OHT management. These include new immunosuppressive drugs such as sirolimus (previously known as rapamycin).[161] Calcium channel blockers such as diltiazem and HMG-CoA reductase inhibitors such as pravastatin may decrease the rate of development of CAV.[161] In addition, coadministering ketoconazole, an inhibitor of cyclosporine metabolism, decreases the cost of cyclosporine therapy and may reduce the incidence of rejection.[161] In the future, agents such as soluble CTLA-4, which invokes T-cell anergy by inhibiting the binding of the CD28 receptor on the T cell to the B-7 receptor on the antigen-presenting cell and, therefore, T-cell activation and clonal expansion, may permit donor heart transplantation without concomitant immunosuppressive drug therapy.[162]

Coronary Artery Revascularization

Because of the prevalence of CAD as a cause for CHF and the growing waiting list for OHT, coronary artery revascularization is an important therapeutic strategy and alternative for selected patients. It is clear that CABG confers an improved survival benefit in patients with moderate to severe LV systolic dysfunction and concurrent symptom-limiting angina pectoris.[39] In addition, CABG surgery can be applied to patients with ischemic cardiomyopathy without angina.[163] After CABG surgery for patients with severe LV dysfunction (LVEF less than 25%), 5-year survival rates range from 73 to 87%.[158] However, it is important to detect and quantify the amount of ischemic but viable myocardium with techniques such as thallium-201 scintigraphy, positron emission tomography, or dobutamine echocardiography to properly select patients with CHF for whom CABG surgery will improve clinical outcomes.[158]

With respect to alternatives to CABG surgery, prospective, comparative studies of percutaneous coronary interventions (PCI) such as percutaneous transluminal coronary angioplasty (PTCA) and CABG surgery are lacking in patients with CHF. However, a clinical history of CHF in conjunction with a decreased LVEF in patients undergoing PCI (principally PTCA) is associated with significant increases in 6-month mortality.[164] Other emerging revascularization techniques for patients with ischemic cardiomyopathy and CHF include transmyocardial or percutaneous myocardial revascularization (TMR or PMR)[165] and intramyocardial angiogenic gene therapy.[166] With the former, channels from the LV cavity to the ischemic myocardium are created by a high-powered CO_2 laser applied either to the heart's epicardial surface (i.e., TMR) using an open chest procedure or to the endocardial surface of the heart (i.e., PMR) via standard femoral arterial access.[165] However, patency of these ventriculomyocardial channels is not maintained chronically, and the sustained improvement in anginal symptoms may occur secondary to the neovascularization that follows the thermal injury induced by the TMR or PMR procedure. PMR appears to be more suitable for patients with severely depressed LV dysfunction caused by CAD.[165] With intramyocardial angiogenic gene therapy, patients receive through a mini-thoracotomy an intramyocardial injection that contains DNA encoding vascular endothelial growth factor (VEGF).[166] VEGF induces neovascularization. A catheter-based system for percutaneous myocardial gene delivery is under investigation and, like PMR, it may hold promise for patients with CHF caused by ischemic cardiomyopathy.

Mechanical and Other Bridges or Alternatives to Orthotopic Heart Transplantation

In addition to OHT and coronary revascularization procedures, other surgical approaches such as dynamic cardiomyoplasty, left ventriculectomy, and mechanical circulatory support devices are being investigated in advanced CHF management.[158,167] With dynamic cardiomyoplasty, the latissimus dorsi muscle, usually the left, while maintaining its blood supply is detached, moved into the chest, and wrapped around the heart. It is then electrically stimulated to convert it from a fast-twitch to slow-twitch muscle to reduce fatigability.[158,167] The electrically stimulated contractions of the latissimus dorsi muscle are intended to assist the systolic function of the heart. The Cardiac–Skeletal Muscle Assist Randomized Trial is under way to determine the role of dynamic cardiomyoplasty in CHF treatment.[167]

Left ventriculectomy, or the Batista procedure, is a direct attempt to surgically reduce ventricular dilation by removing a substantial segment of the LV free wall.[167] Therefore, according to the law of Laplace, ventricular wall stress is reduced. Mitral valve repair or modification is often performed at the time of ventriculectomy. Early single-center results with this procedure report an actuarial 11-month survival of nearly 90%, with a significant reduction in the need for OHT.[167] However, better selection of the most suitable patients is needed before this procedure can be applied more widely.

Several mechanical circulatory support devices are available as transitions to myocardial recovery or as bridges to OHT.[158] These include the intra-aortic balloon pump (IABP), HeartMate LV assist system (LVAS), the Novacor N100 LVAS, the Thoratec ventricular assist device (VAD), the Abiomed VAD, and the CardioWest total artificial heart (TAH).[158] The IABP is intended only for short-term support of acute HF. The LVAS and VAD systems are FDA-approved as bridges to OHT, and the TAH is currently under investigation as a bridge to OHT. In the future, it is highly likely that the LVAS and TAH systems will be used as alternatives to OHT given the mismatch between the number of donor hearts available for OHT and the number of patients needing OHT.

ALTERNATIVE THERAPIES

In addition to the aforementioned conventional or investigational pharmacologic and surgical therapies, several alternative remedies have been studied in patients with CHF. Early open-label and placebo-controlled studies in which coenzyme Q_{10}, an endogenously synthesized provitamin with antioxidant properties that is also involved in mitochondrial ATP synthesis, was administered to patients with CHF showed improvements in LVEF, clinical symptoms, and NYHA status.[168] However, in a recent placebo-controlled crossover study, coenzyme Q_{10}, 100 mg per day for 3 months, did not improve resting LVEF or quality of life in patients with LV systolic dysfunction despite more than a doubling of coenzyme Q_{10} plasma levels.[169]

L-Carnitine is an essential endogenous cofactor that under ischemic conditions enhances carbohydrate metabolism by facilitating β-oxidation of lipids and reduces intracellular accumulation of the toxic metabolites long-chain acylcarnitine and long-chain acyl CoA.[170] Long-chain acylcarnitine can disrupt cell membranes, inhibit sarcolemmal Na^+–K^+–ATPase, impair normal cellular electrophysiology, and inhibit release of endothelium-derived relaxing factor, whereas long-chain acyl CoA uncouples oxidative phosphorylation.[170] In CHF, serum L-carnitine levels are high, but myocardial levels are low.[170] Propionyl-L-carnitine (PLC), an analog of L-carnitine that more rapidly enters into myocytes than L-carnitine and has additional antioxidant properties, when given in a randomized, placebo-controlled trial at dosages of 500 mg three times daily to patients with moderate CHF, significantly increased LVEF and exercise capacity.[170] However, the role of PLC in HF not secondary to carnitine deficiency syndromes remains to be determined.

Creatine and phosphocreatinine play important roles in ATP regeneration in exercising skeletal muscles.[171] In chronic CHF, resting skeletal muscle biopsies have shown reduced creatine concentrations, and magnetic resonance imaging studies have revealed a delay in the resynthesis of phosphocreatine after exercise.[171] In a recent study, patients with chronic CHF were randomized to receive creatine 5 g four times daily for 5 days, or placebo.[171] In the patients receiving creatine supplementation, there was a significant increase in forearm muscle contractions at 75% of maximal contraction and decreases in ammonia and lactate concentrations per contraction. However, sustained benefits and safety of creatine supplementation along with appropriate patient identification must be addressed before creatine can be routinely recommended for patients with CHF.

Other dietary supplements have been administered to patients with CHF. Thiamine deficiency may occur in patients as the result of long-term therapy with loop diuretics.[170] Although thiamine supplementation at dosages of 200 mg/day may significantly improve LVEF, other beneficial outcome measures have not been evaluated.[172] Vitamin C, in dosages of 1 g twice daily for 4 weeks, improved endothelial function by enhancing flow-dependent arterial dilation in patients with CHF via increased availability of nitric oxide.[173] However, as for thiamine, the long-term benefits of vitamin C supplementation remain to be determined. The administration of ω3 fatty acids, 8 g per day for 18 weeks, to a patient with advanced CHF and cardiac cachexia resulted in a decrease in circulating TNF-α and increases in body weight, body fat percentage, and serum albumin.[174]

FUTURE THERAPIES

Several agents that influence a variety of pathophysiologic processes are under development. BNP, a hormone produced by the ventricles, is structurally similar to ANP and has been hypothesized to modulate fluid status in patients with CHF. Intravenous nesiritide, a recently developed synthetic form of BNP, was associated with reductions in pulmonary capillary wedge pressure (PCWP), systemic vascular resistance (SVR), and plasma NE and aldosterone levels.[175,176] A compensatory increase in CI also was observed. Nesiritide represents a new class of agents that may be used to manage acute CHF exacerbations. In addition, several endopeptidase inhibitors, which inhibit the degradation of natriuretic peptides, and combination endopeptidase and ACEIs are currently under development.[177] An improvement in hemodynamics has occurred after both intravenous and oral administration of bosentan, an ET_A and ET_B antagonist.[178] Specific ET_A receptor antagonists and ECE inhibitors also are under investigation. Administering the MMP inhibitor CP-471,474 has attenuated the early LV enlargement after experimental AMI.[179] Levosimendan, a calcium sensitizer, improves the response of myofilaments to calcium by binding troponin C, thereby stabilizing the troponin C conformation and augmenting calcium binding, which improves contractility.[180] Intravenous formulations are currently under investigation for management of acute CHF. Two agents have been studied that antagonize TNF-α.[181,182] Pentoxifylline, which suppresses TNF-α production, has improved NYHA functional class and LVEF.[181] Intravenous infusions of etanercept, a soluble TNF-α receptor two (TNF-R_2) fusion protein that binds TNF-α, has improved quality-of-life scores, 6-minute walk test, and LVEF.[182]

Heart Failure Caused by Diastolic Dysfunction

Diastolic dysfunction, an inadequacy of ventricular relaxation and impaired LV filling, can present with the same signs and symptoms of CHF associated with systolic dysfunction or it can be asymptomatic.[2] Diastolic dysfunction is characterized by a normal or near-normal LVEF (i.e., more than 40 to more than 53%), abnormally elevated ventricular filling pressures, but normal or modestly increased ventricular volumes (Table 40.1).[183] The diagnosis of diastolic dysfunction is one of exclusion in which a patient exhibits clinical criteria for CHF but has preserved systolic function (i.e., normal LVEF) as determined by echocardiography.[183] In addition, radionuclide angiography can be used to evaluate ventricular filling, which is delayed in the setting of diastolic dysfunction.[183] Typical causes of diastolic dysfunction include HTN, aortic stenosis, hypertrophic cardiomyopathies, and CAD, which produce either significant LV hypertrophy, thereby altering the passive elastic properties of the ventricle, or myocardial ischemia, which impairs energy-dependent diastolic relaxation.[183] In some series of patients with CHF, diastolic dysfunction accounts for 14 to 51% of the cases.[183,184] In at least one series, women accounted for 65% of the group with CHF and normal LVEF.[184] Survival rates for patients with symptomatic diastolic dysfunction are about twice those of patients with symptomatic systolic dysfunction.[183,184] However, the mortality risk for patients with CHF and normal LVEF is four times greater than for controls without CHF.[184] Readmission rates for patients with CHF secondary to diastolic dysfunction are similar to those for patients with CHF caused by systolic dysfunction.[183]

The pharmacologic treatment of symptomatic or asymptomatic diastolic dysfunction is empiric because there have been no large-scale, prospective, controlled investigations. Nonetheless, the goals of therapy should parallel those for treating systolic dysfunction, with special attention devoted to managing HTN aggressively to minimize or reverse LV hypertrophy and other remodeling responses, recognizing and treating CAD and myocardial ischemia to improve energy-dependent ventricular diastolic relaxation, relieving congestive symptoms related to increased ventricular filling pressures, and improving diastolic filling by slowing HR.[183] For symptomatic patients (Fig. 40.3), diuretics in conjunction with salt restriction are indicated initially to relieve congestive symptoms. Thereafter, β-adrenergic blockers, calcium channel blockers (e.g., verapamil), or ACEIs, and by extension ARB, may be beneficial. The former two are negative inotropic and negative chronotropic agents. In addition, both agents have anti-ischemic effects that would be beneficial for patients with symptomatic diastolic dysfunction secondary to CAD. All of these agents may promote regression of LV hypertrophy. ACEIs, ARB, and β-adrenergic blockers also have other benefits mediated via antagonism of neurohormonal maladaptive responses. Interestingly, in the DIG study, administering digoxin to a subgroup of patients with preserved systolic function resulted in a reduction in hospitalization for worsening CHF.[121] However, at this time routine digoxin use cannot be recommended. Nitrates plus hydralazine also can be beneficial.[183] Surgical therapy may be indicated for symptomatic diastolic dysfunction secondary to CAD or aortic stenosis.[183] For asymptomatic patients (Fig. 40.4), antihypertensive agents generally reduce LV hypertrophy.[185] The cost of treating CHF secondary to diastolic dysfunction is estimated to be one-fourth of the cost of treating CHF caused by systolic dysfunction.[183]

Acute Heart Failure

Acute HF is a common medical emergency generally occurring in one of two clinical settings. Patients with chronic CHF may acutely decompensate. This condition may result from either a natural progression of CHF associated with a decline in cardiac function or some identifiable cardiovascular precipitating factors such as superimposed ischemia or new-onset atrial fibrillation. Alternatively, systemic or patient-related precipitating factors, including infection or medication or dietary noncompliance, may contribute to CHF decompensation. Acute, new-onset HF also may occur in association with AMI. Although similar agents are used to treat acutely decompensated chronic CHF and acute HF caused by AMI, selection of specific drugs may vary. The following discussion is limited to acute decompensation of chronic CHF.

PATHOPHYSIOLOGY

Acute decompensation of chronic severe CHF is characterized by failure of compensatory mechanisms to maintain adequate perfusion to the vital organs.[186] Most patients exhibit some or all of the following (Fig. 40.1): increased afterload or impedance to LV ejection, as evidenced by increased systemic vascular resistance; increased preload or elevated LV filling pressures and secondary pulmonary congestion; myocardial hypertrophy; sodium retention; peripheral edema; myocardial ischemia; and enhanced neurohormonal activation including the SNS, the RAA system, and vasopressin antidiuretic hormone. Excessive activity of each of these mechanisms contributes to the vicious circle of CHF, ultimately leading to death.

Unlike the earlier stages of HF that may necessitate a multitude of tests for diagnosis, acute, severe decompensation is easily recognized.[186] Classically, hypotension occurs but blood pressure may be maintained by peripheral vasoconstriction. Compensatory tachycardia often is observed and is especially ominous if it persists. The patient's skin may appear cool and pale because of vasoconstriction. However, diaphoresis may be observed occasionally. Skin mottling and cyanosis indicate shunting of blood from the periphery in an effort to maintain perfusion to the heart and brain. Urine output decreases, and in severe failure states inadequate cerebral perfusion alters mental status. Dyspnea and tachycardia often are present. Systemic venous and pulmonary congestion may manifest as peripheral edema, elevated CVP, and pulmonary edema.

Acute cardiogenic pulmonary edema is the most dramatic sign of LV failure.[186] The terrified patient is sitting bolt upright and expectorating pink, frothy sputum. The patient feels as if he or she is drowning. Diaphoresis may be accompanied by cool and ashen skin. Respiratory rate is rapid and accessory muscles are used for respiration. Pulmonary auscultation reveals rhonchi, wheezes, and rales. Although heart sounds may be difficult to hear, an S_3 usually is present. Overt signs of venous congestion usually are evident.

Therapy for patients with acutely depressed LV function is aimed at identifying and removing precipitating causes, reducing elevated LV filling pressure and systemic vascular resistance, and augmenting CO. Overall management depends on the severity of the acute exacerbation and the extent of compensatory mechanism activation. Some patients can be treated as outpatients with medication adjustment, but most patients need hospitalization for more intensive therapy, including parenterally administered diuretics, vasodilators, inotropic agents, and fluids. About 50% of hospitalized patients are admitted to an intensive care unit[187] for frequent patient assessment with the use of continuous ECG and hemodynamic monitoring. The latter is useful for distinguishing between cardiogenic and noncardiogenic causes of acute exacerbations and guiding therapeutic decisions. One-year survival for patients admitted with acute exacerbation of chronic CHF approaches 62%.[187]

HEMODYNAMIC MONITORING

The use of bedside hemodynamic monitoring with flow-directed pulmonary artery (i.e., Swan–Ganz) catheters and systemic arterial catheters remains a state-of-the art tool in critical care medicine. Although placing a pulmonary artery catheter is not risk free and some experts contend that this procedure is overused, there is little disagreement over its value in treating patients with acutely decompensated chronic CHF.[188] However, because the hemodynamic parameters obtained are used to design patient-specific drug regimens, correct interpretation by skilled health care professionals is needed to optimize use of hemodynamic parameters and initiate appropriate therapeutic interventions. Recent data indicate that considerable variability exists in the ability of many health care professionals to assess patient data accurately. Erroneous interpretation and potential complications of right heart catheterization (pulmonary infarction, arrhythmias, thromboembolism, perforation, balloon rupture, and catheter knotting) usually are minimized by careful assessment of all hemodynamic data obtained and placement of the catheter by experienced physicians.

The pulmonary artery catheter is inserted at the bedside, often with the aid of fluoroscopy. A balloon is attached to the tip of the catheter and inserted into the central venous circulation, typically via the subclavian, internal jugular, or femoral vein. The catheter follows antegrade blood flow into the superior vena cava and the right atrium, across the tricuspid valve, and into the right ventricle (Fig. 40.7).[45] The catheter is advanced into the pulmonary artery and is then inflated to obtain the pulmonary artery occlusion pressure (PAOP). The inflated catheter historically has been called a wedged catheter, so the PAOP is most often called the pulmonary capillary wedge pressure (PCWP).

The systemic arterial pressure, obtained via an arterial line, is monitored continuously, but in severe HF states this is not a reliable indicator of tissue perfusion. The PCWP is extremely important because it indicates pulmonary venous pressure and correlates with signs of pulmonary congestion (Table 40.12). It also indirectly measures the filling pressure of the left ventricle or preload. The pulmonary artery diastolic pressure (PADP) is also a valuable index of LV filling pressure. The multilumen construction of the Swan–Ganz catheter also permits simultaneous measurements of right ventricular preload by

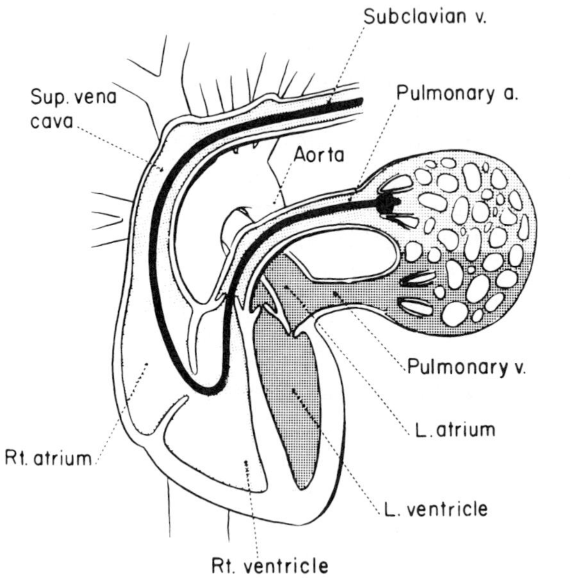

Figure 40.7. Final anatomic positioning of the Swan–Ganz Catheter, depicting balloon inflation in the pulmonary artery. (Reprinted with permission from Bollish SJ, Foster TJ. Swan–Ganz catheter: an important tool for monitoring drug therapy in the critically ill. Hosp Formul 16:99–103, 1980.)

Table 40.12 ▪ Normal Hemodynamic Values

Systemic arterial pressure (systolic/diastolic)	120/80 mm Hg
Mean arterial pressure	70–80 mm Hg
Pulmonary artery pressure (systolic/diastolic)	30/15 mm Hg
Pulmonary capillary wedge pressure	<12 mm Hg
Left atrial pressure	5–12 mm Hg (mean)
Left ventricular end-diastolic pressure	5–12 mm Hg (mean)
Pulmonary vascular resistance	150–250 dynes/sec/cm^5
Systemic vascular resistance	800–1200 dynes/sec/cm^5
Stroke volume	70–130 mL
Right ventricular stroke work	10–15 g·m
Left ventricular stroke work	60–80 g·m
Cardiac output	4–8 L/min
Cardiac index	2.2–4.0 L/min/m^2
Mixed venous oxygen content	13–16 mL/dL
Arterial oxygen content	18–20 mL/dL
Pulmonary capillary oxygen content	20 mL/dL
Arterial–mixed venous oxygen difference	5.0–5.5 mL/dL
Oxygen consumption	22 ± 40 mL/min

Source: Reference 188.

measuring right atrial pressure (RAP), which is equal to the CVP. SVR is a calculated parameter commonly used to estimate ventricular afterload. However, SVR does not accurately reflect the interaction of factors both internal and external to the myocardium. SV is the volume of blood ejected with each heartbeat. CO is the volume of blood ejected by the heart per unit time and usually is expressed in liters per minute. CO varies with body size and is therefore normalized by dividing the value by the patient's BSA, yielding CI. Estimates of CO generally are obtained by thermodilution technique. A thermal indicator (usually cooled sterile D_5W or normal saline) is injected into the right atrium. A thermistor at the end of the catheter measures the change in blood temperature downstream. The CO is then computer calculated using a modification of the Fick principle.

Even though it is not widely used, the arteriovenous oxygen difference is a better indicator of blood flow than is CI.[188] It is fairly constant and independent of BSA, metabolic rate, or oxygen uptake. The arteriovenous oxygen difference assesses the adequacy of CO in relation to the metabolic needs of the tissues. It entails withdrawal of blood samples from the pulmonary and radial arteries. If the patient is not hypoxemic, the mixed venous oxygen content (or saturation) is a good predictor of clinical outcome. A mixed venous oxygen saturation of less than 40% is associated with a very poor prognosis.

TREATMENT

Nonspecific measures designed to decrease pulmonary congestion and improve oxygenation are indicated in all patients with acute failure (Figs. 40.5 and 40.6).[186] In addition, the patient should be evaluated for the presence of precipitating, potentially reversible factors. Supplemental oxygen, perhaps facilitated by mechanical ventilation, improves oxygen delivery. The patient should be seated to minimize respiratory distress. Morphine sulfate administration is beneficial because of its potent venodilatory effect and anxiolytic action. Small dosages (2 to 4 mg) are repeated often until acute pulmonary congestion is relieved or alternative parenteral vasodilator therapy begun. Respiratory depression and systemic hypotension may limit morphine use. Once the Swan–Ganz catheter and arterial line are inserted, patient-specific regimens may be tailored based on the hemodynamic profile and the clinical signs and symptoms.

Diuretics

A mainstay of treatment for acute decompensation and pulmonary edema, intravenous furosemide or another loop diuretic, causes prompt venodilation and reduces PCWP and pulmonary artery pressure (Figs. 40.5 and 40.6).[189] The venodilatory action of intravenous furosemide is observed within several minutes of administration and precedes its natruretic effect.[112] Intravenous furosemide administration should not be delayed due to the immediate unavailability of hemodynamic monitoring because dramatic relief of the signs and symptoms of pulmonary congestion may be obtained.[189,190] Either frequent intermittent intravenous injections or a continuous infusion of the drug can be used (Table 40.8). The latter is superior with respect to enhancing urinary output and avoiding potential ototoxic adverse effects. In either case, after the initial dose, hemodynamic data, urine output, and sustained relief of pulmonary congestion should guide the furosemide dosage. Oral furosemide generally does not exert an acute venodilatory effect. Bumetanide and torsemide are alternative loop diuretics, although furosemide usually is given first.

Vasodilators

By blocking the positive feedback mechanisms of severe HF, parenteral vasodilators may abruptly improve CO and relieve pulmonary congestion.[186] The patient's hemodynamic profile guides selection of specific vasodilators according to their effects on preload and afterload (Fig. 40.6). Sodium nitroprusside often is the first vasodilator used because it acts on both preload and afterload. It has a fast onset of action and short duration of action, so sodium nitroprusside is easily titrated. In many patients, it lowers pulmonary artery pressure, PCWP, and SVR, resulting in increased CO. The initial infusion rate is 0.25 to 0.5 μg/kg/minute and is titrated upward based on hemodynamic and clinical response. Generally blood pressure, pulmonary artery pressures, and urine output are monitored continuously. CO and SVR are determined every 2 to 6 hours to aid in dosage adjustment. The most common hazard of nitroprusside in treating severe HF is hypotension.

Intravenous nitroglycerin is especially useful in acute decompensation because it is easily titrated. Because it predominantly increases venous capacitance (i.e., decreases preload), its effect is primarily to decrease PCWP and pulmonary artery pressures (Fig. 40.6).[186,189] Thus, it provides dramatic relief for patients with severe pulmonary congestion. It may also moderately decrease SVR and thus improve CO. Intravenous nitroglycerin dosages vary widely, but initial therapy may begin at 5 to 10 μg/minute. Dangers of nitroglycerin represent an extension of its pharmacologic action and usually are limited to hypotension and reflex tachycardia.

Positive Inotropic Agents

Inotropic agents improve contractility by increasing intracellular calcium concentrations. In addition, calcium reuptake into the sarcoplasmic reticulum is improved during diastole. Agents used for inotropic support during acute CHF exacerbations include the β-adrenergic agonists and the phosphodiesterase inhibitors. Digoxin is of limited use in managing acute exacerbations. Because severe chronic congestive failure is complicated by overstimulation of the SNS and downregulation of β-receptors, exogenous catecholamine administration generally is reserved for acute exacerbations. Dopamine may be especially useful in patients with mild to moderate hypotension (Fig. 40.6).[144,186] The initial dosage is 0.5 to 1.0 μg/kg/minute and is titrated upward according to filling pressures, CO, and urine output. If hypotension is severe (i.e., 90 mm Hg or less), dopamine dosages in the range of 5 to 20 μg/kg/minute provide the α-adrenergic stimulation necessary to maintain perfusion to the vital organs and improve CO (Fig. 40.6). Dopamine side effects include tachycardia, ventricular arrhythmias, and excessive vasoconstriction, especially at higher dosages. Nevertheless, it remains a valuable agent, especially when used in combination with nitroprusside. Additionally, many clinicians advocate the use of dopamine at dosages of less than 2 μg/kg/minute to improve urine output in patients with renal dysfunction secondary to poor CO (Fig. 40.6).[146] However, objective data to support this indication are lacking.

Dobutamine is a synthetic catecholamine that is a selective β_1-agonist that augments cardiac contractility, HR, and cardiac output.[144,186] The improvement in CO may then cause a reflex decrease in both filling pressures and SVR (Fig. 40.6). Unfortunately, these improvements are achieved at the expense of increasing myocardial oxygen consumption. Careful dosage titration is needed to balance dobutamine's negative effects on myocardial oxygen consumption with the positive effects on CO and myocardial perfusion. Dobutamine infusions are begun at 1 to 2 μg/kg/minute and titrated upward every 10 to 30 minutes, with optimal maintenance infusions generally between 5 and 15 μg/kg/minute. Close monitoring of the patient's HR during the dosage titration is needed to achieve an optimal benefit:risk ratio between effects on CO and myocardial ischemia. Adverse effects usually are limited but may include tachycardia, arrhythmias, headaches, anxiety, and tremor. Combination therapy with dobutamine and either milrinone or amrinone therapy may provide greater improvement in LV performance than either agent alone.

Amrinone and milrinone inhibit phosphodiesterase III and subsequently increase intracellular cyclic adenosine monophosphate. Amrinone and milrinone have both positive inotropic actions and significant vasodilator activity.[144,186] Amrinone is associated with the development of a dose-dependent thrombocytopenia, so milrinone is used more often. In CHF associated with a low CI, milrinone reduces pulmonary and systemic vascular resistances, RAP, and PCWP. CI increases as a consequence of these "unloading" properties and the positive inotropic effect of the drug. Therefore, their indications overlap those for the intravenous vasodilators, nitroglycerin and nitroprusside, and the parenteral sympathomimetics, dopamine and dobutamine (Fig. 40.6). In contrast to nitroglycerin and nitroprusside, milrinone has a long terminal $t_{1/2}$, so the time to peak pharmacodynamic effects is delayed, necessitating the use of a loading dose to achieve rapid hemodynamic effects. Milrinone dosing guidelines incorporate loading doses of 37.5 to 75 μg/kg, followed by maintenance infusions of 0.375 to 0.75 μg/kg/minute. Many clinicians prefer not to administer a loading dose, with the understanding that the peak pharmacologic effects will be delayed. Like other positive inotropic agents, milrinone can evoke tachycardia and precipitate myocardial ischemia. Additionally, milrinone may lead to hypotension through excessive vasodilation. Milrinone is renally cleared and may accumulate in renal failure, warranting close monitoring of renal function. Milrinone may be used as an alternative to dobutamine or in combination with dobutamine in patients who need intravenous inotropic support.

After hemodynamic and clinical stabilization with the use of intravenous diuretics, vasodilators, inotropes, and fluids, usually in combination, the patient is transitioned to an oral regimen.[190] The regimen should minimally consist of an ACEI titrated, if possible, to dosages shown to decrease mortality in clinical trials; loop diuretic dosages or loop diuretic–thiazide diuretic combinations adjusted for Scr (Table 40.8) and symptoms of fluid retention, especially pulmonary congestion; and digoxin dosed to SDC as previously discussed. Dosages of diuretics and ACEIs higher than those targeted in clinical trials may be administered, with titration guided by hemodynamic monitoring of PCWP, with a theoretical target of 15 to 16 mm Hg and RAP of 7 mm Hg or less in the absence of postural hypotension.[191] Normalizing the SVR (i.e., approximately 1000 to 1200 dynes/second/cm^{-5}), maintaining an SBP 80 mm Hg or higher, and maintaining a CI adequate to support life (generally greater than 2.0 L/minute/m^2 and possibly greater than 2.5 L/minute/m^2) are other hemodynamic goals that can be achieved by tailoring vasodilator therapy with ACEIs, either alone or in combination with other vasodilators such as nitrates, hydralazine, or perhaps ARBs.[191] Once the patient is stabilized to a certain NYHA functional class with optimal, conventional medications, then decisions to add new drugs such as β-blockers or to evaluate the patient for additional nonpharmacologic therapies such as OHT must be made (Fig. 40.5).

Conclusion

CHF remains a common clinical syndrome, the prevalence of which is increasing as the population ages. A sound working knowledge of the pathophysiology of CHF and how to implement, monitor, and integrate the various therapies is essential to preventing initiation and progression of CHF and improving the symptoms, quality of life, and longevity of patients with CHF. With the exception of diuretics, which are used to manage symptomatic complaints, current therapy is targeted largely at modifying maladaptive neurohormonal and cytokine-mediated mechanisms, which are initially activated in an attempt to maintain CO. ACEIs remain the cornerstone of CHF therapy. In the future, however, ARBs may supplant ACEIs, given the non-ACE pathways that can synthesize AII. Digoxin and especially β-blockers are additional agents that modulate maladaptive neurohormonal activation. The now-realized clinical importance of β-blockade introduces a new quadruple-drug therapy era in pharmacologic CHF management (Fig. 40.2). However, because clinician use of ACEIs remains suboptimal and because patient compliance decreases as a function of the number of prescriptions, there will be difficulties in implementing this intricate quadruple-drug regimen. In the future, in addition to new pharmacologic treatments, the tailoring of existing pharmacotherapy to patient subsets to simplify treatment must be addressed.

PROGNOSIS

Despite the lack of published information describing the natural history of HF in the absence of treatment, studies in patients receiving some form of pharmacologic treatment have revealed that the overall prognosis is grim. In the Framingham Study the 5-year survival after the diagnosis of CHF was 25% for men and 38% for women.[3] These survival statistics are worse than those reported for the placebo groups in several pharmacologic treatment trials.[192] However, the Framingham Study covered a period before the more widespread use of ACEIs and enrolled older patients. For hospitalized patients the 1-year mortality ranges from 30 to 50%, whereas for patients with less severe chronic stable CHF treated with appropriate therapy, the annual mortality is about 10%.[31] Between 1979 and 1996 deaths from CHF in the United States increased almost 120%.[7] The major causes of death from CHF are progression of disease or sudden death caused by lethal ventricular arrhythmias.

Several clinical variables have been shown to be predictive of prognosis in patients with CHF. Diminished LVEF, especially below 20%, or peak oxygen consumption (Vo_{2max}) during maximal exercise testing 14 mL/minute/kg or less predicts a poor prognosis.[193] Increases in cardiothoracic ratio on chest roentgenogram, severity of symptoms (i.e., higher NYHA class), and plasma NE more than 600 pg/mL also predict a poor prognosis.[193] Elevated plasma levels of ET-1 and its inactive precursor, big ET-1,[194] and increased natriuretic peptide concentrations[31] appear to be of negative prognostic value as well. In some studies,[195] but not others,[196] the presence of nonsustained ventricular arrhythmias (i.e., couplets and triplets or nonsustained ventricular tachycardia) in patients with CHF are independent predictors of a diminished survival. Older patients also exhibit a worse prognosis than younger patients. Even patients who are treated with "life-saving" pharmacologic therapy have an unsatisfactory prognosis.[7,31] In VHeFT-II, for example, the 5-year survival in the enalapril group was approximately 55%. Thus, CHF remains a highly lethal clinical syndrome despite "effective" medical intervention.

PHARMACOECONOMICS

For 1999 the projected figure for health care expenditures for CHF in the United States is $21 billion.[7] This includes

$19.6 billion for direct costs (i.e., hospitalizations, professional fees, medications, and home health care) and $1.4 billion for indirect costs, which consist of lost productivity from morbidity and mortality.[7] Of these costs, hospitalization and nursing home placement are the major component, accounting for $15 billion, or approximately 75% of the direct costs.[7]

Drug therapy costs for CHF for 1999 are estimated to be $1 billion, or about 5% of the direct costs.[7] However, for some drug therapies such as ACEIs and β-adrenergic blockers, the cost per life gained ranges from a cost saving of $2500 over 5 years.[143] These savings result principally from a decrease in hospitalization.[143] ACEIs, β-blockers, and digoxin and perhaps diuretics appear to be cost-effective treatments for CHF.[143]

KEY POINTS

- CHF is a clinical syndrome that progresses to worsening symptoms and death largely as a consequence of maladaptive effects triggered by neurohormones and cytokines.
- CHF can result from abnormalities in either systolic or diastolic dysfunction.
- Participation in cardiac rehabilitation programs can improve exercise tolerance and quality of life and may reduce mortality in patients with CHF.
- In CHF management, patient education is extremely important, especially with respect to facilitating compliance with dietary and medication treatment plans.
- Based on their ability to consistently improve both clinical status and longevity, ACEIs are considered first-line therapy for CHF.
- ACEI therapy should begin with low dosages that are titrated slowly to target dosages.
- Alternative vasodilator therapy such as ARB or the combination of nitrates plus hydralazine should be reserved for patients intolerant of ACEIs. β-Blockers are currently advocated for treating patients with stable NYHA class II to III CHF, based on their ability to reduce mortality and hospitalization rates.
- As with ACEIs, the initiation of β-blocking therapy begins with low dosages that are increased slowly and carefully.
- Diuretics are used to relieve CHF symptoms.
- Digoxin can be used safely in most patients with CHF caused by systolic dysfunction, with target SDCs between 0.7 and 1.2 ng/mL.
- The use of chronic, intermittent, or continuous inotrope infusions should be reserved for severe, refractory CHF.
- Anticoagulant therapy is indicated in patients with CHF and coexisting atrial fibrillation or other conditions that predispose them to thromboembolic conditions.
- ICDs are indicated in patients with a history of sustained ventricular tachycardia.

REFERENCES

1. Consensus Recommendations for the Management of Chronic Heart Failure. Part I. Evaluation of heart failure. Am J Cardiol 83(Suppl A):2A–8A, 1999.
2. Gaasch WH. Diagnosis and treatment of heart failure based on left ventricular systolic or diastolic dysfunction. JAMA 271:1276–1280, 1994.
3. Ho KK, Anderson KM, Kannel WB, et al. Survival after onset of congestive heart failure in Framingham Heart Study subjects. Circulation 88:107–115, 1993.
4. Gheorghiade M, Bonow RO. Chronic heart failure in the United States. A manifestation of coronary artery disease. Circulation 97:282–289, 1998.
5. Feenstra J, Grobbee DE, Remme WJ, et al. Drug-induced heart failure. J Am Coll Cardiol 33:1152–1162, 1999.
6. Coats AJ. Is preventive medicine responsible for the increasing prevalence of heart failure? Lancet 352(Suppl I):39–41, 1998.
7. American Heart Association. 1999 Heart and Stroke Statistical Update. Dallas, TX: American Heart Association, 1998.
8. Colucci WS. Molecular and cellular mechanisms of myocardial failure. Am J Cardiol 80(Suppl L):15L–25L, 1997.
9. Jacob J, Gilbert EM. The sympathetic nervous system in chronic heart failure. Prog Cardiovasc Dis 41(Suppl 1):9–16, 1998.
10. Schmermund A, Lerman Lo, Ritman EL, et al. Cardiac production of angiotensin II and its pharmacologic inhibition: effects on the coronary circulation. Mayo Clin Proc 74:503–513, 1999.
11. Love MP, McMurray JJ. Endothelin in chronic heart failure: current position and future prospects. Cardiovasc Res 31:665–674, 1996.
12. Rohde LE, Ducharme A, Arroyo LH, et al. Matrix metalloproteinase inhibition attenuates early left ventricular enlargement after experimental myocardial infarction in mice. Circulation 99:3063–3070, 1999.
13. Givertz MM, Colucci WS. New targets for heart-failure therapy: endothelin, inflammatory cytokines, and oxidative stress. Lancet 352(Suppl I):34–38, 1998.
14. Stein BC, Levin RI. Natriuretic peptides: physiology, therapeutic potential, and risk stratification in ischemic heart disease. Am Heart J 135:914–923, 1998.
15. Schirger JA, Heublein DM, Chen HH, et al. Presence of Dendroaspis natriuretic peptide-like immunoreactivity in human plasma and its increase during human heart failure. Mayo Clin Proc 74:126–130, 1999.
16. Drexler H. Nitric oxide synthases in failing human heart. A double-edged sword? Circulation 99:2972–2975, 1999.
17. Katz AM. Is the failing heart energy depleted? Cardiol Clin 16:633–644, 1998.
18. Bristow MR. Why does the myocardium fail? Insights from basic science. Lancet 352(Suppl I):8–14, 1998.
19. Floras JS. Clinical aspects of sympathetic activation and parasympathetic withdrawal in heart failure. J Am Coll Cardiol 22(Suppl A):72A–84A, 1993.
20. Kapadia S, Dibbs Z, Kurrelmeyer K, et al. The role of cytokines in the failing human heart. Cardiol Clin 16:645–656, 1998.
21. Francis GS. TNF-α and heart failure. The difference between proof of principle and hypothesis testing. Circulation 99:3213–3214, 1999.
22. The Task Force on Heart Failure of the European Society of Cardiology. Guidelines for the diagnosis of heart failure. Eur Heart J 16:741–751, 1995.
23. Marantz PR, Tobin JN, Wassertheil-Smoller S, et al. The relationship between left-ventricular systolic function and congestive heart failure diagnosed by clinical criteria. Circulation 77:607–612, 1988.
24. Harlan WR, Oberman A, Grimm R, et al. Chronic congestive heart failure in coronary artery disease: clinical criteria. Ann Intern Med 86:133–138, 1977.
25. Economides E, Stevenson LW. The jugular veins: knowing enough to look. Am Heart J 136:6–7, 1998.
26. Butman SM, Ewy GA, Standen JR, et al. Bedside cardiovascular examination in patients with severe chronic heart failure: importance of rest or inducible jugular vein distension. J Am Coll Cardiol 22:968–974, 1993.
27. McGee SR. Physical examination of venous pressure: a critical review. Am Heart J 136:10–18, 1998.
28. Mattelman SJ, Hakki A, Iskandrian AS, et al. Reliability of bedside evaluation in determining left ventricular function and correlation with left-ventricular ejection fraction determined by radionuclide ventriculography. J Am Coll Cardiol 1:417–420, 1983.
29. Fleg JL, Hinton PC, Lakatta EG, et al. Physician utilization of laboratory procedures to monitor outpatients with congestive heart failure. Arch Intern Med 149:393–396, 1989.
30. Packer M, Gottlieb SS, Kessler PD. Hormone-electrolyte interactions in the pathogenesis of lethal cardiac arrhythmias in patients with congestive heart failure. Am J Med 80(Suppl 4A):23–29, 1986.
31. Sharpe N, Doughty R. Epidemiology of heart failure and ventricular dysfunction. Lancet 352(Suppl I):3–7, 1998.
32. McDonagh TA, Robb SD, Murdoch DR, et al. Biochemical detection of left-ventricular systolic dysfunction. Lancet 351:9–13, 1998.

33. AHA Medical Scientific Statement. 1994 revisions to classification of functional capacity and objective assessment of patients with diseases of the heart. Circulation 90:644–645, 1994.
34. Weber KT, Janicki JS. Cardiopulmonary exercise testing for evaluation of chronic cardiac failure. Am J Cardiol 55:22A–31A, 1985.
35. Guyatt GH. Measurement of health-related quality of life in heart failure. J Am Coll Cardiol 22(Suppl A):185A–191A, 1993.
36. Guyatt GH, Sullivan MJ, Thompson PF, et al. The 6-minute walk: a measure of exercise capacity in patients with chronic heart failure. Can Med Assoc J 132:919–923, 1985.
37. Uretsky BF, Pina I, Quigg RJ, et al. Beyond drug therapy: nonpharmacologic care of the patient with advanced heart failure. Am Heart J 135:S264–284, 1998.
38. O'Connor CM, Gattis WA, Swedberg K. Current and novel pharmacologic approaches in the management of advanced heart failure. Am Heart J 135:S250–263, 1998.
39. Winkel E, DiSesa VJ, Costanzo MR. Advances in transplantation. Part 1: advances in heart transplantation. Dis Mon 45:63–87, 1999.
40. Consensus Recommendations for the Management of Heart Chronic Heart Failure. Part II: management of heart failure. Am J Cardiol 83(Suppl A):9A–30A, 1999.
41. Sullivan MJ, Higginbotham M, Cobb FR. Exercise training in patients with chronic heart failure delays ventilation aerobic threshold and improves submaximal exercise performance. Circulation 79:324–329, 1989.
42. Coats AJ, Adamopoulos S, Meyer TE, et al. Effects of physical training in chronic heart failure. Lancet 335:63–66, 1990.
43. Belardinelli R, Georgiou D, Cianci G, et al. Randomized, controlled trial of long-term moderate exercise training in chronic heart failure. Circulation 99:1173–1182, 1999.
44. Pina IL, Fitzpatrick JT. Exercise and heart failure: a review. Chest 110:1317–1327, 1996.
45. Bollish SJ, Foster TJ. Swan–Ganz catheter: an important tool for monitoring drug therapy in the critically ill. Formulary 16:99–103, 1980.
46. Bennett SJ, Huster GA, Baker SL, et al. Characterization of the precipitants of hospitalization for heart failure decompensation. Am J Crit Care 7:168–174, 1998.
47. Silver MA, Conventional treatments for heart failure. In: Success with heart failure. Help and hope for those with congestive heart failure. New York: Plenum, 1994:25–34.
48. Regan TJ. Alcohol and the cardiovascular system. JAMA 264:377–381, 1990.
49. Pavan D, Nicolosi GL, Lestuzzi C, et al. Normalization of variables of left ventricular function in patients with alcoholic cardiomyopathy after cessation of excessive alcohol intake: an echocardiographic study. Eur Heart J 8:535–540, 1987.
50. Miller LG. Herbal medicinals. Arch Intern Med 158:2200–2211, 1998.
51. Ghali JK, Kadakia S, Cooper R, et al. Precipitating factors leading to decompensation of heart failure: trait among urban blacks. Arch Intern Med 148:2013–2016, 1988.
52. Goodyer LJ, Miskelly F, Milligan P. Does encouraging good compliance improve patients' clinical condition in heart failure? Br J Clin Prac 49:173–176, 1995.
53. Stewart S, Pearson S, Horowitz JD. Effects of home-based intervention among patients with congestive heart failure discharged from acute hospital care. Arch Intern Med 158:1067–1072, 1998.
54. Shah NB, Der E, Ruggerio C, et al. Prevention of hospitalization for heart failure with an interactive home monitoring program. Am Heart J 135:373–378, 1998.
55. Rich MW, Brooks K, Luther P. Temporal trends in pharmacotherapy for congestive heart failure at an academic medical center: 1990–1995. Am Heart J 135:67–72, 1998.
56. Rich MW. Heart failure disease management: a critical review. J Card Fail 5:64–75, 1999.
57. Heerdink ER, Leufkens HG, Herings RM, et al. NSAIDs associated with increased risk of congestive heart failure in elderly patients taking diuretics. Arch Intern Med 158:1108–1112, 1998.
58. Kömhoff M, Gröne HJ, Klein T, et al. Localization of cyclooxygenase-1 and 2 in adult and fetal human kidney: implication for renal function. Am J Physiol 272:F460–F468, 1997.
59. Braunwald E. ACE inhibitors: a cornerstone of the treatment of heart failure. N Engl J Med 325:351–353, 1991.
60. American Society of Health-System Pharmacists. ASHP therapeutic guidelines for angiotensin-converting enzyme inhibitors in patients with left ventricular dysfunction. Am J Health Syst Pharm 54:299–313, 1997.
61. Garg R, Yusuf S, for the Collaborative Group on ACE Inhibitor Trials. Overview of randomized trials of angiotensin-converting enzyme inhibitors on mortality and morbidity in patients with heart failure. JAMA 273:1450–1456, 1995.
62. Mason DT, Melmon KL. Effects of bradykinin on forearm venous tone and vascular resistance in man. Circ Res 17:106–113, 1965.
63. Grassi G, Cattaneo BM, Seravalle G, et al. Effects of chronic ACE inhibition on sympathetic nerve traffic and baroreflex control of the circulation in heart failure. Circulation 96:1173–1179, 1997.
64. Parmley WW. Cost-effective management of heart failure. Clin Cardiol 19:240–242, 1996.
65. ACE Inhibitor Myocardial Infarction Collaborative Group. Indications for ACE Inhibitors in the early treatment of acute myocardial infarction. Circulation 97:2202–2212, 1998.
66. McGrae M, Feinglass J, Lee P, et al. Heart failure between 1986 and 1994: temporal trends in drug-prescribing practices, hospital readmissions, and survival at an academic medical center. Am Heart J 134:901–909, 1997.
67. Stafford RS, Saglam D, Blumenthal D. National patterns of angiotensin-converting enzyme inhibitor use in congestive heart failure. Arch Intern Med 157:2460–2466, 1997.
68. Philbin EF, Rocco RA. Use of angiotensin-converting enzyme inhibitors in heart failure with preserved left ventricular systolic function. Am Heart J 134:188–195, 1997.
69. Havranck EP, Abrams F, Stevens E, et al. Determinants of mortality in elderly patients with heart failure. Arch Intern Med 158:2024–2028, 1998.
70. Gattis WA, Larsen RL, Hasselblad V, et al. Is optimal angiotensin-converting enzyme inhibitor dosing neglected in elderly patients with heart failure? Am Heart J 136:43–48, 1998.
71. Packer M, Medina N, Yushak M. Relation between serum sodium concentration and the hemodynamic and clinical response to converting enzyme inhibition with captopril in severe heart failure. J Am Coll Cardiol 3:1035–1043, 1984.
72. Pacher R, Globits S, Bergler-Klein J, et al. Clinical and neurohumoral response of patients with severe congestive heart failure treated with two different captopril dosages. Eur Heart J 14:273–278, 1993.
73. Reigger GA, Effects of quinapril on exercise tolerance in patients with mild to moderate heart failure. Eur Heart J 12:705–711, 1991.
74. Packer M, Poole-Wilson P, Armstrong P, et al. Comparative effects of low and high doses of angiotensin-converting enzyme inhibitor, lisinopril, on morbidity and mortality in chronic heart failure. ATLAS Study Group. Circulation 100:2312–2318, 1999.
75. NETWORK Investigators. Clinical outcome with enalapril in symptomatic chronic heart failure; a dose comparison. Eur Heart J 19:481–489, 1998.
76. Packer M, Lee WH, Yushak M, et al. Comparison of captopril and enalapril in patients with severe heart failure. N Engl J Med 315:847–853, 1986.
77. Levine TB. Effect of angiotensin converting enzyme inhibition on renal function in the treatment of heart failure. Clin Ther 11:495–502, 1989.
78. Bakris GL, Weir MR. ACE inhibitor associated elevations in serum creatinine: is this a cause for concern? Arch Intern Med 160:685–693, 2000.
79. Meissner MD, Wilson AR, Jessup M. Renal artery stenosis in heart failure. Am J Cardiol 62:1307–1308, 1988.
80. Adrejak M, Adrejak MT. Enalapril, captopril and cough. Arch Intern Med 148:249–251, 1988.
81. Varonier HS, Panzoni R. The effect of inhalations of bradykinin in healthy and atopic (asthmatic) children. Int Arch Allergy Appl Immunol 34:293–296, 1968.
82. Pitt B, Segal R, Martinez FA, et al. Randomized trial of losartan versus captopril in patients over 65 with heart failure. Lancet 349:747–752, 1997.
83. Leor J, Reicher-Reiss H, Goldbourt U, et al. Aspirin and mortality in patients treated with angiotensin-converting enzyme inhibitors: a cohort study of 11,575 patients with coronary artery disease. J Am Coll Cardiol 33:1920–1925, 1999.
84. Sander GE, McKinnie JJ, Greenberg SS, et al. Angiotensin-converting enzyme inhibitors and angiotensin II receptor antagonists in the treatment of heart failure caused by left ventricular systolic dysfunction. Prog Cardiovasc Dis 41:265–300, 1999.
85. McKelvie RS, Yusuf S, Pericak D, et al. Comparison of candesartan, enalapril, and their combination in congestive heart failure. Randomized Evaluation of Strategies for Left Ventricular Dysfunction (RESOLVD) Pilot Study. Circulation 100:1056–1064, 1999.
86. Baruch L, Anand I, Cohen IS, et al. Augmented short- and long-term hemodynamic and hormonal effects of an angiotensin receptor blocker added to angiotensin converting enzyme inhibitor therapy in patients with heart failure. Circulation 99:2658–2664, 1999.
87. Tocchi M, Rosanio S, Anzuini A, et al. Angiotensin II receptor blockade combined to ACE inhibition improves left ventricular dilation and exercise ejection fraction in congestive heart failure [abstract]. J Am Coll Cardiol 31:188A, 1998.
88. Hamroff G, Katz S, Mancini D, et al. Addition of angiotensin II receptor blockade to maximal angiotensin-converting enzyme inhibition improves

exercise capacity in patients with severe congestive heart failure. Circulation 99:990–992, 1999.
89. Elkayam U, Karaalp IS, Wani OR, et al. The role of organic nitrates in the treatment of heart failure. Prog Cardiovasc Dis 41:255–264, 1999.
90. Cohn JN, Archibald DG, Ziesche S, et al. Effect of vasodilator therapy on mortality in chronic congestive heart failure. N Engl J Med 314:1547–1552, 1986.
91. Cohn JN, Johnson G, Ziesche S, et al. A comparison of enalapril with hydralazine-isosorbide dinitrate in the treatment of congestive heart failure. N Engl J Med 325:303–310, 1991.
92. Franciosa JA, Weber KT, Levine TB, et al. Hydralazine in the long-term treatment of chronic failure: lack of a difference from placebo. Am Heart J 104:587–594, 1982.
93. Conradson TB, Ryden L, Ahlmark G, et al. Clinical efficacy of hydralazine dosage in refractory heart failure. Clin Pharmacol Ther 27:337–346, 1980.
94. Elkayam U, Shotan A, Mehra A, et al. Calcium channel blockers in heart failure. J Am Coll Cardiol l22(Suppl A):139A–144A, 1993.
95. Scognamiglio R, Rahimtoola SH, Fasoli G, et al. Nifedipine in asymptomatic patients with severe aortic regurgitation and normal left ventricular function. N Engl J Med 331:689–694, 1994.
96. Rothlisberger C, Sareli P, Wisenbaugh T. Comparison of single dose nifedipine and captopril for chronic severe mitral regurgitation. Am J Cardiol 73:978–981, 1994.
97. Packer M, O'Connor CM, Ghali JK, et al. Effect of amlodipine on morbidity and mortality in severe chronic heart failure. Prospective randomized amlodipine survival evaluation study group. N Engl J Med 335:1107–1114, 1996.
98. O'Connor CM, Carson PE, Miller AB, et al. Effect of amlodipine on mode of death among patients with advanced heart failure in the PRAISE Trial. Am J Cardiol 82:881–887, 1998.
99. Cohn JN, Ziesche S, Smith R, et al. Effect of calcium antagonist felodipine as supplementary vasodilator therapy in patients with chronic heart failure treated with enalapril: VHeFT III. Vasodilator Heart Failure Trial (VHeFT) Study Group. Circulation 96:856–863, 1997.
100. Bleske BE, Gilbert EM, Munger MA. Carvedilol: therapeutic application and practice guidelines. Pharmacotherapy 18:729–737, 1998.
101. Waagstein F, Bristow MR, Swedberg K, et al. Beneficial effects of metoprolol in idiopathic dilated cardiomyopathy: Metoprolol in Dilated Cardiomyopathy (MDC) Trial Study Group. Lancet 342:1441–1446, 1993.
102. MERIT-HF Study Group. Effect of metoprolol CR/XL in chronic heart failure: metoprolol CR/XL randomized intervention trial in congestive heart failure (MERIT-HF). Lancet 353:2001–2007, 1999.
103. CIBIS-II Investigators. The cardiac insufficiency bisoprolol study II (CIBIS-II): a randomised trial. Lancet 353:9–13, 1999.
104. Packer M, Bristow MR, Cohn JN, et al. The effect of carvedilol on morbidity and mortality in patients with chronic heart failure. U.S. Carvedilol Heart Failure Study Group. N Engl J Med 334:1349–1355, 1996.
105. Delea TE, Vera-Llonch M, Richner RE, et al. Cost effectiveness of carvedilol for heart failure. Am J Cardiol 83:890–896, 1999.
106. Lechat P, Packer M, Chalon S, et al. Clinical effects of beta-adrenergic blockade in chronic heart failure. Circulation 98:1184–1191, 1998.
107. Kukin ML, Kalman J, Charney RH, et al. Prospective, randomized comparison of effect of long-term treatment with metoprolol or carvedilol on symptoms, exercise, ejection fraction, and oxidative stress in heart failure. Circulation 99:2645–2651, 1999.
108. MacDonald PS, Keogh AM, Aboyoun CL, et al. Tolerability and efficacy of carvedilol in patients with New York Heart Association class IV heart failure. J Am Coll Cardiol 33:924–931, 1999.
109. Vantrimpont P, Rouleau JL, Wun CC, et al. Additive effects of beta-blockers to angiotensin-converting enzyme inhibitors in the Survival and Ventricular Enlargement (SAVE) Study. J Am Coll Cardiol 29:229–236, 1997.
110. Exner DV, Dries DL, Waclawiw MA, et al. Beta-adrenergic blocking agent use and mortality in patients with asymptomatic and symptomatic left ventricular systolic dysfunction: a post hoc analysis of the studies of left ventricular dysfunction. J Am Coll Cardiol 33:916–923, 1999.
111. Cody RJ, Kubo SH, Pickworth KK. Diuretic treatment for the sodium retention of congestive heart failure. Arch Intern Med 154:1905–1914, 1994.
112. Mokrzycki MH. Diuretic treatment of heart failure. Heart Fail 10:181–191, 1994.
113. Krämer BK, Schweda F, Riegger GA. Diuretic treatment and diuretic resistance in heart failure. Am J Med 106:90–96, 1999.
114. Pitt B, Zannad F, Remme WJ et al. The effect of spironolactone on morbidity and mortality in patients with severe heart failure. N Engl J Med 341:709–717, 1999.
115. Barr CS, Lang CC, Hanson J, et al. Effects of adding spironolactone to an angiotensin-converting enzyme inhibitor in chronic congestive heart failure secondary to coronary artery disease. Am J Cardiol 76:1259–1265, 1995.
116. Moser M, Herbert PR. Prevention of disease progression, left ventricular hypertrophy and congestive heart failure in hypertension treatment trials. J Am Coll Cardiol 27:1214–1218, 1996.
117. Antes LM, Fernandez PC. Principles of diuretic therapy. DM 44:254–268, 1998.
118. Brater DC. Diuretic therapy. N Engl J Med 339:387–395, 1998.
119. Ellison DH. The physiologic basis of diuretic synergism: its role in treating diuretic resistance. Ann Intern Med 114:886–894, 1991.
120. The RALES Investigators. Effectiveness of spironolactone added to an angiotensin-converting enzyme inhibitor and a loop diuretic for severe chronic congestive heart failure (The Randomized Aldactone Evaluation Study [RALES]). Am J Cardiol 78:902–907, 1996.
121. The Digitalis Investigation Group. The effect of digoxin on mortality and morbidity in patients with heart failure. N Engl J Med 336:525–533, 1997.
122. Schwinger RH, Wang J, Frank K, et al. Reduced sodium pump α_1, α_3, and β_1-isoform protein levels and Na^+, K^+-ATPase activity but unchanged Na^+–Ca^{+2} exchanger protein levels in human heart failure. Circulation 99:2105–2112, 1999.
123. Krum H, Bigger JT, Goldsmith RL, et al. Effect of long-term digoxin therapy on autonomic function in patients with chronic heart failure. J Am Coll Cardiol 25:289–294, 1995.
124. Hauptman PJ, Garg R, Kelly RA. Cardiac glycosides in the next millennium. Prog Cardiovasc Dis 41:247–254, 1999.
125. Reuning RH, Geraets DR, Rocci ML, et al. Digoxin. In: Evans WE, Shentag JJ, Jusko WJ. Applied pharmacokinetics: principles of therapeutic drug monitoring. 3rd ed. Vancouver, WA: Applied Therapeutics, 1992:20-1–20-28.
126. Magnani B, Malini PL. Cardiac glycosides. Drug interactions of clinical significance. Drug Saf 12:97–109, 1995.
127. Bizjak ED, Mauro VF. Digoxin-macrolide drug interaction. Ann Pharmacother 31:1077–1079, 1997.
128. Hui J, Geraets DR, Chandrasekaran A, et al. Digoxin disposition in elderly humans with hypochlorhydria. J Clin Pharmacol 34:734–741, 1994.
129. Rodriquez I, Abernethy DR, Woosley RL. *P*-glycoprotein in clinical cardiology. Circulation 99:472–474, 1999.
130. Young JB, Gheorghiade M, Packer M, et al. Are low serum levels of digoxin effective in chronic heart failure? Evidence challenging the accepted guidelines for a therapeutic serum level of the drug. J Am Coll Cardiol 21:378A, 1993.
131. Gheorghiade M, Hall VB, Jacobsen G, et al. Effects of increasing maintenance dose of digoxin on left ventricular function and neurohormones in patients with chronic heart failure treated with diuretics and angiotensin-converting enzyme inhibitors. Circulation 92:1801–1807, 1995.
132. Slatton ML, Irani WN, Hall SA, et al. Does digoxin provide additional hemodynamic and autonomic benefit at higher doses in patients with mild to moderate heart failure and normal sinus rhythm? J Am Coll Cardiol 29:1206–1213, 1997.
133. Smith TW, Antman EM, Friedman PL, et al. Digitalis glycosides: mechanisms and manifestations of toxicity. Prog Cardiovasc Dis 26:413–458, 495–540; 27:21–56, 1984.
134. Jones WN, Perrier D, Trinca CE, et al. Evaluation of various methods of digoxin dosing. J Clin Pharmacol 22:543–550, 1982.
135. Koup JR, Jusko WJ, Elwood CM, et al. Digoxin pharmacokinetics: role of renal failure in dosage regimen design. Clin Pharmacol Ther 18:9–21, 1975.
136. Luke DR, Halstenson EC, Opsahl JA, et al. Validity of creatinine clearance estimates in the assessment of renal function. Clin Pharmacol Ther 48:503–508, 1990.
137. Williamson KM, Thrasher KA, Fulton KB, et al. Digoxin toxicity. An evaluation in current clinical practice. Arch Intern Med 158:2444–2449, 1998.
138. Marik PE, Fromm L. A case series of hospitalized patients with elevated digoxin levels. Am J Med 105:110–115, 1998.
139. Kelly RA, Smith TW. Recognition and management of digitalis toxicity. Am J Cardiol 69:108G–119G, 1992.
140. Borron SW, Bismuth C, Muszynski J. Advances in the management of digoxin toxicity in the older patient. Drugs Aging 10:18–33, 1997.
141. Gandhi AJ, Vlasses PH, Morton DJ, et al. Economic impact of digoxin toxicity. Pharmacoeconomics 12:175–181, 1997.
142. Rabetoy GM, Price CA, Findlay JW, et al. Treatment of digoxin intoxication in a renal failure patient with digoxin-specific antibody fragments and plasmapheresis. Am J Nephrol 10:518–521, 1990.
143. Cleland JG. Health economic consequences of the pharmacological treatment of heart failure. Eur Heart J 19(Suppl P):P32–P39, 1998.
144. Chatterjee K, Wolfe CL, DeMarco T. Nonglycoside inotropes in congestive heart failure. Are they beneficial of harmful? Cardiol Clin 12:63–72, 1994.
145. Ewy GA. Inotropic infusions for chronic congestive heart failure. Medical miracles or misguided medicinals? J Am Coll Cardiol 33:572–575, 1999.
146. Leier CV, Binkley PE. Parenteral inotropic support for advanced congestive heart failure. Prog Cardiovasc Dis 41:207–224, 1998.

147. Shakar SF, Abraham WT, Gilbert EM, et al. Combined oral positive inotropic and beta-blocker therapy for treatment of refractory class IV heart failure. J Am Coll Cardiol 31:1336–1340, 1998.
148. Garg RK, Gheorghiade M, Jafri SM. Antiplatelet and anticoagulant therapy in the prevention of thromboemboli in chronic heart failure. Prog Cardiovasc Dis 41:225–236, 1998.
149. Dries DL, Domanski MJ, Waclawiw MA, et al. Effect of antithrombotic therapy on risk of sudden coronary death in patients with congestive heart failure. Am J Cardiol 79:909–913, 1997.
150. Peters NS, Wit AL. Ventricular architecture and arrhythmogenesis. Circulation 97:1746–1754, 1997.
151. Echt DS, Liebson PR, Mitchell LB, et al. Mortality and morbidity in patients receiving encainide, flecainide, or placebo: the Cardiac Arrhythmia Suppression Trial. N Engl J Med 324:781–788, 1991.
152. Doval HC, Nul DR, Grancelli HO, et al. Randomised trial of low-dose amiodarone in severe congestive heart failure. Lancet 344:493–498, 1994.
153. Singh SN, Fletcher RD, Fisher SG, et al. Amiodarone in patients with congestive heart failure and asymptomatic ventricular arrhythmias. N Engl J Med 333:77–82, 1996.
154. Torp-Pedersen C, Møller M, Bloch-Thomsen PE, et al. Dofetilide in patients with congestive heart failure and left ventricular dysfunction. N Engl J Med 341:857–865, 1999.
155. Pinski SL, Fahy GJ. Implantable cardioverter-defibrillators. Am J Med 106:446–458, 1999.
156. Stevenson WG, Ganz LI. Atrial fibrillation in heart failure. Heart Fail 13:22–29, 1997.
157. Dries DL, Exner DV, Gersh BJ, et al. Atrial fibrillation is associated with an increased risk for mortality and heart failure progression in patients with asymptomatic and symptomatic left ventricular systolic dysfunction: a retrospective analysis of the SOLVD trials. J Am Coll Cardiol 32:695–703, 1998.
158. Frazier OH, Myers TJ. Surgical therapy for severe heart failure. Curr Prob Cardiol 23:726–764, 1998.
159. Grossi P, Gasperina DD, Corona A, et al. Preemptive ganciclovir therapy as a strategy for prevention of human cytomegalovirus disease following thoracic organ transplantation: the experience of Pavia, Italy [abstract]. J Heart Lung Transplant 17:51, 1998.
160. Valantine HA, Gao SZ, Menon SG, et al. Impact of prophylactic immediate posttransplant ganciclovir on development of transplant atherosclerosis. A post hoc analysis of a randomized, placebo-controlled study. Circulation 100:61–66, 1999.
161. Valantine HA, Schroeder JS. Recent advances in cardiac transplantation. N Engl J Med 333:660–661, 1995.
162. Schwartz RS. The new immunology: the end of immunosuppressive drug therapy? N Engl J Med 340:1754–1756, 1999.
163. Townsend JN, Pagano D, Allen SM, et al. Results of surgical revascularization in ischaemic heart failure without angina. Eur J Cardiothorac Surg 9:507–510, 1995.
164. Anderson RD, Ohman EM, Holmes DR, et al. Prognostic value of congestive heart failure history in patients undergoing percutaneous coronary interventions. J Am Coll Cardiol 32:936–941, 1998.
165. Kantor B, McKenna CJ, Caccitolo JA, et al. Transmyocardial and percutaneous myocardial revascularization: current and future role in the treatment of coronary artery disease. Mayo Clin Proc 74:585–592, 1999.
166. Losordo DW, Vale PR, Symes JF, et al. Gene therapy for myocardial angiogenesis. Initial clinical results with direct myocardial injection of $phVEGF_{165}$ as sole therapy for myocardial ischemia. Circulation 98:2800–2804, 1998.
167. Kass DA. Surgical approaches to arresting or reversing chronic remodeling of the failing heart. J Card Fail 4:57–66, 1998.
168. Pepping J. Coenzyme Q10. Am J Health Syst Pharm 56:519–521, 1999.
169. Watson PS, Scalia GM, Galbraith A, et al. Lack of effect of coenzyme Q on left ventricular function in patients with congestive heart failure. J Am Coll Cardiol 33:1549–1552, 1999.
170. Arsenian MA. Carnitine and its derivatives in cardiovascular disease. Prog Cardiovasc Dis 40:265–286, 1997.
171. Andrews R, Greenhaff P, Curtis S, et al. The effect of dietary creatine supplementation on skeletal muscle metabolism in congestive heart failure. Eur Heart J 19:617–622, 1998.
172. Leslie D, Gheorghiade M. Is there a role for thiamine supplementation in the management of heart failure? Am Heart J 131:1248–1250, 1996.
173. Hornig B, Arakawa N, Kohler C, et al. Vitamin C improves endothelial function of conduit arteries in patients with chronic heart failure. Circulation 97:363–368, 1998.
174. Ventura HO, Mehra MR, Milani RV. Cardiac cachexia in advanced heart failure: suppression of tumor necrosis factor by omega-3 fatty acids. CHF 4:44–45, 1998.
175. Hobbs RE, Miller LW, Bott-Silverman C, et al. Hemodynamic effects of a single intravenous injection of synthetic brain natriuretic peptide in patients with heart failure secondary to ischemic or idiopathic dilated cardiomyopathy. Am J Cardiol 78:896–901, 1996.
176. Abraham WT, Lowes BD, Ferguson DA, et al. Systemic hemodynamic, neurohormonal, and renal effects of a steady-state infusion of human brain natriuretic peptide in patients with hemodynamically decompensated heart failure. J Card Fail 4:37–44, 1998.
177. Coleman SG, Duff R. Endopeptidase inhibitors. Drugs R&D. 4:339–340, 1999.
178. Sütsch G, Bertel O, Kiowski W. Acute and short-term effects of the nonpeptide endothelin-1 receptor antagonist bosentan in humans. Cardiovasc Drug Ther 10:717–725, 1996.
179. Rohde LE, Ducharme A, Arroyo LH, et al. Matrix metalloproteinase inhibition attenuates early left ventricular enlargement after experimental myocardial infarction in mice. Circulation 99:3063–3070, 1999.
180. Hasenfuss G, Pieske B, Castell M, et al. Influence of the novel inotropic agent levosimendan on isometric tension and calcium cycling in failing human myocardium. Circulation 98:2141–2147, 1998.
181. Sliwa K, Skudicky D, Candy G, et al. Randomized investigation of effects of pentoxifylline on left-ventricular performance in idiopathic dilated cardiomyopathy. Lancet 351:1091–1093, 1998.
182. Deswal A, Bozkurt B, Seta Y, et al. Safety and efficacy of a soluble P75 tumor necrosis factor receptor (Enbrel, etanercept) in patients with advanced heart failure. Circulation 99:3224–3226, 1999.
183. Dauterman KW, Massie BM, Gheorghiade M. Heart failure associated with preserved systolic function: a common and costly clinical entity. Am Heart J 135:S310–S319, 1998.
184. Vasan RS, Larson MG, Benjamin EJ, et al. Congestive heart failure in subjects with normal versus reduced left ventricular ejection fraction. J Am Coll Cardiol 33:1948–1955, 1999.
185. Mosterd A, D'Agostino RB, Silbershatz H, et al. Trends in the prevalence of hypertension, antihypertensive therapy, and left ventricular hypertrophy from 1950 to 1989. N Engl J Med 340:1221–1227, 1999.
186. Smith TW, Braunwald E, Kelly RA. The management of heart failure. In: Braunwald E, ed. Heart Disease: A Textbook Cardiovascular Medicine. 4th ed. Philadelphia: WB Saunders, 1992:464–519.
187. Jaagosild P, Dawson NV, Thomas C, et al. Outcomes of acute exacerbation of severe congestive heart failure. Arch Intern Med 158:1081–1089, 1998.
188. McGrath RB. Invasive bedside hemodynamic monitoring. Prog Cardiovasc Dis 29:129–144, 1986.
189. Nairns RG, Chusid P. Diuretic use in critical care. Am J Cardiol 10:139–145, 1984.
190. Stevenson LW, Massie BM, Francis GS. Optimizing therapy for complex or refractory heart failure: a management algorithm. Am Heart J 135:S293–S309, 1998.
191. Stevenson LW. Therapy tailored for symptomatic heart failure. Heart Fail 11:87–107, 1995.
192. Massie BM, Shah NB. Evolving trends in the epidemiologic factors of heart failure: rationale for preventive strategies and comprehensive disease management. Am Heart J 133:703–712, 1997.
193. Francis GS. Determinants of prognosis in patients with heart failure. J Heart Lung Transplant 13:S113–S116, 1994.
194. Pousset F, Isnard R, Lechat P, et al. Prognostic value of plasma endothelin-1 in patients with chronic heart failure. Eur Heart J 18:254–258, 1997.
195. Doval HC, Nul DR, Grancelli HO, et al. Nonsustained ventricular tachycardia in severe heart failure. Circulation 94:3198–3203, 1996.
196. Singh SN, Fisher SG, Carson PE, et al. Prevalence and significance of nonsustained ventricular tachycardia in patients with premature ventricular contractions and heart failure treated with vasodilator therapy. J Am Coll Cardiol 32:942–947, 1998.

CHAPTER 41

CARDIAC ARRHYTHMIAS

Daniel C. Robinson and Mark A. Gill

Cardiac arrhythmias are disorders of the normal heartbeat. Arrhythmias can arise from a variety of conditions, such as electrolyte disturbances, structural abnormalities, metabolic derangements, and drug toxicity. Treatment of cardiac arrhythmias can include vagal maneuvers, electrical countershock, and drugs. This chapter discusses some of the pharmacologic and nonpharmacologic treatments of cardiac arrhythmias.

The appropriate selection of treatment for any arrhythmia is aided by an understanding of cardiac anatomy and electrophysiology. This chapter reviews the aspects of anatomy and electrophysiology that support an understanding of antiarrhythmic agents. The frequency of serious adverse reactions from antiarrhythmic drugs should be compared with the morbidity associated with the particular disturbance under consideration. This balance, when known, is presented under each type of arrhythmia. Once a drug is chosen, the principles of pharmacokinetics may be applied to tailor the regimen to each patient. This chapter provides examples of equations used to calculate drug dosing regimens.

TREATMENT GOALS: CARDIAC ARRHYTHMIAS

- Restore normal cardiac rhythm.
- Balance therapeutic benefits of antiarrhythmic drugs with the potential for serious adverse reactions, including proarrhythmias.
- Electrical countershock if arrhythmia results in hemodynamic instability.
- Correct any underlying electrolyte or metabolic abnormalities.
- Discontinue any drugs that may exacerbate arrhythmia.
- Consider pharmacotherapy of arrhythmia if clinically indicated.

Overview

ELECTROPHYSIOLOGY

The electrical system of the heart consists of intrinsic pacemakers and conduction tissues. It is convenient to conceptualize the progression of normal cardiac rhythm in anatomic terms (Fig. 41.1). Figure 41.2 correlates the standard electrocardiogram (ECG) with the normal electrical pathway.

The rate of electrical firing of the heart depends on the most rapid pacemaker. Spontaneous electrical firing or automaticity can occur anywhere in the heart under certain conditions. Normally, the sinoatrial (SA) node, located where the superior vena cava meets the right atrium, has the most rapid intrinsic rate (60 to 100 bpm). Therefore, any electrical activity not initiated by a normal impulse generated by the SA node is considered an arrhythmia. Most arrhythmias are labeled by the anatomic location and rate.

SA node firing initiates atrial contraction. The electrical impulse is conducted through the atria via the internodal tracts to the atrioventricular (AV) node near the coronary sinus, between the two atria. The AV node has pacemaker properties but normally coordinates atrial and ventricular contraction. The AV node normally limits excessively rapid atrial rates from activating the ventricles.

The conduction system in the ventricles is more elaborate than that in the atria because the muscle mass is larger. Rapid and effective excitation is critical because the ventricles contribute the most to cardiac output.

Fibers leaving the AV node are called the bundle of His. They separate into the bundle branches, which traverse the septum between the ventricles. Conduction between the AV node and the bundle of His is measured by the P-R interval (Fig. 41.2). The final conducting components of the ventricles are the Purkinje fibers, which emanate from

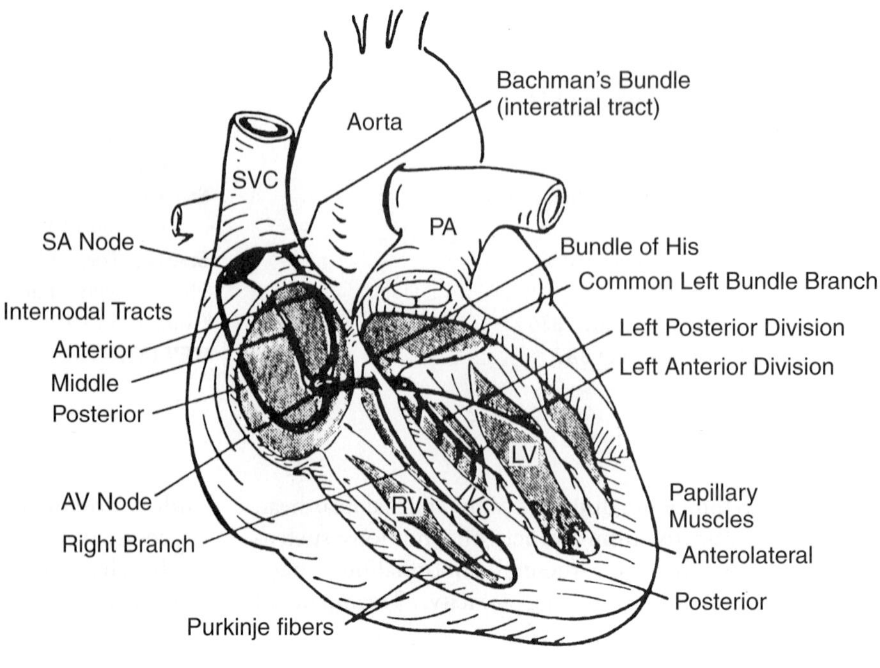

Figure 41.1. Anatomy of the electrical system of the heart. The impulse is generated by the sinoatrial *(SA)* node and is conducted through the atria to the atrioventricular *(AV)* node, which directs the current to the bundle of His, into the bundle branches, and finally to the Purkinje fibers. *PA,* pulmonary artery; *SVC,* superior vena cava.

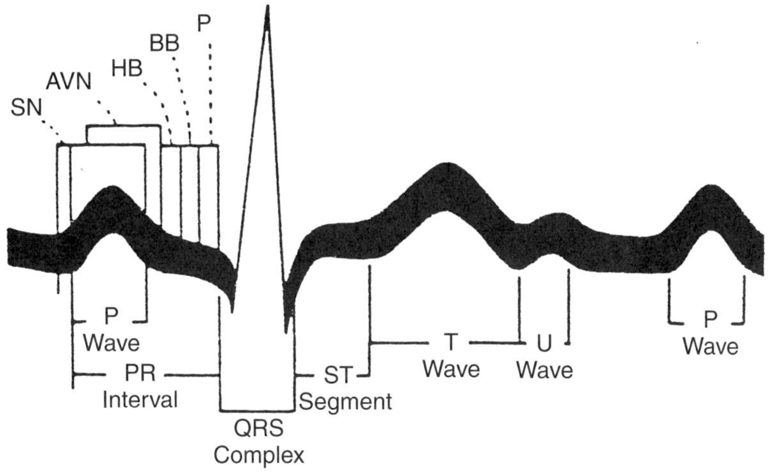

Figure 41.2. The normal electrocardiogram. The P wave is atrial depolarization. The P-R interval (0.12 to 0.20 seconds) is formed from the firing of the SA node *(SN)* and conduction through the AV node *(AVN)*, bundle of His *(HB)*, the bundle branches *(BB)*, and Purkinje fibers *(P)*. The QRS complex (0.05 to 0.10 seconds) is ventricular depolarization. The ST segment is the refractory period. The T wave is ventricular repolarization. The Q-T interval is 0.35 to 0.44 second in duration.

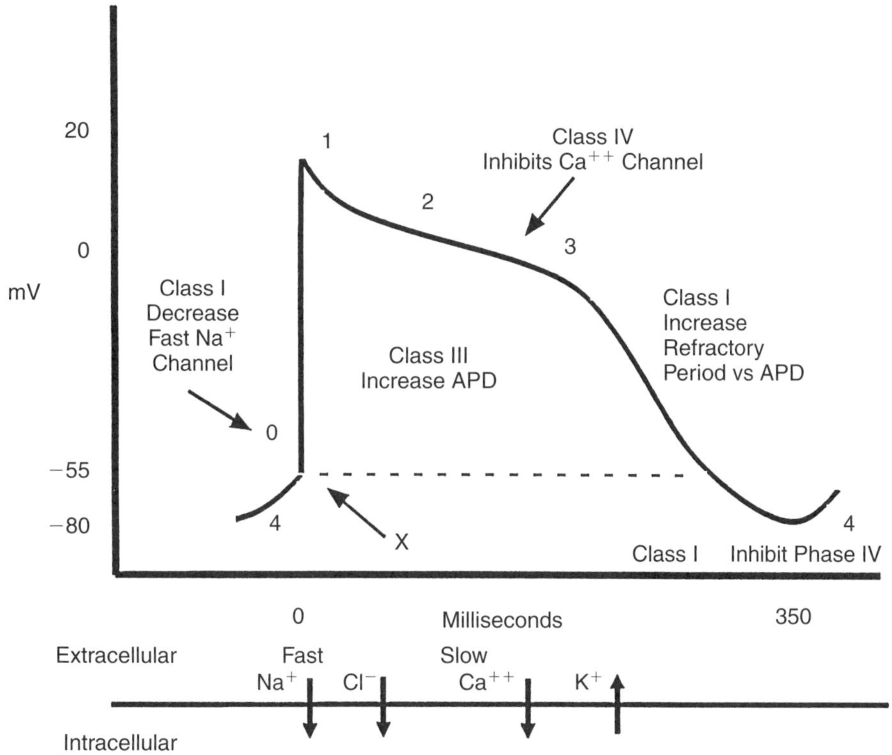

Figure 41.3. The action potential of a cardiac conduction cell correlated with electrolyte shifts. *X* is the threshold potential. The effects of the antiarrhythmic drug classes are noted for the phases of the action potential. *APD,* action potential duration.

the bundle branches to stimulate the ventricular cardiac muscle to contract. The QRS complex measures depolarization of the ventricles. The Q-T interval reflects both ventricular depolarization and repolarization.

ACTION POTENTIAL

Conduction and electrical firing in myocardial cells can be analyzed by measuring the membrane potential of various tissues. The electrical potential of these membranes is established by the flow of ions. When electrodes are placed into these tissues, the characteristic repetitive pattern seen is called an action potential (Fig. 41.3). This action potential may be divided into five phases. Phase 0 is the period of rapid depolarization. It is mediated by two ionic currents. The initial event is the rapid influx of sodium ions into the cardiac cell. As the sodium depolarizes the tissues, the threshold for the slow response is reached. The slow response depends on the transfer of calcium. Phase 1, the rapid repolarization of the tissue, may depend on inactivation of the sodium current and activation of chloride flow. Phase 2 is a plateau phase maintained primarily by calcium flow. Phase 3 is the repolarization of the cells initially begun by calcium flow inhibition. Repolarization is accelerated by potassium flow outward. The rate of fall of phase 3 and its depth determine the membrane responsiveness. Tissues may depolarize only after reaching a particular level of repolarization, at least −50 to −55 mV for normal Purkinje fibers. The tissue cannot be reactivated regardless of the stimulus until it falls below the threshold potential (*X* in Fig. 41.3). This level of repolarization therefore determines the end of the absolute refractory period (ARP). The

ARP varies in length depending on the action potential duration (APD). Phase 4 is the resting membrane potential that results from a combination of ionic currents, primarily the slow inward current carried by sodium.[1] In pacemaker cells the tissue has spontaneous depolarization, also known as automaticity, with a steep rise in Phase 4. The rate of firing of pacemaker cells is related to their automaticity, with SA > AV > Purkinje fibers. Nonpacemaker tissue has a shallow slope of phase 4 and generally requires activation by other tissues.

ARRHYTHMOGENESIS

In general, arrhythmias can be described as abnormalities in electrical development (as in ectopic tachyarrhythmias), electrical conduction (as in reentry arrhythmias), or a combination of both mechanisms.

Abnormalities in electrical development result from automaticity or triggered activity producing ectopic beats.[2] Ectopic beats can develop as pacemaking cells emerge when anoxia, fiber stretch, catecholamine excess, or edema increases the slope of phase 4. Abnormal automaticity can develop at any site in the heart. Generally, the fastest-firing tissue drives the heart. In the normal heart, atrial pacemakers have faster intrinsic rates than ventricular pacemakers. When the sinus node rate falls below the intrinsic rate of another tissue, that tissue then drives the heart. Triggered activity is caused by early after-depolarizations needing a preceding action potential for their induction. After-depolarizations can occur with oscillations in the plateau

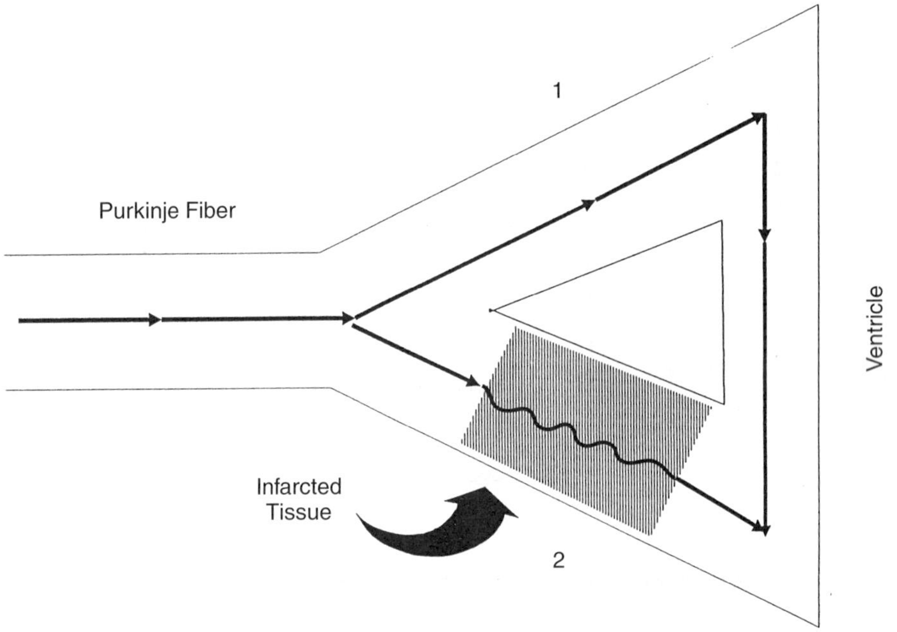

Figure 41.4. Reentry. A conduction fiber that bifurcates into fibers 1 and 2 to stimulate ventricular tissues. The normal pattern is for conduction through fibers 1 and 2 at similar rates. In this figure, fiber 2 is infarcted, which slows conduction until it is blocked by refractory cells. The impulse is impeded along fiber 1. Fiber 2 is activated by the impulse crossing the ventricular muscle tissue. The retrograde impulse finds fiber 2 repolarized and crosses, but at a slow rate. This circuit may be repeated or may terminate if fiber 1 is depolarized.

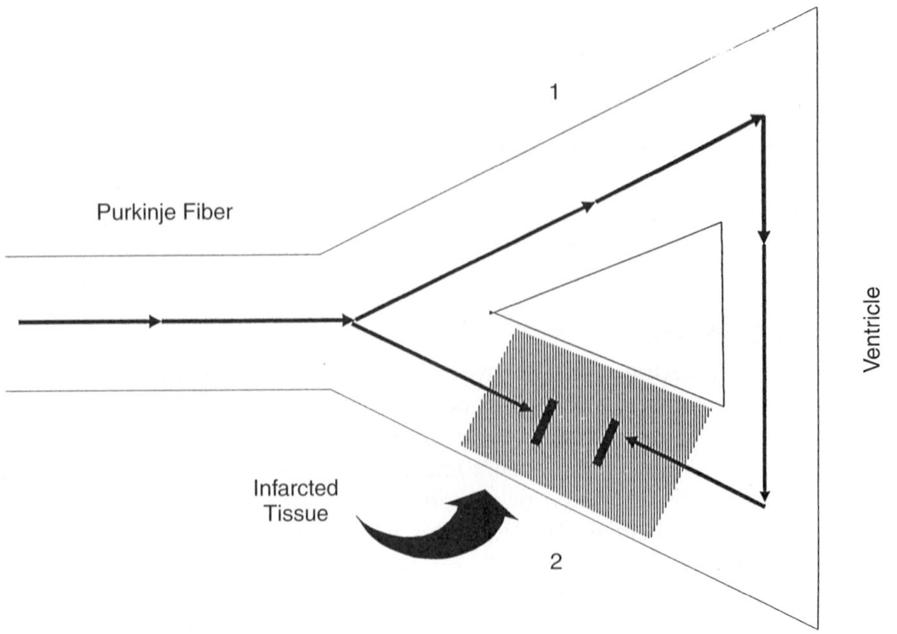

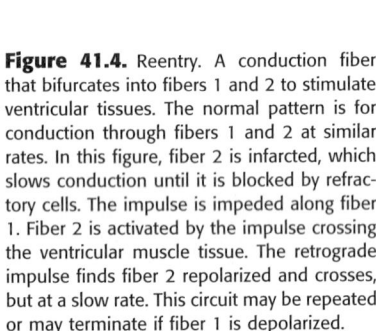

Figure 41.5. Antiarrhythmic drug effect on reentry. Antiarrhythmics may inhibit reentry by slowing conduction in both directions in fiber 2 so that the cells are still refractory when the impulses arrive.

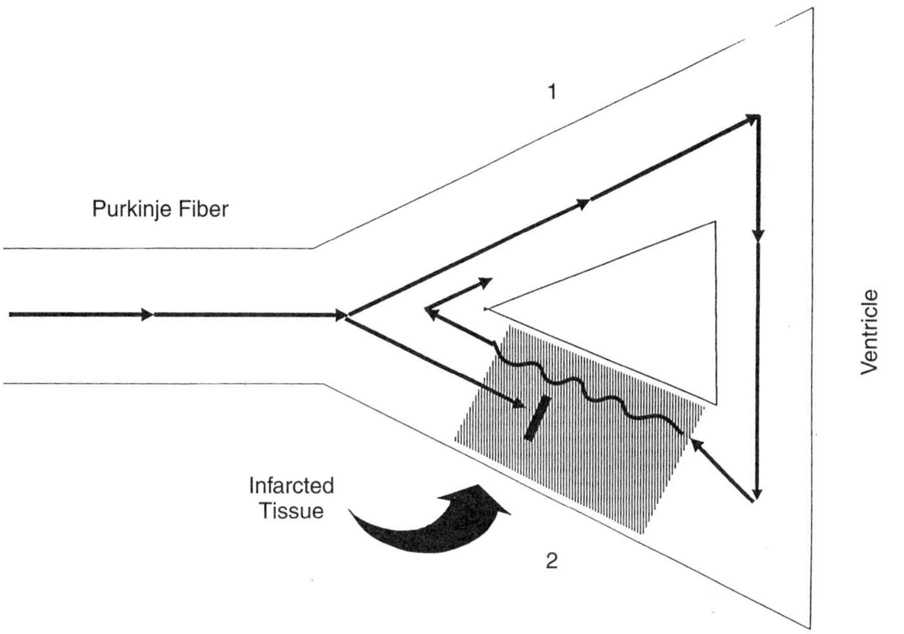

Figure 41.6. Antiarrhythmic drug effect. Another effect enhances conduction in the damaged portion of fiber 2 so that the impulse down fiber 1 finds depolarized fiber and cannot maintain the circuit.

phase of the action potential, leading to a second depolarization before the first is completed. Hypoxia, fiber stretch, catecholamines, high P_{CO_2}, and digitalis overdose can lead to triggered activity.

Reentry arrhythmias depend on different velocities along adjacent fibers and unidirectional block in electrical conduction (Fig. 41.4). This allows continued excitation in a repetitive manner. This circus rhythm may develop as areas of infarcted tissue block or delay conduction. A single circuit of the fibers may induce a premature contraction, whereas continuous cycling of impulses might produce sustained tachycardia. This process may occur in both atrial and ventricular tissue.

Antiarrhythmics have varying effects on reentry mechanics. One effect might be to inhibit membrane responsiveness in fiber 2 so that block is produced in both directions (Fig. 41.5). Another effect might be to enhance conduction in the damaged portion of fiber 2 so that the impulse down fiber 1 finds depolarized fiber and cannot maintain the circuit (Fig. 41.6).

Conduction velocity may be decreased by blocking the fast response and allowing emergence of the slow response, as in infarction or digoxin toxicity. In addition, because ARP depends on the APD, if repolarization is accelerated, cardiac tissue may be more excitable. A measure of this effect is the maximum upstroke velocity of phase 0. Mechanisms (primarily drugs) that prolong the APD also lengthen the ARP and thereby reduce excitability. This prolongation of repolarization is associated with lengthening of the Q-T interval (called QTc when corrected for heart rate; QTc = Q-T/R-R interval) (Fig. 41.2). Prolongation of depolarization also lengthens the QRS duration.

DRUG ACTION

Antiarrhythmic drugs are classified according to their electrophysiologic properties (Table 41.1). Class I drugs depress myocardial membranes, with varying ability to slow the slope of phase 0 through inhibition of sodium transport. This class is further separated into three groups based on differing effects on repolarization and conduction.[3] Class Ia drugs (quinidine, procainamide, and disopyramide) lengthen refractory periods and the duration of action potentials. Prolongation of the P-R and Q-T intervals and widening of the QRS is expected. In contrast, Ib agents (lidocaine, tocainide, mexiletine, and phenytoin) shorten

Table 41.1 ▪ Classification of Antiarrhythmic Agents

Class	P-R Interval	QRS Duration	QTc Duration	Agent
Ia	0, +	+++	+++	Quinidine Procainamide Disopyramide Moricizine[a]
Ib	0	0	0, –	Lidocaine Tocainide Phenytoin Mexiletine
Ic	+	+++	+++	Flecainide Propafenone
II	+++	0	0, –	β-Blockers
III	+	+	+++	Bretylium Amiodarone[b] Sotalol[c] Ibutilide *N*-acetylprocainamide
IV	+++	0	0	Calcium channel blockers

0, no activity; –, slight shortening; +, slight prolongation; +++, significant prolongation.

[a]Moricizine has been placed in various categories (e.g., Ia, Ib).

[b]Amiodarone also has properties of classes I, II, and IV.

[c]Sotalol also has β-blocking properties of class II.

repolarization and the Q-T interval. Conduction and the QRS interval are altered minimally. Finally, Ic antiarrhythmics are the most potent depressants of phase 0 in the class I drugs. Class Ic (flecainide and propafenone) is noted for slowing of conduction, as seen by widening of P-R and QRS intervals with minimal effect on APD or Q-T interval.

Class II includes the β-blocking drugs. Many arrhythmias are produced or exacerbated by hyperactivity of the sympathetic nervous system. Elevated sympathetic tone results in an increase in automaticity and a reduction in refractory period that could induce the activity of reentrant circuits. The clinical effects of class II agents depend on several variables, including the presence or absence of membrane-stabilizing effects (i.e., propranolol, pindolol, and acebutolol act like class I drugs, with a decrease in slope of phase 0) and intrinsic sympathomimetic activity (pindolol or acebutolol), which in theory would counter the bradycardia and AV conduction depression of β-blockade. The effects of class II drugs depend on the underlying sympathetic tone. In states of increased adrenergic activity, such as myocardial infarction, class II drugs decrease the resting membrane potential, decrease slope of phase 0, and slow conduction velocity, whereas in normal sympathetic tone these three parameters are unchanged.

Class III agents include bretylium, *N*-acetylprocainamide (NAPA), amiodarone, sotalol, and ibutilide. These drugs prolong the APD from phase 2 lengthening and, to a similar degree, prolong the refractory period. Bretylium, amiodarone, and sotalol have other differing electrophysiologic effects. For example, bretylium initially increases sympathetic tone followed by a decrease, whereas amiodarone and sotalol are both sympatholytic. In addition, some effects of amiodarone are felt to result from a decrease in thyroid hormone activity. NAPA does not alter QRS duration but does prolong QTc intervals.

Class IV includes the calcium channel blockers verapamil, diltiazem, and bepridil. These agents block the calcium-mediated current passing through the slow channel. The predominant effect is to prolong the APD. They also decrease phase 4 depolarization and increase the threshold potential. The result is a slowing of AV conduction. Bepridil can also depress phase 0 and prolong APD, giving it the properties of class I and class III antiarrhythmics.[3] Because of the broad spectrum of effects bepridil has on cardiovascular electrophysiology, it has been evaluated for treatment in supraventricular and ventricular arrhythmias; however, its use in treating arrhythmias has been limited because of reported cases of agranulocytosis and torsade de pointes.

Some have questioned the utility of this classification system because arrhythmia suppression by an agent within a subclass (e.g., Ic) may not predict positive response from another Ic antiarrhythmic.[4] There is evidence that this disparity exists for other classes (e.g., Ia and Ib).[5,6] In addition, this classification system does not support agents with multiple antiarrhythmic properties, such as moricizine, amiodarone, and sotalol. A more practical approach of characterizing agents by antiarrhythmic action could resolve difficulties with the current classification system.[3,7,8]

HOLTER MONITORING

Isolated and brief evaluation of ECGs has limited prognostic sensitivity. A more appropriate approach for select patients is to use a Holter monitor. This is a technique for long-term, continuous recording of ECG signals on magnetic tape for scanning and selection of significant but brief changes that might otherwise escape notice. Such monitoring can be used to correlate symptoms with episodes of arrhythmias. In addition, Holter monitoring before and after use of antiarrhythmics can be used to judge efficacy.

ELECTROPHYSIOLOGIC STUDY

Electrophysiologic study (EPS) is another technique used to manage arrhythmias. It is performed in a controlled and monitored environment in which the ECG and vital signs are evaluated while the heart is electrically stimulated to produce arrhythmias. Drugs are then used sequentially in attempts to suppress the arrhythmia. In theory, the induced arrhythmia simulates the naturally occurring arrhythmia and guides selection of appropriate chronic therapy.

Types of Cardiac Arrhythmias

Sinus Bradycardia

Sinus bradycardia is defined in adults as a heart rate below 60 bpm, with each impulse originating in the SA node, followed by normal conduction through the AV node and His–Purkinje system. The normal heart rate in children varies according to age. In most cases, sinus bradycardia is a normal physiologic variant. It usually reflects diminished SA node automaticity, although it may also be caused by improper impulse propagation out of the SA node.

SA node automaticity is regulated by underlying autonomic tone (sympathetic and vagal) and is lower during sleep and in trained athletes. Sinus rates as low as 30 bpm and sinus pauses of up to 2.8 seconds with first and second-degree AV block have been observed in completely asymptomatic patients.[9] The slow heart rate results in a longer ventricular filling time and a larger end-diastolic volume. Ventricular wall stretching produces an increased force of contraction by the Frank–Starling mechanism. The higher stroke volume results in an unchanged cardiac output despite the bradycardia. As long as the heart rate increases appropriately in response to elevations in sympathetic tone (e.g., exercise), many patients with resting sinus bradycardia remain asymptomatic. Asymptomatic sinus bradycardia is a benign condition that does not warrant treatment, aside from elimination of underlying factors that may worsen the bradycardia. These include drugs (e.g., β-blockers, digitalis, calcium channel blockers, or cholinergic agents), hypothyroidism, increased intracranial pressure, and certain electrolyte abnormalities.

EPIDEMIOLOGY

Sinus bradycardia is seen in 10 to 41% of patients with acute myocardial infarctions (AMIs), especially the inferior type.[10] It is most often caused by increased vagal tone associated with inferior ischemia or infarction.

CLINICAL PRESENTATION AND DIAGNOSIS

Sinus bradycardia usually is seen in the early hours after infarction and is often asymptomatic. Ischemic sinus node dysfunction may also occur but is less common. Uncomplicated asymptomatic sinus bradycardia does not warrant treatment other than careful observation.

TREATMENT

Therapy is indicated when hypotension, heart failure, chest pain, shortness of breath, ventricular irritability, or decreased level of consciousness is present.[11] Initial treatment should include lower extremity elevation and infusion of volume expanders. Drugs that may further worsen hypotension (e.g., morphine, nitroglycerin) or bradycardia (e.g., β-blockers, calcium channel blockers) should be used carefully. Severe bradycardia may increase ventricular irritability and result in arrhythmias such as premature ventricular contractions (PVCs). These often resolve after correction of the bradycardia and do not warrant conventional antiarrhythmics.

Pharmacotherapy

Atropine

The direct vagolytic action of atropine increases sinus node automaticity and accelerates conduction, usually producing a prompt increase in heart rate and blood pressure. The initial recommended dosage is 0.5 to 1 mg intravenously, repeated as needed to a maximum of 0.04 mg/kg or 3 mg.[11] Low dosages should be avoided because they may produce vagal stimulation with worsened bradycardia or a biphasic response of slowing followed by acceleration in 2 to 3 minutes. Total atropine dosages of 3 mg produce full vagal blockade and may induce unwanted effects.[11] Adverse cardiovascular effects include excessive tachycardia with increased myocardial oxygen consumption, ventricular irritability, and the potential for increasing infarct size.[12] This necessitates caution in patients with AMI. Noncardiac effects include urinary retention, blurred vision, dry mouth, mydriasis, and toxic psychosis. Patients with sinus node disease may exhibit an inadequate response to atropine, whereas patients with denervated hearts after cardiac transplantation have no response to atropine; both need pacemakers.

Isoproterenol

Isoproterenol, a β-adrenergic agonist, is a second-line drug that should be used with extreme caution in an AMI because it increases heart rate, ventricular irritability, and myocardial oxygen consumption. Peripheral vasodilation may exacerbate hypotension, which further limits use. It may be temporarily useful for refractory torsade de pointes and hemodynamically unstable bradycardia until pacemaker therapy can be initiated.[11]

Nonpharmacologic Therapy

Pacemakers

Patients not responding to atropine or those with persistent symptoms need pacemakers. Either the transvenous or transcutaneous route may be used. Transvenous pacing is the most reliable, with ventricular pacing the traditional mode. Atrial pacing gives the best hemodynamic response, but intact and reliable AV conduction is needed. Dual-chamber pacemakers that sequentially pace the atrium and ventricle may be preferred in patients with severe heart failure. In transcutaneous cardiac pacing, a low-density current is passed between two self-adhesive pads located anteriorly and posteriorly over the apex of the heart. This results in a hemodynamic response comparable to that of transvenous pacing and has the advantages of faster, easier, and less invasive implementation.[13] Its primary limitation is a lower reliability, with successful pacing in 40 to 80% of patients.

Sinus bradycardia associated with an AMI usually is transient, so temporary pacemakers generally suffice. It is not associated with a higher incidence of complications or mortality. With proper management, this arrhythmia carries a good to excellent prognosis.

Sick Sinus Syndrome

The sick sinus syndrome (SSS) encompasses a wide spectrum of impulse formation or conduction abnormalities in the SA node, perinodal tissues, atria, and AV node.

EPIDEMIOLOGY

SSS may be idiopathic or seen in patients with cardiac or other diseases such as amyloidosis, collagen vascular diseases, or endocrine imbalances. SSS is more common in older adults and is thought to be caused by a degenerative process associated with an increase in conducting system fibrous tissue.[14]

CLINICAL PRESENTATION AND DIAGNOSIS

The many ECG and electrophysiologic manifestations of SSS include sinus bradycardia with an inadequate chronotropic response to exercise, sinus pauses or arrest, SA node exit block, paroxysmal supraventricular tachyarrhythmias (PSVTs, usually atrial fibrillation [AF] or flutter) alternating with sinus bradycardia (called the tachycardia–bradycardia syndrome), prolonged suppression of SA node activity after conversion from supraventricular tachycardia (SVT), and carotid hypersensitivity, seen as abnormal sinus slowing or pauses after carotid sinus massage.

TREATMENT

Some patients with ECG or electrophysiologic evidence of SSS are asymptomatic, have a good prognosis, and do not need treatment.[15] Others develop a broad spectrum of central nervous system or hemodynamic symptoms, ranging from brief periods of fatigue, irritability, dizziness, and confusion to syncope (Stokes–Adams attacks), seizures, and congestive heart failure (CHF). Angina and palpitations may also be seen in patients with the tachycardia–bradycardia syndrome.

Before treatment is initiated, reversible or transient causes of sinus node dysfunction should be excluded or minimized. Drug-induced causes include digitalis, β-blockers, calcium channel blockers (especially verapamil), class Ia and Ic antiarrhythmics, agents that affect the central nervous system (donepezil or selegiline), and certain antihypertensives (clonidine, guanethidine, or reserpine). Treatment is indicated in symptomatic patients with a documented correlation between inadequate sinus node activity and symptoms.

Pharmacotherapy

Pharmacologic attempts to increase SA node automaticity (e.g., chronic atropine administration) are not effective. Antiarrhythmic drugs likewise are not useful, with the exception of the tachycardia–bradycardia syndrome, where they can be used to treat the tachycardic component.

Nonpharmacologic Therapy

Many patients with tachycardia–bradycardia need concomitant pacemakers because of prolonged pauses when converting from the tachyarrhythmia to sinus rhythm or an exacerbation of the bradycardic episodes caused by the antiarrhythmic. Those with intermittent AF may also benefit from anticoagulants (discussed under Atrial Fibrillation).

Pacemakers

Permanent pacemakers are the therapy of choice for SSS, which accounts for 40 to 50% of the population with pacemakers. Several pacing options are available. Atrial, ventricular, or dual-demand pacemakers sense and pace the atria, ventricle, or both chambers, respectively. Rate-responsive pacemakers respond to various signals (motion sensors, respiratory rate, oxygen saturation, or lactate concentrations) with a faster pacing rate, thereby simulating a more physiologic response to exercise. Recent evidence has shown an association between traditional ventricular demand pacemakers and adverse events, including chronic AF, CHF, and thromboembolism.[16] Causes include a lack of AV synchrony and abnormal retrograde ventriculoatrial conduction. Atrial demand pacemakers are therefore preferable, but patients must first be carefully screened to exclude AV node and His–Purkinje system conduction defects. Drugs with negative AV chronotropic or dromotropic effects must be administered carefully. Pacing relieves symptoms and is generally well tolerated. Previous studies in patients with SSS did not demonstrate improved morbidity or mortality (50% at 5 years),[14,17] possibly because of underlying poor cardiac function. Recognition of the deleterious effects of ventricular demand pacemakers now raises the question of whether they may have offset a trend toward higher survival. Recent studies have shown an improved short-term survival in older adults with atrial pacemakers.[16] Long-term studies in large populations should be performed.

Atrioventricular Block

Abnormalities of AV conduction are classified into three types, based on the extent of impulse transmission across the AV node. The anatomic location of the conduction block determines the clinical significance, prognosis, and therapy.

FIRST-DEGREE ATRIOVENTRICULAR BLOCK

First-degree AV block is defined as a prolongation of the P-R interval to 0.20 seconds or more, with 1:1 atrioventricular conduction of all impulses. This is a common ECG finding, with an incidence of 0.5 to 10%. Conduction delay in the AV node is the most common cause. Both cardiac (AV nodal disease, AMI, myocarditis) and noncardiac (enhanced vagal tone) causes have been identified. Patients are rarely symptomatic, and treatment generally is not needed.[15] Digitalis, β-blockers, calcium channel blockers, and potassium may cause or worsen this pattern. First-degree AV block is not an absolute contraindication to these drugs, but close observation is necessary because they may produce higher-grade block.

SECOND-DEGREE ATRIOVENTRICULAR BLOCK

In second-degree AV block, there is intermittent failure of AV impulse conduction. The anatomic site of block may be the AV node, His bundle, or bundle branch system. This type of block is subdivided into Mobitz types I and II. Mobitz type I, or Wenckebach block, is characterized by a gradual prolongation of AV conduction (P-R interval on ECG) until a sinus impulse (P wave) is not conducted to the ventricles. The cycle then begins anew with a short followed by progressively longer P-R intervals and a nonconducted P wave. EPS usually implicates a conduction abnormality in the AV node proximal to the bundle of His. The presence and extent of Mobitz type I AV block is influenced by underlying autonomic tone. It may be seen in normal subjects (especially athletes) or may be caused by drugs (e.g., digitalis, β-blockers, or verapamil), electrolyte abnormalities, or inflammation. This pattern is also seen in acute inferior myocardial infarction. It usually appears within the first 72 hours after infarction, is transient, and infrequently progresses to higher-grade block.[10]

Many patients with Mobitz type I AV block are asymptomatic, in which case drugs or pacemakers are not needed.[15] Close observation of patients with AMI or digitalis toxicity is warranted. Treatment is indicated when the patient exhibits symptoms (central nervous system or hemodynamic) or ventricular irritability or the ventricular rate persists at less than 40 bpm.[13] Atropine facilitates AV nodal conduction by decreasing the effective and functional refractory periods of the AV node. It often restores 1:1 conduction in patients with Mobitz type I block and normal AV nodes[12] and may be useful in managing digitalis toxicity. However, this effect is unpredictable in patients with AMI, and temporary pacemakers are therefore indicated. β-Blockers, verapamil, and digoxin should be used with caution in these patients.

Mobitz type II block is present when the P-R interval of conducted beats remains constant, with unpredicted intermittent nonconduction of atrial impulses. It reflects a conduction abnormality distal to the bundle of His and is often associated with a wide QRS (bundle branch block) pattern on ECG. This type of block is seen in acute anterior or anteroseptal myocardial infarction, usually during the first 72 hours after infarction. It reflects extensive ischemia and necrosis of the septum, bundle branches, and Purkinje fibers. Almost all patients are symptomatic. Mobitz type II AV block with bundle branch block is an unstable rhythm with an ominous prognosis, often progressing abruptly to complete heart block, severe bradycardia, or asystole. Atropine generally is ineffective. Pacemakers are therefore mandatory and usually permanent.[15] Most AV block rhythms are labeled according to the ratio of P waves to QRS complexes (e.g., 2:1 or 3:1). This information alone is of limited utility without the ventricular rate. A 3:1 block is not always more harmful than a 2:1 block. A 2:1 block is more dangerous if the atrial rate is 70 (leading to a ventricular rate of only 35) than a 3:1 block where the atrial rate is 150 (leading to a ventricular rate of 50).

THIRD-DEGREE ATRIOVENTRICULAR BLOCK

Third-degree AV block occurs when no P waves are conducted to the ventricles. Also known as complete heart block, it reflects a total absence of AV conduction. This results in an escape rhythm, with the AV junction, His bundle, or Purkinje cells acting as the pacemaker. The site of block is related to the symptoms, prognosis, and therapy. When conduction is blocked within the AV node (proximal conducting system), the AV junction or proximal His bundle cells function as the pacemaker. Normal-appearing QRS complexes are seen, reflecting normal ventricular impulse conduction. The physiologic escape rate for the AV junctional cells is 40 to 60 bpm, which increases in response to elevated sympathetic tone. Complete heart block with AV junctional escape may be a congenital rhythm or it may be seen (usually transiently) in acute inferior myocardial infarction. This is a fairly stable rhythm. Normal ventricular conduction along with the ability to increase the rate with exercise allows some patients to remain asymptomatic. Infants and children with congenital proximal complete heart block may tolerate this rhythm well for long periods, needing close observation but no intervention.[9,15] Treatment is indicated in patients with symptoms (hypotension, syncope, persistent chest pain, heart failure), inadequate chronotropic response to exercise, or ventricular arrhythmias. Atropine may be used in emergent situations but is of limited value and is not effective in the long term. Permanent pacemakers are the therapy of choice. Pacemakers are reliable and well tolerated in infants and children with the congenital form of this rhythm. The role of pacemakers in patients with myocardial infarction remains unclear.

Complete heart block in the distal His bundle or Purkinje system (distal conducting system) results in an idioventricular escape rhythm, with wide QRS complexes occurring at a rate of 30 to 40 bpm. This reflects abnormal impulse conduction through the ventricles and the slow intrinsic rate of ventricular pacemaker tissues. This pattern may be seen in AMI and other diseases such as myocarditis, cardiomyopathy, and sarcoidosis. The slow rate coupled with abnormal ventricular conduction usually causes hemodynamic or central nervous system symptoms. In patients with acute anterior or anteroseptal myocardial infarction, this is an unstable rhythm with abrupt progression to asystole or ventricular arrhythmias. Atropine is not effective.[12] Patients with third-degree AV block and an idioventricular rhythm need permanent pacemakers[13,15] regardless of symptoms. The abrupt occurrence of this type of block in the setting of an AMI carries an ominous prognosis and a high risk of sudden death.

Sinus Tachycardia

Sinus tachycardia is characterized by a rate of more than 100 and usually less than 180 bpm, with impulses originating in the SA node and conducted normally to the AV node and His–Purkinje system. In most cases, it reflects increased SA node automaticity. A gradual acceleration and deceleration may allow differentiation from other SVTs. The rate varies with sleep or changes in posture. Sinus tachycardia is a normal physiologic response to myriad conditions, including exercise, anxiety, pain, stress, fright, fever, hypoxia, anemia, hypovolemia, hypotension, early CHF, hyperthyroidism, and pheochromocytoma. It is seen in about one-third of patients with AMI and is attributed to sympathetic overactivity. Drugs with direct or indirect sympathomimetic or vagolytic activity may cause or contribute to sinus tachycardia. Common causes include sympathomimetics, catecholamines, β-agonists, methylxanthines, and anticholinergics.

Most patients with sinus tachycardia are asymptomatic, except perhaps for palpitations. Patients with coronary artery disease may experience angina because of increased myocardial oxygen demand. Those with poor cardiac reserve and sustained episodes of tachycardia may develop CHF.

Sinus tachycardia treatment consists of managing the underlying condition. Treating the tachycardia itself is not necessary and may have deleterious effects because decreasing the heart rate decreases the cardiac output and oxygen delivery to the tissues. In the rare instance (e.g., hyperthyroidism) in which sinus tachycardia is sustained and symptomatic, propranolol or another β-blocker may be given if the patient is not in CHF.

Atrioventricular Nodal Reentry

PSVTs are a group of common arrhythmias often seen in healthy subjects with otherwise normal cardiovascular system. Reentry (sometimes called circus movement tachycardia) is the mechanism for more than 90% of cases. Several variants are seen. AV nodal reentry is sometimes known as PSVT and accounts for 50 to 60% of cases. Reentry using an accessory AV pathway (AV reentry, Wolff–Parkinson–White [WPW] syndrome, or concealed bypass tract conduction, discussed in a separate section) causes 30% of cases. Finally, reentry within the SA node (4%) or atria (4 to 8%) may also occur, primarily in patients with underlying heart disease. Typical features of reentry include abrupt initiation and termination, a regular rate of 150 to 250 bpm (up to 325 in infants), narrow QRS complexes of normal morphology, and 1:1 AV conduction. Abrupt initiation and ventricular rate regularity are specific characteristics of AV nodal reentry, often used as clues in differentiating it from ectopic atrial tachycardia, AF, or atrial flutter.

EPIDEMIOLOGY

AV nodal reentry can be seen at any age from infancy to adulthood. It is a common arrhythmia in infants, children, and young adults. Approximately 50% of patients have no underlying heart disease. Brief runs often are detected on

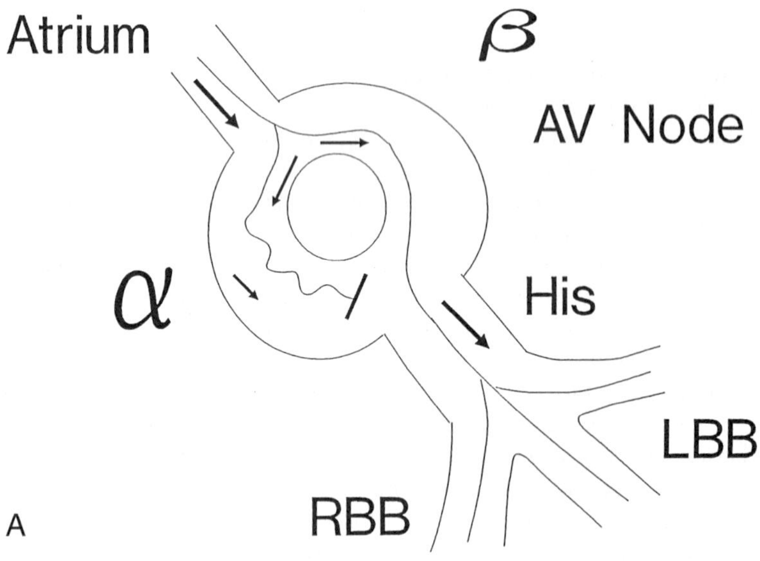

A

Figure 41.7. Atrioventricular (AV) nodal reentry. **A,** Atrioventricular *(AV)* nodal reentry, sinus rhythm. The impulse is blocked in the α-pathway and reaches the ventricles via the β-pathway. *His,* bundle of His; *LBB,* left bundle branches; *RBB,* right bundle branch.

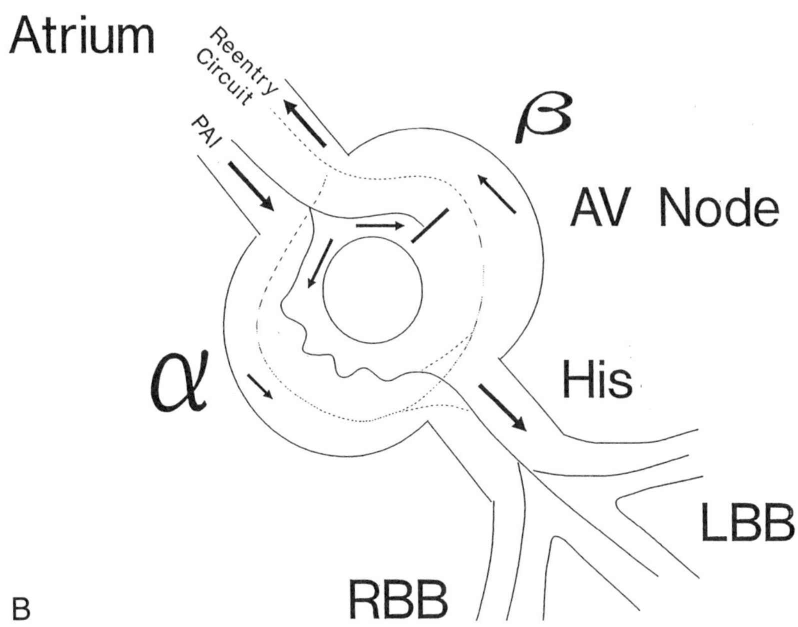

Figure 41.7. B, AV nodal reentry, premature atrial impulse *(PAI, solid line).* The PAI is blocked in the β-pathway and reaches the ventricles via the α-pathway. If the β-pathway is recovered, AV nodal reentry *(dotted line)* may be initiated.

24-hour ECG monitors of asymptomatic patients. Many cases are idiopathic. Noncardiac causes such as fever, infection, or drugs (sympathomimetics, catecholamines, β-agonists) are seen in a minority of patients.

ELECTROPHYSIOLOGY

An understanding of the electrophysiology of reentry is useful in evaluating therapeutic modalities. Under normal conditions, impulses begin in the SA node and terminate in the Purkinje fibers, where the surrounding tissue is refractory. In reentry, the impulse is able to reactivate the conducting system by "hiding" in the heart long enough for the surrounding tissue to regain excitability. Slow conduction in the AV node makes this a likely site for reentry. In AV nodal reentry, there are at least two functional pathways in the AV conducting system, sharing common proximal and distal limbs (Fig. 41.7*A*). The α-pathway has slow conduction velocity and a short refractory period, whereas the β-pathway has fast conduction velocity and a long refractory period. During sinus rhythm, each impulse arrives at the AV junction, travels antegrade (toward the ventricles) down both pathways, reaches the His bundle via the fast β-pathway, and terminates in the His–Purkinje system. Conduction down the slow α-pathway ceases at the His bundle, where the tissue is refractory (Fig. 41.7*A*). The long cycle length in sinus rhythm allows both pathways to recover excitability before the next sinus impulse arrives at the AV junction.

In reentry (Fig. 41.7*B*), a premature impulse enters the AV node at a time when the slow α-path will conduct but the fast β-path is refractory. The impulse travels through the AV junction via the α-pathway. The His–Purkinje system and ventricles are then activated in normal fashion. Additionally, retrograde transmission (toward the atria) occurs up the now recovered β-pathway, creating an atrial echo. If the α-pathway is recovered, the impulse travels antegrade (toward the ventricles), and a reentry circuit is created. The impulse travels antegrade down the slow α-pathway and retrograde up the fast β-pathway, with the atria and ventricles as "innocent bystanders."[2] In AV nodal reentry, the entire circuit is located in the AV junction. Clearly, to induce and sustain reentry, the premature impulse must be critically timed, and a fine balance must exist between conductivity and refractoriness. The impulse must always find excitable tissue in the direction in which it is propagating. If refractory tissue is encountered, the circuit is broken, and the rhythm terminates abruptly. On ECG, the premature atrial beat has a prolonged P-R interval. Subsequent P waves often are buried in the QRS complex, reflecting simultaneous activation of the atria and ventricles. QRS morphology is normal unless there is aberrant conduction or antegrade preexcitation down an anomalous AV connection pathway (WPW syndrome).

CLINICAL PRESENTATION AND DIAGNOSIS

The clinical manifestations depend on the heart rate, the duration of the arrhythmia, and the presence of underlying heart disease. Reentrant rhythms usually are not life-threatening, except in patients with the WPW syndrome. Most patients notice the fast heart rate almost immediately and may complain of dizziness, light-headedness, weakness, or nonspecific chest discomfort. Less common symptoms include dyspnea, syncope, and angina. CHF is uncommon because ventricular (His–Purkinje) conduction remains normal in most patients. However, the shortened ventricular filling time lowers stroke volume and may induce CHF in patients with a tenuous cardiovascular reserve. Infants often have nonspecific symptoms such as fussiness, lethargy, poor feeding, or rapid breathing yet may present with severe CHF and shock.

ACUTE TREATMENT

The goal of treatment for AV nodal reentry is to interrupt the circuit by slowing conduction or prolonging refractoriness in either AV junctional pathway. When the impulse encounters refractory tissue, the tachycardia terminates abruptly. Correctable contributing factors such as fever, infection, hypoxia, anemia, or hyperthyroidism should be treated. The arrhythmia may be terminated using pharmacologic, electrical, or other measures. The immediate treatment is dictated by the hemodynamic status of the patient.

Nonpharmacologic Therapy

Direct Current Cardioversion

In patients with hemodynamic instability (severe hypotension or heart failure, pulmonary edema, myocardial ischemia, acute alteration in mental status), electrical cardioversion is the therapy of choice. Direct current (DC) cardioversion depolarizes a critical number of myocardial cells simultaneously, allowing the sinus node to reestablish dominance as the pacemaker. For conversion of SVTs, lower energies (10 to 50 joules, or 0.5 joules/kg) often are adequate. This is a uniformly effective, immediate method of termination with minimal adverse effects. The only major adverse effect is the induction of ventricular arrhythmias, which can be avoided by synchronizing the electrical discharge to the QRS complex. Myocardial damage is rare with lower energies. Short-acting sedatives may be given before the procedure in older children and adults. Electroconversion is not advised in patients with stable cardiovascular status because other measures are considered less invasive and safer. Moreover, DC cardioversion precludes a direct assessment of the efficacy of various other maneuvers and drugs on the arrhythmia. This information is useful in managing recurrent episodes.

Vagal Maneuvers

In hemodynamically stable patients, interventions to increase vagal tone are performed first. These measures decrease conductivity and increase refractoriness in the AV node and decrease automaticity in the SA node by increasing parasympathetic tone. Used either alone or in conjunction with antiarrhythmic drugs, vagotonic maneuvers terminate 50 to 80% of cases of AV nodal reentrant tachycardia.

The most common vagal measures are carotid sinus massage (or pressure) and the Valsalva maneuver. Carotid sinus massage stimulates the baroreceptors of the carotid artery, which slows the sinus rate, prolongs AV conduction, lowers cardiac output, decreases venous return, and decreases peripheral vascular resistance.[18] Alteration in the critical balance between conduction and refractoriness disrupts the cycle and terminates the rhythm. The Valsalva maneuver (prolonged forced expiration against a closed glottis) may be induced by blowing into a blood pressure manometer tube to maintain a pressure of 30 to 60 mm Hg for 10 to 30 seconds. Conversion to sinus rhythm occurs during the relaxation phase, when a parasympathetic surge induces antegrade AV nodal block. Other vagotonic procedures include deep breathing, gagging, coughing, eyeball pressure, and squatting.

Carotid sinus massage and Valsalva maneuver may not be successful in infants and young children. In these patients, the diving reflex may be initiated by immersing the face in a pan of ice water for 10 to 15 seconds or placing a washcloth soaked in ice water on the face. This causes an acute vagal surge that is more prominent and clinically effective in young patients. A slowing of the tachycardia rate is followed by abrupt conversion to sinus rhythm. The diving reflex may induce asystole and should be used only under monitored conditions.

Background increases in sympathetic tone may attenuate the effectiveness of vagal maneuvers.[19] This may explain the lower efficacy when standing, as compared with the supine position. These measures generally are more effective in the young, probably because of a reduction in overall autonomic tone associated with aging. Vagal maneuvers should be performed as early as possible after arrhythmia initiation, before elevated sympathetic tone reduces efficacy.[19]

Vagotonic procedures should not be used in patients with a history of sinus node dysfunction because prolonged sinus node recovery time may cause sinus arrest after the reentry circuit is terminated. Carotid sinus massage or pressure may cause carotid artery ischemia in patients with preexisting atherosclerotic narrowing or (rarely) ventricular tachyarrhythmias.[18] Pressure to the carotid arteries should never be applied bilaterally. Both carotid arteries should be examined before the procedure, and it should not be attempted in patients with evidence of cerebrovascular insufficiency (e.g., carotid bruits). Because of the prevalence of sinus node and cerebrovascular disease in older adults, vagotonic stimuli should be avoided or used with great caution in this population.

Pharmacotherapy

Adenosine

Adenosine (Adenocard) is an injectable product indicated for conversion of PSVT, including that associated with accessory bypass tracts (WPW). If vagal maneuvers are unsuccessful, adenosine is the drug of choice for terminating AV nodal reentry.[11]

Mechanism

Adenosine is a ubiquitous endogenous purine nucleoside. Its myriad biologic effects include regulating coronary, cerebral, renal, and skeletal blood flow, modulating neurotransmission and immune response, inhibiting platelet aggregation, stimulating gastrin secretion, inhibiting lipolysis, and inducing bronchoconstriction. The actions of adenosine on cardiac tissues include a very transient, powerful negative dromotropic effect on the AV node and a similar negative chronotropic effect in the sinus node, AV junction, and ventricles. In EPSs the primary effects are a lengthening of sinus cycle and a prolongation of the A-H interval (i.e., the time from atrial excitation to the His bundle, which approximates the AV conduction time), followed by complete or partial AV nodal block.[20] Adenosine has no effect on the His–Purkinje interval. Cardiac activity is thought to be related to alterations in calcium and potassium ion currents, but the precise mechanisms are unclear.[21] Adenosine exerts minimal effect on vagal tone.

Adenosine is produced in many tissues and organs, but plasma concentrations are low because of rapid transport and metabolism. Local effects are mediated through interactions with intracellular and extracellular receptors, which may be upregulated, downregulated, supersensitized, and desensitized under different conditions. Analogs with agonist and antagonist activity and variable receptor affinity further modulate the effect. The effects of adenosine depend primarily on binding to the cell surface receptors; therefore, the concentration in the extracellular space correlates directly with the magnitude of the effect. Extracellular fluid concentrations are linked to adenosine production and elimination via multiple pathways.

Adenosine is continuously produced and released by erythrocytes and cells in the liver, heart, skeletal muscle, and endothelium. At physiologic concentrations (0.1 to 1 μmol), it is taken up avidly by erythrocytes and phosphorylated into adenosine monophosphate by adenosine kinase. At higher concentrations, it is deaminated by adenosine deaminase to inosine, which is further metabolized to hypoxanthine and uric acid. These metabolites have no antiarrhythmic effect. The balance between production and elimination is tightly regulated at the local level.

Clinical Use

Adenosine restores sinus rhythm within 10 to 20 seconds in 85 to 100% of adults and children with spontaneous or induced AV nodal reentrant tachycardias.[21–25] Antegrade pathway conduction block occurs in the majority of patients (Table 41.2).[21–25] In patients with sinus node or intra-atrial reentry, AF or atrial flutter, ectopic atrial tachycardia, or ventricular tachycardia (VT), adenosine induces a higher-grade AV block[21,26]; the transiently (less than 20 seconds) slower ventricular rate may allow visualization of P waves and therefore aid in diagnosis, but atrial activity is unchanged, and these arrhythmias are rarely terminated.

In randomized[22,25] and nonrandomized[24,27] comparative trials of adenosine and verapamil, conversion rates are comparable or favor adenosine for patients with AV nodal reentry or AV reentry involving an accessory pathway. Termination of the tachycardia generally is more rapid with adenosine than verapamil, but the clinical importance of this is unclear. Repetitive administration results in consistent conversion at a similar dosage each time or repeated failures.

Pharmacokinetics

Adenosine is not absorbed by the oral route. After intravenous injection, it is rapidly distributed into intracellular, extracellular, and interstitial spaces. It crosses the blood–brain barrier, and a vasodilatory effect on the cerebral vessels may account for the common occurrence of headache. In vitro studies have measured a half-life of less than 10 seconds.[28] Traditional pharmacokinetic studies are hampered by rapid clearance, with ongoing metabolism as specimens are collected. Parameters such as distribution volume and clearance therefore have not been reported.

Table 41.2 ▪ Sites of Primary Drug Action in Atrioventricular Nodal Reentry

AV node antegrade slow conduction pathway
Calcium channel blockers (verapamil, diltiazem)
Digoxin
Adenosine
β-Blockers
Amiodarone
AV node retrograde fast conduction pathway
Class Ia drugs (quinidine, procainamide, disopyramide)
Class Ic drugs (flecainide, propafenone)
Class III drugs (amiodarone, sotalol)
Suppression of atrial ectopy
Class Ia drugs (quinidine, procainamide, disopyramide)
Class Ic drugs (flecainide, propafenone)
β-Blockers
Class III drugs (amiodarone, sotalol)

AV, atrioventricular.

Toxicity

Noncardiac adverse effects occur in 15 to 81% of patients.[20,22,24,25,29] The most common are flushing, dyspnea or a feeling of suffocation, and headache. Chest pain or pressure may mimic angina. Cough, malaise, and nausea have also been observed. Inhaled adenosine has been reported to induce bronchoconstriction in asthmatic patients.[20] The effect of intravenous adenosine in patients with preexisting obstructive airway disease is not known because most clinical trials have excluded asthmatics. Adenosine therefore should be used cautiously in these patients. Adverse effects after intravenous adenosine abate within 1 to 2 minutes and are therefore limited in most patients.

Despite the action of adenosine to reduce systemic vascular resistance, intravenous boluses are well tolerated hemodynamically. Blood pressure remains unchanged or may even increase at the time of conversion to sinus rhythm. Masking of peripheral vasodilation in conscious subjects receiving bolus doses may be the result of autonomic reflexes. The lack of negative inotropic effect gives a theoretical advantage for adenosine in patients with severe heart failure; however, trials in this population are lacking.

Postconversion arrhythmias or conduction disorders occur in up to 60% of patients receiving adenosine. Sinus bradycardia, sinus tachycardia, sinus arrest, and various degrees of AV block last less than 1 to 2 minutes and do not warrant intervention in most patients. However, caution should be exercised in patients with sinus node disease because sinus arrest for up to 4 seconds has been observed.[22] Premature atrial or ventricular impulses after conversion to sinus rhythm occur in 33 to 60% of patients.[22,29] This may reinitiate reentry, an effect that is more common after adenosine than after verapamil.

Interactions

Drug interactions with adenosine may involve alterations in extracellular and intracellular transport as well as receptor affinity. Although many drugs have in vitro or theoretical mechanisms for interaction, systematic clinical trials are lacking. Interactions with dipyridamole and theophylline have the strongest documentation. Dipyridamole blocks the cellular uptake of adenosine, thereby inhibiting its metabolism.[28] This may enhance the negative chronotropic and dromotropic effects of adenosine. Very limited evidence suggests a similar effect with diazepam. Aminophylline and theophylline bind to the extracellular adenosine receptor sites and therefore act as competitive antagonists.[20] Patients receiving these drugs (and possibly caffeine) may exhibit a blunted response to adenosine. Carbamazepine can suppress AV conduction at therapeutic or mildly elevated blood concentrations. In the presence of carbamazepine, conduction inhibition through the AV node by adenosine can be enhanced, producing a higher degree of heart block.[11,26] When using adenosine, patients who are on carbamazepine should be treated cautiously. The possible role of calcium in the pharmacologic effect of adenosine suggests potential interactions with calcium channel blockers and digoxin, but these have not been well studied. The clinical implications of these interactions have not been established. The ultrashort duration of action of adenosine should minimize long-term effects of any drug interactions observed.

Administration

The standard adult dosage of adenosine is 6 mg given by rapid intravenous bolus over 1 to 2 seconds, followed by a normal saline flush. If no response is observed in 2 minutes, 12 mg intravenously may be given. A second 12-mg dose may be given in 1 to 2 minutes if needed. Clinical trials of adenosine in infants and children have used dosages of 0.0375 to 0.25 mg/kg,[23] but the drug is not approved by the U.S. Food and Drug Administration (FDA) for pediatric use. Despite the lack of FDA approval, adenosine is considered by some clinicians the drug of choice (after vagal maneuvers fail) for the acute management of AV nodal reentrant tachycardia in children.[30] The ultrashort half-life of the drug necessitates careful attention to the site and rate of administration. The pharmacologic effect depends on the amount of drug delivered to the heart. A slow administration rate or slow rate of blood flow (e.g., heart failure) may result in significant metabolism before the drug reaches the heart and therefore attenuate the effect of the drug. Conversely, administration into central veins (e.g., femoral vein during EPS) may result in a more marked response. Reflex tachycardia caused by vasodilation has been reported after slow administration. Individual variation in underlying autonomic tone and the administration of other antiarrhythmics may enhance or attenuate adenosine's effect.

The very high efficacy rate of adenosine is comparable to or perhaps even better than that of verapamil. It can restore sinus rhythm more rapidly than verapamil, although the clinical importance of this difference is unclear. The lack of negative inotropic and hypotensive effects makes it especially useful in patients with heart failure or hypotension. However, DC cardioversion remains the treatment of choice in severe hemodynamic instability. The very short half-life allows rapid titration of individual doses, reduces concern about long-lasting or cumulative adverse effects, and minimizes the effects of drug interactions. Adenosine is an ideal drug for studying arrhythmias in the electrophysiology laboratory. However, the short half-life may also be a limitation because of the recurrence of reentry and lack of utility for long-term management. Moreover, the rate of adverse reactions is higher than with verapamil. Verapamil and adenosine share the need for cautious use in patients with sinus node dysfunction, conduction system disease, or WPW syndrome. Adenosine is preferred in patients with hypotension or heart failure, whereas verapamil is favored in patients with obstructive airway disease or those taking dipyridamole or methylxanthines (and possibly benzodiazepines, β-blockers, digoxin, and carbamazepine).

Verapamil

Verapamil inhibits channel-mediated entry of calcium into the cell. Effects are most evident in the SA node, AV node, and cardiac and peripheral vascular smooth muscles because these tissues depend on calcium flux for action potential generation. In contrast, atrial and ventricular myocardium and the His–Purkinje system normally are fast-channel (sodium flux dependent) tissues. This explains the lack of efficacy of verapamil in ventricular arrhythmias.

The net effect of verapamil results from an interplay between direct and indirect effects. Direct actions include depressing automaticity in the SA and AV nodes (negative chronotropic effect), reducing conduction velocity in the AV node (negative dromotropic effect), reducing myocardial contractility (negative inotropic effect), and dilating coronary and peripheral arteries. These effects are modified by reflex sympathetic stimulation evoked by the peripheral arterial dilation. Increased cardiac automaticity and contractility largely offset the negative chronotropic and inotropic effects. The net cardiac effect is a negative dromotropic effect on antegrade conduction through the AV node (Table 41.2). Other effects become important only in diseased hearts (e.g., sinus node disease or CHF).

Among the calcium channel blocking agents, verapamil has the lowest degree of peripheral arterial dilation relative to its effects on the heart. This characteristic is advantageous in treating arrhythmias, but the prominent negative inotropic effect may be a limitation in some patients. In contrast, nifedipine is a much more potent vasodilator, causing marked hemodynamic alteration before conduction effects are seen. Therefore, nifedipine is not useful as an antiarrhythmic. Diltiazem has electrophysiologic and hemodynamic effects comparable to those of verapamil and has demonstrated efficacy and safety in clinical trials.[31,32]

Administration

Intravenous verapamil dosages of 5 to 10 mg or 0.075 to 0.15 mg/kg over 2 minutes (3 minutes in older adults) convert 60 to 90% of adult patients with AV nodal reentry to normal sinus rhythm within 5 to 10 minutes. If there is no response, a second dose of 0.15 mg/kg intravenously may be given 15 to 30 minutes later. Vagal maneuvers should be performed before the second dose.

Pharmacokinetics

After oral administration, more than 90% of the dose is absorbed, but extensive first-pass metabolism limits systemic availability to 20 to 35%.[33,34] Food prolongs the time to peak concentration but not the extent of absorption. Large interpatient and intrapatient variability exists, with serum concentrations after administration of the same dosage varying as much as 10-fold. Verapamil is approximately 90% protein bound to albumin and α_1-acid glycoprotein.[34] The volume of distribution of 4.5 to 7 L/kg in healthy adults is higher in cirrhosis. It is converted rapidly and extensively in the liver to multiple metabolites that are largely inactive. The only active metabolite, norverapamil (the *N*-demethylated derivative), has approximately 20% of the potency of the parent drug. Verapamil undergoes biexponential or triexponential decline, with an elimination phase half-life of 3 to 5 hours after a single dose.[33,34] Long-term administration may result in nonlinear accumulation, with a decreased clearance and prolonged half-life.[34] Seventy percent of an oral or intravenous dose is recovered in the urine in 5 days, almost exclusively as metabolites, with 10 to 15% found in the feces.[35]

Patients with cirrhosis demonstrate a significantly higher bioavailability (52.3% versus 22% for normal subjects) because of a less marked first-pass effect as well as a longer half-life and lower clearance.[33,36] Those with arrhythmias or CHF may have altered hepatic clearance related to hepatic blood flow.

After a single intravenous dose, there is a good relationship between serum concentrations and electrophysiologic effects. However, studies of oral administration have yielded a poor correlation of serum concentrations with clinical efficacy. This is explained in part by stereoselective differences in its pharmacodynamics and pharmacokinetics. Commercially available preparations of verapamil are racemic mixtures of the D- and L-isomers. The L-isomer has more potent negative chronotropic, inotropic, and dromotropic effects.[37] Stereoselective first-pass metabolism after oral dosing results in preferential extraction of the L-isomer. Bioavailability of the L-isomer (20%) is therefore lower than that of the D-isomer (50%).[36] The L-isomer has a distribution volume, clearance, and unbound fraction approximately twice those of the D-isomer.[36] The relative ratios of L- and D-isomers after intravenous and oral administrations are therefore different, with intravenous dosing giving a larger fraction of total verapamil concentration than the more active L-isomer. Serum concentrations needed for a given P-R interval prolongation after intravenous doses are lower than those after oral administration.[34] This may explain the higher efficacy after acute intravenous administration than after chronic oral administration and wide interpatient and intrapatient variability in response to a fixed serum concentration. Another explanation for the discrepancy between the clinical effects of intravenous and oral dosing is preferential myocardial uptake after intravenous administration.[34] Alteration of response by underlying sympathetic tone further disrupts the relationship between serum concentration and drug effect. Conventional assays measuring total verapamil concentration are not useful in assessing efficacy. Analytic methods to isolate the individual enantiomers are not widely available.

Toxicity

Adverse reactions occur in 10 to 14%[35] of patients receiving verapamil but warrant discontinuation in only 1 to 5%. Adverse effects after intravenous administration are an extension of the pharmacologic effect and include hypotension, disturbances in AV conduction, bradycardia or sinus arrest, and CHF. These reflect calcium channel blockade in the vascular smooth muscle, AV node, SA node, and myocardium, respectively. Mild, transient hypotension is the most common adverse reaction. Most patients do not need treatment; in some, the reduction in afterload may even allow an increase in cardiac output. In symptomatic patients, placement in Trendelenburg's position with intravenous fluid administration usually is adequate. Patients with borderline blood pressures before verapamil (systolic pressure 90 to 100 mm Hg or less) may develop severe hypotension. These patients should receive adenosine. Alternatively, pretreatment with 1 g intravenous calcium chloride or gluconate is thought to block the peripheral but not the cardiac receptors.[38,39] Calcium therefore blunts or abolishes the hypotensive effect while preserving AV nodal effect when given either before or after verapamil. Sudden cardiovascular collapse with profound hypotension, bradycardia, apnea, and death has been reported after verapamil administration in neonates and infants.[40] Although verapamil is an excellent drug in older children, it should be avoided in children less than 1 year old.[30,41]

Verapamil is not thought to have a significant proarrhythmic effect but must be used cautiously in patients with preexisting conduction disorders. Premature atrial or ventricular impulses occasionally reactivate reentry. AF and serious ventricular arrhythmias are uncommon. Bradycardia or heart block caused by excessive AV nodal effect may warrant treatment with isoproterenol, atropine, calcium, or pacemakers. Verapamil is contraindicated in patients with preexisting SA nodal disease (SSS) because of high risk of prolonged sinus arrest after termination of the arrhythmia. Verapamil is a first-line drug in most patients, but it is contraindicated in patients with sinus node disease, marked hypotension, or heart failure and in neonates. Adenosine is preferred in these patients.

An important drug interaction occurs between verapamil and β-blockers. Concomitant administration of these drugs results in AV blocking and negative inotropic effects by independent mechanisms. This increases the risk of serious cardiovascular effects such as CHF,[42] high-degree AV block, or hypotension. Serum concentrations of digoxin may be increased by verapamil[43] via an increase in half-life and reduction in distribution volume and total clearance. Furthermore, verapamil should be used with caution in suspected digoxin toxicity because of its additive effects on the AV node.

Monitoring parameters for intravenous verapamil in arrhythmias include cardiac rhythm and rate and blood pressure. Continuous ECG monitoring is strongly advised. Routine serum concentration assessment is not recommended.

Pharmacologic Vagal Stimulation

If vagal maneuvers, adenosine, or verapamil are unsuccessful, pharmacologic vagal stimulation may be attempted. Edrophonium (5 to 10 mg intravenously) inhibits acetylcholinesterase, resulting in a direct vagal effect. Metaraminol (0.5 to 2 mg intravenously), phenylephrine (0.5 mg intravenously), or methoxamine (5 to 15 mg intravenously) transiently raises blood pressure (to a goal of systolic 160 to 170 mm Hg), stimulates the carotid baroreceptors, and induces a reflex increase in vagal tone. These drugs should be preceded and followed by vagotonic maneuvers. They should be used with caution in patients with baseline sinus node dysfunction. Further caution is advised when using edrophonium in patients receiving digoxin and with pressor agents in patients with severe CHF. Although their use in adults has been largely surpassed by adenosine and verapamil, these drugs remain useful in infants and children.

Other Pharmacotherapy

Diltiazem, digoxin, propranolol, quinidine, procainamide, amiodarone, and sotalol can also be used to terminate AV nodal or AV reentry. Diltiazem inhibits antegrade AV nodal conduction with comparable effectiveness to verapamil. Doses of 0.15 to 0.25 mg/kg intravenously over 2 minutes restore sinus rhythm within 2 to 10 minutes in 60 to 100% of patients.[32,44] Repeat doses of 0.35 mg/kg intravenously over 2 minutes, 15 minutes after initial dose, is associated with additional success in initial nonresponders.[32] A potential advantage of diltiazem is a mild negative inotropic effect compared to verapamil,[45] which may allow its use in patients with severe left ventricular impairment.[46]

Digoxin has a lower response rate and a longer onset of action for conversion to sinus rhythm (several hours) than verapamil. It produces direct slowing of AV conduction by a different mechanism (vagal and antiadrenergic effect blocks AV nodal conduction; Table 41.2). Patients who do not respond to other drugs or maneuvers may respond to digoxin, especially children without accessory pathway conduction. Digoxin is also useful in patients with severe left ventricular dysfunction. Specific aspects of digoxin therapy are discussed under Atrial Fibrillation.

Propranolol prolongs antegrade AV conduction and refractoriness and also depresses automaticity at the SA node, AV junction, and His–Purkinje fibers (Table 41.2). Propranolol is not a first-line drug because it is less efficacious than adenosine and verapamil, and it is contraindicated in patients who have received verapamil because of the additive effects on cardiac conduction and contractility. It is used primarily in infants and children who have not received verapamil and when digoxin is not desirable (e.g., accessory pathway conduction). Metoprolol and esmolol have the advantages of cardioselectivity and ultrashort half-life, respectively.

Quinidine, procainamide, flecainide, and propafenone block conduction in the fast (usually retrograde) pathway (Table 41.2). They are not as effective in AV nodal or AV reentry and are reserved for refractory cases. They may be useful in cases in which supraventricular and ventricular tachyarrhythmias cannot be distinguished. Class I antiarrhythmic agents should be used with caution because of their potential for proarrhythmias.

Amiodarone and sotalol suppress ectopic atrial activity. In addition, amiodarone prolongs antegrade and retrograde AV conduction, whereas sotalol prolongs retrograde conduction only (Table 41.2). Both agents are highly effective in terminating supraventricular tachyarrhythmias; however, their use is limited by unfamiliarity with dosing and serious adverse effects.

Other Nonpharmacologic Therapy

Pacemakers

Patients who do not respond to pharmacologic treatment should receive electrical therapy, which may include DC cardioversion (described earlier) or specialized pacing techniques. Pacing techniques include one or two critically timed extra stimuli or a rapid sequence of impulses (burst overdrive pacing).[47] As a rule, burst-pacing techniques are more effective. The goal of pacing is to create a strategically timed region of refractoriness. The paced impulse enters the circuit, collides with the advancing wavefront, blocks the succeeding wavefront, and stops the reentry circuit. Proximity of pacing site to the anatomic origin of the arrhythmia enhances the likelihood of success. Though highly effective, pacing is an invasive technique that entails transvenous or transesophageal catheter placement and EPS for application. Complications include tachycardia acceleration and fibrillation of the paced chambers.

CHRONIC TREATMENT

The need for prophylaxis is dictated by the frequency of episodes, the tachycardia rate, and its hemodynamic effects. In general, the presence and extent of symptoms are related to the rate and duration of the arrhythmia. The benefits of arrhythmia suppression must be balanced carefully against the risks and inconveniences of long-term antiarrhythmic therapy. In the absence of heart disease, most patients have infrequent attacks of short duration without cardiovascular compromise and do not need chronic suppression. Patients with underlying heart disease, frequent attacks, or debilitating symptoms (syncope, angina, hypotension, heart failure) may benefit from prophylaxis.

The goal of chronic prophylaxis is to prevent or minimize the frequency of attacks and their hemodynamic consequences. Complete abolition is not necessary and may be worse than no therapy because of proarrhythmic or other adverse drug effects. Precipitating factors such as sympathomimetics, β-agonists, caffeine, tobacco, or ethanol should be limited or discontinued. Patients with arrhythmias responsive to physical maneuvers such as carotid sinus pressure should be instructed in their proper application. This may obviate pharmacologic prophylaxis.

Electrophysiologic Studies

Ideally, treatment should be guided by EPS. Percutaneously inserted catheters are positioned in the heart to identify the site of origin and mechanism of the arrhythmia, to permit repetitive initiation and termination of arrhythmias, and to evaluate the efficacy of drugs and other maneuvers. Suppression of induced arrhythmias in the laboratory often is a valuable predictor of efficacy for subsequent episodes. Therefore, EPS serves the following functions:

- To accurately characterize the electrophysiologic mechanism of the arrhythmia. This allows more rational drug or technique selection.
- To identify the underlying mechanism before nonpharmacologic options such as pacemakers, surgery, or catheter ablation are implemented.
- To rapidly achieve a therapeutic regimen in patients with hemodynamically serious consequences such as syncope, hypotension, or heart failure. EPSs permit expeditious trials of multiple antiarrhythmic drugs or techniques. Identification of serum concentration–antiarrhythmic effect relationships may allow individualized targeting of drug dosages.
- To identify symptomatic patients with WPW syndrome who are at risk of developing life-threatening arrhythmias.

EPSs are limited by poor predictability of response in as many as one-third of patients. This is sometimes explained by alterations in autonomic tone at the time of spontaneous arrhythmia recurrence; EPSs are performed in the resting, supine state, whereas arrhythmias recur in ambulatory patients. These differences in sympathetic tone alter the electrophysiologic characteristics and response to drugs. Furthermore, EPSs are costly and uncomfortable. Some practitioners therefore prefer to treat patients with well-tolerated arrhythmias empirically, reserving EPSs for patients in whom initial strategies fail.

Strategies for the pharmacologic prophylaxis of AV nodal reentry are not as well established as those for managing acute episodes. Many therapeutic options exist, some or all of which may give a satisfactory outcome. As a rule, patient response is not as predictable and efficacy rates are lower than for acute episodes, with no single drug emerging as the treatment of choice. Initial selections are based on specific patient considerations, dosing intervals, adverse effect profile, cost of drugs and monitoring tests, and physician preference or experience. Treatment can be directed at the antegrade or retrograde pathway. Calcium channel blockers, digoxin, or β-blockers are common initial choices. Quinidine is also efficacious, but hospitalization is needed for the first few days of therapy because of potential proarrhythmic events. Nondrug therapies include antitachycardia pacemakers and surgery to ablate or modify the AV node.

Pharmacotherapy

Verapamil

Despite its excellent intravenous efficacy for acute episodes of AV nodal reentry, oral verapamil has been less successful in the prophylaxis of recurrent arrhythmias. Efficacy varies widely between 40 and 90%. Successful termination with intravenous verapamil does not predict long-term efficacy with oral treatment. Serum concentrations needed for specific AV node conduction effects are higher after oral administration than after intravenous administration.[33,36] The lower potency of oral dosing may result from stereospecific presystemic metabolism of racemic verapamil, which causes preferential hepatic extraction of the more active L-isomer.[36,37] Because the L-isomer accounts for most of the AV nodal effect, this may explain both the more frequent therapeutic failures and the wide variability in serum concentration–response data.[37] Alterations in autonomic tone at the time of arrhythmia recurrence further modulate the efficacy of verapamil.

Initial daily dosages of 120 to 240 mg are titrated to average maintenance dosages of 240 to 480 mg. The sustained-release preparations offer comparable bioavailability, slower absorption with less fluctuation, and more sustained serum concentrations, permitting once- or twice-daily dosing. Observations of significant nonlinear accumulation with a prolonged half-life after chronic oral dosing may permit a longer dosing interval for the conventional tablets as well.[34]

Oral verapamil is very well tolerated in most patients. Smooth muscle relaxation in the gastrointestinal tract may cause constipation. Peripheral edema and headache also can be seen. Verapamil does not aggravate bronchospastic or vasospastic disorders and therefore is safer in patients unable to take β-blockers.

The effectiveness of oral diltiazem for prophylaxis of recurrent reentrant supraventricular arrhythmias is not well defined. Daily dosages of 180 to 360 mg were thought to be effective; however, a recent placebo-controlled trial did not demonstrate a beneficial effect of diltiazem over placebo for suppressing SVT.[48] Larger clinical trials are needed to establish the role of oral diltiazem for this indication.

Monitoring parameters for oral verapamil therapy include cardiac rhythm and rate, constipation, and peripheral edema. Routine serum concentration monitoring is not necessary.

Digoxin

The suppressant effect of digoxin on AV nodal conduction occurs via a mechanism different from that of verapamil. It is particularly useful in infants and children, often as a single agent, after WPW syndrome with antegrade accessory pathway conduction has been excluded. Its positive inotropic effect is unique among the common antiarrhythmics and permits its use in patients with heart failure. The ideal digoxin dosage is one that controls the ventricular rate during the tachyarrhythmia yet does not cause bradycardia while in sinus rhythm. Specific aspects of digoxin therapy are discussed under Atrial Fibrillation.

Quinidine

Quinidine is the leading antiarrhythmic drug in the United States in terms of frequency of use. It was selected by 60 to 80% of U.S. physicians as drug of first choice for maintenance of sinus rhythm after cardioversion of AF.[49] Quinidine is a prototype class Ia drug that differs from digoxin and verapamil in its action on the fast (sodium) channel. Its net effect reflects a modification of its direct action by an indirect vagolytic effect. The direct action is a generalized slowing of both automaticity and conduction velocity in the SA node, AV node, and His–Purkinje systems. Vagolysis overrides many of these effects, resulting in a net increase in sinus rate and AV nodal conduction velocity. His–Purkinje conduction time remains delayed, reflecting minimal autonomic influence in these tissues. The effects of quinidine are minimal in healthy, well-polarized tissues and most marked at rapid heart rates, in ectopic pacemakers, and in hypoxic or ischemic tissues. Peripheral α-adrenergic blockade and relaxation of vascular smooth muscle associated with intravenous administration may further influence cardiac action. Alteration of baseline susceptibility to the direct or indirect action of quinidine may explain interpatient variation in net effect.

The efficacy of quinidine in SVTs results from a decrease in atrial ectopy, which suppresses the inciting premature impulses, and a slowing of conduction in the retrograde fast path (Table 41.2). It is not useful after reentry has begun and may even be deleterious because of an increase in AV nodal conduction velocity. Patients should therefore have adequate AV node slowing (e.g., from digoxin) before quinidine therapy is initiated for supraventricular tachyarrhythmias. Interestingly, controlled studies of quinidine in AV nodal reentry are lacking despite widespread clinical use.

Pharmacokinetics

After oral administration, quinidine demonstrates variable absorption and first-pass effect, resulting in about 70% bioavailability (range 45 to 100%).[50] Peak serum concentrations are seen at 1 to 2 hours for the standard formulation of the sulfate salt and 3 to 5 hours with the sustained-release formulations of the sulfate and gluconate salts. The rate and extent of absorption are lower in patients with heart failure.[51] Quinidine is 80 to 89% protein bound to albumin and α_1-acid glycoprotein. It demonstrates two-compartment kinetics, with average distribution and elimination phase half-lives of 7 minutes and 6 to 7 hours, respectively.[50] The steady-state distribution volume in normal subjects is 3 L/kg.[50] About 85% is metabolized to several active and inactive forms, including 3-hydroxyquinidine, 2-oxoquinidinone, and quinidine-*N*-oxide. Ten to 20% is eliminated unchanged in the urine in 24 hours, primarily by glomerular filtration. Total clearance averaging 4.5 mL/minute/kg is widely variable and may depend on the dosage and route of administration.[50,52]

Quinidine metabolites may contribute to both the antiarrhythmic and proarrhythmic effects.[53] Total serum concentrations of 3-hydroxyquinidine are lower than those of the parent compound, but a higher unbound fraction results in free metabolite concentrations comparable to those of the parent drug.[52] Both quinidine and 3-hydroxyquinidine may accumulate with multiple dosing, resulting in higher serum concentrations and an increase in QTc interval prolongation.[52] Quinidine is metabolized in the liver via cytochrome P-3A4. Quinidine inhibits cytochrome P-3A4, resulting in increased effects of warfarin, β-blockers, disopyramide, procainamide, and propafenone.[54]

Patients with CHF have a lower volume of distribution and total clearance, without alteration in half-life.[51] Increased concentrations of β_1-acid glycoprotein concentration commonly observed after AMI[55] and during paroxysmal AF may result in diminished drug effect because of more extensive protein binding.[55] Patients with cirrhosis demonstrate decreased protein binding, an increased half-life and volume of distribution, and no change in total clearance.[50] A diminished volume of distribution and renal clearance without change in half-life are seen with renal failure.

Quinidine is available in several salts: quinidine sulfate (83% base), quinidine gluconate (62% base), and quinidine polygalacturonate (80% base). Because dosages are expressed as the salt rather than the base, it is important to account for the different potencies when switching forms. The usual daily dosage is 200 to 400 mg of the sulfate salt or its equivalent three to four times daily for the conventional tablets. Dosage should be decreased in CHF and (possibly) cirrhosis. Children and young adults (less than 30 years) may need higher dosages. Dosage adjustment in renal insufficiency is controversial.

Intravenous administration has traditionally been discouraged because of dose- and rate-related hypotension caused by α-adrenergic blockade and a direct peripheral venodilation. Reports suggest that intravenous administration is safe when given no faster than 0.5 mg/kg/minute to a total dosage of 10 mg/kg of quinidine gluconate, with careful blood pressure monitoring.[56] Intramuscular administration is not advised because absorption is erratic, administration is painful, and it may result in sterile abscess formation.

The utility of serum concentration monitoring is hindered by the nonspecificity of common analytic methods. The parent drug, its metabolites, and dihydroquinidine (a known impurity in commercial-grade drug) can be detected to varying degrees. The different pharmacokinetic and pharmacodynamic profiles of these compounds obscure the relationship between serum concentrations and therapeutic or adverse effects. Assays of total (bound and unbound) quinidine are further limited in diseases such as AMI, where the extent of protein binding can vary from day to day. High-performance liquid chromatography is considered the most specific and therefore the reference procedure, with a therapeutic range of 1 to 4 mg/L.[55] The enzyme immunoassay and double-extraction photofluorometric assay have therapeutic ranges of 2 to 5 mg/L. Individualized target serum concentration goals based on clinical or EPS response may be more useful than values based on population parameters. It is also important to recognize that therapeutic range estimates derived from trials of ventricular arrhythmias may not be applicable to SVTs. Serum concentration measurement therefore is useful in suspected noncompliance or toxicity but may not be necessary in well-controlled patients without clinical toxicity.

Toxicity

Adverse effects occur in 18 to 50% of patients taking quinidine, with 9 to 14% patients needing drug discontinuation.[57,58] In the Boston Collaborative Drug Surveillance Program,[57] gastrointestinal reactions, primarily diarrhea with or without nausea, were particularly troublesome and the most common reason for discontinuing therapy, accounting for 7.8%. Fever was seen in 1.7%. Various dermatologic reactions, cinchonism (tinnitus, dizziness, hearing and visual disturbances) and hematologic reactions (thrombocytopenia, hemolytic anemia) each occurred in less than 1% of patients. Hepatotoxicity has been observed particularly early in the use of quinidine. Patients should be monitored for the first 4 to 8 weeks of therapy for unexplained fever and elevation of hepatic enzymes.[54]

The most serious cardiac reaction is exacerbation of arrhythmias. This may manifest as the induction of a new arrhythmia or conversion of an existing stable arrhythmia to an unstable one. Paroxysmal syncope or presyncope is correlated on ECG with intermittent polymorphic VT or fibrillation, often of the torsade de pointes pattern. It typically follows a pause or abrupt decrease in ventricular rate. The first tachycardic QRS complex occurs as a triggered response, emerging from a large postpause U wave. The intervening sinus beats often demonstrate a markedly prolonged QTc interval. Torsade de pointes occurs in 2 to 3% of patients beginning quinidine treatment.[53] Patients with pretreatment Q-T prolongation, bradycardia, hypokalemia, hypomagnesemia, heart block, and heart failure (or possibly those taking digoxin)[43] are at increased risk. Proarrhythmic effects can appear at any time, generally within 3 to 5 days after initiation of therapy or dosage increase. As many as 50% have serum concentrations of less than 2 mg/L, reflecting the idiosyncratic rather than toxic nature of the reaction.[53] In vitro testing suggests that quinidine metabolites or impurities may also contribute to the proarrhythmic effect.[53] Proarrhythmic events are less common in patients with SVTs than are ventricular arrhythmias, possibly because patients with SVTs are more likely to have structurally normal hearts. Most episodes are self-limiting and usually abate 12 to 24 hours after the drug is discontinued. Some patients develop cardiovascular insufficiency or collapse. Treatment is limited to discontinuing the drug, maintaining serum potassium concentrations at or above normal, and administering magnesium, DC cardioversion, or overdrive pacing; most antiarrhythmic drugs are ineffective (see Torsade de Pointes).

Other cardiovascular reactions include bradyarrhythmias or an increased ventricular rate in patients with AF. Hypotension after intravenous administration of quinidine is minimized by slow infusion rates. Symptomatic hypotension is treated by administration of fluids and a reduction in infusion rate.

A recent meta-analysis evaluating the safety and efficacy of quinidine revealed a disturbing threefold higher death rate in patients on maintenance therapy than in patients on placebo over a 1-year period.[58] The percentage of patients dying in the quinidine group was 2.9%, compared with 0.8% in the placebo group; however, the causes of death were not well characterized and included causes other than cardiovascular ones. Death related to chronic quinidine therapy is thought to result from proarrhythmia, a belief that has not yet been clinically documented. Some cardiologists are recommending against using class I agents in favor of low-dose amiodarone.[59]

The interaction of quinidine with digoxin is particularly important in treating SVTs because the concomitant use of digoxin is important to protect the AV node from the vagolytic effects of quinidine. Reduction of digoxin dosage often is necessary. Other drug interactions with quinidine include those with hepatic enzyme inducers (phenobarbital, phenytoin, rifampin) or inhibitors (cimetidine) and warfarin.

Monitoring guidelines for quinidine in AV nodal reentry prophylaxis include heart rate and rhythm, QRS and QTc intervals, and gastrointestinal symptoms. Patients with intolerable gastrointestinal reactions should be evaluated on a different salt form or a sustained-release preparation (at equivalent dosage) before switching to another drug. Administration with food or aluminum hydroxide type antacids may also lessen symptoms. Serum concentrations may be monitored, but the laboratory should be contacted to determine the assay method, its limitations, and the recommended therapeutic range. To facilitate detection and treatment of proarrhythmic events, some recommend that patients be hospitalized for the first 3 to 5 days of therapy. Others point out that the proarrhythmia onset may be delayed despite these precautions.

β-Blockers

Propranolol and the other β-blocking agents have many effects on cardiac conduction and contractility. Their efficacy in SVTs results from a slowing of automaticity in sinus and ectopic pacemakers, a decrease in conduction velocity through the AV node, and an increase in the refractory period of the AV node (Table 41.2). Quinidinelike membrane-stabilizing properties are seen only at very high dosages and do not contribute to arrhythmia control. When successful during EPS evaluation, long-term efficacy is very good. Despite their numerous adverse effects and contraindications, these agents retain their usefulness in the prophylaxis of AV nodal reentry because their mechanism of action differs from that of the other commonly used drugs. They are especially useful in SVTs associated with excessive catecholamine release, as in hyperthyroidism, pheochromocytoma, exercise, or emotional upset. A reduction in exercise tolerance may be bothersome in young patients. In theory, most of the currently available β-blocking drugs should be effective in SVTs, but large-scale studies are lacking. Dosage needs for propranolol and the other β-blockers are difficult to predict because of variation in the response of individual patients to fixed concentrations of drug. Underlying sympathetic tone and variations in pharmacokinetics further influence patient response. Other aspects of β-blockers are discussed under Sudden Death.

Other Drugs

Procainamide, disopyramide, flecainide, sotalol, and amiodarone all have good efficacy in controlling AV nodal reentry. Unfortunately, adverse effects relegate them to a secondary role. The proarrhythmic effects of flecainide are a major limitation. These drugs should be used with careful observation, especially in patients with structural heart disease.

Nonpharmacologic Therapy

Nonpharmacologic therapies for AV nodal reentry include pacemakers, surgical interruption of the reentry circuit, and percutaneous catheter ablation or modification. They are indicated when medical therapy is ineffective or not tolerated. Because these modalities allow patients to remain drug-free, noncompliant patients, younger patients unwilling to comply with lifelong drug treatment, older adults in whom symptoms of the arrhythmia or adverse effects of antiarrhythmic medication may be intolerable, or women desiring pregnancy may also be candidates. Extensive EPSs and cardiac mapping studies are important in maximizing success.

Pacemakers

Permanent pacemakers have been used in the chronic management of AV nodal reentry for many years. They either minimize arrhythmogenesis or terminate tachycardias after they occur. Overdrive pacing at a rate slightly faster than the sinus rate, or programmed atrial and ventricular stimulation, will alter refractoriness in the limbs of the reentrant circuit and therefore prevent the arrhythmia. Techniques for terminating the tachycardia are the same as those discussed under Acute Treatment.[47] The most sophisticated devices are activated automatically by a sensing function, may be programmed both before and after insertion, and have a memory function that remembers and delivers an algorithm of previously successful terminating sequences. Unfortunately, reliable termination of AV nodal reentry entails concomitant antiarrhythmic drug therapy in as many as 50% of patients receiving pacemakers.[47] Adverse effects include precipitation of tachyarrhythmias, syncope, and sudden death, especially in patients with accessory pathways. Additionally, pacemakers must be checked and reprogrammed regularly, may not eliminate symptoms, and are not curative. This last limitation has become more meaningful as surgical methods offering complete cure have evolved. Patients with sinus node disease are ideal candidates because the pacemaker can manage both tachycardic and bradycardic episodes. They are also useful in those who are not candidates for surgery or refuse surgery.

Surgery

Surgical techniques include careful dissection of the perinodal tissue to alter intranodal or accessory pathway conduction, which is especially useful in the WPW syndrome, or cryoablation of atrial fibers around the AV node to abolish extranodal retrograde pathways while preserving antegrade conduction.[60] These procedures have been studied in both adults and children, primarily with AV nodal reentry or AV reentry using an accessory pathway. They are highly successful on short-term evaluation but incur the typical risks and limitations of open chest procedures.

Percutaneous Catheter Modification of the Atrioventricular Node

Recent refinements in technique have allowed selective modification of the AV node using percutaneously placed catheters. Either the antegrade (slow) or retrograde (fast) pathway can be abolished or impaired. The AV node or surrounding tissues are modified by applying DC, laser, or most commonly radiofrequency energy sources. Antegrade pathway conduction modification is now preferred over retrograde conduction because of greater efficacy (more than 90% versus 50 to 90%, respectively) and minimal risk of AV block (less than 2% versus 2 to 8%, respectively).[61,62] Complications other than AV block include thromboembolism, arrhythmias (including inappropriate sinus tachycardia), and valvular damage. Intravenous heparin is infused during the procedure to prevent thromboemboli formation. Post-modification therapy may include 3 to 6 months of aspirin or warfarin therapy and β-blockers for the control of inappropriate sinus tachycardia if it occurs. The benefit of short-term antiplatelet or anticoagulation therapy after the modification procedure has not yet been determined. The percutaneous approach has the advantage of avoiding an open chest procedure with cardiopulmonary bypass. Because of the curative properties, high efficacy, and low potential for adverse effects, percutaneous modification is fast becoming a preferred method of treatment. However, long-term follow-up data about cardiac effects and safety for this treatment modality are needed.

Additional Nonpharmacologic Therapies

Additional nonpharmacologic strategies for treating AV nodal reentry and AV reentry associated with an accessory pathway are evolving rapidly. Their primary use at present is limited to patients who are resistant or intolerant to antiarrhythmic drug therapy. Their expeditious, cost-effective, and curative features are major attributes. As technologies are developed and refined, nonpharmacologic therapy is likely to be useful in a wide spectrum of patients.

Ectopic Atrial Tachycardia

Enhanced automaticity (ability to generate spontaneous impulses) of an ectopic atrial focus may result in an arrhythmia known as ectopic atrial tachycardia. Like reentry, it is initiated by a premature atrial impulse. Unlike reentry, this arrhythmia is characterized by a warmup period with gradual acceleration and termination via a gradual deceleration. The ventricular rate ranges from 100 to 280 bpm. Periods of AV block are common. This arrhythmia is important because ectopic atrial tachycardia with block in a patient taking digitalis is highly suspicious for toxicity. Other acute causes include AMI, trauma, chronic lung disease, or certain metabolic abnormalities.

Multifocal atrial tachycardia (MAT) is a form of ectopic atrial tachycardia thought to be caused by either enhanced automaticity or triggered activity.[63] On ECG, at least three different ectopic P-wave morphologies are seen, representing three or more ectopic foci, with irregular P-R and P-P intervals. The ventricular rate of 130 to 220 bpm is variable ("irregularly irregular") during the tachycardic episodes. This allows differentiation from AV nodal or AV reentry but may result in confusion with AF. MAT is seen in 0.3 to 0.4% of hospitalized patients. It occurs typically in older adults with chronic lung or heart disease who are critically ill with acute pulmonary or cardiac failure or sepsis. It is associated with an elevation in circulating catecholamines and may be precipitated by hypoxia, electrolyte disturbances, acid-base disorders, or drugs such as methylxanthines or β-agonists.

Ectopic atrial tachycardia often is nonresponsive to standard antiarrhythmics or pacing. Vagal maneuvers, verapamil, adenosine, and digoxin commonly initiate or increase AV block, thereby slowing the ventricular rate. However, the atrial rate remains unchanged and the arrhythmia persists. Special care must be exercised in treatment with digoxin because this drug may induce ectopic atrial tachycardia. In cases of suspected digitalis-induced arrhythmia, potassium is the agent of choice because it will counteract the action of digitalis at the cellular level. Phenytoin, lidocaine, propranolol, or digoxin-immune Fab fragments may also be used. DC cardioversion is dangerous in digitalis toxicity because it may precipitate intractable ventricular arrhythmias.

MAT is often difficult to manage. Pharmacologic attempts to block the AV node or decrease ectopic activity are rarely successful. Trials of digoxin, quinidine, procainamide, phenytoin, and lidocaine have been disappointing. Surgery to resect or ablate the ectopic foci, as well as electrical modalities (pacing or DC cardioversion), are also ineffective. Treating the underlying disease is the only reliable therapy. Correcting predisposing factors terminates the arrhythmia in most patients, although recurrence is common. Verapamil[64] and metoprolol[65] have been reported to slow the ventricular rate, reduce atrial ectopy, or reduce abnormal atrial or AV junctional-triggered activity. In one trial, metoprolol was associated with a larger reduction in ventricular rate and higher rate of conversion to sinus rhythm than verapamil.[66] However, the hypotensive and adverse pulmonary effects of these drugs limit their utility. They should be reserved for patients with symptoms of hypoperfusion. The high mortality rate of patients with MAT (40 to 50%) results from the underlying condition, not the arrhythmia. Antiarrhythmics have not been shown to reduce mortality.[63]

Atrial Fibrillation

AF is characterized by rapid, chaotic atrial firing at a rate of 350 to 600 bpm. The AV node blocks most impulses, resulting in random, irregular ventricular conduction averaging 100 to 180 impulses/minute in untreated patients. Ventricular (His-Purkinje) conduction usually is normal.

EPIDEMIOLOGY

AF is thought to be caused by intra-atrial reentry. Uneven refractoriness of adjacent atrial tissues allows the formation of multiple reentrant wavelets. These wavelets become wandering reentry circuits completely dissociated from one another. AF may be chronic, paroxysmal, or a single, isolated occurrence. Transition from paroxysmal to chronic AF depends on the underlying cause and the duration of paroxysmal episodes. AF is the most common sustained arrhythmia and the second most common overall.

The incidence of AF is about 0.4% in people under 60 years old and 2 to 4% for those over 60 years.[67] Paroxysmal or single isolated episodes of AF are seen with cardiac surgery, fever, infection, pulmonary embolism, ethanol intoxication, or drug toxicity (sympathomimetics, β-agonists, methylxanthines). AF is also seen in 10 to 15% of patients with AMI, usually lasting less than 24 hours.[10] Chronic AF is associated with CHF, coronary artery disease, rheumatic heart disease, dilated or hypertrophic cardiomyopathy, hypertensive heart disease, hyperthyroidism, and certain congenital heart diseases. The greatest predictor of chronic AF is left atrial enlargement, which is associated with these conditions. AF without associated cardiovascular disease ("lone AF") occurs in 0.5 to 30%, with the wide range reflecting different definitions and populations.[68]

PATHOPHYSIOLOGY

The principal hemodynamic effects of AF result from a shortened diastolic filling time, leading to decreased left ventricular end-diastolic volume and stroke volume, and a loss of synchronized atrial contraction, resulting in increased mean left atrial pressure in addition to the preceding two effects. Loss of atrial systole causes a 20 to 30% reduction in stroke volume in normal people, which is increased in patients with heart disease. When coupled with incomplete ventricular filling, the net effect is a decrease in cardiac reserve. Elevations in heart rate are initially associated with an increased cardiac output. Once a critical rate is exceeded, ventricular filling time becomes a limiting factor, and further increases in heart rate result in reduced cardiac output.

The nonhemodynamic consequence of AF is embolism resulting from turbulent blood flow through the atria with mural thrombus formation. Embolic risk is highest in the first 2 to 4 weeks after the onset of AF and at the time of transition from paroxysmal to chronic AF. In some patients, the embolic event is the presenting manifestation of previously undetected AF. Embolism to arteries in the cerebral circulation is most common and accounts for about 7% of all strokes.[67] Other locations include the extremities and the mesenteric, coronary, and renal circulations. Framingham study subjects with chronic AF caused by rheumatic mitral valve disease were found to have a 17.6-fold increase in stroke risk, with a 5.6-fold increase for AF of other causes.[69] Risk factors for embolism in chronic AF include a history of emboli or an association with advanced age, CHF, ventricular dysfunction, and left atrial enlargement.[68,70] In patients with lone AF, stroke risk is low in young but probably higher in older patients and those with hypertension.

CLINICAL PRESENTATION AND DIAGNOSIS

The clinical manifestations of AF include the signs and symptoms of CHF, most commonly in the pulmonary system, and exacerbated with exercise. Some patients may develop angina or symptoms of cerebral insufficiency such as confusion, fatigue, or syncope. Palpitations may be especially troublesome in patients with paroxysmal AF. Older adults with AV node dysfunction may have slow ventricular rates at rest but nonetheless have reduced cardiac reserve with exercise or stress. As many as 30% are asymptomatic at the time of diagnosis.[71] Irregular apical and radial pulses result from random impulse transmission through the AV node and are the classic physical signs of AF. ECG findings include a lack of discrete atrial activity, variable R-R intervals, normal-appearing QRS complexes (unless aberrant conduction or bundle branch block is present), and an irregular baseline between QRS complexes.

ACUTE TREATMENT

The primary goal of the acute AF management is to correct the hemodynamic manifestations by increasing cardiac output. This is usually accomplished by pharmacologic slowing of the ventricular rate, which lengthens diastolic filling time and increases stroke volume (Fig. 41.8).[72] Electrical or chemical conversion to sinus rhythm in the acute phase is reserved for patients with hemodynamic instability or ventricular rate more than 150 bpm.[11] The optimal ventricular rate for maximizing cardiac output is unknown. An arbitrary ventricular rate of less than 100 bpm is often chosen as a therapeutic goal. However, the following therapeutic aspects must be emphasized. Strict attention to ventricular rate should not be at the expense of objective and symptomatic relief or of drug intoxication. Underlying factors favoring tachycardia should be considered, especially excess catecholamine release as in infection, hyperthyroidism, or sympathomimetic drug overdose. In these patients, a rate of 100 to 120 bpm may be acceptable as long as the signs and symptoms are controlled. Strict adherence to a goal of less than 100 bpm may result in bradycardia when the underlying problem is corrected. Rate titration should consider the clinical appearance of the patient as well as the anticipated rapidity of catecholamine correction. Aggressive treatment of coexisting conditions such as fever, infection, hypoxia, anemia, or hyperthyroidism is essential.

A review of the role of the AV node in AF is useful in understanding the pharmacologic management. The AV node is not involved in the initiation and perpetuation of AF per se but plays a critical role as a filter of atrial impulses. The AV node is the primary determinant of ventricular rate in AF. In contrast, the SA node determines

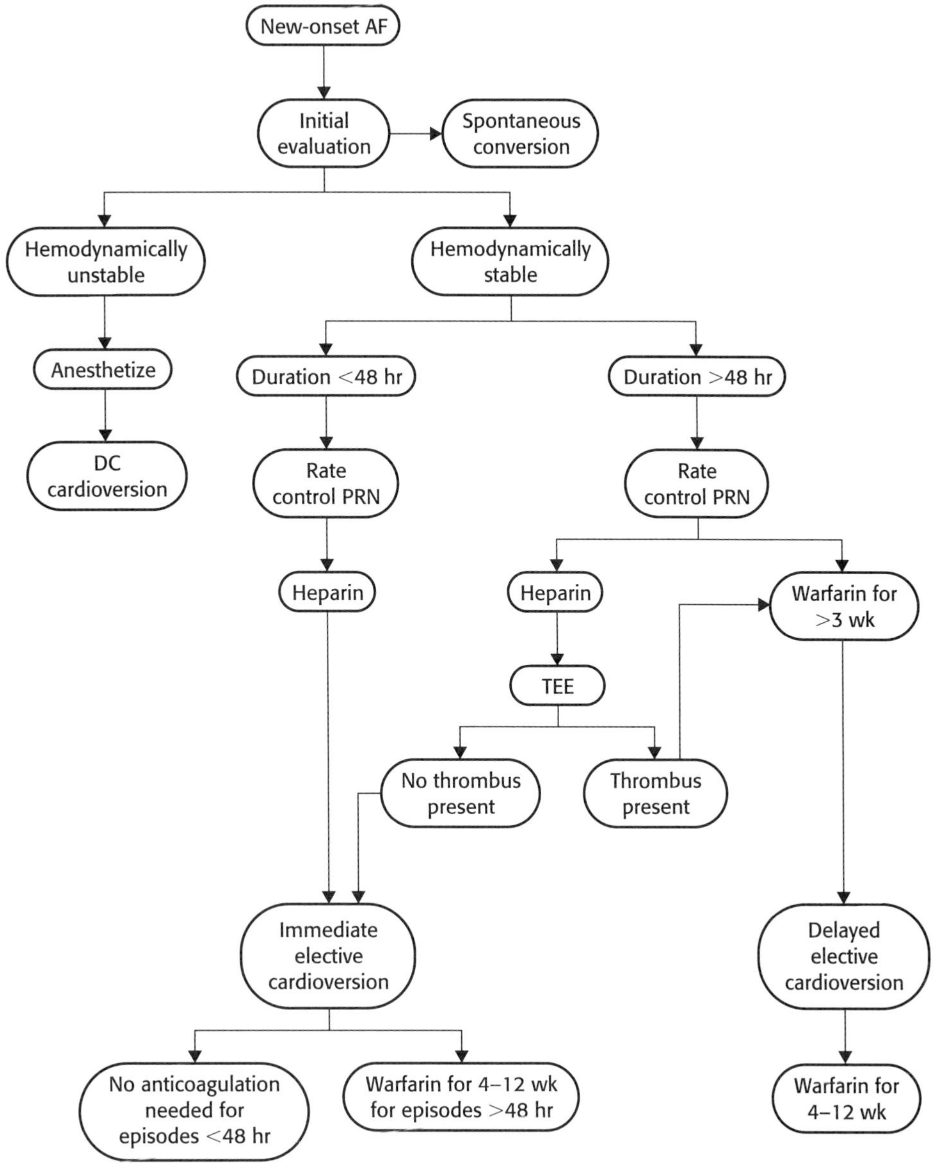

Figure 41.8. Algorithm for short-term management of atrial fibrillation. *AF*, atrial fibrillation; *DC*, direct current; *TEE*, transesophageal echocardiography. (*Source:* Reference 72.)

the rate in sinus rhythm. The intrinsic conductivity of AV nodal tissues and extracardiac factors that may alter conduction (autonomic tone, drugs) have a critical influence on ventricular rate. Vagal stimulation results in increased filtering and less conduction across the AV node. Increased sympathetic tone enhances AV nodal conduction, resulting in an excessive increase in ventricular rate with exercise or stress. Control of ventricular rate both at rest and during exercise is important in maintaining the function of the patient. However, changes in AV nodal conductivity will not terminate the arrhythmia.

Pharmacotherapy

Digoxin

Digitalis has positive inotropic and negative chronotropic and dromotropic properties. The last effect accounts for its efficacy in AF, is seen only at higher dosages, and occurs via a variety of mechanisms. The predominant effect is indirect via vagal stimulation, with direct AV nodal action having a minor role. This vagotonic effect is largely attenuated by catecholamines, explaining the limited ability to control ventricular rates during exercise or stress.[73–75] Digitalis does not suppress ectopy; most patients remain in AF. In fact, digoxin does not prevent recurrence of paroxysmal AF in patients in sinus rhythm. The effect of digitalis on accessory pathways differs from that on the AV node, and it should not be used in patients with AF and the WPW syndrome. Digoxin is no longer considered the drug of choice for AF. Rather, verapamil, diltiazem, or a β-blocker should be used before digoxin.[76] The digoxin–quinidine combination was compared with a verapamil–quinidine combination for paroxysmal AF.[77] Only 45% of patients converted to normal sinus rhythm (NSR) with digoxin, compared with 84% for the verapamil group.

Administration

Optimally, individual digoxin loading doses are determined based on the observed response to initial therapy (Table 41.3).[72] Dosages of 0.5 mg intravenously are followed by 0.125 to 0.25 mg intravenously or orally every 4 to 8 hours until the desired response is seen. The dosage and interval should take into account the time for tissue distribution of 6 to 8 hours. This regimen usually results in rate control in 12 to 24 hours. In a recent prospective observational study, the average total digoxin dosage needed for initial control of ventricular rate was 0.8 mg (range 0.125 to 6.125 mg), and the average time to initial ventricular rate control was 9.5 hours.[78] Intramuscular administration is not advised because of erratic absorption and excessive pain at the injection site. Infants, children, and patients with hyperthyroidism may need higher than estimated dosages, whereas those with coronary artery disease or obstructive airway disease may be especially sensitive to digitalis. Oral maintenance dosages for AF average 0.25 to 0.375 mg daily in adult patients with normal renal function. Calculated dosages may be used as a guideline, but the clinical response of the patient is a better criterion of efficacy.

Monitoring parameters for digoxin use in AF include ventricular rate (apical pulse) and the signs and symptoms of CHF. The radial (peripheral) pulse is not an appropriate monitoring criterion because it may not reflect efficacy in patients with very high apical rates. In these patients, some ventricular contractions may not elicit detectable peripheral pulses, causing a pulse deficit. Renal function and serum electrolytes (especially potassium and magnesium) should also be monitored, along with observation for signs and symptoms of toxicity. Using serum concentrations as a guide to dosing is not advised in managing SVTs such as AV nodal reentry and AF. Correlation between therapeutic response (i.e., ventricular rate) and serum concentrations is poor.[79,80] This is probably because other factors (underlying autonomic tone, exogenous catecholamines, electrolyte concentrations) alter cardiac sensitivity to digitalis independently of serum concentrations. Despite this limitation, serum concentrations may be useful in evaluating patient compliance, suspected toxicity, or drug interactions. Concentrations should be drawn at least 6 to 8 hours after administration to allow tissue distribution.

Table 41.3 ▪ Drug Management of Atrial Fibrillation

Agent	Acute Intravenous Therapy	Chronic Oral Therapy
β-Blockers		
Metoprolol	2.5–5 mg every 2–5 min to a maximum of 15 mg.	50–100 mg BID
Propranolol	0.5–3 mg, repeat in 10 min, then repeat after 4 hr.	10–120 mg TID or 80–320 mg QD for slow release
Esmolol	0.05–0.2 mg/kg/min.	N/A
Atenolol	2.5–5 mg over 5 min; repeat in 10 min	25–100 mg once daily
Calcium channel blockers		
Verapamil	5–20 mg in 5-mg increments every 30 min or 0.005-mg/kg/min infusion.	120–360 mg daily (divided doses or slow release)
Diltiazem	0.25–0.35 mg/kg followed by 5–15 mg/hr.	120–360 mg daily as slow release
Digitalis glycoside		
Digoxin	0.75–1.5 mg in 3 or 4 divided doses over 12–24 hr.	0.125–0.5 mg daily
Miscellaneous		
Ibutilide	0.01 mg/kg over 10 min, repeat if needed.	N/A

Source: Reference 72.
N/A, not applicable.

Interactions

Two drug interactions of digoxin are relevant in supraventricular tachyarrhythmia management. An elevation of serum digoxin concentrations to two to three times baseline occurs in most patients taking digoxin and quinidine concomitantly. Digoxin concentrations increase within hours of quinidine administration, reaching a new steady state in several days. This interaction depends on the serum concentration of quinidine but not that of digoxin and is caused by a decrease in volume of distribution and renal and nonrenal clearance of digoxin by quinidine. Because there is no evidence of an alteration of digoxin receptor site activity or sensitivity, digoxin toxicity may ensue. Dosage reduction by 50% and careful serum concentration monitoring are advised.[43] Serum digoxin concentrations may be increased by a similar mechanism in patients receiving verapamil or diltiazem, with new steady-state digoxin concentrations achieved in 7 to 14 days. The clinical importance of this reaction is not well established, although some have recommended a 50% reduction in digoxin dosage.[43]

Toxicity

The subjective evaluation of patients for digoxin toxicity is difficult because of the nonspecific nature of the symptoms. Anorexia, nausea, vomiting, weakness, and lethargy are the most common symptoms. Vision changes, disorientation, and hallucinations are less common. Elevated serum concentrations may assist in the diagnosis; however, there is overlap between toxic and therapeutic values. Moreover, electrolyte abnormalities (hypokalemia, metabolic alkalosis, hypomagnesemia, or hypercalcemia) or hypoxia may contribute to clinical toxicity even at "nontoxic" serum concentrations. Toxic cardiac effects result from enhanced automaticity, promotion of triggered activity, or a depression of AV nodal conduction. A useful monitoring tool for toxicity in patients with AF is the ECG. The excessive effects of digoxin result in an exaggerated AV nodal block, seen initially as occasional long equal pauses (intermittent junctional escape). Eventually, the ventricular rate becomes regular at 35 to 30 bpm, reflecting complete junctional escape. At higher concentrations, junctional pacemaker firing may accelerate, causing a junctional tachycardia. PVCs caused by enhanced firing of ectopic ventricular foci also are common. As toxicity progresses, essentially any arrhythmias can be seen. Toxicity is managed by discontinuation of the drug, potassium unless contraindicated, antiarrhythmics, or digoxin-immune Fab fragments. Refer to the Digitalis-Induced Premature Ventricular Contractions for management details.

Other aspects of digoxin therapy can be found in Chapter 40, Congestive Heart Failure.

Verapamil

Verapamil exerts a direct effect on the AV node that is not mediated by the autonomic nervous system. Thus, in contrast to digoxin, verapamil retains its usefulness during exercise or stress. Some patients may demonstrate regularization of ventricular rate while remaining in AF; however, this does not augment hemodynamic function.[81] A lack of suppressant effect on ectopic foci results in conversion to sinus rhythm in only 10 to 15% of patients, probably through improved hemodynamic function. Verapamil is prompt, reliable, effective, and safe. The dosage for AF is the same as that for AV nodal reentry: 5 to 10 mg (0.075 to 0.15 mg/kg) intravenously over 2 to 3 minutes, repeated in 30 minutes if needed. It has an onset of action of 5 to 10 minutes and duration of about 30 minutes after a bolus injection. Constant infusions of 5 mg/hour initially, titrated to a ventricular rate less than 100 bpm, a systolic blood pressure more than 90 mm Hg, and a maximum dosage of about 10 mg/hour for up to 7 days have been reported,[82] although this is not an FDA-labeled method of administration. Infusions should be preceded by bolus doses. Because of its rapid onset of action and more predictable effect in patients with high circulating catecholamine concentrations, some practitioners consider verapamil the drug of choice over digoxin in AF.[83] The primary limitation of verapamil is its negative inotropic effect. Downward dosage adjustment should be considered in patients with heart or liver failure because of impaired drug elimination. It should be used cautiously in patients receiving digoxin (because of the previously discussed drug interaction) and patients with WPW syndrome. Monitoring parameters include the ECG, ventricular rate, blood pressure, and signs and symptoms of heart failure. Other aspects of verapamil are discussed in the section Atrioventricular Nodal Reentry.

Diltiazem

AF and atrial flutter can also be treated successfully with intravenous diltiazem.[84] Diltiazem exerts a direct effect on the AV node similar to that of verapamil. Restoration of sinus rhythm with diltiazem occurs infrequently, as with verapamil. The potential advantages of diltiazem over verapamil are its low incidence of hypotension and minimal negative inotropic effect.[84] The diltiazem dosage for AF is 0.25 mg/kg intravenously over 2 minutes followed by 0.35 mg/kg in 15 minutes if the initial response was inadequate. Diltiazem controls ventricular rate in about 5 minutes with continued control for 3 to 10 hours after one or two bolus doses.[44,84] In patients needing ventricular rate control until other methods of arrhythmia suppression can be used (long-term antiarrhythmic therapy or cardioversion), an intravenous infusion can be administered at a rate of 10 to 15 mg/hour.[85] The diltiazem dosage should be reduced in patients with heart or liver failure because of its reliance on hepatic elimination. It should be used cautiously in patients receiving digoxin and patients with WPW syndrome. Diltiazem should not be given in close temporal proximity with intravenous β-blockers. Monitoring parameters include the ECG, ventricular rate, blood pressure, and signs and symptoms of heart failure.

Esmolol

Esmolol (Brevibloc) is approved for rapid control of ventricular rate in patients with AF or atrial flutter when short-term control of ventricular rate is needed. It also is indicated for noncompensatory tachycardia when heart rate must be reversed.

The β-blocker esmolol demonstrates the typical effects of a cardioselective β-blocker without intrinsic sympathomimetic activity or membrane-stabilizing effects and demonstrates the additional unique property of an ultrashort duration of action. This permits its use to slow AV nodal conduction directly, with minimal concern for long-lasting adverse effects. Esmolol is hydrolyzed rapidly by red cell esterases, with distribution and elimination half-lives of 2 and 9 minutes, respectively.[86] The total clearance of 17 to 20 L/kg/hour reflects the largely hepatic elimination to methanol and a metabolite with minimal β-blocking activity.[86,87] Esmolol is initiated with a loading dose of 500 μg/kg over 1 minute, followed by maintenance infusions of 50 to 300 μg/kg/minute. If control is not established, the loading dose is repeated and the infusion rate increased. Dosage adjustments may be made as often as every 5 to 15 minutes. Most patients respond at dosages of 100 μg/kg/minute.

Clinical Use

Clinical trials have shown esmolol to be comparable to propranolol in reducing the ventricular rate in SVTs, with an overall response rate of 64 to 72%, including 6 to 14% who converted to sinus rhythm.[86–88] Comparative studies with verapamil have shown similar reductions in ventricular rate, with a higher number of patients converting to sinus rhythm after esmolol.[89] The onset of action is less than 5 minutes, with a return to baseline heart rate 10 to 20 minutes after discontinuation. Esmolol therefore offers the flexibility to continually and rapidly titrate the dosage to the desired effect. Furthermore, there is an added element of safety if adverse effects occur because the effects subside soon after the infusion is discontinued.

Toxicity

The primary adverse effect is hypotension, occurring in 33 to 44% of patients.[86,88] Hypotension is most common at dosages of 200 μg/kg/minute or more, in postoperative patients or patients over 65 years old, or those with baseline hypotension.[88] Most patients remain asymptomatic and are treated by a reduction in dosage. Severe hypotension may warrant discontinuation, with blood pressure returning to normal in 20 to 30 minutes. Local injection site irritation is concentration and duration related and occurs in up to 8% of patients. This effect is minimized by diluting infusions to concentrations less than 10 mg/mL, but this may hamper use in volume-restricted patients. Limited data support the safety of esmolol in patients with traditional contraindications to β-blockers such as diabetes mellitus or obstructive airway disease.[86,88] In general, however, it should be avoided or used with caution in these patients. Many patients must switch to an alternative agent such as diltiazem, digoxin, or verapamil. One hour after such drugs are started, the esmolol can be tapered by 50%.[54] After the second dose of the alternative drug, esmolol can be discontinued if the heart rate remains controlled.

β-Blockers are particularly useful in AF caused by high circulating catecholamine concentrations, including hyperthyroidism or sympathomimetic overdose, because they pharmacologically attenuate the underlying cause of the arrhythmia. Critically ill perioperative and cardiac patients should be treated with esmolol. β-Blockers may be necessary for only a short time in these patients because correction of the precipitating cause may restore digoxin sensitivity or even allow conversion to sinus rhythm.

Ibutilide

Ibutilide (Corvert) is indicated for the rapid conversion of AF or atrial flutter of recent onset. It is less likely to convert the rhythm to NSR if the duration of the arrhythmia is prolonged. Ibutilide is structurally similar to sotalol. Because it prolongs the APD, ibutilide is a class III agent, but it is unique in activating the slow inward sodium current instead of slowing the potassium rectifier channel seen with other agents in its class.[90] An advantage of ibutilide is its lack of hypotensive or negative inotropic effects. It has dose-related effects in prolonging Q-T intervals that are correlated with its antiarrhythmic activity.[54]

Pharmacokinetics

Ibutilide has been marketed for intravenous use. It has minimal protein binding (40%).[91] It is metabolized largely by systems other than cytochrome P450-3A4 or P450-2D6, so interactions with other antiarrhythmics have not been reported. The elimination half-life varies from 2 to 12 hours (average 6 hours).[90] Ibutilide clearance could be expected to decline with impaired liver function, but age, sex, and renal function have no effect.

Clinical Use

Ibutilide was compared with procainamide in patients with spontaneous, paroxysmal atrial flutter or fibrillation.[91] Ibutilide converted 64% of patients with atria flutter, whereas procainamide did not convert any. Ibutilide converted 32% of patients with atrial fibrillation, whereas procainamide converted only 5%. The low efficacy rates in this study may have been related to the long duration of the arrhythmia.

Toxicity

The most common toxicity to ibutilide is also the most serious: polymorphic VT. It is an expected effect of QTc prolongation seen with other antiarrhythmics (classes Ia and III). Because of the seriousness of this adverse effect, continuous ECG monitoring is needed even up to 4 hours after the drug is given or until the QTc has returned to baseline.[90]

Administration

Serum potassium and magnesium concentrations should be measured and corrected before ibutilide is used.[92] It should not be used with other agents that prolong the QTc. Ibutilide is given as 1 mg (or 0.01 mg/kg) intravenously over 10 minutes. If after 10 minutes the arrhythmia persists, the dose can be repeated.

Nonpharmacologic Therapy

At present, cardiac pacemakers or other devices are not considered first-line treatments in the acute AF management.

CHRONIC TREATMENT

After initial control of ventricular rate, pharmacologic or electrical methods may be used for conversion to sinus rhythm (Fig. 41.9).[72] If conversion is successful, maintenance therapy (generally with the same antiarrhythmic used for conversion) is begun in an attempt to sustain sinus rhythm. Patients who remain in AF or revert shortly after conversion are given drugs to slow the ventricular rate and maximize cardiac output. Patients with chronic AF may also be candidates for long-term anticoagulation. Therapeutic goals in chronic AF include relief of symptoms, reduction in embolic risk, and improvement in overall cardiac function and exercise tolerance.

Conversion to sinus rhythm is desirable because it will improve cardiac performance, relieve clinical symptoms, and decrease the risk of embolism markedly. Patients with AF of recent onset may convert spontaneously to sinus rhythm during initial drug treatment or after the inciting stress is eliminated. Unfortunately, not all patients remain in sinus rhythm. Although conversion to sinus rhythm is crucial for some patients (e.g., those with hemodynamic instability), in others it may be neither practical nor useful. Ideally, an assessment of the likelihood of sustained sinus rhythm should be made before attempted conversion. Higher success rates are seen in patients with a corrected or controlled underlying cause and those with recent arrhythmia onset. Patients likely to revert to AF include those with cardiomegaly (particularly left atrial enlargement), mitral

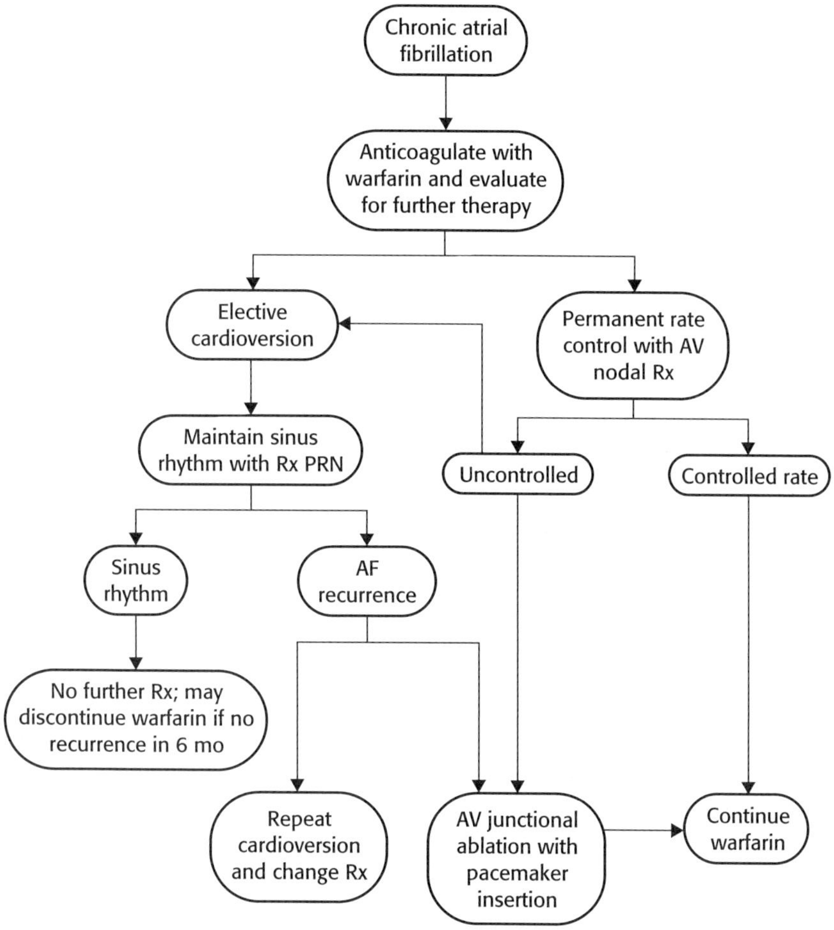

Figure 41.9. Algorithm for long-term management of atrial fibrillation. *AF,* atrial fibrillation. (*Source:* Reference 72.)

valve disease, AF of more than 3 months' duration, and moderate to severe heart failure.[93] A curious finding has been a lack of atrial mechanical function (systole) for several days or weeks after cardioversion despite a return of normal electrical activity in certain patients.[94] This may account for the lack of improvement in exercise tolerance and cardiac output as well as the continued risk of embolism in the period immediately after conversion. In a study of 52 patients who underwent cardioversion (electrical, pharmacologic, or spontaneous), 68% recovered effective mechanical atrial function by day 3 and 76% recovered by day 7.[95] Electrical conversion was more likely to cause a greater degree and longer duration of atrial dysfunction.

Nonpharmacologic Therapy

Direct Current Cardioversion

Cardioversion may be accomplished either electrically or pharmacologically. DC cardioversion depolarizes a critical number of myocardial cells simultaneously, allowing the SA node to reestablish control as the pacemaker. The current should be synchronized with the QRS complex on ECG to avoid delivery during the vulnerable period of ventricular recovery. Lower initial energies are often used, although as much as 400 J may ultimately be needed. An antiarrhythmic (usually quinidine) is initiated 1 to 2 days before cardioversion to help maintain sinus rhythm. Short-acting sedatives or anesthetics are given immediately before the procedure. DC cardioversion is initially successful in 80 to 95% of patients.[71,93,96,97] Any patient may be considered for DC cardioversion, but the best candidates are those without mitral valve disease or significant atrial enlargement and those with recent onset AF.[98] Data compiled from 824 patients demonstrated a 2.4% incidence of complications, including emboli in 1.3%, ventricular arrhythmias in 0.4%, and miscellaneous complications in 0.6%.[93] DC cardioversion should be performed with caution in patients with digitalis toxicity because of the higher risk of ventricular arrhythmias. Generally it is not necessary to withhold digoxin immediately before cardioversion in patients without digitalis toxicity.[99] Patients with known or suspected SSS should be evaluated carefully for possible pacemaker insertion before attempted cardioversion, especially if receiving drugs that exacerbate bradycardia such as calcium channel or β-blockers. Short-term anticoagulation is appropriate to decrease the embolic risk (see Anticoagulants).

Pharmacotherapy

Drugs for Conversion to Sinus Rhythm

Pharmacologic conversion to sinus rhythm, though less invasive than DC cardioversion, is also less successful. Digitalis, verapamil, and diltiazem rarely convert patients with AF to sinus rhythm, probably because of their minimal effects on atrial automaticity.

Quinidine

Quinidine is the most commonly used agent for pharmacologic cardioversion and is also used to maintain sinus rhythm after conversion. Quinidine may have both beneficial and deleterious effects in AF. A decrease in atrial ectopy accounts for its efficacy, whereas its vagolytic effect at the AV node may enhance impulse transmission, resulting in a very rapid ventricular rate. Therefore, patients with AF should have adequate AV nodal slowing before quinidine is administered. Because of the possibility of quinidine-induced long Q-T syndrome or torsade de pointes, all patients should be hospitalized with cardiac monitoring for attempted conversion. Torsade de pointes can also occur with chronic use of quinidine where a trigger such as hypokalemia induces the proarrhythmia.[49] Other risk factors for torsade de pointes include female sex, structural heart disease, concomitant use of digoxin, and hypomagnesemia.

A typical therapeutic strategy is to administer quinidine for several days, then proceed to DC cardioversion if conversion does not occur with quinidine alone. Common dosage regimens for conversion are 300 to 400 mg of the sulfate salt orally every 6 hours. Intravenous quinidine may also be given with close hemodynamic monitoring, as discussed under Atrioventricular Nodal Reentry. The reported success rate with quinidine conversion averages 71%.[93]

After the first successful conversion, the risks and cost of prophylactic antiarrhythmics to sustain sinus rhythm must be weighed against the likelihood of reversion to AF. Patients thought to be at low risk for reversion to AF may be observed off antiarrhythmics, with the understanding that only about 30%[71,96] of untreated patients maintain sinus rhythm for 1 year. If AF recurs, prophylactic antiarrhythmic therapy is initiated. There is no superior drug for maintaining sinus rhythm. Strategies often are influenced by personal experience, local tradition, and theoretical considerations. Quinidine has the strongest literature evidence for efficacy, but adverse effects, including death from proarrhythmic events, are severe limitations. Daily maintenance dosages of 800 to 1600 mg of the sulfate salt (or its equivalent) have yielded success rates of 40 to 60% after 1 year.[57] Subtherapeutic serum concentrations, poor compliance, and inappropriate initial selection of patients for conversion contribute to the lower long-term success.

Other Drugs

Patients who do not convert or do not sustain sinus rhythm with quinidine may be given procainamide or disopyramide in standard dosages. Flecainide is also effective, but reports of proarrhythmic effects in AF patients[100,101] limit use. Trials of amiodarone for induction and maintenance of sinus rhythm have demonstrated efficacy in maintaining sinus rhythm as well as controlling ventricular rate if AF recurs. However, the high response rate must be balanced against its toxicity, which is common and may be severe. Sotalol has also been shown to be effective in terminating AF and maintaining sinus rhythm and serves as an alternative in AF resistant to other agents. The use of sotalol is limited by proarrhythmia, which has been reported in 2% of patients treated for SVT.[102]

Drugs to Control Ventricular Rate

In some patients, conversion is not attempted because the likelihood of sustained sinus rhythm is thought to be low. Others convert initially but revert to AF shortly thereafter. Therapy in these patients is directed at regulating the ventricular rate. The optimal rate for maximizing cardiac output has not been established. A reasonable goal is a ventricular rate of less than 90 bpm at rest and 110 bpm with mild exercise. Most are given digoxin, with or without other agents. As reviewed earlier, sympathetic stimulation may override the effect of digoxin, resulting in an unacceptably high ventricular rate. Trials comparing digoxin with verapamil or diltiazem have yielded conflicting results. Although all have noted better rate control with the calcium channel blocker, some have shown an associated improvement in exercise capacity,[75,103] whereas others have observed no change.[73,74] Therefore, better control of the ventricular rate may not improve cardiac output or exercise tolerance, thus negating any major advantage of calcium channel blockers over digoxin. β-Blockers may be used in patients with excess catecholamine effect but can worsen heart failure and decrease exercise tolerance.[42] Quinidine is not useful in patients with chronic AF and may even be detrimental because of its vagolytic effect.

Monitoring parameters for patients with chronic AF include subjective symptoms such as dyspnea, fatigue, angina, and palpitations as well as objective criteria such as ventricular (or apical) rate. Objective measurements of exercise tolerance and cardiac output may be performed, but they do not always correlate with a subjective sense of improvement.

Anticoagulants

Anticoagulants are used to reduce the embolic risk associated with AF. Recent data from five randomized multicenter trials have refined antithrombotic treatment for stroke prevention in patients with AF.[104–108] The decision to anticoagulate an individual patient with AF is based on the presence of risk factors associated with stroke risk. Cerebral embolism commonly results in large neurologic deficits with severe residual disability, occurs without warning symptoms, is recurrent in about 11% of patients, and carries a mortality of up to 25%.[109] On the other hand, the incidence of major bleeding with anticoagulants at conventional intensities has been estimated at 2 to 5% yearly, with 1% per year suffering intracranial hemorrhage.[109] These values may be even higher in older adults, who make up the majority of patients with AF.

After the onset of AF, several days are needed for thrombus formation. Anticoagulants therefore are not indicated for AF of less than 2 days' duration. Once thrombi are formed, however, several weeks are needed to allow fibrotic organization and adherence to the atrial wall. Moreover, atrial mechanical function (i.e., atrial systole) may be delayed for several weeks after ECG-documented conversion to sinus rhythm.[94] The embolic risk in the Framingham study was 14% within the first year after onset and 5% per year thereafter.[69] Risk is similar after pharmacologic or electric cardioversion. The American College of Chest Physicians (ACCP) recommendations for anticoagulants at the time of cardioversion include the following:[110] For AF of more than 2 days' duration, anticoagulate with warfarin to an international normalized ratio (INR) intensity of 2.0 to 3.0 for 3 weeks before and 4 weeks after cardioversion; use no anticoagulants for AF of less than 2 days' duration, unless other risk factors for embolism are present; for patients needing emergent cardioversion, anticoagulate with heparin on the day of cardioversion if AF is of several days' duration, there is a high risk of recurrence, or other risk factors are present. Risk factors are previous transient ischemic attack or stroke, hypertension, diabetes, thyrotoxicosis, mitral stenosis, and other forms of heart disease. In selected cases the use of transesophageal echocardiography can exclude atrial thrombi and avoid the need for 3 weeks of prior anticoagulation.[111]

Assessment of embolic risk in patients with chronic AF remains an enigmatic clinical problem. Table 41.4[67] is a simplified assessment of embolic risk with suggested management strategies. Consensus exists about the high embolic risk in patients with documented recent embolism, AF associated with older mechanical heart valve prostheses, and mitral valve disease. Patients with a history of stroke, coronary disease, thyrotoxicosis, and modern mechanical valves are at a high but somewhat lower risk. The medium- to low-risk group comprises the largest number of patients, including those with mitral regurgitation, aortic valve disease, heart failure, hypertension, diabetes, advanced age, and bioprostheses. Risk–benefit data for anticoagulants in this group are somewhat limited. Several recent large placebo-controlled trials in patients with chronic nonvalvular AF[104–108] have demonstrated efficacy of warfarin therapy to an international normalized ratio (INR) of 1.4 to 4.5. The overall risk reduction for stroke has been reported to be 68% from pooled data of five of these trials.[112] Aspirin 325 mg/day was also found to be beneficial for preventing stroke associated with AF[106] and is recommended by the ACCP in patients who are poor candidates for anticoagulation.[113] Compared with warfarin, aspirin is less effective but is associated with less hemorrhagic complications.[106,114] Careful assessment of bleeding risk is a critical element in the decision for or against anticoagulant use in individual patients. Underlying risk factors for bleeding associated with warfarin therapy include age 65 years or older, history of gastrointestinal bleeding, stroke, cancer, recent surgery, and hypertension.[115] Patients unable to comply with medication regimens or laboratory follow-up, as well as those with dementia or alcohol abuse, may be poor candidates for anticoagulation regardless of embolic risk. Bleeding risk is also reduced by maintaining anticoagulants in the less intense range (INR 2.0 to 3.0) whenever possible.[115] Scrupulous monitoring is essential and can lower bleeding risk substantially. In the Stroke Prevention in Atrial Fibrillation trial, the annual rate of major hemorrhage for patients anticoagulated with warfarin to an INR of 2.0 to 3.5 was limited to 1.7% by meticulous supervision (compared with 0.9% for aspirin 325 mg orally daily and 1.2% for placebo).[106]

Other Nonpharmacologic Therapy

Patients with intolerable symptoms who are resistant to other therapies can be treated by surgical or catheter ablation of the AV node with permanent pacemaker placement. Ventricular rate is controlled, but fibrillation of the atria continues. A surgical technique known as the maze procedure involves multiple small incisions in the atrium

Table 41.4 ▪ Stratification of Thromboembolic Risk in Atrial Fibrillation

	Thromboembolic Risk (per yr)			
	High (>6%)	**Medium-High (4–6%)**	**Medium-Low (2–4%)**	**Low (<2%)**
Underlying heart disease	Prior embolism Old mechanical prosthesis	Mitral stenosis Thyrotoxicosis	Mitral regurgitation Aortic valve disease	Lone atrial fibrillation (age <60) Isolated mitral valve prolapse
		Coronary artery disease Modern mechanical prosthesis History of stroke or transient ischemic attack	Heart failure Increasing age Hypertension	
			Diabetes Bioprosthesis	
Long-term AC therapy	AC (INR = 2.5–3.5)[a]	AC (INR = 2.0–3.0)[b]	AC (INR = 2.0–3.0)[c]	No therapy

Source: Reference 67.

AC, anticoagulation; *INR,* international normalized ratio of prothrombin time.

[a]In high-risk patients with old mechanical prostheses, dipyridamole may be added to warfarin.

[b]In patients with mechanical prostheses, INR range should be 2.5–3.5.

[c]The decision for anticoagulation should be individualized.

that disrupt the pathways that conduct the reentrant impulses.[116] This surgical technique terminates AF, restores AV synchrony, and preserves atrial transport function with a 93% success rate.[117] Nonpharmacologic therapy is reserved for patients with serious symptoms of AF that cannot be controlled by other methods.

PROGNOSIS

The long-term prognosis in patients with chronic AF is poor, with a yearly cardiovascular mortality (10%) twice that of age-matched controls (5%).[67] Mortality is related to age at onset and the presence and extent of coexisting heart disease.

Wolff–Parkinson–White Syndrome

WPW syndrome is a congenital heart disease characterized by the presence of an anatomically distinct AV connection in addition to the AV nodal tissue. This anomalous pathway, called the accessory AV pathway (or Kent bundle), can be located anywhere in the heart and consists of working myocardium that forms an electrical bridge connecting the atrium and the ventricle. Impulse conduction can occur both antegrade and retrograde. Patients with WPW typically have sinus rhythm at baseline, with PSVTs. While in sinus rhythm, antegrade conduction is over both the AV node and accessory pathway; ventricular activation is thus a fusion of the two impulses. Because the accessory pathway can activate ventricular muscle directly (bypassing all or part of the AV node and His–Purkinje system), early or preexcitation of part of the ventricle occurs (Fig. 41.10).

The accessory pathway and AV node may form reentry circuits that allow SVTs, most commonly AV reentry or AF.[118] AV reentry is distinguished from AV nodal reentry by the use of the accessory pathway as part of the circuit. Accessory pathway conduction in the reentry circuit may be antegrade (called antidromic reentry) or retrograde (orthodromic reentry). Orthodromic reentry is 15 times more common than antidromic. In this form, impulses travel antegrade from the atrium to the ventricle via the AV node and retrograde from the ventricle to the atrium via the accessory pathway (Fig. 41.11). Multiple accessory pathways are seen in 5 to 15% of patients, usually associated with antidromic reentry.

EPIDEMIOLOGY

WPW syndrome is often seen in otherwise healthy infants, children, and young adults. The clinical importance of the arrhythmias varies from benign to life-threatening, depending on the electrophysiologic properties of the accessory pathway and the AV node. Arrhythmias seen in infancy may persist, disappear, or disappear then recur many years later.[119] This is thought to reflect a change in the conduction properties of the accessory pathway over time. Orthodromic AV reentry is the most common SVT. The most feared arrhythmia in WPW is AF with antegrade conduction down an accessory pathway with a short refractory period. In this case, the protective effect of the AV node against ery rapid ventricular rates is lost. Extremely rapid impulse transmission directly from the atrium to the ventricle may lead to ventricular flutter or fibrillation and sudden death.

PATHOPHYSIOLOGY

The classic ECG in sinus rhythm includes a short P-R interval with a δ-wave preceding the QRS complex representing preexcitation. The QRS complex has abnormal morphology because of the fusion of normal conduction down the AV node–His bundle system and preexcitation of the left ventricular free wall. The initiating arrhythmic event usually is a critically timed premature atrial or ventricular impulse. Ventricular rates average 100 to 280 per minute in AV reentry (higher in children) and

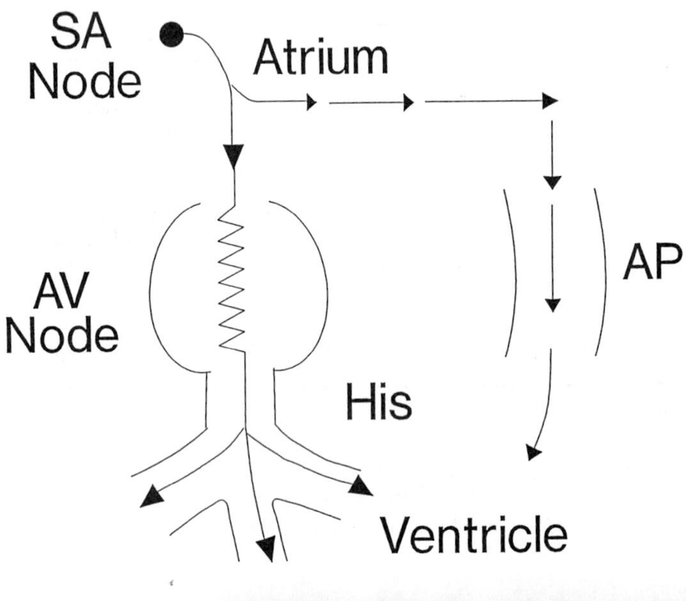

Figure 41.10. Wolff–Parkinson–White syndrome, sinus rhythm. The impulse reaches the ventricles via the atrioventricular *(AV)* node–His–Purkinje system with simultaneous preexcitation via the accessory pathway *(AP)*. *SA*, sinoatrial.

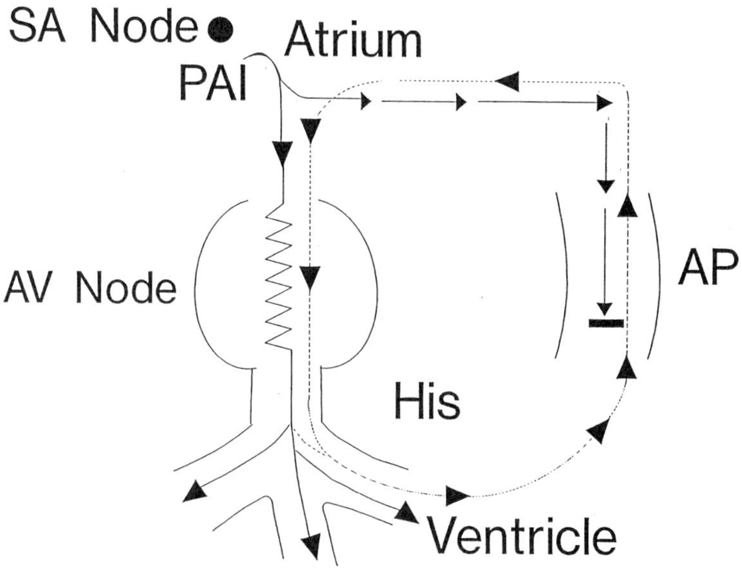

Figure 41.11. Orthodromic atrioventricular reentry. The premature atrial impulse *(PAI, solid line)* is blocked in the accessory pathway *(AP)* and reaches the ventricles via the atrioventricular *(AV)* node–His–Purkinje system. If the AP is recovered, AV reentry *(dotted line)* may be initiated. *SA,* sinoatrial.

140 to 320 per minute in AF. The direction of the reentry circuit (orthodromic or antidromic), variation in mode of ventricular activation, and different accessory pathway anatomies all contribute to marked interpatient and intrapatient ECG variation during SVTs. Detection of WPW syndrome and differentiation of its associated arrhythmias take an experienced ECG interpreter.

CLINICAL PRESENTATION AND DIAGNOSIS

The clinical manifestations and hemodynamic consequences of AV reentry and AF are the same in patients with or without WPW syndrome, ranging from palpitations to syncope and sudden death.

TREATMENT

Patients with WPW may be difficult to treat because the effect of the drug on the accessory pathway is not predicted by effect on the AV node. Moreover, drug action on antegrade conduction may differ from that on retrograde. Underlying autonomic tone may alter conduction independently of drug effect. Therefore, a drug may be beneficial for one patient yet deleterious for another. Management should be individualized by EPS. These studies locate and characterize the accessory pathway, identify the mechanism of the arrhythmia, and evaluate their effects on each anatomic component. Other termination techniques such as atrial pacing also may be evaluated.

As a rule, AV reentry associated with WPW syndrome is readily terminated using traditional maneuvers and drugs, as discussed in the Atrioventricular Nodal Reentry section. In patients with AF, however, great care must be exercised to avoid enhanced AV conduction with subsequent acceleration of ventricular rate and degeneration into ventricular fibrillation. This is a primary consideration in only a small minority of patients (with a short antegrade accessory pathway refractory period). Unfortunately, it is not possible to identify susceptible patients on clinical grounds alone. Some may be entirely asymptomatic yet have electrophysiologic risk for sudden cardiac death. Moreover, the population at risk based on EPS is much larger than that which will ultimately have a fatal arrhythmia. Little is known about the natural history of asymptomatic WPW syndrome. Extensive testing and treatment to prevent sudden death in asymptomatic patients remains controversial.

Pharmacotherapy

After conversion to sinus rhythm, patients with recurrent symptomatic attacks may receive prophylactic therapy to minimize further episodes of SVT. Regimens commonly include class Ia or Ic drugs, sotalol, amiodarone, or β-blockers. Controlled comparative trials have not been performed, and no drug has demonstrated superiority. Drug treatment often is suboptimal because of limited efficacy and excessive toxicity. Preventive therapy is reserved for patients with recurrent disabling arrhythmias.

Drug effect on AV nodal and accessory pathway conduction is summarized in Table 41.5. The type Ia drugs quinidine, procainamide, and disopyramide slow or block antegrade accessory pathway conduction, with a lesser and more variable effect on retrograde conduction. These drugs also block retrograde AV nodal conduction and suppress atrial and ventricular ectopy. The effects of drugs may vary with different accessory pathway refractory periods, emphasizing the importance of EPS.

Digitalis and verapamil maintain their AV nodal effects. However, digitalis may shorten the accessory pathway refractory period. Verapamil generally has minimal effect on the accessory pathway but may also shorten the refractory period. These drugs are very effective first-line agents for terminating and preventing the recurrence of AV reentry. However, in AF or flutter, they may accentuate conduction and accelerate ventricular rate in the (unusual) patients with antegrade accessory pathway conduction. Potentially lethal

Table 41.5 ▪ Sites of Primary Drug Action in Wolff–Parkinson–White Syndrome

AV node antegrade conduction	
	Calcium-channel blockers (verapamil,[a] diltiazem)
	Digoxin[a]
	Adenosine
	β-Blockers
AV node retrograde conduction, accessory pathway antegrade conduction	
	Class Ia drugs (quinidine, procainamide, disopyramide)
AV node and accessory pathway, antegrade and retrograde conduction	
	Class Ic drugs (flecainide, propafenone)
	Class III drugs (amiodarone, sotalol)
Suppression of atrial ectopy	
	Class Ia drugs (quinidine, procainamide, disopyramide)
	Class Ic drugs (flecainide, propafenone)
	β-Blockers
	Class III drugs (amiodarone, sotalol)

[a]Digoxin and verapamil may decrease the accessory pathway antegrade refractory period, a dangerous effect in Wolff–Parkinson–White syndrome with atrial fibrillation.

VT or fibrillation may ensue. Digitalis and verapamil therefore should not be used in AF with documented or suspected preexcitation unless previous EPSs have shown them to be safe.

Most trials of adenosine in AV reentry have shown its primary site of action to be the AV nodal loop of the reentrant circuit, with little or no effect on accessory pathway conduction. Coupled with its lack of hypotensive properties, some investigators believe adenosine is safer than verapamil or digitalis in documented or suspected WPW syndrome.[30,120]

Propranolol and the other β-blockers alter AV nodal conduction but have minimal effect on accessory pathway conduction in either direction. They are not often used as single agents in WPW but are sometimes combined with other drugs such as digoxin or quinidine.

Amiodarone, sotalol, flecainide, and propafenone have additional unique antiarrhythmic mechanisms compared with the older agents. These drugs slow AV nodal and accessory pathway conduction in both directions and lengthen atrial and ventricular refractory periods. Therefore, they can be expected to terminate or control SVTs associated with WPW and also prevent their recurrence by suppressing ectopy. These drugs offer the best antiarrhythmic profile for SVTs associated with accessory pathways. Studies have demonstrated promising results. Unfortunately, the proarrhythmic effects of the class Ic drugs[73] and sotalol[102] and the toxicities of amiodarone limit their use.

Nonpharmacologic Therapy

Because of the unpredictable and often inadequate response to drugs, nonpharmacologic therapy is an important component of treating WPW syndrome.

Direct Current Cardioversion

DC cardioversion retains its near-uniform reliability and efficacy and is the treatment of choice in patients with hemodynamic instability.

Pacing

Atrial pacing may be used in AV reentry, although it may induce transient AF with rapid ventricular rate in patients with rapid antegrade accessory pathway conduction. Permanent ventricular pacing may be necessary in patients needing large dosages of antiarrhythmics or those with sinus node disease (pacing eliminates excessive bradycardia while the patient is in sinus rhythm).

Surgery

Surgical interruption of the accessory pathway is an effective, usually curative treatment. After detailed electrophysiologic and cardiac mapping studies, the accessory pathway is transected or ablated using an endocardial or epicardial approach.[119] AV nodal conduction is preserved. Surgical division of accessory pathways is 90 to 100% effective in experienced centers, with less than 1% mortality in uncomplicated cases and rare early or late recurrences.[60]

Percutaneous Catheter Ablation

A less invasive technique, percutaneous catheter ablation, uses DC cardioversion, lasers, or radiofrequency to modify the AV node or destroy accessory pathways. The success rate and mortality of this procedure are similar to those of surgical ablation; however, this procedure does not entail an open chest or general anesthesia.

Appropriate Patients

Because these procedures are curative, they may be considered the treatment of choice in patients unresponsive or intolerant to antiarrhythmics, those with arrhythmias associated with marked adverse hemodynamic effects, patients with AF with rapid antegrade accessory pathway conduction, young patients who would otherwise need lifelong drug therapy, or women desiring pregnancy.

Premature Ventricular Contractions

PVCs are ectopic beats originating in the ventricular muscle. These beats are not initiated by the SA node but are stimulated by the spontaneous electrical firing of the local tissue.

EPIDEMIOLOGY

PVCs are the most common arrhythmia. Depending on the length of the observation, the frequency of PVCs in otherwise healthy subjects is variable. In one series of 50 male medical students without apparent heart disease, one-half had PVCs on 24-hour monitoring.[121] In most patients, this arrhythmia produces no symptoms whatsoever. However, it is also the most common arrhythmia (40 to 80%) seen with myocardial infarctions, where it may adversely affect survival.

PVCs may be separated into simple and complex arrhythmias. PVCs seen in asymptomatic subjects with no cardiac disease usually are simple in that they are isolated beats, occurring singly, with a wave pattern on the ECG that repeats itself, indicating that the beat originates from the same site (unifocal). These appear to be well tolerated until their frequency compromises ventricular filling. Complex PVCs are uncommon in subjects with no cardiac disease but are common in patients with coronary artery disease. They may be subclassified as multiform or multifocal, which means that the ECG wave form is different between ectopies, suggesting more than one site in the ventricles is showing automaticity. Another complex classification refers to paired PVCs or runs of PVCs. These are consecutive PVCs without intervening sinus beats. The final type of complex PVC is called early R-on-T, referring to the R wave of the PVC interrupting the T wave of the sinus beat. Complex PVCs are highly correlated with sudden death.

Several classes of drugs may induce PVCs. These include the sympathomimetic amines (epinephrine, pseudoephedrine, phenylephrine, phenylpropanolamine, amphetamine), the methylxanthines (caffeine, theophylline), digitalis, cocaine, and certain general anesthetics (cyclopropane and halothane). Type Ia antiarrhythmics, flecainide, and sotalol may also induce PVCs and VT. These drugs should be discontinued, or their dosages should be reduced.

A variety of noncardiac conditions may induce PVCs, such as anemia, surgery, hypoxia, stress, hypokalemia, and hypomagnesemia. Eliminating the precipitating condition should resolve the PVCs and obviate potentially toxic antiarrhythmics.

TREATMENT

The approach to treating PVCs has changed in recent years as a result of the Cardiac Arrhythmia Suppression Trials (CAST I and CAST II).[122,123] These trials attempted to compare the use of encainide, flecainide, moricizine, and placebo in suppressing asymptomatic or mildly symptomatic PVCs to reduce mortality after a myocardial infarction. The trial with encainide and flecainide was suspended after a preliminary analysis revealed higher mortality with these agents than with placebo.[122,123] The use of moricizine yielded results similar to those of encainide and flecainide when compared with placebo.[122–124] The results of these trials indicate that PVC suppression does not decrease sudden cardiac death after a myocardial infarction. Therefore, in an otherwise healthy person, asymptomatic PVCs do not warrant suppression. Some patients may complain of palpitations that, if intolerable, can be treated with a β-blocker. PVC suppression in the presence of other comorbid conditions to reduce sudden death must be balanced against the risk of increased mortality associated with antiarrhythmic therapy and is discussed in the Sudden Death section.

PVCs are an independent risk factor for sudden death; however, even though they may predispose to sudden death, the cause of death is not known. It may be a random event precipitated by the unfortunate timing of PVCs. Procainamide, lidocaine, and quinidine reduce the frequency of PVCs without eliminating them. However, studies evaluating the response to these drugs do not demonstrate a significant decrease in mortality rate. On the other hand, death may be a result of acute ischemia, which is not altered by antiarrhythmic drugs. The agents shown to improve survival rate may act on ischemia, not on the basis of their antiarrhythmic effects.

Digitalis-Induced Premature Ventricular Contractions

PVCs are the most common arrhythmia produced by digitalis. Generally, this arrhythmia resolves when the digitalis is discontinued. For frequent or symptomatic PVCs, potassium replacement in hypokalemic or normokalemic patients may suppress the arrhythmia. For sustained PVCs induced by digitalis, lidocaine or phenytoin has been used successfully. Phenytoin is considered an ideal agent to treat digitalis-induced arrhythmias because it improves AV conduction while it suppresses ventricular irritability. Unfortunately, phenytoin is not nearly as effective in PVCs of different causes. For refractory arrhythmias that are life threatening, especially when an overdose of digitalis has produced hyperkalemia, digoxin-immune Fab (antigen binding fragments to digoxin; Digibind) can be administered intravenously over 30 minutes or intravenous push (IVP) if an arrest is imminent.[125] The use of digoxin-immune Fab is discussed in Chapter 4, Clinical Toxicology.

Ventricular Tachycardia

VT is a rapid (100 to 250 bpm), regular, ectopic rhythm of three or more consecutive ventricular complexes. VT is more serious than PVCs, producing more marked hemodynamic deterioration as a result of decreased diastolic filling and loss of coordinated ventricular contraction with atrial kick. VT is also ominous because it often degenerates into ventricular fibrillation. VT may be seen in the prehospital phase of an AMI as a result of enhanced automaticity. At this stage, the rhythm is somewhat more stable. The third phase of VT seen in ischemic heart disease is noted after several days to weeks.

There are two general types of VT. Nonsustained VT (NSVT) is three or more coupled PVCs occurring at rates greater than 100 bpm and terminating spontaneously in less than 30 seconds. These may warrant only close observation if they are asymptomatic. VT present beyond 30 seconds is considered sustained VT. Sustained VT often is associated with hemodynamic instability. The drug therapy for sustained VT may be defined by laboratory-programmed electrical stimulation of the rhythm to determine the most efficacious drug, dosage, and plasma concentration. This laboratory model is reported to reflect clinical VT and predict appropriate therapy. The successful drug concentration in the acute laboratory situation correlates well with the therapeutic concentration observed chronically for drugs such as quinidine and procainamide but not for propranolol, which depends on prevailing sympathetic tone.[126] Patients whose arrhythmia is not controlled during laboratory-programmed electrical stimulation usually have a relapse of their VT while on chronic suppression therapy. In the patient with VT and hemodynamic instability, the therapy of choice is electrical cardioversion. In patients without a pulse, the rhythm should be treated as with ventricular fibrillation. VT with a pulse but in an unstable patient may be cardioverted with synchronized shock of 100 J.[11] VT in the late hospital phase of an AMI is often asymptomatic, but it is a highly important risk because patients with VT are five times more likely to die within 1 year than those without the arrhythmia.[127] However, whether antiarrhythmics influence the mortality rate is not known. In drug refractory VT, options include surgical or radiofrequency ablative techniques and implantable cardioverter defibrillator (ICD).[128,129]

TREATMENT

Nonpharmacologic Therapy

Implantable Cardioverter Defibrillator

The ICD was developed in the early 1980s. It was intended to protect patients from sudden arrhythmic death. Early experience with ICDs revealed excellent conversion of episodes of VT and ventricular fibrillation (VF). Skeptics were concerned that despite conversion to NSR, the device may not prolong life. An early trial, the Multicenter Automatic Defibrillator Implantation Trial (MADIT) studied unsustained VT in patients with coronary artery disease, still inducible despite intravenous procainamide. Patients were randomized to ICD or conventional antiarrhythmic drugs.[130] The study concluded that ICD resulted in a lower mortality rate (16%) than antiarrhythmic drugs (39%). MADIT was criticized because "conventional therapy" could include class I agents known to result in higher mortality than placebo. Another trial, avoiding class I agents, compared ICD with amiodarone or sotalol.[131] Patients were symptomatic survivors of VF or VT with an ejection fraction (EF) less than 0.40. ICD resulted in a mortality rate 27% lower than that of the antiarrhythmic drugs. Recent American College of Cardiology and American Heart Association consensus guidelines recommend ICD in the following situations:[132]

- Cardiac arrest caused by VF or VT not from a transient or reversible cause
- Spontaneous sustained VT
- Syncope of undetermined origin with symptomatic sustained VT of VF induced at EPS when drugs are ineffective
- NSVT with coronary disease, prior MI, LV dysfunction, and inducible VF or sustained VT at EPS that is not suppressible by a class I drug.

Pharmacotherapy

Lidocaine

Lidocaine is the drug of choice for rapid control of VT and suppression of PVCs when indicated. The therapeutic serum concentration for lidocaine is 1 to 5 mg/L. Lidocaine therapy usually is initiated with an intravenous loading dose to produce rapid arrhythmia control. The loading dose must account for the small central compartment, 0.5 L/kg in normal subjects, reduced to 0.3 L/kg with CHF, and increased to 0.6 L/kg in liver disease.[133] A minimum concentration in the central compartment must be reached because the heart acts as if it belongs in this compartment while limiting the maximum concentration because the brain is considered to be in this compartment. The loading dose (LD) may be calculated to produce a plasma concentration (Cp) of 3 mg/L using the central volume (Vc) of 0.5 L/kg as follows and administered over 1 to 2 minutes:

$$\text{LD} = \text{Cp} \times \text{Vc} = 3\ \text{mg/L} \times 0.5\ \text{L/kg} = 1.5\ \text{mg/kg}$$

Because the loading dose is rapidly distributed away from the heart and the central compartment with an α-phase half-life of about 10 minutes, arrhythmias may recur after the initial dose. Additional boluses, using one-half the initial dosage, may be given after 10 to 20 minutes or when ectopy recurs. Unfortunately, all bolus doses are effective only transiently because of the rapid distribution.

An alternative is to give the initial load, followed by a high-dose infusion of 120 μg/kg/minute for 25 minutes, followed by an appropriate maintenance infusion. The high-dose infusion is intended to avoid the subtherapeutic concentrations produced on a constant infusion of lidocaine for arrhythmia suppression. This constant infusion may be calculated based on the steady-state serum concentration of about 3 mg/L (Cpss) and lidocaine clearance (Cl), which is 15.6 mL/minute/kg in normal male subjects, 20.2 mL/minute/kg in normal female subjects, 5.5 mL/minute/kg in CHF, and 6.0 mL/minute/kg for chronic liver disease,[133] as follows:

$$\text{MD} = \text{Cpss} \times \text{Cl} = 3\ \text{mg/L} \times 6\ \text{mL/min/kg} = 18\ \mu\text{g/kg/min (with liver failure)}$$

Other factors that may reduce lidocaine clearance include advanced age, propranolol, and cimetidine. Only 5% of lidocaine is eliminated unchanged in the urine, and renal failure does not decrease lidocaine clearance. Certain metabolites of lidocaine such as monoethylglycinexylidide (MEGX) and glycinexylidide (GX) are active compounds. GX is cleared by the kidneys and may accumulate in renal impairment. MEGX and GX may contribute to the toxicity of lidocaine when it is administered for extended periods.

Lidocaine serum concentrations may be obtained at any point during the first 12 hours of therapy. There are advocates for early (1 to 2 hours after the start of the infusion) and late (2 to 4 hours) sampling followed by a delayed sample at 8, 12, or 24 hours.[134] Concentrations of 1 to 2 mg/L are rarely effective. Many patients have control of their arrhythmia with concentrations of 3 to 5 mg/L, and neurologic toxicity may limit any further dosage increases. Paresthesias, dizziness, drowsiness, and euphoria may be seen. Resistant arrhythmias may warrant concentrations of 6 to 8 mg/L at the risk of further confusion, nausea, vomiting, dysarthria, and psychoses. Sweating, tremors, and muscle fasciculation may precede seizures, respiratory arrest, and coma. Lidocaine metabolites may contribute to the neurologic toxicity. A serum lidocaine concentration beyond 9 mg/L is rarely justified.

A downward adjustment in lidocaine dosage may be needed after 24 hours or at the onset of signs and symptoms of toxicity. Steady-state concentrations should be expected by approximately four times the normal lidocaine half-life of 100 minutes. In patients with liver disease, steady state may be delayed because of the half-life of 300 minutes.[133] Patients with uncomplicated AMI receiving continuous infusions of lidocaine have developed progressive accumulation after 30 hours. Such patients have a prolonged elimination half-lives of 3 to 4 hours. To avoid the accumulation of lidocaine with prolonged administration, it has been suggested that the infusion rate be reduced by one-half after the first 24 hours of dosing.[135]

Procainamide

Procainamide is an alternative when lidocaine toxicity or arrhythmias resistant to lidocaine develop. Procainamide is a versatile drug that can be administered orally and parenterally, but toxicity, not therapeutic inadequacy, has relegated procainamide to a secondary role. The approved indication for procainamide is in treating documented ventricular arrhythmias (e.g., sustained VT) that are life threatening.[54]

After oral administration, procainamide has a bioavailability of 75%, but certain patients may absorb as little as 10%. In addition, the rate of absorption and time to peak serum concentration vary considerably. First-pass hepatic metabolism may account for some of the reduced bioavailability. Food may delay the absorption. There are various manufacturers of immediate-release and sustained-release procainamide formulations. Switching between generic and proprietary immediate-release procainamide formulation may result in arrhythmia recurrence.[136] Similarly, interchange of the sustained-release procainamide may also result in arrhythmia relapse in certain patients, yet mean data suggest bioequivalence for at least two products.[137] Sustained release of procainamide is accomplished by either a wax matrix or a nondisintegrating core. Generally, the areas under the curve, maximum to minimum serum procainamide concentrations, and steady-state procainamide concentrations for the two types of products are similar; however, the time to maximum serum concentration is delayed for the nondisintegrating matrix.[138] Patients may complain of whole or partial tablets appearing in the stool, but this may not reflect incomplete absorption. Patients should be cautioned not to chew or crush the sustained-release tablets. Drug interactions and altered procainamide concentrations may be observed when procainamide is given along with trimethoprim, quinidine, cimetidine, and ranitidine.

Intravenous procainamide displays two-compartment kinetics similar to those of lidocaine. A rapid distribution phase with a half-life of 5 minutes occurs, with the drug binding extensively to tissues. There is evidence that procainamide does not penetrate well into fat. Thus, total weight should not be used in calculating dosages; ideal weight is preferred. Intravenous bolus doses may be needed for rapid arrhythmia control. The negative inotropic and hypotensive effects of procainamide limit the rate at which the drug may be given. Even in emergency situations, procainamide should not be given at a rate exceeding 30 mg/minute to avoid hypotension. The loading dose (LD) is influenced by the therapeutic range for procainamide (Cp) of 4 to 8 mg/L, the distribution volume (Vdss) of 2 L/kg, and the procainamide content (S) of the hydrochloride salt, 0.82, as follows:

$$LD = Cp \times Vdss/0.82 = 6 \text{ mg/L} \times 2 \text{ L/kg}/0.82 = 14.6 \text{ mg/kg}$$

In renal impairment and CHF, the volume of distribution may be decreased by 25%. Loading doses have been given as small boluses of 50 to 100 mg every 5 minutes until arrhythmia control is seen or toxicity develops. An alternative is a loading infusion of 17 mg/kg over 1 hour, followed by the maintenance dose. The generally accepted therapeutic range for procainamide is 4 to 8 mg/L. However, the indication for the drug may influence the therapeutic range. This range of 4 to 8 mg/L may be appropriate for patients with acute or chronic coronary artery disease with the intent of suppressing PVCs. On the other hand, higher dosages may be needed to suppress VT, producing concentrations in the range of 10 to 20 mg/L.

The selection of procainamide maintenance dosages is intimately related to its metabolic fate. Procainamide may be excreted unchanged in the urine to the extent of 50%. The liver and other sites transform 7 to 24% of procainamide to its major metabolite, NAPA. The rate of acetylation varies between patients, who may be grouped as fast or slow acetylators. Fast acetylators convert a higher percentage of procainamide to NAPA than slow acetylators. About 85% of NAPA is excreted unchanged by the kidneys; thus

NAPA accumulates more than procainamide as renal function deteriorates. It seems that procainamide and NAPA compete for renal tubular secretion. NAPA may thus prolong the procainamide elimination half-life.[139]

The typical patient receiving intravenous procainamide is placed on a dosage of 2 to 4 mg/minute. This may be tailored to the patient, using 2.8 mg/kg/hour as a standard, reduced in cardiac or renal impairment by one-third for moderate impairment and two-thirds for severe impairment.[140] Calculations using population averages of kinetic variables for oral procainamide have not been particularly accurate. In general, patients may be started on 50 mg/kg/day and titrated to response or toxicity. The dosage should be reduced in cardiac or renal impairment by one-third for moderate impairment and two-thirds for severe impairment. In renal impairment, the procainamide half-life may be increased from a normal of 2 to 4 hours to 5 to 10 hours, whereas the NAPA half-life is greatly increased from a normal of 6 hours to as much as 42 hours. Age, independent of renal function, may also affect procainamide.[141] There is evidence that procainamide dosage reduction may not be necessary in patients with chronic stable CHF who are receiving medical therapy.[142]

Although the metabolite NAPA has some antiarrhythmic activity, the two drugs do not have the same electrophysiologic effects, and in patients they may be additive or antagonistic. Thus the use of ratios or sums of the two serum concentrations has met with mixed results. Some clinicians use a minimum sum of 10 mg/L and a maximum of 30 mg/L.[140,143] There is probably more benefit to the use of NAPA concentrations in monitoring for toxicity than for predicting efficacy.

A limiting factor in compliance with procainamide is the dosing interval for the immediate-release product. With normal renal function, the maintenance dosage of 50 mg/kg/day must be given at 3- to 4-hour intervals. The sustained-release formulations allow a 6-hour dosing interval. There is evidence that an 8-hour interval may be appropriate in some cases, although the FDA indication is for 6 hours.[144,145] It is suggested that patients receive the immediate-release product first, for titration, then be converted to a sustained-release product if necessary. The total daily dosage of the immediate-release product should be the initial daily dosage of the sustained-release product. It has been suggested that sustained-release procainamide preparations should be avoided in patients with colostomies or in other rapid gastrointestinal transit states.[146] In 1996 a twice-daily sustained-release formulation was marketed (Procanbid). This product was compared with a four-times-daily extended-release formulation. Procanbid had similar maximum and average steady-state blood concentrations but lower trough concentrations than the four-times-daily product.[147]

Adverse effects commonly seen with procainamide include gastrointestinal distress, weakness, dizziness, nervousness, and blurred vision. These symptoms resolve if the dosage is reduced, but many patients develop tolerance to these effects with continued procainamide use without a dosage reduction. Cardiac toxicity seen with procainamide concentrations greater than 12 mg/L may include progressive lengthening of the QTc interval and QRS complex duration, hypotension, and myocardial depression. However, procainamide may be less likely to exacerbate heart failure than other agents such as disopyramide or tocainide.[148] A lupuslike syndrome may develop in more than 20% of patients taking procainamide. Procainamide lupus differs from systemic lupus erythematosus in that arthritic features are more prominent, whereas dermatologic, hematologic, and renal changes are rare. Symptoms may develop as early as 2 weeks after initiating procainamide or as long as 2 years later. Risk factors include high dosages, high serum concentrations, and slow acetylation status. A hepatic mixed-function oxidase metabolite, procainamide hydroxylamine, has been implicated in causing the lupuslike syndrome.[149] Common signs and symptoms include fever, rash, myalgias, arthralgias, pericarditis, pleuritis, hepatosplenomegaly, and rarely pericardial tamponade. Many more patients have positive serologic tests for lupus than have symptoms (see Chapter 34, Systemic Lupus Erythematosus). Originally, the sustained-release product was reported to produce neutropenia more often than immediate-release procainamide.[150] More recent data suggest that the rate of neutropenia is less than 1% and the risk is independent of formulation.[151] All patients should be monitored for this hematologic complication with frequent white blood cell counts at the beginning of therapy. Patients should be followed for unexplained fevers because of the risk of infection related to the neutropenia. The parenteral procainamide products contain sulfites. The product should be used with caution in asthmatic patients and avoided in cases of known sulfite allergies, which can produce bronchospasm or anaphylaxis.[152]

Disopyramide

Disopyramide currently is available for oral use to treat ventricular arrhythmias (as 100- and 150-mg capsules each in conventional or sustained release). Disopyramide was approved in the United States in 1977. It may be as effective as quinidine in treating AF. Parenteral disopyramide is as effective as lidocaine in treating ventricular arrhythmias but is not yet available in the United States.[153]

Pharmacokinetics

Disopyramide is well absorbed (83%). With the immediate-release product, peak serum concentrations occur in 2 hours. Disopyramide is 50 to 65% protein bound, with the majority bound to alpha$_1$ acid glycoprotein (AAG) and a small amount (5 to 10%) to albumin. The degree of binding is nonlinear. At higher disopyramide concentrations, a greater amount of the drug is free.[154] It is assumed that the free drug is active.[155] The volume of distribution in normal subjects is 0.8 L/kg. Variable amounts of disopyramide (36 to 71%) have been reported to be cleared by the kidney as unchanged drug. The remainder is an *N*-dealkylated metabolite with some antiarrhythmic activity. Healthy subjects have elimination half-lives ranging from 4.4 to 8.2 hours. Renal impairment may prolong the half-life from 8.4 to 53 hours. The half-life may also be prolonged in patients with AMI. There appears to be an interaction with phenytoin and disopyramide: Phenytoin increases the metabolism of disopyramide.[156] Other interactions include erythromycin and rifampin, which can increase or decrease disopyramide serum concentrations, respectively. Macrolide antibiotic–disopyramide interactions have produced life-threatening QTc interval prolongation; new warnings have been placed in the product monograph.[157] The interaction has also been reported with clarithromycin.[158]

The therapeutic range for disopyramide appears to be 3 to 6 mg/L. This therapeutic range may not apply in certain diseases, using the conventional assay measuring total disopyramide. In cirrhosis, the AAG content decreases, and the free disopyramide concentration is higher than in normal subjects.[159] After myocardial infarction, patients show a rise in AAG, with a decrease in free disopyramide concentration.[160] In some studies, atrial arrhythmias responded to lower concentrations than ventricular ectopies. Although steadily increasing the plasma concentration of disopyramide progressively reduces the frequency of ectopy, responders and nonresponders have similar mean concentrations. Therefore, patients should be titrated to response rather than by an arbitrary drug serum concentration.

Administration

Oral disopyramide may be initiated with a loading dose of 300 mg of the immediate-release product (200 mg for moderate renal impairment, moderate liver dysfunction, or decompensated heart failure). Maintenance doses of 100 to 150 mg may be given at 6-hour intervals; the lower dosage is indicated for renal, liver, and cardiac insufficiency. The recommended maximum daily dosage is 800 mg, yet up to 1600 mg has been used with close monitoring. For patients with severe renal impairment, the dosing interval may be prolonged to 12, 24, or 36 hours for creatinine clearances of 15 to 40, 5 to 15, or 1 to 5 mL/minute, respectively.

A sustained-release preparation of disopyramide has been marketed. It has been studied in both normal volunteers and patients with arrhythmias.[161] The dosing interval may be prolonged from 6 hours with the immediate-release to 12 hours with the sustained-release product. A proposed theoretical advantage of the sustained-release product is the avoidance of a transient high-peak serum disopyramide concentration.[162] This, coupled with the potential for higher free drug concentration as a result of the nonlinear protein-binding characteristics of disopyramide, may lead to fewer adverse effects, yet this has not been proved.

Toxicity

Common adverse reactions observed with disopyramide have been anticholinergic symptoms such as dry mouth, blurred vision, constipation, and urinary retention. Disopyramide thus should be avoided in patients with urinary retention (e.g., men with benign prostatic hypertrophy), glaucoma, or myasthenia gravis. Anticholinergic reactions may occur in as many as 45% of patients receiving disopyramide, and 25% may need to discontinue therapy.[163] Acetylcholinesterase inhibitors, such as pyridostigmine, may effectively prevent the anticholinergic effects of disopyramide.[163] Hypoglycemia has been associated with disopyramide with risk factors of advanced age, chronic renal impairment, and malnutrition. Death has resulted from persistent hypoglycemia.[164] Potassium blood concentrations may affect the efficacy of disopyramide. Hypokalemia may decrease the antiarrhythmic effect of disopyramide, and hyperkalemia may increase the risk of disopyramide toxicity. The electrolyte abnormalities should be corrected before disopyramide is used.[54] Like quinidine, disopyramide may prolong the QTc interval and QRS complex duration. Disopyramide has a negative inotropic effect. Initial reports on disopyramide were encouraging, indicating that quinidine produced more frequent adverse effects, yet the reports of acute heart failure developing during chronic disopyramide have dampened enthusiasm for this drug. The risk of developing symptomatic heart failure may be as high as 16%.[165] The drug has been used without complications in patients with heart failure, but such patients are at a much greater risk of decompensation. The onset of symptoms is variable, and there is no apparent correlation with the dosage. Patients developing signs and symptoms of heart failure should discontinue disopyramide. Symptoms usually resolve over a few days, but some patients may need diuretics or digitalis. As with other antiarrhythmics that prolong the QTc interval, disopyramide may cause ventricular arrhythmias, at times with symptoms similar to those of quinidine syncope. Many patients revert after discontinuing the disopyramide; others may need suppression with lidocaine. Disopyramide has warnings against its use in asymptomatic PVCs.[54]

Propafenone

Propafenone (Rhythmol) was approved in the United States in 1989. It has indications for documented life-threatening ventricular arrhythmias (e.g., sustained VT) and was approved in late 1997 for preventing recurrence of paroxysmal AF and PSVT associated with disabling symptoms.[54] In light of the CAST results, using propafenone to suppress ventricular arrhythmias should be restricted to patients in whom the benefit outweighs the risk. Propafenone is a type Ic antiarrhythmic that blocks the fast inward sodium channel, producing a slowed rate of rise of phase 0 of the action potential. Propafenone also has weak β-blocking and calcium channel blocking effects.[166] There is a dose-related increase in P-R interval and QRS duration.

Pharmacokinetics

Currently, propafenone is marketed only in an oral dosage form in the United States (as 150-, 225-, and 300-mg tablets). Absorption is complete (more than 95%) with time to maximal concentration in 1 to 3 hours. The drug is highly protein bound (77 to 95%) and undergoes saturable metabolism, leading to variable absolute bioavailability of 11 to 39%. Propafenone is almost completely cleared by the liver with polymorphic oxidative metabolism via cytochrome P-450.[167] Extensive metabolizers have a half-life of 5.5 hours, whereas poor metabolizers (approximately 7% of the U.S. population) have a half-life of 17.2 hours. The major metabolite of propafenone is 5-hydroxypropafenone, which is active and detectable only in extensive metabolizers. Patients who are poor metabolizers exhibit greater β-blocking effects, possibly because of higher blood concentrations of the parent compound, which tends to accumulate with chronic dosing.

Clinical Use

Propafenone has shown efficacy in supraventricular arrhythmias, including AF and reentrant tachycardia, and is considered by some clinicians to be the antiarrhythmic of choice in WPW syndrome.[54,120] Propafenone was compared to sotalol in symptomatic paroxysmal AF.[168] Each drug was judged as effective and about equal in preventing episodes (79% for propafenone). In another trial, propafenone in similar patients was compared with quinidine. Although this trial was criticized for methodologic problems,[169] the results indicated that propafenone restored sinus rhythm in only 28% of patients, compared to 84% in quinidine. In a prophylactic study of PSVT and paroxysmal AF, propafenone (300 mg twice or three times daily) was compared with placebo.[170] Placebo was 6.8 times more likely to lead to treatment failure than was propafenone 600 mg daily. Higher dosages increased the effectiveness of propafenone at the expense of toxicity.

Toxicity

The most common adverse reaction to propafenone is a metallic or bitter taste that may resolve without a change in dosage. Propafenone may cause central nervous system effects such as dizziness, headache, paresthesias, and fatigue or gastrointestinal effects such as nausea, vomiting, anorexia, and constipation, which can be minimized by decreasing the dosage or increasing the dosing interval.[167] Because of the β-blocking properties of propafenone, the drug should be avoided in patients with chronic bronchitis or emphysema.[54] Propafenone has rarely been associated with liver injury and agranulocytosis. Cardiac adverse effects of propafenone include proarrhythmia, worsening of CHF, and conduction disturbances.[167] Propafenone should be used only when CHF symptoms have been controlled in such patients.

Interactions

Drug interactions with propafenone are likely because of its extensive hepatic metabolism and high protein binding. Cimetidine and quinidine increase serum propafenone serum concentrations through altered hepatic metabolism. Rifampin increases the hepatic metabolism of propafenone, resulting in decreased serum concentrations. Propafenone inhibits warfarin metabolism, resulting in a prolonged anticoagulant response. Propafenone may increase serum digoxin concentrations, warranting adjustment of the digoxin dosage. Similarly, propafenone may increase serum propranolol concentrations; however, dosage adjustment may not be needed because the therapeutic range of propranolol is very wide.[54]

Administration

The starting dosage of propafenone is 150 mg three times a day. The dosage may be increased to a maximum of 300 mg three times a day, with a minimum of 3 to 4 days between increases. Older adults and patients with hepatic dysfunction or renal impairment may need lower dosages. Severe liver dysfunction may lead to greatly increased bioavailability from lessened first-pass hepatic metabolism. Use of 20 to 30% of the normal dosage of propafenone may be appropriate in patients with liver dysfunction. Patients treated chronically must be monitored carefully because of the potential for propafenone to accumulate over time.

Flecainide

Flecainide (Tambocor 50-, 100-, and 150-mg tablets) is a fluorinated analog of procainamide currently available in oral form only. Since the CAST trials, the FDA indications for flecainide have been limited to documented life-threatening arrhythmias, such as sustained VT, and VF. It is also indicated for paroxysmal AF and reentrant tachycardia associated with disabling symptoms. Flecainide should not be used for chronic AF because of an excess development of VT and VF. In addition, flecainide should not be used in patients with a recent myocardial infarction.

Pharmacokinetics

Absorption after oral dosing of flecainide is fairly rapid, with peak serum concentrations occurring in 3 to 4 hours. The bioavailability is nearly 100%. There is no apparent first-pass effect. Food does not affect flecainide absorption. Flecainide has a large volume of distribution, 8 to 10 L/kg, reflecting substantial tissue distribution. The protein binding of flecainide is 37 to 58%. The free fraction of flecainide is proportional to serum albumin and AAG concentrations. In a situation such as the immediate post-AMI period, in which AAG concentrations rise, flecainide is displaced, producing higher free flecainide concentrations. About one-quarter of flecainide is excreted unchanged by the kidneys, and the remainder is primarily conjugated by the liver to inactive metabolites. The normal half-life of flecainide is about 14 hours and is prolonged by ventricular arrhythmias, heart failure, and renal impairment.[171] Flecainide is marketed as a racemic mixture. The enantiomers of flecainide are metabolized with a genetically determined rate showing polymorphism. Patients are classified as poor metabolizers and extensive metabolizers.[172] In patients with liver cirrhosis, the elimination half-life may be significantly longer than expected.[173] Initial dosing should be low, 50 to 100 mg orally twice daily, and increased at 4-day intervals as needed and tolerated. The usual maintenance dosage is 100 to 200 mg twice daily. The therapeutic range for flecainide is 0.3 mg/L (with a reported 50% probability of efficacy) to 0.7 mg/L (with less than 10% probability of cardiovascular toxicity).[174]

Interactions

Interactions with flecainide have been observed with digoxin, amiodarone, cimetidine, and propranolol. Cimetidine and amiodarone may reduce flecainide clearance. Propranolol or verapamil and flecainide may have additive negative inotropic effects. Flecainide may raise serum digoxin concentrations by an apparent decrease in volume of distribution. Smoking may increase flecainide clearance.[54]

Toxicity

Unlike other class I drugs, flecainide does not produce frequent gastrointestinal toxicity. Dizziness and blurred vision may occur. A prolongation of P-R interval and QRS complex duration should be expected, and up to 30% is well tolerated. Flecainide may induce serious arrhythmias that may not be preceded by conduction changes. A history of sustained VT, daily dosages of flecainide greater than 400 mg, high flecainide concentrations (more than 1 mg/L), and reduced EFs may contribute to drug-induced arrhythmias. This proarrhythmic effect of flecainide may occur in 6.6% of patients with sustained VT but only 0.9% with NSVT.[175] The mortality rate of the proarrhythmic events was also higher in sustained VT. Structural heart disease may also predict more proarrhythmias from flecainide. The results of the CAST trial suggest that flecainide and perhaps any class Ic agent should not be used in anything but a life-threatening arrhythmia. Even in such a situation, flecainide may be considered after class Ia and class Ib drugs. In the CAST trial, the mortality rate over 10 months was 5.1% for flecainide and 2.3% for placebo.

Moricizine

Moricizine (Ethmozine in 200-, 250-, and 300-mg tablets) structurally resembles phenothiazines, but the antiarrhythmic does not have antidopaminergic effects. Moricizine cannot be assigned to a subgroup of class I because it has properties of all three. Moricizine prolongs QRS duration, as class Ia drugs do, shortens APD as class Ib agents do, and prolongs the P-R interval, as agents in class Ic do. Moricizine has been described as a membrane stabilizer with anticholinergic properties and the ability to suppress both normal and abnormal automaticity.[176] The current FDA-approved indication for moricizine is life-threatening, sustained VT. It is recommended that therapy be initiated in the hospital.[54]

Pharmacokinetics

Moricizine is completely absorbed after oral administration, with peak blood concentrations occurring at 1 to 3 hours, but bioavailability is limited to 34 to 38% by pronounced first-pass metabolism. Food may lower peak moricizine concentrations, but the extent of absorption is not decreased.[177] Moricizine has a large apparent volume of distribution (300 L) and is highly protein bound (about 95%) to albumin and α_1-acid glycoprotein. Moricizine is metabolized by sulfoxidation, ring hydroxylation, *N*-dealkylation, and glucuronide and sulfate conjugation to at least 26 metabolites. The drug induces cytochrome P-450 activity, causing a decrease in its own elimination half-life with chronic dosing from 1.9 hours (single dose) to 1.4 hours. Drug blood concentrations do not predict response, and in fact the onset of antiarrhythmic action is substantially delayed (about 16 hours) beyond the time to peak concentration of the drug.[178]

Clinical Use

Moricizine may be as effective as quinidine or disopyramide with fewer adverse effects in treating patients with ventricular arrhythmias.[177] In the Cardiac Arrhythmia Pilot Study (CAPS) trial, moricizine was less effective than encainide and flecainide in suppressing PVCs and NSVT.[179] However, in patients with depressed left ventricular function (EF less than 0.45), the agents were similar. In contrast, moricizine continued to be studied in the CAST trial, whereas encainide and flecainide were withdrawn from randomization because of excessive mortality.[180] Subsequently, moricizine was found to produce greater mortality than placebo, and the trial was stopped.[123]

Toxicity

Adverse effects of moricizine are infrequent and include dizziness, nausea, headache, and perioral paresthesia. Moricizine has proarrhythmic effects observed in 3.2 to 15% of patients.[176] The rate of proarrhythmia has been reported in up to 45% of patients with EFs less than 40%.[181] Cimetidine may reduce moricizine clearance, and moricizine may reduce theophylline clearance.

Administration

The starting dosage of moricizine is 200 mg three times a day. There is evidence that twice-a-day dosing is equivalent to three-times-a-day dosing. The dosage may be increased to 300 mg three times a day with small incremental adjustments at 3-day intervals. Lower dosages are recommended in kidney or liver impairment.

Mexiletine

Mexiletine (Mexitil and various others, 150-, 200-, and 250-mg capsules) is a class Ib agent with a structure and mechanism of action similar to those of lidocaine. At present, mexiletine is available in an oral dosage form only, with FDA approval for life-threatening ventricular arrhythmias such as sustained VT.

Pharmacokinetics

Mexiletine is well absorbed orally, with a bioavailability of 80 to 90% in healthy volunteers and peak concentrations occurring at 2 to 4 hours. Absorption may be delayed and incomplete in patients with AMI. Antacids, narcotics, cimetidine, and atropine delay the time to peak concentration but not the serum concentration–time profile for mexiletine. On the other hand, metoclopramide increases the rate of absorption with no effect on the serum concentration–time profile. Intravenously administered mexiletine is thought to exhibit three-compartment kinetics. It has a large volume of distribution, about 5 L/kg, and extensive tissue protein binding, and less than 1% of the drug remains in the blood.[182] Mexiletine is metabolized primarily by the liver, with about 8% of the drug recovered unchanged in the urine in healthy volunteers. Urine excretion is pH dependent, with a more rapid clearance as pH decreases.[182] The elimination half-life of mexiletine is 9.4, 12.1, and 16.7 hours after oral dosing to healthy subjects, patients with arrhythmia, and patients with AMI, respectively. Cigarette smoking may induce mexiletine conjugation, reducing the half-life from 11.1 to 7.2 hours.[183] Phenytoin enhances mexiletine metabolism, with a decrease in mexiletine half-life of about 50%.[182] Renal function does not appear to affect mexiletine clearance, and the drug does not seem to be dialyzable.[184]

Administration

The therapeutic range for mexiletine is 0.75 to 2.0 mg/L. Because of the slow clearance of mexiletine, a loading dose may be needed, but full loading doses rarely are tolerated. A compromise is to give a starting dose of 400 mg once, followed by 200 mg every 8 hours, or 10 to 15 mg/kg/day. There is evidence that a 12-hour regimen with same total daily dosage is as effective as the 8-hour regimen.[185]

Toxicity

There is a high frequency of adverse reactions with loading doses, but with chronic use, it is considered to be comparable to quinidine or procainamide.[186] Adverse effects often limit the mexiletine dosage and reduce the ability to suppress arrhythmias. When this occurs, it may be possible to add other drugs to a tolerated but ineffective dosage of mexiletine. In fact, the combination of quinidine and mexiletine has been more effective than quinidine alone, with fewer adverse effects.[187] An additional benefit is that mexiletine may block the increase in QTc interval produced by quinidine.[188] The additive antiarrhythmic effect is also demonstrated with mexiletine and disopyramide[189] and mexiletine and sotalol.[190] Mexiletine effectively reduces the frequency of PVCs in most patients, even those who do not respond to other agents. Chronic, sustained, recurrent VT does not respond well to mexiletine, but if EPS shows mexiletine to control induced VT, it is usually effective chronically.[191] The incidence of adverse effects may be as high as 54% of patients receiving chronic mexiletine, usually involving neurologic or gastrointestinal effects. Tremor, dizziness, vertigo, paresthesias, nystagmus, diplopia, ataxia, and confusion may occur. Nausea, vomiting, and dyspepsia are common (up to 40% of patients). Cardiovascular effects include hypotension, sinus bradycardia, AV dissociation, and in overdosage, widened QRS complex. In usual dosages, mexiletine does not reduce left ventricular function.

Tocainide

Tocainide (Tonocard, 400- and 600-mg tablets), an amine analog of lidocaine, is indicated for the suppression of life-threatening ventricular arrhythmias. It is especially useful if the arrhythmias responded first to lidocaine.

Pharmacokinetics

Tocainide currently is available only in an oral dosage form. It appears to be absorbed rapidly and completely, but food may decrease the peak plasma concentration without altering the extent of absorption. About one-half the tocainide is cleared unchanged by the kidneys; the rest is glucuronidated by the liver. The normal elimination half-life of 11 hours may be prolonged in patients with chronic arrhythmias, ventricular dysfunction, and renal impairment.[192] The therapeutic range for tocainide concentrations is 3 to 9 mg/L. Toxicity may occur with concentrations above 10 mg/L. Rifampin may induce tocainide metabolism, leading to a shortened tocainide elimination half-life.[193] On the other hand, cimetidine decreases the bioavailability of tocainide.[194]

Clinical Use

Tocainide is indicated for suppressing life-threatening ventricular arrhythmias. It has very limited utility in atrial arrhythmias. Although tocainide may reduce the frequency of PVCs, it may not be as effective or as well tolerated as older drugs such as quinidine.[195] Tocainide may be effective when class Ia drugs have failed.

Toxicity

The utility of tocainide chronically is limited by the high frequency of adverse reactions (up to 70%). Ataxia, tremor, dizziness, paresthesias, night sweats, nausea, and vomiting are common toxicities. Like lidocaine and procainamide, tocainide may produce confusion, psychoses, and seizures. Symptoms may resolve if the drug is administered with meals, which reduces the magnitude of the peak serum concentration without altering the extent of absorption. There are case reports of an association between tocainide use and the development of pulmonary fibrosis and interstitial pneumonitis. The pulmonary toxicity may resolve after tocainide is discontinued.[196] Agranulocytosis has been reported with tocainide, and the mortality rate is high at 25%.[54] Although neutropenia is rare, it may be life threatening. It is suggested that white blood cell counts be monitored frequently, particularly early in therapy because most cases occur during the first 12 months. Rash and fever have also been reported. Cross-reactivity may occur in patients allergic to lidocaine or procainamide.

Sotalol

Sotalol (Betapace in 80-, 120-, 160-, and 240-mg tablets) was FDA approved in 1992 for use in life-threatening ventricular arrhythmias. Sotalol is categorized as a class III agent that also has properties of class II (β-blockade). The marketed product is a racemic mixture of D- and L-sotalol, both with equal effect on lengthening the APD and refractory period. The main difference between the two compounds is the relative lack of β-blocking activity of D-sotalol.

Pharmacokinetics

Oral absorption of sotalol is virtually complete, with a bioavailability of 90 to 100% and no first-pass metabolism. Food and antacids can reduce the bioavailability by about 20%, but this probably is not clinically significant.[197] Peak plasma concentrations occur within 2 to 4 hours of an oral dose. The hydrophilic nature of sotalol prevents much distribution into tissue or protein binding. It has a volume of distribution of 0.9 to 2.4 L/kg. Hepatic metabolism of sotalol is minimal, with no active metabolite formation. The primary route of elimination is renal. The elimination half-life of sotalol depends on renal function and varies as follows: 6 to 18 hours in normal renal function, 24 to 64 hours in moderate renal failure, and 34 to 98 hours in end-stage renal failure.[197] Sotalol is removed by hemodialysis.[198]

Toxicity

The adverse effects of sotalol can be attributed to its β-blocking and Q-T prolongation properties. Fatigue, dyspnea, and bradycardia are the most common reasons for discontinuing sotalol.[102] Other adverse effects include dizziness, headache, bronchospasm, and CHF exacerbation. Proarrhythmia is the most serious adverse effect attributed to sotalol, with an overall occurrence of 4.3%.[102] The most common arrhythmias induced are torsade de pointes and sustained VT or VF. The incidence of proarrhythmia increases with increasing dosages of sotalol; most occur at dosages greater than 320 mg/day.[102] Proarrhythmias are most likely to occur within 7 days of sotalol initiation or dosage increase.

Administration

Initial sotalol dosing should begin with 80 mg twice a day and titrated every 2 to 3 days to the desired therapeutic effect. Most patients respond to dosages between 160 and 320 mg/day; however, some patients may need dosages up to 640 mg/day for arrhythmia suppression.[199] Dosages above 320 mg/day should be used only when the therapeutic benefit outweighs the risk of proarrhythmia.

Clinical Use

The class II and III properties of sotalol allow this drug to be effective in a variety of arrhythmias. Sotalol can suppress atrial and ventricular ectopy, depress reentrant conduction, and block the ventricular response to AF. A trial comparing sotalol with quinidine has shown equal efficacy in maintaining sinus rhythm after DC cardioversion for chronic AF, with better tolerance.[200] In a study comparing seven drugs with antiarrhythmic properties (imipramine, mexiletine, pirmenol, procainamide, propafenone, quinidine, and sotalol) in patients with VT, sotalol was more effective at suppressing arrhythmias and had the least probability of discontinuation because of adverse effects.[201] Sotalol had a lower mortality rate and less proarrhythmic effect than class I agents in the Electrophysiologic Study Versus Electrocardiographic Monitoring (ESVEM) trial.[202] Enthusiasm for sotalol led to the Survival with Oral D-Sotalol[203] (SWORD) trial that studied patients after an MI with poor EF (i.e., less than 0.40). D-Sotalol resulted in a risk of death 20.7 times greater than that of placebo in the subgroup of remote MI and mildly impaired EF. Women appeared to be at greater risk of mortality from sotalol than men. In no subgroup did D-sotalol perform better than placebo.

Torsade de Pointes

Torsade de pointes is a proarrhythmia characterized by rapid series of VT with varying axes on the ECG. Torsade de pointes may or may not be associated with the prolonged Q-T interval. Torsade de pointes may be a result of type Ia antiarrhythmics, sotalol, metabolic derangements, or idiopathic mechanisms. Patients receiving type Ia antiarrhythmics should be monitored closely for QTc prolongation to avoid episodes of torsade de pointes that may impair hemodynamics or lead to malignant ventricular arrhythmias. In the absence of the prolonged Q-T interval syndrome, torsade can be managed as VT. On the other hand, the prolonged Q-T interval syndrome is commonly caused by quinidine and in the past was called quinidine syncope. The syncope most often occurs within 1 to 3 days of initiation of quinidine, although occasionally patients may be receiving the drug for more than a year when symptoms develop. However, this delayed syndrome typically is at or below the therapeutic range. When the syndrome develops in patients receiving quinidine for AF, the VT typically occurs after conversion to sinus rhythm. The frequency of the long Q-T syndrome is higher for quinidine than for the other class Ia agents (disopyramide and procainamide).[204] Unlike with the class Ia agents, the incidence of torsade de pointes induced by sotalol increases with increasing dosage.[205] The therapy of choice for torsade is intravenous magnesium[11] 2 g over 1 minute. Magnesium administration is effective even in normomagnesemic patients. Magnesium may cause hypotension and hypokalemia.[206] An alternative therapy is rapid overdrive pacing. Bretylium has also been used in quinidine-induced VT.[128]

Ventricular Flutter and Fibrillation

Some consider ventricular flutter a separate entity from ventricular fibrillation (VF). Ventricular flutter is a rapid ectopic firing at one or more sites in the ventricles at a fairly regular rate of 150 to 300 bpm. QRS complexes appear to run into each other, obliterating ST segments and P waves, but the wave appears sawtoothed. Classically, VF was a rapid (150 to 500 bpm), disorganized ventricular rhythm. In VF, the ectopic beat does not develop from a single area; instead, the firing is random and changing. Individual fibers or groups of fibers contract independently. When observed, the heart shows areas of twitching. Consequently, there is no effective net contraction and no pumping of blood.

CLINICAL PRESENTATION AND DIAGNOSIS

Almost 50% of patients who develop VF do not have warning arrhythmias (see Premature Ventricular Contractions), especially during the early phase of AMI. Often the period between warning arrhythmias and VF is very short (measured in seconds). In the setting of an AMI, 88% of patients with VF develop it within the first 6 hours of the infarct. If resuscitated, such patients generally have a good prognosis. VF associated with or caused by heart failure may occur at any time after an infarct and is associated with a higher mortality rate because myocardial damage is more extensive.

PREVENTION

Because the criteria for predicting VF are not very accurate, some centers use prophylactic antiarrhythmics to prevent fatal VF. This therapy is highly controversial. Some studies, using low-dose infusions (2 mg/minute), report that lidocaine does not prevent VF, particularly in the first few hours of the infarct.[201] Higher dosages of lidocaine (3 mg/minute) have been shown to prevent VF at the expense of frequent toxicity (15%) in patients less than 70 years old without heart failure or block.[207] This regimen is recommended for the first 24 hours only. Prophylactic lidocaine has come under intense criticism because of unacceptable toxicity (in 51% of patients) and questionable efficacy.[208] Unfortunately, serum lidocaine concentrations provided little help in preventing these adverse reactions. This lack of efficacy was confirmed by meta-analysis of multiple trials, suggesting that prehospital mortality was not decreased with lidocaine and the in-hospital mortality was actually increased by lidocaine.[209]

TREATMENT

Nonpharmacologic Therapy

Electrical Cardioversion

The primary treatment of VF is electrical cardioversion. The likelihood of successful conversion increases if coronary artery perfusion is maintained. In 80% of patients, a single shock is adequate to convert to a more stable rhythm. Nonresponders should receive cardiopulmonary resuscitation with repeated shock therapy, epinephrine, and lidocaine. Lidocaine has been the preferred pharmacologic agent for VF. Bretylium is an effective alternative.

Pharmacotherapy

Bretylium

Bretylium is considered by some to be an alternative for patients resistant to lidocaine, although others advocate bretylium before lidocaine in managing DC conversion–resistant VF. Clearly, a distinction should be drawn in indications for these agents. VF prevention is different from active PVC suppression. To complicate matters further, VF in sudden death syndrome may respond differently from VF in ischemia. Bretylium may have poor to adequate activity in PVC suppression, but it has excellent antifibrillatory activity. Bretylium is taken up by the amine pump in the adrenergic neuron. It displaces norepinephrine, then blocks subsequent release of catecholamines. The temporary period of sympathetic excess may produce hypertension and arrhythmias, particularly in patients with digitalis toxicity. The antiarrhythmic action of bretylium may be independent of its sympatholytic effects. However, The hypertension observed with bretylium correlates well with changes in norepinephrine plasma concentration.[210] The ability of bretylium to reduce the disparity in refractory periods between normal and infarcted tissues may indicate why it is effective in VF, which is felt to be sustained by reentry between these two tissues. Because bretylium does not depress automaticity, PVC frequency is largely unaffected.

Pharmacokinetics

Bretylium exhibits two-compartment kinetics. Bretylium elimination is primarily (70 to 80%) via the kidneys. In normal volunteers, the half-life is 7.8 hours, compared with 33.4 hours in patients with impaired renal function.[211] The antiarrhythmic concentration is not well established; a range of 0.5 to 1.5 mg/L has been suggested.

Administration

Bretylium may produce chemical defibrillation without electric shock when it is given, undiluted, by rapid injection at a dosage of 5 mg/kg. Rapid administration should be reserved for emergency use, as in cardiopulmonary resuscitation. The average time to reversion after bretylium is 9 to 10 minutes. If after 5 to 10 minutes there is no response, 10 mg/kg may be given, up to a maximum of 30 to 35 mg/kg. For less serious arrhythmias, bretylium can be given over 8 to 10 minutes, with 5 to 10 mg/kg as the loading dose. If the arrhythmia persists, the dosage may be repeated at 1-hour intervals up to 30 mg/kg. For chronic suppression, bretylium may be given intramuscularly or by intermittent infusions (over 8 to 10 minutes), every 6 to 8 hours. Bretylium has also been given by constant infusion at 1 to 2 mg/minute.

Toxicity

The common adverse effects of bretylium are related to its adrenergic-blocking actions, producing transient hypertension followed by hypotension, worsened arrhythmias, and angina. Rapid intravenous injection often produces nausea and vomiting. Hyperthermia is an unusual reaction to bretylium. A reported temperature of 108.2°F was ascribed to bretylium infusion.[212] The febrile illness resolved when the infusion was stopped.

Clinical Use

Bretylium was compared with intravenous amiodarone in patients with recurrent, symptomatic VT or VF.[213] Patients were refractory or intolerant to lidocaine and procainamide. Bretylium was more likely to produce toxicity (hypotension, CHF, or diarrhea) than amiodarone. Amiodarone (low-dose group) was at least as effective as bretylium and superior to bretylium when a higher dosage (1000 mg/day) of amiodarone was used. Mortality rates were similar.

Amiodarone

Oral amiodarone (Cordarone) is indicated for recurrent VF or recurrent hemodynamically unstable VT when other agents have failed through ineffectiveness or toxicity. Intravenous amiodarone is indicated for initiating treatment and prophylaxis of frequently recurring VF and hemodynamically unstable VT in patients refractory to other therapy. Amiodarone is a class III agent with properties of classes I, II, and IV. Its use generally is restricted to treating drug-resistant arrhythmias because of serious adverse effects. Amiodarone structurally resembles thyroxine.

Pharmacokinetics

Oral amiodarone bioavailability is poor and erratic, with 22 to 86% absorption.[214] The time to peak absorption is about 6 hours. After absorption, the drug is widely distributed to fat, lung, liver, muscle, and spleen, with a very large volume of distribution (approximately 5000 L). The elimination half-life varies from 26 to 107 days and appears biphasic. Amiodarone is metabolized to its major active metabolite, desethyamiodarone (DEA). The utility of monitoring serum amiodarone concentrations is controversial because of the extensive distribution to tissues and apparent role of DEA in arrhythmia suppression. There is some evidence that arrhythmias may recur if concentrations fall below 1.0 mg/L. Toxicity may occur if serum concentrations exceed 2.5 mg/L. Variable correlations have been made with red cell concentrations of amiodarone. Various dosing schemes have been suggested to avoid the delay in reaching steady-state serum amiodarone concentrations. Up to 1600 mg is given daily for a week, then 800 mg daily for 2 to 4 weeks, and finally the dosage is reduced to the minimally tolerable dosage, usually 200 to 600 mg daily in two divided doses. Intravenous amiodarone is given as a rapid infusion of 150 mg over 10 minutes, then a slow infusion of 1 mg/minute for 6 hours, followed by a maintenance infusion of 0.5 mg/minute.[54] Although patients can be converted from parenteral to oral amiodarone, the products produce different cardiac effects. Intravenous amiodarone does not have antithyroid effects, and the active metabolite does not accumulate in cardiac tissue to produce antiarrhythmic effects. Intravenous amiodarone has more pronounced calcium channel blocking effects and antiadrenergic effects than the oral form.[215] Because of the high risk of phlebitis, intravenous infusions should be delivered via central lines. Surface tension of intravenous amiodarone makes drop counter infusions unreliable, necessitating the use of volumetric devices. Many of the dose-defining clinical trials used polyvinyl chloride tubing that adsorbs amiodarone. Glass or polyolefin should be used when infusions last longer than 2 hours.[54]

Toxicity

A wide range of adverse effects may be encountered with long-term amiodarone use. Corneal deposits are common. In one series, 79% of patients developed microdeposits but no change in visual acuity.[216] Some cardiologists suggest observing only for visual symptoms such as photophobia or blurring, which develop less often than the microdeposits.[217] Abnormal liver enzymes may be encountered in 10 to 20% of patients.[218] The drug appears to concentrate in liver tissue. Although enzymes may rise, typically to two to three times normal, hepatic function may not change, and the drug may be continued with ultimate resolution of the problem. However, severe liver damage and death have been associated with amiodarone.[218] Dermatologic reactions to amiodarone may occur in up to 11.6% of patients[217] and have been described as photosensitivity or blue-gray skin discoloration. Pulmonary abnormalities associated with amiodarone are considered to be a justification for discontinuing therapy. Pulmonary fibrosis, the most severe abnormality, usually is symptomatic and may be reversible on discontinuation with or without glucocorticoid administration. However, pulmonary fibrosis caused by amiodarone may also be fatal. Amiodarone-induced pulmonary abnormalities rarely occur at dosages less than 400 mg/day.[218] The iodine content of amiodarone is 37%, which is thought to be responsible for the occurrence of hypothyroidism or hyperthyroidism. Amiodarone interferes with the metabolism of thyroxine (T_4), resulting in increased serum concentrations of T_4 and decreased serum concentrations of triiodothyronine (T_3). Patients typically are not symptomatic of hyperthyroidism; in fact, thyroid-stimulating hormone concentrations may be increased, which suggests insensitivity to thyroid hormone effect. If symptomatic, patients may notice tremor, myopathy, and sleep disturbance.[218] There is controversy over the predictability of antiarrhythmic response and toxicity with the use of the serum reverse T_3 (rT_3)

concentrations. Very high rT_3 concentrations (greater than 130 ng/dL) have been associated with the development of pulmonary fibrosis, arrhythmogenicity, and sudden cardiac death.[219] Amiodarone-induced hyperthyroidism may warrant dosage reduction or withdrawal and antithyroid therapy. Amiodarone-induced hypothyroidism may present with signs of sinus bradycardia, which can reduce cardiac output or cause constipation. Hypothyroidism treatment includes amiodarone dosage reduction or withdrawal and thyroid hormone replacement therapy. Proarrhythmia associated with amiodarone is rare. A recent evaluation of pooled data from multiple trials of patients treated with amiodarone reported an overall proarrhythmia incidence of 2% and an incidence of less than 1% for torsade de pointes.[220]

Interactions

Amiodarone may produce drug interactions with warfarin, digoxin, procainamide, and quinidine.[221] It has been suggested that the dosage of quinidine or procainamide be reduced by 30 to 50% when amiodarone is added and that Q-T and QRS intervals be monitored for excessive prolongation. Amiodarone inhibits warfarin metabolism. It is suggested that the warfarin maintenance dosage be decreased by one-half when amiodarone is added, and prothrombin times should be monitored carefully. When amiodarone is given to patients receiving digoxin, it is suggested that the digoxin maintenance dosage should be halved and adjusted according to serum digoxin concentrations.

Clinical Use

A wide variety of arrhythmias respond to therapy with amiodarone. It is effective in the maintenance of sinus rhythm after DC cardioversion in patients with AF[222] and in the termination of reentrant arrhythmias, including the WPW syndrome. Intravenous amiodarone also is effective in suppressing ventricular arrhythmias,[223–225] and oral amiodarone appears to decrease cardiac mortality after MI.[225–228] Low-dose amiodarone (200 mg/day) was compared with individualized antiarrhythmics or no therapy in patients with persisting asymptomatic complex arrhythmias after MI. During the first year after an MI, amiodarone resulted in fewer deaths than in the other groups.[229] Amiodarone used after an MI in patients incapable of taking β-blockers found fewer deaths and decreased frequency of ventricular arrhythmias.[227]

Sudden Death

The predominant cause of sudden death is VF, usually preceded by sustained VT or PVCs. In approximately 25% of cases, sudden death (presumably via VF) is not preceded by a history of cardiac symptoms. Thus, preventing VF with chronic antiarrhythmics becomes a question of patient selection. Sudden cardiac collapse from VF in ambulatory patients often (in 55% of cases) is not associated with an AMI. These patients after resuscitation have a very high (three times greater than primary VF with an AMI) mortality rate. Chronic antiarrhythmics have produced mixed results in sudden death. Certain arrhythmias such as sustained VT or symptoms such as syncope have long been viewed as harbingers of future fatal events, suggesting aggressive treatment. Examination of patients entered into the ESVEM trial did not confirm this approach. This study concluded that presenting arrhythmia did not predict the type of arrhythmia recurrence.[230] CHF classified by symptom activity scale (SAS) class and EF were predictors of arrhythmic death or cardiac arrest. The cutoff for risk using EF is considered to be 0.30. To further cloud these issues, Holter monitoring and EPS results may not correspond in predicting future arrhythmias or cardiac arrest.[230]

In the recent years, antiarrhythmic use to prevent sudden death has changed significantly, especially in light of the results of the CAST I and II trials. Drug use has become more conservative and is based on patient risk of sudden death, determined by the degree of underlying heart disease and the type of presenting arrhythmia. One system of classifying arrhythmias based on risk of sudden death has been proposed by Morganroth and Bigger.[231] They classify ventricular arrhythmias as benign, potentially lethal, or lethal based on the type of arrhythmia and the degree of underlying heart disease.

Patients with benign ventricular arrhythmias are characterized as having PVCs or NSVT as the presenting arrhythmia, no hemodynamic symptoms, and no structural heart disease. About 30% of patients with ventricular arrhythmias are classified as having benign arrhythmias. The risk of sudden death in these patients is minimal, so no therapy is recommended. Some patients have intolerable symptoms from the arrhythmia (i.e., palpitations), which, if necessary, can be treated with β-blockers.

Potentially lethal arrhythmias affect about 65% of patients with ventricular arrhythmias and carry a moderate to high probability for sudden death. They are further categorized into two types for treatment purposes. The first type of potentially lethal arrhythmias occurs in patients with PVCs or NSVT, no hemodynamic symptoms, and a moderate degree of structural heart disease (LVEF 40%, no late potentials on signal-averaged ECG). Because of the moderate risk of sudden death in this group, antiarrhythmics are not considered beneficial, and treatment is the same as with benign ventricular arrhythmias.

The second type of potentially lethal ventricular arrhythmia includes patients who have asymptomatic or mildly symptomatic PVCs or NSVT and a moderate to severe degree of structural heart disease (≥10 PVCs per hour, LVEF less than 40%, late potentials on signal-averaged ECG, and decreased heart rate variability). Because the risk of sudden death in these patients is high, treatment is recommended and should include antiarrhythmics guided by EPS.

About 5% of ventricular arrhythmias are considered lethal. These patients have sustained VT and VF with hemodynamic symptoms and have severe underlying cardiac disease (previous MI, LVEF less than 40%, cardiomyopathy, or coronary artery disease). The risk of sudden death is highest in patients with lethal ventricular arrhythmias. The recommended sequence of therapy includes EPS-guided class Ia antiarrhythmics followed by either a class Ib or a combination of Ia and Ib. If the class I agents fail, then amiodarone or sotalol can be considered, with ablative techniques, surgical intervention, or implantable cardiac defibrillators as alternatives.

When considering the choices for chronic VT management and prevention of sudden death, β-blockers also deserve consideration. Unfortunately, a variety of conditions may preclude patients from the potential benefit of β-blockade, such as uncontrolled heart failure, bradycardia, second- or third-degree heart block, SA block, insulin-dependent diabetes mellitus, peripheral vascular disease, and chronic obstructive pulmonary disease.

β-Blockers

The remaining discussion is limited to β-blockers with substantial literature supporting their use in sudden death, AMI, or arrhythmias.

Propranolol

Propranolol has not met with exceptional results in ventricular ectopic suppression. It may not be effective in preventing ectopy after an AMI. In VT treatment, propranolol has been disappointing. However, it may be useful in exercise-induced arrhythmias, ventricular arrhythmias associated with mitral valve prolapse, digitalis-induced arrhythmias, and arrhythmias associated with a long Q-T interval.

Propranolol has been studied in the post-AMI period, with mixed results in lowering the risk of sudden death. The report from the National Heart, Lung and Blood Institute revealed a 26% lower mortality rate for propranolol than for placebo.[232] The site of the infarct, age, and sex had no influence on the response to propranolol. The initial dosage of propranolol, 40 mg three times daily, was adjusted to 60 or 80 mg three times daily depending on the serum propranolol concentrations.

Pharmacokinetics

Propranolol is felt to have the highest membrane-stabilizing potency of the β-blockers. Called a quinidine-like action, it is manifest only in overdose situations, however. Propranolol is a nonselective antagonist to β_1 (cardiac) and β_2 (lungs and blood vessels) receptors. It is well absorbed (more than 90%), but first-pass hepatic extraction may reduce bioavailability to about 30%. Protein binding is about 90%. Propranolol is cleared rapidly by hepatic metabolism, with a half-life of 3.5 to 6 hours. Propranolol may be given intravenously in rare situations, as 0.5 to 0.75 mg repeated every 2 minutes up to a maximum of 0.1 mg/kg. The effective dosage may be repeated at 6- to 8-hour intervals. The oral propranolol dosage is much higher but variable. A typical starting dosage is 10 mg every 6 hours. The dosing interval may not correlate with the short half-life; a twice-daily regimen has been effective.

Toxicity

The most common adverse reactions seen with propranolol involve the central nervous system and include fatigue, hallucinations, weakness, insomnia, and nightmares. These effects may not be related to β-blockade, and differences between the various β-blockers have not been demonstrated. Because it is nonselective, propranolol may exacerbate bronchospasm. Although propranolol may precipitate or worsen CHF, if the arrhythmia is felt to have induced symptoms, propranolol may relieve the symptoms because it suppresses the arrhythmia. The β-blockers with intrinsic sympathomimetic activity may produce less cardiac depression and may be indicated in patients prone to heart failure. Propranolol (by β-blockade) may allow unopposed α-vasoconstriction, producing cold or painful extremities. Claudication, skin necrosis, and gangrene have been observed. Nonselective agents should be avoided after such symptoms develop; cardioselective or high intrinsic sympathomimetic agents are preferred.

Timolol

Timolol is a nonselective antagonist with good absorption (more than 90%) and bioavailability (75%). Protein binding is low (10%). Timolol is cleared primarily by the liver, with slight (20%) renal excretion. The half-life is short (3 to 4 hours). Adverse effects are similar to those of propranolol.

Timolol has been compared with placebo in the chronic prophylaxis against post-AMI sudden death.[232] Patients taking placebo had nearly three times as many arrhythmias that warranted treatment as the timolol group. Besides a decrease in overall mortality rate with timolol, the incidence of sudden death and presumably fatal VF was reduced by approximately one-half. The study used a fixed-dose regimen (5 mg twice daily for 2 days, then 10 mg twice daily), which was associated with a significant reduction in resting heart rate. Whether beneficial effects in mortality might be seen without a decrease in resting heart rate is not known.

Metoprolol

Metoprolol may be considered an alternative to propranolol for arrhythmias because it is more selective for β_1-receptors, and it may be preferred over propranolol for patients with chronic or acute obstructive pulmonary disease. Metoprolol should be used with caution because in high dosages it may also block β_2-receptors.

Metoprolol is well absorbed (more than 95%), with greater bioavailability than propranolol (about 50%). Protein binding is slight (12%). Metoprolol is cleared hepatically, with a half-life of 3 to 4 hours. The typical patient is started at a daily dosage of 100 mg. Metoprolol has adverse effects similar to those of propranolol, with less risk for patients with asthma or peripheral vascular disease.

Metoprolol has been compared with placebo in patients with AMI treated for 90 days.[233] Metoprolol was initiated as 15 mg intravenously, followed by an oral dosage of 100 mg twice daily. It reduced mortality by 36%, with beneficial effects in all age groups.

Other β-blockers of potential usefulness in ventricular arrhythmias include acebutolol, atenolol, bisoprolol, nadolol, and pindolol. As a class, β-blockers appear to be beneficial in treating patients after AMI. The efficacy seems to be independent of intrinsic sympathomimetic activity, β_2-receptor blockade, and membrane-stabilizing properties. However, these properties may aid with individual drug selection in certain patients. The duration of therapy has not been established. The onset of therapy has varied between studies, yet some evidence exists that immediate β-blockade (e.g., within 12 hours after the onset of pain) may limit the enzyme-estimated infarct size.

Summary Topics

PHARMACOECONOMICS

Only a handful of studies have evaluated the economic utility of arrhythmia treatments. In the MADIT trial,[234] the cost of ICDs was compared with that of antiarrhythmic drugs. Initially, ICD is expensive (for acquisition and implantation), but subsequently antiarrhythmics become more costly. Because ICD reduced mortality, the investigators were able to calculate a cost-effectiveness ratio of $27,000 per life-year saved. This figure is comparable to other cardiac-related life-saving modalities. Caution is indicated because MADIT selected only high-risk patients. When less ill subjects are considered, the ratio exceeds $50,000 when compared to amiodarone therapy and could be judged as prohibitive.[235] These studies can be applied only to patients with ventricular arrhythmias. Extrapolations should not be made to atrial or conduction arrhythmias.

CONCLUSION

Cardiac arrhythmias are complex, have various causes and alterations in electrophysiology, differ in severity and prognosis, and warrant individualized treatment with potentially toxic drugs. A thorough understanding of the pharmacology, pharmacodynamics, pharmacokinetics, and adverse reactions for each antiarrhythmic drug is needed for safe and effective treatment of patients with arrhythmias. No single drug is effective for any arrhythmia in all patients, although certain drugs are clearly first-line agents. Dosages of many antiarrhythmics should be calculated using known values for the pharmacokinetic variables. However, these dosages usually are only estimates of the dosage needed for a patient, and adjustments may be needed. Patients must be monitored carefully, which often involves drug concentration monitoring. Many new antiarrhythmics have been marketed. The ultimate question still remains unresolved for most arrhythmias: Will these drugs decrease mortality?

KEY POINTS

- Cardiac arrhythmias can range from benign to lethal.
- Arrhythmias can arise from a variety of causes (e.g., electrolyte disturbances, structural abnormalities, metabolic derangements, drug toxicity).
- Antiarrhythmic drug therapy should be individualized to the patient's response and toxicity.
- Holter monitoring and EPS can be used to assess drug efficacy.
- The risk:benefit ratio of treating each type of VT should be considered before therapy is initiated.
- The use of drugs to suppress ventricular arrhythmias should be limited to life-threatening arrhythmias.

REFERENCES

1. Anonymous. Textbook of cardiovascular medicine. Philadelphia: Lippincott-Raven, 1998:1531.
2. Wit AL. Cellular electrophysiologic mechanisms of cardiac arrhythmias. Cardiol Clin 8:393–409, 1990.
3. Nattel S. Antiarrhythmic drug classifications. A critical appraisal of their history, present status, and clinical relevance. Drugs 41:672–701, 1991.
4. Saini V, Podrid PJ, Slater W, et al. Encainide and flecainide: are they interchangeable? Am Heart J 117:1253–1258, 1989.
5. Wyse DG, Mitchell LB, Duff HJ. Procainamide, disopyramide and quinidine: discordant antiarrhythmic effects during crossover comparison in patients with inducible ventricular tachycardia. J Am Coll Cardiol 9:882–889, 1987.
6. Hession M, Blum R, Podrid PJ, et al. Mexiletine and tocainide: does response to one predict response to the other? J Am Coll Cardiol 7:338–343, 1986.
7. Anonymous. The Sicilian gambit. A new approach to the classification of antiarrhythmic drugs based on their actions on arrhythmogenic mechanisms. Task Force of the Working Group on Arrhythmias of the European Society of Cardiology. Circulation 84:1831–1851, 1991.
8. Wyse DG. Pharmacologic therapy in patients with ventricular tachyarrhythmias. Cardiol Clin 11:65–83, 1993.
9. Dreifus LS, Michelson EL, Kaplinsky E. Bradyarrhythmias: clinical significance and management. J Am Coll Cardiol 1:327–338, 1983.
10. Hindman MC, Wagner GS. Arrhythmias during myocardial infarction: mechanisms, significance, and therapy. Cardiovasc Clin 11:81–102, 1980.
11. Anonymous. Guidelines for cardiopulmonary resuscitation and emergency cardiac care. Emergency Cardiac Care Committee and Subcommittees, American Heart Association. Part VIII. Ethical considerations in resuscitation. JAMA 268:2282–2288, 1992.

12. Schweitzer P, Mark H. The effect of atropine on cardiac arrhythmias and conduction. Part 2. Am Heart J 100:255–261, 1980.
13. Wood M, Ellenbogen KA. Bradyarrhythmias, emergency pacing, and implantable defibrillation devices. Crit Care Clin 5:551–568, 1989.
14. Rodriguez RD, Schocken DD. Update on sick sinus syndrome, a cardiac disorder of aging. Geriatrics 45:26–30, 1933.
15. Dreifus LS, Fisch C, Griffin JC, et al. Guidelines for implantation of cardiac pacemakers and antiarrhythmia devices. A report of the American College of Cardiology/American Heart Association Task Force on Assessment of Diagnostic and Therapeutic Cardiovascular Procedures (Committee on Pacemaker Implantation). J Am Coll Cardiol 18:1–13, 1991.
16. Santini M, Alexidou G, Ansalone G, et al. Relation of prognosis in sick sinus syndrome to age, conduction defects and modes of permanent cardiac pacing. Am J Cardiol 65:729–735, 1990.
17. Sgarbossa EB, Pinski SL, Maloney JD. The role of pacing modality in determining long-term survival in the sick sinus syndrome. Ann Intern Med 119:359–365, 1993.
18. Schweitzer P, Teichholz LE. Carotid sinus massage. Its diagnostic and therapeutic value in arrhythmias. Am J Med 78:645–654, 1985.
19. Mehta D, Wafa S, Ward DE, et al. Relative efficacy of various physical manoeuvres in the termination of junctional tachycardia. Lancet 1:1181–1185, 1988.
20. Parker RB, McCollam PL. Adenosine in the episodic treatment of paroxysmal supraventricular tachycardia. Clin Pharm 9:261–271, 1990.
21. diMarco JP, Sellers TD, Lerman BB, et al. Diagnostic and therapeutic use of adenosine in patients with supraventricular tachyarrhythmias. J Am Coll Cardiol 6:417–425, 1985.
22. diMarco JP, Miles W, Akhtar M, et al. Adenosine for paroxysmal supraventricular tachycardia: dose ranging and comparison with verapamil. Assessment in placebo-controlled, multicenter trials. The Adenosine for PSVT Study Group. Ann Intern Med 113:104–110, 1990.
23. Till J, Shinebourne EA, Rigby ML, et al. Efficacy and safety of adenosine in the treatment of supraventricular tachycardia in infants and children. Br Heart J 62:204–211, 1989.
24. Rankin AC, Rae AP, Oldroyd KG, et al. Verapamil or adenosine for the immediate treatment of supraventricular tachycardia. Q J Med 74:203–208, 1990.
25. Hood MA, Smith WM. Adenosine versus verapamil in the treatment of supraventricular tachycardia: a randomized double-crossover trial. Am Heart J 123:1543–1549, 1992.
26. Chronister C. Clinical management of supraventricular tachycardia with adenosine. Am J Crit Care 2:41–47, 1993.
27. Garratt C, Linker N, Griffith M, et al. Comparison of adenosine and verapamil for termination of paroxysmal junctional tachycardia. Am J Cardiol 64:1310–1316, 1989.
28. Klabunde RE. Dipyridamole inhibition of adenosine metabolism in human blood. Eur J Pharmacol 93:21–26, 1983.
29. Rankin AC, Oldroyd KG, Chong E, et al. Adenosine or adenosine triphosphate for supraventricular tachycardias? Comparative double-blind randomized study in patients with spontaneous or inducible arrhythmias. Am Heart J 119:316–323, 1990.
30. Till JA, Shinebourne EA. Supraventricular tachycardia: diagnosis and current acute management. Arch Dis Child 66:647–652, 1991.
31. Huycke EC, Sung RJ, Dias VC, et al. Intravenous diltiazem for termination of reentrant supraventricular tachycardia: a placebo-controlled, randomized, double-blind, multicenter study. J Am Coll Cardiol 13:538–544, 1989.
32. Dougherty AH, Jackman WM, Naccarelli GV, et al. Acute conversion of paroxysmal supraventricular tachycardia with intravenous diltiazem. IV Diltiazem Study Group. Am J Cardiol 70:587–592, 1992.
33. McAllister RGJ, Kirsten EB. The pharmacology of verapamil. IV. Kinetic and dynamic effects after single intravenous and oral doses. Clin Pharmacol Ther 31:418–426, 1982.
34. Hamann SR, Blouin RA, McAllister RG Jr. Clinical pharmacokinetics of verapamil. Clin Pharmacokinet 9:26–41, 1984.
35. McCall D, Walsh RA, Frohlich ED, et al. Calcium entry blocking drugs: mechanisms of action, experimental studies and clinical uses. Curr Probl Cardiol 10:1–80, 1985.
36. Hoon TJ, Bauman JL, Rodvold KA, et al. The pharmacodynamic and pharmacokinetic differences of the D- and L-isomers of verapamil: implications in the treatment of paroxysmal supraventricular tachycardia. Am Heart J 112:396–403, 1986.
37. Echizen H, Vogelgesang B, Eichelbaum M. Effects of D, L-verapamil on atrioventricular conduction in relation to its stereoselective first-pass metabolism. Clin Pharmacol Ther 38:71–76, 1985.
38. Weiss AT, Lewis BS, Halon DA, et al. The use of calcium with verapamil in the management of supraventricular tachyarrhythmias. Int J Cardiol 4:275–284, 1983.
39. Haft JI, Habbab MA. Treatment of atrial arrhythmias. Effectiveness of verapamil when preceded by calcium infusion. Arch Intern Med 146:1085–1089, 1986.
40. Epstein ML, Kiel EA, Victorica BE. Cardiac decompensation following verapamil therapy in infants with supraventricular tachycardia. Pediatrics 75:737–740, 1985.
41. Garson A Jr. Medicolegal problems in the management of cardiac arrhythmias in children. Pediatrics 79:84–88, 1987.
42. Packer M, Meller J, Medina N, et al. Hemodynamic consequences of combined beta-adrenergic and slow calcium channel blockade in man. Circulation 65:660–668, 1982.
43. Bussey HI. The influence of quinidine and other agents on digitalis glycosides. Am Heart J 104:289–302, 1982.
44. Buckley MM, Grant SM, Goa KL, et al. Diltiazem. A reappraisal of its pharmacological properties and therapeutic use. Drugs 39:757–806, 1990.
45. Bohm M, Schwinger RH, Erdmann E. Different cardiodepressant potency of various calcium antagonists in human myocardium. Am J Cardiol 65:1039–1041, 1990.
46. Heywood JT, Graham B, Marais GE, et al. Effects of intravenous diltiazem on rapid atrial fibrillation accompanied by congestive heart failure. Am J Cardiol 67:1150–1152, 1991.
47. De Belder MA, Malik M, Ward DE, et al. Pacing modalities for tachycardia termination. Pacing Clin Electrophysiol 13:231–248, 1990.
48. Clair WK, Wilkinson WE, McCarthy EA, et al. Treatment of paroxysmal supraventricular tachycardia with oral diltiazem. Clin Pharmacol Ther 51:562–565, 1992.
49. Grace AA, Camm AJ. Drug therapy: quinidine. N Engl J Med 338:35–45, 1998.
50. Ueda CT. Quinidine. In: Applied pharmacokinetics. Spokane: Applied Therapeutics, 1992:1–22.
51. Woosley RL, Echt DS, Roden DM. Effects of congestive heart failure on the pharmacokinetics and pharmacodynamics of antiarrhythmic agents. Am J Cardiol 57:25B–33B, 1986.
52. Wooding-Scott RA, Smalley J, Visco J, et al. The pharmacokinetics and pharmacodynamics of quinidine and 3-hydroxyquinidine. Br J Clin Pharmacol 26:415–421, 1988.
53. Roden DM, Thompson KA, Hoffman BF, et al. Clinical features and basic mechanisms of quinidine-induced arrhythmias. J Am Coll Cardiol 8:73A–78A, 1986.
54. Anonymous. Drug facts and comparisons CD-ROM. St Louis: Kluwer, 1998.
55. Wooding-Scott RA, Darling IM, Slaughter RL. Comparison of assay procedures used to measure total and unbound concentrations of quinidine. Drug Intell Clin Pharm 23:999–1004, 1989.
56. Swerdlow CD, Yu JO, Jacobson E, et al. Safety and efficacy of intravenous quinidine. Am J Med 75:36–42, 1983.
57. Cohen IS, Jick H, Cohen SI. Adverse reactions to quinidine in hospitalized patients: findings based on data from the Boston Collaborative Drug Surveillance Program. Prog Cardiovasc Dis 20:151–163, 1977.
58. Coplen SE, Antman EM, Berlin JA, et al. Efficacy and safety of quinidine therapy for maintenance of sinus rhythm after cardioversion. A meta-analysis of randomized control trials. Circulation 82:1106–1116, 1990.
59. Zehender M, Hohnloser S, Muller B, et al. Effects of amiodarone versus quinidine and verapamil in patients with chronic atrial fibrillation: results of a comparative study and a 2-year follow-up. J Am Coll Cardiol 19:1054–1059, 1992.
60. Ferguson TBJ, Cox JL. Surgical therapy for patients with supraventricular tachycardia. Cardiol Clin 8:535–555, 1990.
61. Manolis AS, Wang PJ, Estes NA. Radiofrequency catheter ablation for cardiac tachyarrhythmias. Ann Intern Med 121:452–461, 1994.
62. Akhtar M, Jazayeri MR, Sra J, et al. Atrioventricular nodal reentry. Clinical, electrophysiological, and therapeutic considerations. Circulation 88:282–295, 1993.
63. Scher DL, Arsura EL. Multifocal atrial tachycardia: mechanisms, clinical correlates, and treatment. Am Heart J 118:574–580, 1989.
64. Hazard PB, Burnett CR. Verapamil in multifocal atrial tachycardia. Hemodynamic and respiratory changes. Chest 91:68–70, 1987.
65. Hazard PB, Burnett CR. Treatment of multifocal atrial tachycardia with metoprolol. Crit Care Med 15:20–25, 1987.
66. Arsura E, Lefkin AS, Scher DL, et al. A randomized, double-blind, placebo-controlled study of verapamil and metoprolol in treatment of multifocal atrial tachycardia. Am J Med 85:519–524, 1988.
67. Stein B, Halperin JL, Fuster V. Should patients with atrial fibrillation be anticoagulated prior to and chronically following cardioversion? Cardiovasc Clin 21:231–247, 1990.

68. Petersen P. Thromboembolic complications in atrial fibrillation. Stroke 21:4–13, 1990.
69. Wolf PA, Kannel WB, McGee DL, et al. Duration of atrial fibrillation and imminence of stroke: the Framingham study. Stroke 14:664–667, 1983.
70. Anonymous. Predictors of thromboembolism in atrial fibrillation: I. Clinical features of patients at risk. The Stroke Prevention in Atrial Fibrillation Investigators. Ann Intern Med 116:1–5, 1992.
71. Lundstrom T, Ryden L. Chronic atrial fibrillation. Long-term results of direct current conversion. Acta Med Scand 223:53–59, 1988.
72. Jung F, DiMarco JP. Treatment strategies for atrial fibrillation. Am J Med 104:272–286, 1998.
73. Lewis RV, Irvine N, McDevitt DG. Relationships between heart rate, exercise tolerance and cardiac output in atrial fibrillation: the effects of treatment with digoxin, verapamil and diltiazem. Eur Heart J 9:777–781, 1988.
74. Lewis RV, Laing E, Moreland TA, et al. A comparison of digoxin, diltiazem and their combination in the treatment of atrial fibrillation. Eur Heart J 9:279–283, 1988.
75. Lang R, Klein HO, Di Segni E, et al. Verapamil improves exercise capacity in chronic atrial fibrillation: double-blind crossover study. Am Heart J 105:820–825, 1983.
76. Anonymous. Drugs for cardiac arrhythmias. Med Lett Drugs Ther 38:75–82, 1996.
77. Innes GD, Vertesi L, Dillon EC, et al. Effectiveness of verapamil–quinidine versus digoxin–quinidine in the emergency department treatment of paroxysmal atrial fibrillation. Ann Emerg Med 29:126–134, 1997.
78. Roberts SA, Diaz C, Nolan PE, et al. Effectiveness and costs of digoxin treatment for atrial fibrillation and flutter. Am J Cardiol 72:567–573, 1993.
79. Beasley R, Smith DA, McHaffie DJ. Exercise heart rates at different serum digoxin concentrations in patients with atrial fibrillation. BMJ 290:9–11, 1985.
80. Goldman S, Probst P, Selzer A, et al. Inefficacy of "therapeutic" serum levels of digoxin in controlling the ventricular rate in atrial fibrillation. Am J Cardiol 35:651–655, 1975.
81. Klein GJ, Twum-Barima Y, Gulamhusein S, et al. Verapamil in chronic atrial fibrillation: variable patterns of response in ventricular rate. Clin Cardiol 7:474–483, 1984.
82. Frisolone JA. Continuous verapamil infusion. Drug Intell Clin Pharm 23:1005–1006, 1989.
83. Klein HO, Kaplinsky E. Digitalis and verapamil in atrial fibrillation and flutter. Is verapamil now the preferred agent? Drugs 31:185–197, 1986.
84. Salerno DM, Dias VC, Kleiger RE, et al. Efficacy and safety of intravenous diltiazem for treatment of atrial fibrillation and atrial flutter. The Diltiazem–Atrial Fibrillation/Flutter Study Group. Am J Cardiol 63:1046–1051, 1989.
85. Ellenbogen KA, Dias VC, Plumb VJ, et al. A placebo-controlled trial of continuous intravenous diltiazem infusion for 24-hour heart rate control during atrial fibrillation and atrial flutter: a multicenter study. J Am Coll Cardiol 18:891–897, 1991.
86. Abrams J, Allen J, Allin D, et al. Efficacy and safety of esmolol vs propranolol in the treatment of supraventricular tachyarrhythmias: a multicenter double-blind clinical trial. Am Heart J 110:913–922, 1985.
87. Anderson S, Blanski L, Byrd RC, et al. Comparison of the efficacy and safety of esmolol, a short-acting beta blocker, with placebo in the treatment of supraventricular tachyarrhythmias. The Esmolol vs Placebo Multicenter Study Group. Am Heart J 111:42–48, 1986.
88. Sung RJ, Blanski L, Kirshenbaum J, et al. Clinical experience with esmolol, a short-acting beta-adrenergic blocker in cardiac arrhythmias and myocardial ischemia. J Clin Pharmacol 26(Suppl A):A15–A26, 1986.
89. Platia EV, Michelson EL, Porterfield JK, et al. Esmolol versus verapamil in the acute treatment of atrial fibrillation or atrial flutter. Am J Cardiol 63:925–929, 1989.
90. Granberry MC. Ibutilide, a new class III antiarrhythmic agent. Am J Health Syst Pharm 55:255–260, 1998.
91. Stambler BS, Wood MA, Ellenbogen KA. Antiarrhythmic actions of intravenous ibutilide compared with procainamide during human atrial flutter and fibrillation: electrophysiological determinants of enhanced conversion efficacy. Circulation 96:4298–4306, 1997.
92. Murray KT. Ibutilide. Circulation 97:493–497, 1998.
93. Morris DC, Hurst JW. Atrial fibrillation. Curr Probl Cardiol 5:1–51, 1980.
94. Lewis RV. Atrial fibrillation. The therapeutic options. Drugs 40:841–853, 1990.
95. Harjai KJ, Mobarek SK, Cheirif J, et al. Clinical variables affecting recovery of left atrial mechanical function after cardioversion from atrial fibrillation. J Am Coll Cardiol 30:481–486, 1997.
96. Karlson BW, Herlitz J, Edvardsson N, et al. Prophylactic treatment after electroconversion of atrial fibrillation. Clin Cardiol 13:279–286, 1990.
97. Dalzell GW, Anderson J, Adgey AA. Factors determining success and energy requirements for cardioversion of atrial fibrillation: revised version. Q J Med 78:85–95, 1991.
98. Anonymous. Textbook of cardiovascular medicine. Philadelphia: Lippincott-Raven, 1998:1686.
99. Mann DL, Maisel AS, Atwood JE, et al. Absence of cardioversion-induced ventricular arrhythmias in patients with therapeutic digoxin levels. J Am Coll Cardiol 5:882–890, 1985.
100. Feld GK, Chen PS, Nicod P, et al. Possible atrial proarrhythmic effects of class 1C antiarrhythmic drugs. Am J Cardiol 66:378–383, 1990.
101. Sihm I, Hansen FA, Rasmussen J, et al. Flecainide acetate in atrial flutter and fibrillation. The arrhythmogenic effects. Eur Heart J 11:145–148, 1990.
102. MacNeil DJ, Davies RO, Deitchman D. Clinical safety profile of sotalol in the treatment of arrhythmias. Am J Cardiol 72:44A–50A, 1993.
103. Roth A, Harrison E, Mitani G, et al. Efficacy and safety of medium- and high-dose diltiazem alone and in combination with digoxin for control of heart rate at rest and during exercise in patients with chronic atrial fibrillation. Circulation 73:316–324, 1986.
104. Petersen P, Boysen G, Godtfredsen J, et al. Placebo-controlled, randomised trial of warfarin and aspirin for prevention of thromboembolic complications in chronic atrial fibrillation. The Copenhagen AFASAK study. Lancet 1:175–179, 1989.
105. Anonymous. The effect of low-dose warfarin on the risk of stroke in patients with nonrheumatic atrial fibrillation. The Boston Area Anticoagulation Trial for Atrial Fibrillation Investigators. N Engl J Med 323:1505–1511, 1990.
106. Anonymous. Stroke Prevention in Atrial Fibrillation Study. Final results. Circulation 84:527–539, 1991.
107. Connolly SJ, Laupacis A, Gent M, et al. Canadian Atrial Fibrillation Anticoagulation (CAFA) study. J Am Coll Cardiol 18:349–355, 1991.
108. Ezekowitz MD, Bridgers SL, James KE, et al. Warfarin in the prevention of stroke associated with nonrheumatic atrial fibrillation. Veterans Affairs Stroke Prevention in Nonrheumatic Atrial Fibrillation Investigators. N Engl J Med 327:1406–1412, 1992.
109. Anonymous. Treatment of atrial fibrillation. Recommendations from a workshop arranged by the Medical Products Agency (Uppsala, Sweden) and the Swedish Society of Cardiology. Eur Heart J 14:1427–1433, 1993.
110. Anonymous. 4th American College of Chest Physicians Consensus Conference on Antithrombotic Therapy. Chest 108:225S–522S, 1995.
111. Mayet J, More RS, Sutton GC. Anticoagulation for cardioversion of atrial arrhythmias. Eur Heart J 19:548–552, 1998.
112. Anonymous. Risk factors for stroke and efficacy of antithrombotic therapy in atrial fibrillation. Analysis of pooled data from five randomized controlled trials. Arch Intern Med 154:1449–1457, 1994.
113. Laupacis A, Albers G, Dunn M, et al. Antithrombotic therapy in atrial fibrillation. Chest 102:426S–433S, 1992.
114. Anonymous. Warfarin versus aspirin for prevention of thromboembolism in atrial fibrillation: Stroke Prevention in Atrial Fibrillation II Study. Lancet 343:687–691, 1994.
115. Levine MN, Hirsh J, Landefeld S, et al. Hemorrhagic complications of anticoagulant treatment. Chest 102:352S–363S, 1992.
116. Pritchett EL. Management of atrial fibrillation. N Engl J Med 326:1264–1271, 1992.
117. Cox JL, Boineau JP, Schuessler RB, et al. Five-year experience with the maze procedure for atrial fibrillation. Ann Thorac Surg 56:814–823, 1993.
118. Berry VA. Wolff–Parkinson–White syndrome and the use of radiofrequency catheter ablation. Heart Lung 22:15–25, 1993.
119. Prystowsky EN. Diagnosis and management of the preexcitation syndromes. Curr Probl Cardiol 13:225–310, 1988.
120. Porter RS. Adenosine: supplementary considerations about activity and use. Clin Pharm 9:271–274, 1990.
121. Brodsky M, Wu D, Denes P, et al. Arrhythmias documented by 24 hour continuous electrocardiographic monitoring in 50 male medical students without apparent heart disease. Am J Cardiol 39:390–395, 1977.
122. Echt DS, Liebson PR, Mitchell LB, et al. Mortality and morbidity in patients receiving encainide, flecainide, or placebo. The Cardiac Arrhythmia Suppression Trial. N Engl J Med 324:781–788, 1991.
123. Anonymous. Effect of the antiarrhythmic agent moricizine on survival after myocardial infarction. The Cardiac Arrhythmia Suppression Trial II Investigators. N Engl J Med 327:227–233, 1992.
124. Anonymous. Preliminary report: effect of encainide and flecainide on mortality in a randomized trial of arrhythmia suppression after myocardial infarction. The Cardiac Arrhythmia Suppression Trial (CAST) Investigators. N Engl J Med 321:406–412, 1989.

125. Riddle K, Lee AJ. Digibind: emergency treatment for digitalis toxicity. J Emerg Nurs 15:266–268, 1989.
126. Horowitz LN, Josephson ME, Farshidi A, et al. Recurrent sustained ventricular tachycardia 3. Role of the electrophysiologic study in selection of antiarrhythmic regimens. Circulation 58:986–997, 1978.
127. Bigger JTJ, Weld FM, Rolnitzky LM. Prevalence, characteristics and significance of ventricular tachycardia (three or more complexes) detected with ambulatory electrocardiographic recording in the late hospital phase of acute myocardial infarction. Am J Cardiol 48:815–823, 1981.
128. Manolis AS, Linzer M, Salem D, et al. Syncope: current diagnostic evaluation and management. Ann Intern Med 112:850–863, 1990.
129. Blanck Z, Dhala A, Deshpande S, et al. Catheter ablation of ventricular tachycardia. Am Heart J 127:1126–1133, 1994.
130. Moss AJ, Hall WJ, Cannom DS, et al. Improved survival with an implanted defibrillator in patients with coronary disease at high risk for ventricular arrhythmia. Multicenter Automatic Defibrillator Implantation Trial Investigators. N Engl J Med 335:1933–1940, 1996.
131. Anonymous. A comparison of antiarrhythmic-drug therapy with implantable defibrillators in patients resuscitated from near-fatal ventricular arrhythmias. N Engl J Med 337:1576–1583, 1997.
132. Gregoratos G, Cheitlin MD, Conill A, et al. ACC/AHA guidelines for implantation of cardiac pacemakers and antiarrhythmia devices: executive summary. A report of the American College of Cardiology/American Heart Association Task Force on Practice Guidelines (Committee on Pacemaker Implantation). Circulation 97:1325–1335, 1998.
133. Pieper JA, Johnson KE. Lidocaine. In: Applied pharmacokinetics. Spokane, WA: Applied Therapeutics, 1992:1–37.
134. Vozeh S, Berger M, Wenk M, et al. Rapid prediction of individual dosage requirements for lignocaine. Clin Pharmacokinet 9:354–363, 1984.
135. LeLorier J, Grenon D, Latour Y, et al. Pharmacokinetics of lidocaine after prolonged intravenous infusions in uncomplicated myocardial infarction. Ann Intern Med 87:700–706, 1977.
136. Grubb BP. Recurrence of ventricular tachycardia after conversion from proprietary to generic procainamide. Am J Cardiol 63:1532–1533, 1989.
137. Hilleman DE, Patterson AJ, Mohiuddin SM, et al. Comparative bioequivalence and efficacy of two sustained-release procainamide formulations in patients with cardiac arrhythmias. Drug Intell Clin Pharm 22:554–558, 1988.
138. Baker BA, Reynolds JR, Gleckel L, et al. Comparative bioavailability of two oral sustained-release procainamide products. Clin Pharm 7:135–138, 1988.
139. Funck-Brentano C, Light RT, Lineberry MD, et al. Pharmacokinetic and pharmacodynamic interaction of *N*-acetyl procainamide and procainamide in humans. J Cardiovasc Pharmacol 14:364–373, 1989.
140. Coyle JD, Lima JJ. Procainamide. In: Applied pharmacokinetics. Spokane, WA: Applied Therapeutics, 1992:1–33.
141. Bauer LA, Black D, Gensler A, et al. Influence of age, renal function and heart failure on procainamide clearance and *N*-acetylprocainamide serum concentrations. Int J Clin Pharmacol Ther Toxicol 27:213–216, 1989.
142. Tisdale JE, Rudis MI, Padhi ID, et al. Disposition of procainamide in patients with chronic congestive heart failure receiving medical therapy. J Clin Pharmacol 36:35–41, 1996.
143. Lima JJ, Goldfarb AL, Conti DR, et al. Safety and efficacy of procainamide infusions. Am J Cardiol 43:98–105, 1979.
144. Kuehl P, Arquin P, Fridahl J. Steady state bioavailability of a sustained release procainamide preparation. Drug Intell Clin Pharm 16:475–476, 1982.
145. Giardina EG, Fenster PE, Bigger JTJ, et al. Efficacy, plasma concentrations and adverse effects of a new sustained release procainamide preparation. Am J Cardiol 46:855–862, 1980.
146. Flanagan AD. Pharmacokinetics of a sustained release procainamide preparation. Angiology 33:71–77, 1982.
147. Yang BB, Abel RB, Uprichard AC, et al. Pharmacokinetic and pharmacodynamic comparisons of twice daily and four times daily formulations of procainamide in patients with frequent ventricular premature depolarization. J Clin Pharmacol 36:623–633, 1996.
148. Gottlieb SS, Kukin ML, Medina N, et al. Comparative hemodynamic effects of procainamide, tocainide, and encainide in severe chronic heart failure. Circulation 81:860–864, 1990.
149. Rubin RL, Curnutte JT. Metabolism of procainamide to the cytotoxic hydroxylamine by neutrophils activated in vitro. J Clin Invest 83:1336–1343, 1989.
150. Ellrodt AG, Murata GH, Riedinger MS, et al. Severe neutropenia associated with sustained-release procainamide. Ann Intern Med 100:197–201, 1984.
151. Meyers DG, Gonzalez ER, Peters LL, et al. Severe neutropenia associated with procainamide: comparison of sustained release and conventional preparations. Am Heart J 109:1393–1395, 1985.
152. Anonymous. AHFS drug information. Bethesda, MD: ASHP, 1998.
153. Sbarbaro JA, Rawling DA, Fozzard HA. Suppression of ventricular arrhythmias with intravenous disopyramide and lidocaine: efficacy comparison in a randomized trial. Am J Cardiol 44:513–520, 1979.
154. Lima JJ, Boudoulas H, Blanford M. Concentration-dependence of disopyramide binding to plasma protein and its influence on kinetics and dynamics. J Pharmacol Exp Ther 219:741–747, 1981.
155. Whiting B, Holford NH, Sheiner LB. Quantitative analysis of the disopyramide concentration–effect relationship. Br J Clin Pharmacol 9:67–75, 1980.
156. Nightingale J, Nappi JM. Effect of phenytoin on serum disopyramide concentrations. Clin Pharm 6:46–50, 1987.
157. Anonymous. MedWatch, the FDA Medical Products Reporting Program. http://www.fda.gov/medwatch/safety/1998/feb98.htm#norpac, Feb. 3, 1998.
158. Paar D, Terjung B, Sauerbruch T. Life-threatening interaction between clarithromycin and disopyramide. Lancet 349:326–327, 1997.
159. Pedersen LE, Bonde J, Graudal NA, et al. Quantitative and qualitative binding characteristics of disopyramide in serum from patients with decreased renal and hepatic function. Br J Clin Pharmacol 23:41–46, 1987.
160. Caplin JL, Johnston A, Hamer J, et al. The acute changes in serum binding of disopyramide and flecainide after myocardial infarction. Eur J Clin Pharmacol 28:253–255, 1985.
161. Capparelli EV, DiPersio DM, Zhao H, et al. Clinical pharmacokinetics of controlled-release disopyramide in patients with cardiac arrhythmias. J Clin Pharmacol 28:306–311, 1988.
162. Zema MJ. Serum drug concentrations and adverse effects in cardiac patients after administration of a new controlled-release disopyramide preparation. Ther Drug Monit 6:192–198, 1984.
163. Teichman S. The anticholinergic side effects of disopyramide and controlled-release disopyramide. Angiology 36:767–771, 1985.
164. Cacoub P, Deray G, Baumelou A, et al. Disopyramide-induced hypoglycemia: case report and review of the literature. Fundam Clin Pharmacol 3:527–535, 1989.
165. Podrid PJ, Schoeneberger A, Lown B. Congestive heart failure caused by oral disopyramide. N Engl J Med 302:614–617, 1980.
166. Lee JT, Kroemer HK, Silberstein DJ, et al. The role of genetically determined polymorphic drug metabolism in the beta-blockade produced by propafenone. N Engl J Med 322:1764–1768, 1990.
167. Bryson HM, Palmer KJ, Langtry HD, et al. Propafenone. A reappraisal of its pharmacology, pharmacokinetics and therapeutic use in cardiac arrhythmias. Drugs 45:85–130, 1993.
168. Lee SH, Chen SA, Tai CT, et al. Comparisons of oral propafenone and sotalol as an initial treatment in patients with symptomatic paroxysmal atrial fibrillation. Am J Cardiol 79:905–908, 1997.
169. Capucci A. Quinidine versus propafenone for conversion of atrial fibrillation to sinus rhythm. Am J Cardiol 81:373–374, 1998.
170. UK Propafenone PSVT Study Group. A randomized, placebo-controlled trial of propafenone in the prophylaxis of paroxysmal supraventricular tachycardia and paroxysmal atrial fibrillation. Circulation 92:2550–2557, 1995.
171. Roden DM, Woosley RL. Drug therapy. Flecainide. N Engl J Med 315:36–41, 1986.
172. Gross AS, Mikus G, Fischer C, et al. Stereoselective disposition of flecainide in relation to the sparteine/debrisoquine metaboliser phenotype. Br J Clin Pharmacol 28:555–566, 1989.
173. McQuinn RL, Pentikainen PJ, Chang SF, et al. Pharmacokinetics of flecainide in patients with cirrhosis of the liver. Clin Pharmacol Ther 44:566–572, 1988.
174. Salerno DM, Granrud G, Sharkey P, et al. Pharmacodynamics and side effects of flecainide acetate. Clin Pharmacol Ther 40:101–107, 1986.
175. Morganroth J, Anderson JL, Gentzkow GD. Classification by type of ventricular arrhythmia predicts frequency of adverse cardiac events from flecainide. J Am Coll Cardiol 8:607–615, 1986.
176. Fitton A, Buckley MT. Moricizine. A review of its pharmacological properties, and therapeutic efficacy in cardiac arrhythmias. Drugs 40:138–167, 1990.
177. Mann HJ. Moricizine: a new class I antiarrhythmic. Clin Pharm 9:842–852, 1990.
178. Nestico PF, Morganroth J, Horowitz LN. New antiarrhythmic drugs. Drugs 35:286–319, 1988.
179. Anonymous. Effects of encainide, flecainide, imipramine and moricizine on ventricular arrhythmias during the year after acute myocardial infarction: the CAPS. The Cardiac Arrhythmia Pilot Study (CAPS) Investigators. Am J Cardiol 61:501–509, 1988.
180. Bigger JT Jr. The events surrounding the removal of encainide and flecainide from the Cardiac Arrhythmia Suppression Trial (CAST) and why CAST is continuing with moricizine. J Am Coll Cardiol 15:243–245, 1990.
181. Clyne CA, Estes NA, Wang PJ. Moricizine. N Engl J Med 327:255–260, 1992.

182. Gillis AM, Kates RE. Clinical pharmacokinetics of the newer antiarrhythmic agents. Clin Pharmacokinet 9:375–403, 1984.
183. Grech-Belanger O, Gilbert M, Turgeon J, et al. Effect of cigarette smoking on mexiletine kinetics. Clin Pharmacol Ther 37:638–643, 1985.
184. Wang T, Wuellner D, Woosley RL, et al. Pharmacokinetics and nondialyzability of mexiletine in renal failure. Clin Pharmacol Ther 37:649–653, 1985.
185. Steen SN, Hughes EM, Sharon G, et al. Efficacy of oral mexiletine therapy at a 12-h dosage interval. Chest 97:358–363, 1990.
186. Singh JB, Rasul AM, Shah A, et al. Efficacy of mexiletine in chronic ventricular arrhythmias compared with quinidine: a single-blind, randomized trial. Am J Cardiol 53:84–87, 1984.
187. Giardina EG, Wechsler ME. Low dose quinidine–mexiletine combination therapy versus quinidine monotherapy for treatment of ventricular arrhythmias. J Am Coll Cardiol 15:1138–1145, 1990.
188. Duff HJ, Roden D, Primm RK, et al. Mexiletine in the treatment of resistant ventricular arrhythmias: enhancement of efficacy and reduction of dose-related side effects by combination with quinidine. Circulation 67:1124–1128, 1983.
189. Kim SG, Mercando AD, Tam S, et al. Combination of disopyramide and mexiletine for better tolerance and additive effects for treatment of ventricular arrhythmias. J Am Coll Cardiol 13:659–664, 1989.
190. Luderitz B, Mletzko R, Jung W, et al. Combination of antiarrhythmic drugs. J Cardiovasc Pharmacol 17(Suppl 6):S48–S52, 1991.
191. diMarco JP, Garan H, Ruskin JN. Mexiletine for refractory ventricular arrhythmias: results using serial electrophysiologic testing. Am J Cardiol 47:131–138, 1981.
192. Roden DM, Woosley RL. Drug therapy. Tocainide. N Engl J Med 315:41-45, 1986.
193. Rice TL, Patterson JH, Celestin C, et al. Influence of rifampin on tocainide pharmacokinetics in humans. Clin Pharm 8:200–205, 1989.
194. North DS, Mattern AL, Kapil RP, et al. The effect of histamine-2 receptor antagonists on tocainide pharmacokinetics. J Clin Pharmacol 28:640–643, 1988.
195. Wasenmiller JE, Aronow WS. Effect of tocainide and quinidine on premature ventricular contractions. Clin Pharmacol Ther 28:431–435, 1980.
196. Feinberg L, Travis WD, Ferrans V, et al. Pulmonary fibrosis associated with tocainide: report of a case with literature review. Am Rev Respir Dis 141:505–508, 1990.
197. Nappi JM, McCollam PL. Sotalol: a breakthrough antiarrhythmic? Ann Pharmacother 27:1359–1368, 1993.
198. Blair AD, Burgess ED, Maxwell BM, et al. Sotalol kinetics in renal insufficiency. Clin Pharmacol Ther 29:457–463, 1981.
199. Hohnloser SH, Woosley RL. Sotalol. N Engl J Med 331:31–38, 1994.
200. Juul-Moller S, Edvardsson N, Rehnqvist-Ahlberg N. Sotalol versus quinidine for the maintenance of sinus rhythm after direct current conversion of atrial fibrillation. Circulation 82:1932–1939, 1990.
201. Mason JW. A comparison of seven antiarrhythmic drugs in patients with ventricular tachyarrhythmias. Electrophysiologic Study Versus Electrocardiographic Monitoring Investigators. N Engl J Med 329:452–458, 1993.
202. Reiffel JE, Hahn E, Hartz V, et al. Sotalol for ventricular tachyarrhythmias, beta-blocking and class III contributions, and relative efficacy versus class I drugs after prior drug failure. Am J Cardiol 79:1048–1053, 1997.
203. Pratt C, Camm AJ, Cooper W, et al. Mortality in the Survival with Oral D-Sotalol (SWORD) trial: why did patients die? Am J Cardiol 81:869–876, 1998.
204. Roden DM. Torsade de pointes. Clin Cardiol 16:683–686, 1993.
205. Lazzara R. Antiarrhythmic drugs and torsade de pointes. Eur Heart J 14(Suppl H):88–92, 1993.
206. Iseri LT, Allen BJ, Brodsky MA. Magnesium therapy of cardiac arrhythmias in critical care medicine. Magnesium 8:299–306, 1989.
207. Chopra MP, Thadani U, Portal RW, et al. Lignocaine therapy for ventricular ectopic activity after acute myocardial infarction: a double-blind trial. BMJ 3:668–670, 1971.
208. Lie KI, Wellens HJ, van Capelle FJ, et al. Lidocaine in the prevention of primary ventricular fibrillation. A double-blind, randomized study of 212 consecutive patients. N Engl J Med 291:1324–1326, 1974.
209. Rademaker AW, Kellen J, Tam YK, et al. Character of adverse effects of prophylactic lidocaine in the coronary care unit. Clin Pharmacol Ther 40:71–80, 1986.
210. Duff HJ, Roden DM, Yacobi A, et al. Bretylium: relations between plasma concentrations and pharmacologic actions in high-frequency ventricular arrhythmias. Am J Cardiol 55:395–401, 1985.
211. Adir J, Narang PK, Josselson J. Nomogram for bretylium dosing in renal impairment. Ther Drug Monit 7:265–268, 1985.
212. Perlman PE, Adams WGJ, Ridgeway NA. Extreme pyrexia during bretylium administration. Postgrad Med 85:111–114, 1989.
213. Kowey PR, Levine JH, Herre JM, et al. Randomized, double-blind comparison of intravenous amiodarone and bretylium in the treatment of patients with recurrent, hemodynamically destabilizing ventricular tachycardia or fibrillation. Circulation 92:3255–3263, 1995.
214. Naccarelli GV, Rinkenberger RL, Dougherty AH, et al. Amiodarone: pharmacology and antiarrhythmic and adverse effects. Pharmacotherapy 5:298–313, 1985.
215. Desai AD, Chun S, Sung RJ. The role of intravenous amiodarone in the management of cardiac arrhythmias. Ann Intern Med 127:294–303, 1997.
216. Heger JJ, Prystowsky EN, Jackman WM, et al. Clinical efficacy and electrophysiology during long-term therapy for recurrent ventricular tachycardia or ventricular fibrillation. N Engl J Med 305:539–545, 1981.
217. Peter T, Hamer A, Mandel WJ, et al. Evaluation of amiodarone therapy in the treatment of drug-resistant cardiac arrhythmias: long-term follow-up. Am Heart J 106:943–950, 1983.
218. Gill J, Heel RC, Fitton A. Amiodarone. An overview of its pharmacological properties, and review of its therapeutic use in cardiac arrhythmias. Drugs 43:69–110, 1992.
219. Kerin NZ, Blevins RD, Benaderet D, et al. Relation of serum reverse T3 to amiodarone antiarrhythmic efficacy and toxicity. Am J Cardiol 57:128–130, 1986.
220. Hohnloser SH, Klingenheben T, Singh BN. Amiodarone-associated proarrhythmic effects. A review with special reference to torsade de pointes tachycardia. Ann Intern Med 121:529–535, 1994.
221. Saal AK, Werner JA, Greene HL, et al. Effect of amiodarone on serum quinidine and procainamide levels. Am J Cardiol 53:1264–1267, 1984.
222. Gosselink AT, Crijns HJ, Van Gelder IC, et al. Low-dose amiodarone for maintenance of sinus rhythm after cardioversion of atrial fibrillation or flutter. JAMA 267:3289–3293, 1992.
223. Herre JM, Sauve MJ, Malone P, et al. Long-term results of amiodarone therapy in patients with recurrent sustained ventricular tachycardia or ventricular fibrillation. J Am Coll Cardiol 13:442–449, 1989.
224. Weinberg BA, Miles WM, Klein LS, et al. Five-year follow-up of 589 patients treated with amiodarone. Am Heart J 125:109–120, 1993.
225. Anonymous. Randomized antiarrhythmic drug therapy in survivors of cardiac arrest (the CASCADE Study). Am J Cardiol 72:280–287, 1993.
226. Cairns JA, Connolly SJ, Gent M, et al. Post-myocardial infarction mortality in patients with ventricular premature depolarizations, Canadian Amiodarone Myocardial Infarction Arrhythmia Trial Pilot Study. Circulation 84:550–557, 1991.
227. Ceremuzynski L, Kleczar E, Krzeminska-Pakula M, et al. Effect of amiodarone on mortality after myocardial infarction: a double-blind, placebo-controlled, pilot study. J Am Coll Cardiol 20:1056–1062, 1992.
228. Pfisterer ME, Kiowski W, Brunner H, et al. Long-term benefit of 1-year amiodarone treatment for persistent complex ventricular arrhythmias after myocardial infarction. Circulation 87:309–311, 1993.
229. Burkart F, Pfisterer M, Kiowski W, et al. Effect of antiarrhythmic therapy on mortality in survivors of myocardial infarction with asymptomatic complex ventricular arrhythmias. Basel Antiarrhythmic Study of Infarct Survival (BASIS). J Am Coll Cardiol 16:1711–1718, 1990.
230. Caruso AC, Marcus FI, Hahn EA, et al. Predictors of arrhythmic death and cardiac arrest in the ESVEM trial. Circulation 96:1888–1892, 1997.
231. Morganroth J, Bigger JT Jr. Pharmacologic management of ventricular arrhythmias after the cardiac arrhythmia suppression trial. Am J Cardiol 65:1497–1503, 1990.
232. Anonymous. The Beta-Blocker Heart Attack Trial. Beta-Blocker Heart Attack Study Group. JAMA 246:2073–2074, 1981.
233. Hjalmarson A, Elmfeldt D, Herlitz J, et al. Effect on mortality of metoprolol in acute myocardial infarction. A double-blind randomised trial. Lancet 2:823–827, 1981.
234. Mushlin AI, Hall WJP, Zwanziger JP, et al. The cost-effectiveness of automatic implantable cardiac defibrillators: results from MADIT. Circulation 97:2129–2135, 1998.
235. Owens DK, Sanders GD, Harris RA, et al. Cost-effectiveness of implantable cardioverter defibrillators relative to amiodarone for prevention of sudden cardiac death. Ann Intern Med 126:1–12, 1997.

CHAPTER 42
ISCHEMIC HEART DISEASE

Kevin M. Sowinski

Angina pectoris is a clinical syndrome of chest discomfort caused by reversible myocardial ischemia that produces disturbances in myocardial function without causing myocardial necrosis. Myocardial ischemia occurs secondary to increased myocardial demand or decreased myocardial oxygen supply. The specific causes of increased demand or decreased supply are discussed. Myocardial ischemia causes several syndromes collectively called ischemic heart disease, which includes stable angina, variant or Prinzmetal's angina, silent myocardial ischemia, and unstable angina. The goals of therapy for the individual syndromes are discussed individually.

Overview

TREATMENT GOALS: ISCHEMIC HEART DISEASE

- Identify and treat cardiovascular risk factors, including lifestyle modifications, medical treatment, and revascularization techniques.
- Reduce the frequency and severity of anginal attacks and increase functional capacity.
- Reduce cardiovascular morbidity and mortality.

EPIDEMIOLOGY

Ischemic heart disease usually is a manifestation of atherosclerotic coronary artery disease, the leading cause of death in the United States. In 1997, coronary artery disease caused approximately 500,000 deaths (1 in every 5 deaths) in the United States.[1,2] The cost of treating coronary artery disease in 1999 was estimated at $118.2 billion.[2] It is difficult to estimate the prevalence of angina in the population as a whole because it is affected by age, gender, and cardiovascular risk factor profile. Prevalence increases with age, is greater in men, and depends on the number of cardiovascular risk factors present. The average annual mortality rate from angina secondary to atherosclerosis is 4%,[3–5] but it is highly variable and is related to coronary artery anatomy, age, gender, other cardiovascular risk factors, anginal functional class, and the ischemic syndrome (e.g., stable angina, unstable angina) with which the patient presents.[3]

PATHOPHYSIOLOGY

Angina pectoris usually is associated with large single-vessel to multivessel atherosclerotic coronary artery disease, coronary artery vasospasm, or both. Approximately 85% of patients with angina pectoris have significant coronary artery disease (defined as more than 75% atherosclerotic reduction in intraluminal area) in one of the major epicardial coronary vessels.[6] The pathogenesis of atherosclerosis is discussed in detail in a recent review.[7,8] The Second Report of the Expert Panel on Detection, Evaluation, and Treatment of High Blood Cholesterol in Adults[9] outlined the following as major risk factors for the development of atherosclerotic coronary artery disease: dyslipidemia (elevated low-density lipoprotein cholesterol or low high-density lipoprotein cholesterol), family history of premature myocardial infarction or sudden death, cigarette smoking, hypertension, diabetes mellitus, men 45 years or older and women 55 years or older or those with premature menopause not receiving estrogen replacement therapy.[9] Recently, the American Heart Association reclassified obesity as a major risk factor for the development of coronary artery disease.[10] In addition to these major risk factors, other factors that may increase cardiovascular risk are sedentary lifestyle, hypertriglyceridemia, small low-density lipoprotein particles, elevated lipoprotein concentrations, elevated serum homocysteine concentrations, abnormalities in coagulation factors, and markers of chronic infection or inflammation.[11,12]

Although most patients with ischemic heart disease have significant occlusions in at least one of the major epicardial coronary arteries, there is little correlation between the extent of atherosclerotic coronary artery disease and the severity of anginal symptoms.[13] Usually, the severity of anginal symptoms tends to be more significant in patients with multivessel coronary artery disease than in patients with single-vessel coronary artery disease, but in any given patient the extent of underlying atherosclerotic coronary artery disease cannot be predicted from the severity, nature, duration, or quality of discomfort. Two common examples of a lack of a correlation between clinical symptoms and underlying pathology are a patient with advanced three-vessel coronary artery disease who does not experience angina but only silent myocardial ischemia or a patient with Prinzmetal's (variant) angina with episodes of excruciating angina yet little or no coronary atherosclerosis.[13] In addition, the severity and duration of anginal symptoms is not necessarily related to prognosis. Prognosis is poorer in patients with left main coronary artery disease or three-vessel coronary artery disease and poor left ventricular systolic function.[3,5,13]

Myocardial ischemia is caused by an imbalance between coronary blood flow (supply) and the metabolic needs of the myocardium (demand). Myocardial ischemia occurs when myocardial oxygen demand exceeds myocardial oxygen supply. It is useful to describe the determinants of myocardial oxygen supply and demand because drug therapy is designed to affect the balance between these variables (Fig. 42.1). The major determinants of myocardial oxygen demand are heart rate, contractility, and left ventricular systolic wall tension.[14] Of the three determinants, heart rate is likely to be the most important, the one most easily adjusted with current drug therapies, and the easiest to assess clinically. Myocardial contractility is the rate of rise in the intraventricular pressure during isovolumetric contraction and is influenced by a number of variables, including the autonomic nervous system, heart rate, blood calcium concentration, and body temperature. Clinical assessment of the beneficial effects of drugs on myocardial contractility is difficult. The third determinant, systolic wall tension, is directly related to the ventricular systolic pressure and ventricular radius and is inversely related to wall thickness. Preload and afterload are important components of these factors. Reducing systolic blood pressure reduces afterload, which ultimately decreases oxygen demand. Reductions in preload reduce left ventricular dimension and ultimately reduce myocardial oxygen demand. One can clinically estimate myocardial oxygen demand by using the double-product (product of heart rate and systolic blood pressure). Although the double-product provides a useful estimate of myocardial oxygen demand, it does not account for contractility as an important factor.

Myocardial oxygen supply is determined by two factors: coronary blood flow and the oxygen-carrying capacity of blood.[14] Although the oxygen-carrying capacity can be affected by certain conditions (e.g., anemia), the most important determinant of myocardial oxygen supply is coronary blood flow. Normally, the arteriolar resistance

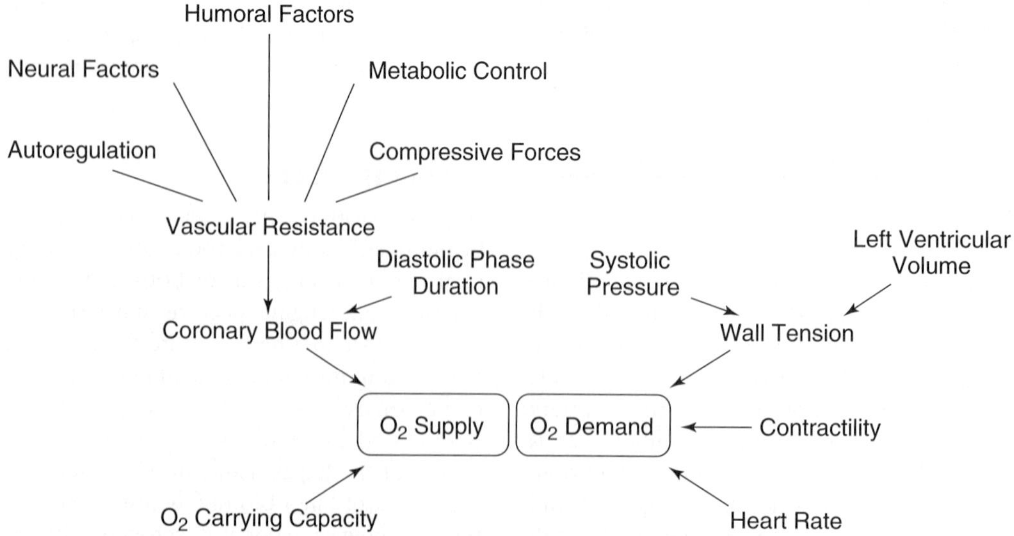

Figure 42.1. Factors affecting myocardial oxygen supply and demand. (Adapted with permission from Ardehali A, Ports TA. Myocardial oxygen supply and demand. Chest 98:699–705, 1990.)

vessels are the most important regulators of coronary blood flow, whereas large epicardial vessels are low-resistance vessels. Myocardial ischemia develops when narrowing of the epicardial vessels by vasospasm or atherosclerosis results in high enough resistance to restrict coronary blood flow. Complex factors that determine coronary blood flow include duration of diastole and coronary vascular resistance. Coronary vascular resistance is determined by metabolic control, autoregulation, extravascular compressive forces, and humoral and neural factors.

Finally, drugs may precipitate ischemia by increasing myocardial oxygen demand or decreasing myocardial oxygen supply. A few examples of these agents are cocaine (increased demand via increased heart rate and blood pressure and decreased supply via coronary vasoconstriction), ergot alkaloids (decreased supply via coronary vasoconstriction), and β-agonists (increased demand via increased heart rate).

CLINICAL PRESENTATION AND DIAGNOSIS

Signs and Symptoms

Chronic stable angina pectoris is called stable because the characteristics of a given patient's anginal history (e.g., frequency, severity, duration of symptoms, time of day) have not changed over the previous 2 months.[1,13] Patients with stable angina often are classified as having either mainly fixed-threshold angina or mainly variable-threshold angina. Anginal syndromes in patients with fixed-threshold angina or exertional angina are precipitated by increased myocardial oxygen demand and tend to occur at some reproducible level of myocardial work. This type of angina is caused by increased myocardial oxygen demand, associated with a fixed obstruction of an epicardial coronary artery by an atherosclerotic plaque. During periods of increased metabolic demand (e.g., physical exertion), delivery of oxygen-carrying blood through the stenotic atherosclerotic coronary artery is insufficient to meet the myocardium's oxygen needs, resulting in myocardial ischemia. Typically, a patient can predict what level of physical activity is likely to produce an anginal attack (e.g., walking up two flights of stairs, walking around the block). On any given day this is fairly reproducible. In contrast, patients with variable-threshold angina have difficulty predicting when or with what level of exertion they will experience an anginal attack. Daily anginal threshold is extremely variable, causing these patients to have good and bad days. The reason for the somewhat variable threshold for causing angina probably is related to a predominance of a vasoconstrictive component, leading to decreased oxygen supply and subsequent myocardial ischemia. Although most people with variable-threshold angina have some degree of atherosclerosis, dynamic narrowing of the coronary vasculature by coronary vasoconstriction is important in the genesis of anginal symptoms. Although it is easy to classify angina into the two extremes of increased demand or decreased supply, most patients fall somewhere in between, with a condition often called mixed angina.[15]

Classically, angina presents as substernal, retrosternal, or transsternal discomfort that radiates, usually to the neck and left arm. Some patients may experience radiation to other areas of the body, including the right arm. The quality of discomfort varies from patient to patient, which reflects wide variability in the way in which patients perceive pain and discomfort. The discomfort usually is a dull rather than a sharp or stabbing pain, and patients may describe it as a strangling or constricting sensation. Patients often use the following descriptors to describe the discomfort: *pressure, heaviness, fullness, squeezing, burning, aching, gas, vise-like,* or *anxiety*. It is important to realize that the severity of discomfort may range from slight discomfort to disabling pain. Anginal discomfort usually has a gradual onset and lasts only a few minutes if the precipitating factor is removed, and relief usually is afforded by rest or sublingual nitroglycerin. Longer durations of angina may imply severe ischemia, coronary vasospasm, unstable angina, or impending or ongoing myocardial infarction. Symptoms lasting for several days are unlikely to be angina. The frequency of anginal attacks ranges from several per day to one per week or month. Anginal frequency determines the specific need for therapy; this is discussed in more detail later. The New York Heart Association or the Canadian Cardiovascular Society functional classification (Table 42.1) for angina often is used to assess the frequency and patterns of angina in a given patient. The classifications are useful in documenting improvements or worsening in patient status. In addition to the functional classifications, patient diaries documenting times and duration of anginal episodes and consumption of sublingual nitroglycerin may be used to classify anginal patterns and to monitor the effectiveness of prophylactic drug therapy. Examples of activities that can be carried out by patients in each functional class are given in Table 42.1. An increase in the consumption of sublingual nitroglycerin or the number or duration of anginal episodes suggests worsening of the disease process or ineffectiveness of prophylactic drug therapy.

Factors associated with provocation of anginal episodes include physical exertion, emotions (e.g., anger, excitation, frustration, anxiety), exposure to cold, heat and humidity, meals, and sexual intercourse. Patients with variable-threshold angina tend to complain of angina evoked by changes in air temperature, emotion, and meals. As described earlier, factors that tend to increase myocardial oxygen demand (exertion, sexual intercourse) precipitate angina in patients with fixed obstructions.

Certain patients may not experience typical symptoms of angina when experiencing myocardial ischemia but rather have anginal equivalents. Anginal equivalents are episodes of myocardial ischemia that result in symptoms of systolic or diastolic left ventricular dysfunction but are not necessarily associated with chest discomfort or other symptoms characteristic of anginal discomfort. Anginal equivalents usually are caused by exertion and are relieved by rest or nitroglycerin. Common symptoms of anginal equivalents include exertional dyspnea, fatigue, and exhaustion.

Table 42.1 ▪ Classification of Angina Pectoris

Class	New York Heart Association Functional Classification	Canadian Cardiovascular Society Functional Classification	Specific Activity Scale
I	Symptoms occur with unusual activity. Minimal or no functional impairment.	Angina does not occur with ordinary physical activity (walking, climbing stairs) but may occur with strenuous, rapid, or prolonged exertion (work, recreation).	Patients can perform to completion any activity involving ≤7 metabolic equivalents (e.g., can carry 24 lb up eight steps, carry objects that weigh 80 lb, do outdoor work (shovel snow, spade soil), do recreational activities (skiing, basketball, squash, handball, jogging or walking 5 mph).
II	Symptoms occur with prolonged or slightly more than usual activity. Mild functional impairment.	Slight limitation of ordinary activity. Angina may occur with walking or climbing stairs rapidly; after meals, in the cold, in the wind, or under emotional stress; with walking uphill; and with walking more than two level blocks and climbing one flight of stairs at a normal pace under normal conditions.	Patients can perform to completion any activity involving ≤5 metabolic equivalents (e.g., have sexual intercourse without stopping, garden, rake, weed, rollerskate, dance foxtrot, walk at 4 mph on level ground) but cannot perform to completion any activity involving ≥7 metabolic equivalents.
III	Symptoms occur with usual activities of daily living. Moderate functional impairment.	Marked limitation of ordinary physical activity. Angina may occur after walking one or two level blocks or climbing one flight of stairs in normal conditions at a normal pace.	Patients can perform to completion any activity involving ≤2 metabolic equivalents (e.g., shower without stopping, strip and make bed, clean windows, walk 2.5 mph, play golf, dress without stopping) but cannot perform to completion any activity involving ≥5 metabolic equivalents.
IV	Symptoms occur at rest. Severe functional impairment.	Inability to carry on any physical activity without discomfort. Angina may be present at rest.	Patients cannot perform to completion any activity involving ≥2 metabolic equivalents.

Source: Adapted with permission from Goldman L, Hashimoto B, Loscalzo A. Comparative reproducibility and validity of systems for assessing cardiovascular functional class: advantages of a new specific activity scale. Circulation 64:1227, 1981. Copyright 1981, American Heart Association.

Many patients also have myocardial ischemia in the absence of any objective signs of angina or anginal equivalents, which is called silent myocardial ischemia. Silent myocardial ischemia is detected by exercise electrocardiogram (ECG) testing (as asymptomatic ST segment depression) and/or by ambulatory ECG testing.[16,17] Patients with silent myocardial ischemia are categorized into three types: patients with coronary artery disease who are totally asymptomatic, patients who have had a myocardial infarction and have asymptomatic ischemia, and patients who experience both symptomatic and asymptomatic ischemia. The incidence of silent myocardial ischemia varies depending on the patient characteristics. In totally asymptomatic patients, the incidence is 4 to 5%, whereas after myocardial infarction it is 30 to 42%.[16,17] Silent myocardial ischemia is extremely common in patients with symptomatic ischemia and ranges from 44 to 88% depending on the series of patients studied.[16,17] The prognosis of silent myocardial ischemia also varies with the type of patient. Asymptomatic patients with coronary artery disease who have abnormal stress ECG tests are at greater risk of coronary events, including myocardial infarction and death, than the general population.[17] The prognosis in patients who have asymptomatic ischemia after myocardial infarction appears to be similar or slightly worse than in other survivors of myocardial infarction with symptomatic ischemia. Finally, patients who have symptomatic and asymptomatic ischemic episodes are likely to have greater risk of myocardial infarction and death than patients with only symptomatic ischemia.[16,17]

Variant angina or Prinzmetal's angina is myocardial ischemia associated with coronary artery vasospasm and is not necessarily associated with atherosclerotic coronary artery disease. Imbalance between myocardial oxygen supply and demand is caused by reduced myocardial oxygen supply due to a critical narrowing of a large epicardial coronary vessel. The clinical manifestations of variant angina are similar to those seen with stable angina, although the pain may be somewhat more intense. The patient's history of angina is usually quite different from chronic stable angina because pain usually occurs at rest, most often between midnight and 8:00 AM.[18]

Circadian rhythms are known to affect anginal occurrence. In fact, the incidence of myocardial infarction, sudden cardiac death, Prinzmetal's angina, silent myocardial ischemia, and myocardial ischemia associated with stable angina is higher in the morning.[19] In addition, the threshold for precipitating anginal attacks tends to be lower in the morning. This phenomenon may lead patients to experience anginal attacks in the morning at lower levels of exertion than would be necessary at other times of day. Patients should be instructed to perform morning activities at a somewhat slower pace to minimize the possibility of provoking myocardial ischemia.

Diagnosis

Clinical Findings

The physical examination may be normal in patients with ischemic heart disease or it may reveal the presence of other risk factors for development of atherosclerotic coronary artery disease. The resting ECG is normal in approximately one-half of patients with chronic stable angina. Abnormal ECG findings include ST segment depression, T-wave inversion, and in patients with Prinzmetal's angina, ST segment elevation.[1] Ambulatory ECG monitoring may be useful in detecting symptomatic and asymptomatic ischemic episodes, as in patients with silent myocardial ischemia.

Exercise Testing

Treadmill or bicycle exercise testing provides a reproducible, objective way to study the relationship between myocardial oxygen supply and myocardial oxygen demand.[20,21] Exercise testing usually is conducted by a specific protocol, such as the Bruce or Naughton protocol.[1,20,21] These protocols allow for incremental increases in exercise work load by increasing the speed and incline of the treadmill. Endpoints measured during exercise testing include duration of exercise, workload achieved, ECG changes, blood pressure, heart rate, and symptoms. As described earlier, the product of heart rate and systolic blood pressure (i.e., the double-product) is used as an index of myocardial oxygen consumption. In patients with known ischemic heart disease (i.e., presence of angina symptoms, previous myocardial infarction), exercise electrocardiography provides important prognostic information.[22] In addition, exercise testing with concomitant ECG monitoring may be useful in patients with an equivocal history of chest pain, for risk stratification, to determine whether medical or surgical treatment is appropriate, and for assessing drug efficacy. Short exercise duration with anginal symptoms, exercise-induced hypotension, and early onset of angina with ST segment depression are all poor prognostic signs for development of cardiovascular events. It should be noted that exercise testing in the presence of drug therapy, notably β-blockers and calcium channel blockers, may complicate the interpretation of exercise testing by reducing the maximum heart rate achieved during exercise.

Radionuclide Imaging

Other techniques are also useful in diagnosing and classifying ischemic heart disease at rest and during exercise.[23–25] Thallium-201 myocardial perfusion scanning can be used in conjunction with exercise testing to provide additional information about reversible and irreversible defects in blood flow to the myocardium. Thallium is a potassium analog that is transported into normal cardiac cells. Thallium is injected at peak exercise, and the patient undergoes a myocardial scanning procedure. Perfusion defects that are detected at this point can represent either infarcted tissue or stress-induced ischemic tissues. Two to three hours later the patient undergoes repeat myocardial scanning and perfusion defects, which are no longer present represent areas of reversible ischemia rather than infarction. Ischemic areas that on the first scan produced defects will now contain thallium. Thallium myocardial perfusion scanning in conjunction with exercise testing appears to be more sensitive and specific in the diagnosis of coronary artery disease but is more expensive than exercise testing alone, cannot usually be performed in a physician's office, and entails radionuclide injection. It should be reserved for special cases and almost always a regular exercise test should be used first.[1,23,24] In patients who are unable to exercise because of certain medical conditions (e.g., advanced age, peripheral vascular disease), alternative tests are available that use pharmacologic agents to simulate the stress of exercise. Pharmacologic stress-testing techniques[25] include dipyridamole- or adenosine-induced vasodilation and dobutamine stress echocardiography in conjunction with thallium myocardial scanning.

Other Diagnostic Techniques

Two-dimensional echocardiography may be useful in detecting myocardial wall motion abnormalities at rest and ischemic-induced wall motion abnormalities during exercise. Echocardiography in conjunction with exercise testing may provide additional information about left ventricular function that would not be provided by exercise testing alone.

Although each of these tests yields important diagnostic and prognostic information in patients with coronary artery disease, definitive diagnosis and assessment of prognosis can be attained only by cardiac catheterization, coronary arteriography, and left ventricular angiography.[26] These methods allow assessment of the severity of coronary anatomy obstruction and assessment of ventricular function. Left heart cardiac catheterization is accomplished by inserting a catheter into the brachial or femoral artery and advancing it into the left ventricle and coronary arteries. During coronary angiography, injections of radiocontrast dye are made into the coronary arteries and the coronary artery anatomy is visualized and extent of coronary obstruction assessed. Because of the cost of this procedure and the risk associated with it, it has been suggested that coronary angiography should be considered only under the certain circumstances. Patients who may benefit from this procedure include those whose angina is unresponsive to maximal medical therapy and who are being considered for revascularization procedures (discussed later in the chapter) or in patients in whom the definitive diagnosis of coronary artery disease cannot be made by less invasive means.

PSYCHOSOCIAL ASPECTS

Alterations in lifestyle are also important in patients with angina because of certain factors that may provoke anginal episodes. Including the patient's family in discussions about lifestyle modifications may help patient compliance, but more importantly it fosters a family understanding of certain limitations that may be placed on the patient. Patients should be counseled to modify their participation in strenuous activities in an attempt to avoid excessive fatigue and exhaustion (e.g., using a golf cart rather than walking while playing golf). Another lifestyle modification would be reducing or eliminating factors known to precipitate an anginal episode. Some patients may know exactly how much exertion they can tolerate before having an anginal attack; other patients may need to learn what the threshold is. In general, patients should perform morning activities at a slower pace and avoid sudden bursts of activity. Patients who are particularly susceptible to heat-precipitated anginal attacks should have air conditioning. A patient who develops angina when going outside when it is very cold should cover his or her mouth and face with a scarf. Eating small meals or napping after meals may help to prevent postprandial anginal attacks. Finally, emotional outbursts (e.g., anger, anxiety, frustration) should be avoided.

THERAPEUTIC PLAN

The management of ischemic heart disease involves five areas: identifying and treating concomitant conditions that may exacerbate or precipitate ischemia, correcting concomitant cardiovascular risk factors, and implementing lifestyle modifications, medical treatment, and revascularization techniques. Treatment strategies for ischemic heart disease syndromes have traditionally been targeted at symptom relief, with nitrates, β-blockers, and calcium channel blockers. However, there is little evidence that this strategy alone reduces cardiovascular mortality. There is considerable evidence that aspirin[27–30] and appropriate lipid-lowering therapy[31–33] reduce cardiovascular morbidity and mortality. Thus, the goals of treatment for ischemic heart disease are to minimize the frequency and severity of angina and increase functional capacity, while causing as few adverse effects as possible, and to reduce cardiovascular morbidity and mortality.

Treatment guidelines for patients with chronic stable angina were developed and published by a joint task force of the American College of Cardiology, American Heart Association, American College of Physicians, and American Society of Internal Medicine in 1999. The guideline is available electronically (http://www.americanheart.org/Scientific/statements/) or can be obtained from the American College of Cardiology (Reprint No. 71-0166).

TREATMENT

Risk Factor Reduction

Because most patients with ischemic heart disease have underlying coronary artery disease, correcting and treating all modifiable cardiovascular risk factors is essential in an effort to reduce the risk of future vascular events. Risk factor reduction should focus on hypertension management, smoking cessation, lipid-lowering therapy, antiplatelet therapy, and cardiac rehabilitation and exercise. Hypertension treatment reduces cardiovascular morbidity and mortality and is the focus of Chapter 39. Blood pressure reduction also reduces myocardial oxygen demand and thus benefits patients with angina. Smoking cessation is especially important in patients with ischemic heart disease. Smoking is associated with increased morbidity and mortality, silent ischemia, arrhythmias, and coronary vasospasm in patients with coronary artery disease.[34] Pharmacologic and nonpharmacologic approaches are available to help patients with smoking cessation. Lipid-lowering drug therapy in patients with angina or prior myocardial infarction with average[33] and elevated serum cholesterol concentrations[31,32] has been shown to reduce cardiovascular morbidity and mortality. A detailed discussion of lipid-lowering therapy is the focus of Chapter 20.

Platelet aggregation is important in the pathogenesis of the acute coronary syndromes but less important in the pathogenesis of stable angina. Data from two studies in patients with chronic stable angina[27,28] show that aspirin reduced the incidence of first myocardial infarction. The mechanism of aspirin's benefit appears to be an inhibition of platelet aggregation and thrombus formation at the site of atherosclerotic plaque disruption. Although the lowest effective dosage is controversial, it is recommended that all patients with angina or clinical or laboratory evidence of ischemic heart disease receive aspirin (160 to 325 mg/day) indefinitely.[29]

Exercise training reduces cardiovascular mortality, improves functional capacity, and attenuates myocardial ischemia and thus is an important lifestyle modification. Exercise programs should adhere to accepted guidelines[35,36] for patients with heart disease. Exercise programs are useful as adjuncts to reducing other coronary risk factors such as obesity, diabetes, and hypertension. Exercise has a beneficial conditioning effect on both skeletal and cardiac muscle and may decrease oxygen demand for any level of exercise. Exercise also favorably effects fat and carbohydrate metabolism, which may reduce cardiovascular risk. Other cardiovascular risk factor reductions should include weight loss if overweight, alcohol use only in moderation,[34] and estrogen replacement therapy in postmenopausal women. Finally, epidemiologic evidence suggests that the increased intake of vitamins (vitamin E, vitamin C, folic acid) is associated with reduced coronary artery disease risk,[37,38] but data from clinical trials are needed before these therapies gain widespread acceptance.

Although risk factor reductions may not reverse existing coronary artery disease, they may aid in the secondary prevention of cardiovascular events. As with any disease or syndrome that increases cardiovascular risk (e.g., hypertension), the first goal of therapy is to decrease cardiovascular risk.

Pharmacotherapy

Pharmacology of Agents Used for Treatment of Ischemic Heart Disease

Nitrates

Mechanism of Action. Organic nitrates are prodrugs and must be converted to their active moiety before they can cause a therapeutic effect. The intracellular mechanism of action of organic nitrates is complex, although organic nitrates are known to be denitrated and liberate nitric oxide. Nitric oxide reacts further with sulfhydryl groups to form S-nitrosothiols. The presence of sulfhydryl groups is necessary for the formation of nitric oxide and S-nitrosothiols and subsequent stimulation of guanylate cyclase.[39,40] Nitric oxide and/or S-nitrosothiols can activate smooth muscle guanylate cyclase, resulting in intracellular cyclic guanosine monophosphate (cGMP) formation. Cyclic guanosine monophosphate decreases intracellular calcium concentrations by increasing calcium extrusion from the cell.[39,40]

Nitrates act as vasodilators in virtually all vascular beds, including veins, arteries, and arterioles. However, higher concentrations are needed for vasodilatory effects in arteries and arterioles than in veins. This is especially true for arterioles, which need concentrations that may not be achieved clinically.[41] Hemodynamically, nitrates cause venodilation and thus reduce venous tone, decrease venous return, and decrease preload, resulting in reductions in myocardial oxygen demand. Additionally, at higher dosages, nitrates may cause arterial vasodilation, causing decreased systolic blood pressure and afterload, resulting in reductions in myocardial oxygen demand. However, because nitrates are such potent vasodilators, they may cause reflex sympathetic discharge, attenuating some of the beneficial effects seen by nitrates.[40,41]

Nitrates may also have several effects on the coronary circulation, including enhancing coronary collateral blood flow, dilating normal coronary arteries in patients with atherosclerosis, and dilating stenotic coronary vessels. Finally, nitrates may reverse coronary vasospasm, making them particularly useful in treating vasospastic angina. These effects may lead to increases in myocardial oxygen supply.

Nitrate Tolerance. A decreased pharmacologic response in the presence of continuously or frequently administered nitrates is well documented and is called nitrate tolerance. Examples of regimens showing the development of tolerance are 24-hour applications of transdermal nitroglycerin, continuous infusions of intravenous nitroglycerin, immediate-release isosorbide dinitrate (ISDN) administered four times daily, sustained-release isosorbide dinitrate (ISDN-SR) administered every 12 hours, and immediate-release isosorbide mononitrate (ISMN) administered every 12 hours. It is likely that all nitrates cause some degree of tolerance and attenuation of pharmacologic effect if used continuously.[42] Both the hemodynamic and antianginal effects are attenuated with continuous administration. The mechanism of nitrate tolerance is complicated. A variety of mechanisms have been proposed, including depletion of sulfhydryl donors, impairing the intracellular formation of nitric oxide and S-nitrosothiols, resulting in decreased formation of cGMP; sympathetic activation after vasodilation, producing reflex vasoconstriction and sodium retention; vascular production of endothelin-1; plasma volume expansion, minimizing the ability of nitrates to decrease left ventricular filling pressures; and increased production of superoxide anion, which leads to degradation of nitric oxide.[40,42]

The prevention of nitrate tolerance via pharmacologic intervention has been attempted with angiotensin-converting enzyme inhibitors, thiazide diuretics, and sulfhydryl donor compounds, although none have been effective clinically.[40,42] Clinically, preventing nitrate tolerance involves the provision of a daily nitrate-free interval. Nitrate-free intervals of at least 10 hours per day with chronic dosing have been shown to reduce the occurrence of nitrate tolerance.[43–45] The time of day for providing a nitrate-free interval usually is at night, but in patients who have nocturnal angina (i.e., most of their attacks at night) it would be prudent to move the nitrate-free interval to the daytime. Although nitrate-free intervals may benefit those who have angina that occurs predictably, patients with severe or unpredictable (occurs day and night) angina would be left unprotected during the nitrate-free interval. In such patients, using either β-blockers (alone or in combination with nitrates) or calcium channel blockers (alone or in combination with nitrates) would be appropriate.

Nitrate Products. Table 42.2 lists the nitrates available for clinical use. Sublingual nitroglycerin is used to treat acute episodes of angina and to prevent an expected anginal episode. It has been shown to be effective at increasing exercise time and relieving acute anginal symptoms and is available as sublingual tablets and aerosol spray. In the event of an acute attack, the patient should be instructed to sit or lie down, place the dose (spray or tablet) under his or her tongue, and not swallow the tablet. Pain relief should occur within 5 minutes. If the pain is not relieved by this time, the process may be repeated until a total of three doses have been given (about 15 minutes), after which time the patient should contact a physician or go to an emergency room. Failure of nitroglycerin to control the pain may be an indication of more serious ischemia or myocardial infarction. Adverse effects seen with sublingual nitroglycerin include light-headedness, dizziness, tachycardia, and headache. Patients may or may not experience burning under the tongue after taking the sublingual dose; the absence of this sensation does not necessarily indicate a lack of potency.

Nitroglycerin is a labile compound that requires special storage and handling. Sublingual tablets should be dispensed in the original, unopened manufacturer's brown bottle. When the bottle is opened the patient should remove the cotton plug and discard it. The tablets should be stored in the manufacturer's brown bottle in a cool, dry place to avoid degradation of the tablets. Patients should be instructed to refill their prescriptions frequently (approximately every 6 months) to ensure adequate potency of the tablets. Because of the storage problems associated with sublingual nitroglycerin, the aerosol spray dosage form has some distinct advantages. Each canister has a shelf life of 3 years, has 200 metered doses, and does not need the same rigid storage conditions as the tablets. The adverse effects and efficacy of each product are similar.[46]

Table 42.2 ▪ Pharmacologic Characteristics of Currently Available Nitrates

Indication Drug and Dosage Form	Route of Administration	Dosage Range	Frequency of Administration (Dosing Interval)
Treating acute anginal attacks			
Nitroglycerin sublingual tablets	Oral, sublingual	0.15–0.6 mg	As needed, repeat dose 1–3 times every 5 min
Nitroglycerin sublingual spray	Oral, sublingual	0.4–0.8 mg	As needed, repeat dose 1–3 times every 5 min
Nitroglycerin buccal tablets	Oral, sublingual	1–3 mg	Once
ISDN chewable tablets	Oral, chewable	2.5–10 mg	Once
ISDN sublingual tablets	Oral, sublingual	5–10 mg	Once
Preventing anginal attacks			
Nitroglycerin tablets	Oral, sublingual	0.15–0.6 mg	2–5 min before activity
Nitroglycerin spray	Oral, sublingual	0.4–0.8 mg	2–5 min before activity
Nitroglycerin tablets	Oral, buccal	1–3 mg	2–5 min before activity or every 4–5 hr while awake
Isosorbide dinitrate tablets	Oral, chewable	5–10 mg	5–10 min before activity
Isosorbide dinitrate tablets	Oral, sublingual	2.5–10 mg	5–10 min before activity
Nitroglycerin SR tablets and capsules	Oral	2.6–13 mg	2–3 times per day; 12-hr dosage free interval[a]
Nitroglycerin ointment	Transdermal	0.5–2 in.	3–4 times per day; 12-hr dosage-free interval[a]
Nitroglycerin patch	Transdermal	0.1–0.8 mg/hr	Once daily; 12-hr dosage-free interval
Isosorbide dinitrate tablets	Oral	5–40 mg	3 times per day; 14-hr dosage-free interval
Isosorbide dinitrate SR capsules and tablets	Oral	40–80 mg	1–2 times per day; 16-hr dosage-free interval[a]
Isosorbide mononitrate tablets	Oral	10–20 mg	2 times per day; 7-hr dosage-free interval
Isosorbide mononitrate SR tablets	Oral	30–240 mg	Once daily

ISDN, isosorbide dinitrate; *SR,* sustained release.

[a]No data are available evaluating the long-term efficacy of these products. The nitrate dosage-free intervals are estimated.

Buccal nitroglycerin tablets provide both immediate and long-term nitroglycerin delivery. The tablet is placed on the gum between the upper teeth and inner lip. A gel forms around the tablet that contains nitroglycerin impregnated in a cellulose matrix. The tablet can stay in place for hours and provides both immediate and sustained nitroglycerin delivery as long as the tablet remains intact, which may be as long as 6 hours in some patients. This is advantageous in that the tablet can provide both acute and prophylactic treatment of anginal episodes. Tolerance to the effects of buccal nitroglycerin is minimal, mainly because the tablet is not in place while the patient sleeps, allowing a nitrate-free interval.

Oral sustained-release formulations of nitroglycerin are available that are administered every 8 to 12 hours. However, there are no data suggesting that chronic efficacy is maintained throughout the dosing interval. Thus, no data are available to determine which dosing regimen would prevent tolerance (Table 42.2).

Nitroglycerin 2% ointment has documented efficacy in patients with angina.[47] It is easy to use but rather inconvenient for patients because of the messiness involved with application of ointment. Patients should be instructed to apply the specified dose (ranges from 0.5 to 2 inches) of ointment to the chest, back, or upper limbs. Patients should rotate the application site daily to reduce skin irritation. Family members or other people applying the ointment to the patient should be instructed to use gloves during the application because of the chance of nitroglycerin absorption through the skin. The ointment can be removed easily by removing the paper containing the ointment and wiping the skin clean of any residual ointment. There will be continued absorption of nitroglycerin for a short time because the skin acts as a reservoir for the drug.

Another form of topically available nitroglycerin, which has become enormously popular since its introduction in 1982, is the nitroglycerin transdermal patch. These patches were designed to deliver a constant amount of nitroglycerin per hour over a specific time period, maintaining nitroglycerin concentrations at steady state. Patients should be instructed to apply a new patch each day to a hairless area of the chest, back, or upper limbs. The site should be rotated daily to prevent local skin irritation. Various factors may increase drug absorption, including physical exercise and high temperatures (e.g., saunas). The ease of administration as compared to nitroglycerin ointment has made these agents very popular with patients. However, rapid development of nitrate tolerance[48,49] necessitates that patients wear the patch no more than 12 hours per day. Provision of a 12-hour nitrate-free period leads to effective exercise improvement in patients with angina.[43,50]

Two oral organic nitrates are available in the United States: ISDN and 5-ISMN. 5-ISMN is a metabolite of ISDN. Both ISDN and 5-ISMN are available as immediate-release and sustained-release preparations. Isosorbide dinitrate is also available as a sublingual and chewable tablet, which can be used to treat and prevent acute anginal episodes. The sublingual tablet has a somewhat slower onset of action and a longer duration of action than sublingual nitroglycerin. The chewable tablet also has a longer duration of action than sublingual nitroglycerin. When patients chew the tablet, particles remain in the mouth and continue to be absorbed.

Isosorbide dinitrate has widely variable bioavailability and a plasma half-life of 1 to 2 hours, whereas 5-ISMN has nearly complete bioavailability and a longer plasma half-life,[51] resulting in more predictable concentrations after oral dosing and allowing once- or twice-daily dosing. Tolerance to the pharmacologic effects of ISDN and 5-ISMN have been described for both agents in the immediate-release and sustained-release preparations.[44,52] ISDN tolerance is avoided by using the immediate-release compound three times daily at 7:00 AM, noon, and 5:00 PM.[44] This regimen provides a nitrate-free interval during the night. Twice-daily dosing schedules of immediate-release 5-ISMN, administered at 8:00 AM and 3:00 PM, enhanced exercise performance for 7 hours after the morning dose and 5 hours after the afternoon dose.[45,53] Sustained-release 5-ISMN has been shown to be effective for up to 12 hours per day when administered once daily, so it is recommended this agent be given once daily.[54]

ADVERSE EFFECTS. Adverse effects caused by all nitrates are an extension of their pharmacologic actions. Headache occurs in most patients and may be described as a throbbing or pulsating sensation. Most patients can take over-the-counter analgesics (e.g., aspirin, acetaminophen) to alleviate this problem. Other adverse effects related to vasodilation include hypotension, dizziness, lightheadedness, and facial flushing. Patients may need lower dosages if these adverse effects occur after sublingual doses of nitroglycerin. Reflex tachycardia may also result from nitrates' potent peripheral vasodilating effects, which causes sympathetic nervous system activation. Patients should be instructed to vary the application site of nitroglycerin ointment and transdermal patches to avoid local skin irritation.

β-Blockers

MECHANISM OF ACTION. β-Adrenergic receptor blockers competitively inhibit the binding of circulating and neurally released catecholamines to the β-adrenergic receptor.[55,56] β-Receptor blockade attenuates the cardiac responses to adrenergic stimulation by catecholamines. β-Blockers have several beneficial effects in ischemic heart disease. First, β-blockers reduce heart rate mainly during times of sympathetic stimulation, which results in reduced cardiac work and thus reduced myocardial oxygen demand. In addition, by slowing heart rate, β-blockers increase diastolic filling time, resulting in increased coronary perfusion and improved oxygen supply. Second, β-blockers reduce myocardial contractility and arterial blood pressure and thereby reduce myocardial oxygen demand. A potential problem with β-blockers is that they may cause coronary vasoconstriction. With blockade of β_2-receptors, which mediate vasodilation, there is unopposed α-receptor–mediated coronary vasoconstriction. This is a particular concern in patients with rest or variant angina, where β-blockers could potentially precipitate an anginal episode.

PHARMACOLOGIC CHARACTERISTICS. The β-blockers differ in their pharmacologic characteristics, including receptor selectivity, pharmacokinetics, lipophilicity, and intrinsic sympathomimetic activity (ISA; Table 42.3).[55,56] β-Adrenergic receptors are classified into at least two subtypes (β_1 and β_2-adrenoceptors) based on the physiologic responses they mediate. β_1-Receptors reside primarily in the myocardium, and their stimulation results in increased heart rate, myocardial contractility, and atrioventricular (AV) nodal conduction. β_2-Receptors also reside in the heart but are the predominant receptors in pulmonary and vascular tissue, where they are responsible for broncho-

Table 42.3 ▪ Pharmacologic Characteristics of the Currently Available β-Blockers

Agent	Receptor Selectivity	ISA	Lipid Solubility	Primary Route of Elimination	Half-Life (hr)	Usual Maintenance Dosage
Acebutolol	β_1	+	Moderate	Renal and hepatic	3–4	200–600 mg BID
Atenolol[a]	β_1	0	Low	Renal	6–9	50–100 mg QD
Betaxolol	β_1	0	Low	Hepatic	14–22	10–20 mg QD
Bisoprolol	β_1	0	Low	Renal	9–12	5–10 mg QD
Carteolol	β_1, β_2	++	Low	Renal	5–6	2.5–10 mg QD
Carvedilol	$\beta_1, \beta_2, \alpha_1$	0	High	Hepatic	2–6	25–50 mg BID
Labetalol	$\beta_1, \beta_2, \alpha_1$	0	Moderate	Hepatic	3–4	200–400 mg BID
Metoprolol[a]	β_1	0	Moderate	Hepatic	3–7	50–100 mg BID
Metoprolol XL[a]						100–200 mg QD
Nadolol[a]	β_1, β_2	0	Low	Renal	14–24	40–80 mg QD
Penbutolol	β_1, β_2	+	High	Hepatic	5	20 mg QD
Pindolol	β_1, β_2	+++	Moderate	Renal and hepatic	3–4	5–20 mg BID
Propranolol[a]	β_1, β_2	0	High	Hepatic	3–5	Variable
Propranolol LA[a]						80–160 mg QD
Timolol	β_1, β_2	0	Moderate	Hepatic	4–5	10–20 mg BID

ISA, intrinsic sympathomimetic activity.
[a]Agents approved by the U.S. Food and Drug Administration to treat chronic stable angina.

dilation and vasodilation. β-Blockers are classified as nonselective or cardioselective, based on the selectivity at blocking β_1-receptors or β_2-receptors. Cardioselective agents (atenolol, metoprolol, and acebutolol) are more selective toward binding to β_1-receptors than to β_2-receptors, where as nonselective agents block both β_1-receptors and β_2-receptors. Theoretically, β_1-selective agents would be more effective at antagonizing the effects of catecholamines at β_1-receptors while causing minimal β_2-receptor blockade. β_1-Selective antagonists have a theoretical advantage in patients with pulmonary disease (e.g., chronic obstructive pulmonary disease, asthma) or when blockade of β_2-receptor is undesirable, as in patients with peripheral vascular disease or insulin-dependent diabetes mellitus. However, cardioselectivity is relative and achievement of high enough plasma concentrations, which can occur within the clinically used dosage range, results in the loss of cardioselectivity. β-Blockers that have ISA, as shown in Table 42.3, produce some degree of β-receptor stimulation at low states of sympathetic activation (e.g., at rest). However, at higher levels of sympathetic activation (e.g., during exercise) these agents act as antagonists. Few data suggest that drugs with ISA are more beneficial than agents without ISA in preventing angina. Because these drugs tend not to lower resting heart rate or cardiac output, they may have theoretical advantages in a patient with already low resting heart rate and cardiac output. Finally, these agents may be detrimental in patients who have had a myocardial infarction or who experience rest angina.

The pharmacokinetic properties of β-blockers are extremely variable and are related to the drug's lipophilicity or hydrophilicity.[57] In general, drugs that are highly lipid soluble tend to be well absorbed from the gastrointestinal tract, are hepatically metabolized, have highly variable oral bioavailability, undergo extensive hepatic first-pass metabolism, and have a short plasma terminal elimination half-life. Table 42.3 lists the lipid solubility of β-blockers. β-Blockers that are more water soluble tend to be incompletely absorbed from the gastrointestinal tract, are eliminated mainly unchanged in the urine, and have less variable oral bioavailability, negligible first-pass hepatic metabolism, and a longer plasma terminal elimination half-life. Although the pharmacokinetics of β-blockers are highly variable, most of these compounds can be dosed once or twice daily to treat angina. The pharmacokinetic properties of a drug and individual patient characteristics should guide the selection of the appropriate agent. For example, if atenolol were to be used in a patient with angina and impaired renal function, a lengthening of the dosing interval may be necessary because atenolol is eliminated mainly by the kidneys.

Regardless of differences in pharmacologic characteristics described here, it should be emphasized that all β-blockers, regardless of differing pharmacologic characteristics, are effective in preventing angina.[58] The efficacy of β-blockers should be determined by their effects on resting and exercise heart rate and on the frequency and severity of anginal syndromes. The β-blocker dosage should be

Table 42.4 ▪ Individualizing Anginal Therapy in Patients with Other Medical Conditions

Indication	Drug Therapy
Compelling indication unless contraindicated	
Prior myocardial infarction	Non-ISA β-blockers
Isolated systolic hypertension	CCB (long-acting DHP)
Systemic hypertension	β-Blockers
Left ventricular systolic dysfunction	Carvedilol
May have favorable effects on comorbid condition	
Sinus bradycardia, second- or third-degree atrioventricular block	DHP CCB, nitrate
Sinus tachycardia, supraventricular tachycardia, atrial fibrillation	β-Blockers, non-DHP CCB
Ventricular arrhythmias	β-Blockers
Severe preexisting headaches	β-Blockers, non-DHP CCB
Hyperthyroidism	β-Blockers
Diabetes mellitus	CCB
Essential tremor	β-Blockers (noncardioselective)
Left ventricular systolic dysfunction	Isosorbide dinitrate
Systemic hypertension	CCB
May have unfavorable effects on comorbid condition	
Sinus bradycardia, second- or third-degree atrioventricular block	β-Blockers,[a] non-DHP CCB[a]
Sinus tachycardia, supraventricular tachycardia, atrial fibrillation	DHP CCB (short acting), nitrate
Left ventricular systolic dysfunction	β-Blockers (except carvedilol); CCB (except amlodipine)
Prior myocardial infarction	ISA β-blockers
Severe preexisting headaches	Nitrates, DHP CCB
Bronchospastic disease (asthma or chronic obstructive pulmonary disease)	β-Blockers[a]
Peripheral vascular disease	β-Blockers
Depression	β-Blockers
Diabetes mellitus	β-Blockers

ISA, intrinsic sympathomimetic activity; *CCB*, calcium channel blockers; *DHP*, dihydropyridine.
[a]Contraindicated.

Table 42.5 ▪ Pharmacologic Characteristics of Currently Available Calcium Channel Blockers

	Major Adverse Effects	Time to Peak Concentration (hr)	Maintenance Dosage
Dihydropyridines	Headache, ankle edema		
Short-acting	Reflex adrenergic and neurohormonal activation (tachycardia, flushing, dizziness)		
Nifedipine[a]		0.5	10–20 mg TID
Nicardipine[b]		0.5–2.0	20–40 mg TID
Medium-acting	Lessened incidence of but still significant reflex adrenergic and neurohormonal activation (tachycardia, flushing, dizziness)		
Nicardipine-SR		1–4	30–60 mg BID
Isradipine		1.5	5–10 mg BID
Long-acting	Subclinical reflex adrenergic and neurohormonal activation		
Amlodipine[a]		6–12	5–10 mg QD
Felodipine-ER		2.5–5	5–10 mg QD
Nifedipine-CC		6	30–60 mg QD
Nifedipine-XL[a]		6	30–60 mg QD
Nisoldipine-ER		6–12	20–40 mg QD
Nondihydropyridines	Bradycardia, AV nodal conduction disturbances, heart failure, headache, dizziness, edema		
Verapamil[a]	Constipation	1–2	60–90 mg TID–QID
Verapamil-SR		1–2	240 mg QD
Bepridil[b]	Proarrhythmia	5	300 mg QD
Diltiazem[a]		2–3	80–120 mg TID
Diltiazem-SR		6–11	60–120 mg BID
Diltiazem-CD[a]		10–14	180–360 mg QD
Diltiazem-XR[b]		4–6	180–540 mg QD

Source: Reference 61.

[a]Approved by the U.S. Food and Drug Administration for treating chronic stable angina and angina associated with coronary artery spasm.

[b]Approved by the U.S. Food and Drug Administration for treating chronic stable angina.

titrated to achieve a resting heart rate of 50 to 60 bpm and maximal exercise heart rate of less than 100 bpm.

Adverse Effects. The adverse effects associated with β-blockers are an extension of their pharmacologic effects and include sinus bradycardia, sinus arrest, AV block, reduced left ventricular function, bronchoconstriction, fatigue, depression, nightmares, sexual dysfunction, and intensification of insulin-induced hypoglycemia.[55,56] Thus, β-blockers should be avoided or used with caution in patients (Table 42.4) with bradyarrhythmias, AV conduction disturbances, asthma or chronic obstructive pulmonary disease, decompensated left ventricular systolic dysfunction, diabetes mellitus, and peripheral vascular disease.

A final issue of clinical importance is the β-blocker withdrawal syndrome. Prolonged therapy with β-receptor antagonists results in an increase in the number of β-receptors. Abrupt withdrawal of β-blockers in these patients may result in an increased number of sensitized receptors available for adrenergic stimulation and possible precipitation of anginal syndromes, unstable angina, and possibly myocardial infarction. For this reason, it is prudent, when discontinuing β-blockers, to decrease the dosage gradually over a 1- to 2-week period.

Calcium Channel Blockers

Mechanism of Action. Calcium channel blockers are a chemically heterogeneous group of agents that block the transmembrane flux of calcium into cardiac and vascular smooth muscle cells by noncompetitive blockade, thereby reducing the rate of calcium entry and intracellular calcium concentrations.[59–61] This reduction in intracellular calcium concentrations results in reduction in the excitation–contraction coupling mechanism responsible for myocardial and smooth muscle contraction.

Pharmacologic Characteristics. Because of the chemical heterogeneity of calcium channel blockers and the existence of three different binding sites (dihydropyridine site, phenylalkylamine site, and benzothiazepine site), these agents exert variable pharmacologic effects.[61] Based on these three binding sites, calcium channel blockers are classified as dihydropyridines, phenylalkylamines, and benzothiazepines, which bind at each respective site. The prototype agents for these three sites are nifedipine, verapamil, and diltiazem, respectively. Table 42.5 lists the available calcium channel blockers and their pharmacologic effects. Because of the different pharmacologic actions of these agents, they are collectively called either dihydropyridines or nondihydropyridines.

Calcium channel blockers have five major physiologic effects: decreased systemic vascular resistance (peripheral vasodilation), decreased coronary vascular resistance (coronary vasodilation), decreased myocardial contractility and slowing of sinus (reduced heart rate), and AV nodal conduction.[60–62] Reductions in systemic vascular resistance, heart rate, and myocardial contractility result in decreased myocardial oxygen demand, whereas decreased coronary vascular resistance increases myocardial oxygen supply. In general, the dihydropyridine agents exhibit greater vascular selectivity, and thus preferentially cause peripheral and coronary vasodilation and have minimal effects on myocardial contractility and sinus and AV nodal conduction. However, because of their rapid and potent vasodilation, short-acting dihydropyridines (Table 42.5) may cause a reflex increase in heart rate, leading to increased myocardial oxygen demand. As listed in Table 42.5, the medium- and long-acting dihydropyridines have lessened effects on neurohormonal activation. On the other hand, the nondihydropyridines are neither vascular nor myocardial selective and thus exhibit all of the pharmacologic effects described here. Given the pronounced differences in the clinical pharmacology of these agents, the selection of an appropriate agent should be based on the characteristics of the drug and the characteristics of the patient being treated.

ADVERSE EFFECTS. Calcium channel blockers are well tolerated. Most of the adverse effects associated with their use are related to their pharmacologic effects. The major adverse effects are illustrated in Table 42.5. The degree or significance of each adverse effect depends on the individual agent. Flushing, headache, and dizziness are related to the vasodilatory effects of calcium channel blockers.[60–62] Dihydropyridines, which are the most potent peripheral vasodilators, tend to cause these adverse effects to the greatest extent. Use of long-acting or extended-release preparations may lessen these adverse effects. Peripheral edema, probably related to arteriolar vasodilation, not sodium and water retention, is also most common in patients treated with dihydropyridines. Depression of myocardial contractility is most common in patients treated with verapamil and diltiazem and to a lesser extent with dihydropyridines. The negative inotropic effects of dihydropyridines typically are masked by the peripheral vasodilation and resulting adrenergic activation. Calcium channel blockers should be used with caution in patients with left ventricular systolic dysfunction, with the exception of amlodipine, which appears to be safe. Bradycardia and AV block can be seen in patients receiving verapamil and diltiazem. These two adverse effects would occur most commonly in patients with baseline sinus bradycardia or AV nodal dysfunction or in patients receiving concomitant β-blockers. Calcium channel blockers may also cause gastrointestinal adverse effects such as nausea and constipation. The latter is caused most commonly by verapamil and may be particularly problematic in older adults. Finally, bepridil, a calcium channel blocker with type I antiarrhythmic effects, can cause proarrhythmia (e.g., ventricular tachycardia, ventricular fibrillation) and thus should be reserved for patients who do not respond adequately to other antianginal drugs.

Pharmacotherapy of Chronic Stable Angina Pectoris

Decisions about when to initiate drug therapy in a particular patient depend on the frequency and severity of anginal attacks. The following recommendations are general and may vary from patient to patient depending on patient preference, severity of angina, and other factors. If angina occurs less than once weekly, using nitroglycerin tablets or spray to treat acute attacks (see Table 42.2 for treatment options) is indicated. The specific dosage administered depends on the patient's hemodynamic response. Sublingual nitroglycerin tablets are available over a wide dosing range, from 0.15 to 0.6 mg, whereas the spray delivers 0.4 mg with each dose. These products are also useful for preventing angina when taken just before the initiation of exertion or some other event that precipitates angina.

If angina occurs more frequently than two to three times per week, chronic prophylactic therapy (see Table 42.2 for treatment options) is necessary.[1] The three drug classes that can be used for this purpose are nitrates, β-blockers, and calcium channel blockers. As discussed earlier, no data suggest that any antianginal medication reduces mortality, so treatment strategies are targeted at symptom relief or ischemia reduction. The only exception is the use of β-blockers in patients post-myocardial infarction and in treating hypertension, in which these agents have been shown to reduce cardiovascular morbidity and mortality (Table 42.4). Initial drug selection for chronic angina treatment should be based on the patient characteristics and concomitant conditions. Long-acting nitrate products used in initial therapy include oral nitroglycerin capsules, transdermal nitroglycerin patches, nitroglycerin ointment, ISDN, and ISMN. The choice of one product over another should be based on patient preference and ease of administration. Patients with heart failure may benefit from the addition of a nitrate because of the reduction in preload and left ventricular filling pressures that accompany their use. All patients treated with nitrates need a 10- to 12-hour nitrate-free period to avoid developing tolerance. Unfortunately, because a nitrate-free period is needed, no nitrate product can provide 24-hour anti-ischemic coverage, thus necessitating additional therapy with β-blockers, calcium channel blockers, or combination therapy. Regardless of which nitrate is selected, it should be started at low dosages to reduce the incidence of adverse effects early in therapy. Subsequent dosage adjustments can be based on incidence of the adverse effects, headache, dizziness, and hypotension. Effectiveness can be assessed by decreased use of sublingual nitroglycerin for acute attacks, improvement in the patient's quality of life (i.e., ability to perform normal activities without experiencing angina), and objective assessment by exercise testing.

All β-blockers are effective in reducing ischemic episodes and may also be used as initial therapy for angina. Patients who would particularly benefit from β-blocker therapy are listed in Table 42.4, most notably those with hypertension. Selecting drug therapy based on concomitant disease states or conditions allows initial treatment of two conditions with one drug. In addition, β-blockers may be used in patients who cannot tolerate nitrate therapy because of adverse effects or failure to suppress angina, especially if the patient has mainly fixed-threshold angina. All β-blockers are effective in managing stable angina, although all are not approved by the U.S. Food and Drug Administration (FDA) for this purpose (see Table 42.3 for approved agents). Selection of an individual agent should be based on the pharmacologic characteristics of a given drug and patient characteristics (e.g., renal function, hepatic function).

Calcium channel blockers are also effective in preventing angina. They are particularly useful in patients with contraindications to β-blockers or patients with mainly variable-threshold angina as well as with conditions listed in Table 42.4. All calcium channel blockers appear to be effective in managing stable angina, although all are not approved by the FDA for this purpose (see Table 42.3 for approved agents). Selection of an individual agent should be based on the pharmacologic characteristics of a given drug and patient characteristics (e.g., renal function, hepatic function). Considerable controversy[63–65] exists about whether calcium channel blockers should be first-line therapy in patients with coronary artery disease. A recent observational study[66] suggests that the short-acting dihydropyridine nifedipine may increase the risk of myocardial infarction in patients with coronary artery disease when used for preventing future cardiovascular events. Thus, it is recommended that short-acting dihydropyridine agents such as the immediate-release formulations of nifedipine or nicardipine be avoided in patients with coronary artery disease.[67] Additional data are needed before this warning is extended to longer-acting agents and sustained-release formulations or nondihydropyridine calcium channel blockers.

Combination drug therapy often is used when monotherapy is unsuccessful in managing anginal episodes. It should be emphasized that combination drug therapy should be reserved for patients who do not benefit or who have intolerable adverse effects with maximized single-drug therapy. Because tolerance develops to chronic therapy with nitrates, β-blockers and calcium channel blockers often are used in combination with nitrates to prevent angina during nitrate-free intervals. The combination of β-blockers and nitrates is used commonly and has therapeutic rationale based on the pharmacology of each drug class. Nitrates offset the β-blockers' potential deleterious increase in left ventricular diastolic pressures and volumes by reducing preload, whereas the β-blockers inhibit nitrate-induced sympathetically mediated reflex tachycardia. Combination therapy with nondihydropyridine calcium channel blockers and nitrates also offers therapeutic benefit, although the combination of dihydropyridines and nitrates may cause excessive hypotension, rebound tachycardia, and headaches.

Therapy with a β-blocker and calcium channel blocker should theoretically reduce myocardial oxygen demand further than could each agent alone. In addition, because β-blockers may increase coronary artery tone, adding a calcium channel blocker may attenuate this potentially detrimental effect.[68] The concern about the use nondihydropyridines with β-blockers is the potential for additive adverse effects, specifically slowing of AV and sinus nodal conduction, hypotension, and systolic function impairment. These concerns can be minimized by selecting patients who are least likely to experience these adverse effects. Patients who are normotensive, have little systolic dysfunction, and have no conduction disturbances are the best candidates for this therapy. The combination of a β-blocker and verapamil should be reserved for patients in whom combination therapy with other agents fails.

Finally, multiple calcium channel blockers have been used in combination. Each class of calcium channel blockers has distinct differences in their effects on cardiac contractility, coronary artery blood flow, sinus and AV nodal conduction, and peripheral vascular resistance. Binding of dihydropyridine compounds to the dihydropyridine receptor is enhanced by diltiazem. The opposite is also true. Conversely, verapamil and dihydropyridines antagonize each other's binding. This suggests that some rationale exists for the use of a combination such as nifedipine and diltiazem to produce beneficial pharmacologic effects. Combination therapy with multiple calcium channel blockers is effective in treating ischemic heart disease,[69,70] but with the limited research experience, the routine use of multiple calcium channel blockers cannot be recommended.

When medical therapy is not effective in reducing the number of anginal syndromes or the underlying coronary artery disease is severe, revascularization therapy with percutaneous transluminal coronary angioplasty (PTCA) or coronary artery bypass graft (CABG) surgery may be an alternative. These topics are discussed later in the chapter.

Pharmacotherapy of Silent Myocardial Ischemia

Therapy for all patients regardless of the type of silent myocardial ischemia should begin with risk factor reduction. The drug therapies used to treat silent myocardial ischemia, though controversial, are similar to those used to treat other types of chronic ischemia, namely nitrates, β-blockers, and calcium channel blockers. Each of these agents reduces the number of ischemic episodes,[16,17,71,72] but their impact on long-term prognosis is not clear. The treatment approach should be individualized depending on whether a patient has totally asymptomatic episodes of ischemia, postinfarction asymptomatic ischemia, or symptomatic and asymptomatic episodes. There is no consensus for therapy of totally asymptomatic patients. Drug therapy should be reserved for patients who have severe and frequent ischemia. In patients with postinfarction asymptomatic ischemia, therapy with β-blockers is logical given the well-established benefits of these agents in preventing reinfarction and death in these patients. Finally, the treatment of patients with asymptomatic and symptomatic ischemic episodes has received the largest attention because this group contains the largest number of patients. Several recent studies have increased our understanding of therapy in these patients. A recent placebo-controlled trial[73] showed that atenolol was effective in asymptomatic and mildly symptomatic patients (with and without previous myocardial infarction) at reducing ischemic episodes and cardiovascular events. A similar patient population was enrolled in a subsequent randomized trial,[72,74] which was designed to investigate three approaches to treating these patients. The three approaches were revascularization with PTCA or CABG, drug therapy targeted at reducing ischemia, and drug therapy targeted at reducing angina. The drug therapies used in this trial were atenolol with or without controlled-release nifedipine or sustained-release diltiazem with or without sustained-release ISDN. Patients who were randomized to the revascularization group had better 2-year survival and experienced fewer cardiac events than either of the medically managed groups. The outcome in the group of patients whose treatment was targeted at reducing ischemia did slightly better than the other medically managed group of patients. The question remains whether suppressing ischemic episodes translates into reducing long-term mortality. The results of these two studies suggest that β-blocker therapy with atenolol reduces ischemia and cardiovascular events, but that revascularization offers a significant advantage to this approach at improving prognosis. Future studies are needed to address these issues further.

Pharmacotherapy of Variant Angina

Sublingual nitroglycerin therapy should be used for acute angina episodes. Calcium channel blockers are effective in the chronic prophylactic management of variant angina. The selection of a particular drug depends mainly on patient characteristics. Nitrates are also effective in these patients, but scheduling a nitrate-free period may not necessarily be best during the sleeping hours. Because most episodes occur during the night or morning, the nitrate-free interval should be scheduled during the day. Nitrate therapy should be reserved for patients with continued symptoms on maximized therapy with calcium channel blockers. Combination therapy with two calcium channel blockers (diltiazem and nifedipine) has been shown to reduce the frequency of angina episodes in patients not receiving full benefit from either agent alone. However, this drug combination was associated with frequent adverse effects.[75] Finally, as described earlier, β-blockers should not be used to treat variant angina because they may exacerbate coronary vasospasm.

Unstable Angina

Unstable angina is a transitory syndrome of ischemic heart disease that is intermediate between chronic stable angina and acute myocardial infarction. The quality of the chest pain is similar to that of chronic stable angina, although the intensity and duration may be greater.

TREATMENT GOALS: UNSTABLE ANGINA

- Prevent myocardial infarction by inhibiting extension of the thrombus.
- Relieve chest pain and reverse ischemia.
- Reduce cardiovascular risk.

PATHOPHYSIOLOGY

The most important pathophysiologic feature of unstable angina is a reduction in myocardial oxygen supply. Three processes contribute to the decreased myocardial oxygen supply in most patients with unstable angina: progression of atherosclerosis, platelet aggregation, and thrombus formation. In some patients, coronary vasospasm or increases in vasomotor tone may also contribute to the decrease in myocardial oxygen supply.

In patients who have either new-onset angina or worsening of previously stable angina, the most likely cause is rapid progression of atherosclerosis. Rapid progression of atherosclerosis probably is caused by fissuring or disruption of the atherosclerotic plaque, leading to platelet aggregation and thrombus formation. As the plaque heals, the thrombus is incorporated and the size of the atherosclerotic plaque increases.[7,8,76] This process is depicted in the lower portion of Fig. 42.2. Pathologic studies suggest that this is a common, recurrent series of events in most patients with unstable angina.

The more common and most severe presentation of unstable angina is rest angina for more than 20 minutes. Plaque disruption, platelet aggregation, and thrombus formation are important pathophysiologic events in this form of unstable angina. In this case, the thrombus causes a partial to nearly complete occlusion of the coronary artery and is responsible for the symptoms. This differs from the pathophysiology of acute myocardial infarction in that acute myocardial infarction usually is associated with total occlusion of the coronary artery.

CLINICAL PRESENTATION AND DIAGNOSIS

Unstable angina has three primary modes of presentation.[1,76,77] The first and usually most severe presentation of unstable angina is rest angina, which is more than 20 minutes in duration. New-onset angina (usually within the previous 1 to 2 months) that occurs with minimal exertion also is classified as unstable angina. Finally, a patient with previously diagnosed chronic stable angina whose angina is increasing in frequency or duration or has a lower threshold for symptom onset is also described as having unstable angina. The ECG changes typically observed in patients with unstable angina are ST segment changes

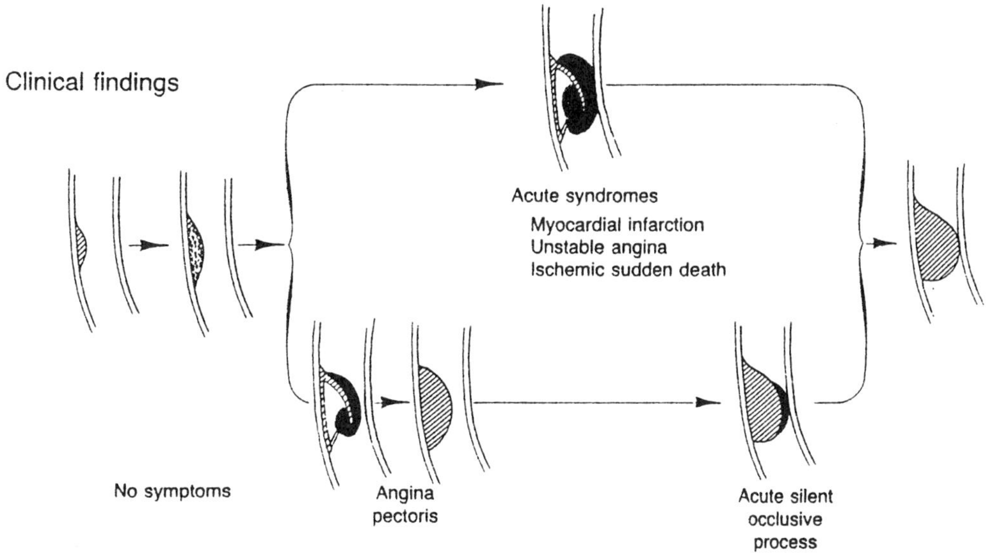

Figure 42.2. Progression of coronary atherosclerosis, according to clinical findings. (With permission from Fuster V, Badimon L, Badimon JJ, et al. The pathogenesis of coronary artery disease and the acute coronary syndromes. N Engl J Med 326:242–250, 1992.)

(elevation or depression) and T-wave inversion. These ECG changes commonly are observed only during the ischemic episode and reverse with relief of chest pain.[1]

A working diagnosis of unstable angina typically is based on the patient's history and chief complaints. Acute myocardial infarction is ruled out by measurement of serial cardiac enzymes (e.g., creatine kinase–MB, troponin). Once the patient's condition is stabilized, the degree of ischemia and underlying atherosclerotic disease usually is assessed by exercise testing or cardiac catheterization.

THERAPEUTIC PLAN

Treatment guidelines for patients with unstable angina were developed and published by the U.S. Public Health Service and the National Heart Lung and Blood Institute in 1994.[77] These guidelines are available electronically (http://text.nlm.nih.gov) or can be obtained from the U.S. Department of Health and Human Services (AHCPR publication no. 94-0602). A summary of the recommendations also has been published.[78]

TREATMENT

Treatment approaches for patients with unstable angina are based on their risk of developing a nonfatal myocardial infarction or death. Patients with new-onset angina or worsening angina are considered low risk and typically are treated as outpatients. Patients with rest pain for longer than 20 minutes are considered intermediate or high risk, depending on several other factors, and are hospitalized.[77]

There are three general goals of therapy for patients with unstable angina. The primary goal is to prevent myocardial infarction by inhibiting extension of the thrombus. The second general goal is to reverse the ischemia and relieve the chest pain by increasing myocardial oxygen supply or decreasing myocardial oxygen demand. The third is to reduce cardiovascular risk.

Pharmacotherapy

Antiplatelet Agents

Patients suspected of having unstable angina or acute myocardial infarction should immediately be given aspirin 160 to 325 mg to chew and swallow, except in the case of a definite contraindication (e.g., documented hypersensitivity, active bleeding). This recommendation is based on data showing that early administration of aspirin is superior to placebo in preventing progression of unstable angina to acute myocardial infarction.[79] Meta-analysis of the trials lasting more than 3 months suggests that aspirin therapy reduces the risk of acute myocardial infarction or death by approximately one-half.[30] Therefore, it is recommended that patients with unstable angina be placed on lifelong aspirin therapy unless there are clear contraindications. The appropriate dosage of aspirin in these patients is the subject of some debate. The data suggest that dosages greater than 325 mg/day are no more effective than 325 mg/day, although the higher dosages are associated with more adverse effects.[30] Dosages of 75 to 160 mg/day seem to have efficacy similar to 325 mg/day.[30] Therefore, it is recommended that all patients with unstable angina take aspirin 75 to 325 mg daily, with the dosage based on clinician or patient preference. Because the lower-dosage forms of aspirin ("baby aspirin") tend to be more expensive, many clinicians choose regular-strength (325-mg) aspirin.

The effects of several other antiplatelet agents on preventing acute myocardial infarction and death have been studied in patients with unstable angina. Dipyridamole plus aspirin has been shown to have efficacy similar to aspirin, suggesting that dipyridamole is an unnecessary addition.[30] Dipyridamole alone has been studied only on a limited basis, and a meta-analysis suggests that it is not significantly better than placebo.[30] Sulfinpyrazone may be more effective than placebo[30] but is inferior to aspirin.[80] Ticlopidine has been shown to reduce the risk of fatal and nonfatal myocardial infarction by 46% over control therapy.[81] Ticlopidine appears to offer no greater benefit than aspirin.[30] The higher cost of ticlopidine and more significant adverse effect profile, notably neutropenia, make aspirin the preferred agent over ticlopidine. Clopidogrel, a thienopyridine derivative like ticlopidine, has been shown to be effective in secondary prevention of cardiovascular events in patients with previous myocardial infarction, stroke, or peripheral vascular disease.[82] Clopidogrel has not been studied in the acute phase of unstable angina. Thus, ticlopidine and clopidogrel appear to be reasonable alternatives for secondary prevention of coronary events in patients who are intolerant to aspirin.

The final common pathway for platelet aggregation involves the platelet glycoprotein IIb/IIIa receptor, which allows fibrinogen binding and platelet aggregation.[83] Glycoprotein IIb/IIIa receptor antagonists inhibit this process and thus reduce the growth of platelet-rich thrombus. Development of these agents represents a major breakthrough in antiplatelet therapy. Several comparative studies[84–87] have shown these agents to be effective in reducing the risk of myocardial infarction and death in patients with unstable angina, with and without percutaneous coronary angioplasty. The specific roles of these compounds in treating unstable angina must be evaluated further. Three glycoprotein IIb/IIIa receptor antagonists are currently available in the United States (abciximab, integrelin, and tirofiban); numerous others are under investigation.

Anticoagulants

Therapy with intravenous unfractionated heparin is indicated in patients with intermediate- to high-risk unstable angina. In this patient group, the primary goal of therapy is to prevent extension of the thrombus and thus prevent acute myocardial infarction. Although aspirin is superior to placebo in these patients, data suggest that unfractionated heparin alone may be superior to aspirin alone.[79,88] In a study of 484 patients with unstable angina, myocardial infarction occurred in 3.7% of aspirin-treated patients and 0.8% of unfractionated heparin–treated patients.[88] Interestingly, some studies have not shown unfractionated heparin to be superior to aspirin or placebo.[89,90] Nonetheless, the expert panel that developed the clinical practice guidelines recommend that unfractionated heparin should be administered immediately when a diagnosis of intermediate- to high-risk unstable angina is made.[77] In most patients, unfractionated heparin is given along with aspirin as described earlier. The recommended dosage regimen is 80 U/kg intravenous bolus followed by a constant-rate infusion of 18 U/kg/hour, adjusted to an activated partial thromboplastin time (aPTT) of 1.5 to 2 times control. In institutions not equipped to administer unfractionated heparin by continuous infusion, the recommended regimen is 5000 U by intravenous bolus every 4 hours.[77] Unfractionated heparin therapy should be continued for 2 to 5 days or until a revascularization procedure, such as CABG or angioplasty, is performed.[77]

Because of the intense monitoring necessary for patients receiving intravenous unfractionated heparin, alternative approaches for providing anticoagulation have been and are being investigated. The most promising of these approaches appears to be the use of low-molecular-weight heparin (LMWH). An extensive review of LMWH is beyond the scope of this chapter, but a detailed review of LMWH has recently been published.[91] LMWH produces a more predictable antithrombotic effect than unfractionated heparin. Laboratory monitoring of aPTT therefore is unnecessary. In addition, these agents have a longer duration of action than unfractionated heparin and can be administered subcutaneously once or twice daily. Currently three agents (ardeparin, enoxaparin, and dalteparin) are available in the United States, although only enoxaparin and dalteparin have been approved by the FDA, for the treatment of unstable angina. Several comparative clinical trials suggest that LMWHs are more effective than placebo and at least as effective as unfractionated heparin in preventing recurrent angina, death, or AMI[92–96] in patients with acute coronary syndromes. The comparative incidence of adverse effects, including bleeding, between LMWHs and unfractionated heparin is similar but somewhat variable among studies. Weight-based unfractionated heparin dosing was not used in any of these trials. Thus, the efficacy of LMWH compared to that of weight-based unfractionated heparin dosing is not known.

Intense investigation also surrounds the use of anticoagulants, such as hirudin, which directly inhibit thrombin. It is thought that these agents may be more efficacious than heparin and may warrant less intensive monitoring. However, several recent comparative studies of hirudin and unfractionated heparin in patients with unstable angina or acute myocardial infarction were stopped prematurely because the rate of intracranial hemorrhage was higher with hirudin than with unfractionated heparin.[97] In addition, in a large comparative trial, an additional beneficial effect of hirudin was observed at 48 hours but dissipated over the ensuing 30 days. As has been observed in previous trials, the incidence of bleeding was higher in the hirudin group.[98] Thus the future role of these agents in treating patients with unstable angina remains to be clarified. Lepirudin, a recombinant DNA hirudin, was recently approved by the FDA for anticoagulant therapy in patients with heparin-induced thrombocytopenia and associated thrombotic complications, not for treating unstable angina.

Thrombolytics

Thrombolytic agents lyse existing clots by activating plasminogen and have been proven to significantly reduce mortality in patients with acute myocardial infarction. Because the primary pathophysiologic abnormality in unstable angina is thrombus formation and because unstable angina can be a precursor to acute myocardial infarction, it seemed reasonable that thrombolytic agents would be beneficial in patients with unstable angina. However, multiple clinical studies conducted with thrombolytic agents in unstable angina have consistently shown that they provide no beneficial effect.[99] In fact, some studies suggest that thrombolytics may be detrimental in patients with unstable angina.[99,100] Thus, thrombolytic therapy in patients with unstable angina is not recommended.

β-Blockers

β-Blockers are effective anti-ischemic and anti-anginal agents that act to decrease myocardial oxygen demand by decreasing heart rate and contractility. It is recommended that all patients with unstable angina receive β-blocker therapy unless there are contraindications.[77] Meta-analysis of randomized, placebo-controlled β-blocker trials in unstable angina suggest that β-blockers decrease the risk of acute myocardial infarction by 13%.[77] Use of β-blockers in unstable angina has not been clearly shown to reduce mortality. However, the mortality-reducing effects of β-blockers in acute myocardial infarction and after myocardial infarction are clear, and these data help form the basis of the recommendation for β-blockers in patients with unstable angina.

β-Blockers should not be given to patients with marked first-degree AV block (ECG P-R interval more than 0.24 seconds), second- or third-degree AV block, a history of asthma, or severe left ventricular dysfunction with congestive heart failure or cardiogenic shock. In patients with bradycardia (heart rate less than 60 bpm) or hypotension (systolic blood pressure less than 90 mm Hg), β-blockers should be withheld until heart rate or blood pressure increases. In patients with chronic obstructive pulmonary disease (who may have a component of reactive airway disease) or diabetes mellitus, β-blockers should be used with caution. A β_1-selective agent may be preferable to a nonselective agent in these patients.

Intravenous β-blocker therapy should be instituted in high-risk patients and oral therapy initiated in intermediate- and low-risk patients. Examples of the most commonly used intravenous β-blocker protocols are metoprolol 5 mg intravenously every 5 minutes for three doses, followed immediately by initiation of metoprolol 50 mg orally every 6 hours; and atenolol 5 mg intravenously, repeated again in 5 minutes, with subsequent initiation of 50 to 100 mg oral atenolol daily. The target resting heart rate for patients with angina treated with β-blockers is 50 to 60 bpm. Oral dosages should be adjusted to achieve this heart rate. β_1-Selective agents are no more effective than nonselective agents. The selection of a specific drug can be based on other issues such as route of elimination, half-life, or cost. It may be prudent to avoid β-blockers with ISA during the acute phase of unstable angina because these agents have been shown to be less effective than other β-blockers in the setting of acute myocardial infarction.

Nitrates

There are few controlled clinical trials evaluating the use of intravenous nitroglycerin in patients with unstable angina. Nonetheless, intravenous nitroglycerin is widely used in clinical practice and it should be given to any patient with unstable angina who continues to have chest pain after administration of three sublingual nitroglycerin doses and initiation of β-blockers.[77] Additionally, intravenous nitroglycerin is recommended for all nonhypotensive patients with high-risk unstable angina. Therapy should be initiated at a dosage of 5 to 10 μg/minute, with 10 μg/minute dosage increases every 5 minutes until chest pain is relieved or the patient develops dose-limiting side effects such as headache or hypotension (systolic blood pressure less than 90 mm Hg or a greater than 30% drop in mean blood pressure). Patients should be converted from intravenous to oral nitrate therapy once they have been symptom free for 24 hours.

Calcium Channel Blockers

Calcium channel blockers should be reserved for patients in whom angina is not controlled with optimal dosages of β-blockers and nitrates or in patients unable to tolerate nitrates or β-blockers.[77] Additionally, calcium channel blockers are recommended for use in patients with a known vasospastic component of their angina. Neither individual studies nor meta-analyses of calcium channel blockers in unstable angina show any beneficial effects on mortality or incidence of myocardial infarction.[101] In fact, short-acting nifedipine has been shown in several studies to increase the risk of myocardial infarction and death when used without concomitant β-blocker therapy in patients with unstable angina.[66,102,103] Therefore, short-acting dihydropyridine calcium channel blockers should be avoided in patients with unstable angina; if they must be used, they should be administered only in combination with a β-blocker.[77]

Revascularization Procedures

Two revascularization procedures, CABG and PTCA, with or without coronary artery stent placement, are widely available for treating ischemic heart disease. These procedures have become widely used in the United States. Because of the risk of morbidity and mortality associated with each procedure, for each patient it must be determined whether the potential benefits of the procedure outweigh the risks. Extensive guidelines for each of these procedures have been published.[104–106]

Coronary Artery Bypass Grafting

CABG is a surgical procedure in which the affected stenosed coronary artery is bypassed in an attempt to reinstitute normal coronary blood flow; two techniques are described here. The first technique involves removing the saphenous vein from the leg, which is then used to bypass the affected vessel. The distal end of the vessel is connected to the aorta, and the proximal end is connected to the coronary artery at a point distal to the obstruction. The second technique involves connecting the distal end of the internal mammary artery beyond the narrowing of the coronary vessel. Expert guidelines[104] recommend the following patients for CABG rather than medical therapy: patients with significant left main coronary artery disease, patients with multivessel coronary artery disease and moderate to severe left ventricular dysfunction, and patients with three-vessel coronary artery disease, which includes severe proximal left anterior descending artery stenosis regardless of left ventricular systolic function. Currently no data suggest better outcome with CABG than with medical therapy in patients with two-vessel (no left anterior descending coronary artery involvement) or single-vessel disease. In these patients, PTCA may be a treatment option.[1]

In patients who have had CABG, stenosis of the bypass graft may occur. Coronary disease of the saphenous vein grafts are thought to occur in three stages: early (within 1 month), intermediate (within 1 year), and late (after 1 year). Occlusion rates of 5 to 15%, 15 to 25%, and up to 50% have been reported for early, intermediate, and late phases, respectively.[107] The role of thrombosis in each of the phases has been documented. The use of antiplatelet therapy with aspirin or ticlopidine or clopidogrel (if the patient is aspirin sensitive) may reduce the rate of occlusion. The late phase of vein graft occlusion probably is related to atherosclerosis of the graft. Late-phase occlusion may be prevented by reducing risks for development of atherosclerosis (e.g., through lipid modifications and smoking cessation). However, antiplatelet therapy should also be continued given its role in the management of ischemic heart disease.

Percutaneous Coronary Intervention

PTCA is an extension of cardiac catheterization that involves passing a balloon-tipped catheter over a guidewire into the coronary artery. The guidewire is slipped past the obstruction, and the balloon-tipped catheter is passed over the wire and positioned at the level of the lesion. The balloon is then inflated, dilating the stenosed vessel. The beneficial actions of PTCA probably are related to arterial intimal disruption, plaque fissuring, and stretching of the arterial wall. Short-term complications from PTCA include abrupt closure of the vessel, ischemia, emergency CABG, myocardial infarction, and death. PTCA is effective (defined as less than 50% obstruction after the procedure) in approximately 90% of patients with nonoccluded, single-vessel disease.[108] The success rate may be lower in patients with unstable angina, older adults, women, and patients with totally occluded vessels. In patients who have undergone successful PTCA, the major concern involves long-term restenosis, which occurs in 40 to 60% of patients, usually within 6 months of the procedure. No interventions have been shown to reduce the risk of restenosis, but given antiplatelet therapy's role in the long-term management of ischemic heart disease, it should be continued over the long term. Coronary artery stents are stainless steel tubes that are inserted into coronary arteries at the site of atherosclerotic plaques to decrease the incidence of restenosis. The use of coronary artery stents is increasing rapidly, and in some cardiac catheterization laboratories more than 50% of patients undergoing angioplasty have coronary artery stents implanted. Because of the thrombogenic nature of a stent and the potential endothelial damage induced by the stent, antithrombotic drug therapy is needed to prevent thrombosis.

Expert guidelines for treating these patients suggest the following for patients receiving coronary artery stents: aspirin (at least 325 mg) initiated more than 2 hours before the procedure and continued indefinitely, intraprocedural heparin administration, or an alternative antithrombotic such as LMWH or ticlopidine or clopidogrel after stent placement. Low-risk patients can be treated effectively with aspirin (given indefinitely) and ticlopidine (250 mg twice daily) or clopidogrel (75 mg daily). The glycoprotein IIb/IIIa receptor antagonists should be considered in these patients. This is a rapidly expanding area in which pharmacotherapy is constantly evolving; future studies will better define the role of other agents in treating these patients.[106,109]

KEY POINTS

- Ischemic heart disease is a manifestation of atherosclerotic coronary artery disease, the leading cause of death in the United States.
- Myocardial ischemia causes several syndromes collectively called ischemic heart disease, including stable angina, variant or Prinzmetal's angina, silent myocardial ischemia, and unstable angina.
- The management of ischemic heart disease involves five areas: identifying and treating concomitant conditions that may exacerbate or precipitate ischemia, correcting concomitant cardiovascular risk factors, and implementing lifestyle modifications, medical treatment, and revascularization techniques.
- The goals of treatment for ischemic heart disease are to minimize the frequency and severity of angina and to reduce cardiovascular morbidity and mortality.
- Drug therapy with nitrates, β-blockers, and calcium channel blockers, alone or in combination, is effective in reducing anginal episodes and reducing the frequency of anginal attacks.
- Revascularization procedures are effective alternatives to medical therapy in certain patients.
- Unstable angina is a syndrome intermediate to chronic stable angina and acute myocardial infarction.
- Unstable angina warrants more intensive management than stable angina.
- General goals of therapy for unstable angina are preventing myocardial infarction and death, reversing ischemia, relieving chest pain, and reducing cardiovascular risk.
- Drug therapy with aspirin, heparin, β-blockers, and nitroglycerin is used in patients with unstable angina.

REFERENCES

1. Gersh BJ, Braunwald E, Rutherford JD. Chronic coronary artery disease. In: Braunwald E, ed. Heart disease: a textbook of cardiovascular medicine. 5th ed. Philadelphia: WB Saunders, 1997:1289–1365.
2. American Heart Association: Heart and stroke facts. 2000 statistical supplement. Dallas, TX: American Heart Association, 2000 (http://www.americanheart.org/statistics/04cornry.html, accessed, March 7, 2000).
3. Kannel WB, Feinleib M. Natural history of angina pectoris in the Framingham study: prognosis and survival. Am J Cardiol 29:154–158, 1972.
4. Participants in the Coronary Artery Surgery Study. Survival of medically treated patients in the coronary artery surgery study (CASS) registry. Circulation 82:562–568, 1982.
5. Alderman EL, Bourassa MG, Cohen LS, et al. Ten-year follow-up of survival and myocardial infarction in the randomized Coronary Artery Surgery Study. Circulation 82:1629–1646, 1990.
6. Lambert CR. Pathophysiology of stable angina pectoris. Cardiol Clin 9:1–10, 1991.
7. Fuster V, Badimon L, Badimon JJ, et al. The pathogenesis of coronary artery disease and the acute coronary syndromes. N Engl J Med 326:242–250, 1992.
8. Fuster V, Badimon L, Badimon JJ, et al. The pathogenesis of coronary artery disease and the acute coronary syndromes. N Engl J Med 326:310–317, 1992.
9. Adult treatment panel II. National Cholesterol Education Program: second report of the Expert Panel on Detection, Evaluation and Treatment of High Blood Cholesterol in Adults. Circulation 89:1333–1445, 1994.
10. Eckel RH, Krauss RM, for the AHA Nutrition Committee. American Heart Association call to action: obesity as a major risk factor for coronary heart disease. Circulation 97:2099–2100, 1998.
11. Grundy SM, Balady GJ, Criqui MH, et al. Primary prevention of coronary heart disease: guidance from Framingham. A statement for healthcare professionals from the AHA task force on risk reduction. Circulation 97:1876–1887, 1998.
12. Danesh J, Collins R, Peto R. Chronic infections and coronary heart disease: is there a link? Lancet 350:430–436, 1997.
13. Shub C. Stable angina pectoris 1. Clinical patterns. Mayo Clin Proc 64:233–242, 1990.
14. Ardehali A, Ports TA. Myocardial oxygen supply and demand. Chest 98:699–705, 1990.
15. Maseri A, Chierchia S, Kaski JC. Mixed angina pectoris. Am J Cardiol 56:30E–33E, 1985.
16. Bleske BE, Shea MJ. Current concepts of silent myocardial ischemia. Clin Pharm 9:339–357, 1990.
17. Cohn PF. Silent ischemia. In: Fuster V, Ross R, Topol EJ, ed. Atherosclerosis and coronary artery disease. Philadelphia: Lippincott-Raven, 1996:1561–1576.
18. Ogawa H, Yasue H, Oshima S. Circadian variation of plasma fibrinopeptide A level in patients with variant angina. Circulation 80:1617–1626, 1989.
19. Muller JE, Tofler GH, Stone PH. Circadian variation and triggers of onset of acute cardiovascular disease. Circulation 79:733–743, 1989.
20. Chaitman BR. Exercise stress testing. In: Braunwald E, ed. Heart disease: a textbook of cardiovascular medicine. 5th ed. Philadelphia: WB Saunders, 1997:153–176.
21. Fletcher GF, Balady G, Froelicher VF, et al. Exercise standards: a statement for healthcare professionals from the American Heart Association. Circulation 91:580–615, 1995.
22. Goldman L, Cook EF, Mitchell N, et al. Incremental value of the exercise test for diagnosing the presence or absence of coronary artery disease. Circulation 66:945–953, 1982.
23. Wackers FJT, Soufer R, Zaret BL. Nuclear cardiology. In: Braunwald E, ed. Heart disease: a textbook of cardiovascular medicine. 5th ed. Philadelphia: WB Saunders, 1997:273–316.
24. Ritchie JL, Bateman TM, Bonow RO, et al. Guidelines for clinical use of cardiac radionuclide imaging: a report of the American Heart Association/American College of Cardiology Task Force on assessment of diagnostic and therapeutic cardiovascular procedures, committee on radionuclide imaging, developed in collaboration with the American Society of Nuclear Cardiology. Circulation 91:1278–1303, 1995.
25. Beller GA. Pharmacologic stress testing. JAMA 265:633–638, 1991.
26. Ellis SG. The role of coronary angiography. In: Fuster V, Ross R, Topol EJ, ed. Atherosclerosis and coronary artery disease. Philadelphia: Lippincott-Raven, 1996:1433–1450.
27. Ridker PM, Manson JE, Gaziano M, et al. Low-dose aspirin therapy for chronic stable angina: a randomized, placebo-controlled clinical trial. Ann Intern Med 114:835–839, 1991.
28. Jull-Moller S, Edvardsson N, Jahnmatz B, et al. Double blind trial of aspirin in primary prevention of myocardial infarction in patients with stable chronic angina pectoris. Lancet 340:1421–1425, 1992.
29. Hennekens CH, Dyken ML, Fuster V. Aspirin as a therapeutic agent in cardiovascular disease. Circulation 96:2751–2753, 1997.
30. Antiplatelet Trialists' Collaboration. Collaborative overview of randomised trials of antiplatelet therapy – I: Prevention of death, myocardial infarction and stroke by prolonged antiplatelet therapy in various categories of patients. BMJ 308:81–106, 1994.
31. Scandinavian Simvistatin Survival Study Group. Randomised trial of cholesterol lowering in 4444 patients with coronary heart disease: the Scandinavian Simvistatin Survival Study (4S). Lancet 344:1383–1389, 1994.
32. Shepherd J, Cobbe SM, Ford I, et al. Prevention of coronary heart disease with pravastatin in men with hypercholesterolemia. N Engl J Med 333:1301–1307, 1995.
33. Sacks FM, Pfeffer MA, Moye LA, et al. The effect of pravastatin on coronary events after myocardial infarction in patients with average cholesterol levels. N Engl J Med 335:1001–1009, 1996.
34. Balady GJ, Fletcher BJ, Froelicher ES, et al. Cardiac rehabilitation programs: a statement for healthcare professionals from the American Heart Association. Circulation 90:1602–1610, 1994.
35. Fletcher GF, Balady G, Froelicher VF, et al. Exercise standards: a statement for health professionals from the American Heart Association. Circulation 91:580–615, 1995.
36. Fletcher GF, Balady G, Blair SN. Statement on exercise: benefits and recommendations for physical activity programs for all Americans. A statement for health professionals by the committee on exercise and cardiac rehabilitation of the Council on Clinical Cardiology, American Heart Association. Circulation 94:857–862, 1996.
37. Omenn GS, Beresford SAA, Motulsky AG. Preventing coronary artery disease: B vitamins and homocysteine. Circulation 97:421–424, 1998.
38. Diaz MN, Frei B, Vita JA, et al. Mechanisms of disease: antioxidants and atherosclerotic disease. N Engl J Med 337:408–416, 1997.
39. Ignarro LJ, Lippton H, Edwards JC, et al. Mechanism of vascular smooth muscle relaxation by organic nitrates, nitrites, nitroprusside and nitric oxide: Evidence for involvement of S-nitrosothiols as active intermediates. J Pharmacol Exp Ther 218:739–749, 1981.
40. Parker JD, Parker JO. Nitrate therapy for stable angina pectoris. N Engl J Med 338:520–531, 1998.
41. Abrams J. Nitrates. Med Clin North Am 72:1–35, 1988.
42. Elkayam U. Tolerance to organic nitrates: evidence, mechanisms, clinical relevance, and strategies for prevention. Ann Intern Med 114:667–677, 1991.
43. DeMots H, Glasser SP. Intermittent transdermal nitroglycerin therapy in the treatment of chronic stable angina. J Am Coll Cardiol 13:789–793, 1989.
44. Parker JO, Farrell B, Lahey KA, et al. Effect of intervals between doses on the development of tolerance to isosorbide dinitrate. N Engl J Med 316:1440–1444, 1987.
45. Thadani U, Maranda CR, Amsterdam E, et al. Lack of pharmacologic tolerance and rebound angina pectoris during twice-daily therapy with isosorbide-5-mononitrate. Ann Intern Med 120:353–359, 1994.
46. Parker JO, Vankoughnett KA, Farrell B. Nitroglycerin lingual spray: clinical efficacy and dose response relation. Am J Cardiol 57:1–5, 1986.
47. Reichek N, Goldstein RE, Redwood DR, et al. Sustained effects of nitroglycerin ointment in patients with angina pectoris. Circulation 50:348–352, 1974.
48. Reichek N, Priest C, Zimrin D, et al. Antianginal effects of nitroglycerin patches. Am J Cardiol 54:1–7, 1984.
49. Parker JO, Fung HL. Transdermal nitroglycerin in angina pectoris. Am J Cardiol 54:471–476, 1984.
50. Chrysant SG, Glasser SP, Bittar N, et al. Efficacy and safety of extended-release isosorbide mononitrate for stable effort angina pectoris. Am J Cardiol 72:1249–1256, 1993.
51. Fung HL. Pharmacokinetics and pharmacodynamics of organic nitrates. Am J Cardiol 60:4H–9H, 1987.
52. Thadani U, Prasad R, Hamilton SF, et al. Usefulness of twice-daily isosorbide-5-mononitrate in preventing development of tolerance in angina pectoris. Am J Cardiol 60:477–482, 1987.
53. Parker JO. Eccentric dosing with isosorbide-5-mononitrate in angina pectoris. Am J Cardiol 72:871–876, 1993.
54. Chrysant SG, Glasser SP, Bittar N, et al. Efficacy and safety of extended-release isosorbide mononitrate for stable effort angina pectoris. Am J Cardiol 72:1249–1256, 1993.
55. Frishman WH. β-Adrenergic blockers. Med Clin North Am 72:37–81, 1988.
56. Sproat TT, Lopez LM. Around the β-blockers, one more time. DICP, Ann Pharmacother 25:962–971, 1991.
57. Kazierad DJ, Schlanz KD, Bottoroff MB. β-Blockers. In: Evans WE, Schentag JJ, Jusko WJ, eds. Applied pharmacokinetics: principles of therapeutic drug monitoring. 3rd ed. Vancouver: Applied Therapeutics, 1992.

58. Thadani U, Davidson C, Singleton W, et al. Comparison of the immediate effects of five β-adrenoceptor-blocking drugs with different ancillary properties in angina pectoris. N Engl J Med 300:750–755, 1979.
59. Weiner DA. Calcium channel blockers. Med Clin North Am 72:83–115, 1988.
60. Opie LH. Calcium channel antagonists in the treatment of coronary artery disease: fundamental pharmacological properties relevant to clinical use. Prog Cardiovasc Dis 36:273–290, 1996.
61. Opie LH. Pharmacological differences between calcium antagonists. Eur Heart J 18:A71–A79, 1997.
62. Frishman WH, Sonnenblick EH. Calcium channel blockers. In: Schlant RC, Alexander RW, eds. The heart arteries and veins. 8th ed. New York: McGraw-Hill, 1994:1291–1308.
63. Opie LH, Messerli FH. Nifedipine and mortality, grave defects in the dossier. Circulation 92:1068–1073, 1995.
64. Yusuf S. Calcium antagonists in coronary artery disease and hypertension: time for reevaluation? Circulation 92:1079–1082, 1995.
65. Kloner RA. Nifedipine in ischemic heart disease. Circulation 92:1074–1078, 1995.
66. Furberg CD, Psaty BM, Meyer JV. Nifedipine, dose-related increase in mortality in patients with coronary heart disease. Circulation 92:1326–1331, 1995.
67. Mancia G, van Zwieten PA. How safe are calcium antagonists in hypertension and coronary heart disease? J Hypertens 7:13–17, 1996.
68. Strauss WE, Parisi AAF. Combined use of calcium-channel and beta-adrenergic blockers for the treatment of chronic stable angina: rationale, efficacy and adverse effects. Ann Intern Med 109:570–581, 1988.
69. Frishman W, Charlap S, Kimmel B, et al. Diltiazem, nifedipine, and their combination in patients with stable angina pectoris: effects on angina, exercise tolerance, and the ambulatory electrocardiographic ST segment. Circulation 77:774–786, 1988.
70. Pucci PD, Pollavini G, Zerauscheck M, et al. Acute effects on exercise tolerance of felodipine and diltiazem alone and in combination, in stable effort angina. Eur Heart J 12:55–59, 1991.
71. Deedwania PC. Is there evidence in support of the ischemia suppression hypotheses? J Am Coll Cardiol 24:21–24, 1994.
72. Knatterud GL, Bourassa MG, Pepine CJ, et al. Effects of treatment strategies to suppress ischemia in patients with coronary artery disease: 12-week results of the asymptomatic cardiac ischemia pilot (ACIP) study. J Am Coll Cardiol 24:11–20, 1994.
73. Pepine CJ, Cohn PF, Deedwania PC, et al. Effects of treatment on outcome in mildly symptomatic patients with ischemia during daily life: the Atenolol Silent Ischemia Study (ASIST). Circulation 90:762–768, 1994.
74. Davies RF, Goldberg AD, Forman S, et al. Asymptomatic Cardiac Ischemia Pilot (ACIP) study two-year follow-up: outcomes of patients randomized to initial strategies of medical therapy versus revascularization. Circulation 95:2037–2043, 1997.
75. Prida XE, Gelman JS, Feldman R, et al. Comparison of diltiazem and nifedipine alone and in combination in patients with coronary artery spasm. J Am Coll Cardiol 9:412–419, 1987.
76. Theroux P, Fuster V. Acute coronary syndromes: unstable angina and non–Q-wave myocardial infarction. Circulation 97:1195–1206, 1998.
77. Clinical practice guideline number 10. Unstable angina: diagnosis and management. U.S. Department of Health and Human Services. AHCPR Publication No. 94-0602.
78. Braunwald E, Jones RH, Mark DB, et al. Diagnosing and managing unstable angina. Circulation 90:613–622, 1994.
79. Theroux P, Ouimet H, McCams J, et al. Aspirin, heparin or both to treat acute unstable angina. N Engl J Med 319:1105–1111, 1988.
80. Cairns JA, Gent M, Singer J, et al. Aspirin, sulfinpyrazone or both in unstable angina. N Engl J Med 313:1369–1375, 1985.
81. Balsano F, Rizzon P, Violi F, et al. Antiplatelet treatment with ticlopidine in unstable angina: a controlled multicenter clinical trial. Circulation 82:17–26, 1990.
82. CAPRIE Steering Committee. A randomized, blinded, trial of Clopidogrel Versus Aspirin in Patients at Risk of Ischaemic Events (CAPRIE). Lancet 348:1329–1339, 1996.
83. Lefkovits J, Plow EF, Topol EJ. Platelet glycoprotein IIb/IIIa receptors in cardiovascular medicine. N Engl J Med 332:1553–1559, 1995.
84. The CAPTURE Investigators. Randomized placebo-controlled trial of abciximab before and during coronary intervention in refractory unstable angina: the CAPTURE trial. Lancet 349:1429–1435, 1997.
85. The platelet receptor inhibition in ischemic syndrome management in patients limited by unstable signs and symptoms (PRISM-PLUS) study investigators. Inhibition of the platelet glycoprotein IIb/IIIa receptor with tirofiban in unstable angina and non–Q-wave myocardial infarction. N Engl J Med 338:1488–1497, 1998.
86. The Platelet Receptor Inhibition in Ischemic Syndrome Management (PRISM) study investigators. A comparison of aspirin plus tirofiban with aspirin plus heparin for unstable angina. N Engl J Med 338:1498–1505, 1998.
87. PURSUIT Investigators. Platelet IIb/IIIa in Unstable Angina: Receptor Suppression Using Integrilin Trial (PURSUIT). N Engl J Med 339:436–443, 1998.
88. Theroux P, Waters D, Qui S, et al. Aspirin versus heparin to prevent myocardial infarction during the acute phase of unstable angina. Circulation 88:2045–2048, 1993.
89. Holdright D, Patel D, Cunningham D, et al. Comparison of the effect of heparin and aspirin versus aspirin alone on transient myocardial ischemia and in-hospital prognosis in patients with unstable angina. J Am Coll Cardiol 24:39–45, 1994.
90. RISC group. Risk of myocardial infarction and death during treatment with low dose aspirin and intravenous heparin in men with unstable coronary artery disease. Lancet 336:827–830, 1990.
91. Spinler SA, Nawarskas JJ. Low-molecular weight heparins for acute coronary syndromes. Ann Pharmacother 32:103–110, 1998.
92. Gurfinkel EP, Manos EJ, Mejail RI, et al. Low molecular weight heparin versus regular heparin or aspirin in the treatment of unstable angina and silent ischemia. J Am Coll Cardiol 26:313–318, 1995.
93. Thrombolysis in Myocardial Infarction (TIMI) 11A trial investigators. Dose-branding trial of enoxaparin for unstable angina: results of TIMI 11A. J Am Coll Cardiol 29:1474–1482, 1997.
94. Klein W, Buchwald A, Hillis SE, et al. Comparison of low-molecular-weight heparin with unfractionated heparin acutely and with placebo for 6 weeks in the management of unstable coronary artery disease: Fragmin in Unstable Coronary Artery Disease study (FRIC). Circulation 96:61–68, 1997.
95. FRISC study group. Low-molecular-weight heparin during instability in coronary artery disease. Lancet 347:561–568, 1996.
96. Cohen M, Demers C, Gurfinkel GP, et al. A comparison of low-molecular-weight heparin with unfractionated heparin for unstable coronary artery disease. N Engl J Med 337:447–452, 1997.
97. Sobel BE. Intracranial bleeding, fibrinolysis, and anticoagulation. Causal connections and clinical implications. Circulation 90:2147–2152, 1994.
98. Gusto IIb Investigators. A comparison of recombinant hirudin with heparin for the treatment of acute coronary syndromes. N Engl J Med 335:775–782, 1996.
99. Waters D, Lan JYT. Is thrombolytic therapy striking out in unstable angina? Circulation 86:1642–1644, 1992.
100. The TIMI IIIB Investigators. Effects of tissue plasminogen activator and a comparison of early invasive and conservative strategies in unstable angina and non–Q-wave myocardial infarction. Results of the TIMI IIIB Trial. Circulation 89:1545–1556, 1994.
101. Held PH, Yusuf S, Furberg C. Calcium channel blockers in acute myocardial infarction and unstable angina: an overview. BMJ 299:1187–1192, 1989.
102. Muller JE, Morrison J, Stone PH, et al. Nifedipine therapy for patients with threatened and acute myocardial infarction: a randomized, double-blind, placebo-controlled comparison. Circulation 69:740–747, 1984.
103. Lubsen J, Tijssen JG. Efficacy of nifedipine and metoprolol in the early treatment of unstable angina in the coronary care unit: findings from the Holland Interuniversity Nifedipine/Metoprolol Trial (HINT). Am J Cardiol 60:18A–25A, 1987.
104. Kirklin JW, Akins CW, Blackstone EH, et al. ACC/AHA guidelines and indications for coronary artery bypass graft surgery, a report of the American College of Cardiology/American Heart Association task force on assessment of diagnostic and therapeutic cardiovascular procedures (subcommittee on coronary artery bypass graft surgery). Circulation 83:1125–1173, 1991.
105. Ryan TJ, Faxon DP, Gunnar RM, et al. Guidelines for percutaneous transluminal coronary angioplasty, a report of the American College of Cardiology/American Heart Association task force on assessment of diagnostic and therapeutic cardiovascular procedures (subcommittee on percutaneous transluminal coronary angioplasty). Circulation 78:486–502, 1988.
106. Pepine CJ, Holmes DR Jr, Block PC, et al. Coronary artery stents. J Am Coll Cardiol 28:782–794, 1996.
107. Pearson T, Rapaport E, Criqui M, et al. Optimal risk factor management in the patient after coronary revascularization, a statement for healthcare professionals from an American Heart Association writing group. Circulation 90:3125–3133, 1994.
108. Landau C, Lange RA, Hillis LD. Percutaneous transluminal coronary angioplasty. N Engl J Med 330:981–993, 1994.
109. Popma JJ, Weitz J, Bittl JA, et al. Antithrombotic therapy in patients undergoing coronary angioplasty. Chest 114:728s–741s, 1998.

CHAPTER 43

ACUTE MYOCARDIAL INFARCTION

Edgar R. Gonzalez and Barbara S. Kannewurf

DEFINITION

Myocardial infarction (MI) is defined as death of myocardial tissue. The extent and location of the infarction depend on the degree of ischemic burden, the availability of coronary collateral blood flow, the rapidity of reperfusion, and the location of the afflicted coronary artery.

TREATMENT GOALS: ACUTE MYOCARDIAL INFARCTION

- Abort the infarction.
- Salvage the area of jeopardized myocardium.
- Increase myocardial oxygen delivery.
- Decrease myocardial oxygen consumption.
- Provide symptomatic relief and reduce anxiety.
- Prevent complications and recurrences.
- Reduce mortality and improve quality of life.

EPIDEMIOLOGY

Every 20 seconds someone in America has an acute myocardial infarction (AMI). Coronary artery disease (CAD), the primary predisposing factor for AMI, affects approximately 13 million Americans of whom 1.5 million have an AMI each year.[1] In the United States, the magnitude of AMI as a public health concern is exemplified by the fact that 1 of 160 Americans has a heart attack. AMI is a frequent cause of emergency hospitalization in community hospitals and university medical centers and is the leading cause of death in the United States. Every hour, an American dies of a heart attack. In 1995, more than 400,000 Americans died from heart attacks; 50% of these patients suffered an out-of-hospital cardiac arrest within the first few hours from the onset of their cardiac symptoms.[2] Mortality among AMI victims ranges from 10 to 15% during the first year, decreasing to 3.5% per year thereafter.[2,3] Survival after AMI is determined partly by the extent of remaining viable myocardium and by the occurrence of complications. Patients with anterior wall infarction, left ventricular dysfunction, and complex ventricular ectopy have the highest 1-year mortality rate after AMI (20%); patients with AMI without these risk factors have a 3% mortality rate.[4]

PATHOPHYSIOLOGY

An increase in myocardial oxygen demand relative to the available myocardial oxygen supply or an acute decrease in myocardial oxygen delivery can precipitate acute myocardial ischemic injury. Episodes of ischemia that last more than 30 minutes usually cause MI. The involved area can be divided into three zones: the zone of infarction, the zone of injury, and the zone of ischemia (Fig. 43.1). The infarction may be limited to the interior of the myocardium (subendocardial MI) or to a visceral layer of the pericardium (epicardial MI) or may extend through the full thickness of the myocardial wall (transmural MI). The most common cause of AMI is atherosclerosis of the coronary arteries, which narrows the coronary lumen and reduces myocardial blood supply. The terms *athero* and *sclerosis* are derived from the Greek words *gruel* and *hard*, respectively. The word *gruel* is similar to the rubbish located at the foundation of most formed plaques. *Hard* corresponds to the fibrotic cap of the lesion. The first noticeable sign of an atherosclerotic lesion is a fatty streak (yellow stripe) that runs parallel to the axis of the vessel.[5] The lesion progresses to form necrotic core composed primarily of lipids and cellular debris. Fibrous caps

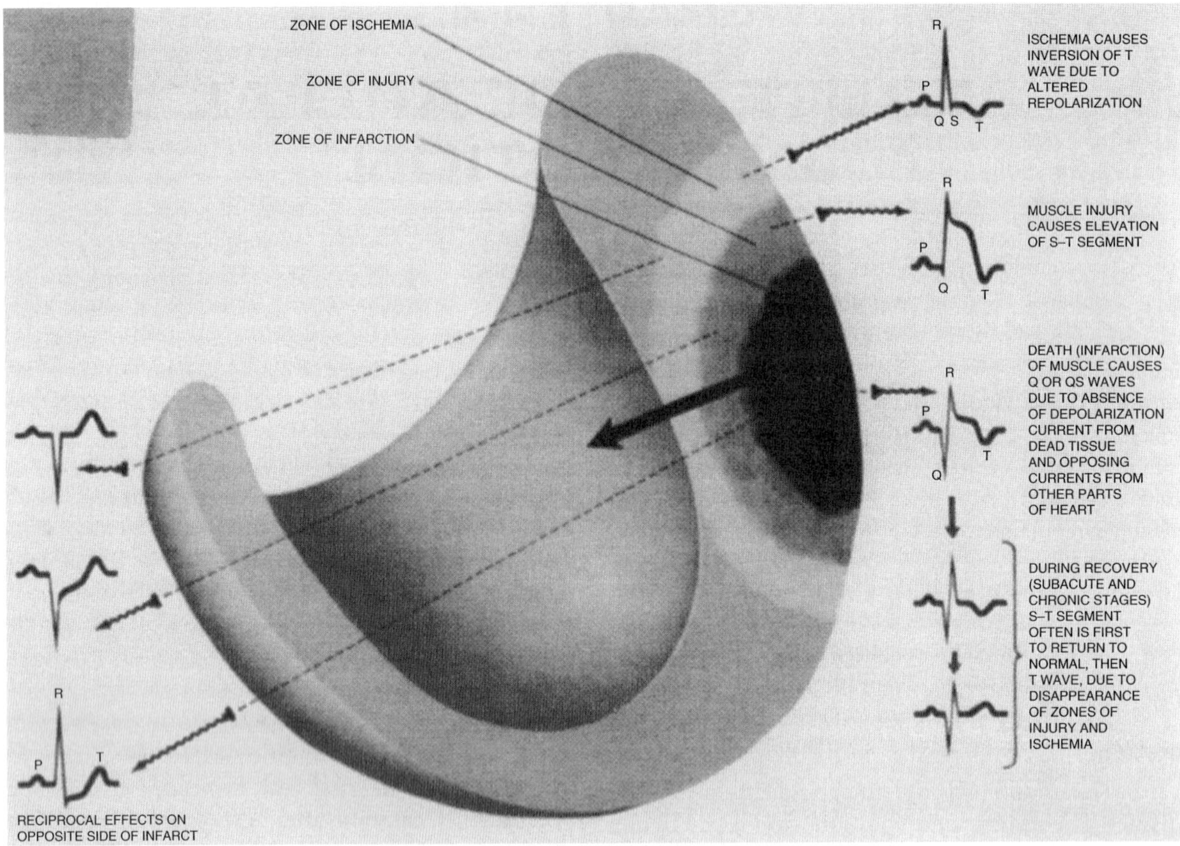

Figure 43.1. Effects of cardiac infarction, injury, and ischemia. (Reprinted with permission from Netter FH. The Netter Collection. In: Yonkman FF, ed. The Ciba collection of medical illustrations: heart. New York: Ciba Pharmaceutical Company, 1969:62.)

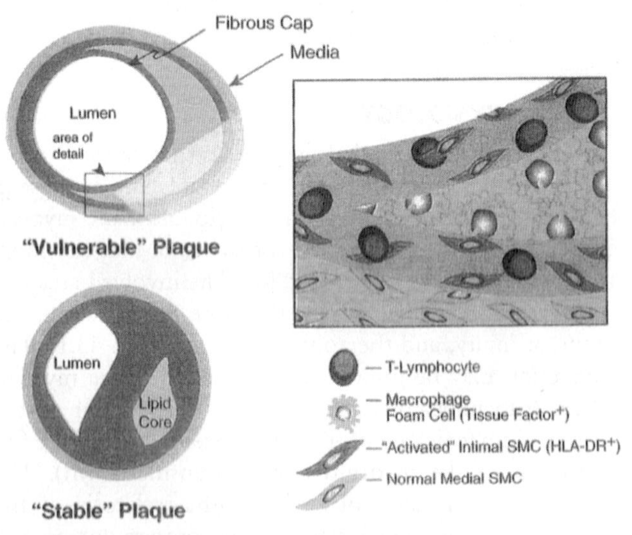

Figure 43.2. Stable and vulnerable plaques. (Reprinted with permission from Libby P. Molecular bases of the acute coronary syndromes. Circulation 91:2844–2850, 1995.)

composed of smooth muscle and collagen cover the fatty streaks leading to "vulnerable" lesions[5] (Fig. 43.2). Ulceration of the vulnerable lesion or regional changes in blood flow trigger platelet aggregation leading to subsequent thrombosis and coronary occlusion.[6,7]

Platelet involvement in thrombus formation begins with vessel wall injury followed by platelet adhesion, activation, and aggregation.[5] After adhesion, platelets become activated through a cascade of steps that involve different agonists, including collagen, thrombin, serotonin, and epinephrine. These agonists trigger the release of agents that foster platelet aggregation (i.e., adenosine diphosphate [ADP] and thromboxane A_2 [TXA_2]). Elevated shear force fosters the formation of atherosclerotic plaques within the intimal lumen. In the presence of disrupted blood flow or vascular insult, arterial thrombi or white clots form in these areas of high shear force.[2] Shear force-induced platelet aggregation is mediated by ADP. ADP and TXA_2 draw new platelets into areas of growing thrombi, leading to arterial thrombus formation. ADP and TXA_2 activate the glycoprotein IIb/IIIa receptor complex to produce a transformational change that allows fibrinogen to bind and links the platelets together. Fibrin strands and erythrocytes coat the platelet-rich area and form thrombus (i.e., red-plug).

Patients at highest risk for suffering an AMI are those with a prior history of AMI, CAD, or malignant arrhythmias.[8] Both modifiable and nonmodifiable risk factors increase the risk of AMI. Nonmodifiable risk factors such as increased age, male sex, and family history identify patients at risk for AMI. Common modifiable risk factors (i.e., cigarette smoking, diabetes mellitus, hyperlipidemia, hypertension, obesity, and physical inactivity) should be identified and, whenever possible, changed.

Diabetes mellitus, high levels of low-density lipoprotein (LDL) cholesterol, increased levels of catecholamines, or other factors affecting blood flow can contribute to the formation of an intravascular clot.[5] Less frequently, coronary vasospasm may precipitate clot formation and lead to complete coronary occlusion. Cocaine abuse has also been implicated as a possible cause of AMI due to complete coronary closure in the absence of coronary atherosclerosis. The morning hours are the peak times for suffering an AMI due to an increase in sympathetic activity that enhances platelet adhesiveness and coronary vasoconstriction. During the early morning hours, there is also an alteration in the plasminogen inhibitor and plasminogen ratio, making existing atherosclerotic plaques more vulnerable to rupture.[8] Antiplatelet agents and β-adrenergic blocking agents reduce the incidence of AMI by attenuating hyperaggregability of platelets and blunting the effects of circulating catecholamines, respectively. Precipitating factors for AMI include vasospasm, physical or emotional stress, hemorrhage, trauma, respiratory failure, hypoglycemia, exogenous sympathomimetics or other vasoactive substances, and hypersensitivity reactions.

Patients with >70% narrowing of the luminal diameter of one or more of the major coronary arteries (right coronary artery [RCA], left main, left anterior descending [LAD], or left circumflex [LCX]) are at greatest risk of ischemic injury (Fig. 43.3). The location of the coronary thrombus determines the anatomic site of the AMI. Occlusion of the LAD artery usually causes an anterior wall infarction that may disrupt function of the left ventricle and may precipitate cardiogenic shock and sudden death. Occlusion of the RCA may produce an inferior wall infarction or a right ventricular (RV) infarction. RV infarction with bradycardia and hypotension may occur in patients with inferior wall MI.[9] Occlusion of the LCX usually results in a lateral wall infarction or a multiple-site infarction (e.g., anterolateral wall infarctions). A posterior wall infarction may also result from occlusion of the LCX, the RCA, or both.[8]

CLINICAL PRESENTATION AND DIAGNOSIS

Signs and Symptoms

The patient's chief complaint and medical history are invaluable in establishing a diagnosis of MI. Chest discomfort (i.e., oppressive, burning, squeezing, choking, or expanding sensation; tightness; or indigestion) is the most common presenting complaint. The discomfort is typically substernal; radiates to the neck, throat, jaw, shoulders, and arms; and may last from 30 minutes to several hours. Substernal chest pain associated with AMI does not subside with rest, is partially relieved by nitroglycerin, and produces a sense of "impending doom." Most patients have prodromal symptoms (e.g., vague chest discomfort, weakness, fatigue, nausea, vomiting, and diaphoresis) before the acute attack.[10] Less commonly, an episode of light-headedness or syncope heralds the onset of AMI. However, approximately 15 to 20% of AMIs are asymptomatic ("silent MI"), and 33% of AMIs go undiagnosed, especially in women with preexisting hypertension, patients with diabetes, and elderly patients.

A detailed medical history may help to differentiate myocardial ischemic pain from noncardiac chest pain and may help uncover medication noncompliance. Review of

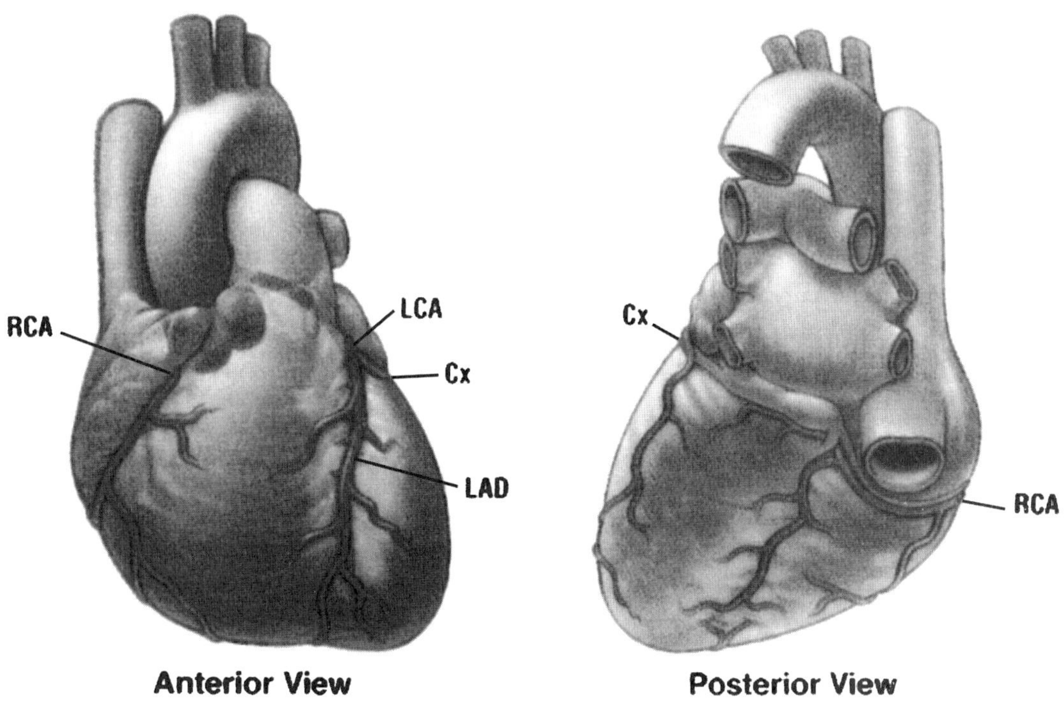

Figure 43.3. Common arteries of the heart: right coronary artery (*RCA*); left coronary artery (*LCA*); left circumflex artery (*Cx*). (*Source:* Reference 8.)

systems may reveal a patient who is anxious, restless, cool, sweaty, and pale. Sinus tachycardia and mild fever are commonly observed. Sinus bradycardia is more common with inferior wall MI because occlusion of the RCA causes sinus node dysfunction. Blood pressure fluctuations are common during AMI. Hypertension may accompany pain and anxiety; whereas hypotension may result from drug-induced vasodilation, left ventricular dysfunction, or hypovolemia. Respirations are often rapid and shallow. Supplemental oxygen increases oxygen delivery and reduces the work of breathing. Heart sounds may be faint or normal; and an atrial gallop (S_4 sound) may be present.

Low-grade fever (i.e., <38° C) may be observed during the first 72 hours after AMI. Other physical findings include hypertensive retinopathy, diabetic nephropathy, and cholesterol-related xanthomas. Nonspecific laboratory abnormalities associated with AMI include polymorphonuclear leukocytosis (12,000 to 15,000/mm^3) that persists for 3 to 7 days and an elevated erythrocyte sedimentation rate, which peaks during the first week. Hypokalemia and hypomagnesemia may be present, especially in patients treated with diuretics, and may precipitate malignant ventricular arrhythmias.

Diagnosis

A detailed history may help differentiate AMI from nonischemic chest pain syndromes (e.g., costochondritis, pericarditis, cardiac tamponade, or gastroesophageal reflux disease). The diagnosis of AMI is confirmed when any two of the following three clinical features are present: ischemic chest pain that lasts longer than 30 minutes and is unrelieved by nitroglycerin; new electrocardiogram (ECG) changes that are consistent with AMI (i.e., ST-segment elevation in two contiguous precordial leads or more than 1- to 2-mm ST-segment elevation in two contiguous limb leads); or the presence of abnormally elevated cardiac enzymes in the bloodstream.

Myocardial necrosis causes the release of intracellular enzymes (e.g, creatinine kinase [CK], lactate dehydrogenase [LDH], and aspartate aminotransferase [AST]), myoglobin, and troponin into the systemic circulation. The temporal pattern of appearance in the systemic circulation after an AMI is of diagnostic importance (Table 43.1). Although the systemic release of CK is increased after skeletal muscle trauma related to surgery, exercise, or intramuscular injections, the MB fraction of CK is released only from heart muscle and its concentration in blood may be used to determine the presence of an AMI. LDH increases more slowly than CK. When assessed within the second and third days postinfarction, LDH has a relatively high specificity (94%) and good clinical sensitivity (85%) for AMI.[3,10] LDH_2 is the major LDH isoenzyme in blood; thus, the normal serum pattern shows more LDH_2 than LDH_1. A change in this relationship is seen after AMI, renal necrosis, and hemolysis. Within 48 hours after AMI, this serum pattern reverses in 80% of patients, who now show higher LDH_1 concentrations than LDH_2 concentrations. Because of poor sensitivity and specificity, the presence of AST is no longer used routinely to diagnose an AMI.

Serum myoglobin (S-Mgb) is an intracellular muscle protein that can serve as another marker for AMI. Because of the small size of S-Mgb size compared with CK, S-Mgb is able to diffuse faster through injured cell membranes. S-Mgb appears at higher than normal levels as early as 1 to 3 hours after the onset of AMI and peaks much more rapidly than either CK or LDH.[11] S-Mgb is of value in the early evaluation of patients with a potential AMI. A rapid rise in S-Mgb and a doubling of the S-Mgb concentration within the first 2 hours of treatment, even if the second level is within normal limits, is highly specific for AMI.[11] Because elevated S-Mgb levels usually return to normal within 12 to 24 hours after the onset of symptoms, an isolated normal S-Mgb or a serial S-Mgb level that does not double does not necessarily rule out AMI.[11]

Studies now suggest that an assay based on monoclonal antibodies against troponin I is a better marker for AMI than CK-MB.[12] Troponin is part of the contractile apparatus of the myocardium. It is a regulatory subunit consisting of I, T, and C subunits.[13] Troponin I, or cardiac troponin, is used in the diagnosis of AMI because of its higher absolute cardiac specificity over the other troponin subunits.[13] Unlike CK and LDH, troponin I is highly specific to cardiac tissue and is not expressed in inflammatory and noninflammatory myopathies, skeletal muscle trauma, or chronic renal insufficiency.[13,14] Troponin I is undetectable in normal healthy adults.[14] The troponin I level peaks within 6 hours of the acute event and may remain elevated for as long as 7 to 10 days. Serial concentrations of troponin I should be measured at 3-hour intervals for the first 6 hours and then every 8 hours for the

Table 43.1 ▪ Myocardial Markers

Parameter	Normal Range	Detectable (hr)	Time to Peak (hr)	Normalization (days)
Total CPK	Varies, 250–400 U/L	6–10	10–24	2–3
CK-MB mass	<8.0 ng/mL	3–6	10–24	3–4
Myoglobin	<76 ng/mL F <92 ng/mL M	1–3	6–9	½–1
Troponin 1	<2.0 ng/mL	4–6	24	3–10

CPK, creatinine phosphokinase; *CK-MB,* MB fraction of creatinine kinase.

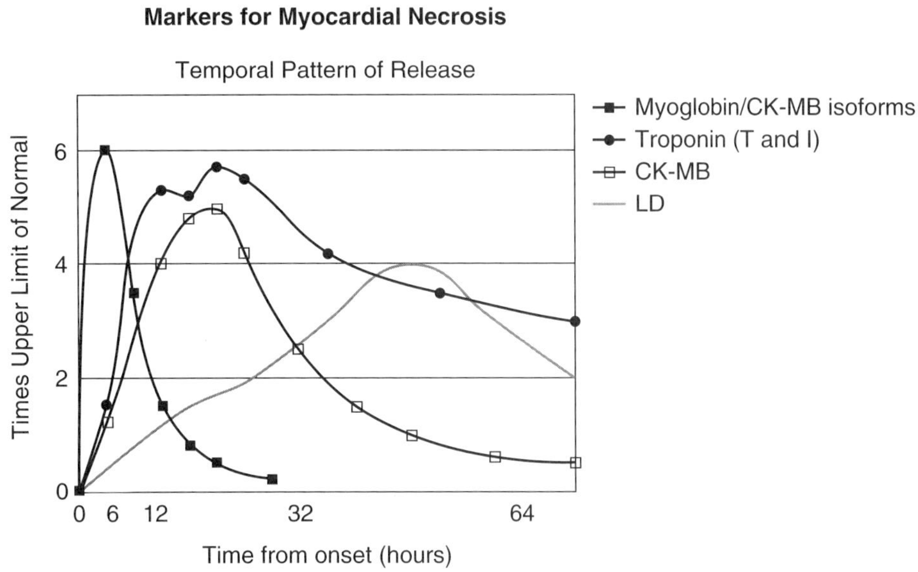

Figure 43.4. Temporal pattern of release of markers for myocardial necrosis. *CK-MB*, MB isoform of creatinine kinase; *LD*, lactate dehydrogenase.

remaining 24 hours (Fig. 43.4). Once an elevated troponin I level is detected, the patient is likely to have myocardial injury. Many medical centers are now using troponin assays in the diagnosis of AMI.

The ECG permits detection of the three pathophysiologic events occurring during an AMI: ischemia (T-wave inversion), injury (ST-segment elevation), and infarction (pathologic Q waves) (Fig. 43.1). The diagnostic feature of MI is a deep, wide Q wave or Q-S pattern (i.e., an initial slight upward deflection followed by a pronounced downward deflection) in the ECG leads corresponding to the area of injury. Although Q waves are seen more commonly in transmural than in nontransmural infarctions, both types may occur with or without Q waves. Therefore, it is more appropriate to use the terms *Q-wave* and *non–Q-wave* infarction.[15] It is important to note that Q waves do not diagnose an infarction. The presence of a Q wave will not be seen on an ECG until approximately 1 day after the event. If a patient is seen in the hospital with Q waves present on an ECG, this is evidence of a previous infarct. Non–Q-wave infarctions are associated with lower in-hospital mortality and complications, but are associated with an increased risk of subsequent events such as another infarction, a reinfarction, ischemia, or even death. Q-wave infarctions are associated with high rates of in-hospital deaths and complications. However, the risk of reinfarction or subsequent events is less.

An anterior wall MI is diagnosed by ST-segment elevations in leads V_1 and V_4 on an ECG strip. An inferior wall infarct results in ST-segment elevation in the inferior leads of an ECG, leads II, III, and aVF. RV infarctions usually cause ST-segment elevation in lead V4R and bradycardia because the RCA serves as the main blood supply to the sinoatrial node. If an inferior wall MI is identified on a left-sided ECG, a right-sided ECG should be done to exclude the possibility of a RV infarction in combination with inferior wall MI. A lateral infarction shows ST-segment elevation in leads I, aVL, V_5, and V_6. ECG changes seen with a posterior infarction are ST-segment depression in leads V_1 and V_2 with tall R waves.

A conduction disturbance of the His bundle fibers (bundle branch block) may conceal the diagnosis of an AMI on an ECG. A bundle branch block distorts the ST segment on an ECG tracing. A left bundle branch block (LBBB) can shadow the diagnosis of an AMI more so than a right bundle branch block (RBBB). Blockage along the LAD can lead to LBBBs; whereas RCA occlusion can lead to RBBBs. A preexisting LBBB or RBBB will not interfere with ECG diagnosis of AMI. To determine if the conduction block is old or new requires previous ECG tracings. In the absence of an old ECG, the presence of either LBBB or RBBB makes the diagnosis of AMI difficult.

Pericarditis is inflammation of the pericardium, the fluid-filled sac that surrounds the heart. Pericarditis may produce chest pain and ECG changes and can confound the diagnosis of AMI. The ECG is useful in distinguishing pericarditis from an AMI based on the shape of the ST-segment elevation. The ST-segment elevation seen in AMI is rounded or concave, whereas pericarditis produces flat or convex ST-segment elevations.[16] In addition to ST-segment elevation seen with pericarditis, the T wave is often above the isoelectric line.

Radionuclide imaging techniques are valuable in assessing myocardial ischemic injury and confirming the suspicion of AMI in patients with atypical clinical presentations. Acute infarct scintigraphic ("hot-spot") imaging with infarct-avid Tc99m-pyrophosphatase aids in localizing and measuring the area of necrosis within 2 to 5 days after the AMI. Myocardial perfusion imaging with thallium-201, which is taken up and concentrated in viable myocardium,

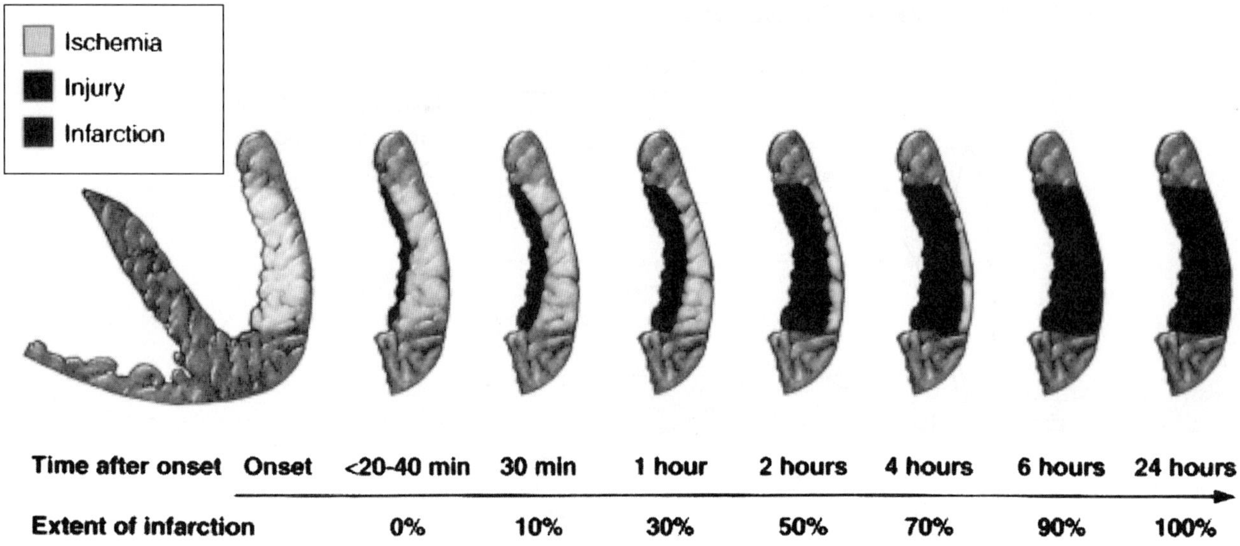

Figure 43.5. Time after onset–damage over time. (*Source:* Reference 8.)

reveals a defect ("cold-spot") within 6 hours after AMI. Radionuclide ventriculography frequently reveals wall motion abnormalities and a reduced ventricular ejection fraction in patients with AMI.

PSYCHOSOCIAL ASPECTS

Time is a crucial factor in the treatment of AMI because thrombolytic therapy within the first hour after the onset of symptoms can salvage myocardial tissue and can abort an evolving AMI. Unfortunately, patients fail to recognize the early signs of AMI and hesitate to seek prompt medical attention. The GISSI (Gruppo Italiano per lo Studio della Sopravvivenza nell'Infarto Miocardico) multicenter study compared 590 patients who were seen more than 12 hours after symptom onset with 600 patients treated within 2 hours and 603 patients treated between 6 and 12 hours.[17] Sixty percent of patients seen within 2 hours received thrombolytic therapy versus 18% of patients admitted more than 12 hours after the onset of symptoms. Factors associated with delayed hospital admission included age older than 65, living alone, diabetes mellitus, mild-to-moderate rather than severe pain, and onset of pain at night or at home.

Patients who are at risk for suffering an AMI as well as family members should be educated about the urgent need to seek help at the initial onset of symptoms and not wait to see if these symptoms abate with time. The classic symptoms as well as prodromal symptoms should be reinforced initially and again at each patient visit. National public awareness campaigns increase knowledge and awareness of the signs and symptoms associated with a heart attack.[18] Unfortunately, the results from these campaigns are disappointing because increased patient awareness appears to taper off several weeks after the end of the public awareness campaigns.[19] These observations suggest the need for patient education.

THERAPEUTIC PLAN

After an AMI, sudden death is likely during the first 24-hours. If the infarction occurs outside the hospital setting, immediate transport to a hospital emergency department (ED) for management is essential. Activation of the 911 system reduces the time interval from ED arrival to definitive treatment and improves the likelihood of myocardial salvage (Fig. 43.5). Once acute therapy has been instituted and the patient's condition has been stabilized, he or she should be transferred to the coronary intensive care unit (CICU) for further observation and care.

Patients are triaged into risk and treatment categories for definitive diagnosis of AMI, for correction of underlying hematologic or electrolyte abnormalities, and for assessment of potential AMI-related complications. For example, a patient with ischemic chest pain that shows ECG changes consistent with an AMI will be rapidly evaluated for thrombolytic therapy. A complete history and physical examination, including rectal examination if not already obtained, should be completed. Routine clinical laboratory studies, including measurements of serum electrolytes and enzymatic markers of cardiac ischemia and injury, are performed. A 12-lead ECG and, if needed, a right-sided ECG should be obtained. Patients should receive oxygen, nitroglycerin, aspirin, and morphine. A chest radiograph with a portable x-ray machine should also be obtained soon after arrival at the ED.

TREATMENT

Pharmacotherapy

Oxygen

Supplemental oxygen reduces the ischemic burden. Hypoxmia usually results from ventilation-perfusion abnormalities, commonly caused by left ventricular dysfunction. Oxygen is administered at a rate of 4 L/min by mask or nasal cannula for the first 24 to 48 hours. Endotracheal intubation and positive airway pressure mechanical ventilation should be used if adequate oxygenation (oxygen saturation >90%) cannot be maintained by mask. High-level, continuous positive airway pressure improves tissue oxygenation and reduces the spontaneous respiratory effort without producing circulatory depression in patients with AMI and with left ventricular dysfunction.[20] Arterial blood gas determinations should be avoided shortly after the administration of thrombolytic therapy to minimize the risk of arterial bleeding. Continuous pulse oximetry monitoring assesses the adequacy of oxygenation and avoids the bleeding risk and discomfort produced by arterial punctures for blood gas monitoring.

Analgesics

Pain relief is an initial therapeutic objective. Prompt pain relief attenuates the sympathetic hyperactivity that increases myocardial oxygen demand and predisposes patients to tachyarrhythmias.[21] Numerous analgesic drugs (morphine, meperidine, and nalbuphine) have been used in AMI. Morphine is the agent of choice except in patients with a well-documented morphine hypersensitivity. In addition to relieving pain and anxiety, the hemodynamic effects of morphine are invaluable in patients with pulmonary edema. Morphine is a potent vasodilator. It increases venous capacitance and decreases systemic vascular resistance.[22] These effects are most pronounced in patients with heightened sympathetic tone. A dose of 2 to 4 mg should be administered intravenously over 1 to 2 minutes and repeated at 5- to 15-minute intervals until the pain is relieved or side effects occur (i.e., hypotension, respiratory depression, or vomiting) that precludes further administration. Adequate hydration and use of the recumbent position help reduce the risk of morphine-induced hypotension.

Concomitant administration of atropine 0.5 mg intravenously may help reverse the vagomimetic effects of morphine on blood pressure and heart rate. Meperidine 25 to 75 mg by slow intravenous injection every 2 to 3 hours as needed for pain control is a suitable alternative in morphine-intolerant patients. The anticholinergic effect of meperidine counteracts the heightened vagal tone in patients with AMI and with either bradycardia or nausea. Tachycardia is a potential adverse effect of meperidine administration. Patients should be monitored for the respiratory-depressant effects of narcotic analgesic.

Nalbuphine hydrochloride is a synthetic opioid analgesic with mixed narcotic agonist and antagonist effects. Results of one study comparing the hemodynamic effects of nalbuphine and morphine in patients with AMI indicate that nalbuphine relieves pain and reduces myocardial oxygen demand without producing hypotension. Nalbuphine is a useful agent in patients with AMI because it produces less respiratory depression, less hypotension, and less vagal stimulation than morphine. Nalbuphine 10 mg is administered intravenously every 3 to 6 hours as needed for pain relief. Although butorphanol, a synthetic opioid agonist-antagonist, does not appear to significantly alter systemic hemodynamics, it should be avoided in patients with AMI because of concerns that this agent may increase systemic vascular resistance and myocardial oxygen demand.[23] Pentazocine and butorphanol should be used with caution in patients with AMI because these agents may increase systemic vascular resistance and myocardial oxygen demand.

Nitrates

Organic nitrates, such as nitroglycerin and nitroprusside, reduce preload and afterload by their venodilatory and arteriodilatory effects, respectively.[24–30] Nitrates reduce myocardial oxygen demand and dilate the epicardial coronary vasculature. Nitroglycerin reduces intramyocardial wall tension, improves myocardial blood flow, and lowers systemic vascular resistance. Sublingual nitroglycerin is tried first unless the patient's systolic blood pressure is less than 90 mm Hg. In the presence of persistent ischemia and hypotension, nitroglycerin paste or intravenous nitroglycerin is preferred over sublingual nitroglycerin because the paste may be applied and removed promptly and the dose of intravenous nitroglycerin may be titrated to prevent further reductions in blood pressure.[24–30]

Nitroglycerin is generally well tolerated. Potential complications of intravenous nitroglycerin include reversible hypotension and bradycardia, hypoxemia due to increased pulmonary ventilation-perfusion mismatch, methemoglobinemia, and headache. Patients with nitroglycerin-induced hypotension usually respond to fluid resuscitation (e.g., 250 to 500 mL of 0.9% saline solution) to maintain adequate cardiac output. Vasopressor agents are seldom required and should be avoided due to their propensity to worsen ischemia by increasing myocardial oxygen demand. Nitroglycerin may trigger a vasovagal reaction. In this situation, patients experience a paradoxical reduction in heart rate after nitroglycerin-induced hypotension.[24–27] These patients require fluid resuscitation and intravenous atropine (0.5 to 1.0 mg).

Nitroglycerin is contraindicated in patients suffering from a right ventricular infarct or those suffering from marked bradycardia (<50 bpm). For patients with right ventricular infarction, the risk of precipitous hypotension with nitroglycerin is substantial because nitroglycerin increases venous capacitance and decreases venous return to the right atrium. These changes decrease left ventricular filling volume and compromise cardiac output. Patients with nitroglycerin-induced hypotension usually respond to fluid resuscitation (e.g., 250 to 500 mL of 0.9% saline solution) to maintain adequate cardiac output. Vasopressor agents are seldom required and should be avoided because of their propensity to worsen ischemia by increasing myocardial oxygen demand.

The persistence of pain over several hours is a bad prognostic sign, usually indicative of continued myocardial ischemia and necrosis. Nitroglycerin effectively relieves refractory angina in most patients. Patients with pulmonary edema derive great benefit from intravenous nitroglycerin because the venodilatory effects of nitroglycerin are directly proportional to preload (i.e., left ventricular end-diastolic pressure).[29] Prompt initiation of intravenous nitroglycerin therapy may reduce infarct size and decrease the incidence of congestive heart failure in patients with AMI.[29] Nitroglycerin infusion decreases both enzymatically assessed infarct size and hospital mortality in patients with AMI and with left ventricular dysfunction.[24]

Intravenous nitroglycerin is an effective adjunct in the management of heart failure associated with MI. It is administered by a continuous intravenous infusion at 10 to 20 μg/min and increased by 5 to 10 μg/min every 5 to 10 minutes until the desired hemodynamic or clinical response occurs. Low doses (30 to 40 μg/min) produce predominantly venodilation; high doses (250 μg/min) lead to arteriolar dilation as well.[25] In cardiogenic shock, the beneficial effects of nitroglycerin are due to systemic vasodilation, which increases cardiac output and lowers oxygen consumption, and to direct vasodilation of the coronary circulation, which increases blood supply to ischemic areas more than nitroprusside.[25,26] The combination of nitroglycerin and an inotrope (dopamine and dobutamine), although not extensively studied, appears to produce marked hemodynamic improvements while reducing the risk of ischemic damage.[26] Overall, patients with the most severe degree of left ventricular failure have the most beneficial hemodynamic effects.

Studies show a difference between nitroglycerin and nitroprusside relative to their effect on myocardial blood flow.[27] Nitroglycerin has a greater vasodilatory effect on venous capacitance vessels than on arterial resistance vessels. In contrast, nitroprusside has a balanced vasodilatory effect on arteriolar resistance vessels and venous capacitance vessels. In patients with AMI, nitroglycerin is preferred over nitroprusside because nitroglycerin is less likely to produce "coronary steal" and worsen myocardial ischemia.[28,29] Coronary steal occurs either when blood is shunted away from the coronary arteries because of a fall in diastolic blood pressure or when blood is shunted away from the coronary collateral circulation because of a reduction in capillary resistance. Nitroglycerin is less likely to produce coronary steal than nitroprusside because nitroglycerin does not reduce coronary resistance, but facilitates blood flow along venous capacitance vessels in the coronary collateral circulation.

In summary, nitroglycerin does not readily relax resistance vessels and is less likely to reduce coronary perfusion pressure or shunt blood away from venous capacitance vessels (e.g., the collaterals) than nitroprusside.[28,29] The risk reduction in mortality in AMI trials with nitroglycerin is 45%; which is greater than the 23% reduction in mortality observed with nitroprusside.[29] These data suggest that intravenous nitroglycerin reduces mortality in AMI.

Antiplatelet Agents

Aspirin inhibits platelet aggregation by irreversible acetylation of cyclooxygenase. Cyclooxygenase is an enzyme involved in the synthesis of TXA_2 and prostaglandin I_2 (PGI_2). TXA_2 is released by platelets, serving as a platelet aggregator as well as a vasodilator.[30] PGI_2 is produced by vascular endothelium and is an inhibitor of platelet aggregation and a vasodilator.[30] Aspirin shifts the balance in favor of PGI_2 because vascular endothelium synthesizes new cyclooxygenase within 6 hours, despite irreversible inactivation of platelet-derived cyclooxygenase.[30] Low-dose aspirin (i.e., 80 to 325 mg/day) inhibits TXA_2 for the lifetime of the platelet (i.e., 7 days).[30] High-dose aspirin (e.g., 1000 mg/day) inhibits PGI_2 as well as TXA_2.[30,31]

Studies have been conducted using aspirin as well as other antiplatelet agents in the prevention of MI in patients with unstable angina.[32,33] Theroux et al.[32] compared aspirin (325 mg twice daily) versus heparin (1000 U/hr) or the combination of both in a double-blind, placebo-controlled trial of 479 patients with unstable angina pectoris. The incidence of MI was 3% with aspirin ($P = .01$), 0.8% with heparin ($P < .001$), and 1.6% with aspirin and heparin ($P = .003$) and 12% with placebo.[32] The mortality rate with active treatment was 0% compared to 1.7% with placebo. Theroux et al.[32] concluded that heparin decreased the incidence of MI; aspirin was also effective but the combination of aspirin and heparin produced a greater number of complications and was no better than heparin alone.

The Second International Study of Infarct Survival Trial (ISIS-II) compared the relative efficacy of intravenous streptokinase (1.5 mU), oral aspirin (160 mg/day), both, or neither in patients with suspected MI.[33] Streptokinase reduced mortality at 5 weeks (9.2% with streptokinase versus 12% with placebo ($P < .0001$). Similar results were observed with aspirin alone (9.4% with aspirin) versus placebo (11.8%) ($P < .00001$). The combination of aspirin and streptokinase was significantly more effective than either agent alone ($P < .0001$). Combination therapy had significantly fewer side effects than either agent did alone. Aspirin was as effective as streptokinase in reducing the risk of death; however, there was more benefit when the agents were used together.[33] Furthermore, aspirin reduced the rate of reinfarction.[33]

Unless contraindicated, the administration of low doses (160 to 325 mg) of aspirin is advocated in all patients suspected of having an AMI. Upon arrival at the ED, patients with unstable angina or AMI should chew two baby aspirin tablets (160 mg total dose) irrespective of the need for thrombolytic therapy.[34]

Ticlopidine and clopidogrel are thienopyridine compounds that selectively bind adenylate cyclase-coupled ADP receptors and irreversibly inhibit platelet aggregation induced by epinephrine, collagen, thrombin, and platelet-activating factor.[35] Thienopyridine compounds reduce fibrinogen levels, platelet deposition on atheromatous plaque, and blood viscosity.[35,36] The antiplatelet effects of thienopyridines occur within 24 to 48 hours and peak after repeated administration around day 5 to 6.[35,36] The recommended dose of ticlopidine is 250 mg administered two times a day. The recommended dose for clopidogrel is 75 mg once a day.

Knudsen et al.[37] compared ticlopidine (250 mg twice daily) with placebo on platelet function in patients with AMI treated within 12 hours of onset of precordial pain. Antiplatelet therapy continued for 3 months after AMI.[36] Acute platelet survival was longer with ticlopidine (8 days) compared with placebo (5 days) ($P < .05$). Three months after the AMI there was no significant difference in platelet survival time between treatment groups. Knudsen et al.[37] concluded that ticlopidine decreased platelet activity and infarct size during AMI.

The CAPRIE study was a randomized, blinded comparative trial of clopidogrel (75 mg once daily) and aspirin (325 mg once daily) in patients at risk for acute ischemia (i.e., stroke, AMI, or peripheral arterial disease).[38] For patients with AMI, the annual reduction in acute ischemic events did not differ between clopidogrel (5.03%) and aspirin (4.84%) ($P = 0.66$). The CAPRIE investigators concluded that clopidogrel and aspirin do not differ with respect to reduction of ischemic events in patients that are seen AMI.[38] The Antiplatelet Trialists' Collaboration reported a 2.4% incidence of neutropenia with ticlopidine.[39] In CAPRIE, the incidence of neutropenia with clopidogrel and aspirin was 0.1% and 0.17%, respectively.[38]

Heparin

Full-dose heparin is administered after thrombolytic therapy to prevent coronary artery reocclusion after successful thrombolysis in patients with AMI. The risk of reocclusion is high immediately after thrombolysis because blood flowing through the newly opened coronary artery is exposed to thrombin bound to fibrin on the residual thrombus. Clinical studies of patients with venous thrombosis and AMI indicate that there is a relation between the anticoagulant response to heparin and clinical efficacy.[40] Patients treated with streptokinase benefit from heparin therapy at relatively small doses (e.g., 12,500 U subcutaneously every 12 hours.). Whereas, this subcutaneous regimen of heparin failed to produce benefit in patients with AMI treated with tissue-type plasminogen activator (t-PA); full-dose heparin (e.g., 5,000 unit bolus followed by 30,000 U/24 hr by continuous infusion) improves patency after coronary thrombolysis with t-PA. A plausible explanation for these apparently contradictory findings is that the lack of systemic lytic effect seen with t-PA requires heparin to be administered early and in high doses compared with heparin requirements after thrombolysis with streptokinase.

The Heparin-Aspirin Reperfusion Trial (HART) compared immediate administration of heparin (5000-unit bolus) followed by a continuous infusion ($n = 106$) of oral aspirin (80 mg) ($n = 99$) as adjunctive therapy to recombinant t-PA (rt-PA) (100 mg over a 6-hour period).[41] Treatment was initiated within 6 hours of symptom onset. The primary endpoints of the study were: (1) patency rates at 7 and 24 hours after rt-PA, (2) ischemic or hemorrhagic complications during hospitalization, and (3) angiography on day 7. Among patients treated with heparin plus aspirin, the infarct-related artery was patent in 82% of patients after the first angiogram compared with 52% in the aspirin group. ($P < .0001$). Of the vessels that were patent initially, 88% were still patent after 7 days in the heparin group, compared with 95% in the aspirin-treated group. This difference; however, failed to reach statistical significance. The number of hemorrhagic complications in the heparin group was 18 compared with 15 in the aspirin-treated group. The number of recurrent events in both groups was similar. The authors concluded that heparin in combination with rt-PA produced a higher patency rate than rt-PA plus aspirin.[41]

The benefits of heparin are proven in unstable angina, but the role of heparin in AMI remains unproven.[42] Current clinical practice is to use subcutaneous heparin for the prevention of venous thromboembolic events in patients with AMI. Heparin is recommended for patients receiving t-PA as well as for patients undergoing percutaneous transluminal coronary angioplasty (PTCA) or surgical revascularization, and those with severe left ventricular dysfunction, mural thrombi, or atrial fibrillation.[42] An intravenous loading dose of 5000 U (approximately 75 U/kg) followed by a continuous infusion of approximately 1000 to 1250 U (approximately 15 to 25 U/kg per hour) is usually given. The partial thromboplastin time (PTT) should be checked no earlier than 4 hours after the initial bolus. Earlier evaluation of PTT may yield extremely high values because of the effect of the initial 5000-U bolus. The infusion rate may be titrated by increments of 100 to 200 U/hr so that the PTT is maintained at 1.5 to 2 times control.

Side effects of heparin include hemorrhage (intracranial or gastrointestinal) and thrombocytopenia. Heparin is contraindicated in patients who have a history of hemorrhage, uncontrolled hypertension, vasculitis, blood dyscrasias, active bleeding, or a bleeding ulcer or who have recently had major surgery. Patients with AMI who do not have contraindications to heparin therapy should receive 5000 U of heparin subcutaneously every 12 hours to decrease the risk of clot formation. Patients who are obese, who suffer from a ventricular aneurysm or cardiogenic shock, or who have a history of thrombophlebitis or arterial or venous embolism are predisposed to thrombus formation and should receive ful anticoagulation. Patients with a transmural anterior MI have a 30 to 40% chance of developing left ventricular thrombi. Anticoagulation of these patients early in the course of therapy will prevent cerebrovascular accidents (CVAs).

Compared with unfractionated heparin, low-molecular-weight heparins (LMWHs) have improved bioavailability, a longer duration of action, a more predictable anticoagulant response, and a decreased risk of bleeding and thrombocytopenia.[42] Gurfinkel et al.[43] evaluated LMWH plus aspirin, unfractionated heparin plus aspirin, or aspirin alone in 219 patients with unstable angina. LMWH reduced the occurrence of recurrent angina compared with unfractionated heparin plus aspirin ($P = .002$) and of nonfatal AMI and urgent revascularization compared with

Table 43.2 ▪ Comparison of Thrombolytic Agents

Agent	Half-life (min)	Dose	Systemic Lytic State	Reperfusion Rate (%)	Reocclusion Rate (%)	Advantages	Disadvantages
APSAC	90	30 U	Yes	60–70	10	Long acting	Antigenicity, expensive
SK	23	1.5 mU	Yes	50–60	15	Inexpensive	Antigenicity
Reteplase	13–16	10 U + 10 U	Minimal	63–85	6	Rapid lysis, clot selective, bolus administration	Expensive, heparin needed
t-PA	6–9	100 mg	Minimal	65–85	20	Clot selective, rapid lysis	Expensive, heparin needed

Source: Reference 4.
APSAC, anisoylated plasminogen streptokinase activator complex; *SK,* streptokinase; *t-PA,* tissue-type plasminogen activator.

aspirin alone ($P = .01$). Gurfinkel et al.[43] did not observe a difference in major bleeding episodes or death between treatment groups.

Klein et al.[44] compared LMWH with unfractionated heparin in 1482 patients with unstable angina or non–Q-wave AMI. All patients received concurrent therapy with aspirin. Klein et al.[44] observed no significant difference with respect to recurrent angina, AMI, death, or adverse effects between LMWH and unfractionated heparin. Additional studies are needed to determine whether LMWHs are more cost-effective than unfractionated heparin in patients with AMI.

Thrombolytic Agents

Thrombolytic therapy can save cardiac muscle in patients with AMI.[45,46] Sustained blood flow to the infarcted area reduces mortality and prevents electrical instability and left ventricular dysfunction. Thrombolytic agents activate both soluble plasminogen and surface-bound plasminogen to plasmin. Plasmin lyses fibrin and dissolves the clot. Fibrin selectivity is dose dependent, and all agents activate circulating plasminogen to different degrees (streptokinase > anisoylated plasminogen streptokinase activator complex [APSAC] > reteplase = t-PA).[47] The activation of circulating plasminogen generates a systemic lytic response, characterized by the conversion of fibrin to fibrin degradation products.[48] The fibrin degradation products have anticoagulant properties that prevent subacute vessel reclosure.

Table 43.2 compares the commercially available thrombolytic agents used in patients with AMI.[4] Streptokinase binds plasminogen to form a complex that activates circulating plasminogen to plasmin. Streptokinase reduces blood viscosity and lowers systemic vascular resistance.[47] Intravenous streptokinase is administered at a dose of 1.5 million U over 30 to 60 minutes. After the administration of streptokinase, patients should receive full-dose heparin for 24 to 72 hours. To reduce the risk of allergic reactions, patients may be given diphenhydramine 25 mg and hydrocortisone 100 mg intravenously before streptokinase infusion.

APSAC is a direct plasminogen activator complex that produces fibrinolysis in 90 to 112 minutes in patients with AMI, and its extended half-life allows a convenient single bolus (30 U) intravenous injection over 4 to 5 minutes. APSAC reduces plasma viscosity and systemic vascular resistance; ease of administration is the main benefit of APSAC.[47] Reperfusion of occluded coronary arteries occurs in 72% of APSAC-treated patients at 90 minutes (range 53 to 91% in individual studies).[49–51] Reocclusion rates vary from 0 to 20%, with an average reocclusion rate of 10%.[52] APSAC improves left ventricular function and survival in patients with AMI.[53]

t-PA produces dose-dependent activation of fibrin-bound plasminogen.[47] Unlike streptokinase and APSAC, t-PA is not antigenic; hematoma and prolonged bleeding at the injection site are the most commonly reported adverse effects.[47] Because the speed of reperfusion is linked to the rate of administration of t-PA, accelerated (90-minute) infusions of t-PA produce more rapid reperfusion without compromising safety.[54,55] To prevent postlytic reocclusion, anticoagulation with full-dose, intravenous unfractionated heparin is required for at least 24 hours. The dose of heparin is adjusted to maintain an activated partial thromboplastin time two times control for at least 24 hours.

Reteplase is a nonglycosylated deletion mutant of t-PA that is produced by expression of an appropriately constructed plasmid in *Escherichia coli.*[56] Reteplase lacks the kringle-1 domain, the finger domain, and the epidermal growth factor domain contained in t-PA.[57] These changes extend the half-life of reteplase (13 to 16 minutes) when compared to t-PA (5 to 6 minutes). The absence of the fibrin-specific finger region and the epidermal growth factor domain affects renal blood flow and fibrin specificity as well as affinity. In addition, reteplase has less affinity for binding fibrin when compared with t-PA.

Reteplase is metabolized in the kidneys, liver, and blood. Renal failure produces a proportional decrease in the clearance of reteplase ($r = 0.713$; $P < .001$).[55,57] Renal dysfunction impairs the elimination of reteplase but not of t-PA.[57] The prolonged half-life and greater activity of reteplase, when compared with those of t-PA, has been demonstrated in animal studies.[53,56–58] Reteplase is 5.3 times more effective than t-PA in lysing jugular venous thrombus after single, intravenous bolus administration.[58] The potential advantages of reteplase over t-PA include more rapid and more complete reperfusion and a longer half-life that allows bolus administration without a continuous infusion.[55,56] The recommended dose of reteplase is two 10-unit intravenous boluses given 30 minutes apart. This convenient regimen is especially valuable in a busy ED.[47]

Thrombolytics reduce morbidity and mortality if given within the first 6 hours after the onset of AMI symptoms.[53,59,60] The goals of thrombolytic therapy are to lyse coronary thrombi during the early phase of AMI, to limit infarct size by reperfusing jeopardized myocardium, and to reduce morbidity and mortality. Patients with recent onset of chest pain (usually less than 12 hours) or persistent ECG abnormalities indicating an evolving transmural AMI are candidates for thrombolytic therapy (Table 43.3).[59]

Treatment within the first hour after the onset of symptoms yields the maximal myocardial salvage in patients with AMI and with ST segment elevation.[61] Pooled data from mortality studies suggest that a 70% reduction in mortality can be achieved when thrombolytic therapy is initiated within 1 hour of symptom onset.[59,60] Afterwards, the incremental benefit of thrombolytic treatment is less, and the degree of myocardial salvage is even further decreased after 3 hours. The Myocardial Infarction Triage and Intervention (MITI) trial showed a 1% mortality rate when thrombolytics are initiated within 70 minutes.[62] A delay in therapy beyond 70 minutes resulted in a 10% mortality rate.[63] Thrombolysis within the first hour of symptoms produces "an abortive effect on AMI" in approximately 40% of patients.[63] Data from the GUSTO-I (Global Utilization of Streptokinase and Tissue Plasminogen Activator for Occluded Coronary Arteries) investigators showed differences between clot-selective and non–clot-selective agents with respect to the open-artery principle.[64] Compared with streptokinase, t-PA opens occluded coronary arteries faster and improves survival if the thrombolytic is administered within 4 hours after symptom onset.[65]

Contraindications to the use of thrombolytic therapy are listed in Table 43.4. An absolute contraindication means that thrombolytic therapy is not to be given regardless of eligibility criteria. However, it is important to consider whether a contraindication is relative or absolute. A relative contraindication means that the clinician must weigh the benefits of giving the thrombolytic versus the risks to patients.

Table 43.3 ▪ Eligibility Criteria for Thrombolytic Therapy

Clinical
Chest pain or chest pain-equivalent syndrome consistent with acute myocardial infarction ≤12 hours from symptom onset with
Electrocardiogram
≥1 mm ST-segment elevation in ≥2 contiguous limb leads
≥2 mm ST-segment elevation in ≥2 contiguous precordial leads
New bundle branch block
Cardiogenic shock
Emergency catheterization and revascularization if possible; consider thrombolysis if catheterization not immediately available.

Table 43.4 ▪ Contraindications to Thrombolytic Therapy

Intracranial neoplasms
Active internal bleeding
Previous history of hemorrhagic stroke
Previous allergic reaction to streptokinase
Suspected aortic dissection
A stroke or other cerebrovascular accident within the last year
Current use of anticoagulants (INR >2–3)
Prolonged and or potentially traumatic cardiopulmonary resuscitation (>10 min)
Severe uncontrolled hypertension upon presentation (blood pressure >180/110)
Recent internal bleeding episode (2–4 weeks)
Pregnancy
Active peptic ulcer
Noncompressible vascular punctures
Prior exposure to streptokinase within the past 2 years
Prior allergic reaction to streptokinase
Major surgery within the last 3 weeks
Menses is not a contraindication to thrombolytic therapy

INR, international normalized ratio.

Bleeding complications are the major concern with thrombolytic agents due to their general interference with hemostatic mechanisms. Thrombolytics do not differentiate between pathologic clots and hemostatic plugs. Lysis of hemostatic plugs can lead to bleeding complications after pharmacologic thrombolysis. Clinical studies show a 5% risk of major bleeding complications from thrombolytic therapy.[53,60] Bleeding complications are minimized by avoiding drugs that affect hemostasis and by avoiding excessive venipunctures. Compared with streptokinase, t-PA appears to be associated with a slightly higher risk of stroke in patients who have an AMI.[66] Data from the GISSI-2 trial suggest that there are 4 additional strokes per 1000 patients treated with t-PA than with streptokinase. Logistic regression analysis on the data from the GISSI-2 trial revealed a significant association between the risk of stroke and older age, female sex, anterior infarction, and more extensive left ventricular dysfunction at the time of admission.[67] In the ISIS-3 study, streptokinase was associated with significantly fewer total strokes and noncerebral bleeding and intracranial bleeding episodes compared with either t-PA or APSAC.[68] When GISSI-2 and ISIS-3 data are combined, t-PA was associated with significantly higher total stroke rates (1.4 versus 1%) (0.6 versus 0.3%) compared with streptokinase.[69] The GUSTO trial showed that t-PA was associated with a significant excessive in hemorrhagic strokes ($P = .03$) when compared with streptokinase.[64]

Allergic reactions are more common with streptokinase and APSAC because these agents are derived from streptococci and act as haptens in the presence of antibodies to streptococcus. Intravenous diphenhydramine and hydrocortisone may reduce the risk of anaphylaxis during administration of these two thrombolytics. Hypotension occurs in approximately 10% of patients treated with streptokinase or APSAC. Once the patient receives streptokinase, that person then is sensitized to the drug and should not receive it again for at least 6 months.[24,52] Other side effects with thrombolytics include angina, flushing, dyspnea, mild febrile reactions, nausea and vomiting, and occasionally, rash, all of which may be symptoms of mild allergic reactions. Allergic reactions and hypotension are rare in patients treated with t-PA.

Clinical trials show that streptokinase, APSAC, and t-PA improve left ventricular function.[54] Studies show that thrombolytics reduce AMI-related mortality compared with placebo. Streptokinase reduces in-hospital mortality by 3.7 to 10% and 1-year mortality by 13.9%. APSAC reduces 1-year mortality by 11.1%; t-PA produces a 3 to 7.2% reduction in prehospital mortality and a 5.9 to 7.3% reduction in 1-year mortality.[48] The International Joint Efficacy Comparison of Thrombolytics (INJECT) trial compared the 35-day mortality rates after treatment with reteplase (10 + 10 U in a bolus regimen) or streptokinase (1.5 mU over 60 minutes) in patients with AMI.[70] Mortality rates did not differ significantly between the reteplase group (9.02%) and the streptokinase group (9.53%) (95% confidence interval, –1.98% to 0.96%).[70]

The Third International Study of Infarct Survival (ISIS-3),[68] The Gruppo Italiano per lo Studio della Sopravvivenza nell'Infarto Miocardico 2 (GISSI-2),[67] The International Group and GUSTO-1[64] confirm the benefits of thrombolytic therapy on AMI-related mortality and morbidity. ISIS-3 assessed the relative efficacy of streptokinase, APSAC, and t-PA.[68] Mortality in all three groups was the same. The GISSI-2 and the International Group compared streptokinase with t-PA and found no difference in mortality between treatment groups.[67,71] However, these trials were criticized because heparin was either withheld or given subcutaneously, a factor that would bias against clot-selective t-PA. The GUSTO-1 trial assessed the importance of intravenous and subcutaneous heparin after administration of streptokinase and t-PA.[64] The results showed one additional life saved per 100 treated patients with t-PA and intravenous heparin compared with streptokinase.[64]

Certain patients appear to benefit most from t-PA.[72] Patients with anterior wall MI have a lower mortality (8.6%) after treatment with t-PA versus streptokinase (10.5%).[64–65] Mortality rates for t-PA versus streptokinase in patients younger than 75 years of age are 4.4 and 5.5%, respectively.[64–65] Neither age equal to or greater than 75 years nor the presence of inferior wall MI affects the relative efficacy of the thrombolytics.[72] Mortality rates are lower with t-PA (5.5%) when compared with streptokinase (6.7%) in patients treated within 2 to 4 hours after the onset of symptoms.[64–65] GUSTO-III compared a 10-U double-bolus dose of reteplase with an accelerated dose of t-PA.[73] All patients received heparin and aspirin. There were no significant differences between the two treatment groups in mortality, stroke, or net clinical benefits.

A recent subanalysis of the MITI project compared in-hospital mortality, long-term mortality, and resource utilization among 3145 patients with AMI; 1050 patients were treated with acute angioplasty and 2095 received thrombolytic therapy. After a 3-year follow-up period, the study showed no differences in acute mortality or long-term mortality rates between treatment groups.[62] However, after 3 years, the mean total cumulative inpatient costs were more than $3,000 higher for patients treated with angioplasty than those patients initially treated with thrombolytic therapy ($25,459 versus $22,163, $P < .001$).[62] As expected, the primary cost drivers were repeat angiograms and repeat angioplasties. The authors concluded that thrombolytic therapy may produce better short-term benefit when compared with angioplasty in patients with AMI.[62]

Successful thrombolytic therapy in AMI depends on more than just the ability to reperfuse the occluded coronary artery. Prevention of reocclusion and subsequent salvage of infarcted myocardium should reduce morbidity and mortality after thrombolytic therapy. Results of early studies that compared reperfusion rates achieved with t-PA and streptokinase suggested that t-PA was twice as effective as streptokinase in establishing reperfusion of acutely occluded coronary arteries.[74,75] In recent trials, myocardial salvage, mortality reduction, or bleeding complications have not differed in patients treated with t-PA versus streptokinase.[76] Clinical experience provides little evidence for the superiority of t-PA over other thrombolytic agents in AMI. The largest trials measuring myocardial function after thrombolytic therapy failed to show that t-PA is more effective than streptokinase,[67,77] or APSAC.[78] Additionally, t-PA is no safer than other thrombolytics.[67,79] The international study of 20,749 patients with AMI showed no difference in mortality rate between t-PA (8.9%) and streptokinase (8.5%).[71] There was also no difference in the incidence of ventricular fibrillation, reinfarction, or heart failure between treatment groups.

Not all patients suspected of having AMI receive thrombolytic therapy. This is unfortunate because mortality is substantially higher among those patients who do not (18%) compared with those who do (2.5%).[72,80,81] Approximately 39% of patients with AMI are treated with thrombolytic therapy.[61] Clinical trials show a 30 to 40% reduction in acute mortality in patients with AMI who receive thrombolytic therapy.[64,82] The primary reason for not receiving thrombolytic therapy is too long a delay between symptom onset and arrival at a treatment facility.[61] Factors responsible for delay in the care of patients with AMI can be grouped into three phases: (1) patient-bystander factors, (2) prehospital factors, and (3) hospital factors.

Thrombolytic treatment initiated within 60 to 90 minutes of symptom onset reduces the size of the AMI and its related mortality. Pharmacists can play a key role as a health care team members to seek ways to ensure that door-to-needle time is reduced from the current 45 to 75 minutes to less than 30 minutes. Thrombolytic agents should be stocked in the ED and the coronary care unit to avoid considerable delays in administration. Pharmacists should help develop critical pathways and treatment guidelines for thrombolytic therapy in AMI.[83,84] Pharmacists can also collect patient outcome data and prescriber compliance information that may be used to make formulary decisions. Information obtained from these evaluations can also be used to implement procedural changes and educational efforts that can significantly reduce hospital delays.[85]

Postreperfusion Management

After successful thrombolysis, the stenotic vessel may reocclude. The rate of reocclusion varies but may be as high as 30%.[59] The likelihood of reocclusion and recovery of regional ventricular function depends on the severity of residual stenosis. After successful thrombolysis, anticoagulation is advocated although there is not consensus on the type, dosage, or duration of therapy. Most often, full-dose heparin is used for 24 to 72 hours. Aspirin (160 or 325 mg/day) is administered for 3 months or longer.[59] There is no role for dipyridamole as an adjunctive antiplatelet agent after thrombolytic therapy.[86–87]

PTCA provides a viable therapeutic alternative in those patients who are seen at a hospital that is capable of performing emergency PTCA. PTCA involves the passing of a balloon-tipped catheter along the venous circulation into the coronary tree to the site of coronary occlusion. Once at the site, the balloon is inflated, causing the occlusive plaque to regress against the vessel wall. The balloon is deflated and reinflated several times until the plaque is reduced and approximately 70% of the arterial caliber has been restored. A major limitation of PTCA is that it requires a skilled team, a fully staffed catheterization laboratory, and a surgical team on stand-by. Potential complications of PTCA include catheter-induced occlusion caused by dissection, vasospasm, or subintimal hematoma and residual stenosis. Routine angioplasty performed within 24 hours of thrombolytic therapy offers no clinical benefit and is associated with an increased incidence of reocclusion and complications.[53] Angioplasty is recommended for patients with ongoing ischemia or pump failure. The use of emergency angioplasty for patients who have AMI may offer several advantages over thrombolytic therapy. PTCA is more effective than thrombolytic therapy in restoring patency and preventing reocclusion and in reducing the risk of death and reinfarction.[88] Angioplasty is associated with significantly less ($P = .05$) risk of hemorrhagic strokes than t-PA.[88] The benefits of angioplasty are especially apparent in patients who are of advanced age, have an anterior infarction, or have tachycardia.[89]

β-Adrenergic Blocking Agents

β-Adrenergic blockade reduces myocardial oxygen consumption by reducing heart rate, contractility, and blood pressure. β-Adrenergic blockers can also reduce catecholamine levels in an ischemic heart and produce favorable redistribution of coronary blood flow.[90–92] Clinical trials with these agents can be divided into those in which treatment was begun early and endpoints such as cardiac enzyme levels, ECG changes, and reinfarction rates are investigated, and those in which treatment was begun later after resolution of the infarct, with mortality rate reduction as the endpoint. There is evidence that intravenous therapy followed by oral administration with atenolol, propranolol, metoprolol, sotalol, or timolol reduces serum CK concentrations.[34] Reduction in ECG abnormalities after AMI has been reported following acute intervention with propranolol, practolol, and metoprolol.[34]

Studies show that β-blockers limit infarct size, reduce the incidence of malignant arrhythmias, and reduce mortality after acute administration in patients with AMI.[53] The Metoprolol in Acute Myocardial Infarction (MIAMI) trial, a multicenter, double-blind, placebo-controlled randomized study in 2877 patients with suspected or definite MI received 5 mg of metoprolol intravenously every 2 minutes for a total of 15 mg within 24 hours of onset of symptoms.[93] Patients were randomly assigned to the study after arrival to the coronary care unit. After intravenous dosing, patients received oral metoprolol 100 mg every 6 hours for the first 2 days beginning 15 minutes after the last intravenous injection. The dose was then decreased to 100 mg every 12 hours for the remaining 13 days of the study. The cumulative mortality for all patients at the conclusion of the 15-day trial was 123 (4.3%) deaths in the treatment groups compared with 142 (4.9%) deaths in the placebo group. This difference did not reach statistical significance. Mortality in patients with definite MI was 120 of 2028 in the metoprolol group versus 137 of 2099 in the placebo group. High-risk patients were found to benefit whereas other subgroups did not benefit.

In the First International Study of Infarct Survival (ISIS-1), a total of 16,207 patients were randomly assigned to receive 5 to 10 mg of atenolol, in 5-mg intravenous doses, or placebo within a mean of 5 hours of onset of suspected MI. Oral dosing in the treatment group followed, with 100 mg of atenolol per day as either a single dose or divided every 12 hours for a total of 7 days. Vascular mortality occurred in 313 of 8037 (3.89%) atenolol-treated patients and 365 of 7990 (4.57%) control patients. The beneficial effect of atenolol in decreasing the incidence of mortality was statistically significant ($P < .04$).[94]

The Thrombolysis in Myocardial Infarction Phase II (TIMI II) study addressed the use of early and late β-adrenergic blocker therapy after t-PA administration.[95] Patients were randomly assigned to one of two groups: immediate β-adrenergic blocker administration (three doses of metoprolol 5 mg intravenously at 2-minute intervals followed by 50 mg orally twice a day for 24 hours, then 100 mg twice a day) and delayed administration (starting on day 6 after MI), consisted of metoprolol 50 mg twice a day for 24 hours, then 100 mg twice daily. The time of entry into the study was less than 4 hours since onset of AMI (mean 2.6 hours). Ejection fraction and early mortality were found to be similar between the two groups; however at day 6, 16 patients in the immediate metoprolol intervention group and 31 patients in the delayed group had nonfatal reinfarctions ($P = .02$). Recurrent ischemic episodes occurred in 107 patients in the early metoprolol intervention group compared to 147 patients in the delayed intervention group ($P = .005$). Mortality at the end of the 6-week study was 5.0% in immediate metoprolol therapy versus 12.1% in the delayed intervention group ($P = .001$).

Based on TIMI II data, intravenous β-blocker therapy reduces mortality and reinfarction rate when administered within 2 hours of the onset of symptoms in patients with AMI receiving thrombolytic therapy.[95] If intravenous β-blocker therapy is initiated within 4 hours of symptom onset, there is a reduction in nonfatal reinfarction and recurrent ischemia.[95] β-Blockers may also reduce the risk of intracranial bleeding in patients with AMI treated with thrombolytics. β-Adrenergic blockers are also valuable in patients with AMI and with atrial tachyarrhythmias or rapid ventricular response rates in atrial fibrillation.[30] Well-designed trials with large numbers of patients show that timolol, metoprolol, and propranolol significantly reduce long-term mortality of AMI.[34] Because these agents were administered after reduction of MI, the decrease in mortality is probably a result of a drop in the incidence of arrhythmias or reinfarction and is not related to infarct size reduction.[34]

Although β-adrenergic blockers are contraindicated in patients with serious myocardial dysfunction, cardiac conduction abnormalities, hypotension, peripheral hypoperfusion, or bronchospastic airway disease, it is reasonable to consider their use in all patients with AMI who have no contraindications, irrespective of concomitant thrombolytic therapy.[53] Recent studies suggest that esmolol infusions at a reduced dosage may be used safely and effectively in thrombolytic-treated patients with AMI who had relative contraindications to β-blocker therapy (e.g., congestive heart failure, pulmonary disease, peripheral vascular disease, bradycardia, or systolic blood pressure less than 100 mm Hg).[96]

Calcium-Channel Blockers

Experimental data in animals suggest that calcium-channel blockers may prevent the progression of ischemia and subsequent necrosis by decreasing myocardial oxygen demand without comprising cardiac output.[10] Recent clinical trials indicate that these agents do not alter outcome in patients with AMI. Verapamil may reduce infarct size, but it does not alter acute mortality.[97] The Danish Multicenter Study Group randomly assigned 100 patients to receive verapamil 0.1 mg/kg intravenously followed by 120 mg orally three times a day or placebo for 6 months.[98] Patients were assigned within 4 hours of onset of symptoms of AMI. Verapamil failed to alter acute mortality, long-term mortality, or reinfarction rate, when compared with placebo.[98]

Studies with nifedipine (20 mg orally every 4 hour for 14 days) failed to show a significant reduction in enzymatically assessed infarct size, compared with placebo.[99] A slight trend for higher mortality was observed in the nifedipine group. The Nifedipine Angina Myocardial Infarction Study (NAMIS) was the first multicenter placebo-controlled trial to assess nifedipine (Procardia) 20 mg every 4 hours, starting 4.6 ± 0.1 hours after the onset of chest pain for 14 days.[99] A total of 171 patients with either a threat of MI or early AMI were admitted into the study. No significant difference in size of infarction, as assessed by CK-MB serum levels, between the two groups was noted. A startling observation was that the nifedipine-treated group exhibited a higher incidence of mortality (7.9% versus 0% in the control group) during the 2-week study period. Long-term mortality at 6-month follow-up was not statistically significant between the nifedipine and placebo groups.

In the Norwegian Nifedipine Multicenter Trial 277 patients were randomly assigned to receive either nifedipine 10 mg five times a day or placebo.[100] Unlike the NAMIS trial, randomization occurred within 12 hours of onset of symptoms. Treatment was initiated within 5.5 ± 2.9 hours of symptom onset and was continued for 6 weeks. Results showed no difference in CK-MB release or 6-week mortality between the two groups.

A placebo-controlled trial of diltiazem in AMI reported a reduction in early recurrent infarction (one-tailed, $P = .03$; two-tailed, $P = .06$) in patients with non–Q-wave MI.[101] This multicenter, double-blind study consisted of 576 patients who were randomly assigned to receive either diltiazem or placebo within 24 to 72 hours of onset of infarction. Diltiazem 90 mg every 6 hours or placebo was continued for 14 days. Reinfarction, defined as a secondary increase in CK-MB during the study period, was observed in 15 of 287 (5.2%) diltiazem-treated patients compared with 27 of 289 (9.3%) control patients ($P = .0297$); however, 61% of the diltiazem patients and 64% of the placebo group were receiving concurrent β-adrenergic blocker therapy and 80% were also receiving long-acting nitrates. Side effects such as heart block, bradycardia (heart rate <40 bpm) and hypotension (systolic blood pressure <90 mm Hg) were more pronounced in the diltiazem group compared with placebo. Although the study concluded that diltiazem was effective in preventing early reinfarction in non–Q-wave MI, no difference in mortality between the two groups was observed during the 14-day study period.[102]

The Multicenter Diltiazem Post-Infarction Trial (MDPIT) evaluated 2466 patients with AMI.[103] Patients received either placebo or diltiazem 60 mg orally twice a day or four times a day. Therapy was initiated between 3 and 15 days after MI. There was no difference in mortality between groups; however there were 11% fewer recurrent cardiac events (e.g., nonfatal reinfarction, death from a cardiac cause) in the diltiazem group. Further analysis of the MDPIT data indicates that diltiazem-treated patients with left ventricular dysfunction (ejection fraction <40%), pulmonary congestion, and acute anterolateral Q-wave MI at baseline had a predictable higher incidence of cardiac death and nonfatal reinfarction.[103] Long-term diltiazem therapy in patients with AMI failed to demonstrate any significant benefit and produced detrimental side effects in patients with left ventricular dysfunction.

Although there is laboratory evidence that calcium-channel blockers reduce infarct size, these results are not observed under clinical conditions.[91] Currently, there is no reason to recommend general treatment with calcium-channel blockers to reduce infarct size. However, patients with documented or suspected vasospastic angina and patients with AMI undergoing emergency angioplasty may benefit from the use of calcium-channel blockers as long as left ventricular function is relatively well preserved.[53]

Angiotensin-Converting Enzyme Inhibitors

Recent studies by Pfeffer et al.[104] show that early and continued use of captopril in patients with symptomatic left ventricular dysfunction after AMI improved survival and reduced morbidity and mortality due to major cardiovascular events.[104] Patients ($n = 2231$) with ejection fractions ≤40% but without overt heart failure or recurrent ischemia were randomly assigned to receive either captopril 50 mg three times daily or placebo within 3 to 16 days after their AMI. Patients were followed for an average of 42 months. Captopril reduced all-cause mortality by 19%, the risk of cardiovascular death was reduced by 21%, the risk of congestive heart failure requiring hospitalization was reduced by 22%, and the risk of recurrent MI was reduced by 25%. These benefits were seen in patients who received thrombolytic therapy, aspirin, and/or β-adrenergic blockers, and in those who did not.[104]

In contrast, the Second Cooperative New Scandinavian Enalapril Survival Study (CONSENSUS II) failed to demonstrate a benefit from the administration of enalapril (up to 20 mg/day) in patients in whom this therapy was initiated within 24 hours after their AMI.[105] A total of 6090 patients were randomly assigned to receive either enalapril or placebo along with conventional therapy with thrombolytics, nitrates, aspirin, β-blockers, diuretics, analgesics, and calcium channel blockers. The trial was prematurely stopped because of the high probability that enalapril was no more effective than placebo in improving 6-month survival.[105]

The Studies of Left Ventricular Dysfunction (SOLVD) Prevention Trial showed that long-term enalapril significantly reduced the incidence of heart failure and the need for hospitalization compared with placebo in patients with asymptomatic left ventricular dysfunction (ejection fraction ≤35%).[106] Approximately 80% of patients in the SOLVD Prevention Trial had suffered an AMI before enrollment in the study. The efficacy of enalapril in preventing the development of heart failure was evident as early as 3 months after the start of treatment.[106] Data produced by the SAVE and SOLVD trials suggest a possible benefit from the early administration of ACE inhibitors to patients with left ventricular dysfunction who are recovering from an AMI. The negative findings of the CONSENSUS II trial may have resulted from too early initiation of angiotensin-converting enzyme (ACE) inhibitor therapy or an inadequate follow-up period.[107] Patients with an anterior wall MI and reduced left ventricular function may benefit from therapy with an ACE inhibitor if it is initiated within the first 2 weeks after the AMI.[72] In patients with left ventricular dysfunction, the use of long-term ACE inhibitor therapy may reduce mortality. These agents attenuate the remodeling process that occurs after an AMI. As a result of the attenuation of remodeling, a reduction in ventricular dilation is observed. The effect of ACE inhibitors on remodeling is probably due to a suppression of endogenous catecholamines. ACE inhibitors prevent the degradation of bradykinin (a vasodilatory substance) that decreases systemic vascular resistance and reduce the workload of the heart. The initiation of ACE inhibitor therapy within the first 2 weeks after MI may save the lives of 5 patients for every 1000 patients with left ventricular dysfunction.[72] Ideal candidates for ACE inhibitor therapy include patients with congestive heart failure or hypertension. For the patient to achieve the greatest benefit from the ACE inhibitor, therapy should be started during the first week after the AMI. However, ACE inhibitor therapy should not be instituted until blood pressure and renal function are assessed and stabilized. In patients with an evolving AMI ACE inhibitor therapy should be started shortly after hospitalization in the absence of hypotension or contraindications. If the patient has impaired left ventricular systolic function (ejection fraction <40%), ACE inhibitor therapy should be continued indefinitely and the dose should be titrated slowly upward to the maximum that can be tolerated. If the patient has no complications and no evidence of left ventricular dysfunction, the ACE inhibitor can be discontinued after 6 weeks of therapy.

The most common side effect associated with the administration of ACE inhibitor is a dry hacking cough. This cough may develop anytime from a few days up to a week after initiation of therapy or an increase in dose. If the patient can tolerate the cough, continuation of the drug is encouraged. If the cough becomes intolerable, therapy can be switched to an angiotensin II (AII) blocker such as valsartan, irbesartan, or losartan. The only problem with the AII blockers is that they have not been shown to decrease mortality like the ACE inhibitors have. Another side effect of ACE inhibitors is angioedema, an anaphylactic reaction that causes severe tongue swelling and can interfere with the patient's breathing. If this occurs, the ACE inhibitor should be discontinued, and the patient should not be given this drug again. However, it is less likely to be a problem with A-II blockers due to the lack of inhibition of bradykinin metabolism.

Magnesium

The effect of hypomagnesemia in cardiac disease is well known.[108,109] Magnesium deficiency is associated with a high frequency of cardiac arrhythmias, symptoms of cardiac insufficiency, and sudden cardiac death.[108–111] Experimental and clinical studies show that magnesium and potassium metabolism are closely linked.[108,112] Diuretics[112,113] usually cause hypomagnesemia, often accompanied by hypokalemia. Transient hypomagnesemia not induced by renal magnesium loss has been observed in patients with AMI.[114] Because hypomagnesemia can precipitate refractory ventricular fibrillation and can hinder the replenishment of intracellular potassium, it must be corrected if present. One or 2 g of magnesium sulfate (2 to 4 mL of a 50% solution) are diluted in 100 mL of dextrose 5% in water (D5W) and administered over 60 minutes.[115] A 24-hour magnesium infusion (8 g $MgSO_4$ in 500 mL of D5W) started on admission to the CICU can significantly lower the incidence of ventricular tachycardia.[114] Magnesium supplementation is a relatively safe method of reducing the incidence of postinfarction ventricular arrhythmias.[111,114] Magnesium toxicity is rare, but side effects from too rapid administration include flushing, sweating, mild bradycardia, and hypotension. Hypermagnesemia may produce depressed reflexes, flaccid paralysis, circulatory collapse, respiratory paralysis, and diarrhea.

Clinical studies on the use of magnesium in AMI have yielded contradictory results. The Leicester Intravenous Magnesium Intervention Trial (LIMIT-2),[116] conducted before the Fourth International Study of Infarct Survival (ISIS-4),[117] suggested that magnesium was highly effective in reducing the odds of death and capable of producing survival benefits comparable to those produced by aspirin and thrombolytic therapy in patients with AMI.[116] The ISIS-4 trial failed to show any benefit from magnesium with respect to mortality reduction after AMI.[117] Important differences in methodological design between LIMIT-2 and ISIS-4 may explain the disparity in response produced by magnesium in patients with AMI. The primary difference is that although in the trials preceding ISIS-4, magnesium was usually administered before or at the time of reperfusion of the infarct-related artery, in ISIS-4, reperfusion was likely to occur in many patients before the administration of magnesium.[117] Considering the proposed mechanisms by which magnesium could improve survival in patients with AMI, administration before reperfusion seems to be of obvious importance. This applies to the postulated preservation of high-energy phosphates and reduction in mitochondrial calcium overload during acute ischemia as well as to a possible role in arrhythmia reduction and reduction in reperfusion injury and myocardial stunning.[118] Furthermore, the low mortality associated with the combined use of thrombolytics, anticoagulants, and antiplatelet drugs may mask the true benefit produced by magnesium.[119] Although further studies are needed to better define the role of early administration of magnesium in patients with AMI receiving thrombolytic therapy, magnesium improves left ventricular function and reduces mortality in patients after AMI, especially those who are not candidates for thrombolytic therapy.[119]

Magnesium should be reserved for those instances of documented hypomagnesemia or hypokalemia. In the ISIS-4 trial[117] there was no decrease in mortality noted, but there was a slight possibility of harm due to drug-induced hypotension. However, one reason for this negative outcome could have been the administration of magnesium after the administration of the thrombolytic agent. When hypokalemia is present, magnesium should be replaced first for magnesium is what drives the K^+ pump.

Potassium

Electrolyte abnormalities, most notably hypokalemia and hypomagnesemia, should be identified and corrected. These electrolyte abnormalities can precipitate malignant ventricular arrhythmias in patients with ischemia, hypertrophied or dilated hearts, or hypoxemia. Hypokalemia is the most common electrolyte abnormality encountered in clinical practice, occurring in 23 to 40% of patients treated with thiazide diuretics.[120] When loop and thiazide diuretics are used in combination, the incidence increases to approximately 100%.[110] Hypokalemia is present in 9 to 25% of patients with AMI and may predispose these patients to ventricular fibrillation.[121] Ornato et al.[122] found a 49% incidence of hypokalemia in their out-of-hospital cardiac arrest victims. Fifty-five percent of all hypokalemic sudden death victims were receiving diuretics without potassium supplementation; hypokalemia occurred in 13% of victims receiving diuretics plus potassium supplementation. Fortunately, hypokalemia is significantly ($P < .001$) less common in patients with uncomplicated AMI (11%) than in sudden death victims (50%).[123] Nonetheless, hypokalemia should be identified and corrected in the AMI setting.

As with magnesium, potassium should not be given to every patient suspected of having an AMI. A documented potassium deficiency should be obtained first. A patient with an AMI should maintain a potassium level no less than 4 mEq/L and no greater than 6 mEq/L. Replacement should be no faster than 10 mEq/hr. The most common side effect associated with the administration of potassium is a burning sensation. If this occurs, the infusion rate may be reduced.

Antirrhythmics

The most common postinfarction complication is disturbance of the normal cardiac rhythm. Pharmacologic manipulation of the cardiac conduction system and the autonomic nervous system, and correction of electrolyte abnormalities reduce the morbidity and mortality associated with cardiac arrhythmias in patients with AMI. Arrhythmias occurring in patients with AMI require vigorous treatment when they produce hemodynamic compromise or an increase in myocardial oxygen demand or predispose to malignant ventricular arrhythmias.

Ventricular fibrillation is the most common cause of death in the early hours after MI and may occur without prior evidence of ventricular premature complexes.[124] Ventricular fibrillation occurs in approximately 11% of patients with AMI and carries a 46% mortality rate.

Approximately 50% of episodes occur within 4 hours and 80% within 12 hours of symptom onset. Although there is no consensus regarding a reduction in morbidity and mortality, routine prophylactic antiarrhythmic therapy was once advocated during the initial 24 hours after MI.[125] Today, the routine use of prophylactic antiarrhythmics in patients with AMI is disputed. Treatment with antiarrhythmics is commonly instituted in patients with warning arrhythmias (i.e., couplets, multifocal premature ventricular contractions, or runs of three or more consecutive premature ventricular contractions). Lidocaine hydrochloride is the prophylactic antiarrhythmic agent of choice in AMI. This agent decreases automaticity, blocks reentry pathways, and elevates the fibrillatory threshold. Lidocaine can reduce the incidence of malignant ventricular arrhythmias during the early phase of AMI but mortality is unchanged.[125] Lidocaine may produce asystole and aggravate myocardial dysfunction, therefore lidocaine is not used very often.

Lidocaine 1.0 mg/kg is administered by intravenous injection over 2 minutes followed immediately by an intravenous infusion of 1 to 4 mg/min (20 to 50 μg/kg/minute). Because of the short distribution half-life (6 to 8 minutes) of lidocaine, an additional 0.5 mg/kg bolus should be given 10 minutes after the initial bolus to maintain adequate plasma lidocaine concentrations. If ventricular arrhythmias persist, 50-mg bolus injections can be repeated to a maximum of 250 mg of lidocaine over a 20-minute period.

Lidocaine is metabolized by the liver and has an elimination half-life of approximately 90 minutes. The metabolism of lidocaine is impaired in the presence of AMI, circulatory shock, hepatic failure, cimetidine, and β-adrenergic blockers. Accumulation of the metabolites of lidocaine may occur in elderly patients and in patients with hepatic and/or renal dysfunction. The dose of lidocaine should be reduced and individualized in such patients because excessive doses of lidocaine can produce central nervous system toxicity and possibly cardiovascular depression. The toxicity of lidocaine is directly related to its concentration in blood. Plasma lidocaine concentrations should be maintained between 1.5 and 5 μg/mL. Patients with AMI may tolerate higher plasma concentrations (8 μg/mL). This may be related to increased binding of lidocaine to α_1-acid glycoprotein, which is released into the systemic circulation in large concentrations after AMI.

Sinus bradycardia is a common finding in patients with inferior wall MI. Transient episodes of bradycardia are often observed during the initial hours after MI and may exert a protective function.[126] If the bradycardia is associated with hypotension or a ventricular arrhythmia, atropine 0.5 to 1 mg should be administered by rapid intravenous injection. Atropine may be repeated at 2- to 4-hour intervals as needed to maintain a heart rate greater than 60 bpm. Asymptomatic bradycardia should not be treated because the risk of increased myocardial oxygen demand outweighs any potential benefit from treatment. Atropine should not be administered in doses less than 0.5 mg because a paradoxical slowing of the heart rate may occur. Electrical pacing is used to manage atropine refractory bradycardia. Intravenous isoproterenol (0.5 to 2.0 μg/min) should be used, if at all, only until a pacemaker can be placed because of the risks of tachyarrhythmias or hypotension.

Sinus tachycardia occurs in 30% of patients with AMI during the first few days postinfarction.[127] Anxiety, pain, fever, and ventricular dysfunction are common causes of this arrhythmia. Young patients with a first anterior wall MI may be seen in a hyperdynamic state with some tachycardia, hypertension, and ventricular ectopy. These patients may benefit from acute therapy with β-adrenergic blockers.[126,128–132] Atrial fibrillation or flutter occurs in up to 20% of patients with AMI and is often associated with left ventricular dysfunction.[127] Because of this association, these rhythms are seen more often with anterior wall MI and are associated with increased mortality. Therapy is indicated if the arrhythmia produces a rapid ventricular response and/or hemodynamic compromise. Restoration of normal sinus rhythm by electrical cardioversion is an immediate priority in the setting of acute hemodynamic instability.

Patients may develop hemodynamic instability from supraventricular tachycardia. Intravenous verapamil 5 mg over 2 minutes and repeated in 30 minutes to a total of 20 mg may be used for conversion to normal sinus rhythm or for control of ventricular response rate. Verapamil should be used with caution, if at all, in patients with left-ventricular dysfunction, hypotension, Wolff-Parkinson-White syndrome, or wide complex tachycardia. Adenosine has the advantage of a shorter half-life and has fewer propensities to produce hypotension than verapamil. The usual dose of adenosine is 6 mg, followed by 12 mg in 3 to 5 minutes if a response is not observed. Total doses greater than 18 mg increase the risk of atrioventricular block, flushing, chest pain, and bronchospasm.

Anticoagulants

All patients with MI should be considered for anticoagulant therapy. According to the Fourth American College of Chest Physicians consensus conference on antithrombotic therapy, if a patient receives warfarin, aspirin should be discontinued. The only recommendation for continuing both warfarin and aspirin is if the patient experiences ischemic episodes with warfarin alone. In these patients, low-dose (81mg) aspirin plus warfarin may be of benefit. Patients with contraindications to aspirin should receive warfarin for 1 to 2 years (international normalized ratio [INR] 2.5 to 3.5). Although administration of anticoagulants to patients with AMI remains controversial, they may be used to prevent systemic and pulmonary embolism formation as well as to halt the progression of infarction. Most patients with uncomplicated AMI do not require full anticoagulation because the low incidence of deep venous thrombosis and pulmonary embolism outweighs the risks of anticoagulation.

Anticoagulation with warfarin for 3 months is recommended after an anterior wall transmural MI. Patients with AMI who are at increased risk for systemic thromboembolic events should be given warfarin for anticoagulation for at least 3 months. A prothrombin time of 1.5 to 2.5 times control (INR 2 to 3) should be the goal of oral anticoagulation.[125,132] Patients with inferior wall MI do not usually develop a left ventricular thrombus formation with resultant CVA. A two-dimensional echocardiogram can be used to assess the presence of a left ventricular thrombus.[125,132] Only those patients with heart failure, atrial arrhythmias, large AMI, old anterior wall MI, or apical dyskinesis or akinesis should receive anticoagulant therapy.

The Warfarin Re-Infarction Study Group[125] randomly assigned 1214 patients with AMI patients within 27 days from onset of symptoms to receive either warfarin to attain a prothrombin time of 1.5 to 2.0 times control or placebo for a mean duration of 37 months (range, 24 to 63 months). Warfarin reduced mortality by 24%, the incidence of reinfarction fell by 34%, and there was a 55% decrease in the incidence of CVA. All differences reached statistical significance. The risk of a major bleeding episode was 0.6% per year. The authors concluded that warfarin therapy after AMI is safe and can significantly affect mortality and morbidity.

The incidence of hemorrhagic side effects from anticoagulation in patients with AMI ranges from 3 to 7%. The mortality rate as a result of hemorrhage is 2 to 4% in warfarin-treated patients and less than 1% in patients receiving heparin.[132] CVAs occur in 2 to 3% and pulmonary embolus in 1 to 2% of patients after MI. On the basis of these observations, only those patients at high risk (i.e., left ventricular hypokinesis and/or mural thrombus), as described earlier, should receive ful anticoagulation.[132] The use of full-dose anticoagulation in patients with AMI must be based on the relative risk and potential benefit derived from anticoagulation. In patients with an absolute contraindication to anticoagulation (e.g., bleeding), the potential benefits of anticoagulation do not justify the risk. In patients with relative contraindications to anticoagulation (history of peptic ulcer disease or recent surgery), the risk of bleeding must be weighed against the risk of embolism. Warfarin is indicated for secondary prevention after MI in patients unable to take aspirin, patients with chronic atrial fibrillation, and patients with a left ventricular thrombus. Warfarin can be administered after MI in patients with extensive wall motion abnormalities and impaired ejection.

Nonpharmacologic Therapy

Treatment for patients with suspected AMI in the intensive care or coronary care unit includes continuous monitoring and prompt response to emergencies. Intramuscular drug administration is avoided because of possible interference with cardiac enzyme determinations, unpredictable drug absorption during episodes of hypoperfusion, and bleeding during anticoagulation. Vital signs, pain relief, body weight, bowel habits, and diet are closely monitored.

Patients should limit their activities to bed rest during the first 24 hours after the acute event. This is done to decrease myocardial oxygen consumption and to prevent extension of infarction during the healing process after an AMI. Activities over the next few days should begin gradually, starting with personal hygiene and in-bed-range-of-motion exercises.

A clear liquid diet is instituted for the first day during the convalescence period.[3,10] Upon discharge from the hospital after MI, a patient should be started on a Step-II diet, which is low in saturated fat and cholesterol (<7% of total calories coming from saturated fat and <200 mg/day of cholesterol). If after diet therapy, the patient's LDL cholesterol is still greater than 130 mg/dL, drug therapy should be started to reduce the LDL cholesterol to a goal of <100 mg/dL. 5-Hydroxymethyl glutaryl coenzyme A (HMG-CoA) reductase inhibitors provide the most effective therapy for lowering LDL cholesterol and raising high-density lipoprotein cholesterol.

ALTERNATIVE THERAPIES

Anxiety may have deleterious effects on the cardiovascular system, especially in patients with AMI. The aim of treatment of anxiety should be to reduce not only the somatic complaints but also the adrenergic hyperactivity often present in MI patients. Three groups of medications can be used to treat cardiac symptoms and anxiety disorder. Antidepressant drugs lower anxiety, but do not suppress adrenergic response and should be avoided in patients with AMI during acute recovery. In contrast, β-blockers blunt the adrenergic response but do not affect anxiety. Benzodiazepines can be used to relax the patient and theoretically decrease catecholamine release secondary to stress.[133,134] Alprazolam and diazepam have been shown to be effective in decreasing anxiety and catecholamine levels in patients with AMI. Once patients are consuming an appropriate diet, stool softeners are often used to decrease isometric stress associated with defecation. Either docusate sodium or docusate calcium 240 mg once or twice daily is satisfactory to soften the stool to avoid straining.

IMPROVING OUTCOMES

Approximately 50% of hospitalized MI patients develop complications.[135] Two general classes of complications have been defined: electrical (arrhythmias) and mechanical (heart failure). ECG monitoring and prompt recognition and treatment of arrhythmias have reduced the in-hospital mortality from MI. Unfortunately, a similarly favorable trend has not been observed with AMI-associated heart failure despite advances in hemodynamic monitoring and inotropic support. Left ventricular failure with subsequent pulmonary congestion is the primary cause of in-hospital death from MI.

Of the 500,000 patients hospitalized yearly for AMI, 400,000 patients survive to hospital discharge.[133] The major mortality risk is within the first 6 months of hospitalization; death is equally distributed between sudden and nonsudden cardiac events.[133,134] The major determinants of death after MI are the extent of jeopardized myocardium and the degree of electrical instability. Anterior infarction, early left ventricular failure, late significant arrhythmias, and poor left ventricular ejection fraction are major predictors of poor prognosis during the peri-infarction period.[133] Although Q-wave infarct patients have twice the initial mortality of patients with non–Q-wave infarction, their 1-year mortality rates are comparable.[136] Factors associated with late mortality after MI include advanced age,[136] history of prior infarction or chronic angina,[137] female sex,[138] hypertension,[139] diabetes mellitus,[139] and continued cigarette smoking.[13]

Considerable effort has been spent on the search for predictors of survival and factors determining the occurrence of reinfarction after AMI.[140] Most patients who survive AMI initially have an uncomplicated event; the pain subsides and there is no evidence of heart failure or arrhythmias. Mortality after MI in unselected groups of patients ranges from 4 to 6% per year.[140] Mortality is higher in patients with moderate impairment of left ventricular function and three-vessel coronary disease. These patients may benefit from elective coronary artery bypass graft after AMI.

Survival after AMI relates to the extent and location of the coronary obstructive lesion and to the adequacy of residual myocardial function. To prevent or retard the progression of atherosclerotic coronary heart disease, conventional coronary risk factor reduction is necessary.[141] Continued cigarette smoking after MI increases the likelihood of reinfarction and coronary death in men and women of all ages. Reduction of excess caloric and cholesterol intake is advisable. Control of systemic hypertension decreases both myocardial oxygen demand and the risk of stroke. Medical management with antianginal drugs reduces myocardial oxygen demand and decreases myocardial ischemia. By decreasing the ischemic burden, chronic therapy with β-adrenergic blockers reduces both the recurrence of MI and the incidence of sudden death for up to 2 years after AMI.[142] Exercise training improves physical work capacity and favorably affects weight control and psychological status.

PHARMACOECONOMICS

Advances in treatment have reduced the death rate from AMI by 30% since 1983; today, 13.5 million Americans have survived a heart attack or unstable angina pectoris.[2] Among those who survive their initial AMI, 31% of women and 23% of men will have another acute ischemic event (i.e., stroke, sudden death, or recurrent AMI) within 6 years.[2] The socioeconomic burden of AMI is substantial. Men with CAD have a 13-year reduction in life expectancy, whereas women have a 12-year reduction in life expectancy.[2,3] Direct costs from AMI (i.e., institutional care, medications, professional visits, home health care, and other medical goods) are $51.1 billion/year.[1] Indirect costs associated with AMI-related loss of income and productivity account for an additional $44.5 billion each year.[1]

Primary prevention measures aim to reduce the occurrence of AMI in disease-free, asymptomatic patients at risk for CAD. Smoking cessation, reduction in LDL cholesterol levels, control of hypertension, regular physical exercise, weight control, and estrogen replacement therapy in postmenopausal women are measures that may reduce the likelihood of AMI in high-risk patients. Secondary prevention aims to abort the occurrence of a second or repeat AMI. Because the number of Americans older than 65 years of age is expected to increase from 34.2 million in 1995 to 60.8 million in 2020 and AMI recurrence is directly proportional to age, secondary prevention is especially important in this age group. In these patients the administration of antiplatelet agents, ACE inhibitors, β-blockers, and HMG-CoA reductase inhibitors reduce the recurrence of AMI.

KEY POINTS

- MI is one of the most common reasons for hospitalization in the Western world.
- Mortality in patients with MI results from both arrhythmias and heart failure.
- The actual mortality rate is about 15%; approximately 10% of patients will die during the first year after their AMI.
- Short-term and long-term survival depends on the extent and location of the coronary obstructive lesions and the prompt correction of post-MI complications.
- The presence or absence of mechanical, electrical, ischemic, and vascular abnormalities provides the necessary information to institute appropriate medical and/or surgical treatment.
- MI evolves over a period of several hours. The extent of myocardial damage is related to the degree of reduction in myocardial tissue perfusion and level of myocardial oxygen consumption.
- Reperfusion of the ischemic myocardium reduces infarct size and improves hemodynamics and functional recovery.
- Thrombolytic therapy, percutaneous balloon angioplasty, and coronary artery bypass surgery are treatment modalities used to achieve prompt reperfusion.
- Adjunctive therapy for MI includes aspirin, β-adrenergic blocking agents, and ACEinhibitors.
- Primary prevention of MI includes smoking cessation, reduction in LDL cholesterol, management of systemic hypertension, exercise, weight control, and estrogen replacement therapy in postmenopausal women.
- Secondary prevention of MI includes the use of antiplatelet agents, ACEinhibitors, β-adrenergic blocking agents, and HMG-CoA reductase inhibitors.
- Advances in the treatment of MI have significantly reduced the death rate from MI.

REFERENCES

1. American Heart Association. 1998 heart and stroke statistical update. Dallas: American Heart Association, 1998.
2. Overmyer RH. Treating atherosclerotic disease: current strategies. Formulary J Managed Care Hosp Decision Makers 33(Suppl 1):S3–S12, 1998.
3. Alpert JS, Braunwald E. Acute : pathological, pathophysiological, and clinical manifestations. In Braunwald, ed. Heart disease. 2nd ed. Philadelphia: WB Saunders, 1984:1262–1270.
4. Gonzalez ER. Thrombolytic therapy for acute myocardial infarction. Hosp Pharm 32:1498–1509, 1997.
5. Gonzalez ER, Kannewurf BS. Atherosclerosis: a unifying disorder with various manifestations. Am J Health Syst Pharm 55(Suppl 1):S4–S7, 1998.
6. Moseri A, L'Abbate A, Bardoldi G, et al. Coronary vasospasm as possible cause of myocardial infarction. A conclusion derived from the study of "preinfarction" angina. N Engl J Med 299:1271–1277, 1978.
7. Epstein SE, Palmeri ST. Mechanisms contributing to precipitation of unstable angina and acute myocardial infarction: implications regarding therapy. Am J Cardiol 54:1245–1252, 1984.
8. Advanced cardiac life support. Dallas: American Heart Association, 1997–1999.
9. Kinch JW, Ryan TJ. Right ventricular infarction. N Engl J Med 330:1211–1217, 1994.
10. Zeller FP, Bauman JL. Current concepts in clinical therapeutics: acute myocardial infarction. Clin Pharm 5:553–572, 1986.
11. Tucker JF, Collins RA, Anderson AJ, et al. Value of serial myoglobin levels in the early diagnosis of patients admitted for acute myocardial infarction. Ann Emerg Med 24:704–708, 1994.
12. Adams JE III, Bodor GS, Davilla-Roman VG, et al. Cardiac troponin-1: a marker with high specificity for cardiac injury. Circulation 88:101–106, 1993.
13. Perviaz S, Anderson FP, Lohmann TP, et al. Comparative analysis of cardiac troponin I and creatine kinase-MB as markers of acute myocardial infarction. Clin Cardiol 20:269–271, 1997.
14. Antman EM, Tanasijevic MJ, Thompson B, et al. Cardiac-specific troponin I levels to predict the risk of mortality in patients with acute coronary syndromes. N Engl J Med 335:1342–1348, 1996.
15. Zelma MJ. Q wave, S-T segment, and T wave myocardial infarction. Am J Med 78:391–398, 1985.
16. Dubin D. Rapid interpretation of EKG's. 5th ed. Tampa: Cover Publishing, 1996.
17. GISSI–Avoidable Delay Study Group. Epidemiology; avoidable delay in the care of patients with acute myocardial infarction in Italy. Arch Intern Med 155:1481–1488, 1995.
18. Blohm MB, Herlitz J, Schroder U, et al. Reaction to a media campaign focusing on delay in acute myocardial infarction. Heart Lung 20:661–666, 1991.
19. Blohm MB, Hartfor M, Karlson BW, et al. An evaluation of the results of media and educational campaigns designed to shorten the time taken by patients with acute myocardial infarction to decide to go to hospital. Heart 76:430–434, 1996.
20. Rasanen J, Vaisanen IT, Heikkila J, et al. Acute myocardial infarction complicated by left ventricular dysfunction and respiratory failure: the effects of continuous positive airway pressure. Chest 87:278–280, 1985.
21. Dole WP, O'Rourke RA. Pathophysiology and management of cardiogenic shock. Curr Probl Cardiol 8(3):1–72, 1983.
22. Lee G, DeMaria AN, Amsterdam EA, et al. Comparative effect of morphine, meperidine, and pentazocine on cardiopulmonary dynamics in patients with acute myocardial infarction. Am J Med 60:341–355, 1976.
23. Stadol. In: Physician's desk reference. Montvale, NJ: Medical Economics Publishing company 1995;49:739–742.
24. Mueller JE, Braunwald E. Can infarct size be limited in patients with acute myocardial infarction? Cardiovasc Clin 69:740–747, 1983.
25. Herling IM. Intravenous nitroglycerin: clinical pharmacology and therapeutic. Chest 1981;73:441–445
26. Roberts R. Intravenous nitroglycerin in acute myocardial infarction. Am J Med 74(6B):45–52, 1983.
27. Swan NA, Evenson MK, Needham KE, et al. Effect of combined nitroglycerin and dobutamine infusion in left ventricular dysfunction. Am Heart J 106:35, 1983.
28. Chiarello M, Gold HK, Leinback RC, et al. Comparison between the effects of nitroprusside and nitroglycerin on ischemic injury during acute myocardial infarction. Circulation 54:766, 1976.
29. Flaherty JT. Comparison of intravenous nitroglycerin and sodium nitroprusside in acute myocardial infarction. Am J Med 74(6B):53–60, 1983.
30. Pitt B, Shae MJ, Romson JL. Prostaglandins and prostaglandin inhibitors in ischemic heart disease. Ann Intern Med 99:83–92, 1983.
31. Hirsh J. The optimal antithrombotic dose of aspirin. Arch Intern Med 145:1582, 1985.
32. Theroux P, Quimet H, McCans J. Aspirin, heparin, or both to treat acute unstable angina. N Engl J Med 313:1369–1375, 1985.
33. ISIS-2 (Second International Study of Infarct Survival) Collaborative Group. Randomized trial of intravenous streptokinase, oral aspirin, both, or neither among 17,187 cases of suspected acute myocardial infarction: ISIS-2. Lancet 2:349–360, 1988.
34. American College of Cardiology/American Heart Association. Guidelines for the management of patients with acute myocardial infarction. Circulation 94:2341–2350, 1996.
35. Gonzalez ER: Antiplatelet therapy in atherosclerotic cardiovascular disease. Clin Ther 20(Suppl B):B42–B53, 1998.
36. McTavish D, Faulds D, Gao KL. Ticlopidine: an updated review of its pharmacology and therapeutic use in platelet-dependent disorders. Drugs 40:239–259, 1990.
37. Knudsen JB, Kjoller E, Skagen K, et al. Randomized trial of prophylactic daily aspirin in British male doctors. Br Med J 296:313–316, 1988.
38. CAPRIE Steering Committee. A randomized, blinded trial of clopidogrel versus aspirin in patients at risk of ischemic events (CAPRIE). Lancet 348:1329–1339, 1996.
39. Antiplatelet Trialists' Collaboration. Collaborative overview of randomized trials of antiplatelet therapy. I. Prevention of death, myocardial infarction, and stroke by prolonged antiplatelet therapy in various categories of patients. Br Med J 308:81–106, 1994.
40. Prins MH, Hirsh J. Heparin as an adjunctive treatment for thrombolytic therapy for acute myocardial infarction. N Engl J Med 323:147–152, 1990.
41. Hsia J, Hamilton WP, Kleiman N, et al. A comparison between heparin and low-dose aspirin as an adjunctive therapy with tissue plasminogen activator for acute myocardial infarction: Heparin-Aspirin Reperfusion Trial (HART) Investigators. N Engl J Med 323:1433–1437, 1990.
42. Trujillo TC, Nolan PE. Unfractionated heparin in acute coronary syndromes: has its time come and gone? Am J Health Syst Pharm 55:2402–2409, 1998.
43. Gurfinkel EP, Manos EJ, Mejail RI, et al. Low molecular weight heparin versus regular heparin or aspirin in the treatment of unstable angina and silent ischemia. J Am Coll Cardiol 26:313–318, 1995.
44. Klein W, Buchwald AB, Hillis SE, et al. Comparison of low molecular weight heparin with unfractionated heparin in the management of unstable coronary disease: Fragmin in Unstable Coronary Artery Disease Study. Circulation 96:61–68, 1997.
45. Bahr RD. Reducing the time to therapy in AMI patients: the new paradigm. Am J Emerg Med 12:501–503, 1994.
46. Julian DG. Time as a factor in thrombolytic therapy. Int J Cardiol 49(Suppl):S17–S19, 1995.
47. Gonzalez ER, Sypniewski E. Acute myocardial infarction: diagnosis and treatment. In: DiPiro J, Talbert R, Hays M, et al., eds. Pharmacotherapy: a pathophysiologic approach. 2nd ed. New York: Elsevier, 1993:231–254.
48. Talley JD. Review of thrombolytic intervention for acute myocardial infarction–is it valuable? J Ark Med Soc 91:70–79, 1994.
49. Monk JP, Heel RC. Anisoylated plasminogen streptokinase activator complex (APSAC). A review of its mechanisms of action, clinical pharmacology and its therapeutic use in acute myocardial infarction. Drugs 34:25–49, 1987.
50. Meinertz T, Kasper W, Schumacher M, et al. The German multicenter trial of anisoylated plasminogen streptokinase activator complex versus heparin for acute myocardial infarction. Am J Cardiol 62:347–351, 1988.
51. AIMS Trial Study Group. Effect of intravenous APSAC on survival after acute myocardial infarction: preliminary report of a placebo controlled clinical trial. Lancet 1:545–549, 1988.
52. Sherry S. Appraisal of various thrombolytic agents in the management of acute myocardial infarction. Am J Med 83(Suppl 2A):31–46, 1987.
53. Gunnar RM, Bourdillon PD, Dixon DW, et al. Guidelines for the early management of patients with acute myocardial infarction: a report of the American College of Cardiology/American Heart Association Task Force on Assessment of Diagnostic and Therapeutic Cardiovascular Procedures. J Am Coll Cardiol 16:249–292, 1990.
54. Carney R. Randomized angiographic trial of recombinant tissue-type plasminogen activator in myocardial infarction. J Am Coll Cardiol 20:17–23, 1992.
55. Chen BP, Chow MS, Kluger J. Perspective on current, future thrombolytic therapy for acute myocardial infarction. Formulary 32:364–385, 1997.
56. Smalling RW, Bode C, Kalbfleisch J, et al. More rapid, complete, and stable coronary thrombolysis with bolus administration of reteplase compared with alteplase infusion in acute myocardial infarction. Circulation 91:2725–2732, 1995.

57. Martin U, Doerge L, Stegmeier K, et al. Influence of the degree of renal dysfunction on the pharmacokinetic properties of the novel recombinant plasminogen activator reteplase in rats. Drug Metab Dispos 24:288–292, 1996.
58. Martin U, Kohnert U, Helerbrand K, et al. Effective thrombolysis by a recombinant *Escherichia coli*-produced protease domain of tissue-type plasminogen activator in rabbit model of jugular vein thrombosis. Fibrinolysis 10:87–92, 1996.
59. Gersh BJ. Role of thrombolytic therapy in evolving myocardial infarction. Mod Concepts Cardiovas Dis 54:13–17, 1985.
60. Schwartz DE, Yamago CC. Thombolysis for evolving myocardial infarction. Ann Intern Med 103;463–469, 1985.
61. National Heart Attack Alert Program Coordinating Committee. Emergency department: rapid identification and treatment of patients with acute myocardial infarction. Ann Emerg Med 23:311–329, 1994.
62. Every NR, Spertus J, Fihn SD, et al. Length of hospital stay after acute myocardial infarction in the Myocardial Infarction Triage and Intervention (MITI) Project registry. J Am Coll Cardiol 28:287–293, 1996.
63. Grines CL, DeMaria AN. Optimal utilization of thrombolytic therapy for acute myocardial infarction: concepts and controversies. J Am Coll Cardiol 16:223–231, 1990.
64. The GUSTO-I Investigators. An international randomized trial comparing four thrombolytic strategies for acute myocardial infarction. N Engl J Med 329:673–682, 1993.
65. The GUSTO Angiographic Investigators. The effects of tissue plasminogen activator, sreptokinase, or both on coronary artery patency, ventricular function, and survival after acute myocardial infarction. N Engl J Med 329:1615–1622, 1993.
66. Maggioni A. The risk of stroke in patients with acute myocardial infarction after thrombolytic and antithrombotic treatment. N Engl J Med 327:1–6, 1992.
67. Gruppo Italiano per lo Studio della Sopravvivenza nell'Infarto Miocardico GISSI-2: A factorial randomised trial of alteplase versus streptokinase and heparin versus no heparin among 12,490 patients with acute myocardial infarction. Lancet 336:65–71, 1990.
68. ISIS-3 (Third International Study of Infarct Survival) Collaborative Group. ISIS-3: a randomised trial of streptokinase vs tissue plasminogen activator vs anistreplase and of aspirin plus heparin vs aspirin alone among 41,299 cases of suspected acute myocardial infarction. Lancet 339:753–770, 1992.
69. Ridker P. Large scale trials of thrombolytic therapy for acute myocardial infarction: GISSI-2, ISIS-3, and GUSTO-I. Ann Intern Med 119:530–532, 1993.
70. International Joint Efficacy Comparison of Thrombolytics. Randomized, double-blind comparison of reteplase double-bolus administration with streptokinase in acute myocardial infarction (INJECT): trial to investigate equivalence. Lancet 346:329–336, 1995.
71. The International Group. In-hospital mortality and clinical course of 20,891 patients with suspected acute myocardial infarction randomized between alteplase and streptokinase with or without heparin. Lancet 336:71–75, 1990.
72. Hochman J. Modern treatment of acute myocardial infarction. Cardiovasc Rev Rep 16:23–35, 1995.
73. GUSTO III. A comparison of reteplase with alteplase for acute myocardial infarction. N Engl J Med 337:1118–1123, 1997.
74. Crabbe SJ, Cloniger CC. Tissue plasminogen activator. A new thrombolytic agent. Clin Pharm 6:373–386, 1987.
75. Sherry S. Recombinant tissue activator (rt-PA): is it the thrombolytic agent of choice of an evolving myocardial infarction. Ann Intern Med 114:417–423, 1991.
76. Sherry S, Marder VJ. Streptokinase and recombinant tissue plasminogen activator (rt-PA) are equally effective in treating acute myocardial infarction. Ann Intern Med 114:417–423, 1991.
77. White HD, Rivers JT, Maslowski AH, et al. Effect of intravenous streptokinase as compared with that of tissue plasminogen activator on left ventricular function after first myocardial infarction. N Engl J Med 320:817–821, 1989.
78. Bassand JP, Cassagnes J, Machecourt T, et al. A multicenter trial of intravenous APSAC versus rt-PA in acute myocardial infarction: assessment of efficacy and safety [Abstract]. J Am Coll Cardiol 13(Suppl A):214A, 1990.
79. Rao AK, Pratt C, Berke A, et al. Thrombolysis in Acute Myocardial Infarction (TIMI) Trial–phase I: hemorrhagic manifestations and changes in plasma fibrinogen and the fibrinolytic system in patients treated with recombinant tissue plasminogen activator and streptokinase. J Am Coll Cardiol 11:1–11, 1988.
80. Gonzalez ER, Katz GM. Coronary thrombolysis: a comparison of intravenous streptokinase and intravenous tissue-type plasminogen activator. Fam Pract Recert 11:109–124, 1989.
81. McGovern PG, Pankow JS, Shaher E, et al. Recent trends in acute coronary heart disease: mortality, morbidity, medical care, and risk factors. N Engl J Med 334:884–890, 1996.
82. Granger CB. Data presented at the American College of Cardiology, 40th Annual Scientific Session. March 16–19, 1997.
83. Cragg DR, Bonemia JD, Jaiyesimi IA, et al. Ineligibility for intravenous [Abstract]. N Engl J Med 335:1253–1260, 1996.
84. Samama MM, Acar J. Thrombolytic therapy: future issues. Thromb Haemost 74:106–110, 1995.
85. Friedman BM. Early interventions in the management of acute myocardial infarction. West Med J 162:19–27, 1995.
86. Klimt DR, Knatterud GL, Stamler J, et al. Persantine-aspirin reinfarction study. Part II. Secondary coronary prevention with persantine and aspirin. J Am Coll Cardiol 7:251–269, 1986.
87. Oates JA, Wood AJ. Dipyridamole. N Engl J Med 316:1247–1257, 1987.
88. Gibbons R. Immediate angioplasty compared with the administration of a thrombolytic agent followed by conservative treatment for myocardial infarction. N Engl J Med 328:685–691, 1993.
89. Lange R, Hillis L. Immediate angioplasty for acute myocardial infarction [Editorial]. N Engl J Med 328:685–691, 1993.
90. May GS, Furbery CD, Eberlein KA, et al. Secondary prevention after myocardial infarction. A review of short-term acute phase trials. Prog Cardiovasc Dis 25:335–359, 1985.
91. Mueller HS, Ayres SM. Propranolol decreases sympathetic necrosis activity reflected by plasma catecholamines during evolution of myocardial infarction in man. J Clin Invest 65:338–346, 1980.
92. Pitt B, Crown P. Effect of propranolol in regional myocardial blood flow in acute ischemia. Cardiovasc Res 4:176–179, 1970.
93. The MIAMI Trial Research Group. Metoprolol in acute myocardial infarction (MIAMI). A randomised placebo-controlled international trial. Eur Heart J 6:199–226, 1985.
94. ISIS-1 (First International Study of Infarct Survival) Collaborative Group. Randomized trial of intravenous atenolol among 16,027 cases of suspected acute myocardial infarction: ISIS-1. Lancet 2:57–66, 1986.
95. The TIMI Study Group. Comparison of invasive conservative strategies after treatment with intravenous tissue plasminogen activator in acute myocardial infarction: results of the Thrombolysis in Myocardial Infarction (TIMI) Phase II trial. N Engl J Med 320:618–627, 1989.
96. Moos AN, Hilleman DE, Mohiudin SM, et al. Safety of esmolol in patients with acute myocardial infarction treated with thrombolytic therapy who have relative contraindications to β-blocker therapy. Ann Pharmacother 28:701–703, 1994.
97. Bussman WD, Seher W, Gresengrus M. Reduction of creatine kinase and creatinine kinase-MB indexes of infarct size by intravenous verapamil. Am J Cardiol 54:1224–1230, 1984.
98. Danish Multicenter Study Group. Verapamil in acute myocardial infarction. Eur Heart J 5:516–528, 1984.
99. Mueller JE, Morrison J, Stone PH, et al. Nifedipine therapy for patients with threatened and acute myocardial infarction. A randomized double-blind, placebo-controlled comparison. Circulation 69:740–747, 1984.
100. Sirnes PA, Overskeid K, Pedersen TR. Evolution of infarct size during the early use of nifedipine in patients with acute myocardial infarction: The Norwegian Nifedipine Multicenter Trial. Circulation 70:638–644, 1984.
101. Gibson RS, Boden WE, Theroux P, et al. Diltiazem and reinfarction in patients with non-Q-wave myocardial infarction. N Engl J Med 315:423, 1986.
102. Gibson RS, Young OM, Boden WE, et al. Prognostic significance and beneficial effect of diltiazem on the incidence of early recurrent ischemia after non-Q wave myocardial infarction: Results from the multicenter diltiazem reinfarction study. Am J Cardiol 60:203–209, 1987.
103. The Multicenter Diltiazem Postinfaction Trial Research Group. The effect of diltiazem on mortality and reinfarction after myocardial infarction. N Engl J Med 319:385, 1988.
104. Pfeffer M, Braunwald E, Moye LA, et al. Effect of captopril on mortality and morbidity in patients with left ventricular dysfunction after myocardial infarction. N Engl J Med 327:669–677, 1992.
105. Swedberg K, Held P, Kjekshus J, et al. Effects of early administration of enalapril on mortality in patients with acute myocardial infarction. N Engl J Med 327:678–684, 1992.
106. The SOLVD Investigators. Effect of enalapril on mortality and the development of heart failure in asymptomatic patients with reduced left ventricular ejection fractions. N Engl J Med 327:685–691, 1992.
107. Cohn J. The prevention of heart failure–a new agenda [Editorial]. N Engl J Med 327:725–727, 1992.
108. Dyckner T, Wester PO. Magnesium in cardiology. Acta Med Scand 666(Suppl):27–31, 1982.

109. Ebel H, Gunther T. role of magnesium in cardiac disease. J Clin Chem Clin Biochem 21:249–265, 1983.
110. Hollifield JW. Potassium and magnesium abnormalities: diuretics and arrhythmias in hypertension. Am J Med 77:28–32, 1984.
111. Rasmussen HS, Norregard P, Lindeneg O, et al. Intravenous magnesium in acute myocardial infarction. Lancet 1:234–235, 1986.
112. Whang R, Flink EB, Dyckner T, et al. Magnesium depletion as a cause of refractory potassium repletion. Arch Intern Med 145:1686–1689, 1985.
113. Whang R, Oei TO, Aikawa JK, et al. Predictors of clinical hypomagnesemia. Arch Intern Med 144:1794–1796, 1984.
114. Rasmussen HS, Aurup P, Hojberg S, et al. Magnesium and acute myocardial infarction. Arch Intern Med 146:872–874, 1986.
115. Ornato JP, Gonzalez ER. Refractory ventricular fibrillation. Emerg Decis 4:35–41, 1986.
116. Long-term outcome after intravenous magnesium sulphate in suspected acute myocardial infarction: the second Leicester Intravenous Magnesium Intervention Trial (LIMIT-2). Lancet 343:816–819, 1994.
117. ISIS-4: (Fourth International Study of Infarct Survival) Collaborative Group. A randomized factorial trial assessing early oral captopril, oral mononitrate, and intravenous magnesium sulphate in 58,050 patients with suspected acute myocardial infarction. Lancet 345:669–685, 1995.
118. Heesch C, Eichhorn EJ. Magnesium in acute myocardial infarction. Ann Emerg Med 24:1154–1160, 1994.
119. Antman E. Randomized trials of magnesium in acute myocardial infarction: when big numbers do not tell the whole story [Editorial]. Am J Cardiol 75:391–393, 1995.
120. Morgan DB, Davidson C. Hypokalemia and diuretics: an analysis of publications. Br Med J 280:905–909, 1980.
121. Kafka, S, Langevin L, Armstron PW. Serum magnesium and potassium in acute myocardial infarction. Arch Intern Med 147:465–469, 1987.
122. Ornato JP, Gonzalez ER, Starke H, et al. Incidence and causes of hypokalemia assciation with cardiac resuscitation. Am J Emerg Med 3:503–506, 1985.
123. Salerno DM, Asinger RW, Elsperger J, et al. Frequency of hypokalemia after successfully resuscitated out-of-hospital cardiac arrest compared with that in transmural acute myocardial infarction. Am J Cardiol 59:84–88, 1987.
124. Wyman MG, Gore S. Lidocaine prophylaxis in myocardial infarction: a concept whose time has come. Heart Lung 12:358–361, 1983.
125. Smith P, Arnesen H, Holme I. The effect of warfarin on mortality and reinfarction after myocardial infarction. N Engl J Med 323:147–152, 1990.
126. Cristal N, Szwareberg J, Gueron M. Supraventricular arrhythmias in acute myocardial infarction: prognostic importance of clinical setting; mechanisms of production. Ann Intern Med 82:35–39, 1975.
127. Singh BN, Venkatesh N. Prevention of myocardial reinfarction and of sudden death in survivors of acute myocardial infarction: role of prophylactic beta-adrenoreceptor blockade. Am Heart J 108:450–455, 1984.
128. Norris RM, Brown MA, Clarke ED, et al. Prevention of ventricular fibrillation during acute myocardial infarction by intravenous propranolol. Lancet 2: 883–886, 1984.
129. Ryden L, Arniego R, Arnman K, et al. A double-blind trial of metoprolol in acute myocardial infarction: effects on ventricular tachyarrhythmias. N Engl J Med 308:614–618, 1983.
130. Mueller H, Ayres SM, Religi A, et al. Propranolol in the treatment of acute myocardial infarction. Circulation 49:1078–1081, 1974.
131. Chadda K, Goldstein S, Byington R, et al. Effect of propranolol after acute myocardial infarction in patients with congestive heart failure. Circulation 73:503–510, 1986.
132. Kaplan K. Prophylactic anticoagulation following acute myocardial infarction. Arch Intern Med 146:595–597, 1986.
133. Hoehn-Saric R, McLeod DR. Cardiac symptoms and anxiety disorders: contributing factors and pharmacologic. Am J Cardiol 60:68j–73j, 1987.
134. Barker PH, Clanachan AS. Inhibition of adenosine accumulation into guinea pig ventricle by benzodiazepines. Eur J Pharmacol 78:241–244, 1982.
135. Rude RE. Acute myocardial infarction and its complications. Cardiol Clin 2:163–171, 1984.
136. Forrester JS, Waters DD. Hospital treatment of congestive heart failure: management according to hemodynamic profile. Am J Med 65:173–180, 1978.
137. Herling IM. Intravenous nitroglycerin: clinical pharmacology and therapeutic considerations. Am Heart J 108:141–149, 1984.
138. Swan NA, Evenson MK, Needham KE, et al. Effect of continuous nitroglycerin and dobutamine infusion in left ventricular dysfunction. Am Heart J 106:35–43, 1983.
139. Parmley WW, Chatterjee K, Charuzi Y, et al. Hemodynamic effect of noninvasive systolic unloading (nitroprusside) and diastolic augmentation (external counterpulsation) in patients with acute myocardial infarction. Am J Cardiol 33:810, 1974.
140. Sanz G, Castaner A, Betrice A, et al. Determinants of prognosis in survivors of myocardial infarction. N Engl J Med 306:1065–1070, 1982.
141. Wenger NK. Uncomplicated acute myocardial infarction: long-term management. Am J Cardiol 52:658–660, 1983.
142. Turi ZG, Braunwald E. The use of beta blockers after myocardial infarction. JAMA 249:2512–2516, 1983.

CHAPTER 44

THROMBOEMBOLIC DISEASE

Christa M. George, Steven R. Kayser, and David S. Adler

DEFINITION

Venous thromboembolism is a serious disorder that can often lead to death. Pulmonary embolism stemming from venous thrombosis is responsible for approximately 60,000 deaths each year.[1] Most patients who die of pulmonary embolism do so during the first hours after the event, making early detection and treatment essential in order to improve patient outcomes.[2]

A deep vein thrombosis is a thrombus composed of cellular material and fibrin, which can form in any vein in the body. Thrombi that occur in the larger leg veins pose a higher risk for pulmonary embolism than do those that occur in the smaller calf veins.[1] A pulmonary embolism is a thrombus that originates from any location in the systemic circulation and becomes lodged in the pulmonary artery, impeding blood flow to the lungs.[3]

TREATMENT GOALS: THROMBOEMBOLIC DISEASE

- The treatment of venous thrombosis should prevent extension of the thrombus, prevent embolism to the lungs, restore normal venous blood flow, and maintain normal venous valve function.
- Specific treatment goals for venous thrombosis include preventing the development of pulmonary embolism, preventing postphlebitic syndrome, reducing morbidity from the initial event, and achieving positive outcomes with minimal adverse events and cost.
- General management of venous thrombosis includes bed rest, elevation of feet, and pain control.
- General management of pulmonary embolism includes administration of oxygen and mechanical ventilation, if necessary. Specific management includes thrombolytic therapy, anticoagulation, embolectomy, or placement of an inferior vena cava filter.[4,5]
- Guidelines for the provision of safe and effective therapy have been published by the American College of Chest Physicians.[6]

EPIDEMIOLOGY

Many conditions may contribute to the development of thromboembolic disease[7] (Table 44.1). In general, any condition or combination of conditions that leads to activation of blood coagulation (hypercoagulability), venous stasis, or damage to the vascular wall puts a patient at risk for the development of a clot. This combination of events is also known as Virchow's triad.

Immobilization and bed rest, with resultant stasis, frequently contribute to thrombosis, especially in elderly and obese people. Prolonged partial occlusion of the veins in any person sitting for prolonged periods may also lead to stasis. A hypercoagulable state existing during the operative period may contribute to clotting. Trauma may initiate clotting; this is a particular problem in patients who have suffered fractures of the hips and pelvis, who may also require prolonged bed rest. Congestive heart failure, ulcerative colitis, myocardial infarction, and other high-risk medical illnesses (e.g., systemic lupus erythematosus) are associated with an increased risk of thrombosis. Carcinomas, particularly pancreatic, bronchogenic, gastric, and prostatic cancers, may produce procoagulant substances that initiate clotting. The increased activity of many clotting factors during pregnancy contributes to an increased risk of thrombosis. Oral contraceptives have been associated with an increased risk of clotting. Less commonly, some unusual blood diseases and hereditary causes have been associated with thrombosis. Deficiencies in protein C, protein S, or antithrombin III have been demonstrated in susceptible patients to be associated with

Table 44.1 ▪ Conditions Associated with Venous Thrombosis

Immobilization
Stasis
Surgery and the postoperative period
Trauma to affected area
High-risk medical illnesses (e.g., congestive heart failure, myocardial infarction)
Malignancies
Pregnancy, oral contraceptives
Heredity
Blood disorders (e.g., protein C or S deficiency, antithrombin III deficiency, factor V Leiden, antiphospholipid antibody syndrome)

thromboembolic complications. Most recently, a genetic mutation in factor V, factor V Leiden, has been discovered to be one of the most common reasons for the hereditary development of venous thrombosis. A rare circulating antiphospholipid antibody has been described in patients with immunologic diseases such as systemic lupus erythematosus. This is associated mostly with arterial thrombosis (Table 44.1).

PATHOPHYSIOLOGY

When injury occurs to the vascular endothelium, platelets adhere to exposed collagen, as well as to other exposed subendothelial tissue. Following platelet adhesion, release of adenosine diphosphate (ADP) by the injured platelets leads to platelet aggregation (Fig. 44.1). Transformation of this temporary platelet plug to a permanent platelet fibrin clot is achieved through activation of the extrinsic or intrinsic blood-clotting system (Fig. 44.2).

Throughout the process of platelet aggregation, a balance is maintained between certain prostaglandins that occur naturally and may be synthesized in vivo. Thromboxane A_2 is found in platelets and is a potent stimulant for platelet aggregation, as well as a potent vasoconstrictor. Prostacyclin, in contrast, is found in vessel walls and is an inhibitor of platelet aggregation, as well as a vasodilator. The balance between prostacyclin and thromboxane may be altered physiologically and also by various drugs (e.g., aspirin), and even by different doses of these drugs.

Each of the clotting factors circulates in the blood as an inactive protein. Before clotting can occur, each clotting factor must be converted to an active or enzymatic form. Exposure of subendothelial collagen, in addition to interaction with platelets, initiates the intrinsic pathway by stimulating the activation of factor XII. Activated factor XII then stimulates the conversion of factor XI to the active form, which then stimulates activation of factor IX. Activated factor IX, in the presence of calcium, phospholipids (platelet factor 3), and factor VIII, stimulates the conversion of factor X to its active form. Activated factor X, in the presence of calcium, phospholipid (platelet factor 3), and factor V, stimulates the conversion of prothrombin to thrombin.

The extrinsic clotting pathway may also stimulate the conversion of prothrombin to thrombin. The release of material that is extrinsic to the blood, such as tissue extract or tissue thromboplastin, activates factor VII, which stimulates the activation of factor X. Factor X thus occupies a central position at the junction of the extrinsic and intrinsic systems; the pathway at this point becomes the common pathway. These two systems act in concert during the evolution of a clot; rarely is one independent of the other.[8]

Thrombin, which is generated by both pathways, stimulates the conversion of fibrinogen to fibrin in the presence of ionized calcium. The initial soluble fibrin clot

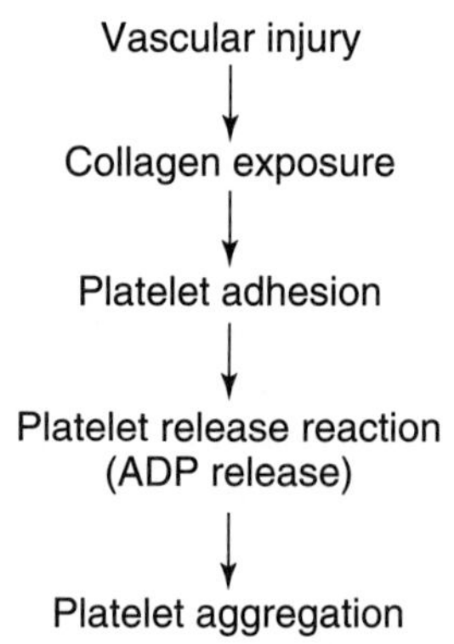

Figure 44.1. Formation of platelet plug.

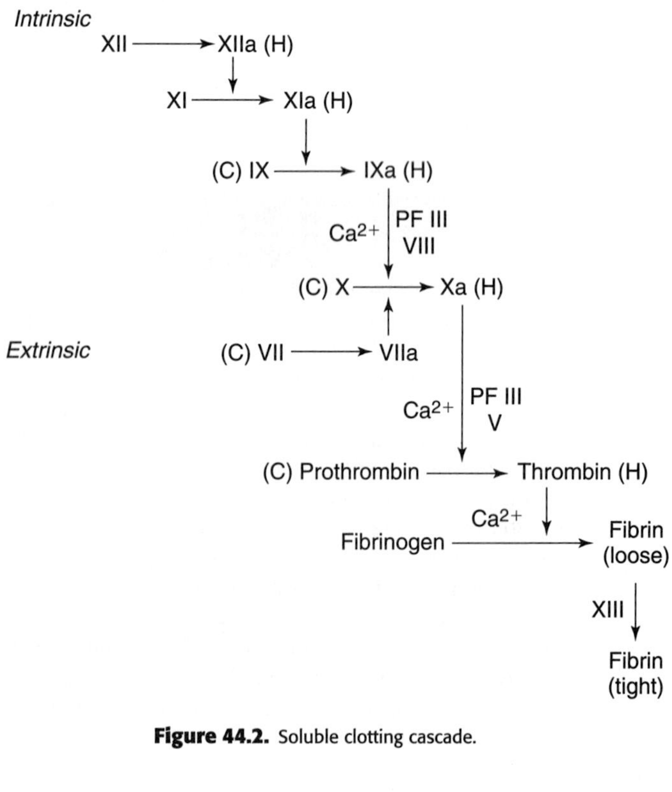

Figure 44.2. Soluble clotting cascade.

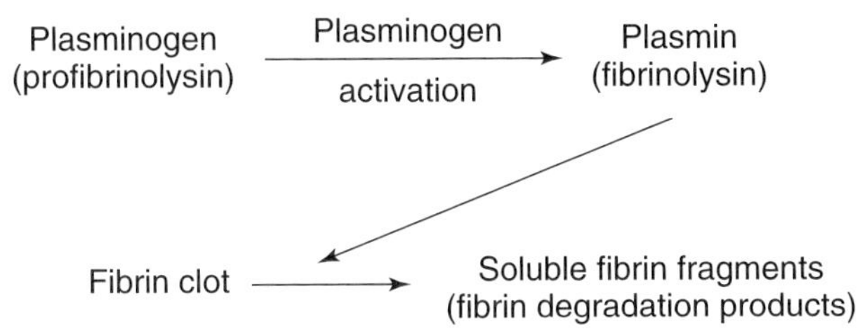

Figure 44.3. Fibrinolysis.

is further converted to an insoluble fibrin polymer when factor XIII is activated by thrombin. In addition to stimulating the conversion of fibrinogen to fibrin, thrombin stimulates platelet aggregation and potentiates the activity of factors V, VIIa, VII, and Xa.

Once thrombin is formed, it is partly removed by absorption into fibrin. This, plus other naturally occurring inhibitors of clotting factors, plays a role in localizing fibrin formation to the sites of injury and in maintaining the fluidity of circulating blood. Agents in normal blood inhibit the activated forms of factors II, X, XI, and XII. Deposition of fibrin also activates plasmin or fibrinolysin, a fibrinolytic enzyme that prevents excessive coagulation (Fig. 44.3).

Two types of thrombi may be formed. "White thrombi," or arterial thrombi, are composed primarily of platelets, although they also contain fibrin and occasionally leukocytes. They generally occur in areas of rapid blood flow and are formed in response to an injured or abnormal vessel wall. "Red thrombi," or venous thrombi, are found primarily in areas of relative stasis, where dilution of activated clotting factors by blood flow is prevented. They are almost completely composed of fibrin and erythrocytes, with a small number of platelets.

The choice of an antithrombotic drug is influenced by the type of thrombus. Heparin and coumarin are used in the treatment of both red and white thrombi. Drugs that affect platelet behavior are most useful for their effects in preventing and treating white thrombi. Fibrinolytic agents dissolve both types of thrombi.

CLINICAL PRESENTATION AND DIAGNOSIS

The clinical diagnosis of venous thrombosis is difficult and frequently misleading, because most venous clots occur without prominent findings.[9] Nevertheless, certain clinical signs are helpful. In 80% of cases of deep vein thrombosis (DVT) reviewed, unilateral ankle edema was present, followed by calf tenderness in 50% and a positive Homans' sign (pain on dorsiflexion of the foot) in only 8%. Increased warmth and calf swelling are also consistent with DVT.[3,10–12]

Deep venous thrombi occur most frequently in the lower extremities, in association with one or more of the previously discussed risk factors. The progression of thrombosis in the calf veins to the iliofemoral system in the thigh is associated with a greater risk of pulmonary embolism. Early recognition and documentation of lower leg thromboses are necessary to reduce the risk of pulmonary embolism.

The most common clinical manifestations of pulmonary embolism are sudden onset of unexplained dyspnea, pleuritic chest pain, tachypnea, and sinus tachycardia. Some patients may have hemoptysis or diaphoresis. Electrocardiographic manifestations may include changes in the ST segment and T waves. Chest radiographs are usually not very helpful. Arterial blood gases generally show a reduced PO_2 and a decreased PCO_2 caused by hyperventilation.

Objectively, the diagnosis of DVT may be confirmed by phlebography, impedance plethysmography, or Doppler ultrasound. Phlebography (venography) is the most reliable for detecting the presence of DVT.[4] Pulmonary embolism may be detected more specifically with the aid of pulmonary perfusion and ventilation scans and pulmonary angiography.

PSYCHOSOCIAL FACTORS

Many psychosocial factors can influence patient attitudes toward an understanding of anticoagulation therapy. These include educational levels, native language, literacy skills, cognitive function, diverse backgrounds, life experiences, family, employment, perceptions of their health status, and society. All of these issues must be addressed in order to enhance patient comprehension and improve outcomes.[13] Specific educational recommendations are discussed later in this chapter.

THERAPEUTIC PLAN

Tables 44.2, 44.3, and 44.4 give general treatment guidelines using unfractionated heparin and low-molecular-weight heparin.[7]

TREATMENT

Pharmacologic Therapy

Unfractionated Heparin

Heparin, a rapid-acting anticoagulant, exerts its antithrombotic effect by accelerating the action of a naturally occurring inhibitor of thrombin, an α_2-globulin, antithrombin III (ATIII). Antithrombin III inhibits activated clotting factors that have a reactive serine residue at their enzymatically active center. Heparin, by binding at the lysine group of ATIII (Fig. 44.4), induces a conformational change in ATIII that allows more ready access of the arginine residue to the serine group on the activated clotting factors.[14–16]

Commercial heparin is obtained from hog mucosa or bovine lung. Unfractionated heparin is a heterogeneous mixture of molecules with an average molecular weight of 12,000 to 15,000 daltons. Heparin must be administered parenterally and is effective following intravenous and subcutaneous administration. It should never be administered intramuscularly because of the risk of hematoma formation.

Standard unfractionated heparin is bound to a number of plasma proteins following administration. This binding in part accounts for the variability in response between patients and the resistance that is occasionally observed. Heparin is metabolized primarily in the liver and reticuloendothelial system and is partly eliminated by excretion into the urine.

The half-life of the anticoagulant effect of heparin in normal individuals and in patients with venous thromboembolism, as measured by changes in the activated partial thromboplastin time (APTT), is approximately 1.5 hour.

Table 44.2 ▪ Guidelines for Anticoagulation: Unfractionated Heparin

Disease suspected:	Obtain baseline APTT, PT, CBC Check for contraindication to heparin therapy Give heparin 5000 U IV and order imaging study
Disease confirmed:	Rebolus with heparin 80 U/kg IV and start maintenance infusion with 18 U/kg IV (see Table 44.3) Check APTT at 6 hr to keep APTT in a range that corresponds to a therapeutic blood heparin level (see Table 44.3) Check platelet count daily Start warfarin therapy on day 1 at 5 mg and adjust subsequent daily dose according to INR; stop heparin therapy after at least 4 to 5 days of combined therapy when INR > 2.0 for 2 consecutive days Anticoagulate with warfarin for at least 3 months at an INR of 2.0 to 3.0 (see Table 44.7)

For dosing of subcutaneous unfractionated heparin, see text.

Source: Reference 7.

APTT, activated partial thromboplastin time; *CBC,* complete blood count; *INR,* international normalized ratio; *PT,* prothrombin time.

The half-life, when plasma heparin activity is measured, depends on the dose and increases with an increased dose. Limited studies show that patients with pulmonary embolism have a greater heparin clearance and shorter half-life than do those with venous thrombosis. This may be due to the continuing thrombin formation on the surface of the embolus, leading to an increased rate of heparin clearance.[17,18]

Therapeutic Indications

Heparin is indicated in the treatment of venous thromboembolism and documented pulmonary embolism and in the prevention of venous thromboembolism.[7,9] It is also indicated for use in early treatment of patients with unstable angina or acute myocardial infarction, during cardiac bypass surgery and vascular surgery, during and after coronary angioplasty, in patients with coronary stents, and in selected patients with disseminated intravascular coagulation.[19] These indications are discussed in other chapters in this text.

Dosing and Administration

Intravenous administration of a large bolus dose of heparin ensures that therapeutic anticoagulation is achieved without delay. There is an unacceptable risk of recurrent thrombosis in patients in whom there is a delay in achieving therapeutic levels of anticoagulation. Conversely, there is a weak relationship between supratherapeutic APTT response and the risk of bleeding.[20]

Traditionally, heparin has been administered starting with an intravenous bolus injection (5000 to 10,000 U) followed by either intermittent intravenous injections (5000 U every 4 to 6 hours) or continuous intravenous infusion (starting at 1000 U/hr). However, numerous approaches have since been developed in order to achieve therapeutic heparin levels more rapidly. These have shown that the development of guidelines aid in achieving therapeutic heparin levels faster and with a lower incidence of recurrent thrombosis and bleeding. Several weight-based dosing nomograms have been developed.[21–23] Tables 44.2 and 44.3 show a commonly used weight-based

Table 44.3 ▪ Body Weight–Based Dosing of IV Heparin[a]

APTT (sec)[c]	Dose Change (U/kg/hr)	Additional Action	Next APTT (hr)
<35 (<1.2 × mean normal)	+4	Rebolus with 80 IU/kg	6
35–45 (1.2–1.5 × mean normal)	+2	Rebolus with 40 IU/kg	6
46–70[b] (1.5–2.3 × mean normal)	0	0	6[d]
71–90 (2.3–3.0 × mean normal)	−2	0	6
>90 (>3 × mean normal)	−3	Stop infusion at 1 hr	6

Source: Reference 7.

[a]Initial dosing; loading 80 IU/kg; maintenance infusion: 18 IU/kg/hr (APTT in 6 hr).

[b]Heparin, 25,000 IU in 250μL D_5W. Infuse at rate dictated by body weight through an infusion apparatus calibrated for low flow rates.

[c]The therapeutic range in seconds should correspond to a plasma heparin level of 0.2 to 0.4 IU/mL by protamine sulfate or 0.3 to 0.6 IU/mL by amidolytic assay. When APTT is checked at 6 hr or longer, steady-state kinetics can be assumed.

[d]During the first 24 hr, repeat APTT every 6 hr. Thereafter, monitor APTT once every morning unless it is outside the therapeutic range.

Table 44.4 ▪ Guidelines for Anticoagulation: Low-Molecular-Weight Heparin

Disease suspected:	Obtain baseline APTT, PT, CBC Check for contraindication to heparin therapy Give unfractionated heparin 5000 U IV and order imaging study
Disease confirmed:	Give LMWH (enoxaparin) 1 mg/kg subcutaneously every 12 hours or 1.5 mg/kg subcutaneously every 24 hours Start warfarin therapy on day 1 at 5 mg and adjust the subsequent daily dose according to INR Consider checking a platelet count between days 3–5 Stop LMWH therapy after at least 4 to 5 days of combined therapy when INR >2.0 for 2 consecutive days Anticoagulate with warfarin for at least 3 months at an INR of 2.0 to 3.0 (see Table 44.7)

Source: Reference 7.
APTT, activated partial thromboplastin time; *CBC,* complete blood count; *INR,* international normalized ratio; *LMWH,* low-molecular-weight heparin; *PT,* prothrombin time.

dosing nomogram that can aid in achieving adequate anticoagulation rapidly.[7]

Heparin may also be given subcutaneously in order to simplify treatment. An initial intravenous loading dose of 3000 to 5000 U should be followed by 15,000 to 17,000 U or 250 U/kg total body weight subcutaneously every 12 hours.[14] The APTT should be performed 4 to 6 hours after the initial dose and once daily during the middle of the dosing interval. The APTT should be maintained above 1.5 times the control value.

Subcutaneous heparin is also used in the prevention of venous thromboembolism and pulmonary embolism in high-risk patients undergoing selected surgical procedures.[9] Table 44.5 lists the risk factors for venous thromboembolic disease. Clinical risk factors include age; prolonged immobility/paralysis; prior venous thromboembolism; cancer; major surgery (especially involving abdomen, pelvis, lower extremities); obesity; varicose veins; congestive heart failure; myocardial infarction; stroke; fractures of the pelvis, hip, or leg; indwelling femoral vein catheter; inflammatory bowel disease; nephrotic syndrome; estrogen use; and hypercoagulable states.[9] Recommendations for prophylaxis are shown in Table 44.6.

Before the initiation of heparin, baseline clotting studies must be performed and should include the prothrombin time (in anticipation of oral anticoagulant therapy), APTT, platelet count, hemoglobin, and hematocrit. Patients should be monitored for any signs and symptoms of bleeding.

Laboratory Assessment

Because the response to a given dose of heparin or warfarin is highly variable, laboratory assessment is considered essential. Recurrence of thromboembolism is much greater when therapeutic anticoagulation is not rapidly achieved. Maintaining the appropriate laboratory test in the therapeutic range helps prevent hemorrhage, as well as the development of recurrent thrombosis.

The activated partial thromboplastin time is the standard test used to monitor heparin therapy. The APTT is primarily a measure of the competence of the intrinsic and common clotting pathways. It is insensitive to factors VII and XIII. It is used in screening for deficiencies of the intrinsic clotting system in patients who are considered to be candidates for oral anticoagulation and in monitoring the response to heparin therapy. The APTT is performed with platelet-poor plasma and so does not reflect the activity of platelets. Normal values for the APTT are between 24 and 36 seconds. Therapeutic heparinization is considered to be an APTT of 1.5 to 2.5 times control.

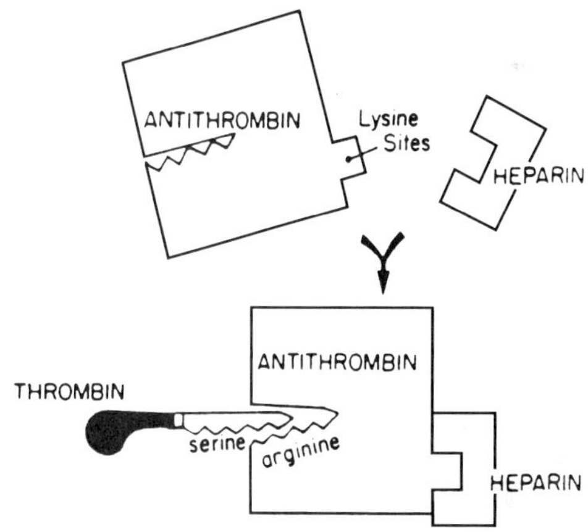

Figure 44.4. Model of heparin-induced confirmation change in antithrombin, resulting in rapid inhibition of thrombin. (*Source:* Reprinted with permission from Rosenberg RD. Actions and interactions of antithrombin and heparin. N Engl J Med 292:146, 1975.)

Table 44.5 ▪ Risk Factors for Venous Thromboembolic Disease

Low	Uncomplicated minor surgery in patients <40 years with no clinical risk factors
Moderate	Any surgery (major and minor) in patients 40–60 years but no additional risk factors; major surgery in patients <40 years but no additional risk factors; minor surgery in patients with risk factors
High	Major surgery in patients >60 years without additional risk factors; major surgery in patients 40–60 years who have additional risk factors; patients with MI and medical patients with risk factors
Highest	Major surgery in patients >40 years plus prior VTE or malignant disease or hypercoagulable state; patients with elective major lower extremity orthopedic surgery, hip fracture, stroke, multiple trauma, or spinal cord injury

Source: Reference 9.
MI, myocardial infarction; *VTE,* venous thromboembolism.

Table 44.6 ▪ Antithrombotic Regimens to Prevent Venous Thromboembolism

Method	Description
LDUH	5,000 U heparin given q8–12hr, starting 1–2 hr before operation
Adjusted-dose subcutaneous heparin	3,500 U heparin given q8hr with postoperative dose adjustments by ±500 U to maintain APTT at high-normal values
LMWH and heparinoids[a]	General surgery Moderate risk: Dalteparin, 2,500 U 1–2 hr before surgery and once daily after surgery Enoxaparin, 2,000 U 1–2 hr before surgery and once daily after surgery Nadroparin, 3,100 U 2 hr before surgery and once daily after surgery Tinzaparin, 3,500 U 2 hr before surgery and once daily after surgery High risk: Dalteparin, 5,000 U 10–12 hr before surgery and once daily after surgery Danaparoid, 750 U 1–2 hr before surgery and twice daily after surgery Enoxaparin, 4,000 U 10–12 hr before surgery and once daily after surgery Enoxaparin, 3,000 U twice daily starting 12–24 hr after surgery Orthopedic surgery Ardeparin, 50 U/kg twice daily starting 12–24 hr after surgery Dalteparin, 5,000 U 8–12 hr before surgery and once daily starting 12 hr after surgery Danaparoid, 750 U 1–2 hr before surgery and twice daily after surgery Enoxaparin, 3,000 U twice daily starting 12–24 hr after surgery or 4,000 U once daily starting 10–12 hr before surgery Nadroparin, 40 U/kg starting 2 hr before surgery and once daily after surgery for 3 days; the dose is then increased to 60 U/kg once daily Tinzaparin, 50 U/kg 2 hr before surgery and once daily after surgery or 75 U/kg once daily starting 12–24 hr after surgery Acute spinal injury Enoxaparin, 3,000 U twice daily Multiple trauma Enoxaparin, 3,000 U twice daily starting 12–36 hr after injury Medical conditions Dalteparin, 2,500 U once daily Danaparoid, 750 U twice daily Enoxaparin, 3,000 U once daily
Adjusted-dose perioperative warfarin	Start daily dose (5 mg) the day of or the day after operation; adjust dose for INR 2–3 by day 5
Preoperative and postoperative two-step warfarin	Start 1–2.5 mg/day 5–14 days before operation, aiming for 2- or 3-sec increase in prothrombin time at time of operation; give 2.5–5 mg/day, aiming for an INR 2–3 in postoperative period
Minidose warfarin	Start 1 mg/days 10–14 days before operation, aiming for INR = 1.5 after operation
IPC/ES	Start immediately before operation, and continue until fully ambulatory

Source: Reference 9.

[a]Dosage expressed in anti-Xa units; use with caution in patients having spinal or epidural anesthesia/analgesia. Ardeparin, enoxaparin, dalteparin, and danaparoid are approved by the FDA.

APTT, activated partial thromboplastin time; *IPC/ES,* intermittent pneumatic compression/elastic stockings; *LDUH,* low dose unfractionated heparin; *LMWH,* low-molecular-weight heparin.

Finger-stick methods are available for the rapid determination of the APTT at the patient's bedside.

The activated clotting time (ACT) of whole blood is sensitive to all clotting factors except factor VII, with undetermined sensitivity to factors V and II. The major advantage of this test is that it is a whole blood test; it does reflect the contribution of platelets in coagulation. The ACT can be performed rapidly at the bedside and is frequently used in dialysis suites, catheterization laboratories, and the operating room to evaluate the degree of heparinization. Normal values are 80 to 130 seconds.

Adverse Reactions

Hemorrhage is the most common adverse reaction to heparin and is generally, but not always, associated with clotting tests outside the recognized therapeutic range. Spontaneous bleeding is rare.

Minor hemorrhage occurs in approximately 4% of courses of anticoagulant therapy, usually into the skin or urine or from the nose. Major hemorrhagic events occur in approximately 2% of courses, usually in the gastrointestinal tract or the central nervous system.

Other adverse effects include thrombocytopenia,[24] osteoporosis, hypoaldosteronism, and generalized hypersensitivity reactions. Two types of heparin-induced thrombocytopenia have been described. The first is mild and transient and occurs early during the course of therapy. It is not immunologically mediated. The second type of thrombocytopenia secondary to heparin appears during the first 3 to 12 days of therapy, is unrelated to dose, and reverses within 3 to 5 days after discontinuation of heparin. It may occur in 5 to 10% of patients and can occur with therapeutic intravenous or prophylactic subcutaneous administration.[19] The incidence is less with low-molecular-weight heparins. One study reported that none of 333 patients and 9 of 332 patients receiving low-molecular-weight heparin and standard heparin, respectively, developed thrombocytopenia.[25] The exact mechanism has not been established, but it appears to be immunologically mediated. Osteoporosis occurs with therapy of more than 10,000 U per day for 6 months or longer. Hypoaldosteronism with resultant hyperkalemia and sodium diuresis is uncommonly associated with heparin therapy.

Drug Interactions

A direct interaction between heparin and nitroglycerin has been proposed as a mechanism for increasing heparin requirements as is seen in some patients who receive both drugs concomitantly. This has not been a universal observation, however, and a controlled trial provides evidence that there is no interference with nitroglycerin doses below 350 μg/min. At doses of nitroglycerin above 350 μg/min, a higher dose of heparin was required to achieve the same prolongation of the APTT. The proposed mechanism is a qualitative antithrombin III abnormality induced by nitroglycerin.[26] Close patient monitoring is required, and any resistance can be overcome with appropriate dosage adjustments. Heparin is physically incompatible with many other drugs, and appropriate sources should be consulted before heparin is mixed with other solutions.

The concomitant administration of heparin along with antiplatelet agents must be directed by the clinical indication. There may be an increased risk of bleeding; however, there may be additional efficacy as well. (See the discussion in the chapter on myocardial infarction.)

Treatment of Overdose

Protamine sulfate, a strongly basic molecule, is a specific antidote that combines with and inactivates heparin. The appropriate dose of protamine depends on the dose of heparin, the time since administration, and the route of administration. If administered immediately after intravenous heparin, 1 mg of protamine is given for every 100 U of heparin. If treatment is delayed, the dose of protamine must be decreased. Response can be assessed with the APTT or ACT.

Although protamine has been reported to exert an anticoagulant effect if it is administered in excessive dosages, this is unlikely to be a problem clinically. Of greater concern are the cardiovascular complications that may be associated with protamine. A decrease in blood pressure and systemic vascular resistance has been observed in humans. This appears to be associated most often with too-rapid administration. Anaphylactoid reactions may occur in 2 to 5% of patients.[27]

In the event of a major hemorrhage, whole blood or fresh frozen plasma should replace lost volume and clotting factors.

Low-Molecular-Weight Heparin

The low-molecular-weight heparins (LMWHs) belong to a class of anticoagulants called the glycosaminoglycans. They differ from unfractionated heparin (UH) in several ways. They have less affinity for thrombin than does UH, while retaining their ability to inactivate factor Xa. The have reduced binding to plasma proteins, reduced binding to macrophages and endothelial cells, reduced binding to platelets, and possible reduced binding to osteoblasts. These properties are responsible for making their dose-response curve more predictable, increasing their plasma half-life, reducing the incidence of heparin-induced thrombocytopenia, and reducing bone loss.[19] They are derived from UH, and the molecular weight ranges from 4000 to 5000. The LMWHs produce their anticoagulant activity through activating antithrombin.

LMWHs have a longer duration of anti–factor Xa activity compared with UH, allowing less frequent dosing intervals. LMWHs are cleared renally and have an increased half-life when administered to patients with renal failure. Dosage adjustments are necessary when LMWHs are administered to these patients. Four LMWHs are approved for use in the United States: enoxaparin, dalteparin, ardeparin, and danaparoid.[28,29]

Therapeutic Indications

Ardeparin, dalteparin, danaparoid, and enoxaparin are indicated for the prophylaxis of venous thromboembolism in patients undergoing selected orthopedic and abdominal surgical procedures. Enoxaparin and dalteparin are indicated for use in patients with unstable angina or non–Q-wave myocardial infarction. Enoxaparin is also indicated for the inpatient treatment of deep venous thrombosis, with or without concomitant pulmonary embolism, and for the outpatient management of deep venous thrombosis without pulmonary embolism.[28]

Dosing and Administration

Low-molecular-weight heparins are administered subcutaneously, usually every 12 to 24 hours. Table 44.6 lists dosing regimens for prevention of DVT.[9] For the inpatient treatment of acute DVT with or without pulmonary embolism (PE), the dose of enoxaparin is 1 mg/kg given subcutaneously every 12 hours or 1.5 mg/kg given subcutaneously every 24 hours (Table 44.3). For the outpatient management of DVT without PE, the enoxaparin dose is 1 mg/kg given subcutaneously every 12 hours for a minimum of 5 days. Warfarin should be started within 72 hours of initiation of enoxaparin.[28]

Laboratory Assessment

The APTT and prothrombin time (PT) are not altered by the LMWHs. The predictable dose response of LMWHs negates any regular laboratory monitoring. When treating established venous thromboembolism, efficacy of anticoagulant activity may be assessed by measuring the drug's anti-Xa activity at the beginning of therapy. However, these values may differ between laboratories, because the anti-Xa assay has not been standardized.[28,29]

Adverse Reactions

The adverse effects associated with LMWHs are similar to those of UH: bleeding and thrombocytopenia. The risk of bleeding during therapy with LMWHs is comparable to that of UH.[28] The incidence of thrombocytopenia is less than that of heparin (0.6% versus 3.5%). LMWHs should not be given to patients with established heparin-induced thrombocytopenia, due to the high incidence of cross-reactivity (almost 100%). The incidence of osteoporosis is less than that of UH (2.6% versus 17.6%).

Other effects associated with LMWHs include delayed hypersensitivity skin reactions at the injection site and elevated serum transaminase levels.[30,31]

Warfarin

Warfarin exerts its pharmacologic effect by interfering with the synthesis of the vitamin K–dependent clotting factors in the liver. These factors are II, VII, IX, and X. Early investigators assumed a competitive antagonism to explain the relationship between warfarin and vitamin K. This has since been disproved. It is now believed that warfarin inhibits the effect of vitamin K at a postribosomal step in the hepatic synthesis of the vitamin K–dependent clotting factors. Vitamin K is required in the conversion of nonactive precursor proteins (precursors of active clotting factors) that lack calcium-binding capacity to active precursor proteins (e.g., prothrombin). This calcium-binding capacity is needed to hold prothrombin onto phospholipid surfaces during its activation to thrombin. Vitamin K accomplishes this activation by carboxylation of glutamyl residues on the precursor protein to form γ-carboxyglutamic acid, which allows for calcium binding. Vitamin K probably carboxylates the glutamyl residues of factors VII, IX, and X as well. During the carboxylation of precursor proteins, vitamin K is converted to vitamin K epoxide. Vitamin K epoxide is then converted back to vitamin K. Warfarin prevents this reaction and thus produces a buildup of inactive precursor proteins. This effect of warfarin can be overcome by the administration of vitamin K.[32,33]

The onset of anticoagulant effect of warfarin depends not only on this interaction with vitamin K, but also on the metabolic clearance of clotting factors that are already present in the blood.

The pharmacokinetics of warfarin has been the most extensively studied of coumarin pharmacokinetics.[34] Warfarin is completely absorbed in the upper gastrointestinal tract, with peak blood levels occurring in 60 to 120 minutes. The volume of distribution of warfarin is 12.5% of body weight. This small volume is consistent with the extensive binding of warfarin to albumin, because it is equivalent to the volume of albumin, 2.6 times the plasma volume.

The mean half-life of warfarin is independent of dose and is 42 hours. Warfarin is 99.5% bound to albumin. No apparent relationship exists between the extent of protein binding of warfarin and the concentration of albumin or total protein in the serum. Furthermore, there appears to be no direct correlation between the effect on PT or international normalized ratio (INR) and the dose of warfarin, because so many variables influence dosing.[35]

Warfarin is metabolized in the hepatic microsomes by mixed-function oxidase enzymes. It is administered as a racemate that contains equal parts of the R and S isomers. The S isomer is approximately five times more potent than the R isomer. The reason why the R and S isomers differ in potency is unclear. The half-life of the R isomer is 45 hours, and the half-life of the S isomer is 33 hours; they have the same volume of distribution. It has been proposed that differences in permeability or affinity to the receptor site account for the differing potencies.

Knowledge of these two isomers is important because drugs may interact with warfarin stereoselectively. For example, metronidazole inhibits the metabolism of the S isomer but has no effect on the R isomer.[36]

Therapeutic Indications

Warfarin is effective in the primary and secondary prevention of venous thromboembolism, as well as in the prevention of systemic embolism in patients with artificial heart valves or with atrial fibrillation. It is also effective in the prevention of acute myocardial infarction in patients with peripheral arterial disease. It is used in the prevention of recurrent infarction, stroke, and death in patients with acute myocardial infarction, and in the prevention of myocardial infarction in men at high risk.[37]

Dosing and Administration

Oral anticoagulant therapy should be initiated without a loading dose.[32,36,38,39] Before the 1980s, clinicians traditionally started therapy with a large initial dose followed by smaller doses over subsequent days. The belief was that therapeutic anticoagulation would be achieved more quickly. Unfortunately, a few clinicians may still initiate warfarin with a loading dose.

The onset of the warfarin effect depends not only on the half-life of the parent drug but also on the half-life of catabolism of the vitamin K–dependent clotting factors. These factors have half-lives of 5 hours for factor VII, 20 to 40 hours for factors IX and X, and up to 60 hours for factor II. Depression of any factor may predispose the patient to bleeding. O'Reilly and Aggeler[39] compared a loading dose of warfarin, 1.5 mg/kg, with two schedules without a loading dose, of 10 mg/day and 15 mg/day. No significant difference was found in the rate of fall of factors II, IX, and X in the different schedules. However, there was a significantly faster decline in factor VII activity with the

Table 44.7 ▪ Duration of Therapy

	Duration
3–6 mo	Reversible or time-limited risk factors[a] and a first event
	Heterozygous activated protein C resistance and a first event
At least 6 mo	Idiopathic etiology and a first event
12 mo to lifetime	Recurrent disease for any reason
	First event with any of the following: Cancer, until resolved; Homozygous activated protein C resistance; Antiphospholipid antibody, until resolved; Deficiency of antithrombin, protein C or S

Source: Reference 7.

[a]Transient immobilization, trauma, surgical operation, or pharmacologic estrogen use. These recommendations are subject to modification by individual characteristics, including age, comorbidity, and likelihood of recurrence.

loading dose compared with the other two regimens. Because the PT is most sensitive to factor VII, a more rapid prolongation of the PT with the loading dose led many to consider this to be proof that loading doses achieve more rapid anticoagulation. Intrinsic coagulation depends most on factors IX and X and less on factor VII. In summary, depression of factor VII offers little if any protection against thromboembolism, and a rapid depression may lead to hemorrhage. Because of the many factors contributing to anticoagulant response, PTs should be obtained daily until therapy is stabilized.[39] In addition, loading doses are dangerous for patients with protein C deficiency or protein S deficiency because of increased risk of warfarin-induced skin necrosis.

To achieve a safe and rapid conversion from heparin to warfarin, it is recommended that both anticoagulants be administered concurrently, beginning from the first day of therapy.[38] Because evidence exists that 5 days of therapeutic heparinization is as effective as 10 days for the treatment of proximal vein thrombosis, this technique may help decrease the hospital stay.[36] Heparin therapy must be sufficient to prolong the APTT into the therapeutic range throughout this shortened period. Heparin treatment should overlap with warfarin for 4 to 5 days. Once the INR has been greater than 2.0 for 2 consecutive days, heparin may be discontinued (Table 44.2). Optimal treatment duration remains to be well established and should be based on risk factors for recurrence of DVT. Table 44.7 lists suggested treatment duration.[7]

When a therapeutic course is concluded, warfarin may be discontinued abruptly with little risk of rebound activation of clotting. Because the half-life of warfarin is prolonged, a tapering effect occurs. A prospective study suggests that in certain patients there is a rebound hypercoagulable state after abrupt discontinuation, but this observation in a small group of patients requires further confirmation.[40]

Laboratory Monitoring

It has generally been recommended that the degree of oral anticoagulant–induced prolongation of the laboratory test should be the same as for heparin, that is, prolongation to 1.5 to 2.5 times normal. The PT is the test that is used to assess warfarin therapy. The PT is prolonged by deficiencies of factors V, VII, X, and II; by low levels of fibrinogen; and by high levels of heparin. The PT thus reflects alterations in the extrinsic and common pathways. A normal PT is approximately 11 seconds. Because of the variability in sensitivity of the thromboplastin reagent that issued in determining the PT, results from different laboratories may differ. The ratio of the patient's PT to the laboratory control will subsequently differ among laboratories. To standardize interpretation of the intensity of anticoagulation, European investigators adopted the INR in 1983. A World Health Organization primary international reference preparation of thromboplastin is used to standardize the commercial source of thromboplastin that is used by a given laboratory. The INR is the preferred standard for assessing the adequacy of anticoagulation with warfarin. The INR is calculated by raising the calculated PT ratio, PT of the patient/PT control from the laboratory, to the power of the international sensitivity index (ISI), which is assigned to each batch of thromboplastin–that is, INR = (PT patient/PT control) raised to the ISI. For example, patient PT of 22 seconds and control PT of 11 seconds, equaling a ratio of 2 when raised to an ISI of 2, is equal to an INR of 4 (i.e., 22/11 raised to the power of 2 = 4). Thromboplastin sources that are less sensitive have lower ISIs. This relationship not only has standardized interpretation of laboratory results but also has led to the appreciation that less intense anticoagulation is often as effective as more intense treatment and is associated with a lower incidence of bleeding.[34] There are several problems with the INR; however, overall it allows for standardization of reporting.[41,42] Table 44.8 shows

Table 44.8 ▪ Relative Intensity of Anticoagulant Therapy[a]

INR 2.0–3.0
Prophylaxis of venous thrombosis (high risk)
Treatment of venous thrombosis/pulmonary embolism
Prevention of systemic embolism associated with tissue heart valves, acute myocardial infarction, atrial fibrillation, valvular heart disease
INR 2.5–3.5
Mechanical heart valves (high risk)
Recurrent systemic embolism (INR 2.0–3.0 may also be effective)

Source: Kayser S. Thromboembolic disease. In: Herfindal ET, Hirshman JL, eds. Clinical pharmacy and therapeutics. 6th ed. Baltimore: Williams & Wilkins, 1996:855.

[a]For more specific recommendations, see reference 6.

recommendations for the intensity of anticoagulation for various indications. The ranges of therapeutic anticoagulation fall within two ranges: an INR of 2.0 to 3.0 and an INR of 2.5 to 3.5. As more experience accumulates, even less intense therapy may be possible and may lead to an even lower incidence of bleeding.

Determinants of Anticoagulant Response

Many factors may alter the response to warfarin (Table 44.9).[43,44]

DIET. Excessive intake of food that is rich in vitamin K may theoretically induce a relative resistance to warfarin. Clinically, this may lead to variations in the INR. Patients may still eat foods such as spinach, kale, cabbage, cauliflower, peas, cereals, and fish; however, they should strive to eat consistent amounts of these foods on a weekly basis. Patients may occasionally be given supplements to improve their nutrition. Although some of these (e.g., Ensure) contain vitamin K, reformulation of these products to decrease the amount of vitamin K has helped minimize the amount of interference with the warfarin response. Changes in consumption of nutritional supplements must be considered when fluctuations in the INR are seen. Some over-the-counter vitamin supplements (e.g., Centrum) contain small amounts of vitamin K, and infrequent or only occasional use must be considered as a possible cause of variability in response to warfarin. Patients should be instructed to avoid these products or to take them all the time.

Conversely, poor nutrition may lead to an increased hypoprothrombinemic response. Fasting or malabsorption may lead to decreased vitamin K absorption and increased warfarin response. Any acute illness that is associated with diarrhea may quickly induce vitamin K deficiency and result in potentiation of warfarin response.

DRUGS. Many drugs may increase or decrease the effect of warfarin. Examples of some drugs that can cause important drug interactions with warfarin are listed in Table 44.10. Despite the relatively small number of drugs that have been well documented to interfere with warfarin, it is necessary to assume that all drugs have the potential for interaction unless proven otherwise.[34,44] An extraordinarily large number of possible interactions have been reported in the literature. With further study, some of the potential interactions may be proven to be clinically relevant.

Table 44.9 ▪ Determinants of Warfarin Response

Diet	Thyroid function
Compliance	Acute illnesses, particularly febrile
Drugs	Hereditary resistance
Liver function	Other

Table 44.10 ▪ Examples of Well-Documented Drug Interactions with Warfarin[a]

Drugs that enhance warfarin effect	*Drugs that decrease warfarin effect*
Amiodarone	Barbiturates
Ciprofloxacin	Cholestyramine
Co-trimoxazole	Nafcillin
Disulfiram	Carbamazepine
Fluconazole	Griseofulvin
Cimetidine	Rifampin
Clofibrate	Vitamin K
Erythromycin	
Metronidazole	
Sulfinpyrazone	

Source: Kayser S. Thromboembolic disease. In: Herfindal ET, Hirshman JL, eds. Clinical pharmacy and therapeutics. 6th ed. Baltimore: Williams & Wilkins, 1996:855.

[a]For further information, see drug interaction texts and primary literature.

LIVER FUNCTION. Because the vitamin K–dependent clotting factors are synthesized in the liver, any disruption of normal liver function may lead to an increased PT, even without warfarin therapy. In the presence of warfarin, this prolongation will be exaggerated.

HYPERMETABOLIC STATES. Fever or hyperthyroidism may result in increased sensitivity to warfarin because of the increased catabolism of the vitamin K–dependent clotting factors. This is the predominant effect, because the kinetics of warfarin appear to be unchanged. The response to warfarin in myxedema is conversely diminished.

HEREDITARY RESISTANCE. A hereditary resistance has been identified in animals and humans. Findings that are consistent with an altered affinity of the receptor for oral anticoagulants or for vitamin K have been reported. This is apparently mediated by a single autosomal gene and is very rare.

OTHER. Many other, less well-documented determinants have been proposed, including climatic changes, smoking, race, age, plasma lipids, congestive heart failure, and renal function.

Adverse Reactions

Hemorrhage, the most important adverse effect of warfarin, is one of the most common reasons for admission to the hospital because of adverse drug reactions. Patients should be informed of the most common sites of bleeding and should look routinely for any signs of bleeding from the gums, nose, throat, skin, gastrointestinal tract, or genitourinary tract.

CUTANEOUS. Warfarin-induced skin necrosis is most likely to be seen in the buttocks, breasts, and thighs. It occurs within the first 10 days of therapy and usually resolves with discontinuation of warfarin but occasionally requires surgical intervention.[32,36] This adverse effect may be due to microvascular thrombosis secondary to protein C deficiency or protein S deficiency. Adequate heparin therapy may help prevent its occurrence in some patients. Other skin lesions that have been reported include urticaria, dermatitis, and the "purple toes" syndrome, a nonhemorrhagic reaction that occurs shortly after initiation of therapy.

TERATOGENIC. Warfarin crosses into the placental circulation and has been reported to cause chondromalacia punctata, or stippling of the bones. Nasal bone deformities have been attributed to maternal consumption of warfarin during the first trimester.[45]

Although heparin does not cross the placenta and may be safer during pregnancy, it is not without maternal risk, and it has also been associated with increased fetal risk.[45]

It appears from limited studies that warfarin does not cross into breast milk.[46]

Drug Interactions

Drugs may interact with warfarin by different mechanisms. Pharmacodynamically, drugs may interfere by antagonizing warfarin at the site of action (e.g., vitamin K) and by altering the synthesis of clotting factors (oral contraceptives), clotting factor catabolism (thyroxine), and the hemostatic process (by inhibiting platelet function). Pharmacokinetically, drugs may interfere with warfarin by altering bioavailability, protein binding, metabolism, and excretion.

It has been proposed for many years that the administration of antibiotics, by suppressing intestinal synthesis of vitamin K by bacteria, would result in enhanced hypoprothrombinemia. It is most likely, however, that dietary sources of vitamin K are more important than the gut production. Nevertheless, patients using antibiotics concurrently with warfarin should have their INR monitored.

Cholestyramine may decrease not only the absorption of warfarin but also the absorption of vitamin K.

Many drugs have been reported to interfere with warfarin absorption, protein binding, and biotransformation. Few drugs actually interact significantly via these mechanisms. Cholestyramine significantly impairs warfarin absorption. The influence of protein displacement should be transient, because the increased free level of drug is metabolized and the levels return to the predisplacement level.

Amiodarone, cimetidine, ciprofloxacin, cotrimoxazole, disulfiram, erythromycin, fluconazole, metronidazole, and sulfinpyrazone most commonly inhibit the metabolism of warfarin, resulting in an enhanced anticoagulant effect. Allopurinol less significantly interferes via this mechanism.

Barbiturates, carbamazepine, griseofulvin, nafcillin, and rifampin reduce the effect of warfarin by increasing its metabolism via induction of microsomal enzymes.[44]

Drugs that affect prothrombin complex concentration may do so by depressing clotting factor synthesis or by increasing the rate of catabolism of clotting factors. Hepatotoxic drugs may potentiate coumarin-induced hypoprothrombinemia by damaging the liver, resulting in decreased synthesis of the vitamin K–dependent clotting factors. Thyroid drugs may increase the response to warfarin secondary to a hypermetabolic state.

Any drug that interferes with hemostasis may increase the risk of therapy with warfarin. Drugs that interfere with platelet function by further impairing hemostasis potentiate the hemorrhagic risk of warfarin and should be avoided. Occasionally, the combination of warfarin with an antiplatelet agent may be useful therapeutically. In these situations, close monitoring is essential.

The selection of a nonsteroidal anti-inflammatory drug (NSAID) is a particularly difficult one because not only may these agents interfere with platelet function and cause gastric irritation, but some (such as phenylbutazone) may interact pharmacokinetically with warfarin as well. Of the available NSAIDs, ibuprofen and naproxen appear to be the safest.

Treatment of Overdose

Excessive hypoprothrombinemia may be reversed with the administration of vitamin K or, if extremely severe, with fresh frozen plasma or whole blood. Prolongation of the PT without evidence of hemorrhage may require no more than withholding further warfarin therapy until the PT returns to the therapeutic range. An alternative approach is to administer small doses of oral vitamin K (e.g., 1 mg or 2.5 mg). This results in a more rapid return to the therapeutic range with little risk of normalization of the PT. If there is evidence of minor bleeding or if the patient is at risk for bleeding, administration of vitamin K is indicated. Vitamin K_1, or phytonadione, is the only vitamin K preparation that should be used, because of its more rapid onset of action. It can be administered intravenously, subcutaneously, or orally; intramuscular administration should be avoided because of the risk of hematoma formation. It should be administered slowly intravenously to prevent cardiorespiratory collapse. Administration of 5 to 10 mg results in a return of the PT to normal in 6 hours after intravenous administration and in 24 hours after oral administration.[47]

Patients who require continued anticoagulation may manifest resistance to subsequent warfarin administration for up to several weeks after vitamin K reversal of warfarin effect.

Management of Surgical Procedures

Patients who are on warfarin or prolonged therapeutic anticoagulation frequently require minor surgical procedures. Therapy may not need to be interrupted for the performance of many minor procedures, and every patient should be evaluated carefully. There are several options for managing these patients. The first is to stop warfarin therapy 4 to 5 days before surgery and use low-dose heparin and warfarin postoperatively for prophylaxis of venous thromboembolism. The second is to stop warfarin therapy 4 to 5 days before surgery and replace it with low-dose heparin therapy (5000 U subcutaneously) or prophylactic dose of LMWH. Postoperatively, low-dose heparin or LMWH and warfarin may be used prophylactically. A third option is to stop warfarin 4 to 5 days before surgery and replace it with full-dose heparin or full-dose LMWH therapy. Another option is to continue warfarin at a lower dose (INR of 1.3 to 1.5) until the day of surgery.[37]

For patients requiring simple dental procedures, tranexamic acid or epsilon amino caproic acid mouthwash may be used without interrupting anticoagulation therapy. The reader is referred to a recent review on managing anticoagulation during dental procedures for a more extensive discussion of this topic.[48]

Fibrinolytic Agents

Fibrinolytic agents play an active role in the dissolution of clots in contrast to heparin and warfarin, which only prevent their occurrence or propagation. Four agents are currently available for clinical use: streptokinase, anistreplase (APSAC), urokinase, and alteplase (rtPA).

These agents activate plasminogen (Fig. 44.3). Urokinase does this by a direct mechanism, streptokinase by first complexing with plasminogen and further activating plasminogen, and alteplase by catalyzing the conversion of plasminogen to plasmin. APSAC is streptokinase bound to plasminogen and protected from subsequent hydrolysis until it is in the bloodstream. Once hydrolyzed, streptokinase is the active agent.

Therapeutic Indications

The use of fibrinolytic agents in the treatment of pulmonary embolism is indicated for the treatment of massive pulmonary embolism without hemodynamic compromise, massive or submassive pulmonary embolism with hemodynamic compromise, anticoagulation treatment failures, submassive pulmonary embolism in patients who cannot tolerate further cardiopulmonary compromise, and extensive proximal venous thrombosis.[49,50]

Fibrinolytic agents should be considered to be contraindicated for patients who have a history of active internal bleeding, a history of cerebrovascular accident or trauma within the last 2 months, known bleeding diathesis, severe uncontrolled hypertension, or any intracranial process such as a neoplasm. Care should be taken, and patients should be evaluated on an individual basis if there is a recent (within 10 days to 2 weeks) history of surgery, organ biopsy, bacterial endocarditis, puncture of noncompressible vessel, pregnancy, minor trauma, acute pericarditis, or severe renal or hepatic disease. There are other conditions in which they may be contraindicated, and the patient must be evaluated to weigh the risks versus the benefits.

Dosing and Administration

Treatment with streptokinase is initiated with a loading dose of 250,000 U administered over 30 minutes, followed by an infusion of 100,000 U per hour for 24 to 72 hours. Urokinase is administered as a loading dose of 4400 U per kilogram over 10 minutes, followed by 4400 U per kilogram per hour for 12 to 24 hours. Tissue plasminogen activator is administered at a dosage of 100 mg over 2 hours. Once thrombolytic therapy has ceased and the thrombin time or APTT has fallen to less than twice the normal values, anticoagulation therapy should be started.[7]

The dose of streptokinase and urokinase for the treatment of deep venous thrombosis is the same as for pulmonary embolism. Treatment should be continued for 72 hours with both agents.

Laboratory Assessment

The hematologic status of the patient should be evaluated before administration of fibrinolytic agents. The thrombin time, PT, APTT, complete blood count, and platelets should be measured. Once it has been established that the patient's baseline coagulation profile is normal, clotting tests are performed to document that a "lytic" state has been achieved. If the thrombin time is prolonged two to five times the normal value, the dosage should not be increased. On the other hand, if there is no prolongation of the thrombin time, especially with streptokinase, one should consider that there is a high concentration of circulating, neutralizing antibodies. This rarely, if ever, occurs with urokinase or alteplase, and they should be used alternatively if there is no response to streptokinase.

Adverse Reactions

The most serious complication following fibrinolytic therapy is hemorrhage, because fibrinolytic agents lyse not only pathologic thrombi but also hemostatic plugs. Despite the reputed greater clot selectivity of rtPA, the incidence of bleeding following use of all agents is similar. Adverse reactions in addition to bleeding include hypotension, allergy, and fever.

Nonpharmacologic Therapy

Nonpharmacologic measures that contribute to the successful prevention or treatment of thromboembolic disease include proper education, use of support garments, and (infrequently) surgery.

Individualized patient education is important in an overall treatment plan. Prevention of stasis by avoiding prolonged sitting, leg crossing, or wearing constricting garments is extremely important. Properly fitted and prescribed elastic stockings and intermittent pneumatic compression devices are also useful. Embolectomy or surgical placement of an inferior vena cava filter (e.g., Greenfield filter) is performed in selected patients.

IMPROVING OUTCOMES

In general, prevention, along with early diagnosis and treatment, is essential to obtaining positive outcomes in the management of venous thrombosis and pulmonary embolism.

Patient Education

Patient education is of special importance during anticoagulation therapy. Topics for patient education include dosing, administration technique, drug and food interactions, monitoring, side effects, indication for therapy, and importance of compliance. Particular attention must be paid to psychosocial factors mentioned earlier in this chapter. Patient education is more effective when the health educator possesses confidence, competence, and good communication skills and is caring.[13]

Methods to Improve Patient Adherence to Drug Therapy

Written, audio, and visual educational materials, dosing calendars, and medication organizers may help improve patient compliance.[51] Involving family members or caregivers in the educational process is often helpful. Self-monitoring of anticoagulation by patients has been proven beneficial as well. Two recent studies have shown that patient self-monitoring can improve accuracy of anticoagulation control and quality of life.[52,53] More studies are needed to determine the effects of self-monitoring on bleeding risk and incidence of thromboembolism.

PHARMACOECONOMICS

LMWHs have been shown to be more cost-effective for the inpatient treatment of venous thromboembolism than UH.[54,55] In a recent economic evaluation, outpatient therapy with LMWHs was shown to be more cost-effective than traditional inpatient-based therapy with UH.[56] Also, there was no difference in clinical outcomes. With regard to quality-of-life assessment, there was a greater improvement in social functioning in the LMWH-treated group when compared with the UH-treated group. Outpatient management with LMWHs requires careful selection of patients. Patients who should be excluded from outpatient management include pregnant women, children, patients with an increased risk of hemorrhage, and those with renal insufficiency.[57]

KEY POINTS

- A venous thrombosis is composed of cellular material that forms in any part of the venous circulation. If left untreated, it may lead to a pulmonary embolus, which is a dislodged thrombus originating from the circulation that impedes blood flow to the lungs.
- Deep vein thrombosis (DVT) and pulmonary embolism (PE) are often clinically silent, making prevention and early detection necessary to achieve optimal patient outcomes.
- Several techniques may be used to diagnose DVT, including ultrasound, impedance plethysmography, and venography. Ventilation/perfusion scanning and pulmonary angiography are used in the diagnosis of PE.
- Treatment goals for DVT include the prevention of pulmonary embolism, prevention of the postphlebitic syndrome, reducing morbidity from the initial event, and achieving positive outcomes with few adverse effects and cost.
- Weight-based nomograms provide guidelines for safe and effective therapy with unfractionated heparin (UH).
- Outpatient use of low-molecular-weight heparin (LMWH) to treat DVT is cost-effective and provides positive clinical and quality-of-life outcomes. Careful patient selection, however, is essential.
- The major complication associated with DVT/PE therapy is bleeding. Careful patient and laboratory monitoring are crucial during therapy.
- The optimal duration of treatment for DVT is not well established. Duration of treatment should be individualized according to risk factors for recurrence of DVT. Generally, however, treatment should last at least 3 months.
- Warfarin has numerous factors, including other drugs, disease, and diet, that affect response to therapy. Careful assessment of these factors and monitoring of the INR is essential.
- Patient education is crucial in achieving positive patient outcomes. This is of particular importance during outpatient therapy.

REFERENCES

1. Hirsh J, Hoak J. Management of deep vein thrombosis and pulmonary embolism: a statement for healthcare professionals. Circulation 93:2212–2245, 1996.
2. Stein PD. Acute pulmonary embolism. Dis Mon 40:467–523, 1994.
3. Weinmann EE, Salzman EW. Deep-vein thrombosis. N Engl J Med 331:1630–1641, 1994.
4. Pearson JD, Lee TH, McCage-Sassan S, et al. Critical pathway to treatment of proximal lower-extremities DVT. Am J Med 100:283–289, 1996.
5. Ansell JE, Buttaro ML, Thomas OV, et al. Consensus guidelines for coordinated outpatient oral anticoagulation therapy management. Ann Pharmacother 31:604–615, 1997.
6. Fifth ACCP consensus conference on antithrombotic therapy. Chest 114:439S–769S, 1998.
7. Hyers TM, Agnelli G, Hull RD, et al. Antithrombotic therapy for venous thromboembolic disease. Chest 114:561S–578S, 1998.
8. Furie B, Furie BC. Molecular and cellular biology of blood coagulation. N Engl J Med 326:800–806, 1992.
9. Clagett GP, Anderson FA, Geerts W, et al. Prevention of venous thromboembolism. Chest 114:531S–560S, 1998.
10. Baker WF, Bick RL. Deep venous thrombosis: diagnosis and management. Med Clin North Am 78:685–712, 1994.
11. Hirsh J. Diagnosis of venous thrombosis and pulmonary embolism. Am J Cardiol 65:45C–49C, 1990.
12. Moser KM. Venous thromboembolism. Am Rev Respir Dis 151:235–249, 1990.
13. Oertel LB. Education curriculum for patients and teaching methods. In: Ansell JE, Oertel LB, Wittkowsky AK, eds. Managing oral anticoagulation therapy: clinical and operational guidelines. Gaithersburg, MD: Aspen, 1999:6A-1.
14. Hirsh J, Dalen JE, Deykin, et al. Heparin: mechanism of action, pharmacokinetics, dosing considerations, monitoring, efficacy, and safety. Chest 102:337S–351S, 1992.
15. Hirsh J, Fuster V. Guide to anticoagulant therapy. Part 1: heparin. Circulation 89:1449–1468, 1994.

16. Hirsh J. Heparin. N Engl J Med 324:1565–1574, 1991.
17. Pineo GF, Hull RD. Classical anticoagulant therapy for venous thromboembolism. Prog Cardiovasc Dis 37:59–70, 1994.
18. Hirsch J, Van Aken WG, Gallus AS, et al. Heparin kinetics in venous thrombosis and pulmonary embolism. Circulation 53:691–695, 1976.
19. Hirsh J, Warkentin TE, Raschke R, et al. Heparin and low-molecular-weight heparin: mechanisms of action, pharmacokinetics, dosing considerations, monitoring, efficacy, and safety. Chest 114:489S–510S, 1998.
20. Hull RD, Raskob GE, Rosenbloom D, et al. Optimal therapeutic levels of heparin therapy in patients with venous thrombosis. Arch Intern Med 152:1589–1595, 1992.
21. Raschke RA, Reilly BM, Guidry JR, et al. The weight-based heparin dosing nomogram compared with a "standard care" nomogram: a randomized controlled trial. Ann Intern Med 119:874–881, 1993.
22. Cruickshank MK, Levine MN, Hirsh J, et al. A standard heparin nomogram for the management of heparin therapy. Arch Intern Med 151:333–337, 1991.
23. Hull Rd, Raskob GE, Rosenbloom D, et al. Optimal therapeutic level of heparin therapy in patients with venous thrombosis. Arch Intern Med 152:1589–1595, 1992.
24. Warkentin TE, Lelton JG. Heparin-induced thrombocytopenia. Prog Hemost Thromb 10:1–34, 1991.
25. Warkentin TE, Levine MN, Hirsh J, et al. Heparin-induced thrombocytopenia in patients treated with low-molecular-weight heparin or unfractionated heparin. N Engl J Med 332:1330–1335, 1995.
26. Becker RC, Corrao JM, Bovill EG, et al. Intravenous nitroglycerin-induced heparin resistance: a qualitative antithrombin III abnormality. Am Heart J 119:1254–1261, 1990.
27. Horrow JC. Protamine: a review of its toxicity. Anesth Analg 64:348–361, 1985.
28. Hovanessian HC. New-generation anticoagulants: the low-molecular-weight heparins. Ann Emerg Med 34:768–779, 1999.
29. Fareed J, Hoppensteadt D, Jeske W, et al. Low-molecular-weight heparins: a developmental perspective. Exp Opin Invest Drugs 6:705–733, 1997.
30. Dunn CJ, Sorkin EM. Dalteparin sodium: a review of its pharmacology and clinical use in the prevention and treatment of thromboembolic disorders. Drugs 52:277–305, 1996.
31. Schiele F, Vuillemenot A, Kramarz P, et al. Use of recombinant hirudin as antithrombotic treatment in patients with heparin-induced thrombocytopenia. Am J Hematol 50:20–25, 1995.
32. Hirsh J. Oral anticoagulant drugs. N Engl J Med 324:1865–1875, 1991.
33. Sheareer MJ. Vitamin K. Lancet 345:229–234, 1995.
34. Hirsh J, Dalen JE, Deykin D, et al. Oral anticoagulants: mechanism of action, clinical effectiveness, and optimal therapeutic range. Chest 102:312S–326S, 1992.
35. Holford NH. Clinical pharmacokinetics and pharmacodynamics of warfarin: understanding the dose-effect relationship. Clin Pharmacokinet 11:483–504, 1986.
36. Hirsh J, Fuster V. Guide to anticoagulant therapy. Part 2: oral anticoagulants. Circulation 89:1469–1479, 1994.
37. Hirsh J, Dalen JE, Anderson DR, et al. Oral anticoagulants: mechanism of action, clinical effectiveness, and optimal therapeutic range. Chest 114:445S–469S, 1998.
38. Hyers TM, Hull RD, Weg JG. Antithrombotic therapy for venous thromboembolic disease. Chest 102:408S–425S, 1992.
39. O'Reilly RA, Aggeler PM. Sutides on coumarin anticoagulant drugs: initiation of therapy without a loading dose. Circulation 38:169–177, 1968.
40. Palareti G, Legnani C, Guazzaloca G, et al. Activation of blood coagulation after abrupt or stepwise withdrawal of oral anticoagulants: a prospective study. Thromb Haemost 72:222–226, 1994.
41. Le DT, Weibert RT, Sevilla BK, et al. The internationalized ratio (INR) for monitoring warfarin therapy: reliability and relation to other monitoring methods. Ann Intern Med 120:552–558, 1994.
42. Hirsh J, Poller L. The international normalized ratio: a guide to understanding and correcting its problems. Arch Intern Med 154:282–288, 1994.
43. O'Reilly RA, Aggeler PM. Determinants of the response to oral anticoagulant drugs in man. Pharmacol Rev 22:35, 1970.
44. Wells PS, Holbrook AM, Crowther NR, et al. Interactions of warfarin with drugs and food. Ann Intern Med 121:676–683, 1994.
45. Hall JG, Pauli RM, Wilson KM, et al. Maternal and fetal sequelae of anticoagulation during pregnancy. Am J Med 68:122–140, 1980.
46. Orme ML, Lewis PJ, DeSwiet MS, et al. May mothers given warfarin breast-feed their infants? Br Med J 1:1564–1565, 1977.
47. Udall J. Don't use the wrong vitamin K. Calif Med 112:65, 1966.
48. Wahl MJ. Dental surgery in anticoagulated patients. Arch Intern Med 158:1610–1616, 1998.
49. Hyers TM, Hull RD, Weg JG. Antithrombotic therapy for venous thromboembolic disease. Chest 108:335S–351S, 1995.
50. Dalen JE, Alpert JS, Hirsh J. Thrombolytic therapy for pulmonary embolism: is it effective? Is it safe? When is it indicated? Arch Intern Med 157:2250–2256, 1997.
51. Carter BL, Jones ME, Waickman LA. Pathophysiology and treatment of deep vein thrombosis and pulmonary embolism. Clin Pharmacokinet 4:279–297, 1985.
52. Sawicki PT. A structured teaching and self-management program for patients receiving oral anticoagulation: a randomized controlled trial. Working group for the study of patient self-management of oral anticoagulation. JAMA 281:145–150, 1999.
53. Kulinna W, Ney D, Wenzel T, et al. The effect of self-monitoring the INR on quality of anticoagulation and quality of life. Semin Thromb Hemost 25:123–126, 1999.
54. Hull RD, Raskob GE, Rosenbloom D, et al. Treatment of proximal vein thrombosis with subcutaneous low-molecular-weight heparin vs intravenous heparin. An economic perspective. Arch Intern Med 157:289–294, 1997.
55. Gould MK, Dembitzer AD, Sanders GD, Garber AM. Low-molecular-weight heparins compared with unfractionated heparin for treatment of acute deep venous thrombosis. A cost-effectiveness analysis. Ann Intern Med 130:789–799, 1999.
56. O'Brien B, Levine M, Willan A, et al. Economic evaluation of outpatient treatment with low-molecular-weight heparin for proximal vein thrombosis. Arch Intern Med 159:2298–2304, 1999.
57. Lindmarker P. Can all patients with deep vein thrombosis receive low-molecular-weight heparin in an outpatient setting? Haemostasis Suppl S1:84–88, 1999.

CHAPTER 45

ALLERGIC AND DRUG-INDUCED SKIN DISEASE

Ann B. Amerson

Allergic and drug-induced skin diseases encompass a wide variety of conditions, both acute and chronic, with varying morphology. The most commonly encountered allergic skin diseases are atopic dermatitis, contact dermatitis, and urticaria. In addition, ingestion of a number of drugs can produce varied dermatologic reactions. A brief review of skin structure and function is provided as a basis for the discussion of the individual conditions. The etiology, pathogenesis, therapeutic interventions, and management of each condition will be discussed. A glossary of common skin manifestations is included in Table 45.1.

OVERVIEW

Skin Structure and Function

The skin, the largest organ of the body, is divided into three (main) distinct layers, the epidermis, the dermis, and the hypodermis (subcutaneous tissue), as indicated in Figure 45.1.[1,2] The epidermis is nonvascular and consists of stratified squamous epithelial cells, which are of two distinct types, keratinocytes and dendritic cells.[2] The dendritic cells are further classified into three types: melanocytes, Langerhans cells, and indeterminate dendritic cells. The epidermis consists of five distinct layers from inside out:

1. stratum germinativum (basal)
2. stratum spinosum (prickle)
3. stratum granulosum (granular)
4. stratum lucidum (lucid)
5. stratum corneum (horny)

The keratinocytes are located in the basal layer and serve as stem cells, which differentiate into other cells in the upper layers of the epidermis. As the keratinocytes migrate toward the surface, they undergo gradual transformation from living cells to dead, thick-walled flat cells that contain

Table 45.1 ▪ Glossary of Common Skin Manifestations

Acanthosis	Increased thickness of the prickle layer of the skin.
Angioedema	An allergic skin disease characterized by patches of circumscribed swelling involving the skin and its subcutaneous layers, the mucous membranes, and sometimes the viscera. Also called angioneurotic edema, giant urticaria.
Bullae	Large vesicles or blisters.
Dermographism	Pressure or friction on the skin gives rise to a transient, raised, usually reddish mark, sometimes white, so that a word traced on the skin becomes visible.
Desquamation	Peeling of skin in the form of scales.
Eczema	Inflammation of the skin characterized by redness, itching, and oozing vesicular lesions that become scaly, crusted, or hardened.
Erythema	Abnormal redness of the skin due to capillary congestion.
Exanthem	An eruptive disease (as measles) or its (exanthematous) symptomatic eruption.
Excoriation	A raw irritated lesion; the act of abrading or wearing off the skin.
Exfoliation	The peeling of the horny layer of the (exfoliative) skin.
Hyperkeratosis	An overgrowth of the horny layer of the epidermis.
Lichenoid	Resembling lichen, which is characterized by the eruption of flat papules.
Macule	A patch of skin that is altered in color but usually not elevated.
Maculopapular	Combining the characteristics of macules and papules.
Morbilliform	Resembling the eruption of measles.
Papule	A small, solid, usually conical elevation of the skin caused by inflammation, accumulated secretion, or hypertrophy of tissue elements.
Plaque	A localized abnormal patch on a body part or surface and especially on the skin.
Pruritus	Localized or generalized itching due to irritation of sensory nerve endings from organic or psychogenic causes.
Urticaria	An allergic disorder marked by raised edematous patches (wheals) of skin or mucous membrane and usually intense itching. Also called hives.
Vesicle	A small abnormal elevation of the outer layer of skin enclosing a watery liquid; blister.
Wheal	Temporary, small, raised area of the skin usually accompanied by itching or burning.

keratin. The basal layer also contains melanocytes, which are the pigment-forming cells.[1,2]

The prickle layer also contains both keratinocytes and melanocytes. The layer is so named because of the cytoplasmic threads called prickles that appear prominently in this layer. The granular layer consists of several thicknesses of flattened cells with protein granules containing keratohyaline. These granules are changed to keratin, a fibrous substance in the outermost layers.

The lucid layer, which appears as a translucent line, is present only in thicker skin such as on the palms and soles. The outermost horny layer or the stratum corneum consists of flat, scaly, dead tissue layers, which are constantly shedding. The horny layer is the dead endproduct while the other four layers are considered the living epidermis. A continual process occurs throughout the sublayers of the epidermis in that new cells from the lower layers push older cells toward the top where they eventually become filled with keratin and die. The epidermis under normal conditions can replicate itself in 3 to 4 weeks.

The dermis or corium consists of connective tissue, cellular elements, and ground substance with a rich blood and nerve supply. The sebaceous glands and shorter hair follicles originate in the dermis, which can be divided into two distinct sublayers, the papillary and reticular units. The papillary layer is adjacent to the epidermis and has a rich supply of blood vessels. The reticular sublayer contains coarser tissue, which connects the dermis and subcutaneous tissue (hypodermis).

The connective tissue of the dermis is composed of collagen fibers, elastic fibers, and reticular fibers, which provide support for and elasticity of the skin. The cellular

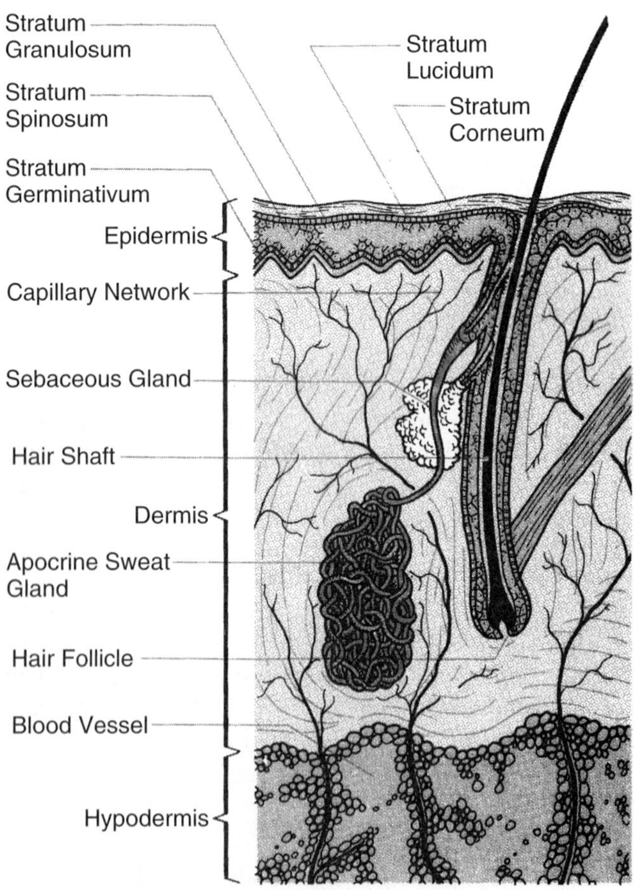

Figure 45.1. Cross section of human skin. (Reprinted from Dermatologic products. Handbook of nonprescription drugs, 11th ed. Washington DC: American Pharmaceutical Association, 1996:538, with permission.)

elements consist of three types of mesodermal cell groups: reticulohistocytes, myeloid, and lymphoid. The reticulohistocyte group consists of fibroblasts, histiocytes, and mast cells with immature cells called reticulum cells. Intracytoplasmic granules containing heparin and histamine are present in mast cells. These cells, normally few in number, are increased in itching dermatoses, such as contact or atopic dermatitis. Histiocytes normally are present in small numbers around blood vessels. In pathologic conditions they migrate in the dermis as monocytes. They may phagocytize bacteria and particulate matter and then are known as macrophages. Fibroblasts form collagen fibers and may serve as precursors for the other connective tissue cells. Polymorphonuclear leukocytes and eosinophils, members of the myeloid group, are common in dermatoses, particularly where an allergic component is involved. Lymphocytes from the lymphoid group are common in inflammatory lesions of the skin.[1,2]

The hypodermis is composed of relatively loose connective tissue. This layer provides pliability to the skin and its thickness varies. In most areas, it contains a unit for formation and storage of fat. The fat layer functions in thermal control, food reserve, and cushioning. The hypodermis supports the blood vessels and nerves that pass from tissues beneath to the dermis. Deeper hair follicles and sweat glands originate in the hypodermis.[1,2]

The skin confines underlying tissue and provides a barrier between the body and environment. It prevents harm from external agents such as ultraviolet radiation, pathogenic organisms, and chemicals. Various factors can alter the effectiveness of the barrier including age, underlying disease states, use of medications (topical or systemic), and integrity of the stratum corneum. Other skin functions involve sensation, temperature control, development of pigment, and synthesis of some vitamins. Moisture regulation is another important function.[1]

Skin appendages are of two types, cornified and glandular.[1,2] Cornified appendages are hair and nails. Glandular appendages are the sebaceous glands and sweat glands, both eccrine and apocrine. Because these appendages are not usually involved in allergic and drug-induced disease, they will not be discussed further.

Nonimmunologic Mechanisms

Although many of the conditions discussed in this chapter are believed to result from allergy, nonimmunologic mechanisms also are postulated to play a role.[3,4] For example, contact dermatitis may be caused through immunologic mechanisms or may result from direct irritant properties. The clinical presentations are essentially identical.[4]

The basic immunologic mechanisms of allergic reactions include four types.[5] Immediate or anaphylactic reactions (type I) result from the production of immunoglobulin (Ig) E antibodies that attach to the surface of basophils or mast cells. With reexposure, the offending substance binds to the antibodies on the cell surface causing release of chemical mediators. These substances may include histamine, serotonin, peptides, leukotrienes, and prostaglandins.[5,6] The clinical effects seen are determined by the interaction of the mediators with the various target organs and may include pruritus, urticaria, bronchospasm, laryngeal edema, and hypotension.

Type II reactions result in antibody-dependent cytotoxicity. The offending substance interacts with surface components of a cell, thus making it appear foreign. Antibodies are produced, which react with the cell-bound substance. The antigen-antibody reaction may trigger the complement system or permit attack by mononuclear killer cells, resulting in cell death as with drug-induced hemolysis.[5]

Type III reactions involve immune complexes. The antigen-antibody complex forms in blood or tissue spaces. IgG or IgM antibodies are usually involved.[6] Inflammation or complement activation may result if these complexes deposit on blood vessel walls or basement membranes. Serum sickness and allergic arteritis are examples of type III reactions.[5]

Type IV reactions are classified as cell-mediated, delayed, or tuberculin type reactions. The offending substance interacts with skin proteins evoking a cell-mediated immune response. Sensitized T lymphocytes release cytokines and lymphokines in response, which cause local edema and inflammation.[5]

Type I (immediate or anaphylactic) and type IV (cell-mediated) reactions are most commonly involved in allergic skin manifestations. In some cases, skin manifestations may occur from circulating immune complexes (type III: serum sickness). Type II reactions (antibody-dependent cytotoxicity) are unlikely to produce cutaneous manifestations.[5,6] In some instances, drug-induced urticaria is an example of a type I reaction, and allergic contact dermatitis is an example of a reaction type IV.

The role of immunologic mechanisms in drug-associated rash is supported by certain clinical features described by Bigby et al.[3] The reaction

1. Occurs in a small percentage of patients.
2. Is not dose-dependent.
3. (Onset of rash) occurs within 1 to 2 weeks after initiation of therapy.
4. Is accompanied by other signs and symptoms, e.g. fever, pruritus, or eosinophilia.
5. Resolves upon withdrawal of agent and recurs if rechallenge is initiated.

The immunologic mechanisms involved will be discussed and the role of nonimmunologic mechanisms for each condition will be identified.

TREATMENT GOALS: ALLERGIC AND DRUG-INDUCED SKIN DISEASE

- Identify and remove the cause of the reaction when possible or eliminate exacerbating factors (atopic dermatitis).
- Identify whether the stage is acute or chronic and then treat symptomatically.

- Use nonfluorinated or low-potency fluorinated topical steroids in conditions needing long-term therapy.
- Use high-potency fluorinated topical steroids for short-term treatment during acute phases.
- Reserve systemic steroids for acute, severe cases with extensive involvement but do not use for longer than 5 to 14 days.
- Relieve symptoms with the use of antihistamines (if histamine is believed to be part of the etiology of the skin problem).
- Treat dry skin with baths and lubricating lotions (atopic dermatitis particularly).
- Educate patients on the proper use of topical measures in treating their condition.
- Educate patients on issues related to their condition to prevent recurrence.

Atopic Dermatitis

DEFINITION

Atopic dermatitis, frequently referred to as eczema, is a chronic pruritic skin disorder that most commonly occurs in persons with a personal or family history of allergic diseases, such as rhinitis, asthma, or conjunctivitis.[7–10]

TREATMENT GOALS: ATOPIC DERMATITIS

- Decrease skin inflammation.
- Eliminate exacerbating factor(s).
- Relieve itch and dry skin.

EPIDEMIOLOGY

Prevalence

The disorder occurs in infants, children, and adults, with an onset usually before 5 years of age. The prevalence is higher in children (3 to 4% in the 1960s compared to 10% or more in the 1990s).[9,10] Estimated cumulative incidence is 10 to 15% in children up to 14 years of age, and the incidence seems to be increasing.[7,9] Heredity plays a role with a possible inherited defect in some bone marrow derived cells.[7,9]

Etiology

The exact cause of atopic dermatitis is unknown. Abnormalities in both immunologic and pharmacophysiologic characteristics occur.[7,8] Several factors support the involvement of immunologic functions: (1) the frequent association of atopic dermatitis with other allergic disorders; (2) substantial elevations of serum IgE; (3) positive wheal and flare reactions to a wide variety of scratch tests; (4) increased susceptibility to bacterial, viral, and fungal infections; and (5) association with immunodeficiency disorders. Pharmacophysiologic abnormalities include evidence of altered adrenergic and cholinergic responses.[7–9]

PATHOPHYSIOLOGY

Immunologic mechanisms receive the most investigation, but the primary event that initiates the reaction is yet to be identified.[7–10] Abnormalities of both humoral and cell-mediated immunity are present. Two of the most important immunologic alterations identified are an impairment of the delayed hypersensitivity response and an increased production of IgE. Identification of cytokines (interferons and interleukins) has allowed further delineation of possible mechanisms and development of possible new treatment strategies. For example, evidence indicates that the mononuclear leukocytes in patients with atopic dermatitis produce lower levels of interferon-γ (IFN-γ) and higher levels of interleukin (IL) 4. IFN-γ mediates delayed hypersensitivity reactions and IL-4 stimulates IgE synthesis.[8] Other interleukins (IL-5, IL-13) also may be involved.[10] IgE apparently is stimulated by specific antigens, attaches to mast cells, and triggers release of mast cell inflammatory mediators (including histamine) that are released upon reexposure to the antigens.[7,8] Other factors, however, must play a role because atopic dermatitis occurs in patients with a deficiency of immunoglobulins, e.g., agammaglobulinemia or Weskott-Aldrich syndrome.

Evidence of cell-mediated factors relates to susceptibility and recurrence of viral infections including herpes simplex, molluscum contagiosum, and warts.[7–9] Patients are frequently resistant to sensitization to poison ivy and dinitrochlorobenzene.[9] The demonstration of decreased numbers of T lymphocytes may indicate lack of sufficient T cells to control B-cell production of immunoglobulin; thus, high levels of IgE are produced.[7,8] In addition, phagocytic capacity is decreased, and chemotaxis of neutrophils and monocytes is impaired.[9]

Another factor supporting an immunologic basis is the demonstration of significant numbers of *S. aureus* bacteria on both the diseased and normal skin of atopic patients.[8,9] Exacerbations of eczema have developed secondary to *S. aureus* skin infections.[9]

Pharmacophysiologic responses in atopic patients involve a number of abnormal cutaneous responses. An exaggerated constrictor response of cutaneous vessels, white dermographism (a white line is produced when the skin is stroked), delayed blanch to cholinergic stimuli, and paradoxical response to application of nicotinic acid are examples.[9] A defect in the β-adrenergic receptor was once theorized when it was demonstrated that cyclic adenosine monophosphate (AMP) responses in atopic patients were subnormal to isoproterenol, prostaglandin E_1, and histamine agents that would normally activate cyclic AMP.[7–9] Decreased cyclic AMP levels have accentuated release of inflammatory mediators from mast cells and basophils.[7] Evidence suggests cyclic AMP phosphodiesterase activity (responsible for degradation of cyclic AMP) is increased accounting for cyclic AMP diminished responsiveness upon challenge. This enzymatic abnormality might be a primary defect in patients with atopic dermatitis and is not dependent on the β-receptor. Chan and Hanifen[8] have reviewed the extensive work in this area, but further study is necessary to unravel the puzzle of atopic dermatitis.

CLINICAL PRESENTATION AND DIAGNOSIS

The diagnostic hallmark is pruritus, often accompanied by erythema and dry skin. The cutaneous features vary greatly depending on age and chronicity of disease. Environmental factors called flare factors that may induce or exacerbate atopic dermatitis are listed in Table 45.2. Laboratory tests and histologic analysis of biopsy do not provide confirmatory information, although an estimated 85% of patients have elevated IgE levels and positive immediate skin tests to foods and inhalant allergens.[7,8] Conditions that should be considered in the differential diagnosis include seborrheic dermatitis, contact dermatitis, nummular dermatitis, scabies, and psoriasis.[7]

A strong relationship exists between food allergy and atopic disease, primarily in children.[7,10] Inhalant allergens, e.g., dust mites, seem to be more of a factor for adults. Foods can exacerbate the dermatitis with evidence that elimination of food allergens results in improvement. The types of foods most commonly involved include eggs, peanuts, milk, soy, wheat, and fish.[7,10]

In infants, atopic dermatitis is most likely to occur around 3 months of age. The eruption generally begins as erythematous patches on the cheeks and spreads to the extensor surfaces of the extremities. The diaper area is usually spared. Intense itching is evident as the infant scratches constantly and rubs against garments and bedding. Many infantile cases resolve over a period of months to years. Some cases continue into childhood or may recur years after resolution of the infantile form.

In children, the flexor surfaces as well as neck, wrists, and ankles are usually involved rather than extensor areas. The eruption is usually either lichenoid consisting of small, discrete, brown or red-brown papules or papular, consisting of larger papules with a central crust. Such lesions tend to be chronic, may disappear around the age of 10 to 12, or may continue into adolescence.[7,9]

In adolescents and adults, papules tend to become confluent forming large lichenified areas. Crusts result from scratching due to intense itching. The lichenoid plaques are poorly marginated and vary in color from bright pink-red to brown or gray-brown. Areas commonly involved are the neck, eyelids, forehead/scalp, anterior chest and wrists. Dorsal areas of the fingers, toes and feet may be affected as well.[7]

The course of atopic dermatitis is quite variable and generally is marked by remissions and exacerbations.[7,9] Most cases begin in infancy but onset may not occur until childhood or after puberty. The reported frequency of persistence varies widely, from 10 to 83%.[9] Part of the variability can be explained by the imprecise diagnostic criteria available. Some factors that suggest an unfavorable prognosis are severe, widespread dermatitis in childhood, a family history of atopic disease, the presence of allergic rhinitis and/or asthma, female sex, and early age of onset (<1 year of age).[9]

Table 45.2 ▪ Flare Factors in Atopic Dermatitis

Dry skin (xerosis)	Heat
Sweating	Cold
Exercise	Temperature change
Infection	Allergic contact dermatitis
Anxiety	Allergies to foods or inhalants
Scratching	Coexisting diseases (e.g., scabies)
Light touch	Greasy ointments
Prickly clothes (wool and acrylic)	

THERAPEUTIC PLAN

Strategies involve a variety of nondrug and drug treatment measures depending on the acuteness or chronicity of the condition. The most common measures include environmental change, skin maintenance care techniques, use of topical corticosteroids, systemic antihistamines, topical or systemic antibiotics, and, selectively, systemic corticosteroids. As noted above, the therapeutic goals are to decrease skin inflammation, to eliminate exacerbating factor(s), and to relieve itch and dry skin.

If environmental factors are identified as contributory, avoidance is advised. This might include avoiding extremes of temperature and humidity, strenuous exercise, rough scratchy clothing, and bathing with harsh soaps and hot water, irritant chemicals, and allergens.[7,10] These factors and others can precipitate or perpetuate the itch-scratch cycle. Stress, anger, or anxiety may contribute to exacerbations of atopic dermatitis in some patients.

Patients often complain of dry skin and pruritus. Topical and systemic therapies are focused on relieving these symptoms, reducing inflammation, and rehydrating the skin.

TREATMENT

Topical Therapy

Several forms of topical therapy are available. Patients with mild or localized atopic dermatitis may require only treatment with a topical corticosteroid ointment or cream. For patients with extensive disease, a combination of topical measures may be necessary.

Baths

Itching can be relieved at least temporarily by tepid baths (showers are less effective). Oatmeal (Aveeno, plain or oilated), bath oils, or tar preparations may be added. Bathing also assists with rehydration of the skin. Using hot water and scrubbing with a washcloth or brush cause irritation and strong soaps should be avoided although mild soaps can be used. A lubricating lotion (Cetaphil, Lubriderm, or Nutraderm) can be used for cleansing instead of soap. To aid dry skin, soaking in lukewarm water then applying a water-in-oil emulsion (e.g., Eucerin) while the skin is still wet assists in rehydrating the keratin layers.[10,11]

Wet Dressings

When lesions are oozing, acute, and possibly infected, the use of wet dressings such as Burow's solution 1:20 or tap water is appropriate. Compresses are applied generally for 20 to 60 minutes three to six times a day. The dressings cool and dry by evaporation, thus stimulating vasoconstriction. In very acute situations, compresses can be applied continuously.

Topical Corticosteroids

These agents are effective in treating many cases of atopic dermatitis. In an acute phase, high-potency topical steroids can be used for 7 to 10 days. Therapy should then be switched to less potent products for up to several more weeks.[10,11] Patients with severe conditions may require chronic use along with lubricants. Nonfluorinated (hydrocortisone 1% or desonide 0.05%) or low-potency fluorinated preparations (triamcinolone 0.025%) are preferred for long-term use.[10,11] Use of fluorinated corticosteroids should be minimized by application only during acute flare reactions, by application only to the most problematic areas, or by once daily or alternate day application. Long-term use of fluorinated corticosteroids, particularly high-potency agents, causes thinning of the skin and can lead to atrophy and telangiectasia particularly on the face and skinfold areas (groin and armpits).[10,11]

Creams or ointments can be used and are best applied within a few minutes after bathing. Patient preference and/or environmental conditions may influence choice. Ointments are most often a better emollient for the dry skin but in a hot, humid region, the ointment may feel occlusive.[12]

Topical Antibacterial Agents

Secondary infection frequently due to *S. aureus* can be treated with topical antibiotics if the skin involvement is somewhat limited.[10,11] Preparations containing erythromycin or bacitracin are preferred because of less sensitization than with agents such as neomycin. Mupirocin is another agent shown to be effective, but the relative cost of various agents should be evaluated.

"Wet" and "dry" methods have been suggested, combining some of the topical approaches.[7] The wet or lubricating method includes the following: short baths or showers in tepid water (hot water stimulates pruritus). Mild soaps can be used but sparingly. After bathing, the skin is lubricated while still wet to help hold water in the stratum corneum. Bath oil, petrolatum, hydrophobic ointment, or topical corticosteroids may be used.[10]

The dry method uses either short showers in tepid water or short baths with oilated oatmeal. Bathing with soap and water is not allowed except for use of a moist cloth to cleanse the arms, groin, and axillae. A nonlipid cleanser is applied to the skin surface twice a day and is gently wiped off. Oily or greasy lubricants are not used. Topical corticosteroids can be applied using products that are in a water/propylene glycol emollient base (Synalar solution).[7] Obviously with either method, a great deal of patient effort and cooperation is necessary.

Systemic Therapy

Agents such as antihistamines, corticosteroids, and antibiotics may be useful under certain circumstances. Two possible benefits from oral administration of antihistamines include relief of pruritus and sedation. Histamine plays some role in atopic dermatitis but probably is not the only mediator involved in pruritus.[1] Mixed opinions exist on the benefits of antihistamines in relieving pruritus.[7,10,11,13] Studies show conflicting results and often have included insufficient numbers of patients.[13] Use of antihistamines may relieve pruritus in some patients[7,13] at least initially,[11] but sedation is seen as the primary benefit by some investigators.[11,12] If sedation is the desired goal, then patients should benefit more from the traditional H_1-blockers.[12]

Oral corticosteroids may be used for acute flare reactions to break the itch-scratch cycle.[10,11] Duration of use should be short term, in the range of 5 to 7 days. Oral corticosteroid therapy generally is discouraged except for refractory episodes.

Systemic antibiotic therapy may be indicated to treat secondary bacterial infections (e.g., folliculitis) that can develop.[10,11] Therapy is directed toward Gram-positive cocci particularly *S. aureus*. A 7-day course of an antistaphylococcal agent (e.g., dicloxacillin, erythromycin, or cephalexin) often is used.[10]

Many patients with atopic dermatitis continue to suffer and may be told by their dermatologists that little more can be done. In patients who are suffering despite state-of-the-art therapies, the first step is to break the cycle of scratching. To help achieve this goal, one approach is a major intervention of a "simulated hospitalization."[14] That is, the patient is required to stop the usual routine of school or work, to have complete bed rest in a semidarkened room for a few days (e.g. Friday PM to Monday AM), and to be given light sedation and a short course (1 week or less) of an oral corticosteroid to reduce inflammation. In addition, if the patient has folliculitis, a course of antibiotics is given.

After these few days of intense therapy to break the cycle of scratching, the major challenge is to keep the skin clear by eliminating the urge to scratch. If the worst scratching occurs during sleep, a higher dose of a sedating antihistamine may be adequate. For instance, if diphenhydramine 25mg is not adequate, try 50 mg or if hydroxyzine 25mg is not adequate, try 50 mg or higher if needed. If sedating antihistamines are not sufficient, other sedating therapies may be considered for a few days or weeks in the most severe cases where quality of life is being affected to a great degree.

Concurrently with a major intervention with medication, another critically important step should be initiated. That intervention involves dealing with the psychology of atopic dermatitis. Details regarding the techniques used to stop scratching are beyond the scope of this chapter. Some options reported[11,14] are as follows:

- "Habit reversal" (scratching can become a habit!)
- Behavioral and cognitive interventions
- Relaxation training
- Learning to express anger and to be assertive

Clearly, emotional stress is a major trigger to scratching in some patients with atopic dermatitis. In children, hostility from a parent or discord between parents can trigger the itch-scratch cycle. Dealing with these factors can obviously be very helpful.

Scratching in some patients remains refractory to these treatments and their various combinations. Other therapies being evaluated in atopic dermatitis include phototherapy with ultraviolet (UV) radiation and agents affecting the immune system (e.g., cyclosporine, thymopentin, and interferon-γ).[10,11,15,16]

Both pruritus and inflammation may be aided by phototherapy with ultraviolet light in all wavelengths (bands A and B).[10,11,15] Studies have shown benefit with UVA, UVB, or combinations of the two wavelengths. Combining oral psoralen with UVA radiation (PUVA) is another option, but response may be slow (up to 2 months). Potential risks with long-term use include accelerated photoaging and increased risk of skin cancer.[10,15] This therapy may be best used short term during periods of severe dermatitis as it is also expensive.

Cyclosporine inhibits T-lymphocyte-dependent immune responses and downregulates cytokine production. Oral cyclosporine in doses of 2.5 to 6.0 mg/kg/day (5.0 mg/kg/day most common) has provided benefit to patients with atopic dermatitis. Improvement usually occurs within 1 to 2 weeks with some continuing improvement over a 6- to 8-week period. Discontinuation results in relapse in a high percentage of patients (50 to 75%). Reduced maintenance doses, ranging from 0.5 to 2 mg/kg/day or 5 mg/kg given every 5 days, have been used successfully in maintaining response.[15] Hypertension, nephrotoxicity, and serious drug interactions are concerns with long-term use.[7,10,15,16] A topical preparation of cyclosporine has been evaluated with mixed results.[10,15] One trial found decreased severity after 2 weeks of treatment with a 10% cyclosporine gel.[16]

Tacrolimus (an inhibitor of T-lymphocyte proliferation) has been used systemically and topically. Most data concern the topical form. A 0.01% tacrolimus ointment results in diminished pruritus within 3 days. Additional study of this approach is needed.[15]

Other investigational approaches involve immunomodulation with cytokines that include IFNs and ILs. Daily subcutaneous injections of IFN-γ (50 to 100 μg) for 12 weeks resulted in more than 50% improvement in 45 to 66% of patients studied. Relief of pruritus occurred in some patients within 2 to 4 days. Relapse within 4 to 7 days occurs in some patients after discontinuation of therapy.[7,8,15] Side effects with this therapy include flu-like symptoms (fever, chills, headache, and myalgia) that respond well to acetaminophen. Leukopenia and thrombocytopenia have been reported but are uncommon. Eosinophil counts are reduced although no significant change occurred in serum IgE levels.

IL-2 has received limited study but did show benefit in one group of six patients with severe disease. Relapse occurred 4 to 6 weeks after discontinuation of therapy. Serum IgE levels were unaffected.[15]

Thymopentin, a synthetic pentapeptide derived from thymic hormone thymopoietin, enhances production of cytokines such as IL-2 and IFN-γ. This agent was used to treat several groups of patients with atopic dermatitis. Doses (50 mg) administered intramuscularly or subcutaneously result in clinical improvement but relapse occurs.[7,15]

Contact Dermatitis

DEFINITION

Contact dermatitis is an inflammatory response of the skin and is divided into two categories based on origin: allergic and irritant. Allergic contact dermatitis is a delayed hypersensitivity reaction with an immunologic basis while irritant contact dermatitis results when a substance has a toxic effect on tissue with no immunologic basis.[4,17]

EPIDEMIOLOGY

Prevalence

The occurrence of contact dermatitis is widespread partly due to the wide variety of substances implicated as causes. (Table 45.3). The prevalence within the general population is not well documented. Some studies have attempted to determine the prevalence of allergy to specific substances

Table 45.3 ▪ Common Causes of Contact Dermatitis

Pharmaceutical agents	Occupational Contactants
Corticosteroids	Chrome
Neomycin	Epoxy glues
"Caine" Anesthetics	Other glues
Merbromin	Formaldehyde
Thimerosal	Nickel
Transdermal Patches	Cobalt
Lubricants	Solvents
Lotions	Resins
Hand creams	Dyes
Face creams	Oils and greases
Bath oils	Solvents and Waterless Cleaners
Cosmetics and Fragrances	Metals
Deodorants	Jewelry
Hair dyes	Surfactants
Make-up	Hand, bath, and shower soaps
Perfumes	Soaps used at work
Rubber Materials	Kitchen and laundry soaps
Gloves	Waterless cleaners
Finger protectors	Plants
Hobby Materials	Poison oak/ivy
Epoxy glues	Algerian ivy
Paints	Chrysanthemums
Solvents	House plants

Source: References 17–19.

in the normal population and positive patch tests have occurred in the following percentages: nickel (5.8%), neomycin (1.1%), ethylenediamine (0.43%), and benzocaine (0.17%).[18] Sex differences are observed for specific allergies. For example, nickel allergy is more frequent in women than in men but this is probably explained by a higher rate of contact through jewelry and clothing.[18] Irritant contact dermatitis accounts for about 80% of the reactions with allergic contact dermatitis responsible for about 20%.[10,19]

Etiology

Causes of allergic contact dermatitis are varied and commonly include metallic salts, plants, rubber compounds (latex), and cosmetics containing preservatives and fragrances.[17,19] Soaps, detergents, petrolatum solvents, acids, and alkalis are frequent offenders in irritant contact dermatitis. Often the dermatitis is related to occupational exposure.[19] The origin, allergic or irritant, usually cannot be differentiated by the clinical presentation.[10,19,20] Irritants may also be allergens.[18]

PATHOPHYSIOLOGY

Allergic contact dermatitis represents a typical delayed hypersensitivity reaction that requires the following:[4]

1. Penetration of the stratum corneum by the allergen
2. Interaction with epidermal or dermal cells
3. Interaction with the immune system
4. Activation of the inflammatory response

Sensitizing agents (haptens) are usually low molecular weight, lipid soluble, and highly reactive.[10] The hapten combines with Langerhans cells that process it and then migrate to regional lymph nodes. The processed hapten interacts with T cells with resulting activation of both the Langerhans cells and T cells. Langerhans cells secrete IL-1 that stimulates the T cells to secrete IL-2. Specific T cells capable of interacting with the antigen proliferate, completing the sensitization phase. A period of 8 to 10 days is generally required for allergy presentation once sensitization has begun.[18]

In the elicitation phase, the T cells then circulate and penetrate into skin. When the skin is exposed to the hapten again, interaction occurs initially with Langerhans cells. The processed hapten interacts with the antigen-specific T cells located in the skin. IL-1 and IL-2 are secreted with further production of antigen specific T cells. The activated T cells also secrete cytokines, INF-γ and tumor necrosis factor B. The former activates the keratinocytes in the skin and starts a complex cascade of interaction with leukocytes and secretion of other cytokines (IL-1, IL-6, and granulocyte–macrophage stimulating factor). Mast cells and macrophages are activated by release of eicosanoids from keratinocytes. The result is the classic inflammatory response.

The histopathologic features include perivascular infiltrates of lymphocytes and monocytes in the upper dermis. Edema is usually present and may involve intracellular and intercellular edema in the epidermis with a condition called spongiosis. Basophils and mast cells are present in the cellular infiltrate and may participate in the inflammatory reaction. Chronically, hyperkeratosis, acanthosis, and a cellular infiltrate in the superficial dermis containing basophils are present.[17]

History-wise, patients may report no problem associated with the previous handling of a material sometimes for prolonged periods (years). The latest exposure results in an eruption, which is called the elicitation dose.[20] An earlier exposure resulted in the initial sensitization. Generally a latent period can be identified.

In the case of irritant contact dermatitis, direct cellular damage occurs with no latent period. Damage is proportional to the toxic properties of the irritant, but may depend on repeated exposure for some substances that are mild irritants. With irritant contact dermatitis, those exposed to the same dose under the same conditions for the same length of time would be expected to react. Reduction of the irritant dose (exposure) often has a good prognosis.[19]

CLINICAL PRESENTATION AND DIAGNOSIS

Contact dermatitis is classified as acute, subacute, or chronic.[10,18] Acute contact dermatitis involves erythema, edema, and formation of papules and vesicles and bullae. The subacute form presents with erythema, tiny superficial vesicles, and less severe symptomatology. In chronic forms, the skin may be cracked and scaly with excoriations and plaque formations.[10,20] Severe itching in the acute phase is prominent and may persist into the other phases. The history and physical examination can provide critical information to establish the diagnosis. An acute dermatitis of the extremities that is of a patchy and streaky nature, coupled with a recent history of outdoor plant exposure, might lead to a diagnosis of poison ivy/oak dermatitis. A dermatitis occurring on the eyelids or face of a woman might be associated with the use of cosmetics, perfumes, or hair sprays. A careful and thorough history regarding general activities, occupation, hobbies, known allergies or previous skin disorders, and family history, along with careful examination of the distribution and extent of the lesions, may suggest possible causes.[10] A listing of common causes of contact dermatitis is provided in Table 45.3, and the substances most likely involved with reactions in certain body areas are indicated in Table 45.4. In many patients, the diagnosis remains unclear, and patch testing may be indicated, particularly for conditions that become chronic or relatively resistant to treatment or that are suspected to be occupationally related.

Table 45.4 ▪ Causes of Contact Dermatitis by Body Region

Scalp	Hair dyes (paraphenylenediamine, a permanent dye), hair lotions, permanents (glyceryl thioglycolate), nickel in hair pins, wig attachments/adhesives
Face	Cosmetics, topical medicaments, plants, preshave and aftershave lotions, airborne allergens
Forehead	Hatbands, any hair products
Eyes	Eyelids affected by cosmetics, face creams, lubricants, hair spray, nail polish; conjunctivitis, thimerosal
Lips and perioral areas	Lipstick, lip protectants, toothpastes, mouthwashes, mangos
Ears	Nickel (earrings), perfume, earplugs, earphones, telephone receiver
Neck	Perfume, nickel (necklace), hair cosmetics, clothing; clothing labels, buttons and zippers
Armpits	Deodorants, depilatories, clothing, perfumes
Hands	Materials encountered at work and/or home, e.g., foods, chemicals, topical medicaments, hand lotions and lubricants, rubber gloves, rubber bands, jewelry, plants
Body (trunk, chest, waist)	Dyes, formaldehyde (fabric finisher), resins, rubber in elastic of clothing, perfumes, scarves
Genitalia	Bubble bath, antiseptic cleansers, condoms, contraceptive creams or jellies, deodorant douches, scented menstrual pads or tampons
Feet	Shoes, shower sandals, fabrics, metal eye holes, sole inserts, adhesives, colorants, athlete's foot remedies

Source: Reference 18.

Patch testing may assist in diagnosis of delayed hypersensitivity contact dermatitis. Standardized methods and concentrations for testing for a variety of substances have been recommended.[18,19] Even with standardized approaches, both false-positive and false-negative reactions may occur.[19,20] For example, an irritant reaction may be difficult to differentiate from a weak allergic reaction. Further discussion of issues related to patch test procedures and interpretation is provided by Beltrani and Beltrani.[19]

TREATMENT

Successful treatment requires the identification and/or removal of the allergen (irritant). This may be accomplished more easily in the case of poison ivy dermatitis than in the case of dermatitis due to industrial exposure.

Specific drug therapy depends more on the stage and the extent of the dermatitis than on the cause.[18] Severe, acute reactions characterized by blistering, swelling, and oozing may require systemic corticosteroids. Various regimens are recommended.[10,18,20] An initial dose of 60 mg of prednisone or equivalent is common (range 40 to 100 mg) or 1 mg/kg in a single daily dose with treatment recommended for periods of 7 to 14 days. Most authors recommend tapering the dose during the treatment period to avoid rebound.[10] Specific doses and duration of treatment are probably best determined by the presentation of the patient. Topical corticosteroids are of little benefit in acute edematous blistering dermatitis because of inadequate penetration. Soothing compresses or baths with water, aluminum acetate, or saline may be beneficial in providing relief at this stage.[10,18] Topical steroid therapy once or twice a day can be instituted once the acute symptoms are controlled and continued after oral therapy is stopped. Ointments are usually preferred because cream preparations have a greater variety of ingredients including fragrances and preservatives that may cause allergy.[20] Oral antihistamines provide little if any benefit other than sedating properties because they do not suppress contact allergy.[10,18] Calamine and other shake lotions, topical antihistamines, and topical anesthetics are best avoided because of lack of benefit and/or potential sensitization.[10,18,19]

For subacute (moderate) or chronic dermatitis, topical corticosteroid therapy is used rather than systemic therapy. A high-potency agent may be applied twice daily in subacute conditions. Often the skin may be dry so that ointment or cream preparations of corticosteroids are preferred over solutions. Compresses and soaks are usually not indicated and other lotions (e.g., Calamine) should be avoided because of a drying effect. In chronic situations, low-, medium-, or high-potency corticosteroid preparations are selected based on the degree of skin thickening (lichenification). Overnight occlusion with plastic enhances penetration of the steroid. Caution should be exercised with high-potency agents because of the potential problem mentioned previously, particularly on the face and in skinfold areas. Lubrication generally is needed with frequent application in a thin layer. White petrolatum is a good choice. If secondary infection is present, systemic antibiotic therapy is usually preferred as topical antimicrobial agents can be sensitizing.[10,18]

About 3% of patients treated with corticosteroids will experience contact allergy to the steroid. The occurrence is sometimes difficult to recognize because of several factors: the anti-inflammatory property of the steroid may mask the allergic reaction; the steroid may have been used topically for some time; and/or the dermatitis may be only slightly worse but just does not improve over time. Budesonide and hydrocortisone are the most frequent offenders with the fewest reactions caused by betamethasone, dexamethasone, and mometasone furoate. Cross-reactivity can occur. Classification of the steroids based on chemical/molecular structure helps identify potential alternative agents, but there is some cross-reactivity even across classes.[20]

PUVA photochemotherapy may be used effectively but is indicated only in carefully selected patients who can comply with and/or do not respond to standard therapy.[19]

Urticaria

DEFINITION

Urticaria and angioedema are edematous vascular reactions of the skin.[10,21] Another name for urticaria is hives. When edema extends into the dermis and hypodermis, it is termed angioedema.

EPIDEMIOLOGY

Prevalence

Urticaria is estimated to occur in 15 to 25% of the population at some time in life.[21,22] All age groups can be affected with acute reactions occurring more often in children and young adults. Chronic urticaria occurs more often in adults, particularly middle-aged women.[22] Urticaria and angioedema occur concurrently in almost half of the patients, another 40% experience only urticaria and around 10% experience angioedema only.[23] Many cases of urticaria are acute, but if the episodes continue for longer than 6 to 8 weeks, the urticaria is termed chronic.[10,22]

Etiology

The etiology of urticaria is varied and often obscure. Urticaria may be associated with or caused by drugs, serums, foods, inhalants, insect bites/stings, contact substances, connective tissue diseases, neoplasms, infections, endocrine disorders, and physical agents.[10,21] The physical agents often include cold, heat, sunlight, pressure, and dermographism.[10,21] The urticaria may be linked to cholinergic or adrenergic factors.[21] Hereditary angioedema, characterized by recurrent, self-limited attacks, is transmitted by autosomal-dominant inheritance with incomplete penetrance.[10] In addition to childhood onset and family history, a specific test for C1-esterase inhibitor, a complement component can be used to confirm the condition. A cause cannot be specifically identified in 70 to 80% of chronic cases and thus the urticaria is termed idiopathic.[10,21]

PATHOPHYSIOLOGY

Five pathophysiologic mechanisms have been proposed for urticaria and/or angioedema: IgE-mediated, complement-mediated, direct mast cell-releasing agents, alteration of arachidonic acid metabolism, and idiopathic.[10,23] Skin biopsies of urticarial lesions show edema in the upper dermis, vascular dilation, and cellular infiltrates in the dermis around the small vessels due to leakage. The histologic nature of the infiltrate may vary and have some relation to clinical course. Some infiltrates are predominately lymphocytic; others are predominantly polymorphonuclear cells (neutrophils, eosinophils, and mononuclear cells). Vasculitis is usually absent with the latter infiltrate. Urticaria characterized by lymphocytic infiltrates generally responds to antihistamine treatment; this constitutes most of patients with chronic urticaria. Cases of urticaria characterized by predominantly polymorphonuclear cell infiltrates tend to be resistant to antihistamines, and the disease exhibits a more severe clinical course.[22] Histamine, an identified mediator in the urticarial response, is produced and stored in dermal mast cells. When activated, the mast cells release histamine as well as other vasoactive substances including kinins, leukotrienes, and prostaglandins. Kinins are vasoactive peptides that may be an important factor in the development of urticaria. They slow smooth muscle contraction, cause vasodilation, and increase vascular permeability. Leukotriene C_4 and prostaglandin D_2 cause urticarial reactions when injected into the skin, but their effects are not blocked by antihistamines.[22] Antibodies of the IgE class can interact with antigen on the mast cell surface, producing histamine release as do complement-fixing antibodies. Direct histamine release may be caused by certain drugs (e.g., radiocontrast media and opiates) and chemicals.[10]

CLINICAL PRESENTATION AND DIAGNOSIS

A careful history that describes the pattern of attacks, the precipitating cause, the duration of wheals, associated symptoms, and atopic background should be taken. As a result, the presence or absence of the following can be established: a relationship to any ingested, inhaled, or injected substance; or a contact reaction, a systemic disease, a hormonal influence, an emotional cause, or infection. While the basic mechanism may still be unknown, the above factors can serve as triggers. For example, in half of patients with idiopathic urticaria, it is made worse by aspirin or nonsteroidal anti-inflammatory drugs (NSAIDs).[22] Thyroid disease, lymphoma, and systemic lupus erythematous have both been linked with urticaria.[10,21]

The skin lesions are circumscribed, elevated, erythematous areas (wheals) of edema that are pruritic.[10,21,23] The size of the wheal can vary from 1 to 2 mm to many centimeters, and groups of lesions may be either localized or generalized. Individual lesions tend to resolve in 24 hours, but new lesions will appear.[10] Patients developing angioedema experience swelling in deep dermal tissue that is not pruritic and can be present with or without the urticarial lesions.[21] The face, lips, eyelids, and tongue are frequently involved in such patients. Some patients may experience respiratory, gastrointestinal, or cardiovascular symptoms.[23] Laboratory and skin testing is of limited value in establishing a diagnosis or cause.[23]

TREATMENT

The best treatment is identification and removal of the cause. As indicated, in the large majority of patients, this approach is unsuccessful because either the cause cannot be identified or multiple factors are involved.[10,23] Treatment then is directed toward the effector cells and inflammatory mediators to either block release or effect. Therapy also may be directed toward receptor sites on target tissues that involve the cutaneous microvasculature and cells.[10]

Antihistamines provide relief in about 65 to 70% of patients with urticaria or angioedema.[13,24] They should be administered on a scheduled basis rather than as needed. Antihistamines are more effective in preventing the actions of histamine rather than reversing the effects.[24] Other mediators are likely to be involved in patients not responding. Of the available H_1-receptor antagonists, they would be expected to be nearly equal in efficacy. Choice can be based on side effects (e.g., is sedation desirable or undesirable?) or pharmacokinetic considerations (see "Antihistamines").[13,23] If one agent is ineffective or not tolerated, a second agent from a different chemical group can be tried. On occasion, a combination of H_1-receptor antagonists can be used (e.g., a nonsedating agent during the day and a sedating agent at night).[13,23] If treatment with H_1-receptor antagonists is successful, the agent should be tapered to prevent flare reactions.[23]

H_2-receptor antagonists such as cimetidine may be combined with H_1-receptor antagonists in treating urticaria.[23–25] Administered alone, the H_2-receptor blockers have little if any demonstrated benefit. Several studies have claimed greater benefit with the combination, but this has not been a consistent observation.[22,25] The H_2-receptor antagonists may be useful only in certain types of urticaria, e.g., cold or angioedema.[25] If the urticaria is refractory, a trial of the combination may be appropriate.[13] Doses of cimetidine have ranged from 400 to 1600 mg/day. Ranitidine has been used in standard oral doses.[24]

The tricyclic antidepressant, doxepin, exhibits H_1 and H_2 histamine receptor blocking activity and is particularly potent against H_1 receptors. Although a benefit has seen in patients with chronic urticaria, sedative effects may limit it to nighttime use, although a dose of 10 mg tid compared to diphenhydramine 25 mg tid produced greater efficacy, less sedation, and more dry mouth.[22,24]

Corticosteroids are not routinely used for chronic urticaria because of the potential length of therapy. Selected patients may benefit from short-term use to control active disease.[22,23] Oral prednisone at doses of 20 to 30 mg/day for 5 days has controlled symptoms. Exacerbation of urticaria occurs upon withdrawal in some patients treated for longer than 5 days.[22]

Other potential treatments include β-adrenergic agonists (e.g., terbutaline) and calcium channel blockers (e.g., nifedipine).[23–25] Patients with chronic idiopathic urticaria have benefited from these treatments, but studies with these agents are limited. Use of these alternate therapies should be limited to refractory cases until further data are available.

Drug-Induced Skin Diseases

Cutaneous reactions to drugs result from immunologic or nonimmunologic mechanisms. Immunologic mechanisms require activation of host pathways and their presence is supported by the clinical features that were noted earlier.[3,6] Sensitization can occur by any route but the greatest risk occurs with topical application and the least risk with oral administration.[26] High-molecular-weight drugs (insulin and antisera) are more likely to cause allergy.

Low molecular-weight drugs are haptens and must combine with protein carriers before an allergic response can occur.

Cutaneous reactions caused by nonimmunologic mechanisms are more common than allergic reactions.[6] Nonimmunologic mechanisms associated with cutaneous drug reactions include activation of effector pathways, overdosage, cumulative toxicity, side effects, drug interactions, metabolic changes, and exacerbation of existing dermatologic conditions.[6] The most relevant of these, the activation of effector pathways, is not antibody dependent, is usually indistinguishable from IgE-mediated reactions, and actually involves at least three different mechanisms. The first involves direct release of mediators, like histamine, from mast cells with presentation as urticaria or angioedema. Drugs implicated in this mechanism are opiates, thiamine, and radiographic contrast media. Radiographic contrast media also have activated complement in the absence of antibody, again resulting in urticaria. The third mechanism involves alteration of arachidonic acid metabolism, the most notable example being anaphylactic-like responses to aspirin and NSAIDs. The other nonimmunologic mechanisms for the most part produce other skin manifestations that are not the focus of this discussion, e.g., bruising with excess warfarin or color changes caused by phenothiazines.[6] Drug-induced skin diseases present through a variety of clinical manifestations as indicated in Table 45.5. The clinical presentation, diagnostic considerations, and time course of each of these will be reviewed briefly.

Drug Exanthem

Drug exanthem is the most common cutaneous reaction, comprising almost half of the skin reactions caused by drugs.[5] It is usually described as a morbilliform or maculopapular eruption, often generalized, but usually starting on the trunk or in areas where pressure and/or trauma occur. The rash is frequently pruritic and symmetric and consists of erythematous macules and papules that may become confluent.[3,6] Fever and eosinophilia may be present. Some agents (ciprofloxacin, vancomycin, and succinylcholine) can cause either IgE-mediated or non–IgE-mediated systemic reactions. A drug-induced exanthem must be differentiated from exanthems of viral origin, although this is difficult because definitive diagnostic tests are lacking. Occurrence usually is within the first week of starting therapy with the offending agent, frequently within the first 3 days. Some antibiotics and allopurinol are considered exceptions. For penicillin, cephalosporins, and cotrimoxazole, exanthems may appear within the first 2 weeks or sometimes later or even after therapy is stopped. With allopurinol, rashes can occur for 3 weeks or more. Most exanthems can be expected to disappear within 1 to 2 weeks after the offending agent is discontinued.

Some characteristics contribute to a higher risk of drug exanthem. Women have a 35% higher risk than men.[26] While estimates have varied from as much as 50 to 80%, clearly, a high percentage of patients with Epstein-Barr virus (including infectious mononucleosis) taking ampicillin (amoxicillin is also implicated) experience a rash.[3,26] Patients with cytomegalovirus infections, chronic lymphocytic leukemia, hyperuricemia, or taking the combination of ampicillin and allopurinol experience a higher frequency of rashes. Patients with acquired immunodeficiency disease (AIDS) taking cotrimoxazole experience more drug exanthems.[3,26]

Table 45.5 ▪ Dermatological Manifestations of Drug-Induced Disease

Exanthematous rashes	Exfoliative dermatitis
Urticaria/angioedema	Photosensitivity (toxicity and allergy)
Fixed drug eruption	Toxic epidermal necrolysis
Erythema multiforme	Vasculitis

Urticaria

Urticaria is responsible for about one-quarter of drug-induced skin reactions, which are described as pruritic, red wheals or as firm erythematous, round or oval plaques of varying sizes. The epidermis overlying appears normal, and no scaling is evident. A lesion generally is present for less than 24 hours but is replaced by new lesions at other sites. Edema of the reticular dermis is a prominent pathologic feature. The term angioedema is used to indicate swelling in deep dermal and subcutaneous tissues often with mucous membrane involvement.[3,6]

If the reaction is IgE dependent, onset can be within minutes but usually within 36 hours. Other systemic signs and symptoms of immediate-type hypersensitivity may occur, including bronchospasm, diaphoresis, hypotension, and eosinophilia. A classic example is urticaria associated with an anaphylactic reaction to penicillin. Urticaria as a component of a serum sickness reaction will occur 4 to 12 days after challenge and will include systemic symptoms such as fever, arthralgias, hematuria, and possibly liver or neurologic symptoms. In some cases the urticaria results from nonimmunologic mechanisms, but it is difficult to differentiate because the time course and presentation resemble the immediate hypersensitivity reaction.[3,6] This reaction is termed pseudoallergic or anaphylactoid.[3]

Discontinuation of the offending agent, if recognized, often results in prompt resolution, although some cases may persist for several weeks after presentation.[3]

Fixed Drug Eruption

Fixed drug eruption is responsible for about 10% of drug-induced skin disorders. It involves the development of a lesion, often solitary, that appears as an erythematous macule and subsequently becomes an edematous plaque.[3,6,27] Vesicles and bullae with desquamation may occur later.[3,27] After resolution of the acute phases, hyperpigmentation remains with colors varying from brown to violet-brown or even black.[27] Lesions most often occur on the face, lip, sacral region, and genitalia. Pruritus and burning may accompany the reaction with the severity reflecting the intensity of the inflammatory response.

Also rare, systemic symptoms may range from malaise to severe prostration.[27] As the name implies, lesions recur in the same place with rechallenge by the offending substance. Symptoms recur usually between half an hour and 8 hours upon reexposure. With repeated exposure, the number of lesions may gradually increase. Drugs most often implicated are phenolphthalein (now removed from over-the-counter laxatives), tetracycline, and oxyphenbutazone.[27,28]

Erythema Multiforme

Erythema multiforme is usually considered an acute, self-limited inflammatory disorder involving skin and mucous membranes although the spectrum can vary widely.[3,6] A prodrome, consisting of malaise, sore throat, and possibly fever with skin lesions developing over 2 to 7 days, may occur. Lesions have a distinctive iris or target appearance and are erythematous plaques with dusky centers with a surrounding ring of edema and a darker erythematous outer border. The plaques are most perfuse peripherally and develop in groups over a period of a few days, fading after one to two weeks. Sites most commonly involved are the backs of the hands, palms, wrists, forearms, feet, elbows, and knees. In the most severe form, the presence of bullous or vesicular lesions accompanied by mucosal involvement and systemic symptoms is termed Stevens-Johnson syndrome (STS). Usually, mucosal and conjunctival lesions occur.[3,26] Drugs cause about 50% of cases with antibacterial sulfonamides, anticonvulsants, NSAIDs, (particularly oxicams), and allopurinol accounting for two-thirds of the reactions.[26,29] Treatment is largely supportive, but early corticosteroid use is recommended to prevent visceral involvement and shorten the intensity and duration.[26] Interestingly, Roujeau et al.[30] have reported an increased risk of occurrence associated with exposure to corticosteroids.

Toxic Epidermal Necrolysis

Toxic epidermal necrolysis (TEN), although uncommon, is a serious skin disorder with significant morbidity and mortality. It is somewhat similar to erythema multiforme but is more acute and catastrophic. A brief prodrome of sore throat, malaise, fever, and chills occurs with skin involvement within 24 hours. Lesions are small, dusky, necrotic macules with early and extensive involvement of periorificial areas and mucous membranes. The lesions progressively enlarge to produce large confluent areas of necrosis with extensive epidermal sloughing within 2 to 5 days. Patients are quite ill with mortality ranging from 30 to 40%.[26] Clinically, TEN may be difficult to distinguish from STS. Treatment is supportive, and steroids are not used.

Staphylococcal scaled skin syndrome, which usually occurs in children or immunocompromised patients, must be considered in the differential diagnosis. Some differentiating factors for staphylococcal scaled skin syndrome are superficial epidermal separation (e.g., intraepidermal, usually the granular layer), absent or mild periorificial and mucous membrane involvement, and no skin pain. Drug-induced TEN generally involves subepidermal separation.[3,29]

Drugs are the most common cause, particularly in adults. The same agents that cause STS are involved in the majority of cases of TEN and include NSAIDs, particularly the butazolodins, sulindac, and piroxicam; sulfonamides (cotrimoxazole); phenytoin; barbiturates; and allopurinol.[6,26,28,29] With allopurinol, TEN with concomitant renal/hepatic failure is often seen in patients with renal insufficiency receiving normal doses. Allopurinol doses should be reduced in patients with renal insufficiency to avoid this reaction.[30]

Exfoliative Dermatitis

Exfoliative dermatitis involves redness of the entire skin with widespread scaling due to exfoliation. Other than in cases of psoriasis, the condition is eczematous. Severe systemic symptoms may accompany and involve hypovolemia, heart failure, intestinal malabsorption, hypoprothrombinemia and hypothermia.[28] Some drugs reported to cause this reaction include gold, carbamazepine, phenytoin, and captopril.[28]

Photosensitivity

Photosensitivity consists of two types, photoallergy and phototoxicity. Most reactions fall into the category of phototoxicity with photoallergy being uncommon.[6,28] Phototoxic reactions can occur with the first exposure to a drug, even within a few hours, and are dose-related. The reaction resembles sunburn and can in some cases progress to blister.[6,28] Removal of the offending agent usually brings resolution. Such reactions will occur in most patients given adequate amounts of drug and adequate exposure to UV light. Chlorpromazine, amiodarone, and doxycycline are examples of drugs implicated in this type of reaction.

Photoallergy involves the combination of the drug, immune system, and light. A delayed hypersensitivity reaction is suspected as the onset is usually delayed and recovery is slow. Such reactions occur in only a small percentage of exposed patients.[3] The rash is usually eczematous but may involve lichenoid, urticarial, bullous, or purpuric lesions. The reaction typically occurs in sun-exposed areas but in severe cases may involve areas that are normally protected. Photoallergic reactions may persist for some time after the drug is withdrawn. Drugs that may cause photoallergic reactions are tetracyclines, thiazide diuretics, sulfonamides, phenothiazines, nalidixic acid, and antihistamines.[3,6,28]

Cutaneous Vasculitis

Cutaneous vasculitis commonly presents as palpable purpura and usually involves the lower extremities although the reaction may be generalized. Other organs such as the liver, kidney, joints, and gastrointestinal tract may become involved. The cutaneous lesions at various times may be macules, papules, urticarial lesions, and, in the most severe cases, hemorrhagic blisters. The origin of the reaction is thought to involve immune mechanisms, but the precise explanation is unknown.[3,6,28] Drugs implicated in causing this reaction include sulfonamides, phenytoin, and phenylbutazone.[3]

Treatment Generalities for Allergic and Drug-Induced Skin Disease

ANTIHISTAMINES

The antihistamines (H_1-receptor antagonists) traditionally have been grouped according to chemical structure: ethanolamines, ethylenediamines, alkylamines, piperazines, piperidines, and phenothiazines.[31,32] However, this classification generally provides little information regarding the expected pharmacodynamic and pharmacokinetic properties. A more useful classification is the terminology of first-generation (classic) and second generation (nonsedating) H_1-receptor antagonists. Comparison in this fashion more clearly distinguishes differences in pharmacodynamic properties. Each group can be examined for desirable pharmacokinetic properties.[13,31,32] Table 45.6 summarizes many of the properties of the H_1-receptor antagonists.

H_1-receptor antagonists are reversible competitive inhibitors of the actions of histamine on H_1-receptors. The antihistamines block the bronchopulmonary and vasoactive effects of histamine, resulting in decreased vascular permeability, decreased pruritus, and relaxation of smooth muscle.[31,32] While differences in potency exist, the antihistaminic activity of the various agents is considered similar when equipotent doses are given.[32] This effect is demonstrated by suppression of the wheal/flare reactions induced by histamine or allergens. The duration of effect varies among agents (Table 45.6).[31,32] In addition, some agents also prevent release of inflammatory mediators from IgE-sensitized mast cells and basophils.[31,32] An effect on calcium either by inhibiting influx across the cell membrane or inhibiting intracellular release is probably responsible. These agents may inhibit late-phase allergic reactions by effects on leukotrienes or prostaglandins.[32]

Classic H_1-receptor antagonists possess anticholinergic activity and produce a central nervous system (CNS) depressant effect. Although sedation is generally undesirable, in many patients with some type of skin disorder (e.g., atopic dermatitis), sedation can be helpful in reducing nocturnal scratching. These effects are clinically apparent at doses used therapeutically. In general, second-generation agents are devoid of clinically apparent anticholinergic activity or CNS effects at therapeutic doses. These agents penetrate poorly into the CNS, and levels are insufficient to block central H_1 or cholinergic receptors. Binding is preferential for peripheral H_1-receptors.[13,31,32]

PHARMACOKINETICS

All of the agents are generally well absorbed after oral administration with peak serum levels reached at around 2 hours.[23,31,35] Most agents undergo metabolism through the cytochrome P-450 system in the liver with clearance and elimination half-lives varying substantially. Active metabolites are formed for some agents such as astemizole. The duration of wheal/flare suppression is related to both dose and the serum elimination half-life. Children usually exhibit shorter half-lives than adults, e.g., chlorpheniramine's half-life is a mean of about 11 hours in children versus about 24 hours in adults and hydroxyzine's half-life is about 7 hours in children compared to 20 hours in adults. Serum half-lives are expected to be prolonged in elderly patients and those with liver disease.[31]

The pharmacokinetic profile of astemizole differs considerably from that of other agents.[31,32] Astemizole and the primary active metabolite, desmethylastemizole, have a half-life of approximately 9 to 10 days after a single dose.[32,36] With once-daily administration of 10 mg, steady-state levels are achieved after 4 to 6 weeks of administration.[32,36] After continued administration, the half-life for astemizole and its metabolites is 18 to 20 days.[32] Inhibition of the wheal/flare response may not be apparent until the second day of administration or later. Initially, use of a loading dose (30 mg) was recommended to decrease the time to onset of effect, but this is no longer recommended. Suppression of the wheal/flare response may be seen for weeks to months compared to a duration of 24 hours or less for most other agents.[32,36]

ADVERSE EFFECTS/DRUG INTERACTIONS

The adverse effect profile of first-generation agents includes CNS and anticholinergic effects. The CNS effects can be divided into depressant, stimulatory, and neuropsychiatric reactions.[31] The primary CNS-depressant effects are sedation, impaired cognitive function, diminished alertness, difficulty in concentrating, dizziness, and tinnitus.[31,32] Sedation or drowsiness occurs in 10 to 25% of antihistamine users. These effects may result in impaired performance as reviewed by Meltzer.[37] Some first-generation agents such as diphenhydramine also cause dystonic reactions.[31,37] Some patients, particularly children, may experience stimulatory effects that involve

Table 45.6 ▪ Antihistamine Activity and Pharmacokinetics

Generic Name (Trade Name)	Chemical Class	T_{max}[32,33] (hr)	$t_{1/2}$[32,33] (hr)	Wheal/Flare[31,33] Suppression (hr)	Sedative[34] Activity[a]	Anticholinergic[34] Activity[a]
First-Generation						
Azatadine (Optimine)	Piperidine	4	9–12	NF	++	++
Brompheniramine (Dimetane)	Alkylamine	3.1 ± 1.1	24.9 ± 9.3	3–9	+	++
Chlorpheniramine (Chlor-Trimeton)	Alkylamine	2.5–3.4	24.4	24	+	++
Clemastine (Tavist)	Ethanolamine	3–5	4–6	12–24	++	+++
Cyproheptadine (Periactin)	Piperidine	6–9	–[b]	NF	+	++
Diphenhydramine (Benadryl)	Ethanolamine	2–3	3–5	NF	+++	+++
Hydroxyzine (Atarax, Vistaril)	Piperazine	2.0	20.0	2–36	++	++
Promethazine (Phenergan)	Phenothiazine	2.7	12.2	NF	+++	+++
Triprolidine (Actidil)	Alkylamine	2.0	2.1	NF	+	++
Tripelennamine (Pyribenzamine)	Ethylenediamine	2–3	–[b]	NF	++	±
Second-generation						
Astemizole (Hismanal)	Piperidine	1–2	10 days	weeks	±	±
Cetirizine (Zyrtec)	Piperazine	0.5–17.4	NF	24	±	±
Fexofenadine (Allegra)	Piperidine	2.6	14.4		±	±
Loratadine (Claritin)	Piperidine	1–2	11.0	24	±	±

NF, not found.
[a]+++, high; ++, moderate; +, low; ±, low to none.
[b]Metabolic and excretory fate not fully elucidated.

appetite or muscles or produce nervousness, insomnia, and irritability. Neuropsychiatric effects reported are anxiety, confusion, depression, and, rarely, hallucinations. The common anticholinergic effects include dry mouth, blurred vision, and urinary retention. Some first-generation agents, such as tripelennamine, cause gastrointestinal symptoms including nausea, vomiting, epigastric distress, diarrhea, or constipation.[31]

The second-generation agents generally are devoid of sedative and anticholinergic effects. The incidence of sedation is similar to that seen with placebo.[31] In some of the skin diseases discussed, sedation may be a desired property and the only benefit in the opinions of some experts.

Drug interactions would be expected with the first-generation agents and other agents that have CNS-depressant effects (alcohol, hypnotics, antianxiety agents, antipsychotics, and analgesics) or anticholinergic activity (antispasmodics, tricyclic antidepressants, antipsychotics, and antiparkinson drugs).[13] These interactions do not occur with second-generation agents.

Since the marketing of second-generation agents, astemizole has been associated with the rare occurrence of the ventricular arrhythmia, torsades de pointes (TDP).[38,39] A prolonged QT interval on an electrocardiogram often precedes TDP, which apparently results from abnormal cardiac repolarization. A prolonged QT interval can be caused by: (1) overdoses of astemizole (two to three times the usual daily dose), (2) liver dysfunction, (3) electrolyte imbalance (hypokalemia or hypomagnesemia), (4) congenital long QT syndrome (rare), or (5) factors that increase the serum levels of astemizole (e.g., drugs that inhibit the cytochrome P-450 enzyme system or liver dysfunction).[38] Terfenadine was removed from the market in 1998 because of similar concerns. The cardiovascular toxicity is due solely to the parent compound. The removal of terfenadine coincided with the availability of fexofenadine, the carboxy metabolite of terfenadine.

To avoid potential problems, patients receiving astemizole should be counseled to avoid increasing their doses above the recommended dosage. The following drugs are contraindicated for concurrent use with astemizole:

ketoconazole, itraconazole, erythromycin, clarithromycin, troleandomycin, mibefradil (removed from the U.S. market in 1998), and quinine. Other antifungal agents (fluconazole, miconazole intravenously, and metronidazole) are not recommended for use with astemizole. Patients also should be cautioned to avoid concurrent use of the following: serotonin reuptake inhibitors, protease inhibitors, grapefruit juice, zileuton, and other potent inhibitors of cytochrome P-450 enzyme CYP3A4.[40] Azithromycin apparently does not affect levels of this enzyme. Patients with significant liver dysfunction or who are receiving concurrent treatment with inhibitors of cytochrome P-450 should be treated with other agents such as loratidine, fexofenadine, or cetirizine.

KEY POINTS

- Allergic and drug-induced skin diseases encompass a varied spectrum of diseases.
- Although allergy is suspected in many cases, the specific allergen may be difficult to identify. Other mechanisms operate in some diseases, but the clinical presentation does not distinguish the etiology.
- Drug-induced conditions tend to be acute and resolve, particularly when the offending agent is removed.
- Atopic dermatitis, contact dermatitis, and idiopathic urticaria tend to be more chronic with exacerbations and remissions.
- Topical corticosteroids, occasional short-term systemic corticosteroids in severe conditions, and antihistamines are the mainstay of drug therapy in addition to other nonspecific topical treatments.

REFERENCES

1. Jacobs MR, Zanowiak P. Topical antiinfective products. In: Feldmann EG, Blockstein WL, eds. Handbook of nonprescription drugs. 9th ed. Washington, DC: American Pharmaceutical Association, 1990:771–773.
2. Sauer GC. Manual of skin diseases. 6th ed. Philadelphia: JB Lippincott, 1991:1–8.
3. Bigby M, Stern RS, Arndt KA. Allergic cutaneous reactions to drugs. Prim Care 16:713–727, 1989.
4. Thestrup-Pedersen K, Larsen CG, et al. The immunology of contact dermatitis. Contact Dermatitis 20:81–92, 1989.
5. Pratt WB. Drug allergy. In: Pratt WB, Taylor P, eds. Principles of drug action: the basis of pharmacology. New York: Churchill Livingstone, 1990:533–548.
6. Wintroub BU, Stern R. Cutaneous drug reactions: pathogenesis and clinical classification. J Am Acad Dermatol 13:167–179, 1985.
7. Rothe MJ, Grant-Kels JM. Atopic dermatitis: An update. J Am Acad Dermatol 35:1–13, 1996.
8. Chan SC, Hanifin JM. Immunologic aspects of atopic dermatitis. Clin Rev Allergy 11:523–541, 1993.
9. Sampson HA. Pathogenesis of eczema. Clin Exp Allergy 20:459–467, 1990.
10. Leung DY, Diaz LA, Deleo V, et al. Allergic and immunologic skin disorders. JAMA 278:1914–1923, 1997.
11. Hanifin JM. Atopic dermatitis. In: Middleton E, et al., eds. Allergy. Principles and practice. 4th ed. St. Louis: Mosby, 1993:1595–1600.
12. Advenier C, Queille-Roussel C. Rational use of antihistamines in allergic dermatological conditions. Drugs 38:634–644, 1984.
13. Hanifin JM. The role of antihistamines in atopic dermatitis. J Allergy Clin Immunol 86(4, Part 2):666–669, 1990.
14. Noren P, Melin L. The effect of combined topical steroids and habit-reversal treatment in patients with atopic dermatitis. Br J Dermatol 121:359–366, 1989.
15. Brehler R, Hildebrand A, Luger TA. Recent developments in the treatment of atopic eczema. J Am Acad Dermatol 36:983–994, 1997.
16. Lim KK, Daniel WP, Schroeter AL, et al. Cyclosporine in the treatment of dermatologic disease: An update. Mayo Clin Proc 71:1182–1191, 1996.
17. Mozzanica N. Pathogenic aspects of allergic and irritant contact dermatitis. Clin Dermatol 10:115–121, 1992.
18. Maibach H, Epstein E. Allergic contact dermatitis. In: Demis DJ, ed. Clinical dermatology. Philadelphia: JB Lippincott, 1988:3(Unit 13-1):1–46.
19. Beltrani VS, Beltrani VP. Contact dermatitis. Ann Allergy Asthma Immunol 78:160–175, 1997.
20. Morren M, Dooms-Goossens A. Contact allergy to corticosteroids. Clin Rev Allergy Immunol 14:199–208, 1996.
21. Lehach JG, Rosenstreich DL. Clinical aspects of chronic urticaria. Clin Rev Allergy 10:281–301, 1992.
22. Tharp MD. Chronic urticaria: pathophysiology and treatment approaches. J Allergy Clin Immunol 98:S325–S330, 1996.
23. Soter NA. Urticaria: Current therapy. J Allergy Clin Immunol 86(6, Part 2):1009–1014, 1990.
24. Kennard CD, Ellis CN. Pharmacologic therapy for urticaria. J Am Acad Dermatol 25(1, Part 2):176–187, 1991.
25. Ormerod AD. Urticaria: recognition, causes and treatment. Drugs 48:717–730, 1994.
26. deShazo RD, Kemp SF. Allergic reactions to drugs and biologic agents. JAMA 278:1895–1906, 1997.
27. Korkij W, Soltani K. Fixed drug eruption. A brief review. Arch Dermatol 120:520–524, 1984.
28. Felix RH, Smith AG. Skin disorders. In: Davies DM, ed. Textbook of adverse drug reactions, 4th ed. Oxford, UK: Oxford University Press, 1991:514–534.
29. Hande KR, Noone RM, Stone WJ. Severe allopurinol toxicity. Am J Med 76:47–56, 1984.
30. Roujeau JC, Kelly JP, Naldi L, et al. Medication use and the risk of Stevens-Johnson syndrome or toxic epidermal necrolysis. N Engl J Med 333:1600–1607, 1995.
31. DuBuske LM. Clinical comparison of histamine H_1-receptor antagonist drugs. J Allergy Clin Immunol 98:S307–S318, 1996.
32. Simons FER, Simons KJ. The pharmacology and use of H_1-receptor-antagonist drugs. N Engl J Med 330:1663–1670, 1994.
33. Antihistamine drugs. In: AHFS drug information 98. Washington, DC: American Society of Hospital Pharmacists. 1998:1–47.
34. Olin BR, ed. Facts and comparisons. St Louis: JB Lippincott Company 1998:188–194c.
35. Paton DM, Webster DR. Clinical pharmacokinetics of H_1-receptor antagonists (the antihistamines). Clin Pharmacokinet 10:477–497, 1985.
36. Simons FER. Recent advances in H_1-receptor antagonist treatment. J Allergy Clin Immunol 86(6, Part 2):995–999, 1990.
37. Meltzer EO. Performance effects of antihistamines. J Allergy Clin Immunol 86(4, Part 2):613–619, 1990.
38. Smith SJ. Cardiovascular toxicity of antihistamines. Otolaryngol Head Neck Surg 111:348–354, 1994.
39. Ament PW, Paterson A. Drug interactions with the nonsedating antihistamines. Am Fam Physician 56:223–230, 1997.
40. Hismanal® Janssen Pharmaceutica. In: Physicians desk reference. Montvale, NJ: Medical Economics, 1999:1425.

CHAPTER 46

COMMON SKIN DISORDERS

Stephan Foster, Christy Lawrence, and Ronald Raspberry

The skin is the largest organ of the body. Its primary functions are to protect the body from the external environment and maintain the homeostatic milieu of the internal environment. The proper function and integrity of the skin are essential to life.

Many disease processes can attack this organ system. In addition, skin manifestations can give important clues to underlying systemic disorders, many of which are discussed elsewhere. In this chapter, we describe some common skin dermatoses that pose therapeutic challenges.

TREATMENT GOALS: COMMON SKIN DISORDERS

- Prevent the development of new acne lesions using topical and systemic medications.
- Differentiate between inflammatory and noninflammatory acne to direct specific treatment toward each.
- Prevent acute and chronic damage to the skin by ultraviolet radiation (UVR).
- Treat warts, or verrucae, to prevent spreading.
- Treat psoriasis, a chronic, inflammatory disorder, aggressively because of its significant morbidity and potential life-threatening complications.

Acne

EPIDEMIOLOGY

Acne vulgaris is a chronic but usually self-limited disorder that, left untreated, can leave physical and emotional scars. It is the most common skin disorder and is estimated to occur to some degree in 85% of adolescents.[1] The incidence of acne is the same in both sexes, with peak occurrence between ages 16 and 19. It resolves in the vast majority of patients by age 25. Girls tend to develop the disorder at an earlier age because of their earlier onset of puberty.[2] Substantial numbers of men and women aged 20 to 40 also are affected by disorder.[3] However, men tend to develop a more severe form of the disease. Genetic factors play a role, particularly for the more severe forms of acne. The high prevalence and the multifactorial origin of the disorder make genetic factors difficult to assess.

PATHOPHYSIOLOGY

The pathogenesis of acne is multifactorial; however, active sebaceous glands are a prerequisite. The development of acne corresponds with the maturing of these glands under hormonal control at puberty. The sebaceous gland is a target of androgens, and hormonal influences play an important role in the multifactorial pathogenesis of acne.[4] This is derived from the testes in males, and the ovaries and adrenal glands in females. Circulating testosterone is converted at the tissue level by 5-α-reductase to dihydrotestosterone, a potent stimulator of sebum production. Sebum is composed of different lipids, including triglycerides and waxes that hydrate the skin. On the average, both male and female patients with acne secrete more sebum than patients without acne, and the level of secretion does correlate with the severity of acne. Acne-prone skin has been shown to have abnormally high 5-α-reductase activity in vitro. In addition, women with more severe acne often have biochemical androgen excess.

Excess sebum plays an important role, through a variety of mechanisms, in the development of an acne lesion. The earliest pathologic change in acne is increased follicular keratinization, resulting in the formation of the comedo.[1] The keratinization is thought to result from hormonal changes, which result in the adherence of keratinocytes to the follicular canal.[5] This mass of material plugs the follicle, causing it to dilate below the surface of the skin. If the follicular opening dilates enough to extrude this material, an open comedo results. The black color is attributed to the impacted keratinous material present, and is not dirt, nor is it likely to be oxidized sebum or melanin, as once thought.[6] An open comedo actually is a mature lesion, not capable of becoming inflammatory. If the follicular opening does not dilate sufficiently, the resultant lesion is a closed comedo. This is the principal site for inflammatory lesion development.

Once the follicle has been occluded, an inflammatory lesion is initiated through an interaction between trapped bacteria, principally *Propionibacterium acnes,* and the retained contents. *P. acnes* is an anaerobe found in high levels in adolescents with acne but in significantly lower concentrations in those without acne. *P. acnes* secretes chemotactic factors for polymorphonuclear leukocytes that can then invade the follicular wall, leading to its disruption and eventual collapse. This results in spillage of its contents into the surrounding dermis, with a subsequent increase of inflammatory response. In addition, *P. acnes* produces lipases that hydrolyze the triglycerides of sebum into glycerol and free fatty acids (FFAs). It uses the glycerol for growth, and the FFAs can further contribute to the inflammatory response. The depth and magnitude of the inflammatory response correspond with the clinical development of pustules, papules, nodules, and cysts. Figure 46.1 demonstrates the three important pathogenic factors in the development of an acne lesion.

A number of exogenous factors can make existing acne worse. Oil-based makeups, pomades, oily soaps, and hair products may occlude the follicle, initiating a comedo. Physical pressure from a headband or hat can induce localized acne. Exposure to excessive heat and humidity can exacerbate acne, but the mechanism is not clear. The ingestion of certain drugs can aggravate acne. Danazol and birth control pills with high progesterone components do this, presumably through increased androgenic activity. Table 46.1 lists other medications that can do this. The mechanism for most of these is not understood. Diet and stress often are implicated, but controlled studies are lacking. Unless a patient implicitly believes a food is aggravating the condition, no food, including chocolate, need be eliminated from the diet.

CLINICAL PRESENTATION AND DIAGNOSIS

Acne lesions occur within the specialized sebaceous hair follicular units found principally on the face and to a lesser

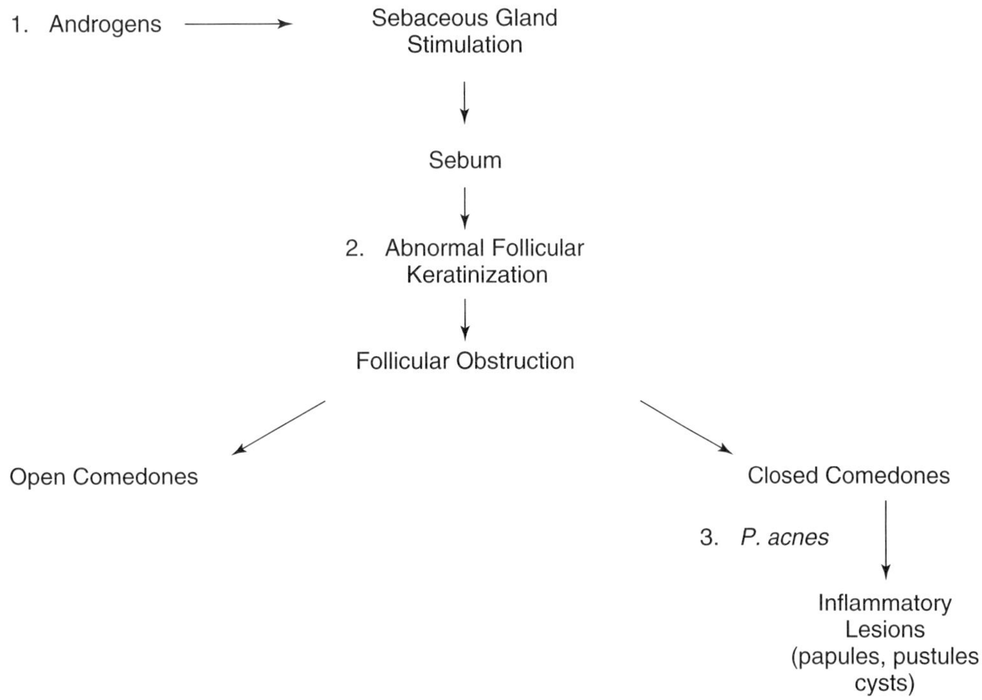

Figure 46.1. Three primary factors in development of acne lesions. Acne treatment is based on reversing these factors, as numbered here.

Table 46.1 ▪ Medications That Aggravate Acne

Hormonal	Nonhormonal *(continued)*
Anabolic steroids	Ethambutol
Danazol	Gold
Gonadotropins	Hydantoin drugs
High–progesterone oral contraceptive pills	Iodides
Prednisone	Isoniazid
Nonhormonal	Lithium
Azathioprine	Maprotiline
Bromides	Quinidine
Cyanocobalamin	Quinine
Disulfiram	Rifampin
	Thiouracil

degree on the chest, shoulders, and back. The two basic lesions are noninflammatory and inflammatory. Noninflammatory lesions consist of open comedones (blackheads) and closed comedones (whiteheads). Comedones develop because of an impaction of keratin and sebum within a dilated follicle and are considered the primary lesions in acne. Mild acne consists of only noninflammatory lesions, but unfortunately most patients progress beyond this point.

Inflammatory lesions are derived from closed comedones. Papules and pustules represent superficial inflammatory lesions, and a preponderance of these lesions constitutes at least moderate acne. Deeper inflammatory lesions include nodules and cysts and are present in the more severe cases of acne. Patients with nodulocystic acne often have extensive involvement of the chest and back. See Table 46.2 for a summary of acne lesions.

Scarring may occur, particularly in the deeper inflammatory forms of acne. It is the most devastating clinical feature prompting early aggressive therapy. The most common scar is the atrophic (ice-pick) form, which is permanent. Hypertrophic, keloidlike scars also occur and are more commonly seen on the trunk. These tend to flatten in time.

Often overlooked is the residual pigmentary alteration seen after inflammatory lesions resolve. This is particularly noticeable in black patients, in whom hyperpigmentation predominates and is often what prompts a visit to the physician. There is no effective treatment for the pigmentary alteration beyond preventing further inflammatory lesions. The majority of the pigmented lesions fade, but it can take 6 months to 1 year for this to occur.

THERAPEUTIC PLAN

Type I, or noninflammatory comedonal acne, is treated with benzoyl peroxide alone or in combination with topical tretinoin. The use of benzoyl peroxide in the morning and tretinoin before bedtime is often effective when monotherapy has failed. If there is an inflammatory component, a topical antibiotic can be added. Type II, or papular acne, is effectively treated with a topical antibiotic along with benzoyl peroxide and tretinoin. One can also consider using combination products. Type III, or pustular acne, warrants oral antibiotics along with the topical therapy used for type II acne. Type IV, or nodulocystic acne, and any other type acne unresponsive to therapy, can be considered for isotretinoin treatment, assuming there are no contraindications to its use. At this stage, referral

Table 46.2 ▪ Acne Lesions

Noninflammatory	Inflammatory
Open comedones (blackheads)	Superficial
Closed comedones (whiteheads) precursor to inflammatory lesions	Papules
	Pustules
	Deep
	Nodules
	Cysts

to a dermatologist may be indicated. Women unresponsive to other treatments can be considered for hormonal therapy.[1]

TREATMENT

The treatment of acne can be difficult and disappointing. Acne is a chronic condition, and at times many months or even years of individualized treatment are needed to achieve control. Nevertheless, if the patient is committed and compliant, it is certainly a treatable disease, and acne control should be expected. Compliance is enhanced if the patient understands both the nature of the disease and the rationale behind the therapy. Virtually all therapy is preventive, with little or no effect on the inflammatory lesions present at the outset. For that reason, maximal efficacy is not reached for several months, even with the most effective treatment. Once acne control is achieved, the patient should understand that maintenance therapy will be needed as long as the tendency to acne persists.

As previously stated, important factors in the pathogenesis of acne are pilosebaceous obstruction by sebum and keratin, androgen-stimulated sebum production, and proliferation of *P. acnes.* Acne therapy is directed at correcting each of these factors. As in other diseases without a single best treatment, many therapies exist, each with specific merits. Many topical therapies are readily available over the counter, and although they are effective in some patients when used properly, they are subject to misuse by uninformed patients. Compliance with a single regimen, whether it be self-initiated or physician-prescribed, should be emphasized for optimal results. A summary of therapeutic agents in acne with their principal mode of activity is shown in Table 46.3.

General Skin Care

There is no evidence that excessive cleansing offers therapeutic benefit; in fact, overcleansing can be an irritant. Additionally, surface sebum and bacteria do not play a role in the development of lesions. When choosing a soap, a patient should avoid one with a high oil content. These are usually reserved for dry, sensitive skin, and can be counterproductive in acne. Expensive medicated soaps usually are not indicated as a supplement to other treatment plans. In noninflammatory acne, a mildly abrasive cleanser may be of some benefit by inducing a superficial exfoliation of the skin. In inflammatory acne or in the patient with dry skin from previous acne therapy, a gentle soap is indicated. Avoidance of all cosmetics is best; however, complete avoidance may be an unrealistic expectation. If cosmetics are to be used, they should be water based. Cosmetics should be removed by soap and water, not by cleansing creams.

Astringents are alcohol-based cleansers that are easy to use and leave the face feeling cool and refreshed. Unfortunately, they are of limited value in treating acne.

Pharmacotherapy

Topical Therapy

Topically applied medications remain the cornerstone of acne therapy. They are often effective alone in mild to moderate acne and are important adjuncts to oral antibiotics in more severe acne. The most widely used topical preparations are benzoyl peroxide and antibiotics, which inhibit the growth of *P. acnes,* and tretinoin, which reverses the abnormal keratinization in the follicles.

Benzoyl Peroxide

Benzoyl peroxide was first formulated for dermatologic use in 1905 and was recognized as useful for acne in 1934. However, the original ointment vehicle was unsuitable for acne therapy. It was not until the mid-1960s that a stable preparation of benzoyl peroxide in a hydrous medium was formulated. Since that time, it has become the most widely used topical medication in acne because of its effectiveness and ready availability, both over the counter and by prescription. When used properly, it can be effective as monotherapy for mild acne and may be used as an adjunct to other therapies in more severe disease.

Table 46.3 ▪ Summary of Therapeutic Agents in Acne and Principal Mode of Activity

Topical Therapy	Oral Therapy
Antimicrobial (*P. acnes*)	Antimicrobial
Benzoyl peroxide	Antibiotics
Antibiotics	Tetracycline
Clindamycin	Minocycline
Erythromycin	Erythromycin
Meclocycline	Trimethoprim–sulfamethoxazole
Tetracycline	Isotretinoin
Azelaic acid	Comedolytic
Sulfur (minor)	Isotretinoin
Salicylic acid (minor)	Decreased sebaceous gland activity
Comedolytic	Isotretinoin (principal action)
Tretinoin	Hormonal therapy
Azelaic acid	Estrogen
Benzoyl peroxide (minor)	Cyproterone acetate
Salicylic acid (minor)	Spironolactone
Resorcin (minor)	
Decreased sebaceous gland activity	
None	

The principal mode of action of benzoyl peroxide is thought to be its bactericidal activity against *P. acnes* and *Staphylococcus aureus* on the skin surface. Subsequently, a decrease of about 40% of the FFAs on the skin surface can be observed. It is metabolized to benzoic acid in the skin, and its lipophilic properties allow it to penetrate better than other topical antimicrobials.[7] Once it penetrates the follicle, the release of nascent oxygen from the peroxide exerts its effect on the bacteria. A total of eleven double-blind clinical trials comparing topical antibiotics with 5% benzoyl peroxide revealed that none of the topical antibiotics were shown to be more effective than benzoyl peroxide against inflamed lesions.[8]

Benzoyl peroxide has also been thought to have comedolytic and exfoliative properties. However, reports of these effects are contradictory, and these actions are considered minor. Benzoyl peroxide has no effect on sebum production or concentration. When the *P. acnes* counts are reduced, FFAs, which contribute to the comedonal plug and inflammation, are also reduced.

Benzoyl peroxide is available over the counter as 2.5, 5.0, and 10.0% creams, lotions, washes, and soaps. It is available in the same concentrations by prescription, usually in various gel vehicles. A 4% formulation in a hydrous medium with good activity but a lower side effect profile has also been introduced. Selecting the appropriate vehicle for each patient is important. Gels are considered more effective vehicles for release of the active substance, but they may be more irritating. Although less effective, a wash or lotion may be all that is tolerated in a patient with more sensitive skin. During the winter, when dry skin can be a problem, switching from the gels to a cream or lotion may be necessary.

There is no difference among the three available concentrations in reducing *P. acnes* numbers in the skin.[1] Therefore, when initiating therapy with benzoyl peroxide, it is reasonable to begin with a low concentration (2.5 to 5.0%) to minimize irritation. Initial therapy should be applied once daily. The patient should apply this sparingly, being careful to avoid the periorbital, perinasal, and perioral skin. Patients may experience mild erythema, burning, or stinging on initial application, and they should be instructed to expect this. If the patient applies the medication at night, the erythema should be minimal by morning. If irritation persists, switching to every-other-night therapy is appropriate.

Tolerance to these side effects usually is achieved as therapy continues. Once tolerance is achieved, the patient should increase the frequency of application to twice a day. Switching to a more potent vehicle or a higher concentration should be initiated only after tolerance is achieved to the lower concentrations without significant improvement in the acne at 4 to 8 weeks. As a general rule, the incidence of side effects increase more than the efficacy with increasing concentrations of benzoyl peroxide.

The most common side effect of benzoyl peroxide is skin irritation, which may in part be responsible for its efficacy. It is known that 1 to 2% of people are allergic to this compound. If patients continue to experience erythema and scaling with low concentrations applied on alternate days, they may have an allergic contact dermatitis. In these cases, stopping the medication is all that is needed, and an alternative therapy is necessary. Patients should be warned that benzoyl peroxide may bleach hair and clothes. Allowing the preparation to completely dry before coming in contact with fabrics can minimize this problem. The question of whether benzoyl peroxide is carcinogenic has been raised. Two earlier studies on rodents have supported this finding, but case-controlled studies in humans have not. To date, it is considered completely safe for use in humans.[9]

Tretinoin

Since being introduced for acne in 1969, this derivative of vitamin A has become the most effective agent in treating acne. It was originally thought that its mode of action was related to its ability to promote erythema and skin peeling. It is now known that its activity is directed at reducing the cohesiveness of keratinocytes within the sebaceous follicle, independent of clinical peeling.[10] This inhibition of the retention hyperkeratosis prevents microcomedo formation. For that reason, tretinoin is superior to all other topical or oral therapies for comedonal acne. Because inflammatory lesions are derived from comedones, tretinoin is an important adjunct to therapy in more severe acne.

The patient should understand that tretinoin can cause mild to severe irritation of the skin, which is more common at initiation of therapy. This is manifested by erythema, dryness, and peeling and is influenced by the formulation used. Tretinoin is now available in a 0.025, 0.05, and 0.1% cream, a 0.01 and 0.025% gel, and a 0.05% lotion. Therapy usually is initiated with the 0.025% cream because the irritation is typically much less and the efficacy is only slightly lower.[7] Tretinoin should not be applied more than once daily initially. It should be applied to completely dry skin because moisture increases the permeability of tretinoin and therefore its irritant potential. The patient should avoid the periorbital, perinasal, and perioral skin. The erythema and dryness are not needed for effectiveness, so if side effects continue to be a problem, using tretinoin every other night or every third night is recommended. As tolerance develops, the frequency can be increased.

Many patients offset the side effects of tretinoin with heavy emollients, but this is counterproductive in acne treatment and should be discouraged. The use of other harsh skin care products such as astringents can increase the irritant potential of tretinoin and should be eliminated if possible. A gentle soap should be used, and a mild lotion if necessary.

Patients may experience a modest exacerbation of their acne on initiation of therapy. This is secondary to the ability of tretinoin to release the retained products of comedones to the skin surface. Patients should understand that this is expected, so that they do not discontinue the therapy unnecessarily. This flare should resolve in 3 to 6 weeks.

Tretinoin decreases the thickness of the stratum corneum, the most superficial layer of the skin.[1] This layer helps protect the skin from solar damage. Patients should be counseled to apply the medication around bedtime and to avoid long exposure to UVR. If exposure is unavoidable, however, patients should use a sunscreen with a sun protection factor (SPF) of at least 15. The thinned stratum corneum also allows better permeability of other topical agents, which is an advantage when used in conjunction with topical antibiotics. Systemic toxicity, as potentially seen with oral retinoids, is not a problem with topical tretinoin even when applied in high concentrations.

The liver rapidly metabolizes the small amount of tretinoin that is absorbed. Although tretinoin has anecdotally been reported in association with congenital birth defects, topical use has not been associated and is classified as a category B drug during pregnancy.[11]

Topical Antibiotics

Topical antibiotics are used in mild to moderate inflammatory acne and as an adjunct in more severe nodulocystic acne. They are not comedolytic, so are not useful alone in noninflammatory acne. The topical most commonly used antibiotics are clindamycin and erythromycin in a variety of vehicles. Meclocycline, a derivative of oxytetracycline, and topical tetracycline also are available. Studies have consistently shown topical antibiotics to be as efficacious as low-dose oral tetracycline in moderate inflammatory disease.[12,13] Topical antibiotics are especially useful when tapering oral therapy.

The principal action of topical antibiotics is their antibacterial effect against *P. acnes*. Clindamycin is more lipophilic than erythromycin and appears to be more effective at reducing *P. acnes* counts.[8] However, when examining clinical efficacy of the different agents, similar results are obtained, implying that other factors may play a role. Topical antibiotics may inhibit *P. acnes* metabolism without killing the organism. This would result in decreased lipase activity, FFAS, and chemotactic factors. Both oral and topical tetracyclines have known anti-inflammatory activities.[1,8]

Topical antibiotics usually are applied twice a day to moist skin after washing with soap and water. As with other topical products, the vehicle is important. Vehicles with a high alcohol content allow better absorption but may be more drying. A cream or ointment may be tolerated better initially in patients with more sensitive skin or during the winter.

A response to topical antibiotics often is evident earlier than that seen with other topical therapies. Improvement is often noted within 2 weeks, although maximal efficacy cannot be determined for at least 12 weeks.

The most common side effect of topical antibiotics is mild erythema and stinging caused by the vehicle. The development of resistant organisms to these antibiotics may occur; however, this has not proven to be clinically significant. Recolonization by susceptible strains of *P. acnes* is seen quickly on discontinuation of therapy.[14] Commercially available topical clindamycin preparations are of the phosphate form and are less readily absorbed through the skin. However, 10% of a daily application does reach the bloodstream, and cases of pseudomembranous colitis have been described with topical use.[15] This is a rare but potential side effect, particularly when clindamycin is applied to large surface areas of skin. Topical meclocycline can impart a faint yellow tint to the skin, which washes off.

Combined Topical Therapies

Combining two topical therapies that are directed at different factors in the pathogenesis of acne makes sense from a practical standpoint. The most commonly used combination is that of tretinoin, with its comedolytic activity, with topical antibiotics or benzoyl peroxide. As stated earlier, by thinning the stratum corneum, tretinoin permits better absorption of the antimicrobials.

The combination of tretinoin and benzoyl peroxide appears to be less irritating than tretinoin alone and is more effective than each used individually. Therapy is initiated with low concentrations of each on an alternate-day basis. When tolerance to the irritant effect is acquired, each may be used daily. The patient usually is instructed to use benzoyl peroxide in the morning and tretinoin at night. This should be followed strictly because the irritant potential is additive when used concurrently. If the patient cannot tolerate benzoyl peroxide, a topical antibiotic may be used.

A commercially available combination of benzoyl peroxide and erythromycin is considered more effective than either alone. Erythromycin is more active than benzoyl peroxide against *P. acnes* but is not lipid soluble. It is thought that benzoyl peroxide somehow carries the more active erythromycin to the target tissue.[7]

Other Topical Therapies

Traditional therapies using salicylic acid (0.5 to 3.0%), sulfur (2 to 10%), or resorcin (2.0 to 6.0%) are no longer commonly used. Their effectiveness is correlated with their ability to induce erythema and desquamation. Salicylic acid is a keratolytic and has some comedolytic activity, but tretinoin is more effective. Sulfur is not comedolytic but appears to hasten the resolution of inflammatory pustular lesions. The combination of sulfur and salicylic acid is synergistic, so they often are compounded together. Each also has weak antimicrobial activity. The combination of benzoyl peroxide 5% and erythromycin 3.0% gel was more effective than erythromycin 4% and zinc 1.2% solution in controlled studies. The anti-inflammatory effect of erythromycin is believed to reduce the irritancy of the benzoyl peroxide.[16]

Some newer topical therapies have been promising in studies and soon may be available commercially. Azelaic acid, a naturally occurring dicarboxylic acid molecule, has been effective for both noninflammatory and inflammatory acne. The dicarboxylic acids initially were found to have a beneficial effect on hyperpigmentary disorders. When patients reported a coincidental improvement in their acne, studies were initiated to investigate this further. A 20% azelaic acid cream was as effective as 0.05% tretinoin cream in reducing comedones, with less irritation.[3,17] The best results with azelaic acid cream were seen in papulopustular acne. Its efficacy is explained by both a strong comedolytic property and a bacteriostatic effect on *P. acnes*. No side effects beyond a local irritation were reported.

There have been a number of attempts to use topical antiandrogens to treat acne. Topical cyproterone acetate was found to be ineffective, and the results of studies with spironolactone cream have been equivocal. A nonsteroidal antiandrogen, inocoterone acetate (RU882), in a 10% solution, exerted a statistically significant but modest (26%) reduction in the number of inflammatory papules and pustules in treated men.[18] However, this compares unfavorably with results expected using established preparations such as benzoyl peroxide or topical antibiotics (50 to 75% reduction in lesions at 2 months).[19] Another topically active antiandrogen, RU58841, has been synthesized. It has been shown to have high affinity for androgen receptors and minimal systemic effects in hamsters.[20]

Systemic Therapy

Antibiotics

Oral antibiotics are used at the outset of therapy for patients with moderate to severe inflammatory acne. They should be used in conjunction with topical benzoyl peroxide, tretinoin, or occasionally topical antibiotics. Tetracycline and its derivative minocycline usually are the drugs of first choice. Erythromycin is a common alternative, and trimethoprim–sulfamethoxazole sometimes is prescribed as a third line of therapy. These agents inhibit *P. acnes,* resulting in decreased chemotactic factor and lipase production. They also exert a direct anti-inflammatory response independent of bacteria. This is more true of tetracycline than of the other antibiotics.

Tetracycline, in dosages of 1 g/day in two to four divided doses, usually is used first. Occasionally, dosages up to 2 g are necessary in nodulocystic acne. Tetracycline is best absorbed if not taken with food, dairy products, iron, or antacids. The patient should be instructed to take the medication 1 hour before or 2 hours after a meal. Tetracycline on an empty stomach may cause nausea in some patients, and in these instances it can be taken with a small amount of food.

Clinical improvement usually is noted within 2 to 4 weeks of therapy. It is clear now that treatment must be continued for at least 5 months, sometimes for 1 or 2 years.[21] Once an adequate response is noted, tapering the dosage by 250-mg increments over several weeks is recommended. The goal is to ultimately discontinue oral therapy while maintaining control with topical therapy alone.

A common side effect of tetracycline is vaginal yeast infection, which can be controlled with topical antiyeast preparations. Tetracycline can also cause photosensitivity eruptions, so patients should wear a sunscreen with an SPF of at least 15 if planning to spend time in the sun. Tetracycline and its derivatives should never be administered during pregnancy because they can cause liver toxicity in the mother and bone and teeth abnormalities in the fetus.

If cost were not a factor, minocycline would be the antibiotic of first choice in acne. It is more lipophilic than tetracycline, allowing it to accumulate more readily in the sebaceous follicle, and its clinical efficacy is better than that of tetracycline.[22] It is better absorbed with food and is less likely to cause nausea than tetracycline. It is also less likely to cause photosensitivity reactions. The usual initial dosage is 50 mg twice a day, so patient compliance is improved.

Minocycline can cause esophagitis secondary to reflux, so it should not be taken just before retiring. A dose-dependent vestibular dysfunction can occur, leading to vertigo, ataxia, nausea, and vomiting. Lowering the dosage can circumvent these effects, but often the medication must be discontinued. A blue-gray pigmentation of skin and mucous membranes is reported with minocycline use. This is more common in sun-exposed areas and may take up to 7 months to resolve. Doxycycline, another derivative of tetracycline, has demonstrated therapeutic equivalence to minocycline but is used less often to treat acne because of a much higher incidence of photosensitivity reactions.

If a patient is unable to take tetracycline, erythromycin is an effective alternative. It is as effective as tetracycline, but the higher incidence of gastrointestinal problems and the more frequent development of resistant strains of *P. acnes* make it the second choice. Advantages of erythromycin include the lower rate of monilial overgrowth, the lack of photosensitivity, and maintenance of efficacy when taken with food. It is considered safe for use during pregnancy; however, consulting with the obstetrician is wise before initiating long-term therapy with any medication during pregnancy. Dosing is the same as for tetracycline.

The safety of long-term antibiotics in treating acne is well established.[23] Concern about possible serious superinfections has not been borne out clinically. There is also concern that broad-spectrum antibiotics can decrease the effectiveness of oral contraceptives.[24] Although this remains controversial, this possibility should be discussed with patients and additional forms of birth control considered.

Isotretinoin

Oral isotretinoin (13 cis-retinoic acid) is the most effective agent in treating acne. This synthetic derivative of vitamin A was introduced in 1982. It was formerly indicated primarily for treating resistant nodulocystic acne, but the majority of treated patients today have therapy-resistant moderate acne. It should also be considered early in the therapy of patients who experience scarring. Dramatic improvement can be seen with isotretinoin, and in contrast to other acne therapies, prolonged remission can be expected. The teratogenicity and multiple potential side effects associated with isotretinoin preclude its use in less severe acne.

The mechanism of action of isotretinoin is multifactorial. It is the only known therapeutic agent that affects all the major factors associated with the pathogenesis of acne.[25] Its most profound effect is on reduction of sebaceous gland size and sebum production. A 50 to 90% reduction in sebaceous gland size can be expected. This inhibition continues in most patients for more than a year after therapy is discontinued. Isotretinoin also normalizes the keratinization process in the follicle. It has no direct antibacterial properties, but isotretinoin reduces *P. acnes* counts indirectly by reducing sebum. Isotretinoin also has direct anti-inflammatory properties as a result of its ability to inhibit the chemotaxis of neutrophils and monocytes.

The usual starting dosage of isotretinoin is 0.5 to 1.0 mg/kg orally per day. The lowest dosage usually is initiated and then gradually increased, based on clinical response and tolerability after 4 to 8 weeks. Therapy is continued for 16 to 20 weeks. Oral antibiotics and topical medications that can further dry the skin should be discontinued before isotretinoin therapy. Improvement usually is noted within 2 months, and continued improvement can be seen for up to 6 months after therapy. Some patients can have relapses after a course of isotretinoin, but they are usually much milder than the initial disease. This is seen more often in those treated with lower dosages. If relapse occurs, a second course can be given, but this is not recommended until 6 months have elapsed because of the delayed improvement that can be seen.

Nearly all patients who receive isotretinoin experience mucocutaneous side effects. These consist primarily of dryness of the skin, eyes, nose, and mouth. Moisturizers can be used to combat the dry skin and cheilitis. An antibiotic ointment is recommended for the nasal passages to prevent cracking, bleeding, and potential colonization by *S. aureus.* Conjunctivitis is common, and corneal opacities can occur, but they usually resolve within 6 weeks after therapy. During this period, patients may be intolerant of contact lenses. Artificial tears can be used to offset this problem.

The most common laboratory abnormality associated with isotretinoin is a dose-related elevation of serum triglyceride levels. Hyperlipidemia occurs in about 25% of patients and is likely to occur in patients with predisposing factors, such as obesity, alcoholism, nicotine use, diabetes, or familial hyperlipidemia, and those receiving concomitant β-blocker, contraceptive, and thiazide therapy. Increased serum triglycerides (19%) are seen more often than increased cholesterol (12%).[3,10,26] Less common is a decrease in high-density lipoprotein levels (15%). This usually is not a problem in the young patient treated for acne, but precautions should be taken. Previous recommendations included a baseline lipid profile, with repeat samples obtained after 1 week of therapy and every 2 weeks until levels stabilize. New guidelines suggest monitoring triglyceride and cholesterol values every 4 weeks for the first 2 to 3 months of therapy, then every 8 weeks thereafter.[10] A low-fat diet and avoidance of alcohol are necessary in mild to moderate elevations. Close monitoring should be done in an obese or diabetic patient. Hyperlipidemia is reversible, with lipid levels returning to baseline within 8 weeks after discontinuing therapy. Less common is an elevation of hepatic enzymes. If elevations appear, isotretinoin treatment should be reduced to 50% or be interrupted.[10] Practically speaking, pretreatment laboratory tests usually are performed to exclude high-risk patients with hyperlipidemia or with diseases such as mononucleosis. These usually are repeated once during the course of therapy. If an elevation in lipid levels is noted after therapy is initiated, the patient is advised to eat a low-fat diet and therapy is continued. Hepatic enzymes rarely become elevated to the extent that therapy discontinuation is necessary.[27] Rarely, a decreased white blood cell count or hypercalcemia is seen. The need for laboratory monitoring of these parameters should be discussed with patients before therapy with isotretinoin.

Synthetic retinoid therapy has been associated with skeletal abnormalities in a small percentage of patients. In patients with acne treated for 20 weeks, significant clinical changes are rare. Most common is muscle and bone discomfort, which respond to mild analgesic therapy. Skeletal hyperostosis, manifested by small spurs along the vertebral bodies, has been noted in 26% of patients with acne in one study. However, 23% of patients had these before therapy, and the significance of this finding during short-term therapy is not known.[28]

Less than 10% of patients notice some hair loss during therapy, usually late in the course. Regrowth is expected. Photosensitivity can occur, and patients should wear an SPF 15 sunscreen before prolonged exposure to the sun. Benign intracranial hypertension is a rare side effect of isotretinoin administration. This is manifested by headache, nausea, vomiting, and visual disturbances. If this occurs, the patient should see a physician immediately.

The most serious potential side effect of isotretinoin is its teratogenicity. Miscarriage and stillbirth are common, and a 25-fold increase in major congenital anomalies is seen.[29] These involve the cranium, face, heart, brain, and thymus during organogenesis. Women must understand the teratogenic potential and the consequences of becoming pregnant while on this medication. A pregnancy test should be performed the week before the start of therapy and monthly throughout treatment. Treatment should start on the second or third day of the next menstrual cycle. Using two methods of contraception is recommended beginning 1 month before therapy and continued without interruption until 1 month after discontinuation.[3] Although teratogenic, isotretinoin is not mutagenic, and future pregnancies should not be affected.[29] The drug has no known effect on spermatogenesis.

Hormonal Therapy

Estrogen therapy has long been noted to improve acne in women. This hormone counteracts the androgenic stimulation of the sebaceous gland, decreasing sebum production. Various combinations of estrogens and progestins in oral contraceptives are effective in treating acne. Higher dosages of estrogens are more effective in reducing sebum production and improving acne but are associated with a higher frequency of estrogen-related side effects. Preparations containing progestins with low androgenic activity and low dosages of estrogens generally should be chosen. A triphasic contraceptive containing norgestimate plus ethinyl estradiol has been approved for treating acne in women.[3] Androgen-dominant oral contraceptive pills containing norgestrel can worsen acne and should be avoided.[4]

Side effects of this therapy are common and include nausea, weight gain, spotting, breast tenderness, and amenorrhea. Less common are brown pigmentation of the skin (chloasma), telangiectasias, allergic reactions, and alopecia. A disadvantage is that it can take several months before noticeable improvement is obtained. Gynecomastia and decreased libido prevent its use in male patients.

Antiandrogens are drugs that prevent androgen activity at the target sites by competing with dihydrotestosterone for the receptor. This therapy is used most commonly in women with hyperandrogenism secondary to polycystic ovarian disease and adrenal hyperactivity manifested by hirsutism and acne. Cyproterone acetate and spironolactone are two antiandrogens that have been used successfully to treat acne.[30]

Excellent results are obtained in women using a combination of low-dose cyproterone acetate (2 mg/day) and ethinyl estradiol (35 μg/day). This combination was twice as effective in reducing acne lesions as OCP alone. The seborrhea improves first, but by the end of 3 months, acne lesions also regress. Beneficial effects are maintained for many months after therapy is withdrawn. A higher dosage of cyproterone acetate (25 to 50 mg/day) may be needed in the resistant patient who also has hirsutism. Side effects of cyproterone are uncommon but include of headache, dizziness, nausea, and menstrual irregularity. These tend to improve with continued therapy. To date, cyproterone acetate is not available in the United States.

Spironolactone is a weak potassium-sparing aldosterone antagonist diuretic with antiandrogenic properties. It has been used alone in dosages of 100 to 200 mg/day, with excellent results achieved in acne regression at 4 to 6 months. Forty percent of cases relapse 6 to 12 months after therapy. It has been used in male patients without development of gynecomastia and decreased libido at these dosages; however, these adverse effects have been seen with spironolactone therapy for other disorders. Potassium levels were not altered at this dosage in subjects of one study; however, spironolactone should be reserved for patients with normal renal function. Periodic evaluation of electrolytes should be done in any patient on long-term spironolactone therapy.

Photodermatoses

Exposure to sunlight plays an essential part in many dermatologic diseases. These effects range from acute damage, including sunburn and photosensitive skin disorders, to chronic skin damage, including photoaging and carcinogenesis. These conditions usually occur on sun-exposed skin, which should be a clue to their recognition by the clinician, who can then proceed with an evaluation to determine the exact cause and appropriate treatment.

Solar Radiation

The sun emits a broad spectrum of electromagnetic radiation, but at the earth's surface, the solar spectrum consists of wavelengths between 290 and 3000 nm. These are divided into UVR (290 to 400 nm), visible radiation (400 to 760 nm), and near-infrared radiation (wavelengths greater than 760 nm), as shown in Table 46.4. UVR is the spectrum that most often affects the skin and is divided into three main categories: UVC (200 to 290 nm), UVB (290 to 320 nm), and UVA (320 to 400 nm).[31]

ULTRAVIOLET C

Wavelengths between 200 and 290 nm are called UVC or germicidal radiation, and they are lethal to microorganisms. Mercury vapor lights and xenon lamps are artificial light sources that produce UVC for bacterial sterilization.[31] UVC is attenuated during its passage through the atmosphere, where it is largely absorbed by the ozone layer. Increased UVC radiation has been detected at various monitoring stations because of ozone depletion. Freons (chlorofluoromethanes) have been targeted as a major cause of ozone depletion; however, numerous pollutants can destroy ozone. Minor changes in the ozone and the loss of its protective effects are damaging to plant and animal life. UVC radiation is carcinogenic.

ULTRAVIOLET B

UVB radiation is often called the sunburn spectrum and includes wavelengths between 290 and 320 nm. This

Table 46.4 ▪ Parts of the Electromagnetic Spectrum

Radiation		Wavelength (nm)
X-rays		
Ultraviolet	UVC	200–290
	UVB	290–320
	UVA	320–400
Visible	Violet	400–760
	Blue	
	Green	
	Yellow	
	Red	
Infrared	Near	760–1,000,000
	Middle	
	Far	
Microwave, radiowave		>1,000,000

spectrum reaches the earth's surface, and on the skin it is largely absorbed within the epidermis. UVB is a strong inducer of erythema or sunburn and can also produce delayed pigmentation or tanning. UVB contributes to chronic sun-damaged skin and skin carcinogenesis. A positive effect of UVB is its importance as a mediator of vitamin D_3 synthesis in the skin. UVB is produced by many artificial light sources for therapeutic purposes and can be blocked by window glass.[32]

ULTRAVIOLET A

Although the amount of UVA (320 to 400 nm) reaching the earth is about 10 times greater than that of UVB, it is 1000-fold less potent than UVB in producing erythema.[33] UVA radiation is subdivided into UVA-1 (340 to 400 nm) and UVA-2 (315 to 340 nm). UVA-1 is less erythemogenic and melanogenic than UVA-2.[31] In artificially high dosages, UVA radiation can produce erythema and immediate pigment darkening of the skin. UVA is the solar spectrum that most often evokes drug photoallergy, phototoxicity, and other photosensitive disorders. It is emitted by numerous therapeutic appliances used to treat dermatologic diseases and is not blocked by untinted window glass. Tanning beds, which emit UVA radiation, have been popular for many years. It has been shown that UVA can damage the skin. In fact, UVA may have carcinogenic and photoaging potential similar to that of UVB radiation.

Acute Effects of Ultraviolet Radiation

The acute effects of UVR on the skin include sunburn, pigmentation, phototoxicity, and photoallergy.

Sunburn

EPIDEMIOLOGY

UVB is the major cause of sunburn and is much more erythemogenic than UVA. Factors that may modify the effects of UVR on the skin include time of day, season, latitude, clouds, surface reflection, and altitude. Skin type is also important in determining the effects of UVR on the skin.[34,35]

PATHOPHYSIOLOGY

Damage to DNA and cell membranes with resulting elaboration of inflammatory mediators is thought to be involved in the skin's response to sun damage. Elevated histamine levels have been detected in blisters, and prostaglandins have been elevated in the skin after UVB irradiation.[33]

CLINICAL PRESENTATION AND DIAGNOSIS

Erythema is the first visible sign of sunburn and may be associated with soreness, swelling, and, in severe cases, blistering, nausea, and vomiting. Erythema produced by UVB occurs 12 to 24 hours after exposure, whereas UVA-induced erythema is more immediate, within the first 6 hours after exposure.[33]

TREATMENT

Generally, a patient with sunburn must suffer through the course of the sunburn. Palliative therapy includes wet dressings, soothing zinc lotions, and spray formulations of topical steroids. Prostaglandin inhibitors such as indomethacin and aspirin have been found to block the earlier phases of erythema when prostaglandin levels are elevated but have been of little use for more delayed effects.[36]

Tanning

There are two components of tanning: an immediate pigment darkening produced by UVA, which occurs immediately after radiation, and delayed pigmentation, stimulated by UVB, which occurs 24 to 72 hours after exposure. Delayed pigmentation enhances melanin content, which can be photoprotective.[32]

Photosensitive Dermatoses

Photosensitivity is an abnormal reaction in skin exposed to sun. It may be provoked by a number of substances that

Table 46.5 ▪ Common Photosensitizers

Oral Photosensitizers		Topical Photosensitizers
Antidiabetics (sulfonylureas)	Antimicrobials *(continued)*	Antiseptics, deodorants, soaps
Chlorpropamide	Nalidixic acid	Halogenated salicylanilides
Tolbutamide	Quinolones	Hexachlorophene
Antihistamines	Sulfonamides	Antifungals
Diphenhydramine	Tetracycline	Buclosamide
Terfenadine	Furocoumarins (drugs)	Fenticlor
Diuretics	Methoxypsoralen	Sunscreens
Chlorothiazide	Trimethylpsoralen	Para-aminobenzoic acid
Furosemide	Antineoplastic	Fragrances
Hydrochlorothiazide	Dacarbazine	Musk ambrette
Phenothiazines	Vinblastine	Coal tar derivatives
Chlorpromazine	Nonsteroidals	Furocoumarins (plants)
Prochlorperazine	Benoxaprofen	Lime, figs, celery, dill, lemon, bergamot, rye, anise, mustard, parsnip, carrot, cow parsley, fennel, masterwort, angelica, buttercup
Promethazine	Ibuprofen	
Thioridazine	Ketoprofen	
Trifluoperazine	Naproxen	
Laxatives	Piroxicam	
Bisacodyl	Miscellaneous	
Sweetener	Amantadine	
Cyclamate	Amiodarone	
Antifungals	Amlodipine	
Griseofulvin	Fenofibrate	
Antimicrobials	Isotretinoin	
Demeclocycline	Nifedipine	
Doxycycline	Quinidine	
Lomefloxacin	Quinine	

come in contact with the skin or are taken internally (see Table 46.5). These are divided into phototoxic, photoallergic, and miscellaneous disorders.

Phototoxic and photoallergic reactions involve the presence of a photosensitizer and UVR to the skin. Phototoxic reactions are nonimmunologic and occur 2 to 6 hours after sun exposure, causing a sunburn type of reaction. Photoallergic reactions occur only in people previously sensitized by a photoallergen and typically occur 24 to 48 hours after sun exposure, producing an eczematoid reaction confined to sun-exposed areas, usually the face, neck, and dorsum of hands. The porphyrias are a class of skin diseases thought to be a photoreaction to a porphyrin product of the host.

Chronic Effects of Ultraviolet Radiation

The chronic effects of UVR on the skin include photoaging and cancer.

PATHOPHYSIOLOGY

Damage to DNA and cell membranes with resulting elaboration of inflammatory mediators is thought to be involved in the skin's response to sun damage. Elevated histamine levels have been detected in blisters, and prostaglandins have been elevated in the skin after UVB irradiation.[33]

Photoaging

Chronic sun exposure changes the appearance of the skin. Photoaged skin is deeply wrinkled, inelastic, coarse, and leathery, with associated pigment changes, freckling, telangiectasias, easy bruising, and ultimately premalignant and malignant skin lesions. Actinic keratoses (solar keratoses) are common sun-induced lesions usually seen in patients with fair complexions who have had excessive sun exposure. They are most prominent in sun-exposed areas of the skin, especially the face and hands. However, the location of actinic keratoses varies according to the location of the sun exposure, and people who sunbathe can develop lesions anywhere. They are small, rough, ill-defined erythematous lesions covered by adherent scales. When these lesions are present on the lip, they are called actinic cheilitis. Actinic keratoses and actinic cheilitis may develop into squamous cell carcinoma in a small percentage of patients.

Photocarcinogenesis

Chronic sun exposure may lead to squamous cell and basal cell skin cancers. These are found more often in sun-exposed areas and are enhanced by the total exposure to UVR. Squamous cell cancers are most commonly shallow ulcers with a raised border, but they may be red, raised, scaling lesions. Basal cell carcinomas are more often nodules on the skin with a pearly, rolled border with prominent telangiectatic vessels on the surface, and they may ulcerate.

The risk of malignant melanoma appears to be increased by intermittent severe sunburn, especially if it occurs during childhood.[37] Malignant melanomas may have different clinical presentations, but any mole that appears to have a blue-black color or variations in color, irregular borders, or a rapid change in size should be evaluated by a dermatologist because these skin cancers can have a grave prognosis if not treated adequately and promptly. The best treatment for most skin cancers is surgical excision.

THERAPEUTIC PLAN

There is strong evidence that sun exposure leads to photoaging and skin cancers, and sun protection should be stressed in the young, in people with fair skin, and in people prone to sun-sensitive disorders. Although the simplest and cheapest way to avoid sun exposure is to avoid outdoor exposure during hours of intense sunlight (10:00 AM to 3:00 PM) and to wear protective clothing and hats, this is not always feasible, and in these circumstances, sunscreens that provide maximal protection must be used.[38]

PREVENTION

The goal of treating photodermatoses is to block one or more steps in their pathogenesis. Although sun avoidance is an obvious solution, this is not always feasible. Protective clothing, including a broad-brimmed hat, will reduce UV exposure. Sunscreens are advocated to prevent sunburn and protect against acute and chronic photodamage.

Sunscreens

Sunscreens are topical preparations that block the effect of UVR on the skin by absorbing, reflecting, or scattering UVR. They are divided into physical sunscreens, which usually are opaque products that reflect and scatter UVR, and chemical sunscreens, which contain agents that absorb UVR, as shown in Table 46.6.

Physical Sunscreens

Physical sunscreens usually are opaque and reflect or scatter UVR. They contain iron oxide, titanium dioxide, talc, zinc oxide, ferric chloride, or ichthammol. They are advantageous in that they absorb a broad spectrum of UVR; however, many people find them cosmetically unacceptable. The recent addition of coloring agents has made them more acceptable, but they can discolor clothes.

Table 46.6 ▪ Sunscreen Chemicals Used in the United States

Chemical	Physical (UVA and UVB)
UVA absorbers	Red petrolatum
Benzophenones (UVA and UVB)	Titanium dioxide
Oxybenzone	Magnesium oxide
Dioxybenzone	Zinc oxide
Sulisobenzone	Magnesium salicylate
Avobenzone (Parsol 1789)	Ferric chloride
Butylmethoxydibenzoylmethane	
Anthranilates	
UVB absorbers	
PABA	
PABA esters	
Padimate-0	
Glyceryl PABA	
Cinnamates	
Salicylates	

UV, ultraviolet; *PABA*, para-aminobenzoic acid.

They are not easily washed off, but they may melt with prolonged heat, necessitating repeated application.[38]

Chemical Sunscreens

The chemical sunscreens contain agents that absorb UVR. They may contain agents that absorb UVA or UVB or a combination of agents to give a broad spectrum of coverage.

Ultraviolet B Absorbers

Para-Aminobenzoic Acid

One of the most widely used chemical agents that absorbs UVB is para-aminobenzoic acid (PABA) and its esters. PABA penetrates the stratum corneum of the skin, where it attaches to proteins, and thus it is not easily washed off after swimming or bathing. It should be applied at least 1 hour before sun exposure to allow adequate time for PABA binding to the skin.

PABA can cause irritation and hypersensitivity reactions. The PABA esters have a lower potential for allergic or irritant reactions and staining. Currently, the most commonly used ester is octyl-dimethyl-PABA, also known as padimate.[39]

Cross-reactivity between PABA and sulfonylureas, sulfonamides, thiazides, and paraphenyldiamine has been shown, and patients with sensitivity to these medications should avoid PABA-containing sunscreens.[40]

Cinnamates

The cinnamates have been increasingly used in the United States for UVB absorption. They have a lower potential for hypersensitivity than the PABA agents and are nonstaining. However, they do not bind the stratum corneum and are easily removed with water. This class of agents includes cinoxate, ethylhexyl *p*-methoxycinnamate, octocryiene, and octyl methoxycinnamate.

Salicylates

The salicylates are UVB absorbers and have been ingredients of sunscreens since the 1920s.

Ultraviolet A Absorbers

The most widely used UVA absorbers are the benzophenone products such as oxybenzone and dioxybenzone. A new compound, butylmethoxydibenzoylmethane (Avobenzone, Parsol 1789), has been found to be a more effective UVA sunscreen than oxybenzone and has been approved in one sunscreen in the United States.[38]

Sun Protection Factor

The concept of SPF was developed by Greiter of Austria[41] and was adopted by the U.S. Food and Drug Administration (FDA) in 1978.[42] Currently, manufacturers specify the SPF on sunscreen labels. The SPF is a quantitative measure of the product to absorb UVB only. The SPF is the ratio of the dosage of UVB energy needed to produce minimal erythema on sunscreen-protected skin compared with the dosage of energy needed to produce minimal erythema on skin without sunscreen protection.[42]

SPF ranges from 2 (minimal protection) to 50 or more. Most sunscreens with SPFs greater than 30 contain at least three different sunscreen agents or greater concentrations of the agents to achieve increased photoprotection; however, this gives them an increased risk of allergic and irritant reactions.[39]

There is controversy about whether superpotent sunscreens are needed. In a study by Kaidbey,[43] sunscreens with SPF of 30 prevented sunburn cell induction in the epidermis when compared with SPF of 15, thus suggesting an advantage of SPF 30 in preventing photodamage.[44] The SPFs of sunscreens are tested indoors and may vary when used outdoors.

Currently, there are no standardized guidelines for labeling the effectiveness of products in UVA protection. It is unclear whether sunscreens protect against melanoma caused by UVA radiation because some high-SPF sunscreens provide some UVA protection.

Substantivity

The substantivity of a sunscreen is a measure of the ability of a sunscreen to adhere to the skin and remain effective despite swimming, bathing, or sweating. A sunscreen is water resistant if it maintains its SPF after two 20-minute immersions in a swimming pool, and it is waterproof if it withstands four such immersions.[45]

Quick-Tanning Lotions

Sunless tanning lotions are becoming more popular to obtain color without sun exposure. These products contain 3 to 5% dihydroxyacetone (DHA) or 0.25% 1,4-dihydroxynaphthoquinone (lawsone). These compounds have no effect on melanocytes, do not stimulate melanin production, and do not give photoprotection unless combined with a traditional sunscreen. DHA becomes oxidized and polymerized to an orange-brown color that adheres to the skin and gives a tan appearance for 7 to 10 days.

Other Considerations

In older adults, it has been thought that the use of sunscreen is more questionable because sunscreens block UV-induced vitamin D synthesis in the skin and may cause an older adult to be more prone to vitamin D deficiency and thus bone fractures. Recent studies have shown this to be false. Studies show that sufficient sunlight is received, probably through the sunscreen itself and the lack of total skin coverage at all times, to allow adequate vitamin D production.[44,46]

Systemic Photoprotective Agents

There is currently no effective, safe systemic photoprotective agent that would circumvent the shortcomings of topical sunscreens. Several agents have shown improvement in specific photosensitive diseases, but they are not as effective as general photoprotectors.

Antimalarials

The aminoquinolines (chloroquine, hydroxychloroquine, quinacrine) are occasionally used to treat several light-sensitive diseases, including systemic lupus erythematosus, polymorphous light eruption, solar urticaria, and porphyria cutanea tarda.

Chloroquine has been shown to have many diverse effects, including enzyme inhibition; protein, DNA, and melanin binding; and antihistaminic and anti-inflammatory effects. It is also an effective absorber of UVR; however, the exact mechanisms of action in the photosensitive disorders are not known.[47] The toxicities of the antimalarials are multiple, and they are not considered the first choice for treating photosensitive disorders. They should be used only after other therapies have failed, and with close supervision.

Ocular toxicity is the greatest limitation of the aminoquinolines. They can cause an irreversible, dose-related retinopathy. To minimize the risk of ocular toxicity, the dosage of chloroquine should not exceed 250 mg/day or hydroxychloroquine 400 mg/day (in a patient weighing more than 100 lb). An ophthalmologic examination should be performed before therapy and every 4 to 6 months during therapy. If any changes in vision occur, such as blurred vision or flashes of light, the drug should be stopped until the patient can be examined by an ophthalmologist.

Other reported side effects include headache, irritability, toxic psychosis, worsening of psoriasis, and leukopenia. They can cause a blue-black pigmentation of the skin, and quinacrine can give a yellow discoloration to the skin. The antimalarials are teratogenic and should be avoided during pregnancy.[48]

Carotenoids

The carotenoids can exert a photoprotective effect in humans and chlorophyl-containing organisms. β-Carotene has been found to absorb light in the visible spectrum (360 to 500 nm); however, some think its photoprotective effect results from its ability to quench single oxygen-derived photochemical reactions.[47] β-Carotene has been effective in treating erythropoietic protoporphyria, a rare hereditary photosensitivity disease caused by a defect in porphyrin metabolism; however, its usefulness in other photosensitivity diseases has been marginal. Oral ingestion should be regulated to keep a blood level between 600 and 800 mg/mL, which usually corresponds to an adult dosage of 150 mg.[47] The main side effect of β-carotene is a slight orange discoloration of the skin, most notable on the palms and soles. Results are not expected until 1 or 2 months of therapy.

TREATMENT

Although sunscreens and sun avoidance are important to prevent photodamage, once chronic photodamage has occurred, treatment that may obviate future surgical intervention may be needed. Recently, several products have been used to treat photodamaged skin.

Topical Tretinoin

Although topical tretinoin is not approved by the FDA to treat photodamaged skin, several studies have supported its beneficial effects. The first suspicion that topical tretinoin may reverse the seemingly irreversible (i.e., fine wrinkling, coarse wrinkling, and hyperpigmented lesions) arose from clinical observations.[49] Clinical improvement is seen during the first 4 to 10 months of treatment. Topical tretinoin is thought to increase collagen levels in photoaged skin, which is the major structural protein of the skin. It not only treats photoaging after it has occurred but is also likely to retard or prevent photoaging before it occurs.

To treat photodamaged skin or precancerous lesions, topical tretinoin usually is initiated at a low strength (0.025% cream or 0.1% cream) and applied at bedtime, avoiding areas close to the eyes. The most significant side effect is irritation, which is readily treated by withholding treatment for 1 to 2 days and decreasing the dosage or changing to alternate-day therapy. The patient should use sunscreens during the day.[1] This treatment should be avoided during pregnancy because it is considered nonessential.

Experience with topical tretinoids is limited, and their long-term effects are unknown. Whether their effects will persist past treatment is unknown. They should be used only in motivated patients who are committed to future sun protection and sun avoidance.

α-Hydroxyacids

α-Hydroxyacids and α-keto acids, including glycolic, pyruvic, and lactic acids, are powerful keratolytic agents and have been used to treat actinic keratosis and wrinkles with some success.[50] There are many different strengths of these acids and different combinations that produce varying degrees of epidermal damage.

Topical Fluorouracil

Topical 5-fluorouracil (5-FU) is an anticancer agent that has been used to treat many precancerous lesions and dermatoses. It is most often used to treat severe actinic keratoses. 5-FU is a structural analog of thiamine and blocks DNA synthesis. Cells that are rapidly growing, such as actinic keratoses, need more DNA and thus accumulate larger amounts of lethal FU, resulting in their death. Normal skin is much less affected by the FU.[51]

FU is available as a 1% cream or solution, 2% solution, and 5% cream or solution. It is usually applied twice daily for 2 to 4 weeks depending on the response. The response includes an inflammatory phase, followed by redness, burning, and oozing, followed by erosion or ulceration that occurs over 1 to 3 weeks depending on the site and strength used. Treatment is stopped when ulceration and crusting appear. The patient must be well informed of this expected response, or there will be many phone calls. Oozing and erosion are expected, and the patient should be given information pamphlets with pictures, which are provided by pharmaceutical companies. If FU is applied with the fingers, the hands should be washed immediately afterward, or gloves can be used during application. FU should not be applied too close to the eyes.

Topical 5-FU is a very effective treatment for actinic keratoses, gives good cosmetic results, and may eliminate the need for surgery. Side effects include an irritant dermatitis, which is difficult to distinguish from the desired effect of 5-FU. If severe, the treatment may have to be interrupted and lubricants or topical steroids used. During therapy, the redness and oozing may be a cosmetic embarrassment, and patients should be forewarned.

The most common local reactions are pain, pruritus, hyperpigmentation, and burning at the site of application. Other rare side effects include photosensitivity, concealment of a cancer, nail changes, telangiectasias, and scarring.[51] Actinic keratoses that do not respond to treatment should be biopsied.

Overall, when used with discretion and with consistent follow-up examinations, 5-FU is an effective and economic treatment for actinic keratoses and gives good cosmetic results.

Masoprocol

Topical masoprocol cream comes in a 10% formulation that has antiproliferative activity against keratinocytes and is reported to be effective in treating solar keratosis. It has not been on the market as long as 5-FU. It should be applied twice a day to the area of solar damage for 28 days. There is a high incidence (10%) of allergic contact dermatitis to this product.

Warts

Warts, also known as verrucae, are caused by human papillomaviruses (HPVs). Their clinical appearance and location commonly classify them. This classification includes verruca vulgaris, or common wart; myrmecia wart, or deep palmoplantar wart; superficial, mosaic-type palmoplantar wart; verruca plana, or flat wart; anogenital wart, or condyloma acuminata; and epidermodysplasia verruciformis. Applying 5% acetic acid for 5 minutes may help reveal inapparent lesions.[52]

TYPES OF WARTS

Verruca Vulgaris (Common Wart)

Approximately 70% of warts are verruca vulgaris, or common warts, which are circumscribed, firm, rough, hyperkeratotic papules that may appear singly or grouped on any skin surface. They occur most commonly on the dorsum of hands and fingers and on the knees of children. Warts can form at sites of trauma, a property known as the Koebner phenomenon. Although they are generally asymptomatic, periungual warts may become fissured, inflamed, and tender and cause local dystrophic nails. Occasionally, warts consist of threadlike, thin, horny projections. This variant, called verruca filiformis, or filiform wart, occurs commonly on the face and scalp.

Myrmecia Wart (Deep Palmoplantar Wart)

Myrmecia, meaning anthills, are deep, dome-shaped nodules often covered with a thick callus and occur most commonly on the palms and soles. They are usually associated with inflammation such as swelling, redness, and considerable tenderness. Although they can be multiple, they generally do not coalesce. Approximately 24% of warts occur on the plantar surfaces, including both the deep and superficial plantar warts. These can be seen on the lateral aspects and tips of fingers and toes.

Superficial, Mosaic-Type Palmoplantar Wart

Superficial palmoplantar warts commonly form at points of pressure, especially the heel and the midmetatarsal area, causing pain with weight bearing. They have a rough, hyperkeratotic surface usually studded with punctate black dots ("seeds"), representing thrombosed capillaries, and a firm, horny peripheral rim. Several lesions may coalesce to form a large plaque, known as a mosaic wart.

Superficial palmoplantar warts may be difficult to distinguish from corns and calluses. Shaving off the keratotic surface may aid in differentiating the two entities; warts have a soft central core with black or bleeding points instead of a horny central core of corn.

Verruca Plana (Flat Wart)

Flat warts, also known as juvenile warts, are smooth, slightly elevated, flat-topped papules that are usually less than 5 mm in diameter. They may be flesh-colored, gray, or brown and are usually multiple on the face, hands, and legs of children. Occasionally, men who shave their beards and women who shave their legs may develop numerous flat warts in the respective areas as a result of autoinoculation. Verruca plana make up approximately 35% of warts.

Anogenital Warts (Condyloma Acuminata)

Condyloma acuminata consist of soft, verrucous or flat papules that can coalesce as cauliflowerlike masses. Malignant degeneration can occur, especially on mucosal surfaces such as the cervix. Before treating external warts in the anogenital region, it is important to find and treat internal adjacent condyloma (do a complete vaginal exam or proctoscopy if indicated).

Epidermodysplasia Verruciformis

Epidermodysplasia verruciformis is a rare, lifelong, persistent disorder characterized by widespread flat warts with a tendency to coalesce into plaques and tinea versicolor–like lesions. An autosomal recessive inheritance pattern has been suggested, and the disease usually begins in childhood. Lesions almost never regress spontaneously, and approximately one-third of patients develop skin cancers in sun-exposed lesions.[53] The lifelong HPV infection in these patients is thought to be caused by an altered immunity. A depressed cell-mediated immunity is found in 90% of these patients.[54] This immune defect may be primary, perhaps leading to the predisposition of HPV infection and oncogenic transformation by these viruses, or it may be secondary to an overwhelming disseminated, chronic infection.

Extracutaneous, mucosal HPV infections also are recognized. Common warts and condyloma acuminata may occur on other mucosal surfaces such as the oral cavity and the larynx, which may lead to respiratory distress.

HPVs have been found in other entities such as focal oral hyperplasia in Native American children and oral hairy leukoplakia.

EPIDEMIOLOGY

The prevalence of warts in the general population is unknown. However, they occur most often in children and young adults, in whom the incidence approaches 10%.[53] Comprehensive surveillance data for HPV is not available, and only estimates of initial visits to physician offices are tracked by the Center for Disease Control and Prevention. Peak numbers occurred in 1987, with an estimated 358,000 initial visits. The estimate for 1997 was approximately 140,000, and the trends are beginning to show a decrease in initial visits.[55] The peak incidence of warts is between ages 12 and 16. Anogenital warts, on the other hand, are the most common viral sexually transmitted disease in the United States. The annual incidence of these warts is 10 to

20% in young adults, with the age of onset ranging from late teens to early thirties.[56] HPV infection is also increased in patients with impaired cell-mediated immunity, as previously mentioned.

The papillomaviruses, which are members of the family Papovaviridae, contain double-stranded, circular, supercoiled DNA enclosed in an icosahedral capsid of 72 capsomers without an envelope. The viral particle has a molecular weight of 5×10^6 Da and is 55 nm in diameter. With the use of DNA hybridization, it became possible to classify the papillomaviruses into different types. If two isolates have less than 50% homology by DNA hybridization, they are considered two different types and are designated numerically. To date, 80 HPV types have been isolated, and each type tends to be associated with different clinical variants.[57] Table 46.7 lists different HPV types correlated with common clinical lesions.[58,59] Potential oncogenic transformation usually occurs in HPV types 3, 5, 8, 9 and 10, associated with epidermodysplasia verruciformis, and HPV types 16, 18, 31, 33, 39, 42–45, 51, 52, and 56, associated with anogenital and cervical condyloma. The incubation period of HPV is variable and ranges from 1 to 20 months. The mode of transmission of cutaneous warts probably is by direct contact and via fomites. It is thought that HPV infection is acquired by inoculation of the epidermis via breaks in the skin. Trauma thus plays a role and may explain the usual distribution of common warts on the hands, fingers, and knees of children. Autoinoculation of the virus may result in new lesions by direct contact. Anogenital warts generally are sexually transmitted, with an approximately 60% chance of infectivity within 9 months in a single sexual contact.[60] The immunologic state of the exposed patients is also an important predisposing factor. More than 40% of kidney transplant recipients with impaired cell-mediated immunity may develop warts.[54]

PATHOPHYSIOLOGY

The histopathologic features of warts generally consist of acanthosis (thickening of the stratum malpighii), papillomatosis (irregular undulation of the epidermis), hyperkeratosis (thickening of the horny layer), intranuclear inclusions, and parakeratosis (retention of nuclei in the horny layer). The distinguishing features of verruca vulgaris include large keratinocytes with a pyknotic nucleus surrounded by a perinuclear clear halo, called koilocytes, located in the upper stratum malpighii; vertical tiers of parakeratosis overlying the crests of papillomatous elevations; and foci of clumped keratohyalin granules in the intervening valleys. Anogenital warts have similar features but lack a granular layer because they occur on or near a mucosal surface. Although flat warts have diffuse koilocytes in the upper epidermis, they tend to lack papillomatosis and parakeratosis. Immunocytochemical studies have detected viral DNA, antigens, and mature virions in keratinocytes at and above the stratum granulosum. Several DNA detection methods are available to identify specific HPV types.[61]

THERAPEUTIC PLAN

The approach to treating warts depends on the patient's age, cooperation, immunologic status, and previous treatments and the location, number, size, duration, and type of the lesions. Studies have shown spontaneous regression of warts in two-thirds of children within 2 years, although new warts may continue to appear.[54] All warts should be treated to prevent spreading to others and on the patients themselves. Sexual partners of patients with anogenital warts should be examined and treated appropriately. During treatment, the patient should be instructed to avoid sexual contact or use condoms. Therapeutic options can be divided into broad categories: chemical destructive therapy, including acids, formalin, glutaraldehyde, and cantharidin; physical destructive therapy, including cryotherapy, electrosurgery, surgical excision, and CO_2 laser; chemotherapeutic agents, including podophyllin, podophyllotoxin, imiquimod, 5-FU, bleomycin, interferons, and retinoids; and immunotherapy (Table 46.8). In general, most forms of wart treatment can be expected to

Table 46.7 ▪ HPV Types and Their Clinical Associations

HPV Types	Most Common Clinical Lesions	Less Common Lesions	Oncogenic Potential
1	Deep palmoplantar warts	Common warts	
2, 4, 7	Common warts	Superficial, mosaic-type palmoplantar warts, anogenital warts	
3, 10, 28, 41	Flat warts		
7	Common warts in butchers		
3, 5, 8–10, 12, 14, 15, 17, 19–29, 36–38, 47, 49	Epidermodysplasia verruciformis		Yes
6, 11, 42–44	Anogenital warts, cervical condyloma (acuminata)	Common warts	Low
16, 18, 31, 33, 35, 39, 42–45, 51, 52, 56, 58, 59, 66–68	Cervical condyloma (acuminata)	Anogenital warts	High

HPV, human papillomavirus.

Table 46.8 ▪ Treatment Modalities for Warts

Chemical destruction	Chemotherapeutic agents *(continued)*
Acids	Podophyllotoxin
Formalin	5-Fluorouracil
Glutaraldehyde	Bleomycin
Cantharidin	Interferons
Physical destruction	Retinoids
Cryotherapy	Immunotherapy
Electrosurgery	Dinitrochlorobenzene
Surgical excision	Squaric acid dibutylester
CO_2 laser	Diphenylcyclopropenone
Chemotherapeutic agents	Inosine pranobex
Podophyllin	

have a 60 to 70% cure rate. Patients should be told that warts may need several treatments, often over a period of several weeks to months. It is often useful to pare the wart down before using many of the aforementioned treatments. In rare instances, a biopsy should be done to help distinguish benign warts from other verrucous-appearing lesions, such as squamous cell carcinoma, deep fungal infections, and verrucous carcinoma.

TREATMENT

Chemical Destructive Therapy

Acids

Salicylic acid in concentrations ranging from 10 to 60% can be used in paints, pastes, gels, or plasters. It is often used for common and palmoplantar warts, including periungual warts. Salicylic acid preparations can be used on all sites of the skin except the face and anogenital area. Other acids often are used in combination with salicylic acid. A popular preparation is equal parts of salicylic acid and lactic acid in four parts of flexible collodion. Monochloroacetic acid crystals compounded with 60% salicylic acid has been found to be effective for plantar warts.[62] Weekly applications of 80 to 90% trichloroacetic acid and, less commonly, bichloracetic acid may be effective for anogenital warts when podophyllin is contraindicated; this acid does not need to be washed off, as does podophyllin. Trichloroacetic acid may be compounded with salicylic acid for treating common and palmoplantar warts.

In general, the acids act as keratolytic agents by physically destroying the keratin layer. Paints are most commonly used and are usually a collodion-based liquid. Treatment consists of soaking the wart in warm water for at least 5 minutes, after which the wart is pared down as far as possible without causing bleeding. A pumice stone may be used if necessary. Next, a drop of the acid solution is applied to just cover the wart and allowed to dry to a white film. The wart is then kept covered for 24 hours, and the procedure is repeated daily until the wart is gone. Salicylic acid plasters are especially suited for treating multiple mosaic plantar warts. After the lesion is pared and moistened with a drop of warm water, the plaster is cut to the size of the wart and applied for 24 to 48 hours, followed by repeated cycles until the wart is gone. A 40% salicylic acid adhesive plaster is a commonly used preparation.

In 1991, the FDA issued a monograph mandating that all salicylic acid–based wart therapy products be changed to nonprescription status with the maximum of 17% concentration of salicylic acid.[63] Lactic acid is no longer allowed as an active agent in over-the-counter products. However, pharmacists may compound these acids, using a higher concentration as necessary.

Formalin

Formalin preparations can be used for plantar or multiple warts. This chemical acts on the affected tissue by its destructive properties. An aqueous solution of 3 to 10% formalin can be used to soak the pared wart for 10 to 30 minutes daily. The surrounding normal skin can be protected with petroleum jelly. Formalin 25% in hydrophilic petrolatum has also been used as a daily application. A potential complication of formalin treatment is the development of allergic contact dermatitis.

Glutaraldehyde

Topical application of 10% glutaraldehyde may be less irritating for palmoplantar warts than formalin preparations. A 1994 study in Japan[64] found a 20% aqueous solution of unbuffered glutaraldehyde to be effective in patients with resistant warts. Glutaraldehyde was applied once a day for 12 weeks. Results showed that 18 of 25 patients (72%) were cured, 5 of whom responded after only 4 weeks of treatment. Pigmentary changes were noted immediately after application; however, after healing, no evidence of scarring or permanent pigmentary change was noted.

Cantharidin

Cantharidin is an extract of the green blister beetle that acts by destroying the epidermis and can dissociate oxidative phosphorylation. A solution containing 0.7% cantharidin in acetone or flexible collodion can be effective in treating common and plantar warts. The vehicle is applied to the pared wart, allowed to dry, and then covered with adhesive tape for 24 hours, after which the process can be repeated weekly. It is not unusual for warts to recur in a doughnut-shaped ring around the original treated wart. It is best used for plantar warts.

Physical Destructive Therapy

Cryotherapy

Although topical medications have the advantage of being painless, cryotherapy is more effective, particularly for anogenital warts, with cure rates up to 90%.[65] It is a popular treatment for many types of warts, including common, palmoplantar, flat, and anogenital warts, especially in pregnant women. Cure rates are slightly less than those of electrosurgery, but cryosurgery is preferred because anesthesia is not needed. Liquid nitrogen (boiling point −196°C) is the most commonly used vehicle, but solid carbon dioxide may also be effective. Cryotherapy causes cell injury by intracellular ice formation, cell shrinkage, and anoxia by intravascular thrombosis.[66]

Before treatment, the wart should be pared down. A cotton-tipped applicator with liquid nitrogen is applied to the wart to create a white "ice ball" extending 1 to 2 mm beyond the visible wart. This process usually takes about 20 to 30 seconds, after which the lesion is allowed to thaw. The procedure is repeated a few times, depending on the size and site of the wart. The object is to produce epidermal necrosis, with the subsequent formation of a small blister. The lesion then dries and peels off together with the wart. This regimen may involve multiple treatments at 1- to 3-week intervals. A common method is a liquid nitrogen spray that delivers liquid nitrogen via a spray canister rather than a cotton applicator. Carbon dioxide can be obtained from sparklet cylinders and mixed with acetone to form a slush. Freezing techniques using a cotton-tipped applicator are similar to those of liquid nitrogen.

Electrosurgery

Electrosurgery is fairly common, but disadvantages include the need for local anesthesia, pain, and greater risk of scarring and infection. Cure rates are slightly higher than those of cryotherapy.[67] The treatment consists of low-current electrodesiccation followed by gentle curettage of the wart to minimize scarring. It should be used only on small warts.

Surgical Excision

In some series, simple surgical excision of anogenital warts has been reported to be more effective than podophyllin application.[68] However, recurrence rates have been reported to be 20 to 30% in other series.[66]

Carbon Dioxide Laser

Cure rates with the carbon dioxide laser are up to 90%, but disadvantages include the high expense and the possible need for general anesthesia and presence of HPV in the laser smoke.[69] It is generally reserved for treating multiple, large, treatment-resistant anogenital, meatal, urethral, or vaginal condylomas.

Chemotherapy

Podophyllin

For many years, podophyllin or podophyllum resin has been used to treat anogenital warts. It is a nonhomogeneous, unstable extract obtained from the plants *Podophyllum peltatum* (found in North America) and *Podophyllum emodi* (found in India, Tibet, and Afghanistan). The resin has four active agents, or lignins: podophyllotoxin, 4-dimethylpodophyllotoxin, α-peltatin, and β-peltatin. The maximal active content is about 40% in *P. emodi,* which consists predominantly of podophyllotoxin and trace amounts of 4-dimethylpodophyllotoxin. *P. peltatum* has a maximal lignin content of approximately 20% and consists of varying quantities of podophyllotoxin and the two peltatins. Podophyllin is most often used as a 20 to 25% solution in compound tincture of benzoin, although other vehicles have been used, such as mineral oil or ethanol. The resin should be stored at room temperature and be replaced at least every 2 years or earlier if it contains precipitates.

Available studies indicate a variable cure rate, ranging from 22 to 98%.[70] Podophyllin provides the best results in patients with a few external, moist condylomas that are new and small. Before treatment, warts should be wiped dry. Podophyllin is then applied to the wart with a sterile cotton-tipped applicator, from which the excess solution is first wrung out. It is recommended that the area of treatment not exceed 3 cm in diameter and the chemical be kept off the normal surrounding skin to avoid local and systemic side effects. Patients are instructed to wash off the podophyllin 4 hours after application with rubbing alcohol or soap and water. The treatment can be repeated at intervals of 1 to 2 weeks and should not exceed 1.0 mL/week.[71]

Podophyllin acts as a strong irritant and arrests mitoses in metaphase by interfering with microtubule formation and causing subsequent epithelial cell death.[72] After the application, an acute inflammatory reaction followed by necrosis usually develops over the treated area. Local irritation may range from erythema, burning, edema, pain, and ulceration. Uncircumcised men may occasionally develop balanitis and phimosis.[72] Severe chemical burns, necrosis, scarring, and fistula formation have been reported with improper use of podophyllin. Thus, podophyllin should not be used as a home remedy but should be applied only by physicians because local and systemic side effects can be severe.

Systemic podophyllin toxicity has been reported in the literature and usually occurs when the chemical has been applied in large volumes over an extensive area of the skin or has been allowed to be in contact with the skin for a long time. Although podophyllin toxicity is multisystemic, neurologic manifestations are the hallmark features and may include mental status change, peripheral neuropathy, seizures, psychosis, and coma. Other clinical presentations include fever, nausea, vomiting, respiratory stimulation, tachycardia, renal failure, ileus, pancytopenia, leukocytosis, marrow suppression, and death.[73] Podophyllin is contraindicated in pregnancy. It is teratogenic in experimental animals, and intrauterine death has been reported after topical application of podophyllin in women.[72] To minimize systemic absorption, podophyllin should not be used in the oral mucosa, vagina, cervix, rectum, or urethra or in infants. Alcohol consumption should be avoided for several hours after treatment because alcohol may facilitate absorption of podophyllin.

Podophyllotoxin (Podofilox)

Podophyllotoxin is the purified and most biologically active agent of podophyllin. Several clinical studies have reported the effectiveness of 0.5% podophyllotoxin on penile warts by self-application. Beutner and von Krogh[74] report a regimen of 0.5% podophyllotoxin applied by the patient twice daily for 3 consecutive days, resulting in a cure rate of 49%. In a subsequent study in which the same preparation was applied by the patient twice daily for 4 and 5 days, they found no significant improvement in efficacy but an increase in local irritation.[74] Edwards et al.[75] compared 0.5% podophyllotoxin applied to penile warts by the patient for 3 consecutive days, with a 4-day drug-free interval, with 20% podophyllin treatment by a physician once a week. Each of these regimens was repeated for up to 6 weeks or cycles. They found an 88% cure rate in the self-treated patients and 63% in the podophyllin-treated patients. Beutner and von Krogh[74] reported a placebo-controlled trial with two to four treatment cycles of 0.5% podophyllotoxin twice daily for 3 days; they noted an 82% clearance in the treated patients, compared to 13% in the placebo group. In these trials, no systemic reactions were reported, and local irritation was considerably less than that induced by podophyllin. Therefore, topical podophyllotoxin is a safe, efficacious, cost-effective treatment for anogenital warts that can be used as a home remedy.

Imiquimod

Imiquimod, an imidozoquinoline amine, is available in a 5% cream for treating condyloma acuminata. It is the second agent available for patient-applied therapy. Experience with this agent is limited, and results of clinical trials are not available.

5-Fluorouracil

5-FU is a fluorinated pyrimidine antimetabolite that interferes with DNA synthesis and to a lesser degree inhibits RNA formation. When applied topically, it has a better penetration in abnormal skin than in normal skin and has a direct immunostimulatory effect on the affected epidermis.[76] It is used most often for managing urethral and vaginal condylomas, but reports of its effectiveness have also been observed in common, plantar, flat, and external genital warts. It has been used as a topical 1 to 5% cream. The patient can apply 5% 5-FU cream to the distal urethra with a cotton applicator after urination. Proximal urethral warts should be treated by a urologist. Applications four times a day for up to 2 weeks may be necessary.[65] Intraurethral suppositories can be made by a pharmacist.[70] Applying 5% 5-FU cream to penile warts for 8 weeks has resulted in an 84% response rate.[76] Daily 5% 5-FU cream application at bedtime for 5 days may be effective for vaginal warts. Gynecologists use 5-FU cream prophylactically to minimize recurrences after laser surgery.[77] A topical 1% solution of 5-FU in 70% alcohol applied twice daily for several weeks has also been used for condylomas.[78] Because 5-FU can cause local inflammation, the vulva and urethra can be protected with zinc oxide or petrolatum.

For common, plantar, and flat warts, 1 to 5% 5-FU cream or ointment can be used as a single agent daily on a wart covered with a waterproof plaster, or it may be compounded with other acids.[79] Five percent 5-FU compounded with salicylic acid has been reported to be effective.[52] α-Hydroxyacids, particularly pyruvic and glycolic acids, have been combined with 5-FU.[50] 5-FU powder dissolved in pyruvic acid to achieve a 1 to 2% solution can be applied to the pared wart with a camelhair brush until the patient feels a burning sensation. Adhesive tape is then applied over the wart for a few hours, after which the chemical is washed off. The procedure can be repeated in 2 to 3 weeks if necessary. A 0.5% 5-fluorouracil in pyruvic acid:ethanol 1:1 preparation can be used as a home remedy. The patient applies the solution two to three times daily for 2 consecutive days, after which the cycle can be repeated in 1 week if needed.

Bleomycin

Bleomycin is an antibiotic produced by *Streptomyces verticillus* with antiviral, antibacterial, and antitumor activity. It binds to DNA and prevents thymidine incorporation and single-stranded scission in DNA. Intralesional bleomycin has been reported to be effective as an alternative form of therapy, particularly for recalcitrant palmoplantar and periungual warts.[80] A tuberculin syringe with a 30-gauge needle is used to inject 0.1 to 1.0 mL of 1 U/mL solution of bleomycin in saline, depending on the size of the wart. The object is to inject intralesionally so that the entire wart blanches. Local pain, erythema, and swelling may persist for 1 to 2 days after treatment. The wart usually blackens, thromboses, forms a eschar, and sloughs off several days after the injection. Cure rates of one or two treatments with a 2-week interval have been reported to be greater than 80%.[80] Complications, usually from intralesional or perilesional infiltration of bleomycin, may include extensive necrosis, permanent nail dystrophy, sclerodermoid changes, joint destruction, and subcutaneous abscesses.[66]

Intralesional bleomycin sulfate therapy using a bifurcated needle puncture technique resulted in a 90% cure rate with a single treatment.[81] The procedure consists of soaking the wart for 10 minutes in warm water, after which the lesion is anesthetized with 2% lidocaine without epinephrine. Bleomycin sulfate solution (1 U/mL in normal saline) is placed onto the wart surface (0.02 mL/5 mm^2). A sterile, stainless steel, bifurcated needle, originally made for smallpox vaccination, is punctured rapidly through the base of the wart about 40 times/5 mm^2 area of the lesion. The warts usually resolve in about 3 weeks. In reducing the amount of bleomycin introduced into the skin, this bifurcated needle carries only 0.001 U and minimizes bleomycin penetration into the dermis. This type of treatment can be performed on many types of warts, except large condylomas, filiform warts, and warts on the loose skin of the penis and eyelid. It is especially suitable for paronychial warts.

Interferons

Interferons are glycoproteins with antiviral activity made by most cells. Current studies show that interferons used alone or in combination with other conventional therapy are effective.[82–89] All three types of interferons, α, β, and γ, have been shown to be effective intralesionally, subcutaneously, and intramuscularly, but only interferon-α is approved for intralesional use in treating genital warts.[90]

Topical treatment has been studied, but with disappointing results.[82] Interferon has an antiproliferative activity that may slow the rapidly dividing keratinocytes in warts, and its immunomodulatory effect may enhance the host's response to HPV infection.[53] Most studies have indicated its effectiveness in condyloma acuminata. Intralesional injection of condyloma with 1×10^6 IU of recombinant interferon-α-2b three times weekly for 3 weeks resulted in a 36% cure rate in one study[83] and 53% in another.[84] A similar study achieved a higher response rate of 62% with intralesional injection of 1×10^6 IU of interferon-α weekly for up to 8 weeks.[85] Systemic administration of interferon either subcutaneously or intramuscularly in to treat genital warts has also been shown to be effective. Dosage comparison studies of systemic interferon have shown that intramuscular injection of 5×10^6 IU/mm^2 of interferon-α for 28 days followed by three times weekly for 2 weeks is highly effective, but the high incidence of systemic side effects makes this dosage unacceptable; low-dose intramuscular injection of 1×10^6 IU/mm^2 for 14 days followed by three times weekly for 1 month appears to be the best tolerated and yet effective regimen.[86]

Interferon-β 1×10^6 IU intralesional injections three times weekly for 4 weeks have been shown to have similar efficacy when compared with recombinant α-2b and lymphoblastoid interferons.[87] In a review of recombinant interferon-γ for treating recalcitrant warts, the optimal dosage of 50 to 100 μg/day subcutaneously resulted in an overall response rate of 50%.[88]

Side effects of interferons are flulike symptoms, including fatigue, malaise, fever, chills, nausea, vomiting, headaches, and transient leukopenia, even with intralesional injections. Relapse rates of interferon therapy are up to 25%.[89] Together with the high cost of this form of treatment, interferon should be used only for very recalcitrant warts.

Retinoids

Retinoids are another mode of therapy for warts under recent investigation. Although the mechanism is unknown, vitamin A derivatives theoretically may block the production of viral particles because these compounds affect cellular differentiation and keratinization, whereas HPV replication appears to be related to keratinocyte differentiation.[53] Retinoids may be capable of preventing malignant transformation, which may be crucial in HPV-induced neoplasia. There are several anecdotal reports of topical and oral retinoids being effective in recalcitrant warts, particularly in immunosuppressive patients. Etretinate 1 mg/kg/day for 2 months improved epidermodysplasia verruciformis with widespread flat wartlike lesions and plaques.[91] Other reports state its effectiveness in recalcitrant plantar warts, but relapses are common and results are not consistent.[92] Topical retinoic acid has been used for flat warts, particularly on the face to minimize scarring.[93]

Immunotherapy

The use of topical sensitizing agents such as dinitrochlorobenzene, squaric acid dibutylester (SADBE), and diphenylcyclopropenone is also popular for recalcitrant large nongenital warts. Immunotherapy usually involves initial sensitization of the patient to an agent, followed by applications of the same chemical to the wart to elicit a contact dermatitis at the base of the wart. The mechanism of contact immunotherapy may be related to induction of type IV hypersensitivity or cell-mediated immunity in the wart-infected tissue, resulting in wart destruction.[94] It probably involves a non–wart antigen specific cell-mediated process. Furthermore, complement-binding wart antibodies in 15% of patients before treatment rose to 43% after therapy.[95]

DNCB has been used frequently in the past. Two percent of DNCB in acetone can be applied to an inconspicuous area on the body for 24 to 48 hours, covered with a bandage, to sensitize the patient.[96] The area then usually becomes erythematous, with blister formation. In 2 weeks after sensitivity develops, 0.1% DNCB in petrolatum is applied to the wart with a cotton-tipped applicator two or three times a week.[96] This procedure may be repeated for an average of 3 to 6 weeks. DNCB therapy has about an 80% cure rate, with low recurrence rates and a low incidence of scarring. It is particularly effective for large, recurrent, recalcitrant periungual, plantar mosaic, and flat warts. Complications may include localized or severe generalized dermatitis and urticaria, pruritus, blistering, and, rarely, secondary infection. DNCB is no longer used in industry, but cross-reaction with other chemicals may occur. There are concerns of the mutagenicity of DNCB in the Ames test, although it has been used safely in the part for wart treatment.

SADBE and diphenylcyclopropenone may be used without concern for mutagenicity, although they are both unstable compounds. SADBE must be refrigerated because of its tendency to undergo hydrolysis, and diphenylcyclopropenone must be stored in both a dark glass and dark place to prevent photodecomposition.[94] A 0.1% diphenylcyclopropenone solution in acetone may be used to sensitize the patient, followed by applications to the wart with a sequence of increasing strengths at weekly intervals. A 0.01% concentration is initiated and followed by 0.025%, 0.1%, 0.5%, and finally, 1.0%.[94]

Cimetidine has been demonstrated to possess immunomodulatory activity and has been reported to be useful in treating warts in children. The mechanism is believed to be increased mitogen-induced lymphocyte proliferation and inhibition of T-suppressor cells. Dosage has ranged from 25 to 40 mg/kg/day, divided into three or four doses. In most patients, little change is seen at 1 month, but it has been reported that at 6 to 7 weeks, warts suddenly start to disappear in more patients.[97] In this study, warts entirely cleared after 2 months in 26 of 30 (81%) children. Cimetidine is not specifically approved for use in children less than 16 years old; nevertheless, no untoward reactions were seen in the study mentioned. Physicians should be aware that cimetidine may interact with other drugs such as phenytoin and theophylline. Recently, efficacy has been reported to be minimal to none.[98]

Seborrheic Dermatitis

DEFINITION

Seborrheic dermatitis is a chronic, inflammatory, erythematous, and scaling eruption.

EPIDEMIOLOGY

Seborrheic dermatitis is a common problem, and the onset is correlated with sebaceous gland activity. During infancy, it is commonly called cradle cap, and spontaneous remission tends to occur by 1 year of age. After this age, the disease is rare until puberty. In infants, seborrheic dermatitis may become generalized to form an exfoliative erythroderma known as erythroderma desquamativum, or Leiner's disease. Infants often have diarrhea, infection, and a failure to thrive. In adults, seborrheic dermatitis has a predilection for men and is more severe in the winter. The disorder is often asymptomatic, but pruritus is not uncommon and at times can be intense.

PATHOPHYSIOLOGY

Seborrheic dermatitis is characterized by an increased epidermal cell turnover. The active ingredient of many antiseborrheic agents, such as coal tar, zinc pyrithione, and selenium sulfide, inhibits mitotic activity. It was once thought that this cytostatic effect was responsible for alleviating the scaling. Although no evidence establishes increased cell turnover as the primary defect, zinc pyrithione, selenium sulfide, and sulfur and salicylic acid preparations all kill yeast. Evidence now suggests that the hyperproliferative state may be secondary to the presence of a lipophilic, pleomorphic fungus, *Pityrosporum ovale*.[99,100] When oral and topical ketoconazole, an imidazole derivative effective against *Pityrosporum*, is used in seborrheic dermatitis, the condition improves.[101] Improvement was correlated with a reduction in the number of yeast organisms. This was confirmed using a precipitated sulfur and salicylic acid preparation.[102] The correlation of seborrheic dermatitis with sebaceous gland activity is thought to result from the importance of sebum on *P. ovale* growth. This observation explains variations in disease activity at certain body sites and the greater prevalence in men because androgens stimulate sebum production. Finally, the pathologic increase in the residual pool of sebum caused by immobility could explain the frequent occurrence of seborrheic dermatitis in patients with a variety of neurologic disorders such as idiopathic and neuroleptic-induced Parkinson's disease.[103]

CLINICAL PRESENTATION AND DIAGNOSIS

Seborrheic dermatitis is recognized by its characteristic distribution on the body. Seborrheic areas include the scalp, eyebrows, glabella, eyelid margins (often with marginal blepharitis and conjunctivitis), cheeks, paranasal areas, nasolabial folds, beard area, presternal area, central back, retroauricular creases, and the external ear canal. Other less commonly involved areas include the axillae, inframammary areas, umbilicus, groin, and intergluteal cleft. Seborrheic dermatitis in the intertriginous areas may exist alone or in conjunction with other seborrheic areas. Similarly, psoriasis may occasionally have an intertriginous distribution, called inverse psoriasis, along with scalp involvement. In this form, it has been designated as seborrhiasis.

The scales of seborrheic dermatitis vary from a dry to thick powdery form, with little to no erythema, to an oily form with greasy or oily scales, and crusts on an erythematous base. The former usually is located on the scalp and is called simple dandruff. The greasier scales are found more commonly on the ears and central face such as the glabella, eyebrows, and nasolabial folds.

TREATMENT

The mainstay of treating seborrheic dermatitis of the scalp is shampoos. Sulfur and salicylic acid (Sebulex), coal tar (Denorex), 1% selenium sulfide (Selsun Blue), and zinc pyrithione (Head and Shoulders) are available over the counter, but the most effective antifungal agents are 2.5% selenium sulfide and 2% ketoconazole, which can be obtained by prescription.[104] The choice of shampoos depends on several factors, including physician and patient preference, cost, and cosmetic appeal to the patient. Depending on the severity of the disease, shampoos can be applied daily to twice weekly. Patients should be reminded that the scalp (not the hair) is being treated, so the patient should allow the shampoo to penetrate for at least 5 minutes before rinsing.

With the exception of accidental oral ingestion, systemic adverse reactions are minimal. Local adverse reactions include skin irritation (usually from the vehicle), occasional reports of hair loss, and discoloration of hair, especially from selenium sulfide and coal tar. As with other shampoos, oiliness or dryness of the hair and scalp may occur. Topical corticosteroid lotions can be added if lesions are very inflammatory and pruritic. A 1% hydrocortisone lotion, applied one to three times daily, is usually safe and effective. Stronger preparations such as 0.025% triamcinolone lotion, 0.01% fluocinolone acetonide solution, 0.05% clobetasol solution, or 0.1% betamethasone valerate lotion may be needed for more severe instances, but they should be used only for very short periods. For thick, crusted, and scaly lesions, a mixture of liquid petrolatum, sodium chloride, and phenol can be applied overnight and rinsed off in the morning. Other preparations that use a similar application schedule include various concentrations of sulfur and salicylic acid in an ointment base.

Other seborrheic areas of the body, including the scalp line, eyebrows, glabella, ears, and nasolabial area, can be treated successfully with 2% ketoconazole cream applied twice a day. Other antifungals, such as terbinafine, have been shown to be effective both topically and orally.[100] Other alternatives include 1 to 2.5% hydrocortisone cream or 0.5% desonide applied two to three times a day. If there is scaling in the auditory meatus, a polymyxin B–hydrocortisone suspension, or 0.5% desonide and 2% acetic acid, four drops three to four times a day is effective. The pruritus that sometimes accompanies the scaling is also relieved. Topical steroids should not be used for seborrheic blepharitis because of the potential to induce glaucoma and cataracts. Hot compresses and gentle debridement and a cotton-tipped applicator and 2% ketoconazole shampoo one or more times daily usually are effective. If the lid margins are severely inflamed, topical antibiotic ointments may be added.

Special considerations must be made for infants with seborrheic dermatitis. Tar preparations should be avoided for fear they will rub it into their eyes. Topical corticosteroids should be limited to 0.5 to 1% hydrocortisone to avoid hypothalamic-pituitary-adrenal (HPA) axis suppression. However, 2% ketoconazole cream should be the treatment of choice for infantile seborrheic dermatitis because of its minimal percutaneous absorption and lack of accumulation in the plasma.[101,105]

Psoriasis

DEFINITION

Psoriasis is an inflammatory disorder characterized by erythematous scaling plaques on virtually any area of the skin surface.

EPIDEMIOLOGY

The disease affects approximately 2% of the general population in the United States. It ranks third after acne and warts as the reason for the most office visits to a dermatologist. Psoriasis occurs with equal frequency in both sexes. It may be symptomatic throughout life and be progressive with age or wax and wane in severity. The condition can be present at birth, and an onset was reported at age 108 years. Most patients develop the initial lesions of psoriasis in the third decade of life. Symptoms appear in men at a mean age of 29 and in women at a mean age of 27. With earlier onset, there is a greater probability of a positive family history of psoriasis.

The morbidity associated with this disease is great. Psoriasis can cause functional impairment, skin disfigurement, and emotional distress. Severe involvement of the hands, feet, and nails may make even routine activities, such as walking or dressing, difficult, particularly in patients with severe psoriatic arthritis. As many as 30% of patients with psoriasis may have arthritis, and 5 to 10% of those patients may experience functional disability. Therefore, psoriasis directly affects the quality of life and may cause difficulty in work performance, problems with social rejection, sexual dysfunction, and depression.

There is no agreement about the cause of psoriasis, but increased epidermal cell proliferation and inflammation have been observed. In psoriatic lesions, cell proliferation is 12 times the normal rate, with a twofold increase in proliferation in uninvolved skin. The increased rate found in uninvolved skin suggests a generalized skin abnormality in psoriasis. As a result of the hyperproliferative state, epidermal turnover and transit times are greatly reduced.

PATHOPHYSIOLOGY

A key feature of newly formed psoriatic lesions is the attraction and migration of inflammatory cells, especially neutrophils. It is now believed that an inflammatory process is the primary cause of the disease.[106] Additional evidence suggests a genetic predisposition linked to chromosome 6P.[107] Many factors have been linked to the exacerbation of psoriasis, including infections; winter weather; drugs such as lithium, β-blockers, antimalarials, nonsteroidal anti-inflammatory drugs, and corticosteroid withdrawal; stress; obesity; alcoholism; and dry, cracked skin.

CLINICAL PRESENTATION AND DIAGNOSIS

Psoriatic lesions are observed most commonly on the scalp, elbows, knees, trunk, and nails. The primary lesion is an erythematous plaque covered with silvery scales. Scale removal may show punctate bleeding points, called Auspitz sign, which help differentiate psoriasis from other chronic dermatoses. Several well-recognized clinical variants involve particular treatment modalities.

Plaque-type psoriasis usually is located on the extensor surfaces of elbows and knees, the lumbar region of the back, and the scalp. Guttate psoriasis, with small, scaly, teardrop-shaped lesions, classically follows group A streptococcal pharyngitis. Inverse psoriasis is a form of psoriasis that often involves exclusively body folds such as the axillae, groin, inframammary folds, navel, intergluteal crease, and glans penis. Palmoplantar differs from plaque-type psoriasis in the variability of erythema, the loss of sharply marginated plaques, and replacement of the characteristic silvery scales by thickened, fissured hyperkeratosis. Erythrodermic psoriasis is an acute inflammatory, erythematous, scaling disorder involving the entire skin surface. Pustular psoriasis can be localized to the palms and soles or be generalized and may appear after withdrawal of corticosteroid therapy given inappropriately for plaque-type psoriasis. Erythrodermic and generalized pustular psoriasis may be life-threatening because of systemic infections or cardiovascular or pulmonary complications. For example, in patients with preexisting cardiovascular disease, the erythroderma may precipitate high-output congestive heart failure or arrhythmia.[108]

THERAPEUTIC PLAN

The hyperproliferative and inflammatory bases of the disease offer two different therapeutic approaches. Most pharmacologic interventions act by modifying one or both of these processes. Therapeutic consideration must also be given to the type of psoriasis, the extent and location of involvement, and the psychological impact of the disease. Because psoriasis varies in its severity, a stepped-care approach can be used (Fig. 46.2). In the first step, side effects are minimal. If treatment resistance is encountered or if the disease is more severe, the second step includes adding or changing to another form of therapy. Each step in the level of care carries an increased risk of side effects. Therefore, the risk:benefit ratio must be assessed before proceeding to the next program. When a patient reaches the highest step in the program, the therapy can be rotated for certain periods of time to minimize life-threatening side effects (Fig. 46.3).

TREATMENT

Pharmacotherapy

Emollients and Keratolytics

Emollient agents hydrate the stratum corneum and prevent the increased transepidermal water loss observed in psoriasis. The hydrating effect softens the stratum corneum and assists in desquamation; the overall effect is moisturizing the skin. An occlusive oily film delivered to the skin surface seals the transepidermal water into the stratum corneum. With water retained in the skin, the stratum corneum becomes more pliable, preventing fissuring and scaling in hyperkeratotic areas. Skin hydration also decreases the binding forces within the stratum corneum and facilitates desquamation.

Most emollient agents are mineral oils and paraffins in an oil-in-water emulsion with emulsifiers, stabilizers, and antimicrobial preservatives. Humectants may be added to the emollient to enhance its water-retaining qualities. These include glycerin, urea, or pyrrolidone carboxylic acid, which hold water within the stratum corneum hygroscopically. Emollients in oil-in-water emulsion can be cosmetically acceptable, but the more oily or occlusive the preparation, the more effective the moisturizer. Some patients may find the oily feeling unacceptable. Therefore, patients should be allowed input into the selection of emollients.

Patients should be instructed to apply the emollients

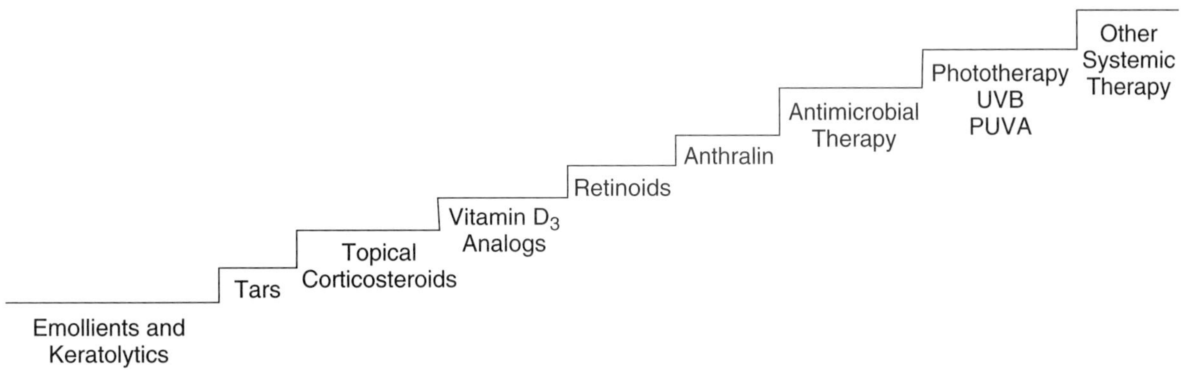

Figure 46.2. Stepped-care approach to psoriasis. Note that as one ascends to each level of therapy, the risk of more serious side effects increases. *PUVA,* psoralen ultraviolet A; *UVB,* ultraviolet B.

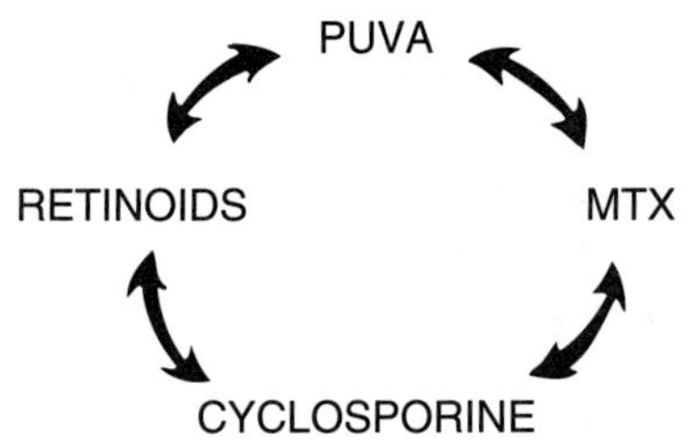

Figure 46.3. Rotation among higher levels of therapy to reduce the incidence of life-threatening side effects. *MTX*, methotrexate; *PUVA*, psoralen ultraviolet A.

three or more times a day. Side effects from frequent application may be acneiform folliculitis or an exacerbation of existing acne from occlusion of the follicular openings. Occlusion of the sweat ducts may produce miliaria, especially in hot and humid climates. Adding urea or lactic acid may produce a stinging sensation, unrelated to any toxic reaction to the skin, whose cause is not known. An occasional problem (as with any topical agent) is allergic contact dermatitis from the contents of the emulsifying agent or its antimicrobial preservatives.

Keratolytic agents promote desquamation of scales. Salicylic acid is the most frequently used keratolytic agent. Concentrations ranging from 2 to 20% are formulated in a variety of ways. For smaller, thinner scaling plaques or for healing patches, a 2% concentration in an ointment base is used. A lotion base, which is excellent for scalp applications, may have up to 6% salicylic acid. Higher concentrations are used for thicker and hyperkeratotic plaques, and concentrations above 6% show marked keratolytic activity. Lactic acid in concentrations of 5 to 12% can also be used to reduce scaling. A popular combination of keratolytics is 6% salicylic acid in 60% propylene glycol with 20% ethyl alcohol. The preparation is applied under occlusion at night to hydrate the skin and remove thick, adherent scales. During the day, topical steroids can be applied to enhance percutaneous penetration and healing. Salicylic acid at concentrations of 2 to 6% is used with tar in creams, ointments, and shampoos. The combination is very efficacious, but preparations are dark gray or brown, may stain clothing, and have an unpleasant smell, causing problems with patient compliance.

Side effects include allergic contact dermatitis to the vehicle and soreness of the treated area. The latter can be alleviated by discontinuing the treatment. Potential side effects of salicylic acid are tinnitus, nausea, and hyperventilation. These systemic side effects are more likely to occur when large areas of damaged skin are exposed to higher concentrations.[109,110]

Tars

The mechanism of action of coal tar is not known. It is currently believed to have antimitotic effects. The initial application of coal tars to normal skin transiently increases epidermal proliferation for the first 2 weeks of treatment. If the coal tar is continued for up to 40 days, a cytostatic effect eventually produces epidermal thinning. Coal tars in combination with UVA light produce photoadducts that inhibit DNA synthesis.

Coal tar is effective monotherapy, and although it takes longer to clear the psoriasis than other treatments, prolonged remission can be expected. Compliance is difficult because of odor, staining, and irritation. To reduce these problems, extracts or refined products of crude coal tar in a 10% concentration with alcohol may be used. This preparation, called liquor carbonis detergens, is incorporated into various cream-based vehicles and bath additives. Coal tar preparations can be applied once or twice a day, but patients should be warned of irritation to the groin, axillae, and periorbital region. Side effects include photosensitivity, acneiform eruptions, and folliculitis.[111] There is potential for an increased risk of skin cancer and internal malignancies with the chronic use of topical coal tars. Mutagenic substances in coal tars are absorbed percutaneously and excreted in urine.[112] The risk of skin carcinoma in patients treated with coal tar does not appear to be higher than in the general population. Reports of combined coal tar and UVR yield mixed results.[113]

Topical Corticosteroids

Topical corticosteroids are the most frequently prescribed medications for psoriasis. They can be used alone or in combination with other agents. Several modes of action probably are important in explaining their antipsoriatic activity. The hyperproliferative response is altered by a reduction in DNA synthesis and epidermal mitoses. There is a reduction in phospholipase A activity, which decreases arachidonic acid production and ultimately affects the production of inflammatory mediators LTB4 and HETE.

Topical corticosteroids also cause vasoconstriction, and the vasoconstrictive properties correlate well with clinical efficacy and are used to rank preparations in order of anti-inflammatory potency (Table 46.9).[114] The broad range of potency results in part from chemical modifications of hydrocortisone. When the molecule is esterified with valerate, dipropionate, or acetonide groups, the potency increases dramatically from increased penetration to the skin. Penetration can also be increased 10- to 100-fold by an occlusive dressing. However, HPA axis suppression is more common when a potent preparation is used. The potency of a corticosteroid preparation can be altered by its vehicle. Gels generally are more effective than ointments, and ointments have greater biological activity than the same corticosteroid in creams or lotions. Creams generally are more effective than lotions.

Ointments can be used on thick, scaly plaques, but they should be avoided in the axillae and groin, where folliculitis may develop secondary to rubbing and maceration. In the intertriginous areas, creams are a better choice. For the scalp and other hairy areas, gels, lotions, or sprays are preferable to ointments and creams.

Table 46.9 ▪ Potency Ranking of Topical Corticosteroids

Superpotent	Augmented betamethasone dipropionate 0.05% ointment
	Clobetasol propionate 0.05% cream and ointment
	Diflorasone diacetate 0.05% ointment
	Halobetasol propionate 0.5% cream and ointment
Potent	Amcinonide 0.1% cream, lotion, and ointment
	Augmented betamethasone dipropionate 0.05% cream
	Betamethasone dipropionate 0.05% cream and ointment
	Betamethasone valerate 0.1% ointment
	Desoximetasone 0.25% cream, ointment, and 0.05% gel
	Diflorasone diacetate 0.05% cream and ointment (emollient base)
	Fluocinolone acetonide 0.2% cream
	Fluocinonide 0.5% cream, ointment, and gel
	Halcinonide 0.1% cream and ointment
	Triamcinolone acetonide 0.5% cream and ointment
Midstrength	Betamethasone benzoate 0.025% cream, gel, and lotion
	Betamethasone dipropionate 0.025 lotion
	Betamethasone valerate 0.1% cream
	Clocortolone pivalate 0.1% cream
	Desoximetasone 0.05% cream
	Fluocinolone acetonide 0.025% cream and ointment
	Flurandrenolide 0.025 and 0.05% cream and ointment and 0.05% lotion
	Fluticasone propionate 0.05% cream and 0.005% ointment
	Hydrocortisone butyrate 0.1% ointment and solution
	Hydrocortisone valerate 0.2% cream and ointment
	Mometasone 0.1% cream, ointment, and lotion
	Triamcinolone acetonide 0.025% and 0.1% cream, ointment, and lotion
Mild	Alclometasone dipropionate 0.05% cream and ointment
	Betamethasone valerate 0.05% lotion
	Desonide 0.05% cream
	Dexamethasone 0.01% and 0.04% aerosol
	Dexamethasone sodium phosphate 0.1% cream
	Fluocinolone acetonide 0.01% cream and solution
	Hydrocortisone, dexamethasone, flumethasone, prednisolone, methylprednisolone in all vehicles

Topical corticosteroids usually are applied twice a day. Applications once or twice a day are as effective as multiple applications, and less frequent applications prevent tachyphylaxis and other side effects.

The incidence of side effects is increased by use of high-potency preparations; application to areas of thin skin such as the face, scrotum, vulva, or intertriginous areas; application to areas where the skin barrier is compromised; and the use of occlusive dressings. Children and patients with renal failure are more susceptible to side effects. To lessen both local and systemic side effects, a weaker potency should be used on the face or in intertriginous areas. On areas of the body that need higher-potency corticosteroids, the preparation should be reduced to a lower strength after plaque clearing begins. Local side effects include striae and atrophy, skin fragility producing bruising, poor wound healing, telangiectasia, acneiform eruptions, pigmentary abnormalities, and allergic contact dermatitis.

Topical steroids can mask clinically inapparent dermatophyte infections. Fluorinated corticosteroids and hydrocortisone butyrate and acetate used on the face commonly result in perioral dermatitis and acne rosacea–like eruptions. As in the systemic administration of corticosteroids, withdrawing potent topical preparations can change a stable plaque-type psoriasis to a pustular form. On the other hand, chronic use can precipitate an erythrodermic flare, especially if topical steroids have been applied to extensive areas of the body surface.

Applications to large areas are more likely to produce systemic side effects, including HPA axis suppression on dosages as small as 2 g/day, glucose intolerance, and (rarely) Cushing's syndrome. HPA axis suppression is reversible after short-term use of potent preparations. Topical corticosteroids should be used with caution around the eyes. Systemic absorption at this site can produce glaucoma, cataracts, or an exacerbation of an ocular infection.[115]

Vitamin D_3

Calcitriol (1,25-dihydroxycholecalciferol) is the active form of vitamin D_3. The skin has receptors for circulating calcitriol, and when bound, keratinocyte proliferation is inhibited and basal cells are induced to differentiate to squamous cells. In vitro, cultured cells from psoriatic skin exhibit a partial resistance to these effects of calcitriol, which is overcome by large increases in calcitriol concentrations. Clinical studies have confirmed the effectiveness of both topical and systemic calcitriol. Unfortunately, the limiting factor is hypercalcemia from systemic administration. However, topical therapy has been well tolerated, with few or no side effects in treating localized psoriasis.[116]

A synthetic analog of calcitriol, calcipotriol, is an effective topical alternative to corticosteroids for psoriasis, without changes in serum levels of ionized calcium. Like calcitriol, calcipotriol shows receptor binding and effects on cell differentiation, but calcipotriol is 100 times less potent in its effect on calcium metabolism.[117] A thin layer of the ointment preparation is applied to the affected areas twice daily for 8 weeks; improvement usually begins after 2 weeks. Patients should be instructed to use no more than 100 g/week. Adverse reactions include burning, itching, and skin irritation in 10 to 15% of patients. Erythema, dry skin, and worsening of psoriasis, including development of face and scalp psoriasis, have been reported in 1 to 10% of patients. Less than 1% of patients develop hypercalcemia. Calcipotriene is the newest topical vitamin D_3 analog on the market.

Retinoids

Two synthetic analogs of vitamin A, etretinate and acitretin, have been used to treat psoriasis. Etretinate, an aromatic retinoid, has been available for clinical use in the United States since 1986. Acitretin is an acid metabolite of etretinate with different pharmacokinetics. Acitretin has a shorter half-life and is not stored in subcutaneous fat like etretinate. The exact mechanism of action on psoriasis is not known, but its various effects on cellular differentiation may cause normalization of keratinization and proliferation. Retinoids also have an anti-inflammatory effect by reducing the levels of leukotriene and HETE. Because adverse side effects are greater than those from topical therapies, UVB, and psoralen UVA (PUVA), retinoids should be reserved for psoriasis recalcitrant to these treatments. The usual starting dosage is 0.75 to 1.0 mg/kg/day in divided doses. A maximum dosage of 1.5 mg/kg/day is recommended, and after 8 to 16 weeks of therapy, a maintenance dosage of 0.5 to 0.75 mg/kg/day is needed.[118] Side effects are similar to those seen with hypervitaminosis A syndrome. Among the major side effects are the embryotoxic and teratogenic effects on animal models and humans. Women of childbearing age must use contraception, which should be continued for 2 years after completing treatment. Acitretin may be of more benefit than etretinate in these patients. Other side effects include elevation of triglyceride or cholesterol levels, mucocutaneous changes such as cheilitis, hepatotoxicity, and musculoskeletal changes.[119] Tazarotene is a new topical retinoid approved for use in the United States. It is dosed once daily and is marketed as a 0.05% and 0.1% gel. It probably should be used in combination with high-potency topical corticosteroids to increase efficacy and reduce irritation. Systemic retinoids should be reserved for psoriasis recalcitrant to topical therapy.[120]

Anthralin

Anthralin, or dithranol, is a topical treatment that has not achieved the popularity in the United States that it has in Britain and Europe. The compound, 1,8-tri-hydroxy-anthracene, has several modes of action, but inhibition of mitochondrial DNA synthesis and various cellular enzymes may be the main reasons for its clinical effectiveness. The overall effect is antiproliferative on the epidermis, which decreases mitoses to normalize the epidermal architecture.[111]

Commercial preparations of anthralin ointment and creams are available in concentrations of 0.1 to 1%. Anthralin is oxidized easily by exposure to air. Salicylic acid in concentrations ranging from 0.2 to 0.4% often is added to a preparation called Lassar's paste to increase its shelf life. Lassar's paste consists of anthralin in concentrations ranging from 0.1 to 5% mixed into zinc oxide paste, with paraffin as a hardener and salicylic acid. This stiff paste is used in the Ingram method for treating large, chronic, plaque-type psoriasis. The treatment program begins with a tar bath and UVB phototherapy, followed by Lassar's paste application to the plaques. Talc or cornstarch is applied to the paste, which sets the paste and absorbs excess moisture, to prevent smearing. This is to prevent local irritation when anthralin comes in contact with normal skin. A soft, loose garment such as pajamas or a sweatsuit can be worn over the paste. The paste is left on for 4 to 12 hours and often can be left on overnight. It is removed with a cloth and light mineral oil or baby oil, and the excess is washed off in a shower or bath with soap. Lower concentrations of anthralin, from 0.1 to 1%, are used initially, but higher concentrations of up to 5% are needed as the psoriasis improves.

As the skin barrier is restored with clinical improvement, higher concentrations of anthralin are needed to provide adequate levels in the epidermis for continued therapeutic efficacy. This clinical observation and the fact that anthralin penetrates more rapidly through the altered stratum corneum of psoriasis led to short-contact therapy. Low concentrations of anthralin ointment (0.1 to 0.5%) are left on for 60 minutes or more, whereas higher concentrations (1%) may be left on for only 10 to 20 minutes. Anthralin is then removed with mineral oil, followed by a shower with soap and water. Short-contact anthralin therapy is effective for well-motivated, intelligent patients and can be used daily on an outpatient basis. Improvement is expected to occur in approximately 3 weeks. The advantages of short-contact therapy over the Ingram method are reductions in both irritation and staining of clothing because earlier washings reduce penetration and irritation in nonlesional skin. Penetration of anthralin through the plaques is far greater and peaks much earlier than in normal skin, maintaining clinical efficacy.[121] The inflammation and staining of clothing can be eliminated by the application of 10% triethanolamine in an aqueous cream. This is applied immediately after short-contact therapy, without interfering with the therapeutic effect.[122]

Anthralin should not be used on the face because of the potential for eye irritation. Intertriginous areas, especially the antecubital and popliteal fossae, axillae, retroauricular, and inguinal folds, as well as the inner thighs should be avoided. Hair and nails may show discoloration, but low anthralin concentrations, short exposure time, and pretreatment with neutral henna to coat the hair prevent anthralin penetration into the hair shaft. Nail polish can prevent anthralin penetration of the nail plate. No systemic toxic effects are associated with topical anthralin use, and contact allergy is rare.[110]

Antimicrobial Therapy

Antimicrobial therapy has been included in the American Academy of Dermatology revised guidelines for treating psoriasis.[123] Antimicrobial psoriasis treatment includes oral and topical antifungals and antibacterials. This therapy is based on accumulating evidence suggesting that psoriasis is aggravated by cutaneous or systemic microbial infections or colonization and that the inflammatory and hyperproliferative response is a direct result of microbial products activating the alternate complement pathway. Patients with psoriasis are believed to inherit a heightened immune responsiveness to the alternate complement pathway to produce their disease.[124] Over the years, the literature has cited frequent associations of psoriasis with streptococcal infections. The most common association is the guttate variant seen in children and young adults. Patients with throat culture or serologic evidence of group A streptococcus have good to excellent clearing of their disease when treated with rifampin in combination with oral penicillin or erythromycin.[125]

Other indications for antimicrobial treatment include various topical imidazole and nystatin antifungal agents for *Candida albicans*–associated diaper psoriasis in infants, oral ketoconazole for scalp psoriasis, and topical 2% erythromycin ointment for inverse psoriasis, especially in the gluteal fold. Detailed accounts of the approach to antimicrobial treatment of psoriasis are outlined in another text.[126]

Phototherapy

Phototherapy, either alone or in combination with other treatments, can be used for moderate to severe psoriasis. The UV spectrum is of interest in psoriasis. Within the UV spectrum, UVB (290 and 320 nm, and particularly 313 nm) is beneficial in healing psoriasis. The UVA spectrum (320 to 400 nm), by itself, is not effective, but when used with psoralen (PUVA), either orally or topically, it is effective. This combination is called photochemotherapy.

Phototherapy is indicated in patients who do not respond to topical therapy or when psoriasis is widespread. Patients should be selected carefully for phototherapy and excluded if they have psoriasis that is worsened by sunlight or a history of photosensitizing disorder or if they are taking drugs that are known to photosensitize. Phototherapy can be used on an outpatient basis to produce long-lasting remission. UVB can also be used at home, but PUVA therapy should be supervised by a dermatologist familiar with photochemotherapy.[127]

Ultraviolet B

If UVB is used as monotherapy, the best results are obtained when erythemogenic dosages are used on nonlesional skin. In calculating the initial dosage, the patient's skin type is considered. This is estimated on the patient's ability to sunburn and tan and is called the minimal erythema dosage (MED), expressed in meters per square centimeter. A test grid is performed on the back using the initial dosage, and the skin is examined 24 hours later. If the skin does not show a pink outline of the grid, the dosage of light is increased by 15 to 20% of the initial dosage. The dosage that causes minimal erythema at 24 hours produces the optimal effect in clearing psoriasis. From the MED, time spent in the UVB cabinet can be calculated. In addition to time spent exposed to UVB, the dosage is determined by the intensity of radiation. Intensity varies with the inverse square of the distance from the radiation source, so the distance between the patient and the light source must be considered. Although this may not be a problem in UVB cabinets because of physical constraints, some patients use UVB fluorescent tubes at home where the patient's distance from the light source affects the therapeutic response. Various protocols have been developed, but the most common outpatient protocol is three times a week using variable exposure increments of MED with the application of emollients. Most patients clear with 18 treatments using this protocol.[127]

UVB combined with crude coal tar is more effective than either agent alone. This combination, known as the Goeckerman regimen, uses crude coal tar at concentrations of 1 to 5% applied during the evening. Because the tar layer prevents the UV light from reaching the skin, it should be removed in the morning using mineral oil before exposure to a suberythemogenic dosage of UVB. It was once thought that the UVB would act on the tar to produce photoadducts, but (as previously stated) the photosensitizing wavelength of tar is in the UVB spectrum. Furthermore, UVB does not enhance the tar-induced suppression of DNA synthesis by epidermal cells, so the reason for its synergy is not known.

A more popular treatment regimen used in the United Kingdom and in continental Europe is the Ingram method, in which the tar bath and UVB radiation are followed by the application of anthralin in Lassar's paste directly onto the plaques. There are no advantages to adding anthralin to the UVB therapy, and with the potential for irritation and staining of clothing, this may be a reason the Goeckerman regimen is used more often in the United States.

A major side effect of UVB therapy is burning from excessive exposure. Sunscreen, zinc oxide, or cloth can be applied to the affected areas to prevent further burning. To prevent UV-induced conjunctival erosions, protective goggles are worn during treatment. Although premature aging of the skin is dose dependent, tar and UVB used in the described manner seem to show no increase in skin cancers.[128]

Photochemotherapy

Photochemotherapy consists of an oral dose of a photoactive drug (a psoralen), followed 2 hours later by exposure to UVA. The psoralens are thought to produce photoadducts from the absorption of UVA. The photochemically induced covalent binding of the psoralen to the pyrimidine bases in DNA inhibits its synthesis and cell replication. Psoralen belongs to the furocoumarin class of compounds. The two derivatives currently available in the United States are 8-methoxypsoralen (methoxsalen, 8-MOP) and 4,5′,8-trimethylpsoralen (trioxsalen, TMP). The third psoralen, 5-methoxypsoralen (bergapten, 5-MOP), is being investigated for clinical use in the United States but is available in Europe.

8-MOP is more potent in causing suppression of DNA synthesis than the other compounds and is the main psoralen in dermatologic use at this time. 8-MOP is administered in a dosage of 0.3 to 0.6 mg/kg. When 8-MOP is administered orally, the blood levels peak at 2 hours, producing maximum sensitivity to UVA. Blood levels can be increased by a low-fat meal. The highest tissue concentrations are found in the gastrointestinal tract, liver, blood, and skin. In the blood, 84% is bound to serum albumin, and tolbutamide can displace the drug from the binding sites to increase the free fraction of 8-MOP. As a result of the displacement, the free fraction of 8-MOP, can produce photosensitivity. 8-MOP is metabolized through the liver by several pathways, including hydroxylation, glucuronide formation, epoxidation, and hydrolysis.

The patient's skin type guides selection of the starting dosage of UVA. Treatment is administered once every other day because the erythema induced by PUVA may not be evident for up to 48 hours after exposure. In general, the dosage of UVA is increased by 1.5 J/cm^2 for each consecutive treatment. Unlike with UVB therapy, the time to produce clearing with UVA is longer, usually after 10 to 20 treatments over 4 to 8 weeks. Once clearing has been achieved, the UVA dosage is held constant. Maintenance therapy must be used because PUVA is only a palliative treatment. The same dosage of UVA that induced clearing is used, but the frequency of treatment is reduced gradually to twice a month.[129]

Topical psoralens combined with UVA, known as bathwater PUVA, is a very popular method in Scandinavia. It can be effective for both extensive plaque-type psoriasis and selected parts of the body, such as the hands and feet. This method avoids the gastric side effects of oral psoralens and is ideal for patients with hepatic impairment. The patient soaks in a bath containing a very low concentration of psoralen before exposure to UVA. TMP usually is used because it has less percutaneous absorption than 8-MOP, but this method carries a greater risk of photosensitivity. To reduce the amount of UVA exposure and the number of treatments, oral retinoid agents, such as etretinate, can be used along with PUVA. Although the mechanism of synergism is not known, it does not seem to involve the increased photosensitivity seen with the retinoid agents.[129] Aside from the erythema and blistering, other acute side effects include pruritus and nausea. Shielding with a drape or sunscreens during subsequent UVA exposure prevents further erythema, and the duration of UVA exposure can be reduced. Pruritus can be controlled with emollients or topical steroids. Dividing the psoralen into two doses given 1 hour apart can reduce the incidence of nausea. A less desirable alternative, especially for severe refractory nausea, is to reduce the dosage and increase the UVA exposure. A potential chronic complication of PUVA therapy is the development of cataracts. The renal excretion of psoralens usually is completed within 8 hours, but eliminating a psoralen from the lens of the eye takes about 24 hours. When UVA from natural sunlight reaches psoralens in the lens, there is a theoretical possibility of binding to the protein and DNA of the lens. Although the risk is small, this complication can be nearly eliminated by wearing UVA-blocking wraparound glasses for 12 to 24 hours after ingesting psoralen. Other more common chronic side effects include a dose-dependent increased incidence of squamous cell carcinoma and lentigines.[129,130]

Systemic Corticosteroid Therapy

Systemic corticosteroid therapy for psoriasis is included here to emphasize that it is not the treatment of choice because of the many side effects associated with prolonged administration and because of the potential severe rebound side effect. There is a potential for conversion of stable plaque-type psoriasis into a pustular flare after withdrawal of corticosteroid therapy.[131]

Methotrexate

Methotrexate (MTX) is a folic acid antagonist that inhibits dihydrofolate reductase, blocking key steps in DNA and RNA synthesis. Initially, MTX was thought to reduce the rapid keratinocyte proliferation that occurs in psoriasis, but it now appears that the primary effect of the drug is on cutaneous inflammation.[132] MTX taken orally is rapidly absorbed through the gastrointestinal tract, but peak levels occur more slowly than in intramuscular or intravenous routes. It is excreted through the kidneys almost unchanged, and the clearance of MTX correlates with endogenous creatinine clearance. However, a small amount is excreted by active tubular secretion. MTX is 50 to 70% bound to albumin and may be displaced by acidic drugs such as phenylbutazone, sulfonamides, salicylates, tetracycline, chloramphenicol, and phenytoin. A potential for toxicity exists when these are used in combination with MTX, especially if renal excretion is impaired. Weak organic acids such as salicylates, probenecid, ketoprofen, and phenylbutazone can compete with MTX to prolong its active tubular secretion. Furthermore, direct renal toxicity occurs with the concomitant use of MTX and indomethacin. Therefore, both agents should be used cautiously in patients with psoriatic arthritis who have poor renal function.[133]

The FDA has approved MTX for use in severe, recalcitrant psoriasis. However, patient selection for MTX should take into account not only the characteristics of the disease, but also the socioeconomic impact to the patient and absolute and relative contraindications. The only absolute contraindications are pregnancy and lactation. Relative contraindications can be waived only when the probable benefits of therapy outweigh the potential risks. One relative contraindication that needs further elaboration is alcohol abuse. With chronic MTX administration, hepatotoxicity resulting in fibrosis and cirrhosis is a serious concern. Alcoholism significantly increases the risk of hepatotoxicity, and MTX should not be used in patients who abuse alcohol.

The usual oral dosage of MTX is 10 to 20 mg in either a single weekly dose or divided into three doses given 12 hours apart once weekly. A test dose of 5 to 10 mg is given, and a compete blood count and liver function test are done 7 days later. In general, 75 to 80% of patients with psoriasis respond within 4 weeks. If no response occurs, the dosage is increased by 2.5 to 5.0 mg/week. Although the most common route of administration is oral, it may be given intramuscularly at dosages of 10 to 25 mg/week. The total dosage rarely exceeds 30 mg. Higher intramuscular dosages are allowed because of the more rapid renal clearance. When the psoriasis is in control, MTX may be tapered by 2.5 mg/week until the lowest possible dosage is found that provides disease control.[134]

Common acute side effects of MTX are nausea and gastrointestinal upset related to dosing. MTX can also produce a phototoxic reaction similar to sunburn. If MTX is used with phototherapy, patients should omit their phototherapy treatments on the days MTX is administered. More serious long-term side effects include hepatotoxicity and bone marrow suppression. The hepatotoxicity seems to be related to the cumulative MTX dosage. Liver function tests are unreliable screening methods for MTX-induced hepatotoxicity, so liver biopsy is currently the only means of monitoring changes attributed to MTX. This has been recommended after a 1.5-g cumulative dosage, and subsequent biopsies should be performed following further 1.0- to 1.5-g cumulative dosages. Guidelines for monitoring MTX toxicity have been published elsewhere.[135] Folinic acid is the treatment of choice for accidental overdose. Leucovorin rescue, as this is called, bypasses the step in folic acid reduction that is blocked by MTX.[133]

Hydroxyurea

Hydroxyurea is a hydroxylated molecule of urea that affects cell proliferation by inhibiting DNA synthesis. The exact mode of action is incompletely understood in psoriasis. Although not approved by the FDA for treating psoriasis, it has been reported to be effective. It is less effective than MTX; the response is slower (6 to 8 weeks), and the response is not as complete (the annular areas of psoriasis persist). A good and rapid response can be achieved with pustular psoriasis. Response to the drug ranges from a favorable response in 45 to 63% of patients to an excellent response in 18 to 38% of patients. This variation may reflect different dosages, varying time intervals, and different criteria for evaluating disease activity. Although this medication is not a first-line agent, it may benefit patients with high alcohol intake because of the low prevalence of hepatotoxicity. A major disadvantage is the frequent occurrence of bone marrow suppression.[136]

Cyclosporine

Cyclosporine is an 11–amino acid cyclic peptide often used to facilitate organ transplantation. Although the precise mechanism of action is not known, the inhibition of lymphokine secretion by activated T cells may play a central role. Because of the cost and toxicity associated with the drug, it is currently recommended only in patients with severe psoriasis that is unresponsive to more conventional therapies. Cyclosporine appears to be as effective as PUVA, UVB, MTX, or retinoid therapy in treating chronic severe plaque psoriasis but less effective in pustular psoriasis. Clearing with cyclosporine occurs more rapidly than with other systemic modalities, but relapse is common after therapy is withdrawn. A rebound phenomenon, such as those seen in systemic corticosteroid withdrawal, usually is not seen. Dosages needed for transplantation (1 5 mg/kg/day) are not appropriate, but lower dosages (2.5 to 5 mg/kg/day) lead to a good response within 4 to 8 weeks. Therapeutic response is faster and more complete with higher dosages, but there is a dose-dependent increased incidence of nephrotoxicity and hypertension. These side effects are reported to be reversed after the dosage is lowered. Other side effects include hepatotoxicity, neurologic abnormalities, gingival hyperplasia, hypertrichosis, and an increased incidence of lymphoma. Because of the many potentially life-threatening side effects, it has been recommended that patients with hypertension, evidence of compromised renal function, concurrent immunosuppression, or history of malignancy, pregnancy, or infection avoid this medication. To date, little is known about the safety and efficacy of long-term maintenance therapy. One study showed hypertension and renal dysfunction to be a problem, but this was corrected with dosage reduction or therapeutic intervention. To reduce the daily dosage, combination with UVB, PUVA, or etretinate has been suggested. Phototherapy may not be a desirable combination in view of cyclosporine's immunosuppression and the potential for carcinogenic effects with phototherapy. High-dose etretinate allowed only a modest reduction in cyclosporine dosage.[137,138]

In conclusion, although systemic cyclosporine is efficacious in clearing psoriasis, several life-threatening side effects limit its use. Because of the toxicity of systemically administered cyclosporine, current investigations focus on topical preparations and intralesional cyclosporine.

Clinical Variants and Specific Treatment Modalities

As mentioned previously, several clinical variants of psoriasis have been recognized that will determine the type of treatment modality. The following discussion summarizes specific treatment modalities for these clinical variants. Children and adults with guttate psoriasis usually are given systemic antimicrobial treatment, based on either cultures or antibody titers showing group A streptococcal infection. For both erythrodermic and generalized pustular psoriasis, MTX and etretinate have been successful monotherapies in controlling these eruptions. Localized psoriasis of the palms and soles responds well to PUVA treatments concentrated in these areas, and adding etretinate to PUVA is reported to be more effective than PUVA alone. Seborrhiasis distributed over the scalp, central chest, and groin may respond to oral ketoconazole. Localized psoriasis of the scalp can be treated with 2% ketoconazole shampoo or other antiseborrheic preparations. Inverse psoriasis of the body folds with associated group B streptococcus colonization has been reported to respond to 2% erythromycin ointment. Finally, the choice of treatment for plaque-type psoriasis depends on the extent of body surface involvement. For more localized disease, topical corticosteroids or anthralin may be used. If more than 50% of the body surface is involved, then phototherapy, photochemotherapy, or systemic therapy should be considered. The two most commonly used forms of systemic monotherapies for plaque-type psoriasis are MTX and retinoids, but the latter is less effective and is usually used in combination with other treatments.[131,139]

CONCLUSION

In summary, seborrheic dermatitis and psoriasis are cutaneous eruptions in which disease expression is based on genetic and environmental factors. The pathophysiology of both diseases involves epidermal cell proliferation and inflammation. Therapies for seborrheic dermatitis and psoriasis are directed at these two pathologic features. Seborrheic dermatitis can be treated with shampoos or with topical antifungals and corticosteroids in areas not involving the scalp. However, psoriasis treatment depends not only on the location, but also on its clinical presentation. Because a wide range of therapies are available for psoriasis, consideration must be given to side effects. The ideal choice is a regimen that provides adequate therapeutic efficacy without compromising the patient's quality of life.

Rosacea

Rosacea, also called middle-age acne or acne rosacea, is a chronic inflammatory disease. It is most common after the age of 30 and more prevalent in people of Celtic and northern European heritage.

EPIDEMIOLOGY

Although many factors have been associated with rosacea, a definite cause is still unknown.[140] Some studies previously suggested that *Helicobacter pylori* may play a role, but this is yet unproven.[141]

PATHOPHYSIOLOGY

Pathologic findings in rosacea include dilation of blood vessels in the papillary dermis and sebaceous hyperplasia.

CLINICAL PRESENTATION AND DIAGNOSIS

The disease begins with a gradual onset of transient flushing and erythema. Patients may notice flares secondary to emotional stress, alcoholic or hot drinks, and hot or spicy foods. Sun damage is commonly associated with rosacea. It occurs mainly over the forehead, nose, and cheeks, although other areas of the face and neck may be involved. Over a period of months to years, persistent erythema with telangiectasias and eventually erythematous papules and pustules, resembling acne, may develop. Unlike in acne, open comedones are never seen in rosacea. The final stage of rosacea, which occurs in severe, chronic cases, is rhinophyma. This is the irreversible soft tissue hypertrophy of the nose, producing the "W.C. Fields nose," which is more common in men.[142] Ocular rosacea may occur in 30 to 50% of the patients with symptoms of dry eyes, blepharitis, conjunctivitis, styes, and possible corneal damage.[141]

TREATMENT

Patients should be instructed to avoid stimuli that may provoke rosacea. Early rosacea, consisting primarily of vasodilation, is difficult to treat. Topical treatment, such as metronidazole twice a day or clindamycin twice a day, may be effective when inflammatory lesions are present. The treatment for resistant rosacea involves 4 to 6 weeks of oral antibiotics, including tetracycline 250 mg four times a day, doxycycline 100 mg twice a day, minocycline 100 mg twice a day, metronidazole 200 mg twice a day, or erythromycin 250 mg four times a day. Antibiotic therapy is effective, but the disease often recurs. Systemic isotretinoin, at dosages of 0.5 to 1 mg/kg/day for 4 to 8 months, can be used for severe disease.[140,141]

The only effective treatments for rhinophyma include cold steel, hot wire loop surgery, laser surgery, and dermabrasion.[143]

KEY POINTS

- Acne treatment is directed at preventing new lesions, not treating existing lesions.
- Acne is a chronic condition and therapy is long term.
- Topical antibiotics are not useful in noninflammatory acne. They are most useful in mild to moderate inflammatory acne and as an adjunct in severe nodulocystic acne.
- Topical tretinoin is a superior agent for comedonal acne.

- Tetracycline and its derivatives and erythromycin are antibiotics of choice for moderate to severe inflammatory acne; however, therapy must be continued for at least 5 months and sometimes up to 2 years.
- Oral isotretinoin is the most effective agent for treating acne; however, potential teratogenicity and side effects warrant close patient monitoring.
- Blocking photodermatoses with protective clothing and sunscreens helps prevent chronic problems of photoaging and cancer. Treatment of these conditions is not as effective as prevention.
- Treatment options for warts are divided into chemical destructive therapy (acids, formalin, glutaraldehyde, cantharidin), physical destruction (cryotherapy, electrosurgery, surgical excision), chemotherapeutic agents (podophyllin, podophyllotoxin, 5-FU, bleomycin, interferons, retinoids), and immunotherapy (dinitrochlorobenzene, SADBE, inosine pranobex).
- Therapies for seborrheic dermatitis include shampoos, topical antifungals, and corticosteroids.
- Psoriasis varies greatly in severity, and treatment must be based on a risk:benefit ratio.
- The selection of therapy for psoriasis depends on the location and clinical presentation.
- There is a wide range of therapies for psoriasis, and treatment must take into account the patient's quality of life.

REFERENCES

1. Baur DA, Butler RCD. Current concepts in the pathogenesis and treatment of acne. J Oral Maxillofac Surg 56:651–655, 1998.
2. Lucky A. A review of infantile and pediatric acne. Dermatology 196:95–97, 1998.
3. Brown SK, Shalita AR. Acne vulgaris. Lancet 351:1871–1876, 1998.
4. Beylot C, Doutre MS, Beylot-Berry M. Oral contraceptives and cyproterone acetate in female acne treatment. Dermatology 196:148–152, 1998.
5. Habif TP. Clinical dermatology. 3rd ed. St Louis: Mosby, 1996:148–180.
6. Nguyen QH, Kim YA, Schwartz RA. Management of acne vulgaris. Am Fam Physician 50:89, 1994.
7. Shalita AR, Leyden JJ. New insights into pathogenesis of acne. 15 Symposium Digest 3(4):25–32, 1991.
8. Toyoda M, Moreohashi M. An overview of topical antibiotics for acne treatment. Dermatology 196:130–134, 1998.
9. Liden S, Lindelof B. Is benzoyl peroxide carcinogenic? Br J Dermatol 123:129–130, 1990.
10. Orfanos CE, Zouboulis C. Oral retinoids in the treatment of seborrhea and acne. Dermatology 196:140–147, 1998.
11. Monga M. Vitamin A and its congeners. Semin Perinatol 21(2):135–142, 1997.
12. Lever L, Marks R. Current views on the aetiology, pathogenesis and treatment of acne vulgaris. Drugs 39(5):681–692, 1990.
13. Eady EA, Joanes DN, Cunliffe WJ. Topical antibiotics for the treatment of acne vulgaris: a critical evaluation of the literature on their clinical benefit and comparative efficacy. J Dermatol Treat 1:215–256, 1990.
14. Eady EA. Bacterial resistance in acne. Dermatology 196:59–66, 1998.
15. Trexler MF, Fraser TG, Jones MP. Fulminant pseudomembranous colitis caused by clindamycin phosphate vaginal cream. Am J Gastroenterol 92(11):2112–2113, 1997.
16. Chu A, Huber FJ, Plott RT. The comparative efficacy of benzoyl peroxide 5%/erythromycin 3% gel and erythromycin 4%/zinc 1.2% solution in the treatment of acne vulgaris. Br J Dermatol 136:235–238, 1997.
17. Gibson JR. Azelaic acid 20% cream (Azelex) and the medical management of acne vulgaris. Dermatol Nurs 9(5):339–344, 1997.
18. Lookingbill DP, Abrams BB, Ellis CN, et al. Inocoterone and acne. Arch Dermatol 128:1197–1200, 1992.
19. Burke B, Early EA, Cunliffe WJ. Benzoyl peroxide versus topical erythromycin in the treatment of acne vulgaris. Br J Dermatol 108:199–204, 1983.
20. Bathman T, Bonfils A, Branck C, et al. RU58841, a new specific topical antiandrogen. J Steroid Biochem Molec Biol 48:55–60, 1994.
21. Meynadier J, Alirezai M. Systemic antibiotics for acne. Dermatology 196:135–139, 1998.
22. Gottlieb A. Safety of minocycline for acne. Lancet 349:374, 1997.
23. Driscoll MS, Rothe MJ, Abrahamian L, et al. Longterm oral antibiotics for acne; Is laboratory monitoring necessary? J Am Acad Dermatol 28:595–602, 1993.
24. Hugh BR, Cunliffe WJ. Interactions between the oral contraceptive pill and antibiotics. Br J Dermatol 122:717, 1990.
25. Meigel WN. How safe is oral isotretinoin? Dermatology 195(Suppl 1):22–28, 1997.
26. Barth JH, Macdonald SP, Mark J, et al. Isotretinoin therapy for acne vulgaris: a re-evaluation of the need for measurements of plasma lipids and liver function tests. Br J Dermatol 129:704–707, 1993.
27. Meigel WN. Discussion on acne. Dermatology 195(Suppl 1):38–40, 1997.
28. Margolis DJ, Attie M, Leyden JJ. Effects of isotretinoin on bone mineralization during routine therapy with isotretinoin for acne vulgaris. Arch Dermatol 132:769–774, 1996.
29. Pochoi PE. The pathogenesis and treatment of acne. Ann Rev Med 41:187–198, 1990.
30. Sciarra F, Toscano V, Concolino G, et al. Antiandrogens: clinical applications. J Steroid Biochem Molec Biol 37(3):349–362, 1990.
31. Pathak MA, Fitzpatrick TB, Greiter F, et al. Preventive treatment of sunburn, dermatoheliosis, and skin cancer with sunprotective agents. In: Fitzpatrick TB, Eisen AZ, Wolff K, et al., eds. Dermatology in general medicine. 4th ed. New York: McGraw-Hill, 1993:1689–1717.
32. Braun-Falco O, Plewig G, Wolff HH, et al. Dermatology. 3rd ed. Berlin: Springer-Verlag, 1991.
33. Soter NA. Acute effects of ultraviolet radiation on the skin. In: Maibach HI. Seminars in dermatology. Philadelphia: WB Saunders, 1990;9(1):1–15.
34. Young AR. Cumulative effects of ultraviolet radiation on the skin. Cancer and photoaging. In: Maibach HI. Seminars in dermatology. Philadelphia: WB Saunders, 1990;9(1):25–31.
35. Diffey BL. Human exposure to ultraviolet radiation. In: Maibach HI. Seminars in dermatology. Philadelphia: WB Saunders, 1990;9(1):2–10.
36. Morrison WL, et al. The effects of indomethacin on ultraviolet-induced delayed erythema. J Invest Dermatol 68:130, 1971.
37. Elwood JM, Jopson J. Melanoma and sun exposure: an overview of published studies. Int J Cancer 73:198–203, 1997.
38. Taylor CR, Stern RS, Leyden JJ, et al. Photoaging/photodamage and photoprotection. J Am Acad Dermatol 22:1–15, 1990.
39. Lowe NJ. Sunscreens and the prevention of skin aging. J Dermatol Surg Oncol 16:936–938, 1990.
40. Boger J, Araugo OE, Flowers F. Sunscreen efficacy, use, and misuse. South Med J 77:1421–1427, 1984.
41. Pathak MA. Sunscreens: topical and systemic approaches for protection of human skin against harmful effects of solar radiation. J Am Acad Dermatol 7:285–312, 1982.
42. Federal Register. Sunscreen drug products for over-the-counter human drugs: proposed safety, effective, and labeling conditions. Washington, DC: Department of Health, Education and Welfare, Food and Drug Administration, Aug 25, 1978;43(166):38206–38269.
43. Kaidbey RH. The photoprotective potential of the new superpotent sunscreens. J Am Acad Dermatol 22:449–452, 1990.
44. Naylor MF, Farmer KC. The case for sunscreens: a review of their use in preventing actinic damage and neoplasia. Arch Dermatol 133:1146–1154, 1997.
45. Lowe NJ. Photoprotection. In: Maibach HI. Seminars in dermatology. Philadelphia: WB Saunders, 1990;9(1):78–83.
46. Marks R, Foley PA, Jolley D, et al. The effect of regular sunscreen use on vitamin D levels in a Australian population. Arch Dermatol 131:415–421, 1995.
47. Black HS. Systemic photoprotective agents. Photodermatology 4:187–195, 1987.
48. Swanbeck G. Aminoquinolones. In: Fitzpatrick TB, Eisen AZ, Wolff K, et al., eds. Dermatology in general medicine. 4th ed. New York: McGraw-Hill, 1993:2869–2871.
49. Kang S, Fisher GJ, Voorhees JJ. Photoaging and topical tretinoin: therapy, pathogenesis, and prevention. Arch Dermatol 133:1280–1284, 1997.
50. Van Scott EJ, Yu RJ. Alpha hydroxyacids. Can J Dermatol 1:108–112, 1989.
51. Goette DR. Topical chemotherapy with 5-fluorouracil. J Am Acad Dermatol 4:663–649, 1981.

52. Arnold HL, Odom RB, James WD. Warts. In: Andrews' diseases of the skin. 8th ed. Philadelphia: WB Saunders, 1990:468–475.
53. Cobb MW. Human papillomaviruses infection. J Am Acad Dermatol 22:547–566, 1990.
54. Lowy DR, Androphy EJ. Warts. In: Fitzpatrick TB, ed. Dermatology in general medicine. 3rd ed. New York: McGraw-Hill, 1987:2355–2372.
55. Centers for Disease Control and Prevention. Sexually transmitted disease surveillance 1997. Atlanta: CDC Publication, September 1998.
56. Koutsky L. Epidemiology of genital human papillomavirus infection. Am J Med 102(5A):3–8, 1997.
57. Beutner KR, Tyring S. Human papillomavirus and human disease. Am J Med 102(5A):9–15, 1997.
58. Penneys N. Diseases caused by viruses. In: Elder D, Elenitsas R, Jaworsky C, et al., eds. Lever's histopathology of the skin. 5th ed. Philadelphia: Lippincott-Raven, 1997:569–589.
59. Verden ME. Issues in the management of human papillomavirus genital disease. Am Fam Physician 55(5): 1813–1820, 1997.
60. Highet AS. Viral warts. Semin Dermatol 7(1):53–57, 1988.
61. Trofatter KF. Diagnosis of human papillomavirus genital tract infection. Am J Med 102(5A):21–27, 1997.
62. Steele KS, Shirodaria P, O'Hare M, et al. Monochloroacetic acid and 60% salicylic acid as a treatment for simple plantar warts: effectiveness and mode of action. Br J Dermatol 118:537–544, 1988.
63. Food and Drug Administration Health and Human Services. Wart removal drug products for over the counter human use: final monograph. 21 CFR, part 358, 1991.
64. Hirose R. Topical treatment of resistant warts with glutaraldehyde. J Dermatol 21:248–253, 1994.
65. Silva PD, Micha JP, Silva DG. Management of condyloma acuminatum. J Am Acad Dermatol 13:457–463, 1985.
66. Mroczkowski TF, McEwen C. Warts and other human papillomavirus infections. Postgrad Med 78(7):91–98, 1985.
67. Stone KM, Becker TM, Hadgu A, et al. Treatment of external genital warts: a randomized clinical trial comparing podophyllin, cryotherapy, and electrodesiccation. Genitourinary Med 66:16–19, 1990.
68. Jensen SL. Comparison of podophyllin application with simple surgical excision in clearance and recurrence of perianal condyloma acuminata. Lancet 2:1146–1148, 1985.
69. Rapini RP. Venereal warts. Prim Care 17(1):127–144, 1990.
70. Marcus J, Camisa C. Podophyllin therapy for condyloma acuminatum. Int J Dermatol 29(10):693–698, 1990.
71. Campbell BJ. The treatment of warts. Prim Care 13(3):465–476, 1986.
72. Miller RA. Podophyllin. Int J Dermatol 24:491–498, 1985.
73. Cassidy DE, Drewry J, Fanning SD. Podophyllum toxicity: a report of a fatal case and a review of the literature. J Toxicol Clin Toxicol 19(1):35–44, 1982.
74. Beutner KR, von Krogh G. Current status of podophyllin for the treatment of genital warts. Semin Dermatol 9(2):148–151, 1990.
75. Edwards A, Atma-Ram A, Thin RN. Podophyllotoxin 0.5% vs podophyllin 20% to treat penile warts. Genitourinary Med 64:263–265, 1988.
76. Rosemberg SK. Sexually transmitted papillomaviral infections. V. Prophylactic use of topical 5-fluorouracil in refractory infection in the male. Urology 34(2):86–88, 1989.
77. Ferenczy A. Comparison of 5-fluorouracil and CO_2 laser for treatment of vaginal condyloma. Obstet Gynecol 64:773–778, 1984.
78. Boyd AS. Condyloma acuminata in the pediatric population. Am J Dis Child 144:817–824, 1990.
79. Hursthouse MW. A controlled trial on the use of topical 5-fluorouracil on viral warts. Br J Dermatol 92:93–99, 1975.
80. Shumer SM, O'Keefe EJ. Bleomycin in the treatment of recalcitrant warts. J Am Acad Dermatol 9:91–96, 1983.
81. Shelley WB, Shelley ED. Intralesional bleomycin sulfate therapy for warts. Arch Dermatol 127:234–236, 1991.
82. Keay S, Teng N, Eisenberg M, et al. Topical interferon for treating condyloma acuminata in women. J Infect Dis 158(5):934–939, 1988.
83. Eron LJ, Judson F, Tucker S, et al. Interferon therapy for condyloma acuminata. N Engl J Med 315(17):1059–1063, 1986.
84. Vance JC, Bart BJ, Hanser RC, et al. Intralesional recombinant alpha-2 interferon for the treatment of patients with condyloma acuminatum or verruca plantaris. Arch Dermatol 122:272–276, 1986.
85. Friedman-Kien AE et al. Natural interferon alfa for treatment of condyloma acuminata. JAMA 259(4):533–538, 1988.
86. Weck PK, Buddin DA, Whisnant JK. Interferons in the treatment of genital human papillomavirus infections. Am J Med 85(Suppl 2A):159–164, 1988.
87. Reichman RC. Treatment of condyloma acuminatum with three interferons administered intralesionally. Ann Int Med 108:675–679, 1988.
88. Mahrle G, Schulze HJ. Recombinant interferon-gamma in dermatology. J Invest Dermatol 95(Suppl 6):132s–137s, 1990.
89. Kirby P. Interferon and genital warts: much potential, modest progress. JAMA 259(4):570–572, 1988.
90. Buetner KR, Ferenczy A. Therapeutic approaches to genital warts. Am J Med 102(5A):28–37, 1997.
91. Lutzner MA. Oral retinoid treatment of human papillomavirus type 5-induced epidermodysplasia verruciformis. N Engl J Med 302(19):1091, 1980.
92. Gross G, Pfister H, Hagedorn M, et al. Effect of oral aromatic retinoid (Ro 10-9359) on human papillomavirus induced common warts. Dermatologica 166:48–53, 1983.
93. Bolton RA. Nongenital warts: classification and treatment options. Am Fam Physician 43(6):2049–2056, 1991.
94. Naylor MF, Neldner KH, Yarbrough GK, et al. Contact immunotherapy of resistant warts. J Am Acad Dermatol 19:679–683, 1988.
95. Eriksen K. Treatment of the common wart by induced allergic inflammation. Dermatologica 160:161–166, 1980.
96. Sanders BB, Smith KW. Dinitrochlorobenzene immunotherapy of human warts. Cutis 27:389–392, 1981.
97. Orlow S. Cimetidine therapy for multiple viral warts in children. J Am Acad Dermatol 28(5):794–796, 1993.
98. Karabulut AA, Sahin S, Eksioglu M. Is cimetidine effective for non-genital warts: a double-blind, placebo-controlled study. Arch Dermatol 133(4):533–534, 1997.
99. Shuster S. The etiology of dandruff and the mode of action of therapeutic agents. Br J Dermatol 1:235–242, 1984.
100. Faergeman J, Jones TC, Hettler O, et al. *Pityrosporum ovale* as the causative agent of seborrhoeic dermatitis: new treatment options. Br J Dermatol 134(Suppl 46):12–15, 1996.
101. Peter RU, Richarz-Barthauer U. Successful treatment and prophylaxis of seborrheic dermatitis and dandruff with 2% ketoconazole shampoo: results of a multi-centre, double-blind, placebo-controlled trial. Br J Dermatol 132(3): 441–445, 1995.
102. Heng MC, Henderson BA, Barker BA, et al. Correlation of *Pityrosporum ovale* density with clinical severity of seborrheic dermatitis as assessed by a simplified technique. J Am Acad Dermatol 23:82–86, 1990.
103. Cowley NC, Farr PM, Shuster S. The permissive effect of sebum in seborrhoeic dermatitis: an explanation of the rash in neurological disorders. Br J Dermatol 122:71–76, 1990.
104. Brown M, Evans TW, Tooley PJH. The role of ketoconazole 2% shampoo in the treatment and prophylactic management of dandruff. J Dermatol Treat 1:177–179, 1990.
105. Taieb A, Legrain V, Palmier C, et al. Topical ketoconazole for infantile seborrhoeic dermatitis. Dermatologica 181:26–32, 1990.
106. Feldman SR, Clark AR. Psoriasis. Med Clin North Am 82(5):1135–1144, 1998.
107. Burden AD, Javed S, Bailey M, et al. Genetics of psoriasis: paternal inheritance and a locus on chromosome 6P. J Inv Dermatol 110(6):958–960, 1998.
108. Christophers E, Sterry W. Psoriasis. In: Fitzpatrick TB, Eisen AZ, Wolff K, et al., eds. Dermatology in general medicine. 4th ed. Philadelphia: WB Saunders, 1993:489–514.
109. Felscher Z, Rothman S. The insensible perspiration of the skin in hyperkeratotic conditions. J Invest Dermatol 6:271–278, 1945.
110. Marks R. Topical therapy for psoriasis: general principles. Dermatol Clin 2:383–388, 1984.
111. Lowe NJ, Ashton R. Anthralin and coal tar therapy for psoriasis. Dermatol Clin 2:389–396, 1984.
112. Wheeler L, Lowe NJ. Mutagenicity of urines from patients undergoing coal tar therapy for psoriasis. J Int Dermatol 77:181–185, 1981.
113. Schmid MH, Korting HC. Coal tar, pine tar and sulfonated shale oil preparations: comparative activity, efficacy and safety. Dermatol 193(1):1–5, 1996.
114. Drug facts and comparisons, 1998 ed. St Louis: Facts and Comparisons, 1998:3136.
115. Trozak DJ. Topical corticosteroid therapy in psoriasis vulgaris. Cutis 46:341–349, 1990.
116. Kragballe K. Treatment of psoriasis by the topical application of the novel cholecalciferol analogue calcipotriol (MC 901). Arch Dermatol 125:1647–1652, 1989.
117. Kragballe K, Wildfang IL. Calcipotriol (MC903), a novel vitamin D_3 analogue simulates terminal differentiation and inhibits proliferation of cultured human lymphocytes. Arch Dermatol Res 282:164–167, 1990.
118. Wolverton SE. Retinoids. In: Wolverton SE, Wilkins JK. Systemic drugs for skin diseases. Philadelphia: WB Saunders, 1991:187.
119. Ellis CN, Voorhees JJ. Etretinate therapy. J Am Acad Dermatol 12:267–291, 1987.

120. Abramowicz M, ed. Two new retinoids for psoriasis. Med Lett 39(1013):105–106, 1997.
121. Fiore M. Practical aspects of anthralin therapy. Cutis 46:351–354, 1990.
122. Ramsay B, Lawrence CM, Bruse JM, et al. The effect of triethanolamine application on anthralin-induced inflammation and therapeutic effect on psoriasis. J Am Acad Dermatol 23:73–76, 1990.
123. Guidelines of care for psoriasis. AAD Bulletin 9:10–15, 1991.
124. Rosenberg EW, Belew PW. Microbial factors in psoriasis. Arch Dermatol 118:143–144, 1982.
125. Rosenberg EW, Noah PW, Zanolli ME, et al. Use of rifampin with penicillin and erythromycin in the treatment of psoriasis. J Am Acad Dermatol 14:761–764, 1986.
126. Rosenberg EW, Skinner RB Jr, Noah PW. Antimicrobial treatment of psoriasis. In: Roenigk H, Maibach HA. Psoriasis. 2nd ed. New York: Marcel Dekker, 1990:815.
127. Paul BS, Lark GO, Swanbeck G, Parrish JA. Therapeutic photomedicine: phototherapy. In: Fitzpatrick TB, Eisen AZ, Wolff K, et al. Dermatology in general medicine. 4th ed. Philadelphia: WB Saunders, 1993:1717–1727.
128. Stern RS, Thibodeau LA, Kleinerman RA, et al. Psoriasis and susceptibility of nonmelanoma skin cancer. J Am Acad Dermatol 12:67–73, 1985.
129. Skinner RB Jr. Psoralens. In: Wolverton SE, Wilkins JK. Systemic drugs for skin diseases. Philadelphia: WB Saunders, 1991:219.
130. Wolff K. Side-effects of psoralen photochemotherapy (PUVA). Br J Dermatol 122(Suppl 36):117–125, 1990.
131. Zanolli MD. Psoriasis and Reiter's disease. In: Sams WM, Lynch PJ, eds. Principles and practice of dermatology. New York: Churchill Livingstone, 1990:307.
132. Zanolli MD, Sherertz EF, Hedberg AE. Methotrexate: anti-inflammatory or antiproliferative? J Am Acad Dermatol 22:523–524, 1997.
133. Olsen EA. The pharmacology of methotrexate. J Am Acad Dermatol 25:306–318, 1991.
134. Tung JP, Maibach HI. The practical use of methotrexate in psoriasis. Drugs 40:697–712, 1990.
135. Roenigk HH, Auerbach R, Maibach HI, et al. Methotrexate in psoriasis: revised guidelines. J Am Acad Dermatol 19:145–156, 1988.
136. Boyd AS, Neldner KH. Hydroxyurea therapy. J Am Acad Dermatol 25:518–524, 1991.
137. Griffiths CE. Systemic and local administration of cyclosporine in the treatment of psoriasis. J Am Acad Dermatol 23:1242–1246, 1990.
138. Guenther L. Cyclosporine. In: Wolverton SE, Wilkins JK. Systemic drugs for skin diseases. Philadelphia: WB Saunders, 1991:167.
139. Matsunami E, Takashima A, Mizumo N, et al. Topical PUVA, etretinate, and combined PUVA and etretinate for palmoplantar pustulosis: comparison of therapeutic efficacy and the influences of tonsillar and dental focal infections. J Dermatol 17:92–96, 1990.
140. Bleicher PA, Charles JH, Sober AJ. Topical metronidazole for rosacea. Arch Dermatol 123:609–614, 1987.
141. Webster GF. Acne and rosacea. Med Clin North Am 82(5):1145–1154, 1998.
142. Plewig G. Rosacea. In: Fitzpatrick TB, Eisen AZ, Wolff K, et al. Dermatology in general medicine. 4th ed. New York: McGraw-Hill, 1993:727–735.
143. Greenbaum SS, Krull EA, Watnick K. Comparison of CO_2 laser and electrosurgery treatment of rhinophyma. J Am Acad Dermatol 18:363–368, 1988.

CHAPTER 47

BURNS

Ted L. Rice

Skin, the largest organ of the body, performs five major functions. It provides protection from the environment, sensory perception, vitamin production, excretion of water and some wastes, and regulation of body temperature. When the skin is damaged, bacteria are no longer prevented from invading, pain is produced (unless superficial sensory nerves are destroyed), and both fluid and heat are lost through the damaged area.

Extensive skin loss or damage requiring hospitalization can occur by many different mechanisms that produce similar effects: thermal injury from hot liquids (scalds), flames, or extreme cold (frostbite) and injury from chemicals, radiation (sunburn), electricity, or trauma (abrasion). In addition, patients with extensive exfoliative dermatoses (e.g., the Stevens-Johnson syndrome or toxic epidermal necrolysis) are treated in burn centers.

Fire victims can suffer severe injury or death without significant body surface burns. A classic demonstration of this is the 1942 Coconut Grove Nightclub fire in which 75 of the 114 deaths were a result of smoke inhalation. Carbon monoxide (CO) poisoning is a frequent cause of death. CO binds preferentially to hemoglobin, displacing oxygen and shifting the oxyhemoglobin dissociation curve to the left, resulting in tissue hypoxia. Although a function of the material burning, smoke contains toxins other than CO, such as cyanide, acrolein, benzine, and phosgene.[1,2]

Outcome after thermal injury is determined by a combination of patient and burn factors. The very young, very old, and previously ill have a poorer prognosis than healthy, young adults after a similar injury. Scoring systems for injury severity include the Thermal Injury Organ Failure Score, which correlates with outcome and the Burn Specific Health Scale to accurately assess the impact of nonfatal burn injury.[3,4] One method for estimating the probability of death after burn injury found that the three risk factors with the strongest predictive value for death were age older than 60 years, extent of burn, and inhalation injury.[5] The importance of inhalation injury is illustrated by a recent review of 100 patients that documents pulmonary complications, e.g., adult respiratory distress syndrome and pneumonia, account for 77% of deaths in patients with burns who also have inhalation injury.[6]

TREATMENT GOALS: BURNS

- Provide appropriate resuscitation.
- Preserve physical function.
- Promote wound healing and optimal cosmetic results.
- Minimize pain and anxiety.
- Provide adequate nutrition.
- Prevent or aggressively treat complications.

PATHOPHYSIOLOGY: WOUND ASSESSMENT

Burn factors determining patient outcome include depth, extent, and body surface location.[7] A list of burn severity criteria is provided in Table 47.1. The important distinction in depth of burn is that partial-thickness injuries heal by cell regeneration; full-thickness injuries, unless very small, require skin grafting. Small full-thickness burns heal by contraction and reepithelialization from progenitor cells at the edges of the wound.

Traditionally, the depth of burns is described in degrees of injury as listed in Figure 47.1. As the depth of injury increases, the number for degree of injury increases. A first-degree burn is very shallow and involves only the epidermis. A second-degree burn involves complete destruction of the epidermis and variable portions of the underlying dermis. When destruction to the dermis is limited to the upper third or less, it is called a superficial second-degree burn. Conversely, a deep second-degree burn has tissue destruction below the top one-third, but not completely through the dermis. A third-degree, or full-thickness, burn has destruction of the entire epidermis and dermis. The terms fourth-degree burn and fifth-degree burn have been used to describe tissue destruction through subcutaneous fat and through muscle, respectively.[8]

CLINICAL PRESENTATION AND DIAGNOSIS

The typical first-degree burn is easily identified. It is painful, erythematous, and blanches to pressure. A superficial second-degree burn is painful, forms blisters, and blanches to pressure. A third-degree burn is usually not painful because superficial nerve endings are destroyed, its appearance is white, leather-like, or black (charred), and it contains thrombosed blood vessels. This dead tissue is called eschar. Unfortunately, sometimes even the most experienced clinician cannot differentiate a partial-thickness from a full-thickness injury. In addition, flame injuries are typically mixtures of full- and partial-thickness injuries. This classic presentation as depicted in Figure 47.2 was described as a target or bulls-eye where the deepest injury is in the center, followed by increasingly superficial injury at increasing distance from the center. Early attempts to improve the accurate assessment of injury depth included histologic staining, injection of radioactive compounds or dyes such as bromphenol blue, and fiberoptic perfusion fluorometry. These methods were invasive, cumbersome, labor intensive, and inaccurate. Although sensitive to variations in positioning and temperature, the laser Doppler has better than 90% accuracy compared to histologic analysis of burn wound depth. The laser Doppler documents a reduction in blood cell velocity in a burn wound, establishing the necessity for surgical excision and grafting.[9] Clinicians must remain cognizant of the need for confirmation of initial assessments of burn depth. Reassessment is necessary because of the changing nature of deep partial-thickness injuries,

Table 47.1 ▪ Burn Injury Severity Classification[a]

	Percent of Body Surface Affected (TBSA)					
	Minor Injury		Moderate Injury		Major Injury	
Depth of Burn	Adult	Child	Adult	Child	Adult	Child
Partial-thickness						
First-degree	<50	<10	50–75	10–20	>75	>20
Second-degree	<15	<10	15–25	10–20	>25	>20
Full-thickness						
Third-degree	<2	<2	2–10	2–10	>10	>10

TBSA, total body surface area.

[a]Irrespective of burn extent, injuries are classified as major when they involve areas of special importance such as the eyes, ears, hands, feet, or genitals. Injuries are major when burns occur in conjunction with other major trauma (e.g., fractures) or inhalation injury.

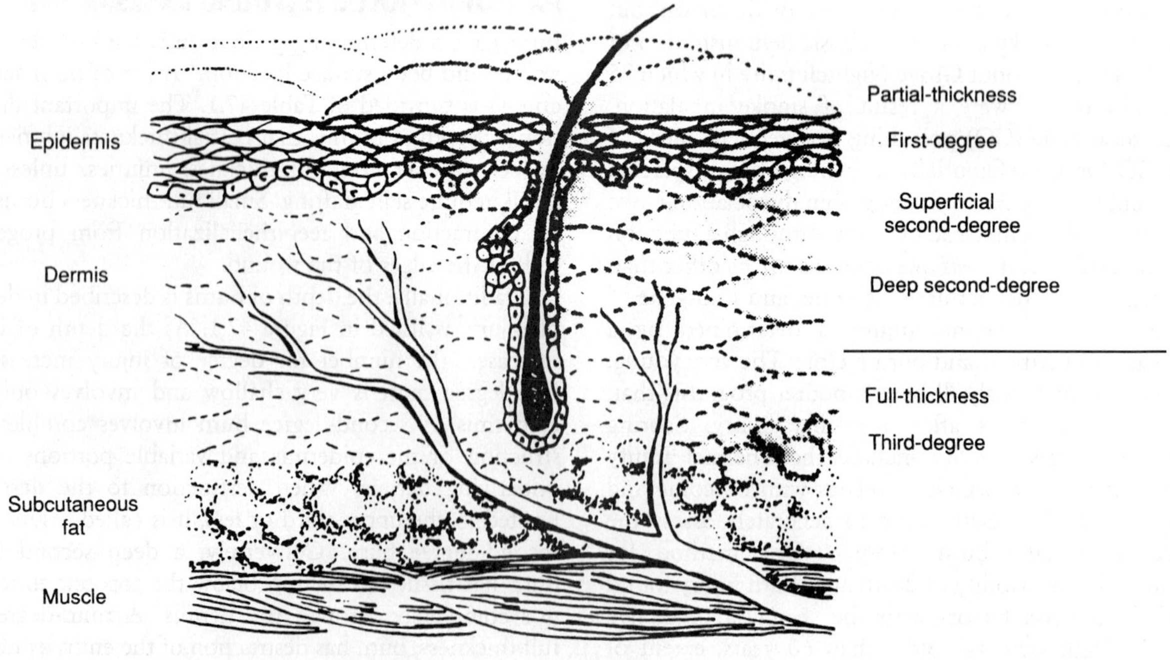

Figure 47.1. Diagram of burn depth in gross skin histology.

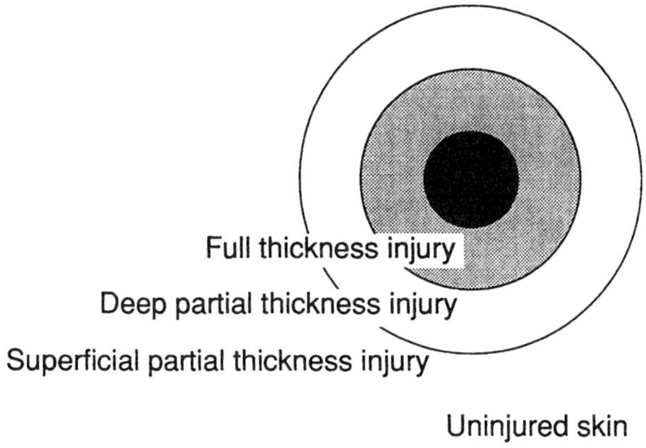

Figure 47.2. Typical pattern of injury following flame burn.

which may become full-thickness because of inadequate resuscitation or infection.[10]

A number of systems are used to calculate the relative percentage of total body surface area (TBSA) burned. The rule of nines is a simple system that can be used to estimate the extent of burn in adults. It represents regions of the body surface as 9% or multiples of 9%, e.g., the head and arms each represent approximately 9% TBSA, the torso 36%, each leg 18%, and the perineum 1%. For burns with an uneven distribution, the patient's hand is a useful measuring tool. One side of the patient's complete hand, i.e., the palm and fingers, is about 1% TBSA.[11] Because the head of infants and children represents a larger TBSA than that of adults, the rule of nines does not hold. A more accurate assessment of TBSA can be made using the Lund-Browder chart. The chart used at the University of Michigan Burn Center is reproduced in Figure 47.3.

TREATMENT

Wound Closure

When a large portion of the skin sustains full-thickness damage or destruction, the current surgical approach is staged eschar excision (debridement) and placement of autologous skin grafts.[12] Split-thickness skin grafts (STSG) approximately 0.06 mm thick are harvested (using a dermatome), expanded by a ratio of 1.5:1 (using a meshing device), and applied to the wound after removal of devitalized tissue and achievement of hemostasis. An important detrimental problem during these operative procedures is coagulopathy, which is produced by hypothermia. To prevent or attenuate hypothermia, the ambient temperature of the operating room is maintained above 37°C, the amount of debridement is limited, and intravenous fluids are warmed up to 40°C. Although appearing hazardous, a pilot study in eight patients demonstrated that intraoperative intravenous fluids can safely be heated to 60°C when administered through a central venous catheter.[13]

Once adherent and vascularized, the STSG from the patient's own noninjured skin (autograft or isograft) permanently closes the wound.[14] Unfortunately, the amount of noninjured skin available for STSGs often cannot completely cover the open wound. A number of skin substitutes can be used to cover the open wound temporarily while waiting for donor site healing and reharvesting of autograft. Commonly used biologic skin substitutes include cadaver skin (allograft or homograft) and animal skin (xenograft or heterograft). Less frequently used biologic skin substitutes are amniotic membranes and tissue-derived collagen. Synthetic skin substitutes include polyurethane films (e.g., OpSite) and petrolatum-impregnated fine-mesh gauze (e.g., scarlet red and Xeroform). Biosynthetic skin substitutes have been developed that are combinations of biologic and synthetic materials, such as Biobrane, which combines collagen with a synthetic membrane.[15] Skin substitutes adhere to the wound; minimize pain; decrease protein, water, and electrolyte loss; and simulate many important skin functions such as providing a barrier to bacteria. Although these skin substitutes provide important functions, they must eventually be replaced by autologous skin.

Recent advances in tissue bioengineering have focused on development of a true dermal replacement or substitute. One approach is the in vitro production of new skin by culture of autologous epidermis. Since the first successful transplantation of cultured autologous epidermis in 1981, keratinocyte growth techniques have been so improved that current methods allow a several thousand-fold expansion of skin specimens within 3 to 4 weeks.[16] However, engraftment of cultured epidermis continues to be inconsistent and should be considered experimental.[17] Another strategy provides a dermal matrix attached to a silicon polymer membrane.[18] Finally, the availability of a "living skin equivalent" composed of either bovine collagen and allogeneic cells (cultured from human neonatal foreskin) or human diploid fibroblasts on a polymer scaffold is an exciting albeit costly strategy for wound healing.[19,20]

Healing of burn wounds can often result in scars that impair normal range of motion and are cosmetically unpleasant. Hypertrophic scars are associated with contractures and are raised, erythematous, and pruritic. Keloid scars extend beyond the original wound and rarely regress. A new therapeutic strategy is the use of silicone sheets and gels.[21]

Pain Management

Effective pain management in patients with burns requires an understanding of both the physiologic responses to injury and the interrelationships between anxiety, depression, and pain. The extent of burn is a significant predictor of pain but only in the first week after the injury. Pain varies greatly from patient to patient and undergoes wide fluctuations over time in each patient. The greatest pain is usually experienced during therapeutic procedures such as hydrotherapy with wound debridement and dressing changes.[22] Patients with high levels of anxiety or depression tend to report more pain when at rest.

LOCATION DATE SERVICE

Reg. No. Class

Name

Address

UNIVERSITY OF MICHIGAN HOSPITALS

BURN CENTER

ESTIMATION OF SIZE OF BURN BY PERCENT

1 COLOR IN THE BURN

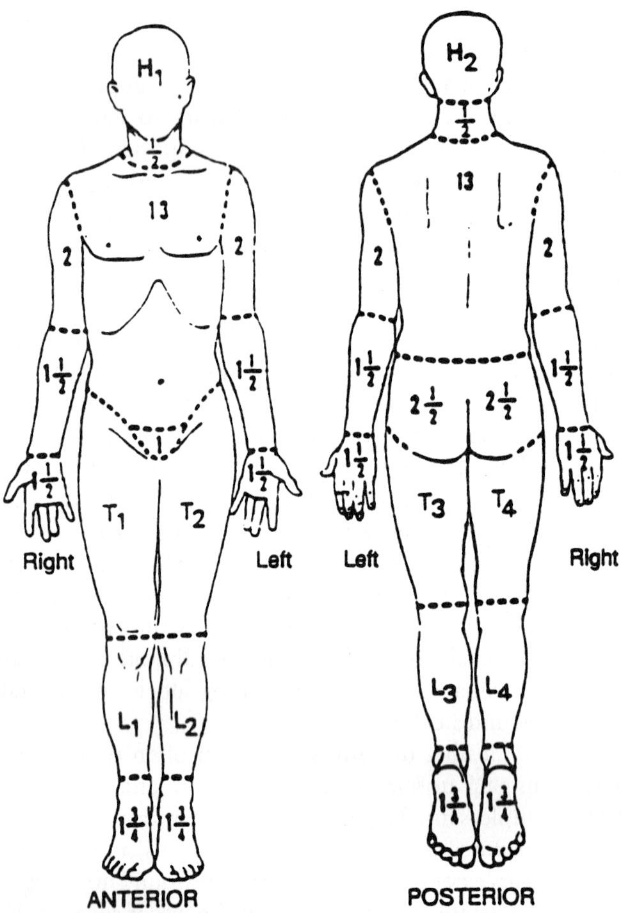

3 CALCULATE EXTENT BURN

	ANTERIOR	POSTERIOR
Head	H_1 ______	H_2 ______
Neck	______	______
Rt. Arm	______	______
Rt. Forearm	______	______
Rt. Hand	______	______
Lt. Arm	______	______
Lt. Forearm	______	______
Lt. Hand	______	______
Trunk	______	______
Buttock	______	______
Perineum	______	______
Rt. Thigh	T_1 ______	T_4 ______
Rt. Leg	L_1 ______	L_4 ______
Rt. Foot	______	______
Lt. Thigh	T_2 ______	T_3 ______
Lt. Leg	L_2 ______	L_3 ______
Lt. Foot	______	______
SUB TOTAL	______	______

% PARTIAL THICKNESS ______ %

& FULL THICKNESS ______ %

% TOTAL AREA BURNED ______ %

2 CIRCLE AGE FACTOR

PERCENT OF AREAS AFFECTED BY GROWTH

	AGE 0	1	5	10	15	ADULT
H (1 or 2) = 1/2 of the head	9 1/2	8 1/2	6 1/2	5 1/2	4 1/2	3 1/2
T (1,2,3, or 4) = 1/2 of a thigh	2 3/4	3 1/4	4	4 1/4	4 1/2	4 3/4
L (1,2,3, or 4) = 1/2 of a leg	2 1/2	2 1/2	2 3/4	3	3 1/4	3 1/2

H-2053949-DS Rev. 3/89 | MEDICAL RECORD | University of Michigan Medical Center | ESTIMATION OF SIZE OF BURN BY PERCENT

Figure 47.3. University of Michigan Hospital Burn Center's estimation of size of burn by percentage.

Historically, pain management practices for patients with burns have not been optimal, with some centers reporting that no analgesics or psychotropic drugs were administered to children during wound debridement.[23] To the observant clinician, careful evaluation of signs such as heart rate, blood pressure, facial expressions, body movement and position, and the quality of an infant's cries is sufficient to evaluate the intensity of pain and guide the need for and administration of analgesics. In addition, maintaining analgesic plasma levels within the ranges established for good analgesia may be beneficial in centers with rapid access to drug analysis laboratories.[24] Currently, a variety of pharmacotherapeutic agents are used in pain management, such as ketamine, propofol, and nitrous oxide.

The amount of opioid necessary to achieve pain control in patients with burns can be substantial, with morphine sulfate self-administered rates of 108 mg/hr reported.[25] This also demonstrates that large doses of morphine sulfate can be administered safely without undue fear of hypoventilation; indeed, a dose of 1650 mg/hr has been reported.[26] Another important contribution to the improved use of opioid analgesics is the allaying of unrealistic fears of producing narcotic addiction in hospitalized patients. The Boston Collaborative Drug Surveillance Program reported only four cases of reasonably well-documented addiction from 11,882 patients who received at least one narcotic preparation.[27]

Rather than conventional analgesic therapy such as intermittent intravenous morphine injections, the use of patient-controlled analgesia in both adult and pediatric patients with burns is gaining popularity.[28,29] However, because of situations such as the need for neuromuscular blockade, many patients with acute burns are not suitable candidates for patient-controlled analgesia.[30]

Nonpharmacologic methods or adjuncts to pain management include hypnotherapeutic intervention; distraction therapy, in which video programs of scenic beauty accompanied by music are used in combination with analgesics; and cognitive-behavioral therapies such as explanation, personal control, altering the meaning of pain, relaxation, imagery, distraction, and self-hypnosis.[31–35]

Fluid Resuscitation

Fluid Loss

Damaged skin loses the ability to serve as a barrier to percutaneous water loss. Evaporative water loss can be substantial.[36] In contrast to the normal vapor pressure of approximately 3 mm Hg, the vapor pressure of full-thickness burns is about 30 mm Hg. The amount of water loss in milliliters per hour can be estimated using the following formula:

$$\text{Evaporative loss (mL/hr)} = (25 + \text{TBSA}) \times \text{BSA}$$

where BSA is body surface area in square meters. In addition, injury to capillaries in the burn wound causes them to leak a protein-rich fluid into the interstitial space, producing edema and blisters. Blood vessels are generally thought of as solid-walled tubes like plumbing, when in fact they are made up of individual cells. When injured or under the influence of cytokines or inflammatory mediators these cells swell apart and produce small "holes" in the vessel wall. The problem resolves within 24 hours, but until then large macromolecules (molecular weights up to 80,000) can leak out of the intravascular space. When the TBSA burned exceeds 25%, a generalized "capillary leak" is produced throughout the body, and fluid exudes from unburned vessels into tissue and organs. The exact pathophysiology of this phenomenon is not clear, but the effects of leukotrienes, prostaglandins, arachidonic acid, and oxygen-derived free radicals have been implicated.

Fluid Requirements

The treatment or resuscitation of the burned patient in shock has been the subject of much interest, research, and controversy. Focused interest was generated in the 1940s because hypovolemic shock was the leading cause of death in patients with burns who survived their initial injury. The goal of initial fluid resuscitation is to restore and maintain tissue perfusion while minimizing edema formation.[37,38] The success of fluid administration is judged primarily by urine production at a rate of 0.5 to 1.0 mL/kg/hr. In addition, clinical observation of the adequately resuscitated patient should reveal a pulse rate less than 120 (adults) and a clear sensorium.[39] Use of a physiologic salt solution (crystalloid) such as lactated Ringer's solution is recommended.

The major controversy related to fluid resuscitation of the burn victim is the necessity for colloid infusion.[40–44] *Colloid* is a general descriptive term for nondiffusible, large-molecular-weight molecules that affect osmotic pressure. Available colloid suspensions include fresh frozen plasma, plasma protein fraction, albumin, dextrans, hetastarch, and pentastarch. Clinicians who routinely use colloids suggest that they are more physiologic and can reduce edema of nonburned tissue. Proponents of crystalloids caution that administered colloids can escape from the intravascular space until the capillary leak is sealed. Although no definitive answer is available, it seems reasonable to exclude colloid infusion from resuscitation fluids for the first 12 hours. Representative resuscitation guidelines are listed in Table 47.2.

A second controversy related to administration of colloid is the use of supplemental albumin to prevent or treat hypoalbuminemia in the postresuscitative phase. In two similar studies of pediatric patients, it was demonstrated that albumin administration did not improve pulmonary function, gastrointestinal tract function, wound healing, or outcome.[45,46] In addition, a recent meta-analysis of albumin administration in critically ill patients concluded that the risk of death was increased in the albumin-treated group.[47]

Fluid requirements after the first 24-hour postburn

Table 47.2 ▪ Resuscitation Formulas for Fluid Requirements During the First 24 Hours After a Burn[a]

Formula	Crystalloid	Colloid	Free Water
Adults			
Parkland	Lactated Ringer's 4 mL/kg/TBSA (%) ½ in first 8 hr ¼ in next 8 hr ¼ in last 8 hr	None	None
Evans	Lactated Ringer's 1 mL/kg/TBSA	1 mL/kg/TBSA	2000 mL/m^2
Brooke	Lactated Ringer's 1.5 mL/kg/TBSA	1 mL/kg/TBSA	2000 mL/m^2
Modified Brooke	Lactated Ringer's 2 mL/kg/TBSA	None	None
Children			
Graves	Lactated Ringer's 3 mL/kg/TBSA	None	Maintenance

TBSA, total body surface area.

[a]Maintenance fluid requirements are 100 mL/kg/day for the first 10 kg body weight, 50 mL/kg/day for the second 10 kg body weight, and 20 mL/kg/day for weight in excess of 20 kg.

period are determined in the usual fashion, with consideration of fluids lost through the burn wound and nasogastric suction. The main benefit of published guidelines is to alert the clinician unfamiliar with burn care that unusually large volumes of fluids and rates of administration are required for patients with severe injuries.[48] Almost every author has acknowledged that patient variability prohibits development of a strictly calculated volume of resuscitative fluid and rate of administration.

In severe injuries, release of free hemoglobin from destroyed red cells and myoglobin from damaged muscle (especially after electrical injury) leads to destruction of renal tubules, acute renal failure, and possibly death.[49] Binding of the free pigments to the renal tubules can be prevented by establishing a brisk urine flow using resuscitation fluids and diuretics such as furosemide or mannitol and alkalinizing the urine (pH ≥6.5) with parenteral sodium bicarbonate. An important consideration is that patients with burns and with rhabdomyolysis have estimated fluid requirements of 7 mL/kg/TBSA (%), almost twice as large as the Parkland formula estimate.[49]

Pharmacokinetic Considerations

The characteristic biphasic metabolic response to injury of an initial short ebb or shock phase (hypometabolic) followed by a flow phase (hypermetabolic) was described by Cuthbertson in 1930. A burn injury that exceeds 10 to 15% TBSA causes pathophysiological alterations in the cardiovascular, gastrointestinal, renal, and hepatic systems. The plasma proteins responsible for drug binding either increase or decrease in concentration, resulting in decreased or increased unbound drug concentrations, respectively. Finally, the movement of drugs into and out of the circulation is increased through the burn wound. The pharmacokinetics and pharmacodynamics of many drugs are changed after thermal trauma.

Cardiovascular Changes

Cardiac output has been demonstrated to decrease by as much as 50% within 6 hours of severe thermal injury. This reduction in output has been attributed to hypovolemia, increased blood viscosity, increased peripheral vascular resistance, and the presence of a cardiotoxic protein termed *myocardial depressant factor*.[50] Theoretically, intravenous drugs have a slower rate of distribution and elimination during this initial 48-hour period.

After resuscitation, the hyperdynamic or recovery phase of injury is associated with increases of cardiac output from one and one-half to three times normal. This may not occur in the patient with preexisting myocardial disease. This increase in tissue perfusion is associated with an increased rate of drug distribution and elimination after intravenous administration.[51]

Gastrointestinal Considerations

Acute stress-related mucosal damage of the stomach and duodenum after severe burns is extremely common and is presumably related to increased acid secretion.[52] The first case of acute gastroduodenal ulcer associated with thermal injury was reported by Swan in 1823. After the 1842 report on a series of 12 patients by Curling, the syndrome was established and named Curling's ulcer. Prophylaxis and treatment of stress-related mucosal damage includes enteral feeding and administration of sucralfate, omeprazole, or H_2-receptor antagonists (H_2RAs).[53] Cimetidine appears to be unique among the H_2RAs in that, after burns, it reduces resuscitative fluid requirements and has increased clearance. A study in burned children demonstrated a reduced cimetidine pharmacodynamic response, in addition to an altered pharmacokinetic profile. The absorption of orally administered drugs may be either increased or decreased, depending upon the drug pK_a and whether intragastric pH has been modified by antacids or H_2RAs.

Renal Function

The initial renal insults after a severe burn injury are general hypoxia and reduced perfusion. After severe injury, liberation of free hemoglobin or myoglobin may result in acute renal failure. These problems can be reversed rapidly with resuscitative efforts and establishment of adequate urine flow. During the postburn hypermetabolic phase, renal blood flow and glomerular filtration rate are increased, although tubular secretion may be impaired. This suggests that the elimination of freely filterable drugs such as the aminoglycosides and vancomycin increases after burn injury. This effect was demonstrated in a study of 20 patients with burns, which reported abnormal increases for both glomerular filtration rate and tobramycin elimination in 13 of 20 patients.[54] The need for increased dosage of gentamicin in patients with burns has been demonstrated in numerous studies of both adults and children.[55–59] There are conflicting results about increased renal elimination of vancomycin after burn injury, but a need for increased dosing is commonly observed.[60,61]

Hepatic Function

The hepatocyte is the most important site for drug metabolism, and in general it produces a metabolite that is more water soluble (facilitates urinary excretion) and of greater molecular weight (facilitates biliary secretion). The chemical reactions are classified into phase I and phase II biotransformations, which may occur in series. Phase I reactions include addition of a polar group (hydroxylation) or deletion of a nonpolar group (N-demethylation). Phase II conjugation with endogenous compounds such as glucuronic acid may follow phase I reactions. The most important enzymes catalyzing these reactions make up the microsomal enzyme oxidation system and include cytochrome P-450 and cytochrome P-450 reductase.

Although the mechanism is not completely clear, burn injury is associated with a marked depression of phase I reactions, while phase II reactions are unaffected. There is some evidence that decreased enzyme activity is due to oxygen-derived free radical damage to the hepatocyte. This discrepancy is evident in the postburn metabolism of diazepam and lorazepam.[50] The phase I metabolism of diazepam is impaired, while the phase II metabolism of lorazepam (glucuronidation) does not differ from normal.[62]

Plasma Protein Binding

Although problems associated with changes in unbound drug concentration associated with inverse changes in plasma protein concentrations are theoretically possible, clinically important examples are few. The two proteins that account for most drug serum protein binding are albumin and α_1 acid glycoprotein (AAG).[63]

Albumin is a large molecule (approximately 69,000 daltons) capable of binding acidic, neutral, and basic drugs. Despite its large molecular weight, albumin is not confined to the intravascular space, 30% of total exchangeable albumin is in extravascular fluid. The postburn serum albumin concentration is commonly reduced by 50% and often reaches critical levels of 10 g/L (1 g/dL) (normal: 3.5 to 4.9 g/dL in adults). The free fractions of diazepam, phenytoin, and salicylic acid increase after burn injury, which has been attributed to a decreased serum albumin concentration.

AAG is an acute-phase reactant that has a high affinity but low capacity for basic drugs and may be saturated at therapeutic concentrations (e.g., lidocaine). The concentration of AAG may increase to as much as 300% of normal during the first postburn week and not return to normal for 4 to 6 weeks. The free fractions of imipramine, lidocaine, meperidine, and propranolol decrease after the first postburn week, presumably in response to an increased AAG concentration.

The critically important breakpoint for drug serum protein binding is approximately 90%. When binding is less than 90%, the pharmacokinetic parameters change little after pathophysiologic changes in binding. Oral administration of drugs with a high hepatic extraction ratio (such as propranolol) would be affected little by changes in plasma protein binding, because of the first-pass effect. Although the potential for problems is low, the clinician monitoring a patient receiving agents that have low therapeutic indices or steep dose-response curves should consider the effect of altered protein binding when evaluating drug toxicity or suboptimal response.

The efficacies of the nondepolarizing neuromuscular blocking agents tubocurarine chloride, metocurine iodide, pancuronium bromide, and atracurium besylate are reduced after the first postburn week, which implies that increased plasma protein binding to AAG is responsible.[64,65] Although increased binding does occur, the relatively small increase cannot explain the sometimes dramatic decrease in response. Investigations of the mechanism for this resistance have ruled out changes in drug clearance or volume of distribution. The decreased potency of these agents may be due to an unidentified substance in the plasma of patients with burns.

Drug Movement Through Burn Wounds

Destruction of the normal barriers to percutaneous absorption occurs with burn injury. The diffusion resistance to water movement through injured skin can be less than one-tenth that of normal skin. Gentamicin is absorbed readily after topical application of a 0.1% cream, and absorbed to a smaller extent with a 0.1% ointment.[66] Eschar penetration has also been demonstrated in vitro for mafenide acetate, nitrofurazone, povidone-iodine, silver nitrate, and silver sulfadiazine.[67]

Drug penetration of the burn wound is not unidirectional. Historically, it has been assumed that eschar penetration by systemically administered drugs was prevented by the avascular nature of the wound. However, systemically administered gentamicin and tobramycin both penetrate burn eschar.[68] Drug loss through the burn wound may add substantially to total drug clearance.

Treatment of Infection

Infection in Patients with Burns

Despite therapeutic advances, infection in burned patients remains the most important cause of death in those who survive initial resuscitation.[69–71] Administration of tetanus immune globulin and/or tetanus toxoid when the patient's tetanus immunization history is not known should be based on the American College of Surgeons guidelines. Colonization of the burn wound has been demonstrated even when the patient is cared for in a laminar-flow room. Explanations for this phenomenon are that endogenous bacteria translocate from the gastrointestinal tract, bacteria are iatrogenically transmitted, and normal skin flora proliferate.[72] In 15 patients with ≥20% TBSA evaluated within 24 hours of burn injury, the gastrointestinal barrier was compromised as evidenced by increased absorption of lactulose and mannitol.[73] However, the potential consequences of bacterial translocation are still debated.[74]

Burn Wound Infection

The methods and materials used in the treatment of burn wound infection have undergone significant changes.[75] Although the importance of bacteria in the burn wound has been recognized, the terminology describing the association between wound bacteria and systemic manifestations of infection is confusing. Moncrief and Teplitz[76] suggested that "burn wound sepsis" be used to describe the events associated with bacterial proliferation to 100,000 colony-forming units per gram of burn wound tissue and subsequent invasion of adjacent nonburned tissue. Unfortunately, this number of bacteria per gram of tissue is not diagnostic of an invasive burn wound infection, and a complex classification scheme ranging from surface contamination to microvascular invasion (I, II, III, IV, V, VIa, VIb, and VIc) has been suggested by Pruitt.[77]

Whether or not the bacteria are localized to the burn or are disseminated, a rational method for selecting from the available topical antimicrobials is necessary. Similar to the Kirby-Bauer method of determining bacterial susceptibility to systemic agents, Nathan et al.[78] first reported on the agar-well diffusion method for determining susceptibilities to topical antimicrobials.[78] Support for this method was supplied by Heggers et al.[79] who demonstrated that the agar-well diffusion test was more reliable than minimum inhibitory concentration determination for predicting bacterial susceptibility.[79]

Topical Antimicrobials

Silver nitrate. The "modern" use of silver nitrate began in the late 1800s with the prevention of ophthalmia neonatorum. Substantial improvement in the treatment of large burns by the use of continuously applied 0.5% silver nitrate solution was reported in 1965.[80] The characteristics that make 0.5% silver nitrate a useful topical antibacterial agent are its safety, water solubility, prolonged antibacterial action, lack of toxicity to viable skin, lack of antigenicity, and ease of preparation. Problems associated with its use include hypochloremia from formation of silver chloride salts, water intoxication because of the hypotonicity of the solution, and hyponatremia or hypokalemia from diffusion into the wet dressings. Other problems are a requirement for bulky dressings that restrict joint motion and ambulation and black staining of everything that comes into contact with the solution.

Silver sulfadiazine. The use of silver sulfadiazine (SSD) in burns was first reported in both a murine burn model and 16 patients.[81] SSD is unique among the usual topical antibacterial agents in that it effectively inhibits *Candida albicans*. The exact antimicrobial mechanism of action of SSD has not been clearly elucidated, but it is attributed to silver inhibition of DNA replication or cell membrane modification. Two studies imply that the sulfadiazine component is not necessary for in vitro bacterial sensitivity. In addition, clinical efficacy may be associated with a reversal of injury-induced suppression of lymphocyte natural killer cell cytotoxicity rather than strict antibacterial effects.

SSD is the topical agent of choice worldwide because of its safety and efficacy.[82–84] Toxicity associated with SSD application is infrequent and associated predominantly with the propylene glycol component of the cream base. The potential for allergic hypersensitivity is shown by circulating sulfadiazine antibodies (predominantly IgG) in the serum of treated patients. Although SSD-associated leukopenia has been reported, it is probably an artifact of the physiologic response to burn injury of white blood cell margination and/or diapedesis (movement through vessels) from the intravascular space.[85] Clinicians continue to apply SSD to patients who develop leukopenia.

Because of its demonstrated efficacy, SSD has been incorporated into a number of biologic and synthetic dressings or skin substitutes, to take advantage of its benefits and eliminate the inconvenience of dressing changes with reapplication of cream. Another method used to improve upon SSD is the addition of other agents such as nitrofurazone, gentamicin, fluoroquinolones, and cerium nitrate. The most successful combination is with chlorhexidine; Silvazine (Smith & Nephew, Clayton, Australia), a commercially available combination, has been used in Australia for over 10 years.

Mafenide Acetate and Nitrofurazone. Although causing pain upon application, mafenide acetate is a useful topical antimicrobial for the treatment of subeschar burn wound infections because of its ability to penetrate the burn wound. Mafenide is often used on burned ears to prevent chondritis. Although closely related chemically, mafenide is not a sulfonamide. The primary metabolite (*p*-carboxybenzene sulfonamide) is a sulfonamide, and it may cause allergic reactions in patients with sulfonamide hypersensitivity. When applied to large TBSA burns, mafenide can produce systemic metabolic acidosis secondary to carbonic anhydrase inhibition.[86] Another disadvantage of mafenide is its high cost, approximately four times that of SSD. The antimicrobial usefulness of nitrofurazone has been demonstrated since the mid-1940s.[87] Its primary use has been in prophylaxis of infection after skin grafting.

Systemic Antimicrobials

The use of prophylactic penicillin during the first postburn week was common during the 1950s and 1960s because of a justified concern of infection by *Streptococcus pyogenes*. This organism produced rapid conversion of partial-thickness to full-thickness wounds and fatalities. However, current laboratory methods for monitoring the burn wound and close clinical monitoring of patients allow the rapid recognition of infection. Recent prospective clinical trials have demonstrated no benefit for prophylactic penicillin. Indeed, subsequent wound cultures in penicillin-treated patients have a greater incidence of resistant organisms.

The choice of antibiotics for systemic infections in patients with burns should be the same as for other patients.[88] However, because the pathophysiologic changes after burn trauma are dynamic, the dosing of systemic antimicrobials must be individualized when possible.[89] Increased requirements for aminoglycosides and vancomycin have been demonstrated in patients with burns (as discussed under "Pharmacokinetic Considerations").

Nutritional Support

The intimate relationship between nutrition and wound healing has been described.[90] The injury-associated hypermetabolic response with altered nutritional requirements including vitamins and micronutrients are discussed.

Metabolic Response to Trauma

The hypermetabolism after trauma was initially explained as a physiologic response to increased heat loss. The rationale was that burned skin allows increased water loss that lowers the skin/wound temperature when it evaporates. However, the precise relationship between evaporative water loss and postburn hypermetabolism is unclear, because conflicting results have been reported from similar investigations.

Similarly, it has been assumed that increased thermogenesis was necessary to compensate for heat loss in a cold environment, because damaged skin cannot respond with decreased perspiration and cutaneous vasoconstriction. However, postburn hypermetabolism is not attenuated, even when the environmental temperature is increased above thermal neutrality. A resetting of the hypothalamic thermal regulatory setpoint is suggested by a study comparing patients with burns to normal control subjects, in which the patients with burns selected a significantly higher environmental temperature when placed in a metabolic chamber.

Metabolic rate may be reduced after relief of pain, although the degree of reduction is not well defined.[91] Historically, pain management of hospitalized patients with opioids has been suboptimal because of unnecessary fears of addiction. Morphine requirements of patients with burns can be substantial, exceeding 60 mg/hr before development of tolerance.[92]

Other contributors to postburn hypermetabolism are prostaglandins, interleukins, components of the complement cascade, and the catabolic neurohumoral milieu of elevated serum cortisol, growth hormone, catecholamines, and glucagon levels.[93,94] Initial insulin secretion inhibition is usually followed by normal or supernormal plasma insulin levels. Despite this insulin recovery, hyperglycemia persists, secondary to insulin resistance at the tissue insulin receptor.

The fuel stores that are mobilized to sustain postburn hypermetabolism include hepatic and muscle glycogen; visceral, plasma, and muscle protein; and fat. Because the major metabolic source of adenosine triphosphate provided to the burn wound is anaerobic glycolysis, the obligatory glucose requirement is increased. Production of glucose from glycogenolysis is relatively short lived because stores only approximate 100 to 200 g and endogenous glucose production exceeds 400 g/day. Significant endogenous glucose is provided by efficient recycling of pyruvate and lactate via the Cori cycle and the glucose-alanine cycle. Catabolism of muscle protein and direct oxidation of amino acids provide approximately 15 to 20% of the total caloric expenditure in the fasting injured patient. The body adapts to using fat as its main energy source and can mobilize abundant energy from the typical fat stores of approximately 160,000 kcal.

Pharmacologic interventions that have been attempted to ameliorate the catabolic state after burn injury include anabolic steroids and human growth hormone. A small ($n = 13$) prospective, randomized trial of the anabolic steroid oxandrolone found a significantly increased rate of weight gain and muscle function than in control subjects.[95] Although a number of studies have demonstrated clinical benefits from adjunctive growth hormone treatment, recent data implicate growth hormone administration as a risk for premature mortality.[96,97]

The specific cause of postburn hypermetabolism is not clear but appears to be multifactorial. Completely arresting postburn hypermetabolism is not currently possible. A reasonable approach is to provide the patient with a warm environment, adequate pain relief, early enteral nutrition, and aggressive wound coverage. In addition, an attempt should be made to minimize endogenous protein catabolism by providing exogenous protein and nonprotein calories.

Nutrient Administration

Patients with less than 20% TBSA burns can usually be maintained on a normal diet, unless there is an associated condition such as severe preburn malnutrition or an injury that prevents mastication. Patients with larger burns are often unwilling or unable to consume enough high-protein and caloric-dense food to fulfill requirements. For these patients, nutritional requirements can be met by insertion of a small-bore nasoenteric feeding tube and administration of commercially available enteral feeding formulations such as Osmolite HN, TwoCal HN, TraumaCal, and Replete. Enteral nutrition is preferred to parenteral nutrition because it is more physiologic, less costly, and avoids complications associated with parenteral nutrition such as catheter-related sepsis.

In contrast to historical recommendations that focused on parenteral nutrition, current guidelines call for early enteral feeding.[98] Even in severely burned patients with absent bowel sounds, feeding into the small intestine through a nasoenteric tube is still possible, because postburn ileus is confined primarily to the stomach.[99] In these severely injured patients, a nasogastric tube is inserted and connected to suction for 2 to 3 days until gastric function returns. Experimental evidence favoring early enteral feeding demonstrated a reduction in catabolism and the hypermetabolic response in a guinea pig burn model. Another beneficial effect of early enteral feeding is the maintenance of gut mucosal mass. Improved gut wall homeostasis may prevent the increased intestinal permeability that allows translocation of enteric bacteria.

Macronutrient Needs

The metabolic demands associated with severe burns exceed those of any other hospitalized patient. The postburn energy expenditure increases with increasing burn size. However, there is an upper limit to required calories. This upper limit is approximately twice the calculated basal energy expenditure (BEE) using the Harris-Benedict equation. Numerous methods are available to calculate the burn patient's daily energy requirement, and representative formulas are listed in Table 47.3.

Although mathematical calculation to predict energy requirements is convenient, determination of the patient's specific caloric needs is desirable.[100] A complex metabolic chamber is necessary to specifically measure energy expenditure, but a reasonably accurate estimation can be performed at the bedside using indirect calorimetry.[101] Metabolic carts measure the respiratory gas exchange of oxygen (VO_2) and carbon dioxide (VCO_2) to indirectly measure energy expenditure (via the reverse Fick equation).

Carbohydrate Requirements

Energy liberated by oxidation of enterally administered carbohydrate is approximately 4 kcal/g. The carbohydrate commonly administered parenterally is hydrous dextrose, which liberates 3.4 kcal/g when completely oxidized. The optimal amount of administered carbohydrate minimizes gluconeogenesis without exceeding energy requirements and being stored as triglycerides.

The utilization of glucose for energy by patients with burns has limits. When glucose is oxidized to liberate energy, equimolar concentrations of oxygen are consumed and carbon dioxide produced (respiratory quotient [RQ] = 1). The normal, fed RQ is approximately 0.84, and it rises when the rate of administered glucose exceeds the maximum rate of use. When glucose is converted into fat, more than eight times as much carbon dioxide is released for each mole of oxygen (RQ >1). Excretion of this extra carbon dioxide could be difficult for a burned patient with an associated inhalation injury. An additional negative aspect of lipogenesis is that it is an energy-consuming process. An elegant study of intravenous glucose, using isotopic tracers, demonstrated that the maximum rate of oxidation is approximately 5 mg/kg/minute. At faster rates of glucose administration, the RQ rapidly increased above 1.0, suggesting lipogenesis. For a 70-kg patient, this maximum rate of glucose utilization translates into 2 L of 25% dextrose-containing total parenteral nutrition solution (500 g) per day.[102]

Fat Requirements

Fat is an efficient provider of energy at 9 kcal/g, but it is vital only for supplying essential fatty acids to prevent essential fatty acid deficiency syndrome. The amount of fat necessary in patients with burns is not known, but fat should provide a minimum 2% of total calories. Fat is an essential component of cell membranes, functions as a carrier for the fat-soluble vitamins, and is important for wound healing.

Patients with severe thermal injury may have reduced lipolytic capacity, especially after parenteral administration of fat emulsion. It appears that parenteral administration of long-chain triglycerides is associated with hepatomegaly, impaired clotting, and decreased resistance to infection. Preliminary evidence indicates that lipids high in linoleic acid (e.g., safflower or soybean oil) are associated with immunosuppression. This is presumably because linoleic acid is the precursor of arachidonic acid, which is the principle substrate for prostaglandins (PGE_1 and PGE_2) and certain leukotrienes. Another advantage of enteral administration is that medium-chain triglycerides are absorbed without the need for bile, and at the cellular level, they are transported into mitochondria without the need for carnitine.

Because of the constraint on the rate of carbohydrate administration, fat must usually be provided in substantial quantities as an energy source. Although not often important clinically, fat has a specific advantage over glucose in patients with pulmonary dysfunction, when a reduced carbon dioxide production for an equivalent amount of oxygen consumed is useful. The optimal fatty

Table 47.3 ▪ Various Formulas Used to Estimate Energy Requirements in Patients with Burns[a]

Adults
1. Harris-Benedict equation (BEE)
   Male : BEE (kcal) = 66 + (13.7 × W) + (5 × H) − (6.8 × A)
   Female : BEE (kcal) = 665 + (9.6 × W) + (1.7 × H) − (4.7 × A)
2. Burke and Wolfe
   kcal/day = 2 × BEE
3. Curreri
   kcal/day = 25 × W + (40 × TBSA)
4. Davies and Liljedahl
   kcal per day = 20 × W + (70 × TBSA)

Children
1. Wolfe
   kcal/day = 2 × BEE
2. Curreri Junior
   kcal per day = {0–1 years} BEE + (15 × TBSA)
   {1–3 years} BEE + (25 × TBSA)
   {3–15 years} BEE + (40 × TBSA)

BEE, basal energy expenditure; *W*, weight in kg; *H*, height in cm; *A*, age in years; *TBSA*, total body surface area.

acid chain length and exact dietary fat requirements for patients with burns remain to be determined.

Protein Requirements

Protein loss across burn wounds is considerable and is greatest in the first 3 postburn days. Although early protein loss across full-thickness burns is greater than that in partial-thickness burns, the rates become approximately the same after postburn day 3. The rate of protein loss is reduced by application of either antimicrobial creams or skin substitutes. Using the average protein loss during the first postburn week (0.5 $mg/cm^2/hr$) a formula that estimates the daily protein loss (g) across the burn wound can be devised: 1.2 × body surface area (m^2) × total body surface area burn (%). Protein loss across the burn wound during the second postburn week occurs at approximately half this rate.

The recommended daily allowance of protein for healthy adults is 0.8 g/kg. The optimal amount of protein required by patients with burns to prevent catabolism of protein stores and promote wound healing is not well defined. The importance of protein-sparing by providing energy must be considered, but some clinicians advocate a high-protein diet aimed at achieving a 100:1 nonprotein calorie to nitrogen ratio in contrast to the standard 150:1 ratio. In clinical practice, approximately 1.5 to 2 g/kg/day (using lean body weight) of protein is provided initially. Nitrogen-balance studies then determine the adequacy of this regimen. Although the nitrogen balance calculation appears simple, [Nitrogen balance = N(in) – N(out)], there is potential error in assessment of both N(in) and N(out). N(in) is the number of grams of nitrogen ingested or infused, and it is common practice to multiply the number of grams of protein or amino acid by 0.16 to estimate grams of nitrogen. This calculation assumes that the protein is made up of 16% nitrogen, but the percentage nitrogen in available parenteral amino acid products varies from 11.1 to 16.9%.[103] The N(out) is calculated by adding the urinary urea nitrogen (UUN) from a 24-hour urine collection to an estimate of nitrogen excretion other than that measured as urine urea. This estimate comprises non-UUN (ammonia, uric acid, creatinine) and nonurinary nitrogen loss (fecal and skin). A commonly used estimate for non-UUN losses is 4 g. One group advocates the measurement of total urinary nitrogen rather than using an inaccurate estimate.[104] As described above, significant quantities of protein (nitrogen) are lost through open burn wounds and must be included when using an estimate.

The branched-chain amino acids (BCAAs) leucine, isoleucine, and valine are unique in that skeletal muscle can oxidize them directly for energy. In contrast, the other amino acids are metabolized almost wholly by the liver. Under ordinary circumstances, only 6 to 7% of the daily energy expenditure is provided through BCAA oxidation by skeletal muscle. The administration of supplemental BCAAs, especially leucine, to patients with burns should (theoretically) reduce protein catabolism in skeletal muscle and increase protein synthesis. However, conclusive evidence of beneficial effects for BCAA-enriched solutions in patients with burns has not been demonstrated, and further studies are needed.[105]

Another strategy to improve outcome in patients with burns is the administration of beneficial nutrients that may reduce inflammation or enhance immunity. Unfortunately, the benefits of these expensive diets have yet to be definitively demonstrated. One trial of a specialized diet that contains arginine, Ω-3 fatty acids, and RNA failed to identify an advantage over a less expensive, high-protein enteral formula.[106]

Measurement of serum proteins such as albumin, prealbumin, transferrin, and retinol-binding protein is often regarded as a reliable index of nutritional status. However, because of surgical excision and grafting of wounds, associated blood loss and transfusions, and administration of exogenous albumin, changes in serum protein concentrations as an indication of nutrition regimen adequacy must be viewed with caution. Nitrogen-balance studies are probably the best assessment of protein status, despite the limitations described previously.

Micronutrient Needs

In contrast to the extensive information about macronutrient requirements, little information is available about the micronutrient needs of patients with burns. There is evidence that micronutrient needs are increased after burns, although the exact amounts have not been defined.[107,108]

Vitamins

At a minimum, patients with burns should receive vitamin supplements based on the Recommended Dietary Allowances (RDA) for enteral administration or the American Medical Association Nutrition Advisory Group (AMA) for parenteral administration. In the absence of preexisting deficiency, there is little indication to administer increased amounts of fat-soluble vitamins. Vitamin C is often supplemented to 5 × RDA because it has little inherent toxic potential and has an important role in collagen deposition and wound healing. Because of their role as cofactors in metabolism and potential increased losses through the wound and urine, the B vitamin group is supplemented to 2 × RDA.

Trace Elements

In the acute-phase reaction to trauma, plasma concentrations of zinc, iron, and copper are markedly diminished.[109] Like vitamin C, zinc is thought to promote wound healing, and it is supplemented to 2 × RDA. Aggressive iron supplementation must be undertaken with some caution because of the potential for increased bacterial growth owing to plasma unbound iron. Deficiency syndromes of copper, selenium, chromium, iodine, manganese, and molybdenum occur in patients receiving long-term total parenteral nutrition, but no cases of deficiency appear to have been reported as a direct result of burn trauma. These trace elements are administered according to RDA or AMA guidelines.

KEY POINTS

- The complex clinical management and rehabilitation of a patient with severe burns requires a multidisciplinary team including surgeons, nurses, a pharmacist, dietitian, physical therapist, occupational therapist, respiratory therapist, and social worker.
- A large TBSA full-thickness burn requires surgical excision and split-thickness skin grafting.
- Fluid requirements during the initial postburn period are surprisingly large, and guidelines for fluid resuscitation have been devised by experienced clinicians.
- The pharmacist must be aware that the postburn hyperdynamic and hypermetabolic phase produces multiple pharmacokinetic and pharmacodynamic changes.
- The nutritional requirements of patients with burns can be substantial, with energy needs often approaching twice those of other hospitalized patients.
- A number of methods are available for estimating energy requirements by mathematical calculation, but determination of the patient's specific caloric needs by indirect calorimetry is desirable.
- The amount of dietary protein required by patients with burns to promote wound healing, replace losses, and prevent catabolism of protein stores is not well defined. Usually, intravenous amino acids or enteral protein at 1.5 to 2 g/kg per day is provided, and nitrogen-balance studies are performed.
- Current guidelines call for the preferential use of enteral (rather than parenteral) nutrition.
- Prevention and treatment of infection in the patient with burns is of paramount importance, because it is the most common cause of death in those who survive initial resuscitation.
- Treatment of systemic infection in patients with burns is similar to methods used for other patients, with dose individualization by antimicrobial serum-concentration monitoring when possible.
- Microbial growth in the burn wound can be substantial after colonization by endogenous or exogenous organisms.
- The availability of topical antimicrobial agents has dramatically improved the control of burn wound infections.

REFERENCES

1. Arturson MG. The pathophysiology of severe thermal injury. J Burn Care Rehabil 6:129–146, 1985.
2. Silverman SH, Purdue GF, Hunt JL, et al. Cyanide toxicity in burned patients. J Trauma 28:171–176, 1988.
3. Blalock SJ, Bunker BJ, DeVellis RF. Measuring health status among survivors of burn injury: revisions of the burn specific health scale. J Trauma 36:508–515, 1994.
4. Saffle JR, Sullivan JJ, Tuohig GM, et al. Multiple organ failure in patients with thermal injury. Crit Care Med 21:1673–1683, 1993.
5. Ryan CM, Schoenfeld DA, Thorpe WP, et al. Objective estimates of the probability of death from burn injuries. N Engl J Med 338:362–366, 1998.
6. Darling GE, Keresteci MA, Ibanez D, et al. Pulmonary complications in inhalation injuries with associated cutaneous burn. J Trauma 40:83–89, 1996.
7. Punch JD, Smith DJ, Robson MC. Hospital care of major burns. Postgrad Med 85:205–215, 1989.
8. Wachtel TL. Major burns. Postgrad Med 85:178–196, 1989.
9. Schiller WR, Garren RL., Bay RC, et al. Laser Doppler evaluation of burned hands predicts need for surgical grafting. J Trauma 43:35–40, 1997.
10. Robson MC, Smith DJ, Heggers JP. Innovations in burn wound management. Adv Plast Reconstr Surg 4:149–176, 1987.
11. Perry RJ, Moore CA, Morgan BDG, et al. Determining the approximate area of a burn: an inconsistency investigated and re-evaluated. Br Med J 312:1338, 1996.
12. Wong L, Munster AM. New techniques in burn wound management. Surg Clin N Am 73:363–71, 1993.
13. Gore DC, Beaston J. Infusion of hot crystalloid during operative burn wound debridement. J Trauma 42:1112–1115, 1997.
14. Demling RH. Burns. N Engl J Med 313:1389–1398, 1985.
15. Nowicki CR, Sprenger CK. Temporary skin substitutes for burn patients: a nursing perspective. J Burn Care Rehabil 9:209–215, 1988.
16. Teepe RGC, Kreis RW, Koebrugge EJ, et al. The use of cultured autologous epidermis in the treatment of extensive burn wounds. J Trauma 30:269–275, 1990.
17. Williamson JS, Snelling CFT, Clugston P, et al. Cultured epithelial autograft: five years of clinical experience with twenty-eight patients. J Trauma 39:309–319, 1995.
18. Lorenz C, Petracic A, Hohl HP, et al. Early wound closure and early reconstruction. Experience with a dermal substitute in a child with 60 per cent surface area burn. Burns 23:505–508, 1997.
19. Muhart M, McFalls S, Kirsner R, et al. Bioengineered skin. Lancet 350:1142, 1997.
20. Naughton G, Mansbridge J, Gentzkow G. A metabolically active human dermal replacement for the treatment of diabetic foot ulcers. Artif Organs 21:1203–10, 1997.
21. Ahlering PA. Topical Silastic gel sheeting for treating and controlling hypertrophic and keloid scars: case study. Dermatol Nurs 7:259–257, 1995.
22. Choiniere M, Melzack R, Rondeau J, et al. The pain of burns: characteristics and correlates. J Trauma 29:1531–1539, 1989.
23. Perry S, Heidrich G. Management of pain during debridement: a survey of U.S. burn units. Pain 13:267–280, 1982.
24. Osgood PF, Szyfelbein SK. Management of burn pain in children. Pediatr Clin North Am 36:1001–1113, 1989.
25. Wermeling DP, Record KE, Foster TS. Patient-controlled high-dose morphine therapy in a patient with electrical burns. Clin Pharm 5:832–835, 1986.
26. Donahue SR. Morphine sulfate intravenous dose of 1650 mg per hour. Hosp Pharm 24:311, 1989.
27. Porter J, Jick H. Addiction rare in patients treated with narcotics. N Engl J Med 302:123, 1980.
28. Choiniere M, Grenier R, Paquette C. Patient-controlled analgesia: a double-blind study in burn patients. Anaesthesia 47:467–472, 1992.
29. Gaukroger PB, Chapman MJ, Davey RB. Pain control in paediatric burns–the use of patient-controlled analgesia. Burns 17:396–399, 1991.
30. Rovers J, Knighton J, Neligan P. Patient-controlled analgesia in burn patients: a critical review of the literature and case report. Hosp Pharm 29:106, 108–111, 1994.
31. Patterson DR, Questad KA, de Lateur BJ. Hypnotherapy as an adjunct to narcotic analgesia for the treatment of pain for burn debridement. Am J Clin Hypn 31:156–163, 1989.
32. Miller AC, Hickman LC, Lemasters GK. A distraction technique for control of burn pain. J Burn Care Rehabil 13:576–580, 1992.
33. Beyer JE, Levin CR. Issues and advances in pain control in children. Nurs Clin North Am 22:661–676, 1987.
34. Pal SK. Cortiella J. Herndon D. Adjunctive methods of pain control in burns. Burns 23:404–412, 1997.
35. Reilly M. Music distraction in burn patients: influencing postprocedure recall. Semin Perioper Nurs 6:242–245, 1997.
36. Rubin WD, Mani MM, Hiebert JM. Fluid resuscitation of the thermally injured patient. Current concepts with definition of clinical subsets and their specialized treatment. Clin Plast Surg 13:9–20, 1986.

37. Demling RH. Fluid replacement in burned patients. Surg Clin North Am 67:15–30, 1987.
38. Graves TA, Cioffi WG, McManus WF, et al. Fluid resuscitation of infants and children with massive thermal injury. J Trauma 28:1656–1659, 1988.
39. Aikawa N, Ishibiki K, Naito C, et al. Individualized fluid resuscitation based on haemodynamic monitoring in the management of extensive burns. Burns 8:249–255, 1982.
40. Horton JW, White DJ, Baxter CR. Hypertonic saline dextran resuscitation of thermal injury. Ann Surg 211:301–311, 1990.
41. Gunn ML, Hansbrough JF, Davis JW, et al. Prospective, randomized trial of hypertonic sodium lactate versus lactated Ringer's solution for burn shock resuscitation. J Trauma 29:1261–1267, 1989.
42. Ross AD, Angaran DM. Colloids vs. crystalloids–a continuing controversy. Drug Intell Clin Pharm 18:202–212, 1984.
43. Waters LM, Christensen MA, Sato RM. Hetastarch: an alternative colloid in burn shock management. J Burn Care Rehabil 10:11–16, 1989.
44. Bowser BH, Caldwell FT. The effects of resuscitation with hypertonic vs. hypotonic vs. colloid on wound and urine fluid and electrolyte losses in severely burned children. J Trauma 23:916–923, 1983.
45. Greenhalgh DG, Housinger TA, Kagan RJ, et al. Maintenance of serum albumin levels in pediatric burn patients: a prospective, randomized trial. J Trauma 39:67–74, 1995.
46. Sheridan RL, Prelack K, Cunningham JJ. Physiologic hypoalbuminemia is well tolerated by severely burned children. J Trauma 43:448–452, 1997.
47. Cochrane Injuries Group Albumin Reviewers. Human albumin administration in critically ill patients: systematic review of randomised controlled trials. Br Med J 317:235–240, 1998.
48. Milner SM, Hodgetts TJ, Rylah LA. The burns calculator: a simple proposed guide for fluid resuscitation. Lancet 342:1089–1091, 1993.
49. Lazarus D, Hudson DA. Fatal rhabdomyolysis in a flame burn patient. Burns 23:446–450, 1997.
50. Martyn J. Clinical pharmacology and drug therapy in the burned patient. Anesthesiology 65:67–75, 1986.
51. Bonate PL. Pathophysiology and pharmacokinetics following burn injury. Clin Pharmacokinet 18:118–130, 1990.
52. Czaja AJ, McAlhany JC, Pruitt BA. Acute duodenitis and duodenal ulceration after burns. Clinical and pathological characteristics. JAMA 232:621–624, 1975.
53. Cioffi WG, McManus AT, Rue LW, et al. Comparison of acid neutralizing and non-acid neutralizing stress ulcer prophylaxis in thermally injured patients. J Trauma 36:541–547, 1994.
54. Loirat P, Rohan J, Baillet A, et al. Increased glomerular filtration rate in patients with major burns and its effect on the pharmacokinetics of tobramycin. N Engl J Med 299:915–919, 1978.
55. Zaske DE, Sawchuk RJ, Gerding DN, et al. Increased dosage requirements of gentamicin in burn patients. J Trauma 16:824–828, 1976.
56. Glew RH, Moellering RC, Burke JF. Gentamicin dosage in children with extensive burns. J Trauma 16:819–823, 1976.
57. Zaske DE, Bootman JL, Solem LB, et al. Increased burn patient survival with individualized dosages of gentamicin. Surgery 91:142–149, 1982.
58. Zaske DE, Chin T, Kohls PR, et al. Initial dosage regimens of gentamicin in patients with burns. J Burn Care Rehabil 12:46–50, 1991.
59. Hollingsed TC, Harper DJ, Jennings JP. Aminoglycoside dosing in burn patients using first dose pharmacokinetics. J Trauma 35:394–398, 1993.
60. Garrelts JC, Peterie JD. Altered vancomycin dose vs. serum concentration relationship in burn patients. Clin Pharmacol Ther 44:9–13, 1988.
61. Brater DC, Bawdon RE, Anderson SA, et al. Vancomycin elimination in patients with burn injury. Clin Pharmacol Ther 39:631–634, 1986.
62. Martyn J, Greenblatt DJ. Lorazepam conjugation is unimpaired in burn trauma. Clin Pharmacol Ther 43:250–255, 1987.
63. Bloedow DC, Hansbrough JF, Hardin T, et al. Postburn serum drug binding and serum protein concentrations. J Clin Pharmacol 26:147–151, 1986.
64. Thompson DF. Neuromuscular blocking agents in burn patients. DICP 23:1006–1008, 1989.
65. Dwersteg JF, Pavlin EG, Heimbach DM. Patients with burns are resistant to atracurium. Anesthesiology 65:517–520, 1986.
66. Stone HH, Kolb LD, Pettit J, et al. The systemic absorption of an antibiotic from the burn wound surface. Am Surg 34:639–643, 1968.
67. Stefanides MM, Copeland CE, Kominos SD, et al. In vitro penetration of topical antiseptics through eschar of burn patients. Ann Surg 183:358–364, 1976.
68. Polk RE, Mayhall CG, Smith J, et al. Gentamicin and tobramycin penetration into burn eschar. Arch Surg 118:295–302, 1983.
69. McManus WF. Patterns of infection over the past ten years: historical patterns. J Burn Care Rehabil 8:32–35, 1987.
70. Gelfand JA. Infections in burn patients: a paradigm for cutaneous infection in the patient at risk. Am J Med 76(suppl 5A):158–165, 1984.
71. Luterman A, Dacso CC, Curreri PW. Infections in burn patients. Am J Med 81(suppl 1A):45–52, 1986.
72. Ziegler TR, Smith RJ, O'Dwyer RT, et al. Increased intestinal permeability associated with infection in burn patients. Arch Surg 123:1313–1319, 1988.
73. Deitch EA. Intestinal permeability is increased in burn patients shortly after injury. Surgery 107:411–416, 1990.
74. Barber A, Inner H, Shires GT. Bacterial translocation in burn injury. Semin Nephrol 13:416–419, 1993.
75. Ryan CM, Tompkins RG. Topical therapy, II. Burns. In Chernow, B, ed. The pharmacologic approach to the critically ill patient. 3rd ed. Baltimore: Williams & Wilkins, 1994:830–843.
76. Moncrief JA, Teplitz C. Changing concepts in burn sepsis. J Trauma 4:233–245, 1964.
77. Pruitt BA. The diagnosis and treatment of infection in the burn patient. Burns Incl Therm Inj 11:79–91, 1984.
78. Nathan P, Law EJ, Murphy DF, et al. A laboratory method for selection of topical antimicrobial agents to treat infected burn wounds. Burns Incl Therm Inj 4:177–187, 1978.
79. Heggers JP, Velanovich V, Robson MC, et al. Control of burn wound sepsis: a comparison of in vitro topical antimicrobial assays. J Trauma 27:176–179, 1987.
80. Moyer CA, Brentano L, Gravens DL, et al. Treatment of large human burns with 0.5% silver nitrate solution. Arch Surg 90:812–867, 1965.
81. Fox CL. Silver sulfadiazine–A new topical therapy for *Pseudomonas* in burns. Arch Surg 96:184–188, 1968.
82. Monafo WW, West MA. Current treatment recommendations for topical burn therapy. Drugs 40:364–373, 1990.
83. Rice TL. Topical antibacterials. Hosp Pharm 27:1099–1108, 1992.
84. Sawhney CP, Sharma RK, Rao KR, et al. Long-term experience with 1 per cent topical silver sulphadiazine cream in the management of burn wounds. Burns Incl Therm Inj 15:403–406, 1989.
85. Thomson PD, Moore NP, Rice TL, et al. Leukopenia in acute thermal injury: evidence against silver sulfadiazine as the causative agent. J Burn Care Rehabil 10:418–420, 1989.
86. Liebman PR, Kennelly MM, Hirsch EF. Hypercarbia and acidosis associated with carbonic anhydrase inhibition: a hazard of topical mafenide acetate use in renal failure. Burns 8:395–398, 1982.
87. Hooper G, Covarrubias J. Clinical use and efficacy of furacin: a historical perspective. J Int Med Res 11:289–293, 1983.
88. Dacso CC, Luterman A, Curreri PW. Systemic antibiotic treatment in burned patients. Surg Clin North Am 67:57–68, 1987.
89. Mason AD, McManus AT, Pruitt BA. Association of burn mortality and bacteremia. A 25-year review. Arch Surg 121:1027–1031, 1986.
90. Meyer NA, Muller MJ, Herndon DN. Nutrient support of the healing wound. New Horiz 2:202–214, 1994.
91. Mackersie RC, Karagianes TG. Pain management following trauma and burns. Anesthesiol Clin North Am 7:211–227, 1989.
92. Wermeling DP, Record KE, Foster TS. Patient-controlled high-dose morphine therapy in a patient with electrical burns. Clin Pharm 5:832–835, 1986.
93. Drost AC, Burleson DG, Cioffi WG. Plasma cytokines following thermal injury and their relationship with patient mortality, burn size and time post burn. J Trauma 35:335–339, 1993.
94. DeBrandt JP, Chollet-Martin S, Hernvann A, et al. Cytokine response to burn injury: relationship with protein metabolism. J Trauma 36:624–628, 1994.
95. Demling RH, DeSanti L. Oxandrolone, an anabolic steroid, significantly increases the rate of weight gain in the recovery phase after major burns. J Trauma 43:47–51, 1997.
96. Jenkins RC, Ross RJM. Growth hormone therapy for protein catabolism. Q J Med 89:813–819, 1996.
97. Maison P, Balkau B, Simon D, et al. Growth hormone as a risk for premature mortality in healthy subjects: data from the Paris prospective study. Br Med J 316:1132–1133, 1998.
98. Enzi G, Casadei A, Sergi G, et al. Metabolic and hormonal effects of early nutritional supplementation after surgery in burn patients. Crit Care Med 18:719–721, 1990.
99. Garrel DR, Davignon I, Lopez D. Length of care in patients with severe burns with or without early enteral nutritional support. A retrospective study. J Burn Care Rehabil 12:85–90, 1991.
100. Cunningham JJ, Hegarty MT, Meara PA, et al. Measured and predicted calorie requirements of adults during recovery from severe burn trauma. Am J Clin Nutr 49:404–408, 1989.
101. Saffle JR, Medina E, Raymond J, et al. Use of indirect calorimetry in the nutritional management of burned patients. J Trauma 25:32–39, 1985.

102. Bell SJ, Blackburn GL, Nutritional support of the burn patient. In Martyn JAJ, ed. Acute management of the burned patient. Philadelphia: WB Saunders, 1990:138–158.
103. Miller SJ. The nitrogen balance revisited. Hosp Pharm 25:61–65, 1990.
104. Konstantinides FN, Radmer WJ, Becker WK, et al. Inaccuracy of nitrogen balance determinations in thermal injury with calculated total urinary nitrogen. J Burn Care Rehabil 13:254–260, 1992.
105. Oki JC, Cuddy PG. Branched-chain amino acid support of stressed patients. DICP 23:399–408, 1989.
106. Saffle JR, Wiebke G, Jennings K et al. Randomized trial of immune-enhancing enteral nutrition in burn patients. J Trauma 42:793–802, 1997.
107. Pasulka PS, Wachtel TL. Nutritional considerations for the burned patient. Surg Clin N Am 67:109–131, 1987.
108. O'Neil CE, Hutsler D, Hildreth MA. Basic nutritional guidelines for pediatric burn patients. J Burn Care Rehabil 10:278–284, 1989.
109. Shewmake KB, Talbert GE, Bowser-Wallace BH, et al. Alterations in plasma copper, zinc, and ceruloplasmin levels in patients with thermal trauma. J Burn Care Rehabil 9:13–17, 1988.

CHAPTER 48

COMMON EYE DISORDERS

Sharon D. Solomon

A number of disorders can affect the structures of the eye, with outcomes ranging from moderate discomfort to significant loss of vision. The health care provider should be familiar with the signs and symptoms of common eye disorders and understand the decision-making process behind treatment. This chapter reviews common eye disorders by anatomic location and by medication classification. The clinical presentations of these disorders, the principles of treatment, and a review of the mechanisms and profiles of commonly used ophthalmic medications are provided.

Figure 48.1 provides an anatomic depiction of the various structures of the eye.

TREATMENT GOALS: COMMON EYE DISORDERS

- Identify and differentiate vision-threatening from non-vision-threatening disorders.
- Differentiate periorbital disorders, such as contact dermatitis, from actual orbital disorders, such as orbital cellulitis.
- Recognize acute infectious and chronic inflammatory disorders of the eye.
- Identify and treat bacterial and viral conjunctivitis.
- Recognize vision-threatening disorders of the anterior segment, such as corneal ulcers and herpes keratitis.
- Recognize and treat corneal abrasions.
- Become familiar with the use of common topical ophthalmic medications, such as antibiotic drops and ointments, and educate the patient on use of these medications.

DISORDERS OF THE EYELID AND LACRIMAL GLAND

The often nonspecific signs of eyelid swelling, diffuse tenderness to palpation, erythema, and increased tearing on presentation should elicit a differential diagnosis of causes ranging from chronic, benign disorders of the lid and lacrimal system to more acute conditions that warrant immediate intervention. The history and examination aid in narrowing the differential diagnosis. The following are common, treatable conditions easily identified in an acute care setting.

Hordeolum and Chalazion

An external hordeolum, or stye, is a small abscess resulting from an acute infection of a lash follicle and its associated sebaceous gland (gland of Zeiss) or sweat gland (gland of Moll). Because *Staphylococcus* is the pathogenic organism, such styes can also develop in patients with chronic, underlying staphylococcal blepharitis. On examination, a visible or palpable discrete swelling in the lid margin may

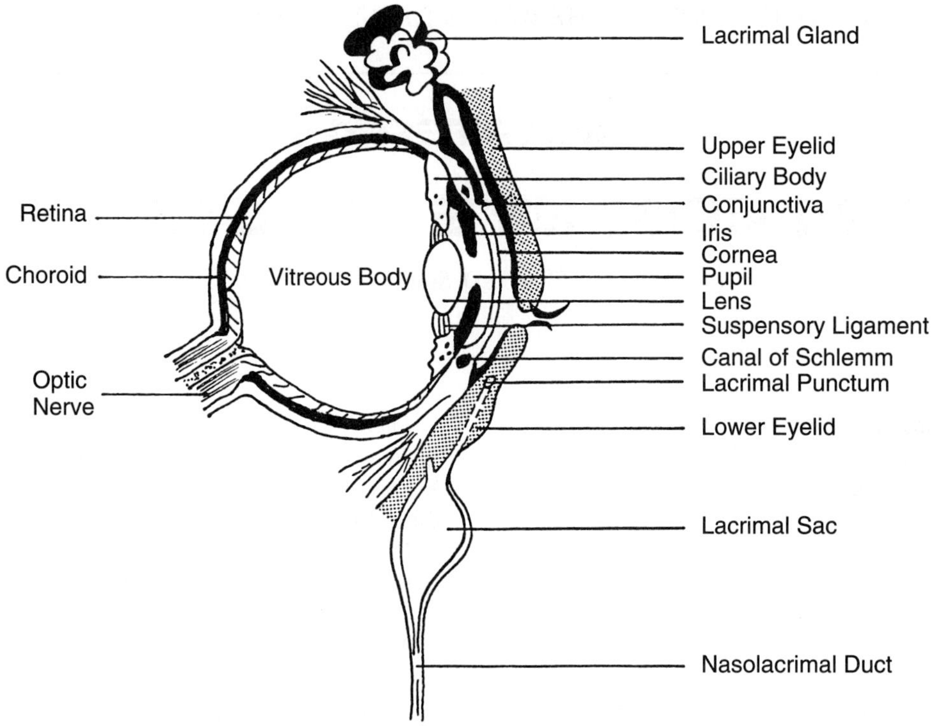

Figure 48.1. Cross-section of the eyeball and lacrimal passages.

be appreciated. The patient may also report a history of previous episodes of stye formation.

An internal hordeolum is a small abscess caused by an acute staphylococcal infection of the glands on the conjunctival aspect of the lid, the meibomian glands. Everting the eyelid on examination may allow better visualization of the yellowish nodule.

Despite causing a moderate degree of discomfort to the patient, external and internal hordeola often resolve spontaneously. Application of warm compresses to the affected lid for 15-minute intervals four times a day often provides symptomatic relief. Coadministration of topical bacitracin or erythromycin ointment to the lid margin twice a day tends to result in more rapid resolution of the lesion. Patients should be advised that it may take up to 4 weeks before the lesion resolves completely.[1]

A chalazion is a chronic, focal inflammation of the eyelid secondary to obstruction of the ducts of the sebaceous meibomian glands. These glands are located in the firm layer of the eyelid, the tarsal plate, and produce the lipid layer of the tear film. When the gland is obstructed and its contents stagnate within the duct, a painless, round, firm nodule forms. During the acute, inflammatory phase of formation of this meibomian cyst, the treatment regimen is similar to that for hordeola. Warm compresses for 15 minutes four times a day, in addition to gentle massage over the lesion, may help to express the contents. Again, the patient should be informed that resolution occurs over weeks. If the chalazion persists for more than 4 weeks, the patient should be referred to an ophthalmologist for either steroid injection into the lesion or surgical incision and curettage of the lesion.[2] The latter is the more common method of treatment because it definitively decompresses the lesion and can be performed in an office setting under local anesthesia. Steroid injections of triamcinolone may need to be repeated for complete resolution of the lesion and may lead to permanent depigmentation of the skin around the injection site.[2]

Blepharitis and Meibomitis

Blepharitis is a chronic condition marked by red, crusty, thickened eyelids with engorged blood vessels at the margins. Patients often complain of itching, burning, and excessive tearing from foreign-body sensation. Lid crusting waxes and wanes but is often worse in the mornings. Infection with *Staphylococcus* at the base of the lashes is believed to have an important role in the genesis of this external eye disorder. Collarettes, hard scales at the lash bases, are associated with *Staphylococcus* infection of the lid margins and contribute to epidermal ulceration. In long-standing cases, patients may suffer from loss of lashes (madarosis) and in-turning of lashes (trichiasis). Proper lid hygiene is the mainstay of alleviating the symptoms of blepharitis. The patient should be advised to scrub the eyelid margins with a mild baby shampoo twice a day, followed by a thin application of an antibiotic ointment, such as bacitracin or erythromycin, to the lid margin.[3] Frequent use of artificial tears relieves dry eye symptoms. Treatment is chronic, with relief of symptoms occurring over 2 to 3 weeks, but the infection is seldom completely eradicated. Patients must resume a more intensive course of similar treatment when the symptoms recur.

Meibomitis, or posterior blepharitis, is characterized by

inspissated oil glands at the eyelid margins. Patients present with symptoms of burning and excessive tearing. About two-thirds of patients have acne rosacea as an underlying disorder. Lid hygiene and cool compresses may help to alleviate symptoms, and the inflammation often is quieted with a course of systemic antibiotics. Oral tetracycline, 250 mg four times daily for 6 weeks, or doxycycline, 100 mg twice daily, have been shown to be efficacious in treating recurrent meibomitis.[1] Pregnant or lactating women and children younger than 12 years should receive oral erythromycin 250 mg four times daily instead because tetracycline and doxycycline are contraindicated in these patients.[1]

Contact Dermatitis

In a patient with the sudden onset of a periorbital rash with eyelid swelling and a mild, watery discharge who denies fever and tenderness to palpation, the diagnosis of contact dermatitis should be considered. A thorough history should be taken to elicit the recent use of a new ophthalmic drop or ointment, cosmetic, facial soap, or shampoo that could be the offending allergen. In some cases, patients may have used a particular ophthalmic drop for a significant length of time before developing a delayed hypersensitivity response to the drug. This is seen commonly in patients with glaucoma, who may receive a number of eyedrops chronically. Treatment involves avoiding the offending agent, which can be identified by stopping one medication at a time. Cool compresses four times a day for 15-minute intervals offer symptomatic relief. For severe itching, an oral antihistamine, such as oral Benadryl 25 to 50 mg up to four times daily for several days should be considered. In particularly severe cases, a mild steroid cream, such as dexamethasone 0.05%, applied to the affected area twice daily for several days may be an option.[4]

Preseptal Cellulitis

Preseptal cellulitis must be considered in the patient presenting with mild fever, tightness of the eyelid skin, and bogginess (chemosis) of the conjunctiva of the eye, in addition to the signs of eyelid edema, erythema, and tenderness. This infection of the eyelid and periorbital structures anterior to the orbital septum usually is the result of inoculation from a puncture wound or laceration or from an adjacent area of infection, such as the sinuses. In adults, the most likely causative organisms are *Staphylococcus aureus* and streptococci. *Haemophilus influenzae* should be considered in children under 5 years, who typically are affected by bacteremic spread from an otitis media or pneumonia.[5] A viral cause, such as herpes, should be considered in patients with an associated skin rash. A severe, acute hordeolum may also predispose to a preseptal cellulitis.

To distinguish a preseptal cellulitis from the more serious orbital cellulitis (discussed later), thorough examination must assess ocular motility, visual acuity, and pupillary reactions, all of which should be normal. Even though the eyelids may be extremely edematous, the eye itself should not be proptotic. There should be no pain with eye movements.

Treatment entails systemic antibiotics and daily monitoring of the infection for regression. For a mild, preseptal cellulitis in a patient older than 5 years, amoxicillin–clavulanate or cefaclor provides good coverage and should be continued for a 10-day course.[6] For a moderate to severe preseptal cellulitis or in a patient less than 5 years old, hospital admission may be required for intravenous ceftriaxone and vancomycin.[5] An orbital computed tomography (CT) scan may also be obtained to rule out orbital cellulitis.

Dacryocystitis and Dacryoadenitis

Dacryocystitis is an acute infection of the lacrimal sac resulting from blockage of the nasolacrimal duct. The obstruction prevents normal drainage of tears from the lacrimal sac into the nose and promotes stasis, predisposing the patient to secondary infection with bacteria. The patient presents with pain, redness, and swelling over the most nasal aspect of the lower lid, where the lacrimal sac is located. In addition to tearing, there may be a mucopurulent discharge readily expressed from the punctum when pressure is applied to the lacrimal sac. These patients should be referred promptly to an ophthalmologist for an ocular examination assessing extraocular motility and proptosis, for Gram stain and culture of expressed discharge, and for systemic antibiotic treatment. Mild cases in both children and adults usually respond to amoxicillin–clavulanate in combination with topical antibiotics, such as trimethoprim–polymyxin.[7] Warm compresses with gentle massage over the lacrimal sac may help to relieve the obstruction. More severe cases of acute dacryocystitis may necessitate hospital admission for intravenous antibiotics and a CT scan to rule out orbital cellulitis.

Dacryoadenitis is an acute infection of the lacrimal gland. Patients present with pain, redness, and swelling over the outer one-third of the upper eyelid. Gently lifting the upper lid may expose a prolapsed palpebral lobe of the lacrimal gland. The infecting bacteria tend to be *S. aureus, Neisseria gonorrhoeae,* and streptococci.[1] There may also be a viral cause, and mumps, infectious mononucleosis, and herpes zoster should be considered. For this reason, patients should also be referred promptly to an ophthalmologist for ocular examination, culture, and treatment with systemic antibiotics.

DISORDERS OF THE ORBIT

Orbital Cellulitis

Orbital cellulitis is one of the few true ocular emergencies necessitating immediate medical attention. Therefore, it is important to be aware of the signs and symptoms of this soft tissue infection, which extends behind the orbital septum. The patient may present with a red eye, blurred vision, fever, purulent discharge, and pain with eye movement. Critical signs include eyelid edema and conjunctival chemosis and injection. The eye may actually be proptotic, with restricted movement in the various directions of gaze.

The infection itself usually occurs secondarily, with

direct extension from the adjacent ethmoid sinuses (ethmoiditis).[8] However, it may also occur after a localized orbital infection, such as dacryoadenitis or dacryocystitis, after eye surgery, or after trauma to the eye. The most common causative organisms are *S. aureus, Streptococcus* species, and *H. influenzae*.[6] A fungal cause, such as *Mucor* mycosis, should be considered in diabetic or immunocompromised patients. Potential complications from orbital cellulitis include extension of the infection into the central nervous system, causing meningitis or brain abscess.

The patient should immediately undergo a complete ophthalmic examination to assess possible afferent pupillary defects, proptosis, and restricted eye movements, and undergo a CT scan of the orbits and sinuses to confirm the diagnosis. Gram stain and cultures of any discharge should be collected before broad-spectrum intravenous antibiotics, usually ceftriaxone and vancomycin, are started.[1] In an uncomplicated case of orbital cellulitis that responds to treatment, a 14-day course of antibiotics usually is needed.

Thyroid Ophthalmopathy

Thyroid ophthalmopathy is the most common cause of unilateral or bilateral proptosis in adults.[9] Patients typically present with double vision, foreign body sensation, and retraction of the eyelids, especially on downgaze. The proptosis, if long-standing, may predispose the patient to corneal exposure with ulcer formation. The disorder occurs in conjunction with Graves' disease, an autoimmune process marked by excessive secretion of thyroid hormones. Women are affected much more often than men. Although the majority of patients have a history of thyroid disease, approximately 16% of women and 34% of men have no evidence of an underlying thyroid disorder.[8]

These patients need medical management of their systemic thyroid disorder and referral to an ophthalmologist to screen for developing exposure keratopathy and optic nerve compression.[1] Exposure keratopathy can be treated with a regimen of frequent artificial tears during the day (every 1 to 6 hours) and lubricating ointment at night. If optic nerve compression, secondary to extraocular muscle enlargement at the orbital apex, is suspected, formal visual field examinations should be performed.

DISORDERS OF THE CONJUNCTIVA AND SCLERA

Conjunctivitis is one of the most commonly treated disorders of the eye. Patients typically present with a red eye and discharge, which may range from mild to copious, clearish to mucopurulent. Vision may be affected because of excessive tearing and irritation. The time of onset of symptoms, type of discharge, and laterality of the infection can aid in differentiating an acute from chronic bacterial or viral conjunctivitis.

Bacterial Conjunctivitis

Bacterial conjunctivitis is characterized by the acute onset of redness, foreign body sensation, mucopurulent discharge, and excessive eyelid crusting upon waking. Typically, both eyes are involved, and the patient gives a history of one eye preceding the other by a day or so in the onset of symptoms. Examination is remarkable for conjunctival hyperemia, mucopurulent discharge, a papillary reaction along the palpebral conjunctiva, and the absence of preauricular lymphadenopathy. The most common causative organisms of a bacterial conjunctivitis are *S. aureus, S. epidermidis, Streptococcus pneumoniae,* and *H. influenzae*.[8]

Simple bacterial conjunctivitis is self-limiting; even without treatment, symptoms resolve in 10 to 14 days. However, it is common practice to treat the infection and hasten the alleviation of symptoms for patient comfort. A conjunctival swab on blood, chocolate, and mannitol media should be sent for routine culture and sensitivities before treatment begins. The mainstay of therapy is 5 to 7 days of topical antibiotics, such as trimethoprim–polymyxin or ciprofloxacin four times daily, in combination with an antibiotic ointment (erythromycin or bacitracin) at bedtime.[1]

Gonococcal conjunctivitis should be high on the differential diagnosis in any patient presenting with a hyperacute (onset within 12 hours), extremely profuse mucopurulent discharge with marked chemosis and papillary reaction. Examination may also reveal preauricular lymphadenopathy as well as pseudomembrane formation. Immediate Gram stain, to detect intracellular Gram-negative diplococci, and conjunctival scrapings for culture and sensitivity are essential. Treatment consists of ceftriaxone 1 g in a single intramuscular dose.[10] In particularly severe presentations with evidence of early peripheral corneal ulcer formation, the patient should be hospitalized for intravenous antibiotics (ceftriaxone 1 g every 12 to 24 hours) and close observation.[8] The eye should be irrigated frequently with sterile saline to clear the discharge and topical erythromycin or bacitracin ointment applied four times daily. Concomitant infection with chlamydia should be suspected and the patient should also receive oral tetracycline 250 to 500 mg four times daily or doxycycline 100 mg twice daily for 2 to 3 weeks.[10]

Viral Conjunctivitis

Viral conjunctivitis usually presents acutely with the onset of a watery mucous discharge, conjunctival hyperemia, and lid edema. Examination often shows a palpebral follicular response, preauricular lymphadenopathy, and, in severe cases, subconjunctival hemorrhages and pseudomembrane formation. Adenovirus is the most common causative organism.[11] In particular, serotypes 8 and 19 are implicated in epidemic keratoconjunctivitis, a severe and highly contagious form of viral conjunctivitis that can cause a concomitant keratitis in up to 80% of cases.[8] In patients with a history of ocular herpes simplex or in whom herpetic vesicles along the skin of the eyelid margin or in the V_1 distribution can be seen, herpes simplex conjunctivitis should be considered.

In general, adenoviral conjunctivitis is a self-limiting condition with spontaneous resolution over 2 to 3 weeks. Symptomatic discomfort may be treated with artificial tears every 3 to 4 hours during waking hours. Cool compresses at 15-minute intervals four times daily can help relieve lid swelling and itching. Although most patients have bilateral involvement by the time they present, they should still be educated on the importance of hand-washing, not sharing towels or linens, and modifying behavior likely to result in the spread of the infection.

Herpes simplex conjunctivitis, unlike adenovirus, tends to be unilateral. Patients should be referred to an ophthalmologist to rule out corneal involvement, which can be vision-threatening. In an isolated conjunctivitis, topical antiviral therapy such as 1% trifluorothymidine (Viroptic) may be used 5 times a day for 7 to 10 days.[1] Cool compresses and artificial tears may also provide symptomatic relief.

Chronic Conjunctivitis

A chronic conjunctivitis is defined by the duration of symptoms, including discharge, conjunctival hyperemia, and general irritation for more than 4 weeks.[8] Adult inclusion conjunctivitis, or chlamydial conjunctivitis, is a chronic conjunctivitis typically affecting sexually active teenagers and young adults.[12] The patient presents with unilateral, mucopurulent discharge, a prominent palpebral and in some cases bulbar follicular reaction, and preauricular lymphadenopathy. A history of a concomitant urethritis or cervicitis may be elicited.

Diagnosis is made from conjunctival smears with direct monoclonal fluorescent antibody microscopy. Treatment is directed at both the ocular and genital infection and consists of oral tetracycline 250 to 500 mg four times daily or oral doxycycline 100 mg twice daily for 3 weeks.[1] Both the patient and the asymptomatic sexual partner should be treated. Oral erythromycin 250 to 500 mg four times daily for 3 weeks should be administered instead of tetracycline in children younger than 12 years and in pregnant or lactating women.[1] A topical ointment, such as erythromycin or tetracycline, should be used three times daily for 3 weeks in combination with systemic treatment.

Allergic Conjunctivitis

Hayfever, or seasonal allergic conjunctivitis, is a type I hypersensitivity immune response in which the binding of antigen–immunoglobulin E antibody complexes to mast cells causes the release of histamine and other inflammatory mediators.[13] The inciting antigen usually is airborne pollen, and the allergic response consists of a conjunctivitis marked by a watery discharge, pruritus, eyelid edema, conjunctival chemosis, and a palpebral conjunctival papillary reaction. The patient often has a history of allergies, and symptoms are worse during a particular season.

Treatment should involve avoiding the inciting agent. In addition, topical mast cell stabilizers, such as 4% cromolyn sodium, may be prescribed 4 to 6 times per day to prevent degranulation of mast cells and the release of histamines and leukotrienes, which would ultimately decrease the duration of most symptoms.[8] Though effective, cromolyn sodium must be used consistently for 7 to 10 days to achieve the desired effect. A topical antihistamine, such as levocabastine 0.05%, may be used four times daily, in combination with a mast cell stabilizer, to offer immediate relief of itching and burning.[1] Olopatadine (Patanol), a newly available combination topical mast cell stabilizer and antihistamine, is highly effective in relieving allergic symptoms and is used only twice daily. The antihistamine component provides immediate symptom relief, and the mast cell stabilizer provides long-term protection from the onset of symptoms.

Subconjunctival Hemorrhage

A ruptured blood vessel in the subconjunctival layer can cause blood to collect beneath the conjunctiva in a sectoral or diffuse pattern. The patient may first notice the extremely red eye after coughing or straining, as during a Valsalva maneuver. The appearance of the eye usually is more disturbing to the patient than any physical discomfort or irritation. Subconjunctival hemorrhage may also result from trauma, and a careful history should be taken to assess the possibility of more serious ocular damage, such as a ruptured globe. In addition, underlying high-blood pressure or a bleeding diathesis may also rarely be the cause of a subconjunctival hemorrhage. A medication history should inquire about chronic use of medications such as Coumadin. On examination, the presence of a conjunctival lesion as the source of the bleed should be ruled out and intraocular pressure should be checked.[1]

This condition usually clears spontaneously over 2 to 3 weeks, and no treatment is needed. Artificial tears can be prescribed as needed for mild irritation. A patient with a history of recurrent subconjunctival hemorrhage should be referred to an internist for a complete workup, including bleeding time, prothrombin and partial thromboplastin time, and complete blood count with platelets.[1]

Episcleritis and Scleritis

Episcleritis is a benign and self-limited disorder that often presents in young adults as an acutely red eye in a sectoral pattern. The patient may complain of mild discomfort in the affected eye, with some tenderness to palpation over the hyperemic area and excessive tearing; however, vision is not affected. On examination, the small vessels beneath the conjunctiva, the episcleral vessels, appear prominent and engorged. Both eyes may be involved, and the pattern of hyperemia may also be diffuse. The patient may have a history of prior attacks.

Most cases of episcleritis are idiopathic and not associated with an underlying systemic disorder.[14] However, an attempt should be made to elicit a history of symptoms suggestive of rheumatoid arthritis, systemic lupus erythematosus, or other collagen vascular diseases in a patient with recurrent bouts of episcleritis. Treatment is directed toward alleviating ocular irritation and decreasing redness of the eye. In mild cases, artificial tears used frequently during the day in combination with short-term use of a topical vasoconstrictor, such as 0.1% naphazoline twice daily, may be adequate therapy.[1] The patient should be warned against excessive or prolonged use of topical vasoconstrictors because they may result in rebound vasodilation and chronic redness. In more severe cases of episcleritis, topical nonsteroidal anti-inflammatory drugs (NSAIDs), such as 0.5% ketorolac, or mild topical steroids, such as fluorometholone, may be used four times daily to provide relief.[8] In rare cases of unresponsiveness, oral NSAIDs, such as ibuprofen 200 to 600 mg three times daily, can be taken in combination with topicals. Patients should be advised to take their medication with meals.

Scleritis is a severe inflammatory condition of the scleral layer of the eye that typically presents with a severe, boring eye pain, sectoral or diffuse redness, tearing, and photophobia. The deeper lying scleral vessels are dilated and, unlike the superficial engorged vessels seen in episcleritis, do not blanch when topical phenylephrine is applied. The patient's eye should be observed grossly under natural lighting conditions for the characteristic bluish hue of the sclera and for the presence of scleral nodules.

Unlike episcleritis, scleritis often is associated with an underlying systemic disease; rheumatoid arthritis is the most common.[15] The disorder tends to be recurrent and may be associated with vision-threatening conditions such as anterior and posterior uveitis, keratitis, cataract, scleral or corneal thinning and risk of perforation with minor trauma, and exudative retinal detachments. In addition to being under the care of an ophthalmologist, the patient should receive a rheumatologic workup to screen for other disorders such as Wegener's granulomatosis, ankylosing spondylitis, and systemic lupus erythematosus.

Treatment of the ocular disorder initially consists of oral NSAIDs, such as ibuprofen 400 to 600 mg four times daily or indomethacin 50 mg twice daily for a course of 1 to 2 weeks.[1] If there is no response to NSAIDs or if the presentation is particularly severe, systemic steroids, such as oral prednisone 60 to 100 mg daily for 2 to 3 days followed by a slow taper, may be needed to quiet the inflammation.[8] Steroid-resistant cases may respond to other immunosuppressive agents, such as cyclophosphamide or azathioprine, but such treatment should be prescribed in coordination with an internist or rheumatologist.

DISORDERS OF THE CORNEA AND ANTERIOR SEGMENT

Corneal Infiltrate and Corneal Ulcer

Contact lens wear is the most common predisposing factor in the development of a corneal infiltrate and its progression to a corneal ulcer.[16] Typically, the patient presents with a red eye, tearing or discharge, a significant degree of ocular pain, photophobia, and foreign body sensation, as well as decreased vision. Examination reveals an infiltrate, or localized, white opacification of the corneal stroma, that may or may not be associated with an overlying epithelial defect. The presence of an epithelial defect and evidence of decreased stromal thickness by slit-lamp examination is diagnostic of a corneal ulcer.[1] Anterior chamber inflammation ranging from mild cell and flare to frank hypopyon may also be seen on examination. A history of less than meticulous contact lens hygiene and overuse of extended-wear soft contact lenses may be elicited.

Bacterial keratitis is the most common form of corneal infection. *Pseudomonas aeruginosa,* in particular, is the most common causative bacterial organism.[17] *S. aureus* and *S. pneumoniae* bacterial keratitis are less common. Fungal keratitis should be considered in patients who have sustained a traumatic corneal injury, especially involving vegetable matter, such as a scrape from a plant leaf.[8] These infiltrates appear suppurative, as in bacterial presentations, but tend to have feathery borders and may have small, adjacent satellite lesions. *Aspergillus* or *Fusarium* spp. are commonly the causative organisms after ocular trauma, whereas infection by *Candida* typically occurs in a baseline debilitated cornea.[8] Corneal infection by the protozoan *Acanthamoeba* should be suspected in soft contact lens wearers with a history of poor lens hygiene (i.e., swimming with contact lenses or using homemade instead of commercially processed cleaning solutions) who have negative bacterial, fungal, and viral cultures and are not responding to conventional treatment.[18] A ring-shaped infiltrate may be appreciated on examination in *Acanthamoeba* keratitis. Herpes simplex virus can also predispose to corneal infection and should be considered in any patient with a history of ocular herpes or in a patient presenting with eyelid vesicles or dendritic epithelial defects that stain with fluorescein.

Referral to an ophthalmologist once a corneal infiltrate or ulcer is suspected is essential because this condition can be sight-threatening. The ophthalmologist must document the dimensions of the infiltrate and the patient's visual acuity, intraocular pressure, and anterior chamber reaction daily to assess whether the condition is responding appropriately to therapy. Before antimicrobial therapy is started, cultures are taken routinely on blood and chocolate agar for bacterial pathogens and Sabouraud's dextrose agar for fungal pathogens. If there is a high index of suspicion for *Acanthamoeba,* cultures can be sent on nonnutrient agar inoculated with *Escherichia coli.*[18] The contact lenses, cases, and cleaning solutions should be cultured as well. The patient should be warned of the serious complications that may arise, namely prolonged infection and risk of corneal perforation, if contact lens wear is resumed too early in the course of treatment.

If culture results are unavailable, treatment usually is directed toward broad-spectrum coverage of Gram-negative and Gram-positive bacteria, unless the history or examination is suspicious for a fungal, viral, or protozoan cause. In a patient with a small corneal infiltrate not associated with an overlying epithelial defect and with minimal discharge and anterior chamber reaction, ciprofloxacin drops every 2 hours while awake, supplemented with tobramycin ointment at bedtime, may be adequate therapy.[1] For larger infiltrates associated with an epithelial defect and moderate to severe anterior chamber inflammation, fortified tobramycin (15 mg/mL) and fortified cefazolin (50 mg/mL) should be used every hour around the clock until the infection begins to show signs of regression.[1] A cycloplegic, such as scopolamine 0.25% twice daily, can be used to prevent scarring of the iris during this acute phase of inflammation and to provide symptomatic relief from ciliary body spasm.

If the patient is not responding to fortified antibiotics or cultures are positive for fungus, natamycin 5% (50 mg/mL) drops may be used every waking hour and every 2 hours at night.[8] All topical or systemic steroid use should be tapered rapidly. It may be necessary to add amphotericin B 0.15% (1.5 mg/mL) drops every hour or oral fluconazole for a fungal keratitis slow to respond to treatment or for one involving the deep stroma and threatening corneal perforation.[1]

Culture-positive *Acanthamoeba* keratitis is treated with a combination of polymyxin–neomycin–gramicidin (Neosporin) and propamidine isethionate 0.1% (Brolene) drops every hour.[1]

Hospitalization may be needed to ensure adequate treatment in patients who are noncompliant with the medical regimen or in whom topical therapy has failed and systemic treatment is needed. As a last resort, a corneal transplant may be needed to restore vision if medical therapy fails.[8]

Herpes Simplex Virus: Corneal Epithelial Disease and Keratitis

As in bacterial keratitis, the patient presenting with herpes simplex infection of the cornea has a red, painful eye with photophobia, tearing, and decreased vision. A periorbital skin rash may be present, and the patient often gives a history of previous episodes of "painful red eye." On examination, corneal sensitivity should be evaluated with a cotton-tipped applicator before topical anesthetic is instilled because corneal sensation may be decreased in the presence of a herpes infection of the cornea. A dendritic or branching epithelial defect usually is appreciated when the corneal surface is stained with fluorescein. A deeper infection of the corneal stroma may present with an intact epithelium but with a disc-shaped area of stromal edema that may later predispose the patient to postherpetic corneal scarring.[8]

Herpes simplex corneal epithelial disease is treated with trifluorothymidine 1% drops (Viroptic) nine times a day for a course of 10 to 14 days.[1] If inflammation of the anterior chamber accompanies the epithelial disease, the patient should be given a cycloplegic agent, such as scopolamine 0.25% twice daily. Any concomitant topical steroid use is contraindicated. The patient should be followed closely, every 2 to 3 days, to evaluate the size of the epithelial defect and the thickness of the corneal stroma. Once the lesion has healed, the topical antivirals should be tapered over the course of a week.

Anterior Uveitis

Uveitis is a term used to describe general inflammation of the structures that make up the uveal tract: the iris, ciliary body, and choroid. Anterior uveitis may consist simply of inflammation of the iris (iritis) or of inflammation of both the iris and ciliary body (iridocyclitis). *Intermediate, posterior,* and *panuveitis* are other categories in the anatomic classification of uveitis; however, because these types of inflammation occur in the deeper structures of the eye and optical lenses are needed for assessment, this discussion is limited to anterior uveitis, which can be assessed with slit-lamp examination.

The patient presenting with acute anterior uveitis complains of photophobia, redness, excessive tearing, and perhaps mildly decreased vision. On examination, the hallmark is white blood cells, ranging from scant to too numerous to count, floating in the anterior chamber. Fine deposits of white cells may be appreciated on the inner aspect, or endothelial surface, of the cornea in the nongranulomatous type of uveitis. In the granulomatous variety, larger "mutton-fat" deposits of white cells on the corneal endothelium and nodules on the iris surface may be appreciated.

There are many causes of anterior uveitis, including trauma, human lymphocyte antigen (HLA) B27 positivity (associated with ankylosing spondylitis and Reiter's syndrome, especially in young men), herpes simplex, sarcoidosis, syphilis, and tuberculosis.[19] The patient's history of underlying systemic conditions and previous episodes of iritis or uveitis is important in determining a course of treatment for the ocular manifestations. Regardless of the suspected cause of the uveitis, the patient should be referred promptly to an ophthalmologist for a complete eye examination to assess whether inflammation exists in the more posterior structures of the eye and to assess intraocular pressure. For a bilateral, granulomatous, or recurrent uveitis, an initial workup would include a complete blood count, a rapid plasma reagin (RPR) and a fluorescent treponemal antibody absorption test to rule out syphilis, a purified protein derivative test for tuberculosis, and an HLA-B27 test for Reiter's syndrome or ankylosing spondylitis.[19] If the history is suspicious for sarcoidosis, a chest radiograph should be ordered.

Despite the underlying cause of the uveitis, the initial treatment plan often consists of a topical steroid, such as 1% prednisolone acetate every 1 to 6 hours depending on the severity of the anterior chamber reaction, and a cycloplegic agent, such as homatropine 5% twice daily.[1] In addition, any detected systemic disorder should be treated. Patients should be seen every 1 to 7 days initially until it is evident that the anterior chamber reaction is subsiding and the intraocular pressure is stable. In addition, patients with chronic uveitis on long-term topical or systemic steroids should be seen frequently to detect an elevated eye pressure secondary to steroid-induced glaucoma.

COMMON EYE DISORDERS SEEN IN THE EMERGENCY ROOM

Corneal Abrasion

A corneal abrasion should be suspected in any patient presenting with foreign body sensation who gives a history of minor trauma to the eye, as a scratch to the eye, or who wears contact lenses. The patient complains of pain and perhaps photophobia and has excessive tearing. The conjunctiva may be diffusely hyperemic. Vision is mildly to moderately decreased if the cornea becomes edematous or if the abrasion lies primarily over the visual axis. On slit-lamp exam, an epithelial staining defect is detected under cobalt blue light with a drop of fluorescein in the eye. The upper and lower eyelid both should be everted to ensure that no retained foreign body exists that could cause more mechanical trauma to the eye. While the epithelial defect is stained with fluorescein, its dimensions and location on the corneal surface should be recorded.

In a patient who does not wear contact lenses, treatment consists of applying an antibiotic ointment (erythromycin) to the eye prophylactically and then pressure patching the eye overnight to allow the epithelium to grow in over the defect. If the abrasion was caused by a contaminated object, such as a baby's fingernail or the leaf of a plant, or if the patient wears contact lenses, and the eye is at high risk for infection, pressure patching should be avoided.[8] Instead, topical antibiotics, such as ciprofloxacin 0.35%, should be administered every 2 to 6 hours, with erythromycin at bedtime.[8] In either case, the patient should be seen in 24 hours to check vision and the size of the epithelial defect and to look for any evidence of anterior chamber inflammation or early evidence of a corneal infiltrate. Topical antibiotics, with or without pressure patching, should be continued until the epithelium has regrown completely and covers the area of the previous defect. Contact lens wear should not be resumed for at least 1 week after the epithelial defect resolves.

Retained Corneal Foreign Body or Rust Ring

Despite the similar presentation of painful foreign-body sensation, photophobia, tearing, and blurred vision, perhaps even with an epithelial defect visible on exam, any patient who gives a history of a foreign body forcibly striking the eye should be dilated and examined thoroughly. The nature of the trauma should be clear: Were glasses or safety glasses being worn? Was the foreign body generated from metal striking metal?[1] Was there an immediate change in the level of vision?

The vision should be documented before any attempt is made to retrieve a surface or intraocular retained foreign body. On examination, the upper and lower eyelids should be everted to rule out any remnant of a foreign body. The corneal surface should be stained with fluorescein to detect an epithelial defect where the foreign body may have entered, and the anterior chamber should be examined carefully for signs of an intraocular retained body. The eye should then be dilated for a careful examination of the vitreous and retina.

A foreign body on the corneal surface can be removed in the office with topical anesthetic (proparacaine 0.5%) using a 25-gauge needle under magnification at the slit-lamp. Often a rust ring remains on the corneal surface where a metal foreign body may have struck the eye and remained adherent to the cornea before being washed out of the eye by irrigation or tearing. The rust ring also can be removed with the use of a topical anesthetic and an ophthalmic drill. The eye should then be treated with topical antibiotics (ciprofloxacin 0.35% every 2 to 6 hours) prophylactically and erythromycin at bedtime until the epithelial defect has healed.[1]

Chemical Burn

Chemical injury to the eye is a true ocular emergency necessitating immediate and constant irrigation even before an examination is performed.[1] Normal saline solution or sterile water, rather than a neutralizing agent, should be used to flush the eye for at least 30 minutes. During irrigation, the fornices and the undersurfaces of the lids should be swept with a cotton-tipped applicator to ensure that globules of the chemical are not being sequestered and continuing to damage ocular tissue. These areas should also be bathed in the irrigating solution. In general, irrigation is continued until the pH of the eye, as measured with litmus paper to the ocular surface, is neutral.

The patient should be seen by an ophthalmologist to assess the severity of the surface damage, including extent of corneal epithelial loss, degree of perilimbal ischemia, and intraocular pressure. Treatment ranges from a topical antibiotic (erythromycin) with pressure patching for an epithelial defect in mild cases to topical steroids and antiglaucoma medications for moderate to severe cases.

COMMON OPHTHALMIC MEDICATIONS

Most ocular medications are solutions, suspensions, or ointments that are administered topically, reaching therapeutic levels in the anterior segment without usually causing systemic side effects. To ensure the delivery of an adequate concentration of topical drug to the anterior segment, patients can be instructed to perform maneuvers such as closing the eye after administration of a drop

Table 48.1 ▪ Single-Agent Antibacterials

Drug	Dosage Form	Strength	Frequency of Dosing
Bacitracin	Ointment	500 U/g	BID–QID
Chloramphenicol	Ointment	0.5%, 1.0%	BID–QID
Ciprofloxacin	Solution	0.35%	1 drop q1–6hr
Erythromycin	Ointment	0.5%	BID–QID
Gentamicin	Ointment	0.3%	BID–QID
	Solution	0.3%	1 drop q1–6hr
Norfloxacin	Solution	0.3%	1 drop q1–6hr
Ofloxacin	Solution	0.35%	1 drop q1–6hr
Sulfacetamide	Ointment	10%	BID–QID
	Solution	10%, 15%, 30%	1 drop q1–6hr
Tobramycin	Ointment	0.3%	BID–QID
	Solution	0.3%	1 drop q1–6hr

Source: Reference 25.

Table 48.2 ▪ Combination Antibacterials

Drug	Dosage Form	Frequency of Dosing
Neomycin + bacitracin + polymyxin B (Neosporin)	Ointment Solution	BID–QID 1 drop q1–6hr
Polymyxin B + bacitracin (Polysporin)	Ointment	BID–QID
Polymyxin B + trimethoprim (Polytrim)	Solution	1 drop q3hr up to 6 drops/day

Source: Reference 25.

Table 48.3 ▪ Antiviral and Antifungal Agents

Drug	Dosage Form	Strength	Frequency of Dosing
Antiviral			
Idoxuridine	Solution	0.1%	1 drop q1hr
Trifluridine	Solution	1%	1 drop 9 times/day
Vidarabine	Ointment	3%	0.5 inch 5 times/day
Antifungal			
Natamycin	Solution	5%	1 drop q1–6hr

Source: Reference 25.

(to increase ocular absorption and decrease systemic absorption of the drug), waiting 5 minutes between drops (so that one medication doesn't simply wash out the other), and occluding the punctum after a drop (to decrease drainage of the medication with tears through the lacrimal system).[20] In addition, the traditional qualities of the drug itself, such as its lipid solubility, viscosity, and concentration, determine how much of the drug is absorbed from the ocular surface. Patients who wear contact lenses should remove them before administering topical medications, some of which may alter the clarity of the lenses.

Antimicrobial Agents

Topical ophthalmic antimicrobial agents (Tables 48.1–48.3) have the same mechanisms of action, coverage, and potential for side effects as their systemic counterparts. Therefore, a possible history of adverse reactions to these drug classes, ranging from local rash to anaphylaxis, should be elicited from the patient.

Bacitracin is an antibiotic that inhibits cell wall synthesis and is active against most Gram-positive cocci, *Neisseria,* and *H. influenzae.* It is available as a single agent or in combination with neomycin and polymyxin B.

Chloramphenicol is a broad-spectrum bacteriostatic agent that inhibits bacterial protein synthesis. It provides good coverage against anaerobic bacteria, *H. influenzae,* and *Neisseria.* The topical form has been reported to rarely precipitate an aplastic anemia in patients.

The fluoroquinolones, ciprofloxacin, ofloxacin, and norfloxacin, are highly effective antimicrobial agents with broad-spectrum activity against both Gram-positive and Gram-negative organisms. These agents interfere with the bacterial enzymes for replication and DNA repair. Ciprofloxacin, in particular, has a lower minimum inhibitory concentration than the aminoglycosides, gentamicin and tobramycin, but inhibits up to 90% of common bacterial pathogens infecting the cornea.[21] As a class, the fluoroquinolones are also less toxic to the corneal epithelium than are the aminoglycosides.

Erythromycin belongs to the macrolide class of antibiotics and works by inhibiting bacterial protein synthesis. It is effective against Gram-positive cocci and bacilli and *Neisseria gonorrhoeae.*

Gentamicin and tobramycin belong to the class of aminoglycosides, which are bactericidal agents that interfere with the initiation of bacterial protein synthesis. These agents are effective against aerobic, Gram-negative bacilli such as *P. aeruginosa,* a common corneal pathogen. They also provide coverage against Gram-positive cocci such as *S. aureus* and *S. epidermidis.*

Sulfacetamide is a bacteriostatic drug that belongs to the sulfonamide class of inhibitors of bacterial folic acid synthesis. It is effective against *S. pneumoniae, Corynebacterium diphtheriae, H. influenzae,* and *Chlamydia trachomatis.* As with its systemic counterparts, the topical form has been implicated in cases of severe sensitivity reactions such as Stevens–Johnson syndrome.

Of the three topical antiviral agents for treating herpes simplex keratitis, trifluridine has the best corneal penetrance and the highest efficacy.

Natamycin is active against a range of filamentous fungi such as *Aspergillus, Fusarium,* and the yeast *Candida albicans.*

Anti-Inflammatory and Antiallergy Agents

The class of anti-inflammatory agents (Tables 48.4–48.7) known as glucocorticoids or steroids work on the efferent

Table 48.4 ▪ Antibacterial and Corticosteroid Combinations

Drug	Dosage Form	Frequency of Dosing
Neomycin + polymyxin + hydrocortisone 1% (Cortisporin)	Ointment Suspension	BID–QID 1 drop q3–4hr
Dexamethasone + neomycin + polymyxin (Maxitrol)	Ointment Solution	BID–QID 1 drop q1–6hr
Neomycin + dexamethasone (Neo-Decadron)	Ointment Solution	BID–QID 1 drop q1–6hr
Tobramycin + dexamethasone (TobraDex)	Ointment Solution	BID–QID 1 drop q1–6hr
10% Sulfacetamide + 0.2% prednisolone acetate (Blephamide)	Ointment Solution	BID 1 drop q1–4hr

Source: Reference 25.

limb of the immune response, decreasing the cellular response of macrophages and T-lymphocytes to sites of inflammation.[22] Thus, these drugs have been highly effective in treating anterior and posterior segment inflammation as well as suppressing corneal graft rejection and preventing scarring in filtration procedures. However, though useful for all the aforementioned reasons, topical steroids have potentially serious adverse effects. Ocular complications include steroid-induced glaucoma, posterior subcapsular cataracts, ptosis, and exacerbation of infection, especially when there is a herpetic cause.[8] In patients who are steroid responders, the intraocular pressure spike rarely occurs before 2 weeks of chronic use of the medication. However, a pressure spike may occur any time during the course of treatment, and even patients on topical steroids for months or years need periodic pressure checks.[22] Discontinuation of the steroid if it has been used for less than 1 year usually results in a return to baseline pressures. Dexamethasone, the most potent steroid agent, also tends to cause the greatest intraocular pressure spikes.[8] Combination antibacterial–steroid agents are available to treat mild conjunctival infections associated with inflammation, especially in the postoperative setting.

The NSAIDs work though the cyclooxygenase pathway to inhibit the production and inflammatory effects of prostaglandins.[23] Diclofenac is a topical NSAID used for the treatment of ocular inflammation. It is also effective in treating cystoid macular edema, a specific type of retinal inflammation that can occur after cataract surgery.[8]

The antihistamines and mast cell stabilizers work on the afferent limb of the immune response to decrease the cascade effect of histamines, prostaglandins, and leukotrienes in causing the itching and hyperemia of allergic and atopic conjunctivitis.[24] Cromolyn sodium blocks histamine release indirectly and must be used prophylactically for several weeks to alleviate symptom onset. Mast cell stabilizers, such as lodoxamide, also take several weeks to alleviate symptoms. The newer histamine receptor antagonists, such as levocabastine, have an onset of action within minutes and last for at least 4 hours.

Mydriatics and Cycloplegics

This class of medications (Table 48.8) is used primarily in an office setting to perform a dilated fundoscopic examination. In cases of moderate to severe postoperative inflammation or in cases of uveitis with significant anterior chamber inflammation, these agents are used to prevent permanent scarring of the pupil. The mydriatic agents dilate the pupil, and the cycloplegic agents paralyze the ciliary muscle to prevent painful spasm and to cause paralysis of accommodation. Atropine has the longest duration of any of these agents, causing dilation for as long as 2 weeks.

Table 48.5 ▪ Corticosteroids

Drug	Dosage Form	Strength	Frequency of Dosing
Dexamethasone	Ointment	0.05%	BID–QID
	Solution	0.1%	1 drop q1–6hr
Fluorometholone	Solution	0.1%, 0.25%	1 drop q1–6hr
Prednisolone	Suspension	1%	1 drop q1–6hr
Rimexolone	Suspension	1%	1 drop q1–6hr

Source: Reference 25.

Table 48.6 ▪ Nonsteroidal Anti-Inflammatory Agents

Drug	Dosage Form	Strength	Frequency of Dosing
Diclofenac	Solution	0.1%	1 drop QID
Ketorolac	Solution	0.5%	1 drop QID

Source: Reference 25.

Table 48.7 ▪ Antiallergy Agents

Drug	Dosage Form	Strength	Frequency of Dosing
Cromolyn sodium	Solution	4%	1 drop 4–6 times/day
Levocabastine	Solution	0.05%	1 drop QID
Lodoxamide	Solution	0.1%	1 drop QID
Naphazoline	Solution	0.1%	1 drop BID–QID, PRN
Naphcon-A	Solution		1 drop BID–QID, PRN
Olopatadine	Solution		1 drop BID

Source: Reference 25.

Table 48.8 ▪ Mydriatics and Cycloplegics

Drug	Dosage Form	Strength	Frequency of Dosing	Duration	Effect
Atropine	Solution	0.5%, 1%, 2%	1 drop QD–TID	Max 7–14 days	C, M
Cyclopentolate	Solution	0.5%, 1%, 2%	1 drop QD–TID	Max 2 days	C, M
Homatropine	Solution	2%, 5%	1 drop QD–TID	Max 3 days	C, M
Phenylephrine	Solution	2.5%, 10%	1 drop QD–TID	Max 5 hr	M
Tropicamide	Solution	0.5%, 1%	1 drop QD–TID	Max 6 hr	M

Source: Reference 25.

C, cycloplegia; *M*, mydriasis.

Table 48.9 ▪ Artificial Tears

Drug	Frequency	Viscosity (centistokes)[a]
Dry Eye Therapy	1 drop PRN	0.7
HypoTears	1 drop PRN	1.2
Refresh Plus	1 drop PRN	2.0
Refresh	1 drop PRN	2.8
Tears Plus	1 drop PRN	2.8
Tears Naturale	1 drop PRN	3.7
Tears Naturale II	1 drop PRN	4.0
Tears Naturale Free	1 drop PRN	4.3
Bion Tears	1 drop PRN	4.5
OcuCoat PF	1 drop PRN	46
Celluvisc	1 drop PRN	170

Source: Reference 25.
[a]Water = 0.7 centistoke.

Artificial Tears

A wide range of agents are available to lubricate the eye and to prevent desiccation of the corneal surface (Table 48.9). These emollients vary in their viscosity; most are more viscous than water. The topical drops, which are up to seven times as viscous as water, are applied frequently during the day, every 30 minutes to 1 hour if necessary, and the lubricating ointments, such as Celluvisc, which is more than 20 times as viscous as water, are used before bedtime.

KEY POINTS

- When treating a patient with a common eye disorder, elicit a thorough description of the patient's symptoms, including decreased vision, pain with eye movement, discharge, and photophobia.
- Assess whether the patient has experienced an acute change from his or her baseline vision or whether the symptoms have been chronic and progressive.
- Be systematic in the examination of the periorbital structures, such as the lid and lacrimal gland, as well as the structures of the eye, such as the conjunctiva, sclera, cornea, and anterior chamber.
- If a vision-threatening disorder, such as orbital cellulitis or a corneal ulcer, is suspected, contact an ophthalmologist immediately.
- Send routine cultures for suspected bacterial conjunctivitis before initiating treatment.
- If a gonococcal conjunctivitis is suspected, the patient should receive systemic as well as topical medication. An ophthalmologist should be consulted.
- Consider a rheumatologic workup in patients with recurrent ocular inflammatory disorders, such as scleritis.
- Know the indications and relative contraindications of the various topical antibiotic, antiviral, and anti-inflammatory agents.

REFERENCES

1. Cullom RD Jr, Chang B. The Wills eye manual: office and emergency room diagnosis and treatment of eye disease. 2nd ed. Philadelphia: JB Lippincott, 1994.
2. Epstein GA, Putterman AM. Combined excision and drainage with intralesional corticosteroid injection in the treatment of chronic chalazion. Arch Ophthalmol 106:514–516, 1988.
3. McCulley JP, Dougherty JM, Deneau DG. Classification of chronic blepharitis. Ophthalmology 89:1173–1180, 1982.
4. Theodore FH, Bloomfield SE, Mondino BJ. Clinical allergy and immunology of the eye. Baltimore: Williams & Wilkins, 1983.
5. Weiss A, Friendly D, Eglin K, et al. Bacterial periorbital and orbital cellulitis in childhood. Ophthalmology 90:195–203, 1983.
6. Harris G. Subperiosteal inflammation of the orbit. A bacterial analysis of 17 cases. Arch Ophthalmol 106:947–952, 1988.
7. Berlin AJ, Rath R, Rich L. Lacrimal system dacryoliths. Ophthalmology 11:435–436, 1980.
8. Kanski JJ. Clinical ophthalmology. 3rd ed. Boston: Butterworth-Heinemann, 1994.
9. Sergott RC, Glaser JS. Graves' ophthalmopathy. A clinical and immunologic review. Surv Ophthalmol 26:1–21, 1981.
10. Haimovici R, Roussel TJ. Treatment of gonococcal conjunctivitis with single intramuscular ceftriaxone. Am J Ophthalmol 107:511–514, 1989.
11. Pettit TH, Holland GN. Chronic keratoconjunctivitis associated with ocular adenovirus infection. Am J Ophthalmol 88:748–751, 1979.
12. Schachter J. Chlamydiae. Am Rev Microbiol 34:285–309, 1980.
13. Butrus SI, Abelson MB. Laboratory evaluation of ocular allergy. Int Opthalmol Clin 28:324, 1988.
14. Watson PG. Diseases of the sclera and episclera. In: Tasman W, Jaeger EA, eds. Duane's clinical ophthalmology. Philadelphia: JB Lippincott, 1992;4.
15. Foster CS, Forstot SL, Wilson LA. Mortality rate and rheumatoid arthritis patients developing necrotizing scleritis or peripheral ulcerative keratitis: effects of systemic immunosuppression. Ophthalmology 91:1253–1263, 1984.
16. Poggio EC, Glynn RJ, Schein OD, et al. The incidence of ulcerative keratitis among users of daily-wear and extended-wear soft contact lenses. N Engl J Med 321:779–783, 1989.
17. Schein OD, Glynn RJ, Poggio EC, et al. The relative risk of ulcerative keratitis among users of daily-wear and extended-wear soft contact lenses. N Engl J Med 321:773–778, 1989.
18. Larkin DFP, Kilvington S, Dart JKT. Treatment of *Acanthamoeba* keratitis with polyhexamethylene biguanide Ophthalmology 99:185–191, 1992.
19. Wakefield D, Montanaro A, McCluskey P. Acute anterior uveitis and HLA-B27. Surv Ophthalmol 36(3):223–232, 1991.
20. Zimmerman TJ, Kooner KS, Kandarakis AS, et al. Improving the therapeutic index of topically applied ocular drugs. Arch Ophthalmol 102:551–553, 1984.
21. Leibowitz HM. Antibacterial effectiveness of ciprofloxacin 0.3% ophthalmic solution in the treatment of bacterial conjunctivitis. Am J Ophthalmol 112:29S–33S, 1991.
22. Tripathi BJ, Millard CB, Tripathi RC. Corticosteroids induce a sialated glycoprotein (Cort-GP) in trabecular cells in vitro. Exp Eye Res 51:735–737, 1990.
23. Flach AJ. Nonsteroidal anti-inflammatory drugs. In: Zimmerman TJ, Kooner KS, eds. Ophthalmologic clinics of North America. Philadelphia: WB Saunders, 1989.
24. Bito LZ. Prostaglandins: old concepts and new perspectives. Arch Ophthalmol 105:1036–1039, 1987.
25. Green SM. Pocket pharmacopoeia. Loma Linda, CA: Tarascon, 1997.

CHAPTER 49

COMMON EAR DISEASES

Michael A. Oszko

The ear is a complex structure consisting of bone and cartilage, sensory and nervous tissue, and fluid. In addition to facilitating the sense of hearing, the structures of the ear are intimately involved in the maintenance of balance and equilibrium. Because of its anatomical complexity, wide ranges of conditions can alter normal ear function. This chapter describes two of the most common disease states that are likely to be encountered by the pharmacist: otitis media; and otitis externa.

Otitis Media

DEFINITION

The term *otitis media* commonly denotes an inflammation of the middle ear. It can be more precisely described by its duration, the presence or absence of infection, and the presence or absence of an effusion.[1] *Acute suppurative* otitis media refers to a clinically identifiable infection of the middle ear in which the symptoms appear suddenly (over several hours) and resolve completely within 3 weeks. If the inflammatory process persists for more than 3 weeks but less than 3 months, it is termed *subacute.* A middle ear discharge that persists for more than 3 months is termed *chronic* otitis media. If middle ear inflammation occurs in the absence of an identifiable infectious etiology, it is considered to be *nonsuppurative. Recurrent* otitis media denotes three distinct episodes of otitis media in the past 6 months or four episodes in the past 12 months.

Otitis media is frequently associated with an effusion in the tympanic cavity. *Secretory* otitis media (also known as *otitis media with effusion*) is the term used if the effusion is located behind an intact tympanic membrane. The effusion may be further characterized as bloody, serous (i.e., serum-like, thin), mucoid (mucus-like, thick), or purulent (pus-like). A patient with secretory otitis media may be either symptomatic or asymptomatic.

Myringitis refers to an inflammation of the tympanic membrane and is not necessarily indicative of the presence of otitis media.

TREATMENT GOALS: OTITIS MEDIA

Because acute otitis media is frequently a self-limiting condition, with greater than 80% of cases resolving spontaneously without pharmacotherapy,[2] consider careful observation of the patient without the use of antimicrobial therapy (i.e., "watchful waiting").[3,4] When a decision is made to treat otitis media with drug therapy:

- Treat the symptoms (primarily pain and fever) of otitis media.

- Sterilize the middle ear effusion.
- Prevent complications (e.g, mastoiditis and impaired language development due to impaired hearing).
- Prevent recurrence of infection.
- Minimize or avoid adverse drug reactions.

EPIDEMIOLOGY

Otitis media is a common disease of early childhood, with the vast majority of children experiencing one or more episodes within the first 2 years of life.[5–7] It is one of the primary reasons that children see a physician, and it is estimated that this condition costs 3.5 billion dollars in direct and indirect health care costs.[8] Despite the high prevalence rate, a number of risk factors for the development of otitis media have been identified[1,5,6,9–11] (Table 49.1). On the other hand, breastfeeding has been shown to be protective against the development of otitis media, presumably because of the transfer of maternal immunoglobulins in the breast milk to the child.

Table 49.1 ▪ Risk Factors for the Development of Otitis Media

First episode <18 months of age	Exposure to second-hand smoke
Male sex	Bottle feeding
Positive family history of otitis media	Use of a pacifier
Sibling history of recurrent otitis media	Child care outside the home
Previous episode of otitis media	Preceding upper respiratory infection

PATHOPHYSIOLOGY

The ear can be divided anatomically into three sections: the outer (or external), middle, and inner (or internal) ear (Fig. 49.1).

The middle ear consists of the tympanic membrane (ear drum) and an air-filled tympanic cavity that houses three tiny bones known collectively as ossicles (Fig. 49.1). The middle ear is a relatively closed system, with a pressure approximately equal to atmospheric pressure. Pressure in the middle ear is maintained by the eustachian tube, which connects the tympanic cavity with the nasopharynx.

Pathogenesis

The pathogenesis of otitis media is not completely understood, but is thought to be the result of two primary factors:[10,12,13] eustachian tube dysfunction; and introduction of infectious material (i.e., viruses and/or bacteria) into the middle ear.

The eustachian tube equalizes the pressure between the tympanic cavity and the atmosphere. Cilia located in the eustachian tube continuously sweep mucus and debris toward the nasopharynx and away from the middle ear. Obstruction of the eustachian tube may result from either mucous membrane edema (secondary to allergy or an upper respiratory tract infection) or blockage by a foreign body, tumor, or lymphatic (e.g., adenoid) tissue. In addition, developmental differences between children and adults with respect to anatomical positioning, length, and functional patency of the eustachian tube may predispose children, but not adults, to eustachian tube dysfunction.[11]

Once an obstruction occurs, a negative pressure (relative to the atmosphere) develops in the tympanic cavity. This

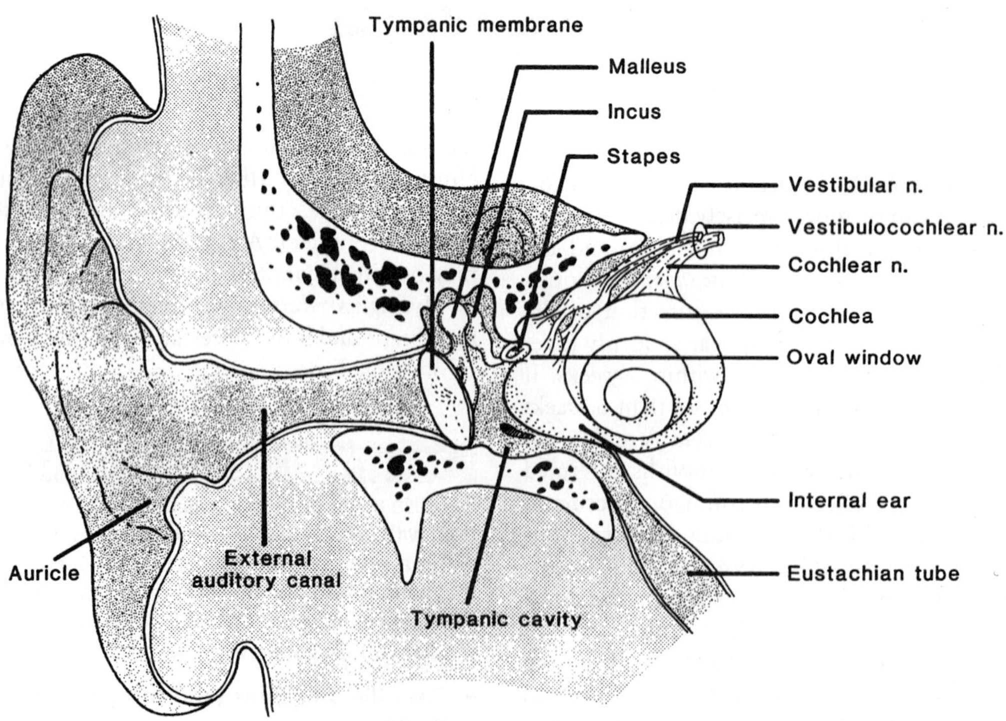

Figure 49.1. Anatomy of the ear.

negative pressure is caused by the absorption of gases through the epithelial lining of the eustachian tube and tympanic cavity. If the obstruction is suddenly relieved, nasopharyngeal mucus and bacteria may be insufflated (i.e., injected directly) into the tympanic cavity. Alternatively, a strong positive pressure originating in the nasopharynx (e.g., nose-blowing) may also force nasopharyngeal contents into the middle ear.

The role of viruses in the pathogenesis of otitis media is being increasingly recognized. Viruses were identified in 6 to 42% of patients with otitis media[14–16] with respiratory syncytial virus being the most commonly detected.[15,16] Whether or not viruses are directly involved in the development of otitis media is unclear, but they may predispose the patient to develop a secondary bacterial infection.

Other etiologic factors for otitis media include trauma, immunoglobulin deficiencies (particularly IgG-class antibodies against bacterial capsular polysaccharides),[17] human immunodeficiency virus (HIV) infection,[18] and, possibly, a genetic predisposition.[19]

Microbiology

Although viruses appear to play a concomitant role in the development of otitis media, the major etiologic pathogens are bacteria. In acute otitis media, the organisms most commonly isolated from the middle ear fluid are *Streptococcus pneumoniae, Haemophilus influenzae,* and *Moraxella catarrhalis.*[20] These organisms commonly colonize the nasopharynx of young children (<2 years), but are less frequently found in older children (>11 years).[21] In infants less than 6 weeks old, *Escherichia coli* and group B streptococci are common pathogens. Other less common organisms include staphylococci (both coagulase positive and negative), *Streptococcus pyogenes*, group A streptococci, other Gram-negative rods, *Chlamydia trachomatis*, and anaerobes. In chronic suppurative otitis media, the predominant organisms are *Staphylococcus aureus*, *Pseudomonas aeruginosa*, and *Klebsiella pneumoniae.*[22]

Up to 50% of *H. influenzae* and 100% of *M. catarrhalis* strains produce β-lactamases.[20] Resistant strains of *S. pneumoniae* (an organism that was once exquisitely sensitive to penicillins) are now appearing with increasing frequency in the United States.[23,24] Because of the increasing prevalence of drug-resistant *S. pneumoniae,* high-dose amoxicillin (80 to 90 mg/kg/day) has been advocated for high-risk patients.[24a]

CLINICAL PRESENTATION AND DIAGNOSIS

Signs and Symptoms

The classical presentation of acute suppurative otitis media is that of an acute (within hours) onset of unilateral otalgia (ear pain), fever, and nasal discharge. Symptoms of otitis media displayed by neonates and small children include excessive fussiness, irritability, and/or tugging at the affected ear. Older children may complain of a sore throat and/or a sense of "fullness" or "pressure" in the ear. These symptoms may be associated with a decrease in hearing acuity. Less frequent symptoms include dizziness, lethargy, headache, anorexia (or reduced feeding in neonates), nausea, vomiting, diarrhea, and otorrhea. It is important to note that all of these signs and symptoms are relatively nonspecific (i.e., many patients presenting with these signs or symptoms do not have otitis media).[25]

Diagnosis

The clinical diagnosis of otitis media is based largely on the patient's signs and symptoms. Otoscopic examination of the ear may reveal an erythematous tympanic membrane that is opaque or dull in appearance. The membrane is frequently bulging, and infrequently, it may be perforated and draining pus. The appearance of the tympanic membrane is highly variable, however, and otitis media is frequently overdiagnosed.[25] Tympanometric testing of the eardrum may reveal reduced compliance, but its diagnostic usefulness is limited in that up to 25% of healthy children will have asymptomatic middle ear effusions.[26]

Isolation of the causative organism may be accomplished by aspirating fluid from the middle ear (tympanocentesis). This procedure is invasive and is only performed when the specific causative organism must be identified. Unfortunately, cultures may be negative in one-third of patients with acute otitis media and two-thirds of patients with recurrent or secretory otitis media.[27,28] While colonization of the nasopharynx by the responsible bacteria appears to be a prerequisite for infection of the middle ear,[29] cultures of the nasopharynx are a poor predictor of the causative organism.[30]

PSYCHOSOCIAL ASPECTS

While otitis media is obviously uncomfortable for the child, this condition takes its toll on the parent(s) or caregiver(s) as well. The fussiness, inconsolability, and lack of appetite that many children experience during an episode of acute otitis media causes many parents to flee to the physician for "something" to alleviate the condition. Frequently, this involves the potentially inappropriate prescribing of antibiotics. Although antibiotic therapy has been shown to have only a modest effect on the overall course of the disease,[2] it may shorten the duration of symptoms[31] and, for this reason, may be appropriate in selected patients.

TREATMENT

Pharmacotherapy

The treatment of otitis media with drug therapy can be divided into three categories: supportive therapy with analgesics and antipyretics; systemic antimicrobial therapy; and adjunctive therapy

Analgesic and Antipyretic Therapy

Two of the most prominent symptoms of acute otitis media are pain and fever. Both of these symptoms can be effectively treated with acetaminophen (10 to 15 mg/kg q4–6hr; maximum 60 mg/kg/day) or ibuprofen (5 to 10 mg/kg q6hr; maximum 40 mg/kg/day). Aspirin should be avoided owing to the potential risk of life-threatening Reye's syndrome.

Systemic Antimicrobial Therapy

Perhaps the most controversial aspect of the pharmacotherapy of acute otitis media is the use of systemic antimicrobial therapy. Despite the consensus that acute otitis media is primarily of bacterial etiology, there is disagreement on three issues: whether or not this condition should be treated with oral antibiotics; the duration of antibiotic therapy; and the endpoint by which antibiotic efficacy should be assessed.

In most patients, the symptoms of acute otitis media resolve spontaneously without treatment within 24 to 72 hours, with resolution of the effusion within 2 weeks. Moreover, meta-analyses of clinical trials of antibiotic therapy in acute otitis media indicates that antibiotics produce only modest short-term improvement in the overall course of the disease.[2,31,32] Thus, it has been suggested that antibiotic therapy should be reserved for those whose condition does not improve within 48 to 72 hours.[33] Unfortunately, it is impossible to identify a priori patients whose otitis media will not resolve spontaneously, and antimicrobial therapy continues to be recommended to reduce the risk of suppurative complications, even though these complications are rare.

Because, in most cases, the causative organism is not isolated before treatment is initiated, the choice of antibiotic is based on its efficacy against the most common pathogens reported in published studies in which microbiological specimens were obtained. Table 49.2 lists antibiotics that are commonly used to treat otitis media.

Selection of an antibiotic to treat otitis media should take into account the drug's pharmacokinetic and pharmacodynamic profile with respect to efficacy and toxicity, as well as other factors (e.g, palatability, route of administration, and cost). Ideally, an antibiotic used to treat otitis media should have several characteristics. It should (1) have excellent oral bioavailability; (2) readily distribute into the middle ear fluid in high concentrations for antibiotics that exhibit concentration-dependent killing or achieve concentrations that exceed the pathogen's minimum inhibitory concentration (MIC) for a significant portion (40 to 50%) of the dosing interval for antibiotics that exhibit time-dependent killing; (3) be bactericidal at low MICs; (4) have a long half-life; (5) be devoid of drug-drug or drug-food interactions that are more common in children; and (6) have little or no toxicity at therapeutic doses.[34,35] Fortunately, all of the antibiotics that are commonly used to treat otitis media reasonably satisfy these criteria.

Figure 49.2 presents an algorithm for treating acute otitis media. For most patients, oral amoxicillin is an appropriate first choice. It is effective against the most likely causative organisms, relatively free of serious side effects (rash and diarrhea are the most common), and inexpensive. If a patient is allergic to penicillins, either trimethoprim-sulfamethoxazole or erythromycin-sulfisoxazole is an effective alternatives. Both of these contain a sulfonamide, but the incidence of side effects is low (<5%) and hematologic toxicity is rare at the dose required to treat otitis media. Alternatively, careful observation of the patient (>2 years of age) while withholding the use of antibiotics can be considered.[33]

Because both *H. influenzae* and *M. catarrhalis* are capable of producing β-lactamases, an antibiotic that is stable against these enzymes should be considered if therapy with amoxicillin appears to be ineffective or if the prevalence of these organisms in a particular geographic area is high. Amoxicillin combined with potassium clavulanate (a β-lactamase inhibitor), second- or third-generation cephalosporins, trimethoprim-sulfamethoxazole, or erythromycin-sulfisoxazole is equally effective. The initial, empiric use of broad-spectrum, β-lactamase-stable antibiot-

Table 49.2 ▪ Antibiotics Used in the Treatment of Otitis Media

Antibiotic	Pediatric (<12 yr) Dose	Comments
Amoxicillin	40–45 mg/kg/day in 3 divided doses	80–90 mg/kg/day in high-risk, penicillin-resistant pneumococci patients
Amoxicillin/potassium clavulanate	40 mg/kg/day in 3 divided doses	Dose based on amoxicillin content
Azithromycin	5 mg/kg/day	Day 1: 10 mg/kg ("loading dose")
Cefaclor	40 mg/kg/day in 3 divided doses	
Cefixime	8 mg/kg/day in 1-2 divided doses	
Cefpodoxime proxetil	10 mg/kg/day in 2 divided doses	
Cefprozil	30 mg/kg/day in 2 divided doses	
Ceftibuten	9 mg/kg/day	
Ceftriaxone	50 mg/kg	Administered intramuscularly; single-dose
Clarithromycin	15 mg/kg/day in 2 divided doses	
Cefuroxime axetil	10 mg/kg/day in 1–2 divided doses	
Erythromycin/sulfisoxazole	50 mg/kg/day in 3–4 divided doses	Dose based on erythromycin content
Loracarbef	30 mg/kg/day in 2 divided doses	
Trimethoprim/sulfamethoxazole	8 mg/kg/day in 2 divided doses	Dose based on trimethoprim content

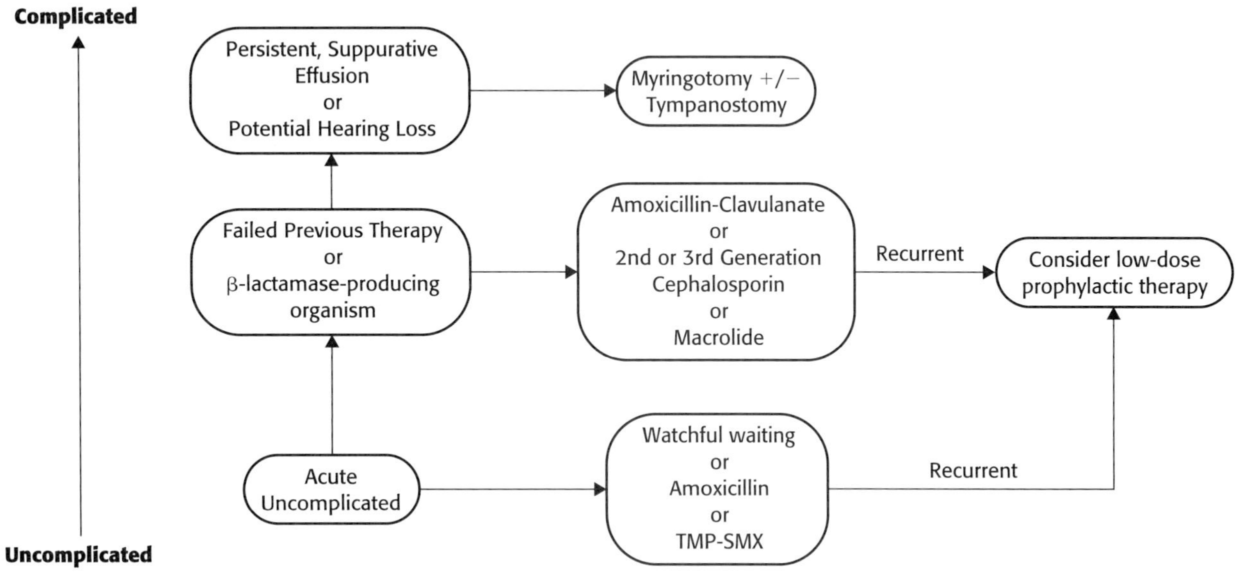

Figure 49.2. Algorithm for treating otitis media. *TMP-SMX,* trimethoprim-sulfamethoxazole.

ics is unwarranted because they do not improve efficacy rates or reduce the incidence of suppurative complications. Furthermore, the newer agents are considerably more expensive than amoxicillin or trimethoprim-sulfamethoxazole, and their broad spectrum may contribute to the development of resistant strains of bacteria.

The traditional length of antibiotic therapy in acute otitis media has been 10 days. However, shorter courses of therapy (i.e., 5 days) have been shown to be equally effective.[36] In addition, a single intramuscular dose of ceftriaxone is as effective as 10 days of treatment with oral amoxicillin,[37] amoxicillin-clavulanate,[38] and trimethoprim-sulfamethoxazole[39] in uncomplicated acute otitis media in children. While this modality has drawbacks (i.e., it is painful, more expensive, and may unnecessarily expose the patient to broad-spectrum therapy), it may be appropriate when a child is unable (or unwilling) to take oral medication, or when noncompliance is a documented problem. Moreover, parents prefer single-dose therapy because of its simplicity.[40] Longer-term therapy (i.e., 10 days) may still be appropriate for children <2 years old.[41]

If the patient's clinical response is unsatisfactory, an additional course of therapy with another antibiotic may be tried. This is unnecessary in most patients. Middle ear effusion will persist for several days to several months in a small number of patients, although in most children the condition will not progress to chronic or recurrent otitis media.

Adjunctive Therapy

In addition to analgesics, antipyretics, and antibiotics, a number of other pharmacologic interventions have been tried. Decongestants, antihistamines, mucolytics, surfactants, and bacterial vaccines have been used to treat otitis media. None of these agents has been shown to improve the outcome of otitis media. The use of oral corticosteroids is controversial, but is currently not recommended.[3] When used in combination with antibiotics, they provide marginal benefit. Intranasal beclomethasone may be a useful adjunct in the treatment of chronic otitis media if there is an allergic component.[42] Monthly administration of immune globulin to children with HIV infection was associated with a significant reduction in the frequency of bacterial infections, including otitis media.[43]

Nonpharmacologic Therapy

In some children with complicated otitis media, it may be necessary to perform a bilateral myringotomy to place tympanostomy tubes. This allows the effusion to drain and the middle ear to be ventilated. This procedure is invasive (requiring general anesthesia) and is associated with a number of complications (otorrhea, granuloma formation, cholesteatoma, and tube obstruction).[44] Despite these drawbacks, myringotomy with tympanostomy tube placement should be considered in children with recurrent otitis media or otitis media with effusion lasting longer than 3 months and in children with evidence of hearing loss and or language delay.[3,44]

IMPROVING OUTCOMES

Although otitis media is a relatively benign process in most patients, there are a number of educational interventions that can prevent future episodes, modify the course of an existing episode, and prevent complications from occurring.

Patient Education

Table 49.1 lists risk factors for otitis media; a number of these factors can be modified by the parent or caregiver. Avoidance of passive cigarette smoke, keeping the child out of day care centers, and limiting exposure to children with upper respiratory infections may reduce the risk of developing otitis media. Minimizing these risk factors is particularly important for children who are prone to develop otitis media.

Parents should be made aware of the fact that antibiotic therapy has only a small impact on the overall course of acute otitis media and their expectation of receiving a prescription for an antibiotic should be modified accordingly. When antibiotic therapy is prescribed, the importance of compliance and of recognizing potential treatment failure must be emphasized. Also, parents should be aware that adjunctive therapies commonly used in upper respiratory infections (antihistamines and decongestants) are ineffective in otitis media but may nonetheless cause side effects.[45]

Methods to Improve Patient Adherence to Drug Therapy

In general, the antibiotics listed in Table 49.2 are equally safe and effective for treating otitis media. With regard to compliance, three factors may distinguish these drugs from one another: simplicity, cost, and palatability.

With regard to cost, amoxicillin and trimethoprim-sulfamethoxazole are the least expensive antibiotics. Newer, more expensive antibiotics are not necessarily more effective or less toxic.

With regard to simplicity, the fewer the number of doses of a medication that must be given, the more likely it is that the regimen will be adhered to. Amoxicillin, though inexpensive, must be administered 3 times daily. This may be problematic if the child is going to a day-care facility, where someone other than the parent must be depended upon to administer the midday dose. In this case, trimethoprim-sulfamethoxazole or another drug that can be administered in 1 to 2 daily doses may be more appropriate.

Finally, the palatability of the antibiotic contributes to compliance as well. The use of oral syringes to deliver the medication to the back of the mouth may be helpful in administering bad-tasting antibiotic suspensions.

PHARMACOECONOMICS

Although otitis media is responsible for an estimated 3.5 billion dollars in health care costs annually, only a small percentage of this is attributable to pharmacotherapy.[3,46] Nonetheless, the fact that only a small short-term improvement is seen with antimicrobial therapy calls into question the cost-benefit of its use. Perhaps more importantly, the potential development of bacterial resistance to antibiotics may, in the long run, prove to be far more costly from a public health standpoint. In addition, the financial impact of noncompliance with and the adverse effects of drug therapy must be considered.[47] Pharmacists and other health care professionals must be cognizant of these issues when evaluating and using antibiotic therapy in the treatment of otitis media.

Otitis Externa

DEFINITION

Otitis externa is an infectious condition of the external ear canal. Although it may be associated with chronic otitis media, it is more frequently an independent condition that affects patients of all ages. One particularly severe form of this condition, *malignant* otitis externa, is characterized by extensive bacterial (predominantly *P. aeruginosa*) invasion into the surrounding bone, soft tissue, and nerve structures and is potentially life threatening.[48]

TREATMENT GOALS: OTITIS EXTERNA

- Facilitate an environment in the external ear canal that promotes healing of the inflamed, infected tissue.
- Dry the ear canal and treat the infection.

PATHOPHYSIOLOGY

The external ear consists of two structures, the auricle and the external auditory canal (Fig. 49.1). The purpose of these structures is to collect and transmit sound waves to the middle ear.

Two conditions produce an environment that is favorable for the development of otitis externa: the introduction of a sharp object (e.g., toothpick or hairpin) into the external auditory canal, which disrupts the integrity of the lining of the canal and permits the growth of bacteria or fungi; and the introduction and accumulation of moisture in the canal. Moisture not only softens the lining of the canal but also provides a medium for the growth of bacteria or fungi. Otitis externa commonly occurs when the ear is frequently exposed to water (e.g., swimming) and for this reason is sometimes referred to as "swimmer's ear."

The two most common organisms that are isolated in otitis externa are *P. aeruginosa* and *S. aureus*.[49] Fungi, primarily *Aspergillus* and *Candida*, are found in about 10% of cases.

CLINICAL PRESENTATION AND DIAGNOSIS

Signs and Symptoms

Otitis externa is characterized by pain, swelling, maceration, and breakdown of the skin and subcutaneous tissues of the external ear canal. Normally, the infection is limited to the external ear. However, it can spread to the surrounding soft tissue or bone.

Diagnosis

The diagnosis of otitis externa is based on the clinical presentation of the patient. Additionally, culture and sensitivity data from the affected ear confirm the diagnosis

Table 49.3 ▪ Selected Topical Preparations for Treating Otitis Externa

Drug Product	Antibiotic	Antibacterial Antifungal	Corticosteroid	Analgesic	Local Anesthetic
Auralgan Otic				Antipyrine 5.4%	Benzocaine 1.4%
Coly-Mycin S Otic	Neomycin SO_4 3.3 mg/mL, colistin SO_4 3 mg/mL		Hydrocortisone 1%		
Cortisporin Otic	Neomycin SO_4 5 mg/mL, polymyxin B SO_4 100 kU/mL		Hydrocortisone 1%		
Floxin Otic	Ofloxacin 0.3%				
Otic Tridesilon		Acetic acid 2%	Desonide 0.05%		
Tympagesic[a]				Antipyrine 5%	Benzocaine 5%
Vosol HC Otic		Acetic acid 2%	Hydrocortisone 1%		

[a]Also contains phenylephrine 0.25%.

and assist in the selection of antimicrobial therapy.[49] With malignant otitis externa, a number of diagnostic criteria have been proposed[48] and may require the assistance of diagnostic imaging (e.g., computed tomography or magnetic resonance imaging) to confirm the diagnosis.

TREATMENT

The goal of treatment of otitis externa is to produce an environment in the external ear canal that promotes healing of the inflamed, infected tissue. This includes drying the ear canal and treating the infection. Table 49.3 lists those drugs commonly found in otic preparations used to treat otitis externa.

Antibiotics

Although antibiotics are found in many otic preparations, they may cause contact dermatitis, permit the overgrowth of resistant organisms (including fungi), and result in local (e.g., neomycin) or systemic (e.g., chloramphenicol) toxicities and are generally not recommended. Ofloxacin available as an otic solution and is as effective as bacitracin-polymyxin B-hydrocortisone.[50] It remains to be seen whether or not this agent exhibits the same potential problems as the older topical antibiotics. Oral antibiotics are indicated only if the infection has spread to the surrounding soft tissue. For malignant otitis externa, a prolonged course of therapy with an antipseudomonal antibiotic, administered intravenously, is usually necessary.[48]

Other Agents

Corticosteroids possess anti-inflammatory, antipruritic, and vasoconstrictive activity and, when applied topically, may be useful in reducing swelling and inflammation in the external ear canal. A few drops of isopropyl alcohol 70% can serve as an excellent drying agent, but it should be used sparingly to prevent excessive drying and subsequent pruritus. Acetic acid may be combined in a 1:1 mixture with isopropyl alcohol to decrease the pH of the solution.

IMPROVING OUTCOMES

For topical therapy to be effective, the otic solution must be properly delivered to the site of infection. Proper technique is particularly important if the patient is going to self-administer the solution. This, along with proper attention to aural hygiene, will bring about resolution of the condition in most patients in 5 to 7 days.

In treating otitis externa, 3 to 4 drops of the desired solution should be instilled into the ear canal four times daily. To prevent the solution from escaping from the ear canal, the otic drops may be placed on a cotton or gauze wick, which is then inserted into the ear canal and left in place. In addition to keeping the solution in contact with the affected tissues, the wick also prevents occlusion of the ear canal due to swelling.

In a small number of patients, the condition becomes chronic and is characterized by dry, scaly, sometimes weeping skin covering the auricle and external ear canal. Again, meticulous aural hygiene, combined with the application of a topical steroid cream (e.g., hydrocortisone) 3 to 4 times daily, will manage the patient's symptoms.

KEY POINTS

- Otitis media is a very common, yet relatively benign, condition of infancy and early childhood.
- Treatment is aimed at preventing acute (e.g., mastoiditis) or chronic complications (e.g., impaired language development secondary to hearing loss) as a result of chronic or recurrent infections.
- Due to the self-limiting nature of the disease and the potential for inducing bacterial resistance, antimicrobial therapy should be reserved for acute episodes in children <2 years of age, or in children with chronic or recurrent infections.
- Adjunctive therapies, such as antihistamines and decongestants, are of little value in the management of otitis media, but they are nonetheless capable of causing side effects.

- Education of the parent or caregiver and judicious selection and use of antimicrobial therapy will improve the outcome of otitis media.
- Otitis externa is an infection of the external auditory canal that affects both children and adults.
- Treatment of otitis externa involves meticulous aural hygiene in addition to topical pharmacotherapy.
- Patient education on the administration of otic preparations is essential, especially if the patient is going to self-administer the medication.
- Malignant otitis externa is severe, potentially life-threatening, and requires aggressive, prolonged therapy with intravenous antibiotics.

REFERENCES

1. Klein JO, Tos M, Hussl B, et al. Recent advances in otitis media: definition and classification. Ann Otol Rhinol Laryngol 139(suppl):10, 1989.
2. Rosenfeld RM, Vertrees JE, Carr J, et al. Clinical efficacy of antimicrobial drugs for acute otitis media: meta-analysis of 5400 children from thirty-three randomized trials. J Pediatr 124:355–367, 1994.
3. Stool SE, Berg AO, Berman S, et al. Clinical practice guideline number 12: otitis media with effusion in young children. Rockville, MD: US Public Health Service, Agency for Health Care Policy and Research, 1994:67–9. AHCPR publication 94-0622.
4. Froom J, Culpepper L, Jacobs M, et al. Antimicrobials for acute otitis media? A review from the International Primary Care Network. Br Med J 315:98–102, 1997.
5. Teele DW, Klein JO, Rosner B, et al. Epidemiology of otitis media during the first seven years of life in children in greater Boston: a prospective cohort study. J Infect Dis 160:83–94, 1989.
6. Paradise JL, Rockette HE, Colborn DK. Otitis media in 2253 Pittsburgh-area infants: prevalence and risk factors during the first two years of life. Pediatrics 99:318–333, 1997.
7. Schappert SM. Office visits for otitis media: United States 1975–1990. Hyattsville, MD: US Public Health Service, 1992. DHHS publication PHS 92-1250.
8. Kaplan B, Wandstrat TL, Cunningham JR. Overall cost in the treatment of otitis media. Pediatr Infect Dis J 16:S9–S11, 1997.
9. Uhari M, Mäntysaari K, Niemelä M. A meta-analytic review of the risk factors for acute otitis media. Clin Infect Dis 22:1079–1083, 1996.
10. Fireman P. Otitis media and eustachian tube dysfunction: connection to allergic rhinitis. J Allergy Clin Immunol 99:S787–S797, 1997.
11. American Academy of Pediatrics Committee on Environmental Health. Environmental tobacco smoke: a hazard to children. Pediatrics 99:639–642, 1997.
12. Bluestone CD, Ostfeld EJ, Bakaletz LO, et al. Eustachian tube and middle ear physiology and pathophysiology. In: Recent advances in otitis media: report of the fifth research conference. Ann Otol Rhinol Laryngol 103(Suppl 164): 13–19, 1994.
13. Yücetürk AV, Ünlü HH, Okumuşs M, et al. The evaluation of eustachian tube function in patients with chronic otitis media. Clin Otolaryngol 22:449–452, 1997.
14. Ruuskanen O, Arola M, Heikkinen T, et al. Viruses in acute otitis media: increasing evidence for clinical significance. Pediatr Infect Dis J 10:425–427, 1991.
15. Arola M, Ruuskanen O, Ziegler T, et al. Clinical role of respiratory virus infection in acute otitis media. Pediatrics 86:848–855, 1990.
16. Heikkenin H, Thint M, Chonmaitree T. Prevalence of various respiratory viruses in the middle ear during acute otitis media. N Engl J Med 340:260–264, 1999.
17. Yamakana N, Hotomi M, Shimada J, et al. Immunological deficiency in "otitis-prone" children. Ann NY Acad Sci 830:70–81, 1997.
18. Chen AY, Ohlms LA, Stewart MG, et al. Otolaryngologic disease progression in children with human immunodeficiency virus infection. Arch Otolaryngol Head Neck Surg 122:1360–1363, 1996.
19. Klein JO, Tos M, Casselbrant ML: Epidemiology and natural history. In: Recent advances in otitis media: report of the fifth research conference. Ann Otol Rhinol Laryngol 103(Suppl 164):9–12, 1994.
20. Block SL. Causative pathogens, antibiotic resistance, and therapeutic considerations in acute otitis media. Pediatr Infect Dis J 16:449–456, 1997.
21. Stenfors LE, Räisänen S. Occurrence of middle ear pathogens in the nasopharynx of young individuals: a quantitative study in four age groups. Acta Otolaryngol 109:142–148, 1990.
22. Wintermeyer SM, Nahata MC. Chronic suppurative otitis media. Ann Pharmacother 28:1089–1099, 1994.
23. Roger G, Carles P, Thien HV, et al. Management of acute otitis media caused by resistant pneumococci in infants. Pediatr Infect Dis J 17:631–638, 1998.
24. Klein JO. Clinical implications of antibiotic resistance for management of acute otitis media. Pediatr Infect Dis J 17:1084–1089, 1998.
24a. Dowell SF, Butler JC, Giebink GS, et al. Acute otitis media: management and surveillance in an era of pneumococcal resistance–a report from the Drug-resistant *Streptococcus pneumoniae* Therapeutic Working Group. Pediatr Infect Dis J 18:1–9, 1999.
25. Weiss JC, Yates GR, Quinn LD. Acute otitis media: making an accurate diagnosis. Am Fam Physician 53:1200–1206, 1996.
26. Klein JO. Persistent middle ear effusions: natural history and morbidity. Pediatr Infect Dis J 1:S1–S11, 1982.
27. Qvarnberg Y, Kantola O, Valtonen H, et al. Bacterial findings in middle ear effusion in children. Otolaryngol Head Neck Surg 102:118–121, 1990.
28. Karma P: Secretory otitis media: infectious background and its implications for treatment. Acta Otolaryngol 449(Suppl):47–48, 1988.
29. Ogra PL, Barenkamp SJ, Mogi, et al. Microbiology, immunology, biochemistry, vaccination. In: Recent advances in otitis media: report of the fifth research conference. Ann Otol Rhinol Laryngol 103(Suppl 164):27–43, 1994.
30. Groothuis JR, Thompson J, Wright PF: Correlation of nasopharyngeal and conjunctival cultures with middle ear fluid cultures in otitis media. Clin Pediatr 25:85–88, 1986.
31. Del Mar C, Glasziou P, Hayem M. Are antibiotics indicated as initial treatment for children with acute otitis media? A meta-analysis. Br Med J 314:1526–1529, 1997.
32. Williams RL, Chalmers TC, Stange KC, et al. Use of antibiotics in preventing recurrent otitis media and in treating otitis media with effusion: a meta-analytic attempt to resolve the brouhaha. JAMA 270:1344–1351, 1993.
33. Culpepper L, Froom J. Routine antimicrobial treatment of acute otitis media: is it necessary? JAMA 278:1643–1645, 1997.
34. Blumer JL. Implications of pharmacokinetics in making choices for the management of acute otitis media. Pediatr Infect Dis J 17:565–570, 1998.
35. Craig WA. Choosing an antibiotic on the basis of pharmacodynamics. Ear Nose Throat J 77(6 Suppl):7–11, 1998.
36. Kozyrsky AL, Hildes-Ripstein GE, Longstaffe SE, et al. Treatment of acute otitis media with a shortened course of antibiotics: a meta-analysis. JAMA 279:1736–1742, 1998.
37. Green SM, Rothrock SG. Single-dose intramuscular ceftriaxone for acute otitis media in children. Pediatrics 91:23–30, 1993.
38. Varsano I, Volovitz B, Horev Z, et al. Intramuscular ceftriaxone compared with oral amoxicillin-clavulanate for the treatment of acute otitis media in children. Eur J Pediatr 156:858–863, 1997.
39. Barnett ED, Teele DW, Klein JO, et al. Comparison of ceftriaxone and trimethoprim-sulfamethoxazole for acute otitis media. Pediatrics 99:23–28, 1997.
40. Bauchner H, Adams W, Barnett E, et al. Therapy for acute otitis media: Preference of parents for oral or parenteral antibiotic. Arch Pediatr Adolesc Med 150:396–399, 1996.
41. Paradise JL. Short-course antimicrobial treatment for acute otitis media: not best for infants and young children. JAMA 278:1640–1642, 1997.
42. Tracy JM, Demain JG, Hoffman KM, et al. Intranasal beclomethasone as an adjunct to treatment of chronic middle ear effusion. Ann Allergy Asthma Immunol 80:198–206, 1998.
43. Olopoenia L, Young M., White D, et al. Intravenous immunoglobulin in symptomatic and asymptomatic children with perinatal HIV infection. J Natl Med Assoc 89:543–547, 1997.
44. Pizzuto MP, Volk MS, Kingston LM. Common topics in pediatric otolaryngology. Pediatr Clin North Am 45:973-991, 1998.
45. Mandel EM, Rockette HE, Bluestone CD, et al. Efficacy of amoxicillin with and without decongestant-antihistamine for otitis media in children. N Engl J Med 316:432–437, 1987.
46. Mainous AG, Hueston WJ. The cost of antibiotics in treating upper respiratory tract infections in a Medicaid population. Arch Fam Med 7:45–49, 1998.
47. Wandstrat TL, Kaplan B. Pharmacoeconomic impact of factors affecting compliance with antibiotic regimens in the treatment of acute otitis media. Pediatr Infect Dis J 16:S27–S29, 1997.
48. Amorosa L, Modugno GC, Pirodda A. Malignant ecternal otitis: review and personal experience. Acta Otolaryngol Suppl (Stockh) 521:3–16, 1996.
49. Bojrab DI, Bruderly T, Abdulrazzak Y. Otitis externa. Otolaryngol Clin North Am 29:761–782, 1996.
50. Jones RN, Milazzo J, Seidlin M. Ofloxacin otic solution for treatment of otitis externa in children and adults. Arch Otolaryngol Head Neck Surg 123:1193–1200, 1997.

CHAPTER 50

GLAUCOMA

J. Douglas Wurtzbacher, Dick R. Gourley, and Constance McKenzie

DEFINITION

Glaucoma is a group of diseases of the eye characterized by damage to the ganglion cells and the optic nerve. If left untreated, these effects may lead to various degrees of loss of vision and blindness. Increased intraocular pressure (IOP) remains the most important risk factor for the development of glaucoma, but is no longer included as a part of the definition of disease. Glaucoma is typically classified as either open-angle or angle-closure (closed-angle), based upon causes of increased IOP.[1,2]

TREATMENT GOALS: GLAUCOMA

Current therapy remains targeted to reducing IOP, either medically or surgically. Studies have shown that reduction in IOP, even in patients with normal IOP (normal tension glaucoma), prevents progression of optic nerve damage and visual field loss.[3,4]

- Initiate immediate medical attention to reduce IOP in cases of acute angle closure glaucoma.
- Avoid medical therapy that may worsen the patient's glaucoma.
- Establish a target IOP to prevent initial or worsening ocular damage.
- Reduce IOP using topical medications with few systemic effects.
- Use combination therapy only after monotherapy proves unsuccessful.
- Provide patient education to improve administration technique to reduce systemic adverse effects and to improve compliance.
- Monitor effectiveness and perform surgical correction if medical therapy is not tolerated or the target IOP is not maintained.

EPIDEMIOLOGY

Prevalence

Glaucoma, defined as damage to the optic nerve and ganglion cells, affects approximately 67 million persons worldwide and 4 million Americans. There may be as many as 15 million Americans who have elevated IOP or ocular hypertension, without clinical signs and symptoms of glaucoma, and have an increased risk of developing disease and having end-organ damage.[5]

Glaucoma usually manifests itself after age 35, but can occur in younger people as well. The prevalence of glaucoma increases with increasing age. Two percent of the population older than 40 years of age and 5 to 9% of those older than 65 years of age have glaucoma. Although there are more men with open-angle glaucoma, sex predilections for the disease are not clinically apparent. Open-angle

Table 50.1 ▪ Glaucoma Classified According to Etiology

A. Primary glaucoma
   1. Open-angle glaucoma
      a. Primary open-angle glaucoma (chronic open-angle glaucoma, chronic simple glaucoma)
      b. Normal-pressure glaucoma (low-pressure glaucoma)
   2. Angle-closure glaucoma
      a. Acute
      b. Subacute
      c. Chronic
      d. Plateau iris

B. Congenital glaucoma
   1. Primary congenital glaucoma
   2. Glaucoma associated with other developmental ocular abnormalities
      a. Anterior chamber cleavage syndromes
         Axenfeld's syndrome
         Sieger's syndrome
         Peter's anomaly
      b. Aniridia
   3. Glaucoma associated with extraocular developmental abnormalities
      a. Sturge-Weber syndrome
      b. Marfan's syndrome
      c. Neurofibromatosis
      d. Lowe's syndrome
      e. Congenital rubella

C. Secondary glaucoma
   1. Pigmentary glaucoma
   2. Exfoliation syndrome
   3. Due to lens changes (phacogenic)
      a. Dislocation
      b. Intumescence
      c. Phacolytic
   4. Due to uveal tract changes
      a. Uveitis
      b. Posterior synechiae (seclusio pupillae)
      c. Tumor
   5. Iridocorneoendothelial (ICE) syndrome
   6. Trauma
      a. Hyphema
      b. Angle contusion/recession
      c. Peripheral anterior synechiae
   7. Postoperative
      a. Ciliary block glaucoma (malignant glaucoma)
      b. Peripheral anterior synechiae
      c. Epithelial downgrowth
      d. After corneal graft surgery
      e. After retinal detachment surgery
   8. Neovascular glaucoma
      a. Diabetes mellitus
      b. Central retinal vein occlusion
      c. Intraocular tumor
   9. Raised episcleral venous pressure
      a. Carotid-cavernous fistula
      b. Sturge-Weber syndrome
   10. Steroid-induced

D. Absolute glaucoma: The end result of any uncontrolled glaucoma is a hard, sightless, and often painful eye.

Source: Reprinted with permission from Vaughan D, Asbury T, Riordan-Eva P. General ophthalmology. 14th ed. Norwalk, CT: Appleton & Lange, 1995.

glaucoma is relatively more common in Whites and Blacks than in American Indians and Asians.

Glaucoma may be classified in a variety of ways (Table 50.1), which describe causative factors, when known. Glaucoma is usually described as either angle-closure or open-angle glaucoma. These terms are based upon the mechanism of obstruction of outflow of aqueous humor and help clinicians develop treatment strategies. Open-angle glaucoma occurs in 80 to 90% of cases.[6] Angle-closure glaucoma is usually a more acute form of disease and is seen in 5 to 10% of all patients. A third type is congenital glaucoma, which results from developmental ocular abnormalities and occurs in less than 2% of patients. Finally, glaucoma may be secondary to other ocular disorders, systemic disorders, or trauma, or may be seen with medication usage, or after intraocular surgery. Of these, this chapter will discuss open- and closed-angle glaucoma and medication-related glaucoma and refer the reader to other sources[1,7] for a more detailed description.

Open-angle glaucoma can be further described as either high-tension or normal-tension (also known as low-tension) glaucoma. An estimated 25 to 30% of Americans and up to 70% of Asian patients with optic nerve damage characteristic of glaucoma have normal IOP, described as normal-tension glaucoma. Long-term studies examining the effects of medical management of normal-tension glaucoma have recently been completed[3,4] and will be discussed further in this chapter.

Glaucoma is the second leading cause of irreversible blindness in the United States. Approximately 150,000 Americans have varying degrees of blindness caused by glaucoma.[6] However, medical treatment can decrease the risk of blindness secondary to glaucoma. Long-term surveillance studies of patients treated for glaucoma demonstrated that 27% of patients are likely to become blind unilaterally and 9% bilaterally over a 20-year period. In patients whose disease was not diagnosed or treated early, this estimate increased to 54 and 22%, respectively.[8] Therefore, early detection and control of IOP is important in managing long-term outcomes of the disease.

Etiology

Optic nerve damage caused by the different types of glaucoma is a result of a variety of initiating factors. Genetic predisposition, physical changes, systemic diseases, or medications may increase a person's risk of developing damage that may be broadly classified as IOP-dependent (most commonly) or IOP-independent.

Increased IOP remains the major etiologic risk factor for the development of glaucoma. Myopia may be an additional risk factor, especially in younger patients.[9,10] A summary of known risk factors associated with an increase in risk of glaucoma is listed in Table 50.2.

The familial relationship of glaucoma has been well established. A study by Wolfs et al.[11] determined the prevalence of glaucoma in families of patients with glaucoma and in control patients. The results of this population-based study found 10.4% of siblings of patients and 1.1% of offspring of patients had glaucoma compared to 0.7 and 0% in families of control patients, respectively. At least three different genes have been identified that, when mutated, may be causally linked to the development of glaucoma.[12]

Glaucoma can occur as a secondary manifestation of systemic disorders or trauma. A list of systemic diseases associated with increased IOP is shown in Table 50.3. In addition, the detection and recognition of drug-induced glaucoma as a potential cause of disease is important. Drugs that have autonomic effects produce several types of ocular changes. Of great significance is the effect of anticholinergic agents on angle-closure glaucoma. Several factors appear to be associated with drug-induced glaucoma (Table 50.4). Specific agents known to increase risk of glaucoma will be discussed in detail subsequently.

PATHOPHYSIOLOGY

Shields et al.[1] describe five stages in the pathogenesis of glaucoma: (1) a variety of initial events, causing (2) changes in aqueous outflow, resulting in (3) increased IOP, which leads to (4) optic nerve atrophy, and finally, (5) progressive loss of vision. This description highlights the importance of aqueous humor production and elimination in the progression of glaucoma and subsequent complications.

Aqueous Humor Production and Elimination

The relative production and elimination of aqueous humor physiologically determines IOP. Increased IOP usually is the result of decreased elimination, but may also be caused by increased production of aqueous humor or both.[13]

Table 50.2 ▪ Risk Factors Associated with Glaucoma

Family history of glaucoma	Regular, long-term steroid/cortisone use
High intraocular pressure	Previous eye injury
African or Asian descent	High blood pressure
Diabetes	
Myopia (nearsighted)	

Table 50.3 ▪ Systemic Conditions Associated with Secondary Glaucoma

Congenital rubella	Lowe's syndrome
Diabetes mellitus	Marfan's syndrome
Down's syndrome	Melanoma (intraocular tumors)
Hallermann-Streiff syndrome	Neurofibromatosis (von Recklinghausen's)
Homocystinuria	Turner's syndrome
Hypertension	Uveitis (secondary)
Idiopathic infantile hypoglycemia	

Source: Modified from Scheie HG, Edwards DL, Yanoff MC. Clinical and experimental observations using alpha chymotrypsin. Am J Ophthalmol 59:469, 1965.

Table 50.4 ▪ Factors Implicated in Potential Drug-Induction of Angle-Closure Glaucoma

Age—usually older than 30 yr	Convexity of the iris—flattened
History—familial, genetic basis	Dose and duration of the offending drug used
Race—usually white	Duration of effect on eye—longer duration
Sex—usually female	Route of administration—topical more than systemic
Anterior chamber angle—shallow and narrow	
Vision—hyperopia, hypermetropia	

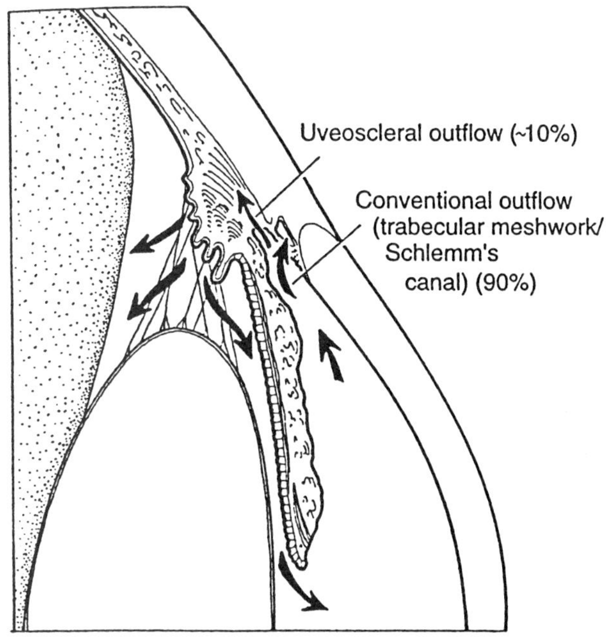

Figure 50.1. Aqueous humor is actively secreted by the ciliary epithelium into the posterior chamber, flows through the pupil into the anterior chamber, and drains through the conventional and unconventional pathways. (Reprinted with permission from Chandler PA, Grant WM, Epstein DL, et al. Chandler and Grant's glaucoma. 4th ed. Baltimore: Williams & Wilkins, 1997.)

Aqueous humor is secreted by the ciliary processes into the posterior chamber of the eye (Fig. 50.1), where it flows to the trabecular meshwork and through the canal of Schlemm. Owing to diurnal variability in aqueous humor production, IOP measurements vary depending upon the time of day. Many patients with open-angle glaucoma have the greatest IOP in the morning and the lowest IOP during the sleeping hours. Because a decrease in the outflow facility of aqueous humor is the primary mechanism for producing an increase in IOP, anatomic changes associated with open-angle and angle-closure glaucoma are important.

Open-Angle Glaucoma

In open-angle glaucoma, a physical blockage occurs within the trabecular meshwork that retards elimination of aqueous humor. The obstruction is presumed to be between the trabecular sheet and the episcleral veins, into which the aqueous humor ultimately flows.

The impairment of aqueous drainage elevates the IOP to between 25 and 35 mm Hg (normal IOP is 10 to 20 mm Hg), indicating that the obstruction is usually partial. This increase in IOP is sufficient to cause progressive cupping of the optic disk and eventually visual field defects. As the trabecular spaces become more involved, detachment of the cornea and formation of bullae may develop. Because visual acuity remains largely unaffected until late in the disease, areas of visual field disturbances or blind spots must be regarded as an indication for medical therapy.

Angle-Closure Glaucoma

In angle-closure glaucoma, increased IOP is caused by pupillary blockage of aqueous humor outflow and is more severe. The basic requirements leading to an acute attack of angle closure are a pupillary block, a narrowed anterior chamber angle, and a convex iris. The sequence of events leading to increased IOP is depicted in Figure 50.2. When a patient has a narrow anterior chamber (Fig. 50.2*A*) or a pupil that dilates to a degree where the iris comes in greater contact with the lens (Fig. 50.2*B*), there is interference with the flow of aqueous humor from the posterior to the anterior chamber. Because aqueous humor is continually secreted, pressure from within the posterior chamber forces the iris to bulge forward (Fig. 50.2*C*). This may progress to complete blockage (Fig. 50.2*D*).

The pathologic complications of angle-closure and open-angle glaucoma include the formation of cataracts, adhesion of the iris to the cornea, atrophy of the optic nerve and retina, complete blockage of aqueous outflow, and ultimately, blindness.

Congenital Glaucoma

Congenital glaucoma is a rare disorder in which IOP is increased as a result of developmental abnormalities of the ocular structures in the newborn or infant. It may occur in association with other congenital abnormalities and anomalies such as homocystinuria and Marfan's syndrome. Congenital glaucoma should be considered in newborns and infants who have sensitivity to light or exhibit excessive tearing or spasm of the eyelids.

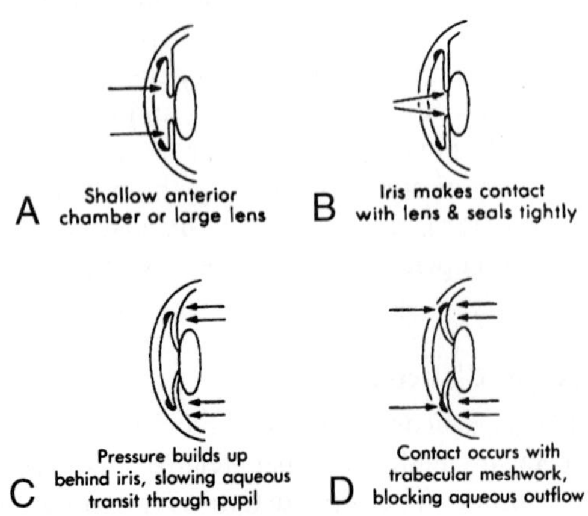
A Shallow anterior chamber or large lens
B Iris makes contact with lens & seals tightly
C Pressure builds up behind iris, slowing aqueous transit through pupil
D Contact occurs with trabecular meshwork, blocking aqueous outflow

Figure 50.2. Abnormal eye with development of pupillary block.

Normal-Tension Glaucoma

The etiology and pathogenesis of normal-tension glaucoma remain to be completely understood. Normal-tension glaucoma is thought to be related, at least in part, to decreased blood flow to the optic nerve. This may eventually cause neuronal damage. In addition, these eyes appear to be more susceptible to pressure-related damage within the normal or high-normal range, and therefore a pressure lower than normal is often necessary to prevent further visual loss.[14]

Drug-Induced Glaucoma

Several therapeutic classes of drugs, such as those with anticholinergic, adrenergic, or corticosteroid effects, have been implicated in inducing or worsening glaucoma.

Medications affect open-angle and closed-angle glaucoma differently. Drugs that dilate the pupil, for instance, may precipitate an acute attack of angle-closure glaucoma but usually do not produce harmful effects in those with open-angle glaucoma. Dilation of the pupil in angle-closure glaucoma may cause the peripheral iris to bulge forward, blocking the trabecular meshwork. The aqueous humor is prevented from reaching the outflow channels, which results in increased IOP. Because excessive resistance to outflow in open-angle glaucoma is caused primarily by changes within the trabecular outflow channels, dilation of the pupil usually will not increase the IOP.

Topical administration of some drugs (Table 50.5) is known to elevate IOP in various patients with glaucoma, and it has been assumed that systemic administration of such medications will have a similar effect. In patients with mild or controlled open-angle glaucoma, it is unwarranted to prohibit the use of systemic sympathomimetic, anticholinergic, and other atropine-like drugs because the evidence that they exacerbate the condition is not well documented.[10,15]

Anticholinergics

In patients with normal eyes, topically instilled anticholinergics such as atropine, scopolamine, and cyclopentolate produce no significant elevation in IOP. However, in patients older than 30 years of age who have abnormally shallow anterior chambers, there is a risk of precipitating acute attacks of angle-closure glaucoma. The incidence has been estimated to be nearly 1 in 4000.[16] Atropine and scopolamine have a profound effect on the eye because of their longer durations of action compared to other agents with anticholinergic effects such as phenothiazines, tricyclic antidepressants, and antihistamines. These locally instilled agents cause mydriasis and cycloplegia that may persist for as long as 2 weeks. In some patients with open-angle glaucoma, they produce a slight increase in IOP (less than 6 mm Hg) when instilled into the eyes. Other mydriatics, however, do not appear to have this effect.[17]

Conventional doses of atropine systemically administered for preanesthesia have little ocular effect; in contrast,

Table 50.5 • Ability of Drugs to Induce Glaucoma

Drug	Route	Glaucoma Type	
		Open-Angle	Angle-Closure
Anticholinergics			
Atropine	Topical	Rare	Frequent
Scopolamine	Topical	Rare	Frequent
Belladonna	Topical	Rare	Frequent
Propantheline	Systemic	Rare	Rare
Adrenergics			
Phenylephrine 10%	Topical	Never	Occasional
Epinephrine	Systemic	Never	Rare
Miotics			
Pilocarpine 4–8%	Topical	Never	Occasional
Echothiophate	Topical	Never	Occasional
Isoflurophate	Topical	Never	Occasional
Carbonic anhydrase inhibitors			
Acetazolamide	Systemic	Never	Rare
Antihypertensives	Systemic	Never	Never
β-Chymotrypsin	Topical	Rare	Occasional
Prochlorperazine	Systemic	Never	Never
Promethazine (high doses)	Systemic	Never	Rare
Ganglionic blocking agents	Systemic	Rare	Occasional
Amphetamines	Systemic	Rare	Occasional
Tricyclic antidepressants	Systemic	Rare	Occasional
Corticosteroids (at equipotent doses)			
Betamethasone	Topical	Frequent	Never
Dexamethasone	Topical	Frequent	Never
Hydrocortisone	Topical	Occasional	Never
Prednisolone	Topical	Occasional	Never
Triamcinolone	Topical	Occasional	Never
Dexamethasone	Systemic	Occasional	Never
Hydrocortisone	Systemic	Occasional	Never
Prednisolone	Systemic	Occasional	Never

equivalent therapeutic doses of scopolamine can cause definite pupillary dilation.[18] Prolonged use of anticholinergics can exacerbate open-angle glaucoma to some extent, but studies have shown that oral atropine at a dose of 0.6 mg every 4 hours for 1 week produces only slight elevations of IOP.[19] In another study, the administration of proprietary cold remedies containing 0.2 mg of belladonna alkaloids (given twice daily for 4 days) caused no changes in IOP in 27 normal volunteers and 37 patients with glaucoma (including 18 patients with chronic angle-closure glaucoma).[20]

Propantheline, a commonly used anticholinergic, produces no significant elevation in IOP in patients with either normal-tension or angle-closure glaucoma. Anticholinergics, in fact, can deepen the anterior chamber by inhibiting the contraction of the ciliary body and produce cycloplegia, which widens rather than narrows the anterior chamber angle, making angle closure less likely to occur. No recent reports of exacerbations of glaucoma with diazepam or amitriptyline have appeared in the literature although the manufacturers of these drugs contraindicate their use in patients with this disorder. Very high doses of phenothiazines given for schizophrenia have produced slight elevations of IOP.[21] Treatment with miotics easily overcame the effect.

In summary, withholding systemic anticholinergics for fear of inducing open-angle glaucoma is not justified. This is true especially with parenteral atropine or scopolamine given before general anesthesia. Sensitivity of the eye to systemic drugs is relatively low. Although these agents can induce angle closure in rare instances, the concomitant use of parasympathomimetic miotics prevents any of the effects of IOP. However, ocularly instilled potent anticholinergics, such as atropine, scopolamine, cyclopentolate, and homatropine, should not be used in patients with a diagnosis of or predisposition to development of angle-closure glaucoma.

Sympathomimetics

Adrenergic agents commonly found in cough and cold preparations, appetite suppressants, bronchodilators, central nervous stimulants, and vasoconstrictors produce slight pupillary dilation. No adverse effects in patients with open-angle glaucoma have been reported. After systemic administration of these agents, the frequency of deleterious effects in patients with angle-closure glaucoma has been extremely small. Adrenergic agents such as epinephrine and phenylephrine have been used ocularly to treat open-angle glaucoma. These agents, however, elevate the IOP by narrowing the anterior chamber angle when instilled into the eyes of patients with angle-closure glaucoma.

General anesthetics producing parasympathetic and sympathetic imbalance may cause pupillary block. Topical pilocarpine 1% may be instilled into the eye before inducing anesthesia to prevent this complication.

Cardiovascular Drugs

There is no convincing evidence that vasodilators significantly aggravate glaucoma even though subconjunctival injection of strong vasodilators such as isoxsuprine and tolazoline can induce transient elevations in IOP, particularly in patients with chronic open-angle glaucoma. Nitrates, nitrites, aminophylline, and cyclandelate can be used safely.[16,21] Antihypertensives decrease intraocular blood flow, which can lead to loss of small visual fields in patients with a high IOP. Therefore, it is best to decrease blood pressure gradually in patients with angle-closure glaucoma. If it is necessary to decrease blood pressure rapidly, one should either increase the patient's miotic medication or simultaneously lower the IOP rapidly with an agent such as acetazolamide.

Corticosteroids

Corticosteroid-induced glaucoma is well documented. This form of glaucoma is usually without pain, physical findings in the eye, or visual field defects. The lesion probably occurs in the trabecular meshwork and severely decreases the outflow facility. After topical therapy, the glaucomatous change occurs in the eye instilled with the drug. This ocular hypertensive effect is usually fully reversible within 1 month after discontinuation of the medication.

The increase in IOP is approximately 10 mm Hg for patients with preglaucomatous anterior chambers and 5 mm Hg in normal persons. In some cases, irreversible eye damage occurs if ocular tension persists for 1 to 2 months or even longer. In addition, cupping of the optic disk and defects of the visual field may develop a few months after topical administration of corticosteroids is begun. Therefore, patients receiving chronic topical steroid therapy should have tonometric examinations every 2 months.

The degree of increase in pressure appears to be associated with the anti-inflammatory potency of the agents involved and is most marked with dexamethasone and betamethasone.[22] Equivalent doses of ophthalmic prednisolone and triamcinolone used four times daily induced elevations of IOP similar to those of betamethasone instilled only once daily. The duration of corticosteroid treatment and the age of the patient influenced the degree of ocular hypertension experienced. In some instances, topical epinephrine or systemic carbonic anhydrase inhibitors can maintain the ocular tension within normal limits. On other occasions, it may be necessary to reduce the frequency of administration, substitute a less potent steroid, or withdraw therapy.

The ocular hypertensive effect induced by topical steroids can be categorized for three groups of patients in the general population in whom glaucoma has not been diagnosed.[23] Two-thirds of the general population (group 1) respond with an average IOP increase of 1.6 mm Hg after 4 weeks of 0.1% dexamethasone three times daily. A second group (29%) responds with an average increase of 10 mm Hg. Finally, a third group (5%) responds with an increase greater than 16 mm Hg. For each group, the rate of IOP increase differs significantly. The clinical implication is that patients who are receiving corticosteroid for at least 1 month and who have tonometric pressures less than 21 mm Hg are unlikely to have glaucomatous complications. In addition, because approximately one-third of the general population will have a group 2 or group 3 response to topical steroids, tonometric monitoring should be performed after the first month of therapy, then every 2 months while receiving therapy.

Miscellaneous Agents

Amphetamines, tricyclic antidepressants, monoamine oxidase inhibitors, indomethacin, and cocaine produce slight degrees of mydriasis, but the likelihood of inducing angle closure with these drugs is very low. Strong miotics such as pilocarpine 4 to 8% and indirect-acting nonreversible cholinesterase inhibitors may lead to pupillary block and inhibition of aqueous humor outflow. This may result in vascular congestion of the peripheral part of the iris so that the swollen iris blocks the canal of Schlemm and prevents the outflow of aqueous humor.[21]

Polarizing neuromuscular blocking agents, such as succinylcholine, used as adjuvants to general anesthesia can cause a marked rise in IOP if the patient is not adequately anesthetized. These agents should not be used in glaucomatous patients. A nondepolarizing neuromuscular blocking agent, such as atracurium, is effective in preventing the rise in IOP.

Other medications, such as the serotonin-specific reuptake inhibitors fluoxetine and paroxetine have also been implicated in case reports as causes of glaucoma.[24–27] Relative to the large number of patients using these medications, the incidence of these problems is low and there is no reason to discourage therapy in patients with glaucoma. Rather, the clinician should closely monitor for potential drug-induced disease in patients who may benefit from either of these agents.

Summary of Drug-Induced Glaucoma

Table 50.5 lists drugs that can induce glaucoma. The following factors must be considered in assessing the problem of drug-induced glaucoma: topically administered drugs induce glaucoma more frequency than those given systemically; conditions under which any drugs are contraindicated are specific for the type of glaucoma and the method of treatment for it; seldom, if ever, does the warning against use of a particular agent in glaucoma specify the type of glaucoma; and patients with chronic open-angle glaucoma that is adequately controlled by therapy are not at risk when treated with either systemic anticholinergics or sympathomimetics.

Finally, acute angle-closure glaucoma is an emergency, and any agent that might precipitate an attack must be used cautiously. Unfortunately, patients who are predisposed to angle-closure glaucoma are not accurately identified without a gonioscopic examination of the anterior angle. Additionally, patients in whom angle-closure glaucoma has been diagnosed and who have had a corrective surgical procedure are not at risk for another episode of angle-closure glaucoma.[28]

CLINICAL PRESENTATION AND DIAGNOSIS

Signs and Symptoms

Glaucoma is insidious in onset and often produces no symptoms or only minor symptoms of discomfort, such as headache or "tired eyes." Many patients do not seek medical attention or do not adhere to medical therapy because of this lack of symptoms. Fortunately, optic nerve and retinal damage are late findings of end-stage disease and can be minimized with effective medical treatment. Symptoms such as persistent headache and eye pain usually cause patients to seek medical assistance before these serious consequences develop.[15]

Open-Angle Glaucoma

The common findings of open-angle glaucoma may be minimal and do not appear immediately. As time progresses, the signs become more marked until they finally restrict vision. The common findings are increased IOP, visual field loss, optic disk changes, decreased outflow facility, and gonioscopically open angles.

An increased IOP can have several interpretations. Most persons have pressures of 21 mm Hg or less. However, some patients may experience pressure-independent glaucomatous damage. This can occur with pressures less than 20 mm Hg, termed normal-tension glaucoma. In general, pressure readings in the high 20s are suspicious, and those greater than 30 are cause for serious concern. Patients between the ages of 50 and 75 with pressures greater than 30 mm Hg as the only sign of glaucoma should be treated medically because decreased vascular perfusion in the elderly can damage the optic nerve. Younger patients with similar readings may require assessment for changes in the optic disk or visual fields at less frequent intervals. There is no universally accepted cutoff IOP that can be used to diagnose glaucoma; the health care provider must judge whether to medically or surgically lower IOP based upon the patient's risk factors, diagnostic findings, and signs of existing optic nerve damage.[6,9,10,15]

Angle-Closure Glaucoma

Acute angle-closure glaucoma usually presents with signs and symptoms of blurred vision (often with colored halos around light), severe ocular pain, and nausea with occasional vomiting. Acute angle-closure glaucoma should be considered a medical emergency. The eye typically appears red, the cornea is cloudy, the pupil is mid-dilated, the anterior chamber is narrow, and the IOP is frequently greater than 50 mm Hg. Visual acuity is reduced by corneal changes or edema. Bullae may be present on the cornea if the acute attack is prolonged. Colored halos result from diffraction of light by the edematous cornea.[9,10,15] Ocular pain may vary from moderate to severe. The oculovagal reflex is thought to produce nausea, vomiting, bradycardia, and sweating that may accompany an acute attack. With very high IOPs, the pupil may become fixed in mid-dilation and eventually damaged. In severe cases, the pupil changes from a round to an oval shape and may resist constriction by topical parasympathomimetic agents.

Chronic angle-closure glaucoma is a less severe form than acute angle-closure glaucoma; the symptoms may range from none to intermittent severe ocular pain along with halo formation and ocular congestion. Synechiae do not form without ocular congestion, which may be evident only with a moderately high pressure reading.

Table 50.6 describes and differentiates clinical findings of patients with open-angle or angle-closure glaucoma.

Diagnosis

Four common tests may be performed that allow diagnosis of glaucoma before visual loss occurs. Direct ophthalmoscopy, also known as slit-lamp examination, allows the physician to observe changes in the optic nerve head. Slit lamp examination is a routine test performed by ophthalmologists to examine the cornea, anterior chamber depth, iris, and the vitreous. Changes such as optic nerve cupping or hemorrhage may be evident upon examination. Photographs of the optic disk may be obtained, which allow physicians to observe and compare changes over time from repeat photographs. Problems with using direct ophthalmoscopy are that it requires a great amount of training and there is considerable interobserver variability. In addition, it is not commonly available in most primary care settings.[6]

Tonometry measures IOP and may be useful as a screening test. Several different devices, such as Goldmann's tonometer, Schiøtz indentation tonometer, or electrical strain gauges measure how much force is required to flatten the central cornea (applanation of the cornea). As previously discussed, some patients with normal IOP may still develop glaucomatous damage. In addition, as many as 70% of patients with ocular hypertension never develop visual problems due to glaucoma.[6] Therefore, many physicians use tonometry in combination with other diagnostic tests.

Table 50.6 ▪ Clinical Findings and Symptoms of Primary Glaucoma

Glaucoma	Onset	Early Findings and Symptoms	Late Findings and Symptoms
Open-angle	Insidious	Asymptomatic slight rise in IOP: decreased rate of aqueous humor outflow, optic disk changes (symptoms may be marginal or absent)	Gradual loss of peripheral vision (over months to years); persistent elevation of IOP; optic nerve degeneration; retinal nerve atrophy; edema of the cornea; cataracts; trabecular meshwork degeneration
Angle-closure	Sudden	Blurred vision; severe ocular pain and congestion; conjunctival redness; cloudy cornea; moderately dilated pupil; poor pupil response to light; IOP markedly elevated; nausea and vomiting	Complete blindness in 2–5 days if not treated

IOP, intraocular pressure.

A third screening method is perimetry. Perimetry measures visual field defects by producing visual stimuli in various locations of the patient's field of vision. Because defects in the visual field and loss of vision are made apparent by perimetry, it is currently considered the "gold standard" diagnostic procedure. Unfortunately, perimetry is too time-consuming and expensive to be a practical screening tool; it should be reserved for those patients who have detectable optic nerve damage by other tests.[2,6]

Finally, gonioscopy is a procedure that allows quantitative measurement of the angle of the anterior chamber. Gonioscopy requires considerable training and is usually only performed by ophthalmologists.

Table 50.7 lists recommended initial diagnostic procedures for open-angle and angle-closure glaucoma, and Table 50.8 describes these procedures in further detail.

PSYCHOSOCIAL ASPECTS

It is estimated that 23 to 43% of patients in whom glaucoma has been diagnosed do not adhere to drug therapy regimens.[29–31] It is important for clinicians to recognize and appropriately assess several psychosocial factors when designing, implementing, and evaluating a therapeutic plan. First, as previously mentioned, most patients have few or no symptoms of disease. Second, open-angle glaucoma should be considered a chronic controllable disease. Finally, some patients may have difficulty with proper medication administration technique or experience adverse effects from medications. All of these aspects can lead to nonadherence to medication therapy. Methods to educate the patient and minimize psychosocial barriers that may affect management of disease will be discussed further throughout the chapter.

Table 50.7 ▪ Recommended Initial Diagnostic Procedures for Open-Angle and Angle-Closure Glaucoma

Open-Angle Glaucoma	Angle-Closure Glaucoma
▪ Family history	▪ Family history
▪ Physical examination of pupil	▪ Physical examination of the cornea and central and peripheral anterior chamber depth using slit-lamp procedure
▪ Measurement of intraocular pressure	▪ Measurement of angle using gonioscopy
▪ Physical examination of the cornea and central and peripheral anterior chamber depth using slit-lamp procedure	
▪ Measurement of angle using gonioscopy	
▪ Dilation of pupil and visualization of optic disk and nerve fiber layer	
▪ Photography or detailed drawing of optic nerve appearance	
▪ Examination of the fundus	
▪ Evaluation of visual field	

Source: Adapted from the Medical Specialty Society, Primary Angle-Closure Glaucoma and Glaucoma Panel, Preferred Practice Patterns Committee. Primary open-angle glaucoma. San Francisco, American Academy of Ophthalmology, 1996.

THERAPEUTIC PLAN

Open-Angle Glaucoma

Conservative medical treatment can successfully control most cases of chronic open-angle glaucoma. The stage or severity of the disease as evidenced by the condition of the optic disk and the quality of the visual field should be the major factors in choosing the treatment. Mild elevations of IOP (less than 30 mm Hg) in the presence of a normal optic disk and visual field are not an absolute indication for therapy. These patients should have routine periodic examinations to detect any optic changes because such changes can be detected long before permanent visual field impairment. There is no absolute level of IOP that must be maintained to assure therapeutic success. The IOP should be maintained at a level that prevents further deterioration of the optic disk and impairment of visual field. If the disk is normal on gonioscopic examination, an IOP in the high 20s is not as important clinically as the same IOP when there is concurrent disk involvement or abnormal visual field. The former situation may warrant only close periodic follow-up, whereas in the latter, appropriate medical treatment should be started. If there is the slightest indication of disk pathologic changes, the IOP should be maintained at 20 mm Hg or even lower by medical management. In patients with considerable disk degeneration and visual field loss, vigorous treatment should be undertaken to obtain a level of 15 mm Hg or lower. The target IOP reduction is therefore variable, depending upon the patient's level of preexisting damage or risk of damage.

In situations where advanced cupping of the optic disk and visual loss are not apparent in the presence of high IOP (greater than 30 mm Hg), medical therapy should be initiated. The aim of therapy is to lower the IOP enough to interrupt the course of the disease. Problems common to antiglaucoma therapy must be considered before reducing IOP with drugs. The expense and inconvenience of the medications should be considered as well as whether the side effects and toxicities of the drugs constitute a greater risk to the patient than the increased level of IOP.

Trials of topical agents involving a single eye may be useful to determine the amount of IOP reduction attributable to medication. The effects of therapy on the IOP can be determined within 1 week or more. β-Blocker therapy is the most widely prescribed drug therapy for the treatment of glaucoma.[9,32] If patients do not respond to β-blocking agents, other therapeutic classes of medications

Table 50.8 ▪ Diagnostic Studies for Glaucoma

Procedures	Comments
Tonometry	Measures intraocular tension. Because of diurnal variation, repeated readings should be done before definite diagnosis. Between acute attacks of angle-closure glaucoma, the intraocular tension may be normal. Applanation tonometry measures the force applied per unit area, whereas indentation tonometry uses a plunger to produce a pit in the cornea, which serves as a measure of intraocular pressure.
Gonioscopy	Differentiates the type of glaucoma. Gonioscopic appearance of narrowed anterior chamber angle is usually diagnostic of angle-closure glaucoma.
Tonography	May reveal impaired facility of aqueous humor outflow. Early open-angle glaucoma can be detected by this technique. Tonometer is applied to the eye and the resultant reduction in the intraocular tension is measured as an indicator of outflow facility.
Water-drinking test	Rise in intraocular tension after rapid ingestion of a quart of water is significant indication of glaucoma. Positive result occurs in 30% of patients with open-angle glaucoma. Negative result does not rule out glaucoma. Tonography and water-drinking test reveal open-angle glaucoma with 90% reliability.
Ophthalmoscopy	Glaucomatous excavation or cupping of the optic disk is found in chronic primary open-angle and congenital glaucomas. Glaucomatous changes of optic disk and/or occlusion of the central retinal vein in absence of elevated intraocular tension should arouse suspicion of glaucoma in early stage.
Visual field examination	Isolated areas of impaired vision surrounded by normal areas in a visual field are indicative of open-angle glaucoma; visual field changes are irreversible and parallel optic disk changes.
Corticosteroid instillation	Striking differences in ocular tension between patients with primary open-angle glaucoma and normal subjects are produced by topically instilled corticosteroids. Steroid provocative test is used to evaluate genetic predisposition for glaucoma. Response of patients with primary angle-closure glaucoma to corticosteroid instillation is similar to that of normal subjects.
Dark room test	Intraocular tension is assessed in patient before and after being placed in a dark room. In patients with chronic angle-closure glaucoma, a considerable rise in the intraocular tension is observed after being in the dark.

should be tried instead of another β-blocker or before using combination therapy. The place in therapy for newer agents, such as latanoprost or topical carbonic anhydrase inhibitors, is not well defined. Until well-designed cost-effectiveness studies or other pharmacoeconomic evaluations are completed, these agents should probably be reserved as second-line monotherapy for patients who do not tolerate or respond to less expensive topical therapy.

Miotic agents should be used at the lowest effective concentration and at intervals no more frequent than necessary to maintain a satisfactory level of IOP. The IOP should be measured before therapy is begun. If the reduction of IOP is not satisfactory, the concentration of the miotic agent should be increased, keeping in mind, however, that there is little advantage to using concentrations of pilocarpine solutions greater than 4% or its equivalent.

Refractoriness often occurs after prolonged use of cholinergic miotics. Rather than increase the frequency of instillation or strength used, an alternative agent should be selected. Responsiveness to the cholinergic miotics often is restored after their replacement for a brief period by an anticholinesterase miotic. Various combinations of glaucoma medications are often given together to potentiate their therapeutic effects. However, not all combinations produce an additive pharmacologic response.

Addition of an agent from another class of antiglaucoma drugs is preferred to substitution or addition of an agent from the same group. Progression of the glaucoma should always be ruled out. The storage condition of the medication, expiration date, and method of administration (including observation of nasolacrimal occlusion) should be assessed when a patient experiences diminished effects from the eye drops. Figure 50.3 summarizes an approach that may be useful in the treatment of open-angle glaucoma.

Angle-Closure Glaucoma

Acute angle-closure glaucoma is a medical emergency that must be treated surgically. Before peripheral iridoplasty or laser iridotomy, one or more of the following agents may be administered to eliminate pupillary block and decrease inflammation: hyperosmotic agents, carbonic acid inhibitors, miotics, and corticosteroids. Figure 50.4 presents a diagrammatic overview of medical and surgical approaches to patients with acute angle-closure glaucoma.

Normal-Tension Glaucoma

Results of the Collaborative Normal-Tension Glaucoma Study[3] were recently made available. In this study, 145 patients from 24 study sites were enrolled. The investigators randomly selected one eye from each patient to either receive medical therapy that would reduce IOP 30% from baseline or to serve as a control. The endpoints included

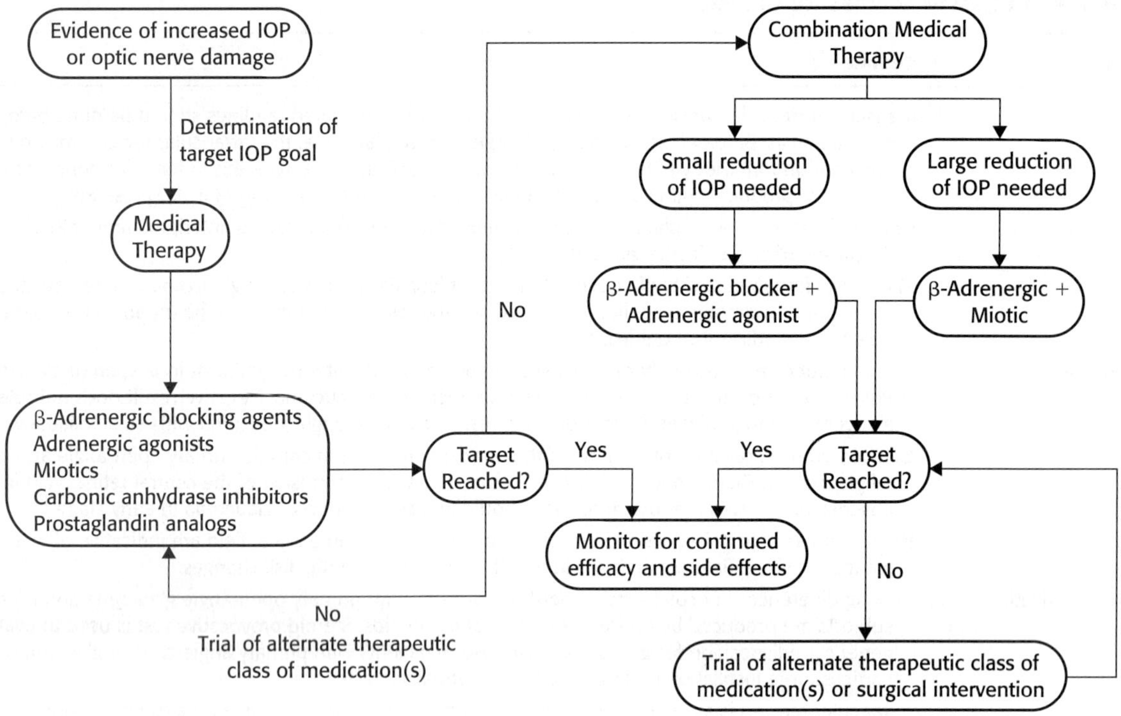

Figure 50.3. Algorithm for the medical management of open-angle glaucoma.

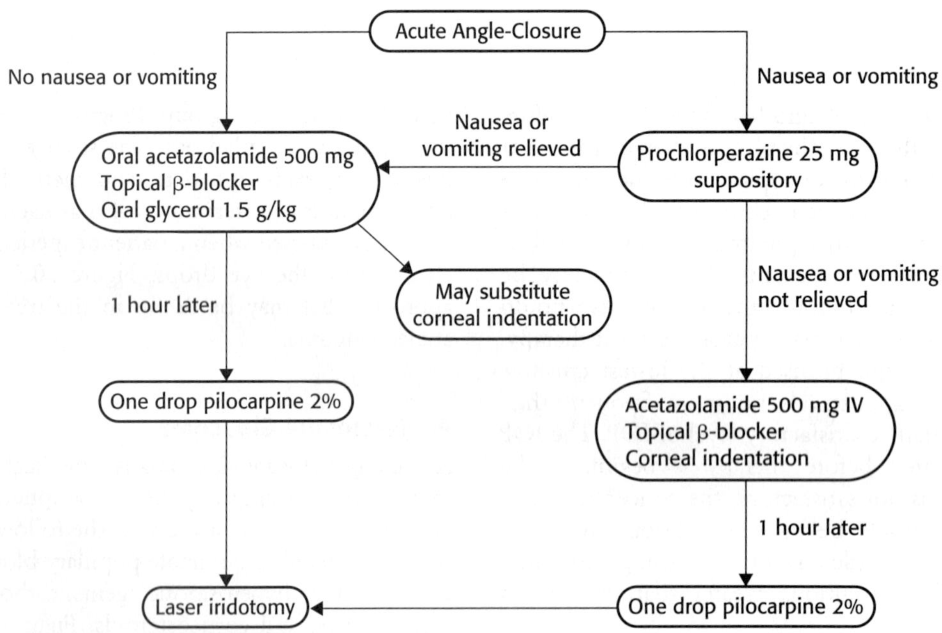

Figure 50.4. Algorithm for the management of acute angle-closure glaucoma. (Adapted with permission from Eskridge JB, Bartlett JD. The glaucomas. In Bartlett JD, Jaanus SD, eds. Clinical ocular pharmacology. Woburn, MA Butterworth-Heinemann, 1988:743.)

strictly defined criteria of progression of optic disk damage or visual field loss.

The study demonstrated that 35% of control eyes versus 12% of treated eyes (p value not stated) reached these endpoints. Additionally, a survival analysis compared the proportion of patients within the two groups and found a significant difference favoring treatment when examining (1) any defined endpoint suggesting glaucomatous damage ($p < 0.0001$) and (2) those patients who reached four of five defined endpoints of glaucomatous damage ($p = 0.01$). Interestingly, patients who were treated had a higher risk of cataracts. Eleven of a total of 34 cataracts occurred in the control group versus 23 in treatment group ($p = 0.0011$). These differences were statistically different when examining treatment patients who received surgical treatment compared to control patients ($p = 0.0001$) but not when comparing medically treated patients and control patients ($p = 0.18$).

In light of these studies of IOP lowering in normal tension glaucoma, it is now thought that patients with normal IOPs who are at risk of developing optic nerve damage should be routinely examined for progression and, if present, treated with agents that effectively reduce baseline IOP by 25 to 30%.[3]

TREATMENT

Pharmacotherapy

The goal of glaucoma therapy is the immediate and sustained reduction of IOP to prevent deterioration of the optic nerve and loss of vision. Medications used in the treatment of glaucoma may be classified as those that increase the elimination of aqueous humor and those that decrease its formation. The five major classes of medications used for the management of glaucoma include β-adrenergic blocking agents, miotics, adrenergic agonists, topical and oral carbonic anhydrase inhibitors, and prostaglandin analogs. Additionally, hyperosmotic agents are used for the short-term rapid decrease of IOP necessary in the management of acute angle-closure glaucoma. Table 50.9 summarizes these therapeutic classes of medications used in the treatment of glaucoma, differentiated by their mechanism of action.

β-Blockers

β-Blockers are the most widely prescribed drugs for the treatment of glaucoma[32] and may be used alone or in combination with other agents. The ocular hypotensive effect caused by β-blockers is probably due to suppression of aqueous humor formation by blockage of the β-adrenoreceptors in the ciliary body.[32,33] β-Blockers decrease aqueous humor production by approximately one-third.[34] All of the agents are available as solutions and are usually administered one to two times daily. Additionally, timolol maleate is available in a gel formulation, which may be given once daily.

Table 50.9 ▪ Medications Used in the Treatment of Glaucoma

Drug Class/Name	Mechanism of IOP-Lowering Effect	Duration of Activity (hr)	Pregnancy Category
β-Blockers	Increase aqueous humor outflow		
Timolol		12–24	C
Levobunolol		12–24	C
Betaxolol		12	C
Metipranolol		12–24	C
Carteolol		12	C
Miotics, direct acting	Increase aqueous humor outflow		
Pilocarpine			C
Solution		4–8	
Gel		18–24	
Ocular insert		1 week	
Carbachol		6–8	C
Miotics, cholinesterase inhibitors	Increase aqueous humor outflow		
Physostigmine		12–36	C
Demecarium		Days/weeks	X
Echothiophate		Days/weeks	C
Sympathomimetics	Decrease aqueous humor formation and increase aqueous humor outflow		
Apraclonidine		7–12	C
Epinephrine		12	C
Dipivefrin		12	B
Brimonidine		12	B
Carbonic anhydrase inhibitors	Decrease aqueous humor formation		
Acetazolamide		8–12	C
Tablets			
ER capsules			
Injectable			
Dichlorphenamide		6–12	C
Methazolamide		10–18	C
Dorzolamide		8	C
Brinzolamide		8	C

ER, extended release.

Historically, reports of propranolol use for the treatment of glaucoma appear as early as 1967.[35] However, because of side effects such as ocular anesthesia, the use of β-blockers was limited until timolol maleate was available.[36] β-Blockers that are commonly used for the treatment of open-angle glaucoma include timolol maleate, betaxolol HCl, levobunolol HCl, carteolol, and metipranolol (Tables 50.10 and 50.11). In addition, timolol was approved by the U.S. Food and Drug Administration (FDA) as a combination product with the carbonic anhydrase inhibitor dorzolamide in 1995. The main clinical difference among the available topical β-blocking agents is the agents' β-receptor selectivity. Betaxolol is the only currently available agent that is selective for the β_1 receptor.[37]

Timolol is a potent, short-acting, nonselective β-blocker. It is available as 0.25 and 0.5% solutions and a longer-acting gel-forming solution. For patients who are sensitive to preservatives, timolol is also available as a preservative-free solution. This dosage form must be used immediately upon opening. The usual starting dose is 1 drop of 0.25% in the affected eye(s) once to twice a day. If this does not control the glaucoma, the dose may be increased to 0.5% solution, 1 drop twice a day.[38,39] When

Table 50.10 ▪ β-Blockers Used in the Management of Glaucoma

Drug (Year Approved)	β-Receptor Selectivity	Dosage[a]	Comments
Timolol (1978)	β_1 and β_2	0.25 and 0.5% drops	Instill 1 drop in affected eye qd or q12hr
		0.25 and 0.5% gel	Instill 1 drop qd. Patients should be instructed to shake the container once before administration and to wait at least 10 min after using the gel before instilling another ophthalmic agent.
Betaxolol (1985)	β_1	0.25 and 0.50% drops	Instill 1 drop qd or q12hr. It may be advantageous over other β-blockers in patients with respiratory diseases due to generally good bronchopulmonary tolerability.
Levobunolol (1986)	β_1 and β_2	0.25 and 0.50% drops	Instill 1 drop qd or q12hr.
Metipranolol (1990)	β_1 and β_2	0.3% drops	Instill 1 drop qd or q12hr.
Carteolol (1992)	β_1 and β_2	1% drops	Instill 1 drop qd or q12hr. Use of carteolol may avoid addition of miotic agents for glaucoma refractory to β-blockers alone. It is the only β-blocker with ISA and has most potent β-blockade activity.

ISA, intrinsic sympathomimetic activity.
[a]For open-angle glaucoma.

Table 50.11 ▪ Selected Pharmacodynamic and Pharmacokinetic Properties of Ocular β-Adrenergic Blockers

Property	Timolol	Carteolol	Betaxolol	Levobunolol	Metipranolol
Relative β-blockade potency (propranolol = 1)	6	10	4	6	2
β_1 selectivity	0	0	++	0	0
ISA	0	++	0	0	0
Local anesthetic effect	0	0	+	0	
Stinging, burning	++	+/–	+++	++	+
Heart rate decrease	++	+	+/–	++	++
Bronchoconstriction	++	+	+/–	++	++
Dyslipidemia	+	0	?	?	?
Ocular perfusion	+/–	+/–	+/–	?	?
Serum half-life (hr)	3–5	3–7	12–20	6	2

ISA, intrinsic sympathomimetic activity.
Reprinted with permission from Zimmerman TJ. Topical ophthalmic β blockers: A comparative review. J Ocul Pharmacol 9:373-384, 1993.

used alone, timolol can produce mean reductions in IOP of approximately 31 to 33%. Timolol may also be used combination with agents such as epinephrine, pilocarpine, carbachol, dorzolamide, or acetazolamide. The addition of timolol to these agents significantly reduced IOP further than either agent alone.[34,38,40–43] A combination product containing timolol maleate and dorzolamide may be useful in increasing compliance compared to administering the agents separately.

If 1 drop of timolol (0.5% solution) twice a day is not effective, switching to another therapeutic category or concomitant therapy with other agents is warranted. When timolol is added to another medication, the other agent should be continued as well. The other agents may be discontinued or its doses adjusted on the following day, depending on the therapeutic response of the patient.

Stabilization of timolol therapy may take several weeks. A reevaluation should take place 2 and 4 weeks after therapy is begun. If the IOP is maintained, the schedule may be decreased to 1 drop once a day because of the daily variations in IOP. Tonometer readings should be performed at different times of the day.[36,44–46] Contraindications for timolol include obstructive pulmonary disease and congestive heart failure.[39]

Timolol is also available in combination with dorzolamide. Studies have shown that the combination product, when given two times daily, produces a similar additional reduction in IOP and adverse event profile as administering the two agents as separate products. This combination may reduce the number of times a patient needs to administer his or her medication from 5 times daily to twice daily.[47–50]

Betaxolol, a β_1 selective adrenergic blocking agent, is available as a 0.5% solution and a 0.25% suspension that is instilled into the eye every 12 hours. In a double-blind randomized study,[51] betaxolol (0.5%) was compared with timolol (0.5%). Both drugs had similar efficacy in reducing IOP. The most frequently reported side effects were mild discomfort and tearing on administration, but side effects were not sufficient to cause discontinuation of therapy. Betaxolol, unlike timolol, offers the advantage of little or no effect[52] on pulmonary disease, but it should still be used with caution in patients with preexisting disease.[32,53,54] Because of its selective β-adrenergic activity, betaxolol produces a greater additive effect than timolol when administered concomitantly with epinephrine. However, betaxolol, like other β-blockers, should not be administered to patients with heart failure.[55] Finally, betaxolol may cause more stinging and burning upon instillation than other available agents.[37]

Levobunolol is available as a 0.25 and 0.5% solution that can be given once or twice a day. Levobunolol is metabolized by the liver to an active metabolite, dihydrolevobunolol, which usually allows for extended dosing periods.[56] Wandel et al.[57] compared once-a-day dosing of levobunolol 0.5 or 1% and timolol 0.5% in 92 patients. Both levobunolol 0.5 and 1% were found to have an overall greater effect on IOP than timolol (7, 6.5, and 4.5 mm Hg, respectively). If IOP is not controlled with a single dose of levobunolol, the frequency of administration should be increased to twice a day. In this case, levobunolol offers no advantage over timolol.[32,37]

Metipranolol is available as a 0.3% solution. Its relative β-blockage potency is the lowest of the β-blockers. Metipranolol has been shown to be as effective as timolol and levobunolol and is an inexpensive choice among the available topical β-blockers. However, metipranolol may cause an increased risk of granulomatous anterior uveitis, resulting in iris nodules and precipitates.[37] Additionally, metipranolol has been reported to cause more stinging and burning upon administration than other agents.[37] Metipranolol has been discontinued in the United Kingdom because of these potential toxicities.

Carteolol is a nonselective β-adrenergic blocker that is available as a 1% solution. It is the most potent of the β-blockers and is the only agent with intrinsic sympathomimetic activity (ISA). Unfortunately, this has not been shown to decrease systemic cardiovascular or pulmonary side effects.[32,37,58]

Side effects of the topical β-blockers include burning or pain after instillation, blurring of vision, and dilated pupils (with epinephrine combinations). Systemic side effects include cardiovascular problems (bradycardia, palpitations, hypertension, and congestive heart failure), central nervous system disturbances (headaches, dizziness, drowsiness, anxiety, and depression), and pulmonary system side effects, including deaths due to precipitation or exacerbation of existing bronchospasm.[32,44–46] Patients with diabetes should also use topical β-blockers with caution because of potential loss of symptoms of hypoglycemia.

The topical β-blockers cause only small changes in pupil size and accommodation. Additionally, blurred vision and night blindness associated with the use of miotic agents are less likely with β-blocking agents. β-Blockers should never be used without concomitant instillation of a topical miotic in patients with angle-closure glaucoma.

In summary, the available agents all typically reduce IOP approximately 25% from baseline. Apparent advantages of one agent over another are limited to side effect profile, dosing schedule, or cost per effective dose. Levobunolol or timolol gel may allow for once-daily dosing. Betaxolol may be a safer alternative in patients with pulmonary disease. The ISA effect of carteolol has not been shown to reduce its side effect profile. Therefore, currently timolol is considered the standard agent against which others must be judged.[37]

Miotics

Miotics act via either direct cholinergic stimulation or as cholinesterase inhibitors. The resulting parasympathetic activity of either of these classes of medication facilitates the outflow of aqueous humor from the anterior chamber of the eye (Table 50.12). This is accomplished primarily by

Table 50.12 ▪ Miotic Drugs Used in the Management of Glaucoma

Drug	Dosage[a]	Comments
Direct-acting		
Pilocarpine hydrochloride, pilocarpine nitrate	0.25–10%	Instill 1 or 2 drops in affected eye q6–8hr to as often as q4hr. Onset of IOP-lowering effect is rapid with a 4–6 hr duration; although strengths >4% are available, there is little advantage to using them.
Pilocarpine gel	4% gel	Apply to affected eye hs. The gel dosage form is used as an adjunct to daytime medications.
Pilocarpine sustained release delivery system	Pilo-20 (20 μg/hr) and Pilo-40 (40 μg/hr)	Place into the affected eye once a week. For ≤2% solution, 20 μg/hr is generally used; for greater strengths, use 40 μg/hr.
Carbachol	0.75–3%	Instill 1 or 2 drops in affected eye q8–10hr to as often as q4hr. Response varies with dose. More require frequent administration may be needed for weaker solutions than usually suggested. It is a suitable alternative when other miotics cannot be used because of allergy or side effects. It has poor corneal penetration, is contraindicated in presence of corneal injury, and is longer acting than pilocarpine.
Short-acting cholinesterase inhibitors		
Physostigmine sulfate	0.25%	Apply 0.25% ointment at bedtime. Onset of IOP-lowering effect is similar to pilocarpine. It is considered to be stronger miotic than pilocarpine.
Long-acting cholinesterase inhibitors		
Demecarium bromide	0.125–0.25%	Instill 1 or 2 drops in affected eye q12hr. It is potent and long-acting and should be used only when shorter-acting miotics do not give the desired result. Duration of miosis is prolonged.
Echothiophate Iodide	0.03–0.25%	Instill 1 drop in affected eye no more than q12hr. It is unstable in solution. It is potent and long-acting with maximum effects seen in 10–20 hr and persisting for several days and should be used when shorter-acting miotics are inadequate. It is contraindicated before filtering surgery and before cataract extraction.

IOP, intraocular pressure.
[a]For open-angle glaucoma.

their action on the musculature of the iris and the ciliary body, which pulls the peripheral iris away from the trabecular meshwork. The trabecular meshwork and veins peripheral to the canal of Schlemm also may be dilated, thereby facilitating the outflow of aqueous humor. Miotics can lower IOP directly by stimulating the postfunctional effector cells innervated by the cholinergic fibers. Structurally, these agents are similar to acetylcholine. Acetylcholine is used during surgery for rapid miosis, but it is not useful in the chronic treatment of glaucoma because it is rapidly hydrolyzed by acetylcholinesterase.[2]

Cholinergic miotics are therapeutically beneficial for treatment of open-angle glaucoma and for preoperative preparation for surgery in angle-closure glaucoma. Their disadvantage is their short duration of action, requiring frequent administration.

Direct-Acting Miotics

Pilocarpine is the cholinergic agent most commonly used for the treatment of glaucoma.[2,9,10,15,28] It is available as a solution, gel, and sustained-release delivery system. Dosage must be titrated to patient response; however, there is little additional benefit to using solutions greater than 4% pilocarpine.[59]

Pilocarpine penetrates the cornea after ocular instillation, with miosis and decreases in IOP reaching their maximum levels in 30 to 40 minutes. The duration of IOP lowering is 4 to 8 hours. The usual frequency of instillation is two or three times daily, but pilocarpine may be given as often as every 2 hours.[10,60]

Pilocarpine gel is useful as an adjunct to the solution when used at bedtime. Because the patient is sleeping, typical side effects such as myopia and fixed pupils occur during the night. This may add to patient acceptance and compliance with medical therapy.[61]

The pilocarpine extended-release delivery system consists of a disk impregnated with pilocarpine, which is placed into the eye. Slightly larger than a contact lens and containing pilocarpine solution in its core, it is worn in the conjunctival sac of the eye where the drug diffuses out at a constant rate of either 20 μg/hr (Pilo-20) or 40 g/hr (Pilo-40). Patients previously using 0.5 or 1% drops are usually given Pilo-20; those using 2 to 4% drops require Pilo-40. The delivery system is replaced every 7 days. Advantages of the extended-release dosage form include a constant rate of drug released, decreased pupillary constriction and myopia, and improved compliance. Disadvantages of the delivery system include expense and irritation (foreign body sensation), which occasionally results in the patient having to return to pilocarpine drops.[62]

Carbachol is an unsubstituted carbamyl ester with a direct action like that of pilocarpine on parasympathetic receptors. It is totally resistant to hydrolysis by cholinesterase or acetylcholinesterase and therefore has a longer duration of action than pilocarpine in comparable strengths for IOP control. Solutions are available in strengths of 0.75 to 3%. In the treatment of open-angle glaucoma, 1 drop is instilled, usually two or three times daily. Response varies with the dose, and the weaker strength solutions require more frequent administration than usually suggested. When pilocarpine and other miotics cannot be used because of either allergy or intolerable side effects, carbachol may be a suitable alternative. However, if the glaucoma is uncontrollable with pilocarpine, it is doubtful that carbachol would yield much, if any, therapeutic improvement.

Diurnal fluctuations of IOP are diminished more effectively by carbachol than by pilocarpine. The major disadvantage of carbachol is its poor corneal penetration. In addition, it must be prepared in a vehicle such as methylcellulose to ensure prolonged contact with cornea or with a wetting agent such as benzalkonium chloride to enhance corneal penetration.[63]

Acetylcholine chloride (Miochol) is only used during surgical procedures. The solution is unstable and must be prepared immediately before the procedure. Additionally, pilocarpine or another miotic agent must be administered before placing the surgical dressing if continued miosis postoperatively is desired.

Methacholine bromide is very similar pharmacologically to acetylcholine, except that it is hydrolyzed more slowly by acetylcholinesterase and is almost totally resistant to cholinesterase. However, poor corneal penetration and instability in solution make it an unsuitable miotic for clinical use in glaucoma.

If IOP is not controlled with direct-acting miotics, more potent agents such as cholinesterase inhibitors may be used.[2]

Cholinesterase Inhibitors

A different method to increase parasympathetic activity is to inhibit the enzyme cholinesterase, thereby permitting the accumulation of acetylcholine and prolonging activity on the effector end organs of the eye. The key pharmacologic difference between the available compounds is the relative irreversibility or permanency of their parasympathomimetic activity. Physostigmine and neostigmine are reversible agents with short durations of effect. These agents are rarely used clinically for the treatment of glaucoma. Organophosphate compounds such as demecarium, echothiophate, and isoflurophate are irreversible compounds that have long durations of action.

Anticholinesterase miotics are therapeutically beneficial for the treatment of primary open-angle glaucoma; they are not indicated for the treatment of angle-closure glaucoma or congenital glaucoma. Because these agents act indirectly by inhibiting cholinesterase activity and prolonging the effects of endogenous acetylcholine, parasympathetic fibers to the pupil must be functional. The anticholinesterases are not effective if given after retrobulbar injections of anesthesia (e.g., during cataract extraction) because liberation of acetylcholine is impaired.

Physostigmine lowers IOP by facilitating the outflow of aqueous humor. It has a longer duration of action and is considered to be a stronger miotic than pilocarpine. Physostigmine is available as a 0.25% ointment that may be applied up to three times a day. Reduction in IOP usually occurs within 10 to 30 minutes, reaching its maximal effect within 1 to 2 hours and lasting 4 hours or more after application. The miotic effects may persist much longer. Aqueous solutions of physostigmine are unstable, and they should not be used if the solution becomes discolored. Physostigmine ointment should be reserved for bedtime use because the intense miosis produced soon after application causes less discomfort for the patient while asleep. The prolonged duration of increased aqueous humor outflow facilitation is ideal and convenient because the patient need not be interrupted from sleeping to administer miotics.[64]

Neostigmine is more stable but less effective than physostigmine because of poorer corneal penetration. Because of this, neostigmine is not clinically useful for the treatment of glaucoma. Demecarium is chemically similar to neostigmine, with miotic and IOP-lowering activity comparable to that of the irreversible agents echothiophate and isoflurophate. Demecarium is commercially available in concentrations of 0.125 and 0.25%. In contrast to the organophosphates, the inhibition of cholinesterase activity by demecarium 0.06 to 0.25% instilled every 12 to 48 hours has beneficial effects on IOP lasting from 12 hours to several days. Maximal reduction of IOP with demecarium is seen in 24 to 36 hours. The rapidity of the onset and duration of miosis is directly related to the concentrations used. Tolerance and refractoriness to demecarium occur earlier than with echothiophate and isoflurophate.[2,63]

Echothiophate has a slow onset but is a long-acting cholinesterase inhibitor.[65] Aqueous solutions of 0.03 to 0.25% instilled 1 drop every 12 to 24 hours for open-angle glaucoma can produce miosis within 10 to 15 minutes although its maximal effect on IOP is not seen until 10 to 20 hours later and may persist for 96 hours or longer. Instillation of the 0.25% solution more often than twice daily does not appear to enhance the reduction in IOP.[66]

The advantage of echothiophate is its long duration of action, requiring fewer installations and better control of

IOP on a daily basis. Glaucoma in some patients may be managed using 1 drop instilled every other day. The intense miosis can produce a pupillary block and resultant shallowing of the anterior chamber of the eye. Therefore, in the presence of subacute narrow angles or angle-closure glaucoma, echothiophate should not be used. In addition, initial tonometric monitoring to ensure that increased IOP does occur after administration has been suggested.[67] Aqueous solutions of echothiophate are unstable and must be prepared just before dispensing. The patient should be advised to refrigerate the prepared solution and discard it after 6 months. Echothiophate should be reserved for use in chronic open-angle glaucoma when the shorter-acting miotics or β-blockers have not successfully reduced IOP.

The side effect profiles of the parasympathetic miotic agents differ based upon pharmacologic activity. A direct- and short-acting miotic such as pilocarpine can produce local conjunctival irritation as a result of frequent instillations. Allergic sensitivity or refractoriness to pilocarpine develops after prolonged use. Frequent instillation of the short-acting miotics can exacerbate chronic allergic conjunctivitis or blepharitis.

Miotics can produce additional annoying side effects such as transient headaches, ocular and periorbital pain, twitching of the eyelids, ciliary congestion, and spasms.[68] The long-acting agent echothiophate produces the most severe symptoms, including discomfort associated with bright lights and close-up work. The affected eye is extremely myopic. This is particularly intense in younger patients who have active accommodation and are initially myopic. Patients should be reassured that these difficulties usually diminish within a week. After intense and prolonged administration of the stronger miotics, pupillary cysts can occur.[69] These are seen more commonly in children, but the reason is not known.

Anticholinesterase miotics may also produce vitreous hemorrhaging, contact dermatitis, and allergic conjunctivitis. Retinal detachment and cataracts have been associated with the use of anticholinesterase miotics; however, their role is probably as a contributing factor secondary to underlying retinal pathologic changes.

Systemic absorption of antiglaucoma drugs after ocular instillation may result in undesirable effects.[70,71] These are seen more commonly after administration of the indirect- and longer-acting anticholinesterase agents. Gastrointestinal disturbances such as nausea, diarrhea, and abdominal pain, as well as muscle spasm and weakness, sweating, lacrimation, salivation, hypotension, bradycardia, bronchial constriction, and respiratory failure have been experienced.[65,70] Most systemic effects reverse rapidly after discontinuation of the drug. For severe cholinergic toxicity, atropine sulfate 2 mg or pralidoxime chloride 25 mg/kg intravenously or subcutaneously can be given without affecting control of the glaucoma.

Any potent long-acting miotic agent should be used with caution when a patient has asthma, Parkinsonism, peptic ulcer disease, or other gastrointestinal disease because anticholinesterase systemic effects can exacerbate the clinical course of these conditions.

When known sensitivities to these agents exist, they should not be used. Considerable inhibition of plasma cholinesterase can be produced by prolonged topical anticholinesterase therapy.[72] A patient receiving these agents must be monitored closely for prolongation of apnea when given succinylcholine chloride during surgery.[72]

Patients who may be exposed to organophosphate pesticides, such as professional gardeners, farmers, or workers in industries that produce these chemicals, should be made aware of the potential problems and risks associated with prolonged topical anticholinesterase exposure.[67] There is an additive and cumulative effect on the parasympathetic nervous system. Systemically administered cholinergic agents such as ambenomium, neostigmine, or physostigmine used in disorders such as myasthenia gravis can potentiate the action of the anticholinesterase miotics.

Glaucoma secondary to ocular inflammation may be exacerbated by these agents owing to further vascular disruption. Lens opacities have been reported in patients treated with anticholinesterase miotics. Cataractogenic lens changes appear to be related to the drug, the concentration the patient is receiving, and the duration of treatment. Cataract formation does not appear to be directly associated with glaucomatous eyes; patients treated with miotics other than the anticholinesterase miotics are less likely to develop lens opacity. The lens changes may be partly reversible when the drug is discontinued. Progressive worsening of the cataract may occur, however, necessitating surgical extraction.

Miosis itself can produce decreased night vision.[68] Poor vision in dim light and blurring of vision from pupillary constriction and accommodative myopia are particularly troublesome for some patients. It is likely that the elderly patient already has diminished visual acuity and therefore should be made aware of the effect of the drug. This problem can be further complicated in aged patients who have cataracts in addition to impairment of vision.

Undesirable side effects from these agents can be minimized by proper instillation of their lowest effective concentrations at reasonable intervals. Patients should be instructed to either tightly close their eyes or occlude the nasolacrimal duct by pressing on the area between the inside corner of the eye and nose for approximately 5 minutes after administration (see also "Patient Education").

Sympathomimetics

Reduction of IOP in open-angle glaucoma may be accomplished successfully by ocular instillation of sympathomimetics. These agents act as agonists at either or both α- and β-adrenergic receptor sites. Catecholamines, including epinephrine, norepinephrine, and dopamine, may act at many levels of aqueous humor production and elimination. Sympathomimetic medications have a complex role in decreasing IOP; their mechanism of action includes both decreased production and increased outflow of aqueous humor.[73]

Epinephrine, 1 to 2% solution instilled every 8 to 24 hours, can reduce IOP in open-angle glaucoma.[74] The rate of aqueous secretion is initially decreased, probably by adrenergic stimulation at receptor sites in the ciliary epithelium. Improved facility of outflow is not immediate but may be seen after several months of epinephrine therapy. The probable mechanism suggested is α-adrenergic response to epinephrine at the trabecular meshwork. The pressure-lowering effect of epinephrine (3 to 15 mm Hg) occurs in 6 to 8 hours and lasts from several hours to days. Patient response appears to be highly variable. Epinephrine is seldom used alone for open-angle glaucoma but is usually used with miotics.[75,76] Epinephrine does not disturb accommodation and is especially beneficial in overcoming the disabling miosis induced by the parasympathomimetics. When used in combination, it should be given 5 to 10 minutes after the miotic has been instilled. Comparative effects of epinephrine bitartrate 2% and epinephrine borate 1% have been studied; no statistical difference in ability to reduce IOP in glaucomatous eyes can be found between individual preparations.[43] The commercial borate salt is buffered to enhance corneal penetration and is perhaps better tolerated than the others.

Dipivefrin, a prodrug of epinephrine, is produced by the addition of two pivalyl side chains to epinephrine. Dipivefrin has better lipid solubility than epinephrine, and thus corneal penetration is better (approximately 17 times better). Studies have shown no significant difference in 0.1% dipivefrin (when compared with 2% epinephrine) in lowering IOP. Kass et al.[75] and Kohn et al[76] compared 0.1% dipivefrin with 2% epinephrine for their effect on lowering IOP and increasing pupil size and the frequency of side effects. Both studies found that these agents lowered IOP significantly. Although dipivefrin was less effective in lowering IOP than epinephrine, fewer systemic side effects were reported in patients receiving dipivefrin.[76] Dipivefrin has caused similar ocular side effects, however.

Dipivefrin is available in a patented dosage form, the C-cap Compliance Cap B.I.D.[77] The dropper top is designed to display the number of doses the patient has taken in an effort to improve medication compliance.

Apraclonidine was the first commercially available selective α_2 receptor agonist. It is structurally similar to the antihypertensive agent clonidine; the addition of an amide group causes apraclonidine to be a more polar molecule. At first it was used only as an adjunctive agent during or immediately after surgical procedures.[73] Recent studies have shown when used in this manner, apraclonidine is effective after procedures such as cataract removal[78,79] and argon laser trabeculoplasty.[80]

Apraclonidine may also be used for long-term control of IOP. When given at 0.5% three times a day, it has been shown to decrease IOP by approximately 3 to 5 mm Hg.[81] Apraclonidine may also be added to other therapy.[82,83] In a randomized trial to determine whether apraclonidine 0.5% or 1% added to timolol 0.5% produced additional benefit, an additional 2.5 to 3.3 mm Hg (10.3 to 13.6%) reduction was apparent at 8 AM, indicating improved control during sleeping hours. At 3 hours after apraclonidine administration, an additional reduction of 4.7 to 5.2 mm Hg (20.0 to 21.7%) was produced.[82] There was no significant difference between those patients receiving 0.5% or 1% apraclonidine.

A separate study examined the addition of apraclonidine 0.5% or placebo instilled three times daily in patients with inadequate IOP control despite receiving maximal medication therapy. A total of 174 patients who were scheduled to undergo surgery continued their current regimen and also were given apraclonidine (86 patients) or placebo (88 patients). More patients receiving apraclonidine than placebo were able to maintain adequate IOP and avoid surgery (60 and 32%, respectively [$p < 0.01$]).

Apraclonidine's side effect profile limits its use as an initial agent for the treatment of glaucoma.[73] Frequently it causes follicular conjunctivitis. It may also cause dry nose and mouth. Because of ocular and nonocular side effects, 21 to 25% of patients in the trial by Stewart et al.[82] discontinued therapy.

Apraclonidine is metabolized by the liver to an active metabolite and its systemic effects may be increased in those patients with either liver or kidney damage. Although apraclonidine is thought to cause minimal cardiovascular effects in normal persons, the manufacturer recommends close cardiovascular monitoring in patients with decreased liver or kidney function.[84]

Brimonidine is a selective α_2 receptor agonist approved for use in the United States in October 1996. Brimonidine is available as a 0.2% solution and its usual dose is 1 drop three times daily.

In separate trials,[85–87] brimonidine 0.2% given twice daily has been compared to timolol 0.5% twice daily. In the first study, 186 patients were randomly assigned to receive brimonidine and 188 patients received timolol for 1 year. Both agents significantly lowered IOP compared to baseline (6.5 mm Hg for brimonidine versus 6.1 mm Hg for timolol). The level of IOP lowering was significantly better for brimonidine only at week 2 and month 3; levels at all other evaluations throughout the 1-year period were not significantly different. The adverse effect profile for brimonidine was noteworthy for dry mouth (33% of patients versus 19.4% in the timolol group) and burning and stinging (28.1% versus 41.9%, respectively). Additionally, ocular allergy was reported in 9% of brimonidine patients.[87] The remaining two studies both found brimonidine to produce a greater peak effect but a lower mean decrease in IOP.[85,86] The adverse effect profiles for these studies were comparable to those observed in the trial by Schuman et al. Importantly, fewer than 3% of patients in either group in the study by Katz[85] withdrew owing to adverse effects.

In contrast to timolol, brimonidine did not cause significant decreases in heart rate. Brimonidine and apraclonidine are both contraindicated in combination with monoamine oxidase inhibitors because of a potential increase in their effects.

Appreciable local and systemic side effects are experienced by patients who use ocular sympathomimetics for long periods.[76] Local side effects include melanin deposits on the conjunctiva and cornea, hyperemia and corneal edema, and allergic blepharoconjunctivitis.[76] Headache, periorbital pain, and lacrimation with intermittent visual blurring and distortion are common complaints. Although the frequency is relatively low, cardiac irregularities and elevations of blood pressure after ocular administration of epinephrine have been reported.[88] Side effects, both local and systemic, are promptly relieved after the epinephrine is discontinued. Closer supervision and caution should be exercised for patients who are receiving anesthetics in preparation for surgery because the reported rate of systemic side effects of the ocular sympathomimetic is higher in such patients. Gonioscopic examinations are advised before the ocular instillation of a sympathomimetic mydriatic to rule out asymptomatic or subacute angle-closure glaucoma. Sympathomimetics are contraindicated in patients with angle-closure glaucoma before peripheral iridectomy. After iridectomy is performed, ocular epinephrine can be useful, especially if aqueous humor outflow is impaired. It should not be used if IOP can be adequately managed by miotics alone.

Carbonic Anhydrase Inhibitors

The lowering of IOP can be achieved by topical or systemic administration of carbonic anhydrase inhibitors.[89] Of the systemic carbonic anhydrase inhibitors, acetazolamide is the most widely used for the treatment of glaucoma. Systemic agents are indicated when patients fail to respond or cannot tolerate topical glaucoma therapy. The addition of the topical agents dorzolamide and brinzolamide has largely replaced the use of systemic agents owing to fewer side effects.[2]

Carbonic anhydrase catalyzes the reversible conversion of carbon dioxide to bicarbonate. In the eye, large concentrations of carbonic anhydrase are found in the ciliary process and retina. Bicarbonate flow into the posterior chamber is controlled by carbonic anhydrase and is decreased upon addition of carbonic anhydrase inhibitors. A result of bicarbonate decrease is a reduction in sodium and water movement into the posterior chamber.[2,90,91]

Topical Agents

The early use of systemic agents topically was not effective because of the high concentrations that were necessary and consequent pH that caused irritation. The introduction of dorzolamide and brinzolamide renewed interest in the use of carbonic anhydrase inhibitors as first-line therapy in selected patients.

Dorzolamide is available as a 2% solution (alone or in combination with timolol maleate) as is indicated for monotherapy or in combination with other agents. When administered three times a day, dorzolamide lowers IOP by 4 to 6 mm Hg at peak and 3 to 4.5 mm Hg at trough (8 hours post-dose). A study by Adamsons et al.[92] examined the use of dorzolamide 2% administered three times daily as monotherapy or add-on therapy with timolol and/or pilocarpine when necessary. Of 304 patients enrolled, 164 (53.9%) continued to receive dorzolamide as monotherapy after 2 years. The IOP-lowering effects of dorzolamide compared to combination therapy were 22.8 and 31 to 36%, respectively. Therapy was generally well tolerated; the most common adverse effects included burning or stinging of the eyes, conjunctivitis, follicular conjunctivitis, and eyelid edema.[92]

A separate study by Kimal Arici et al.[93] examined the addition of latanoprost to dorzolamide therapy. Two groups of 15 patients received either latanoprost (group 1) or dorzolamide (group 2) for 10 days, followed by combination therapy with both agents for an additional 10 days. Both groups had significant decreases in IOP at day 10 (30% decrease for group 1, 19.4% group 2). An additional 15% decrease in IOP was observed in group 1 patients when dorzolamide was added to therapy, and an additional 24.1% decrease in group 2. The authors concluded that these agents, when used together, were more effective in lowering IOP than either agent alone.

Brinzolamide is available as a 1% suspension and is typically administered three times daily. When brinzolamide was given either twice daily or three times daily and compared to dorzolamide 2% or timolol 0.5% over a 3-month period, Silver[48] demonstrated three of the four regimens to be equivalent, based upon mean IOP reductions (3.8 to 5.7 mm Hg with brinzolamide bid, 4.2 to 5.6 mm Hg with brinzolamide tid, 4.3 to 5.9 mm Hg with dorzolamide tid, and 5.2 to 6.3 mm Hg with timolol bid). Timolol 0.5% given twice daily was statistically superior to the other three regimens (p value not reported). Brinzolamide produced fewer complaints of stinging and burning than dorzolamide. Patients receiving brinzolamide should be reminded that the suspension must be shaken before administration to ensure proper dosing.

Systemic Agents

The systemic drug of choice is usually acetazolamide. Acetazolamide is available as 125- and 250-mg tablets and 500-mg sustained-release capsules. Intravenous acetazolamide may also be useful for rapidly reducing IOP. A single dose of oral acetazolamide can reduce IOP for 8 to 12 hours. The maximum effect is seen about 2 hours after oral administration. After intravenous administration, the maximum effect is attained within 15 minutes, and the duration of effect is approximately 4 to 5 hours.[89]

Acetazolamide can reduce aqueous inflow approximately 40 to 60% and IOP by 25 to 40%. Dichlorphenamide and methazolamide have similar effects and only differ by potency and side effect (Table 50.13). These agents are more likely to cause side effects leading to discontinuation of therapy and are rarely used.

Table 50.13 ▪ Carbonic Anhydrase Inhibitors Used to Manage Glaucoma

Drug and Dosage Form	Dose	Onset	Duration (hr)	Comment
Acetazolamide tablets 125 and 250 mg	125–250 mg qid	1/2–1 hr	4–6	
Acetazolamide sequels 500 mg	500 mg bid	1–2 hr	10–18	May be better tolerated than immediate-release formulation
Acetazolamide 500 mg vials	500 mg IV	1 min	4	Useful for rapid decrease in IOP
Methazolamide tablets 25 and 50 mg	25–50 mg bid titrated to 50-100 mg bid to tid	1 hr	10–14	50 mg is equivalent to 250 mg of acetazolamide; dose-response for adverse effects and amount of IOP reduction
Dichlorphenamide tablets 50 mg	25–50 mg bid, tid, or qd	1/2 hr	6–12	Metabolic acidosis occurs less frequently with dichlorphenamide than with other carbonic anhydrase inhibitors; used with patient intolerance or refractory to acetazolamide; anorexia nausea, paresthesias, dizziness, or ataxia and tremor should alert patients or clinicians to the possibility of toxicity
Dorzolamide 2% solution	1 drop affected eye(s) tid		8	
Brinzolamide 1% suspension	1 drop affected eye(s) tid		8	Suspension must be shaken before administration

IOP, intraocular pressure.

Source: Adapted from Flach AJ. Topical acetazolamide and other carbonic anhydrase inhibitors in the current medical therapy of the glaucomas. Glaucoma 8:20–27, 1986.

Unfortunately, 50% of patients are unable to tolerate systemic carbonic anhydrase therapy.[89,94] Acetazolamide sustained-release capsules are somewhat better tolerated than the immediate-release tablets, but approximately 40% of patients cannot tolerate acetazolamide in this dosage form. A study of compliance with acetazolamide therapy in 87 patients demonstrated that 56% of patients were either not taking medication (30 patients) or not taking medication as frequently as prescribed (19 patients).[95]

Older patients appear to be more intolerant to the carbonic anhydrase inhibitors than younger patients.[89,96] Patients who have sulfa allergies should not take systemic or topical carbonic anhydrase inhibitors because these agents contain a sulfonamide group. Fatalities have occurred, although rarely, as a result of severe reactions to sulfonamides including Stevens-Johnson syndrome, toxic epidermal necrolysis, fulminant hepatic necrosis, agranulocytosis, aplastic anemia, and other blood dyscrasias. A baseline complete blood count (CBC) should be performed. For patients continuing therapy, periodic monitoring should include CBCs and measurement of serum electrolytes.

The most common side effects of the systemic carbonic anhydrase inhibitors include malaise, fatigue, weight loss, depression, and anorexia. Additional side effects, such as nausea, vomiting, intestinal colic, diarrhea, and paresthesia of the face and extremities may also appear. Transient myopia is an unusual and rare occurrence.

Acetazolamide produces hyperglycemia in prediabetic and diabetic patients receiving oral hypoglycemic agents. Hyperuricemia has occurred after treatment with carbonic anhydrase inhibitors. Prolonged use of these drugs can lead to urinary and renal colic secondary to formation of calcium calculi.[97,98] Alkalinization of the urine by acetazolamide results in an enhanced renal tubular reabsorption of drugs such as quinidine, amphetamine, and tricyclic antidepressants. Alkalinization of the urine can also decrease the acid-dependent antibacterial activity of methenamine. Carbonic anhydrase inhibitors are not recommended in patients with hemorrhagic glaucoma, hepatic or renal dysfunction, or renocortical hypofunction or a history of prior sensitivities to the drug.

The use of carbonic anhydrase inhibitors in chronic angle-closure glaucoma should be discouraged because symptoms of progressive angle narrowing can easily be obscured.

Prostaglandin Analogs

Prostaglandins are produced in the body by the action of the enzyme cyclooxygenase on arachidonic acid. The use of nonsteroidal anti-inflammatory agents (NSAIDs) blocks this activity, reducing the many known effects of prostaglandins throughout the body. Prostaglandins are known to cause increased IOP and inflammation when injected into animal models. Initial studies demonstrated that high doses of prostaglandins increased IOP.[99] However, some animal models react differently from humans, and when given to human subjects in low concentrations, prostaglandin $F_{2\alpha}$ ($PGF_{2\alpha}$) effectively lowers IOP. The mechanism is thought to be via increased uveoscleral outflow of aqueous humor.[2,99] Latanoprost is the only prostaglandin analog currently clinically available.

Latanoprost is a 17-phenyl substituted $PGF_{2\alpha}$ available as a 0.005% solution. It was approved by the U.S. FDA in August 1996 for the reduction of elevated IOP in patients with open-angle glaucoma and ocular hypertension who are either insufficiently responsive to or intolerant of other IOP-lowering medications.[100]

Latanoprost is a prodrug and must be hydrolyzed to its active acid form in the cornea. After topical administration, peak levels in the cornea appear after approximately 2 hours. Latanoprost is metabolized in the liver via fatty acid β-oxidation. Due to rapid elimination, levels of latanoprost and its metabolites (1,2-dinor and 1,2,3,4-tetranor) are detectable in the plasma for only 1 hour.

After hepatic β-oxidation, the metabolites are mainly eliminated via the kidneys. Approximately 88% of the topical dose is recovered in the urine.

Safety and efficacy studies have demonstrated that latanoprost may decrease IOP as much as 25 to 35%.[101] In three multicenter trials in the United States, Scandinavia, and the United Kingdom, latanoprost 0.005% given once daily significantly lowered IOP at least as much, and in some cases,[102] more than timolol 0.5% given twice daily. One-year analyses in a subgroup of 198 patients showed that a decrease in IOP of 32% regardless of age, sex, race, or eye color was maintained.

Additionally, latanoprost may be used in combination with other agents. In separate studies, a further reduction in IOP of 2.5 to 9 mm Hg (15 to 35%) was seen with latanoprost added to timolol 0.5% given twice daily.[99] It is important to note that the mechanisms of action of latanoprost and miotic agents are antagonistic. Therefore, patients should not receive these agents together, and any miotic agent should be discontinued before adding latanoprost.

Latanoprost has been well tolerated in the majority of trials. The most common adverse effects have been local ocular effects such as blurred vision, burning and stinging, conjunctival hyperemia, foreign body sensation, itching, increased pigmentation of the iris, and punctate epithelial keratopathy (all in 5 to 15% of patients during clinical trials).[100]

Latanoprost has a unique adverse effect of darkening the iris by increasing the number of melanosomes (pigment granules) in melanocytes in about 7% of patients. Additionally, some patients may experience lengthened or darkened eyelashes. Patients who only treat a single eye may notice increased pigmentation in the treated eye and therefore experience heterochromia.[100] This effect may be permanent.

In summary, excellent clinical efficacy has been seen with latanoprost 0.0005% given as 1 drop daily in the evening. To ensure maximal benefit and minimize adverse effects, it is important to discuss the possible effects on pigmentation with patients. In addition, patients should be aware that latanoprost has been shown to be less effective if amounts greater than 1 drop per eye given daily are used. Latanoprost should be used with caution in patients with liver or kidney dysfunction.

Hyperosmotic Agents

Hyperosmotic agents lower the IOP by creating an osmotic gradient between the plasma and aqueous humor from the anterior chamber of the eye (Table 50.14). Given systemically, these agents draw fluids from the anterior chamber of the eye into the plasma. Hyperosmotic agents are most useful in the preoperative management of

Table 50.14 ▪ Hyperosmotic Agents Used in the Management of Glaucomas

Drug	Dosage (g/kg)	Route	Comments
Ascorbic acid	0.4–1.0	IV/oral	Gastric distress and diarrhea with oral administration; seldom used because more effective agents are available
Glycerin (50% solution)	1.0–1.5	Oral	Nausea, vomiting, hyperglycemia can occur; caution in diabetic patients; as effective as produced
Isosorbide	1–2	Oral	Can be given to diabetic patients; tension comparable to those of intravenous hyperosmotics; diarrhea frequently experienced
Mannitol (20% solution)	1.0–2.0	IV	Requires larger volumes than other hyperosmotics; used in diabetic patients; less irritating and free of tissue necrosis when solution extravasates; not contraindicated in patients with renal disease; monitor for cellular dehydration, hypokalemia, cardiac irregularities, urinary output, and chest pain; more effective for glaucoma with inflammation than urea or glycerol; avoid excessive use
Urea (30% solution)	1.0–1.5	IV	Given IV over 30 min; unstable; side effects are sloughing, phlebitis, headaches, nausea, vomiting hemolysis "rebound diuresis"; contraindicated in nephrotic patients; caution in hepatic impairment; use freshly made solution only; maximal effect 1 hr

primary acute angle-closure glaucoma. The degree of IOP lowering depends on the tension elevation and the osmotic gradient induced. The greatest effect of rapid changes in plasma osmolarity is on the eye, with very profound pressure elevations. The most commonly used hyperosmotics are mannitol, urea, and glycerol.

Mannitol can effectively reduce acutely elevated IOPs when given slowly by the intravenous route as a 20% solution to adults and a 10% solution to children.[101,102] The ocular hypotensive effect is produced in 30 to 60 minutes and lasts from 4 to 6 hours. The effectiveness of the hyperosmotic agents depends on the rate of administration. Mannitol is preferred in the management of secondary glaucoma accompanied by hyperemia or uveitis because it penetrates the eye less readily, which is an advantage when inflammatory processes are active. Agents that enter the eye rapidly produce a lower osmotic gradient and a shorter duration of action than those that do so slowly or not at all. Inflammation greatly increases the ocular permeability of agents such as urea. Therefore, it is less desirable under those circumstances. There is relatively less local tissue irritation, thrombophlebitis, and necrosis occurring with mannitol than with urea when given intravenously. Renal disease does not contraindicate the use of mannitol.

Excessive thirst is a common sensation experienced by patients after infusion of hyperosmotic agents. However, these patients should not be given fluids during the period of osmotic dehydration. Secondary rises in IOP occur after administration of fluids, diminishing the therapeutic effects of the hyperosmotics. Headache is also a common complaint, but it can be minimized simply by bed rest. Symptoms of cellular dehydration, hypokalemia, and cardiac irregularities secondary to mannitol therapy should be monitored. On rare occasions, disorientation and severe agitation may be observed. Pulmonary edema and congestive heart failure may be precipitated in the elderly, especially with mannitol infusions. Potassium deficiency can accompany diuresis after hyperosmotic infusion, and patients with hepatic, renal, or cardiac disorders should be cautiously monitored. Mannitol is not absorbed and is ineffective when given orally.

Urea given by the intravenous route as a 30% solution reduces elevated IOP within 30 to 40 minutes. Miotics and carbonic anhydrase inhibitors are used concomitantly with urea in the management of acute glaucoma before surgery. Nausea, vomiting, confusion, disorientation, and anxiety may be seen. Severe headache, a common complaint, can begin soon after the initiation and continue for the duration of the intravenous infusion. The patient's head should not be elevated during this time.

Although urea produces less cellular dehydration because of its ease of penetrability into the cell, a "rebound phenomenon" can occur as the plasma level of the hyperosmotic agent drops below that of the vitreous fluid. As the urea is cleared from the circulation rapidly with diuresis, the osmolality of the blood declines. The hyperosmotic vitreous in turn draws fluid into the eye, resulting in increased IOP or pressure "rebound" effect.[103]

Ascorbic acid successfully reduces IOP in rabbits with glaucoma. For refractoriness to acetazolamide and miotics, ascorbic acid given intravenously can lower the ocular hypertension. A 20% solution of sodium ascorbate at a pH of 7.2 to 7.4 can produce normal ocular tension in 60 to 90 minutes.

Oral hyperosmotic agents effectively reduce elevated IOP and are useful where the rapid-action infused preparations are not required. Glycerol is a convenient hyperosmotic agent when given as a 50 or 75% solution.[104] The ocular penetration of glycerol is poor; therefore, a substantial osmotic gradient can be produced between the plasma and aqueous humor. IOP reduction is as effective as with hyperosmotic agents given by intravenous infusion. IOP normally returns to pretreatment levels within 5 to 6 hours. Hyperglycemia and glycosuria can occur after glycerol, and it should be used with particular caution in patients with labile diabetes.[104] Acute diabetic ketoacidosis has been reported after treatment with glycerol. Nausea, diarrhea, and headache are also common complaints after oral glycerol.

The reduction of IOP with isosorbide is comparable to that with intravenous mannitol, urea, or oral glycerol. Given as a 50% solution orally, its absorption is rapid, and it is primarily unchanged on excretion in the urine. Effective reduction in IOP occurs within 30 minutes after ingestion and remains for 1 to 2 hours or more depending on the dose. Side effects include transient headaches and diarrhea. Other gastrointestinal disturbances such as nausea are usually less of a problem with isosorbide than with glycerol.[105]

Nonpharmacologic Therapy

Surgery

Surgical management of open-angle glaucoma should be reserved for patients in whom single-drug and combination therapy has not been tolerated or maximal efforts have been unsuccessful in maintaining an acceptable level of IOP and preventing progressive changes of the optic disk or the visual field. The surgical procedure, peripheral iridectomy, involves creating a collateral drainage from the anterior chamber.

Laser Therapy

Laser trabeculoplasty, an alternative to peripheral iridectomy, is the most often used nonpharmacologic treatment for chronic open-angle glaucoma. Laser iridotomy, in most cases, is recommended rather than traditional surgery for angle-closure glaucoma. Remis et al.[106] reported that laser surgery can reduce the IOP by 7 to 13 mm Hg in more than 80% of patients.

Argon Laser Trabeculoplasty

Using the argon laser coupled to a high-magnification biomicroscope, the surgeon places approximately 50 to

100 lesions in an evenly spaced sequence on the inner surface of the trabecular meshwork. Histopathologic studies by scanning electron microscopy have shown that laser light energy produces fibrosis at the treatment site. It is theorized that these laser "burns" cause localized shrinkage, which in turn produces tension on the adjacent, untreated trabecular beams. The previously collapsed spaces between the beams are then pulled open, allowing aqueous humor to pass more easily and resulting in a reduction in IOP.

At least 1 hour before argon laser trabeculoplasty (ALT), apraclonidine hydrochloride 1% is instilled into the operated eye for control of IOP. Apraclonidine is used in conjunction with trabeculoplasty to prevent an acute elevation in IOP, which can occur after ALT. Its onset of action is seen within 1 hour of instillation, and its maximal effect is seen within 3 to 5 hours. It is used 1 hour before ALT, and a second drop is instilled immediately after completion of the laser surgical procedure.[107,108] Apraclonidine hydrochloride has replaced pilocarpine as the agent of choice before ALT. A topical anesthetic is instilled before the procedure, and then the patient is seated at the slit-lamp laser photocoagulator.

Laser Iridotomy

Laser iridotomy is the treatment of choice for pupillary block or angle-closure glaucoma. In most cases, laser surgery is recommended rather than traditional surgery and is performed on an outpatient basis. One hour before laser iridotomy surgery, topical apraclonidine hydrochloride 1% is instilled in the eye, along with pilocarpine drops. The pilocarpine causes pupillary constriction, which thins the iris, making laser puncture much easier. At the time of laser surgery, a topical anesthetic is instilled. An opening measuring approximately 50 to 100 μ in diameter is created in the peripheral iris that releases the pupillary block component of angle-closure glaucoma (F. Reid, personal communication, 1991).

Complications of laser treatment of glaucoma include intraocular inflammation in the form of uveitis, intraocular bleeding, elevated IOP, diplopia, pigment dissemination, and lens injury (F. Reid, personal communication, 1991).

Recently, a study demonstrated that black and white patients may respond differently to surgical procedures.[109] In this study, patients received either ALT followed by trabeculectomy and a second trabeculectomy, if needed (group 1, ATT) or trabeculectomy, ALT, and a second trabeculectomy, if needed (group 2, TAT).

The two groups were followed for 7 years. Visual loss was assessed at the end of the study. The results of the study showed that 35 and 28% of black patients assigned to groups 1 and 2, respectively, had a reduced rate of visual field loss. In contrast, 31 and 35% of white patients assigned to groups 1 and 2, respectively, had reduced visual field loss after 7 years. Some of the results varied, depending upon the length of follow-up. Overall, the authors concluded that all black patients should receive surgical procedures in the sequence of group 1 (ATT) and white patients without life-threatening health problems should receive surgical procedures in the order of group 2 (TAT). Additional studies may help clarify reasons why this difference occurred.

ALTERNATIVE THERAPIES

The one alternative therapy that has received widespread attention is the use of marijuana to lower IOP. Historically, accounts of the use of marijuana to decrease IOP appear as early as 1971.[110] The National Institutes of Health in the United States sponsored studies from 1978 through 1984 that demonstrated decreased IOP when marijuana was inhaled or taken orally or intravenously. Unfortunately, topical administration was not shown to be effective, and serious adverse effects were present in doses that were useful clinically. These included increased heart rate, decreased blood pressure, and dry eyes.[111]

Although there are limitations to the clinical utility of marijuana for the treatment of glaucoma, research based upon the active chemical component or components of marijuana (including tetrahydrocannabinol) may be valuable. Many unanswered questions remain regarding the safe and effective use of marijuana for glaucoma. The Institute of Medicine,[111] American Academy of Ophthalmology,[112] and the National Eye Institute of the National Institutes of Health[113] all support continued research into the safety and effectiveness of various delivery systems for the use of marijuana in glaucoma.

FUTURE THERAPIES

There are currently at least 21 different agents being tested in various clinical stages of development for the treatment of glaucoma.[114] Included are β-blocking agents (adaprolol), N-methyl-D-aspartate antagonists (dexanabinol), NSAIDs (diclofenac), prostaglandin analogs (unoprostone), and neuroprotective agents (memantine). Additionally, improved delivery systems using submicron emulsions or other extended-release systems are being examined. Finally, agents that act via their effect on the ocular vasculature such as verapamil are being investigated as potential therapies to prevent the neuronal damage of glaucoma. It is hoped that these agents will lead to an ideal agent with improved safety, efficacy, and ease of administration that will lead to improved clinical outcomes.

IMPROVING OUTCOMES

The successful outcome of glaucoma treatment depends greatly on the patient's proper use of medications. Methods to improve the use of medication can include patient education and determination of patient compliance with therapy.

Patient Education

An asymptomatic patient who does not understand why expensive and inconvenient eyedrops are required will be less inclined to use them according to prescribed instructions. The blurring of vision and occasional discomfort or other adverse effects associated with the use of these medications further enhance noncompliance. The patient with glaucoma should understand the nature of the disorder and appropriate expectations for the drugs being used to control it.

Patients should be instructed on the proper technique for administering eyedrops. This includes several steps such as handwashing, checking the solution for any discoloration and the expiration date, shaking vials if the medication is in suspension, not touching the dropper tip to the skin, tilting back the head, pulling down the lower lid, and administering the correct number of drops. It is important to stress (1) that the patient either close the eye or place an index finger over the tear duct for 3 to 5 minutes (termed nasolacrimal occlusion) to minimize the amount of medication that reaches the systemic circulation, and (2) that drops of differing types of medication be spread apart by at least 10 minutes. Ideally, the health care provider can also observe the patient after instruction to verify the patient's understanding and manual dexterity.

Some authors[2] recommend educating patients to take their medications based upon the colors of the vial lid. This practice could potentially lead to medication errors if vial lids are accidentally interchanged or if the patient has other medications that appear similar. Pharmacists should remind patients to always check the instructions on the prescription label. If a patient cannot read the label because of loss of eyesight or if the patient is not literate, large print instructions, the use of other caregivers, or other methods such as nontextual pictograms can help ensure proper medication technique.

Methods to Improve Patient Adherence to Drug Therapy

Optimal therapeutic results can occur only in an environment of mutual cooperation and understanding between patients and the health care providers responsible for their care. Physicians should assess compliance whenever IOP appears to be uncontrolled before suggesting increases in medication strength or other changes in therapy.

Methods to improve medication compliance in patients with glaucoma should be attempted and can include education about the importance of disease screening and progression of disease, direct observation of administration technique, and modification to therapeutic plans to simplify medication regimens or overcome adverse effects, when necessary.

Pharmacists are in a unique position to help clinicians monitor for compliance. If patients who are typically noncompliant take their medication before office visits, their IOP may appear normal. A laboratory value that measures long-term IOP control is not available. Pharmacists, however, can monitor refill activity of patients receiving medications at one site. In addition, managed health plans having prescription drug claims for payment purposes may also be able to monitor for patients who do not receive refills within a certain time period. Those patients may be targeted for educational interventions and resulting changes in their use of refills.

Disease Management Strategies to Improve Patient Outcomes

The strategies to improve compliance with therapy already discussed should be expected to improve IOP control, and ultimately, patient outcomes.

PHARMACOECONOMICS

Relatively few economic studies have been performed regarding the different agents available for the treatment of glaucoma. Part of this is due to the difficulty in assigning an appropriate short-term outcome that reliably and accurately results in improved outcomes. The use of IOP as an endpoint may not be appropriate in all patients, as there is no standard IOP target. Therefore, some patients only require a decrease of 3 to 5 mm Hg while others require a much greater effect. A cost-effectiveness analysis that examines a cost per mm Hg lowering effect may therefore be misleading. Because of differing side effect profiles of the various classes of medication, a cost minimization analysis, which assumes equal outcomes, often is inappropriate. Finally, because of the chronic nature of glaucoma, cost utility analyses that examine blindness as an outcome will take many years to complete and may not be feasible.

Despite these problems, some rather extensive economic evaluations have recently been completed.[115,116]

A study by Stewart et al.[115] examined daily cost of therapy with the six commercially available β-blockers. For the purposes of the study, the authors assumed equal efficacy and safety among the available agents.

The protocol used 10 subjects to administer, per their normal techniques, 1 drop from each of 10 differing β-blocker preparations (differing pharmaceutical formulations and generic equivalents, when available, of timolol, levobunolol, carteolol, betaxolol, and metipranolol). The authors then calculated drop size and total bottle volume to determine amounts that would be wasted or used by the patients. Sixty random pharmacies throughout the United States were then surveyed for the cost of the medications. Using these data, the authors found a daily range of costs (based only upon usable administered drops) of $0.55 to $1.35 (U.S.). Interestingly, the amount wasted, as calculated from drop size, ranged from 27 to 54% of the stated dropper volume. This study was the first to highlight the importance of drop size using volunteers to administer medication as well as to examine the use of generic equivalent medications. Unfortunately, the assumption of equal efficacy and safety may not be valid for all patients.

A cost-utility analysis comparing dorzolamide and pilocarpine was completed by Rocchi and Tingey.[116] The authors assumed a governmental payor perspective (Canadian Provincial Ministry of Health) and assessed costs and consequences of the alternatives over a 10-year period. A decision-analysis model, using published as well as expert panel estimates of the cost and probabilities of outcomes, was completed. Quality adjusted life years (QALYs) were calculated for adverse outcomes and an incremental cost/QALY was calculated for the two alternatives. The results of the model demonstrated that patients receiving dorzolamide had higher costs and higher QALYs. The incremental cost/QALY for a patient receiving dorzolamide was $9,390 (CAN) more than that for pilocarpine. The authors noted that a cost/QALY less than $20,000 (CAN) is usually considered worthwhile dollars spent in health care. Sensitivity analysis changing the adverse event rate and cost of medication did not change the overall calculated cost/QALY threshhold of $20,000. The authors concluded that dorzolamide should be reimbursed by provincial formularies, based upon these results.

More economic studies of this type should help providers initiate medical therapy for glaucoma as efficiently as possible in appropriate patients and groups of patients.

KEY POINTS

- Increased IOP is the most important risk factor for progression of glaucomatous damage to the optic nerve.
- Glaucoma is typically classified as open-angle (most common) or angle-closure glaucoma. Treatment strategies differ by glaucoma type.
- Immediate medical attention is required to reduce IOP in patients with acute angle closure glaucoma.
- Pharmacists should evaluate a patient's complete medical regimen to avoid medical therapy, which may worsen the patient's glaucoma.
- A target IOP is established based upon the patient's current IOP and risk factors for progression of end-organ damage with the goal to prevent initial or worsening ocular damage.
- Reduction of IOP should be attempted using topical medications with low systemic effects. Typically, β-blocking agents are the agents first chosen, unless otherwise contraindicated.
- Other medication classes, such as miotics, sympathomimetics, carbonic anhydrase inhibitors, and prostaglandin analogs have all been used to decrease IOP. Each medication class has unique properties and side effect profiles that should be considered before initiating therapy.
- The patient should only use combination therapy after monotherapy proves unsuccessful or is not tolerated.
- One of the most important factors in successful glaucoma therapy is compliance with medical regimens. Health care providers should educate the patient in the proper administration technique to reduce systemic adverse effects and to improve compliance.
- Health care providers should monitor for effectiveness and adverse events.
- Surgical correction should be attempted only if medical therapy is not tolerated or is unsuccessful in maintaining the target IOP.

REFERENCES

1. Shields MB, Ritch R, Krupin T. Classifications of the glaucomas. In: Ritch R, Sheilds MB, Krupin T, eds. The glaucomas: clinical science. 2nd ed. St. Louis: Mosby, 1996:717–725.
2. Alward WL. Medical management of glaucoma. N Engl J Med 339:1298–307, 1998.
3. Comparison of glaucomatous progression between untreated patients with normal-tension glaucoma and patients with therapeutically reduced intraocular pressures. Collaborative Normal-Tension Glaucoma Study Group. Am J Ophthalmol 126:487–497, 1998.
4. The effectiveness of intraocular pressure reduction in the treatment of normal-tension glaucoma. Collaborative Normal-Tension Glaucoma Study Group. Am J Ophthalmol 126:498–505, 1998.
5. The Glaucoma Foundation. Available at: http://www.glaucoma-foundation.org. Accessed March 21, 1999.
6. Screening for glaucoma. In: DiGuiseppi C, Atkins D, Woolf SH, et al. Guide to clinical preventive services (CPS). 2nd ed. Alexandria, VA: National Library of Medicine, 1996.
7. Chandler PA, Grant WM, Epstein DL, et al. Chandler and Grant's glaucoma. 4th ed. Baltimore: Williams & Wilkins, 1997.
8. Hattenhauer MG, Johnson DH, Ing HH, et al. The probability of blindness from open-angle glaucoma. Ophthalmology 105:2099–2104, 1998.
9. Danyluk AW, Paton D. Diagnosis and management of glaucoma. Clin Symp 43:2–32, 1991.
10. Vaughan D, Asbury T, Riordan-Eva P, et al. General ophthalmology. 13th ed. Norwalk, CT: Appleton & Lange, 1992.
11. Wolfs RC, Klaver CC, Ramrattan RS, et al. Genetic risk of primary open-angle glaucoma. Population-based familial aggregation study. Arch Ophthalmol 116:1640–1645, 1998.
12. Alward WL, Fingert JH, Coote MA, et al. Clinical features associated with mutations in the chromosome 1 open-angle glaucoma gene (GLC1A) [see comments]. N Engl J Med 338:1022–1027, 1998.
13. Epstein DL. Practical aqueous humor dynamics. In: Chandler PA, Grant WM, Epstein DL, et al., eds. Chandler and Grant's glaucoma. 4th ed. Baltimore: Williams & Wilkins, 1997:670.
14. Doctor, I have a question: about glaucoma. Available at: http://www.glaucoma-foundation.org/dihaq. Accessed March 21, 1999.
15. Newell FW. Ophthalmology: principles and concepts. 8th ed. St. Louis: Mosby, 1996.
16. Grant WM. Ocular complications of drugs. Glaucoma. JAMA 207:2089–2091, 1969.
17. Harris LS. Cycloplegic-induced intraocular pressure elevations: a study of normal and open-angle glaucomatous eyes. Arch Ophthalmol 79:242–246, 1968.
18. Mehra KS, Chandra P, Khare BB. Ocular manifestations of parenteral administration of scopolamine (hyoscine). Br J Ophthalmol 49:557–558, 1965.
19. Lazenby GW, Reed JW, Grant WM. Anticholinergic medication in open-angle glaucoma. Long-term tests. Arch Ophthalmol 84:719–723, 1970.
20. Mulberger RD. Effect of a common cold product containing belladonna on intraocular pressure. Eye Ear Nose Throat Mon 47:61–64, 1968.
21. Fraunfelder FT, Meyer SM. Drug-induced ocular side effects and drug interactions. 2nd ed. Philadelphia: Lea & Febiger, 1982.
22. Smith CL. "Corticosteroid glaucoma": a summary and review of the literature. Am J Med Sci 252:239–244, 1966.
23. Pappa K. Corticosteroid drugs. In: Munger T, Craig E, eds. Havener's ocular pharmacology. 6th ed. St. Louis: Mosby, 1994:364–428.

24. Eke T, Bates AK. Acute angle closure glaucoma associated with paroxetine. Br Med J 314:1387, 1997.
25. Kirwan JF, Subak-Sharpe I, Teimory M. Bilateral acute angle closure glaucoma after administration of paroxetine. Br J Ophthalmol 81:252, 1997.
26. Lewis CF, DeQuardo JR, DuBose C, et al. Acute angle-closure glaucoma and paroxetine. J Clin Psychiatry 58:123–124, 1997.
27. Ahmad S. Fluoxetine and glaucoma [letter]. DICP 25:436, 1991.
28. Hiatt RL, Fuller IB, Smith L, et al. Systemically administered anticholinergic drugs and intraocular pressure. Arch Ophthalmol 84:735–740, 1970.
29. Levy R. Improving compliance with prescription medications: an important strategy for containing health-care costs. Med Interface Mar:34–41, 1989.
30. Gurwitz JH, Glynn RJ, Monane M, et al. Treatment for glaucoma: adherence by the elderly. Am J Public Health 83:711–716, 1993.
31. Gurwitz J, Yeomans S, Glynn R, et al. Patient noncompliance in the managed care setting: the case of medical therapy for glaucoma. Med Care 36:357–369, 1998.
32. Zimmerman TJ. Topical ophthalmic β blockers: a comparative review. J Ocul Pharmacol 9:373–384, 1993.
33. Coakes RL, Brubaker RF. The mechanism of timolol in lowering intraocular pressure in the normal eye. Arch Ophthalmol 96:2045–2048, 1978.
34. Dailey RA, Brubaker RF, Bourne WM. The effects of timolol maleate and acetazolamide on the rate of aqueous formation in normal human subjects. Am J Ophthalmol 93:232–237, 1982.
35. Phillips CI, Howitt G, Rowlands DJ. Propranolol as ocular hypotensive agent. Br J Ophthalmol 51:222–226, 1967.
36. Boger WPD, Steinert RF, Puliafito CA, et al. Clinical trial comparing timolol ophthalmic solution to pilocarpine in open-angle glaucoma. Am J Ophthalmol 86:8–18, 1978.
37. Sorensen SJ, Abel SR. Comparison of the ocular β-blockers. Ann Pharmacother 30:43–54, 1996.
38. Timoptic in the management of chronic open-angle glaucoma. West Point, PA: Merck Sharp & Dohme, 1979.
39. Timolol maleate. In: Mosby's GenRx. 9th ed. 1999. Available at: http://www.mdconsult.com. Accessed March 15, 1999.
40. Kass MA. Efficacy of combining timolol with other antiglaucoma medications. Surv Ophthalmol 28(Suppl):274–279, 1983.
41. Korey MS, Hodapp E, Kass MA, et al. Timolol and epinephrine: long-term evaluation of concurrent administration. Arch Ophthalmol 100:742–745, 1982.
42. Keates EU, Stone RA. Safety and effectiveness of concomitant administration of dipivefrin and timolol maleate. Am J Ophthalmol 91:243–248, 1981.
43. Cyrlin MN, Thomas JV, Epstein DL. Additive effect of epinephrine to timolol therapy in primary open angle glaucoma. Arch Ophthalmol 100:414–418, 1982.
44. β blockers for glaucoma. Lancet 1:1064–1065, 1979.
45. Phillips CI, Bartholomew RS, Kazi G, et al. Penetration of timolol eye drops into human aqueous humour. Br J Ophthalmol 65:593–595, 1981.
46. LeBlanc RP, Krip G. Timolol. Canadian multicenter study. Ophthalmology 88:224–228, 1981.
47. Strohmaier K, Snyder E, DuBiner H, et al. The efficacy and safety of the dorzolamide-timolol combination versus the concomitant administration of its components. Dorzolamide-Timolol Study Group. Ophthalmology 105: 1936–1944, 1998.
48. Silver LH. Clinical efficacy and safety of brinzolamide (Azopt), a new topical carbonic anhydrase inhibitor for primary open-angle glaucoma and ocular hypertension. Brinzolamide Primary Therapy Study Group. Am J Ophthalmol 126:400–408, 1998.
49. Boyle JE, Ghosh K, Gieser DK, et al. A randomized trial comparing the dorzolamide-timolol combination given twice daily to monotherapy with timolol and dorzolamide. Dorzolamide-Timolol Study Group. Ophthalmology 105:1945–1951, 1998.
50. Clineschmidt CM, Williams RD, Snyder E, et al. A randomized trial in patients inadequately controlled with timolol alone comparing the dorzolamide-timolol combination to monotherapy with timolol or dorzolamide. Dorzolamide-Timolol Combination Study Group. Ophthalmology 105:1952–1959, 1998.
51. Stewart RH, Kimbrough RL, Ward RL. Betaxolol vs timolol. A six-month double-blind comparison. Arch Ophthalmol 104:46–48, 1986.
52. Schoene RB, Abuan T, Ward RL, et al. Effects of topical betaxolol, timolol, and placebo on pulmonary function in asthmatic bronchitis. Am J Ophthalmol 97:86–92, 1984.
53. Lesar TS. Comparison of ophthalmic β-blocking agents. Clin Pharm 6:451–463, 1987.
54. Allen RC, Hertzmark E, Walker AM, et al. A double-masked comparison of betaxolol vs timolol in the treatment of open-angle glaucoma. Am J Ophthalmol 101:535–541, 1986.
55. Betaxolol. Mosby's GenRx. 9th ed. 1999. Available at: http://www.mdconsult.com. Accessed March 15, 1999.
56. Levobunolol. Mosby's GenRx. 9th ed. 1999. Available at: http://www.mdconsult.com. Accessed March 15, 1999.
57. Wandel T, Charap AD, Lewis RA, et al. Glaucoma treatment with once-daily levobunolol. Am J Ophthalmol 101:298–304, 1986.
58. Diggory P, Cassels-Brown A, Fernandez C. Topical β-blockade with intrinsic sympathomimetic activity offers no advantage for the respiratory and cardiovascular function of elderly people. Age Ageing 25:424–428, 1996.
59. Harris LS, Galin MA. Dose response analysis of pilocarpine-induced ocular hypotension. Arch Ophthalmol 84:605–608, 1970.
60. Pilocarpine. online. Mosby's GenRx. 9th ed. 1999. Available at: http://www.mdconsult.com. Accessed March 15, 1999.
61. Goldberg I, Ashburn FS Jr, Kass MA, et al. Efficacy and patient acceptance of pilocarpine gel. Am J Ophthalmol 88:843–846, 1979.
62. Pearson DC. Complications with the use of Ocusert [Letter]. Arch Ophthalmol 94:168, 1976.
63. Nardin G, Zimmerman T. Ocular cholinergic agents. In: Ritch R, Shields M, Krupin T, eds. The glaucomas. 2nd ed. St. Louis: Mosby, 1996:1399–1407.
64. Sugrue MF. The pharmacology of antiglaucoma drugs. Pharmacol Ther 43:91–138, 1989.
65. Leopold IH. Cholinesterases and the effects and side-effects of drugs affecting cholinergic systems. Am J Ophthalmol 62:771–777, 1966.
66. Kellerman L, King A. Echothiophate iodide in glaucoma. Am J Ophthalmol 62:278, 1966.
67. Echothiophate. Mosby's GenRx. 9th ed. 1999. Available at: http://www.mdconsult.com. Accessed March 18, 1999.
68. Taniguchi T, Kitazawa Y. A risk-benefit assessment of drugs used in the management of glaucoma. Drug Saf 11:68–74, 1994.
69. Everitt DE, Avorn J. Systemic effects of medications used to treat glaucoma. Ann Intern Med 112:120–125, 1990.
70. Ellis PP. Systemic reactions to topical therapy. Int Ophthalmol Clin 11:1–11, 1971.
71. Ellis P. Systemic effects of locally applied anticholinesterase agents. Invest Ophthalmol 5:146, 1966.
72. Eilderton TE, Farmati O, Zsigmond EK. Reduction in plasma cholinesterase levels after prolonged administration of echothiophate iodide eyedrops. Can Anaesth Soc J 15:291–296, 1968.
73. Gieser S, Juzych M, Robin A, et al. Clinical pharmacology of adrenergic drugs. In: Ritch R, Shields M, Krupin T, eds. The glaucomas. 2nd ed. St. Louis: Mosby, 1996:1425–1448.
74. Obstbaum SA, Kolker AE, Phelps CD. Low-dose epinephrine. Arch Ophthalmol 92:118–120, 1974.
75. Kass MA, Mandell AI, Goldberg I, et al. Dipivefrin and epinephrine treatment of elevated intraocular pressure: a comparative study. Arch Ophthalmol 97:1865–1866, 1979.
76. Kohn AN, Moss AP, Hargett NA, et al. Clinical comparison of dipivalyl epinephrine and epinephrine in the treatment of glaucoma. Am J Ophthalmol 87:196–201, 1979.
77. Package insert. Propine (dipivefrin). Markham, Ontario, Canada: Allergan, 1996.
78. Simsek S, Demirok A, Yasar T, et al. Effects of 0.5% and 0.25% apraclonidine on postoperative intraocular hypertension after cataract extraction. Eur J Ophthalmol 8:67–70, 1998.
79. Sterk CC, Renzenbrink-Bubberman AC, van Best JA. The effect of 1% apraclonidine on intraocular pressure after cataract surgery. Ophthalmic Surg Lasers 29:472–475, 1998.
80. Threlkeld AB, Assalian AA, Allingham RR, et al. Apraclonidine 0.5% versus 1% for controlling intraocular pressure elevation after argon laser trabeculoplasty. Ophthalmic Surg Lasers 27:657–660, 1996.
81. Toris CB, Tafoya ME, Camras CB, et al. Effects of apraclonidine on aqueous humor dynamics in human eyes. Ophthalmology 102:456–461, 1995.
82. Stewart WC, Ritch R, Shin DH, et al. The efficacy of apraclonidine as an adjunct to timolol therapy. Apraclonidine Adjunctive Therapy Study Group. Arch Ophthalmol 113:287–292, 1995.
83. Robin AL, Ritch R, Shin DH, et al. Short-term efficacy of apraclonidine hydrochloride added to maximum- tolerated medical therapy for glaucoma. Apraclonidine Maximum-Tolerated Medical Therapy Study Group. Am J Ophthalmol 120:423–432, 1995.
84. Package insert. Iopidine (apraclonidine). Fort Worth: Alcon Laboratories, 1998.
85. Katz LJ. Brimonidine tartrate 0.2% twice daily vs timolol 0.5% twice daily: 1-year results in glaucoma patients. Brimonidine Study Group. Am J Ophthalmol 127:20–26, 1999.
86. LeBlanc RP. Twelve-month results of an ongoing randomized trial comparing brimonidine tartrate 0.2% and timolol 0.5% given twice daily in patients with

glaucoma or ocular hypertension. Brimonidine Study Group 2. Ophthalmology 105:1960–1967, 1998.
87. Schuman JS, Horwitz B, Choplin NT, et al. A 1-year study of brimonidine twice daily in glaucoma and ocular hypertension. A controlled, randomized, multicenter clinical trial. Chronic Brimonidine Study Group. Arch Ophthalmol 115:847–852, 1997.
88. Carlstedt B, Stanaszek W. Glaucoma. US Pharmacist 12:7690, 1987.
89. Lippa E. Carbonic anhydrase inhibitors. In: Ritch R, Shields M, Krupin T, eds. The glaucomas. 2nd ed. St. Louis: Mosby, 1996:1463–1481.
90. Maren TH. The rates of movement of Na^+, Cl^-, and HCO_3^- from plasma to posterior chamber: effect of acetazolamide and relation to the treatment of glaucoma. Invest Ophthalmol 15:356–364, 1976.
91. Zimmerman TJ, Garg LC, Vogh BP, et al. The effect of acetazolamide on the movement of sodium into the posterior chamber of the dog eye. J Pharmacol Exp Ther 199:510–517, 1976.
92. Adamsons IA, Polis A, Ostrov CS, et al. Two-year safety study of dorzolamide as monotherapy and with timolol and pilocarpine. Dorzolamide Safety Study Group. J Glaucoma 7:395–401, 1998.
93. Kimal Arici M, Topalkara A, Guler C. Additive effect of latanoprost and dorzolamide in patients with elevated intraocular pressure [In Process Citation]. Int Ophthalmol 22:37–42, 1998.
94. Lichter PR. Reducing side effects of carbonic anhydrase inhibitors. Ophthalmology 88:266–269, 1981.
95. Alward PD, Wilensky JT. Determination of acetazolamide compliance in patients with glaucoma. Arch Ophthalmol 99:1973–1976, 1981.
96. Shrader CE, Thomas JV, Simmons RJ. Relationship of patient age and tolerance to carbonic anhydrase inhibitors. Am J Ophthalmol 96:730–733, 1983.
97. Pepys MB. Acetazolamide and renal stone formation. Lancet 1:837, 1970.
98. Parfitt AM. Acetazolamide and sodium bicarbonate induced nephrocalcinosis and nephrolithiasis: relationship to citrate and calcium excretion. Arch Intern Med 124:736–740, 1969.
99. Camras C. Prostaglandins. In: Ritch R, Shields M, Krupin T, ed. The glaucomas. 2nd ed. St. Louis: Mosby, 1996:1449–1461.
100. Latanoprost. Mosby's GenRx. 9th ed. 1999. Available at: http://www.mdconsult.com. Accessed March 15, 1999.
101. Weiss D, Shaffer R, Harrington D. Treatment of malignant glaucoma with intravenous mannitol infusion. Arch Ophthalmol 69:154, 1963.
102. Adams R. Ocular hypotensive effect of intravenously administered mannitol. Arch Ophthalmol 69:55, 1963.
103. Kolker AE. Hyperosmotic agents in glaucoma. Invest Ophthalmol 9:418–423, 1970.
104. McCurdy D, Schneider B, Scheic H. Oral glycerol: the mechanism of intraocular hypotension. Am J Ophthalmol 61:1244–1249, 1966.
105. Krupin T, Kolker AE, Becker B. A comparison of isosorbide and glycerol for cataract surgery. Am J Ophthalmol 69:737–740, 1970.
106. Remis LL, Epstein DL. Treatment of glaucoma. Annu Rev Med 35:195–205, 1984.
107. Apraclonidine. Mosby's GenRx. 9th ed. 1999. Available at: http://www.mdconsult.com. Accessed January 19, 1999.
108. Pollack IP, Brown RH, Crandall AS, et al. Prevention of the rise in intraocular pressure following neodymium-YAG posterior capsulotomy using topical 1% apraclonidine. Arch Ophthalmol 106:754–757, 1988.
109. The Advanced Glaucoma Intervention Study (AGIS): 4. Comparison of treatment outcomes within race. Seven-year results. Ophthalmology 105: 1146–1164, 1998.
110. Hepler RS, Frank IR. Marihuana smoking and intraocular pressure. JAMA 217:1392, 1971.
111. Marijuana and medicine: assessing the Science Base [prepublication copy]. Available: http://bob.nap.edu/html/marimed/. Accessed April 21, 1999.
112. The use of marijuana in the treatment of glaucoma. Available: http://www.eyenet.org. Accessed April 28, 1999.
113. NEI statement. The use of marijuana for glaucoma. Available: http://nei.nih.gov. Accessed April 28, 1999.
114. Kamal D, Hitchings R. Normal tension glaucoma–a practical approach. Br J Ophthalmol 82:835–840, 1998.
115. Stewart WC, Sine C, Cate E, et al. Daily cost of β-adrenergic blocker therapy [see comments]. Arch Ophthalmol 115:853–856, 1997.
116. Rocchi A, Tingey D. Economic evaluation of dorzolamide vs. pilocarpine for primary open-angle glaucoma. Can J Ophthalmol 32:414–418, 1997.

CHAPTER 51

HEADACHE

Mary L. Wagner, Mary M. Sotirhos, and Stephen D. Silberstein

DEFINITION

The International Headache Society (IHS) divides headaches into primary and secondary headache disorders. These are further subdivided into 13 subcategories (Table 51.1). The primary headache disorders include migraine headache, tension-type headache (TTH), and cluster headache. Migraine is subdivided into migraine without aura (common migraine) and migraine with aura (classic migraine). TTH is subclassified as either episodic TTH (ETTH) or chronic TTH (CTTH). Cluster headache is similarly divided into the episodic and chronic varieties. Although chronic daily headache (CDH) is a commonly used term, it is not recognized by the IHS as a separate entity.[1,2] Headaches that are a symptom of another disease are known as secondary headaches. This chapter discusses only primary headaches.

TREATMENT GOALS: HEADACHE

- Acute treatment should alleviate headache pain and associated symptoms.
- Preventive treatment should reduce the frequency and severity of anticipated attacks and improve the quality of life of persons with headache.
- Lifestyle adjustments and behavior modification should reduce the need for medication.
- The choice for headache treatment should take into account any comorbid conditions and achieve maximum efficacy with minimal side effects.

EPIDEMIOLOGY

Migraine Headache

Migraine occurs in 18% of women, 6% of men, and 4% of children in the United States.[3,4] It usually begins in the first three decades of life, and is most prevalent during the fifth decade.[4,5] Organic causes (secondary headache) must be considered when headaches begin after age 50. Most migraineurs have a family history of migraine, and most also have TTH.[4] Contrary to the findings of clinic-based studies, the American Migraine Study found that migraine was more prevalent in families of lower socioeconomic class. Despite 10 million physician visits each year, migraine is still underdiagnosed and undertreated. Most persons with migraines do not see a physician. Medications are prescribed for only about a third of patients with headaches, and about half of these will discontinue

Table 51.1 ▪ International Headache Society Classification of Headache

A. Primary headache disorders
  1. Migraine
  2. Tension-type headache
  3. Cluster headache and chronic paroxysmal hemicrania
  4. Miscellaneous headaches not associated with structural lesions

B. Secondary headache disorders
  5. Headache associated with head trauma
  6. Headache associated with vascular disorders
  7. Headache associated with nonvascular intracranial disorders
  8. Headache associated with substances or their withdrawal
  9. Headache associated with noncephalic infections
  10. Headache associated with metabolic disorders
  11. Headache or facial pain associated with disorders of the cranium, neck, eyes, ears, nose, sinuses, teeth, mouth, or other facial or cranial structures
  12. Cranial neuralgias, nerve trunk pain, and deafferentation pain
  13. Headache not classifiable

Source: Reference 2.

their medications because of dissatisfaction with treatment results.[3]

Tension-Type Headache

TTH is the most common headache type, with a lifetime prevalence of 69% in men and 88% in women. Only patients with more severe or chronic headaches, unresponsive to over-the-counter preparations, seek medical attention. TTH can begin at any age, but onset during adolescence or young adulthood is most common. Forty percent of patients have a family history of TTH.[4] Headache prevalence declines with increasing age; severity decreases in women who continue to report headaches but does not change in men.[6] Twenty-five percent of patients with TTH also have migraine. Patients with ETTH are no different from control subjects in terms of stress, depression, anxiety, emotional conflicts, sleeping problems, and fatigue, but CTTH is often complicated by coexisting conditions, such as migraine, depression, and drug overuse.

Cluster Headache

Cluster headache is less common than migraine or TTH, with a prevalence of 0.01 to 0.4% in various populations.[2] Prevalence is higher in men and in African Americans. A family history of cluster headache is rare. Ninety percent of patients are seen with episodic cluster headaches. Cluster headaches can begin at any age, but they most commonly begin in the late 20s and only 10% of patients develop cluster headaches in their 60s.[4,6–8] Cluster events may be associated with high altitudes, sleep apnea, seasonal changes, or rapid eye movement sleep. These headaches may last throughout the patient's life. Drug therapy may help change patients' headaches from chronic to episodic cluster[4,6,8]; however, cure is rare.

Chronic Daily Headache

Many clinicians do not agree on a definition for CDH. Most simply, CDH is a headache that occurs daily for more than 15 days a month for at least a month. Primary CDH has been subclassified into headaches lasting >4 hours (CTTH, transformed migraine, new daily persistent headache, and hemicrania continua) or <4 hours (cluster headache, chronic paroxysmal hemicrania, hypnic headache, or idiopathic stabbing headache). Intermittent headaches are characterized by frequent but brief attacks, whereas CDH are more pervasive and continuous. Primary headaches (migraine, tension-type, and cluster headaches) and various secondary headache disorders can develop into CDH. Approximately 40% of patients evaluated in headache clinics suffer from CDH. Patients often develop CDH because of acute medication (opioids, simple analgesics, ergot alkaloids, and triptans) overuse. These individuals may also not respond as well to prophylactic therapy.[2]

PATHOPHYSIOLOGY

General Pain Theory

Pain control systems are involved in all headache types and play an important role in the perception of headaches. Peripheral pain receptors transmit sharp, localized pain via myelinated A-fibers and aching, burning pain via unmyelinated C-fibers to the dorsal horn of the spinal cord. Substance P (SP) and excitatory amino acids are believed to be the neurotransmitters for the peripheral pain transmission system. In the spinal cord, enkephalins and γ-aminobutyric acid (GABA) modulate pain transmission. From the dorsal horn, two ascending pathways carry pain sensations to the somatosensory cortex (neothalamic pathway) and to the limbic forebrain and other areas (paleothalamic pathway).[9]

The brainstem sites responsible for craniovascular pain are being mapped using *fos*-immunohistochemistry, a method for investigating activated cells. The trigeminal nucleus extends beyond the traditional nucleus caudalis to the dorsal horn of the high cervical region in a functional continuum that could be called the trigeminal nucleus cervicalis. This group of cells is the site for referral of head pain and may account for the pain distribution in migraine and other forms of headache. Information is transmitted to the trigeminocervical neurons in the caudal brainstem and high cervical spinal cord and then relayed to the thalamus. The thalamus passes information on to the cortex. Pain localization occurs in the somatosensory cortex, and emotional or affective responses occur in the frontal cortex, anterior cingulate, and insula cortex.

The central nervous system (CNS) modulates pain, in part, by the serotonergic and adrenergic pain-control systems. The descending serotonergic system originates in the periaqueductal gray of the midbrain and, via the raphe magnus in the medulla, connects with the dorsal horn of the spinal cord. Analgesia is produced, in part, by serotonin (5-hydroxytryptamine or 5-HT) interacting with enkephalin-containing neurons. The ascending serotonergic system innervates the cerebral blood vessels, the thalamus, the hypothalamus, and the cortex. It is involved in the regulation of cerebral blood flow (CBF), sleep, and neuroendocrine control. Both ascending and descending noradrenergic pathways originate in the locus ceruleus of the pons. The ascending noradrenergic pathway innervates the microcirculation and the cerebral cortex. The descending noradrenergic pathway terminates in the dorsal horn of the spinal cord. Analgesia may be produced by interaction with GABA-containing interneurons.[9]

The brain itself is insensitive to pain, but other structures, such as the skin of the scalp, the head and neck muscles, the great venous sinuses, the meningeal and cerebral arteries, parts of the fifth, ninth, and tenth cranial nerves, and parts of the dura mater, are pain sensitive. Pain impulses from these sites are transmitted to the spinal cord and brainstem. Direct connections between the primary sensory neurons (e.g., the trigeminal nerve) and the cerebral blood vessels have been detected.[9]

The trigeminal nerve contains calcitonin gene-related peptide (CGRP), SP, and neurokinin A (NKA). Stimulation of the trigeminal nerve leads to release of these mediators from unmyelinated sensory fibers in the dural vasculature. CGRP mediates vasodilation, whereas SP and NKA induce vascular leakage with extravasation of plasma proteins, platelet aggregation, and mast cell degranulation, resulting in neurogenic inflammation (inflammation and dilation of cephalic vessels) and pain. Ergots and triptans block the release of these substances by stimulating 5-HT$_{1B/D}$ heteroreceptors on the trigeminal nerve endings.[4]

Genetics

In addition to environmental and neurologic disturbances initiating migraine, individuals' genetic characteristics may lower their headache threshold, making some of them more susceptible to headaches. An epidemiologic survey found that first-degree relatives of migraineurs had a 1.5- to 1.9-fold greater risk of developing migraine.[10] Familial hemiplegic migraine was the first migraine to be mapped to a chromosome, predominantly chromosome 19 (55%), with the remainder mapped to chromosome 1 (15%) or to an unknown chromosome (30%). The defect in this gene alters P-Q-type neuronal calcium channels, lowers the threshold for migraine, and predisposes the patient to more frequent and severe migraines.[2] Further studies are warranted to establish the true relationship between headaches and genetics.

Migraine Headache

Any migraine theory must explain the prodrome, aura, headache, and associated symptoms. Wolff's vascular theory (reactive vasodilation) and Heyck's theory (reduced arteriovenous oxygen content) have largely been replaced by the comprehensive neurovascular theory that is based on CBF, magnetic resonance spectroscopy, and magnetoencephalography research. According to this theory, neuronal dysfunction, with subsequent vascular changes, is responsible for the onset and propagation of migraine headaches (Fig. 51.1).[2,4]

The hypothalamus and limbic system affect both afferent and efferent 5-HT and adrenergic pathways. Disturbances here may hasten the onset of migraine prodrome. A wave of decreased CBF, spreading forward from the occipital cortex, precedes the aura and persists into the headache phase. This change in CBF is associated with cortical spreading depression, a short-lasting wave of neuronal depolarization. Cortical spreading depression, a proposed cause of aura, may be initiated by an intracellular magnesium deficiency, mediated in part by N-methyl-D-aspartate (NMDA) and modulated by hypothalamic and limbic 5-HT and adrenergic pathways. Subsequently, the trigeminal nucleus caudalis, a major relay nucleus for pain in the brainstem, may be activated, possibly, by cortical spreading depression or a biochemical dysfunction affecting the trigeminal nerve. Stimulation of the trigeminal nerve results in release of SP and NKA leading to neurogenic inflammation. Release of CGRP and nitric oxide alters blood flow in adjacent microcirculatory blood vessels. After the aura phase, regional CBF increases and eventually returns to normal. The pain of migraine headaches with aura may be caused and propagated by cortical spreading depression, activation of the trigeminal nucleus caudalis, and subsequent neurogenic inflammation. An imbalance between facilitatory and inhibitory neurons to the trigeminal nucleus caudalis may render it more sensitive to input that normally would not trigger firing. This may explain why patients with migraines have an increased susceptibility to head pain even during migraine-free periods.[2,4,6]

Serotonin may play an important role in the pathogenesis of migraine headaches. Increased 5-HT metabolism and decreased platelet 5-HT concentrations are associated with migraines. Reserpine, which depletes brain stores of 5-HT and catecholamines, promotes migraine headaches, whereas intravenous 5-HT aborts migraine headaches.[2] Interestingly, migraine headaches may decrease with age, possibly due to a decrease of 5-HT receptors in the brain. In addition, platelet concentrations of 5-HT are lower in patients with migraines who abuse analgesics versus those who do not abuse analgesics or people without headaches, possibly explaining CDH.[11] At least seven families of 5-HT receptors (5-HT$_1$, 5-HT$_2$, 5-HT$_3$, 5-HT$_4$, 5-HT$_5$, 5-HT$_6$, and 5-HT$_7$), many with subtypes (5-HT$_{1[A,B,D,E,F]}$, 5-HT$_{2[A,B,C]}$, and 5-HT$_{5[A,B]}$) have been identified. It is believed that activation of the 5-HT$_{1A}$ receptor causes nausea, while activation of the 5-HT$_{1B}$ receptor produces vasoconstriction. Activation of 5-HT$_{1D}$ receptors decreases the release of 5-HT, norepinephrine, acetylcholine, CGRP, and SP. The inhibitory 5-HT$_{1D}$ and perhaps the 5-HT$_{1F}$ heteroreceptor on trigeminal nerve terminals block neurogenic inflammation by inhibiting the release of neuroactive peptides. In addition, activation may block pain transmission in the trigeminal system. Most drugs used to abort migraine, such as ergots and triptans, are agonists at the

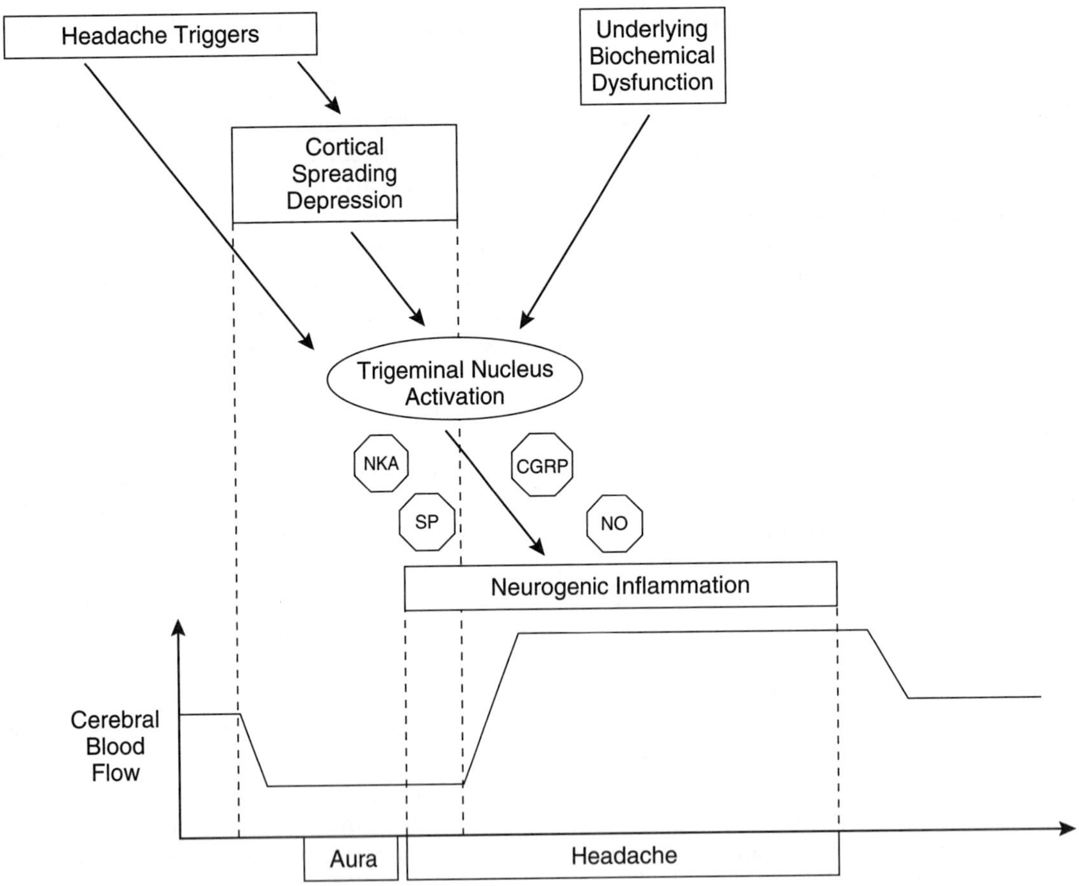

Figure 51.1. Pathophysiology of migraine headaches. The Comprehensive Neurovascular theory predicts relationships between neuronal events and cerebrovascular changes. Activation of the trigeminal nucleus complex results in the release of substance P (*SP*), neurokinin A (*NKA*), calcitonin gene related peptide (*CGRP*), and nitric oxide (*NO*), which initiate neurogenic inflammation, alter cerebral blood flow, and propagate headache. Adapted from references 2 and 4.

5-HT_{1D} receptor; they also display affinity for the 5-HT_{1A}, 5-HT_{1B}, and perhaps the 5-HT_{1F} receptors. 5-HT_2 stimulation results in bronchoconstriction, platelet aggregation, gastrointestinal smooth muscle contraction, and neuronal depolarization in the CNS. Most drugs that prevent migraines are 5-HT_2 antagonists. 5-HT_3 stimulation causes nausea, vomiting, and activation of autonomic reflexes. Metoclopramide, a 5-HT_3 antagonist, is useful in the treatment of migraine-induced nausea.[2,4,6]

Other neurotransmitters and mediators, such as histamine, catecholamines, vasoactive peptides, endogenous opioids, prostaglandins, free fatty acids, and steroid hormones, are also implicated in the pathogenesis of migraine. Migraineurs have increased plasma catecholamine levels before and during the migraine attack. Norepinephrine produces vasoconstriction via the postsynaptic α_1-receptors and promotes release of serotonin from platelets. Dopaminergic hyperactivity may also play a major role in migraine pathogenesis.[12] Increased dopamine concentrations may be partially responsible for the nausea and other symptoms during a migraine attack. Estrogens modulate 5-HT_1 and 5-HT_2 receptors and are implicated in the development of menstrual migraine. A rapid fall in estrogen, which increases prostaglandin and prolactin levels, may be responsible for the initiation of the migraine attack. Migraine often worsens during the first trimester of pregnancy, but then remits thereafter owing to sustained high estrogen levels.[4]

Migraineurs may have an altered blood-brain barrier during the headache phase. The locus ceruleus, a noradrenaline-containing cell group, may affect brain blood flow and blood-brain barrier permeability.[2] The efficacy of antimigraine drugs is dependent on access to the receptor site, but an altered blood-brain barrier may inhibit the delivery of drug to the site of action, thus diminishing its efficacy.

Tension-Type Headache

Physical or psychologic stress or nonphysiologic working conditions may trigger ETTH. CTTH may be associated with a perceived increase in stressful life events. Tension headaches may also be precipitated by menstruation.[4] Diminished sympathetic activity, decreased concentrations of 5-HT, and elevated concentrations of SP have been observed in the plasma of patients with TTH. Reduced CNS 5-HT levels may be responsible for abnormal pain modulation, producing the decreased pain thresholds observed in most patients with CTTH. Serotonin levels vary above or below normal in patients suffering from ETTH.[2]

Although many patients with TTH have muscle tenderness, TTH is not the result of sustained contraction of the pericranial muscles. Muscle ischemia is not present during headache and muscle blood flow is normal. Increased nociception from strained muscles or reduced antinociception from emotional stress may modulate TTH. Central pain facilitatory neurons in the ventromedial medulla may produce supraspinal facilitation of the trigeminal nucleus caudalis, which also receives peripheral input from the cephalic blood vessels and the pericranial muscles. An imbalance between the facilitatory and inhibitory neurons to the trigeminal nucleus caudalis may produce central sensitization. Similar to migraine, CTTH may present with a neuron hypersensitivity in the trigeminal nucleus caudalis neurons secondary to supraspinal facilitation and a general increase in nociception.[2]

Cluster Headache

The pathogenesis of cluster headaches has not been well defined. Any pathogenesis theory must explain the unilateral periorbital pain distribution, the severity, the autonomic symptoms, and the circadian rhythm of the attack. Cluster headache had been attributed to an inflammatory process in the cavernous sinus, which injures the pericarotid sympathetic nerves. This theory cannot explain the circadian rhythms of the attack, and, in fact, recent positron emission tomographic (PET) data establish that blood flow changes in the cavernous sinus region are not limited to cluster headache. PET studies of a provoked attack of cluster headache have shown activation of the ipsilateral hypothalamus. Unlike migraine, there was no brainstem activation. This suggests that the pathophysiology of cluster and migraine headaches is driven from different areas of the central nervous system.[13]

Cluster events may be related to alterations in the circadian pacemaker. Attacks increase after time changes, or when there is a loss of circadian rhythm for blood pressure, temperature, and hormones, including prolactin, melatonin, cortisol, and endorphins. The remarkable half-yearly, yearly, or even biennial cycling of the bouts is one of the most fascinating processes of human biology. Cluster headache may be regarded as a dysfunction of neurons in the pacemaker or clock regions of the brain (posterior hypothalamus), which allows activation of a trigeminal-autonomic loop in the brainstem. Both migraine and cluster headaches may share a final common pathway: the trigeminal vascular system. Activation results in the release of vasoactive peptides and neurogenic inflammation. The hypothalamus projects to the triennial motor, but not sensory, nuclei. It could directly activate brainstem autonomic nuclei, which could lead to changes in the cavernous sinus. The hypothalamus could also have a direct effect on the descending pain control system.[14] Plasma 5-HT metabolism may also be increased.[15]

CLINICAL PRESENTATION AND DIAGNOSIS

The IHS established formal criteria for headache diagnosis in 1988, distinguishing between primary headache disorders and those due to a secondary cause (Table 51.1). There are both medical and pharmacologic causes of headache (Table 51.2). A complete history is needed for diagnosis and should include the following information: (1) age at headache onset, (2) time of headache onset (day or season), (3) description of the pain (location, severity, and type), (4) attack frequency (including any change in frequency), (5) associated symptoms, (6) precipitating factors, (7) methods of palliation used, (8) the patient's sleep habits, and (9) family history. In addition, a complete medication history should be taken to evaluate the dose, duration of use, and effectiveness of previous headache medications and to determine if any medications being used could exacerbate headaches. Table 51.3 summarizes the diagnostic characteristics of headache disorders.

Migraine Headache

A diagnosis of migraine without aura requires the patient to have at least five headache attacks, each lasting 4 to 72 hours, and two of the following characteristics: unilateral location, pulsating quality, moderate or severe intensity, or aggravation by routine physical activity. At least one of the following should occur during the attack: nausea/vomiting or photophobia and phonophobia.[4]

A diagnosis of migraine with aura requires the patient to have at least two attacks with at least three of the following characteristics: (1) one or more fully reversible aura symptoms; (2) at least one aura symptom developing gradually over more than 4 minutes or two or more symptoms occurring in succession; (3) no single aura symptom lasting more than 60 minutes; and (4) headache after aura with a free interval of less than 60 minutes. If the aura lasts longer than 1 hour but less than 1 week, the migraine is called migraine with prolonged aura (Table 51.4).[4]

Table 51.2 ▪ Pharmacologic Causes of Headache

Amantadine	Histamine H_2-antagonists
Analgesics[a]	Isometheptene[a]
Barbiturates	Sumatriptan[a]
Caffeine[a]	Sympathomimetics (amphetamines, dopamine, fenfluramine, theophylline)
Cannabis	Tetracycline
Corticosteroids and their withdrawal	Trimethoprim
Digitalis	Vasodilators (captopril, dipyridamole, hydralazine, nifedipine, nitrates[b], prazosin, reserpine)
Ergotamine and its withdrawal[a]	
Estrogens and oral contraceptives	
Fluoxetine	
Ethanol[b]	

Source: Reference 2.
[a]Cause rebound headaches when used too frequently.
[b]Most common headache triggers.

Table 51.3 ▪ Differential Diagnosis by Presentation of Selected Headache Disorders

Headache Type	Age of onset (yr)	Location	Duration	Frequency/Timing	Severity	Quality	Associated Features
Migraine	10–40	Hemicranial	Several hours to 3 days	Variable	Moderate to severe	Throbbing > steady ache	Nausea, vomiting, photo/phono/osmophobia, scotomata, neurologic deficits
Tension type	20–50	Bilateral	30 min–7+ days	Variable	Dull ache may wax/wane	Vise-like, band-like pressure	Generally none
Cluster	15–40	Unilateral, peri-retro-orbital	30–120 min	1–8 times per day, nocturnal attacks	Excruciating	Boring, piercing	Ipsilateral conjunctival injection, lacrimation, nasal congestion, rhinorrhea, miosis, facial sweating
Mass lesion	Any	Any	Variable	Intermittent, nocturnal, upon arising	Moderate	Dull steady/throbbing	Vomiting, nuchal rigidity, neurologic deficits
Subarachnoid hemorrhage	Adult	Global, often occipitonuchal	Variable	Not applicable	Excruciating	Explosive	Nausea, vomiting, nuchal rigidity, loss of consciousness, neurologic deficits
Trigeminal neuralgia	50–70	2nd–3rd > 1st division's trigeminal nerve	Seconds, occur in volleys	Paroxysmal	Excruciating	Electric shock-like	Facial trigger points, spasm of muscles ipsilaterally (tic)
Giant cell arteritis	>55	Temporal, any region	Intermittent, then continuous	Constant, +/– worse at night	Variable	Variable	Tender scalp arteries, polymyalgia rheumatica, jaw claudication

Source: Reprinted with permission from Silberstein SD, Lipton RB, Goadsby PJ. Headache in clinical practice. Oxford: Isis Medical Media, 1998.

Migraine may consist of three phases: (1) premonitory, (2) the attack [subdivided into (2a) the aura, and (2b) the headache], and (3) the postdrome[2,4,6] (Table 51.4). Premonitory (prodrome) symptoms occur in about 60% of patients. Symptoms begin hours to days before the headache and can continue into the aura and headache phases.

Table 51.4 ▪ Migraine Headache Symptoms

1. Premonitory Phase (Prodrome)	
Mental	General
Depression	Stiff neck
Euphoria and hyperactivity	Cold feeling
Irritability	Sluggishness
Restlessness	Thirst
Mental slowness or poor concentration	Polyuria
Fatigue and drowsiness	Anorexia or food cravings
Neurologic	Diarrhea or constipation
Photophobia	Fluid retention
Phonophobia	
Hyperosmia	
Dysphasia	

2a. Attack Phase: Aura	
Visual field changes (20–35%)	Sensory (33%)
Photopsia (flashing lights)	Paresthesias (numbness or tingling in the extremities and face)
Scotomata (flashes, specks, geometric forms)	Motor disturbances and aphasia (20%)
Scintillations (fluorescent flashes of light)	Monoparesis or hemiparesis
Teichopsia (alternating light and dark lines)	Difficulty speaking
Visual distortions	Difficulty understanding language
Hallucinations	

2b. Attack: Headache (Pain Description and Associated Symptoms)	
Headache	Neuropsychologic
Location (bilateral 40%, unilateral 60%)	Persistence of prodromal symptoms
Throbbing quality (40–60%)	Photophobia
Scalp tenderness (66%)	Phonophobia
Short-lived "ice-pick" pain jabs (40%)	Osmophobia
Gastrointestinal	Lightheadedness
Anorexia	Mood and mental changes
Food cravings	Other
Nausea and vomiting (86%)	Edema and polyuria
Constipation	Nasal stuffiness (10–20%)
Diarrhea (16%)	Rhinorrhea

3. Postdrome Phase	
Neuropsychologic	Others
Fatigue or listlessness	Muscle weakness and aching
Irritability or mood changes	Anorexia or food cravings
Impaired concentration	Scalp tenderness

Sources: References 2, 4, 6.

During this time, patients may experience various psychologic, sensory, constitutional, or autonomic symptoms. These symptoms may be hard to diagnose because they may occur by themselves or with mild headaches.[2]

The attack phase consists of the aura and the headache. The aura, occurring in about 20% of migraineurs, consists of visual, sensory, motor, brainstem, or language disturbances. It develops over 5 to 20 minutes and lasts less than 1 hour. Symptoms may accompany the headache or occur up to an hour before the headache. Sometimes the aura may occur without the headache.[2,16]

The headache can begin at any time during the day. The pain usually develops gradually and then subsides after 4 to 72 hours in adults and 2 to 48 hours in children. If the headache lasts longer than 72 hours, it is labeled status migrainosus. The pain is usually located in the temples, but can occur anywhere in the face or head and may radiate down the neck and shoulder. The pain is moderate to severe in intensity and usually described as throbbing or pulsating with a unilateral distribution; however, the symptoms may begin as, or become, bilateral.[2,16] Most patients experience associated gastrointestinal and neuropsychologic symptoms, with nausea being the most common. Photophobia and phonophobia cause patients to seek relief in a dark, quiet room to decrease sensory stimulation. Most patients experience between one and four headaches a month.[2,6]

After the headache phase, the postdrome, or recovery, phase may occur and last up to 24 hours. During this phase, some patients may feel alert or tired, euphoric or depressed, or refreshed or worn out, and others may complain of poor concentration, food intolerance, or scalp tenderness.[2]

Tension-Type Headache

The diagnosis of TTH requires that patients experience at least 10 previous headaches, each lasting 30 minutes to 7 days, with at least two of the following characteristics: a pressing or tightening (nonpulsating) quality, mild to moderate intensity, bilateral location, and no aggravation with physical activity. In addition, patients should not have nausea or vomiting. They may have either photophobia or phonophobia but not both. ETTH occurs less than 15 days a month, whereas CTTH occurs 15 or more days a month for at least 6 months. Patients with CTTH may have one of the following: nausea, photophobia, or phonophobia.[2,4,6]

Patients describe the onset of the headache as gradual, often occurring during or after stress. Headaches last 30 minutes to a week, with a median of 12 hours. The headache is typically worse later in the day. The pain is usually bilateral, may be located in the forehead, the temples, or the back of the head, and may radiate to the neck and shoulders. Patients describe the steady, nagging, persistent, dull, aching pain as a tightness, a soreness, a squeezing sensation, or a constricting, vise-like pressure. They may say, "it's as if a band were wrapped around my head,"[4] or complain of scalp tenderness, rigid neck muscles, and jaw discomfort. Unlike migraine, there is no prodrome or associated autonomic or gastrointestinal symptoms. Some patients complain of anorexia.

Cluster Headache

The diagnosis of cluster headache requires the patient to have at least five untreated attacks of severe, unilateral, orbital, supraorbital, and/or temporal pain lasting 15 to 180 minutes. At least one of the following associated symptoms must occur: conjunctival injection, lacrimation, nasal congestion, rhinorrhea, facial sweating, miosis, ptosis, or eyelid edema. Headache frequency during a cluster attack varies from one every other day to eight per day. Episodic cluster headaches are distinguished by headache periods of 1 week to 1 year with remission periods lasting at least 14 days, whereas chronic cluster headaches have no remission periods or remissions lasting less than 14 days. Episodic cluster headaches can evolve into chronic cluster headaches.[7]

Cluster attacks may begin with slight discomfort that rapidly increases (within 15 minutes) to excruciating pain. The attacks often occur at the same time each day and frequently awaken patients from sleep. Untreated, the attacks generally last for 30 to 90 minutes, but can persist up to 180 minutes. The pain is described as unilateral, deep, constant, boring, pressing, piercing, or burning in nature and located behind or around the eye. It may radiate to the forehead, temples, jaws, nostrils, ears, neck, or shoulder. Patients may say, "it's like driving a hot poker into my eye."[4] Some patients cannot describe the pain, and 30% describe it as throbbing or pulsating. Patients are usually pain-free between cluster periods, with remissions lasting 6 months to 2 years; however, isolated, mild, brief attacks may occur between cluster periods. During an attack, patients often feel agitated or restless and feel the need to isolate themselves and move around. Cluster headaches have, by definition, one or more associated symptoms of autonomic dysfunction. Lacrimation is reported by about 83% of patients. Gastrointestinal symptoms are uncommon. Most patients have one or two cluster periods a year that last 2 to 3 months, with one to two attacks per day.[7]

PSYCHOSOCIAL ASPECTS

Children and adults with headaches experience more physical complaints, stress, psychologic symptoms, and decreased quality of life than do those without headaches. They also exhibit more absenteeism from school and work.[17,18] These patients are more likely to experience depression and anxiety.[19] They live in fear that their headaches will affect their ability to meet obligations to family, co-workers, and friends.[2] People who express resentment over having to make sacrifices to accommodate the needs of headache patients may reinforce these feelings.

THERAPEUTIC PLAN

Migraine Headache

The treatment algorithm is based on the patient's headache severity, concurrent symptoms, comorbid conditions and the efficacy-adverse effect ratio and cost of the medications (Fig. 51.2). Generally, the agents with the highest efficacy/adverse effect ratio and lowest cost are used first. The route of administration depends on patient preference, prior response to that route of administration, and the presence of certain migraine-associated symptoms. For example, patients with severe nausea and vomiting should be treated with parenteral, rectal, or intranasal (IN) medications. Patients with mild to moderate headache pain should be treated with analgesics with or without caffeine. If these fail in the same or prior attacks, move on to triptans, dihydroergotamine (DHE), mixed analgesics, or opioids. Patients with severe pain should start treatment with combination analgesics, opoioids, triptans, or DHE. Nonpharmacologic and adjunctive medications for associated headache symptoms are also used concurrently.[2]

After the acute attack is treated, patients should be educated about their disease, medications, how to monitor their symptoms with a diary, and the possible need for preventive therapy. Nonpharmacologic treatments may minimize the need for medications.

Tension-Type Headache

Patients with TTH usually self-medicate with over-the-counter analgesics, rarely seek medical attention, and may be at increased risk for CDH from medication overuse. First-line treatment consists of nonpharmacologic treatments followed by over-the-counter analgesics. Prescription analgesics may be used if the former fail.[2] Preventive therapy is rarely needed but should be administered when a patient has frequent (more than two per week), long (more than 3 hours) headaches that produce disability or the need for frequent acute therapy. Based on clinical experience, antidepressants are preferred in these patients.[2]

Cluster Headache

Most oral agents are absorbed too slowly to be effective in the acute treatment of cluster headaches. Effective acute treatments that provide rapid onset of action include oxygen inhalation, SC sumatriptan, IM/IV DHE, or IN lidocaine. Opioids are not usually indicated in the acute treatment of cluster headache, because their efficacy is limited and frequent use may lead to addiction.[2,7]

Most patients with cluster headaches require preventive treatment because each attack is too short in duration and too severe in intensity to treat adequately with acute administration of medication. Furthermore, failure to stop the headache quickly may result in months of suffering or overuse of medications. Preventive therapies for episodic cluster headaches, in order of preference, include verapamil or ergotamine, methysergide, lithium or valproic acid, and topical capsaicin. Preferred choices for chronic cluster

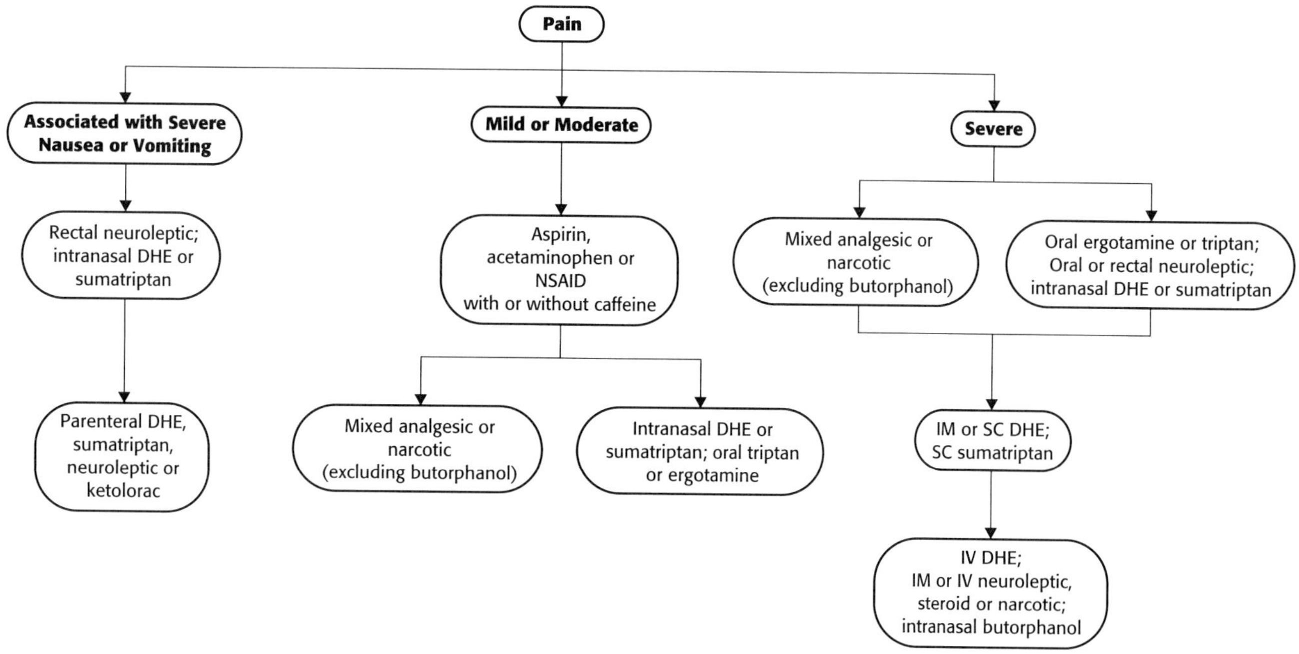

Figure 51.2. Algorithm for the pharmacologic treatment of migraine headaches. Pharmacologic treatment is based on the patient's headache severity, concurrent symptoms, comorbid conditions and the efficacy/adverse effect ratio and cost of medications. Parenteral, intranasal, or rectal preparations are also preferred when the pain intensifies in less than 1 hour. *DHE,* dihydroergotamine; *NSAID*, nonsteroidal anti-inflammatory drug. Adapted from reference 2.

headaches include verapamil, lithium, or valproic acid. If single-drug therapy fails, dual therapy with two of these agents or with methysergide may be used. If headaches still persist, triple therapy, including ergotamine, may be tried.

Corticosteroids are used to break a cluster cycle while waiting for other drugs to take effect or to treat a refractory chronic cluster headache. To maximize effectiveness, medications should be started early in a cluster period, continued until the patient is headache free for 2 weeks, and discontinued as a slow taper until needed for the next cluster period.[2]

TREATMENT

Pharmacotherapy

Pharmacologic treatments should be added when nonpharmacologic treatments alone fail to provide adequate headache relief. Avoiding headache triggers augments the efficacy of all medications for achieving pain relief. Therapy for headaches is divided into acute (abortive) and preventive treatment. The aim of acute treatment is to relieve headache pain and associated symptoms. It should be limited to two to three times a week. Preventive therapy should reduce the frequency and severity of anticipated attacks, but acute treatment is still needed for breakthrough attacks.

Drugs used for the acute treatment of headache include analgesics (alone or in combination with caffeine or barbiturates), opioids (alone or in combination with other drugs), isometheptene combinations, selective serotonin agonists, ergotamine derivatives, corticosteroids, neuroleptics, and antiemetics. Agents that prevent headaches include β-blockers, antidepressants, calcium channel blockers, serotonin antagonists, anticonvulsants, and lithium. Dosing guidelines and indications for these agents are described in Table 51.5 and Table 51.6.

Some acute agents only provide analgesia, while others directly stop the migraine process. These agents are available in various of routes of administration and the choice of an agent should be individualized. A nonoral route of administration is a more appropriate choice if the time between headache onset and peak intensity is less than 1 hour, or nausea and vomiting are present. The quick relief achieved by these agents may lead to overuse or abuse, possibly leading to CDHs. The clinician should consider preventive treatments if excessive use of these agents occurs.

The decision to begin preventive treatment includes: (1) two or more attacks a month that produce disability that lasts 3 or more days; (2) contraindication to, or ineffectiveness of, symptomatic medications; (3) the use of acute medication more than twice a week; or (4) special circumstances, such as hemiplegic migraine or rare headache attacks producing profound disruption or risk of permanent neurologic injury. Preventive medication is usually given daily for months or years; however, treatment can be episodic, subacute, or chronic. It may be administered episodically when there is a known headache trigger, such as exercise or sexual activity. In such situations, patients are instructed to pretreat before exposure or activity. Patients who are undergoing a time-limited exposure to a trigger (high altitude ascent) or a reduced migraine threshold (menstruation) can be treated sub-acutely by having them medicate before and during the exposure.[21] Patients with

Table 51.5 ▪ Acute Pharmacotherapy

Agent	Usual Adult Dose	Maximum Daily Dose	Time to Onset of Action	Headache	Comments
Ergot alkaloids					
DHE	0.25–1 mg IM/IV; may repeat every 1 hr 1 mg SC, repeat in 1 hr 2 mg IN (0.5 mg each nostril and repeat in 15 min)	3 mg IM/IV 3 mg SC 3 mg IN	<10 min (IV) 15–30 min (IM) 30 min (SC) 30 min (IN)	M, C	Fewer adverse effects than ergotamine. Total parenteral dose should not exceed 6 mg/wk. IN dosage form requires education about assembly and priming. Discard unused spray after 8 hr.
Ergotamine	1–2 mg PO/SL/PR, may repeat every 30 min	6 mg PO/SL/PR	30 min (PO)	M, C	Do not use in patients with ischemic heart disease, uncontrolled hypertension, or cerebrovascular disease. May need to pretreat with antiemetic. Do not exceed 10 mg/wk.
Selective serotonin agonists					
Sumatriptan	6 mg SC, may repeat once after 1 hr 25–100 mg PO, may repeat once in 2 hr 5–20 mg IN, may repeat in 2 hr	12 mg SC 300 mg PO 40 mg IN	10–15 min (SC) 30–60 min (PO) 15–20 min (IN)	M, C M M	Good for patients with nausea. Should be used with caution in patients with cardiovascular disease. Limit to twice a week. IN administration: no need to prime, each canister delivers one dose. Better administration may minimize ADRs.
Zolmitriptan	2.5–5.0 mg PO, may repeat once in 2 hr	10 mg	45 min	M	Disintegrating tablet pending approval.
Naratriptan	1–2.5 mg PO, may repeat once in 4 hr	5 mg 2.5 mg in renal dysfunction	60–180 min	M	
Rizatriptan	5–10 mg PO, may repeat twice, each time separated by 2 hr	30 mg	30–120 min	M	Disintegrating tablet formulation may benefit patients suffering from nausea and vomiting. Reduce dose in patients taking propranolol.
Opioid analgesics					
Butorphanol	1 mg IN, may repeat in 60–90 min 2 mg IM, may repeat 3–4 hr	8 mg 4 mg	15 min	M	Has less abuse potential than other opioids. Limit use to 4 doses/day and 2 days/wk.
Hydromorphone	2–4 mg PO	16 mg	15–30 min	M	Has abuse potential.
Meperidine	75–100 mg parenteral 300 mg PO	400 mg	Peak analgesia 60 min (PO) 30–50 min (IM) 20 min (IV)	M	Has abuse potential.
Morphine	5–10 mg parenteral 30–60 mg PO	60 mg	Peak analgesia 60 min (PO) 20–60 min (PR) 30–60 min (IM) 20 min (IV)	M	Has abuse potential.

(continued)

infrequent attacks are unlikely to receive sufficient benefit to justify the cost, side effects, and inconvenience of preventive treatment.[22]

Drug choice depends on several factors, including the patient's headache type, comorbid conditions, and medication history, as well as each drug's pharmacologic profile. Monotherapy is preferred, but carefully planned combination therapy may be necessary when several comorbid conditions or severe refractory migraines exist. Analgesics or ergot derivatives may compete for the same peripheral receptor site as the preventive therapy, so to ensure maximal benefit from preventive medication these agents should not be abused. Furthermore, oral contraceptives, hormone replacement therapy, or vasodilating drugs (nifedipine or nitroglycerin) may induce migraine or interfere with preventive drugs. Women of childbearing age should

Table 51.5 *(continued)*

Agent	Usual Adult Dose	Maximum Daily Dose	Time to Onset of Action	Headache	Comments
Nonopioid analgesics					
Aspirin	325–650 mg PO, 300–600 mg PR, repeat every 4 hr prn	1000 mg	30 min	M, T	Enteric and rectal forms have slower onset and effervescent form has faster onset.
Acetaminophen	325–650 mg PO/PR, repeat every 4 hr prn	4000 mg	60 min	M, T	Limit to 2–3 times/wk.
Ibuprofen	400–600 mg PO, repeat every 6 hr prn	2400 mg	60 min	M, T	Ibuprofen may have fewer gastrointestinal side effects than other NSAIDs.
Ketorolac	10 mg PO, repeat every 6 hr prn 30–60 mg IM	40 mg PO 90 mg IM	60 min	M, T	Need to monitor renal function. Limit use to 5 days total. As good as chlorpromazine 25 mg IV.
Naproxen	250–500 mg PO, repeat every 8 hr prn	1500 mg	60 min	M, T	May cause drowsiness.
Naproxen sodium	275–550 mg PO, repeat every 8 hr prn	1650 mg		M, T	Is more rapidly absorbed than naproxen.
Neuroleptics					
Chlorpromazine	25–50 mg IV/IM, repeat every 4 hr prn 50–100 mg PR, repeat every 6–8 hr prn	400 mg	10–20 min 60 min	M, T	Has antiemetic effect. Monitor for orthostatic hypotension when administering IV/IM.
Prochlorperazine	5–10 mg IV/IM, repeat every 4 hr prn 25 mg PR, repeat every 8–12 hr prn	40 mg IV/IM 75 mg PR	10–20 min 60 min	M, T	Has antiemetic effect. Monitor for dizziness and drowsiness.
Thiothixene	5 mg PO/IM	20 mg		M	
Corticosteroids					
Dexamethasone	4–8 mg PO; repeat in 60 min	32 mg		M, C	
Prednisone	40–100 mg PO	200 mg		M, C	Administer in short courses then rapidly taper over 2–3 wk.
Miscellaneous agents					
Lidocaine	1 mL of 4% IN solution every 15 min		15–30 min	M, C	Proper administration is imperative to get full benefit.
Oxygen	7–10 L/min for 15–30 min IH		5–10 min	C	Is more effective when given at maximum pain intensity.
Clonidine	0.2 mg	0.6 mg		M	Is adjunct for drug detoxification.
Metoclopramide	10 mg PO 5–10 min before or with simple analgesics		30 min	M	Is a gastrokinetic agent. Limit use to no more than 3 days/wk.

Sources: References 2, 4, 6, 7, 20, 21, 23.

IM, intramuscular; *IV,* intravenous; *IN,* intranasal; *IH,* inhalation; *PO,* oral; *PR,* rectal; *SC,* subcutaneous; *M,* migraine headaches; *C,* cluster headaches; *T,* tension-type headaches; *ADRs,* adverse drug reactions; *NSAIDs,* nonsteroidal anti-inflammatory agents.

be aware of the teratogenic potential of some of these preventive agents and be advised to take adequate contraceptive measures. The medication selected should be started at a low dose and gradually increased to a dose necessary to achieve headache control or to the maximum recommended dose. Patients with migraine often respond to a lower dose of a drug than that recommended for other conditions, but they may also be more sensitive to the drug's adverse effects.[2] An adequate trial of preventive treatment may require 2 to 6 months before any relief is noticed. Once headache control has been achieved for 9 to 12 months, attempts should be made to slowly taper the drug over weeks and discontinue it if possible.[23] Patients may continue to experience relief after discontinuing treatment; however if they need to restart therapy, headache relief may be achieved with lower doses.

Nonopioid Analgesics

Aspirin, acetaminophen, and nonsteroidal anti-inflammatory drugs (NSAIDs) are used for acute and preventive treatment of migraine and TTH. Aspirin and acetaminophen are recommended by the IHS for the treatment of mild to moderate migraines; however, many patients suffering from mild to moderate migraines prefer

Table 51.6 ▪ Preventive Pharmacotherapy

Drug	Starting dose (mg/day)	Maximum dose (mg/day)	Headache	Efficacy/ADR Ratio[a]	Comments
β-Blockers					
Atenolol	25	150	M, T	4/2	Maximal benefit may be delayed for 2–3 months. Begin with low doses and increase gradually. β-blockers are good for patients with hypertension and angina. Avoid β-blockers with ISA.
Metoprolol	50	300	M, T	4/2	
Nadolol	20	240	M, T	4/2	
Propranolol	40	320	M, T	4/2	
Timolol	20	60	M, T	4/2	
Calcium channel blockers					
Verapamil	120	720	M, T, C	2/1	Higher doses needed for cluster headaches. Calcium channel blockers are good for patients with prolonged aura.
Nimodipine	120	360	C	2/2	
Diltiazem	90	360	M, C	1/1	
Serotonin antagonists					
Cyproheptadine	2	32	M	3/2	Very commonly used in children; antihistamine activity.
Methysergide	1 mg q 3d	14	M, T, C	4/4	Very effective drug with poor side effect profile; fibrotic changes, requires drug holidays.
Antidepressants					
Amitriptyline	10	300	M, T	4/2	Amitriptyline is the only TCA with well-established efficacy in migraine treatment. Antidepressants are good for patients with depression and pain syndromes
Doxepin	10	150	M, T	3/2	
Imipramine	10	200	M, T	3/2	
Nortriptyline	10	125	M, T	3/2	
Phenelzine	30	90	M, T	3/4	Requires close medical supervision and dietary restrictions.
Fluoxetine	10	80	M, T	2/1	Has fewer anticholinergic effects, causes more insomnia, and is a good option for patients who cannot tolerate TCAs.
Anticonvulsants					
Valproic acid/divalproex	250	3000	M, T,C	4/2	Use with caution in children. Has fewer gastrointestinal effects than valproic acid.
Nonopioid analgesics					
Ibuprofen	800	2400	M	1/1	Use for menstrual migraine.
Naproxen	500	1500	M	2/2	Use for menstrual migraine.
Corticosteroids					
Prednisone	40	100	C	3/3	Use for episodic cluster headaches. Taper dose over 1–2 wk.
Ergot alkaloids					
Ergotamine	2	4	C	3/3	Avoid in M and chronic C because of rebound headache risk.
Methylergonovine	0.6	2	M, C	2/4	
Miscellaneous agents					
Calcitonin	100 IU IM 200 IU IN		M	2/3	Has risk for antibody formation.
Lithium	600	1800	MC	3/3	C_p = 0.4–0.8 mEq/L for cyclic migraine.
Riboflavin	400		M	2/1	

Sources: References 2, 4, 6, 7, 20, 21.

IM, intramuscular; *IN*, intranasal; *M*, migraine headaches; *C*, cluster headache; *T*, tension-type headaches; *ISA*, intrinsic sympathomimetic activity; *TCA*, tricyclic antidepressants; C_p, plasma clearance.

[a]Efficacy rating (1 = low efficacy and 4 = high efficacy). ADR = adverse drug effect rating (1 = low ADR risk and 4 = high ADR risk).

NSAIDs.[2] Patients not responding to one agent may respond to another. Nonopioid analgesics most likely decrease neurogenic inflammation and headaches by prostaglandin synthesis inhibition.

NSAIDs are particularly useful in patients with menstrual migraine and those with concomitant arthritis. The more lipid-soluble NSAIDs, such as indomethacin or ketoprofen, may be more efficacious owing to greater CNS penetration.[24] Long-acting NSAIDs may have less risk of rebound headaches[25] and may be useful for treating patients who abuse ergotamine.[6] Ibuprofen and naproxen are significantly more effective than placebo and may be more effective than aspirin or acetaminophen.[2] NSAIDs should not be taken continuously for more than 1 week for menstrual migraine (ketorolac must be limited to 5 days in any situation), and otherwise they should be limited to three times per week.

Adverse reactions to nonopioid analgesics include gastrointestinal (GI) upset, GI bleeding, peptic ulcers, abdominal pain, dizziness, fluid retention, sedation, and tinnitus. Aspirin should be avoided in patients with peptic ulcer disease, in those with hematologic disorders, and in children less than 15 years of age. NSAIDs should be avoided in patients experiencing nausea and vomiting[21] and are relatively contraindicated in patients with gastritis, peptic ulcer disease, or kidney disease. Indomethacin and aspirin suppositories or ketorolac injections may be used in patients with nausea or vomiting. Patients should be told to take NSAIDs with meals to minimize adverse GI effects. They should be monitored for potential GI blood loss, renal dysfunction, worsening of hypertension, and aggravation of colitis. Large quantities (more than 50 g/mo) of simple analgesics may cause migraine headaches to transform into CDH.[3]

Opioid Analgesics

Opioids are useful for patients with intractable menstrual migraine, for those who have contraindications to other migraine medications or for whom these medications fail, and for those who require rescue medication, especially in the middle of the night. Although these agents are not first-line agents for acute cluster headache therapy, nonparenteral opioid analgesics play a small role in relieving cluster headaches, particularly in patients who cannot use ergots or sumatriptan. Opioids should not be used more than an average of 2 days/wk.[2] Dependence and risk for rebound headaches after abrupt opioid discontinuation occurs within 2 to 3 weeks of regular use; therefore, doses should be slowly reduced when therapy is discontinued. Combination preparations containing nonopioid analgesics, caffeine, and intermediate-acting barbiturates possess a similar abuse and rebound potential.[26] The analgesic action of the opioids is related to their action at the μ, κ, and δ opioid receptors located on neurons at supraspinal and spinal levels. Opioids may also produce peripheral analgesia by modulating neuropeptide release from receptor endings.[27]

The efficacy of opioid analgesics in headache treatment is poorly documented in the literature. In a retrospective trial, only 29% of patients with an acute migraine attack experienced relief from an intramuscular combination of meperidine and promethazine. DHE/metoclopramide was superior to meperidine/hydroxyzine and butorphanol in an open-label study. A double-blind trial with intramuscular butorphanol showed dose-dependent relief of acute migraine, but 21 and 42% of patients required pain and antiemetic relief medication, respectively. The nasal formulation of butorphanol is more effective than placebo and has a faster onset of action than intramuscular methadone in patients with moderate to severe migraine headaches.[6,28] The effect of mixed agonist-antagonists on rebound headache is unclear; however, they have a lower abuse potential than pure agonists.[2]

The most common adverse effects of opioids are sedation, nausea, and vomiting; however, psychiatric reactions have been reported.[27] Butorphanol has an adverse effect profile similar to that of most other opioids and sedation may occur in 43% of patients.[29] In general, opioids should not be used in patients with a history of abuse potential.

Combination Preparations

Combination products are used when patients do not respond to simple analgesics. The ingredients of these products may have synergistic activity, thus allowing lower doses to be used and adverse effects to be minimized. Prudent use of combination analgesics is very effective in stopping or reducing the severity of TTH. Patients with a history of coronary artery disease or transient ischemic attacks have limited choices for migraine relief and combination analgesics are a good choice for these individuals.[2] Overuse of combination analgesics may lead to addiction and rebound headaches, so it is recommended that their use be limited, on average, to 2 days/wk.[21]

Aspirin and acetaminophen are often combined with butalbital, caffeine, and other opioids (codeine, propoxyphene, dihydrocodeine, hydrocodone, or oxycodone). Butalbital helps reduce anxiety and aids in sleep, whereas caffeine enhances drug absorption and may enhance analgesia.[30] More than 200 mg of caffeine per day may lead to caffeine withdrawal headaches after drug discontinuation.[20] A combination product containing acetaminophen, aspirin, and caffeine was superior to placebo in the treatment of migraine headaches.[31] The combination treatment statistically improved nausea, photophobia, and phonophobia as well as headaches at 30 minutes. Adverse events associated with the combination treatment were comparable to the adverse events seen with the acetaminophen, aspirin, or caffeine alone. Acute use of acetaminophen should be limited to 4000 mg/day for less than 10 days, and chronic use should be limited to less than 2600 mg/day. In addition, some clinicians limit acetaminophen use to less than two to three times per week. Adverse effects of opioids include drowsiness and dizziness.

Selective Serotonin Agonists (Triptans)

There are currently four triptan agents available in the United States: sumatriptan, zolmitriptan, naratriptan, and rizatriptan. Eletriptan, almotriptan, and frovatriptan are awaiting Food and Drug Administration (FDA) approval. Triptans are indicated for the treatment of acute migraine; however, SC sumatriptan is also indicated for the treatment of cluster headaches.[32] All agents are available in tablet formulations, but sumatriptan is also available in SC injection, IN, and rectal dosage forms (Europe). Rizatriptan is also available as a rapidly dissolving oral wafer.

Sumatriptan is a serotonin receptor agonist with a high affinity for $5\text{-HT}_{1B/D}$ receptors, relative selectivity for 5-HT_{1D} receptors, and a low affinity for 5-HT_{1A} receptors.[32] Zolmitriptan, naratriptan, and rizatriptan also have a high affinity for 5-$HT_{1B/1D}$ receptors. There are slight differences between the agents in their affinity for the other 5-HT receptor subtypes.

The pharmacokinetic properties of triptans are shown in Table 51.7. Triptans exhibit variable oral absorption with naratriptan being the most bioavailable. The rizatriptan and zolmitriptan wafer contents are not absorbed through the buccal cavity, but rather swallowed with the saliva and absorbed later in the GI system. Triptans are not highly protein bound and with the exception of sumatriptan, all penetrate the CNS. The significance of CNS penetration is unknown and apparently does not relate to drug efficacy or to the incidence of adverse neurologic events. All triptans undergo hepatic biotransformation. Zolmitriptan and rizatriptan have active metabolites that achieve plasma concentrations 66 and 14%, respectively, of those of the parent drugs. Unlike other triptans, naratriptan does not undergo metabolism via monoamine oxidase (MAO_A) but rather via cytochrome P-450. More than half of the triptan metabolites are excreted into the urine with 50% of the naratriptan dose being excreted unchanged in the urine. The half-life of naratriptan is approximately twice that of the other agents.

Some drugs, but not food, affect the pharmacokinetic properties of oral triptans. Oral contraceptives increase plasma naratriptan concentrations whereas smoking decreases plasma naratriptan concentrations. Propranolol increases the plasma concentrations of rizatriptan (limiting the dose) and zolmitriptan. Cimetidine increases zolmitriptan concentrations. Pharmacodynamic drug interactions with triptans are also important. Triptans should not be administered within 24 hours of treatment with another triptan, ergot alkaloid, or methysergide. Serotonin syndrome (weakness, hyperreflexia, and poor coordination) may very rarely occur when triptans and selective serotonin reuptake inhibitors (SSRIs) are coadministered. Triptan therapy (except naratriptan) should also commence no sooner than 2 weeks after MAO_A inhibitor treatment discontinuation.[32–35]

SC sumatriptan offers the fastest onset of pain relief. Headache relief starts within 10 minutes after injection, and migraine pain is reduced or completely relieved in 70% of patients within 1 hour and in 86% of patients within 2 hours. SC sumatriptan also ameliorates nausea, vomiting, photophobia, and phonophobia and is effective in the treatment of perioperative migraine, menstrual migraine, and early morning migraine. Smaller doses (2 to 4 mg) provide headache relief in 70% of patients with TTH with coexistent migraine, albeit with a slower onset of action (60 minutes). SC sumatriptan also effectively relieves cluster headaches, often producing benefit 5 to 7 minutes after administration.[32]

Orally administered sumatriptan is almost equivalent in migraine efficacy to SC sumatriptan, but has a longer onset time (30 to 60 minutes versus 10 minutes).[36] The oral formulation exhibits a dose-dependent efficacy profile that plateaus at 50 to 100 mg above, which the incidence of adverse effects increases significantly.[6]

IN sumatriptan, an alternative to SC administration, has a slightly delayed onset of action (15 to 20 minutes) with maximum effect achieved by 2 hours. Two hours after sumatriptan administration, the efficacy of a 20-mg nasal spray (62 to 78%) is slightly better than that of a 100-mg oral tablet (51 to 69%), comparable to that of a 25-mg suppository (68%), and equivalent to that of a 6-mg SC injection (62 to 85%).[32]

Many patients who initially respond to sumatriptan report a return of headache symptoms within 24 to 48 hours after dosing. Naratriptan has a lower headache recurrence rate, perhaps owing to its longer half-life. Approximately half of patients, however, who take an oral triptan for migraine headaches may require an additional dose or other relief medication 24 hours after the initial dose. Repeated administration of SC sumatriptan is not recommended for those with no response, although those with a partial response may receive an additional dose within a 24-hour interval. An intranasal sumatriptan dose may be repeated once in 2 hours if the headache persists. A dose-related increase in migraine relief is seen with doses up to

Table 51.7 ▪ Comparisons of Oral Triptans

	Sumatriptan	Naratriptan	Zolmitriptan	Rizatriptan
Bioavailability (%)	14	70	40	45
T_{max} during headache (hr)	1.5–2.5	3–4	2–3	1–1.5[a]
Volume of distribution (L/kg)	2.4	2.5	7.0	2.0
Half-life (hr)	2.5	6	3	2–3
Metabolism	MAO_A	CYP450	CYP450, MAO_A	MAO_A
Active metabolite	No	No	Yes	Yes
Renally excreted unchanged (%)	3	50	8	14
Responding at 2 hr (%)[b]	51–69	48	60–67	71
Responding at 4 hr (%)[b]	71–79	60–66	77	NA

Sources: References 2, 32–35.

T_{max}, time to maximum concentration; *MAO_A*, monoamine oxidase; *CYP450*, cytochrome P-450; *NA*, not available.

[a]Wafer form 1.6–2.5 hr.

[b]Percentage of patients reporting headache relief.

40 mg, suggesting a ceiling effect or saturation of the nasal mucosa. The safety of treating more than four headaches with IN sumatriptan within a 30-day period has not been established; the maximum daily dose is 40 mg.[32,37]

SC sumatriptan has the highest incidence of adverse effects, while all oral triptans have a similar incidence of adverse effects. Less than 10% of patients receiving zolmitriptan, naratriptan, or rizatriptan discontinue treatment after a year as a result of adverse effects. Note that triptans can cause coronary artery vasospasm and should be used cautiously in patients with coronary artery disease (CAD), peripheral vascular disease (PVD), or uncontrolled hypertension, in patients at risk for these disorders, or in those older than 40 years of age. Physicians should carefully monitor patients with risk factors for CAD for adverse effects after administration of the first triptan dose and perform an electrocardiogram (ECG) in the rare event that angina-like symptoms occur.[2] Other adverse events include atypical sensations (paresthesia or warm feelings), pain sensations (neck, jaw, or chest pressure, pain, or tightness), GI symptoms (dry mouth and nausea), and neurologic symptoms (dizziness or somnolence). IN administration of sumatriptan may lead to taste disturbances, nausea, and nasal discomfort, while SC sumatriptan causes injection site pain.[32]

Nonselective Serotonin Agonists

Ergots are used for both acute and preventive treatment of migraine and cluster headaches. These agents effectively reduce the intensity and duration of attacks and are used to treat moderate to severe migraines when simple analgesics fail.[2] Preventive ergot use, however, should be reserved for patients with menstrual migraine and cluster headaches at the beginning of a cycle. Ergotamine is available as sublingual, oral, or suppository dosage forms. The sublingual route of administration is the least effective, and the rectal route is the most effective.[2,6] Ergotamine is also available in combination with caffeine.

DHE, an ergot derivative, is generally preferred over ergotamine because it causes less nausea (except when given IV) and rarely causes rebound headaches. DHE can be administered by SC, IM, or IV injection and IN. Although the parenteral forms of DHE are slightly more effective than the IN formulation, they cause more adverse effects.[2]

In contrast to the triptans, ergot alkaloids are nonspecific serotonergic (5-HT_{1A}, 5-HT_{1B}, 5-HT_{1C}, 5-HT_{1D}, and 5-HT_{1F}), adrenergic (α agonist and antagonist), and dopaminergic receptor agonists.[2,3] Ergots also cause arterial and venous vasoconstriction, decrease platelet aggregation, and decrease neurogenic inflammation. DHE, a less potent vasoconstrictor, also inhibits the baroreceptor circulatory reflex and has a greater effect on venous capacitance vessels than on arterial resistance vessels.[6]

Ergotamine has been available for many years and is used as a reference standard in controlled trials with newer agents. However, it has been compared, in controlled trials, to the newer agents. One of the first efficacy studies reported headache relief in 41% of patients taking 2 mg orally every hour up to 8 mg and in 89% of patients taking IV ergotamine 0.5 mg. Oral ergotamine (1 to 6 mg) was equivalent or superior to placebo, aspirin (500 mg), isometheptene (130 to 390 mg), and various NSAIDs, but not as good as sumatriptan (100 mg orally). It is not clear whether ergotamine should be avoided during the aura phase of migraine.[6]

Open-label trials indicate that parenteral DHE aborts 75% of migraine attacks. One double-blind study found that IV DHE with metoclopramide was superior to placebo, meperidine with hydroxyzine, and butorphanol. Another study found that DHE was superior to lidocaine but inferior to chlorpromazine.[6] Repetitive IV DHE is 90% effective in treating daily headache, status migrainosus, and cluster headache.[38] DHE can also be self-administered via SC injection, and 45% of patients interviewed after 2 to 3 years of self-administered IM DHE had at least a 50% response.[39] SC DHE has a slower onset of action but is as effective as SC sumatriptan with less headache recurrence.[40]

IN DHE is as effective as oral ergotamine tartrate with caffeine but inferior to SC sumatriptan in relieving migraine attacks.[41] DHE nasal spray may not be as good as IV DHE in relieving acute cluster headache, and higher doses of the nasal spray may be needed.[7] About 27% of patients respond to IN DHE after 30 minutes[42] and 35 to 71% of patients experience headache reversal after 30 minutes.[6,43] Increasing the dose beyond 2 mg does not increase efficacy.[42]

Ergotamine absorption is more complete and less erratic with rectal administration than with oral.[44] The absorption of DHE is most erratic with SC injection.[4,45] The bioavailability of DHE is 100% after IM administration, but only 40% after IN administration and less than 1% after oral, owing to extensive first-pass hepatic metabolism.[6,46] Ergotamine and DHE are primarily metabolized in the liver with a clearance about equal to hepatic blood flow. Ergotamine's elimination half-life is 3 hours with a terminal half-life of approximately 21 hours. DHE's half-life is approximately 10 hours, and it has an active metabolite that is present at plasma concentrations 5 to 7 times higher than those of the parent drug. Dosage schemes are individualized for each patient, starting with the lowest dose and increasing to the highest dose that does not cause nausea.[4,6] Oral or rectal administration of antiemetics 15 to 30 minutes before ergotamine administration decreases the associated nausea.

The adverse effects of ergotamine include nausea, vomiting, abdominal discomfort, peripheral vasoconstriction, thirst, pruritus, vertigo, muscle cramps, and paresthesias. Chronic ergotamine use can lead to vasospasm, anorectal ulcers, ischemic neuropathy, fibrotic disorders, and drug-induced headache.[6] Ergotamine overuse can also cause rebound headaches in migraineurs, and clinicians often restrict its use to fewer than two doses a week except in patients with cluster headache, who may use ergots nightly at the beginning of a cycle, as a preventive measure.[2] Overdose or prolonged use can cause ergotism and cyanosis, claudication, or gangrene of limbs. Symptoms of ergotism include nausea, confusion, drowsiness, postural hypotension, vasospasm, distal paresthesias, and coldness of the extremities. Ergotism should be treated with a vasodilator for 24 hours.[6] Both ergotamine and DHE should be used with caution in patients with CAD, PVD, or uncontrolled hypertension. They are contraindicated for use in pregnant patients or in patients with sepsis, renal failure, or hepatic failure.[47]

Adverse effects of DHE include burning at the injection site, dizziness, paresthesias, abdominal cramps, and chest tightness. IN DHE may cause nausea, a bitter taste, and local irritation of the nose and throat.[4] Patients with cardiac risk factors or who are older than 40 years old should undergo ECG testing before receiving the first ergot dose.[2]

The risk of ergot-induced adverse events may be increased with concurrent use of methysergide, β-blockers, dopamine, erythromycin derivatives, and sumatriptan.[6] To avoid excessive vasoconstriction, patients should wait at least 6 hours after a sumatriptan dose before taking an ergot preparation.

Corticosteroids

Corticosteroids may decrease perivascular inflammation and are used in episodic and chronic cluster headaches as well as status migrainosus. Intravenous corticosteroids may be used in combination with neuroleptics, opioids, metoclopramide, or DHE to treat refractory migraine headaches. Parenteral corticosteroids may be beneficial as monotherapy when ergot preparations are contraindicated or have failed.[21] Steroids are believed to be effective even when patients have had symptoms for a few days and have not responded to other migraine medications.

Corticosteroids are the fastest acting of the cluster headache therapies, with responses occurring in 1 to 2 days. They are only used as initial therapy for less than a month to break the cluster headache cycle before other medications with slower onset of action can take effect. The most commonly used steroids for episodic cluster headaches are prednisone (up to 100 mg/day) and dexamethasone (4 mg twice daily) administered for 2 to 3 weeks in tapering doses. Prednisone produces marked relief in 77% of episodic cluster headache patients and partial improvement in another 12%. Steroids improve chronic cluster headaches in 40% of patients.

Adverse effects include insomnia, mood changes, hyponatremia, hyperglycemia, osteoporosis, and gastric ulcers. Episodic and chronic cluster headaches may recur when steroids are discontinued. Steroids are relatively contraindicated in patients with hypertension, peptic ulcer disease, diabetes, and diverticulosis.[4,7] Additional information regarding corticosteroid pharmacotherapy and monitoring is described in Chapter 13, Rheumatoid Arthritis.

Neuroleptics

Phenothiazines are the neuroleptics most commonly used to treat acute migraine, TTH, and status migrainosus. These agents antagonize dopamine, decrease 5-HT reuptake, produce anticholinergic effects, and block α-adrenergic receptors (which induces orthostatic hypotension). The dopaminergic blockade is responsible for the drug's beneficial antiemetic effect and undesirable extrapyramidal symptoms. Intravenous injections of chlorpromazine or prochlorperazine are 70 to 90% effective in relieving migraine headaches.[6] Although this route of administration is more effective than intramuscular or rectal doses, it carries a greater risk for orthostatic hypotension.[48] The pharmacokinetics of neuroleptic agents are very similar to those of the antidepressants and some (chlorpromazine, thioridazine, and haloperidol) also have active metabolites. Droperidol, a neuroleptic related to haloperidol, has been shown in open trials to be an effective antimigraine agent when given IM or IV.[49]

Up to 80% of patients may experience adverse effects after parenteral injections of phenothiazines, with drowsiness being the most common. Akathisia is seen less frequently, and dystonic reactions are rare. Additional information regarding neuroleptic pharmacotherapy and monitoring is described in Chapter 57, Schizophrenia.

β-Blockers

Preventive use of β-blockers is 60 to 80% effective in producing a 50% reduction in migraine attack frequency and severity. It is unclear how β-blockers prevent migraine, but their action is most likely related to the inhibition of β_1-receptors with secondary effects on serotonin.[50] β-Blockers with intrinsic sympathomimetic activity (ISA), such as pindolol and acebutolol, are less effective in the treatment of migraine.[6] β-Blockers are particularly useful in patients with hypertension or angina. The relative efficacy between the agents in this class (propranolol, metoprolol, timolol, nadolol, and atenolol) has not been clearly established, so the choice should be based on β_1-selectivity, lack of ISA, idiosyncratic adverse effects, and comorbid conditions. The use of long-acting formulations may improve compliance and if one agent does not work, the patient may respond to a different β-blocker. Patients with both migraine and TTH may benefit from a combination of a β-blocker and a tricyclic antidepressant.[51] β-Blockers are contraindicated in pregnant patients or those who have asthma, depression, hypotension, congestive heart failure, Raynaud's disease, or diabetes. Approximately 10 to 15% of patients experience adverse effects; the most common involve the CNS (fatigue, sedation, sleep abnormalities, depression, memory impairment, and hallucinations), but patients may also complain of GI upset, impotence, and cardiovascular effects (orthostasis, bradycardia, and decreased exercise tolerance).[6] β-Blockers may precipitate ergotism when taken with an ergot preparation.[52] Additional information regarding β-blocker pharmacotherapy and monitoring is described in the Cardiovascular Disorders section.

Antidepressants

Antidepressants are 40 to 70% effective in reducing the frequency of migraine and TTH. Tricyclic antidepressants inhibit norepinephrine and serotonin reuptake. The atypical antidepressants (fluoxetine, fluvoxamine, sertraline, and paroxetine) are SSRIs. The monoamine oxidase inhibitors (MAOIs) block the degradation of catecholamines. The lack of a temporal relationship between reuptake inhibition (within hours), prophylactic headache response (3 to 10 days), and antidepressant action (2 to 3 weeks) indicates that antinociceptive efficacy may be unrelated to antidepressant action. Antidepressant plasma concentrations do not correlate with headache efficacy. The antinociceptive activity of antidepressants may be related to decreases in β-receptor density and norepinephrine-mediated cyclic AMP response, upregulation of $GABA_B$-receptors, and downregulation of 5-HT_2-receptors. Of these, inhibition of the 5-HT_2-receptors and 5-HT reuptake inhibition may be most crucial. Antidepressants are useful in patients with concurrent depression, anxiety, insomnia, or pain disorders. Generally the MAOIs and tricyclic antidepressants (TCAs) are more effective than the SSRIs but they have a greater risk of adverse effects.[2,4,6]

Amitriptyline, nortriptyline, and doxepin are the most commonly used TCAs, but only amitriptyline has been proven effective in a double-blind, placebo-controlled trial.[22] Low doses of TCAs, administered 1 hour before bedtime, are usually sufficient.[25] SSRIs have gained popularity due to their positive theoretical effect on migraine and good safety profile. Fluoxetine has varying results in preventing migraine[25] but improves chronic daily headache.[2] Venlafaxine may be effective, but has not been studied in patients with headaches. Trazodone, a serotonin-specific antidepressant, should be avoided because it is metabolized to *m*-chlorophenylpiperazine, a 5-HT_{1A} and 5-$HT_{2A/C}$ receptor agonist and migraine precipitant.[53]

Adverse effects of TCAs occur in 10 to 20% of patients and include anticholinergic effects, cardiovascular effects, sexual dysfunction, and weight gain. These agents are contraindicated in patients with narrow-angle glaucoma and urinary retention and should be used with caution in patients with cardiac disease or seizure disorders. Although SSRIs are less likely to produce sedation, weight gain, and cardiovascular changes, they may induce headaches, insomnia, and sexual dysfunction. The adverse effect profile of the MAOIs is similar to that of the TCAs, but concurrent ingestion of tyramine-containing foods, meperidine, or sympathomimetic agents, including isometheptene, may precipitate a hypertensive crisis. The concurrent use of fluoxetine and MAOIs has resulted in fatalities, and several weeks must elapse before one agent can be initiated after discontinuation of the other.[4] Additional information regarding antidepressant pharmacotherapy and monitoring is described in Chapter 56, Mood Disorders.

Calcium Channel Blockers

These agents are used primarily in the prevention of migraine and cluster headaches,[2,6] but some parenteral or sublingual formulations may be used acutely. Calcium channel blockers decrease the frequency of the attacks, have minimal effect on headache severity and are, generally, not as effective as other agents. In addition, the vasodilatory action of some calcium channel blockers may induce or worsen migraine attacks.[21] They are particularly useful in patients who have a prolonged aura phase, a migrainous infarction, are unable to take β-blockers, or have hypertension or angina.[2]

The mechanism of action of calcium channel blockers is unclear but excessive levels of intracellular calcium under ischemic conditions can produce neuronal damage and cell death. Calcium enters the cell primarily by slow voltage-sensitive channels and NMDA-linked receptor channels. Calcium channel blockers affect slow voltage-sensitive calcium channels, of which there are three subtypes, L, T, and N. L-type calcium channels are present in cardiovascular smooth muscle as well as endocrine cells and some neurons. T-type channels are also found in cardiac tissue, whereas N-type channels only affect neurons and mediate system neurotransmitter release. Most calcium channel blockers used in the treatment of headaches affect the L-type channel.[54] Flunarizine exhibits nonspecific antagonism to sodium as well as primarily T- and N-type calcium channels and may therefore have an advantage in terms of cerebral cell protection and lack of cardiovascular effects.[55] The antimigraine effect of flunarizine does not appear to correlate with its dopaminergic blockade.[56] The high lipid solubility of calcium channel blockers, in particular nicardipine, is important for drug penetration into the lipid bilayer of neuronal cells and the site of action.

Studies with calcium channel blockers in headache have focused primarily on three agents: verapamil, nimodipine, and flunarizine. Parenteral (20 mg) or sublingual (10 mg) flunarizine may be useful in treating acute migraine attacks.[4] Oral verapamil prophylaxis is only 40% effective in reducing migraine frequency by 50%.[57] Nifedipine is not considered effective in migraine prophylaxis, usually causing a dull persistent headache, and nimodipine shows limited efficacy only in the prevention of migraine with aura.[6] Small uncontrolled studies with diltiazem and nicardipine support their use in the preventive treatment of migraine.[6,58] Flunarizine appears to be the most efficacious and is comparable to β-blockers in this respect.[6] Nimodipine and verapamil are 50 to 80% effective in reducing cluster headache symptoms.[7] An adequate trial of therapy may require at least 2 months because of a delayed onset of action, which can increase a patient's frustration and decrease compliance.[25]

The most common adverse effects include dizziness, depression, tremor, constipation, peripheral edema, hypotension, and bradycardia. Flunarizine may cause weight gain, sedation, extrapyramidal symptoms, and depression. Calcium channel blockers are relatively contraindicated in patients with significant heart block, congestive heart failure, hypotension, and sick sinus syndrome.[21] Additional information regarding calcium channel blocker pharmacotherapy and monitoring is described in the Cardiovascular Disorders section.

Serotonin Antagonists

Methysergide

Methysergide is a semisynthetic ergot 5-HT_{1D} receptor agonist and 5-HT_{2A}, 5-HT_{2B} and 5-HT_{2C} receptor antagonist used to prevent migraine and cluster headaches. Methysergide may prevent migraines by decreasing platelet aggregation, inhibiting neurogenic plasma extravasation and inflammation, and producing vasoconstriction in the carotid vascular bed. It has an active metabolite, methylergometrine, with dopamine agonist activity. Methylergonovine (methylergometrine) is effective in migraine prophylaxis, but it has not been well studied.[21] In open-label trials, methysergide (6 to 16 mg/day) decreased headache frequency by more than 50 in 64% of migraineurs. Methysergide may be less effective in migraine with aura (53%) than without aura (76%). Several controlled trials have shown methysergide (3 to 6 mg/day) to be superior to cyproheptadine and comparable to pizotifen, lisuride, propranolol, and flunarizine in the prophylaxis of migraine.[2,4,6]

Methysergide is about 70% effective in the prevention of cluster headaches. It may be the drug of choice for preventing episodic cluster headaches in patients less than 30 years of age because these headaches usually last less than 4 months. It is less effective in chronic cluster headaches.[2] Cluster cycles are usually less than 3 months in duration and the development of long-term adverse effects is less of a concern. Tachyphylaxis with chronic use may be seen.[4,7]

The oral bioavailability of methysergide is only 13% due to extensive hepatic first-pass metabolism. Peak blood concentrations occur within an hour and the drug crosses the blood-brain barrier and distributes into breast milk. The elimination half-lives of methysergide and methylergometrine are 60 and 220 minutes, respectively.[6]

Methysergide is used as a last resort in headache prevention because the risk of serious adverse effects is greater than that for other medications, with 20% of patients discontinuing therapy.[6] Initial adverse effects, which often decrease with time, include muscle aches, hallucinations, abdominal discomfort, and nausea/vomiting. Concomitant administration of food or antacids or dividing the daily dose decreases GI effects. Other adverse effects include peripheral arterial insufficiency, peripheral edema, and weight gain. Of most concern is retroperitoneal, pulmonary, or endocardial fibrosis, a rare and chronic complication (1:2500). A 1-month drug holiday every 6 months to minimize these adverse effects has been suggested, but this approach has not been proven to be useful.[2,4,6] When a drug holiday is initiated, the dose should be tapered down over at least a week to minimize rebound headaches. During the drug holiday, patients will require other prophylactic treatment. Fibrotic changes may be detected with a chest radiograph, an echocardiogram, or magnetic resonance imaging of the abdomen.[7] Patients should be told to contact their doctor if they experience any coldness or pain in their fingers or toes, flank pain, chest pain, or dysuria. Fortunately, fibrotic changes usually regress after drug discontinuation. Methysergide use is contraindicated in patients with cardiovascular disease, cerebrovascular disease, severe hypertension, peripheral vascular disease, peptic ulcer disease, pregnancy and familial fibrotic disorders. Methysergide, combined with ergotamine or sumatriptan, can cause severe vasoconstriction.[6]

Cyproheptadine

Cyproheptadine is a 5-HT_{2A}, 5-HT_{2B}, and 5-HT_{2C} antagonist with antihistaminic and anticholinergic activity. It is often used for migraine prophylaxis in childhood migraine or hormonally mediated migraines. Open-label studies indicate that cyproheptadine improves migraine in 43 to 65% of patients, but comparative trials indicate that it is inferior to methysergide. Adverse drug reactions are considered to be fewer than with methysergide and include drowsiness, dizziness, dry mouth, increased appetite, and weight gain. Cyproheptadine is contraindicated in patients with glaucoma. Administering the majority of the dose at bedtime may minimize daytime drowsiness.[2,4,6]

Anticonvulsants

Carbamazepine and phenytoin have shown some effectiveness in decreasing headache pain; however, valproic acid is the most commonly used preparation in patients with migraine, CDH, or cluster headaches. Lamotrigine has been studied for migraine prophylaxis, with conflicting results.[59] Gabapentin has decreased migraine and CDH in open trials, and controlled trials are currently in progress. Valproic acid is the drug of choice for migraine patients with concurrent manic-depressive disorders, epilepsy, paroxysmal electroencephalograms (EEGs) or anxiety disorders.[2]

Valproic acid's efficacy is comparable to that of β-blockers and flunarizine.[60] It is, however, more effective in reducing duration, severity, and frequency of attacks in severe migraines than in mild to moderate migraine.[61] Headache frequency decreases by 50% in 48% of migrainures.[60,62,63] Patients with cluster headaches also showed improvement with valproic acid (600 to 2,000 mg/day) in one small, open-label study.[7] Patients with TTH do not improve with valproic acid.[60] If a partial response is noted with a low dose, increasing the dose may improve efficacy; however, if no response is noted at the low dose, increasing the dose will not be beneficial. Some clinicians, however, may increase the dose of valproic acid to achieve a trough level of 120 mg/ml in nonresponders.[2] The most common adverse effects reported in these trials were nausea, dyspepsia, fatigue, increased appetite, and weight gain. Other adverse effects include sedation, tremor, transient hair loss, increased bleeding time, and thrombocytopenia. Hepatotoxicity is rare, but baseline liver function tests should be obtained. Using divalproex, a delayed-release valproic acid derivative, may minimize nausea. Valproic acid is relatively contraindicated in patients with liver disease or bleeding disorders and in children younger than 10 years of age.

Lamotrigine and gabapentin do not alter the metabolism of other drugs. Valproic acid decreases the metabolism of many drugs. Phenytoin and carbamazepine increase the metabolism of many drugs. Thus, the efficacy and toxicity of any concomitant therapy should be evaluated when these antiepileptic drugs are added or discontinued. Additional information regarding anticonvulsant pharmacotherapy and monitoring is described in Chapter 52, Seizure Disorders.

Lithium Carbonate

Lithium is used in the treatment of both cyclic migraine and cluster headaches. The mechanism of action of lithium is unclear, but it may alter circadian rhythms, reduce rapid eye movement sleep, or decrease neuronal activity by depleting inositol. More patients with chronic (78%) than episodic (63%) cluster headache respond to preventive lithium and, in nearly 20% of patients receiving lithium, chronic cluster headaches change to episodic cluster headaches. Lithium improves headaches by 60 to 90% in 42% of patients with episodic cluster headaches and by more than 90% in 54% of patients with chronic cluster headaches. Triple therapy (lithium, verapamil, and ergotamine) has improved episodic cluster headaches in 90% of patients. Lithium has a half-life of approximately 24 hours, and a therapeutic response onset may take 1 to 2 weeks. Some patients may develop tolerance to lithium's effects. Serum concentrations should be monitored weekly during the titration phase and every 3 months thereafter.[4,6,7]

Common adverse effects include tremor, polyuria, nausea, muscle weakness, and ankle edema. Long-term adverse effects include hypothyroidism, renal failure, ECG changes, leukocytosis, and diabetes insipidus. Therefore, baseline monitoring should include thyroid function, urinalysis, ECG, leukocyte measurements, and electrolytes. Adverse effects can be minimized by maintaining lithium serum concentrations less than 1 mEq/L. Caution should be used when lithium is administered in conjunction with verapamil, because lithium doses will most likely need to be reduced. Changes in the patient's dietary salt intake or initiation of diuretic therapy will affect renal lithium elimination.[4] Additional information on lithium pharmacotherapy and monitoring is found in Chapter 56, Mood Disorders.

Lidocaine

Lidocaine, a local anesthetic that prevents the conduction of nerve impulses, effectively relieves cluster headaches[64,65]; however, its role in migraine is unclear.[66,67]

IV administration gives a faster onset of action, but a shorter duration, than IM administration. IN lidocaine is less than 50% bioavailable, and the concentrations of its metabolites (monoethylglycinexylidide and glycinexylidide) are undetectable.[68] Lidocaine plasma concentration monitoring is not useful in the treatment of headaches.

When administering IN lidocaine, patients should hyperextend their head and rotate their head toward the side of the headache, place the drops in the ipsilateral nostril, and remain recumbent to assure proper drug absorption. This procedure may be repeated once after 15 minutes. Adverse effects include taste alterations and burning sensations in the nasopharyngeal and ocular areas.[2,64,65]

Oxygen

Oxygen inhalation provides acute relief from cluster headaches, although in some attacks it may delay rather than abort the attack. The key to a successful response is high oxygen flow and content as well as sufficient time for inhalation. Administered through a mask, hyperbaric oxygen effectively relieved cluster attacks within 5 minutes in nearly 70% of patients.[2] Another trial with hyperbaric oxygen relieved cluster attacks in 86% of patients. In a preliminary report, 90% of patients treated with hyperbaric oxygen for 40 minutes had near-total migraine relief.[69]

Adjunctive Therapy

Many acute migraine medications relieve headache pain, but some have minimal or no effect on the associated symptoms of nausea, vomiting, and delayed GI emptying (gastric stasis). Gastric stasis may interfere with drug absorption.[21] Metoclopramide decreases nausea and vomiting but also enhances drug absorption by decreasing gastric stasis. Adjunctive therapy is most effective when administered at symptom onset.[2,70] Drowsiness and dizziness are the most common adverse effects, but dystonic reactions may occur rarely. If patients cannot tolerate the side effects of metoclopramide, ondansetron (a selective 5-HT_3 receptor antagonist) or neuroleptics will relieve associated symptoms.[2] Caffeine co-administration may also improve drug absorption and analgesia. Clonidine decreases autonomic withdrawal symptoms in patients who discontinue chronic or high opioid doses. The patch formulation may be helpful as adjunctive therapy for detoxification in patients who have headaches from excess analgesic or ergotamine use.[4,6]

Miscellaneous/Investigational Agents

Calcitonin, magnesium, α_1-adrenergic antagonists, and riboflavin are being evaluated for their role in migraine prophylaxis. Calcitonin, a polypeptide hormone secreted by the thyroid, may be effective in preventing migraine headaches.[4] Commercially available products use calcitonin extracted from salmon or synthesized to resemble human calcitonin. An injectable human calcitonin preparation is under development. Serum and cerebrospinal fluid levels of magnesium appeared low in patients experiencing migraine, leading to the hypothesis that magnesium supplementation would lower the incidence of migraine. Magnesium, however, did not reduce the incidence or the intensity of migraine headaches compared to placebo, but caused a higher incidence of diarrhea.[71] The duration and intensity of menstrual migraine and the severity of premenstrual syndrome symptoms, however, were reduced by oral magnesium in a small study.[2] Preliminary results with α_1-adrenergic antagonists are promising because low- to mid-range doses reduce the frequency and intensity of migraines.[72] Riboflavin at a dose of 400 mg/day was significantly more effective than placebo in decreasing headache frequency.[73]

IN capsaicin may abort cluster headaches. It reduces the frequency of headaches by 67% and provides complete relief in approximately half of the patients treated. Patients with episodic cluster headaches respond better to capsaicin than those with chronic cluster headaches.[28]

Nonpharmacologic Therapy

Some patients may have an inherited predisposition to headaches triggered by various habits, foods, hormones, or environmental factors[2,4] (Table 51.8). Identifying the trigger can be a difficult task for the patient. The patient should keep a diary of headache incidences, and record the time, place, meals, weather, presence of menses, amount of sleep or related habits that may be associated with the attack. Once a reproducible trigger has been determined, avoidance of the trigger may lessen attacks.

Nonpharmacologic treatments for migraine and TTH include relaxation techniques, hypnosis, psychotherapy, biofeedback, physical therapy, and acupuncture.[1,20,74] These techniques also may be used alone or in combination with drug therapy. Physical therapy helps patients relieve stress and muscle tension via massage, stretching exercises, aerobic exercises, ultrasound treatments, electric stimulation, and hot or cold pack therapy. Cold compresses to the affected area provided relief in 65 to 70% of TTH patients. Biofeedback teaches patients to control bodily functions including heart rate, blood pressure, and muscle tension by receiving feedback by visual, auditory, or electromyographic instruments and may decrease headaches in 65 to 85% of patients. Learning methods to release muscle tension, induce relaxation, and regulate breathing during daily activities helps alleviate headache pain. Dry needling or injection of local anesthetics or corticosteroids into trigger points may also relieve pain.

Treatment for Special Populations

Pregnant Patients

The true incidence of migraine during pregnancy is uncertain; however, headache symptoms improve in approximately 60 to 70% of migraineurs during pregnancy.[2] Tension headaches are rarely affected by pregnancy, although a slight increase may occur before delivery.[75]

Many conditions may mimic the clinical presentation of migraines and a thorough examination to establish a diagnosis is warranted when migraines occur for the first time during pregnancy. Neurodiagnostic tests should not be avoided if they are needed and if other methods cannot provide adequate information. Computed tomography of the head is considered safe.[2]

Nonpharmacologic treatments (reassurance, coping-skill development, ice, massage, and biofeedback) should be attempted before or in conjunction with medication use. Many medications cross the placenta, and pharmacologic treatment should be used for symptomatic relief of headache only when other means have failed. The use of some headache-relieving drugs is contraindicated or should be avoided during pregnancy.

For acute attacks, NSAIDs, acetaminophen (alone or with codeine), codeine alone, or other opioids can provide relief of symptoms. Aspirin may, when given in large doses near term, induce maternal or fetal bleeding. Barbiturate and benzodiazepine use should be limited, and all ergots are absolutely contraindicated owing to their known embryotoxicity. There are insufficient data on use of the triptans during pregnancy; however, the manufacturers of sumatriptan and naratriptan have a pregnancy registry to enroll pregnant women using triptans and monitor fetal outcomes.[76] Metoclopramide, trimethobenzamide, chlorpromazine, prochlorperazine, and promethazine can be used safely for intractable nausea and vomiting. Mild nausea can be treated with phosphorylated carbohydrate solution or doxylamine succinate and vitamin B_6 (pyridoxine).

Preventive therapy should be used only when the fetus is at risk, i.e., when excessive nausea and vomiting may result in malnutrition of the fetus. The patient needs to be informed of the risks involved in taking preventive treatment and evaluate the benefits versus risks in consultation with a caregiver. Methysergide is contraindicated in pregnancy. Barbiturates, phenytoin, and carbamazepine can impair folate absorption and reduce red cell folate levels, which has been associated with spontaneous abortions, fetal malformations, or neural tube defects in newborns. Valproic acid is teratogenic and should be discontinued 1 to 2 months before planned conception. Lithium may have a teratogenic risk and should be used cautiously in pregnancy. Fluoxetine and amitriptyline probably have the lowest teratogenic risk among the prophylactic agents.[2]

Table 51.8 ▪ Headache Triggers

Habits	Food	Hormonal	Environmental
Irregular sleep	Tyramine food	Menses	Bright lights, glare
Irregular exercise	Alcohol	Pregnancy	Stress
Irregular meals	Caffeine withdrawal	Menopause	Altitude changes
Smoking	Monosodium-glutamate		Extreme cold/heat
Alcohol			Loud noises
			Odors

Sources: References 2, 4.

After delivery, the transfer of maternal drug to the baby via breast-feeding is of concern because many drugs are secreted into breast milk. The clinical significance of this is questionable, however, because the drug concentration in breast milk may be low. Drugs that are compatible with breastfeeding are acetaminophen, opioids, β-blockers, adrenergic blockers, calcium channel blockers, carbamazepine, valproic acid, and corticosteroids. A breastfeeding migraineur should avoid bromocriptine, ergotamine, and lithium. Bromocriptine inhibits lactation, as does excessive or prolonged use of ergots. In addition, ergots are also secreted into breast milk and may cause signs of ergotism (nausea and vomiting) in the child. Lithium is also extensively secreted into breast milk (50% maternal concentration) and should only be used if the benefits outweigh the risks.[28] Triptans, benzodiazepines, antidepressants, and neuroleptics should be used cautiously, and barbiturates may cause excessive sedation in the nursing infants.[2] If the mother desires to use a triptan, she should express and discard her breast milk for 8 hours after the dose.[32]

Pediatric Patients

Acute treatment begins with analgesics and family reassurance. Acetaminophen should be used instead of aspirin because of the risk of Reye's syndrome. Because sudden changes in daily routine may cause headaches in children, an attempt should be made to maintain a regular daily schedule. The safety of ergots in children has not been established, and they should be avoided in young children; however, DHE can be used alone or in combination with metoclopramide or promethazine. Combination therapy can achieve an 80 to 90% improvement of intractable headaches. Two studies evaluating naratriptan and sumatriptan in children found both agents to be less effective in children than in adults,[77,78] and triptans are currently not indicated or recommended for children. Pediatric prophylactic drug therapy does not differ from that used in adult patients. The most commonly used medications are propranolol (1 to 3 mg/kg/day) and cyproheptadine (0.2 to 0.4 mg/kg/day). Tricyclic antidepressants may be used as adjunctive therapy or in patients with difficult-to-control headaches. A drug taper or holiday should be considered if a child has been headache-free for 3 months.[4]

Geriatric Patients

Headaches presenting after the age of 65 require a complete diagnostic examination to identify or exclude secondary etiologies, such as cerebrovascular disease, mass lesions, giant cell arteritis, trigeminal neuralgia, or medication-induced headaches (Tables 51.1 and 51.3). Nitrates are common pharmacologic triggers for migraine and cluster headaches. Therefore, treatment should primarily address the comorbid condition or trigger and/or provide symptomatic pain relief. Once secondary etiologies have been excluded, the primary headache disorder should be identified and treated accordingly. Nonpharmacologic treatment is preferred in older adults, because many of them have decreased renal or hepatic function, are more sensitive to side effects, and may receive concomitant medications that can interact with treatment. Preventive medicines should be reserved for patients with frequent or debilitating headaches. Ergots and serotonin agonists can cause vasoconstriction, leading to ischemia or exacerbation of hypertension, and should be used cautiously in older adults. Sedatives should be avoided. Older adults are also more prone to NSAID-induced peptic ulcer disease as well as extrapyramidal and anticholinergic effects of antiemetic agents and TCAs. The choice of a pharmacologic agent is very patient specific; all agents should be started at a low dose and titrated up very slowly until optimal relief with minimal side effects is achieved.[2]

ALTERNATIVE THERAPIES

Alternative therapies, such as acupuncture, chiropractic manipulation, herbal medicine, and aromatherapy, may be used alone or as adjunctive treatment.[79] Patients should consult a physician or pharmacist before trying these therapies, because some of them may present more risk than benefit. Most of these treatments induce relaxation, alleviate stress, and may be more beneficial for TTH or stress-related migraines.

Acupuncture is recognized by the World Health Organization as a treatment for more than 100 conditions, and acupuncturists are licensed in more than 30 states across the United States. Special needles are placed at acupuncture pressure points to restore a balance in the flow of energy within the body and prevent headaches. Several studies have reported a decrease in the frequency and severity of headaches after acupuncture treatments.[79]

Chiropractic treatment of headaches focuses on spinal manipulation to correct subluxations and reduce muscle tension. Spinal manipulation probably provides little benefit,[80] and patients who report no headache relief after 6 weeks should be reevaluated.[79]

St John's wort (*Hypericum perforatum*) upregulates 5-HT_{1A} and 5-HT_{2A} receptors,[81] and feverfew (*Tanacetum parthenium*) may inhibit platelet aggregation and serotonin secretion.[82] Clinical data supporting the efficacy of these herbal remedies for headache are lacking.

The unique scent of essential oils used in aromatherapy may induce relaxation and relieve tension headaches or stress-related migraines. Patients inhale the vapors of chamomile, cardamom, lavender, marjoram, peppermint, and rosemary arising from a bowl of water or a bath. Many chiropractors, acupuncturists, and masseuses incorporate aromatherapy in their practice.

IMPROVING OUTCOMES

Patient Education

Patients should be educated about their headaches and their medications and about how to monitor their progress. They should be reassured that headaches are not life threatening and that headache frequency may be controlled but headaches may not completely disappear with treatment. Good sources of information include the National Headache Foundation (800-843-2256 or http://www.headaches.org) and the American Council for Headache Education (800-255-ACHE or http://www.achenet.org).

The response to medications is often idiosyncratic. A medication may provide relief without side effects in some patients but not be tolerated by others. Medication counseling should focus on the appropriate administration and monitoring of the prescribed medication. Patients should not adjust doses without consulting their physician or pharmacist. Medication overuse (excessive increases in dose or administration frequency) may be a sign of ineffective treatment, addiction, or tolerance and may lead to CDH. Patients need to be aware of common medication-related adverse effects and the need to let their physician know when they occur. Patients receiving IN DHE should be told how to assemble the applicator, and those receiving IN sumatriptan should be told that they do not need to prime the applicator, because each canister delivers only one dose. Patients receiving SC sumatriptan should be taught how to load the autoinjector and how to discard the empty syringes. When using the autoinjector syringe, the patient should inject the contents into the deltoid muscle or the lateral part of the thigh. Recent evidence, however, suggests that the upper lateral quadrant of the gluteal area is a more appropriate injection site for muscular patients who lack adipose tissue in the thigh.[83]

Patients need to take an active role in their treatment to ensure resolution and relief of headaches. A diary helps patients be more aware of what triggers and controls their headaches. The diary should record the date and time of day of an attack as well as possible precipitating and relieving factors. Patients should also document medications taken and any positive or negative effects of these medications. Personal feelings experienced during headache attacks should also be recorded in the diary to help monitor changes in quality of life. The diary will aid the patient's physician in making medication adjustments and improving outcomes with less trial and error.

Health Care Provider Education

Health care providers need to be better educated about headache etiology and treatment. The incidence of CDH may be reduced if clinicians obtain a complete medication history and maintain periodic updates to rule out medication overuse. The patient diary should be reviewed to see if there are also any changes between office visits and especially after medication changes. This makes the patient more aware of the disease process and helps the physician or pharmacist monitor for compliance and evaluate the effectiveness and adverse effects of treatment.

PHARMACOECONOMICS

The economic burden of headaches includes both direct and indirect costs. In a study comparing health care resource utilization in a managed care organization, migraineurs spent 64% more on health care resources and incurred greater direct costs, such as physician or emergency department visits, additional medications (2.8 times more), and diagnostic procedures (6 times more), than nonmigraineurs.[84] Migraineurs also incur greater indirect costs, such as lost wages and decreased productivity. Adults spend 3 million days bedridden each month, children miss 3.2 million days per school year, and employers lose U.S. $5 to 17 billion per year from decreased productivity and missed workdays because of migraines.[85,86]

About 65% of patients suffering from headaches do not receive proper medical care and often self-medicate their condition with poor results.[18] Prescription drugs for headaches are expensive, and proper monitoring involves use of health care resources. Nevertheless, cost-effective care can significantly decrease the financial impact of headaches on society. Although preventive treatment increases treatment cost, it can decrease headache frequency and the cost of acute treatment and emergency department visits. Thus, cost-effective management of migraine headaches consists of appropriate use of nonpharmacologic and pharmacologic treatments to improve the patient's quality of life while minimizing overall cost. Proper management should optimize drug efficacy while reducing inappropriate drug usage and adverse effects.

Analgesics are the least expensive acute treatment option. Enteric-coated sustained release or nasal formulations cost more. Generally, the ergots are less expensive than the triptans, but this benefit is offset by the cost of adjunctive medications for nausea. The cost of all the oral triptans is comparable. Nasal sprays are more expensive than oral formulations but less expensive than injectable formulations. Health-related quality-of-life scores improved and workplace productivity increased by 12.1 to 89.8 hours/yr for patients receiving sumatriptan, which was greater than for other antimigraine therapies (aspirin, NSAIDs, opioids, barbiturates, caffeine, and ergot alkaloids).[32] The costs of the first-line agents (β-blockers and antidepressants) for prophylactic treatment of headaches are comparable.

KEY POINTS

- Proper headache classification is essential in choosing the appropriate therapy.
- All secondary causes of headache must be ruled out.
- Inappropriate management of headaches has a significant economic impact on worker productivity, quality of life, and health care costs.
- The goal of treatment is to reduce the frequency and severity of attacks and improve quality of life.
- Treatment involves both pharmacologic and nonpharmacologic measures, and their effects may be synergistic.

- Acute treatment should be limited to two to three times a week to avoid the development of rebound or chronic daily headache.
- Preventive therapy may not eliminate all headaches, and acute treatment may still be needed for breakthrough attacks.

REFERENCES

1. Silberstein SD. Tension-type and chronic daily headache. Neurology 43:1644–1649, 1993.
2. Silberstein SD, Lipton RB, Goadsby PJ. Headache in clinical practice. Oxford: Isis Medical Media, 1998.
3. Cady RK, Shealy CN. Recent advances in migraine management. J Fam Pract 36:85–91, 1993.
4. Dalessio DJ, Silberstein SD. Wolff's headache and other head pain. 6th ed. New York: Oxford University Press, 1993.
5. Lipton RB, Silberstein SD, Stewart WF. An update on the epidemiology of migraine. Headache 34:319–328, 1994.
6. Olesen J, Tfelt-Hansen P, Welch KMA. The Headaches. New York: Raven Press, 1993.
7. Silberstein SD. Pharmacological management of cluster headache. CNS Drugs 2:199–207, 1994.
8. Mathew NT. Cluster headache. Neurology 42(Suppl 2):22–31, 1992.
9. Bonica JJ. The management of pain. 2nd ed. Philadelphia: Lea & Febiger, 1990.
10. Russell MB, Iselius L, Olesen J. Migraine without aura and migraine with aura are inherited disorders. Cephalalgia 16:305–309, 1996.
11. Srikiatkhachorn A, Maneesri S, Govitrapong P, et al. Derangement of serotonin system in migrainous patients with analgesic abuse headache: clues from platelets. Headache 38:43–49, 1998.
12. Peroutka SJ. Dopamine and migraine. Neurology 49:650–656, 1997.
13. May A, Bahra A, Buchel C, et al. Lancet 352:275–278, 1998.
14. Schoenen J. Cluster headaches–central or peripheral in origin? Lancet 352:253–255, 1998
15. D'Andrea G, Granella F, Alecci M, et al. Serotonin metabolism in cluster headache. Cephalalgia 18:94–96, 1998.
16. Olesen J. Headache Classification Committee of the International Headache Society. Classification and diagnostic criteria for headache disorders, cranial neuralgia, and facial pain. Cephalalgia 8(Suppl 7):1–96, 1988.
17. Carlsson J, Larsson B, Mark A. Psychosocial functioning in schoolchildren with recurrent headaches. Headache 36:77–82, 1996.
18. Rapoport AM, Adelman JU. Cost of migraine management: a pharmacoeconomic overview. Am J Manag Care 4:531–545, 1998.
19. Spierings ELH, van Hoof MJ. Anxiety and depression in chronic headache sufferers. Headache Q 7:235–238, 1996.
20. Trachtenbarg DE. Tension headaches. Postgrad Med 95:44–56, 1994.
21. Silberstein SD. Preventive treatment of migraine: an overview. Cephalalgia 17:67–72, 1997.
22. Noble SL, Moore KL. Drug treatment of migraine: part II. Preventive therapy. Am Fam Physician 56:2049–2054, 1997.
23. Capobianco DJ, Cheshire WP, Campbell JK. An overview of the diagnosis and pharmacological treatment of migraine. Mayo Clin Proc 71:1055–1066, 1996.
24. Bannwarth B, Netter P, Pourel J, et al. Clinical pharmacokinetics of nonsteroidal anti-inflammatory drugs in the cerebrospinal fluid. Biomed Pharmacother 43:121–126, 1989.
25. Baumel B. Migraine: a pharmacological review with newer options and delivery modalities. Neurology 44(Suppl 3):S13–S17, 1994.
26. Markley HG. Chronic headache: appropriate use of opiate analgesics. Neurology 44(Suppl 3):S18–S24, 1994.
27. Jaffe JH, Martin WR. Opioid analgesics and antagonists. In Goodman LS, Gilman A, Rall TW, et al., eds. The pharmacological basis of therapeutics. ed. 8. New York: McGraw-Hill, 1990:485–521.
28. Kumar KL. Recent advances in the acute management of migraine and cluster headaches. J Gen Intern Med 9:339–348, 1994.
29. Upmalis DH. Stadol NS [Letter]. Headache 33:394, 1993.
30. Migliardi JR, Armellino JJ, Friedman M, et al. Caffeine as an analgesic adjuvant in tension headache. Clin Pharmacol Ther 56:576–586, 1994.
31. Lipton RB, Stewart WF, Ryan RE, et al. Efficacy and safety of acetaminophen, aspirin, and caffeine in alleviating migraine headache pain. Arch Neurol 55:210–217, 1998.
32. Perry CM, Markham A. Sumatriptan. An updated review of its use in migraine. Drugs 55:889–922, 1998.
33. Package insert. Zomig® (zolmitriptan) tablets. Wilmington, DE: Zeneca Pharmaceuticals, November 1997.
34. Package insert. Amerge® (naratriptan hydrochloride) tablets. Research Triangle Park, NC: Glaxo Wellcome, January 1998.
35. Package insert. Maxalt® (rizatriptan benzoate) orally disintegrated tablets. West Point, PA: Merck & Co, June 1998.
36. Packheiser A, Levien T. Features of available triptans [Document 140809]. Pharmacist's Lett 14:1–4, 1998
37. Salonen R, Ashford E, Dahlof C, et al. Intranasal sumatriptan for the acute treatment of migraine. J Neurol 241:463–469, 1994.
38. Silberstein SD, Schulman EA, Hopkins MM. Repetitive intravenous DHE in the treatment of refractory headache. Headache 30:334–339, 1990.
39. Weisz MA, El-Raheb M, Blumenthal HJ. Home administration of intramuscular DHE for the treatment of acute migraine headache. Headache 34:371–373, 1994.
40. Winner P, Ricalde O, Le Force B, et al. A double-blind study of subcutaneous dihydroergotamine vs subcutaneous sumatriptan in the treatment of acute migraine. Arch Neurol 53:180–184, 1996.
41. Touchon J, Bertin L, Pilgrim AJ, et al. A comparison of subcutaneous sumatriptan and dihydroergotamine nasal spray in the acute treatment of migraine. Neurology 47:361–365, 1996.
42. Gallagher RM. Acute treatment of migraine with dihydroergotamine nasal spray. Dihydroergotamine Working Group. Arch Neurol 53:1285–1291, 1996.
43. The dihydroergotamine nasal spray multi-center investigators. Efficacy, safety, and tolerability of dihydroergotamine nasal spray as monotherapy in the treatment of acute migraine. Headache 35:177–184, 1995.
44. Sanders SW, Haering N, Mosberg H, et al. Pharmacokinetics of ergotamine in healthy volunteers following oral and rectal dosing. Eur J Clin Pharmacol 39:331–334, 1986.
45. Schran HF, Tse FLS. Pharmacokinetics of dihydroergotamine following subcutaneous administration in humans. Int J Clin Pharmacol Ther Toxicol 23:1–4, 1985.
46. Silberstein SD. The pharmacology of ergotamine and dihydroergotamine. Headache 37(Suppl 1):S15–S25, 1997.
47. Rall TW. Drugs affecting uterine motility. In Goodman LS, Gilman A, Rall TW, et al., eds. The pharmacological basis of therapeutics. ed. 8. New York: McGraw-Hill, 1990:933–953.
48. Thomas SH, Stone CK, Ray VG, et al. Intravenous versus rectal prochlorperazine in the treatment of benign vascular or tension headache: a randomized, prospective, double-blind trial. Ann Emerg Med 24:923–927, 1994.
49. Wang SJ, Silberstein SD, Young WB. Droperidol treatment of acute refractory migraine and status migrainosus. Headache 37:377–382, 1997.
50. Przegalinski E, Tataczynska E, Chojnacka-Wojcik E. The role of hippocampal 5-HT_{1A} receptors in the anticonflict activity of β adrenoceptor antagonists. Neuropharmacology 34:1211–1217, 1995.
51. Pfaffenrath V, Kellhammer U, Pöllmann W. Combination headache: practical experience with a combination of a β-blocker and an antidepressive. Cephalalgia 6(Suppl 5):25–32, 1986.
52. Venter CP, Joubert PH, Buys AC. Severe peripheral ischaemia during concomitant use of β blockers and ergot alkaloids. Br Med J 289:288–289, 1984.
53. Brewerton TD, Murphy DL, Mueller EA, et al. Induction of migraine like headaches by the serotonin agonist m-chlorophenylpiperazine. Clin Pharmacol Ther 43:605–609, 1988.
54. Triggle DJ. Calcium antagonists. History and perspective. Stroke 21(Suppl 12):IV49–IV58, 1990.
55. Pauwels PJ, Leysen JE, Janssen PA. Ca^{++} and Na^{+} channels involved in neuronal cell death. Protection by flunarizine. Life Sci 48:1881–1893, 1991.
56. Wober C, Brucke T, Wober-Bingol C, et al. Dopamine D_2 receptor blockade and antimigraine action of flunarizine. Cephalalgia 14:235–240, 1994.
57. Solomon GD. Verapamil in migraine prophylaxis–a five-year review. Headache 29:425–427, 1989.
58. Roumeau BJ. Nicardipine in the prevention of migraine headaches. Clin Ther 14:672–677, 1992.
59. Steiner TJ, Findley LJ, Yuen AW. Lamotrigine versus placebo in the prophylaxis of migraine with and without aura. Cephalalgia 17:109–112, 1997.
60. Jensen R, Brinck T, Olesen J. Sodium valproate has a prophylactic effect in migraine without aura: a triple-blind, placebo-controlled, crossover study. Neurology 44:647–651, 1994.
61. Kumar KL, Cooney TG. Headaches. Med Clin North Am 79:261–282, 1995.
62. Hering R, Kuritzky A. Sodium valproate has a prophylactic effect in migraine: a double-blind study vs placebo. Cephalalgia 12:81–84, 1992.
63. Rothrock JF, Kelly NM, Brody ML, et al. A differential response to treatment with divalproex sodium in patients with intractable headache. Cephalalgia 14:241–244, 1994.

64. Kittrelle JP, Grouse DS, Seybold ME. Cluster headache local anesthetic abortive agents. Arch Neurol 42:496–498, 1985.
65. Robbins L. Intranasal lidocaine for cluster headache. Headache 35:83–84, 1995.
66. Kudrow L, Kudrow DB, Sandweiss JH. Rapid and sustained relief of migraine attacks with intranasal lidocaine: preliminary findings. Headache 35:79–82, 1995.
67. Maizels M, Scott B, Cohen W, et al. Intranasal lidocaine for treatment of migraine. JAMA 276:319–321, 1996.
68. Scavone JM, Greenblatt DJ, Fraser DG. The bioavailability of intranasal lidocaine. Br J Clin Pharmacol 28:722–724, 1989.
69. Myers DE, Myers RA. A preliminary report on hyperbaric oxygen in the relief of migraine headache. Headache 35:197–199, 1995.
70. Albibi R, McCallum RW. Metoclopramide: pharmacology and clinical application. Ann Intern Med 98:86–95, 1983.
71. Pfaffenrath V, Wessley P, Meyer C, et al. Magnesium in the prophylaxis of migraine–a double blind, placebo controlled study. Cephalalgia 16:436–440, 1996.
72. Vatz KA. Alpha 1-Adrenergic blockers: do they have a place in the prophylaxis of migraine? Headache 37:107–108, 1997.
73. Schoenen J, Jacquy J, Lenaerts M. Effectiveness of high-dose riboflavin in migraine prophylaxis. A randomized controlled trial. Neurology 50:466–470, 1998.
74. Adler CS, Adler SM. Biofeedback-psychotherapy for the treatment of headache. Headache 16:189–191, 1976.
75. Scharff L, Marcus DA, Turk DC. Headache during pregnancy and in the postpartum: a prospective study. Headache 37:203–210, 1997.
76. Package insert. Imitrex® (sumatriptan) injection. Research Triangle Park, NC: Glaxo Wellcome, December 1997.
77. Hamalainen ML, Hoppu K, Santavuori P. Sumatriptan for migraine attacks in children: a randomized placebo controlled study. Neurology 48:1100–1103, 1997.
78. Rothner A, Edwards K, Kerr L, et al. Efficacy and safety of naratriptan tablets in adolescents in migraine. J Neurol Sci 150:S106, 1997.
79. Fox A, Fox B. Alternative healing: headaches. Franklin Lakes, NJ: Career Press, 1996.
80. Bove G, Nilsson N. Spinal manipulation in the treatment of episodic tension-type headache–a randomized controlled trial. JAMA 280:1576–1579, 1998.
81. Teufel-Mayer R, Gleitz J. Effects of long-term administration of hypericum extracts on the affinity and density of the central serotonergic 5-HT1A and 5-HT2A receptors. Pharmacopsychiatry 30(Suppl 2):113–116, 1997.
82. Groenwegen WA, Heptinstall S. A comparison of the effects of an extract of feverfew and parthenolide, a component of feverfew, on human platelet activity in-vitro. J Pharm Pharmacol 42:553–557, 1990.
83. Frid A, Hardebo JE. The thigh may not be suitable as an injection site for patients self-injecting sumatriptan. Neurology 49:559–561, 1997.
84. Clouse JC, Osterhaus JT. Healthcare resource use and costs associated with migraine in a managed healthcare setting. Ann Pharmacother 28:659–664, 1994.
85. Stang PE, Osterhaus JT. Impact of migraine in the United States: data from the National Health Interview Survey. Headache 33:29–35, 1993.
86. Osterhaus JT, Gutterman DG, Plachetka JR. Healthcare resource and lost labor costs of migraine headache in the United States. Pharmacoeconomics 2:67–76, 1992.

CHAPTER 52

SEIZURE DISORDERS

Brian K. Alldredge

Seizure Disorders

DEFINITION

A *seizure* is defined as the clinical manifestation of excessive or hypersynchronous activity of neurons within the cerebral cortex.[1] Although the term often connotes an event characterized by an abrupt loss of consciousness, with generalized muscle contraction and jerking (i.e., a generalized tonic-clonic or grand mal seizure), the clinical manifestations of various seizure types are quite heterogeneous. The specific signs and symptoms that accompany the event depend on the functional area of the brain that is involved and may include various degrees of motor, sensory, or cognitive dysfunction. The word *epilepsy* comes from the Greek word meaning *to seize* and is used to describe a disorder of recurrent seizures due to a chronic, underlying cause. Patients who experience isolated seizures due a correctable cause (e.g., drug toxicity, alcohol abuse, or metabolic abnormalities) do not necessarily have epilepsy.

TREATMENT GOALS: SEIZURE DISORDERS

- Accurately diagnose the patient's seizure type and epilepsy syndrome.
- Identify and eliminate patient-specific seizure precipitants.
- Select optimal antiepileptic drug therapy based on seizure type, epilepsy syndrome, patient age, sex, and concomitant medical conditions.
- Adjust antiepileptic drug therapy to attain complete control of seizures.
- Monitor for clinical and laboratory evidence of adverse effects of drug therapy.
- Minimize the use of poly-drug therapy and sedating antiepileptic drugs whenever possible.
- Address patient concerns regarding the effect of seizures (and antiepileptic drugs) on daily activities, employment, and social interactions.
- Recognize when patients should be referred to a comprehensive epilepsy center for evaluation of other therapeutic modalities, such as surgery, vagus nerve stimulation, or ketogenic diet.

EPIDEMIOLOGY

The lifetime prevalence of epilepsy is approximately 3%.[2] The incidence is highest in the first 10 years of life and declines thereafter through the age of 50 until the elderly years, when the incidence increases again. Epilepsy begins before the age of 18 in more than 75% of patients.[1] It is estimated that 1 of every 11 people in the United States will experience a seizure at some time during life.[2]

Seizures may result from primary or acquired disturbances of central nervous system (CNS) function, metabolic derangements, or a variety of systemic disorders. Some of the common causes of new-onset seizures are listed in Table 52.1. Common causes of seizures vary according to patient age. For example, fever is only a common cause of seizures during late infancy and early childhood. Similarly, inherited forms of epilepsy usually begin in childhood or adolescence. In adulthood, acquired causes of seizures and epilepsy such as stroke, CNS tumor, CNS infection, and drug and alcohol toxicity, are more common.

Identification of the cause of seizures is of primary importance in the determination of subsequent management. If precipitating factors are identified that are amenable to therapeutic intervention (e.g., metabolic disorders or CNS infection), then specific treatment modalities should be instituted to correct the underlying cause. Rarely is there a need for chronic antiepileptic drug (AED) therapy. Conversely, when no cause of seizures can be identified by history, physical examination, laboratory investigation, or neuroimaging studies, the seizure disorder is termed *idiopathic*, and if seizures recur, long-term AED therapy is warranted.

Drugs are a particularly common cause of new-onset seizures. In most instances, drug-induced seizures are dose-related and occur either with an overdose or when doses are not adjusted in patients with impaired drug elimination capacity.[3] Persons with a history of seizures, epilepsy, or organic brain disease are more susceptible to drug-induced seizures. Table 52.2 lists drugs that have caused seizures.

Table 52.1 ▪ Common Causes of New-Onset Seizures

Primary or acquired neurologic disorders
Febrile seizures of childhood
Genetic or developmental disorders
Idiopathic
Head trauma
Cerebrovascular disease
Brain tumor
Central nervous system infection
Alzheimer's disease or other neurodegenerative diseases
Systemic or metabolic disorders
Anoxia or ischemia
Drug overdose or toxicity (see Table 52.2)
Hyponatremia
Hypocalcemia
Hypoglycemia
Hypomagnesemia
Hepatic failure
Renal failure
Alcohol abuse and withdrawal
Eclampsia
Porphyria

Table 52.2 ▪ Drugs That Can Cause Seizures

Antimicrobials
β-Lactams and related compounds
Quinolones
Isoniazid
Antivirals
Acyclovir
Ganciclovir
Psychotropic agents
Antidepressants
Antipsychotics
Lithium
Theophylline
Class 1B antiarrhythmic agents
Radiographic contrast agents
Drugs of abuse
Amphetamine
Cocaine
Methylphenidate
Sedative-hypnotic drug withdrawal
Alcohol
Barbiturates (short-acting)
Benzodiazepines (short-acting)
Miscellaneous
Cyclosporine
Flumazenil
OKT3
Tramadol

PATHOPHYSIOLOGY

Seizures are caused by a perturbation in the normal balance of excitatory and inhibitory influences within the brain. Synchronized, high-frequency bursts of action potentials are the initiating event of a seizure. These bursts are caused by an influx of extracellular calcium followed by opening of voltage-dependent sodium channels. This depolarization phase is followed by a hyperpolarization phase that is mediated by the inhibitory neurotransmitter γ-aminobutyric acid (GABA) or by potassium channels. Most AEDs suppress seizures by altering ion flux through membrane channels or by altering neurotransmitter activity within the CNS.

CLINICAL PRESENTATION AND DIAGNOSIS

Whereas an etiologic diagnosis of seizures is needed to establish whether chronic AED therapy is necessary, the classification of epileptic seizures by their clinical and electrophysiologic manifestations is necessary to determine which AED is most likely to be effective. In most circumstances the seizure can be classified after a complete patient history in which the patient describes the events that occurred during the attack. This should include questions about any symptoms that warn the patient of an impending seizure (i.e., the aura), the specific ictal manifestations, and any postictal abnormalities. Throughout this process, the patient should be discouraged from labeling the attacks but rather should be guided to relate the events as they were experienced or as they were described by observers. The current scheme that is used for the classification of epileptic seizures and syndromes was established by the International League Against Epilepsy.[4,5] A modified version of this classification is presented in Table 52.3.

Classification of Seizure and Epilepsy Types

Seizures are classified as being either generalized or partial on the basis of their clinical and electroencephalographic features. Generalized seizures are those that begin in both hemispheres of the brain. Previously, these seizures were subdivided into convulsive and nonconvulsive generalized seizures according to the severity of associated motor disturbances. Nonconvulsive generalized seizures included absence (petit mal), myoclonic, and atonic seizures. Clonic and tonic-clonic seizures were previously referred to as grand mal seizures.

Table 52.3 ▪ International Classification of Epileptic Seizures and Syndromes

- Partial seizures (focal, local)
  - Simple partial seizures (consciousness preserved)
    - With motor signs (jacksonian)
    - With somatosensory or special sensory symptoms
    - With autonomic symptoms or signs
    - With psychic symptoms
  - Complex partial seizures (consciousness impaired)
    - Simple partial onset followed by impaired consciousness
    - Impaired consciousness at onset
  - Secondarily generalized seizures
    - Simple partial seizures evolving to generalized tonic-clonic seizures
    - Complex partial seizures evolving to generalized tonic-clonic seizures
    - Simple partial seizures evolving to complex partial seizures evolving to generalized tonic-clonic seizures
- Generalized-onset seizures (convulsive or nonconvulsive)
  - Tonic-clonic seizures
  - Absence seizures
    - Typical absence seizures
    - Atypical absence seizures
  - Myoclonic seizures
  - Tonic seizures
  - Atonic seizures
- Localization-related (focal) epilepsies
  - Idiopathic
    - Benign epilepsy of childhood
  - Symptomatic
    - Temporal lobe epilepsy
    - Extratemporal epilepsy
- Generalized epilepsy
  - Idiopathic
    - Benign neonatal convulsions
    - Childhood absence epilepsy
    - Juvenile myoclonic epilepsy
    - Other
  - Idiopathic and/or symptomatic
    - Infantile spasms (West syndrome)
    - Lennox-Gastaut syndrome
    - Myoclonic epilepsies
- Special syndromes
  - Febrile seizures

Source: References 4, 5.

Generalized Seizures

Generalalized Tonic-Clonic Seizures

Generalized tonic-clonic seizures are characteristic of maximal involvement of neurons of both hemispheres of the brain. Typically, these seizures begin with tonic (rigid) flexion of the extremities followed by extension. During this phase, air is forced from the larynx to produce an audible cry. The tonic phase of the seizure usually lasts 15 to 20 seconds and is quickly followed by the clonic (jerking) phase, during which there are spasms of the trunk and extremities and often biting of the tongue. The clonic phase usually lasts 20 to 30 seconds and is followed by a postictal state, during which the patient may sleep or awaken confused and disoriented. There is then a gradual return of consciousness and orientation over a period of 15 to 30 minutes, after which the patient has no recall of the event. Increases in blood pressure and heart rate, incontinence of urine or feces, and a brief interruption of normal breathing with cyanosis commonly accompany this type of seizure. Generalized tonic-clonic seizures may begin in both hemispheres of the brain (referred to as primarily generalized seizures) or begin in a localized area of the cortex (a partial seizure) and subsequently spread to involve both hemispheres (referred to as secondarily generalized tonic-clonic seizures).

Absence Seizures

Absence (petit mal) seizures occur primarily during childhood and are characterized by an abrupt interruption of consciousness followed by a fixed stare. Automatisms (coordinated involuntary movements such as lip smacking, chewing, or grimacing) or mild clonic movements may also occur. During the seizure there is no loss of postural tone. The seizure usually lasts several seconds and ends as abruptly as it begins with the patient immediately regaining full alertness. Absence seizures may occur as often as hundreds of times a day and are often initially perceived by family or teachers as daydreaming. This seizure type is characterized by a classic pattern on the electroencephalogram of bilateral 3-Hz spike-wave discharges. Absence seizures usually have their onset between the ages of 4 and 12 years and remit during adolescence or early adulthood in 60 to 70% of patients. In the remainder, generalized tonic-clonic seizures usually develop. Atypical absence seizures differ from traditional absence seizures in having a longer duration, focal motor manifestations, and a greater association with developmental delay.

Atonic Seizures

Atonic seizures are characterized by a sudden loss of muscle tone. Because the patient may fall abruptly, injuries are common, and it is often necessary to protect the patient's head by prescribing the use of a helmet during the daytime. Myoclonic seizures are characterized by jerking movements of a single or multiple muscle groups. Tonic seizures are similar to generalized tonic-clonic seizures except that they lack the usual clonic phase.

Partial Seizures

Partial seizures begin in an area of the brain that is limited to one hemisphere and are often indicative of some underlying focal brain lesion (e.g., perinatal injury, trauma, stroke, or brain tumor). Partial seizures are differentiated according to whether or not consciousness is impaired during the event. Complex partial seizures are associated with impairment of consciousness; simple partial seizures are not.

Simple Partial Seizures

Simple partial seizures are characterized by either motor manifestations (e.g., clonic jerking of one limb) or sensory symptoms (e.g., a foul odor or visual distortions). In some patients with motor symptoms the seizure may spread to contiguous areas of the cortex, resulting in the recruitment of additional muscle groups ("jacksonian march"). Autonomic symptoms such as piloerection or pupillary dilatation or psychic symptoms such as feelings of deja vu or fear may also accompany simple partial seizures; however, they are less common. In all cases, patients can respond to their environment throughout the attack.

Complex Partial Seizures

Complex partial seizures (psychomotor or temporal lobe seizures) are characterized by impaired consciousness and a heterogeneous group of abnormal symptoms or behaviors. Although the variety of symptoms associated with complex partial seizures is wide, each individual usually reports stereotypical attacks. Auras precede complex partial seizures in many patients. Unusual epigastric sensations are the most common, although various motor, sensory, or psychic symptoms (as described for simple partial seizures) may occur. Consciousness is then impaired for an average of about 2 minutes. During this time, patients may exhibit automatisms such as lip smacking, buttoning or unbuttoning of clothing, or wandering behavior. Less often, the behavioral abnormalities include violent outbursts, crying, or sexual actions. Either simple or partial complex seizures may spread to involve both hemispheres of the brain (usually as a generalized tonic-clonic seizure). These events are termed partial seizures with secondary generalization.

Epilepsy Syndromes

In some cases the seizure classification, etiologic diagnosis, patient age, and coexistent medical conditions can be used to define a specific epileptic syndrome. An epileptic syndrome is a constellation of signs and symptoms that tend to occur together. Identification of epileptic syndromes may provide useful information that is not necessarily implied by either the etiologic diagnosis or the seizure classification, such as a specific choice of AED, the anticipated duration of AED therapy, and patient prognosis. Not all patients who have epilepsy can be classified as having an epileptic syndrome. Examples of epileptic syndromes include childhood absence epilepsy, juvenile myoclonic epilepsy, and Lennox-Gastaut syndrome.

Febrile Seizures

Febrile seizures are defined as generalized tonic-clonic seizures associated with temperatures greater than 38°C that occur in the absence of other identifiable causes. Febrile seizures are the most common form of epilepsy in children, occurring in 2 to 5% of this population. Affected children are usually between the ages of 3 months and 5 years and are otherwise neurologically and developmentally normal. Febrile seizures are classified as either simple or complex. Complex febrile seizures are prolonged (>15 minutes), occur in series (two or more seizures in 24 hours), or have associated focal features. The remainder are classified as simple febrile seizures. Simple febrile seizures are usually benign, self-limited, and associated with only a 2 to 3% risk of recurrent, nonfebrile seizures in later life.[6] The risk of epilepsy is approximately 4% in children who have complex febrile seizures.

Because most febrile seizures are self-limited and are not associated with acute or long-term neurologic sequelae, aggressive treatment is not required. Most febrile seizures occur within 24 hours of the onset of a febrile episode and can be prevented by promptly instituting antipyretic measures as soon as the fever is evident. Parents should be instructed to sponge the child with tepid water for 10 to 15 minutes and to administer acetaminophen every 4 hours for a temperature greater than 38°C. Acute treatment with AEDs is usually not necessary unless the seizure continues for longer than 10 or 15 minutes. In this case, diazepam by intravenous or rectal administration is usually effective. Chronic administration of AEDs to children with a history of simple febrile seizures is not indicated.

Children with complex febrile seizures, preexisting neurologic abnormalities, or a family history of nonfebrile epilepsy are at greater risk for the development of epilepsy in later life. Drug therapy for the prevention of febrile seizures should be considered for these patients, although there is no evidence that the risk of nonfebrile epilepsy is reduced. Phenobarbital is effective for the treatment of febrile seizures; however, it must be administered continuously to ensure adequate drug levels at the onset of a febrile episode. Initiating oral phenobarbital at the onset of febrile illness is not appropriate. Rectal administration of diazepam (using the parenteral solution) results in rapid absorption and provides rapid protection from febrile seizures.[6] Rectal diazepam gel (Diastat) may also be effective. Many clinicians prefer intermittent treatment with rectal diazepam, because it avoids chronic medication adverse effects and the need for continuous administration.

Diagnosis

Table 52.4 outlines the features of a comprehensive evaluation for patients with new-onset seizures. The diagnosis of epilepsy and proper classification of epileptic

Table 52.4 ▪ Workup for the Patient with New-Onset Seizures

- Patient history
  - Seizure description
    - Preictal phenomena (aura)
    - Ictal manifestations (including level of consciousness)
    - Postictal state
    - Provocative factors
  - Perinatal and developmental history
  - History of febrile seizures
  - History of head trauma
  - History of central nervous system infection
  - Family history of epilepsy
- Physical examination
- Laboratory evaluation
  - Complete blood count
  - Electrolytes
  - Glucose
  - Cerebrospinal fluid
  - Blood urea nitrogen
  - Osmolality
  - Toxicology screen
- Electroencephalogram
- Brain imaging study
  - Computed tomography
  - Magnetic resonance imaging

seizures are based primarily on the patient's history and witnessed accounts of the events. Although a complete evaluation usually includes other laboratory and diagnostic studies, a diagnosis of epilepsy can be clearly established only when an accurate and unambiguous history is obtained. Most patients and witnesses can give a clear account of generalized tonic-clonic seizures. However, more careful questioning is often necessary to elicit the subtle manifestations that accompany partial, absence, and other less dramatic seizure types.

Once it is apparent that a seizure has occurred, subsequent efforts should be directed toward establishing the cause. A thorough evaluation including a medical history and physical and laboratory examinations should focus on the variety of primary, metabolic, and systemic factors that may cause new-onset seizures (Table 52.1). Seizures that are a result of a reversible cause (e.g., acute metabolic or systemic disorder) must be differentiated from those that are related to a primary CNS disorder. Even with extensive workup, the etiology of epilepsy remains unidentified in 60 to 70% of patients. A genetic cause is suggested when the age at seizure onset is less than 25 years and there is a family history of epilepsy.[7]

The electroencephalogram (EEG) is useful as a tool for both the diagnosis and classification of seizures. Spike and wave discharges on the EEG in conjunction with a clinical history of spontaneously recurring seizures can usually establish the diagnosis of epilepsy. Although epileptiform abnormalities on the EEG are usually seen during a seizure, most EEG recordings are made between seizures (interictal EEG). Absence of EEG abnormalities on an interictal recording can rarely rule out the diagnosis of epilepsy. Epileptiform abnormalities are found in only about 50% of epileptic patients after a single interictal recording. Recording the EEG after sleep deprivation increases the diagnostic yield of the study. The yield also can be improved with repeated recordings; however, in 15% of epileptic patients no EEG abnormalities are ever found.[7] Just as the diagnosis of epilepsy is rarely excluded on the basis of a normal interictal EEG, the presence of EEG abnormalities, in and of itself, is not diagnostic for epilepsy. EEG abnormalities are seen in 10 to 15% of the nonepileptic population and are not indicative of epilepsy unless strong evidence from the patient history supports the diagnosis.[7]

Computed tomography (CT) and magnetic resonance imaging (MRI) scans are particularly useful when evidence from the history or neurologic examination suggests a structural lesion of the brain (e.g., focal neurologic abnormalities or a history that is suggestive of partial seizures), although they are often used in the initial evaluation of patients with new-onset seizures, regardless of the seizure type. MRI is more likely to detect lesions that are associated with partial epilepsy and is preferred over CT.[1] Positron emission tomography (PET), an advanced imaging technique that allows more precise localization of areas of abnormal blood flow or metabolism, is useful for evaluation of patients for whom surgical intervention is considered. However, its availability is limited by high equipment costs.

Finally, in some patients, seizure-like activity may be a manifestation of some other nonepileptic condition (Table 52.5). The misdiagnosis of these events as seizures can result in unnecessary and potentially harmful therapy.

Table 52.5 ▪ Disorders That May Mimic Epilepsy

- Gastroesophageal reflux
- Breath-holding spells
- Migraine
  - Confusional
  - Basilar
  - With recurrent abdominal pain and cyclic vomiting
- Sleep disorders (especially parainsomnias)
- Cardiovascular events
  - Pallid infantile syncope
  - Vasovagal attacks
  - Vasomotor syncope
  - Cardiac arrhythmias
- Movement disorders
  - Shuddering attacks
  - Paroxysmal choreoathetosis
  - Nonepileptic myoclonus
  - Tics and habit spasms
- Psychological disorders
  - Panic disorder
  - Hyperventilation attacks
  - Pseudoseizures
  - Rage attacks

Source: Reprinted with permission from Scheuer ML, Pedley TA. The evaluation and treatment of seizures. N Engl J Med 323:1468–1474, 1990.

Accordingly, the diagnosis of epilepsy should be reevaluated whenever the seizure-like events fail to respond to the usual treatments.

PSYCHOSOCIAL ISSUES

In addition to the medical issues that accompany the diagnosis of epilepsy, patients often experience anxiety and fear with the confirmation that they have a disorder that is chronic, affects the brain, and is accompanied by a loss of control over their body and consciousness. Patients may experience an impaired sense of independence owing to the necessity for regular interactions with the health care system and the need for chronic, daily medication. Additionally, persons with epilepsy are often subject to driving restrictions and a need to report their condition on applications for insurance and employment. A comprehensive approach to the treatment of persons with epilepsy should include attention to medical, psychosocial, and environmental (or behavioral) factors because these issues significantly affect the patient's quality of life.

When a diagnosis of epilepsy is made, some alteration of the patient's usual activities may be required depending on the timing and clinical manifestation of seizures. For example, patients who are affected by seizures associated with loss of consciousness or normal muscle control should restrict activities that place them or others at risk of injury. This may include partial or complete restriction of driving privileges and avoidance of activities such as swimming unattended, working at heights, and operating potentially dangerous machinery. Common sense should be the ultimate guide in the determination of specific lifestyle limitations that the patient's epileptic condition necessitates.

Certain changes in daily activities may reduce the occurrence of seizures by avoiding patient-specific risk factors. Conditions that are occasionally identified by patients as seizure precipitants include stress, exercise, alcohol or caffeine consumption, altered sleep schedules, and missed meals. When these or other precipitating conditions are identified, the patient and health care provider should work cooperatively to establish guidelines that minimize these risks yet do not unnecessarily encumber the patient's daily routine.

TREATMENT

Pharmacotherapy

AED pharmacotherapy is the mainstay of epilepsy treatment. The goals of AED treatment are to completely control seizures and to minimize drug-related adverse effects. Specific therapeutic endpoints must be individualized for each patient. The choice of AED should be based on the seizure type, the age and sex of the patient, concurrent medical conditions, potential adverse effects, and the pharmacokinetic and pharmacodynamic features of the individual drugs. When these factors are considered and the guiding principles of AED therapy (discussed later) are followed, good to excellent seizure control can be attained in most patients. However, some patients may continue to suffer from recurrent seizures despite appropriate drug treatment.

Principles of Antiepileptic Drug Selection and Usage

Preference for Monotherapy with Nonsedating Agents

Monotherapy is preferred to polytherapy with AEDs because of lower costs associated with medications and blood level monitoring, reduced potential for adverse reactions and undesirable drug interactions, and improved medication compliance with a more simplified drug administration schedule. Furthermore, evidence indicates that polytherapy offers no advantage over monotherapy for the majority of patients with epilepsy. For patients in whom single drug therapy does not provide sufficient seizure control, polytherapy may be necessary to achieve the goals of treatment.

In addition to selecting the minimum effective number of AEDs, it is important to choose agents on the basis of their adverse-effect profile. The specific adverse effects of each drug are discussed later; however, the use of sedating AEDs should be minimized or avoided. Phenobarbital and benzodiazepines are examples of sedating AEDs; other drugs covered in this chapter are not. Sedation and decreased mentation are particularly common on initiation of therapy with barbiturate and benzodiazepines. Over time, however, an adaptive process occurs during which these effects become less noticeable. Despite the development of tolerance to the overt sedative effect of these drugs, evidence suggests that subtle effects on intelligence, memory, complex motor skills, and behavior often persist during treatment. In some cases these changes are noted by patients or their families only after the drug is discontinued.[8] In this regard, therapy with nonsedating agents is preferred when possible, and the relative place of sedating AEDs has been reconsidered. For example, phenobarbital is as effective as phenytoin and carbamazepine for the treatment of generalized tonic-clonic seizures, but the latter agents are preferred because of their relative lack of CNS-depressant effects.

When possible, therapy should begin with one of the nonsedating AEDs such as phenytoin, carbamazepine, valproate, or ethosuximide. Phenobarbital and benzodiazepines should be reserved until nonsedating alternatives have failed. Nitrazepam and clobazam are benzodiazepines, which may have advantages over clonazepam in terms of sedation-related adverse effects. However, these drugs are not available for use in the United States. In summary, sedating AEDs should be avoided when possible, and in many cases, the substitution of nonsedating alternatives can result in noticeable improvement in cognitive, motor, and behavioral function.

Drug Selection Based on Seizure Classification

Once the diagnosis of epilepsy has been made, the choice of AED therapy is guided by considering the relative

Table 52.6 ▪ Antiepileptic Drugs of Choice Based on Seizure Classification

		Generalized Seizures		
	Partial Seizures[a]	Generalized Tonic-Clonic	Absence	Myoclonic, Atonic, Atypical Absence
Drugs of choice	Carbamazepine Phenytoin Valproate	Valproate Carbamazepine Phenytoin	Ethosuximide Valproate	Valproate
Alternatives	Lamotrigine Gabapentin[b] Topiramate[b] Tiagabine[b] Primidone Phenobarbital	Lamotrigine Topiramate Primidone Phenobarbital	Clonazepam Lamotrigine	Clonazepam Lamotrigine Topiramate Felbamate

[a]Simple-partial, complex-partial, and secondarily generalized tonic-clonic seizures.
[b]Used primarily as adjunctive therapy.

efficacy and toxicity of each agent. Proper classification of the patient's seizure type or epilepsy syndrome is the most important step in choosing the appropriate agent. Table 52.6 lists the preferred AEDs for the treatment of different seizure types. Table 52.7 offers a cost comparison of some of the common first-line AEDs as well as newer agents that are marketed for the treatment of medically refractory epilepsy.

Partial Seizures. Carbamazepine, phenytoin, phenobarbital, and primidone are equally effective for the treatment of partial seizures, including simple-partial, complex-partial, and secondarily generalized partial seizures.[9] However, carbamazepine and phenytoin are usually tolerated better. Phenytoin has a long half-life that allows for once-daily dosing and carbamazepine is available in two extended-release dosage forms, which allow for twice-daily dosing. These products are preferred for patients who are unlikely to comply with a chronic regimen requiring multiple daily doses. However, phenytoin is associated with cosmetic changes that make it less desirable for the treatment of epilepsy in children, adolescents, and women. Valproate is also useful for the treatment of partial seizures, but carbamazepine provides better seizure control and fewer long-term adverse effects.[10] Gabapentin, lamotrigine, felbamate, tiagabine, and topiramate are new AEDs that are effective for treating partial seizures. Lamotrigine is effective as monotherapy and appears to be better tolerated than carbamazepine monotherapy.[11] The other new agents are most useful as adjunctive therapy if standard AED therapy has failed or for patients who are intolerant of standard AEDs (e.g., carbamazepine, phenytoin, and valproate). Although prospective clinical trials have not been conducted to compare the relative efficacy of the new AEDs, a recent systematic review found no significant differences between gabapentin, lamotrigine, tiagabine, and topiramate as adjunctive therapy.[12] Overall, partial seizures do not respond to treatment as well as seizures that are generalized from their onset. Approximately 65% of patients with partial seizures attain complete control of seizures with AED monotherapy.[13] In the remaining patients, a trial of adjunctive therapy is warranted.

Table 52.7 ▪ Cost Comparison of Innovator-Brand Antiepileptic Drug Therapy

Drug	Sample High-Dose Regimen	Cost/Month[a]
Tegretol[b] (carbamazepine)	600 mg TID	$126
Tegretol-XR (extended release carbamazepine)	600 mg TID	$117
Carbatrol (extended release carbamazepine)	600 mg TID	$117
Dilantin[b] (phenytoin)	400 mg QD	$ 34
Depakene[b] (valproic acid)	750 mg TID	$397
Depakote (divalproex sodium)	750 mg TID	$225
Neurontin (gabapentin)	900 mg TID	$290
Lamictal (lamotrigine)	300 mg TID	$252
Gabatril (tiagabine)	16 mg TID	$167
Topamax (topiramate)	200 mg BID	$199

Source: Data from Drug Topics Red Book 1999.
[a]Cost for 30 days of treatment (rounded to the nearest dollar) according to wholesale price (AWP) listings.
[b]Generic drug product also available.

Generalized Tonic-Clonic Seizures. Carbamazepine, phenytoin, and valproate are the drugs of choice for the treatment of generalized tonic-clonic seizures. Valproate is often considered the drug of choice for the treatment of primarily generalized tonic-clonic seizures. Approximately 75 to 85% of patients achieve complete seizure control during monotherapy with this agent.[2] Carbamazepine or phenytoin is preferred for the treatment of children younger than 2 years of age because of the higher risk of valproate-associated hepatotoxicity in these patients. However, carbamazepine and phenytoin can exacerbate seizures in children with primary generalized epilepsy syndromes. These children should be monitored closely for worsened seizures or the emergence of a new seizure type. Although not approved for the treatment of primarily generalized tonic-clonic seizures, some studies have found lamotrigine and topiramate to be effective for this seizure type. Phenobarbital and primidone are also effective against generalized tonic-clonic seizures, but because of their adverse effects, they are usually reserved for use as alternative second- or third-line agents.

ABSENCE SEIZURES. Ethosuximide and valproate are equally effective for the treatment of absence seizures. Ethosuximide is preferred over valproate when only absence seizures are involved because it is associated with fewer serious adverse effects. Valproate is preferred if generalized tonic-clonic seizures also occur.[1] The response to these agents is usually dramatic. In controlled trials, 70 to 90% of patients who were treated with ethosuximide or valproate experienced cessation or a dramatic reduction in absence seizures.[14] The combination of ethosuximide and valproate is often effective when monotherapy fails to yield adequate results. Clonazepam is also effective against absence seizures. However, because of frequent dose-related adverse effects and the development of tolerance to the antiepileptic effect of this drug, it should be reserved for patients in whom ethosuximide and valproate fail. Carbamazepine is ineffective for the treatment of absence seizures and may even exacerbate these and other seizure types when used for the treatment of children with mixed seizure disorders.[3]

MYOCLONIC, ATONIC, AND ATYPICAL ABSENCE SEIZURES. Valproate is effective for the treatment of myoclonic, atonic, and atypical absence seizures and is the initial drug of choice for patients with mixed types. Valproate effectively controls myoclonic seizures in 75 to 90% of patients with generalized idiopathic and juvenile myoclonic epilepsy. Myoclonic seizures after anoxic encephalopathy are more resistant to treatment. Clonazepam is also effective as monotherapy or in combination with valproate when either drug alone does not provide adequate seizure control. Lamotrigine, topiramate, and felbamate have activity against a broad range of seizure types including myoclonic, atonic, and atypical absence seizures.

Initiating Antiepileptic Drug Therapy

AEDs are more frequently associated with adverse effects during initiation of therapy; therefore, treatment should begin with low doses and the dose should be gradually escalated according to the patient's clinical status. When therapy is initiated too aggressively, patients may experience uncomfortable adverse effects and are often unwilling to continue treatment with that agent despite a reduction in dosage. Patients should be told to report adverse effects so that an adjustment in therapy can be made as soon as possible. Phenytoin and phenobarbital are usually tolerated well when they are initiated near the usual maintenance dosage (e.g., 300 and 90 mg daily, respectively, in adults). Upon initiation of therapy, patients should understand the goal of treatment and the time course over which seizure control is anticipated. The importance of strict compliance with the prescribed regimen should also be emphasized.

Adjusting and Monitoring Antiepileptic Drug Therapy

There is great interpatient variability in the dose-response relationship for all of the AEDs that are in common use. Therefore, after therapy is initiated, the optimal drug dose for each patient should be determined. This necessitates the titration of therapy until the desired clinical response is achieved or the patient experiences unacceptable dose-related adverse effects.

The determination of acceptable seizure control requires input from both patient and clinician. Although complete control of seizures is always desirable, patients may choose to continue therapy that allows minimal interruption of their lifestyle even though seizures occasionally recur. The clinician must assess the temporary disability and potential for harm (to both the patient and others) that may accompany a seizure and use this information, with input from the patient, to determine whether dosage adjustments should be made.

If the first agent does not achieve the desired therapeutic goal, then an alternative AED that is appropriate for the patient's seizure type should be gradually substituted rather than added. The first drug is usually removed once a therapeutic effect (or blood level) of the new agent is attained. When removed, AEDs should always be tapered gradually. Abrupt discontinuation of AEDs may exacerbate seizures and is rarely necessary. The rate of drug tapering is empiric. Most practitioners gradually discontinue therapy over 1 to 3 months. Only after monotherapy has failed (usually with two or three agents) should multiple AED treatments be tried.

AED therapy fails for many reasons. Although various drugs may demonstrate equal efficacy in large populations of patients, an individual may respond better to one agent than to others. Additional factors that should be considered include poor medication compliance, erroneous diagnosis or seizure classification, progressive neurologic disease, and lifestyle factors that compromise the efficacy of treatment (e.g., recreational drug or alcohol abuse). Noncompliance with treatment is probably the most common cause of AED therapy failure, and this possibility should be carefully investigated. Common reasons for noncompliance include complicated dosing regimens, fear about chronic adverse effects of AED therapy, and denial of the need for epilepsy therapy. Patients who report a change in the character of their seizures (e.g., seizures are now preceded by an aura, whereas previously there was no warning) or frequent seizures after a long period of complete control should be referred for a thorough medical evaluation to rule out other neurologic disease (e.g., brain tumor).

Blood Levels

The widespread availability of blood level monitoring of AED therapy has had a dramatic effect on the use of these agents. For example, combination AED regimens were frequently begun (e.g., phenytoin and phenobarbital) before clinicians had the ability to individualize the doses for either agent. On the basis of past experience in which a single drug was occasionally ineffective and above-average doses sometimes led to toxicity, it was assumed that most patients would benefit if multiple drugs were used. Blood level monitoring and knowledge of the pharmacokinetic properties of AEDs, are now used to maximize efficacy and minimize adverse effects.

The therapeutic range of plasma concentrations is a useful guide for titrating therapy. Within this range, many patients achieve seizure control without unacceptable side effects. However, it is also common to observe an adequate therapeutic response at concentrations less than the usual therapeutic range, and some patients tolerate and indeed require blood levels above the upper limit of the therapeutic range to maintain seizure control. Thus, although these limits are useful as guides to therapy, the clinician should strive to determine the optimum AED plasma concentration for each individual patient rather than relying on published ranges.[15]

Plasma-concentration monitoring of AEDs is most useful under the following conditions: (1) to document the blood level associated with good seizure control, (2) to document therapeutic failures, (3) to evaluate noncompliance or drug malabsorption, (4) to guide subsequent dosage adjustments that are required on a clinical basis, and (5) to evaluate possible drug-related adverse effects. The timing of blood sampling for drug level determination is important, particularly during therapy with AEDs that have a short half-life (e.g., carbamazepine and valproate). For these agents, blood levels can fluctuate significantly over the course of the dosing interval. Comparisons between drug levels may be inaccurate unless the blood is sampled at a consistent time relative to the dose. For most patients it is recommended that blood samples be taken in the morning, before the first daily dose of medication. An exception is patients with repeated, transient symptoms that are suggestive of dose-related drug toxicity. For these patients, blood sampling should coincide with the adverse experience so that the contribution of the drug level can be assessed.

Plasma-level monitoring of AEDs is often both overused and misused.[15] It is common (and arguably appropriate) to document drug levels on an occasional basis in patients whose epileptic condition is well controlled (e.g., every 12 months). However, other drug-level determinations should not be done unless there is clinical indication of their necessity. Likewise, there is often a tendency to adjust AED therapy on the basis of the level without taking into account the patient's clinical status. For example, it may be tempting to decrease the drug dose when the reported blood level is above the usual therapeutic range. However, some patients require higher concentrations than usual to achieve the desired therapeutic effect. Likewise, patients whose seizures are controlled with levels less than the therapeutic range neither need a dose increase nor should be assumed to no longer require AED treatment. In his editorial regarding the use of AED blood level monitoring, W. Edwin Dodson wrote that "[c]hanging an antiepileptic drug dose based only on the drug level is like driving a car looking only at the speedometer and not out the window. Wrecks are inevitable and frequent."[15]

Antiepileptic Drugs

Clinical pharmacokinetic features of the common AEDs are summarized in Table 52.8.

Carbamazepine

Carbamazepine is a highly lipophilic iminostilbene compound that is structurally related to the tricyclic antidepressant agent imipramine. Carbamazepine is very effective for the treatment of generalized tonic-clonic and partial seizures, but it is not effective against myoclonic or absence seizures. The antiepileptic effect of carbamazepine is probably related to its effects on sodium channels to limit sustained, repetitive firing and alter synaptic transmission.

Carbamazepine (Tegretol and generic) is available as oral (200-mg) and chewable (100-mg) tablets and as a suspension (100 mg/5 mL). Two controlled-release oral dosage forms are also available: Tegretol-XR in 100-, 200-, and 400-mg tablets and Carbatrol in 200- and 300-mg capsules. Advantages of these products include twice-daily dosing and reduced fluctuations between peak and trough plasma concentrations (compared with immediate release products). The extended-release characteristics of Tegretol-XR are lost if the tablet is broken or chewed. Patients should be counseled to swallow the tablet whole and told that the tablet shell may appear in the stool. Carbatrol is formulated in a bead-filled capsule that can be emptied onto food. No parenteral formulation of carbamazepine is available for commercial use. Therapy with carbamazepine is usually initiated at a dose of 100 to 200 mg twice daily with gradual dose titration, in 200-mg increments, every 3 to 7 days. Although the manufacturer recommends that daily doses of carbamazepine not exceed 1200 mg, daily doses of 2000 mg and above are occasionally required for optimal therapy. Because of gastric disturbances, loading doses of carbamazepine are not recommended for usual outpatient therapy. However, single carbamazepine doses of 8 mg/kg (using either tablets or suspension) are useful for inpatients for whom rapid attainment of a therapeutic level is desired.[16]

Absorption of carbamazepine from the gastrointestinal tract is slow and erratic and often does not follow first-order kinetics. The time to peak plasma levels after oral administration may vary from an average of 4 to 8 hours to as long as 24 hours. Although prolonged absorption of the drug may be due to slow dissolution of

Table 52.8 ▪ Clinical Pharmacokinetics of Antiepileptic Drugs

	Carbamazepine	Phenytoin	Valproate	Ethosuximide
Adult daily dose	600–2400 mg	300–400 mg	750–2250 mg	1000–2000 mg[a]
Initial dose	100–200 mg BID	300 mg QD	125–250 mg BID–TID	500 mg QD
Dosage schedule	BID–QID	QD–BID	BID–TID	QD–TID
Bioavailability (%)	75–85	85–95	100	
Time to peak absorption (hr)	4–8	4–8	2–8	1–7
Volume of distribution (L/kg)	0.8–1.6	0.5–0.7	0.09–0.17	0.6–0.9
Protein binding (%)	75–78	90–93	88–92	0
Plasma half-life (hr)	24–45 (single dose) 8–24 (chronic therapy)	9–40	6–16	20–60
Therapeutic plasma levels				
(μg/mL)	4–12	10–20	50–150	40–100
(μmol/L)	16–48	40–80	200–400	283–708

	Gabapentin	Lamotrigine	Topiramate	Tiagabine	Felbamate
Adult daily dose	900–3600 mg	200–500 mg	200–400 mg	32–56 mg	3600 mg
Initial dose	300 mg QD	50 mg QD[b] or 25 mg QOD[c]	25–50 mg QD	4 mg QD	400 mg TID
Dosage schedule	TID	BID	BID	BID–QID	TID–QID
Bioavailability (%)	60	98	80	90	90
Time to peak absorption (hr)	2–3	2–4	3–4	1–1.5	2–4
Volume of distribution (L/kg)	0.7–0.8	0.9–1.2	0.6–0.8	0.8–1.2	0.75–0.85
Protein binding (%)	0	55	13–17	96	25
Plasma half-life (hr)	5–7	14–27	22–24	7–9	14–23
Therapeutic plasma levels (μg/mL) (μmol/L)	Not determined	Not determined	Not determined	Not determined	Not determined

	Phenobarbital	Primidone	Clonazepam	Clorazepate
Adult daily dose	100–200 mg	750–1500 mg	6–18 mg	22.5–90 mg
Initial dose	90 mg QD	125–250 mg BID	0.5-1 mg QD	7.5 mg TID
Dosage schedule	QD–BID	BID–QID	QD–TID	QD–TID
Bioavailability (%)	95–100	90–100	80–90	—
Time to peak absorption (hr)	1–4	1–3	1–4	0.5–2[d]
Volume of distribution (L/kg)	0.51–0.57	0.4–0.8	2.1–4.3	1–1.9[d]
Protein binding (%)	48–54	20–30	80–90	95–98[d]
Plasma half-life (hr)	72–144	5–18	30–40	55–100[d]
Therapeutic plasma levels				
(μg/mL)	10–40	5–15	5–70 ng/mL	Not determined
(μmol/L)	43–172	23–69	16–220 nmol/mL	

[a]The daily dose for children is 20–40 mg/kg.
[b]Starting dose for patients taking enzyme-inducing antiepilepsy drugs only.
[c]Starting dose for patients taking enzyme-inducing antiepilepsy drugs in combination with valproate.
[d]Pharmacokinetic values for *N*-desmethyldiazepam, the active metabolite of clorazepate.

the drug from tablet form, the suspension is also absorbed erratically. Food has no consistent effect on the bioavailability of carbamazepine.

Carbamazepine is almost exclusively cleared by hepatic metabolism. Oxidation of the parent drug to carbamazepine 10,11-epoxide (CBZ-E) is the major metabolic pathway for elimination. The remainder is glucuronidated, sulfur-conjugated, or oxidatively metabolized by other routes. Only 2% of the dose is recovered unchanged in the urine. The half-life of the drug after a single dose may range from 24 to 45 hours. With chronic administration the half-life of carbamazepine is reduced, and interindividual differences in clearance are enhanced. Increased clearance of carbamazepine occurs during the first few weeks of therapy because of autoinduction of the CYP3A4 isoenzyme of the cytochrome P-450 system. This causes an increase in oxidation to CBZ-E. This metabolic conversion is also enhanced by other enzyme-inducing drugs, such as phenytoin, phenobarbital, and primidone. Thus, the metabolic clearance and half-life may vary significantly, depending on the duration of treatment and concomitant drug therapy. It is not uncommon to observe a reduction in the half-life of carbamazepine from 30 hours after a single dose to 12 hours with chronic therapy and a further reduction to 8 hours during polytherapy with other AEDs. Larger daily doses (<1200 mg) and more frequent administration (three or four times a day) of carbamazepine are often necessary to minimize plasma level fluctuations and the attendant risk of breakthrough seizures or transient adverse effects. In this situation, extended-release carbamazepine products are useful to simplify the dosing regimen and enhance compliance.

Because of the large interindividual variability in carbamazepine absorption and clearance, the time-dependent alterations in metabolism, and the potential for fluctuations in drug concentrations over a dosage interval, careful plasma-level monitoring is often needed to determine optimal therapy. Steady-state concentrations of carbamazepine are reached within several days after therapy is initiated, although levels may decline by as much as 50% during the first month of therapy because of autoinduction of metabolism. After 1 month, autoinduction is complete, and plasma levels vary predictably with changes in dosage.

Adverse Effects. Initial, dose-related adverse effects of carbamazepine are common and include dizziness, drowsiness, anorexia, and nausea. Although tolerance to these effects develops within the first few weeks of therapy, their occurrence can be minimized or avoided by gradual dose titration. Persistent gastrointestinal upset may be relieved by giving the drug with meals. Reversible, dose-related symptoms of carbamazepine toxicity include diplopia (commonly the initial manifestation of toxicity), nausea, headache, dizziness, and ataxia. Because of fluctuations in the blood level of carbamazepine over the course of a usual dosage interval, dose-related toxicities may occur transiently at times of peak drug plasma concentrations. Extended-release carbamazepine products are often useful for ameliorating these symptoms.

Other dose-related neuropsychiatric adverse effects of carbamazepine include depression, irritability, mental sluggishness, and impairment of concentration and short-term memory. However, these adverse effects are less common than with phenobarbital and primidone. Furthermore, in several clinical epilepsy trials, patients with personality and behavioral disorders who were treated with carbamazepine had significant improvement during therapy.[17] When dose-related adverse effects persist throughout the day, the total daily dose of carbamazepine should be decreased; when they are transient and occur 2 to 4 hours after a dose, an adjustment in the dosing schedule may suffice. Unusual movement disorders and carbamazepine-induced seizures can occur acutely after an overdose.

Rash occurs in approximately 5% of patients treated with carbamazepine, usually between the first and second week of therapy. Benign, maculopapular, urticarial, and morbilliform reactions are the most common adverse effects, but exfoliative dermatitis and Stevens-Johnson syndrome may also occur. In some cases, rash may be accompanied by fever, generalized lymphadenopathy, hepatomegaly, splenomegaly, and, less commonly, nephritis and vasculitis. Symptoms are reversible on drug discontinuation, and corticosteroids may hasten recovery. Cross-reactivity between carbamazepine and other aromatic AEDs (e.g., phenytoin and phenobarbital) may complicate the subsequent management of these patients. In such cases, valproate is usually well tolerated.[18] Other idiosyncratic adverse reactions include hepatitis and systemic lupus erythematosus (SLE). Hepatitis usually occurs within the first few weeks of therapy and may coincide with eosinophilia and other symptoms of drug hypersensitivity. Carbamazepine may also cause a mild elevation of liver enzyme levels in fewer than 10% of patients, which appears to have no adverse clinical consequence. Carbamazepine-induced SLE is delayed, usually occurring after 6 to 12 months of therapy.

Among the most worrisome of idiosyncratic adverse reactions associated with carbamazepine is aplastic anemia. Although rare, this condition is fatal in about one-half of affected patients. The incidence of carbamazepine-associated aplastic anemia is estimated to be 0.5 per 100,000 treatment-years.[19] Neither patient age nor daily or total dosage significantly affects this risk. Carbamazepine is also associated with a dose-independent transient leukopenia, which occurs in about 10% of patients. In most cases the leukopenia is mild and resolves, despite continuation of treatment. However, in about 2% of patients, leukopenia persists until the drug is removed.[19] Carbamazepine-induced leukopenia does not appear to be a risk factor for aplastic anemia. While aplastic anemia can develop at any time during the first year of carbamazepine treatment, leukopenia is most commonly seen within the first month. The risk of serious hematologic reactions to carbamazepine can be minimized by patient education and laboratory monitoring. When therapy is initiated, patients should be counseled to seek immediate medical attention for abrupt onset of high fever, infection, petechiae, or unusual fatigue. If the diagnosis of aplastic anemia is confirmed, carbamazepine should be discontinued immediately, and the patient should not be given the drug again. Laboratory monitoring should include complete blood counts before initiation of treatment and every 2 weeks for the first 2 months of therapy. If no abnormalities are detected, hematologic monitoring should continue either at intervals of 3 months or when the patient develops signs or symptoms of myelosuppression. If mild leukopenia develops, complete blood counts should be evaluated at 2-week intervals until they return to baseline values. Therapy should be discontinued if the absolute neutrophil count drops below 1500/mm^3 or if infection occurs.

Carbamazepine may also cause hyponatremia and water retention, probably by increasing antidiuretic hormone secretion. This effect appears to be dose-related, as it is most often associated with blood levels of carbamazepine above the therapeutic range and often responds to a reduction in dose. At low serum sodium concentrations (<120 mEq/L), patients may report headache, confusion, dizziness, or loss of seizure control. Treatment consists of water restriction and/or reduction or discontinuation of carbamazepine therapy. Treatment with demeclocycline may be effective for patients who require continued carbamazepine therapy. Carbamazepine can cause cardiac conduction disturbances, primarily in older patients. Cardiotoxicity may be more common with higher doses and in patients with an underlying cardiac abnormality. A thorough history and baseline electrocardiogram should precede the initiation of carbamazepine therapy in older patients.

Drug Interactions. Carbamazepine, a potent inducer of drug metabolism, enhances the clearance of drugs metabolized by uridine diphosphate glucuronosyltransferase (UGT) as well as the CYP2C and CYP3A isoenzymes of the cytochrome P-450 system.[20] Increased elimination has been demonstrated for theophylline, doxycycline, haloperidol, warfarin, corticosteroids, valproate, clonazepam, ethosuximide, lamotrigine, felbamate, and various hormones. Thus, the potential for reduced effectiveness of these agents should be considered when carbamazepine therapy is begun. Because the failure rate of oral contraceptives is increased 4- to 5-fold during coadministration with carbamazepine and other enzyme-inducing AEDs (e.g., phenytoin, phenobarbital, and primidone), patients should be monitored for breakthrough bleeding. Use of an oral contraceptive with a higher estrogen content or an alternative form of birth control should be considered. The effect of carbamazepine on plasma levels of phenytoin, phenobarbital, and primidone is inconsistent and probably reflects various degrees of enzyme induction and inhibition. Routine monitoring of blood levels is recommended when carbamazepine is added to the regimen of any patient who is receiving AED therapy.

Drug interactions that affect CYP 3A4 (the P-450 isoenzyme mainly responsible for carbamazepine metabolism) are common. Danazol, dextropropoxyphene, erythromycin, clarithromycin, isoniazid, verapamil, and diltiazem can inhibit carbamazepine metabolism and induce clinical symptoms of toxicity. Cimetidine may inhibit the metabolism of carbamazepine, but ranitidine has no effect. Carbamazepine levels can also be affected by concomitant therapy with other AEDs. Phenytoin, phenobarbital, and primidone may increase the metabolism of carbamazepine and lead to a reduction in the steady-state plasma concentration. However, in some patients, addition of phenytoin can result in an increase in carbamazepine levels. Carbamazepine blood levels may increase, decrease, or remain the same when valproate is added. This may reflect the variable effects of valproate displacement of carbamazepine from protein-binding sites and valproate-mediated inhibition of carbamazepine metabolism.

Phenytoin and Fosphenytoin

Phenytoin, a diphenyl-substituted hydantoin derivative, was introduced for the treatment of epilepsy in 1938. It soon became one of the most widely prescribed AEDs because it possessed anticonvulsant activity at nonsedative doses. Phenytoin is effective for the treatment of partial and generalized tonic-clonic seizures, but it has no activity against absence and febrile seizures. Other hydantoin derivatives, including ethotoin and mephenytoin, also have anticonvulsant activity, but their clinical utility is limited. Phenytoin blocks neuronal sodium and calcium conductance, as well as calcium-mediated excitatory neurotransmission, which probably is involved in its ability to regulate neuronal excitability under abnormal conditions. The specific mechanism of the anticonvulsant effect of phenytoin is unknown.

Phenytoin (Dilantin and generic) is available as the free acid in suspension (30 and 125 mg/5 mL) and 50-mg chewable tablets. The sodium salt of phenytoin is contained in phenytoin capsules (30 and 100 mg) and phenytoin injectable (50 mg/mL); for these dosage forms, phenytoin content is expressed in milligrams of sodium phenytoin. Because of the difference in molecular weight between the acid and salt forms of the drug, the capsule and parenteral dosage forms contain 8% fewer phenytoin acid equivalents than the suspension and chewable tablets do. This difference in drug content should be accounted for when changing products.

In adults, phenytoin can be initiated at a dose of 300 mg daily. The usual effective maintenance dose is 300 to 400 mg daily. Only extended-release phenytoin capsules (e.g., Dilantin Kapseals), are approved for once-daily maintenance dosing. The suspension and parenteral dosage forms should be given in divided daily doses. Loading doses of phenytoin help patients who require rapid attainment of a therapeutic level. The usual loading dose of phenytoin is 15 to 18 mg/kg. Oral loading doses of phenytoin can be given as a single dose or divided into individual increments of 200 to 400 mg separated by 2 to 4 hours. Previously, it was recommended that phenytoin loading doses be administered in small increments separated by several hours to enhance the rate of drug absorption. However, recent evidence suggests that single-dose loading with phenytoin is well tolerated and results in a shorter delay in the attainment of a therapeutic plasma level than the split-dose technique.[21] By either method, phenytoin is absorbed slowly after oral administration, and the resultant peak plasma concentration is approximately half that achieved after an equivalent intravenous loading dose. When given by the intravenous route, phenytoin should be administered at a maximal rate of 50 mg/min to reduce the risk of hypotension and cardiac arrhythmias.

These adverse effects are at least partially related to the 40% propylene glycol diluent that is used in the parenteral formulation of the drug; however, phenytoin itself also has active cardiovascular effects. Blood pressure, heart rate, and the electrocardiogram should be monitored periodically when large doses of phenytoin are administered intravenously.

Phenytoin is poorly water-soluble at acidic pH. Very little drug exists in solution in the stomach, and phenytoin absorption takes place primarily in the proximal part of the small intestine. Because the rate of drug dissolution in intestinal fluid is dose-dependent, the time to peak drug concentration after an oral loading dose of phenytoin may be delayed. The bioavailability of phenytoin approaches 100% for most well-formulated products, but it is prudent to avoid changing dosage forms and products because small changes in bioavailability can result in large changes in serum concentration (and seizure control).

Additional complications of the low water solubility of phenytoin are evident after intramuscular administration. Phenytoin crystallizes when it is injected into muscle, resulting in a depot of drug that is both potentially damaging to local tissue and slowly and erratically absorbed from the injection site. For these reasons, phenytoin should not be given intramuscularly.

Fosphenytoin (Cerebyx), a water-soluble prodrug of phenytoin for intravenous or intramuscular administration, is available for the acute treatment of seizures and for the treatment or prevention of seizures in patients unable to take medication by the oral route. Because fosphenytoin is less hydrophobic than phenytoin, it does not require propylene glycol as a diluent, and it is compatible with most common intravenous solutions (including those containing dextrose). Fosphenytoin is rapidly converted to phenytoin by circulating phosphatases with a half-life of 15 minutes. Advantages of fosphenytoin over phenytoin include less venous irritation and discomfort after intravenous administration, more reliable absorption after intramuscular administration and improved admixture compatibility. However, fosphenytoin is significantly more expensive than parenteral phenytoin, and it can cause burning, itching, or paresthesias in groin and facial areas during intravenous administration. These symptoms are usually mild and resolve by stopping the infusion or reducing the infusion rate. Doses of fosphenytoin are expressed as phenytoin equivalents (PE), which are the milligram amounts of phenytoin released by the action of phosphatases on the parent drug. For example, a fosphenytoin dose of 500 mg PE releases 500 mg of phenytoin in the presence of phosphatases. Doses of fosphenytoin should be checked carefully to ensure that they are written as intended. Fosphenytoin can be administered intravenously at infusion rates up to 150 mg PE per minute.[22]

Under normal conditions, phenytoin is approximately 90% bound to plasma proteins, primarily albumin. Conditions that can alter protein binding include renal failure, a lowered plasma albumin concentration, and the presence of displacing drugs. In each case these factors result in a decrease in phenytoin binding and an increase in the free fraction and volume of distribution. However, despite alterations in the free fraction, the free concentration of phenytoin is not changed significantly. Because the free drug exerts the therapeutic and toxic effects at receptor sites, the clinical response to a given dose of phenytoin is unchanged by altered protein binding. However, careful interpretation of the total (bound and unbound) phenytoin concentration is warranted. Equation 52.1 approximates the concentration of phenytoin that would be observed if the albumin concentration were normal (C_{normal}) from the total (bound and unbound) concentration ($C_{observed}$) and the patient's albumin concentration (Alb) in grams per deciliter[23]:

$$C_{normal} = \frac{C_{observed}}{0.2 \cdot Alb + 0.1} \quad (52.1)$$

In patients with end-stage renal disease (creatinine clearance <10 mL/min), the affinity of albumin for phenytoin is reduced by approximately 50%, and Equation 52.2 should be used[23]:

$$C_{normal} = \frac{C_{observed}}{0.1 \cdot Alb + 0.1} \quad (52.2)$$

Free (unbound) concentrations are also available from many clinical laboratories.

Phenytoin is eliminated primarily by hepatic metabolism. The major metabolic route involves *para*-hydroxylation of the parent compound to yield 5-(*p*-hydroxyphenyl)-5-phenylhydantoin. This metabolite is then glucuronidated and excreted primarily in the urine. Other hydroxylated metabolites are also generated during phenytoin metabolism, and all metabolites are inactive. Less than 5% of the drug is eliminated unchanged in the urine.

Unlike many drugs that are cleared from the body by a first-order elimination process, the clearance of phenytoin varies over the range of plasma levels that are clinically useful for the treatment of seizures. At very low plasma levels, phenytoin clearance is first-order, and small dosage changes result in a proportional change in the level. However, as the phenytoin concentration approaches the therapeutic range, the maximal capacity for phenytoin metabolism is approached, and a change in dosage can result in a disproportionately large change in the steady-state level. Thus, phenytoin dosage adjustments must be made cautiously. Also, the time required to attain a steady-state level of phenytoin can vary from several days to several weeks. The Michaelis-Menten model of saturable enzyme kinetics has been used to characterize the relationship between phenytoin dose and plasma level at steady state. By using Equation 52.3, the rate of phenytoin administration (in milligrams per day) can be calculated from the desired steady-state plasma level. Population estimates of V_{max} (maximal rate of phenytoin metabolism = 7 mg/kg/day in adults) and K_m (phenytoin concentration at which V_{max} is half-maximum = 4 mg/L in adults) can be used if patient-specific data are not available[23]:

$$R_i = \frac{V_{max} \cdot Cp_{ss}}{K_m + Cp_{ss}} \quad (52.3)$$

Adverse Effects. Acute, dose-related adverse effects of phenytoin include ataxia, diplopia, dizziness, drowsiness, encephalopathy, and involuntary movements. These symptoms usually occur at phenytoin levels greater than 30 mg/mL and are reversible when phenytoin is discontinued or the dose is reduced. Involuntary movements during phenytoin intoxication may include dyskinesias of the limbs, trunk, or face and are similar to those encountered with long-term antipsychotic drug therapy except that they are completely reversible upon drug discontinuation. Phenytoin has also been reported to exacerbate seizures at toxic levels, but this is rare. Nystagmus is a dose-related effect that may occur at plasma levels within the therapeutic range and does not necessitate a reduction in dosage.

Adverse effects associated with long-term therapy include gingival hyperplasia, facial coarsening, peripheral neuropathy, and vitamin deficiencies. Gingival hyperplasia is a dose-related effect that occurs in more than 40% of adult patients taking phenytoin. It usually begins within the first 3 months and may progress during the first year of phenytoin therapy. Patients who are at risk for gingival hyperplasia include children and those with poor oral hygiene. Patients taking phenytoin should be counseled to brush and floss their teeth regularly and to have regular dental checkups. Mild gingival hyperplasia may respond to improved dental and periodontal care or a reduction in phenytoin dosage. In advanced cases, gum resection surgery may be required. Alternative AED therapy should be considered for these patients. Chronic phenytoin therapy is also associated with dysmorphic changes in the lips, nose, brow, and other facial structures as well as other cosmetic changes, including hirsutism and acne. These adverse effects are a major limitation to the use of phenytoin for the treatment of children, adolescents, and young women.

Peripheral neuropathy with decreased deep tendon reflexes and sensory deficits may also occur during long-term phenytoin therapy. These symptoms are most common during polytherapy with phenytoin and phenobarbital and are not reversible. Phenytoin-induced megaloblastic anemia with folic acid deficiency occurs in fewer than 1% of patients and responds to folic acid supplementation. Prophylactic folic acid supplementation is unnecessary and may alter phenytoin metabolism. Alterations of bone density, mass, and mineral content have been associated with phenytoin, usually when it is given in combination with other enzyme-inducing AEDs. Although most patients with AED-related bone disease are asymptomatic, clinically apparent osteomalacia and osteoporosis may occur and requires appropriate treatment. Whether patients without clinical evidence of bone disease should receive prophylactic vitamin D and calcium supplementation is not known. Certainly, patients with known risk factors for metabolic bone disease (e.g., inadequate diet, sunlight, or exercise) should be monitored closely. AED-induced acceleration in vitamin D metabolism to less active products and impaired absorption of calcium may cause or contribute to this complication of chronic therapy.

Idiosyncratic adverse reactions usually occur within the first 8 weeks of phenytoin therapy, including rash, hepatitis, lymphadenopathy, and hematologic alterations. Skin rashes, which occur in fewer than 10% of patients, usually manifest within the first 14 days of phenytoin therapy and may be accompanied by hepatitis, lymphadenopathy, and fever. The rash is usually morbilliform but may progress to Stevens-Johnson syndrome, erythema multiforme, or toxic epidermal necrolysis. Phenytoin should be discontinued if the rash involves mucous membranes or is accompanied by fever or pain. Hepatitis occurs rarely and usually in the presence of fever, rash, and lymphadenopathy. It usually occurs during the first 3 weeks of therapy (but may be delayed by 1 year from initiation) and necessitates the immediate discontinuation of phenytoin. Although drug discontinuation optimizes the chance of recovery, some patients' conditions continue to deteriorate, and (rarely) phenytoin-induced hepatic injury leads to encephalopathy, coma, and death. Hematologic adverse reactions during phenytoin therapy include a modest, transient depression in leukocytes and, very rarely, aplastic anemia or agranulocytosis. Patients with severe idiosyncratic reactions to phenytoin should not be given the drug again. Also, the potential for cross-reactivity with other aromatic AEDs should be considered (see "Adverse Effects" for carbamazepine).

Drug Interactions. Like carbamazepine, phenytoin is a potent inducer of hepatic microsomal enzymes and it increases the metabolism of drugs that are metabolized by CYP2C, CYP3A4, and UGT. Phenytoin can reduce the therapeutic effect of oral contraceptives, warfarin, corticosteroids, cyclosporine, theophylline, and other AEDs. Phenytoin increases the metabolism of carbamazepine, valproate, felbamate, lamotrigine, topiramate, tiagabine, and clonazepam, resulting in a decrease in plasma concentrations and a potential reduction in the clinical anticonvulsant effect. Phenytoin also may increase the ratio of primidone to phenobarbital concentrations when it is administered to patients whose conditions are stabilized with primidone. Although phenytoin may enhance warfarin metabolism with long-term use, the effect is complicated, particularly early after the addition of phenytoin. Phenytoin can enhance the effect of warfarin initially, an effect probably caused by displacement of warfarin from protein binding sites and competition between the two drugs for metabolism. Both phenytoin and the S-isomer of warfarin are metabolized by CYP2C9 isoenzymes. After 1 to 2 weeks, the metabolic induction properties of phenytoin predominate, and the clinical effect of warfarin may decline.[20] An increase in warfarin dosage may be needed to maintain a consistent anticoagulant effect. For these reasons, warfarin therapy should be monitored closely during phenytoin coadministration.

Drug interactions affecting phenytoin may involve alterations in phenytoin absorption, metabolism, or protein binding. Antacids and nutritional formulas have been shown to reduce plasma levels of phenytoin, but in neither case is the interaction predictable. Steady-state phenytoin levels may fall during coadministration with aluminum- and magnesium-containing antacids, but the magnitude of the effect is variable. Given the potential for an interaction, it is reasonable to space antacid and phenytoin doses by 2 to 3 hours. Phenytoin levels drop after institution of nasogastric feedings, but the mechanism of this interaction is unclear. With flushing of the nasogastric tube, phenytoin adsorption to the apparatus is probably minimal. Concurrent administration with Isocal and Osmolite, but not Ensure, may reduce phenytoin levels.[24] Patients' phenytoin levels should be monitored closely when enteral feedings are initiated or stopped and if the formula is changed.

Heparin, phenylbutazone, tolbutamide, and valproate displace phenytoin from plasma protein-binding sites. Many drugs alter the metabolism of phenytoin. It is important to be aware of these interactions, because small changes in phenytoin clearance can have a large effect on the steady-state plasma level. Folic acid, alcohol, and rifampin can increase the metabolism of phenytoin. Drugs that can reduce the metabolism of phenytoin include valproate, isoniazid, amiodarone, cimetidine, fluconazole, ketoconazole, omeprazole, fluoxetine, ticlopidine, disulfiram, sulfonamides, and chloramphenicol.[20]

Valproate

Valproate is a unique AED because of its chemical structure and its broad activity against both partial and generalized seizures. Unlike most other AEDs, which have a substituted heterocyclic ring structure, valproate is a short, branched-chain fatty acid. Many clinicians consider valproate to be the drug of choice for the treatment of primary generalized epilepsies including tonic-clonic and absence seizures.[25] Ethosuximide and valproate are equally effective against absence seizures. Valproate is as effective as carbamazepine for the treatment of secondarily generalized tonic-clonic seizures, but carbamazepine is more effective against complex partial seizures.[10] Valproate is also effective as monotherapy for treating patients who have a combination of generalized tonic-clonic seizures and absence or myoclonic seizures. The mechanism of action of valproate has not been completely elucidated but probably involves blockade of voltage-dependent sodium channels as well as potentiation of GABA, the primary inhibitory neurotransmitter within the CNS.

Valproate is available as valproic acid (Depakene) in soft gelatin capsules (250 mg) and syrup form (250 mg/5 mL) and as divalproex sodium (Depakote) in enteric-coated tablets (125, 250, and 500 mg) and sprinkle capsules (125 mg) that may be emptied onto food. Divalproex sodium dissociates into valproate in the gastrointestinal tract. A parenteral dosage form is also available for intravenous administration in patients who cannot take medication by the oral route. Intramuscular administration of parenteral valproate is not well tolerated. In adults, valproate should be initiated at a dose of 125 to 250 mg two or three times a day with gradual dose titration in 250-mg increments every 3 to 7 days. The usual effective daily dose of valproate is 750 to 1500 mg. Twice-daily dosing can be used in some patients; however, TID dosing is recommended when valproate is given concomitantly with enzyme-inducing AEDs. An extended-release dosage form of valproate is likely to be approved for use in the near future.

The bioavailability of valproate is close to 100% for all oral dosage forms, but the rate of absorption may vary. Peak levels occur within 2 hours after administration of valproate syrup and capsules. Enteric-coated tablets were developed to minimize the gastric distress associated with the plain capsule by prolonging the rate of drug dissolution. Consequently, the time to peak levels is delayed and may vary from 3 to 8 hours. Although food has no significant effect on the absorption of the soft gelatin capsules, the rate of valproate absorption from enteric-coated tablets is delayed.

Valproate is highly bound to plasma proteins, so the volume of distribution is small. The extent of protein binding varies and depends highly on the dose and plasma level of the drug. At concentrations less than 75 mg/L, valproate is approximately 90% bound to plasma proteins, primarily albumin. As the total concentration of valproate increases greater than 100 mg/L, albumin binding sites become saturated, and the free fraction of the drug may increase by up to 50%. The distribution and protein binding of valproate can be affected by a variety of other factors, including albumin and free fatty acid concentrations, pregnancy, age, and the presence of displacing drugs (e.g., phenytoin).

The relationship between the dose and steady-state plasma levels of valproate is curvilinear. Thus, with increasing dosage a less-than-proportional change in the plasma concentration occurs. Because only the unbound fraction of drug is available for metabolic transformation, this curvilinear relationship may be explained by the increase in valproate clearance that would be expected when free valproate concentrations increase as a consequence of saturable protein binding. Valproate is eliminated almost exclusively by hepatic metabolism with a half-life of 12 to 16 hours in healthy volunteers. The half-life may be reduced during concomitant therapy with other AEDs. Oxidation of valproate at the β and γ positions and glucuronide conjugation of the parent and metabolites are the primary routes of metabolism. The major metabolites of valproate are eliminated slowly and may also be active. This may explain the fact that the maximal response to valproate can be delayed by several weeks beyond the time required to achieve steady-state plasma levels of the parent drug. Also, the anticonvulsant effect during valproate therapy outlasts its presence in plasma, further supporting the hypothesis that metabolites contribute to the antiepileptic effect of the drug.

ADVERSE EFFECTS. The most common adverse effects during valproate therapy are gastrointestinal. As many as 35% of patients who are treated with either capsules or syrup report nausea, vomiting, anorexia, or other symptoms of gastrointestinal discomfort. Patient tolerance can be improved by using the enteric-coated products (tablets or sprinkles), and most patients prefer them.

The dose-related neurologic adverse effects that are seen with valproate are like those seen with other AEDs. Fine tremor, a reversible, dose-related adverse effect, occurs frequently. When tremor occurs transiently during the day, adjustment of the drug regimen to minimize plasma level fluctuations may alleviate the problem. Otherwise, a reduction in the total daily dose of valproate or concomitant treatment with a low dose of propranolol or primidone may be necessary. Cognitive adverse effects of valproate are similar to those of phenytoin.[26]

Other dose-related adverse effects include weight gain, loss or thinning of hair, altered platelet function, and increases in hepatic enzyme levels. Weight gain occurs in up to 50% of patients and probably reflects a reduction in energy use. Hair thinning or alopecia is transient and usually occurs on initiation of therapy. Reduction of valproate dosage may help. Valproate causes a dose-related reduction in platelet count and impairment of platelet function leading to an increase in bleeding time.[27] These effects may be significant for patients with high plasma levels of valproate or those undergoing surgical procedures. Approximately 40% of patients will experience a dose-related increase in serum transaminases during valproate therapy. This abnormality is usually asymptomatic and rapidly responds to a reduction in dose or discontinuation of the drug. Practitioners should discontinue valproate in the following instances: (1) an elevation in hepatic enzymes three times above baseline, (2) abnormalities in laboratory tests of hepatic synthesis or metabolism (e.g., elevated bilirubin or prothrombin time or decreased serum albumin concentration), or (3) the development of clinical signs or symptoms of hepatitis. Baseline laboratory values, including liver enzymes and hepatic function tests, should be determined before therapy with valproate is initiated.

Valproate has also been associated with fulminant hepatotoxicity leading to coma and death. Although the overall incidence of fatal hepatotoxicity is very low (1 of 49,000 treated patients), certain patients are particularly at risk. Specific risk factors include age less than 2 years, AED polytherapy, and developmental delay.[28] The risk of fatal hepatotoxicity is exceedingly low in patients older than 10 years of age who are receiving monotherapy. When it occurs, fulminant hepatotoxicity is usually seen during the first 6 to 12 months of therapy. Gastrointestinal distress, anorexia, or sudden loss of seizure control may precede the development of fulminant hepatic failure, so patients should be counseled at the start of therapy to report these or other clinical signs or symptoms of hepatitis as soon as they develop. The prognosis may be improved if therapy is discontinued quickly.

Dreifuss et al.[28] suggest the following guidelines for minimizing the risk of fatal valproate hepatotoxicity:

> (a) avoid administering valproate as part of anticonvulsant polytherapy in children younger than age 3 years, unless monotherapy has failed or the potential benefits of polypharmacy outweigh the risks; (b) avoid administering valproate to patients with preexisting liver disease or a family history of childhood hepatic disease; (c) administer valproate in the lowest possible dose that is consistent with seizure control; (d) avoid concomitant administration of valproate and salicylates, and avoid fasting in children with intercurrent illnesses; (e) monitor clinically for such symptoms as nausea, vomiting, headache, lethargy, edema, jaundice, or seizure breakthrough, especially after febrile illness.

Greater recognition of patients who are at risk for valproate hepatotoxicity is probably responsible for the significant decrease in the number of hepatic fatalities despite the overall increased use of the drug.[1]

DRUG INTERACTIONS. Metabolic interactions between valproate and other AEDs are common. Unlike phenytoin, carbamazepine, phenobarbital, and primidone, valproate is not an enzyme-inducing drug. Conversely, valproate inhibits the metabolism of drugs that are biotranformed by CYP2C9, epoxide hydrolase and UGT enzymes. This inhibition has been implicated in valproate interactions with phenobarbital and phenytoin (both metabolized by CYP2C9), as well as lamotrigine and lorazepam (both metabolized by glucuronidation).[20] Valproate inhibits the oxidative metabolism of phenobarbital, leading to an average increase in phenobarbital levels of 80%. However, because of variability in this increase (0 to 200%), routine adjustment of the dose of phenobarbital is not recommended. Rather, blood levels of phenobarbital should be monitored, with appropriate adjustment of the dose if necessary. The interaction between phenytoin and valproate is complex and probably involves both enzyme inhibition and protein binding displacement. Phenytoin levels commonly fall after initiation of valproate therapy, probably owing to displacement of phenytoin from protein-binding sites and an attendant increase in phenytoin clearance and volume of distribution. The free fraction of phenytoin may increase further with subsequent increases in valproate dosage. During continued therapy with valproate, phenytoin levels may remain low or rise to the preadministration level or above. Regardless of the subsequent change in phenytoin levels, the free fraction of phenytoin probably remains elevated during polytherapy and may increase further with increasing doses of valproate. Thus, total plasma levels of phenytoin should be interpreted cautiously. Monitoring of unbound phenytoin levels may be useful during concomitant valproate therapy.

The metabolism of valproate is susceptible to induction by other AEDs, including phenobarbital, carbamazepine, phenytoin, and primidone. Serum levels of valproate decrease by an average of 30 to 40%, and the half-life is reduced to 6 to 9 hours. Because of the difficulty of maintaining consistent, therapeutic concentrations of valproate in patients who are taking other AEDs, monotherapy with valproate is highly recommended.

Antipyretic doses of aspirin may displace valproate from protein-binding sites and competitively inhibit β-oxidation. Unlike other AEDs, valproate does not increase the failure rate of oral contraceptives. However, because of potential neural tube effects, women of childbearing age should use this agent cautiously and routine supplementation of folic acid is recommended.

Ethosuximide

Ethosuximide is a member of the succinimide class of antiepileptic agents, which includes phensuximide and methsuximide. The latter agents share similar antiepileptic effects with ethosuximide, but they are rarely used in the treatment of seizures because they are less effective and their use is associated with more significant adverse effects. Ethosuximide is as effective as valproate for the treatment of absence seizures, but ethosuximide is often preferred for young children because of the potential for valproate-associated hepatotoxicity. Ethosuximide has no activity against partial and generalized tonic-clonic seizures. Although the mechanism of ethosuximide's antiepileptic effect is unknown, the drug may suppress seizures by alteration of calcium flux in the thalamus or by the depletion of excitatory neurotransmitter stores within the CNS.

Ethosuximide (Zarontin) is available as capsules (250 mg) and syrup (250 mg/5 mL) for oral use. The initial dose of ethosuximide is 250 mg daily for children 3 to 6 years of age and 500 mg for children 6 years and older. The dose should be increased at weekly intervals in 250-mg increments as necessary. Infants require larger doses on a weight basis than adolescents and adults do. Despite the long half-life of ethosuximide, the drug is often given in divided doses to minimize gastrointestinal distress.

Ethosuximide is metabolized hepatically to inactive hydroxylated products that are then excreted. Approximately 20% of a given dose is excreted in the urine unchanged. Serum level monitoring helps to guide therapy, but the upper end of the therapeutic range is loosely defined. Many patients tolerate levels greater than 100 mg/mL, and plasma concentrations of 150 mg/mL or greater are occasionally required for optimal treatment.

Adverse Effects. Sedation, nausea, anorexia, and headache are the most common adverse effects reported on initiation of ethosuximide therapy. Tolerance to these symptoms usually develops within the first weeks of treatment, and they can be minimized by reducing the dose or by introducing the drug gradually as outlined above. Behavioral disturbances, including irritability, depression, and frank psychosis, occur independent of the drug dose. These symptoms are rare and usually occur in children or adolescents who have a history of behavioral or psychiatric problems. Discontinuation of the drug is usually required. In most patients, ethosuximide has no detrimental effect on intellectual function. Idiosyncratic reactions during ethosuximide therapy include mild, transient leukopenia, rare pancytopenia, rash, and SLE. Periodic complete blood counts should be performed during the first 6 to 12 months of therapy, and the patient should be observed for the development of clinical symptoms, suggesting serious bone marrow suppression.

Drug Interactions. Ethosuximide is not an enzyme inducer or inhibitor and has no important effect on the disposition of most other AEDs. Ethosuximide levels may be reduced by carbamazepine and increased by valproate, presumably by enzyme induction and inhibition, respectively. Phenytoin, phenobarbital, and primidone have no clinical effect on ethosuximide levels.

Gabapentin

Gabapentin is a chemically unique cyclohexane derivative of GABA that was synthesized to cross the blood-brain barrier and mimic the inhibitory effects of this neurotransmitter on the CNS. Gabapentin increases occipital lobe brain GABA levels; however, it is not known if this contributes to the drug's anticonvulsant effect.[29] Gabapentin is effective as adjunctive (add-on) therapy for patients with partial and secondarily generalized tonic-clonic seizures. In clinical trials, gabapentin reduces the frequency of these seizures by 50% or more in 25% of patients. By comparison, only 10% of placebo-treated patients experienced a similar reduction in seizures. The drug is not approved for children or as monotherapy. The drug has little or no activity against primarily generalized tonic-clonic and absence seizures. In addition to its use for epilepsy, gabapentin is also prescribed for the treatment of pain and psychiatric disorders.[30,31] U.S. Food and Drug Administration (FDA) approval for these indications is pending.

Gabapentin (Neurontin) is available as oral capsules in 100-, 300-, and 400-mg strengths and as oral tablets in 600- and 800-mg strengths. Therapy with gabapentin can be titrated to an effective dose rapidly, giving 300 mg on the first day, 300 mg twice on the second day, and 300 mg three times on the third day. Many practitioners now initiate gabapentin at a dose of 300 mg TID and find this to be well tolerated. Thereafter, therapy should be titrated according to patient response. Daily doses of 3600 mg and above have been well tolerated and are sometimes required. For daily doses of 3600 mg or less, gabapentin should be given on a TID schedule. Daily doses above 3600 mg should be divided into four doses to improve absorption.

The bioavailability of gabapentin is approximately 60% after oral administration of doses between 900 and 1800 mg daily, but further dosage increases result in less than proportional increases in plasma concentrations. This lack of dose proportionality appears to be caused by saturation of the large neutral amino acid transport mechanism (system L transporter) that is responsible for gabapentin absorption across the intestinal membrane. The time to peak absorption of gabapentin is 2 to 3 hours. Food is reported to have no effect on the rate and extent of absorption; however, one study found an increase in peak plasma concentrations when gabapentin was given with a high-protein meal.[32]

Unlike other AEDs, gabapentin is neither metabolized nor bound to plasma proteins. The drug is excreted unchanged in the urine at a rate that is directly proportional to creatinine clearance. Reduction of gabapentin dosage is indicated when creatinine clearance is less than 60 mL/min. In patients with normal renal function, the half-life of gabapentin is approximately 5 hours and does not change with chronic dosing. Although some studies have suggested that gabapentin is more effective at higher plasma concentrations, a therapeutic range of plasma concentrations has not yet been defined.

Adverse Effects. Overall, gabapentin is well tolerated and is associated with mild adverse effects, primarily affecting the CNS. In premarketing studies of gabapentin as adjunctive therapy, adverse effects included somnolence (19%), dizziness (17%), ataxia (12%), and fatigue (11%). These adverse effects appear to be dose-related and can be managed by adjustments of gabapentin dosage or the doses of concomitant agents. Rash appears in fewer than 1% of patients, a rate that compares favorably with those of other AEDs. Additional adverse effects may include weight gain (usually less than 10% of the baseline weight), movement disorders (dystonia or myoclonus), and lower extremity edema. Routine laboratory monitoring is not required during gabapentin therapy.

Drug Interactions. Because gabapentin is neither metabolized nor bound to plasma proteins, it has a much lower potential than do other AEDs to interact with other drugs. Indeed, gabapentin does not affect the plasma levels of carbamazepine (including its epoxide metabolite), phenytoin, phenobarbital, or valproate. Likewise, these AEDs do not alter the disposition of gabapentin. Aluminum/magnesium hydroxide antacids (given concomitantly or 2 hours after gabapentin) and cimetidine have been shown to reduce gabapentin plasma levels by 12 to 20%, but these interactions are not likely to be clinically significant.

Lamotrigine

Lamotrigine was originally synthesized in a drug development program to exploit the antiepileptic effect of novel antifolate agents. Lamotrigine has weak antifolate properties, but its efficacy as an AED is unrelated to this property. Rather, lamotrigine inhibits voltage-dependent sodium channels, resulting in a decreased release of excitatory neurotransmitters such as aspartate and glutamate. In this regard, its mechanism of action is similar to that of carbamazepine and phenytoin. Lamotrigine is approved as monotherapy in adults and as adjunctive therapy in adults and adolescents for partial and secondarily generalized tonic-clonic seizures. Approximately 25% of patients experience a 50% or greater reduction in partial-onset seizures when lamotrigine is added to existing AED therapy. Lamotrigine is also effective for seizures associated with the Lennox-Gastaut syndrome. Preliminary evidence suggests that lamotrigine also has activity against primary generalized epilepsies (including juvenile myoclonic epilepsy).

Lamotrigine (Lamictal) is available as oral tablets in 25-, 100-, 150-, 200-, and 250-mg strengths. It is also available in dispersible tablets (5-, 25-, and 100-mg) that can be chewed, swallowed, or dispersed in liquid. Because lamotrigine disposition is significantly affected by other AEDs, the dosage of this agent needs to be adjusted according to concomitant therapy. When administered with enzyme-inducing AEDs (carbamazepine, phenytoin, phenobarbital, and primidone), lamotrigine should be initiated at a dose of 50 mg daily for 2 weeks and increased to 50 mg twice a day for 2 more weeks. Thereafter, the lamotrigine dose may be increased weekly in increments of 100 mg/day to a maintenance dose of 300 to 500 mg daily (divided twice a day). Some patients may benefit from doses up to 700 mg/day. For patients who are receiving enzyme-inducing AEDs with valproate, lamotrigine should be initiated at a dose of 25 mg every other day for 2 weeks and increased to 25 mg/day for 2 more weeks. Thereafter, the lamotrigine dose can be increased every 1 to 2 weeks in increments of 25 mg/day to a maintenance dose of 100 to 200 mg/day (divided twice a day). When given with valproate alone, lamotrigine doses should be reduced further, but more specific recommendations are not available.

The oral bioavailability of lamotrigine is 98%, and peak plasma levels occur 2 to 4 hours after administration. Food has no significant effect on absorption. Lamotrigine is 55% bound to plasma proteins, making clinically significant protein-binding interactions unlikely. Lamotrigine is metabolized by glucuronic acid conjugation to an inactive product. The half-life of lamotrigine is approximately 24 hours during monotherapy, but other AEDs significantly affect the rate of elimination. Concomitant therapy with enzyme-inducing AEDs enhances lamotrigine metabolism and reduces the half-life to approximately 14 hours. The half-life is approximately 27 hours in patients who are taking valproate and enzyme-inducing AEDs. The half-life is increased to 59 hours in patients who are taking valproate without enzyme-inducing AEDs. No clear relationship exists between plasma concentrations of lamotrigine and clinical effect. In clinical trials, trough serum levels of lamotrigine ranged from 1 to 3 mg/L.

Adverse Effects. Adverse effects during lamotrigine therapy are usually mild or moderate and resolve with dosage reduction. Pooled data from placebo-controlled add-on studies found that the most common side effects involved the CNS and included dizziness (38%), headache (29%), diplopia (28%), ataxia (22%), and somnolence (14%). Approximately 10% of patients who received lamotrigine developed a skin rash, and it was the most common reason for drug discontinuation (3%). The rash usually develops in the first 4 to 6 weeks of therapy and is more common in patients who are receiving an AED regimen that includes valproate. The incidence of rash also increases with higher starting doses and a faster rate of dosage escalation. Potentially life-threatening skin rashes, including Stevens-Johnson syndrome and toxic epidermal necrolysis, have been reported in as many as 1 of 50 to 1 of 100 children and 1 of 1000 adults. Patients should be counseled to report the occurrence of a skin rash to their health care provider immediately, and lamotrigine should be discontinued at the first sign of rash.

Drug Interactions. As was indicated above, lamotrigine metabolism can be significantly affected by other AEDs. These interactions are clinically significant and should be considered during the initiation and titration of lamotrigine therapy. Acetaminophen can increase the clearance of lamotrigine but the mechanism of this interaction is unknown. Lamotrigine is a weak inducer of UGT and causes a small increase in its own metabolism; however, it does not have a significant effect on the elimination of carbamazepine, phenytoin, phenobarbital, primidone, or oral contraceptives. Lamotrigine causes a modest decrease in valproate concentrations. There are conflicting reports on the effect of lamotrigine on CBZ-E concentrations. One study reported that lamotrigine had no effect on CBZ-E concentrations; however, another study reported that CBZ-E concentrations increased by a mean of 45% during lamotrigine administration. After addition of lamotrigine to carbamazepine, some patients experience diplopia, dizziness, or somnolence without any evident change in carbamazepine or CBZ-E concentrations, suggesting a pharmacodynamic interaction between these two agents.[20]

Felbamate

Felbamate is a chemically unique carbamate derivative that is structurally related to the sedative-hypnotic meprobamate. It was approved by the FDA in August 1993 and rapidly became a popular agent for several reasons: (1) it was the first new AED that had been marketed in the United States since valproate in 1978; (2) it was the first drug that was brought to the market through the Antiepileptic Drug Development Program, a program established by the National Institutes for Neurological Disease and Stroke to facilitate the preclinical and clinical evaluation of new chemical entities for the treatment of epilepsy; (3) the drug was shown to be effective as monotherapy and adjunctive therapy for adults with partial seizures (with and without secondary generalization) and as adjunctive therapy for children with partial or generalized seizures associated with the Lennox-Gastaut syndrome; and (4) the drug seemed to be very well tolerated in clinical trials. In other preliminary studies, felbamate also was shown to have activity against absence, atypical absence, and juvenile myoclonic seizures. The mechanism of felbamate's antiepileptic effects is unknown.

One year after the introduction of felbamate, an association with potentially life-threatening hematologic and hepatic adverse effects was reported (see "Adverse Effects" below). These reports have caused reconsideration of the relative risks and benefits of felbamate therapy, and the drug is currently recommended only for "patients who respond inadequately to alternative treatments and whose epilepsy is so severe that a substantial risk of aplastic anemia and/or liver failure is deemed acceptable in light of the benefits conferred by its use."[33] Research is ongoing to identify the mechanism of these adverse effects with the hope that patients at high risk can be identified before drug exposure.

Felbamate (Felbatol) is available as oral tablets in 400- and 600-mg strengths and as an oral suspension (600 mg/5 mL). Therapy with felbamate can be initiated at 1200 mg/day (given three or four times a day) and increased at weekly intervals by 1200 mg/day to a dose of 3600 mg/day. Some patients may require higher doses for maximal benefit. The dosages of concomitant AEDs should be reduced by 20 to 30% on initiation of felbamate therapy, and further reductions may be required during titration of therapy (see "Drug Interactions" below).

Felbamate is at least 90% absorbed after oral administration, and its bioavailability is unaffected by food or antacids. The drug is 25% bound to plasma proteins (primarily to albumin), so clinically significant protein-binding interactions are unlikely. Felbamate is eliminated by hydrolysis and cytochrome P-450-mediated metabolism to inactive products (50%) and by renal excretion of unchanged drug (50%). The half-life is 20.5 hours and is not affected by chronic administration. Plasma concentrations of felbamate have not been correlated with clinical efficacy.

Adverse Effects. At the time of FDA approval in 1993, felbamate was shown to be well tolerated in many premarketing clinical trials. When administered as adjunctive therapy to adults with partial seizures, felbamate was associated with headache (37%), nausea (34%), somnolence (19%), anorexia (19%), dizziness (18%), insomnia (17%), and fatigue (17%). The incidence of these adverse effects was reduced by approximately one-half when felbamate was used as monotherapy, suggesting that concomitant AEDs were at least partly responsible for these symptoms. Weight loss was reported in 4% of adults and 6% of children receiving felbamate.

Felbamate had been evaluated in approximately 1700 patients in controlled clinical trials at the time of its introduction to the U.S. market. As is the case with rare idiosyncratic reactions, it was not until felbamate was used in a much larger population that the risks of the drug became known. On August 1, 1994 (after approximately 100,000 patient exposures), Wallace Laboratories announced that felbamate had been associated with 10 cases of aplastic anemia, and the FDA recommended the immediate withdrawal of the drug unless drug discontinuation would pose a more serious risk to the patient. Subsequently, additional cases have been reported (a total of 34 cases worldwide), and it is estimated that the risk of felbamate-associated aplastic anemia is more than 100-fold greater than that seen in the untreated population. The estimated incidence of aplastic anemia is approximately 1 in 4000.[34] For comparison, the risk of aplastic anemia with chloramphenicol is estimated to be approximately 1 of 40,000. The risk of aplastic anemia is highest within the first year of therapy and does not appear to be related to felbamate dosage. The mortality has been approximately 30%.

Felbamate has also been associated with 23 cases of acute hepatic failure worldwide. The period of highest risk appears to be during the first year of therapy, and there is no clear correlation with felbamate dosage. The estimated incidence of felbamate-associated hepatotoxicity is 1 of 26,000 to 34,000. For comparison, the incidence of fulminant hepatic failure associated with valproate is 1 of 10,000 to 49,000 exposures.[34]

In addition to amending the prescribing information for felbamate, the manufacturer has included a patient information/consent form with the package insert. The use of this or some other consent form and the interpretation of the appropriate criteria for felbamate use vary widely among different centers and individual prescribers. The use of laboratory monitoring of hematologic and hepatic function also varies. The manufacturer recommends that liver function tests be performed at baseline and at 1- to 2-week intervals while treatment continues. No guidelines for hematologic monitoring are given. At the Northern California Comprehensive Epilepsy Center we order a complete blood count with differential, platelet count, serum iron, reticulocyte count, alanine transaminase, aspartate transaminase, and bilirubin concentrations at baseline, every 2 weeks for months 1 and 2 of felbamate therapy, every month for months 3 through 12, and every 6 months thereafter. However, the value of these monitoring guidelines has not been established. Felbamate should probably be avoided for patients with a history of autoimmune disorders, previous blood dyscrasias, or hepatic abnormalities.

Drug Interactions. Felbamate is an inhibitor of β-oxidation and CYP2C19 metabolism. Thus, addition of felbamate requires a reduction in the dosages of phenytoin, phenobarbital (both CYP2C19 substrates), and valproate (metabolized by β-oxidation). The effect of felbamate on steady-state plasma concentrations of phenytoin and valproate is dose-related. At felbamate doses of 1200 mg/day, phenytoin concentrations increase by an average of 23%. Felbamate doses of 1800 mg/day increase phenytoin concentrations by an average of 47% above baseline. An initial reduction in phenytoin dosage of 20 to 30% on initiation of felbamate is usually sufficient to prevent symptoms of phenytoin toxicity. However, further phenytoin dosage reductions may be required as the dosage of felbamate is increased. Valproate dosages should be reduced by approximately 30% on initiation of felbamate, and further dose reductions may be required during the titration of felbamate therapy. Felbamate has no significant effect on the protein binding of valproate.

Felbamate induces CYP3A4 metabolism, causing a decrease in mean carbamazepine concentrations by 20 to 30%; however, CBZ-E concentrations increase by 30 to 55%.[35] To prevent dose-related symptoms of toxicity such as diplopia, drowsiness, and ataxia, carbamazepine doses should be reduced by approximately 30% when felbamate therapy is begun.

Felbamate concentrations can also be affected by other AEDs. Phenytoin and carbamazepine reduce steady-state concentrations of felbamate by 40 to 50%. However, because there is no consistent correlation between felbamate levels and clinical effect, no adjustment in felbamate dosage is required. Valproate does not have a significant effect on plasma concentrations of felbamate.

Topiramate

Topiramate is a monosaccharide derivative that is distinct from other AEDs, both in terms of chemical structure and mechanism of action. The drug has several pharmacologic properties that may contribute to its anticonvulsant effect: it inhibits voltage-sensitive sodium channels; enhances GABA-mediated chloride flux across neuronal membranes; and it inhibits binding of kainate to a specific subtype of the excitotoxic glutamate receptor. Topiramate is also a weak inhibitor of carbonic anhydrase although this probably does not contribute to the drug's anticonvulsant properties. Topiramate is approved as adjunctive treatment for partial, secondarily generalized tonic-clonic, and primary generalized tonic-clonic seizures in adults and children. Approximately 45% of patients with refractory partial epilepsy experience a 50% or greater reduction in seizures when topiramate is used as adjunctive treatment. In preliminary studies, topiramate has also been effective for generalized-onset seizures, seizures associated with the Lennox-Gastaut syndrome, infantile spasms, and as monotherapy.[35]

Topiramate (Topamax) is available as oral tablets in 25-, 100-, and 200-mg strengths and in 15- and 25-mg sprinkle capsules that can be poured onto food. The manufacturer's recommended starting dose for adults is 50 mg daily, increasing by 50 mg/day at weekly intervals to 200 to 400 mg daily in two divided doses. Some patients may experience improved tolerability (with regard to CNS adverse effects) when topiramate is introduced at a slower rate. For example, some practitioners prefer to begin topiramate at 25 mg daily, increase weekly by 25 mg/day until a dose of 50 mg BID is reached, and then continue by escalating the dose in 50 mg/day increments at weekly intervals. Most patients do not experience additional benefit from doses greater than 400 mg/day, however, occasionally higher doses are required for optimal treatment (as high as 1000 mg/day or more).

The oral bioavailability of topiramate is 80%, and peak plasma levels occur 3 to 4 hours after administration. Food delays the absorption of topiramate, but the extent of absorption is unaffected. Topiramate is 15% bound to plasma proteins and protein-binding interactions have not been reported. Urinary excretion of the unchanged drug is the predominant route of elimination (70%). However, enzyme-inducing AEDs increase the proportion of topiramate clearance due to metabolism and cause a 40 to 50% decrease in topiramate concentrations. The half-life of topiramate is 24 hours after a single dose to healthy adults. There is a lack of correlation between topiramate plasma concentrations and clinical effect. Therefore, routine monitoring of topiramate concentrations is not necessary.

Adverse Effects. Common adverse effects during topiramate therapy are usually mild or moderate and are minimized by using a conservative dose-escalation schedule. Pooled data from placebo-controlled trials of topiramate as adjunctive therapy indicate that the most common adverse effects are somnolence (30%), dizziness (28%), ataxia (21%), psychomotor slowing (17%), and problems with speech, such as word-finding difficulty (17%). Other adverse effects include difficulty with concentration or attention, confusion, weight loss, and tremor. Difficulty concentrating and psychomotor slowing are the most common reasons for discontinuation. A recent comparative study in healthy adults found more significant cognitive effects associated with topiramate than with gabapentin and lamotrigine.[36] Kidney stones occur in 1.5% of patients, and patients should be counseled to maintain adequate fluid intake during topiramate treatment.

Drug Interactions. As mentioned above, topiramate metabolism is enhanced by enzyme-inducing AEDs such as carbamazepine, phenytoin, and phenobarbital. Topiramate can reduce the clearance of phenytoin. However, the magnitude of the effect is variable with phenytoin concentrations, increasing from 0 to 25%. Topiramate has no significant effect on the metabolism of other AEDs. Ethinyl estradiol concentrations are reduced during concomitant therapy with topiramate and women should be monitored closely for breakthrough bleeding. Consideration should be given to using an oral contraceptive with a higher estrogen content (e.g., ≥35 μg of ethinyl estradiol).[20]

Tiagabine

Tiagabine, a nipecotic acid derivative with a chemical structure unique among AEDs, inhibits the reuptake of GABA into presynaptic neurons and glial cells. This is thought to be the mechanism of its anticonvulsant effect. The drug is approved as adjunctive therapy in adults with partial and secondarily generalized tonic-clonic seizures. In clinical trials, approximately 25% of patients treated with tiagabine demonstrate a 50% or greater reduction in partial-onset seizures.

Tiagabine (Gabatril) is available as oral tablets in 4-, 12-, 16-, and 20-mg strengths. When administered with enzyme-inducing AEDs, tiagabine should be initiated at a dose of 4 mg daily and increased in 4 mg/day increments at weekly intervals. Usual maintenance dosages of tiagabine are 32 to 56 mg/day given in two to four divided doses. With doses greater than 32 mg/day, TID or QID dosing is often necessary to minimize transient adverse effects associated with peak blood levels. More conservative dose titration is usually needed when tiagabine is used with noninducing AEDs such as valproate, gabapentin, or lamotrigine.

The oral bioavailability of tiagabine is 90%. Tiagabine is absorbed quickly with peak blood levels occurring 1 hour after administration of the drug with a meal. The extent of drug absorption is not affected by food. Tiagabine is 96% bound to plasma proteins, primarily albumin and α_1-acid glycoprotein. However, clinically significant protein-binding interactions are minimal (see "Drug Interactions" below). Drug elimination is primarily by metabolism via CYP3A4 and glucuronidation enzymes. The half-life of tiagabine is 7 to 9 hours in healthy volunteers after a single dose, and it is shortened by 50 to 65% when coadministered with enzyme-inducing AEDs. There is no clear relationship between tiagabine blood levels and clinical response.

Adverse Effects. Common adverse effects reported during placebo-controlled, adjunctive therapy trials with tiagabine include dizziness (27%), lack of energy (20%), somnolence (18%), nausea (11%), and nervousness (10%). These adverse effects are usually dose-related and respond to a reduction in dosage or slowing of the rate of dose escalation. Other adverse effects that occur occasionally include tremor, generalized muscle weakness, and difficulty with concentration or attention.

Drug Interactions. Tiagabine does not induce or inhibit the metabolism of other AEDs. Although tiagabine is highly protein-bound, it does not appear to displace other highly bound drugs such as phenytoin, valproate, or warfarin.[37] However, tiagabine itself is displaced from protein binding sites by naproxen, valproate, and salicylates. The clinical significance of tiagabine displacement interactions is unknown. Because tiagabine is metabolized by CYP3A4, inhibitors of this isoenzyme would be expected to reduce its metabolism. However, the effect of erythromycin (a CYP3A4 inhibitor) on tiagabine metabolism is inconsistent. Until further data are available, erythromycin, ketoconazole, and other inhibitors of CYP3A4 should be used cautiously with tiagabine.[20] As mentioned above, enzyme-inducing AEDs enhance the metabolism of tiagabine by 50 to 65%.

Phenobarbital

All barbiturates have anticonvulsant activity, but only phenobarbital and primidone are used commonly for the chronic treatment of epilepsy, because they are effective at subhypnotic doses. Phenobarbital was first used for the treatment of seizures in 1912, and it continues to be prescribed widely. However, because of adverse effects on the CNS, this agent is now used primarily as an alternative when monotherapy with first-line agents has failed. Phenobarbital is most useful for the treatment of partial and generalized tonic-clonic seizures. Phenobarbital elevates the seizure threshold and prevents the spread of electrical seizure activity. Although the precise mechanism of action is unknown, these effects may be related to the ability of phenobarbital to modulate the inhibitory action of GABA or to attenuate the postsynaptic effects of excitatory neurotransmitters such as glutamate.

Phenobarbital is available as the sodium salt in a variety of dosage forms, including oral capsules and tablets (various strengths), elixir (20 mg/5 mL), and injectable preparations (various concentrations). The usual maintenance dose of phenobarbital for adults is 1 to 3 mg/kg/day. In neonates and children the usual daily dose is 3 to 4 mg/kg. Phenobarbital is usually given as a single daily dose at bedtime to avoid peak sedative effects during the day. Although food may delay absorption, the absolute bioavailability of phenobarbital is unchanged. The long half-life of phenobarbital (approximately 4 days) may cause a delay of 2 to 3 weeks until steady-state levels are achieved. Therefore, a loading dose should be administered when a prompt therapeutic effect is needed. The usual loading dose of phenobarbital is 15 mg/kg. When it is given intravenously, the rate of administration should not exceed 100 mg/min. Oral loading doses may also be used. The oral loading doses of phenobarbital should be divided into three equal increments and separated by 24 hours. Patients should be monitored for the attendant sedation and incoordination that may occur.

Phenobarbital is nearly completely absorbed after oral and intramuscular administration, with peak concentrations occurring in less than 4 hours. Phenobarbital is 45 to 60% bound to plasma proteins, and for this reason, clinically significant protein binding interactions are rare. Phenobarbital is eliminated by a first-order process. Thirty to 50% of phenobarbital is metabolized by the liver to inactive products that are glucuronidated or sulfated and excreted in the urine. Approximately 25% of the dose is excreted in the urine unchanged. Excretion of phenobarbital is enhanced significantly in alkaline urine and during forced diuresis.

Adverse Effects. CNS adverse effects during phenobarbital therapy are generally dose-related and include sedation, nystagmus, dizziness, and ataxia. Mild drowsiness is common on initiation of therapy, but tolerance to this effect usually develops within the first several weeks. Occasionally, sedation will persist during chronic treatment, and for these patients the dose should be reduced. Of greater concern are the subtle effects of phenobarbital on behavior, mood, and cognition. Reversible hyperactivity and insomnia occur in up to 40% of children who are treated with phenobarbital, and paradoxical excitation has been reported in older patients as well. These behavioral changes usually occur within the first few months of therapy and are more prevalent in patients with organic brain disease. A noticeable improvement in behavior may be seen when phenobarbital is replaced with valproate or carbamazepine. Phenobarbital may also cause depression and lack of interest or ambition that are recognized by others or appreciated only after discontinuation of the drug. Although the cognitive effects of phenobarbital are not well characterized, several investigations have found a dose-related impairment of memory, performance on intelligence and vigilance tests, work performance, and performance of complex verbal and nonverbal tasks. These changes probably persist despite the development of tolerance to the sedative effects of the drug.

Serious adverse effects of phenobarbital are uncommon, and, in general, this drug is associated with fewer idiosyncratic adverse effects than is phenytoin or carbamazepine.[9] Morbilliform rash is the most common idiosyncratic reaction, occurring in 1 to 3% of patients. Rarely, the rash may progress to Stevens-Johnson syndrome or exfoliative dermatitis or may occur in conjunction with symptoms of hepatitis or bone marrow suppression. The potential for cross-reactivity between phenobarbital and other aromatic AEDs (e.g., carbamazepine and phenytoin) should be considered in changing therapy for these patients. Megaloblastic anemia with folic acid deficiency occurs in fewer than 1% of phenobarbital-treated patients and responds to folic acid supplementation. Like phenytoin, phenobarbital is associated with bone disorders (e.g., osteomalacia) during chronic therapy.

Drug Interactions. Most drug interactions with phenobarbital are characterized by alterations of metabolism. By increasing the synthesis and retarding the degradation of hepatic enzymes, phenobarbital accelerates the metabolism of many agents that are metabolized by the mixed-function oxidase system, including theophylline, warfarin, cyclosporine, chloramphenicol, valproate, felbamate, lamotrigine, chlorpromazine, haloperidol, and tricyclic antidepressants. The degree of enzyme induction and alteration of drug metabolism varies greatly among patients and is to some extent under genetic control. Enzyme induction usually last for 2 to 3 weeks after phenobarbital is discontinued. Carbamazepine levels may remain unchanged or decline during phenobarbital coadministration. Phenobarbital can also inhibit the metabolism of some drugs, presumably by competition for similar metabolic pathways. The effect of phenobarbital on plasma levels of phenytoin is unpredictable because both induction and inhibition of metabolism probably occur (both phenytoin and phenobarbital are substrates for

CYP2C9). Phenytoin levels may modestly rise, decline, or (as in most cases) show no change. Valproate often causes a clinically important reduction in the metabolism of phenobarbital, with resultant symptoms of phenobarbital toxicity (see "Drug Interactions" for valproate). The effect of phenytoin on phenobarbital plasma levels is unpredictable, and in most cases, clinically important alterations are not seen.

Primidone

Primidone is structurally related to the barbiturates, and like phenobarbital, it is effective for the treatment of partial and generalized tonic-clonic seizures. Primidone is an active anticonvulsant agent, as are its two major metabolites, phenobarbital and phenylethylmalonamide. Although the clinical use of primidone is similar to that of phenobarbital, adverse effects are more commonly a limiting factor during long-term primidone therapy. Some patients may respond to primidone therapy despite the failure of phenobarbital to control seizures.

Primidone (Mysoline and generic) is available as oral tablets (50 and 250 mg) and as an oral suspension (250 mg/5 mL). Primidone should be initiated slowly, to allow the development of tolerance to the acute gastrointestinal and sedative effects of the parent drug. For adults, therapy can be started at a dose of 125 to 250 mg twice a day with gradual dosage increases every 4 to 7 days in 125- to 250-mg increments until the effective dose is reached.

Metabolic transformation of primidone to phenobarbital and phenylethylmalonamide occurs by oxidative metabolism and pyrimidine ring cleavage, respectively. Primidone and its metabolites are also excreted by the kidney to a significant extent. Because the half-life of primidone is relatively short, the drug is usually given in divided doses to maintain more consistent plasma levels of the parent drug and reduce the likelihood of transient side effects at times of peak primidone levels. Pharmacokinetic monitoring of primidone therapy includes routine assessment of both primidone and phenobarbital levels. Samples should be drawn at a consistent time relative to the dose. Whereas primidone reaches steady-state concentrations quickly, there is usually a delay of 2 to 3 weeks before plateau concentrations of phenobarbital are attained. During chronic treatment, plasma concentrations of phenobarbital are approximately one to three times higher than those of primidone. This fact is sometimes useful in monitoring compliance.

Adverse Effects. The adverse effects of primidone are similar to those of phenobarbital. Thus, the potential for primidone-related neurotoxicity is of concern during long-term therapy. In addition, primidone itself is frequently associated with initial dose-related adverse effects, including sedation, dizziness, and nausea. Decreased libido and impotence appear to be more common during primidone therapy than with other AEDs. Serious adverse effects during primidone therapy are rare.

Drug Interactions. The metabolism of primidone or its metabolites can be affected by other AEDs, including phenytoin and valproate. Phenytoin increases phenobarbital levels during coadministration with primidone. The result is an approximate doubling of the phenobarbital: primidone concentration ratio. Primidone levels do not appear to be significantly affected during phenytoin therapy. Valproate can reduce the metabolic clearance of metabolically derived phenobarbital and produce signs of barbiturate intoxication during primidone therapy. Valproate has a negligible effect on the plasma concentrations of primidone. Carbamazepine may increase the metabolism of primidone, although in many patients this interaction is not clinically important.

Benzodiazepines

Diazepam, lorazepam, clonazepam, and clorazepate are the only benzodiazepine agents that are FDA-approved for the treatment of seizures. Diazepam and lorazepam have little utility in the chronic treatment of epilepsy, but they are frequently used intravenously for the termination of status epilepticus. In general, benzodiazepines are more effective in suppressing generalized epileptiform activity than focal discharges, and these agents limit the spread of epileptic discharges without suppressing the primary seizure focus. Nonetheless, clinical use of clonazepam and clorazepate for the chronic treatment of epilepsy includes both generalized and partial seizure types. Although the precise mechanism of the anticonvulsant effect of these agents is unknown, the benzodiazepines are thought to facilitate inhibitory neurotransmission in the CNS by enhancing the postsynaptic effects of GABA.

Clonazepam

Clonazepam is useful, alone or as an adjunct to other agents, for the treatment of Lennox-Gastaut syndrome and akinetic and myoclonic seizures. The drug is also useful for the treatment of absence seizures that fail to respond to valproate or ethosuximide. Clonazepam is not approved for the treatment of partial or generalized tonic-clonic seizures, and experience in its use for the treatment of these seizure types is limited.

Clonazepam (Klonopin) is available as oral tablets in strengths of 0.5, 1, and 2 mg. An intravenous preparation is available for use in Europe, but it is not available in the United States. Clonazepam should be initiated at low doses (0.5 mg three times a day for adults; 0.01 to 0.03 mg/kg divided twice or three times a day for infants and children) and gradually titrated upward at 3- to 7-day intervals. The maximum recommended daily dose is 20 mg for adults and 0.1 to 0.2 mg/kg for infants and children. Although the half-life of clonazepam is long enough to allow once-daily dosing for many patients, the drug is often administered in divided doses. This is particularly important for patients who are intolerant of the transient sedative effects that occur after peak absorption and for infants and children, in whom the drug's half-life may be shortened.

Clonazepam is eliminated primarily by reduction of the nitro group to form 7-amino clonazepam, an inactive metabolite. Although loss of efficacy may occur during chronic therapy (see "Adverse Effects" below), clonazepam does not induce its own metabolism. There is wide variation in the relationship between the dose and plasma levels of clonazepam. There is also significant overlap between the plasma levels that are associated with the antiepileptic effect of the drug and those that are associated with dose-related adverse effects. For these reasons the therapeutic range of clonazepam levels is imprecisely defined, though many references cite a therapeutic range of 13 to 72 μg/mL. However, therapeutic monitoring of clonazepam concentrations during routine therapy is not often used.

Adverse Effects. Adverse effects are common during clonazepam treatment and necessitate drug discontinuation in up to one-third of patients. Dose-related adverse effects are particularly common and include drowsiness and ataxia. Although tolerance of the overt sedative effects of clonazepam and other benzodiazepines usually develops during the first few weeks of therapy, mild impairment of cognitive and motor skills may persist throughout treatment. In other patients, dose-related adverse effects are not tolerable, and clonazepam therapy must be discontinued. Clonazepam can also cause behavioral disturbances, including hyperactivity, irritability, restlessness, and aggressive or violent behavior. Children are affected more frequently than adults are. Dosage reduction may be attempted, but it does not always alleviate behavioral changes. Other noteworthy adverse effects include excessive salivation, bronchial hypersecretion, weight gain, and, rarely, exacerbation of seizures. Abrupt discontinuation of clonazepam may precipitate seizures or status epilepticus. Therefore, clonazepam should be gradually withdrawn when treatment is to be terminated.

The long-term clinical utility of clonazepam is limited by the development of tolerance to the antiepileptic effect. Approximately one-third of patients who initially benefit from clonazepam therapy experience some loss of efficacy, usually within the first 6 months of treatment. Although the antiepileptic effect may be restored by increasing the dose, as many as 30% of patients who develop tolerance do not regain adequate seizure control.

Drug Interactions. Clinically important drug interactions with clonazepam are uncommon. Clonazepam has no significant effect on the pharmacokinetic disposition of phenytoin, carbamazepine, or primidone. However, phenytoin, carbamazepine, and phenobarbital can reduce the steady-state concentrations of clonazepam, presumably by the induction of hepatic metabolism. The combined use of clonazepam and valproate has been reported to exacerbate absence seizures. Although the simultaneous use of these agents is not a strict contraindication, caution should be observed.

Clorazepate

Clorazepate dipotassium is approved for use as an adjunct to other agents for the treatment of partial seizures. Clorazepate is a prodrug that is rapidly decarboxylated in the acidic medium of the stomach to yield *N*-desmethyldiazepam (DMD), the primary active metabolite. This metabolite is responsible for the antiepileptic effect of the parent compound.

Clorazepate (Tranxene) is available as a prompt-release oral tablet (3.75, 7.5, and 15 mg) and as an extended-release oral tablet (11.5 and 22.5 mg) for once-daily dosing. Therapy with clorazepate should be initiated with the prompt-release form at a dose of 7.5 mg three times a day for adults and 7.5 mg twice a day for children (ages 9 to 12 years). The dose should be increased at 7-day intervals, in increments of 7.5 mg or less, to a maximum daily dose of 90 mg for adults and 60 mg for children. Transient dose-related adverse effects may be minimized and compliance may be improved by a change to the extended-released dosage form for patients whose seizures are controlled with clorazepate.

DMD and its hydroxylated metabolites (including oxazepam) are conjugated and excreted in the urine. Plasma level monitoring is of little use in the management of patients who are taking clorazepate.

Adverse Effects. Adverse effects of clorazepate are similar to those of clonazepam and include sedation, dizziness, hypersalivation, and behavioral changes. Tolerance to the antiepileptic effect of clorazepate has been reported, but it does not seem to be as common, or to develop as quickly, as with clonazepam.

Drug Interactions. Concurrent antacid administration may significantly slow the rate of conversion from clorazepate to DMD, as can other disease states that are characterized by an increase in gastric pH. However, during prolonged administration, steady-state DMD levels are not significantly reduced. Smoking and concurrent AED therapy with enzyme-inducing agents can accelerate the metabolism of clorazepate. Clorazepate has no known effect on the disposition of other AEDs.

Treating the Pregnant Woman Who Has Epilepsy

There is much controversy about the treatment of pregnant women who have epilepsy. Central issues are the risk of fetal malformations that are attributable to individual seizures and to the epileptic diathesis, the degree of additional risk that is attributable to AED therapy, and the antiepileptic agent of choice for minimizing the risk of fetal malformations. Although a detailed discussion of these topics is beyond the scope of this chapter, several important principles should be considered. The reader is referred to other reviews for additional discussion of this topic[38,39] and to Chapter 100, Drug Use in Pregnancy and Lactation.

Therapeutic considerations that are unique during pregnancy include (1) changes in maternal seizure control, (2) the choice of antiepileptic agents, (3) alteration of AED pharmacokinetics, and (4) the potential for AED-associated coagulopathy in the newborn. Approximately 60% of women with epilepsy will have no change in seizure frequency during pregnancy.[38] Among the remaining patients, worsening of seizures occurs in approximately one-third of pregnant women.[39] This may be attributable to several factors, including reduced medication compliance caused by maternal fears that the medication may injure the developing fetus, pharmacokinetic changes in AED disposition, and sleep deprivation.

Overall, the incidence of fetal abnormalities in children of epileptic mothers is approximately 6%, roughly twice that found in the general population. Although there is considerable controversy about which AED has the lowest teratogenic risk, there is a clear association between some AEDs and fetal malformations. Trimethadione is clearly associated with a syndrome of anomalies, and this drug should be avoided during pregnancy. Affected infants may have craniofacial abnormalities, including microcephaly, and ocular defects, cardiac abnormalities, intrauterine growth retardation, short stature, and developmental delay. Currently, there is no conclusive evidence on which to base a preference for the use of carbamazepine, phenobarbital, phenytoin, or valproate during pregnancy,[39] and the safety of newer AEDs (gabapentin, lamotrigine, topiramate, and tiagabine) has yet to be established. Neural tube defects have been associated with maternal use of valproate (1 to 2%) and carbamazepine (0.5 to 1%) during pregnancy. Phenytoin has been associated with a constellation of anomalies including craniofacial malformations, mental retardation, deficiencies in growth, and mental or motor performance, and limb defects that have been grouped as the fetal hydantoin syndrome. However, similar abnormalities have been associated with other AEDs. The mechanism of teratogenesis caused by AEDs is unknown but may be related to folic acid deficiencies or to arene oxide intermediates that are generated during the metabolism of aromatic AEDs. All women with childbearing potential who have epilepsy should receive folic acid supplementation. The optimal dose is unknown but most practitioners use 1 to 2 mg daily. Because no AED is clearly less teratogenic than the others, the preferred AED during pregnancy is the drug that best controls the patient's seizures. Also, it is clear that AED polytherapy is associated with a greater risk of fetal malformations. Correspondingly, it is recommended that monotherapy (with the lowest effective dose) be used whenever possible.

Pregnancy is associated with significant changes in the pharmacokinetic properties of AEDs. These changes include acceleration of hepatic drug metabolism, increased apparent volume of distribution, and alterations in plasma protein binding. The result is a decline in plasma AED concentrations and, in some patients, loss of seizure control. Consequently, AED plasma levels and the clinical status of the patient should be monitored regularly during pregnancy. Monitoring of unbound plasma concentrations of phenytoin, valproate, and carbamazepine, is recommended due to protein binding changes associated with pregnancy. Drug concentrations should be determined approximately every 3 months during pregnancy. After delivery, AED plasma concentrations should be determined weekly, and appropriate dosage adjustments should be made.

Approximately 50% of the infants who are born to mothers taking phenytoin, phenobarbital, and primidone during pregnancy are deficient in vitamin K-dependent clotting factors at birth. Although neonatal hemorrhage is uncommon, infants should be treated with vitamin K 1 mg intramuscularly immediately at birth. Clotting should then be monitored every 2 to 4 hours, and repeat doses of vitamin K should be administered as needed. Preferably, coagulopathy can be prevented by treating the mother with vitamin K 10 mg orally each day for 4 weeks before delivery.

All AEDs are excreted in breast milk to some degree. The ratio of breast milk to serum concentration is 80 to 100% for ethosuximide, 40 to 50% for phenobarbital, 40% for carbamazepine, 18 to 20% for phenytoin, and 1 to 10% for valproic acid.[39] Although most epileptic mothers may safely breastfeed their infants, the potential effect of drug transfer to the baby should be considered, especially if the infant appears to be lethargic or irritable, or feeds poorly.

Despite the concern of parents and clinicians about the risks of epilepsy and AED therapy during pregnancy, it is important to realize that more than 90% of epileptic women have normal children. However, epileptic women of childbearing age must understand the value of prepregnancy planning and, once pregnant, be made aware of the risks for fetal abnormalities, the potential consequences of medication noncompliance, and the need for close therapeutic monitoring during pregnancy and for several weeks after childbirth.

Withdrawal of Antiepileptic Drug Therapy

Several community-based studies have shown that among patients with epilepsy who are followed for more than 10 years, more than half attain a 2- to 5-year remission from seizures during drug therapy. Remission rates tend to be highest for patients who have primary generalized seizures and range from 60% for those with tonic-clonic seizures to 80% for children with typical absence attacks.

In general, patients who remain free of seizures for 2 years or more may be considered candidates for AED withdrawal. The potential benefits of drug withdrawal include avoidance of the cognitive and behavioral adverse effects of AED therapy, reduction in the risk of adverse drug reactions and drug interactions, and a return by the patient to a lifestyle that is unencumbered by the need for chronic medication. However, the decision to withdraw AED therapy is complex, both medically and socially, and requires clear explanation to the patient of both the risks and benefits.

Medical factors that appear to affect the risk of seizure recurrence after AED drug withdrawal are summarized in Table 52.9. In particular, it is important to consider the age at onset of epilepsy, seizure type, EEG abnormalities, and

Table 52.9 ▪ Factors That Affect the Risk of Seizure Recurrence After Antiepileptic Drug Withdrawal

Favorable Prognosis	Unfavorable Prognosis
Childhood-onset epilepsy	Adult-onset epilepsy
Longer seizure-free interval before drug withdrawal	Frequent seizures before remission
Absence seizures	Partial-onset seizures
Primary generalized tonic-clonic seizures	EEG abnormalities at time of drug withdrawal
Normal or improved EEG at time of drug withdrawal	Abnormal neurologic examination and subnormal IQ
Normal neurologic examination and normal IQ	Abrupt withdrawal of benzodiazepine or barbiturate antiepileptic drugs
	Atypical febrile seizures
	Juvenile myoclonic epilepsy

EEG, electroencephalogram.

rate of drug withdrawal in assessing the risk of seizure recurrence. Relapse rates after AED withdrawal in patients who have been free of seizures for 2 years or more are approximately 30% for children and 40% for adults with epilepsy.[40] Thus, 60 to 70% of patients will remain free of seizures when AED therapy is withdrawn after a 2-year remission. The risk of seizure recurrence is highest during the period of AED reduction and within the first year after drug withdrawal.

The rate of drug withdrawal may also affect seizure recurrence. Gradual withdrawal of AEDs is preferred and most practitioners discontinue therapy over a period of 1 to 3 months, depending upon the patient and the drug. Abrupt withdrawal is a risk factor for status epilepticus. Furthermore, rapid removal of AED therapy itself may precipitate seizures due to drug withdrawal (as distinct from a recurrence of seizures due to the underlying epileptic condition). Seizures during withdrawal are most common with benzodiazepine or barbiturate AEDs. Because there are no means to determine reliably whether recurrent seizures are truly epileptic in origin, the need for continued drug therapy is unclear unless the rate of taper is long enough to effectively rule out a drug-withdrawal phenomenon.

Any decision to withdraw AED therapy on the basis of a favorable medical prognosis must also include a careful assessment of the patient's work and social environments. Not only should patients clearly understand the risks and benefits of drug withdrawal, they must also be encouraged to participate actively in the decision. Patients who have been seizure-free for long intervals often have valid concerns about the possible recurrence of seizures at home, at work, or while driving. During AED withdrawal it is often recommended that the patient not drive for several months. Furthermore, in some areas a recurrent seizure during this period may result in the suspension of driving privileges until AED therapy is restarted and adequate control is demonstrated. These and other patient-specific social factors should be discussed with each individual for whom AED withdrawal is considered.

Nonpharmacologic Therapies

Vagus Nerve Stimulation

Approved in 1997, the vagus nerve stimulator is the first device approved for the treatment of epilepsy. The device consists of a fully implantable pulse generator and an electrode that attaches to the left vagus nerve. Stimulation parameters are adjusted according to patient tolerance and seizure control. Usually the device is programmed for stimulations lasting 30 seconds, followed by 5 minutes of off time, with this pattern repeating continuously while the device is in operation. There is also a hand-held magnet that can be used to manually activate the device to deliver stimulation. This latter feature is used by some patients to abort seizures at the time their seizure aura begins. The vagus nerve stimulator is approved for use in adults and adolescents as adjunctive treatment (with AED therapy) for partial-onset seizures that do not respond to drug therapy. In clinical trials, use of the vagus nerve stimulator reduces the frequency of seizures by 50% or more in 25% of patients. This response is comparable to many of the newer AEDs such as gabapentin and tiagabine. Therapeutic benefits from vagus nerve stimulation are maintained for up to 5 years (and possibly longer) with continued use of the device. Preliminary evidence also supports the efficacy of vagus nerve stimulation in children and in patients with medically refractory generalized-onset seizures; however, more study is needed to confirm these observations. The most common adverse effects associated with use of the vagus nerve stimulator are hoarseness, coughing, and throat discomfort during the stimulation burst.[41]

Surgery

Approximately 20 to 35% of persons with epilepsy will have persistent seizures despite treatment with AEDs. Many of these patients may benefit from surgical intervention; however, only a small percentage of candidates are referred for evaluation at one of the many epilepsy-surgery centers that exist in the United States.[42] Patients who are most likely to benefit from surgery are those with partial-onset seizures whose symptoms remain intractable despite optimal medical therapy. The degree to which seizures and drug toxicity impair the functional abilities of the patient must also be considered. Presurgical evaluation includes intensive medical and neurologic testing to localize the lesion. MRI, PET, and single-photon emission computed tomography scans, as well as simultaneous EEG and video telemetry monitoring, are very useful in this regard. Neuropsychologic testing is used to assess the potential effects of epilepsy surgery on memory and language function. Resection of a seizure focus from the anterior temporal lobe is the most common surgical procedure performed. After temporal lobectomy, approximately 65% of patients are rendered free of seizures for at least 2 years and 20 to 25% experience a significant reduction.[42]

ALTERNATIVE THERAPIES

Ketogenic Diet

The ketogenic diet, introduced in the 1920s, is a high-fat, low-carbohydrate, low-protein diet that has recently experienced a resurgence in popularity because of enhanced public interest. The mechanism of the diet's benefit is unknown but is thought to be related to ketosis and its effect on the brain. Children younger than 10 years of age are most likely to benefit for two reasons: they are more prone to ketosis and because the diet is unpalatable, children are more likely to comply with the diet when they depend on a parent or care-provider to prepare their meals. The diet has been used to treat patients with both partial-onset and generalized-onset seizures and 33 to 67% of patients experience a benefit in terms of reduced seizure frequency or intensity.[43] A 3-month trial is usually sufficient to determine if the diet will benefit the patient. The effect of the ketogenic diet on the clearance of AEDs has not been adequately studied; therefore, drug concentrations should be monitored during implementation of the diet. Also, acetazolamide (occasionally used for its anticonvulsant effects) should be discontinued when the diet is initiated to prevent the development of metabolic acidosis. Acetazolamide may be reintroduced several weeks after ketosis has been established.

Behavioral Therapies

Psychologic techniques for control of epileptic seizures are often successful for patients with seizures triggered by flashing lights or visual patterns, reading, or listening to music (referred to as reflex epilepsies). In these patients, behavioral conditioning has been used with success. The role of behavioral therapies in other types of epilepsy remains limited; however, some patients report benefit from relaxation and biofeedback therapies.

FUTURE THERAPIES

Several novel drugs are currently under investigation for possible use as AEDs in the United States, including oxcarbazepine, zonisamide, and vigabatrin. Oxcarbazepine (Trileptal) is a 10-keto analog of carbamazepine with a similar spectrum of anticonvulsant effect and an improved tolerability profile over carbamazepine. Oxcarbazepine is metabolized by reductase enzymes to a monohydroxy derivative that is pharmacologically active; no epoxide metabolites of oxcarbazepine are formed. An advantage of oxcarbazepine is that the drug is less likely to induce hepatic drug metabolism than carbamazepine. An IV formulation is also being studied. Zonisamide (Excegran) is a novel investigational AED that appears to have a broad spectrum of activity against both partial and generalized-onset seizures. Potential advantages of zonisamide include a broad spectrum of anticonvulsant effect (including activity against progressive myoclonic epilepsies), a long half-life, and minimal effect on the disposition of other AEDs. Vigabatrin (Sabril) is an investigational AED that has been extensively evaluated in the United States. The drug irreversibly inhibits GABA transaminase, resulting in an increase in brain and cerebrospinal fluid GABA levels. Although this drug is effective for adjunctive treatment of partial-onset seizures, recent reports of vigabatrin-related visual field defects (primarily loss of peripheral vision) are of concern and have delayed the approval of this drug in the United States. The cause of these visual disturbances is unknown.

IMPROVING OUTCOMES

In addition to pharmacologic and nonpharmacologic therapies, patients with epilepsy (and their families) often benefit from education regarding their condition and reinforcement of the importance of compliance to prescribed therapeutic regimens. Psychiatric comorbidity (such as anxiety, mood, or thought disorders) also may complicate the treatment of patients with epilepsy. Whether these conditions arise as a consequence of the psychosocial issues related to epilepsy or are caused by neurochemical features related to epilepsy itself is unknown. When present, these problems require both detection and proper management.

Patient Education

The Epilepsy Foundation of America (4351 Garden City Drive, Landover, Maryland 20785) and its local affiliates also have available a wide range of client services and brochures to help patients (and their families) understand epilepsy and its treatment and to deal with the problems and psychosocial implications of seizures. Advocacy information is also available, including legal rights as they relate to employment, insurance, and education, as well as information on driving restrictions by state. The Epilepsy Foundation of America can also be reached by telephone (1-800-EFA-1000) or via the Internet (http://www.efa.org/).

Methods to Improve Patient Adherence to Drug Therapy

Noncompliance with AED therapy is a common cause for recurrent seizures in patients with epilepsy. Reasons for noncompliance with AEDs include high drug costs, adverse effects of drug therapy, fears regarding potential medical or psychologic effects of medication, memory deficit, and various lifestyle issues. An understanding of the factors that affect adherence to drug therapy is necessary to develop effective strategies to improve compliance. Patients should be questioned about these and other factors that affect their ability to take medication as prescribed. Education is often the most important intervention to improve adherence–as long as it is targeted appropriately to the patient's specific problems or concerns. Materials available from the Epilepsy Foundation of America (see above) are often useful as educational aids. Reducing the number of divided daily doses that must be remembered by the patient may also improve compliance. Because consistency in medication blood levels is important for maintaining seizure control, use of extended- or sustained-release products help in this regard. Various other compliance aids are available, including medication alarms and pill containers divided into daily compartments.

Disease Management Strategies to Improve Patient Outcomes

Given the high costs associated with epilepsy care (see "Pharmacoeconomics" below), and the complexity of care as it relates to diagnosis, treatment selection, and therapy adjustment, some institutions have instituted disease management strategies to improve the quality and cost efficiency of care. Patients with uncontrolled seizures and those who are high users of health care resources are often the target of such programs that focus on confirmation of a correct diagnosis, patient education, compliance education, and evaluation of appropriate drug selection and dosing. However, the utility of such disease-management programs has yet to be validated.

PHARMACOECONOMICS

It is estimated that the total cost of epilepsy to the United States, including direct and indirect costs, is approximately $12.5 billion per year.[44] Indirect costs of epilepsy associated with lost productivity account for approximately 60% of total costs. AED treatment accounts for 40% of the total direct costs associated with treatment, making it the single most costly component of direct patient care and exceeding the costs of emergency services, inpatient hospital costs and outpatient physician visits combined.[45] However, there have been very few cost-effectiveness studies on AED therapy, and most of the research in this regard has been sponsored by pharmaceutical companies with a financial interest in the study results. In a 1996 review of the pharmacoeconomic considerations of drug treatment for epilepsy, Oliver Cockerell stated: "At present, there are no good cost-utility or cost-benefit analyses available for epilepsy. This situation needs urgent correction."[46]

Despite the lack of good pharmacoeconomic studies in epilepsy treatment, it is likely that patient-specific considerations in drug selection, monitoring, and therapy adjustments will improve seizure control and reduce the total costs of epilepsy care. Use of the least expensive AED may not equate to optimally cost-effective care. For example, in the treatment of a patient with medically refractory epilepsy, addition of an expensive, new AED as adjunctive therapy may well result in a reduction in total costs by reducing either direct costs (e.g., clinic or emergency room visits), indirect costs (e.g., missed work days), or both. Nonetheless, additional pharmacoeconomic studies are required to distinguish the relative cost-effectiveness of various treatment alternatives for patients with both easily controlled and treatment-resistant seizures.

Status Epilepticus

OVERVIEW

Status epilepticus (SE) is a medical emergency that requires prompt, effective treatment to minimize permanent neurologic damage and death. In adults, SE is defined as a seizure lasting 5 minutes or longer or the occurrence of two or more seizures without recovery of consciousness between events.[47] Morbidity and mortality after SE are related primarily to the condition that precipitated the episode and to neuronal injury from continuous electrical and convulsive seizure activity. Patient prognosis is more likely to be poor when SE lasts longer than 90 minutes and when the event is caused by acute CNS injury such as stroke, anoxia, CNS infection, or head injury. The mortality associated with SE is approximately 20% in adults, even with aggressive anticonvulsant drug therapy.

The most common cause of SE in patients with a history of epilepsy is noncompliance with AED therapy. Additionally, the various factors listed in Table 52.1 that can cause seizures are also potential causes of SE. The initial workup for patients should include a thorough medical and neurologic evaluation to identify the cause of the patient's seizures. Potentially treatable causes of SE, such as CNS infection and metabolic abnormalities, should be identified and treated as soon as possible.

TREATMENT GOALS: STATUS EPILEPTICUS

- Terminate seizures as quickly as possible
- Identify and treat any potentially reversible causes
- Medically manage systemic complications that arise from prolonged convulsive seizures (e.g., hyperthermia or hypoxia).

TREATMENT

During SE, patients should receive oxygen supplementation and should be monitored for hyperthermia. Passive cooling measures should be used to minimize the potentially damaging effects of fever during prolonged convulsions. The electroencephalogram should be monitored in any patient who receives a paralytic agent and in patients who remain unconscious after the seizures have been controlled. In these situations, seizures may continue even in the absence of convulsive muscle movements.

Figure 52.1 outlines the timeline, sequence of drug administration, and dosing for drugs commonly used in the management of SE in adults. Lorazepam is the agent of choice for the initial treatment of SE. Benzodiazepines, such as diazepam and lorazepam terminate SE in 80 to 90% of patients, usually within 3 to 5 minutes after intravenous administration. The usefulness of diazepam is limited by its short duration of anticonvulsant effect (15 minutes to 2 hours). This drug is highly lipophilic and quickly redistributes out of the brain to other fat stores in the body. Lorazepam has a longer duration of action and is preferred over diazepam for this reason. Phenytoin and fosphenytoin are effective for the treatment of SE; however, since the peak anticonvulsant effects of both drugs are delayed by approximately 20 minutes from the start of drug administration, they are usually administered after lorazepam. Phenytoin (and fosphenytoin) provide additional long-lasting protection from recurrent seizures. Phenobarbital is usually reserved for use as a second-line agent for SE that does not stop after lorazepam and phenytoin. Like phenytoin, the peak effect of phenobarbital is delayed and because of the drug's sedative effect, phenobarbital can confound the assessment of mental status after seizures are terminated. High-dose, continuous infusions with anesthetic doses of either propofol or midazolam are the treatments of choice for SE that does not respond to the drugs discussed above.[48] Patients with

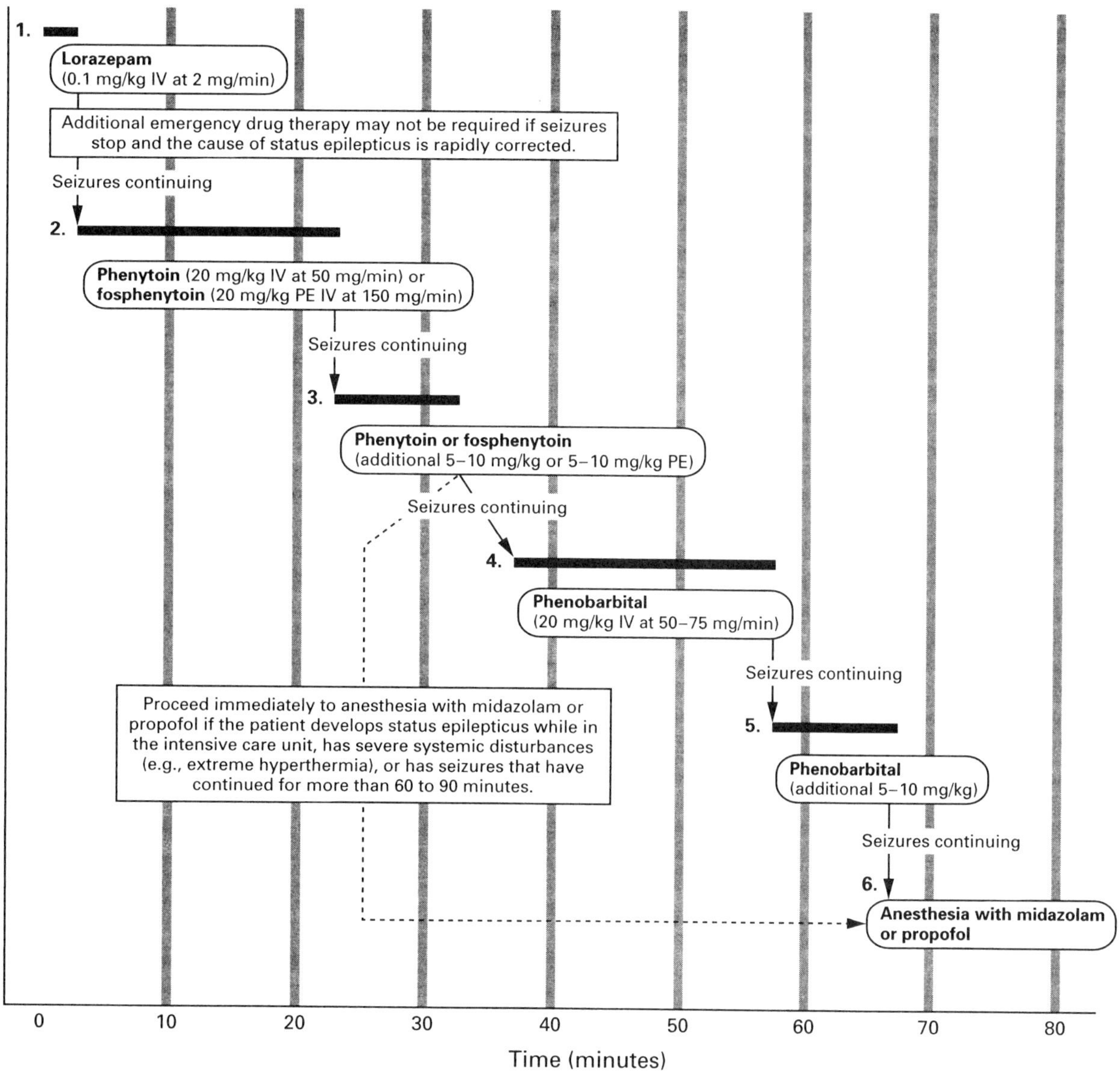

Figure 52.1. Antiepileptic drug therapy for status epilepticus. *IV* intravenous; *PE*, phenytoin equivalents. The horizontal bars indicate the approximate duration of drug infusions. (Reprinted with permission from Lowenstein DH, Alldredge BK. Status epilepticus. N Engl J Med 338:970–976, 1998.)

refractory SE usually require admission to an intensive care unit for ventilatory support and continuous monitoring of the EEG and vascular hemodynamics.

KEY POINTS

- An accurate diagnosis of the patient's seizure type and epilepsy syndrome is required for successful management.
- Patient-specific seizure precipitants should be identified and eliminated.
- Select optimal AED therapy based on seizure type, epilepsy syndrome, patient age, sex, and concomitant medical conditions.
- Adjust AED therapy to attain complete control of seizures with minimal or no adverse effects.
- Monitor for clinical and laboratory evidence of adverse effects of drug therapy.
- Minimize the use of poly-drug therapy and sedating AEDs whenever possible.
- Carbamazepine and phenytoin are the drugs of choice for initial therapy of patients with partial-onset seizures.
- Valproate is the drug of choice for patients with primarily generalized tonic-clonic seizures and patients who experience both tonic-clonic and absence seizures.
- Ethosuximide is the drug of choice in patients who experience only absence seizures.
- Periodic monitoring of AED blood levels may be useful for guiding subsequent dosage adjustments (for phenytoin in particular), and for monitoring medication compliance, adverse effects, and the effects of drugs or conditions that alter AED clearance.
- The clinical status of the patient should be the ultimate guide regarding the necessity for dosage adjustment.
- In patients who have persistent seizures despite titration of therapy to the maximal tolerated dosage, another AED should be gradually substituted for the original medication.
- When sequential monotherapy with two or three AEDs fails to control seizures, consideration should then be given to adjunctive therapy with one of the new AEDs (e.g., gabapentin, lamotrigine, topiramate, or tiagabine).
- Recognize when patients should be referred to a comprehensive epilepsy center for evaluation of other therapeutic modalities (e.g., surgery, vagus nerve stimulation, or ketogenic diet).
- Patients and their families require education and support regarding epilepsy, its treatment, and its effect on daily activities.

REFERENCES

1. Theodore WH, Porter RJ. Epilepsy: 100 elementary principles. 3rd ed. London: WB Saunders, 1995.
2. Scheuer ML, Pedley TA. The evaluation and treatment of seizures. N Engl J Med 323:1468–1474, 1990.
3. Alldredge BK, Simon RP. Drugs that can precipitate seizures. In: Resor SR, Kutt H, eds. The medical treatment of epilepsy. New York: Marcel Dekker, 1992:497–523.
4. Commission on Classification and Terminology of the International League Against Epilepsy. Proposal for revised clinical and electroencephalographic classification of epileptic seizures. Epilepsia 22:489–501, 1981.
5. Commission on Classification and Terminology of the International League Against Epilepsy. Proposal for classification of epilepsies and epileptic syndromes. Epilepsia 26:268–278, 1985.
6. Knudsen FU. Febrile seizures–treatment and outcome. Brain Dev 18:438–449, 1996.
7. Chadwick D. Diagnosis of epilepsy. Lancet 336:291–295, 1990.
8. Theodore WH, Porter RJ. Removal of sedative-hypnotic antiepileptic drugs from the regimens of patients with intractable epilepsy. Ann Neurol 13:320–324, 1983.
9. Mattson RH, Cramer JA, Collins JF, et al. Comparison of carbamazepine, phenobarbital, phenytoin, and primidone in partial and secondarily generalized tonic-clonic seizures. N Engl J Med 313:145–151, 1985.
10. Mattson RH, Cramer JA, Collins JF, et al. A comparison of valproate with carbamazepine for the treatment of complex partial seizures and secondarily generalized tonic-clonic seizures in adults. N Engl J Med 327:765–771, 1992.
11. Reunanen M, Dam M, Yuen AWC. A randomised open multicentre comparative trial of lamotrigine and carbamazepine as monotherapy in patients with newly diagnosed or recurrent epilepsy. Epilepsy Res 23:149–155, 1996.
12. Marson AG, Chadwick DW. New antiepileptic drugs: a systematic review of their efficacy and tolerability. Br Med J 313:1169–1174, 1996.
13. Devinsky O. Patients with refractory seizures. N Engl J Med 340:1565–1570, 1999.
14. Sato S, White BG, Penry JK, et al. Valproic acid versus ethosuximide in the treatment of absence seizures. Neurology 32:157–163, 1982.
15. Dodson WE. Level off. Neurology 39:1009–1010, 1989.
16. Cohen H, Howland MA, Luciano DJ, et al. Feasibility and pharmacokinetics of carbamazepine oral loading doses. Am J Health-Syst Pharm 55:1134–1140, 1998.
17. Dalby MA. Behavioral effects of carbamazepine. In: Penry JK, Dalby DD, eds. Advances in neurology. New York: Raven Press, 1975;11:331–343.
18. Alldredge BK, Knutsen AP, Ferriero D. Antiepileptic drug hypersensitivity syndrome: in vitro and clinical observations. Pediatr Neurol 10:169–171, 1994.
19. Hart RG, Easton JD. Carbamazepine and hematological monitoring. Ann Neurol 11:309–312, 1982.
20. Anderson GD. A mechanistic approach to antiepileptic drug interactions. Ann Pharmacother 32:554–563, 1998.
21. Tuchman AJ, Zisfein J, Paccione M, et al. Single- versus divided-dose oral phenytoin loading: a controlled study [Abstract]. Neurology 44(Suppl 2):A295, 1994.
22. Boucher BA. Fosphenytoin: a novel phenytoin prodrug. Pharmacotherapy 16:777–791, 1996.
23. Winter ME, Tozer TN. Phenytoin. In: Evans WE, Schentag JJ, Jusko WJ, eds. Applied pharmacokinetics: principles of therapeutic drug monitoring. 3rd ed. Vancouver: Applied Therapeutics, 1992:25.1–25.44.
24. Nation RL, Evans AM, Milne RW. Pharmacokinetic drug interactions with phenytoin (part II). Clin Pharmacokinet 18:131–150, 1990.
25. Brodie MJ, Dichter MA. Antiepileptic drugs. N Engl J Med 334:168–175, 1996.
26. Meador KJ, Loring DW, Moore EE, et al. Comparative cognitive effects of phenobarbital, phenytoin, and valproate in healthy adults. Neurology 45:149–1499, 1995.
27. Gidal B, Spencer N, Maly M, et al. Valproate-mediated disturbances of hemostasis: relationship to dose and plasma concentration. Neurology 44:1418–1422, 1994.
28. Dreifuss FE, Langer DH, Moline KA, et al. Valproic acid hepatic fatalities. II: US experience since 1984. Neurology 39:201–207, 1989.
29. Petroff OAC, Rothman DL, Behar KL, et al. The effect of gabapentin on brain gamma-aminobutyric acid in patients with epilepsy. Ann Neurol 39:95–99, 1996.
30. Wetzel CH. Use of gabapentin in pain management. Ann Pharmacother 31:1082–1083, 1997.
31. Letterman L, Markowitz JS. Gabapentin: a review of published experience in the treatment of bipolar disorder and other psychiatric conditions. Pharmacotherapy 19:565–572, 1999.
32. Gidal BE, Maly MM, Budde J, et al. Effect of a high-protein meal on gabapentin pharmacokinetics. Epilepsy Res 23:71–76, 1996.
33. Felbatol product information. Cranbury, NJ: Wallace Laboratories, February 1999.
34. Pellock JM, Brodie MJ. Felbamate: 1997 update. Epilepsia 38:1261–1264, 1997.
35. Sachdeo RC. Topiramate. Clinical profile in epilepsy. Clin Pharmacokinet 34:335–346, 1998.

36. Martin R, Kuzniecky R, Ho S, et al. Cognitive effects of topiramate, gabapentin, and lamotrigine in healthy young adults. Neurology 52:321–327, 1999.
37. Brodie MJ. Tiagabine pharmacology in profile. Epilepsia 36:S7–S9, 1995.
38. Zahn CA, Morrell MJ, Collins SD, et al. Management issues for women with epilepsy: a review of the literature. Neurology 51:949–956, 1998.
39. Morrell MJ. Guidelines for the care of women with epilepsy. Neurology 51(Suppl 4):S21–S27, 1998.
40. Report of the Quality Standards Subcommittee of the American Academy of Neurology. Practice parameter: a guideline for discontinuing antiepileptic drugs in seizure-free patients-summary statement. Neurology 47:600–602, 1996.
41. Schachter SC, Saper CB. Vagus nerve stimulation 39:677–686, 1998.
42. Engel J. Surgery for seizures. N Engl J Med 334:647–652, 1996.
43. Bainbridge JL, Gidal BE, Ryan M. The ketogenic diet. Pharmacotherapy 19:782–786, 1999.
44. Epilepsy: a report to the nation. Landover, MD: Epilepsy Foundation of America, 1999.
45. Begley CE, Annegers JF, Lairson DR, et al. Cost of epilepsy in the United States: a model based on incidence and prognosis. Epilepsia 35:1230–1243, 1994.
46. Cockerell OC. Pharmacoeconomic considerations in the drug treatment of epilepsy. CNS Drugs 6:450–461, 1996.
47. Lowenstein DH, Alldredge BK. Status epilepticus. N Engl J Med 338:970–976, 1998.
48. Alldredge BK, Lowenstein DH. Status epilepticus: new concepts. Curr Opin Neurol 12:183–190, 1999.

CHAPTER 53

PARKINSONISM

Jack J. Chen and Sam K. Shimomura

"Some turn this sickness yet might take,
Ev'n yet." But he: "What drug can make
A wither'd palsy cease to shake?"
"The Two Voices," 1842
Alfred Lord Tennyson

DEFINITION

In 1817, Dr. James Parkinson published a case series describing six patients afflicted with the "shaking palsy" (paralysis agitans), a chronic and progressive neurologic disorder (Table 53.1).[1] Since then, the term *parkinsonism* has been used to describe any clinical syndrome associated with the four cardinal features of tremor, rigidity, bradykinesia, and postural instability. Even today, very little can be added to Parkinson's keen observation of "involuntary tremulous motion, with lessened muscular power, in parts not in action and even when supported; with a propensity to bend the trunk forwards, and to pass from a walking to a running pace; the senses and the intellects being uninjured."[1] However, we now know that the risk of developing dementia is almost twice that in normal controls. Parkinson also recognized the development of several secondary symptoms (e.g., constipation, drooling, dysphagia, speech and sleep disturbances), the profound adverse impact on quality of life, and the importance of caregiver support.

Parkinsonism can be classified based on etiologic factors and clinical characteristics (Table 53.2). The majority of parkinsonism cases are of the idiopathic type, which we will call Parkinson's disease (PD). Other types can be classified as secondary parkinsonisms, multisystem Parkinson plus syndromes, or hereditary parkinsonisms.

Since the 1950s, drug-induced parkinsonism has been the second most common form of parkinsonism (Table 53.3).[10,11] The two major types of parkinsonism-inducing agents are those that deplete central stores of dopamine (e.g., reserpine and methyldopa) and those that antagonize central dopaminergic receptors. Overall, agents that block central dopamine receptors (e.g., phenothiazines, butyrophenones, metoclopramide) are responsible for 70 to 80% of worldwide drug-induced cases. Interestingly, administering potent anticholinergic agents (e.g., diphenhydramine, trihexyphenidyl) provides relief, whereas levodopa is ineffective. In a case-controlled study of older adults, metoclopramide users were three times more likely to be on the antiparkinson drug levodopa than non–metoclopramide users. This finding suggests that drug-induced parkinsonism may often be misdiagnosed and treated as idiopathic PD.

Multisystem Parkinson plus syndromes are characterized by the presence of parkinsonian features along with other unique autonomic, neurologic, and psychiatric abnormalities. Several variants have been characterized and include corticobasal degeneration, progressive supranuclear palsy, multiple-system atrophies, and dementia with Lewy body disease. In general, these atypical parkinsonisms are unresponsive or, at best, transiently responsive to antiparkinson therapy.

TREATMENT GOALS: PARKINSONISM

- Because there is no cure for PD, direct therapy at relieving symptoms and improving or maintaining quality of life. Initiate symptom-relieving therapy when functional impairment is evident.
- Before initiating therapy, consider patient's level of functional and cognitive impairment and age.
- Adapt treatment to patient's specific functional impairment and quality of life issues. For example, rigidity may endanger the livelihood of a surgeon or professional pianist, and bradykinesia would impair the quality of life for a retiree who enjoys square dancing.

Table 53.1 ▪ Historical Landmarks

1817	James Parkinson publishes "An Essay on the Shaking Palsy."[1]
1860s	Belladonna alkaloids recognized for antiparkinson activity.
1912	First published neurosurgical operation for relief of parkinsonism.[2]
1912	Lewy bodies described.[3]
1919	Depigmentation of the substantia nigra described.[4]
1960	Parkinsonism attributed to striatal dopamine depletion.[5]
1970	Levodopa FDA approved.
1973	Amantadine FDA approved.
1975	Carbidopa–levodopa and carbidopa FDA approved.
1978	Bromocriptine FDA approved for parkinsonism.
1983	MPTP-induced parkinsonism (the "frozen addicts") discovered.[6]
1988	Pergolide FDA approved.
1988	First fetal nigral tissue transplant for parkinsonism.[7]
1989	Selegiline FDA approved.
1991	Carbidopa–levodopa sustained-release tablets introduced.
1996	α-Synuclein gene mutation discovered.[8]
1997	Pramipexole and ropinirole FDA approved.
1998	Tolcapone FDA approved.
1999	Entacapone FDA approved.

Source: Modified with permission from Chen JJ. Parkinson's disease: pharmacological aspects and practical issues. Los Angeles: Taiwanese-American Parkinson's Association, 1997.

FDA, U.S. Food and Drug Administration; *MPTP,* 1-methyl-4-phenyl-1,2,3,6-tetrahydropyridine.

- If cognitive impairment or dementia is present at baseline, give preference to carbidopa/levodopa over direct dopamine agonists, anticholinergics, amantadine, or selegiline because the latter agents tend to exacerbate underlying dementia more than levodopa.
- Initiate neuroprotective therapy as early as possible.
- Because younger patients face a greater duration of disease and are more likely to develop levodopa-related motor complications, give preference to neuroprotective agents and levodopa-sparing strategies.
- Consider nonpharmacologic modalities such as education, physical therapy, speech therapy, and dietary modification, which can play an important role in improving quality of life.

EPIDEMIOLOGY

In the United States, approximately 1 million people have PD, with a slight predominance toward men and Caucasians. Overall, the mean age at diagnosis ranges from 55 to 60 years and the crude incidence is approximately 20 to 30 per 100,000 person-years. However, when stratified according to age, the incidence increases dramatically to 115 per 100,000 person-years (65 to 74 years) and 255 per 100,000 person-years (75 to 84 years).[10] Similarly, the prevalence estimate also increases with age.[15] Less than 30% of cases are diagnosed before age 55 and less than 10% before age 40. The term *juvenile parkinsonism* is used if symptoms occur before age 21 and the term *young-onset* if symptoms occur between 21 and 40 years.[16] Case-controlled studies have reported a hereditary pattern in approximately 10% of cases and a two to three times greater risk of PD in first-degree relatives.[17,18] Results from a large twin study suggest that genetic factors may play a greater role in patients with symptoms beginning at or before age 50.[19] Recent epidemiologic data report a mortality risk of two to five times expected rates.[15,20] This risk is strongly related to the presence of gait disturbance and dementia.

PATHOPHYSIOLOGY

PD is characterized by progressive degeneration of the substantia nigra, with subsequent depletion of striatal

Table 53.2 ▪ Classification of Parkinsonism

Primary parkinsonisms
- Idiopathic Parkinson's disease
- Juvenile parkinsonism

Secondary parkinsonisms
- Drugs (phenothiazines, metoclopramide, reserpine, flunarizine, cinnarizine)
- Infections (postencephalitic, human immunodeficiency virus–associated, subacute sclerosing panencephalitis)
- Other (brain neoplasm, normal-pressure hydrocephalus, parathyroid abnormalities, hypothyroidism, hepatocerebral degeneration, syringomesencephalia)
- Toxins (MPTP, carbon monoxide, manganese, methanol, organophosphates)
- Head trauma ("punch drunk" syndrome)
- Neurovascular (multi-infarct, Binswanger's disease)

Multisystem Parkinson plus syndromes
- Corticobasal degeneration
- Multiple system atrophies
  - Olivopontocerebellar atrophy
  - Shy–Drager syndrome
  - Striatonigral degeneration
- Progressive supranuclear palsy (Steele–Richardson–Olszewski syndrome)
- Dementia syndromes
  - Alzheimer's with parkinsonism
  - Guamanian amyotrophic lateral sclerosis–parkinsonism dementia ("lytico-bodig")
  - Diffuse Lewy body disease
  - Pick's disease

Hereditary parkinsonisms
- Autosomal dominant
  - Chromosome 2p
  - Chromosome 4q (α-synuclein mutation)
  - Chromosome 19q (rapid-onset dystonia parkinsonism)
  - Huntington's disease (juvenile-onset)
  - Neuroacanthocytosis
- Autosomal recessive
  - Chromosome 6q (autosomal recessive juvenile parkinsonism)
  - Hallervorden–Spatz disease
  - Wilson's disease
- X-linked
  - Lubag (Filipino dystonia parkinsonism)
  - Waisman syndrome (X-linked parkinsonism with mental retardation)

MPTP, 1-methyl-4-phenyl-1,2,3,6-tetrahydropyridine.

dopamine and disequilibrium of the extrapyramidal motor circuits (Fig. 53.1). In normal adults, the rate of dopaminergic cell loss occurs linearly, with a 5% decline per decade. In PD, cell loss accelerates exponentially, with a 45% decline during the first decade after diagnosis. It is estimated that parkinsonian symptoms do not appear until a critical threshold of 80% loss of striatal dopamine concentration has occurred.[22] Imbalances of other neurotransmitters (e.g., acetylcholine, γ-aminobutyric acid [GABA], glutamate, norepinephrine, serotonin) and degeneration within the locus ceruleus, hypothalamus, and cortex are also characteristic.[23,24] The defining histopathologic hallmark is the Lewy body, a spherical, eosinophilic inclusion found in the cells of the substantia nigra. The formation of Lewy bodies may be a protective mechanism in response to the accumulation of oxidative and ubiquitinated protein waste products.[25,26] On autopsy, Lewy bodies are also found in people without symptoms of PD and are suggestive of preclinical PD, which may precede the onset of symptoms by 5 or more years.[21]

The cause of PD remains obscure, but multiple factors such as age-related neurodegeneration, genetic constitution, and toxin exposure may play a role (Fig. 53.2).[23]

Table 53.3 ▪ Drugs That May Produce or Exacerbate Parkinsonism

- Antiepileptics
  - Valproic acid
  - Vigabatrin
- Antidepressants
  - Amoxapine
  - Lithium
  - Selective serotonin reuptake inhibitors (fluoxetine, fluvoxamine, paroxetine, sertraline)
- Butyrophenones
  - Droperidol
  - Haloperidol
- Calcium channel blockers
  - Amlodipine, diltiazem, verapamil
  - Cinnarizine and flunarizine[a]
- Centrally acting antihypertensives
  - α-Methyldopa
  - Reserpine (*Rauwolfia serpentina*)
- Cholinesterase inhibitors
  - Donepezil
  - Tacrine
- Phenothiazines
  - Chlorpromazine
  - Fluphenazine
  - Perphenazine
  - Prochlorperazine
  - Thiethylperazine
  - Thioridazine
  - Thiothixene
  - Trifluoperazine
  - Triflupromazine
- Miscellaneous
  - Amiodarone
  - Disulfiram
  - Metoclopramide
  - Phenytoin
  - Pimozide

[a]Atypical calcium channel blockers; not marketed in the United States.

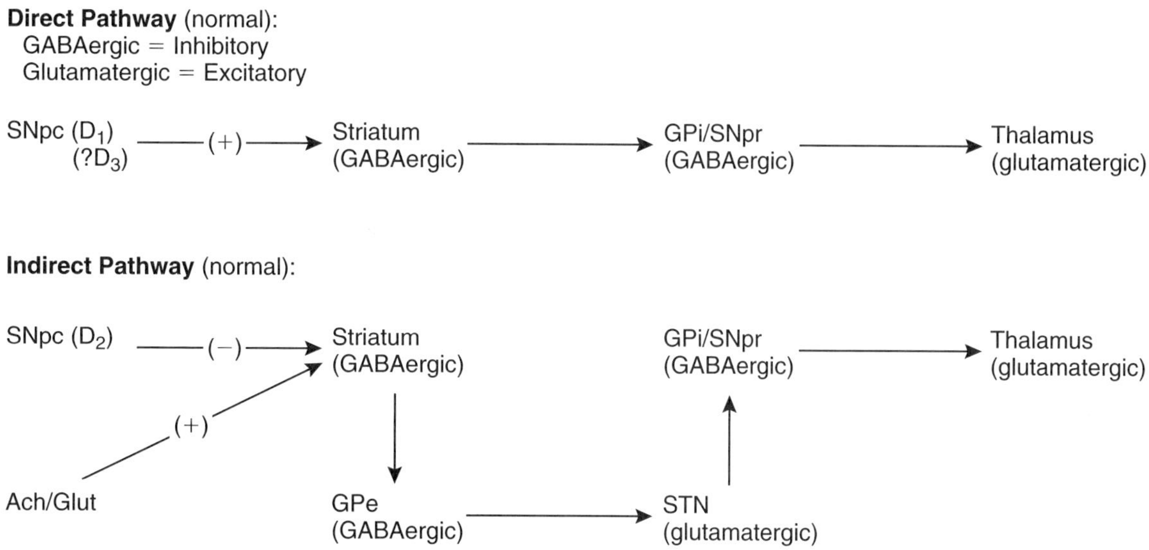

Figure 53.1. Normal motor circuit: direct and indirect pathways. Learned movement is regulated by a complex motor circuit involving the extrapyramidal motor system, which is composed of the basal ganglia (caudate nucleus, putamen, and globus pallidus) and the substantia nigra. The caudate nucleus and putamen are also known collectively as the striatum. The substantia nigra, which contains about 80% of the dopamine-producing cells in the brain, has two regions. The pars compacta *(SNpc)* produces dopamine and is rich in neuromelanin, an insoluble byproduct of dopamine auto-oxidation. The pars reticulata *(SNpr)* produces the inhibitory transmitter γ-aminobutyric acid *(GABA)* and is not pigmented. The presynaptic SNpc neurons synthesize, store, and transport dopamine to the striatum. Striatal neurons then communicate with neurons of the thalamocortical pathway (subthalamic nucleus *(STN)*, thalamus, and cerebral cortex) via direct and indirect pathways. The direct pathway is linked to striatal D_1 receptors and the indirect pathway to striatal D_2 receptors. D_1 and D_2 receptor activation results in stimulation and inhibition, respectively. The internal capsule of the globus pallidus *(GPi)* and the GABAergic SNpr exert an inhibitory influence and act as the final common gateway to the thalamus. In Parkinson's disease, decreased striatal dopamine results in less inhibition of the direct pathway with resultant thalamic overinhibition caused by excessive GABA activity. The indirect pathway is less stimulated, resulting in subthalamic nucleus disinhibition and overinhibition of the thalamus from glutaminergic overactivity. The result of these complex interactions is inhibition of learned movement. *Ach,* acetylcholine; *Glut,* glutamate; *GPe,* globus pallidus externa.

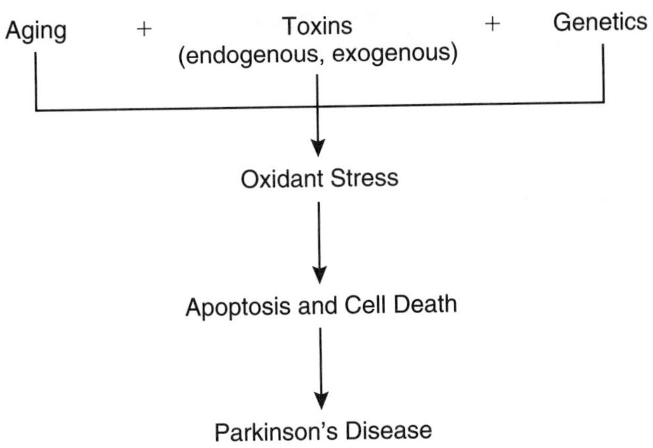

Figure 53.2. Causes of Parkinson's disease.

In the early 1980s, young addicts were developing severe parkinsonism within 24 hours after injecting a designer meperidine analog. After much investigative effort, Langston et al.[6] discovered that the drug samples had been heavily contaminated with 1-methyl-4-phenyl-1,2,3,6-tetrahydropyridine (MPTP), a byproduct of the synthetic process. MPTP was soon characterized as a protoxin converted by monoamine oxidase type B (MAO-B) to MPP^+ (1-methyl-4-phenylpyridine), a potent neurotoxin. Interestingly, MPP^+ is chemically related to paraquat. Subsequently, population-based, case-controlled studies have demonstrated a higher risk of parkinsonism associated with occupational exposure to various herbicides (e.g., paraquat) and insecticides and consumption of naturally occurring exotic neurotoxins.[27–30]

Whether caused by toxin exposure or genetic susceptibility, evidence suggests that subsequent oxidant stress and apoptosis play a major role in promoting neurodegeneration.[31,32] In the parkinsonian brain, concentrations of protective reductants (e.g., glutathione) are reduced and reactive oxidants (e.g., O_2^-, ^-OH, Fe^{3+}) are elevated. Additionally, defects of mitochondrial respiration and xenobiotic-metabolizing enzymes (e.g., glutathione transferase, cytochrome P-450 2D6, *N*-acetyltransferase) may also contribute to free radical generation and oxidant stress.[33,34]

CLINICAL PRESENTATION AND DIAGNOSIS

Signs and Symptoms

Because the definitive diagnosis of PD entails pathologic confirmation of Lewy bodies, clinical diagnosis relies on physical examination. The cardinal clinical features of PD are tremor at rest, rigidity, akinesia or bradykinesia, and postural instability (represented by the acronym *TRAP*). Individually, these physical findings are nonspecific, but as a whole, they constitute parkinsonism.

Initially, motor features develop unilaterally and then spread to contralateral extremities.[35] A rhythmic, pill-rolling tremor of the hand and upper extremities is the most visible yet least disabling symptom. This tremor generally occurs at rest and is of slower frequency (3 to 6 Hz) and greater amplitude than tremor associated with alcoholism, hyperthyroidism, or nervousness. The resting tremor often disappears during sleep and is exacerbated by stress. Patients may also demonstrate postural tremor (occurs when arms are outstretched) or action tremor (occurs when an object is held). In contrast to the other cardinal features, tremor severity generally remains stable over time.[36]

A cogwheel rigidity is common with passive flexion of the elbow or wrist, and the presence of facial, truncal, and lower-extremity rigidity often manifests as a lack of facial expression (masked facies), stooped posture, and turning en bloc, respectively. The masking of facial expression often is an early symptom of PD and may be misinterpreted as apathy, unfriendliness, or depression. Common problems associated with rigidity include impairment of basic activities of daily living (e.g., buttoning a shirt, putting on earrings), difficulty arising from a chair, and inability to turn over in bed.

Akinesia and bradykinesia are the absence and slowness of movement, respectively. Difficulty in initiating and executing learned movements contributes substantially to functional impairment (e.g., worsening of gait, significant interference with employability, ability to manage household and business affairs, and basic activities of daily living). The combination of bradykinesia and rigidity often contributes to a characteristic slow, shuffling gait, micrographia, and reduced arm swing.

Postural instability or poor balance is a disabling symptom of advanced disease. Often a slow, shuffling gait is transformed into a rapid, festinating gait with a tendency to fall forward. Retropulsion with a tendency to fall backward also occurs. As a result, patients are at greater risk for injuries. Pharmacologic intervention generally is ineffective. Walking aids and protective headgear are useful for preventing injury, and in severe cases, chronic wheelchair use may be needed.

Although not considered a cardinal feature, "freezing," or a sudden, episodic inhibition of motor function, is not uncommon and also contributes to falls. Patients may report that their "feet are stuck to the floor" and that they have difficulty initiating steps (start hesitation) or turns (turn hesitation). Freezing often is exacerbated by anxiety or when perceived obstacles (e.g., doorways, turnstiles) are encountered. A variety of environmental, physical, and sensory cues are used to reduce the occurrence of freezing episodes.[37]

In addition to the primary motor features, nonmotor symptoms are also very common and significantly impair quality of life. Examples include bladder incontinence, constipation, dementia, depression, drooling, dysphagia, erectile dysfunction, olfactory deficit, orthostatic hypotension (OH), paresthesias, seborrheic dermatitis, sleep disturbances, sweating, and temperature intolerances. Because nonmotor symptoms can be pharmacologically exacer-

Table 53.4 ▪ Modified Hoehn and Yahr Staging

Stage 0	No signs of disease
Stage 1	Unilateral disease
Stage 1.5	Unilateral with axial involvement
Stage 2	Bilateral disease without balance impairment
Stage 2.5	Mild bilateral disease with recovery on pull test
Stage 3	Mild to moderate bilateral disease, some postural instability; physically independent
Stage 4	Severe disability; unable to live alone independently
Stage 5	Unable to walk or stand without assistance

bated, clinicians should routinely screen for drug–disease interactions.

Diagnosis

Biochemical or genetic markers that can accurately detect PD are unavailable. Neuroimaging techniques, such as magnetic resonance imaging, single-photon emission computed tomography, and fluorodopa positron emission tomography are useful for differentiating idiopathic PD from some forms of atypical parkinsonism but are not universally incorporated into the diagnostic workup.[38] A careful drug history and clinical diagnosis are essential because the treatment and prognosis of idiopathic PD differ markedly from those of drug-induced parkinsonism or multisystem Parkinson plus syndromes. Even when drug-induced parkinsonism is ruled out, misdiagnosis occurs in 25% of cases.[39] However, a clinical diagnosis of PD can be made with high probability if the patient presents with bradykinesia and either rest tremor or rigidity; motor features are initially unilateral; motor features are progressive; there is absence of early falls, dementia, or cerebellar (e.g., ataxia) or pyramidal (e.g., spasticity) signs; and there is an excellent and sustained symptomatic response to dopaminergic therapy.[40]

Once a clinical diagnosis of PD is made, assessment scales are useful for monitoring disease progression. Hoehn and Yahr[41] have developed a user-friendly, multistaging system based on the presence and severity of postural instability (Table 53.4). However, the modified United Parkinson's Disease Rating Scale (UPDRS) is a more sensitive method for evaluating functional status, disease progression, and effectiveness of antiparkinson therapy.[42] The Schwab & England Activities of Daily Living scale is also a very useful tool for assessing quality-of-life parameters (e.g., speech, salivation, swallowing, handwriting, cutting food, handling utensils, dressing, grooming, turning in bed, walking, and pain).

PSYCHOSOCIAL ASPECTS

Typically, early-stage PD is associated with minimal adverse psychosocial consequences. However, as the disease progresses, the psychosocial impact on patients and family members may be profound. Neurobehavioral changes, such as depression, are common and can be a manifestation of disease-related biochemical imbalances or psychological withdrawal.[43] Social avoidance may arise from personal embarrassment or from a fear of falling outside the house. Patients may have difficulty adjusting to gradual loss of autonomy (e.g., loss of employment or driving privileges). Likewise, family caregivers often experience greater levels of stress, frustration, anxiety, and depression, especially as the patient becomes increasingly dependent on them for assistance with activities of daily living.[44] The adverse psychosocial impact of PD can be minimized by fostering a positive attitude and initiating psychoeducational interventions. Toward this end, support groups are an excellent source of educational, emotional, and social support for patients and caregivers. Groups specific to the patient's demographic characteristics (e.g., age, ethnicity, gender) may offer greater appeal to some patients. Additional information can be obtained from organizations such as the National Parkinson Foundation (800-327-4545, www.parkinson.org) and the American Parkinson Disease Association (800-223-2732, http://www.apdaparkinson.com). International associations can be contacted through the World Parkinson Disease Association (www.wpda.com).

THERAPEUTIC PLAN

Guidelines and algorithms for managing PD have been published and are updated periodically (Fig. 53.3).[45,46]

TREATMENT

Pharmacotherapy

Common pharmacologic agents and dosing regimens are listed in Table 53.5. The three basic tenets of antiparkinson therapy are as follows: Initiate therapy with gradual dosage titration ("start low and go slow"), maintain therapy at the lowest effective dosage, and, if needed, discontinue therapy with a gradual taper.

Anticholinergics

Before the advent of levodopa, centrally acting anticholinergic agents such as benztropine, trihexyphenidyl, biperiden, and procyclidine were the mainstays of therapy. In general, symptomatic improvement is modest and favors tremor control. Because of troublesome side effects, therapy generally is short-lived, particularly in older adults. The most suitable candidates are young patients with tremor-predominant disease. Interestingly, patients may respond to one anticholinergic but not to another. Common side effects include blurred vision, dry eyes, dry mouth, drowsiness, confusion, memory impairment, tachycardia, constipation, and urinary retention. If therapy is to be discontinued, downward dosage titration is recommended because abrupt withdrawal may result in severe agitation and confusion. In older adults or patients experiencing intolerable side effects, the use of a centrally acting, nonselective

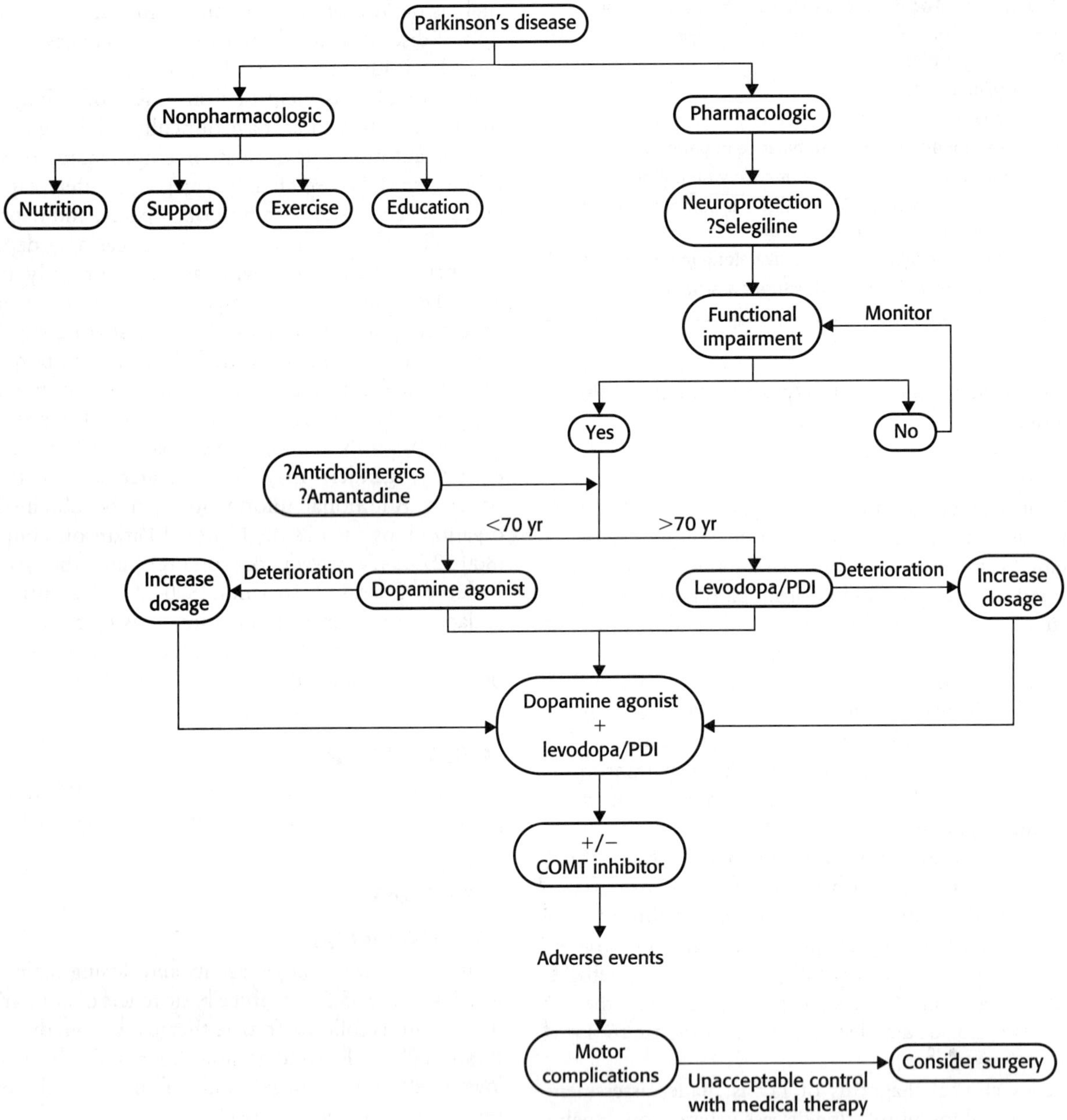

Figure 53.3. Algorithm for managing Parkinson's disease. *COMT,* catechol-O-methyltransferase; *PDI,* peripheral decarboxylase inhibitor. (Adapted with permission from Neurology 50(Suppl 3):S1–S57, 1998.)

β-blocker, such as propranolol, may be effective for tremor control.[47]

Amantadine

Amantadine hydrochloride (Symmetrel) is an antiviral agent that was serendipitously found to have antiparkinson activity.[48] The mechanism of antiparkinson activity remains unknown but may involve potentiation of neuronal dopamine release, blockade of dopamine reuptake, or antagonism of cholinergic or glutamatergic receptors.[49] Rimantadine, a methyl derivative of amantadine, also has antiparkinson properties.[50]

Within days of initiation, modest improvements in bradykinesia, rigidity, and, to a lesser extent, tremor can be expected. With amantadine monotherapy, tachyphylaxis occurs after 4 to 8 weeks in some patients, but discontinuation for a few weeks often restores responsiveness. When it is combined with levodopa, a synergistic benefit may occur. Amantadine is also useful as an add-on agent for alleviating levodopa-induced dyskinesias.[51]

In general, side effects are mild. Central side effects include confusion, nightmares, hallucinations, hyperexcitability, insomnia, and dizziness. Peripheral side effects include nausea, OH, and dry skin or eczema. Patients may also develop a benign and reversible form of livedo reticularis, a vascular cutaneous reaction characterized by a reddish-purple, fishnet-patterned mottling of the upper or lower extremities, often accompanied by ankle edema.[52]

Therapy is initiated at 100 mg per day with breakfast for the first week and then 100 mg twice a day with breakfast and lunch thereafter. Doses administered in the late afternoon may cause insomnia. The dosage may be increased to a maximum of 400 mg/day. Abrupt discontinuation of therapy should be avoided because of the risk of withdrawal encephalopathy.[53] Because amantadine is renally excreted as unchanged drug and high plasma levels may precipitate toxic delirium, stepwise dosage reduction is recommended for patients with creatinine clearance less than 50 mL/minute/1.73 m^2.[54]

Levodopa

For more than 30 years, levodopa has been the most effective and enduring form of antiparkinson therapy. Levodopa is the L-isomer of the amino acid dihydroxyphenylalanine and is a natural precursor for all catecholamine neurotransmitters. The D-isomer is therapeutically obsolete because it is not converted to dopamine in vivo and is associated with granulocytopenia. After entry into the peripheral circulation, levodopa crosses the blood–brain barrier (BBB), where it is taken up by the dopaminergic neurons of the substantia nigra and converted to dopamine by the enzyme dopa decarboxylase (Fig. 53.4). The dopamine is then stored, transported, and eventually released to act on dopamine receptors in the striatum. In essence, levodopa therapy is a form of neurotransmitter replacement analogous to insulin as a form of hormone replacement therapy. In recent years, in vitro experiments have demonstrated that levodopa can be either neurotoxic or neurotrophic, depending on the experimental conditions.[55,56] The results of ongoing clinical trials may shed more light on these laboratory findings.

Carbidopa (α-methyldopa hydrazine) is a reversible, peripheral dopa decarboxylase inhibitor (PDI) that does not cross the BBB. When administered in the absence of a PDI, levodopa undergoes significant peripheral metabolism to dopamine. This is therapeutically undesirable because dopamine cannot cross the BBB and is also highly emetogenic because it stimulates the chemoreceptor trigger zone, which is outside the BBB. With the addition of carbidopa, central levodopa bioavailability is increased from 1% to 5 to 10%. In addition, peripherally mediated side effects, such as nausea and vomiting, are reduced, allowing more rapid induction of therapy. Traditionally, it

Table 53.5 ▪ Antiparkinson Drugs

Drug	Dosage
Anticholinergics	
Benztropine (Cogentin) 0.5-, 1-, 2-mg tablets	Initially 0.5–1 mg at bedtime with gradual titration to 3–6 mg/day in 2–4 divided doses.
Trihexyphenidyl (Artane) 2- and 5-mg tablets, 5 mg time-released capsules, 2-mg/5-mL elixir	Initially 1 mg daily at mealtime with titration to 6–10 mg/day in 3 or 4 divided doses. Time-released = twice–daily dosing.
Dopaminergics	
Amantadine (Symmetrel) 100-mg capsules or tablets, 50-mg/5-mL syrup	Initially 100 mg with breakfast. Increase to 100 mg with breakfast and lunch.[a] Maximum dosage 400 mg/day.
Carbidopa/levodopa (Sinemet) 10/100-mg, 25/100-mg, 25/250-mg tablets	Initially 25/100 mg/day with breakfast. Increase to 25/100 mg 3 times daily. Titrate up to 250/1000 mg/day in 4 or more divided doses.
Carbidopa/levodopa sustained-release (Sinemet CR) 25/100-mg, 50/200-mg tablets	Initiate at 25/100 mg/day with breakfast. Increase to 50/200 mg 2–4 times daily.
Bromocriptine (Parlodel) 2.5-mg tablets and 5-mg capsules	Initially 1.25 mg twice a day with meals. Increase by 2.5 mg/day every 2–4 wk. Target dosage 10–50 mg/day in 2 or 3 divided doses.
Pergolide (Permax) 0.05-, 0.25-, 1-mg tablets	Initially 0.05 mg/day for 2 days. Increase by 0.1–0.15 mg/day every third day for 12 days. Then increase by 0.25 mg/day to 1 mg 3 times daily.
Pramipexole (Mirapex) 0.125-, 0.25-, 1-, 1.5-mg tablets	Initially 0.125 mg/day; titrate weekly to target dosage of 3–4.5 mg in 3 divided doses.[b]
Ropinirole (Requip) 0.25-, 0.5-, 1-, 2-, 4-, 5-mg tablets	Initially 0.25 mg/day; titrate weekly to 6–9 mg in 3 divided doses. Maximum dosage 24 mg/day.
Enzyme inhibitors	
Carbidopa (Lodosyn) 25-mg tablets	25 mg to be taken 30 min before carbidopa–levodopa doses.
Selegiline (Eldepryl, Carbex, Atapryl) 5-mg tablets or capsules	Initially 5 mg with breakfast. Increase to 5 mg with breakfast and lunch.
Entacapone (Comtan) 200-mg tablets	200 mg with each dose of immediate-release carbidopa–levodopa. Maximum dosage 1800 mg/day.
Tolcapone (Tasmar) 100- and 200-mg tablets	Initially 100 mg with the first dose of carbidopa–levodopa. Titrate to 100–200 mg 3 times daily (taken at 6-hr intervals).

[a]Amantadine: 100 mg once daily if creatinine clearance (CrCl) = 40–50 mL/min/1.73 m^2; 200 mg twice weekly if CrCl = 30–40 mL/min/1.73 m^2.

[b]Pramipexole: Twice-daily dosing if CrCl = 35–59 mL/min; once-daily dosing if CrCl = 15–34 mL/min.

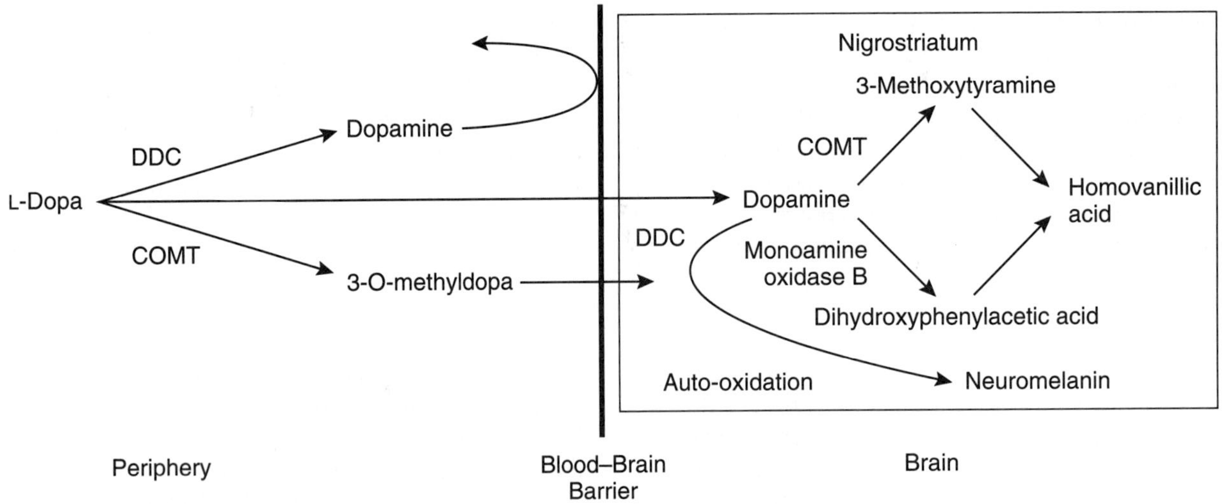

Figure 53.4. Levodopa metabolic pathways. *COMT*, catechol-O-methyltransferase; *DDC*, dopa decarboxylase.

has been stated that 75 to 100 mg per day of carbidopa is needed for maximal enzyme inhibition. However, some patients may need additional supplementation.[57] The carbidopa and levodopa combination product is marketed under the proprietary name Sinemet ("without emesis" or "without metabolism"). Carbidopa is also available as a single-drug product (Lodosyn). In some countries, a different PDI, benserazide, is combined with levodopa and marketed as Madopar.

Significant improvement in bradykinesia, rigidity, and, to a lesser extent, tremor can be expected. Improvements in postural instability are minimal. The effects of a missed dose in patients with early, mild disease often go unnoticed. Overall, motor function can be improved 50% or more in about two-thirds of patients. Patients should be advised that physical activities (e.g., dancing, walking, sports) should be resumed gradually to minimize falls and associated morbidity.

Therapy is initiated with one-half to one tablet of 25 mg carbidopa and 100 mg levodopa (Sinemet 25/100) administered once a day and titrated weekly to 25/100 mg three times a day. Many patients can tolerate more rapid titration. Because diet-derived large neutral amino acids compete with levodopa for transport across the BBB, carbidopa/levodopa should be taken on an empty stomach (i.e., 30 minutes before or 1 to 2 hours after a meal) and with a glass of water to improve bioavailability.[58] However, in early disease, this drug–food interaction may not be clinically significant and patients often need administration with food to help alleviate gastrointestinal discomfort. Periodic dosage titration, either up or down, is expected and determined by the rate of disease progression, adjustments of other antiparkinson drugs, and severity of side effects. In patients who are responding, most neurologists do not titrate beyond 800 mg per day. If minimal response occurs at 1000 mg per day, an alternative diagnosis (e.g., atypical parkinsonism) must be considered. Levodopa is contraindicated in patients with narrow-angle glaucoma but may beused safely in wide-angle glaucoma if intraocular pressure is monitored carefully. Because dopamine is a melanin intermediate, levodopa is contraindicated in patients with malignant melanoma. However, critical reviews of the literature suggest that melanoma progression is not influenced by levodopa.[59,60] If discontinuation of therapy is needed, abrupt withdrawal should be avoided to reduce the risk of neuroleptic malignant–like syndrome characterized by confusion, rigidity, respiratory arrest, and fever.[61]

Sinemet CR is a sustained-release tablet designed to maintain constant plasma levels of levodopa. In mild to moderate disease, Sinemet CR compares favorably with standard Sinemet, and less frequent dosing is needed.[62,63] Additionally, conversion to the CR formulation is a cost-effective method for alleviating peak dose dyskinesias and wearing-off phenomenon.[64] Peripheral levodopa bioavailability with the CR formulation is less than that of standard Sinemet (71% versus 99%, respectively).[65] Accordingly, a 10 to 30% higher total daily levodopa dosage may be needed for comparable therapeutic effects. Additionally, levodopa absorption occurs gradually over 4 to 5 hours and results in sustained plasma levels. Dosing intervals should be reduced by 30 to 50% when converting from standard Sinemet. Patients must be advised that Sinemet CR should not be chewed, crushed, or liquefied. Unlike the standard formulation, Sinemet CR should be taken with food to improve bioavailability. Food increases gastric retention and allows greater tablet erosion and thus more release of levodopa from the CR matrix. The latency time from dose administration to onset of motor improvement is approximately 60 minutes (in contrast to 30 minutes for standard Sinemet). Patients should be assured that the lack of a "surge" does not reflect medication failure, and patients with moderate to advanced disease may need a small booster dose of standard Sinemet in the morning. Additionally, the CR formulation does not produce the euphoriant effects or levodopa surge associated with standard Sinemet.

Levodopa Side Effects

GASTROINTESTINAL. Nausea, vomiting, and anorexia are most common during therapy initiation or dosage increases and are alleviated by administration with food or the addition of supplemental carbidopa. Antiemetics that can be used include trimethobenzamide, serotonin ($5HT_3$)-receptor blockers (e.g., ondansetron), and the peripheral dopamine receptor blocker domperidone. Antiemetic agents with central antidopaminergic activity (e.g., droperidol, metoclopramide, prochlorperazine) should be avoided. Prokinetic agents such as cisapride are useful for symptoms associated with gastroparesis. Other side effects include abdominal pain, constipation, diarrhea, and dry mouth. Uncommonly, mild elevations of liver function tests, peptic ulcer, and gastrointestinal bleeding may occur.

CARDIOVASCULAR. OH is a common feature of advanced PD and may be exacerbated by any dopamimetic agent. When symptomatic, OH significantly impairs ambulation and increases the risk of falls. Symptoms include syncope, dizziness, light-headedness, and fatigue. Cerebral hypoperfusion and reflex tachycardia may precipitate cognitive changes and adverse myocardial events. Pharmacologic interventions include the use of fludrocortisone with salt supplementation or the addition of midodrine, an α-receptor agonist. Dosages of other OH-exacerbating agents including amantadine, direct dopamine agonists, selegiline, tricyclic antidepressants, and antipsychotics should be reduced or eliminated. A variety of nonpharmacologic interventions also are available (e.g., elastic stockings).

NEUROPSYCHIATRIC. Patients may experience neuropsychiatric manifestations such as agitation, confusion, euphoria, inappropriate behavior, hallucinosis, psychosis, and, uncommonly, hypersexuality. The hallucinosis generally is associated with benign visual imagery (e.g., of people or animals) and is associated with preserved insight. Less commonly, an auditory, olfactory, or tactile component may be present. Unlike hallucinosis, dopa-induced psychosis is characterized by frightening visions and paranoid delusions (e.g., of persecution or spousal infidelity). Ultimately, psychosis may result in nursing home placement and increased mortality.[66] In addition to levodopa, dosages of adjunctive medications (anticholinergics, selegiline, amantadine, direct dopamine agonists) should be reduced or eliminated in a stepwise manner. If dosage reduction results in unacceptable worsening of parkinsonism, the atypical antipsychotics clozapine and quetiapine can be used safely and effectively.[67,68] Butyrophenone and phenothiazine antipsychotic agents (Table 53.3) exacerbate parkinsonism and should be avoided.

Levodopa-Related Motor Complications

After 3 to 5 years of levodopa therapy, 20 to 75% of patients develop some type of motor complication or oscillation, which can occupy up to 50% of the waking day.[62,69,70] Younger patients are particularly susceptible.[71] The exact mechanism of motor complications is unknown but probably arises from complex interactions between ongoing neurodegeneration, levodopa pharmacokinetics, and pharmacodynamic changes at the receptor level.[72] The key to managing motor complications is appropriate identification of the various subtypes. Toward this end, the use of a patient diary is highly recommended and is very useful for analyzing the relationships between drug administration and motor oscillations.

WEARING-OFF PHENOMENON. The term *wearing-off* or *motor fluctuation* refers to a levodopa benefit lasting less than 4 hours. This postdose effect is predictable and is related to the waning of levodopa levels. Wearing-off symptoms include both motor and nonmotor manifestations. Motor symptoms include dystonia (involuntary, sustained cramping) and worsening parkinsonism. Nonmotor symptoms include a wide range of autonomic, sensory, and mental changes. Patients may experience shortness of breath, fatigue, tachycardia, pallor, facial flushing, pain (musculoskeletal, radicular, or neuropathic), gastrointestinal hypomotility (abdominal pain, bloating, belching), vasomotor abnormalities (limb edema, temperature changes), profuse sweating, urinary frequency, apathy, episodic depression, and disabling panic attacks. Therapeutic strategies include more frequent administration of carbidopa/levodopa, sup-

Table 53.6 ▪ Levodopa Drug Interactions

Drug	Comments
Butyrophenones Droperidol (Inapsine) Haloperidol (Haldol)	Antagonistic at central dopamine receptors.
Inhalational anesthesia Cyclopropane Halothane	Sensitizes myocardium and increases risk of levodopa-induced tachyarrhythmias.
Iron supplements	Binds to levodopa in the stomach. Administer at least 2 hr apart.
Monoamine oxidase inhibitors (nonselective) Phenelzine (Nardil) Tranylcypromine (Parnate)	Risk of "cheese" effect. Discontinue 2 wk before initiating levodopa.
Methyldopa	Inhibits the central conversion of levodopa to dopamine.
Phenothiazines Chlorpromazine (Thorazine) Fluphenazine (Prolixin) Mesoridazine (Serentil) Perphenazine (Trilafon) Prochlorperazine (Compazine) Thioridazine (Mellaril) Thiothixene (Navane) Trifluoperazine (Stelazine) Triflupromazine (Vesprin)	Antagonistic at central dopamine receptors.
Miscellaneous Amoxapine (Asendin) Metoclopramide (Reglan) Pimozide (Orap)	Antagonistic at central dopamine receptors.

plementation with a long-acting agent (e.g., Sinemet CR or direct agonist), or addition of a levodopa extender (e.g., catechol-O-methyltransferase [COMT] inhibitor, selegiline). Some patients are more sensitive to dietary protein–levodopa interactions, and elimination of excess protein or a trial of protein redistribution may be worthwhile.[73,74] Nocturnal "off" symptoms such as painful calf dystonias are common and are relieved by clonazepam or small dosages of carbidopa/levodopa.

Dyskinesias. Dyskinesias are involuntary choreiform movements involving the head, neck, torso, and extremities. Peak-dose dyskinesias or dystonias are predictable and are correlated with peak levodopa levels in the brain. Therapeutic management strategies are aimed at reducing peak levodopa levels. Some patients may alternate between "off" and "on" with dyskinesias, with few normal "on" periods in between (i.e., "yoyoing"). Other less common dyskinesias include square-wave dyskinesia and diphasic dyskinesia.[70]

On–Off Phenomenon. On–off oscillations are unpredictable, sudden transitions between "on" and "off" states and appear to be unrelated to the timing of drug administration. The duration of "on" and "off" periods ranges from minutes to hours. Management is difficult and includes more frequent administration of carbidopa/levodopa, use of long-acting agents, or the addition of a levodopa extender. For severe cases, liquid carbidopa/levodopa can be used to allow finer dosage titration. The liquid form must be compounded and is administered very frequently (e.g., every 1 to 2 hours) or by continuous enteral infusion.[75,76]

Drug Interactions

Several drugs may adversely affect the therapeutic activity of levodopa (Table 53.6). Pyridoxal-5-phosphate, the active form of pyridoxine, acts as a coenzyme to dopa decarboxylase and catalyzes the peripheral deactivation of levodopa. However, with the development of carbidopa, this interaction has become clinically insignificant, and pyridoxine restriction is unnecessary in patients receiving combination carbidopa/levodopa.

Laboratory Abnormalities and Assay Interference

With high-dose levodopa, a positive Coombs' test with or without frank hemolysis, similar to that reported with methyldopa, may be noted after 3 to 12 months of therapy.[77,78] Levodopa may interfere with the following laboratory tests and give rise to false-positive results: serum and urine uric acid readings measured by the colorimetric method (but not by the more specific ultraviolet uricase method);[79] urine catecholamine, metanephrine, and vanillylmandelic acid; Labstix or Ketostix (used to detect urine ketones);[80] and Phenistix (used to test for phenylketonuria).

Drug Holidays

Levodopa-induced psychosis and motor complications have been attributed to alterations in dopamine receptor sensitivities or expression. A drug holiday is a complete withdrawal of levodopa to allow dopamine receptors to re-equilibrate. Drug holidays lasting up to 2 weeks have been associated with reductions in subsequent levodopa needs and reductions in drug-related motor and psychiatric complications. However, benefits usually are short-lived, and, more importantly, drug holidays predispose patients to complications such as deep vein thrombosis, pulmonary embolism, aspiration, and depression. Most neurologists believe that the benefits of a drug holiday do not outweigh the risks.[81]

Direct Dopamine Agonists

Worldwide, many direct agonists are available for managing PD: apomorphine, bromocriptine, cabergoline, lisuride, pergolide, piribedil, pramipexole, and ropinirole. Unlike levodopa, these agents directly stimulate striatal dopamine receptors and do not involve enzymatic activation. Additional pharmacologic and clinical differences are listed in Table 53.7. Apomorphine, lisuride, and piribedil are not marketed in the United States. Cabergoline (Dostinex), a synthetic, long-acting ergoline, is available in the United States but is not approved by the U.S. Food and Drug Administration (FDA) for treating parkinsonism. The remaining four direct agonists (bromocriptine, pergolide, pramipexole, ropinirole) are commonly used in the United States and produce improvements in tremor, rigidity, and bradykinesia but not postural instability.

For decades, clinical dogma has been to reserve direct agonists as add-on therapy for patients experiencing motor complications while on levodopa. However, recently published evidence-based consensus guidelines emphasize levodopa-sparing pharmacotherapy, that is, the preferential use of direct agonists in patients with early, uncomplicated PD.[45,46,82,83] The rationale for this approach is multifactorial. First, clinical data demonstrate that direct agonists are

Table 53.7 ▪ Major Differences Between Levodopa and Direct Dopamine Agonists

Levodopa	Direct Dopamine Agonists[a]
Most effective symptomatic therapy.	Generally less effective than levodopa.
May improve mortality.	Effect on mortality not well studied.
Motor complications predominate over neuropsychiatric complications.	Neuropsychiatric complications predominate over motor complications.
Short half-life results in fluctuations of striatal levels.	Long half-life results in fewer fluctuations of striatal levels.
Clinical activity influenced by changes in enzymatic activity and dietary LNAA intake.	Clinical activity not influenced by enzymatic activity or dietary factors.
Dependent on functional nigral neurons for conversion to dopamine.	Directly stimulates striatal dopamine receptors.

LNAA, large, neutral amino acid (histidine, isoleucine, leucine, methionine, phenylalanine, tryptophan, tyrosine, valine).

[a]Bromocriptine, pergolide, pramipexole, ropinirole.

as effective as levodopa and well-tolerated when initiated in patients with early-stage disease.[84,85] However, as the disease progresses, the efficacy of direct agonists tends to wane and adding levodopa becomes essential. Second, initiating therapy with a direct agonist is associated with a significantly lower risk of developing disabling dyskinesias than is levodopa therapy.[86] For younger patients, levodopa-sparing management strategies are particularly prudent because the emergence of disabling motor complications can have profound adverse effects on economic and social productivity. Third, in vitro experiments demonstrate that direct agonists exhibit neuroprotective properties.[87,88]

Dosing guidelines for the direct agonists are listed in Table 53.5. Because successful therapy in agonist-naive patients depends on careful and slow dosage titration, patients should be informed that benefits may not be obtained for several weeks and, if used in patients with a history of dementia, the initial dosage should be reduced by 50%. If patients are not responding or are intolerant of one agonist, another agonist may be used successfully. In agonist-experienced patients, rapid conversion to another agonist may be performed safely and effectively.[89] Abrupt discontinuation of therapy should be avoided because of the risk of neuroleptic malignant syndrome.

As a class, the direct agonists share similar dopaminergic side effects, many of which are dose-related. Peripheral effects include nausea, vomiting, constipation, OH, and edema. Of particular importance, patients should be monitored for first-dose hypotension. Central side effects include dizziness, somnolence, insomnia, confusion, yawning, visual hallucinations, and psychosis. Hypersexual behavior may also occur.[90] Unlike with levodopa, monotherapy with direct agonists uncommonly induces dyskinesias.[91] Other side effects that differentiate each agonist are described in the following sections.

Bromocriptine

Bromocriptine (Parlodel) is an ergot-derived agonist that stimulates D_2 receptors and mildly antagonizes D_1 sites. Although originally indicated for disorders of hyperprolactinemia, bromocriptine was the first direct agonist to be FDA approved for PD management (Table 53.1). Although bromocriptine is beneficial in all stages of PD, comparative studies demonstrate that it is less effective than pergolide, pramipexole, and ropinirole.[92–95] As an adjunct to levodopa, bromocriptine allows an overall reduction of 20% or more in daily levodopa dosage.

Because of its ergotlike structure, bromocriptine also exerts agonist activity at α-receptors and serotonin receptors. This may contribute to other side effects such as vasoconstriction, rhinitis, erythromelalgia (a painful, reddish skin rash), peptic ulcers, livedo reticularis, pleuropulmonary disease (PPD), and retroperitoneal fibrosis. Bromocriptine-induced PPD is reversible and occurs in about 2 to 5% of patients after 5 years of therapy. Patients receiving dosages greater than 20 mg/day for more than 6 months may be at increased risk.[96] A baseline chest radiograph is recommended before initial therapy.

Drugs that are potent inhibitors of the cytochrome P-450 3A4 enzyme (e.g., erythromycin, clarithromycin, nefazodone) may increase plasma bromocriptine levels severalfold.[97]

Pergolide

Pergolide (Permax) was the second agonist approved by the FDA for treating PD. Pergolide is a semisynthetic ergot derivative with strong D_2 receptor agonism. Unlike bromocriptine, pergolide also stimulates D_1 receptors. The therapeutic equivalency ratio of pergolide to bromocriptine is about 1 : 10.[89] Pergolide is also effective in all stages of PD. As an adjunct to levodopa, pergolide allows an overall reduction of approximately 40% in daily levodopa dosage.[93,98,99]

Although pergolide has a long half-life (27 hours), the duration of clinical activity is about 6 hours, and multiple daily doses are needed. Side effects are common but generally less frequent than with bromocriptine. Although pergolide has been associated with abnormal cardiac rhythms, the drug can be used safely in patients with stable cardiac disease.[100,101] As with bromocriptine, retroperitoneal fibrosis and other ergotaminelike side effects may occur.

Pramipexole

Pramipexole (Mirapex) is considered a second-generation agonist and was the third direct agonist approved by the FDA for treating PD. Pharmacologically, pramipexole differs from the first-generation agonists, bromocriptine and pergolide, in several respects. First, pramipexole is a nonergot agonist, and ergotamine-related side effects, such as retroperitoneal fibrosis, are not to be expected. Second, pramipexole is very specific for the D_3-subtype receptor (which belongs to the D_2 receptor family). The clinical effects caused by this specificity remain speculative but may include improved efficacy and antidepressant or mood-elevating activity.[102] Third, pramipexole is excreted renally as unchanged drug and exhibits no significant inhibition of hepatic cytochrome P-450 enzymes.[103]

Pramipexole is effective in all stages of PD and, when added to a levodopa regimen, allows a 25 to 30% reduction in daily levodopa dosage. During dosage titration, patients should be warned of the potential for sudden daytime somnolence ("sleep attacks"), which may prove hazardous, especially while driving or operating heavy equipment.[104] In patients with a creatinine clearance less than 60 mL/minute, a dosage decrease is recommended.

Ropinirole

Ropinirole (Requip) is a nonergot second-generation agonist that exhibits high affinity for D_2 and D_3 receptor subtypes with minimal activity at nondopaminergic receptor sites (i.e., α, histaminic, cholinergic, serotonergic). Like other direct agonists, ropinirole is beneficial in all stages of PD and, when added to a levodopa regimen, allows a 30% reduction in daily levodopa dosage.[105]

Side effects are similar to those of pramipexole. However, the prevalence of somnolence and hallucinations may be less and that of dizziness and OH may be greater. The maximum recommended daily dosage of ropinirole is 24 mg. Unlike pramipexole, ropinirole dosage adjustments are not needed for renal function. Ropinirole is metabolized in part by the cytochrome P-450 1A2 isoenzyme, and inhibitors of this enzyme (e.g., ciprofloxacin, ethinyl estradiol) may increase plasma ropinirole levels. Additionally, ropinirole and its major metabolites inhibit the cytochrome P-450 2D6 isoenzyme in vitro.

Enzyme Inhibitors

Dopa decarboxylase, COMT, and MAO-B are three major enzymes involved in levodopa and dopamine metabolism (Fig. 53.4). As discussed previously, carbidopa is used as an adjunct to enhance levodopa pharmacokinetics. Enzyme inhibitors specific for MAO-B and COMT are also commonly used to treat PD and are discussed in the following sections.

Seligiline

Selegiline (L-deprenyl, Eldepryl, Carbex, Atapryl) is an irreversible enzyme inhibitor with relative selectivity for MAO-B. Clinically, selegiline produces mild symptom-relieving effects by virtue of its ability to inhibit central dopamine metabolism. However, laboratory experiments also demonstrate that selegiline and its metabolite, *N*-desmethylselegiline, protect against free radical–induced neurotoxicity and apoptosis.[106] Although definitive evidence of clinical neuroprotection remains elusive, pathologic samples from brains of selegiline-treated patients have been shown to contain more nigral neurons and fewer Lewy bodies than brains of selegiline-naive patients.[107]

As monotherapy in early PD, selegiline is associated with a delay in the need for levodopa, slowed symptom progression, and extended employability.[108,109] In moderate to advanced disease, adjunctive selegiline reduces the need for levodopa and attenuates wearing-off symptoms.[110] However, the role of selegiline is complicated by clinical data suggesting that it increases the risk of mortality (when used in combination with levodopa)[111] and by the introduction of COMT inhibitors as an alternative for managing wearing-off symptoms. Although numerous studies have failed to confirm an adverse effect on mortality,[112,113] it may be prudent to avoid selegiline in patients with a history of dementia, frequent falls, and postural hypotension.[111]

Side effects are mild and include insomnia, dizziness, headache, benign cardiac arrhythmias, dry mouth, and nausea. Many patients may also report an increased sense of well-being. Uncommonly, exacerbation of peptic ulcer disease and elevations in liver enzymes may occur. Because insomnia or vivid dreaming may result from levoamphetamine metabolites or increased central dopaminergic activity, patients should be instructed to take doses no later than noon.

Because of the risk of serotonin syndrome, concomitant use of selegiline and meperidine is contraindicated, and caution is urged with concomitant use of serotonin reuptake inhibitors, imipramine, clomipramine, lithium, sibutramine, and high-dose dextromethorphan. Additionally, at dosages greater than 20 mg/day, selectivity for MAO-B is compromised and patients may be at greater risk for the "cheese" effect.[112] This potentially fatal reaction, characterized by hypertension, vomiting, tachycardia, and headache, results from the ingestion of tyramine-containing products (e.g., aged, fermented, pickled, smoked foods including cheeses, meats, fish, and red wines), sympathomimetic-containing preparations (e.g., over-the-counter remedies with ephedrine, phenylpropanolamine, pseudoephedrine), or levodopa-containing products.

Catechol-O-Methyltransferase Inhibitors

The highly selective, reversible, nitrocatechol-structured COMT inhibitors (entacapone [Comtan] and tolcapone [Tasmar]) are yet another means of extending the therapeutic activity of levodopa. In the presence of a PDI, such as carbidopa, levodopa metabolism is shifted toward the COMT pathway (Fig. 53.4). COMT then metabolizes levodopa to 3-O-methyldopa (3-OMD), an inactive byproduct that competes with levodopa for passage across the BBB and may contribute to the development of motor fluctuations.[114] With the coadministration of a COMT inhibitor, the bioavailability of levodopa to the brain is increased and levels of 3-OMD are reduced. Because levodopa area under the concentration–time curve (AUC) and elimination half-life are increased, the dosage and frequency of levodopa administration can be reduced. Levodopa absorption pharmacokinetics, peak plasma concentrations (C_{max}), and the time of peak occurrence (T_{max}) are minimally altered.

ENTACAPONE. Entacapone is a peripherally acting COMT inhibitor that, when coadministered with levodopa and PDI formulations, is useful for reducing wearing-off symptoms.[115] Generally 200 mg is administered with each dose of immediate-release levodopa and PDI and is associated with a 50% increase in levodopa half-life and AUC.[114] In clinical studies, patients have tolerated up to 2000 mg, or 10 doses per day.[116] Because entacapone is eliminated primarily via biliary excretion, mild to moderate hepatic impairment increases bioavailability twofold, so the dosage should be halved.[115]

Patients should be informed that dopaminergic side effects (e.g., dyskinesias, gastrointestinal disturbances, dizziness, hallucinations) may occur and can be alleviated with downward titration of levodopa or entacapone. Nondopaminergic side effects include dry mouth, intensification of urine coloration (caused by nitrocatechol metabolites), and diarrhea. The diarrhea often occurs after 1 to 3 months after initiation of therapy, is usually self-limiting, and responds to antidiarrheal agents.

Entacapone is associated with few specific laboratory abnormalities. In clinical studies, the incidence of significant liver enzyme elevations was low (less than 1%). Nevertheless, periodic liver enzyme monitoring may be prudent until long-term surveillance data are available. Clinically significant decreases in hemoglobin levels have been noted, and periodic monitoring of red blood cell indices may also be prudent.[117]

An increased risk of adverse cardiovascular reactions may be associated with concurrent administration of nonselective MAO inhibitors.[118] However, concurrent use with selegiline is well tolerated.[119] COMT inhibitors may also inhibit the metabolism of other drugs with catechol structures, including epinephrine, isoproterenol, apomorphine, dobutamine, fenoldopam, methyldopa, and nadolol. Like other catechol-structured molecules (e.g., levodopa), entacapone chelates iron in vitro, and administration with oral pharmaceutical iron preparations should be separated by at least 2 hours.[120]

TOLCAPONE. Tolcapone is a broad-spectrum (i.e., centrally and peripherally acting) COMT inhibitor that, when coadministered with levodopa and PDI formulations, is useful in all stages of PD. Benefits include improvements in "on" time and reductions in "off" time and total daily levodopa intake.[121–123] However, because of reports of fatal, fulminant liver failure, tolcapone should be reserved only for patients with motor fluctuations who are not adequately responding to or are intolerant of other adjunctive therapies.[124] In contrast to entacapone, tolcapone is administered according to a fixed-interval schedule of 100 to 200 mg three times a day (Table 53.5) and is associated with increases of levodopa half-life and AUC of up to 100%.[114] However, some patients derive benefit at lower dosages or with less frequent dosing.

In general, common side effects are similar to those of entacapone. Because of the risk of hepatocellular injury, measurement of serum alanine aminotransferase–aspartate aminotransferase (ALT/AST) levels is recommended at baseline, every 2 weeks during the first year of therapy, every 4 weeks for the next 6 months, and then every 8 weeks thereafter. Because hepatotoxicity appears to be dose related, this laboratory protocol must be repeated after each dosage increase. Tolcapone should be discontinued if ALT/AST levels exceed the upper limit of normal, if patients report signs and symptoms of liver failure (e.g., persistent nausea, lethargy, anorexia, jaundice, dark urine, clay-colored stools, pruritus, and abdominal tenderness), or if patients do not experience a significant symptomatic benefit after 3 weeks of therapy. The drug interaction profile of tolcapone is similar to that of entacapone.

Nonpharmacologic Therapy

Optimal PD management entails an integrated multidisciplinary approach and involves a variety of nonpharmacologic interventions such as education, physical therapy, speech therapy, and nutrition. Although discussed briefly in this chapter, more detailed information on nonpharmacologic interventions is readily available from organized public resources.

Education should be appropriately selective and problem oriented because disease progression and severity, presence of motor and nonmotor symptoms, and response to drug therapy differ for each patient. Patients and family members should understand how symptoms can affect personal and social activities and that lifestyle adjustments are needed. For example, activities of daily living may take more time to perform.

Consultation with a physical or occupational therapist is often very helpful for developing exercise routines and for improving the safety of work and living quarters. In addition to improving task performance, other benefits of exercise include improvements in functional status, mood, quality of mobility provided by drugs, and mortality.[125,126]

Several forms of speech treatment are available, but not all produce long-lasting results. However, an intensive outpatient program known as the Lee Silverman Voice Treatment can provide long-term benefits.[127]

Consultation with a dietician and a speech pathologist may be helpful because patients often experience difficulty with preparing, chewing, or swallowing food. Additionally, demented patients may be difficult to feed or uncooperative. Preventive nutrition is also important. Adequate calcium intake and sunlight exposure (at least 15 minutes/day) can help reduce the long-term risk of osteoporosis and bone fractures.[128]

Surgery

An increased understanding of neuroanatomy coupled with improved neuroimaging and stereotactic techniques has rekindled interest in surgical interventions. Targets include the ventrointermediate thalamic nucleus (Vim), the internal capsule of the globus pallidus (GPi), and the subthalamic nuclei (Fig. 53.1). After target localization, either electrothermal tissue ablation or high-frequency deep brain stimulation (DBS) is performed. DBS has become the favored technique and is associated with advantages such as preservation of neural tissue and ease of adjusting stimulation parameters to provide optimal control. For patients with drug-refractory disabling tremors, thalamotomy or DBS of the Vim is the preferred procedure.[129] Afterward, medication is still needed to manage bradykinesia and rigidity. For young, nondemented patients with refractory akinetic–rigid disease or dopa-induced dyskinesias, pallidotomy or DBS of the GPi results in significant motor improvements.[130,131] However, patients often remain on antiparkinson therapy for optimal control. As an alternative to GPi-targeted techniques, DBS of the subthalamic nucleus appears very promising.[132]

Grafting or transplantation of human embryonic mesencephalon tissue into the striatum has received much attention. However, despite impressive results, this technique remains experimental.[133] Alternatively, xenotransplantation with embryonic porcine mesencephalon tissue is under investigation.[134]

ALTERNATIVE THERAPIES

α-Tocopherol (vitamin E) has antioxidant properties and was studied as a potential neuroprotective agent in a large number of patients.[109] Although dosages of 1000 IU twice daily are associated with a 70% increase in cerebral spinal fluid levels of vitamin E, the effects of the antioxidant were no different from those of placebo.[135] Agents that promote energy metabolism, such as coenzyme Q10, have been studied, but preliminary clinical results have been disappointing.[136] Additional clinical studies are ongoing.

The pods of the broad bean, *Vicia faba*, are a source of naturally occurring levodopa, and ingestion of *Vicia faba* pods has been shown to improve parkinsonian symptoms.[137] A 100-g serving of *Vicia faba* pods contains approximately 250 mg of levodopa.[138] Other natural sources of levodopa include the velvet bean (*Stizolobium* spp.) and the beans of *Mucuna pruriens*, a medicinal plant native to India.[139,140] However, ingesting large quantities of naturally occurring levodopa preparations induces nausea and vomiting unless taken with carbidopa or domperidone. As a botanical alternative for nausea and vomiting, ginger (*Zingiberis officinalis*), sweetened for palatability or brewed as a liquid decoction, may also be effective.

FUTURE THERAPIES

Rasagiline (TV-1012) is an irreversible MAO-B inhibitor that is in advanced stages of clinical trials. Laboratory studies indicate that rasagiline rescues dying neurons and also has dopaminergic effects.[141] Unlike selegiline, the metabolite of rasagiline, 1-(R) aminoindan, does not have amphetaminelike properties. Remacemide, an antiglutamatergic agent, is also under investigation as a neuroprotective agent.[142] In laboratory and animal studies, trophic factors such as glial-derived neurotrophic factor and GM1 ganglioside have produced encouraging results, but clinical data are limited.[143] A novel D_2 agonist, N-0923, is undergoing clinical studies and is a promising agent for transdermal delivery systems.[144]

IMPROVING OUTCOMES

Aside from appropriate pharmacologic management, several nonpharmacologic interventions are essential for achieving treatment goals. Multidisciplinary education and intervention are vital and should involve family members and caregivers. Educational pamphlets are readily available from various nonprofit organizations.

PHARMACOECONOMICS

PD is an expensive neurologic condition to treat. The annual drug expenditure for treatment in the United States has been estimated to range from $208 million to $279 million.[145,146] In one study, mean annual direct costs including drugs, inpatient hospitalizations, and formal care for patients with moderate-stage disease were approximately $10,200 per patient, as compared to $4700 per patient without PD.[147] However, when indirect costs (e.g., quality of life, loss of productivity, economic impact on family caregivers) are included, the adverse economic impact of PD may be profound. Factors that influence the cost of illness include age of symptom onset; level of disability; presence of motor complications, falls, and dementia; and nursing home placement.[145,148] Although prospective data are lacking, interventions that slow disease progression (e.g., neuroprotection) and reduce motor complications (e.g., levodopa sparing regimens) would be expected to relieve the economic burden of PD.

KEY POINTS

- PD belongs to a family of clinical entities characterized by the presence of tremor, rigidity, akinesia and bradykinesia, and postural instability as well as mental and autonomic changes. The resulting symptoms have profound effects on quality of life for both patients and caregivers.
- The causes of PD remain obscure. However, age-related changes, toxin exposure, and genetic predisposition are believed to play a role in promoting oxidant stress, with subsequent neurodegeneration and depletion of nigrostriatal dopamine.
- Appropriate treatment can delay the onset of functional impairment, provide significant symptomatic relief, and improve quality of life. Toward this end, successful management depends on proper diagnosis, familiarity with pharmacologic and nonpharmacologic modalities, and individualized treatment.
- Levodopa with PDI remains the most efficacious form of pharmacotherapy, but the development of late-stage motor and neuropsychiatric complications remains problematic.
- Current recommendations favor the selective use of anticholinergic agents for young patients with tremor-predominant disease, direct dopamine agonists for young patients with akinetic-rigid disease, and levodopa and PDI for older adults. Additionally, early initiation of selegiline should be considered as a means of delaying the onset of functional impairment.
- For medically refractory cases, surgical intervention may be needed.
- Ultimately, as stated by Schwab and England more than 50 years ago, "the secret to success with [PD] is complete adaptability to it,"[149] and toward this end, multidisciplinary involvement is essential.

REFERENCES

1. Parkinson J. An essay on the shaking palsy. London: Sherwood, Neely, and Jones, 1817.
2. Speelman JD, Bosch DA. Resurgence of functional neurosurgery for Parkinson's disease: a historical perspective. Mov Disord 13:582–588, 1998.
3. Lewy FH. Paralysis agitans. I. Pathologische anatomie. In: Lewandowsky M, ed. Handbuch der neurologie. Berlin: Springer-Verlag, 1912:920–933.
4. Tretiakoff C. Contribution a l'étude de l'anatomie pathologique du locus niger de soemmering avec quelques deductions relatives a la pathogenie des troubles de tonus musculaire et de la maladie de Parkinson. Paris: Thesis, 1919.
5. Ehringer H, Hornykiewicz O. Verteilung von Noradrenalin und Dopamin (3-Hydroxytyramin) im Gehirn des Menschen und ihr Verhalten bei

Erkrankungen des extrapyramidalen Systems. Klin Wschr 38:1236–1239, 1960. Republished in English translation in Parkinsonism and Related Disorders 4:53–57, 1998.
6. Langston JW, Ballard P, Tetrud JW, et al. Chronic parkinsonism in humans due to a product of meperidine-analog synthesis. Science 219:979–980, 1983.
7. Lindvall O, Rehncrona S, Brundin P, et al. Human fetal dopamine neurons grafted into the striatum in two patients with severe Parkinson's disease. A detailed account of methodology and a 6-month follow-up. Arch Neurol 46:615–631, 1989.
8. Polymeropoulos MH, Higgins JJ, Golbe LI, et al. Mapping of a gene for Parkinson's disease to chromosome 4q21–q23. Science 274:1197–1199, 1996.
9. Marder K, Tang MX, Cote L, et al. The frequency and associated risk factors for dementia in patients with Parkinson's disease. Arch Neurol 52:695–701, 1995.
10. Rajput AH, Offord KP, Beard CM, et al. Epidemiology of parkinsonism: incidence, classification, and mortality. Ann Neurol 16:278–282, 1984.
11. Bower JH, Maraganore DM, McDonnell SK, et al. Incidence and distribution of parkinsonism in Olmstead County, Minnesota, 1976–1990. Neurology 52:1214–1220, 1999.
12. Errea-Abad JM, Ara-Callizo JR, Aibar-Remon C. Drug-induced parkinsonism. Clinical aspects compared with Parkinson's disease. Rev Neurol 27:35–39, 1998.
13. Mamo DC, Sweet RA, Keshavan MS. Managing antipsychotic-induced parkinsonism. Drug Saf 20:269–275, 1999.
14. Avorn J, Gurwitz JH, Bohn RL, et al. Increased incidence of levodopa therapy following metoclopramide use. JAMA 274:1780–1782, 1995.
15. Bennett DA, Beckett LA, Murray AM, et al. Prevalence of parkinsonian signs and associated mortality in a community population of older people. N Engl J Med 334:71–76, 1996.
16. Quinn N, Critchley P, Mardsen CD. Young onset Parkinson's disease. Mov Disord 2:73–91, 1987.
17. Golbe LI. The genetics of Parkinson's disease: a reconsideration. Neurology 40(Suppl 3):7–14, 1990.
18. Marder K, Tang MX, Mejia H, et al. Risk of Parkinson's disease among first-degree relatives: a community-based study. Neurology 47:155–160, 1996.
19. Tanner CM, Ottman R, Goldman SM, et al. Parkinson disease in twins. An etiologic study. JAMA 281:341–346, 1999.
20. Louis ED, Marder K, Côté L, et al. Mortality from Parkinson's disease. Arch Neurol 54:260–264, 1997.
21. Fearnley JM, Lees AJ. Ageing and Parkinson's disease: substantia nigra regional selectivity. Brain 114:2283–2301, 1991.
22. Bernheimer H, Birkmayer W, Hornykiewicz O, et al. Brain dopamine and the syndromes of Parkinson and Huntington. Clinical, morphological and neurochemical correlations. J Neurol Sci 20:415–455, 1973.
23. Lang AE, Lozano AM. Parkinson's disease (first of two parts). N Engl J Med 339:1044–1053, 1998.
24. Duvoisin RC. Cholinergic–anticholinergic antagonism in parkinsonism. Arch Neurol 17:124–136, 1967.
25. Jenner P, Olanow CW. Understanding cell death in Parkinson's disease. Ann Neurol 44(Suppl 1):S72–S84, 1998.
26. Mezey E, Dehejia A, Harta G, et al. Alpha synuclein in neurodegenerative disorders: murderer or accomplice? Nat Med 4:755–757, 1998.
27. Liou HH, Tsai MC, Chen CJ, et al. Environmental risk factors and Parkinson's disease: a case-control study in Taiwan. Neurology 48:1583–1588, 1997.
28. Gorell JM, Johnson CC, Rybicki BA, et al. The risk of Parkinson's disease with exposure to pesticides, farming, well water, and rural living. Neurology 50:1346–1350, 1998.
29. Caparros-Lefebvre D, Elbaz A, and the Caribbean Parkinson Study Group. Possible relation of atypical parkinsonism in the French West Indies with consumption of tropical plants: a case-control study. Lancet 354:281–286, 1999.
30. Spencer PS, Nunn PB, Hugon J, et al. Guam amyotrophic lateral sclerosis-parkinsonism with dementia linked to a plant excitant neurotoxin. Science 237:517–522, 1987.
31. Olanow CW. An introduction to the free radical hypothesis in Parkinson's disease. Ann Neurol 32:S2–S9, 1992.
32. Mardsen CD, Olanow CW. The causes of Parkinson's disease are being unraveled and rational neuroprotective therapy is close to reality. Ann Neurology 44(Suppl 1):S189–S196, 1998.
33. Swerdlow RH, Parks JK, Miller SW, et al. Origin and functional consequences of the complex I defect in Parkinson's disease. Ann Neurol 40:663–671, 1996.
34. Riedl AG, Watts PM, Jenner P, et al. P450 enzymes and Parkinson's disease: the story so far. Mov Disord 13:212–220, 1998.
35. Poewe WH, Wenning GK. The natural history of Parkinson's disease. Ann Neurol 44(Suppl 1):S1–S9, 1998.
36. Louis ED, Tang MX, Cote L, et al. Progression of parkinsonian signs in Parkinson's disease. Arch Neurol 56:334–337, 1999.
37. Mizuno Y, Kondo T, Mori H. Various aspects of motor fluctuations and their management in Parkinson's disease. Neurology 44(Suppl 6):S29–S34, 1994.
38. Brooks DJ. Advances in imaging Parkinson's disease. Curr Opin Neurol 10:327–331, 1997.
39. Hughes AJ, Daniel SE, Kilford L, et al. Accuracy of clinical diagnosis of idiopathic Parkinson's disease: a clinico-pathological study of 100 cases. J Neurol Neurosurg Psychiatry 55:181–184, 1992.
40. Litvan I. Parkinsonian features. When are they Parkinson's disease? JAMA 280:1654–1655, 1998.
41. Hoehn MM, Yahr MD. Parkinsonism: onset, progression and mortality. Neurology 17:427–442, 1967.
42. Fahn S, Elton RL, UPDRS Committee. Unified Parkinson's disease rating scale. In: Fahn S, Marsden CD, Calne DB, et al., eds. Recent developments in Parkinson's disease. Florham Park, NJ: Macmillan Health Care Information, 1987;2:153–164.
43. Cote L. Depression: impact and management by the patient and family. Neurology 52(Suppl 3):S7–S9, 1999.
44. Dura JR, Haywood-Niler E, Kiecolt-Glaser JK. Spousal caregivers of persons with Alzheimer's and Parkinson's disease dementia: a preliminary comparison. Gerontologist 30:332–336, 1990.
45. Koller WC, Silver DE, Lieberman A. An algorithm for managing Parkinson's disease. Neurology 44(Suppl 1):S1–S52, 1994.
46. Olanow CW, Koller WC. An algorithm (decision tree) for the management of Parkinson's disease: treatment guidelines. Neurology 50(Suppl 3):S1–S57, 1998.
47. Koller WC, Herbster G. Adjuvant therapy of parkinsonian tremor. Arch Neurol 44:921–923, 1987.
48. Schwab RS, England AC, Poskanzer DC, et al. Amantadine in the treatment of Parkinson's disease. JAMA 208:1168–1170, 1969.
49. Danysz W, Parsons CG, Kornhuber J, et al. Aminoadamantines as NMDA receptor antagonists and antiparkinsonian agents: preclinical studies. Neurosci Biobehav Rev 21:455–468, 1997.
50. Evidente VG, Adler CH, Caviness JN, et al. A pilot study on the motor effects of rimantadine in Parkinson's disease. Clin Neuropharmacol 22:30–32, 1999.
51. Verhagen Metman L, Del Dotto P, van den Munckhof P, et al. Amantadine as treatment for dyskinesias and motor fluctuations in Parkinson's disease. Neurology 50:1323–1326, 1998.
52. Silver DE, Sahs AL. Livedo reticularis in Parkinson's disease patients treated with amantadine hydrochloride. Neurology 22:665–669, 1972.
53. Factor SA, Molho ES, Brown DL. Acute delirium after withdrawal of amantadine in Parkinson's disease. Neurology 50:1456–1458, 1998.
54. Horadam VW, Sharp JG, Smilack JD, et al. Pharmacokinetics of amantadine hydrochloride in subjects with normal and impaired renal function. Ann Intern Med 94:454–458, 1981.
55. Melamed E, Offen D, Shirvan A, et al. Levodopa toxicity and apoptosis. Ann Neurol 44(Suppl 1):S149–S154, 1998.
56. Mena MA, Davila V, Sulzer. Neurotrophic effects of L-dopa in postnatal midbrain dopamine neuron/cortical astrocyte cocultures. J Neurochem 69:1398–1408, 1997.
57. Durso R, Josephs E, Evans JE, et al. Carbidopa doses in current clinical practice do not maximize inhibition of peripheral levodopa decarboxylation. Neurology 52(Suppl 2):A214, 1999.
58. Leenders KL, Poewe WH, Palmer AJ, et al. Inhibition of L-[^{18}F]fluorodopa uptake into human brain by amino acids demonstrated by positron emission tomography. Ann Neurol 20:258–262, 1986.
59. Weiner WJ, Singer C, Sanchez-Ramos JR, et al. Levodopa, melanoma, and Parkinson's disease. Neurology 43:674–677, 1993.
60. Woofter MJ, Manyam BV. Safety of long-term levodopa therapy in malignant melanoma. Clin Neuropharmacol 17:315–319, 1994.
61. Cunningham MA, Darby DG, Donnan GA. Controlled-release delivery of L-dopa associated with nonfatal hyperthermia, rigidity and autonomic dysfunction. Neurology 41:942–943, 1991.
62. Block G, Liss C, Reines S, et al. Comparison of immediate-release and controlled release carbidopa/levodopa in Parkinson's disease. A multicenter 5-year study. Eur Neurol 37:23–27, 1997.
63. Linazasoro G, Grandas F, Martínez-Martin PM, et al. Controlled release levodopa in Parkinson's disease: influence of selection criteria and conversion recommendations in the clinical outcome of 450 patients. Clin Neuropharmacol 22:74–79, 1999.
64. Hempel AG, Wagner ML, Maaty MA, et al. Pharmacoeconomic analysis of using Sinemet CR over standard Sinemet in parkinsonian patients with motor fluctuations. Ann Pharmacother 32:878–883, 1998.

65. Yeh KC, August TF, Bush DF, et al. Pharmacokinetics and bioavailability of Sinemet CR: a summary of human studies. Neurology 39(Suppl 2):25–38, 1989.
66. Goetz CG, Stebbins GT. Mortality and hallucinations in nursing home patients with advanced Parkinson's disease. Neurology 45:669–671, 1995.
67. Parkinson Study Group. Low-dose clozapine for the treatment of drug-induced psychosis in Parkinson's disease. N Engl J Med 340:757–763, 1999.
68. Juncos JL, Arvanitis L, Sweitzer D, et al. Quetiapine improves psychotic symptoms associated with Parkinson's disease. Neurology 52(Suppl 2):A262, 1999.
69. Miyawaki E, Lyons K, Pahwa R, et al. Motor complications of chronic levodopa therapy in Parkinson's disease. Clin Neuropharmacol 20:523–530, 1997.
70. Djaldetti R, Melamed E. Management of response fluctuations: practical guidelines. Neurology 51(Suppl 2):S36–S40, 1998.
71. Kostic V, Przedborski S, Flaster E, et al. Early development of levodopa-induced dyskinesias and response fluctuations in young-onset Parkinson's disease. Neurology 41:202–205, 1991.
72. Sage JI, Mark MH. Basic mechanisms of motor fluctuations. Neurology 44(Suppl 6):S10–S14, 1994.
73. Juncos JL, Fabbrini G, Mouradian MM, et al. Dietary influences on the antiparkinsonian response to levodopa. Arch Neurol 44:1003–1005, 1987.
74. Riley D, Lang AE. Practical application of a low-protein diet for Parkinson's disease. Neurology 38:1026–1031, 1988.
75. Pappert EJ, Goetz CG, Niederman F, et al. Liquid levodopa/carbidopa produces significant improvement in motor function without dyskinesia exacerbation. Neurology 47:1493–1495, 1996.
76. Syed N, Murphy J, Zimmerman T, et al. Ten year's experience with enteral levodopa infusions for motor fluctuations in Parkinson's disease. Mov Disord 13:336–338, 1998.
77. Cotzias GC, Papavasiliou PS. Autoimmunity in patients treated with levodopa. JAMA 207:1353–1354, 1969.
78. Territo MC, Peters RW, Tanaka KR. Autoimmune hemolytic anemia due to levodopa therapy. JAMA 226:1347–1348, 1973.
79. Cawein MJ, Hewins JP. False rise in serum uric acid after L-dopa. N Engl J Med 28:1489–1490, 1969.
80. Cawein MJ, Williamson MA, Ebenezer C, et al. Levodopa and tests for ketonuria. N Engl J Med 283:659, 1970.
81. Mayeux R, Stern Y, Mulvey K, et al. Reappraisal of temporary levodopa withdrawal ("drug holiday") in Parkinson's disease. N Engl J Med 313:724–728, 1985.
82. Olanow CW, Obeso JA. Dopamine agonists in early Parkinson's disease. Kent, UK: Wells Medical, 1997.
83. Bhatia K, Brooks DJ, Burn DJ, et al. Guidelines for the management of Parkinson's disease. The Parkinson's Disease Consensus Working Group. Hosp Med 59:469–480, 1998.
84. Tolosa E, Blesa R, Bayes A, et al. Low-dose bromocriptine in early phases of Parkinson's disease. Clin Neuropharmacol 10:169–174, 1987.
85. Rascol O, Brooks DJ, Brunt ER, et al. Ropinirole in the treatment of early Parkinson's disease: a 6-month interim report of a 5-year levodopa-controlled study. Mov Disord 13:39–45, 1998.
86. Rascol O, Brooks DJ, Korczyn AD, et al. Ropinirole reduces risk of dyskinesias compared to L-dopa when used in early Parkinson's disease [abstract]. XIII International Congress on Parkinson's Disease, Vancouver, Canada, July 24–28, 1999.
87. Yamamoto M. Do dopamine agonists provide neuroprotection? Neurology 51(Suppl 2):S10–S12, 1998.
88. Olanow CW, Jenner P, Brooks D. Dopamine agonists and neuroprotection in Parkinson's disease. Ann Neurol 44(Suppl 1):S167–S174, 1998.
89. Goetz CG, Blasucci L, Stebbins GT. Switching dopamine agonists in advanced Parkinson's disease. Is rapid titration preferable to slow? Neurology 52:1227–1229, 1999.
90. Rascol A, Montastruc JL, Guiraud-Chaumeil B, et al. Bromocriptine as the first treatment of Parkinson's disease: long-term results. Rev Neurol (Paris) 138:401–408, 1982.
91. Utti RJ, Tanner CM, Rajput AH, et al. Hypersexuality with antiparkinsonian therapy. Clin Neuropharmacol 12:375–383, 1989.
92. Pezzoli G, Martignoni E, Pacchetti C, et al. Pergolide compared with bromocriptine in Parkinson's disease: a multicenter, crossover, controlled study. Mov Disord 9:431–436, 1994.
93. Wolters EC, Tissingh G, Bergmans PLM, et al. Dopamine agonists in Parkinson's disease. Neurology 45(Suppl 3):S28–S34, 1995.
94. Korczyn AD, Brunt ER, Larsen JP, et al. A 3-year randomized trial of ropinirole and bromocriptine in early Parkinson's disease. Neurology 53:364–370, 1999.
95. McElvaney NG, Wilcox PG, Churg A, et al. Pleuropulmonary disease during bromocriptine treatment of Parkinson's disease. Arch Intern Med 148:2231–2236, 1988.
96. Nelson MV, Berchou RC, Kareti D, et al. Pharmacokinetic evaluation of erythromycin and caffeine administered with bromocriptine. Clin Pharmacol Ther 47:694–697, 1990.
97. Olanow CW, Fahn S, Muenter M, et al. A multicenter double-blind placebo-controlled trial of pergolide as an adjunct to Sinemet in Parkinson's disease. Mov Disord 9:40–47, 1994.
98. Pezzoli G, Canesti M, Pesenti A, et al. Pergolide mesylate in Parkinson's disease treatment. J Neural Transm 45(Suppl 1):203–212, 1995.
99. Olanow CW, Fahn S, Muenter M, et al. A multicenter double-blind placebo-controlled trial of pergolide as an adjunct to Sinemet in Parkinson's disease. Mov Disord 9:40–47, 1994.
100. Tanner CM, Chablani R, Goetz CG, et al. Pergolide mesylate: lack of cardiac toxicity in patients with cardiac disease. Neurology 35:918–921, 1985.
101. Wynalda MA, Wienkers LC. Assessment of potential interactions between dopamine receptor agonists and various human cytochrome P450 enzymes using a simple in vitro inhibition screen. Drug Metab Dispos 25:1211–1214, 1997.
102. Lieberman A, Ranhosky A, Korts D. Clinical evaluation of pramipexole in advanced Parkinson's disease: results of a double-blind, placebo-controlled, parallel-group study. Neurology 49:162–168, 1997.
103. Guttman M for the International Pramipexole–Bromocriptine Study Group. Double-blind comparison of pramipexole and bromocriptine treatment with placebo in advanced Parkinson's disease. Neurology 49:1060–1065, 1997.
104. Frucht SJ, Rogers J, Greene PE, et al. Falling asleep at the wheel: a serious side effect of pramipexole and ropinirole. Neurology 52(Suppl 2):A409, 1999.
105. Lieberman A, Olanow CW, Sethi K, et al. A multicenter trial of ropinirole as adjunct treatment for Parkinson's disease. Neurology 51:1057–1062, 1998.
106. Olanow CW, Mytilineou C, Tatton W. Current status of selegiline as a neuroprotective agent in Parkinson's disease. Mov Disord 13:55–58, 1998.
107. Rinne JO, Röyttä M, Paljärvi L, et al. Selegiline (deprenyl) treatment and death of nigral neurons in Parkinson's disease. Neurology 41:859–861, 1991.
108. Tetrud JW, Langston JW. The effect of deprenyl (selegiline) on the natural history of Parkinson's disease. Science 245:519–522, 1989.
109. Parkinson Study Group. Effects of tocopherol and deprenyl on the progression of disability in early Parkinson's disease. N Engl J Med 328:176–183, 1993.
110. Myllylä VV, Sotaniemi K, Mäki-Ikola O, et al. Role of selegiline in combination therapy of Parkinson's disease. Neurology 47(Suppl 3):S200–S209, 1996.
111. Ben-Shlomo Y, Churchyard A, Head J, et al. Investigation by Parkinson's Disease Research Group of the United Kingdom into excess mortality seen with combined levodopa and selegiline treatment in patients with early, mild Parkinson's disease: further results of randomised trial and confidential inquiry. Br J Med 316:1191–1196, 1998.
112. Heinonen EH, Myllylä V. Safety of selegiline (deprenyl) in the treatment of Parkinson's disease. Drug Saf 19:11–22, 1998.
113. Olanow CW, Myllylä VV, Sotaniemi KA, et al. Effect of selegiline on mortality in patients with Parkinson's disease. A meta-analysis. Neurology 51:825–830, 1998.
114. Bonifati V, Meco G. New, selective catechol-*O*-methyltransferase inhibitors as therapeutic agents in Parkinson's disease. Pharmacol Ther 81:1–36, 1999.
115. Holm KJ, Spencer CM. Entacapone: a review of its use in Parkinson's disease. Drugs 58:159–177, 1999.
116. Rinne UK, Larsen JP, Siden Å, et al. Entacapone enhances the response to levodopa in parkinsonian patiens with motor fluctuations. Neurology 51:1309–1314, 1998.
117. Comtan product monograph. Novartis Pharma, Switzerland, May 1999.
118. Illi A, Sundberg S, Ojala-Karlsson P, et al. The effect of entacapone on the disposition and haemodynamic effects of intravenous isoproterenol and epinephrine. Clin Pharmacol Ther 58:221–227, 1995.
119. Davis TL, Roznoski M, Burns RS. Effects of tolcapone in Parkinson's patients taking L-dihydroxyphenylalanine/carbidopa and selegiline. Mov Disord 10: 349–351, 1995.
120. Orama M, Tilus P, Taskinen J, et al. Iron (III)-chelating properties of the novel catechol-O-methyltransferase inhibitor in aqueous solution. J Pharm Sci 86:827–831, 1997.
121. Adler CH, Singer C, O'Brien C, et al. Randomized, placebo-controlled study of tolcapone in patients with fluctuating Parkinson disease treated with levodopa-carbidopa. Arch Neurol 55:1089–1095, 1998.
122. Kurth MC, Adler CH, St. Hilaire M, et al. Tolcapone improves motor function and reduces levodopa requirement in patiens with Parkinson's disease experiencing motor fluctuations: a multicenter, double-blind, randomized, placebo-controlled trial. Neurology 48:81–87, 1997.

123. Rajput AH, Martin W, Saint-Hilaire MH, et al. Tolcapone improves motor function in parkinsonian patients with the "wearing-off" phenomenon. Neurology 49:1066–1071, 1997.
124. Assal F, Spahr L, Hadengue A, et al. Tolcapone and fulminant hepatitis. Lancet 352:958, 1998.
125. Schenkman M, Donovan J, Tsubota J, et al. Management of individuals with Parkinson's disease: rationale and case studies. Phys Ther 69:944–955, 1989.
126. Kuroda K, Tatara K, Takatorige T, et al. Effect of physical exercise on mortality in patients with Parkinson's disease. Acta Neurol Scand 86:55–59, 1992.
127. Ramig LO, Countryman S, O'Brien C, et al. Intensive speech treatment for patients with Parkinson's disease: short- and long-term comparison of two techniques. Neurology 47:1496–1504, 1996.
128. Sato Y, Kikuyama M, Oizumi K. High prevalence of vitamin D deficiency and reduced bone mass in Parkinson's disease. Neurology 49:1273–1278, 1997.
129. Benabid AL, Pollack P, Gao D, et al. Chronic electrical stimulation of the ventralis intermedius nucleus of the thalamus as a treatment of movement disorders. J Neurosurg 84:203–214, 1996.
130. Lang AE, Lozano AM, Montgomery E, et al. Posteroventral medial pallidotomy in advanced Parkinson's disease. N Engl J Med 337:1036–1042, 1997.
131. Pawha R, Wikinson S, Smith D, et al. High-frequency stimulation of the globus pallidus for the treatment of Parkinson's disease. Neurology 49:249–253, 1997.
132. Limousin P, Krack P, Pollak P, et al. Electrical stimulation of the subthalamic nucleus in advanced Parkinson's disease. N Engl J Med 339:1105–1111, 1998.
133. Lindvall O. Neural transplantation: a hope for patients with Parkinson's disease. Neuroreport 8:iii–x, 1997.
134. Deacon T, Schumacher J, Dinsmore J, et al. Histological evidence of fetal pig neural cell survival after transplantation into a patient with Parkinson's disease. Nat Med 3:350–353, 1997.
135. Vatassery GT, Fahn S, Kuskowski MA, et al. Alpha tocopherol in CSF of subjects taking high-dose vitamin E in the DATATOP study. Neurology 50:1900–1902, 1998.
136. Shults CW, Beals FM, Fontaine D, et al. Absorption, tolerability, and effects of mitochondrial activity of oral coenzyme Q10 in parkinsonian patients. Neurology 50:793–795, 1998.
137. Rabey JM, Vered Y, Shabtai H, et al. Improvement of parkinsonian features correlate with high plasma levodopa values after broad bean (*Vicia faba*) consumption. J Neurol Neurosurg Psychiatry 55:725–727, 1992.
138. Kempster PA, Wahlqvist ML. Dietary factors in the management of Parkinson's disease. Nutr Rev 52:51–58, 1994.
139. Miller ER. Dihydroxyphenylalanine, a constituent of the velvet bean. J Biol Chem 44:481–486, 1920.
140. Damodaran M, Ramaswarmy R. Isolation of L-3,4-dihydroxyphenylalanine from the seeds of *Mucana pruriens*. Biochem J 31:2149–2152, 1937.
141. Finberg JP, Lamensdorf I, Commissiong JW, et al. Pharmacology and neuroprotective properties of rasagiline. J Neural Transm 48(Suppl):95–101, 1996.
142. Greenamyre JT, Eller RV, Zhang Z, et al. Antiparkinsonian effects of remacemide hydrochloride, a glutamate antagonist, in rodent and primate models of Parkinson disease. Ann Neurol 35:655–661, 1994.
143. Kordower JH, Palfi S, Chen EY, et al. Clinicopathological findings following intraventricular glial-derived neurotrophic factor treatment in a patient with Parkinson's disease. Ann Neurol 46:419–424, 1999.
144. Calabrese VP, Lloyd KA, Brancazio P, et al. N-0923, a novel soluble dopamine D2 agonist in the treatment of parkinsonism. Mov Disord 13:768–774, 1998.
145. West R. Parkinson's disease. London: Office of Health Economics, 1991.
146. Dodel RC, Singer M, Köhne-Volland R, et al. The economic impact of Parkinson's disease. Pharmacoeconomics 14:299–312, 1998.
147. Rubenstein LM, Chrischilles EA, Voelker MD. The impact of Parkinson's disease on health status, health expenditures, and productivity. Pharmacoeconomics 12:486–498, 1997.
148. LePen C, Wait S, Moutard-Martin F, et al. Cost of illness and disease severity in a cohort of French patients with Parkinson's disease. Pharmacoeconomics 16:59–69, 1999.
149. Schwab RS, England AC. Parkinson's disease. J Chron Dis 8:488–509, 1958.

CHAPTER 54

PAIN MANAGEMENT

Lori A. Reisner

Divinum est opus sedare dolorem.
(Divine is the effort to conquer pain.)
–Hippocrates

DEFINITION

Pain is defined as "an unpleasant sensory and emotional experience associated with actual or potential tissue damage, or described in terms of such damage."[1] Pain is always subjective, and there are no specific tests that can quantitatively or qualitatively measure pain. Tests such as a pain scales can be used by the clinician in an attempt to measure pain objectively, as can observations of grimacing, limping, and tachycardia, but these are crude methods at best and can only be used to support rather than identify a patient's report of pain.

Acute pain arises from an injury or trauma to or spasm or disease of the skin, muscles, somatic structures, or viscera of the body. It is perceived and communicated via the peripheral mechanisms identified as classic pain pathways, i.e., the A-δ and C fibers (see "Pathophysiology"). The intensity of acute pain is usually proportional to the degree of damage, and it serves a biologic purpose in causing an organism to withdraw from or avoid a noxious stimulus. It is characterized by limited duration and diagnosis is not difficult. Acute pain decreases in intensity as the damaged area heals and tissue repair takes place.[2]

Chronic pain persists beyond what would be expected from a precipitating injury or tissue insult and is separated into cancer (malignant) pain and nonmalignant (or benign) pain. The term *benign* is a misnomer, however, because persons with nonmalignant pain often suffer a great deal of physical and psychologic damage. Chronic pain is further characterized by its location: it may arise from visceral or myofascial (muscle and connective tissue) locations or from neurologic causes such as herpes zoster infection or diabetic neuropathy.

TREATMENT GOALS: PAIN

- Decrease subjective intensity and duration of the pain complaint.
- Decrease the potential for conversion of acute pain to chronic persistent pain syndromes.
- Decrease suffering and disability associated with pain.
- Decrease psychologic and socioeconomic sequelae associated with undertreatment of pain.
- Minimize adverse reactions or intolerance to pain management therapies.
- Optimize drug therapy to avoid drug-drug interactions.
- Improve the patient's quality of life and optimize ability to perform activities of daily living.

EPIDEMIOLOGY

Pain is the most common symptom that provokes people to seek medical attention. Despite this, the epidemiology of pain is not as well documented as is the incidence of many chronic diseases. Comparatively little research has been done on the rate of occurrence of acute pain, because it is a natural consequence of trauma or surgery and by definition is self-limiting. Studies evaluating the prevalence of pain in the community offer ranges of 7 to 64%, and the variation is due to sampling methods.[3] One survey estimated recurrent pain as affecting 37% of persons sampled, while 8% of these reported severe and persistent pain, and fewer than 3% had severe and persistent pain lasting longer than 6 days.[4] Backache is an example of a common pain complaint, with a point prevalence of 15 to 30%, a 1-month prevalence of 30 to 40%, and a lifetime prevalence of about 60 to 80%.[5] Pain from osteoarthritis is thought to affect approximately half of the U.S. population older than age 70,[6] and headache is also a relatively common pain phenomenon. Both of these syndromes may be under-reported due to the availability of over-the-counter analgesic medications. Although epidemiologic studies are scarce and variable in their conclusions, chronic pain has a significant number of societal implications, and estimates of its economic impact due to medical treatments, disability, and lost work days have been attempted. Such estimates yield a cost to the U.S. economy of approximately $100 billion annually. Back pain, arthritis and fibromyalgia are believed to be the greatest contributors to the economic burden of chronic pain. However, economic figures have the same statistical problems that plague prevalence estimates and therefore should be evaluated critically.

PATHOPHYSIOLOGY

During the 1960s Melzack and Wall proposed the "gate control" theory of pain, in which it was thought that a painful stimulus acted upon pain-sensitive receptors and caused an electrochemical nerve impulse to travel to the brain, which then initiated the physical and psychologic responses to pain. Although certain key details of the gate control theory have since been revised, it is still widely accepted to explain the way pain signals are collected, transmitted, and interpreted within the central nervous system (CNS), as it allows for the existence of specific pain receptors as well as for the role of the nervous system in pain mediation. Essentially, the gate control mechanism occurs as follows: afferent C fibers and A-δ nerve fibers transmit pain signals to an area known as the substantia gelatinosa, located in the dorsal horn of the spinal cord (Fig. 54.1). Cells within the dorsal horn collect and interpret these signals, and send them to transmission cells with terminals projecting to distant sites outside of the dorsal horn. Some of the C fibers and the A-δ fibers terminate in the dorsal root horn, whereas others form a complex known as the lateral spinothalamic tract. Pain impulses travel up along this tract to the thalamus and from there to the cerebral cortex of the brain.[7] Competing nerve impulses (i.e., stimulus from a different nerve branch) can block pain signals at the nervous system "gates," diminishing the intensity of the pain-relaying messages. Other controls that descend from the brain to inhibit firing of responsive neurons in the dorsal horn exist and therefore blunt or halt pain signals.[8]

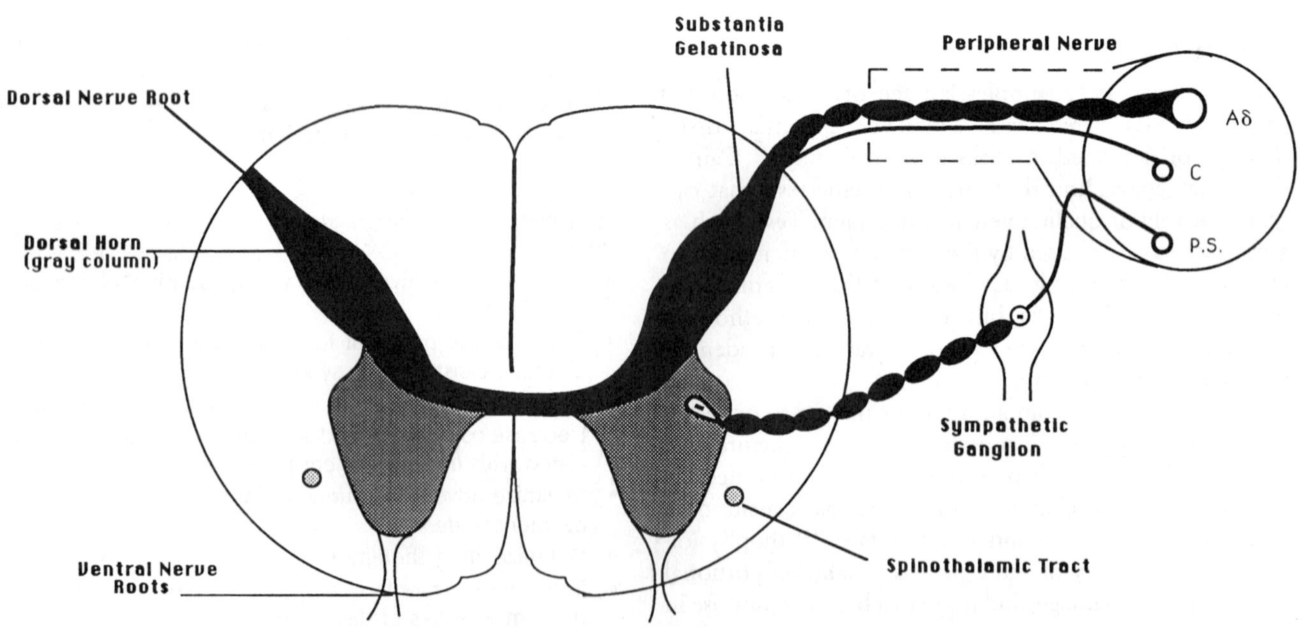

Figure 54.1. Transverse section of the spinal cord with peripheral nerve section illustrating two different types of axons: A-δ fibers and C fibers with cell bodies in the dorsal root and sympathetic fibers with cell bodies in the sympathetic ganglion. A-δ fibers and preganglionic sympathetic fibers are myelinated, whereas both C fibers and postganglionic sympathetic (*P.S.*) fibers are unmyelinated. The myelinated fibers carry impulses at a faster rate. Sympathetic fibers are thought to mediate some of the body's response to pain signals traveling along the peripheral nerve to the spinal cord and may also be involved in neurogenic inflammation. (*Source:* Adapted from Fields HL. Pain. New York: McGraw-Hill, 1987; and Clemente CD. Gray's anatomy, 30th ed. Philadelphia: Lea & Febiger, 1985).

Peripheral Pain Sensory System

When a painful (noxious) stimulus is applied to a sensitive area such as the skin, a series of events occur that are ultimately identified as a painful sensation. Sensitive tissues are those that contain pain receptors, also called nociceptors. Nociceptors are primary afferent nerves with terminals outside of the spinal cord that respond to noxious stimuli. Two phenomena occur via the nociceptors.[9] The first is receptor activation or transduction, in which chemical, thermal, or mechanical energy is translated to an electrochemical nerve impulse in the primary afferent nerve. The second event is transmission of the impulse as coded electrochemical information to structures in the CNS that interpret the signal as pain. Transmission occurs initially in the spinal cord, where neurons relay messages from the nociceptors to the brain. The messages elicit many responses, such as a withdrawal reflex or a subjective perceptual event (exclaiming, "Ouch!"). The majority of nociceptors conduct their signals in two velocity ranges. Larger diameter, myelinated A-δ, or rapid-firing fibers include muscle receptors, among other primary afferents, and constitute most of the known myelinated nociceptors. These A-δ fibers are most sensitive to stimulation by heat and by sharp, pointed instruments; hence they are known as mechanothermal or mechanical nociceptors. A third type of A-δ fiber may exist, which is sensitive to irritant chemicals. A-δ fibers have the property of sensitization, that is, repeated application of a noxious stimulus produces increased sensitivity of these receptors.[10]

The unmyelinated axons are known as C, or slow-firing fibers, and make up about 75% of the primary afferents in peripheral nerve. They have a smaller diameter than their fast conducting counterparts and are sensitive to noxious thermal, mechanical, and chemical stimuli. As with the A-δ fibers, C fibers also sensitize with repeated application of painful stimuli, although they may be less sensitive immediately after a stimulus.[9]

Evidence of the role of both A-δ and C fibers in pain perception is found in observations that brief, intense stimuli applied to a limb produce two distinct sensations: an early sharp, localized "pricking" pain of brief duration followed by a dull, diffuse, and prolonged unpleasant sensation.[11] By using compression to selectively block A-δ fibers, the initial sharp pain is abolished. Likewise, blockade of the C fibers by local anesthetics such as lidocaine leads to abolition of dull prolonged pain.[12,13]

How a pain sensation is perceived depends upon the size of the area stimulated, the frequency of stimulus application, and duration and location of the stimulus.[14] Although pain is a definite and singular experience based upon activity in specific receptors, any single nociceptor's activity is influenced by simultaneous activity at nearby nociceptors. Thus the pain experience is a composite of concurrent inputs at multiple receptors.[9]

When tissue injury occurs, the nociceptors undergo depolarization, leading to generation (transduction) of a nerve impulse. Depolarization is followed by pain and hypersensitivity lasting from minutes to days. Persistent pain can result from ongoing tissue damage or lingering chemical irritants released by cells during the initial insult. Other possibilities include a lasting change in the integrity of the receptor itself or even in the CNS.[9] Such changes are examples of neuroplasticity, which has garnered great interest in recent pain research. Neuroplasticity may explain the transformation of acute to more chronic pain states after some injuries or traumatic events.

Stimulus intensity that exceeds a nociceptor's pain threshold results in visible signs of tissue damage. More extensive injuries lead to local increased sensitivity to mild stimuli (hyperesthesia). Hyperesthesia causes injured tissues to develop tenderness, so that normally innocuous stimuli produce pain. This hyperalgesia is paralleled by changes in the activity of the nociceptors, including sensitization. After superficial injury to the skin, an intense vasodilation occurs at the injury site (Fig. 54.2). This is rapidly followed by edema (a wheal) and secondary vasodilation that produces reddening (flare) which spreads into adjacent, uninjured skin. The hypersensitive region progressively enlarges with time and depends mainly on the activity of the C fibers, because both the flare and remote sensitization are blocked by local anesthetics. Thus, activity in C fibers causes vasodilation and sensitizes adjacent C fibers. The long-lasting changes that occur after injurious stimuli may play a major role in determining both intensity and quality of clinically important pain.[9]

Central Pain Transmission

The cell bodies of the nociceptors are located in the dorsal root ganglion, and most of their axons terminate in the dorsal horn of the spinal cord. Some afferents project to the spinal cord through a ventral root as well, and both roots are thought to be important for pain transmission.

There may exist different pain-transmitting pathways, including the spinothalamic, spinoreticular, spinocervical, and dorsal column tracts. Animal models of pain transmission have failed to precisely define the human pain pathways because of species differences, but it is understood that the various nociceptive pathways of the human, primate, cat, and rat reach their destination in the thalamus of the brain.[15]

The lateral spinothalamic tract is thought to be the dominant spinal cord pathway for signaling pain in humans, as lesions of this tract result in the absence of pain below the lesion. In addition, stimulation of this tract induces pain in humans.[16] The termination zone of the spinothalamic tract and that of some dorsal column nuclei appear to overlap in the thalamus, and low-threshold stimulation of the dorsal column either by electrical or chemical means can interrupt the flow of pain signal transmission. This "gating" provides the basis for the use of transcutaneous electrical nerve stimulation (TENS) and dorsal column electrical stimulators in the treatment of chronic pain.[17]

CNS opioid receptors have been identified in high concentration in the dorsal horn. They have also been

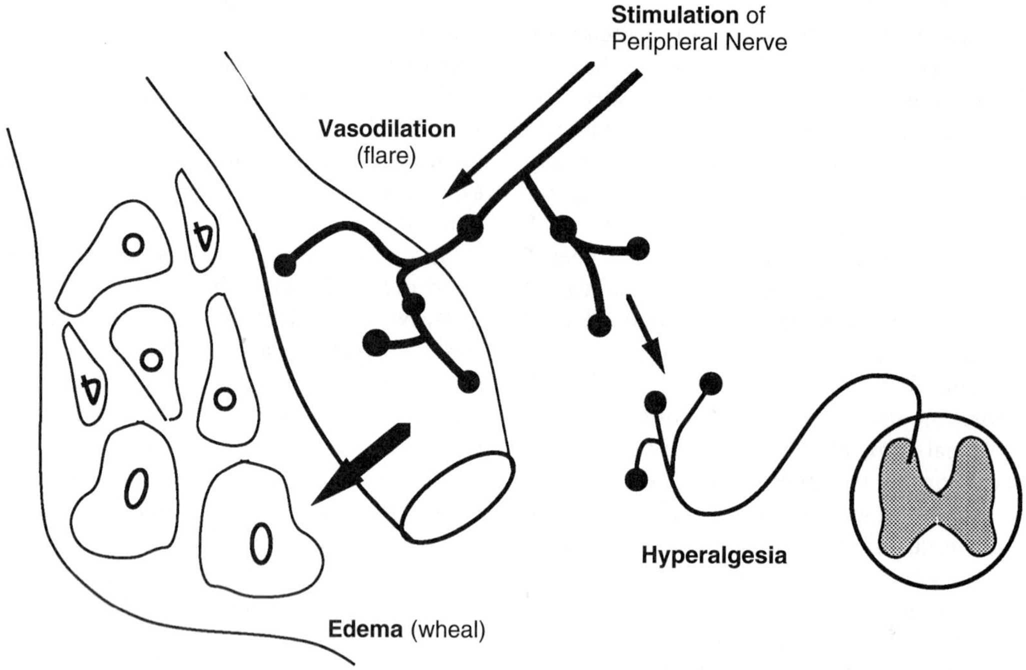

Figure 54.2. Events occurring after an insult to the peripheral nerve. Stimulation of the nerve ending produces a stimulus to vessel walls at the site of injury or trauma. Histamine, bradykinin, and other chemical mediators lead to vasodilation, then edema. Electrochemical signals across nociceptive synapses transmit the pain sensation to pathways in the spinal cord and ultimately to the brain, specifically the thalamus. (*Source:* From Fields HL. Pain. 2nd ed. New York: McGraw-Hill, 1997, with permission.)

Table 54.1 ▪ Chemicals That Are Active in Nociceptive Transduction

Substance	Source	Enzyme Mediator	Potency
Nociceptor activators			
Histamine	Released from mast cells	None known	+
Potassium	Released from damaged cells	None known	++
Bradykinin	Plasma proteins	Kallikrein	+++
Nociceptor sensitizers			
Prostaglandins	Arachidonic acid released by damaged cells	Cyclooxygenase	+/−
Leukotrienes	Arachidonic acid released by damaged cells	Lipooxygenase	+/−
Substance P	Primary afferent	None known	+/−

Source: Reference 9.

localized in the brainstem, medulla, pons, amygdala, and cerebrum, including the limbic system. In humans, administration of morphine into the brain's ventricles produces potent pain relief in patients with terminal cancer.[18] The mechanism of opioid analgesia is discussed later in this chapter.

Pain-Producing Substances

Several chemical compounds accumulate near nociceptors after tissue injury. They may arise from cell leakage, from synthesis by local substrates released via enzymes induced by damage, or from release by the nociceptor itself[9] (Table 54.1).

Among the substances released when tissue is damaged are histamine from mast cells and potassium, both of which excite nociceptors and produce pain upon injection into human skin. Adenosine triphosphate may also exhibit this effect. These compounds either act alone or in combination to sensitize nociceptors.[19]

One substance known to produce pain is bradykinin, a polypeptide produced by cleavage of plasma proteins after tissue injury. Actions of bradykinin include both low-concentration indirect production of hyperalgesia and high-concentration direct stimulation of nociceptors.[20]

Other compounds synthesized in the area of tissue damage are the byproducts of arachidonic acid metabolism, including prostaglandins and leukotrienes. These chemicals are present in high concentrations in inflammatory fluids and are potent mediators of inflammation. Prostaglandins are formed from arachidonic acid via the enzyme cyclooxygenase; of these, prostaglandin E_2 (PGE_2) is the most potent. Prostacyclin (PGI_2) is also a potent inducer of pain and hyperalgesia. PGE_2 is thought to produce hyperalgesia by direct action on the nociceptors, but prostaglandins may also sensitize nociceptors via coupling to a cyclic adenosine monophosphate system.[21] Other prostaglandins contribute to nociceptor activation by their interaction with additional chemical mediators. For example, prostaglandin E_1 produces pain only when injected with either bradykinin or histamine. Similarly, norepinephrine may produce peripheral hyperalgesia via enhanced production of prostacyclin. Aspirin and other nonsteroidal anti-inflammatory drugs (NSAIDs) have analgesic activity due to their inhibition of cyclooxygenase.[22] Bradykinin-induced hyperalgesia may occur by stimulation of specific PGE_2 production and can be blocked by the NSAIDs.[23]

Leukotrienes are produced from arachidonic acid by the enzyme lipoxygenase. Like prostaglandins, these agents produce hyperalgesia. However, leukotrienes are not notably blocked by cyclooxygenase inhibitors, but by depletion of polymorphonuclear leukocytes. Both prostaglandins and leukotrienes may exert their hyperalgesic effects by mediation of other pain-eliciting compounds.[24]

In contrast to substrates released in the region of injury, nociceptors themselves discharge pain-enhancing substances. Substance P, a polypeptide, is liberated from some C fibers and excites pain transmission pathways in the dorsal horn. In experimental arthritis, intramuscular gold sodium thiomalate, a neurotoxin, causes substance P depletion by decreasing the number of C fibers in adjacent peripheral nerves. Substance P is a potent vasodilator and leads to release of histamine from mast cells, explaining its role in the immunomodulation as well as the pain of arthritis. Histamine itself also activates nociceptors and produces vasodilation.[25]

Modulation and Interruption of Central Pain Processing

Opioid Receptors

Opioids, also called narcotics, administered into the spinal fluid reduce nearly all manifestations of clinical pain in humans. Subpopulations of opioid receptors are characterized by their sensitivity to selective opioid agonists.[26] Specific receptors in the CNS and peripheral tissues are responsible for modulating the effects of opioids and they are subdivided into four types: the mu (μ), delta (δ), kappa (κ), and epsilon (ϵ) receptors. Sigma (ς) receptors were once considered part of the class of opioid receptors, but are now classified as a distinct receptor type. The μ- and κ-receptors both produce analgesia, whereas the μ-receptor is responsible for the habituating and withdrawal effects of the opioids. Mu-Receptors, located primarily in pain-modulating areas of the CNS, induce central analgesia and respiratory depression.[27] Kappa-Receptors are responsible for analgesia at the levels of the spinal cord and the brain and are found in greatest concentration in the cerebral cortex and in the substantia gelatinosa of the dorsal horn. Because they are thought to produce analgesia without inducing opioid habituation, there is great interest in the development of κ-specific receptor agonists. Although experimental κ-agonists such as spiradoline have shown low dependence and abuse liability, they are not ideal analgesics because of their psychotomimetic (hallucinogenic) and dysphoric effects. New evidence suggests that sex differences may exist with regard to receptor sensitivity. It has been suggested experimentally that men may derive better analgesia from μ-receptor activation, whereas κ-agonists may produce a greater analgesic response in women.[28] Delta-Receptors are located in the limbic area of the brain and in the spinal cord and may play a role in the euphoria that selected opioids produce. Evidence also exists that implicates them in analgesia at the spinal cord level. Some researchers consider δ-receptors to be a subpopulation of the μ-receptors, or as mediators of μ-receptors. The function of ϵ-receptors has not yet been elucidated, whereas ς-receptors, although not true opioid receptors, are believed to produce the psychotomimetic and dysphoric effects of some opioid agonists and partial agonists such as butorphanol and pentazocine.[29]

Endogenous opioids known as endorphins, enkephalins, and dynorphins are found in varying concentrations in the CNS.[30] Their roles are not completely understood, but dynorphins and enkephalins appear to be responsible for intrinsic regulation of pain perception within the medulla, while endorphins and enkephalins probably serve this function within the substantia gelatinosa. Each of the endogenous opioids has greater preference for a particular receptor type: β-endorphin and enkephalins are potent at μ- and δ-receptors, while the κ-receptor is the target site for the dynorphins.[31]

The site of action of opioids depends upon the method of administration. Systemically injected or ingested opioids produce high brain opioid concentrations with relatively low spinal concentrations. The reverse occurs with spinal administration of the drug, i.e., intrathecal (into the subarachnoid space) or epidural injection. At the spinal level, opioids are thought to inhibit pain signals carried by the A-δ and C fibers at their synapses in the substantia gelatinosa.

Opioids exert at least part of their analgesic action by inhibiting substance P release in the central and peripheral nervous systems. They also interfere with the actions of prostaglandins at peripheral sites, particularly μ-receptor-specific opioids which inhibit PGE_2 hyperalgesia in a dose-dependent fashion.[32] It is speculated that opioids produce analgesia by causing adenosine release, because methylxanthines such as caffeine can antagonize the effects of morphine.[33,34]

Opioids may exert their inhibitory actions via hyperpolarization of neurons through altered conductance of potassium or calcium. However, evidence exists that they also cause in vitro excitatory actions at the nerve terminals.

This bimodal action is dose-dependent and helps explain the mechanisms of opioid tolerance and dependence.[35]

Tolerance and tachyphylaxis probably result from repeated exposure of receptors to high doses of opioid analgesics.[27] Continuously administered low-dose opioids can slow the development of tolerance. Patient-controlled analgesia (PCA), in which a controlled amount of drug is infused continuously, with bolus or "rescue" doses for breakthrough pain, produces less tolerance than intermittent high doses of an opioid. A second potential approach to delay tolerance is use of agents that are analgesic at a specific receptor; thus far, however, κ- or δ-receptor specific agents are investigational only. Owing to varying degrees of affinity for different receptors, narcotics do not produce complete cross-tolerance. In general, greater cross-tolerance exists among opioids with high affinity to the same receptor, but less cross-tolerance is seen between opioids acting at different receptors. Because most available opioids have some affinity for each receptor type, the extent of cross-tolerance is variable and unpredictable.[36] When changing a patient's medication from one opioid agonist to another, half the calculated equianalgesic dose may be used initially and then the dose titrated upward as required.[37]

In addition to their analgesic effects, opioids produce drowsiness, sedation, mood changes, and disorientation and memory impairment. Respiratory depression occurs by a direct action on the medullary respiratory and ventilation centers to reduce their responsiveness to carbon dioxide tension (P_{CO_2}), and by depression of brain centers responsible for the rate and rhythm of respirations. Studies comparing morphine to other opioids have shown that equianalgesic doses of these agents do not differ significantly in their ability to depress respiration. Nausea and vomiting occur by opioid stimulation of dopamine release in the chemoreceptor trigger zone of the medulla. Opioid-induced emesis is treated with antiemetics that exert dopamine-blocking action, e.g., droperidol or prochlorperazine. Dopaminergic actions are also involved in the euphoria experienced with opioids.[38] Miosis occurs through a stimulatory effect on the oculomotor nerve, and pinpoint pupils are pathognomonic for opioid toxicity. Central stimulation by opioids can also induce skeletal muscle rigidity or convulsions, which may not be suppressed by anticonvulsant agents.[39]

Opioid receptors have been localized outside of the nervous system. In the gastrointestinal tract, opioids increase smooth muscle tone in portions of the stomach, duodenum, ileum, and large intestine, leading to decreased motility and spasm. Morphine reduces secretion of hydrochloric acid and pancreatic enzymes and inhibits mucosal transfer of fluids and electrolytes across the intestinal epithelium. Digestion and propulsion of food are delayed, and absorption of oral drugs may be slowed. These properties have led to the development of the piperidine opioid congeners diphenoxylate and loperamide to treat hypersecretory diarrhea.

Therapeutic doses of morphine, codeine, or their analogs can lead to increased pressure in the common bile duct with elevations of serum lipase or amylase. Spasm and constriction of the sphincter of Oddi are probably responsible for this effect. Methadone, meperidine, fentanyl, or narcotic agonist-antagonist combinations do not raise biliary pressure to the same degree as other opioids and can be used to treat pain from biliary colic or pancreatitis.[40]

In the cardiovascular system, opioids produce orthostatic hypotension by peripheral arteriolar and venous dilation. This is either a direct effect or the result of opioid-stimulated histamine release. Vasodilation can be reversed partially by histamine-receptor (H_1) blocking agents and completely by opioid antagonists such as naloxone. Patients with coronary artery disease or evolving myocardial infarction may experience reduced myocardial oxygen consumption, but effects on the normal heart are insignificant. Opioid-induced respiratory depression can result in cerebrovascular dilation and increased intracranial pressure, effects that are hazardous in patients with cor pulmonale or in persons with cerebrovascular compromise who may experience further damage from increased cerebrospinal fluid (CSF) pressure. A second factor that discourages use of opioids is depression of cognitive function and masking of cerebral damage secondary to pathophysiologic events such as strokes.

In the smooth muscle of the bladder and ureter, opioids increase the tone of the ureter and the vesical sphincter, leading to urinary hesitancy or retention. Such bladder effects can be reduced by administration of prazosin or similar α_1-adrenergic antagonists. In the uterus, morphine reverses oxytocin-stimulated hyperactivity, leading to prolonged labor. Opiates also depress respiration in the infant, as all narcotics cross the placenta. Epidurally administered opioids are often used during parturition to reduce systemic effects. Preferred intravenous agents for use in obstetrics are the opioid agonist-antagonists butorphanol and nalbuphine, because of their "ceiling effect" on respiration, i.e., higher doses do not increase the degree of neonatal respiratory depression.[41]

Cutaneous blood vessels dilate with opioids, making the skin flushed and warm. Histamine release is partly responsible for these effects and for the pruritus and sweating that often follow narcotic administration. Urticaria is particularly problematic after spinal administration of opioids, but can be relieved with naloxone.[38]

Other Pain-Responsive Receptors

Table 54.2 lists the receptors that are involved in modulation of pain pathways. The adrenergic agonists norepinephrine and clonidine, an α_2 agonist, produce significant analgesia in humans when administered into the spinal fluid, highlighting the role of adrenergic modulation of pain. Although it can produce peripheral hyperalgesia by enhancing prostacyclin production, norepinephrine acts centrally on the dorsal horn via descend-

Table 54.2 ▪ Receptors That Are Involved in Modulation of Pain Pathways

Receptor	Subtypes	Agonist	Action	Location	Antagonist
Opioid	μ, δ, κ	Morphine	Analgesia	Brain and spinal cord	Naloxone
Adrenergic	α_1		Reduction in sympathetic nervous system output	Dorsal column	Prazosin
	α_2	Clonidine		Dorsal column	Yohimbine
	α and β	Norepinephrine		Dorsal column	Yohimbine
Serotonergic	Type I	Tricyclic antidepressants Sumatriptan		Spinothalamic tract	Cyproheptadine
Cholinergic		Acetylcholine	Antinociception	Dorsal horn	Atropine
GABAergic	A		Inhibits firing of nociceptors	Peripheral	
	B	Baclofen		Dorsal horn	

ing impulses from the brain to inhibit pain. The antinociceptive actions of both clonidine and norepinephrine can be reversed in a dose-dependent manner with adrenergic antagonists such as yohimbine.[42,43]

Serotonin receptors are found along the spinothalamic tract. Serotonin appears to reduce pain centrally by modulating descending impulses from the brain. This forms the basis for treatment of neuropathic pain syndromes with antidepressants that block presynaptic reuptake of serotonin.[44] However, noradrenergic systems are likely also involved in this phenomenon, because selective serotonin reuptake inhibitors (e.g., fluoxetine) do not appear to be as effective in treating neurogenic pain as the tricyclic antidepressants (TCAs), which block reuptake of both serotonin and norepinephrine.[45]

Cholinergic binding sites have been discovered in the dorsal horn. Application of the muscarinic agonist acetylcholine produces analgesia, which can be reversed by atropine. Such antinociceptive effects are not reduced by opioid antagonists.[46]

Gamma-aminobutyric acid (GABA) receptors (GABAergic receptors) are divided into two types: $GABA_A$ receptors are sensitive to muscimol and $GABA_B$ receptors to baclofen. Of known GABAergic compounds, only baclofen has been shown to produce analgesia, although nonspecific GABA agonists such as clonazepam may also be useful for some painful conditions.[47] $GABA_B$ agonists inhibit firing of the nociceptors, particularly the C fibers. Unlike opioids, baclofen does not inhibit substance P release in the spinal column. Baclofen is administered orally or intrathecally to treat central pain syndromes resulting from injury to the spinal cord, especially if consequent muscle spasms are involved.[48,49]

CLINICAL PRESENTATION AND DIAGNOSIS

Signs and Symptoms

Acute pain may be accompanied by signs of autonomic nervous system activity–tachycardia, hypertension, diaphoresis, mydriasis, and pallor–that mimic those of anxiety, which often coexists with acute pain. Chronic pain is rarely accompanied by autonomic symptoms. Persons who report chronic pain often fail to show objective evidence of an ongoing pathologic event upon physical or radiologic examination, although patients who have undergone multiple surgical procedures can develop fibrotic (scar) tissue which may be apparent in imaging studies.

Superficial pain is derived from the skin or underlying subcutaneous and mucous tissues. It is characterized by local throbbing, burning, or pricking. It may be associated with tenderness, allodynia (pain from a stimulus that normally does not provoke pain), or hyperalgesia. Visceral pain presents as diffuse, dull, aching pain that is poorly localized and is noticed at the onset or early stages of disease. It may be associated with nausea and other autonomic symptoms. Deep somatic pain is dull and aching in nature and can be localized, although there may be radiating components. Injury or disease of deep somatic structures produces the same response as does injury to the skin or viscera.[50]

Diagnosis and Evaluation

In addition to physical examination, a simple "PQRST" mnemonic can aid the practitioner in evaluating pain. P represents the palliative or precipitating factors associated with the pain, such as diet, stress, or physical exertion. Q represents the quality of the pain, i.e., whether it is sharp, dull, constant, aching, shooting, etc. R stands for "region" or "radiation" and is used to locate the pain. S is the subjective description by the patient of the pain's severity, and its effects on daily habits and lifestyle. For example, does pain cause waking or appetite loss? Finally, T represents the temporal, or time-related nature of the pain. It is useful to ask the patient whether the pain is worse in the evening or the morning, whether it is related to any habitual daily activity, or other questions designed to detect diurnal, weekly, or monthly patterns. Women may experience differences in pain at various points in their menstrual cycles, as estrogen induces hyperalgesia.[51]

In addition to knowing how, where, and when the pain began and what leads to its continuation, other pertinent facts about a patient's lifestyle are germane to accurate pain assessment. A pain questionnaire aids in the evaluation and treatment of the patient with chronic pain in the ambulatory care setting.[52]

Detailed information about the pain should be gathered to supplement the more general PQRST scale. It is necessary to determine what help the patient requests and whether his or her goals are consistent with the treatment offered. Patients with chronic pain cannot expect to be pain-free, as underlying degenerative pathophysiologic or neuroplastic changes in the CNS are often permanent. Changes in aspects of lifestyle such as exercise and exertion, employment, and emotional approaches to living with chronic pain may reduce its dominance in one's life, however.

Location of the pain is ascertained with anatomical drawings on which the patient marks areas where it is worse. For pain intensity, a visual analog scale (VAS) is a reproducible method to objectively measure and quantify pain. The VAS is a 10-cm line without subdivision marks. On the left extreme of the line "no pain" is written. On the rightmost extreme of the line, "worst pain imaginable" is written (Fig. 54.3) A subject is asked to draw a hash mark on the line at the point best corresponding to his or her pain. Successive VAS scales are compared over time to evaluate response to therapy.

An important portion of any questionnaire involves the past medication history as well as current pain medication and other treatments. From this portion of the evaluation, proper selection of analgesics, analgesic adjuncts, and patient compliance can be assessed. Patients who are compulsive in their consumption of pain medications, or those receiving subtherapeutic doses of appropriate medication can be identified.

Finally, a checklist of problems related to major organ systems should be included. Patients who complain of multiple somatic symptoms along with pain may be experiencing depression or another affective disorder. Correction of the underlying depression may lead to remission of pain and somatic complaints.

Assessing pain in pediatric patients is more difficult than with adults, as young children are often unable to adequately verbalize descriptors of pain intensity and quality. In children, a modified visual scale, the Faces Pain Scale (Fig. 54.4) can be used.[53]

Some researchers believe that human pain response can be divided into two categories: pain-sensitive (PS) or pain-tolerant (PT) subjects, who differ in aspects of pain behavior. PS subjects experience pain with qualitative differences, which depend more on psychologic variables than with PT subjects. These experiences can be measured by electroencephalography devices. Because of the role stress plays in response to pain and their higher observed stress level, PS subjects demonstrate a lower pain threshold.[54] Further research will determine additional criteria for classifying pain response and whether these two categories can be generalized to include a broad range of painful stimuli.

PSYCHOSOCIAL ASPECTS

Intensity of pain varies with each individual, with pain perception being determined by a person's psychologic background in addition to physiologic factors. Because pain is multifactorial in nature, it can be classified on emotional, social, spiritual and physical spheres (Figure 54.5). Emotional pain consists of isolation, depression and fear, factors that can reinforce each other. Social pain comprises strained or broken relationships as well as financial problems resulting from disability. Spiritual pain includes feelings of guilt, regret, or worthlessness, and physical pain encompasses disease and debilitation. Chronic pain can dull normal autonomic responses to stress, e.g., hypertension and sweating. Signs of depression most often manifest as sleep disturbance and irritability. Delayed sleep onset and frequent waking may occur, with patients reporting exhaustion from lack of sleep and from the inability to tolerate the stresses imposed by continuous pain. Chronic pain often leads to anxiety and depression, which in turn exacerbate the pain. This cycle can ultimately induce adoption of a "pain lifestyle" in which polypharmacy and polysurgery become over-represented

Figure 54.3. Visual analog scale. The subject is asked to draw a hash mark at a point on the line corresponding to his or her pain. The line is usually 100 mm in length, and a ruler is used to measure the placement of the mark, with a corresponding number value (i.e., millimeters) assigned to the measurement. Subsequent visual analog scale measurements can indicate improvement or worsening of pain severity.

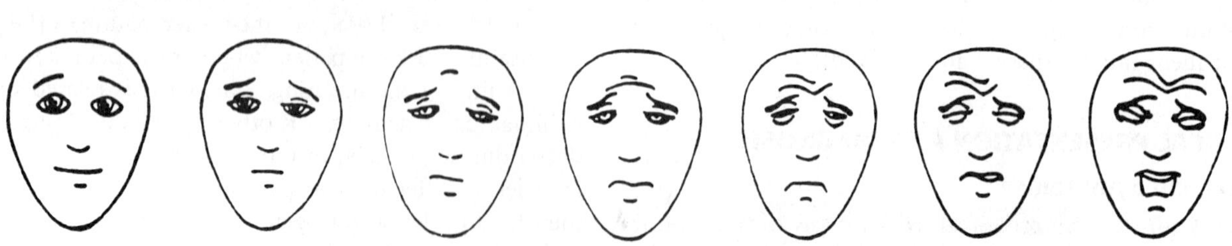

Figure 54.4. The Faces Pain Scale for assessment of pain in pediatric patients. Children are asked to point to the face that best describes the way they feel. (*Source*: From Bieri D, Reeve RA, Champion GD, et al. The faces pain scale for the self-assessment of the severity of pain experienced by children: development, initial validation, and preliminary investigation for ratio scale properties. Pain 41:139–150, 1990, with permission.)

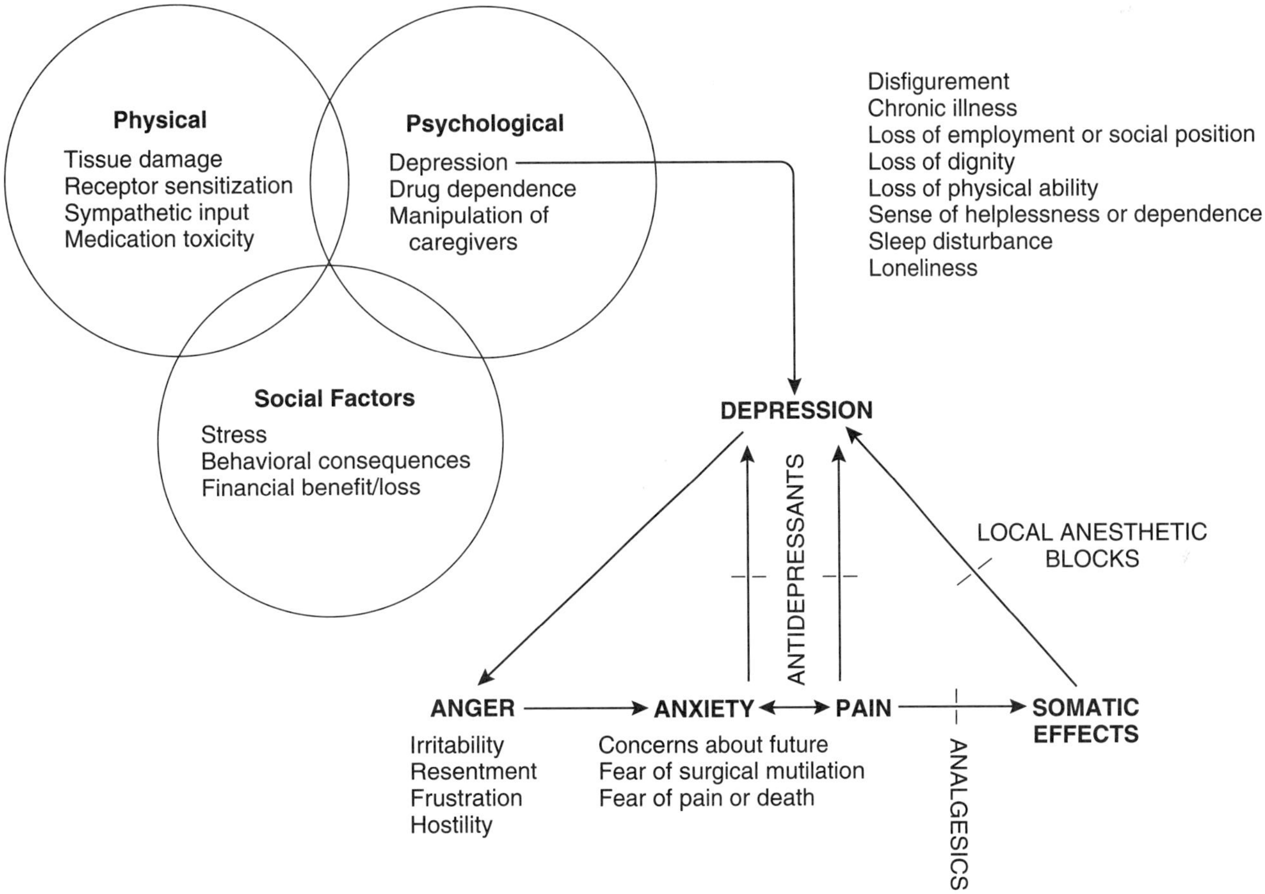

Figure 54.5. Determinants and modifiers of pain response and behavior. Portions of the pain, depression, and anger relationships can be interrupted by the pharmacologic interventions shown.

in a patient's medical history. If secondary gain such as increased attention from family members or financial reward becomes an issue, there is less incentive to recover from a pain syndrome. Pain may also mask underlying psychologic or physical abuse and can present itself as a symptom of emotional need.[55]

A distinction can usually be made between the "pain patient" and the patient in pain. The patient in pain exhibits findings seen more often with acute pain such as pacing, grimacing, or alterations in heart rate and blood pressure. These persons will probably have a full psychologic recovery from the painful episode once adequate pain control is achieved. Even in many such patients with chronic pain, reliance on medications is stable at a minimal level, and the patient demonstrates a high degree of self-dependence in overcoming a pain-related disability. Interaction with health care providers is not extensive, and the patient exhibits self-motivation in returning to a premorbid lifestyle.

The pain patient, on the other hand, is an individual who has suffered pain for a period of time long enough to produce notable changes in lifestyle, such as a discharge from employment and heavy reliance on family members or the health care system to offer relief. These patients may be tearful and anxious and may also exhibit symptoms of acute pain which abate when the patient is distracted. Patients with extreme pain behaviors visit and/or call their health care providers often and may manipulate their medication regimens without the advice of a health care provider. Patients who use their medications more often than directed may be required to "contract" with their providers, a system in which they are given a specific quantity of medicines for a predetermined period of time. Pain patients may have difficulty establishing realistic goals for their therapy and request a "cure" for their pain syndrome, although none is likely to exist.

THERAPEUTIC PLAN

Focus of Treatment

Treatment of acute pain focuses upon superficial or deep location of pain and its origin and is directed toward the underlying etiology. Effective management involves the use of agents that target short-term symptomatic relief, and the goal is to mollify pain impulses during the period of tissue healing. Opiates such as morphine, hydromorphone, or fentanyl are used acutely in postsurgical pain treatment, but other important agents are the NSAIDs, because they can limit pain, swelling, and erythema at the site of trauma, enhancing patient comfort and possibly shortening the duration of the pain syndrome.

Treatment of chronic pain is focused not only on symptoms, but also on the suffering and disability produced. Symptoms of depression–hopelessness, helplessness, weight loss, and sleep disturbance–may accompany chronic pain, and must be treated concomitantly.[2] Pain arising from cancer or other malignant disease exhibits characteristics of both acute and chronic pain. It may be constant or intermittent in nature. A definable etiology such as tumor recurrence is usually present. Similar to chronic nonmalignant pain, therapy is composed of psychologic and disability interventions along with analgesics in effective and tolerable doses.

In the treatment of chronic pain, doses of narcotic or nonopioid analgesics should be given on an around-the-clock basis, as there is no evidence that such pain will abate abruptly. Pain initially perceived as minor can increase to intolerable levels within a few hours. Once this phenomenon occurs, a larger dose of analgesic will be required to overcome pain-associated anxiety and bring the pain below the threshold of patient tolerance. For malignant pain, habituation is not a concern, as pain modulates the body's response to opioids and tolerance is slow to develop.

Approach to Therapy

Pain therapy is begun with non-narcotic analgesics where possible, followed by the step-wise addition of opioids and analgesic adjuncts (Figure 54.6).

An algorithm for medication selection in various pain syndromes is illustrated in Figure 54.7. Cancer pain arises at the primary site as a result of tumor expansion, nerve compression or infiltration by the tumor, malignant obstruction, or infection of malignant ulcers. It may also occur at distant metastatic sites. Furthermore, treatment for tumors such as radiation therapy may lead to mucositis and subsequent pain. Some of the more commonly encountered symptoms of cancer pain occur in the musculoskeletal tissue and in the nervous system. Although the majority of bony metastases do not produce pain, infiltration of bone is the most common cause of cancer pain. A constant, unpleasant, burning sensation often indicates compression of somatic nerves by tumor. This pain can also be accompanied by an intermittent lancinating pain.[56]

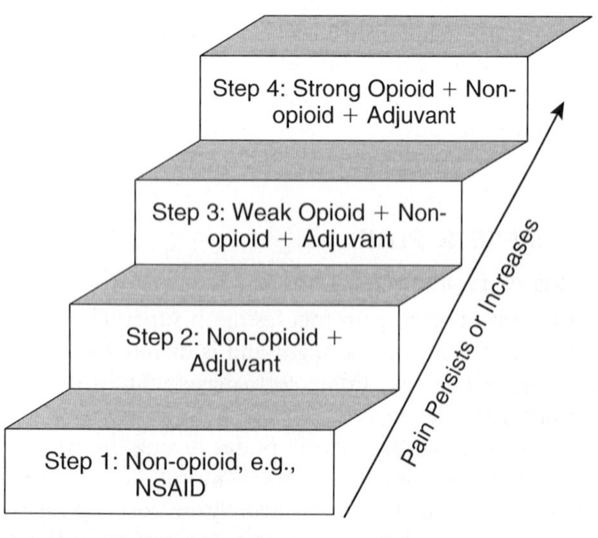

Figure 54.6. Analgesic stepladder for chronic pain management. (*Source:* Reference 62.)

For cancer pain, analgesics should be given at regular intervals and in adequate doses (Table 54.3). Medication should never be prescribed on an "as needed" (prn) basis, as the objective is to maintain maximum possible patient comfort at all times through maintenance of therapeutic levels. Oral medication is preferred, especially long-acting drugs, unless factors prohibit such administration. These include malignant bowel obstruction or severe nausea from emetogenic chemotherapeutic agents. Sublingual narcotic administration has also been studied, with the more lipophilic agents providing better analgesia than the less lipophilic morphine, presumably due to improved absorption. An alkaline pH also enhances the sublingual absorption of most opioids. Rectal administration of suppositories may suffice, although this method is less reliable owing to variable absorption of drugs from the rectal mucosa. Parenteral infusion is a dependable method of analgesic delivery, and can be used in the home setting as well as the hospital environment with portable, programmable infusion pumps. Many such pumps are now available with syringe drivers or medication cassettes that require infrequent refills. Medication can thus be prepared by a home health care agency and supplied to the patient on a regular basis.[57,58]

Treatment of mild to moderate cancer pain should begin with non-narcotic analgesics; when these drugs alone are ineffective, they are combined with intermediate potency opioid agonists such as codeine or its derivatives. NSAIDs are effective in relieving many symptoms of bone-associated cancer pain, as are corticosteroids. However, the extensive adverse effect profile of the corticosteroids should be considered. Bony metastases release PGE_2, which sensitizes peripheral nociceptors. NSAIDs and corticosteroids act by inhibiting the elaboration of PGE_2. In addition to relieving pain, these drugs reduce stiffness, swelling, and tenderness.[59] Other effective treatments for bony metastatic pain include bisphosphonates such as pamidronate, bone-seeking isotopes such as strontium-99, and radiation therapy.[60,61]

Finally, potent opioid agonists such as morphine or methadone should be used in the pain management regimen.[62] A common agent for treatment of advanced cancer pain is morphine, because of its potency and dosing flexibility. It is generally well tolerated by patients with a terminal illness. Alternatives include hydromorphone, methadone, and levorphanol. Diacetylmorphine (heroin) is not available in the United States, and does not possess

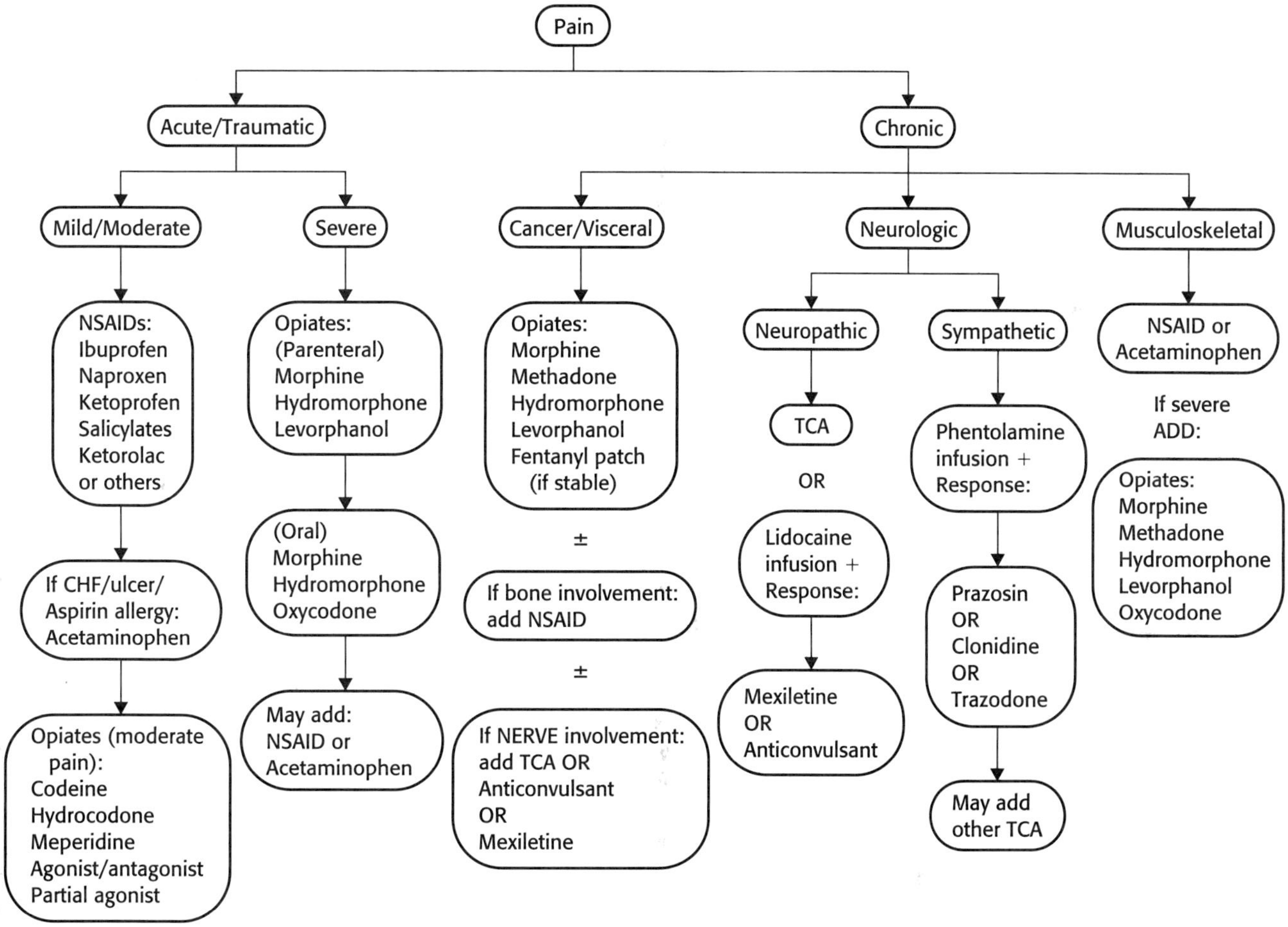

Figure 54.7. Algorithm for medication selection in the treatment of pain. *CHF,* congestive heart failure; *NSAIDs,* nonsteroidal anti-inflammatory drugs; *TCA,* tricyclic antidepressant.

Table 54.3 ▪ Principles of Analgesia for Cancer Pain

1. Choose appropriate analgesic(s).
2. Determine the dose by individual requirement.
3. Time doses to regular schedule (not prn).
4. Anticipate pain; do not "chase" it.
5. Minimize sedation or other untoward effects.
6. Utilize the oral route whenever feasible.
7. Treat nausea and constipation early.
8. Use adjuvant medications whenever necessary.
9. Tolerance and dependence are not problems.

any advantages for treating pain, because it is hepatically metabolized in vivo to morphine, its active analgesic component. Heroin has a slightly faster onset of action, but a shorter duration of analgesia than morphine. It is more soluble, allowing use via the intramuscular route; however, methadone is an appropriate alternative to morphine.[63]

Analgesic adjuvants such as tricyclic antidepressants may be added to the drug regimen for cancer pain, particularly if neural involvement occurs. The benefits of analgesia may be enhanced by the psychotropic effects of the drugs upon depression. Other adjuncts include antihistamines, phenothiazines, anticonvulsants, and amphetamines.[62,64]

Neuropathic pain can arise from either discrete or generalized sites of nerve injury or may be idiopathic in nature. Two common neuropathic pain syndromes are postherpetic neuralgia ("shingles") and peripheral neuropathies arising from various causes such as diabetes mellitus or acquired immune deficiency syndrome; less common are neuropathies induced by agents such as the antiretroviral drugs zidovudine (AZT), didanosine and zalcitabine or the vinca alkaloids. Neuropathic pains are most often sharp, lancinating, burning, hot, electrical, shocking, or searing. They can be intermittent or constant and may involve paresthesias manifested by tingling or numbness of a limb. Neuropathic pain is relatively unresponsive to opioids, but this may be a function of inadequate dosing and underlying patient variables rather than the pharmacology of the opioids.[65]

Postherpetic neuralgia (PHN) is a persistent pain syndrome resulting from infection with varicella-zoster virus (herpes zoster). The infection is initially manifested by fever, headache, lymphadenopathy, and malaise. It is followed by increasing pain or itching over a local area known as a dermatome, which is innervated by a specific nerve branch. Treatments for acute herpes zoster infection include systemic corticosteroids, antiviral agents, interferon, adenine arabinoside, and cimetidine. More invasive procedures, including somatic and sympathetic nerve blocks with local anesthetics and/or corticosteroids have proven efficacious.[66] Rarely, herpes zoster can leave an elderly or immunocompromised patient with permanent nerve damage resulting in persistent pain characterized as lancinating, burning, or itching. Common dermatomes affected by PHN include the cervical, cranial/trigeminal, thoracic, and lumbar regions. Herpes zoster is a reactivation of a latent virus originally acquired through acute varicella ("chickenpox") infection. The afferent nerve pathways undergo degeneration and interruption, causing deafferentation followed by nerve reorganization.[67] The cornerstone of treatment of PHN is the use of TCAs. In addition to their pain-remitting effects, TCAs can also treat the vegetative signs of depression such as sleep disturbance or anorexia.[68] Anticonvulsants are also used: carbamazepine and valproic acid have been given in doses of 600 to 1200/ or 500 to 1500 mg/day, respectively. Gabapentin, in doses ranging from 2400 to 4800 mg/day or more, has also been used.[69] The anticonvulsants reduce complaints of lancinating pain. They are gradually adjusted upward from low starting doses, particularly in older patients.[70] Topical local anesthetics also help reduce pain on the affected dermatome.[71] A cream containing capsaicin, a purified derivative of the red chili pepper, can be applied directly to the area of itching and inflammation. Studies comparing this agent to placebo show a favorable response; however, its use is accompanied by 1 or more days of intense burning, because it acts as a nerve ending counterirritant by stimulating and then desensitizing afferent C fibers.[72] Other topical agents such as aspirin and clonidine may also be useful.[73,74] Intravenous administration of lidocaine (5 mg/kg) has also been beneficial in PHN, as has its oral congener mexiletine. Sympatholytic agents such as systemically administered clonidine may prove beneficial as well. Baclofen is also useful for refractory PHN pain of the trigeminal distribution.[75,76]

Diabetic neuropathy is usually reported as distal sensorimotor loss and is a long-term complication of diabetes mellitus. Like PHN, diabetic neuropathies respond well to the TCAs or anticonvulsants. Intravenous lidocaine has been administered with encouraging results, and mexiletine may also prove useful for this condition. Aldose reductase inhibitors, which counteract hyperglycemia-induced metabolic changes at peripheral nerve sites, show promise for reversing early changes associated with functional nerve loss.[77,78]

Phantom limb pain has been described variously as burning, tingling, throbbing, shooting, and stabbing. Neurosurgical procedures are not permanently successful in reducing pain. Biofeedback has a role in increasing temperature and blood perfusion and in reducing discomfort at the amputation site. Anticonvulsants are helpful in reducing paroxysms of pain, as are TCAs.[79] Calcitonin may also play a role in the treatment of phantom limb pain.[80]

A syndrome known as sympathetically maintained pain, reflex sympathetic dystrophy (RSD), causalgia, complex regional pain syndrome, or post-traumatic spreading neuralgia, predominates in areas of the extremities innervated by thoracolumbar branches of the nervous system. It may coexist with other forms of neuropathic pain. Causalgia is marked by burning pain, allodynia, and hyperpathia and occurs in a hand or foot after nerve injury. RSD is continuous pain in a portion of an extremity after injury, and is associated with sympathetic hyperactivity.[1] Causes include multiple fractures or surgery to a localized area without involvement of a major nerve. Manifestations of RSD, in addition to burning pain stimulated by activity of the extremity, include vascular phenomena of coldness, numbness, or pain with changes in skin color. Trophic changes such as shiny, hairless skin or loss of bone mass may occur later. RSD may be lifelong. Treatment involves vasoactive agents such as prazosin as well as analgesic medications. Initial episodes usually respond to local corticosteroid injections; episodes refractory to corticosteroid treatment respond to regional sympathetic blockade with local anesthetics or instillation of a sympatholytic agent such as guanethidine. Topical application of clonidine or capsaicin to the affected area also shows promise.[81,82]

Myofascial pain arises from the muscles (myalgias), bones, joints (arthralgias), or connective tissue. Like a neuropathy, it can be idiopathic, iatrogenic, or injurious in origin. Muscle pain arising from exertion or strain is easily treated with NSAIDs, as is bone pain after dental or orthopedic procedures. Idiopathic musculoskeletal pain includes myositis and fasciitis, which are treated with local injections of anesthetics. Inflammatory diseases of muscle include polymyositis, dermatomyositis, and polymyalgia rheumatica. Flares may respond to low-dose intermittent steroids, e.g., prednisone 10 to 60 mg/day tapered over a 2 week period.[83] Fibromyalgia is a condition characterized by diffuse musculoskeletal aching with tender points and is often accompanied by poor sleep and symptoms of depression. Current theories about its pathogenesis involve CNS sensitization and hyperexcitability following persistent peripheral input from nociceptors in muscle.[84] Though standard treatments for fibromyalgia do not exist, TCAs have been used with variable results. Serotonin-selective reuptake inhibitors appear to be less useful.[85]

Examples of iatrogenic, or drug-induced musculoskeletal pains include those arising from the use of zidovudine (AZT), an agent used in treatment of acquired immune deficiency syndrome, and amphetamine or phencyclidine overdose leading to rhabdomyolysis and myoglobinuria.[86] In 1989, an illness associated with consumption of L-tryptophan for insomnia was reported which included myalgia, eosinophilia, weakness, fever, arthralgia, dyspnea, rash, extremity edema, and pneumonia. The acute phase was notable for severe myalgia followed by proximal muscular weakness. Sensory and motor neuropathy were late complications, and it mimicked rheumatic diseases such as systemic sclerosis, polymyalgia rheumatica or fibrositis. A contaminant of L-tryptophan was suspected. Patients did not respond adequately to nonsteroidal anti-inflammatory agents, hydroxychloroquine sulfate, or penicillamine. High-dose corticosteroids produced a modicum of success, though these drugs were often discontinued due to severe muscle cramping. Intramuscular injections of local anesthetic and steroid combinations (e.g. lidocaine/triamcinolone or bupivacaine/hydrocortisone) produced short-term reduction of myalgic pain. In extreme cases, the pain was opioid-responsive.[87]

Sickle cell disease results in acute infarctions and necrosis of organs secondary to vaso-occlusive episodes or "crises." Painful episodes are attributed to tissue injury from obstruction of blood flow by the deformed erythrocytes; however, a small population of persons affected with sickle cell disease report constant pain that persists between such episodes. Similarly, hemophilia may cause spontaneous bleeding into joints (hemarthroses) during flares of the disorder. Nonsteroidal anti-inflammatory agents and acetaminophen are the mainstay of therapy for mild to moderate pain from sickle cell disease. Opiate analgesics such as meperidine, morphine or hydromorphone are reserved for severe acute episodes, and are dosed according to duration of action and relative potency. Consideration of hepatic or renal dysfunction due to venoocclusion of these organs is required. When a crisis begins to abate, narcotic tapering is instituted, with pharmacologic emphasis placed on the nonopioid drugs.[88] Other treatments include vasodilators such as dihydropyridine calcium-channel blockers.[89]

TREATMENT

Pharmacotherapy

Opioid Analgesics

Opioids include natural and synthetic agents. They reduce moderate to severe pain and are unique in their ability to do this without producing loss of consciousness. All opioids have the potential for tolerance, habituation, and addiction. There are three classes of opioids: the phenanthrene derivatives, which include morphine, codeine, hydromorphone, levorphanol, oxymorphone, oxycodone, hydrocodone, dihydrocodeine, and opium; the phenylpiperidine derivatives, which include meperidine (pethidine), fentanyl, sufentanil, alfentanil, and remifentanil; and the diphenylheptane derivatives, which include methadone, levomethadyl, and propoxyphene (Table 54.4). Several agonist/antagonist combinations and partial opioid agonists are also available that are weaker than their pure agonist counterparts and are thus purported to be less habituating.

Potent Opiates

Morphine and other potent opioids are used to treat severe acute, chronic, or terminal malignant pain. They can be given orally, rectally, as continuous subcutaneous or intravenous infusions, intramuscularly, or directly into the CNS via epidural or intrathecal administration. The CNS route allows minute doses without sensory, motor, or sympathetic dysfunction. Newer methods of administration include transdermal, intranasal, and buccal routes.

Required doses of opioids vary according to a patient's prior exposure, severity of pain, hepatic or renal function, and route of administration. The oral:parenteral morphine ratio is approximately 5:1, owing to a large first-pass effect. Oral preparations include short-acting tablets and elixirs as well as extended-release tablets. Conversion from short-acting to longer duration formulations requires consideration of active drug and metabolite accumulation. One approach is to reduce the total daily dose by 25%, divide this amount by three or four, and then administer the resulting amount every 8 or 6 hours, respectively. When increasing the dose, an extra tablet is initially added at night to eliminate daytime somnolence, followed by the addition of subsequent tablets until effective analgesia is noted.

Morphine and hydromorphone exert major pharmacodynamic effects on μ-and κ-receptors. Large doses of morphine can reduce systemic vascular resistance, producing a transient fall in blood pressure. Hydromorphone has less potential to produce nausea, vomiting, constipation, sedation, or euphoria than morphine and can be used as a substitute when these adverse effects warrant a therapeutic alternative. Concentrated parenteral preparations are useful for opioid-tolerant patients with cancer in whom high narcotic requirements have posed a problem because of the volume of drug required for administration. Although high-dose infusions of morphine or hydromorphone are associated with muscle rigidity and spasm, all narcotics can cause muscular rigidity, presumably by accumulation in the sensitive regions of the brain.[90]

Oral morphine is variably absorbed, with a bioavailability of approximately 20 to 30%. It is also absorbed rectally. Peak analgesia occurs about 20 to 60 minutes after a dose, and lasts longer in opioid-naive individuals. The major metabolite of morphine is morphine-3-glucuronide, which is inactive. Minor active metabolites include morphine-6-glucuronide and normorphine, with a small amount biotransformed to codeine. Approximately 90% of morphine is excreted unchanged by the kidneys, with most of the remaining 10% excreted via biliary elimination.[91]

Parenteral hydromorphone and levorphanol are about five times as potent as morphine, with oral:parenteral ratios of 5:1 and 2:1, respectively. Both are available as tablets and as parenteral formulations for intravenous, intramuscular, or subcutaneous use. Hydromorphone can also be administered intraspinally or rectally.[92] Hydromorphone, a semisynthetic opioid, has a more rapid onset and shorter duration of action than morphine. Hydromor-

Table 54.4 ▪ Centrally Acting Analgesic Characteristics

	IM Dose (mg)[a]	Oral Eq.[a]	Routes	Onset (min)	Duration (hr)	$t_{1/2}$ (hr)	Notes
Opioid agonists for severe pain							
Phenanthrenes							
Morphine (various)	10	60[b]	PO, SC, IV, IM, PR	IV: 5, PO: 60	3–6	2–3	
Hydromorphone (Dilaudid)	1.5	7.5	PO, SC, IV, IM, PR	See morphine	3–6	2–4	
Levorphanol (Levo-Dromoran)	2	4	PO, SC, IM	30–90	4–6	4–12	Accumulates
Oxymorphone (Numorphan)	1.5	6	PO, SC, IV, IM	10–90	3–6	3–4	
Phenylpiperidines							
Fentanyl (Sublimaze)	0.1	N/A	IV, spinal, buccal, patch	10	1–2	3–4	
Sufentanil (Sufenta)	10 μg	N/A	IV, IM, SC, intraspinal	10	2–4		Duration dose-related?
Diphenylheptanes							
Methadone (Dolophine)	10	10	PO, SC, IM	SC, IM = 60	6–8	21–25	Accumulates
Opioids for mild to moderate pain							
Phenanthrenes							
Codeine (various)	120	200	PO, SC, IV, IM	See morphine	3–6		
Hydrocodone (various)	N/A	30	PO	30–60	3–4		
Oxycodone (various)	N/A	20	PO	30–60	4–6		
Dihydrocodeine (various)	N/A	30	PO	30–60	4–6		
Phenylpiperidines							
Meperidine (Demerol)	100	400	PO, SC, IV, IM	15–60	1–3	3–4	Can provoke seizures
Pentazocine (Talwin)	30–60	150	PO, SC, IV, IM	10	3–4	2–4	Dysphoric
Diphenylheptanes							
Propoxyphene (Darvon)	N/A	65–130	PO	60–90	4–6	6–12	Hepatotoxic
Partial agonists/antagonists							
Buprenorphine (Buprenex)	0.3	N/A	SC, IV, IM	15	4–6	2–3	Not naloxone reversible
Butorphanol (Stadol)	2	N/A	SC, IV, IM, intranasal	15–45	3–4		Dysphoric
Nalbuphine (Nubain)	10	N/A	SC, IV, IM	15	4–6	2–3	Respiratory ceiling
Dezocine (Dalgan)	10–15	N/A	SC, IV IM	15	3–6	4–6	
Opioid antagonists							
Naloxone (Narcan)	0.4–0.8	N/A	IV	10	2–3	1–1.5	
Naltrexone (Trexan)	N/A	50	PO	30–60	24–72	9–17	Duration dose-dependent

Eq., equivalents.

[a]Based on single doses.

[b]Multiple dose conversion = 30 mg oral morphine to 10 mg IM morphine.

phone is converted mainly to a glucuronide metabolite, with urinary excretion.[93] Levorphanol is a potent, semisynthetic opioid agonist for moderate to severe pain, including intractable pain in terminally ill patients. It produces more sedation and smooth muscle stimulation than does morphine in equianalgesic doses and has the same potential for habituation or addiction as naturally occurring opioids. Like methadone, it has a long half-life and a longer duration of action than morphine, meperidine, or hydromorphone. Levorphanol is well absorbed and like hydromorphone, undergoes hepatic metabolism to a glucuronide conjugate excreted by the kidneys. Peak analgesia occurs approximately 20 to 90 minutes after intravenous or subcutaneous injection, respectively. Duration of analgesia may be shorter in opioid-tolerant individuals.[94] It is often used as a substitute when large requirements lead to the need for frequent morphine dosing.

Meperidine is used for moderate traumatic or postoperative pain, and like morphine is given for pain from myocardial infarction or for sedation in patients with pulmonary edema. However, caution is advised in patients with atrial flutter or supraventricular tachycardia, because meperidine can increase systemic vascular resistance and heart rate. Parenteral meperidine reduces rigors associated with amphotericin-B administration, and is used as a premedication for patients receiving this antifungal agent. Some preparations contain metabisulfite preservatives, which produce anaphylaxis or hypersensitivity reactions, especially in asthmatic patients. Parenteral meperidine has one-tenth the potency of morphine. Because it is so poorly absorbed, oral doses are 25 to 30% as effective as parenteral doses. Meperidine is available as tablets, an oral solution, and an injectable preparation. It is metabolized to meperidinic acid, which is excreted by the kidneys as a glucuronide metabolite. Of greater importance is normeperidine, which can accumulate in patients with renal impairment to induce central nervous stimulation and tonic-clonic seizures. Approximately one-third of meperidine is converted to this *N*-demethyl metabolite, which has twice the convulsant activity and a fraction of the analgesic potency of meperidine and a half-life of 12 to 16 hours. Meperidine is shorter-acting than morphine and produces the same degree but a shorter duration of respiratory depression. It is often administered during labor, owing to its less extensive placental penetration, which reduces respiratory and CNS depression in the newborn infant.[95] Oral combinations with promethazine or acetaminophen and parenteral combinations with promethazine or atropine also exist, although there is little rationale for using such fixed-dose combinations because patient-specific dosing is preferred. Combination products are more expensive than individual constituents and can produce additive side effects without providing additional benefit.

Methadone is useful for treatment of terminal painful conditions, as its longer duration of action allows for less frequent dosing. Methadone has unique pharmacokinetic properties: oral absorption is nearly complete, and the half-life is 13 to 47 hours, with an average of 25 hours. Its analgesic duration increases from 4 to 6 hours for a single dose to 6 to 8 hours after repeated administration. However, CNS depression persists up to 36 hours after overdose, an important factor in reversing the effects with the opioid antagonist naloxone. The half-life of naloxone is about 60 to 90 minutes, so a patient requires naloxone by continuous infusion until the risk period has ended.[92]

Methadone is equivalent to morphine on a single-dose basis; however, with repeated administration accumulation in CNS and lipid tissues occurs. The total dose can be decreased 10% per day until a stable analgesic regimen is obtained. In detoxifying opioid-dependent patients with chronic pain, a "blind taper" can be used in which methadone oral solution is mixed with acetaminophen elixir or cherry syrup. The methadone dose is thus decreased gradually while maintaining the same total volume administered to the patient. Methadone is available as tablets, oral solution, and parenterally for intramuscular use.

Fentanyl is a synthetic opioid derivative of the 4-anilinophenyl-piperidine class and is approximately 100 times more potent than morphine. It is used clinically as an analgesic administered either intraspinally or intravenously, and as a preoperative anesthetic agent because of its potency, rapid onset, and short duration of action. Recently, a buccal preparation of fentanyl was made available for preoperative sedation when the parenteral route is undesirable. Fentanyl is a highly lipophilic agent, leading to rapid uptake and elimination, but orally the drug undergoes extensive first-pass metabolism. Parenteral administration has therefore been the typical route, but large initial doses required to sustain analgesia lead to a risk of overdose. Stable levels can be achieved through continuous intravenous administration when the infusion rate matches the plasma elimination rate. Transdermal administration has widened the clinical use of this agent because it also supplies the drug at a stable rate. Transdermal fentanyl is available in four strengths, with patches releasing 25, 50, 75, or 100 μg/hr. These patches are most applicable in the treatment of stable terminal cancer pain. Each patch lasts approximately 72 hours, but several days are required to reach steady-state concentrations. Supplemental doses of a short-acting analgesic should be used as needed during the initial 24 hours after application to relieve breakthrough pain, until the patch reaches maximal effect. Similarly, the drug is not rapidly eliminated if the patch must be removed due to untoward effects. Transdermal patches are noninvasive and offer an advantage in facilitating patient mobility. Conversion to an oral opioid can be done easily if such conversion becomes feasible. Sufentanil, another synthetic phenylpiperidine derivative which is approximately 10 times more potent than fentanyl and more lipophilic, may also be administered by this novel route in the future.[39] Unlike previous permeability studies with other drugs, percutaneous penetration of these weak bases depends on pH but not on anatomical location of the patch.[96]

Narcotic Analgesics for Mild to Moderate Pain

Codeine (methylmorphine) is a natural opioid derivative related to morphine. It is a less potent analgesic, as are its derivatives hydrocodone and dihydrocodeine. Oxycodone, a third codeine derivative, exhibits intermediate potency. Propoxyphene is also less potent than its structural analog methadone. All of these drugs are effective for mild to moderate pain. Codeine is biotransformed to morphine, and medications such as fluoxetine which diminish this conversion via inhibition of cytochrome P-450 (2D6) pathways reduce the opioid's efficacy. Practitioners should carefully evaluate response of a patient given concomitant codeine and fluoxetine who reports suboptimal analgesia and consider an alternative opiate.

Tramadol is a "bimodal" agent that possesses activity at both opioid and monoaminergic (serotonergic) pathways in the CNS. An active metabolite demonstrates weak opioid receptor affinity, particularly at the μ-receptors. Tramadol has been used in place of more potent opioid analgesics for treatment of moderate to moderately severe acute pain[97] and may also have use for treating chronic pain syndromes such as low back pain and neuropathic conditions. Advantages of tramadol include lower abuse liability and reduced potential for respiratory depression. Disadvantages include adverse effects such as dizziness, dry mouth, sedation, and constipation. At high doses it may induce seizures, but this effect is rare and most often associated with inadvertent or intentional overdose.[98] Typical doses for tramadol are 50 to 100 mg orally every 6 hours, to a maximum of 400 mg/day. Therapy for older patients should be started at lower doses, as they may be more sensitive to dizziness and other untoward effects. Accumulation can occur in older patients and in patients with renal or hepatic impairment; therefore, a recommended starting dose in such patients is 50 mg every 12 hours.[92]

Agonist/Antagonists

Agonists and antagonists have varying effects at different opioid receptors, and their affinity for any particular receptor is dose-related. A characteristic of agonist/antagonist combinations is a "ceiling" effect with regard to analgesia and respiratory depression.[27] This means that doses above the threshold or ceiling do not increase the degree of analgesia or the potential for respiratory failure. Butorphanol, a synthetic opioid agonist-antagonist, is available parenterally and as an intranasal spray. Pentazocine, a benzomorphan derivative, does not decrease propulsive activity of the intestines in therapeutic doses.[39] It is contraindicated in myocardial infarction because it may increase blood pressure and systemic vascular resistance, and has been combined with naloxone in oral preparations to discourage its abuse. Nalbuphine may have less psychotomimetic effects than either butorphanol or pentazocine.[99]

Partial Agonists

Buprenorphine and dezocine have less reported abuse liability than morphine but can precipitate withdrawal in narcotic-addicted patients. Dezocine is a nonscheduled opioid analgesic approved for parenteral administration, whereas buprenorphine has been administered parenterally and sublingually. Both agents are indicated for postoperative or post-traumatic acute pain. Like other opioids, they are metabolized by glucuronidation. In addition, dezocine appears to have a sulfate metabolite. Side effects of these agents include constipation or diarrhea, hyper- or hypotension, nausea, vomiting, anxiety, and sedation. Dezocine reportedly has high μ-receptor affinity, moderate δ- and α-affinity, and low ς-affinity. The threshold dose of dezocine for respiratory depression is 30 mg.[100]

Narcotic Antagonists

Naloxone is a short-acting, specific opioid receptor antagonist used to reverse the untoward side effects of narcotics, such as pruritus and respiratory depression. It is a competitive saturable inhibitor of the opioid receptor and is usually administered in doses of 0.1 to 0.2 mg as needed. Care should be taken not to administer an excessive amount, because large doses also reverse opioid analgesia and may precipitate abstinence symptoms.[92] Naltrexone is an oral opioid antagonist, and because of its extended duration of action, doses may be given as infrequently as twice weekly. It is most often used in treatment of opioid habitués.

Nonopioid Analgesics: NSAIDs and Acetaminophen

Aspirin and other NSAIDs are useful for the treatment of pain from injury, surgery, trauma, arthritis, or cancer. The NSAIDs are especially effective in the management of bone pain.[101] Acetaminophen, although not possessing anti-inflammatory properties, is the most commonly used nonprescription pain reliever. NSAIDs differ from opioid analgesics in several ways: an analgesic ceiling exists for these agents, they are antipyretics, and they do not induce tolerance or physical or psychologic dependence. In addition, their actions occur partly through inhibition of cyclooxygenase. Cyclooxygenase acts as a catalyst in the formation of prostaglandins, which sensitize nociceptors to the effects of pain-eliciting substances such as bradykinin. Because of predominant action in the peripheral nervous system, the NSAIDs and acetaminophen work synergistically with the centrally acting opioids. NSAIDs also have central effects which contribute to their analgesic activity, and have demonstrated a reduction in C-fiber activity in the thalamus.[102,103]

The NSAIDs are approximately equipotent, and no structure-activity relationship exists for these agents. Some of the NSAIDs have been studied more extensively with regard to the pharmacokinetics of synovial and joint penetration. Patient response varies considerably, so if a patient does not obtain therapeutic efficacy with one drug at a maximum dose, an alternative NSAID should be tried.[48]

Absorption of the NSAIDs occurs in the stomach and duodenum. The rate of absorption increases with slower gastric emptying or decreases when food or antacids are present in the stomach, although the total amount of drug absorbed is unchanged. The extent of absorption can be affected by the salt formulation. Currently, two products are available in the salt form: naproxen sodium and diclofenac potassium. Both agents are rapidly absorbed and thus are believed to reduce dyspepsia associated with gastric residence time. In addition, they possess a rapid onset of action, making them useful for treatment of migraine headache and other acute pain syndromes in the ambulatory setting. NSAIDs are eliminated primarily through biotransformation in the liver, with metabolites excreted by the kidney. Some may undergo enterohepatic recirculation.[104]

The propionic acid class of agents includes ibuprofen, naproxen, fenoprofen, flurbiprofen, ketoprofen, and oxaprozin. Ketoprofen is unique in that it also inhibits the lipoxygenase enzyme, which results in decreased leukotriene production. Whether this has clinical relevance is unknown. Ketoprofen is as effective in treating cancer pain as an acetaminophen and codeine combination in single dose comparisons.[105]

Ketorolac is a pyrrolacetic acid structurally related to zomepirac, tolmetin, and indomethacin and possesses potent analgesic with moderate anti-inflammatory activity. For postoperative pain, ketorolac is as effective as morphine, meperidine, or pentazocine, although the onset of action occurs slightly later. Like other NSAIDs, it inhibits platelet aggregation and can prolong bleeding time, induce gastric ulceration, or decrease renal function. The most common side effects are somnolence and other central effects such as nausea and dizziness. Available for intramuscular and intravenous administration, it is well absorbed with a time to maximum effect of approximately 45 minutes. The major metabolite is a glucuronide, and elimination is mostly renal, with approximately 90% excreted in the urine. The usual intramuscular dose is 30 to 60 mg as a single dose or 30 mg every 6 hours as needed. The maximum daily dose should not exceed 120 mg/day. Doses should be reduced by half for intravenous administration, older patients, those with decreased creatinine clearance, or patients who weigh less than 110 pounds (50 kg). The major role of ketorolac is acute postoperative analgesia when opioids are undesirable, because it is nonhabituating and does not appear to decrease respiratory drive.[106] It has also proven to be effective in managing pain due to biliary or renal colic.[107] There is little rationale to support the use of ketorolac in a patient tolerating oral medications or in one for whom intramuscular narcotics are appropriate, and conversion to an oral NSAID such as ibuprofen or naproxen is indicated. Oral ketorolac is also available for the treatment of acute pain, with a recommended maximum therapeutic duration of 5 days.

Anthranilic acids are also called fenamates, and although mefenamic acid is reported to have greater prostaglandin inhibition at the myometrium, it does not provide greater analgesia than other NSAIDs. Frequently reported adverse effects, such as diarrhea and CNS impairment have limited its use.

Piroxicam has an extended plasma half-life and is given once daily.[108] Other once-daily NSAIDs include oxaprozin, nabumetone (a nonacidic prodrug that is metabolized to an acetic acid), and sustained-release ketoprofen. However, these drugs are unsuitable for treatment of acute or chronic pain, as plasma levels drop below the analgesic threshold before the end of the dosing interval. They are useful for treatment of rheumatologic conditions, because anti-inflammatory action persists beyond the duration of analgesia, and once-daily dosing enhances patient compliance.

New "cyclooxygenase-2" selective NSAIDs, including celecoxib and rofecoxib are available. These drugs are promoted as NSAIDs that disrupt inflammatory prostaglandin synthesis via inhibition of a specific subtype of cyclooxygenase (COX-2), but not the production of prostaglandins required for "housekeeping" or homeostatic functions in the body such as gastrointestinal mucosal protection. Therefore, they are believed to have minimal propensity to cause gastrointestinal ulceration or interfere with platelet function and may represent a significant clinical advancement over traditional NSAIDs for pain associated with osteoarthritis flares or rheumatoid arthritis.[109]

Analgesic Adjuncts

Antidepressants

Human response to pain includes the "fight or flight" reaction mounted against physical or emotional stresses. Two simultaneous phenomena occur: corticoadrenal and sympathetic responses. The first results in production of endogenous glucocorticoid steroids to mobilize energy sources and inhibit prostaglandins. The sympathetic response induces an outpouring of norepinephrine, a catecholamine, and serotonin, an indoleamine, within neuronal synaptic junctions. TCAs, which inhibit the reuptake and storage of these neurogenic amines, have analgesic properties related to their ability to increase pain tolerance (Table 54.5).[110,111] This effect occurs in the absence of depression and the onset of analgesia is often more rapid than the antidepressant effect.[112] It has been proposed that TCAs also possess local anesthetic properties, which helps explain their more rapid antinociceptive effect.[113] In addition, vegetative symptoms associated with chronic pain such as sleep disturbance and depression are reduced by central serotonin enhancement. Serotonergic processes are an integral part of endogenous pain inhibitory mechanisms, so TCAs have proven useful as adjuncts in chronic pain management.[114] Patients should be

Table 54.5 ▪ Antidepressants That Are Used as Analgesic Adjuvants

			Receptor Blockade				
Medication	**Trade Name(s)**	**Daily Dose (mg)**	**Cholinergic (Dry Mouth, Constipation)**	**Histaminergic (Weight Gain, Sedation)**	**Adrenergic (Orthostatic Hypotension)** α_1	α_2	**Notes**
Tricyclic tertiary amines							
Amitriptyline	Elavil	25–150	Very high	Very high	High–very high	Moderate	
Doxepin	Sinequan	25–150	Moderate	Very high	High–very high	Moderate	+ Sleep effects
Imipramine	Tofranil	25–150	Moderate–high	Moderate	High	Insignificant	↑ Cardiac risks
Tricyclic secondary amines							
Desipramine	Norpramin	25–150	Slight	Slight	Moderate	None–slight	Often activating
Nortriptyline	Pamelor	25–100	Moderate	Moderate	Slight–moderate	Insignificant	
Heterocyclic[a]							
Nefazodone	Serzone	100–200	None–slight	None–slight	Moderate	Insignificant	+ Sleep effects
Trazodone	Desyrel	50–300	None–slight	Moderate	Very high	Moderate	+ Sleep effects
Venlafaxine	Effexor	75–225	Slight	None–slight	Unknown	Unknown	

[a]Pain relief with these agents is unproven or controversial.

instructed that 1 to 3 weeks or more are typically required before such antinociception occurs.[115]

The antidepressants include several classes of agents, which can be organized into three categories: the TCAs, the monoamine oxidase inhibitors (MAOIs), and newer heterocyclic compounds. Clinical effects include improvement in mood and sleep, anxiolysis, and a decreased perception of pain. The tricyclic agents are commonly used in the management of neurogenic pain conditions. The MAOIs have been used infrequently for treatment of painful conditions and are reserved for patients with conditions refractory to TCAs. Some clinicians prefer them for migraine headache management. However, MAOIs are more difficult to use because of food and drug interactions, and their benefits in treating pain have not been well-documented. Newer nontricyclic agents include serotonin selective reuptake inhibitors (SSRIs), venlafaxine, mirtazepine, and bupropion, an aminoketone, which like MAOIs is reserved for persons with refractory depression. None of these have been thoroughly studied for their effects on chronic pain.

The most commonly used antidepressant for painful conditions is amitriptyline in doses of 50 to 300 mg/day. Persons with chronic pain usually have poor sleep habits, making this drug useful in overcoming insomnia or nighttime waking. An agent with fewer anticholinergic effects such as nortriptyline may be substituted for amitriptyline. Desipramine, an active metabolite of imipramine, is also less sedating and has fewer anticholinergic effects than its parent compound.

Analogs of fluoxetine with shorter half-lives prevent their accumulation in slow metabolizers such as the elderly. Paroxetine is an SSRI modeled after the prototype agent zimeldine. It significantly decreases symptoms of painful diabetic neuropathy without withdrawal effects or changes in nerve function measurements. Paroxetine at 40 mg/day is also devoid of autonomic side effects, which frequently limit the use of TCAs.[116]

Neuroleptics

Of the neuroleptics, fluphenazine potentiates the effects of amitriptyline in patients with diabetic neuropathies and central (poststroke) pain. It also aids sleep onset and is typically given in small doses of 1 mg at bedtime, up to a maximum of 3 mg/day in divided doses or all at bedtime.[117] Methotrimeprazine is available as a treatment for mild to moderate pain. Its duration of action is equal to that of morphine, and it possesses analgesic equivalence to morphine or meperidine, without similar habituating/addictive potential or likelihood of respiratory depression. It has been underutilized in chronic pain management because of sedative and anticholinergic effects, which decrease patient tolerance. The use of other neuroleptics is controversial because of risk of extrapyramidal adverse effects, and phenothiazine analgesia is unproven with the exception of the above agents.[118]

Anticonvulsants

The mechanism of action of carbamazepine and valproate is suppression of spontaneous neuronal firing. Lancinating, burning pains are best treated by these drugs, which are typically long-acting, but can induce their own metabolism. Carbamazepine and valproate are prescribed for tic douloureux (trigeminal neuralgia), cranial nerve disorders, neural invasion by cancerous tumor, radiation fibrosis, surgical scarring, deafferentation, and other neuralgic syndromes. Doses of carbamazepine and valproate are the same as those used for treatment of convulsive disorders. Plasma levels should be monitored, because side effects may include bone marrow suppression, ataxia, diplopia, nausea, lymphadenopathy, and hepatic dysfunction. Periodic liver function tests, blood counts, and serum drug levels should be obtained for patients receiving chronic therapy.[119] Gabapentin has been used successfully in a broad range of pain states, including neuropathy, multiple sclerosis, and migraine headache.[120] The dose range varies by response and patient tolerance and may range from 1200 to 4800 mg or more per day. Because of its cost, it is not always a first-line consideration. Recently released agents such as lamotrigine and topiramate may offer some utility in the treatment of chronic neurogenic pain states in patients whose treatment with antidepressants or other anticonvulsants is unsuccessful.

Other Medications

Lidocaine is also given for neuropathic syndromes, and like all local anesthetics, enters the CNS after intravenous administration. Mexiletine has been used in lidocaine-responsive patients requiring a longer acting agent, because the effects of lidocaine are short-lived. Both agents reduce neuronal firing through stabilization of sodium-conducting channels in nerve cell membranes. When administered systemically, they diffuse into the peripheral nerves. Analgesic doses of mexiletine are the same as those needed for antiarrhythmic effects, i.e., approximately 10 mg/kg/day to produce plasma levels of 0.75 to 2.0 μg/ml. The use of tocainide, an oral lidocaine analog, is not advised owing to a higher incidence of serious adverse effects such as aplastic anemia. Side effects of both lidocaine and mexiletine include dizziness, lightheadedness, ataxia, nausea, and vomiting. High doses of these agents can lead to tremor and convulsions. The gastrointestinal effects of mexiletine can be reduced by taking the medication with food or antacids.[121]

Intrapleural administration of bupivacaine has been performed in patients with rib fractures and in patients with abdominal and thoracic pain after surgery. It exemplifies the many newer modalities available to the practitioner.[122]

Two centrally acting α_2 agonists, clonidine and guanethidine, are also used for pain management. They reduce sympathetic outflow from the CNS by presynaptic inhibition of norepinephrine release. Clonidine may interact with opioid receptors by inducing the release of the endogenous peptide dynorphin and has been used with some success in suppressing the symptoms of opioid withdrawal attributed to a hyperadrenergic state, including agitation, diarrhea, and sweating. This drug may also be used during surgery to reduce inhalation and opioid anesthetic requirements, as it potentiates morphine analgesia. Unlike morphine, however, clonidine is not reversed by naloxone, although its actions can be blocked by κ-specific antagonists. Clonidine may also prove useful in patients with spinal cord injury and neuropathic and sympathetically mediated pain syndromes. It is available as an oral tablet or as a patch, which provides constant blood levels of the drug for 5 to 7 days, thus increasing compliance. It is also available for intrathecal administration. Clonidine may produce orthostatic hypotension, so a candidate for therapy should first receive a baseline evaluation of blood pressure.[123,124] With a mechanism of action similar to that of clonidine, guanethidine is also used in patients with sympathetic pain. Guanethidine produces significant vasodilation, counteracting the vasoconstriction due to sympathetic hyperactivity, with resultant warming of an affected extremity and a reduction in pain. Guanethidine holds promise in the treatment of pain associated with rheumatoid arthritis, as patient response to regional guanethidine blockade has been favorable.[125]

Prazosin is an agent used for the relief of sympathetically mediated pains such as reflex sympathetic dystrophy. It has high specificity and affinity for the α_1-adrenergic receptor. Like clonidine, it produces vasodilation with significant orthostasis. Prazosin should be dosed initially at bedtime to reduce the risk of syncope owing to a precipitous drop in blood pressure. Doses can be gradually increased according to patient response and tolerance of side effects. Other agents used to relieve sympathetically mediated pain include intravenous phentolamine and oral phenoxybenzamine. However, these agents are nonselective for the α_1 receptor and also produce α_2 adrenergic effects. A test infusion of phentolamine can be used to predict guanethidine or prazosin response.[126]

Benzodiazepines such as diazepam are used for skeletal muscle relaxation and anxiolysis in the treatment of acute pain, whereas clonazepam has been used in the management of neuropathic and atypical facial pain. Side effects include sedation, cognitive impairment, and sometimes profound depression, all of which decrease activity of the patient with pain, and some researchers believe benzodiazepines may even exacerbate pain. In addition, they produce habituation and serious withdrawal reactions including seizures. Older adults are more susceptible to these effects. Therefore, TCAs are more rational choices for relieving the insomnia and anxiety that accompanies chronic pain.[127]

Antihistamines such as hydroxyzine and promethazine have been used to augment the sedative or anxiolytic effects and reduce the itching associated with opioids. They may have some analgesic activity, although this is controversial.

Dextroamphetamine 5 to 10 mg/day can be used in patients with cancer pain to overcome the sedation of opioids. It also relieves some vegetative effects of depression that often accompany a terminal diagnosis.[128] Methylphenidate 5 to 10 mg/day has also been used for these purposes.

Innovative Methods of Drug Delivery

PCA devices take advantage of intravenous bolus injections to produce rapid analgesia along with slower infusion to produce steady-state opioid concentrations for sustained pain control. Typical agents used include morphine, hydromorphone, and fentanyl. Because opioid kinetics vary greatly between patients, the rates of infusion must be tailored. Many computerized PCA devices are available, which rely on the same principle of a baseline infusion plus optional bolus and "rescue" doses. Boluses are self-administered and can be controlled by a predetermined lockout period. PCA is popular for acute postoperative pain relief, owing to its wide dosing flexibility. PCA is also useful for patients with chronic malignant pain, allowing patient independence. Many PCA devices are compact enough to be worn on a belt or carried in a pocket.[129]

Opiates administered into the spinal fluid are used for patients with malignant pain, acquired tolerance to systemic opioids, and sudden exacerbations of pain (e.g., surgical amputees) and for patients in whom neurolytic techniques have failed. Morphine was the first opioid used in this manner. Unfortunately, spinal opioids may produce a greater degree of urinary retention, biphasic respiratory depression, urticaria, pruritus, nausea, and vomiting than opioids administered parenterally or orally. Agents that undergo significant migration up the spinal column toward the brain are most often associated with these side effects, as drug polarity influences such cephalad migration. Morphine is more polar than meperidine and undergoes a greater degree of migration, leading to delayed respiratory depression. It reaches the respiratory center approximately 3 hours after administration. Because of this, efforts have been made to reduce the severe side effects through combinations of opioids and local anesthetics such as bupivacaine as well as combinations with clonidine. By taking advantage of analgesic synergism via different mechanisms of action, smaller doses of each drug may be administered. Several other analgesic opioid and nonopioid drugs have been studied since the introduction of intraspinal morphine. Spinally infused opioids have the potential for precipitating abstinence syndrome when withdrawn, but it is not clear if intraspinal opioids produce differences in the development of narcotic tolerance when compared to oral administration. Changes in opioid receptor number and/or drug-receptor affinity owing to chronic occupation of the opioid receptors is believed to account for the tolerance phenomenon, but removal of opioid for a period of 7 to 14 days can result in recovery of drug efficacy. Long-term spinal infusion of opioids does not cause permanent sensory or motor functional loss or histophysiologic changes, although it may lead to mild dorsal column degeneration. Disadvantages include risk of infection or puncture of the dura mater and catheter displacement.[130,131]

The entire volume of CSF turns over approximately every 5 hours. Any drug placed into the CSF is rapidly distributed and eliminated into systemic circulation. Bulk flow of CSF toward the head causes a lumbar injection of an opioid to reach the brainstem, leading to effects such as drowsiness and vomiting within 2 to 4 hours. A bolus causes concentrated drug to reach the brainstem, whereas a continuous infusion pump allows a steady state to be reached after five drug half-lives. Distribution across the dura from epidural administration occurs within 10 to 40 minutes. More lipid-soluble agents, such as methadone or fentanyl, distribute along the spinal cord in a very limited manner due to rapid crossing of the dura and consequent migration out of the CSF.[132]

The action of opioids in the spinal cord makes them ideal for powerful and relatively selective inhibition of pain information processing. Repeated bolus administration and continuous infusion of narcotics into the epidural space for terminal cancer pain both have utility and efficacy. An implantable pump allows continuous infusion of opioids or other agents into the spinal space without requiring an external port. Spinal morphine or fentanyl has the advantage of providing adequate pain relief in patients when other forms of these drugs are not tolerated. Cancer patients receiving highly emetogenic antineoplastic drugs, for example, may lose significant amounts of oral drug by vomiting. A third advantage of this method of drug delivery is facilitation of ambulation, allowing a patient to leave the hospital. Epidural administration of narcotics or other analgesic agents has also been useful in the postoperative and obstetrical settings for short-term pain relief (2 to 5 days) after surgical procedures.[133,134]

Intrathecal opioid administration has received widespread attention. In vitro and in vivo data suggest a strong inverse relationship between intrathecal potency and lipophilicity for morphine, normorphine, methadone, meperidine, fentanyl, and buprenorphine. This can be explained by the rapid migration of highly lipophilic agents out of the CSF. Generalizations about relative intravenous or intramuscular narcotic efficacy do not correlate to intrathecal or epidural potency, and specific δ-receptor agonists may prove useful for spinal infusion with minimal μ-receptor cross-tolerance. Similarly, clonidine via intrathecal administration can produce analgesia without morphine cross-tolerance.[135] Hormones as diverse as somatostatin and calcitonin have been administered intraspinally for analgesia. Intrathecal baclofen is used for treatment of intractable pain and spasm caused by spinal injury. Like clonidine, baclofen can potentiate morphine analgesia or produce analgesic effects alone. Intrathecal methadone 5, 10, and 20 mg has been used for patients after orthopedic surgery; however, because of its higher side effect profile and lower efficacy when compared with morphine, it is not widely used via the intraspinal routes.[136–137]

Morphine can be administered directly into the brain's cerebral ventricles for treatment of cancer pain. Morphine administered in this fashion is effective and naloxone-reversible. The disadvantages of this technique are risk of meningitis, nausea, vomiting, and pruritus.[138]

Special Considerations in Analgesic Pharmacotherapy

Narcotics exert anticholinergic effects that can be compounded by the concomitant use of anticholinergic agents such as diphenhydramine, hydroxyzine, tertiary TCAs, or atropine. The most serious consequence of combined use of these drugs is precipitation of an anticholinergic crisis, manifested by psychosis, tachycardia, cardiac conduction abnormalities with possible first, second, or third degree heart block, coma, and death by cardiorespiratory failure.

Alcohol is often used by patients with chronic pain to decrease suffering. They may drink themselves into a stupor to achieve pain relief through decreased consciousness. Combining analgesics and ethanol produces additive CNS depression with mood changes, depression of respiratory drive, and the danger of lethal overdose. Alcohol in combination with NSAIDs can lead to increased CNS side effects of the NSAIDs, such as disorientation and dizziness, as well as increased gastric irritation and ulceration.

As with alcohol and antihistamines, opiates can potentiate the effects of barbiturates, meprobamate, or benzodiazepines, including transient delirium and respiratory failure. Of particular concern is the interaction between fentanyl and midazolam, an ultra-short-acting benzodiazepine used in preoperative anesthetic "cocktails." This combination produced a few deaths from cardiorespiratory failure until lower doses of midazolam with more judicious perioperative monitoring of the patient were instituted.[139]

Patients with obstructive respiratory diseases such as asthma and emphysema or structural abnormalities like kyphoscoliosis are at greater risk of respiratory-drive depression with opioids. Half of the usual starting dose should be prescribed, titrating upward with careful attention to respiratory rate and oxygen saturation. Narcotic suppression of the cerebellar chemoreceptor response to carbon dioxide can have catastrophic consequences in patients whose response to carbon dioxide is already blunted from chronic respiratory disease.

Patients with hepatic failure are at potential risk for drug-induced sequelae when given opioids or NSAIDs, because of the inability of the liver to glucuronidate these agents for renal excretion. In addition, many NSAIDs have been shown to induce hepatocellular damage.[140] Acetaminophen is an agent commonly combined with centrally acting opioids. In patients with hepatic dysfunction secondary to alcoholic cirrhosis or hepatitis, chronic doses can precipitate hepatic failure. Cirrhosis also affects the disposition of opioids, as meperidine, pentazocine, and propoxyphene all exhibit increased bioavailability and decreased clearance.[141,142]

Most of the opioids are conjugated and demethylated in the liver to form nor-metabolites as well as glucuronide metabolites, both of which are excreted by the kidneys. In renal impairment, these metabolites accumulate and produce side effects that last longer than the biologic half-lives of the parent compounds. This is particularly true of morphine, dihydrocodeine, propoxyphene, and meperidine. Methadone appears safe to use in renal dysfunction when administered at 12- or 24-hour intervals.[143,144]

Nonpharmacologic Therapy

Surgery

Cordotomy is a method of severing the sympathetic chains that emanate from the spinal cord. Indications for such intervention are short life expectancy and specific unilateral or focal pain. In percutaneous cordotomy, a lesion is produced in the spinothalamic tract, most often at level of the first or second cervical vertebrae. This method has virtually replaced open cordotomy, in which a quadrant of the spinal cord is almost completely severed at the cervical or thoracic level. Pain relief by either technique is transient, rarely lasting more than 2 years. The advantage of cordotomy includes analgesia without significant loss of motor function or touch sensation.[145]

Neuroablative Blocks and Neurolysis

Chemical destruction of nerves (neurolysis) is used at spinal nerve roots and is a relatively simple and painless procedure, which can be done with minimal equipment. It is shorter-acting than cordotomy, but unlike this procedure, can be done in the elderly and those with poor general health. Agents used include absolute alcohol and phenol.

Central and Peripheral Nervous System Stimulators

Various types of central and peripheral nervous system stimulators are used for neurogenic, neuropathic, and ischemic pain syndromes. Dorsal column stimulators (DCS) operate on a principle similar to that of TENS, because both produce analgesia by inducing partial depolarization of neurons. DCS consists of an electrode placed in the epidural space and attached to a programmable continuous-pulse pacemaker implanted into a subcutaneous pocket in the abdomen. A sensory thalamic stimulator (STS) consists of an electrode placed into the thalamus of the brain. DCS and STS are used in cases of intractable neurogenic pain unresponsive to medications or other therapies. Peripheral nerve stimulators are implantable devices that are most successful in pain syndromes caused by injury to a peripheral nerve. Newer stimulators are taking the form of thermal, vibrotactile, and magnetic stimulators, although these methods have not evolved sufficiently for widespread use in pain management.[146]

Physical Therapy

Physical and rehabilitative therapies have been used to treat acute pain resulting from sports injuries as well as chronic pain. The goals of physical therapy exercises and training are increased mobility, strength, and function and a decrease in symptoms of pain or discomfort. Often, an additional goal is a return to employment.

ALTERNATIVE THERAPIES

Acupuncture

Acupuncture is a technique of specialized needle insertion along specific nerve tracts to alter electrochemical flow in nerve pathways and to reduce pain. It has been practiced in China and other Asian countries for centuries and has gained popularity in the United States during the past few decades. Systemic effects are extremely rare, making it an alternative for patients with medical contraindications to drug therapies such as TCAs. It can also be used in conjunction with pharmacologic therapies to improve response. With increasing acceptance of this practice, many health insurance companies now offer acupuncture as a covered benefit for their members. However, response is variable and unpredictable.[147]

Herbal Medications and Dietary Supplements

A variety of herbal medications have been used to treat pain arising from different regions of the body. Many of these herbal medicines contain volatile oils such as camphor and other compounds such as sesquiterpene lactones and flavonoids. Feverfew (*Tanacetum parthenium*) contains all of these chemical entities and has been used for headache and rheumatic diseases (e.g., arthritis). It is thought to impede platelet aggregation and prostaglandin synthesis as well as release of antihistamines and other inflammatory mediators. Comfrey (*Symphytum officinale*), marigold (*Calendula officinalis*), peppermint (*Mentha piperita*), and primrose (*Primula elatior*) are a few examples of other herbals used for relief of muscle and neurogenic pain syndromes. It is difficult to find controlled clinical trials of these agents in humans, although some have undergone animal trials to identify their active components and the pharmacology of these components. Opium poppy (*Papaver somniferum*) is used as a natural analgesic in other parts of the world and gave rise to modern-day opioids such as morphine.[148] Marijuana (*Cannabis sativa*) is currently under investigation for analgesic properties using methods to evaluate the effects of cannabinoid receptors in mammals, but definitive trials are not yet documented. The reader is referred to more extensive references for a complete review of herbal medications used for pain symptom relief.

Glucosamine and chondroitin sulfates are dietary supplements under investigation in clinical trials for relief of symptoms of osteoarthritis in weight-bearing joints such as the knee. Both are components of glycosaminoglycans. Glucosamine is also required for biosynthesis of glycoproteins, proteoglycans, and hyaluronate, all structural components of joint connective tissue. Limited studies comparing their use to NSAIDs are available, but more extensive trials are as yet unpublished.[149] The National Institutes of Health is currently investigating these agents.

Psychologic Interventions

Counseling, biofeedback, and stress management training as well as cognitive-behavioral techniques have been used to assist patients in reducing their symptoms of chronic pain. Self-hypnosis and self-relaxation are other methods used for this objective. In addition, such interventions can enhance coping skills and reduce disability and social isolation associated with long-term or lifelong painful conditions.[147]

FUTURE THERAPIES

N-Methyl-D-aspartate (NMDA) is an excitatory amino acid in the CNS, which has been discovered to produce hyperalgesia of CNS origin. Glutamate may play a similar role in activating pain systems. Research into NMDA receptor antagonists has offered an exciting hint at the future of pharmacologic agents for pain management. Such antagonists may prevent acute pain from transforming into chronic pain, and they may also attenuate opioid receptor tolerance when administered concomitantly.[150,151] Amantadine, an antiviral drug also used in the treatment of Parkinson's disease, may show efficacy in managing neuropathy.[152] Ketamine, a commercially available anesthetic, is also an NMDA antagonist. Unfortunately, it is only available parenterally and produces occasional adverse reactions, such as dysphoria and hallucination. Dextrorphan, the demethylated metabolite of dextromethorphan, although not yet commercially available, is another agent undergoing investigation. Studies with combinations of dextromethorphan and morphine are ongoing.[153,154]

Cholecystokinin antagonists have gained attention for their role in analgesia based on observations that morphine-induced analgesia can be antagonized in vivo by cholecystokinin. Administration of proglumide, an investigational agent, potentiates morphine-induced analgesia in both animals and humans. Calcium-channel blockers may also potentiate morphine analgesia by modulation of calcium availability to the cell. These drugs, like proglumide, are devoid of any analgesic activity when given alone. Tizanidine, an α_2-adrenergic agonist with muscle relaxant properties, also offers hope for treating pain associated with myofascial dysfunction. Although chemically similar to clonidine, it is less potent in lowering blood pressure.

Endogenous opioid peptides (endorphins, dynorphins, and enkephalins) have not proven superior to exogenous opioids in the management of pain. Their analgesic effects are short in duration, and they produce the same side effects as drugs like morphine. Other nonopioid endogenous peptides have been suggested for their roles in pain modulation. Specific δ-receptor agonists have risen to the forefront of opioid research. Recent evidence suggests they may produce analgesia without inducing habituation. Opioid peptides also show promise as therapeutic agents, because they differ from opioids in several ways. Peptide analogs of enkephalins undergo degradation by placental enzymes, inhibiting or preventing their transfer across placental membranes. This would make them ideal agents in obstetrics by placing the fetus at less risk. Moreover, no δ-receptors have yet been demonstrated in fetal brain tissue, increasing the safety margin of future δ-specific peptides. A third advantage the peptides may have over their opioid counterparts is degradation to constituent amino acids instead of active and possibly toxic metabolites. There is less potential for renal or hepatic damage with such peptides. Fourth, peptide δ-agonists, as mentioned, are likely to have less dependence and abuse liability than μ- or κ-agonists. Patients who have become tolerant to μ-agonists such as morphine may benefit from little or no analgesic cross-tolerance with the δ-opioid peptides.[155]

IMPROVING OUTCOMES

Patient Education

The pharmacist has a unique role in developing useful medicinal tools to ease suffering brought on by acute or chronic pain. Through rational drug prescribing habits and education of both patients and caregivers, effective regimens can be designed to increase pain control while decreasing untoward drug side effects. The pharmacist can assist in implementing such regimens to reduce drug dependence and overall drug use while increasing patient activity. A movement toward pharmacist involvement with pain management teams is gaining momentum, as government and third-party insurers seek ways to reduce the financial burden of chronic pain in terms of dollars spent and work days lost due to disability. Specific patient education points should include the expected benefit of the drug(s), appropriate dose and schedule for administration, potential adverse reactions and drug-drug or drug-disease interactions, and self-monitoring techniques for assessing response to therapy. Patients can be encouraged to maintain pain diaries documenting their pain levels and medication use throughout the day to assist health care providers in designing the most effective regimens. Pharmacist education regarding tapering or titration schedules is fundamental to optimal pain management, and written instructions should be provided along with verbal explanations of dosing schedules. The consequences of nonadherence should be emphasized.

Methods to Improve Patient Adherence to Drug Therapy

In acute pain management, time-contingent dosing should be used initially to prevent escalating pain, with downward tapering of the analgesic doses as pain severity allows. This can usually take place 1 to 2 days after the precipitating event. As above, written instruction will prevent confusion and ensure appropriate analgesic use. Chronic pain management should also involve time-contingent dosing regimens, and patients require education regarding expectations for nonopioid analgesics. In particular, patients should be instructed not to use medications with latency to onset (e.g., TCAs) on a "prn" basis. They should be informed of the delay in obtaining therapeutic efficacy to avoid premature discontinuation or escalation of medications. Patients should also have another caregiver, such as a family member, who understands the medication regimen and can assist in monitoring for beneficial as well as deleterious effects of drug therapy. This is particularly true of older adults, who may become forgetful if they are taking medications that produce cognitive impairment (opioids, antidepressants, neuroleptics, benzodiazepines, or muscle relaxants), which may lead to over- or under-compliance with the specified regimen. The pharmacist should offer himself or herself as a source of information and instruction and encourage patients to return if any problems with drug therapy develop.

Disease Management Strategies to Improve Patient Outcomes

Multidisciplinary methods of pain management are the focus of effective treatment for complex chronic pain syndromes. The goal of centers using these methods is not to "cure" pain, as this is often unachievable, but to ease the suffering of patients with chronic pain and to reduce their reliance on opioids and other analgesics. These centers strive to improve pain control and improve both psychologic and physical functioning and conditioning by involving specialists in the fields of anesthesia, neurology/neurosurgery, clinical pharmacy, physical therapy, physiatry, psychiatry, psychology, and nursing.

The pharmacist's role in researching nontraditional medicines for pain relief is also integral. In studies involving the use of lidocaine, antidepressants, and anticonvulsants for relief of chronic pain, pharmacists have served as co-investigators. Even in the areas of traditional pain management, they can monitor medication compliance and efficacy. In the multidisciplinary setting, the pharmacist can provide counseling and guidance to patients who are adjusting their intake of antidepressants, anticonvulsants, or other nonopioid medications as well as monitor rational opioid use. A lucid understanding of pharmacology and pharmacokinetics is invaluable in this setting, since opioid habituation, abstinence, and narcosis are highly undesirable and counterproductive. Many clinic settings allow the pharmacist to see patients on a regular basis, documenting pain relief scores, monitoring side effects, determining when and by how much medication doses should be increased or decreased, selecting alternatives to nontolerated medications, and obtaining pharmacokinetic data or other laboratory parameters. The pharmacist's knowledge of real or potential drug interactions can assist in designing regimens that will be most useful in treating patients with acute or chronic debilitating pain syndromes.

PHARMACOECONOMICS

NSAIDs account for about $500 million annually of U.S. drug expenditures, while opioids and adjunctive medication therapies are associated with lower expenditures. However, clinically significant gastrointestinal events (e.g., gastrointestinal hemorrhage) attributed to NSAIDs may cause as many as 15,000 or more deaths in the United

States each year and account for large expenditures related to hospitalization. Addition of misoprostol or antiulcer therapies can also increase the therapeutic costs of using NSAIDs. It is unknown at this time if the newer COX-2-specific NSAIDs will have an impact on these expenditures, because long-term postmarketing surveillance is required to make such a determination.

Lost work days, frequent contacts with medical personnel, disability insurance premiums, and disability payments owing to chronic pain also have a significant effect on the economy, although the global impact can only be estimated. Intangible factors, such as diminished quality of life, psychologic changes (e.g., depression), and social isolation produced by chronic pain cannot be adequately measured.

The pharmacist can play a key role in reducing such economic burdens by educating patients and caregivers about the potential for adverse drug reactions and drug-drug interactions and can assist in screening patients who are at high risk for such untoward events. In addition, the pharmacist can help design medication regimens that minimize pharmacologic overlap and optimize synergistic or additive effects of analgesics with different mechanisms of action.

KEY POINTS

- Pain continues to be an enigmatic entity, but advances in molecular biology research are providing clues to more specific mechanisms of pain generation and chronicity. With better targeted therapies, patients should be able to expect adequate pain relief with a minimum of adverse events.
- Therapy should be focused on decreasing the subjective intensity and duration of the pain complaint, decreasing the potential for conversion of acute pain to chronic persistent pain syndromes, decreasing suffering and disability associated with pain, decreasing psychologic and socioeconomic sequelae associated with undertreatment of pain, and minimizing the adverse reactions or intolerance to pain management therapies.
- Successful therapeutic strategies optimize drug therapy to avoid drug-drug interactions and improve the patient's overall quality of life and ability to perform activities of daily living.
- The pharmacist should use his or her unique understanding of drug mechanisms to develop effective treatment regimens in collaboration with other members of the patient's health care team.
- The pharmacist should provide relevant and specific knowledge about opioids, NSAIDs, and other adjunctive medications for pain relief and be willing to contrast the costs and benefits of any therapies under consideration.
- The pharmacist should also function as the primary provider of patient and physician education and should assist in monitoring the outcome of pharmacologic interventions.
- The pharmacist can provide comparative information on the pharmacoeconomics of various drug therapies, to minimize the cost burdens of pain to society and to the individual patient.

REFERENCES

1. Merskey H, ed. IASP Committee on Taxonomy, Classification of chronic pain: descriptions of chronic pain syndromes and definitions of pain terms. Pain Suppl 3:S28–S217, 1986.
2. American Pain Society. Principles of analgesic use in the treatment of acute pain and chronic cancer pain, 2nd ed. Clin Pharm 9:601–611, 1990.
3. Crombie IK. Epidemiology of persistent pain. In Jensen TS, Turner JA, Wiesenfeld-Hallin Z, eds. Proceedings of the 8th World Congress on Pain, progress in pain research and management. Seattle: IASP Press, 1997;8:53–55.
4. Von Korff M, Dworkin SF, Le Resche L. Graded chronic pain status: an epidemiologic evaluation. Pain 40:279–291, 1990.
5. Clinical Standards Advisory Group. Epidemiology review: the epidemiology and cost of back pain. Annex to the CSAG Report on Back Pain. London: HMSO, 1994:1–72.
6. Lawrence JS, Bremner JM, Bier F. Osteoarthrosis, prevalance in the population and relationship between symptoms and x-ray changes. Ann Rheum Dis 25:1–24, 1966.
7. Ganong WF. Review of medical physiology. Los Altos, CA: Lange Medical Publications, 1985:105.
8. Wall PD. Presynaptic control of impulses at the first central synapse in the cutaneous pathway. In: Physiology of spinal neurons. Progress in brain research. Amsterdam: Elsevier, 1964:12:92–118.
9. Fields HL. Pain. New York: McGraw-Hill Book Company, 1987:13–28.
10. Adriaensen H, Gybels J, Handwerker HO, et al. Response properties of thin myelinated A-δ fibers in human skin nerves. J Neurophysiol 49:111–122, 1983.
11. Price DD, Hu JW, Dubner R, et al. Peripheral suppression of first pain and central stimulation of second pain evoked by noxious heat pulses. Pain 3:57–68, 1977
12. Torebjork HE. Afferent C units responding to mechanical, thermal and chemical stimuli in human non-glabrous skin. Acta Physiol Scand 92:374–390, 1974.
13. Torebjork HE, Hallin RG. Perceptual changes accompanying controlled preferential blocking of A and C fibre responses in intact human skin nerves. Exp Brain Res 16:321–332, 1973
14. Wall PD, McMahon SB. Microneuronography and its relation to perceived sensation: a critical review. Pain 21:209–229, 1985.
15. Willis WD. The origin and destination of pathways involved in pain transmission. In: Wall PD, Melzack R, eds. Textbook of pain. 2nd ed. New York: Churchill Livingstone, 1989:112–123.
16. Vierck CJ, Luck MM. Loss and recovery of reactivity to noxious stimuli in monkeys with primary spinothalamic cordotomies, followed by secondary and tertiary lesions of other cord sectors. Brain 102:233–238, 1979.
17. Wall PD, Sweet WH. Temporary abolition of pain in man. Science 155:108–109, 1967.
18. Yaksh TL, Aimone LD, The central pharmacology of pain transmission. In: Wall PD, Melzack R, eds. Textbook of pain. 2nd ed. New York: Churchill Livingstone, 1989:190.
19. Perl ER, Sensitization of nociceptors and its relation to sensation. In: Bonica JJ, Albe-Fessard D, eds. Advances in pain research and therapy. New York: Raven Press, 1976;1:17–28.
20. Beck PW, Handwerker HO. Bradykinin and serotonin effects on various types of cutaneous nerve fibres. Pfluegers Arch 347:209–222, 1974.
21. Taiwo YO, Bjerknes LK, Goetzl EJ, et al. Mediation of primary afferent peripheral hyperalgesia by the cAMP second messenger system. Neuroscience 32:577–580, 1989.
22. Ferreira SH. Prostaglandins, aspirin-like drugs, and analgesia. Nature 240:200–203, 1972.
23. Taiwo YO, Levine JD. Characterization of the arachidonic acid metabolites mediating bradykinin and noradrenaline hyperalgesia. Brain Res 458:402–406, 1988.
24. Levine JD, Lau W, Kwiat G, et al. Leukotriene B_4 produces hyperalgesia that is dependent on polymorphonuclear leukocytes. Science 225:743–745, 1984.
25. Levine JD, Moskowitz MA, Basbaum AI. The effect of gold, an anti-rheumatic therapy, on substance P levels in rat peripheral nerve. Neurosci Lett 87:200–202, 1988.

26. Yaksh TL. Multiple opioid receptor systems in brain and spinal cord: parts 1 and 2. Eur J Anaesth 1:171–243, 1984.
27. DiFazio CA. Pharmacology of narcotic analgesics. Clin J Pain 5(Suppl 1):S5–S7, 1989.
28. Gear RW, Gordon NC, Heller PH, et al. Gender difference in analgesic response to the kappa-opioid pentazocine. Neurosci Lett 205:207–209, 1996.
29. Millan MJ. Kappa opioid receptors and analgesia. Trends Pharmacol Sci 11:70–76, 1990.
30. Carmody JJ. Opiate receptors: an introduction. Anaesth Intensive Care 15:27–37, 1987.
31. Goldstein A, James IF. Multiple opiate receptors: criteria for identification and classification. Trends Pharmacol Sci 5:503–505, 1984.
32. Ferreira SH, Nakamura M. II. Prostaglandin hyperalgesia: the peripheral analgesic activity of morphine, enkephalins, and opioid antagonists. Prostaglandins 18:191–200, 1979.
33. Levine JD, Taiwo YO. Involvement of the mu-opiate receptor in peripheral analgesia. Neurosci 32:571–575, 1989.
34. DeLander GE, Hopkins CJ. Spinal adenosine modulates descending antinociceptive pathways stimulated by morphine. J Pharmacol Exp Ther 239:88–93, 1986.
35. Duggan AW, North RA. Electrophysiology of opioids. Pharmacol Rev 35:219–282, 1983.
36. Martin WR. A homeostatic and redundancy theory of tolerance to and dependence on narcotic analgesics. Res Publ Assoc Res Nerv Ment Dis 46:206–225, 1968.
37. Foley KM. Treatment of cancer pain. N Engl J Med 313:84–95, 1985.
38. Bozarth MA, Wise RA. Anatomically distinct opiate receptor fields mediate reward and physical dependence. Science 224:516–517, 1984.
39. Jaffe JH, Martin WR, Opioid analgesics and antagonists. In: Gilman AG, Goodman LS, Rall TW, et al., eds. The pharmacological basis of therapeutics. 7th ed. New York: Macmillan, 1985:491–531.
40. Chisholm RJ, Davis FM, Billings JD, et al. Narcotics and spasm of the sphincter of Oddi. A retrospective study of operative cholangiograms. Anaesthesia 38:689–691, 1983.
41. Romagnoli A, Keats AS. Ceiling effect for respiratory depression by nalbuphine. Clin Pharmacol Ther 27:478–485, 1980.
42. Tamsen A, Gordh T. Epidural clonidine produces analgesia. Lancet 1:231–232, 1984.
43. Howe JR, Wang JY, Yaksh TL. Selective antagonism of the antinociceptive effect of intrathecally applied alpha-adrenergic agonists by intrathecal prazosin and intrathecal yohimbine. J Pharmacol Exp Ther 224:552–558, 1983.
44. Schmauss C, Hammond DL, Ochi JW, et al. Pharmacological antagonism of the antinociceptive effects of serotonin in the rat spinal cord. Eur J Pharmacol 90:349–357, 1983.
45. Max MB, Lynch SA, Muir J, et al. Effects of desipramine, amitriptyline, and fluoxetine on pain in diabetic neuropathy. N Engl J Med 326:1250–1256, 1992.
46. Post C, Gordh T Jr, Jansson I, et al. Interactions between spinal noradrenergic and cholinergic mechanism of anti-nociception [Abstract]. Pain Suppl 4:S408, 1987.
47. Bartusch SL, Sanders BJ, D'Alessio JG, et al. Clonazepam for the treatment of lancinating phantom limb pain. Clin J Pain 12:59–62, 1996.
48. Panerai AE, Sacerdote P, Bianchi M, et al. In: Lipton S, Tunks E, Zoppi M, eds. Advances in pain research and therapy. Vol 13. The pain clinic. New York: Raven Press, 1990:41–44.
49. Dickenson AH, Brewer CM, Hayes NA. Effects of topical baclofen on C-fibre evoked neuronal activity in the rat dorsal horn. Neuroscience 14:557–562, 1985.
50. Bonica JJ. The management of pain. 2nd ed. Philadelphia: Lea & Febiger, 1990:1.
51. Levine JD, Taiwo, YO. β-Estradiol induced catecholamine-sensitive hyperalgesia: a contribution to pain in Raynaud's phenomenon. Brain Res 487:143–147, 1989.
52. Fields HL. The Medical Center at the University of California, San Francisco, pain questionnaire, © 1988.
53. Bieri D, Reeve RA, Champion GD, et al. The Faces Pain Scale for the self-assessment of the severity of pain experienced by children: development, initial validation, and preliminary investigation for ratio scale properties. Pain 41:139–150, 1990.
54. Peters ML, Schmidt AJ. Human pain responsivity. Pain 41:117–121, 1990.
55. Sternbach RA. Clinical aspects of pain. In: Sternbach RA, ed. The psychology of pain. 2nd ed. New York: Raven Press, 1986:223–239.
56. Foley KM. Cancer pain syndromes. J Pain Symptom Manage 2:T3–T7, 1987.
57. Ferrer-Brechner T. Rational management of cancer pain. In Raj PP, ed. Practical management of pain. Chicago: Year Book, 1986:312–328.
58. Inturrisi CE. Newer methods of opioid drug delivery. In IASP refresher course on pain management: book of abstracts. Hamburg, Germany: International Association for the Study of Pain, 1987:27–39.
59. Bennett A. The role of biochemical mediators in peripheral nociception and bone pain. Cancer Surv 7:55–67, 1988.
60. Vinholes JJ, Purohit OP, Abbey ME, et al. Relationships between biochemical and symptomatic response in a double-blind randomised trial of pamidronate for metastatic bone disease. Ann Oncol 8:1243–1250, 1997.
61. Baziotis N, Yakoumakis E, Zissimopoulos A, et al. Strontium-89 chloride in the treatment of bone metastases from breast cancer. Oncology 55:377–381, 1998.
62. World Health Organization. Cancer pain relief. Geneva: World Health Organization, 1986.
63. Inturrisi CE, Max MB, Foley KM, et al: The pharmacokinetics of heroin in patients with chronic pain. N Engl J Med 210:1213–1217, 1984.
64. Halpern LM. Psychotropics and ataractics and related drugs. Adv Pain Res Ther 2:275–283, 1979
65. Portenoy RK, Foley KM, Inturrisi CE. The nature of opioid responsiveness and its implications for neuropathic pain: new hypotheses derived from studies of opioid infusions. Pain 43:273–286, 1990.
66. Satterthwaite JR. Acute herpes zoster: diagnosis and treatment. Pain Manage 3:17–28, 1990.
67. Portenoy RK, Duma C, Foley KM. Acute herpetic and postherpetic neuralgia: clinical review and current management. Ann Neurol 20:651–664, 1986.
68. Loeser JD. Postherpetic neuralgia: a review of pathophysiology and treatment. Presented at the Annual Meeting of the American Pain Society, Washington, DC, November 8, 1986.
69. Segal AZ, Rordorf G. Gabapentin as a novel treatment for postherpetic neuralgia. Neurology 46:1175–1176, 1996.
70. Davis EH. Clinical trials of Tegretol in trigeminal neuralgia. Headache 9:77–82, 1969.
71. Litman SJ, Vitkun SA, Poppers PJ. Use of EMLA cream in the treatment of post-herpetic neuralgia. J Clin Anesth 8:54–57, 1996.
72. Bernstein JE, Korman NJ, Bickers, DR, et al. Topical capsaicin treatment of chronic postherpetic neuralgia. J Am Acad Dermatol 21:265–270, 1989.
73. De Benedittis G, Lorenzetti A. Topical aspirin/diethyl ether mixture versus indomethacin and diclofenac/diethyl ether mixtures for acute herpetic neuralgia and postherpetic neuralgia: a double-blind crossover placebo-controlled study. Pain 65:45–51, 1996.
74. Abadir AR, Kraynack BJ, Mayda J 2nd, Gintautas J. Postherpetic neuralgia: response to topical clonidine. Proc West Pharmacol Soc 39:47–48, 1996.
75. Chabal C, Russell LC, Burchiel KJ. The effect of intravenous lidocaine, tocainide and mexiletine on spontaneously active fibers originating in rat sciatic neuromas. Pain 38:333–338, 1989.
76. Max MB, Schafer SC, Culnane M, et al. Association of pain relief with drug side effects in postherpetic neuralgia: a single-dose study of clonidine, codeine, ibuprofen, and placebo. Clin Pharmacol Ther 43:363–371, 1988.
77. Bach FW, Jensen TS, Kastrup J, et al. The effect of intravenous lidocaine on nociceptive processing in diabetic neuropathy. Pain 40:29–34, 1990.
78. Masson EA, Boulton AJ. Aldose reductase inhibitors in the treatment of diabetic neuropathy. A review of the rationale and clinical evidence. Drugs 39:190–202, 1990.
79. Sherman R, Sherman C, Gall N. A survey of current phantom-limb pain treatment in the United States. Pain 8:85–99, 1980.
80. Jaeger H, Meier C. Calcitonin in phantom limb pain: a double-blind study. Pain 48:21–27, 1992.
81. Fine PG. The pharmacologic management of sympathetically maintained pain. Hosp Formul 23:796–808, 1988.
82. Davis KD, Campbell JN, Raja SN, et al. Topical application of an α-2 agonist relieves hyperalgesia in sympathetically-maintained pain [Abstract]. Pain Suppl 5:S421, 1990.
83. Currie S. Inflammatory myopathies. Polymyositis and related disorders. In: Walton JN, ed. Disorders of voluntary muscle. 4th ed. Edinburgh: Churchill Livingstone, 1981:525–568.
84. Sorenson J, Graven-Nielsen T, Henriksson KG, et al. Hyperexcitability in fibromyalgia. J Rheumatol 25:152–155, 1998.
85. Wolfe F, Cathey MA, Hawley DJ. A double-blind placebo controlled trial of fluoxetine in fibramyalgia. Scand J Rheumatol 23:255–259, 1994.
86. Lane RJM, Mastaglia FL. Drug-induced myopathies in man. Lancet 2:562–566, 1978.
87. Criswell LA, Sack KE. Tryptophan-induced eosinophilia myalgia syndrome. West J Med 153:269–274, 1990.
88. Shapiro BS. The management of pain in sickle cell disease. Pediatr Clin North Am 36:1029–1055, 1989.
89. Ellory JC, Culliford SJ, Smith PA, et al. Specific inhibition of Ca-activated K channels in red cells by selected dihydropyridine derivatives. Br J Pharmacol 111:903–905, 1994.

90. Melzacka M, Neelhut T, Havemann U, et al. Pharmacokinetics of morphine in striatum and nucleus accumbens: relationship to pharmacological actions. Pharmacol Biochem Behav 23:295–301, 1985.
91. Hoskin PJ, Hanks GW, Aherne GW, et al. The bioavailability and pharmacokinetics of morphine after intravenous, oral and buccal administration in healthy volunteers. Br J Clin Pharmacol 27:499–505, 1989.
92. AHFS drug information. Bethesda, MD: American Society of Hospital Pharmacists, 1998:1671–1720.
93. Reidenberg MM, Goodman H, Erle H, et al. Hydromorphone levels and pain control in patients with severe chronic pain. Clin Pharmacol Ther 44:376–382, 1988.
94. Foley KM. Controversies in cancer pain: medical perspectives. Cancer 63:2257–2265, 1989.
95. Kaiko RF, Foley KM, Grabinsky PY, et al. Central nervous system excitatory effects of meperidine in cancer patients. Ann Neurol 13:180–185, 1983.
96. Roy SD, Flynn GL. Transdermal delivery of narcotic analgesics: pH, anatomical, and subject influences on cutaneous permeability of fentanyl and sufentanil. Pharm Res 7:842–847, 1990.
97. Stamer UM, Maier C, Grond S, et al. Tramadol in the management of post-operative pain: a double-blind, placebo- and active drug-controlled study. Eur Acad Anaesth 14:646–654, 1997.
98. Lee RC, McTavish D, Sorkin EM. Tramadol–a preliminary review of its pharmacodynamic and pharmacokinetic properties, and therapeutic potential in acute and chronic pain states. Drugs 46:313–340, 1993.
99. Meyers FJ, Meyers FH. Management of chronic pain. Am Fam Physician 36:139–146, 1987.
100. O'Brien JJ, Benfield P. Dezocine: a preliminary review of its pharmacokinetic properties, and therapeutic efficacy. Drugs 38:226–248, 1989.
101. Stambaugh JE. The use of nonsteroidal anti-inflammatory drugs in chronic bone pain. Orthop Rev 18:54–60, 1989.
102. McCormack K. The spinal actions of nonsteroidal anti-inflammatory drugs and the dissociation between their anti-inflammatory and analgesic effects. Drugs 47(Suppl 5):28–45, 1994.
103. Jurna I, Brune K. Central effect of the non-steroid anti-inflammatory agents, indomethacin, ibuprofen, and diclofenac, determined in C fibre-evoked activity in single neurones of the rat thalamus. Pain 41:71–80, 1990.
104. Harris RH, Vavra I. Ketoprofen. In: Rainsford KD, ed. Anti-inflammatory and anti-rheumatic drugs. Vol II. Newer anti-inflammatory drugs. Boca Raton, FL: CRC Press, 1985:151–170.
105. Sunshine A, Olson NZ. Analgesic efficacy of ketoprofen in postpartum, general surgery, and chronic cancer pain. J Clin Pharmacol 28:S47–S54, 1988.
106. Buckley MMT, Brogden RN. Ketorolac. A review of its pharmacodynamic and pharmacokinetic properties, and therapeutic potential. Drugs 39:86–109, 1990.
107. Gillis JC, Brogden RN. Ketorolac. A reappraisal of its pharmacodynamic and pharmacokinetic properties and therapeutic use in pain management. Drugs 53:139–188, 1997.
108. Wiseman EH. Pharmcologic studies with a new class of nonsteroidal anti-inflammatory agents–the oxicams–with special reference to piroxicam (Feldene). Am J Med 72:2–8, 1982.
109. Masferrer JL, Isakson PC, Seibert K. Cyclooxygenase-2 inhibitors: a new class of anti-inflammatory agents that spare the gastrointestinal tract. Gastroenterol Clin North Am 25:363–372, 1996.
110. Krishnan KR, France RD. Antidepressants in chronic pain syndromes. Am Fam Physician 4:233–237, 1989.
111. Lee R, Spencer PS. Antidepressants and pain: a review of the pharmacological data supporting the use of certain tricyclics in chronic pain. J Int Med Res 5(Suppl 1):146–156, 1977.
112. Feinmann C. Pain relief by antidepressants: possible modes of action. Pain 23:1–8, 1985.
113. Bryson HM, Wilde MI. Amitriptyline. A review of its pharmacological properties and therapeutic use in chronic pain states. Drugs Aging 8:459–476, 1996.
114. Messing RB, Lytle LD. Serotonin-containing neurons: their possible role in pain and analgesia. Pain 4:1–21, 1977.
115. Magi G. The use of antidepressants in the treatment of chronic pain. Drugs 42:730–748, 1991.
116. Sindrup SH, Gram LF, Brøsen K, et al. The selective serotonin reuptake inhibitor paroxetine is effective in the treatment of diabetic neuropathy syndromes. Pain 42:135–145, 1990.
117. Davis JL, Lewis SB, Gerich JE, et al. Peripheral diabetic neuropathy treated with amitriptyline and fluphenazine. JAMA 238:2291–2292, 1977.
118. McGee JL, Alexander MR. Phenothiazine analgesia: fact or fantasy. Am J Hosp Pharm 36:633–650, 1979.
119. Hatangdi VS, Boas RA, Edwards EG. Postherpetic neuralgia: management with antiepileptic and tricyclic drugs. Adv Pain Res Ther 1:583–587, 1976.
120. Rosenberg JM, Harrell C, Ristic H, et al. The effect of gabapentin on neuropathic pain. Clin J Pain 13:251–255, 1997.
121. Chabal C, Russell LC, Burchiel KJ. The effects of intravenous lidocaine, tocainide and mexiletine on spontaneously active fibers originating in rat sciatic neuromas. Pain 38:333–338, 1989.
122. Rocco A, Reiestad F, Gudman J, et al. Intrapleural administration of local anesthetics for pain relief in patients with multiple rib fractures. Reg Anaesth 12:10–14, 1987.
123. Crawley JN, Laverty R, Roth RH. Clonidine reversal of increased norepinephrine metabolite levels during morphine withdrawal. Eur J Pharmacol 57:247–250, 1979.
124. Maze M, Segal IS, Bloor BC. Clonidine and other $alpha_2$ adrenergic agonists: strategies for the rational use of these novel anesthetic agents. J Clin Anesth 1:146–157, 1988.
125. Levine JD, Fye K, Heller P, et al. Clinical response to regional intravenous guanethidine in patients with rheumatoid arthritis. J Rheumatol 13:1040–1043, 1986.
126. Exton JH. Mechanisms involved in α-adrenergic phenomena. Am J Physiol 248:E633–E647, 1985.
127. King SA, Strain JJ. Benzodiazepines and chronic pain. Pain 40:3–4, 1990.
128. Forrest WH, Brown BW, Brown CR, et al. Dextroamphetamine with morphine for the treatment of postoperative pain. N Engl J Med 296:712–715, 1977.
129. Barkas G, Duafala ME. Advances in cancer pain management: a review. Patient-controlled analgesia. J Pain Symptom Manage 3:150–160, 1988.
130. Magora F. The spinal route. In: Lipton S, Tunks E, Zoppi M, eds. Advances in pain research and therapy. Vol. 13. The pain clinic. New York: Raven Press, 1990:309–314.
131. Max MB, Inturrisi CE, Kaiko RF et al. Epidural and intrathecal opiates: cerebrospinal fluid and plasma profiles in patients with chronic cancer pain. Clin Pharmacol Ther 38:631–641, 1985.
132. Gourlay GK, Cherry DA, Plummer JL, et al. The influence of drug polarity on the absorption of opioid drugs into CSF and subsequent cephalad migration following lumbar epidural administration: application to morphine and pethidine. Pain 31:297–305, 1987.
133. Rawal N, Arner S, Gustaffson LL, et al. Present state of extradural and intradural opioid analgesia in Sweden. A nationwide follow-up survey. Br J Anaesth 59:791–799, 1987.
134. Onofrio BM, Yaksh TL. Long-term pain relief produced by intrathecal morphine infusion in 53 patients. J Neurosurg 72:200–209, 1990.
135. Coombs DW, Saunders RL, Fratkin JD, et al. Continuous intrathecal hydromorphone and clonidine for intractable cancer pain. J Neurosurg 64:890–894, 1986.
136. Dickinson AH, Sullivan AF, McQuay HJ. Intrathecal etorphine, fentanyl and buprenorphine on spinal nociceptive neurones in the rat. Pain 42:227–234, 1990.
137. Jacobson L, Chabal C, Brody MC, et al. Intrathecal methadone: a dose-response study and comparison with intrathecal morphine 0.5 mg. Pain 43:141–148, 1990.
138. Yaksh TL, Stevens CW. Properties of the modulation of spinal nociceptive transmission by receptor-selective agents. In: Dubner R, Gebhart GF, Bond MR, eds. Proceedings of the Fifth World Congress on Pain. Amsterdam: Elsevier, 1988:417–435.
139. Forster A, Morel D, Bachmann M, et al. Respiratory depressant effects of different doses of midazolam and lack of reversal with naloxone–a double-blind randomized study. Anesth Analg 62:920–924, 1983.
140. Masubuchi Y, Saito H, Horie T. Structural requirements for the hepatotoxicity of nonsteroidal anti-inflammatory drugs in isolated rat hepatocytes. J Pharmacol Exp Ther 287:208–213, 1998.
141. Seeff LB, Cuccherini BA, Zimmerman HJ, et al. Acetaminophen hepatotoxicity in alcoholics. Ann Intern Med 104:399–404, 1986.
142. Neal EA, Meffin PJ, Gregory PB, et al. Enhanced bioavailability and decreased clearance of analgesics in patients with cirrhosis. Gastroenterology 77:96–102, 1979.
143. Wolfert AI, Sica DA. Narcotic usage in renal failure [Editorial]. Int J Artif Organs 11:411–415, 1988
144. Kreek MJ, Schecter AJ, Gutjahr CL, et al. Methadone use in patients with chronic renal disease. Drug Alcohol Depend 5:197–205, 1980.
145. Siegfried J, Neurosurgical treatment of neurogenic pain. In: Lipton S, Tunks E, Zoppi M, eds. Advances in pain research and therapy. Vol. 13. The pain clinic. New York: Raven Press, 1990:207–215.
146. McGlone FP, Marsh D. Stimulators for treatment of pain. In: Lipton S, Tunks E, Zoppi M, eds. Advances in pain research and therapy. Vol. 13. The pain clinic. New York: Raven Press, 1990:79–82.
147. Justins DM. Management strategies for chronic pain. Ann Rheum Dis 55:588–596, 1996.

148. Gruenwald J, Brendler T, Jaenicke C, eds. PDR for herbal medicines. Montvale, NJ. Medical Economics Company, Inc., 1998:704, 712, 971, 1064, 1163, 1171.
149. Kelly GS. The role of glucosamine sulfate and chondroitin sulfates in the treatment of degenerative joint disease. Altern Med Rev 3:27–39, 1998.
150. Kolkehar R, Meller ST, Gebhart GF. Characterization of the role of spinal N-methyl-D-aspartate receptors in the nociceptor in the rat. Neuroscience 57:385–395, 1993.
151. Øye I, Paulsen O, Maurset A. Effects of ketamine on sensory perception: evidence of a role of N-methyl-D-aspartate receptors. J Pharmacol Exp Ther 260:1209–1213, 1992.
152. Pud D, Eisenberg E, Spitzer A, et al. The NMDA receptor antagonist amantadine reduces surgical neuropathic pain in cancer patients: a double-blind, randomized, placebo-controlled trial. Pain 75:349–354, 1998.
153. Wiesenfeld-Hallin Z. Combined opioid-NMDA antagonist therapies. What advantages do they offer for the control of pain syndromes? Drugs 55:1–4, 1998.
154. Elliott KJ, Brodsky BS, Hyanansky BA, et al. Dextromethorphan shows efficacy in experimental pain (nociception) and opioid tolerance. Neurology 45(Suppl 8):S66–S68, 1995.
155. Rapaka RS, Porreca F. Development of delta opioid peptides as nonaddicting analgesics. Pharm Res 8:1–8, 1991.

[illegible]

CHAPTER 55

ANXIETY DISORDERS

Patricia L. Canales, Marshall Cates, and Barbara G. Wells

DEFINITIONS

Anxiety is an unpleasant feeling of apprehension or fearful concern. It can be a normal, reasonable, and expected response to a stressful situation or perceived danger, or it may be an excessive, irrational state that signifies a mental disorder. The distinction between the two may be difficult to make. Generally in the former, anxiety serves adaptive purposes, and in the latter, it is clearly maladaptive. Anxiety disorders covered in this chapter include generalized anxiety disorder (GAD), panic disorder (PD), obsessive-compulsive disorder (OCD), posttraumatic stress disorder (PTSD), and social phobia (SP). Each anxiety disorder presents differently with regard to clinical symptoms, onset, course, treatment, and response to treatment.[1]

TREATMENT GOALS: ANXIETY DISORDERS

- Because anxiety disorders generally are chronic and recurring and are often associated with other psychiatric disorders and chronic medical illnesses, complete remission of symptoms often is difficult to achieve. Nevertheless, combination treatment approaches should be used to improve patients' functioning and quality of life.
- Treatment for GAD should focus on decreasing psychic and somatic anxiety.
- Management of PD should be targeted at decreasing not only the frequency of panic attacks, but also the levels of anticipatory anxiety and phobic avoidance, with attention to reducing the physical symptoms associated with panic attacks; treatment for OCD should be aimed at decreasing time spent carrying out compulsive behaviors and minimizing obsessive thoughts.[2–4]
- Because patients with PTSD experience varying symptoms over the course of their illness, treatment should minimize the current target symptoms using combinations of antidepressants, anxiolytics, and mood stabilizers.[5,6]
- Treatment goals for SP include reducing the feelings of fear and avoidance, as well as managing physical sequelae of anxiety.

EPIDEMIOLOGY

The National Comorbidity Survey (NCS) supported by the United States Alcohol, Drug Abuse, and Mental Health Administration provides the most recent information on the epidemiology of anxiety disorders.[7] The lifetime incidence of anxiety disorders is 24.9%. In the 12 months before the NCS survey, 17.2% of the population experienced an anxiety disorder. These data suggest that anxiety disorders are more chronic than affective or substance use disorders.

PD, with or without agoraphobia (phobic avoidance behaviors), has a lifetime incidence of 5% in women and 2% in men.[7] The lifetime incidence of GAD is 5.1%, and the diagnosis of this disorder is somewhat more common in women.[7] OCD has a lifetime incidence of 2.3%.[8] Although the lifetime incidence of PTSD for the general population is about 1%, traumatized populations such as combat veterans and refugees can have a lifetime incidence of 30 to 50% and a current rate of 10 to 38%.[9] SP is the most common anxiety disorder, with a lifetime incidence of 13.3%, and it is somewhat more common in women than men.[7]

Comorbidity is a major factor in determining adequate treatment and outcome. One study reported that 28% of patients with PD and 21% of those with SP had a history of major depression.[10] The NCS study revealed that comorbidity generally is associated with a more serious course and that one-sixth of the population has a lifetime history of three or more mental disorders. Uncomplicated PD has a lifetime rate of suicide attempts of 7%, whereas comorbid PD has a rate of 26.3%.[11] These can be compared to the lifetime rate of 1% in people without a mental disorder.

PATHOPHYSIOLOGY

Various psychodynamic, psychoanalytic, behavioral, cognitive, genetic, and biologic theories have been proposed to explain anxiety disorders. Several anxiety disorders have a familial pattern suggestive of a genetic component.[12] However, the anxiety disorders discussed in this chapter are heterogeneous and may have no single cause.

Neurotransmitter systems involved in anxiety generation include the serotonergic, noradrenergic, dopaminergic, adenosinergic, and benzodiazepine (BZD)–γ-aminobutyric acid (GABA) systems. The biologic theories best understood are the noradrenergic model, BZD–GABA receptor model, and serotonergic hypothesis.

It is clear that patients with anxiety disorders, particularly PD, exhibit symptoms of peripheral autonomic hyperactivity including tremulousness, palpitations, and hyperventilation.[1] According to the noradrenergic model, the autonomic nervous system of patients with anxiety disorders becomes oversensitive to various stimuli, responding with excess amounts of norepinephrine. The locus ceruleus (LC) is a brainstem nucleus that contains 70% of the noradrenergic neurons in the brain. It has extensive projections to the limbic system, cerebral cortex, and cerebellar cortex. When presented with uncontrollable and threatening stimuli, the LC is stimulated to release norepinephrine. Evaluating the effects of agents used to treat anxiety leads to further support of the noradrenergic model. Drugs with anxiolytic or antipanic efficacy, such as the tricyclic antidepressants (TCAs) and BZDs, decrease neuronal firing in the LC.[13] Alprazolam decreases corticotropin-releasing factor (CRF) concentrations in the LC.[14] Drugs that stimulate LC activity (e.g., caffeine and yohimbine) usually are anxiogenic, and patients with anxiety disorders are often more susceptible to the anxiogenic effects of these drugs.[15]

GABA is the major inhibitory neurotransmitter. Two types of GABA receptors have been described: $GABA_A$ receptors, which are coupled to chloride channels, and $GABA_B$ receptors, which are coupled to calcium and possibly cyclic adenosine monophosphate (cAMP). When GABA interacts with the $GABA_A$ receptor, this facilitates opening of the chloride channel linked to the receptor. The result is augmentation of chloride ion influx intraneuronally (hyperpolarization), making depolarization less likely.[16] BZDs facilitate the actions of GABA by binding to $GABA_A$ receptors and inducing a conformational change that increases the affinity of the receptor for GABA.[17]

Serotonin, a neurochemical that is found predominantly in the amygdala and frontal cortex, has been proposed to play a role in anxiety disorders. Animal studies have shown that stimulation of the areas of the brain that are highly serotonergic leads to symptoms of anxiety.[18,19] Some researchers hypothesize that serotonergic input at the amygdala is responsible for the anticipatory anxiety and avoidance behaviors seen in PD. There is also some evidence that serotonergic innervations at the periaqueductal gray area may be involved in the panic response.[18,19]

Pharmacologic challenges and interventions have led to further support for serotonin involvement in anxiety disorders. The selective serotonin reuptake inhibitors (SSRIs), such as fluoxetine, are now widely used to treat anxiety disorders.[3] Treatment with SSRIs has reversed the abnormalities found in positron emission tomography (PET) studies in some anxiety disorders.[20] The only medications that are effective in OCD are highly selective serotonin reuptake inhibitors.[20] Serotonin reuptake inhibition seems to be necessary for the antipanic effect of antidepressant medications.[21] Buspirone has a partial agonist effect on the $5\text{-}HT_{1A}$ serotonin receptor and is used in treating various anxiety disorders.[17]

The hypothalamic–pituitary–adrenal axis (HPA) also plays a role in anxiety disorders. Perceived threat or stress activates the HPA axis and one of its components, CRF. CRF plays an important role in generating anxiety by activating the LC. CRF released by hypothalamic neurons eventually leads to the release of cortisol from the adrenal gland, and the cortisol interacts with the HPA axis to inhibit CRF production. Evidence suggests that CRF is responsible for integrating the endocrine, autonomic, and behavioral responses of an organism to stress. Cortisol levels are low in one type of anxiety disorder (PTSD), and it is postulated that these patients are more sensitive to the feedback inhibition of the HPA axis by cortisol.[14,22]

CLINICAL PRESENTATION AND DIAGNOSIS

Evaluation of the anxious patient must be thorough, and medical and psychiatric illnesses must be considered carefully. A physical examination, psychiatric examination (including the mental status examination), appropriate laboratory testing, and an understanding of the patient's history, including a drug history, are essential. It is also important to determine whether the symptoms of anxiety represent situational anxiety or an anxiety disorder. Situational anxiety is a normal response to a stressful situation and usually lasts only 2 to 3 weeks. Short-term treatment with an antianxiety agent may be helpful, but more prolonged therapy usually is not necessary.

A variety of medical conditions may cause anxiety symptoms (Table 55.1). In this case, the anxiety may be labeled as anxiety disorder due to a general medical condition, as outlined in the *Diagnostic and Statistical Manual of Mental Disorders, Fourth Edition* (*DSM-IV*).[1]

Table 55.1 ▪ Medical Disorders Associated with Anxiety

Cardiovascular	Gastrointestinal
Arrhythmias	Ulcerative colitis
Angina	Peptic ulcer disease
Myocardial infarction	Irritable bowel syndrome
Hypertension	Metabolic
Mitral valve prolapse	Vitamin B_{12} deficiency
Congestive heart failure	Porphyria
Respiratory	Inflammatory
Chronic obstructive pulmonary disease	Rheumatoid arthritis
Pulmonary embolism	Lupus erythematosus
Pneumonia	Neurologic
Hyperventilation	Neoplasms
Endocrine	Encephalitis
Hyperthyroidism	Miscellaneous
Hypothyroidism	Chronic infections
Hypoglycemia	Malignancies
Pheochromocytoma	

Furthermore, knowledge that one has a chronic and perhaps disabling medical illness can precipitate anxiety, which may complicate treatment and rehabilitation.[23]

Anxiety may also be a symptom of an underlying primary psychiatric disorder. Almost all major psychiatric illnesses may be associated with symptoms of anxiety. These include schizophrenia, major depression, dysthymia, mania, delirium, dementia, and substance-related disorders.[24] Anxiety related to substance abuse is categorized in the *DSM-IV* as substance-induced anxiety disorder.

When symptoms of anxiety are secondary to an underlying medical or psychiatric illness, the primary illness is treated first. Short-term use of an antianxiety agent may also be necessary.

Several pharmacologic agents are known to produce anxious symptoms, most notably central nervous system (CNS) stimulants and depressants. The most common CNS stimulants that cause symptoms of anxiety include albuterol, amphetamines, cocaine, fenfluramine, isoproterenol, and methylphenidate. Nonprescription drugs well known to cause anxiety include caffeine, nicotine, and decongestants (e.g., ephedrine, pseudoephedrine, oxymetazoline, phenylephrine, phenylpropanolamine, and naphazoline).[25] Older adults and patients with PD may be especially sensitive to the anxiety-producing effects of these agents. CNS depressants (e.g., alcohol, narcotic analgesics, barbiturates, meprobamate, BZDs) may cause anxiety and agitation as a paradoxical reaction, particularly in children and older adults. More commonly, however, anxiety associated with the use of these agents is seen when these agents are abruptly discontinued after chronic use.[24]

The official classification of anxiety disorders, according to the American Psychiatric Association, is detailed in the *DSM-IV* (Table 55.2).[1] This manual also specifies the diagnostic criteria and differential diagnosis for each disorder.

The *DSM-IV* specifies criteria for panic attack separate from the disorders because panic attacks occur in the context of several different anxiety disorders. A panic attack is a discrete period of intense fear or discomfort that is accompanied by at least four somatic or cognitive symptoms (Table 55.3). Panic attacks have a sudden onset, intensify quickly, and usually reach their apex in 10 minutes or less. Patients often report feeling a sense of impending doom or feeling that they are about to die, are having a heart attack, or are "going crazy."[1]

Generalized Anxiety Disorder

The essential feature of GAD is excessive and unrealistic worry about several life situations that has been present for 6 months or longer. The anxiety must be difficult to control and must be accompanied by at least three of the following six symptoms: restlessness, fatigability, difficulty concentrating, irritability, muscle tension, and disturbed sleep. The course of GAD is chronic but fluctuating.[1] Many patients with GAD also experience somatic symptoms (e.g., headache, irritable bowel syndrome) and depressive symptoms. This disorder often exists concurrently with mood disorders, other anxiety disorders, and substance abuse or dependence.

Panic Disorder

The essential criterion of this disorder is recurrent, unexpected panic attacks followed by at least one month

Table 55.2 ▪ *DSM-IV* Classification of Anxiety Disorders

Panic disorder	Acute stress disorder
With agoraphobia	Generalized anxiety disorder
Without agoraphobia	Anxiety disorder due to a general medical condition
Agoraphobia without history of panic disorder	Substance-induced anxiety disorder
Specific phobia	Anxiety disorder not otherwise specified
Social phobia	
Obsessive–compulsive disorder	
Posttraumatic stress disorder	

Table 55.3 ▪ Symptoms Associated with a Panic Attack

Palpitations or tachycardia	Feelings of dizziness, light-headedness, or fainting
Sweating	Feelings of unreality or feelings of being detached from oneself
Trembling or shaking	Fear of losing control or going crazy
Sensations of shortness of breath or smothering	Fear of dying
Feeling of choking	Numbness or tingling sensations
Chest pain	Chills or hot flashes
Nausea or abdominal distress	

Source: Reference 2.

of persistent concern with the possibility of experiencing further attacks, worry about the possible implications or consequences of the episodes, or a significant change in the patient's behavior secondary to the attacks. Unexpected panic attacks are those that occur without a specific stimulus. The patient must have at least two unexpected attacks for the diagnosis, but most patients have more than two and have other attacks that are related to anticipating an attack or being in a situation that generates fear.[1,26] The frequency of the attacks is quite variable. Patients with PD may experience daily attacks for a week or weekly attacks or may be free of attacks for weeks or months.[1]

Many patients with PD also develop symptoms of agoraphobia, a fear of having a panic attack in a place or situation where help may be unavailable or where escape might be difficult or embarrassing. As a result, patients often avoid these situations, placing travel restrictions on themselves or venturing out only in the presence of a companion. Common agoraphobic situations include being away from home alone, being in crowds or long lines, being on bridges, and traveling in a bus, train, or car. PD with agoraphobia is associated with significant social and occupational impairment. In severe cases, patients may be unable to leave the house alone.[1]

PD is often a chronic, relapsing illness that may warrant lifetime treatment. Fifty to 65% of patients with PD have a comorbid diagnosis of major depressive disorder, with the depression preceding the PD in one-third of the cases.[1] Between 8 and 30% of patients with PD have another comorbid anxiety disorder.[1]

Obsessive–Compulsive Disorder

The essential feature of OCD is recurrent obsessions or compulsions that cause marked distress, are time consuming, or interfere significantly with normal occupational functioning, social activities, or relationships.[1]

Obsessions are persistent ideas, thoughts, impulses, or images that are experienced as distressing, intrusive, and senseless. Examples include recurrent thoughts of harming a loved one, recurrent blasphemous thoughts, or recurrent thoughts of contamination. The obsessions are not simply excessive worries about real-life problems, and the person recognizes that the obsessions are the product of his or her own mind. Compulsions are repetitive, intentional behaviors performed in response to an obsession. The compulsion is excessive and may not realistically be connected with the obsession it is designed to neutralize. Usually the person recognizes that the behavior is inappropriate or unreasonable. Although the behavior provides some alleviation of anxiety, patients with OCD do not derive pleasure from carrying out the compulsion. Examples of common compulsions are repetitive hand washing, counting, checking, and touching. When these patients resist a compulsion or are prevented from performing the compulsive behavior, there is a sense of mounting anxiety.[1]

Patients with OCD are often moderately to severely impaired. Avoidance behavior caused by obsessions is common, and, in some cases, acting on compulsions may become the major life activity. Complications of OCD include abuse of alcohol or antianxiety agents.[1]

Posttraumatic Stress Disorder

PTSD may develop when a person experiences or witnesses an event that involves actual or threatened death or serious injury, or a threat to the physical integrity of self or others. As a response to the event, the person reacts with intense fear, helplessness, or horror.[1]

Directly experienced traumatic events associated with the development of PTSD include military combat, violent personal assault, being kidnapped or taken hostage, being a prisoner of war, incarceration in a concentration camp, natural or human-made disasters, and severe automobile accidents. Witnessing the serious injury or death of another or learning about such events that occur to a family member or close friend may also induce PTSD.[1]

The person with PTSD persistently reexperiences the traumatic event through recurrent, intrusive thoughts or images, recurring nightmares, or flashbacks in which the actual event seems to be occurring. They tend to avoid situations in which they are reminded of the traumatic event. People with PTSD have a numbing of general responsiveness, which includes diminished interest in activities previously enjoyed, feelings of detachment or estrangement from others, and the inability to develop closeness or loving feelings toward others. They often have a sense they will not live long, have a career, get married, or have children (sense of foreshortened future). Patients with PTSD often are unable to recall an important aspect of the traumatic event.[1] Symptoms of dissociation are quite common and may include a sense of losing time, finding oneself somewhere but not knowing how one got there, being outside of one's body, and being confused about who or where one is.[27]

Another distinguishing aspect of PTSD is extensive and persistent symptoms of increased arousal, including difficulty sleeping, irritability or outbursts of anger, difficulty concentrating, hypervigilance, and an exaggerated startle response.[1]

Extensive comorbidity is associated with this disorder, and the vast majority of patients with PTSD also experience other anxiety disorders, major depressive disorder or dysthymia, or substance-related disorders (most commonly alcohol abuse).[7]

The more severe and violent the trauma, the more likely the person is to develop PTSD and the more likely it is to be persistent, with significant comorbidity. Some patients with PTSD improve, have very mild symptoms, and do well over time; however, others have a more persistent symptomatic course or have waxing and waning symptoms.[7]

Social Phobia

SP is characterized by a persistent fear of social or performance situations in which embarrassment may occur. The anxiety may be associated with a variety of situations (generalized SP) or may be more specific (discrete SP). When exposed to the social or performance situation, the patient experiences an immediate anxiety response (e.g., palpitations, tremors, sweating, gastrointestinal discomfort, diarrhea, muscle tension, blushing, confusion) that may take the form of a situationally bound or situationally predisposed panic attack. The social situation or performance usually is avoided or endured with severe distress. Adults with SP usually perceive their fears as unreasonable.[1]

To avoid embarrassment, people with SP may avoid eating, drinking, or writing in public for fear that others will see them tremble. They may avoid using public lavatories or speaking in public. The main cognitive characteristic is fear of negative evaluation. They often are hypersensitive to criticism or rejection, have difficulty being assertive, have low self-esteem, and have poor social skills.[1]

Comorbidity with other anxiety disorders, substance abuse, and depression is very common.[28] Diagnosis of SP is made only if there is significant impairment of the person's daily routine, occupational functioning, or social interactions.[1]

TREATMENT

Pharmacotherapy

Commonly used antianxiety medications include BZDs, buspirone, β-blockers, TCAs, monoamine oxidase inhibitors (MAOIs), and SSRIs.

Benzodiazepines

Currently available BZD antianxiety agents are alprazolam (Xanax), chlordiazepoxide (Librium), clonazepam (Klonopin), clorazepate (Tranxene), diazepam (Valium), halazepam (Paxipam), lorazepam (Ativan), oxazepam (Serax), and prazepam (Centrax). All of these agents are approved by the U.S. Food and Drug Administration (FDA) for treating anxiety except clonazepam, which is technically an anticonvulsant. As a class, BZDs are very widely prescribed; they account for approximately 5% of prescriptions written in the United States.[16] The most common indication for BZD therapy is GAD. Double-blind, randomized clinical trials have shown that BZDs clearly reduce the symptoms of GAD more effectively than placebo.[29] Approximately three-fourths of GAD patients treated with BZDs have at least moderate improvement.[16]

Many controlled trials have established the efficacy of alprazolam as an antipanic agent.[30] A daily dosage of 2 to 6 mg usually is sufficient for most patients with PD taking alprazolam.[31] However, there is evidence that total daily BZD dosages in PD tend to be much higher than those in GAD.[31] For instance, some patients with PD need 10 mg/day or more of alprazolam, 6 mg/day clonazepam, 60 mg/day diazepam, or 16 mg/day lorazepam for optimal therapeutic effectiveness.[31,32] A switch from alprazolam to clonazepam has been deemed beneficial for patients experiencing interdose symptom breakthrough, presumably because of clonazepam's longer half-life.[32] In addition, patients who do not respond to one BZD may respond to another.[31]

The high-potency BZDs are effective for SP, with onset of response occurring within 2 weeks. Clonazepam was reported to significantly improve 85% of patients with long-term treatment, despite gradual dosage reduction during the study period.[33] Typical effective dosages are 1.5 to 2 mg/day. Alprazolam is another BZD considered effective for SP and typically is effective at 3 mg/day.[3]

BZDs have not been well studied in treating PTSD. Alprazolam failed to improve PTSD-specific symptoms in a double-blind, placebo-controlled crossover study.[34]

BZDs may exert antianxiety effects by potentiating the inhibitory neurotransmitter GABA. BZD binding sites have been identified in cortical and limbic forebrain areas in the CNS. These receptors are linked to GABA receptors. When BZDs interact at the BZD receptor, the affinity of the GABA receptor for GABA increases. This amplifies the GABA-mediated chloride ion influx intracellularly, with resulting hyperpolarization and inhibition of firing in the LC.[16,20]

The pharmacokinetics of the BZD antianxiety agents are summarized in Table 55.4. Subtle differences in the pharmacokinetic profiles may aid clinicians in selecting the most appropriate agent. When immediate effects are desired, as in acute anxiety treatment or as-needed anxiety treatment, it is important to select an agent with rapid onset. In treating more chronic anxiety with more prolonged dosing, this becomes less important. Similarly, if panic attacks occur between alprazolam doses, it may be helpful to switch the patient to clonazepam because the longer half-life of elimination seems to be associated with a more sustained duration of action.[30]

The highly lipophilic BZDs, diazepam and clorazepate, are rapidly absorbed and distributed into the CNS. As a result, an anxiolytic effect can be anticipated within 1 hour of dosing with these agents. This rapid entry into the CNS may be associated with a rush in some patients that may contribute to the likelihood of abuse. Similarly, the highly lipophilic agents are rapidly distributed peripherally to inactive storage sites (adipose tissue). This accounts for the short duration of action seen with single dosing of clorazepate and diazepam.[35] Lorazepam and oxazepam are less lipophilic. This results in a slower onset of antianxiety effect but a more prolonged effect than might be expected based on half-life because extensive tissue distribution does not occur.[36]

Clorazepate and prazepam are prodrugs and do not have antianxiety activity until they are converted to the metabolite *N*-desmethyldiazepam (N-DMDZ). Clorazepate is converted rapidly in the acidic gastric environment to N-DMDZ by a pH-dependent process. Antacid administration may elevate the pH of the stomach and decrease the rate of N-DMDZ formation. Conversion of prazepam to N-DMDZ is a much slower process because transformation occurs in the liver. Consequently, several hours are needed to achieve peak plasma concentrations of N-DMDZ after prazepam administration. Prazepam would not be an appropriate drug to choose when acute (rapid) antianxiety effects are desired.

In the unusual circumstance that an intramuscular preparation is to be used, lorazepam provides the most predictable absorption. Diazepam and chlordiazepoxide intramuscular injections can be painful and are absorbed erratically.[35]

With chronic dosing, the rate and extent of accumulation depend on clearance and half-life of the parent compound and active metabolites. The BZDs are biotransformed by two primary metabolic processes: hepatic microsomal oxidation (*N*-dealkylation and aliphatic hydroxylation) and glucuronide conjugation. Oxidation may be impaired by aging, liver disease, and concurrent administration of drugs that inhibit oxidative processes. In this situation, greater plasma concentrations and total body stores at steady state would be expected.[35] Conjugation is not affected by these factors.

As shown in Table 55.4, several BZDs are converted to *N*-DMDZ, which is an active metabolite with a half-life of 36 to 200 hours. Further oxidation converts N-DMDZ to oxazepam, which is then conjugated and excreted. Extensive accumulation of N-DMDZ at steady state provides a long duration of antianxiety effects, allowing once- or twice-daily dosing. In the presence of impaired oxidation, prolonged half-life and increased accumulation may be associated with excessive sedation and ataxia in some patients.[35]

Alprazolam, oxazepam, and lorazepam have short to intermediate half-lives of elimination, so a shorter time is needed to achieve steady-state accumulation and plasma concentrations. Alprazolam is oxidized to α-hydroxyalprazolam, which is present in small amounts and probably does not contribute substantially to clinical efficacy. Oxazepam and lorazepam do not undergo oxidation; they are simply glucuronidated and excreted.[35] For this reason, oxazepam and lorazepam are considered good choices for the patient suspected of having impaired oxidative processes.

Patients with hypoalbuminemia may have a significantly greater free (pharmacologically active) fraction of those BZDs that are highly protein bound. For these patients, lorazepam or alprazolam would be a rational choice because of its lower percentage of protein binding.

BZDs with long half-lives of elimination may be dosed once daily at bedtime, thereby providing hypnotic effects and daytime antianxiety effects (Table 55.5). Agents with shorter half-lives (oxazepam, lorazepam, alprazolam) usually are administered in divided daily doses. Patients should be started on low dosages and titrated upward to the lowest effective dosage. Treatment duration should be as brief as possible.

All of the BZDs have similar efficacy in treating GAD if appropriate dosages are used. Approximate equivalent dosages, relative to diazepam 5 mg, are alprazolam 0.25 mg, clonazepam 0.25 mg, lorazepam 1 mg, clorazepate 7.5 mg, chlordiazepoxide 10 mg, prazepam 10 mg, oxazepam 15 mg, and halazepam 20 mg.

Overall, BZDs are very well tolerated by most patients (Table 55.6). By far the most common adverse effects of BZDs involve CNS depression. Side effects such as sedation, ataxia, and incoordination tend to be more

Table 55.4 ▪ Pharmacokinetic Profile of the Benzodiazepine Antianxiety Agents

Generic Name	Time to Peak Plasma Concentration (hr)	Elimination Half-Life[a] (hr)	Protein Binding (%)	Metabolic Pathway	Clinically Important Metabolites
Alprazolam	1–2	12–15	80	Oxidation	None
Chlordiazepoxide	1–4	5–30	96	Oxidation	Desmethchlor-diazepoxide Demoxepam N-DMDZ Oxazepam
Clonazepam	1–4	20–50	85	Nitro reduction	None
Clorazepate	1–2	Prodrug	97	Oxidation	N-DMDZ Oxazepam
Diazepam	0.5–2	20–80	98	Oxidation	N-DMDZ Oxazepam
Halazepam	1–3	7–14	97	Oxidation	3-Hydroxy-halazepam N-DMDZ Oxazepam
Lorazepam	2–4	10–20	85	Conjugation	None
Oxazepam	2–4	5–20	97	Conjugation	None
Prazepam	6	Prodrug	97	Oxidation	3-Hydroxy-prazepam N-DMDZ Oxazepam

Source: Reference 40.

N-DMDZ, N-Desmethyldiazepam; half-life = 36–200 hr.

[a]Parent compound.

Table 55.5 ▪ Dosing of Antianxiety Medications[a]

Antianxiety Agent	Initial Dosage[b]	Titration[b]	Maximum Dosage[c]
Benzodiazepines			
Alprazolam	0.25 mg TID	0.25–0.5 mg/day q2–4d	1 mg QID
Chlordiazepoxide	5 mg TID	5–10 mg/day q2–4d[d]	100 mg QHS
Clonazepam	0.5 mg BID	0.5–1.0 mg/day q2–4d[d]	3 mg BID
Clorazepate	7.5 mg BID	3.75–7.5 mg/day q2–4d[d]	60 mg QHS
Diazepam	5 mg BID	2–5 mg/day q2–4 d[d]	40 mg QHS
Lorazepam	1 mg TID	0.5–1.0 mg/day q2–4d	5 mg BID
Oxazepam	10 mg TID	10–15 mg/day q2–4d	30 mg TID
Buspirone	5 mg TID	5 mg/day q2–3d	20 mg TID
β-Blockers			
Atenolol	25 mg QAM	25 mg/day q3–4d	100 mg QAM
Propranolol	10 mg TID	20–40 mg/day q2–3d	120 mg TID
Tricyclic antidepressants			
Clomipramine	25 mg QHS	25 mg/day q2–4d	250 mg QHS
Imipramine[e]	25–50 mg QHS	25 mg/day q2–4d	300 mg QHS
Nortriptyline	25 mg QHS	25 mg/day q2–4d	150 mg QHS
Monoamine oxidase inhibitors			
Phenelzine	15 mg QAM	15 mg/day q3–4d[f]	45 mg BID
Tranylcypromine	10 mg QAM		30 mg BID
Selective serotonin reuptake inhibitors			
Fluoxetine	20 mg QAM	20 mg/day q2–4wk	80 mg QAM
Fluvoxamine	50 mg QHS	50 mg/day q1wk	150 mg BID
Paroxetine	20 mg QAM	10 mg/day q1wk	50 mg QAM
Citalopram	20 mg QAM	20 mg/day q1wk	40 mg QAM
Sertraline	50 mg QAM	50 mg/day q1wk	200 mg QAM

[a]These are intended as general guidelines only. Older adults usually need approximately one-half the dosages needed for younger adults.
[b]Patients with panic disorder treated with selective serotonin reuptake inhibitors or tricyclic antidepressants need lower initial dosages and slower titrations.
[c]Benzodiazepine-treated patients with panic disorder may need higher dosages.
[d]After initial response, titrate q1–2wk because of long half-life.
[e]Similar dosing strategies for amitriptyline, desipramine, and doxepin.
[f]Until 60 mg/day, then increase further only if there is no improvement after 8–12 wk.

common during the initial phase of therapy and diminish with continued treatment. Older adults, debilitated patients, and patients with hepatic or renal disease are more likely to experience CNS adverse effects.[37] Impaired memory reported with BZD use is called anterograde amnesia because loss of memory is for events occurring after drug ingestion. In addition, a paradoxical reaction involving excitement, aggressiveness, and confusion may occur, especially in older adults.[36]

Drug interactions involving BZDs are shown in Table 55.7. Caution is recommended when combining alcohol, opioid analgesics, or other CNS depressants with BZDs because of additive or synergistic CNS depression. Many drug interactions involve the induction or inhibition of BZD oxidative metabolism; these interactions are of little concern when BZDs such as lorazepam or oxazepam are used.

Physiologic dependence is defined as the emergence of withdrawal symptoms upon discontinuation of therapy. BZD dependence is well documented, and a mild withdrawal syndrome occurs in up to 44% of patients receiving therapeutic dosages of BZDs for 4 to 6 weeks.[38] Mild withdrawal symptoms include anxiety, insomnia,

Table 55.6 ▪ Common or Serious Adverse Effects of Antianxiety Medications

Benzodiazepines: drowsiness, weakness or fatigue, ataxia, slurred speech, confusion or disorientation, incoordination, impaired memory, paradoxical agitation or excitement, dizziness, nausea

Buspirone: nausea, dizziness, headache, insomnia, agitation, drowsiness, dysphoria

β-Blockers: depression, nightmares, insomnia, weakness or fatigue, lethargy, hypotension, bradycardia, dizziness, heart failure, bronchospasm, exacerbation of peripheral vascular disease or Raynaud's disease, masking of hypoglycemic symptoms in diabetics

Tricyclic antidepressants: sedation, orthostatic hypotension, dry mouth, blurred vision, constipation, urinary retention, weight gain, slowed atrioventricular conduction, tremor, seizures, sexual dysfunction

Monoamine oxidase inhibitors: orthostatic hypotension, dry mouth, constipation, drowsiness, insomnia, overstimulation, agitation, sexual dysfunction, edema, weight gain, dizziness, hypertensive crisis

Selective serotonin reuptake inhibitors: nausea, anxiety, insomnia, nervousness, diarrhea, anorexia, dizziness, weight loss, dry mouth, headache, tremor, sweating, sexual dysfunction

Table 55.7 ▪ Drug Interactions with the Benzodiazepine Antianxiety Agents[a]

Drug	Effect
Antacids	Decreased rate of diazepam and chlordiazepoxide absorption; decreased rate and extent of N-DMDZ conversion from clorazepate.
β-Blockers	Propranolol and metoprolol cause a small reduction in oxidative metabolism of diazepam and DMDZ.
Cimetidine	Decreased oxidative metabolism of most BZDs.
Digoxin	Elevated digoxin serum concentrations with signs and symptoms of toxicity reported with addition of alprazolam or diazepam.
Disulfiram	Decreased oxidative metabolism of BZDs.
Erythromycin	Inhibition of oxidative metabolism of triazolam and possibly other BZDs.
Ethanol	Inhibition of BZD metabolism; additive or synergistic CNS depression.
Hydantoins	Increased and decreased phenytoin serum concentrations reported with addition of diazepam or chlordiazepoxide; increased oxazepam elimination.
Isoniazid	Decreased oxidative metabolism of diazepam and triazolam.
Levodopa	Worsening of parkinsonian symptoms.
Oral contraceptives	Decreased clearance of diazepam, chlordiazepoxide, triazolam, and perhaps alprazolam; metabolism of oxazepam, lorazepam, and temazepam may be increased.
Probenecid	May increase lorazepam levels by decreasing clearance.
Rifampin	Increased oxidative metabolism of diazepam and N-DMDZ.
Theophylline	Antagonism of CNS depressant effects of BZDs.
Valproic acid	Decreased oxidative metabolism of diazepam; protein binding of diazepam may also be altered.

Source: Reference 42.

N-DMDZ, N-desmethyldiazepam; *BZDs,* benzodiazepines; *CNS,* central nervous system.

[a]This is not intended to be an all-inclusive list.

irritability, anorexia, diaphoresis, and sensitivity to light and sound. In more severe cases, withdrawal may include confusion, depersonalization, myoclonus, nausea, delirium, and psychosis. The onset of withdrawal usually occurs 1 to 2 days after discontinuing (or reducing the dosage of) short- to intermediate-half-life BZDs and 5 to 10 days after discontinuing (or reducing the dosage of) the long-half-life entities. Although prominent withdrawal symptoms generally subside within 1 to 3 weeks, mild symptoms may persist for several months.[16] Withdrawal is more likely to occur and to be severe if the duration of therapy has been long and if high dosages have been used. Withdrawal may also be more severe after drugs with shorter half-lives, such as lorazepam, oxazepam, and alprazolam, are used.[36]

Two other discontinuation syndromes may be confused with withdrawal. Relapse is simply the return of the original symptoms of anxiety, which may occur weeks to months after drug discontinuation. Rebound is a return of the original symptoms but with greater intensity. This may occur hours to days after drug discontinuation, and it is followed by recovery to pretreatment status.[16]

BZDs should be discontinued gradually, by one-eighth to one-fourth of the total dosage every few weeks to allow careful monitoring and to reduce the risk of withdrawal or rebound. Substituting a long-half-life BZD for a short- to intermediate-half-life drug before downward tapering may reduce the severity of withdrawal symptoms.[16] Alprazolam may not be cross-tolerant with other BZDs, but clonazepam has been substituted for alprazolam successfully.[39]

It is crucial to recognize that abuse is a separate issue from dependence. Abuse is persistent or sporadic excessive drug use inconsistent with or unrelated to acceptable medical practice. Patients with a history of alcohol or other drug abuse are at greatest risk of becoming BZD abusers. In patients without this history, BZD abuse is unusual.[40] Diazepam, followed by alprazolam and lorazepam, has been judged to have the greatest potential for abuse among the BZDs.[16]

Although tolerance develops to the sedative, muscle relaxant, and anticonvulsant properties of the BZDs, tolerance does not appear to develop to the antianxiety or antipanic effects in most patients.[41] Consequently, most patients are unlikely to attempt to increase the dosage.

Buspirone

Buspirone is a member of a unique chemical class called the azapirones. It is structurally dissimilar to previously marketed agents and exhibits no cross-tolerance with the BZDs. It is approved for managing anxiety and for short-term relief of anxiety symptoms. However, it lacks anticonvulsant, muscle relaxant, and hypnotic properties. Several double-blind studies in GAD have demonstrated that buspirone has antianxiety activity superior to that of placebo and equal to that of BZDs.[42,43]

Buspirone was found to be as effective as clomipramine in treating obsessive–compulsive and depressive symptoms in patients with OCD in a 6-week, double-blind, controlled study.[44] However, studies examining buspirone as adjunct therapy for OCD have yielded mixed results.

Nine of 11 patients with SP completing an 8-week open trial of buspirone showed moderate to marked improvement.[45] Buspirone has not been well studied in PTSD treatment, and it is commonly considered to be ineffective in treating PD.

The mechanism of action of buspirone in exerting antianxiety effects is poorly understood, but it clearly does not interact with benzodiazepine receptors and may increase rather than decrease brain noradrenergic and dopaminergic activity. Buspirone is a 5-HT_{1A} partial agonist and reportedly stimulates presynaptic 5-HT_{1A} receptors and blocks postsynaptic 5-HT_{1A} receptors.[46–49] Because 5-HT has a complex role in anxiety and interacts in many ways with other neurotransmitters, the effect of buspirone in treating anxiety may involve multiple neurotransmitter systems in the midbrain, hence the term *midbrain modulator*.[16]

Buspirone is absorbed rapidly and undergoes extensive first-pass metabolism. After oral administration, plasma concentrations of unchanged buspirone are low. Peak plasma concentrations of 1 to 6 ng/mL occur 40 to 90 minutes after a single oral dose of 20 mg. Food may decrease the presystemic clearance of buspirone, resulting in an increased area under the plasma concentration–time curve and an increased peak plasma concentration. Buspirone demonstrates nonlinear pharmacokinetics. Therefore, a dosage increase may result in a greater increase in steady-state plasma concentrations than would have been predicted. Buspirone is approximately 95% protein bound. It is metabolized primarily by oxidative mechanisms, producing several hydroxylated metabolites, one of which is active: 1-pyrimidinylpiperazine (1-PP). 1-PP probably contributes little or nothing to antianxiety effects. The mean half-life of elimination of unchanged buspirone after a single dose of 10 to 40 mg is 2 to 3 hours. Although not studied extensively, clearance appears to be unaffected by age, but it decreases markedly in patients with cirrhosis and to a lesser extent in patients with renal impairment.[50]

Because of its short half-life, buspirone generally is given in 3 divided doses per day. The most common maintenance range is 20 to 30 mg/day,[51] but many clinicians now advocate the use of 30 to 60 mg/day to achieve optimal response (Table 55.5).[3]

Unlike with BZDs, at least 1 to 2 weeks are needed before onset of antianxiety activity, and maximal effects may take up to 6 weeks.

In general, buspirone causes less sedation and fewer psychomotor difficulties than BZDs (Table 55.6). Dizziness, nausea, and headache occur in more than 5% of patients.[51] Drowsiness can be seen with dosages greater than 20 mg/day, and dysphoria has been reported with dosages greater than 30 mg/day.

Concurrent use of buspirone and MAOIs is not recommended because blood pressure may increase. Concurrent trazodone and buspirone administration has been reported to cause a threefold to sixfold elevation in alanine aminotransferase levels; however, the combination is often used clinically with little difficulty. Buspirone may displace digoxin from plasma proteins. Serum haloperidol concentrations may be increased by buspirone. Buspirone metabolite levels may be increased by cimetidine.[16] Unlike the BZDs, buspirone lacks a pharmacokinetic interaction with alcohol and does not potentiate the impairment in psychomotor performance caused by alcohol.[36]

Unlike BZDs, buspirone does not produce physical dependence, withdrawal symptoms, or abuse.[16]

β-Adrenergic Blockers

Propranolol is considered to be a less effective antianxiety agent than BZDs. Propranolol may be considered useful in selected patients with GAD with prominent cardiovascular symptoms of anxiety, such as tachycardia, palpitations, and tremor.[16]

Single-dose β-blocker treatment is likely to be effective for performance anxiety.[52] Atenolol appeared to be more helpful in discrete SP than in generalized SP in a placebo-controlled study; however, the sample size of the subtype was too small to draw definitive conclusions.[53]

Propranolol-treated patients with PTSD were reported to have fewer intrusive thoughts and nightmares and to experience less explosiveness and autonomic instability.[54] β-Blocker therapy for PD is considered controversial. Thus far, two controlled trials evaluating propranolol in PD have offered conflicting results.[32]

Propranolol is almost completely absorbed after oral administration but undergoes extensive first-pass metabolism. Propranolol is highly lipid soluble and highly bound to plasma proteins. The elimination half-life is approximately 3 to 5 hours.[55]

Atenolol is about 50% absorbed after oral administration and exhibits minimal hepatic metabolism. Lipid solubility and protein binding are considered to be very low. Atenolol is eliminated primarily unchanged in the urine, and the half-life is about 6 to 7 hours.[55]

Propranolol usually is dosed every 8 hours, whereas atenolol can be dosed once daily. Propranolol dosages used to treat most anxiety symptoms are 40 to 360 mg/day, although standard dosages have not been established firmly (Table 55.5).[37] For treating SP, 40 to 120 mg/day of propranolol is recommended, and for performance anxiety, 10 to 20 mg as a single dose, taken 1 hour before the performance, may be effective.[37]

Several problems exist with respect to β-blocker dosing. First, the dosage must be titrated against common side effects as well as efficacy. Many patients cannot be titrated upward to sufficient anxiolytic dosages because of bradycardia or hypotension. Second, β-blockers should not be discontinued abruptly but rather gradually tapered to prevent adverse cardiovascular effects and rebound anxiety.[56]

β-Blocker therapy generally is well tolerated if patients are well selected (Table 55.6). They are contraindicated in patients with sinus bradycardia, greater than first-degree atrioventricular block, congestive heart failure, and bronchial asthma. β-Blockers can worsen Raynaud's syndrome and other peripheral vascular diseases. In addition, β-blockers can mask symptoms of hypoglycemia in diabetics. CNS side effects, such as depression and nightmares, are more likely to be seen with propranolol than atenolol because of differences in lipid solubility and

CNS penetration. Common side effects such as bradycardia and hypotension necessitate careful monitoring of the patient's vital signs.

When given along with oral hypoglycemics or insulin, β-blockers may impair glycemic control and may mask symptoms of hypoglycemia. When taken with sympathomimetics having both α- and β-adrenergic effects, β-blockade results in unopposed α-adrenergic activity, which can lead to significant elevations in blood pressure and excessive bradycardia. β-Blockers can potentiate the antihypertensive effects of other hypotension-producing drugs. β-Blockers can inhibit the hepatic metabolism of theophylline, and mutual inhibition of therapeutic effects is possible with this drug combination.[55]

Tricyclic Antidepressants

TCAs are not traditionally considered to be treatments for GAD; however, results from several placebo-controlled studies have confirmed their efficacy. One such study revealed comparable efficacy of imipramine, trazodone, and diazepam in treating patients with GAD who did not have comorbid major depression or PD. Although diazepam-treated patients showed the most improvement during the first 2 weeks of treatment, imipramine exhibited somewhat better anxiolytic efficacy than diazepam during the last 6 weeks of treatment.[57]

Imipramine is the most widely studied TCA in treating PD, and its efficacy is now well established. More recently, clomipramine has been reported by some investigators to be superior to imipramine in PD treatment, and one study reported efficacy at dosages as low as 25 mg/day.[3]

Clomipramine is well-documented in several double-blind trials to be effective in treating OCD, and it is currently one of only four drugs with FDA approval for this indication.

The TCAs have the most solidly established efficacy in treating core intrusive PTSD symptoms. Imipramine and amitriptyline have produced positive results in placebo-controlled studies involving veterans with PTSD.[58]

TCAs are rapidly and completely absorbed after oral administration, but bioavailability is limited by first-pass metabolism. Plasma levels vary widely between patients because of genetic differences in hepatic metabolism, lipid solubility, and extent of protein binding.[55]

TCAs are very lipid soluble, and protein binding is more than 90%. TCAs are metabolized primarily by the liver to active metabolites. Amitriptyline and imipramine are demethylated to nortriptyline and desipramine, respectively. Doxepin and clomipramine also have demethylated active metabolites. Many TCAs also have hydroxylated metabolites.[55]

The elimination half-life varies widely between various TCAs and among patients but is considered approximately 24 hours for most agents.[55]

In low to moderate dosages, the entire dosage of a TCA usually can be administered once daily at bedtime to take advantage of its sedative effect (Table 55.5). Ordinarily, TCA therapy for PD is initiated at a low dosage (imipramine 10 to 25 mg/day) and increased gradually to maximize compliance and minimize side effects, especially a hyperstimulatory reaction. Patients treated with TCAs for PTSD, GAD, and PD respond to a wide range of dosages, although typically the antidepressant dosing range of the TCA (50 to 300 mg/day) is needed. Patients treated with clomipramine for OCD usually need 150 to 250 mg/day.

The most common side effects seen with TCAs include sedation, orthostatic hypotension, and anticholinergic effects (Table 55.6). Twenty percent of patients with PD taking TCAs experience a hyperstimulatory reaction characterized by intensification of anxiety symptoms, agitation, tachycardia, and insomnia. Medication compliance suffers in many patients who manifest this side effect.[59] Patients who experience this side effect need low initial dosages and very gradual upward titration.

Concurrent use of MAOIs with TCAs has resulted in hypertensive crisis, hyperpyretic episodes, convulsions, and death. The combination has been used safely when both drugs are cautiously initiated simultaneously or when the MAOI is gradually added to the TCA; however, a TCA should never be added to an existing MAOI regimen. It is recommended that TCA–MAOI combination therapy be undertaken only under the supervision of a clinician experienced in prescribing this combination. TCAs can antagonize the antihypertensive action of clonidine and guanethidine. Concurrent use of sympathomimetics with TCAs may potentiate cardiovascular effects, possibly resulting in arrhythmias, tachycardia, or severe hypertension. Medications that can increase plasma TCA levels, possibly resulting in toxicity, include cimetidine, phenothiazines, fluoxetine, sertraline, and paroxetine.[55]

Monoamine Oxidase Inhibitors

Many placebo-controlled trials have shown the MAOIs, particularly phenelzine, to be effective antipanic agents. In one open trial, phenelzine blocked panic attacks in 100% of patients with PD and 95% of agoraphobic patients.[60] Despite this established efficacy, the side effect profile and dietary restrictions preclude the routine use of MAOIs in most patients with PD.

Seventy-four patients with SP completed an 8-week double-blind, randomized, placebo-controlled study comparing phenelzine and atenolol. The overall response rates were 64% for phenelzine, 30% for atenolol, and 23% for placebo. Patients with generalized SP were preferentially responsive to phenelzine.[53]

Several open studies suggested possible effectiveness of phenelzine in treating PTSD. The efficacy of phenelzine was confirmed in an 8-week, double-blind, randomized trial in 34 veterans comparing imipramine, phenelzine, and placebo. Patients in both active treatment groups improved. Treatment-responsive symptoms included nightmares, flashbacks, and intrusive recollections but not avoidance.[61]

MAOIs are rapidly and completely absorbed from the gastrointestinal tract, undergo rapid oxidative metabolism in the liver, and are renally eliminated.[55] MAOIs usually are administered on a twice-daily schedule (Table 55.5). The usual therapeutic dosage range for phenelzine in treating anxiety disorders is 45 to 90 mg/day.

Common adverse effects of MAOIs include weight gain, orthostatic hypotension, edema, and sexual dysfunction (WOES; Table 55.6). Drowsiness is more common with phenelzine, whereas tranylcypromine tends to cause overstimulation. Compared with TCAs, MAOIs cause fewer anticholinergic effects but more problematic orthostatic hypotension.[62] Because of this side effect profile as well as dietary and drug restrictions, patients generally prefer other antianxiety medications to MAOI therapy.

The serotonin syndrome and hypertensive crisis are potentially lethal reactions attributed to drug interactions with MAOIs. The serotonin syndrome is a hyperserotonergic state manifested by confusion, restlessness, myoclonus, hyperreflexia, diaphoresis, shivering, tremor, diarrhea, and fever. Drugs such as clomipramine (and other TCAs), meperidine, SSRIs, tryptophan, dextromethorphan, and trazodone can cause the serotonin syndrome when taken concurrently with MAOIs. Hypertensive crisis, manifested by hypertension, severe headache, stiff or sore neck, nausea, and vomiting, can be caused by using MAOIs with sympathomimetics (ephedrine, pseudoephedrine, amphetamines, phenylephrine, phenylpropanolamine, levodopa), tyramine-containing foods, and TCAs.[63]

Selective Serotonin Reuptake Inhibitors

Currently available SSRIs include fluoxetine, sertraline, paroxetine, fluvoxamine, and citalopram. Drugs with clearly established efficacy in treating OCD have serotonin reuptake inhibiting properties. Fluoxetine, fluvoxamine, sertraline, and paroxetine are approved by the FDA for OCD treatment. Controlled studies have revealed positive effects of fluoxetine, sertraline, paroxetine, and fluvoxamine on OCD symptoms. Various double-blind studies comparing SSRIs and clomipramine have shown that SSRIs are as effective as clomipramine and have fewer adverse effects.[64–68]

The SSRIs have been used successfully to treat PD, but only recently have there been placebo-controlled studies to support their efficacy. Fluvoxamine has been evaluated in two 8-week placebo-controlled trials and was shown to produce a panic-free state in up to 73% of patients.[69,70] Citalopram, in dosages of 20 to 30 mg/day, was shown to be as effective as clomipramine in one 8-week placebo controlled study of 475 patients with PD.[71] In one study of 243 patients, fluoxetine 20 mg/day was shown to be more effective than placebo in reducing panic attacks and phobic symptoms.[72] Sertraline 50 to 200 mg/day has been evaluated in two 10-week placebo controlled trials and one 12-week placebo controlled trial. All resulted in significant reductions in the frequency of panic attacks after sertraline therapy.[73–75] Paroxetine is the most well-studied SSRI in PD and has been shown to be more effective than placebo and comparable to clomipramine in producing a panic-free state.[76,77]

A significant reduction in symptoms occurred when patients with PTSD who took fluoxetine in a double-blind, placebo-controlled study. Of particular interest is the apparent ability of the SSRIs to treat the avoidance and numbing symptoms of PTSD in trials thus far.[58]

Three open trials have examined fluoxetine's efficacy in SP, and all yielded moderately effective results.[78]

The SSRIs are generally well absorbed orally, although the rate of absorption is slow (t_{max} = 5 to 8 hours). Food may decrease the rate, but not extent, of the absorption of fluoxetine, whereas it may increase the C_{max} and bioavailability of sertraline. All of the SSRIs are highly protein bound (more than 95%) except fluvoxamine, which is only 77% protein bound.[79]

The SSRIs undergo extensive hepatic metabolism. Fluoxetine and sertraline are metabolized to the active metabolites norfluoxetine and desmethylsertraline, respectively. It should be noted, however, that desmethylsertraline retains only a fraction of the pharmacologic activity of the parent drug. Paroxetine and fluvoxamine have no active metabolites. The half-lives of fluoxetine and norfluoxetine are 2 to 3 days and 7 to 9 days, respectively. The half-lives of sertraline and desmethylsertraline are 26 hours and 62 to 104 hours, respectively. The half-life of paroxetine is approximately 10 to 16 hours, and that of fluvoxamine is 15 hours. After multiple administration of fluoxetine or paroxetine, $t_{1/2}$ and AUC values are greatly increased, possibly because these drugs inhibit their own metabolism. Sertraline exhibits linear pharmacokinetics over its clinically relevant dosage range.[79]

SSRIs generally are dosed once daily in the morning to avoid insomnia; however, fluvoxamine is initiated as a single daily dose at bedtime, with daily dosages greater than 100 mg given in two divided doses. One must bear in mind that changes in the fluoxetine dosage are not fully reflected in the plasma for several weeks because of the long elimination half-life of both parent drug and active metabolite.[39] However, sertraline, paroxetine, and fluvoxamine can have dosages adjusted at weekly intervals.

In treating most patients with anxiety disorders, typical antidepressant dosages of the various SSRIs are needed. Starting dosages are lower (fluoxetine 5 mg/day, sertraline 25 mg/day) and titration is more gradual in treating PD because of possible hyperstimulatory reactions.

SSRIs are free of anticholinergic, orthostatic, and sedative effects. Sexual dysfunction, nausea, headache, nervousness, and insomnia are common side effects of SSRIs and are the most common reasons for discontinuation of SSRIs (Table 55.6).[39] There have also been reports of akathisia, tremors, and dystonic reactions with SSRIs.[80–82] Like TCAs, SSRIs can cause a hyperstimulatory reaction in patients with PD. There has been increasing evidence over the last few years that patients abruptly discontinuing SSRI therapy may experience discontinuation symptoms that include dizziness, insomnia, fatigue, anxiety, nausea, headache, and sensory disturbances. It is recommended that SSRIs be tapered rather than abruptly discontinued whenever possible.[83]

SSRIs should not be used concurrently with MAOIs because of the risk of precipitating the serotonin syndrome. A sufficient washout phase should be observed after discontinuation of either medication before therapy is initiated with the other. A full 5 weeks should lapse after fluoxetine is discontinued before an MAOI is initiated. Concurrent use with tryptophan can result in agitation, restlessness, and gastrointestinal distress.[57] All SSRIs, especially fluoxetine, can increase TCA levels to possible toxicity.[79] Fluvoxamine inhibits the metabolism of propranolol, warfarin, theophylline, and carbamazepine. Fluoxetine inhibits the metabolism of carbamazepine and diazepam. Paroxetine reduces digoxin clearance and prolongs bleeding time in patients receiving warfarin. Sertraline inhibits the metabolism of diazepam and warfarin.[79]

Nonpharmacologic Therapy

Just as the last decade has brought psychopharmacologic advances in treating anxiety disorders, there have been significant gains in the effectiveness of nonpharmacologic interventions. Cognitive therapy and behavior therapy have been well researched and have often been combined to treat the various anxiety disorders.

The effectiveness of cognitive–behavioral therapy in PD has been reported to be as high as 80%, with the effect lasting up to 2 years.[84,85] In long-term PD treatment, cognitive–behavioral therapy may be very helpful.[86] This type of treatment focuses on coping with the fear of symptoms of anxiety. Patients often make catastrophic interpretations of the meaning of panic symptoms (e.g., "I am having a stroke"; "I am about to go insane"), and these thoughts induce a high level of anticipatory anxiety and may cue the next panic attack. The therapy is aimed at eliminating this fear of symptoms and the associated anxiety and avoidance. Also, stepwise exposure to feared bodily sensations, combined with cognitive restructuring, help patients decrease detrimental misinterpretations of somatic symptoms of panic.[86] Therapist-guided or instructed exposure to phobic situations is an important aspect of this therapy.[26] Alprazolam may interfere with cognitive–behavioral therapy because it may prevent the controlled elicitation of anxiety during therapy sessions.[87] According to Taylor,[88] however, the thoughtful integration of cognitive–behavioral therapy and pharmacotherapy produces an optimal outcome. He suggests that many patients need some medication before they can undertake intensive exposure therapy and that psychological interventions can facilitate medication withdrawal and prepare patients for long-term treatment.

SP is felt to respond to the combination of cognitive–behavioral therapy and pharmacotherapy.[89] Cognitive–behavioral therapy, applied relaxation therapy, and traditional psychodynamic psychotherapy have been found to be helpful for patients with GAD.[88,90,91] OCD is a particularly difficult anxiety disorder to treat, but combining pharmacotherapy with other interventions probably is the most effective approach. Combining either clomipramine or fluoxetine with the behavioral treatments of exposure and response prevention (not allowing the compulsion to occur) was associated with a 75% rate of significant improvement in one study.[92] PTSD usually warrants both pharmacotherapy and nonpharmacologic interventions, which may include individual, group, and family psychotherapies.[93,94]

IMPROVING OUTCOMES

Disease State Management Strategies

Generalized Anxiety Disorder

Pharmacotherapy of GAD should be used as part of a comprehensive treatment plan that includes nondrug approaches, such as psychological and behavioral therapies.[16] The BZDs, buspirone, TCAs, and to a lesser extent the β-blockers are the most appropriate pharmacologic alternatives (Table 55.8).

All BZDs are considered to be effective antianxiety

Table 55.8 ▪ Efficacy of Various Drug Classes in Treating Anxiety Disorders

	Generalized Anxiety Disorder	Obsessive–Compulsive Disorder	Panic Disorder	Posttraumatic Stress Disorder	Social Phobia
Benzodiazepines	X		X[a]		X[a]
Buspirone	X				
β-Blockers					X
Tricyclic antidepressants	X	X[b]	X	X	
Monoamine oxidase inhibitors			X	X	X
Selective serotonin uptake inhibitors		X	X	X	X

[a]High potency (i.e., alprazolam, clonazepam).
[b]Clomipramine.

agents, and selection of one agent over another usually is based on pharmacokinetic properties and the patient's clinical situation, medical status, and history of response and tolerability. Predictors of response include acuteness of symptoms, presence of a precipitating stress, high level of psychic and somatic anxiety, low level of depression and interpersonal problems, lack of previous treatment or good response to previous treatment, expectation of recovery, desire for medications, awareness that symptoms are psychological, and improvement during the first week of treatment.[16]

In treating GAD, the lowest effective BZD dosage for the shortest possible period should be used. Periodic attempts at drug discontinuation should be made after patients' needs are assessed. Many clinicians try to discontinue BZDs gradually after several months of therapy. For patients who relapse, intermittent treatment (lasting weeks to months) coinciding with the fluctuating nature of the illness often is effective. Some patients may need to continue long-term medication because of frequent relapses, persistent stresses, inability to resolve conflict, or risk of physical harm from chronic anxiety.[16] Major risks associated with long-term use (e.g., dependence and impaired psychomotor function) must be weighed against the benefits of BZD therapy.[16]

Buspirone therapy has several advantages over BZD therapy. Because buspirone carries no obvious risk for abuse, dependence, or withdrawal, it is an appropriate choice for patients with GAD and a history of drug abuse and patients likely to need long-term treatment. Buspirone causes fewer CNS side effects such as sedation and psychomotor and cognitive impairment and does not enhance sedation or psychomotor impairment by alcohol or other CNS depressants. The major disadvantage of buspirone is that it takes several weeks before a significant effect occurs, whereas BZDs exert their effects quickly. Thus, buspirone is not an appropriate choice for patients who need immediate anxiety relief. Also, buspirone must be taken continuously to exert anxiolysis, so it cannot serve as an as-needed medication. Buspirone dosing is more cumbersome because generally a three-times-daily schedule is needed.[3]

Response rates achieved with buspirone are comparable to those seen with BZDs.[31] However, evidence suggests that the psychological symptoms of anxiety respond to buspirone better than the physical symptoms of anxiety.[95] Furthermore, it is a common belief that former users of BZDs may respond less well to buspirone.[31] A potential reason for this peculiarity is that the subjective effect of buspirone compares unfavorably with the sedative–euphoric effects of BZDs.[95] Another explanation is that patients recently withdrawn from BZDs and placed on buspirone experience BZD withdrawal, which goes unblocked by the non–cross-tolerant azapirone.[95] Finally, patients who have previously experienced rapid anxiety relief with a BZD may be dissatisfied with the delayed onset of antianxiety effects associated with buspirone. When switching a patient from a BZD to buspirone, it is appropriate to add buspirone to BZD treatment for 2 to 4 weeks before the BZD taper begins.[16]

Results from several well-controlled studies suggest that TCAs may have a significant role in GAD treatment.[3] Antidepressants are useful for chronic subpanic anxiety and anxiety associated with depression.[16] The inherent concerns associated with chronic BZD use make TCA therapy a particularly attractive alternative for long-term GAD management. In terms of cost, generic preparations of the TCAs are considerably less expensive than buspirone.[31] A disadvantage of TCA therapy is a greater incidence of side effects that may be problematic for anxious patients.[31] TCA therapy should be initiated with small dosages and titrated upward gradually to minimize these effects.[3] The onset of the anxiolytic action is gradual, and the effectiveness of the TCA tends to increase.[3]

Combination strategies have been used in cases of treatment-resistant anxiety. Although not systematically examined, selected patients may benefit from various combinations involving BZDs, buspirone, TCAs, and β-blockers.[31]

Panic Disorder

Psychopharmacologic agents with proven efficacy in treating patients with PD are shown in Table 55.8. The efficacy of BZDs and antidepressants is not limited to panic attacks but includes other components of the disorder such as anticipatory anxiety, depression, and phobic avoidance.[32]

Alprazolam is the BZD traditionally used to treat PD, but other high-potency agents considered effective include clonazepam, lorazepam, and diazepam.[3] One advantage of BZD therapy in PD is the rapid onset of effect, which typically occurs within 1 to 2 weeks.[31] Also, the BZDs have an overall favorable side effect profile[3] and are better tolerated than antidepressants.[32] However, sedation is a troublesome side effect that affects a substantial number of patients with PD taking BZDs, especially early in treatment.[32] Another disadvantage of BZD therapy is the difficulty in discontinuing treatment caused by withdrawal and reemergence of panic.[31] Whereas dependence and withdrawal are realistic concerns, patients with PD rarely abuse BZDs, and abuse is more likely to occur among patients with a personal or family history of drug or alcohol abuse.[2] It should be noted that comorbidity of PD and alcoholism is not uncommon.[32] There is no evidence of tolerance to the antipanic effects of BZDs, so it is not necessary to increase the dosage with long-term PD treatment.[3]

Advantages of antidepressants relative to BZDs include lack of concern over dependence, withdrawal, or abuse and antidepressant efficacy as well as antipanic efficacy.[3] Disadvantages of antidepressants include a delayed onset of effects (4 to 6 weeks) and hyperstimulatory reactions, which complicate therapy and affect compliance.[3] Antidepressants should be chosen for patients with a history of substance abuse, those with prominent depression, or those who do not tolerate BZDs.[2]

Imipramine and clomipramine are the two TCAs most studied for PD, but other TCAs, such as desipramine and nortriptyline, probably are effective as well.[3] TCAs have the advantage of once-daily dosing but have the disadvantage of causing side effects that prevent dosage increases to optimal levels in a substantial portion of patients with PD.[3] Recent research conducted to examine therapeutic plasma levels of TCAs in PD and agoraphobia has revealed that imipramine levels of approximately 125 to 150 ng/mL and desipramine levels above 125 ng/mL may be optimal.[3]

Some clinicians believe that MAOIs may have superior efficacy, particularly in treatment-resistant patients.[31] However, the potential dangerous side effects and drug interactions of MAOIs limit their use in PD.[30] MAOIs should be reserved for the most severely ill or treatment-refractory patients.[2]

SSRIs share the aforementioned advantages of antidepressants over BZDs, and they have a favorable side effect profile compared to TCAs and MAOIs. Thus, many clinicians now consider SSRIs to be first-line treatment for PD.[3,31] Hyperstimulatory reactions occur in some patients, but fluoxetine is well tolerated by most patients when treatment is initiated at 5 mg/day and titrated cautiously.[3]

Various clinical scenarios have dictated combined BZD and antidepressant use in PD. Antidepressants can be added when depressive symptoms emerge during BZD monotherapy.[3] Combination therapy may also be used in cases of treatment-resistant PD.[31] Finally, combination therapy early in treatment followed by a taper of the BZD has been used as a strategy to avoid the long-term use of BZDs and to circumvent the slow onset of action of antidepressants.[32]

PD is a chronic illness, but some patients enjoy periods without panic attacks.[32,35] A treatment period of 6 to 12 months followed by a gradual discontinuation phase has been suggested for BZDs.[32] One-year maintenance treatment with imipramine can be protective against relapse, even with a much lower dosage than needed during acute treatment.[3] However, many patients with PD may need several years of drug therapy; some patients may need indefinite therapy.[2]

Behavioral treatment also is effective for PD. The combination of behavioral treatment and drug treatment may be optimal for many patients with PD. Unfortunately, nearly one-half of patients with PD continue to experience some degree of symptoms during the course of their illness despite treatment.[3]

Obsessive–Compulsive Disorder

Drugs that inhibit serotonin reuptake, such as clomipramine and the SSRIs, are clearly beneficial in OCD treatment (Table 55.8). These drugs can decrease the devastating symptoms and improve the patient's quality of life.[96] However, there are caveats concerning OCD pharmacotherapy. First, these drugs may be more effective for obsessions than for compulsions.[96] Second, only an approximately 40 to 60% reduction in symptoms is seen with pharmacotherapy alone, so many patients continue to be symptomatic enough to meet criteria for the diagnosis of OCD even after adequate trials of medications.[3] Superior response may be seen with the combination of pharmacotherapy and behavior therapy, such that 80% of patients experience at least moderate improvement with the combined modalities.[4] Also, behavior therapy may quicken the response to medications and reduce the likelihood of relapse after medication discontinuation.[3]

Clomipramine may be slightly more effective than the SSRIs, but clomipramine therapy is more problematic than SSRI therapy because of its typical TCA side effect profile, seizure risk, and toxicity in overdose.[4] Patients may respond differentially to the various SSRIs, so sequential trials may be worthwhile in light of nonresponse to a particular agent.[3]

To minimize side effects, starting dosages of these agents should be low and dosage escalation should be gradual.[4] The SSRIs are more likely than clomipramine to cause an initial hyperstimulatory effect.[4] Up to 250 mg/day of clomipramine may be needed for maximum effect, and the dosage ranges for the SSRIs are comparable to those used to treat depression. Although individual patients may preferentially respond to higher dosages of the SSRIs, comparable efficacy can generally be achieved with lower dosages.[3] Dosages can be reduced in the maintenance phase once a response has been achieved.[4]

Response of OCD symptoms to pharmacotherapy occurs slowly, such that improvement may be noted after about 3 to 4 weeks and a graded improvement continues up to 10 to 12 weeks.[4] Duration of treatment is debated; however, most practitioners agree that drug treatment should be continued for at least 1 year before gradual discontinuation is considered.[4] Relapse may be a likely consequence of medication discontinuation.[96]

Treatment-resistant patients may respond to augmentation with agents such as lithium or buspirone. These agents may act by enhancing serotonin function.[97] Although they have been said to be effective in case reports and open trials, the augmentation potential of these agents has been disappointing in controlled studies. Nevertheless, in refractory patients augmentation strategies are justified because individual patients may experience beneficial results.[3]

Posttraumatic Stress Disorder

Pharmacotherapeutic studies have demonstrated that the symptoms of PTSD respond to medication (Table 55.8), but it is also clear that most patients receiving pharmacotherapy experience limited gains and continue to meet the diagnostic criteria for PTSD even after successful treatment. The treatment plan should be broadly based, including various combinations of psychopharmacologic, psychodynamic, and behavioral treatments.[58] Furthermore, pharmacotherapy may enhance the efficacy of the other forms of treatment.[58]

The goals of pharmacotherapy in PTSD include reducing intrusive symptoms, improving avoidance symptoms, reducing hyperarousal, relieving depression, controlling impulsivity, controlling psychotic features, and facilitating psychotherapy.[5]

Placebo-controlled studies have shown both positive and negative outcomes with pharmacotherapy for core PTSD symptoms. Although there have been few such studies, several conclusions have been drawn about factors that differentiate positive from negative trials. First, positive trials have involved drugs with prominent serotonergic effects, such as amitriptyline, imipramine, phenelzine, and fluoxetine. Two of the three negative trials involved the nonserotonergic agents alprazolam and desipramine. Next, positive trials have tended to use high drug dosages, whereas negative trials have used lower dosages. Finally, positive trials have had a treatment duration of up to 8 weeks, whereas negative trials have had a treatment duration of only 4 to 5 weeks.[5]

Patients with PTSD often do not respond to a single medication because of persistent core symptoms and comorbid symptoms. Silver et al.[98] proposed the popular therapeutic strategy of using an antidepressant for initial pharmacologic treatment, assessing response after an adequate trial, then addressing comorbid symptoms with combination drug therapy. The TCAs appear to be effective for intrusive symptoms and for anxiety and depressive symptoms, but not as effective for avoidance symptoms.[58] The SSRIs may differ from other medications by improving avoidance and numbing symptoms in addition to intrusive symptoms.[58] The MAOIs largely have been relegated to a treatment-resistant role, for reasons previously discussed. Hyperarousal symptoms, often persistent despite antidepressant therapy, and impulsive symptoms are best treated with propranolol or the mood-stabilizing drugs lithium, carbamazepine, or valproic acid. BZD therapy should be used cautiously because of the prevalence of substance abuse in this patient population as well as the ability of BZDs to induce depression and cause behavioral disinhibition.

It may take 8 weeks or longer before beneficial effects of pharmacotherapy are evident in PTSD symptoms,[58] and maximum effects may take several months. Patients with chronic PTSD may need to continue pharmacotherapy for years.[6]

Many pharmacotherapeutic questions remain unanswered at this time. These include whether medication response varies with the type of trauma, determination of the mechanisms of action of various drugs, rates of relapse after drug discontinuation, and efficacy of drug therapy relative to psychotherapy.[58]

Social Phobia

Cognitive–behavioral techniques are recognized as being effective for SP,[31] and recently pharmacologic therapy has shown utility as a primary treatment.[99] The goal of drug treatment is to decrease the fear and avoidance associated with SP. Drugs of choice in treating SP are listed in Table 55.8.

Typical effective dosages are 1.5 to 2 mg/day of clonazepam or 3 mg/day of alprazolam.[31] The long-term benefits of BZD therapy appear to be maintained over time with no obvious tolerance and minimal adverse effects.[3] However, high relapse rates after BZD discontinuation and potential BZD abuse in a population with a high comorbidity of alcoholism are worrisome.[31,78] β-Blockers clearly are effective for performance anxiety (discrete type of SP) when given about 1 hour before the feared event.[31] β-Blockers probably are of little benefit in treating generalized SP, but a trial for acute and maintenance therapy of discrete SP is worthwhile.[3]

Phenelzine has the best demonstrated efficacy in SP treatment, and MAOIs are especially effective for patients with generalized SP.[3] Eight weeks of treatment may be needed for full therapeutic effects, but approximately two-thirds of patients eventually respond to MAOI therapy.[31] Of significance is the fact that a large proportion of patients maintain clinical improvement after discontinuation of MAOI therapy.[99] MAOI therapy is complicated, unfortunately, by troublesome side effects and dietary restrictions.

Fluoxetine has been touted as a particularly effective SP treatment in open trials; however, double-blind, placebo-controlled trials are sorely needed to assess the utility of the SSRIs in this disorder. It has been suggested that patients with either generalized or discrete SP are likely to respond to fluoxetine treatment.[99] Interestingly, investigators have not noted hyperstimulatory effects in the early stages of SSRI treatment of SP, in contrast to what is seen often in PD.[78]

Additional study is needed to further delineate the efficacy of different drug treatments, determine the optimal duration of drug therapy, and examine the potential role of combined psychotherapeutic interventions.[99]

Patient Education

Patients should be told about the expected benefits, expected length of therapy, common side effects, and precautions to be observed with any medications they are taking. Detailed patient education information can be found in the USP-DI published by the United States Pharmacopeial Convention.[55] Patients should be told that although they probably will experience some antianxiety or antipanic effects during the first weeks, they should maintain regular contact with the prescriber as long as they are taking this medication. The prescriber should regularly assess side effects and determine the need to continue drug therapy. If depression emerges or becomes more pronounced, the prescriber should be notified.[55]

Patients should be told that BZDs can cause drowsiness and decrease coordination. Patients should be warned against driving a car or operating dangerous machinery until they know how the drug affects them.

Patients should understand that with continued dosing, their medication can cause a physical dependence and that stopping the medication abruptly may result in withdrawal side effects. Therefore, they should not discontinue medication abruptly without first checking with the prescriber, who may elect to taper the dosage gradually before discontinuing it.[55]

Women of childbearing potential should understand that taking BZDs during pregnancy can be associated with risks, including birth defects (if taken during the first trimester), physiologic dependence in the baby, and other selected problems in the newborn, such as drowsiness, slow heartbeat, and difficulty breathing.[55]

As with most medications, patients taking buspirone should inform the clinician if they are pregnant, plan to become pregnant, or are breastfeeding. Patients should be advised to not drive or engage in other potentially hazardous activities until they know how the medication affects them. Patients should be well educated on buspirone's low sedative profile (relative to BZDs) and on the delayed onset of therapeutic effects. If patients are educated on the lack of potential for causing physiologic dependence, they are more likely to willingly sacrifice immediate sedative and antianxiety effects and comply with treatment.[55]

Patients initiated on β-adrenergic blocker therapy should be counseled on its potential for causing dizziness secondary to hypotension. If dizziness occurs, patients should be advised to stand up slowly from a sitting or lying position and to grab hold of the bed, railing, or wall to prevent loss of balance or falls.[55]

Patients starting TCA therapy should be informed of its potential to cause transient worsening of anxiety and insomnia, which generally persist during the first 2 to 3 weeks of therapy. Chronic side effects may include sedation, dry mouth, urinary retention, blurred vision, and weight gain.[55]

Counseling for patients taking an MAOI includes warning of adverse effects and drug–drug and drug–food interactions. Patients should be warned of orthostatic hypotension, insomnia, potential weight gain, edema, and sexual dysfunction. Patients should be advised to see a physician or pharmacist before taking any over-the-counter agents, particularly preparations for weight loss and colds. In addition, written information about absolute and relative dietary restrictions should be provided.[55]

Patients receiving SSRI therapy should be informed of the potential for transient side effects that include headache, nervousness, restlessness, and insomnia. Side effects that may persist include nausea and sexual dysfunction. Patients should be advised that abrupt discontinuation of an SSRI may cause a withdrawal phenomenon that is characterized by insomnia, worsened anxiety, headache, and dizziness.[39,83]

KEY POINTS

- Patients with anxiety disorders have significant morbidity, and some patients can be profoundly disabled by their illness.
- Accurate diagnosis is crucial to selecting the most rational pharmacotherapy for anxiety disorders.
- Nonpharmacologic treatment can improve response to antianxiety medications in patients with anxiety disorders.
- Drug therapy for anxiety should be designed around patient-specific factors such as lifestyle issues, financial resources, comorbidities, drug adverse effects, and past treatment response.
- Initial therapy for anxiety disorders should be an adequate trial of monotherapy, and if there is no improvement, the clinician should consider switching to an alternative agent.
- BZDs are considered first-choice agents for treating GAD and PD. When selecting a BZD, the clinician should consider differences in onset of effect, duration of action, the presence of active metabolites, protein binding, and available dosage forms.
- Nonbenzodiazepine alternatives, such as buspirone, should be considered for patients with a history of substance abuse or dependence or burdened by daytime sedation. Furthermore, if the patient has significant depressive symptoms, treatment with a TCA is a good choice.
- An SSRI is useful in patients with PD who must remain awake and alert during the day, whereas a TCA may be more appropriate for patients who may benefit from its sedative properties.
- SSRIs are first-choice agents for OCD management.
- PTSD should be managed initially with a trial of a TCA or an SSRI with persistent symptoms such as depression, impulsivity, aggression, hyperarousal, or psychotic symptoms managed with the addition of a mood stabilizer, a β-adrenergic blocker, a BZD, or an antipsychotic.
- BZDs are effective short-term treatment for SP, and for chronic therapy a trial of an SSRI is a desirable alternative.
- Patients with anxiety disorders who do not experience complete symptom remission may have improved functioning and quality of life using combinations of anxiolytics, antidepressants, and mood stabilizers.

REFERENCES

1. American Psychiatric Association. Diagnostic and statistical manual of mental disorders, DSM-IV. Washington, DC: American Psychiatric Association, 1994:393–444.
2. Shelton RC. Pharmacotherapy of panic disorder. Hosp Comm Psychiatry 44:725–726, 1993.
3. Brawman-Mintzer O, Lydiard RB. Psychopharmacology of anxiety disorders. Psychiatr Clin North Am, Annual of Drug Therapy 1:51–79, 1994.

4. Rasmussen SA, Eisen JL, Pato MT. Current issues in the pharmacologic management of obsessive compulsive disorder. J Clin Psychiatry 54(Suppl 6):4–9, 1993.
5. Vargas MA, Davidson J. Post-traumatic stress disorder. Psychiatr Clin North Am 16:737–748, 1993.
6. Davidson J. Drug therapy of post-traumatic stress disorder. Br J Psychiatry 160:309–314, 1992.
7. Kessler RC, McGonagle KA, Zhao S, et al. Lifetime and 12-month prevalence of DSM-III-R psychiatric disorders in the United States. Arch Gen Psychiatry 51:8–19, 1994.
8. Weissman MM, Bland RC, Canino GJ, et al. The cross national epidemiology of obsessive compulsive disorder: the cross national collaborative group. J Clin Psychiatry 55(Suppl 3):5–10, 1994.
9. Tomb DA. The phenomenology of post-traumatic stress disorder. Psychiatr Clin North Am 17:237–250, 1994.
10. Swinson RP, Cox BJ, Woszczyna BA. Use of medical services and treatment for panic disorder with agoraphobia and for social phobia. Can Med Assoc J 147:878–883, 1992.
11. Johnson J, Weissman MM, Klerman GL. Panic disorder, comorbidity, and suicide attempts. Arch Gen Psychiatry 47:805–808, 1990.
12. Weissman MM. Family genetic studies of panic disorder. J Psychiatr Res 27(Suppl 1):69–78, 1993.
13. Charney DS, Heninger GR. Noradrenergic function and the mechanism of action of antianxiety treatment. I. The effect of long-term alprazolam treatment. Arch Gen Psychiatry 42:458–467, 1985.
14. Owens MJ, Vargas MA, Nemeroff CB. The effects of alprazolam on corticotropin-releasing factor neurons in the rat brain: implications for a role for CRF in the pathogenesis of anxiety disorders. J Psychiatr Res 27(Suppl 1):209–220, 1993.
15. Charney DS, Heninger GR, Breier A. Noradrenergic function in panic anxiety. Arch Gen Psychiatry 41:751–763, 1984.
16. Dubovsky SL. Generalized anxiety disorder: new concepts and pharmacologic therapies. J Clin Psychiatry 51(Suppl):3–10, 1990.
17. Hyman SE, Nestler EJ. The Molecular Foundations of Psychiatry. Washington, DC: American Psychiatric Press, 1993:150–157.
18. Graeff FG, Guimeras TS, De Andrade TG. Role of 5-HT in stress, anxiety and depression. Pharmacol Biochem Behav 54:129–141, 1996.
19. Lucki I. Serotonin receptor specificity in anxiety disorders. J Clin Psychiatry 57(Suppl 6):5–10, 1996.
20. Insel TR, Winslow JT. Neurobiology of obsessive compulsive disorder. Psychiatr Clin North Am 15:813–824, 1992.
21. Humble M, Wistedt B. Serotonin, panic disorder and agoraphobia: short-term and long-term efficacy of citalopram in panic disorders. Int Clin Psychopharmacol 6(Suppl 5):21–39, 1992.
22. Southwick SM, Bremner D, Krystal JH, et al. Psychobiologic research in post-traumatic stress disorder. Psychiatr Clin North Am 17:251–264, 1994.
23. Schuckit MA. Anxiety related to medical disease. J Clin Psychiatry 44:31–36, 1983.
24. Hayes PE, Dommisse CS. Current concepts in clinical therapeutics: anxiety disorders, part I. Clin Pharm 6:140–147, 1987.
25. Cameron OG. The differential diagnosis of anxiety: psychiatric and medical disorders. Psychiatr Clin North Am 8:3–23, 1985.
26. Agras WS. The diagnosis and treatment of panic disorder. Annu Rev Med 44:39–51, 1993.
27. Bremner JD, Steinberg M, Southwick SM, et al. Use of the structured clinical interview for DSM-IV dissociative disorders for systematic assessment of dissociative symptoms in posttraumatic stress disorder. Am J Psychiatry 150:1011–1014, 1993.
28. Rosenbaum JF, Pollock RA. The psychopharmacology of social phobia and comorbid disorders. Bull Menninger Clin 58(Suppl A):A67–A83, 1994.
29. Bradwejn J. Benzodiazepines for the treatment of panic disorder and generalized anxiety disorder: clinical issues and future directions. Can J Psychiatry 38(Suppl 4):S109–S113, 1993.
30. Tesar GE. High-potency benzodiazepines for short-term management of panic disorder: the U.S. experience. J Clin Psychiatry 51(Suppl 9):4S–10S, 1990.
31. Roy-Byrne P, Wingerson D, Cowley D, et al. Psychopharmacologic treatment of panic, generalized anxiety disorder, and social phobia. Psychiatr Clin North Am 16:719–735, 1993.
32. Rosenberg R. Drug treatment of panic disorder. Pharmacol Toxicol 72:344–353, 1993.
33. Davidson JRT, Ford SM, Smith RD, et al. Long-term treatment of social phobia with clonazepam. J Clin Psychiatry 52(Suppl 11):16–20, 1991.
34. Braun P, Greenberg D, Dasberg H, et al. Core symptoms of posttraumatic stress disorder unimproved by alprazolam treatment. J Clin Psychiatry 51:236–238, 1990.
35. Greenblatt DJ, Shader RI, Abernethy DR. Current status of benzodiazepines, part I. N Engl J Med 309:354–358, 1983.
36. Dommisse CS, Hayes PE. Current concepts in clinical therapeutics: anxiety disorders, part II. Clin Pharm 6:196–215, 1987.
37. Guze B, Richeimer S, Szuba M. The psychiatric drug handbook. St Louis: Mosby, 1992:2, 4, 7.
38. Power KG, Jerrom DWA, Simpson RJ, et al. Controlled study of withdrawal and rebound anxiety after six week course of diazepam for generalized anxiety. BMJ 290:1246–1248, 1985.
39. Perry PJ, Alexander B, Liskow BI. Psychotropic drug handbook. 6th ed. Cincinnati: Harvey Whitney, 1991:289.
40. Busto U, Seller EM, Naranjo CA, et al. Patterns of benzodiazepine abuse and dependence. Br J Addict 81:87–94, 1986.
41. Pollack MH. Long-term management of panic disorder. J Clin Psychiatry 51(Suppl 5):11S–13S, 1990.
42. Rickels K. Buspirone in clinical practice. J Clin Psychiatry 51(Suppl 9):51S–54S, 1990.
43. Strand M, Hetta J, Rosen A, et al. A double-blind controlled trial in primary care patients with generalized anxiety: a comparison between buspirone and oxazepam. J Clin Psychiatry 51(Suppl 9):40–45, 1990.
44. Pato MT, Pigott TA, Hill JL, et al. Controlled comparison of buspirone and clomipramine in obsessive–compulsive disorder. Am J Psychiatry 148:127–129, 1991.
45. Munjack DJ, Bruns J, Baltazar PL, et al. A pilot study of buspirone in the treatment of social phobia. J Anxiety Disord 5:87–98, 1991.
46. de Montigny C, Blier P, Chaput Y. Electrophysiologically identified serotonin receptors in the rat CNS. Neuropharmacology 23:1511–1520, 1984.
47. Sharp T, Bramwell SR, Grahame-Smith DG. 5-HT_1 agonists reduce 5-hydroxytryptamine release in rat hippocampus in vivo as determined by brain microdialysis. Br J Pharmacol 96:283–290, 1989.
48. Smith LM, Peroutka SJ. Differential effects of 5-hydroxytryptamine selective drugs on the 5-HT behavioral syndrome. Pharmacol Biochem Behav 24:1513–1519, 1986.
49. Lucki I, Wieland S. 5-hydroxytryptamine receptors and behavioral responses. Neuropsychopharmacology 3:481–493, 1990.
50. Gammans RE, Mayol RF, Labudde JA. Metabolism and disposition of buspirone. Am J Med 80:41S–51S, 1986.
51. Mead Johnson Pharmaceutical Division/Bristol Myers. Buspar package insert. Evansville, IN, 1990.
52. Agras WS. Treatment of social phobias. J Clin Psychiatry 51(Suppl 10):52S–55S, 1990.
53. Liebowitz MR, Schneier F, Campeas R, et al. Phenelzine vs atenolol in social phobia. Arch Gen Psychiatry 49:290–300, 1992.
54. Kolb LC, Burris BC, Griffiths S. Propranolol and clonidine in the treatment of post traumatic stress disorder of war. In: van der Kolk BA, ed. Post traumatic stress disorders psychological and biological sequelae. Washington, DC: American Psychiatric Press, 1984:29–42.
55. United States Pharmacopeial Convention. USP-DI. 14th ed. Rockville, MD: United States Pharmacopeial Convention, 1994.
56. Noyes R. Beta-adrenergic blocking drugs in anxiety and stress. Psychiatr Clin North Am 8:119–132, 1985.
57. Rickels K, Downing R, Schweizer E, et al. Antidepressants for the treatment of generalized anxiety disorder: a placebo-controlled comparison of imipramine, trazodone, and diazepam. Arch Gen Psychiatry 50:884–895, 1993.
58. Sutherland SM, Davidson JRT. Pharmacotherapy for posttraumatic stress disorder. Psychiatr Clin North Am 17:409–423, 1994.
59. Noyes R, Garvey MJ, Cook BL, et al. Problems with tricyclic antidepressant use in patients with panic disorder or agoraphobia: results of a naturalistic follow-up study. J Clin Psychiatry 50:163–169, 1989.
60. Buigues J, Vallejo J. Therapeutic response to phenelzine in patients with panic disorder and agoraphobia with panic attacks. J Clin Psychiatry 48:55–59, 1987.
61. Frank JB, Kosten TR, Giller EL, et al. A randomized clinical trial of phenelzine and imipramine for posttraumatic stress disorder. Am J Psychiatry 145:1289–1291, 1988.
62. Rabkin J, Quitkin FM, Harrison W, et al. Adverse reactions to monoamine oxidase inhibitors. Part I. A comparative study. J Clin Psychopharmacol 4:270–278, 1984.
63. Maxmen JS. Psychotropic drugs fast facts. New York: WW Norton, 1991:104.
64. Freeman CPL, Timble MR, Deakin JFW, et al. Fluvoxamine versus clomipramine in the treatment of obsessive compulsive disorder: a multicenter, randomized, double-blind, parallel group comparison. J Clin Psychiatry 55:301–305, 1994.
65. Koran LM, McLeroy SL, Davison JRT, et al. Fluvoxamine versus clomipramine for obsessive compulsive disorder: a double blind comparison. J Clin Psychopharmacol 16:121–129, 1996.

66. Zohar J, Judge R. Paroxetine versus clomipramine in the treatment of obsessive–compulsive disorder. Br J Psychiatry 169:468–474, 1996.
67. Bisserbe JC, Lane RM, Filament MF, et al. A double-blind comparison of sertraline and clomipramine in outpatients with obsessive–compulsive disorder. Eur Psychiatry 12:82–93, 1997.
68. Pigott TA, Pato MT, Bernstein SE, et al. Controlled comparisons of clomipramine and fluoxetine in the treatment of obsessive–compulsive disorder. Arch Gen Psychiatry 47:926–932, 1990.
69. Hoehn-Saric R, McCleod DR, Hipsley PA. Effect of fluvoxamine on panic disorder. J Clin Psychopharmacol 13:321–326, 1993.
70. Black DW, Wesner R, Bowers W, et al. A comparison of fluvoxamine, cognitive therapy, and placebo in the treatment of panic disorder. Arch Gen Psychiatry 50:44–50, 1993.
71. Wade AG, Lepola U, Koponen HJ, et al. The effect of citalopram in panic disorder. Br J Psychiatry 170:549–553, 1997.
72. Michelson D, Lydiard RB, Pollack MH, et al. Outcome assessment and clinical improvement in panic disorder: evidence from a randomized controlled trial of fluoxetine and placebo. The Fluoxetine Panic Disorder Study Group. Am J Psychiatry 155:1570–1577, 1998.
73. Pollack MH, Otto MW, Worthington JJ, et al. Sertraline in the treatment of panic disorder: a flexible-dose multicenter trial. Arch Gen Psychiatry 55:1010–1016, 1998.
74. Londborg PD, Wolkow R, Smith WT, et al. Sertraline in the treatment of panic disorder. A multi-site, double-blind, placebo-controlled, fixed-dose investigation. Br J Psychiatry 173:54–60, 1998.
75. Pohl RB, Wolkow RM, Clary CM. Sertraline in the treatment of panic disorder: a double-blind multicenter trial. Am J Psychiatry 155:1189–1195, 1998.
76. Lecrubier Y, Judge R, and the Collaborative Paroxetine Panic Study Investigators. Long-term evaluation of paroxetine, clomipramine, and placebo in panic disorder. Acta Psychiatr Scand 95:153–160, 1997.
77. Ballenger JC, Wheadon DE, Steiner M, et al. Double-blind, fixed-dose, placebo-controlled study of paroxetine in the treatment of panic disorder. Am J Psychiatry 155:36–42, 1998.
78. Liebowitz MR. Pharmacotherapy of social phobia. J Clin Psychiatry 54(Suppl 12):31–35, 1993.
79. van Harten J. Clinical pharmacokinetics of selective serotonin reuptake inhibitors. Clin Pharmacokinet 24(3):203–220, 1993.
80. Coulter DM, Pillans PI. Fluoxetine and extrapyramidal side effects. Am J Psychiatry 152:122–125, 1995.
81. Lipinski JF, Mallya G, Zimmerman P, et al. Fluoxetine-induced akathisia: Clinical and theoretical implications. J Clin Psychiatry 50:339–342, 1989.
82. Leo RJ. Movement disorders associated with the serotonin selective reuptake inhibitors. J Clin Psychiatry 57:449–453, 1996.
83. Zajecka J, Tracy KA, Mitchell S. Discontinuation symptoms after treatment with serotonin reuptake inhibitors: a literature review. J Clin Psychiatry 58:291–297, 1997. United States Pharmacopeial Convention: USP-DI. 14th ed. Rockville, MD: United States Pharmacopeial Convention, 1994.
84. Margraf J, Barlow DH, Clark DM, et al. Psychological treatment of panic: work in progress on outcome, active ingredients, and follow-up. Behav Res Ther 31:1–8, 1993.
85. Beck AT, Sokol L, Clark DA, et al. A crossover study of focused cognitive therapy for panic disorder. Am J Psychiatry 149:778–783, 1992.
86. Otto MW, Gould RA, Pollack MH. Cognitive–behavioral treatment of panic disorder: considerations for the treatment of patients over the long term. Psychiatr Ann 24:307–315, 1994.
87. Sanderson WC, Wetzler S. Observations on the cognitive behavioral treatment of panic disorder: impact of benzodiazepines. Psychotherapy 30:125–132, 1993.
88. Taylor CB. Psychopharmacologic treatment of anxiety disorders. In: The American Psychiatric Press textbook of psychopharmacology. Washington, DC: American Psychiatric Press, ch. 32.
89. Barlow DH. Comorbidity in social phobia: implications for cognitive–behavioral treatment. Bull Menninger Clin 58(Suppl A):A43–A57, 1994.
90. Borkovec TD, Costello E. Efficacy of applied relaxation and cognitive–behavioral therapy in the treatment of generalized anxiety disorder. J Consult Clin Psychol 61:611–619, 1993.
91. Durham RC, Allan T. Psychological treatment of generalized anxiety disorder: a review of the clinical significance of results in outcome studies since 1980. Br J Psychiatry 163:19–26, 1993.
92. Munford PR, Hand I, Liberman RP. Psychosocial treatment for obsessive-compulsive disorder. Psychiatry 57:142–152, 1994.
93. McFarlane AC. Individual psychotherapy for post-traumatic stress disorder. Psychiatr Clin North Am 17:393–408, 1994.
94. Allen SN, Bloom SL. Group and family treatment of posttraumatic stress disorder. Psychiatr Clin North Am 17:425–437, 1994.
95. Sussman N. The uses of buspirone in psychiatry. J Clin Psychiatry 12:3–19, 1994.
96. Jackson CW, Morton A, Lydiard RB. Pharmacologic management of obsessive-compulsive disorder. South Med J 87:310–320, 1994.
97. McDougle CJ, Goodman WK, Price LH. The pharmacotherapy of obsessive-compulsive disorder. Pharmacopsychiatry 26(Suppl):24–29, 1993.
98. Silver JM, Sandberg DP, Hales RE. New approaches in the pharmacotherapy of posttraumatic stress disorder. J Clin Psychiatry 51(Suppl 10):33–38, 1990.
99. Social phobia: an overview of treatment strategies. J Clin Psychiatry 54:165–171, 1993.

CHAPTER 56

MOOD DISORDERS

Glen L. Stimmel

DEFINITION

The predominant feature of all four primary mood disorders is a disturbance in mood, but they must be distinguished from the more brief syndromes of sadness that may be part of many other conditions or temporary reactions to life stressors and from bereavement in response to a major loss. The primary mood disorders include major depression, dysthymia, bipolar disorders, and cyclothymia.

TREATMENT GOALS: MOOD DISORDERS

- Base treatment on chronic and recurrent nature of mood disorders.
- Eliminate acute symptoms in manic and depressive episodes.
- Apply maintenance therapy to prevent relapse (return of original symptoms) and recurrence (future manic or depressive episodes).

EPIDEMIOLOGY

The lifetime prevalence of major depression is 17%, spread fairly evenly over the age groups from 15 to 54 years, being twice as common in women as in men.[1] Among older adults living in the community, the prevalence of major depression is 3%, but it is 15 to 25% for those living in nursing homes, who have a 13% annual incidence of new episodes.[2] Dysthymia has a lifetime prevalence of 6% and is two to three times more common in women. Bipolar disorders appear in 1.3% of the population (0.8% bipolar I and 0.5% bipolar II), and cyclothymia occurs in 0.4 to 1.0%. Bipolar I disorder and cyclothymia are equally common in men and women, whereas bipolar II disorder is more common in women.[3]

PATHOPHYSIOLOGY

Although much is known about the mechanism of action of various antidepressant drugs and mood-stabilizing drugs, the exact etiology of mood disorders is not known. The most clearly established biologic fact regarding mood disorders is the existence of a genetic substrate, with genetic loading greatest in bipolar illness. At least two-thirds of patients with bipolar disorder have a positive family history of mood disorder. A compelling convergence of information from computed tomography, magnetic resonance imaging, positron emission tomography, and single-photon emission computed tomography studies of patients with depression suggest that this disorder is associated with regional brain dysfunction, particularly changes in blood flow and/or metabolism in the frontal-temporal cortex and caudate nucleus.[4]

There are many drugs reported to cause depression, but establishing a direct causative relationship is very difficult. No drug has been shown to be causally related to depression with as high a frequency as depression that occurs naturally. These drugs include many antihypertensives (reserpine, propranolol, methyldopa, and clonidine), hormones (estrogen and progesterone), corticosteroids, and antiparkinson drugs (levodopa and amantadine).[5]

CLINICAL PRESENTATION AND DIAGNOSIS

The diagnostic criteria and symptoms of the four major mood disorders are listed in Table 56.1.[3]

Major Depressive Disorder

Patients with major depressive disorder either have experienced one episode of depression or have recurrent depressive episodes. This disorder is commonly referred to as unipolar. The frequency of episodes is quite variable, with some patients having episodes separated by many years of normal functioning, whereas others have frequent clusters of episodes. Most patients with one major depressive episode will have more in the future. Of patients who recover from one depressive episode, 28% experience a recurrence within 1 year, 62% within 5 years, and 75% within 10 years. Only 18% who recover from the index episode remain free of depressive episodes throughout the subsequent 10 years.[6] The risk of completed suicide in patients with major depression is 15%, which is about 30 times the risk in the general population. Several subtypes of major depression, each requiring somewhat different treatment approaches, are listed in Table 56.2.[3] Double depressions present clinically as major depression, and only a careful history will detect the preexisting dysthymia. Successful treatment of psychotic depression requires use of an antipsychotic drug for several weeks to months in combination with the antidepressant drug. Electroconvulsive therapy remains the most effective treatment for psychotic depression.[7] Atypical depression presents with a reversal of the usual depressive symptoms, such as increased sleep and appetite. Monoamine oxidase inhibitors (MAOIs) have been shown to be more effective than tricyclic antidepressants (TCAs) for atypical depression. The newer antidepressants have not yet been compared to MAOIs for treatment of these depressions.[8] Seasonal affective disorder is unique in being responsive to sessions of bright light (2500 lux), given 1 to 2 hours each day.[9]

Table 56.1 ▪ Symptoms and Diagnostic Criteria for Mood Disorders

Major depressive episode: five or more of the following symptoms present nearly every day for 2 weeks:
- Depressed mood most of every day[a]
- Marked decreased interest or pleasure in most all activities (anhedonia)[a]
- Appetite or weight change (>5% body weight in 1 month)
- Insomnia or hypersomnia
- Psychomotor agitation or retardation
- Fatigue or loss of energy
- Worthlessness, excessive guilt
- Decreased ability to think or concentrate, indecisiveness
- Recurrent thoughts of death, suicidal ideation or attempt

Dysthymia: depressed mood most of the day, more days than not, for 2 years. When depressed, two of more of the following symptoms cause significant distress or impaired social or occupational functioning:
- Poor appetite or overeating
- Insomnia or hypersomnia
- Low energy or fatigue
- Low self-esteem
- Poor concentration or indecisiveness
- Feelings of hopelessness

Manic episode: distinct period of persistently elevated, expansive or irritable mood lasting at least 1 week characterized by at least 3 of the following:
- Inflated self-esteem or grandiosity
- Decreased need for sleep
- More talkative than usual; pressure to keep talking
- Flight of ideas; subjective experience that thoughts are racing
- Distractibility
- Increase in goal-directed activities; psychomotor agitation
- Excessive involvement in pleasurable activities that have a high potential for painful consequences (sexual, illegal, financial)
- Marked impairment in occupational functioning or usual social activities, or necessity to hospitalize to prevent harm to self or others, or psychotic symptoms

Hypomania: same symptoms as mania but last at least 4 days, without impaired social or occupational functioning and no psychotic symptoms or need to hospitalize

Cyclothymia: for at least 2 years, the presence of numerous periods of hypomanic symptoms and numerous periods of depressive symptoms that do not meet full criteria for mania or major depression

[a]One of these two symptoms must be present.

Table 56.2 ▪ Subtypes of Major Depression

Double depression: dysthymia with a superimposed major depressive episode

Major depression with psychotic features: most common psychotic symptom is delusions

Major depression with atypical features: depression characterized by mood reactivity, in which mood brightens in response to a positive event, plus two of the following:
- Increased appetite and weight gain
- Hypersomnia
- Leaden paralysis (heavy leaden feeling of arms and legs)
- Interpersonal rejection sensitivity (long-standing)

Major depression with seasonal pattern: episodes begin in fall or winter, remit in spring; 2 years of seasonal pattern necessary

Dysthymia

Dysthymia is different from the other three primary mood disorders in that it is characterized by chronic depressive symptoms rather than episodes of mood disturbance. As a chronic mild depression, dysthymia is most commonly encountered in primary care settings, is less often diagnosed and treated, and yet causes significant social and occupational dysfunction. Antidepressant drugs now have established efficacy in the treatment of dysthymia. A common clinical mistake is to give patients with dysthymia a lower dose of antidepressant because their depressive symptoms are less severe. For antidepressant drug treatment of dysthymia to be successful, full doses are necessary, just as if a major depression were being treated.[10,11]

Bipolar Disorder

Two types of bipolar disorder have been described, depending upon the severity of the manic episode. Bipolar

I disorder is characterized by full manic episodes and major depressive episodes, while bipolar II disorder has hypomanic and major depressive episodes (Table 56.1). The diagnosis of bipolar disorder requires only one episode of mania. Depression is not necessary for the diagnosis, but it is inevitable later in the course of the illness. After experiencing one manic episode, more than 90% of patients will have future episodes. The onset of mania is usually sudden and dramatic. Frequently manic patients do not recognize they are ill and resist treatment. Lability of mood is common, in which the mood can rapidly shift from one mood state to another. Many patients with bipolar disorder have an excellent work history between episodes, making prevention of relapse of critical importance. Mixed mania is a common type of bipolar illness in which manic and major depressive symptoms are present simultaneously. Rapid cycling is a term used for patients who experience four or more mood episodes in 1 year. Secondary mania is a term used to describe other causes for mania or hypomanic symptoms. Antidepressant drugs can precipitate a manic or hypomanic episode in patients with bipolar disorder, particularly when mood-stabilizing medication is not used in combination with the antidepressant. Glucocorticoids, such as prednisone, stimulant drugs, and hyperthyroidism are other examples of factors that cause secondary mania. Suicide attempts occur in about 25% of patients with bipolar disorder, with suicide completion rates of about 15%.[12]

Cyclothymia

Cyclothymia is a milder form of bipolar illness. It is a chronic mood disturbance of longer than 2 years characterized by numerous episodes of hypomania and depressions (Table 56.1).[2] Cyclothymia differs from bipolar type II disorder in that the depressive episodes in cyclothymia never meet the criteria for major depression. Cyclothymia is frequently found in relatives of patients with bipolar disorder, as if the patient with cyclothymia has the genetic potential for bipolar disorder but the full syndrome never develops. Patients with cyclothymia seldom require drug therapy, but when necessary, mood stabilizers are effective.

PSYCHOSOCIAL ASPECTS

Despite the primary role pharmacotherapy plays in the treatment of mood disorders, the psychosocial aspects of mood disorders must be identified and incorporated into a total treatment plan. At best, pharmacotherapy will eliminate symptoms of a manic or depressive episode, but the patient's day-to-day coping skills and strained relationships with family, friends, and work colleagues that result from the disorder must be addressed with supportive therapy.

THERAPEUTIC PLAN

Two national practice guidelines for treatment of major depression were published in 1993,[13,14] a consensus statement for depression in late life was updated in 1997,[15] and a practice guideline for bipolar disorders was published in 1994.[16] Two key concepts are fostered in the practice guidelines for major depression. The first is the need for continuation therapy for all patients and lifelong maintenance therapy for some patients (Table 56.3). Second, doses for continuation and maintenance therapy must be the same as the acute dose effective for eliminating depressive symptoms. When patients are given lower maintenance doses, their risk of relapse is much greater than when doses are maintained at acute dose levels. For example, patients successfully treated with paroxetine 40 mg daily given a 20-mg maintenance dose had a 52% recurrence of depression over 2 years compared to 24% recurrence with a maintenance dose of 40 mg daily.[17]

A growing concern is the undertreatment of major depression, both in its recognition in primary care settings and the often inadequate dose and duration of treatment when recognized.[18] Undertreatment of depression is a result of many factors that involve the patient, the provider, and health care systems. The shift toward primary care management of depression and away from specialty treatment raises concerns about quality of care and patient outcomes. Whereas the ideal pharmacotherapy for depression (Table 56.3) suggests that antidepressants can be effective in at least 70% of patients, the reality of care falls far short of that ideal. It is estimated that only 5 to 10% of patients with depression are effectively treated over the course of their lifetime.[19]

The key concept of the bipolar treatment guidelines is to decrease the frequency, severity, and psychosocial consequences of episodes and to improve psychosocial functioning between episodes. Inadequate treatment or delay in treatment of manic episodes may lead to substantial and prolonged financial, legal, and social consequences.

TREATMENT

Depressive Disorders

Pharmacotherapy

The many drug treatment options and effective dose ranges for depression in nonelderly adults are listed in Table 56.4. After three decades of use of TCAs, the last

Table 56.3 ▪ Ideal Dose and Duration of Antidepressant Therapy for Major Depression

Acute phase: 6–8 weeks at full therapeutic doses with the aim to reduce and eliminate symptoms

Continuation phase: all patients receive 4–9 months more at full therapeutic dose with the aim to prevent relapse and return of depressive symptoms

Maintenance phase

- For patients with history of 3 or more depressive episodes, maintain at full therapeutic dose for an additional 1–2 years
- For patients with a history of more than 2 episodes within 5 years, maintain at full therapeutic dose lifelong
- Aim is to prevent recurrence of future depressive episodes

Table 56.4 ▪ Effective Dosage Ranges of Antidepressant Drugs

Drug	Dose Range
Selective serotonin reuptake inhibitors (SSRIs)	
Fluoxetine (Prozac)	10–60
Sertraline (Zoloft)	50–200
Paroxetine (Paxil)	20–50
Fluvoxamine (Luvox)	100–200
Citalopram (Celexa)	20–60
Serotonin norepinephrine reuptake inhibitor	
Venlafaxine (Effexor)	225–375
Serotonin antagonist reuptake inhibitor	
Trazodone (Desyrel)	200–600
Nefazodone (Serzone)	300–600
Norepinephrine-dopamine reuptake inhibitor	
Bupropion (Wellbutrin)	300–450
Noradrenergic and specific serotonergic antidepressant	
Mirtazepine (Remeron)	15–45
Tricyclic antidepressants (TCAs)	
Amitriptyline (Elavil)	150–300
Clomipramine (Anafranil)	150–300
Desipramine (Norpramin)	50–150
Doxepin (Sinequan)	150–300
Imipramine (Tofranil)	150–300
Nortriptyline (Pamelor)	50–150
Protriptyline (Vivactil)	20–60
Trimipramine (Surmontil)	150–300
Monoamine oxidase inhibitors (MAOIs)	
Phenelzine (Nardil)	45–90
Tranylcypromine (Parnate)	20–50

decade has seen a continuing evolution in the development of unique drug treatment options, which have virtually eliminated TCAs as first-line therapy.

Clinical Relevance of Antidepressant Mechanisms

Selecting an antidepressant drug for a patient, as well as rational combination drug therapy, can now be based upon the unique differences in mechanism offered by the available antidepressants. Antidepressants began as pharmacologically "dirty" drugs, with the TCAs blocking reuptake of norepinephrine and to some extent serotonin (5-HT), but also having prominent antagonistic effects on muscarinic, histaminic, and adrenergic receptors. These latter effects caused the many adverse effects and toxicity of TCAs and led to frequent noncompliance with therapy. More recently, the TCAs have mostly been replaced by the "cleaner," more specific selective serotonin reuptake inhibitors (SSRIs), which selectively enhance serotonin. Thus, SSRIs have few to none of the cardiovascular, anticholinergic, and sedative effects so common with TCAs. But by increasing serotonin in every serotonin pathway and at each of the dozen or more receptor subtypes, the therapeutic benefits are accompanied by unwanted anxiety, insomnia, sexual dysfunction, and gastrointestinal disturbances. The most recent phase in the evolution of antidepressants was the return to multiple mechanisms but ones selected to reduce unwanted effects while maintaining efficacy. Venlafaxine is a potent SSRI, but it also blocks reuptake of norepinephrine. Although its adverse effect profile is similar to that of the SSRIs, its dual neurotransmitter effect is suggested to offer enhanced efficacy. Nefazodone has selective serotonergic effects, but has an added mechanism of blocking postsynaptic 5-HT_2 receptors, preventing the sexual dysfunction so common with SSRIs. Finally mirtazepine, through α_2 adrenergic blockade, has the dual effect of enhancing both norepinephrine and serotonin, plus postsynaptically blocking both the 5-HT_2 and 5-HT_3 receptors, preventing the sexual dysfunction, anxiogenic, and gastrointestinal adverse effects. This continuing evolution in antidepressant mechanisms allows the clinician to select and modify drug regimens to meet the needs of individual patients.[20–22]

Tricyclic Antidepressants

TCAs are very effective antidepressants but with an adverse effect profile that limits their use in both acute and maintenance phases of treatment (Table 56.5). One advantage TCAs have over newer antidepressants is that plasma levels can be used to determine an effective TCA dose. TCAs with a well-established correlation of plasma level range with antidepressant efficacy include nortriptyline (50 to 150 ng/mL), desipramine (100 to 160 ng/mL), amitriptyline (75 to 175 ng/mL), and imipramine (>200 ng/mL).[23]

Table 56.5 ▪ Common Adverse Effect Profiles of Antidepressants

Drug	Sedation	Anticholinergic	Orthostatic Hypertension
Amitriptyline	High	High	High
Imipramine	Moderate	Moderate	High
Clomipramine	High	High	High
Doxepin	High	High	High
Nortriptyline	Moderate	Moderate	Moderate
Desipramine	Low	Low	Low
Phenelzine	Moderate	Low	Very high
Tranylcypromine	Low	Low	Very high

Drug	Activation	Gastrointestinal	Sexual Dysfunction
Fluoxetine	High	High	High
Sertraline	Moderate	High	High
Paroxetine	Low	High	High
Fluvoxamine	Sedation	High	High
Citalopram	Very low	High	High
Venlafaxine	Moderate	High	High
Bupropion	High	Moderate	Very low
Nefazodone	Sedation	Low	Very low
Mirtazepine	Sedation	Very low	Very low

Nortriptyline is unique in having a curvilinear response, or therapeutic window, in which clinical efficacy declines as the level exceeds 150 ng/mL. Plasma level monitoring is not routine, but indicated when there is a lack of response at therapeutic doses, significant adverse effects at lower doses, suspected noncompliance, or the stopping or starting of known enzyme inhibitors or inducers, and in older adults. Initial common, dose-related adverse effects include sedation, anticholinergic effects, and orthostatic hypotension. With maintenance therapy, weight gain is the most common adverse effect and is often responsible for discontinuation of therapy. A major disadvantage of TCAs is the lethality of overdoses. Overdoses of more than 2000 mg (a 10-day supply) of a TCA alone can be fatal.

Monoamine Oxidase Inhibitors

MAOIs are effective antidepressants and are particularly indicated for atypical depression and treatment-resistant depression. Phenelzine and tranylcypromine are equal in efficacy with similar adverse effects; phenelzine is more likely to be sedating while tranylcypromine is more likely to be activating. It is their orthostatic hypotensive effects that limit the initial dose and rate of dose titration. Severe hypertensive reactions after ingestion of foods containing high concentrations of tyramine is rare, but the risk can be minimized by careful monitoring and individually targeted dietary assessment and education. The severity of the reaction depends upon many factors. Six milligrams of tyramine produces mild elevation of blood pressure, 10 mg has a marked pressor effect, and 25 mg can result in a severe hypertensive crisis. The patient first becomes aware of a sudden-onset, painful, throbbing, occipital headache that, if severe, may progress to profuse sweating and palpitation. The foods for the patient to absolutely avoid include all aged cheeses and meats, concentrated yeast extracts, sauerkraut, and broad bean pods (fava beans). Most patients can safely continue their MAOI drug therapy and eat in moderation many foods that are listed on MAOI diets. Although foods have received most of the attention, several drugs are more dangerous than foods in combination with MAOIs. These include sympathomimetics (ephedrine and phenylpropanolamine), stimulants (amphetamines and cocaine), levodopa and meperidine, buspirone, venlafaxine, and SSRIs.[24]

Stimulants

Controversy continues about whether psychostimulant drugs have any value in the treatment of mood disorders. Nine of 10 placebo-controlled trials do not support their use in outpatients with mild to moderate depression. Stimulants have no place in the treatment of major depression. They were shown to be effective as brief, low-dose therapy for apathetic institutionalized geriatric patients, with the expectation that depressed mood would improve partially at best. Methylphenidate 20 to 30 mg/day for 2 to 4 weeks is usually tolerated well, with exacerbation of preexisting anxiety the only consistent adverse effect.[25]

Selective Serotonin Reuptake Inhibitors

The widespread acceptance and prescribing of SSRIs coupled with the declining use of TCAs in the 1990s are a result of their lesser lethality with overdoses, relative lack of cardiovascular and anticholinergic effects, and convenience because dosage titration is often unnecessary. An effective SSRI dose for depression is generally lower than that necessary to treat other disorders such as obsessive-compulsive disorder, panic disorder, and bulimia. The initial dose of fluoxetine should be 10 mg once daily in the morning, most patients require 20 mg daily, with 40 mg occasionally being necessary. Sertraline is given initially at 50 mg followed by dose titration in most patients to an effective dose of 100 to 150 mg daily. Paroxetine can be initiated at either 10 to 20 mg at bedtime, with most patients requiring doses of 20 to 40 mg.[26] Fluvoxamine should begin at 50 mg at bedtime, increased to 100 to 150 mg daily. Citalopram can begin at its minimally effective dose of 20 mg, with some patients requiring 30 to 40 mg daily. All five SSRIs can be given once daily.

As a group, the SSRIs cause the same common adverse effects, namely some degree of activation and insomnia, gastrointestinal (GI) distress, and sexual dysfunction (Table 56.5). There is no consistent evidence that the likelihood of GI effects or sexual dysfunction will differ among the five SSRIs if given in equivalent doses.[27–31] The expected degree of activation versus sedation does differ, with fluoxetine being the most likely to be activating, whereas paroxetine and fluvoxamine are the least activating, with some patients even experiencing mild sedation. These differences suggest a recommendation of either morning or bedtime daily dosing. Extrapyramidal-like movement disorders have been reported with SSRIs, probably caused by increased serotonergic input to dopaminergic pathways.[32] Fluoxetine has been associated with 75% of all reported cases, although it has been the most commonly prescribed SSRI, and in half of the reported cases, use of other medication may have played a causative role in the movement disorders.

The most likely sexual dysfunction caused by serotonergic agonists is delayed ejaculation in men and anorgasmia in women. Current estimates are that at least 20 to 30% of patients taking SSRIs, venlafaxine, or clomipramine experience sexual dysfunction, with some reports indicating 67 to 96%.[33] TCAs and MAOIs commonly cause sexual dysfunction as well but at a slightly lower frequency. Only bupropion, nefazodone, and mirtazepine are relatively free of sexual dysfunction effects and represent the best alternative antidepressants when treatment must be changed. For patients who are responding well to their SSRI but for whom sexual dysfunction threatens compliance, either nefazodone 150 mg or mirtazepine 15 mg, adjunctively owing to their 5-HT_2 blockade, will treat the sexual dysfunction and allow continuation of the effective antidepressant. Although a dose-related effect, sexual dysfunction should not be managed by decreasing the dose of the antidepressant because continuation and maintenance doses should be the same as the acute dose. Serotonin antagonists such as cyproheptadine have also been used, but may interfere with the antidepressant effect of the SSRI. Yohimbine and sildenafil are not effective for SSRI-induced delayed ejaculation or anorgasmia, but are useful for erectile dysfunction.[34]

When SSRIs are discontinued, they must be gradually tapered rather than abruptly stopped. A gradual taper allows monitoring for signs of relapse, with a prompt resumption of drug therapy if seen. An SSRI discontinuation syndrome has recently been defined, which includes symptoms of dizziness, problems with balance, insomnia, fatigue, nausea, irritability, anxiety/agitation, flu-like chills, and headache.[35,36] It is more common with the shorter half-life SSRIs (paroxetine and fluvoxamine); symptoms may last up to 3 weeks but are rapidly reversed upon resumption of the original medication.

All SSRIs must be used cautiously in patients receiving other serotonin agonists, because fatalities have been reported from a serotonin syndrome. The drugs of greatest concern are the MAOIs, with caution also necessary with bupropion and other serotonergic antidepressants.[21,37] Common symptoms of serotonergic syndrome include fever, diaphoresis, myoclonus, tremor, confusion, and diarrhea. Cardiovascular collapse, coma, and death are rare but possible.

Four of the SSRIs are potent inhibitors of cytochrome P-450 isoenzymes, creating the potential for drug interactions with other drugs that rely on these isoenzymes for their metabolism. Citalopram is unique as the one SSRI without significant effect on cytochrome P-450 isoenzymes, while the other four SSRIs and nefazodone are potent inhibitors. Venlafaxine, bupropion, and mirtazepine also have no clinically important effects on these isoenzymes. Table 56.6 lists a representative sample of potential drug-drug interactions of concern in which inhibition of the metabolism of substrate drugs may lead to increased blood levels and adverse effects.[38,39] Information on drug-drug interactions as listed in Table 56.6 is constantly changing, so it should not be viewed as comprehensive or completely correct after its date of writing. The clinical outcome of such interactions is highly variable and unpredictable–some drugs that interact may be used together if there is adequate monitoring and adjustment of dosage.

Table 56.6 ▪ Antidepressants and Cytochrome P-450 Drug Interactions

CYP Isozyme	Inhibitors	Substrate Drugs of Concern
1A2	Fluvoxamine	Theophylline, caffeine, warfarin, tacrine, haloperidol, acetaminophen, TCAs, clozapine, olanzapine
2D6	Paroxetine, fluoxetine, sertraline	Propranolol, timolol, metoprolol, desipramine, nortriptyline, risperidone, codeine, dextromethorphan, phenothiazines, type 1C antiarrhythmics (encainide, flecainide), venlafaxine, bupropion
3A4	Fluvoxamine, nefazodone	Terfenadine, astemizole, cisapride, steroids, triazolobenzodiazepines (alprazolam, triazolam, midazolam), erythromycin, nifedipine, diltiazem, verapamil, zolpidem, cyclosporine, tamoxifen, indinavir, ritonavir, saquinavir, warfarin

CYP, cytochrome P-450; *TCAs,* tricyclic antidepressants.

Venlafaxine

Venlafaxine causes potent serotonin reuptake blockade as well as reuptake blockade of norepinephrine. Unlike SSRIs, it requires dose titration and must be given in divided doses unless the extended-release formulation is used. Initial recommended doses of 37.5 mg BID result in many patients experiencing nausea, so 18.75 mg BID is a better tolerated initial dose.[26] Most patients require 225 mg daily, with some needing up to 375 mg. The extended-release formulation allows once daily dosing, but offers no distinct advantage in terms of GI adverse effects.[40] Venlafaxine has an adverse effect profile similar to that of the SSRIs (Table 56.5), with a unique effect of sustained increased diastolic pressure at higher doses. In doses up to 225 mg, venlafaxine has virtually no effect on blood pressure, but at 375 mg daily, the mean increase in diastolic blood pressure was 7.5 mm Hg.[41] Regular blood pressure monitoring is necessary for venlafaxine. It has no clinically important inhibitory effect on cytochrome P-450 isoenzymes.

Nefazodone and Trazodone

Nefazodone has SSRI activity coupled with potent postsynaptic 5-HT_{2A} antagonism. Its most common adverse effects include initial sedation and orthostatic hypotension, so initial doses must be lower and divided. An initial dose of 50 mg in the morning and 100 mg at bedtime can be titrated upward to the minimum effective dose of 150 mg BID as quickly as tolerated by the patient. Once an effective dose is established, nefazodone can be given once daily at bedtime.[26] Nefazodone has established efficacy for severe depression, which is a continuing controversy for SSRIs possibly being less effective for more severe depression. Nefazodone shares with bupropion the unique effect of increasing rapid eye movement (REM) sleep and normalizing sleep architecture while TCAs and SSRIs decrease REM sleep and worsen sleep architecture.[42,43] Its 5-HT_{2A} blocking effect is responsible for nefazodone not causing the sexual dysfunction so commonly seen with other serotonergic antidepressants. Nefazodone is a potent inhibitor of cytochrome P-450 3A4, giving it the potential for different drug interactions compared to SSRIs (Table 56.6).

Trazodone is an effective antidepressant, but because of its sedative and orthostatic hypotensive effects it is difficult for most patients to achieve a therapeutic daily dose of 300 to 600 mg. Trazodone has undergone a resurgence of use as an adjunctive treatment with SSRIs or bupropion and as a hypnotic drug in doses of 50 to 100 mg at bedtime.[44] A rare but serious adverse effect of trazodone requiring patient counseling is priapism. Trazodone is responsible for more than 80% of all drug-induced cases of priapism, and the mechanism is thought to be related to unopposed α-adrenergic blockade. Sustained painful penile erection, if untreated, leads to permanent impotence in most patients. Immediate treatment is required, involving intracavernosal α-adrenergic agonists. Priapism has occurred with single doses of trazodone as low as 50 mg, so all male patients receiving trazodone must be counseled about this rare but potentially serious adverse effect.[34] Nefazodone, although similar in mechanism, has only 5% of trazodone's α-adrenergic blocking effect and has not caused priapism.[45,46]

Bupropion

Bupropion is an activating antidepressant with a unique mechanism of action that essentially lacks cardiovascular, anticholinergic, and sexual dysfunction effects.[47] The finding of high seizure rates among bulimic patients treated with bupropion resulted in eventual marketing with limitations on the rate of dose escalation and maximum dosage. This complex dosing schedule, coupled with concern regarding seizures, limited the use of bupropion as a first-line agent. Development of a subsequent sustained-release preparation has simplified the dosing schedule. Although daily doses of up to 450 mg are associated with a 0.4% risk of seizures, the risk dropped to 0.1% with sustained-release bupropion up to 300 mg daily.[26] Sustained-release bupropion can be given in a maximum single dose of 200 mg, so its therapeutically effective dose of 300 mg/day must be given in a BID schedule. Immediate-release bupropion can be given in a maximum of 150 mg/dose, so TID dosing is necessary if the dose exceeds 300 mg/day.[48] Bupropion has a mild dopamine agonist effect, meaning it may worsen preexisting psychotic symptoms. Bupropion has developed the reputation that it is less likely to cause patients with bipolar depression to switch into mania, so it has become a commonly used antidepressant in patients with bipolar disorder.[49]

Mirtazepine

Mirtazepine provides both serotonin and norepinephrine agonist effects coupled with postsynaptic blockade of $5\text{-}HT_2$ and $5\text{-}HT_3$ receptors. This unique mechanism maintains clinical efficacy for depression while minimizing the activating, GI, and sexual dysfunction effects so common with SSRIs.[50] Its common adverse effects include sedation and weight gain, both of which are inversely related to dose. Thus, in contrast to what would normally be expected, if these symptoms occur, the dose should be increased rather than lowered. The initial dose is 15 mg at bedtime, with an effective dose range of 15 to 45 mg. To minimize sedation and increased appetite, it is possible to begin therapy with 30 mg at bedtime.[26] In addition to its use as a single agent for depression, mirtazepine has been used as an adjunct to SSRIs to treat the GI and sexual dysfunction effects.

Nonpharmacologic Therapy

Electroconvulsive Therapy

Electroconvulsive therapy (ECT) remains the most effective treatment available for psychotic depression and treatment-resistant depressions. It is more effective and has a more rapid onset of effect than drug therapy. Disadvantages of ECT include frequent relapse after treatment termination, temporary cognitive impairment, a significant social stigma concerning its use, and in many states, legal barriers to its use. After a successful course of ECT, there is a 50% risk of relapse within the next 12 months unless maintenance antidepressant drug therapy is given. Although ECT was misused and overused before the 1970s, modification of ECT by anesthesia and neuromuscular blocking drugs make it a safe and humane treatment option. A series of two to three ECT treatments weekly for 2 to 3 weeks is usually effective. Although the use ECT often is more a political or legal issue than a therapeutic issue, it should be viewed as a treatment option that can be life-saving for patients who otherwise would not recover from their depressive illness.[51,52]

Psychotherapy

A variety of psychotherapies are available as either a sole treatment or as an adjunct to antidepressant medication. Interpersonal psychotherapy, cognitive-behavioral therapy, behavioral therapy, brief dynamic therapy, and marital therapy have all been used in the treatment of depression. These psychotherapies have been shown to often be effective for mild to moderate depression, but studies of continuation or maintenance therapy are lacking. Whereas medication at best can eliminate the symptoms of depression, psychotherapy is best at assisting the patient develop day-to-day coping skills that may assist in preventing relapse. Thus, a combination of medication and psychotherapy yields the best results.[14,53]

Alternative Therapies

It is often assumed that herbal medicines are either effective and completely safe or completely ineffective. Neither is true regarding St. John's wort (*Hypericum perforatum*). A meta-analysis of 23 randomized trials in mild to moderate depression found St. John's wort to be more effective than placebo. Comparison to standard antidepressants in fewer trials found an equal reduction of symptoms, but antidepressant doses were inadequate, and no information is available regarding efficacy in more severe depression.[54,55] Hypericin, a reddish pigment, has been the focus of attention as the likely active antidepressant compound in St. John's wort. Although initially thought to have MAOI activity, pure hypericin lacks MAO activity, and other flavanoid components may be responsible for its antidepressant activity. Doses of hypericin have ranged from 0.2 to 1.0 mg or total plant extract of 2 to 4 g. Thus, there is no established effective dose range, and standardization of *Hypericum* extracts for hypericin content is no guarantee of pharmacologic equivalence.[56] In the meta-analysis, 20% of patients taking St. John's wort reported side effects, which included GI symptoms, photosensitivity and allergy, and fatigue. The uncertainty of the MAO inhibition mechanism raises the potential for food and drug interactions, but none has yet been reported. Combinations of SSRIs and St. John's wort should be used cautiously until the potential for interaction is understood.

Bipolar Disorders

The goal of treatment of bipolar disorders is to reestablish euthymia by acutely treating episodes of mania, hypomania, or depression, and further, to prevent future episodes with maintenance drug therapy. At any one time, a patient with bipolar disorder may be manic, hypomanic, depressed, or euthymic. Mood stabilizers, including lithium and several anticonvulsant drugs, are used in all phases of the disorder in both the acute and maintenance phase of therapy. Treatment of bipolar disorder is characterized by the use of multiple medications rather than monotherapy. Mood stabilizers are very commonly used in combination with antipsychotic drugs or benzodiazepines for manic episodes, and in combination with antidepressants for depressive episodes.[57] Treating a depressive episode in a patient with bipolar disorder is the same as treatment of a major depressive disorder as discussed earlier, with the exception that a mood stabilizer should be used along with the antidepressant. Use of an antidepressant alone carries a great risk of pharmacologically switching the patient abruptly from depression to mania. An expert consensus guideline for treatment of depression in bipolar disorder suggests that either bupropion or SSRIs are the preferred antidepressants in combination with a mood stabilizer. A common belief is that bupropion is the least likely among antidepressants to cause a switch into mania based upon its unique mechanism of action[58] and that there is a greater risk with TCAs than with SSRIs. A number of cases of induction of mania with bupropion and SSRIs have been reported, however, suggesting the need for a mood stabilizer even with these antidepressants.[59,60]

Lithium

The fact that a simple chemical element of nature can have such a profound clinical effect in treating bipolar disorder is amazing. The introduction of lithium in the United States in 1970 provided for the first time an effective treatment for mania, replacing the marginally effective use of chlorpromazine at 2000 to 6000 mg/day or excessive doses of sedative-hypnotics. Lithium was also the first drug with proven prophylactic value as maintenance therapy for patients with bipolar disorder. Lithium was very slow to gain acceptance, however, because lithium chloride was used in the 1940s as a salt substitute in cardiac patients, resulting in many instances of serious toxicity and deaths.

Lithium has proven efficacy for acute treatment of manic episodes and in the prevention of recurrent manic and depressive episodes in patients with bipolar disorder.[16] In addition, lithium is equal to antidepressants as maintenance therapy to prevent recurrence in unipolar major depression. Finally, lithium is the most effective of all adjunctive treatments to add to an antidepressant for treatment-resistant depression.[61] Lithium is effective in 60 to 90% of patients with an acute manic episode, but much less effective for patients with mixed mania and those who experience rapid cycling.[62] Lithium's mechanism of action is still unknown despite many hypotheses. Current investigations are focusing on lithium's subcellular effects of decreasing the increased G protein activity observed in patients with bipolar disorder and lithium's ability to decrease second messenger activity, including cyclic adenosine monophosphate and phosphatidylinositol.[63]

PHARMACOKINETICS. Lithium carbonate is almost completely absorbed from the GI tract within 8 hours of oral administration, with peak blood levels achieved in 2 to 4 hours. Peak concentration from a single 600-mg dose is 0.45 to 0.85 mEq/L. The initial distribution volume corresponds to the extracellular fluid space, with a final volume of distribution of 0.8 to 1.2 L/kg. Lithium is not bound to proteins or metabolized, but is excreted unchanged in the urine. Lithium is freely filtered through the glomerulus, with about 80% being reabsorbed in the proximal tubule, competing with sodium. Its average plasma elimination half-life is 18 to 24 hours.[64,65] Compared to younger patients, older adults eliminate lithium more slowly from a smaller volume of distribution. The elimination half-life of lithium in older adults is about 25% longer than in younger patients, typically ranging up to 36 hours. Older patients require one-third to one-half less lithium doses than younger patients.[66]

There is very good correlation of clinical response and adverse effects to lithium levels. For acute mania, levels of 0.9 to 1.2 mEq/L are often adequate, whereas levels as high as 1.5 mEq/L are occasionally necessary. Maintenance levels of 0.6 to 0.8 mEq/L are effective for most patients, but relapse rates are lower if levels are maintained at 0.6 to 1.2 mEq/L[67] (Table 56.7). Levels greater than 1.5 mEq/L are regularly associated with signs of toxicity, and levels greater than 2.0 mEq/L result in serious toxicity. The narrow range between therapeutic and toxic levels make plasma level monitoring mandatory for all patients receiving lithium. A 12-hour interval between the last dose

Table 56.7 ▪ Therapeutic Dose and Levels of Mood Stabilizers

Drug	Oral Dose Range (mg/day)	Plasma Level
Lithium		
Acute	1500–2400	0.8–1.2 mEq/L
Chronic	900–1500	0.6–0.8 mEq/L
Valproate	750–4000	50–120 mg/L

Table 56.8 ▪ Lithium Steady-State Prediction

Day	Lithium Received (mg)	Plasma Level (mEq/L)
1	900	
2	900	0.51
3	900	

Blood is drawn on morning of Day 3 before lithium administration, so 0.51 represents 2 days of 900 mg. Assuming a 24-hour half-life, 0.51 represents 75% of the steady-state (ss) level.

Estimated ss level at 900 mg/day = 100/75 x 0.51 = 0.68 mEq/L.

For each 300 mg/day added, the new ss level will increase 0.15 to 0.35 mEq/L. Thus, to reach the desired level of 1.0 mEq/L, the dose should increase by 300 mg:

Estimated ss level at 1200 mg/day = (0.68 + 0.15) to (0.68 + 0.35) = 0.83 to 1.03 mEq/L.

and drawing the blood sample in a patient receiving the same divided daily dose for at least 1 week yields a standardized lithium level that is reproducible.

Dosing. For acute manic episodes, a daily dose of 1500 to 2400 mg is usually necessary to achieve a plasma level near 1.0 mEq/L. The initial dose must be smaller and divided to assess tolerance to the initial adverse effects. A typical starting dose of 300 mg TID is conservative and can be increased by 300-mg increments every 2 to 3 days. More aggressive dosing titration may be necessary for some inpatients whose manic symptoms are severe and whose past history indicates the need for higher doses. A plasma level measured 2 to 3 days after initiation of therapy can be used to calculate the steady-state level at that dose, with subsequent 300-mg dose increments yielding a plasma level increase of 0.15 to 0.35 mEq/L (Table 56.8).[68] A loading dose of 30 mg/kg of slow-release lithium given in three divided doses over 6 hours has been shown to accurately predict a 12-hour level of 1.0 mEq/L without adverse effects.[69] Once a patient has reproducible blood levels at the same dose and is on maintenance therapy, monthly blood levels are sufficient. Initiation of lithium for outpatient prophylaxis should be done very conservatively because the patient is not symptomatic and adverse effects may affect compliance. A reasonable starting dose is 300 mg BID, with weekly 300-mg dose increments. An oral daily dose of 900 to 1500 mg usually yields lithium plasma levels within the maintenance range of 0.6 to 0.8 mEq/L. For most patients, the acute phase dose and blood level can be reduced by about one-third for maintenance therapy.[70] Before lithium is begun, a physical examination and history should focus on detection of cardiovascular, endocrine, and renal disease. Baseline tests should include serum creatinine, blood urea nitrogen, complete blood count, urinalysis, thyroid function tests, electrolytes, serum calcium, pregnancy test in women of childbearing age, and an electrocardiogram if the patient is older than 40 or has cardiovascular disease.

Lithium Adverse Effects. Adverse effects and their relationship to therapeutic or toxic lithium levels, as well as non–dose-related adverse effects are listed in Table 56.9. Although the list is long, many patients with a carefully monitored and adjusted plasma level experience few if any significant adverse effects. The most common adverse effects are polyuria, polydipsia, and weight gain. The most bothersome effects that lead to noncompliance, however, are weight gain, confusion, and mental slowness.[71] Most of the dose-related effects are related to peak plasma levels, so use of a slow release preparation or bedtime dosing often minimizes these effects. The most common renal effect of lithium is impaired concentrating capacity owing to reduced renal response to antidiuretic hormone, manifested as polyuria and secondary polydipsia. The mild polyuria seen early in treatment resolves in most patients, with few patients being troubled by persistent polyuria. Persistent polyuria can be mild and well tolerated, but may progress to nephrogenic diabetes insipidus, characterized by urine output of greater than 3 L/day and urine specific gravity as low as 1.002 to 1.005. Polyuria may be managed by changing to once-daily dosing and lowering the dose as low as clinically possible, and in severe cases, addition of either hydrochlorothiazide 25 to 50 mg or amiloride 5 to 20 mg/day. Use of amiloride is preferred because it does not affect lithium levels or potassium levels.[16] Much concern has been raised about the long-term renal effects of lithium. Although 10 to 20% of patients display morphologic renal changes, there is no reduction in glomerular filtration rate or development of renal insufficiency. There are reports of a few patients developing a rising serum creatinine after 10 years of lithium therapy.[16]

Table 56.9 ▪ Lithium Adverse Effects

Dose-related	
Therapeutic levels	Nausea, diarrhea, polyuria, polydipsia, cognitive impairment, fine hand tremor (intention tremor), muscle weakness
Signs of toxicity	Coarse hand tremor, persistent nausea, diarrhea, slurred speech, confusion, seizures, increased deep tendon reflexes, irregular pulse, hypotension, coma
Non–dose-related	Nephrogenic diabetes insipidus, goiter, hypothyroidism, hypercalcemia, weight gain, macropapular or acneiform reactions, benign leukocytosis

GI effects are most apparent during the first week of therapy or after a dosage increase and are directly related to peak plasma levels. Taking lithium with food and a switch to the slow-release formulation successfully manages the nausea. Cognitive impairment is usually manifest as dulling, impaired memory, poor concentration, confusion, and mental slowness. It is difficult to detect while a patient manifests either manic or depressive symptoms, but becomes more problematic during maintenance therapy. A fine hand tremor is seen in up to 50% of patients initially and may persist. Lithium tremor is not a resting tremor, is not extrapyramidal based, and is usually noticeable upon voluntary movement. Most patients are unaware of the tremor; it becomes noticeable only when delicate movements are attempted such as drinking coffee or eating soup. Management of tremor includes dose reduction if possible, reduction of caffeine intake, and as a last resort, addition of a β-blocker. Propranolol 40 to 80 mg/day or metoprolol 50 to 100 mg/day is an effective treatment option.

Lithium toxicity is usually seen when plasma levels exceed 1.5 mEq/L, although signs of toxicity have been frequently reported with therapeutic levels in older adults. Signs and symptoms of toxicity include worsening of many of the effects seen at therapeutic levels (marked tremor, severe nausea, and diarrhea), plus central effects of slurred speech, vertigo, and increased confusion. Both patients and family members should be counseled about recognizing the signs of toxicity and instructed to contact their prescriber immediately if these effects are seen. Lithium intoxication represents a serious medical emergency. Mild intoxication can quickly become severe if the patient continues lithium but stops eating because of worsening GI effects. Several days of fasting coupled with diarrhea means significant sodium loss, leading to increased lithium reabsorption and even higher levels. Hemodialysis is indicated when the lithium level exceeds 4.0 mEq/L, if the patient has renal failure, or if electrolyte and fluid balance cannot be maintained. Fatalities are uncommon and are usually a result of renal failure or cardiovascular collapse, whereas persistent neurologic and renal sequelae are more common.[16,72]

Lithium's endocrine and metabolic effects include the potential for a diffuse nontender goiter in 5% of patients, with an equal number becoming hypothyroid. Lithium inhibits the synthesis and release of thyroid-stimulating hormone (TSH) and inhibits the action of TSH. The most consistent laboratory finding is an elevated TSH level seen in about 30% of patients. A persistent elevated TSH for more than 3 months indicates replacement therapy with L-thyroxine. Thyroid function should be evaluated every 6 to 12 months, along with regular examination of the patient's neck for signs of goiter and eyes for exophthalmos. In the first year of lithium therapy, patients gain an average of 4 kg, with 20% gaining more than 10 kg. Intake of high-caloric fluids is common owing to polydipsia, so patients should be counseled to drink water rather than sodas or juices.

Lithium may aggravate preexisting dermatologic conditions, especially acne and psoriasis. Leukocytosis during lithium therapy is secondary to neutrophilia accompanied by lymphocytopenia. The mean white blood cell increase is 3000 to 4000/mm^3 and is without the shift to the left seen in an infectious process. Although this is a benign effect, it is useful to obtain a baseline complete blood count before starting lithium.

Drug Interactions. There are relatively few drug-drug interactions of concern, but even a small increase in a lithium level can lead to severe adverse effects and toxicity. Thiazide diuretics reduce lithium clearance within several days, causing lithium levels to rise as much as 50%. The combination of drugs can be used, but lithium dosage must be reduced and plasma level monitoring increased. Nonsteroidal anti-inflammatory drugs, particularly indomethacin, naproxen, and ibuprofen, decrease lithium clearance and may increase lithium levels by 20 to 60% after 3 to 7 days of concurrent use. Sulindac and aspirin do not significantly affect lithium levels. Angiotensin-converting enzyme inhibitors and calcium channel blockers may also substantially increase lithium levels by as much as 100 to 200%. Although all of these combinations may be used together, adjustment of the lithium dose and closer plasma level monitoring are indicated.[73]

Lithium and Pregnancy. Any woman of childbearing age should be using a contraceptive method while taking lithium and a pregnancy test is mandatory before starting lithium therapy. The teratogenicity of lithium is well established, with demonstrated malformations of the heart and large vessels in 4 to 12% of babies born to lithium-treated mothers versus 2–4% in untreated comparison groups.[74,75] Because the cardiovascular system is formed during weeks 3 to 9 after conception, lithium is contraindicated during the first trimester of pregnancy. Because other mood stabilizers such as valproate are also best avoided in the first trimester, symptomatic treatment with antipsychotic or antidepressant drugs is preferred if any drug treatment is necessary. Lithium may be used if absolutely necessary during the second and third trimesters, but should be discontinued or the dosage reduced by 50% several weeks before the due date. The dehydration associated with labor and fluid shifts during delivery may lead to toxicity in the mother otherwise. Lithium should be resumed a few days after delivery with a reduced dose to counteract the increased risk of postpartum mania and depression. Infants breast fed by mothers taking lithium have serum concentrations 10 to 50% of the mother's level, causing most clinicians to advise against breastfeeding while taking lithium.[16,75]

Valproate

Only valproate's use as a mood stabilizer is reviewed in this chapter. Valproate is now considered an equally effective first-line mood stabilizer compared to lithium. Valproate is equal in efficacy to lithium for classic mania, and more effective than lithium for patients who experience rapid cycling, patients with bipolar disorder with comorbid substance abuse, and patients with mixed mania.[62] Because patients with mixed mania represent 40 to 50% of acutely manic patients, these efficacy differences suggest that valproate will supplant lithium as the most commonly used mood stabilizer. Valproate has minimal antidepressant activity, and is more effective in preventing manic than depressive episodes.[16,76]

Valproate may be initiated in low divided doses, such as 250 mg TID, to minimize the initial GI adverse effects. The dose can be titrated upward by 250 to 500 mg/day every several days based upon tolerance to adverse effects, to reach the target level of 50 to 120 mg/L (Table 56.7).[57] For patients with acute mania, valproate can be safely given in a loading dose of 20 mg/kg/day in a divided schedule to achieve levels of at least 50 mg/L within 24 hours.[77] In patients responsive to valproate, onset of clinical effect occurred within the first 3 days of therapy. Because 7 to 10 days are typically required for onset of lithium's clinical response, this difference may be of both clinical and pharmacoeconomic importance.[78] Once an optimal dose has been achieved, the total daily dose may be given at bedtime to maximize compliance and convenience.

Other Mood Stabilizers

Because some patients may not respond to or tolerate lithium and valproate, there is a need for alternatives to these two first-line mood stabilizers. Carbamazepine has a long history of evaluation and use as a mood stabilizer, but is best considered an adjunctive treatment rather than an effective single agent mood stabilizer.[16,79] Newer anticonvulsants have recently become more commonly used as alternatives to lithium and valproate. Controlled clinical trials in bipolar disorder are underway for both lamotrigine and gabapentin.[79] Lamotrigine has been shown in open trials and case series to be effective in rapid cycling bipolar disorder and refractory bipolar disorder.[80,81] Gabapentin, in open trials and case series, has shown efficacy for both mood stabilizing and antidepressant activity in patients with bipolar disorder.[82] It is premature to suggest effective doses or levels for treatment of bipolar disorder.

Acute Manic Episode

The decision to use lithium or valproate depends upon presenting symptomatology as discussed above, as well as past history of response or adverse effects and concurrent medical problems. Lithium is usually initiated in divided doses of 15 mg/kg/day, increased every 3 to 4 days up to a target plasma level of 1.0 mEq/L. Because lithium has a lag time in the onset of its clinical effect, adjunctive medication is often necessary. If the patient is psychotic, an antipsychotic drug is indicated, but patients whose symptoms include only psychomotor agitation and sleep difficulty benefit most from an adjunctive benzodiazepine. High-potency antipsychotic drugs are preferred to minimize concerns of excessive sedation and cardiovascular effects commonly seen with low-potency antipsychotic drugs. Haloperidol has been shown to be an effective adjunct, and doses seldom should exceed 10 mg/day.[83] Clonazepam and lorazepam, both in divided daily doses of 2 to 6 mg, are the preferred benzodiazepine adjuncts to lithium.[57] After symptoms have resolved for 2 to 6 weeks, an attempt to taper and discontinue the adjunctive antipsychotic or benzodiazepine should begin so the patient eventually is taking only the mood stabilizer.

Valproate can be given in a loading dose as described above, with the potential of an earlier onset of effect and decreased need for adjunctive medication. A target level of 45 to 60 mg/L is often effective without significant adverse effects. Vomiting, nausea, and weakness are all more likely if levels are greater than 125 mg/L.[84]

Maintenance Therapy with Mood Stabilizers

Bipolar disorder is usually recurrent, with a mean episode frequency of about 4 episodes in 10 years. Because this is highly variable, some patients may not have a second episode for years after their first. Patients with one manic episode, with good insight and a good support system, should be treated with a mood stabilizer for at least 1 year and then considered for discontinuation of drug therapy. For patients with one manic episode with an acute onset, psychotic symptoms, or very disruptive symptoms, long-term maintenance therapy is recommended.[85] Patients who had two bipolar episodes should receive long-term maintenance therapy.

Lithium has established long-term efficacy in preventing both manic and depressive episodes, although a high drop-out rate from maintenance therapy limits its long-term value.[86,87] Controlled studies for valproate as maintenance therapy have not yet been done. For patients who respond to valproate acutely, however, maintenance therapy with valproate should be continued. With discontinuation of lithium maintenance therapy the patient returns to the underlying episode frequency, whereas continuing lithium reduces the frequency and severity of bipolar episodes. There is some evidence suggesting lithium discontinuation refractoriness, in which patients who discontinue effective lithium prophylaxis develop a more severe and subsequent treatment resistance to lithium.[85] The occurrence of an episode of mania or depression during maintenance therapy does not suggest treatment failure. No mood stabilizer is effective in preventing all future episodes. Severe or repeated breakthrough episodes, however, suggest the need to reevaluate the drug regimen and consider alternative treatment options.[16]

FUTURE THERAPIES

There are currently no major advances in pharmacotherapy for depressive disorders on the near horizon. One new class of antidepressants scheduled for approval and marketing by the year 2000 is represented by reboxetine, a selective noradrenergic reuptake inhibitor lacking the typical TCA adverse effects.[88] For mood stabilizers, the success of valproate has led to evaluation of other newer anticonvulsants for mood disorders whose role has yet to be established.

IMPROVING OUTCOMES

Methods to Improve Patient Adherence to Antidepressants

The ideal drug therapy for depression described in Table 56.3 is rarely achieved but should form the basis for counseling patients about proper use, dose, and duration of treatment. The delay of several weeks in onset of effect must be understood by patients. Because adverse effects may begin on the first day and noticeable improvement in mood may take 1 to 2 weeks, patients may reasonably conclude that the drug is not working, only making them feel worse and leading to premature discontinuation. Likewise, patients must understand the need to continue drug therapy for at least 4 to 9 months after symptoms resolve to prevent recurrence. Counseling regarding adverse effects should be guided by Table 56.5 so the common effects expected are discussed, including comments about management of each adverse effect mentioned. Use of alcohol should be discouraged primarily owing to the concern that alcohol may worsen the patient's mood. With the newer antidepressants essentially lacking sedative and orthostatic hypotensive effects, there are no significant pharmacologic-based interaction concerns. Telling a patient never to drink while taking an antidepressant will more likely result in noncompliance with the medication to prevent the interaction, while a focus on the warning of potential consequences of drinking allows the informed patient to make reasonable decisions.[89]

Methods to Improve Patient Adherence to Mood Stabilizers

The nature of manic episodes, characterized by euphoria, inflated self-esteem, and lack of insight often interferes with mood stabilizer medication compliance. Few patients choose to take medication that will eliminate their hypomania or manic symptoms unless they understand the negative consequences of their illness. Patient counseling that focuses on the medication's ability to prevent future episodes, especially the unwanted depressive episodes, and the negative financial, legal, and social consequences of manic episodes, is more effective than trying to convince a patient that a mood stabilizer will treat their euphoria, excessive optimism, and decreased need for sleep. Few patients are bothered by their manic or hypomanic symptoms. In a 5 year follow-up study in a lithium clinic, about one-fourth of patients discontinued lithium on their own initiative. The most common reasons for patients to stop lithium included perceived inefficacy, adverse effects, and the conviction that medication was no longer required because symptoms were gone.[87] Other studies in patients with bipolar disorder report medication noncompliance owing to a denial of illness and lack of control over one's life.[90] Patient counseling can address these reasons for discontinuation. An evaluation of a lithium education program using a videotape, written handout, and follow-up visit was found to increase patients' knowledge level about bipolar disorder and treatment as well as compliance with lithium therapy.[91] An 8-page education guide for patients and families has been published, which provides educational material about bipolar illness, mood stabilizers, management of adverse effects, support groups, and a reading list of books by people with bipolar disorder or depression.[92] One comparison of compliance with lithium and valproate found full compliance with valproate to be significantly better.[90]

PHARMACOECONOMICS

Since the introduction of SSRIs, there have been a number of studies suggesting that effective treatment of depression lowers the overall cost of care for depressed patients and that SSRIs are less costly due to greater compliance and fewer dropouts because of adverse effects compared to TCAs.[93] Failure to complete acute and continuation therapy is more costly overall than a completed course of antidepressant therapy.[94] SSRIs and nefazodone have been shown to decrease the total cost of care compared to TCAs despite their higher drug cost owing to fewer hospitalizations, the much higher cost of treating TCA overdose, and a greater TCA discontinuation rate.[95,96]

KEY POINTS

- Mood disorders are characterized by episodes of mood disturbance, and for most patients are recurrent, necessitating long-term maintenance drug therapy.
- All patients with major depression require a minimum of 6 to 12 months of drug therapy at the full acute dose, and patients with a history of three or more episodes will benefit from lifelong maintenance drug therapy.
- An understanding of the unique differences of the mechanisms of antidepressants allows the most rational drug selection and rational combination drug therapy to maximize therapeutic benefit and minimize adverse effects.
- TCAs are no longer first -line antidepressants because of their significant adverse effect profile, lethality in overdose, and high discontinuation rate by patients.
- SSRIs have supplanted TCAs as first-line agents because of their greater tolerability and safety in overdose.
- Venlafaxine, nefazodone, bupropion, and mirtazepine each have unique advantages and disadvantages compared to SSRIs that allow an individualization of drug selection.
- St. John's wort is an effective treatment only for mild to moderate depression, but its efficacy for major depression and dose range remain to be established.
- ECT remains an effective treatment option for severe depression when drug therapy fails.
- Patient counseling regarding antidepressants must include discussion of their delayed onset of effect, the need for a minimum of 4 to 9 months of treatment after

symptoms resolve, as well as common expectable adverse effects and their management.

- SSRIs have demonstrated superiority in reducing the total cost of care compared to TCAs.
- Valproate has equivalent efficacy compared to lithium for bipolar disorder, superior efficacy for patients who experience rapid cycling and those with mixed mania, but minimal antidepressant activity.
- Use of loading doses of valproate for acute mania allows more rapid onset of clinical effect.
- All mood stabilizers are commonly used in combination with antipsychotic drugs or benzodiazepines for acute mania and antidepressants for bipolar depression.

REFERENCES

1. Blazer DG, Kessler RC, McGonagle KA, et al. The prevalence and distribution of major depression in a national community sample: the national comorbidity survey. Am J Psychiatry 151:979–986, 1994.
2. Reynolds CF. Treatment of depression in late life. Am J Med 97(Suppl 6A):39S–46S, 1994.
3. American Psychiatric Association. Diagnostic and statistical manual of mental disorders. 4th ed. Washington, DC: American Psychiatric Association, 1994:317–391.
4. Cummings JL. The neuroanatomy of depression. J Clin Psychiatry 54(Suppl 9):14–20, 1993.
5. Rush DR, Stimmel GL. When drugs cause psychiatric symptoms. Patient Care 23:57–75, 1989.
6. Hirschfeld RMA. Guidelines for the long-term treatment of depression. J Clin Psychiatry 55(Suppl 12):61–69, 1994.
7. Schatzberg AF, Rothschild AJ. Psychotic (delusional) major depression: should it be included as a distinct syndrome in DSMIV? Am J Psychiatry 149:733–745, 1992.
8. Stewart JW, Tricamo E, McGrath PJ, et al. Prophylactic efficacy of phenelzine and imipramine in chronic atypical depression: likelihood of recurrence on discontinuation after 6 months' remission. Am J Psychiatry 154:31–36, 1997.
9. Lafer B, Sachs GS, Labbate LA, et al. Phototherapy for seasonal affective disorder: a blind comparison of three different schedules. Am J Psychiatry 151:1081–1083, 1994.
10. Shelton RC, Davidson J, Yonkers KA, et al. The undertreatment of dysthymia. J Clin Psychiatry 58:59–65, 1997.
11. Lapierre YD. Pharmacological therapy of dysthymia. Acta Psychiatr Scand 89(Suppl 383):42–48, 1994.
12. Schatzberg AF. Bipolar disorder: recent issues in diagnosis and classification. J Clin Psychiatry 59(Suppl 6):5–10, 1998.
13. AHCPR Depression Guideline Panel. Clinical Practice Guideline No. 5. Depression in primary care. Vol. 1: detection and diagnosis. Vol. 2: treatment of major depression. AHCPR Publication No. 93-0550 and 93-0051. Rockville, MD: US Department of Health and Human Services, Public Health Service, April 1993.
14. American Psychiatric Association. Practice guideline for major depressive disorder in adults. Am J Psychiatry 150(Suppl):1–26, 1993.
15. Lebowitz BD, Pearson JL, Schneider LS, et al. Diagnosis and treatment of depression in late life. Consensus statement update. JAMA 278:1186–1190, 1997.
16. American Psychiatric Association. Practice guideline for the treatment of patients with bipolar disorder. Am J Psychiatry 151:1–36, 1994.
17. Franchini L, Gasperini M, Perez J, et al. Dose-response efficacy of paroxetine in preventing depressive recurrences: a randomized, double-blind study. J Clin Psychiatry 59:229–232, 1998.
18. Hirschfeld RMA, Keller MB, Panico S, et al. The national depressive and manic-depressive association consensus statement on the undertreatment of depression. JAMA 277:333–340, 1997.
19. Docherty JP. Barriers to the diagnosis of depression in primary care. J Clin Psychiatry 58(Suppl 1):5–10, 1997.
20. Stahl SM. Basic psychopharmacology of antidepressants, part 1: antidepressants have seven distinct mechanisms of action. J Clin Psychiatry 59(Suppl 4):5–14, 1998.
21. Stahl SM. Serotonin: it's possible to have too much of a good thing. J Clin Psychiatry 58:520–521, 1997.
22. Frazer A. Pharmacology of antidepressants. J Clin Psychopharmacol 17(Suppl 1):2S–18S, 1997.
23. Preskorn SH. Pharmacokinetics of antidepressants. J Clin Psychiatry 54(Suppl 9):14–34, 1993.
24. Sweet RA, Brown EJ, Heimberg RG. Monoamine oxidase inhibitor dietary restrictions: what are we asking patients to give up? J Clin Psychiatry 56:196–201, 1995.
25. Satel SL, Nelson JC. Stimulants in the treatment of depression: a critical overview. J Clin Psychiatry 50:241–249, 1989.
26. Sussman N, Stimmel GL. New dosing strategies for psychotropic drugs. Prim Psychiatry 4:24–30, 1998.
27. Stokes PE. Fluoxetine: a five-year review. Clin Ther 15:216–243, 1993.
28. Murdoch D, McTavish D. Sertraline: a review of its pharmacodynamic and pharmacokinetic properties. Drugs 44:604–624, 1992.
29. Nemeroff CB. The clinical pharmacology and use of paroxetine, a new selective serotonin reuptake inhibitor. Pharmacotherapy 14:127–138, 1994.
30. Kiev A, Feiger A. A double-blind comparison of fluvoxamine and paroxetine in the treatment of depressed outpatients. J Clin Psychiatry 58:146–152, 1997.
31. Noble S, Benfield P. Citalopram. CNS Drugs 8:410–431, 1997.
32. Leo RJ. Movement disorders associated with the serotonin reuptake inhibitors. J Clin Psychiatry 57:449–454, 1996.
33. Segraves RT. Antidepressant-induced sexual dysfunction. J Clin Psychiatry 59(Suppl 4):48–54, 1998.
34. Gutierrez MA, Stimmel GL. Management of and counseling for psychotropic drug-induced sexual dysfunction. Pharmacotherapy 19:823–831, 1999.
35. Schatzberg AF, Haddad P, Kaplan EM, et al. Serotonin reuptake inhibitor discontinuation syndrome: a hypothetical definition. J Clin Psychiatry 58(Suppl 7):5–10, 1997.
36. Zajecka J, Tracy KA, Mitchell S. Discontinuation symptoms after treatment with serotonin reuptake inhibitors: a literature review. J Clin Psychiatry 58:291–297, 1997.
37. Brown TM, Skop B, Mareth TR. Pathophysiology and management of the serotonin syndrome. Ann Pharmacother 30:527–533, 1996.
38. Jefferson JW. Drug interactions–friend or foe? J Clin Psychiatry 59(Suppl 4):37–47, 1998.
39. Ereshefsky L. Drug-drug interactions involving antidepressants: focus on venlafaxine. J Clin Psychopharmacol 16(Suppl 2):37S–53S, 1996.
40. Cunningham LA. Once-daily venlafaxine extended release (XR) and venlafaxine immediate release (IR) in outpatients with major depression. Ann Clin Psychiatry 9:157–164, 1997.
41. Feighner JP. The role of venlafaxine in rational antidepressant therapy. J Clin Psychiatry 55(Suppl 9):62–68, 1994.
42. Thase ME. Depression, sleep, and antidepressants. J Clin Psychiatry 59(Suppl 4):55–65, 1998.
43. Dopheide JA, Stimmel GL, Yi DD. Focus on nefazodone. Hosp Formulary 30:205–212, 1995.
44. Nierenberg AA, Adler LA, Peselow E, et al. Trazodone for antidepressant-associated insomnia. Am J Psychiatry 151:1069–1072, 1994.
45. Banos JE, Bosch F, Farre M. Drug-induced priapism. Med Toxicol 4:46–58, 1989.
46. Pecknold JC, Langer SF. Priapism: trazodone versus nefazodone [Letter]. J Clin Psychiatry 57:547–548, 1996.
47. Preskorn SH. Comparison of the tolerability of bupropion, fluoxetine, imipramine, nefazodone, paroxetine, sertraline, and venlafaxine. J Clin Psychiatry 56(Suppl 6):12–21, 1995.
48. Davidson JRT, Connor KM. Bupropion sustained release: a therapeutic overview. J Clin Psychiatry 59(Suppl 4):25–31, 1998.
49. Zarate CA, Tohen M, Baraibar G, et al. Prescribing trends of antidepressants in bipolar depression. J Clin Psychiatry 56:260–264, 1995.
50. Stimmel GL, Dopheide JA, Stahl SM. Mirtazepine: an antidepressant with noradrenergic and specific serotonergic effects. Pharmacotherapy 17:10–21, 1997.
51. Lerer B, Shapiraa B, Calev A, et al. Antidepressant and cognitive effects of twice versus three times weekly ECT. Am J Psychiatry 152:564–570, 1995.
52. Welch CA. Electroconvulsive therapy. In: Treatment of psychiatric disorders. Washington DC: American Psychiatric Association, 1989;3:1803–1813.
53. Weissman MM, Markowitz JC. Interpersonal psychotherapy: current status. Arch Gen Psychiatry 51:599–606, 1994.
54. Linde K, Ramirez G, Mulrow CD, et al. St John's wort for depression–an overview and meta-analysis of randomised clinical trials. Br Med J 313:253–258, 1996.
55. Volz HP. Controlled clinical trials of hypericum extracts in depressed patients–an overview. Pharmacopsychiatry 30(Suppl 2):72–76, 1997.
56. deSmet PAGM, Nolen WA. St John's wort as an antidepressant: longer term studies are needed before it can be recommended in major depression [Editorial]. Br Med J 313:241–242, 1996.

57. Sachs GS. Bipolar mood disorder: practical strategies for acute and maintenance phase treatment. J Clin Psychopharmacol 16(Suppl 1):32S–47S, 1996.
58. Frances AJ, Kahn DA, Carpenter D, et al. The expert consensus guidelines for treating depression in bipolar disorder. J Clin Psychiatry 59(Suppl 4):73–79, 1998.
59. Fogelson DL, Bystritsky A, Pasnau R. Bupropion in the treatment of bipolar disorders: the same old story? J Clin Psychiatry 53:443–446, 1992.
60. Howland RH. Induction of mania with serotonin reuptake inhibitors. J Clin Psychopharmacol 16:425–427, 1996.
61. Rouillon F, Gorwood P. The use of lithium to augment antidepressant medication. J Clin Psychiatry 59(Suppl 5):32–39, 1998.
62. Bowden CL. Predictors of response to divalproex and lithium. J Clin Psychiatry 56(Suppl 3):25–30, 1995.
63. Ownby RL, Goodnick PJ. Lithium. In: Goodnick PJ. Mania: clinical and research perspectives. Washington, DC: American Psychiatric Press, 1998: 241–262.
64. Amdisen A. Serum level monitoring and clinical pharmacokinetics of lithium. Clin Pharmacokinet 2:73–92, 1977.
65. Ward ME, Musa MN, Bailey L. Clinical pharmacokinetics of lithium. J Clin Pharmacol 34:280–285, 1994.
66. Hardy BG, Shulman KI, Mackenzie SE, et al. Pharmacokinetics of lithium in the elderly. J Clin Psychopharmacol 7:153–158, 1987.
67. Gelenberg AJ, Kane JM, Keller MB, et al. Comparison of standard and low serum levels of lithium for maintenance treatment of bipolar disorder. N Engl J Med 321:1489–1493, 1989.
68. Gutierrez MA, Walker NR, Kramer BA. Evaluation of a new steady-state lithium prediction method. Lithium 2:57–59, 1991.
69. Kook KA, Stimmel GL, Wilkins JN, et al. Accuracy and safety of a priori lithium loading. J Clin Psychiatry 46:49–51, 1985.
70. Bowden CL. Key treatment studies of lithium in manic-depressive illness: efficacy and side effects. J Clin Psychiatry 59(Suppl 6):13–19, 1998.
71. Gitlin MJ, Cochran SD, Jamison KR. Maintenance lithium treatment: side effects and compliance. J Clin Psychiatry 50:127–131, 1989.
72. Rose SR, Klein-Schwartz, Oderda GM, et al. Lithium intoxication with acute renal failure and death. Drug Intell Clin Pharmacol 22:691–694, 1988.
73. Sarid-Segal O, Creelman WL, Ciraulo DA, et al. Lithium. In: Ciraulo DA, Shader RI, Greenblatt DJ, et al. Baltimore: Williams & Wilkins, 1995:175–213.
74. Cohen LS, Friedman JM, Jefferson JW, et al. A reevaluation of risk of in utero exposure to lithium. JAMA 271:146–150, 1994.
75. Llewellyn A, Stowe ZN, Strader JR. The use of lithium and management of women with bipolar disorder during pregnancy and lactation. J Clin Psychiatry 59(Suppl 6):57–64, 1998.
76. McElroy SL, Keck PE, Pope HG, et al. Valproate in the treatment of bipolar disorder: literature review and clinical guidelines. J Clin Psychopharmacol 12(Suppl 1):42S–52S, 1992.
77. Keck PE, McElroy SL, Tugrul KC, Bennett JA. Valproate oral loading in the treatment of acute mania. J Clin Psychiatry 54:305–308, 1993.
78. Keck PE, Nabulsi AA, Taylor JL, et al. A pharmacoeconomic model of divalproex vs lithium in the acute and prophylactic treatment of bipolar I disorder. J Clin Psychiatry 57:213–222, 1996.
79. Keck PE, McElroy SL, Strakowski SM. Anticonvulsants and antipsychotics in the treatment of bipolar disorder. J Clin Psychiatry 59(Suppl 6):74–81, 1998.
80. Fatemi SH, Rapport DJ, Calabrese JR, et al. Lamotrigine in rapid-cycling bipolar disorder. J Clin Psychiatry 58:522–527, 1997.
81. Fogelson DL, Sternbach H. Lamotrigine treatment of refractory bipolar disorder [Letter]. J Clin Psychiatry 58:271–273, 1997.
82. Young LT, Robb JC, Patelis-Siotis I, et al. Acute treatment of bipolar depression with gabapentin. Biol Psychiatry 42:851–853, 1997.
83. Rifkin A, Doddi S, Karajgi B, et al. Dosage of haloperidol for mania. Br J Psychiatry 165:113–116, 1994.
84. Bowden CL. Dosing strategies and time course of response to antimanic drugs. J Clin Psychiatry 57(Suppl 13):4–9, 1996.
85. Dunner DL. Lithium carbonate: maintenance studies and consequences of withdrawal. J Clin Psychiatry 59(Suppl 6):48–55, 1998.
86. Tondo L, Baldessarini RJ, Hennen J, et al. Lithium maintenance treatment of depression and mania in bipolar I and bipolar II disorders. Am J Psychiatry 155:638–645, 1998.
87. Maj M, Pirozzi R, Magliano L, Bartoli L. Long-term outcome of lithium prophylaxis in bipolar disorders: a 5 year prospective study of 402 patients at a lithium clinic. Am J Psychiatry 155:30–35, 1998.
88. Gutierrez MA, Stimmel GL, Yi DD. Reboxetine: A selective norepinephrine reuptake inhibitor. Formulary 34:909–919, 1999.
89. Stimmel GL. How to counsel patients about depression and its treatment. Pharmacotherapy 15(6 Part 2):100S–104S, 1995.
90. Weiss RD, Greenfield SF, Najavits LM, et al. Medication compliance among patients with bipolar disorder and substance use disorder. J Clin Psychiatry 59:172–174, 1998.
91. Peet M, Harvey NS. Lithium maintenance: a standard education programme for patients. Br J Psychiatry 158:197–200, 1991.
92. Kahn DA, Ross R, Rush J, et al. Expert consensus treatment guidelines for bipolar disorder: a guide for patients and families. J Clin Psychiatry 57(Suppl 12A):81–88, 1996.
93. Saklad SR. Pharmacoeconomic issues in the treatment of depression. Pharmacotherapy 15(6 Part 2):76S–83S, 1995.
94. McCombs JS, Nichol MB, Stimmel GL, et al. The cost of antidepressant drug therapy failure: a study of antidepressant use patterns in a Medicaid population. J Clin Psychiatry 51(Suppl 6):60–69, 1990.
95. Revicki DA, Brown RE, Keller MB, et al. Cost-effectiveness of newer antidepressants compared with tricyclic antidepressants in managed care settings. J Clin Psychiatry 58:47–58, 1997.
96. Sclar DA, Robison LM, Skaer TL, et al. Antidepressant pharmacotherapy: economic evaluation of fluoxetine, paroxetine, and sertraline in a health maintenance organization. J Int Med Res 23:395–412, 1995.

CHAPTER 57
SCHIZOPHRENIA

Glen L. Stimmel

DEFINITION

Schizophrenia is a chronic thought disorder in which characteristic psychotic symptoms are seen during the acute phase of the illness with either partial or full resolution of symptoms between psychotic episodes, coupled with a deterioration from a previous level of social and occupational functioning. Schizophrenia is not synonymous with psychosis. The term *psychosis* is broader and includes infectious, metabolic, endocrine, and drug-induced causes for psychotic symptoms such as delusions and hallucinations. Many psychiatric and neurologic disorders also may include psychotic symptoms, such as mania, major depression, and the dementias. Schizophrenia is not a split personality, Dr. Jekyll–Mr. Hyde syndrome, or multiple personality disorder. Although patients with schizophrenia may at times be psychotic and exhibit bizarre behavior, between psychotic episodes they often remain in total control of their behavior, feelings, and thoughts.

TREATMENT GOALS: SCHIZOPHRENIA

- Goals and strategies of treating a patient with schizophrenia vary according to the phase and severity of illness.
- In the acute phase, reduce or eliminate psychotic symptoms and improve role functioning.
- During stabilization, provide support to decrease the risk of relapse, increase the patient's adaptation to life in the community, and consolidate remission of symptoms.
- In the stable phase, ensure that the patient maintains and improves his or her level of functioning and quality of life, treat any reemerging psychotic symptoms, and continue adverse effect monitoring and management.[1]

EPIDEMIOLOGY

Schizophrenia affects an estimated 1% of the U.S. population, with about 300,000 acute episodes occurring annually. The prevalence rate appears to be constant across different countries and cultures. The age of onset is typically between the late teens and mid-30s, with men and women affected in roughly equal numbers. A later age of onset is more common in women and is associated with less cognitive impairment and better outcome. Both genetic and environmental factors are important in the etiology of schizophrenia. Whereas the risk in the general population is about 1%, the risk for first-degree relatives is 10%. Substantial discordance rates in monozygotic twin studies (only 40 to 50% risk) indicate that environmental factors are also important.[2]

PATHOPHYSIOLOGY

Schizophrenia is best viewed as a syndrome with a large continuum of pathophysiologic disruptions. The older hypothesis of overactive dopaminergic pathways is much too simplistic to explain schizophrenia. Thus far, the pathophysiology of dopaminergic and serotonergic systems is best understood. Overactivity of mesolimbic and mesocortical dopaminergic pathways to the temporolimbic region and frontal cortex are believed to explain the positive symptoms of schizophrenia, whereas the relative lack of dopaminergic function in the prefrontal cortex has been suggested to explain the negative symptoms of schizophrenia. Much of this work is based upon an understanding of the mechanisms of action of antipsychotic drugs and their relative efficacy for specific symptoms. Dopamine blockade is associated with efficacy for positive symptoms, whereas serotonergic blockade enhances dopaminergic activity in the prefrontal cortex to decrease negative symptoms. Furthermore, dopaminergic systems can be modulated by a variety of other systems–adrenergic, cholinergic, and peptidergic. Although the clinical effects of drugs with well-known neurotransmitter mechanisms is evident, understanding the exact pathophysiology of schizophrenia remains indirect and undetermined.[3,4]

CLINICAL PRESENTATION AND DIAGNOSIS

Signs and Symptoms

Symptoms are classified as either positive or negative, correlating with differences in pathophysiology and responsiveness to drug therapy (Table 57.1).[2,5] The positive symptoms are most likely to lead to hospitalization and family disruption, but the negative symptoms interfere with patients being able to have close friends, maintain employment, relate to their families, and become integrated into their community. Negative symptoms contribute the most to the morbidity and economic costs of schizophrenia.

Positive Symptoms

A disturbance in perception is termed a hallucination, in which one has a sensory awareness in the absence of an external stimulus. The most common example is auditory hallucinations, in which voices or noises are perceived as coming from outside one's head when in fact no voices are present. Visual and tactile hallucinations are possible in schizophrenia, but are more characteristic of drug-induced psychoses. Delusions represent the most common disturbance in thought content, defined as a fixed false belief. Delusions can vary in theme and content, but are typically bizarre or terrifying. Persecutory or paranoid delusions are most common, in which the person believes he or she is being followed, spied on, or tormented. Referential delusions are also common, in which a person believes song lyrics, another person's gesture, or television reports are specifically directed at him or her. Beliefs that one's thoughts are being inserted or withdrawn by an outside force, one's thoughts are being broadcast aloud, or one's body or actions are being controlled by an outside force are additional common delusions. False beliefs or concerns that are not firmly held are termed "ideation" (e.g., paranoid ideation, and ideas of reference). Disorganized thinking and speech is described as "loose associations" or "derailment" in which the patient may shift from one topic to another with no awareness that the topics are unrelated. More severe thought disorder can be manifest as "word salad" in which unrelated words or phrases are strung together in speech. "Concrete thinking" is the loss of an ability to think in abstract terms. Bizarre behavior may be manifest as disheveled or unusual dress or grooming, poor hygiene, inappropriate sexual behavior, and odd mannerisms.

Table 57.1 ▪ Symptoms of Schizophrenia

Positive symptoms (distorted functions)
Hallucinations (e.g., hearing voices, seeing things)
Delusions (fixed false belief not shared by culture)
Disorganized speech, thought, language
Disorganized bizarre behavior
Negative symptoms (diminished functions)
Alogia (decreased fluency of thought or speech)
Affective blunting of emotional expression
Avolition (lack of drive, motivation)
Anhedonia/asociality (decreased ability to feel pleasure/form relationships)
Attention impairment (decreased ability to focus attention)

Negative Symptoms

Alogia, or poverty of speech, is manifest by very brief, empty responses to questions related to a lack of thoughts, not a resistance to speak. Affective blunting is typically described as constricted affect, or at its worst, flat affect. There is an unchanging facial expression, decreased spontaneous movements, poverty of gestures, poor eye contact, and lack of vocal inflection. These symptoms may be interpreted by family as apathy, laziness, or indifference, and must also be distinguished from drug-induced pseudoparkinsonism and depressed mood. Avolition, or the lack of self-initiated goal-directed activity, directly interferes with psychosocial training programs and the potential for adequate social and occupational functioning.

Diagnosis

In addition to the presence of the characteristic symptoms described above, the diagnosis of schizophrenia requires continuous signs of the disturbance for at least 6 months with at least 1 month of active symptoms, plus a marked decline in social or occupational functioning. Diagnostic criteria require two or more of the following symptoms during the 1 month of active symptoms: delusions, hallucinations, disorganized speech, grossly disorganized behavior, and negative symptoms. When all criteria are met except symptoms have been present for only 1 to 6 months, a diagnosis of schizophreniform disorder is given. Acute onset of psychotic symptoms lasting less than 1 month is termed a brief psychotic disorder. Schizoaffective disorder is a distinct and separate psychotic mood disorder, which meets the diagnostic criteria for both schizophrenia and either a manic episode or a major depressive episode. Although many acutely psychotic patients often exhibit some mood disturbance, upon follow-up, most will be found to have either schizophrenia or a primary mood disorder. Schizoaffective disorder is a diagnosis that must be validated over time, because precision in diagnosis is needed to ensure that patients receive the most appropriate pharmacotherapy for their disorder.[2]

PSYCHOSOCIAL ASPECTS

Because the diagnosis of schizophrenia requires a marked decline in social or occupational functioning over time, psychosocial factors are of critical importance in effective treatment. Drug therapy at its best will eliminate psychotic symptoms, still leaving the patient with significant financial, social, occupational, and family difficulties.

THERAPEUTIC PLAN

Two national professional organizations published practice guidelines for schizophrenia in 1997–the American Psychiatric Association, with plans to revise and update every 3 to 5 years,[1] and the American Pharmaceutical Association.[6] In both cases, the proposed treatment algorithms do not include the newer atypical antipsychotic drugs, which will alter their recommended treatment decisions.

TREATMENT

Pharmacotherapy

Once referred to as major tranquilizers, antipsychotic drugs have a selective specific effect in eliminating or at least minimizing psychotic symptoms. They are not supersedatives or tranquilizers and are most properly called antipsychotic drugs. The appearance of the newer atypical antipsychotic drugs, with their minimal potential for causing extrapyramidal side effects (EPS), has led to the abandonment of the term "neuroleptic" to refer to antipsychotic drugs.

Available Antipsychotic Drugs

Antipsychotic drugs can be classified chemically or pharmacologically, the latter having the most clinical relevance. Table 57.2 lists commonly used drugs using a classification of low- and high-potency typical and atypical antipsychotic drugs. This classification groups the drugs based upon similar adverse effect profiles and therapeutic efficacy. The typical drugs are potent dopamine-2 receptor blockers, while the atypical drugs have less dopaminergic blockade but greater serotonin-2 receptor blockade. The low-potency drugs additionally have potent antihistaminic, antimuscarinic, and α_1 adrenergic blockade effects. In general, the typical drugs effectively treat positive symptoms while the atypical drugs treat both positive and negative symptoms and have minimal risk for EPS. Low-potency drugs are more likely to cause sedation and anticholinergic and cardiovascular effects with fewer EPS, whereas the primary adverse effects of the high-potency drugs are EPS.[7]

Table 57.2 ▪ Available Antipsychotic Drugs

- Typical antipsychotics
  - Low potency
    - Chlorpromazine (Thorazine)
    - Thioridazine (Mellaril)
    - Mesoridazine (Serentil)
  - High potency
    - Fluphenazine (Prolixin)
    - Perphenazine (Trilafon)
    - Trifluoperazine (Stelazine)
    - Thiothixene (Navane)
    - Haloperidol (Haldol)
    - Loxapine (Loxitane)
    - Molindone (Moban)
- Atypical antipsychotics
  - Clozapine (Clozaril)
  - Risperidone (Risperdal)
  - Olanzapine (Zyprexa)
  - Quetiapine (Seroquel)

Treatment of Acute Psychotic Episode

When a patient presents to an emergency room in an acutely psychotic state, the many medical and drug-induced causes for psychosis must first be ruled out. If a patient is experiencing an acute exacerbation of schizophrenia, the degree of agitation and hostility versus psychotic symptomatology dictates the pharmacotherapy decisions. The use of rapid titration of high-dose antipsychotic drugs (e.g., haloperidol 5 mg IM every hour) was common practice 10 to 15 years ago, but a more rational moderate antipsychotic dose with benzodiazepines is now recommended. Doses higher than 10 to 15 mg of haloperidol acutely were found not to be any more effective and only to cause worse adverse effects. Although most antipsychotic drugs have no clinically useful correlation of plasma levels to clinical response, haloperidol has been suggested to have a therapeutic window, with an optimal plasma level range of 5 to 15 ng/mL, achievable in most patients when given doses of 4 to 10 mg/day.[8,9] Acute agitation and hostility are best treated by talking with the patient and using physical restraints first, then giving either a benzodiazepine and/or an antipsychotic drug.[10] Benzodiazepines, such as lorazepam 2 mg PO or IM every 30 minutes for three doses, can effectively reduce agitated behavior, reducing the dosage of the antipsychotic drug necessary for the psychotic symptoms, and thus reducing the potential for adverse effects. Benzodiazepines are not recommended in older adults, brain-damaged patients, patients intoxicated with sedative-hypnotics, or those with a history of a paradoxical reaction to benzodiazepines. The psychotic symptoms require an antipsychotic drug, which can safely be given in combination with the benzodiazepine. High-potency antipsychotic drugs (e.g., haloperidol) are preferred, and low-potency drugs should be avoided because of their sedative and cardiovascular effects. Atypical drugs are not yet considered first-line drugs for acute psychosis. Their potential for orthostatic hypotensive effects and the decreased dopaminergic effects necessary to control acute positive psychotic symptoms still make high-potency drugs the preferred choice.[10]

For a patient with acute psychotic symptoms without significant agitation, the choice of the antipsychotic drug depends upon presence or absence of negative symptoms, past history of response and adverse effects, the patient's attitude toward drugs used in the past, and the desired adverse effect profile. When drug therapy is initiated, the lower end of the daily dosage range is given in divided doses initially (e.g., haloperidol 2 mg BID or risperidone 1 mg BID), allowing assessment of initial adverse effects before titrating upward within the therapeutic dosage

Table 57.3 ▪ Oral Dosage Ranges and Potency

Drug	Acute Dose (mg/day)	Maintenance Dose (mg/day)	Potency[a]
Chlorpromazine	400–1000	100–300	100
Thioridazine	400–800	100–200	100
Fluphenazine	10–60	3–20	2
Perphenazine	8–64	4–32	8
Trifluoperazine	20–80	5–20	5
Thiothixene	20–80	5–30	4
Haloperidol	10–60	3–20	2
Loxapine	40–160	20–80	10
Molindone	50–200	20–100	10
Clozapine	300–600	150–400	–[b]
Risperidone	4–6	2–4	–[b]
Olanzapine	10–20	5–50	–[b]
Quetiapine	300–600	150–300	–[b]

[a]Chlorpromazine 100 mg has equal antipsychotic activity to haloperidol 2 mg based upon dopaminergic blockade.

[b]–, potency of atypical drugs cannot be compared to that of typical drugs.

range (Table 57.3). The ranges listed in Table 57.3 are usual effective dose ranges, so occasionally patients require higher doses, and others may be effectively maintained on doses lower than those listed in the table.

Table 57.3 also lists the relative potency of the typical antipsychotic drugs. Potency bears no relationship to effectiveness, but refers only to milligram equivalency of antipsychotic effect based upon dopaminergic activity. These potency relationships allow conversion from an equivalent dose of one typical drug to another, although differences in the adverse effect profile must also be considered when switching. For example, haloperidol 15 mg is equivalent to chlorpromazine 750 mg. Although this is an equivalent antipsychotic dose, such a switch could not be done directly because of the significant sedation, orthostatic hypotension, and anticholinergic effects of chlorpromazine. No potency equivalents can be stated for atypical drugs because their mechanism is not primarily based upon dopamine blockade.

Maintenance Therapy

Many different strategies have been evaluated to minimize the risk of relapse in patients with schizophrenia. When patients discontinue their antipsychotic drug, they have a substantial risk for relapse. The efficacy of maintenance antipsychotic drugs in preventing relapse is well established. The clinical decisions regarding maintenance dose and length of therapy involve how to minimize the risk of relapse and adverse effects while maximizing treatment adherence. Virtually all patients with schizophrenia not treated with antipsychotic medication will have a relapse within about 3 years.[11] Across studies, the 1-year relapse rate after drug discontinuation averages 70%, while continuous use of antipsychotic maintenance therapy reduces the relapse rate to 23%.[12] Use of intermittent treatment only when patients exhibit prodromal signs or frank psychotic symptoms, although an appealing concept, works about as well as placebo in preventing relapse.[11] The most effective method to prevent relapse is continuous drug therapy at lower maintenance doses, usually 50% less than the acute dose after 1 year (Table 57.3).[12,13] The atypical drugs offer a minimal risk of EPS and tardive dyskinesia with maintenance therapy, which should enhance treatment adherence. Use of depot antipsychotic drugs has also been shown to significantly decrease relapse compared to use of oral medication, although those studies did not include the newer atypical antipsychotic drugs.[11]

Dosing Strategies

Once an effective dose is found after initial upward titration of dosage, most patients benefit from once-daily dosing. For sedating drugs, bedtime dosing minimizes daytime sedation and minimizes the need for an additional hypnotic drug. Once-daily dosing increases medication compliance and simplifies drug regimens. Only those patients unable to tolerate the adverse effects of once-daily dosing should remain on divided dosing schedules.

Depot Formulations

The use of fluphenazine decanoate (FD) or haloperidol decanoate (HD) represents a unique option for maintenance drug therapy. The advantages of these formulations is that a patient can be given an IM injection every 2 to 4 weeks rather than ingesting daily oral medication. A depot antipsychotic is indicated for patients who respond well to acute PO drug therapy but are consistently noncompliant or refuse oral medication. Depot therapy should not be used acutely, owing to the variable and delayed onset of effect compared to oral medication. Treatment of acute symptoms requires the flexibility of dose titration offered by oral or nondepot IM preparations. Depot therapy should be given only after the PO dose has stabilized at an effective level, and the patient can be converted to the depot formulation. Studies of relapse rates find an average difference of 15% favoring depot to oral maintenance medication. Whereas depot therapy is used in 40 to 60% of European countries, it is estimated that in the United States only 10 to 20% of patients receive depot therapy.[14]

FD and HD are equally effective and have virtually identical adverse effect profiles.[15] Because HD can be given once monthly and FD requires twice monthly administration, all new candidates for depot therapy should be given HD. The effective dose range for FD is 12.5 to 50 mg IM every 2 weeks and for HD is 100 to 450 mg IM every month. To convert a patient's medication from oral haloperidol, the initial HD dose IM should be 10 to 20 times the oral daily dose. The first injection should not exceed 100 mg, so the balance of the initial dose can be given in a second injection 3 to 7 days later. Thus, a patient receiving haloperidol 20 mg PO would receive HD 100 mg IM initially followed in 3 to 7 days by 300 mg IM for a total monthly dose of 400 mg. The usual monthly maintenance dose range is 10 to 15 times the oral daily dose. Thus, the dosage in a patient initially given HD 400 mg/month with psychotic symptoms stabilized should be slowly reduced by 25% each month toward a target maintenance dose of 200 to 300 mg monthly. The total monthly dose should not exceed 450 mg, and the maximum volume per injection should not exceed 3 mL. With HD, peak haloperidol concentrations occur between 3 to 9 days, with an apparent elimination half-life of 3 weeks, and a steady-state level with multiple dosing is reached after 12 to 16 weeks.[16,17]

Adverse Effects and Their Management

Extrapyramidal Side Effects

EPS represent the most common and troublesome adverse effects of antipsychotic drugs, being the primary cause of noncompliance. There are three categories of EPS: acute dystonias, pseudoparkinsonism, and akathisia. The definitions and symptoms are listed in Table 57.4. EPS are commonly caused by the typical antipsychotic drugs with dopaminergic blocking properties, but may also be seen with the atypical drugs with dopaminergic and serotonergic blocking effects.[18]

Table 57.4 ▪ Manifestations of Extrapyramidal Effects and Tardive Dyskinesia

Dystonic reactions (painful spasm of a muscle or muscle group)
Oculogyric crisis—fixed upward stare
Torticollis—neck twisting
Trismus—clenched jaw
Opisthotonus—arching of back
Laryngospasm—difficulty breathing, speaking, swallowing
Pseudoparkinsonism
Akinesia
Rigidity and immobility
Stiffness and slowness of voluntary movement
Mask-like facial expression
Drooling (sialorrhea)
Stooped posture
Shuffling, festinating gait
Slow, monotone speech
Tremor
Regular rhythmic oscillations of extremities, especially hands and feet
Pill-rolling movement of fingers
Akathisia (subjective inner feeling of restlessness, anxiety plus motor restlessness)
Inability to sit still, constant pacing
Continuous agitation and restless movements
Rocking and shifting of weight while standing
Shifting of legs, tapping of feet while sitting
Tardive dyskinesia
Mouth—rhythmical involuntary movements of tongue, lips, jaw; protrusion of tongue, puckering of mouth, chewing movements
Choreiform—involuntary irregular purposeless quick movements of arms/legs; jerky, flailing movements
Athethoid—continuous worm-like slow movements of arms
Axial hyperkinesis—to and fro clonic movements of spine

Dystonic reactions are usually seen within the first 72 hours of treatment with a dopamine-blocking drug and are seen most frequently in young men. High-potency drugs are most likely to cause dystonia (e.g., 65% of patients given haloperidol).[19] Fortunately, dystonic reactions are usually brief, and among all EPS, are most responsive to treatment. Anticholinergic agents, such as benztropine 2 mg IM or diphenhydramine 50 mg IM, will usually be effective within 10 to 30 minutes. Because laryngospasm can represent a medical emergency, IV benztropine or diphenhydramine should be used. After acute treatment, oral benztropine should be continued with the antipsychotic drug. Controversy remains regarding automatic use of anticholinergic agents prophylactically when antipsychotic drugs are begun in an attempt to prevent EPS. A decision regarding prophylaxis should be based upon the relative risk factors present for EPS. Prophylaxis is indicated when one or more of the following risk factors are present: patients with a past history of EPS (particularly if noncompliant), patients given a high-potency antipsychotic drug, and young men. Use of benztropine 1 mg BID prophylactically is effective and can be tapered and discontinued after 1 to 2 months if no EPS occur.[18]

Pseudoparkinsonism, resulting from dopaminergic blockade in the striatum, mimics Parkinson's disease in its symptomatology. Symptoms may develop weeks to several months after an antipsychotic drug is started. The most common and reliable rating scale used for pseudoparkinsonism is the Simpson-Angus scale. Although less responsive to treatment than dystonic reactions, pseudoparkinsonism symptoms can usually be effectively treated. Use of dopaminergic agents is not effective owing to blockade of receptors, so anticholinergic agents are first-line treatment. Benztropine 1 to 6 mg PO daily is preferred over trihexyphenidyl 5 to 15 mg daily because its longer half-life allows once-daily dosing. Because EPS movements disappear during sleep, benztropine is best given in the morning. Amantadine 100 to 400 mg daily offers a second-line choice for patients not responsive to anticholinergic drugs or who cannot tolerate their adverse effects (dry mouth, blurry near vision, constipation, urinary retention, and memory impairment).[18,20]

Akathisia is the most common EPS and is least responsive to treatment. It is often difficult to distinguish akathisia from psychotic agitation, which is crucial because treatment of each is very different. The most common and reliable rating scale used to evaluate akathisia is the Barnes Akathisia Scale. Akathisia is rarely responsive to anticholinergic agents and is best treated with either propranolol 40 to 160 mg daily or benzodiazepines (e.g., lorazepam 1.5 to 5 mg daily or clonazepam 0.5 to 2 mg daily).[18,21] The severity of akathisia is often greater with the depot drugs—discontinuing depot fluphenazine or haloperidol because of intolerable and untreatable akathisia and switching to an atypical antipsychotic is common.

Table 57.5 ▪ Relative Adverse Effect Profiles[a]

Drug	Sedation	EPS	Anticholinergic	Postural Hypotension
Haloperidol	1	5	1	1
Fluphenazine	1	5	1	1
Thiothixene	2	4	2	1
Trifluoperazine	2	4	2	1
Molindone	1	3	1	1
Loxapine	2	3	2	2
Chlorpromazine	4	2	3	4
Thioridazine	4	2	4	4
Clozapine	4	0–1	4	4
Risperidone	1	1–2	1	2
Olanzapine	2	1	2	1
Quetiapine	2	0–1	1	2

EPS, extrapyrimidal side effects.
[a]1 = low; 5 = high.

The approximate frequency of EPS in patients receiving thioridazine is 10 to 15%, chlorpromazine 20 to 25%, and fluphenazine and haloperidol 40 to 50% (Table 57.5). One of the major advantages of atypical drugs is their relative lack of EPS compared to typical antipsychotic drugs. Clozapine is the least likely antipsychotic drug to cause EPS and the incidence with risperidone is more than with clozapine but much less than with the typical antipsychotic drugs.[22] More head-to-head comparison trials are needed to accurately place olanzapine and quetiapine among the atypical drugs, but they both are unlikely to cause EPS.

Tardive Dyskinesia

Tardive diskinesia (TD) is a late-appearing antipsychotic drug-induced movement disorder that looks like an EPS but whose etiology and treatment are very different. For most patients, the movements of TD are restricted to the mouth area and are mild and not bothersome (Table 57.5). Unlike EPS, TD typically appears upon antipsychotic dosage reduction or discontinuation, improves when the antipsychotic dose is increased, worsens with administration of anticholinergic drugs, and may persist for months or years after antipsychotic drugs are discontinued. All typical antipsychotic drugs are capable of causing TD owing to their prominent dopaminergic blockade in the striatum. The atypical antipsychotic drugs have a much lower risk of TD because of their serotonergic effects and much lesser striatal dopaminergic blocking effect. The prevalence of TD cannot be precisely stated because there are so many variables when considering an effect that develops after years of treatment. The risk of persistent TD based on prospective studies in all age groups is suggested to be 20% after 5 years of cumulative typical antipsychotic drug exposure, with an incidence of about 4% per year for the first 5 years.[23] In older populations the rate is even higher. Once a patient develops TD, symptoms tend to remain constant and usually do not worsen with continued antipsychotic drug therapy.[24] One-month drug holidays or intermittent rather than continuous maintenance therapy was once believed to help prevent TD. It is now known that the risk for TD is three times greater if antipsychotic drug therapy is interrupted more than two times. Continuous low-dose antipsychotic drug therapy is most effective in preventing relapse and reducing the risk of TD with typical antipsychotic drugs.[25]

TD is believed to result from long-term blockade of striatal dopaminergic receptors with resultant hypersensitivity of those receptors. There are no drug treatment options effective for TD despite case reports and open trials of more than 60 different agents. Management of a patient with TD should consist of discontinuing any anticholinergic agent and lowering the antipsychotic dose as low as clinically possible. Although the needed long-term studies have not been done, drug therapy in patients is rationally being switched to atypical drugs to spare the striatal dopaminergic system. Because treatment of TD is so disappointing, prevention is most important. All patients given antipsychotic drugs should be regularly monitored for early signs of TD (movements on the surface of the tongue, facial tics such as frequent blinking, and choreoathetoid finger or toe movements). The Abnormal Involuntary Movement Scale (AIMS) is the most commonly used screening tool for TD.

Anticholinergic Effects

Peripheral anticholinergic effects are commonly experienced by patients taking chlorpromazine, thioridazine, and clozapine. In addition, patients taking high-potency drugs often require anticholinergic agents for EPS, so they too are often bothered by dry mouth, blurred near vision, and constipation. These effects are dose-related and additive. Anticholinergic effects can be minimized by switching to once-daily bedtime dosing or by decreasing dosage when possible. Dry mouth and blurred vision are usually worse in the first 2 weeks; then some tolerance develops even if the same dose is maintained. Constipation can be a more serious concern if left untreated, leading to impaction and ileus. The reduction in gastrointestinal motility and secretions results in a hard, dry stool that is best treated with increasing fluid intake, diet and exercise counseling, and stool softeners. Docusate 100 to 500 mg daily will usually be effective within 2 to 3 days, and treatment can be on an interrupted basis for 4 to 7 days at a time.

More serious anticholinergic effects include urinary hesitancy and retention and cognitive impairment. Either effect requires immediate dosage reduction or switching to a less anticholinergic drug regimen. These two effects are magnified in intensity and severity in patients with prostatic hypertrophy, older patients, or patients with dementia.

Cardiovascular Effects

The most frequent cardiovascular effect caused by both typical and atypical drugs is orthostatic hypotension (Table 57.5). It is dose-related and is most prominent in the first 2 weeks of therapy or after a dose increase. After several weeks, there is usually tolerance to the subjective dizziness, while the actual postural drop in blood pressure persists. The elderly and patients taking other drugs with hypotensive effects are at most risk for orthostatic hypotensive effects. Although easily prevented with patient education, orthostatic hypotension in uncounseled patients can lead to falls, fractures, and subsequent noncompliance.

Thioridazine in doses above 300 mg daily and to a lesser extent chlorpromazine may induce electrocardiogram (ECG) changes, T-wave abnormalities in particular. High-potency antipsychotic drugs have the potential for ECG changes only with parenteral administration. Haloperidol and droperidol parenterally in doses greater than 50 mg/24 hr should be monitored, because the QT_c interval may be increased by 25% over baseline.[26]

Neuroleptic Malignant Syndrome

Neuroleptic malignant syndrome (NMS) is an uncommon but serious adverse effect that occurs in 1 to 2% of patients receiving typical antipsychotic drugs. NMS is characterized by (1) fever, (2) severe EPS such as lead pipe rigidity, trismus, and other dystonias, (3) signs of autonomic instability such as tachycardia, labile hypertension, diaphoresis, and incontinence, and (4) fluctuating levels of consciousness. In the 1980s, the mortality rate was 22%, which has now dropped to less than 5% due to earlier recognition and treatment. NMS typically occurs after 3 to 9 days of antipsychotic therapy with symptoms rapidly progressing over 24 to 72 hours and persisting 5 to 10 days after the antipsychotic drug is discontinued.[27] The etiology was once thought to be overwhelming dopaminergic blockade effects, because most instances of NMS were seen in patients receiving high doses of high-potency drugs. This has been recently challenged by the reports of NMS with clozapine and risperidone.[28] Treatment of NMS consists of discontinuation of the antipsychotic drug, parenteral hydration, and control of fever. If no marked improvement is seen after 1 to 2 days, dantrolene 240 to 600 mg/day and/or bromocriptine 7.5 to 30 mg/day can be considered, because recovery times have been reported to be shorter for drug-treated patients than for those receiving only supportive care.[29]

Endocrine and Sexual Function Effects

The most common endocrine effects of antipsychotic drugs include menstrual irregularities and galactorrhea in up to 30% of women, and gynecomastia in men.[30,31] These effects are a result of dopaminergic blockade causing prolactin levels to increase. No specific treatment is necessary beyond assuring the patient that it is a reversible benign effect. Because ovulation may continue despite irregular or missed menstrual periods, continued contraception must be encouraged. Increased prolactin levels in men decrease libido and erectile function. Both decreased libido and erectile dysfunction are commonly reported with antipsychotic drugs. Clozapine, olanzapine, and quetiapine are the least likely antipsychotic drugs to cause endocrine effects because they do not elevate prolactin levels. Ejaculatory difficulty and difficulty achieving orgasm are also common complaints in 30 to 40% of men, most likely due to α-adrenergic blockade along with the elevated prolactin levels.[31] Retrograde ejaculation, in which semen flows backward into the bladder upon ejaculation, is most often reported with thioridazine, due to its α-adrenergic blockade.

Seizures

Clozapine is the antipsychotic drug most likely to cause a seizure, followed by chlorpromazine, with haloperidol being the least likely.[32] Seizures are dose related, being more likely with a rapid rate of upward dose titration and higher doses. With usual doses, seizures with antipsychotic drugs except clozapine occur in less than 0.5% of patients. Seizures occur in 1 to 2% of patients given clozapine in doses less than 300 mg/day, but reach 5% when doses exceed 600 mg/day.[33]

Weight Gain

With the exception of molindone, all antipsychotic drugs may cause weight gain of as much as 5 to 15% of body weight. Weight gain of 20 to 30 pounds over 1 to 2 months has become a primary reason for noncompliance with atypical antipsychotic drugs. Clozapine has been associated with a mean 12-kg weight increase, with 20% of patients gaining more than 10% of their body weight. The exact mechanism of weight gain is unknown, but it involves both antihistaminic and serotonergic blockade effects. Molindone is unique in having a central anorexigenic effect via serotonin agonist activity coupled with its low affinity for histamine receptors. No effective treatment for weight gain has been identified beyond nutrition counseling, exercise, and dietary modification.[33,34]

Drug Interactions

Most all drug interactions with antipsychotic drugs are predictable based upon known pharmacologic and pharmacokinetic information. Common drug interactions include additive sedative and hypotensive and anticholinergic effects. For example, alcohol enhances both the sedative and hypotensive effects of chlorpromazine and clozapine. All antipsychotics are extensively hepatically metabolized through microsomal oxidation and conjugation reactions, making them susceptible to enzyme inducers and inhibitors. The cytochrome P-450 enzyme(s) responsible for metabolism of antipsychotic drugs are 1A2 (clozapine), 2D6 and 1A2 (phenothiazines), 1A2 and 2D6 (minor) (haloperidol), 2D6 (risperidone), 1A2 and 2D6 (minor) (olanzapine), and 3A4 (quetiapine).[35,36] Cigarette smoking has been shown to increase the clearance of many antipsychotic drugs by 50 to 150%.[37]

Unique Features of Atypical Antipsychotic Drugs

The atypical antipsychotic drugs as a group offer major advantages to patients compared to the typical antipsychotic drugs. The atypical drugs only infrequently cause EPS, carry a much lower risk of TD, offer unique efficacy for negative symptoms and cognitive dysfunction, provide efficacy for some patients whose positive symptoms are refractory to typical antipsychotics, have shown cost-effectiveness for total cost of care despite the higher drug cost, and have very different and complex receptor-binding profiles. These differences revolutionized the treatment of schizophrenia in the mid-1990s, with atypical drugs virtually replacing the typical drugs except for those patients already stabilized and doing well on the typical drugs and for treatment of agitated acute psychotic episodes.[38,39]

Recent evidence indicates that cognitive dysfunction may be a core symptom of schizophrenia for some patients and that the degree of cognitive impairment predicts outcome better than other symptoms. Anticholinergic agents (e.g., benztropine) have long been recognized to have a profound negative effect on learning and memory functions. As a result of EPS from high-potency drugs, patients must often be given doses of anticholinergic drugs that impair cognition. Likewise, the low-potency drugs, along with clozapine and to a lesser extent olanzapine, have potent anticholinergic effects that may also impair learning and memory functions. Risperidone and quetiapine offer a low risk of EPS coupled with the least inherent anticholinergic effects.

Clozapine

Clozapine was the first atypical antipsychotic drug to be marketed that offered major advantages but unique and serious adverse effects as well. Its unique efficacy for treatment-resistant patients and negative symptoms, as well as the fact that it rarely causes EPS, is related to its greater affinity to block serotonergic and dopamine-4 receptors than dopamine-2 receptors.[40] Frequent adverse effects include sedation, orthostatic hypotension, anticholinergic effects, and excessive salivation, while persistent sedation and prominent weight gain complicate long-term therapy. Seizures, as discussed above, are dose related and are 5 to 10 times more likely to occur than with other antipsychotic drugs. Agranulocytosis is the major adverse effect of concern, occurring in 0.4 to 2% of patients. Clozapine agranulocytosis is characterized by a white blood cell (WBC) count of less than 2000 cells/mm^3, a polymorphonuclear leukocyte count of less than 500 cells/mm^3, and relative lymphopenia. WBC count monitoring is a mandatory component of treatment, and despite weekly monitoring, 12 deaths (3.1% of cases) have been reported due to complications of clozapine agranulocytosis.[41] Early presenting symptoms of agranulocytosis include lethargy, weakness, fever, and sore throat. Because most cases occur within the first 6 months of therapy, weekly WBC count monitoring is required for 6 months, then less frequently thereafter. If the WBC count falls below 3000/mm^3 or the absolute neutrophil count is below 1500/mm^3, clozapine therapy should be immediately interrupted. The initial dose of clozapine must be very low and titrated upward slowly due to its significant adverse effect profile–12.5 to 25 mg/day increased by 25 to 50 mg/day over 2 weeks. Most patients who respond require 200 to 400 mg/day, although doses up to 900 mg/day may be necessary. Optimal plasma levels are 200 to 350 ng/mL.[33,42] Because several other atypical antipsychotic drugs are now available that offer the benefits of efficacy for negative symptoms and rarely cause EPS without the concern of seizures and agranulocytosis, clozapine is now reserved only for the most treatment-resistant patients.

Risperidone

Risperidone is a potent serotonin-2 (5-HT_2) receptor blocking agent with weaker but dose-dependent dopamine-2 (D_2) receptor blockade. This mechanism supports its efficacy for negative symptoms and a lower risk of causing EPS.[43] Although clozapine still has the best established efficacy for treatment-resistant patients, risperidone thus far has shown equal efficacy in this population.[44] The effective dose range for most patients is 2 to 6 mg/day. Risperidone is not sedating for most patients and may even cause initial insomnia with bedtime dosing. Common adverse effects include insomnia, agitation, orthostatic hypotension, and weight gain. The risk of EPS is dose-related: rare at 1 to 2 mg/day but increasing as the dose exceeds 6 mg/day.[45]

Olanzapine

Olanzapine is a serotonin and dopamine receptor antagonist with receptor effects similar to clozapine. It is effective for the negative symptoms of schizophrenia, EPS are rare, and seizures and blood dyscrasias have not been reported. Common adverse effects include sedation and weight gain, although orthostatic hypotensive and anticholinergic effects are possible. Over several months of therapy, 56% of patients gain more than 7% of their baseline weight. The initial dose is either 5 or 10 mg once daily at bedtime, and most patients optimally respond to 10 mg/day.[46,47]

Cigarette smokers, due to CYP4501A2 enzyme induction, may require at least 20 mg/day.

Quetiapine

Among the four atypical antipsychotic drugs quetiapine has the least affinity for dopamine receptors and thus should be the least likely to cause EPS and elevations in prolactin levels. Unlike most antipsychotic drugs, its metabolism relies primarily upon cytochrome P-450 enzyme 3A4 rather than 1A2 or 2D6. Common adverse effects include sedation and weight gain, with initial orthostatic hypotension possible. The initial dose is 25 mg BID, increasing by 25 to 50 mg every 1 to 2 days up to a target range of 300 to 600 mg/day on a BID schedule.[48,49]

Nonpharmacologic Therapy

Although antipsychotic drugs can eliminate or minimize psychotic symptoms, psychologic, vocational, and social therapies are necessary to facilitate day-to-day coping skills and improve the long-term outcome of patients with schizophrenia. Before the availability of atypical antipsychotics, many patients remained socially isolated and dysfunctional because of their negative symptoms. Now that both positive and negative symptoms can often be successfully treated, psychosocial treatment programs are even more necessary to assist patients in achieving their full social and occupational potential. If patients with schizophrenia only receive medication, their treatment is inadequate.

ALTERNATIVE THERAPIES

For significant psychotic disorders such as schizophrenia, there are no alternative therapies or herbal remedies.

FUTURE THERAPIES

The success of the first few atypical antipsychotic drugs is leading to the development of additional antipsychotic drugs with complex mechanisms involving many neurotransmitter systems. Strategies to treat schizophrenia include the development of dopamine antagonists with high selectivity for different subtypes of dopamine receptors, dopamine partial agonists, antagonists at different serotonin receptor subtypes, drugs with mixed pharmacologic profiles, and drugs that modify transmission via amino acids or peptides in the brain.[50]

IMPROVING OUTCOMES

A principal reason to counsel patients taking antipsychotic drugs is to increase the likelihood of their compliance with maintenance therapy. The prevalence of medication noncompliance among patients with schizophrenia is 50% 1 year after discharge and 75% at 2 years. The factors most responsible for noncompliance with antipsychotic drugs include adverse effects (especially EPS), forgetfulness and cognitive deficits of schizophrenia, lack of insight and denial of illness, complexity of the drug regimen, and unsupportive family beliefs.[51] Patient and family education about the illness and appropriate expectations regarding treatment response, coupled with adequate monitoring and management of adverse effects can increase compliance and outcome.[52,53] It is critical for patients and family members to understand that antipsychotic drugs are primarily useful in preventing return of symptoms, so maintenance therapy is necessary after symptoms are gone. Support groups such as the National Alliance for the Mentally Ill (NAMI), with numerous local chapters, are very effective sources of information about schizophrenia for family members. Antipsychotic drugs are best described to patients and family members as medicine for "thinking," useful in treating such symptoms as hearing voices, confused or frightening thoughts, or fears of being around other people. After mentioning some positive aspects of the medication, then common adverse effects should be mentioned along with what to do if they occur. Merely listing the possible adverse effects alone may scare the patient and provides no help in their knowing what to do about adverse effects that do occur. Table 57.5 suggests which adverse effects should be mentioned in counseling. For example, haloperidol counseling should focus on EPS ("muscle side effects"), whereas quetiapine counseling should focus on initial orthostatic hypotension and sedation.

PHARMACOECONOMICS

A survey in the United Kingdom found that 75% of the cost of treating schizophrenia was hospital and community-based care, whereas only 5% was drug cost, and 97% of the total direct cost of treating schizophrenia is incurred by less than half the patients.[54] Drug treatment, although initially expensive, which can successfully help this subgroup of patients and reduce the total cost of care will be a rational and cost-effective decision. Cost-benefit studies with both clozapine and risperidone have shown that their higher drug costs are easily offset after 1 to 2 years due to decreased rates of rehospitalization or less time spent in the hospital.[55] An unknown cost factor involving improved outcome with atypical antipsychotic drugs, however, is the fact that as more patients' negative symptoms are successfully treated, there will be an increased need for psychosocial treatment programs to build or restore social and occupational skills.

KEY POINTS

- Schizophrenia is a chronic disorder requiring maintenance treatment to prevent relapse.
- A distinction between positive and negative symptoms influences the drug of choice along with consideration of adverse effect profiles and past history of response.
- Prudent use of a combination of a benzodiazepine with an antipsychotic drug is preferred over high-dose antipsychotic drug therapy when treating acute episodes.

- Without maintenance medication, 70% of patients have a relapse within 1 year.
- Continuous low-dose maintenance antipsychotic drug therapy is recommended because intermittent treatment does not prevent relapse as well and increases the risk of TD.
- Depot antipsychotic drugs are underutilized in the United States as depot drugs lower the relapse rate compared to oral medication.
- EPS and TD represent the most common and serious adverse effects from typical antipsychotic drugs and are the primary causes of noncompliance with treatment.
- Weight gain is the most troublesome long-term adverse effect, seen commonly with both typical and atypical antipsychotic drugs.
- Atypical antipsychotic drugs revolutionized the treatment of schizophrenia in the mid-1990s–for the first time, negative symptoms can be effectively treated, EPS are rare, and approximately 50% of previously treatment-resistant patients hospitalized for decades can now be successfully treated and discharged to the community.
- Clozapine opened the door to this new era, but its use is severely limited because it may cause agranulocytosis and seizures.
- Risperidone, olanzapine, and quetiapine represent the beginning of a new generation of atypical drugs, which have become first-line treatment for schizophrenia.
- Effective treatment of negative symptoms has allowed many more patients to be able to benefit from occupational and psychosocial skills training programs.
- The total cost of care for schizophrenia can be reduced by using the newer atypical drugs despite their higher costs relative to typical antipsychotic drugs.

REFERENCES

1. Herz MI, Liberman RP, Lieberman JA, et al. APA practice guideline for the treatment of patients with schizophrenia. Am J Psychiatry 154(Suppl 4):1–63, 1997.
2. American Psychiatric Association. Diagnostic and statistical manual of mental disorders. 4th ed. Washington, DC: American Psychiatric Association, 1994: 273–315.
3. Ereshefsky L, Tran-Johnson TK, Watanabe MD. Pathophysiologic basis for schizophrenia and the efficacy of antipsychotics. Clin Pharm 9:682–707, 1990.
4. Buchanan RW, Brandes M, Breier A. Treating negative symptoms: pharmacological strategies. In: Breier A. The new pharmacotherapy of schizophrenia. Washington, DC: American Psychiatric Press, 1996:179–204.
5. Anonymous. Current concepts in schizophrenia: international symposia report new standards for assessment and treatment. J Clin Psychiatry 56:214–225, 1995.
6. American Pharmaceutical Association. APhA guide to drug treatment protocols–management of schizophrenia. Washington, DC, June 1997.
7. Zavodnick S. A pharmacological and theoretical comparison of high and low potency neuroleptics. J Clin Psychiatry 39:332–336, 1978.
8. Palao DJ, Arauxo A, Brunet M, et al. Haloperidol: therapeutic window for schizophrenia. J Clin Psychopharmacol 14:303–310, 1994.
9. Coryell W, Miller DD, Perry PJ. Haloperidol plasma levels and dose optimization. Am J Psychiatry 155:48–53, 1998.
10. Hillard JR. Emergency treatment of acute psychosis. J Clin Psychiatry 59 (Suppl 1):57–60, 1998.
11. Davis JM, Kane JM, Marder SR, et al. Dose response of prophylactic antipsychotics. J Clin Psychiatry 54(Suppl 3):24–30, 1993.
12. Carpenter WT. Maintenance therapy of persons with schizophrenia. J Clin Psychiatry 57(Suppl 9):10–18, 1996.
13. Gilbert PL, Harris J, McAdams LA, et al. Neuroleptic withdrawal in schizophrenic patients. Arch Gen Psychiatry 52:173–188, 1995.
14. Glazer WM, Kane JM. Depot neuroleptic therapy: an underutilized option. J Clin Psychiatry 53:426–433, 1992.
15. Chouinard G, Annable L, Campbell W. A randomized clinical trial of haloperidol decanoate and fluphenazine decanoate in the outpatient treatment of schizophrenia. J Clin Psychopharmacol 9:247–253, 1989.
16. Jann M, Ereshefsky L, Saklad SR. Clinical pharmacokinetics of the depot antipsychotics. Clin Pharmacokinet 10:315–333, 1985.
17. Ereshefsky L, Toney G, Saklad SR, et al. A loading-dose strategy for converting from oral to depot haloperidol. Hosp Community Psychiatry 44:1155–1161, 1993.
18. Holloman LC, Marder SR. Management of acute extrapyramidal effects induced by antipsychotic drugs. Am J Health-Syst Pharm 54:2461–2477, 1997.
19. Remington GJ, Voineskos G, Pollock B, et al. Prevalence of neuroleptic-induced dystonia in mania and schizophrenia. Am J Psychiatry 147:1231–1233, 1990.
20. Tonda ME, Guthrie SK. Treatment of acute neuroleptic-induced movement disorders. Pharmacotherapy 14:543–560, 1994.
21. Sachdev P, Kruk J. Clinical characteristics and predisposing factors in acute drug-induced akathisia. Arch Gen Psychiatry 51:963–974, 1994.
22. Miller CH, Mohr R, Umbricht D, et al. The prevalence of acute extrapyramidal signs and symptoms in patients treated with clozapine, risperidone, and conventional antipsychotics. J Clin Psychiatry 59:69–75, 1998.
23. Morgenstern H, Glazer WM. Identifying risk factors for tardive dyskinesia among long-term outpatients maintained with neuroleptic medications. Arch Gen Psychiatry 50:723–773, 1993.
24. Gardos G, Casey DE, Cole JO, et al. Ten-year outcome of tardive dyskinesia. Am J Psychiatry 151:836–881, 1994.
25. van Harten PN, Hoek HW, Matroos GE, et al. Intermittent neuroleptic treatment and risk for tardive dyskinesia: Curacao Extrapyramidal Syndromes Study III. Am J Psychiatry 155:565–567, 1998.
26. Lawrence KR, Nasraway SA. Conduction disturbances associated with administration of butyrophenone antipsychotics in the critically ill: a review of the literature. Pharmacotherapy 17:531–537, 1997.
27. Gurrera RJ, Chang SS, Romero JA. A comparison of diagnostic criteria for neuroleptic malignant syndrome. J Clin Psychiatry 53:56–62, 1992.
28. Sachdev P, Kruk J, Kneebone M, et al. Clozapine-induced neuroleptic malignant syndrome: review and report of new cases. J Clin Psychopharmacol 15:365–371, 1995.
29. Gelenberg AJ. The best treatment for NMS is: (A) dantrolene (B) bromocriptine (C) the combination (D) none of the above. Biol Ther Psychiatry News 15:13, 16, 1992.
30. Zito JM, Sofair JB, Jaeger J. Self-reported neuroendocrine effects of antipsychotics in women: a pilot study. DICP 24:176–180, 1990.
31. Segraves RT. The effects of minor tranquilizers, mood stabilizers, and antipsychotics on sexual function. Prim Psychiatry 4:46–48, 1997.
32. Stimmel GL, Dopheide JA. Psychotropic drug-induced reductions in seizure threshold. CNS Drugs 1:37–50, 1996.
33. Lieberman JA. Maximizing clozapine therapy: managing side effects. J Clin Psychiatry 59(Suppl 3):38–43, 1998.
34. Doss FW. The effect of antipsychotic drugs on body weight: a retrospective review. J Clin Psychiatry 40:528–530, 1979.
35. Preskorn SH. Clinically relevant pharmacology of selective serotonin reuptake inhibitors. Clin Pharmacokinet 32(Suppl 1):1–21, 1997.
36. DeVane CL. Drug interactions and antipsychotic therapy. Pharmacotherapy 16(Part 2):15S–20S, 1996.
37. Goff DC, Baldessarini RJ. Drug interactions with antipsychotic agents. J Clin Psychopharmacol 13:57–67, 1993.
38. Stahl SM. Awakening from schizophrenia: intramolecular polypharmacy and the atypical antipsychotics. J Clin Psychiatry 58:381–382, 1997.
39. Lieberman JA. Understanding the mechanism of action of atypical antipsychotic drugs. Br J Psychiatry 163(Suppl 22):7–18, 1993.
40. Meltzer HY. An overview of the mechanism of action of clozapine. J Clin Psychiatry 55(Suppl 9B):47–52, 1994.
41. Honigfeld G, Arellano F, Sethi J, et al. Reducing clozapine-related morbidity and mortality: 5 years of experience with the Clozaril national registry. J Clin Psychiatry 59(Suppl 3):3–7, 1998.
42. Conley RR. Optimizing treatment with clozapine. J Clin Psychiatry 59(Suppl 3):44–48, 1998.
43. Cohen LJ. Risperidone. Pharmacotherapy 14:253–265, 1994.

44. Bondolfi G, Dufour H, Patris M, et al. Risperidone versus clozapine in treatment-resistant chronic schizophrenia: a randomized double-blind study. Am J Psychiatry 155:499–504, 1998.
45. Curtis VA, Kerwin RW. A risk-benefit assessment of risperidone in schizophrenia. Drug Saf 12:139–145, 1995.
46. Bever KA, Perry PJ. Olanzapine: a serotonin-dopamine receptor antagonist for antipsychotic therapy. Am J Health-Syst Pharm 55:1003–1016, 1998.
47. Nemeroff CB. Dosing the antipsychotic medication olanzapine. J Clin Psychiatry 58(Suppl 10):45–49, 1997.
48. Casey DE. Seroquel (quetiapine): preclinical and clinical findings of a new atypical antipsychotic. Exp Opin Invest Drugs 5:939–957, 1996.
49. Small JG, Hirsch SR, Arvanitis LA, et al. Quetiapine in patients with schizophrenia. Arch Gen Psychiatry 54:549–557, 1997.
50. Fleischhacker WW. New drugs for the treatment of schizophrenic patients. Acta Psychiatr Scand 91(Suppl 38):24–30, 1995.
51. Marder SR. Facilitating compliance with antipsychotic medication. J Clin Psychiatry 59(Suppl 3):21–25, 1998.
52. Kemp R, Kirov G, Everitt B, et al. Randomised controlled trial of compliance therapy. Br J Psychiatry 172:413–419, 1998.
53. Fleischhacker WW, Meise U, Gunther V, et al. Compliance with antipsychotic drug treatment: influence of side effects. Acta Psychiatr Scand 89(Suppl 382):11–15, 1994.
54. Davies LM, Drummond MF. Economics and schizophrenia: the real cost. Br J Psychiatry 165(Suppl 25):18–21, 1994.
55. Hargreaves WA, Shumway M. Pharmacoeconomics of antipsychotic drug therapy. J Clin Psychiatry 57(Suppl 9):66–76, 1996.

CHAPTER 58

SLEEP DISORDERS

Michael Z. Wincor

DEFINITION

On average, we spend one-third of our lives sleeping, yet many of us take this psychophysiologic phenomenon for granted. Only when it becomes disturbed, do we pay some attention to it; even then, we probably heed the warnings of daytime fatigue less than we should. We do not know why, but we definitely need to sleep, and the exact sleep need varies a great deal among people. It has been found in various national surveys that during the course of a year 25 to 35% of the adult population have some complaint concerning sleep.[1] Up to 17% of the population experience serious insomnia. Patients with serious insomnia tend to be older women with high levels of psychic distress and somatic anxiety as well as multiple health problems. Between 2 and 4% of those surveyed use hypnotics or other psychotherapeutic agents to promote sleep. The vast majority of hypnotic users take these drugs for short periods (1 day to 2 weeks); only 11% (0.3% of all adults) report using the drugs regularly for a year or more.[2] An additional 3 to 4% use nonprescription sleep aids. However, a small survey of community pharmacists indicated little involvement in counseling patients about over-the-counter sleep aids.[3] Although insomnia and daytime sleepiness are two of the most common human complaints, most patients with serious insomnia (85%) do not receive treatment with either prescription or nonprescription hypnotics. With a fundamental understanding of sleep disorders, the clinician can make an important contribution not only in encouraging patients to seek proper evaluation, but also in educating the patient about prescription medications and nonpharmacologic approaches and advising patients on selection of over-the-counter sleep aids as well.

TREATMENT GOALS: SLEEP DISORDERS

- Treat any of the sleep disorders by normalizing sleep and, perhaps more importantly, improving daytime functioning and preventing the adverse consequences of disturbed sleep.
- Give any sleep complaint the same meticulous attention as that afforded to a complaint of chest pain, flank pain, or coughing up blood.
- Make a distinction between excessive daytime sleepiness, insomnia, and phenomena associated with specific sleep stages or sleep-wake transitions when assessing the sleep complaint.
- For excessive daytime sleepiness, consider obstructive sleep apnea and narcolepsy, as well as self-imposed sleep deprivation.
- Avoid all central nervous system (CNS) depressants in the management of sleep apnea.
- For pharmacologic treatment of narcolepsy focus on the excessive daytime sleepiness (e.g., CNS stimulants, modafinil) and the cataplexy (e.g., protriptyline, selective serotonin reuptake inhibitors [SSRIs]).
- For insomnia, distinguish between short-term and chronic types and identify the etiology; both drug (e.g., CNS stimulants, CNS depressant withdrawal, and ethanol) and non-drug factors (e.g., psychiatric disorders, medical disorders, circadian rhythm disorders, and poor sleep hygiene) must be considered.
- If a treatable cause of insomnia is identified (e.g., major depression), give specific treatment appropriate for that problem (e.g., antidepressant).
- Aim for improved sleep and improved daytime functioning in treatment of insomnia, including nondrug approaches (e.g., improved sleep hygiene).

- In general, treat short-term, not persistent, insomnias with hypnotics. Drugs of choice are the benzodiazepines (BZDs) (e.g., flurazepam, temazepam, triazolam, quazepam, and estazolam) and the BZD_1 receptor-specific nonbenzodiazepines (e.g., zolpidem and zaleplon); selection of an agent is based on differences in pharmacokinetic profiles and the needs of the individual patient.
- Use antihistamines (e.g., hydroxyzine, diphenhydramine, and doxylamine) for mild, short-term insomnia with due caution in light of their strong anticholinergic properties and high incidence of "morning hangover."
- Consider trazodone and other sedating antidepressants to improve sleep in patients with major depression who are being treated with stimulating selective serotonin reuptake inhibitors; patients must be monitored for possible orthostatic hypotension and, in the case of the tricyclics, anticholinergic side effects.
- Consider melatonin for patients with circadian rhythm disorders (e.g., jet lag).
- Use kava kava and valerian only with recognition that quality assurance is sometimes less than adequate and that more information is needed with respect to appropriate indications, optimal dosing, short- and long-term adverse effects, and potential interactions.

EPIDEMIOLOGY

Parasomnias

Of the more than 20 parasomnias, only sleepwalking (somnambulism), sleep terrors (pavor nocturnus), and nightmares are discussed in detail here. Both sleepwalking and sleep terrors are phenomena occurring in delta sleep with a peak prevalence between 4 and 12 years of age. At least one episode of sleepwalking is seen in about 15% of children and in 2 to 5% of adults. Sleep terrors (pavor nocturnus or night terrors) are seen in approximately 3% of children and less than 1% of adults, as they typically resolve during adolescence. It is estimated that 10 to 50% of children between 3 and 6 years of age have enough nightmares to disturb the parents. Approximately 50% of the adult population admit to having at least an occasional nightmare, and perhaps 1% experience frequent nightmares (one or more per week).[4]

Sleep Apnea

Sleep apnea generally has an onset in adulthood, usually after age 30, with a probable prevalence of 1 to 4% of the population, and, in the case of obstructive sleep apnea, is at least eight times more prevalent in men than in women. Although the incidence is high in older adults, many are asymptomatic (i.e., they have no complaints that would have brought this condition to the attention of a physician or sleep disorders specialist).[5]

Narcolepsy

Narcolepsy, along with obstructive sleep apnea, is a major cause of excessive daytime sleepiness and is found in approximately 0.1% of the population. Its onset is often during adolescence.[6,7]

Insomnia

As stated earlier, up to 35% of all adults will have insomnia in a given year. Some surveys estimate that this is the percentage of people who have a sleep problem at any given time.[1] The results of a prevalence study of randomly selected elderly (aged 65 and older) persons indicate that sleep apnea can be found in 24% and periodic limb movements during sleep can be found in 45%, with 10% showing both.[8,9]

The largest analysis of patients studied objectively in sleep disorders centers found that the most prevalent diagnosis for a complaint of insomnia was insomnia associated with psychiatric disorders (35%). Approximately half of these patients had a major affective disorder and half had personality disorders; less than 5% had major psychoses. Psychophysiologic insomnia (15%) was the second most frequent diagnosis, followed by drug and alcohol dependence (12.4%). Nearly 9% of people with complaints of insomnia had no significant sleep pathologic disorder. Sleep apnea syndromes accounted for 6.2% of insomnia. Circadian rhythm disorders were diagnosed in only 2.9% of the patients; however, this category may be underrepresented because of a lesser awareness at that time.[10]

The results, unfortunately, may not be representative of the population at large because they are findings from sleep disorders centers. Most persons with a sleep problem probably do not seek medical attention. No adequate, large-scale epidemiologic study has yet been done in the general population (i.e., persons seen in a primary care practice or in a community pharmacy). The most common sleep disorders may be adjustment sleep disorder (i.e., transient situational insomnia), insomnia associated with anxiety disorders, psychophysiologic insomnia, inadequate sleep hygiene, insomnia associated with mood disorders, obstructive sleep apnea syndrome, delayed or advanced sleep phase syndromes, shift work sleep disorders, alcohol/hypnotic/stimulant-dependent sleep disorders, and periodic limb movement disorder.

PATHOPHYSIOLOGY

Sleep Physiology

Sleep has been studied in various ways. Behaviorally, one can observe changes in body position, decreased responsiveness to external stimuli, and eyelid closure. Anatomically, sleep-regulating centers in the brainstem have been identified. Neurochemically, various neurotransmitters are involved in sleep mechanisms. Not long ago, we simply pointed to norepinephrine as being involved in wakefulness and dreaming sleep and serotonin as involved in nondreaming sleep. Then it became clear that there is an interaction between the cholinergic systems and the noradrenergic systems. In the future, contributions of other neurotransmitters and various endogenous peptides will likely be elucidated.[11,12]

Electrophysiology and Sleep Stages

Currently, the standard method for observing and measuring sleep is electrophysiologic.[13] In the laboratory, sleep is recorded polygraphically, with electroencephalograms (EEGs), electro-oculograms (EOGs) from each of the two eyes, and electromyograms (EMGs) generally of the mentalis and submentalis muscles. Two EOGs, one EEG, and one EMG would be the minimal recordings used for scoring sleep stages. A number of other physiologic variables may be needed to identify specific sleep disorders, as will be discussed. The entire recording process is often referred to as polysomnography. Today, by means of portable devices, such recordings are possible in the patient's home.

By means of these recordings, sleep can be divided into nonrapid eye movement (NREM) sleep that is further subdivided into stages 1 through 4 and rapid eye movement (REM) sleep. Wakefulness is characterized by a low-voltage, fast EEG; high muscle tone; and various types of eye movements, including blinks. Stage 1 sleep is characterized by a low-voltage, mixed-frequency EEG; slightly decreased muscle tone; and slow, rolling eye movements. The subjective experience of this transition stage varies widely among people, some experiencing it as wakefulness, others as drowsiness, and yet others as sleep. Stage 2 is characterized by sleep spindles and K-complexes in the EEG and is recognized as unequivocal sleep. Stages 3 and 4 are characterized by high-amplitude, slow activity in the EEG known as delta waves; hence, these two stages together are often referred to as delta sleep. Delta sleep appears to be the deep, restorative sleep that most people (especially patients with insomnia) think of when they visualize sleep.

REM sleep is characterized by a low-voltage, mixed-frequency EEG, in many ways quite similar to that seen in stage 1, but with very low muscle tone and bursts of bilaterally conjugate rapid eye movements. It appears as though the sleeper is watching a movie or actively observing some activity. Classical dreaming occurs in REM sleep; dream reports can be obtained 80 to 90% of the times that subjects are awakened during or at the end of REM periods. Brain and autonomic activity may be greater and more variable than during relaxed wakefulness.

Physiologic Changes During Sleep

Physiologically, much activity occurs during sleep. Although heart rate and respiratory rate are slow and regular during NREM sleep, they, along with blood pressure, become irregular with rapid changes in REM sleep. In the male, erections occur regularly during REM sleep. In fact, this phenomenon of nocturnal penile tumescence is often used in an attempt to distinguish between psychologic and physiologic etiologies of impotence. Body temperature descends to its lowest in the early morning, while, during REM sleep, the sleeper is poikilothermic (cold-blooded). Cortisol levels are lowest at sleep onset, while growth hormone is released during delta sleep. Melatonin secretion increases in sleep and can be suppressed by bright light.

Function of Sleep

Although the function of sleep is not clearly understood, it is believed that NREM sleep serves to restore, rejuvenate, and revitalize the body. Slow-wave sleep seems to play an important role in thermoregulation and tissue repair. Metabolic rate decreases during sleep, with a fall not only in body temperature, but also a decrease in glucose consumption and production of catabolic hormones. On the other hand, along with the increase in growth hormone seen in delta sleep, there is an increase in skeletal muscle protein synthesis during sleep. Slow-wave sleep may have a role in maintaining immune function. It would appear, then, that adequate sleep is critical for growing children and persons with healing wounds or infections.

REM sleep may be needed to sort through short-term memory stores, deleting unnecessary data and laying down important information in long-term memory. REM sleep may also play a role in maintaining noradrenergic receptor sensitivity. Whatever its role, REM sleep appears to be of vital physiologic importance in that REM deprivation leads to a dramatic REM rebound during recovery sleep.[14]

Sleep Cycle

The architecture of sleep in the normal young adult is cyclic. The sleeper quickly passes from wakefulness through stages 1 and 2, spending a moderate block of time in delta sleep. Some 90 minutes after sleep onset, the sleeper enters the first REM period of the night, which may last only 5 to 7 minutes. The cycle is repeated four to five times each night. As the night progresses, less time is spent in delta sleep, with most delta sleep occurring in the first half of the night. REM periods become longer and more intense, both physiologically and psychologically, as the night goes on. The final REM period of the night may last as long as 30 to 60 minutes. Most persons who recall a dream in the morning are waking from this REM period and remembering the dream's content. In general, one spends approximately 75% of the night in NREM sleep and the remaining 25% of the night in REM sleep.

In older adults, however, the typical sleep architecture described here may be quite different, with a considerable decrease in delta sleep, an increase in light sleep, an increase in awakenings during the night, and a generally more disrupted night of sleep. There may be a slight decrease in total sleep time during the night, compared with young adults, but how much daytime napping and specific sleep pathologic conditions (e.g., sleep apnea and periodic limb movements) contribute to this apparent decrease is unclear. Even in randomly selected, noncomplaining, elderly persons, the incidence of sleep apnea and periodic limb movements is as high as 58%.[8,9,15]

The parameters that can be measured objectively in the sleep laboratory, which are of particular interest with respect to insomnia and drug effects on sleep, are listed in Table 58.1. Latency to sleep onset (or sleep latency) is defined as the length of time taken to fall asleep after getting into bed. The number of awakenings and number of stage shifts during the night are indications of how disrupted sleep has been. REM intensity, or the frequency of bursts of rapid eye movements, may at times be a subtler indicator of changes in REM sleep than simply the total number of minutes spent in REM sleep during the night. Finally, other physiologic measurements may include electrocardiogram, respiration, oxygen saturation, and activity of the anterior tibialis muscles.

Sleep Apnea

Sleep apnea is often described as obstructive, central, or mixed. Obstructive sleep apnea is caused by something obstructing the airway. The problem may be the tongue falling back across the airway, enlarged tonsils, or some other craniofacial abnormality. Respiratory effort continues as is demonstrated by strain gauge recordings around the thorax and abdomen in the absence of nasal/oral airflow (measured by a device attached to the face below the nostrils). In central sleep apnea, respiratory effort ceases, indicating a problem in the respiratory centers of the brain, with a resultant absence of nasal and oral airflow. In mixed sleep apnea, there seems to be a cessation of central respiratory effort, followed by an obstructive event, and then even when respiratory effort resumes, there is no airflow. In any of these cases, as oxygen saturation falls (which can be measured with an earlobe oximeter) and carbon dioxide levels rise, the brain automatically produces a "mini-arousal" resulting in resumption of breathing. Whether the patient complains of insomnia or excessive daytime sleepiness is subjective, but obstructive sleep apnea seems to be more highly associated with complaints of excessive daytime sleepiness, whereas central sleep apnea appears to be more closely associated with complaints of insomnia.[5,6]

Narcolepsy

Sleep laboratory findings strongly suggest that narcolepsy involves a dysregulation of REM sleep. In addition to cataplexy and sleep paralysis (which represent the loss of muscle tone in REM sleep), narcoleptic patients have sleep-onset REM periods (i.e., instead of the normal latency of 90 minutes after sleep onset to the first REM period, they can make a transition from wakefulness immediately to REM sleep). The genetic basis of the disorder is supported by an association between the human leukocyte antigen-DR2 phenotype and narcolepsy.[16]

Table 58.1 ▪ Sleep Parameters

Latency to sleep onset
Total sleep time
Sleep stage durations
Sleep stage percentages of total sleep time
Number of awakenings during the night
Number of stage shifts during the night
Rapid eye movement intensity
Other physiologic measurements

CLINICAL PRESENTATION AND DIAGNOSIS

Historical Perspective

In the 1970s, a group of clinically oriented sleep researchers developed an organization, the Association of Sleep Disorders Centers, as well as a scheme for classifying sleep disorders.[17] Simply stated, disorders of initiating and maintaining sleep were equivalent to insomnia, the disorders of excessive somnolence were equivalent to excessive daytime sleepiness, the disorders of the sleep-wake schedule involved disturbances of biologic rhythms, and the parasomnias included a number of miscellaneous disorders associated with sleep, sleep stages, or partial arousals. There was a considerable amount of overlap in possible etiologies among the major categories of disorders, with the exception of the parasomnias. In fact, the determining factor in applying a label to the patient was often the nature of the subjective complaint (e.g., "Doctor, I'm not sleeping well at night" versus "Doctor, I'm always sleepy").

As sleep disorders clinicians worked with this classification scheme over the years, an international effort for revision and modification began. The result was *The International Classification of Sleep Disorders* (ICSD),[18] a very extensive listing and description of the sleep disorders (as outlined in Table 58.2). It was published by what was called the American Sleep Disorders Association, in cooperation with the European Sleep Research Society, the Japanese Society of Sleep Research, and the Latin American Sleep Society. Concurrently, but separately, a committee of the American Psychiatric Association was revising its official *Diagnostic and Statistical Manual of Mental Disorders*, 4th edition (DSM-IV). The result was a somewhat abbreviated nomenclature for the sleep disorders most likely to be encountered in a psychiatric practice.[19] It is outlined in Table 58.3 for the sake of completeness; however, because the ICSD is the more exhaustive, international classification, it will serve as the basis of this discussion. Eighty-four specific sleep disorders are described in the ICSD. It is beyond the scope of this chapter to cover each of them in detail; however, examples in each of the major categories are listed in Table 58.2 to provide the reader with an idea of the progress made in the past 20 years in identifying and classifying sleep disorders.

The entire field of sleep disorders medicine is in its infancy, at most approaching adolescence. For many of the sleep disorders, both etiology and prevalence are as yet unclear (in instances where these are established or even postulated, such information will be mentioned). The remaining discussion is focused on the disorders that have been best studied, are seen most often, or are most likely to

Table 58.2 ▪ International Classification of Sleep Disorders (ICSD): Framework and Examples

1. Dyssomnias: disorders that are characterized by difficulty in initiating or maintaining sleep or by excessive sleepiness
   A. Intrinsic sleep disorders: developing within the body or from causes within the body

307.42-0	Psychophysiologic insomnia
347	Narcolepsy
780.53-0	Obstructive sleep apnea syndrome
780.51-0	Central sleep apnea syndrome
780.51-1	Periodic limb movement disorder
780.52-5	Restless legs syndrome

   B. Extrinsic sleep disorders: developing from causes outside of the body

307.41-1	Inadequate sleep hygiene
780.52-6	Environmental sleep disorder
780.52-0	Hypnotic-dependent sleep disorder
780.52-1	Stimulant-dependent sleep disorder
780.52-3	Alcohol-dependent sleep disorder

   C. Circadian rhythm sleep disorders: related to the timing of sleep in the 24-hour day

307.45-0	Time zone change (jet lag) syndrome
307.45-1	Shift work sleep disorder
780.55-0	Delayed sleep phase syndrome

2. Parasomnias: undesirable physical phenomena occurring predominantly during sleep, including disorders of arousal, partial arousal, and sleep stage transition
   A. Arousal disorders: Disorders of impaired arousal from slow wave (delta) sleep

307.46-0	Sleepwalking
307.46-1	Sleep terrors

   B. Sleep-wake transition disorders

307.47-2	Sleep starts
307.47-3	Sleep talking
729.82	Nocturnal leg cramps

   C. Parasomnias usually associated with REM sleep

307.47-0	Nightmares
780.56-2	Sleep paralysis
780.59-0	REM sleep behavior disorder

   D. Other parasomnias

306.8	Sleep bruxism
780.56-0	Sleep enuresis
780.53-1	Primary snoring

3. Medical/psychiatric sleep disorders
   A. Associated with mental disorders

292-299	Psychoses
296-301	Mood disorders
300	Anxiety disorders
300	Panic disorder
303	Alcoholism

   B. Associated with neurological disorders

331	Dementia
332-333	Parkinsonism

   C. Associated with other medical disorders

490-494	Chronic obstructive pulmonary disease
493	Sleep-related asthma
530.1	Sleep-related gastroesophageal reflux
531-534	Peptic ulcer disease
729.1	Fibrositis syndrome

4. Proposed sleep disorders: disorders for which insufficient or inadequate information is available to substantiate their unequivocal existence

780.54.3	Menstrual-associated sleep disorder
780.59-6	Pregnancy-associated sleep disorder
307.47-4	Terrifying hypnagogic hallucinations

Source: Reference 18.

Table 58.3 ▪ DSM-IV Classification of Sleep Disorders

Primary sleep disorders	
Dyssomnias	
307.42	Primary insomnia
307.44	Primary hypersomnia
347	Narcolepsy
780.59	Breathing-related sleep disorder
307.45	Circadian rhythm sleep disorder
307.47	Dyssomnia not otherwise specified
Parasomnias	
307.47	Nightmare disorder
307.46	Sleep terror disorder
307.46	Sleepwalking disorder
307.47	Parasomnia not otherwise specified
Sleep disorders related to another mental disorder	
307.42	Insomnia related to...
307.44	Hypersomnia related to...
Other sleep disorders	
780.xx	Sleep disorder due to...(a medical condition)
———	Substance-induced sleep disorder

Source: Reference 19.

have a pharmacotherapeutic component to treatment. Particular emphasis is placed on insomnia and the use of hypnotics.

Parasomnias

Somnambulism

Typically, the sleepwalker sits up, gets out of bed, walks around, and returns to bed. The person appears to be navigating well, but critical skills and reactivity are impaired (e.g., if you were to rearrange the furniture in the house, the sleepwalker would probably stumble over it).[4]

Sleep Terrors

Sleep terrors are characterized by extreme vocalizations, motility, and autonomic variability. Recall of frightening content is minimal or absent. Hence, the phenomenon may be more disturbing to others in the house than to the child experiencing it. The parents of the child may hear a "blood-curdling" scream; run into the sleeper's bedroom; and find the child wet from perspiration, breathing forcefully, and experiencing tachycardia. Fortunately, the absence of frightening content results in nothing psychologic with which to associate the event. Generally, there is amnesia for the event.[4]

Nightmares

Unlike sleep terrors, nightmares ("bad dreams") occur in REM sleep (in about 5% of the general population) and are associated with elaborate and frightening content. There is less motility and autonomic variability than in sleep terrors.[4]

Sleep Apnea

Sleep apnea, a sleep-induced respiratory impairment, is a condition characterized by episodes of cessation of breathing.[5] Each apneic episode, often lasting 20 to 30 seconds, is terminated by a brief arousal from sleep during which breathing resumes. There may be as many as several hundred of these "mini-arousals" during a single night, but the patient may not be aware of their occurrence. The patient may instead complain of morning headache, irritability, and general difficulty with daytime functioning. Often, the bed partner is the best source of information, reporting that the patient snores very loudly or has periods in which breathing stops followed by gasps for air. Often there is a recent history of weight gain associated with onset of symptoms. Common complications of sleep apnea include arrhythmias, systolic or diastolic hypertension, and signs of pulmonary arterial hypertension and right-sided heart failure.

Narcolepsy

Patients with narcolepsy are extremely sleepy throughout the day and find themselves falling asleep at inopportune moments. There are four classic features: excessive daytime sleepiness, cataplexy, sleep paralysis, and hypnagogic hallucinations. Cataplexy is described as brief (lasting only seconds to minutes) episodes of muscle weakness that may result in the patient collapsing. They are often precipitated by emotionally charged stimuli (e.g., laughter, anger, or excitement). Sleep paralysis, which occurs during the transition either between wakefulness and sleep or between sleep and wakefulness, involves inhibition of the musculature. This is particularly frightening because the patient is aware of the paralysis. Hypnagogic hallucinations, which occur during the transition between wakefulness and sleep, are brief dreamlike events but perhaps more fragmented and bizarre than a typical dream.[6,7]

Insomnia

Insomnia is a problem that 95% of all adults have experienced at least once in their lives. It must be defined in terms of both amount of sleep and its perceived quality. No absolute number of hours of sleep per se constitutes insomnia because sleep need among persons is highly variable. The person who sleeps 5 hours per night, only needs 5 hours per night, and functions in his or her daily activities at peak performance does not have insomnia. However, the person who needs 8 hours per night, sleeps only 7 with a perception of fragmented sleep, and complains of daytime impairment may indeed be suffering from insomnia. Hence, insomnia must be seen as a perceived relative decrease in the quantity and/or quality of sleep along with some perceived consequences in waking life. These perceptions take the form of a subjective complaint by the patient. In many respects, the sleep of patients with insomnia is not that dramatically different from that of good sleepers, but they perceive it as poor sleep. Unfortunately, at present, there is no definitive way to measure the quality of sleep in the sleep laboratory; however, it appears likely that fragmentation of sleep (as indicated by arousals, stage shifts, and perhaps subtle findings in EEG frequencies) is most closely associated with perceived quality.[4,20]

Insomnia can be viewed from various perspectives. The severity (i.e., from mild to severe) clearly has implications with respect to treatment decisions. Whether the insomnia is transient or chronic is important in both diagnosis and treatment. Finally, the pattern of a typical night may be characterized by difficulty falling sleep, difficulty staying asleep (numerous awakenings during the night), early morning awakening (3 to 4 hours earlier than expected, with an inability to return to sleep), or some combination of these problems.

The actual neurochemical or pathophysiologic bases for the various types of insomnia are, in general, unknown. There are numerous "causes" for insomnia. Many of the drug and nondrug factors associated with insomnia are listed in Tables 58.4 and 58.5. Medical causes include pain of various types (e.g., arthritis, pruritus, or duodenal ulcer). Pain not only interferes with the ability to fall asleep but also may lead to increased nocturnal arousals and a generally "lighter" sleep. Nocturia may be part of a medical disorder or a result of a dose of a diuretic taken too late; the result in either case is fragmentation of sleep. Psychologic or psychiatric causes of insomnia can be as common as worry or excitement (e.g., over an important examination or job interview). Almost everyone is familiar with an occasional bout of insomnia associated with emotional arousal. In addition, it is almost certain that some type of sleep disturbance will accompany an acute episode of any of the major psychiatric disorders (e.g., schizophrenia, major depression, or mania), and often the sleep disturbance is one of the diagnostic criteria. Other causes may include disruption of circadian rhythms (e.g., jet lag or work shift

Table 58.4 ▪ Nondrug Factors Associated with Long-Term Insomnia

Psychiatric disorders	Medical/neurologic disorders *(continued)*
Mood disorders	Asthma
Anxiety disorders	Bronchitis
Somatoform disorders	Chronic obstructive pulmonary disease
Eating disorders	Chronic liver failure
Personality disorders	Chronic renal failure
Chronic pain	Congestive heart failure
Alcohol/substance abuse	Cystic fibrosis
Sleep disorders	Dementia
Sleep apnea	Epilepsy
Periodic limb movement disorder	Gastroesophageal reflux
Restless legs syndrome	Head injury
Delayed sleep phase syndrome	Hyperthyroidism
Psychophysiologic conditioning	Hypoglycemia
Shift work	Malignancy
Medical/neurologic disorders	Menopause
Angina	Parkinson's disease
Arthritis	Peptic ulcer disease

Table 58.5 ▪ Drugs Associated with Insomnia

Alcohol	Corticosteroids	Oral contraceptives
Amphetamines	Decongestants	Phenytoin
Antipsychotics	Diuretics	Quinidine
Appetite suppressants	Hypnotics (chronic use)	Reserpine
β-Agonists/ blockers	Levodopa	Selective serotonin reuptake inhibitors
Bupropion	Methyldopa	Theophylline
Caffeine	Methysergide	Thyroid preparations
Clonidine	Monoamine oxidase inhibitors	Tricyclic antidepressants
Cocaine	Nicotine	

change), change of environment (e.g., sleeping for the first night or two in a hotel room in a strange city), sleep apnea, periodic limb movements, stimulant drugs, drug dependence, and drug withdrawal.

Often it is useful to classify insomnia as transient, short-term, or persistent (also called long-term or chronic). This distinction is valuable for both diagnosis and treatment decisions. Transient insomnia occurs in an otherwise normal sleeper, has a duration of only several days, and is often associated with an acute stress or disruption of the biologic clock (e.g., jet lag or change in work schedule). Short-term insomnia is very similar to transient insomnia except that its duration is several weeks. It too is often associated with some situational stress (e.g., loss of a loved one, family conflict, or work conflict) or serious medical illness.

Persistent insomnia lasts longer than several weeks and is often associated with psychiatric or medical conditions. Sleep apnea syndrome and the association of insomnia with psychiatric disorders have already been discussed. Periodic limb movement disorder (also called periodic leg movements, nocturnal myoclonus, or PMS [periodic movements during sleep]) is characterized by periodic (every 20 to 40 seconds), stereotypic, myoclonic movements of the anterior tibialis or other limb muscles during sleep, resulting in arousals. Like the arousals of sleep apnea, the patient may experience several hundred per night and yet not be aware of them the following day. Often, as with sleep apnea, the bed partner will voice the complaint, in this case about the sleeper's "kicking" throughout the night. The condition is age-related, showing a marked increase in incidence after 40 years of age. A related condition that can affect the ability to fall asleep is restless legs syndrome. This is characterized by uncomfortable sensations in the legs at rest, which can be relieved by movement; hence, the patient feels the need to get out of bed and move around.

A number of biologic rhythm disorders can be associated with a complaint of persistent insomnia, for example, delayed sleep phase syndrome.[21] Patients want to fall asleep at 11:00 PM and awaken at 7:00 AM. They get into bed at 11:00 PM and find that they cannot fall asleep for 4 or 5 hours. When they wake up (usually with the help of an alarm or two) at 7:00 AM to meet their and society's daily demands, they feel unrefreshed and tired. This pattern is repeated night after night. If patients are asked how late they would sleep if they did not have to get out of bed at 7:00 AM, they would probably say 11:00 AM or noon; hence, they could indeed sleep 8 hours. The patient's ability to sleep simply does not coincide with the period set aside for sleep; the body (i.e., his or her internal biologic clock) is not sleepy at the time that he or she wants to be sleeping.

Drugs and alcohol can be associated with insomnia in numerous ways. Any drug with stimulant properties can disrupt sleep, especially if taken late in the day. The use of CNS depressants, including alcohol, can lead to dependence; then, on withdrawal, it is common to see more disturbed, restless sleep. Even within a single night, alcohol can disrupt sleep. Although it may make the individual feel more relaxed and able to fall asleep, the short duration of action may allow a mild withdrawal in the middle of the night, associated with more disrupted sleep and increased dreaming due to a REM rebound (i.e., early in the night, the alcohol suppresses REM sleep and, as the effect of the alcohol wears off, there is a tendency to make up the lost REM sleep later in the night).

Psychophysiologic insomnia may be transient, short-term, or persistent. It is a conditioned or learned insomnia that the sleeper has associated with the bed, bedroom, or sleep process. The harder the patient tries, the more difficult it becomes to sleep. The patient becomes more and more focused on the inability to sleep and the resultant daytime impairment. Interestingly, such persons sleep remarkably well in the laboratory or in a strange hotel room, away from the conditions with which insomnia is associated, or at times when they are not thinking about trying to fall asleep (e.g., while watching TV or reading).

Finally, sleep-related gastroesophageal reflux, characterized by regurgitation of gastric contents or fluid into the esophagus during sleep, can awaken the patient from sleep, with heartburn or a sour taste in the mouth.

PSYCHOSOCIAL ASPECTS

Insomnia and the other sleep disorders can be crippling for many people. As life becomes more complex, it would not be surprising to see an increase in the incidence of transient insomnia. Seventy percent of those with difficulty sleeping never discuss the problem with a physician. Another 24% discuss their problem but only as a secondary issue during a physician visit. Only 6% seek the help of a physician as a primary reason for their office visit.[22] To what extent this represents embarrassment, denial, stoicism, or underestimation of the significance of the problem on the part of patients versus inadequate exploration on the part of clinicians is uncertain. Nonetheless, impaired cognitive functioning, decreased job performance, increased absenteeism, and decreased quality of life have all been associated with insomnia.[23]

TREATMENT

Pharmacotherapy

Parasomnias

Medications that may exacerbate or induce sleepwalking (e.g., thioridazine, chloral hydrate, lithium, fluphenazine, perphenazine, and desipramine) should be discontinued if possible. Theoretically, sleepwalking could be reduced by suppressing delta sleep. Most BZDs suppress delta sleep, and in an adult with frequent episodes, especially with a history of injury to self or others, a BZD may be a very appropriate and efficacious intervention. However, in the case of childhood sleepwalking, the benefit of treatment over simply protecting the individual from injury is questionable in light of the unknown risks of long-term exposure of the child's developing CNS to BZDs. The same reservations about use of delta sleep suppressants apply to sleep terrors as well.[4]

Sleep Apnea

The single most important pharmacologic intervention in the treatment of any type of sleep apnea is the careful avoidance of all drugs that have CNS depressant activity. These include anxiolytics, hypnotics, narcotics, and alcohol. Any agent that can interfere with the ability of the brain to produce an apnea-terminating mini-arousal is potentially lethal. Even CNS depressants that appear to have little or no effect on respiration during wakefulness must be avoided because some evidence indicates differential effects during sleep. Although some data indicate that a subset of patients with central sleep apnea may experience improved sleep quality from triazolam, increased total sleep time, and decreased apneic episodes,[24] it remains safest to avoid CNS depressants in all patients with sleep apnea. Active pharmacologic intervention in treating sleep apnea has shown mixed, fairly unimpressive results. Tricyclic antidepressants, particularly protriptyline, have been used in both obstructive and central sleep apnea. Protriptyline may act by decreasing REM sleep or by increasing oropharyngeal muscle tone.[25] Respiratory stimulants, such as medroxyprogesterone[26] and acetazolamide,[27] show only limited efficacy with no studies demonstrating long-term effectiveness.

Narcolepsy

Pharmacologic treatment of narcolepsy is focused on the excessive daytime sleepiness on the one hand and the cataplexy on the other.[7] CNS stimulants are used for the sleepiness. Hesitation in prescribing amphetamines (due to concerns over abuse, tolerance, and dependence) has led to the more common use of methylphenidate starting at 2.5 mg twice daily. Rarely, pemoline is started at a dose of 18.75 mg/day. Most recently, modafinil, which is not an amphetamine, was approved by the U.S. Food and Drug Administration (FDA) for treatment of excessive daytime sleepiness associated with narcolepsy. Given as a single 200-mg dose each morning modafinil produces increased alertness. Although potentially less likely to be abused, it may not be as effective as methylphenidate or D-amphetamine.[28] For the cataplexy, imipramine (in the past) and, more recently, the less sedating protriptyline (at an initial dose of 5 mg titrated up to 60 mg daily) have been used; in addition, SSRIs are now more commonly being used.

General principles of pharmacologic management include using the lowest effective dose possible, with gradual titration and careful monitoring for therapeutic and adverse effects (particularly the anticholinergic and hypotensive effects of the tricyclic antidepressant), and temporarily withdrawing the stimulant when tolerance has developed. It is ideal if the temporary withdrawal can be scheduled at a time when a return of daytime sleepiness will have the least impact on the general functioning of the patient (e.g., during a vacation break from work or school).

Insomnia

Treatment of insomnia depends highly upon the type. Again, an extremely important distinction exists between persistent or chronic and transient or short-term insomnia. Hypnotics are reserved primarily for transient or short-term insomnia. The persistent insomnias often have other specific interventions of choice. The persistent insomnias associated with major psychiatric disorders are most appropriately treated with the specific class of agents targeted for the particular disorder. For example, the patient with a major depressive disorder should be receiving an antidepressant as the primary drug treatment. The sleep disturbance, one symptom of the depressive episode, will be one of the first target symptoms to respond to the treatment. For the psychotic patient, selection and titration of an antipsychotic would be the most appropriate treatment. If the insomnia is associated with drug dependence or drug withdrawal, gradual tapering of the offending agent or the equivalent amount of a cross-tolerant long-acting agent is the primary treatment. If the insomnia is associated with a stimulant, in many cases the agent should simply be discontinued abruptly.

In the case of insomnia associated with medical disorders, adjunctive, short-term use of a hypnotic to promote sleep may be reasonable, while a specific treatment is used for the primary problem. Further, there are times when a patient is best served by education. The elderly patient whose sleep has become more fragmented or the "short sleeper" whose sleep need is small and shows no daytime impairment may both simply need assurance that he or she is sleeping normally.

Periodic limb movements of sleep, a persistent insomnia, is an exception to the general rule of not using hypnotics for chronic insomnias because it is occasionally treated with these agents. Originally treated with clonazepam, it appears that an equivalent response can be obtained with

Table 58.6 ▪ Hypnotics: Classification and Dosages

Generic Name	Trade Name	Dose Range
Barbiturates		
Pentobarbital	Nembutal	100–200 mg
Secobarbital	Seconal	100–200 mg
Amobarbital	Amytal	100–200 mg
Nonbarbiturate nonbenzodiazepines		
Ethchlorvynol	Placidyl	0.5–1.0 g
Glutethimide	Doriden	0.5–1.0 g
Chloral hydrate	Noctec	0.5–2.0 g
Antihistamines		
Diphenhydramine	Benadryl, Sominex-2	25–100 mg
Doxylamine	Unisom	25–100 mg
"Natural" products		
L-Tryptophan	Trofan	1.0–4.0 g
Melatonin		0.3–5 mg
Benzodiazepines		
Flurazepam	Dalmane	15–30 mg
Temazepam	Restoril	15–30 mg
Triazolam	Halcion	0.125–0.25 mg
Quazepam	Doral	7.5–15 mg
Estazolam	ProSom	1.0–2.0 mg
BZD_1 receptor-specific nonbenzodiazepines		
Zolpidem	Ambien	5–10 mg
Zaleplon	Sonata	5–10 mg

any BZD.[29] The BZDs do not significantly reduce the number of movements, but patients report improved quality of sleep and feeling more refreshed in the morning. For restless legs syndrome, codeine and related compounds (e.g., oxycodone) or carbamazepine, typically one Percodan tablet or 200 mg of carbamazepine given at bedtime, have helped some patients. More recently, considerable success has been demonstrated using levodopa/carbidopa at bedtime for patients with both periodic limb movements and restless legs syndrome.[30,31]

Hypnotics

The Ideal Hypnotic. It is helpful to describe the ideal hypnotic. Although it does not exist, keeping the ideal characteristics in mind helps to place the existing agents into perspective. Ideally, the drug should induce sleep rapidly after ingestion. It should maintain sleep for the entire duration expected, without lasting so long that it produces a "morning hangover" and impaired daytime performance. It should not induce development of tolerance or dependence when used over a number of consecutive nights, and abrupt discontinuation should not result in a drug-withdrawal or rebound insomnia. It should have a wide margin of safety, and it should make abnormal sleep normal, while not making the sleep of a normal sleeper abnormal. Finally, it should have no potential for drug-drug interactions.

Classification and Pharmacology of Selected Agents. Many of the more commonly used hypnotic agents are presented in Table 58.6. Note that for older adults, dosing should begin at or below the low end of the dosage ranges shown. The older barbiturates lost popularity as a result of their narrow margin of safety, moderately high abuse potential, potential drug-drug interactions as a result of liver enzyme induction, suppression of delta and REM sleep, with a REM rebound after abrupt discontinuation, and loss of efficacy in inducing and maintaining sleep within 14 consecutive nights of use at a consistent dose.[32]

The older nonbarbiturate nonbenzodiazepines were thought to be superior to the barbiturates because of their lack of the barbiturate structure. However, with the exception of chloral hydrate, they share many of the disadvantages of the barbiturates, and they have additional ones as well. For instance, methaqualone, which is no longer available, was found to have an even higher abuse potential than the barbiturates. Glutethimide, in an overdose situation, presents the emergency room staff not only with a CNS depressant overdose but also with anticholinergic toxicity. In several European countries agents such as ethchlorvynol and glutethimide are not available. Although there has been controversy over their availability in the United States for the past 25 years, they remain on the market. Chloral hydrate, an exception, lacks some of these disadvantages, but it does displace other protein-bound drugs (e.g., warfarin), it causes gastrointestinal irritation in some patients, and at the higher doses (1 to 2 g) needed for some patients, it may lose its effectiveness in inducing and maintaining sleep at least as rapidly as the barbiturates.[33]

The antihistamines, primarily diphenhydramine and doxylamine, are used by taking advantage of their sedative side effects. Some would argue that this drug class is a good choice for patients with a high potential for abusing the BZDs (i.e., those with a history or current problem of substance abuse). Unfortunately, little research into the hypnotic efficacy of these drugs has been done in the sleep laboratory. By subjective report, patients assess the soporific effect of diphenhydramine 50 mg to be equivalent to pentobarbital 60 mg.[34] Increasing the dose of diphenhydramine does not produce a linear increase in hypnotic effect, but it does produce greater anticholinergic side effects, which can be particularly troublesome in elderly patients. Not only are they bothered by constipation, urinary retention, dry mouth, and blurred near vision, but they are particularly sensitive to the central anticholinergic effects of confusion, disorientation, impaired short-term memory, and, at times, visual and tactile hallucinations. In addition, morning hangover is often experienced. Hence, the patient should be monitored for and counseled about these side effects as well as drug interactions with other CNS depressants.

The more sedating antidepressants, amitriptyline, doxepin, and trazodone, have been used in relatively low doses as hypnotics in recent years. Like the antihistamines, they are being used to take advantage of their sedative side effects. All three of these agents can produce significant orthostatic hypotension; in addition, amitriptyline and doxepin are highly anticholinergic. No systematic studies have been conducted to assess efficacy in nondepressed patients with insomnia. On the other hand, trazodone, given in doses of 50 to 150 mg at bedtime, has been shown to improve sleep in patients with major depression who are being treated in the morning with the SSRIs[35]; there is no indication, however, that the depression is relieved any faster than with the SSRI alone.

The BZDs have come closest to the ideal hypnotic. Indeed, this was one of several major conclusions of the Consensus Development Conference on Drugs and Insomnia at the National Institute of Mental Health in November 1983.[36] Three conclusions of significance to this discussion were that (1) hypnotics should be used primarily in the treatment of transient or short-term insomnia (e.g., situational, jet lag, and work shift change), (2) when pharmacotherapy is indicated, a BZD is generally the drug of choice (although if this conference were held at present, zolpidem and zaleplon would most likely be included as well), and (3) selection of the specific agent should be based on its pharmacokinetic and pharmacodynamic characteristics in relation to the individual patient and situation.

Flurazepam was the first of the BZDs marketed as a hypnotic. Its favorable profile, compared with the barbiturates and the nonbarbiturate nonbenzodiazepines, includes a wider margin of safety, lower abuse potential, and fewer drug-drug interactions. In addition, it produces little or no REM suppression at lower doses (15 mg), and even at higher doses (30 mg) REM suppression is not followed by a REM rebound upon abrupt discontinuation of the drug, probably because of the slow elimination of its long-acting active metabolite, *N*-desalkylflurazepam. Whether it demonstrates no withdrawal is unclear; one may need to look at sleep patterns several weeks beyond discontinuation of the drug. It has the additional advantage of remaining effective at a consistent dose for at least 28 consecutive nights of use. It does suppress delta sleep, and the long-acting metabolite (with an elimination half-life of 47 to 100 hours) accumulates over time. This can cause impaired daytime functioning, especially in elderly patients, leading to falls resulting in injuries.[37] Peak plasma levels are achieved within 30 to 60 minutes.

Temazepam offers the advantage of a short-to-intermediate elimination half-life of 9.5 to 12.4 hours. However, it can be as long 20 to 30 hours in elderly patients, so one must watch for possible accumulation and morning hangover with repeated use. It shares many of the properties of flurazepam with respect to effects on sleep. In doses of 15 to 30 mg, it increases total sleep time and decreases the frequency and duration of nocturnal awakenings in insomniac patients. It suppresses delta sleep, and, although there is a decrease in REM sleep during the first half of the night, there is a corresponding increase in the second half. However, there is an ongoing question about its ability to shorten sleep latency significantly in the patient who has difficulty falling asleep because it can take 1 to 2 hours to work. Initial studies of the drug included two dosage forms, a hard gelatin capsule with a powder inside (available in the United States) and a soft gelatin capsule containing a solution of the drug in polyethylene glycol. With the soft gelatin capsule, the drug appears to be absorbed more quickly. This formulation issue has yet to adequately addressed by the manufacturer.

Triazolam, a triazolobenzodiazepine, is unique in that it is ultrashort to short acting, with an elimination half-life of 2 to 3 hours (5.5 at the most). Peak plasma levels are achieved within 30 to 80 minutes. Triazolam appears to be absorbed about as quickly as flurazepam, but eliminated much more rapidly. Although it suppresses REM sleep in the first half of the night, there appears to be compensation for this in the second half (probably as drug levels are decreasing). It seems to have little effect on delta sleep, which distinguishes it from flurazepam, temazepam, and other benzodiazepines. It is least likely of the BZDs to produce morning hangover. Indeed, at the 0.25-mg dose, the effect is equal to that with placebo. Like flurazepam and temazepam, it increases the general quality of sleep, decreases nocturnal awakenings, and increases total sleep time.[38–42]

There has been some concern among clinicians and the public that triazolam is more likely to produce psychomotor impairment, psychologic adverse effects, and anterograde amnesia than other BZDs. However, rather than a unique risk of triazolam, this may be a function of the dose and pattern of use, potency, combination with other CNS depressants, and the mechanism of adverse drug reaction reporting, rather than a unique risk of triazolam.[43]

Some of the concern over triazolam has been associated with "traveler's amnesia." This is the situation in which an individual flying across a number of time zones decides to force sleep during the flight with a short-acting hypnotic, perhaps having ingested some ethanol on the plane as well. Later the traveler has little or no recall for a number of hours after ingestion of the drug (e.g., arrival at the airport and subsequent activities). Until we fully understand this form of anterograde amnesia, it may simply be safer to readjust the internal biologic clock after arriving at our destination. Whatever the actual incidence of psychomotor impairment, psychologic adverse affects, and anterograde amnesia may be (as yet still unclear), especially at the lower doses currently being recommended and used, it is prudent to carefully monitor and counsel patients using triazolam.

Quazepam and estazolam are the two BZDs most recently marketed as hypnotics in the United States. Estazolam, the second triazolobenzodiazepine hypnotic, appears to decrease sleep latency and nocturnal awakenings, while increasing total sleep time and improving depth of sleep and sleep quality.[44] Peak plasma levels are achieved within 0.5 to 4 hours, although with the doses generally used, the onset of action appears to be similar to that seen with flurazepam and triazolam. The half-life of elimination is 8 to 28 hours. Based on its onset of action and elimination half-life, it may be a "faster-acting temazepam." This would place it in the position of being an agent that can significantly decrease sleep latency (a distinct advantage over temazepam) and provide a duration of action intermediate between flurazepam and triazolam. However, results of objective, sleep laboratory studies are mixed with respect to estazolam's ability to significantly decrease latency to sleep onset.

Although quazepam has an intriguing specificity for the BZD_1 receptor subtype, the clinical significance of this property is unclear. Indeed, although the parent compound has a 39-hour half-life of elimination, one of its metabolites, *N*-desalkyl-2-oxoquazepam, is identical to *N*-desalkylflurazepam, which is the long-acting active metabolite of flurazepam. Therefore, one would expect that, clinically, its properties would be very similar to those of flurazepam. It is doubtful that it offers any advantages over flurazepam. Peak plasma levels are achieved in 1 to 2 hours.[45]

Zolpidem is an imidazopyridine compound with a number of intriguing characteristics. It is not a benzodiazepine; however, the molecule is designed in such a way that it binds selectively to the BZD_1 receptor. Its specificity distinguishes it from all the other currently marketed BZD hypnotics except quazepam, and the fact that it does not have any nonspecific, BZD receptor binding metabolites distinguishes it from quazepam.

Pharmacologically, zolpidem's BZD_1 receptor specificity seems to account for its strong hypnotic activity with minimal anxiolytic, muscle relaxant, and anticonvulsant activity even at higher doses than recommended for insomnia (although at extremely high doses, the specificity appears to be lost). This is certainly advantageous in a hypnotic; however, theoretically, one would exercise extreme caution in attempting to switch a patient from long-term and/or high-dose use of a BZD to zolpidem. Zolpidem would not be expected to protect the patient from withdrawal symptoms of increased anxiety, muscle disturbances, or convulsions. In addition, in patients for whom a single bedtime dose of a sedative-hypnotic is desired to help the patient sleep at night and have a carryover anxiolytic effect throughout the day, zolpidem would not appear to be appropriate.

Zolpidem is rapidly absorbed, resulting in a rapid onset of action. It has a mean plasma elimination half-life of 2.3 hours in healthy subjects, 2.9 hours in elderly patients, and close to 10 hours in patients with hepatic cirrhosis. It is metabolized to three major pharmacologically inactive metabolites.

With respect to specific effects on sleep, zolpidem decreases latency to sleep onset (sleep occurring within 20 to 30 minutes after ingestion), increases total sleep time, decreases the number of awakenings during the night, and subjectively improves the quality of sleep. Although some evidence exists for a slight suppression of REM sleep when higher-than-recommended doses are used, in most studies the drug appears to have little effect on this stage of sleep. Unlike most BZDs, zolpidem does not suppress delta sleep; in fact, in one study delta sleep was increased in healthy, young adults.

Zolpidem, in lower doses (5 to 10 mg), appears to provide a full night of sleep with little or no daytime impairment or effects on memory. It appears to have a lower abuse potential than the BZDs. In fact, at very high doses, it produces nausea, dizziness, anxiety, and dysphoria; such effects would discourage many recreational drug users. Rebound insomnia has been minimal or absent after abrupt discontinuation of zolpidem. In a sleep laboratory study lasting 4 weeks, no evidence of tolerance was seen polysomnographically. Subjectively, patients receiving zolpidem for 5 weeks or longer report no significant changes in efficacy over time.

Adverse effects associated with zolpidem (in doses of 10 mg or less) have primarily been headache, drowsiness, dizziness, lethargy, nausea, myalgia, and sinusitis. The incidence of headache and drowsiness seems to be age-related, and drowsiness, nausea, and anterograde amnesia appear to be dose-related, increasing significantly at a dose of 20 mg. Falls and confusion can be seen in elderly patients if they are treated with doses in excess of 10 mg (which is twice the recommended starting dose for this population). Except for what appears to be additive CNS depressant effects when zolpidem is used in combination with chlorpromazine or imipramine, no drug interactions have been noted with haloperidol, cimetidine, ranitidine, warfarin, or digoxin.[46]

Zaleplon, a BZD_1 receptor-specific pyrazolopyrimidine, appears to be similar to zolpidem in its dosing, onset of action, effects on sleep stages, and profile of side effects. The major difference is in duration of action, in that it has an elimination half-life of about 1 hour. This property may make it most useful for sleep initiation problems and less likely to significantly increase total sleep time or decrease nocturnal awakenings. Whether it has a lower incidence of psychomotor impairment, amnesia, and rebound insomnia than zolpidem has yet to be established.[47]

Drug-Withdrawal Insomnia and Rebound Insomnia. When barbiturates were used more commonly for the treatment of insomnia, drug-withdrawal insomnia was described as a phenomenon associated with the abrupt discontinuation of the hypnotic after long-term use.[48] After chronic REM suppression, discontinuation led to a REM rebound, accounting for as much as 40% of total sleep time. This REM rebound was accompanied by very intense and frightening dreams as well as a generally disrupted night of sleep. The patient, not understanding the nature of the phenomenon, was likely to immediately return to chronic, high-dose use. With gradual tapering of the drug or an equivalent amount of a longer-acting agent and patient education regarding the possibility of temporarily increased dreaming and decreased quality of sleep, patients are better able to tolerate discontinuation of their hypnotics.

More recently, rebound insomnia has been described as a phenomenon associated with the abrupt discontinuation of the shorter-acting BZDs (e.g., temazepam and triazolam).[49] It involves a worsening of sleep, even beyond what it was like before the patient started taking the drug. The exact incidence of the phenomenon is unclear, but it is prudent to warn the patient about a possible transient worsening of sleep immediately after the drug is stopped. Gradual tapering of the drug, rather than abrupt discontinuation, may lessen the severity of these withdrawal symptoms.[50] As an example, a patient taking 0.25 mg of triazolam every night for several weeks could reduce the dose by half (to 0.125 mg) for 3 nights, by half again (to one half of a 0.125-mg tablet) for the next 3 nights, and then finally discontinue the medication.

PROBLEMS AND CONTROVERSIES. Two important issues with insomnia and hypnotics are that no one drug is ideal for every patient with insomnia and that not all patients with insomnia should be treated with hypnotics. As previously stated, hypnotics are to be used almost exclusively for the treatment of transient or short-term insomnia. The implication is that a thorough assessment will be made of every patient with a complaint of insomnia. Although hypnotic-induced sleep may be unnatural in some respects, an ultimate measure of efficacy must be seen as optimal daytime performance.[51,52]

Some prescribers and patients believe that all hypnotics should be avoided because of the possible development of dependence. If they are used appropriately–for brief periods and at low doses–the risk is low. Also, drug-dependence insomnia, in which sleep worsens with long-term use of hypnotics even while the patient continues to take the drug, should not be a problem. In many respects, our society has been responsible for many of the transient insomnias (e.g., jet lag, work shift change, and situational) and must take responsibility, either pharmacologically or nonpharmacologically, for dealing with the problem.

GENERAL CLINICAL GUIDELINES. A careful diagnostic assessment is necessary before treating any insomnia. See Table 58.7 for ideas on what types of questions to ask in screening a patient. Do not allow your own experiences to interfere with your assessment. Unfortunately, because most of us have had at least an occasional bout of insomnia, we may too easily assume that everyone else's problem is similar to our own. Clarify the complaint and do a drug history. Assess the possibility that the problem is drug-induced. Look for stimulating drugs such as sympathomimetic decongestants or caffeine. Look for CNS depressant withdrawal such as moderate-to-heavy ethanol intake at dinner time. Assess the contribution of street drugs. In addition, look for sedating drugs as causes of excessive daytime sleepiness. Finally, find out what, if anything, has worked for the same problem in the past. Ask if the problem is one of insomnia or excessive daytime sleepiness. Patients may be excessively sleepy if they have obstructive sleep apnea or narcolepsy. If it is a case of self-induced sleep deprivation (e.g., studying for examinations), caffeine tablets may be appropriate short-term, but evaluate possible drug-disease interactions (e.g., hypertension) and tell the patient about sleep hygiene. If the complaint is of insomnia, determine if it is transient or chronic. If transient, a nonprescription sleep aid containing doxylamine or diphenhydramine may be worth a try for a few nights, but tell the patient about anticholinergic effects and possible morning hangover and consider alternatives if the antihistamine is either ineffective or intolerable. If the insomnia is chronic, the patient deserves as meticulous an evaluation as the patient who comes in with a complaint of chronic stomach pain or unremitting, chronic headache. There are many reasons for chronic insomnia, and a number of them are treatable. Finally, be prepared for appreciation and praise. If a treatable and responsive insomnia is identified in only one patient a year, the change in quality of life will make that patient forever grateful.

Table 58.7 ▪ Important Questions to Ask in Assessing a Sleep Complaint

- How long have you had this problem?
- What is your normal bedtime/sleep pattern and has it changed recently?
- How long do you usually sleep? Do you go to sleep at about the same time each night? Do you take daytime naps?
- How long does it take you to fall asleep? How often do you wake up during the night? What time do you wake up? Are you able to fall back to sleep?
- Have you been experiencing pain, worry, stress, work or family problems recently that could be associated with your sleep problem?
- Do you suffer from any emotional or physical illness?
- Do you consume any drugs, alcohol, or caffeine-containing foods or beverages?
- Has your bed partner observed any snoring or unusual movements?
- How do you feel upon awakening and during the day: tired, depressed, sleepy, irritable?
- Do any of your relatives suffer from poor sleep?
- Does anything help your sleep: sleeping pills, exercise, or sleeping in another room?

Until recently, if a decision has been made to treat insomnia pharmacologically, BZDs have been the treatment of choice; pharmacokinetic differences play a major role in selecting which benzodiazepine to use. Zolpidem offers one more option. Zaleplon may offer yet another. Drug selection must take into account onset of action and duration with respect to single versus multiple dosing and past history of response. If possible daytime impairment associated with accumulation of long-acting active metabolites (especially in elderly patients) is a concern, avoid flurazepam and quazepam; choose one of the shorter-acting BZDs, zolpidem, or zaleplon. Also, recall that accumulation becomes a much greater concern with continuous use over several nights than with infrequent use as needed (in which drug action is terminated as quickly as it can be redistributed out of brain tissue). If the possible delayed onset of action of temazepam is a concern, choose the more rapidly acting flurazepam, triazolam, zolpidem, zaleplon, or, perhaps, estazolam. If possible anterograde amnesia is a concern, use very low doses, caution the patient, and consider avoiding hypnotic use in situations in which the drug effect may not have worn off by the time the individual needs to be awake, alert, and fully functioning. The choices do not always have to be limited to the agents specifically marketed as hypnotics. For instance, diazepam is superior to flurazepam in onset of action and yet shares the property of accumulation of a long-acting active metabolite under multiple-dosing conditions. In general, the choice of drug depends upon pharmacokinetic profile and benefits sought.

The hypnotics should be avoided in patients with sleep apnea, patients who use alcohol or other CNS depressants heavily, pregnant patients, and patients in whom alert nighttime performance is mandatory (e.g., firemen or pilots). Although the BZDs are relatively safe, one must be cautious in giving them to patients with a high risk for suicide. Patients who overdose often use combinations of agents, often washing down everything with alcohol. Combination of BZDs with alcohol can be fatal. Most likely, an additive or synergistic mechanism is the basis for the interaction, resulting in impaired psychomotor functioning and excess sedation. Acute ethanol ingestion appears to enhance BZD absorption, decrease the volume of distribution, and impair elimination (as a result of hepatic enzyme inhibition). Zolpidem has additive, not synergistic, effects when combined with alcohol, and it is recommended that the two not be taken in combination.

The benefit that the patient is seeking must be determined. Ideally, the patient is looking for both improved sleep and improved daytime functioning. Simply increasing the number of hours of sleep is generally not a sufficient reason for prescribing hypnotics. Once the hypnotic is chosen, the lowest effective dose to achieve a clear-cut benefit is used. This requires periodic follow-up with the patient, quantification of the results, and educating the patient about the need to begin with a low dose and give it an adequate trial. For flurazepam, this is 15 mg. With triazolam in an elderly patient, the dose is 0.125 mg or perhaps even half a 0.125-mg tablet. For zolpidem, the dose is 5 mg in an elderly patient and 10 mg in the healthy adult. The importance of starting with a low dose cannot be overstated. For instance, with flurazepam the optimal effect may not be experienced for 2 to 3 days; this may be due to slow accumulation of *N*-desalkylflurazepam. In addition, especially in elderly patients, daytime sequelae must be monitored. These are important educational and monitoring roles for the pharmacist. Questions that should be asked of patients when monitoring hypnotic effects and side effects are listed in Table 58.8. Drug-drug and drug-disease interactions should be identified and avoided. Examples of drug-drug interactions include additive CNS depression when the hypnotics are combined with other CNS depressants and accumulation of flurazepam, quazepam, and their long-acting metabolite *N*-desalkylflurazepam in the presence of cimetidine (which interferes with oxidative metabolic processes). A primary drug-disease interaction is the use of an agent requiring oxidative metabolic transformation (e.g., flurazepam and quazepam) in the presence of liver disease or old age. If one of the older nonbenzodiazepines is being prescribed, the effect of liver enzyme induction must be kept in mind, in addition to additive effects with other CNS depressants. With zolpidem, recall that the elimination half-life is increased approximately fourfold in the presence of hepatic cirrhosis.

Table 58.8 ▪ Important Questions to Ask in Monitoring Hypnotic Therapy

Is your sleep improved?
Are you taking the medication as it was prescribed?
Have you increased your dose or taken a second dose at night?
Are you experiencing undesirable sleepiness in the morning or during the day?
Are you awakening early?
Have you noticed changes in your mood, behavior, or memory?
Are you more nervous, irritable, or anxious than usual?
Are you having problems with dizziness, unsteadiness, or lightheadedness?

The issue of use of hypnotics for chronic insomnia is complex. Few data are available regarding the efficacy and safety of hypnotics when taken for more than 1 to 2 months. In addition, there is no evidence to indicate that chronic hypnotic use produces lasting, objective improvement in sleep and daytime function in the persistent insomnias. Therefore, if hypnotics are prescribed, the goal with chronic insomnia should be pulsed, intermittent treatment and periodic medical reevaluation. Indeed, for many patients with chronic insomnia, the underlying problem is a psychiatric condition, drug or alcohol dependence, sleep apnea, or delayed sleep phase syndrome. Treatments specific to the disorder and nonpharmacologic approaches should be tried first. If psychiatric and medical disorders have been ruled out and nonpharmacologic approaches have failed, referral to a sleep-disorders center would be appropriate. In the rare instances in which a thorough sleep evaluation has been done and a hypnotic is used to treat a chronic insomnia (e.g., periodic limb movement disorder), the patient should be evaluated often for improvement in both sleep and daytime functioning, as well as for the persistence of the therapeutic effect at a constant dose. The reason for this, at least with the typical BZDs, is that longer-term use carries an increased risk of dependence, tolerance with resulting escalation of dose, and difficult withdrawal.

Patient education should include emphasis on short-term use, discussion of possible daytime sedation and impairment with the longer-acting agents, the importance of avoiding other CNS depressants, and, again at least with the typical BZDs, the risks of tolerance and dependence if used for too long and/or at excessively high doses. If hypnotics are to be used for extended periods of time, it may be useful to suggest skipping a night or two occasionally. This allows the patient to see if the drug is still really needed, and perhaps it can reduce the development of tolerance. When the drug is discontinued–ideally in a gradual, tapered way–the patient must be told about possible temporary withdrawal phenomena.

Nonpharmacologic Therapy

Parasomnias

Fortunately, both somnambulism and sleep terrors are usually "outgrown." Treatment of sleepwalking consists primarily of protecting the individual from harm. This may include locking doors and windows at night and giving the sleepwalker a first-floor bedroom. Again, for sleep terrors, treatment consists primarily of waiting for the disorder to be "outgrown." With respect to nightmares, after REM suppressant drug withdrawal is ruled out as the cause, psychologic intervention is the usual treatment. This may be as simple as a parent providing comfort and reassurance to a child with an occasional nightmare or as complex as intensive psychotherapy for an adult with frequent, highly disturbing nightmares.[4]

Sleep Apnea

Treatment varies with the type of sleep apnea under consideration. For obstructive sleep apnea, sometimes simple weight loss or removal of enlarged tonsils may solve the problem. Sometimes preventing the patient from sleeping on his or her back, by sewing a tennis ball to the back of the nightshirt, can lead to a significant decrease in apneic episodes. When life-threatening complications of repeated episodes of hypoxemia (e.g., arrhythmias, pulmonary hypertension, or right ventricular failure) are present, aggressive intervention should be considered. A rather elegant plastic surgical procedure performed in some patients is the uvulopalatopharyngoplasty; it involves major reconstruction of the pharyngeal airspace. Unfortunately, in many cases, long-term follow-up has been lacking. Other, less dramatic surgical procedures–some involving laser surgery–have been performed more recently. A helpful and commonly used approach is continuous positive airway pressure.[53] A small device sits beside the bed that is connected by a tube to a facial mask worn by the patient throughout the night. The device, initially calibrated during one or two nights in a sleep disorders center, provides a continuous flow of air, which keeps the airway open. For many patients who are appropriately counseled and learn to tolerate the noise, mucosal drying, and minor discomfort of the facial mask, the technique can have a major impact on the quality of sleep and resultant daytime functioning. Adhesive strips designed to spread open the nostrils may be of benefit, but probably only to those patients whose primary problem is characterized by constricted nasal passages having the potential for such mechanical opening. Finally, various dental appliances designed to pull the tongue forward and maintain an open airway can be used.

Narcolepsy

Nonpharmacologic treatment of narcolepsy consists of several interventions. The patient and family members must be educated about the disorder to dispel the misconception that the patient is simply a lazy, unmotivated, nonproductive person. There are local and national support groups available. In addition, careful scheduling of daytime naps can be particularly helpful. The patient may feel fairly refreshed for up to several hours after a 15- or 20-minute nap.

Insomnia

Some general rules of sleep hygiene that can be recommended for both persistent and transient insomnias are presented in Table 58.9. In addition, other nonpharmacologic approaches are available. These include desensitization, meditation, biofeedback, stimulus control, and others.[54] Delayed sleep phase syndrome can be treated by chronotherapy or light therapy.[21,55] Because the patient with delayed sleep phase syndrome can sleep but is sleepy at the wrong time of the 24-hour day, chronotherapy is a means of adjusting the internal clock by 2- to 3-hour blocks each day until sleep occurs at the desired time.

ALTERNATIVE THERAPIES

One amino acid, L-tryptophan, became popular as a natural hypnotic because it is a precursor to serotonin, a neurotransmitter that seems to be significantly involved in NREM sleep. L-Tryptophan had never been approved by the FDA as a hypnotic; it was sold as a food supplement. The overall efficacy of this agent is unclear. Positive response is unpredictable as the predictors of response have not been identified.[56] Some 1500 cases (including 24 fatalities) of an eosinophilia-myalgia syndrome associated with the use of L-tryptophan were reported to the U.S. Centers for Disease Control and Prevention (CDC) in Atlanta.[57] The CDC defines this L-tryptophan-associated eosinophilia-myalgia syndrome as (1) an increase in eosinophils to counts greater than $1000/mm^3$, (2) myalgia that interferes with daily activities, and (3) the absence of some other identifiable cause (e.g., parasites or leukemia). Although the nature of this association is unclear (for instance, there has been strong speculation that some contaminant was accidentally introduced through use of a new strain of bacillus in the production process into the bulk supplies shipped from overseas), the FDA and CDC recommended that people stop using the agent and that physicians stop prescribing it. If it should come back into use, it should be noted that it not a totally innocuous substance. Most commonly, people are bothered by its gastrointestinal irritation, which women who have been pregnant compared to morning sickness. In addition, chronic use has been associated with both niacin and pyridoxine deficiencies. The combination of L-tryptophan and a monoamine oxidase inhibitor (e.g., phenelzine, isocarboxazid, or tranylcypromine) or fluoxetine can

Table 58.9 ▪ Sleep Hygiene: Suggestions for Improved Sleep

1. Set a regular time to go to bed and a regular time to wake up. Regularity is a key component to improving sleep. You must set these times and adhere to them as diligently as possible. At least as important as a regular bedtime is the establishment of a regular wake-up time. No matter how long it took to fall asleep, no matter how little sleep you have had, and no matter how flexible your morning schedule is, there should be no "sleeping in." This would only further confuse and disorganize the internal biologic clock (i.e., the circadian pacemaker).
2. Engage in regular, moderate exercise early in the day; do not exercise vigorously in the evening. Heavy exercise too late in the evening can lead to a worsening of sleep in all but the best-conditioned athlete; therefore, for most of us, heavy exercise should be scheduled earlier in the day.
3. Generally avoid daytime naps. The idea is to consolidate sound, solid sleep through the night. Satisfying some of your sleep need during the day may prevent this. The exception is the person who routinely takes a daytime nap (e.g., the "siesta"); such a person generally has a somewhat shorter than average night of sleep.
4. Eat a light snack or beverage before bedtime if hungry; do not eat heavy or spicy food in the evening, and do not eat late evening meals or drink large quantities of liquids in the evening. A heavy meal late in the evening can severely disrupt sleep in the patient with gastroesophageal reflux (e.g., "heartburn"). Too much liquid can result in multiple awakenings to go to the bathroom.
5. Make the bedroom as comfortable and secure as possible. You should attempt to see that the bedroom is dark and quiet and is neither too hot nor too cold. Although minor fluctuations in room temperature and firmness of the mattress probably have little impact on sleep, extremes can be disturbing. A sense of security can also be quite important.
6. Use the bedroom only for activities associated with sleep. Although many of us, while in bed, use the bedroom for watching television, preparing work for the following day, eating snacks, and paying bills, the individual with a sleep problem needs to set the bedroom aside for sleep only. (Sexual activity may be an exception.) In addition, just as warm milk and cookies become a ritual for some children before bedtime, some adults must develop a similar relaxing ritual that can be a part of the stimulus for a sleep response.
7. If not asleep within 30 minutes, move to another room and engage in a boring or relaxing activity. Get out of bed, leave the bedroom, and do something nonstimulating; for some, this would be watching a late night talk show on television and for others it might be reading one's professional journals. After some 30 to 60 minutes, another attempt should be made to fall asleep. The idea is to not spend too much time in bed awake; an association between the bed and an inability to fall sleep can simply compound the problem.
8. Sleep only as much as needed to feel refreshed and alert during the day. Sleep need varies considerably among individuals. Discover for yourself what your sleep need is and satisfy it. Spending extra time in bed awake, thinking that you need to sleep more, may associate the bedroom with wakefulness rather than sleep.
9. Avoid or minimize use of caffeine (coffee, tea, and soft drinks), alcohol, and tobacco. Each person must discover how late such use can be tolerated. However, for the very sensitive, caffeine intake may need to be discontinued each day by noon. Although alcohol is often used as a self-treatment for relaxation and sleep induction, its rapid elimination during the first half of the night may result in some degree of withdrawal, characterized by increased dreaming and nightmares as well as a general disruption of sleep during the latter half. In addition, nicotine may be stimulating in some persons.
10. Avoid routine use of hypnotics. Although hypnotics can be very effective for short-term treatment of a variety of insomnias, long-term use may result in a type of drug-dependence insomnia, characterized by sleep that is even worse than it was before use of the drug. If the sleep difficulty persists despite following the preceding suggestions and perhaps even a brief trial of nonprescription hypnotics, discuss the problem with a physician or pharmacist. Consider learning relaxation techniques or hypnosis. Some people simply need to be able to relax sufficiently to allow sleep to occur. Consider psychotherapy; because at least 35% of all patients seen in sleep disorders centers for complaints of insomnia have an identifiable psychiatric or psychologic cause, some form of psychotherapy or psychiatric treatment may be helpful.

produce a "serotonin syndrome," characterized by disorientation, agitation, hyperthermia, hyperreflexia, diaphoresis, ocular oscillations, and myoclonic jerking. Finally, low doses have been associated with changes in liver ultrastructure in normal rats and have been lethal in rats with adrenal insufficiency.

Melatonin, endogenously synthesized from serotonin and secreted by the pineal gland, has now become a popular "natural" self-treatment for a variety of disorders. Exogenous melatonin products have not been approved by the FDA but are available in health food stores. Limited studies of doses generally ranging from 0.3 to 5 mg demonstrate efficacy in treating insomnia and jet lag.[58] Large controlled trials are still needed as long-term efficacy is unclear and little is known about adverse effects. In addition, the sources and purity of the products sold in health food stores are uncertain.

Other natural products include valerian and kava kava. Like BZDs, both have been used in the treatment of anxiety and insomnia, appear to act through central γ-aminobutyric acid systems, and, at least in the case of kava kava, can interact with other CNS depressants (e.g., ethanol and alprazolam).[47,59] Until more systematic studies have been conducted, as is also true for melatonin, patients should be cautioned with respect to what we do not know regarding safety, efficacy, purity, and sources.

IMPROVING OUTCOMES

As discussed earlier (see "General Clinical Guidelines"), clinicians can improve outcomes in patients with sleep disorders by first assuring that a careful and thorough assessment of the sleep complaint is completed. Once this is accomplished, therapy should be as specific as possible for the disorder identified. In all cases, it should be remembered that insomnia is a symptom, not a disorder. Helping the patient to understand the nature of the disorder, the goals of treatment, and the importance of compliance and practicing good sleep hygiene all contribute to positive outcomes. Lastly, monitoring both therapeutic and adverse effects should be frequent and comprehensive.

PHARMACOECONOMICS

The significant impact of sleep disturbances on the many aspects of our lives is becoming increasingly clear. The U.S. Department of Transportation estimates that up to 10% of automobile accidents are directly related to sleepiness, accounting for a cost of $29 billion in fatalities and disabling injuries.[60] It is estimated that of the 25% of Americans who perform shift work, at least 60% have a chronic sleep disorder. Sleep disorders are estimated to be responsible for 52% of work-related accidents at a cost of $24 billion.[61] The relatively small cost of treatment far outweighs the cost of not treating insomnia and other sleep disorders.

CONCLUSION

Sleep is a fascinating psychophysiologic phenomenon that is cyclic and can be measured electrophysiologically. Much is now known about sleep and its disorders, but sleep disorders medicine is still in its infancy. Millions of our patients have a variety of sleep disorders. They are a heterogeneous group of disorders capable of producing major social and/or occupational disability; disturbed sleep can be crippling for many people. With appropriate assessment and treatment, the transient insomnias can be managed to improve both nighttime sleep and daytime performance. Although there may be no cures for many persistent insomnias such as sleep apnea, increased understanding of these disorders is leading to prevention of harm to patients by inadequate assessment or inappropriate use of hypnotics. Further, with better assessment and increased referral by pharmacists, many patients with some of the persistent insomnias (e.g., psychiatric disorders and delayed sleep phase syndrome) can be helped significantly.

Sleep complaints deserve the same meticulous assessment and concern as complaints of chest pain, flank pain, or coughing up blood. Disorders of excessive daytime sleepiness (obstructive sleep apnea and narcolepsy), insomnia (transient as well as persistent types), and unusual behaviors and mental activity during sleep (sleepwalking, sleep terrors, and nightmares) have been described. Not all sleep complaints should be treated with hypnotics; indeed, some of the sleep disorders may be worsened by hypnotics or other drugs.

Use of hypnotics is generally most appropriately reserved for the treatment of transient or short-term insomnias. Although a number of hypnotics are available, the BZDs and BZD_1 receptor-specific nonbenzodiazepines are currently accepted as the drugs of choice; selection within the group is based primarily on differences in pharmacokinetic profiles. The clinician has the opportunity to play an important role in assessing the disorder, recommending treatment, or recommending further evaluation for the many patients with complaints of insomnia or excessive daytime sleepiness. In addition, the pharmacist can play a major role in educating the patient about therapy and monitoring for therapeutic and adverse effects. With careful diagnosis and treatment tailored to the patient and his or her particular problem, more people will be sleeping better and also performing considerably better in their daily activities.

KEY POINTS

- Treatment of any of the sleep disorders is focused on normalizing sleep and, perhaps more importantly, improving daytime functioning and preventing the adverse consequences of disturbed sleep.
- Any sleep complaint deserves the same meticulous attention as that afforded a complaint of chest pain, flank pain, or coughing up blood; in assessing the sleep complaint, a distinction should be made between excessive daytime sleepiness, insomnia, and phenomena associated with specific sleep stages or sleep-wake transitions.
- Sleep is an active, cyclic, psychophysiologic phenomenon, the function of which is unclear, but the need for which is certain.
- The parasomnias include delta sleep phenomena (e.g., sleepwalking or sleep terrors) and REM-sleep phenomena (e.g., nightmares).
- In the case of excessive daytime sleepiness, consideration should be given to obstructive sleep apnea (characterized by repeated episodes of cessation of breathing, each terminated by a brief arousal, and often associated with loud snoring) and narcolepsy (characterized by excessive daytime sleepiness, cataplexy, sleep paralysis, and hypnagogic hallucinations), as well as self-imposed sleep deprivation.
- A key guideline in the management of sleep apnea is to avoid all CNS depressants.
- Pharmacologic treatment of narcolepsy is focused on the excessive daytime sleepiness (e.g., CNS stimulants or modafinil) and the cataplexy (e.g., protriptyline or SSRIs).
- Insomnia is a symptom, not a disease, and, therefore, requires an attempt to distinguish between short-term and chronic types and to identify the etiology; both drug (e.g., CNS stimulants, CNS depressant withdrawal, and ethanol) and nondrug factors (e.g., psychiatric disorders, medical disorders, circadian rhythm disorders, and poor sleep hygiene) must be considered. If a treatable cause is identified (e.g., major depression), the specific treatment appropriate for that problem (e.g., antidepressant) should be primary.
- The goal of treatment of insomnia, including nondrug approaches (e.g., improved sleep hygiene), should be to improve both sleep and daytime functioning.

- In general, the short-term insomnias are most appropriately treated with hypnotics, and the drugs of choice are the BZDs (e.g., flurazepam, temazepam, triazolam, quazepam, and estazolam) and the BZD_1 receptor-specific nonbenzodiazepines (e.g., zolpidem and zaleplon); selection of an agent is based on differences in pharmacokinetic profiles and the needs of the individual patient.
- Antihistamines (e.g., hydroxyzine, diphenhydramine, and doxylamine) may be used for mild, short-term insomnia with due caution in light of their strong anticholinergic properties and high incidence of "morning hangover."
- Trazodone and other sedating antidepressants may improve sleep in patients with major depression who are being treated with stimulating SSRIs; patients must be monitored for possible orthostatic hypotension and, in the case of tricyclic antidepressants, anticholinergic side effects.
- Melatonin may be considered in patients with circadian rhythm disorders (e.g., jet lag).
- Kava kava and valerian, similar to BZDs, appear to act upon central γ-aminobutyric acid systems; however, like melatonin, they should be used only with recognition that quality assurance is sometimes less than adequate and that more information is needed with respect to appropriate indications, optimal dosing, short- and long-term adverse effects, and potential interactions.

REFERENCES

1. Bixler EO, Kales A, Soldatos CR, et al. Prevalence of sleep disorders in the Los Angeles metropolitan area. Am J Psychiatry 136:1257–1262, 1979.
2. Mellinger GD, Balter MB, Uhlenhuth EH. Insomnia and its treatments. Arch Gen Psychiatry 42:225–232, 1985.
3. Wincor MZ, Johnson KA. Non-prescription hypnotics: purchase and pharmacist-patient interaction in the community pharmacy. Presented to the 14th European Symposium on Clinical Pharmacy. Stockholm, October 1985.
4. Kales A, Soldatos CR, Kales JD. Sleep disorders: insomnia, sleepwalking, night terrors, nightmares, and enuresis. Ann Intern Med 106:582–592, 1987.
5. Strollo PJ, Rogers RM. Current concepts: obstructive sleep apnea. N Engl J Med 334:99–104, 1996.
6. Kales A, Vela-Bueno A, Kales JD. Sleep disorders: sleep apnea and narcolepsy. Ann Intern Med 106:434–443, 1987.
7. Aldrich MS. The clinical spectrum of narcolepsy and idiopathic hypersomnia. Neurology 46:393–401, 1996.
8. Ancoli-Israel S, Kripke DF, Klauber MR, et al. Sleep-disordered breathing in community-dwelling elderly. Sleep 14:486–495, 1991.
9. Ancoli-Israel S, Kripke DF, Klauber MR, et al. Periodic limb movements in sleep in community-dwelling elderly. Sleep 14:496–500, 1991.
10. Coleman R, Roffwarg H, Kennedy S, et al. Sleep–wake disorders based on a polysomnographic diagnosis: a national cooperative study. JAMA 247:997–1003, 1982.
11. Hobson JA, Lydic R, Baghdoyan HA. Evolving concepts of sleep cycle generation: from brain centers to neuronal populations. Behav Brain Sci 9:371–448, 1986.
12. Siegel JM. Mechanisms of sleep control. J Clin Neurophysiol 7:49–65, 1990.
13. Rechtschaffen A, Kales A, eds. A manual of standardized terminology, techniques and scoring system for sleep stages of human subjects (pub. no. 204, Public Health Service Publications). Washington, DC: US Government Printing Office, 1968.
14. Karni A, Tanne D, Rubenstein BS, et al. Dependence on REM sleep of overnight improvement of a perceptual skill. Science 265:679–682, 1994.
15. Bliwise DL. Sleep in normal aging and dementia. Sleep 16:40–81, 1993.
16. Inoko H, Ando A, Tseuji K, et al. HLA-DQ chain DNA restriction fragments can differentiate between healthy and narcoleptic individuals with HLA-DR2. Immunogenetics 23:126–128, 1986.
17. Sleep Disorders Classification Committee, Association of Sleep Disorders Centers. Diagnostic classification of sleep and arousal disorders. Sleep 2:1–137, 1979.
18. Diagnostic Classification Steering Committee of the American Sleep Disorders Association (Thorpy MJ, Chair). International classification of sleep disorders:diagnostic and coding manual. Rochester, MN: American Sleep Disorders Association, 1990.
19. American Psychiatric Association. Diagnostic and statistical manual of mental disorders. 4th ed. Washington, DC: American Psychiatric Association, 1994.
20. Carskadon MA, Dement WC, Mitler MM, et al. Self reports versus sleep laboratory findings in 122 drug-free subjects with complaints of chronic insomnia. Am J Psychiatry 133:1382–1388, 1976.
21. Regestein QR, Monk TH. Delayed sleep phase syndrome: a review of its clinical aspects. Am J Psychiatry 152:602–608, 1995.
22. The Gallup Organization for the National Sleep Foundation. Sleep in America: 1995. Princeton, NJ: The Gallup Organization, 1995.
23. Zammit GK, Weiner J, Damato N, et al. Quality of life in people with insomnia. Sleep 22(Suppl 2):S379–S385, 1999.
24. Bonnet MH, Dexter JR, Arand DL. The effect of triazolam on arousal and respiration in central sleep apnea patients. Sleep 13:31–41, 1990.
25. Whyte KF, Gould GA, Airlie MA. Role of protriptyline and acetazolamide in the sleep apnea/hypopnea syndrome. Sleep 11:463–472, 1988.
26. Strohl KP, Hensley MJ, Saunders NA, et al. Progesterone administration and progressive sleep apneas. JAMA 245:1230–1232, 1981.
27. Tojima H, Kunitomo F, Kimura H, et al. Effects of acetazolamide in patients with the sleep apnea syndrome. Thorax 43:113–118, 1988.
28. US Modafinil in Narcolepsy Study Group. Randomized trial of modafinil for the treatment of pathological somnolence in narcolepsy. Ann Neurol 43:88–97, 1998.
29. Mitler MM, Browman CP, Menn SJ, et al. Nocturnal myoclonus: treatment efficacy of clonazepam and temazepam. Sleep 9:385–392, 1986.
30. Trenkwalder C, Walters AS, Hening WA. Periodic limb movements and restless legs syndrome. Neurol Clin 14:629–650, 1996.
31. Hening W, Allen R, Earley C, et al. The treatment of restless legs syndrome and periodic limb movement disorder. Sleep 22:970–999, 1999.
32. Kales AK, Bixler EO, Kales JD, et al. Comparative effectiveness of nine hypnotic drugs: sleep laboratory studies. J Clin Pharmacol 17:207–213, 1977.
33. Kales A, Allen C, Scharf MB, et al. Hypnotic drugs and their effectiveness: all night EEG studies of insomniac subjects. Arch Gen Psychiatry 23:226–232, 1970.
34. Teutach G, Mahler DL, Brown CR, et al. Hypnotic efficacy of diphenhydramine, methapyrilene, and pentobarbital for nighttime sedation. Clin Pharmacol Ther 17:195–201, 1975.
35. Nierenberg AA, Adler LA, Peselow E, et al. Trazodone for antidepressant-associated insomnia. Am J Psychiatry 151:1069–1072, 1994.
36. National Institute of Mental Health, Consensus Development Conference. Drugs and insomnia: the use of medications to promote sleep. JAMA 251:2410–2414, 1984.
37. Ray WA, Griffin MR, Downey W. Benzodiazepines of short and long elimination half-life and the risk of hip fracture. JAMA 262:3303–3307, 1989.
38. Ashton H. Guidelines for the rational use of benzodiazepines: when and what to use. Drugs 48:25–40, 1994.
39. Wincor MZ. Insomnia and the new benzodiazepines. Clin Pharm 1:425–432, 1982.
40. Kales A, Kales JD. Sleep laboratory studies of hypnotic drugs: efficacy and withdrawal effects. J Clin Psychopharmacol 3:140–150, 1983.
41. Rickels K. Clinical trials of hypnotics. J Clin Psychopharmacol 3:133–139, 1983.
42. Greenblatt DJ, Harmatz JS, Englehardt N, et al. Pharmacokinetic determinants of dynamic differences among three benzodiazepine hypnotics. Arch Gen Psychiatry 46:326–332, 1989.
43. Bunney WE, Azarnoff DL, Brown BW, et al. Report of the Institute of Medicine committee on the efficacy and safety of Halcion. Arch Gen Psychiatry 56:349–352, 1999.
44. Pierce MW, Shu VS. Efficacy of estazolam: the United States clinical experience. Am J Med 88(Suppl 3A):6–11, 1990.
45. Kales A. Quazepam: hypnotic efficacy and side effects. Pharmacotherapy 10:1–12, 1990.
46. Langtry HD, Benfield P. Zolpidem: a review of its pharmacodynamic and pharmacokinetic properties and therapeutic potential. Drugs 40:291–313, 1990.
47. Wagner J, Wagner ML, Hening WA. Beyond benzodiazepines: alternative

pharmacologic agents for the treatment of insomnia. Ann Pharmacother 32:680–691, 1998.
48. Kales A, Bixler E, Tan T, et al. Chronic hypnotic-drug use: ineffectiveness, drug-withdrawal insomnia, and dependence. JAMA 227:513–517, 1974.
49. Kales A, Scharf M, Kales J. Rebound insomnia: a new clinical syndrome. Science 201:1039–1041, 1978.
50. Schweizer E, Rickels K, Case G, et al. Long-term therapeutic use of benzodiazepines: II. Effects of gradual taper. Arch Gen Psychiatry 47:908–915, 1990.
51. Gillin JC, Byerley WF. The diagnosis and management of insomnia. N Engl J Med 322:239–247, 1990.
52. Everett DE, Avorn J, Baker MW. Clinical decision-making in the evaluation and treatment of insomnia. Am J Med 89:357–362, 1990.
53. Handelsman H, Carter E. Continuous positive airway pressure for the treatment of obstructive sleep apnea in adults. (Health Technology Assessment Reports 1986, no. 3.) Rockville, MD: National Center for Health Services Research and Health Care Technology Assessment, 1986.
54. Morin CM, Culbert JP, Schwartz SM. Nonpharmacological interventions for insomnia: a meta-analysis of treatment efficacy. Am J Psychiatry 151:1172–1180, 1994.
55. Czeisler CA, Kronauer RE, Allan JS, et al. Bright light induction of strong (type O) resetting of the human circadian pacemaker. Science 244:1328–1333, 1989.
56. Schneider-Helmert D, Spinweber CL. Evaluation of L-tryptophan for treatment of insomnia: a review. Psychopharmacology 89:1–7, 1986.
57. Raphals P. Disease puzzle nears solution. Science 249:619, 1990.
58. Wincor MZ. Melatonin and sleep: a balanced view. J Am Pharm Assoc 38:228–229, 1998.
59. Almeida JC, Grimsley EW. Coma from the health food store: interaction between kava and alprazolam. Ann Intern Med 125:940–941, 1996.
60. The involvement of sleep in motor vehicle crashes. National Highway Traffic Safety Administration memorandum. Washington, DC: U.S. Department of Transportation, National Highway Traffic Safety Administration, U.S. Government Printing Office, November 22, 1995.
61. Leger D. The cost of sleep-related accidents: a report of the national commission on sleep disorders research. Sleep 17:84–93, 1994.

CHAPTER 59

ATTENTION-DEFICIT/ HYPERACTIVITY DISORDER (ADHD)

Collin A. Hovinga and Stephanie J. Phelps

Attention-deficit/hyperactivity disorder (ADHD) is characterized by persistent patterns of inattention, hyperactivity, and impulsivity.[1] Although all children may occasionally exhibit inattentive and restless behavior, a person with ADHD displays inattention and/or hyperactivity to a degree that is both debilitating and more pronounced than that seen in other persons at a similar level of development.

The first official diagnostic criteria, for what we now call ADHD, were published in 1980. Like most psychiatric disorders, ADHD is a clinical diagnosis that relies on patient history, physical assessment, neurologic examination, and behavioral evaluation. Unfortunately, the diagnosis does not currently involve laboratory assessment or radiologic confirmation. While early DSM criteria focused on hyperactivity,[2] the revised criteria were broadened to include and emphasize inattention and impulsivity.[3] The current DSM-IV criteria allow a clinician to subtype a child's disorder as predominantly hyperactive, predominantly inattentive, or a combination of both.[1] The DSM-IV diagnostic criteria are limited because they fail to consider the developmental nature of the disorder; hence ADHD may go undetected in many adults.

Approximately 65% of children with ADHD also have at least one comorbid disorder. These include learning disabilities, behavioral disorders, and/or psychiatric conditions. Each of these may impair a child's academic performance, affect the child's self-image, and alter the ability to interact with peers and family members. When left untreated, these comorbid factors may increase a person's risk of a serious psychopathologic disorder later in life.[4] Overall, children with ADHD have a 25-fold greater risk of institutionalization for delinquent behaviors, a 10-fold greater risk of developing antisocial personality disorders, and a 5-fold greater risk of drug abuse.[5]

During the 1970s and 1980s, media debates focused on the "labeling" of children with ADHD and on the use of stimulants to treat this disorder. Allegations by some suggested that the diagnosis of ADHD was either a "myth" or was merely applied to control children who displayed unwanted behaviors. Most now agree that ADHD is one of the best-studied disorders in medicine, and the data on its validity are more compelling than those for many other disorders.[4,6] To date, more than 170 studies involving more than 6000 school-aged children with ADHD have been published.[4]

Whereas most believe that ADHD has a neurobiologic foundation, its pathophysiology remains elusive. Recent advances in molecular biology have given us a better understanding of the genetic basis for ADHD. Likewise, a new imaging technique (i.e., functional magnetic resonance imaging [fMRI]) has suggested a possible neuroanatomical basis for the disorder. Obviously, there has been increased interest in these areas and their possible utility in the diagnosis and treatment of ADHD.

The management of ADHD is complex and requires a multimodal approach that uses both nonpharmacologic and pharmacologic therapies. Once comorbid factors are considered, optimal treatment is individualized based on the clinician's recommendation and the family's preferences.

Pharmacotherapy for ADHD originated approximately 60 years ago. Today the ability of medications to ameliorate the core effects of ADHD is well established. Certain drugs including stimulants (i.e., methylphenidate, dextroamphetamine, pemoline, and Adderall), tricyclic antidepressants (TCAs), and clonidine are used more frequently. Other agents (i.e., monoamine oxidase inhibitors, bupropion, venlafaxine, fluoxetine, and carbamazepine) are reserved for patients with more refractory disorders.

TREATMENT GOALS: ADHD

- Ensure an accurate diagnosis of ADHD in a child or an adult, using DMS-IV criteria.
- Establish treatment goals jointly with the patient and the family.
- Address patient concerns and misconceptions about ADHD with emphasis on how the disorder has an impact on a person's behaviors, academic performance, and social interactions.
- Identify core symptoms that can be used to monitor positive and negative responses to therapy.
- Select optimal drug therapy after consideration of any preexisting comorbidities.
- Improve the person's academic or work performance and enhance his or her social skills without producing intolerable or significant adverse effects.
- Educate and counsel patients, parents, and teachers about ADHD and drug therapy.
- Tailor drug therapy (dose and interval) based on patient response and tolerance.
- Monitor for clinical or laboratory evidence of side effects.
- Recognize when and how to discontinue therapy.

EPIDEMIOLOGY

Prevalence

Today, ADHD is the most common neurobehavioral disorder of childhood.[4] Although reports of its occurrence in children range from as low as 1.7% to as high as 16%,[4] the DSM-IV notes that prevalence rates in the United States are approximately 3 to 5% (i.e., greater than 2 million children).[1] However, these figures probably underestimate the true incidence, because they do not include preschool, adolescent, or adult patients. Historically, the incidence in males has been four to nine times higher than that noted in females[4,5]; however, the disorder is now being diagnosed more frequently in girls so that the male:female ratio is now 2:1.[7] ADHD accounts for 50% of referrals to child neurologists, neuropsychologists, behavioral pediatricians, and child psychiatrists.[8] Although one usually associates ADHD with preschool or school-aged children, 70 to 80% of children with ADHD will continue to exhibit some symptoms into adolescence or will qualify for the diagnosis of a full disorder.[6] Approximately 65 to 80% will have the full disorder in late adolescence (16 to 19 years of age). Only a small percentage (3 to 8%) of hyperactive children will retain the disorder into adulthood when the DSM-IV criteria are applied.[6] However, when developmentally referenced and empirically based definitions are used and parents serve as a source of information, 68% of subjects continue to exhibit symptoms of the disorder into adulthood.[6]

Etiology

Although many factors correlate with an increased risk of ADHD, most relationships are extremely weak and nonspecific. Several items including dietary (i.e., sugar consumption, food additives and dyes, vitamin deficiencies, or food allergies), environmental factors (i.e., lead poisoning or high voltage wiring), poor prenatal care (i.e., alcohol and nicotine exposure), birth complications (i.e., brain damage), and poor parenting have been considered in the etiology of ADHD. For years, there has been speculation that minimal brain damage or minimal brain dysfunction may be associated with ADHD. Recently, it was suggested that hypoxia and hypotension in utero could selectively damage neurons located in anatomical regions important in ADHD.[9] The above causes are supported largely by anecdotal information. Hence, there is little if any controlled evidence to support their role and they have been largely discounted.

Many family, twin, and adoption studies have suggested a genetic link in ADHD.[10] Studies in adopted children show that siblings of children with ADHD have two to three times the risk of developing ADHD than normal control subjects. Furthermore, the diagnosis of ADHD is more frequently shared in full siblings than in half siblings. The strongest support for a familial link for the disorder comes from the finding that twins sharing the same genetic material (monozygotic twins) have a higher probability of experiencing ADHD than nonidentical (dizygotic) twins.

Recently, molecular biologic techniques have attempted to define a specific DNA sequence associated with ADHD. Although a causative gene has not been definitively identified, two possible candidates have been proposed. Current hypotheses suggest that specific alleles of either the dopamine transporter (*DAT1*) gene[11] and/or the dopamine receptor D_4 (*DRD4*) gene[12] may result in altered dopamine transmission.

PATHOPHYSIOLOGY

Few patients with ADHD undergo invasive studies that allow for any direct examination of neuropathology. Likewise, noninvasive studies (i.e., routine neuroimaging and electroencephalogram [EEG]) are usually normal and are therefore noncontributory. Hence, many indirect lines of evidence (i.e., fMRI) have led to our current understanding of the pathophysiology of ADHD. The indirect approach begins with the observed inability of the child with ADHD to maintain attention and compares this to what is currently speculated about attention mechanisms in the brain.

One current theory maintains that the posterior regions of the brain allow a person to switch from one activity to another, whereas the frontal regions of the brain allow a person to maintain a specific activity. The posterior brain regions (i.e., parietal cortex, a region of the brain where sensory stimuli converge) switch attention to a new activity and then "hand-off" to the frontal brain regions (i.e., anterior cingulate gyrus and prefrontal cortex) that maintain the attention to the new activity. In particular, the region of the frontal lobes of the brain referred to as the "prefrontal cortex" seems to be important in maintaining attention and "working memory." Working memory is felt to be a person's ability to maintain subject matter in the mind continuously and to manipulate the subject matter intellectually. Examples of working memory include adding or subtracting numbers in one's head or naming all the states that begin with the letter "M."

Indirect evidence suggests that children with ADHD may have problems activating the frontal lobe regions that manage working memory. Persons with documented neuroanatomical damage to the frontal lobes, and particularly to the right frontal lobe, demonstrate behavior that is similar to that of children with ADHD (e.g., short attention span, impulsivity, and hyperactivity). Damage to the inferior right frontal lobe (orbitofrontal cortex) seems to be associated more with impulsivity and hyperactivity, whereas damage to the lateral right frontal lobe (laterofrontal cortex) seems to be associated with difficulties in maintaining attention. A magnetic resonance imaging (MRI) study noted that children with ADHD have 10% smaller right frontal lobes than do matched-control children.[13] Likewise, Filipek et al[14] reported that a group of children with ADHD had brain volumes about 10% smaller than normal in the anterior superior and anterior inferior regions.[14]

Neuropsychologic tests have been developed that are sensitive to neuroanatomical damage in the frontal lobes and to damage in the parietal lobes. These same tests suggest that children with ADHD have problems with measures of frontal lobe function, but perform normally on measures of parietal lobe function. Positron emission tomography (PET) scans of normal adults given tasks that should require use of working memory show a relative increase in metabolism in the frontal lobes during the task. Adults with ADHD persisting from childhood, but not currently on medication, show a relative decrease in frontal lobe metabolism by PET scan on the same tasks. Those adults, when given stimulant medication, show a "normalization" of the PET scan with increased frontal lobe activity during the tasks.

Animal studies support the contention that the attention mechanisms are modulated by neurotransmitter input from several regions of the brainstem. The ventral tegmental area of the upper brainstem supplies dopaminergic and noradrenergic neurotransmitter input to the orbitofrontal and laterofrontal cortex (prefrontal cortex). The dorsal raphe in the brainstem activates the ventral tegmental gray and also provides serotonergic neurotransmission diffusely to the cerebral hemispheres, especially to the anterior cingulate gyrus. The locus ceruleus in the brainstem inhibits the dorsal raphe and provides noradrenergic neurotransmitter input to the parietal cortex and laterofrontal cortex (prefrontal cortex). The noradrenergic receptors in the prefrontal cortex are primarily α_2-adrenergic.

One hypothesis is that the locus ceruleus may periodically activate the parietal cortex and allow for a change of attention to a new stimulus. When the activity of the locus ceruleus subsides, the dorsal raphe is able to activate the ventral tegmental gray, which then releases dopamine to the prefrontal cortex to maintain attention. Animal studies have shown that the activation of the prefrontal cortex inhibits the parietal cortex and the locus ceruleus, thus decreasing the effect of new, but distracting, sensory stimuli. Another hypothesis is that in children with ADHD, the locus ceruleus activates the parietal cortex, allowing the child to change attention to new stimuli, but that the transition to activation of the ventral tegmental gray and prefrontal cortex is deficient. Thus, the child with ADHD does not properly activate frontal lobe working memory and does not inhibit new sensory information arriving by way of the parietal cortex.

Stimulant medications such as methylphenidate and amphetamine are thought to improve attention in children with ADHD by increasing dopamine and noradrenaline in the prefrontal cortex by both activating working memory and inhibiting distraction from new stimuli. Clonidine, an α_2-adrenergic stimulant, is thought to improve attention primarily by action at the α_2-adrenergic postsynaptic receptors of the laterofrontal regions in prefrontal cortex.

Current studies do not clearly elucidate what role the dorsal raphe and serotonin may play in disorders of attention. However, there is a subset of children with ADHD and obsessive compulsive behavioral features that seem to improve when given serotonergic medications and become worse with dopaminergic/adrenergic medications.

CLINICAL PRESENTATION AND DIAGNOSIS

Signs and Symptoms

Patients with ADHD display persistent patterns of inattention, hyperactivity, and impulsivity. The inattention associated with ADHD can be manifest in various ways. Although these patients are physically present during a school lesson, their minds seem to be elsewhere, making them literally unavailable to learn. Homework, if done or not lost, is often messy and incomplete, and appears to have been done in a haphazard manner. These patients lack organizational ability and poorly grasp time/task management skills. It is common for them to fail to follow through on requests and to partially complete or ignore chores. They often make careless mistakes, pay little attention to details or instruction, and give partial effort to many tasks instead of completing one entire assignment. Patients with ADHD are easily distracted and quickly abandon current tasks to focus on even the most trivial stimuli. This is especially true as the complexity or difficulty of a task increases. In social settings, they appear bored, quickly lose interest in conversation and switch from one topic to the next. They have difficulty following prescribed rules of conduct, as well as game rules during play time.

The hyperactive person appears to have an endless source of energy that can seldom be repressed. Generally, an active curious child is considered healthy in our society; however, the child with ADHD exhibits hyperactivity to a degree that is problematic. Children with ADHD are often described as being constantly "on the go" or "driven by a motor." They have trouble remaining seated for any length of time and constantly squirm and fidget. Hyperactivity is also manifested by an inability to play quietly when expected, by running or playing raucously when inappropriate, and by excessive talking. These children are often unable to get through "quiet time" without incident. Their disruptive classroom behavior frequently draws disciplinary actions. As a child with ADHD develops, the presentation of hyperactivity changes. Before 3 years of age, activity increases. After 3 years of age, activity begins a downward trend, so that hyperactivity is generally not present by adolescence. Awareness of this pattern is important for successful therapy because one might wrongfully assume that a patient who is no longer hyperactive does not need continued treatment.

Impulsivity often causes a child to be labeled disruptive or disrespectful. It can manifest itself as impatience and the immediate expression of thought without regard to setting (e.g., blurting out answers, comments, and emotions). Impulsive children often interrupt conversations and show extreme frustration when they are not allowed to talk. These patients grab inappropriate objects (e.g., a hot skillet or fragile items), intrude into other people's space or tamper with others' possessions, and act without regard for consequences.

Because the presentation varies with age, it is important to consider age when assessing clinical presentation. Because most parents describe their "normal" preschool children as inattentive and hyperactive, a diagnosis of ADHD is difficult in this age group. The preschool child with ADHD generally has additional symptoms such as temper tantrums, argumentative behavior, and aggressive or fearless behavior. They may also exhibit sleep disturbances.

During the school-age years cognitive work becomes increasingly difficult. Although they may have above average intelligence, they may seem immature for their age. Their school performance is affected by difficulty concentrating or focusing on assigned tasks. Hence, these children have greater school failure and grade-repeating rates. A combination of low self-esteem and impulsivity, hyperactivity, and/or inattention may lead to difficulty in peer relationships. During this time, elementary school children may also begin to exhibit comorbid symptoms (i.e., reading difficulty).

Previously, it was thought that children with ADHD outgrew the disorder by puberty; however, we now know that this is not true. The presentation of ADHD in adolescents has not been well established. Symptoms may change with increasing age such that fewer symptoms are considered indicative of ADHD. Because students no longer have one teacher for all subjects or are not in one class all day, their symptoms may go unnoticed. Their inattention and cognitive difficulties may lead to poorly organized approaches to schoolwork. Failing to complete independent academic work is a hallmark of ADHD in the adolescent. These adolescents are generally 2 academic years behind their contemporaries.[15] Unfortunately, there is no evidence that early treatment with psychostimulants alters their later academic achievement. During these years, adolescents want greater independence and desire both same-sex and opposite-sex peer relationships. However, patients with antisocial behaviors secondary to ADHD may have difficulty developing and maintaining relationships. These patients may also begin to display risky behaviors including higher rates of accidents (e.g., auto and bike), suicide attempts, teen pregnancy, violence, and substance abuse.[6]

It is now known that 30 to 70% of children with ADHD will continue to display some symptoms as adults.[3] On average, symptoms diminish by about 50% every 5 years between the ages of 10 and 25 years. Hyperactivity declines more quickly than impulsivity or inattentiveness.[16] The presence of disorganization continues to have an impact in the workplace and frequently requires the person to keep an extensive list of activities as reminders. These persons may feel that they "never get their act together." Poor concentration and procrastination may persist into adulthood, leading to shifting activities (e.g., moving from one activity to another), endless unfinished projects, and frequent job changes. They may also have problems sustaining long-term relationships. The presence of intermittent explosive outbursts may be related to comorbid symptomatology or may be a special type of ADHD associated with labile mood. Perhaps because the early diagnostic criteria focused on hyperactivity, a vast majority of adult patients with no childhood evaluation or treatment are female. Women in whom ADHD was undiagnosed in childhood may display a high incidence of mood disorders (e.g., anxiety).

Prospective studies have described three potential outcomes in children with ADHD.[17] The first outcome, "developmental delay," occurs in 30% of subjects. These persons no longer manifest any functional impairment. The second outcome is called "continual display" and occurs in

40% of subjects. These persons continue to have functionally impairing symptoms into adulthood. Additionally, they may have a variety of different types of social and emotional difficulties. The third outcome occurs in 30% of patients and is called "developmental decay." Although these persons continue to exhibit the core symptoms of ADHD, they also develop serious psychopathologic disorders such as alcoholism, substance abuse, and antisocial personality disorder.

Comorbid Disorders

For years clinicians have noted an association between certain comorbid disorders and ADHD. In fact, approximately 65% of children with ADHD have at least one comorbid disorder that includes a learning disability (i.e., reading disability or dyslexia) and/or psychiatric conditions.[4] Estimates of reading disability in patients with ADHD range from as low as 9%[18] to as high as 92%.[19] Children with ADHD are also more likely to perform below expectations in both reading and arithmetic.[20]

Although we do not currently understand why these comorbid disorders are associated with ADHD, several theories have been suggested. Some believe that ADHD is actually a consequence of a learning disability, reflecting the cumulative effects of a lack of motivation and disinterest in school.[21] Other groups believe that a reading disorder does not reflect a true comorbidity. They feel that an attention disorder is a cognitive problem that many children with reading disorders have and that inattention does not represent the symptom complex associated with ADHD.[22] A third group contends that there are separate cognitive deficits in reading disorders and ADHD. For example, children with reading disorders had difficulty with tasks involving confrontation naming and rapid automatized naming, while children with ADHD had difficulty with word list learning and recall.[23] The fourth group simply postulates that reading disorders and ADHD represent separate diagnostic entities that frequently occur in the same patient.[24]

A number of psychiatric conditions occur with ADHD. Between 10 and 20% of children in both community and clinical studies have mood disorders, 20% have conduct disorders, and up to 40% have oppositional defiant disorders.[25] Bipolar disorder is being increasingly recognized in patients with ADHD.[26] Only about 7% of those with ADHD have tics or Tourette's syndrome, but 60% of those with Tourette's syndrome have ADHD.[4]

Diagnosis

Table 59.1 outlines the current diagnostic criteria for ADHD.[1] Over the years, an evolving understanding of the disorder has contributed to the dynamic nature of the criteria. The *Diagnostic and Statistical Manual of Mental Disorders*, 2nd ed. (DSM-II) characterized "hyperkinetic reactions of childhood" as a disorder caused by suppression or internalization of interpersonal problems.[27] Ten years later, the DSM-III classified the disease as *attention deficit disorder* (ADD), with or without hyperactivity.[2] In the DSM-III-R the symptom criteria were further modified to stress the importance and core inclusion of hyperactivity. The qualifier with or without hyperactivity was deleted and the term *attention-deficit/hyperactivity disorder* (ADHD) was born.[3] Additionally, the new criteria broadened the definition to provide an increased emphasis on attention problems.[1,4] To reduce the number of false-positive diagnoses, the current DSM-IV criteria require that symptoms begin before the age of 7, be present in at least two settings (e.g., home and school), and be continuously present for at least 6 months.[1] When applied correctly, the criteria result in high interrater reliability, good validity, and high predictability of prognosis and medication effectiveness. Unfortunately, the current criteria fail to address the developmental nature of this disorder. Because a patient's clinical presentation changes with age, ADHD remains undiagnosed in many adults.

The essential feature for diagnosis is a consistent and persistent pattern of hyperactivity, impulsivity, and/or

Table 59.1 ▪ DSM-IV Diagnostic Criteria for Attention-Deficit/Hyperactivity Disorder

A. Six (or more) symptoms of either inattention or hyperactivity for longer than 6 months

Inattention

1. Often fails to give close attention to details or makes careless mistakes in schoolwork, work, or other activities
2. Often has difficulty sustaining attention in tasks or play activities
3. Often does not seem to listen when spoken to directly
4. Often does not follow through on instructions and fails to finish assignments
5. Often has difficulty organizing task and activities
6. Often avoids or dislikes tasks that require sustained mental effort
7. Often loses things necessary for tasks or activities (e.g., toys, books, assignments)
8. Is often easily distracted by extraneous stimuli
9. Is often forgetful in daily activities

Hyperactivity-impulsivity

1. Often fidgets with hands or feet or squirms in seat
2. Often leaves seat in classroom or situations in which remaining seated is expected
3. Often runs or climbs about excessively when inappropriate
4. Often has difficulty playing quietly
5. Is often "on the go" or acts as if "driven by a motor"
6. Often talks excessively
7. Often blurts out answers before questions have been completed
8. Often has difficulty waiting turn
9. Often interrupts or intrudes on others

B. Symptoms present before age 7

C. Impairment from symptoms is present in two or more distinct settings (e.g., school, home, work)

D. Clear evidence of significant impairment in social, academic, or occupational functioning

Source: Adapted with permission from American Psychiatric Association. Diagnostic and statistical manual of mental disorders. 4th ed. (DSM-IV). Washington, DC: American Psychiatric Association, 1994.

inattention that is maladaptive and more pronounced than that seen in subjects at a comparable stage of development. Symptoms must be severe enough to cause decreased productivity and interpersonal difficulties between the patient and parent, peer, or teacher groups.

Like most mental disorders, diagnosis involves patient history and behavioral assessment. Because a definitive diagnostic test (biochemical, physiologic, anatomical, genetic, radiologic, etc.) is not available currently, the diagnosis of ADHD is a clinical one. A number of diagnostic tools including parent, teacher, and child interviews, observation of the parent and child, physical and neurologic examinations, developmental testing, behavior rating scales, and psychologic evaluations are used to develop a diagnosis.

A patient's history is essential to a correct diagnosis. It is composed of both parent and teacher observations of the child's behavior within the home, school, and social environments. The clinician should obtain information about both acceptable and unacceptable behaviors, when they first appeared, and what factors the parents or teacher believes may exacerbate a particular behavior. It is also important to determine what coping methods have been attempted and if any method has been successful. School records and grades should be reviewed in hopes of identifying performance or behavior trends. For example, things such as a recent change in grades, performance in select subjects, performance based on class size, and grade differences in classes before and after lunch should be assessed. If a noticeable pattern can be identified, the parents and teacher should be further questioned about contributing factors (i.e., class scheduling, class size, etc.).

The child should also be observed and interviewed. Evaluation should include assessment of language and motor functioning, social skills, and emotional maturity. It is important to determine if the child is maintaining the expected social skills. Likewise, one should gain some appreciation of the child's perception of school and family or home structure. Although one announced visit to the classroom may not provide conclusive information, when possible the child should be observed in the classroom environment.

The child's symptoms can be assessed systematically and quantified using parent or teacher questionnaire scales (i.e., the Conners Teacher's Rating Scale, or the Attention Deficit Disorder Evaluation Scale). Although a number of rating scales and psychologic testing instruments may be given, no single test should be used to make or refute the diagnosis.[4] In clinical practice, scales such as the Conners, SNAP-IV, and Disruptive Behavior Disorder Scale are more helpful in assessing and monitoring treatment than in making a diagnosis.[4]

The physical examination is intended to identify any abnormal features or underlying health problems that might mimic ADHD or its comorbid factors. Growth measurements should be noted and assessed. There should also be an emphasis on hearing and vision testing. Standard blood and urine chemistry analyses should be obtained to rule out other diseases that may mirror ADHD. Because alterations in serum magnesium, zinc, or iron have been associated with ADHD, some practitioners check serum magnesium, zinc, and iron levels. If suggested by patient history, a thyroid profile and lead levels should be obtained. Additionally, approximately 25% of children with symptoms consistent with ADHD actually suffer from sleep disorders. The influence of medication should be considered in the evaluation of any child before the diagnosis of ADHD is made. Many medications (e.g., phenobarbital, gabapentin, theophylline, and albuterol) can effect cognition and behavior.[28]

A thorough neurologic examination including an evaluation of mental status, reflexes, general sensation, and cranial nerve and motor function should be performed. Although some children may have "soft" signs suggestive of neuromaturational delays, the examination is usually normal in children with ADHD. Because EEGs are generally normal, they are not usually obtained.

After completion of the above, the patient is referred for psychologic testing. Neuropsychologic tests that focus on sustained attention (i.e., Continuous Performance Task, the Wisconsin Card-Sorting Test, Test of Variables of Attention, the Matching Familiar Figures Test, and the Wechsler Intelligence Scale for Children-Revised) are not diagnostic for ADHD; however, they may evaluate specific impairments associated with the disorder.[4] Although patients with ADHD can be very intelligent and creative, their scores in arithmetic, digit span, and coding are typically lower than average.

Finally, the differential diagnosis must rule out the presence of other conditions that may mimic ADHD. Neurobiologic factors affecting brain development (i.e., chromosomal or genetic abnormalities such as Tourette's syndrome, sickle-cell anemia, or Turner's syndrome) should be excluded. Likewise, medical disorders such as hyperthyroidism, head trauma, seizure disorder, meningitis, and toxin-associated (i.e., lead poisoning, fetal alcohol syndrome, uterine cocaine exposure) disorders should be ruled out. Additionally, processing disorders (i.e., language and learning disorders), cognitive impairment, and mental retardation should be eliminated. Finally, environmental factors such as an abusive home, a dysfunctional family, and school placement should be considered as potential causes for the child's behavior.

Because a brief interview with a child, parent, or teacher may result in a false-positive or false-negative diagnosis, the diagnosis of ADHD requires extensive interaction and assessment. Both parent and teacher rating scales (i.e., Conners Parent's and Teacher's Rating Scales, Parent/Teacher Child Behavior Checklist, and Barkley Home/School Situations Questionnaire) may provide valuable information about core symptoms of ADHD, as well as possible comorbid conditions. These scales may also serve to evaluate the efficacy of any treatment.

PSYCHOSOCIAL ASPECTS

The impact of ADHD on the patient, family, society and the health care system is enormous. Careful diagnosis of ADHD in the young child is important because the social stigma at this level of development can be particularly cruel and debilitating. The negative effects on the patient's self-esteem, the stress to families, the financial cost, and the impact on academic and vocational activities cannot be understated.

Effect on the Patient

Approximately 65% of children with ADHD have at least one comorbid learning disability (e.g., reading disorders and subnormal intelligence) and/or psychiatric conditions (e.g., mood, conduct, or oppositional defiant disorders). Each of these may impair a child's academic performance, which usually has a negative impact on the child's self-image. Conversely, a recent study noted that some children with ADHD compensate for skill deficits through an inflated or exaggerated self-image.[29] These alterations in self-image affect a patient's ability to interact with both peers and family members. Perhaps the most devastating impact of ADHD is the tendency for these children to be rejected by their peers. Even administration of medication in school can be difficult for children and may enhance ridicule by their peers. Unfortunately, peer rejection in childhood is a predictor of negative long-term outcomes including school drop out, delinquency, substance abuse, and adult mental health problems.[5,6] Additionally, patients with ADHD experience higher rates of accidental injury secondary to aggressive behavior patterns.[5,6]

The pressure to perform well academically may persist into high school and college. To gain entrance into the "right" college or graduate school, students must maintain a high grade-point average. Hence, "B's and C's" have become unacceptable to many families. Typically, a student with ADHD is provided "special" circumstances to ensure their "optimal" performance. For instance, a student may be given more time for a college entrance examination (e.g., SAT), course examinations, or board examination (e.g., NAPLEX) after graduation. As patients get older, there is greater competition for fewer choice jobs. The pressures of the work environment may make it difficult for an adult to concentrate. For these reasons, employers are being asked to make exceptions in the workplace for persons with ADHD. Unfortunately, ADHD has become so common that a doctor's diagnosis may no longer be sufficient for special consideration.

Effect on the Patient's Family

Families of children with ADHD experience an increasing levels of parenteral frustration, marital discord, and divorce. Whether ADHD is the effect or cause of these problems remains controversial. Interestingly, 41% of parents feel that ADHD is caused by a genetic influence, 12% of parents attribute the disease to poor parenting, and 13.4% believe that it is the result of marital conflicts or family problems.[30] The cost of health care may be substantial and can also place additional stress on the family.

Increased societal pressures on family life may result in a misdiagnosis of ADHD. Because an increasing number of single parents or both parents are in the workforce, there is an increasing number of children in preschool. The preschool environment places younger children in a more organized and less flexible social schedule. While many children do well and thrive in this environment, some children are not developmentally or socially ready for the structure that exists. Had these children remained at home until they were older, their seemingly "abnormal" behavior may not have come to the attention of teachers and physicians.

Effect on Society

Persons with ADHD consume an inordinate amount of resources and attention from schools, the criminal justice system, and other social services. Declining Federal and State funds may indirectly contribute to a diagnosis of ADHD. Although ADHD is not recognized as a separate category of special education, schools have officially encouraged the U.S. Department of Education to provide services for children with ADHD under the existing special education categories (e.g., learning disabilities, emotional disturbances, and other health impairments). Although special education services are available, the qualification criteria are stringent. For example, to qualify with a learning disability a student must exhibit a substantial difference between intellectual ability and academic performance. Although children with ADHD may have low reading or math skills these may not be low enough to meet the requirement. Similarly, existing criteria for an emotional disturbance are not always interpreted to include children with ADHD. If it is estimated that approximately 2 million school children have ADHD, only 45% of all children with ADHD appear to be in special education classes. Although less than half of children with ADHD receive special academic services because of their disorder, the financial cost is significant. In fact, in 1995, students with ADHD accounted for $3.2 billion dollars of additional national public school expenditures.[31]

Persons with disabilities (i.e., ADHD) cannot legally face discrimination and are entitled to special services under the Individuals with Disabilities Education Act of 1990 and Section 504 of the 1973 Rehabilitation Act. Unfortunately, parents may discover that the only way to obtain assistance is to have their child labeled with a "disorder." Section 504 accommodations are usually requested only when children are denied eligibility for special education. Federal legislative funding has not been fully appropriated with this law, leaving states to provide funding for these entitlements. Additionally, courts have forced schools to allocate funds to provide services for the disabled.

Effect on the Health Care System

ADHD also affects physicians and the health care system in general. In a survey of pediatrician practices regarding ADHD, 53% reported they spend more than 1 hour with a patient with ADHD. Interestingly, whereas 63% reported setting aside special amounts of time to care for patients with ADHD, 39.7% felt that the time required for care was problematic. In addition, only 13% of pediatricians felt they were adequately compensated for treating patients with ADHD and about 9% suggested that better insurance compensation would change the care of these children.[30] Thus, when presented with a child with a potentially complex behavioral problem, it may be tempting to simply prescribe a medication rather than address the emotional issues, family relationships, or school environment.

Even with a multimodal evaluation and treatment plan, little else may be done at the primary care level. Although most pediatricians would contact the school, only 18.7% would refer children with ADHD to a psychiatrist, psychologist, educational therapist, school social worker, or some other person in a related discipline.[30] Although specialists (i.e., behavioral-developmental pediatricians and child psychiatrists) need to be involved with resolving the intricacies of the child, family, and school situation, cost-containment measures associated with managed care increasingly permit referrals only when medication has been considered for the child. These conditions may contribute to the use of medications rather than working with a dysfunctional family, decreasing the size of the classroom, or augmenting funding for special education services. Because stimulants such as methylphenidate work "more" quickly, they are more attractive to families, physicians, managed care companies, and financially strapped educational systems.

Cost barriers and lack of insurance coverage may prevent an appropriate diagnosis and treatment of ADHD. This, combined with the observed lack of integration with special educational services, can represent considerable long-term cost to society.

THERAPEUTIC PLAN

Although there has been a National Institute of Health (NIH) consensus conference on the treatment of ADHD, no guidelines resulted from the meeting. Currently, there is no universally agreed upon method to treat this disorder. Based upon a review of the literature, the authors recommend the algorithm in Figure 59.1.

TREATMENT

Pharmacotherapy

Stimulants

In 1937, Bradley first reported the efficacy of a racemic mixture of amphetamine sulfate in the treatment of children with a variety of disruptive behaviors.[32] Medication played a relatively minor role in the management of ADHD until 1955. At this point, methylphenidate became available and began to replace amphetamine as the preferred drug in the treatment of ADHD.[4,31,33] Because of fears of abuse, in the 1970s the Drug Enforcement Agency classified methylphenidate and amphetamines as schedule II controlled substances. This began the practice of monitoring the amounts of each substance produced in the United States.[31] Treatment of ADHD with stimulants increased dramatically from 1971 to 1987 as use doubled every 4 to 7 years. An anti-Ritalin law suit and negative media campaigns curtailed the use of stimulants until 1990.[33] Subsequently, methylphenidate use has continued to rise, particularly because of (1) greater public and physician awareness and acceptance of stimulants in treating ADHD, (2) a broadening of the diagnostic criteria that lessened the focus on hyperactivity, (3) a greater understanding of the outcomes associated with unmanaged ADHD, (4) decreased concerns regarding the long-term side effects, and (5) the continued use of stimulants into adolescence and adulthood.[4] Estimates of the use of methylphenidate use vary in the range of 1.5 to 2.6 million or 2.8% of U.S. children and adolescents receiving the drug in 1995.[31,33]

Currently, stimulants are the most frequently used agents in the management of ADHD with methylphenidate accounting for greater than 90% of stimulants used in the United States.[4] The other stimulants include dextroamphetamine, pemoline, and most recently Adderall, a racemic mixture of amphetamine salts (75% dextroamphetamine and 25% levoamphetamine). Although the exact mechanism of action of the stimulants is unknown, it is believed that they modulate function of central catecholamines (dopamine and norepinephrine).[34] Methylphenidate has been shown to act as a competitive antagonist at striatal dopamine transporters, increasing the amounts of synaptic dopamine.[35]

In contrast to most drugs for which there is limited knowledge in pediatrics, stimulants have been extensively studied. Their beneficial effects have been well documented in more than 6000 school-aged children enrolled in greater than 170 studies.[4,36–38] Stimulants significantly improve ADHD core symptoms of inattention, hyperactivity, and impulsivity. In addition, these drugs facilitate short-term improvements in academic performance and social behavior. Unfortunately, their influence on scholastic and peer interactions is highly variable with many children failing to reach normal levels of functioning.[38–41]

Although most of our current knowledge about the stimulants has been derived from latency age (6 to 12 years) male children, similar efficacy has been observed in female children and adolescents.[37,42] The benefits of stimulants in preschoolers with ADHD are limited and inconsistent.[37] Furthermore, this age group seems more predisposed to stimulant-induced adverse effects. Original studies in adults with ADHD suggested that stimulants were less effective.[37] Response rates in this population averaged 50%, a rate much lower than the 70% observed in children. However, a more recent study, using methylphenidate, supports the efficacy of stimulants in adults provided adequate doses are administered.[43]

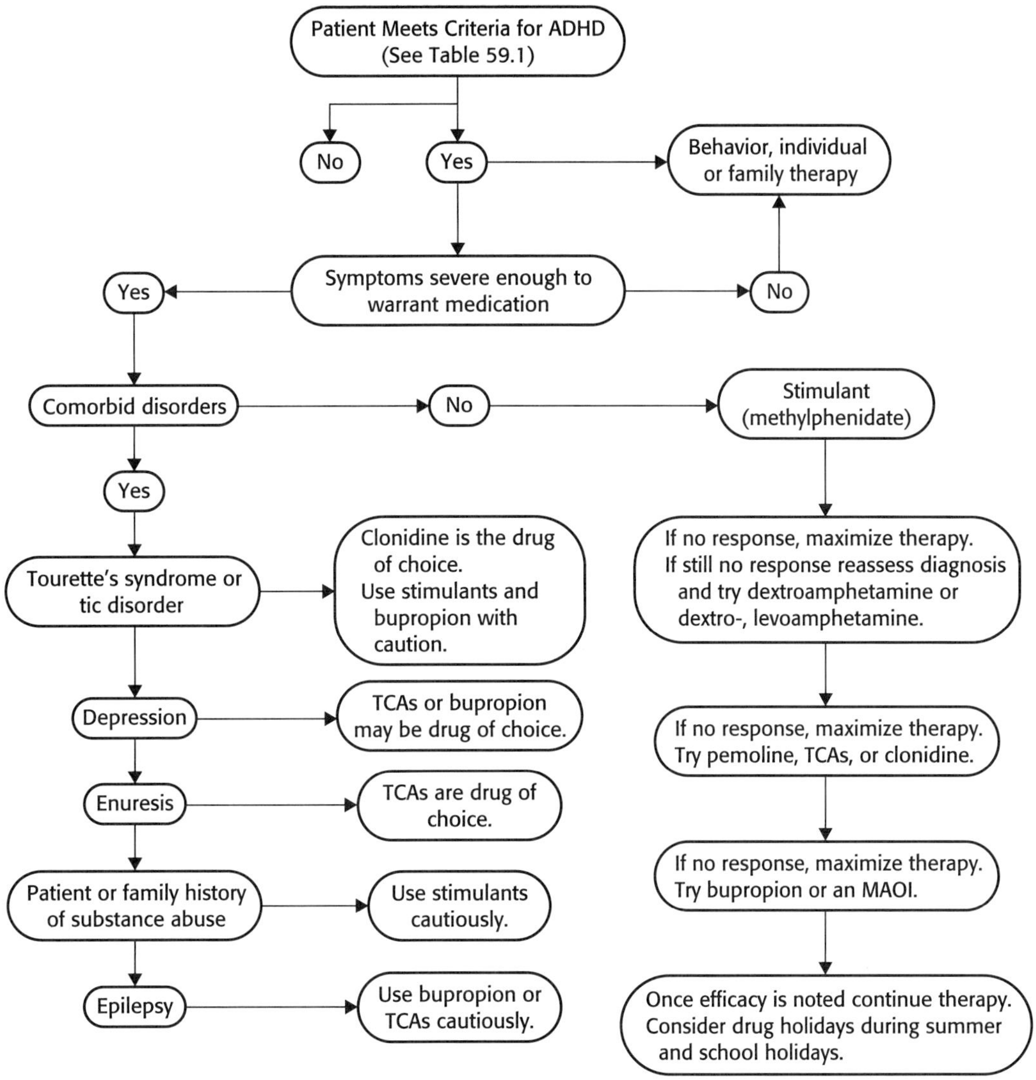

Figure 59.1. Algorithm for the treatment of attention-deficit/hyperactivity disorder (ADHD). *MAOIs*, monoamine oxidase inhibitors; *TCAs*, tricyclic antidepressants.

Stimulants have been used in children in whom both ADHD and other comorbid conditions were diagnosed.[37] In contrast to popular belief, stimulants rarely increase aggression in patients with ADHD/conduct disorder. These children show similar improvements with marked decreases in both aggressive (physical and verbal) and antisocial behaviors. Stimulants seem to produce less of a response in children with ADHD plus depression-anxiety. Current studies in this population are limited and fail to address comorbid depression or anxiety symptoms.[37] Mixed findings have been observed in mentally handicapped children. Stimulants seem more effective in those with mild to moderate retardation, but inconsistent responses are seen in those with more severe degrees of impairment. Interestingly, the best predictor of treatment response is not age, IQ, or general disruptive behavior but the presence of clearly defined ADHD symptoms (hyperactivity, inattentiveness, and impulsivity).[37]

In general, the stimulant's onset of action is rapid with effectiveness noted after an initial dose.[44,45] Studies have shown that each individual agent has comparable efficacy.[38,40,46] If doses are titrated appropriately, approximately 70% of children with ADHD will show symptomatic improvement with a single stimulant. Caution is warranted in judging a response too quickly. Children with ADHD may fail to respond to an individual stimulant, but may respond to an alternative drug in this class. Response rates increase up to 96% when two agents are tried.[36] Another concern is the belief that stimulants induce a "clinically specific" or what has been described as a "paradoxical" response in children with ADHD. Response to a stimulant is not diagnostic of ADHD. Normal children given dextroamphetamine or methylphenidate will display decreased motor activity with improved attention, including faster reaction time, superior memory, and more vigilance.[47,48] No patient-specific variable has been shown to be predictive of response.

Despite the fact that the short-term benefits of stimulants have been well documented, their long-term impact in children with ADHD is less impressive. Many of the original gains in academic and social interactions have been attributed to increases in attention and concentration with associated decreases in impulsivity.[38,40] In comparing stimulant-treated and untreated children with ADHD, no differences in number of grades failed, retention of subject material, achievement test scores, or college enrollment have been noted in follow-up. Similar results have been observed in examining psychological adjustment and delinquent behaviors requiring institutionalized placement.[38,40] It has been suggested that long-term outcomes may be more positive with combination therapy, which includes both stimulants and behavioral modification or academic assistance.[49]

There are few data directly comparing the efficacy of stimulants and other drugs used to treat ADHD, nor has combination pharmacotherapy been extensively evaluated. One report concluded that methylphenidate was superior to imipramine, whereas, a second study showed clonidine to be as effective as methylphenidate.[50,51] The concurrent use of methylphenidate and desipramine has been shown to result in greater behavioral inhibition and increased complex problem-solving ability than either agent used alone.[52]

The dosing of stimulants has undergone much debate. Traditionally, as with most pediatric medications, the stimulants were dosed on a mg/kg basis. This practice has fallen out of favor with the finding that body mass and drug plasma concentrations fail to predict beneficial clinical responses.[53–56] This is consistent with the fact that methylphenidate and its metabolite (ritalinic acid) are highly polar with little disposition into adipose tissue. Early studies suggested that specific doses of methylphenidate improved select ADHD symptoms. Lower doses (0.3 mg/kg) were found to be optimal for learning, whereas larger doses (1 mg/kg) proved most efficacious in behavioral improvements.[57] Subsequently, methylphenidate's dose-response curve has been proven to be linear, with improvements in behavior, learning, and social interactions occurring with increasing doses.[39,53,58] Although this finding is generally true, individual children respond differently to the same dose of stimulant with some ADHD symptoms being more influenced than others.[53]

Each stimulant has different pharmacokinetic characteristics (Table 59.2), which influence individual stimulant dosing frequency. Although methylphenidate and dextroamphetamine are both considered short-acting compounds, the latter has a slightly longer duration of action. Using either agent, clinical response is noted within 30 to 60 minutes, and peak effects are observed 1 to 4 hours after a given dose. The pharmacokinetics and pharmacodynamics of the dextro- and levoamphetamine combination are influenced by dose. As doses increase, the drug's effects peak later and exhibit a longer duration of action.[59]

Dosing schedules for the stimulants are given in Table 59.3. Typically, these agents are administered every 4 to 6 hours. The starting dose for methylphenidate in school-aged children (>6 years) is 5 mg before breakfast, repeated at lunch. Doses may be increased weekly by 5 to 10 mg, based on clinical response and appearance of side effects. Typically, doses range from 0.3 to 0.8 mg/kg/dose with a maximum of 60 mg administered per day. Doses used in adolescents and adults may be lower on a mg/kg basis, but studies in adults suggest doses as high as 1 mg/kg/dose may be necessary to produce a desired response.[43] These larger doses have not increased the incidence or severity of side effects. Initial doses and the titration schedule for dextroamphetamine and the dextro- and levoamphetamine product are similar to that of methylphenidate with the usual and maximal therapeutic doses being about one-half to two-thirds that of methylphenidate.[60]

In contrast to the other stimulants, in which clinical benefits peak during the oral absorptive phase and subside

Table 59.2 ▪ Pharmacokinetics of the Central Nervous System Stimulants

Parameter	Methylphenidate	Dextroamphetamine	Dextro- and Levoamphetamine Combination	Pemoline
Elimination half-life (hr)	2–3	6–7	11.1 (7.4–15.4)	2–12 (7–8.6 in children)
Time to peak T_{max} (hr)	IR: 1–3 SR: 4.7 (1.3–8.2)	IR: 3–4 SR: 8–10	2.9 (1.5–8) dose dependent	2–4
Onset of action (hr)	IR: 1 SR: >2	IR: 1 SR: >2	2.4 (1.5–3) dose dependent	~2 (2–3 weeks in some individuals)
Duration of action (hr)	IR: 2–4 SR: 2–8 (erratic)	IR: 3–5 SR: 5–9	5–7 dose dependent	8–24
Metabolite	Ritalinic acid (active)	Benzoic/hippuric acid (inactive)	Undetermined	Pemoline dione (active)
Excretion	Urinary	Urinary	Urinary	Urinary/fecal

Table 59.3 ▪ Dosing Schedule for Central Nervous System Stimulants

Medication	Age Group	Initial Dose (mg)	Between Dose Interval (hr)	Titration (mg)	Usual Maximal Dose (mg/kg/dose)
Methylphenidate: tablets (scored), 5, 10,	Child (> 6 yr)	5	3–4	5	0.3–0.8 (60 mg/day)
15, 20 mg	Adults	5	2–3		40–90 mg/day
Methylphenidate: extended release	Child (>6 yr)	Not to be used as initial therapy	8	NA	0.3–0.8 (60 mg/day)
(wax matrix), 20 mg	Adults				40–80 mg/day
Dextroamphetamine:	Child (>6 yr)	5	4–6	5	0.2–0.5
tablets (scored),	Child (3–5 yr)	2.5		2.5	(40 mg/day)
5, 10 mg	Adult	5	3–4	5	20–45 mg/day
Dextroamphetamine:	Child (>6 yr)	5	8	5	0.2–0.5
extended release	Child (3–5 yr)	2.5		2.5	(40 mg/day)
(sprinkles), 5, 10, 15 mg	Adult	5		5	20–45 mg/day
Dextro, levoamphetamine:	Child (>6 yr)	5	4–6	5	0.15–0.4
tablets (double scored),	Child (3–5 yr)	2.5		2.5	(40 mg/day)
5, 10, 20, 30 mg	Adult	5		5	30 mg/day
Pemoline: tablets (scored),	Child (>6 yr)	37.5	24	18.75	1–2 (112 mg/day)
18.75, 37.5, 75 mg; chewable tablet, 37.5 mg	Adult	18.75		18.75	37.5–150 mg/day

faster than their plasma concentrations, pemoline has a much more variable time course of effect. Although pemoline's half-life tends to be shorter in children and may increase with multiple dosing,[61] its duration of action is at least 7 hours, which still permits once daily dosing.[62–64] Initial doses of 37.5 mg are administered each morning. Then, doses are increased by 18.75 mg weekly with average therapeutic doses ranging from 1 to 2 mg/kg/day. Pemoline is the only stimulant that has an absolute maximum pediatric daily dose (112.5 mg). Initial dose for adults are 18.75 mg/day, titrated weekly to average doses ranging from 37.5 to 150 mg/day. Traditionally, it was believed that 2 to 4 weeks were necessary for pemoline to reach its full effect. However, studies involving children with ADHD have shown this to be false, with marked symptomatic improvements noted 2 hours after a given dose.[45,61,64]

Tolerance to the stimulants has been rarely reported.[65] Children experiencing a late afternoon reoccurrence of ADHD symptoms or rebound (e.g., increased irritability, crankiness, aggression, overactivity, or crying) may benefit from an additional dose given 4 hours after the noontime dose.[66] Contrary to popular belief, late afternoon doses of methylphenidate have failed to increase insomnia.[66] Alternatively, a longer acting agent (pemoline, or possibly the dextro- and levoamphetamine combination) or a sustained-release product may be used. Unfortunately, the sustained-release forms of methylphenidate have a variable duration of action and may prove less effective in improving certain behaviors.[64,67,68] In attempts to overcome a lag in stimulant effects, combinations of immediate release and sustained-release products have been used.[68]

Stimulants are considered to be among the safest of drugs used in the treatment of ADHD. A summary of the side effects associated with stimulants can be found in Table 59.4. The most common side effects are decreased appetite, stomachache, insomnia, irritability, and headache.[69–71] These side effects tend to be of mild to moderate severity, respond to dose reduction, or subside while drug therapy continues. Other adverse effects mistakenly attributed to these agents may actually decrease once treatment begins (i.e., staring, anxiety, nail biting, and unhappiness/sadness).[69,71] Thus, it is important to inquire about the frequency and severity of these symptoms before initiation of a stimulant. Rarely, stimulants produce blood dyscrasias, dysphoria, or induce compulsive behaviors (i.e., picking of the nose or skin). When these drugs are administered in higher doses, they may produce overfocusing (i.e.,"zombification"), severe agitation, tremors, euphoria, or cardiac abnormalities (tachycardia, palpitations, and hypertension). At near toxic doses, these agents may induce fatigue, mental depression, psychosis, convulsions, paranoia, hallucinations, hyperpyrexia, respiratory depression, and coma. Although rare, stimulants may prove lethal.[60]

The effects of stimulants on growth are controversial. Original studies showed long-term treatment with stimulants resulted in significant reductions in height.[72,73] This led to the practice of drug holidays during the summer in which catch up growth could occur.[74] Later, it was shown that once stimulants were discontinued in childhood, ultimate adult height remained uncompromised.[75] Currently, it is believed that children with ADHD may have either a temporary delay in their growth spurt or a slower

Table 59.4 ▪ Side Effects of Medications for Attention Deficit/Hyperactivity Disorder

Medication	Adverse Effects
Stimulants	Insomnia, decreased appetite, weight loss, agitation, irritability, increased heart rate or blood pressure Rarely: Growth suppression, dysphoria or compulsive behaviors, blood dyscrasias, choreform, movements (pemoline), hepatotoxicity (pemoline), behavioral exacerbation with sudden withdrawal
Tricyclic antidepressants (TCAs)	Anticholinergic (dry mouth, constipation, blurred vision, urinary retention), weight gain, sedation, orthostatic hypotension (adults), hypertension (children and adolescents) Rarely: cardiac arrhythmias or conduction disturbances, flulike symptoms (headache, lethargy) after abrupt withdrawal
Clonidine	Sedation, dry mouth, hypotension, depression, rebound hypertension with sudden withdrawal, dermatitis associated with patch therapy Rarely: nightmares, weight gain, headache
Monoamine oxidase inhibitors (MAOIs)	Dietary restrictions, weight gain, drowsiness, insomnia, hypertensive crisis if tyramine-containing foods are consumed, stimulants, specific serotonin reuptake inhibitors, or TCAs consumed during therapy with MAOIs
Bupropion	Dry mouth, gastrointestinal upset, headache, nonspecific rash, seizures (if induction dose >150 mg or daily dose >450 mg)

Source: Reference 60.

rate of height increase.[75] This phenomenon seems independent of stimulant use and occurs in children with and without continuous drug exposure.

Traditionally, there has been concern about the use of stimulants in children with ADHD and with Tourette's syndrome or other tic disorders. This belief resulted from early case reports suggesting that stimulants exacerbated Tourette's symptoms in predisposed children.[76] Thus, stimulants became contraindicated in this patient population. Subsequent studies have shown that stimulants used in moderate doses (0.1 to 0.5 mg/kg) fail to exacerbate motor tics and may actually decrease the frequency of vocal tics.[77,78] If stimulant treatment is initiated, it still seems prudent to monitor tic symptoms in children with Tourette's syndrome, other tic disorders, or a family history of either condition.

The ability of amphetamine and methylphenidate to induce euphoria has labeled them as potentially abusable drugs. Although there are only two reports of patients with ADHD using their methylphenidate illicitly, there is concern that cases of abuse may be underdetected or that stimulants may serve as the "gateway" to the abuse of other substances.[79,80] Neither of these seems to be true. Both retrospective and longitudinal studies fail to demonstrate a specific pattern of abuse in children with ADHD with or without comorbid substance abuse.[69,81] Findings in adults suggest that marijuana, not the stimulants, is the most frequently abused illicit compound in adults regardless of ADHD symptoms.[82] There has been more concern over diversion of medications from the patient with ADHD to parents, siblings, or peers. This fact is particularly true for adolescents who are increasingly using stimulants obtained without a doctor's order.[83] Pemoline does not have the same abuse potential and may be an attractive option if diversion or illicit stimulant use is suspected. Alternatively, a nonstimulant ADHD medication may be tried.

Although a rare occurrence, pemoline has been associated with choreoathetoid movements and transient hepatitis. In most patients, both conditions are reversible with drug discontinuation. However, there have been 13 cases of pemoline-induced acute hepatic failure reported to the Food and Drug Administration (FDA).[60] Typically, the time to onset is variable, is not dose related, and is hepatocellular in nature.[84] It most commonly presents with elevations in liver enzymes (aspartate aminotransferase and alanine aminotransferase), nausea, vomiting, lethargy, malaise, and more rarely jaundice. Currently, there is no way to differentiate between the reversible and fatal forms of hepatotoxicity. Pemoline is contraindicated in patients with a history of coexisting liver disorder or in those receiving medications that may potentially harm liver function (i.e., macrolides, antiepileptics, and antifungals). Although of questionable benefit, liver function tests should be performed before starting pemoline and monitored periodically thereafter. More importantly, patient and parents should contact their clinicians immediately if they experience nausea, vomiting, lethargy, malaise, jaundice, or persistent upper abdominal pain (>2 weeks) or suddenly produce dark-colored urine.[60]

Although methylphenidate is usually the first stimulant tried, dextroamphetamine and the dextro- and levoamphetamine combination are also reasonable options as initial treatment of ADHD. Because of its association with hepatotoxicity, pemoline is considered a second-line agent. Regardless of which stimulant is chosen, an initial medical history should be taken and should include questions about any conditions that might contraindicate use of stimulant therapy (e.g., hypertension and/or cardiovascular disease, psychotic or agitated states, seizure disorder, hyperthyroidism, glaucoma, tic disorder, or hepatic disease). In patients with any of the above conditions, careful monitoring or use of an alternative class of medications is advised.

A medication history should be obtained to identify any potential drug interactions resulting from the addition of a stimulant. Concurrent use of stimulants and monoamine oxidase inhibitors (MAOIs) may cause hypertensive crisis and stroke secondary to excessive adrenergic stimulation.[60] This combination should be avoided and 14 days should pass between the discontinuation of an MAOI and the initiation of a stimulant.[60] Other interactions are not well substantiated. There have been reports of stimulants increasing the pharmacologic effects of warfarin and elevated serum concentrations of imiprimine and antiepileptic drug (e.g., phenobarbital, phenytoin, and primidone). Rare cases of cardiac toxicity have resulted from the coadministration of methylphenidate and clonidine.[5] If stimulants are added to any of the mentioned medications, dose reduction may be warranted.

At baseline and at follow-up, height, weight, blood pressure, sleep history, and ADHD symptomology should be recorded. A side effect questionnaire may be used (i.e., Barkley Side Effects Questionnaire [BSEQ]) to differentiate baseline behavior from drug-induced side effects. In addition, laboratory studies (i.e., complete blood count and liver function tests) should be performed.

Careful dosing titration is necessary to prevent treatment failure. Initially low doses are started and administered daily (including weekends) for the first 3 to 4 weeks. This allows sufficient time for patients, teachers, and caregivers to evaluate the positive and negative effects of stimulant therapy. Early in treatment, dysphoria has occurred rarely. If any unusual mood changes are noted, the dose of stimulant should be reduced or an alternative agent (stimulant or antidepressant) should be tried.[5] Because no single indicator can adequately assess response to treatment, multiple measures from a variety of sources should be used.[5] This is an important consideration when deciding on dosage increases. Doses are increased weekly until improvement in a patient's ADHD is noted. Once a proper stimulant dose is achieved, therapy may be interrupted periodically (weekends, summertime, or the end of the school year) to evaluate the need for additional treatment. These interruptions may also be important if significant drug-induced side effects are suspected. Exceptions to this practice include those patients with severe hyperactivity or aggression.[5] Patients are judged to be nonresponders if they receive the maximally recommended dose with minimal or no improvement in ADHD symptoms or when side effects become too severe to warrant continuation of therapy. In such cases, a trial of an alternative stimulant may prove successful.

Proper selection of a stimulant dosage form may help contribute to successful treatment of ADHD. Trade name products should be used because of the unreliable absorption characteristics associated with many generic products. Unfortunately, no liquid forms of stimulants exist. Children unable to swallow pills may use immediate-release products (methylphenidate, dextroamphetamine, and the dextro- and levoamphetamine combination), or pemoline (37.5-mg chewable tablet). These dosage forms may be crushed and added to food, making them easier to ingest. Many of these products are scored, which permits easier dosage titration.

A long-acting product may be a preferred option for children or adults uncomfortable with or unable to receive stimulants at school or work. Similarly, these products may increase compliance in certain patients (i.e., forgetful patients, those with conduct disorder, or rebellious adolescents). Patients should be counseled not to crush or chew these products, because this will result in immediate exposure to the entire day's dose and possible adverse effects. The dextroamphetamine sustained-release capsules may be opened and the beads sprinkled on food (e.g., applesauce) without altering the sustained-release properties of the drug.

Tricyclic Antidepressants

Although not approved by the FDA for the treatment of ADHD, the TCAs (e.g., imipramine, desipramine, and nortriptyline) are the second-line agents for the 10 to 30% of patients who fail to respond to stimulant medications or who cannot tolerate the side effects associated with stimulants. Many practitioners would consider the TCAs more effective than stimulants in patients who are highly anxious or who have concurrent mood disorders. They may also have particular benefit for children who have comorbid affective disorders, nocturnal enuresis, or sleep disturbances or when there is a history of substance abuse. Although the exact mechanism of action of the TCAs in ADHD is unknown, they do affect brain amines (e.g., norepinephrine, dopamine, and serotonin) by blocking presynaptic reuptake and subsequent inactivation at the nerve terminal. TCAs have several advantages over the stimulants including a longer duration of action, single daily dosing, no risk of insomnia or symptoms of rebound, and no potential for abuse or addiction. Unlike the stimulants, tolerance to the TCAs generally develops after 2 to 3 months of treatment.[10]

Twenty-nine studies have been performed to establish the efficacy of the TCAs in children or adults with ADHD. Several reviews have evaluated these studies.[37,85] Open investigations have generally noted an 80 to 90% response rate, while the response rate ranges from 48 to 68% in controlled studies. Numerous well-controlled studies have documented that the TCAs are superior to placebo, especially with regard to behavioral measures; however, the TCAs are less effective than the stimulants on both behavioral and cognitive measures. Importantly, the TCAs are particularly effective in patients with ADHD who have concomitant depression, conduct disorders, or tic disorders. This finding suggests that these patients may represent a subpopulation of patients with ADHD.[86] Furthermore, the ability of TCAs to decrease symptoms of anxiety and depression may indirectly contribute to their observed efficacy in this set of patients. Hopefully, future diagnostic criteria may prospectively identify these patients, leading to improved treatment modalities for this subclass of patients.

One of the major controversies surrounding the use of TCAs in ADHD is which TCA is better for use in ADHD. Although imipramine has been the most studied and more commonly prescribed TCA, one should not assume that it is more efficacious than the other TCAs. In fact, all of the TCAs are effective in ADHD.[85] The discriminating factors in selection of a TCA may be side effect profile (e.g., cardiovascular with desipramine) and limited studies (e.g., nortriptyline).

The TCAs are rapidly and completely absorbed after oral administration with peak plasma levels occurring between 2 and 8 hours. They are highly lipophilic and protein-bound substances; hence, medications that compete for protein binding can alter the amount of TCA that penetrates into the central nervous system (CNS). TCAs are hepatically metabolized with an initial removal of a methyl group. In the case of the tertiary amines, an active compound is formed. For example, the active metabolite of imipramine is desipramine. The TCAs are further hydroxylated and subsequently conjugated to inactive compounds. It is important to remember that 5 to 10% of children and adolescents are "slow hydroxylators" of TCAs. This genetic variation can cause significantly prolonged half-lives and increase the peak serum TCA concentrations. Hepatic clearance of the TCAs can be increased by the barbiturates and cigarette smoking. Conversely, hepatic clearance can be decreased by quinidine, cimetidine, neuroleptics (e.g., phenothiazines), selective serotonin reuptake inhibitors (SSRIs) (e.g., fluoxetine, sertraline, and paroxetine), phenytoin, and oral contraceptives. Unlike the slow onset noted when TCAs are used for depression, the onset of action in ADHD is apparent within 2 to 3 days.[87] Although the TCAs are often given once a day, some patients with rapid metabolism may require twice a day dosing. Because of the relatively long half-lives of the TCAs, they are not associated with rebound of symptoms between doses.

Because patients have varying degrees of conduct disorder, anxiety, and depressive symptoms, it is likely that the TCAs may affect hyperactivity, inattention, conduct problems, aggressiveness, and affective symptoms in different ways at different doses. Currently, a controversy exists regarding the dosage of TCAs required to produce the maximal benefit in ADHD. There is only limited evidence that low-dose TCAs are superior to high-dose TCAs in ADHD. There is no evidence to support the use of doses less than 1 mg/kg/day. Because only recent studies have reported doses in mg/kg/day and there are also no dose finding studies, the question of the "ideal" dose in ADHD remains unknown. To reduce the severity of potential side effects, the initial dose of imipramine or desipramine is 10 mg twice daily. Once the patient demonstrates that he or she can tolerate these agents, the dosing can be changed to once daily, usually at bedtime. Doses can be increased by 25 to 50 mg weekly until a positive response is evident. Doses of 75 to 200 mg/day are commonly used. Most drug references suggest that total daily doses should not exceed 2.5 mg/kg/day of imipramine or its equivalent, recent studies suggest that up to 5 mg/kg/day may be required for efficacy.[86] Although there is no relationship between plasma concentration and efficacy, routine serum concentration monitoring and maintenance of concentrations within the therapeutic range may minimize toxicity.

Overall, side effects are more prevalent with the TCAs than with the stimulants (Table 59.4). The most common, predictable, short-term effects are anticholinergic (e.g., dry mouth, constipation, blurred vision, and urinary hesitancy) in nature. These mild adverse effects do not usually require termination of therapy and can generally be treated with symptomatic intervention or dosage adjustment. Decreased saliva production can cause tooth decay; hence, patients taking TCAs should have routine dental care. Anticholinergic effects are more prominent with tertiary amines (e.g., imipramine) than with secondary amines (e.g., desipramine and nortriptyline); therefore, a secondary amine should be considered when anticholinergic effects from another TCA become bothersome.

With the exception of desipramine, excessive weight gain has also been noted in the TCAs; therefore, baseline and periodic weight should be assessed. Although sedation associated with the TCAs is usually transient, the dose can be given once daily at bedtime to minimize this effect. Because of their ability to lower the seizure threshold, TCAs should be used cautiously in patients with a history of seizures or recent head trauma. Some patients may display what is termed "behavioral toxicity," which mimics the symptoms of ADHD (i.e., irritability, agitation, forgetfulness, anger, and confusion). Obtaining a TCA serum concentration may be necessary to elucidate the etiology of these symptoms.

Common cardiovascular effects include orthostasis, hypertension, and tachycardia. Unlike adults, who tend to have hypotensive reactions, adolescents and probably children have a greater risk for the development of hypertension.[87] Although rare, more serious cardiovascular side effects including arrhythmias (e.g., prolonged-QT interval) and heart block have occurred.[87] While no relationship has been noted between dose and change in the electrocardiogram (ECG), a relationship between decreased cardiac conduction and plasma TCA concentrations has been observed. Imipramine and desipramine concentrations that approach 250 ng/mL have been shown to be associated with more serious cardiac effects.[88] Therefore, exceeding concentrations of 300 ng/mL of imipramine and desipramine is not recommended.

Five reports of medically unexplained sudden deaths secondary to the acute onset of cardiac arrhythmias in children (8–15 years) receiving normal doses of desipramine have been published.[87,89] All patients had serum desipramine concentrations within the acceptable range. After reviewing all of the available information, the Special Commission of the Heart, Lung and Blood Institute of the NIH found no effect of desipramine in the death of these children.[90] The commission concluded that if the occurrence was more than a coincidence, the phenomenon is likely idiosyncratic.

TCA use should be preceded by a complete history and physical including determination of baseline blood pressure and heart rate. Because no evidence indicates that such monitoring can help clinicians identify a patient at risk for sudden death, the routine monitoring of ECG in patients on TCAs is controversial. Although the American Academy of Pediatrics does not recommend routine ECG monitoring at this time,[91] the American Academy of Child and Adolescent Psychiatry[10] recommends a baseline ECG, another ECG within days of a dosage increase, and another when steady state at maximal doses is achieved. Although the benefits of ECG monitoring are questionable, it would seem advisable to follow the more conservative guidelines until more is known about the etiology of the cardiovascular effects.

These agents are contraindicated for children who have a history of acquired or congenital cardiac disease or murmurs or have a family history of cardiomyopathy or diastolic hypertension. If a previously normal ECG becomes abnormal (e.g., persistent tachycardia, significant intraventricular conduction delays, or QT_c of more than 460 msec), the practitioner should reassess response to the TCAs. If the TCA has been beneficial, one might reduce the TCA dose in hopes of maintaining efficacy and restoring a normal ECG. If the ECG abnormality persists despite a reduction in dose, another TCA or an alternative agent should be tried. Because the active metabolites of nortriptyline may be less cardiotoxic than those of other TCAs, it may have some advantage in these patients. If the ECG abnormalities continue or if cardiac symptoms occur, the TCA should be slowly discontinued, and the patient should wear a Holter monitor for 24 hours and be referred to a cardiologist.[89]

Unlike stimulants, TCAs should not be discontinued on weekends, and at no time should the medication be rapidly withdrawn. When discontinued, the TCA should be tapered over 2 to 3 weeks to prevent rebound hyperactivity and other withdrawal effects (e.g., flulike syndrome with gastrointestinal upset, headache, and lethargy).

Monoamine Oxidase Inhibitors

Because stimulants have been shown to weakly inhibit the enzyme monoamine oxidase, several monoamine oxidase inhibitors (MAOIs) including tranylcypromine, clorgyline, moclobemide, and selegiline have been used in ADHD. One study comparing the efficacy of two MAOIs to that of dextroamphetamine noted that all agents improved behavior and reduced hyperactivity.[92] In a placebo-controlled crossover study that investigated selegiline in patients with ADHD and Tourette's syndrome, 90% of the children and adolescents showed significant improvement.[93] However, two patients experienced an aggravation of their tic symptoms. The MAOIs exhibited an onset of action that was significantly shorter than that noted in the treatment of depression. Mild side effects including fatigue, drowsiness, and appetite suppression were noted (Table 59.4). Although results have been positive with the MAOIs, they are rarely used because of the need to maintain a low-tyramine diet with the nonspecific MAOIs (i.e., tranylcypromine and clorgyline). Similarly, hypertensive crisis may occur after ingestion of tyramine in patients using higher doses of the selective MAOIs (i.e., moclobemide and selegiline). This makes these agents unattractive for use in ADHD. These agents may be considered in highly treatment-resistant or drug-intolerant adults, but their use is discouraged in patients with prominent impulsivity.[87]

Bupropion

Bupropion is an atypical, structurally novel, antidepressant that exhibits primarily dopaminergic activity. Although its mechanism of action is unclear, bupropion does not significantly inhibit the reuptake of either serotonin or norepinephrine. Peak plasma concentrations after a single dose occur in 2 hours, and the elimination half-life averages 14 hours.[94] Although it does not cause cardiac conduction abnormalities or have the potential for abuse, it has been associated with the exacerbation of tics secondary to its strong dopaminergic effects.[95] This makes it a poor choice for patients with ADHD and a comorbid tic disorder. Bupropion has also been reported to induce a rash (maculopapular, urticarial, and pruritic) in 17% of patients (Table 59.4).

Bupropion was removed from the market in the mid-1980s because of a high incidence of epileptic seizures. Reintroduction of the agent in 1989 was accompanied by dosage guidelines and strict warnings regarding the effects of bupropion on seizure threshold. This side effect is generally noted in patients receiving greater than 450 mg/day and with individual doses greater than 150 mg.[5] Additionally, patients with preexisting neurologic abnormalities or eating disorders may be at increased risk for bupropion-induced seizures. Several double-blind, placebo-controlled studies have noted that bupropion is effective in treating children with ADHD.

The largest study was a multicenter, randomized, double-blind, placebo-controlled trial involving 109 children (72 bupropion-treated and 37 placebo).[96] Significant reduction in hyperactivity and impulsivity and improvement in cognition were noted within 3 days in patients receiving 3 to 6 mg/kg/day of bupropion divided in three daily doses. Bupropion has also been shown to be effective in adult patients with ADHD.[97] Bupropion is administered in two or three daily doses, beginning with a low dose of 37.5 or 50 mg twice a day.[10] The dose is titrated every 2 weeks to a usual maximum dose of 250 mg/day (300 to 400 mg in adolescents).[10]

Venlafaxine

Although venlafaxine is structurally similar to the amphetamines, it is considered an antidepressant and possesses both serotonergic and noradrenergic activity. To date, there are no controlled studies of this agent in ADHD; however, the open studies in adults[98–100] and children appear promising.[101,102] In adult studies, overall response rates have been impressive with as many as 20 to 80% of patients showing improvement.[98–100] In the pediatric studies, 75% of patients with newly diagnosed ADHD responded.[101] In addition, 20% of patients who failed to respond to prior drug treatment responded to venlafaxine. It should be noted that the dropout rate because of side effects (e.g., increased hyperactivity in children or sedation in adults) exceeded 20% in both adults and children.

Selective Serotonin Reuptake Inhibitors

There is limited literature on the use of SSRIs in the treatment of ADHD. SSRIs have been noted to be effective in one open label pediatric study (fluoxetine),[103] one case report in a young child (fluoxetine),[104] and one in an adult (sertraline).[105] Currently, these limited reports do not support the usefulness of SSRIs in treating the core symptoms of ADHD. These agents may be more effective in addressing comorbid mood and anxiety disorders associated with ADHD. For a more extensive discussion of the controversy over use of SSRIs in ADHD, the reader is referred to a review by Popper.[86]

Clonidine or Guanfacine

Clonidine and guanfacine, antihypertensive medications, are also used in the treatment of ADHD. These drugs act as α_2-agonists and bind to CNS presynaptic or postsynaptic receptors to cause site-specific decreases or increases in noradrenergic neural transmission, respectively. Although their exact mechanism of action in ADHD is unknown, clonidine and guanfacine are believed to ameliorate adrenoreceptor dysfunction present in those with ADHD.

Although studies are limited and treatment groups are small, clonidine has been effective in some children with ADHD.[51,106] It is comparable to methylphenidate in efficacy and lacks the negative adverse effects (e.g., irritability, tics, or anorexia) associated with stimulates. Although a third-line agent, clonidine should be used in patients who are unresponsive to or intolerant of stimulants or antidepressants. It may also be useful in patients with sleep disturbances (i.e., insomnia secondary to stimulants),[107] those with tics associated with Tourette's syndrome,[108,109] or those with more severe aggressive/hyperactive symptoms. In contrast, this agent is less effective in patients with primarily inattentive symptoms. Although clonidine is frequently used in combination with the stimulants, there are limited studies evaluating the concurrent use of methylphenidate and clonidine. Combination therapy has resulted in the ability to use lower doses of stimulants or prevent rebound symptoms associated with the stimulants.[10]

To minimize the drug's side effects, initial doses are started low and the first dose is administered at bedtime. Initial doses are 0.05 mg/day at bedtime with subsequent increases of 0.05 mg/wk as tolerated. Average maintenance doses of 3 to 5 μg/kg/day (0.15 to 0.3 mg/day) are divided into three or four doses. Once a patient reaches a stable maintenance dose, the clonidine transdermal patch (Catapres-TTS) may be used to increase patient compliance and reduce fluctuations in serum concentrations of the drug.[5] Catapres-TTS comes in 0.1, 0.2, and 0.3 mg/day strengths, which may be cut into sections to meet a patient's dosage needs. Typically, children need to change the patch more frequently (every 3 to 5 days) than adults (every 7 days). Patients should be advised to periodically rotate the patch's site of placement to minimize contact dermatitis. If a rash develops, topical steroid creams have been used.

Side effects of clonidine are listed in Table 59.4. Major limitations associated with the use of clonidine are its gradual onset of action and ability to produce pronounced dose-related sedation. Typically after 2 to 3 weeks of treatment, effectiveness is noted as the drowsiness subsides.[106] Hypotension and bradycardia may also occur. Rebound hypertension, increased incidence of tics, and hyperactivity have been reported if clonidine is abruptly discontinued; therefore, clonidine must be tapered slowly (0.5 mg every 1 to 3 days). Various ECG abnormalities have been noted and five unexplained sudden deaths have occurred in children receiving clonidine.[110] These rare reports of cardiotoxicity are usually associated with combined clonidine and methylphenidate therapy. Although the mechanism is unclear, current recommendations suggest that the dose of methylphenidate be reduced by 40% when it is used in combinations with clonidine.[5]

Compared to clonidine, guanfacine seems attractive because of its longer duration of action and more favorable side effect profile. However, there has been less experience with this drug in the treatment of ADHD. One small open-label study in children and adolescents reported positive effects on both hyperactivity and attention.[106]

Anticonvulsants

Although carbamazepine is extensively used in Europe for the treatment of ADHD, it is not FDA approved for this indication; hence, its use in the United States is limited. Because carbamazepine has a tricyclic structure and is used as a mood-stabilizing agent, intuitively one might expect it to have some efficacy in ADHD. Overall, some therapeutic effects have been noted in approximately 70% of children.[111] Although rare, the hematologic and hepatotoxic effects of carbamazepine make it less ideal than the TCAs. No studies have evaluated the effects of phenytoin or valproate in patients with ADHD.

Other Agents

Antipsychotics (e.g., chlorpromazine, haloperidol, and thioridazine) reduce hyperactivity; however, they do not improve cognition or attention span.[112] They are less effective than either the stimulants or TCAs and are associated with significant adverse reactions including extrapyramidal effects and tardive dyskinesia. In larger doses the antipsychotics decrease cognitive function and impair learning. For these reasons, this class of medications should be given in the lowest possible doses, and use should be limited to patients with severe ADHD unresponsive to other agents.

Benzodiazepines and barbiturates are ineffective and worsen ADHD by causing paradoxical excitement and agitation.[28,113] Amanatadine,[114] caffeine,[115] fenfluramine,[116] and lithium[117] are also ineffective.

Nonpharmacologic Therapy

Psychosocial treatment of ADHD originated from the belief that it may overcome the limitations associated with pharmacologically based therapy. Although medications have been shown to improve the core symptoms of ADHD, they fail to result in normalization of a person's functioning.[38,40,41] The benefits of medication tend to be short-lived and reverse upon drug withdrawal. In addition, medications may produce unpleasant side effects and lower self-esteem.[69,71] Psychosocial interventions focus upon the development of functional skills (academic/social) and adaptive behaviors that patients with ADHD lack. These therapies come in a variety of forms, which may be combined to meet the specific needs of the individual patient. Generally, greater success has been observed using more intensely structured programs (clinical behavioral or summer treatment programs), which encompass various environments (home, classroom, and play) and involve parents, teachers, and children.[118] Unfortunately, these modalities have consistently proven less effective than medications when used alone.[5,119]

Cognitive-behavioral therapy (self-instructional training, cognitive modeling, cognitive/interpersonal problem solving, self-monitoring, and self-reinforcement) may be taught to an individual patient or in groups. These interventions attempt to teach ADHD patients self-control skills and internal problem-solving techniques that will ultimately decrease impulsivity and improve both behavior and academic performance.[119] Although mechanistically attractive, this modality has proven ineffective in children with ADHD. Although initial improvements are noted, they quickly subside because of a lack of generalization to new environments and because the child is not motivated to apply the newly learned techniques.

Behavioral therapies (behavior modification, contingency management, and operant conditioning) involve the identification of a patient's undesirable behaviors and the environmental conditions that elicit and maintain them.[5] Ultimately, behavioral changes are produced using either positive or negative reinforcers. One example is the token economy, in which children earn or lose stars, points, etc. for displaying appropriate or inappropriate behaviors. These tokens may be traded for things the child likes (toys or privileges). Time out is a similar approach in which negative behaviors are discouraged by putting the child in a nonstimulating environment. These tools may be used by both parents and teachers to encourage positive behaviors at home and at school. Although behavioral therapies are generally considered more efficacious than cognitive treatments, they suffer from the same inability to be generalized to new situations. Despite the short-term academic and social improvements, normalization in inattention, hyperactivity, and impulsivity rarely occurs.[5,120]

Patients with ADHD often require additional interventions tailored to their specific needs. Social skills training helps facilitate interactions between parents, siblings, students, and peers. Group social training is preferred because patients with ADHD lack self-monitoring skills In addition, this setting allows practice and modeling of newly learned behaviors. Academic skills training involves instruction in proper study habits, note and test taking, organizational/time management skills, and the ability to follow directions. It is particularly important that education occur in an environment with minimal distractions where careful attention can be paid to any specific learning disabilities. Individual psychotherapy may be a useful adjunct for patients with ADHD who have low self-esteem or comorbid depression or in those with difficulty coping with the ADHD symptoms. Therapists may also assist in increasing medication compliance using contingency-contracting. Family psychotherapy is indicated for families with prior dysfunction or for those with problems stemming from raising a child with ADHD. This may also serve as a means to reinforce or implement behavioral interventions. Therapeutic recreation uses participation in sports or play activities to improve peer interactions and self-image.

The concept of multimodal therapy has become popular because no single treatment modality (medication or psychosocial) has succeeded in producing long-term normalization across all areas affected by ADHD. Although combined therapy and medication-only treatments perform similarly for most measures, this is not a universal finding.[6,49,121] Some studies suggest combined therapy may produce additional clinical gains in selected patients.[121] Likewise, it may prevent the reappearance of certain ADHD-associated behaviors once medications are discontinued.[122] In other studies, multimodal therapy has permitted the use of lower doses of medications.[123] Although the conclusions drawn from these studies are limited due to sample size, design flaws, or short duration, multimodal treatment may be an attractive option for some patients (e.g., those with dose-related side effects, incomplete responses to medications, or certain comorbid conditions).

ALTERNATIVE THERAPIES

Alternative therapies include any nonprescription or behavior therapies. Over the years elimination diets, macronutritional and micronutritional supplements, antifungal and thyroid treatments, deleading procedures, and herbal therapies have been administered. Additionally, acupuncture, and EEG and electromyogram biofeedback have been performed.

Elimination Diets

The simple elimination of sugar and candy from the diet of children does not appear to affect symptoms in children with ADHD. Several controlled studies have reported either significant improvement compared with placebo or deterioration of condition with a placebo substituted for the offending substance. At this time it is not known what percentage of the ADHD population has diet-associated ADHD. Preliminary evidence suggests that these patients are middle or upper class preschool-aged patients with atopy and prominent irritability and sleep disturbances. They also have physical as well as behavioral symptoms. If an offending agent can be identified, it may be possible to successfully desensitize the patient.

Nutritional Supplements

A variety of nutritional supplements have been used to treat ADHD. Both macronutrients (amino acids, essential fatty acids, and carbohydrates) and micronutrients (vitamins and minerals) have been used. Although patients with ADHD may have low levels of amino acids including serotonin, supplementation with tryptophan, tyrosine, or phenylalanine has not produced long-term benefits.[6]

Children with ADHD have lower total serum free fatty acid concentrations. Specifically, both the *n*-3 and *n*-6 series of fatty acids are lower in children with ADHD than in control patients. Because neuronal membranes are composed of polyunsaturated fatty acids (i.e., *n*-3 and *n*-6 series) a deficiency of these essential nutrients may affect development. Likewise, aggression has been inhibited in young adults given docosahexaenoic acid of the *n*-3 series. Two double-blind placebo-controlled studies involving administration of a *n*-6 series fatty acid had varied results.[6]

Several studies have evaluated the supplementation of vitamins and minerals in patients with ADHD. Both megavitamin cocktails and megadoses of select vitamins have proven ineffective.[6] Studies have also investigated the supplementation of iron, zinc, and magnesium in patients with ADHD. Supplementation of iron to nonanemic patients with ADHD resulted in improved parent scores but not teacher ratings on the Conners Parent and Teacher Rating Scales. Furthermore, improvements in verbal learning and memory, and a decrease in hyperactivity have been noted. Although several animal studies and anecdotal human experience suggest that zinc deficiency is associated with hyperactivity, no prospective studies have been performed to support routine zinc supplementation in patients with ADHD. However, one group of investigators did suggest that response to stimulants may be dependent on adequate intake of zinc.[6] Another report noted that 95% of children with ADHD are deficient in magnesium.[6] While no placebo-controlled trials have been conducted, one study reported that Conners ratings were significantly decreased in patients receiving magnesium.[6]

Deleading

Animal and human data suggest that lead toxicity can cause neuropsychiatric symptoms. Lead serum concentrations as low as 10 μg/dL have been associated with behavioral and cognitive problems. Some have advocated that patients with ADHD and elevations in serum lead concentrations should be treated with penicillamine (calcium disodium edetate, if allergic to penicillin).[6]

Herbal Treatments

A few open label studies have been conducted in China using combinations of Chinese herbs or herbal liquors or syrups.[6] Although these reports have noted positive results, placebo-controlled double-blind studies are warranted. To date, no studies have been reported on gingko biloba, Calmplex, or Defendol.

FUTURE THERAPIES

Although the stimulants have proven their short-term effectiveness in numerous studies of ADHD, future research is attempting to develop new, safe, effective, and nonaddictive medications. The discoveries of the potential site of action of stimulants and a genetic loci possibly responsible for ADHD symptoms have directed focus on agents that modulate the dopaminergic and noradrenergic systems. Such agents include noradrenergic-specific compounds (tomoxetine), nicotinic analogs, and cholinergic agents. Tomoxetine, a noradrenergic uptake inhibitor has shown some promising results in adults with ADHD.[124] New diagnostic techniques such as fMRI may better define the neurologic basis of ADHD, and assist in objective diagnosis, and provide additional directions in which to target new therapies.

IMPROVING OUTCOMES

Patient Education

There are a variety of drug classes used in the treatment of ADHD, each with various side effects and monitoring parameters. Faced with managed care cost containment and increased patient loads, physicians often do not discuss issues related to drug therapy with patients. This leaves unanswered questions, which may result in patient frustration and unsuccessful therapy. Unlike many medical conditions, patient counseling must address both the proper use of the medications (Table 59.5) and the social stigma tied to many of the agents (i.e., stimulants and antidepressants) used to treat ADHD. Teaching about medication and treatment follow-up may include the patient, parent, and teacher. Many patients with ADHD have reading and/or learning impairments; thus counseling should include both easy-to-understand verbal and written instructions. In addition, the health care professional should provide a phone number for questions that may arise once the patient has left the clinic or pharmacy. This is particularly important for patients who are unable to pay attention while discussing their medications.

Patients may receive multiple medications, which may prove confusing to the patient or parent. Polytherapy also provides increased probability of drug interactions. The health care practitioner should inquire about use of any concurrent medications (prescription, over-the-counter, or

Table 59.5 ▪ Attention-Deficit/Hyperactivity Disorder (ADHD) Medication Counseling Tips

Medication	Counseling Advice
Stimulants	• This medication is the most common medication used to treat ADHD. It is very effective with rapidly noticeable benefits (increased attention, decreased impulsity/hyperactivity). • Take this medication with meals to avoid upset stomach. If weight loss is noted, then the dose may need to be decreased. Some ADHD patients perform unusual behaviors while taking this medication, if this occurs the dose may need to be lowered or the medication stopped. • This medication may worsen certain health conditions. Consult your doctor/pharmacist if you have a history of heart disease, another mental disorder (psychosis or mania), or a movement/tic disorder (Tourette's syndrome). • This medication may increase the blood levels/effects of some other medications (warfarin, phenobarbital, phenytoin, primidone, tricyclic antidepressants, and clonidine). This is why it is important to notify your pharmacist/doctor of any current (or changes in your) medications (over-the-counter/prescription). • If your doctor has prescribed pemoline, your doctor may have to do routine blood tests. Contact your doctor/pharmacist if you experience unusual tiredness, upper abdominal pain (2 weeks), nausea, vomiting, or dark-colored urine. • Sustained-release products should not be crushed or chewed. If your doctor has prescribed Dexadrine Spansules, the capsules may be opened and the contents placed in food (applesauce) to ease swallowing.
Tricyclic antidepressants (TCAs)	• Although this medication is used for depression, it does not mean you have the diagnosis of depression. This drug is also used to improve symptoms associated with ADHD. • The most common side effects of this drug include dry mouth, constipation, urinary retention, weight gain, changes in blood pressure, and sedation. Occasionally, this medication worsens behaviors. Doses should be taken at bedtime to decrease their sedative effect. Regular dental visits and good dental hygiene are particularly important while taking this medication. In general, these side effects decrease while taking the medication or respond to dose reduction; if not contact your doctor/pharmacist. • It is important that you do not stop taking this medication abruptly. Slow tapering is necessary to prevent withrawal symptoms (flulike symptoms). • The effects of this medication may be increased by some other medications (cimetidine, phenothiazines, phenytoin, oral contraceptives, quinidine, selective serotonin reuptake inhibitors, and stimulants). Other medications/habits decrease their effect (phenobarbital and smoking). This is why it is important to tell your pharmacist/doctor of any current (or changes in your) medications (over-the-counter/prescription). • This medication may worsen some medical conditions; tell your doctor if you have a history of heart disease, glaucoma, or seizure disorder/epilepsy. • Your doctor may routinely monitor your heart while on this medication. Contact your doctor/pharmacist if you notice any unusual changes in heart rate, shortness of breath, or pain/tightening in the chest.
Monoamine oxidase inhibitors (MAOIs)	• Although this medication is used for depression, it does not mean you have the diagnosis of depression. This drug is also used to improve symptoms associated with ADHD. • The effects of this medication may take time to appear. Some patients do not notice rapid improvements in ADHD symptoms. • The most common side effects of this medication include weight gain, drowsiness, or insomnia. Taking initial doses at bedtime and eating smaller, more frequent meals may help minimize these effects. • This medication may result in toxicity when used with some other medications (merperidine, antidepressants, stimulants, sympathomimetics). This is why it is important to notify your pharmacist/doctor of any current (or changes in your) medications (over-the-counter/prescrption). • While taking this medication you need to be on a tyramine-free diet. This means avoiding eating certain foods (aged cheeses, wine, and certain processed meats). Consult your doctor/dietician for a comprehensive list of these foods. • This medication may worsen some medical conditions; tell your doctor if you have a history of heart disease or pheochromocytoma (norepinephrine-secreting tumor). • This medication has significantly increased blood pressures (hypertensive crisis) in some individuals. Contact your doctor/pharmacist if you experience any increase in heart rate, heartbeat pounding of the chest (palpitations), unusual sweating, or dizziness.
Bupropion	• Although this medication is used for depression, it does not mean you have the diagnosis of depression. This drug is also used to improve symptoms associated with ADHD. • The most common side effects of this medication are mild and include dry mouth, stomach upset, rash, and headache. • Rarely do seizures occur. Tell your doctor if you have a history of a seizure disorder/epilepsy or an eating disorder. If one dose of medication is missed, contact your doctor/pharmacist before taking two doses. • Although this medication has been used safely in patients with a tic disorder, it may increase the severity of tics in certain predisposed persons. Tell your doctor if you have a history of a tic disorder, Tourette's syndrome, or if while on this medication you experience a change in the frequency/severity of tic symptoms. • Notify your doctor/pharmacist if you are taking or have recently taken (within 14 days) a monoamine oxidase inhibitor. Concurrent use has been associated with a sudden increase in blood pressure.

(continued)

Table 59.5 *(continued)*

Medication	Counseling Advice
Clonidine	• The effects of this medication may take time to appear. Some patients do not notice rapid improvements in ADHD symptoms. • The most common side effects include sedation, dry mouth, nightmares, and decreases in blood pressure. These effects should decrease while on the medication. Taking the first dose at bedtime will help minimize its sedative effect. • Some individuals become increasingly sad (depressed) while taking this medication. Contact your doctor/pharmacist if this occurs. • It is important that this medication is not stopped abruptly because sudden increases in blood pressure may occur. • If your doctor has prescibed the clonidine patch for you, you need to (1) wash and dry the area before application, (2) change the patch every 3 to 5 days, and (3) alternate the site of application to prevent a rash from occurring. Notify your doctor/pharmacist if one appears. • This medication may worsen symptoms of heart disease. Tell your doctor/pharmacist if you have a heart condition or are taking any heart/blood pressure medications.

herbal substances). In addition to potential interactions, responses may identify untreated comorbid conditions, drug contraindications (i.e., TCA with cardiac disease), or drug effects that may mimic the symptoms of ADHD.

In initial counseling and in follow-up, a side effect questionnaire (i.e., the BSEQ) should be used. This enables the health care professional to discern whether a side effect is drug-related or an effect of the disorder itself. As with all medications, patients and parents should be cautioned on the proper and safe storage of medications. This is particularly true for patients with prescriptions for agents with abuse or overdose potential (stimulants and TCAs). Next, the frequency of administration should be discussed. For example, typically methylphenidate is administered at breakfast, lunch, and possibly late afternoon. In contrast, the TCAs and pemoline can be administered once daily. Many patients with ADHD cannot be relied upon to take their own medications. Careful coordination with multiple caregivers may be necessary to ensure that each dose is given. The health care provider may need to provide "reminders" or easy routines for the patient, parent, or teacher to follow (pill boxes, dose alarms, administration of medications at meals or after school). Some schools require that medication be kept in a professionally labeled bottle. This may require the clinician to provide a second labeled bottle for this purpose. Various members of the health care team may also need to inform the patient or parent or initiate any clinical or laboratory monitoring needed for a particular agent.

Methods to Improve Patient Adherence to Drug Therapy

Adherence to drug therapy may be a particular problem with patients who have ADHD. Both clinical symptoms and environmental influences may decrease compliance. For example, a patient's inattention may result in forgotten doses. Patients with ADHD/oppositional disorder may refuse to take medications. In addition, patients with ADHD may have dysfunctional families in which the parent cannot be relied upon to administer medications either because of the primary dysfunction or the diversion of medications to other family members. Because ADHD does not produce physical morbidity, patients may fail to realize the importance of taking their medications. Other patients may dread being labeled with a mental disorder (ADHD) or being perceived as a drug abuser. In addition, patients may worry about potential adverse effects. These concerns may make the patient hesitant to take medications in certain environments, if at all.

In addition to the above-mentioned medication reminders, the health care practitioner may need to dispel any patient concerns (i.e., "Stimulants used for ADHD rarely produce addiction, or growth suppression"). Further assurance can be gained by mentioning means in which therapy will be monitored and implementation of ways to minimize side effects (i.e., slow dosage titration, taking initial doses at bedtime [TCAs or clonidine], or after meals [stimulants]). In skeptical or oppositional patients, the health care provider may need to discuss the importance of ADHD medications or contact parents or other health care workers about the need to incorporate medication compliance into behavioral modification programs. In patients reluctant to take medications at school or work or for those who frequently forget, a sustained-release product or an agent with a longer half-life (TCAs, clonidine, pemoline, or the dextro- and levoamphetamine product) may prove beneficial.

Many children and some adults cannot swallow pills. Selection of an appropriate dosage form may make adherence to therapy more likely. Many of the ADHD medications can be crushed or opened and placed in food or are chewable. Older patients may find the clonidine patch an attractive option.

Disease Management Strategies to Improve Patient Outcomes

Once the diagnosis of ADHD is made, successful treatment hinges on tailoring therapy to a patient's preexisting conditions and impairments (Fig. 59.1). Specific or troublesome symptoms should be identified and used as guides or endpoints in therapy. Establishing these references may require input from the patient, parent, teachers, and other health care professionals. Because medication effects are often short-lived and fail to improve all the manifestations of ADHD, nonpharmacologic interventions (behavioral modification, individual/family psychotherapy, and/or academic/social skills training) are essential for positive patient outcomes. This is particularly important for younger patients (>6 years) in whom therapy may prove less effective, in patients predisposed to medication-induced adverse effects, and in those with severe academic, social, or functional deficits.

If a patient's ADHD symptoms are severe enough to warrant pharmacotherapy, comorbid diseases should guide selection of an initial ADHD medication. Because of its proven efficacy, rapid onset, and lower severity of side effects (less than amphetamine-containing products), methylphenidate is the first medication tried in the majority (those without specific comorbidities) of patients with ADHD. After an adequate trial (~1 month) with appropriate maintenance dosing, an alternative stimulant (dextroamphetamine or the dexto- and levoamphetamine combination) may be tried. If the next agent fails, second-line agents (TCAs, clonidine, or pemoline) may be considered. In patients with refractory ADHD, bupropion or an MAOI may prove effective.

Although stimulants are most commonly used, these agents may not be optimal for certain patients with ADHD. For example, clonidine has proven effective in decreasing both tics and ADHD symptoms making it the drug of choice in patients with Tourette's syndrome or tic disorders. Because of their potential (actual or perceived) ability to increase tic severity, bupropion and the stimulants are avoided in those with movement disorders. Initial treatment in patients with comorbid depression or enuresis should be a TCA or possibly bupropion. Both drugs have the ability to decrease the seizure threshold and should be avoided in patients with epilepsy. The ability of stimulants (e.g., methylphenidate, dextroamphetamine, and the dexto- and levoamphetamine combination) to produce euphoria makes them a possible source of abuse; hence, in if substance abuse is suspected (patient or family) pemoline or another class of medications is preferred. Combination therapy is an attractive option for patients with refractory ADHD and those prone to troublesome side effects. Polypharmacy may permit the use of lower doses of both medications or counteract the adverse effects of either agent. One example is the use of methylphenidate and clonidine for patients with persistent insomnia.

Because the severity of ADHD symptoms is influenced by multiple factors, a variety of measurement tools should be used to determine both dosage titration and clinical response. Initially, drugs should be administered daily. Once a given patient's target symptoms show consistent improvement, the dose is held constant and drug holidays (i.e., weekends, summer time, and holidays) are encouraged. This assesses the further need for continued drug therapy, minimizes adverse effects, and may improve self-esteem.

PHARMACOECONOMICS

Although ADHD is frequently diagnosed, there is limited information about the amount of services received and the actual expense required for its treatment. Current data suggest that ADHD has a significant effect upon the nation's economy and that the monetary demands of the disorder are growing. Many factors seem to contribute to the observed increase in expenditures. The use of diagnostic, mental health, and counseling services has consistently increased from 1989 to 1996. Children with ADHD seem to require a greater number of outpatient services (both primary care and mental health) than children with or without other psychosocial problems.[6] As a result of these clinical visits, a greater percentage of patients with ADHD receive prescription medications. Medicaid studies note that polypharmacy has increased 7.5% each year over a 7-year period. Interestingly, family practitioners seem more likely to prescribe stimulants than either pediatricians or psychiatrists.

Children and Adults With Attention Deficit Disorders (CHADD)[6] has conducted a survey evaluating the health care coverage for patients with ADHD. Results suggest that the majority of patients with ADHD have health care coverage with the greatest percentages belonging to preferred provider organizations (PPOs) and health maintenance organizations (HMOs). Despite this coverage, half of patients with ADHD felt that their health care plan did not offer the necessary access to professionals required to ensure proper treatment of the disorder. Approximately 62% of patients had to pay out-of-pocket expenses to receive this care. Among the 90% of patients receiving medications for ADHD, approximately 80% had to pay some amount for these medications. The cost of medications for ADHD can also result in a significant financial burden for families already paying for other health-related expenses.

KEY POINTS

- The optimal management of ADHD is contingent on a reliable and accurate diagnosis using DSM-IV criteria.
- Treatment goals should be established jointly with the patient and the family.
- Treatment of ADHD must address multiple aspects of the child's disorder and should not be reduced to the use of medication alone.
- The majority of patients will respond to one of the available stimulants (i.e., methylphenidate, dexamphetamine, dextro- and levoamphetamine combination or pemoline). Although few differences have been found among the stimulants, methylphenidate is the most studied and most used drug.
- Most randomized clinical trials have assessed short-

term (i.e., up to 3 months) use of stimulants. There are no long-term studies evaluating stimulants or psychosocial therapy use over several years. Likewise, there are no long-term outcome studies assessing the effect of medication-treated ADHD on educational and occupational achievements, involvement with the judicial system, or other areas of social dysfunction.

- Treatment with stimulants does not "normalize" behavior problems. Although there is improvement in core symptoms there is little improvement in long-term academic performance or social skills.
- Decreased appetite, insomnia and irritability are common with the stimulants. High doses of stimulants may cause CNS damage, cardiovascular damage, hypertension, and possibly motor disorders.
- The TCAs are the drugs of choice for the 30% of patients who fail to respond to stimulant medications or who cannot tolerate the side effects associated with stimulants. There is some evidence to suggest that patients who display greater anxiety, depression, or mood disturbances in conjunction with their ADHD may respond better to TCAs than to stimulants. Likewise, some believe that the condition of patients who exhibit aggression may deteriorate with TCAs.
- Medically unexplained sudden death has been reported in children receiving normal doses of desipramine. For this reason, imipramine is preferred over desipramine in children and adults with ADHD. Although the American Academy of Pediatrics does not recommend routine ECG monitoring at this time, the American Academy of Child and Adolescent Psychiatry recommends a baseline ECG, one within days of a dosage increase, and another once steady-state at maximal doses is achieved. Although the benefits of ECG monitoring are questionable, it would seem advisable to follow the more conservative guidelines.

REFERENCES

1. American Psychiatric Association. Diagnostic and statistical manual of mental disorders. 4th ed (DSM IV). Washington, DC: American Psychiatric Association, 1994.
2. American Psychiatric Association. Diagnostic and statistical manual of mental disorders. 3rd ed (DSM III). Washington, DC: American Psychiatric Association, 1982.
3. American Psychiatric Association. Diagnostic and statistical manual of mental disorders. 3rd ed (DSM III-R). Washington, DC: American Psychiatric Association, 1987.
4. Goldman LS, Genel M, Bezman RJ, et al. Diagnosis and treatment of attention-deficit/hyperactivity disorder in children and adolescents. JAMA 279:1100–1107, 1998.
5. American Academy of Child and Adolescent Psychiatry. Practice parameters for the assessment and treatment of children, adolescents, and adults with attention-deficit/hyperactivity disorder. J Am Acad Child Adolesc Psychiatry 36:85S–121S, 1997.
6. NIH Consensus Development Conference. Attention deficit hyperactivity disorder. National Institutes of Health Continuing Medical Education. November 16–18, 1998.
7. Swanson JM, Lerner M, Williams L. More frequent diagnosis of attention deficit hyperactivity disorder. N Engl J Med 333:944, 1995.
8. Cantwell DP. Attention deficit disorder: a review of the past 10 years. J Am Acad Child Adolesc Psychiatry 35:978–987, 1996.
9. Lou HC. Etiology and pathogenesis of attention-deficit hyperactivity disorder (ADHD): significance of prematurity and perinatal hypoxic-hemodynamic encephalopathy. Acta Paediatr 85:1266–1271, 1996.
10. Working Group on Quality Issues. American Academy of Child and Adolescent Psychiatry. Summary of the pediatric parameters for the assessment and treatment of children, adolescents, and adults with ADHD. J Am Acad Child Adolesc Psychiatry 36:1311–1317, 1997.
11. Cook EH, Stein MA, Krasowski CD, et al. Association of attention deficit disorder and the dopamine transporter gene. Am J Hum Genet 56:993–998, 1995.
12. LaHoste GJ, Swanson JM, Wigal SB, et al. Dopamine D4 receptor gene polymorphism is associated with attention deficit hyperactivity disorder. Mol Psychiatry 1:121–124, 1996.
13. Castellanos FX, Giedd JN, March WI, et al. Quantitative brain magnetic resonance imaging in attention-deficit hyperactivity disorder. Arch Gen Psychiatry 53:607–616, 1996.
14. Filipek PA, Semrud-Clikeman M, Steingard RJ, et al. Volumetric MRI analysis comparing subjects having attention-deficit hyperactivity disorder with normal controls. Neurology 48:589–601, 1997.
15. Woolf AD, Suckermann BS. Adolescence and its discontents: attentional disorders among teenagers and young adults. Pediatrician 13:119–127, 1986.
16. Hill JC, Schoener EP. Age dependent decline of attention deficit hyperactivity disorder. Am J Psychiatry 153:1143–1146, 1996.
17. Cantwell DP. Hyperactive children have grown up. What have we learned about what happened to them? Arch Gen Psychiatry 42:1026–1028, 1985.
18. Halperin JM, Gittelman R, Klein DF, et al. Reading disability hyperactive children: a distinct subgroup of attention deficit disorder with hyperactivity? J Abnorm Child Psychol 12:1–14, 1984.
19. Silver L. The relationship between learning disabilities, hyperactivity, distractibility, and behavioral problems. J Am Acad Child Adolesc Psychiatry 20:385–397, 1981.
20. Cantwell DP, Satterfield JH. The prevalence of academic underachievement in hyperactive children. J Pediatr Psychol 3:168–171, 1978.
21. McGee R, Share DL. Attention deficit disorder-hyperactivity and academic failure: which comes first and what should be treated? J Am Acad Child Adolesc Psychiatry 27:318–325, 1988.
22. Pennington BF, Groddirt D, Welsh MC. Contrasting cognitive deficits in attention deficit hyperactivity disorder versus reading disability. Dev Psychol 29:511–523, 1993.
23. Felton RH, Wood FB, Brown IS, et al. Separate verbal memory and naming deficits in attention disorder and reading disability. Brain Lung 31:171–184, 1987.
24. Shaywitz BA, Fletcher JM, Holahan JM, et al. Cognitive profiles of reading disability: interrelationships between reading disability and attention deficit-hyperactivity disorder. Child Neuropsychol 1:170–186, 1995.
25. Wilens TE. Update on attention deficit hyperactivity disorder, I. Curr Affect Illness 15:5–12, 1996.
26. Biederman J, Faerone SV, Mick E, et al. Attention deficit hyperactivity disorder and juvenile mania an overlooked comorbidity? J Am Acad Child Adolesc Psychiatry 35:997–1008, 1996.
27. American Psychiatric Association. Diagnostic and statistical manual of mental disorders. 2nd ed (DSM II). Washington, DC: American Psychiatric Association, 1968.
28. American Academy of Pediatrics. Committee on Drugs. Behavioral and cognitive effects of anticonvulsants therapy. Pediatrics 96:538–540, 1995.
29. Diener MB, Milich R. Effects of positive feedback on the social interactions of boys with attention deficit hyperactivity disorder: a test of self-protective hypothesis. J Clin Child Psychol 26:256–265, 1997.
30. Kwasman A, Tinsley BJ, Lepper HS. Pediatricians' knowledge and attitudes concerning diagnosis and treatment of attention deficit and hyperactivity disorder. A national survey approach. Arch Pediatr Adolesc Med 149:1211–1216, 1995.
31. Diller LH. The run on Ritalin: attention deficit disorder and stimulant treatment in the 1990's. Hastings Center Report 26:12–18, 1996.
32. Bradley C. The behavior of children receiving Benzedrine. Am J Psychiatry 94:577–585, 1937.
33. Safer DJ, Zito JM, Fine EM. Increased methylphenidate usage for attention deficit disorder in the 1990's. Pediatrics 98:1084–1088, 1996.
34. Zametkin AJ, Rapoport JL. Neurobiology of attention deficit disorder with hyperactivity: where have we come in 50 years? J Am Acad Child Adolesc Psychiatry 26:676–686, 1987.
35. Volkow ND, Ding Y, Fowler JS, et al. Is methylphenidate like cocaine? Arch Gen Psychiatry 52:456–463, 1995.
36. Elia J. Drug treatment for hyperactive children: therapeutic guidelines. Drugs 46:863–871, 1993.
37. Spencer T, Biederman J, Wilens T, et al. Pharmacotherapy of attention-deficit

hyperactivity disorder across the life-cycle. J Am Acad Child Adolesc Psychiatry 35:409–432, 1996.
38. Barkley RA. A review of stimulant drug research with hyperactive children. J Child Psychol Psychiatry 18:137–165, 1977.
39. Rapport MD, Denny C, DuPaul GJ, et al. Attention deficit disorder and methylphenidate: normalized rates, clinical effectiveness, and response prediction in 76 children. J Am Acad Child Adolesc Psychiatry 33:882–893, 1994.
40. Jacobvitz D, Sroute LA, Stewart M, et al. Treatment of attentional and hyperactivity problems in children with sympathomimetic drugs: a comprehensive review. J Am Acad Child Adolesc Psychiatry 29:677–688, 1990.
41. Whalen CK, Henker B, Buhrmester D, et al. Does stimulant medication improve the peer status of hyperactive children? J Consult Clin Psychol 57:545–549, 1989.
42. Pelham WE, Walker JL, Sturges J, et al. Comparative effects of methylphenidate on ADD girls and boys. J Am Acad Child Adolesc Psychiatry 28:773–776, 1989.
43. Spencer T, Wilens T, Biederman J, et al. A double-blind, crossover comparison of methylphenidate and placebo in adults with childhood-onset attention deficit hyperactivity disorder. Arch Gen Psychiatry 52:434–443, 1995.
44. Buitelaar JK, Vander Gaag RJ, Swaab-Barneveld H, et al. Prediction of clinical response to methylphenidate in children with attention-deficit hyperactivity disorder. J Am Acad Child Adolesc Psychiatry 34:1025–1032, 1995.
45. Pelham WE, Swanson JM, Bender Furman M, et al. Pemoline effects on children with ADHD. a time-response by dose-response analysis on classroom measures. J Am Acad Child Adolesc Psychiatry 34:1504–1513, 1995.
46. Pelham WE, Aronoff H, Midlam J, et al. A comparison of Ritalin and Adderall: efficacy and time-course in children with attention-deficit/hyperactivity disorder, Pediatrics 103:e43, 1999.
47. Rapoport JL, Buchsbaum MS, Zahn TP, et al. Dextroamphetamine: cognitive and behavioral effects in normal prepubertal boys. Science 199:560–563, 1978.
48. Peloquin LJ, Klorman R. Effects of methylphenidate on normal children's mood, event-related potentials, and performance in memory scanning and vigilance. J Abnorm Psychol 95:88–98, 1986.
49. Satterfield JH, Satterfield BT, Schell AM. Therapeutic interventions to prevent delinquency in hyperactive boys. J Am Acad Child Adolesc Psychiatry 26:56–64, 1987.
50. Rapoport JL, Quinn PO, Bradbard G, et al. Imipramine and methylphenidate treatments of hyperactive boys. Arch Gen Psychiatry 30:789–793, 1974.
51. Hunt RD. Treatment effects of oral and transdermal clonidine in relation to methylphenidate: an open pilot study in ADD-H. Psychopharmacol Bull 23:111–114, 1987.
52. Rapport MD, Carlson GA, Kelly KL, et al. Methylphenidate and desipramine in hospitalized children: I. Separate and combined effects on cognitive function. J Am Acad Child Adolesc Psychiatry 32:333–342, 1993.
53. Rapport MD, Stoner G, DuPaul GJ, et al. Methylphenidate in hyperactive children: differential effects of dose on academic, learning, and social behavior. J Abnorm Child Psychol 13:227–244, 1985.
54. Rapport MD, DuPaul GJ, Kelly KL. Attention deficit hyperactivity disorder and methylphenidate: the relationship between gross body weight and drug response in children. Psychopharmacol Bulletin 25:285–290, 1989.
55. Rapport MD, Denny C. Titrating methylphenidate in children with attention deficit/hyperactivity disorder: is body mass predictive of clinical response? J Am Acad Child Adolesc Psychiatry 36:523–530, 1997.
56. Brown GL, Ebert MH, Mikkelsen EJ, et al. Behavior and motor activity response in hyperactive children and plasma amphetamine levels following a sustained release preparation. J Am Acad Child Psychiatry 19:225–239, 1980.
57. Sprague RL, Sleator EK. Methylphenidate in hyperkinetic children: differences in dose effects on learning and social behavior. Science 198:1274–1276, 1977.
58. Pelham WE, Bender ME, Caddell J, et al. Methylphenidate and children with attention deficit disorder. Arch Gen Psychiatry 42:948–952, 1985.
59. Swanson JM, Wigal S, Greenhill LL, et al. Analog classroom assessment of Adderall in children with ADHD. J Am Acad Child Adolesc Psychiatry 37:519–526, 1998.
60. McEvoy GK, ed. American Hospital Formulary Service drug information 98. Bethesda, MD: American Society of Hospital Pharmacists, 1998.
61. Sallee FR, Stiller RL, Perel JM. Pharmacodynamics of pemoline in attention deficit disorder with hyperactivity. J Am Acad Child Adolesc Psychiatry 31:244–251, 1992.
62. Sallee FR, Perel J, Bates T. Oral pemoline kinetics in hyperactive children. Clin Pharmacol Ther 37:606–609, 1985.
63. Collier CP, Soldin SJ, Swanson JM, et al. Pemoline pharmacokinetics and long term therapy in children with attention deficit disorder and hyperactivity. Clin Pharmacokinet 10:269–278, 1985.
64. Pelham WE, Greenslade KE, Vodde-Hamilton M, et al. Relative efficacy of long-acting stimulants on children with attention deficit-hyperactivity disorder: a comparison of standard methylphenidate, sustained-release methylphenidate, sustained-release dextroamphetamine, and pemoline. Pediatrics 86:226–237, 1990.
65. Safer DJ, Allen RP. Absence of tolerance to the behavioral effects of methylphenidate in hyperactive and inattentive children. Pediatric Pharmacol 115:1003–1008, 1989.
66. Stein MA, Blondis TA, Schnitzler ER, et al. Methylphenidate dosing: twice daily versus three times daily. Pediatrics 98:748–756, 1996.
67. Pelham WE, Sturges J, Hoza J, et al. Sustained release and standard methylphenidate effects on cognitive and social behavior in children with attention deficit disorder. Pediatrics 80:491–501, 1987.
68. Fitzpatrick PA, Klorman R, Brumaghim JT, et al. Effects of sustained release and standard preparations of methylphenidate on attention deficit disorder. J Am Acad Child Adolesc Psychiatry 31:226–234, 1992.
69. Barkley RA, McMurray MB, Edelbrock CS, et al. Side effects of methylphenidate in children with attention deficit hyperactivity disorder: a systemic, placebo-controlled evaluation. Pediatrics 86:184–192, 1990.
70. Ahmann PA, Waltonen SJ, Olson KA, et al. Placebo controlled evaluation of ritalin side effects. Pediatrics 91:1101–1106, 1993.
71. Efron D, Jarman F, Barker M. Side effects of methylphenidate and dexamphetamine in children with attention deficit hyperactivity disorder: a double-blind, crossover trial. Pediatrics 100:662–666, 1997.
72. Safer DJ, Allen R, Barr E. Depression of growth in hyperactive children on stimulant drugs. N Engl J Med 287:217–220, 1972.
73. Safer DJ, Allen RP. Factors influencing the suppressant effects of two stimulant drugs on the growth of hyperactive children. Pediatrics 51:660–667, 1973.
74. Gittelman Klein R, Landa B, Mattes JA, et al. Methylphenidate and growth in hyperactive children: a controlled withdrawal study. Arch Gen Psychiatry 45:1127–1130, 1988.
75. Spencer TJ, Biederman J, Harding M, et al. Growth deficits in ADHD children revisited: evidence for disorder-associated growth delays? J Am Acad Child Adolesc Psychiatry 35:1460–1469, 1996.
76. Lowe TL, Cohen DJ, Detlor J, et al. Stimulant medications precipitate Tourette's syndrome. JAMA 247:1168–1169, 1982.
77. Castellanos FX, Giedd JN, Elia J, et al. Controlled stimulant treatment of ADHD and comorbid Tourette's syndrome: effects of stimulant and dose. J Am Acad Child Adolesc Psychiatry 36:589–596, 1997.
78. Gadow KD, Nolan EE, Sverd J. Methylphenidate in hyperactive boys with comorbid tic disorder: II. Short-term behavioral effects in school settings. J Am Acad Child Adolesc Psychiatry 31:462–471, 1992.
79. Jaffe SL. Intranasal abuse of prescribed methylphenidate by an alcohol and drug abusing adolescent with ADHD. J Am Acad Child Adolesc Psychiatry 30:773–775, 1991.
80. Goyer PF, Davis GC, Rapoport JL. Abuse of prescribed stimulant medication by a 13 year-old hyperactive boy. J Am Acad Child Adolesc Psychiatry 18:170–175, 1979.
81. Horner BR, Scheibe KE. Prevalence and implications of attention-deficit hyperactivity disorder among adolescents in treatment for substance abuse. J Am Acad Child Adolesc Phsychiatry 36:30–36, 1997.
82. Biederman J, Wilens T, Mick E, et al. Psychoactive substance use disorders in adults with attention deficit hyperactivity disorder (ADHD): effects of ADHD and psychiatric comorbidity. Am J Psychiatry 152:1652–1658, 1995.
83. Drug Enforcement Administration, Office of Diversion Control. Conference report: stimulant use in the treatment of ADHD. Washington DC, 1996.
84. Berkovitch M, Pope E, Phillips J, et al. Pemoline-associated fulminant liver failure: testing the evidence for causation. Clin Pharmacol Ther 57:696–698, 1995.
85. Pliszka SR. Tricyclic antidepressants in the treatment of children of children with attention deficit disorder. J Am Acad Child Adolesc Psychiatry 26:127–132, 1987.
86. Biederman J, Baldessarini RJ, Wright V, et al. A double-blind controlled study of desipramine in the treatment of ADD: I. Efficacy. J Am Acad Child Adolesc Psychiatry 28:777–784, 1989.
87. Popper CW. Antidepressants in the treatment of attention-deficit/hyperactivity disorder. J Clin Psychiatry 58:14–29, 1997.
88. Biederman J, Baldessarini RJ, Wright V, et al. A double-blind placebo controlled study of desipramine in the treatment of ADD: II. Serum drug levels and cardiovascular findings. J Am Acad Child Adolesc Psychiatry 28:903–911, 1989.
89. Daly JM, Wilens T. The use of tricyclic antidepressants in children and adolescents. Pediatr Clin North Am 45:1123–1135, 1998.
90. Biederman J, Thisted RA, Greenhill L, et al. Estimation of the association between desipramine and the risk of sudden death in 5- to 14-year-old children. J Clin Psychiatry 56:87–93, 1995.
91. Committee on Children with Disabilities and Committee on Drugs. American

Academy of Pediatrics. Medication for children with attentional disorders. Pediatrics 98:301–304, 1996.
92. Zametkin A, Rapoport JL, Murphy DL, et al. Treatment of hyperactive children with monoamine oxidase inhibitors: I. Clinical efficacy. Arch Gen Psychiatry. 42:962–966, 1985.
93. Feigin A, Kurlan R, McDermott MP, et al. A controlled trial of deprenyl in children with Tourette's syndrome and attention deficit hyperactivity disorder. Neurology 46:965–968, 1996.
94. Casat CD, Pleasants DZ, Schroeder DH, et al. Bupropion in children with attention deficit disorder. Psychopharmacol Bull 25:198–201, 1989.
95. Spencer T, Biederman J, Steingard R, et al. Bupropion exacerbates tics in children with attention-deficit hyperactivity disorder and Tourette's syndrome. J Am Acad Child Adolesc Psychiatry 32:211–214, 1993.
96. Conners CK, Casat CD Gualtieri CT, et al. Bupropion hydrochloride in attention deficit disorder with hyperactivity. J Am Acad Child Adolesc Psychiatry 35:1314–1321, 1996.
97. Wender PH, Reimherr FW. Bupropion treatment of attention-deficit hyperactivity disorder in adults. Am J Psychiatry 148:1018–1020, 1990.
98. Adler LA, Resnick S, Kunk M, et al. Open-label trial of venlafaxine in adults with ADD. Psychopharmacol Bull 31:785–788, 1995.
99. Hedges D, Reoherr FW, Rogers A, et al. An open trial of venlafaxine in adult patients with attention deficit hyperactivity disorder. Psychopharmacol Bull 31:779–783, 1995.
100. Findling RL, Schwartz MA, Flannery DL, et al. Venlafaxine in adults with attention-deficit/hyperactivity disorder. J Cln Psychiatry 57:184–189, 1996.
101. Olvera RL, Pliszka SR, Luh J, et al. An open trial of venlafaxine in the treatment of attention-deficit/hyperactivity disorder in children and adolescents. J Child Adolesc Psychiatry 6:241–250, 1996.
102. Pleak RR, Gormly LJ. Effects of venlafaxine for treatment of ADHD in a child [Letter]. Am J Psychiatry 152:1099, 1995.
103. Barrickman L, Noyes R, Kuperman S, et al. Treatment of ADHD with fluoxetine: a preliminary trial J Am Acad Child Adolesc Psychiatry 30:762–767, 1991.
104. Campbell NB, Tamburrino MB, Evans CL, et al. Fluoxetine for ADHD in a young child. J Am Acad Child Adolesc Psychiatry 34:1259–1260, 1995.
105. Frankenburg FR, Kando JC. Sertraline treatment of ADHD and Tourette's syndrome. J Clin Psychopharmacol 14:359–360, 1994.
106. Hunt RD, Mineraa RB, Cohen DJ. Clonidine benefits children with attention deficit disorder and hyperactivity: report of a double-blind placebo-crossover therapeutic trial. J Am Acad Child Psychiatry 24:617–629, 1985.
107. Wilens TE, Beiderman J, Spencer T. Clonidine for sleep disturbances associated with attention-deficit hyperactivity disorder. J Am Acad Child Adolesc Psychiatry 33:424–426, 1994.
108. Steingard R, Biederman J, Spencer T, et al. Comparison of clonidine response in the treatment of attention-deficit hyperactivity disorder with and without comorbid tic disorders. J Am Acad Child Adolesc Psychiatry 32:350–353, 1993.
109. Singer HS, Brown J, Quaskey S, et al. The treatment of attention-deficit hyperactivity disorder in Tourette's syndrome: a double-blind placebo-controlled study with clonidine and desipramine. Pediatrics 95:75–81, 1995.
110. Clonidine for treatment of attention-deficit/hyperactivity disorder. Med Lett Drug Ther 38:109–110, 1996.
111. Silva RR, Munoz DM, Alpert M. Carbamazepine use in children and adolescents with features of attention-deficit hyperactivity disorder: a meta-analysis. J Am Acad Child Adolesc Psychiatry 35:352–358, 1996.
112. Winsberg BG, Yepes LE. Antipsychotic (major tranquilizers, neuroleptics). In: Werry JS, ed. Pediatric psychopharmacology: the use of behavior modifying drugs in children. New York: Brunner Mazel, 1978:234–274.
113. Millichap J. Drugs in the management of minimal brain dysfunction. Ann NY Acad Sci 205:321–324, 1973.
114. Mattes J, Gittelman R. A pilot trial of amantadine in hyperactive children. Presented at the New Clinical Drug Evaluations Unit (NCDEU) meeting. Key Biscayne, FL, May 1979.
115. Firestone P, Davey J, Goodman JT, et al. The effects of caffeine and methylphenidate on hyperactive children. J Am Acad Child Adolesc Psychiatry 17:445–456, 1978.
116. Donnelly M, Rapoport JL, Potter WZ, et al. Fenfluramine and dextroamphetamine treatment of childhood hyperactivity; clinical and biochemical findings. Arch Gen Psychiatry 46:205–212, 1989.
117. Greenhill LL, Reider RO, Wender PH, et al. Lithium carbonite in the treatment of hyperactive children. Arch Gen Psychiatry 28:636–640, 1973.
118. Pelham WE, Wheeler T, Chronis A. Empirically supported psychosocial treatments for ADHD. J Clin Child Psychol 27:189–204, 1998.
119. Abikoff H. Cognitive training in ADHD children: less to it than meets the eye. J Learn Disabil 24:205–209, 1991.
120. Abikoff H, Gittelman: Does behavior therapy normalize the classroom behavior of hyperactive children? Arch Gen Psychiatry 41:449–454, 1984.
121. Klein RG, Abikoff H. Behavior therapy and methylphenidate in the treatment of children with ADHD. J Atten Disord 2:89, 1997.
122. Ialongo NS, Horn WF, Pascoe JM, et al. The effects of a multimodal intervention with attention-deficit hyperactivity disorder children: a 9-month follow-up. J Am Acad Child Adolesc Psychiatry 32:182–189, 1993.
123. Carlson CL. Pelham WE, Milich R, et al. Single and combined effects of methylphenidate and behavior therapy on the classroom performance of children with ADHD. J Abnorm Child Psychol 20:213–231, 1992.
124. Spencer T, Biederman J, Wilens T, et al. Effectiveness and tolerability of tomoxetine in adults with attention deficit hyperactivity disorder. Am J Psychiatry 155:693–695, 1998.

CHAPTER 60

OBESITY AND EATING DISORDERS

Delbert L. Mandl and Jason L. Iltz

Obesity

Leave gourmandizing, know that the grave doth gape for thee thrice wider than for other men.
—William Shakespeare, 16th century

Despite these perceptive words, Shakespeare and his contemporaries admired an ample form. Suppleness denoted a person graced by God and was the hallmark of the opulent and idly rich. Rubens would certainly have scoffed at the idea of Twiggy as a model of beauty. It took the industrial revolution to give obesity a bad reputation. Mechanization caused voluntary or forced reduction in average activity without a decrease in caloric intake, and obesity became the single most prevalent metabolic disorder in the United States.

DEFINITION

Obesity can be defined as a condition occurring from the sum total of environmental, emotional, and familial factors that have as the lowest common denominator an abnormal energy balance usually resulting from excessive caloric intake and inadequate caloric loss. In simplest terms, obesity exists when there is excess energy stored as body fat. More specifically, body mass index (BMI), the parameter frequently used to characterize body weight, is a value that normalizes a patient's weight based on height. It can be calculated by dividing the patient's weight in kilograms by the patient's height in meters squared (kg/m^2). Using nonmetric measurements the BMI can be calculated using the following formula:

$$BMI = [\text{weight (in pounds)}/\text{height (in inches)}^2] \times 704.5$$

The Clinical Guidelines on the Identification, Evaluation, and Treatment of Overweight and Obesity in Adults define overweight and obesity as persons with a BMI of 25 to 29.9, and ≥ 30, respectively.[1]

TREATMENT GOALS: OBESITY

- Through the concerted efforts of many practitioners, obesity is now considered a chronic disease. Like hypertension, it is a silent disease resulting in many complications if not addressed continually. Therefore, address treatment at reducing body weight or at least preventing further gain and maintaining the weight loss long term.

- By facilitating weight loss, abate the complications associated with obesity, for example, decrease blood pressure in obese hypertensive patients, decrease blood glucose in patients with type II diabetes, decrease low-density lipoprotein cholesterol and triglycerides, and increase high-density lipoprotein cholesterol in obese patients with hyperlipidemia.
- Achieve desired weight loss through the combined efforts of the individual and practitioners using low-calorie diets (LCD), physical activity, behavior therapy, and if necessary pharmacotherapy and surgery.
- Focus initial weight loss efforts on a realistic goal of a 10% weight reduction from baseline. This equates to approximately a 1- to 2-pound weight loss per week over 6 months.
- Continue support throughout treatment, with a reevaluation at 6 months to determine success, and assess further the need for additional weight loss.
- Because of high rates of rebound weight gain, continue efforts to maintain weight loss to decrease morbidity and mortality accompanying obesity.

EPIDEMIOLOGY

Currently it is estimated that close to 97 million adults in the United States have some degree of obesity,[1] making it the second leading cause of preventable death.[2] Broken down by sex, 59.4% of men and 50.7% of women older than 20 years of age are overweight or obese, with an all-inclusive 54.9% for both women and men.[3] On average, approximately 25% of adults in the United States, at a given time, are attempting to lose weight through some type of weight reduction program.[4]

The incidence of obesity appears to be increasing over time. The percentage of overweight persons in the United States has risen from 30.5% in 1960 to 32% in 1994, astonishingly though, the population classified as obese has increased from 12.8% to 22.5% in the same time period.[1] Not only is obesity a problem in the adult population, but it is also becoming prominent in children and adolescents. An estimated 13.7% of children (aged 6 to 11 years) and 11.5% of adolescents (aged 12 to 17 years) are overweight.[5] Age, sex, race, and extent of physical activity influence the degree of body fat.

At the start of life, adipose tissue comprises approximately 12% of body weight and rapidly increases to an average of 25% at 6 months of age. During early adulthood, the percentage of body fat in males is 15 to 18%, and 20 to 25% in females. A gradual increase in body fat occurs with age, approaching an average of 30 to 40% in adult men and women.[6]

Differences in racial background and socioeconomic status appear to influence body fat, but it is often difficult to accurately distinguish the individual effect that each of the factors has. Reports demonstrate a greater prevalence of obesity in black versus white women; however, the reverse is true with men—obesity is more likely to occur in white rather than black men.[3] Furthermore, persons in lower socioeconomic classes tend to have a higher rate of obesity relative to their middle and upper class counterparts. This relationship holds true particularly in females and does not appear as pronounced in males.[6]

As one might expect, an inverse relationship exists between level of physical activity and development of obesity. Persons with sedentary lifestyles or a physical handicap that restricts activity are prone to obesity. Increasing the degree of physical exercise is associated with a reduction in body fat as lean body mass increases; however, this relationship is rapidly reversed upon discontinuation of the energy expenditure.

PATHOPHYSIOLOGY

Pathogenesis

In a small percentage of patients, obesity has an identifiable organic cause.[7] Weight gain in excess of 1 kg/day invariably implies fluid retention and is frequently a signal of cardiovascular, renal, or hepatic disorders.[8] Medications can also produce weight gain by inducing fluid retention in susceptible persons, either through direct (steroids and related drugs) or indirect (medicinals high in sodium) mechanisms. Only rarely is obesity a symptom of a specific endocrinopathy, such as insulinoma or Cushing's disease. Their peculiar fat distribution, attendant symptoms, and history of sudden appetite changes easily differentiate these uncommon disorders.

Idiopathic obesity is a complex interplay of physiologic, hereditary, psychologic, and metabolic influences which have, as their ultimate manifestation, chronic dietary indiscretion.

Physiologic Factors

Since the discovery nearly 80 years ago that obesity can be induced surgically in animals, a great deal of interest has developed in the relationship between abnormal appetite and possible aberrations within the hypothalamus. Lesions in the ventromedial nucleus of the hypothalamus (satiety center) result in hyperphagia, whereas lesions in the lateral hypothalamic areas (feeding center) result in cessation of eating.[9,10] Factors controlling these centers are unknown but have been associated with endocrine and metabolic determinants.

Obese persons exhibit behavior that might indicate a derangement in the satiety center. When obese and nonobese persons are allowed to ingest freely, the nonobese regulate food intake based on internal cues, such as hunger sensations and caloric density of the food, whereas, obese persons regulate food intake by external cues such as time and environment, regardless of the caloric density of the food.[11]

In the first year of life, the number of existing fat cells is relatively fixed. Increasing the size of adipose cells (hypertrophic) accommodates storage of excess energy. Before adolescence, the number of adipose cells multiply as young children grow. In obese children, this rate of multiplication is greater than in nonobese children, resulting in a larger number of adipose cells (hypercellular) throughout life. In contrast, adult-onset obesity is primarily the result of hypertrophic obesity.[12]

Weight loss is more rapid and prolonged in persons with hypertrophic obesity compared to hypercellular obesity. Attempts to reduce weight to norms in hypercellular patients are very difficult and can result in extreme hunger symptoms similar to those seen with starvation and also psychologic and physical disability.[13]

Because evidence favors the increased likelihood of overweight children becoming obese adults,[14] preventative measures are important. These measures include avoiding overfeeding of infants, encouraging the use of unsugared foods, keeping junk foods and snacks out of the house, and encouraging activity.

Genetic Factors

The role of heredity in obesity is a matter of great speculation and research. Oftentimes environmental factors pertaining to food intake greatly confound this issue, making it difficult to determine the true impact of genetics on obesity. Studies involving adopted children and twins have been performed in an attempt to overcome these environmental influences. Results reflect little correlation in relative body weight between adopted children and their adoptive parents; however, definite trends do exist when the weights of the children are compared to those of their biologic parents.[15] Furthermore, the body weights of twin siblings appear to correlate well, identical twins showing greater correlation than fraternal twins.[16] These observations lend support to a genetic component of obesity.

Statistically, when both parents are of normal weight, the incidence of having an obese child is approximately 9%. If one or both parents are obese, there is a 50 and 80% incidence of obese offspring, respectively.[15]

Psychologic Factors

Familial and cultural eating habits are implanted at an early age. As a society, we place great emphasis on food–to most one of life's enduring pleasures is a rich, hearty meal. The obese patient carries this gratification to an extreme level.

Obese persons often exhibit an immense appetite for psychologic reasons. Overeating may be a manifestation of anxiety or depression, where the pleasures of food serve as a substitute for the satisfactions missed from other sources. As a result, the obese characteristically dine until the food is completely gone or until they are overtly uncomfortable, while the nonobese usually stop eating when their hunger is gone.

Because obesity is often associated with neurotic traits, overeating is commonly considered to be a behavioral defect. In the pathologically obese, where no distinct underlying problem exists, psychologic factors undoubtedly play a major role. Obviously, obesity is a complicated mix of psychologic, genetic, and metabolic influences, which manifest as abnormal appetite and resultant overweight.

Metabolic Factors

Insulin refractoriness is the most significant metabolic deviation in obesity because insulin regulates the major pathways for fat accumulation and storage. Insulin-induced lipogenesis is an attractive hypothesis to explain the cause of obesity, but current evidence suggests that insulin refractoriness is more a result, rather than a cause, of obesity.

Adrenal overactivity is a common finding in massively obese patients. This is reflected by elevated urinary corticosteroids, mild hirsutism, borderline hypertension, and glucose intolerance.[17] Again, these abnormalities are most likely the result, rather than the cause of obesity, seeing that they develop in nonobese subjects after gorging and disappear as weight returns to normal.

Metabolic enzyme deficiency may also result in abnormalities in thermogenic dissipation of calories in obese patients. Cellular enzyme systems account for much of thermogenic calorie loss, and there is evidence that the obese may have inefficient catalytic rates.[18] Impaired hormonal control by catecholamines and insulin may be involved, but this hypothesis is controversial.[19]

DIAGNOSIS AND COMPLICATIONS

Diagnosis

Patients with massive obesity, peculiar fat distribution, or sudden, rapid weight gain require extensive evaluation. However, common idiopathic obesity does not usually demand elaborate evaluation techniques.

Quantifying obesity is not difficult. The patient who is 136 kg (300 lb) overweight is readily recognized as obese. Moderate obesity is easily diagnosed using standard height-weight charts and calculating BMI. Other possibly more accurate methods to determine total body fat, such as bioelectrical impedance and dual-energy X-ray absorptiometry, offer no significant advantage over BMI, are limited in clinical practice, and are expensive. However, calculating BMI is not without deficiencies, because it can overestimate body fat in muscular persons and underestimate body fat in older adults who have lost muscle mass. The easiest and most accurate method of quantifying body fat involves measuring triceps, subscapular, or suprailiac skinfold thickness with constant pressure calipers. Skinfold thickness measurements coupled with height-weight data give a convenient and accurate evaluation of the degree of obesity.

Abdominal obesity is an independent predictor of risk and morbidity. Although more accurately measured by magnetic resonance imaging and computed tomography, practicality and expense limit the clinical usefulness of these methods. A high risk of developing concomitant disease states is associated with a waist circumference of >102 cm (40 inches) in men and >88 cm (35 inches) in women.[1] Waist circumference should be measured and used with BMI to assist in determining the degree of obesity, associated risks, and morbidity.

Complications

Many serious disorders are associated with severe obesity (Table 60.1). Significant excess weight is clearly detrimental to longevity and a definite statistical link exists between obesity and hypertension, diabetes, cardiovascular disease, and gastrointestinal (GI) disorders (Fig. 60.1). This link pertains primarily to moderate and severe obesity, because the longevity of marginally or slightly obese persons compares favorably to that of nonobese persons. In addition, significantly underweight persons are also at risk for digestive and pulmonary disease.

Obesity during pregnancy is associated with a 7-fold increase in diabetes, a 4-fold increase in essential hypertension, and a 2-fold risk of pregnancy-induced hypertension.[20] Increased rates of perinatal mortality from 37 per 1000 deliveries involving lean women to 121 per 1000 deliveries among obese women have also been reported.[21]Substantial excess weight is also associated with altered pharmacokinetics of certain drugs.[22,23]

Table 60.1 ▪ Disorders Associated with Obesity

Hypertension
Congestive heart failure
Diabetes
Cerebrovascular disease
Gallbladder disease
Hyperlipidemia
Respiratory distress syndrome (Pickwickian)
Obstetric complications
Osteoarthritis
Varicose veins
Flat feet
Hiatus hernia
Intertriginous dermatitis

Despite evidence of the detrimental effects of obesity on health, the prevalent factor motivating most people to lose weight is not health but cosmetic ideals.

TREATMENT

Successful approaches to the management of obesity are often difficult and pose a significant challenge to persons interested in reducing their weight. There is no "standard treatment" that is effective in most or even a large fraction of obese patients, and weight reduction programs must be designed to fit the personality, lifestyle, and health status of each patient. Success depends on the person's motivation, behavioral modification, and the establishment of reasonable goals and expectations. Crash programs and demands for extreme alterations from established lifestyles are uniformly unsuccessful in the long run and potentially dangerous.

A comprehensive weight reduction program incorporates components of caloric restriction, exercise, behavioral modification, and possibly pharmacologic and invasive approaches. The critical factor is that caloric expenditures exceed caloric demands and that a permanent change in caloric intake must be achieved to maintain desired weight.

Increasing numbers of overweight and obese persons are making this one of the nation's leading health problems. In fact, direct costs associated with obesity account for almost 6% of the national health expenditure in the United States[24] Health risks and complications resulted in a total cost of $99.2 billion in 1995, with a little over half ($51.6 billion) coming from direct medical costs of obesity-associated diseases.[1] Diet foods, products, and programs result in more than $30 billion spent annually.[25] Because of these factors the National Institutes of Health (NIH) and National Heart Lung and Blood Institute (NHLBI) formed a panel of experts to establish guidelines to assist the health care provider in recognizing and treating this chronic problem.

As mentioned earlier, the guidelines released by this panel suggest that the first step is to assess the individual's

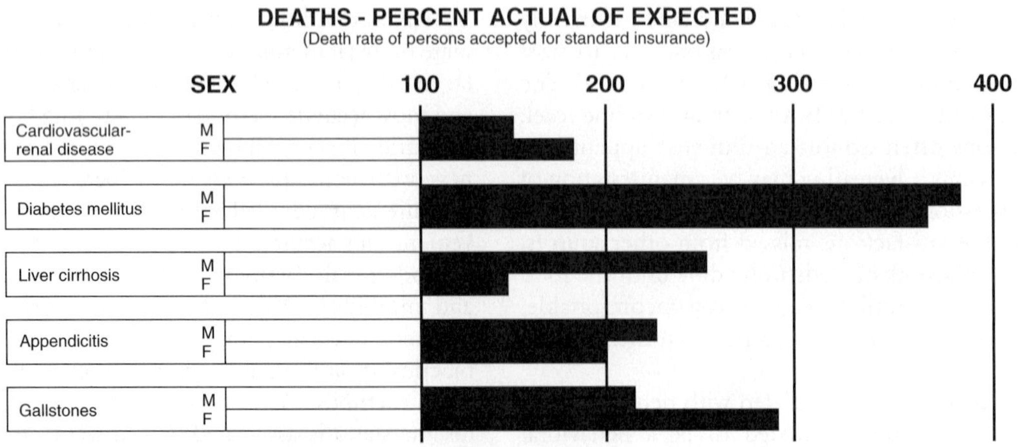

Figure 60.1. Relationship between obesity and serious medical disorders. (Reprinted with permission from the Metropolitan Life Insurance Company.)

Table 60.2 ▪ Classification of Overweight and Obesity by Body Mass Index (BMI), Waist Circumference, and Associated Disease Risk[a]

	BMI (kg/m²)	Obesity Class	Disease Risk[a] Relative to Normal Weight and Waist Circumference	
			Men ≤102 cm (≤40 in) Women ≤88 cm (≤35 in)	>102 cm (>40 in) >88 cm (>35 in)
Underweight	<18.5			
Normal[b]	18.5–24.9			
Overweight	25.0–29.9		Increased	High
Obesity	30.0–34.9	I	High	Very high
	35.0–39.9	II	Very high	Very high
Extreme obesity	≥40	III	Extremely high	Extremely high

Source: Adapted from reference 26.

[a]Disease risk for type II diabetes, hypertension, and cardiovascular disease.

[b]Increased waist circumference can also be a marker for increased risk even in persons of normal weight.

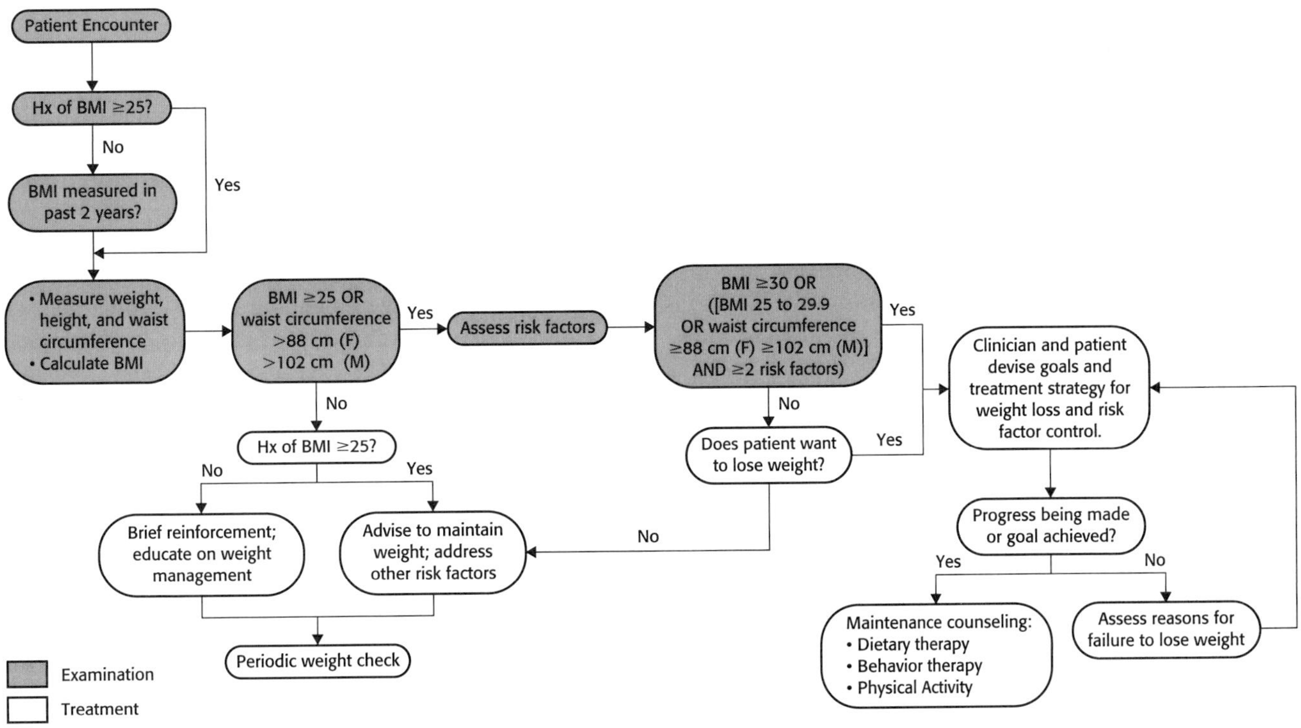

Figure 60.2. Obesity treatment algorithm. The algorithm applies only to the assessment for overweight and obesity and subsequent decisions based on that assessment. It does not reflect any initial overall assessment for other conditions and diseases that the physician may wish to do. *BMI*, body mass index; *Hx*, history. (Adapted with permission from National Institutes of Health/National Heart, Lung, and Blood Institute. Clinical guidelines on the identification, evaluation, and treatment of overweight and obesity in adults: the evidence report. June 17, 1998: 1–228.)

weight status and risk factors (Table 60.2).[26] An algorithm was established to address only the treatment of overweight and obesity, recognizing that treatment for these conditions also encompasses treatment of cardiovascular risk factors (Fig. 60.2). Again, the initial goal of weight loss should be a reduction of baseline weight by 10%. Achievement of this goal can be attained by a slow 1 to 2 lb/wk weight loss over a 6-month period, with routine evaluation and encouragement. Weight loss requires a combination of therapeutic modalities including dietary therapy, exercise, behavior therapy, and, if necessary, pharmacotherapy and surgery.

Regulation of Caloric Intake

Modest reduction of caloric intake through dieting and setting realistic goals and expectations is the most palatable and easily available method of treatment. A good diet prevents the patient from becoming too hungry and noncompliant. The importance of learning good eating habits and familiarity with the caloric content of various foods should be strongly emphasized.

The primary goal of any diet is to reduce the caloric intake below expenditure so excess energy stored in the form of fat can be used. Weight loss should not exceed 1 kg (2 lb) per week unless close medical supervision is involved. Any program resulting in weight loss of more than 0.3 kg (0.7 lb) per day usually involves more fluid than tissue loss. Obligatory water loss accounts for the accelerated weight loss frequently observed during the initial weeks of dieting. Although use of diuretics for weight reduction exploits this phenomenon, this practice is both illusory and hazardous.[27]

In obese subjects, approximately a 3500-calorie deficit is required to lose 0.5 kg (1 lb) of tissue. To achieve this deficit, a bewildering array of diets have been advocated, each differing in ratios of carbohydrate, fat, and protein and each claiming superiority over all the others. Easy weight loss diets tend to exploit the obese individual who is not ready for a permanent level of change and discipline. Items like dietary drinks offer easy, short-term solutions, but their simplicity and convenience merely put off the essential need to learn about food and food values. Diet books appear with great regularity, and despite their guarantees and initial effectiveness, few induce the permanent solutions of discipline and lifestyle changes.

"Crash diets" are dangerous in susceptible persons when applied to extremes. Diets involving limited foods, such as the "Beverly Hills Diet," promote nutritional misinformation and can result in severe health problems.[28,29] Very low calorie diets (VLCDs) consisting of ≤800 kcal/day are designed to cause a calorie deficit while preserving lean body mass. One such diet, the "Last Chance Diet," resulted in dozens of fatalities related to cardiovascular abnormalities caused by negative nitrogen balance and consequent protein tissue loss.[30] The Cambridge and Optifast diets are other VLCDs that incorporate higher quality protein sources (egg albumin, casein, or soy) and adequate nutritional content; however, concern persists that such diets are inherently dangerous when used as sole nutritional sources.[31] The use of VLCDs should be restricted to patients with moderate to severe obesity who are under close medical supervision, with special attention to cardiovascular monitoring.[32] Although these diets appear to be effective in rapidly reducing weight short-term, even when supplemented with other treatment modalities, their effectiveness as long-term maintenance therapy is modest.

With all VLCDs, fluid and electrolyte abnormalities, arrhythmias, dehydration, ketoacidosis, hyperuricemia, alopecia, and teratogenesis are potential complications. These diets are contraindicated in patients with diabetes, cardiovascular disorders, kidney and liver disease, and pregnancy.

Diets based on starvation represent an extreme form of caloric restriction with intake less than 200 kcal/day. Starvation diets are associated with very rapid and significant reductions in body weight; however, their use is limited because of potential side effects, the need for extremely close medical supervision, and the high percentage of weight regain that occurs after discontinuation of the diet.

To assist with weight loss, patients are instructed to decrease daily caloric intake, especially calories obtained from fat. Low-fat diets are highly encouraged, but decreased palatability produces poor compliance. Various fat substitutes have been used by manufacturers, most of which are carbohydrate or protein-based. Recently, olestra, a fat-based substitute, gained approval from the Food and Drug Administration (FDA) as a food additive. Olestra is advantageous because of its stability at higher temperatures, allowing use in baked and fried foods, and it is nonabsorbable, rendering no caloric value.[33] The nonabsorbable property also has detrimental effects causing adverse GI effects such as bloating, diarrhea, loose stools, flatulence, anal leakage, and decreased absorption of fat-soluble vitamins A, D, E, and K.[33]

Exercise

The inclusion of physical exercise in a weight reduction program can be a valuable supplement to dieting. Regular exercise increases the degree of energy expenditure, favoring adipose tissue reduction and prolonged maintenance of weight loss. Because of reductions in caloric intake associated with dieting, persons may experience a compensatory decrease in total energy expenditure of 15% more than the percentage reduction in body weight (i.e., 25% after 10% decrease in weight, 35% after a 20% decrease).[34] Regular exercise generates an increase in basal metabolic rate, which counteracts this adaptive response to dieting.

For exercise to be useful, it must be regular, of high quality, and consistent with the patient's lifestyle. Aggressive exercise should be avoided at the onset owing to the lack of conditioning and potential for injury. Depending on the person, a regimen of thrice weekly exercise sessions starting at 10 minutes per outing, and building up to 30 to 45 minutes of more intense exercise at least 5 days a week, if not everyday, should be initiated.[35] The selection of an activity of moderate intensity and longer duration is preferred because the longer time frame favors usage of fat stores. In mild to moderate obesity patients, exercise results in a significant reduction in adipose tissue; however, in some instances overall body weight may not change significantly owing to increases in lean body mass.

Unfortunately, quality exercise is not acceptable to many obese patients. They often turn to "effortless" weight reduction devices, such as mechanical vibrators, inflatable weight-reducing clothing, or "spot reducers." As one author noted, these devices are little better than doing nothing, and the primary reduction often occurs in the exerciser's wallet.[6]

Increases in technology promote more sedentary work environments. This, coupled with the "fast-paced" world we are a part of, does not always allow adequate time for aerobic exercise. Therefore, conscious efforts need to be made by patients to increase energy expenditure by all possible means, for instance, walking the stairs instead of taking an elevator or escalator.

Behavior Modification

Behavior therapy can also facilitate weight reduction, especially in the long-term management of massively obese patients who require assistance in accepting the seriousness of their problem. The primary goal of behavioral treatment is to modify behaviors that are associated with or promote eating.[37] Therapy can be divided into three separate components. First, self-monitoring forces obese patients to record on a daily basis the type of food items eaten and when and where they were eaten. The purpose of daily record keeping is to increase the individual's awareness and identify specific eating patterns or behaviors. Once these patterns are identified, the second phase of behavioral therapy focuses on breaking the relationship between repetitive patterns or events (external cues) and actual ingestion of the meal. Oftentimes this is done through assigning specific times and places in which meals can be eaten, chewing food a specific number of times, or taking sips of water between each bite. Finally, behavioral modification incorporates a system of positive self-feedback to reinforce and maintain an optimal attitude toward weight reduction. The majority of studies evaluating the effectiveness of behavioral therapy on weight reduction indicate a greater duration or maintenance of weight loss than with programs that lack a behavioral modification component.[38]

A number of self-help programs such as Weight Watchers, NutriSystems, Overeaters Anonymous, and Take Off Pounds Sensibly (TOPS), provide obese persons with important psychologic support and motivation to bring about permanent weight control measures. Membership in these programs is enormously large with Weight Watchers alone claiming several million active members.

Pharmacotherapy

Incorporating drug therapy into a weight loss regimen is accomplished via three different mechanisms: (1) reduction of food intake, (2) inhibition of nutrient/fat absorption, and (3) increased energy expenditure.[25] However, drug therapy is generally used as one component of a comprehensive weight loss program in patients with BMI ≥30 with no obesity-related risk factors or diseases, or for patients with BMI ≥27 with obesity-related risk factors or diseases.[1]

Appetite Suppressants

Obese patients who are adequately instructed on dietary management and are treated with appetite suppressants tend to lose more weight on average than patients on a diet alone. In a review of more than 200 studies of appetite suppressants involving 10,000 patients, pooled data demonstrated an average loss of 0.25 kg (0.56 lb) per week more versus placebo.[39] However, because these drugs are typically labeled for a duration of 2 to 4 weeks only, the average patient will lose only 1 additional kg when they are used as recommended. When appetite suppressants are used, it becomes critical for the patient to realize that improved dietary compliance is the goal of therapy and diet, not the drug, is responsible for weight loss. Drug use is only temporary, and restoration of drug-free dieting through behavior change is the desired outcome.

Unfortunately, the routine use of appetite suppressants in the initial phases of a weight reduction program may detract from the importance of dietary/behavioral measures and provide a psychologic escape from the need to change lifelong eating habits. A comparison of patients treated with either pharmacotherapy or behavioral therapy indicates that, while pharmacotherapy produces more weight loss, the benefits are short-lived and weight is rapidly regained when the drug is discontinued. At the end of a 1-year follow-up, patients treated with behavioral therapy alone weighed significantly less than patients treated with drugs alone. Also, combined pharmacotherapy and behavioral therapy produce results inferior to those with behavioral therapy alone.[40]

Appetite suppressants should be reserved for use in situations where (1) a reducing diet has been established and an unsatisfactory response has been observed; (2) a plateau is reached after initial success with dieting alone; or (3) a relapse is encountered after a prolonged period of progress. Unfortunately, many physicians prescribe appetite suppressants early in therapy because they cannot resist the pressures placed on them by patients who have invariably experienced failure with do-it-yourself dieting and come to the physician expecting more. Better long-term results could be realized if physicians would lend their esteem and credibility to dietary/behavioral approaches, including vigorous monitoring for compliance, rather than undermining the importance of self-motivated dieting by prescribing appetite suppressants in the initial stages. However, some of the newer agents have shown promise in long-term management, and it may be appropriate to use these agents in the initial stages of therapy.

Pharmacology

Appetite suppressants are thought to exert their effect directly on the hypothalamic satiety center, which is under adrenergic control. Most suppressants augment brain catecholamine action, except fenfluramine, dexfenfluramine, fluoxetine, and sertraline, which act specifically on serotonin (5-HT). Sibutramine, which recently received FDA approval, inhibits the reuptake of both norepinephrine (NE) and 5-HT. Thus, appetite suppressants can be broken into three classes: (1) adrenergic agents, (2) serotonergic agents, and (3) adrenergic/serotonergic agents (Table 60.3).

Conventional wisdom holds that tolerance develops rapidly to the anorectic effects of these agents, as evidenced by the decelerating weight loss curves with continued use. This belief has led to recommendations that appetite suppressants be limited to short-term use. However, most appetite suppressants appear to maintain weight loss for the duration of administration and discontinuation after long-term use results in a rapid rebound of increased appetite and weight regain. Therefore, tolerance to the appetite suppressant effects may not be significant at the doses usually used, and long-term treatment may be plausible for selected patients. Studies involving the combination of fenfluramine/phentermine (fen/phen), and dexfenfluramine alone established efficacy of long-term pharmacotherapy.[41,42] These drugs were commonly prescribed until July 1997 when researchers from the Mayo Clinic reported 24 cases of cardiac valve abnormalities.[43] Additional cases of cardiovascular problems were reported, which prompted the FDA to request the voluntary withdrawal of fenfluramine and dexfenfluramine on September 15, 1997.[33] With fenfluramine and dexfenfluramine withdrawn from the market, phentermine and sibutramine are the agents most commonly prescribed.

The antidepressants fluoxetine and sertraline, which are selective inhibitors of 5-HT reuptake, are currently being evaluated for the management of obesity. Study results suggest modest rates of effectiveness over a 6-month period, with some studies reporting regained weight with continued treatment.[25] Fluoxetine and sertraline are approved by the FDA for the treatment of depression. However, their use in the treatment of obesity has not yet been approved. The low abuse potential and their ability to effectively reduce weight make serotonergic agents a welcomed addition to the potential agents used to treat obesity. Excellent reviews of the various drug therapies for the treatment of obesity have recently been published.[33,44]

Abuse Potential

Because several of the available agents are reinforcing (i.e., euphorigenic) central nervous system stimulants, their misuse potential is high. However, misuse of these agents is not typically associated with anorectic use in motivated, obese patients. Misuse is more a result of indiscriminate prescribing with subsequent diversion for nonmedical, "recreational" use. Among the anorectic drugs, amphetamines account for the greatest number of abuse episodes, with estimates that more than 10% of the legitimately manufactured amphetamines wind up in the hands of abusers.[45] Therefore, stimulants in controlled substance class II are no longer used in the treatment of obesity.[46]

In December 1978, the Advisory Review Panel on OTC Miscellaneous Internal Drug Products found the nonprescription ingredient, phenylpropanolamine (PPA), safe and effective for weight control. The widespread promotion of PPA as the "ultimate diet pill" and its close association with prescription ingredients (e.g., Dexatrim, Dex-A-Diet, Acutrim, etc.) led to special problems of misuse. PPA is the most common ingredient in "look-alike" counterfeit drugs, which are packaged in tablets and capsules to look virtually identical to amphetamines and sold as "legal stimulants."

Drug Selection

No superiority has been shown for the appetite-suppressant effects of any of these agents. Aside from physician preference, product selection is primarily determined by trial and error, using the entire spectrum of available agents (Table 60.3). Patients who cannot tolerate an agent from one chemical class may benefit from agents in another class. Restlessness, insomnia, tremors, tachycardia, nausea, diarrhea, constipation, dry mouth, and mydriasis are commonly reported side effects. In susceptible patients, elevated blood pressure and cardiac arrhythmias may occur especially with sibutramine. Once again,

Table 60.3 ▪ Appetite Suppressants Used to Treat Obesity

Category	Generic Name	Brand Name	Dosage and Frequency	DEA Class
Adrenergic agents	Benzphetamine	Didrex	25–50 mg QD to TID	III
	Phendimetrazine	Bontril, Plegine, Prelu-2, X-Trozine	105 mg QD	III
	Phentermine			IV
	Hydrochloride	Adipex-P, Fastin, Oby-trim	18.75–37.5 mg QD	
	Resin	Ionamin	15–30 mg QD	
	Diethylpropion			IV
	Immediate-release	Tenuate	25 mg TID	
	Controlled-release	Tenuate Dospan	75 mg QD	
	Mazindol	Sanorex, Mazanor	1–3 mg QD to TID	IV
	Phenylpropanolamine	Dexatrim, Acutrim	75 mg QD	OTC
Serotonergic agents	Fenfluramine[a]	Pondimin	20–40 mg QD to TID	IV
	Dexfenfluramine[a]	Redux	15 mg BID	IV
	Fluoxetine[b]	Prozac	10–20 mg QD	
	Sertraline[b]	Zoloft	25–50 mg QD	
Adrenergic/serotonergic agent	Sibutramine	Meridia	10–15 mg QD	IV

DEA, Drug Enforcement Agency.
[a]Withdrawn from the U.S. market in September 1997.
[b]Not approved by the Food and Drug Administration for the treatment of obesity.

agents acting on 5-HT (fluoxetine and sertraline) are an exception, producing fewer adverse effects than other drugs, but they can cause headaches, sleep disturbances, decreased libido, and sexual dysfunction.[44]

The duration of action can also help determine the best anorectic agent for a given patient. If overeating occurs in the evening, little benefit is derived from morning doses. Likewise, long-acting agents are irrational choices when dietary indiscretion is limited to a particular time of day. In both instances, short-acting agents are preferred. Combinations of anorectic agents with other ingredients, such as barbiturates or phenothiazines, probably possess no greater efficacy and exhibit an expanded array of side effects.

Persons receiving appetite suppressants should be advised about stimulant side effects, dry mouth, and possible insomnia. Sucking on sugarless hard candy minimizes dry mouth. Taking the dose early in the day can minimize insomnia from long-acting agents. Patients receiving serotonergic agents should be warned about possible drowsiness and additive depressant effects with ethanol or other sedatives. Drug interactions can occur with all of these agents, and caution should be exercised when they are used concomitantly with monoamine oxidase inhibitors, antihypertensives, tricyclic antidepressants (TCAs), and caffeine. Sibutramine should not be prescribed for persons taking other agents affecting 5-HT, such as fluoxetine and other selective serotonin reuptake inhibitors (SSRIs), sumatriptan and other 5-HT agonists for migraine, and dextromethorphan. Lithium toxicity has been reported to be precipitated by mazindol.[47]

Appetite suppressants should also be dispensed with caution to pregnant patients. In studies involving amphetamines and morpholines, an increased incidence in oral clefts was noted when the drug was taken during the first 56 days of pregnancy.[48]

Lipase Inhibitors

Orlistat, a lipase inhibitor, was approved by the FDA on April 23, 1999 as an adjunct to weight loss methods. It is indicated for weight loss and weight maintenance when used in conjunction with a reduced caloric diet and indicated to reduce the risk of weight gain after prior weight loss. Orlistat appears to block the absorption of about 30% of consumed dietary fat. A dosage range of 100 to 400 mg TID appears to be optimal for most patients.[49] Inhibition of fat absorption encountered with orlistat results in numerous GI related side effects including loose and oily stools, fecal incontinence, abdominal cramping, and nausea. These side effects do not appear to be dose related, but may in part be related to the amount of dietary fat ingested.[49] The absorption of fat soluble vitamins is also decreased.

Bulk-Forming Agents

Bulk-forming agents are indigestible hydrophilic colloids that swell when hydrated to give a sense of repletion. Results of clinical studies have been contradictory, and bulk can be easily obtained through dietary means with the addition of high fiber fruits and vegetables. These are less expensive and more palatable and should become a part of the patient's lifelong diet anyway.

Thermogenic Agents

Use of thyroid hormone has been advocated for the treatment of obesity because of its thermogenic properties. Its early use was based on the incorrect observation that an abnormally low basal metabolic rate (BMR) accompanied obesity. This observation was later shown to be an artifact owing to the poor correlation between body surface area and BMR in grossly obese patients.[8] Currently, advocates claim that thyroid hormone may prevent the compensatory drop in BMR caused by caloric restriction. Critics argue that very substantial doses of thyroid hormone are required (390 to 910 mg) to even slightly increase BMR, and these pharmacologic doses can have deleterious cardiovascular effects in obese patients already predisposed to heart problems. In view of the risks, use of thyroid hormone in obese patients should be avoided unless there is clear evidence of thyroid deficiency.[50]

Additional drugs that appear to enhance thermogenesis include ephedrine, caffeine, nicotine, growth hormone, and investigational β-agonists.[38,51] Furthermore, a synergistic thermogenic effect has been documented when a combination of ephedrine and caffeine is administered.[51] A limited number of studies have evaluated these agents and, despite an apparent effect on increased energy expenditure, associated side effects tend to limit the usefulness of these agents.

Invasive Treatment Approaches

At the extreme end of the treatment continuum, more invasive approaches to obesity are available and include mandibular fixation, vagotomy, surgical manipulation of the GI tract and liposuction. Use of these methods should be restricted to morbidly obese patients (BMI ≥40 or ≥35 with comorbid conditions) whose obesity is refractory to the previously mentioned approaches.[1]

Limited data suggest that fixation of the mandible (jaw wiring) can effectively reduce weight by restricting solid food intake. Although this particular procedure is associated with significant weight reduction, rapid weight regain is encountered in almost all patients after removal of the wires.[52] Truncal vagotomy is another approach involving surgical interruption of the vagal nerve in an attempt to reduce the stimuli responsible for triggering eating. Unfortunately, the additional side effects associated with such a procedure limit its usefulness.[52]

Jejunoileal and gastric surgery involves bypassing a significant portion of the small intestine and stomach, respectively. Weight loss with either proceeds slower than with fasting and, unfortunately, may stop quite short of ideal weight. Jejunoileal bypass works by inducing a malabsorptive state and is associated with significant digestive discomfort, nutrient malabsorption, polyarthritis, fatty liver degeneration, oxalate nephrolithiasis, and tuberculosis.[52,53] Gastric bypass surgery produces a decreased gastric reservoir, which results in epigastric distress or vomiting when the capacity is exceeded. Gastric bypass may have fewer long-term complications but is technically more difficult and is associated with a higher incidence of early postoperative complications. Nevertheless, despite these many complications, surgery remains the only viable solution in selected patients to avoid permanent disability or death.

Liposuction should be viewed as more of a cosmetic method for body contouring, rather than a means of weight reduction. A frequent misunderstanding about liposuction is that significant amounts of adipose tissue can be eliminated with this procedure. Oftentimes, if excessive tissue is extracted, serious complications such as blood loss, nerve damage, infection, and disfiguration of the skin contour may occur. Furthermore, successful operations tend to involve younger persons in whom the elasticity of the skin structure is intact.[52] Therefore, the number of obese patients potentially able to benefit from the procedure is limited. For the above-mentioned reasons, liposuction should not be advocated for managing obesity.

ALTERNATIVE THERAPIES

Much of the population elects to self-medicate, leading to an increase in the use of herbal and homeopathic remedies. Of these, chromium has received most of the attention for weight loss and blood glucose control. The beneficial effects of chromium supplementation are attributed to its essential necessity for insulin function. Many of the reports have been contradictory, allowing for indecisiveness with chromium supplementation recommendations. A study in young obese females reported a significant increase in weight gain with a daily supplementation of 400 μg chromium picolinate over a 9-week period. No change in weight was noted in the groups with exercise only or taking chromium picolinate and exercise. However, subjects taking chromium nicotinate and exercising demonstrated a significant weight loss.[54] Yet, caution must be advised when recommending chromium picolinate for weight loss. Chronic renal failure in the form of interstitial nephritis caused by heavy metal exposure[55] was reported a 49-year-old woman ingesting 600 μg daily for six weeks. Without a regulatory agency, safety and efficacy data of homeopathic therapies are unknown, requiring clinicians to rely on case reports to guide recommendations. Future studies may continue to help delineate the effects of chromium on weight loss.

FUTURE THERAPIES

Many new areas of drug development are occurring as a result of the recognition of morbidity and costs associated with overweight and obesity-related conditions. Since approval of sibutramine, little progress has been made in the area of appetite suppressants. Nevertheless, advances in thermogenic agents, digestive inhibitors, and hormonal manipulation are being made.

Understanding the mechanisms for thermogenic control has led to the development of β_3-agonists. These agonists mediate thermogenesis peripherally, whereas the sympathetic nervous system is responsible for central mediation.[56] An increased tendency for weight gain was noted in persons with a gene mutation for the β_3-adrenergic receptor.[57] As expected, the main adverse effects observed involve tremor and shaky hands. Fortunately, no cardiovascular effects are noted owing to the specificity for the β_3-adrenergic receptor. Overwhelming success has been lacking with the many different β_3-agonist compounds studied. Still, much is being learned and research in the area continues.

The hypothalamus regulates energy balance by signaling feelings of hunger or satiety after receiving neural, hormonal, and nutrient messages from areas of the body. This complex system is the target for much research. Neuropeptide Y is a potent appetite stimulant, which also decreases energy expenditure via suppression of the sympathetic nervous system.[58] Obviously studies are focused on the ability to develop an antagonist to the neuropeptide Y receptor. Galanin is another peptide with actions similar to those of neuropeptide Y, whereas cholecystokinin opposes these hormones by signaling the body to decrease food intake.[33] Again, research in the treatment of overweight and obesity is targeting receptors of these regulatory hormones. Finally, cloning of the *ob* gene from adipose tissue has been reported.[59] This gene encodes for the protein leptin, which is secreted by adipocytes in response to increased energy stores, and functions to suppress food intake and increase energy expenditure.[33,58] Most of the current research is focused on this complex hormonal regulation of feeding behavior.

SUMMARY

In virtually all patients, obesity can be preventable. When it occurs, the cure is uniquely simple and noninvasive. Despite this, a significant fraction of the population is suffering from what can be depicted as a "human energy crisis." This is due largely to the insensitivity of our society to the unfavorable health outcomes associated with sustained obesity and the unwillingness of obese persons to undertake lifetime treatment (i.e., good dietary habits). Our acceptance of obesity as a benign condition leads to poor motivation and poor patient compliance.

Health care professionals play an important role in the management of obesity. As has been emphasized, the use of drugs, although temporarily beneficial, can detract from the attainment of permanent solutions. The health care professional is in an important position to put the many components of treatment into perspective, and with educational and reinforcing techniques, assist the obese patient to achieve lasting results.

Eating Disorders

The two classic eating disorders (EDs) are anorexia nervosa (AN) and bulimia nervosa. AN is a syndrome characterized by self-starvation, extreme weight loss, excessive exercise, body image disturbance, and an intense fear of becoming obese, despite being grossly underweight.[60] The first modern account of AN was by Sir William Gull in the late 19th century.[61] Bulimia nervosa has only recently been recognized as a psychiatric problem, with the first scientific citation appearing in 1979.[62] Bulimia nervosa is characterized by binge eating usually followed by some form of purging, such as self-induced vomiting, medication-induced vomiting (ipecac), laxative abuse, or associated behaviors such as diuretic use, diet pill use, or compulsive exercising.[59,63] Almost half of those with AN have bulimic symptoms, and one-third of those with bulimia have a history of anorexia or a major depressive disorder.[64] Some investigators recognize two separate subgroups of AN based on the presence of bulimic symptoms.[65,66] Bulimic AN refers to a subset of patients with AN who restrict their intake, but also purge with the use of vomiting.[62] Thus, most patients with eating disorders fall on a spectrum between purely food restrictive (AN) and binge-and-purge (bulimia).[67]

TREATMENT GOALS: EATING DISORDERS

- Due to the secretive nature and broad mistrust associated with EDs, it is vital that health care professionals are able to recognize the typical signs, symptoms, and behaviors often portrayed by individual patients.
- Prevent, treat, and delay the progression of various secondary complications associated with EDs.
- Psychotherapy, the mainstay of treatment for EDs, is designed to help patients overcome the denial associated with their disorder, reconstruct self-identity, and build self-confidence.
- The acute treatment for AN should be aimed at restoration of normal body weight.
- Pharmacotherapy is often prescribed in an effort to further diminish or eliminate the characteristic anorectic or binge-and-purge behaviors associated with EDs.
- Multidisciplinary goals associated with long-term treatment of EDs should focus on preventing noncompliance and relapse.

EPIDEMIOLOGY

An intense preoccupation with food, eating, body shape and size, and fear of weight gain is common to both anorectics and bulimic patients. Bulimia is characterized by mild or marked weight fluctuations, whereas severe weight loss is found in AN. The weight of a bulimic patient does not typically fluctuate to the dangerously low levels seen in AN. The most common type of ED is normal-weight bulimia, which involves patients who are within 10% of ideal weight despite purging.[68] A normal weight, coupled with characteristic secretiveness regarding binge-and-purge behavior, makes these patients very difficult to detect.

This preoccupation with food and eating stems in part from the cultural value Western society places on thinness and the thoughts that fat is disgusting and that weight gain means one is bad or out of control. Susceptible persons have an unfettered drive to achieve society's ideal figure. AN usually begins between the ages of 8 years and the mid-30s, but most commonly first appears in females in their early teens with a bimodal pattern of onset usually occurring at 13 to 14 and 17 to 18 years.[57] Commonly, the teenager perceives a real or imagined weight problem, and progresses from a modest effort to lose weight to a compulsive preoccupation with food restriction. "Anorexia" is a misnomer because most patients do not lose their appetites.

Bulimia has a similar pattern of onset. It begins later in adolescence, and usually after a period of being overweight. Unsuccessful attempts to diet, coupled with self-imposed or family pressure to lose weight, leads the individual, either accidentally or through a friend, to the discovery that self-induced vomiting or laxative use is a convenient way to reduce weight. This ultimately escalates into the binge-and-purge bulimic behavior.

Approximately 95% of patients with AN and 80% of patients with bulimia are female, often white, and from middle or upper class backgrounds.[57,62,65] Five to 10% of adolescent girls and young women are affected to some degree, and it is estimated that the incidence of AN and bulimia nervosa has doubled over the past two decades.[69,70] Up to 2% of teenage girls from upper socioeconomic backgrounds develop AN, and 3 to 5% of college women suffer from bulimia. The lifetime prevalence rate for AN in women is 1%, whereas bulimia nervosa has a lifetime incidence of 4% in women.[58,59] The prevalence of ED in men is approximately one-tenth that in women.[71] Twenty percent of patients with EDs have a history of alcohol or other drug abuse.[65]

DIAGNOSIS AND COMPLICATIONS

Diagnosis

EDs are classified as psychiatric illnesses. Diagnostic criteria from the fourth edition of the American Psychiatric Association's *Diagnostic and Statistical Manual of Mental Disorders* (DSM-IV)[72] are presented in Table 60.4.

The generalized secretiveness and denial of signs and symptoms associated with EDs often makes these illnesses very difficult to detect. Most patients with EDs do not

Table 60.4 ▪ DSM IV Criteria for Anorexia Nervosa and Bulimia Nervosa

Anorexia nervosa

A. Refusal to maintain body weight at or above a minimal normal weight for age and height (e.g., weight loss leading to maintenance of body weight 15% below that expected or failure to make expected weight gain during period of growth, leading to body weight 15% below that expected).

B. Intense fear of gaining weight or becoming fat, even though underweight.

C. Disturbance in the way in which one's body weight, size, or shape is experienced; undue influence of body weight or shape on self-evaluation or denial of the seriousness of the current low body weight.

D. In females, absence of at least three consecutive menstrual cycles when otherwise expected to occur (primary or secondary amenorrhea). (A woman is considered to have amenorrhea if her periods occur only after hormone [e.g., estrogen] administration.)

Specify type

Restricting type: During the episode of anorexia nervosa the person does not regularly engage in binge eating or purging behavior (i.e., self-induced vomiting or the misuse of laxatives or diuretics).

Binge eating/purging type: During the episode of anorexia nervosa, the person regularly engages in binge-eating or purging behavior (i.e., self-induced vomiting or the misuse of laxatives or diuretics)

Bulimia nervosa

A. Recurrent episodes of binge eating. An episode of binge eating is characterized by both of the following:
1. Eating, in a discrete period of time (e.g., within any 2-hour period), an amount of food that is definitely larger than most people would eat during a similar period of time and under similar circumstances.
2. A sense of lack of control over eating during the episode (e.g., a feeling that one cannot stop eating or control what or how much one is eating).

B. Recurrent inappropriate compensatory behavior to prevent weight gain, such as self-induced vomiting; misuse of laxatives, diuretics, or other medications; fasting; or excessive exercise.

C. The binge-eating and inappropriate compensatory behaviors both occur, on average, at least twice a week for 3 months.

D. Self-evaluation is unduly influenced by body shape and weight.

E. The disturbance does not occur exclusively during episodes of anorexia nervosa.

Specify type

Purging type: The person regularly engages in self-induced vomiting or the misuse of laxatives or diuretics.

Nonpurging type: The person uses other inappropriate compensatory behaviors, such as fasting or excessive exercise, but does not regularly engage in self-induced vomiting or the misuse of laxatives or diuretics.

come forward voluntarily to the health care clinician; instead they are most often referred by external sources such as friends, teachers, coaches, companions, or family members.[57] Once referred by the external source, the patient usually denies symptoms, is petulant, and is highly secretive, deeply distrustful, and unwilling to reveal personal thoughts, behaviors, or routines. Health care professionals can play an important role in recognizing and counseling patients with EDs. Patients with EDs exhibit typical signs, symptoms, and behaviors, which are listed in Table 60.5. Based on these signs, symptoms, and behaviors, rapid judgments may need to be made about whether a patient is suffering from one of these serious, potentially life-threatening disorders. Because many of the drugs misused by bulimic patients are purchased without a prescription, pharmacists can monitor and restrict repeated sales of stimulant laxatives, enemas, appetite suppressants, and syrup of ipecac to young women. Suspicious use of diuretic agents, such as furosemide or thiazides, in apparently healthy young women should also be questioned. In one study of 275 bulimic patients, 34% admitted to using a prescription diuretic for weight control.[73] Finally, the health care professional must be knowledgeable about community services available to help patients with EDs once they are identified. Appropriate referrals to other health care providers and regional or local support groups can be extremely helpful for getting these patients the proper and necessary care.

Complications

The complications of AN are mainly those of starvation. The most consistent medical findings, aside from cachexia, are amenorrhea and estrogen deficiency.[74] Thirty percent of anorexic teenage girls do not menstruate until their 30s.[75] Decreased fertility has also been observed in both men and women with AN. In extreme cases, every physiologic system may be disturbed, including the endocrine, cardiovascular, renal, gastrointestinal, hematologic, metabolic, musculoskeletal, and central nervous

Table 60.5 ▪ Recognizing Patients with Eating Disorders

- Female in early to late teens who (1) exhibits weight loss or no significant weight gain during development (AN) or (2) exhibits frequent significant weight fluctuations (bulimia)
- Young women fitting the ED stereotype who repeatedly purchase laxatives, enemas, appetite suppressants, syrup of ipecac, or diuretics and who typically cover themselves with baggy, nonconforming clothing to conceal their illness
- Complaints of irregular menstrual cycles or amenorrhea
- History of depression or alcohol/other drug use or abuse
- Other nonspecific complaints: swollen parotid glands, constipation, frequent sore throats from vomiting; abdominal complaints from laxative abuse, etc.
- Physical characteristics: Russell's sign, hypertrophied salivary glands, poor dentition, dehydration, edema, decreased subcutaneous fat, atrophic breasts, dry skin with lanugo-like hair, yellowing of skin due to carotenemia, sunken eyes, possible alopecia, bradycardia, hypotension, hypothermia, and abdominal bloating
- Laboratory screening: electrolyte imbalances, acidosis or alkalosis, anemia, leukopenia, thrombocytopenia, low plasma protein, hypoglycemia, and elevated liver enzymes; urine and stool samples to detect diuretic or laxative abuse
- Other signs: impulsivity (shoplifting, promiscuity), poor self-esteem, post-trauma symptoms, personality disorders, cognitive distortions, suicidal ideation/attempts, self-destructive or self-mutilating behaviors.

systems.[57,58,76] Cardiac complications are the most common cause of death.[58] Vital signs reveal hypotension with systolic blood pressure as low as 70 mm Hg and sinus bradycardia with rates in the 30s to 40s.[58] Postural hypotension is observed in roughly 60% of patients.[71] Sinus bradycardia and cardiac arrhythmias, including supraventricular premature beats and ventricular tachycardia, may be precipitated by a diminished heart muscle mass, decreased contractile force, hypokalemia, or other severe electrolyte imbalance.[57,58,77] Mortality associated with AN, excluding suicide, ranges from 5 to 9% percent.[57,78] Suicide may account for an additional 2 to 5% of deaths.[74] In untreated or poorly treated patients, the mortality rate approaches 20%.[71] Long-term follow-up after treatment reveals that approximately 70% of patients with AN have at least moderate symptomatic improvement and 20 to 30% of patients are left chronically ill.[57]

Complications associated with bulimia tend to be less severe and involve the consequences of chronic bingeing and purging. Unlike the anorectic patient, whose emaciation attracts attention, the bulimic patients may be at or near ideal weight, making it easier to conceal the disorder. If weight loss is substantial, menstrual irregularities are common.[73] Subtle changes in serum electrolytes may be seen in patients who vomit chronically, and laxative and diuretic abuse further contributes to hypokalemia with muscle weakness and fasciculations. Frequently, bulimic patients have a characteristic "chipmunk face" secondary to parotid gland swelling. Increased susceptibility to infections, complaints of frequent sore throats, and poor dentition are also characteristic findings in bulimia nervosa. Subtle hand changes, called Russell's sign, are often present in patients who vomit chronically. These changes include skin lesions on the dorsum of the hand overlying the index and middle finger metacarpophalangeal joints, primarily on the dominant hand.[79] These lesions, caused by repeated contact of the patient's incisors to the dorsum of the hand during self-induced emesis, range from abrasions or excoriations to callous-like papules or nodules.[75] Some bulimic patients have vomited so much that they no longer need stimulation to induce emesis. These patients who have lost their gag reflex are at an increased risk for aspiration pneumonia, especially after the use of central nervous system depressants, such as alcohol. A particularly dangerous practice is the repeated induction of vomiting with syrup of ipecac. Chronic absorption of ipecac can lead to potentially fatal cardiac, GI, and neuromuscular toxicity.[61,80] Complications associated with AN and bulimia are reviewed and compared in Table 60.6.

TREATMENT

The treatments of AN and bulimia require a multidisciplinary approach, often incorporating psychotherapy and pharmacotherapy. Health care providers should rarely embark on the task of treating patients single-handedly. Instead, clinicians with expertise in specialty areas, who are versed in the treatment of EDs should be consulted and used. Multidisciplinary teams often consist of the primary care physician, a specialized physician, psychiatrist, dietitian, and mental health professional (e.g., psychologist, social worker, or nurse). Clinical pharmacy specialists also play a major role in patient education and in the recommendation, selection, and monitoring of prescription and nonprescription medication. Treating EDs is virtually always a long-term process and requires considerable clinical skill, patience, and compassion to build an effective, trusting relationship with the patient.

Psychotherapy

Psychotherapy is the mainstay of treatment for EDs. Psychotherapy includes individual, group, family, supportive, cognitive-behavioral, and insight-oriented therapy, with the primary objective of helping patients to overcome denial of the problem and to reconstruct self-identity and self-confidence. Although psychotherapy is largely completed on an outpatient basis, the use of residential treatment programs, halfway houses, hospitalization, and day-hospital treatment programs is always an option for patients with more severe or hard-to-manage disease.

Pharmacotherapy

Despite several trials with a number of different pharmacologic agents, optimal and overwhelmingly successful drug therapies have not been identified. To complicate matters, anorectic patients and their families tend to deny the existence and severity of the illness and fail to obtain adequate medical and psychiatric care.[73] Bulimia nervosa patients are more likely to seek treatment, but have a low tolerance for extended compliance leading to a high relapse rate.[81] Although successful treatment with drug therapy occurs in all types of patients with ED, it is most often successful in patients with binge-and-purge behaviors.

Antidepressants

Several different antidepressants have been studied in the treatment of EDs. Numerous published trials involving antidepressants have confirmed a benefit in the management of EDs. In successful treatment of bulimia with antidepressants alone, most patients had a relapse after the drug was stopped, emphasizing that drugs are only a part of a multifocal strategy. The optimal duration of therapy is unknown. However, bulimic patients have been successfully treated with antidepressants for 2 years or more.[82] Some studies have suggested a possible link between EDs and major depressive illness, including a blunted dexamethasone suppression test[72] and lowered urinary metabolites of NE.[83] In addition, AN and bulimia are associated with changes in noradrenergic, serotonergic, and opioid systems, which are thought to perpetuate pathologic eating behavior.[84] Thus, drugs modifying activity of these neurotransmitters may potentially be useful in the treatment of EDs.

Fluoxetine, a SSRI, has been one of the most widely studied agents in recent years for the treatment of EDs.[85–87] The Fluoxetine Bulimia Nervosa Collaborative

Table 60.6 ▪ Complications of Anorexia Nervosa and Bulimia Nervosa

Organ System	Anorexia Nervosa	Bulimia Nervosa
Endocrine/Metabolic	Amenorrhea Decreased norepinephrine secretion Decreased somatomedin C Low or erratic vasopressin secretion Hypercarotenemia Low gonadotropins, estrogens, testosterone Sick euthyroid syndrome Raised cortisol and positive dexamethasone suppression test Raised growth hormone Abnormal temperature regulation (hypothermia) Dehydration, electrolyte disturbances (hypokalemia, hypomagnesemia, hypocalcemia, hyponatremia, hypophosphatemia) Hypercholesterolemia Hypoglycemia Raised liver enzymes Refeeding syndrome	Menstrual irregularities Metabolic acidosis Electrolyte disturbances
Cardiovascular	Bradycardia Hypotension Arrhythmia Prolonged QT interval Decreased heart mass Attenuated response to exercise Pericardial effusion Superior mesenteric artery syndrome	Ipecac toxicity Arrhythmia Cardiomyopathy Orthostatic hypotension
Renal	Acute and chronic renal failure Increased blood urea nitrogen Partial diabetes insipidus Polyuria Peripheral edema	Electrolytes disturbances (hypokalemia, diuretic-induced) Renal failure Proteinuria Hematuria
Gastroenterological	Decreased gastric emptying and motility Decreased lipase, lactose Constipation Bowel obstruction Elevated amylase Pancreatitis Irritable bowel syndrome Elevated hepatic enzymes	Sore throat Swelling of parotid gland (chipmunk face) Acute gastric dilation, rupture, tearing Esophagitis Stomatitis Hematemesis Diarrhea Constipation Steatorrhea Dental carries, erosion of tooth enamel Decreased gastric emptying and motility Laxative dependence Hypokalemia (diuretic induced) Rectal bleeding Gastric/duodenal ulcer Ipecac toxicity
Hematological	Anemia Leukopenia Thrombocytopenia Hypocellular bone marrow Low plasma protein	
Pulmonary		Aspiration pneumonia
Musculoskeletal	Cramps, tetany Muscle weakness Stress fractures Osteopenia Osteoporosis	Muscle weakness Fasciculations
Immunological	Impaired immune function Low complement levels Impaired T-cells Granulocyte abnormalities Bacterial infections	

(continued)

Table 60.6 *(continued)*

Organ System	Anorexia Nervosa	Bulimia Nervosa
Neurological	Impaired autonomic activity Seizures Abnormal electroencephalogram Nerve compressions Peripheral neuritis Cerebral atrophy	Ipecac toxicity
Dermatological	Dry, scaly skin Brittle hair and nails Increased lanugo-like body hair Easy bruising	Russell's sign Easy bruising

Source: References 60, 61, 64, 77, 79, 89, 102.

Study Group compared two dose ranges for fluoxetine (60 mg/day versus 20 mg/day) over an 8-week period and found a statistically significant decrease in binge-eating episodes with the higher dosage.[88] Reduced 5-HT and tryptophan activity in the central nervous system coupled with low NE plasma and cerebrospinal fluid levels have been proposed as possible contributors to bulimia nervosa.[59] Reduced 5-HT activity has resulted in increased food intake in animal models.[59] Therefore, binge eating could be at least in part related to a failure of 5-HT to inhibit the NE activation of feeding.[59] Given this information, the success of SSRIs in the treatment of bulimia nervosa is understandable. Although fluoxetine is the only SSRI with an indication for bulimia nervosa, virtually all SSRIs (including paroxetine, sertraline, and fluvoxamine) have been used in clinical practice. The recommended starting dose for fluoxetine is 60 mg/day. Slow upward dose titration over several days is advisable to decrease the incidence and severity of side effects often associated with the initiation of therapy, including nausea, anxiety, and insomnia. Although most patients require 60 mg/day maintenance doses of fluoxetine, it is advisable to use the lowest possible effective maintenance dose and periodically reassess the need for continued treatment. Starting and maintenance doses for the other available SSRIs have not been agreed upon in clinical practice but are generally higher than those recommended for the treatment of depressive disorders.

Fluoxetine and other SSRIs have also been used in the treatment of AN. Although success rates lag behind those seen in patients with bulimia, improvement has been noted. Doses of 20 mg/day have been recommended.[89] The unlabeled dosage range for fluoxetine in the treatment of AN is 20 to 80 mg/day. Slow upward dose titration over several days is again advisable in these patients to decrease the severity and incidence of the early, unwanted side effects previously mentioned.

SSRIs are given once daily and are tolerated very well by most patients. Persistent side effects patients complained most about in clinical practice included dry mouth, increased sweating, decreased libido, and sexual dysfunction.

Various TCAs, including desipramine, imipramine, and amitriptyline have been used to treat patients with EDs. All three agents have unlabeled uses for the treatment of EDs. As with SSRIs, bulimia nervosa responds more favorably to pharmacotherapy with TCAs than does AN.

Desipramine and imipramine are the most extensively researched TCAs and are the preferred TCAs for treatment of bulimia nervosa.[85] One of the best studies demonstrating the effectiveness of desipramine in bulimia carefully excluded subjects with major depressive disorder,[90] suggesting that the drug may have a direct antibulimic effect. The dosage range reported in the literature for desipramine and imipramine in the treatment of EDs is 150 to 300 mg/day.

In another study, amitriptyline produced disappointing results compared to control groups, but suboptimal amitriptyline doses (150 mg/day) and mixed therapy, including psychotherapy for both study and control groups, may have confounded the results.[91] Amitriptyline has been used successfully in clinical practice for both AN and bulimia.

Doses for the above TCAs are essentially the same as those used for major depressive disorders and are administered for at least 6 to 8 weeks. TCAs should be chosen with caution because of their potential for unwanted adverse events. TCAs may potentially increase the risk of cardiac arrhythmia and severe hypotension, especially in those in whom purging and vomiting has led to dehydration and cardiac dysfunction.[86] Other potential side effects include worsened constipation, increased risk of seizures, dry mouth, blurred vision, nausea, and sedation.

A double-blind controlled study with phenelzine, a monoamine oxidase inhibitor (MAOI), produced a striking reduction in bingeing behavior in bulimic patients.[92] Phenelzine has an unlabeled indication for the treatment of bulimic patients who show characteristics of atypical depression. Other classes of antidepressants such as SSRIs and TCAs are preferred to MAOIs such as phenelzine because of overall patient acceptability and because they preclude dietary restriction problems in patients with diet-indiscreet illness. Other potentially deleterious or bothersome adverse effects include orthostasis, constipation, altered seizure threshold, palpitations, dry mouth and blurred vision.

Open studies of trazodone, another serotonergic antidepressant, produced mixed results and even worsening of bulimic behavior.[93,94] As with its use in major depressive episodes, therapeutic doses of trazodone can rarely be achieved because of unwanted side effects. These include orthostasis, arrhythmia, palpitations, dizziness, and blurred vision.

In 1986, a trial of bupropion in a bulimic population resulted in a relatively high incidence of seizures, forcing the temporary withdrawal of bupropion from the market[95] Although the risk of seizure can be managed effectively by three times daily dosing (about every 8 hours) and limiting the maximum individual doses to150 mg/dose (450 mg/day), many patients with EDs have altered seizure thresholds resulting from their illness, making bupropion an unsuitable choice for many patients.

St. John's wort, an over-the-counter herbal antidepressant product, may potentially be useful in patients with EDs owing to its reuptake inhibition of 5-HT and NE. Although no clinical studies regarding its use in patients with EDs have been identified, it offers a viable option to patients who prefer natural or holistic remedies rather than currently available prescription products.

Other Agents

A number of other drug modalities have been used in patients with EDs. In a double-blind study of 72 patients with AN, cyproheptadine in high doses (32 mg/day) produced modest weight gain compared to amitriptyline and placebo.[96] The anticonvulsants phenytoin, carbamazepine, and valproic acid have all been studied in the treatment of bulimic patients.[97–99] Results have been generally disappointing, but there have been isolated patients with symptomatic improvement. There may be a subgroup of binge eaters, whose behavior is secondary to a neurologic disorder analogous to epilepsy, who may be more likely to respond to an anticonvulsant agent.[100] In addition, the opiate antagonists naloxone and naltrexone, lithium, and other agents have been studied.[89] Clearly, further controlled studies in larger numbers of patients are warranted to establish the safety and specific role of these agents in the management of EDs.

Combination Psychotherapy and Pharmacotherapy

Oftentimes the patient and health care professional desire quick and easy solutions and reach for medication in place of much needed interpersonal therapy for treating EDs. As previously mentioned, psychotherapy is the mainstay of treatment and should not be replaced, overlooked, or downplayed when medication therapy is decided upon. Instead, both measures should be used together to give the patient every chance for successful treatment. Only a handful of studies have been completed showing the relative efficacy of combining psychotherapy and pharmacotherapy in the treatment of bulimia nervosa.[101] Results from these trials in bulimic patients are mixed, and there is little scientific evidence to suggest that psychotropic medications offer significant advantages to patients with AN already receiving behavioral therapy.[89,98] The mainstay of acute therapy for AN should therefore be a focus on restoration of normal body weight. Even if patients with AN show signs of depression, progressive weight gain tends to correct underlying depression without the need for antidepressants. Therefore, antidepressants play a somewhat limited role in the management of AN.

SUMMARY

AN and bulimia nervosa are serious, potentially fatal EDs found most commonly in young persons during adolescence. Patients with AN and bulimia nervosa are predominantly female, outnumbering male patients by an incidence of 10:1. Current evidence suggests a relationship between depression or other neurotransmitter abnormalities and EDs, particularly bulimia. Recognition of EDs is often very difficult because of the highly secretive nature of the patient's illness. Early detection and diagnosis often help facilitate treatment and can prevent many of the serious and life-threatening complications often associated with EDs. Successful treatment of EDs involves a multidisciplinary approach, often incorporating psychotherapy and pharmacotherapy. Although psychotherapy remains the cornerstone of treatment for both AN and bulimia nervosa, medication therapy is commonly used. In general, bulimia nervosa responds more favorably to medication therapy than does AN. Antidepressants, specifically SSRIs and TCAs, have been used successfully in the treatment of EDs and appear to provide symptomatic relief in patients who are not clinically depressed. At the present time, a trial of antidepressants is considered appropriate in patients with EDs if behavioral therapy needs augmentation or is proving unsuccessful. In all cases, medication should compliment psychotherapy rather than take the place of.

It must be remembered that patients are often noncompliant and tend to misuse and overuse drugs. Relapses are heralded by excessive purchases of laxatives, syrup of ipecac, and over-the-counter weight control products, and surreptitious diuretic use.

Through vigilant monitoring of patient compliance to psychotherapy and pharmacotherapy interventions and observing for evidence of relapses, health care professionals play an important role in the multidisciplinary management of patients with EDs.

KEY POINTS

- The incidence of obesity is increasing, not only in the adult population, but also in children and adolescents, and has become the second leading cause of preventable death.
- Obesity occurs from a complex interplay of physiologic, hereditary, psychologic, and metabolic influences.
- Skinfold thickness measurements coupled with BMI give a convenient measurement and accurate evaluation of the degree of obesity.

- Waist circumference should be measured and used with BMI to assist in determining the degree of obesity, associated risks, and morbidity.
- Many serious disorders (hypertension, diabetes, cardiovascular disease, and GI disorders) are associated with obesity and are detrimental to the longevity of the patient.
- Treatment of obesity should involve dietary therapy, exercise, behavior therapy, and, if necessary, pharmacotherapy and surgery.
- Pharmacotherapy provides a temporary means of weight loss and must be used in combination with other treatment modalities to gain lasting results.
- The two classic EDs are AN and bulimia nervosa. AN is a syndrome characterized by self-starvation, extreme weight loss, excessive exercise, body image disturbance, and an intense fear of becoming obese, despite being grossly underweight. Bulimia nervosa is characterized by binge eating usually followed by some form of purging, such as self-induced vomiting, medication-induced vomiting (ipecac), laxative abuse, or associated behaviors such as diuretic use, diet pill use, or compulsive exercising.
- The most common type of ED is normal-weight bulimia, which involves patients who are within 10% of ideal weight despite purging.
- EDs are classified as psychiatric illnesses. Diagnosis is based on criteria from the fourth edition of the American Psychiatric Association's *Diagnostic and Statistical Manual of Mental Disorder* (DSM-IV).
- Complications associated with AN can affect virtually every physiologic organ system.
- A particularly dangerous practice is the repeated induction of vomiting with syrup of ipecac. Chronic absorption of ipecac can lead to potentially fatal cardiac, GI, and neuromuscular toxicity.
- The treatments of AN and bulimia require a multidisciplinary approach, often incorporating psychotherapy and pharmacotherapy. Psychotherapy is the mainstay of treatment for EDs and should not be replaced, overlooked, or downplayed when medication therapy is decided upon. In general, bulimia nervosa responds more favorably to medication therapy than does AN.
- Antidepressants, specifically SSRIs and TCAs, have been successful in the treatment of EDs and appear to provide symptomatic relief in patients who are not clinically depressed. Other pharmacotherapeutic modalities such as cyproheptadine, anticonvulsants, and opiate antagonists have also been studied.

REFERENCES

1. National Institutes of Health/National Heart, Lung, and Blood Institute. Clinical guidelines on the identification, evaluation, and treatment of overweight and obesity in adults: the evidence report. June 17, 1998:1–228. http://www.nhlbi.nih.gov/guidelines/obesity/ob_home.htm.
2. McGinnis JM, Foege WH. Actual causes of death in the United States. JAMA 270:2207–2212, 1993.
3. Flegal KM, Carroll MD, Kuczmarski RJ, et al. Overweight and obesity in the United States: prevalence and trends, 1960–1994. Int J Obes Relat Metab Disord 22:39–47, 1998.
4. Edwards KI. Obesity, anorexia, and bulimia. Med Clin North Am 77:899–910, 1993.
5. Update: prevalence of overweight among children, adolescents, and adults–1988–1994. MMWR Morb Mortal Wkly Rep 46:198–202, 1997.
6. Bray GA, Gray DS. Obesity. Part 1–pathogenesis. West J Med 149:429–441, 1988.
7. Tan T, Handford HA, Soldatos CR. Current therapy of eating disorders. II: obesity. Ration Drug Ther 18:1, 1984.
8. Foster DW. Gain and loss in weight. In: Isselbacher KJ, Braunwald E, Wilson JD, et al. Harrison's principles of internal medicine. 13th ed. New York: McGraw-Hill, 1994:222.
9. Anand BK. Nervous regulation of food intake. Physiol Rev 41:667–672, 1961.
10. Celesia GG, Archer CR, Chung HD. Hyperphagia and obesity, relationship to medial hypothalamic lesions. JAMA 246:151–153, 1981.
11. Schacter S. Obesity and eating: internal and external values differentially affect the eating behavior of obese and normal subjects. Science 161:751–756, 1968.
12. Knittle JL, Timmers K, Ginsberg-Fellner F, et al. The growth of adipose tissue in children and adolescents. J Clin Invest 63:239–246, 1979.
13. Stunkard A, Rush J. Dieting and depression reexamined–a critical review of reports of untoward responses during weight reduction for obesity. Ann Intern Med 81:526–533, 1974.
14. Guo SS, Roche AF, Chumlea WC, et al. The predictive value of childhood body mass index values for overweight at age 35 years. Am J Clin Nutr 59:810–819, 1994.
15. Price RA, Cadoret RJ, Stunkard AJ, et al. Genetic contributions to human fatness: an adoption study. Am J Psychiatry 144:1003–1008, 1987.
16. Stunkard AJ, Foch TT, Hrubec A. A twin study of human obesity. JAMA 256:51–54, 1986.
17. Danowski TS. The management of obesity. Hosp Pract 11(April):39–46, 1976.
18. Bondy PK. Metabolic obesity? N Engl J Med 303:1057–1058, 1980.
19. Newsholme EA. A possible metabolic basis for the control of body weight. N Engl J Med 302:400–405, 1980.
20. Abrams B, Parker J. Overweight and pregnancy complications. Int J Obes 12:293–303, 1988.
21. Naeye RL. Maternal body weight and pregnancy outcome. Am J Clin Nutr 52:273–279, 1990.
22. Skertis I, Lesar T, Zaske DE, et al. Effect of obesity on gentamicin pharmacokinetics. J Clin Pharmacol 21:288–293, 1981.
23. Cheymol G. Clinical pharmacokinetics of drugs in obesity. An update. Clin Pharmacokinet 25:103:114, 1993.
24. Wolf AM, Colditz GA. The cost of obesity: the U.S. perspective. Pharmacoeconomics 5:34–37, 1994.
25. National Task Force on the Prevention and Treatment of Obesity: Long-term pharmacotherapy in the management of obesity. JAMA 276:1907–1915, 1996.
26. Obesity: preventing and managing the global epidemic. Report of the WHO Consultation of Obesity. Geneva: World Health Organization, June 3–5, 1997.
27. Van Itallie TB, Yang M. Diet and weight loss. N Engl J Med 197:1158–1161, 1977.
28. Mazel J. The Beverly Hills diet. New York: Macmillan, 1981.
29. Mirkin GB, Shore RN. The Beverly Hills diet: dangers of the newest weight loss fad. JAMA 246:2235–2237, 1981.
30. Protein diets. FDA Drug Bull 8:2, 1978.
31. Wadden TA, Stunkard AJ, Brownell KD, et al. The Cambridge diet–more mayhem? JAMA 250:2833–2834, 1983.
32. National Task Force on the Prevention and Treatment of Obesity. Very low-calorie diets. JAMA 270:967–974, 1993.
33. Cerulli J, Lomaestro BM, Malone M. Update on the pharmacotherapy of obesity. Ann Pharmacother 32:88–102, 1998.
34. Leibel RL, Rosenbaum M, Hirsch J. Changes in energy expenditure resulting from altered body weight. N Engl J Med 332:621–628, 1995.
35. NIH Consensus Conference. Physical activity and cardiovascular health. JAMA 276:241–246, 1996.
36. Franklin BA, Rubenfire M. Losing weight through exercise. JAMA 244:377–379, 1980.
37. Aronne LJ. Obesity. Med Clin North Am 82:161–181, 1998.
38. Bray GA, Gray DS. Obesity. Part II–treatment. West J Med 149:555–571, 1988.
39. Scovill BA. Review of amphetamine-like drugs by the Food and Drug Administration: clinical data and value judgments. In: Bray GA, ed. Obesity in perspective. Washington, DC: US Government Printing Office, 1976: 441–443.

40. Craighead LW, Stunkard AJ, O'Brien RM. Behavior therapy and pharmacotherapy for obesity. Arch Gen Psychiatry 38:763–768, 1981.
41. Weintraub M. Long term weight control: The National Heart, Lung, and Blood Institute funded multimodal intervention study. Clin Pharmacol Ther 51(Suppl):581–633, 1992.
42. Guy-Grand B, Apfelbaum M, Crepaldi G, et al. International trial of long term dexfenfluramine in obesity. Lancet 2:1142–1144, 1989.
43. Connolly HM, Crary JL, McGoon MD, et al. Valvular heart disease associated with fenfluramine-phentermine. N Engl J Med 337:581–588, 1997.
44. Blackburn GL, Miller D, Chan S. Pharmaceutical treatment of obesity. Nurs Clin North Am 32:831–848, 1997.
45. The Green Sheet. Dec. 5, 1977.
46. Bray GA. Use and abuse of appetite suppressant drugs in the treatment of obesity. Ann Intern Med 119(Part 2):707–713, 1993.
47. Hendy MS, Dove AF, Arblaster PG. Mazindol-induced lithium toxicity. Br Med J 280:684–685, 1980.
48. Milkovich R, van den Berg BJ. Effects of antenatal exposure to anorectic drugs. Am J Obstet Gynecol 129:637–642, 1977.
49. Drug facts and comparisons. Loose-leaf ed. St Louis: Facts and Comparisons, 1999.
50. Bray GA. Drug treatment of obesity. Am J Clin Nutr 55(Suppl 2):538S–544S, 1992.
51. Astrup A, Toubro S, Cannon S, et al. Thermogenic synergism between ephedrine and caffeine in healthy volunteers. A double blind placebo controlled study. Metabolism 40:323–329, 1991.
52. Greenway FL. Surgery for obesity. Endocrinol Metab Clin North Am 25:1005–1027, 1996.
53. Bruce RM, Wise L. Tuberculosis after jejunoileal bypass for obesity. Ann Intern Med 87:574–576, 1977.
54. Grant KE, Chandler RM, Castle AL, et al. Chromium and exercise training: effect on obese women. Med Sci Sports Exerc 29:992–998, 1997.
55. Wasser WG, Feldman NS, D'Agati VD. Chronic renal failure after ingestion of over-the-counter chromium picolinate. Ann Intern Med 126:410, 1997.
56. Astrup A, Toubro S, Christensen NJ, et al. Pharmacology of thermogenic drugs. Am J Clin Nutr 55(Suppl):246S–824S, 1992.
57. Clement K, Vaisse C, Manning BSJ, et al. Genetic variation in the β_3-adrenergic receptor and an increased capacity to gain weight in patients with morbid obesity. N Engl J Med 333:352–354, 1995.
58. Wilding J. Science, medicine, and the future of obesity treatment. Br Med J 315:997–1000, 1997.
59. Zhang Y, Proenca R, Maffei M, et al. Positional cloning of the mouse *obese* gene and its human homologue. Nature 372:425–432, 1994.
60. Beresin EV. Anorexia nervosa. Compr Ther 23:664–671, 1997.
61. Mehler PS, Gray MC, Schulte M. Medical complications of anorexia nervosa. J Womens Health 6:533–541, 1997.
62. Weltzin TE, Fernstrom MH, Kaye WH. Serotonin and bulimia nervosa. Nutr Rev 52:399–408, 1994.
63. Muscari ME. Primary care of adolescents with bulimia nervosa. J Pediatr Health Care 10:17–25, 1996.
64. Newman MM, Halmi KA. The endocrinology of anorexia nervosa and bulimia nervosa. Neurol Clin 6:195, 1988.
65. Gidwani GP, Rome ES. Eating disorders. Clin Obstet Gynecol 40:601–615, 1997.
66. Walsh BT, Devlin MJ. The pharmacologic treatment of eating disorders. Psychiatr Clin N Am 15:149, 1992.
67. Brotman AW, Rigotti N, Herzog DB. Medical complications of eating disorders: outpatient evaluation and management. Compr Psychiatry 26:258, 1985.
68. Mickley D. Evaluating common eating disorders–ten questions to ask your patient. Female Patient 13:33, 1988.
69. Pope HG, Hudson JI, Yurgelun-Todd D, et al. Prevalence of anorexia nervosa and bulimia in three student populations. Int J Eat Disord 3:45, 1984.
70. Pope HG, Hudson JI, Yurgelun-Todd D. Anorexia nervosa and bulimia among 300 women shoppers. Am J Psychiatry 141:292, 1984.
71. Jimerson DC, Herzog DB, Brotman AW. Pharmacologic approaches in the treatment of eating disorders. Harv Rev Psychiatry 1:82–93, 1993.
72. American Psychiatric Association. Diagnostic and statistical manual of mental disorders. 4th ed revised. Washington, DC: American Psychiatric Association, 1994.
73. Russell G. Bulimia: an ominous variant of anorexia nervosa. Psychol Med 9:429, 1979.
74. Warren MP, Vande Weile RL. Clinical and metabolic features of anorexia nervosa. Am J Obstet Gynecol 117:435, 1975.
75. Giannini AJ, Newman M, Gold M. Anorexia and bulimia. Am Fam Physician 41:1169, 1990.
76. Weiner H. The physiology of eating disorders. Int J Eat Disord 4:347, 1985.
77. Herzog DB, Copeland PM. Eating disorders. N Engl J Med 313:295, 1985.
78. Seidensticker JF, Tzagournis M. Anorexia nervosa–clinical features and long term follow-up. J Chronic Dis 21:361, 1968.
79. Daluiski A, Rahbar B, Meals RA. Russell's sign: subtle hand changes in patients with bulimia nervosa. Clin Orthop 343:107–109, 1997.
80. Adler AG, Walinsky P, Krall RA, et al. Death resulting from ipecac syrup poisoning. JAMA 243:1927, 1980.
81. Mitchell JE, Davis L, Goff G. The process of relapse in patients with bulimia. Int J Eat Disord 4:457, 1985.
82. Mitchell PB. The pharmacological management of bulimia nervosa: a critical review. Int J Eat Disord 7:29, 1988.
83. Biederman J, Herzog DB, Rivinus T, et al. Urinary MHPG in anorexia nervosa patients with and without a major depressive disorder. J Psychiatr Res 18:149, 1984.
84. Fava M, Copeland PM, Schweiger U, et al. Neurochemical abnormalities of anorexia nervosa and bulimia nervosa. Am J Psychiatry 146:963, 1989.
85. Fichter MM, Leibl K, Rief W, et al. Fluoxetine versus placebo: a double-blind study with bulimic in patients undergoing intensive psychotherapy. Pharmacopsychiatry 24:1–7, 1991.
86. Fluoxetine Bulimia Nervosa Collaborative Study Group: Fluoxetine in the treatment of bulimia nervosa: a multicenter, placebo-controlled, double-blind trial. Arch Gen Psychiatry 49:139–147, 1992.
87. Marcus MD, Wing RR, Ewing L, et al. A double-blind, placebo-controlled trial of fluoxetine plus behavior modification in the treatment of obese binge-eaters and non-binge eaters. Am J Psychiatry 147:876–881, 1990.
88. Wolfe BE. Dimensions of response to antidepressant agents in bulimia nervosa: a review. Arch Psychiatr Nurs 9:111–121, 1995.
89. Beumont, PJV, Russell JD, Touyz SW. Treatment of anorexia nervosa. Lancet 341:1635–1640, 1993.
90. Pope HG Jr, Hudson JI, Jonas JM, et al. Bulimia treated with imipramine: a placebo-controlled, double-blind study. Am J Psychiatry 140:554, 1983.
91. Mitchell JE, Groat R. A placebo-controlled, double-blind trial of amitriptyline in bulimia. J Clin Psychopharmacol 4:186, 1984.
92. Walsh BT, Stewart JW, Roose SP, et al. Treatment of bulimia with phenelzine; a double-blind, placebo-controlled study. Arch Gen Psychiatry 41:1105, 1984.
93. Wold P. Trazodone in the treatment of bulimia. J Clin Psychiatry 44:275, 1983.
94. Pope HG, Hudson JI, Jonas JM. Antidepressant treatment of bulimia: preliminary experience and practical recommendations. J Clin Psychopharmacol 3:274, 1983.
95. Carson SW. Bupropion, is it here to stay? DICP Ann Pharmacother 23:704, 1989.
96. Halmi KA, Eckert E, LaDu TJ, et al. Anorexia nervosa: treatment efficacy of cyproheptadine and amitriptyline. Arch Gen Psychiatry 43:177, 1986.
97. Wermuth BM, Davis KL, Hollister LE, et al. Phenytoin treatment of the binge-eating syndrome. Am J Psychiatry 134:1249, 1977.
98. Kaplan AS, Garfinkle PE, Darby PL, et al. Carbamazepine in the treatment of bulimia. Am J Psychiatry 140:1225, 1983.
99. Herridge PL, Pope HG Jr: Treatment of bulimia and rapid cycling bipolar disorder with sodium valproate: a case report. J Clin Psychopharmacol 5:229, 1985.
100. Moore SL, Rakes SM. Binge eating–therapeutic response to diphenylhydantoin: case report. J Clin Psychiatry 43:385, 1982.
101. Crow SJ, Mitchell JE. Integrating cognitive therapy and medications in treating bulimia nervosa. Psychiatr Clin North Am 19:755–760, 1996.
102. Woodside DB. A review of anorexia nervosa and bulimia nervosa. Curr Probl Pediatr 25:67–89, 1995.

CHAPTER 61

ALCOHOLISM

Jerry R. Phipps Jr., Jeffrey N. Baldwin, and Theodore G. Tong

DEFINITION

Alcoholism is a primary, chronic disease with genetic, psychosocial, and environmental factors influencing its development and manifestations. Alcoholism is often progressive and fatal and characterized by continuous or periodic impaired control over drinking, preoccupation with the drug alcohol, use of alcohol despite adverse consequences, and distortions in thinking, most notably denial.[1]

Alcohol abuse involves persistent patterns of heavy alcohol consumption with associated health or social consequences. Alcoholism is differentiated from abuse by the presence of craving, tolerance, and physical dependence, which result in behavioral changes and loss of control over drinking. Persons who are alcoholic experience both psychologic and physical dependency and tolerance. Psychologic dependency is perhaps the single most important factor and involves the compulsive use of and craving for a drug. Physical dependency is characterized by a series of physiologic events that occur when the drug is discontinued, including the withdrawal or abstinence syndrome. Tolerance develops when the continued use of a drug is required and increasing doses are needed to produce the same effect.

Although the most important feature of addictive disorders is the psychologic dependency, it is the least understood. A person may be made physically dependent on alcohol, but abuse may not be recognized or diagnosed as such until behavioral effects secondary to psychologic dependence are present. Many persons consume alcoholic beverages but relatively few develop physical and psychologic dependency on the drug. A commonly held belief is that if someone does not drink daily or only drinks alcoholic beverages with relatively low alcohol content, such as wine or beer, they cannot be alcoholic. The quantity, type, and frequency of alcohol consumption are relatively unimportant; loss of control over consumption once initiated and continued use despite clear evidence of adverse consequences (social, physical, or legal) are more important in the diagnosis of alcoholism.

TREATMENT GOALS: ALCOHOLISM

- Address treatment of alcohol abuse and alcoholism both acutely and chronically.
- Established treatment goals jointly with the patient.
- Maintain and support vital functions in patients with acute alcohol intoxication.
- Convert the acutely agitated and alcohol-impaired patient with toxic psychosis symptoms to a calm, but arousable and responsive patient using drug therapy.
- Rule out alternative causes of intoxication in the unconscious patient, including hypoglycemia, physical injury, and other drugs.
- Avoid pharmacologic attempts to accelerate the metabolism or clearance of alcohol from the body of the intoxicated patient.
- Ensure withdrawal and detoxification of ethanol followed by subsequent interventions to maintain abstinence.
- Ensure detoxification from alcohol by substitution with and slow withdrawing of a longer-acting sedative-hypnotic medication.

- Individualize patient-specific drug regimens and doses in treatment of acute alcohol withdrawal with consideration given to underlying conditions and concurrent polydrug abuse.
- Use nonpharmacologic factors to enhance the treatment of many clinical problems that accompany the acute detoxification from alcohol process.
- Encourage patient motivation to stop drinking and participation in recovery support programs.

EPIDEMIOLOGY

Alcohol is the most misused drug in the United States today. Approximately 10% of American adults and 3% of adolescents in the United States are addicted to alcohol or other drugs.[2] Moreover, of the 100 million adult Americans who use alcohol, 10 to 15% are estimated to be alcoholic.[3] This rate increases to 30 to 50% when close relatives are alcoholic.[4] Alcoholism is one of America's major health problems, contributing to 100,000 deaths annually, making it the third leading cause of preventable mortality in the United States, after tobacco and diet/activity patterns.[5] In two separate evaluations, men consuming either two or three drinks daily had an increased mortality.[6,7] Moreover, women who drank more than 2.5 alcoholic drinks per day had increased mortality.[8]

Alcoholism is a condition far more common than generally perceived, with only 3 to 5% of the country's alcoholic population classified as the "skid row" or public inebriate type. Alcoholics come from all levels of our society; the majority are found in the working and homemaking population. However, within industrialized countries the prevalence of excessive drinking is higher among men from lower socioeconomic groups whereas women do not have a direct relationship from socioeconomic standing with alcohol consumption.[9] The largest percentage of American alcoholics is between the ages of 35 and 50 years. Professionals and business people have high rates of alcohol consumption and alcoholism. Alcohol use in the younger school-aged population and "problem drinking" among women have increased and appear to be continuing trends.[10,11] Although the prevalence of alcohol misuse among older adults is lower, detection of the problem is difficult, and it is often unrecognized. Vulnerability of the older alcoholic to the harmful effects of alcohol is much greater.[12]

Alcoholism is an illness that can shorten one's life span considerably; it has an impact on our entire society. About 40% of medical and surgery patients have an alcohol-related problem, and 15% of the total national health expenditure for hospital care is spent on alcohol-related illness.[13,14] In a 1996 analysis on the prevalence of alcohol involvement in crime, alcohol was involved in 40% of all traffic fatalities and homicides as well as 30% of sexual assaults.[15]

Alcoholism is a treatable illness when diagnosed in its early stages. However, death rates from alcohol abuse in the major-risk age groups, such as young men, are more than twice those for the general population. Unfortunately, there is a serious deficit of accessible and high-quality alcoholism treatment services because the majority of the services available are designed to deal with only the later stages of alcoholism. Alcoholism, like other diseases such as hypertension and diabetes mellitus, can be considered a biologic disease with a genetic predisposition, which is activated by environmental factors.[16,17] Thus, a "biopsychosocial" approach is usually used in the identification, treatment, and ongoing recovery support systems for alcoholics. Difficulty in differentiating between alcohol abuse and alcoholism (alcohol dependence) may be cited by some as a reason for questioning the disease concept. However, other diseases such as hypertension may be equally difficult to define when borderline. A telephone survey found that about 89% of the surveyed population considered alcoholics to be ill, yet 47% also felt that the alcoholic person was morally weak.[18] This reveals a fairly strong public sentiment that alcoholism represents "willful misconduct" and is an important societal impediment in the identification and treatment of the disease.

In 1951, Amark first introduced the theory of genetic transmission of alcoholism. Ever since there have been numerous reports supporting this theory. Male relatives of alcoholics have a 25% prevalence rate of alcoholism compared to the population prevalence of approximately 5%. Female relatives of alcoholics are 50 times more likely to be alcoholics than their peers without alcoholic relatives.[19,20] In addition, there have been several studies in twins that support a genetic link in alcoholism by finding that monozygotic twins have higher rates of alcoholism than dizygotic twins. Moreover, sons of alcoholic biologic parents adopted at birth were four times more likely to become alcoholics than were sons of nonalcoholic fathers.[21]

PATHOPHYSIOLOGY

Alcohol is a psychoactive agent that can be characterized pharmacologically as a sedative-hypnotic drug. At low doses, the action of alcohol is an excitatory and stimulatory effect as a result of its depression of inhibitory centers in the brain. In a dose-response relationship, at sufficient doses, alcohol produces a depressant action. Although alcohol is able to provide relief of anxiety and sedation at one dose level, it produces sleep and depression of the central nervous system and respiratory system at higher levels.

Alcohol is present in a variety of popular beverages: beer and ale are products of the fermentation of cereal grains and contain 3 to 6% alcohol; wine results from the fermentation of yeast on sugars present in fruits and contains 11 to 20% alcohol; brandy is produced from the distillation of wine products and usually contains 40% alcohol; hard liquors are the distillates of fermented products such as grain and are available as gin, rye, bourbon, scotch, and vodka and contain approximately 40 to 50% alcohol. Hard liquors are commonly labeled with a proof number that is twice the alcohol concentration by volume. Nonalcoholic ("N.A.") beers and wines rarely are alcohol free; they often contain up to 1% alcohol.

Alcohol is efficiently and rapidly absorbed by the stomach and small intestine in 30 to 120 minutes after ingestion. Absorption is direct and complete by simple (passive) diffusion; alcohol distributes freely in body tissues and fluids. Its volume of distribution ranges from 0.58 to 0.70 L/kg of body weight. The concentration of alcohol in the brain rapidly approaches that in the blood.

Factors that modify alcohol absorption are volume, dilution, rate of ingestion, and presence of food in the stomach. Protein and water both slow absorption of alcohol whereas carbonation facilitates it. The level of gastric alcohol dehydrogenase (ADH), which is involved in gastric metabolism of alcohol, is about 80% higher in nonalcoholic males than females, whereas chronic alcoholism results in a decrease of about 40% in men and 15% in women. This may help to explain why blood alcohol levels in females, corrected for size, are relatively higher than in males and may partially explain the greater susceptibility to and early onset of liver and brain damage in female alcoholics.[22] Alcohol crosses the placenta and may be found in the milk of lactating mothers.

The liver is the main site of the first step in the oxidation of ethyl alcohol. Ethanol is oxidized by ADH to acetaldehyde, which subsequently is oxidized by acetaldehyde dehydrogenase to acetate. These reactions convert nicotinamide adenine dinucleotide (NAD) to reduced NAD (NADH). Excess NADH causes metabolic disorders such as hyperlactacidemia, hyperuricemia, hypoglycemia, and hyperlipidemia.[23] Acetaldehyde inhibits repair of alkylated nucleoproteins, reduces mitochondrial oxygen use, and promotes cell death by depletion of reduced glutathione, increasing lipid peroxidation, and increasing toxic effects of free radicals.[24–26] Long-term consumption of alcohol induces the microsomal ethanol-oxidizing system (MEOS), particularly cytochrome P-4502E1.[27] This induction contributes to metabolic tolerance to alcohol in alcoholics and increases the metabolism of a number of drugs, such as pentobarbital, propranolol, warfarin, and diazepam.[23] Unfortunately, cytochrome P-4502E1 converts many foreign substances into highly toxic metabolites; most notable among these are cocaine and acetaminophen. Therapeutic amounts (e.g., 2.5 to 4 g/day) of acetaminophen can cause hepatic injury in alcoholics.[24] Conversely, short-term use of alcohol may inhibit metabolism of such drugs by direct competition for cytochrome P-4502E1.[23]

Although most drugs are known to be metabolized or cleared from the body in a fixed percentage ("first-order") of the dose taken, alcohol is unique in that nonlinear or saturation elimination kinetics is followed, and, therefore, it is removed from the blood in a fixed amount ("zero order") over time. Most of the ingested dose of alcohol is eliminated by liver metabolism. In a 70-kg (approximately 150-lb) person, the rate of alcohol metabolism is approximately 7 g/hr. At this rate of metabolism, the blood alcohol level will decline at a rate of nearly 15 mg/100 ml/hr. An average "shot" of distilled spirit, 86 proof, contains about 15 g of ethyl alcohol; because body water is approximately 65% of body weight in a 70-kg person, the blood ethyl alcohol content after one shot will be 15 g/50 L, or 30 mg/dL, with 50 L being the approximate volume of total body water calculated from the percentage of weight. If taken in one swallow, it will take approximately 2 hours for the blood ethyl alcohol level to return to zero. Within 1 hour after drinking any of the following: five 12-oz cans of beer, four 4-oz glasses of table wine, five 1-oz glasses of liqueur, five 1-oz shots of distilled spirits, or three 3-oz martinis, a 70-kg person would have a blood ethanol concentration of 100 mg/dL (the amount legally defined as intoxication in many states; some now use 50 to 80 mg/dL). There is, however, wide variability observed in individual ethanol metabolism, so blood ethanol concentrations may vary considerably among persons who consume these amounts. Ethanol elimination by the kidneys and lungs and through sweat is minimal with approximately 2 to 10% cleared by these routes depending on the amount of alcohol ingested.

Alcohol affects almost every organ system in the body. The more important and known medical complications and pathologic consequences from excessive alcohol consumption are summarized in Table 61.1.[28]

Cardiovascular System

Cardiac dysfunction may account for up to 50% of the difference between normal death rates and those in alcohol-abusing or alcohol-dependent persons. Alcohol may serve as the primary cause of as many as 24% of cases of hypertension. Blood pressure elevation occurs with acute intoxication and often parallels the severity of alcoholism with chronic use. Modest to moderate consumption of alcohol (up to two drinks per day) may reduce the risk for myocardial infarction and death, possibly by increasing the level of high-density lipoprotein cholesterol and antithrombotic activity.[41–43] Although there seems to be little doubt that alcohol can exert a protective effect against coronary heart disease, consumption of well beyond two drinks per day is associated with an increasing occurrence of coronary heart disease. Along with cigarette smoking, chronic excessive drinkers are at higher risk for hypertension, ischemic heart disease, and stroke.

Recognition of alcoholic cardiomyopathy has been made difficult by its similarity to two other types of alcohol-related cardiomyopathies.[29,30] Nutritional deficiency in thiamine can lead to an unusual type of cardiac disorder ("wet beriberi heart disease"), which is characterized by a state of high output failure, fluid retention, and cardiac dilatation. Another cause of cardiomyopathy has

Table 61.1 ▪ Complications of Alcoholism

Complication	Usual Onset	Comments
Increased morbidity and mortality	Chronic	Most common causes are cirrhosis, cancers of respiratory and gastrointestinal tracts, accidents, suicide, and ischemic heart disease.
Fluid and electrolyte abnormalities	Acute	Alcohol has diuretic action as blood alcohol concentration increases. Stable or decreasing blood alcohol concentrations result in antidiuresis. Hyperosmolarity, hypokalemia, hypophosphatemia, and hypomagnesemia are common. Mild lactic acidemia may contribute to asymptomatic elevation of uric acid owing to interference with renal secretion of uric acid.
Hypoglycemia	Acute or chronic	Alcohol depletes liver glycogen stores and decreases gluconeogenesis; blood glucose may drop precipitously. Stupor and coma, apart from the direct effects of alcohol on the nervous system, are experienced. This is a dramatic but relatively uncommon complication.
Hyperglycemia	Acute	During early phases of alcohol withdrawal, blood glucose may be elevated because of increased release of catecholamines. Alcoholic pancreatitis and decreased peripheral glucose use are contributing factors.
Hyperketonemia	Acute	Alcoholic patients often develop hyperketonemia and metabolic acidosis in the absence of hyperglycemia. Often the patient is hypoglycemic and without glycosuria. This is presumably caused by alcohol-induced starvation ketosis. Insulin is not administered.
Hypothermia	Acute	Occurs often as a result of prolonged exposure to cold (not uncommon in unconscious or stuporous state); pancreatitis and meningitis may also contribute.
Liver disease		Best known sequela of chronic alcoholism and a leading cause of morbidity. Three common liver diseases are often associated with alcoholism: acute fatty liver, alcoholic hepatitis, and alcoholic cirrhosis. Individual sensitivity is variable and the degree of liver dysfunction does not appear to be related only to the amount of alcohol ingested. Nutritional status, genetic composition, and immunologic factors appear to interact in the development of alcoholic liver disease.
Acute fatty liver	Acute	Develops in nearly all who ingest alcohol excessively (defined by some as an intake of at least 70 g of ethyl alcohol daily) even for only a few days. Treatment: stop drinking and give a diet with adequate vitamin and protein replacement.
Alcoholic hepatitis	Acute or chronic	Apparently a toxic inflammatory response of the liver in 10–30% of chronic or acute alcoholics. A high percentage of those with alcoholic hepatitis who continue to drink develop cirrhosis within 5–10 years. Most patients require 8–12 weeks to show improvement from the acute stage. Treatment is supportive: an adequate diet, vitamin supplements, bed rest, and stopping drinking. In severe cases, liver failure (hepatic coma), variceal bleeding, and hepatorenal syndrome often are present. Clinical features are similar to those of other forms of toxic or viral liver injury. Hepatomegaly, jaundice, splenomegaly, fever, and ascites are common. Corticosteroids may be of benefit in fulminant cases, but their exact role in treatment of this disorder is still being investigated. Some studies have failed to show any benefit from their use.
Alcoholic or Laennec's cirrhosis	Chronic	Symptoms are often nonspecific in character, e.g., fatigue, weight loss, lethargy. Other physical signs include slight hepatomegaly, splenomegaly, ascites, gynecomastia, spider angiomas, and palmar erythema. About 10–30% of alcoholics develop alcoholic cirrhosis, usually after drinking heavily for 10–15 years. The three most common causes of death with alcoholic cirrhosis are bleeding esophageal varices, liver failure (encephalopathy and coma), and infection. The only treatment is to stop drinking or seek a liver transplant.
Portal hypertension	Acute or chronic	A sequela of hepatitis. Return of blood from abdominal viscera to the heart is impaired as pressure rises and collateral blood vessels enlarge. All abdominal organs become congested; splenomegaly and ascites result.
Ascites	Acute or chronic	Seen often in patients with portal hypertension and may be worsened by alcoholic liver disease and a low serum albumin level. A low sodium diet, spironolactone, and sometimes diuretics are helpful. As liver disease improves, ascites often resolves. Careful monitoring of electrolytes must be done when diuretics and aldosterone antagonists are used.

(continued)

Table 61.1 *(continued)*

Complication	Usual Onset	Comments
Esophageal varices	Acute	These thin-walled, collateral blood vessels of the portal system are prone to hemorrhaging. Hemorrhage usually occurs when the portal pressure rises because of expanded plasma volume, worsening liver involvement, or increased intraabdominal pressure. Thin walls and accompanying esophagitis are also contributing causes.
Encephalopathy	Acute	The central nervous system is depressed by toxins, e.g., ammonia that reaches it through shunted blood that has bypassed liver. The patient is usually lethargic, has "flapping tremor" and deterioration of fine movement, and is unable to perform any purposeful activity before lapsing into coma. The central nervous system is more sensitive than usual to anoxia, sedative-hypnotics, opiates, or tranquilizers. Coma is often precipitated by gastrointestinal hemorrhage, hypokalemia, infection, or large amounts of nitrogen from dietary sources such as proteins.
Gastrointestinal problems, e.g., pancreatitis, gastritis, peptic ulcer	Acute or chronic	Acute pancreatitis occurs more commonly in alcoholics and is most often seen in persons who have been drinking heavily for 8–10 years or more. Often no characteristic clinical picture except for abdominal pain is present. Nausea and vomiting are common. It is one of the more frequent causes for hospitalization of alcoholics after a drinking bout. Other manifestations of this condition include shock, hypocalcemia, hyperglycemia, marked fluid loss, or dehydration. Acute gastritis, often hemorrhagic, is common in alcoholics and is worsened by the chronic use of aspirin. The incidence of peptic ulcer is probably higher in alcoholics than in nonalcoholics. Tearing of the gastroesophageal mucosa (Mallory-Weiss syndrome) with severe bleeding may occur as consequence of vomiting; this should be considered a medical and surgical emergency.
Malabsorption	Chronic	Changes in gastrointestinal morphology and decreased enzyme activity in the intestinal tract have been observed in chronic alcoholic patients, even with an adequate diet. Thiamine, vitamin B_{12}, folate, xylose, iron, and fat malabsorption occur. Alcohol consumption and poor diet are major contributors to malabsorption.
Hyperlipidemia	Acute or chronic	Alcohol ingestion induces an elevation of serum triglycerides in persons with type IV hyperlipoproteinemia. Because alcoholic liver disease begins with fatty infiltrates, hypertriglyceridemia may be an early contributory factor to the hepatic and cardiac disorders from alcohol.
Cardiomyopathies	Acute or chronic	Alcohol presumably affects the heart by depressing ventricular activity, reducing myocardial uptake of free fatty acids, enhancing uptake of triglycerides, and causing myocardial cell injury. Direct toxic effects of alcohol on the myocardium, multiple vitamin deficiencies, inadequate protein intake, and electrolyte disturbances are all contributory.
Myopathy	Acute or chronic	Generalized and occasionally focal muscle weakness develops during or after a heavy drinking bout. Muscle edema, pain, and cramps are common and may be accompanied by tenderness and edema. Elevated muscle enzymes (creatine phosphokinase and aldolase) may be present. In severe cases, myoglobulinuria can occur. Mortality is high (50%) when alcoholic myopathy occurs concomitantly with hyperkalemia and renal failure.
Infection	Acute or chronic	Acute and chronic alcohol ingestion decreases resistance to bacterial infection, especially in the respiratory tract. Most pulmonary infections in alcoholics are caused by *Pneumococcus*. Susceptibility to *Klebsiella* and *Haemophilus* organisms is also greater. Because they are debilitated, alcoholics have a higher risk of reactivated tuberculosis; it has been claimed that 20% of patients with active tuberculosis are alcoholics. Aspiration pneumonia is also a major complication. Absence of elevation of white blood cell counts or temperature should not preclude the possibility of infections in an alcoholic.
Hematologic disorders, e.g., anemia, leukopenia, thrombocytopenia	Chronic	Four major factors contribute to hematologic disorders: poor diet, blood loss, liver disease, and alcohol itself. Folate deficiency is probably the most important hematologic abnormality in alcoholics. Good diet alone cannot protect against the bone marrow toxicity of alcohol if a major portion of calories are ingested as ethanol. Stopping of alcohol, a nutritious diet including folic acid and multivitamins, and treatment of other medical complications nearly always reverse hematologic abnormalities.

(continued)

Table 61.1 *(continued)*

Complication	Usual Onset	Comments
Neurologic disorders, polyneuropathy	Chronic	A degenerative process of nerve and brain tissues secondary to nutritional deficiency is common with a long history of alcoholism. Clinical and pathologic features of polyneuropathy are almost identical with those of beriberi. Subjective sensory disturbances and loss of reflexes and motor activity occur. Recovery is slow and often incomplete, even with complete alcohol abstinence.
Wernicke's disease	Acute or chronic	The clinical presentation includes ocular disturbances (e.g., nystagmus), muscle weakness or paralysis, diplopia, ataxia, disorientation, and confusion often accompanying signs of thiamine deficiency. It can be treated by thiamine.
Korsakoff's psychosis	Acute or chronic	More apparent disturbances in this disorder are cognitive defect and personality changes. Memory may be affected to exclusion of other components of mental function. Recent memory is affected the most. Other clinical features often are confusion and confabulation. Recovery is slow and usually incomplete, despite treatment with thiamine and other vitamins and cessation of drinking.
Amblyopia	Chronic	A disorder of the optic nerve occurring alone or in conjunction with other neuropathies, manifested by blurred vision.
Skin disorders	Chronic	Skin disorders are common (30–50%) in alcoholic patients and can result from vitamin deficiency diseases such as scurvy or pellagra. Neglected skin disorders often result in secondary infections; seborrhea, lacerations, abrasions, acne, scabies, and pediculosis are also frequent. When common skin conditions (e.g., psoriasis, eczema) are not responding to the usual treatment measures, alcoholism may play a role.
Teratogenesis	Chronic	Multiple congenital defects, prenatal growth retardation, and delay in development are fetal abnormalities that result from heavy alcohol abuse during pregnancy.
Neonatal intoxication and withdrawal	Chronic	Ethanol crosses the placental barrier freely. The clearance rate of alcohol is reduced in premature infants. Substantial impairment of motor activity, alertness, and respiration are reported in neonates after ethanol infusion just before delivery.
Sexual impotence, loss of libido	Chronic	Experienced often by male alcoholics. Endocrine effects of alcohol, characteristics of hypogonadism (i.e., gynecomastia), loss of facial hair, spider angiomata, and testicular atrophy, and testosterone deficiency are seen.
Cancer	Chronic	Excessive use of alcohol combined with tobacco has been implicated in greater risks for cancers, particularly of the head, neck, mouth, pharynx, larynx, esophagus, and liver. Alcohol may activate cocarcinogens through induction of cytochrome P-4502E1.

Source: References 26, 28–40.

been associated with excessive consumption of beer containing cobalt, an added foaming agent. There are patients with a history of alcoholism who have heart disease that is unrelated to either of these possible causes. Evidence that alcohol is metabolized in the heart to fatty acid ethyl esters, which interfere with mitochondrial function to cause cardiomyopathy, have been suggested. With continued abstinence, alcohol-induced cardiomyopathy may be reversible in some patients.[44,45]

Hematopoietic System

The association of anemia, macrocytosis, and alcoholism was long held to be attributable to nutritional deficiencies. Studies have shown that there is a direct role of alcohol on suppression of folate metabolism, depletion of folate from body stores, and malabsorption of folate. The direct toxicity of alcohol on erythropoiesis is demonstrated by vacuolation of erythroid and myeloid precursors.[31,32] A sideroblastic or "iron-loading" anemia can result from the impairment by alcohol of iron incorporation and metabolism in the red blood cell. Alcohol affects iron absorption by increasing jejunal absorption of iron, as reflected in hemochromatosis and a rise in serum iron levels. Iron deficiency anemia due to gastritis and to gastrointestinal bleeding also can occur. Alcoholic thrombocytopenia occurs in 25 to 30% of acutely ill alcoholics; platelets often have shorter than normal life spans, and thrombopoiesis is ineffective because of marrow suppression and folate deficiency.

Hepatic System

There are three distinct histologic patterns of alcohol-induced liver disease. All three may coexist simultaneously and do not represent a single progression. Cirrhosis may occur in the absence of prior hepatitis.[46] The risk of developing alcoholic liver disease is related to the quantity and duration of alcohol consumption. Factors such as genetics, nutritional state, and environment also predispose to the development of alcoholic liver disease.[33] Alcoholic "fatty liver" disease is the most common alcohol-induced hepatic abnormality, occurring in 90 to 100% of chronic alcoholics.

The postulated mechanism for fatty accumulation in the liver is that an increase in the NADH:NAD ratio during ethanol oxidation is responsible for accumulation of hepatic triglycerides. Uncomplicated fatty liver disease is usually asymptomatic or presents as nausea, vomiting, and right upper quadrant abdominal pain, rarely presenting with the usual signs of liver disease such as ascites, jaundice, or splenomegaly. Mild, usually reversible, elevation of liver enzymes is the most frequent laboratory finding. Not as relatively benign as once believed, fatty liver disease can progress to liver failure and occasionally death.

Alcoholic hepatitis is a much more serious disorder; 10 to 30% of alcoholics develop this complication, usually after years of excessive drinking or after an abrupt increase in alcohol intake. Liver injury results from the degenerative effects of alcohol on subcellular structures. The clinical course of alcoholic hepatitis ranges from acute or chronic asymptomatic, mild, severe, and fulminant forms. It is often an incidental diagnosis when hepatomegaly and mild elevations in liver function study results are detected during a physical examination. Some patients who develop the fulminant course will rapidly develop liver failure. The death rate in patients with severe alcoholic hepatitis is substantial.

The pathogenesis of alcoholic cirrhosis has not been determined completely. Although approximately half of the survivors from alcoholic hepatitis subsequently experience cirrhosis of the liver, this condition may develop in the absence of any previously documented hepatitis. The liver is characterized as being finely nodular or grossly deformed, which may be smaller or larger than normal. Laboratory findings include hyperbilirubinemia, hypoalbuminemia, and prolonged prothrombin time. Complications from cirrhosis include encephalopathy, portal hypertension with bleeding at the esophageal varices, portal vein thrombosis, and hepatorenal syndrome.

CLINICAL PRESENTATION AND DIAGNOSIS

Signs and Symptoms

Acute Alcohol Intoxication

The relationship between blood ethyl alcohol concentration and clinical signs and symptoms of intoxication are variable and depend on the rate of ingestion, amount consumed, alterations in absorption, metabolism, excretion, and chronicity of exposure (Table 61.2). The correlation of the blood alcohol concentration to behavioral effects has obvious important medical and legal importance. As a consequence of tolerance, higher blood alcohol concentrations may be required to produce clinical effects in alcoholics than in occasional drinkers. There are drinkers who exhibit such extreme degrees of tolerance to alcohol that they appear sober even with blood alcohol concentrations two to three times higher than the limit permitted by law for driving an automobile. The lethal blood alcohol level is variable but in the range of 400 to 700 mg/dL. The lethal level may be substantially lowered when opiates, neuroleptics, or other sedative-hypnotics are taken along with an excessive amount of alcohol.

Acute Intoxication from Alcohol Substitutes

Occasionally, alcohol substitutes such as methanol, ethylene glycol, isopropyl alcohol, or paraldehyde are ingested. Often the availability and low cost of products containing alcohol substitutes by comparison to alcoholic beverages, make it convenient for persons intent on drinking alcohol to seek out these products. Many of these products are readily found around the home; they are sweet smelling and pleasant tasting, often colorless, and appear innocuous enough to young children who might be attracted to them. Many of these products are packaged in an attractive manner and not in child-resistant containers, thus contributing to risks of accidental ingestion. There are differences in the clinical manifestations after ingestion of these agents which distinguishes each (Table 61.3).

Methanol

After ingestion, methanol is rapidly absorbed and distributed throughout the total body water, similarly to ethanol. The toxic dose is extremely variable; as little as 4 mL has been reported to cause blindness, whereas no permanent impairment was demonstrated after an alleged 500 mL had been consumed. Methanol is metabolized by ADH enzymes in the liver to formaldehyde and formic acid. The rate of this process is independent of the dose and blood concentration and is approximately one-seventh the rate for ethanol metabolism. Formic acid accumulation is associated with the clinical symptoms experienced.

Methanol produces slight central nervous system depression; unlike ethanol, inebriation is not often observed. Optic nerve and retinal injury from the toxic metabolites develops within 12 to 24 hours after acute exposure. An

Table 61.2 ▪ Blood Ethanol Concentrations and Clinical Effects in the Nontolerant Adult Drinker

Blood Ethanol Level (mg/100 mL)	Clinical Effects
20–99	Slight changes in mood and feelings progressing to muscular incoordination, impaired sensory function, personality and behavioral changes (talkative, noisy, morose)
100–199	Marked mental impairment, incoordination, clumsiness and unsteadiness in standing or walking, ataxia, prolonged reaction time, gross intoxication
200–299	Nausea, vomiting, diplopia, marked ataxia
300–399	Hypothermia, severe dysarthria, amnesia, stage 1 anesthesia
400–700	Coma, respiratory failure, and death

Table 61.3 ▪ Toxicities of Alcohol Substitutes

Substance	Sources	Signs and Symptoms	Management
Methanol (methyl alcohol "denatured alcohol")	Found in solvents, denaturant, antifreeze; toxic amounts attained through inhalation and ingestion	Intractable metabolic acidosis and optic nerve injury can result in 12–24 hr after ingestion. Toxic metabolites: formic acid and formaldehyde. Find both metabolites in urine.	Approximate lethal dose: 1–4 mL/kg in adult. Treat by administering intravenous ethanol to block the generation of toxic metabolites by alcohol dehydrogenase. Administer sodium bicarbonate. Peritoneal dialysis and hemodialysis can be useful.
Isopropanol (isopropyl alcohol)	Found in rubbing alcohol, solvents; toxic amounts attained through inhalation and ingestion	Severe hypoglycemia, acidosis, and coma; hypothermia and convulsions also occur. Infants and children are at risk of hypoglycemia. Gastrointestinal irritant. Acetone on breath, in urine, and serum in absence of hyperglycemia or glycosuria.	Approximate lethal dose: 250 g for adult. Alkalinization to correct metabolic acidosis may be helpful. Manage primarily with support.
Ethylene glycol	Found in antifreeze	Clinical abnormalities of the central nervous and cardiopulmonary systems. Oxidation of ethylene glycol by alcohol dehydrogenase to oxalic acid and calcium oxalate, which precipitate in kidney. Oliguria and acute renal failure can occur.	Approximate lethal dose: 100 mg for adult. In children, much lower doses are associated with renal, cardiac, and central nervous system toxicity. Treat by administration of intravenous ethanol. Alkalinization to correct metabolic acidosis and to solubilize calcium oxalate is useful. Hemodialysis has been successful in removing ethylene glycol.

asymptomatic period of up to 1 day may follow acute methanol poisoning before the onset of headache, nausea, and vomiting. Severe abdominal pain, occasionally presumed mistakenly to be the result of ethanol-induced pancreatitis, is experienced. Central nervous system depression, coma, and respiratory failure take place late in the course. The breath odor of alcohol or methanol is often not present. In the later stages of the intoxication, the breath odor of formalin and Kussmaul respiration may be noticed. Visual disturbances occur. They range in severity from mild diminished vision to total blindness, very often accompanied by photophobia, pain, and conjunctival changes. Eye examination shows dilated, nonreactive pupils with optic disk hyperemia and retinal edema. The early recognition of the clinical presentation of acute methanol intoxication is commonly hampered by the effects of concomitant excessive ethanol ingestion.

Laboratory findings in acute methanol intoxication usually include metabolic acidosis, with a large anion gap and moderate ketonemia. The serum amylase level is often markedly elevated. A significant leukocytosis is also part of this poisoning. Urine analysis yields albuminuria with slight to moderate acetonuria. Differential diagnostic considerations would include diabetic ketoacidosis, lactic acidosis, uremic acidosis, and acute intoxication from ethylene glycol, paraldehyde, isoniazid, or salicylates. Detection of methanol and formic acid in the urine would confirm methanol poisoning.

Early diagnosis and vigorous treatment of methanol poisoning can be sight- and life-saving. A methanol blood level can be obtained. It is estimated that for each 40 mg/dL of methanol in blood, there is an accompanying rise in plasma osmolality of 15 mOsm/kg of H_2O. Sodium bicarbonate to reverse the metabolic acidosis and ethanol, either intravenously or orally, should be administered. Ethanol with its greater affinity for ADH can competitively inhibit the generation of the toxic metabolites of methanol. Blood ethanol levels of 100 mg/dL or higher are required to saturate the liver enzyme ADH. A loading dose of ethanol of 0.6 g/kg of body weight, or about 40 g for a 70-kg person, is needed to achieve this desired concentration in the blood. This dose can be given conveniently by mouth with four 1-oz shots of 80-proof whiskey or intravenously as 500 mL of a 10% ethanol solution. Maintenance doses of ethanol should average 7 to 10 g/hr or 109 mg/kg/hr. Hemodialysis is an effective method to treat methanol poisoning and should be initiated promptly where the blood methanol level is greater than 50 mg/dL. The rapidity of blood methanol level reduction appears to be critical for a favorable outcome. Doses of ethanol required to maintain a blood level of 100 mg/dL should be increased to 237 mg/kg/hr. Therefore, a total of 17 g of ethanol must be given hourly during dialysis for a 70-kg person to satisfactorily maintain the desired ethanol blood level. Blood levels of ethanol should be monitored often until the methanol has been cleared from the blood.[47] If acute ingestion of methanol has taken place several minutes to a few hours before initiation of treatment, further gastrointestinal absorption should be decreased with activated charcoal and removal by emesis or lavage. Respiratory and circulatory support should be established and maintained. Forced diuresis does not enhance elimination of either methanol or its metabolites.

Ethylene Glycol

The initial symptoms of acute ethylene glycol poisoning are similar to those for acute ethanol intoxication except for differences in their onset and duration. The earliest sign of ethylene glycol intoxication is inebriation. A breath odor of alcohol is conspicuously absent in persons who have ingested only ethylene glycol. Central nervous system depression and gastrointestinal distress are experienced early in the course. During the first 12 hours, hypertension and leukocytosis are often seen. Symptoms may progressively worsen until pulmonary edema, convulsions, respiratory failure, and coma occur.[34] Ethylene glycol itself is relatively nontoxic, but its metabolic products are responsible for considerable toxicity. Severe metabolic acidosis, similar to that experienced with acute methanol poisoning, is seen. Glyoxylic acid, oxalic acid, and hippurate are the acid breakdown products of ethylene glycol that cause this profound acidosis. The overproduction and accumulation of lactate and other organic acids also contribute to the acidosis. Acute oliguric renal failure can occur. This is usually severe and believed to be irreversible, although survival from this condition has occurred. There are marked renal pathologic changes, including focal hemorrhagic necrosis, oxalate crystals in the convoluted renal tubules, and epithelial cell destruction. Calcium oxalate crystals, considered an important diagnostic marker for ethylene glycol poisoning, are often but not always seen on urinalysis. Urinalysis normally shows albumin, red blood cells, and casts.

Myopathy is another common feature of ethylene glycol poisoning. Searching for signs of ethylene glycol is not often helpful for establishing an early diagnosis. The blood ethylene glycol level, if rapidly available, is more useful. Serum osmolality can be used to provide an estimation of the toxic ethylene glycol concentration. For every 50 mg/dL of ethylene glycol, the plasma osmolality is increased by 10 mOsm/kg of H_2O. A high anion and osmolal gap with metabolic acidosis is characteristic of this poisoning. Treatment of acute ethylene glycol poisoning is focused on preventing the metabolism to the toxic metabolites and enhancing its elimination from the body. Ethanol inhibits the metabolism of ethylene glycol by competitively competing for ADH. The monitoring and pharmacokinetic considerations of ethanol administration, which have been described for methanol are applicable for ethylene glycol also. The necessity for rapid treatment in ethylene glycol poisoning cannot be overstated. Because the half-life of ethylene glycol is approximately 3 hours, ethanol administration should be initiated promptly. Alkalinization should be attempted with consideration for risks of volume overload and exacerbation of existing electrolyte imbalance.

Hemodialysis readily eliminates ethylene glycol and its metabolites from the body. Blood ethylene glycol levels should be closely monitored because redistribution of the alcohol from tissue to the body water often occurs after dialysis. Repeated dialysis may be necessary to completely clear the ethylene glycol. Support of vital functions such as ventilation, perfusion, and volume are important as in all acute overdoses involving the alcohols.

Isopropyl Alcohol

Isopropyl alcohol is rapidly absorbed after ingestion. Peak plasma levels with distribution throughout body fluids and tissues may be reached within 1 hour. Inhalation of isopropyl alcohol vapors can produce considerable systemic absorption. With the exception of children, skin absorption is minimal. Children bathed with excessive amounts of rubbing alcohol have experienced coma. Isopropyl alcohol is metabolized in the liver by ADH enzymes to form acetone. Only 15% of this alcohol, when consumed, is eliminated as acetone via the saliva, lungs, and kidneys. The remainder is further converted to acetate, formate, and carbon dioxide. The rate of isopropyl alcohol metabolism to acetone is slower than that of ethanol. Both isopropyl alcohol and acetone are central nervous system depressants. Tolerance to the toxic levels of both is experienced similarly to the ethanol tolerance seen in chronic alcoholics. Toxic symptoms can occur with an ingestion of at little as 20 mL. Deaths from ingestion of 4 to 8 oz of 70% isopropyl alcohol have been reported. The symptoms of acute isopropyl alcohol intoxication are similar to those of acute ethanol intoxication except for the absence of any early stimulatory phase. Dizziness, headache, confusion, a flushing sensation, ataxia, stupor, hypothermia, and hypotension may be felt. Nausea, vomiting, diarrhea, and severe gastritis occasionally accompanied by bleeding are frequent. Children are often hypoglycemic. Respiratory failure and death can occur within a few hours after sufficient ingestion of isopropyl alcohol. Marked hypotension, renal dysfunction, and hepatic dysfunction are ominous predictors of outcome on such occasions.

Volume for volume, the toxicity of isopropyl alcohol is considered to be twice that of ethanol. Toxic symptoms are noticed when blood isopropyl alcohol levels reach 50 mg/dL. In children, symptoms are likely to occur at even lower levels. Coma is associated with levels greater than 120 mg/dL. The range of blood isopropyl alcohol levels between fatal and severe nonfatal intoxication is narrow. Acetonuria and acetonemia in the absence of glucosuria, hyperglycemia, or acidemia in an acutely intoxicated patient should arouse suspicion of acute isopropyl alcohol poisoning. Unlike ethanol, there is no fixed relationship between the concentration of isopropyl alcohol in the blood and urine; therefore, blood level determination in such circumstances is necessary.

There is no specific treatment for an acute isopropyl alcohol overdose. Methods for preventing further and continuous absorption and giving symptomatic and supportive treatment to maintain vital function should be used. Forced diuresis is of little value. Hemodialysis has been shown to be life-saving in patients with severe and unresponsive isopropyl alcohol poisoning. Repeated gastric lavage to prevent continued reabsorption of isopropyl alcohol has been reported to successfully reverse severe acute toxic symptoms. Use of serial activated charcoal may be effective in removing this alcohol. Many manufacturers of rubbing alcohol have begun to substitute ethanol for isopropyl alcohol, presumably because it is less toxic. Whenever dealing with a history of acute rubbing alcohol ingestion, one should determine which of these alcohols is in the product before treatment.

Chronic Alcohol Abuse/Alcoholism

Common early physical signs and symptoms of alcoholism include hypertension, gastritis, diarrhea or irritable colon, burns, bruises, red face, puffy face and eyes, enlarged nose with prominent veins, reddened conjunctiva, obesity, insomnia, or impotence.

Malnutrition is commonplace among alcoholics.[48] Chronic alcohol consumption results in impaired digestion and absorption of essential nutrients. Nearly all alcoholics have diminished food intake while drinking because alcohol presumably suppresses appetite. Alcohol represents "empty calories" lacking in nutritive value. Taken in excess, alcohol also prevents adequate gastrointestinal absorption of nutrients and contributes to debilitated and malnourished conditions. Nutritional problems that alcoholics are most susceptible to are deficiencies of protein, water-soluble vitamins, and minerals (Table 61.4). Accumulation of fluids with resultant ascites is a frequent complication of alcoholic cirrhosis. It is secondary to nutritional, endocrine, and metabolic disorders resulting from alcoholism. The basis of management is to supply a normal or fortified diet with restricted sodium intake to replace only daily losses. "Hidden sources" of sodium such as intravenously administered fluids including plasma and drugs may be responsible for unexpected reaccumulation of fluids in these patients. Careful monitoring for problems that are related to nutritional balance of the hospitalized alcoholic patient is essential for successful management and care.

Acute Alcohol Abstinence (Withdrawal) Syndrome

An acute abstinence, or withdrawal, syndrome is a common problem experienced by the alcoholic when alcohol is discontinued abruptly; delirium tremens (DTs) is the most severe form. The severity of the withdrawal syndrome cannot always be predicted on the basis of the quantity or duration of alcohol ingestion. Although most patients experience only minor and moderate symptoms, described often as a "hangover," it is difficult to rule out the possibility that progressively more severe and even life-threatening withdrawal reactions may occur. There is a wide variability in the severity and duration of this syndrome; in 5 to 6% of those undergoing this experience it will progress to the most severe stage: delirium tremens.

The early physiologic and behavioral effects of acute alcohol abstinence experienced (8to 36 hours after cessation of drinking) include anorexia, tremors ("shakes"), flushing, increased blood pressure, pulse, respiration rate and temperature, intermittent hallucinations, seizures ("rum fits"), sleep disturbance, and sweating. Mild to moderate withdrawal may stimulate the alcoholic to resume drinking to reverse the symptoms. A common finding in the later progression of alcoholism is the use of morning drinks ("eye openers") to reduce these effects from drinking the previous night. Late effects, experienced 2 to 6 days after cessation of drinking, may include severe tremors, marked agitation, profound disorientation, excitation, persistent visual and auditory hallucinations, marked sleep disturbances, fever, tachycardia, and other life-threatening complications. Patients experiencing major alcohol withdrawal symptoms or DTs, estimated to occur in 5% of hospitalized withdrawing alcoholics, are seriously ill. Patients with DTs are febrile, disoriented, and agitated and often have an accompanying concurrent medical problem such as infection or coma. Although the mortality rate for this condition has decreased during the past 50 years, deaths from DTs still occur (variously estimated at 5 to 20%), particularly in patients with underlying or alcohol-associated conditions such as pancreatitis, cirrhosis, gastrointestinal bleeding, pneumonia, or sepsis. It should not be taken for granted that the intoxicated or bizarre behavior in alcoholics is an effect of alcohol; hypoxia, hyperosmolarity, hypomagnesemia, or hypoglycemia may be contributing to it.[49]

The exact pathophysiologic mechanism for the acute alcohol withdrawal syndrome is uncertain. With hyperventilation and respiratory alkalosis, a corresponding rise in arterial pH and fall in serum magnesium takes place. Central nervous system excitability, altered sleep patterns, and other signs of withdrawal are experienced, probably as a result of decreased cerebral blood flow and oxygen delivery to the brain and electrolyte imbalance.

Fetal Alcohol Syndrome

The relationship between heavy alcohol consumption in pregnancy and fetal abnormalities has been suspected since antiquity. In 1973, Jones and his colleagues described a unique clustering of fetal defects in offspring of mothers with chronic alcoholism as the fetal alcohol syndrome.[44] Clarren and Smith[35] characterized this pattern of malformation as follows: (1) prenatal and postnatal growth deficiency; (2) central nervous system dysfunction including physiologic depression, hypotonia, irritability and jitteriness, mental retardation, poor coordination and hyperactivity during childhood; (3) craniofacial abnormalities including short palpebral fissures, short upturned nose, hypoplastic philtrum, flat mid-face and thinned upper lip; and (4) other major organ system defects such as abnormalities of the eyes, ears, and mouth, heart murmurs,

Table 61.4 ▪ Nutritional Problems Associated with Alcoholism

Source	Signs and Symptoms	Comments
Protein	Fatty liver and hypoalbuminemia may be result of deterioration of liver function or low protein intake. Others seen: hypocholesterolemia, edema, normocytic anemia.	Association of alcohol with liver disease complicates the interpretation of many clinical signs of protein deficiency. Alcoholic liver disease is not prevented by eating well or limiting alcohol consumption only to certain types of beverages. Administration of protein to patients with severe active alcoholic cirrhosis can precipitate hepatic coma. When protein is poorly tolerated or the patient becomes progressively disoriented, showing asterixis or flapping tremors, administration of protein should be discontinued.
Water-soluble vitamins, vitamin B complexes, thiamine	Signs and symptoms are variable depending on severity of the deficiency: ophthalmoplegia, sixth-nerve palsy, nystagmus, weakness, ataxia, peripheral neuropathies, confusion, amnesia, coma, heart failure, Wernicke's syndrome, "beriberi" heart disease, sudden death.	Most common deficiency in alcoholics. Polyneuropathy is the mildest and most common form of thiamine deficiency. Depressed tendon reflexes, muscle cramps, weakness, paresthesias, and pain develop. The lower extremities are most often affected. Prognosis is grave; deficiency must be recognized early. Treatment is to give thiamine. Administration of glucose without thiamine may further deplete stores of thiamine. Thiamine deficiency-induced heart failure does not respond well to digitalis or diuretics. Animal studies suggest that thiamine deficiency reduces myocardial oxygen consumption due to deficiency of the coenzyme thiamine pyrophosphate. Average thiamine requirement for an adult is 1.5–2 mg/day. Alcoholics often require more; 100–200 mg results in dramatic reversal of signs and symptoms.
Niacin	Weakness, photosensitive dermatitis, stomatitis, gastritis, diarrhea, peripheral neuropathy, dementia, encephalopathy	Alcoholic pellagra is the result of the lack of dietary nicotinic acid or its precursor, tryptophan. Niacin contributes to formation of specific coenzyme nucleotides (NAD), which participate in intracellular metabolism and cell respiration. Replacement dose is 200 mg niacinamide three times a day.
Riboflavin	Weakness, photosensitive dermatitis, stomatitis, gastritis, diarrhea, peripheral neuropathy, dementia, encephalopathy	Riboflavin deficiency usually accompanies alcoholic pellagra. Riboflavin is an essential constituent of coenzymes responsible for oxidative and electron transport processes. Replacement dose is 10 mg/day.
Pyridoxine	Irritability, anemia, insomnia, peripheral neuropathy, ataxia, skin lesions	Pyridoxine is responsible for a variety of enzymatic activities particularly related to nitrogen metabolism.
Ascorbic acid	Anorexia, petechial ecchymoses, gingivitis and bleeding gums, dry mouth, loss of hair, perifollicular hemorrhages, purpuric lesions, ecchymoses, itchy dry skin, weakness, lethargy	Ascorbic acid is a coenzyme involved in the metabolism of amino acids. Usual amount recommended is 10 mg/day.
Folic acid	Macrocytic anemia, reticulocytosis	Deficiency of folic acid is the primary cause of macrocytic anemia in chronic alcoholics. Alcohol directly affects the hematopoietic activity and interferes with utilization of folic acid. Must discontinue alcohol. Usual amount recommended for replacement is 1.0 mg daily.
Magnesium	Lethargy, muscle weakness, coarse athetoid movements, gross tremors of hands and tongue, mental changes, convulsions, stupor, coma	Alcohol promotes the renal excretion of magnesium. Renal effect and inadequate diet cause significant depletion. Symptoms of acute alcohol withdrawal are often complicated by coexisting magnesium depletion. The total body magnesium deficits are not reflected by serum magnesium levels.
Potassium	Weakness, lethargy	Poor dietary intake of potassium and loss by diuresis, vomiting, and diarrhea contribute to hypokalemia.

septal defects, genitourinary abnormalities, hemangiomas, and musculoskeletal problems such as hernias. Longitudinal studies show that these children experience immunodeficiency. No "catch-up" seems to occur in terms of either behavior or intellect in the impaired child with the fetal alcohol syndrome.

The reported incidence of fetal alcohol syndrome is rare, affecting 1:300 to 1:2000 infants. Estimates of the proportion of women who drink heavily during pregnancy range from 2 to 13%, depending on the population studied and survey methodologies.

Many factors may influence the phenotypic outcome of pregnancy in the alcoholic mother, including variable dose exposure at variable gestational periods as well as the genetic background of the individual fetus. Alcohol, like other teratogens, does not uniformly affect all those exposed to it. Rather, there seems to be a continuum of effects of alcohol on the fetus with increasingly severe outcomes generally associated with higher intakes of alcohol by the mother.[35] It should also be noted that alcohol readily enters breast milk, thereby providing alcohol to the nursing infant. There appears to be no established safe amount of alcohol or a safe time to drink it during pregnancy and lactation.

Diagnosis

Acute Intoxication

The severity of the acute intoxication depends on the blood alcohol level and individual tolerance. Levels below 50 mg/dL, or 0.05%, rarely produce significant effects in adults. In children, signs of alcohol intoxication are often prominent at this level. The presence or absence of the odor of alcohol on a patient's breath cannot be used to establish a diagnosis of alcohol intoxication. Unique odors should still be noted since they may offer a diagnostic clue as to the overall clinical condition of an intoxicated patient. The plasma osmolality can be a useful indicator since the relationship of osmolality with plasma alcohol is linear. A rise of approximately 25 to 30 mOsmol/kg of H_2O reflects a 100 mg/dL, or 0.1%, increase in plasma alcohol. Concomitant conditions such as trauma, blood loss, infection, multiple drug use, and hypoglycemia often complicate the recognition and assessment of an intoxicated patient; therefore, the measurement or estimate of the blood alcohol level or comparable analysis of urine, saliva, and expired air is valuable for confirming alcohol intoxication and to establish an appropriate treatment plan.[49]

Other toxicologic tests, particularly for barbiturates and other sedative drugs and also salicylates may be indicated to detect suspected commonly occurring polydrug toxicity. In addition, specific laboratory studies for liver function, renal function, serum electrolytes with particular attention to the potassium, magnesium, and phosphate levels and the anion gap, arterial blood gases, blood ketones, and glucose should be performed routinely. The urine should be examined for the appearance of any crystal-like material or myoglobin. After a prolonged drinking binge, myoglobinuria, hyperkalemia, and increased serum creatine kinase levels secondary to alcohol myopathy may occur. An electrocardiogram should be performed, and changes characteristic of abnormal calcium, magnesium, and potassium levels or the presence of hypoxia or hypothermia should be recognized. An abdominal x-ray examination (kidney, ureters, and bladder) may offer useful clues to the identity of materials ingested in any possible multiple overdose involving an acutely alcohol-intoxicated patient. Some common drugs often taken in suicide attempts such as phenothiazines, tricyclic antidepressants, heavy metals including iron, arsenic, and halides, iodides and bromides, chloral hydrate, and enteric-coated tablets are radiopaque. X-ray films of the skull and chest are also advisable at the time of initial examination.

Alcohol Abuse and Alcoholism

The diagnosis of alcoholism is difficult because of the societal stigmatization of the disease, denial, and imprecise diagnostic criteria. The clinical signs and subtleties of the condition are varied, elusive, and without reliable parameters. Objective laboratory verification of the diagnosis is often unavailable or incomplete. Although a specific genetic marker for alcoholism has been recently suggested, this is not universally accepted and likely represents only one of a number of factors (e.g., multiple gene loci, environment, gender, and ethnicity) that affects predisposition.[50] Reliable biochemical or genetic markers for diagnosing alcoholism are not available. Much depends on the experience and motivation of the observer in deciding whether a patient is suffering from alcoholism or not. Unfortunately, many physicians and other health professionals are poorly educated concerning the diagnosis of alcoholism, resulting in the underdiagnosis and mismanagement of alcohol-related problems. The first recognition of alcoholism often occurs during a hospitalization when an advanced manifestation of alcoholism, such as ascites or cirrhosis, is being treated. Many patients with unrecognized alcoholism probably experience minor withdrawal symptoms, such as agitation and insomnia, during the course of hospital stays or when admitted to nursing homes.

Early identification of an existing alcohol problem is important because the prognosis with treatment is much more promising when the difficulty is recognized early in its course. Clues that provide early recognition are found in the demographic, social, familial, and cultural characteristics of those who consume alcohol.[51] Frequent episodes of drinking to the point of intoxication, an inability to control the intake of alcohol, alcoholic "blackout" periods (loss of memory while intoxicated, not passing out), drinking despite strong social contraindications such as job loss, legal problems such as drunk driving arrests, or family or marital discord resulting from pathologic drinking are signs of the presence of this condition. There are several alcoholism screening tests in common use (Michigan Alcoholism Screening Test [MAST], the brief MAST [BMAST], CAGE [*c*ut down drinking, *a*nnoyed by criticism of drinking, guilty about drinking, and *e*ye openers], AUDIT [*a*lcohol *u*se *d*isorders *i*dentification *t*est], and TWEAK [*t*olerance, others *w*orry about your drinking, *e*ye opener, *a*mnesia, c(*k*)ut down drinking]); the CAGE is applied more often because of its brevity, relative reliability, and ease of administration.[52]

Diagnostic criteria for alcohol abuse and alcoholism are often difficult and subjective; however, the *Diagnostic and*

Statistical Manual of Mental Disorders, 4th edition (DSM-IV) criteria established by the American Psychiatric Association can serve as a convenient starting point for the diagnosis of alcohol dependence.[53] Alcohol abuse is characterized by a maladaptive pattern of alcohol use leading to clinically significant impairment. Within a 2-month period, one or more of the following criteria must be met: (1) negative effects on school or job performance, (2) neglect of household or child care responsibilities, (3) alcohol-related absences from either school or work, (4) use of alcohol in physically hazardous conditions, and (5) legal difficulties as a result of alcohol use.[53] Persons may continue to consume alcohol despite knowing that continuation may result in social or interpersonal problems. Therefore, a single situation can fulfill several of the diagnostic criteria for alcohol abuser. For example, a person who is arrested for the second instance of driving under the influence (DUI) of alcohol after consuming alcohol to the extent of intoxication fulfills several of the criteria. At minimum, the person has used alcohol in physically hazardous conditions by operating an automobile and will face legal difficulties as a result of the DUI arrest. Moreover, the person would not be able to return to work that afternoon and may not be able to fulfill childcare responsibilities such as picking up a child at daycare.

In alcohol dependence, the maladaptive pattern of alcohol use is manifested by at least three of the following during a 1-year period: (1) tolerance, (2) withdrawal, (3) total alcohol consumption increase or length of alcohol use longer than intended, (4) persistent desire or successful effort to increase control or decrease consumption of alcohol, (5) much time spent to obtain or drink alcohol or recover from its affects, (6) social, occupational, or recreational activities discontinued or reduced as a result of drinking alcohol, and (7) alcohol use continued despite the knowledge of having a physical or psychologic problem from alcohol use. Tolerance can be manifested by either a need for increased amounts of alcohol to achieve intoxication or the desired effect or diminished effect with the continued use of the same amount of alcohol. Withdrawal is characterized by either of the following categories: (1) two or more of the following are present: autonomic hyperactivity (i.e., tachycardia or diaphoresis), hand tremor, insomnia, nausea or vomiting, hallucinations, psychomotor agitation, anxiety, or grand mal seizures; or (2) alcohol or other substances are taken to relieve or avoid withdrawal.[53]

PSYCHOSOCIAL ASPECTS

Alcoholism affects every aspect of personal and family life of the alcoholic. Employment, financial problem, family problems, and social isolation are only a few effects of chronic alcohol abuse. Specific psychosocial attributes are not easily identified as positive indicators of alcoholism. In an evaluation of Danish patients, lower educational levels were associated with an increased incidence of excessive alcohol consumption in men.[9] Among people 65 years or older, a positive association has been shown between volume of alcohol consumed and poorer psychosocial well-being; however, drinking frequency was not related to psychosocial status.[12]

The challenge for the alcoholic and the clinician is to identify a cause-effect relationship between the psychosocial effects and alcoholism. For example, the alcoholic states that he or she drinks as a result of financial problems. However, the alcoholism then exacerbates the financial problems by the direct cost of alcohol and indirect effects such as missed work. The resultant potentiation of financial difficulty places the alcoholic in a viscous cycle. Parental alcoholism often disrupts family life; therefore, the effects of alcoholism on the children of alcoholics must also be addressed. A prominent negative effect of alcoholism is the disturbance of family rituals such as holidays, vacations, or school events. These disruptions can result in the children perceiving themselves as either the cause of the disruption or as abnormal compared to their peers. The effects of such feeling of inadequacy can present social challenges for the child that include problematic family rituals when the child reaches adulthood. However, the maintenance of family rituals in light of heavy periods of drinking in an alcoholic parent is correlated with lower incidence of alcoholism in the children of alcoholics.[21]

Higher levels of family conflict have been reported in families of alcoholics.[54] Families of alcoholics have been characterized by a lack of parenting, poor home management, and a lack of family communication skills.[55] Moreover, a multitude of problems have been associated with alcoholism, including emotional or physical violence, decreased family cohesion, decreased family organization, martial strain, financial problems, and frequent family relocations.[21] Each of these, as well as other family problems, have consequences that extend the scope of involvement with alcohol and result in the development of additional family dysfunctions that adds to the complexity of alcoholism.

THERAPEUTIC PLAN

The consensus diagnosis and treatment plans for alcoholism are summarized and addressed in this chapter. However, the criteria found in DSM-IV established by the American Psychiatric Association serve as the gold standard for the diagnosis of alcoholism as well as other mental disorders.[53] The Agency for Health Care Policy and Research has recently released an evidence-based report on the "Pharmacotherapy of Alcohol Dependence" to address drug therapy treatment for alcoholism.[56]

TREATMENT

Pharmacotherapy

Acute Intoxication

The basic treatment for acute alcohol intoxication is to maintain and support vital functions (i.e., maintain a patent airway and adequate blood pressure and avoid aspiration) until no longer needed during the detoxification process, which takes from 7 to 10 days.[57,58] In the comatose patient, particularly if this involves accidental ingestion of alcohol by a child, acute alcoholic hypoglycemia and other possible causes of coma such as subdural hematoma should be ruled out. Central nervous system stimulants should not be used. The major problems encountered in the management of acute alcohol intoxication are (1) pneumonia, a leading cause of morbidity; (2) overhydration; and (3) complications from unnecessary therapeutic maneuvers.

The possible presence of alcohol should not be overlooked when evaluating a suspected acute case of drug intoxication. One study revealed that almost one of every five patients with an acute drug overdose in whom the presence of alcohol was unsuspected or thought to be irrelevant was found to have high blood levels of alcohol. The notion that acute alcohol intoxication is benign should be dispelled. Diagnosis of any drug intoxication should include a blood ethanol determination in addition to other laboratory tests.

Alcoholic coma is a life-threatening situation that usually responds well to supportive treatment. Establishment of a clear airway and assisted ventilation are essential in patients with this condition. Oxygenation and volume replacement with intravenous fluids generally improves the hypotension. Patients who are experiencing protracted vomiting may have substantial fluid deficits. If alcoholic hypoglycemia is suspected or if the blood glucose level is at 70 mg/dL or lower, 50 to 100 mL of 50% glucose should be given intravenously. Thiamine 100 mg given to prevent the possible exacerbation of the Wernicke-Korsakoff syndrome should be administered before or along with the glucose. If recent ingestion of drugs is suspected, gastric lavage can be carefully performed in the unconscious patient with appropriate guarding of the airway to avoid the risk of aspiration. Emetics, such as syrup of ipecac, given to prevent the further absorption of drugs taken in an overdose should be used with great caution in any acutely intoxicated conscious alcoholic patient because tearing of the gastroesophageal mucosa may occur as a life-threatening consequence of ipecac-induced protracted vomiting.

The use of 10 and 40% solutions of fructose given either orally or intravenously in attempts to accelerate the metabolism of ethanol is not recommended. The minimal benefits from such an effort are outweighed by the disadvantages. Adverse effects from fructose include nausea, vomiting, hyperuricemia, worsening of metabolic acidosis, and volume depletion. Increasing the rate of clearance of alcohol from the body also leads to more rapid development of the alcohol withdrawal symptoms.[59] Administration of naloxone to reverse alcohol-induced coma has been reported to produce some antagonistic effects in patients with acute alcohol intoxication. In cases described, the responses were quite variable; in some patients, improvement was only slight. Difficulties encountered when trying to exclude concomitant opiate use in those patients reported to have responded and failed attempts to reproduce these findings in the laboratory have left this issue of naloxone use as an antagonist to alcohol-induced coma unresolved.[60,61,]

Treatment of hepatic encephalopathy precipitated by alcohol is to reverse the precipitating factors and lower serum ammonia levels. The immediate approach to bleeding esophageal varices is blood replacement, possible administration of vasopressin, and use of a Sengstaken-Blakemore tube if necessary. Sclerosant solutions can be injected for bleeding varices of the esophagus. Sodium morrhuate and sodium tetradecyl sulfate are available variceal sclerosing agents. Reduction of increased blood flow in the portal collateral system and increased intrahepatic resistance with vasoconstrictors, such as vasopressin and somatostatin, or β-adrenergic blockers , are beneficial in lowering variceal pressures. Surgery may be required to further decompress the varices by shunting the flow of the hepatic portal circulation after the patient's condition has stabilized. Hepatic encephalopathy is further characterized by sodium retention, progressively worsening oliguria, and eventually azotemia.

A toxic psychosis associated with acute alcohol intoxication occasionally presents as an emergency situation. It is characterized by a markedly impaired sensorium with confusion, amnesia, and disorientation. There is often a sudden onset of aggressive and hostile behavior with associated psychotic symptoms including hallucinations and delusions. The treatment of this agitated phase can be accomplished with sedation to produce a calm, but still arousable, condition. Benzodiazepines and haloperidol can be used judiciously in these circumstances.

A number of considerations should be kept in mind when treating and caring for the patient acutely intoxicated or overdosed with alcohol. The symptoms of both acute alcohol intoxication and response to treatment vary among patients. Factors such as age, weight, tolerance, and concomitant ingestion of other drugs must be considered. Polydrug abuse in the adult with alcohol intoxication should be suspected and withdrawal from barbiturates or opiates may be a further complication. In children, the toxicologic effects of ingredients contained in alcoholic solutions that are used for cough and colds, for pain and allergic symptoms, or for sleep should be considered. Medical and surgical illnesses may contribute to the toxicologic problems of acute alcohol poisoning. The basis of treatment should be to maintain and support vital functions and to individualize all aspects of care and treatment.[49]

Acute Alcohol Abstinence (Withdrawal) Syndrome

The primary objective of detoxification is to remove alcohol from the body with as few withdrawal symptoms as possible.[62] This process involves the substitution and slow withdrawing of a long-acting sedative-hypnotic drug for the shorter-acting one, alcohol. Some patients in mild withdrawal may not require drugs for relief. In the past 30 years, many different drugs and drug combinations have been described in the medical literature for the treatment of acute alcohol withdrawal. In a like manner, a 1995 national survey of 176 inpatient treatment facilities reported great diversity in pharmacologic management of alcohol withdrawal. The most common drugs used in decreasing order were chlordiazepoxide, diazepam, barbiturates, phenytoin, clonidine, and oxazepam.[63] A review of the studies that investigated the effectiveness of drugs in treating the withdrawal syndrome suggests that many such studies were poorly controlled and lack objective comparisons of effects. In carefully conducted studies, some drugs have not been shown to be necessarily or universally much more effective than placebos. The major benefit of the antianxiety agents may be, in many instances, for the nursing and medical staff as the patient is made more manageable.

Benzodiazepines

The benzodiazepines, such as diazepam, chlordiazepoxide, clorazepate, oxazepam, and lorazepam, are longer-acting and safer, do not produce gastritis, and have antiseizure activity compared with other sedative-hypnotics. They are used also because of the convenient dosage forms available. Diazepam and chlordiazepoxide can be administered by oral and intravenous routes, often in gradually tapering doses. Lorazepam is available in oral and parenteral dosage forms. Clorazepate and oxazepam are available in the oral form. The usual therapeutic endpoint in the management of acute alcohol withdrawal symptoms is to produce a calmed but awake patient, using whatever doses are required to achieve this endpoint.[64,65,]

The pharmacokinetics of these drugs in patients undergoing alcohol withdrawal or in patients with mild liver impairment has aroused a great deal of clinical and research interest. The elimination half-lives of oxazepam, lorazepam, chlordiazepoxide, clorazepate, and diazepam are 8, 16, 16, 24, and 32 hours, respectively, with wide individual variations existing. In patients with alcohol cirrhosis, the elimination of diazepam from the body is presumably decreased because of decreased clearance by the liver and increased tissue distribution. Because the major metabolites of benzodiazepines, with the exception of oxazepam and lorazepam, are also psychoactive, accumulation of effects during chronic administration of these drugs should be evaluated carefully in patients with cirrhosis. There is no evidence to suggest that any one of the benzodiazepines is better than another for use in acute alcohol detoxification. Most studies on the use of benzodiazepines in this situation have been conducted with chlordiazepoxide. Oxazepam and lorazepam might be considered the drugs of choice, particularly in patients with liver disease who are likely to have impaired metabolism of these drugs.

Dose requirements of these drugs for detoxification are quite variable. The usual range for diazepam is 30 to 200 mg during the first 24 hours, but a few patients may require 1000 mg or more. It should be remembered that withdrawing alcoholics may require higher doses of sedative-hypnotic drugs than other agitated patients, probably because of tolerance and decreased sensitivity.[66] Some alcoholic patients are only calmed by doses that would be severely depressive in nonalcoholic patients. Because dose requirements are variable, no fixed dose schedule can be predicted for a given patient. In a patient undergoing a mild-to-moderate withdrawal syndrome, an initial oral dose of diazepam 20 mg can be administered orally, followed by 10 to 20 mg every 2 to 3 hours. However, elderly patients should receive only 10 mg initially, followed by doses every 4 to 6 hours if needed. If chlordiazepoxide is the preferred drug, 25 to 100 mg can be given every 2 to 6 hours, depending on symptoms. A total dose of 400 to 600 mg may be needed by extremely tolerant patients with severe symptoms. In the elderly patient, 50 mg two to four times a day should be sufficient for symptom relief. Treatment with benzodiazepines can even be successfully used for patients experiencing mild withdrawal symptoms without coexisting illnesses.[67]

Every patient should be reevaluated and drug requirements reassessed every few hours until initial sedation is achieved and then at least daily during the maintenance phase. Standing orders for repetitive doses are not advisable. Predetermined, fixed dosing regimens contribute often to unnecessary oversedation of the patient undergoing withdrawal. For severe withdrawal, intravenous diazepam should be cautiously administered in a dose of 10 to 30 mg every 30 or more minutes until the patient is calm. Then a maintenance regimen of 10 to 20 mg can be given intravenously or orally as needed during the day and in the evening to enable sleep. Because of the risks of hypotension and respiratory depression, the patient should be assessed before and periodically after every intravenous dose of a sedative-hypnotic drug. Intramuscular administration of the benzodiazepines should be avoided because of their slow and erratic absorption. With the shorter-acting benzodiazepines, loading doses are not required; however, to maintain blood levels sufficient to sustain relief from withdrawal symptoms, doses of oxazepam and lorazepam at 15 to 30 mg and 1 to 4 mg, respectively, need to be given at 6- to 8-hour intervals. Withdrawing these drugs during the detoxification process should be accomplished by lowering their dose rather than by lengthening their administration interval beyond 8 hours.

Phenothiazines

The major neuroleptics have not been shown to be any more effective than the sedative-hypnotic drugs and should not be used. They can result in increased seizures, impaired thermoregulation, extrapyramidal effects, and postural hypotension. The syncope and arrhythmias that can result from these drugs can produce serious consequences in the acutely withdrawing alcoholic. At high doses, delirium can occur as a result of their anticholinergic effects.

Butyrophenones

Haloperidol in oral doses of 5 to 10 mg or 5 mg intramuscularly has been advocated for use in treating hallucinations and acute agitation associated with alcohol. Producing less sedation, hypotension, and hypothermia compared to the phenothiazines, haloperidol, like other dopamine antagonists, however, may cause extrapyramidal and centrally mediated anticholinergic reactions. Extreme caution should be exercised with the use of this drug since the central nervous system depression from the concomitant alcohol may be additive or potentiated.

Clonidine

Clonidine, a centrally acting inhibitor of adrenergic vasomotor centers used in the treatment of hypertension, has been compared with benzodiazepines in the management of acute alcohol withdrawal. Used successfully to treat opiate withdrawal, clonidine can also relieve the tremors, tachycardia, systolic hypertension, and diaphoresis secondary to alcohol withdrawal and appears to be as effective as chlordiazepoxide. Because the ability of clonidine to protect against withdrawal seizures is uncertain, the role of the drug should remain limited to situations where the risks of seizures and serious medical or psychiatric complications are minimal.[65]

Carbamazepine

Carbamazepine has been shown to prevent alcohol withdrawal in animal studies and does not potentiate central nervous system or respiratory depression caused by alcohol. It has been widely used for alcohol withdrawal in Europe and has been shown to be comparable to oxazepam in treating mild to moderate withdrawal. Its role in treatment of alcohol withdrawal in the United States remains to be determined.[62]

Phenytoin

The seizures associated with acute alcohol withdrawal (rum fits) are usually self-limiting and often do not require anticonvulsant medication. The episode is brief, consisting usually of a single grand mal-like seizure and only occasionally appears as repeated seizures. Seizures usually occur in patients with a history of traumatic epilepsy or seizure onset in childhood or adolescence. In the postictal period after alcohol withdrawal seizures, very few patients show electroencephalographic abnormalities. In the acute situation during status epilepticus, small doses (2 to 4 mg) of intravenous diazepam can be administered. Patients who are seen with or are suspected to have alcohol withdrawal seizures require careful observation and thorough evaluation for traumatic, infectious, or metabolic causes. Withholding anticonvulsant medications over a 6- to 12-hour period may permit an opportunity to characterize any subsequent seizure that might occur.[68]

Long-term antiepileptic drug therapy is unproven and is not indicated for alcohol withdrawal seizures. Focal seizures suggest a central nervous system lesion and are not alcohol related. Patients with status epilepticus or focal seizures may experience greater risks for seizures during alcohol withdrawal.

Propranolol

Theoretically, a β-adrenergic blocking drug such as propranolol should be beneficial in preventing the adrenergic overactivity that occurs during alcohol withdrawal. The alcohol withdrawal syndrome is likely to be mediated in part by the autonomic system.[69] Few clinical studies on the use of β-blockers in alcohol withdrawal have been published. A trial comparing atenolol, a β-blocker, with placebo in a large group of hospitalized patients withdrawing from alcohol, showed that the drug had an ameliorating effect on the symptoms experienced. Because β-blockers lack anticonvulsant activity, both groups also received oxazepam 15 or 30 mg QID. The results showed a shorter duration of hospital stay, a reduced need for benzodiazepines during hospitalization, and a more rapid return of vital signs to normal in the atenolol-treated patients.[70] Propranolol has been shown to be effective in reducing tremor, blood pressure, heart rate, and urinary and total catecholamine levels in patients withdrawing from alcohol.

Potential hazards include the precipitation of congestive heart failure, asthmatic attacks, and peripheral vascular insufficiency and the masking of symptoms of hypoglycemia. Benefits from the use of β-adrenergic blockers should, nevertheless, be weighed carefully in each case against the risks before they can be considered as therapeutic agents for acute alcohol withdrawal syndrome.

Paraldehyde

Paraldehyde was once used widely in the treatment of alcohol withdrawal. A major complication of this drug is its ability to produce an acidosis from its acetaldehyde and acetic acid metabolites, further complicating an already altered acid-base status. Oral or rectal administration in an acutely agitated alcoholic is impractical and causes local irritation of mucous membranes.

Ethanol

The use of alcohol in the management of acute alcohol withdrawal symptoms is hazardous because of its short duration of action and the risk of continuing the metabolic, endocrine, and neurologic disturbances and pathologic changes.

Thiamine (Vitamin B_1)

The most serious consequences of thiamine deficiency experienced by chronic alcoholics are neuromuscular effects. Wernicke's syndrome and Korsakoff's syndrome, characterized by ophthalmoplegia, ataxia, peripheral neuropathy, and progressive confusion, are manifestations of the deficiency.[71,72] Thiamine is routinely administered intravenously (100 to 200 mg) to withdrawing alcoholics as a preventative measure. Because glucose solutions are invariably administered to such patients, deficient stores of thiamine may be further depleted as a result.

Vitamin K

Vitamin K is used particularly in patients with alcoholic hepatitis or cirrhosis because prothrombin production is often impaired.

Folic Acid

The moderate to severe anemia seen in alcoholics is usually of the megaloblastic type caused by folic acid deficiency. A combined megaloblastic anemia and microcytic anemia indicating iron deficiency usually results from blood loss in addition to nutritional deficits.[73]

Fluids, Glucose, and Electrolytes

It is important to correct the fluid and electrolytes imbalances, particularly sodium, potassium and magnesium, that accompany acute withdrawal.[74,75] In some patients, water is retained and renal resorption of sodium, potassium, and chloride is increased contrary to the notion that all acutely withdrawing alcoholics are dehydrated from the diuresis produced by alcohol.[76] An observation common in patients with severe alcohol withdrawal is hypomagnesemia with serum levels ranging from 0.7 to 1.4 mEq/L. Because symptoms of withdrawal such as tremor, hyperreflexia, and seizures are similar to those associated with this condition, the administration of magnesium is thought to aid in reducing the severity and even preventing some of these symptoms.

Summary

The following considerations should be kept in mind when treating and caring for the alcoholic patient in the acute withdrawal phase. The acute alcohol withdrawal syndrome and response to treatment varies among alcoholic patients. Polydrug abuse occurs in the chronic alcoholic and withdrawal from barbiturates or opiates would further complicate therapy. An opiate-dependent person who is also dependent on alcohol is generally detoxified from the alcohol while being maintained on methadone. Benzodiazepines are the drugs of choice for treating the acute alcohol withdrawal syndrome because they are distinctly safer than other medications. Patient variables may influence the pharmacokinetics of benzodiazepines, the dose, and the route of administration. The doses of the medication used to treat withdrawal symptoms should be tapered to avoid delayed withdrawal symptoms. Complete eradication of withdrawal symptoms may indicate overmedication. Medical and surgical illness may worsen the acute withdrawal syndrome. Nonpharmacologic factors such as staff attitude and ward environment can be effective in helping with the anxiety, insomnia, depression, and other problems that often occur during acute detoxification. There is no evidence that drug therapy during acute alcohol detoxification modifies the outcome of long-term treatment of alcoholism. Detoxification is the first, not the final, step in therapy for alcoholism. The most important factors in successful treatment of and recovery from alcoholism are the motivation of the patient to stop drinking and ongoing participation in recovery support programs, such as Alcoholics Anonymous (AA).

Chronic Alcoholism

Although the period of detoxification is relatively short, it may take months for the physiologic processes to return to normal. Maintaining a prolonged alcohol-free period after detoxification enhances treatment of the chronic alcoholic. It is commonly thought that alcoholism is primarily a manifestation of underlying psychiatric problems, and most methods of treatment and dealing with those problems will not succeed while the patient continues to drink. A variety of pharmacotherapeutic approaches are available for management of chronic alcoholism including use of medications either alone or in combination with behavior modification techniques. Whereas some recovering alcoholics feel that recovery requires total abstinence from any medication, successful recovery maintenance for some depends upon pharmacotherapy under the direction of a physician or pharmacist experienced in addiction disorders.

Disulfiram

Disulfiram is considered best used in the context of a close physician-patient or therapist-patient relationship with attempts to modify behavior.[77] Despite the fact that disulfiram has been available and used for more than 40 years, a consensus on its therapeutic utility has still not been developed. This is due to methodologic problems inherent in studies in which there is a lack of accurate definitions for the stages of the disorder and an absence of a method to assess compliance. Nevertheless, a meta-analysis of the literature reported that study results involving oral disulfiram were variable; however, there was modest evidence of a reduction in drinking frequencies without a significant increase in abstinence. Data for disulfiram implants are also inconsistent, but positive evidence exists that disulfiram decreases the number of drinking days.[78]

When administered alone, disulfiram is relatively nontoxic, but in the presence of alcohol it alters alcohol metabolism. Disulfiram causes an increase in the blood acetaldehyde levels by interfering with acetaldehyde dehydrogenase action, producing an acetaldehyde syndrome. It also inhibits dopamine β-hydroxylase leading to the release and depletion of norepinephrine stores. The patient becomes flushed and develops a scarlet appearance; as the vasodilation continues, palpitations, chest pain, hyperventilation, headache, tachycardia, weakness, hypotension, and syncope occur. Respiratory difficulty, nausea, vomiting, blurred vision, and vertigo may also occur. The reaction may be produced by as little as a few milliliters of alcohol and can last from 30 minutes to several hours. The action of disulfiram may last up to 10 days after the patient's last dose. At higher blood alcohol levels, more marked symptoms including cardiac arrhythmias, heart failure, and death are experienced.

The usual initial dosage of disulfiram is 250 to 500 mg/day for 5 to 7 days. The dosage may then be reduced to 125 to 250 mg/day. Disulfiram is rapidly absorbed from the gastrointestinal tract; it achieves full pharmacologic action in approximately 12 hours. Disulfiram is eliminated slowly; approximately 20% still remains in the body after a week. Although disulfiram is relatively safe for most patients, it can cause acneform eruptions, fatigue, tremor, restlessness, impotence, and a garlicky or metallic taste in the mouth. With large doses, psychologic depression occurs, probably as a result of interference in dopamine β-hydroxylase activity in the brain. Disulfiram has also been shown to retard the metabolism of oral anticoagulants, isoniazid, and other drugs. Any patient receiving disulfiram should be warned to avoid medications that contain alcohol, particularly over-the-counter preparations such as some cough and cold medicines, tonics, antihistamines, body and after-shave lotions, colognes, mouthwashes, and alcohol sponges.

The intensity and duration of the disulfiram-alcohol reaction symptoms are related to the disulfiram dosage, the amount of alcohol consumed, and individual sensitivity. Blood alcohol levels as low as 5 to 10 mg/dL can cause a mild reaction. Although the disulfiram-alcohol reaction is usually short-lived and without major sequelae, death can occur. In many fatalities, the disulfiram dose was excessive, but in others there was no apparent explanation. In these inexplicable fatalities, the causes of death were intracranial hemorrhage, acute myocardial infarction, pulmonary edema, and cerebral edema.[79]

There are reports of antidotal treatment of the disulfiram-alcohol reaction with ascorbic acid, iron salts, or antihistamines, but the results are not definitive. Intravenous administration of ascorbic acid (0.5 to 2.0 g) is based on experimental evidence that ascorbic acid appears to reverse the disulfiram inhibition of cellular oxidation. However, nonspecific supportive measures such as placing the patient in the Trendelenburg posture, administration of oxygen, infusion of fluids and solutes, and (if needed) vasopressor agents are more beneficial than the unproved use of these questionable antidotes. Table 61.5 summarizes the special factors to be considered in the use of disulfiram.

Naltrexone

Naltrexone, an opiate antagonist, was approved for use in the treatment of alcohol dependence in 1994. It attenuates the reinforcing but not the negative effects of alcohol consumption; feelings of intoxication and craving are reduced when alcohol is consumed by patients receiving naltrexone. It appears to be most effective when combined with support counseling in patients who experience heightened craving and high levels of somatic distress.[80] Patients must be motivated to comply with the once-daily oral regimen of this drug. Product cost may be a major deterrent to its wider use.

Naltrexone can precipitate narcotic withdrawal syndromes in patients dependent on opiates. It is also contraindicated in patients with active hepatitis or liver failure because high doses have caused hepatotoxicity. Baseline and every 3 months follow-up determinations of transaminase and bilirubin levels are recommended. Nausea is the most frequent side effect, coinciding with peak levels, which occur 90 minutes after administration. This attenuates over time. The recommended oral dose is 50 mg daily taken in the morning. Initiation of treatment at 25 mg/day for the first 2 days of therapy has been reported to minimize side effects of the drug.[81]

Table 61.5 ▪ Considerations in Use of Disulfiram

Assessment	Management	Evaluation
Assess for informed consent, motivation, social stability.	Adequate blood level may take up to 4 days, although effect begins within 12 hr. The effect may last up to a week after discontinuation of disulfiram.	Check for side effects (usually transient, lasting 2 wk), drowsiness, fatigue, impotence, acneform eruption, metallic taste.
Persons with moderate to severe hypertension, psychiatric problems, or suicidal ideation should not receive this drug.	Metallic taste may cause anorexia; good oral hygiene may decrease taste.	Nausea and vomiting, dizziness, hypotension, headache, syncope, and flushed face in disulfiram-alcohol reaction are seen.
Interview patient.	Tell patient to avoid alcohol; give list of over-the-counter drugs and foods containing alcohol. Paraldehyde may cause reaction and should not be given. Give with caution concurrently with central nervous system depressants; it may potentiate their effects.	Check for other medications being taken, i.e., phenytoin, barbiturates, isoniazid, metronidazole, or warfarin. Disulfiram can potentiate their therapeutic or toxic effects.
	Patient should carry appropriate medical alert identification with this drug.	

Sedative-Hypnotic Drugs

Anxiety, depression, and insomnia are common in chronic alcoholics. Under most circumstances, these symptoms can be treated supportively, without psychotropic medications. The indiscriminate prescribing of antianxiety agents is all too frequent, and they have a high potential for abuse in the alcoholic population. There is no evidence to support outpatient use of psychotropic drugs in the long-term treatment of alcoholism. The use of placebos for relief of anxiety may be worthwhile when basic behavioral problems are dealt with concomitantly.

Antidepressants

Antidepressants for patients in need of therapy for chronic and severe depression should be considered only after careful evaluation of the patient. Antidepressant drugs are too often a convenient means of suicide in the depressed alcoholic patient. When antidepressants are prescribed for an alcoholic patient, the patient should be warned that the concomitant use of alcohol or other central nervous system-depressing agents with these drugs will produce severe impairment of motor and sensory function. One study in alcoholic patients with comorbid depression demonstrated a decrease in the amount and frequency of drinking compared with those receiving placebo.[82] The newer antidepressants have a lower potential for acute toxicity and may present less risk to a recovering depressed alcoholic. Therefore, antidepressants may be beneficial in the treatment of depressed alcoholics, but further investigation is needed.

Lithium

There are studies suggesting that lithium, which is indicated for manic-depressive disorders, may prevent the progress of primary alcoholism; however, results of these investigations indicate that a comprehensive evaluation of lithium for further evidence of its efficacy is needed.[83] The dual diagnosis of another psychiatric illness accompanying alcoholism has been increasing, with manic-depressive illness being a frequent diagnosis. In such patients, lithium therapy may support recovery and might affect the course of alcoholism.

Nonpharmacologic Therapy

Equally important in obtaining assistance for the alcoholic is getting them to agree to be evaluated for the problem. Denial is a common characteristic of chemical dependency and is often associated with alcoholism. Although some patients may respond to a personal expression of concern from a friend, employer, or physician, many patients require a formal intervention to get help. A formal intervention is a carefully planned confrontation of the alcoholic during which those who have observed alcohol-related behaviors report these in objective terms and present an ultimatum that the person get help or suffer consequences such as loss of job, family, friends, or other significant support. A person such as a counselor normally coordinates interventions; and some professions provide trained interveners from within the profession to facilitate interventions. Normally, the person is encouraged to obtain formal evaluation or enter treatment as soon as possible, preferably that day. The goal initially is to break through denial systems and help the alcoholic to realize that alcoholism is a disease that can be treated. Recovery from alcoholism is a lifelong process. Relapse is only one drink away for alcoholics; they usually consider themselves "recovering" rather than "recovered" alcoholics.

Several techniques for behavioral modification are used with the chronic alcoholic. Individual psychotherapy is useful in those patients who are intelligent, well motivated, and financially secure. Group psychotherapy allows for interaction among alcoholics to deal with difficulties they have in common. An estimated success rate of 80 to 90% of health professionals and 70% of employed people who participate in a full recovery program for at least 2 years can be contrasted with a 4-year sobriety rate of less than 5% for skid row alcoholics. In managing the chronic alcoholic, the goal is to achieve and maintain sobriety or prolong the periods of sobriety to give the patient time to learn to identify and avoid factors that may promote drinking, or so-called "slips."

The preferred full-recovery program includes (1) education about the disease of alcoholism, (2) abstinence from alcohol and other psychoactive substances (not forever, but "one day at a time," as is recommended by AA), and (3) group therapy (regular attendance at AA meetings or the equivalent; formal, interactive group therapy, preferably for at least 2 years; and family therapy, including participation of family members in Al-Anon or similar support group meetings). Initially, treatment usually involves intensive outpatient therapy for a number of weeks, then regular "after-care" meetings, usually through the treatment provider. Difficult cases may require inpatient therapy.

Employee assistance programs are available through most major employers; these programs often require employees to sign a recovery agreement. Such agreements assure understanding of the terms of continued employment, encourage ongoing sobriety, and provide employers with assurance of compliance. Random drug screening at employee expense is often a stated condition of the agreement.

For patients who have inadequate support systems in place at home to assure sobriety during outpatient therapy or early in the recovery process after such therapy, "half-way" houses may be used. These provide a community living environment with fairly rigid rules, ongoing group therapy, and requirements, such as maintaining employment, that encourage responsibility and social adaptation during sobriety. Half-way houses are most often used by persons recovering from drug addictions other than alcohol and by those with multiple addictions.

The group support approach of AA takes a more structured and evangelistic attitude in dealing with alcoholics and is reported to have returned many alcoholics to sobriety and maintenance of ongoing recovery. The basic tenants of AA's 12 steps are acceptance of the disease nature of alcoholism, acceptance of an external locus of control in life, "cleaning house" (guilt reduction through the process of confession and maintenance of ongoing honesty), and helping other alcoholics. AA is a private organization whose members offer mutual support to each other to remain free of alcohol. Meetings occur regularly in most communities, and, globally, in most countries. Alcoholics in early recovery are often encouraged to attend 90 AA meetings in 90 days; this encourages alcoholics to maintain frequent contact with a support system and forces them to attend a number of different meetings. Because AA meetings vary in format and character, the recovering alcoholic can eventually identify meetings that meet their specific needs and schedules. Other similar groups such as the Salvation Army also have help groups for assisting in recovery of alcoholics. Alcoholism resources listed in the yellow pages of telephone books can identify these and other treatment and support resources in the community. Many support groups exist for specific populations, such as lawyers, physicians, pharmacists, and nurses. These exist to provide support for problems unique to recovery for each group and are not intended to replace participation in other support groups, such as AA.

ALTERNATIVE THERAPIES

There is a prevailing notion that alcohol may have some usefulness in the treatment of a variety of disorders and conditions. Clinical evidence, however, is not encouraging about the role of alcohol in therapy, and it may actually worsen many conditions for which its use has been suggested (Table 61.6).

Intravenous administration of 10% v/v alcohol has been used with some success to delay premature labor and prolong gestation. The efficacy of this method has been compared with ritodrine to delay premature labor by inhibiting uterine contractions. Ritodrine, a synthetic sympathomimetic amine, was considered more effective. Blood alcohol levels of 100 to 150 mg/dL are required to inhibit uterine contractions. Studies of placenta and cord blood alcohol levels after delivery showed they were slightly less than that of the mother. In fact, neonatal depression of respiratory and circulatory activity after administration of alcohol before delivery has been reported.

Table 61.6 ▪ "Therapeutic" Use of Alcohol

Proposed Use	Actual Effect
Relief of anxiety	Anxiety often worsens when blood alcohol level falls, as in withdrawal.
Bedtime sedation	Sleeplessness is less common as blood alcohol level declines.
Improvement of nutrition	Blood glucose levels become more labile; although each gram of alcohol = 7.1 calories on oxidation, "empty" calories are gained. Overall nutrition is not improved with alcohol because vitamins, minerals or other essential dietary materials are absent in alcoholic beverages.
Diuresis of edema	Diuretic response to alcohol occurs when blood alcohol level is on the rise; antidiuresis, hyperosmolarity, and fluid retention occur as blood alcohol concentration falls.
Anemia	Iron metabolism and bone marrow function are affected, and folate antagonism contributes to anemia despite the frequent presence of iron in wines.
Lowering of blood glucose in diabetics	Lowering of blood glucose is negligible. In fact, alcohol produces more labile blood glucose levels.
Heart disease	The alcohol metabolite acetaldehyde is toxic to myocardium and not effective as a coronary vasodilator. Alcohol is a myocardial depressant. Although alcohol enhances coronary blood flow, myocardial oxygen consumption simultaneously increases.
Anti-infective	Chronic alcoholism predisposes to systemic infections.

FUTURE THERAPIES

The major advances in the treatment of alcoholism have been within the identification of the disease by health care professionals and in psychologic treatment. At least one of the atypical neurolyptics (tiapride) has demonstrated potential for use in the treatment of alcoholism. Tiapride, a selective dopamine receptor antagonist, has been used in the treatment of tardive dyskinesis, and Tourette syndrome. The management of the hyperaroused patient is the proposed place for this therapy. Tiapride has been shown to facilitate the management of acute alcohol withdrawal but has not demonstrated efficacy in severe reactions such as hallucinations and seizures.[84] One of the key advantages to tiapride is the lack of either physical or psychologic dependence. Tiapride does have the potential to cause neuroleptic malignant syndrome, which limits its usefulness in the treatment of alcoholism.[85]

IMPROVING OUTCOMES

Patient Education

The health care professional is presented with a variety of unique patient education opportunities with the alcoholic patient. Because approximately 70 to 80% of adults consume alcoholic beverages, it is almost inevitable that medications either prescribed by a physician or bought over-the-counter will be taken concomitantly with alcohol or while alcohol is still in the body. Alcohol may be present in some preparations and interact with prescribed medications to produce untoward effects in the unsuspecting patient.[83] Alcoholics should be encouraged to seek advice before taking over-the-counter medications and to avoid taking psychoactive substances.

In general, a practitioner experienced in addiction medicine should manage therapy with any psychoactive medication. This does not mean that a recovering alcoholic or addict cannot receive controlled substances for specific, short-term uses, such as severe pain; the physician must limit the amount prescribed to no more than the amount required by most patients. The experienced practitioner must recognize the possibility that the recovering alcoholic may lose control fairly rapidly and may attempt to obtain additional medication beyond the normal period of use.

Preventing Drug–Alcohol Interactions

Alcohol administration in high concentrations results in increased metabolism by MEOS, with concurrent inhibition of metabolism of drugs that undergo microsomal degradation. The repeated administration of alcohol has been shown to cause nonspecific hepatic microsomal enzyme induction, resulting in increased clearance of both alcohol and microsomally metabolized drugs, such as barbiturates.[86–88] After withdrawal of alcohol, enhanced hepatic metabolism of drugs may persist for some time, requiring higher doses of affected drugs. Metabolic pathways such as *N*-desmethylation of the longer-acting benzodiazepines and oxidation and glucuronidation are inhibited by acute alcohol intake. With chronic use, however, metabolism increases. This explains partially the "tolerance" to the action of sedatives observed in some chronic alcoholics. Warfarin, phenytoin, tolbutamide, procainamide, and isoniazid are nonpsychoactive drugs subject to hepatic microsomal enzyme activity. The plasma half-lives of these drugs are markedly decreased in some chronic and heavy users of alcohol as a result of their increased rate of clearance. Clinical reports of problems from such interactions, however, are few. Variable and unpredictable response to drugs in the alcoholic should suggest the possibility of some metabolic alteration of drug kinetics. It has become increasingly evident that toxicity to certain drugs and chemicals is enhanced in chronic alcoholics as a result of this mechanism. The hepatotoxic risk with acetaminophen usage or with carbon tetrachloride ingestion is increased in chronic alcoholics because of increased formation of toxic metabolites of these chemicals caused by MEOS induction.

Alcohol is primarily a central nervous system depressant. When combined with other drugs with similar depressing action on the central nervous system, an additive or synergistic effect occurs. This is the most important type of interaction between alcohol and other drugs. Moreover, cimetidine, ranitidine, and nizatidine, but not famotidine, have been shown to decrease gastric ADH activity, resulting in increased alcohol absorption and effects.[89,90]

Alcoholics taking tolbutamide and other antidiabetic drugs, chloramphenicol, griseofulvin, quinacrine, or metronidazole have reported a mild "disulfiram-like" reaction. Alcohol consumption during ceforanide, cefotetan, or cefoperazone therapy may precipitate a disulfiram-like reaction. Some alcoholic beverages such as Chianti wines contain appreciable amounts of tyramine so that when ingested by patients using monoamine oxidase (MAO)-inhibiting drugs (i.e., procarbazine and pargyline), they cause an acute hypertensive episode. Interference with tyramine metabolism by the MAO inhibitors results in the release of norepinephrine from the sympathetic nerve terminal. A summary of selected drug-alcohol interactions is presented in Table 61.7.

Disease Management Strategies to Improve Patient Outcomes

To improve patient outcomes, a therapeutic alliance should be formed with the patient. If at any time in the treatment process the patient feels as though the provider is judgmental, that alliance can be broken resulting in a decrease in trust and possible therapeutic setback. Therefore, it is imperative that the provider set goals with the patient at the initiation of treatment and assist the patient in attaining these goals. If the therapeutic goals are agreed upon at the onset and trust is built, then the provider is given more flexibility in straightforward discussions that are necessary. In addition, the practitioner should always remain cognizant of the psychosocial and patient confidentiality issues that accompany alcoholism.

PHARMACOECONOMICS

Estimates of the cost of alcohol abuse and alcoholism in the United States increased from $148 billion in 1992 to more than $166 billion in 1995.[56,91] As a component of total care cost, alcohol-related treatment costs exceeded $18 billion in 1992 with therapy for comorbid health problems accounting for $13 billion. Specialized detoxification and rehabilitation services accounted for $4 billion to provide care for the 1.8 million patients while prevention costs reached nearly $2 billion.[92] Alcohol-related premature deaths exceeded 107,000 in 1992, resulting in cost estimates of $31 billion. Moreover, a decrease in potential productivity was estimated at $67 billion for the same period.

Total health care costs of alcoholic patients are significantly higher than those for nonalcoholics. The 4-year average family monthly medical costs were reported to be twice those of families with no apparent alcoholic members. However, the increase in costs was not due totally to alcoholic treatment. The monthly medical cost for alcoholics began to rise 6 months before detoxification, peaking at 13 times the average for the month before treatment.[93] There has not been a difference noted between males and females in cost of care.[94] For younger alcoholics medical costs have been reported to have

Table 61.7 ▪ Summary of Selected Alcohol-Drug Interactions

Drugs Interacting with Alcohol	Mechanism	Effect	Significance
Anticoagulants (oral): warfarin	Metabolism enhanced with chronic alcohol abuse	Diminished anticoagulant effect	Moderate
	Metabolism reduced with acute alcohol intoxication	Increased anticoagulant effect	Moderate
Antihistamines	Additive	Increased central nervous system depression	Moderate
Aspirin (and other salicylates)	Additive	Increased occult blood loss and damage to gastric mucosa	Moderate
Acetaminophen	Metabolism enhanced in chronic alcohol abuse	Increase risk for hepatotoxicity	Moderate
	Metabolism reduced in acute alcohol intoxication	Reduce risk for hepatotoxicity	Moderate
Anticonvulsants: phenytoin (Dilantin) and others	Metabolism enhanced with chronic alcohol abuse	Diminished anticonvulsant effect	Moderate
	Metabolism reduced with acute alcohol intoxication	Increased anticonvulsant effect	Moderate
Antimicrobials			
Isoniazid	Metabolism enhanced in chronic alcohol abuse	Diminished isoniazid effect	Moderate
		Increased incidence of isoniazid hepatitis	Not established
Cefoperazone, metronidazole, chloramphenicol, griseofulvin	Metabolism of alcohol reduced	Disulfiram-like reaction	Minor/moderate

returned to averages for nonalcoholics after treatment while patients older than 50 years of age continued to have elevated health care costs posttreatment.[94] The increase in costs for care in older patients emphasizes the importance of both early detection and treatment.

CONCLUSION

The treatment goal for the alcoholic is long-term abstinence from alcohol use. Much confusion has arisen though in the midst of a widely publicized 1976 report by the Rand Corporation on alcoholism, which seems to imply that some alcoholics can return to social drinking.[95] Nevertheless, the medical and psychology professions have long advocated the opposing viewpoint. For instance, AA considers abstinence as the only goal for anyone with an alcohol problem. Careful evaluation of data from the Rand Report does not support the notion that alcoholics can safely return to drinking. What it did point out was that after an 18-month period, relatively few alcoholics were practicing long-term abstinence despite an impressive improvement rate (70%). Most had intermittent periods of abstinence interspersed with "controlled" drinking. Relapse to uncontrolled drinking by those who continued to drink in a controlled manner and those who continued abstinence were found to be no different. Major methodologic problems are suggested by the large number (more than 80%) of subjects lost to follow-up at the end of the 18-month study period. The same investigators in a 1980 follow-up report sharply modified their original claims; however, this has accomplished little to discourage the many and vocal advocates of "controlled drinking" for alcoholics.[96]

The use of pharmacotherapy and chemical intervention to enhance efforts to abstain from alcohol use and prevent relapse is receiving considerable attention currently as reports of promising experience with opiate antagonists, serotonergic drugs, and agents such as acamprosate (calcium acetyl homotaurinate) emerge from among the treatment community.[78] The effectiveness studies involving these and other prospects will require careful systematic and comparative review of the evidence and outcome.

Abstinence from alcohol should not be a goal for treatment but rather a means to an end. The treatment of alcoholism is best accomplished if conducted in a relationship of understanding and trust with others. This can be a concerned and interested friend or spouse or a professional person such as a pharmacist, therapist, physician, or a member of a therapeutic or rehabilitation group. Dependence on alcohol is no different in any significant way from dependence on other addictive drugs such as opiates and barbiturates. Although there are differences in social attitudes toward drinking and drug abuse, many features of alcohol and "hard drug" addiction are remarkably similar. The similarities and differences should be appreciated and understood by those who are involved in the treatment, care, and rehabilitation of alcohol-dependent patients.

KEY POINTS

- The treatment of alcohol dependence relies on a two-step approach that deals with withdrawal and detoxification followed by subsequent interventions to maintain abstinence.
- The maintenance and support of vital functions are basic to the treatment strategy for acute alcohol intoxication.
- The unconscious alcohol intoxicated or poisoned patient should have causes such as alcohol hypoglycemia, physical (subdural or head trauma) and other chemicals (drugs) ruled out.
- Pharmacologic attempts to accelerate the metabolism or clearance of alcohol from the body of the intoxicated patient are not recommended.
- The goal of treatment for an acutely agitated and alcohol-impaired patient with toxic psychosis symptoms is to produce a calm, but still arousable and responsive condition.
- The detoxification from alcohol involves a process of substitution with and slow withdrawing of a longer acting sedative-hypnotic medication for ethanol.
- The doses and regimens of medications used to treat acute alcohol withdrawal should be tailored to response, the presence of underlying conditions and concurrent polydrug abuse.
- Nondrug factors can be effective in helping with the treatment of many clinical problems that accompany the process of acute detoxification from alcohol.
- Successful treatment for and recovery from chronic alcoholism is dependent on the patient's motivation to stop drinking and participation in recovery support programs.

REFERENCES

1. Morse RM, Flavin DK. The definition of alcoholism. The Joint Committee of the National Council on Alcoholism and Drug Dependence and the American Society of Addiction Medicine to Study the Definition and Criteria for the Diagnosis of Alcoholism. JAMA 268:1012–1014, 1992.
2. US Department of Health and Human Services. Eighth special report to the US Congress on alcohol and health. Rockville, MD: US Department of Health and Human Services, 1993.
3. West LJ, Maxwell DS, Noble EP, et al. Alcoholism. Ann Intern Med 100:405–416, 1984.
4. Cotton NS. The familial incidence of alcoholism. J Stud Alcohol 40:89–116, 1979.
5. McGinnis JM, Foege WH. Actual causes of death in the United States. JAMA 270:2207–2012, 1993.
6. Camargo CA Jr, Hennekens CH, Gaziano JM, et al. Prospective study of moderate alcohol consumption and mortality in US male physicians. Arch Intern Med 157:79–85, 1997.
7. Boffetta P, Garfinkel L. Alcohol drinking and mortality among men enrolled in an American Cancer Society prospective study. Epidemiology 1:342–348, 1990.
8. Fuchs CS, Stampfer MJ, Colditz GA, et al. Alcohol consumption and mortality among women. N Engl J Med 332:1245–1250, 1995.
9. Droomers M, Schrijvers CT, Stronks K, et al. Educational differences in excessive alcohol consumption: the role of psychosocial and material stressors. Prev Med 29:1–10, 1999.
10. American Academy of Pediatrics Committee on Substance Abuse. Alcohol use and abuse: a pediatric concern. Pediatrics 95:439–442, 1995.
11. Blume LN, Nielsen NH, Riggs JA. Alcoholism and alcohol abuse among women: report of the council on scientific affairs. J Womens Health 7:861–871, 1998.
12. Graham K, Schmidt G. Alcohol use and psychosocial well-being among older adults. J Stud Alcohol 60:345–351, 1999.
13. US Department of Health and Human Services. Ninth special report to the US Congress on alcohol and health. Washington, DC: US Department of Health and Human Services, 1997.
14. Broadening the base of treatment for alcohol problems: report of a study by a committee of the Institute of Medicine. Washington, DC: National Academy Press, 1990.
15. US Department of Justice. Alcohol and crime: an analysis of national data on the prevalence of alcohol involvement in crime. Washington, DC: US Department of Justice, 1998.
16. US Department of Health and Human Services. Seventh special report to the US Congress on alcohol and health. Rockville, MD: US Department of Health and Human Services, 1990.
17. Wallace J. The new disease model of alcoholism. West J Med 152:502–505, 1990.
18. Blum TC, Roman PM, Bennett N. Public images of alcoholism: data from a Georgia survey. J Stud Alcohol 50:5–14, 1989.
19. Goodwin DW. Is alcoholism hereditary? New York: Oxford University Press, 1976.
20. Goodwin DW. Alcoholism and genetics: the sins of the fathers. Arch Gen Psychol 42:171–174, 1985.
21. Johnson JL, Leff M. Children of substance abusers: overview of research findings. Pediatrics 103:1085–1099, 1999.
22. Frezza M, di Padora C, Pozzata G, et al. High blood alcohol levels in women. N Engl J Med 322:95–99, 1990.
23. Lieber CS, ed. Medical and nutritional complications of alcoholism: mechanisms and management. New York: Plenum, 1992.
24. Espina N, Lima V, Lieber CS, et al. In vitro and in vivo inhibitory effect of ethanol and acetaldehyde on O-methylguanine transferase. Carcinogenesis 9: 761–766, 1988.
25. Lieber CS, Baraona E, Hernandez-Munoz R, et al. Impaired oxygen utilization: a new mechanism for the hepatotoxicity of ethanol in sub-human primates. J Clin Invest 83:1682–1690, 1989.
26. Lieber CS. Medical disorders of alcoholism. N Engl J Med 333:1058–1065, 1995.
27. Lieber CS, DeCarli LM. Hepatic microsomal ethanol-oxidizing system: in vitro characteristics and adaptive properties in vivo. J Biol Chem 245:2505–2512, 1970.
28. Eckardt MJ, Harford TC, Kaelbar CT, et al. Health hazards associated with alcohol consumption. JAMA 246:648–666, 1981.
29. Segel LD, Klausner SC, Harney-Gnadt JJ, et al. Alcohol and the heart. Med Clin North Am 68:147–161, 1984.
30. Demakis JG, Proskey A, Rahimtoola SH. The natural course of alcohol cardiomyopathy. Ann Intern Med 80:293, 1974.
31. Eichner ER. The hematologic disorder of alcoholism. Am J Med 54:621, 1973.
32. Larkin EC, Watson-Williams EJ. Alcohol and blood. Med Clin North Am 68:105–120, 1984.
33. Pimstone NR, French SW. Alcoholic liver disease. Med Clin North Am 68:39–56, 1984.
34. Scully RE, Galdabini JJ, McNeely BU. Case records of the Massachusetts General Hospital: case 38-1979: ethylene glycol poisoning. N Engl J Med 301:650–657, 1979.
35. Clarren SK, Smith DW. The fetal alcohol syndrome. N Engl J Med 298:1063, 1978.
36. Nakada T, Knight RT. Alcohol and the central nervous system. Med Clin North Am 68:121–131, 1984.
37. Haller RG, Knochel JP. Skeletal muscle disease in alcoholism. Med Clin North Am 68:91–103, 1984.
38. Adams HG, Jordan C. Infections in the alcoholic. Med Clin North Am 68:179–201, 1984.
39. Kaysen G, Noth RH. The effects of alcohol on blood pressure and electrolytes. Med Clin North Am 68:221–246, 1984.
40. Williams HE. Alcoholic hypoglycemia and ketoacidosis. Med Clin North Am 68:33–38, 1984.
41. Altura BM. Introduction to the symposium and overview. Alcoholism (NY) 10:557–559, 1986.
42. Klatsky AL. Epidemiology of coronary heart disease: influence of alcohol. Alcohol Clin Exp Res 18:88–96, 1994.

43. Rubin R, Rand ML. Alcohol and platelet function. Alcohol Clin Exp Res 18:105–110, 1994.
44. Lange LG, Kinnunen PM. Cardiovascular effects of alcohol. Adv Alcohol Subst Abuse 6:47–52, 1987.
45. Klatsky AL. The cardiovascular effects of alcohol. Alcohol Alcohol 22(Suppl 1):117–124, 1987.
46. Lieber CS. Alcohol and the liver: 1984 update. Hepatology 4:1243–1260, 1984.
47. McCoy HG, Cipolle RJ, Ehlers SM, et al. Severe methanol poisoning: application of a pharmacokinetic model for ethanol therapy and hemodialysis. Am J Med 67:804–807, 1979.
48. Leevy C, Baker H. Vitamins and alcoholism. Am J Clin Nutr 21:1325, 1968.
49. Purdie FR, Honigman B, Rosen P. Acute organic brain syndrome: a review of 100 cases. Ann Emerg Med 10:455–461, 1981.
50. Blum K, Noble EP, Sheridan PJ, et al. Allelic association of human dopamine D_2 receptor gene in alcoholism. JAMA 263:2055–2060, 1990.
51. Ewing JA. Detecting alcoholism: the CAGE questionnaire. JAMA 252:1905–1907, 1984.
52. Schorling JB, Buchsbaum DG. Screening for alcohol and drug abuse. Med Clin North Am 81:845–865, 1997.
53. American Psychiatric Association. Diagnostic and statistical manual of mental disorders. 4th ed. Washington, DC: American Psychiatric Association, 1994.
54. Moos RH, Billings AG. Children of alcoholics during the recovery process: alcohol and matched control families. Addict Behav 7:155–164, 1982.
55. Patterson GR, Stoughamer-Loeber M. The correlation of family management practices and delinquency. Child Dev 33:1299–1307, 1984.
56. Pharmacotherapy for alcohol dependence. Summary, evidence report/technology assessment: number 3. Rockville, MD: Agency for Health Care Policy and Research, 1999.
57. Sellers EM, Kalant H. Alcohol intoxication and withdrawal. N Engl J Med 294:757–762, 1976.
58. Khantzian EJ, McKenna GJ. Acute toxic withdrawal reactions associated with drug use and abuse. Ann Intern Med 90:361, 1979.
59. Thompson WL, Johnson AD, Maddrey WC. Diazepam and paraldehyde for treatment of severe delirium tremens. Ann Intern Med 82:175–180, 1975.
60. Lyon LJ, Antony J. Reversal of alcoholic coma by naloxone. Am Intern Med 96:464–465, 1982.
61. Mattila MJ, Nuotto E, Seppala T. Naloxone is not an effective antagonist of ethanol. Lancet 1:775–776, 1981.
62. Mayo-Smith MF. Pharmacological management of alcohol withdrawal: a meta-analysis and evidence-based practice guideline: American Society of Addiction Medicine Working Group on Pharmacological Management of Alcohol Withdrawal. JAMA 278:144–151, 1997.
63. Saitz R, Friedman LA, Mayo-Smith MF. Alcohol withdrawal: a nation wide survey of impatient treatment practices. J Gen Intern Med 10:479–487, 1995.
64. Sellers EM, Kalant H. Alcohol intoxication and withdrawal. N Engl J Med 294:757–762, 1976.
65. Baumgartner GR, Rowen RC. Clonidine versus chlordiazepoxide in the management of acute alcohol withdrawal syndrome. Arch Intern Med 147:1223, 1987.
66. Kloz UA, Avant GR, Hoyumpia A, et al. The effects of age and liver disease on the disposition and elimination of diazepam in adult man. J Clin Invest 55:347, 1975.
67. Hayashida M, Alterman AL, McClellan AT, et al. Comparative effectiveness and cost of inpatient and outpatient detoxification of patients with mild to moderate alcohol withdrawal syndrome. N Engl J Med 320:358–365, 1989.
68. Brown CG. The alcohol-withdrawal syndrome. West J Med 138:579–581, 1983.
69. Mendelson JH. Propranolol and behavior of alcohol addicts after acute alcohol ingestion. Clin Pharmacol Ther 15:571, 1974.
70. Kraus ML, Gottlieb LD, Horwitz RI, et al. Randomized clinical trial of atenolol in patients with alcohol withdrawal. N Engl J Med 313:905–909, 1985.
71. Nakada T, Knight RT. Alcohol and the central nervous system. Med Clin North Am 68:121–131, 1984.
72. Victor M, Adams RD. On the etiology of the alcoholic neurologic diseases with special reference in the role of nutrition. Am J Clin Nutr 9:379, 1961.
73. Segel LD, Klausner SC, Harney-Gnadt JJ, et al. Alcohol and the heart. Med Clin North Am 68:147–161, 1984.
74. Vetter WR, Cohn LH, Reichgott M. Hypokalemia and electrocardiographic abnormalities during acute alcohol withdrawal. Arch Intern Med 120:536, 1967.
75. Beard JD, Knott DH. Fluid and electrolyte balance during acute withdrawal in chronic alcoholic patients. JAMA 204:135, 1968.
76. Kaysen G, Noth RH. The effects of alcohol on blood pressure and electrolytes. Med Clin North Am 68:221–246, 1984.
77. Fuller RK, Branchey L, Brightwell DR, et al. Disulfiram treatment of alcoholism: a Veterans Administration Cooperative study. JAMA 256:1449–1455, 1986.
78. Garbutt JC, West SL, Carety TS, et al. Pharmacological treatment of alcohol dependance. JAMA:281:1318–1325,1999.
79. Elenbaas RM, Ryan JL, Robinson WA, et al. On the disulfiram-like activity of moxalactam. Clin Pharmacol Ther 32:347–355, 1982.
80. O'Malley SS, Jaffe A, Chang G, et al. Naltrexone and coping skills therapy for alcohol dependence: a controlled study. Arch Gen Psychiatry 49:881–887, 1992.
81. Saitz R, O'Malley SS. Pharmacotherapies for alcohol abuse. Med Clin North Am 81:81–907, 1997.
82. Cornelius JR, Salloum IM, Ehler JG, et al. Fluoxetine in depressed alcoholics: a double blind, placebo-controlled trial. Arch Gen Psychiatry 54:700–705, 1997.
83. Dorus W, Ostrow DG, Anton R, et al. Lithium treatment of depressed and nondepressed alcoholics. JAMA 262:1646–1652, 1989.
84. Peters DH, Faulds D. Tiapride: a review of its pharmacology and therapeutic potential in the management of alcohol dependence syndrome. Drugs 47:1010–1032, 1994.
85. Shaw GK, Majumdar SK, Waller S, et al. Tiapride in the long-term management of alcoholics of anxious or depressive temperament. Br J Psychiatry 150:164–168, 1987.
86. Lane EA, Guthrie S, Linnoila M. Effects of ethanol on drug and metabolite pharmacokinetics. Clin Pharmacokinet 10:228–247, 1985.
87. Hoyumpa AM, Schenker S. Ethanol-drug interaction. Annu Rev Med 33:113–149, 1982.
88. Lieber CS. Interaction of ethanol with drugs, hepatotoxic agents, carcinogens and vitamins. Alcohol Alcohol 25:157–176, 1990.
89. Caballeria J, Baraona E, Rodamilans M, et al. Effects of cimetidine on gastric alcohol dehydrogenase activity and blood ethanol levels. Gastroenterology 96:388–392, 1989.
90. Caballeria J, Baraona E, Rodamilans M, et al. Cimetidine and alcohol absorption. Gastroenterology 97:1067–1068, 1989.
91. Harwood H, Fountain D, Livermore G, et al. Economic costs of alcohol and drug abuse in the United States: 1992. Report to the national Institute on Drug Abuse and the National Institute on Alcohol Abuse and Alcoholism. Fairfax, VA: The Lewin Group, 1998.
92. Harwood HJ, Fountain D, Livermore G. Economic costs of alcohol abuse and alcoholism. Recent Dev Alcohol 14:307–330, 1998.
93. Holder HD. The cost offsets of alcoholism treatment. Recent Dev Alcohol 14:361–374, 1998.
94. Blose JO, Holder HD. The utilization of medical care by treated alcoholics: longitudinal patterns by age, gender, and type of care. J Subst Abuse 3:13–27, 1991.
95. Armour DJ, Polich JM, Stambul HB. Alcoholism and treatment. The Rand Corporation, R-1739-NIAAA. New York: Wiley, 1978.
96. Polich JM, Armour DJ, Braiker HV. The course of alcoholism four years after treatment. The Rand Corporation, R-2433-NIAAA. New York: Wiley, 1980.

CHAPTER 62

SUBSTANCE ABUSE

Stephen C. Cooke, Bob L. Lobo, and James C. Eoff III

Overview of Substance Abuse

Mankind's struggle with intoxicating substances dates back to our earliest recorded history. That humans have always used and misused substances for the purposes of pain relief, escape, pleasure, and self-abuse is a telling commentary. Sumerian texts from 4500 BC describe cannabis intoxication and the societal repercussions of drunkenness. Egyptian sources from the time of the great pharaohs detail a process for fermentation and the Bible advocates against drunkenness.

Before the turn of the century and the implementation of federal product standards via the Harrison Narcotic Act of 1914, lay persons could order heroin, cocaine, cannabis, and opium for personal use through wholesale and retail companies. The years following the U.S. Civil War found America inundated with thousands of middle class narcotic addicts whose drug of choice was an opium-containing preparation known as laudanum. Coca-Cola, one of the nation's most recognizable products, originally contained the cocaine alkaloid. Sigmund Freud experimented with cocaine, both personally and for his patients. Early pharmacologic interventions in psychiatry used the prototypical hallucinogen, lysergic acid (LSD), as a purported window into the soul.

Even though this problem is universal, a great deal of myth and misunderstanding still surrounds the nature of substance abuse. At its simplest level, psychoactive compounds are substances that alter perception and state of mind. More complex, however, are the psychosocial complications that these psychoactive agents produce, both in the individual and society alike.

The widespread availability of abusable agents, including new synthetic compounds and analogs of existing substances has contributed to the worldwide epidemic of substance abuse. Surveys conducted by the National Institute on Drug Abuse (NIDA) have shown a small, but generalized downward trend in usage across all drug classes compared to historically high levels in the early and mid 1970s.[1] These data, although hopeful, are misleading because the actual total numbers of people engaging in drug abuse and misuse are higher now than in the mid-1970s because of the increased national census. Although the incidence of drug use may be declining in some areas, the societal complications arising from drug abuse are still very much apparent. Drug-related visits to emergency rooms in 1995 totaled 531,000; half of which were due to drug overdose. Substance abusers suffer from higher rates of mortality and morbidity and account for a disproportionate share of total health care costs.[2] The United States has appointed a "drug czar" and spends billions of dollars annually on programs of education, arrest, drug eradication, and national border integrity. The merits and associated efficacy of this expense are a matter of ongoing debate. Interestingly, the most dangerous drug, in terms of addictability, mortality, and associated costs, nicotine, has legalized status in the United States. Although completely legal for adults, nicotine is responsible for three times as many deaths every year as alcohol, heroin, and cocaine combined.[3]

A study prepared by the Institute for Health Policy at Brandeis University for The Robert Wood Johnson Foundation estimated the total economic cost of drug abuse at $67 billion in 1990, up $23 billion from 1985. The White House Office of National Drug Control Policy (ONDCP) conducted a study to determine how much money is spent on illegal drugs that otherwise would support legitimate spending or savings by the user in the overall economy. ONDCP found that between 1988 and 1991 the annual retail trade in illicit drugs amounted to between $45 and $51 billion. In 1991, Americans spent about $49 billion on these drugs, broken down as follows: $30 billion on cocaine, $9 billion on heroin, $8 billion on marijuana, and $2 billion on other illegal drugs and on the misuse of legal drugs. Another recent government study found that state and local governments spent $15.9 billion on drug control activities in fiscal year 1991, an increase of nearly 13% over the 1990 figure. The total Federal budget for drug control activities in that same year was $11 billion.[4]

A great deal of societal misunderstanding surrounds the proper use of terms such as substance abuse, intoxication, dependence, and withdrawal. Therefore, the use of a standardized guide is necessary to minimize confusion and to provide proper diagnostic reliability. The accepted standard in psychiatry is the *Diagnostic and Statistical Manual of Mental Disorders,* 4th ed. (DSM-IV).[5] As found in the DSM-IV, Substance Related Disorders include disorders that are not only related to exposure to a drug of abuse, but also to the side effects of medications and to toxin exposure (e.g., volatile inhalants). Substances of abuse are divided into 11 separate classes and include alcohol, amphetamines, cannabis, caffeine, inhalants, hallucinogens, cocaine, opioids, phencyclidines, nicotine, and sedatives, hypnotics, or anxiolytics.

As defined by the DSM-IV, *substance intoxication* is a reversible syndrome, specific to a particular substance and secondary to recent ingestion or overexposure to a substance. Maladaptive and clinical behaviors are directly related to the pharmacologic effects (or side effects) of the specific substance. *Substance abuse* is defined as a maladaptive pattern of substance use that results in significant adverse consequences. Consequences may include absenteeism, legal problems, social and interpersonal difficulties, and repeated failure to fulfill obligations. *Substance dependence* (Table 62.1) is characterized by a maladaptive pattern of use leading to adverse cognitive, behavioral, and psychologic symptoms. This pattern of repeated self-administration typically leads to tolerance, withdrawal, and compulsive use of the substance. *Substance withdrawal* is evidenced by the development of substance-specific psychologic and cognitive changes that occur secondary to cessation or reduction in prolonged substance use. The development of this syndrome is accompanied by significant distress and obvious reduction in important areas of life functioning.

The phrase *drug abuse treatment* is somewhat misleading, as *drug abuse rehabilitation* is a more accurate description of

Table 62.1 ▪ Diagnostic Criteria for Substance Dependence

A. Maladaptive pattern of substance use
B. Use leads to social, professional impairment
C. Tolerance, as defined by
   1. Increased doses needed to achieve desired effect
   2. Diminished effect with same dose
D. Presence of withdrawal
E. Substance taken in larger amounts over time
F. Unsuccessful attempts to decrease use
G. Large amounts of time spent to acquire, use, or recover from substance
H. Responsibilities abandoned for substance
I. Substance use continues despite adverse consequences

Source: Reference 5.

the ideal process. The overall goal of treatment or rehabilitation is to allow persons dependent on substances of abuse to learn to live effectively and comfortably without the use of alcohol or other drugs. The first phase of treatment is focused on restoring physical health and usually entails medical supervision of withdrawal and concomitant treatment of any associated medical problems. This first phase is necessary as a foundation for future treatment success. The second phase of treatment focuses on education, patient acceptance of illness, and aftercare.

TREATMENT GOALS: SUBSTANCE ABUSE

- Detoxify and medically stabilize the patient.
- Provide a rationale for sobriety through education and examples of success.
- Ensure that the patient understands the biologic basis of his or her illness through group and/or individual education.
- Help the patient to develop the ability to identify and avoid potential triggers for continued drug use.
- Encourage the patient's active participation in aftercare programs with organizations such as Narcotics, Cocaine, or Alcoholics Anonymous.
- Advise the patient to develop new social circles that involve sober or non-drug using friends and peers.
- Emphasize that total abstinence is the ultimate goal and indicative of treatment success.

EPIDEMIOLOGY

Substance abuse and dependence is more common in males than in females and is also more common in the unemployed and in certain minorities.[6] A worrisome trend noted over the last 20 years is the continually decreasing age at first drug use. Substance use and dependence are also more common in heath care professionals than in nonmedical professionals with an equivalent amount of education and training. High levels of professional stress and ease of access have been suggested as possible explanations for this phenomenon. Substance-specific epidemiologic trends are discussed later in this chapter.

The dual diagnosis of a major psychiatric disorder along with substance abuse is a common occurrence. As many as 75% of men and 65% of women with a substance use disorder meet the criteria for an additional psychiatric diagnosis. The most common comorbidity is an additional substance of abuse. Other associated comorbidities include major depression, anxiety disorders, and personality disorders. The presence of an additional psychiatric disorder is typically indicative of poor prognosis, a greater degree of impairment, and an increased risk of suicide and/or mortality.

PATHOPHYSIOLOGY

Several factors causing the progression of substance use to substance abuse or dependence have been suggested. Although no one theory is universally accepted in the medical community, a comprehensive etiologic theory must take into account biologic, social, and psychologic factors. Genetic studies have shown rates of substance abuse that are 3 to 4 times higher in identical twins than in dizygotic twins.[7] Children of drug dependent parents are 4 times more likely to become dependent on a substance of abuse. Adopted children from non-substance-abusing parents who are placed in homes of drug-abusing stepparents show a higher rate of eventual drug dependence. This suggests that although genetics are involved, so too is the environment in which a person develops.

A great deal of research over the past decade has attempted to identify a specific biologic marker for substance abuse and dependence. Researchers have noted abnormalities in neurotransmitter functioning in the brains of addicts, especially related to the neurotransmitter most affected by the addict's substance of choice. Additionally, the continuous abuse of a substance over time leads to modulation of neurotransmitter-receptor systems, thus requiring the presence of the substance of abuse to maintain homeostasis. Recent studies have moved past a simple neurotransmitter model and are now focusing on second-messenger systems and gene regulation.

Behavioral models focus on four main attributes of substance abuse. These include positive reinforcement, adverse effects, substance discrimination, and environmental cues. First, most drug abusers relate a positive or pleasurable experience after ingesting a substance for the first time, thus resulting in positive reinforcement. Second, substances are also usually associated with negative effects, which can result in behavior modification through decreased use or the consumption of another substance in an attempt to minimize adverse effects of the first substance. Third, substance abusers are able to discriminate their substance of abuse from pharmacologically similar substances. Benzodiazepines and phenothiazines possess similar pharmacologic properties, yet benzodiazepines are much more likely to be abused than chlorpromazine. Last, almost all drug users report triggers or cues that they permanently associate with substance use. The removal of a patient from these environmental cues is often one of the first steps suggested during substance abuse treatment.

PSYCHOSOCIAL ASPECTS

Perhaps no other medical disorder causes as pronounced a "ripple effect" as substance abuse. Just as the name implies, the ripple effect relates to the ever-broadening influence that substance abuse exerts. Initially, only the substance user is involved. Shortly thereafter, the immediate family becomes entangled. Employers may then begin to feel the effects of absenteeism or errors in the workplace. Decreased productivity, increased crime and violence, disproportionate health care costs, and increased mortality all affect the stability and quality of our society. Familial support is encouraged through family counseling or involvement in organizations such as Al-Anon and Al-Teen. Family therapy seeks to teach acceptance of the substance abuser without endorsing the substance abuse. This type of psychotherapy provides a nonthreatening, supportive environment for families to work through the negative consequences of substance abuse. The optimal role of psychosocial treatments, which broadly encompass psychotherapies such as cognitive, behavioral, or supportive therapy, counseling, skills training, and family therapy, has not been determined. Although commonly used, empirical research into the effectiveness and efficacy of these models is scarce.

PHARMACOECONOMICS

Adequate pharmacoeconomic evaluation and/or comparison of the various treatment options for patients with drug abuse have not been conducted. Whether these much needed trials will be conducted in the near future remains an unknown. Research funding for this area is not currently a national priority. The vast majority of monies spent in the area of drug abuse are now directed into law enforcement efforts; including prevention through community education, criminalization, and extended incarceration for recidivistic drug offenders, and international/national eradication of drug supplies and sources.

One economic truth that exists is the dearth of integrated inpatient-outpatient treatment facilities for all but the very affluent. Top-of-the-line treatment facilities can cost as much as $800 to $1000 per treatment day with a standard program length averaging 28 days.[8] Obviously, a $25,000 per treatment event cost is prohibitive for most persons. Middle-income addicts also face economic blockade from employers and insurance companies that have pared mental health and addiction benefits in an effort to reduce short-term costs. These persons are often trapped between the extremes of ineligibility for public assistance and an inability to pay out-of-pocket expenses associated with treatment. Programs sponsored by Medicaid and Medicare for the economically disadvantaged have undergone radical changes in the face of recent funding cutbacks and lowered reimbursement. Average length of stay at these programs has dropped to an average of 5 days compared to 10 days just over 2 years ago. Many times, in an effort to minimize costs, programs for lower- or no-income addicts only offer services such as detoxification and medication management while peripheral services such as vocational rehabilitation and dual diagnosis treatment are eliminated.

Opioids

The terms opioids or opiates come from the word *opium* which is the dried crude extract of the unripe poppy pod, *Papaver somniferum*. This pod contains approximately 20 alkaloids of opium. Opioids generally fall into three categories based upon their natural occurrence (Table 62.2). The first group are the naturally occurring opioids and consist of morphine and codeine. The second group are the semisynthetic chemical derivatives of the naturally occurring opioids such as diacetylmorphine (heroin), hydromorphone, and hydrocodone. The final group are the synthetic opioids consisting of meperidine, fentanyl, methadone, and others. Another related class of drugs are the opioid antagonists. These are drugs that have been synthesized for use in the treatment of opioid overdose and dependence. Included in this group of drugs are naloxone and naltrexone. A few synthetic opioids possess both agonist and antagonist activity at opioid receptors, such as pentazocine, buprenorphine, and butorphanol.

Heroin is the most commonly abused drug of the opioid class.[9] Most of the heroin available for sale in the United States is smuggled in from South America, Mexico, and Asia. Analysis of price, purity, seizure data, and other intelligence and abuse indicators revealed that there are currently two general, but distinct, heroin markets in the United States, roughly divided geographically by the Mississippi River. In the first 6 months of 1996, at least 90% of all identifiable Domestic Monitor Program heroin purchases made in Boston, Newark, New York City, and Philadelphia were of South American origin. In the West, black tar heroin and brown powder heroin from Mexico predominate.[10]

The opioids can rapidly produce tolerance and dependence. Doses of opioids given for long periods of time must be gradually tapered because of severe withdrawal. This withdrawal syndrome is also seen in abusers of opioids who are unable to obtain their drug of choice.

EPIDEMIOLOGY

In 1991 an estimated 1.3% of the United States population had used heroin at least once. There are more than 500,000 persons with opioid dependence in the United States. Half of those are in New York City alone. Males outnumber females by three to one. Most persons with opioid dependence are in their thirties and forties but report first use during their twenties.[6] Injection continues to be the number one method of heroin administration. However, the number of patients using injection as their primary means of administration has decreased from 93% in 1989

Table 62.2 ▪ Narcotics and Related Compounds

Naturally occurring and derivatives
Opium
Morphine
Codeine
Tincture of opium
Camphorated tincture of opium
Semisynthetic derivatives
Heroin (diacetylmorphine)
Oxycodone (Percodan, Percocet, Tylox)
Hydrocodone (various)
Oxymorphone (Numorphan)
Hydromorphone (Dilaudid)
Synthetic agents
Meperidine (Demerol)
Loperamide (Imodium)
Diphenoxylate (Lomotil)
Anileridine (Leritine)
Fentanyl (Innovar, Sublimaze)
Methadone (Dolophine)
L-Acetylmethadol (LAAM)
Propoxyphene (Darvon)
Pentazocine (Talwin)
Butorphanol (Stadol)
Nalbuphine (Nubain)

to 77% in 1995.[10] The majority of this decrease in injection as the main route of administration is a result of the increase in the purity of heroin found on the streets, which allows snorting and/or smoking as the primary means of administration for many abusers. Although the number of opioid-dependent persons is commonly estimated to be approximately 500,000, the number of persons abusing opioids approaches a figure nearer to 2 million people in the United States.[11]

PATHOPHYSIOLOGY

The opioids as a class are drugs that bind to opioid receptors. Multiple opioid receptors designated as μ, δ, κ, ς, and ϵ have been identified.[12] The μ receptor is the primary receptor for morphine. The μ receptor is also highly sensitive to the antagonistic effects of naloxone. The μ receptor mediates many of the effects of opioids such as analgesia, euphoria, sedation, miosis, hypothermia, bradycardia, respiratory depression, and increased release of prolactin and growth hormone. δ receptors are more sensitive to endogenous enkephalins. Opioids such as pentazocine and butorphanol, which are more selective for the κ receptor, produce analgesia with less risk of respiratory depression and euphoria.[13] It has been demonstrated that the chronic administration of morphine results in the sensitization of specific brain regions, especially the nucleus accumbens and the locus ceruleus.[14] Activity of the locus ceruleus decreases as a result of acute opioid administration and increases upon opioid withdrawal. Parenteral administration of opioids results in an increase in the extracellular dopamine concentrations in the nucleus accumbens.[6]

Intravenous injection of an opioid causes a warm flushing of the skin and a lower abdominal sensation often described as being similar to sexual orgasm. Because tolerance to the effects of opiates develops rapidly, it is often difficult for the user to recreate this initial first dose high. After the initial rush, there is a period of apathetic detachment for a few hours until the effect of the drug wears off.[15] The essential features of opioid intoxication are initial euphoria followed by apathy as described above, dysphoria, psychomotor agitation or retardation, impaired judgment, or impaired social or occupational functioning which develops during or shortly after use of an opioid. This intoxication is accompanied by pupillary constriction, except in the case of severe overdose, and drowsiness or even coma, slurred speech, and impairment in attention or memory. These symptoms should not be attributable to a general medical condition or another mental disorder.[5]

COMPLICATIONS

The abuse of opioids can lead to a wide array of medical complications beyond the obvious risk of overdose and withdrawal symptoms. Most of the complications are indirect and depend more on the method of use than on the direct effects of the drugs (Table 62.3). Repeated use of unsterilized needles and syringes may cause acute viral hepatitis, bacterial endocarditis, aseptic abscesses, embolism, thrombophlebitis, and cellulitis.[15] The incidence of acquired immunodeficiency syndrome (AIDS) in IV opioid addicts was as high as 60% in one study.[16] Contributing to the spread of human immunodeficiency virus (HIV) is the high rate of intravenous drug abuse, needle sharing, and sexual contact among this population. An estimated 25% of all persons with AIDS abuse intravenous drugs.[6] Approximately 90% of persons with opioid dependence have an additional psychiatric diagnosis (most commonly major depressive disorder, alcohol related disorders, antisocial personality disorder, and anxiety disorders). An estimated 15% of opioid-dependent persons will attempt suicide at least once during their life.[6] The death rate among young opioid-dependent persons is increased as much as 20-fold by infections, homicides, suicides, overdoses, and AIDS.[6]

CLINICAL PRESENTATION, DIAGNOSIS, AND TREATMENT

Recognition and Management

In general, the signs and symptoms that suggest the presence of opioid intoxication are altered mood, psychomotor retardation, drowsiness, slurred speech, and impaired memory and attention.[6] Whereas intoxication by opioids may cause distinctive pinpoint pupils, opioids taken in amounts resulting in an overdose may cause dilated pupils secondary to anoxia caused by respiratory depression. Other symptoms of opioid overdose are marked unresponsiveness, coma, slow respiration, hypothermia, hypotension, and bradycardia. Respiratory depression is the most

Table 62.3 ▪ Medical Complications of Intravenous Drug Abuse

System	Complication
Skin	Abscesses, cellulitis, edema, emboli, excoriation, jaundice, macules, nodules, purpura, "tracks," ulcers
Lymph nodes	"Addict's lymphadenopathy," lymphatic hyperplasia
Eyes	Emboli from talc and cornstarch, quinine amblyopia, scleral icterus
Mouth	Poor dental hygiene
Pulmonary	Infections secondary to aspiration, bronchiectasis, atelectasis, septic emboli, tuberculosis, pulmonary hypertension, decreased vital capacity, asthma, noncardiogenic pulmonary edema
Cardiovascular	Arrhythmias, endocarditis complicated by systemic and pulmonary emboli, vasculitis, gangrene
Hematologic	Anemia, hemolysis, malaria, neutropenia
Neurologic	Subarachnoid hemorrhage, neuropathies, meningitis, central and peripheral emboli, nerve damage
Gastrointestinal	Hepatomegaly, hepatitis, splenic abscess, portal hypertension, constipation, bowel obstruction, hemorrhoids
Genitourinary	Heroin nephropathy, vasculitis, glomerulonephritis secondary to hepatitis or infection, myoglobinuria from muscle destruction, acute tubular necrosis, acute renal failure
Extremities	Phlebitis, edema, arthritis, rhabdomyolysis, tetanus
Immunologic	False-positive VDRL, rheumatoid factor, hypergammaglobinemia, serologic abnormalities, increased risk for acquired immunodeficiency syndrome (AIDS)
"Cotton fever"	Pyrogenic reaction, shaking chills, headache, vomiting, gastrointestinal pain, leukocytosis shortly after intravenous administration subsiding in 1 or 2 hours

dangerous side effect of opioid overdose and may result in death if not promptly treated. For those persons suspected to have opioid intoxication or overdose, administration of naloxone should reverse the effects of the opiate. Treatment usually begins with the administration of 0.4 mg intravenously and should be repeated four to five times within the first 30 to 45 minutes as necessary. In addition, the patient's airway should be maintained and vital signs should be carefully observed. Naloxone possesses a short duration of action; therefore, the patient may lapse back into unresponsiveness after seeming to recover from the overdose. The administration of excessive amounts of opioid antagonists, may also result in the signs and symptoms of opioid withdrawal.

Opioid withdrawal involves the emergence of three or more of the following: dysphoric mood, nausea or vomiting, muscle aches, lacrimation or rhinorrhea, pupillary dilation, sweating, piloerection, diarrhea, yawning, fever, or insomnia within several days of cessation of opioid use that has been heavy or prolonged or within minutes of administration of an opioid antagonist such as naloxone. (Table 62.4). With short-acting drugs such as heroin, withdrawal symptoms occur within 6 to 24 hours after the last dose in dependent persons, peak within 1 to 3 days, and gradually subside during a period of 5 to 7 days. Symptoms may take as long as 2 to 4 days to emerge in the case of longer-acting opiates such as methadone.[9] Less acute symptoms and craving may persist for weeks to months. Although opioid withdrawal is clinically significant, it is typically not life threatening. Treatment of opioid withdrawal involves detoxification of the patient from the effects of the opioid. Detoxification may be accomplished by allowing the withdrawal syndrome to take its natural course while treating the patient for subjective complaints or by administering an opioid and beginning a process of slow tapering until discontinued. Alternatively, patients may be given maintenance doses of opioid substitutes for extended periods so that they may function responsibly in society.

Conventionally, drug therapy for opiate withdrawal has been with the synthetic opioid methadone. The lowest effective dose of methadone possible to stop the signs and symptoms of withdrawal should be administered. Initial doses of methadone 20 to 30 mg given orally every 24 hours are typical. In the inpatient setting, additional doses may be given if symptoms of withdrawal reemerge within 2 to 16 hours after the initial dose. However, in the outpatient setting, these additional doses are impossible to administer; therefore, the practitioner should use extreme caution in evaluating the patient's need for opiate replacement. Patients should not be given doses greater than 30 mg in a single dose unless the appropriate level of physiologic dependence is well documented. After the initiation of a detoxification program, doses of methadone may be decreased by 5 to 10 mg/day until discontinuation is reached. Observation of the patient for 1 to 2 days after the complete discontinuation of methadone is necessary to evaluate the patient's stability. Detoxification with

Table 62.4 ▪ Narcotic Withdrawal/ Abstinence Symptoms

Dilated pupils	Vomiting
Elevation of pulse rate	Diarrhea
Elevation of blood pressure	Dehydration
Elevation of temperature	Weakness
Elevation of respiratory rate	Chills
Muscle aches	Rhinorrhea
Irritability	Lacrimation
Twitching	Gooseflesh
Tremulousness	Yawning
Nausea	Restlessness

methadone should be followed by psychosocial therapy to maximize treatment success.

An alternative to methadone treatment in the opioid dependent patient is clonidine, an α-adrenergic agonist with inhibitory action primarily at the locus ceruleus. Clonidine has been used to depress the overactivity of the sympathetic nervous system that is seen in patients who are withdrawing from opioids.[17] Clonidine has been found to be 80 to 90% effective in decreasing opiate withdrawal signs and symptoms among inpatient populations. Advantages of detoxification with clonidine include a somewhat more rapid detoxification and an absence of the euphoria sometimes observed with methadone.[18] Initial doses of clonidine are usually started at 6 μg/kg/day, in three divided doses. Doses can be increased as necessary to a maximum of 17 μg/kg/day. The same dosage is maintained for 7 days, then tapered and discontinued over the next 3 days.[9] The most common side effect requiring monitoring with clonidine therapy is orthostatic hypotension. Doses should be held if the patient's blood pressure drops significantly. Clonidine also offers the potential advantage of a transdermal dosage form. however, this route has not been well studied in the treatment of opioid withdrawal.

Maintenance Therapy

Methadone maintenance has been the mainstay of pharmacotherapy for opioid dependence since its introduction by Dole and Nyswander.[19] Methadone maintenance treatment programs are regulated by the U.S. Food and Drug Administration (FDA) and the Drug Enforcement Administration. To be eligible for a methadone maintenance program, an abuser must be at least 18 years of age and have been physiologically dependent upon opioids for at least 1 year. Careful screening procedures must be used to establish physiologic dependence and rule out drug-seeking behavior. Programs may set their own guidelines within state and federal regulations. Each program obtains urine samples for drug screens from their enrollees, but the frequency with which these screens are performed may vary from program to program. Programs must provide counseling to patients in addition to opioid replacement. Counseling is essential to the success of the patient in a maintenance program.[8] Methadone maintenance is a controversial subject because some view this as a way for abusers to swap an illegal high for one that is legal. Patients in treatment have shown up to an 85% decrease in criminal behavior during methadone maintenance and employment rates that are 40 to 80% higher.[20]

Since the 1970s, levo-α-acetylmethadol (LAAM), a long-acting congener of methadone, has been used experimentally for opioid maintenance.[9] LAAM received approval in 1993 for the maintenance treatment of opioid dependence. There is extensive literature on the safety and efficacy of LAAM in the treatment of opioid dependence. The major difference between methadone and LAAM is the duration of action of the two drugs, which is based on their metabolism.[20] Whereas methadone is metabolized to inactive compounds, LAAM is metabolized into two active congeners that possess more opioid agonist activity than LAAM itself. LAAM may be given on a 3 days a week schedule instead of the daily schedule required for methadone.

Buprenorphine is a partial agonist of the μ opioid type and is a clinically effective analgesic agent with an estimated potency 25 to 40 times that of morphine.[10] Chronic dosing with buprenorphine blocks the effect of other opioids and suppresses the self-administration of heroin by opioid abusers.[21] Detoxification from heroin dependence using buprenorphine may be as effective as that with methadone or clonidine.[21] Buprenorphine, much like methadone, must be administered daily.

Special Populations

The incidence of obstetric complications in women maintained on methadone is less than the incidence in heroin users.[22] It has been well documented that treating opiate-dependent pregnant women with methadone as part of a comprehensive program, including prenatal care, can reduce the incidence of obstetric and fetal complications and associated neonatal morbidity and mortality. Withdrawing pregnant women from opiate treatment is not recommended before the 14th week of gestation because of the risk of spontaneous abortion and after the 32nd week because of the possibility of withdrawal-induced stress. Breastfeeding can be considered for the mother receiving methadone maintenance who is not abusing other drugs owing to the small amounts of methadone detected in breast milk. The immunologic and bonding benefits of breastfeeding are of great importance to both the recovering mother and newborn.[22]

Neonatal abstinence is a generalized disorder characterized by central nervous system (CNS) signs and symptoms of hyperirritability, gastrointestinal dysfunction, respiratory distress, and vague autonomic symptoms that include yawning, sneezing, mottling, and fever. The onset of these withdrawal symptoms can range from within hours of birth to 2 weeks postpartum. The majority of these symptoms are present within the first 72 hours after birth. Neonatal abstinence can be treated with detoxification pharmacotherapy without any undue effects on the infant. In addition to assessing the neonate for abstinence, overall comfort should be maintained by swaddling, use of a pacifier for excessive sucking, frequent diaper changes, the use of soft sheets or sheepskin to decrease excoriation, and positioning to reduce aspiration.[22]

There are very few guidelines or protocols to treat or prevent withdrawal symptoms in pediatric patients.[23] When physical dependence has been established, sudden discontinuation of an opioid produces a withdrawal syndrome within 24 hours of drug cessation. Symptoms reach their peak within 72 hours and include abdominal cramps, vomiting, diarrhea, tachycardia, hypertension, diaphoresis, restlessness, insomnia, movement disorders, reversible neurologic abnormalities, and seizures.[24] Pediatric treatment regimens are derived primarily from the experience developed in the neonatal intensive care unit in treating infants born to opioid-addicted mothers and from extrapolation from the adult literature. Techniques include nonpharmacologic methods such as swaddling and decreased environmental stimulation to pharmacologic means using opioids, barbiturates, benzodiazepines, phenothiazines, α_2-adrenoceptor agonists, and chloral hydrate.[25] The goal of pharmacologic therapy is to decrease the severity and duration of the abstinence syndrome.[23] After a regimen has been established in the pediatric patient, doses of opioid replacement drugs may be reduced by 10 to 20% daily until discontinuation. For breakthrough symptoms of withdrawal, clonidine 2 to 4 µg/kg every 4 to 6 hours is of benefit.

Sedatives, Hypnotics, and Anxiolytics

Sedatives are drugs that reduce subjective tension and induce mental calmness. The term sedative is virtually synonymous with the term anxiolytic, which is a drug that reduces anxiety. Hypnotics are drugs that are used to induce sleep.[24] Drugs commonly associated with this classification are the benzodiazepines (Table 62.5), barbiturates (e.g., phenobarbital and pentobarbital), and barbiturate-like drugs (e.g., methaqualone and meprobamate). All drugs of this type are cross-tolerant with alcohol and may be lethal when combined with alcohol. In particular, overdoses of benzodiazepines alone are relatively benign but small amounts of benzodiazepines when combined with other CNS depressants, especially alcohol, can cause fatal reactions.

EPIDEMIOLOGY

CNS depressants are among some of the most prescribed substances in the United States. A recent survey reported that approximately 15% of the U.S. population has had a benzodiazepine prescribed by a physician.[6] Other surveys report that approximately 10% of adults have taken a benzodiazepine during the last year. A community survey conducted in the United States in 1991 reported that about 4% of the population sampled had at some time used sedatives for nonmedicinal purposes; approximately 1% had such use in the last year, and 0.4% in the last month. For antianxiety agents, approximately 6% of the population had at some time used them for nonmedical purposes; almost 2% had such use in the last year and 0.5% in the last month.[5]

Table 62.5 ▪ Short- and Long-Acting Benzodiazepines

Short-Acting Agents	Long-Acting Agents
Triazolam (Halcion)	Chlordiazepoxide (Librium)
Oxazepam (Serax)	Diazepam (Valium)
Temazepam (Restoril)	Halazepam (Paxipam)
Lorazepam (Ativan)	Clorazepate (Tranxene)
Alprazolam (Xanax)	Prazepam (Centrax)
	Clonazepam (Klonopin)
	Flurazepam (Dalmane)

PATHOPHYSIOLOGY

Benzodiazepines, barbiturates, and barbiturate-like substances all have their primary effects on the γ-aminobutyric acid type A ($GABA_A$) receptor complex, which contains a chloride ion channel, a binding site for GABA, and a well-defined binding site for benzodiazepines.[24] When one of these substances binds to the complex, it increases the affinity of the receptor for its endogenous neurotransmitter, GABA. This results in increased flow of chloride ions through the channel into the neuron. The influx of negatively charged ions into the neuron induces an inhibitory effect, because it hyperpolarizes the neuron relative to the extracellular space. After prolonged use of benzodiazepines, the stimulation of $GABA_A$ receptors results in less influx of chloride ions than before the period of benzodiazepine use.[25] In short, there is a downregulation of the GABA receptor response.

The effects of benzodiazepines, barbiturates, and barbiturate-like drugs relate to their CNS depressant actions. Chronic CNS depressant abuse may lead to neuropsychologic impairment.[26] Use of sedatives, hypnotics, or anxiolytics may result in slurred speech, incoordination, unsteady gait, nystagmus, impairment in attention or memory, and stupor or coma.

Benzodiazepines are used medically for their anxiolytic, hypnotic, anticonvulsant, and antispastic effects.[27] All benzodiazepines exhibit these effects when given in equipotent doses. The primary differences between the individual benzodiazepines lie in the variance of kinetic parameters, specifically half-life and onset of action. All benzodiazepines appear to have an equal likelihood of producing physical dependence.[28]

COMPLICATIONS

Studies indicate that 84% of primary CNS depressant abusing patients had resumed use of CNS depressants 4 to

Table 62.6 ▪ Signs and Symptoms of Central Nervous System Depressant Withdrawal

Neuropsychiatric symptoms	Symptoms of hyperexcitability
Ataxia	Agitation
Depersonalization	Anxiety
Depression	Hyperactivity
Fasciculations	Insomnia
Formications	Gastrointestinal symptoms
Headache	Abdominal pain
Hyperventilation	Constipation
Malaise	Diarrhea
Myalgia	Nausea
Paranoid delusions	Vomiting
Paresthesias	Cardiovascular symptoms
Pruritus	Chest pain
Tinnitus	Flushing
Tremors	Palpitations
Visual hallucinations	Genitourinary symptoms
	Incontinence
	Loss of libido
	Urinary urgency, frequency

6 years after hospital discharge. Physical signs of alcoholism had developed in 22 and 8% had committed suicide.[29] These figures are indicative of how difficult it is to maintain a drug-free life for abusers of sedative-hypnotics.

The signs and symptoms of depressant withdrawal are listed in Table 62.6. Withdrawal from shorter-acting sedatives appears within 24 hours and reaches a peak in 2 to 3 days. With longer-acting sedatives, signs and symptoms of withdrawal may not be present until 2 or 3 days after the last dose of drug and withdrawal symptom severity peaks more slowly than faster-acting drugs.

CLINICAL PRESENTATION, DIAGNOSIS, AND TREATMENT

Recognition and Management

The diagnosis of intoxication with a sedative-hypnotic substance may be aided by the use of a urine toxicology screen for the suspected substance. The clinical signs and symptoms of intoxication involve the recent use of a sedative-hypnotic substance, clinically significant maladaptive behavioral or psychologic changes (inappropriate sexual or aggressive behavior, mood lability, impaired judgment, and impaired social or occupational functioning), which develop during or shortly after substance use and may also include slurred speech, incoordination, unsteady gait, nystagmus, impairment in attention or memory, and stupor or coma.[5]

The treatment of acute CNS depressant intoxication must involve the determination as to whether the patient is dependent on the substance or not. Hospitalization in an intensive care unit is usually warranted in the early stages of overdoses from sedative-hypnotics. Patients not tolerant to the effects of the substance should be observed closely and monitored for maintenance of airway, breathing, and blood pressure. Within the first few hours of ingestion, gastric lavage may be considered as a means to prevent any further absorption. After gastric lavage, oral doses of activated charcoal may also be given. The ratio between the lethal to effective dosage ranges with most barbiturates is between 3:1 and 30:1. For benzodiazepines, the lethal to effective ratio is nearly 200:1, making lethal overdosage on benzodiazepines rare.[6] The use of CNS stimulants to counteract the effects of the depressants is not recommended and may increase mortality.

CNS depressant withdrawal is characterized by autonomic hyperactivity, increased hand tremor, insomnia, nausea and vomiting, transient visual, tactile, or auditory hallucinations or illusions, psychomotor agitation, anxiety, and reduction of the seizure threshold. Treatment of CNS-depressant dependence typically involves detoxification. Benzodiazepines or phenobarbital are both used to detoxify patients dependent on CNS depressants. The important step in beginning a detoxification program is to determine the amount of substance the patient has been using. Patient drug histories are valuable in this determination, but abusers frequently overestimate the amount they normally abuse. To compute the initial starting dose of phenobarbital, the patient's average daily use of the abused CNS depressant is correlated to an equivalent dose of phenobarbital (Table 62.7).[30] Alternatively, the patient may be given doses of the detoxification drug until mild intoxication occurs. Some clinics orally administer 120-mg doses of phenobarbital hourly until sedative effects and/or nystagmus appear, and this total dose is then given in divided daily doses.[31] The patient should be stabilized on

Table 62.7 ▪ Phenobarbital Withdrawal Equivalents

Medication	Trade Name	Dose Equivalent to 30 mg of Phenobarbital for Withdrawal (mg)
Benzodiazepines		
Alprazolam	Xanax	1
Clonazepam	Klonopin	2
Clorazepate	Tranxene	7.5
Diazepam	Valium	10
Flurazepam	Dalmane	15
Lorazepam	Ativan	2
Oxazepam	Serax	10
Temazepam	Restoril	15
Triazolam	Halcion	0.25
Barbiturates		
Amobarbital	Amytal	100
Butalbital	Butisol	100
Pentobarbital	Nembutal	100
Secobarbital	Seconal	100
Others		
Chloral hydrate	Noctec	500
Ethchlorvynol	Placidyl	500
Glutethimide	Doriden	250
Meprobamate	Miltown	1200
Zolpidem	Ambien	5

the new drug and monitored for signs and symptoms of intoxication or withdrawal. After stabilization, the total daily dose of phenobarbital is decreased 30 mg/day.[32] If signs and symptoms of withdrawal appear during detoxification, the daily dose of phenobarbital should be increased by 50%, and the patient should be stabilized again before restarting the 30 mg/day reduction in dosage. Generally speaking, the clinician should not use the same drug that patients abuse to detoxify them because the connection between the drug of choice and the pattern of abuse are too difficult to break.

Most benzodiazepine abusers also abuse other substances. Benzodiazepines may be used to either enhance the effects of other substances or to manage some of the unpleasant side effects of other substances of abuse. Psychotherapy is an important part in the treatment of sedative-hypnotic-dependent patients. Therapists can help patients realize how dependence is interfering with relationships and undermining their ability to function.[30]

Special Populations

Benzodiazepine use during pregnancy is associated with congenital anomalies including cleft palate; however, the absolute rate is low.[33] Additionally, benzodiazepines taken in the third trimester may cause withdrawal symptoms in the infant after birth.[34]

Elderly patients may be more sensitive to the CNS-depressant effects of these agents, especially the longer-acting benzodiazepines. Falls in elderly patients can be prevented by giving sedative-hypnotics when patients are unlikely to be walking or by avoiding them entirely in the older adults.

Central Nervous System Stimulants

Cocaine

Cocaine is a naturally occurring alkaloid found in the leaves of the coca plant *Erythroxylon coca.* Cocaine in the hydrochloride salt form is commercially available and occurs as colorless crystals or as a white, crystalline powder. The hydrochloride salt form has a characteristic saline, slightly bitter taste and is soluble in both water and alcohol. Cocaine has been used by the Indians of South America in the form of the coca leaf for more than 2000 years. Coca plants are indigenous to Peru, Bolivia, Ecuador, and Colombia. Coca leaves were reportedly used by the Peruvian society in the 16th century in religious and social rituals. Humans were given cocaine as an analgesic during a procedure in which holes were drilled into the skull to allow evil spirits out. Coca leaves are also used as a source of the vitamins B_1, C, and riboflavin and as a folk remedy for physical maladies.[35]

The chemical isolation of cocaine from the coca plant occurred in the late 1800s and has been attributed to German chemist Albert Newman. Cocaine was used originally for its anesthetic properties in surgery. The extract of cocaine could be found in the original Coca-Cola product, but in 1903, cocaine was replaced by caffeine. By 1906, the Pure Food and Drug Act had prohibited the addition of cocaine to beverages or foods. As public awareness grew and increased mortality, mental problems, and addiction were linked to cocaine, Federal control of the substance became necessary. The Harrison Narcotic Act of 1914 declared cocaine to be an illegal narcotic and prohibited its nonmedical uses. As the availability of cocaine decreased, its abuse was reduced significantly. A resurgence of cocaine's use occurred in the 1960s. The Drug Abuse Prevention and Control Act of 1970 made cocaine a schedule II controlled substance because of its high potential for abuse. During the 1970s, the affluent of society were the primary group of users because of the high cost of the drug.[36]

EPIDEMIOLOGY

A 1991 National Household Survey on Drug Abuse (NHSDA) found an 11.5% prevalence of lifetime cocaine use in persons 12 years of age and older; 3% of the population had used cocaine in the past year, with 0.9% using within the past month. The age group of 26 to 34 years had the highest prevalence rate of 25.8% for cocaine use, followed by the younger age group of 18 to 25 years with a 17.9% rate. The highest rates of current cocaine use occurred in the unemployed among the groups aged 18 to 25 and 26 to 34 years old. Among those 12 years and older, males had a higher usage rate than females, using cocaine at twice the rate in both the past year and past month. There was no difference in lifetime use of cocaine among whites, African Americans, or Hispanics.[37] The 1996 NHSDA found that about 1.7 million Americans were current (at least once per month) users of cocaine. The rate of current cocaine use was highest among Americans aged 18 to 25 (2.0%). This was an significant increase of 0.7% from the previous year's survey.[38]

The University of Michigan's Institute for Social Research has been conducting an ongoing study known as the Monitoring the Future Study (MTF) since 1975. MTF is an annual survey on drug use and attitudes of America's adolescents. The 1997 survey showed that the proportion of high-school seniors who used cocaine at least once in their lifetimes peaked in 1985 (17.3%), and decreased to 5.9% in 1994. By 1997, use had increased to 8.7%.[39]

PATHOPHYSIOLOGY

Cocaine is a local anesthetic that blocks initiation or conduction of nerve impulses after local application. It is also a potent vasoconstrictor when applied topically to mucous membranes. By interfering with the uptake of norepinephrine by adrenergic nerve terminals, cocaine produces an indirect adrenergic effect and potentiates the effects of catecholamines. Vasoconstriction, mydriasis, hypertension, tachycardia, and hyperthermia are a result of the adrenergic effects of cocaine.[24] Dopamine reuptake inhibition increases extracellular dopamine concentration in mesolimbic and mesocortical reward pathways of the brain and is thought to be the cause of cocaine-induced euphoria and psychotic symptoms associated with abuse.[40] The mesolimbic area of the brain is responsible for our state of hunger, sex drive, memory, and reward. Cocaine also blocks the reuptake of serotonin, but its effects in relation to cocaine abuse are not well understood.[41]

The major routes of administration of cocaine are sniffing or snorting, injecting, and smoking (including free-base and crack cocaine).[42] Snorting or sniffing is the process of inhaling cocaine powder through the nose where it is absorbed into the bloodstream through the nasal tissues. The onset of effect is 2 to 3 minutes when the drug is snorted, and the duration of action ("high") may last 15 to 30 minutes. Injecting the drug directly into the bloodstream results in an onset of effect in less than 1 minute.

Smoking involves inhaling cocaine vapor or smoke into the lungs where absorption into the bloodstream is rapid and occurs in about 8 to 10 seconds. The high from this route of administration may only last 5 to 10 minutes and may be the reason why users want to repeat the use of this drug within 20 to 30 minutes after the first dose. Craving may lead to binges lasting up to 3 or 4 days, resulting in the development of tolerance. The average plasma half-life of cocaine is about 75 minutes, with peak plasma concentrations occurring between 30 and 60 minutes, depending on the route of administration. Cocaine is highly metabolized by the liver to two primary inactive metabolites, ecgonine methyl ester and benzoylecgonine, and then excreted by the kidneys.[24]

Smoking has become the most common route of administration of cocaine because the smoked form of cocaine (crack) is easily manufactured and is available at a lower cost. It is also preferred because it allows extremely high doses to reach the brain very quickly and results in an intense and immediate high. Crack is manufactured when the hydrochloride form is dissolved in water with sodium bicarbonate (baking soda) or ammonia and heated to remove the hydrochloride component. Once the freebase precipitates out and is dried, a "rock" is formed. The term "crack" refers to the crackling sound heard when the mixture is heated (smoked) in a glass or metal pipe.[43,44]

Acute ingestion of cocaine can produce significant central nervous stimulation manifested as an elated or elevated mood, talkativeness, mydriasis, restlessness, or irritability, nausea or vomiting, sudden headache, cold sweats or tremors. Circulatory effects may include an initial decrement in pulse rate, then tachycardia, increased blood pressure, or skin pallor due to vasoconstriction. Respiratory effects include increased respiratory rate or dyspnea. Psychologic symptoms may include increased self-confidence and alertness, increased energy, and enhanced libido, resulting in potentially dangerous sexual behavior, impaired judgment, and grandiosity in the perception of increased physical and mental abilities. Severe intoxication may result in serious medical consequences.[24]

Cocaine withdrawal or a postintoxication depression (crash) occurs within a few hours to days after cessation or reduction in cocaine use that has been heavy and prolonged. Dysphoric mood and several physiologic changes such as fatigue, vivid, unpleasant dreams, insomnia or hypersomnia, increased appetite, psychomotor retardation, or agitation occur after the use of the drug has stopped. Anhedonia and craving for cocaine that can be intense may also be part of the withdrawal process. Depression and suicidal thoughts may be serious complications that require immediate attention. The withdrawal symptoms can last up to a week depending on the amount of cocaine that was used. Persons experiencing cocaine withdrawal symptoms may self-medicate with alcohol, benzodiazepines, sedatives, or hypnotics.

COMPLICATIONS

Adverse effects from cocaine may occur after acute or chronic use (Table 62.8). Cardiovascular complications are the leading causes of morbidity and mortality associated with cocaine use. Myocardial infarction directly related to cocaine use has been widely documented and is not related to dose or route of administration. Life-threatening arrhythmias, hypertensive crisis, endocarditis, thrombosis, and rupture of the ascending aorta are other serious cardiovascular complications seen with cocaine use. Pulmonary complications have been on the rise with the increased usage of the smoked forms of cocaine.[45-47] "Crack lung" is being seen more in the cocaine abuser and presents as a productive cough, bronchospasm, severe chest pain, hemoptysis, difficulty breathing, and hyperthermia. Pneumonia, pulmonary edema, pneumothorax, and respiratory arrest are other complications seen.[48,49] CNS complications include stroke, hemorrhage, hyperpyrexia, dysphagia, and dysarthria. Cocaine-induced psychotic disorder, mood disorder, anxiety disorder, sexual dysfunction, and sleep disorder are all complications of cocaine abuse/use that may occur.[5]

Table 62.8 ▪ Medical Complications of Cocaine Use

System or Condition	Complication Examples
Cardiovascular	Myocardial infarction, premature ventricular contraction, ventricular tachycardia, ventricular fibrillation, congestive heart failure, chest pain, endocarditis, hypertension, pneumopericardium, rupture of ascending aorta, thrombosis, thrombophlebitis
Central nervous	Stroke, subarachnoid hemorrhage, intracranial hemorrhage, cerebral vasculitis, hyperpyrexia, dysphagia, dysarthria
Respiratory	Alveolar hemorrhage (crack lung), pneumonia, pneumomediastinum, pulmonary edema, pneumothorax, respiratory arrest
Ophthalmic	Retinopathy, central retinal artery occlusion
Pregnancy	Abrupt placenta fetal hypoxemia, fetal death in utero, spontaneous abortion, preterm labor, convulsions in breast feeding baby, feeding disorder, teratogenicity
Psychiatric	Panic disorder, psychosis and violence
Miscellaneous	Renal artery thrombosis, midline granuloma, subcutaneous emphysema, nasal problems, rhabdomyolysis, sexual dysfunction, various infectious diseases and other complications with IV drug use (Table 62.3)

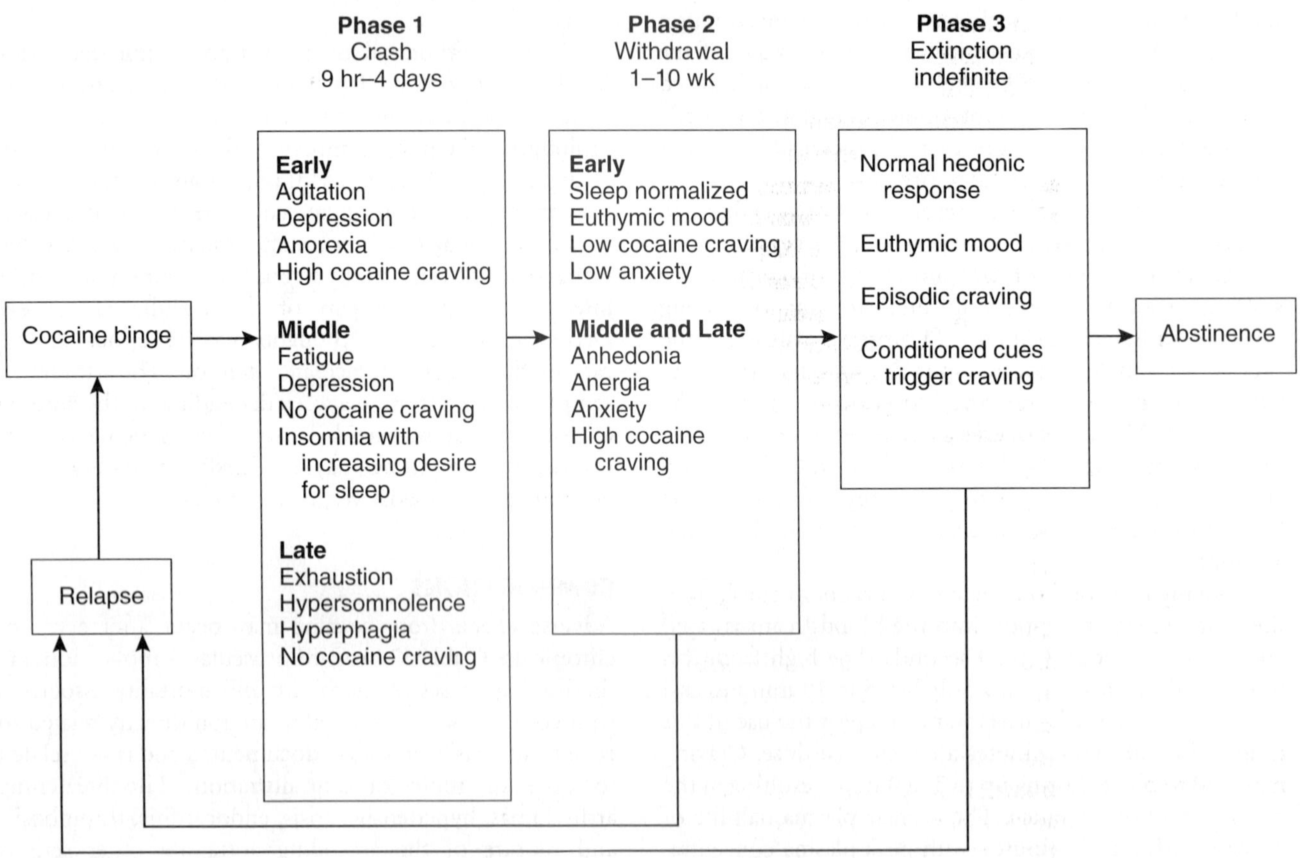

Figure 62.1. Phases of cocaine abstinence. (*Source:* Reference 51.)

CLINICAL PRESENTATION, DIAGNOSIS, AND TREATMENT

Recognition and Management

Cognitive, behavioral, and physiological symptoms are exhibited in cocaine-dependent persons.[50] There is a definite pattern of withdrawal after cocaine bingeing (Fig. 62.1).[51] Large amounts of money may be spent to support binges, and the user may become involved in illegal activities to obtain cocaine. Work and childcare responsibilities may be neglected, and social or recreational activities abandoned or reduced. Paranoia, aggressive behavior, anxiety and agitation, depression, and weight loss may also occur. Continuous use despite the knowledge of a complication that may be life-threatening is often reported. Cocaine abuse is differentiated from cocaine dependence in that the intensity and frequency of use are less in cocaine abuse.[5] Criteria for abuse include neglect of obligations to family or employer, repeated use in hazardous situations, legal problems, and recurrent social or interpersonal problems. Episodes of abuse may occur around payday or special occasions.

Management of cocaine abuse and dependence focuses on two primary goals: (1) the initiation of abstinence through disruption of binge cycles and (2) the prevention of relapse. The initial assessment should determine the level of care needed for the user. Other psychiatric or medical conditions of the user must be included in the assessment. Abstinence is described as a three-phase syndrome: crash, withdrawal, and extinction (Fig. 62.1). The crash is characterized by exhaustion after a binge. Initial depression, agitation, and anxiety are followed by craving for sleep. Clinical management includes observation for increased thoughts of suicide. The symptoms resemble those of major depression. The withdrawal phase is characterized by decreased energy, lack of interest, and anhedonia. This is a very volatile state for the user when vivid memories of cocaine-induced euphoria are intense. It is during this time that the abuser is most likely to relapse. Symptoms usually decrease over 2 to 10 weeks if the user maintains abstinence from cocaine. The extinction phase is an indefinite period during which cravings for cocaine continue to occur. The user is still at an increased risk to relapse. Cravings may be evoked by moods, people, locations, or objects associated with cocaine use that act as cues to conditioned associations with drug use. In time, it is hoped that the cues will lose their potency, and cravings will become progressively less.

Psychotherapy is the mainstay for cocaine abuse treatment.[52] It is composed of three major components: (1) relapse prevention therapy is based on cognitive-behavioral principles and deals with the serious problem of relapse through development of self-control strategies; (2) lifestyle modification incorporate supportive group therapies and self-help groups into the development of a system that will promote the maintenance of abstinence; and (3) systematic cue exposure addresses the relapse-producing factors that are problematic in the user's everyday life. These include pharmacologic, social, occupational, medical, legal, and family factors, and psychiatric disorders.[5]

Pharmacotherapy for the treatment of cocaine abuse is generally reserved for the patient whose addition has been refractory to the nonpharmacologic approaches to cocaine abuse. Pharmacotherapy may be considered in three categories of patients: (1) patients with comorbid psychiatric disorders, (2) patients identified with significant general medical illnesses or risks from continued cocaine use, and (3) patients in whom heavy cocaine use has resulted in neuroadaption (neurotransmitter deficits and alterations in receptor numbers). There are no agents approved by the U.S. Food and Drug Administration for the treatment of cocaine abuse, and controlled trials are lacking in this area. Several agents have been investigated as potential therapeutic options. Amantadine increases dopaminergic transmission and has been reported to reduce craving initially, but after 3 weeks of treatment, it was no more effective than placebo.[53] Bromocriptine is a dopamine agonist, which has also been studied with equivocal results.[54] Desipramine, a tricyclic antidepressant, has been hypothesized to reverse cocaine-induced supersensitivity through its reduction of postsynaptic dopaminergic receptor sensitivity.[55] However, because of its delayed onset of action, minimal positive effects have been noted. Studies of methylphenidate are also disappointing because tolerance occurs and eventually leads to a continued craving for cocaine.[56] Carbamazepine has been investigated as a possible treatment because of its ability to produce an alteration of dopamine receptors. One study reported that cocaine taken concurrently with carbamazepine was associated with significant increases in heart rate and blood pressure, so its use is not recommended.[57]

Cocaine overdose is potentially life-threatening and a medical emergency (Table 62.9). Along with general supportive care and following vital signs, the potential for hyperadrenergic crisis should be monitored closely. Cardiac arrhythmias are the major cause of death owing to cocaine toxicity, so careful monitoring of cardiac function is indicated. Cocaine-induced hypertension may be treated with nitroprusside, phentolamine, or a calcium channel blocker; hypotension should be treated with norepinephrine; and cardiac ischemia may be treated with nitroglycerin. Seizures are treated with either diazepam or lorazepam, and if refractory seizures occur then phenobarbital or phenytoin should be used.

Urinalysis is an accepted means of determining recent cocaine use and is widely used in the workplace to identify an employee who is using cocaine. The major metabolites of cocaine, benzoylecognine and ecgonine methyl ester, can be found in the urine for up to 36 hours after the last use of the drug. However, false-negative results with the immunoassay test are possible. Cocaine can also be measured in saliva and hair. The smoking of cocaine base produces a pyrolysis product that can be detected in the urine and thereby serve as a marker for use of cocaine by the smoking route.

Special Populations

A major public health concern is the use of cocaine by women during pregnancy.[53] The fetus exposed to cocaine in utero is at risk for spontaneous abortion, congenital deformities, microencephaly, and other prenatal complications. Postdelivery complications include low birth weights and withdrawal symptoms in the infant. Efforts should focus on the long-term outcomes of exposure to cocaine in utero as well as reducing subsequent exposure to a drug-using lifestyle.

Table 62.9 ▪ Signs and Symptoms of Cocaine Toxicity

Phase	CNS	Circulatory	Respiratory
I (early stimulation)	Euphoria/elation Mydriasis Talkativeness Excited/flighty Restless/irritable Nausea/vomiting Vertigo Sudden headache Cold sweats Tremor/twitching (especially face, fingers) Generalized tics Preconvulsive movements Pseudohallucinations Verbalization of impending doom	Initial decreased pulse rate, then increased Increase in blood pressure Skin pallor (vasoconstriction) Premature ventricular contractions	Increased respiratory rate Dypsnea
II (advanced stimulation)	Decreased responsiveness to stimuli Generalized hyperflexia	Increased pulse rate Increased blood pressure initially followed by decreased blood pressure owing to decreased cardiac output with ventricular arrhythmias	
	Increased deep tendon reflexes Incontinence Convulsions, status epilepticus Malignant encephalopathy possible Gasping, rapid or irregular respiratory rate	Rapid pulse, weak and irregular Peripheral then central cyanosis Cheyne-Stokes progressive hypoxia	
III (depressive)	Flaccid paralysis of muscle coma Pupils fixed and dilated Loss of reflexes Loss of vital support functions	Ventricular fibrillation Circulatory failure Ashen gray cyanosis No palpable pulse	Agonal gasps Respiratory failure Gross pulmonary edema Paralysis of medullary brain center Death
	Paralysis of medullary brain center Death	Cardiac arrest Paralysis of medullary brain center Death	

Amphetamines

In 1887, amphetamine was synthesized for the first time and was introduced into clinical practice by 1932 as an over-the-counter inhaler to treat nasal congestion and asthma. A tablet form of amphetamine was produced in 1937 for the treatment of narcolepsy, depression, lethargy, and ultimately obesity. The licit and illicit use of amphetamine increased until the Federal Controlled Substances Act of 1970 was put into place to more strictly regulate its use. Although amphetamine has been used in the past for the treatment of obesity, rapid tolerance to its effects and the potential for abuse limit its usefulness.[59] Indications for amphetamines include attention-deficit/hyperactivity disorder and narcolepsy.

Methamphetamine is the stimulant of choice by users because of its potent CNS effects and availability.[60] In 1996, the Drug Enforcement Agency seized 879 methamphetamine laboratories across the United States with the majority of these primarily in the West and Southwest. Street methamphetamine is called by many names including speed, meth, and crank. Methamphetamine hydrochloride is a white crystalline powder. The freebase of methamphetamine (ice) consists of white chunky crystals resembling ice, which can be inhaled by smoking. Analyses of samples seized in the United States have shown purity levels of 90 to almost 100%.

EPIDEMIOLOGY

The MTF study reported that in 1997, 4.4% of high school seniors had used crystal methamphetamine at least once in their lifetimes, an increase from 2.7% in 1990.[39] The Community Epidemiology Work Group Study, which assesses the current epidemiology of drug abuse among 20 major U.S. metropolitan areas and selected foreign countries reported in 1996 that methamphetamine was the dominant illicit drug problem in San Diego. The report also showed San Francisco and Honolulu to have substantial methamphetamine-using populations. Other cities that showed patterns of increasing use were Denver, Los Angeles, Minneapolis, Phoenix, Seattle, and Tucson. New trafficking patterns through some states such as Missouri, Nebraska, and Iowa have led to an increased availability and potential increase in use. The NHSDA, according to its 1996 findings, showed that 2.3% of the population (aged 12 and older) had tried methamphetamine at least once in their lifetime.[38]

PATHOPHYSIOLOGY

Amphetamines are sympathomimetic agents that produce stimulation of the CNS. They increase the activity of catecholamine transmitters (e.g., norepinephrine and dopamine) by blocking reuptake, increasing release, and reducing degradation.[24] They increase heart rate, blood pressure, body temperature, and respiratory rate. They also produce euphoria, increased alertness, a sense of increased energy, tremors, and decreased appetite. Higher doses result in irritability, aggressive behavior, anxiety, excitement, auditory hallucinations, and paranoia. Violent behavior is often seen in the abuser. Mood may change from friendly to hostile very rapidly. Hyperthermia, convulsions, stroke, arrhythmias, and myocardial infarction can result in death.[61,62] Other long-term effects of methamphetamine include respiratory complications and extreme anorexia or malnourishment. Low birth weight, small head circumference, early gestational age, and growth retardation have all been noted in the offspring of pregnant women who have used amphetamines.[63]

The metabolism of methamphetamine is very slow compared to that of cocaine. When taken orally, it is rapidly absorbed and the peak effects are seen within 2 to 3 hours. Methamphetamine is taken orally or intranasally (snorting), is injected, and is also smoked. Immediately after smoking or injection, the user experiences an intense sensation, called a "rush" or "flash," that lasts only a few minutes and is described as extremely pleasurable. Oral or intranasal use produces a euphoric high, but not a rush. Animal research has shown that high doses of methamphetamine damage neuronal endings. Dopamine- and serotonin-containing neurons do not die after methamphetamine use, but their nerve endings are cut back and regrowth appears to be limited.

Table 62.10 ▪ Common Signs and Symptoms of Acute Amphetamine Intoxication

Restlessness	Paranoia
Anxiety	Delusional thoughts
Tremor	Visual hallucinations
Muscle tension	Auditory hallucinations
Repetitious body movement	Physical malnutrition
Facial grimacing	Needle tracks and abscesses
Dystonia	Hypertensive crisis
Temporary amnesia	Cardiac arrhythmias

CLINICAL PRESENTATION, DIAGNOSIS, AND TREATMENT

Common signs and symptoms of amphetamine intoxication are listed in Table 62.10.[5] Therapy for amphetamine intoxication is similar to that for cocaine as discussed previously. Amphetamine withdrawal symptoms usually peak in 2 to 4 days and improve in about 1 week. The "crash" after intoxication may result in anxiety, tremulousness, lethargy, fatigue, headaches, nightmares, profuse sweating, muscle or stomach cramps, and increased hunger. The most severe withdrawal symptom is depression and associated suicidal ideation.

Treatment of amphetamine dependence and abuse is similar to that for cocaine in that supportive measures are the mainstay of therapy.[64] Multiple therapeutic modalities (individual, group, and family psychotherapy) can help the abuser to remain abstinent from the substance. Specific amphetamine-induced symptoms should be treated individually. Haloperidol, a typical antipsychotic agent, may be prescribed for the first few days to relieve the hallucinations, delusions, or paranoia that may appear. Users may consume the drug continuously for up to several days without sleep, commonly called binging. This generally drives the user into a period of worsening paranoia, belligerence, and aggression known as tweaking. The user often collapses from exhaustion, only to awaken and repeat the cycle unless treatment is provided. The user may also be treated with an oral benzodiazepine to calm agitation or hyperactivity.[65]

Hallucinogens

Hallucinogens (psychedelics, entactogens) have been used for centuries in some cultures. Stone sculptures of hallucinogenic mushrooms carved with gods and demons dating to before 500 BC have been found in parts of Mexico and Central America. Peyote, a hallucinogenic cactus, has been used by Mexican Indians for centuries and is considered a sacrament by the Native American Church of the United States.

Modern society's experience with hallucinogenic substances began in 1943 with the synthesis of lysergic acid diethylamide (LSD) by Albert Hoffmann. While working on the purification of LSD in his laboratory at the Sandoz

Drug Company, Hoffmann accidentally ingested some of the drug. He reported that he was overcome by unusual sensations, which forced him to interrupt his work and go home, where he experienced a "dreamlike state consisting of fantastic pictures, extraordinary shapes, and an intense, kaleidoscopic play of colors." Shortly thereafter, Sandoz investigated LSD in humans. Although early investigators were enthusiastic about the potential role of LSD as an adjunct to psychotherapy, controlled studies failed to demonstrate beneficial effects.

Hallucinogenic mushrooms are most commonly *Psilocybe cubensis*, although there are three different genera. Psilocybin and psilocin are the psychoactive components. The majority of street samples of hallucinogenic mushrooms do not contain psilocybin, but instead contain LSD, phencyclidine (PCP), or no psychoactive drug. Signs and symptoms of psilocybin intoxication occur within 1 hour and last at least several hours.[66]

Peyote is a small, spineless cactus native to the Rio Grande valley of Texas and Mexico. Peyote is ingested in the form of "mescal buttons," which are dried crowns of the cactus. Each button may contain 50 to 100 mg of the active constituent, mescaline. Mescaline tablets found on the street may be either synthetic mescaline or ground peyote compressed into a tablet. Analysis of street samples indicates that less than 20% of samples actually contain mescaline. The pharmacologic effects of mescaline are seen within 1 hour, peak after several hours, and usually last 4 to 6 hours.[66]

The hallucinogenic drug 3,4-methylenedioxymethamphetamine (MDMA), or "ecstasy," is an amphetamine derivative with hallucinogenic as well as stimulant properties. Originally used as an appetite suppressant and prescribed to soldiers in World War I, its use became prevalent in the 1980s as an adjunct to psychotherapy and as a drug of abuse. There are several other amphetamine analogs with hallucinogenic properties, all of which are illegal. These are often called "designer drugs" and are usually distributed as a powder, pill, or capsule. The most common dose of MDMA ingested is 50 to 150 mg. Street samples often contain adulterants or other drugs. Effects are seen within 1 hour and may persist for 8 hours.

EPIDEMIOLOGY

Among students, the abuse of LSD and other hallucinogens is increasing.[67] In 1991, lifetime use of LSD was reported by 8.8% of seniors and by 1997 13.6% of seniors had tried LSD. The widespread abuse of MDMA may be traced to British teens attending dance parties known as "raves,"[68] where they may dance vigorously and continuously to loud, synthesized rock music while under the influence of MDMA. By the 1990s, raves had spread to large coastal cities in the United States.[69] Data indicate that MDMA abuse is increasing.[70] A survey of undergraduate students at Tulane University in 1990 indicated that 24% of students had tried MDMA.[71]

PATHOPHYSIOLOGY

Hallucinogens bear a close structural resemblance to serotonin, norepinephrine, or dopamine. There is no standard method of classification for hallucinogens. Substances such as LSD, psilocin, psilocybin, dimethyltryptamine (DMT), dipropyltryptamine (DPT), and bufotenine contain an indole ring similar to serotonin and are called indole alkaloid derivatives. LSD is the prototype of indole alkaloids. Mescaline, MDMA, 2,5-dimethoxy-4-methylamphetamine (STP), and other amphetamine congeners are called phenethylamine derivatives. Like LSD, these agents also have hallucinogenic properties, but are not as potent.

LSD is a synthetic derivative of lysergic acid, a substance found naturally on wheat and rye infected with the fungus *Claviceps purpurea*. LSD is available on the street in a variety of dosage forms for oral use. Most commonly, the drug is available on impregnated blotting paper or postage stamps. In contrast to hallucinogenic mushrooms and mescaline, the majority of LSD sold on the street actually contains LSD. The mechanism of action of hallucinogenic drugs is unclear.[72,73] There are few data on the human pharmacokinetics of LSD. Several metabolites have been identified. Excretion into the bile accounts for 80% of the administered dose. The half-life of LSD is approximately 5 hours. Profound pharmacologic effects occur with doses as low as 20 to 50 μg orally. Intoxication occurs within 1 hour, peaks in several hours, and lasts 6 to 8 hours.

COMPLICATIONS

Intoxication with LSD and other indole alkaloid hallucinogens produces a plethora of autonomic, psychologic, and perceptual changes (Table 62.11). Increased heart rate, blood pressure, body temperature, flushing, piloerection, tremor, muscle weakness, and rhythmical dilation and constriction of pupils may be seen.[74] Euphoria, increased arousal, uncontrollable laughter, dysphoria, anxiety, violence, or panic may occur, and experienced users often premedicate with benzodiazepines to reduce the risk of anxiety and "bad trips." Other adverse psychologic effects may include fear of going insane, paranoia, and impaired judgment. Perceptual changes that are sought by the user include intensification of perceptions, illusions, synesthesia, and hallucinations. Intoxication with MDMA results in psychologic and sympathomimetic effects; the hallucinogenic effects are much less intense than those seen with LSD. Users often experience tachycardia, mydriasis, muscle tension, and jaw-clenching.[75] Reasons cited for MDMA use include enhanced sociability, affability, and feelings of closeness to friends.

Ingestion of LSD may result in unpredictable effects. Bad trips are not uncommon and consist of severe anxiety, withdrawal, fear of impending death, or agitation. Although the drug itself may be relatively nontoxic, death

Table 62.11 ▪ Signs and Symptoms of Hallucinogenic Reactions

Sensory	Psychologic	Cognitive	Physiologic
Altered perception of color, objects, size, and shape	Anxiety	Impaired memory, recall, attention	Dilated pupils
Distortion of time, direction, and distance	Panic	Reduced mental performance	Tremor
Synesthesias (e.g., "seeing sounds," "hearing colors")	Depression	Difficulty with problem solving	Piloerection ("gooseflesh")
	Mood alterations Paranoid ideation Hallucinations (when sufficiently large doses are taken		Sweating Dizziness Weakness
			Paresthesias Ataxia Blurred vision Hyperreflexia Elevated blood pressure Hyperactivity Coma Elevated temperature Nausea Vomiting Hunger Tachycardia Bleeding (in massive LSD overdoses; thought to be evidence of platelet dysfunction) Clonic movements Blood pressure decline (in severe overdoses)

LSD, lysergic acid diethylamide.

due to accidents, suicides, and homicides are well described. Some users may experience prolonged psychotic reactions, and it is thought that schizophrenia may be precipitated in susceptible persons. However, evidence that permanent psychotic disorders may be caused by hallucinogens is weak.

A potential consequence of LSD ingestion is the hallucinogen persisting perception disorder, commonly called "flashbacks."[74] Symptoms of this disorder include recurrent visual disturbances, which recur long after the drug is eliminated from the body. Symptoms include flashes of color, trails of moving images, transient hallucinations, and other effects that are similar to those experienced while under the influence of the drug. The presence of this disorder suggests that hallucinogens may cause persistent or permanent changes to parts of the brain involved in vision.

MDMA ingestion may be followed by serious complications including hyperthermia, hypertension, cardiac arrhythmia, hyponatremia, rhabdomyolysis, delirium, seizures, coma, and death.[76] MDMA has been shown to be neurotoxic in every animal model studied, and evidence is mounting that MDMA abuse may cause permanent damage to serotonergic neurons in humans.[77] Serotonin syndrome has been reported after single-dose, recreational ingestion.[78] Because serotonin plays an important role in mood and memory, repeated MDMA abuse could lead to depression and memory impairment.[79]

Tolerance to many of the pharmacologic effects of hallucinogens occurs after only several days of use. Thus, hallucinogen abusers ingest hallucinogens only sporadically. For this reason, dependence is very unlikely. Cross-tolerance between LSD, mescaline, and psilocybin has been demonstrated in animal models. There is no known hallucinogen withdrawal syndrome, but users may feel "washed out" for several days after abusing hallucinogens.

CLINICAL PRESENTATION, DIAGNOSIS, AND TREATMENT

Recognition and Management

Treatment of bad trips associated with hallucinogen ingestion should be supportive. Patients should be reassured that they are safe and will recover uneventfully. In cases of severe agitation benzodiazepines may be useful. Antipsychotic drugs should be avoided, because they are not effective and may actually intensify the experience. There is no specific treatment for flashbacks. There are numerous uncontrolled reports of drugs that may be effective. In most cases the symptoms disappear over months or years.

Youth who attend raves are known to ingest drinks fortified with electrolytes to replenish fluids lost from dancing and to prevent dehydration. Emergency management of MDMA abuse may require supportive care with particular attention to fluid and electrolyte status and cardiovascular function. Hallucinogen abusers should be informed regarding the risks of hallucinogen intoxication. There is widespread belief among those using hallucinogens, especially MDMA that they are safe.

Special Populations

The adolescents who attend raves are at greatest risk for MDMA abuse. Other indicators of potential abuse include worsening school performance, use of other licit and illicit drugs, and poor interpersonal relationships with parents. Youth who become involved with hallucinogens should receive comprehensive treatment.[80]

Phencyclidine

Phencyclidine was developed in the 1950s as a general anesthetic for veterinary and human use under the trade name of Sernyl. Although it was approved and marketed for human use for a short period of time, the postoperative delirium and unpleasant side effects resulted in withdrawal of the drug from the market in 1965. Phencyclidine was then marketed for veterinary use only in 1967 as Sernylan, until 1978 when it was classified as a schedule I controlled substance and removed from the market. Parke Davis continues to market a similar arylcycloalkylamine compound, ketamine (Ketalar), which causes similar adverse effects to PCP in a few patients and has also appeared with increasing frequency on the street scene as "monkey morphine" or vitamin K. PCP appeared on the street scene in the late 1960s under the street names of "hog, PeaCe Pill, crystal, flakes, and angel dust." Its popularity increased in the mid-1970s, frequently as a substitute for less-available drugs such as tetrahydrocannabinol (THC), peyote, mescaline, psilocybin, and LSD. Publicity about serious adverse effects led to a decline in PCP use in the late 1980s.[81] PCP can be used orally, injected, or snorted, but it is most commonly smoked to allow users to monitor the dosage more carefully. PCP can be applied to tobacco, parsley, or marijuana (laced or dusted joint, or killerweed). It is also sold in combination with a variety of other drugs and many times substituted for street drugs that are difficult to obtain, such as THC, peyote, mescaline, or LSD.

PATHOPHYSIOLOGY

In small doses PCP produces intoxication, with staggering gait, ataxia, slurred speech, numbness of the extremities, and a dissociative feeling. Horizontal and/or vertical nystagmus is often present. Muscular rigidity, sweating, apathy, and a blank stare may develop. Users report feelings of depersonalization and disordered thoughts. The effects of PCP generally last 4 to 6 hours depending upon the dosage. With doses in excess of 5 mg, a more pronounced analgesic effect is noticed. Hostile or unusual behavior is possible as doses are increased.[82] The patient may show agitation, combativeness, and psychosis. Users perceive a superhuman strength, invulnerability, and body image distortions. Blood pressure is likely to be increased along with heart rate. Increased salivation, fever, repetitive movements, and muscular rigidity have also been reported. With increasing doses, analgesia is increased. Users do not perceive pain. Anesthesia, stupor, or coma and convulsions may occur, although the eyes may remain open. With higher doses, prolonged coma, muscle rigidity, opisthotonic posturing, and convulsions may occur. Nystagmus may or may not be present at toxic doses. Respiratory depression, seizures, acidosis, and rhabdomyolysis are also possible.[83] Hypoglycemia, increased creatinine phosphokinase, aspartate aminotransferase, alanine aminotransferase, and increased uric acid levels may be noted. Isolation of patients from external stimuli to the degree compatible with support of vital functions and control of self destructive or violent behavior is recommended. Recovery is usually rapid, although some reports of overdosage include symptoms that last for several weeks. Mental status may take several days to weeks to return to normal. A psychotic phase has been reported for several weeks in some patients after a single dose of PCP.

COMPLICATIONS

Serious neurologic and psychologic disorders have been reported with chronic PCP use, ranging from personality changes and confusional states to psychotic states that may be long lasting. Patients with schizophrenia may be especially vulnerable to the psychotogenic effects of PCP. Other disorders that have been commonly reported with chronic PCP use are anxiety, nervousness, paranoia, delusions, memory disturbances, speech problems, anxiety, and mood swings ranging from social withdrawal and isolation to highly aggressive violent behavior that may last up to 1 year after cessation of drug use. Psychotic states have been reported to last several weeks after a single dose of PCP. Flashbacks have been reported to recur over a period of up to 2 months after discontinuing PCP use.

Chronic use of PCP can lead to both psychologic and physical dependence. Monkeys with implanted catheters will not administer LSD to themselves, but they do self-administer PCP.[84] Chronic users have reported continued difficulty with memory, speech, and visual disturbances lasting up to 1 year after discontinuing the drug.

Severe depression, nervousness, and personality changes are often resistant to treatment. The recovery phase of users discontinuing PCP is often marked with severe depression, stimulating recurrent drug abuse.

CLINICAL PRESENTATION, DIAGNOSIS, AND TREATMENT

Treatment of bad trips or an overdose of PCP often requires emergency care. Benzodiazepines are used to calm the patient. Attempts to talk-down the patient are generally ineffective and may often trigger violent behavior. Hostile and combative patients may require haloperidol to protect the patient and others from violent behavior. Chlorpromazine is not recommended because of possible hypotensive effects and augmentation of the anticholinergic actions of PCP.[85] Treatment of overdosage is symptomatic and focused on supporting vital functions.[86] Hypersalivation may require suction, respiratory depression may require artificial ventilation, convulsions have been successfully treated with diazepam, and hypertension has been treated with hydralazine, sublingual nifedipine, nitroprusside, or phentolamine. Anticonvulsants should be used to prevent seizures and excessive muscle contractions, because these along with hyperthemia may aggravate rhabdomyolysis.

Marijuana

Marijuana (cannabis) has been used as a medicine or euphoriant in Asia and the Middle East since antiquity. Western cultures have used cannabis medicinally for at least several hundred years. Tinctures, extracts, and packaged cannabis products for oral use were available in American and British pharmacies throughout the 19th century. These products were recommended for migraine headaches, pain, insomnia, and epilepsy.

The medicinal use of cannabis declined in the early 20th century as a result of the availability of more effective drugs and the stigma associated with marijuana smoking. By the time *Reefer Madness* was filmed in 1936, cannabis had lost its reputation as a useful remedy and had become widely known as a dangerous substance of abuse. Although opposed by the American Medical Association, the Marijuana Tax Act of 1937 effectively banned marijuana in the United States. Marijuana use did not become prevalent in the United States again until the 1960s.

Cannabis is usually smoked in the form of marijuana, which is the chopped and dried leaves, stems, and flowering buds of *Cannabis sativa*. Hashish (hash) is made from the dried resin of the flowering buds. Marijuana may be smoked in the form of a cigarette (joint) or with a water pipe (bong). Hashish is generally more potent than marijuana and is smoked from a pipe or bong or mixed with tobacco and smoked like a cigarette. Smokers typically inhale deeply and hold their breath to maximize alveolar THC absorption.

EPIDEMIOLOGY

Marijuana is the most commonly abused illicit drug in most age groups in the United States. Its use appears to be increasing, especially among the nation's youth.[39] Data from the 1997 NHSDA indicated that 9.4% of children between 12 and 17 years of age reported prior cannabis use compared with 7.1% in 1996. In 1997, 11 million Americans (5%) were current users of marijuana.[39]

Data from the NIDA's MTF indicates that from 1979 to 1992 there was a significant downward trend in marijuana use among high school seniors. Lifetime use in 12th graders was at an all time high of 60% in 1979, and subsequently dropped to 32.6% in 1992.[87] Since 1992, lifetime use has increased every year.[86] Among 12th graders surveyed in 1998, 49% reported prior use, compared with 22% of 8th graders.[87] The perceived risk of smoking marijuana appears to be decreasing among students.[87] This is an alarming trend, since current use may be a function of perceived risk.

Adding to the confusion regarding the perceived risk of marijuana use is the ongoing controversy over the potential role of marijuana as medicine. Prominent physicians within the United States and abroad continue to debate the merits versus risk of making marijuana available to patients. Britain's House of Lords Science and Technology Committee has recommended that cannabis be reclassified as a schedule II drug, allowing research and prescription. In the United States, the federal ban on use of marijuana has been challenged by the states of Florida, Ohio, Washington, Idaho, California, and Arizona. In these states, physicians may recommend marijuana for patients with AIDS, cancer, anorexia, pain, and other medical conditions. Although marijuana may not be legally purchased in these states, patients with a legal "prescription" may invoke the law if arrested for possession of the substance. In addition, underground "cannabis buyers clubs" may be found in some states where these laws have been passed. An unfortunate consequence of the uncertain medical role of marijuana may be that young people are receiving a mixed message about the health risks of marijuana abuse.

PATHOPHYSIOLOGY

More than 60 cannabinoids have been isolated from marijuana. The euphoric and psychoactive effects may be due to a combination of several of them. However,

Δ-9-THC is the primary psychoactive component believed to produce most of the characteristic effects. THC is an effective antiemetic and appetite stimulant and is commercially available as dronabinol.

Attempts are being made to separate the potential therapeutic effects from the psychoactive effects of cannabinoids.[88] Congeners of THC may be developed as analgesics, antiemetics, immunosuppressants, or other potentially useful drugs without adverse effects on cognition.

THC is absorbed immediately into the bloodstream and distributed to lipophilic tissues where it redistributes slowly. Accumulation in fatty tissues can result in detection of THC for many weeks after chronic use.[89] The bioavailability of smoked marijuana is approximately 20%, depending on the technique used.[90] Because of a high first-pass effect, the oral bioavailability is very low. Thus, most cannabis users smoke the drug, rather than ingest it orally. The elimination half-life is approximately 20 to 30 hours.[89] THC is extensively metabolized to several inactive metabolites that are excreted in the feces and urine.[89]

Early research on cannabinoids suggested that nonspecific effects on membranes were responsible for their pharmacologic effects. More recent work indicates that THC acts at specific receptor sites, called cannabinoid receptors.[91,92] Two of these receptors have been identified and cloned and are designated CB1 and CB2. CB1 receptors are present in high concentrations in the CNS, especially the olfactory bulb, basal ganglia, hippocampus, amygdala, and cerebellum. Evidence suggests that CB1 activation may modulate neurotransmitter release. CB1 receptors are also located in spleen and immune effector cells. CB2 receptors are not found in the brain, but in spleen, macrophages, peripheral nerve terminals, and immune cells. The presence of CB receptors in the immune system is consistent with studies demonstrating immune system effects of cannabinoids.[93,94]

The experienced user seeks a pleasant, dreamy state of euphoria, relaxation, perceptual alterations, and intensification of ordinary sensory experiences. Infectious laughter may occur. After several hours, the user may be tired and hungry. Impaired motor coordination, impaired judgment, and social withdrawal may occur with cannabis intoxication.[95] Unpleasant anxiety and dysphoric reactions may occur in inexperienced users and may be a common reason for discontinuation of use.[96]

The immediate physiological effects of cannabis smoking include dry mouth, tachycardia, peripheral vasodilation, bronchodilation, conjunctival blood vessel engorgement, reduced lacrimation, and decreased intraocular pressure. Some of these side effects suggest antagonist effects at the acetylcholine receptor, although this is not well established.

COMPLICATIONS

The possibility of acute toxicity from marijuana use is remote. The LD50 in rodents is extremely high, and there are no confirmed reports of death as a result of marijuana smoking. Epidemiologic studies have not demonstrated increased mortality in marijuana smokers.[97] However, it is likely that short-term studies underestimate the health risks, since it may take two to three decades of abuse (as with tobacco) before complications are seen. Marijuana smoking results in significant impairment of psychomotor functioning, which may affect the user's ability to operate machinery or drive a motor vehicle. It is clear that marijuana intoxication impairs driving skills, but the impairment is less profound and more difficult to quantitate than that seen with alcohol consumption. Marijuana and alcohol are often consumed together, resulting in even more severe impairment of driving performance than either agent alone. Automobile accidents may be the most serious personal and public health consequence of acute cannabis consumption.

Adverse psychiatric effects such as delusions, hallucinations, panic reactions, agitation, and confusion have been associated with smoking marijuana.[98] These reactions are more likely to be seen in novice users, or those who consume large doses. It has been reported that schizophrenia may be exacerbated after smoking marijuana, but it is highly unlikely that marijuana is a specific cause of schizophrenia.

Cannabinoids probably affect the same reward systems as alcohol, cocaine, nicotine, and opioids.[99] Partial tolerance to the psychoactive and physiologic effects of repeated cannabis administration occurs after a few doses.[96] Some users report mild withdrawal symptoms upon cessation, which may include insomnia and anxiety. In contrast to nicotine, alcohol, and opiate dependence, cannabis withdrawal does not seem to be the motivating factor in those with a pattern of chronic abuse. As with other substances of abuse, some users will continue to use the drug despite adverse consequences. In contrast to alcohol, cocaine, and opiate addiction, it is uncommon for patients dependent upon marijuana alone to be seen for detoxification or withdrawal. In practice, many patients with cocaine and opiate addiction also abuse marijuana.

Studies demonstrate that chronic, daily abuse of marijuana produces subtle impairments in memory, attention, and the ability to learn complex material.[100] Sensitive tests show that heavy users may have difficulty sustaining attention, as well as registering, processing, and using information.[100] The longer cannabis is used, the more significant the cognitive impairment. It is unknown whether these effects are persistent, or if they are reversible upon discontinuation of the drug.

Another unresolved question concerning chronic marijuana smoking is the potential to cause an "amotivational syndrome." This syndrome describes youth who lack initiative, reduce social contacts, and drop out of school. Although marijuana abuse may be seen in students who are poor performers and high school dropouts, cause and effect have not been established.

Marijuana smoking is associated with a variety of potentially serious adverse effects on the respiratory tract.

Because cannabis users tend to inspire more deeply and hold their breath longer than tobacco users, the average joint has been estimated to be equivalent to 4 to 5 tobacco cigarettes in carboxyhemoglobin concentration and tar content.[89] Chronic use of marijuana is clearly associated with bronchitic symptoms including coughing, wheezing, and increased sputum production.[89] Marijuana and tobacco have additive effects on histopathologic abnormalities and bronchitic symptoms. Marijuana smoking may produce decrements in pulmonary function, and the prevalence of respiratory symptoms is similar to that seen with tobacco smokers.[89] For these reasons, chronic obstructive pulmonary disease is a probable, although at this time, an unproven consequence of chronic marijuana smoking. Because tobacco smoking is unequivocally associated with cancers of the respiratory tract and head and neck, it is plausible that chronic cannabis use may also predispose patients to these cancers.

In vitro studies demonstrate that THC exerts multiple adverse effects on the immune system, especially cell-mediated immunity. It is unclear whether these effects are clinically significant in humans. Nonetheless, there is some evidence to suggest that marijuana smoking may predispose patients to recurrent bronchitis, sinusitis, and herpes simplex infections.[90] Immunocompromised patients may be at risk for invasive aspergillosis from marijuana contaminated with *Aspergillus fumigatus*.[101] Clinical research into the immune system effects of cannabis is warranted, especially since many of the patients using "medical marijuana" have cancer or AIDS, and would be at higher risk for opportunistic infections.

CLINICAL PRESENTATION, DIAGNOSIS, AND TREATMENT

Recognition and Management

Reassurance should be the first-line treatment for severe anxiety reactions or paranoia associated with acute intoxication. Withdrawal symptoms are not a clinically significant issue. Patients who report regular cannabis consumption should be informed about the potential risk of immune system impairment, upper respiratory symptoms, and cognitive decrements. In addition, they should be informed that marijuana smoke contains many of the same constituents as tobacco smoke, and thus may be carcinogenic. Lastly, they should be warned about the detrimental effects of cannabis ingestion on driving performance.

Special Populations

There is controversy about the potential role of marijuana as a "gateway" drug that leads to use of more dangerous illicit drug substances. It is commonly observed that children and adolescents who smoke marijuana are more likely to take risks and become users of other illicit substances. It has not been established that marijuana itself is a cause of this pattern, but it seems clear that social interaction with other marijuana smokers may lead to increased access to other illicit drugs. Students who are addicted to marijuana should be educated about the risks, should be required to sever ties with other drug using friends, and should receive comprehensive treatment for substance dependence.

Marijuana smoking may reduce fertility in male and female animals, but the effects in humans are unclear. Cannabis reduces birth weight in animals, but to a lesser degree than tobacco smoke. Studies in humans are inconclusive, but some suggest reduced birth weight.[102] Epidemiologic evidence suggests that it is unlikely that cannabis use during pregnancy causes birth defects.[103] Some have suggested that an increased risk of cancer (leukemia, rhabdomyosarcoma, and astrocytoma) may be seen in children born to mothers who used cannabis during pregnancy. Further study should be performed to confirm or refute these initial observations. THC is found in the breast milk of lactating women who smoke marijuana. Women who are pregnant or lactating should be informed that the fetus or newborn will be exposed to THC during marijuana smoking, and this may have adverse effects that are as yet undetermined.

Nicotine

The use of tobacco was introduced in France in 1560 by a French diplomat named Jean Nicot–from whom tobacco receives its botanical name, *Nicotiana*. He believed tobacco to possess some medicinal value. The production of tobacco began in North America in 1612 after tobacco seeds were brought from South America to Virginia. In 1828, Posselt and Reiman isolated nicotine from the leaves of tobacco. Smoking cigarettes was not a very popular pastime until the invention of the first practical cigarette-making machine in the early 1880s. During the 1500s, European physicians thought that tobacco should be used only for medicinal purposes. The American Puritans thought it to be a dangerous narcotic. In the 1960s, scientists studied the effects of tobacco on the body and determined that tobacco use–especially cigarettes–could cause lung cancer and heart disease. Since 1966, manufacturers have been required to have a health warning on all packages and cartons of cigarettes. In 1971, a law was put into place that banned all radio and television commercials advertising cigarettes. In 1972, manufacturers agreed to include a health warning in all cigarette advertising. In 1989, the U.S. Surgeon General issued a report concluding that cigarettes and other forms of tobacco, such as cigars, pipe tobacco, and chewing tobacco, are addictive and that nicotine is the drug in tobacco that causes addiction. This report also stated that smoking was a major cause of stroke and the third leading cause of death in the United States.[24]

EPIDEMIOLOGY

The 1997 MTF study showed that prevalence rates for smoking among young people remain high, despite the demonstrated health risk associated with smoking.[39] Students surveyed who admitted to ever using cigarettes in the past were: 47.3% of 8th graders, 60.2% of 10th graders, and 65.4% of 12th graders. Since 1975, cigarettes have consistently been the substance the greatest number of high school students use daily. From 1991 to 1996, the number of students who reported having smoked in the past month increased steadily among 8th, 10th, and 12th graders. In 1997, these rates decreased slightly among 8th and 10th graders, to 19.4 and 29.8%, respectively, but increased from 34.0 to 36.5% among 12th graders. In 1997, about 3.5% of 8th graders, 8.6% of 10th graders, and 14.9% of 12th graders said they smoked half a pack of cigarettes or more per day. In 1997, smokeless tobacco (chew or snuff) was used in the past month by 5.5% of 8th graders, 8.9% of 10th graders, and 9.7% of 12th graders.[104] In 1995, among college students, 39.3% had smoked cigarettes within the past year and 26.9% within the past month. Of those 1 to 4 years beyond high school but not in college, 39.0% had smoked cigarettes within the past year and 29.7% within the past month.[39]

The NHSDA, a study conducted by the Office of Applied Studies, Substance Abuse and Mental Health Services Administration in 1995, found that of Americans ages 12 to 17 who had smoked marijuana in their lifetime, 74% had tried cigarettes before marijuana. In 1996 the survey showed that current smokers are more likely to be heavy drinkers and illicit drug users. Among smokers, the rate of heavy alcohol use was 12.8% and the rate of illicit drug use was 14.7%. Among nonsmokers, only 2.5% were heavy drinkers and 2.6% were illicit drug users.[38]

PATHOPHYSIOLOGY

Nicotine is a tertiary amine and one of the few natural liquid alkaloids. Of the two isomers, the levorotatory form, (*S*)-nicotine, is the more pharmacologically active. It is a weak base and is both water- and lipid-soluble. The most toxic, addictive, and widely used vehicle for nicotine delivery is the cigarette. Cigarette smoke is mildly acidic and therefore must be inhaled to be effectively absorbed. Most cigarettes contain 6 to 8 mg of nicotine, with the acute lethal dose being 60 mg. Nicotine is absorbed quickly in the alveoli of the lungs as well as through oral and gastrointestinal mucosa and the skin. Smoke inhalation mimics the effects of an intravenous injection and exposes the heart and brain to concentrations of nicotine within a matter of 7 to 9 seconds, which then dissipate within a few minutes. More than 90% of nicotine inhaled in smoke is absorbed. The half-life of nicotine is about 2 hours. Nicotine and its metabolites are rapidly eliminated by the kidney.

Cigarette smoking produces arousal and relaxation, improves attention, learning, reaction time, and problem solving, and produces some degree of euphoria. Nicotine causes ganglionic stimulation by depolarization when consumed in low doses and causes ganglionic blockade at high doses. Nicotine freely penetrates into the CNS where it stimulates and then depresses the vital medullary and respiratory centers.[105] Central respiratory paralysis and severe hypotension caused by medullary depression result with high doses of nicotine. Peripheral effects caused by the use of nicotine are complex and include increases in blood pressure and cardiac rate and increased peristalsis and secretions. The blood pressure falls as a result of ganglionic blockade at higher doses along with decreased activity in both the gastrointestinal tract and the bladder. In small doses, blood vessels may be constricted and flow may be impaired. Problems could then arise for patients with peripheral vascular disease, angina, or high blood pressure. Through both its central and peripheral actions, nicotine improves mood and decreases anxiety. It also has been shown to decrease distress in response to stressful stimuli and decrease aggression. Smokers have also noted a decreased appetite for simple carbohydrates, a decrease in stress-induced eating, and an increase in the resting metabolic rate.

COMPLICATIONS

Continued use of nicotine-containing products produces the development of tolerance and physiologic dependence.[106] Several studies have shown that nicotine is just as capable of producing dependence as heroin, cocaine, or alcohol.[107,108] A withdrawal syndrome occurs when the user tries to quit. The onset of withdrawal occurs within a few hours of the last cigarette. Symptoms include an increased craving, anxiety, irritability, and increased appetite. A decrease in cognitive capabilities is seen, as well as a decrease in heart rate. These symptoms are generally most severe within the first 1 to 3 days and may continue for 3 to 4 weeks or longer. The severity of these symptoms is related to prior intake of nicotine–frequency and amount being the two most important factors. The withdrawal symptoms are unpleasant and lead to relapse even before the syndrome begins to subside. Most persons resume smoking within 3 days and so abstinence is generally short-lived. It is estimated that nearly 20 million smokers make a serious attempt to stop smoking each year. Less that 7% of these smokers achieve a 1-year abstinence.[109]

Tobacco is second only to alcohol as the most commonly used recreational drug in the United States. It is estimated that approximately 71% of the adult population have smoked tobacco, and that about 62 million Americans aged 12 and older (29%) are current cigarette smokers. The leading cause of preventable illness in the United States can be attributed to tobacco use.[110,111] In 1990, 419,00 deaths were related to tobacco use (Table 62.12).[110] Approximately $50 billion per year are spent on medical expenses directly attributed to cigarette smoking.[112,113]

CLINICAL PRESENTATION, DIAGNOSIS, AND TREATMENT

Treatment principles include providing the user with medications to reduce or eliminate drug use, alleviate withdrawal symptoms, and prevent relapse. Both nonpharmacologic and pharmacologic interventions are used as a means of treatment. In 1996, the Agency for Health Care Policy and Research (AHCPR) released guidelines to aid clinicians in delivering effective intervention for smoking cessation.[114] The guidelines recommend the following: (1) offer every smoker a treatment plan; (2) determine the tobacco-use status of every patient; (3) at least a minimal intervention should be provided to every patient who uses tobacco; (4) establish the treatment plan according to the dose and intensity of the tobacco use, remembering that the more intense the treatment, the more effective it will be in producing long-term abstinence, and (5) three key treatment elements are effective and at least one or more should be included in the smoking cessation intervention plan: nicotine replacement therapy, social support (i.e., support groups, programs offered by the American Cancer Society, American Lung Association, or American Heart Association, or clinician-provided encouragement and assistance), and skills training/problem solving.

The most frequent unassisted cessation method used is "cold turkey," when the patient simply decides to quit. This method is used by more than 80% of smokers attempting to quit. Other unassisted methods include intake limitation, brand changing (reduced tar), and nonprescription aids.[115,116] For others, nicotine replacement introduces a measured amount of nicotine into their system that gradually tapers down until they are past the withdrawal phase.[117] There are several forms of nicotine replacement available including polacrilex gum, the transdermal patch, and nasal spray (Table 62.13). Recent data indicate that treatment with nicotine patches doubles or triples long-term smoking cessation rates.[118] Manufacturers recommend wearing the patches for 4 to 12 weeks, but the optimal duration of patch use is unknown; 8 weeks' treatment appears to be as effective as a longer duration. Nicotine in gum (nicotine polacrilex) is available in 2- and 4-mg doses. Manufacturers recommend using nicotine gum for 4 to 6 months, but the optimal duration is unknown.[119] Patches are generally better tolerated and easier to use than nicotine gum. Skin irritation is the most frequently reported adverse effect with the nicotine patch. The gum may cause flatulence, indigestion, nausea, an unpleasant taste, hiccups and a sore mouth, throat, and jaw.

Recently the FDA approved sustained-release bupropion as an agent for smoking cessation. Other agents such as buspirone, a nonbenzodiazepine antianxiety drug and various antidepressants have also been used as aids to smoking cessation. Further research is needed to define the role of these agents in the treatment of nicotine dependence, either alone or in combination with nicotine replacement therapy.

Nicotine dependence is difficult to treat, but effective use of available options can greatly enhance a smoker's chances of quitting. All smokers should be educated about the risks of tobacco use and the benefits of quitting and should be advised to quit.

Table 62.12 ▪ Smoking-Related Deaths in the United States in 1990

Cause of Death	No. of Deaths
Cardiovascular disease	179,820
Lung cancer[a]	119,920
Cancer other than lung cancer	31,402
Respiratory disease	84,475
Disease in infants[b]	1,711
Burns	1,362

Source: Data from Centers for Disease Control and Prevention.
[a]Includes deaths associated with exposure to environmental tobacco smoke.
[b]Persons less than 1 year of age.

Table 62.13 ▪ Nicotine Replacements on the Market

Product	Dose
Nasal solution	
Nicotrol NS	0.5 mg/metered spray
Oral inhalation	
Nicotrol Inhaler	10 mg/cartridge
Topical/transdermal	
Nicotrol	15 mg/16 hr
Habitrol	7 mg/24 hr
	14 mg/24 hr
	21 mg/24 hr
Nicoderm CQ	7 mg/24 hr
	14 mg/24 hr
	21 mg/24 hr
Prostep	11 mg/24 hr
	22 mg/24 hr
Buccal/transmucosal	
Nicorette	2 mg/piece sugarless gum
Nicorette DS	2 mg/piece sugarless gum

Inhalants

Inhalant abuse (volatile substance abuse, solvent abuse) is the intentional inhalation of a volatile substance for the purpose of intoxication. Volatile nitrates have been abused for decades, especially among homosexual men seeking euphoria, reduction of inhibitions, and relaxation of anal sphincter tone. Amyl nitrate was available without a prescription until 1969. Nitrous oxide has long been a substance of abuse for dentists and other health care professionals with access to a supply of the drug. Inhalant abuse became widespread in the 1950s and 1960s when model airplane glue sniffing became popular, especially among children and teenage boys of low socioeconomic class. The problem of inhalant abuse later spread to older and middle-income youth. More recently, the media has sensationalized fatal cases of inhalant abuse, especially cases associated with autoeroticism.

A wide array of volatile substances may be intentionally inhaled for the purpose of intoxication (Table 62.14). Most of the abused inhalants contain aliphatic, aromatic, or halogenated hydrocarbons. In fact, almost all pressure-aerosolized products contain a volatile hydrocarbon propellant, and thus may be abused. Model airplane glue and rubber cement contain several volatile substances, including *n*-hexane, toluene, and aliphatic acetates.[120] Other liquid inhalants may include paint thinner, lacquers, and gasoline. Aerosols include air fresheners, deodorants, hair spray, cooking spray, butane, and other household products, most of which contain toluene, acetates, trichloroethylene, or tetrachloroethylene.[120] Volatile solvents are highly lipid soluble and easily cross the alveoli into the bloodstream where they are taken up by red blood cells and distributed throughout the body. Distribution to the CNS occurs rapidly and is followed by redistribution to secondary sites.[120]

A variety of techniques are used to deliberately concentrate and inhale volatile solvents. "Sniffing" is the practice of inhaling fumes directly from the container. "Huffing" is a technique whereby the substance is applied to a cloth that is placed over the nose and mouth, allowing for more direct inhalation and more intense effects. The greatest concentration of vapors is achieved by "bagging" the substance. This popular technique involves spraying/pouring the substance into a bag, placing the bag over the mouth, and inhaling deeply. Reports of death from anoxia or aspiration of vomitus have occurred in users who placed the bag over their head.[121]

Table 62.14 ▪ Commonly Abused Solvent Products

Glue	Toluene, xylene, acetone, benzene, *n*-hexane
Cleaning fluids	Trichloroethylene, toluene, carbon tetrachloride, tetrachlorethylene, 1,1,1-trichloroethane
Petrochemicals (gasoline)	Hydrocarbons, lead
Aerosols	Fluorocarbons
Lighter fluid	Butane
Acrylic paint	Toluene
Paints, varnishes, thinning lacquers	Trichloroethane, methylene chloride, T toluene, alcohols, ketones
Cements	Acetone, toluene, hydrocarbons, trichloroethylene, hexane
Dyes	Acetone, methylene chloride
Nail polish remover	Acetone, amyl acetate, alcohol

Nitrous oxide is commonly used as a propellant in whipping cream canisters. Nitrates may be obtained at outdoor rock concerts in the form of "whippets," which are balloons or small plastic bags containing nitrous oxide. In addition, butyl nitrate may be obtained on the street in ready-to-use containers with brand names such as "Rush," "Locker Room," or "Bolt." Many of these products were formerly available legally in "head shops."

EPIDEMIOLOGY

Easy access to a wide assortment of common household products that can be deliberately inhaled has facilitated a worldwide epidemic of inhalant abuse. Because of the tremendous variety of substances classified as inhalants, it can be difficult to quantitate the extent of abuse. Whereas nitrate abuse has been a problem for decades, the recent increase in inhalant abuse is mostly due to non-nitrate volatile substance abuse. Since the MTF began surveying 8th graders in 1991, they have consistently been more likely than upperclassmen to abuse inhalants.[39] Lifetime use in high school students has generally averaged between 15 and 20% of students. Lifetime use peaked in 1995, when 21.6% of 8th graders reported having abused inhalants. The frequency of inhalant abuse has decreased (very slightly) from 1996 to 1998. This trend may be due to increasing public awareness of the problem of inhalant abuse.

Although inhalant abuse may begin in 6- to 8-year-old children, the peak age of inhalant abuse is 14 or 15 years of age. As students grow older, abuse of inhalants tends to decrease, in part because of a stigma associated with the practice. Older students may be more likely to view the practice as "immature." Risk factors for inhalant abuse may include low socioeconomic class, ethnicity, male sex, and delinquency.[80] Evidence suggests that inhalant abuse has become more common among youth of all socioeconomic levels than is recognized by the public.[122]

PATHOPHYSIOLOGY

Volatile solvents are general CNS depressants and are pharmacologically related to the anesthetic gases (Table 62.15). Thus, the effects resemble those seen with early

Table 62.15 ▪ General Effects of Inhaled Volatile Solvents

Common Side Effects	Rare Dangers
Euphoria	"Sudden sniffing death"
Drowsiness	Suffocation
Headache	
Nausea	
Partial amnesia	
Visual disturbance	
Hallucination	
Ataxia	
Impaired judgment	
Reduced muscle and reflex control	
Tolerance	
Metabolic acidosis	
High anion gap	
Hypokalemia	

stages of anesthesia. After inhalation, an initial excitatory phase occurs, which is associated with euphoria and disinhibition.[120] Transient visual and auditory hallucinations, ataxia, nausea, vomiting, increased salivation, and dizziness may occur during this phase. The second phase is associated with CNS depression, which is rarely severe. Slurred speech, seizures, delirium, anger, and depression may occur during the depressive phase. Clinical effects may resemble ethanol intoxication, but a more rapid onset of effect and a much shorter duration of effect is seen with inhalants.[123]

Organic nitrates such as amyl and butyl nitrates produce smooth muscle relaxation and vasodilation (Table 62.16). These substances can produce a feeling of "rush," flushing, and dizziness. When inhaled, nitrous oxide (laughing gas) produces euphoria, giddiness, analgesia, and sedation. The effects of volatile nitrates are very short-lived, so doses must be repeated frequently.

COMPLICATIONS

Significant medical consequences can result from inhalant abuse, the most serious of which is sudden death.[120] Sudden deaths may be caused by reflex vagal inhibition of the heart, anoxia, respiratory depression, or cardiac arrhythmias. Vagal inhibition of the heart may occur when cool propellants stimulate the larynx. Anoxia may occur when the inhalant abuser places the bag over their head. Respiratory depression is unusual with inhalants.

At least one-half of deaths associated with inhalant abuse are caused by cardiac arrhythmia. The probable mechanism of arrhythmia is hydrocarbon-induced sensitization of the myocardium to catecholamines. When the user experiences sympathetic nervous system activation (e.g., when caught abusing) the surge of catecholamines may trigger the fatal heart rhythm.[124] This phenomenon has gained significant media attention and is sometimes called "sudden sniffing death syndrome." Victims of sudden sniffing death syndrome typically cannot be resuscitated. Sudden death may occur in any inhalant abuser, whether novice or experienced. Other common causes of death related to inhalant abuse include trauma after accidents and suicide.

Tolerance may develop with daily use of inhalants, and symptoms resembling sedative-hypnotic withdrawal can emerge after chronic abuse.[120] Inhalants have reinforcing effects in laboratory animals, and abuse in humans may lead to dependence. Medical as well as psychosocial complications can result from inhalant abuse. Chronic use of inhalants is associated with school failure, delinquency, depression, and difficulties with social adjustment.[125,126] Chronic inhalant abuse may cause persistent cerebellar damage, resulting in tremor and ataxia.[127] Symptoms consistent with subcortical dementia such as apathy, memory and intellectual impairment, headaches, emotional instability, depression, weakness, and tremor may be seen.[128] Computed tomographic scanning has demonstrated cerebral atrophy as evidenced by widened cerebral and cerebellar sulci and ventricular enlargement. Magnetic resonance imaging studies indicate that white matter changes may be irreversible.[129] Thus, damage to the CNS is a well-established consequence of inhalant dependence.

Peripheral nervous system damage has also been documented in chronic inhalant abusers.[130] Symptoms of proximal or distal muscle weakness, muscle wasting, high stepping gait, decreased deep tendon reflexes, and distal paresthesias are all consistent with neuropathy. Inhalant-associated neuropathy can be confused with Guillain-Barré syndrome. Peripheral neuropathy is associated specifically with inhalants containing *n*-hexane and methyl *n*-butyl ketone. In addition, nitrous oxide abuse has also been associated with peripheral neuropathy. Other toxicities may be associated with inhalant dependence, including cardiotoxicity, pulmonary toxicity, nephrotoxicity, and

Table 62.16 ▪ Organic Nitrites Effects

Physiologic Effects	Adverse Effects
Vasodilation	Giddiness
Venous pooling	Headache
Hypotension	Nausea
Reflex tachycardia	Vomiting
Reduced cerebral blood flow	Flushing
Tissue hypoxia	Dermatitis
Sphincter relaxation	Methemoglobinemia
Tolerance	Weakness
	Dizziness
	Syncope
	Shortness of breath
	Chest pain
	Tracheobronchitis
	Increased intraocular pressure

hepatotoxicity.[11] Solvent abuse in early pregnancy may be teratogenic. Use later in pregnancy may result in depression of CNS function in the neonate.

CLINICAL PRESENTATION, DIAGNOSIS, AND TREATMENT

Recognition of inhalant abuse may be possible in school-aged children who emit the odor of volatile substances and who are obviously intoxicated.[123] Other signs may include perioral eczema, glue or solvent stains, poor grooming, social isolation, or deviant behaviors. Parents should be highly suspicious of inhalant abuse if volatile substances are discovered where children sleep or play. Urine drug screens are not useful for the detection of inhalant abuse.

The treatment of inhalant abusers is difficult, because many adolescents who abuse inhalants are poly substance abusers. As with dependence on other substances, abstinence should be the primary goal. Another goal is rehabilitation that addresses concurrent psychologic and social problems. The American Academy of Child and Adolescent Psychiatry has developed guidelines for treatment of substance use disorders that can be applied to inhalant dependence.[131] They recommend that treatment should be intensive and of sufficient duration to achieve changes in attitudes and behavior regarding substance abuse. Also, treatment should include family involvement, group therapy, and should encourage a drug-free lifestyle for the user and all family members. Students should be required to sever ties with drug-abusing friends. Treatment should be sensitive to the cultural and socioeconomic realities of the user and family.[8,122]

Prevention of inhalant abuse should be a priority, since abuse and dependence are associated with serious consequences. Limiting the availability of volatile substances is impractical, since these products have legitimate uses and are ubiquitous. It is questionable whether large warning labels would reduce abuse, because the label may actually make products containing volatile substances more easy for children to identify. Education may be the most appropriate strategy to reduce inhalant abuse, especially if initiated before the age of experimentation. The American Academy of Pediatrics advocates a progressive, school-based inhalant curriculum beginning in kindergarten with developmentally appropriate modules throughout elementary school in areas where inhalant abuse is prevalent.[124] The benefit of other interventions, such as the provision of role-models and alternative recreation, is unproven.

KEY POINTS

- Substance abuse dates to our earliest recorded history and yet continues to plague modern society. Despite billions of dollars spent on education, eradication, property seizure and law enforcement, substance abuse and dependence still continue at epidemic levels.
- Substance abuse is associated with disproportionate health care costs, increased mortality, and disease comorbidity and destroys families and individual lives when left untreated.
- Although substance abuse is universally prevalent, a great deal of misunderstanding is associated with the biologic basis for dependence and its effective treatment.
- Substance abuse and dependence are prevalent medical illnesses that require professional assistance to treat.
- Treatment for substance abuse includes a pretreatment phase, which includes medical detoxification or withdrawal and the rehabilitative phase, which includes education, abstinence, and aftercare.
- Substance abuse and dependence result in increased mortality, absorb a disproportionate share of total health care costs, and are associated with increased disease comorbidity, especially other psychiatric disorders.
- Substance dependence is characterized by a maladaptive pattern of substance use that leads to adverse cognitive, behavioral, and psychologic symptoms. Repeated self-administration occurs despite adverse effects. Tolerance, withdrawal, and compulsive substance use are characteristic of dependence.
- Etiologic theories are inconclusive but probably entail a combination of behavioral, genetic, and biologic components.
- Heroin supplies in the United States currently have a higher level of purity than in the past two decades, which has allowed ingestion via smoking or snorting, as opposed to the traditional intravenous method of administration.
- Opioid withdrawal is usually medically benign. Agents such as methadone, LAAM, and buprenorphine are effective treatment options during narcotic detoxification.
- Sedatives and anxiolytic drugs are some of the most commonly used medications, with almost 15% of the U.S. population having had a benzodiazepine prescribed by a physician. Anxiolytic/sedative withdrawal is accomplished through gradual tapering of a cross-tolerant medication and provision of supportive care and emergency symptomatic treatment.
- Cocaine abuse, especially in the smokable form of crack, is epidemic in certain segments of the United States. Crack is cheap, is readily available, produces an immediate and profound high, and is very addictive.
- Current levels of amphetamine abuse in the United States are being fueled by the relatively easy synthesis and production of synthetic supplies in small "meth labs," more than 800 of which were seized and destroyed in 1996 alone.
- Plant source hallucinogen use dates to 500 BC in some cultures. Synthetic hallucinogens became available in the 1940s with the synthesis of LSD. Addiction to

hallucinogens is rare and users seldom report for medical assistance, except in the case of "bad trips" or severe paranoia.

- Marijuana is the most commonly used illicit drug in the United States. Patients requesting detox or medical assistance for marijuana abuse alone is rare. Samples of marijuana in the United States have gradually increased in percentage of THC, the psychoactive compound found in marijuana, over the last three decades.
- Inhalant abuse is associated with younger patients. Techniques such as "huffing" or "bagging" are associated with increased mortality.

REFERENCES

1. Johnston LD, O'Malley JD, Bachman JG. National survey results on drug use from the monitoring the future study, 1975–1995: volume I, secondary school students. Rockville, MD: National Institute on Drug Abuse, 1996.
2. Zook CJ, Moore FD. High-cost users of medical care. N Engl J Med 302:996–1001, 1980
3. McGinnis JM, Foege WH. Actual causes of death in the United States. JAMA 207:2207–2212, 1993.
4. White House Office of National Drug Control Policy. 1994 drug control strategy. Washington, DC, 1995.
5. Substance related disorders. In: Diagnostic and statistical manual of mental disorders. 4th ed (DSM-IV). Washington, DC: American Psychiatric Association, 1994:175–272.
6. Substance-related disorders. In: Kaplan HI, Saddock BJ, eds. Concise textbook of clinical psychiatry. Baltimore: Williams &Wilkins, 1996:75–119.
7. Kosten TR. Generic substance and polydrug use disorders. In: Tasman, A, Kay J, Lieberman JA, eds. Psychiatry. 1st ed. Philadelphia: WB Saunders, 1997:743–754.
8. Cost and therapeutics. The Economics of Neuroscience 1:22–23, 1999.
9. Woody GE, McNichokis LF. Opioid related disorders. In: Tasman A, Kay J, Lieberman JA, eds. Psychiatry, 1st ed. Philadelphia: WB Saunders Company, 1997:867–80.
10. Supply of illicit drugs to the U.S., the 1997 NNICC report. Arlington, VA: US Drug Enforcement Administration, 1998.
11. Opioids. In: Bloom FE, Kupfer DR, eds. Psychopharmacology: The fourth generation of progress. New York: Raven Press, 1995:1731–1744.
12. Reisine T, Paasternak G. Opioid analgesics and antagonists. In: Hardman JG, Limbird LE, Molinoff PB, et al., eds. Goodman & Gilman's the pharmacological basis of therapeutics. 9th ed. New York: McGraw-Hill, 1996:521–555.
13. Alcohol and other psychoactive substance use disorders. In: Textbook of psychiatry. 2nd ed. Washington, DC: American Psychiatric Press, 1994: 355–410.
14. Biology of psychoactive substance dependence disorders: opiates, cocaine, and ethanol. In: textbook of psychopharmacology. Washington, DC: American Psychiatric Press, 1995:537–556.
15. Jaffe JH. Opiates: clinical aspects. In: Lowinson, JF, Ruiz, P, Millman, RB, et al., eds. Substance abuse: a comprehensive textbook. 2nd ed. Baltimore: Williams & Wilkins, 1992:186–194.
16. Steel PM, Haverkos HW. Epidemiologic studies of HIV/AIDS and drug abuse. Am J Drug Alcohol Abuse 18:167–175, 1992.
17. Gold MS, Pottach AC, Sweeney DR, et al. Opiate withdrawal using clonidine. JAMA 243:343–346, 1980.
18. Gold MS, Redmond DE, Kleber HD. Noradrenergic hyperactivity in opiate withdrawal supported by clonidine reversal of opiate withdrawal. Am J Psychiatry 136:100–102, 1979.
19. Dole VP, Nyswander ME. A medical treatment for diacetylmorphine (heroin) addiction. JAMA 193:646–650, 1965.
20. Strain EC, Stitzer ML, Liebson IA, et al. Buprenorphine versus methadone in the treatment of opioid dependence: self reports, urinalysis, and addiction severity index. J Clin Psychopharmacol 16:58–67, 1996.
21. Treatment of substance related disorders. In: Textbook of psychopharmacology. Washington, DC: American Psychiatric Press, 1995:707–724.
22. Kaltenbach K, Berghella V, Finnegan L. Opioid dependence during pregnancy: effects and management. Obstet Gynecol Clin North Am 25:139–151, 1998.
23. Yaster M, Kost-Byerly S, Berde C, et al. The management of opioid and benzodiazepine dependence in infants, children, and adolescents. Pediatrics 98:135–140, 1996.
24. O'Brien, CP. Drug addiction and drug abuse. In: Hardman JG, Limbird LE, Molinoff PB, et al., eds. Goodman & Gilman's the pharmacological basis of therapeutics. 9th ed. New York: McGraw-Hill, 1996:557–577.
25. Anand KJ, Arnold JH. Opioid tolerance and dependence in infants and children. Crit Care Med 22:334–342, 1994.
26. Bergman H, Borg S, Holin L. Neuropsychological impairment and exclusive abuse of sedatives or hypnotics. Am J Psychiatry 137:215–217, 1980.
27. Abuse and therapeutic use of benzodiazepines and benzodiazepine-like drugs. In Psychopharmacology: the fourth generation of progress. New York: Raven Press, 1995:1777–1791.
28. Shader RI, Greenblatt DJ. Use of benzodiazepines in anxiety disorders. N Engl J Med 328:1398–1405, 1993.
29. Allgulander CS, Ljungberg L, Fisher LD. Long term prognosis in addiction on sedative and hypnotic drugs analyzed with the regression model. Acta Psychiatr Scand 75:521–531, 1987.
30. Sedative, hypnotic, or anxiolytic use disorders. In: Tasman, A, Kay J, Lieberman JA, eds. Psychiatry. 1st ed. Philadelphia: WB Saunders, 1997: 881–891.
31. Robinson GM, Sellers EM, Janecek E. Barbiturate and hypnosedative withdrawal by a multiple oral phenobarbital loading dose technique. Clin Pharmacol Ther 30:71, 1981.
32. Martin PR, Kapen BM, Whiteside EA. Intravenous phenobarbital therapy in barbiturate and hypnosedative withdrawal reactions: a kinetic approach. Clin Pharmacol Ther 26:856–864, 1979.
33. Chasnoff IJ, Laundress HJ, Barrett ME. The prevalence of illegal drug use or alcohol use during pregnancy and discrepancies in mandatory reporting in Pinellas County, Florida. N Engl J Med 322:1202–1206, 1990.
34. Yaster M, Kost-Byerly S, Berde C, et al. The management of opioid and benzodiazepine dependence in infants, children, and adolescents. Pediatrics 98:135–140, 1996.
35. Nicholi AM. Historical perspective: the long and colorful history of Erythoxylon coca. J Am Coll Health 32:252–257,1984.
36. Gawin FH. New uses of antidepressants in cocaine abuse. Psychosomatics 27(11 Suppl):24, 1986.
37. NHSDA National Household Survey on Drug Abuse: main findings 1991. Rockville, MD: Substance Abuse and Mental Health Services Administration, 1993. DHHS Publication No. SMA 93–1980.
38. NHSDA. Main findings 1996. Rockville, MD: Substance Abuse and Mental Health Services Administration. 1998. DHHS Publication No. SMA 97-3149.
39. National survey results on drug use from the monitoring the future study 1975–1997. Washington, DC: National Institute on Drug Abuse. Government Publication No. 97-4139.
40. Woolverton WL, Johnson KM. Neurobiology of cocaine abuse. Trends Pharmacol Sci 13:193, 1992.
41. Roberts DC, Corchran ME, Fibiger HC. On the role of ascending catecholaminergic systems in the intravenous self-administration of cocaine. Pharmacol Biochem Behav 6:615–620, 1977.
42. Manschreck TC. The treatment of cocaine abuse. Psychiatr Q 64:183, 1993.
43. Siegel RK. History of cocaine smoking. J. Psychoactive Drugs 14:277, 1992.
44. Siegel RK. Cocaine smoking. N Engl J Med 300:373, 1979.
45. Isner JM, Estes NA III, Thompson PD, et al. Acute cardiac events temporally related to cocaine abuse. N Engl J Med: 315:1438–1443, 1986.
46. Gradman A. Cardiac effects of cocaine: a review. Yale J Biol Med 61:137–147, 1988.
47. Cregler LL, Mark H. Medical complications of cocaine abuse. N Engl J Med 315:1495–1500, 1986.
48. Kissner DG, Lawrence WD, Selis JE, et al. Crack lung: pulmonary disease caused by cocaine abuse. Am Rev. Respir Dis 136:1250–1252, 1987.
49. Forrester JM, Steele AW, Waldron JA, et al. Crack lung: an acute pulmonary syndrome with a spectrum of clinical and histopathologic findings. Am Rev Respir Dis 142:462–467, 1990.
50. Withers NW, Pulvirenti L, Koob GF, et al. Cocaine abuse and dependence. J Clin Psychopharmacol 15:63–78, 1995.
51. Hall WC. Tolbert RC, Ereshefsky L. Cocaine abuse and its treatment. Pharmacotherapy 10:47–65, 1990.
52. Higgins ST, Budney AJ, Bickel WK, et al. Achieving cocaine abstinence with a behavioral approach. Am J Psychiatry 150:763–769, 1993.
53. Morgan CH, Kosten TR, Gawin FH, et al. A pilot trial of amantadine for cocaine abuse. NIDA Res Monogr 81:81–85, 1988.
54. Tennant FS, Sagherian AA. Double-blind comparison of amantadine and bromocriptine for ambulatory withdrawal from cocaine dependence. Arch Intern Med: 147:109–112, 1987.

55. Weddington WW, Brown BS, Haertzen CA, et al. Comparison of amantadine and desipranine combined with psychology for treatment of cocaine dependence. Am J Drug Alcohol Abuse 17:137–152, 1991.
56. Gawin FH, Riordan CA, Koeber HD. Methylphenidate use in non-ADD cocaine abusers-a negative study. Am J Drug Alcohol Abuse 11:193–197, 1985.
57. Hatsukami D, Keenan R, Halikas J, et al. Effects of CBZ on acute responses to smoking cocaine-base in human cocaine users. Psychopharmacology (Berl) 104:120–124, 1991.
58. Lutiger B, Grahan K, Einarson TR, et al. Relationship between gestational cocaine use and pregnancy outcome: a meta-analysis. Teratology 44:405–414, 1991.
59. Inaba DS, Cohen WE. Uppers, downers and all arounders. 2nd ed. Ashland, OR: CNS Publications, 1993:49–78.
60. Beebe DK, Walley E. Smokable methamphetamine ("ice"): an old drug in a different form. Am Fam Physician 51:449, 1995.
61. Jackson JG. Hazards of smokable methamphetamine. N Engl J Med 321:907, 1989.
62. Ragland AS, Ismail Y, Arsura EL. Myocardial infarction after amphetamine use. Am Heart J. 125:247–249, 1993.
63. Morgan JP. Controlled substance analogues: current clinical and social issues. In: Lowinson JH, Ruiz P, Millman RB, et al., eds. Substance abuse: a comprehensive textbook. 2nd ed. Baltimore: Williams & Wilkins, 1992.
64. Jaffe JH. Amphetamine (or amphetamine-like)-related disorder. In: Kaplan, HI, Sadock BJ, eds. Comprehensive textbook of psychiatry. 6th ed. Williams & Wilkins, Baltimore, 1995.
65. Koelega HS. Stimulant drugs and vigilance performance: a review. Psychopharmacology 111:1–16,1993.
66. Spoerke DG, Hall AH. Plants and mushrooms of abuse. Emerg Med Clin North Am 8:579–593, 1990.
67. Schwartz RH. LSD: Its rise, fall, and renewed popularity among high school students. Pediatr Clin North AM 42:403–413, 1995.
68. Randall T. Ecstasy-fueled "rave" parties become dances of death for English youths. JAMA 268:1505–1506, 1992.
69. Schwartz RH, Miller NS. MDMD (ecstasy) and the rave: a review. Pediatrics 100:705–708, 1997.
70. Cuomo MJ, Dyment PG, Gammino VM. Increasing use of "ecstasy" (MDMA) and other hallucinogens on a college campus. J Am Coll Health 42:271–274, 1994.
71. Ropero-Miller JD, Goldberger BA. Recreational drugs: current trends in the 90s. Clin Lab Med 18:727–745, 1998.
72. Glennon RA. Do classical hallucinogens act as 5-HT2 agonists or antagonists? Neuropsychopharmacology 3:509–517, 1990.
73. Garratt JC, Alreja M, Aghajanian GK. LSD has high efficacy relative to serotonin in enhancing the cationic current: intracellular studies in rat facial motoneurons. Synapse 13:123–123, 1993.
74. Leikin JB, Krantz AJ, Zell-Kanter M, et al. Clinical features and management of intoxication due to hallucinogenic drugs. Med Toxicol Adverse Drug Exp 4:324–350, 1989.
75. Green AR, Cross AJ, Goodwin GM. Review of the pharmacology and clinical pharmacology of 3,4-methylenedioxymethamphetamine (MDMA or "ecstasy"). Psychopharmacology 119:247–260, 1995.
76. McCann UD, Slate SO, Ricaurte GA. Adverse reactions with 3,4-methylenedioxymethamphetamine (MDMA; 'ecstasy'). Drug Saf 15:107–115, 1996.
77. McCann UD, Szabo A, Scheffel U, et al. Positron emission tomographic evidence of toxic effect of MDMA ('ecstasy') on brain serotonin neurons in human beings. Lancet 352:1433–1437, 1998.
78. Mueller PD, Korey WS. Death by "ecstasy": The serotonin syndrome? Ann Emerg Med 32:377–380, 1996.
79. Bolla KI, McCann UD, Ricaurte GA. Memory impairment in abstinent MDMA ('ecstasy') users. Neurology 51:1532–1537, 1998.
80. American Academy of Child and Adolescent Psychiatry Work Group on Quality Issues. Practice parameters for the assessment and treatment of children and adolescents with substance use disorders. J Am Acad Child Adolesc Psychiatry 36:140S–156S, 1997.
81. Davis BL. The PCP epidemic: a critical review. Int J Addict 17:1137–1155, 1982.
82. McCarron MM, Schulze BW, Thompson GA. Acute phencyclidine intoxication: incidence of clinical findings in 1000 cases. Ann Emerg Med 10:237–242, 1981.
83. Patel R, Connor G. A review of thirty cases of rhabdomyolysis associated renal failure among phencyclidine users. Clin Toxicol 23:547–556, 1986.
84. Nabeshima T, Fukaya H, Yamaguchi K, et al. Development of tolerance and supersensitivity to phencyclidine in rats after repeated administration of phencyclidine. Eur J Pharmacol 135:23–33, 1987.
85. Giannini AJ, Eighan MS, Loiselle RH. Comparison of haloperidol and chlorpromazine in the treatment of phencyclidine psychosis. J Clin Pharmacol 24:202–204, 1984.
86. Aronow R, Miceli JN, Done AK. A therapeutic approach to the acutely overdosed PCP patient. J Psychedelic Drugs 12:259–267, 1980.
87. Marijuana update. National Clearinghouse for Alcohol and Drug Information. SAMHSA. September 1997. Drug Abuse Warning Network Series: D-3.
88. Hirst RA, Lambert DG, Notcutt WG. Pharmacology and potential therapeutic uses of cannabis. Br J Anaesth 81:77–84, 1998.
89. Simpson D, Braithwaite RA, Jarvie DR, et al. Screening for drugs of abuse (II): cannabinoids, lysergic acid diethylamide, buprenorphine, methadone, barbiturates, benzodiazepines, and other drugs. Ann Clin Biochem 34:460–510, 1997.
90. Van Hoozen BE, Cross CE. Marijuana: respiratory tract effects. Clin Rev Allergy Immunol 15:243–269, 1997.
91. Devane WA, Hanus L, Breuer A, et al. Isolation and structure of a brain constituent that binds to the cannabinoid receptor. Science 258:1946–1949, 1992.
92. Abood ME, Martin DR. Neurobiology of marijuana abuse. Trends Pharmacol Sci 13:201, 1992.
93. Friedman H, Klein TW, Newton C, et al. Marijuana, receptors and immunomodulation. Adv Exp Med Biol 373:103, 1995.
94. Nahas G, Latour C. The human toxicity of marijuana. Med J. Aust 156:495, 1992.
95. Woody GE, MacFadden W. Cannibis-related disorders. In: Kaplan HI, Scdock BJ, eds. Comprehensive textbook of psychiatry. 6th ed. Baltimore: Williams & Wilkins, 1995.
96. Hall W, Solowij N. Adverse effects of cannabis. Lancet 352:1611–1616, 1998.
97. Sidney S, Beck JE, Tekawa IE, et al. Marijuana use and mortality. Am J Public Heath 87: 585–590, 1997.
98. Chopra GS, Smith JW. Psychotic reactions following cannabis use in East Indians. Arch Gen Psychiatry; 30:24–27, 1974.
99. Wickelgren I. Marijuana: harder than thought? Science 276:1967–1968, 1997.
100. Pope HG, Yurgelun-Todd D. The residual cognitive effects of heavy marijuana use. JAMA 275:521–527. 1996.
101. Hamadeh R, Ardehali A, Locksley RM, et al. Fatal aspergillosis associated with smoking contaminated marijuana in a marrow transplant recipient. Chest 94:432–434, 1988.
102. Fried PA. Prenatal exposure to tobacco and marijuana: effects during pregnancy, infancy, and early childhood. Clin Obstet Gynecol 36:319–336, 1993.
103. Zuckerman B, Frank D, Hingson R, et al. Effects of maternal marijuana and cocaine on fetal growth. N Engl J Med 320:762–768, 1989.
104. Gottlieb A, Pope SK, Rickert VI. Patterns of smokeless tobacco use by young adolescents. Pediatrics 91:75–78, 1993.
105. Grenhoff J, Svensson R. Pharmacology of nicotine. Br J Addict 84:477–492, 1989.
106. Benowitz NL. Cigarette smoking and nicotine addiction. Med Clin North Am 76:415–437, 1992.
107. Fiore MC. Trends in cigarette smoking in the US. The epidemiology of tobacco use. Med Clin North Am 76:289–303, 1992.
108. Henningfield JE, Clayton R, Pollin W. The involvement of tobacco in alcoholism and illicit drug use. Br J Addict 85:217–292, 1990.
109. Henningfield JE, Cohen C, Slade JD. Is nicotine more addictive than cocaine? Br J Addict 86:545–569, 1991.
110. Cigarette smoking-attributable mortality and years of potential life lost–United States, 1990. MMWR Morb Mortal Wkly Rep 42:645–649, 1993.
111. Cancer facts and figures–1993. New York: American Cancer Society, 1993.
112. Bartecchi CE, MacKenzie TD, Schrier RW. The human costs of tobacco use (1). N Engl J Med 330:907–912, 1994.
113. MacKenzie TD, Bartecchi CE, Schrier RW. The human costs of tobacco use (2). N Engl J Med 330:975–980, 1994.
114. Fiore MC, Bailey WC, Cohen SJ, et al. Smoking Cessation: Clinical Practice Guideline No 18: Rockville, MD: US Department of Health and Human Services, Public Health Service, Agency for Health Care Policy and Research, April 1996. AHCPR Publication 96-0692.
115. Sachs DPL. Advances in smoking cessation treatment. In: Simmons D, ed. Current pulmonology. Chicago: Year Book Medical Publishers, 1991:12: 139–198.
116. The health benefits of smoking cessation: a report of the Surgeon General. Rockville, MD: US Department of Health and Human Services, Office on Smoking and Health, 1990. Publication No. (CDC) 90–8416.
117. Use of nicotine to stop smoking. Med Lett 37:6–8,1995.
118. Fiore MC, Smith SS, Jorenby DE. The effectiveness of the nicotine patch for smoking cessation–a meta-analysis. JAMA 271:1940–1947, 1994.

119. Fagerstrom KO. Effects of nicotine chewing gum and follow-up appointments in physician-based smoking cessation. Prev Med 13:517–527, 1984.
120. Inhalant abuse: its dangers are nothing to sniff at. Bethesda, MD: NIDA, 1994. NCADI Publication No. PHD675.
121. Marelich GP. Volatile substance abuse. Clin Rev Allergy Immunol 15:271–289, 1988.
122. Committee on Substance Abuse and Committee on Native American Child Health. Inhalant abuse. Pediatrics 97:420–423, 1996.
123. Espeland K. Identifying the manifestations of inhalant abuse. Nurs Pract 20:49,1995.
124. Meadows R, Verghese A. Medical complications of glue sniffing. South Med J 89:455–462, 1996.
125. Prasher VP, Corbett JA. Aerosol addiction. Br J. Psychiatry 157:922–924, 1990.
126. Gossett JT, Lewis JM, Phillips VA. Extent and prevalence of illicit drug use as reported by 56,745 students. JAMA 216:1464–1470, 1971.
127. Davies B, Thorley A, O'Connor D. Progression of addiction careers in young solvent misusers. Br Med J 290:109–110, 1985.
128. Hormes JT, Filley CM, Rosenberg NL. Neurological sequelae of chronic solvent vapor abuse. Neurology 36:698–702, 1986.
129. Filley CM, Heaton RK, Rosenberg NL. White matter dementia in chronic toluene abuse. Neurology 40:532–534, 1990.
130. Caldemeyer KS, Pascuzzi RM, Moran CC, et al. Toluene abuse causing reduced MR signal intensity in the brain. AJR 161:1259–1261, 1993.
131. Lolin Y. Chronic neurological toxicity associated with exposure to volatile substances. Hum Toxicol 8:293–300, 1989.

CHAPTER 63

SMOKING CESSATION

Daniel T. Kennedy and Ziba Gorji Chang

The pharmacist is in an ideal position to promote smoking cessation because of the number of patients seen in pharmacy practice as well as the availability of nonprescription nicotine replacement therapies (NRTs). The Agency for Health Care Policy and Research (AHCPR) has concluded that any health care professional who has access to and interest in patients along with knowledge about NRTs can be pivotal in the smoking cessation process.[1] The AHCPR has stated that a dose-response relationship exists between the amount of time that a health care professional spends with an individual patient and the success of sustained smoking cessation. One-on-one interventions of as little as 3 minutes may lead to smoking cessation rates of 11% while counseling sessions of greater than 10 minutes may lead to smoking cessation rates of 19%.[1] Sustained smoking quit rates of even 10% are considered successful.[2] A health care professional's advice to a patient to quit smoking may raise cessation rates by up to 30%.[3]

TREATMENT GOALS: SMOKING

- Describe the morbidity, mortality, and economic impact of smoking on both the individual and environment.
- Educate patients on the benefits of smoking cessation.
- Select a patient-specific method of smoking cessation to optimize outcomes.

BACKGROUND ON SMOKING AND SMOKING CESSATION

Morbidity, Mortality, and Economic Impact

The morbidity, mortality, and economic impact of cigarette smoking in the United States are staggering. Smokers have an increased risk of cerebrovascular disease, chronic obstructive pulmonary disease, and heart disease.[4] Some acute health risks of smoking include shortness of breath, impotence, infertility, increased serum carbon monoxide concentration, and aggravation of asthma.[1] Cigarette smoking contributes to 30% of all cancer deaths and to 87% of lung cancer deaths annually.[5] Cancer of the oral cavity, esophagus, kidney, bladder, stomach, cervix, pancreas, and hematopoietic system has been linked to cigarette smoking. The prevalence of smoking is higher in American men than in women (27 and 23%, respectively).[1] Currently, approximately 24.7% of adults in the United States smoke, for an estimated total of 47 million people.[3] Smoking is more common among adults living below the poverty level than among others (32.5 versus 23.8%) and far less common among college-educated adults than high school dropouts (14 versus 37.5%).[3] Smoking is less prevalent among Asians/Pacific Islanders and Hispanics, 16.6 and 18.3%, respectively, and more prevalent among Native American/Native Alaskan populations (36.2%).[3] More than 400,000 Americans die each year as a result of smoking-related illness, and this number continues to increase.[6] It has been estimated that smokers of one to two packs of cigarettes a day lose anywhere from 4.4 to 6.8 years of life.[7] One of every five deaths in this country can be directly associated with cigarette smoking. In 1993, the estimated direct cost of medical care for smoking-related illnesses in the United States was $50 billion and the annual cost of lost productivity and earnings associated with smoking-related disability was approximately $47 billion.[8] Direct and indirect costs due to smoking amount to approximately $2.59 for each pack of cigarettes sold. Overall cigarette smoking has declined from 42% of Americans in 1965 to 25.5% in 1994.[2] Teen use of marijuana and tobacco is now on the rise after a downward trend in the use of these substances ended between 1992 and 1993.[9] Approximately 1 million children in the United States become smokers annually with 3000 new young people initiating the habit each day.[1,4] The tobacco industry's massive marketing plan has had a substantial effect on children.[10] The recognition rate of Old Joe Camel (the cartoon character promoting Camel cigarettes) has been reported to be as high as 91.3% among 6-year-old children.[11]

Environmental Tobacco Smoke

Environmental tobacco smoke (ETS), which is also known as "second-hand smoke," consists of the smoke inhaled and exhaled by the smoker, the smoke issued from the end of the cigarette between puffs, and vapor-phase components that diffuse through cigarette paper into the environment.[12] The risks of ETS have been widely publicized and substantiated in the literature. Household members exposed to ETS have a higher risk of lung cancer than those not exposed to ETS.[1] Breathing second-hand smoke has been associated with an increased risk of ischemic heart disease, increasing a person's risk by 25%.[13] Children who are exposed to ETS have a higher incidence of health-related problems, such as asthma, bronchitis, pneumonia, and otitis media.[1,4] Of special concern is the 20 to 25% of women who continue to smoke while pregnant, resulting in an increased risk of sudden infant death syndrome, spontaneous abortion, and fetal growth retardation.[14]

Health Benefits of Smoking Cessation

The Surgeon General and the AHCPR have substantiated the following statements supporting the health benefits of smoking cessation.[1,6,15–17] First, smoking cessation has major and immediate health benefits for men and women of all ages. Benefits apply to those with and without smoking-related disease. Second, former smokers live longer than continuing smokers. For example, those who quit smoking before the age of 50 will have only half the risk of dying in the next 15 years as those who continue to smoke. Third, smoking cessation decreases the risk of lung cancer, other cancers, heart attack, stroke, and chronic lung disease. For example, in 1 year, the excess risk of coronary heart disease in a patient who stops smoking is half that of a smoker. In 5 years, the risk of cancer of the mouth, throat, and esophagus is half that of a smoker's. In 10 years, the death rate from lung cancer is similar to that of a nonsmoker. Fourth, women who stop smoking before pregnancy or during the first 3 to 4 months of pregnancy reduce their risk of having a low birth weight baby to that of women who never smoked. Fifth, those parents who stop smoking will decrease the exposure risk of ETS on both the unborn fetus and on those in the household. Finally, the health benefits of smoking cessation far outweigh the risks of weight gain which often accompany quitting. Most people attempting to quit will gain less than 4.5 kg (10 lb), but others will gain substantially more weight. Because weight gain often causes relapse, it is vital for the clinician to stress the importance of this final point and to be honest with the patient making an attempt to quit smoking.

PATHOPHYSIOLOGY OF NICOTINE

Pharmacologic and Physiologic Effects

Nicotine is a tertiary amine and is the addictive component found in cigarette smoke. It is capable of affecting the actions of the sympathetic and parasympathetic nervous systems via activation of nicotinic receptors.[14] Nicotine acts on these receptors in the brain, autonomic ganglia, adrenal medulla, neuromuscular junctions, and other organs.[6] This wide distribution of nicotinic receptors in the body accounts for many of the physiologic effects experienced by smokers.

Most of the effects of nicotine on the central nervous system are due to direct actions on brain receptors, leading to the release of acetylcholine, norepinephrine, dopamine, serotonin, vasopressin, growth hormone, adrenocorticotropin, and β-endorphin.[18] Release of specific neurotransmitters has been speculatively linked to the reported reinforcing effects of nicotine.[19] The release of norepinephrine and dopamine may be associated with pleasure and anorexia. Release of acetylcholine may be associated with improved cognition and behavioral task performance. Smokers attribute arousal and/or relaxation to the central nervous system effects of smoking and purport the benefits of improved attention; enhanced problem-solving skills; and reduced anger, tension, and stress.[14]

Smoking a cigarette or an infusion of nicotine activates the sympathetic nervous system, resulting in increased heart rate, blood pressure, and cardiac stroke volume and output.[18] Nicotine may also activate chemoreceptors in the aortic and carotid bodies, causing vasoconstriction and tachycardia. Peripheral vascular changes include cutaneous vasoconstriction, associated with a decrease in skin temperature.[18] This often contributes to the cold extremities of the chronic smoker and may potentiate complications of other disease states affecting the peripheral vasculature such as diabetes. Hematologic effects of nicotine include increased platelet activation and increased thromboxane A_2 release.[6] Endocrine and metabolic effects of nicotine include a negative impact on the lipid profile (increased low-density lipoprotein and decreased high-density lipoprotein), early onset of menopause and an increased risk of osteoporosis in women due to decreased estrogen levels, and an increased metabolic rate leading to decreased body weight.

Pharmacokinetics

Nicotine is a weak base with a pK_a of 8.0 that is soluble in both water and lipids.[19] The nicotine found in most commercially available forms of tobacco is acidic; therefore, minimal buccal absorption of nicotine from cigarette smoke occurs, even when the smoke is held in the mouth. Nicotine that is inhaled into the lungs is readily absorbed into the systemic circulation due to the huge alveolar surface area, thin epithelial and endothelial layers, and extensive capillary bed.[19] Once absorbed, the nicotine is rapidly distributed to all organs of the body via the arterial circulation. It has been estimated that it takes 19 seconds or less from the start of a puff from a cigarette for nicotine to reach the brain.[20] Nicotine is primarily metabolized by the liver, with small amounts being metabolized by the lungs or excreted unchanged in the kidneys. The half-life of nicotine averages 2 hours, although there is considerable variation (range, 1 to 4 hours).[18] The primary inactive metabolites of nicotine are cotinine and nicotine-*N*-oxide. Although there is variation on the amount of nicotine contained in different brands of cigarettes, all those commercially available deliver adequate amounts of nicotine to establish and maintain dependence.[21]

Nicotine Dependence

Nicotine effects related to dependence are sustained by the physiologic and psychologic activities resulting from cigarette smoking. These effects increase the compulsion to smoke by producing positive and negative reinforcement.[6] The effects of positive reinforcement include arousal, relaxation, reduced stress, enhanced vigilance, improved cognitive function, elevated mood, and decreased body weight.[14] The effects of negative reinforcement refer to the relief of withdrawal symptoms, including irritability, restlessness, drowsiness, anxiety, hunger, weight gain, sleep disturbances, and difficulty concentrating.[14] When an attempt to stop smoking is initiated, withdrawal symptoms reach maximal intensity 1 to 2 days after cessation and gradually decrease in intensity over a period of 2 weeks.[19] However, the desire to smoke may persist for a lifetime in the patient who has successfully stopped smoking. The Fagerstrom Test for Nicotine Dependence (FTND) is a six-item questionnaire designed to assist the health care professional in determining nicotine dependence (Fig. 63.1).[22] A score of greater than 6 (maximum score of 10) on the FTND indicates a high level of nicotine dependence. The FTND, along with a history of prior attempts to quit, is a valuable tool in determining a course of action for smoking cessation. The patient with a high level of nicotine dependence who is attempting smoking cessation may have difficulty overcoming the initial withdrawal symp-

Questions and Possible Answers	Score
How soon after you wake up do you smoke your first cigarette?	
≤5 min	3
6–30 min	2
31–60 min	1
≥61 min	0
Do you find it difficult to refrain from smoking in places where it is forbidden (e.g. in church, at the library, in a cinema)?	
Yes	1
No	0
What cigarette would you hate most to give up?	
The first in the morning	1
Any other	0
How many cigarettes per day do you smoke?	
≤10	0
11–20	1
21–30	2
≥31	3
Do you smoke more frequently during the first hours after waking than during the rest of the day?	
Yes	1
No	0
Do you smoke if you are so ill that you are in bed most of the day?	
Yes	1
No	0
Total Score:	______

Figure 63.1. The Fagerstrom test for nicotine dependence. (*Source:* Reference 22.)

toms and may greatly benefit from pharmacotherapy to aid cessation. Even the person with a low-to-moderate level of nicotine dependence (FTND score of 6 or less) may benefit from NRT or bupropion to aid in smoking cessation. The decision to use pharmacotherapy or the "cold turkey" method should be based on the FTND, previous attempts to quit, and patient preference.

Effects of Smoking on Drug Therapy

Cigarette smoke may interact with medications through pharmacokinetic and/or pharmacodynamic mechanisms.[23] These types of interactions may lead to adverse events or undesirable patient outcomes. Smoking-drug interactions must be considered not only in those who are currently smoking, but also when a smoking cessation attempt is initiated. A group of chemicals in cigarette smoke known as the polycyclic hydrocarbons (PAHs) are principally responsible for enhancing drug metabolism through induction of the cytochrome P-450 enzymes in the liver, specifically the CYP1A2 isoenzyme.[14] This differs from the past hypothesis that nicotine was primarily responsible for enhancing drug metabolism. PAHs, which are the product of incomplete combustion of organic matter such as wood, coal, tobacco, crude oil, and gasoline, are found in appreciably large amounts in cigarette smoke.[23] Induction of the CYP1A2 isoenzyme may enhance the metabolism of theophylline, imipramine, amitriptyline, tacrine, acetaminophen, caffeine, clomipramine, and clozapine.[6,23,24] Smokers may require a higher dosage of these medications to obtain a therapeutic response. Also, upon smoking cessation, dosage adjustments may be necessary. For example, a 25 to 33% reduction in the dosage of theophylline may be required when a patient stops smoking to avoid toxicity.[24,25] However, normalization of hepatic enzymes after smoking cessation is variable; therefore, dosage adjustments should be based on monitoring of theophylline serum concentrations.[26]

Components of cigarette smoke have inherent pharmacologic properties that may potentiate pharmacodynamic interactions. Examples include decreased therapeutic effect of certain antihypertensive and antianginal agents; increased risk of myocardial infarction, stroke, and thromboembolic disease in women who smoke and take an estrogen-containing oral contraceptive; decreased sedative effect of diazepam and chlordiazepoxide; decreased rate of insulin absorption, leading to hyperglycemia; decreased response to histamine (H_2)-receptor antagonists; and increased risk of development and recurrence of a peptic ulcer.[6,14] Increased doses of pentazocine and propoxyphene may be required in smokers to achieve the same analgesic effects seen in nonsmokers for reasons that are not fully understood.[23] Smokers may also require higher doses of furosemide, thiazide diuretics, flecainide, and heparin than nonsmokers to achieve a similar clinical response. The pharmacodynamic interactions described above are often subtle, but demand constant attention from the health care professional. For example, an insulin-dependent smoker may need higher doses of insulin to maintain glycemic control and lower doses if smoking cessation is attempted.[6] The clinician must encourage strict patient monitoring (via fingerstick blood glucose testing) to guide drug therapy. Patient signs and symptoms of efficacy and toxicity related to drug therapy must also be closely monitored in the diabetic patient who smokes.

THE PHARMACIST'S ROLE IN SMOKING CESSATION

Ask, Advise, Identify, Assist, and Arrange Strategy

A major goal of Healthy People 2000 is to reduce smoking prevalence by the year 2000 to 15%.[27] Pharmacists can play an integral role in achieving this goal because they are some of the most easily accessible health care professionals as well as the most trusted.[28,29] Unlike other health care professionals, pharmacists can address smoking cessation with a greater population because many persons without any past medication history enter a pharmacy to purchase nonprescription items such as vitamins. The AHCPR emphasizes that pharmacists, as well as other health care professionals, should use the ask, advise, identify, assist, and arrange (AAIAA) strategy, a five-step strategy for smoking cessation (Fig. 63.2).[1,6,14]

Step 1: Pharmacists should *ask* each patient about tobacco use. Documentation of the patient's smoking status is a necessity. Repeat assessments are not necessary for adults who have never smoked.[15] However, some may

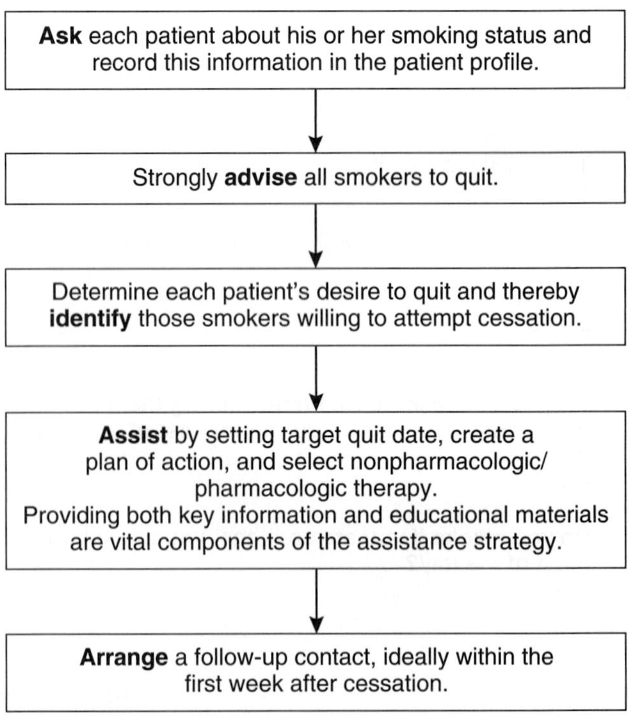

Figure 63.2. Agency for Health Care Policy and Research (*AHCPR*) model strategies. (*Source:* Reference 6.)

Precontemplation	Contemplation	Preparation	Action	Maintenance
Smoker currently has no intent to quit	Smoker is considering quitting in the next 6 months, but has no specific plans.	Smoker plans on qutting in the next month and may have attempted to quit during the previous year.	Smoker has abstained from smoking for 1 day to 6 months.	Smoker has abstained from smoking for at least 6 months.

Figure 63.3. Transtheoretical model stages of change. (*Source:* Reference 6.)

argue that a smoking inquiry should occur at each patient encounter, regardless whether a patient previously informed the pharmacist of no tobacco use. The primary reason for this argument is that patients may start tobacco use after the initial assessment.

Step 2: Pharmacists should *advise* all smokers to quit smoking. Health risks associated with smoking should be mentioned to the patient in a clear, strong, and personalized manner.

Step 3: Pharmacists should *identify* patients willing to make an attempt to quit. Pharmacists can do this by using the transtheoretical model (TTM) to categorize patients into one of five stages. The TTM will be discussed later in this chapter. Pharmacists should focus on patients in the preparation phase because these smokers are ready to quit within a 30-day period.

Step 4: Pharmacists must *assist* patients with a plan to quit. This requires setting up quit date, determining a method of cessation, giving key advice on successful quitting, and providing educational materials.

Step 5: Pharmacists must *arrange* for follow-up contact. This is the most important step. Contact can be either in person or via phone. The first follow-up after a patient's quit date should be done within the first week. During follow-up, patients should be provided with encouragement and positive support. Also, if NRT or another pharmacologic agent is being used for cessation, proper use should be reviewed and any problems that may have arisen should be addressed. Finally, for patients who have relapsed, emphasis must be made that relapse is not a sign of failure. Patients must be reminded that relapse can be used as a learning experience and the average smoker attempts to quit several times before sustained abstinence is attained.[30] For patients who relapse, the importance of recommitment to total abstinence must be stressed.

Transtheoretical Model

Identification of smokers who are ready to quit is an important step in the AAIAA strategy. The TTM allows pharmacists to categorize smokers into one of the following five stages of change: precontemplation, contemplation, preparation, action, and maintenance.[6,14,30] As smokers go through this continuum, they also experience several processes of change (Fig. 63.3 and Table 63.1).[30]

- *Precontemplation*: Smokers in the precontemplation stage are unwilling to consider an attempt to quit. Pharmacists should approach these smokers with information about the negative consequences of smoking. However, these patients are not usually convinced the negative effects of smoking outweigh the positive. Before moving along the continuum of stages, smokers in the precontemplation stage must undergo the process of social liberation. Smokers undergoing this process become more aware of other smokers attempting to quit and the increasing number of public places designated as smoke-free.
- *Contemplation*: Patients in this stage are receptive to information about smoking cessation. They are considering quitting usually within the next 6 months; however, it is common for patients to remain in this stage for a lengthy period of time. Processes of change that peak in this stage include dramatic relief, helping relationships, consciousness-raising, and environmental reevaluation. Pharmacists can aid smokers in this stage by offering suggestions about stimulus control or counterconditioning as well as emotional support.
- *Preparation*: At this stage, smokers have usually made one attempt to quit in the past year and are ready to make another attempt in the next 30 days. Pharmacists can be a great benefit to patients in this stage by helping the patient establish goals, providing positive support, and discussing a possible plan of action.
- *Action*: Patients in the action phase have quit smoking within the past 6 months. To decrease the likelihood of relapse, patients may use techniques such as reinforcement management, self-reevaluation, and stimulus control. Pharmacists can offer a tremendous amount of help to these patients by providing counter-conditioning tips, providing support, and identifying reasons for relapse if it occurs.
- *Maintenance*: Patients in this stage have abstained from smoking for at least 6 months. Relapse is possible even if patients have reached this stage; therefore, pharmacists can emphasize avoiding stimuli that may lead to relapse.

METHODS OF SMOKING CESSATION

Pharmacists are a vital resource for smokers attempting to quit. Not only can they provide positive support and prepare patients for their quit date, they can also help the patient to select an appropriate method of cessation.

Several methods of cessation are available for smokers

Table 63.1 ▪ Processes and Stages of Change in Smoking Behavior

Processes of Change	Peak Stage of Change
Social liberation Noticing that others in one's environment are quitting smoking and that increasingly more public places are becoming designated as smoke-free	Precontemplation
Dramatic relief Becoming upset or emotional in response to information about the hazards of smoking	Contemplation
Helping relationships Recognizing the existence of meaningful or salient others who provide support for one's smoking cessation efforts	Contemplation
Consciousness raising Gaining and thinking about information that is relevant to one's smoking	Contemplation
Environmental reevaluation Recognizing the harmful effects of smoking on the physical and social environments	Contemplation
Reinforcement management Rewarding oneself or being rewarded by others for not smoking	Action
Self-reevaluation Cognitively evaluating one's attitudes toward one's smoking and cigarette dependency	Action
Stimulus control Altering or manipulating the environment to remove cues that trigger smoking and introducing cues to facilitate cessation	Action
Counterconditioning Developing and engaging in new behaviors to take the place of smoking	Maintenance
Self-liberation Realizing that one is capable of successfully abstaining from cigarettes if one chooses to	Maintenance

Source: Reference 2.

desiring to quit. To select an appropriate method, many patient factors must be considered including number of cigarettes smoked per day, duration of smoking history, level of nicotine dependence (FTND), previous quit attempts, and other drugs or disease states. Once a method is selected, patients should be instructed on proper use, if applicable, and what to expect.

Nicotine Pharmacotherapy

Nicotine-Replacement Therapy

NRT may be considered advantageous for several reasons. First, based on the number of cigarettes smoked per day, NRT may provide less daily amounts of nicotine than cigarettes. In addition, NRTs may result in less suffering from withdrawal symptoms associated from the cold turkey method of cessation. Second, unlike smoking cigarettes, patients are not exposed to carcinogens while using NRT. Lastly, NRTs provide slower and less variable plasma concentrations of nicotine, resulting in a reduction of the reinforcing effects of smoking.[21,31,32] In addition, the highest abstinence rates are produced with combined individualized NRT and nonpharmacologic interventions.[33]

Currently there are four methods of NRT: the nicotine transdermal patch, nicotine gum, nicotine nasal spray, and the nicotine oral inhaler (Tables 63.2 and 63.3). These are all indicated by the Federal Drug Administration (FDA) as aids for smoking cessation to alleviate nicotine withdrawal symptoms.

Nictotine Transdermal Patches

Currently, there are four nicotine patches available on the market. Nicotrol and Nicoderm CQ patches are available on a nonprescription status whereas Habitrol and Prostep patches require a prescription.

The Nicotrol patch is available only as a 15 mg/16 hr patch. The manufacturer's dosing recommendations are the simplest of all the nicotine patches. It is applied daily upon awakening and is removed at bedtime for 6 weeks. Additionally, no tapering is required.[1,8,15,34]

The Nicoderm CQ™ patch is available in the following three strengths: 21, 14, and 7 mg/24 hr patches. Although these are designed to deliver nicotine over a 24-hour period, they can also be used for a 16-hour period. The Nicoderm CQ™ 21 mg/24 hr patch applied for 16 hours is comparable to the Nicotrol 15 mg/16 hr patch in that they both release approximately 0.9 mg of nicotine per hour. Recommended dosing is based on the number of cigarettes smoked daily. For persons who smoke less than 10 cigarettes a day, one 14 mg/24 hr patch should be applied daily for 6 weeks followed by one 7 mg/24 hr patch daily for 2 weeks. For persons who smoke greater than 10 cigarettes a day, the recommendation is to start with one 21 mg/24 hr patch daily for 6 weeks followed by one 14 mg/24 hr patch daily for 2 weeks and then one 7 mg/24 hr patch daily for 2 weeks.[1,8,15,34]

The Habitrol patch is also available as 21, 14, and 7 mg/24 hr patches. For persons who smoke fewer than 10 cigarettes per day, weigh less than 100 pounds, or have cardiovascular disease, the following regimen is recommended: one 14 mg/24 hr patch daily for 4 to 8 weeks followed by one 7 mg/24 hr patch daily for 2 to 4 weeks. For those not meeting any of the above criteria, the 21 mg/24 hr patch should be used for 4 to 8 weeks, then the 14 mg/24 hr patch for 2 to 4 weeks, and lastly the 7 mg/24 hr patch for 2 to 4 weeks.[1,8,15,34,35]

The Prostep patch is available in two doses: the 22 mg/24 hr patch and the 11-mg/24-hour patch. Dosing is based on patient's weight. For persons who weigh less than 100 pounds, the 11 mg/24 hr patch should be used for 4 to 8 weeks. Persons weighing at least 100 pounds should start with the 22 mg/24 hr patch for 4 to 8 weeks followed by the 11 mg/24 hr patch for 2 to 4 weeks.[1,8,15,36]

Several points must be addressed concerning duration of therapy and the use of the 24-hour versus the 16-hour nicotine patch. First, recommended duration of therapy for the Nicotrol patch is 6 weeks with no tapering, whereas the other nicotine patches recommend tapering, which can result in duration of therapy up to 16 weeks. However, evaluation of the literature showed no increased efficacy with tapering and/or extending treatment beyond 8 weeks.[37] Regarding the issue of using the 24-hour versus the 16-hour nicotine patch, studies have shown both to be equally efficacious.[37] However, the increased incidence of adverse drug effects (ADEs) associated with the use of the

Table 63.2 ▪ Smoking Cessation Therapies

Cessation Method	Dosing	Taper	Pharmacokinetics
Patch Rx (Habitrol, Prostep) Non-Rx (Nicotrol, Nicoderm CQ)	Nicotrol (patients smoking >10 cigarettes): 15 mg/day for 6 wk Nicoderm CQ (21, 14, 7 mg/24 hr) Light smokers (≤10 cigarettes/day): one 14 mg/24 hr patch for 16 or 24 hr/day for 6 wk, then one 7 mg/24 hr patch for 16 or 24 hr/day for 2 wk Heavier smokers (>10 cigarettes/day): one 21 mg/24 hr patch for 16 or 24 hr/day for 6 wk, then one 14 mg/24 hr patch for 16 or 24 hr/day for 2 wk, then one 7 mg/24 hr patch for 16 or 24 hr/day for 2 wk Habitrol (21, 14, 7 mg/24 hr) Healthy patients: 21 mg/day for 4–8 wk, then 14 mg/day for 2–4 wk, then 7 mg/day for 2–4 wk Other patients[a] : 14 mg/day for 4–8 wk, then 7 mg/day for 2–4 wk Prostep (22 or 11 mg/24 hr) Patients ≥100 lb: 22 mg/day for 4–8 wk, then 11 mg/day for 2–4 wk Patients <100 lb: 11 mg/day for 4–8 wk	Not necessary	Nicotrol, Nicoderm CQ 21 mg/24 hr; Habitrol 21 mg/24 hr; Prostep 22 mg/24 hr deliver 0.9–1.0 mg/hr
Gum (Non-Rx) Nicorette (2 mg, 4 mg) Nicorette Mint (2 mg, 4 mg)	2 mg (4 mg for highly dependent patients, patients who request it, or those for whom 2 mg failed) chewed and "parked" between the cheek and gum intermittently over 30 min every 1–2 hr for 6 wk, then every 2–4 hr for 3 wk, then every 4–8 hr for 3 wk Do not exceed 30 pieces/day (20 pieces/day for 4-mg strength)	Yes	Peak plasma concentrations reached in approximately 30 min Acidic saliva will decrease nicotine absorption (coffee, soda) 0.9 mg of nicotine per 2-mg dose
Nasal spray (Rx) Nicotrol NS 10 mg/mL	One or two 1-mg doses (each dose is two 0.5-mg sprays, one in each nostril) per hour initially, increased as needed Do not exceed 5 doses/hr or 40 doses/day Full dose for up to 8 wk, then gradually decrease dose over 4–6 wk	Yes	Peak plasma concentrations reached within 5–15 min Less absorption if patient has rhinitis or cold
Oral inhaler (Rx) Nicotrol Inhaler 10-mg nicotine cartridges—4 mg delivered	Place the nicotine cartridge into the mouthpiece and push the two pieces of the inhaler together, breaking a seal on each end of the cartridge Initial use is 6–16 cartridges/day Patient controls the depth and frequency of inhalation Optimal effects have been reported with continuous puffing over 20 minutes Begin tapering after 12 wk of therapy	Yes	Peak plasma concentrations reached within 10–15 min One puff of the inhaler is equal to 1/10 to 1/8 nicotine content in one cigarette puff
Bupropion (Rx) Zyban	Start therapy 2 wk before quit date; begin with 150 mg daily for 3 days If tolerated, dose can be increased to 150 mg twice daily Continue for 7–12 wk	No	$T_{1/2} \approx 21$ hr

Sources: References 15, 24.

Rx, pharmacologic; *Non-Rx*, nonpharmacologic.

[a]Patients who smoke <10 cigarettes/day, those who weigh less than 100 lb, or those with cardiovascular disease.

Table 63.3 ▪ Patient Information for Smoking Cessation Therapies

Cessation Method	Adverse Drug Effects	Cautions	Patient Information[a]
Patch Rx (Habitrol, Prostep) Non-Rx (Nicotrol, Nicoderm CQ)	Skin irritation (pruritus, erythema), insomnia (more common with 24-hr patch)	Pregnancy Heart disease (post-MI, arrhythmias, severe angina, uncontrolled hypertension)	Apply patch to hairless area between neck and waist Rotate sites (do not use the same site within 7 days) Hydrocortisone or triamcinolone cream may be used for skin irritation Dispose of the patch properly (away from children and pets) No benefit with using patch >8 wk has been established
Gum (Non-Rx) Nicorette (2 mg, 4 mg) Nicorette Mint (2 mg, 4 mg)	Mouth irritation, sore jaw, dyspepsia, nausea, hiccups	Denture wearers Pregnancy Heart disease (post-MI, arrhythmias, severe angina, uncontrolled hypertension)	Use on a scheduled basis Avoid eating or drinking anything except water 15 min before, during, and after using the gum Start tapering after 2–3 mo of use Do not use longer than 6 mo Dispose of the gum properly
Nasal spray (Rx) Nicotrol NS 10 mg/mL	Rhinitis, throat irritation, sneezing, coughing	Rhinitis Common cold Pregnancy Heart disease (post-MI, severe angina, arrhythmias, uncontrolled hypertension)	Do not use longer than 6 mo Reserved for patients who fail to quit with the patch or gum Tilt head back slightly and insert bottle tip into nostril Do not sniff while spraying into nostril
Oral inhaler (Rx) Nicotrol Inhaler 10 mg nicotine cartridges—4 mg delivered	Dyspepsia, coughing, oral burning, mouth irritation	COPD Asthma Pregnancy Heart disease (post-MI, severe angina, arrhythmias, uncontrolled hypertension)	Do not use longer than 6 mo Do not use if patient has menthol allergy This product may have psychologic advantage for patients requiring the "hand-to-mouth" ritual Each cartridge is effective for 24 hr after it is pierced by the mouth-piece
Bupropion (Rx) Zyban	Headache, insomnia, dry mouth	DI: weak inducer of the P-450 enzymes (phenytoin, phenobarbital, carbamazepine), MAOIs Conditions: seizures, bulimia, anorexia, CNS disorders, chronic alcohol use	Start 1–2 wk before quit date Doses should be separated by at least 8 hr

Sources: References 15, 24.

Rx, pharmacologic; *Non-Rx*, nonpharmcologic; *MI*, myocardial infarction; *COPD*, chronic obstructive pulmonary disease; *DI*, drug interactions; *MAOIs*, monoamine oxidase inhibitors; *CNS*, central nervous system.

[a]Patients using nicotine replacement therapies should not smoke cigarettes.

24-hour patch makes the 16-hour patch a desirable option for many patients. The 24-hour patch may be beneficial for patients who initiate smoking within the first few minutes after awakening or those who find it necessary to smoke during sleeping hours.

All nicotine transdermal systems are self-adhesive and consist of the following layers: an impermeable backing layer, a drug-containing reservoir, an adhesive layer, and a removable protective layer.[38] The higher strength patches deliver approximately 0.9 to 1.0 mg of nicotine per hour. Absorption of nicotine from the transdermal systems is gradual. A major difference compared to cigarettes is that there is no immediate uptake of nicotine to the brain. Therefore, patients do not experience the immediate positive benefits that they would after initiating smoking a cigarette. After the 24-hour nicotine patch is started, steady-state levels are achieved within 2 to 3 days.[38,39] Nicotine absorption does not significantly vary between nicotine patch administration on the back, arm, and chest.[38,40,41] Nicotine concentrations decrease within 1 to 3 hours upon cessation of patch use.[31,32] Ten to 12 hours after patch removal, nicotine plasma concentrations become undetectable.[42]

One of the most common ADEs of the patches is skin irritation, which can be manifested as pruritus, burning, or erythema.[21,31,38,40,43–45] It can occur in up to 50% of patients using the nicotine patch.[31,40] The incidence is lower with the use of the 16-hour patch than with the

24-hour patch.[46] These usually minor ADEs disappear within 24 hours after discontinuing the use of the nicotine patch.[1] Nonprescription products that may help alleviate the skin irritation include hydrocortisone cream, triamcinolone cream, or oral diphenhydramine.[1,43] Additionally, rotation of the application site can help minimize skin irritation.[31,40,43–45] Sleep disturbances such as insomnia and vivid dreams have also been experienced by persons using the nicotine patch.[21,31,38,40,43–45] These are more common with the 24-hour patch versus the 16-hour patch.[31,46] Removal of the nicotine patch before bedtime helps to minimize sleep disturbances.[1,31] Other less frequent ADEs reported with the transdermal patches include gastrointestinal effects, headache, and dizziness.[38,45]

Many studies have assessed the efficacy of the nicotine patch. Fiore et al.[37] performed a meta-analysis that evaluated 17 double-blind, placebo-controlled nicotine patch studies which assessed abstinence rates at the end of treatment and at 6 months. The authors concluded that patients are twice as likely to abstain from smoking with patch use than with placebo. Moreover, the authors concluded from their evaluation that (1) the 16-hour and the 24-hour nicotine patches were equally efficacious, (2) extending the duration of therapy beyond 8 weeks did not increase efficacy, and (3) tapering off the nicotine patch did not demonstrate greater efficacy.[37,47] Other transdermal nicotine patch studies have evaluated abstinence rates at greater than 6 months.[48–50] Richmond et al.[49,50] assessed abstinence rates at 1 year and 3 years after quit date. Treatment with the nicotine patch more than doubled the abstinence rates compared to placebo. In terms of safety, the nicotine patch has been proven not to cause worsening of myocardial ischemia or arrhythmia in patients with coronary heart disease.[51] However, any patient with heart disease attempting cessation should be monitored closely by a physician as well as by a pharmacist. Overall, the nicotine transdermal patch is considered first-line therapy for patients requiring a pharmacologic method of cessation.

Patients starting the nicotine patch should be informed about several issues. First, the nicotine patch should be applied to a hairless area on the body between the neck and the waist after awakening. It should not be applied to the same site within 7 days. Patients using the nicotine patch for a 16-hour period should remove it before bedtime. After the nicotine patch is removed, it should be disposed of properly because it contains a sufficient amount of nicotine to cause serious harm to pets and children. Proper disposal must be emphasized for all NRTs.

The nicotine patch will not restrict patients from their daily activities and can be worn in the shower or pool. If the nicotine patch falls off during the day, waterproof or cloth tape can be used keep it on the skin. Patients should also be warned not to smoke while using the nicotine patch. Those who do smoke while using the nicotine patch may experience signs and symptoms of nicotine toxicity.[52]

Nicotine Gum

Nicotine polacrilex gum is available without a prescription in a 2- and 4-mg dose in regular (Nicorette) and mint flavor (Nicorette Mint).[31,34] Recommended dosing is one piece every 1 to 2 hours for 6 weeks, then one piece every 2 to 4 hours for 3 weeks, and then one piece every 4 to 8 hours for 3 weeks.[31,34]

Nicotine is released as the gum is chewed.[44] Absorption occurs through the buccal mucosa and is decreased at a lower pH.[21,44] Approximately half the dose is absorbed systemically from a piece of nicotine gum.[31] Because nicotine plasma concentrations peak about 30 minutes after the patient starts to chew the nicotine gum, it should be used on a scheduled basis, not on an as-needed basis.[44]

Adverse drug reactions associated with nicotine gum include injury to the oral mucosa, jaw aches, hiccups, dyspepsia, belching, throat irritation, and nausea.[21,46] Patients with dentures, recent dental work, or temporomandibular joint disease should be cautious with the use of nicotine gum as a method of cessation.

In terms of efficacy, clinical trials have shown better abstinence rates with nicotine gum than with placebo.[21,31] Nicotine gum demonstrated 12-month abstinence rates approximately 1.4 to 1.6 times that of placebo.[31] The 4-mg dose may be a better option than the 2-mg dose for patients who smoke more than 24 cigarettes a day, have a high level of nicotine dependency, or have failed to quit using the 2-mg gum. Overall, the nicotine gum is considered a second-line agent. Although there have been no studies comparing the nicotine gum to the nicotine patch, the nicotine patch is preferred because it is easier to use than the nicotine gum and requires less patient education.

Patients using nicotine gum should be informed about several issues. First, it must be emphasized that nicotine gum should not be chewed like regular chewing gum. Patients should be instructed to chew nicotine gum until a peppery taste emerges and then "park" it between the cheek and gum. This routine should be repeated intermittently over a period of 30 minutes. Additionally, because of decreased absorption at a low pH, patients should be instructed to avoid acidic beverages such as coffee, soda, and juices 15 minutes before and while chewing nicotine gum. Patients should also be informed that nicotine gum should not be used as an indefinite substitute for cigarettes. Use of nicotine gum should not be continued beyond 4 to 6 months of therapy.[31] Lastly, patients should dispose of the nicotine gum properly.

Combination use of the nicotine patch and nicotine gum has been studied.[53,54] Several studies have demonstrated that combination use significantly decreases withdrawal symptoms and increases abstinence rates than use of either dosage form alone.[53,54] This combination may be recommended to patients who relapse after attempting to quit with the gum or the patch. However, the nicotine patch and bupropion combination may be a better option because patients will not be absorbing as much nicotine systemically and fewer adverse effects may be seen.

Nicotine Nasal Spray

Nicotine nasal spray is another option for smoking cessation; however, a prescription is required. Initial dosing for the nicotine nasal spray is one or two doses per hour; each dose consists of one 0.5-mg spray into each nostril. Patients can increase frequency as needed, but should not exceed 5 doses per hour or 40 doses per day. Once an optimal dose is achieved, the patient should maintain this scheduled dose for up to 8 weeks and then gradually taper over 4 to 6 weeks.[31,34,55,56] No specific tapering regimen is recommended; however, strategies include decreasing the frequency of the nicotine nasal spray or decreasing the dose to half the usual dose by spraying into only one nostril over a period of 1 to 2 months.

Nicotine from the nasal spray dosage is absorbed rapidly through the nasal mucosa. The rate of absorption is faster than with any other NRT, with peak plasma concentrations achieved within 5 to 15 minutes.[55] Approximately one-half to two-thirds of the nicotine is absorbed into the systemic circulation from the nasal spray.[31]

Adverse effects of the nicotine nasal spray make it one of the less popular methods. The most common adverse effects are nasal irritation, sneezing, watery eyes, and coughing.[55,57,58] At least 75% of patients have experienced at least one of the above side effects.[31] However, these adverse effects often subside with continued use.[56]

Several studies have evaluated the efficacy of nicotine nasal spray.[59–61] All studies demonstrated that nicotine nasal spray was more effective than placebo when evaluating short-term and long-term success rates. This dosage form may be an option for the patient who has relapsed after attempting to quit with the nicotine patch or the nicotine gum. Additionally, because of its quick onset of action, nicotine nasal spray may be beneficial for patients requiring more prompt alleviation of withdrawal symptoms.

Patients should be informed of several issues regarding use of nicotine nasal spray. Patients may become dependent with this dosage form because of the quick onset of action.[31] Therefore, patients should not use this product for longer than 6 months. Proper use should also be emphasized. The nicotine nasal spray should not be used like other nasal sprays. The patient should tilt the head back slightly and insert the bottle tip into the nostril. Next, the patient should breathe in through the mouth and hold a breath. Then, the patient should press the bottom of the nasal spray to release one spray. Unlike other nasal sprays, patients should not sniff or inhale through the nose but should instead breathe through the mouth to enhance absorption via the nasal mucosa.

Nicotine Inhaler

The nicotine inhaler is a recent innovation in NRT and is available by prescription only. It consists of a separating mouthpiece into which a nicotine cartridge is placed. Doses should be individualized specifically for the patient. The highest abstinence rates were seen in patients using between 6 and 16 cartridges per day.[62] Patients control the rate and depth of inhalation; however, optimal effects were noted in patients who inhaled continuously over a 20-minute period.[62] Treatment should be continued for a period of 3 months followed by gradual tapering over another 6 to 12 weeks.[62]

Most of the nicotine released from the inhaler is absorbed within the lining of the mouth and the upper esophagus. Less than 5% reaches the lower respiratory tract. Each 10-mg cartridge delivers only 4 mg of nicotine; however, usually only half (2 mg) is systemically absorbed.[62] Each puff from the inhaler is comparable to one-tenth to one-eighth the amount of nicotine taken in by a cigarette puff. After inhalation, peak plasma concentrations are achieved within about 15 minutes.[62]

Adverse effects are often experienced with this NRT.[62] The most common is local irritation.[31,34,62–64] Up to 40% of patients using the nicotine inhaler have experienced mouth and throat irritation.[62] Additionally, coughing and rhinitis occurred more often for persons using the nicotine inhaler than placebo.[62] It should be noted that these local effects did subside with continued use of the nicotine inhaler. Other ADEs include dyspepsia, hiccups, nausea, and diarrhea. Patients with bronchospastic disease such as asthma or chronic obstructive pulmonary disease should use the nicotine inhaler under direct supervision of a health care professional.

Studies evaluating the efficacy of the nicotine inhaler have noted different results regarding long-term efficacy. Schneider et al.[59] showed significantly higher abstinence rates at 3 months with the nicotine inhaler group versus placebo; at 6 and 12 months, no significance was noted for either group. Other studies have shown significant long-term abstinence rates with the nicotine inhaler compared to placebo.[64,65] Overall, further analysis is needed to determine long term efficacy of this dosage form. The nicotine inhaler may be beneficial for patients who cannot forego the hand-to-mouth ritual of smoking.

Patients should be instructed on proper use of the nicotine inhaler. The nicotine cartridge is placed into the mouthpiece and the two pieces are pushed together, piercing the nicotine cartridge. Once the cartridge is placed into the mouthpiece, it is effective for up to 24 hours. After 24 hours, the delivery system is ineffective and the cartridge must be disposed of properly. In addition, patients should be informed not to use the nicotine inhaler longer than 6 months. As with other NRTs, patients should keep the nicotine cartridges away from children and pets.[55]

Non-Nicotine Pharmacotherapy

Bupropion (Zyban) is an antidepressant with noradrenergic and dopaminergic activity.[31,52,66] Its benefit as a smoking cessation agent became apparent when health care providers noticed increased smoking quit rates in patients treated with bupropion for depression.[52] It is speculated that its noradrenergic activity plays a role with nicotine withdrawal whereas the dopaminergic activity reduces the reinforcing properties of nicotine.[34] Bupropion is the first non-nicotine drug therapy approved for smoking cessation and is currently available only with a prescription.

Bupropion has a half-life of 21hours; therefore, it can take up to a week to reach steady state, and patients must be informed to set their quit date at least 1 week after starting the drug.[66] Proper dosing administration is as follows: 150 mg/day for 3 days to monitor for ADEs, followed by 150 mg twice a day for 7 to 12 weeks. Doses should be separated by at least 8 hours. Patients should not exceed doses greater than 300 mg/day because of increased potential for seizures. Tapering of the medication is not necessary after the 7- to 12-week treatment period.[66]

Bupropion is usually well-tolerated. ADEs that have been noted include insomnia, dry mouth, tremors, and rashes.[66,67] Insomnia and dry mouth have an incidence rate of greater than 5% whereas tremors and rash, although not common, have been associated with discontinuation of the drug.[66,67]

Several contraindications of bupropion prohibit its use in certain patients. Because of the drug's potential to decrease seizure threshold, patients with central nervous system disorders or those currently taking bupropion (Wellbutrin) for depression should not duplicate therapy with bupropion (Zyban). Likewise, patients with a history or concurrent diagnosis of bulimia or anorexia nervosa also should not receive the drug because of the increased seizure risk. Lastly, concomitant use of bupropion and monoamine oxidase inhibitors (MAOIs) is contraindicated. Animal studies suggest that concomitant use of bupropion and MAOIs may enhance bupropion toxicity.[68] At least 14 days must elapse after discontinuation of a MAOI before initiating bupropion therapy.[66]

Bupropion is primarily metabolized by the cytochrome P-450 enzyme system, specifically the 2B6 isozenzyme.[66] Therefore, potential drug interactions may exist between bupropion and cyclophosphamide as well as orphenadrine. Other drugs that may interact with bupropion include carbamazepine, phenobarbital, phenytoin, and cimetidine. Cimetidine may inhibit the metabolism of the drug while carbamazepine, phenobarbital, and phenytoin may induce the metabolism of bupropion. Bupropion should be used cautiously with other agents or drug therapies that may lower seizure threshold such as antipsychotics, antidepressants, theophylline, systemic steroids, or abrupt discontinuation of benzodiazepines.[66]

The efficacy of bupropion for smoking cessation was evaluated by Hurt et al.[67] They performed a double-blind, placebo-controlled trial comparing abstinence rates with several doses of sustained-released bupropion (10, 150, and 300 mg/day) compared to placebo. Results showed that abstinence rates at 1 year were significantly higher in the 150 and 300 mg/day groups compared to placebo. Although the two doses lead to comparable quit rates, 300 mg/day is recommended over 150 mg/day for two reasons. First, an inverse relationship between bupropion dose and weight gain was noted in the study. Mean weight gain in the 150 mg/day group and 300 mg/day group was 2.3 and 1.5 kg, respectively. Additionally, patients in the 300 mg/day group had a significantly better rate of continuous abstinence from the target quit date through the end of therapy.

Jorenby et al.[69] evaluated the efficacy of bupropion, a nicotine patch, a combination of both, or placebo for smoking cessation. The investigations concluded that treatment with bupropion alone or in combination with the nicotine patch resulted in higher long-term cessation rates compared to placebo or the nicotine patch alone. However, the conclusions of this study should be accepted with caution. Abstinence rates of the placebo group and nicotine patch group were comparable in this study. Previous literature does not support this result.[37] Future studies are needed to substantiate bupropion's superiority over the nicotine patch.

Other Pharmacotherapies

Other pharmacologic agents for smoking cessation have been reported in the literature. Among these are clonidine, buspirone, doxepin, and silver acetate. Clonidine, a central α_2-agonist, is primarily used as an antihypertensive agent.[70] Several studies have evaluated clonidine's efficacy for smoking cessation.[71–80] Several researchers found clonidine to be superior to placebo for smoking cessation.[31,72] However, this conclusion was limited to women. Davison et al.[73] also evaluated clonidine for smoking cessation and found no significant difference compared to placebo at 12 weeks. The AHCPR conducted a meta-analysis of oral clonidine use for smoking cessation and determined that clonidine should not be recommended for smoking cessation treatment because of insufficient evidence and a high discontinuation rate related to ADEs such as dry mouth and drowsiness.[1,31] Buspirone, an anxiolytic agent, is speculated to reduce withdrawal symptoms. Short-term trials have demonstrated this.[81] However, other studies have not been able to validate this conclusion.[81] The AHCPR does not recommend buspirone because of the lack of data.[1] Antidepressants have also been evaluated as possible smoking cessation agents, specifically the tricyclic antidepressant doxepin.[82,83] Although efficacy was noted with this agent, it should not be recommended because of notable nonadherence primarily related to ADEs.[83] The AHCPR did not review any of these studies on doxepin because they did not meet the selection criteria for review.[1] Nortriptyline has also been evaluated for smoking cessation.[84] Significant improvements were noted regarding withdrawal symptoms and cessation rates compared to placebo. However, ADEs such as dry mouth and dysgeusia are often experienced with nortriptyline, thereby making the drug intolerable for many patients. Finally, silver acetate was also reviewed by the AHCPR as a smoking cessation agent. The mechanism of this drug as a smoking cessation agent is its unpleasant taste created by interacting with the sulfides in tobacco smoke. The committee concluded that no significant benefit was seen with the use of silver acetate for smoking cessation.[1] Rare cases of silver poisoning have been reported; therefore, the FDA prohibits the use of this agent as a smoking cessation aid.[31]

Nonpharmacologic Methods

Cold turkey should be considered as a method of cessation in patients who smoke 10 cigarettes or less a day.[1,14] This method is also considered a first-line approach in pregnant and/or lactating women. Although cold turkey is the least costly method of cessation, patients are more likely to experience withdrawal symptoms. Additionally, abstinence after 1 year of cessation using the cold turkey method is approximately 5%.[14]

Persons attempting to quit cold turkey often use certain behavioral therapies to reinforce their quitting efforts. Techniques include self-management, relapse prevention, nicotine fading, and aversion conditioning.[43] Self-management includes methods such as self-monitoring and stimulus control, which serve to increase patients' awareness of their smoking habits. Self-monitoring requires patients to keep a record of their smoking habits whereas stimulus control promotes avoidance of smoking in the presence of certain triggers or cues.

Relapse prevention is beneficial for patients who go back to smoking after a quit attempt.[43] Techniques used for relapse prevention include avoidance of situations leading to relapse, coping strategies, and contingency management. Coping strategies include methods such as deep breathing or listening to relaxation tapes. Contingency management uses a reward or punishment system for the purpose of maintaining the patient's motivation to abstain from smoking.

Nicotine fading is an attempt to gradually taper the amount of nicotine a smoker absorbs by either switching to cigarettes with less nicotine or decreasing the number of cigarettes per day. However, the efficacy of this method is limited because patients can compensate for the decrease in the amount of nicotine by inhaling cigarettes for a longer period of time.[43]

Aversion techniques have also been used as a method for smoking cessation. The theory behind this method is that exposure to the unpleasant effects of high, quick doses of nicotine prevent patients from returning to smoking. The process involves a patient smoking about one puff every 6 seconds until the cigarette is finished or the patient experiences nausea. However, patients may not abstain from smoking after using this technique because of the smoker's awareness of previous positive effects experienced with smoking.[31]

CONCLUSION

Encouraging and assisting smokers to quit is one of the most important tasks any health care professional can accomplish. The deleterious effects of smoking on the economic and overall health status of those in the United States are well documented, as are the benefits of smoking cessation. The pharmacist, because of drug expertise and availability, is recognized as a health care professional who can have a substantial impact on the prevalence of smoking. The pharmacist should ask each patient about smoking and tobacco use and assist those ready to make a quit attempt. Providing patient education on both behavioral modification and available pharmacotherapeutic options for smoking cessation is a vital role of the pharmacist. Most importantly, after the initial consultation, the pharmacist must follow-up with persons attempting smoking cessation to ensure success.

KEY POINTS

- The pharmacist is in an ideal position to promote smoking cessation because of the number of patients seen in pharmacy practice as well as the availability of nonprescription NRTs.
- Currently, approximately 24.7% of adults in the United States smoke–an estimated total of 47 million people.
- The risks of ETS for both children and adults have been widely publicized and substantiated in the literature.
- Smoking cessation has major and immediate health benefits for men and women of all ages.
- Nicotine is the addictive component found in cigarette smoke. It is capable of affecting the actions of the sympathetic and parasympathetic nervous systems via activation of nicotinic receptors.
- Although there is variation on the amount of nicotine contained in different brands of cigarettes, all those commercially available deliver adequate amounts of nicotine to establish and maintain dependence.
- A group of chemicals in cigarette smoke known as the PAHs are principally responsible for enhancing drug metabolism through induction of the P-450 enzymes in the liver, specifically the CYP1A2 isoenzyme.
- The AHCPR emphasizes that pharmacists, as well as other health care professionals, should use the "AAIAA" strategy (ask, advise, identify, assist, arrange), a five step strategy for smoking cessation.
- The TTM allows pharmacists to categorize smokers into one of the following five stages of change: precontemplation, contemplation, preparation, action, and maintenance.
- Several methods of cessation are available for smokers desiring to quit. To select an appropriate method, many patient factors must be considered including number of cigarettes smoked per day, duration of smoking history, level of nicotine dependence, previous quit attempts, and other drugs or disease states.
- Cold turkey should be considered as a method of cessation in persons who smoke 10 cigarettes or less a

day. For those who smoke more than 10 cigarettes per day or who demonstrate a high level of nicotine dependence, NRT and/or bupropion may be used.

- Overall, the nicotine transdermal patch is considered first-line therapy for patients requiring a pharmacologic method of cessation.

REFERENCES

1. Fiore MC, Bailey WC, Cohen SJ, et al. Smoking cessation. Clinical Practice Guideline No. 18. Rockville, MD: US Department of Health and Human Services, Public Health Service, Agency for Health Care Policy and Research, April 1996. AHCPR Publication 96-0692.
2. Telepchak JM. Smoking cessation: new strategies and opportunities for pharmacists. Am Druggist Jan:48–55, 1997.
3. Cigarette smoking among adults–United States 1995. Morb Mortal Wkly Rep 46:1217–1220, 1997.
4. American Cancer Society. Cancer facts and figures–1996. Atlanta, GA: American Cancer Society.
5. Garnett WR. The vital role of the pharmacist in patient management for OTC smoking cessation products. Pharm Times 1A–28A, 1996.
6. Wongwiwatthananukit S, Jack HM, Popovich NG. Smoking cessation: part 1–an overview. J Am Pharm. Assoc 38:58–70, 1998.
7. Rogot E. Smoking and the life expectancy among U.S. veterans. Am J Pub Health 68:1023–1225, 1978.
8. Nunn-Thompson C, Barr CC, Tommasello AC, et al. APhA special report: a review of the new smoking cessation strategies from the Agency of Health Care Policy and Research. Washington, DC:American Pharmaceutical Association, 1996.
9. Federal figures show teen drug use up sharply in 1995. Am J Health Syst Pharm 53:2255, 1995.
10. Sargent JD, Dalton MA, Beach M, et al. Cigarette promotional items in public schools. Arch Pediatr Adolesc Med 151:1189–1196, 1997.
11. Fischer PM, Schwartz MP, Richards JW, et al. Brand logo recognition by children aged 3 to 6 years: Mickey Mouse and Old Joe the Camel. JAMA 266:3145–3148, 1991.
12. Byrd JC. Environmental tobacco smoke: medical and legal issues. Med Clin North Am 76:377–398, 1992.
13. Law MR, Morris JK, Wald NJ. Environmental tobacco smoke exposure and ischaemic heart disease: an evaluation of the evidence. Br Med J 315:973–980, 1997.
14. Kennedy DT, Goode JVR, Small RE. Smoking and the role of the community pharmacist in cessation. Am Pharmacist May:49–54, 1998.
15. Fiore MC, Bailey WC, Cohen SJ, et al. The Agency for Health Care Policy and Research smoking cessation clinical practice guideline. JAMA 275:1270–1280, 1996.
16. Samet JM. The health benefits of smoking cessation. Med Clin North Am 76:399–414, 1992.
17. US Department of Health and Human Services. The health benefits of smoking cessation: a report of the Surgeon General, 1990. Rockville, MD: US Department of Health and Human Services, 1990. DHHS Publication No. (CDC) 90-8416.
18. Benowitz NL. Pharmacologic aspects of cigarette smoking and nicotine addiction. N Engl J Med 319:1318–1330, 1988.
19. Benowitz NL. Cigarette smoking and nicotine addiction. Med Clin North Am 76:415–437, 1992.
20. Benowitz NL. Pharamacology of nicotine: addiction and therapeutics. Ann Rev Pharmacol Toxicol 36:597–613, 1996.
21. Henningfield JE. Nicotine medications for smoking cessation. N Engl J Med 333:1196–1203, 1995.
22. Heatherton TF, Kozlowski LT, Frecker RC, et al. The Fagerstrom test for nicotine dependence: a revision of the Fagerstrom tolerance questionnaire. Br J Addict 86:1119–1127, 1991.
23. Schein JR. Cigarette smoking and clinically significant drug interactions. Ann Pharmacother 29:1139–1148, 1995.
24. Miller LG. Cigarettes and drug therapy: pharmacokinetic and pharmacodynamic considerations. Clin Pharm 9:125–135, 1990.
25. Lee BL, Benowitz NL, Jacob P. Cigarette abstinence, nicotine gum, and theophylline disposition. Ann Intern Med 106(4):553–555, 1987.
26. Hunt SN, Jusko WJ, Yurchak AM. Effect of smoking on theophylline disposition. Clin Pharmacol Ther 19(5 Part 1):546–551, 1976.
27. US Public Health Service. Healthy People 2000: National health promotion and disease prevention objectives. Washington, DC: Department of Health and Human Services, Public Health Service, 1994. DHHS Publication No. (PHS) 96012.
28. Smith MD, McGhan WF, Lauger G. Pharmacist counseling and outcomes of smoking cessation. Am Pharm NS35(8):20–32, 1995.
29. 1993 Gallup Poll. Princeton, NJ: The Gallop Organization, 1993.
30. Hudmon KS, Berger BA. Pharmacy applications of the transtheoretical model in smoking cessation. Am J Health Syst Pharm 52:282–287, 1995.
31. Wongwiwatthananukit S, Jack HM, Popovich NG. Smoking cessation: part II–pharmacologic approaches. J Am Pharm Assoc 38:339–353, 1998.
32. Henningfield JE, Keenan RM. Nicotine delivery kinetics and abuse liability. J Consult Clin Psychol 61:743–50, 1993.
33. Thompson GH and Hunter DA. Nicotine replacement therapy. Ann Pharmacother 32(10):1067–75, 1998.
34. Kennedy DT, Goode JR, Small RE. Smoking cessation therapies. Am Pharmacist June:65–70, 1998.
35. Habitrol® package insert. Summit, NJ: Novartis Consumer Health, Inc., August 1993.
36. Prostep® package insert. Philadelphia: Wyeth-Ayerst, August 1996.
37. Fiore MC, Smith SS, Jorenby DE, et al. The effectiveness of the nicotine patch for smoking cessation: a meta-analysis. JAMA 271:1940–1947, 1994.
38. Palmer KJ, Buckley MM, Faulds D. Transdermal nicotine: a review of its pharmacodynamic and pharmacokinetic properties, and therapeutic efficacy as an aid to smoking cessation. Drugs 44:498–529, 1992.
39. Gorsline J, Gupta SK, Dye D, et al. Steady-state pharmacokinetics and dose relationship of nicotine delivered from Nicoderm® (nicotine transdermal system). J Clin Pharmacol 33:161–168, 1993.
40. Gora ML. Nicotine transdermal systems. Ann Pharmacother 27:742–750, 1993.
41. Gorsline J, Okerholm RA, Rolf CN, et al. Comparison of plasma nicotine concentrations after application of Nicoderm (nicotine transdermal system) to different skin sites. J Clin Pharmacol 32:576–581, 1992.
42. Fincham, Lender D, Hughes J, et al. American Pharmaceutical Association new product bulletin: NICODERM CQ. Washington, DC: American Pharmaceutical Association. 1996.
43. Haxby DG. Treatment of nicotine dependence. Am J Health Syst Pharm 52:265–281, 1995.
44. Lee EW, D'Alonzo GE. Cigarette smoking, nicotine addiction, and its pharmacologic treatment. Arch Intern Med 53:34–48, 1993.
45. Greenland S, Satterfield MH, Stephan FL. A meta-analysis to assess the incidence of adverse effects associated with the transdermal nicotine patch. Drug Saf 18:297–308, 1998.
46. McEvoy GK, ed. AHFS drug information 97. Bethesda, MD: American Society of Health-System Pharmacists 1049–1061, 1997.
47. Hilleman DE, Mohiuddin SM, Delcore MG. Comparison of fixed-dose transdermal nicotine, tapered-dose transdermal nicotine, and buspirone in smoking cessation. J Clin Pharmacol 34:222–224, 1994.
48. Hurt RD, Dale LC, Fredrickson PA, et al. Nicotine patch therapy for smoking cessation combined with physician advice and nurse follow-up. JAMA 271:595–600, 1994.
49. Richmond RL, Kehoe L, Cesar de Almeida Neto A. Effectiveness of a 24-hour transdermal nicotine patch in conjunction with a cognitive behavioural programme: one year outcome. Addiction 92:27–31, 1997.
50. Richmond RL, Kehoe L, Cesar de Almeida Neto A. Three year continuous abstinence in a smoking cessation study using the nicotine transdermal patch. Heart 78:617–618, 1997.
51. Tzivoni D, Keren A, Meyler S, et al. Cardiovascular safety of transdermal nicotine patches in patients with coronary artery disease who try to quit smoking. Cardiovasc Drug Ther 12:239–244, 1998.
52. Goldstein MG. Bupropion sustained-release and smoking cessation. J Clin Psychiatry 59(4): 66–72, 1998.
53. Fagerstrom KO. Combined use of nicotine replacement products. Health Values 18:15–20, 1994.
54. Fagerstrom KO, Schneider NG, Lunell E. Effectiveness of nicotine patch and nicotine gum as individual versus combined treatments for tobacco withdrawal symptoms. Psychopharmacology 111:271–277, 1993.
55. Nicotrol®NS package insert. Fort Washington, PA: McNeil Consumer Products Co., March 1996.
56. Nunn-Thompson C, Brideau DJ, Shapiro J, et al. American Pharmaceutical Association new product bulletin: Nicotrol NS™. Washington, American Pharmaceutical Association, 1996.
57. Hurt RD, Dale LC, Croghan GA, et al. Nicotine nasal spray for smoking cessation: pattern of use, side effects, relief withdrawal symptoms, and cotinine levels. Mayo Clin Proc 73:118–125, 1998.
58. Schuh KJ, Schuh LM, Henningfield JE. Nicotine nasal spray and vapor inhaler: abuse liability assessment. Psychopharmacology 130:352–361, 1997.

59. Schneider NG, Lunell E, Olmstead RE, et al. Clinical pharmacokinetics of nasal nicotine delivery. Clin Pharmacokinet 31(1):65–80, 1996.
60. Blondal T, Franzon M, Westin A. A double-blind randomized trial of nicotine nasal spray as an aid in smoking cessation. Eur Respir J 10:1585–1590, 1997.
61. Stapleton JA, Sutherland G, Russell AH. How much does relapse after one year erode effectiveness of smoking cessation treatments? Long term follow up of randomized trial of nicotine nasal spray. Br Med J 316:830–831, 1998.
62. Nicotrol® Inhaler package insert. Fort Washington, PA: McNeil Consumer Products Co., May 1997.
63. Schneider NG, Olmstead R, Nilsson F, et al. Efficacy of a nicotine inhaler in smoking cessation: a double-blind placebo-controlled trial. Addiction 91:1293–1306, 1996.
64. Hjalmarson A, Nilsson F, Sjostrom L, et al. The nicotine inhaler in smoking cessation. Arch Intern Med 157:1721–1728, 1997.
65. Tonnesen P, Norregaard J, Mikkelsen K, et al. A double-blind trial of a nicotine inhaler for smoking cessation. JAMA 269:1268–1271, 1993.
66. Zyban® Package Insert. Research Triangle Park, NC: GlaxoWellcome Inc., May 1997.
67. Hurt RD, Sachs DP, Glover ED, et al. A comparison of sustained-release bupropion and placebo for smoking. N Eng J Med 337:1195–1202, 1997.
68. McEvoy GK, ed. AHFS drug information 98. Bethesda, MD: American Society of Health System Pharmacists, 1998:1819.
69. Jorenby DE, Leischow SJ, Nides MA, et al. A controlled trial of sustained-release bupropion, a nicotine patch, or both for smoking cessation. N Engl J Med 340:685–691, 1999.
70. Nunn-Thompson CL, Simon PA. Pharmacotherapy for smoking cessation. Clin Pharm 8:710–720, 1989.
71. Nana A, Praditsuwan R. Clonidine for smoking cessation. J Med Assoc Thai 81:87–93, 1998.
72. Glassman AH, Stetner F, Walsh BT, et al. Heavy smoker, smoking cessation, and clonidine. Results of double-blind, randomized trial. JAMA 259:2863–2866, 1988.
73. Davison R, Kaplan K, Fintel D, et al. The effect of clonidine on the cessation of cigarette smoking. Clin Pharmacol Ther 44:265–267, 1988.
74. Franks P, Harp J, Bell B. Randomized, controlled trial of clonidine for smoking cessation in a primary care setting. JAMA 262:3011–3013, 1989.
75. Appel D. Clonidine helps cigarette smokers stop smoking. Am Rev Respir Dis 135(Suppl):354, 1987.
76. Villagra VG, Rosenberger JL, Girolami S. Transdermal clonidine for smoking cessation: a randomized, double blind, placebo controlled trial. Circulation 80(Suppl 11):58, 1989.
77. Hilleman D, Mohiuddin SM, Malesker MA, et al. Double-blind placebo-controlled evaluation of transdermal clonidine in smoking cessation. Chest 96(Suppl):208S, 1989.
78. Murray KM, Cappello C, Baez SA. Lack of efficacy of transdermal clonidine in a smoking cessation class. Am Rev Respir Dis 189(Suppl):A338, 1989.
79. Hao W, Derson Y. Effect of clonidine on cigarette cessation and in the alleviation of withdrawal symptoms. Brit J Addict 83:1221–1226, 1988.
80. Covey LS, Glassman AH. A meta-analysis of double-blind placebo-controlled trials of clonidine for smoking cessation. Br J Addict 86:991–998, 1991.
81. Hughes JR. Non-nicotine pharmacotherapies for smoking cessation. J Drug Dev 6:197–203, 1994.
82. Edwards NB, Simmons RC, Rosenthal TL, et al. Doxepin in the treatment of nicotine withdrawal. Psychosomatics 29:203–206, 1988.
83. Edwards NB, Murphy JK, Downs AD, et al. Doxepin as an adjunct to smoking cessation: a double-blind pilot study. Am J Psychiatry 146:373–376, 1989.
84. Prochazka AV, Weaver MJ, Keller RT, et al. A randomized trial of nortripyline for smoking cessation. Arch Intern Med 158:2035–2039, 1998.

CHAPTER 64

INFECTIOUS DISEASES: INTRODUCTION

Erika J. Ernst

Selecting and monitoring antimicrobial therapy requires an understanding of the interrelations among the patient, microbiology laboratory, and pharmacological factors (Fig. 64.1). Some patient factors, such as immune status, affect both potential pathogens (bug) and the antimicrobial agents selected to treat them (drug). The selection process for an appropriate antimicrobial regimen involves several steps (Table 64.1). First, the need for antimicrobial therapy must be established. Unfortunately, this important first step is not always accomplished, leading to inappropriate use of antimicrobials. It has been estimated that 50 to 75% of physician office visits for colds, bronchitis, and upper respiratory tract infections result in prescriptions for antibiotics. These prescriptions largely represent inappropriate use of antibiotics, because over 90% of these infections are caused by viruses and antibiotics have little clinical impact on their resolution.[1]

ESTABLISHING INFECTION

Establishing the presence of a bacterial infection is not easy and requires piecing together clinical and laboratory clues of infection. Clinically, an infection is suspected when a patient displays the hallmark signs of inflammation, fever, pain, swelling, and redness. A fever, described as an increase in the body's temperature, which normally fluctuates between 36.2 and 37.2°C (97.5–98.9°F), is generally defined as an elevated body temperature of greater than or equal to 37.7°C (99.9°F).[2] This symptom can be misleading, however, because not all febrile responses are infectious in origin. For example, many collagen vascular disease manifestations also may include fever. There are many other clinical signs of infection, some of which may be more specific for a particular pathogen or site of infection. For example, a "stiff neck" is an important sign of meningitis. The disease-specific signs and symptoms of infection are discussed elsewhere in this volume.

The hallmark sign of infection on laboratory analysis is an increased white blood cell count (WBC). The body upregulates the release of white blood cells into the circulation in response to invasion of microbial pathogens, resulting in a higher than usual percentage of immature neutrophils called bands. This laboratory finding is sometimes referred to as a shift to the left. Other laboratory signs of infection include an increased erythrocyte sedimentation rate (ESR) and increased liver transaminase enzyme tests (LFTs). The elevated ESR and LFTs are nonspecific results and also may be the result of noninfectious medical problems. When the collection of clinical and laboratory signs and symptoms in a particular patient suggests infection, the next step in the antimicrobial selection process is to attempt to establish the causative pathogen.

IDENTIFYING THE PATHOGEN

In the case of suspected infection, culture specimens are obtained from the suspected site in an attempt to identify the pathogen(s) responsible. The type of specimen differs depending on the site of infection and patient characteristics. For example, one obtains sputum when pneumonia or a lung infection is suspected, a urine culture for cystitis or pyelonephritis, and cerebrospinal fluid (CSF) for meningitis. The Gram stain is a useful test for rapid characterization of an organism by cell wall structure and cell morphology. It is performed on sputum, urine, CSF, and wound specimens; however, it is not performed on blood samples because of the large sample volume (~20 mL) that is usually necessary for successful growth of organisms

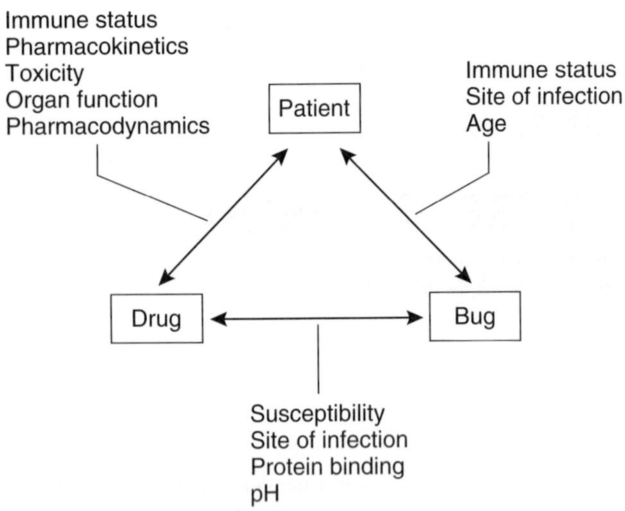

Figure 64.1. Interrelations of patient, microbiological, and pharmacological factors.

Table 64.1 ▪ Antimicrobial Drug Therapy Selection Process

Step 1	Establish the need for antimicrobial therapy.
Step 2	Attempt to identify the pathogen.
Step 3	Select empiric antimicrobial therapy.
Step 4	Monitor therapy for efficacy and toxicity.
Step 5	Refine antimicrobial therapy for definitive identification of pathogen or infection.

from the blood.[3] The Gram stain results are reported by the staining characteristics of the organism (Gram-positive or Gram-negative) and the cell morphology (cocci or bacilli [rods]). Additional characterization using bacterial oxygen tolerance (i.e., aerobic versus anaerobic) also is useful (Table 64.2). Not all bacterial organisms can be seen or are distinguishable using Gram staining, particularly organisms that grow intracellularly or do not have peptidoglycan-containing cell walls (Table 64.3). Determining an organism's Gram staining characteristics narrows the potential pathogens and may assist in directing initial empiric therapy. For example, if a patient suspected of having pneumonia has Gram-negative rods in his or her sputum, then penicillin, which is often used for treating pneumonia, is an inappropriate selection in this situation because it is not active against most Gram-negative rods. In addition to Gram staining, other tests that are commonly used for rapid identification of organisms include the acid fast bacilli (AFB) stain for mycobacteria, India ink for *Cryptococcus* spp., and potassium hydroxide (KOH) for other fungal pathogens. Antibody staining and detection methods are sometimes employed, as well as DNA probes using polymerase chain reaction (PCR) amplification techniques, which are being widely developed.

Culture and sensitivity testing is the next step after staining techniques. It is limited by the time required to complete the testing process, which varies depending on the organism, but requires at least 48 hours. Three general types of susceptibility testing methods are used clinically: (1) disk diffusion testing, (2) broth microdilution testing, and (3) Etest methods. Other susceptibility testing methods exist, namely, agar dilution and macrodilution; however, they are used mainly for drug development because they are more labor intensive.

The disk diffusion test is performed by placing disks, each impregnated with different antibiotics, on an agar plate that has been "streaked" or inoculated to completely cover the surface with organism. This test also is

Table 64.2 ▪ Categorization of Organisms by Gram Staining Characteristics and Oxygen Tolerance

Gram-positive Cocci	**Gram-negative Cocci**
Aerobic	Aerobic
Staphylococcus aureus	*Neisseria gonorrhoeae*
Staphylococcus epidermidis	*Neisseria meningitidis*
Streptococcus pyogenes	*Moraxella catarrhalis*
Streptococcus pneumoniae	
Viridans Streptococci	
Enterococcus faecalis	
Enterococcus faecium	
Anaerobic	
Peptostreptococcus spp.	
Peptococcus spp.	
Gram-positive Bacilli	**Gram-negative Bacilli**
Aerobic	Aerobic
Listeria monocytogenes	*E. coli*
Bacillus anthracis	*Klebsiella pneumoniae*
Corynebacterium diptheriae	*Proteus mirabilis*
Corynebacterium jeikeium (group JK)	*Serratia marcescens*
Rhodococcus spp.	*Pseudomonas aeruginosa*
Anaerobic	*Enterobacter* spp.
Clostridium difficile	*Haemophilus influenzae*
Clostridium perfringens	*Legionella pneumophila*
Clostridium tetani	Anaerobic
Propionibacterium acnes	*Bacteroides fragilis*
Actinomyces spp.	*Fusobacterium* spp.

Table 64.3 ▪ Microorganisms Not Seen on Gram Stain

Bacterial organisms
Chlamydia spp., including *C. pneumoniae*
Mycoplasma spp., including *M. pneumoniae*
Legionella pneumoniae
Listeria monocytogenes
Mycobacteria such as *M. tuberculosis* and *M. avium intracellulare*
Rickettsiae including *R. rickettsii* and *Coxiella burnetii*
Spirochetes such as *Treponema pallidum*
Viral organisms
Influenza A and B
Hepatitis viruses
Cytomegalovirus (CMV)

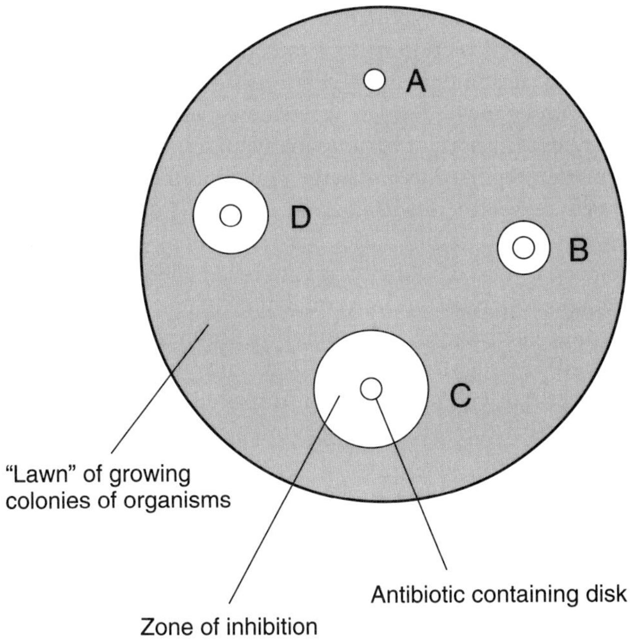

Figure 64.2. Schematic of a disk diffusion susceptibility test. Antibiotic containing disks (A–D) are placed on a plate of media containing a "lawn" of organisms. Following a period of incubation, the plate is inspected and zones of inhibition measured. The disk containing antibiotic A displays no apparent zone of inhibition, indicating the organism is resistant to this antibiotic. Disks B–D display varying zone sizes that may be sensitive or resistant depending on the breakpoint value for each antibiotic.

referred to as the Kirby-Bauer test, after the authors who first described this method.[4] After a period of incubation, during which the antibiotic has diffused into the agar, the plates are inspected for growth in the circumference zone surrounding the disk. Zones of inhibition and results are reported as sensitive or resistant, depending on the size of the zone of inhibition (Fig. 64.2). Broth microdilution testing employs the use of a microtiter tray with each row containing serial twofold dilutions of a particular antibiotic. The organism under study is added to each well in the tray and allowed to incubate before it is inspected for growth. The minimum inhibitory concentration (MIC) is defined as the well containing the lowest concentration of antibiotic that inhibited growth of the organism as determined by visual inspection of the wells (Fig. 64.3). The Etest (AB Biodisk Solna, Sweden) is a method that combines the disk diffusion and microdilution methods. A strip is impregnated with an antibiotic but contains a concentration gradient as opposed to a single concentration. This strip is placed on an agar plate containing a "lawn" of organism. The MIC is the point on the test strip at which the zone of inhibition intersects the test strip (Fig. 64.4).[5]

An organism is considered susceptible or resistant to an antimicrobial based on standardized results of breakpoint values for the MIC or zone of inhibition depending on the testing method and the particular microorganism, as well as the drug. These breakpoint values are determined by the National Committee on Clinical Laboratory Standards (NCCLS), an organization that develops and recommends laboratory testing methods.[6] Several criteria influence the breakpoint determinations, including a drug's pharmacokinetics, tissue penetration, protein binding, and the general susceptibility of a microorganism to antibiotics.

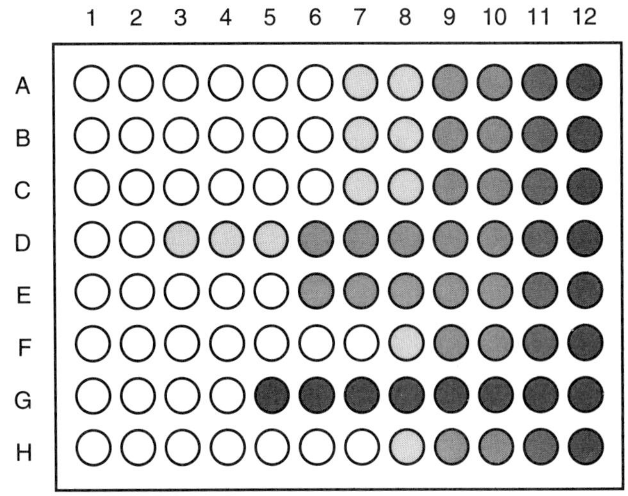

Figure 64.3. Schematic of microtiter tray for MIC testing. Individual antibiotics are tested in each row (A–H) at doubling concentrations in each well from high (column 1) to low (column 11) with a column containing no antibiotic (column 12) serving as a growth control. The MIC for each antibiotic is the concentration in the first well containing no visual growth. For example, the MIC for the drug in row D is the concentration in well 2, whereas the MIC for drugs F and H is the concentration in well 7, which may be different for each drug depending on the concentrations tested.

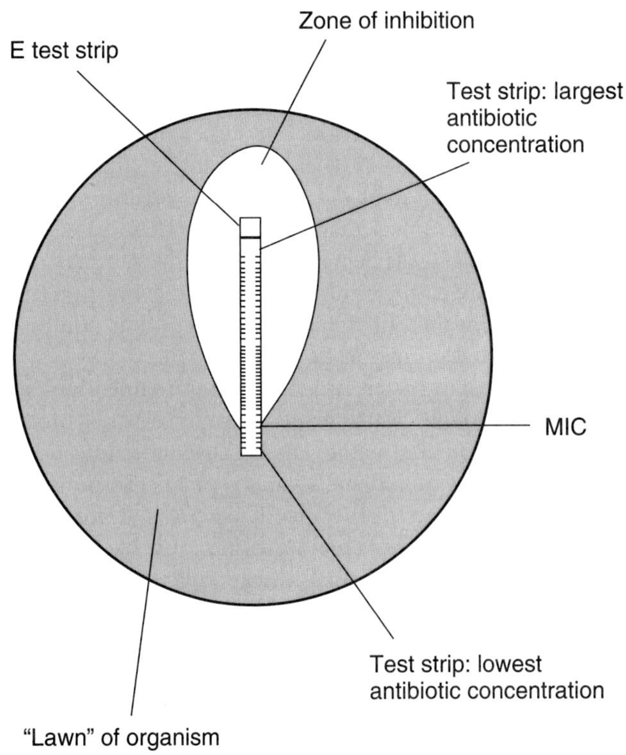

Figure 64.4. Schematic of Etest method. An Etest strip is placed on a media plate containing growing organism. After a period of incubation, the MIC is determined by the point at which the zone of inhibition intersects the test strip. The concentrations at each point are printed on the test strip.

SELECTING ANTIMICROBIAL THERAPY

Establishing the causative pathogen through laboratory testing is not always possible because of limitations in specimen collection and handling. Generally, empiric antibiotics, directed at potential pathogens, are begun before the results of culture and sensitivity tests are available. Gram stain results may or may not be more quickly available in order to guide empiric therapy. Waiting to administer antibiotics until after these results are available is not advisable in most cases and may potentially result in worsening of the patient's condition, or death in the case of serious infections such as meningitis. Patient characteristics such as age, immune status, and comorbid diseases, as well as the site of infection are factors that influence potential pathogens. Infections generally are caused by groups of common pathogens that are specific colonizers of a particular body site, but may differ depending on patient characteristics. For example, the most common organisms that cause meningitis in neonates are *E. coli, S. agalactiae, Listeria* monocytogenes, and *Klebsiella* spp., whereas the likely infecting organisms in adults are *S. pneumoniae* and *N. meningitidis*.[7–9] Cellulitis, an infection of the skin, commonly is caused by group A streptococci, which usually are found on the skin, but do not cause infection unless the mucosal barrier is compromised. In contrast, patients with diabetes mellitus or peripheral vascular disease develop lower limb cellulitis, which more often is caused by enteric Gram-negative bacilli or anaerobic organism.[10]

It is often a difficult task for clinicians to distinguish bacterial colonization from active infection. For example, patients with chronic obstructive pulmonary disease often are found to have large numbers of organisms in their sputum that may or may not be indicative of pneumonia. Likewise, some specimens may contain organisms that are not responsible for infection but rather are a result of contamination, such as a blood sample that grows coagulase-negative staphylococci. This organism is a common skin colonizer that may have contaminated the blood sample as it was being obtained. If the skin was not properly cleansed, the venipuncture needle can pick up organisms from the skin when it is pierced, thus resulting in bacterial contamination of the specimen.

Empiric therapy often is necessary before microbiological information is available; it generally treats a broad spectrum of potential pathogens because most infectious diseases may be caused by a variety of microorganisms. Definitive or directed therapy is determined for each patient when the pathogenic organisms have been identified and their antimicrobial susceptibility patterns are known. After the infecting organism has been identified, and its susceptibility pattern determined, directed therapy is useful. Directed therapy is important because it is a more patient-specific regimen and is perhaps narrower in spectrum.

Patient Factors Influencing Empiric Drug Selection

Antimicrobial therapy should be selected to maximize efficacy and minimize toxicity. To accomplish this, it is important to consider patient factors such as allergy, renal and hepatic function, site of infection, concomitant drug therapy, and underlying conditions such as chronic illness and pregnancy. Proper assessment of reported drug allergies is important because many undesirable side effects are often reported as an allergy that should not necessarily preclude treatment with a given antibiotic.[11] For example, erythromycin often causes gastrointestinal upset, which may be reported by the patient to be an allergy. Renal and hepatic function are important patient characteristics to consider before drug selection, because these are the main routes of drug elimination; thus, toxicity may result if dosages are not adjusted for impaired organ function. Furthermore, preexisting organ impairment may influence drug selection for drugs that are toxic to the kidney (e.g., the aminoglycosides) or liver (e.g., isoniazid).[12,13] Concomitant drugs may interact with some antimicrobial agents; fluconazole may be a better choice than ketoconazole in a patient taking an H_2-blocker such as ranitidine, because ketoconazole absorption is influenced by gastric pH, whereas fluconazole is not.[14,15] Pregnancy and other conditions may influence antibiotic selection. Sulfonamide antibiotics are not recommended in the last trimester of pregnancy because they can cause kernicterus (increased bilirubin leading to brain damage) in infants; suitable alternative agents should be selected for pregnant patients.[16]

Pharmacological Factors Influencing Drug Selection

In addition to patient factors, drug factors such as pharmacokinetic and pharmacodynamic characteristics of antibiotics should be considered during the selection process. Pharmacokinetic factors such as maximal serum concentration (C_{max}), half-life ($t_{1/2}$), and area under the concentration time curve (AUC) influence selection. A drug with a longer half-life may be selected to enhance compliance. Tissue penetration and protein binding are important factors because a drug cannot be effective if adequate concentration is not achieved at the site of infection. For example, many antimicrobial agents, β-lactams included, although achieving high concentrations in the urine, do not adequately penetrate the prostate to optimally treat prostatitis. Therefore, when selecting an antimicrobial agent for the treatment of prostatitis, the penetration of potential drug therapies into this tissue must be evaluated. Similarly, when treating meningitis it is imperative to evaluate drug penetration into the CSF. Generally, drugs that are highly protein bound do not penetrate well enough into the CSF to achieve adequate bactericidal concentration.[17] The area of antimicrobial pharmacodynamics–the relationship between drug concentration and the rate and extent of microbial killing–is becoming more important for drug therapy selection.

Antimicrobial pharmacodynamics generally investigate the pharmacokinetics of the drug (AUC, C_{max}) in relationship to the MIC of a pathogen. For the aminoglycoside and quinolone antibiotics, the factor associated with a successful outcome in animal models is maximizing the ratio of C_{max} or AUC relative to the MIC.[18,19] This means achieving a higher peak concentration in the body relative to the MIC of the organism is associated with successful eradication of the organism. This is termed concentration-dependent activity, increasing activity with increasing concentrations.

Antibiotics also have a postantibiotic effect (PAE), which is the period of time an antibiotic continues to suppress growth of an organism after the antibiotic has been removed from the in vitro culture medium. PAE is generally drug–organism specific pharmacodynamic effect. Most antimicrobials display a PAE against Gram-positive cocci, whereas the aminoglycosides and fluoroquinolones also produce PAE in Gram-negative bacilli. The clinical importance of PAE is not clearly defined, although animal studies suggest that antimicrobials, which produce PAE, may be administered to allow the serum drug concentration to fall below the MIC of the infecting organism.[20]

Antibiotics, which display concentration-dependent activity and an extended PAE, may be given less frequently than anticipated by their half-life.[21] In order to take advantage of the pharmacodynamic properties of the aminoglycosides, single daily dosing instead of the traditional multiple daily doses has been studied extensively and shown to be effective and safe in many patient populations.[22] This application of the pharmacodynamic properties of the aminoglycosides may actually reduce the incidence of drug-induced renal toxicity while maintaining positive clinical outcomes. By comparison, cell wall active antibiotics such as the β-lactams do not display concentration-dependent activity or a prolonged PAE. Rather, they display concentration-independent (or time-dependent) microbiological activity. This means that as long as the serum or tissue drug concentration remains at or above the MIC of the organism, the activity of the drug is maximized.[23] Therefore, the β-lactams may be given as small, frequent doses or as a continuous infusion (which may be impractical) to maximize its pharmacodynamic properties.[21,24] This area of research offers an opportunity for the application of the interrelations among the bug, drug, and patient factors associated with successful treatment.

Selecting Combination Therapy

Combination therapy may be necessary on many occasions. First, more than one antimicrobial may be required in order to treat a number of potential pathogens. For example, aerobic and anaerobic coverage is needed in patients with peritonitis, and only a few antimicrobial agents have both aerobic and anaerobic activity. Second, combination therapy may be selected to take advantage of synergistic properties of the antimicrobials. Synergy occurs when two drugs given in combination are more active together than either drug alone.[25] β-lactam antibiotics in combination with aminoglycosides display synergy in vitro against a variety of pathogens, including *Enterococcus* spp. and *P. aeruginosa*, and are often given together.[26] Combination therapy may be selected to decrease the potential for resistance development during therapy. This is the case with the treatment of tuberculosis, which is always treated with at least three drugs to prevent the development of resistance.[27] Some disadvantages of combination therapy include the increased cost associated with administering more than one antibiotic, the potential for increased frequency of side effects, and possible antagonistic combinations. The combination of the antifungal agents fluconazole and amphotericin B have been shown in vitro to display antagonism.[28,29] Other potentially antagonistic combinations include the induction of β-lactamases by double β-lactam therapy.[30] It is difficult to document antagonistic combinations in humans; however, combinations shown to be antagonistic in vitro generally are avoided in vivo to avoid the potential for therapeutic failure.

MONITORING RESPONSE

The next step in the drug selection process is monitoring therapy to determine if any changes are necessary. Monitoring antimicrobial drug therapy is important for ensuring successful and safe outcomes. Symptomatic improvement is a hallmark sign of effective antibiotic therapy and generally is considered a clinical cure if maintained after completion of therapy. Microbiological cure is the documentation of eradication of the infecting organism. Microbiological cure generally is used in research studies and is applicable outside this setting for certain severe infections such as endocarditis and meningitis. Interestingly, some patients judged to be cured clinically may represent a microbiological failure. That is, they appear to be symptomatically improved but the infecting organism was not completely eradicated with treatment, as with the case of many pulmonary or skin and soft tissue infections. Microbiological cure, therefore, is not an expected treatment goal for many infections. Therapeutic (clinical) failure occurs when a patient fails to improve clinically on a given antibiotic. This may occur because of bacterial resistance, inadequate dosage, noncompliance, or superinfection with another organism. In certain cases, antibiotic administration alone is inadequate for cure and a surgical debridement or repair procedure is necessary for a successful outcome. For example, a person with an abscess may need to have it drained surgically, or infected devices such as a prosthetic joint may need to be removed for resolution of osteomyelitis.

Antibiotic toxicity is the other main area for therapy monitoring. Complications may be minimized if side effects are evaluated early and dosages are adjusted or medications are changed. A patient's renal function should be closely monitored because many antimicrobials are eliminated by the kidneys and drug accumulation with resultant toxicities is possible. Changes in renal function may require alterations in the dosage or dosing schedule of the antibiotic. Serum levels of certain antibiotics, such as aminoglycosides, may be measured to ensure an adequate dosage regimen and to avoid potentially toxic levels.

For patients receiving antibiotics in the outpatient setting, patient and family education is important for successful treatment. Patients should be informed about food–drug and drug–drug interactions and proper storage and handling of their antibiotics. Some antibiotics, such as penicillin, should be taken on an empty stomach, whereas others need to be taken with food. Many antibiotic suspensions used for children need to be shaken well and stored in the refrigerator. The need for compliance and the importance of completing the entire course of antibiotics as prescribed should always be emphasized to avoid the emergence of bacterial resistance. Relapse may occur if the infection is not treated for an adequate length of time.

REFINING ANTIMICROBIAL THERAPY

The final step in the drug therapy selection process is to refine empiric therapy based on the results of identification and susceptibility tests. The MIC results should be reviewed to ensure that the causative pathogen is sensitive to the antibiotic selected. Ideally, the least expensive yet effective agent is selected. A pediatric patient with meningitis may be started on cefotaxime for empiric therapy. When the culture and sensitivity report results reveal *S. pneumoniae* to be sensitive to penicillin, therapy may be changed to the less expensive and narrower spectrum agent. Several factors other than the medication cost influence the cost effectiveness of a selected regimen. Costs of therapy include not only nursing administration, pharmacy preparation, and storage costs, but also costs associated with monitoring therapy, such as laboratory tests to monitor for toxicities (i.e., serum creatinine, LFTs, etc.) or more expensive serum drug concentrations. An expensive medication that is given once daily and has relatively no monitoring expenses may be associated with less overall cost compared with an inexpensive antibiotic that is given multiple times a day or has expensive monitoring costs. The antimicrobial drug therapy selection process requires careful consideration of several steps. At each step the interrelations of patient, bug, and drug factors need to be fully evaluated to ensure a successful outcome.

REFERENCES

1. Gonzalez R, Steiner JF, Sande MA. Antibiotic prescribing for adults with colds, upper respiratory tract infections, and bronchitis by ambulatory care physicians. JAMA 278:901–904, 1997.
2. Gelfand JA, Dinarello CA, Wolff SM. Fever, including fever of unknown origin. In: Isselbacher KJ, Brawnwald E, Wilson JD, et al., eds. Harrison's principles of internal medicine. 13th ed. New York: McGraw-Hill, 1994:81.
3. Woods GL, Washington JA. The clinician and the microbiology laboratory. In: Mandel GL, Bennett JE, Dolin R, eds. Mandel, Douglas and Bennett's principles and practice of infectious diseases. 4th ed. New York: Churchill Livingstone, 1995:169.
4. Bauer AW, Kirby MM, Sherris JC, et al. Antibiotic susceptibility testing by a standardized, single-disk method. Am J Clin Pathol 45:493–496, 1966.
5. Thornsberry C. Forward to ETEST symposium. Diag Microbiol Infect Dis 15:459–463, 1992.
6. National Committee for Clinical Laboratory Standards. Performance standards for autimicrobial susceptibility testing. In: Sixty informational supplement: NCCLS document M100–S6. Wayne, PA: NCCLS, 1995.
7. Schuchat A, Robinson K, Wenger JD, et al. Bacterial meningitis in the United States in 1995. N Engl J Med 337:970–976, 1997.
8. Durand ML, Calderwood SB, Weber DJ, et al. Acute bacterial meningitis in adults. A review of 493 episodes. N Engl J Med 328:21–28, 1993.
9. Rockowitz J, Tunkel AR. Bacterial meningitis. Practical guidelines for management. Drugs 50:838–853, 1995.
10. Fox HR, Karcmer AW. Management of diabetic foot infections, including the use of home intravenous antibiotic therapy. Clin Podiatric Med Surg 13:671–681, 1996.
11. Weiss ME. Drug allergy. Med Clin North Am 76:857–882, 1992.
12. Kahlmeter G, Dahlager JI. Aminoglycoside toxicity–a review of clinical studies published between 1975 and 1982. J Antimicrob Chemother 13(Suppl A):9–23, 1984.
13. Salpeter SR. Fatal isoniazid-induced hepatitis: its risk during chemoprophylaxis. West J Med 159:560–564, 1993.
14. Van Der Meer JW, Keuning JJ, Scheijgrond HW, et al. The influence of gastric acidity on the bioavailability of ketoconazole. J Antimicrob Chemother 6:552–554, 1980.
15. Albengres E, Le Louet H, Tillement JP. Systemic antifungal agents. Drug interactions of clinical significance. Drug Safety 18:83–97, 1998.
16. Cockerill FR 3d, Edson RS. Trimethoprim-sulfamethoxazole. Mayo Clin Proc 62:921–929, 1987.
17. Lutsar I, McCracken GH Jr, Friedland IR. Antibiotic pharmacodynamics in cerebrospinal fluid. Clin Infect Dis 27:1117–1127, 1998.
18. Lacy MK, Nicolau DP, Nightingale CH, et al. The pharmacodynamics of aminoglycosides. Clin Infect Dis 27:23–27, 1998.
19. Lode H, Borner K, Koeppe P. Pharmacodynamics of fluoroquinolones. Clin Infect Dis 27:33–39, 1998.
20. Shibl AM, Pechere JC, Ramadan MA. Postantibiotic effect and host-bacteria interactions. J Antimicrob Chemother 36:885–887, 1995.
21. Drusano GL. Role of pharmacokinetics in the outcome of infections. Antimicrob Agents Chemother 32:289–297, 1988.
22. Preston SL, Briceland LL. Single daily dosing of aminoglycosides. Pharmacotherapy 15:297–316, 1995.
23. Soriano F, Garcia-Corbeira P, Ponte C, et al. Correlation of pharmacodynamic parameters of five beta-lactam antibiotics with therapeutic efficacies in an animal model. Antimicrob Agents Chemother 40:2686–2690, 1996.
24. Eliopoulos GM, Moellering RC. Antimicrobial combinations. In: Lorian V. Antibiotics in laboratory medicine. 4th ed. Baltimore: Williams & Wilkins, 1996:330.
25. Drusano GL. Human pharmacodynamics of beta lactams, aminoglycosides and their combination. Scand J Infect Dis Suppl 74:235–248, 1990.
26. Craig WA, Ebert SC. Continuous infusion of beta-lactam antibiotics. Antimicrob Agents Chemother 36:2577–2583, 1992.
27. Iseman MD. Treatment of multidrug-resistant tuberculosis. N Engl J Med 329:784–791, 1993.
28. Lewis RE, Lund BC, Klepser ME, et al. Assessment of antifungal activities of fluconazole and amphotericin B administered alone and in combination against *Candida albicans* by using a dynamic in vitro mycotic infection model. Antimicrob Agents Chemother 42:1382–1386, 1998.
29. Sugar AM, Liu X. Interactions of itraconazole with amphotericin b in the treatment of murine invasive candidiasis. J Infect Dis 177:1660–1663, 1998.
30. Hopefl AW. Overview of synergy with reference to double beta-lactam combinations. DICP 25:972–977, 1991.

CHAPTER 65

IMMUNIZATION THERAPY

Emily B. Hak and Maureen P. McColl

OVERVIEW

Immunization for disease prevention was used by the late 1790s, when inoculation with cowpox was used to provide immunity against smallpox. Using immunization-induced immunity has successfully controlled and even eliminated disease.[1] In 1972 the World Health Organization (WHO) declared that smallpox had been eradicated by the worldwide vaccination program. The last case of wild-type polio in the Western hemisphere was reported in 1991, and worldwide polio eradication is imminent with the current aggressive vaccination program. As part of the Healthy People 2000 initiative, programs have been designed to enhance the immunization status of people of all ages.[2]

Passive or temporary immunity is provided by exogenous antibodies in the form of immunoglobulin G (IgG). In addition to antibody replacement, IgG is effective in other types of diseases, primarily those that are autoimmune. Many specific immune globulin products are now available and more are being studied.

The American Academy of Pediatrics Committee on Infectious Diseases *Red Book* presents revised recommendations for treatment of infectious diseases.[3] As they occur, changes in recommendations are published in *Pediatrics, The Journal of the American Medical Association* (*JAMA*), and the *Morbidity and Mortality Weekly Review* (*MMWR*). The Centers for Disease Control and Prevention (CDC) provides online immunization information at www.cdc.gov/nip and pediatric immunization information at www.cdc.gov/nip/vfc.

ACTIVE IMMUNIZATION

Immunization stimulates an endogenous immunologic response using an attenuated live or inactivated microorganism or antigenic products from a microorganism. A single injection may not be sufficient to stimulate the desired response, and a series of primary injections may be needed. In some cases, booster immunizations are provided at scheduled intervals throughout life to retain an adequate antibody response.

To improve quality of life through disease prevention, immunizations are being offered in a variety of settings, including pharmacies, businesses, and community settings. Those who provide immunizations should have a protocol that outlines procedures that will be taken in emergency situations, be trained in management of acute events such as cardiopulmonary resuscitation, and have emergency management supplies available.

Ontogenic Events

The immune system begins to develop early in fetal life. At 7 weeks gestation, small lymphocytes appear in the circulation, and at 9 weeks B cells primarily involved in the humoral immune response are seen in fetal liver. At term birth, all of the components of the immune system are present and functional, but immunoglobulin production is low. However, active transport of maternal IgG across the placenta results in IgG serum concentrations in term neonates that are 5 to 10% greater than in the mother. Although neonates can produce all classes of immunoglobulins, they cannot produce specific antibodies against all antigens. At birth, there is no immunologic memory, complement concentrations are low, opsonin activity is poor, and neutrophil chemotaxis and phagocytosis are reduced. By 1 year of age, complement concentrations in the classic and alternative pathways are at adult values. By 2 years of age, the memory response to polysaccharide antigen is present, immune-complex diseases begin to appear, and immunoglobulin M (IgM) concentrations reach adult values. Secretory immunoglobulin A (IgA) peaks by 2 to 4 years; however, the capacity for specific IgA antibody production slowly matures until puberty. Adult IgG concentrations are reached by 4 to 6 years of age.

The age at which an infant can respond appropriately to a specific immunization depends on the disappearance of transplacentally acquired antibodies and the maturity of the immune system to respond to specific antigens. The presence of maternally derived antibodies may prevent an appropriate response for the first year of life; therefore, immunization against these antigens is delayed. Children less than 2 years of age have a poor response to polysaccharide antigens. The diphtheria toxoid dosage used to immunize those less than 7 years of age is three to four times greater than the dosage used in older individuals, perhaps related to persistent maternal antibody in infants. The presence of disease, allergies, immunosuppression, dialysis, pregnancy, travel, and epidemics may require modification of an immunization schedule or dosage and consideration of the immunization type (live or inactivated) or other components. Travel to countries where a specific infectious disease is endemic may require immunization or prophylactic measures to prevent infection.

Differences Among Immunizing Agents

Toxoids are modified nontoxic products of microorganisms or exotoxins that retain the ability to stimulate an immunologic response. Immunity is not permanent, and scheduled boosters are required to continue immunity. Vaccines are derived directly from the microorganisms and can be killed, inactivated, live attenuated, polysaccharide, or composed of a component of the microorganism that is antigenic (referred to as acellular). The response induced by many vaccines confers long-lasting and, in many cases, permanent immunity. Attenuated live vaccines stimulate an immunologic response similar to natural infection (e.g., IgA with oral polio vaccine) and usually result in lifelong immunity. However, live vaccines have the risk, albeit small, for development of disease that is even greater in those who are immunosuppressed. Recombinant DNA technology allowed the development of vaccines with low risk for disease transmission. Acellular pertussis vaccines result in a much lower febrile response; thus, the risk for febrile seizures is lower. In general, polysaccharide vaccines are less immunogenic than other types of vaccines and elicit only a minimal response in those less than 2 years of age. Conjugation of the polysaccharide to proteins stimulates an adequate antigenic response even in infants as young as 6 weeks of age.

Other Immunization Components

Immunizations contain products that are either added to enhance immunogenicity, to preserve the product, to stabilize the product, or are residual from the antigenic detoxifying process. Aluminum phosphate, aluminum hydroxide, or calcium phosphate are used as adjuvants to delay absorption and increase antigenicity. Thimerosal, a mercury derivative, and 2-phenoxyethanol may be added as preservatives. Possible other ingredients include lactose, sucrose, gelatin, sorbitol, neomycin, and streptomycin. Many vaccines are grown in chick embryos and one, hepatitis B, is raised in yeast. Some vaccines are treated with formaldehyde during antigenic processing. Immunizations, their components, and preferred route of administration are listed in Tables 65.1 and 65.2.

Route of Administration

Although a few vaccines are given orally, and intranasal spray vaccines are being tested, most are given parenterally as subcutaneous, intramuscular, or intradermal injections. Immunizations should be administered according to the recommended route, or the desired immunologic response may not occur. Products containing aluminum should be given intramuscularly because of increased risk of tissue irritation with subcutaneous administration. Intramuscular injections should be given in the anterolateral aspect of the thigh in infants and deltoid muscle in children or older individuals. Injections in the buttocks should be avoided because the presence of fat can interfere with absorption, there is potential for damaging the sciatic nerve, and the gluteal muscles are not developed in infants. Immunizations administered subcutaneously should be given in the anterolateral aspect of the upper arm or thigh.

Patients at risk for bleeding, including those with hemophilia or those who are anticoagulated, require special consideration for immunizations given intramuscularly. Patients with hemophilia can be given intramuscular injections right after factor replacement using a ≤23-gauge needle and application of direct pressure at the injection site for 2 minutes.

Table 65.1 ▪ Routine Pediatric Immunizations

Disease	Immunization Type	Antigenic Components and Amount	Other Components[a]	Route[b]	Brand Name	Marketed By	Location
Diphtheria	Toxoid	*Corynebacterium diphtheriae* endotoxin					
		6.7 floculating units (Lf)	A, T	i.m.	DTP	Connaught	Swiftwater, PA
		6.7 Lf	A, T	i.m.	DT	Connaught	
		12.5 Lf	A, T, F	i.m.	Tri-Immunol	Wyeth-Lederle	Philadelphia, PA
		12.5 Lf	A, T, F	i.m.	TETRAMUNE	Lederle-Praxis	Wayne, NJ
		9 Lf	A, T, F, G, P	i.m.	Acel-Imune	Wyeth-Lederle	
		6.7 Lf	A, T, F, G, P	i.m.	Tripedia	Connaught	
		25 Lf	A, F, P, Pe	i.m.	Infarix	SmithKline Beecham	Philadelphia, PA
		1.5–2 Lf	A, T	i.m.	Td	Connaught	
		15 Lf	A, T, F, fetuin	i.m.	Certiva	North American Vaccine	Columbia, MD
Tetanus	Toxoid	*Clostridium tetani* endotoxin					
		5 Lf			DTP		
		5 Lf			DT		
		5 Lf			Tri-Immunol		
		5 Lf			TETRAMUNE		
		5 Lf			Acel-Imune		
		5 Lf			Tripedia		
		10 Lf			Infarix		
		5 Lf			Td		
		6 Lf			Certiva		
Pertussis	Whole cell vaccine	Inactivated *Bordetella pertussis*					
		4 mouse protective units			DTP		
		4 mouse protective units			Tri-Immunol		
		4 mouse protective units			TETRAMUNE		
	Acellular vaccine	86% FHA, 8% PT, 4% pertactin			Acel-Imune		
		40–60 μg pertussis antigen (Takeda)					
		PT (23.4 μg), FHA (23.4 μg) (BIKEN)			Tripedia		
		PT (25 μg), FHA (25 μg), pertactin (8 μg)			Infarix		
		40 μg pertussis toxoid			Certiva		
Polio	Attenuated, live virus vaccine	Types 1, 2, 3 polio virus (>10^5 infectivity titers of each)	S, N, St	oral	ORIMUNE	Lederle	Pearl River, NY
	Inactivated virus vaccine	Types 1, 2, 3 polio virus 40 D antigen units of type 1, 8 D antigen units of type 2, 32 D antigen units of type 3	F, Pe, N, St, Px	i.m. s.c.	IPOL	Connaught	

(continued)

Antibody Response to Immunization

The response begins soon after immunization, but adequate protection against disease may not be achieved for weeks. In some cases, the response to the first dose is insufficient to protect against disease or the initial response wanes with time; thus, complete vaccination may require a series of doses given at least 1 month apart. Immunization against several diseases can be accomplished at the same time, either with an approved combination product or with multiple injections at different sites. Administering a live immunization within 1 month of another may interfere with the antibody response.

DELAYED OR MISSED IMMUNIZATIONS

It is not necessary to repeat immunizations that have already been given, should a child less than 7 years of age fail to receive all recommended immunizations on time. Rather, the immunizations that have not been given should be administered at the recommended intervals. Unimmunized children 15 months to 5 years of age can be given diphtheria, tetanus, acellular pertussis (DTaP), diphtheria, tetanus whole-cell pertussis (DTwP); oral polio vaccine (OPV), inactivated polio vaccine (IPV); measles, mumps, rubella (MMR); hepatitis B virus (HBV) vaccine; varicella; and any one of the *Haemophilus influenza*

Table 65.1 *(continued)*

Disease	Immunization Type	Antigenic Components and Amount	Other Components[a]	Route[b]	Brand Name	Marketed By	Location
Hepatitis B	Inactivated virus vaccine	Hepatitis B surface antigen (HbsAg) adw subtype produced in yeast cells using reombinant DNA technology (10–40 μg/mL)	T, F, A, YP	i.m.	Recombivax HB[d]	Merck and Co.	West Point, PA
			T, A, YP	i.m.	Engerix-B	SmithKline Beecham	
			F, A, YP	i.m.	COMVAX[d]	Merck and Co.	
Haemophilus influenza type b (Hib)	Polysaccharide (PRP) vaccine	Hib PRP (25 μg) conjugated to diphtheria toxoid (18 μg)	T	i.m.	ProHIBiT	Connaught	
		Hib PRP (10 μg) conjugated to 24-μg tetanus toxoid	S	i.m.	ActHIB	Connaught	
			S	i.m.	OmniHIB	SmithKline Beecham	
		Hib PRP (10 μg) conjugated to diphtheria CRM_{197} protein (25 μg)	T[c]	i.m.	HibTITER TETRAMUNE	Wyeth Lederle	
		Hib PRP (15 μg) conjugated to 250-μg *Neisseria meningitidis* outer membrane protein complex of the B11 strain	A, T, L	i.m.	PedvaxHIB	Merck and Co.	
			A, L	i.m.	COMVAX		
Measles	Attenuated, live virus vaccine	1,000 tissue culture infectious doses ($TCID_{50}$) of Enders attenuated Edmonston strain	N, G, S, Ch	s.c.	MMRII	Merck and Co.	
					ATTENUVAX	Merck and Co.	
Mumps	Attenuated, live virus vaccine	20,000 $TCID_{50}$ of Jeryl Lynn strain	N, G, S, Ch	s.c.	MMRII		
					MUMPSVAX	Merck and Co.	
Rubella	Attenuated, live virus vaccine	10,000 $TCID_{50}$ of Wistar RA 27/3 strain	N, G, S, Ch	s.c.	MMRII		
					MERUVAX	Merck and Co.	
Varicella	Attenuated, live virus vaccine	≥1,350 plaque forming units (PFU) of Oka/Merck	N, G, S	s.c.	Varivax	Merck and Co.	

[a] *A*, aluminum; *T*, thimerosal; *F*, <0.02% formaldehyde; *G*, gelatin; *P*, polysorbate; *Pe*, 2-phenoxyethanol; *FHA*, filamentous hemagglutinin antigen; *PT*, pertussis toxin; *S*, sorbitol; *N*, neomycin; *St*, streptomycin; *Px*, polymixin B; *YP*, yeast protein; *L*, lactose; *Ch*, produced in chick embryo cell lines.
[b] *i.m.*, intramuscular; *s.c.*, subcutaneous; *i.d.*, intradermal.
[c] In multidose vials.
[d] The pediatric formulations of these vaccines are being reformulated to remove the thimerosal preservative.

type B (Hib) vaccines at the same time.[3] Children more than 5 years of age should be given all the named immunizations except the Hib vaccine. The second DTaP (DTwP, DT), HBV vaccine, and OPV or IPV should be given 2 months after the initial immunization, and the third HBV vaccine and DTaP (DTwP, DT) 2 months after the second doses. Six to 12 months after the third DTaP (DTwP, DT), a second dose of MMR and booster doses of DTaP (DTwP, DT) and OPV or IPV should be given.[3]

Unimmunized children more than 7 but less than 18 years of age should be immunized with tetanus toxoid and the lowest dose of diphtheria toxoid (Td), OPV or IPV, HBV vaccine, and MMR with these repeated in 2 months. A single varicella vaccination will suffice in those less than 13 years of age; however, older children require a second varicella vaccination that can be given more than 1 month after the first. A third immunization with Td, OPV or IPV, and HBV vaccine is given after 6 to 12 months. All individuals should receive Td every 8 to 10 years.

VACCINE-RELATED ADVERSE EVENTS REPORTING

All immunizations can produce adverse effects that are predominantly mild and self-limiting. Although rare, certain adverse events temporally associated with immunization have resulted in severe permanent injury or death. Serious side effects temporally related to immunization must be reported to the U.S. Department of Health and Human Services through the Vaccine Adverse Event Reporting System (VAERS).[3] VAERS functions as the system for monitoring and tracking suspected serious adverse events after immunization.[4]

Table 65.2 ▪ Immunizations for Special Groups and Travel

Disease	Immunization Type	Antigenic Components and Amount	Other Components[a]	Route[b]	Brand Name	Marketed By	Location
Cholera	Killed vaccine	8 units each of Ogawa and Inaba serotypes of *Vibrio cholerae* per mL (dose ranges 0.2–0.5 mL depending on age)	Ph	i.m. s.c. i.d.	cholera vaccine	Wyeth Laboratories	Marietta, PA
Hepatitis A	Inactivated virus vaccine	Hepatitis A viral strain HM175, 360 and 720 ELISA (EL) units for children; 1440 EL units for adults	A	i.m.	Havrix	SmithKline Beecham	Philadelphia, PA
		Hepatitis A virus antigen, 50 unit/mL	A, F	i.m.	VAQTA	Merck and Co.	West Point, PA
Influenza	Activated virus vaccine	Two type A viral antigens and one type B based on epidemiologic data 6 to 9 months before the next influenza season	T, F, P, Ch	i.m.	FluShield	Wyeth Laboratories	
			T, F, G, Ch	i.m.	Fluzone	Connaught	Swiftwater, PA
Japanese encephalitis	Inactivated virus vaccine	Japanese encephalitis virus Nakayama-NIH strain	S, T, G, F, MP	s.c.	JE-VAX	Connaught	
Lyme disease	Acellular	30-μg outer surface lipoproteiin (OspA) of *Borrelia burgdorferi*	A, Pe	i.m.	LYMErix	SmithKline Beecham	
Neisseria meningitidis	Polysaccharide vaccine	Polysaccharide from 4 types (50-μg each) of Groups A, C, Y and W-135 meningococcus	T, L	s.c.	MENOMUNE	Connaught	
Rabies	Inactivated virus vaccine	Wistar rabies virus strain PM-1503-3M, 2.5 IU of rabies antigen/mL	N, P, alb	i.m.	Imovax	Connaught	
			N, P, alb	i.d.	Imovax Rabies I.D.	Connaught	
	Inactivated	Kissling strain of Challenge Virus Standard rabies virus	A	i.m.	Rabies Vaccine Adsorbed	BioPort Corp.	Michigan
	Inactivated	Flury LEP grown in chicken fibroblast culture		i.m.	RabAvert	Chiron Corp	
Streptococcus pneumoniae	Polysaccharide vaccine	Polysaccharide from 23 types (25 μg each) of pneumococcus	T	i.m.	PNU-IMUNE 23	Lederle	Pearl River, NY
			Ph	s.c.	PNEUMOVAX 23	Merck and Co.	
Tuberculosis	Live, attenuated Virus	Bacillus of Calmette and Guerin [BCG] strain of *Mycobacterium bovis* (TICE) 1 to 8×10^8 colony forming units	gly, L	per	BCG vaccine, USP	Organon Inc.	West Orange, NJ
Typhoid	Killed vaccine	*Salmonella typhosa* (Ty-2 strain) ≤1000 million/mL (dose is 0.25 or 0.5 mL)	Ph	s.c.	typhoid vaccine	Wyeth Laboratories	
	Polysaccharide vaccine	polysaccharide from *Salmonella typhi* Ty-2 strain, 25 μg/0.5 mL dose	Ph	i.m.	Typhim Vi	Connaught	
	Live, attenuated virus	*Salmonella typhi* Ty 21a, 2 to 6×10^9 colony forming units	S, L, As	oral	Vivotif Berna	Berna Products Corp.	Coral Gables, FL
Yellow fever	Live virus vaccine	17 D strain of yellow fever virus 5.04 $\log_{10}$ plaque forming units (PFU)	S, G, Ch	s.c.	YF-VAX	Connaught	

[a]*A*, aluminum; *T*, thimerosal; *F*, <0.02% formaldehyde; *G*, gelatin; *P*, polysorbate; *Pe*, 2-phenoxyethanol; *S*, sorbitol; *N*, neomycin; *St*, streptomycin; *Px*, polymixin B; *YP*, yeast protein; *L*, lactose; *Ch*, produced in chick embryo cell line; *Ph*, phenol; *A*, albumin; *MP*, mouse serum protein; *As*, ascorbic acid; *gly*, glycerin.

[b]*i.m.*, intramuscular; *s.c.*, subcutaneous; *i.d.*, intradermal; *per*, percutaneous using a multiple puncture disc; *p.o.*, per os (oral).

NATIONAL CHILDHOOD VACCINE COMPENSATION ACT

The large amount of money awarded in the courts for vaccine-associated adverse effects forced some manufacturers to suspend production of vaccines and toxoids and threatened the viability of the national immunization program. The National Childhood Vaccine Compensation Act was passed to provide financial assistance to children with serious adverse reactions that were temporally related to vaccination, in turn relieving the manufacturers of significant financial burden. To develop this program, the government appropriated funds for 5 years and placed a tax on each vaccine, with the amount of tax directly related to the possibility of severe adverse reaction.[5] As of March 1997, immunizations that are covered include diphtheria, tetanus, whole-cell pertussis, acellular pertussis, measles, mumps, rubella, oral polio, inactivated polio, hepatitis B, Hib, and varicella. It is expected that as vaccines are added to the recommended pediatric schedule, they will also be covered. Funds are available to provide treatment and rehabilitation costs that are not covered by private insurance, and damages up to $250,000 have been awarded for pain and suffering. If this route of compensation is used, the right to institute legal proceedings against the manufacturer or individuals who prescribed or administered the vaccine is relinquished.[6] Reportable adverse events are not necessarily eligible for compensation. For example, a febrile seizure should be reported but is not compensable unless encephalopathy occurs within 72 hours.

ROUTINE PEDIATRIC IMMUNIZATIONS

The American Academy of Pediatrics (AAP), the American Medical Association (AMA), and the American Academy of Family Practice (AAFP) make recommendations for routine pediatric immunizations (Table 65.3). States have immunization requirements for day care and school enrollment that may be less stringent than AAP, AMA, and AAFP recommendations; however, many states are increasing their requirements to comply with federal mandates.

Misconceptions regarding contraindications and precautions to immunization result in a significant number of missed opportunities for vaccination. Sound clinical judgment under those conditions–viewed as precautions and strict adherence to absolute contraindications–should minimize missed vaccination opportunities and avoidable adverse events. In general, routine pediatric immunizations begin when an infant is 6 to 8 weeks of age. Healthy preterm infants should begin immunizations at the same chronological age as term infants, and the full dosage should be used to ensure an adequate response.[3,7,8]

Routine pediatric immunizations include those for diphtheria, tetanus, pertussis, *Haemophilus influenza* type b, hepatitis B, polio, measles, mumps, rubella, varicella, and

Table 65.3 ▪ Usual Pediatric Immunization Schedule

Age	Hepatitis B[a]	Polio[b]	Diphtheria, Tetanus, Pertussis[c]	H. influenza type b[d]	Measles, Mumps, Rubella	Varicella
Birth	HBV (1)					
2 months	HBV (1,2)	IPV	DTaP	Hib (1,2)		
4 months	HBV (2)	IPV	DTaP	Hib (1,2)		
6 months	HBV (1,2)		DTaP	Hib (1)		
12 months		IPV		Hib (1,2,3)[e]	MMR[e]	var[e]
15 months			DTaP[e]			
4–6 Years		IPV	DTaP			
11–12 Years					MMR	
14–16 Years			Td[f]			var[g]

[a]HBV may be given in either of two schedules:
(1) (a) Hepatitis B surface antigen (HBsAg) + mother: within 12 hr birth (with 0.5 mL HBIG at separate site), 1–2 months, 6 months
(b) HBsAg unknown status mother: within 12 hr birth (status of mother should be determined and if positive, 0.5 mL HBIG given with the first week of life), 1–2 months, 6 months
(2) Hepatitis B surface antigen (HBsAg) – mother: 2 months, 4 months 6–18 months.

[b] The third polio vaccine given as IPV should be at least 6 months after the second.

[c]DTwP can be substituted.

[d]Schedule for Hib conjugate immunization depends on the product chosen:
(1) HibTITER, ActHIB, or OmniHIB, (2) PedvaxHIB, (3) ProHIBiT should only be used as a booster.

[e]To decrease the number of office visits required for immunizations, polio, Hib, MMR, and var can be deferred until 15 months or DTaP can be given at 12 months as long as 6 months have elapsed since the previous DTaP immunization; Tripedia. (Connought's DTaP can be mixed in the same syringe with ActHIB and administered as a single injection as the booster dose at ≥15 months of age.)

[f]Td given to children >7 and adults, repeat every 10 years throughout life.

[g]Adolescents without a history of vaccination or chickenpox require two doses >1 month apart.

Table 65.4 ▪ Diseases Prevented by Routine Pediatric Immunizations

Causative Agent	Disease Manifestations	Disease Complications or Long-Term Sequela	Comments
Corynebacterium diphtheriae (diphtheria)	Local inflammation and necrosis of mucous membranes resulting in the formation of plaquelike membranes	Cardiomyopathy, neuropathy, hepatic necrosis	Treated with diphtheria antitoxin and antibiotics. Disease does not induce immunity. Vaccination is required.
Bordetella pertussis (whooping cough)	1 to 2 wk catarrhal stage with upper respiratory tract symptoms, followed by 3 weeks of severe paroxysmal coughing (whoops). Recovery is wks to months.	Severe coughing can produce asphyxia, cerebral anoxia, seizures, coma. Permanent neurological damage or death can occur.	Most severe in young. Adolescents and adults may only have persistent severe cough and may be a reservoir for infection. Immunity duration after disease is unknown.
Clostridium tetani tetanus (lockjaw)	Pain, generalized muscle rigidity, and spasm that can be progressive	Airway obstruction, cyanosis asphyxiation	Treatment is supportive with tetanus immunoglobulin, antitoxin, and tetanus toxoid. Disease does not result in immunity.
Poliomyelitis enterovirus (spinal or bulbar polio)	90% of cases are asymptomatic. Minor infection: fever, malaise, headache, nausea	Paralysis, neurologic weakness	Only cases in U.S. are associated with OPV.
Morbillivirus (measles, rubeola)	Prodrome (1–2 wks): Koplik spots on buccal/pharyngeal mucosa, fever, cough, conjunctivitis, photophobia, coryza. Later: high fever, macularpapular rash on face and neck that spreads downward.	Otitis media, croup, diarrhea, thrombocytopenic purpura, death (3 in 1,000 cases), encephalitis (1 in 1,000 cases)	Highly contagious, active infection results in lifelong immunity.
Paramyxovirus (mumps, epidemic parotitis)	Fever, neck muscle pain, malaise, and headache, unilateral or bilateral parotid gland swelling	Orchitis or epididymitis (45% in postpubertal males that can result in sterility, 7% postpubertal females), encephalitis (1 in 6,000)	Repeat cases can occur.
Rubella (German measles, 3-day measles)	Mild catarrhal symptoms, erythematous discrete rash, low grade fever, cervical lymphadenopathy	Congenital rubella (50–80% during 1st trimester), 10–20% (2nd trimester), arthritis and neuritis more common in older females	Congenital rubella may result in low birth weight, hepatomegaly, splenomegaly, congenital heart disease, cataracts, hearing loss, or mental retardation.
Haemophilus influenza type b	Meningitis, epiglottitis, pneumonia, septic arthritis, osteomyelitis, cellulitis, otitis media, pericarditis	Hearing loss, mental retardation, death	Disease in those >2 years old results in permanent immunity. Index case and close contacts need rifampin prophylaxis.
Hepatitis B virus	Acute hepatitis, jaundice, fatigue, hepatomegaly	Chronic hepatitis, cirrhosis, hepatocellular carcinoma. Asymptomatic carriers are a reservoir and transmit disease.	Spread through direct contact with body fluids. 90% of infants born to infected mothers become carriers or develop infection.
Rotavirus	Emesis, diarrhea, low-grade fever	Severe dehydration, electrolyte abnormalities, acidosis, death	Transmission is fecal–oral. The virus has been found on toys and hard surfaces. Most common cause of diarrhea in those <2 years.
Varicella virus (chickenpox)	Fever, macularpapular rash with characteristic vesicular pruritic lesions	Group A streptococcal secondary infection, necrotizing fascitis, encephalopathy, pneumonia	Active infection usually results in permanent immunity. Reactivation of latent virus results in zoster or shingles.

rotavirus.[9] The etiologic agent, disease manifestations, and complications are briefly reviewed in Table 65.4.

Diphtheria, Tetanus, Pertussis

In developing countries, unsanitary conditions at birth result in 400,000 deaths annually owing to neonatal tetanus.[10] In the United States, 142 cases of tetanus were reported between 1995 and 1997; they occurred most frequently in unimmunized adults.[11] The annual number of cases of diphtheria in the United States is ≤5, and, as with tetanus, occurs most often in the unimmunized. Active infection with diphtheria or tetanus does not necessarily confer immunity, and immunization during convalescence is required. All individuals should be immunized against diphtheria and tetanus every 7 to 10 years throughout life.[3,7]

In 1934, the incidence of pertussis was more than 250,000, with 7,500 deaths.[12] The number of cases of pertussis dramatically decreased with vaccination, although it continues to exceed 5,000 documented cases annually; the actual number of cases is probably much higher. Pertussis in adolescents and adults often goes unrecognized because the symptoms are often atypical, and a severe persistent cough may be the only overt symptom of infection.[13–16] Newer evidence suggests that active infection with pertussis may not provide lifelong immunity.[14,15] The number of cases increased during the 1980s despite attainment of greater than 90% vaccination rates, perhaps owing to vaccine failures or a gradual decrease in immunity by 3 years after vaccination.[16] A review of 1996 cases in Vermont found that 68% of those who had pertussis, most of which was culture confirmed, had received four pertussis vaccinations.[17]

Immunization against diphtheria, tetanus, and pertussis, originally formulated with a whole-cell (w) pertussis vaccine (DTwP), can be accomplished with a single injection. The pertussis vaccine component believed to be the cause of many of the adverse reactions is the endotoxin produced by the *Bordetella pertussis*. A febrile response to DTwP is common; it results in an increased risk for seizure in children with a preexisting neurologic disorder or provides the first pyrogenic stimulus for a febrile seizure.[12] In a prospective trial, seizures occurring after DTwP immunization were similar to febrile seizures in control patients and were usually uncomplicated.[18] Permanent neurologic injury associated with DTwP occurs but is rare. Unfortunately, congenital or other preexisting serious neurological disease becomes obvious during the first year of life and coincides with the time routine pediatric immunizations are being administered. This coincidence, coupled with the desire to establish a cause for serious neurologic disease in infants, has influenced the linkage of pertussis vaccine to serious central nervous system (CNS) sequelae.

Common adverse events associated with DTwP vaccination include fever, mild local swelling and inflammation at the injection site, increased fussiness, crying, and drowsiness.[19] The incidence of seizures and hypotonic-hyporesponsive episodes associated with DTwP is 1 in 1750 doses, fever greater than 40.5°C (104.9°F) within 48 hours is 1 in 330 injections, and severe persistent crying is approximately 1 in 100 cases.[3] These events are self-limited and without sequelae in most cases. DTwP was postulated as a cause of Sudden Infant Death Syndrome (SIDS); however, no controlled study has found a relationship.[20] Those more than 7 years of age should not be given the whole-cell pertussis vaccine because of the increased risk for adverse effects.

Acellular pertussis vaccines were developed because the whole-cell pertussis vaccine is responsible for most adverse effects with DTwP.[13,21] Combination vaccines with acellular pertussis antigens (DTaP) have at least equal immunogenicity to DTwP and contain less or no endotoxin; thus, the incidence of adverse effects is decreased.[22,23] DTaP is preferred over DTwP and should be used for all children who require pertussis vaccination.[3] Pertussis immunity wanes with time, and it is possible that acellular pertussis vaccination will be recommended throughout life along with diphtheria and tetanus toxoids.[24]

Anaphylactic reactions are rare (2 per 100,000 doses of DTwP) and the incidence is unknown for DTaP. Any child who experiences an immediate reaction to either DTwP or DTaP should not receive further doses of either until the allergic component has been identified. Development of encephalopathy within 7 days of vaccination should preclude the child from receiving further doses of any pertussis vaccine. DT can be given to complete the primary series for tetanus and diphtheria.[3]

Precautions for the use of DTwP and DTaP include the development of any of the following after a previous dose: persistent uncontrollable crying or screaming for ≥3 hours within 48 hours, hypotonic-hyporesponsive state, a fever more than 40.5°C (104.9°F) not attributable to another cause, or seizure occurring within 72 hours of immunization. Parents should be questioned about reactions to previous vaccinations before repeat doses are given. If previous immunizations were associated with these adverse events, and the benefit of pertussis vaccination is felt to outweigh the risk, DTaP should be used to complete the series.[11] Whole-cell pertussis vaccine should be avoided in children with neurological disorders or a history of seizures, and DTaP should be considered if benefits outweigh risks. In most cases of progressive or unstable neurological status unrelated to vaccine administration, vaccination should be delayed until the disorder has been treated or defined.[7,11] Pretreatment with an acetaminophen (10–15 mg/kg) at the time of and 4 to 8 hours after immunization decreases the risk of adverse effects.[25]

Polio

In 1954 Jonas Salk developed an inactivated polio vaccine (IPV) that did not confer long-term immunity, nor did it provide mucosal (IgA) immunity. In 1961 Albert Sabin developed a live, attenuated oral polio vaccine (OPV) that protects against polio and induces gastrointestinal (GI) immunity. OPV results in lifelong immunity and is inexpensive and easy to administer. Since 1979 the only cases of polio in the United States have been vaccine-associated or imported from other countries where polio remains endemic. OPV immunization has virtually eradicated naturally occurring polio from the United States, and its continued use worldwide is considered important in the global eradication of polio.

OPV has been preferred since its introduction in the 1960s owing to its high efficacy, low cost, ease of use, and resultant mucosal immunity. After OPV is given, the virus replicates and is present in the oral pharynx and GI tract for 6 to 8 weeks. Because of this, OPV should not be given at intervals less than 8 weeks, and at least two OPV doses are needed to provide mucosal immunity. Also, live virus shed in stool from vaccinated individuals enhances immunization rates by exposing unimmunized persons to the vaccine virus, thereby resulting in indirect immunization.[3,26]

Rarely, vaccine associated paralytic polio (VAPP) occurs with OPV, most commonly with the first dose, in approximately one case per 760,000.[3] Those at increased risk include individuals with unknown immunodeficiency disorders at the time of vaccination and close contacts who are underimmunized or immunocompromised. In 1988, an improved and enhanced potency inactivated vaccine was licensed and replaced the Salk vaccine.[27] Viral shedding does not occur with IPV, and VAPP has not been attributed to its use. Disadvantages with this vaccine are that it is more expensive, is administered by injection, and does not provide mucosal immunity.

Because the only cases of polio in the United States have been associated with OPV or have been imported, the Advisory Committee on Immunization Practices (ACIP) of the CDC and AAP Committee on Infectious Diseases revised the recommendations for childhood polio vaccination. In 1997, three strategies for polio immunization were suggested: (1) all four doses of IPV; (2) two doses of IPV followed by two doses of OPV; or (3) all four doses of OPV. Interestingly, the 1999 recommendations did not include all four doses of OPV because the risk for VAPP is greatest with OPV as the first dose; and with increased time after birth, unrecognized immunodeficiency may be diagnosed prior to OPV administration.[9] Immunocompromised patients, including those receiving immunosuppressants (e.g., steroids, chemotherapy), and their household contacts should receive IPV only because they are at greater risk for VAPP from exposure to the live attenuated virus.[28] Children living in households with inadequately immunized adults should only receive IPV. The AAP has recommended that only the IPV be used in the United States beginning January 2000.

Haemophilus influenzae Type B

Polysaccharide vaccines are weakly immunogenic. In infants the polysaccharide *Haemophilus influenzae* type b (Hib) vaccine did not produce immunity in children younger than 24 months of age, the age of most frequent disease occurrence. The complexing of the polysaccharide to proteins (tetanus toxoid, diphtheria toxoid, OMP-meningococcus) resulted in an adequate stimulation of the immune system in young infants and decreased the incidence of invasive disease in those at highest risk by 95%.[3,29,30] The tetanus and diphtheria carrier proteins are chemically and immunologically similar to the diphtheria and tetanus toxoids contained in DTwP and DTaP, and concurrent vaccination for diphtheria or tetanus may be required to elicit an optimal antibody response. Therefore, if the DTwP, DTaP, or DT vaccine is not given concurrently, the OMP-meningococcus conjugate should be used to immunize those younger than 24 months of age. The same Hib vaccine should be used to complete the primary series; however, this is not an absolute requirement. Any of these vaccines can be used as the booster. DTwP or DTaP/Hib combination vaccines can be used as booster doses between 12 and 15 months of age. Hib conjugate vaccines do not provide immunity against diphtheria, tetanus, or meningococcal disease.[3,7] Otitis media and upper respiratory tract infections in children are frequently caused by nontypeable *Haemophilus influenzae* and the vaccine is not effective against these organisms.

Hib disease in an infant or child younger than 2 years of age does not result in immunity; vaccination should be started 1 month after the onset of illness. All previous Hib doses should be ignored and the full immunizing series given. In addition, a child with Hib disease requires rifampin prophylaxis in order to eradicate nasopharyngeal carriage. For a discussion of rifampin prophylaxis with Hib, see Chapter 73, Central Nervous System Infections.

Children with human immunodeficiency virus (HIV) infection, immunoglobulin deficiency, functional or anatomic asplenia, Hodgkin's disease, sickle-cell disease, or who are recipients of a bone marrow transplant or who are receiving chemotherapy may have a decreased response to Hib conjugate vaccination. Children with solid tumor have a 50% response rate to the diphtheria conjugate Hib vaccine compared to children with leukemia, who have an 80% response rate.[31] The response to the OMP-meningococcus vaccine in preterm neonates is less than in term infants.[32] Recent reports show that infants and children with sickle cell disease and those after bone marrow transplant have a good response to Hib vaccination.[33,34]

Few adverse effects are associated with Hib vaccines. Approximately 25% of recipients experience pain and local redness or swelling at the site of injection. These reactions generally are mild and resolve in 24 hours. Systemic effects such as fever or irritability occur infrequently. When Hib is administered at the same time as DTwP or DTaP, the incidence of these effects is not greater than with either DTwP or DTaP alone. Children more than 5 years of age do not require Hib vaccine because they have probably developed immunity and are at low risk for invasive disease. Hib vaccine is recommended for older children and adults with functional asplenia (anatomic or surgical) or immunosuppression (HIV infection, chemotherapy, or IgG2 subclass deficiency).

Hepatitis B

Infection with hepatitis B virus (HBV) is a significant cause of morbidity and mortality owing to acute and chronic hepatitis, cirrhosis, and hepatocellular carcinoma. Chronic carriers may be asymptomatic and provide a reservoir for viral transmission. Universal immunization against HBV must be achieved to decrease HBV transmission and eradicate the disease.[35] For a thorough discussion of hepatitis B, see Chapter 28, Hepatitis, Viral and Drug Induced.

The risk of becoming chronically infected is inversely related to age at the time of infection; the youngest patients are at highest risk. Because of concerns about possible accumulation of mercury in young and low birth weight infants, the AAP recommends the use of hepatitis B vaccine that does not contain thimerosal for infants less than

6 months of age. However, thimerosal-containing vaccine should be used for high-risk infants if a nonthimerosal-containing vaccine is not available. If not treated, 80 to 90% of infants born to hepatitis B surface antigen (HBsAg)-positive mothers will become infected. The carrier state can be prevented in approximately 90% of infants who are given the vaccine and hepatitis B immune globulin (HBIG) within 12 hours of birth. Thus, identification of HBsAg-positive mothers is important. This measure also may identify other contacts of the mother who are at risk of infection so they can be treated. Other groups at high risk include hemodialysis patients, those who receive blood products frequently, or those who are exposed to infected body fluids.

Hepatitis B vaccine is recommended for all infants and children before starting school. Those on hemodialysis or who are immunosuppressed may require larger dosages to induce antibody concentrations that are considered protective. Long-term followup in children and adults indicates that immune memory remains for 5 to 9 years despite the fact that antibody titers decline.[35] Currently booster doses of HBV vaccine are not recommended; however, the CDC surveillance of HBV infection will confirm that vaccine-induced immunity continues.

Most people who become infected acquire the disease as adolescents or adults. Health care workers, hospital staff, clients or staff of institutions for the mentally retarded, recipients of clotting factors, household contacts of HBV carriers, hemodialysis patients, homosexually active males, persons with multiple heterosexual partners, and intravenous drug abusers are at increased risk for HBV infection and require preexposure hepatitis B vaccine. Persons requiring postexposure hepatitis B vaccine include infants born to carrier mothers, people with accidental percutaneous or permucosal exposure to infected blood, sexual partners of persons with acute HBV infection, and household contacts of persons with acute HBV infection.[3]

Routine serologic testing of vaccine recipients is not indicated. People who should have HB antibody concentrations measured 1 to 2 months after the third vaccine dose include hemodialysis patients; immunosuppressed patients with HBV exposure risk, including those with HIV; and patients being treated postexposure. Additional doses should be given for titers less than 10 mIU/mL.[3]

Between 1 and 6% of patients report injection site pain and temperature greater than 37.7°C (99.9°F). Allergy to the vaccine is reported rarely and anaphylaxis has been reported to occur in about one in 600,000 doses. There has been no evidence of an association with HBV vaccine and Guillain-Barré syndrome since the introduction of the recombinant hepatitis B vaccines. Furthermore, recombinant HBV vaccines have no potential for contamination with HIV. The plasma-derived HBV vaccine is no longer produced in the United States; however, it can be obtained from Merck for individuals with yeast allergy.

A noted association between hepatitis B vaccination and the diagnosis of CNS demyelinating diseases such as multiple sclerosis provided the impetus for a technical consultation among recognized experts in public health and regulatory authorities, academia, the pharmaceutical industry, and the WHO in September of 1998.[36] The data available for review and discussion were insufficient to demonstrate either a causal or stimulatory effect of the hepatitis B vaccines on CNS disease development; thus, this association may be coincidental.[36] Epidemiologic and immunologic studies will continue to evaluate this issue.

Measles, Mumps, Rubella

The number of measles cases reported drastically declined from the previous low incidence of 309 cases in 1995 to 135 cases in 1997 following the institution of the two-dose MMR vaccination regimen.[37] The incidence of mumps and rubella have remained low and continue to decline.[2] The incidence of congenital rubella syndrome parallels the incidence of rubella and is amplified when outbreaks occur in unvaccinated populations of women who are of childbearing age.[38] Although individuals immunized with MMR can shed virus in the saliva and tears, there is no risk for disease transmission.

Several factors related to the MMR vaccine must be considered before administration. People who were born before 1957 likely had the disease and do not require immunization. MMR and the individual vaccines are live virus vaccines and should not be administered to immunosuppressed individuals, with the exception of young children with HIV infection. Individuals who are to receive immunosuppressive doses of steroids, chemotherapy, or radiation should be immunized either 2 weeks before or 3 months after therapy.[7,28] For those who receive immune globulin for measles prophylaxis, MMR can be given 5 months after a 0.25-mL/kg dose in healthy individuals, or 6 months after a 0.5-mL/kg dose in immunosuppressed individuals.[39] The immunoglobulin dosage determines the length of time after immunoglobulin infusion that MMR immunization will elicit an appropriate antibody response.[39]

Adverse events related to these vaccines are primarily clinical symptoms of mild disease. Symptoms consistent with subclinical measles infection occur from 6 to 11 days after immunization and include a transient rash, fever up to 39.4°C (102.9°F), headache, cough, sore throat, photophobia, and malaise. Although rare, seizures have been reported during the febrile episode, particularly in children fewer than 2 years of age. Arthralgias and joint pain have been reported in up to 25% of susceptible adult females 2 to 6 weeks after receiving rubella vaccines. Self-limited thrombocytopenia occurring within 2 months of vaccination is rare (one case per 30,000–40,000 doses).

Measles and mumps viruses used in the vaccine are grown in chick embryo cell culture, which raises a concern for patients with hypersensitivity to eggs. One strategy to vaccinate these individuals has been to perform scratch and prick tests to determine sensitivity, and to vaccinate using a desensitization protocol. A recent study evaluated MMR vaccination in children with hypersensitivity to egg protein and found that a positive skin test occurred in only three of 17.[40] Subsequent administration of MMR resulted in no immediate or delayed hypersensitivity.[40] The chance of reaction is remote because of the small amounts of egg cross-reacting protein present in the vaccine. Furthermore, skin testing for reactivity to vaccine is not predictive of allergic reactions. Current recommendations are to observe MMR vaccinees with egg hypersensitivity for 90 minutes after vaccination with the standard dosage. The vaccine should be given only in an environment with emergency equipment and appropriate personnel to treat anaphylaxis.[3]

Varicella

Chickenpox, as primary infection with the varicella zoster virus (VZV) is commonly known, is a highly contagious, usually self-limited childhood infection with an attack rate of more than 90% in susceptible individuals.[41] Between 1988 and 1996, 10,000 children were hospitalized with varicella or varicella complications; 90% of the deaths that occurred were in children without high risk for severe infection.[42] Much of the societal cost associated with varicella is related to the time parents lose from work to care for children who are not allowed to go to school or day care while the lesions remain.[43] Children who are immunocompromised have more severe disease, prolonged recovery, or potential serious sequelae, and those who become infected for the first time as adults may also have a more difficult course. Reactivation of the latent virus results in herpes zoster or "shingles," and it involves the thoracic, cervical, lumbar, or sacral nerves. Shingles occurs most often in persons older than 10 years of age.

The vaccine was first developed from a virus isolated from a child in Japan in the early 1970s. Protective efficacy of the vaccine is about 86% for any infection but almost 100% in preventing severe disease in immunocompetent individuals with close contact.[44] Although one immunization results in protection in 95% of healthy children, it is less effective in adolescents, adults, and children with acute lymphoblastic leukemia (ALL) in remission.[41] Vaccination should be avoided for at least 5 months following administration of immunoglobulin.

Adverse effects associated with varicella vaccination include transient pain, tenderness, or redness at the injection site in 20 to 35% of vaccinees. Within 1 month, 8% develop a mild maculopapular or varicelliform rash with a few lesions. Vaccinees who develop breakthrough varicella have milder cases and shorter duration of lesions than those who contract varicella naturally. Vaccinated children with leukemia who develop a rash may transmit the vaccine virus to susceptible contacts; however, the virus rarely has been recovered from these lesions in immunocompetent individuals.[45] Viral transmission from vaccinees who develop a varicella rash to immunocompromised contacts is not a sufficient reason to withhold vaccination. The effects of varicella immunization on the later occurrence of zoster is of concern. The occurrence of zoster appears to be directly related to the number of lesions (or vesicles); thus those who have few lesions are at less risk for zoster. The full effect of varicella vaccination on adult varicella infection and cases of zoster in the future remains to be seen.

The varicella vaccine is an attenuated live virus vaccine; it is contraindicated in immunocompromised persons (including those receiving high dosages of corticosteroids) with the exception of children with leukemia, who would have serious complications with natural varicella.[45]

Rotavirus

Rotavirus is the leading cause of dehydrating diarrheal disease in children less than 5 years of age; transmission is fecal-oral. Each year, rotavirus infection accounts for 70,000 hospital admissions and 100 deaths in the United States.[46]

The live virus oral vaccine consists of serotypes 1, 2, 3, and 4, which are responsible for the majority of human disease. Serotype 3 is a rhesus rotavirus that is cross-reactive with human rotavirus serotype 3, and types 1, 2, and 4 are rhesus-human reassortant viruses that contain the human serotype-specific viral protein 7. In clinical trials, a three-dose vaccine regimen reduced rotavirus diarrhea by at least 50% and decreased the severity of disease in those who did develop rotavirus diarrhea.[47,48] After vaccine administration, the virus replicates in the GI tract and approximately one-half of those vaccinated have virus present in a stool up to 5 days after dosing. Transmission of the vaccine virus has occurred, but the vaccine does not cause human rotavirus disease.

Initially, vaccine related adverse effects after the first dose included fever of more than 38°C (100.4°F) up to 5 days after the dose (21 versus 6% in the placebo group), decreased appetite (17 versus 11%), irritability (41 versus 32%), and decreased activity (20 versus 13%).[49] Because the vaccine was live and could be transmitted, immunocompromised infants were not to be given the vaccine and contact with vaccines was to be avoided for 4 weeks.[49]

Shortly after the vaccine was recommended to be routinely administered to infants at 2, 4, and 6 months of age, a relationship between the vaccine and development of intussusception was noted. The manufacturer withdrew the vaccine from the market.

IMMUNIZATIONS FOR SPECIAL GROUPS

Vaccines for special groups are listed in Table 65.2.

AIDS Vaccine

It has been difficult to develop a vaccine effective against AIDS, primarily because the human immunodeficiency virus (HIV) mutates rapidly in vivo. During 1998, a bivalent AIDS vaccine comprised of Gp120 proteins located in the viral envelope from two different HIV strains, AIDSVAX (VaxGen, San Francisco, California), moved into a planned 3-year period of phase III testing in volunteers at high risk for HIV infection.[50]

Hepatitis A

Hepatitis A, or infectious hepatitis, is a highly contagious disease transmitted by the fecal–oral route. In the United States, 143,000 individuals contract hepatitis A, and

80 individuals die at an estimated cost of $200 million annually.[51] Worldwide, 1.4 million cases are reported each year; it is believed that the actual number of cases are several times that number. Chapter 28 provides a thorough discussion of hepatitis A.

Individuals who should receive hepatitis A vaccine include those who plan to travel to an endemic area or who live in an area experiencing an outbreak. The efficacy of hepatitis A vaccination was demonstrated in Thai children living in an area with an outbreak rate of 119 cases per 100,000 population.[52] Antibody titers were increased for 4 years, and authors suggested that protection may be as long as 20 years.[52]

The vaccine should be given at least 2 weeks prior to expected hepatitis A exposure; the number of injections required depends on the product. Children from 2 to 18 years of age who are given Havrix 360 ELISA (EL) units should receive a second dose 1 month after the first and a booster 6 to 12 months after the second dose. In children 2 to 18 years old who receive VAQTA or Havrix 720 EL units and adults who receive Havrix 1440 EL units, an initial injection is given followed by a booster in 6 to 12 months (Table 65.2). Adverse effects, primarily pain at the injection site, occur more often with hepatitis A vaccine compared with HBV vaccine.[52]

During hepatitis A outbreaks, immune globulin may be given concurrently with vaccination. In these cases, antibody titers are lower than in individuals who receive the vaccine alone; a booster may be required.[53]

Influenza

Influenza viruses are orthomyxoviruses of three antigenic types, A, B, and C. Types A and B cause disease. Influenza is spread by direct contact and is characterized by the sudden onset of fever, headache, malaise, muscle aches, and cough. Later, respiratory symptoms become more prominent, and nausea and vomiting may occur.[3] Specific symptoms vary widely among people with influenza, as does symptom severity. Influenza type A is subclassified by hemagglutinin (H), which can be subtype H1, H2, or H3, and neuraminidase (N), which can be subtype N1 or N2. Antigenic shifts are major variations in either the H or N antigens. Antigenic drifts are minor variations within the same subtype. Antigenic shifts and drifts are the primary reasons that new variants of influenza occur.[3,54]

The anticipated patterns of influenza are evaluated in March and April of each year, and the vaccine is formulated based on the influenza strains that are expected to be prevalent in the upcoming influenza season. At least 6 months are required for production, quality control, and distribution. The vaccine is available as an inactivated, whole-virus vaccine and split (subvirion) virus vaccine made from two type A and one type B virus strains.

Individuals older than 6 months of age who require regular medical followup or who have been hospitalized during the previous year for chronic pulmonary diseases including asthma, significant cardiac disease, immunosuppression (including drug therapy), HIV infection, sickle cell anemia, and diseases that require long-term aspirin therapy should be vaccinated. Other children, adolescents, and adults at increased risk from influenza include those with chronic cardiovascular disease, renal disease, diabetes mellitus, hemoglobinopathies (sickle cell disease), or pulmonary disorders (e.g., cystic fibrosis, bronchiectasis, obstructive pulmonary disease, asthma, and class 3 tuberculosis). All individuals older than 65 years of age and those in chronic care facilities should be immunized.[54] Pregnant women in the second or third trimester should receive influenza vaccine. Close contacts, including children, of those at risk for serious sequela from influenza should also be vaccinated each year.

Generally, the vaccine is given in the autumn 1 month before the expected influenza season begins. From 2 weeks to 6 months after vaccination, antibody concentrations should be protective. Since immunity declines after 6 months, annual revaccination is necessary.

Children between the ages of 6 months and 13 years of age are at increased risk for adverse effects from the whole-virus vaccine and should be immunized using either the subvirion vaccine or purified surface-antigen vaccine, referred to as the split-virus vaccines. Children less than 3 years of age should be given one-half the usual dosage. Children younger than 8 years old do not have an adequate immunologic response after the first exposure to influenza vaccine, and require two doses of the vaccine given 1 month apart the first time influenza immunization is given. Only one dose is required for subsequent influenza immunizations.

The most common adverse effects include pain, induration, and erythema at the injection site. Flulike symptoms such as fever, chills, myalgia, and malaise may begin within 12 hours and are more common in children given the whole-virus vaccine. Febrile seizures have been reported. Adverse effects can be minimized by acetaminophen given at the time of immunization and at 4, 8, and 12 hours after. Dosages of 650 mg were more effective than 325 mg in a placebo-controlled trial in hospital employees vaccinated against influenza.[55]

Influenza antigens are grown in chick embryo cultures and individuals with anaphylactic hypersensitivity to eggs are at increased risk for serious adverse effects. A desensitization protocol can be used to decrease the risk for adverse effects; however, it may be more appropriate to use chemoprophylaxis with amantadine or rimantadine instead of vaccination.[3]

Influenza and pneumococcal vaccines can be administered concurrently at different sites, thereby increasing compliance. Conversely, the influenza vaccine should not be given within 3 days of the whole-cell pertussis immunization because both can cause fever. Children older than 15 months of age can receive the DTaP and the influenza vaccine at the same time.[3]

The federally funded influenza immunization program through Medicare has been successful in increasing influenza immunization rates from about 40 to 60% in those more than 65 years of age. Immunization rates tend to be higher in older individuals with other risk factors, such as diabetes or heart disease, and in those who are more educated. Important reasons that the elderly fail to receive influenza immunizations are the lack of awareness of the Medicare program and lack of transportation to obtain the immunization. Individuals who have had adverse effects from previous "flu shots" also tend to avoid reimmunization.[56]

Lyme Disease

The causative agent for Lyme disease is *Borrelia burgdorferi,* a spirochete that uses the hard tick as its primary vector. Most cases are reported in the mid-Atlantic, northeastern, and midwestern United States; however, cases have been reported from 45 states. An initial local reaction, termed erythema migrans, occurs at the site of the tick bite and may be accompanied by fever, headache, and arthralgia. The initial lesion can expand over days to weeks to include an area more than 5 cm in diameter with vesicular or necrotic areas. Multiple erythema migrans occurs 3 to 5 weeks later and includes multiple lesions that are smaller than the initial rash. During this period, cranial nerve palsies, meningitis, and conjunctivitis can occur in addition to arthralgia, myalgia, headache, and fatigue. Later disease occurs up to 1 year after exposure and is characterized by chronic arthritis, and, in certain cases, encephalopathy and neuropathy.

The vaccine consists of the *Borrelia burgdorferi* outer surface lipoprotein A (OspA) and is manufactured using recombinant technology. Immunization stimulates the formation of endogenous antibodies that are transferred to the attached tick and kill the spirochetes present in the tick midgut, thus preventing transfer of the spirochete into the human. Susceptible individuals between the ages of 15 and 70 years of age should receive three doses, the second 1 month after the first and the third 1 year after the first. Vaccine efficacy after the first dose was 49 or 68% and after the third dose was 76 or 92%.[57,58] Adverse effects that occur within 30 days of immunization include local reactions at the injection site, chills, fever, muscle aches, and flulike symptoms.

Meningococcal Disease

Neisseria meningitidis is a Gram-negative diplococcus that causes meningococcemia with or without meningitis. The onset of fever, chills, malaise, and the characteristic rash is abrupt and progression to disseminated intravascular coagulation, shock, coma, and death can occur within a few hours. Infection occurs most often in children less than 5 years of age, with most disease occurring in those 6 to 12 months of age. Although nine serotypes have been identified, groups B, C, Y, and W-135 are the most common causes of disease in the United States. Disease transmission is by aerosolized droplets from close personal contact with symptomatic individuals or asymptomatic colonized carriers. Approximately 3% of households with an index case will have more than one secondary case.

The vaccine contains polysaccharide antigens for serotypes A, C, Y, and W-135; therefore, the immunologic response is generally poor in those less than 2 years of age.[59] In addition, serotype B, the major cause of disease in children, is not included in the vaccine. However, the vaccine is very effective in preventing disease secondary to serotype A in children more than 3 months of age.[60] In addition, a child with meningococcal disease requires rifampin prophylaxis in order to eradicate nasopharyngeal carriage. See Chapter 73, CNS Infections, for a discussion of rifampin prophylaxis.

Meningococcal vaccination is routinely performed in the military. People more than 2 years of age who have functional or anatomic asplenia or complement deficiency should be vaccinated. During an epidemic, infants 3 to 18 months of age should be given two doses 3 months apart. After vaccination, duration of immunity for serotype A in children less than 4 years of age is probably less than 3 years.[3] Adverse effects seen with meningococcal vaccine include mild local and systemic effects. Fever is more common in younger children but is rarely greater than 38.5°C (101.3°F).[59] See Chapter 64, Infectious Diseases, for a discussion of rifampin prophylaxis of exposed individuals.

Pneumococcal Disease

Streptococcus pneumoniae, the leading pathogen in community-acquired pneumonia, is the second most common cause of meningitis in the United States. It is the etiologic agent for otitis media in more than one million infants and children each year. An estimated 40,000 individuals die each year from pneumococcal pneumonia and meningitis.[61] Although there are more than 80 pneumococcal serotypes worldwide, most disease is caused by 10 serotypes. Emerging pneumococcal resistance increases the importance of immunization in individuals at high risk for the disease.

In 1983 the 14-valent pneumococcal vaccine was replaced by the 23-serotype vaccine, which covered 85 to 98% of disease isolates worldwide. These serotypes are responsible for approximately 88% of adult bacteremia and meningitis, 85% of acute otitis media, and nearly 100% of pediatric bacteremia and meningitis.[62] As with other polysaccharide vaccines, this vaccine is poorly immunogenic, with efficacy ranging from 48 to 70%. The duration of immunity conferred by vaccination is unknown. Increasing immunogenicity by conjugating the polysaccharide with different protein carriers such as diphtheria or tetanus toxoids, as was done with Hib protein conjugate vaccines, is being investigated.[63,64] One vaccine is comprised of five pneumococcal serotypes conjugated to CRM197, which is one of the conjugating proteins used in Hib vaccine (HibTITER). In children with HIV, the seroconversion rate was twice as great for the five serotypes administered as a conjugate as that seen with the unconjugated vaccine.[65]

Vaccination is indicated in individuals older than 2 years of age at high risk for acquiring serious pneumococcal infection, including sickle cell anemia, anatomic or functional asplenia, chronic renal failure, nephrotic syndrome, Hodgkin's disease, and immunosuppression, incorporating children with HIV and healthy individuals older than 65 years of age.[3,61] Patients should be vaccinated 2 weeks before elective splenectomy or beginning immunosuppressive medications.[3] If this is not possible, the vaccine can be given 3 months after the completion of therapy. Influenza and pneumococcal vaccines can be administered concurrently at different sites.

The need for repeat vaccination with the pneumococcal vaccine has been debated for years. Children less than 10 years of age at high risk for severe pneumococcal disease should be revaccinated within 3 to 5 years of previous immunization. Older children and adults with severe risk for pneumococcal disease should be revaccinated 6 years after the initial vaccination.[3]

Few serious adverse effects are associated with initial immunization with the pneumococcal vaccine. Discomfort, induration, and erythema at the injection site occur in 40 to 90% of patients. Systemic effects occur less frequently, but include fever, weakness, muscle aches, chills, headache, nausea, and photophobia. Patients with immune thrombocytopenia have experienced exacerbations of disease following pneumococcal immunization.

Tuberculosis

Tuberculosis (TB) is a necrotizing bacterial infection caused by *Mycobacterium tuberculosis*. Occasionally, *Mycobacterium bovis* has caused human disease in the United States. After many years of decline, the incidence of TB in the United States has increased because patients with AIDS develop secondary TB. In addition to an increased incidence, there has been an increase in multiple drug-resistant TB.[66] Screening for TB exposure and infection is done through skin testing. Children should receive either the multiple puncture or the Mantoux TB skin test at about 15 months of age (concurrent with first MMR), before school entry, and during adolescence (14 to 16 years of age). Individuals in high-risk groups, including those who are contacts of adults with TB or those with HIV, immunosuppression, Hodgkin's disease, lymphoma, diabetes mellitus, chronic renal failure, and malnutrition, should receive annual TB skin tests.[3] See Chapter 68 for a complete discussion of tuberculosis.

The TICE strain of Bacillus Calmette-Guérin (BCG) of *Mycobacterium bovis* is used for this live vaccine. Administration is percutaneous using a multiple puncture disk. Small red papules appear at the site within 10 to 14 days of immunization and reach maximum intensity after 4 to 6 weeks. A tuberculin skin test is applied 2 to 3 months after immunization. If negative, a second dose of the vaccine should be given. Usually, the site has completely healed and faded by 6 months; however, some persons may have a residual scar. Because vaccination should result in a positive TB skin test, this test is not useful for identifying TB in BCG vaccinees. Adverse effects include skin ulceration at the site, regional adenitis, and occasionally, lupoid reactions. Osteitis has been reported from 4 months to 2 years after BCG vaccination in neonates; the incidence varies according to country, which may relate to product.[67]

A meta-analysis evaluated the occurrence of TB in those vaccinated with BCG found the incidence was decreased by 50%.[66] The duration of protection is not known, but sensitivity to tuberculin skin testing has persisted for 7 to 10 years. Routine vaccination with BCG vaccine is not recommended. Candidates for vaccination include children in close contact with infected patients who are untreated, ineffectively treated, or resistant to treatment, and may include other groups that have an excessive new infection rate.[68] Because of the risk for development of disease, BCG is contraindicated in patients who are immunosuppressed or who have burns, symptomatic HIV, or skin infections.[3]

Rabies

Rabies is caused by an RNA virus of the rhabdovirus group that affects the CNS. Known natural reservoirs include skunks, foxes, raccoons, and bats, but all mammals can be affected. Transmission is primarily by infected secretions, usually saliva, that are transmitted by a bite. Initially, the virus remains close to the wound; however, migration along a neuronal pathway to the CNS ultimately occurs. The incubation period is between 20 and 60 days, but may be more than 6 months. Rabies has occurred secondary to corneal transplant from a donor who unknowingly had rabies. The clinical manifestations of rabies can be divided into three stages: (1) a nonspecific prodrome, (2) an acute encephalitis, and (3) a profound dysfunction of brainstem centers. Recovery without intervention is rare and occurs slowly.

The most effective effort in decreasing rabies in humans is the extensive rabies vaccination program conducted in domestic animals.[69] From 1980 to 1994 in the United States, 20 cases of rabies were reported in humans; half of these were imported, a few were associated with an animal bite, and most were diagnosed at autopsy. As a result of these 20 cases, more than 800 individuals who were exposed to rabies required prophylaxis that cost $850,000.[69]

The original vaccine was a suspension of fragments of rabies virus from infected spinal cords that was modified several times because of the significant adverse effects. Work in the early 1960s led to the development of the human diploid-cell rabies vaccine (HDCV) that is more immunogenic and has fewer side effects than previous vaccines. Since then, two more rabies vaccines have been developed. One is grown in fetal rhesus lung cell culture, inactivated and adsorbed to aluminum, rabies vaccine absorbed (RVA) and the other is grown in purified chick embryo cell culture and inactivated (PCEC).[70] Both RVA and PCEC must be given by intramuscular injection.

Preexposure Prophylaxis

Individuals who have a high risk for exposure to rabies, such as veterinarians and dog catchers, should receive preexposure prophylaxis against rabies. For preexposure immunization, injections are given on days 0, 7, and 28 (three doses) and intradermal injections (HDCV) may be appropriate. Routine serologic testing is recommended only for those who are immunosuppressed. RVA or HDCV should be administered intramuscularly for preexposure rabies prophylaxis in individuals receiving chloroquine or mefloquine for malaria prophylaxis. In this situation, intradermal injection of rabies vaccine may not result in an appropriate antibody response.

Postexposure Prophylaxis

Unimmunized individuals who are acutely exposed should be immunized with the appropriate product given intramuscularly on days 0, 3, 7, 14, and 28.[3] Intradermal injections should not be used. RIG 20 IU/kg should be given as soon as possible, but no longer than 8 days after exposure, infiltrating as much of the dose around the bite as possible and the remainder given intramuscularly at a site distant to vaccine administration.

Persons who are previously immunized should receive two intramuscular doses of vaccine, one immediately and one 3 days later. Rabies immune globulin (RIG) should not be given to individuals who have been immunized preexposure.

Vaccination causes local discomfort, swelling, erythema, and induration in up to 90% of individuals, and usually subsides in 1 to 3 days. Up to 10% of patients have systemic reactions that include nausea, vomiting, abdominal pain, headache, malaise, and low-grade fever. An immune complexlike reaction characterized by urticaria with or without arthralgia, arthritis, or angioedema has been reported in up to 7% of individuals receiving boosters.[3,70] Anaphylactic reactions have been reported rarely. Once initiated, rabies prophylaxis should not be discontinued because of local or mild systemic reactions to the vaccine.

VACCINATION FOR TRAVEL

Travel to developing countries may expose the traveler to diseases that are endemic in other areas of the world. Immunization or prophylactic measures decrease the likelihood of contracting these diseases. Before traveling to areas outside the United States, the CDC should be contacted regarding information about immunizations required for entrance into individual countries or prophylactic medications and other measures that are advised. This should be done as early as possible before anticipated travel to be sure there is time to complete the immunization series for all required vaccinations.[71,72]

Cholera

Cholera is problematic in areas where conditions are unsanitary. Cholera vaccine results in adequate immunity in only 40 to 60% of vaccinees, the duration of effect is relatively short, and the vaccine is not effective against the most common serotype now responsible for disease. For these reasons, cholera vaccination is no longer recommended and no country requires documentation of cholera vaccination prior to entry. Experimental attenuated live oral cholera vaccines are more effective and have fewer side effects; however, none are approved for use. The CDC should be consulted for appropriate precautions to decrease the risk for cholera, which include water purification and safe food handling.

Japanese Encephalitis

Japanese encephalitis is a mosquito-borne viral disease that frequently is fatal. The disease rarely occurs on the main islands of Japan or in Hong Kong, but is common in rural Asian rice growing areas where the infected mosquitoes thrive. The vaccine can be used in individuals more than 1 year of age, and a three-dose schedule is recommended with the first two immunizations given 1 week apart and the third dose given 1 or 3 weeks (preferable) after the second. Length of immunity is likely more than 1 year. Allergic reactions, including urticaria and angioedema, have occurred as late as 17 days after vaccination, and individuals should remain in an area where there is easy access to medical care for 10 days after vaccination. Thus, the immunization series must be completed more than 10 days before travel.

Typhoid

Typhoid fever is caused by ingestion of water and food contaminated by *Salmonella typhi*. Vaccination is recommended for individuals who travel to rural areas of tropical countries or to areas where there are unsanitary conditions and an increased risk for disease exposure. Although immunization results in antibody production in 50 to 90% of individuals, the degree of immunity is not great and can be readily overcome with a large inoculum.

Three vaccines are available, including two administered parenterally (inactivated and capsular polysaccharide) and one that is given orally (attenuated, live). A fourth vaccine is provided by the U.S. government for military use. The primary series of the inactivated typhoid vaccine consists of two doses given more than 4 weeks apart. A booster is required every 3 years if reexposure is expected and is better tolerated if given by the intradermal route.

The primary immunization with the polysaccharide vaccine should be followed by a booster dose every 2 years if reexposure to typhoid is expected. This vaccine is not recommended for use in children less than 2 years of age.[73] The primary immunization series with Vivotif Berna, the oral typhoid vaccine, consists of one capsule every other day for four doses. Capsules are stored in the refrigerator and should be taken with cool water about 1 hour before a meal. This vaccine is contraindicated in children less than 6 years old, those with an acute febrile illness or acute GI illness, and in individuals receiving sulfa drugs or antibiotics. The same dosage and schedule is repeated every 5 years if reexposure to typhoid is expected.

The inactivated vaccine contains significant quantities of endotoxin and often results in 1 to 2 days of discomfort at the injection site, fever, malaise, and headache. Although rare, the occurrence of serious systemic adverse reactions can be decreased using intradermal administration. The incidence of fever and headache are the same between the live and polysaccharide vaccines. Nausea, vomiting, abdominal cramps, and urticarial rash are frequent with the oral vaccine. Adverse effects with the live and polysaccharide vaccines are less than with the inactivated vaccine and overall are least with the attenuated, live oral vaccine.[73]

Yellow Fever

Urban yellow fever is transmitted from infected humans by the *Aedes aegypti* mosquito, which has been controlled or eliminated in many African and South American countries. Jungle yellow fever also is transmitted by mosquito vectors, and it is responsible for most yellow fever reported today. Those who will be traveling to rural endemic areas or laboratory workers who may be exposed to the virus should be vaccinated.[72,74] A single dose induces immunity that persists for more than 10 years. Infants less than 4 months of age should not be vaccinated because of the increased risk of encephalitis, and vaccination of infants from 4 to 9 months of age should be based on estimates of risk of exposure to yellow fever.[71] The vaccine is available only in Yellow Fever Vaccination Centers where the Yellow Fever Vaccination Certificates, required for entrance into some countries, are issued.

Up to 10% of vaccinees have mild headaches, myalgia, or low-grade fever from 5 to 10 days after immunization. Immediate hypersensitivity reactions are rare. Yellow fever vaccine is a live virus vaccine grown in chick embryo culture; it should not be given to those who are immunocompromised or experience anaphylactic reactions to eggs. In these cases, an immunization waiver stating the contraindication may be sufficient to gain entrance into countries that require Yellow Fever Immunization Certificates. If the risk for yellow fever is high and immunization necessary, skin testing may be performed to determine the vaccine allergic potential. If skin tests are positive, a desensitization protocol can be accomplished by subcutaneous injection of 0.05 mL of a 1:10 dilution of vaccine followed by increasing amounts of full strength vaccine of 0.05, 0.1, 0.15, and 0.2 mL every 15 to 20 minutes with appropriate emergency equipment and qualified personnel available.[3]

Cholera and yellow fever vaccines should be given at least 3 weeks apart because of reported decreases in antibody response to both vaccines with concomitant administration. However, if time constraints do not permit, the ACIP recommends they be administered at the same time but at different sites.[74]

Malaria

Transmission of *Plasmodium* spp. parasites by *Anopheles* mosquitoes is responsible for malaria. Although it is not a problem in the United States, worldwide at least one million children die from malaria each year.[75] *Plasmodium falciparum* and *vivax* are becoming more resistant to chloroquine and resistance to newer antimalarials is increasing.[75] The first antimalarial vaccine, SPf66, was tested in Thailand and Latin America. Vaccination of Thai children resulted in no protection from malaria; however, an efficacy rate of ≥35% was reported in Latin Americans, which was felt to be promising.[76,77] Although the same vaccine type was used, they were from two different manufacturers, and it was felt that this may account for the differences in study results. Research in this area is ongoing.

Malaria prevention is based primarily on decreasing exposure to mosquitoes and chemoprophylaxis, with the agent chosen dependent on expected organism exposure. Standard therapy is with chloroquine, started 1 week before travel and continuing for 4 to 6 weeks after exposure.[71,72,78] Associated adverse effects include dizziness, headache, GI problems, and pruritus. For individuals using chloroquine prophylactically, three tablets of pyrimethamine-sulfadoxine should be available in the event that a febrile illness occurs when professional medical care is not available. Those with a history of hypersensitivity to sulfonamides, pregnant women near term, and infants less than 2 months of age should not take pyrimethamine-sulfadoxine. Therapy should be discontinued immediately on appearance of a rash because of the rare association with Stevens-Johnson syndrome. An alternative agent for nonpregnant individuals more than 8 years of age is doxycycline, started 1 to 2 days before travel and continuing for 4 to 6 weeks after exposure. Doxycycline causes photosensitivity and may be upsetting to the GI tract.

Individuals traveling to areas with chloroquine-resistant malaria should receive mefloquine beginning 1 week before departure and continue with weekly doses until 4 weeks after exposure.[78] Children less than 15 kg, pregnant women in the first trimester, individuals with epilepsy, and those with severe psychiatric disorders should not receive mefloquine. In addition, individuals receiving β-blockers, calcium-channel blockers, chloroquine, quinidine or quinine, or valproic acid should not receive mefloquine because of the risk for drug interactions. With mefloquine, GI disturbances and dizziness are reported. Occasionally, hallucinations and seizures have been reported; however, these are more frequent with higher dosages than those used for malaria prophylaxis. An alternative to mefloquine is doxycycline.

Travelers to areas endemic for *Plasmodium vivax* or *Plasmodium ovale* should be aware of the risk for relapse after infection with these organisms. To prevent relapse in individuals who have prolonged exposure to malaria, primaquine is taken daily for 14 days, or a larger dosage can be taken once a week for 8 weeks beginning the last 2 weeks of chloroquine prophylaxis after leaving the malarious area. The CDC should be consulted for the appropriateness of therapy and for an acceptable method to deliver primaquine in small dosages. Primaquine is contraindicated in pregnancy and may cause hemolysis in individuals with G6PD deficiency.

PASSIVE IMMUNIZATION

Direct administration of nonspecific (e.g., immunoglobulin) or specific (e.g., antitoxin) antibodies results in short-term immunity. After the exogenous antibodies are metabolized, the immunity disappears and reexposure can result in infection. This is a prophylactic measure and duration of protection is limited and dose-related.

In most cases immune globulin should not be given until 2 weeks after immunization because of interference with the antibody response. In general, immunization with a live virus vaccine should be delayed for at least 3 months after immune globulin is given. When concomitant dosing of immune globulin and a live virus vaccine occurs, the immunization should be repeated in 3 months unless seroconversion is documented. Exceptions include OPV and yellow fever vaccines because there is no interference with the antibody response. Both immunoglobulin administration and concurrent immunization are warranted with rabies and perinatal hepatitis B exposure, but the products are given at contralateral sites.

Immune Globulin

Immune globulin is used to provide exogenous antibodies to individuals who have immunodeficiency, certain autoimmune or infectious diseases, or who are exposed to certain infectious diseases. Immune globulin products are prepared from more than 1000 donors to ensure a broad spectrum of antibodies; however, this results in a potential for viral contamination. To minimize this potential, all donor units are tested for viral contamination before fractionation. Furthermore, newer fractionation techniques are effective in removing or inactivating HIV in donor units spiked with the virus. The risk for transmission of HIV from immune globulin remains theoretical, and no cases of HIV infection have been directly attributed to infusion of immune globulin.

However, several cases of hepatitis C were associated with two brands of immunoglobulin for intravenous use (IGIV), which were voluntarily withdrawn from the market.[79] The manufacturing process was since modified to include a solvent detergent treatment designed to inactivate viruses. Other viral inactivation procedures being used now include incubation at low pH, enzyme addition, and pasteurization. A different type of concern was the discovery that individuals who died with Creutzfeldt-Jakob disease (CJD), a rare, slowly progressive neurologic disease caused by prions, had donated blood that was used in the preparation of IGIV products. Although the risk of transmitting CJD through IGIV infusion is theoretical, the FDA recommended withdrawal of IGIV that contained plasma from donors: (1) subsequently diagnosed with CJD, (2) with blood relatives who have CJD, (3) who received pituitary-derived human growth hormone, or (4) who received a dura mater transplant. This withdrawal resulted in a significant shortage of blood products, including IGIV.

Because IGIV is a purified immune globulin product that is infused intravenously, larger dosages of immune globulin can easily be given. IGIV is produced by a variety of manufacturers and varies in immune globulin concentrations, IgA content, manufacturing techniques, additives, product form, storage requirements, and FDA-approved indications.

IGIV is used primarily to treat immunodeficiency syndromes resulting from a lack of or impaired function of immunoglobulin. In patients with IgG subclass deficiency, IGIV is reserved for those who have recurrent infections. Other approved indications include infection prophylaxis in bone marrow transplant patients more than 17 years of age, children with HIV, and patients with chronic lymphocytic leukemia. IGIV treatment prevents or reduces the number of infections in people with immunodeficiency. An IgG concentration less than 200 mg/dL (normal ≥1500 mg/dL) is associated with an increased risk for sudden, overwhelming bacterial infection. Increasing serum concentrations to more than 400 mg/dL is sufficient in most cases.[80] Although the lowest effective dosage is 150 mg/kg, an IGIV dosage of 200 to 400 mg/kg per month is used in most patients.[80] In addition to use in immunodeficiencies, IGIV is approved for use in treating idiopathic thrombocytopenic purpura (ITP) and Kawasaki disease. Although the precise mechanism for efficacy in these diseases is not known, it is likely owing to immunomodulation.

IGIV has been used to treat many other diseases. The University Hospital Consortium Expert Panel made recommendations for off-label use of IGIV that included patients with Guillain-Barré syndrome, severe posttransfusion purpura, and chronic inflammatory demyelinating polyneuropathy.[81] IGIV also has been used in patients with burns, multiple myeloma, cytomegalovirus infection, and neonatal sepsis; however, its routine use in these conditions is not recommended.[80,81]

Up to 10% of patients who receive IGIV have nausea, vomiting, chills, fever, malaise, fatigue, dizziness, headache, urticaria, tightness in the chest, flushing, dyspnea, and pain in the chest, hip, or back. These effects are usually related to the rate of infusion and can be managed by stopping the infusion until the symptoms subside and restarting the infusion at a lower rate. Pretreatment with acetaminophen, diphenhydramine, or glucocorticoids can decrease side effects. Patients with IgA deficiency are at risk for developing anaphylaxis owing to anti-IgA antibody formation; they should receive products with the lowest IgA concentration.

The protein content of immune globulin for intramuscular use (IGIM) is about 165 mg/mL. IGIM is used to provide passive immunity to individuals within 2 weeks of exposure to hepatitis A, non-A non-B hepatitis, measles, and rubella. A dose of 0.02 mL/kg given before or within 2 weeks of exposure to hepatitis A is 80 to 90% successful in preventing infection.[3] For exposure to measles, a dose of 0.25 mL/kg in healthy individuals or 0.5 mL/kg in immunosuppressed or immunodeficient individuals, but not to exceed a 15 mL total dose, given within 6 days of exposure can decrease morbidity or prevent the disease. Measles vaccination should be deferred 5 months in those who receive 0.25 mL/kg and 6 months in those receiving 0.5 mL/kg.[39] Because of the large volume, the dosage may need to be divided and administered at multiple sites. Associated adverse effects are primarily pain at the injection site, and less commonly, flushing, headache, chills, and nausea.[3] IGIM should not be infused intravenously.

Hyperimmune Globulins

Immune globulin products with high concentrations of specific antibodies are used to provide immunity against specific diseases. These products are made from the serum of individuals with increased concentrations of the specific antibody. All plasma used to prepare hyperimmune globulin products is negative for HBsAg. Hyperimmune globulin products include cytomegalovirus (CMVIG), hepatitis B (HBIG), tetanus (TIG), rabies (RIG), Rhesus (RhIG), varicella zoster (VZIG), and respiratory syncytial virus (RSV-IGIV).[3,35,82–88] CMVIG and RSV-IGIV are administered intravenously, whereas the other products are given intramuscularly. The use of these products is reviewed in Table 65.5. The usual adverse effects are local pain and tenderness at the site of injection for products given intramuscularly; however, fever, rash, and, rarely, anaphylactic shock may occur. Other hyperimmune globulin products are being studied and may find a place in therapy for specific indications such as *Pseudomonas aeruginosa* immune globulin in cystic fibrosis. In addition to hyperimmune globulins, a monoclonal antibody for RSV, palivizumab, has been developed. Palivizumab is administered intramuscularly to children at high risk during RSV season and the problem with fluid overload seen with RSV-IGIV is avoided.[89]

Table 65.5 ▪ Hyperimmune Globulins

Product[a]	Indication and Use
CMVIG	Used in renal, liver, and bone marrow transplant patients. Some controversy remains as to whether or not the benefits of CMVIG outweigh the increased cost over IVIG.[82,83]
HBIG	Postexposure to hepatitis B. Should be given within 24 hours of percutaneous exposure and within 14 days of sexual contact. Neonates born to HBsAg positive or unknown status mothers are given HBIG and the first dose of hepatitis B vaccine within 12 hours of birth.[3,35]
RIG	Postexposure to rabies given concurrently with vaccine. RIG should be administered within 8 days of initiation of the vaccination schedule. Not to be used in individuals previously vaccinated.[3,69]
RhIG	1. Rh-negative mother following delivery of a Rh-positive fetus to prevent subsequent infant deaths from erythroblastosis fetalis.[3,81] Ideally, given within 72 hours of delivery but it may given up to 28 days after. Should be given regardless of the duration of pregnancy. 2. Rh-positive children with acute and chronic idiopathic thrombocytopenic purpura (ITP) and adults with chronic ITP. Doses vary depending on patient's hematocrit. In vivo hemolysis can occur and result in anemia.[85,86]
RS IVIG	Prevention of RSV infections in high-risk premature infants and children <24 months with bronchopulmonary dysplasia. Infusions are given once a month during RSV season. Fluid overload is problematic. Not indicated in those with congenital heart disease.[88]
TIG	Postexposure for tetanus-prone wounds and active tetanus infection. Administer with Td: (1) if minor wound and >10 years since Td; (2) if major wound and >5 years since Td; and (3) if Td primary immunization series incomplete.[3]
VZIG	Postexposure to high-risk individuals including those: (1) <15 years old who have not had varicella; (2) who are immunocompromised; (3) infants born to mothers who develop varicella 5 days before or 2 days after delivery; and (4) premature infants <28 weeks' gestation. Administer within 48 hours for maximum benefit and no later than 96 hours following exposure.[3,87]

[a]*CMVIG*, cytomegalovirus immune globulin; *HBIG*, hepatitis B immune globulin; *RIG*, rabies immune globulin; *RhIG*, Rh (rhesus) immune globulin; *RS IVIG*, respiratory syncytial virus immune globulin; *TIG*, tetanus immune globulin; *VZIG*, varicella zoster immune globulin.

Antitoxins

Antitoxins are derived from equine serum; therefore, the risk for severe allergic reactions including anaphylaxis is increased, and special precautions must be taken prior to administration. First, a careful history of past allergic responses (especially to animals) should be elicited because these individuals may be extremely sensitive to antitoxins. Then a scratch test or "eye test" should be performed to determine an individual's sensitivity, and if negative, a small amount of very dilute antitoxin is injected intradermally.[3] A negative response to the intradermal test dose does not rule out the possibility of a systemic reaction. Indications for the use of antitoxins are very limited, and these products should be used only in the presence of an appropriately trained individual with the necessary emergency equipment available. Usually antitoxin is given intramuscularly; however, in some cases, intravenous infusion may be used. The risk for a systemic reaction with intravenous infusion is increased; thus, doses should be dilute, infused very slowly, and the patient monitored closely. Antitoxins are available through the CDC for the treatment of diphtheria, tetanus, and botulism.

IMMUNOCOMPROMISED HOST

The antibody response to immunization in immunocompromised individuals is less than in healthy individuals; however, usually the response is adequate. In some situations, as with hepatitis B vaccination, it is prudent to measure antibody concentrations and give boosters if antibody concentrations fall. Because endogenous immunity is not intact in these individuals, live vaccines may have enhanced or prolonged viral replication, resulting in systemic disease.

Patients who are immunosuppressed because of disease (e.g., malignancy, immune deficiency syndromes) or who are receiving immunosuppressants (e.g., high-dose steroids, chemotherapy, irradiation) should not be given live virus vaccines (OPV, MMR, varicella, oral typhoid, BCG, and yellow fever) because of the risk for development of active disease, with the exception that children with HIV should receive MMR. Immunosuppressed individuals are at risk for the development of VAPP should they come in contact with an individual recently immunized with OPV who is shedding live virus in stool. Infants and children who are close contacts of immunosuppressed individuals should be immunized against polio using IPV.

Individuals with asymptomatic HIV infection should receive inactivated vaccines. The AAP and ACIP recommend that children with HIV receive routine pediatric immunizations (DTaP, IPV, MMR, Hib) regardless of symptoms.[3] In addition, the AAP and ACIP recommend immunizing children with symptomatic HIV infection against pneumococcal infection and influenza.[3,90] Varicella vaccination is not recommended in children with HIV.[3]

Cancer patients may be immunosuppressed owing to the malignancy, nutritional status, or anticancer therapy (e.g., irradiation, chemotherapy). Patients with active malignant disease should not be given live vaccines. Although killed vaccines and toxoids may be given, the degree of immune response to the immunization depends on the chemotherapeutic agent being used and may be inadequate to confer immunity. Whenever possible, vaccines should be given before radiation or chemotherapy. Patients more than 2 years old with Hodgkin's lymphoma should be immunized with pneumococcal and Hib vaccines 10 to 14 days before therapy is started. Patients who have not received chemotherapy for 3 to 4 weeks may have an adequate antibody response to influenza vaccine. Live virus vaccines, such as varicella, can be given to patients who are in remission from leukemia when 3 months have lapsed since the last chemotherapy was administered.

After immunosuppressive therapy has been discontinued, a quantitatively normal immunologic response usually develops 3 to 12 months later. Corticosteroids given as replacement therapy (e.g., Addison's disease); topical steroid therapy; long-term alternate-day therapy with low to moderate doses of short-acting steroids; or single-dose intraarticular, bursal, or tendon injections are not usually immunosuppressive and live virus vaccine administration is not contraindicated in patients receiving this.[3] Those who receive equivalent prednisone dosages of 2 mg/kg or ≥20 mg (in those >10 kg) a day or every other day for ≤14 days can be given a live virus vaccine immediately after discontinuation of the glucocorticoid; however, some clinicians advocate waiting 2 weeks. Patients receiving equivalent prednisone dosages of 2 mg/kg, or more than 20 mg (in those >10 kg) a day or every other day for >14 days should not receive live virus vaccine until they have been off glucocorticoids for at least 1 month.[3]

Individuals with functional (e.g., sickle cell disease) or anatomic asplenia have an increased risk of infection from encapsulated microorganisms, which appears to be greatest in children. Pneumococcus is the most common encapsulated pathogen in splenectomized individuals. Immunization with the pneumococcal, meningococcal, and Hib vaccines are recommended for all asplenic individuals more than 2 years of age. Because the response to pneumococcal vaccine is poor, prophylactic penicillin is recommended for sickle cell patients less than 5 years of age. It is not clear at what age penicillin prophylaxis can be stopped.

PREGNANCY AND LACTATION

The consequences of natural infection and the likelihood of exposure must be balanced against the risk of immunization for both the mother and baby during pregnancy and lactation.[7,91] The decision to immunize must be made with limited or no data available regarding the risk for congenital anomalies or other adverse outcomes. Active immunizations that are needed should be administered during the third trimester whenever possible. The ACIP and AAP publish recommendations for managing difficult situations. In general, passive immunization with immune globulin is considered safe for pregnant women.[3,7]

Active immunization with toxoids is safe when performed in the third trimester. It is desirable to update those who have not received a Td booster within the previous 10 years or to fully immunize previously unimmunized pregnant women against tetanus and diphtheria, preferably during the third trimester of pregnancy.[3,7]

Immunization with the MMR live, attenuated virus vaccine is contraindicated in pregnancy. Because of the potential risk of fetal rubella infection, women who are of childbearing age who are vaccinated with these agents should be counseled to avoid conception for 3 months following immunization. Although immunization with MMR should be avoided immediately before and during pregnancy, published findings of women who inadvertently received the rubella vaccine within 3 months of conception reported no evidence that the vaccination was responsible for congenital rubella syndrome.[3,92] Congenital varicella is associated with significant fetal abnormalities; therefore, varicella vaccine should not be given within 1 month of a planned pregnancy or during pregnancy.[3] A pregnant parent is not a reason to defer vaccination in children.

Inactivated viral and bacterial vaccines present less risk than live vaccines because these organisms do not replicate in vivo. Women who are more than 14 weeks pregnant should be immunized for influenza at the appropriate time of year.[3,54] The risks of pneumococcal immunization to the fetus are unknown; therefore, the risk of infection in a high-risk mother must be weighed against the potential harm to the fetus.[7]

An unimmunized and pregnant woman who anticipates travel outside the United States and exposure to wild-type polio virus should be immunized with OPV or IPV.[3] If travel to an area with a high risk for contracting yellow fever cannot be postponed, the yellow fever vaccine should be given.[7,74] Malaria prophylaxis with chloroquine or hydroxychloroquine is not contraindicated in pregnancy. However, travel to areas with *P. falciparum* that is resistant to chloroquine or hydroxychloroquine should be avoided, because both mefloquine and doxycycline are contraindicated in pregnancy.[71]

The postpartum period is thought to be a good time to review immunization status and update any necessary immunizations. Breast feeding is not adversely affected by immunizations in the infant or mother, and lactation is not a contraindication to immunization with any agent.[3] Most live viruses from vaccines are not transferred to breast milk. Although there may be transfer of antibody to the infant who is fed with human milk, this is not associated with any difficulties. Infants who are breast fed should be immunized according to the usual schedule.

PHARMACY CONSIDERATIONS

Knowing about the preparation of individual vaccines and immunoglobulin preparations including manufacturing techniques, excipients, storage recommendations, and reconstitution is essential to minimize vaccine adverse reactions and maximize patient response. The package insert should be consulted for specific product information.

Vaccine associated allergic reactions are generally related to: (1) viral vaccines grown in chick embryo culture, (2) antibiotics or preservatives, (3) stabilizers, or (4) antitoxin or antisera of animal origin. Although rare, individuals who experience anaphylactic reactions to eggs may experience a similar reaction to a vaccine grown in chick embryo culture. MMR can generally be safely given to patients with an egg allergy. Desensitization or a graded protocol can be used successfully for other vaccines grown in chick embryo cultures, such as yellow fever, to immunize individuals with egg allergies. New recommendations for influenza are to use antivirals as a prophylaxis against influenza rather than immunize with this vaccine, which is grown in chick embryo culture. Trace amounts of antibiotics (e.g., neomycin, streptomycin) or preservatives (e.g., thimerosal) added to immunobiologics may be responsible for hypersensitivity reactions. Delayed minor reactions attributed to neomycin or streptomycin have been reported between 48 and 96 hours after immunization with MMR. Anyone with a history of anaphylactic reaction to neomycin or streptomycin should not receive vaccines that contain these antibiotics. No vaccine contains penicillin. Mercury, from thimerosal, may accumulate in individuals who receive repeated courses of IGIM. People who are sensitive to mercury may experience a reaction; however, no specific causal relationship has been reported.

Antisera or antitoxins of animal origin are likely to cause allergic reactions. Horse serum is used to produce diphtheria, tetanus, and botulism antitoxins; equine antirabies serum; and antivenins. Biologicals of equine origin are inherently immunogenic; thus, all patients should undergo a scratch test or eye test using a dilution of the product to be administered before treatment to determine the intensity of precautions to be taken during administration.

Safe handling and storage of vaccines and immunobiologics is essential to ensure vaccine potency and to prevent vaccine failure.[93] Pharmacists should be familiar with the usual appearance of lyophilized and reconstituted products to help validate that product integrity was maintained during transport, and to ensure that product degradation did not occur during storage. The shelf-life should be validated and expiration dates noted, and the appropriate storage conditions should be maintained. Care must be taken to ensure timely reconstitution before immunization to maintain potency and prevent vaccine failure.

Pharmacies are unique settings for immunizations because they are conveniently located and readily accessible. In addition, most systems are computerized and linked; therefore, information can easily be shared. According to changes in many pharmacy practice acts, many pharmacists are becoming credentialed to direct immunization programs and administer immunizations. This requires an understanding of the state board of pharmacy regulation, education, new skill development (e.g., cardiopulmonary resuscitation, immunization techniques), documentation of the program, patient evaluation for immunizations, specialized record keeping, and required reporting to the VAERS system.

FUTURE IMMUNIZATION THERAPY

A renewed commitment to disease prevention has focused attention on developing safer and more efficacious immunizations, simplifying schedules, increasing vaccine supplies, developing more combination vaccines, expanding locations for vaccine administration, and producing new immunizations for diseases that currently are not preventable.[94] To enhance the immunogenicity of influenza vaccine, a live cold-adapted vaccine for intranasal administration is being studied in adults and children.[95,96] Several manufacturers have various combinations of diphtheria, tetanus, acellular pertussis, hepatitis B, Hib, and IPV, as well as meningococcal and pneumococcal protein conjugate vaccines under evaluation.

Immunizations of the future may be derived from a component of an organism that stimulates the immunologic response. They also may be an "empty" viral particle or they may be manufactured using recombinant DNA technology. Different administration routes are being explored, including intranasal aerosols or nose drops/spray and time-release capsules. The further development of safer, more effective vaccines will have a positive impact on decreasing infectious diseases, provided immunizations are administered to the appropriate target population.

PSYCHOSOCIAL

Psychosocial issues surrounding the use of immunizations and immune globulins are multifactorial. Some individuals believe that immunizations are unnecessary because the incidence of some vaccine-preventable diseases is low. Certain religious groups object to the use of any immunizations or products that are of human source. Outbreaks of disease have been directly attributed to failure to vaccinate for religious reasons. Media presentations on adverse effects temporally related to immunization were directly responsible for a dramatic increase in the numbers of lawsuits against vaccine manufacturers, which in turn threatened the viability of the national pediatric immunization initiative. In addition, parents refused pertussis immunization for their children, resulting in a significant increase in pertussis. Other reasons parents and physicians refuse or defer immunization is because of the pain associated with injection. This problem should be minimized as more combination vaccines are introduced and other routes for vaccine administration are being tested.

PHARMACOECONOMICS

The economic benefits of universal routine pediatric immunizations and immunizing targeted groups at increased risk for influenza and pneumococcal disease is unquestioned. As more immunizations are developed, however, the economic impact of the disease will be considered.

KEY POINTS

- Immunization prevents potentially devastating disease in infants, children, adolescents, and adults of all ages.
- Strategies include universal immunization against diseases that significantly threaten all individuals and the targeting of specific groups for immunization against diseases that cause significant morbidity and mortality in those groups.
- Adverse effects associated with immunizations are related to the type of immunization. In general, adverse effects associated with inactive or killed vaccines are related to the injection site, and consist of redness and soreness. Fever also can occur soon after injection. Immunization with live vaccines results in subclinical infection in immunocompetent individuals and the adverse effects mimic those seen with the disease. Individuals who are immunocompromised should not receive live vaccines.
- Recommendations regarding who should be immunized with which vaccines are updated periodically, and current information can be obtained from the CDC or local health department.
- Immune globulins provide passive general or specific immunity for a defined period of time. Immune globulins can be used to treat disease or prevent disease after exposure. In most cases immune globulins interfere with the antibody response to active immunization.
- Antitoxins are animal in origin and are potentially associated with significant adverse effects.

REFERENCES

1. Anonymous. Certification of poliomyelitis eradication–the Americas, 1994. MMWR 43(39):720–722, 1994.
2. Anonymous. Reported vaccine-preventable diseases–United States, 1993, and the Childhood Immunization Initiative. MMWR 43(4):57–60, 1994.
3. American Academy of Pediatrics. 1997 Red Book Report of the Committee on Infectious Diseases. 24th ed.
4. Braun MM, Ellenberg SS. Descriptive epidemiology of adverse events after immunization: reports to the Vaccine Adverse Event Reporting System (VAERS), 1991–1994. J Pediatr 131:529–535, 1997.
5. Bartell LA, Charney SA. National vaccine injury compensation act: a viable alternative to litigation? J Pharm Pract 2:36–44, 1989.
6. Clayton EW, Hickson GB. Compensation under the National Childhood Vaccine Injury Act. J Pediatr 116:508–513, 1990.
7. General recommendations on immunization. Recommendations of the Advisory Committee on Immunization Practices (ACIP). MMWR 43(RR-1):1–38, 1994.
8. Bernbaum J, Draft A, Samuelson J, et al. Half-dose immunization for diphtheria, tetanus, pertussis: response of preterm infants. Pediatrics 83:471–476, 1989.
9. American Academy of Pediatrics Committee on Infectious Diseases. Recommended childhood immunization schedule–United States, January–December 1999. Pediatrics 103:182–185, 1999.
10. Dietz V, Galazka A, van Loon F, et al. Factors affecting the immunogenicity and potency of tetanus toxoid: implications for the elimination of neonatal and non-neonatal tetanus as public health problems. Bull WHO 75:81–93, 1997.
11. Bardenheier B, Prevots DR, Khetsuriani N, et al. Tetanus surveillance–United States, 1995–97. MMWR 47(SS-2):1–13, 1998.
12. Diphtheria, tetanus, and pertussis: recommendations for vaccine use and other preventive measures. Recommendations of the ACIP. MMWR 40(RR-10):1–28, 1991.
13. Edwards KM. Acellular pertussis vaccines–a solution to the pertussis problem? J Infect Dis 168:15–20, 1993.
14. Halperin SA, Bortolussi R, MacLean D, et al. Persistence of pertussis in an immunized population: results of the Nova Scotia enhanced pertussis surveillance program. J Pediatr 115:686–693, 1989.
15. Cromer BA, Goydos J, Hackell J, et al. Unrecognized pertussis infection in adolescents. Am J Dis Child 147:575–577, 1993.
16. Aoyama T, Takeuchi Y, Goto A, et al. Pertussis in adults. Am J Dis Child 146:163–166, 1992.
17. Pertussis outbreak–Vermont, 1996. MMWR 46(35):822–826, 1997.
18. Blumberg DA, Lewis K, Mink CAM, et al. Severe reactions associated with diphtheria–tetanus–pertussis vaccine: detailed study of children with seizures, hypotonic–hyporesponsive episode, high fevers, and persistent crying. Pediatrics 91:1158–1165, 1993.
19. Cody CL, Baraff LJ, Cherry JD, et al. Nature and rates of adverse reactions associated with DTP and DT immunizations in infants and children. Pediatrics 68:650–660, 1981.
20. Griffin MR, Ray WA, Livengood JR, et al. Risk of sudden infant death syndrome after immunization with the diphtheria–tetanus–pertussis vaccine. N Engl J Med 319:618–623, 1988.
21. Cherry JD. Acellular pertussis vaccines–a solution to the pertussis problem. J Infect Dis 168:21–24, 1993.
22. Pichichero ME, Deloria MA, Rennels MB, et al. A safety and immunogenicity comparison of 12 acellular pertussis vaccines and one whole-cell pertussis vaccine given as a fourth dose in 15- to 20-month old children. Pediatrics 100:772–788, 1997.
23. Edwards KM, Meade BD, Decker MD, et al. Comparison of 13 acellular pertussis vaccines: overview and serologic response. Pediatrics 96:548–557, 1995.
24. Edwards KM, Decker MD, Graham BS, et al. Adult immunization with acellular pertussis vaccine. JAMA 269:53–56, 1993.
25. Ipp MM, Gold R, Greenberg S, et al. Acetaminophen prophylaxis of adverse reactions following vaccination of infants with diphtheria–pertussis–tetanus toxoids-polio vaccine. Pediatr Infect Dis J 6:721–725, 1987.
26. McBean AM, Modlin FJ. Rationale for the sequential use of inactivated poliovirus vaccine and live attenuated poliovirus vaccine for routine poliomyelitis immunization in the United States. Pediatr Infect Dis J 6:881–887, 1987.
27. Adenyl-Jones SC, Faden H, Ferdon MB, et al. Systemic and local immune responses to enhanced-potency inactivated poliovirus vaccine in premature and term infants. J Pediatr 120:686–689, 1992.
28. Use of vaccines and immune globulins in persons with altered immunocompetence. Recommendations of the Advisory Committee on Immunization Practices. MMWR 42(RR-4):1–18, 1993.
29. Schoendorf KC, Adams WG, Kiley JL, et al. National trends in *Haemophilus influenzae* meningitis mortality and hospitalization among children, 1980 through 1991. Pediatrics 93:663–668, 1994.
30. Anonymous. Progress toward elimination of *Haemophilus influenzae* type b disease among infants and children–United States, 1987–1993. Current Trends MMWR 43:144–148, 1994.
31. Shenep JL, Feldman S, Gigliotti F, et al. Response of immunocompromised children with solid tumors to a conjugated vaccine for *Haemophilus influenza* type b. J Pediatr 125:581–584, 1994.
32. Washburn LK, O'Shea TM, Gillis DC, et al. Response to *Haemophilus influenzae* type b conjugate vaccine in chronically ill premature infants. J Pediatr 123: 791–794, 1993.
33. Newcome W, Santosham M, Bengston S, et al. Immunogenicity of *Haemophilus influenzae* type b polysaccharide and *Neisseria meningitidis* outer membrane protein complex conjugate vaccine in infants and children with sickle cell disease. Pediatr Infect Dis J 12:1026–1027, 1993.
34. Guinan EC, Molrine DC, Antin JH, et al. Polysaccharide conjugate vaccine responses in bone marrow transplant patients. Transplantation 57:677–684, 1994.
35. American Academy of Pediatrics Committee on Infectious Diseases. Universal hepatitis B immunization. Pediatrics 89:795–800, 1992.
36. Halsey NA, Duclos P, van Damme P, et al. Hepatitis B vaccine and central nervous system demyelinating diseases. Pediatr Infect Dis J 18:23–24, 1999.
37. Quarterly Immunization Table. MMWR 47(3):67, 1998.
38. Anonymous. Rubella and congenital rubella syndrome–United States, January 1, 1992–May 7, 1994. MMWR 43(21):391–401, 1994.
39. American Academy of Pediatrics Committee on Infectious Diseases. Recom-

mended timing of routine measles immunization for children who have recently received immune globulin preparations. Pediatrics 93:682–685, 1994.
40. James JM, Burks AW, Roberson P, et al. Safe administration of the measles vaccine to children allergic to eggs. N Engl J Med 332:1262–1266, 1995.
41. Drawl-Klein LA, O'Donovan CA. Varicella in pediatric patients. Ann Pharmacother 27:938–949, 1993.
42. Anonymous. Varicella related deaths among children–United States, 1997. MMWR 47(8):365–368, 1998.
43. Lieu TA, Cochi SL, Black SB, et al. Cost-effectiveness of a routine varicella vaccination program for US children. JAMA 271:375–381, 1994.
44. Izurieta HS, Strebel PM, Blake PA. Postlicensure effectiveness of varicella vaccine during an outbreak in a child care center. JAMA 278:1495–1499, 1997.
45. Gershon AA, Steinberg SP, Gelb L, et al. Live attenuated varicella vaccine use in immunocompromised children and adults. Pediatrics 78(suppl):757–762, 1986.
46. Ho M-S, Glass RI, Pinsky PF, et al. Rotavirus as a cause of diarrheal morbidity and mortality in the United States. J Infect Dis 158:1112–1116, 1988.
47. Joensuu J, Koskenniemi E, Pang XL, et al. Randomised placebo-controlled trial of rhesus-human reassortant rotavirus vaccine for prevention of severe rotavirus gastroenteritis. Lancet 350:1205–1209, 1997.
48. Rennels MG, Glass RI, Dennehy P, et al. Safety and efficacy of high-dose rhesus-human reassortant rotavirus vaccines–report of the national multicenter trial. Pediatrics 97:7–13, 1996.
49. Wyeth Laboratories Inc. Rotavirus Vaccine, Live, Oral Tetravalent RotaShield package insert. Marietta, PA: August 1998.
50. Stephenson J. AIDS vaccine moves into phase 3 trials. JAMA 280:7–8, 1998.
51. Hadler SC. Global pattern of hepatitis A virus infection changing patters. In: Hollinger FB, Lemon SM, Margolis H, eds. *Viral hepatitis and liver disease.* Baltimore: Williams & Wilkins, 1991:14–20.
52. Innis BL, Snitbhan R, Kunasol P, et al. Protection against hepatitis A by an inactivated vaccine. JAMA 271:1328–1334, 1994.
53. Green MS, Cohen D, Lerman Y. Depression of the immune response to an inactivated hepatitis A vaccine administered concomitantly with immune globulin. J Infect Dis 168:740–743, 1993.
54. Prevention and control of influenza: part I, vaccines. Recommendations of the ACIP. MMWR 43(RR-9):1–13, 1994.
55. Aoki FY, Yassi A, Cheang M, et al. Effects of acetaminophen on adverse effects of influenza vaccination in health care workers. Can Med Assoc J 139:1425–1430, 1993.
56. Nichol KL, Lofgren RP, Gapinski J. Influenza vaccination. Knowledge, attitudes and behavior among high-risk outpatients. Arch Intern Med 152:106–110, 1992.
57. Steere AC, Sikand VK, Meurice F, et al. Vaccination against Lyme disease with recombinant *Borrelia Burgdorferi* outer-surface lipoprotein A with adjuvant. N Engl J Med 339:209–215, 1998.
58. Sigal LH, Zahradnik JM, Lavin P, et al. A vaccine consisting of recombinant *Borrelia Burgdorferi* outer-surface protein A to prevent Lyme disease. N Engl J Med 339:216–222, 1998.
59. Peltola H, Safary A, Kayhty H, et al. Evaluation of two tetravalent ($ACYW_{135}$) meningococcal vaccines in infants and small children: a clinical study comparing immunogenicity of O-acetyl-negative and O-acetyl-positive group C polysaccharide. Pediatrics 76:91–96, 1985.
60. Greenwood BM, Hassan-King M, Whittle HC. Prevention of secondary cases of meningococcal disease in household contacts by vaccination. Br Med J 1:1317–1319, 1978.
61. Butler JC, Breiman RF, Campbell JF, et al. Pneumococcal polysaccharide vaccine efficacy. JAMA 270:1826–1831, 1993.
62. Klein JO. The epidemiology of pneumococcal disease in infants and children. Rev Infect Dis 3:S246–S253, 1981.
63. Musher DM, Watson DA, Domingues EQ. Pneumococcal vaccination: work to date and future prospects. Am J Med Sci 300:45–52, 1990.
64. Dintzis RZ. Rational design of conjugate vaccines. Pediatr Res 32:376–385, 1992.
65. King JC, Vink PE, Farley JJ, et al. Comparison of the safety and immunogenicity of a pneumococcal conjugate with a licensed polysaccharide vaccine in human immunodeficiency virus and non-human immunodeficiency virus-infected children. Pediatr Infect Dis J 15:192–196, 1996.
66. Colditz GA, Brewer TF, Berkey CS, et al. Efficacy of BCG vaccine in the prevention of tuberculosis. JAMA 271:698–702, 1994.
67. Advisory Council for the Elimination of Tuberculosis and the ACIP. The role of BCG vaccine in the prevention and control of tuberculosis in the United States. MMWR 45(RR-4):1–18, 1996.
68. Smith KC, Green HL. A case for *Bacillus Calmette-Guérin* vaccine in United States-born children. Pediatr Infect Dis J 18:15–17, 1999.
69. Fishbein DB, Robinson LE. Rabies. N Engl J Med 329:1632–1638, 1993.
70. Human rabies prevention–United States, 1999, Recommendations of the Advisory Committee on Immunization Practices (ACIP). MMWR 48(RR-1):1–21, 1999.
71. Hill DR, Pearson RD. Health advice for international travel. Ann Intern Med 108:839–852, 1988.
72. Wolfe MS. Vaccines for foreign travel. Pediatr Clin North Am 37:757–769, 1990.
73. Typhoid Immunization. Recommendations of the Advisory Committee on Immunization Practices (ACIP). MMWR 43(RR-14):1–7, 1994.
74. Advisory Committee on Immunization Practices. Yellow fever. MMWR 39(RR-6):1–6, 1990.
75. Krishna S. Malaria. Br Med J 315:730–732, 1997.
76. Nosten F, Luxemburger C, Kyle DE, et al. Randomised double blind placebo-controlled trial of SPf66 malaria vaccine in children in northwestern Thailand. Lancet 348:701–707, 1996.
77. Valero MV, Amador LR. Galindo C, et al. Vaccination with SPf66, a chemically synthesized vaccine, against Plasmodium falciparum malaria in Colombia. Lancet 341:705–710, 1993.
78. Advisory Committee on Immunization Practices. Recommendations for the prevention of malaria among travelers. MMWR 39(RR-3):1–10, 1990.
79. Schneider L, Geha R, Magnuson WG. Outbreak of hepatitis C associated with intravenous immunoglobulin administration–United States, October 1993–June 1994. MMWR 43(28):505–509, 1994.
80. Phelps SJ, Reynolds MA, Tami JA, et al. ASHP therapeutic guidelines for intravenous immune globulin. ASHP Commission on Therapeutics. Clin Pharmacol 11:117–136, 1991.
81. Ratko TA, Burnett DA, Foulke GE, et al. Recommendations for off-label use of intravenously administered immunoglobulin preparations. JAMA 273:1865–1870, 1995.
82. Snydman DR, Werner BG, Dougherty NN, et al. A further analysis of the use of cytomegalovirus immune globulin in orthotopic liver transplant patients at risk for primary infection. Transplant Proc 26(Suppl 1):23–27, 1994.
83. Glowacki LS, Smaill FM. Meta-analysis of immune globulin prophylaxis in transplant recipients for the prevention of symptomatic cytomegalovirus disease. Transplant Proc 25:1408–1410, 1993.
84. Duerbeck NB, Seeds JW. Rhesus immunization in pregnancy: a review. Obstet Gynecol 48:801–810, 1993.
85. Andrew M, Blanchette VS, Adams M, et al. A multicenter study of the treatment of childhood chronic idiopathic thrombocytopenic purpura with anti-D. J Pediatr 120:522–527, 1992.
86. Blanchette V, Imbach P, Andrew M, et al. Randomised trial of intravenous immunoglobulin G, intravenous anti-D, and oral prednisone in childhood acute immune thrombocytopenic purpura. Lancet 344:703–707, 1994.
87. Advisory Committee on Immunization Practices. Recommendations on varicella-zoster immune globulin for the prevention of chickenpox. MMWR 33:84–100, 1984.
88. American Academy of Pediatrics Committee on Infectious Diseases. Respiratory syncytial virus immune globulin intravenous: indications for use. Pediatrics 99:645–650, 1997.
89. Welliver RC. Respiratory syncytial virus immunoglobulin and monoclonal antibodies in the prevention and treatment of respiratory syncytial virus infection. Semin Perinatol 22:87–95, 1998.
90. Onorato IM, Markowitz LE, Oxtoby MJ. Childhood immunization, vaccine-preventable diseases, and infection with human immunodeficiency virus. Pediatr Infect Dis J 7:588–595, 1988.
91. Saballus MK, Lake KD, Wager GP. Immunizing the pregnant woman. Postgrad Med 81:103–113, 1987.
92. Bart SW, Stetler HC, Preblud SR, et al. Fetal risk associated with rubella vaccine: an update. Rev Infect Dis 7(Suppl 1):S95–S102, 1985.
93. Casto DT, Brunell PA. Safe handling of vaccines. Pediatrics 87:108–112, 1991.
94. Ellis RW, Douglas RG. New vaccine technologies. JAMA 271:929–931, 1994.
95. Palese P, Zavala F, Muster T, et al. Development of novel influenza virus vaccines and vectors. J Infect Dis 176(Suppl 1):S45–S49, 1997.
96. King JC Jr, Lagos R, Bernstein DI, et al. Safety and immunogenicity of low and high doses of trivalent live cold-adapted influenza vaccine administered intranasally as drops or spray to healthy children. J Infect Dis 177:1394–1397, 1988.

CHAPTER 66

UPPER RESPIRATORY INFECTIONS

David E. Nix

The Common Cold

The common cold is not a single infectious disease, but rather a group of self-limiting viral upper respiratory infections (URIs) producing a similar clinical syndrome. The average preschool child contracts approximately 6 to 10 colds per year, and the average adult has 2 to 4 colds annually. Roughly 23 million lost work days and 26 million missed school days are the result of the common cold each year.[1] Many more persons continue their usual activities with lower productivity and uncomfortable symptoms. Furthermore expenditures for products used to treat cold symptoms exceed $2.5 billion annually after adjusting for inflation.[2,3] The common cold is generally regarded as a mild condition that rarely causes significant morbidity. However, serious exacerbations of underlying disease may occur in patients with asthma or preexisting obstructive lung disease.[4] Patients with the common cold are also more susceptible to acquiring otitis media and sinusitis.[5–7]

EPIDEMIOLOGY

The common cold is caused by a number of viruses including rhinovirus, coronavirus, respiratory syncytial virus (RSV), parainfluenza virus, adenovirus, enterovirus, influenza A virus, and influenza B virus. Rhinovirus is by far the most common, isolated in 52 to 53% of patients with cold-like symptoms.[8,9] There are more than 100 different antigenic types of rhinovirus.[10] Influenza A virus and coronavirus were isolated from 5 to 9% of patients. Occasionally, more than one viral agent was isolated (5%)

or viral agents were isolated along with potential bacterial pathogens (3%) including *Chlamydia pneumoniae*, *Mycoplasma pneumoniae*, *Streptococcus pneumoniae*, and *Haemophilus influenzae*.[9] With state of the art diagnostic methods in one study, the etiology could not be established in 30% of patients with cold-like symptoms.

Rhinovirus is present year round; however, the incidence of infection peaks in the early spring (April and May) and fall, reaching the highest incidence in the fall.[9,11] The incidence of infection from coronavirus, the second most common viral agent, peaks in the early summer and again in the autumn to early winter. Coronavirus has been detected in up to 30% of upper respiratory infections.[12] The pattern of RSV infection is similar to that for rhinovirus; however, the peak incidence is slightly later in the spring (April through June) and fall (October through November). The isolation of influenza A virus from patients with cold-like symptoms is indicative of a mild influenza illness, and the incidence is expected to follow trends in influenza illness within a community. Parainfluenza virus type 3 is present in summer months and is associated with annual outbreaks or epidemics.[13] Isolation of adenovirus is fairly constant throughout the year.[9]

Transmission of the common cold may occur by direct contact with nasopharyngeal secretions or by inhalation of small and large airborne particles.[14–16] Viruses can be isolated from the hands of patients with the common cold. Transmission may occur with a simple touch or handshake.[16] In addition, viruses can remain viable in nasal secretions for several hours after being deposited on inanimate objects (e.g., door handles or faucets). The uninfected individual acquires the virus on his or her hands, then inoculates the mucosal surfaces by touching the face, nose, or eyes.[15] Prevention of transmission is possible by washing hands frequently with disinfectants, by using of virucidal tissues, and perhaps by avoiding facial and eye contact with the hands. However, these methods are not very practical. One study suggested that aerosol transmission is the chief mode of transmission in adults.[16]

CLINICAL PRESENTATION AND DIAGNOSIS

Signs and Symptoms

The incubation period for the common cold after exposure varies by specific etiology. The symptoms of rhinovirus infection may begin as early as 16 hours after inoculation. The incubation period for coronavirus is 24 to 48 hours, whereas RSV and parainfluenza viruses have an incubation period of 72 hours. Signs and symptoms of the common cold include sore throat, nasal obstruction, nasal stuffiness, mild fever, sneezing, watery eyes, hoarseness, cough, headache, malaise, myalgia, sinus pain, and postnasal discharge. Tyrrell et al.[17] reported signs and symptoms of volunteers who were infected experimentally with rhinovirus ($n = 71$), RSV ($n = 11$), or coronavirus ($n = 34$). The signs and symptoms were similar despite differences in the viral etiology, although cough and hoarseness were more prevalent and nasal obstruction less common with one of the three strains of rhinovirus. The average percentage of patients experiencing a particular symptom is provided in Table 66.1. Typically, the common cold begins as a sore "scratchy" throat and progresses to include nasal stuffiness and nasal obstruction. The pharynx may be slightly red with signs of postnasal drainage; however, marked redness and exudate suggest pharyngitis rather than the common cold. With the common cold, sore throat generally resolves within 24 to 72 hours. The nasal discharge is initially thin, but becomes thicker within a day or so. Infection caused by adenoviruses and enteroviruses is more often associated with fever, pharyngitis, and systemic symptomatology.[18] Usually, influenza presents with high fever (>38.5°C), pronounced malaise, prostration, and myalgia. However, mild cases of influenza may mimic cold-like symptoms. The common cold may last between 2 and >14 days; however, about 7 to 10 days is most common.

Table 66.1 ▪ Average Percentage of 116 Volunteers Exhibiting Various Symptoms After Experimental Infection with Cold Viruses (Rhinovirus, RSV, or Coronavirus)

Symptom	%	Symptom	%
Nasal stuffiness	95	Sinus pain	21
Nasal obstruction	91	Chills	18
Sore throat	80	Myalgia	14
Sneezing	72	Postnasal discharge	12
Headache	40	Evening fever	7
Malaise	39	Morning fever	6
Watery eyes	30	Cervical adenitis	3
Cough	25	Sputum production	3
Hoarseness	25		

Source: Reference 17.

Diagnosis

The common cold is diagnosed based on clinical signs and symptoms and exclusion of more serious illnesses. Because of the self-limiting nature of the common cold and the lack of effective treatment, there is no indication for performing viral cultures or other specific diagnostic testing. In very young children common cold symptoms may precede croup or bronchiolitis. In young adults and children older than 4 years, the cold-like symptoms need only to be distinguished from allergies and vasomotor rhinitis. Because influenza results in more serious complications and carries a significant risk of mortality in elderly patients, this disease must be distinguished from the common cold. Knowing the patterns of URIs within a region is helpful to distinguish the common cold from influenza and other infections. The presence of lower respiratory symptoms such as wheezing can, in most cases, be used to exclude the common cold. However, infection with cold viruses in patients with asthma and underlying obstructive pulmonary disease may exacerbate the underlying illness.

After about 3 days of symptoms, the common cold should not progress further in terms of severity. Most patients will only exhibit rhinitis, nasal congestion and obstruction, and possibly mild cough. Significant worsening of symptoms after 3 days or the presence of conjunctivitis, laryngitis, pharyngitis, muscular aches, or lower respiratory signs should bring the diagnosis of the common cold into question.[18] Wheezing in patients without a history of asthma is also of concern. However, patients with asthma or airway hyperresponsiveness may experience increases in wheezing, particularly in response to exercise, for weeks after having the common cold.

TREATMENT

There is no widely accepted specific therapy for the common cold. Use of interferon nasal spray,[19] zinc gluconate lozenges,[20] high-dose vitamin C,[21] and investigational antiviral drugs[22–27] has shown limited or no benefit in shortening the duration of symptoms and/or reducing viral shedding. High-dose vitamin C (at least 1 g/day) may provide a small benefit; however, this benefit is controversial.[21] In addition, several of the treatments (interferon, zinc gluconate, and antiviral drugs) are associated with significant side effects. Zinc gluconate lozenges are unpalatable. A nasal spray containing soluble intercellular adhesion molecule 1 (ICAM-1) was shown to reduce cold symptoms by almost 50% when used before or within 12 hours after experimental rhinovirus infection. ICAM-1 is responsible for binding of rhinovirus to susceptible nasopharyngeal cells, permitting virus entry. Soluble ICAM-1 is a competitive inhibitor of this binding. It is likely that this therapy will be expensive if it becomes available. Moreover, it is not clear if treatment given beyond 12 hours after exposure to rhinovirus would be effective.[28]

Current therapy for the common cold focuses on symptomatic relief and includes analgesics, systemic and topical decongestants, and antihistamines. Aspirin and acetaminophen suppress the development of antibodies and prolong the duration of viral shedding.[29] These agents reduce fever that may be a protective response to infection. However, fever is only present in a small minority of patients. Aspirin and acetaminophen may be useful to reduce headache, malaise, and muscle aches if they are present. These agents should not be used routinely for the common cold. The association of aspirin use and Reye's syndrome in children with influenza warrants further caution in the routine use of aspirin.[30] This association has not been described in association with the common cold. However, influenza can sometimes mimic the common cold and Reye's syndrome has been reported, although rarely, with adenoviruses and parainfluenza viruses. Ibuprofen and naproxen have no detrimental effect on serum antibody response and virus shedding and appear effective for relieving some cold symptoms.[29,31]

The use of antihistamines to relieve cold symptoms is controversial. Histamine does not appear to play a significant role in the pathogenesis of the common cold. Some antihistamines possess anticholinergic action, which may reduce nasal secretions. The use of a sustained release formulation of brompheniramine was effective for reducing sneezing, rhinorrhea, and cough after experimentally induced rhinovirus colds.[32] In patients with natural colds, clemastine provided some symptomatic relief of rhinorrhea and sneezing, but the effects appeared less prominent.[33] A review of studies before 1996 concluded that antihistamines do not have major effects on overall cold symptoms, although some attenuation of sneezing and rhinorrhea may occur.[34] These minor benefits must be weighed against the potential for side effects, primarily somnolence and dry mouth and throat. Intranasal ipratropium bromide, an anticholinergic agent, is efficacious for reducing rhinorrhea and sneezing.[35]

Systemic and topical decongestants have been widely used to relieve nasal congestion. Topical solutions of oxymetazoline, xylometazoline, and phenylpropanolamine are rapidly effective in relieving congestion and improving nasal airflow.[36] With xylometazoline, this effect persists for 6 hours. These agents are only indicated for short-term use (<3 days) because rebound congestion can occur with more prolonged use. Systemic decongestants including pseudoephedrine and phenylpropanolamine also are effective for symptomatic relief. A recent study showed that oral pseudoephedrine is more effective than placebo for relieving nasal congestion.[37]

Intranasal and inhalation formulations of sodium cromoglycate (cromolyn sodium), used every 2 hours for the first 2 days, then four times daily thereafter, provide symptomatic relief of cold symptoms compared to placebo. The duration of cold symptoms was significantly shortened and symptoms decreased in the final 3 days.[38]

Cough associated with the common cold is usually related to postnasal drainage and throat irritation and is under voluntary control. Antitussive agents such as codeine are not effective for this type of cough.[39,40] Codeine may be useful for chronic cough based on a reflex mechanism that occurs in some patients after resolution of the cold. Antihistamines and decongestants may be effective in relieving cough associated with acute upper respiratory infection.

Considerable interest in the effectiveness of echinacea for prevention and treatment of the common cold has evolved in recent years. A double-blind placebo-controlled study showed no benefit of using echinacea for preventing the common cold or respiratory infection.[41] The relative risk of acquiring an URI was 0.88 (95% confidence interval [CI] of 0.60 to 1.22) with treatment. Once a cold occurred, the median duration of symptoms was 4.5 days in the echinacea group and 6.5 days in the placebo group (not significant). It remains possible that a very small effect would be detected in a larger trial; however, the clinical significance remains questionable. Variations in the source and chemical makeup of various echinacea products could explain why other sources claim efficacy with echinacea for the treatment of the common cold. There is no role for the use of antibacterial drugs in the treatment of the common cold.[42] Antibiotics may be required only to manage complications such as acute otitis media or acute rhinosinusitis.

Acute Rhinosinusitis

Acute rhinosinusitis is an extremely common URI, accounting for 16 to 25 million physician visits annually. Although the costs of managing acute rhinosinusitis are uncertain, expenditures of $200 million for prescription drugs and more than $2 billion for over-the-counter drugs have been estimated.[43,44] History and physical examination are the most practical methods used to diagnose acute rhinosinusitis; however, the clinical presentation is nonspecific. A limited computed tomography (CT) scan provides the most definitive information for diagnosing sinusitis.[45] Since most cases of sinusitis are not serious and are self-limited, a CT scan is not cost effective. Standard sinus radiographs are difficult to interpret and are not very sensitive or specific. Antimicrobial therapy is considered appropriate for the treatment of acute rhinosinusitis[46]; however, the benefits of such treatment have recently been questioned.[47–49]

EPIDEMIOLOGY

The most common bacterial pathogens isolated from sinus aspirates in adults are *S. pneumoniae* (41%), *H. influenzae* (35%), and *Moraxella catarrhalis* (4%). Various streptococcal species and anaerobes from oral flora comprised 14% of the isolates, and *Staphylococcus aureus* accounted for 3%. The isolation of oral flora from the paranasal sinuses may be associated with periodontal disease. Bacteria were not isolated in 41% of the patients with presumed acute maxillary sinusitis.[50,51] Many of these patients with negative bacterial cultures are considered to have viral sinusitis associated with the common cold.[5] In children with acute maxillary sinusitis, *S. pneumoniae* (41%) is the most common cause, followed by *H. influenzae* (19%) and *M. catarrhalis* (19%). *M. catarrhalis* is isolated more frequently in children younger than 5 years of age.[51,52] As in adults, no bacteria could be recovered in almost 40% of children with acute maxillary sinusitis. Causative agents in neonates include *Listeria monocytogenes* and Gram-negative enteric bacteria in addition to the organisms listed for adults and children. The same is true for immunocompromised patients in whom fungi and Gram-negative bacteria are more likely present.

CLINICAL PRESENTATION AND DIAGNOSIS

Signs and Symptoms

Acute rhinosinusitis presents as sinus tenderness, cough, sinus pressure, nasal obstruction, headache, postnasal drainage, discolored nasal discharge, and sore throat. Halitosis, malaise, fever, chills, maxillary toothache, and periorbital swelling occur less commonly.[53] Signs and symptoms of acute sinusitis are nonspecific and also may occur with allergic rhinitis and viral URIs. Allergic rhinitis and viral URI often precede the development of acute rhinosinusitis. In fact, 39 to 87% of patients with the common cold have radiographic evidence of sinusitis on day 7 of their illness.[5,54] Obstruction of the nasal or sinus passages caused by septal spurs, nasal polyps, tumors, foreign bodies, and mucosal hypertrophy also predispose an individual to acute rhinosinusitis. Sinusitis can be classified according to the duration of symptoms: acute (2 to 4 weeks), subacute (2 to 4 weeks to 2 to 3 months), and chronic (>2 to 3 months).[55]

The most common presentation occurs in persons with initial cold-like symptoms. Colored nasal discharge, nasal obstruction, facial pressure, and cough persist or worsen by 8 to 10 days after the onset of symptoms. Although symptoms of the common cold may persist for 14 days or longer, improvement should occur by the end of the first week.[56] A lack of improvement or worsening after 1 week could indicate acute rhinosinusitis. A second presentation, occurring in fewer patients, includes fever (temperature >38°C), chills, facial pain, and marked tenderness, erythema, or swelling.

The maxillary sinuses are most frequently involved in acute rhinosinusitis followed by the frontal sinuses.[56] Infection involving the frontal, ethmoid, and sphenoid sinuses has been most commonly associated with intracranial complications, although such complications are rare.[57,58] Maxillary sinusitis is most often associated with pain over one cheekbone, under the eye, or resembling a maxillary toothache. Moderate to severe frontal headache and tenderness above the eyebrows and nose are consistent with frontal sinusitis. The ethmoid sinuses are located on each side of the nasal cavity. Ethmoid sinusitis is associated with pain at the inner corner of the eye, periorbital or temporal headache, and tenderness over the lacrimal fossa. The sphenoid sinuses are located posterior to the nasal pharynx just below the cranial cavity. Patients with sphenoid sinusitis may have multifocal headache involving the occipital, frontal, temporal, and retroorbital regions.

Diagnosis

It is not cost-effective to use radiologic and invasive procedures for the diagnosis of acute rhinosinusitis in most patients.[46] A careful history and physical examination are sufficient for presumptive diagnosis of acute rhinosinusitis. The nasal mucosa should be examined using an otoscope with nasal speculum after the use of a topical decongestant. The presence of thick, colored, mucopurulent secretions is consistent with acute rhinosinusitis. The presence of clear, watery secretions is more consistent with allergic rhinitis, particularly in patients with a history of seasonal allergic disorders. Sinus tenderness, sinus pressure, and postnasal discharge are often used as criteria for diagnosing sinusitis; however, these findings have not been shown to be sensitive and specific for identifying acute rhinosinusitis.[53] Characteristics associated with greater than 70% sensitivity include colored nasal discharge, cough, and sneezing. The specificities of these three characteristics were only 52, 44, and 34%, respectively. The presence of a maxillary toothache and painful chewing were quite specific (93 and 84%, respectively), but were present in only 11 to 15% of patients. Failure to improve after use of decongestants was 80% specific, but was only present in 28% of the patients.[59] These data are often used to discredit the accuracy of clinical examination in diagnosing sinusitis.[56] It is important to use groups of characteristics rather than single characteristics. When maxillary toothache, colored nasal discharge, poor response to decongestants, abnormal transillumination, and purulent nasal secretions on examination are considered, the predicted probability of sinusitis was 9, 21, 40, 63, 81, or 92% if 0 to 5 of the above factors are present, respectively.[59] The major problem with these data is that sinus radiographs were used to establish the diagnosis of sinusitis. Clearly, the results would be more certain if CT was used. Transillumination is a technique in which a strong light source is directed toward the lacrimal area and the light transmitted through the sinus is observed. If there is normal transmission of light, the sinus is probably not infected. Transillumination has poor sensitivity and specificity when used by itself.[60,61]

Sinus radiography is the most common imaging technique used to evaluate patients with sinusitis. Opacification, mucosal thickening, polyps, or air-fluid levels in patients with a history compatible with acute rhinosinusitis are regarded as evidence for the diagnosis. The ethmoid sinuses cannot be evaluated using sinus radiographs. In addition, there is considerable controversy on the true value of sinus radiographs because of the high frequency of false-positive and false-negative results.[46]

A CT scan is considered the gold standard for evaluating sinusitis. However, because of the limited availability and high expense, this procedure is most commonly used for immunocompromised patients, patients with suspected intracranial complications, patients with periorbital extension (swelling or edema), or patients with refractory disease. A limited CT scan of the sinuses is becoming more economical and more widely available, leading many specialists to recommend abandoning sinus radiographs in favor of a CT scan. Surgical decompression and sinus cultures also should be considered in these patients.[56] A CT scan may also be useful in patients with recurrent acute rhinosinusitis in whom structural abnormalities are suspected. Magnetic resonance imaging (MRI) scans are comparable to CT scans for evaluating soft tissue abnormalities; however, MRI is not useful for evaluation of bony abnormalities.

The definitive method for establishing the etiology of infection is sinus puncture, aspiration, and culture. This invasive technique is only warranted for neonates, immunocompromised patients, patients who fail to improve after treatment, and patients with suppurative complications such as periorbital cellulitis, meningitis, or intracranial abscess. Sinus cultures are also used in clinical trials of antimicrobial agents and in studies to examine the etiology of acute rhinosinusitis.

TREATMENT

The scope of this review is limited to the treatment of nonimmunocompromised children older than 2 years of age and adults. The management of patients with severe pain and/or focal neurologic signs or evidence of meningitis is also beyond the scope of this review. The first question to be addressed is whether antimicrobial therapy is warranted for uncomplicated acute rhinosinusitis. Many studies have involved patients referred to ear-nose-throat specialists for evaluation and treatment. These patients are more likely to have severe or recurrent disease or failure to initial treatment. Without any antimicrobial treatment, resolution of symptoms occurs in 70 to 80% of patients with presumed acute rhinosinusitis.[47–49] In a recent double-blind, randomized controlled trial, the efficacy of amoxicillin was not superior to that of placebo after a 7-day treatment period. Cure or substantial improvement was noted in 83% of patients given amoxicillin and 77% of patients given placebo ($P = .01$). Adverse effects, including gastrointestinal complaints and skin rash, were significantly more common in the treatment group (28% versus 9%, respectively).[47] Patients eligible for entry into the study had to be previously referred for sinus radiographs. The radiographs were then used as part of the enrollment criteria. Sinus radiographs are not sensitive or specific for the diagnosis of acute rhinosinusitis. In addition, many clinicians do not regard amoxicillin as a first-line agent for treatment of acute rhinosinusitis. A similar study failed to show a significant benefit of doxycycline compared to placebo.[48] A review of all placebo controlled trials between 1966 and 1996 revealed numerous methodologic problems and concluded that the effectiveness or lack thereof of antibiotics in acute rhinosinusitis is not based on sufficient evidence.[49]

Despite any controversy, antibiotic therapy is considered appropriate for acute rhinosinusitis when symptoms are severe or persist for longer than 8 to 10 days.[46,56] The later criterion is important to avoid treating patients who simply have a common cold. Early therapy of acute rhinosinusitis may reduce mucosal damage and scarring that may lead to recurrent acute rhinosinusitis or chronic sinusitis. Once the decision to use antimicrobial therapy is made, the choice of specific agents is a controversial issue. A recent meta-analysis found only small differences between different antibiotics based on clinical efficacy.[62] β-Lactam agents that are resistant to β-lactamases fared better than other β-lactam agents. Penicillins as a whole were less efficacious than sulfonamides and macrolides, and cephalosporins were associated with less adverse effects than penicillins. Interpretation is difficult since the groupings of antimicrobial drugs were heterogeneous with respect to spectrum of activity.

Penicillin-susceptibility serves as a major classification for isolates of *S. pneumoniae.* The incidence of isolates characterized by intermediate susceptibility or resistance to penicillin is increasing. Susceptibility surveillance studies involving isolates from the United States and Canada between 1996 and 1997 revealed intermediate susceptibility to penicillin (minimum inhibitory concentration [MIC] 0.1 to 1 μg/mL) in 20 to 28% and resistance (MIC >2 μg/mL) in 8.4 to 16% of isolates among more than 12,000 isolates.[63,64] Among the oral β-lactam agents, amoxicillin remains the most active drug when nonsusceptibility to penicillin is encountered. Oral cephalosporins are generally inactive against strains with nonsusceptibility to penicillin. Later-generation cephalosporins including ceftibuten and cefixime have reduced activity against even penicillin-susceptible strains of *S. pneumoniae.* Penicillin-resistant *S. pneumoniae* isolates are often characterized by multiple resistance to macrolides and sulfonamides. Alternative treatments include short-course parenteral ceftriaxone,[65,66] which has been used for otitis media, and fluoroquinolones.[67] The use of fluoroquinolones is limited in children owing to concerns about cartilage and tendon damage.

Approximately 30 to 37% of isolates of *H. influenzae* are expected to be resistant to amoxicillin due to β-lactamase production.[63] This type of resistance is reversed by the use of the combination amoxicillin/clavulanate. Only 0.1% of strains are resistant to amoxicillin and are β-lactamase negative. Many strains are resistant to early-generation cephalosporins including cephalexin, cephradine, and cefaclor and macrolides. Of the second-generation cephalosporins, cefuroxime axetil is active against >95% of *H. influenzae* isolates. The third-generation oral cephalosporins, including cefprozil, cefdinir, ceftibuten, cefixime, and cefpodoxime, are effective against essentially 100% of *H. influenzae* strains. Of the macrolides, azithromycin appears to be the most active while erythromycin has minimal activity. Clarithromycin by itself also has very limited activity against *H. influenzae;* however, the active metabolite, 25-hydroxyclarithromycin may increase the activity in vivo. There are also differences in the pharmacokinetics in that azithromycin undergoes extensive intracellular accumulation and has lower serum and interstitial fluid concentrations. These differences were counterbalancing, and the efficacies of azithromycin and clarithromycin were similar in an experimental model of lower respiratory infection.[68] More than 90% of *M. catarrhalis* isolates produce a penicillinase and are resistant to amoxicillin. These organisms are susceptible to all oral cephalosporins and amoxicillin/clavulanate.[63]

Therapy of acute rhinosinusitis is almost always empiric in children older than 6 months of age and in nonimmunocompromised patients. Because the predominant pathogens are all inhibited by amoxicillin/clavulanate, this combination agent is considered the standard to which other agents should be compared. Other first-line antimicrobial drugs include amoxicillin and sulfamethoxazole-trimethoprim.[46] Of particular importance is the continuing increase in penicillin MICs against *S. pneumoniae* and the multiple resistance found in penicillin-resistant isolates. Increasing penicillin resistance in *S. pneumoniae* mandates more rigorous investigation of which patients with acute rhinosinusitis may benefit from antimicrobial therapy and which patients may not. This will allow more limited use of antimicrobial therapy. Penicillin resistance in *S. pneumoniae* is not mediated through β-lactamase production; consequently, clavulanic acid adds no benefit for treatment of this pathogen. Adverse effects, particularly diarrhea, are perhaps more common with amoxicillin/clavulanate than with other oral penicillins and cephalosporins. Gastrointestinal complaints are also common with erythromycin and sulfamethoxazole-trimethoprim. The newer fluoroquinolones may offer advantages in terms of coverage; however, other issues, including cost and clinical utility (limitations of the use in children) need further consideration.

Some general comments can be made about the selection of antimicrobial drugs for treatment of acute rhinosinusitis. First, comparative trials of different antimicrobial agents usually do not show superiority of one agent over another. Studies conducted before 1990 and even in the early 1990s probably had few cases of patients infected with penicillin-resistant *S. pneumoniae,* and this may affect the outcome of therapy. Sample sizes are typically planned without considering the rate of spontaneous resolution. If a study is conducted with 100 patients in each of two treatment groups and the spontaneous resolution rate is 70%, then one is effectively comparing 30 patients in each treatment group. This makes it more difficult to conclude that true differences exist.

The following drugs (dose) have been compared to amoxicillin/clavulanate (500 mg every 8 hours) in randomized trials: azithromycin (500 mg once daily × 3 days), levofloxacin (500 mg once daily), cefprozil (500 mg every 12 hours), roxithromycin (150 mg every 12 hours), ceftibuten (400 mg every day), cefdinir (300 mg every 12 hours and 600 mg once daily), clarithromycin (500 mg every 12 hours), cefuroxime axetil (250 mg every 12 hours), and loracarbef (400 mg every 12 hours).[69–78] Amoxicillin 750 to 1500 mg/day every 8 to 12 hours was the reference treatment for the following drugs (dose): cefpodoxime axetil (200 mg every 12 hours), cefaclor (500 mg every 8 hours), clarithromycin (500 mg every 12 hours), cefixime (400 mg once daily), azithromycin (500 mg, then 250 mg once daily × 4 days), cefuroxime axetil (250 mg every 12 hours), and minocycline (100 mg twice daily).[79–86] Finally, cefuroxime axetil (250 mg twice daily) served as the reference treatment in comparative trials including sparfloxacin (400 mg, then 200 mg/day × 5 days) and ciprofloxacin (500 mg twice daily).[87,88] All of the treatments were administered for 8 to 10 days unless otherwise stated. The clinical effectiveness was not significantly different between treatments in any of the studies; however, a few of the studies had sample sizes less than 100 patients. The only study concluding superiority of a treatment involved a comparison between cefpodoxime and cefaclor. Cefpodoxime was more effective with cure in 84% compared to 68% with cefaclor.[89] Other trials were performed but are not discussed here due to the lack of a reference or use of a nonstandard reference drug. Better tolerance was concluded in eight studies in which amoxicillin/clavulanate served as the reference drug. Amoxicillin/clavulanate typically causes a greater frequency of gastrointestinal complaints, especially diarrhea. No comparative studies involving children younger than 12 years of age were found.

Adjunctive (symptomatic) treatment with topical and systemic decongestants is commonly used for acute rhinosinusitis. These agents relieve symptoms of nasal congestion; however, there is no evidence that they promote sinus drainage. Oral phenylpropanolamine was shown not to improve maxillary sinus drainage assessed by CT scan in one study.[90] In another study, treatment with topical oxymetazoline and an oral antihistamine-decongestant combination (brompheniramine and phenylpropanolamine) were no more effective than placebo in children with acute rhinosinusitis.[91] Although documentation of efficacy is poor, decongestants should be used to provide symptomatic relief of nasal congestion.[56] Antihistamines may be useful in patients who have allergic rhinitis concurrently. Because allergic rhinitis is a predisposing condition for sinusitis, the effects of intranasal corticosteroids as adjunctive therapy for acute rhinosinusitis has been studied. Intranasal flunisolide and budesonide provide some relief of symptoms (facial pain and tenderness, turbinate swelling, and global assessment) and somewhat faster resolution of abnormal radiographic findings.[92,93] These agents are particularly useful in patients with underlying allergic rhinitis. Rarely, surgical decompression using sinus puncture or fiberoptic rhinoscopy is required to manage an infected sinus and prevent suppurative complications.[46]

Table 66.2 provides a list of antimicrobial drugs that are approved by the U.S. Food and Drug Administration (FDA) for the treatment of sinusitis. Antimicrobial drugs that are well-established treatments for acute sinusitis based on published studies, but are not approved by the FDA are also included. Amoxicillin, for example, is not approved for the treatment of acute rhinosinusitis; however, it is frequently used as a reference treatment. The fluoroquinolones are relatively contraindicated for use in children. These drugs should not be used except for serious infections for which other agents are believed to be inferior. Sinusitis, therefore, would not be an indication except in immunocompromised patients with a documented pathogen resistant to other readily available drugs. Other sources of information should be consulted for antibiotic use and dosing in children younger than 2 years of age. Many of the manufacturers' dose recommendations do not cover children younger than the ages of 2 months to 2 years.

Table 66.2 ▪ Antimicrobial Agents Approved by the U.S. Food and Drug Administration for Treating Acute Sinusitis in Children and Adults

Drug	Approved Dosage for Children	Approved Dosage for Adults
Amoxicillin/ clavulanate (dosage based on amoxicillin)	14–15 mg/kg Q8hr or 20–22 mg/kg Q12hr	250–500 mg Q8hr
Cefuroxime axetil	Not approved	250 mg Q12hr
Cefprozil	7.5–15 mg/kg Q12hr	250–500 mg Q12hr
Loracarbef	Not approved	200–400 mg Q12hr
Cefpodoxime	5 mg/kg Q12hr	200 mg Q12hr
Cefdinir	7 mg/kg Q12hr or 14 mg/kg Q24hr	300 mg Q12hr or 600 mg Q24hr
Sulfamethoxazole/ trimethoprim	(40 mg/8 mg)/kg Q12hr	(800 mg/160 mg) Q12hr
Clarithromycin	7.5 mg/kg Q12hr	250–500 mg Q12hr
Ciprofloxacin	Not approved[a]	500 mg Q12 h
Levofloxacin	Not approved[a]	500 mg Q24hr

Use and dosage should be confirmed in official references for children younger than 2 years of age.

[a]Fluoroquinolones are relatively contraindicated in children except in serious infections where alternative treatments are not available.

COMPLICATIONS

Serious complications resulting from acute rhinosinusitis are uncommon. In one large public hospital, 12 patients with suppurative intracranial infections with a sinogenic source were identified over a 10-year period.[94] Of patients requiring hospital admission for sinusitis, 3.7% had intracranial infection. The most common infectious complications included cerebral abscess, meningitis, epidural abscess, and subdural abscess. Other complications including periorbital cellulitis are occasionally reported. It appears that intracranial complications are more common with chronic sinusitis than with acute rhinosinusitis.[95] In children, cerebral abscess, extra-axial abscess, and meningitis were reported; however, only 13 cases were found over 10 years in a large pediatric hospital.[96] Clearly, surveillance of these infrequent complications is necessary to ensure that the risk is not substantially increased with more limited use of antimicrobial drugs.

Otitis Media

Infection of the middle ear may present as acute otitis media (AOM) or as otitis media with effusion (OME or serous otitis media). AOM is extremely prevalent in young children, occurring in the majority of children at least once within the first 6 years of life. Many of these children also develop chronic OME, which may be associated with hearing impairment and learning disability. Care of otitis media is estimated to account for approximately 24.5 million physician office visits annually.[97] Tympanostomy for the management of OME has become the most common surgical procedure in the United States. The prevalence of otitis media decreases with age, and it is considerably less common in adults.

EPIDEMIOLOGY

As early as 6 months of age, 48% of infants experience at least one episode of AOM. By 1 year of age 62 to 79% of infants experience one or more episodes of otitis media and almost 20% have had three or more episodes. The frequency of at least one occurrence of otitis media further increases to 83 to 92% by 2 to 3 years of age. The peak incidence for AOM is between the age of 6 months and 1 year.[98,99] The most important risk factors for development of otitis media are lower socioeconomic status and contact with large number of other children (common in day-care settings).[99] The risk of AOM and OME appears to be more common in infants who are not breastfed, Blacks, children who live in urban environments, males, and children exposed to second-hand smoke. Children who contract AOM early in life are more likely to have recurrent otitis media.

The eustachian tube connects to the middle ear at a 10-degree angle at birth, and the angle increases up to about 45 degrees in adulthood. The eustachian tube also lengthens to about double its original length by adulthood. Because of the acute angle in young children, there is greater risk of obstruction leading to fluid accumulation.[100] The presence of a viral respiratory tract infection or seasonal allergic rhinitis may also contribute to eustachian tube dysfunction. Once the eustachian tube is blocked, conditions are excellent for bacterial proliferation. Neonates and infants lack a fully mature immune system, and this contributes to the higher incidence of AOM. Breastfeeding reduces susceptibility to AOM, possibly by contributing passive immunity.

Increases in the incidence of AOM are noted throughout the fall season. The incidence peaks in the winter and gradually decreases in the spring and summer months, coinciding with the peak times for viral URIs.[100] Exposure to smoking and other irritants is a risk factor for developing AOM and OME. Many children develop OME after an episode of AOM; however, OME may occur in children without such history. OME may be associated with the same bacterial pathogens that are found with AOM.

The pathogens involved in otitis media are essentially the same as those involved in acute rhinosinusitis. *S. pneumoniae*, *H. influenzae*, and *M. catarrhalis* account for approximately 30 to 47, 14 to 35, and >14% of the identified pathogens, respectively.[101–102] About one-third (26 to 43%) of the cultures are sterile, and some of these may involve viral agents. Penicillin-resistant *S. pneumoniae* is an increasing problem in children with AOM, particularly in children who attend daycare centers. In Costa Rica, a study involving 398 children found that penicillin-resistant and penicillin-intermediate strains of *S. pneumoniae* represented 2.2 and 17% of the 46 isolates, respectively.[101] The percentage of penicillin-resistant and intermediate strains in the United States was somewhat higher, 5 and 26%, respectively.[103] Infection with penicillin-resistant *S. pneumoniae* is a risk factor for recurrent otitis media and is associated with long-term antimicrobial use. Less commonly, *Streptococcus pyogenes*, *Staphylococcus aureus*, and *Peptostreptococcus* spp. are isolated. In neonates, the list of potential pathogens also includes Enterobacteriaceae, Group B streptococci, and *Pseudomonas aeruginosa*.[104]

CLINICAL PRESENTATION AND DIAGNOSIS

Signs and Symptoms

AOM is characterized by acute onset of ear pain, fever, and middle-ear effusion. Irritability, anorexia, vomiting, and diarrhea are common in young children. OME is associated with more insidious onset and a relatively chronic course. This disease is characterized by excessive fluid in the middle ear, mild symptoms including ear pain and discomfort, and a hearing deficit. Spontaneous rupture of the tympanic membrane, discharge in the external ear canal, and vertigo may occur.[105] Many cases of OME are detected only after routine otologic examination or after a child fails a routine audiometric examination.

Diagnosis

In infants, the most common symptoms are irritability/lethargy (69%), fever (52%), cough (36%), vomiting (21%), diarrhea (20%), tachypnea (20%), and anorexia (18%).[106] The most common symptoms associated with AOM in children include earache, sore throat, night restlessness, and fever.[105] Diagnosis of AOM is made on the basis of acute symptoms and examination using pneumatic otoscopy. The pneumatic otoscope introduces a puff of air while the movement of the tympanic membrane is observed. If the membrane is resistant to movement then the middle ear in considered to contain excess fluid. The tympanic membrane is typically bulging, and loss of the ossicular landmarks and light reflex is noted. Erythema and pronounced vascularity may also be observed.[107] Tympanometry is another technique that may be used.[108] The instrument produces a sound and the movement response of the tympanic membrane is observed. Both techniques require that the patient remain still during the examination.

Most patients with AOM are managed empirically based on the most probable pathogens. In certain patients, a culture may be obtained by puncturing the tympanic membrane and aspirating fluid. This procedure is known as a diagnostic tympanocentesis. Tympanocentesis is indicated for children who are critically ill or who have sepsis syndrome, patients who have a poor response to antimicrobial therapy, neonates, immunocompromised patients, and patients with suspected suppurative complications.[109]

TREATMENT

Early treatment of AOM with antimicrobial drugs has been routinely used in the United States; however, other countries (e.g., the Netherlands) have adopted a wait for 3 days policy. There is no evidence that the outcomes differ between the early treatment and the more conservative approach. Recently, because of the increasing incidence of drug-resistant bacteria, delayed antimicrobial therapy is being discussed in the United States.[110] Untreated AOM is associated with a spontaneous resolution rate of approximately 81%. Antimicrobial therapy can increase the resolution rate, but only by about 14%. Thus, only 14 of 100 patients treated would benefit from antimicrobial therapy.[111] Antimicrobial therapy may cause adverse effects (e.g., diarrhea and skin rashes) that offset the potential benefits of therapy. The cost of therapy and potential promotion of drug-resistant bacteria must also be considered.

In the United States, an expert panel convened to develop principles for managing AOM and OME and a summary of their recommendations follows.[97] Otitis media should be classified as AOM or OME based on the presence or absence of symptoms of acute infection. Antimicrobial treatment is indicated for AOM. In uncomplicated occurrences in children older than 2 years of age, treatment with a 5- to 7-day course of antimicrobials may be used in place of the traditional 10-day course. Persistent OME after treatment of AOM is common and does not require additional treatment. In contrast, antimicrobial treatment is not indicated in children with OME unless the effusion persists for greater than 3 months. After 3 months, treatment is optional. Three meta-analyses show a small (14%) benefit of antimicrobial therapy in resolving middle ear effusions.[111] However, there appears to be no effect of treatment when assessed longer than 1 month after treatment. Based on these findings, some experts recommend not treating OME with antimicrobial agents at all.[97]

Amoxicillin is the drug of choice selected by consensus.[110] This therapy is inexpensive, and clinical trials have not shown any of the newer antimicrobial agents to be more effective. The same issues of antimicrobial resistance discussed for acute rhinosinusitis apply for AOM and OME. Because the incidence of penicillin-resistant *S. pneumoniae* has risen in recent years, studies performed more than 5 years earlier may not be representative of cases of AOM seen today. Meta-analyses were conducted in the early 1990s evaluating the efficacy of antimicrobial drugs for treating both AOM and OME. For OME, a meta-analysis included results from 5400 children from 33 randomized controlled trials.[112] Antimicrobial therapy was marginally effective compared to placebo with resolution occurring an average of 13.7% (95% CI, 8.2 to 19.2%) more often with treatment. There was no evidence that extended spectrum drugs (amoxicillin/clavulanate, sulfamethoxazole/trimethoprim, erythromycin/sulfasoxazole, penicillin/sulfasoxazole, or any cephalosporin) performed better than standard spectrum drugs (amoxicillin, penicillin, or erythromycin). The drugs grouped as extended spectrum would be expected to have differing spectrums against *H. influenzae* and penicillin-resistant *S. pneumoniae*. Because of this grouping, this study fails to answer whether amoxicillin/clavulanate, cefuroxime axetil, or cefpodoxime, β-lactam drugs that provide the best overall time above the MIC,[113] are more effective than amoxicillin. In addition, the rate of isolation of penicillin-resistant *S. pneumoniae* affects the time above the MIC and clinical response.

Because of the increased prevalence of penicillin resistant *S. pneumoniae*, higher doses of amoxicillin (80 mg/kg/day) are now recommended. It is reasonable to use amoxicillin/clavulanate or a second- or third-generation cephalosporin in patients who fail to respond to amoxicillin. Oral cephalosporins that are effective for most strains of *H. influenzae* and *M. catarrhalis* include cefuroxime axetil and cefprozil (second-generation agents) and cefpodoxime, cefdinir, cefixime, and ceftibuten (third-generation against). These agents are not active against strains of *S. pneumoniae* that are resistant to high-dose amoxicillin. For patients with refractory disease where penicillin-resistant *S. pneumoniae* is proven or suspected, treatment with intramuscular ceftriaxone, 50 mg/kg daily, for 3 days should be considered.[65] In adult patients, one of the newer fluoroquinolones (e.g., moxifloxacin or gatifloxacin) with improved *S. pneumoniae* coverage may be used.

The duration of treatment for AOM was investigated in a separate meta-analysis.[114] Several trials have evaluated short-course therapy (3 to 5 days) versus standard therapy (8 to 10 days). The results were affected by the time in which the outcome assessment was made. If the outcome assessment was performed at 8 to 19 days, an advantage was observed in favor of the standard treatment duration (odds ratio 1.52, 95% CI of 1.17 to 1.98). Stated another way, a child would be 1.52 times more likely to have continued symptoms on days 8 to 19 if treated with short-course therapy compared to 8 to 10 days. This small difference diminished when the assessment of efficacy was made at 20 to 30 days (odds ratio 1.22, 95% CI of 0.98 to 1.54) or 31 to 40 days (odds ratio 1.16, 95% CI of 0.87 to 1.55). Similar results were obtained in a recent double-blind randomized clinical trial.[115] However, short-course therapy is not recommended for children younger than 2 years of age.[97]

A meta-analysis to evaluate the role of antimicrobial therapy for the treatment of OME was performed using published studies from 1980 to 1990.[116] This study pooled data from 1325 children from 10 different trials. Antimicrobial therapy resulted in an additional 22.8% increase in the resolution of middle ear effusion compared to no antimicrobial treatment. Studies that reported the lowest spontaneous resolution rate tended to have higher relative differences with antimicrobial treatment.

Table 66.3 lists drugs currently approved for the treatment of otitis media in children and adults and their respective doses. Although amoxicillin is considered the gold standard, agents that exhibit stability to β-lactamases are commonly used.

Table 66.3 ▪ Oral Antimicrobial Agents Approved by the U.S. Food and Drug Administration for Treating Otitis Media in Children and Adults

Drug	Approved Dosage for Children	Approved Dosage for Adults
Amoxicillin	13 mg/kg Q8hr 25–30 mg/kg Q8hr[a]	500 mg Q8hr
Amoxicillin/ clavulanate (dosage based on amoxicillin)	13–15 mg/kg Q8hr or 20–22 mg/kg Q12hr	500 mg Q8hr
Cephalexin	19–25 mg/kg Q6hr	250–500 mg Q6hr
Cephradine	19–25 mg/kg Q6hr or 38–50 mg/kg Q12hr	250 mg Q6h or 500 mg Q12hr
Cefaclor	13–20 mg/kg Q8hr	250 mg Q8hr
Cefuroxime axetil	15 mg/kg Q12hr (suspension)	250–500 mg Q12hr
Cefprozil	15 mg/kg Q12hr	250–500 mg Q12hr
Loracarbef	15 mg/kg Q12hr	Not approved
Cefpodoxime	5 mg/kg Q12hr	200 mg Q12hr
Cefdinir	7 mg/kg Q12hr or 14 mg/kg Q24hr	Not approved
Cefixime	4 mg/kg Q12hr or 8 mg/kg Q24hr	400 mg Q24hr
Ceftibuten	9 mg/kg Q24hr	400 mg Q24hr
Sulfamethoxazole/ trimethoprim	(40 mg/8 mg)/kg Q12hr	(800 mg/160 mg) Q12hr
Erythromycin	10 mg/kg Q6hr	250–500 mg Q6hr
Azithromycin	10 mg/kg × 1 dose, then 5 mg/kg Q24hr × 4 doses	Not approved
Clarithromycin	7.5 mg/kg Q12hr	Not approved
Erythromycin/ sulfasoxazole	12.5/37.5 mg/kg Q6hr	400/1200 mg Q6hr

Use and dosage should be confirmed in official references for children younger than 6 months of age.

[a]High dose regimen is recommended in areas where penicillin-nonsusceptible-*S. pneumoniae* is prevalent (see text).

COMPLICATIONS

Otogenic complications of AOM include tympanic membrane perforation, cholesteatoma (middle ear cyst), ossicular fixation or destruction, labyrinthitis, and chronic otitis media. Because of persistent hearing loss associated with OME, impairment of speech/language acquisition and delayed cognitive development may result. Additional complications include cervical abscess, temporal osteomyelitis, facial paralysis, mastoiditis, brain abscess, meningitis, subdural or epidural abscess, lateral sinus thrombosis, and hydrocephalus.[117] The incidence of intracranial complications after AOM is estimated to be 0.04 to 0.15%. Acute mastoiditis was the most common serious complication in the preantibiotic era. This infection is typically caused by *S. pneumoniae* and more than 60% of patients require surgery (mastoidectomy) for management.[118] There is concern that more restrictive use of antimicrobial agents may lead to increased frequency of complications; however, this has not been observed to date.

Pharyngitis

Acute pharyngitis is a common infectious disease, particularly in children. This infection may be caused by a variety of viral and bacterial pathogens.[119] Most cases of acute pharyngitis are self-limited, and specific treatment is needed only for pharyngitis caused by group A β-hemolytic streptococci (*S. pyogenes*). Rare causes of bacterial pharyngitis that also require treatment include *Neisseria gonorrhoeae, Francisella tularensis, Yersinia pestis*, and *Corynebacterium diphtheriae*.[119] Identification of these latter pathogens necessitates special laboratory testing which is only necessary in limited clinical settings.

EPIDEMIOLOGY

The most important cause of pharyngitis or tonsillitis in terms of the need for treatment and frequency of occurrence is *S. pyogenes*. Acute bacterial pharyngitis may also be caused by group C and G streptococci, *Arcanobacterium hemolyticum*, and possibly *M. pneumoniae* and *Chlamydia pneumoniae*. In addition, viral causes include rhinovirus, coronavirus, adenovirus, parainfluenza virus, herpes simplex virus, influenza virus, coxsackievirus, Epstein-Barr virus, and cytomegalovirus.[119] The occurrence of sore throat is associated with more than 10% of primary care physician visits, yet less than 20% of patients with a sore throat actually visit a heath care provider.[120]

Nearly all common causes of pharyngitis are self-limiting, with symptoms lasting from 2 to 7 days. Pharyngitis caused by group A β-hemolytic streptococci (GABHS) is sometimes associated with rheumatic fever, which is considered a nonsuppurative sequela. Because of the potential seriousness of rheumatic fever, identification and therapy of GABHS infection is warranted.[119] In the first half of the twentieth century, acute rheumatic fever (ARF) was a relatively common complication of GABHS infection. Many patients who developed ARF went on to develop rheumatic heart disease, requiring long-term antimicrobial prophylaxis and heart valve replacements.[120] In a study of military recruits, ARF occurred in 4.1% of patients with group A β-hemolytic streptococcal pharyngitis who were not treated with an antimicrobial drug.[121] The endemic risk of ARF after untreated streptococcal pharyngitis in the second half of the twentieth century has ranged from 0.3 to 0.4%.[120] Epidemics or outbreaks of ARF have occurred sporadically and the incidence of ARF may approach 3% during these outbreaks. Cases of GABHS infection in the United States are most commonly associated with M serotypes M1, M2, M4, and M12. Serotypes M1, M3, and M18 appear more commonly in patients with suppurative complications, and M3 and M18 appear to be more commonly associated with ARF.[122]

CLINICAL PRESENTATION AND DIAGNOSIS

Signs and Symptoms

Classically, group A β-hemolytic streptococcal GABHS is characterized by an acute-onset sore throat with fever, tonsillar exudate, and swollen, tender anterior cervical lymph nodes. Numerous studies have demonstrated that GABHS cases are difficult to differentiate from other causes of acute pharyngitis based on symptoms alone, even by experienced clinicians. The throat is usually quite erythematous with patches of purulent exudate (white to gray in color) on the tonsils and posterior pharynx. Erythema of the uvula and tongue is sometimes present. Fever is typically greater than 38°C, although the clinical course is highly variable.[119]

Diagnosis

The only reliable method to diagnose GABHS infection is to perform a throat culture or rapid antigen detection test (RADT). A throat culture is performed by swabbing the posterior pharynx and then plating the specimen on sheep blood agar followed by incubation for at least 18 to 24 hours. Recovery may be higher if the plate is incubated for 36 to 48 hours before the final determination of the presence or absence of GABHS. GABHS colonies produce surrounding β-hemolysis, which is recognized earlier when they are incubated in an anaerobic environment. Routine cultures may be set up with a glass cover slip placed over the area of inoculation. Alternatively, a stab culture can be prepared by inoculating the specimen under the surface of the agar to create a reduced oxygen environment. Culture is considered to be more than 90% sensitive and highly specific.[119]

The development of a RADT allows the immediate testing of patients during an office visit. A RADT is performed from a throat swab, and the test requires less than 5 minutes to complete. Although a RADT is very specific for GABHS, the sensitivity is only 60 to 90% compared to culture.[119] For this reason, patients with a negative RADT should have a culture performed for confirmation. Patients with a positive RADT should be treated with an antimicrobial agent without the need for a follow up culture.

Except in limited circumstances (epidemic), treatment of suspected streptococcal pharyngitis should not be started without a positive culture or positive RADT. There is some controversy regarding who should have a culture or RADT performed. The extreme view is that a culture needs to be performed in any patient with pharyngitis because GABHS cannot be distinguished from other causes of acute pharyngitis on clinical grounds. Fewer than 10 to 20% of patients with pharyngitis actually seek medical care; however, the incidence of ARF remains low. This prompted a Canadian group to develop four criteria to establish the risk of GABHS infection.[123] The criteria are absence of cough, history of temperature greater than 38°C, tonsillar exudate, and swollen, tender anterior cervical nodes. The probability of having GABHS infection was 2 to 3% if none of the criteria were present, 3 to 7% if one criterion was present, 8 to 16% if two criteria were present, 19 to 34% if three criteria were present, and 41 to 61% if all four criteria were present. The group suggested that no culture or therapy should be provided for low-risk patients with one or fewer criteria. Patients with two to three of the criteria should have throat cultures performed and then be treated only if the culture results are positive. In specific situations, patients with all four of the above criteria could be treated empirically, before culture results are obtained, to reduce the symptoms and potential transmission to others. The latter suggestion is most rational when there is evidence of a local epidemic. Epidemiologic factors should be considered when deciding to treat for GABHS. The occurrence of sore throat in patients who have been in close contact with an individual with known streptococcal pharyngitis suggests GABHS as the etiology. Increased probability of GABHS infection is also associated with the occurrence of sore throat in the winter and early spring in children between the ages of 5 and 15 years.

TREATMENT

Treatment for streptococcal pharyngitis may be initiated to reduce the duration of symptoms, limit spread, and prevent ARF. Because of the self-limited nature of streptococcal pharyngitis, the primary goal of treatment is not to hasten resolution of symptoms; however, if antimicrobial therapy is initiated within the first 24 to 36 hours of symptoms, some benefit in the resolution time may occur.[120,124] Occasionally, epidemics or clusters of pharyngitis caused by GABHS occur in military bases, schools, and other places where large groups congregate. If therapy is initiated early, within 24 to 36 h of symptom onset, the time of contagiousness is shortened. The primary reason for treating patients with streptococcal pharyngitis is the prevention of ARF. Antimicrobial treatment appears effective in preventing ARF if administered as late as 7 to 9 days after onset of symptoms.[117]

Only one study, conducted in 1950, assessed the effect of antibiotic treatment on the risk of ARF. Procaine penicillin G, 300,000 U intramuscularly every other day for three doses, resulted in a reduction in the incidence of ARF from 4.1% with placebo to 0.39%.[121] Oral penicillin V, 250 mg two to four times daily for 10 days, was later substituted for procaine penicillin G. The risk of ARF after streptococcal pharyngitis appeared to be falling even before therapy was shown to be beneficial. Today, the true risk of rheumatic fever is unknown, but appears to be much lower.[119]

Penicillin therapy in patients with streptococcal pharyngitis may be harmful because of the eradication of α-hemolytic streptococci and other bacteria that comprise the normal pharyngeal flora. The presence of commensal organisms may provide some protection against infections with pathogenic bacteria. In addition, unnecessary use of antimicrobial drugs may contribute to the emergence of drug-resistant bacteria, cause adverse drug effects, and increase the risk of recurrent pharyngitis.[120] The latter observation may be a result of a dampened immune response to infection.

Penicillin treatment is associated with a 15 to 20% failure to eradicate GABHS from the pharynx. The significance of this finding remains unclear, but some clinicians believe that this represents clinical failure in terms of the ability to prevent ARF.[121] Repeat throat cultures at the end of therapy are not recommended for asymptomatic patients.[119] The failure of penicillin to eradicate GABHS may be due to the presence of commensal organisms such as *H. influenzae* and *M. catarrhalis*. These organisms produce β-lactamase in the local environment, which may result in destruction of penicillin.[121] Treatment with β-lactamase-stable antimicrobial agents such as amoxicillin/clavulanate, cephalosporins, and macrolides results in higher eradication rates of GABHS in some studies. However, it remains unproven whether the improved eradication rate translates to a lower risk of ARF.

Erythromycin is the recommended alternative for treating penicillin-allergic patients with GABHS pharyngitis.[119] Recommended regimens include 20 to 40 mg/kg/day of erythromycin estolate or 40 mg/kg/day of erythromycin ethylsuccinate administered in three to four divided doses per day for 10 days.[125] Although all strains of *S. pyogenes* are susceptible to penicillin, low rates of resistance to erythromycin have been noted in the United States and resistance is more frequent in Europe. Also, erythromycin is inactive against *H. influenzae* and *M. catarrhalis,* which may be copathogens in some patients with streptococcal pharyngitis. Many patients are unwilling to complete a 10-day regimen of erythromycin because of gastrointestinal adverse effects.[125] For this reason, clarithromycin or azithromycin is often used in place of erythromycin. Both of these agents have the benefit of less frequent dosing (twice daily for clarithromycin and once daily for azithromycin). In addition, a shorter course (5 days) is recommended with azithromycin (12 mg/kg/day). Clarithromycin (15 mg/kg/day) and azithromycin achieve greater eradication rates of GABHS than the standard penicillin V treatment and cause fewer gastrointestinal effects than erythromycin.[125,126]

Amoxicillin/clavulanate contains an inhibitor of β-lactamases, and this agent would be expected to have advantages when β-lactamases are present, due to copathogens or commensal organisms. There is no evidence from clinical studies that amoxicillin/clavulanate is more effective than penicillin. Penicillin V therapy was associated with a 9.6% persistence rate of GABHS, whereas amoxicillin/clavulanate treatment was associated with a 3.8% persistence rate (difference not significant), although β-lactamase activity was detected in 74% of patients in whom the organism persisted at the end of treatment.[127]

Several oral cephalosporins have been studied and used for the treatment of streptococcal pharyngitis. Many of the studies concluded that higher eradication rates of GABHS were seen with oral cephalosporins than with penicillin V.[126] Cephalosporins appear to eradicate GABHS in chronic carriers much more effectively than penicillin V. Many patients may be chronic carriers of GABHS with infection due to a virus or other pathogen. It is not possible to distinguish colonization from infection in these patients. Thus, there is controversy whether the lower eradication rate for penicillin V is clinically important. Oral cephalosporins are better tolerated than amoxicillin/clavulanic acid and erythromycin; however, they are considerably more expensive.

Table 66.4 provides a listing of antimicrobial agents that are approved for the treatment of acute streptococcal pharyngitis.

Table 66.4 ▪ Antimicrobial Agents Approved by the U.S. Food and Drug Administration for Treating Acute GABHS Pharyngitis in Children and Adults

Drug	Approved Dosage for Children	Approved Dosage for Adults
Benzathine penicillin G (single IM dose)	300,000–600,000 U (<27 kg) 900,000 U (>27 kg)	1.2 million U
Penicillin V	20 mg/kg/day div Q8–12hr (<50 kg) 15 mg/kg/day div Q8–12hr (>50 kg)	250 mg Q8–12hr
Amoxicillin	20–40 mg/kg/day div Q8hr	250–500 mg Q8hr
Cephalexin	25–50 mg/kg/day div Q12hr	1 g/day div Q6 or Q12hr
Cephradine	25–50 mg/kg/day div Q6–12hr	1 g/day div Q12–24hr
Cefadroxil	30 mg/kg/day div Q12–24hr	1 g/day div Q12–24hr
Cefaclor	20 mg/kg/day div Q12hr	375 mg Q12hr
Cefuroxime axetil	25 mg/kg/day div Q12hr (suspension)	250 mg Q12hr
Cefprozil	15 mg/kg/day div Q12hr	500 mg Q24hr
Loracarbef	15 mg/kg/day div Q12hr	200 mg Q12hr
Cefpodoxime	10 mg/kg/day div Q12hr	100 mg Q12hr
Cefdinir	14 mg/kg Q24hr	600 mg/day div Q12–24hr
Cefixime	8 mg/kg/day div Q12–24hr	400 mg div Q12–24hr
Ceftibuten	9 mg/kg Q24hr	400 mg Q24hr
Erythromycin (dosage of erythromycin base)	20–50 mg/kg/day div Q6hr	250–500 mg Q6hr
Azithromycin	12 mg/kg Q24hr × 5 days	500 mg, 250 mg Q24hr × 4
Clarithromycin	15 mg/kg/day div Q12hr	250 mg Q12hr

Use and dosage should be confirmed in official references for children under the age of 6 months.

COMPLICATIONS

Complications of acute group A β-hemolytic streptococcal pharyngitis can be divided into suppurative complications, toxin-mediated complications, and nonsuppurative complications. Suppurative complications involve contiguous spread of infection including peritonsillar abscess, retropharyngeal abscess, cervical lymphadenitis, otitis media, sinusitis, and mastoiditis.[117,118] Recent reports include an apparent increase in streptococcal bacteremia, and some of these cases were related to primary pharyngitis.[128] Lemierre's syndrome or postanginal sepsis originates as acute pharyngitis which progresses to septic thrombophlebitis of the internal jugular vein. Septic thrombi then disseminate to the lung, liver, and other organs and usually involve *Fusobacterium* sp. This pathogen is present as normal pharyngeal flora and gains access to the bloodstream as a result of pharyngeal inflammation.[129] Scarlet fever is the classic toxin-mediated complication that resulted in substantial mortality in the preantibiotic era. This syndrome is currently termed streptococcal toxic shock-like syndrome (TSLS).[128] TSLS typically occurs after necrotizing fasciitis or myositis with toxin-producing strains of *S. pyogenes*. Approximately 10 to 20% of cases resulted from primary pharyngitis. TSLS presents as hypotension, multisystem organ failure, and erythematous rash or desquamation. The incidence of TSLS appears to have increased since 1988.[128]

Nonsuppurative complications of GABHS infection include ARF and acute glomerulonephritis. ARF is an autoimmune disorder that results in carditis (heart valve destruction), polyarthritis, chorea, and less frequently erythema marginatum and subcutaneous nodules.[128,130] Several outbreaks of ARF have been reported since 1984. The most serious sequela of ARF is heart valve damage, which worsens with subsequent infections involving GABHS. Rheumatic heart disease is an important cause of cardiovascular mortality and morbidity in underdeveloped countries; however, it is infrequent in developed regions.[128]

Acute glomerulonephritis (AGN) is an inflammatory disorder that follows pharyngeal or cutaneous infection with nephrogenic strains of GABHS. Approximately 10 to 15% of patients infected with such strains develop AGN. AGN typically occurs in young children, approximately 10 days after GABHS infection, and presents as edema, hypertension, acute renal failure, and rust-colored urine. The inflammation is believed to result from immune complex deposition in glomerular tissue. Most patients recover from AGN without serious sequelae.[117] The treatment of streptococcal pharyngitis with antimicrobial agents does not appear to prevent AGN as it does ARF.

Acute Laryngotracheobronchitis (Viral Croup)

Viral croup is a common, usually self-limiting illness of young children. The disease is characterized by noisy breathing (inspiratory stridor) and a dry bark-like cough. The cough and abnormal breathing sounds result from inflammation and edema of the tracheal walls and impaired mobility of the vocal cords. In the most severe forms, the inflammation is extensive enough to obstruct the airway.

EPIDEMIOLOGY

Viral croup occurs in children between 1 and 6 years of age with the highest incidence during the second year of life.[131] Up to 5% of children contract viral croup between their first and second birthday. The peak incidence occurs in the late fall and winter months, and males are affected at a disproportionately higher rate than females. Although most cases of viral croup are caused by the parainfluenza virus, croup may also be caused by adenovirus, respiratory syncytial virus, and influenza A virus.

CLINICAL PRESENTATION AND DIAGNOSIS

Signs and Symptoms

Viral croup usually begins with mild cold-like symptoms including rhinorrhea, mild pharyngitis, cough, and low-grade fever. As inflammation and edema of the tracheal wall develop, the lumen narrows, thereby restricting airflow. Inspiratory stridor occurs due to air passing though the narrowed opening, and this is often audible from a distance. The child's speech will be hoarse because of the swelling and altered mobility of vocal cords. Expiratory stridor and wheezing may also be present; however, lung breath sounds are normal. Most children show improvement after 1 to 2 days and resolution of symptoms by 3 to 7 days.

Diagnosis

Viral croup must be differentiated from spasmodic croup, acute epiglottitis, bacterial tracheitis, and a variety of other conditions that lead to tracheal edema and obstruction. Foreign bodies lodged in the trachea must also be considered.[131] Most children with viral croup have normal oxygen saturation as determined by pulse oximetry. The presence of hypoxia and low oxygen saturation indicates severe obstruction and the need for immediate treatment. Radiological studies including a radiograph of the neck and a limited CT scan may support the clinical diagnosis. A CT scan provides the most sensitive and specific confirmation; however, the procedure is not routinely necessary. Laryngoscopy is particularly helpful when a foreign body or acute epiglottitis is suspected. However, this procedure should not be performed in children with hypoxia or severe respiratory distress.

TREATMENT

The management of viral croup should focus on assessment of airway obstruction and maintenance of the open airway. Emergency airway management and hospital admission may be required in severe cases. Symptomatic treatment may include analgesics (acetaminophen or ibuprofen) and adequate hydration. Cool mist therapy has been used to elevate humidity, which is believed to decrease the viscosity of mucus secretions and soothe inflamed mucosa. The mist should be delivered by aerosol, although even sitting in a bathroom with the shower running is effective.[131] Some experts feel that current data do not support the use of humidified air or especially "croup tents."[132] Drinking liquids may also provide symptomatic benefit.

Aerosolized epinephrine delivered by nebulizer should be used in children with moderate to severe airway narrowing as assessed by decreased oxygen saturation, labored breathing, and failure to respond to cool mist (if used) and analgesics. The epinephrine decreases swelling and edema through α-receptor stimulation and constriction of small arterioles. Caution is advised in children with tachycardia and underlying congenital heart disease. Aerosolized epinephrine may reduce the need for intubation and tracheostomy.

Corticosteroids (e.g., dexamethasone 0.6 mg/kg) are recommended in children with severe croup. More recent studies demonstrate that nebulized budesonide (2 mg) is equivalent to oral or intramuscular dexamethasone for moderate to severe viral croup.[133,134] Corticosteroids reduce the need for intubation, shorten the time to improvement and duration of emergency room or hospital stay, and reduce the need for repeated aerosol epinephrine administration.

Acute Epiglottitis

Acute epiglottitis was a topic in the previous edition of this book. This disease is a very serious condition involving cellulitis and swelling of the epiglottis. Children with acute epiglottis are at significant risk for acute airway obstruction and death if endotracheal intubation or emergency tracheostomy is not performed. Acute epiglottis is usually caused by infection with *H. influenzae*, type B. Fortunately, the availability and widespread use of *Haemophilus* type B vaccine in children has almost eliminated acute epiglottis, and this topic will not be discussed further in this chapter.

KEY POINTS

The Common Cold

- Symptoms may overlap with bacterial causes of URI.
- Antimicrobial agents are not effective and should not be used.
- Symptomatic treatment is with acetaminophen and a decongestant.

Acute Rhinosinusitis

- Differentiate acute rhinosinusitis from viral URI (more severe or persistent symptoms).
- Alternatives for treatment include amoxicillin/clavulanate, selected oral cephalosporins, trimethoprim/sulfamethoxazole, newer macrolides, and fluoroquinolones (adults only).
- Five-day treatment regimens are as effective as 10-day regimens for some agents in children older than 2 years of age and adults.

Otitis Media

- Differentiate AOM from OME.
- Antimicrobial treatment is indicated for AOM.
- Antimicrobial treatment is optional for OME if symptoms persist >3 to 6 months.
- First-line treatment with amoxicillin is recommended by consensus groups; however, the potential for resistance is increasing.

Pharyngitis

- Definitive diagnosis by RADT and/or culture.
- Treatment of patients with GABHS with oral penicillin V.
- Alternative treatment is oral erythromycin; however, oral cephalosporins, newer macrolides, and amoxicillin clavulanate are also effective.

Acute Laryngotracheobronchitis (Viral Croup)

- Differentiate viral croup from other causes of acute airway obstruction.
- Treatment involves analgesics and possibly cool mist to increase humidity.
- Treat moderate to severe disease with aerosolized epinephrine and oral dexamethasone.
- Anti-infective therapy is not recommended.

Acute Epiglottitis

- Usually caused by type B *Haemophilus influenzae.*
- Acute epiglottitis is now rare due to widespread use of *H. inluenzae* type B vaccine in children.

REFERENCES

1. Turner RB. The treatment of the common cold. J Infect Dis Pharmacother 1:21–34, 1995.
2. Tompkins RK, Wood RW, Wolcott BW, et al. The effectiveness and cost of acute respiratory illness medical care provided by physicians and algorithm-assisted physicians' assistants. Med Care 15:991–1003, 1977.
3. Rosenthal I. Expense of physician care spurs OTC, self-care market. Drug Top 132:62–63, 1988.
4. Busse WW. The role of the common cold in asthma. J Clin Pharmacol 39:241–245, 1999.
5. Puhakka T, Mäkelä MJ, Alanen A, et al. Sinusitis in the common cold. J Allergy Clin Immunol 102:403–408, 1998.
6. Moody SA, Alper CM, Doyle WJ. Daily tympanometry in children during the cold season: association of otitis media with upper respiratory tract infections. Int J Pediatr Otorhinolaryngol 45:143–150, 1998.
7. Elkhatieb A, Hipskind G, Woerner D, et al. Middle ear abnormalities during natural rhinovirus colds in adults. J Infect Dis 168:618–621, 1993.
8. Monto AS, Sullivan KM. Acute respiratory illness in the community. Frequency of illness and the agents involved. Epidemiol Infect 110:145–160, 1993.
9. Mäkelä MJ, Puhakka T, Ruuskanen O, et al. Viruses and bacteria in the etiology of the common cold. J Clin Microbiol 36:539–542, 1998.
10. Pitkäranta A, Hayden FG. Rhinoviruses: important respiratory pathogens. Ann Med 30:529–537, 1998.
11. Arruda E, Pitkäranta A, Witek TJ Jr, et al. Frequency and natural history of rhinovirus infections in adults during autumn. J Clin Microbiol 35:2864–2868, 1997.
12. Isaacs D, Flowers D, Clarke JR, et al. Epidemiology of coronavirus respiratory infections. Arch Dis Child 58:500–503, 1983.
13. Easton AJ, Eglin RP. Epidemiology of parainfluenza virus type 3 in England and Wales over a 10 year period. Epidemiol Infect 102:531–535, 1989.
14. Gwaltney JM Jr, Moskalski PB, Hendley JO. Hand-to-hand transmission of rhinovirus. Ann Intern Med 88:463–467, 1978.
15. Gwaltney JM Jr, Hendley JO. Transmission of experimental rhinovirus by contaminated surfaces. Am J Epidemiol 116:828–833, 1982.
16. Dick EC, Jennings LC, Mink KA, et al. Aerosol transmission of rhinovirus colds. J Infect Dis 156:442–448, 1987.
17. Tyrrell DAJ, Cohen S, Schlarb JE. Signs and symptoms in common colds. Epidemiol Infect 111:143–156, 1993.
18. Kirkpatrick GL. The common cold. Prim Care 23:657–675, 1996.
19. Sperber SJ, Levine PA, Sorrentino JV, et al. Ineffectiveness of recombinant interferon-beta serine nasal drops for prophylaxis of natural colds. J Infect Dis 160:700–705, 1989.
20. Macknin ML, Piedmonte M, Calendine C, et al. Zinc gluconate lozenges for treating the common cold in children. JAMA 279:1962–1967, 1998.
21. Hemila H. Vitamin C supplementation and common cold symptoms: problems with inaccurate reviews. Nutrition 12:804–809, 1996.
22. Hayden F, Hipskind GJ, Woerner DH, et al. Intranasal pirodavir (R77,975) treatment of rhinovirus colds. Antimicrob Agents Chemother 39:290–294, 1995.

23. al Nakib W, Higgins PG, Barrow GI, et al. Suppression of colds in human volunteers challenged with rhinovirus by a new synthetic drug (R61837). Antimicrob Agents Chemother 33:522–525, 1989.
24. Zerial A, Werner GH, Phillpotts RJ, et al. Studies on 44 081 R.P., a new antirhinovirus compound, in cell cultures and in volunteers. Antimicrob Agents Chemother 27:846–850, 1985.
25. Miller FD, Monto AS, DeLong DC, et al. Controlled trial of enviroxime against natural rhinovirus infections in a community. Antimicrob Agents Chemother 27:102–106, 1985.
26. Phillpotts RJ, Higgins PG, Willman JS, et al. Evaluation of the antirhinovirus chalcone Ro 09-0415 given orally to volunteers. J Antimicrob Chemother 14:403–409, 1984.
27. Phillpotts RJ, Wallace J, Tyrrell DA, et al. Failure of oral 4′,6-dichloroflavan to protect against rhinovirus infection in man. Arch Virol 75:115–121, 1983.
28. Turner RB, Wecker MT, Pohl G, et al. Efficacy of tremacamra, a soluble intercellular adhesion molecule 1, for experimental rhinovirus infection: a randomized clinical trial. JAMA 281:1797–1804, 1999.
29. Graham NM, Burrell CJ, Douglas RM, et al. Adverse effects of aspirin, acetaminophen, and ibuprofen on immune function, viral shedding, and clinical status in rhinovirus-infected volunteers. J Infect Dis 162:1277–1282, 1990
30. Brown AK, Fikrig S, Finberg L. Aspirin and Reye syndrome. J Pediatr 102:157–158, 1983.
31. Sperber SJ, Hendley JO, Hayden FG, et al. Effects of naproxen on experimental rhinovirus colds. A randomized, double-blind, controlled trial. Ann Intern Med 117:37–41, 1992.
32. Gwaltney JM Jr, Druce HM. Efficacy of brompheniramine maleate for the treatment of rhinovirus colds. Clin Infect Dis 25:1188–1194, 1997.
33. Turner RB, Sperber SJ, Sorrentino JV, et al. Effectiveness of clemastine fumarate for treatment of rhinorrhea and sneezing associated with the common cold. Clin Infect Dis 25:824–830, 1997.
34. Luks D, Anderson MR. Antihistamines and the common cold. A review and critique of the literature. J Gen Intern Med 11:240–244, 1996.
35. Hayden FG, Diamond L, Wood PB, et al. Effectiveness and safety of intranasal ipratropium bromide in common colds. A randomized, double-blind, placebo-controlled trial. Ann Intern Med 125:89–97, 1996.
36. Smith MB, Feldman W. Over-the-counter cold medications. A critical review of clinical trials between 1950 and 1991. JAMA 269:2258–2263, 1993.
37. Taverner D, Danz C, Economos D. The effects of oral pseudoephedrine on nasal patency in the common cold: a double-blind single-dose placebo-controlled trial. Clin Otolaryngol Allied Sci 24:47–51, 1999.
38. Aberg N, Aberg B, Alestig K. The effect of inhaled and intranasal sodium cromoglycate on symptoms of upper respiratory tract infections. Clin Exp Allergy 26:1045–1050, 1996.
39. Freestone C, Eccles R. Assessment of the antitussive efficacy of codeine in cough associated with common cold. J Pharm Pharmacol 49:1045–1049, 1997.
40. Curley FJ, Irwin RS, Pratter MR, et al. Cough and the common cold. Am Rev Respir Dis 138:305–311, 1988.
41. Grimm W, Muller HH. A randomized controlled trial of the effect of fluid extract of *Echinacea purpurea* on the incidence and severity of colds and respiratory infections. Am J Med 106:138–143, 1999.
42. Dowell SF, Schwartz B, Phillips WR. Appropriate use of antibiotics for URIs in children: part II. Cough, pharyngitis and the common cold. The Pediatric URI Consensus Team. Am Fam Physician 58:1335–1342, 45, 1998.
43. Kankam CG, Sallis R. Acute rhinosinusitis in adults: difficult to diagnose, essential to treat. Postgrad Med 102:253–258, 1997.
44. Josephson GD, Gross CW. Diagnosis and management of acute and chronic sinusitis. Compr Ther 23:708–714, 1997.
45. Duvoisin B, Landry M, Chapuis L, et al. Low dose CT and inflammatory disease of the paranasal sinuses. Neuroradiology 33:403–406, 1991.
46. Joint Council of Allergy, Asthma and Immunology. Sinusitis practice parameters. J Allergy Clin Immunol 102(Suppl):S107–S144, 1998.
47. van Buchem FL, Knottnerus JA, Schrijnemaekers VJJ, et al. Primary-care based randomized placebo-controlled trial of antibiotic treatment in acute maxillary sinusitis. Lancet 349:683–687, 1997.
48. Stalman W, van Essen GA, van der Graaf Y, et al. The end of antibiotic treatment in adults with acute rhinosinusitis-like complaints in general practice? A placebo-controlled double-blind randomized doxycycline trial. Br J Gen Pract 47:794–799, 1997.
49. Stalman W, van Essen GA, van der Graaf Y, et al. Maxillary sinusitis in adults: an evaluation of placebo-controlled double-blind trials. Fam Pract 14:124–129, 1997.
50. Gwaltney JM, Scheld WM, Sande MA, et al. The microbial etiology and antimicrobial therapy of adults with acute community-acquired sinusitis: a 15 year experience at the University of Virginia and review of other selected studies. J Allergy Clin Immunol 90:457–462, 1992.
51. Wald ER. Microbiology of acute and chronic sinusitis in children and adults. Am J Med Sci 316:13–20, 1998.
52. Wald ER. Microbiology of acute and chronic sinusitis in children. J Allergy Clin Immunol 90:452–460, 1992.
53. Hueston WJ, Ebertein C, Johnson D, et al. Criteria used by clinicians to differentiate sinusitis from viral upper respiratory tract infection. J Fam Pract 46:487–492, 1998.
54. Gwaltney JM Jr, Phillips CD, Miller RD, et al. Computer tomographic study of the common cold. N Engl J Med 330:25–30, 1994.
55. Wald ER, Byers C, Guerra N, et al. Subacute sinusitis in children. J Pediatr 115:28–32, 1989.
56. Gwaltney JM Jr. Acute community acquired sinusitis. Clin Infect Dis 23:1209–1225, 1996.
57. Giannoni CM, Stewart MG, Alford EL. Intracranial complications of sinusitis. Laryngoscope 107:863–867, 1997.
58. Clayman GL, Adams GL, Paugh DR, et al. Intracranial complications of paranasal sinusitis: a combined institutional review. Laryngoscope 101:234–239, 1991.
59. Williams JW Jr, Simel DL, Roberts L, et al. Clinical evaluation for sinusitis. Making the diagnosis by history and physical examination. Ann Intern Med 117:705–710, 1992.
60. Otten FW, Grote JJ. The diagnostic value of transillumination for maxillary sinusitis in children. Int J Pediatr Otorhinolaryngol 18:9–11, 1989.
61. Spector SL, Lotan A, English G, et al. Comparison between transillumination and the roentgenogram in diagnosing paranasal sinus disease. J Allergy Clin Immunol 67:22–26, 1981.
62. de Ferranti SD, Ioannidis JPA, Lau J, et al. Are amoxycillin and folate inhibitors as effective as other antibiotics for acute sinusitis? A meta-analysis. BMJ 317:632–637, 1998.
63. Thornsberry C, Ogilvie P, Kahn J, et al. Surveillance of antimicrobial resistance in *Streptococcus pneumoniae, Haemophilus influenzae,* and *Moraxella catarrhalis* in the United States in 1996–1997 respiratory season. Diagn Microbiol Infect Dis 29:249–257, 1997.
64. Doern GV, Pfaller MA, Kugler K, et al. Prevalence of antimicrobial resistance among respiratory tract isolates of *Streptococcus pneumoniae* in North America: 1997 results from the SENTRY antimicrobial surveillance. Clin Infect Dis 27:764–770, 1998.
65. Leibovitz E, Piglansky L, Raiz S, et al. Bacteriologic efficacy of a three-day intramuscular ceftriaxone regimen in nonresponsive acute otitis media. Pediatr Infect Dis J 17:1126–1131, 1998.
66. Varsano I, Volovitz B, Horev Z, et al. Intramuscular ceftriaxone compared with oral amoxicillin–clavulanate for treatment of acute otitis media in children. Eur J Pediatr 156:858–863, 1997.
67. Doern GV, Pfaller MA, Erwin ME, et al. The prevalence of fluoroquinolone resistance among clinically significant respiratory tract isolates of *Streptococcus pneumoniae* in the United States and Canada: 1997 results from the SENTRY Antimicrobial Surveillance Program. Diagn Microbiol Infect Dis 32:313–316, 1998.
68. Alder JD, Ewing PJ, Nilius AM, et al. Dynamics of clarithromycin and azithromycin efficacies against experimental *Haemophilus influenzae* pulmonary infection. Antimicrob Agents Chemother 42:2385–2390, 1998.
69. Klapan I, Culig J, Oreskovic K, et al. Azithromycin versus amoxicillin/clavulanate in the treatment of acute sinusitis. Am J Otolaryngol 20:7–11, 1999.
70. Adelglass J, DeAbate CA, McElvaine P, et al. Comparison of the effectiveness of levofloxacin and amoxicillin–clavulanate for the treatment of acute sinusitis in adults. Otolaryngol Head Neck Surg 120:320–327, 1999.
71. Adelglass J, Bundy JM, Woods R. Efficacy and tolerability of cefprozil versus amoxicillin/clavulanate for the treatment of adults with severe sinusitis. Clin Ther 20:1115–1129, 1998.
72. Chatzimanolis E, Marsan N, Lefatzis D, et al. Comparison of roxithromycin with co-amoxiclav in patients with sinusitis. J Antimicrob Chemother 41(Suppl B):81–84, 1998.
73. Sterkers O. Efficacy and tolerability of ceftibuten versus amoxicillin/clavulanate in the treatment of acute sinusitis. Chemotherapy 43:352–357, 1997.
74. De Abate CA, Perrotta RJ, Dennington ML, et al. The efficacy and safety of once-daily ceftibuten compared with co-amoxiclav in the treatment of acute bacterial sinusitis. J Chemother 4:358–363, 1992.
75. Gwaltney JM Jr, Savolainen S, Rivas P, et al. Comparative effectiveness and safety of cefdinir and amoxicillin–clavulanate in treatment of acute community-acquired bacterial sinusitis. Cefdinir Sinusitis Study Group. Antimicrob Agents Chemother 41:1517–1520, 1997.
76. Dubois J, Saint-Pierre C, Tremblay C. Efficacy of clarithromycin vs. amoxicillin/clavulanate in the treatment of acute maxillary sinusitis. Ear Nose Throat J 72:804–810, 1993.
77. Camacho AE, Cobo R, Otte J, et al. Clinical comparison of cefuroxime axetil

and amoxicillin/clavulanate in the treatment of patients with acute bacterial maxillary sinusitis. Am J Med 93:271–276, 1992.
78. Sydnor TA Jr, Scheld WM, Gwaltney J Jr, et al. Loracarbef (LY 163892) vs amoxicillin/clavulanate in bacterial maxillary sinusitis. Ear Nose Throat J 71:225–232, 1992.
79. von Sydow C, Savolainen S, Soderqvist A. Treatment of acute maxillary sinusitis: comparing cefpodoxime proxetil with amoxicillin. Scand J Infect Dis 27:229–234, 1995.
80. Huck W, Reed BD, Nielsen RW, et al. Cefaclor vs amoxicillin in the treatment of acute, recurrent, and chronic sinusitis. Arch Fam Med 2:497–503, 1993.
81. Wald ER, Reilly JS, Casselbrant M, et al. Treatment of acute maxillary sinusitis in childhood: a comparative study of amoxicillin and cefaclor. J Pediatr 104:297–302, 1984.
82. Calhoun KH, Hokanson JA. Multicenter comparison of clarithromycin and amoxicillin in the treatment of acute maxillary sinusitis. Arch Family Med 2:837–840, 1993.
83. Edelstein DR, Avner SE, Chow JM, et al. Once-a-day therapy for sinusitis: a comparison study of cefixime and amoxicillin. Laryngoscope 103:33–41, 1993.
84. Casiano RR. Azithromycin and amoxicillin in the treatment of acute maxillary sinusitis. Am J Med 91(Suppl 3A):27S–30S, 1991.
85. Brodie DP, Knight S, Cunningham K. Comparative study of cefuroxime axetil and amoxycillin in the treatment of acute sinusitis in general practice. J Int Med Res 17:547–551, 1989.
86. Mattucci KF, Levin WJ, Habib MA. Acute bacterial sinusitis. Minocycline vs amoxicillin. Arch Otolaryngol Head Neck Surg 112:73–76, 1986.
87. Klein GL, Whalen E, Echols RM, et al. Ciprofloxacin versus cefuroxime axetil in the treatment of adult patients with acute bacterial sinusitis. J Otolaryngol 27:10–16, 1998.
88. Gehanno P, Berche P. Sparfloxacin versus cefuroxime axetil in the treatment of acute purulent sinusitis. Sinusitis Study Group. J Antimicrob Chemother 37(Suppl A):105–114, 1996.
89. Gehanno P, Depondt J, Barry B, et al. Comparison of cefpodoxime proxetil with cefaclor in the treatment of sinusitis. J Antimicrob Chemother 26(Suppl E):87–91, 1990.
90. Aust R, Drettner B, Falck B. Studies of the effect of peroral fenylpropanolamin on the functional size of the human maxillary ostium. Acta Otolaryngol 88:455–458, 1979.
91. McCormick DP, John SD, Swischuk LE, et al. A double-blind, placebo-controlled trial of decongestant-antihistamine for the treatment of sinusitis in children. Clin Pediatr 35:457–460, 1996.
92. Meltzer EO, Orgel HA, Backhaus JW, et al. Intranasal flunisolide spray as an adjunct to oral antibiotic therapy for sinusitis. J Allergy Clin Immunol 92:812–823, 1993.
93. Ovarnberg Y, Kantola O, Salo J, et al. Influence of topical steroid treatment on maxillary sinusitis. Rhinology 30:103–112, 1992.
94. Giannoni CM, Stewart MG, Alford EL. Intracranial complications of sinusitis. Laryngoscope 107:863–867, 1997.
95. Clayman GL, Adams GL, Paugh DR, et al. Intracranial complications of paranasal sinusitis: a combined institutional review. Laryngoscope 101:234–239, 1991.
96. Giannoni C, Sulek M, Friedman EM. Intracranial complications of sinusitis: a pediatric series. Am J Rhinology 12:173–178, 1998.
97. Dowell SF, Marcy SM, Phillips WR, et al. Otitis media: principles of judicious use of antimicrobial agents. Pediatrics 101(Suppl):165–171, 1998.
98. Teele DW, Klein JO, Rosner B. Epidemiology of otitis media during the first seven years of life in children in greater Boston: a prospective cohort study. J Infect Dis 160:83–94, 1989.
99. Paradise JL, Rochette HE, Colborn DK, et al. Otitis media in 2253 Pittsburg-area infants: prevalence and risk factors during the first two years of life. Pediatrics 99:318–333, 1997.
100. Haddad J Jr. Treatment of acute otitis media and its complications. Otolaryngol Clin North Am 27:431–441, 1994.
101. Arguedas A, Loaiza C, Perez A, et al. Microbiology of acute otitis media in Costa Rican children. Pediatr Infect Dis J 17:680–689, 1998.
102. Brook I, Gober AE. Microbiologic characteristics of persistent otitis media. Arch Otolaryngol Head Neck Surg 124:1350–1352, 1998.
103. McLinn S, Williams D. Incidence of antibiotic-resistant Streptococcus pneumoniae and beta-lactamase–positive *Haemophilus influenzae* in clinical isolates from patients with otitis media. Pediatr Infect Dis J 15(Suppl):S3–S9, 1996.
104. Shurin PA, Howie VM, Pelton SI, et al. Bacterial etiology of otitis media during the first six weeks of life. J Pediatr 92:893–896, 1978.
105. Faden H, Duffy L, Boeve M. Otitis media: back to basics. Pediatr Infect Dis J 17:1105–1113, 1998.
106. Tetzlaff TR, Ashworth C, Nelson JD. Otitis media in children less than 12 weeks of age. Pediatrics 59:827–832, 1977.
107. Pelton SI. Otoscopy for the diagnosis of otitis media. Pediatr Infect Dis J 17:540–543, 1998.
108. Brookhouser PE. Use of tympanometry in office practice for diagnosis of otitis media. Pediatr Infect Dis J 17:544–551, 1998.
109. Hoberman A, Paradise JL, Wald ER. Tympanocentesis technique revisited. Pediatr Infect Dis J 16(Suppl 2):S25–S26, 1997.
110. Culpepper L, Froom J. Routine antimicrobial treatment of acute otitis media: is it necessary? JAMA 278:1643–1645, 1997.
111. Rosenfeld RM. What to expect from medical treatment of otitis media. Pediatr Infect Dis J 14:731–738, 1995.
112. Rosenfeld RM, Vertrees JE, Carr J, et al. Clinical efficacy of antimicrobial drugs for acute otitis media: metaanalysis of 5400 children from thirty-three randomized trials. J Pediatr 124:355–367, 1994.
113. Craig WA, Andes D. Pharmacokinetics and pharmacodynamics of antibiotics in otitis media. Pediatr Infect Dis J 15:255–259, 1996.
114. Kozyrskyj AL, Hildes-Ripstein E, Longstaffe SEA, et al. Treatment of acute otitis media with a shortened course of antibiotics: a meta-analysis. JAMA 279:1736–1742, 1998.
115. Cohen R, Levy C, Boucherat M, et al. A multicenter, randomized, double-blind trial of 5 versus 10 days of antibiotic therapy for acute otitis media in young children. J Pediatr 133:634–639, 1998.
116. Rosenfeld RM, Post JC. Meta-analysis of antibiotics for the treatment of otitis media with effusion. Otolaryngol Head Neck Surg 106:378–386, 1992.
117. Gooch WM III. Potential infectious disease complications of upper respiratory tract infections. Pediatr Infect Dis J 17(Suppl):S79–S82, 1998.
118. Barry B, Delattre J, Vie F, et al. Otogenic intracranial infection in adults. Laryngoscope 109:483–487, 1999.
119. Bisno AL, Gerber MA, Gwaltney JM Jr, et al. Diagnosis and management of Group A streptococcal pharyngitis: a practice guideline. Clin Infect Dis 25:574–583, 1997.
120. McIsaac WJ, Goel V, Slaughter PM, et al. Reconsidering sore throats. Part 1: problems with current clinical practice. Can Fam Physician 43:485–493, 1997.
121. Pichichero ME. Streptococcal pharyngitis: is penicillin still the right choice? Compr Ther 22:782–787, 1996.
122. Johnson DR, Stevens DL, Kaplan EL. Epidemiologic analysis of group A streptococcal serotypes associated with severe systemic infections, rheumatic fever, or uncomplicated pharyngitis. J Infect Dis 166:374–382, 1992.
123. McIsaac WJ, Goel V, Slaughter PM, et al. Reconsidering sore throats. Part 2: alternative approach and practical office tool. Can Fam Physician 43:495–500, 1997.
124. Dagnelie CF, van der Garaaf Y, De Melker RA. Do patients with sore throat benefit from penicillin? A randomized double-blind placebo-controlled clinical trial with penicillin V in general practice. Br J Gen Pract 46:589–593, 1996.
125. Tarlow MJ. Macrolides in the management of streptococcal pharyngitis/tonsillitis. Pediatr Infect Dis 16:444–448, 1997.
126. Shulman ST. Evaluation of penicillins, cephalosporins, and macrolides for therapy of streptococcal pharyngitis. Pediatrics 97:955–959, 1996.
127. Dykhuizen RS, Golder D, Reid TMS, et al. Phenoxymethyl penicillin versus co-amoxiclav in the treatment of acute streptococcal pharyngitis, and the role of β-lactamase activity in saliva. J Antimicrob Chemother 37:133–138, 1996.
128. Shulman ST. Complications of streptococcal pharyngitis. Pediatr Infect Dis J 13(Suppl):S70–S74, 1994.
129. Williams A, Nagy M, Wingate J, et al. Lemierre syndrome: a complication of acute pharyngitis. Int J Pediatr Otorhinolaryngol 45:51–57, 1998.
130. Dajani AS. Current status of nonsuppurative complications of Group A streptococci. Pediatr Infect Dis J 10(Suppl):S25–S27, 1991.
131. Rosekrans JA. Viral croup: current diagnosis and treatment. Mayo Clin Proc 73:1102–1107, 1998.
132. Orlicek SL. Management of acute laryngotracheo-bronchitis. Pediatr Infect Dis J 17:1164–1165, 1998.
133. Johnson DW, Jacobson S, Edney PC, et al. A comparison of nebulized budesonide, intramuscular dexamethasone, and placebo for moderately severe croup. N Engl J Med 339:498–503, 1998.
134. Klassen TP, Craig WR, Moher D, et al. Nebulized budesonide and oral dexamethasone for treatment of croup: a randomized controlled trial. JAMA 279:1629–1632, 1998.

CHAPTER 67

PNEUMONIA

J. Edwin Underwood Jr.

Overview

DEFINITION

Pneumonia is defined as an inflammation of the lung caused by bacteria, viruses, or less commonly, noninfectious agents such as drugs or chemicals. The principal site of infection is the alveolus and the surrounding interstitial tissues.[1] Community-acquired pneumonia (CAP) is an infection that occurs outside of the institutionalized setting. CAP can occur during any time of the year, but it is most often encountered during late fall through late spring. Nosocomial pneumonia occurs in the institutionalized patient or may occur during the peri-institutionalized period.

Pneumonia has long been recognized as a serious and historically fatal infectious disease. In the early 1900s bacterial pneumonia was referred to as the "Captain of the men of death."[2] Today, despite the availability of numerous broad-spectrum antibiotics and improved diagnostic methods, pneumonia remains an infectious disease responsible for significant morbidity and mortality. The biggest challenge confronting clinicians is identifying the etiology of the infection and selecting the appropriate treatment. Initial antibiotic therapy, as well as complete treatment, is often empiric. Therefore, the clinician must have a thorough understanding of the body's defenses and of the etiology, pathogenesis, clinical presentation, and pharmacotherapy of pneumonia to effectively treat this disease.

TREATMENT GOALS: PNEUMONIA

- Obtain an accurate patient history and determine the need for hospitalization.
- Determine the relevance of concomitant disease states and other pertinent patient characteristics.
- Select the most appropriate and cost-effective antibiotic.
- Streamline antibiotic therapy once a specific pathogen is identified.
- Achieve clinical improvement and eradicate the pathogen.
- Ensure good outcomes and minimize costs.

EPIDEMIOLOGY

Pneumonia is the sixth most common cause of death and the most common cause of death from and infectious disease in the United States.[3] The annual incidence of CAP in the United States is 2 to 4 million cases with as many as 20 to 25% of patients requiring hospitalization.[4–6] Most patients with CAP can be treated in the ambulatory setting with oral antibiotics, and the mortality rate is less than 5%. In contrast, the mortality rate for patients with CAP requiring hospitalization is as high as 25% and accounts for a significant amount of hospital resources.[4,6] Nosocomial pneumonia occurs in approximately 300,000 patients annually, is the second most common hospital-acquired infection, and is the leading cause of death among the nosocomial infections.[7–9] Mortality rates for nosocomial pneumonia range between 20 and 50% depending on the population being studied. Patients who have had surgery and those in the intensive care unit (ICU) who are receiving mechanical ventilation are at greatest risk.[7] Consequently, nosocomial pneumonia increases total costs of care by prolonging hospitalization and requiring expensive antibiotic and supportive therapy. It is estimated that this infection lengthens hospital stay by an additional 7 to 9 days, costing an additional $2 billion annually.[10] The total cost of treating community- and hospital-acquired pneumonia is estimated to be as high as $23 billion each year ($14 billion in direct care costs and $9 billion in lost wages).[3]

PATHOPHYSIOLOGY

Host Defenses and Pathogenesis

The body's defense mechanisms against lower respiratory tract (LRT) infections comprise a complex and integrated system. Intact defense mechanisms help maintain a nearly sterile environment from the larynx to the terminal airways and can be divided into four groups: (1) mechanical, (2) phagocytic, (3) immunologic, and (4) secretory. A delicate balance exists between host defenses and exposure to infectious pathogens. Pneumonia occurs when this balance is disrupted. Specifically, infection occurs when there is a defect in the host defenses, exposure to a particularly virulent organism, exposure to an overwhelming number of organisms, or a combination of any of these events. Four pathologic mechanisms are involved in the development of pneumonia: (1) aspiration of oropharyngeal secretions, (2) inhalation of aerosolized organisms, (3) hematogenous spread, and, less commonly, (4) contiguous spread by direct extension of infections from adjacent tissues.

The lung defenses originate in the upper respiratory tract (URT), which consists of the anterior nares, nasopharynx, oropharynx, and larynx. The basic hemodynamic design of the URT provides the initial, important filtration barrier against potential pathogens and foreign material. Large particles are filtered and trapped by the hair and mucus in the nares. Swirling air currents in the URT cause impaction of smaller particles that penetrate through the nares, get trapped on the mucous membranes of the nasopharynx, and are then expelled or swallowed. The lungs consist of branching airways (bronchi) that ultimately terminate into thin-walled sacs called alveoli. The surface of the LRT is lined with mucus-secreting cells interspersed among ciliated columnar epithelial cells and makes up the mucociliary transport system. This transport system, which terminates before reaching the alveoli, consists of millions of cilia that beat approximately 1000 times/min, creating an efficient transport system for foreign material, macrophages, and lung secretions away from the smaller airways.[11] Smaller particles escaping the initial filtration defense mechanisms of the URT are removed by the mucociliary transport system into the oropharynx where they are coughed up and swallowed or expectorated. Dysfunction of the mucociliary transport system results in the inability to effectively remove matter, including microorganisms, from the lower airways and may be caused by several factors (Table 67.1). Chronic lung disease, aging, and smoking create a disproportionate ratio of mucus-secreting cells to ciliated epithelial cells, overwhelming the mucociliary transport system with excessive secretions that hinder efficient function. This situation provides an environment for bacterial overgrowth called colonization. Subsequently, colonization with pathogenic organisms occurs, making these persons more susceptible to the development of pneumonia. Particles >1 μm may escape the mucociliary transport system and reach the alveoli. Alveolar macrophages are the predominant resident phagocytic cells found in the alveoli, interstitial spaces, and surfaces of the airways.[11] Their primary responsibility is to handle foreign material and microorganisms that have successfully passed through the mucociliary transport system. Low numbers of microorganisms reaching this level are easily removed by alveolar macrophage ingestion (phagocytosis) in the immunocompetent host (Fig. 67.1).[12] Encapsulated bacteria such as *Streptococcus pneumoniae* and certain types of *Haemophilus influenzae* must be opsonized before phagocytosis can take place. Phagocytes containing bacteria remnants are removed by way of the mucociliary transport system and expectorated or swallowed. It has been estimated that as many as 5 million macrophages leave the lung by this route every hour.[13] If the host is challenged by a virulent pathogen or a high number of organisms, alveolar macrophages and the few available pulmonary polymorphonuclear neutrophils (PMNs) are unable to resolve the insult. When this occurs, chemotactic agents and immunoglobulins recruit extrapulmonary PMNs via the alternative and classical pathways of the complement system (Fig. 67.1). The outcome of this recruitment is a more intense inflammatory response that causes exudation and edema and results in the classic pathogenic condition of pneumonia. Numerous factors may interfere with the phagocytic activity of alveolar macrophages, recruitment of PMNs, or host immunity and predispose the patient to the development of pneumonia (Table 67.2). Pulmonary secretions in the mucosal airway and alveoli consist of surfactant, transferrin, immunoglo-

Table 67.1 ▪ Factors That Diminish Mucociliary Transport of Cellular and Bacterial Debris from the Lower Airways

Smoking	Cystic fibrosis
Chronic bronchitis	Viral infection
Immotile cilia syndrome	Aging
Chronic obstructive pulmonary disease	Inhalation of toxic substances
Asthma	Hyperoxia

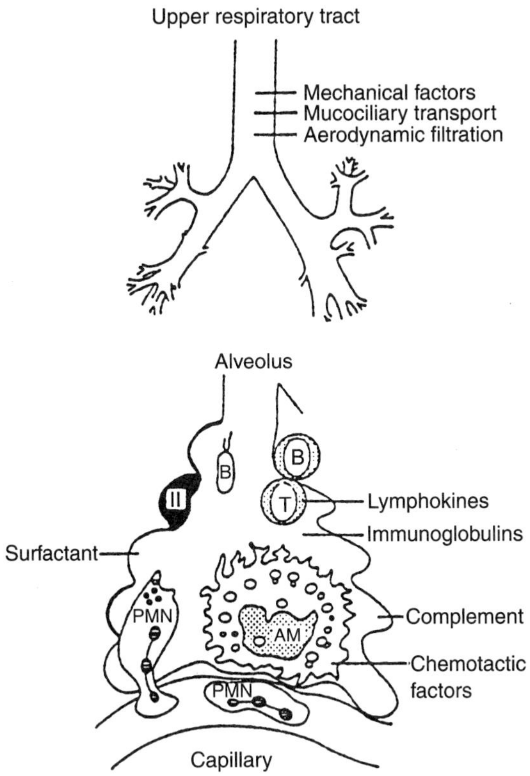

Figure 67.1. Defense mechanisms of the lung. (Reprinted with permission from Reynolds HY. Host defense impairments that may lead to respiratory infections. Clin Chest Med 8[3]:344, 1987.)

bulins, complement, and free fatty acids that are bacteriocidal and contribute to host defenses.[11]

Viruses compromise ciliary function and impair alveolar macrophage activity. In addition, interactions may occur between respiratory viruses and bacteria that increase either the severity or the likelihood of bacterial pneumonia.[11] Patients who become infected with the influenza A virus are at a higher risk for development of a secondary bacterial pneumonia, predominantly by *Staphylococcus aureus* and *S. pneumoniae*.

Cell-mediated immunity is an important host defense mechanism that enhances phagocytosis in response to cytokine production, but it may also result in lung injury leading to pneumonia. T cells are important in eliminating pathogens such as *Mycobacterium* sp., *Mycoplasma pneumoniae*, *Legionella* sp., and fungi that can survive inside the macrophage. In addition to being susceptible to pneumonia secondary to defects in cellular immunity, persons with acquired immunodeficiency syndrome (AIDS) are also more susceptible to pneumonia caused by encapsulated organisms such as *S. pneumoniae* and *H. influenzae* because of defects in humoral immunity. The reader should refer to Chapter 77 for a more detailed discussion of pneumonia in patients with AIDS.

The oropharynx contains a consistent variety of microbial flora including both aerobic and anaerobic Gram-positive and Gram-negative organisms called normal flora (Table 67.3). Normal oral secretions contain approximately 10^8 aerobic organisms/mL and 10 times as many anaerobic organisms, which present a large bacterial challenge to the LRT daily.[14] Oropharyngeal anaerobic organisms help maintain a normal and healthy bacterial homeostasis, which resists overgrowth of other potentially pathogenic organisms.[15] In the immunocompetent host, IgA, lysozyme, and glycoproteins found in saliva and on mucosal surfaces inhibit bacterial adherence and abnormal proliferation. Thus, in the normal host, few pathogenic Gram-negative bacteria are able to colonize the mucosa of the oropharynx or upper airways. Bacterial colonization is an important and critical first step for the development of hospital-acquired (nosocomial) pneumonia and also for the development of CAP in chronically ill or elderly patients. These patients and patients who have had surgery exhibit a higher incidence of colonization with pathogenic Gram-negative organisms, including *Pseudomonas aeruginosa*, because of a lack of these protective oropharyngeal factors.[11] The balance of oropharyngeal normal flora and the beneficial effects of resistance to colonization exerted by mouth anaerobes can also be disturbed by the administration of antibiotics.[15] Any factor that disrupts oropharyngeal bacterial homeostasis may predispose the host to colonization and, ultimately, pneumonia.[11] In contrast, the prevalence of Gram-negative pathogens in the oropharynx of normal subjects is very low, even when they are exposed to a hospital environment.[13] Table 67.4 lists risk factors that may increase oropharyngeal bacterial colonization.

Table 67.2 ▪ Factors Associated with Diminished Alveolar Macrophage Activity and Chemotaxis

Chronic	Acute
Alcohol ingestion	Bacterial endotoxin
Advanced age	Hypoxemia
Diabetes mellitus	Metabolic acidosis
Sickle cell disease	Pulmonary edema
Malnutrition	Uremia
Immunosuppressive drugs	Hyperoxia
Corticosteroid treatment	Mechanical obstruction
Hypogammaglobulinemia	Viral infection
Chronic obstructive pulmonary disease	
Acquired immune deficiency syndrome	
Malignancies	
Cystic fibrosis	

Table 67.3 ▪ Normal Flora of the Oropharynx

Streptococcus pneumoniae	*Haemophilus influenzae*
Streptococcus *pyogenes*	*Neisseria* spp.
Streptococcus viridans	Corynebacteria
Staphylococcus aureus	Lactobacillaceae
Moraxella (*Branhamella*) *catarrhalis*	Various anaerobes

Table 67.4 ▪ Factors That Increase Gram-Negative Bacterial Colonization

Malnutrition	Prolonged hospitalization
Chronic illness	Antacids
Advanced age	H_2 blockers
Nursing home residence	Antibiotic use
Surgery	Ventilator assistance
Cigarette smoking	Intensive care unit stay

Source: References 7, 8, 11, 18.

Mechanisms of Pathogenesis

Aspiration of oropharyngeal contents is the most common route for microbial access to the LRT and is the most frequent mechanism responsible for the development of both community-acquired and nosocomial pneumonia. Microaspiration of oral secretions is a normal physiologic phenomenon that occurs in 70% of healthy subjects during sleep[8] and rarely leads to infection in the normal host with intact defense mechanisms. Normal epiglottic closure and cough reflex resulting in expulsion from the lung are important pulmonary defense mechanisms that aid in preventing aspiration. Coughing allows aspirated material, excessive secretions, and foreign material in the trachea or major bronchi to be removed quickly from the airways. Factors that compromise epiglottic closure and the ability to cough are associated with a higher incidence of pneumonia (Table 67.5).

There is strong evidence for a causal relationship between gastric colonization with Gram-negative bacilli and the development of nosocomial pneumonia due to aspiration or translocation of these organisms.[16] Normal gastric pH and gastrointestinal (GI) motility serve as protective factors against overgrowth of endogenous and exogenous sources of bacteria in the stomach. Upper GI bleeding due to stress ulcers is a significant cause of morbidity and mortality among critically ill hospitalized patients.[9] However, the use of antacids and H_2 antagonists in the ICU for stress ulcer prophylaxis is associated with gastric colonization with Gram-negative organisms. A direct relationship exists between the increase in gastric pH and the number of Gram-negative organisms isolated from the stomach.[16] The significance of this finding is still being studied. In a prospective randomized trial, Driks et al.[17] observed a lower rate of pneumonia and a significantly lower mortality rate for patients receiving mechanical ventilation in the ICU treated with sucralfate than for patients treated with H_2 antagonists combined with antacids for stress ulcer prophylaxis. However, the lower rate of pneumonia observed in this study did not reach statistical significance. Despite the established efficacy of sucralfate in preventing stress ulcers, further studies are needed that clearly establish its superiority over other antiulcer agents in preventing nosocomial pneumonia in critically ill patients receiving stress ulcer prophylaxis.

There is additional evidence that supports the reduction or elimination of Gram-negative bacteria in the GI tract to minimize the occurrence of nosocomial pneumonia in the ICU setting.[18] Selective decontamination of the digestive tract has been used as an effective means of preventing nosocomial pneumonia in patients receiving mechanical ventilation in the ICU.[16] However, results from these trials should be accepted with caution because of study flaws and legitimate concerns regarding bacterial resistance.[9,16]

Inhalation of aerosolized organisms is a less common pathogenic mechanism responsible for pneumonia. However, for organisms such as *Legionella pneumophila* and *Mycobacterium tuberculosis*, this is a primary means of access to the LRT to cause infection. In addition, airborne transmission of viral agents, such as respiratory syncytial virus (RSV) and influenza A, is the most common cause of nosocomial pulmonary infections in pediatric wards and possibly in other hospital settings as well.[13] Improperly cleaned respiratory devices, particularly those that deliver aerosols, provide a potential source of microorganisms when used in the hospital setting. Nosocomial pneumonia may occur by this mechanism in any hospitalized patient. However, when these devices are used for patients receiving mechanical ventilation support, the URT defense mechanisms and cough reflex are bypassed by the endotracheal tube, allowing microorganisms direct access into the LRT. Some researchers refer to occurrence of pneumonia resulting from the use of these devices as direct inoculation.[13] Proper cleaning of respiratory equipment and good infection control procedures are essential and are associated with a reduced incidence of nosocomial pneumonia in the hospital and ICU setting.[19] The Centers for Disease Control and Prevention (CDC) and the American Thoracic Society have published extensive and comprehensive guidelines for the prevention of nosocomial pneumonia.[19,20]

Hematogenous seeding of the lungs and contiguous spread by direct extension of infections from adjacent tissues are pathogenic mechanisms that rarely cause pneumonia. Right-sided endocarditis and septic pelvic thrombophlebitis are infections that may cause pneumonia when the infecting organism from these respective sites travels through the bloodstream and seeds the lung tissue. Hematogenous spread may also be a unique mechanism

Table 67.5 ▪ Factors That Decrease the Cough Reflex and Increase the Risk of Aspiration, Leading to Pneumonia

Delayed gastric emptying	General anesthesia
Supine position during enteral feeding	Drugs that impair mental status
Alcohol intoxication	Nasogastric intubation
Seizure	Endotracheal intubation
Stroke	Tracheostomy

Source: References 13, 15.

causing pneumonia due to *Escherichia coli* in the patient with urosepsis.[13] Contiguous spread is very uncommon, but has occurred in patients with hepatic abscess.[21]

CLINICAL PRESENTATION AND DIAGNOSIS

Signs and Symptoms

An adequate history is helpful and should be obtained from all patients. Mandell[1] recommends that the history should attempt to define (1) the clinical setting of the pneumonia, (2) any defects in host defense mechanisms that may predispose the patient to the development of pneumonia, and (3) exposure to specific pathogens. The age of the patient and any underlying diseases should be noted. Factors predictive of a more severe course and death due to CAP should be recognized and include advanced age, absence of pleuritic chest pain, tachypnea, hypotension, confusion, elevated blood urea nitrogen level, leukopenia, and digoxin toxicity.[3] Patients having one or more of these should be considered for hospitalization. The physical examination is an essential component in evaluating the patient with pneumonia. Abnormal vital signs include fever, tachypnea, and tachycardia. The pulse usually increases by 10 bpm for every degree centigrade of temperature elevation.[22] Bradycardia may suggest pneumonia caused by *M. pneumoniae, Chlamydia* sp., *Legionella* sp., or infection with a viral agent.[22] Although tachypnea and tachycardia may be present in many patients with pneumonia, these are the most sensitive but least specific signs of pneumonia in older adults.[23] Auscultation of the lung usually reveals fine crackling rales and diminished breath sounds over the affected area. In the presence of pleural effusion, breath sounds may appear diminished or may even be absent. In the presence of a consolidated pneumonia, sound transmission may be improved, have a more tubular quality, and have a more pronounced expiratory phase.[24] Sound transmission can also be assessed without auscultation. Spoken or whispered sounds transmitted through a consolidated area of lung result in bronchophony and whispered pectoriloquy, respectively.[24] Egophony is a nasal or bleating sound that may be present in the patient with pneumonia. Egophony is evident when the sound of a spoken "E" is heard by the examiner to sound like an "A." Percussion dullness and lack of normal resonance are evident in approximately 30% of patients and indicate the presence of consolidation.[3] The patient may exhibit restricted movement on the affected side and obtain relief by lying on that side.[25] Cyanosis due to hypoxia occurs secondary to poor ventilation and may suggest severe pneumonia and the need for hospitalization and oxygen supplementation.

Laboratory evaluation usually reveals an elevated white blood cell (WBC) count with an increased number of immature banded neutrophils (left shift). Approximately 20 to 30% of patients will have positive blood cultures and isolation of a pathogen from this source strongly suggests the etiology of the pneumonia.[4,26] Blood samples for arterial blood gases and routine chemistry should be obtained from the patient who has severe symptoms, dehydration, or cyanosis, or who requires hospitalization. Classic symptoms of bacterial pneumonia include rapid onset, fever, chills, pleuritic chest pain, and cough that is productive of purulent sputum. Ten to 30% of patients with bacterial pneumonia also complain of headache, nausea, vomiting, abdominal pain, diarrhea, myalgia, and arthralgia.[3] In 1938, Reimann first separated pneumonia syndromes into "typical" and "atypical" based on observations of the clinical presentation.[6] He recognized that some patients failed to exhibit the classic symptoms of bacterial pneumonia (fever, rapid onset of infection, purulent sputum production, and elevated WBC count), while others were observed to atypically have a milder fever, a more insidious onset of infection, cough without production of purulent sputum, a normal WBC count, and an overall milder infection. Atypical presentations are sometimes associated with more nonspecific extrapulmonary manifestations such as abdominal pain, diarrhea, and confusion. Consequently, diagnosis of pneumonia is sometimes more difficult in patients who exhibit atypical symptoms. Pneumonia caused by *M. pneumoniae, Chlamydia* sp., *Legionella* sp., viruses, and others account for some of these atypical presentations.

A number of studies have found that distinguishing between typical and atypical clinical presentations lacks utility.[6] For example, elderly patients and those who are chronically ill, both of whom represent a large proportion of patients with pneumonia, often do not demonstrate the classic symptoms of pneumonia described above, despite being infected with a typical bacterial pathogen. Pneumonia in elderly patients is more often associated with a lower incidence of fever or productive cough and a higher incidence of mental status changes, tachypnea, tachycardia, bacteremia, and death.[27] Therefore, caution should be exercised when interpreting the presenting signs and symptoms as being "typical" or "atypical." Nevertheless, the reader should be knowledgeable of the distinctions between them because they can be helpful when assessing some patients, and the terms are widely accepted and used in clinical settings, albeit sometimes incorrectly.

Diagnosis

Diagnosis of pneumonia is based on clinical, radiologic, laboratory, and microbiologic findings. No single test is capable of determining the cause of pneumonia. A lateral and posterior-anterior chest radiograph is one of the most important tools used to diagnose pneumonia.[22,28–30] The chest roentgenogram also serves to establish a baseline to gauge therapeutic response to antimicrobial therapy and to assess complications.[28] Complications of pneumonia usually require hospitalization and include pleural effusion, abscess, empyema, and cavitation. If significant pleural effusion is present, a diagnostic thoracentesis for culture and sensitivity information should be performed. The classic pneumonia chest radiograph usually reveals an infiltrate (area of consolidation) in one or more lobes of the lung, either unilaterally or bilaterally.[12] Often, however, the radiograph displays a pattern of nonlobar or diffuse involvement termed bronchopneumonia. Underlying illnesses, especially exacerbation of congestive heart failure (CHF), malignancy, chronic obstructive pulmonary disease (COPD), and adult respiratory distress syndrome (ARDS) increase the difficulty of radiologic interpretation, thereby sometimes obscuring the diagnosis of pneumonia in these patients.[31] Patients who are dehydrated at initial presentation may be less likely to have evidence of pneumonia on the chest radiograph. Despite this purported observation, it has not consistently been demonstrated in animal and human models and is only validated from a few case reports.[3,31] Although certain radiologic patterns may be observed that suggest the presence of a specific pathogen, an etiologic diagnosis cannot be reliably made by the chest radiograph appearance alone. The chest radiograph is also useful in distinguishing those with bronchitis from those with pneumonia.[32]

Despite controversy over the reliability of microscopic examination of the sputum Gram stain, it remains the primary tool for determining the etiology of pneumonia and should be obtained from all patients with CAP.[28] The Gram stain of an adequate sputum sample allows the clinician to make a presumptive diagnosis of the cause of the pneumonia and promptly initiate the appropriate antibiotic. Much of the controversy surrounding reliability of the Gram stain is its reported lack of sensitivity and specificity in some clinical trials. Strict criteria have been established and should be used when microscopically examining the Gram stain. An adequate sample contains >25 PMNs and <10 squamous epithelial cells per low power field and a predominating pathogen.[33] When these criteria are used and proper technique is followed, contamination with oropharyngeal flora is less likely and sensitivity can be as high as 85% in determining the etiology of the pneumonia.[22,30] Specimens meeting these criteria are also suitable for culture, allowing antibiotic sensitivities to be established. Unfortunately, children, older adults, and uncooperative patients are not always able to elicit a deep enough cough to produce an adequate sputum sample, hindering the identification of a pathogen. In such cases, an induced sputum collection using nebulized albuterol, saline, or hypertonic saline may be helpful. Proper technique in the procurement of the sputum sample is very important as well. Improper collection or transport to the laboratory will result in culture contamination that represents normal oropharyngeal flora and can lead to false-positive or false-negative culture results that do not represent the organism at the site of infection. Experts recommend that the ideal sputum specimen be produced from a deep cough obtained before initiation of antibiotics, then rapidly transported, and properly processed in the laboratory within 1 to 2 hours after collection.[34] Pneumonia caused by atypical pathogens (*Legionella* sp., *Chlamydia* sp., *M. pneumoniae*, or viral agents) may be suggested in an alert and cooperative patient who fails to cough up purulent sputum or has a Gram stain with high numbers of PMNs and low numbers of squamous epithelial cells but without bacteria.[28,32]

When an adequate sputum sample cannot be obtained, invasive diagnostic procedures may be used to determine the etiology of the pneumonia. Invasive procedures are generally reserved for those who are severely ill or for the patient with unresolving pneumonia. Transtracheal aspiration (TTA) is an invasive procedure in which a 14-gauge needle is inserted through the cricothyroid membrane into the trachea below the level of the larynx, but not reaching the lower peripheral airways.[26,28] At this position, the tracheobronchial tree is normally sterile and the isolation of a pathogen usually indicates the cause of the pneumonia.[13] TTA is particularly helpful in diagnosing pneumonia caused by anaerobic pathogens.[12,13] However, the popularity of TTA has decreased, and it is used less often because of the risk of complications and need for expertise in performing this procedure. Sputum Gram stain meeting the criteria of >25 PMNs and <10 squamous epithelial cells per low power field closely reflected specimens obtained by TTA from similar patients in one study.[33] Hence, collection of an adequate sputum sample may supersede the need for TTA in most patients. In addition, TTA is an unreliable tool in the diagnosis of nosocomial pneumonia because of the presence of colonizing organisms in the area being sampled, resulting in a higher incidence of false-positive bacterial cultures.

Fiberoptic bronchoscopy is another invasive procedure used for diagnosing the presence and etiology of pneumonia. It is a relatively safe procedure, but is not without risks of complications. Therefore, it is usually reserved for critically ill or immunocompromised patients and the patient with nosocomial pneumonia who is receiving mechanical ventilation. Fiberoptic bronchoscopy provides the experienced pulmonologist direct access to the lower airways with the ability to visualize and sample tissues and secretions. Protected specimen brush (PSB) and bronchoalveolar lavage (BAL) are two diagnostic procedures used with fiberoptic bronchoscopy. If correctly performed, both have high sensitivity and specificity for determining the cause of pneumonia. A potential advantage of BAL over PSB is its ability to sample a larger area of the lung, allowing the clinician to microscopically examine the specimen after the procedure.[26] Samples obtained using either PSB or BAL are suitable for culture using quantitative techniques.

Transthoracic needle aspiration is an invasive procedure that is seldom used in the diagnosis of pneumonia due to its risks of serious complications and the evolution of safer fiberoptic bronchoscopy techniques. Open lung biopsy provides the least contaminated specimens. However, because of the risk of complications and controversy over its benefits, it is usually reserved for diagnosing complicated or unresolving pneumonia in patients with AIDS and in other immunosuppressed patients.[26]

Immunoassays and serologic tests used for the identification of antibodies or bacterial and viral antigens of various bodily fluids and surfaces include compliment fixation, microimmunofluorescence, polymerase chain reaction (PCR), DNA probes, cold agglutination, counterimmunoelectrophoresis (CIE), direct fluorescent antibody (DFA), and enzyme-linked immunosorbent assay.[23,35] CIE has been used to detect antigens in various body fluids including urine, serum, sputum, and pleural fluid.[12] Currently, because of their high expense, variable specificity and sensitivity, need for specialized medical technologists, and lack of U.S. Food and Drug administration (FDA) approval, many of these tests are used primarily to confirm a clinical diagnosis or for clinical trial purposes[22] and have yet to find their niche in identifying the causative organism of pneumonia in everyday clinical settings. An exception can be made for the *Legionella* urinary antigen detection kit, which is rapid, accurate, routinely used, and readily available in most hospital and reference laboratories. Serologic titers using immunofluorescence may be performed but, because of their delayed response, are more helpful for epidemiologic purposes than for acute diagnosis of pneumonia.

Types of Pneumonia

Community-Acquired Pneumonia

THERAPEUTIC PLAN

The treatment of CAP involves selection of the appropriate antibiotic(s) and the provision of supportive care if required. The patient's age, coexisting diseases, and the setting in which the pneumonia occurs often suggest the most likely infecting organism and, therefore, the most logical empiric therapy. Many antibiotics are currently available and are effective in the treatment of pneumonia. Antibiotic choice should be individualized for the patient and take into consideration the spectrum of activity, pharmacokinetics, adverse effects, clinical efficacy, patient outcomes, and cost. The need for hospitalization and whether the patient's condition necessitates parenteral antibiotic therapy must also be considered.

Investigators from the pneumonia Patient Outcomes Research Team have developed and validated a reliable model to distinguish those patients with CAP at risk of death.[36] Their prediction rule takes into account 5 patient stratifications and 19 variables using a cumulative point system (Fig. 67.2).[34,36] Such a model can be used to help physicians make more consistent and reliable hospital admission decisions regarding patients with CAP but should not be used in lieu of good clinical judgment. Other factors that influence the decision to hospitalize include availability of home support, reliability of antibiotic compliance, and availability of alternative settings for supervised care.[34]

TREATMENT

Empiric treatment of CAP should always be effective for the most common pathogen, *S. pneumoniae*. Many clinicians also prefer to cover the "atypical" pathogens empirically as well (*Legionella* sp., *Chlamydia* sp., and *M. pneumoniae*). The reader should recognize that many guidelines for the empiric treatment of CAP have been published. Sometimes these guidelines are influenced by both personal preference and scientific data and may even differ slightly based on geographic location. The Infectious Diseases Society of America (IDSA) has established guidelines for the management of CAP in immunocompetent adults.[34] These guidelines appear to be more straightforward compared to previous published guidelines.[4] A modified version of these guidelines can be found in Table 67.6 and serves as a reasonable approach to empiric therapy for CAP. Table 67.7 lists treatment of pneumonia according to pathogen once it is reliably identified.[34]

Generally, antibiotics chosen for initial empiric therapy should have a reasonably broad spectrum of activity against the most likely pathogens. Factors that influence the selection of empiric therapy include Gram stain results, comorbidity necessitating a need to protect against a broader spectrum of pathogens, drug allergies, severity of the pneumonia, the setting of treatment (inpatient or outpatient), antibiotic cost, patient convenience as it relates to compliance, and geographic location. These factors comprise an important and individualized role in the initial selection of an empiric antibiotic. The most cost-effective agent should be chosen. This decision should include consideration of length of hospital stay, if the patient is to be hospitalized, and patient outcome. In some instances, the most cost-effective therapy may be a more expensive antibiotic that prevents the need for hospitalization or gets the patient out of the hospital faster. Such a choice may serve to cut total costs of care more than using a less expensive antibiotic.

Every effort should be made to obtain sputum specimens, blood cultures, and other appropriate diagnostic specimens for culture before initiation of antibiotics. In

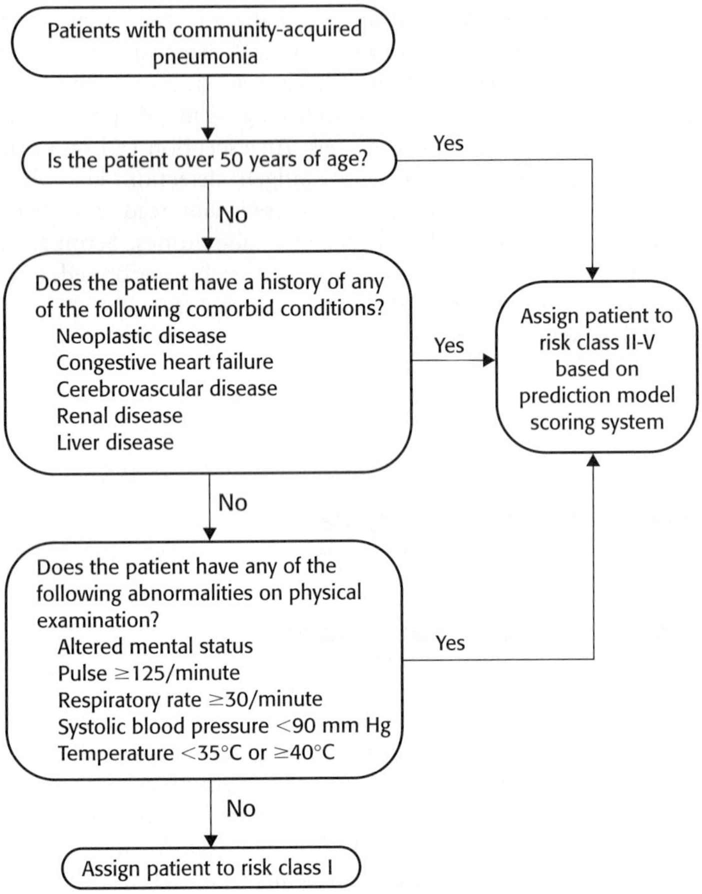

Scoring System

Patient Characteristic	Points Assigned[a]
Demographic factors	
Age: males	age (in yrs)
females	age (in yrs) −10
Nursing home resident	+10
Comorbid illnesses	
Neoplastic disease	+30
Liver disease	+20
Congestive heart failure	+10
Cerebrovascular disease	+10
Renal disease	+10
Physical examination findings	
Altered mental status	+20
Respiratory rate ≥30/minute	+20
Systolic blood pressure <90 mm Hg	+20
Temperature <35°C or ≥40°C	+15
Pulse ≥125/minute	+10
Laboratory findings	
pH <7.35	+30
BUN >10.7 mmol/L	+20
Sodium <130 mEq/L	+20
Glucose >13.9 mmol/L	+10
Hematocrit <30%	+10
PO_2 <60 mm Hg[b]	+10
Pleural effusion	+10

[a] A risk score (total point score) for a given patient is obtained by summing the patient age in years (age −10 for females) and the points for each applicable patient characteristic.

[b] Oxygen saturation <90% also was considered abnormal.

Stratification of Risk Score

Risk	Risk Class	Based on
Low	I	Algorithm
	II	≤70 total points
	III	71–90 total points
Moderate	IV	91–130 total points
High	V	>130 total points

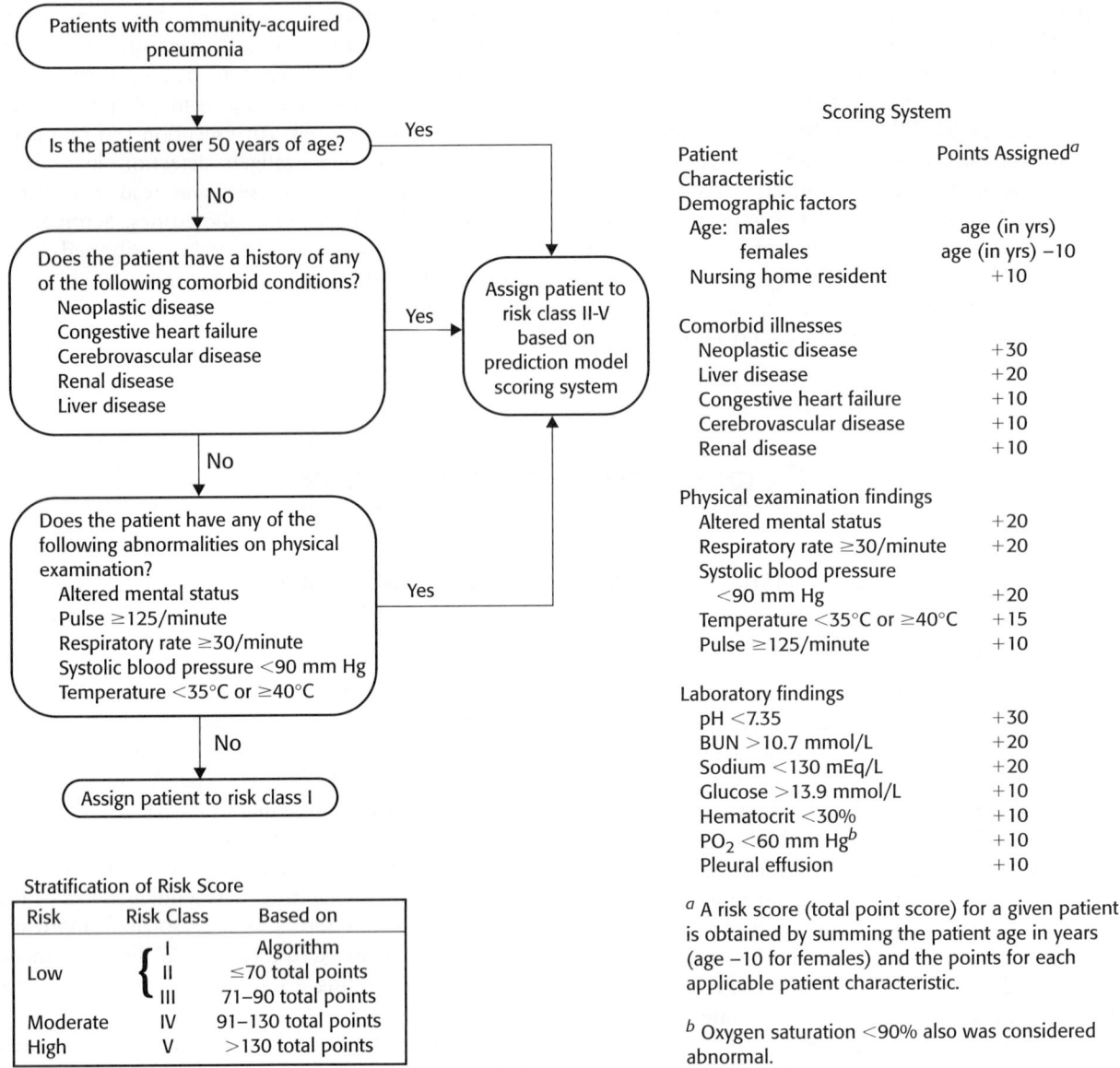

Figure 67.2. Prediction model for identifying and stratifying patient risk for persons with community-acquired pneumonia. (Reprinted with permission from Barlett JG, Breiman RF, Mandell LA, et al. Community-acquired pneumonia in adults: guidelines for management. Clin Infect Dis 26:811–838, 1998.)

the outpatient setting, the clinician may only obtain a sputum specimen for Gram staining and culture. In the hospitalized patient, blood cultures should be drawn from two separate sites 10 or more minutes apart.[34] Obtaining pretreatment specimens should not significantly delay the first dose of antibiotic, especially in elderly or critically ill patients. Meehan et al.[37] found that elderly patients who received the first dose of antibiotic longer than 8 hours after admission to the hospital had a higher mortality than those patients who received antibiotics sooner. Antibiotic therapy should be initiated promptly after diagnosis, and subsequent doses should be given on time until therapy is completed. Likewise, the ambulatory patient should be counseled to complete the full course of antibiotic despite achievement of physical improvement.

The sputum Gram stain results can and should aid in the selection of empiric therapy. However, in some clinical settings, a pathogen is not identified in up to 50% or more of patients with pneumonia,[6] necessitating the use of empiric therapy throughout the clinical course. If the Gram stain is equivocal or not available, empiric therapy must be based on the most likely organisms and patient characteristics (Table 67.6). Therefore, adequate knowledge of the most likely pathogens is essential to initiate treatment with the appropriate antimicrobial agent. Once the causative organism has been reliably identified by culture and antibiotic sensitivities are established, a narrow-spectrum agent can be and should be substituted. Such a substitution is clinically sound, saves money, and reduces the likelihood of resistance. This type of substitution can be easily made in the hospital setting but is perceived to be impractical in the ambulatory setting and typically does not occur there. Approximately 75% of patients with CAP will be treated as outpatients.[34] In actual practice, ambulatory patients may or may not have a sputum culture performed and will be given a full course of antibiotics during the initial presentation. Furthermore, ambulatory patients may not return to the provider before antibiotics are completed unless a clinical response is not achieved. This underscores the importance of appropriate empiric antibiotic selection, especially in the outpatient setting where the antibiotic is not likely to be changed based on culture results.

Generally, patients admitted to the hospital will receive intravenous antibiotics initially. However, there are no pneumonia studies that have proven a superior outcome for parenteral antibiotics compared to oral antibiotics with good bioavailability.[34] Oral antibiotic therapy can be considered in the initial management of the hospitalized patient with CAP when the drug has adequate oral bioavailability and activity[34] and the patient does not have a malabsorption syndrome, cannot tolerate oral therapy, or is not critically ill. Table 67.8[38] lists examples of antibiotics with good oral bioavailability. Because the majority of patients hospitalized for CAP are managed initially with relatively expensive intravenous antibiotics, emphasis has been placed on the appropriate time to switch to oral therapy. The IDSA recommends that a switch to oral therapy is appropriate when the patient's condition is clinically improving and the patient is hemodynamically stable, able to take medication by mouth, and has a functioning GI tract.[34] In general, most patients who respond to initial therapy meet these criteria by day 3 of therapy, and the switch to oral therapy is made at that time.[34] Other experts state that a change to oral therapy should only be made when the patient's clinical condition has stabilized and fever has subsided.[4] Percutaneous endoscopic gastrostomy tube or nasogastric feeding tube administration may also be considered in patients meeting the above criteria, barring drug-nutrient interactions.

Once antibiotic therapy is initiated, it should not be changed during the first 72 hours unless the patient exhibits significant clinical deterioration, experiences adverse effects, or unless specific diagnostic information, such as culture and sensitivity data, become available, permitting an appropriate change.

Table 67.6 ▪ Guidelines for the Selection of Empiric Antibiotic Therapy for Patients with Community-Acquired Pneumonia

Outpatients
- Generally preferred: macrolide,[a] quinolone,[b] or doxycycline
- Modifying factors
  - Suspected penicillin resistant *Streptococcus pneumoniae:* quinolone[b]
  - Suspected aspiration: clindamycin *OR* amoxicillin/clavulanate
  - Young adult (>17–40 years): doxycycline

Hospitalized patients
- General medical ward
  - Generally preferred: third-generation cephalosporin[c] with or without a macrolide[a] *OR* a quinolone[b] (alone)
  - Alternatives: cefuroxime with or without a macrolide[a] *OR* azithromycin (alone)
- Intensive care unit
  - Generally preferred: erythromycin or azithromycin *PLUS* cefotaxime, ceftriaxone, or ampicillin/sulbactam. *ADD* clindamycin or metronidazole if anaerobes (aspiration) suspected unless ampicillin/sulbactam selected
  - Alternatives[d]: levofloxacin *PLUS* clindamycin
- Modifying factors
  - Structural disease of the lung: antipseudomonal penicillin, cefepime, or a carbapenem[e] *PLUS* an aminoglycoside or a quinolone[b] *PLUS* a macrolide[a]
  - β-Lactam allergy: a quinolone[b]
  - Suspected or witnessed aspiration: levofloxacin *PLUS* either clindamycin or metronidazole, *OR* β-lactam/β-lactamase inhibitor combination[f] (alone)

Source: References 4, 34.

[a]Erythromycin, azithromycin, or clarithromycin. Erythromycin and azithromycin are available in oral and intravenous dosage form. Erythromycin is the least expensive of these agents.

[b]Levofloxacin, grepafloxacin, sparfloxacin, or other new quinolones with enhanced activity against *Streptococcus pneumoniae*. Levofloxacin is available in oral and intravenous dosage forms.

[c]Cefotaxime or ceftriaxone.

[d]These alternatives may be a more desirable choice if there is high suspicion of penicillin-resistant *S. pneumoniae.*

[e]Imipenem or meropenem.

[f]Ampicillin/sulbactam, piperacillin/tazobactam, or ticarcillin/clavulanate.

Pharmacokinetic Considerations

A tenet of successful antibiotic treatment of infectious diseases requires that the agent reach an effective concentration at the site of infection. To date, there are no reliable studies proving that intrapulmonary concentration measurement from any lung tissue site is a better predictor of efficacy than serum concentrations in the treatment of pneumonia.[39] However, it is logical to assume that concentration at the site is relevant and is an area that merits further study, specifically as it relates to clinical outcome. Lung epithelial lining fluid (ELF) concentrations of antimicrobial agents probably represent the most clinically relevant measurement for treating pneumonia.[39] However, determination and interpretation of ELF concentrations may sometimes be methodologically flawed and in need of standardization.[39] Most antibiotics reach the infected lung tissue by passive diffusion across the blood-bronchoalveolar barrier. Diffusion is dependent on the degree of ionization, concentration gradient, and pharmacokinetic properties of the drug (size, lipid solubility, and protein binding).[40] Antibiotics that are un-ionized and lipophilic penetrate into lung tissue most readily, and inflamed lung tissue may enhance the permeability of drugs as well.[40] Because albumin is too large to gain access into the lung by passive diffusion through pulmonary capillary pores, a high affinity for protein binding may

Table 67.7 ▪ Treatment of Pneumonia According to Pathogen

Pathogen	Preferred Antimicrobial	Alternative Antimicrobial
Streptococcus pneumoniae Penicillin-susceptible (MIC, <0.1 μg/mL)	Penicillin G or penicillin V, amoxicillin	Cephalosporins,[a] macrolides,[b] clindamycin, fluoroquinolones,[c] doxycycline
Intermediately penicillin-resistant (MIC, 0.1–1 μg/mL)	Parenteral penicillin G, ceftriaxone or cefotaxime, amoxicillin, fluoroquinolones[c]; other agents based on in vitro susceptibility test results	Clindamycin, doxycycline, oral cephalosporins[a]
Highly penicillin-resistant[d] (MIC, ≥2 μg/mL)	Agents based on in vitro susceptibility results, fluoroquinolones,[c] vancomycin	
Empirical selection	Fluoroquinolones[c]; selection based on susceptibility test results in community[e]	Clindamycin, doxycycline, vancomycin
	Penicillin[f]	Cephalosporins,[a] macrolides,[b] amoxicillin, clindamycin
Haemophilus influenzae	Second- or third-generation cephalosporins, doxycycline, β-lactam/β-lactamase inhibitor, fluoroquinolones[c]	Azithromycin, TMP-SMZ
Moraxella catarrhalis	Second- or third-generation cephalosporins, TMP-SMZ, amoxicillin/clavulanate	Macrolides,[b] fluoroquinolones,[c] β-lactam/β-lactamase inhibitor
Anaerobes	Clindamycin, penicillin plus metronidazole, β-lactam/β-lactamase inhibitor	Penicillin G or penicillin V, ampicillin/amoxicillin with or without metronidazole
Staphylococcus aureus[d] Methicillin-susceptible	Nafcillin/oxacillin with or without rifampin or gentamicin[d]	Cefazolin or cefuroxime, vancomycin, clindamycin, TMP-SMZ, fluoroquinolones[c]
Methicillin-resistant	Vancomycin with or without rifampin or gentamicin	Requires in vitro testing; TMP-SMZ
Enterobacteriaceae (coliforms: *Escherichia coli, Klebsiella, Proteus, Enterobacter*)[d]	Third-generation cephalosporin with or without an aminoglycoside, carbapenems[g]	Aztreonam, β-lactam/β-lactamase inhibitor, fluoroquinolones[c]
Pseudomonas aeruginosa[d]	Aminoglycoside plus antipseudomonal β-lactam: ticarcillin, piperacillin, mezlocillin, ceftazidime, cefepime, aztreonam, or carbapenems[g]	Aminoglycoside plus ciprofloxacin, ciprofloxacin plus antipseudomonal β-lactam
Legionella species	Macrolides[b] with or without rifampin, fluoroquinolones[c]	Doxycycline with or without rifampin
Mycoplasma pneumoniae	Doxycycline, macrolides,[b] fluoroquinolones[c]	
Chlamydia pneumoniae	Doxycycline, macrolides,[b] fluoroquinolones[c]	
Chlamydia psittaci	Doxycycline	Erthromycin, chloramphenicol
Nocardia species	Sulfonamide with or without minocycline or amikacin, TMP-SMZ	Imipenem with or without amikacin, doxycycline or minocycline
Coxiella burnetii[h]	Tetracycline	Chloramphenicol
Influenza A	Amantadine or rimantadine	
Hantavirus	None[i]	

Source: Reprinted with permission from Bartlett JG, Breiman RF, Mandell LA, et al. Community-acquired pneumonia in adults: guidelines for management. Clin Infect Dis 26:811–838, 1998.

MIC, minimum inhibitory concentration; *TMP-SMZ*, trimethoprim-sulfamethoxazole.

[a]Intravenous: cefazolin, cefuroxime, cefotaxime, ceftriaxone; oral: cefpodoxime, cefprozil, cefuroxime.

[b]Erythromycin, clarithromycin, or azithromycin.

[c]Levofloxacin, sparfloxacin, grepafloxacin, trovafloxacin, or another fluoroquinolone with enhanced activity against *S. pneumoniae*; ciprofloxacin is appropriate for *Legionella* species, fluoroquinolone-susceptible *S. aureus*, and most Gram-negative bacilli.

[d]In vitro susceptibility tests are required for optimal treatment; for *Enterobacter* species, the preferred antibiotics are fluoroquinolones and carbapenems.

[e]High rates of high-level penicillin resistance, susceptibility of community strains unknown, and/or patient is seriously ill.

[f]Low rates of penicillin resistance in community and patient is at low risk for infection with resistant *S. pneumoniae*.

[g]Imipenem and meropenem.

[h]Agent of Q fever.

[i]Provide supportive care.

decrease the ability of the drug to penetrate lung tissue.[1] It is important to consider all of the pharmacokinetic and pharmacodynamic properties of a drug when evaluating its appropriateness for the treatment of pneumonia. Specific bacteriologic properties may also influence antibiotic choice. Pneumonias caused by intracellular pathogens (*M. pneumoniae, Chlamydia* sp., *Legionella* sp.) respond more favorably to antibiotics that achieve therapeutic intracellular concentrations. If the patient has coexisting bacteremia, serum drug concentration is equally important.

Monitoring Response to Therapy

The expected response to antimicrobial therapy depends on the severity of the pneumonia, the pathogen being treated, host factors, chest radiographic findings, and antibiotic choice.[34] After initiation of appropriate antibiotic therapy, defervescence usually occurs within 48 to 72 hours and is generally the first sign of improvement. Complete defervescence can take as long as 5 to 7 days in patients who are immunosuppressed, have concurrent bacteremia, are elderly, or have Legionnaires' disease.[34] Most patients will show signs of subjective and objective improvement within 3 to 5 days as evidenced by a diminishing WBC count, normalization of oxygen saturation, and less dyspnea. Chest radiographic abnormalities are usually the last signs of pneumonia to resolve. In fact, some patients may exhibit a worsening of the radiographic appearance during the first several days of therapy. This is an expected occurrence and should not be interpreted as deterioration unless accompanied by clinical worsening as well. Most younger patients (<50 years old) and those without underlying disease states show complete resolution of chest radiographic abnormalities by 4 weeks.[34] In contrast, elderly patients or those with underlying diseases, particularly alcoholism and COPD, show radiographic clearing much more slowly.[34] Serial follow-up chest radiographs performed on the hospitalized patient are probably overused and unnecessary for resolution assessment, but may be appropriately used to detect complications and check the placement of intravenous lines or endotracheal tube.[34]

Follow-up blood or sputum cultures are not necessary for those who respond to therapy.[34] For those who do not respond to therapy, repeat culture information will usually reveal equivocal results that offer little help.

Pathogen-Specific Treatment

Table 67.7 shows treatment of pneumonia according to specific pathogen.

Pneumococcal Pneumonia

S. pneumoniae is the most common cause of CAP. It accounts for 10 to 25% of all cases of CAP[28,41] and may actually be responsible for more than 60% of cases.[31,34] Patients with classic pneumococcal pneumonia have abrupt onset of fever, a severe chill or rigor, pleuritic chest pain, and a cough productive of purulent, rust-colored sputum. Exceptions include elderly or chronically ill patients who may present with only tachypnea, tachycardia, and mental status changes. Gram stain of the sputum classically reveals many PMNs, few epithelial cells, and many lancet-shaped Gram-positive diplococci. Physical examination and chest radiograph are consistent with evidence of bacterial pneumonia. A unique finding in up to 40% of patients is evidence of herpes simplex (fever blisters).[22] Laboratory evaluation reveals an elevated WBC count of 10,000 to 35,000 cells/mm^3 with an increased number of immature banded neutrophils.

In the United States the drug of choice for pneumococcal pneumonia caused by penicillin-susceptible (minimum inhibitory concentration [MIC] <0.1 μg/mL) and intermediately susceptible (MIC 0.1 to 1.0 μg/mL) strains of *S. pneumoniae* is still penicillin. However, because of increased incidence of organisms resistant to penicillin in this country, it can no longer be safely recommended as empiric therapy for CAP. Historically, a higher incidence of pneumococcal resistance to penicillin has been seen in other countries such as New Guinea, Spain, Israel, Poland, Japan, and South Africa. Up to 62% of isolates in these countries have exhibited MICs for penicillin ranging from intermediately sensitive (MIC 0.1 to 1.0 μg/mL) to highly resistant (MIC ≥2.0 μg/mL).[41] In the United States, penicillin resistance has increased markedly during the last decade.[42] The CDC recently reported penicillin resistance in 6.6% of pneumococcal isolates in the United States.[43] In the recent multinational SENTRY antimicrobial resistance surveillance program only 56.2% of 845 *S. pneumoniae* isolates were susceptible to penicillin (MIC <0.1 μg/mL).[44] Despite this dramatic increase in resistance, no clinical failures have been documented in penicillin-treated patients with pneumonia attributed to *S. pneumoniae* exhibiting in vitro penicillin resistance.[34] Because of the lack of reported treatment failures despite an increasing resistance pattern, this phenomenon appears to be more of a penicillin tolerance, which will most likely over time continue to push MICs higher and higher. At present, appropriate empiric drug selection and the clinical correlation of in vitro resistance of *S. pneumoniae* to penicillin is not clear. Another troublesome observation is that other antibiotics that have historically been effective against *S. pneumoniae* (trimethoprim/sulfamethoxazole [TMP/SMZ], macrolides, and oral cephalosporins) are also becoming less effective against penicillin-resistant strains. In contrast, the newest generation of quinolones (levofloxacin, gatifloxacin, sparfloxacin, and trovafloxacin) exhibit good in vitro activity against penicillin- and multidrug-resistant strains of *S. pneumoniae*.[45] Resistance of *S. pneumoniae* to penicillin will continue to be a dynamic area of research, and the reader is encouraged to keep abreast of the current literature.

Appropriate empiric therapy for suspected pneumococcal pneumonia should take into account the geographic pattern of penicillin resistance, especially in children or others who have been exposed to many antibiotics. Severe

Table 67.8 ▪ Antibiotics with Excellent Oral Bioavailability and Equivalent to Intravenous Bioavailability

Trimethoprim/sulfamethoxazole	Ciprofloxacin
Clindamycin	Ofloxacin
Azithromycin	Levofloxacin
Metronidazole	Minocycline
Chloramphenicol	Doxycycline

Source: Reference 38.

concomitant infections, such as pneumococcal bacteremia or meningitis, must also be considered. Penicillin G should not be used for treatment of penicillin-resistant pneumococcal meningitis.[46] Patients seen with suspected pneumococcal CAP in regional settings where there is an increased prevalence of *S. pneumoniae* strains with high in vitro penicillin resistance (MIC ≥2.0 μg/mL) should probably receive empiric therapy with alternative agents such as vancomycin or one of the new generation fluoroquinolones (levofloxacin 500 mg PO every day or gatifloxacin or sparfloxacin).[34] In general practice, it may be reasonable to select an antibiotic that is likely to be effective for intermediately or highly resistant penicillin pneumococci until the sputum culture proves otherwise. This approach does present a dilemma to clinicians in the outpatient setting where patients may return only after antibiotics are completed or when no culture has been done or results are equivocal. Unfortunately with this approach, the potentially harmful consequences of using empiric broad-spectrum antibiotics in the ambulatory setting will continue to be present. When possible, empiric broad-spectrum therapy chosen initially should be appropriately changed to a more narrow spectrum agent when accurate culture and sensitivity information is available. Uncomplicated, mild pneumococcal pneumonia having a documented in vitro susceptibility or intermediate susceptibility to penicillin can usually be treated in the outpatient setting with amoxicillin 500 mg PO tid or penicillin V 1 to 2 g given in four divided doses for 7 to 10 days. Some clinicians may opt to give a single IM injection of 600,000 U of procaine penicillin G followed by oral therapy. Hospitalized patients with severe or complicated pneumococcal pneumonia exhibiting a documented in vitro susceptibility or intermediate susceptibility can be effectively treated with aqueous penicillin G 5 to 10 million Units daily in divided doses.[22] Erythromycin 1 to 2 g daily, azithromycin, and most parenteral first- and second-generation cephalosporins are effective alternatives in the penicillin-allergic patient. However, up to 15% of penicillin-allergic patients are also allergic to cephalosporins, and their use should be guided by the severity of the penicillin allergy and history of previous exposure to cephalosporins. In general, cephalosporins should be avoided in those who have experienced anaphylaxis to penicillin. Despite widespread use, excellent lung tissue penetration, and increased effectiveness for Gram-positive bacteria of ofloxacin over ciprofloxacin, older-generation quinolone antibiotics are not good choices because of unreliable pneumococcal sensitivities and reported treatment failures. The new generation of quinolones (levofloxacin, gatifloxacin, sparfloxacin) offers enhanced effectiveness for Gram-positive bacteria while maintaining good activity against Gram-negative bacteria. In addition, these agents have so far remained effective against penicillin-resistant strains of *S. pneumoniae,* and they effectively cover atypical pathogens that can be significant causes of CAP as well. Aminoglycosides are not effective and are unreliable for treatment of *S. pneumoniae.*

When appropriate therapy is initiated, a favorable response and defervescence are usually seen within 48 to 72 hours. As a general rule, a switch from IV to oral therapy may be made at this time to complete the full course of therapy. Chest film abnormalities may persist for up to 4 to 6 weeks, especially in elderly patients or patients with underlying pulmonary disease. Those who develop complications such as pneumococcal meningitis, endocarditis, bacteremia, or arthritis should receive 20 million units of aqueous penicillin G intravenously per day in divided doses. In geographic regions with a high prevalence of penicillin resistance or documented resistance, high-dose vancomycin in combination with cefotaxime has been advocated for the patient with pneumococcal meningitis.[43] Significant risk factors for the development of pneumococcal pneumonia include age >50 years old, smoking, residence in a nursing home, neutropenia, seizure disorder, and asplenia or splenic dysfunction. Other high-risk groups include patients with cardiovascular disease, COPD, diabetes mellitus, AIDS, chronic renal or hepatic failure, Hodgkin's disease, sickle cell disease, those receiving chemotherapy or immunosuppressive therapy, and alcoholics. Patients with these risk factors or who fall into high-risk groups have an increased likelihood of pneumonia complications, higher mortality rates, and a greater need for hospitalization due to pneumococcal pneumonia[47] and should receive active immunization with the polyvalent pneumococcal vaccine. The vaccine consists of 23 types of purified, capsular polysaccharide antigens, which represent the majority of *S. pneumoniae* types responsible for pneumococcal infections in the United States. Efficacy is dependent on the recipient's ability to produce antibodies in response to the vaccine. Despite controversy over its reduced efficacy in immunocompromised and elderly patients, it is generally accepted that its benefits outweigh the risks of not receiving the vaccination. The vaccine is clearly of benefit in high-risk persons who are otherwise immunocompetent and is most effective when given early in chronic disease.[48,51] Likewise, the influenza vaccine is also recommended for high-risk patients to reduce complications and the potential for secondary bacterial pneumonia.

Haemophilus influenzae

H. influenzae makes up a portion of the normal flora of the URT in virtually all persons older than 1 year of age.[50] Approximately 5% of *H. influenzae* exist as the encapsulated form, whereas 95% are nonencapsulated. *H. influenzae* type B is responsible for most childhood URT infections and meningitis. Vaccination against this type has become increasingly important and has resulted in fewer cases of childhood meningitis caused by this pathogen.[46] *H. influenzae* has long been recognized as a significant pathogen for LRT infections in adults, especially among alcoholics, persons with AIDS, older adults, and those with chronic pulmonary diseases like COPD. Three-quarters of adult patients affected are seen with a worsening cough, tachypnea, and a low-grade fever, which may indicate acute exacerbation of chronic bronchitis and not pneumonia. In these patients, the sputum Gram stain is unreliable because colonization with *H. influenzae* and other Gram-negative pathogens is common. A smaller percentage of patients have a more sudden onset of symptoms, fever, purulent sputum production, and pleuritic chest pain, which indicates pneumonia rather than bronchitis. Sputum Gram stain shows many PMNs and a predominance of Gram-negative coccobacilli indicative of *H. influenzae*. A chest radiograph may reveal lobar involvement and a high percentage of patients will have blood cultures positive for the organism, which confirms the etiology.

Ampicillin and amoxicillin were once considered the drugs of choice for treatment of LRT infections caused by *H. influenzae* and are still considered alternatives for URT infections in some patients. Ampicillin resistance caused by plasmid-mediated β-lactamase production is being encountered more frequently in the community and hospital setting. For the hospitalized patient, the empiric antimicrobial should be reasonably broad; choices may include a second-generation cephalosporin such as cefuroxime 750 mg IV every 8 hours or the third-generation cephalosporins cefotaxime 1 g IV every 8 hours or ceftriaxone 1 g IV every 24 hours. Ampicillin/sulbactam 1.5 g IV every 6 hours may also be considered when β-lactamase-producing *H. influenzae* is suspected. Antimicrobial therapy should be later streamlined based on culture and sensitivity information. A variety of other agents are effective against ampicillin-resistant strains, which include TMP/SMX, and most of the new and old systemic quinolones. Azithromycin, now available intravenously as well as orally, is approved for the treatment of mild to severe CAP caused by *H. influenzae*, *S. pneumoniae*, and atypical pathogens in a dose of 500 mg intravenously every day for 3 to 5 days followed by 250 mg to 500 mg orally every day to complete the full course. Because of its activity against common pathogens, *S. pneumoniae*, *H. influenzae*, and atypical pathogens (*M. pneumoniae*, *Chlamydia* sp., *Legionella* sp.), azithromycin may offer an advantage of single-drug therapy in some patients requiring empirical treatment for CAP of unknown etiology. The MIC of erythromycin is not sufficient to treat most infections caused by *H. influenzae* and should, therefore, not be used. This agent is added to cefuroxime and other β-lactam antibiotics to empirically treat infection due to atypical pathogens. Despite additive or synergistic activity of clarithromycin and its 14-hydroxy metabolite, this agent has failed to eradicate *H. influenzae* in some patients with CAP and bronchitis when given in an oral dose of 500 mg twice a day.[51] The clinical significance of these findings has been minimal. If oral therapy is indicated, clarithromycin may be used alternatively for treatment of mild LRT infections caused by *H. influenzae*, and its activity against this organism is superior to that of erythromycin. Combination agents containing a β-lactam and a β-lactamase inhibitor such as amoxicillin/clavulanic acid, ticarcillin/clavulanic acid, ampicillin/sulbactam, or piperacillin/tazobactam are also effective against β-lactamase-producing strains of *H. influenzae*. Ticarcillin/clavulanic and piperacillin/tazobactam are seldom necessary in these instances because of their broad spectrum of activity and availability of more cost-effective agents. Amoxicillin/clavulanic acid, TMP/SMX, cefuroxime axetil, cefpodoxime, cefixime, or the new generation quinolones are suitable for ambulatory patients and for switching from intravenous to oral therapy, if β-lactamase-producing strains are causing the infection. Cefixime should be avoided if *S. aureus* or pneumococci cannot be ruled out. Newer oral cephalosporins, loracarbef and cefprozil, and the older second-generation cephalosporin, cefaclor, may be considered secondary alternatives for ambulatory patients but are usually not justified due to lack of cost-effectiveness and availability of more appropriate therapies. The new generation of quinolones (levofloxacin, gatifloxacin, sparfloxacin, and trovafloxacin) maintain good activity against *H. influenzae*. Like azithromycin, the new quinolones are effective for common pathogens causing CAP (*S. pneumoniae*, penicillin-resistant *S. pneumoniae*, *H. influenzae*, *M. pneumoniae*, *Chlamydia* sp., and *Legionella* sp.) and also offer an advantage of single-drug therapy for empiric treatment of CAP. In addition, these agents have outstanding oral bioavailability and tissue penetration. Levofloxacin and gatifloxacin are available in both parenteral and oral dosage forms. The intravenous dosage strength is equivalent to the oral dosage form for both agents, thus making conversion less troublesome for some clinicians. Because of its broader spectrum of activity, trovafloxacin should be reserved for patients in whom anaerobes are strongly suspected or cannot be ruled out, such as those in whom aspiration pneumonia is possible. However, in light of recent postmarketing findings and FDA restrictions, the benefits of trovafloxacin use should outweigh the risks. Trovafloxacin use has been associated with serious liver toxicity in some patients.

Moraxella (Branhamella) catarrhalis

M. catarrhalis is part of the normal flora of the URT and was once considered to be nonpathogenic. It is now recognized as a relatively common cause of exacerbation of bronchitis, sinusitis, otitis media, and pneumonia. Patients with underlying pulmonary disease appear to be more prone to infection with this organism. Up to 15% of CAP may be attributed to this pathogen.[28] Smoking, COPD, chronic corticosteroid use, and viral illness may allow overgrowth of this organism, potentially leading to the development of pneumonia. Patients usually present with mild to moderate symptoms, which are sometimes indistinguishable from those of bronchitis. Chills, fever, and pleuritic chest pain are present in less than 33% of patients, but evidence of pneumonia on chest radiograph may be as high as 43%.[52] WBC counts may be mildly elevated and bacteremia is uncommon. Sputum Gram stain, if obtainable, may show a predominance of Gram-negative, kidney bean-shaped diplococci.[53] There is evidence that β-lactamase production by these organisms has increased in recent years,[52] which may account, in part, for the fact that *M. catarrhalis* has become a legitimate pathogen. Historically, ampicillin and amoxicillin were considered effective antibiotics against *M. catarrhalis*. Today, β-lactamase-producing strains are resistant to both agents regardless of the MIC.[52] Antibiotics used to treat infections caused by β-lactamase-producing strains of *M. catarrhalis* include TMP/SMX, amoxicillin/clavulanic acid, cefuroxime and most other second-generation cephalosporins, systemic quinolones, and third-generation cephalosporins. Ampicillin is the drug of choice for non-β-lactamase-producing strains. Erythromycin, clarithromycin, and azithromycin are alternative agents. When available, culture and sensitivity information should be used to guide therapy.

Atypical Pneumonia

Atypical pathogens are suspected to be common causes of CAP.[35] These pathogens are sometimes more commonly associated with physical and clinical findings that differ from the classic presenting signs and systems of pneumonia caused by "typical" bacterial pathogens such as *S. pneumoniae*. Atypical presentations are sometimes associated with more extrapulmonary symptoms, especially GI complaints. As previously stated, because the clinical presentation of CAP can vary substantially from patient to patient, a true etiologic pathogen cannot be reliably identified based on clinical findings alone. Pneumonia caused by *M. pneumoniae, Chlamydia* sp., and viruses account for many of these atypical presentations. *L. pneumophila* may cause an atypical presentation at first (during the first 24 to 48 hours) but the presentation becomes more classic or "typical" after the early onset period. *Legionella* infection is associated with a more pronounced leukocytosis than *M. pneumoniae* or *Chlamydia pneumoniae*. Other less common causes of atypical CAP syndromes include *Chlamydia psittaci* (psittacosis), *Coxiella burnetii* (Q fever), *Francisella tularensis* (tularemia), *M. tuberculosis*, fungi, and respiratory viruses (influenza A and B, adenovirus, parainfluenza, and RSV).

Legionella pneumophila

L. pneumophila is a Gram-negative bacillus that causes pneumonia in adults more commonly than in children. It is often grouped with other atypical pathogens, but it is capable of causing severe, life-threatening pneumonia with a mortality rate of up to 14%.[35] Legionnaires' disease is a rapidly progressive and severe form of pneumonia caused by this organism, whereas Pontiac fever is a nonpneumonia acute febrile illness caused by the same organism. *L. pneumophila* is ubiquitous in aquatic environments, and outbreaks of pneumonia have been associated with excavation, construction, cooling towers, ventilation systems, and shower heads. Institutional outbreaks causing nosocomial pneumonia have been associated with contaminated water supplies. In a small study conducted by the Allegheny County (PA) Health Department, five of six hospitals tested were found to have *Legionella* sp. growing in cultures from a variety of institutional water sources.[54] Three of the participating institutions also documented cases of nosocomially acquired Legionnaires' disease during the study period.[54] These researchers recommend that environmental cultures for *Legionella* sp. in the water distribution systems should be performed routinely in an effort to prevent nosocomially acquired infection.[54]

L. pneumophila serogroup 1 is responsible for the majority of cases of Legionnaires' disease. In the community, peak incidence occurs between late summer and early fall and may be as high as 30% in some geographic locations, but it is encountered less often in most areas.[55] The organism is not spread from person to person. Specific predispositions to infection include smoking, age older than 60, alcoholic liver disease, and high-dose corticosteroid use in institutionalized patients. Patients are often seen in the early stages with abrupt onset of high fever, anorexia, myalgia, headache, confusion, diarrhea, and cough with a small amount of nonpurulent sputum production. Extrapulmonary symptoms appear to be relatively common and may represent the only clinical findings that distinguish Legionnaires' disease from classic bacterial pneumonia. Contrary to previous reports, bradycardia is no longer felt to be a distinguishing clinical finding.[35] The combination of high fever, hyponatremia, central nervous system manifestations, and a lactate dehydrogenase level >700 U/mL strongly suggests Legionnaires' disease.[35] Other laboratory tests commonly reveal an elevated WBC count, and, occasionally, hypophosphatemia and elevated liver enzymes. If a sufficient sputum specimen is available, identification of the organisms is possible by direct immunofluorescence. Serologic indirect immunofluorescent antibody determination may also be used to detect *L. pneumophila*. Unfortunately, most patients do not become seropositive until the third to sixth week of convalescence, making this test impractical for guiding acute therapy. Serologic titers are more useful for epidemiologic purposes. The diagnostic hallmark is *Legionella* culture.[35] However, this evaluation is not available in most clinical laboratories and requires technical expertise and specialized medium for growth of *Legionella*.[35] A very sensitive, specific, and rapid radioimmunoassay that detects *L. pneumophila* serogroup 1 antigen in the urine is routinely available and may be used to rapidly diagnose pneumonia caused by *L. pneumophila*.

Intravenous erythromycin lactobionate 30 to 60 mg/kg/day divided every 6 hours is the treatment of choice for *Legionella* pneumonia.[35] When clinical improvement occurs, intravenous therapy may be switched to oral erythromycin 500 mg four times a day to complete a 14-day course. Immunocompromised patients should receive therapy for 21 days.[35] In patients with severe Legionnaires' disease, the addition of oral rifampin in a dose of 300 to 600 mg every 12 hours may be helpful,[55] although rifampin should never used alone. Intravenous azithromycin 500 mg every day may be used as first-line therapy in those patients who are at risk or who develop phlebitis, which is often associated with intravenous erythromycin. However, venous irritation associated with intravenous erythromycin can be minimized by adequately diluting the solution and lengthening the infusion time. If the patient cannot tolerate oral erythromycin, alternatives include azithromycin, clarithromycin, tetracycline, doxycycline, or the new generation systemic quinolones. Azithromycin, which has fewer GI side effects than clarithromycin, may be the most helpful agent for patients who cannot tolerate the GI side effects of erythromycin. However, GI side effects associated with erythromycin can also be minimized by using enteric coated dosage forms or oral preparations that can be taken with food. The estolate salt of erythromycin should be avoided because of a higher incidence of liver toxicity. Anecdotally, the new generation quinolones (levofloxacin, gatifloxacin, and sparfloxacin) may be the preferred first-line agents in immunocompromised patients with *L. pneumophila*,[35] presumably because of their excellent tissue and intracellular penetration. *Legionella* sp., including *L. pneumophila*, are not susceptible to β-lactam antibiotics.

Mycoplasma pneumoniae

M. pneumoniae is one of the smallest free-living organisms known to man.[56] It does not have a cell wall and shares properties of both viruses and bacteria. *M. pneumoniae* is more likely to cause pharyngitis or a self-limiting URT infection than pneumonia. However, atypical CAP due to this organism is common, accounting for up to an estimated 20 to 30% of pneumonia cases in adults younger than 30 years of age and up to 50% of cases in persons who live in close quarters.[56,57] Endemic outbreaks of *Mycoplasma* pneumonia have been observed in college dormitories and military installations. Historically, acquisition of this organism was thought to occur primarily in young adults. Contrary to previous reports of *Mycoplasma* pneumonia being relatively uncommon in elderly patients,[58] the Ohio study reported a significant increase in the number of cases and an increased need for hospitalization in those older than 64 years of age.[59] The incidence of *Mycoplasma* pneumonia varies from year to year and generally peaks every 4 years.[57] It is most prevalent in the fall, but may occur during any time of the year. The organism is transmitted person to person through respiratory secretions. *Mycoplasma* pneumonia may manifest from a mild self-limiting influenza-type illness to severe life-threatening pneumonia requiring intensive care in the hospital. It should be emphasized that some persons who acquire *Mycoplasma* may experience a self-limited respiratory infection, fully recover without sequelae, and never seek medical attention or receive antibiotic therapy. For others, a lengthy incubation period of up to 3 weeks is followed by the gradual onset of pneumonia. Patients can be seen with a variety of complaints including a worsening sore throat, nonproductive cough that is worse at night, headache, low-grade fever, general malaise, myalgia, and earache. Although a rare finding, *M. pneumoniae* infection should be strongly suspected in the patient with erythema multiforme and atypical pneumonia symptoms.[55] The chest radiograph most commonly reveals a pattern of bronchopneumonia. Definitive microbiologic diagnosis of *M. pneumoniae* is routinely difficult, but can be made by isolation of the organism or demonstration of an appropriate antibody response.[56] Elevated cold agglutinin titers greater than 1:64 occur in a majority of patients during the second to third week of illness. DFA can detect the presence of IgG and IgM antibodies, making this test sensitive but not reliably specific for acute infection. Thus, determination of *M. pneumoniae* as the causative pathogen is often impractical, and therapy is usually presumptive based on clinical evaluation and history. The lack of rapid, practical, and accurate diagnostic tests for *M. pneumoniae* probably accounts for why it is not documented more often as a cause of CAP.[35] PCR kits are available for the rapid detection of this organism. Their use is limited by cost, underavailability, and lack of FDA approval. Other diagnostic techniques using new technology will continue to gain popularity in the future.

Most persons with *Mycoplasma* pneumonia can be treated as outpatients with oral erythromycin 500 mg every 6 hours for 14 days. Tetracycline 500 mg every 6 hours or doxycycline 100 mg twice a day for 14 days is also an effective treatment. More expensive and broader spectrum alternative regimens include clarithromycin 250 to 500 mg every 12 hours, azithromycin 500 mg on day 1 followed by 250 mg for 4 days, or any of the new generation quinolones (levofloxacin, gatifloxacin, or sparfloxacin). β-Lactam antibiotics are not effective because *M. pneumoniae* does not have a cell wall.

Chlamydia pneumoniae

C. pneumoniae is an obligate intracellular Gram-negative pathogen that causes atypical pneumonia. It is transmitted through close human to human contact and has a lengthy incubation period of 2 to 4 weeks.[35] Its prevalence increases through adolescence to adulthood, and it accounts for up to at least 10% of all CAPs.[56] In general populations, its seroprevalence is 50% by age 20 and continues to increase, reaching approximately 75% in older adults.[35] *C. pneumoniae*, which is often acquired early in life, may persist in some individuals and cause recurrent infections throughout life. Reports have emerged describing the persistence of this organism and *M. pneumoniae* in respiratory secretions despite achievement of a clinical response with appropriate therapies.[60] Epidemiologic evidence also suggests an association between *C. pneumoniae* and the development of atherosclerosis, leading to coronary artery disease in men.[61] Further study of this association and the role of antibiotics is warranted before recommendations can be made. In addition, a relation between infection with *C. pneumoniae* and the development of asthma has been suggested.[35]

Pneumonia caused by *C. pneumoniae* is usually mild to moderate in severity but may be severe in some, especially in older adults or those who are chronically ill. Fatal infections have been reported in patients with underlying COPD and CHF.[56] *C. pneumoniae* may also cause sinusitis, pharyngitis, or bronchitis rather than pneumonia. When pneumonia does occur, many patients have reported severe pharyngitis and hoarseness in the previous 1 to 3 weeks.[56] Patients generally are seen with a low-grade fever, nonproductive cough, and a normal WBC count. The chest radiograph may show a diffuse process and consolidation is uncommon. One clue to the presence of *C. pneumoniae* as the causative pathogen is a low-grade eosinophilia.[55] The two most common serologic tests for *C. pneumoniae* are IgM complement fixation and microimmunofluorescence. Etiologic diagnosis is usually presumptive based on clinical findings and history. Because there is no reliably specific, practical, and cost-effective microbiologic test and because standard "atypical" antibiotic regimens usually are effective for *C. pneumoniae*, the true incidence of this organism may be under-recognized. Furthermore, because of its self-limiting nature, many patients do not seek treatment or develop pneumonia. The treatment of choice for pneumonia caused by *C. pneumoniae* has traditionally been tetracycline 500 mg by mouth every 6 hours or doxycycline 100 mg every 12 hours for 14 to 21 days. Lengthy courses with these agents are necessary to prevent relapse. Alternatives include azithromycin 1.5 g over 5 days, clarithromycin 500 mg bid for 10 days, or any of the new generation quinolones (levofloxacin, gatifloxacin, or sparfloxacin) for 7 to 14 days. Any of these alternative regimens may be preferred, despite increased cost, because of the shorter treatment duration without loss of efficacy and the ease of once or twice daily dosing compared to tetracycline dosing. No firm guidelines exist for erythromycin dosing. If erythromycin is used, care should be taken to avoid underdosing and premature discontinuation (no less than 3 weeks of therapy) to prevent relapse.

Nosocomial Pneumonia

PATHOPHYSIOLOGY

Despite advances in the development of antimicrobial therapy, nosocomial or hospital-acquired pneumonia still occurs with high frequency and causes significant morbidity and mortality. Pathogens arise primarily from overgrowth of the patient's endogenous flora or from exogenous sources via respiratory equipment and the hands of hospital personnel. In general, the etiology of nosocomial pneumonia is influenced by the underlying illness of the patient, the type of unit in which care is being provided, unit and institutional antibiotic usage, and the hospital's microbial flora and antibiotic sensitivity patterns. Patients cared for in the ICU and those who are receiving mechanical ventilation support are at greatest risk for the development of nosocomial pneumonia. The highest postoperative nosocomial pneumonia rates involve patients who have undergone thoracic or abdominal surgery.[7] Among nursing home patients, nosocomial pneumonia is one of the most common reasons for hospitalization. Risk factors for the development of nosocomial pneumonia, as well as predictors of a more severe course, are listed in Table 67.9.

The basic mechanisms involved in the pathogenesis of pneumonia previously discussed also apply in the hospital setting. However, it should be recognized that most of the nosocomial pneumonias involve patients who are immunocompromised due to other acute illnesses or surgery. In this state, normal immune processes and defenses are more likely to be overwhelmed when exposed to pathogenic bacteria. Colonization of the oropharyngeal cavity, trachea, or the upper GI tract with pathogenic bacteria is the first step involved in the development of most nosocomial pneumonias. Table 67.4 lists factors associated with Gram-negative bacteria colonization of the oropharyngeal cavity. The degree of colonization with pathogenic Gram-negative organisms and *S. aureus* increases proportionally to the severity of the patient's illness.[62] Colonization occurs in as many as 40% of patients in the ICU within 3 days, increasing the risk of these patients developing nosocomial pneumonia rather quickly in this setting.[10] The ICU typically serves the sickest patients. Therefore, the most resistant organisms are usually found there because of routine use of broad-spectrum antibiotics, further complicating the prevention and treatment of nosocomial pneumonia. After colonization has taken place, the patient subsequently microaspirates these organisms, which overwhelms the weakened immune system

Table 67.9 ▪ Risk Factors for the Development of Nosocomial Pneumonia and Predictors of a More Severe Course

Acute or Chronic Illnesses	Others
Central nervous system dysfunction	Prolonged hospitalization
Chronic obstructive lung disease	Thoracic or abdominal surgery
Diabetes mellitus	Prolonged postoperative period
Hypotension	Corticosteroid use
Metabolic acidosis	Cigarette smoking history
Coma	Advanced age
Malnutrition	Macroaspiration
Alcoholism	
Azotemia	
Cancer	
Acquired immunodeficiency syndrome (AIDS)	

Source: References 20, 69.

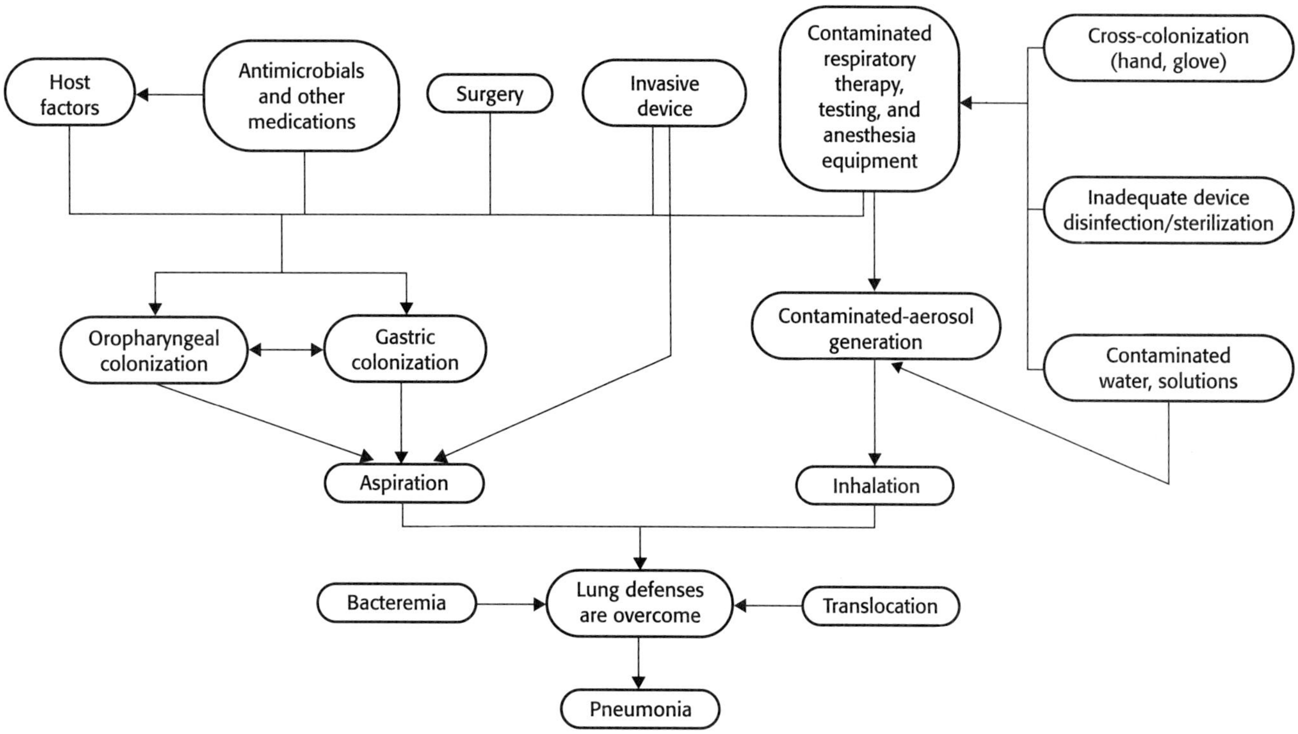

Figure 67.3. Pathogenesis of nosocomial bacterial pneumonia. (*Source:* Reference 19.)

and lung defenses. For patients receiving mechanical ventilation, contaminated oropharyngeal and tracheal secretions may leak past the endotracheal cuff, drain into the upper bronchioles, and ultimately cause pneumonia. Another common cause of nosocomial pneumonia is inhalation of aerosolized organisms via respiratory equipment. Hematogenous spread and translocation from other infectious sources to the lungs do occur, but are less common. Figure 67.3 shows an algorithm that describes the pathogenesis of nosocomial pneumonia.[19]

Approximately 60% of nosocomial pneumonias are caused by aerobic Gram-negative bacilli, whereas the remaining 40% are attributable to Gram-positive organisms, primarily *S. aureus*, polymicrobial sources, or anaerobic pathogens.[13,63] A review of 15,499 isolates in the National Nosocomial Infection Study revealed that *Pseudomonas aeruginosa*, *Enterobacter* spp., *Klebsiella pneumoniae*, and *S. aureus* were the most common pathogens associated with nosocomial pneumonia in the participating institutions.[64] *Legionella* spp. are also becoming a more recognized nosocomial pathogen.[10,19]

CLINICAL PRESENTATION AND DIAGNOSIS

Diagnosis of nosocomial pneumonia is usually made by the recognition of new or progressive infiltrates on chest radiograph, new onset of fever, leukocytosis, and cough or tracheal secretions containing purulent material. Sputum Gram stain and culture may be less reliable because of the presence of upper airway and oropharyngeal colonization with many different and potentially causative bacteria. Blood, pleural fluid, and sputum for culture and Gram stain all may be used to determine the etiology and guide antimicrobial therapy. Etiologic diagnosis of the patient receiving mechanical ventilation is even more challenging and may require the use of invasive procedures such as bronchoscopy using BAL or PSB or open lung biopsy in the immunosuppressed patient. The use of invasive procedures in the diagnosis of pneumonia has been discussed previously in this chapter.

Table 67.10 ▪ Individual Criteria Defining Severe Nosocomial Pneumonia

Admission to the intensive care unit
Respiratory failure (mechanical ventilation or FiO_2 >35% to keep O_2 saturation >90%)
Rapid radiographic progression, multilobar involvement, cavitation, or other lung complication
Evidence of true Gram-negative septic shock with or without end-organ dysfunction
Vasopressor administration >4 hr
Urine output <20 mL/hr or <80 mL over 4 hr
Acute renal failure requiring dialysis

Source: Reference 10.

THERAPEUTIC PLAN

Nosocomial pneumonia may be defined as mild, moderate, or severe (Table 67.10). The American Thoracic Society has grouped nosocomial pneumonias according to severity (mild, moderate, or severe), onset (early or late), and risk factors present.[20] Early onset is defined as nosocomial pneumonia occurring within 5 days of admission and involves fewer pathogenic organisms than nosocomial pneumonia of late onset (longer than 5 days after admission).[20] Empiric antibiotic treatment for nosocomial pneumonia requires a clinical knowledge of the different spectrum of pathogens versus those causing CAP. Table 67.11 categorizes nosocomial pneumonia and provides recommendations for reasonable empiric antibiotic therapy.

Empiric treatment may incorporate use of a broad-spectrum cephalosporin with or without an aminoglycoside or broad-spectrum monotherapy. Aminoglycosides have been favored for empiric treatment of nosocomial pneumonia because of synergism with β-lactam antibiotics, rapid killing rate, postantibiotic effect, and activity against Gram-negative pathogens, including *P. aeruginosa*. Monotherapy with aminoglycosides should be avoided in the treatment of any pneumonia for the following reasons. The lower physiologic pH of infected lung tissues and acidic secretions have a negative effect on the activity of aminoglycosides.[1] In addition, aminoglycosides are water soluble and do not readily pass into lung tissue. Both factors require that therapeutic peak serum concentrations of gentamicin or tobramycin, in a multidose day regimen, be maintained above 6 mg/L to ensure satisfactory lung

Table 67.11 ▪ Empiric Antibiotic Regimens for Nosocomial Pneumonia Based on Likely Pathogen, Severity, and Concurrent Illness

Group 1[a]	Group 2[b]	Group 3[c]
Core pathogens:	Core pathogens:	Core pathogens:
Haemophilus influenzae		
Streptococcus pneumoniae		
Staphylococcus aureus	PLUS:	PLUS:
Enteric Gram-negative bacilli		
Klebsiella sp.	Anaerobes	*Pseudomonas aeruginosa*
Enterobacter sp.[d]	*Legionella* sp.	*Acinetobacter* sp.[d]
Escherichia coli	*Pseudomonas aeruginosa*[e]	MRSA
Proteus sp.		
Serratia marcescens		
Empiric treatment:	Empiric treatment[f]:	Empiric treatment:
Second-generation cephalosporin	Add IV vancomycin (if MSRA is suspected)	Antipseudomonal penicillin (piperacillin/tazobactam)
OR		OR
Nonpseudomonal third-generation cephalosporin	Add clindamycin of ampicillin/sulbactam (if anaerobes are suspected)	Antipseudomonal cephalosporin (ceftazidime, cefepime)
Cefotaxime or		OR
Ceftriaxone		Aztreonam[g]
OR		Imipenem/cilastatin
Fourth-generation cephalosporin	Add erythromycin ± ripampin OR new generation quinolone (if *Legionella* sp. is suspected)	PLUS
Cefepime		Aminoglycoside (gentamicin or tobramycin)
OR		OR
β-Lactam/β-lactamase inhibitor		Systemic quinolone (ciprofloxacin, trovafloxacin)
Ampicillin/sulbactam or		Add IV vancomycin (if MSRA is suspected)
Piperacillin/tazobactam		
OR		
Systemic quinoline[h]		
Ciprofloxacin[h] or		
Levofloxacin		

Source: References 20, 69.

MRSA, methicillin-resistant *Staphylococcus aureus*.

[a]Group 1 includes those with early-or late-onset mild to moderate pneumonia without risk factors and early-onset severe pneumonia without risk factors (early onset <5 days since admission; late onset >5 days since admission).

[b]Group 2 includes those with early- or late-onset mild to moderate pneumonia with risk factors. (Refer to Table 66.9 for risk factors.)

[c]Group 3 includes those with late-onset severe pneumonia without risk factors and all other severe pneumonias with risk factors regardless of onset. (Refer to Table 66.10 for criteria defining severe pneumonia.)

[d]Cefepime or systemic quinolones may be preferred over other cephalosporins if this organism is suspected.

[e]Treat as severe pneumonia in Group 3.

[f]Empiric therapy includes antibiotics listed in group 1 plus those listed as indicated.

[g]Aztreonam is only effective for Gram-negative organisms.

[h]Includes levofloxacin, trovafloxacin, and ciprofloxacin. Avoid ciprofloxacin if *S. pneumoniae* is strongly suspected.

penetration and improved patient outcomes.[65,66] These shortcomings have prompted research in the area of aerosolized and endotracheal administration of aminoglycosides to overcome their pharmacokinetic disadvantages. Both methods attempt to provide a greater concentration of drug at the site of infection while limiting systemic adverse effects. Despite these theoretical advantages, the role of these methods of administration in clinical practice remains controversial but deserves continued study.[67] Empiric monotherapy may be acceptable with some antimicrobial agents and a wide array of selections are possible. It is imperative that one be familiar with the institution's microbial flora and susceptibility patterns before choosing the empiric agent. The institution's antibiogram should be used in making empiric therapeutic decisions in the treatment of nosocomial pneumonia.

TREATMENT

Pathogen-Specific

Gram-Negative Bacillary Pneumonia

A multitude of Gram-negative organisms have been implicated as the cause of nosocomial pneumonia including the *Enterobacteriaceae* (*Klebsiella* sp., *Enterobacter* sp., *Escherichia coli*, *Proteus* sp., *Morganella* sp., *Serratia marcescens*, and *Providencia* sp.) and *P. aeruginosa*, *Acinetobacter* sp., and *Xanthomonas maltophilia*. *P. aeruginosa* is more common in patients with COPD and those receiving mechanical ventilation support.[68] *P. aeruginosa* colonization has also been recognized to occur more often in those who are both mechanically ventilated and malnourished.[69]

Because of the aggressive nature of the Gram-negative pathogens, the clinician must initiate empiric therapy before the pathogen is identified. Empiric treatment of Gram-negative bacillary pneumonia should take into account patient history, diagnostic information, and the institution's antibiogram in an attempt to provide effective coverage for all likely pathogens (Table 67.11). Microbial susceptibility patterns differ among institutions and may differ from unit to unit within the same institution. Therefore, one must recognize that no single antibiotic or combination of antibiotics is suitable for every clinical situation encountered. If *P. aeruginosa* alone is suspected, antipseudomonal β-lactam antibiotics such as ticarcillin, piperacillin, cefepime, or ceftazidime plus an aminoglycoside such as gentamicin or tobramycin are acceptable first-choice regimens. Amikacin should generally be reserved for those organisms resistant to gentamicin and tobramycin. Regimens that include an antipseudomonal β-lactam antibiotic plus an aminoglycoside decrease the development of resistance and achieve a synergistic bactericidal effect. Because of the high mortality rate associated with *P. aeruginosa* pneumonia, therapy should be aggressive. Gentamicin or tobramycin may be administered as a 2 to 3 mg/kg loading dose[70] followed by a maintenance dosage to achieve peak serum concentrations of at least 6 mg/L and trough serum concentrations >2 mg/L. The aminoglycoside maintenance dose should be based on the patient's weight, renal function, and serum concentration data. Alternatively, larger doses (e.g., 5 to 6 mg/kg) of aminoglycosides given over an extended interval (e.g., every 24 to 48 hours versus every 8 to 12 hours) are appealing because they achieve high therapeutic peak serum concentrations while allowing trough serum concentrations to fall below 2 mg/L before the next dose is administered. This dosage scheme also takes advantage of the postantibiotic effect that aminoglycosides exhibit against Gram-positive and Gram-negative bacteria. Several studies described equal efficacy and less nephrotoxicity in a once-a-day gentamicin dosing regimen versus an every 8 to 12 hour regimen.[71–74] Other antipseudomonal regimens include a systemic quinolone combined with an antipseudomonal β-lactam antibiotic, imipenem/cilastatin, aztreonam, or an aminoglycoside. Quinolones and carbapenems (imipenem/cilastatin or meropenem) should not be used as monotherapy against *P. aeruginosa* because resistance may develop rather quickly. Among the quinolones, ciprofloxacin has the highest in vitro activity against *P. aeruginosa*, but resistance is not uncommon and other systemic quinolones exhibit clinical efficacy against this organism. However, cross-resistance by *P. aeruginosa* and other Gram-negative organisms to the quinolones as a class does occur.[75] Because of the varying degrees of *P. aeruginosa* in vitro susceptibility among regions and institutions, the hospital's antibiogram and clinical experience should be used to guide the selection of the most reliable systemic quinolone against this organism. An antipseudomonal β-lactam antibiotic plus a systemic quinolone combination is an appropriate alternative, but these drugs are not always synergistic. This combination may be preferable to an aminoglycoside plus systemic quinolone combination because the former exerts activity at different bacterial sites while achieving adequate bactericidal concentrations. Double β-lactam antibiotic combinations are undesirable when treating *P. aeruginosa* because they do not achieve synergy and may induce β-lactamase production that inhibits both agents, causing multidrug resistance.[69] The addition of the β-lactamase inhibitors clavulanic acid and tazobactam to ticarcillin and piperacillin, respectively, does not enhance their intrinsic activity against *P. aeruginosa*. Clavulanic acid and tazobactam lack affinity for the β-lactamase produced by this organism. Therefore, ticarcillin/clavulanic acid or piperacillin/tazobactam are unnecessary when treating infections caused only by *P. aeruginosa*. However, these agents can be useful when treating nosocomial pneumonia caused by other β-lactamase-producing Gram-negative bacilli, and those that are polymicrobial, especially when anaerobic coverage is also desired. Third-generation cephalosporins such as cefotaxime or ceftriaxone are acceptable choices for Gram-negative organisms unless *Enterobacter* sp., *P. aeruginosa*, or anaerobes are suspected. Pneumonia caused by *Enterobacter* sp. can usually be treated with a systemic quinolone alone, with an extended-spectrum penicillin such as piperacillin plus an aminoglycoside, or with β-lactamase inhibitor combinations such as piperacillin/tazobactam. Drug resistance of this organism is increasing in many hospitals and third-generation cephalosporins, especially ceftazidime, should be avoided when *Enterobacter* sp. are suspected. Cefepime is a new fourth-generation cephalosporin that appears to be superior to other cephalosporins against *Enterobacter* sp. and may have a therapeutic niche against this organism. When reliable culture and sensitivity information is available, it should be used to guide antimicrobial therapy.

Staphylococcus aureus

S. aureus is a coagulase-positive Gram-positive coccus that appears in clusters on the Gram stain. It has been implicated in up to 14% of nosocomial pneumonias[67] and usually results from either aspiration or hematogenous spread. It is most commonly seen in comatose patients and those with head trauma[69] but may occur in any hospitalized patient. Pneumonia caused by *S. aureus* also occurs in the community setting after recovery from influenza. Patients typically exhibit an abrupt onset of fever, chills, dyspnea, pleuritic chest pain, cough productive of purulent sputum, and an elevated WBC count and approximately 20% of patients are bacteremic.[29] Chest radiogram reveals multilobar infiltrates or bilateral involvement.[29] Release of extracellular toxins by this organism can result in extensive lung tissue destruction, causing cavitation or a necrotizing pneumonia. Many strains of *S. aureus* produce penicillinase, which inactivates penicillin, necessitating the use of an antistaphylococcal penicillin. Intravenous nafcillin 2 g every 4 to 6 hours for 10 to 14 days is an effective first choice. If necrotizing pneumonia is present, therapy for up to 6 weeks may be necessary. Methicillin is not recommended because of an increased risk of interstitial nephritis. An intravenous first-generation cephalosporin such as cefazolin 1 g every 8 hours is also an appropriate first choice when the level of staphylococcal resistance to methicillin is low or when culture and sensitivity information indicate sensitivity to methicillin.[22] When oral therapy becomes appropriate, nafcillin should be avoided because of its poor absorption. Dicloxacillin, cloxacillin, cephalexin, or cephradine may be used when oral therapy is desired. None of the penicillins, cephalosporins, or quinolones are clinically active against methicillin-resistant *S. aureus* (MRSA). Intravenous vancomycin may be used in penicillin- and cephalosporin-allergic patients and should be the first choice when MRSA is cultured or strongly suspected. If MRSA is often found in a particular setting, the clinician may opt to use intravenous vancomycin empirically until culture and sensitivity information proves otherwise. Increasingly, vancomycin is the initial empiric choice for nosocomial pneumonia when *S. aureus* is suspected. Nevertheless, prudence is necessary with the use of this agent primarily because of the emergence of vancomycin-resistant enterococci. The usual intravenous vancomycin dose is 1 g every 12 to 24 hours, but should be based on the patient's weight, renal function, and serum concentration data when deemed necessary. Oral vancomycin is not well absorbed and is not effective for the treatment of systemic infections.

Aspiration Pneumonia and Lung Abscess

Aspiration of large amounts of oropharyngeal or gastric contents (macroaspiration) can introduce a significant number of pathogens to the lower airways causing "aspiration" pneumonia. This event is termed macroaspiration as opposed to microaspiration, which is the primary cause of other pneumonias. Due to the high incidence of anaerobic organisms, the terms "aspiration pneumonia" and "anaerobic pneumonia" are often used synonymously to describe these infections. Patients with seizure disorders, neurologic disorders, and lung cancer, stroke victims with dysphagia, alcoholics, drug abusers, debilitated elderly patients, and intubated patients, especially in the setting of periodontal disease, are at greatest risk for the development of aspiration pneumonia (Table 67.5). In addition, medications that cause sedation, reduce consciousness, or inhibit the cough reflex may predispose patients to macroaspiration, leading to pneumonia. Aspiration pneumonia may occur in either the community or hospital setting and is usually a polymicrobial infection involving a variety of anaerobic and aerobic organisms. In the community setting a mixture of normal mouth anaerobic organisms predominate in as many as 88% of cases, whereas as few as 35% of anaerobic organisms are identified in nosocomial aspiration pneumonia.[76] Unless there are clear risk factors for aspiration or aspiration is witnessed, the role of anaerobes as the cause of CAP may be overlooked. This oversight may be attributed to the similarity of presentation and Gram stain appearance for atypical and anaerobic pneumonia,[77] and the inability of most clinical laboratories to grow anaerobes from sputum specimens. In the hospital setting, several pathogens may be present, including *S. aureus*, Gram-negative bacilli, and anaerobes, or the infection may be polymicrobial. Aspiration pneumonia has an insidious onset, and most ambulatory patients do not seek medical attention until later in the course after the development of complications.[77] Complications of aspiration pneumonia may be serious and include empyema or abscess, resulting in necrosis of lung tissue. Outpatients usually present with low-grade fever, moderately increased WBC count, weight loss, and anemia. Cough becomes productive with putrid, foul-smelling sputum in up to 60% of patients later after the development of abscess or empyema.[77] The appearance on a chest radiograph may reflect the position of the patient at the time of the aspiration event and may also reveal abscess or cavitation. Involvement of the posterior segments of the upper lobes is usually consistent with aspiration in the recumbent position and lower lobe involvement generally indicates aspiration in the upright position.[77] Sputum Gram stain reveals many PMNs and a variety of Gram-positive and Gram-negative organisms, usually representing the patient's normal flora. Pneumonia from anaerobic organisms should be strongly suspected in the patient who is seen with a slow onset of pneumonia symptoms and has a high risk for aspiration. The etiologic diagnosis of aspiration pneumonia is usually made on a presumptive basis because of difficulty in obtaining appropriate specimens and the inability of most laboratories to perform antibiotic sensitivity testing for anaerobic organisms. Historically aspiration pneumonia has responded to therapy when the appropriate empiric agent is selected. Several studies have identified *Fusobacterium* sp., *Bacteroides melaninogenicus*, and *Peptostreptococcus* sp. as the three most common pathogens associated with aspiration pneumonia.[76–79] Definitive etiologic diagnosis in these studies was made from uncontaminated specimens obtained using a variety of invasive procedures. Other anaerobic organisms and microaerophilic and aerobic streptococci also play an important role in these infections and should also be considered when empiric therapy is chosen. Treatment of aspiration pneumonia involves the appropriate antibiotic and drainage of the abscess or empyema when present. Penicillin V is effective for most anaerobes existing above the diaphragm and aerobic and microaerophilic streptococci that cause aspiration pneumonia. Early trials showed that oral penicillin V 3 g/day was as effective as aqueous penicillin G and established penicillin as the drug of choice for aspiration pneumonia.[77] More recently, up to 55% of *Fusobacterium* sp. and *B. melaninogenicus* have been identified in vitro to produce β-lactamase and exhibit resistance to penicillin.[77] Clindamycin is active against most staphylococci, streptococci, and anaerobes, including β-lactamase-producing *Bacteroides fragilis* and other *Bacteroides* sp., thus making it a more attractive treatment choice for anaerobic pneumonia. Several studies have demonstrated a higher number of treatment failures and relapses with penicillin than with clindamycin.[78,79] For these reasons, intravenous clindamycin 600 mg every 8 hours or 300 mg every 6 hours followed by 300 to 450 mg every 6 hours orally has become the first-choice regimen for most clinicians. Metronidazole is also very effective against anaerobic pathogens, including β-lactamase-producing pathogens. However, treatment failures have been encountered with this agent most likely because it is not effective for microaerophilic and aerobic streptococci. Hence, if metronidazole is used, it should be combined with penicillin to cover these additional organisms. Lung abscess and empyema are usually treated initially with parenteral agents and surgical drainage until the patient is afebrile. A prolonged course of 4 to 6 weeks with oral clindamycin or metronidazole plus penicillin V is necessary until complete resolution of the abscess or empyema or stable appearance of the chest radiograph, which may take longer than 10 weeks.[77] Patients should be counseled that adequate duration of and compliance with treatment are important to prevent relapse. In the patient with nosocomial aspiration pneumonia, empiric antibiotic therapy should be effective for anaerobes and Gram-negative bacilli. Logical empiric treatment options would be a third-generation cephalosporin such as cefepime, ceftriaxone, or cefotaxime plus clindamycin. Alternatively, levofloxacin 500 mg PO daily plus PO metronidazole or clindamycin offers good broad coverage for the patient with nosocomial aspiration pneumonia. Intravenous vancomycin should be added if there is a high prevalence of MRSA in the setting where the patient develops aspiration pneumonia.

KEY POINTS

- Despite the availability of new antibiotics and improved diagnostic methods, pneumonia remains an infectious disease that causes significant morbidity and mortality.
- The biggest challenge confronting the clinician is identification of the causative organism and selection of the appropriate antibiotic.
- An adequate history is important in guiding empiric therapy and should take into account the clinical setting of the pneumonia, any host defense defects, and any exposure to specific pathogens.
- The chest radiograph and sputum Gram stain along with clinical and laboratory signs and symptoms are the primary tools used for diagnosing pneumonia and determining the cause.
- Empiric antibiotic therapy should be broad enough in spectrum to be effective for the most likely pathogens and should be individualized based on the setting in which the pneumonia occurs, the setting where treatment will occur, the history of the present illness, pertinent patient characteristics expected to have an impact on therapy, and concomitant disease states of the patient.
- Factors that should be taken into consideration include the spectrum of activity, pharmacokinetic properties, pharmacodynamic properties, adverse effects, clinical efficacy, and cost.
- Once the causative organism is reliably identified through culture and sensitivity testing, therapy may be

streamlined to a narrow spectrum, more cost-effective agent.

- In the hospitalized patient, a conscious effort should be made to select an effective antibiotic that can possibly decrease the length of stay.
- Other important goals of therapy include achievement of good patient outcomes through symptomatic improvement and eradication of the causative organism at a reasonable cost.

REFERENCES

1. Mandell LA. Antibiotics for pneumonia therapy. Med Clin North Am 78:997–1014, 1994.
2. Osler W. The principles and practice of medicine. 4th ed. New York: D. Appleton, 1901:108.
3. Marrie TJ. Community acquired pneumonia. Clin Infect Dis 18:501–515, 1994.
4. American Thoracic Society. Guidelines for the initial management of adults with community acquired pneumonia: diagnosis, assessment of severity, and initial antimicrobial therapy. Am Rev Respir Dis 148:1418–1426, 1993.
5. Paz HL, Wood CA. Pneumonia and chronic obstructive pulmonary disease. Postgrad Med 90:77–86, 1991.
6. Campbell GD. Overview of community acquired pneumonia: prognosis and clinical features. Med Clin North Am 78:1035–1047, 1994.
7. Winter JH. The scope of lower respiratory tract infection. Infection 19(Suppl 7):359–364, 1991.
8. Craven DE, Steger KA, Barat LM, et al. Nosocomial pneumonia: epidemiology and infection control. Intensive Care Med 18(Suppl):3–9, 1992.
9. Scheld WM, Mandell GL. Nosocomial pneumonia: pathogenesis and recent advances in diagnosis and therapy. Rev Infect Dis 13(Suppl 9):43–51, 1991.
10. McEarchern R, Campbell GD. Hospital-acquired pneumonia: epidemiology, etiology, and treatment. Infect Dis Clin North Am 12:761–780, 1998.
11. Busse WW. Pathogenesis and sequelae of respiratory infections. Rev Infect Dis 13(Suppl 6):477–485, 1991.
12. Mullenix TA, Prince RA. Lower respiratory tract infections. In: Herfindal ET, Gourley DR, Hart LL, eds. Clinical pharmacy and therapeutics. 5th ed. Baltimore: Williams & Wilkins, 1992:1080–1091.
13. Stratton CW. Bacterial pneumonias: an overview with emphasis on pathogenesis, diagnosis, and treatment. Heart Lung 15:226–244, 1986.
14. Johanson WG. Overview of pneumonia. In: Wyngaarden JB, Smith LH, Bennett JC, eds. Cecil textbook of medicine. 19th ed. Philadelphia: WB Saunders, 1992:409–413.
15. Thompson R. Prevention of nosocomial pneumonia. Med Clin North Am 78:1185–1195, 1994.
16. Heyland D, Mandell LA. Gastric colonization by Gram-negative bacilli and nosocomial pneumonia in the intensive care unit patient. Evidence for causation. Chest 101:187–192, 1992.
17. Driks MR, Craven DE, Celli BR, et al. Nosocomial pneumonia in intubated patients given sucralfate as compared with antacids or histamine type 2 blockers. N Engl J Med 317:1376–1382, 1987.
18. Hamer DH, Barza M. Prevention of hospital-acquired pneumonia in critically ill patients. Antimicrob Agents Chemother 37:931–938, 1993.
19. Centers for Disease Control and Prevention. Guidelines for prevention of nosocomial pneumonia. MMWR 46(RR-1):1–79, 1997.
20. American Thoracic Society. Hospital-acquired pneumonia in adults: diagnosis, assessment of severity, initial antimicrobial therapy, and preventative strategies. A consensus statement. Am J Respir Crit Care Med 153:1711–1725, 1995.
21. Gorbach SL, Bartlett JG, Blacklow NR. Infectious diseases. Philadelphia: WB Saunders, 1992.
22. Donowitz GR, Mandell GL. Acute pneumonia. In: Mandell GL, Douglas RG, Bennett JE, eds. Principles and practice of infectious diseases. 4th ed. New York: Churchill Livingstone, 1995;1:619–632, 1769.
23. Stein D. Managing pneumonia acquired in nursing homes: special concerns. Geriatrics 45(3):39–47, 1990.
24. Fauci AS, Braunwald E, Isselbacher KJ, et al. Harrison's principles of internal medicine. 14th ed. New York: McGraw-Hill, 1998.
25. Cluff LE, Johnson JE. Pneumonia. In: Cluff LE, Johnson JE, eds. Clinical concepts of infectious diseases. Baltimore: Williams & Wilkins, 1972.
26. Lode H, Schaberg T, Raffenberg M, et al. Diagnostic problems in lower respiratory tract infections. J Antimicrob Chemother 32(Suppl A):29–37, 1993.
27. Whitson B, Campbell GD. Community-acquired pneumonia: new outpatient guidelines based on age, severity of illness. Geriatrics 49:24–36, 1994.
28. Brown RB. Community-acquired pneumonia: diagnosis and therapy of older adults. Geriatrics 48:43–50, 1993.
29. Marrie TJ. Pneumonia. Clin Geriatr Med 8:721–734, 1992.
30. Levy M, Dromer F, Brion N, et al. Community-acquired pneumonia: importance of initial noninvasive bacteriologic and radiologic investigations. Chest 92:43–48, 1988.
31. Fein AM, Niederman MS. Severe pneumonia in the elderly. Clin Geriatr Med 10:121–142, 1994.
32. Plouffe JF, McNall C, File TM. Value of noninvasive studies in community acquired pneumonia. Infect Dis Clin North Am 12:689–699, 1998.
33. Murray PR, Washington JA. Microscopic and bacteriologic analysis of expectorated sputum. Mayo Clinic Proc 50:339–344, 1975.
34. Barlett JG, Breiman RF, Mandell LA, et al. Community-acquired pneumonia in adults: guidelines for management. Clin Infect Dis 26:811–838, 1998.
35. File TM, Tan JS, Plouffe JF. The role of atypical pathogens *Mycoplasma pneumoniae, Chlamydia pneumoniae,* and *Legionella pneumophila* in respiratory infections. Infect Dis Clin North Am 12:569–592, 1998.
36. Fine MJ, Auble TE, Yealy DM, et al. A prediction rule to identify low-risk patients with community acquired pneumonia. N Engl J Med 336:243–250, 1997.
37. Meehan TP, Fine MJ, Krumholz HM, et al. Quality of care, process and outcomes in elderly patients with pneumonia. JAMA 278:2080–2084, 1997.
38. Cunha BA. Intravenous-to-oral antibiotic switch therapy. Postgrad Med 101:111–128, 1997.
39. Nix DE. Intrapulmonary concentrations of antimicrobial agents. Infect Dis Clin North Am 12:631–646, 1998.
40. Aoun M, Klastersky J. Drug treatment in the hospital: what are the choices? Drugs 42:962–973, 1991.
41. Marrie TJ. New aspects of old pathogens of pneumonia. Med Clin North Am 78:987–993, 1994.
42. Doern GV, Brueggemann A, Cetron MS, et al. Antimicrobial resistance of *Streptococcus pneumoniae* recovered from outpatients in the United States during the winter months of 1994 to 1995: results of a 30 center national surveillance study. Antimicrob Agents Chemother 40:1208–1213, 1996.
43. Centers for Disease Control and Prevention. Resistant *Streptococcus pneumoniae:* Kentucky and Tennessee. MMWR 43:23–31, 1994.
44. Doern GV, Pfaller MA, Kugler K, et al. Prevalence of antimicrobial resistance among respiratory tract isolates of *Streptococcus pneumoniae* in North America: 1997 results from the SENTRY antimicrobial surveillance program. Clin Infect Dis 27:764–770, 1998.
45. Barry AL, Fuchs PC, Brown SD. In vitro activities of five quinolone compounds against strains of *Streptococcus pneumoniae* with resistance to other antimicrobial agents. Antimicrob Agents Chemother 40:2431–2433, 1996.
46. Bradley JS, Scheld WM. The challenge of penicillin-resistant *Streptococcus pneumoniae* meningitis: current antibiotic therapy in the 1990s. Clin Infect Dis 24(Suppl 2):S213–S221, 1997.
47. Hedlund JU, Kalin ME, Ortqvist AB, et al. Antibody response to pneumococcal vaccine in middle-aged and elderly patients recently treated for pneumonia. Arch Intern Med 154:1961–1965, 1994.
48. Sims RV, Steinmann WC, McConville JH, et al. The clinical effectiveness of pneumococcal vaccine in the elderly. Ann Intern Med 108:653–657, 1988.
49. Shapiro ED, Berg AT, Austrian R, et al. The protective efficacy of polyvalent pneumococcal polysaccharide vaccine. N Engl J Med 325:1453–1460, 1991.
50. Moxon ER, Wilson R. The role of *Haemophilus influenzae* in the pathogenesis of pneumonia. Rev Infect Dis 13(Suppl 6):518–526, 1991.
51. McEvoy GK, Litvak K, Welsh OH, et al. AHFS drug information. Bethesda, MD: American Society of Hospital Pharmacists, 1994:208.
52. Verghese A, Berk SL. *Moraxella (Branhamella) catarrhalis.* Infect Dis Clin North Am 5:523–535, 1991.
53. Hampson NB, Woolf RA, Springmeyer SC. Oral antibiotics for pneumonia. Clin Chest Med 12:395–407, 1991.
54. Goetz AM, Stout JE, Jacobs SL, et al. Nosocomial Legionaire's disease discovered in community hospitals following cultures of the water system: seek and ye shall find. Am J Infect Control 26:8–11, 1998.
55. Cunha BA. Atypical pneumonias: clinical diagnosis and empirical treatment. Postgrad Med 90:89–101, 1991.
56. Martin RE, Bates JH. Atypical pneumonia. Infect Dis Clin North Am 5:585–601, 1991.
57. Clyde WA Jr. Clinical overview of typical *Mycoplasma pneumoniae* infections. Clin Infect Dis 17(Suppl 1):32–36, 1993.
58. Lynch JP. Community-acquired pneumonia: what new trends mean in practice. J Respir Dis 13:1619–1643, 1992.
59. Marston BJ, Plouffe JF, File TM, et al. Incidence of community-acquired pneumonia requiring hospitalization: results of a population-based active surveillance study in Ohio. Arch Intern Med 157:1709–1718, 1997.

60. Hammerschlag MR, Chirgwin K, Roblin PM, et al. Persistent infection with *Chlamydia pneumoniae* following acute respiratory illness. Clin Infect Dis 14:178–182, 1992.
61. Saikku P. The epidemiology and significance of *Chlamydia pneumoniae*. J Infect 25(Suppl I):27–34, 1992.
62. Johanson WG, Pierce AK, Sanford JP. Changing pharyngeal bacterial flora in hospitalized patients. N Engl J Med 281:1137–1140, 1969.
63. Meduri GU. Diagnosis of ventilator-associated pneumonia. Infect Dis Clin North Am 7:295–325, 1993.
64. Horan T, Culver D, Jarvis W, et al. Pathogens causing nosocomial infections. CDC: Antimicrob Newslett 5:65–67, 1988.
65. McCormack JP, Jewesson PJ. A critical re-evaluation of the "therapeutic range" of aminoglycosides. Clin Infect Dis 14:320–339, 1992.
66. Moore RD, Smith CR, Lietman PS. Association of aminoglycoside plasma levels with therapeutic outcome in Gram-negative pneumonia. Am J Med 77:657–662, 1984.
67. Reed MD, Witte MK. Lower respiratory tract infections. In: DiPiro JT, Talbert RL, Hayes PE, et al., eds. Pharmacotherapy: a pathophysiological approach. 2nd ed. Norwalk, CT: Appleton & Lange, 1993:1543–1559.
68. Silver DR, Cohen IL, Weinberg PF. Recurrent *Pseudomonas aeruginosa* pneumonia in an intensive care unit. Chest 101:194–198, 1992.
69. Niedderman MS. An approach to empiric therapy of nosocomial pneumonia. Med Clin North Am 78:1123–1139, 1994.
70. Chelluri L, Warren J, Jastremski MS. Pharmacokinetics of a 3 mg/kg body weight loading dose of gentamicin in critically ill patients. Chest 95:1295–1297, 1995.
71. Prins JM, Buller HR, Kuijper EJ, et al. Once versus thrice daily gentamicin in patients with serious infections. Lancet 341:335–339, 1993.
72. Nicolau DP, Belliveau PP, Nightingale CH, et al. Implementation of a once-daily aminoglycoside program in a large community teaching hospital. Hosp Pharm 30:674–676, 679–680, 1995.
73. Hatala R, Tuan D, Cook D. Once daily aminoglycoside dosing in immunocompetent adults: a meta-analysis. Ann Intern Med 124:717–725, 1996.
74. Barza M, Ioannidis JP, Cappelleri JC, et al. Single or multiple daily doses of aminoglycoside: a meta-analysis. BMJ 312:338–344, 1998.
75. Hooper DC. Expanding uses of fluoroquinolones: opportunities and challenges. Ann Intern Med 129:908–910, 1998.
76. Lorber B, Swenson RM. Bacteriology of aspiration pneumonia: a prospective study of community- and hospital-acquired cases. Ann Intern Med 81:329–331, 1974.
77. Bartlett JG. Anaerobic bacterial infections of the lungs and pleural space. Clin Infect Dis 16(Suppl 4):248–255, 1993.
78. Gudiol F, Manresa F, Pallares R, et al. Clindamycin versus penicillin for anaerobic lung infections: high rate of penicillin failures associated with penicillin-resistant *Bacteroides melaninogenicus*. Arch Intern Med 150:2525–2529, 1990.
79. Levison ME, Mangura CT, Lorber B, et al. Clindamycin compared with penicillin for the treatment of anaerobic lung abscess. Ann Intern Med 98:466-471, 1983.

CHAPTER 68

TUBERCULOSIS

Caroline S. Zeind, Greta K. Gourley, and Dawn M. Chandler-Toufieli

Tuberculosis (TB) is currently responsible for more deaths worldwide than any other infectious disease.[1] The human immunodeficiency virus (HIV) epidemic is causing an increased incidence of TB cases worldwide, particularly in areas such as sub-Saharan Africa.[2] HIV infection is the most powerful risk factor for the activation of latent *M. tuberculosis* infection.[3] TB has been declared a public health emergency by the World Health Organization (WHO).[4] In 1998, more people died of TB than in any other year in history.[5] If TB controls are not strengthened, the WHO estimates that, by 2020, 70 million more people will die from TB. The emergence of multidrug-resistant tuberculosis (MDR-TB) is a worldwide problem, and threatens efforts to control the disease.[6,7] In the United States, outbreaks of MDR-TB in patients infected with HIV have been characterized by delayed diagnoses, inadequate treatment regimens, high mortality, and significant rates of nosocomial transmission.[8] The true global magnitude of MDR-TB is not well described, although several countries with high prevalence rates have been identified.[6,7] Adherence to the recommendations for the treatment of TB among adults and children that were provided in a joint statement of the American Thoracic Society (ATS) and the Centers for Disease Control and Prevention (CDC) will help to prevent the development of more cases of MDR-TB, reduce the occurrence of treatment failure, and reduce the transmission of tuberculosis.[9]

TREATMENT GOALS: TUBERCULOSIS

- Cure individuals with tuberculosis disease.
- Impede transmission within the community.
- Isolate individuals during the infectious period and initiate appropriate treatment.
- Prevent the emergence of MDR-TB by selecting appropriate antituberculosis regimens and ensuring patient adherence to therapy.
- Adjust the patient's therapy if MDR-TB is detected.
- Evaluate the patient's response to therapy by evaluation of sputum cultures.
- Implement directly observed therapy (DOT) to improve patient adherence to prescribed regimens.
- Consider preventive therapy and initiate treatment if warranted for those patients infected with TB, but without active disease.

EPIDEMIOLOGY

Etiology

Mycobacterium tuberculosis, or the tubercle bacillus, is a member of the genus Mycobacteriaceae, order Actinomycetales. It, along with *M. bovis* and *M. Africanum,* which are also species of this order, causes TB in humans. Currently, disease owing to *M. bovis* or *M. Africanum* is rare in the United States.[10,11] *M. tuberculosis* infects humans, other primates, and other mammalians that are in contact with humans. The only reservoir of the organism, however, is humans.[10]

Mycobacteria are slow growing (4 to 6 weeks) aerobic rods.[11] The bacilli contain surface lipids that render them acid fast, because they resist decolorization with acid alcohol after staining. Heat or detergents are usually required for primary staining because of the lipid characteristics of these organisms.[11]

M. tuberculosis contains many immunoreactive substances, such as surface lipids and water-soluble components of cell wall peptidoglycan, that appear to exert their effects through primary actions on host macrophages. Mycobacteria contain several protein and polysaccharide antigens that are involved in the pathogenesis of disease. Cell-mediated hypersensitivity, which is characteristic of TB, is discussed later in this chapter.[11]

Incidence

The incidence of TB in the United States in 1997 was 19,855 cases (7.4 cases per 100,000 population). This represented a 26% decrease from 1992 (26,673; 10.5 cases per 100,000), when the number of cases peaked, marking the resurgence of TB in the United States. The 1997 rate represents the lowest number of TB cases since 1953, when national reporting was started. Although the rates in California, Florida, Illinois, New Jersey, New York, and Texas have declined substantially since 1992, 57% of all TB cases were reported by these states in 1997. Regional analysis revealed that 40% of all TB cases were reported from 64 major cities, reflecting the continued concentration of TB in urban areas of the United States.[12]

The demographics of sex and age group are similar to previous reports. Males are reported to contract the disease at a rate two times higher than that of females. During 1996, the risk of contracting TB was lowest in the 0- to 14-year-old age group and highest in individuals 65 years of age or older. The case rates were highest among Asian/Pacific Islanders (41.6 cases per 100,000) and non-Hispanic blacks (22.3 cases per 100,000), and lowest for non-Hispanic whites (2.8 cases per 100,000).[13]

The fifth consecutive year of decreased TB cases in the United States primarily reflects a decline in cases of individuals of all ages who were born in the United States. During the same time period, the cases among foreign-born individuals increased by 6%, with 39% of all 1997 TB cases being reported in this patient population. The TB case rate for foreign-born individuals remains at least four to five times higher than for U.S.-born individuals.[12]

In 1993 the CDC began monitoring antituberculosis (anti-TB) drug resistance through a national surveillance system in order to track anti-TB drug-susceptibility in the United States. During 1997, 84% of the initial *M. tuberculosis* isolates were tested for drug susceptibility. Of the 42 states that reported susceptibility data for at least 75% of culture-positive cases, 7.6% of the isolates were resistant to at least isoniazid and 1.3% were resistant to at least isoniazid and rifampin (MDR-TB). At least one MDR-TB case was reported in 27 of the 42 states. Of interest, 47% of all MDR-TB cases were reported in New York and California.[12]

The overall decline of reported TB cases in the United States is attributed to stronger TB-control programs that focus on prompt identification of individuals with TB, initiation of appropriate therapy, and assurance of completion of therapy.[12] Although the number and rate of reported TB cases in the United States continues to decrease, TB remains a major global public health problem.

TRANSMISSION AND PATHOPHYSIOLOGY

M. tuberculosis is acquired by inhalation of infectious airborne particles, called droplet nuclei, that are small enough (1–5 μm) to reach the alveolar air spaces.[11] Patients with active pulmonary or laryngeal TB expel these airborne droplets primarily by coughing, sneezing, or vocalizing; the particles can remain suspended in the air for several hours, allowing exposure to a susceptible person (contact). Factors that determine the probability of infection are the intensity of exposure and probably the effectiveness of innate host defenses.[14] Transmission of infection can be reduced by adequate ventilation and ultraviolet lighting.[11]

On entry of the tubercle bacilli into the lungs, a nonspecific acute inflammatory response occurs, which is usually accompanied by little or no symptoms.[11] The tubercle bacilli are then ingested by alveolar macrophages and transported to regional lymph nodes. If the spread of the organism is not contained at the level of regional lymph nodes, the bacilli reach the bloodstream, causing widespread dissemination (Fig. 68.1). The majority of lesions of disseminated TB heal, although they remain potential foci of later reactivation.

During the 2 to 10 weeks after primary infection, while bacilli continue to replicate in their intracellular environment, a cell-mediated immune response occurs in the infected host.[11,14] This immunologic response is characterized by complex interactions as lymphocytes enter areas of infection and release chemotactic factors, interleukins, and lymphokines. These lymphokines in turn recruit circulating monocytes, inducing their transformation into macrophages, and subsequently into specialized cells, which become organized into granulomas. Further multiplication and spread usually are confined by the immunologic response, although mycobacteria may persist within macrophages as dormant organisms for several years.[11,14] Healing then occurs, often accompanied by late calcification of the granulomas, which sometimes leaves a residual lesion that is visible on chest radiography.[11]

The cell-mediated response is characterized by the delayed-type hypersensitivity (DTH) reaction of the purified protein derivative (PPD) skin test. Most people who are infected with TB will have a positive reaction to the PPD skin test within 2 to 8 weeks after infection, a condition known as latent infection.[11] Cell-mediated immunity effectively contains the infection in 90 to 95% of immunocompetent people, and no clinical disease develops. These individuals undergo complete healing of primary TB lesions with no subsequent evidence of disease. Of the remaining 5 to 10%, one-half will develop disease within the first year or two because of ineffective immunity, and the other half will develop disease later in life.[11] Clinical disease results from failure to control the mycobacterial replication that followed initial infection (progressive pri-

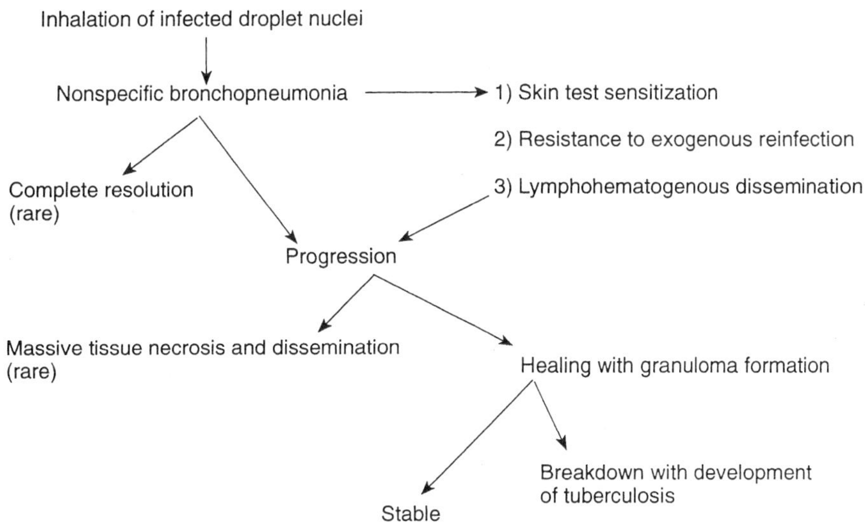

Figure 68.1. Results of infection with *M. tuberculosis.* (From Glassroth J, Robbins AG, Snider DE Jr. Medical progress: tuberculosis in the 1980's. N Engl J Med 302[2]:1442, 1980.)

mary TB) or when latent organisms overcome immunologic control (reactivation TB).[14]

HIV infection has dramatically altered the natural history of TB because of its profound effects on cell-mediated immunity. The CD4+ T-lymphocyte depletion results in a defective immunologic response to *M. tuberculosis*.[15,16] People infected with HIV with recently acquired *M. tuberculosis* are at a high risk of progressive primary TB and those with latent *M. tuberculosis* infection are at a high risk of reactivation TB.[15,16] In comparison to the 10% lifetime risk among people who have TB infection without HIV infection, people infected with HIV develop reactivation disease at a rate of 5 to 12% per year.[17–19] As a result, pulmonary TB was added to the list of indicator diseases in the 1993 acquired immunodeficiency syndrome (AIDS) surveillance case definition.

Studies using DNA fingerprinting to distinguish recently acquired infections from remote latent infections have suggested that perhaps one-third of recent cases of TB in New York City and San Francisco were owing to recently transmitted infections.[20,21] In addition, rapid progression from recent *M. tuberculosis* infection to active TB (progressive primary TB) has been observed in people infected with HIV exposed to *M. tuberculosis* during institutional outbreaks.[22–24] People infected with HIV are so vulnerable to the development of active TB that clinical disease may occur within weeks of exposure to *M. tuberculosis*. In those patients with advanced HIV infection, previous *M. tuberculosis* infection is not always protective, and exogenous reinfection can occur with a different infecting strain of the organism.[25]

SCREENING AND IDENTIFYING INDIVIDUALS WITH TUBERCULOSIS INFECTION

Clinicians should use the following strategies to prevent and control TB.[9,26]

1. Identify and completely treat those persons who have active TB.
2. Conduct thorough contact investigations (find and evaluate persons who have had contact with TB patients, and determine if they have infection or active disease and treat appropriately).
3. Screen high-risk populations to identify persons infected with TB and provide appropriate therapy to prevent the infection from progressing to active TB.

The Mantoux tuberculin skin test (TST) is the standard method for screening and identifying individuals with *M. tuberculosis* infection; an intradermal injection of 5 tuberculin units (5 TU) of PPD of killed tubercle bacilli is usually administered on the inner forearm.[26] The DTH response to the Mantoux test should be examined and interpreted by a trained health care provider 48 to 72 hours after the injection for induration.[11] By gentle palpation of the indurated area, the transverse diameter of the induration is measured; erythema should be excluded from the measurement.

Criteria endorsed by the ATS and CDC for a positive TST are summarized in Table 68.1. These criteria are intended for use as a guide to identify individuals at high risk for TB who are candidates for preventive therapy (once active disease is excluded).[9,26,27]

A negative reaction to the TST does not rule out TB infection or disease. There are circumstances in which DTH response may be absent owing to cell-mediated deficiency, a term known as anergy. This condition may occur in immunosuppressed persons including those with HIV infection, those with overwhelming miliary or pulmonary TB, or those with other conditions.[11,28] Anergy skin testing can be performed to assess the response to skin-test antigens to which a cell-mediated, DTH response is expected. In 1991, the CDC published guidelines recommending that anergy skin testing in conjunction with PPD-tuberculin skin testing be performed for HIV-infected persons being evaluated for latent infection with *M. tuberculosis*.[29] Companion or "control" antigens (mumps and *Candida*) placed by using the

Table 68.1 ▪ Summary of Interpretation of Tuberculin Skin-Test Results

Tuberculin Reaction	Criteria
≥5 mm of induration: Considered positive for the highest-risk groups	Includes persons who have had close contact with a person with infectious TB, people with HIV infection or risk factors for HIV infection but unknown HIV status, and persons who have chest radiographs that are consistent with previous TB.
≥10 mm of induration: Considered positive for other high-risk groups	Includes persons who have several medical conditions that increase the risk that TB will progress to disease. Such conditions include diabetes mellitus, silicosis, prolonged high-dose corticosteroid therapy and other immunosuppressive therapy (including bone marrow and organ transplantation), some hematologic disorders (leukemias and lymphomas), other specific malignancies (i.e., carcinoma of the head or neck), chronic renal failure, gastrectomy, jejunoileal bypass, or low body weight (≥10% below ideal body weight). Other high-risk groups are injecting drug users who are known to be HIV seronegative; foreign born people who recently arrived from countries that have high-prevalence or incidence of TB; residents and employees of high-risk congregate settings and homeless shelters; medically underserved, low-income populations, including high-risk racial and ethnic groups; local populations who have been identified as high-prevalence groups (such as homeless people or migrant farm workers); and children <4 years of age or infants, children, and adolescents exposed to adults in high-risk categories.
≥15 mm of induration: Considered positive for persons who do not meet criteria listed above	Routine screening is not recommended for populations at low risk for infection with *Mycobacterium tuberculosis.*

Source: Reference 26.

Mantoux method of intradermal injection in conjunction with PPD testing was recommended to provide additional information about a person's ability to mount a DTH response. The DTH antigens, mumps and *Candida*, are FDA approved for intradermal DTH testing to assess cell-mediated immunity.[28] When interpreting skin testing results, a positive DTH response (≥5 mm of induration measured within 48–72 hours), in conjunction with a negative PPD response, has been interpreted as evidence that the negative PPD test is a true negative and that the person is not infected. Lack of DTH response, in conjunction with a negative PPD response, has been interpreted as evidence that the individual is unable to mount a positive response to PPD even if infected with TB.[29]

Since the publication of the 1991 guidelines, limitations in the usefulness of anergy testing in public health TB screening programs have been documented. Factors that limit the usefulness of anergy skin testing for decision making regarding TB-preventive therapy for persons infected with HIV in the United States include the following:[28,29]

1. Problems regarding the standardization and reproducibility of anergy skin-testing methods
2. The variable risk for TB associated with a diagnosis of anergy
3. Lack of documented benefit of anergy skin testing as part of screening programs for *M. tuberculosis* infection among HIV-infected persons

Revised recommendations by the CDC no longer routinely recommend the inclusion of anergy testing in conjunction with PPD-tuberculin skin testing in screening programs for *M. tuberculosis* infection among persons infected with HIV.[28] However, in selected situations, DTH evaluation may be useful in guiding individual decisions regarding preventive therapy.

CLINICAL PRESENTATION AND DIAGNOSIS

As previously mentioned, screening programs can (1) identify infected persons who are at high risk for disease and who would benefit from preventive therapy, (2) identify persons who may have clinical disease and need treatment, and (3) exclude those who have a history of adequate treatment for TB infection. Individuals with a positive TST should have a chest radiograph, which is a useful tool for both diagnosis and evaluation of TB.[8,11] In pulmonary TB, the most typical lesion is a multinodular infiltration in the apical posterior segments of the upper lobes and superior segments of the lower lobes.[11] Persons with HIV infection and TB may have a chest radiograph that shows a classic reactivation pattern, an "atypical" (i.e., pleural effusion) pattern, or evidence of past infection (i.e., calcified lymph node or lung nodule).[14] If the chest radiograph is normal, the diagnosis of TB should not be excluded on the basis of this evidence alone because radiographic findings may lag behind the rapid evolution of active TB.[30,31]

The patient evaluation should include a medical history, including assessing whether the patient has medical conditions, especially HIV infection, that increase the risk for TB disease. If HIV infection is recognized for the first time, a TST should be performed.[32] If the result is positive (≥5 mm of induration), the patient should undergo chest radiography and clinical evaluation for the exclusion of active TB. If symptoms suggestive of TB are present in an individual infected with HIV, the patient should undergo chest radiography and clinical evaluation regardless of his or her TST status.[32]

The diagnosis can be established most readily by sputum examination and culture for the majority of patients with pulmonary TB.[11] However, lack of positive acid-fast smears does not rule out presumptive TB, because smears may be negative. In 40 to 67% of patients infected with HIV who have TB, acid-fast bacilli (AFB) were found on microscopic examination of sputum specimens, and *M. tuberculosis* was recovered from 74 to 95% in culture.[33–35] Specialized stains enable the visualization of the organism; however, determinations of the type of mycobacteria seen and the determination of drug susceptibility requires culturing of the specimen.[11] Because *M. tuberculosis* is slow growing, the conventional culturing technique takes approximately 4 weeks, with several additional weeks for susceptibility testing. Newer systems, such as the BACTEC radiometric system, speed up this process, reducing culturing time by 2 weeks.[11] Antimicrobial susceptibility testing of initial *M. tuberculosis* isolates from all patients should be performed because of the rising incidence of MDR-TB. Radiometric testing usually yields results 4 to 7 days following initial detection of mycobacterial growth.[36]

A recently introduced method of diagnosis, the Mycobacteria Growth Indicator Tube (MGIT), appears to be a rapid, easy-to-use system with a high accuracy for detecting mycobacteria directly from clinical specimens.[37] This system uses a traditional broth medium and a novel fluorescent indicator for the recovery of mycobacteria from patient specimens. The fluorescence in the MGIT is readily visible without elaborate instrumentation, enabling large numbers of cultures to be read quickly. Other newer methods of diagnosis that appear promising include serologic tests that use enzyme-linked immunosorbent (ELISA) techniques and gene amplification by the polymerase chain reaction (PCR).[11]

When extrapulmonary TB is suspected, a variety of clinical specimens other than sputum (e.g., urine, cerebrospinal fluid [CSF], pleural fluid, pus, or biopsy specimens) may be needed for examination.[10]

The CDC recommends that a patient suspected of having or known to have TB should be placed in an AFB isolation room, which has negative pressure meeting appropriate criteria.[38] Respiratory isolation should be discontinued only when patients are receiving effective therapy, when clinical improvement is observed, and when three consecutive sputum samples, collected on different days, are AFB-smear negative.

Before the recognition of HIV infection, the majority of cases of TB were pulmonary.[11] However, extrapulmonary TB either alone or in combination with pulmonary TB may occur in up to two-thirds of patients infected with HIV who have TB.[11] The extent of pulmonary disease varies from minimal clinical illness that is barely discernible on chest radiographs to major involvement with extensive cavitation and debilitating symptoms.[11] The symptoms of pulmonary TB include a productive cough, chest pain, and hemoptysis. Systemic symptoms include fever, night sweats, chills, easy fatigability, anorexia, and weight loss. Extrapulmonary TB may involve sites such as lymph nodes, genitourinary tract, bones and joints, meninges, peritoneum, and pleura.[11] Hematogenous dissemination to virtually any organ system is possible in individuals infected with HIV. TB should be suspected in persons infected with HIV who have unexplained fever; cough; pulmonary infiltrates; lymphadenopathy; brain abscess; meningitis; pericarditis; pleural effusions; or intraabdominal, musculoskeletal, or cutaneous abscesses.[14] Because the clinical features of HIV-infected patients with TB are many times nonspecific, diagnosis can be difficult. Failure to suspect TB and order the appropriate diagnostic studies can lead to diagnostic delays. In light of the rapidly progressive nature of TB in persons infected with HIV, the diagnosis should be pursued expeditiously. Patients infected with HIV who have TB have increased dissemination of TB, increased number and severity of symptoms, and rapid progression to death unless treatment is begun.[39] Patients with disseminated disease may experience shaking chills, hypotension, and acute respiratory distress.[39,40] The local signs and symptoms experienced in persons infected with HIV will depend on the organs involved as well as coexisting HIV-related complications.[39]

MULTIDRUG-RESISTANT TUBERCULOSIS

MDR-TB is defined as a case of TB caused by a strain of *M. tuberculosis* that exhibits resistance to at least isoniazid and rifampin.[6,7] Microbial resistance to anti-TB agents may be classified as either primary or acquired.[6] Primary drug resistance occurs in patients without histories or other evidence of prior treatment. Various risk factors for primary resistance include coming from a country with a high prevalence of drug-resistant TB, exposure to a patient with drug-resistant TB, and greater than 4% primary resistance to isoniazid within the community.[9] Acquired drug resistance occurs in patients who have been treated with anti-TB agents for at least 1 month, including those with treatment failures and relapses.[6] The quality of TB treatment programs affects the development of both types of resistance. Inadequate treatment programs allow the emergence of resistant organisms, producing acquired drug resistance in patients who are inadequately treated. Once these organisms are transmitted and TB disease develops, the infected person has "primary" resistant disease. It is estimated that the average cost for treating a case of MDR-TB is $180,000, which is much more costly than treating a case caused by a drug-susceptible strain ($12,000).[41,42] The management of patients with drug-resistant TB is discussed later in this chapter.

Although the exact magnitude of worldwide drug resistance is unknown, recent surveillance of the prevalence of resistance in 35 countries suggests that this is a global problem.[6] In 1994 the Global Project on Anti-Tuberculosis Drug Resistance Surveillance was initiated by the WHO and the International Union against Tuberculosis and Lung Disease (IUATLD). The purpose of this study was to use standardized methods to measure the prevalence of resistance to anti-TB drugs in countries throughout the world.[6] The results of the first 4 years of the project were published and contained information on drug resistance to isoniazid, rifampin, ethambutol, and streptomycin in 35 countries or regions on five continents. Results of the study revealed that primary multidrug resistance was observed in every country surveyed except Kenya, and the median prevalence was 1.4% (range, 0–14.4%). In persons with acquired drug resistance the median prevalence of multidrug resistance was 13% (range, 0–54%), much higher than the rate owing to primary resistance. The overall prevalence of MDR-TB was 2.2% (range 0–22.1%). Although the overall prevalence of MDR-TB reported is low, the high prevalences in the former Soviet Union, Asia, the Dominican Republic, and Argentina are concerning. A recent reversal of previously declining rates of TB in Eastern Europe and in particular, the former Soviet Union, probably is because of an irregular supply of drugs and nonstandardized regimens; other contributing factors may include nosocomial infection and outbreaks in prisons.[6,43,44] The relationship between drug resistance and the quality of TB control programs is complex; however, there may be a link between the quality of TB control programs and levels of drug resistance.[6]

PSYCHOSOCIAL ASPECTS

From a psychosocial perspective, treatment of TB should take the following into consideration:

- Individualize treatment to meet the specific needs of each patient.
- It is essential to provide compassionate care and offer support services to patients.
- Also offer support services to care givers and family members who will be involved with the care of the patient.
- Identify if depression, anxiety, fear, or feelings of isolation are present and refer patient to a clinical specialist and support groups.
- Since TB may have negative connotations, educate patients about the disease and assure them that having TB should not be viewed as shameful.
- Provide information regarding infectivity that will allow the individual to know when he or she can return to daily activities.

THERAPEUTIC PLAN

The availability of anti-TB agents has revolutionized the prognosis of patients with TB and TB infection.[45] Streptomycin (STM) was introduced for the management of TB during the 1940s. It soon became apparent that STM monotherapy frequently resulted in treatment failure that was associated with in vitro resistance to the drug.[46,47] In the 1950s and 1960s, isoniazid (INH) and paraaminosalicylic acid (PAS) were combined with STM in a regimen that cured TB in nearly all patients. Treatment programs were very successful because they were carried out in hospitals, where patient adherence to therapy could be ensured. As a consequence, acquired drug resistance was uncommon. During the late 1960s, therapy was shifted to the outpatient setting. Unfortunately, reduced adherence to anti-TB regimens in the outpatient setting has led to rising rates of treatment failure, relapse, and acquired drug resistance.[48–53]

Most patients with TB can be cured with adherence to therapeutic regimens.[45] The goal of drug therapy of active TB is twofold: to cure the sick and to impede the transmission of tubercle bacilli in the community. In people with TB infection, INH therapy prevents disease in the treated person while sparing others the potential of becoming infected from contact with that person.[9] On the basis of controlled clinical trials, three basic principles for the treatment of TB (disease) have evolved: (1) regimens for treatment of disease must contain multiple drugs to which the organisms are susceptible, (2) the drugs must be taken regularly, and (3) drug therapy must continue for a sufficient period of time.[9,54] The aim of therapy is to provide the most efficacious regimen with the least toxicity possible for the shortest period of time.

Three subpopulations of the tubercle bacilli can potentially coexist during an infection.[10] Anti-TB agents are targeted toward various sites of mycobacterial growth in the body (Table 68.2).[55] The most numerous population consists of extracellular bacteria; these organisms are killed most readily by INH and STM and to a lesser extent by rifampin (RMP). The second population is composed of organisms that seek out the acidic environment of caseating granulomas. RMP exhibits the greatest activity in killing these organisms. The final population of organisms exists within the activated macrophages (intracellular). Because of the acidic environment within macrophages, the activity of most anti-TB agents is inhibited. Pyrazinamide (PZA) possesses the greatest activity against this population.

Current anti-TB regimens use combinations of agents to eliminate extracellular organisms from the sputum, decrease infectivity, and destroy slowly dividing organisms within granulomas and macrophages.[56–58] By combining various agents, regimens as short as 6 months' duration can be used while minimizing drug resistance.

Table 68.2 ▪ Principal Activity and Site of Action of the Major Antituberculous Agents

Agent	Activity	Site of Action
Isoniazid (INH)	Bactericidal	Intracellular bacilli, extracellular bacilli, bacilli in caseous lesions
Rifampin (RMP)	Bactericidal	Intracellular bacilli, extracellular bacilli, bacilli in caseous lesions
Pyrazinamide (PZA)	Bactericidal	Intracellular bacilli
Streptomycin (STM)	Bactericidal	Extracellular bacilli
Ethambutol (EMB)	Bacteriostatic	Intracellular bacilli, extracellular bacilli

Source: Reference 55.

Table 68.3 ▪ Regimen Options for the Preferred Treatment of Children and Adults: Tuberculosis Without HIV Infection

Option 1[a]	Option 2[a]	Option 3[a]
Administer daily INH, RMP, and PZA for 8 weeks followed by 16 weeks of INH and RMP daily or 2–3 times/week[b] If INH resistant rate is not <4%, EMB or STM should be added to the initial regimen until susceptibility to INH and RMP is demonstrated.[c]	Administer daily INH, RMP, PZA and STM, or EMB for 2 weeks followed by 2 times/week[b] administration of the same drugs for 6 weeks (by DOT), and subsequently, with 2 times/week administration of INH and RMP for 16 weeks (by DOT).[c]	Treat by DOT, 3 times/week[b] with INH, RMP, PZA, and EMB or STM for 6 months.[c]

Source: Reference 61.

[a]For patients with tuberculosis and HIV infection, refer to reference 78.

[b]Any regimen administered 2 times/week or 3 times/week should be monitored by DOT for the duration of therapy.

[c]With any of the options, consult a TB medical expert if the patient is symptomatic or smear or culture positive after 3 months.

Directly Observed Therapy

A proven strategy to ensure patient adherence to anti-TB medications is the use of directly observed therapy (DOT).[59] In DOT the patient is observed by a health care provider or other responsible person as the patient ingests the anti-TB medications. In addition, DOT provides the opportunity for patient education and also enables earlier detection of adverse effects.[60] DOT may be administered to patients in a clinical setting, as well as in the patient's home, place of employment, school, or other mutually agreed-on setting.[9] Anti-TB medications can be administered with DOT daily or two or three times a week; this has proven to be highly successful in a wide variety of settings.[9,61] The involvement of pharmacists throughout the world in DOT programs will be beneficial for several reasons. Not only can pharmacists ensure patient adherence to therapy, but they also can provide drug information to patients and monitor for drug-induced adverse effects.[60] The risk of acquired drug resistance can be minimized by pharmacists and other health care providers who implement DOT programs.

The cost of implementing DOT is more than offset by the savings that result from the decreased risk of treatment failure, relapse, drug resistance, and secondary spread.[9,59] This patient-centered approach appears to be effective in a variety of high-risk groups such as the homeless, refugees, the unemployed, substance abuse patients, and patients with HIV infection.[62] In addition, this strategy appears effective regardless of the country or community where the program is implemented. DOT should be considered in all patients who are treated for TB and is strongly recommended in patients with HIV infection; there appears to be a reduced degree of safety in treating patients with HIV infection, and patient adherence to anti-TB therapy is crucial. The various regimen options that are available for administration with DOT are listed in Table 68.3.[61] Although these specific regimens have not been studied in children, the results achieved in adults suggest potential benefits in children.

Patients with Multidrug-Resistant Tuberculosis

Managing patients with MDR-TB is extremely challenging; "hot zones" of ongoing transmission have been identified in several countries. In areas where MDR-TB is a problem, establishment of DOT therapy alone for short-course therapy is insufficient because short-course therapy does not cure MDR-TB.[63] A strategy that includes DOT, along with specific provisions for treating MDR-TB, has been proposed by a group of TB experts.[63] This approach has been termed "DOTS-plus" and is designed to triage patients with MDR-TB to individualized treatment regimens or, if possible, into empirical retreatment schemes appropriate to the local epidemiology.[63] A community-based approach to treating MDR-TB in Peru utilizing "DOTS-plus" obtained successful results.[63] This recently introduced strategy holds great promise for utilization by other areas with outbreaks of MDR-TB.

TREATMENT

Antituberculous Agents Currently in Use

Isoniazid

Since its introduction in 1952, isonicotinicyl hydrazine (INH) has been the most widely used anti-TB agent.[9] The drug exhibits many qualities of an ideal agent; it is bactericidal, relatively nontoxic, inexpensive, and well absorbed orally or parenterally.

Although the mechanism of action is unknown, INH appears to inhibit the biosynthesis of mycolic acids, which are important constituents of the mycobacterial cell wall.[64] The drug is actively transported into the bacterium, where it acts to kill rapidly multiplying extracellular bacteria and inhibits the growth of dormant organisms existing within macrophages and in caseating granulomas.[65]

INH generally is administered as a single dose of 300 mg for adults and 10 to 20 mg/kg (maximum 300 mg) for children.[61] Rapid and complete absorption occur following oral administration, achieving peak concentrations of 3 to 5 μg/mL after a 3- to 5-mg/kg dose.[66] When INH is administered orally with food, a reduction in the extent of absorption and peak plasma concentration of INH may occur. Aluminum-containing antacids may decrease gastrointestinal (GI) absorption of INH.[67] The drug is widely distributed throughout the body; significant quantities have been detected in the pleural, ascitic, and cerebrospinal fluid; caseous material; saliva; skin; and muscle.[9,68]

Metabolism via the hepatic P450 mixed oxidase system accounts for 70 to 90% of the elimination of INH. Several metabolic pathways are involved, with acetylation being the major pathway.[69,70] After acetylation by the liver, the drug is excreted as a metabolite by the kidneys; it appears unchanged in the urine, along with other metabolites, including hydrazones.[45] The relative fractions of INH, acetylisoniazid, and hydrazones in the urine differ considerably among patients. The rate of acetylation of INH is genetically controlled.[71] Individuals are categorized as either fast or slow acetylators, depending on the rate of acetylation of INH in the liver. Approximately 45 to 65% of the American and northern European populations are classified as slow acetylators. Inuit (Eskimos) and Asians primarily are rapid acetylators. The elimination rate of INH depends on acetylator phenotype; half-lives of approximately 0.5 to 2 hours are observed in the fast acetylators and 2 to 5 hours in slow acetylators.[65] Patients who are slow acetylators may be more susceptible to the side effects related to higher concentrations, such as peripheral neuropathy.[45] It has been postulated that hepatotoxicity is more common in rapid acetylators, owing to the production of larger amounts of the metabolite acetylhydrazine.[72] The acetylhydrazine metabolite is thought to be involved in the development of INH-induced hepatotoxicity.[70] More recent data suggest that rapid acetylators are not at increased risk for hepatitis from INH and that the rate of acetylation is unlikely to be of therapeutic significance.[73,74]

Only a small amount of INH is eliminated unchanged by the kidneys. Therefore, dosage adjustments in patients with renal dysfunction are necessary only for individuals who are slow acetylators with a creatinine clearance less than 10 mL/min.[75,76] A reduction of the daily dose by 50% is recommended for these individuals, as well as for those with severe hepatic disease, to prevent accumulation of the drug and to reduce the potential for hepatotoxicity. In patients who are undergoing dialysis, significant amounts of INH are removed from the blood by hemodialysis and peritoneal dialysis. Dosage adjustments may be necessary.

Peripheral neuropathy appears to be a dose-dependent adverse effect of INH.[9,65] It is uncommon at a dose of 5 mg/kg, occurring in 2% of patients receiving INH. At higher dosages, peripheral neuropathy may develop in 10 to 20% of the patients. Peripheral neuropathy is most likely caused by INH-induced depletion of pyridoxine stores or competitive inhibition with pyridoxine in its role as a cofactor in the synthesis of synaptic neurotransmitters.[77] Pyridoxine (15–50 mg/day) should be given with INH to people who have conditions in which neuropathy is common (e.g., diabetes, uremia, alcoholism, or malnutrition).[9,65] Persons with HIV infection who are undergoing TB treatment with INH also should receive supplementation with pyridoxine (25–50 mg daily or 50–100 mg twice a week) to reduce the occurrence of INH-induced side effects in both the central and peripheral nervous system.[78] For pregnant women and persons who have a seizure disorder, it is recommended that pyridoxine be given with INH. As was previously mentioned, patients with slow acetylation may be more susceptible to the development of peripheral neuropathy.[45]

Hepatotoxicity associated with the use of INH occurs in approximately 1 to 2% of patients.[69,70] In the majority of cases, transaminase values return to pretreatment values despite continuation of INH; however, in rare cases progressive liver dysfunction, jaundice, bilirubinuria, and severe and even fatal hepatitis have occurred. Although the mechanism of hepatitis is unknown, it is probably associated with hepatic metabolites.[70] Age appears to be the most significant factor in determining the risk of INH-induced hepatotoxicity. A U.S. Public Health Service Surveillance Study evaluated the toxicity of INH in 13,838 patients.[79] The results of this study indicated that the rate of hepatitis increased directly with increasing age to 65 years. The rate of hepatitis was 0% in patients who were less than 20 years old; 0.3% in patients 20 to 34 years old; 1.2% in patients 35 to 49 years old; and 2.3% in patients 50 to 64 years old. However, recent studies have demonstrated that hepatitis may occur in approximately 4% of patients older than 65 years of age who are receiving the drug.[80] Excessive or chronic alcohol consumption, chronic liver disease, intravenous drug use, and being a postpubertal African-American or Hispanic female have also been identified as risk cofactors.[9,77]

Baseline measurement of liver enzyme levels should be performed for patients receiving INH and should be monitored periodically.[11] In patients older than 35 years of age, a transaminase measurement, such as aspartate aminotransferase (AST, SGOT), should be obtained before initiation of therapy and monthly thereafter.[9] Patients also should be questioned monthly for signs and symptoms of liver disease and should be instructed to report to their physician any of the prodromal symptoms of hepatitis (e.g., malaise, fatigue, weakness, anorexia, or nausea). Should these symptoms appear or if the signs that are suggestive of hepatic damage occur (e.g., liver enlargement with tenderness, jaundice, or dark urine), prompt discontinuation of INH is warranted; this usually prevents progression (Table 68.4).[9] Some clinicians recommend discontinuation of INH if transaminase values exceed three to five times the normal levels.[45]

Other rare adverse effects that are reported with INH administration include various central nervous system (CNS) toxicities (i.e., hallucinations, convulsions), dermatologic (i.e., acne, allergic rashes), hematologic (i.e., aplastic anemia), and GI effects.[65]

Several drug interactions have been reported with the use of INH in combination with other agents.[65,81] INH is

Table 68.4 ▪ Signs and Symptoms of Hepatic Damage or Other Adverse Effects

Unexplained anorexia
Nausea
Vomiting
Dark urine
Icterus
Rash
Persistent paresthesias of hands and feet
Persistent fatigue
Weakness or fever of >3 days
Abdominal tenderness (especially right upper quadrant)

Source: Reference 9.

an inhibitor of several cytochrome P450-dependent microsomal pathways.[82,83] Acetylation is the major pathway; therefore, acetylator phenotyping may be a factor to consider in the interaction on INH with various agents.[83,84] INH inhibits the metabolism of several agents, including phenytoin, disulfiram, carbamazepine, warfarin, benzodiazepines, and vitamin D; increased serum concentrations may occur with concomitant use of INH.[81]

Results of studies examining the interaction between INH and phenytoin indicate that phenytoin intoxication occurs mainly in slow acetylators of INH.[83–85] It is necessary to monitor phenytoin serum levels in patients who are receiving INH and phenytoin concomitantly, especially slow acetylators of INH. A reduction in the dosage of phenytoin is warranted for patients who are exhibiting clinical symptoms of phenytoin intoxication or toxic serum phenytoin levels.

As was mentioned previously, concomitant administration of INH and food results in impaired absorption of INH; the peak concentration, the mean concentration, and the total amount of drug are reduced.[86,87] Because aluminum-containing antacids may decrease GI absorption of INH, administering INH at least 1 hour before taking antacids is recommended.[67] More studies evaluating INH absorption with antacids and laxatives are necessary.[67,88]

INH is also an inhibitor of monoamine and diamine oxidase.[89] Adverse reactions such as skin flushing, palpitations, headache, nausea and vomiting, and itching have been reported in patients who are receiving INH and ingesting foods with high histamine or tyramine content.[89–99] These reactions were attributed to monoamine and diamine oxidase inhibition by INH. Patients should be counseled to take INH on an empty stomach and to avoid foods with high histamine or tyramine content (e.g., selected fishes, cheeses, and wines).[81]

INH may possibly exhibit enzymatic induction of certain agents.[81] In patients who are receiving INH, RMP, and ketoconazole concomitantly, decreases in ketoconazole concentrations have been reported; this interaction appears to involve an additive affect of INH and RMP to reduce ketoconazole concentrations.[100,101]

The potential interaction between INH and theophylline has been examined in various European and U.S. studies.[102–104] In studies using INH at dosages of 400 mg per day or 10 mg/kg per day, a reduction in theophylline clearance was observed.[102,103] A study in the United States that used INH at a dosage of 300 mg per day reported a mean 16% increase in theophylline clearance.[104] On the basis of the results of these studies, it appears that INH at dosages of 300 mg per day does not cause clinically significant decreases in theophylline clearance.[105] In patients who are receiving larger daily doses of INH (e.g., 400 or 600 mg), or possibly in underweight individuals who are receiving 300 mg per day, this interaction may be significant. A summary of clinically significant INH interactions is provided in Table 68.5.[81] Included are INH interactions that require further study and should be considered in monitoring therapy.

Rifamycins: Rifampin, Rifabutin, and Rifapentine

Rifampin (RMP) is a semisynthetic derivative of rifamycin B that is an antibiotic produced by *Streptomyces mediterranei;* this agent exhibits a broad spectrum of activity that includes activity against *Neisseria, Staphylococcus, Haemophilus,* most streptococci, and several species of *Enterobacteriaceae.*[65] The drug is bactericidal for *M. tuberculosis,* with most strains being inhibited in vitro by concentrations of 0.5 μg/mL. Its mechanism of action entails inhibition of DNA-dependent RNA polymerase of mycobacteria and other microorganisms, preventing chain initiation. RMP exhibits greater activity than INH against slower or intermittently growing organisms that are present in macrophages.[106] RMP is unique in its ability to destroy the organisms in semisolid caseous material. When it is used in combination with INH, synergy is obtained, thus enabling the duration of treatment for TB to be shortened from 18 to 24 months to 6 to 9 months.[107]

RMP generally is administered as a single dose of 600 mg one time a day or biweekly for adults and 10 to 20 mg/kg (maximum 600 mg) for children. The drug is well absorbed from the GI tract, and peak serum concentrations of approximately 7 μg/mL are achieved within 2 to 4 hours. However, because of considerable interpatient variation, peak plasma concentrations of the drug may range from 4 to 32 μg/mL.[108–111] Although the peak plasma concentrations may be slightly reduced when RMP is administered with food, this difference is not known to be clinically significant.[45] The drug is 60 to 90% protein-bound and penetrates well into the tissues, including the CNS, liver, lungs, bone, saliva, and tears.[112,113] RMP, as well as the other rifamycin derivatives, rifabutin and rifapentine, may impart an orange discoloration to the urine, feces, sputum, tears, and sweat. Soft contact lenses may be permanently discolored; patients should be counseled accordingly.[65,114–117]

Following absorption from the GI tract, RMP is eliminated in the bile, where it undergoes enterohepatic circulation.[65] At this time, the drug is deacetylated to desacetylri-

Table 68.5 ▪ Isoniazid (INH) Interactions

Agent	Comments	Clinical Management
Acetaminophen[a]	Combined with INH, hepatotoxicity is more likely to occur.	Monitor patients for signs and symptoms of hepatotoxicity and periodic monitoring of liver enzymes.
Antacids (aluminum hydroxide)	May delay and decrease absorption of INH.	Give INH at least 1 hour before antacids.
Anticoagulants	Increased effect reported at INH dose of 9 mg/kg/day; unlikely to occur at lower doses.	Monitor INR; decrease in anticoagulant dosage may be necessary.
Benzodiazepines	Rifampin's effect if given concomitantly should be considered.	Decrease in dosage of select benzodiazepines may be necessary.
Carbamazepine[b]	Increased carbamazepine levels and toxicity possible.	Monitor serum carbamazepine levels; decrease in carbamazepine dosage may be necessary.
Cheese, fish, wine[b]	Avoid foods with high histamine or tyramine content.	Monitor patients for flushing, palpitations, headache, itching, nausea, and vomiting.
Food[b]	May delay and decrease absorption of INH.	Take INH on an empty stomach.
Ketoconazole[b]	INH has an additive effect with rifampin to decrease ketoconazole concentrations.	Monitor; adjust dosage if necessary.
Phenytoin[b]	Mainly occurs in slow acetylators of INH. If rifampin given concurrently, phenytoin levels decrease (i.e., induction effects outweighs INH's inhibitory effect).	Monitor serum phenytoin levels; decrease in phenytoin dosage may be necessary.
Theophylline	Potential decrease in theophylline clearance appears to occur at INH doses greater than 300 mg daily. If rifampin is given concurrently, theophylline levels decreased (i.e., induction effect outweighs INH's inhibitory effect).	Monitor serum theophylline levels.
Vitamin D	Further study necessary.	Monitor vitamin D levels as well as calcium and phosphate levels in select patients.

Source: Reference 81.

[a]O'Shea D, Kim RB, Wilkinson GR. Modulation of CYP 2E1 activity by Isoniazid in rapid and slow *N*-acetylators. Br J Clin Pharmacol 43:99–103, 1997. Chien JY, Peter RM, Nolan CM, et al. Influence of polymorphis *N*-acetyltransferase phenotype on the inhibition of acetaminophen bioactivation with long-term isoniazid. Clin Pharm Ther 61(No. 1):24–34, 1997.

[b]Clinical significance established.

fampin, a metabolite with antibacterial activity similar to that of the parent compound. Intestinal reabsorption is decreased by deacetylation; thus, metabolism promotes elimination of the drug. The serum half-life of RMP initially ranges from 1.5 to 5 hours. Because RMP is a potent inducer of hepatic microsomal enzymes, it induces its own metabolism, thus shortening its half-life to 2 to 3 hours. The half-life of RMP may be increased in the presence of hepatic dysfunction, and dosage adjustments may be necessary. In patients with renal impairment, adjustment of dosage is not necessary.

In recommended doses, RMP generally is well tolerated.[114,115] Significant adverse reactions occur in fewer than 4% of patients with TB. The most common adverse effects are GI upset (i.e., nausea and vomiting [1.5%], rash [0.8%], and fever [0.5%]). Although uncommon in recommended doses, an influenzalike syndrome may occur with intermittent administration of doses of RMP greater than 10 mg/kg.[118] The patient may complain of fever, chills, malaise, arthralgias, and headache. The syndrome also may include interstitial nephritis, acute renal failure, eosinophilia, thrombocytopenia, hemolytic anemia, and shock. Patients receiving RMP should be monitored for changes in renal function and skin appearance. Adherence to the prescribed dosing regimen is important because interrupted therapy may cause an increase in the incidence of toxicity.

Elevations in hepatic enzymes occur in approximately 10 to 15% of patients when RMP is administered alone.[119] In combination with INH, elevations in serum transaminases may occur in 20 to 30% of patients.[120] This usually occurs within the first 8 weeks of therapy. The development of hepatitis in patients with normal hepatic function is rare. Alcoholism, chronic liver disease, and advanced age may increase the risk of hepatotoxicity with the administration of RMP alone or in combination with INH. Whether the combination of INH and RMP increases the incidence of hepatotoxicity remains controversial. As with INH, patients should be monitored for signs of hepatotoxicity.

The rifamycins are inducers of hepatic microsomal enzymes.[78] Of the three available rifamycins, RMP is the most potent CYP450 inducer, whereas rifabutin has significantly less activity as an inducer; rifapentine, the most recently approved rifamycin derivative, has intermediate activity as an inducer.[78] RMP may enhance the elimination of several drugs, including theophylline, warfarin, oral contraceptive agents, phenytoin, cyclosporine, glucocorticoids, methadone, ketoconazole, and oral sulfonylureas.[121–123] These interactions may result in decreased efficacy of these agents, such as reduced efficacy of oral contraceptives, including several reports of unplanned pregnancy.[124,125] Rifabutin and rifapentine also may enhance the elimination of various drugs; these agents, like RMP, also may reduce the efficacy of oral contraceptives, and alternative forms of birth control should be recommended.[116,117] Potentially clinically significant RMP drug interactions that have been reported more recently include interactions with haloperidol, several antiarrhythmics, diltiazem, fluconazole, and select benzodiazepines.[123]

Over the past few years several antiretroviral agents have been FDA approved for the management of HIV disease. Because mycobacterial infections such as TB are common in patients infected with HIV, drug interactions must be carefully assessed to ensure efficacy and to avoid toxicity.[78] Two major classes of antiretroviral agents, the HIV protease inhibitors (PIs) and the non-nucleoside reverse transcriptase inhibitors (NNRTIs), are extensively biotransformed via cytochrome P450 (oxidative) metabolism; agents within these classes exhibit substantial drug interactions with the rifamycins. The PIs are CYP450 inhibitors, ritonavir being the most potent inhibitor. The NNRTIs have diverse effects on CYP450; nevirapine is an inducer, delavirdine is an inhibitor, and efavirenz is both an inducer and an inhibitor. Rifamycin-related CYP450 induction reduces the serum levels of agents in both of these classes.

In 1996 the CDC established guidelines to assist clinicians in making therapeutic decisions regarding treatment of TB in patients with HIV infection.[126] Recently, the CDC revised these guidelines to include more recent data from studies that evaluated alternative therapies for managing patients infected with HIV with drug-susceptible TB and infection.[78] The updated guidelines no longer recommend discontinuation of PI therapy to allow the use of RMP for TB treatment for patients with HIV-related TB. The revised guidelines provide treatment options for those patients who are taking antiretroviral agents that are extensively metabolized via the cytochrome P450 system, thus enabling continued antiretroviral therapy during treatment of TB. As mentioned previously, rifabutin exhibits fewer induction effects than RMP and is a reasonable alternative to RMP in TB treatment regimens in patient with HIV infection.[78] The use of RMP to treat active TB in a patient who is taking a PI or NNRTI is contraindicated because RMP substantially lowers serum concentrations of agents within these classes. Rifabutin, which is FDA approved for the prevention of disseminated *Mycobacterium avium* complex (MAC) disease in patients with advanced HIV infection, has been studied both in HIV-infected and non–HIV-infected patients with TB; recent data in patients coinfected with TB and HIV support the role of rifabutin as an alternative to RMP in TB regimens.[78] Current guidelines by the CDC recommend rifabutin as an alternative to RMP in treating TB in patients with HIV infection who are also receiving PIs (with the exception of ritonavir or hard-gel capsule saquinavir [Invirase]) or with the NNRTIs nevirapine or efavirenz (but not delavirdine). Another alternative regimen recommended by the CDC for patients who are receiving PI or NNRTIs is a streptomycin-based regimen that does not contain a rifamycin. The treatment of TB without a rifamycin requires a longer duration of therapy (at least 9 months). Updated information that includes antiretroviral drug interactions with RMP and other rifamycin derivatives are available.[127,128] Table 68.6 provides a summary of RMP interactions with recommendations for management.[78,123,127]

Rifapentine is the first anti-TB drug to be FDA approved in over 25 years.[117] The United States is the first country to approve this agent. Rifapentine has a longer half-life than RMP, providing a longer duration of action. In studies, rifapentine was used in combination with agents such as INH, PZA, and EMB. The use of rifapentine enables the reduction in the number of pills that a patient must take to cure pulmonary TB. In studies in South Africa, the use of this agent enabled patients to take their medications just once a week during the last 4 months of therapy. This simplification of anti-TB regimens holds promise for achieving higher adherence rates and lower drug resistant rates. Because this agent was recommended by the FDA for accelerated approval, ongoing trials are underway to access various combination therapies. The combinations studied include simplified regimens such as weekly rifapentine and INH compared with RMP and INH administered three times a week for 4 months following the conventional 2 months of intensive four-drug therapy.[129] Further study will elucidate rifapentine's role in anti-TB therapy. Presently, rifapentine is not recommended as a substitute for RMP in TB treatment regimens because the safety and efficacy of this agent for the treatment of patients with HIV-related TB have not been established.

Ethambutol

Ethambutol (EMB) is a synthetic antimycobacterial agent that generally is considered to be tuberculostatic in the recommended doses.[65] Its precise mechanism of action is unknown, although the drug has been shown to inhibit the incorporation of mycolic acid into the mycobacterial cell wall.[130] Inhibition of mycobacterial growth requires approximately 24 hours. In vivo activity of EMB appears to be targeted toward actively dividing mycobacteria. Most strains of *M. tuberculosis* are inhibited in vitro by concentrations of 1 to 5 μg/mL.[9] The peak plasma concentration 2 to 4 hours after a 15 mg/kg oral dose is approximately 5 μg/mL.[65]

Approximately 75 to 85% of EMB is absorbed from the GI tract.[65] Administering the drug with food does not interfere with absorption. Either single daily doses of 15 to 25 mg/kg or a 50 mg/kg twice weekly regimen may be chosen. Although EMB penetrates well into most tissues and fluids, CSF concentrations are low, even in the presence of meningeal inflammation. About two-thirds of an oral dose of EMB is eliminated in the urine; approximately 50% is excreted unchanged via glomerular filtration and

Table 68.6 ▪ Rifampin (RMP) Drug Interactions[a]

Agent	Comments	Clinical Management
Antacids	Further study necessary.	May need to space apart RMP and aluminum hydroxide doses.
Anticoagulants, oral[b]	Decreased effect may occur.	Increase anticoagulant dose based on monitoring of INR.
Atovaquone	Atovaquone concentration may be subtherapeutic.	Monitor clinical response; increased dosage may be required.
Beta-blockers	Decreased effect may occur.	May need to increase propranolol or metoprolol dose.
Chloramphenicol	Chloramphenicol concentration may be subtherapeutic.	Monitor serum chloramphenicol concentration; if necessary increase dosage.
Clarithromycin	Further study necessary.	Monitor signs and symptoms of infection.
Contraceptives, oral[b]	Document patient counseling. Unplanned pregnancy may occur.	Use alternative forms of birth control.
Cyclosporine[b]	Cyclosporine levels may be subtherapeutic.	Monitor serum cyclosporine concentration; increase in dosage is likely.
Dapsone	Further study is necessary when used for *Pneumocystis carinii* prophylaxis.	Monitor for hematologic toxic effects.
Diazepam	A 300% increase in diazepam oral clearance has been reported.	Monitor clinical response; increase diazepam dose if necessary.
Digitoxin[b]	Decreased effect may occur.	Monitor serum digitoxin concentration; monitor for arrhythmia control and signs and symptoms of heart failure. Increase dose if necessary.
Digoxin	Interaction is most likely to be significant in patients with renal impairment.	Monitor serum digoxin concentrations; monitor for arrhythmia control and signs and symptoms of heart failure.
Diltiazem	Alternative agent recommended because even a very large increase in oral diltiazem dose may not be sufficient (similar interaction with verapamil).	Use an alternative agent if possible.
Disopyramide	Initial study reported a reduction in disopyramide serum half-life by about 50%.	Monitor arrhythmic control; increase dose if necessary.
Doxycycline	Doxycycline concentration may be subtherapeutic.	Monitor clinical response and serum doxycycline concentrations; increased dosage may be needed.
Fluconazole	A 22% decrease in fluconazole serum half-life was reported in one trial in healthy subjects.	May need to increase fluconazole dosage; monitor signs and symptoms of infection.
Glucocorticoids[b]	Decreased effect may occur.	Increase glucocorticoid dosage twofold to threefold.
Haloperidol	Initial study indicates that serum concentrations and half-life are decreased by about 50%.	Monitor serum haloperidol levels; change dosing regimen if necessary.
Itraconazole	Decreased effect may occur.	Monitor clinical response; dosage increase is likely.
Ketoconazole[b]	Avoid combination if possible.	If utilized, monitor serum ketoconazole concentrations; increase dosage if necessary.

(continued)

tubular secretion. Hepatic metabolism occurs through oxidation, and two inactive metabolites are formed. Up to 15% of the drug is excreted in the urine in the form of these inactive metabolites.[131] About 20% is excreted as unchanged drug in the feces. The serum half-life is approximately 4 hours in patients with normal renal function and may increase to 7 hours or longer in patients with renal failure.[65] Dosage adjustment is required for patients who have renal impairment.[132]

EMB is a relatively safe drug and produces very few adverse effects when the recommended dosages are used.[65] The most toxic effect of EMB is retrobulbar neuritis, which is characterized by decreased visual acuity, loss of red-green color vision, and central scotomata.[133] This appears to be a dose-related phenomenon that is more common at doses above 50 mg/kg per day. The occurrence is reported to be 5% in patients who are receiving daily doses of 25 mg/kg and less than 1% in patients who are being treated with 15 mg/kg per day.[65] In patients with renal impairment, the frequency of ocular toxicity is increased because of accumulation of the drug. Baseline examination of visual acuity should be performed before initiation of EMB therapy, followed by monthly eye examinations. Patients should be instructed to report any changes in visual acuity and seek medical attention immediately if changes do occur. Caution should be exercised in prescribing EMB for children who are too young for assessment of visual acuity and red-green color discrimination. The use of possible alterna-

Table 68.6 *(continued)*

Agent	Comments	Clinical Management
Methadone[b]	Decreased effect may occur.	Increase methadone dose; control withdrawal symptoms.
Midazolam	Decreased effect may occur.	Monitor for decreased efficacy; increase dose as necessary.
Nifedipine	Alternative class of drugs should be considered.	Monitor clinical response; increase in dosage may be necessary.
Non-nucleoside reverse transcriptase inhibitors (NNRTIs)[b]	Decreased effect occurs; refer to revise guidelines provided by CDC.[78]	Use of RMP to treat active TB in a patient who is taking a NNRTI (or PI) is contraindicated. Substitution of rifabutin for RMP in TB treatment regimens is one proposed option (for specific NNRTIs that can be used with rifabutin); another option is the use of a STM-based regimen that does not contain a rifamycin.[78]
Nortriptyline	Decreased effect may occur.	Monitor clinical response and serum nortriptyline concentrations.
Pefloxacin	Awaiting further study.	Moderate RMP induction effect; no dosage adjustment recommended.
Phenytoin[b]	Phenytoin levels may be subtherapeutic	Monitor phenytoin serum levels; increase dose if necessary.
Propafenone	Decreased effect may occur.	Monitor arrhythmic control and serum propafenone levels; increase dose if necessary.
Protease inhibitors (PIs)[b]	Decreased effect occurs; refer to revise guidelines provided by CDC.[78]	Use of RMP to treat active TB in a patient who is taking a PI (or NNRTI) is contraindicated. Substitution of rifabutin for RMP in TB treatment regimens is one proposed option (for specific PIs that can be used with rifabutin); another option is the use of a STM-based regimen that does not contain a rifamycin.[78]
Quinidine[b]	Quinidine levels may be subtherapeutic.	Monitor arrhythmic control and serum quinidine levels; increase dose if necessary.
Sulfonylureas	Monitor blood glucose on discontinuation of RMP.	Monitor blood glucose control; increase sulfonylurea dose if necessary.
Tacrolimus	Decreased effect may occur.	Monitor serum tacrolimus concentrations and clinical response; increase in dosage may be necessary.
Theophylline[b]	Theophylline levels may be subtherapeutic.	Monitor serum theophylline levels; dosage increase is likely.
Tocainamide	Approximately 30% decrease in tocainamide serum half-life was reported in one trial in healthy subjects.	Monitor arrhythmic control; increase dose it necessary.
Triazolam	Decreased effect may occur.	Monitor for decreased efficacy; increase dosage as necessary.
Verapamil[b]	Alternative agent recommended because even a very large increase in oral verapamil dose may not be sufficient.	If utilized, monitor serum verapamil levels; monitor clinical response.
Zidovudine	Decreased effect may occur.	Monitor clinical response and viral load; increase in dosage may be necessary.

Source: References 78, 123, 127. See references 121 and 122 for further information.

[a]For each interaction, when rifampin is discontinued, enzyme induction effect is slowly reduced over 1 to 2 weeks.

[b]Major clinical significance is well established.

tive agents should be considered. Other adverse effects of EMB include hypersensitivity reactions, neuritis, GI intolerance, headache, and hyperuricemia. Increased concentration of urate in the blood is most likely owing to decreased clearance of renal urate.[134]

Pyrazinamide

Pyrazinamide (PZA), a synthetic pyrazine analog of nicotinamide, exhibits bactericidal activity against mycobacteria in an acid environment.[65] Although its precise mechanism is unknown, the drug is slowly bactericidal against the slow-growing bacilli within the acidic pH of the macrophages.[135] The unique intracellular activity of the drug has led to the incorporation of PZA into the initial phase of therapy. The drug has been used recently in short-course regimens with INH and RMP for the treatment of TB.[136] The minimum inhibitory concentration (MIC) in an acid environment is 20 μg/mL against *M. tuberculosis*, although the tubercle bacilli within the monocytes are killed by concentrations of 12.5 μg/mL.[65] PZA is well absorbed from the GI tract, peak serum concentrations occurring approximately 2 hours after ingestion. Following doses of 20 to 25 mg/kg, peak serum concentrations range from 30 to 50 μg/mL. The drug is widely distributed throughout the body, including the CSF. PZA is primarily excreted by glomerular filtration, but it is also hydrolyzed and hydroxylated. In people with normal renal function, the elimination half-life is 9 to 10 hours. When a patient has renal impairment, minor dosage adjustments may be required. The usual dosage is 15 to 30 mg/kg per day (maximum 2 g), 50 to 70 mg/kg two times a week (maximum 4 g), or 50 to 70 mg/kg three times a week (maximum 3 g).

The most common and toxic effect of PZA is dose-dependent hepatotoxicity.[65] In early studies using high doses of 3 g per day (40 to 50 mg/kg), a 15% incidence of hepatotoxicity was reported. Transient, asymptomatic elevations of serum transaminase levels are the earliest abnormalities produced by the drug. Initial 2-month regimens consisting of INH, RMP, and PZA, which use PZA at a dosage of 15 to 30 mg/kg, do not indicate a significant increase in hepatotoxicity.[137,138] Other adverse effects include hypersensitivity reactions, photosensitivity, GI intolerance, dysuria, malaise, fever, and arthralgias.[65] Salicylates usually provide symptomatic relief of PZA-related arthralgias.[9] PZA may cause elevations in prothrombin time (by decreasing prothrombin concentration or activity) and serum bilirubin levels.[65] Because PZA inhibits renal tubular secretion of uric acid, hyperuricemia occurs frequently.[139] Acute gout is uncommon. However, acute gouty attacks may be problematic in individuals with a history of gout precipitation. In these cases, discontinuation of the drug may be warranted.

Streptomycin

Streptomycin (STM), an aminoglycoside antibiotic, was the first clinically effective drug to become available for the treatment of TB.[65] The drug is bactericidal in an alkaline environment and acts by inhibiting protein synthesis. The manufacturer recommends that STM (and capreomycin) be administered only intramuscularly. Difficulty arises when patients require treatment but lack sufficient body mass to tolerate intramuscular injections. Because aminoglycosides are poorly absorbed from the GI tract, the intravenous route has been used as an alternative route. The National Jewish Center for Immunology and Respiratory Medicine has published their policy for administering STM and capreomycin by the intravenous route.[140]

STM is highly effective within the extracellular environment; however, it diffuses poorly into granulomas and macrophages and lacks activity in the intracellular environment. The majority of strains of *M. tuberculosis* are inhibited in vitro at a concentration of 8 μg/mL. Following an intramuscular dose of 15 mg/kg, peak serum concentration levels averaging approximately 40 μg/mL are achieved. Excretion is primarily renal, with the majority of drug being excreted unchanged in the urine. The half-life in blood ranges from 2 to 5 hours in individuals with normal renal function. In patients with renal insufficiency, the dosage should be reduced.[76] STM has moderate tissue penetration.

Ototoxicity is the major toxic effect of STM.[9] This usually results in vertigo and ataxia, although hearing loss also may occur. Other adverse effects include hypersensitivity and fever. Nephrotoxicity occasionally occurs, although STM has fewer adverse effect on the kidneys than do kanamycin and capreomycin. The risk of nephrotoxicity may be increased in patients receiving other nephrotoxic drugs concomitantly or in patients with preexisting renal insufficiency. It is recommended that a total cumulative dose of no more than 120 g be given unless there are no other therapeutic options. In individuals who are older than 60 years of age, both ototoxicity and nephrotoxicity are more common. All patients who are receiving STM should have baseline hearing and renal function tests, as well as periodic monitoring for changes. Several drug interactions are possible with concomitant administration of STM. As with other aminoglycosides, STM interacts with neuromuscular blocking agents, which may result in prolonged respiratory depression.[141]

Paraaminosalicylic Acid

Paraaminosalicylic acid (PAS) is a tuberculostatic agent that is rarely used in current anti-TB regimens.[65] It is a structural analog of paraaminobenzoic acid (PABA); thus, its mechanism of action appears to be similar to that of sulfonamides, competitive antagonism of PABA. Most strains of *M. tuberculosis* in vitro are inhibited at concentrations of 1 μg/mL. The usual dosage in adults and children is 150 mg/kg by mouth (maximum 10 to 12 g/day), administered in divided doses. The drug is well absorbed from the GI tract and distributes throughout the total body water, achieving high concentrations in the pleural fluid and caseous tissue. However, concentration levels in the CSF are low, possibly because of active transport outward.[142] Following a single 4-g oral dose, plasma concentrations ranging from 75 to 100 μg/mL are achieved within 1 to 2 hours. The high dosages are necessary because the drug has an elimination half-life of about 1 hour.[65] More than 80% of the drug is eliminated in the urine; approximately 50% is in the form of an acetylated compound. The dosage should be reduced in patients with renal dysfunction. A significant sodium load is present in a dose when the tablet preparation is used.[9] If the delayed-release granule formulation is used, the dose should be administered with acidic food or drink.

The frequency of adverse effects associated with the use of PAS ranges from 10 to 30%.[65] The most frequent complaint is GI upset (i.e., nausea, vomiting, anorexia, diarrhea, and epigastric pain), which may contribute to patient nonadherence to therapy. Other adverse effects include hypersensitivity reactions in 5 to 10% of patients, thrombocytopenia, and rarely hepatitis. Probenecid blocks the renal excretion of PAS, resulting in increased plasma concentrations of PAS. Caution should be exercised with this combination because of the possibility of PAS toxicity. Patients should be counseled about the importance of adherence to therapy. The drug should be administered in two to four equally divided doses with meals to minimize gastric irritation.[65]

Ethionamide

Ethionamide is an oral agent that is structurally similar to INH but has less activity.[65] It is used as a second-line agent in combination with other anti-TB agents following failure with the primary regimens. Its precise mechanism of action is unknown, although it appears to involve protein synthesis inhibition. The majority of *M. tuberculosis* strains are inhibited by concentrations of 0.6 to 2.5 μg/mL. The activity of this agent may be either tuberculostatic or tuberculocidal, depending on the susceptibility of the organism and drug concentration at the site of infection. Rapid resistance occurs in vitro, and cross-resistance occurs between ethionamide and INH. The recommended daily dose is 15 to 20 mg/kg, with a maximum dosage of 1 g per day.[9] Absorption is rapid from the GI tract following oral administration.[65] Peak concentrations of approximately 20 μg/mL are achieved in 3 hours following a 1-g dose. The serum half-life is approximately 3 hours. Ethionamide is evenly distributed into the blood and various organs. Metabolism is predominantly hepatic.

The most common adverse effects of ethionamide are anorexia, nausea, and vomiting. For most patients it is necessary to gradually increase the dose to the full amount. A useful approach to maintaining treatment is administering ethionamide at bedtime with an antiemetic drug taken 30 minutes before the dose and occasionally a hypnotic.[9] Other adverse effects include arthralgias, impotence, photosensitivity dermatitis, gynecomastia, hypothyroidism, hepatitis, and a metallic taste in the mouth. The frequency of hepatitis associated with ethionamide does not appear to be greater than that associated with PZA. Patients should have hepatic enzymes monitored monthly. The drug should be discontinued if the hepatic enzymes reach five times normal levels, even in the absence of symptoms.

Cycloserine

Cycloserine is an anti-TB agent that is an analog of the amino acid D-alanine. Like ethionamide, the drug is limited to certain situations.[9] Most strains of *M. tuberculosis* are inhibited by concentrations of 5 to 20 μg/mL, and the drug is considered to be bacteriostatic.[65] Cycloserine inhibits the processes that incorporate D-alanine in bacterial cell wall synthesis. The drug is available in 250-mg capsules. Following the usual dose of 15 to 20 mg/kg per day, the drug is rapidly absorbed from the GI tract. Cycloserine distributes into most body fluids and tissue, including the CSF. The most common adverse effects of the drug involve the CNS. Emotional and behavioral disturbances, including psychosis, have been reported. These reactions tend to appear within the first 2 weeks of therapy and usually disappear on discontinuation of the drug. Manifestations of the CNS effects of cycloserine are more likely to occur in patients who have a history of psychological problems or a chronic psychiatric condition. The mental status of these patients should be assessed regularly to monitor for these adverse effects. Other adverse effects include convulsions and peripheral neuropathy, especially when the drug is used in combination with INH. Thus, 150 mg per day of pyridoxine should be administered with cycloserine. Cycloserine inhibits the hepatic metabolism of phenytoin, especially when it is taken with INH.[9] If necessary, the dosage of phenytoin should be reduced. Cycloserine is contraindicated in individuals with a history of epilepsy, depression, or severe anxiety.[65] The risk of CNS effects may be increased with concurrent use with ethionamide, INH, and alcohol.

Capreomycin and Kanamycin

Capreomycin and kanamycin are injectable aminoglycoside antibiotics that may be used in combination with other effective anti-TB drugs.[9] Concurrently administering more than one aminoglycoside should be avoided. Capreomycin and kanamycin both inhibit protein synthesis and are tuberculostatic. Capreomycin is available in 1-g vials; kanamycin is available in 75-mg, 500-mg, and 1-g vials. The usual daily dosage of both agents is 15 to 30 mg/kg given intramuscularly, with a maximum daily dosage of 1 g. The frequency of renal toxicity is similar, and regular monitoring of serum creatinine is necessary. Auditory toxicity appears to be more common with kanamycin than with streptomycin and capreomycin. Monthly audiometry is recommended in patients who are receiving kanamycin. Vestibular toxicity is uncommon. Capreomycin may produce damage to the eighth cranial nerve, resulting in high-frequency loss before vestibular dysfunction occurs. Recommendations with these agents include an audiogram performed at baseline and repeated at least every other month while the patient is receiving therapy, and periodic examinations for vestibular function. In older patients the maximal daily dosage of capreomycin should be limited to 750 mg.

Thiacetazone

Thiacetazone is an anti-TB agent that is biochemically related to INH.[9] The drug is not available in the United States. However, it is used in many resource-poor developing countries because limited funds have often forced administrators of TB control programs to use suboptimal treatment regimens. Its activity is bacteriostatic, and it is more toxic than INH. Standard therapy in a large part of sub-Saharan Africa has consisted of the use of INH, thiacetazone, and streptomycin for 2 months and then INH and thiacetazone for 10 months.[14] The failure rate of this regimen is more than 10% in fully adherent HIV-seronegative patients with TB and is even less effective for HIV-infected patients.[14,143,144] Moreover, cutaneous hypersensitivity reactions have occurred in 10 to 20% of patients infected with HIV; these reactions may be severe and occasionally have been fatal.[145,146] Consequently, the WHO is seeking resources that would enable the use of supervised short-course chemotherapy with RMP-including regimens in countries in which the prevalence of HIV and TB is high.[147] The vestibular toxicity associated with the use of streptomycin may be potentiated by the concurrent use of thiacetazone.[9]

Potentially Effective Antituberculous Agents

New agents that have been evaluated in children or adults for anti-TB activity include amikacin, quinolones, clofa-

Table 68.7 ▪ Drugs for the Initial Treatment of Tuberculosis in Children and Adults

Drug	Daily Dose		Two Times a Week		Three Times a Week	
	Children	Adults	Children	Adults	Children	Adults
First-line agents:						
Isoniazid, mg/kg	10–20, max 300 mg	5, max 300 mg	20–40, max 900 mg	15, max 900 mg	20–40, max 900 mg	15, max 900 mg
Rifampin, mg/kg	10–20, max 600 mg	10, max 600 mg	10–20, max 600 mg	10, max 600 mg	10–20, max 600 mg	10, max 600 mg
Pyrazinamide, mg/kg	15–30, max 2 g	15–30, max 2 g	50–70, max 4 g	50–70, max 4 g	50–70, max 3 g	50–70, max 3 g
Streptomycin, mg/kg	20–40, max 1 g	15, max 1 g	25–30, max 1.5 g	25–30, max 1.5 g	25–30, max 1.5 g	25–30, max 1.5 g
Ethambutol, mg/kg	15–25, max 2.5 g	15–25, max 2.5 g	50, max 2.5 g	50, max 2.5 g	25–30, max 1.5 g	25–30, max 1.5 g
Second-line agents:						
p-Aminosalicylic acid, mg/kg	150, max 12 g	150, max 12 g				
Ethionamide, mg/kg	15–20, max 1 g	15–20, max 1 g				
Cycloserine, mg/kg	15–20, max 1 g	15–20, max 1 g				
Capreomycin, mg/kg; Kanamycin, mg/kg	15–30, max 1 g	15–30, max 1 g				

Source: Reference 61.

zimine, and β-lactams.[9] Although these agents have not been tested in multidrug regimens for treating TB, the increase in the number of MDR-TB cases may create more situations in which the usefulness of these agents must be considered. Because these agents have not yet been fully evaluated in well-designed, randomized trials for TB treatment or prophylaxis, they should not be used to replace any of the previously recommended agents until efficacy is established. The following agents discussed either are licensed or are available through an investigational new drug (IND) request in the United States. Recommendations for dosage regimens of these drugs as anti-TB agents have not been established, and consultation with TB experts is necessary, especially if these agents are used in infants and children.

Amikacin is tuberculocidal against *M. tuberculosis* in vitro.[9] The drug is administered intramuscularly as a single daily dose of 15 mg/kg five times a week. If the drug is administered intravenously, a single daily dose of 15 mg/kg is given over 30 minutes. One hour after intramuscular administration of a 7.5-mg/kg single dose, the average peak serum concentration is 21 μg/mL.[148] The MIC for amikacin is about 4 to 8 μg/mL for a broad range of strains of *M. tuberculosis.*[149]

Several fluoroquinolones, such as ciprofloxacin, ofloxacin, and sparfloxacin, exhibit in vitro activity against *M. tuberculosis.*[150,151] A newer agent, levofloxacin, which is the L-isomer of ofloxacin, is twice as active in vitro against *M. tuberculosis* than the racemic mixture.[152] Data concerning the use of these agents for the treatment of TB appear promising, although data are limited.[150–152]

Clofazimine is an oral phenazine dye that is weakly bactericidal against *M. leprae.*[45] The drug exerts in vitro and in vivo activity against mycobacteria, including *M. tuberculosis*. The efficacy of clofazimine in the treatment of TB has not been established.[152]

Amoxicillin is an aminopenicillin with a broad spectrum of antibacterial activity against many Gram-positive and Gram-negative microorganisms. The in vitro activity against *M. tuberculosis* is greatly enhanced by the addition of a β-lactamase inhibitor to amoxicillin.[153] The β-lactamase inhibitors (e.g., clavulanic acid) lack intrinsic antimycobacterial activity; however, they inhibit the enzyme that is partially responsible for the resistance of *M. tuberculosis* to β-lactam antibiotics. A recent 7-day study compared the activity of amoxicillin/clavulanate, ofloxacin, and INH by measuring the effects on recovery of *M. tuberculosis* colony forming units from sputum of patients with smear-positive TB.[154] The results of early bactericidal activity of amoxicillin/clavulanate was comparable to the activity reported for anti-TB agents other than INH. Further studies are necessary to define the role of β-lactam antibiotics as anti-TB agents.

Other agents that are currently under investigation include sulfonamides, macrolides, folate antagonists, and interferon-γ administered via aerosolization.[53,155]

Initial Treatment Regimens

Tables 68.3 and 68.7 provide initial treatment regimens and dosages for children and adults. Over the past 45 years, many studies evaluating the use of anti-TB regimens have provided specific information about the use of combination therapy. On the basis of the results of these studies, the CDC and ATS provide several important generalizations.[9]

- INH should be used in any treatment regimen for the entire duration of therapy unless contraindications are present or the organisms are resistant to the drug.
- Although there are some reports of good results with 4-month regimens, in general, relapse rates are unacceptably high. An exception is the adult who is carefully evaluated and found to have sputum-culture-negative pulmonary TB. For such adults the success rate with 4-month regimens has been high.
- RMP and INH should be used for the entire duration of therapy when 6-month regimens are chosen.
- In treatment regimens of less than 9 months' duration, efficacy is enhanced by administering PZA during the initial phase of therapy.
- The efficacy of a regimen is decreased when EMB or STM, in the recommended dosages, is substituted for PZA in the initial phase of therapy.
- Following an initial daily phase of treatment as short as 2 weeks, intermittently administering appropriately adjusted doses of the anti-TB agents provides results that are similar to those of daily administration. Four-drug regimens that are administered three times a week throughout the duration of treatment provide equally good results in adults. Data are not available concerning three times a week regimens in children. Experience with other intermittent regimens suggests that equal efficacy may be achieved with three times a week regimens in children.

These guidelines are applicable only when the TB is caused by organisms that are susceptible to the standard anti-TB agents. Community rates of initial resistance to INH have remained low–less than 4% in some areas of the United States.[9] Local data are useful in determining whether the population in general is at low risk for drug resistance or whether specific subgroups in the population can be defined that are at low risk.[156] In areas in which rates of initial resistance to anti-TB drugs are low, continued surveillance of drug susceptibility patterns is necessary to ensure that low rates of drug resistance continue.

In several outbreaks of MDR-TB, organisms were resistant to both INH and RMP and frequently to EMB, as well as to other agents.[157] In these situations the response to treatment with standard initial regimens is poor. Because most cases of MDR-TB have occurred among adults infected with HIV, there has been transmission of infection and progression to disease among their contacts.

When initiating therapy for TB, clinicians should be aware of the prevalence of drug resistance in their communities, as well as the epidemiologic features of people who are most likely to be carrying these organisms.[9] Patients with newly diagnosed TB should have drug susceptibility testing performed on the organisms that were initially isolated. The earliest identification of growth can be achieved by radiometric or colorimetric detection techniques. If performance of full drug susceptibility studies is not possible, testing for resistance to RMP can identify strains that are likely to have multiple drug resistance. The minimal duration of treatment for all children and adults with culture-positive TB is 6 months, which should include an initial phase of INH, RMP, and PZA for a 2-month period.[157] The initial regimen also should include EMB (or STM in children who are too young to be monitored for visual acuity) until the results of drug susceptibility studies are available, unless there is a low likelihood of drug resistance (i.e., primary resistance to INH in the community is less than 4% and the patient has no known exposure to a drug-resistant case, is not from a country where the prevalence of drug resistance is high, and has not received prior therapy with anti-TB agents). Following the initial phase of a 2-month period of therapy, a second phase of treatment consisting of INH and RMP should last for 4 months. If the clinical response to therapy is slow or suboptimal, treatment should be prolonged.

Efficacy also has been achieved with 9-month regimens using INH and RMP.[158] Initial drug regimens also should include EMB or STM (STM in children who are too young to be monitored for visual acuity) until the results of drug-susceptibility studies are available, unless there is little possibility of drug resistance. Following an initial 1 or 2 months of daily therapy, INH and RMP may be administered two times a week.[159]

In adults with sputum-smear-negative and sputum-culture-negative active pulmonary TB, a shorter duration of therapy is possible.[9] In these patients, 4-month therapy with INH and RMP, preferably with PZA for the first 2 months, provides results that are equivalent to those for patients with culture-positive disease who are treated with longer regimens.[160,161] This regimen also is recommended for adult tuberculin reactors who have silicosis and are sputum-smear-negative and sputum-culture-negative or for adult reactors with a chest radiograph that is suggestive of old, healed TB.[9] An acceptable alternative therapy is a regimen of INH therapy for 12 months.

Drug-Monitoring Parameters

Baseline measurements of hepatic enzymes, bilirubin, serum creatinine, a complete blood count, and a platelet count are required for adults who are treated for TB.[9] A serum uric acid level should be measured if PZA is used. Baseline examination of both visual acuity and red-green color perception is necessary for patients who are to be treated with EMB. Baseline tests are useful in detecting abnormalities that may complicate a regimen; adjustments in dosages may be necessary on the basis of these values. They also provide a means of comparison with measurements obtained during therapy if an adverse reaction is suspected. For children, baseline tests, except for visual acuity, are not necessary unless a complicating condition exists or is clinically suspected.

All patients, adults and children, who are receiving anti-TB therapy should be monitored clinically for adverse drug effects and should be instructed to look for symptoms that are associated with common adverse effects of their medications.[9] Medical personnel should follow patients at least monthly during therapy and ascertain whether symptoms suggesting drug toxicity are present. In general, routine laboratory monitoring for toxicity in patients with normal baseline tests is not necessary. Should symptoms suggest drug toxicity, appropriate laboratory testing should be performed to confirm or exclude such toxicity.

Evaluation of Response to Therapy

Management of Patients with Positive Pretreatment Sputum

Patients with positive bacteriology (*M. tuberculosis* identified in sputum) should be evaluated by repeated examinations of sputum following initiation of anti-TB therapy.[9] Sputum examinations should be performed at least at monthly intervals until sputum conversion is documented. More than 85% of patients with positive pretreatment cultures should convert to negative after 2 months of therapy with regimens consisting of INH and RMP.

Patients in whom sputum cultures do not convert to negative following 2 months of therapy should be reevaluated, and drug susceptibility tests should be repeated.[9] If drug resistance is not demonstrated, the treatment should be continued with DOT. If resistant organisms are present, modification of the treatment regimen is necessary and must include at least two drugs to which the organisms are susceptible. Administration of the modified regimen should be provided with DOT. Bacteriologic evaluations should be performed at least at monthly intervals thereafter until cultures convert to negative.

Patients whose sputum converts to negative following 2 months of therapy require at least one further sputum smear and culture performed at the completion of therapy.[9] Chest radiographs during therapy are not as useful as sputum examination; on completion of therapy a chest radiograph provides a baseline for comparison with future radiographs. Routine follow-up is not necessary for patients with susceptible organisms who exhibit a prompt and adequate bacteriologic response following therapy with regimens containing INH and RMP.

Management of Patients with Negative Pretreatment Sputum

Extensive efforts, including induction of sputum by inhalation of hypertonic saline, should be made to establish a microbiologic diagnosis for adults with radiographic abnormalities that are consistent with TB.[9] Consideration should be given to bronchoscopy and bronchoalveolar lavage for patients who are not able to produce a satisfactory sputum specimen. If another diagnosis is not established, presumptive therapy for TB may be warranted. Response to therapy in these patients can be provided by clinical evaluation and chest radiograph. A chest radiograph that shows no improvement after 3 months of anti-TB therapy implies that the abnormality is owing to another process or is the result of previous (not current) TB. If the TST is positive and other diagnoses have been ruled out, INH and RMP therapy can be continued for a total duration of 4 months. If TB is suspected in a child, microbiologic data can be obtained from early morning gastric aspirates or urine. Aggressive efforts should be made to establish a diagnosis in children with pneumonia that is unresponsive to standard treatments or in children with HIV infection. When culture and susceptibility information is not available from the adult contact, specimens for smear, culture, and susceptibility tests should be obtained from children.

Management of Patients Whose Treatment Has Failed or Who Have Relapsed

Patients whose sputum does not convert to negative after 5 to 6 months of anti-TB therapy are considered treatment failures.[9] A current sputum specimen should be obtained, and susceptibility testing should be performed at this time. The currently used regimen may be continued while the results are pending, or at least three drugs that are not part of the current regimen can be added. Once the results of the susceptibility testing are available, the regimen should be adjusted accordingly and DOT should be used.

Unlike patients who are treatment failures, patients who relapse after completion of a regimen containing INH and RMP with organisms that are susceptible to the drugs at the start of therapy usually maintain susceptibility to these agents.[162] In general, the management of these patients involves reinstitution of the regimen that was previously used with DOT. If drug susceptibility testing reveals resistant organisms, the regimen must be modified and reinstituted.

Management of Patients Who Have Drug-Resistant Disease

In managing patients who have organisms that are resistant to one or more drugs, the basic principle is to administer at least two drugs for which susceptibility has been demonstrated.[9] For patients who demonstrate INH resistance, the recommended 6-month, four-drug regimen is effective.[163] On documentation of isolated INH resistance, INH should be discontinued, and PZA should be continued throughout the entire 6-month duration of therapy. For patients who are receiving the 9-month regimen without PZA, INH should be discontinued on documentation of isolated INH resistance. If the initial regimen included EMB, treatment consisting of RMP and EMB should be continued for a 12-month minimum.[164] If EMB was not included in the initial regimen, drug susceptibility tests should be repeated, INH should be discontinued, and two new agents (e.g., EMB and PZA) should be added. Adjustments to this regimen can be made, if necessary, once the results of the susceptibility tests are available.

Good data are not available on the efficacy and duration of therapy of various regimens that are used for patients with organisms that are resistant to both INH and RMP.[9] On discovery of drug resistance, it is likely that many patients will demonstrate resistance to other first-line agents. It is recommended that at least three new agents be used to which the organism is susceptible, with continuation of this regimen until sputum conversion is documented; completion of therapy with at least 12 months of two-drug therapy is necessary. Anti-TB therapy for a total duration of 24 months is sometimes given empirically. Although the role of the new agents mentioned previously is unknown, these agents are being used in such cases. Surgery may provide substantial benefit and improvement in cure rate in patients in whom the majority of disease can be resected.[165]

Special Treatment Circumstances

Children and Adolescents

Treatment principles for TB in children and adolescents are essentially the same as those for adults.[166] A high rate of success has been observed with 9-month regimens that include INH and RMP.[167] Six-month regimens with three-drug therapy consisting of INH, RMP, and PZA have also shown success.[55,168] Dosing of these drugs should be based on body weight.[55] The daily, twice-weekly, and thrice-weekly doses that are used for children are noted in Table 68.7.[61] Follow-up evaluations on successful completion of treatment are the same as those described for adults.[9]

Guidelines for TB treatment in children infected with HIV are provided by the CDC.[78] Treatment should be initiated without delay. Ethambutol generally should be included as part of the initial regimen, unless the infecting strain of *M. tuberculosis* is known or suspected of being susceptible to INH and RMP.

In addition to the basic pharmacotherapy, seven treatment considerations delineated in the ATS treatment recommendations include the following:[9]

- Greater dissemination occurs in individuals who are younger than 4 years of age. This heralds the need for prompt and vigorous therapy once diagnosis is suspected.
- Generally, treatment of primary intrathoracic TB is identical to treatment of pulmonary TB. An exception to this recommendation is applicable in the case of drug nonresistance. When this is true, RMP and INH for 6 months supplemented with PZA in the first 2 months is sufficient.
- Sputum specimens are less helpful in diagnosis. Dependence on the culture and sensitivity from the adult case source may be necessary. If drug resistance is suspected and adult isolates are unavailable, early morning gastric aspirates, bronchoalveolar lavage, or tissue diagnosis may be required.
- Bacteriologic examinations are less reliable in response evaluation. Clinical and radiologic examinations are of greater importance in evaluation. Hilar adenopathy may require 2 to 3 years of complete radiographic resolution so that a normal chest radiograph is not a necessary criterion for halting therapy.
- Ocular toxicity is difficult to monitor. STM and PZA are useful alternatives to EMB.
- Bone and joint disease, disseminated disease, and meningitis require 12 months of treatment, compared with other extrapulmonary TB (including cervical adenopathy), that can be treated the same as pulmonary TB.
- Management of the newborn whose mother (or other household contact) has TB is based on individual considerations. Separation of the mother and infant should be minimized.

Pregnant and Lactating Patients

The benefits outweigh the risks that are involved in the treatment of TB in pregnant women. Also, TB during pregnancy does not warrant a therapeutic abortion. Treatment should include the use of INH, RMP, and EMB (unless primary INH resistance is likely). Pyridoxine is recommended when INH is used. Because of inadequate teratogenic data, PZA is not recommended. Other drugs that should be avoided include STM, kanamycin, capreomycin, cycloserine, and ethionamide. Of these, STM is the only one with documented teratogenic effects (i.e., interference with ear development and congenital deafness).[9,169,170]

Pregnant women infected with HIV should be treated without delay, and treatment regimens that are recommended include a rifamycin; guidelines are available to assist clinicians. The particular antiretroviral regimen that a pregnant woman with HIV infection is receiving should be considered when selecting a TB regimen.[78]

Small concentrations of anti-TB drugs are present in breast milk. Nursing should not be abandoned, because this does not cause toxicity in the newborn; nor should it be considered an effective treatment for prevention in the nursing infant.[9,171] In cases in which both the infant and the mother are receiving anti-TB drugs, breastfeeding should probably be discontinued.[55]

PREVENTIVE THERAPY

Treatment of Tuberculosis Infection

Treatment of TB in people who are infected is termed "preventive therapy." It does not include treatment of individuals with active disease or those who have been exposed but are not yet infected. Preventive therapy refers to the reduction or eradication of the bacterial population in "healed" or radiographically nonvisible lesions. Effectiveness of a 12-month regimen of INH for preventive therapy for those with a positive TST lasts for 20 years; in the absence of reinfection this coverage is believed to last for life. For primary prophylaxis (the person has been exposed but is not yet infected), INH is effective only while the patient is receiving the drug.[9,172] The risk of inducing INH resistance is enhanced when INH alone is used in a person with current disease; therefore, the recommended regimens for treatment (combination therapy) are indicated until the diagnosis is clarified. If current disease is ruled out, combination treatment can be stopped after 4 months in adults and after 6 months in children.[9,161]

Specific evaluations must be completed before institution of INH preventive therapy for the individuals cited in the preceding section. These evaluations include determining whether preventive therapy is warranted, ruling out active disease, and identifying if contraindications to INH therapy exist.

INH alone is given for prevention in a once-daily dose of 300 mg per day for adults and 10 to 15 mg/kg body weight per day, not to exceed 300 mg per day for children.[9] Adherence to therapy for at least 6 months is strongly advised. The ATS and CDC have previously recommended that individuals infected with HIV receive 12 months of treatment.[9] Data from more recent studies indicate that the optimal duration of preventive therapy with INH in persons with HIV infection should be greater than 6 months; INH therapy for 9 months appears to be sufficient; therapy beyond 12 months does not appear to provide further protection.[78] A 9-month regimen of INH can be administered either daily or twice a week in HIV-infected adults; if a twice a week schedule is chosen, directly observed preventive therapy (DOPT) should be used.

In many developing countries, resources are lacking to screen all individuals for HIV-1 and TB, and to provide preventive therapy for several months duration for HIV-1 infected individuals with a positive tuberculin skin test. Interestingly, a prospective, randomized unmasked trial conducted in Haitian adults compared the efficacy of 6 months of twice a week INH therapy with 2 months of twice a week RMP and PZA for prevention of TB in HIV-1 seropositive and PPD-positive individuals.[173] The results of the study were promising, with similar efficacy demonstrated in both groups; ongoing studies are assessing the efficacy of similar short-course regimens for preventive therapy. More recent data, summarized in recommendations by the CDC, indicate that in the United States, a regimen of RMP and PZA administered daily for 2 months is a reasonable option for preventive therapy for adults with HIV infection who are not receiving PIs or NNRTIs.[78] For those patients who are receiving antiretroviral regimens that include PIs (with the exception of ritonavir, and hard-gel saquinavir [Invirase]) or NNRTIs (with the exception of delavirdine), a 2-month regimen of rifabutin and PZA can be administered daily. According to the American Academy of Pediatrics, children should receive 9 months of therapy. For children infected with HIV who are candidates for preventive therapy, the American Academy of Pediatrics recommends a 12-month regimen of INH administered once a day.

Situations Warranting the Use of Alternative Preventive Therapy

Close Contacts of INH-Resistant Cases

Child contacts and high-risk individuals (e.g., immunocompromised hosts) should be treated with RMP when INH resistance is apparent. Some clinicians would support adding a second drug, such as EMB. Administration of standard therapeutic doses for 6 months in adults and 9 months in children is recommended.[9]

High Probability of Multidrug-Resistant Infection

If organisms are resistant to both INH and RMP, except in cases of high risk, ongoing observation without preventive therapy is recommended.[174] Consideration should be given to preventive treatment using EMB and PZA daily for 6 months at the usual therapeutic dosages in high-risk cases (e.g., HIV infection). When resistance to EMB is present, PZA plus a fluoroquinolone (ofloxacin or ciprofloxacin, which are FDA-approved only for patients who are older than 18 years of age) is recommended for 6 months.[9]

Intolerance to INH

When INH intolerance is known, RMP in standard therapeutic dosages for 6 months for adults and 9 months for children is recommended. Some clinicians may add a second drug such as EMB.[9]

Use of Bacille Calmette-Guérin Vaccine

Bacille Calmette-Guérin (BCG) vaccines are live vaccines derived from an attenuated strain of *Mycobacterium bovis*.[11,175] The vaccine was first administered to humans in the early 1920s. BCG vaccination is usually administered by the intradermal method and often results in local adverse effects; serious or long-term complications are rare.[175] The health care provider should refer to the package labeling prior to administration for the specified dosage and route indicated because there are many different BCG vaccines available worldwide that are derived from the original strain. The vaccines vary in efficacy and estimates of efficacy rates have ranged from 0 to 80% in randomized, placebo-controlled trials and in case control studies.[11,175] Higher rates of efficacy in the protection of young children have been observed in prevention of more serious forms of TB, such as TB meningitis and miliary TB.[11,175]

In the United States, the risk for TB infection in the overall population is low and a national policy is not indicated for BCG vaccination.[175] Furthermore, the use of BCG vaccine is limited because its efficacy is uncertain in preventing infectious forms of TB and the reactivity to tuberculin that occurs after vaccination interferes with the management of persons who are possibly infected with TB.[175] Therefore, the use of BCG vaccine in the United States is reserved for situations in which select individuals meet the following specific criteria:

- Consideration should be given to infants and children who reside in high-risk settings provided that no other options are available (i.e., removing the child from the source of infection).
- Consideration should be given to health care providers who work in settings in which the likelihood of transmission and infection with MDR-TB is high and the TB control precautions have failed.

Although BCG is an alternative to preventive therapy in cases discussed in the preceding section, it should not be used in cases in which there is other active infection, depressed host immunity (e.g., HIV infection, therapy with immunosuppressive drugs), or pregnancy.[9,175]

Because many developing countries lack the ability to diagnose HIV infection in newborns and because TB transmission to children is common in these countries, it is recommended by WHO that all infants in Africa without symptomatic HIV infection continue to receive BCG vaccine.[176] The benefits of BCG outweigh the risk in infants without HIV infection and possibly infants infected with HIV who are not yet immunocompromised; however, as previously mentioned, the BCG vaccination is contraindicated in adults infected with HIV.[32]

CONCLUSION

Unfortunately, TB is not a conquered disease of the past. The resurgence of TB and the rising prevalence of MDR-TB worldwide indicate that the battle is being lost.[59] Several factors have been identified that are contributing to the deteriorating situation regarding TB. Inadequate implementation of preventive TB measures delays the diagnosis of TB, which facilitates transmission to others. Other factors include the problems of homelessness, poverty, substance abuse, and the HIV epidemic.[59] In addition, insufficient funding of TB control programs and lack of accessibility to anti-TB medications in various countries requires further exploration and commitment by government agencies, the pharmaceutical industry, and health care providers.

Drug therapy continues to be the cornerstone of an effective TB treatment plan, enabling TB to be a curable and preventable disease.[9] Future advancements in drug development, including a more effective vaccine, will further assist in the elimination of TB. Of equal importance, rapid patient identification and isolation are necessary components of TB control programs. Various strategies have been developed by the CDC/ATS to ensure effective therapy of TB.[9] DOT will eliminate noncompliance by patients and can be administered two or three times a week. The overall clinical and social management of patients with TB and their contacts is the ultimate goal. In this setting, the success of therapy is achievable.

KEY POINTS

- TB is a global public health problem.
- TB is transmitted by aerosolized droplet nuclei.
- Transmission can be reduced by adequate ventilation and ultraviolet lighting.
- Close contacts are highly susceptible.
- Contact investigation is an important component of TB prevention and control.
- Cell-mediated immunity is manifested by DTH response to PPD skin test.
- There are two types of MDR-TB: primary and acquired.
- Drug therapy goals include curing the sick and impeding transmission to others.
- A primary aim is to provide the most efficacious anti-TB regimen with the least toxicity for the shortest period of time.
- Treatment of active TB requires combination therapy.
- Implementation of DOT is encouraged in all settings.

REFERENCES

1. Dolin PJ, Raviglione MC, Kochi A. Global tuberculosis incidence and mortality during 1990-2000. Bull WHO 72:213–220, 1994.
2. Narain JP, Raviglione MC, Kochi A. HIV-associated tuberculosis in developing countries: epidemiology and strategies for prevention. Tubercle Lung Dis 73:311–321, 1992.
3. Rose DN, Schecter CB, Sacks HS. Preventive medicine for HIV infected patients: an analysis of isoniazid prophylaxis for tuberculin reactors and for anergic patients. J Gen Intern Med 7:589–594, 1992.
4. TB: A Global Emergency. Geneva, Switzerland: World Health Organization, 1994.
5. World TB Day marked by hundreds of organizations. Press Release. Geneva, Switzerland: World Health Organization, 23 March 1998.
6. Pablos-Mendez A, Raviglione MC, Laszlo A, et al. Global surveillance for antituberculosis drug resistance, 1994–1997. N Engl J Med 338:1641–1649, 1998.
7. Cohn DL, Bustreo F, Raviglione MC. Drug-resistant tuberculosis: review of the worldwide situation and the WHO/IUATLD global surveillance project. Clin Infect Dis 24:S121–130, 1997.
8. Dooley SW, Jarvis WR, Martone WJ, et al. Multidrug-resistant tuberculosis (editorial). Ann Intern Med 117:257–259, 1992.
9. American Thoracic Society. Treatment of tuberculosis and tuberculosis infection in adults and children. Am J Respir Crit Care Med 149:1359–1374, 1994.
10. Des Prez RM, Heim CR. *Mycobacterium tuberculosis.* In Mandell GL, Douglas RG, Bennett JE, eds. Principles and practice of infectious diseases. 3rd ed. New York: Churchill Livingstone, 1990:1877–1906.
11. Raviglione MC, O'Brien RJ. Tuberculosis. In: Fauci AS, Braunwald E, Isslebacher KJ, et al, eds. Harrison's principles of internal medicine. 14th ed. New York: McGraw-Hill, 1998:1004–1014.
12. CDC. Tuberculosis morbidity–United States, 1997. MMWR 47(13):253–257, 1998.
13. CDC. Tuberculosis morbidity–United States, 1996. MMWR 46(30):695–700, 1997.
14. Shafer RW, Edlin BR. Tuberculosis in patients infected with Human Immunodeficiency Virus: perspective on the past decade. Clin Infect Dis 22:683–704, 1996.
15. Saltini C, Amicosante M, Girardi E, et al. Early abnormalities of the antibody response against *Mycobacterium tuberculosis* in human immunodeficiency virus infection. J Infect Dis 168:1409–1414, 1993.
16. Zhang M, Gong J, Iyer DV, et al. T cell cytokine responses in persons with tuberculosis and human immunodeficiency virus infection. J Clin Invest 94:2435–2442, 1994.
17. Selwyn PA, Hartel D, Lewis VA, et al. A prospective study of the risk of tuberculosis among intravenous drug users with human immunodeficiency virus infection. N Engl J Med 320:545–550, 1989.
18. Guelar A, Gatell JM, Verdejo J, et al. A prospective study of the risk of tuberculosis among HIV-infected patients. AIDS 7:1345–1349, 1993.
19. Antonucci G, Girardi E, Raviglione MC, et al. Risk factors for tuberculosis in HIV-infected persons: a prospective cohort study. JAMA 247:143–148, 1995.
20. Small PM, Hopewell PC, Singh SP, et al. The epidemiology of tuberculosis in San Francisco: a population-based study using conventional and molecular methods. N Engl J Med 330:1703–1709, 1994.
21. Alland D, Kalkut GE, Moss AR, et al. Transmission of tuberculosis in New York City: an analysis by DNA fingerprinting and conventional epidemiologic methods. N Engl J Med 330:1710–1716, 1994.
22. Daley CL, Small PM, Schecter GF, et al. An outbreak of tuberculosis with accelerated progression among persons infected with the human immunodeficiency virus: an analysis using restriction-fragment-length polymorphisms. N Engl J Med 326:231–235, 1992.
23. Edlin BR, Tokars JI, Grieco MH, et al. An outbreak of multidrug-resistant tuberculosis among hospitalized patients with the acquired immunodeficiency syndrome. N Engl J Med 326:1514–1521, 1992.
24. Coronado VG, Beck-Sague CM, Hutton MD, et al. Transmission of multidrug-resistant *Mycobacterium tuberculosis* among persons with human immunodeficiency virus infection in an urban hospital: epidemiologic and restriction fragment length polymorphism analysis. J Infect Dis 168:1052–1055, 1993.
25. Small PM, Shafer RW, Hopewell PC, et al. Exogenous reinfection with multidrug-resistant *Mycobacterium tuberculosis* in patients with advanced HIV infection. N Engl J Med 328:1137–1144, 1993.
26. CDC. Screening for tuberculosis and tuberculosis infection in high-risk populations. MMWR 44(No. RR-11):19–34, 1995.
27. American Thoracic Society/CDC. Diagnostic standards and classification of tuberculosis. Am Rev Respir Dis 142:725–735, 1990.
28. CDC. Anergy skin testing and preventative therapy for HIV-infected persons: revised recommendations. MMWR 46(suppl RR-15):1–11, 1997.
29. CDC. Purified protein derivative (PPD)-tuberculin anergy and HIV infection: guidelines for anergy testing and management of anergic persons at risk of tuberculosis. MMWR 40(suppl RR-5):27–33, 1991.
30. Greenberg SD, Frager D, Suster B, et al. Active pulmonary tuberculosis in patients with AIDS: specifics of radiographic findings (including a normal appearance). Radiology 193:115–119, 1994.

31. Pedro-Botet J, Gutierrez J, Miralles R, et al. Pulmonary tuberculosis in HIV-infected patients with normal chest radiographs. AIDS 6:91–93, 1992.
32. Centers for Disease Control and Prevention. 1999 USPHS/IDSA guidelines for the prevention of opportunistic infections in persons infected with human immunodeficiency virus: US Public Health Service (USPHS) and Infectious Diseases Society of America (IDSA). MMWR 48 (No. RR-10): 12–13, 1999.
33. Klein NC, Duncanson FP, Lenox TH III. Use of mycobacterial smears in the diagnosis of pulmonary tuberculosis in AIDS/ARC patients. Chest 95:1190–1192, 1989.
34. Long R, Scalcini M, Manfreda J, et al. The impact of HIV on the usefulness of sputum smears for the diagnosis of tuberculosis. Am J Public Health 81:1326–1328, 1991.
35. Elliot AM, Namaambo K, Allen BW, et al. Negative sputum smear results in HIV-positive patients with pulmonary tuberculosis in Lusaka, Zambia. Tuber Lung Dis 74:191–194, 1993.
36. Traub SL. Basic skills in interpreting laboratory data. Bethesda, MD: American Society of Health-System Pharmacists, 1996:359–360.
37. Casal M, Gutierrex J, Vaquero M. Comparative evaluation of the mycobacteria growth indicator tube with the BACTEC 460 TB system and Lowenstein-Jensen medium for isolation of mycobacteria from clinical specimens. Int J Tuberc Lung Dis 1(1):81–84, 1997.
38. CDC. Guidelines for preventing the transmission of *M. tuberculosis* in health-care facilities, 1994. MMWR 43(suppl RR-13):1–132, 1994.
39. Shafer RW, Kim DS, Weiss JP, et al. Extrapulmonary tuberculosis in patients with human immunodeficiency virus infection. Medicine (Baltimore) 70:384–97, 1991.
40. Vadillo M, Corbella X, Carratala J. AIDS presenting as septic shock caused by *M. tuberculosis*. Scand J Infect Dis 26:105–106, 1994.
41. Mahmoudi A, Iseman MD. Pitfalls in the care of patients with tuberculosis: common errors and their association with the acquisition of drug resistance. JAMA 270:65–68, 1993.
42. Cohen ML. Epidemiology of drug resistance: implications for a post-antibiotic era. Science 257:1050–1055, 1992.
43. Connix R, Pfyffer GE, Mathieu C, et al. Drug resistant tuberculosis in prisons in Azerbaijan: case study. Br Med J 316:1423–1425, 1998.
44. Raviglione MC, Rieder HL, Styblo K, et al. Tuberculosis trends in Eastern Europe and the former USSR. Tuberc Lung Dis 75:400–416, 1994.
45. Van Scog RE, Wilkowske CJ. Antituberculous agents. Mayo Clin Proc 67:179–187, 1992.
46. Mitchison DA. Development of streptomycin resistant strains of tubercle bacilli in pulmonary tuberculosis: results of simultaneous sensitivity tests in liquid and on solid media. Thorax 5:144–1461, 1950.
47. Canetti G. Present aspects of bacterial resistance in tuberculosis. Am Rev Respir Dis 92:687–703, 1965.
48. Hobby GL. Primary drug resistance in tuberculosis: a review. Am Rev Respir Dis 86:839–846, 1962.
49. Hobby GL. Primary drug resistance in tuberculosis: a review. Am Rev Respir Dis 87:29–36, 1963.
50. Doster B, Caras CJ, Snider DE. A continuing survey of primary drug resistance in tuberculosis, 1961 to 1968: a U.S. Public Health Service cooperative study. Am Rev Respir Dis 113:419–427, 1976.
51. Kopnoff DE, Kilburn JO, Glassroth JL, et al. A continuing survey of tuberculosis primary drug resistance in the United States: March 1975 to November 1977: a United States Public Health Service cooperative study. Am Rev Respir Dis 118:835–842, 1978.
52. Snider DE, Cauthen GM, Farer LS, et al. Drug-resistant tuberculosis. Am Rev Respir Dis 144:732, 1991.
53. Iseman MD. Treatment of multidrug-resistant tuberculosis. N Engl J Med 329(11):784–791, 1993.
54. Perez-Stable EJ, Hopewell PC. Chemotherapy of tuberculosis. Semin Respir Med 9:459, 1988.
55. Hooker KD, Jost PM. Tuberculosis. In: Herfindal ET, Gourley DR, Hart LL, eds. Clinical pharmacy and therapeutics. 5th ed. Baltimore: Williams & Wilkins, 1992:1092–1108.
56. Aquinas SM. Short-course therapy for tuberculosis. Drugs 24:118–132, 1982.
57. Angel JH. The case for short-course chemotherapy of pulmonary tuberculosis. Drugs 27:1–8, 1983.
58. Stratton MA, Reed MD. Short-course drug therapy for tuberculosis. Clin Pharmacy 5(12):977–987, 1986.
59. Iseman MD, Cohn DL, Sbarbaro JA. Directly observed treatment of tuberculosis: we can't afford not to try it. N Engl J Med 328(8):576–578, 1993.
60. Ebert SC. ASHP Therapeutic position statement on strategies for preventing and treating multi-drug resistant tuberculosis. Am J Health Syst Pharmacy 54:428–431, 1997.
61. CDC. Initial therapy for tuberculosis in the era of multidrug resistance. Recommendations of the advisory council for the elimination of tuberculosis. MMWR 42(suppl RR-7):1–8, 1993.
62. Chaulk CP, Kazandjian VA for the Public Health Tuberculosis Guidelines Panel. Directly observed therapy for treatment completion of pulmonary tuberculosis. Consensus statement of the public health tuberculosis guidelines panel. JAMA 279(12):943–947, 1988.
63. Farmer P, Kim JY. Community based approaches to the control of multidrug resistant tuberculosis: introducing "DOTS-plus." Br Med J 317:671–674, 1998.
64. Takayama K, Schnoes HK, Armstrong EL, et al. Site of inhibitory action of isoniazid in the synthesis of mycolic acids in *Mycobacterium tuberculosis*. J Lipid Res 16:308–317, 1975.
65. Mandell GL, Petri WA. Drugs used in the chemotherapy of tuberculosis, *Mycobacterium avium* complex disease, and leprosy. In Hardman JG, Limbird LE, Molinoff PB, et al., eds. The pharmacologic basis of therapeutics. 9th ed. New York: Macmillan, 1996:1155–1174.
66. Dickinson JM, Aber VR, Mitchison DA. Bactericidal activity of streptomycin, isoniazid, rifampin, ethambutol, and pyrazinamide alone and in combination against *Mycobacterium tuberculosis*. Am Rev Respir Dis 116:627–635, 1977.
67. Hurwitz A, Schlozman DL. Effect of antacids on gastrointestinal absorption of isoniazid in rat and man. Am Rev Respir Dis 109:41–47, 1974.
68. Holdiness MR. Cerebrospinal fluid pharmacokinetics of antituberculous antibiotics. Clin Pharmacokinet 10:532–534, 1985.
69. Maddrey WC, Boitnott JK. Isoniazid hepatitis. Ann Intern Med 79:1–12, 1973.
70. Mitchell JR, Zimmerman HJ, Ishak KG. Isoniazid liver injury: clinical spectrum, pathology and probable pathogenesis. Ann Intern Med 84:181–192, 1976.
71. Evans D, Manley KA, McKusick VA. Genetic control of isoniazid metabolism in man. Br Med J 2:485–491, 1960.
72. Mitchell JR, Thorgeirsson UP, Black M, et al. Increased incidence of isoniazid hepatitis in rapid acetylators: possible relation in hydrazine metabolites. Clin Pharmacol Ther 18:70–79, 1975.
73. Alexander MR, Louie SG, Guernsy BG. Isoniazid-associated hepatitis. Clin Pharmacy 1:148–153, 1982.
74. Martinez-Roig A, Cami J, Llorens-Terol J, et al. Acetylation phenotype and hepatotoxicity in the treatment of tuberculosis in children. Pediatrics 77:912–915, 1986.
75. Anderson RJ, Gambertoglio JG, Schrier RW. Clinical use of drugs in renal failure. Springfield, IL: Charles C Thomas, 1976.
76. Bennett WM, Aronoff GR, Morrison G, et al. Drug prescribing in renal failure: dosing guidelines for adults. Am J Kidney Dis 3:155–193, 1983.
77. Girling DJ. Adverse effects of antituberculous drugs. Drugs 23:56–74, 1982.
78. CDC. Prevention and treatment of tuberculosis among patients infected with human immunodeficiency virus: principles of therapy and revised recommendations. MMWR 47 (RR20):1–51, 1998.
79. Kopanoff DE, Snider DE Jr, Caras GJ. Isoniazid-related hepatitis: a U.S. Public Health Service cooperative surveillance study. Am Rev Respir Dis 117:991–1001, 1978.
80. Stead WW, To T. The significance of the tuberculin skin test in elderly persons. Ann Intern Med 107:837–842, 1987.
81. Baciewicz AM, Self TH. Isoniazid interactions. South Med J 78(6):714–718, 1985.
82. Maukkassah SF, Bidlack WF, Yang WCT. Mechanism of the inhibitory action of isoniazid on microsomal drug metabolism. Biochem Pharmacol 30:1651–1658, 1981.
83. Kutt H, Brennan R, Dehejia H, et al. Diphenylhydantoin intoxication. Am Rev Respir Dis 101:377–384, 1970.
84. Brennan RW, Dehejia H, Kutt H, et al. Diphenylhydantoin intoxication attendant to slow inactivation of isoniazid. Neurology 20:687–693, 1970.
85. Miller RR, Porter J, Greenblatt DJ. Clinical importance of the interaction of phenytoin and isoniazid. Chest 75:356–358, 1979.
86. Melander A, Danielson K, Hanson A, et al. Reduction of isoniazid bioavailability in normal men by concomitant intake of food. Acta Med Scand 200:93–97, 1976.
87. Mannistro P, Mantyla R, Klinge R, et al. Influence of various diets on the bioavailability of isoniazid. J Antimicrob Chemother 10:427–434, 1982.
88. Mattila MJ, Takki S, Jussila J. Effects of sodium sulphate and castor oil on drug absorption from the human intestine. Ann Clin Res 6:19–24, 1974.
89. Hauser MJ, Baier H. Interactions of isoniazid with foods. Drug Intell Clin Pharmacol 16:617–618, 1982.
90. Smith CK, Durack DT. Isoniazid and reaction to cheese. Ann Intern Med 78:520–521, 1978.
91. Lejonc JL, Gusmini D, Brochard P. Isoniazid and reaction to cheese [Letter]. Ann Intern Med 91:793, 1979.
92. Uragoda CG, Lodha SC. Histamine intoxication in a tuberculous patient after ingestion of cheese. Tubercle 60:59–61, 1979.

93. Lejonc JL, Schaeffer A, Brochard P, et al. Hypertension arterielle paroxystique provoquee sous isoniazide par l'ingestion de gruyere: deux cas. Ann Med Interne 131:346–348, 1980.
94. Uragoda CG, Kottegoda SR. Adverse reactions to isoniazid on ingestion of fish with a high histamine content. Tubercle 58:83–89, 1977.
95. Senanayake N, Vyravanathan S, Kanagasuriyam S. Cerebrovascular accident after a "skipjack" reaction in a patient taking isoniazid. Br Med J 2:1127–1128, 1978.
96. Uragoda CG. Histamine poisoning in tuberculous patients after ingestion of tuna fish. Am Rev Respir Dis 121:157–159, 1980.
97. Aloysius DJ, Uragoda CG. Histamine poisoning on ingestion of tuna fish. J Trop Med Hyg 86:13–15, 1983.
98. Uragoda CG. Histamine poisoning in tuberculosis patients on ingestion of tropical fish. J Trop Med Hyg 81:243–245, 1978.
99. Uragoda CG. Histamine intoxication with isoniazid and a species of fish. Ceylon Med J 23:109–110, 1978.
100. Brass C, Galgiani JN, Blaschke TF, et al. Disposition of ketoconazole, an oral antifungal in humans. Antimicrob Agents Chemother 21:151–158, 1982.
101. Englehard D, Stutman HR, Marks MI. Interaction of ketoconazole with rifampin and isoniazid. N Engl J Med 74:18–47, 1983.
102. Hoglund P, Nillson LG, Paulsen O. Interaction between isoniazid and theophylline. Eur J Resp Dis 70:110–116, 1987.
103. Samigun M, Santoso B. Lowering of theophylline clearance by isoniazid in slow and rapid acetylators. Br J Clin Pharmacol 29:570–573, 1990.
104. Thompson JR, Buckart GJ, Self TH, et al. Isoniazid-induced alterations of theophylline pharmacokinetics. Curr Ther Res 32:921–925, 1982.
105. Thompson JR, Self TH. Theophylline and isoniazid. Br J Clin Pharmacol 30:909, 1990.
106. Thornsberry C, Hill BC, Swenson JM, et al. Rifampin: spectrum of antibacterial activity. Rev Infect Dis 5:S412–417, 1983.
107. Wehrli W. Rifampin: mechanisms of action and resistance. Rev Infect Dis 5:S407–411, 1983.
108. Fox W. Whether short-course chemotherapy? Br J Dis Chest 75:331–357, 1981.
109. Kucer A, Bennett N. The use of antibiotics: a comprehensive review with clinical emphasis. 3rd ed. Philadelphia: Lippincott, 1979.
110. Koup JR, Williams-Warren J, Viswanathan CT, et al. Pharmacokinetics of rifampin in children. II: oral bioavailability. Ther Drug Monit 8:17–22, 1986.
111. Council on Drugs. American Medical Association. Evaluation of a new antituberculosis agent. JAMA 220:414–415, 1972.
112. McCracken GH, Ginsberg CM, Zweighaft TC, et al. Pharmacokinetics of rifampin in infants and children: relevance to prophylaxis against *Haemophilus influenzae* type b disease. Pediatrics 66:17–21, 1980.
113. Sippel JE, Mikhail IA, Girgis NI, et al. Rifampin concentrations in cerebrospinal fluid of patients with tuberculosis meningitis. Am Rev Respir Dis 109:579–580, 1974.
114. Furesz S. Clinical and biological properties of rifampicin. Antibiot Chemother 16:316–351, 1970.
115. Grosset J, Leventis S. Adverse effects of rifampin. Rev Infec Dis 5:S440–446, 1983.
116. Pharmacia & Upjohn Company. Rifabutin (Mycobutin) product information, 1996.
117. Hoechst Marion Roussel. Rifapentine (Priftin) product information, 1998.
118. Flynn CT, Rainford DJ, Hope E. Acute renal failure and rifampicin: danger of unsuspected intermittent dosage. Br Med J 2:428, 1974.
119. Girling DJ, Hitze HL. Adverse reactions to rifampicin. Bull WHO 57:45–49, 1979.
120. Gronhagen-Riska C, Hellstrom PE, Froseth B. Predisposing factors in hepatitis induced by isoniazid-rifampin treatment of tuberculosis. Am Rev Respir Dis 118:461–466, 1978.
121. Baciewicz AM, Self TH. Rifampin drug interactions. Arch Intern Med 144:1167, 1984.
122. Baciewicz AM, Self TH, Bakemeyer WB. Update on rifampin drug interactions. Arch Intern Med 147:565, 1987.
123. Borcherding SM, Baciewicz AM, Self TH. Update on rifampin drug interactions II. Arch Intern Med 152:711–715, 1992.
124. Gupta KC, Joshi JV, Anklesria PS, et al. Plasma rifampicin levels during oral contraception. J Assoc Phys India 36:365–366, 1988.
125. Skolnick, JL, Stoler BS, Katz DB, et al. Rifampin, oral contraceptives, and pregnancy. JAMA 236(12):1382, 1976.
126. CDC. Clinical update: impact of HIV protease inhibitors in the treatment of HIV-infected tuberculosis patients with rifampin. MMWR 45(42):921–925, 1996.
127. Strayhorn VA, Baciewicz AM, Self TH. Update on rifampin drug interactions, III. Arch Intern Med 157:2453–2458, 1997.
128. Burman WJ, Gallicano K, Peloquin C. Therapeutic implications of drug interactions in the treatment of human immunodeficiency virus-related tuberculosis. Clin Infect Dis 28:419–430, 1999.
129. Tam CM, Chan SL, Lam, CW, et al. Rifapentine and isoniazid in the continuation phase of treating pulmonary tuberculosis. Am J Respir Crit Care Med 157:1726–1733, 1998.
130. Takayama K, Armstrong EL, Kunugi KA. Inhibition by ethambutol of mycolic acid transfer into the cell wall of *Mycobacterium smegmatis*. Antimicrob Agents Chemother 16:240, 1979.
131. Peets EA, Sweeney WM, Place VA. The absorption, excretion and metabolic fate of ethambutol in man. Am Rev Respir Dis 91:51–58, 1965.
132. Holdiness MR. Clinical pharmacokinetics of the antituberculous drugs. Clin Pharmacokinet 9:511–544, 1984.
133. Liebold JE. The ocular toxicity of ethambutol and its relation to dose. Ann NY Acad Sci 135:904–909, 1966.
134. Postlethwaite AE, Bartel AG, Kelly WN. Hyperuricemia due to ethambutol. N Engl J Med 286:761–762, 1972.
135. Mackandess GB. The intracellular activity of pyrazinamide and nicotinamide. Am Rev Tuberc 74:718–728, 1956.
136. Zierski M, Bek E. Side effects of drug regimens used in short course chemotherapy for pulmonary tuberculosis: a controlled study. Tubercle 61:41–49, 1980.
137. Pilheu JA, De Salvo MC, Koch O, et al. Liver alterations in antituberculosis regimens containing pyrazinamide. Chest 80:720–724, 1981.
138. Steele MA, Des Prez RM. The role of pyrazinamide in tuberculosis chemotherapy. Chest 94:845, 1988.
139. Cullen JH, Early LJA, Fiore JM. The occurrence of hyperuricemia during pyrazinamide-isoniazid therapy. Am Rev Tuberc Pulm Dis 74:289–292, 1956.
140. Peloquin CA. Comment: intravenous streptomycin. Ann Pharmaocother 27:1546–1547, 1993.
141. Hansten PD, Horn JR. Drug interactions analysis and management. Vancouver: Applied Therapeutics, 1997.
142. Spector R, Lorenza WV. The active transport of para-aminosalicylic acid from the cerebrospinal fluid. J Pharmacol Exp Ther 185:642–648, 1973.
143. Perriens JH, Colebunders RL, Karahunga C, et al. Increased mortality and tuberculosis treatment failure rate among human immunodeficiency virus (HIV) seronegative patients with pulmonary tuberculosis treated with "standard" chemotherapy in Kinshasa, Zaire. Am Rev Respir Dis 144:750–755, 1991.
144. Okwera A, Whalen C, Byekwaso F, et al. Randomized trial of thiacetazone and rifampicin-containing regimens for pulmonary tuberculosis in HIV-infected Ugandans. Lancet 344:1323–1328, 1994.
145. Nunn P, Kibuga D, Gathua S, et al. Cutaneous hypersensitivity reactions due to thiacetazone in HIV-1 seropositive patients treated for tuberculosis. Lancet 337:627–630, 1991.
146. Chintu C, Luo C, Bhat G, et al. Cutaneous hypersensitivity reactions due to thiacetazone in the treatment of tuberculosis in Zambian children infected with HIV-1. Arch Dis Child 68:665–668, 1993.
147. Raviglione MC, Narain JB, Kochi A. HIV-associated tuberculosis in developing countries: clinical features, diagnosis, and treatment. WHO 70:515–526, 1992.
148. Peloquin CA. Antituberculous drug pharmacokinetics. In: Heifets LB, ed. Drug susceptibility in the chemotherapy of mycobacterial infections. Boca Raton, FL: CRC Press, 1991.
149. Berning SE, Madsen L, Iseman MD, et al. Long-term safety of ofloxacin and ciprofloxacin in the treatment of mycobacterial infections. Am J Respir Crit Care Med 151:2006–2009, 1995.
150. Peloquin CA. Levofloxacin for drug-resistant *Mycobacterium tuberculosis*. Ann Pharmacother 32:268–269, 1998.
151. Mor N, Vanderkolk J, Heifets L. Inhibitory and bactericidal activities of levofloxacin against *Mycobacterium tuberculosis* in vitro and in human macrophages. Antimicrob Agents Chemother 38:1161–1164, 1994.
152. Cynamon MH, Klemens SP. New antimycobacterial agents. Clin Chest Med 10:355–364, 1989.
153. Wong CS, Palmer GS, Cynamon MH. *In vitro* susceptibility of *Mycobacterium tuberculosis, Mycobacterium bovis,* and *Mycobacterium kansasii* to amoxycillin and ticarcillin in combination with clavulanic acid. J Antimicrob Chemother 22:863–866, 1988.
154. Chambers HF, Kocagoz T, Sipit T, et al. Activity of Amoxicillin/Clavulanate in patients with tuberculosis. Clin Infect Dis 26:874–877, 1998.
155. Condos R, Rom WN, Schluger NW. Treatment of multidrug-resistant pulmonary tuberculosis with interferon-γ via aerosol. Lancet 349:1513–1515, 1997.
156. CDC. Nosocomial transmission of multidrug-resistant TB in health-care workers and HIV-infected patients in an urban hospital: Florida. MMWR 39:718, 1990.

157. Combs DL, O'Brien RJ, Geiter LJ. USPHS tuberculosis short-course therapy trial 21: effectiveness, toxicity, and acceptability. The report of final results. Ann Intern Med 112:397, 1990.
158. Slutkin G, Schecter GF, Hopewell PC. The results of 9-month isoniazid-rifampin therapy for pulmonary tuberculosis under programs in San Francisco. Am Rev Respir Dis 138:1622, 1988.
159. Dutt AK, Moers D, Stead WW. Short-course chemotherapy for tuberculosis with mainly twice-weekly isoniazid and rifampin: community physicians' seven-year experience with mainly outpatients. Am J Med 77:223, 1984.
160. Hong Kong Chest Service/Tuberculosis Research Centre, Madras/British Medical Research Council: A controlled trial of 3-month, 4-month and 6-month regimens of chemotherapy for sputum-smear negative pulmonary tuberculosis: results at 5 years. Am Rev Respir Dis 139:871, 1989.
161. Dutt AK, Moers D, Stead WW. Smear- and culture-negative pulmonary tuberculosis: four-month short course chemotherapy. Am Rev Respir Dis 139:867, 1989.
162. Snider DE, Long MW, Cross FS, et al. Six-months isoniazid-rifampin therapy for pulmonary tuberculosis. Am Rev Respir Dis 129:573, 1984.
163. Singapore Tuberculosis Service/British Medical Research Council. Clinical trial of six-month and four-month regimens of chemotherapy in the treatment of pulmonary tuberculosis. Am Rev Respir Dis 119:579–585, 1979.
164. Zierski M. Prospects of retreatment of chronic resistant pulmonary tuberculosis: a critical review. Lung 154:91, 1977.
165. Iseman MD, Madsen L, Goble M. Surgical intervention in the treatment of pulmonary disease caused by drug-resistant *Mycobacterium tuberculosis*. Am Rev Respir Dis 141:623, 1990.
166. American Academy of Pediatrics. Report of the committee on infectious diseases. 22nd ed. Elk Grove, IL: American Academy of Pediatrics, 1991: 487–508.
167. Abernathy AS, Dutt, Stead WW, et al. Shortcourse chemotherapy for tuberculosis in children. Pediatrics 72:801, 1983.
168. Starke JR. Multidrug chemotherapy for tuberculosis in children. Pediat Infect Dis J 9:785–793, 1990.
169. Briggs GG, Freeman RK, Yaffeb SJ. Drugs in pregnancy and lactation. 4th ed. Baltimore: Williams & Wilkins, 1994:460–461, 745, 768–769, 790–791.
170. Snider DE, Layde RM, Johnson MW, et al. Treatment of tuberculosis during pregnancy. Am Rev Respir Dis 122:65, 1980.
171. Snider DE, Powell KE. Should women taking antituberculosis drugs breastfeed? Arch Intern Med 144:589, 1984.
172. Comstock GW, Gaum C, Snider DF. Isoniazid prophylaxis among Alaskan Eskimos: a final report of the Bethel isoniazid studies. Am Rev Respir Dis 119:827–830, 1979.
173. Halsey NA, Coberly JS, Desormeaux J, et al. Randomized trial of isoniazid versus rifampicin and pyrazinamide for prevention of tuberculosis in HIV-1 infection. Lancet 351:786–792, 1998.
174. CDC. Management of persons exposed to multidrug-resistant tuberculosis. MMWR 41:59–71, 1992.
175. CDC. The role of BCG vaccine in the prevention and control of tuberculosis in the United States. MMWR 45(RR-4):1–15, 1996.
176. World Health Organization. BCG immunization and paediatric HIV infection. Wkly Epidemiol Rec 67:129–132, 1992.

CHAPTER 69

URINARY TRACT INFECTIONS

Cinda Christensen

DEFINITION

Infections can develop throughout the urinary tract but most frequently involve the bladder (cystitis) or kidney (pyelonephritis). In men, the prostate, epididymis, and testis can also become infected by bacteria originating from the urinary tract.[1] The presence of bacteria or fungi in the urine is termed bacteriuria and funguria, respectively. However, the detection of bacteria or fungi in the urine does not always imply infection or a clinically significant condition. Bacteria in the urine without signs and symptoms of infection is termed asymptomatic bacteriuria.

Urinary tract infections (UTIs) are classified as either uncomplicated or complicated. This distinction is important because management strategies often differ between these two groups. Uncomplicated UTIs include acute cystitis and pyelonephritis in previously healthy individuals. These patients have the lowest risk of complications or treatment failure. Complicated infections can be acute or chronic, and occur in a diverse mix of patients with metabolic, functional, or structural abnormalities of the urinary tract or kidneys.[2,3] Metabolic factors include diabetes mellitus, renal failure, and kidney transplantation. Examples of functional abnormalities are neurogenic bladder and vesicoureteral reflux. Structural abnormalities result from stones, tumors, strictures, or foreign objects such as catheters, stents, and other forms of instrumentation.[3]

Patients with complicated UTIs have a higher risk of severe infection, treatment failure, or recurrent infection.[4] Anatomic or functional disorders of the urinary tract are associated with an increased incidence of UTI and lower cure rates. Conversely, inflammatory or immunological defects often result in similar infection rates, but instead may result in more severe infections when they do occur.[5]

Recurrent infection in a patient with a previous UTI can be owing to either a relapse or reinfection. Relapses are caused by the same microorganism as in the preceding infection, and usually occur within 2 to 4 weeks after treatment has ended.[6] Reinfections typically occur after a greater length of time, and may be owing to a new strain or species. Patients who never improve or who immediately relapse following completion of treatment have persistent infection.[5,7]

Urosepsis is a serious condition wherein the bacterial species found within the urinary tract is also recovered from the patient's blood in conjunction with the clinical picture of sepsis. Patients who develop urosepsis are usually physically debilitated or have an underlying immunodeficiency.

TREATMENT GOALS: URINARY TRACT INFECTIONS

- Eradicate completely clinical disease-causing microorganisms and ameliorate all associated symptoms. This is a reasonable expectation in most uncomplicated infections, but for some patients with uncorrectable abnormalities of the urinary tract, complete resolution may not be achievable. In the latter circumstance, the goals may be to decrease the frequency and severity of infections and to preserve renal function.[2]
- Eradicate pathogenic strains of bacteria or fungi from the urinary tract (i.e., microbiologic cure).
- Resolve or alleviate associated symptoms (i.e., achieve clinical cure).
- Limit extent and severity of infection so as to prevent significant morbidity or mortality.
- Achieve successful clinical outcome with a treatment regimen that is cost effective, has minimal risk of adverse reactions, and is not prohibitive to patient compliance.

- Minimize alterations of microbial flora that may result in vaginal candidiasis, *C. difficile* colitis, or the emergence of resistant organisms within the urinary tract or other body sites.
- Prevent recurrent infection by either patient education, prophylaxis, or suppressive therapy.
- Ensure patient comprehension of how to take medications, the possible side effects of therapy, and how to avoid relevant drug–drug interactions.
- Prevent infection relapse with adequate duration of appropriate therapy.

EPIDEMIOLOGY

Prevalence

UTIs necessitate more than 7 million outpatient visits and are associated with 1 million hospitalizations in the United States annually.[7,8] As the most common occurring infectious disease, UTIs have a significant financial and humanistic public health impact. Each year, an estimated 1 billion dollars is spent in the United States diagnosing and treating acute bladder infections in young women alone. Additionally, such women will typically experience 6.1 days of symptoms and lose 1.2 days of work or school.[9]

Urinary tract infections can occur in essentially all members of the population, but are most prevalent among young and middle-aged women. The prevalence patterns of bacteriuria varies for men and women at different ages (Table 69.1).[1] In infancy, boys are more likely to develop bacteriuria and UTIs than are girls, owing to the greater incidence of congenital genitourinary tract abnormalities in boys. Among older children and throughout early and middle adulthood, women far outnumber men in the development of UTIs. UTIs are very rare in healthy younger men unless the urinary tract has undergone instrumentation such as cystoscopy. As men reach their older years, the prevalence of bacteriuria increases dramatically, almost equaling that of women. This is primarily caused by prostatic hypertrophy and functional debility associated with advanced age.

In women, the prevalence of bacteriuria steadily rises with increasing age.[10] Poor functional status further increases the prevalence of bacteriuria.[11] The development of symptomatic urinary tract infection occurs in 25 to 35% of women between the ages of 20 and 40 years. As many as 20% of women with an initial episode will experience a recurrent infection, and 12% will recur within 1 year of the initial episode.[6,9] For those women with two preceding UTIs, 47% will have another recurrence within a year.[6] In otherwise healthy women, most of these recurrences are reinfections.

Table 69.1 ▪ Prevalence of Bacteriuria in Various Populations[a]

Population	Male (%)	Female (%)
Community-based		
Infants	2	0.5
Young children	0.1	1.5
College students	<0.01	5
Adults (30–65 years old)	0.1	10
Elderly persons		
65–85 years old	5	15
>85 years old	15	25
Patient-based		
Adults (medical clinic)	4	6
Adults (urology clinic)	8	N/A
Adult inpatient		
<70 years old	7.5	30
>70 years old	25	30
Institutionalized elder persons	>30	>30
Patients after instrumentation		
Urethral catheterization	5	5
Transurethral procedures	20	40

Source: Adapted with permission from Lipsky BA. Urinary tract infections in men: epidemiology, pathophysiology, diagnosis, and treatment. Ann Intern Med 110(2):138–150, 1989.

[a]Percentages are approximations derived from a wide range of values from many studies in diverse settings; in these studies, specimens were obtained by various methods, and different definitions of bacteriuria were used.

Morbidity and Mortality

Although recurrent infections can significantly alter a patient's quality of life, most UTIs do not result in long-term morbidity or mortality. Studies have demonstrated that chronic asymptomatic bacteriuria does not contribute to renal impairment, nor does frequent recurrent cystitis.[11–13] With effective treatment, acute uncomplicated pyelonephritis usually results in only minimal renal scarring that is clinically insignificant.[2]

There are notable exceptions to the usually benign course of most UTIs. Urinary tract infections can contribute to renal scarring and failure in infants and children with anatomic anomalies such as vesicoureteral reflux. The uncommon development of chronic pyelonephritis also can lead to irreversible renal dysfunction. Asymptomatic bacteriuria in pregnant women has been shown to increase the risk of infant mortality and low birth weight.[2,10] Patients at highest risk for UTI-associated mortality are bacteremic patients with multiple comorbidities or long-term catheterization.[14,15]

Risk Factors

Multiple risk factors exist that can predispose an individual to the development of UTIs (Table 69.2). Among healthy young women, the most common risk factor is sexual activity, with the highest risk occurring within 48 hours of intercourse.[16] This increased risk is possibly owing to enhanced movement of organisms from the vaginal introitus to the urethra.[2] Also, the use of a diaphragm with spermicide or spermicide-coated condoms results in a twofold to threefold increase in risk of acquiring a UTI.[17,18] The spermicide, usually nonoxnol-9, appears to alter vaginal flora such that urinary pathogens can colonize the vaginal introitus more easily. Lower estrogen levels in postmenopausal women and recent antibiotic use can also alter vaginal flora and predispose to bacteriuria and UTI.[11,19]

Table 69.2 ▪ Risk Factors for Developing Bacteriuria and Urinary Tract Infections

Children	Congenital anomalies such as vesicoureteral reflux, male sex
Healthy young or middle-aged women	Sexual activity, diaphragm or condom use with spermicide, history of UTI in childhood, prior adult UTI, prior administration of antibiotics
Healthy young or middle-aged men	Instrumentation of the urinary tract, lack of circumcision, anal intercourse
Elderly	Uterine prolapse and low estrogen in women, prostatic hypertrophy, decreased antimicrobial activity of prostatic secretions in men, diabetes, functional debility (bedridden), bowel incontinence
All ages	Catheterization, other instrumentation, neurogenic bladder, nephrolithiasis, obstructive tumors and strictures, certain blood groups, renal failure, kidney transplantation

Source: References 1, 7, 8, 17–19, 21 22, 29, 64.

Additional risk factors are associated with the development of pyelonephritis. Pregnancy-induced changes, such as decreased peristalsis and dilation of the ureters, allow bacteria greater access to the kidneys during the later stages of pregnancy.[10] In diabetics, decreased neutrophil function, renal microangiopathy, neurogenic bladder, and glucosuria, which are often associated with diabetes, may contribute to the greater frequency of upper tract involvement.[20,21] Obstruction of the ureters by stones, strictures, or tumors also increases susceptibility to pyelonephritis. Some individuals have a genetic predisposition related to blood grouping that increases their risk for recurrent UTIs and pyelonephritis. The vaginal and urinary epithelial lining of these individuals exhibit enhanced affinity for uropathogenic organisms, thus creating favorable conditions for colonization and persistence.[21,22]

PATHOPHYSIOLOGY

The entry of organisms into the urinary tract can occur through either an ascending route from the urethra, a descending route via the kidneys from the blood, or possibly via the lymphatics.[19] The organisms infecting via the ascending route originate almost exclusively from the bowel. These organisms spread to the perineum and, in women, colonize the vaginal introitus and vagina. Once the vaginal introitus and periurethral area are colonized, bacteria can readily gain entry to the urethra and bladder. Since vaginal colonization with potential urinary pathogens is an important intermediate step in pathogenesis, changes in vaginal flora or pH that promote colonization of urinary pathogens dramatically increase the risk of developing a UTI.[17,19] In healthy adult males, UTIs are very uncommon because of the greater distance organisms must travel from the perineum to the urethra. Also, the longer urethra in males further discourages entry into the bladder.[1,2]

After bacteria (or fungi) reach the bladder, the balance between host defenses and bacterial virulence will determine if the bacteria will be able to survive and replicate efficiently and invade the bladder mucosa. Most bacteria introduced into the bladder of healthy individuals are normally cleared by host defenses within 2 to 3 days. However, if patients have high postvoid residuals, alterations in urine flow from stones or strictures, or prolonged urethral catheterization, bacteriuria may never spontaneously resolve. Chronic or intermittent bacteriuria may remain asymptomatic if the organisms are not able to attach to and invade bladder mucosa. Mucosal invasion attracts neutrophils to the bladder lining, and white blood cells (WBCs) can then be found in the urine (pyuria). With the onset of this local inflammatory response, the patient may then experience the symptoms of infection. Systemic responses such as fever or leukocytosis rarely occur with uncomplicated cystitis. Spontaneous resolution of infection may occur in 70% of previously healthy females within 30 days.[2]

Pyelonephritis results when bacteria successfully ascend the ureters and infect one or both kidneys. The entire kidney is rarely involved; instead patchy areas of necrosis and scarring are found adjacent to normal tissue.[2] Local inflammation occurs with neutrophil invasion, and the systemic response results in leukocytosis, cytokine release, and immunoglobulin M (IgM) and immunoglobulin G (IgG) elevations. A significant number of patients will be bacteremic, and urosepsis may develop in those with comorbidities.[23] Full recovery and sterilization of the kidney tissue may take as long as 6 to 10 weeks, even in previously healthy patients.[2]

Acquisition of a UTI from the descending route appears to account for only 3% of all UTIs. Bacteremia or fungemia from a nonurinary tract source rarely results in clinically significant kidney infection. The exception is for organisms with a special affinity for kidney tissue such as *Staphylococcus aureus* or *Candida* spp.[2] Complete ureteral obstruction or preexisting renal injury substantially increases the risk of kidney infection in the presence of bacteremia.[21] Once the kidney(s) is infected, bacteria or fungi can enter the urine stream and proceed to the bladder, where bacteriuria may then be detected.

Host Defenses

The host defenses that deter bacteria from colonizing and infecting the urinary tract are primarily mechanical, not immunological. Urination washes out microorganisms that have entered the urethra and bladder. Since normal postvoid bladder residuals are only 0.09 to 2.4 mL, the vast majority of colonizing organisms are physically removed with each void.[2] The peristaltic action of the ureters and the one-way vesicoureteral valve at the junction with the bladder prevents pathogens from ascending from the bladder to the kidneys.[10]

Other host defenses discourage replication or attachment of microorganisms. Certain antibacterial substances in the bladder mucosa can deter microorganism attachment. Glycoproteins and oligosaccharides in urine act as false ligands for bacterial attachment, leaving fewer bacteria to attach to the mucosa. In men, prostatic secretions contain compounds with antibacterial properties. The pH and osmolarity of urine can alter bacterial growth because both very dilute urine and concentrated, low pH urine can inhibit growth.[21]

Individuals with abnormal urine dynamics are at greater risk of UTI. For example, patients with neurogenic bladder have higher postvoid residual urine volumes and, therefore, are less efficient at removing bacteria with urination. Also, the dilated ureters of women in the later stages of pregnancy cannot effectively prevent organisms from reaching the kidneys. In healthy people therefore, an uncomplicated UTI results when the virulence of the pathogen is sufficient to overcome normal host defenses. Conversely, a complicated UTI results from the inadequacy of host defenses to prevent even low-virulence organisms from establishing infection. The immune system has no significant role in preventing UTIs, but is activated only after infection has occurred. The primary role is to limit the severity and spread of infection. Therefore, patients who are immunocompromised do not have a greater incidence of UTI, but are at higher risk of severe forms of infection when they do occur.[4,5]

Microbiology

Enteric bacteria are the most common organisms causing UTIs. This is, in part, owing to the anatomic proximity of bowel flora to the urethra, particularly in women. More important is the pathogenicity specific to the urinary tract that certain species of enteric organisms have acquired. Such organisms are called uropathogens for their ability to cause infection even in the healthy host. The most prevalent causative agent is *Escherichia coli* among all patient groups in both upper and lower tract infections (Table 69.3).

Different strains of *E. coli* have different degrees of virulence. Those strains with the greatest capacity for attachment to uroepithelial receptors succeed more frequently in establishing infection.[22,23] Strong affinity for urinary tract epithelium also correlates with bacterial persistence within the vagina and periurethral area in women. Subsequently, the same strain can be responsible for recurrent UTIs in women if therapy is not effective against organisms harbored outside the urinary tract.[6] The most pathogenic strains of *E. coli* are those that have filamentous cellular structures termed p-pili or p-fimbriae. *E. coli* with p-pili are responsible for almost all cases of bacteremic pyelonephritis in previously healthy patients.[5]

In uncomplicated UTIs in women, *Staphylococcus saprophyticus* is the next most common causative organism. *Staphylococcus saprophyticus* is a coagulase-negative staphylococci that does not originate from the bowel. This organism causes cystitis and pyelonephritis clinically similar to *E. coli*.[24] Identified risk factors for UTIs owing to *S. saprophyticus* include: use of spermicide coated condoms, young age, previous UTI, multiple sexual partners, and possibly the season of the year.[25]

Other bacteria known to cause UTIs in a small but significant number of patients are *Klebsiella pneumoniae* and *Proteus mirabilis*.[24,26] These enteric organisms are often difficult to eradicate from the urinary tract, particularly when the kidney is involved. The formation of magnesium ammonium phosphate calculi has been associated with *P. mirabilis* infection. These stones can provide a continuous nidus for infection and treatment failure.[2]

In complicated UTIs, a broader spectrum of microbial species is encountered. A greater variety of organisms can cause infection because the requisite degree of microbial virulence is less in patients with structural or functional abnormalities of the urinary tract. Many of these patients have had multiple courses of antimicrobial therapy and have become colonized with microorganisms that are intrinsically resistant or have acquired resistance to usual treatment regimens.[3] Although *E. coli* is most frequently identified as the causative agent in complicated UTI, other organisms such as *Candida* spp., *Pseudomonas aeruginosa*,

Table 69.3 ▪ Prevalence of Organisms Causing Urinary Tract Infections

Causative Organism	Cystitis*	Pyelonephritis	Complicated	Catheterized
E. coli	80	85	37	21
S. saprophyticus	10	5		
Coag. neg. staphylococci			5	8
Klebsiella spp.	3	5	8	6
Proteus spp.	2	3	5	6
Candida spp.			1	20
P. aeruginosa			15	10
Enterococci			15	11
Enterobacter spp.			6	6
Other	5	2	8	32

Source: References 3, 15, 24, 26, 27, 36, 65.
*Numbers are percentages (%).

enterococci, *Enterobacter* spp., and other Gram-negative aerobic bacilli are common pathogens in this patient population.[7,9,27] Fungal UTIs are common among hospitalized patients, particularly those with diabetes mellitus, urinary catheterization, malignancy, recent broad spectrum antibacterial therapy, and kidney transplantation.[28] In addition to *S. aureus* and *Candida* spp., *Mycobacterium tuberculosis* and *Salmonella* spp. can also infect the urinary tract via dissemination from the bloodstream. Pseudomonal UTI may be acquired via the bloodstream or the urethra.[2]

Asymptomatic bacteriuria and funguria usually are owing to a variety of relatively nonvirulent bacteria or fungi. Patients with functional or structural defects often harbor organisms intermittently or chronically. These nonpathogenic strains do not invade or attach to uroepithelium; therefore, an immune response and subsequent clinical symptoms do not develop.[23] The presence of these nonpathogenic organisms may actually protect against infection by more virulent bacteria.[29]

CLINICAL PRESENTATION AND DIAGNOSIS

Signs and Symptoms

Acute Uncomplicated Cystitis

The vast majority of patients diagnosed with acute uncomplicated cystitis are young to middle-aged women. The majority of women experience the typical symptoms of pain or burning on urination (dysuria), frequent voiding of small amounts of urine (frequency), and the need to urinate immediately (urgency).[20] Suprapubic tenderness or low back pain may be reported in some individuals. Very few patients experience systemic symptoms such as fever or chills, even though 20 to 30% have "silent" involvement of the kidney.[9,26] On gross visual examination, the urine may look cloudy or blood-tinged. On urinalysis, nearly all patients have pyuria and 40% have hematuria.[7,9,30]

Making the diagnosis of acute cystitis is relatively straightforward in patients presenting with typical symptoms and pyuria, especially if the patient reports sexual activity within the previous 24 to 48 hours.[26] However, only 65% of women presenting to medical care with symptoms possibly referable to the urinary tract actually have a UTI.[31] Other diagnoses to exclude are infections of the vagina, such as candidiasis; bacterial vaginosis; and trichomoniasis.[9] Sexually transmitted infections such as chlamydial urethritis can mimic bacterial cystitis. Patients with cystitis associated with sexual activity with a new partner should be screened for sexually transmitted diseases because coinfection is not uncommon.[32]

The presence of the characteristic symptoms of dysuria, frequency, and urgency, in addition to a positive dipstick or microscopic urinalysis for pyuria, usually are sufficient to make the diagnosis of uncomplicated cystitis in otherwise healthy patients. These patients can be started on antimicrobial treatment without further workup.[7] To assist in making the diagnosis, individuals with unclear symptoms or a negative urinalysis should have a urine sample collected for culture and sensitivity testing. Owing to the possibility of atypical or resistant organisms, a urine culture also is indicated for patients recently receiving antimicrobial therapy. A microscopic urinalysis should be performed in any symptomatic patient when the less sensitive dipstick result is negative for pyuria. Older women, children (particularly infants), men of all ages, diabetics, and patients with early relapse of UTI, are at risk for possible complicated or upper tract UTI and should have a more extensive history and physical examination performed. Also, these patients often have a broader range of possible pathogens and should have a urine culture performed.[1,9]

According to the Infectious Diseases Society of America guidelines, a midstream urine culture of greater than or equal to 10^3 CFU/mL of a single uropathogen is indicative of cystitis in patients with pyuria and symptoms consistent with lower tract infection.[26] However, for unspeciated coagulase-negative staphylococci, greater than or equal to 10^5 CFU/mL is used as a cutoff because of the potential for contamination by these organisms. In a symptomatic patient with pyuria, a midstream urine culture with less than 10^2 CFU/mL can be seen in patients with chlamydial urethritis, infections due to other fastidious organisms, early infection, partially treated infection, and candidal or bacterial vaginitis. Significant hematuria can exclude vaginal or urethral sources of symptoms because the bladder or higher urinary structures are usually the source of the red blood cells.[2,20] In symptomatic patients without pyuria, a culture showing less than 10^5 CFU/mL probably does not represent UTI. If the same patient has greater than or equal to 10^5 CFU/mL of a single Gram-negative enteric organism and other likely diagnoses have been ruled out, treatment for UTI would be indicated. Although rare, lack of pyuria may represent early infection before an inflammatory response has been mounted.[29] For patients without risks for complicated UTI, any urine culture result with mixed organisms or with a nonuropathogen is probably owing to contamination.

Many women with acute uncomplicated cystitis experience recurrent infections, the majority of which are reinfections with the same bacteria. A more extensive history and physical examination along with a microscopic urinalysis and urine culture is indicated at least once for these patients. If no complicating factors are subsequently uncovered, invasive diagnostic procedures rarely uncover abnormalities.[9] Future episodes are given minimal diagnostic workup and are treated with standard regimens. Approaches to lowering the frequency of recurrent infection may include changing the contraceptive method for patients using a diaphragm with spermicide, encouraging postcoital voiding, treating the partner of patients with recurrent *S. saprophyticus* infection, and systemic or topical estrogen replacement therapy in postmenopausal women.[16,33] Reliable patients may benefit from self-initiated therapy in which a supply of appropriate antimicrobial therapy is kept ready by the patient, and treatment is initiated when the typical symptoms recur. With more frequent recurrences, antimicrobial prophylaxis

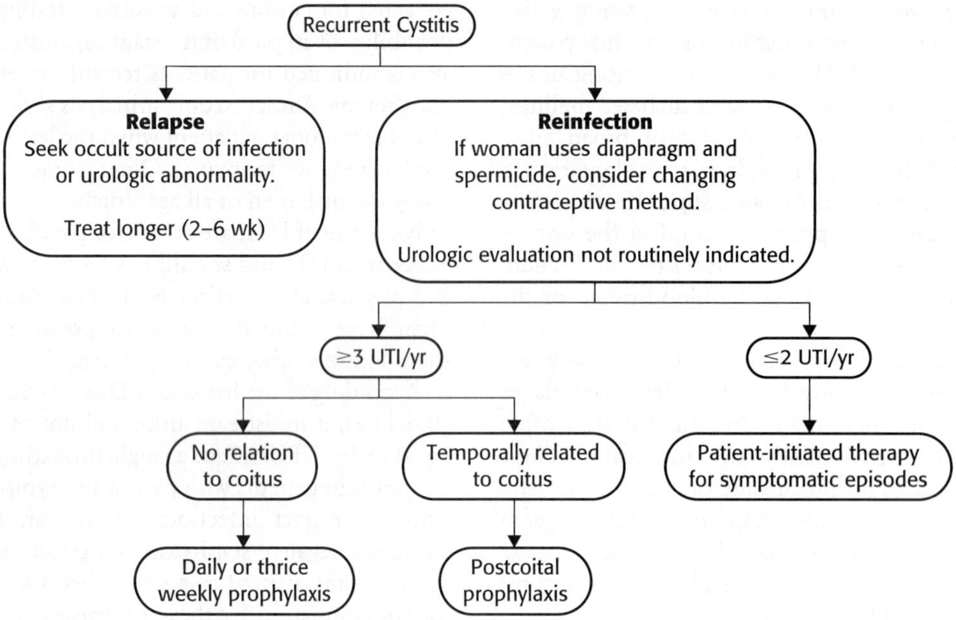

Figure 69.1. Algorithm for managing recurrent cystitis in women. (Adapted with permission from Stamm WE, Hooton TM. Management of urinary tract infections in adults. N Engl J Med 329:1331, 1993.)

may be beneficial in decreasing the number of episodes (Fig. 69.1).[9,34]

Acute Uncomplicated Pyelonephritis

Acute uncomplicated pyelonephritis can range from relatively benign to a severe, destructive infection of the kidneys. At presentation, some patients merely complain of mild fever or flank pain, whereas others may experience the full range of symptoms such as fever, chills, nausea, vomiting, flank pain, costovertebral angle tenderness, weakness, malaise, or headache.[35] Symptoms of cystitis may not always precede the development of pyelonephritis. Notably, patients at either age extreme may present with mild, nonspecific symptoms in the face of significant kidney involvement.[26]

The initial workup of the patient with presumptive pyelonephritis includes a complete blood count, urinalysis, urine Gram stain, and urine culture. Blood cultures also should be obtained in patients with severe symptoms, because 15 to 30% of patients are bacteremic.[23] Most individuals have a leukocytosis with increased band cells (often termed a left shift). On urinalysis, substantial pyuria is almost always present, and hematuria, proteinuria, and white blood cell casts may also be seen.[30] The causative agent is primarily *E. coli*, although strains associated with upper tract disease usually exhibit greater pathogenicity and virulence.[7] Urine bacterial counts of greater than or equal to 10^5 CFU/mL are detected in 80 to 95% of patients. A higher cutoff of greater than or equal to 10^4 CFU/mL is generally recommended for the diagnosis of acute pyelonephritis because low bacterial counts are so infrequently associated with pyelonephritis as compared to cystitis.[9] Symptomatic patients with lower bacterial counts may have urinary tract obstruction or a perinephric abscess. The Gram stain may be useful in directing initial treatment, whereas culture and antimicrobial susceptibilities are essential for the redirection of therapy in patients who are unresponsive to or intolerant of initial treatment.[30]

The decision to hospitalize a patient is primarily based on the severity of symptoms. Patients with persistent nausea and vomiting cannot take oral antimicrobials; therefore, they require parenteral therapy. Adjunctive care, such as intravenous fluid replacement or parenteral pain medications, may also necessitate hospitalization. Others who are deemed at high risk for noncompliance or who might fail to return for followup should also be hospitalized.

Most hospitalized patients improve significantly within 72 hours of starting treatment and can be discharged home in 3 to 4 days. Culture results are available by this time and an appropriate oral home regimen can be selected. For both inpatients and outpatients, failure to improve on effective antimicrobials after 72 hours, or an early relapse, warrants further diagnostic testing to rule out possible renal abscess or obstruction.[26] Approximately 12% of outpatients treated for pyelonephritis with standard regimens return to medical care for persistent symptoms.[36] All patients should have a repeat urine culture performed approximately 1 week after the end of treatment to identify those few uncured patients.[8,30]

Complicated Urinary Tract Infections

Complicated UTIs occur in a diverse mix of patients who have an increased risk of either acquiring a UTI or experiencing a severe or persistent UTI. This category includes patients with mild lower tract disease as well as those with significant kidney infection and urosepsis. The clinical presentation may include the hallmark symptoms of dysuria, frequency, and urgency; however, vaguer symptoms of fatigue, headache, temperature instability, and irritability may be the only clues.[4] Immunosuppressed persons may not exhibit the usual symptoms because of their dampened inflammatory response to infection. An important example of this is the debilitated elderly, who may have UTI-associated bacteremia with neither a fever nor leukocytosis.[14] Men with prostatic enlargement and UTI may complain only of obstructive symptoms, but with further questioning, symptoms referable to the UTI can be revealed.[1] Therefore, the clinician must hold a greater degree of suspicion for possible UTI in these at-risk individuals because treatment delays may lead to more serious infections.[37]

An extensive workup may be indicated initially in the patient not previously known to have urinary abnormalities, to delineate the abnormality and to determine if it is correctable. Without amelioration of the underlying problem, relapses or reinfections are to be expected.[3,7] Some infections may never be cured without corrective action, as with infection in the presence of kidney stones or urinary stents.[4]

For patients with known or suspected complicated UTIs, a urinalysis, urine culture, blood count, and serum creatinine should be performed. For those who are more ill or are immunocompromised, blood culture and imaging studies of the upper tract may be indicated to determine the extent and severity of infection.[26] Diabetics in particular have an increased risk of perinephric abscess or emphysematous pyelonephritis.[38] Pyuria is expected, but is less specific, because the primary urinary abnormality may be responsible for the presence of white blood cells.[26] An appropriately obtained urine culture is crucial to effective treatment because a multitude of nonuropathogens can infect the urinary tract in individuals who have hampered host defenses.

Antimicrobial susceptibility testing also is requisite because multiple antimicrobial courses for prior UTIs often lead to resistant strains that cause subsequent infections.[2,3] Colony counts usually are greater than or equal to 10^5 CFU/mL; the most prevalent organism is *E. coli* followed by other Gram-negative bacilli, *Pseudomonas aeruginosa*, enterococci, and coagulase-negative staphylococci other than *S. saprophyticus*.[1,2] Negative culture results may necessitate further testing for fastidious organisms. It may be reasonable to wait for culture and sensitivity results to return before initiating treatment in the stable patient because the causative organism can be unpredictable. Because persistence and relapse of infection are common, a repeat urine culture is recommended 1 or 2 weeks after therapy.[7]

Hospitalization is indicated for patients who cannot take oral medications, need other intravenous therapy, have probable kidney involvement, or possible urosepsis. The diagnosis of urosepsis is made when bacteremia from a urinary source is associated with fever, tachycardia, hypotension, and general decompensation.[37] Urosepsis occurs most frequently in the debilitated elderly, immunocompromised persons, and individuals with chronic urinary obstruction.[2]

Nosocomial and Catheter-Associated Urinary Tract Infections

UTIs occurring in patients with indwelling urinary catheters are considered complicated; they pose unique management problems. Most catheter-associated UTIs are nosocomially acquired because urinary catheterization most often occurs in the institutional setting. Also, UTIs are one of the most common nosocomial infections. Mortality rates increase almost threefold among catheterized patients who develop a nosocomial UTI.[14,15] Confounding factors in nosocomial UTIs are: the severity of the underlying illness causing hospitalization; antimicrobial therapy for other infections, which increases the risk for resistant or unusual organisms; the administration of multiple medications, which may interact with UTI treatment; and possibly, the inability of the patient to describe symptoms of UTI because of altered mental status. Management of catheter-associated UTIs varies considerably, depending on whether catheterization is short-term or chronic.

Even with good insertion and maintenance techniques, the incidence of bacteriuria among catheterized patients increases with time at a rate of 3 to 10% per day of catheterization. Thus, a large percentage of patients are bacteriuric after 1 week and virtually all are bacteriuric after 1 month of catheterization. The organisms are believed to gain entry via the space between the catheter and the urethral mucosa. The biofilm that develops on catheters may allow organisms within it to elude leukocytes and antimicrobials.[7,39] The organisms found on culture are similar to those associated with other complicated UTIs except that yeasts, primarily *Candida albicans*, and enterococci are more prevalent.[15,28] Patients with long-term catheters often have polymicrobial bacteriuria.[39]

Differentiating between infection and colonization can be difficult, because bacteriuria is nearly assured for catheterized patients. Symptoms may not be clearly referable to the urinary tract, because hospitalized patients may have other reasons for lower abdominal discomfort, leukocytosis, and fevers. Also, the usual symptoms of dysuria, hesitancy, and urgency are not seen in catheterized patients. Overall, only 30 to 50% of infected patients undergoing short-term catheterization experience symptoms.[39,40] For those patients who have symptoms, a urinalysis, urine, and blood culture should be obtained. Screening for bacteriuria in asymptomatic individuals is generally discouraged because antimicrobial treatment in this situation usually leads to recolonization with more resistant strains. Owing to the high risk of severe infection, antimicrobial prophylaxis may be indicated in kidney transplant and granulocytopenic patients with short-term catheterization.[39]

Antimicrobial treatment of catheter-associated UTIs has a relatively high failure and relapse rate.[7] Removal of the catheter usually increases cure rates; however, for patients who require chronic catheterization, replacement with a new catheter does not always improve the odds for success. Recurrence rates in patients chronically catheterized may be improved with suprapubic bladder catheterization, because bacterial colonization on the abdominal wall is less than in the periurethral area.[39]

Diagnosis

Diagnostic testing procedures are used when the clinical presentation or physical examination does not yield a clear diagnosis. The most frequently used tests are dipstick urinalysis, urine microscopy with or without Gram stain, and quantitative urine culture with antimicrobial susceptibility. Such tests help to determine whether the patient's symptoms are consistent with UTI and to identify the possible infecting organism. Other diagnostic procedures include localization tests such as bilateral ureteral catheterization, bladder wash-out techniques, and antibody-coated bacteria assays.[30] These procedures are used to differentiate upper tract from lower tract infection, but are rarely necessary in the management of most patients. Ultrasound and computerized tomography (CT) studies may help to identify renal abscesses or structural abnormalities of the kidneys. Intravenous pyelograms are performed less frequently now, but also may help to assess possible structural defects and urine flow patterns.

Collecting the urine specimen correctly is important to ensure the accuracy of the results for both urinalysis and urine culture procedures. In noncatheterized patients, urine is collected in a sterile container midway through urination. Using a midstream voided urine sample is preferred because any contaminating elements from the urethra are washed out prior to the specimen collection. Although rarely done in routine cases, specimens obtained via catheterization or suprapubic bladder aspiration have the lowest risk of contamination.

Urinalysis

A complete urinalysis consists of a biochemical dipstick test of fresh urine and a microbiologic examination of the urine sediment. Urine dipsticks have multiple reagent pads that undergo color changes when dipped in the urine sample. The pad colors are then compared to a standardized color reference. Most dipsticks can determine pH and a quantitative value for red blood cells, protein, nitrites, and leukocyte esterase.[30] Leukocyte esterase is an enzyme produced by activated leukocytes, and is used as a marker for the presence of leukocytes in the urine sample.[29] The dipstick urinalysis is often the only diagnostic test used by the office practitioner or clinic-based practitioner to confirm the clinical diagnosis of uncomplicated cystitis.[7] On microscopic examination of the urine sediment, the number of leukocytes, erythrocytes, bacteria, fungi, and other solid elements can be quantified.

The most important aspects of the urinalysis in diagnosing urinary tract infections are pH, the presence of blood (hematuria), bacteria (bacteriuria), fungi (funguria), and particularly leukocytes (pyuria) or WBC casts.[9,30] A high pH may indicate the presence of urea-splitting organisms such as *Proteus* spp. In nonmenstruating patients, the presence of hematuria can often localize the problem to the urinary tract. Finding microorganisms on urinalysis may assist in making the diagnosis of UTI, but may also represent contamination from mixed organisms residing in the distal urethra or periurethral area.

The leukocyte count is of primary importance when determining the significance of bacteriuria and confirming UTI as the cause of dysuria.[30,41] Pyuria usually is defined as greater than or equal to eight leukocytes per mm^3, which correlates to two to five leukocytes per high power field.[7] However, most patients with UTIs have 20 or more leukocytes/mm^3. Pyuria in the absence of bacteriuria or positive urine culture can occur in patients with vaginal infections or urethritis owing to chlamydia or other fastidious organisms.[41]

Urine Culture

Several culture techniques are available, but the biplate method is used most commonly. With the biplate method, selective media on one side of the culture dish are used to isolate possible Gram-negative urinary pathogens, whereas the other side usually contains nonselective culture media. Use of the selective culture media often allows for more rapid identification of potential uropathogens. The microorganism colony count is determined using the nonselective side of the plate. The number of colonies can be correlated to the number of organisms or colony-forming units (CFU) per milliliter in the original urine sample. Using the standard inoculum size, this method can detect bacterial concentrations of greater than or equal to 10^3 CFU/mL. Antibacterial susceptibility testing is then performed on the patient's predominant organism(s) recovered from the biplate.

In the office or clinic setting, the dipslide culture method can be useful. A plastic paddle coated with the two different culture media is dipped into the urine sample and placed in a container for incubation. The density of colony growth on the nonselective side is compared to photographs of control specimens to estimate the microorganism count in the original specimen.[20,30] Antibacterial susceptibility testing cannot be done in the clinic setting with this method.

Traditionally, a single species microorganism count of greater than or equal to 10^5 CFU/mL from a midstream urine specimen was considered indicative of infection. Multiple studies have demonstrated, however, that as few as greater than or equal to 10^2 CFU/mL in a symptomatic patient with pyuria is representative of true infection.[41] As many as half of all young women with true uncomplicated cystitis have bacterial counts of 10^2 to 10^4 cfu/mL.[31] In symptomatic women without pyuria, greater than or equal to 10^5 CFU/mL is still required for the diagnosis of UTI. Any sample with greater than or equal to 10^2 CFU/mL obtained by suprapubic bladder aspiration or urethral catheterization is considered significant.[42]

Urine cultures are not routinely performed for presumed cases of uncomplicated lower UTIs because the causative agent is reliably *E. coli* and occasionally *S. saprophyticus*. The finding of typical clinical symptoms in patients with pyuria or hematuria usually is sufficient to make the diagnosis and start empiric treatment.[7,30] However, with unclear symptoms, complicated cases, treatment failure, or pyelonephritis, a urine culture should be performed to confirm the diagnosis and to ensure effective treatment. Also, patients with urinary tract symptoms who do not demonstrate pyuria by urinalysis should have a urine culture performed.[3,8] A Gram stain completed before culture may be useful to guide initial treatment for complicated UTIs.

THERAPEUTIC PLAN

Once the diagnosis and classification of UTI is made, a therapeutic plan is formed from a consideration of patient factors, microbiologic factors, and clinical outcome data. Table 69.4 summarizes the commonly recommended therapeutic regimens. The summary recommendations are applicable in the majority of circumstances; however, recognizing situations where the usual treatment is not appropriate is of considerable importance.

Patient factors such as pregnancy, organ dysfunction, potentially serious drug interactions, and drug allergies may preclude the use of standard regimens. Other factors, such as patient acceptability of the dosage form (e.g., liquid versus tablet), the potential for noncompliance, and drug costs or insurance coverage, must also be considered.

Standard guidelines for treatment may not be applicable when antimicrobial resistance patterns in the local community or in individual patients differ from national or regional patterns. This is most important for patients at risk for progressive or serious infection.

Published clinical outcome data can demonstrate superior or comparable efficacy between treatment regimens while controlling for patient and microbiologic factors. Such data are most usefully applied to individual cases when the study and treatment cases are similar.

Table 69.4 ▪ Treatment Regimens for Bacterial Urinary Tract Infections

Condition	Characteristic Pathogens	Mitigating Circumstances	Recommended Empirical Treatment
Acute uncomplicated cystitis in healthy women	*E. coli, S. saprophyticus, P. mirabilis, Klebsiella pneumoniae*	None	3-day regimen: oral trimethoprim-sulfamethoxazole, trimethoprim, norfloxacin, ofloxacin, lomefloxacin, or enoxacin
		Diabetes, symptoms for >7 days, recent urinary tract infection, use of diaphragm, age >65 years	Consider 7-day regimen: oral trimethoprim-sulfamethoxazole, trimethoprim, norfloxacin, ofloxacin, lomefloxacin, or enoxacin
		Pregnancy	Consider 7-day regimen: oral amoxicillin, macrocrystalline nitrofurantoin, cefpodoxime proxetil, or trimethoprim-sulfamethoxazole
Acute uncomplicated pyelonephritis in healthy women	*E. coli, P. mirabilis, K. pneumoniae, S. saprophyticus*	Mild to moderate illness, no nausea or vomiting—outpatient therapy	Oral trimethoprim-sulfamethoxazole, norfloxacin, ciprofloxacin, ofloxacin, lomefloxacin, or enoxacin for 10–14 days
		Severe illness or possible urosepsis—hospitalization required	Parenteral trimethoprim-sulfamethoxazole, ceftriaxone, ciprofloxacin, ofloxacin, or gentamicin (with or without ampicillin) until fever gone; then oral trimethoprim-sulfamethoxazole, norfloxacin, ciprofloxacin, ofloxacin, lomefloxacin, or enoxacin for 14 days
		Pregnancy—hospitalization recommended	Parenteral third generation cephalosporin, gentamicin (with or without ampicillin), aztreonam, or trimethoprim-sulfamethoxazole until fever gone; then oral amoxicillin, a cephalosporin, or trimethoprim-sulfamethoxazole for 14 days
Complicated urinary tract infection	*E. coli, Proteus* spp., *Klebsiella* spp., *Pseudomonas* spp., *Serratia* spp., enterococci, staphylococci	Mild to moderate illness, no nausea or vomiting—outpatient therapy	Oral norfloxacin, ciprofloxacin, ofloxacin, lomefloxacin, or enoxacin for 10–14 days
		Severe illness or possible urosepsis—hospitalization required	Parenteral ampicillin and gentamicin, ciprofloxacin, ofloxacin, ceftriaxone, aztreonam, or imipenem-cilastatin until fever gone; then oral trimethoprim-sulfamethoxazole, norfloxacin, ciprofloxacin, ofloxacin, lomefloxacin, or enoxacin for 10–14 days

Source: Adapted with permission from Stamm WE, Hooton TM. Management of urinary tract infections in adults. N Engl J Med 329:1329, 1993.

TREATMENT

Pharmacotherapy

The ideal agent for the treatment of UTIs should have the following characteristics:

- Bactericidal activity (bacteristatic may be sufficient) against the most common uropathogens
- High, sustained concentrations in both urine and urinary tract tissue (e.g., kidney, prostate)
- Effective elimination of uropathogens from the vagina and bowel without significantly altering the normal flora of these areas
- Effective via oral administration with few doses per day
- Safety for use in children and pregnant women
- Minimal and mild adverse reactions
- Relatively low expense

Table 69.5 lists some pharmacologic comparisons of available agents. Antimicrobials currently considered first-line treatment, namely trimethoprim/sulfamethoxazole (TMP/SMX) or the fluoroquinolones, have most of the listed characteristics. TMP/SMX has been the drug of choice for most UTIs for many years because of these preferred qualities; however, decreasing antibacterial activity against *E. coli* and other Gram-negative bacilli has led some clinicians to limit its use to low-risk patients or to documented susceptible pathogens.[7]

Although clinically efficacious, fluoroquinolones are expensive, some have significant drug–drug interactions, and excessive use has been shown to increase bacterial resistance to this valuable class of antimicrobials. Fluoroquinolones are also relatively contraindicated in young children and pregnant women because of reports of cartilage abnor-

Table 69.5 ▪ Pharmacological Data and Oral Treatment Doses for Uncomplicated Cystitis

Drug	Adult Dose	Adjustment for RF[a]	Pediatric Dose[b]	Urine Conc[c]	Adverse Reactions[d]	Significant Drug Interactions
Amoxicillin	500 mg TID × 7 days	500 mg Q12–24 hours	10 mg/kg TID	>500	Allergic rxn Diarrhea	Probenecid, allopurinol, oral contraceptives
Cephalexin/ Cephradine	500 mg BID × 7 days	250 mg BID	10 mg/kg TID	2000	Allergic rxn	
Cefaclor	250 mg TID × 7 days	None	10 mg/kg TID	>600	Allergic rxn	
TMP/SMX	1 DS BID × 3 days	Not recommended	4 mg TMP/kg BID	>30/>40	Allergic rxn, nausea, photosensitivity	Warfarin, cyclosporin, phenytoin, sulfonylureas, methotrexate
Trimethoprim	100 mg BID × 7–10 days	Not recommended	2–3 mg/kg BID	30–180	Rash, nausea	Phenytoin
Ciprofloxacin	250 mg BID × 3 days	250 mg QD	Not recommended	>200	Headache, rash, nausea, photosensitivity	Antacids, sucralfate, Ca, Mg, Fe, warfarin, theophylline, caffeine
Norfloxacin	400 mg BID × 7 days	400 mg QD	Not recommended	>200	Same as cipro	Like ciprofloxacin, less effect on warfarin, methylxanthines
Ofloxacin	200 mg BID × 3–7 days	100 mg QD	Not recommended	>200	Insomnia, same as cipro	Like ciprofloxacin, less effect on warfarin, methylxanthines
Levofloxacin	250 mg QD × 3–7 days	250 mg QOD	Not recommended	>100	Same as cipro	Like ciprofloxacin, less effect on warfarin, methylxanthines
Lomefloxacin	400 mg QD × 3–7 days	200 mg QD	Not recommended	>300	Same as cipro, photosensitivity	Like ciprofloxacin
Nitrofurantoin (macrocrystal)	50–100 mg QID × 7 days	Not recommended	1.5 mg/kg QID	50–150	Nausea, headache	Urine alkalinizing agents, probenecid
Fosfomycin	3 g × 1 (mixed in water)	None	Not recommended if <12 years	>1000	Diarrhea, headache	Metoclopramide
Gatifloxacin	400 mg × 1 OR 200 mg QD × 3 days	N/A	Not recommended	N/A	Same as cipro, dizziness	Antacids, Mg, Fe, Zn, digoxin

[a] *RF*, renal failure; creatinine clearance <10 mL/min.
[b] For children >2 months of age.
[c] Peak concentration in μg/mL.
[d] Adverse reactions associated with short-term use.

malities in studies on immature animals. Fluoroquinolones may be preferred in the treatment of prostatitis because of their excellent penetration into prostatic tissues.

Although inexpensive, well-tolerated, and very active against most uropathogens in vitro, the oral first-generation cephalosporins and nitrofurantoin have higher relapse and reinfection rates. This is attributed to tissue concentrations inadequate to treat silent kidney infection and eliminate the reservoir of uropathogens in the vagina.[2,7] Owing to high resistance rates and low tissue concentrations, amoxicillin is considered unreliable except for the treatment of enterococcal UTI. β-lactam antimicrobials also have been associated with higher rates of posttreatment candidal vaginitis.[9,34]

Single-agent trimethoprim meets most of the desired criteria, but antibacterial activity has also decreased over time. Gentamicin has long demonstrated clinical efficacy, but the risk of renal toxicity and ototoxicity, and obligatory parenteral administration has limited its usage to upper tract or nosocomial UTIs. Oral carbenicillin indanyl and methenamine mandelate are no longer used for UTI treatment, but may occasionally be used for prophylactic therapy.[34]

Uncomplicated Cystitis

Most antimicrobials that are approved for use in women with uncomplicated UTIs achieve a greater than 80% success rate with at least 7 days of therapy. Clinical outcome results may vary, however, because of differences in study population, patient exclusion criteria, and length of followup.[43] Overall susceptibility rates for organisms isolated from study patients with uncomplicated UTIs are greater than 90% for fluoroquinolones, cephalosporins, and nitrofurantoin. Trimethoprim and TMP/SMX are active against 85 to 90% of isolates, whereas less than 70% remain susceptible to ampicillin or amoxicillin.[44,45]

Interest in decreasing treatment duration has led to studies of 3-day and single-dose regimens. Single-dose regimens generally have produced success rates lower than either 3-day or 7-day regimens. Although associated with fewer adverse reactions, single-dose treatment also results in higher relapse and reinfection rates.[43] These recurrences have been attributed to insufficient treatment of uropathogens residing in the vagina and possible upper tract disease.[2] UTIs caused by *S. saprophyticus* in particular have significantly higher failure rates with single-dose therapy.[46,47]

Trimethoprim given as a large single dose, yields long-term cure rates of 71% versus 87% for the usual 7-day regimen.[47] TMP/SMX given as a single dose (2 DS tablets) versus 10 days of standard twice-daily dosing resulted in 76 and 95% success rates, respectively, at early followup.[48] Single-dose fluoroquinolone treatment has been associated with 78 to greater than 90% success rates, with use of norfloxacin producing the poorest results.[49–51] Fosfomycin, a drug approved only for single-dose treatment, has demonstrated an 80 to 90% cure rate.[52] Patients without a history of recurrent UTIs and those expected to be poorly compliant with standard regimens are the best candidates for single-dose treatment.[48]

Success rates found with 3-day courses of fluoroquinolones or TMP/SMX have been approximately 82 to 90%, and appear to be nearly as effective as longer courses.[51,53,54] Most authors recommend 3-day regimens when using a fluoroquinolone (other than norfloxacin) or TMP/SMX due to similar clinical efficacy as 7-day treatments. Three-day regimens are also associated with fewer adverse reactions, vaginitis, and cost.[8] Short-course regimens of cephalosporins, amoxicillin, and nitrofurantoin are associated with significantly lower success rates and therefore are not recommended.[54]

Uncomplicated Pyelonephritis

Because the causative organisms are similar in pyelonephritis to lower UTIs, the preferred antimicrobials are similar as well. Fluoroquinolones and TMP/SMX are the mainstays of treatment and can be given orally in stable outpatients or intravenously in hospitalized patients. Oral β-lactam antimicrobials and nitrofurantoin are not appropriate owing to inadequate tissue concentrations.[7] Parenterally administered cephalosporins achieve adequate tissue concentrations, but third-generation cephalosporins often achieve greater serum concentration/MIC ratios. Although not preferable, the standard regimen of gentamicin, with or without ampicillin, is still used in many institutions.

Hospitalized patients can be switched to an oral treatment regimen once clinical improvement is seen and nausea has resolved. Urine culture results should be available by then to guide oral antimicrobial selection. Dosing for TMP/SMX is the same as for cystitis, but fluoroquinolone doses should be increased to systemic infection treatment doses.[7] Cure rates of greater than or equal to 90% have been demonstrated with 2-week total treatment with TMP/SMX; similar rates could be expected with fluoroquinolone treatment. Longer treatment has not been shown to improve cure rates in uncomplicated cases.[55] In milder outpatient cases, 10 days of therapy may be curative.[1]

Complicated Urinary Tract Infections

Making generalized recommendations for the treatment of complicated UTIs is difficult because of the diversity of underlying defects that give rise to these infections. Due to the wider range of possible causative agents and the higher risk of treatment failure or relapse, broad spectrum antimicrobials with good tissue penetration generally are preferred for empiric therapy. Table 69.6 lists pooled susceptibility data for urinary isolates from hospitalized patients across North America. TMP/SMX should be used cautiously, or only after susceptibility results are available, in areas with known high TMP/SMX resistance rates.[7,56] Most fluoroquinolones produce short-term cure rates of 65 to 90% with systemic treatment doses, but recurrences are expectantly high.[56,57] There are no convincing data, however, that one drug or class of drugs is more effective

Table 69.6 ▪ In Vitro Antimicrobial Susceptibilities of Urinary Isolates from Hospitalized Patients in North America

Organism	Oflox	Cipro	Norflox	Amp	Cef	CTX	Gent	Nitro	TMP/SMX
Escherichia coli	>99	>99	100	58–66	71–91	>99	98	95	>99
Klebsiella spp.	95	92–96	96	2	81–84	93–99	93–95	58	>99
Enterococcus spp.	40–70	24–66	60	90–97	13	9	NT	96	NT
Pseudomonas spp.	69–73	82–91	91	0	1	15–44	84	1	93
Proteus spp.	98–100	94–100	99	89–94	91–94	98	94–97	0	100
Enterobacter spp.	94–100	93–100	100	5–12	9–12	70–82	94–97	43	100
Coagulase-negative staphylococci	70–81	69–80	80	17–57	52–72	46–61	60	99	NT

Source: References 66, 67, 68.

Oflox, ofloxacin; *Cipro,* ciprofloxacin; *Norflox,* norfloxacin; *Amp,* ampicillin; *Cef,* cefazolin; *CTX,* ceftriaxone; *Gent,* gentamicin; *Nitro,* nitrofurantoin; *TMP/SMX,* trimethoprim/sulfamethoxazole.

than another for these patients, in whom relapse rates are often as high as 50%.[3,6]

Mild to moderate complicated UTIs usually can be treated with oral medications; however, for hospitalized patients with significant illness or those who cannot take oral medications, parenteral therapy may be needed. For possible enterococcal infections, ampicillin and gentamicin is reasonable for most patients requiring intravenous therapy. Empiric antipseudomonal therapy may be appropriate for some individuals with nosocomial UTIs or prior history of pseudomonal UTIs.[7] Antipseudomonal cephalosporins, aztreonam, extended spectrum penicillin/β-lactamase inhibitors, carbapenems, aminoglycosides, and most fluoroquinolones could be used for these patients. Two-drug regimens may be necessary for upper tract infection with *Pseudomonas* spp. Once clinical improvement is seen, oral antimicrobials can be used to finish therapy in suitable patients.[7]

The recommended length of treatment for most complicated UTIs is usually 10 to 14 days, but infections in men with prostatitis or patients with persistent nidus of infection might require several additional weeks of treatment for cure. Patients with chronic indwelling urinary catheters are persistently colonized with microorganisms; therefore, the goal of therapy in these individuals should be resolution of symptoms, not absence of bacteriuria.[3]

Treatment of fungal UTIs can also be problematic in that most occur in catheterized patients. Removal of the catheter, improved control of blood sugar in diabetics, and discontinuance of antibacterial agents may improve outcomes. Bladder irrigation with amphotericin B at 5 to 50 mg/L for a few days has been shown to be effective for fungal cystitis in patients who require continued catheterization.[58] However, fluconazole 100 mg orally or intravenously daily for 5 days also has been relatively successful in eradicating *Candida* spp. from the bladder in 73 to 77% of patients.[28]

Prophylactic and Suppressive Therapy

Patients with frequent recurrences of uncomplicated cystitis may benefit from either intermittent or postcoital prophylaxis. Intermittent therapy is given either daily or a few days per week at dosages lower than those used for treatment.[7] Table 69.7 lists the agents and dosages used for continuous prophylaxis. In women whose recurrent infections are associated with sexual activity, single-dose postcoital prophylaxis may be appropriate. Postcoital prophylaxis with ciprofloxacin 125 mg has been shown to be as effective as daily prophylaxis.[59] Other effective regimens for postcoital prophylaxis include TMP/SMX 40/200 mg, cephalexin 250 mg, and nitrofurantoin 50 mg as single doses.[3]

Table 69.7. ▪ Continuous Antimicrobial Prophylactic Regimens for Recurrent Urinary Tract Infection

Antimicrobial Agent[a]	Daily Dose	Infections/ Patient-Year	Vaginal Flora Effect
Trimethoprim/sulfamethoxazole	40 mg/200 mg	0–0.15	+
Trimethoprim	100 mg	0–0.15	+
Norfloxacin	200 mg	0–0.15	+
Nitrofurantoin	50–100 mg	0.1–0.8	
Nitrofurantoin-Macrodantin	50–100 mg	0.3	–
Cephalexin	125–250 mg	N/A	–
Cefaclor	250 mg	0.3	–
Cephradine	250 mg	N/A	–

Source: Adapted with permission from Stapleton A, Stamm WE. Prevention of urinary tract infection. Infect Dis Clin NA 11:719–733, 1997.

[a]Agents are generally given at bedtime, daily, or three times per week. Those that have an effect on reducing vaginal colonization with uropathogens are indicated.

N/A, not assessed; +, reduces vaginal colonization with uropathogens; –, no reduction in vaginal colonization with uropathogens.

Reliable patients with less frequent recurrences may do well with self-initiated therapy. These patients keep a ready supply of antimicrobials at home and when the typical symptoms recur, they can begin treatment immediately. Treatment is usually a single dose or 3-day regimen.[7] Figure 69.1 shows the usual management of recurrent cystitis in women.

Few patients with recurrent complicated UTIs benefit from long-term prophylactic therapy because treatment of patients with uncorrectable underlying abnormalities merely results in colonization with more resistant organisms.[2,3] This is particularly true of chronically catheterized patients. Some patients, however, never clear their infection with treatment, and chronic suppressive therapy may be appropriate to control symptoms and prevent further degradation in kidney function. Although regimens vary for suppressive therapy, an antimicrobial agent active against the infecting pathogen is used at doses reduced from treatment doses yet higher than those used for prophylaxis.[3]

Pregnant women with recurrent cystitis or pyelonephritis, and infants with congenital abnormalities such as vesicoureteral reflux (VUR), also benefit from antimicrobial prophylaxis.[2,34] Pregnant women with significant bacteriuria have a significantly higher incidence of pyelonephritis, low birth weight infants, premature delivery, and infant mortality; therefore, treatment is indicated for pregnant women with bacteriuria even in the absence of symptoms. Prophylaxis is given to patients with either recurrent bacteriuria or UTI. Antimicrobial prophylaxis also is indicated for infants with VUR, because recurrent infection is common in these patients and has been associated with permanent renal damage.[2]

Adjunctive Therapy

Some patients may benefit from adjunctive therapy with phenazopyridine, a urinary analgesic, to decrease the discomfort associated with bladder spasms. Acetaminophen or nonsteroidal antiinflammatory drugs (NSAIDs) can be used to alleviate fevers, aches, and pains.

Therapy for Postmenopausal Women

In postmenopausal women with recurrent cystitis, estrogen replacement therapy may normalize the vaginal milieu, thereby discouraging colonization by uropathogens.[11]

Nonpharmacologic Therapy

To decrease the incidence of recurrent infections, regular postcoital voiding, increased fluid intake, and drinking cranberry juice have been useful in some patients. Originally, the acidity of cranberry juice was believed to decrease recurrences, but studies have concluded that the amount of cranberry juice needed to be consumed to significantly decrease urinary pH would be prohibitive to patient compliance. It is now believed that cranberry juice contains a compound(s) that inhibits bacterial adherence to urinary epithelium.[34]

IMPROVING OUTCOMES

For most UTIs, clinical cure is an obtainable goal. A multitude of regimens are effective, so the clinician must weigh the risks and benefits of a given regimen for each patient. Obtaining a complete drug history should identify possible risks for adverse drug and hypersensitivity reactions. Assessment of potential patient compliance is a major factor in improving outcomes. A less effective regimen in clinical study participants, such as single-dose therapy, may be the best therapy in chronically noncompliant individuals.

Appropriate followup also is important so that patients who fail therapy or relapse early can be assessed quickly for possible complicating factors, some of which may be correctable. Any patient who fails therapy or relapses should be questioned about adherence to the prescribed treatment because noncompliance is a common explanation for treatment failure.

All patients receiving antimicrobial therapy should be informed of possible adverse reactions and drug–drug interactions, and how best to avoid or manage them. Mild antimicrobial associated diarrhea may be tolerable, but severe diarrhea requires a call to the prescriber. Photosensitivity reactions are common with TMP/SMX as well as with some fluoroquinolones, and patients should be cautioned about sun exposure and the use of sunscreens. Patients prescribed ciprofloxacin or enoxacin should be warned to decrease or eliminate caffeine from their diets, particularly if they are sensitive to the effects of caffeine. Patients should also be informed to avoid taking fluoroquinolones with antacids or iron supplements, and are variably affected by dairy products, thereby preventing treatment failure owing to decreased absorption of the drug.

An explanation of the risks of noncompliance, such as treatment failure or relapse, is also appropriate. However, since treatment of most UTIs is relatively short, compliance is less of a factor than for other illnesses, although with long-term prophylactic therapy, the benefits of compliance should be clearly stated. Self-initiated therapy requires education about potential drug interactions, because the patient may be taking new medications the next time UTI treatment is started. The patient should also be warned not to self-initiate therapy if she suspects or knows she has become pregnant, because both TMP/SMX and fluoroquinolones are relatively contraindicated in the first trimester of pregnancy.

PHARMACOECONOMICS

A limited number of studies have analyzed the cost effectiveness of the commonly recommended approaches to UTI treatment. It has been recommended that diagnostic studies such as urine culture, urine microscopy, and even dipstick urinalysis should be reserved for complicated UTIs and pyelonephritis. Many practitioners treat empirically without any laboratory workup because the majority of women with uncomplicated UTIs will experience typical clinical signs and symptoms. This practice has been found to be cost effective in these patients, although one-third may be treated unnecessarily.[60] Over-the-counter antibiotic treatment of UTIs may provide easier access to treatment, quicker symptom relief, and reduced physician office charges. However, this approach was not projected to be cost effective owing to the long-term costs associated with increased bacterial resistance.[61]

Antimicrobial choice and duration of treatment can significantly impact the overall cost of therapy. TMP/SMX has been used successfully and inexpensively for many years, but current trends of increasing bacterial resistance with subsequent treatment failures may eventually make other options more cost effective.[62] First-generation cephalosporins and nitrofurantoin are relatively inexpensive and active against most uropathogens, but higher relapse rates and poorer patient compliance with the required 7- to 10-day treatment regimen may lead to greater costs associated with retreatment. Success rates with fluoroquinolone therapy are excellent with even 3-day regimens, but higher drug costs and risk of eventual bacterial resistance with overuse prevent fluoroquinolones from becoming the preferred agents for all patients.

Patients with severe UTIs have traditionally been given parenteral antimicrobials for initial treatment. However, oral administration of highly bioavailable antimicrobials, such as TMP/SMX and the fluoroquinolones, can achieve similar clinical outcomes at substantially lower cost. Ciprofloxacin has been shown to be equally effective given either intravenously or orally to patients with severe pyelonephritis or complicated UTI, including those patients with concomitant bacteremia.[63] Patients experiencing nausea or vomiting may need to receive parenteral antimicrobials until oral tolerability returns.

KEY POINTS

- UTIs can involve the bladder (cystitis), the kidney (pyelonephritis), or other urinary structures, and the severity can vary substantially between patients.
- The highest prevalence of UTIs is in young to middle-aged women.
- Uncomplicated UTIs occur in otherwise healthy persons, whereas complicated UTIs occur in persons with structural, functional, or immunologic abnormalities.
- Uropathogens originate primarily from the bowel, with *E. coli* the most prevalent pathogen.
- The most common symptoms associated with cystitis are dysuria, frequency, and urgency.
- Pyelonephritis is often associated with fever, chills, nausea, and leukocytosis.
- Pyuria and bacteriuria with greater than or equal to 10^3 CFU/mL is generally considered indicative of UTI in symptomatic patients.
- Therapy with TMP/SMX or a fluoroquinolone is recommended for 3 days in healthy women with uncomplicated cystitis, 7 to 10 days for complicated cystitis, and 10 to 14 days for pyelonephritis.
- Oral cephalosporins, trimethoprim, nitrofurantoin, and amoxicillin are associated with higher failure rates.
- Individualization of therapy is dictated by illness severity, allergy history, drug interactions, microbiologic susceptibility, compliance potential, and cost.
- Recurrent uncomplicated UTIs can be managed with prophylactic or self-initiated therapy.
- Prostatitis treatment requires prolonged antimicrobial administration with an agent that achieves good concentrations in prostatic fluid (such as fluoroquinolones).

REFERENCES

1. Lipsky BA. Urinary tract infections in men: epidemiology, pathophysiology, diagnosis, and treatment. Ann Intern Med 110:138–150, 1989.
2. Rubin RH, Cotran RS, Tolkoff-Rubin NE. Urinary tract infection, pyelonephritis, and reflux nephropathy. In: Brenner BM. Brenner and Rector's The Kidney. 5th ed. Philadelphia: Saunders, 1997:1597–1654.
3. Nicolle LE. A practical guide to the management of complicated urinary tract infection. Drugs 53:583–592, 1997.
4. Ronald AR, Harding GKM. Complicated urinary tract infections. Infect Dis Clin North Am 11:583–591, 1997.
5. Tolkoff-Rubin NE, Rubin RH. Urinary tract infection in the immunocompromised host. Lessons from kidney transplantation and the AIDS epidemic. Infect Dis Clin North Am 11:707–717, 1997.
6. Ikaheimo R, Slitonen A, Heiskanen T, et al. Recurrence of urinary tract infection in a primary care setting: analysis of a 1-year follow-up of 179 women. Clin Infect Dis 22:91–99, 1996.
7. Stamm WE, Hooton TM. Management of urinary tract infections in adults. N Engl J Med 329:1328–1334, 1993.
8. Wisinger DB. Urinary tract infections. Current management strategies. Postgrad Med 100:229–236, 1996.
9. Hooton TM, Stamm WE. Diagnosis and treatment of uncomplicated urinary tract infection. Infect Dis Clin North Am 11:551–581, 1997.
10. Patterson TF, Andriole VT. Detection, significance, and therapy of bacteriuria in pregnancy. Update in the managed health care era. Infect Dis Clin North Am 11:593–607, 1997.
11. Nicolle LE. Asymptomatic bacteriuria in the elderly. Infect Dis Clin North Am 11:647–661, 1997.
12. Nicolle LE, Henderson E, Bjornson J, et al. The association of bacteriuria with resident characteristics and survival in elderly institutionalized men. Ann Intern Med 106:682–686, 1987.
13. Abrutyn E, Mossey J, Berlin JA, et al. Does asymptomatic bacteriuria predict mortality and does antimicrobial treatment reduce mortality in elderly ambulatory women? Ann Intern Med 120:827–833, 1994.
14. Ackermann RJ, Monroe PW. Bacteremic urinary tract infection in older people. J Am Geriatr Soc 44:927–933, 1996.
15. Platt R, Polk BF, Murdock B, et al. Mortality associated with nosocomial urinary-tract infection. N Engl J Med 307:637–642, 1982.
16. Strom BL, Collins M, West SL, et al. Sexual activity, contraceptive use, and other risk factors for symptomatic and asymptomatic bacteriuria. A case control study. Ann Intern Med 107:816–823, 1987.
17. Fihn SD, Latham RH, Roberts P, et al. Association between diaphragm use and urinary tract infection. JAMA 254:240–245, 1985.
18. Fihn SD, Boyko EJ, Normand EH, et al. Association between use of spermicide-coated condoms and *Escherichia coli* urinary tract infections in young women. Am J Epidemiol 144:512–520, 1996.
19. Smith HS, Hughes JP, Hooton TM, et al. Antecedent antimicrobial use increases the risk of uncomplicated cystitis in young women. Clin Infect Dis 25:63–68, 1997.
20. Kunin C. Urinary tract infections: detection, prevention, and management. 5th ed. Baltimore: Williams & Wilkins, 1997.
21. Sobel JD. Pathogenesis of urinary tract infection. Role of host defenses. Infect Dis Clin North Am 11:531–549, 1997.
22. Lomberg H, Hanson LA, Jacobsson B, et al. Correlation of P blood group, vesicoureteral reflux, and bacterial attachment in patients with recurrent pyelonephritis. N Engl J Med 308:1189–1192, 1983.
23. Svanborg C, Godaly G. Bacterial virulence in urinary tract infection. Infect Dis Clin North Am 11:513–529, 1997.
24. Latham RH, Running K, Stamm WE. Urinary tract infections in young adult women caused by *Staphylococcus saprophyticus*. JAMA 250:3063–3066, 1983.
25. Fihn SD, Boyko EJ, Chen CL, et al. Use of spermicide-coated condoms and other risk factors for urinary tract infection caused by *Staphylococcus saprophyticus*. Arch Intern Med 158:281–287, 1998.
26. Falagas ME, Gorbach SL. Practice guidelines: urinary tract infections. Infect Dis Clin Practice 4:241–257, 1995.

27. Kollef MH, Sharpless L, Vlasnik J, et al. The impact of nosocomial infections on patient outcomes following cardiac surgery. Chest 112:666–675, 1997.
28. Jacobs LG. Fungal urinary tract infections in the elderly. Treatment guidelines. Drugs Aging 8:89–96, 1996.
29. Hoberman A, Wald ER. Urinary tract infections in young fertile children. Pediatr Infect Dis J 16:11–17, 1997.
30. Komaroff AL. Urinalysis and urine culture in women with dysuria. Ann Intern Med 104:212–218, 1986.
31. Stamm WE, Counts GW, Running KR, et al. Diagnosis of coliform infection in acutely dysuric women. N Engl J Med 307:463–468, 1982.
32. Berg E, Benson DM, Haraszkiewicz P, et al. High prevalence of sexually transmitted disease in women with urinary infections. Acad Emerg Med 3:1030–1043, 1996.
33. Griebling TL, Nygaard IE. The role of estrogen replacement therapy in the management of urinary tract incontinence and urinary tract infection in postmenopausal women. Endocrinol Metab Clin NA 26:347–360, 1997.
34. Stapleton A, Stamm WE. Prevention of urinary tract infection. Infect Dis Clin North Am 11:719–733, 1997.
35. Johnson JR, Stamm WE. Urinary tract infections in women: diagnosis and treatment. Ann Intern Med 111:906–917, 1989.
36. Pinson AG, Philbrick JT, Lindbeck GH, et al. ED management of acute pyelonephritis in women: a cohort study. Am J Emerg Med 12:271–278, 1994.
37. Pewitt EB, Schaeffner AJ. Urinary tract infection in urology, including acute and chronic prostatitis. Infect Dis Clin North Am 11:623–645, 1997.
38. Patterson JE, Andriole VT. Bacterial urinary tract infections in diabetes. Infect Dis Clin North Am 11:735–750, 1997.
39. Warren JW. Catheter-associated urinary tract infections. Infect Dis Clin North Am 11:609–621, 1997.
40. Beaujean DJMA, Blok HEM, Vandenbroucke-Grauls CMJE, et al. Surveillance of nosocomial infections in geriatric patients. J Hosp Infect 36:275–284, 1997.
41. Kunin CM, VanArsdale White L, Hua Hua T. A reassessment of the importance of "low count" bacteriuria in young women with acute urinary symptoms. Ann Intern Med 119:454–460, 1993.
42. Stark RP, Maki DG. Bacteriuria in the catheterized patient. What quantitative level of bacteriuria is relevant? N Engl J Med 311:560–564, 1984.
43. Rubin RH, Shapiro ED, Andriole VT, et al. Evaluation of new anti-infective drugs for the treatment of urinary tract infection. Clin Infect Dis 15(Suppl): S216, 1992.
44. Spencer RC, Moseley DJ, Greensmith MJ. Nitrofurantoin modified release versus trimethoprim or co-trimoxazole in the treatment of uncomplicated urinary tract infection in general practice. Brit Soc Antimicrob Chemother 33(Suppl A):121–129, 1994.
45. Amyes SGB, Baird DR, Crook DW, et al. A multicentre study of the in-vitro activity of cefotaxime, cefuroxime, ceftazidime, ofloxacin, and ciprofloxacin against blood urinary pathogens. J Antimicrob Chemother 34:639–648, 1994.
46. Arav-Boger R, Leibovici L, Danon YL. Urinary tract infections with low and high colony counts in young women. Arch Intern Med 154:300–304, 1994.
47. Osterberg E, Aberg H, Hallander HO, et al. Efficacy of single-dose versus seven-day trimethoprim treatment of cystitis in women: a randomized double-blind study. J Infect Dis 161:942–947, 1990.
48. Fihn SD, Johnson C, Roberts PL, et al. Trimethoprim-sulfamethoxazole for acute dysuria in women: a single dose or 10-day course. A double-blind, randomized study. Ann Int Med 108:350–357, 1988.
49. Jardin A, Cesana M, and the French Multicenter Urinary Tract Infection–Rufloxacin Group. Randomized, double-blind comparison of single-dose regimens of rufloxacin and pefloxacin for acute uncomplicated cystitis in women. Antimicrob Agents Chemother 39:215–220, 1995.
50. Hooton TM, Johnson C, Winter C, et al. Single-dose and three-day regimens of ofloxacin versus trimethoprim-sulfamethoxazole for acute cystitis in women. Antimicrob Agents Chemother 35:1479–2483, 1991.
51. Saginur R, Nicolle LE, Canadian Infectious Diseases Society Clinical Trials Study Group. Single-dose compared with 3-day norfloxacin treatment of uncomplicated urinary tract infection in women. Arch Intern Med 152:1233–1237, 1992.
52. Elhanan G, Tabenkin H, Yahalom R, et al. Single-dose fosfomycin trometamol versus 5-day cephalexin regimen for treatment of uncomplicated lower urinary tract infections in women. Antimicrob Agents Chemother 38:2612–2614, 1994.
53. Iravani A, Tice AD, McCarty J, et al. Short-course ciprofloxacin treatment of acute uncomplicated urinary tract infection in women. The minimum effective dose. Arch Intern Med 155:485–494, 1995.
54. Hooton TM, Winter C, Tiu F, et al. Randomized comparative trial and cost analysis of 3-day antimicrobial regimens for treatment of acute cystitis in women. JAMA 273:41–45, 1995.
55. Stamm WE, McKevitt M, Counts GW. Acute renal infection in women: treatment with trimethoprim-sulfamethoxazole or ampicillin for two or six weeks. Ann Intern Med 106:341–345, 1987.
56. Nicolle LE, Louie TJ, Dubois J, et al. Treatment of complicated urinary tract infections with lomefloxacin compared with that with trimethoprim-sulfamethoxazole. Antimicrob Agents Chemother 38:1368–1373, 1994.
57. Frankenschmidt A, Naber KG, Bischoff W, et al. Once-daily fleroxacin versus twice-daily ciprofloxacin in the treatment of complicated urinary tract infections. J Urol 158:1494–1499, 1997.
58. Jacobs LG, Skidmore EA, Cardoso LA, et al. Bladder irrigation with amphotericin B for treatment of fungal urinary tract infections. Clin Infect Dis 18:313–318, 1994.
59. Melekos MD, Werner Asbach H, Gerharz E, et al. Post-intercourse versus daily ciprofloxacin prophylaxis for recurrent urinary tract infections in premenopausal women. J Urol 157:935–939, 1997.
60. Barry HC, Ebell MH, Hickner J. Evaluation of suspected urinary tract infection in ambulatory women: a cost analysis of office-based strategies. J Fam Pract 44:49–60, 1997.
61. Rubin N, Foxman B. The cost-effectiveness of placing urinary tract infection treatment over the counter. J Clin Epidemiol 49:1315–1321, 1996.
62. Plumridge RJ, Golledge CL. Treatment of urinary tract infection. Clinical and economic considerations. Pharmacoeconomics 9:295–306, 1996.
63. Mombelli G, Pezzoli R, Pinoja-Lutz G, et al. Oral vs intravenous ciprofloxacin in the initial empirical management of severe pyelonephritis or complicated urinary tract infections. Arch Intern Med 159:53–58, 1999.
64. Hooton TM, Scholes D, Hughes JP, et al. A prospective study of risk factors for symptomatic urinary tract infection in young women. N Engl J Med 335:468–474, 1996.
65. National Nosocomial Infections Surveillance (NNIS) Report. Data Summary from October 1986–April 1997, Issued May 1997. Am J Infect Control 25:477–487, 1997.
66. Jones RN, Kehrberg EN, Erwin ME, et al. Prevalence of important pathogens and antimicrobial activity of parenteral drugs at numerous medical centers in the United States. Study on the threat of emerging resistances: real or perceived? Diagn Microbiol Infect Dis 19:203–215, 1994.
67. Hoban DJ, Jones RN, The Canadian Ofloxacin Study Group. Canadian ofloxacin susceptibility study: a comparative study from 18 medical centers. Chemother 41:34–38, 1995.
68. Gillenwater JY, Clark M. Tentative direct antimicrobial susceptibility testing in urine. J Urol 156:149–153, 1996.

CHAPTER 70

INTRAABDOMINAL INFECTIONS

Marjorie Robinson

DEFINITION

Intraabdominal infections present serious clinical problems because they are difficult to diagnose and successfully treat. Such infections generally occur after leakage of bacteria from the gastrointestinal (GI) tract into the sterile environment of the peritoneal cavity. The peritoneal cavity is the cavity below the diaphragm extended to the floor of the pelvis. The resulting infections may be diffuse peritonitis or localized abscesses.

Intraabdominal infections are defined in this chapter as primary peritonitis, secondary peritonitis, tertiary peritonitis, and intraabdominal abscesses. Primary peritonitis may seemingly occur spontaneously; therefore, it is sometimes referred to as spontaneous bacterial peritonitis (SBP). Primary peritonitis or SBP as initially described in childhood is caused by *Streptococcus pneumoniae* and is usually found in adult patients who have a history of alcoholic cirrhosis and ascites.[1,2] Primary peritonitis is also associated with postnecrotic liver disease, nephrosis, and peritoneal dialysis. Secondary peritonitis is usually associated with one or a combination of processes such as abdominal trauma; surgery; or intrinsic obstructive, neoplastic, or inflammatory GI disease. Tertiary peritonitis is defined as a later stage in the disease, when clinical peritonitis and systemic signs of sepsis (e.g., fever, tachycardia, tachypnea, hypotension, elevated cardiac index, low systemic vascular resistance, leukopenia, leukocytosis, and multiorgan failure) persist after treatment for secondary peritonitis.[3] These patients are usually immunocompromised (e.g., patients with AIDS, organ transplant recipients, and patients receiving cancer treatment or steroids for neoplasms). Intraabdominal abscess may be associated with primary, secondary, or tertiary peritonitis.

TREATMENT GOALS: INTRAABDOMINAL INFECTIONS

- Manage—both pharmacologically and nonpharmacologically.
- Maintain general homeostatic support, including management of hemodynamic, respiratory, and intestinal integrity; analgesia; sedation; and nutritional support for the patient.
- Prevent bacteremia.
- Select an antimicrobial agent for pharmacologic treatment that targets the suspected organism (facultative Gram-negative organisms and obligate anaerobes).
- Treat the cellulitis and/or peritonitis that surround the perforated gut.
- Initiate surgical drainage or radiologic alternatives to remove septic collections.
- Prevent treatment failures in the development of tertiary peritonitis or intraabdominal abscess.[4]

EPIDEMIOLOGY

Primary peritonitis refers to a spontaneous invasion of bacteria into the peritoneal cavity. This occurs predominantly in infants, young children (10 to 20%), and immunocompromised and cirrhotic patients (who usually have ascites [25%]). Secondary peritonitis refers to a peritoneal infection secondary to perforation, bowel necrosis, or a penetrating infectious process. Perforation of a hollow viscus accounts for 60 to 80% of the etiology of secondary peritonitis. Tertiary peritonitis refers to persistent or recurrent intraabdominal infections seen in immunocompromised patients, usually postoperative secondary peritonitis.[5]

The microbiology of intraabdominal infections is a critical factor in the epidemiology of this infection. *Enterobacteriaceae* and anaerobes originating from the GI tract cause the great majority of intraabdominal infections. In general, however, the normal GI tract bacterial flora is of low virulence. The number of bacterial species and the colony counts increase as one traverses down along the GI tract from the mouth to the colon. This flora is stable early in childhood and, for the most part, does not differ with geographic location, race, diet, or increasing age. In a human stomach there is usually less than 10^4 colony-forming units/mL (CFU/mL) of aerobic and anaerobic microflora. Acidity and normal GI motility are factors that inhibit bacterial growth in this region.[6] Trauma or diseases of the stomach and duodenal region may compromise these protective factors. Thus, medical conditions such as a gastric ulceration, achlorhydria, obstructing duodenal ulcer, carcinoma, an upper GI bleed, or certain drug therapies may result in the abnormal proliferation of the local flora (e.g., anaerobic streptococci, *Streptococci viridans*, lactobacilli, and yeast).

The microflora of the proximal small bowel is similar to that observed in the stomach, although increased numbers of *Enterobacteriaceae* and *Bacteroides* spp. may be found. Peristalsis is most rapid in the jejunum and upper ileum, which in part explains the low bacterial counts relative to the distal ileum. Injury or disease of this upper portion of the GI tract results in relatively low bacterial inocula into the peritoneal cavity. Thus, the number and severity of clinical infections related to such injuries would be fewer compared with injuries of the large bowel. Between the proximal and terminal ileum is a bacterial transition zone where the composition of organisms changes toward greater numbers of aerobic and anaerobic Gram-negative bacilli, and counts are up to 10^8 CFU/mL.

The highest concentration of microorganisms in the GI tract is in the colon. As many as 10^{11} CFU/g of organisms are present and account for roughly one-third of the total weight of the GI contents. Anaerobes outnumber aerobes by a ratio of 1:100 to 1:1000, with *Bacteroides* spp. being the predominant bacteria.[7] Under the usual conditions within the lumen of the GI tract, anaerobic organisms behave as harmless commensals, but when introduced into surrounding host tissues and the peritoneal cavity they express their pathogenic potential. Certain underlying clinical conditions, such as compromised vascular supply or tissue necrosis, may predispose a patient to anaerobic infections. Such clinical situations are associated with confined tissue spaces with a low oxidation-reduction potential and hypoxia, and thus provide an environment for uncontrolled anaerobic proliferation. Although more than 400 species of anaerobes reside in the colon and 200 in the oral cavity, only a few produce the majority of clinical anaerobic infections. *Bacteroides fragilis* accounts for only approximately 5% of the colonic microflora, yet causes many times the incidence of clinical infection, compared with any other *Bacteroides* spp.

The bacteria isolated from the ascitic fluid in patients with SBP are usually those of the normal intestinal flora. More than 92% of all cases of SBP are monomicrobial, with aerobic Gram-negative bacilli being responsible for more than two-thirds of all cases. *Escherichia coli* organisms account for nearly half of these cases, followed by *Klebsiella* spp. and other Gram-negative bacteria. In contrast, secondary peritonitis infections usually involve mixed microflora, both aerobic and anaerobic bacteria. Within this setting of mixed bacteria, there appears to be the potential for synergism. *Enterobacteriaceae* have been demonstrated to lower oxygen tension or redox potential within the peritoneal cavity, thus promoting growth of obligate anaerobes. Conversely, there is some evidence that the presence of low virulence anaerobic organisms enhance the pathogenicity of aerobic Gram-negative bacilli, such as *E. coli, Klebsiella* spp., and *Proteus mirabilis*. A variety of obligate anaerobes have been observed to interfere with intracellular bacterial killing by polymorphonuclear leukocytes (PMNs), as well as PMN chemotaxis and phagocytosis.[8] The bacteria of tertiary peritonitis are considered innocuous colonizers and not true pathogens; they may be organisms with low intrinsic virulence, such as *Staphylococcus epidermidis*, *Candida* spp., or *Enterococcus faecium*. In addition, inducible β-lactamase producing Gram-negative bacilli, such as *Enterobacter* sp., *Serratia* sp., *Citrobacter* sp., *Acinetobacter* sp., and *Pseudomonas aeruginosa* are also seen in this population.

Results from observations in humans and in the animal model of intraabdominal sepsis reveal a biphasic disease process. After intraabdominal inoculation of intestinal flora, animals initially developed acute peritonitis, predominantly from aerobic Gram-negative bacilli and less frequently from enterococci.[9] This phase was associated with a 40% mortality rate. Surviving animals later developed intraabdominal abscesses that were culture-positive most often for obligate anaerobes. However, in this model when a large inoculum of a single strain of bacteria was used (5×10^7 CFU/mL), no strain alone, aerobic or anaerobic, was able to induce abscesses. This evidence reaffirms the significance of synergism for abscess formation.

The microbiology of peritonitis in patients receiving continuous ambulatory peritoneal dialysis (CAPD) reveals that most cases are caused by the aerobic organisms commonly residing on skin. Most episodes (70%) are caused by Gram-positive cocci (*S. aureus*, *S. epidermidis*, and various streptococci). Less frequently (25%) *Enterobacteriaceae* cause infection, and infrequently (5%) anaerobes, mycobacteria, and fungi are the cause. It is thought that anaerobic organisms rarely cause infection in this group of patients because of the high oxygen tension present in the dialysate.

PATHOPHYSIOLOGY

The pathogenesis of primary peritonitis is not well understood and may result from bacterial spread from hematogenous or lymphatic sources, or from microperforation (e.g., intestinal transmural migration) of an otherwise intact GI tract. Secondary peritonitis from traumatic injury or GI disease results in the following situations when the first-line host defense mechanisms become overwhelmed: when the infecting inoculum is very large, when the bacterial contamination is caused by mixed flora that act synergistically to evade the first-line defenses, and in the presence of a foreign body (e.g., CAPD catheter) when host defenses are not efficient and intraleukocytic sequestration of organisms occurs.[2,10]

The concept of "mixed bacterial infection" is especially relevant to secondary and tertiary peritonitis and intraabdominal abscesses.[11] As many as 400 anaerobic and aerobic species of microorganisms have been found to be present as part of the normal intestinal flora. Thus, when infection occurs after GI content spillage, multiple organisms may be responsible. However, the mere presence of an organism (i.e., on culture) does not guarantee its pathogenicity. *Enterobacteriaceae* are able to produce endotoxins and thus can trigger septic shock. *Bacteroides* spp. have a virulence factor, the polysaccharide capsule, that explains in part their pathogenicity. The presence of other organisms, such as *Enterococcus* spp., has not reproducibly caused morbidity or mortality.

Even after identification of the pathogens, clinical outcome may be influenced by other factors. They include the bacterial load at the site of infection (i.e., the inoculum size) and immunologic variables relating to local host defenses, as well as the general systemic immune response, the progression, or severity of the underlying intrinsic GI disease. Most important are the success of surgical interventions performed, and whether the antimicrobial agents administered penetrate to the site of infection and are pharmacologically active in that environment. All of these factors should be considered before the selection of therapy, as well as when assessing clinical response.

A general understanding of anatomic relationships within the peritoneal cavity is important for determining the possible sources of intraabdominal infection, as well as anticipating the extent and routes of spread of infection. The peritoneal cavity in males is a completely closed space, whereas in females the free ends of the fallopian tubes perforate it. This distinction is important because pelvic peritonitis often accompanies pelvic inflammatory disease (PID), especially if infection of the fallopian tubes is severe. Organs found within the peritoneal cavity include the stomach, jejunum, ileum, transverse and sigmoid colon, cecum, liver, gallbladder, pancreas, spleen, and appendix. The peritoneal cavity has various pouches and recesses into which bacteria or infected exudate may potentially collect and become loculated. The peritoneal cavity is lined by a serous membrane that consists of a mesothelial cell monolayer beneath which are lymphatics, blood vessels, and nerve endings. The peritoneal space usually contains sufficient fluid to maintain surface moistness, which facilitates movement of the viscera. This moist peritoneal membrane is also highly permeable so that solutes and water are quickly transported in a bidirectional manner.

Host defense mechanisms generally combat bacterial invasion of the peritoneal cavity. Humoral and cellular immune defense mechanisms form the initial response to bacterial contamination, and the regional lymphatic circulation clears the bacterial debris. Intraabdominal infection results when these first-line host defenses are overwhelmed because the infecting inoculum is very large; the bacterial contamination is caused by mixed bacterial flora (i.e., anaerobic and aerobic), which act synergistically to evade host defenses; or a foreign body renders host defenses inefficient. The peritoneal membrane is next to respond by exuding a fluid containing opsonins, antibodies, complement, PMNs, and macrophages into the peritoneal cavity. This inflammatory response is presumably facilitated by means of local vasodilation and increased vascular permeability. Inflammation increases the membrane's permeability so that the transport of large molecules and protein is enhanced. This may additionally improve an antimicrobial agent's ability to penetrate into the peritoneal cavity during peritonitis.

CLINICAL PRESENTATION AND DIAGNOSIS

Signs and Symptoms

General malaise, prostration, nausea, vomiting, diarrhea, fever, dehydration, leukocytosis with a left shift, and electrolyte imbalance are systemic symptoms that may be observed in patients with intraabdominal infections. Intraabdominal abscesses may often "smolder" for long periods of time without symptoms or with inconsistent symptoms.

Aerobic and anaerobic Gram-negative bacteria may release endotoxin, a lipopolysaccharide from the bacterial cell wall into the bloodstream, which is responsible for some of the serious clinical symptoms observed. These symptoms are septic shock, adult respiratory distress syndrome (ARDS), and disseminated intravascular coagulation (DIC). However, none of these clinical findings is specific to intraabdominal infections, and they may occur to a varying degree in patients or may not be observed at all. Hypotension may also be exacerbated by reduced intravascular volume secondary to the massive influx of fluid from the vascular space into the peritoneum during peritonitis.

Abdominal pain and tenderness may be localized or general.[12] Specific abdominal pain on respiration or coughing and rebound tenderness or tenderness on gentle percussion are signs of acute peritonitis. The musculature that is overlying the area of inflamed peritoneum may become spastic. Involuntary muscle rigidity of the entire abdominal wall (i.e., "guarding") may develop with diffuse peritonitis. This muscle rigidity, however, is frequently absent or difficult to elicit in patients in the latter stages of peritonitis, patients who are obese, or patients with significant third-spacing of fluid (e.g., ascites).

Diagnosis

The serous fluid in the peritoneal cavity is normally clear yellow with a low specific gravity (<1.016) and has low protein concentration (usually <3 g/mL), with albumin being the predominant protein. Fibrinogen is not normally present. Solute concentrations are similar to those observed in plasma. A few leukocytes (<300 g/mL) and desquamated serosal cells also may be found.

Infected peritoneal fluid is visibly cloudy. Measurements used for immediate diagnosis include pH below 7.34 and PMN count above 500/mL. Other predictive measures include a fluid lactate concentration above 25 mg/dL and a fluid glucose concentration below 60 mg/dL. Diagnostic sensitivity improves when multiple parameters are used to establish the diagnosis.[13]

Specimens from the infected tissue or fluid should be obtained during surgery or by needle aspirate and directly cultured for both anaerobic and aerobic bacteria. Gram stain of specimens also may help to identify pathogens more quickly, so that empiric antimicrobial therapy can be tailored to the patient. The Gram staining procedure is especially important in situations where the patient has been on antibiotics before obtaining the specimen, when cultures may never turn positive.

The diagnosis of intraabdominal abscesses has been improved, particularly with the use of computed tomography (CT) scans.[14] Isotope scans and ultrasonography are much less useful because of nonspecific and false-positive results. Also, CT-guided needle aspiration procedures or placement of percutaneous drains is established as one of the most significant surgical adjuncts in the management of intraperitoneal infection developed in the last decade.

PSYCHOSOCIAL ASPECTS

Patients with intraabdominal infections represent a broad spectrum of psychological and social strata. Primary peritonitis in adults is often associated with alcoholic patients.[15] Secondary peritonitis is associated with a broad range of patients. Infections are related to perforations, ulcerations, and malignancies; therefore, patients may have received these injuries from motor vehicle accidents, domestic violence, or gang-related activity. Tertiary peritonitis is associated with immunocompromised patients, such as patients infected with the human immunodeficiency virus (HIV) or patients with cancer. The attitudes of patients toward pharmacotherapy play a pivotal role in their acceptance of therapy.

THERAPEUTIC PLAN

A Surgical Infection Society Policy Statement has been developed for the selection of antibiotics in the treatment of intraabdominal infections. This policy statement is based on in vitro activity, animal models, and documented efficacy clinical trials. In addition, these guidelines include pharmacokinetics, mechanism of action, microbial resistance, and safety information (Fig. 70.1).[16]

General guidelines for evaluating new antiinfective drugs for the treatment of intraabdominal and pelvic infections are outlined by the Infectious Disease Society of America and endorsed by the Surgical Infection Society. These guidelines classify infections as complicated (requiring an operative procedure), uncomplicated (managed pharmaceutically), and postoperative wound (operative procedure should be curative, but antiinfective drugs are used to prevent further infection at the site).[17]

TREATMENT

Pharmacotherapy

Selection of empiric antimicrobial therapy should follow a careful thought process that considers first the suspected site(s) and source of infection, along with the most likely pathogens. Empiric therapy should be chosen to include,

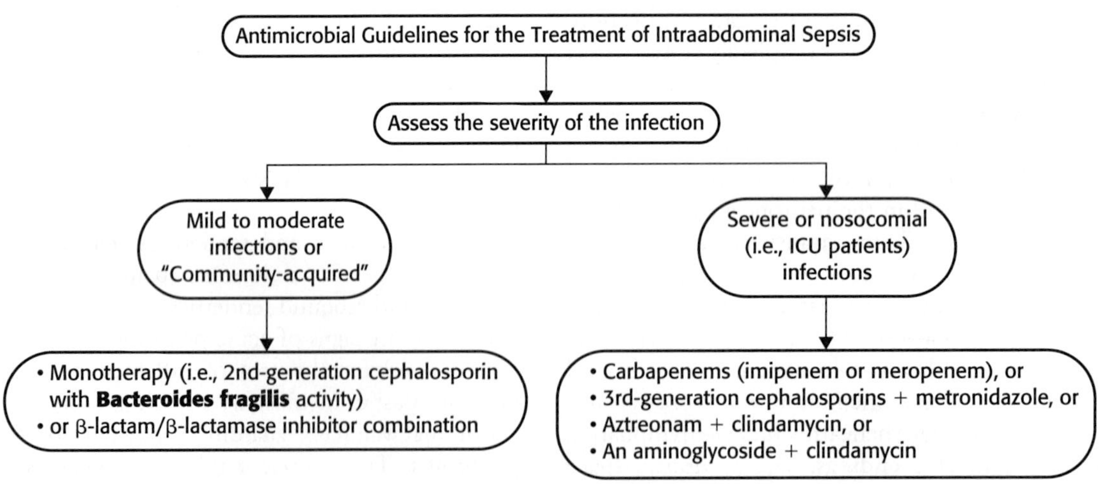

Figure 70.1. Algorithm of antimicrobial guidelines for the treatment of intraabdominal sepsis. (*Source:* Based on recommendations from the Antimicrobial Agents Committee of the Surgical Infections Society. Bohnen JMA, Solomkin JS, Dellinger EP, et al. Guidelines for clinical care: anti-infective agents for intraabdominal infection—a surgical infection society policy statement. Arch Surg 127:83–88, 1992.)

Table 70.1 ▪ Antimicrobials for Empiric Therapy of Intraabdominal Infections: Description of Spectrum of Activity

Generic Name (Trade Name)	Usual Adult[a] Daily Dosage	Activity Against *Bacteroides fragilis*	Activity Against Enterobacteriaceae	Activity Against *Enterococcus* spp.
Metronidazole (Flagyl)	500 mg q8h	Yes	No	No
Clindamycin (Cleocin)	600–900 mg q8h	Yes	No	No
Chloramphenicol (Chloromycetin)	50 mg/kg/day, divide q6h	Yes	Yes	No
Cefuroxime (Zinacef, Kefurox)	750 mg or 1.5 g q8h	No	Yes	No
Cefotetan (Cefotan)	1–2 g q12h	Yes	Yes	No
Cefoxitin (Mefoxin)	1–2 g q6–8h	Yes	Yes	No
Cefmetazole (Zefazone)	1–2 g q6–8h	Yes	Yes	No
Cefotaxime (Claforan)	1–2 g q6–8h	Some	Yes	No
Ceftizoxime (Ceftizox)	1–2 g q6–8h	Yes	Yes	No
Ceftazidime (Fortaz, Tazidime, Tazicef)	1–2 g q8h	No	Yes	No
Ceftriaxone (Rocephin)	1–2 g q24h	No	Yes	No
Cefepime (Maxipime)	1–2 g q12–8h	No	Yes	No
Ampicillin and Sulbactam (Unasyn)	1.5–3 g q6h	Yes	Yes	Yes
Ticarcillin and Clavulanic Acid (Timentin)	3.1 g q4h	Yes	Yes	Some
Piperacillin and Tazobactam (Zosyn)	4.5 g q6h	Yes	Yes	Yes
Imipenem (Primaxin)	500 mg q6–8h	Yes	Yes	No
Gentamicin or Tobramycin	5–10 μg/mL peak <2 trough	No	Yes	No
Vancomycin (Vancocin)	1 g q12h (trough 5–10 μg/mL)	No	No	Yes
Penicillin G	1–2 mg q4–6h	No	No	Yes
Ampicillin	1–2 g q4–6h	No	Some	Yes
Mezlocillin (Mezlin)	4 g q6h	Some	Yes	Yes
Piperacillin (Pipracil)	4 g q6h	Some	Yes	Yes
Ticarcillin (Ticar)	3 g q4h	Some	Yes	Some
Aztreonam (Aztactam)	1 g q6–8h	No	Yes	No
Ofloxacin (Floxin)	400 mg q12h	No	Yes	No
Ciprofloxacin (Cipro)	400 mg q12h	No	Yes	No
Levofloxacin (Levaquin)	500 mg q24h	No	Yes	No
Trovafloxacin (Trovan)	300 mg q24h	Yes	Yes	Yes
Quinupristin and Dalfopristin (Synercid)[b]	7.5 mg/kg q8h	No	No	Yes

[a]Not adjusted for renal impairment.
[b]For Vancomycin-resistant *Enterococcus faecium*.

as narrowly as possible, only those suspected organisms. It is helpful to classify the infection as either community acquired or nosocomial, and appropriate susceptibility data should then be applied to the antibiotic selection process. Using the antibiotic(s) with the narrowest spectrum possible additionally reduces the incidence of secondary drug resistance, superinfection, and confusion when assessing clinical response.

Next, the unique pharmacologic properties of each potential antimicrobial must be considered with regard to its ability to penetrate to the site of infection; its inoculum effect (stability toward β-lactamases produced by a large Gram-negative bacterial inocula); and its activity in infection environments–those of low metabolic activity (as in abscesses), those of lower pH, and in more anaerobic conditions.

Last are the considerations of potential adverse reactions, dosing, and costs, which enter the schema for final antimicrobial selection. Table 70.1 includes antimicrobial agents that have been used either as monotherapy or in combination with one another to treat intraabdominal infection. The drug dosage in adults is provided as well as a description of the spectrum of activity.

There are an extensive number of acceptable antibiotic monotherapy regimens or combination regimens for the treatment of intraabdominal infections.[18,19] All regimens must include coverage for *Enterobacteriaceae* and *B. fragilis*. Each reasonable regimen has subtle advantages or disadvantages in a specific patient. The following descriptions of antibiotic therapies will not give exact recommendations for therapy, but will provide a necessary framework and some important details for the formulation of patient-specific therapy (Table 70.1). Controversy still arises regarding the need for empiric coverage of *Enterococcus* spp. organisms; most experts still think that this coverage is not necessary. Exceptions to this recommendation are patients exhibiting signs of septic shock or situations in which the blood or peritoneal fluid Gram stain reveals a predominance of Gram-positive cocci. Empiric therapy that includes antistaphylococcal and antipseudomonal activity is not routinely necessary unless there are known predisposing factors.

Penicillin or ampicillin can be used to provide antibacterial coverage for aerobic–anaerobic Gram-positive cocci from the oropharyngeal or upper GI regions. Cephalosporins also are active against these organisms as well as against *Enterobacteriaceae*. In addition, some of the second- and third-generation cephalosporins have broader antibacterial activity including many anaerobic Gram-negative bacilli.

Aminoglycosides are often used to provide specific antimicrobial activity against aerobic Gram-negative bacilli that are found in the GI tract. However, if traditionally dosed, these agents have a narrow therapeutic-toxic serum concentration range that makes dosage adjustments and monitoring more complicated. Single, daily dosing (i.e., once-daily) may make these drugs more useful. Aminoglycosides are highly active in vitro against most strains of facultative aerobes, which are important in producing bacteremia and early mortality in intraabdominal infections. This efficacy was illustrated in an animal model of intraabdominal sepsis and has since been a component of the standard of therapy.[20] Aztreonam has a similar narrow spectrum of activity.

Various extended spectrum penicillin and second- and third-generation cephalosporins have been used more recently instead of aminoglycosides because their activity against most aerobic Gram-negative bacilli is comparable. Fourth-generation cephalosporin, cefepime, has a wider spectrum and greater potency than third-generation cephalosporins. The combination of a penicillin plus an aminoglycoside compares to cefoxitin, with regard to susceptibility of aerobic Gram-negative bacilli and anaerobic–aerobic Gram-positive streptococci, and it includes enterococci. The toxicity issue for aminoglycosides remains their limiting factor. The incidence of aminoglycoside-induced nephrotoxicity in patients being treated for intraabdominal infections has been reviewed.[21] There is growing interest in the routine use of aminoglycosides as once-daily large doses (using a single high dose 5 to 7 mg/kg with therapeutic peaks of 18 to 24 μg/mL and troughs <0.3 μg/mL).[22] This dosage scheme is thought to have less potential for ototoxicity and nephrotoxicity because this regimen does not allow drug accumulation in patients who have normal renal function.[23]

No cephalosporin has antimicrobial activity against enterococci. Penicillins (penicillin, ampicillin, mezlocillin, piperacillin) and vancomycin, when given alone, are bacteriostatic for this organism. The combination of one of these latter agents plus an aminoglycoside is bactericidal against enterococci, which is another reason such combinations are used when treating intraabdominal sepsis with septic shock.

Fluoroquinolones, such as ciprofloxacin and levofloxacin, have excellent abdominal penetration and superior Gram-negative aerobic activity compared with cephalosporins. The extended-spectrum quinolone, trovafloxacin, in addition to superior Gram-negative and Gram-positive activity, also has anaerobic activity. Adverse effects associated with trovafloxacin include serious liver injury resulting in liver transplantation and/or death. Trovafloxacin should be reserved for patients in a hospital or long-term care facility with a serious life-threatening infection for which no safer alternative is available.

Antimicrobial agents with good activity against obligate anaerobes reduce the incidence of abscesses, a later complication of intraabdominal infections. This coverage is needed in addition to, not instead of, therapy for aerobes. Chloramphenicol has a broad spectrum of activity against anaerobes, but few studies have evaluated its efficacy.[24] In addition, the potential for serious toxicity (e.g., aplastic anemia and bone marrow suppression) has minimized its usefulness as a first-line drug.

Clindamycin has been used successfully for treatment of abdominal abscesses. The value of clindamycin has been reduced, however, by the problems of drug-induced diarrhea, pseudomembranous colitis, and emerging clindamycin-resistant *B. fragilis*, which has been reported to be higher than 20% in some regions.[25] Metronidazole has been directly compared with clindamycin for the treatment of serious intraabdominal infections owing to anaerobic organisms and demonstrated equal efficacy and probably better safety. Metronidazole is bactericidal with a narrow spectrum of antianaerobic bacterial activity. If possible, metronidazole should be avoided during pregnancy and lactation because of concerns of teratogenicity.

Cefoxitin was the first of the β-lactams to show in vitro activity against *B. fragilis* and is still very useful.[26] It has been shown to be safe and effective for the treatment of community-acquired mixed flora intraabdominal infections, whether given alone or with an aminoglycoside. Caution must be taken, though, because not all of the second- and third-generation cephalosporins are appropriate for single-drug therapy. Each has its own problems: cefuroxime, ceftazidime, ceftriaxone, and cefepime are only active against *Enterobacteriaceae*; cefmetazole lacks widespread acceptance (the methyl-tetrazole ring infers potential toxicity); and cefotetan, cefotaxime, and ceftizoxime have only moderate *B. fragilis* activity.

Imipenem and meropenem are very potent carbapenems that are stable against many types of β-lactamases and have excellent activity against all suspected Gram-negative organisms (aerobic and anaerobic). However, both are expensive and potentially neurotoxic, and therefore are often reserved for short-term empiric therapy in seriously ill patients thought to have multiple resistant pathogens.

Primary peritonitis (SBP) is usually caused by a single pathogen, and in 80 to 85% of cases three organisms have been responsible–*E. coli*, streptococci, and *Klebsiella* spp. Ampicillin plus an aminoglycoside can be used for empiric treatment for SBP. Ototoxicity and nephrotoxicity are associated with the addition of aminoglycosides in any therapy. Hypersensitivity to ampicillin is also a consideration. A single agent, such as a second- or third-generation cephalosporin, is a reasonable alternative if nephrotoxicities or ototoxicities are a consideration. The risks and benefits must be evaluated in each patient. In fact, SBP has been prevented by antimicrobial prophylaxis in high-risk cirrhotic patients (gastrointestinal bleeding, ascitic fluid protein levels of <1 g/dL, and patients recovering from a previous episode of primary peritonitis). Selective decontamination of the gut with oral norfloxacin (400 mg daily) or trimethoprim/sulfamethoxazole (one double-strength tablet daily for 5 days every week) has been shown to reduce the incidence of primary peritonitis.[3,27]

Effective treatment of secondary peritonitis is directed toward Gram-negative and anaerobic organisms. Clindamycin plus gentamicin remains the gold standard of therapy. The nephrotoxicity and ototoxicity associated with gentamicin and the enterocolitis associated with clindamycin have resulted in alternative therapies. Third-generation cephalosporins can be substituted for the aminoglycosides and metronidazole can be substituted for clindamycin. Metronidazole should be combined with an agent active against microaerophilic Gram-positive cocci. These organisms, although sensitive to clindamycin, are resistant to metronidazole. Monotherapy includes agents with activity against aerobes and anaerobes, such as imipenem, meropenem, and β-lactams/β-lactamase combinations including ampicillin/sulbactam, ticarcillin/clavulanate, and piperacillin/tazobactam. Second-generation cephalosporins such as cefotetan and cefoxitin have demonstrated high *B. fragilis* resistance. Tertiary peritonitis occurs in immunocompromised patients who present with resistant Gram-negative organisms such as *Enterobacter* sp., *Serratia* sp., *Citrobacter* sp., *Acinetobacter* sp., and *Pseudomonas aeruginosa*. These patients should be treated with a regimen that includes imipenem, meropenem, cefepime, fluoroquinolones, or an aminoglycoside. Amphotericin B is the gold standard for invasive *Candida* infections. However, this drug is complicated by its nephrotoxicity. Fluconazole and itraconazole are less toxic, but are intrinsically resistant to *Candida krusei, Candida tropicalis,* and *Torulopsis glabrata. Enterococcus faecium* organisms are potential pathogens when isolated in tertiary peritonitis and are pathogenic when isolated from urine or bile. Antibiotic selections are extremely limited in vancomycin-resistant enterococcus. Chloramphenicol, doxycycline, and dalfopristin/quinupristin are used in these instances with variable success.[28,29]

Table 70.2 ▪ Summary of Culture Results from Intraabdominal Infection Studies

Aerobic Organism	Study 1 (*n* = 161)	Study 2 (*n* = 144)	Study 3 (*n* = 48)	Study 4 (*n* = 162)
Enterococcus spp.	19	17	6	23
Streptococci	14	33	6	36
Staphylococci	7	24	8	10
E. coli	99	67	40	57
Proteus spp.	9	10	8	6
Enterobacter spp.	5	0	2	14
Klebsiella spp.	30	13	0	15
Pseudomonas spp.	15	10	2	15
Miscellaneous aerobes	22	14	2	9
Candida spp.	0	4	4	9
Streptococci	0	1	13	4
Peptococci	0	4	19	4
Peptostreptococci	8	6	17	0
Fusobacterium	35	3	4	6
Clostridium spp.	29	36	31	18
Bacteroids fragilis	100	66	52	23
Other *Bacteroids* spp.	19	36	58	21
Miscellaneous anaerobes	0	25	8	22

Source: Data are from blood and peritoneal cultures; reported in references 24, 31–34.

Note: Percentages in each study do not add up to 100% because each culture may have been positive for more than one organism. Percentage (%) positive cultures by organism.

Antibiotics directed against only aerobic organisms were used before the technical improvements made in anaerobic culturing and sensitivity methods, which revealed the true incidence of anaerobic abscess infections.[30] Now, parenteral therapy for both anaerobic and aerobic organisms of the GI flora is recommended based on observations in animal models of intraabdominal sepsis and clinical experience. Data from five clinical studies spanning the last 17 years have been compiled (Table 70.2) to give a snapshot of how often and what types of mixed infection pathogens are recovered from patients with varying intraabdominal infections.[24,31–34] In the patient with intraabdominal sepsis, the crucial therapy modality is prompt, adequate surgical intervention. Parenteral antibiotics also are used to decrease the incidence of bacteremia and abscess formation. By necessity, the empiric antimicrobial regimen is selected based on clinical considerations. Thus, every clinician must be aware of the differences of the microflora at various levels of the GI tract, along with their usual antimicrobial susceptibility. Empiric therapies are then formulated using these data. Therapy usually includes antimicrobial coverage for the aerobic Gram-negative bacilli, *Enterobacteriaceae*, that cause early infection morbidity, as well as coverage for *B. fragilis*, which causes late infection morbidity.

Special considerations must be taken into account

when considering intraperitoneal drug administration in patients who receive dialysis via continuous ambulatory peritoneal dialysis (CAPD).[35] Studies have shown a loss of activity of some antibiotics in dialysis fluid owing to the low pH and high osmolarity of the dialysate solution. Aminoglycosides specifically have shown reduced bactericidal activity when the test media pH is lowered to pH 5.5, which simulates the pH of infected dialysate solution. Also, combining β-lactams and aminoglycosides in the same peritoneal dialysis bag should not be routinely performed because there may be significant inactivation of the aminoglycoside depending on the β-lactam employed. These are important considerations when CAPD patients treated with aminoglycosides do not clinically respond as expected. These patients are reported to have a high incidence of infection arising from bacterial contamination caused during the technical aspects of CAPD. The advantages of CAPD compared with hemodialysis have been tempered by this constant risk of peritonitis. Therefore, successful treatment of intraabdominal infections in these patients holds a separate significance.

Nonpharmacologic Therapy

Surgical management of intraabdominal infections is initially based on any necessary operative procedures to repair GI perforations or injury. Equally important are debridement procedures for removal of any necrotic material and infectious foci. This includes drainage of abscesses and debridement of infected, necrotic tissue or bowel. The goal of surgical procedures is to debulk the infection and devitalized tissue, which then allows antibiotics and host defenses to have an impact. Surgical intervention has little place in primary peritonitis but may exist in exploratory laparotomy to achieve diagnosis. Surgical intervention for secondary peritonitis is directed to the primary cause. Surgery prevents peritoneal soiling and recurrence, and allows drainage of purulent exudate.

Treatment for intraabdominal abscess is the same as treatment for secondary peritonitis. Antimicrobial therapy is secondary to drainage. Antibiotics are used to control systemic complications of sepsis and are ineffective if appropriate drainage is not achieved. Deaths do occur from undrained intraabdominal abscesses.[36]

Surgery may be a therapeutic plan in CAPD patients to remove an infected catheter. The indication for Tenckhoff catheter removal in CAPD patients with peritonitis has not been established. It is believed by some physicians that continuing regular CAPD in patients with peritonitis improves outcome because infectious exudate can be physically removed by each dialysis. Others feel that it is important to remove the catheter (thus losing dialysis access) because curing an infection that involves a foreign body (i.e., the catheter) is extremely difficult. If a patient has not responded to therapy alone within 5 days, a conservative recommendation would be to consider removal of the Tenckhoff catheter. Experience with fungal and *Pseudomonas peritonitis* in CAPD suggests that early catheter removal is indicated.

ALTERNATIVE THERAPIES

Alternative therapies are not recommended because of the increase mortality rates (80%) for penetrating intraabdominal traumas before surgical and pharmacological intervention.

FUTURE THERAPIES

Advances in the treatment of intraabdominal infections are contingent on the development of broad-spectrum antibiotics. These antibiotics also need to have excellent intraabdominal penetration and be more stable in the acidic medium of an abscess. Other extended-spectrum quinolones, such as trovafloxacin,[37] with aerobic and anaerobic activities as well as a less toxic profile are in development. New fourth-generation cephalosporins including cefpirome, cefoselis, cefepime, cefclidin, cefozopram, and cefluprenam offer promise, as well. Of these new cephalosporins, only cefepime has been approved in the United States.[38] Oral agents that are well absorbed may be used early to decrease the patient's length of hospital stay.[39]

Monoclonal antibodies may enhance host response and improve tissue injury associated with the inflammatory process. The role of monoclonal antibodies has yet to be defined in the treatment of intraabdominal infections. In addition to antimicrobial therapy, future advances must include improved radiographic methods for early diagnosis of septic foci.[40]

IMPROVING OUTCOMES

Spontaneous bacterial peritonitis (SBP) in adults with cirrhosis and ascites is reported to occur in as many as 8 to 27% of patients and has a resulting mortality rate of approximately 50%. The overall mortality rate in these patients may be as high as 95% because SBP is often accompanied by severe hepatic failure.

Most patients with secondary peritonitis can be placed in one of three categories: (1) penetrating abdominal trauma, (2) appendicitis, or (3) other.[41] Generally, patients are young males and have a very low rate of morbidity and mortality, although the prognosis of secondary peritonitis is closely associated with early diagnosis and prompt surgical intervention. A mathematical equation has been derived to predict the risk of posttrauma infection in patients with penetrating abdominal trauma. Factors entering into the equation are age, ostomy formation (performed for all left colonic injuries), shock, number of organs injured, and amount of blood or blood products administered before the time of surgery.[42] Postoperative complication rates also have been associated with the extent of organ failure or numbers of organs affected, duration and stage of illness, adequacy of surgical procedures, and presence of other chronic underlying illnesses, including immunosuppression. An important outcome indicator is length of hospital stay, which has been measured to be 7 to 14 days for most intraabdominal infections, although in patients with complications it can be a great deal longer.

Patient Education

Patients with intraabdominal infections must be educated on their disease presentation and treatment. Patients at high risk for primary peritonitis should be placed on prophylactic therapy and must be counseled on the benefits of prophylaxis. Patients who are alcoholic must be referred to the necessary treatment and support centers for abstinence from alcohol. In addition, patients should be educated on nutritional status and proper diet. All patients must be educated on the potential complications that can occur if medical and pharmacological treatment are not observed.

Patients should be educated on potential adverse effects of their treatment, such as GI distress, headaches, and dizziness. Furthermore, patients need to be counseled on potential drug and food interactions with their respective medications, prior to discharge. (Fluoroquinolones should not be taken concomitantly with food or multivitamins, with iron supplements, or with divalent ions and products such as antacids.)

Methods to Improve Patient Adherence to Drug Therapy

Patients with intraabdominal infections are primarily treated in an acute hospital setting. On discharge, oral agents may be given; at this time steps should be taken to counsel patients on appropriate adherence.

Prevention of recurrence of primary peritonitis requires prophylactic therapy. Patients should be educated on the benefits of treatment. Lifestyle modifications can be made to assist patients in their adherence to regimens. Such modifications can involve marking on a calendar or the use of a pill box with daily markings. Suggestions to associate daily activities with dosing, such as brushing teeth, also can be used.

Disease Management Strategies to Improve Patient Outcomes

Support of intravascular volume with fluid therapy is essential to maintain adequate blood pressure and renal perfusion. The use of so-called volume expanders, such as albumin and hetastarch, has not been shown to be essential in this setting, and in addition, they are expensive. Electrolyte imbalances and metabolic acidosis should be corrected with intravenous therapy.

Oral intake of foods should be temporarily discontinued and nasogastric (NG) suction started as soon as peritonitis is suspected to prevent GI distension. Suction should be continued until peristaltic activity returns and the patient begins to pass flatus. NG suction may contribute to the patient's overall fluid loss and dehydration, as well as acid-base and electrolyte problems.

Administration of oral medications should be discontinued in patients receiving NG suctioning. The GI absorption of oral medications under such circumstances may be erratic owing to changes in pH and motility. The drug may also be inadvertently removed from the GI tract by the suctioning procedure.

Therapy of patients with paralytic ileus consists of GI tract rest, NG suction, and treatment of the underlying GI disease. Adynamic or paralytic ileus occurs to some extent with any peritoneal injury or surgery, including peritoneal inflammation. Early in the course of peritoneal irritation the intestine may have a transient period of hyperperistalsis, but soon after, motility decreases or is even absent to the point of obstruction. Severity and duration depend on the type of insult, but usually lasts from 2 to 3 days, even in an uncomplicated surgical case. Studies indicate that the pathogenesis of this condition involves neurogenic, hormonal, and local factors. The adrenergic response to intraabdominal inflammation stimulates the sympathetic pathways of the intestine, resulting in the slowing of peristalsis. The accumulation of gas and fluids within the bowel lumen distends the intestinal wall to the point at which intraluminal pressure exceeds capillary perfusion pressure, causing bowel ischemia.

Symptoms of paralytic ileus include progressive abdominal distension and vomiting of pooled gastric contents and biliary secretions. Localized pain and profuse vomiting only occur if there is complete bowel obstruction and strangulation.

Patients with abdominal adhesions require surgical treatment, which is necessary to free these attachments. As a normal host defense, the body attempts to isolate infections of the abdomen into localized pockets. The peritoneum exudes large quantities of fibrin into the peritoneal fluid while fibrinolytic activity is reduced. The result is the formation of a network of fibrinous strands between the loops of bowel and the adjacent visceral surfaces. If the fibrin is not reabsorbed, the strands are invaded by fibroblasts and develop a blood supply. Fibrin strands transform into firm adhesive bands. The absence of peristalsis allows these adhesions to form more easily.

Surgical intervention also is required for patient improvement. Proper drainage is required to remove foreign and purulent masses from affected areas. Surgical correction of perforations as well as the underlying pathology of the infection are also required. Newer radiological methods, ultrasonography, and CT scanning impact on early diagnosis and greatly improve patient outcome. In addition, support of vital organs and proper nutrition can greatly impact the improvement of recovering patients. Patients requiring mechanical or other measures to support vital organs may have reduced nutritional intake.

Multiple complications that affect patient outcome also may arise. Organ failures may occur owing to shock and/or infections. These complications must be managed individually to improve patient outcome.

PHARMACOECONOMICS

Pharmacoeconomics of intraabdominal infections require stratification of the severity of the infections, from mild to moderate infections (community-acquired) in which a single agent can be used, versus severe or nosocomial intraabdominal infections, in which two or more agents usually are used. Various pharmacoeconomic studies have compared monotherapies (second-generation cephalosporins versus β-lactase inhibitors versus imipenem/meropenem).[43,44] Treatment failures, clinical cure, number of adverse events, number of antibiotic doses, and duration of antibiotic therapy are all pharmacoeconomic outcome measures. Severe or nosocomial intraabdominal infections are inherently more expensive because of the potential complications that may arise in immunocompromised patients.[34,45] Furthermore, treatment cost increases with the number of laboratory tests ordered and the length of hospital stay (usually intensive care units). Direct drug cost is outweighed by the cost of adverse drug effects and the cost of treatment failures. Length of hospital stay continues to be an important outcome indicator and is one of the determinants of treatment cost.

KEY POINTS

- It is important to maintain homeostatic support when managing intraabdominal infections.
- Surgical intervention, when appropriate, is critical in the management of intraabdominal infections.
- The goal of treatment is to prevent bacteremia.
- Empiric therapy must target the suspected organisms in each individual infection.
- Monotherapy can be considered in mild to moderate community-acquired intraabdominal infections.
- In the treatment of primary peritonitis, ampicillin plus an aminoglycoside is the usual standard of care. However, a single second-generation or third-generation agent is a reasonable alternative if nephrotoxicities or ototoxicities are considerations. Evaluate based on risks and benefits.
- Clindamycin plus gentamicin remains the gold standard in the treatment of secondary peritonitis.
- Third-generation cephalosporins may be substituted for clindamycin.
- Metronidazole may be substituted for clindamycin.
- Metronidazole should be combined with an agent active against microaerophilic Gram-positive cocci.
- Resistance may emerge with third-generation cephalosporins among inducible β-lactamase producing Gram-negative bacilli. Treat with imipenem, meropenem, cefepime, fluoroquinolones, or aminoglycosides.
- Second-generation cephalosporins, such as cefotetan and cefoxitin, are active against aerobic Gram-positive bacilli, Gram-negative bacilli, and anaerobes. Recently they have demonstrated high *B. fragilis* resistance.
- Tertiary peritonitis occurs primarily in immunocompromised patients.
- Intraabdominal abscess treatment is the same as treatment for secondary peritonitis; anaerobes predominate, and antimicrobial therapy is secondary to drainage.
- Direct drug cost is outweighed by the cost of adverse drug effects and the cost of treatment failures.

REFERENCES

1. Bhuva M, Ganger D, Jensen D. Spontaneous bacterial peritonitis: an update on evaluation, management, and prevention. Am J Med 97:169–175, 1994.
2. Such J, Runyon BA. Spontaneous bacterial peritonitis. Clin Infect Dis 27:669-676, 1998.
3. Johnson CC, Baldessarre J, Levison ME. Peritonitis: update on pathophysiology, clinical manifestations, and management. Clin Infect Dis 24:1035–1047, 1997.
4. Sherlock DJ, Benjamin IS. Clinical aspects of intraabdominal infection. In: Gorbach SL, ed. Pharmanual: the pharmacotherapy of intraabdominal infections. Quebec: Pharmalibri Publishers, 1997:5–32.
5. Farthmann EH, Schoffel U. Epidemiology and pathophysiology of intraabdominal infections (IAI). Infection 26(5):329–334, 1998.
6. Nichols RL. Intraabdominal sepsis: characterization and treatment. J Infect Dis 135:S54–S57, 1977.
7. Hentges DJ. The anaerobic microflora of the human body. Clin Infect Dis 16(Suppl 4):S175–S180, 1993.
8. Ingham HR, Tharagonnet D, Sisson PR, et al. Inhibition of phagocytosis in vitro by obligate anaerobes. Lancet 2:1252–1254, 1977.
9. Onderdonk AB, Shapiro ME, Finberg RW, et al. Use of a model of intraabdominal sepsis for studies of the pathogenicity of *Bacteroides fragilis*. Rev Infect Dis 6:S91–S95, 1984.
10. Buggy BP, Schaberg DR, Swartz RD. Intraleukocytic sequestration as a cause of persistent *Staphylococcus aureus* peritonitis in continuous ambulatory dialysis. Am J Med 76:1035–1039, 1984.
11. Dougherty SH. Antimicrobial culture and susceptibility testing has little value for routine management of secondary bacterial peritonitis. Clin Infect Dis 25(Suppl 2):S258–S261, 1997.
12. Levison ME, Bush LM. Peritonitis and other intraabdominal infections. In: Mandell GL, Bennett JE, Dolin R, eds. Mandell, Douglas and Bennett's principles and practice of infectious diseases. 4th ed. New York: Churchill Livingstone, 1995:705–740.
13. Garcia-Tsao G, Conn HO, Lerner E. The diagnosis of bacterial peritonitis: comparison of pH, lactate concentration and leukocyte count. Hepatology 5:91–96, 1985.
14. Wilson SE. A critical analysis of recent innovations in the treatment of intraabdominal infection. Surg Gynecol Obstet 177(Suppl):11–17, 1993.
15. Peteet JR, Brenner S, Curtiss D, et al. A stage of change approach to addiction in the medical setting. Gen Hosp Pschiatr 20(5):267–273, 1998.
16. Bohnen JMA, Solomkin JS, Dellinger EP, et al. Guidelines for clinical care: anti-infective agents for intraabdominal infection–a surgical infection society policy statement. Arch Surg 127:83–88, 1992.
17. Solomkin JS, Hemsell DL, Sweet R, et al. General guidelines for the evaluation of new anti-infective drugs for the treatment of intraabdominal and pelvic infections. Clin Infect Dis 15(Suppl 1):S33–S42, 1992.
18. DiPiro JT, Cue JI. Single-agent versus combination antibiotic therapy in the management of intraabdominal infections. Pharmacotherapy 14:266–272, 1994.
19. Bohnen JM. Antibiotic therapy for abdominal infection. World J Surg 22(2):152–157, 1998.
20. Nichols RL, Smith JW, Fossedal EN, et al. Efficacy of parenteral antibiotics in the treatment of experimentally induced intraabdominal sepsis. Rev Infec Dis 1:302–312, 1979.
21. Ho JL, Barza M. Role of aminoglycoside antibiotics in the treatment of intraabdominal infection. Antimicrob Agents Chemother 31:485–491, 1987.
22. Kapusnik JE, Hackbarth CJ, Chambers HF, et al. Single-large daily dose versus conventional intermittent dosing of tobramycin for the treatment of guinea pigs with *Pseudomonas aeruginosa* pneumonia. J Infect Dis 158:7–12, 1988.
23. Gilbert DN. Once daily aminoglycoside therapy. Antimicrob Agents Chemother 35:339–345, 1991.
24. Harding GKM, Buckwold FJ, Ronald AR, et al. Prospective, randomized, comparative study of clindamycin, chloramphenicol, and ticarcillin, each in combination with gentamicin in therapy for intraabdominal and female genital tract sepsis. J Infect Dis 142:384–393, 1980.
25. Rasmussen BA, Bush K, Tally FP. Antimicrobial resistance in *Bacteroides*. Clin Infect Dis 16(Suppl 4):S390–S400, 1993.
26. Johnson CC. Susceptibility of anaerobic bacteria to beta-lactam antibiotics in the United States. Clin Infect Dis 16(Suppl 4):S371–S376, 1993.
27. Singh N, Gayowski T, Yu VL, et al. Trimethoprim-sulfamethoxazole for the prevention of spontaneous bacterial peritonitis in cirrhosis: a randomized trial. Ann Intern Med 122:595–598, 1995.

28. Nathens AB, Rotstein OD, Marshall JC. Tertiary peritonitis: clinical features of a complex nosocomial infection. World J Surg 22(2):158–163, 1998.
29. Davis JH, Huycke MM, Wells CL, et al. Surgical Infection Society position on vancomycin-resistant enterococcus. Arch Surg 131(10):1061–1068, 1996.
30. Wexler HM. Susceptibility testing of anaerobic bacteria–the state of the art. Clin Infect Dis 16(Suppl 4):S328–S333, 1993.
31. Lau WY, Teoh-Chan CH, Fan ST, et al. The bacteriology and septic complication of patients with appendicitis. Ann Surg 200:576–581, 1984.
32. Jones RC, Thal ER, Johnson NA, et al. Evaluation of antibiotic therapy following penetrating abdominal trauma. Ann Surg 201:576–585, 1985.
33. Solomkin JS, Dellinger EP, Christou NV, et al. Results of a multicenter trial comparing imipenem/cilastatin to tobramycin/clindamycin for intraabdominal infections. Ann Surg 212:581–591, 1990.
34. Barie PS, Vogel SB, Patchen Dellinger EP, et al. A randomized, double-blind clinical trial comparing cefepime plus metronidazole with imipenem-cilastatin in the treatment of complicated intraabdominal infections. Arch Surg 132:1254–1302, 1997.
35. Horton MW, Deeter RG, Sherman RA. Treatment of peritonitis in patients undergoing continuous ambulatory peritoneal dialysis. Clin Pharmacol 9:102–118, 1990.
36. Fry DE, Garrison RN, Heitsch RC, et al. Determinants of death in patients with intraabdominal abscess. Surgery 88:517–522, 1980.
37. Donahue PE, Smith DL, Yellin AE, et al. Trovafloxacin in the treatment of intra-abdominal infections: results of a double-blind, multicenter comparison with imipenem/cilastatin. Trovafloxacin Surgical Group. Am J Surg 176 (Suppl 6A):53S–61S, 1998.
38. Garau J. The clinical potential of fourth-generation cephalosporins. Diagn Microbiol Infect Dis 31:479–480, 1998.
39. Solomkin JS, Dellinger EP, Bohnen JM, et al. The role of oral antimicrobials for the management of intraabdominal infections. New Horizons 6(Suppl 2):S46–S52, 1998.
40. Schein M, Wittman DH, Holzheimer R, et al. Hypothesis: compartmentalization of cytokines in intraabdominal infection. Surgery 119:694–700, 1996.
41. DiPiro JT. Considerations for therapy of mixed infections: focus on intraabdominal infection. Pharmacotherapy 15:15S–21S, 1995.
42. Nichols RL, Smith JW. Risk of infection, infecting flora and treatment considerations in penetrating abdominal trauma. Surg Gynecol Obstet 177(Suppl):50–54, 1993.
43. Messick CR, Mamdani M, McNicholl IR, et al. Pharmacoeconomic analysis of ampicillin-sulbactam versus cefoxitin in the treatment of intraabdominal infections. Pharmacotherapy 18(1):175–183, 1998.
44. Jaccard C, Troillet N, Harbarth S, et al. Prospective randomized comparison of imipenem-cilastatin and piperacillin-tazobactam in nosocomial pneumonia or peritonitis. Antimicrob Agents Chem 42(11):2966–2972, 1998.
45. Collins MD, Dajani AS, Kim KS, et al. Comparison of ampicillin/sulbactam plus aminoglycoside vs. ampicillin plus clindamycin plus aminoglycoside in the treatment of intraabdominal infections in children. The Multicenter Group. Pediat Infect Dis 17(Suppl 3):S15–18; Discussion S20–S21, 1998.

CHAPTER 71

GASTROINTESTINAL INFECTIONS

Shawn R. Akkerman

Gastroenteritis (GE) remains a major cause of morbidity and mortality worldwide, particularly among children, in whom 1.5 billion episodes of diarrhea and 4 million associated deaths occur each year.[1] In the United States, children under 5 years of age experience 20 to 35 million episodes of diarrhea, 10% of which result in doctor visits; more than 200,000 hospitalizations and 300 deaths occur annually.[2,3] Studies have also demonstrated significant GE-associated morbidity and mortality, especially among older adults, for adults in developed countries.[4,5]

This chapter focuses on the epidemiologic, pathophysiologic, and clinical characteristics of the predominant viral and bacterial GE pathogens and the appropriate drug and nondrug therapies for the management of GE.

TREATMENT GOALS: GASTROINTESTINAL INFECTIONS

- Because the most common symptom of acute infectious GE is diarrhea, focus treatment on delivering adequate and appropriate oral fluid and electrolyte rehydration, nutrition management, and maintenance therapy based on patient's degree of dehydration.
- Assess need for intravenous fluid therapy or hospitalization based on duration and severity of GE symptoms, degree of dehydration, patient's age, and patient's ability to maintain oral intake.
- Provide supportive care and institute refeeding following rehydration with breast milk or a balanced, mixed diet.
- Evaluate appropriateness of antidiarrheal therapy given likely pathogen, expected duration of disease, clinical presentation, and potential side effects.
- Evaluate need for and choice of antibiotic therapy based on duration of disease, likely pathogen, potential side effects, and concern of presence or development of antimicrobial resistance.

EPIDEMIOLOGY

Viruses are the leading cause of GE around the world; the most common are rotavirus and Norwalk virus. Bacterial GE is less frequent and is caused by *Salmonella*, *Shigella*, *Campylobacter*, *Yersinia*, *Vibrio*, and *Escherichia coli*. Parasites, such as *Giardia lamblia*, *Entamoeba histolytica*, and *Cryptosporidium*, may also be associated with diarrheal diseases; these are discussed with other intestinal parasites in Chapter 79, Parasitic Infections. Additionally, the reader is referred to other references for information about GE in immunocompromised patients, other viral infections, overgrowth of normal flora, antibiotic-induced *Clostridium difficile* colitis, and agents that cause diarrhea through food poisoning.[6–13]

Viruses

The primary human GE viruses are rotavirus, enteric adenovirus, Norwalk virus, calicivirus, and astrovirus.[14,15] These viruses may be predominantly associated with an endemic disease pattern (rotavirus, enteric adenovirus) or an epidemic or outbreak disease pattern (Norwalk, calicivirus, astrovirus).

Rotavirus is the single most important cause of dehydrating diarrhea in both developed and developing countries.[16] Rotavirus GE is believed to be seasonal, first appearing in the fall in the western United States, moving eastward, and reaching the Northeast by late winter and spring.[15,17] It primarily affects infants and children between 3 and 24 months of age, but adults may become infected after close contact with an infected child.[18] Although usually considered an endemic disease, outbreaks of rotavirus GE can occur and are common, especially in day-care centers.[18,19] The virus is transmitted by the fecal-oral route and is excreted in the feces throughout the illness. The incubation period is approximately 2 days. Diarrhea may be severe and is often accompanied by vomiting and fever. The duration of illness may range from 3 to 8 days.[15,18,19]

Enteric adenoviruses are specific strains (serotypes 40 and 41) that, unlike other adenoviruses, do not cause conjunctivitis or respiratory tract symptoms. Endemic adenoviral GE is not seasonal, primarily affects children under age 2, and is the second most common cause of severe viral diarrhea in children.[18] It is transmitted via the fecal-oral route and has an 8- to 10-day incubation period. The presentation is one of watery diarrhea followed by 2 or 3 days of low-grade fever and vomiting. The illness often lasts for 5 to 12 days, longer than other forms of viral GE.[15,18]

Norwalk virus is one of the viruses in the calicivirus family and is often associated with outbreaks of GE. Such outbreaks occur in families, camps, schools, nursing homes, hospitals, cafeterias, and sports teams, and on cruise ships. The virus may be acquired by the fecal-oral route or airborne transmission or may result from consumption of contaminated drinking or swimming water or inadequately cooked shellfish. Although Norwalk virus is also known as "winter vomiting disease," infection can occur year-round, usually affecting adults and older children but not infants or younger children.[15] The incubation period is 12 to 48 hours, followed by the abrupt onset of nausea and vomiting with or without diarrhea. The duration of illness is usually brief (1 or 2 days).[18]

Astroviral and other caliciviral GE occur most commonly in infants and young children but with less frequency than other viral GE pathogens. Both have been associated with outbreaks in day-care centers and nursing homes and with the ingestion of contaminated water or shellfish.[14,18,20] The important clinical and epidemiologic characteristics of viral GE pathogens are summarized in Table 71.1.

Bacteria

Salmonella species are Gram-negative bacilli of the Enterobacteriaceae family and can be divided into nontyphoidal and typhoidal (*Salmonella typhi*, the causative agent of typhoid fever) species. *Salmonella enteritidis* is the predominant nontyphoidal species, has many serotypes, and is responsible for the majority of cases of *Salmonella*-induced GE. Infection is usually caused by ingestion of contaminated water or food, particularly meat, poultry, or dairy products.[16,21] Other sources include eggs and egg-containing products and certain domestic animals, such as turtles, whose commercial sale in the United States has been prohibited because of their common carriage of this organism.[21] Transmission occurs via the fecal-oral route, and the incubation period is approximately 6 to 48 hours after ingestion. *Salmonella* GE causes watery diarrhea, which often contains blood and mucus and usually abates within 3 to 7 days. Infants less than 6 months of age, human immunodeficiency virus–infected persons, and patients with sickle cell disease are particularly susceptible to disseminated disease following GE. Sequelae can include meningitis, osteomyelitis, myocarditis, and pneumonia.[16,21,22] Chronic carriage of the organism is common, especially in children.[23]

Shigella species are Gram-negative rods that are known to cause GE in humans that is also called bacillary dysentery. Four types of *Shigella* have been implicated: *Shigella sonnei* (most prevalent in industrialized countries), *Shigella flexneri* (most important in the 1920s and 1930s), *Shigella boydii* (uncommon), and *Shigella dysenteriae* (the most virulent, and not commonly seen in developed countries since early in the twentieth century). Because *Shigella* is acid resistant and requires a very small inoculum to cause disease, it is easily transmitted from person to person via the fecal-oral route.[16] *Shigella* infections occur more often in the summer and fall and are the primary cause of bacterial GE in day-care centers.[21,22] Shigellosis tends to be more common in children from 6 months to 10 years of age but can also affect older patient populations.[22,24] Following transmission, the incubation period is 24 to 48 hours. The patient with shigellosis initially has high fever, abdominal cramping, and profuse, watery diarrhea, which lasts about 24 hours. After this period, the diarrhea becomes less frequent and may contain blood and mucus. Illness duration is approximately 4 or 5 days. The most common complication is neurotoxicity with seizures, which occurs in 10 to 40% of infected children.[21]

Campylobacter species are spiral-shaped Gram-negative bacilli known to cause systemic and gastrointestinal illnesses. *Campylobacter jejuni* is the most common species associated with acute GE in humans and is one of the organisms implicated as a cause of traveler's diarrhea.[21] Animal reservoirs of this organism include cattle, sheep,

Table 71.1 ▪ Clinical and Epidemiologic Characteristics of Viral Gastroenteritis

Virus	Epidemiology	Transmission	Incubation	Symptoms	Duration
Rotavirus	Winter peak, endemic/ epidemic	Fecal-oral, food, water	2 days	Watery diarrhea, fever, vomiting	3–8 days
Adenovirus	Year-round; epidemic	Fecal-oral	8–10 days	Diarrhea, fever, vomiting, respiratory symptoms	5–12 days
Norwalk virus	Year-round with winter peak; epidemic	Fecal-oral, shellfish, water	12–48 hours	Nausea, vomiting, with or without diarrhea	1–2 days
irus	Winter peak; epidemic	Fecal-oral, shellfish, water	1–2 days	Mild diarrhea, fever, vomiting	2–3 days
s	Year-round; epidemic	Fecal-oral, shellfish, water	1–4 days	Mild diarrhea, fever, vomiting	4–5 days

swine, fowl, cats, and dogs. *Campylobacter* GE is more common in the summer and has a bimodal infection frequency, occurring mostly in children less than 1 year old and in young adults.[16,21] Outbreaks have been associated with contaminated water, raw meat, poultry, clams, and unpasteurized dairy products or contact with young dogs or cats.[24] Transmission is by the fecal-oral route followed by an incubation period of 1 to 7 days. Initial symptoms are fever, headache, and myalgias that last for 12 to 24 hours. Acute GE symptoms ensue with abdominal cramping, fever, and a secretory diarrhea that may contain mucus and blood.[16,22] Symptoms often resolve within 5 to 7 days but in severe cases may persist for several weeks.

Escherichia coli is a Gram-negative rod that is a common inhabitant of the human gastrointestinal tract. GE can be caused by five different types of the organism. There are different virulence properties among the types, some of which may overlap. The primary types are enterotoxigenic *E. coli* (ETEC) and enterohemorrhagic *E. coli* (EHEC). Less common, but equally important, are enteropathogenic *E. coli* (EPEC), enteroaggregative *E. coli* (EaggEC), and enteroinvasive *E. coli* (EIEC).[26]

ETEC is the predominant cause of traveler's diarrhea in adults and infantile diarrhea in developing countries. It has also been associated with outbreaks caused by ingestion of contaminated food or water. Both ETEC and *Shigella* were responsible for the majority of GE cases experienced by U.S. troops during Operation Desert Shield.[27] ETEC symptoms such as low-grade fever, abdominal cramping, and watery diarrhea follow a 1- to 3-day incubation period.[28] Illness usually remits in approximately 3 to 5 days.

EHEC may cause diarrhea, hemorrhagic colitis, hemolytic uremic syndrome (HUS), and postdiarrheal thrombotic thrombocytopenic purpura. *Escherichia coli* O157:H7 is the best-described strain in this class to date. Since its discovery in 1983, it has received much public and scientific attention as a result of several deaths in outbreaks linked to ingestion of contaminated hamburger meat and contaminated swimming water.[29,30] The incubation period is 3 to 4 days, at which time patients experience some abdominal pain and fever. Within 1 or 2 days, nonbloody diarrhea follows and may be accompanied by vomiting. The diarrhea becomes bloody within 1 or 2 more days and usually lasts about 4 to 10 days. Approximately 10% of *E. coli* O157:H7 infections in children less than 10 years old progress to HUS. If it occurs, HUS will develop within 1 week after the onset of diarrhea. Complications of HUS include seizures, stroke, renal failure, hypertension, glucose intolerance, and death.[26]

Yersinia enterocolitica is another Gram-negative coccobacillus that causes GE in both children and adults. It is a major cause of bacterial GE in Europe and Canada with a preference for colder climates. It is thought to be an important but underrecognized pathogen in the United States as well. Modes of transmission include ingestion of contaminated foods (particularly pork and pork products), water, and unpasteurized milk. Symptoms of *Yersinia* GE are abdominal pain, vomiting, fever, and blood-streaked diarrhea. The illness may last 7 to 21 days, with continued excretion of the organism for weeks after symptoms subside.[31,32]

Other miscellaneous Gram-negative organisms have been reported to cause clinical GE in certain patient groups. *Vibrio* species are a cause of GE in the United States and around the world. The primary pathogenic species are *Vibrio cholerae* (the causative agent of cholera) and *Vibrio parahaemolyticus*. Of interest and great concern is the significant emergence of cholera on the North American and particularly the South American and Indian continents.[33] Noncholera *Vibrio*, *Aeromonas*, and *Plesiomonas* species share an association with water. Infection due to these organisms is usually linked with the ingestion of raw or undercooked seafood, often shellfish, or contaminated water.[31,34] The important clinical and epidemiologic characteristics of bacterial GE pathogens are summarized in Table 71.2.

Other Pathogens

Other organisms such as *Isospora*, *Cyclospora*, and *Aerobacter* have emerged as potential human GE pathogens. These organisms may be transmitted fecally or via contaminated water or food and will often cause more severe and symptomatic disease in immunocompromised individuals.[35–37] Although agents such as *Campylobacter upsaliensis* and Torovirus have been associated with GE illness in humans, their true role as enteropathogens remains to be determined.[38,39]

PATHOPHYSIOLOGY

Host Defenses

There are four well-established host defense mechanisms against enteric pathogens: (1) gastric acidity, (2) peristalsis, (3) resident microflora, and (4) immune response. Most pathogens do not reach the intestine because of the highly acidic environment of the stomach. They may survive if they are acid resistant (e.g., *Shigella*) or if a large inoculum of organism is ingested.[16] Food, achlorhydria, gastric resection, or iatrogenic factors, such as antacids, H_2 antagonists, or H^+/K^+ ATPase inhibitors, may reduce gastric pH and increase the risk of GE in certain patients. Slowed intestinal motility may allow colonization and increased contact time of enteropathogens with the intestinal mucosa. Motility may be impaired by antiperistaltic compounds such as diphenoxylate or loperamide or by underlying diseases such as stroke or diabetes.[40] Antibiotics (especially broad-spectrum compounds) decrease normal flora of the gastrointestinal tract and allow overgrowth of pathogenic or colonizing nosocomial organisms known to cause GE.

Finally, immature or compromised immune status predisposes patients to enteric infections. Conversely, active or passive immunity (e.g., antibodies in breast-milk) aids in the prevention of GE.[41,42] Immune responses to GE organisms have been and continue to be the focus of

Table 71.2 ▪ Clinical and Epidemiologic Characteristics of Bacterial Gastroenteritis

Bacteria	Transmission	Incubation	Symptoms	Duration	Complications
Salmonella spp.	Fecal-oral; eggs, milk, meat, turtles	6–48 hours	Watery, mucoid, bloody diarrhea	3–7 days	Osteomyelitis, meningitis, pneumonia, myocarditis
Shigella spp.	Fecal-oral; food, water	24–48 hours	Fever, diarrhea, cramping	4–5 days	Seizures, HUS
Campylobacter spp.	Fecal-oral; water, dairy, meat, pets	1–7 days	Fever, cramping, secretory diarrhea	5–7 days	None (with *C. jejuni*)
ETEC	Fecal-oral; food, water	1–3 days	Watery diarrhea, cramping	3–5 days	None
EHEC	Fecal-oral; hamburger, waste	3–4 days	Fever, vomiting, bloody diarrhea	4–10 days	HUS, TTP, seizures, renal failure, stroke
Yersinia spp.	Fecal-oral; water, milk, pork	2–11 days	Fever, diarrhea, abdominal pain	1–3 days	Bacteremia, ileitis, arthritis
Vibrio cholerae	Fecal-oral; water, shellfish	6–48 hours	Profuse, watery diarrhea	5–7 days	Renal failure, acidosis, hypoglycemia

EHEC, enterohemorrhagic *Escherichia coli; ETEC,* enterotoxigenic *Escherichia coli; HUS,* hemolytic uremic syndrome; *TTP,* thrombotic thrombocytopenic purpura.

Table 71.3 ▪ Pathogenic Mechanisms of Enteric Organisms

	Rotavirus	Norwalk	*Salmonella* spp.	*Shigella* spp.	*Escherichia coli*	*Vibrio* spp.	*Campylobacter* spp.
Increased secretion							
Enterotoxins			+		+	+	
Prostaglandins			+			+	
Crypt proliferation	+	+					
Decreased absorption							
Villi destruction	+	+			+	+	
Cytotoxins				+	+		+
Epithelial invasion			+	+		+	+
Altered transit		+?	+	+	+		+

Source: References 47, 48, 49.

intense research efforts to develop effective and inexpensive methods of prophylaxis against GE illnesses. The reader is referred to several excellent articles on the subject of vaccine use and development for bacterial and viral enteric pathogens.[43–46]

Virulence Mechanisms of Enteropathogens

One of the main functions of the small intestine and colon is the absorption and secretion of fluids, ions, and nutrients. These processes take place in the villus-crypt units that line the small intestinal mucosa. GE pathogens impair absorption, increase secretion, or both. The result is too much water in the stool or diarrhea.[47]

Water absorption occurs passively and is linked to two pathways of active sodium transport. The first pathway involves an Na^+/Cl^- cotransport mechanism that is inhibited by cyclic adenosine monophosphate (cAMP) or GMP. Some GE pathogens produce toxins that lead to elevated cAMP levels. The result is reduced Na^+ and water absorption and increased Cl^- secretion and, ultimately, more water and electrolyte volume in the stool and diarrhea.[47,48] The second pathway involves an Na^+/nutrient (e.g., glucose, amino acids) cotransport mechanism, which is very important in understanding the treatment of diarrhea. Administering a glucose-containing solution promotes sodium and water absorption via this pathway and aids in rehydration of the patient with diarrhea.[47]

Other means by which GE pathogens are able to cause diarrhea include (1) destruction of intestinal surface villi that results in increased secretion of water and electrolytes; (2) production of enterotoxins and secretogogues (e.g., prostaglandins, interleukins), which stimulate secretion; (3) damage and ulceration of the intestinal epithelium with leakage of serous fluid, blood, and cells into the lumen; and (4) altered intestinal myoelectric activity and transit secondary to enterotoxins, cytotoxins, or organism invasion.[47,48] A summary of the organisms with their associated pathogenic mechanisms is provided in Table 71.3.

CLINICAL PRESENTATION AND DIAGNOSIS

Signs and Symptoms

GE syndromes can be classified as either inflammatory or noninflammatory. Inflammatory GE is characterized by fever and abdominal cramping with small-volume, bloody, mucoid diarrhea. Microscopic stool examination often reveals the presence of numerous fecal leukocytes. This is indicative of cytotoxin-induced damage and organism invasion of the colonic mucosa that causes blood, serous fluid, and white blood cells to leak into the lumen.[16,47] Inflammatory diarrheal illnesses often are more severe and may cause systemic symptoms such as vasculitic rashes, arthritis, and bacteremia.[47,49,50]

Noninflammatory GE is characterized by low-grade fever; nausea and vomiting; and large-volume, watery diarrhea. In contrast to inflammatory GE, diarrhea is the result of nondestructive pathogenic mechanisms (e.g., enterotoxin, altered transit) that primarily affect absorptive and secretory processes. Therefore, no cellular components, such as red or white blood cells, should be present on microscopic stool examination because of the lack of intestinal epithelial damage.[16,47]

Diagnosis

A careful history, including recent travel, medications (including antibiotic use), family or other contact illnesses, weight loss, recent food or water ingestion, and underlying diseases, should be obtained. Evaluation of the appearance, quantity, and duration of the diarrhea is also important. Direct examination of a stool specimen for blood, mucus, and leukocytes is preferable to a description of the stool by the patient. With these data and knowledge of the epidemiology and setting of likely GE organisms, a presumptive causative agent can usually be identified. Stool cultures may be useful in diagnosis but should be reserved for unresponsive diarrheal illness, immunocompromised patients, or patients with signs of inflammatory or systemic disease. The presence of leukocytes, lactoferrin, or blood in the stool may be helpful in predicting a positive culture result as well.[4] Stool cultures are costly and should be appropriately requested in order to isolate suspected pathogens that require special media and procedures.[16] Studies have shown that the positivity rate of stool cultures is 2% or less, resulting in a cost of between $900 and $1200 for each pathogen detected.[4] The only commercially available viral diagnostic tool is a rapid group A rotaviral antigen test.[19] Testing for other viral enteropathogens must be performed in a research or specialty laboratory.

Because fluid and nutritional therapies are the cornerstone of GE management, physical assessment of signs of dehydration and electrolyte abnormalities is crucial. In children and some adults, evaluation of the degree of dehydration includes assessment of objective signs (skin turgor, mucous membranes, sunken eyes or fontanelle, pulse, blood pressure, urine output, capillary refill time, absent tears) and subjective signs (mental status, thirst, lethargy, extremities).[51] Table 71.4 lists the physical signs associated with differing degrees of dehydration. It is important to note that the signs and symptoms of dehydration in older adults may be vague, or even absent. Such factors as underlying mental status, concomitant medications (i.e., antihypertensives, anticholinergics), and poor intake can confound evaluation of clinical signs such as skin turgor, pulse, and blood pressure.[52] The health care provider should know when other diagnostic procedures, such as radiologic or endoscopic evaluations, are necessary and refer patients quickly to the appropriate medical source. Information on the differential diagnosis of infectious and noninfectious diarrhea can be found elsewhere.[6]

TREATMENT

Nonpharmacologic Therapy

The cornerstone of treatment for all types of infectious GE is fluid and electrolyte replacement. Therapy consists of two phases: (1) the rehydration phase, in which water and electrolytes are given to replace existing losses, and (2) the

Table 71.4 ▪ Clinical Assessment and Management of Diarrhea in Children

Degree of Dehydration	Signs[a]	Rehydration Therapy (within 4 hours)	Replacement of Stool Fluid Losses	Dietary Therapy[b]
Mild (3–5%)	Slightly dry buccal membranes, slightly increased thirst	ORS[c] 50 mL/kg	10 mL/kg or ½ to 1 cup of ORS for each diarrheal stool	Breast milk, half- or full-strength milk or formula
Moderate (6–9%)	Sunken eyes or fontanelle, poor skin turgor, dry buccal membranes, increased thirst	ORS 100 mL/kg	Same as above	Same as above
Severe (≥10%)	Signs of moderate dehydration with one of the following: rapid thready pulse, cyanosis, cold extremities, rapid breathing, lethargy, coma	IV fluids (Ringer's lactate), 20 mL/kg/hr until pulse, perfusion, and mental status return to normal; then 50–100 mL/kg of ORS	Same as above	Same as above

Source: Reference 51.

[a]If patient exhibits no signs of dehydration, rehydration therapy is not indicated. Begin maintenance therapy and replacement of stool losses.

[b]Early refeeding is recommended. Children who tolerate solid food can continue their usual diet, but foods high in simple sugars and fats should be avoided.

[c]Oral rehydration solution.

maintenance phase, which includes both replacement of ongoing fluid and electrolyte losses and adequate dietary intake.[51] Fluid may be given by the oral or intravenous (IV) route. The degree of dehydration and the patient's age and ability to maintain oral intake determine the method of fluid repletion to be used.

Oral rehydration therapy (ORT) is preferred in all cases of mild to moderate dehydration and for the prevention of subsequent dehydration.[16] ORT is as effective in achieving rehydration and provides several advantages compared with IV therapy.[22] ORT is less invasive, less costly, and less likely to result in overhydration, and it allows for rapid institution of therapy in the home setting.[18,53,54] It has revolutionized the management of infectious GE in endemic areas but, for reasons that are unclear, remains greatly underused in developed countries such as the United States.[16,55] Possible explanations for this reluctance include caregiver or health provider inconvenience, risk of iatrogenic hypernatremia, presence of vomiting, and lack of third-party reimbursement for home or office-based ORT versus IV hydration and hospitalization.[56]

Indications for the use of IV hydration are severe dehydration (10% or greater fluid deficit), hypovolemic shock, or inability to take oral therapy (e.g., coma, uncontrolled vomiting, ileus). Less than 2% of community cases and less than 10% of patients requiring medical attention meet the criteria for IV therapy.[16] Two populations are at greatest risk from dehydration and may require IV hydration more frequently: infants, who have a higher surface area to fluid volume ratio, and older adults, who may experience more serious sequelae as a result of concomitant atherosclerotic disease.[22,40] When indicated, IV therapy should consist of an isotonic solution (such as Ringer's lactate) and be infused within 4 to 6 hours.[16] Sodium, potassium, and bicarbonate should be carefully monitored and replaced appropriately based on measured losses and serum concentrations. Table 71.4 indicates the clinical signs and appropriate treatments associated with different degrees of dehydration for patients with GE.

The choice of which oral rehydration solution (ORS) to use in the management of GE-induced diarrhea is an important one. The optimal ORS should be isotonic and contain adequate amounts of water, sodium, potassium, and bicarbonate. Glucose is also a necessary component to enhance sodium and water absorption via mucosal glucose/sodium cotransport mechanisms. Other carbohydrates, such as fructose and sucrose, can also be used but may be less effective.[57] In 1975, the World Health Organization (WHO) and the United Nations International Children's Emergency Fund (UNICEF) developed a single ORS formula for use in treating diarrhea.[51] This ORS contains (in mmol/L): sodium, 90; potassium, 20; chloride, 80; citrate, 30; and glucose, 111 (2%). It is available in packets for easy mixture; it has been shown to be effective in the management of diarrhea; and it has dramatically reduced the number of dehydration-related deaths in developing countries since its institution. Several premixed oral rehydration solutions are commercially available and are listed in Table 71.5. The American Academy of Pediatrics (AAP) recommends that solutions used for rehydration contain 75 to 90 mEq/L of sodium and those for hydration maintenance or prevention of dehydration contain 40 to 60 mEq/L of sodium, to prevent hypernatremia.[54] An ORS with 75 to 90 mEq/L should always be used in the setting of highly purging diarrhea (e.g., greater than 10 mL/kg/hr) and, when used for maintenance, should be administered with other low-sodium fluids (e.g., breast milk, formula, water).[51] It should be noted that "clear liquids" often found in the home, such as cola, ginger ale, fruit juice, chicken broth, and Gatorade, are not recommended for treatment. These solutions often contain excess sugar and inadequate

Table 71.5 ▪ Comparison of Oral Rehydration Solutions

Oral Rehydration Solution	Carbohydrate Concentration (g/L)	Carbohydrate Source	Sodium (mEq/L)	Potassium (mEq/L)	Chloride (mEq/L)	Base (mEq/L)
WHO-ORS	20	Glucose	90	20	80	30
Rehydralyte	25	Glucose	75	20	65	30
Pedialyte	25	Glucose	45	20	35	30
Infalyte	30	Rice syrup	50	20	40	34
Lytren	20	Glucose	50	25	45	30
Ricelyte	–	Starch polymers	50	25	45	34
Hydra-Lyte	12	Glucose	84	10	59	20
Generic pediatric solution	25	Glucose	45	20	35	30
Resol	20	Glucose	50	20	50	34
Rice based	50	Starch (rice)	60–90	20	80	30

Source: References 16, 22, 40.

WHO-ORS, World Health Organization's oral rehydration solution.

bicarbonate and electrolytes and can cause osmotic diarrhea.[51,55] However, they can be used for prevention of dehydration and in milder cases of diarrhea. Free water alone should always be avoided, because this may result in hyponatremia. If compliance related to poor palatability (very salty) of the ORS formulations is a problem, practical solutions include feeding in small amounts, adding flavoring agents, or freezing the solution in an ice-pop form.[54]

Other substrates have been investigated for use in ORS formulas. Cereal-based oral rehydration solutions deliver larger amounts of carbohydrates to the lumen than glucose-based solutions and are able to further increase fluid absorption without an increase in osmotic load. Rice-based solutions have been found to be equally effective, with reduced duration and volume of diarrhea.[16,58] Early reinstitution of feeding after rehydration can provide similar benefits.[54] Health care providers should be familiar with the different available ORS products and their appropriate uses and should encourage parents of young children to have a supply of ORS at home at all times for early use when diarrhea occurs.[51]

Although the past standard of practice has been to withhold food until diarrhea is resolved, recommendations now are to institute feeding within the first 24 hours of the onset of diarrhea or as soon as possible after rehydration.[54] Data suggest that early feeding reduces the severity and duration of diarrhea, aids in intestinal mucosa repair, and prevents malnutrition.[54,59] For infants, breast milk or full-strength formula can be used. In fact, breast milk is preferred because of its lower osmolality and enzyme, hormonal, and antimicrobial content.[60] For older children, a regular diet should be resumed consisting of frequent but small amounts of complex carbohydrates (cereal, rice, potatoes, bread), lean meats, yogurt, vegetables, and fresh fruits.[51,54] In general, sorbitol-containing foods, caffeine, and foods high in simple sugars or fat should be avoided. It is necessary to avoid lactose-containing liquids or foods only if lactose intolerance is known, because full-strength milk is tolerated by 80% or more of children with acute diarrhea. A balanced, mixed diet is preferred over more restrictive diets such as the frequently recommended bananas, rice, apple sauce, and toast (BRAT) diet, which is low in energy, protein, and fat.[54,59]

Pharmacotherapy

Antidiarrheal Agents

In general, there are few data to support the utility of the antidiarrheal agents in the management of infectious GE in adults or children. The benefits and risks of antidiarrheal therapy in treating infectious GE depend on the particular product, the infectious agent, and the age of the patient. Indeed, it could be argued that diarrhea is itself a host defense mechanism, designed to expel the pathogen, and should not be suppressed. Use of antidiarrheal agents, when indicated, should in no way interfere with or shift the focus from appropriate fluid, electrolyte, and nutritional therapy.

Antimotility agents such as tincture of opium, diphenoxylate-atropine, and loperamide may reduce the frequency of stool in milder cases of GE seen in adults and older children in developed countries. However, risks associated with these agents include side effects (atropinism, sedation, lethargy), ileus, toxic megacolon, and increased bowel wall invasion and organism excretion.[47,61] Antimotility agents should not be given to infants, older adults, or any patient with an inflammatory, bloody diarrhea, usually indicating infection with an invasive pathogen.[40,61] In cases of mild to moderate diarrhea, particularly traveler's diarrhea, loperamide may be useful in reducing the duration of symptoms. When indicated, the regimen to be used is loperamide 4 mg as a single dose, then 2 mg after each loose stool, not to exceed 16 mg/day. Loperamide is available over the counter in liquid, capsule, and tablet forms and is preferred over, and generally better tolerated than, other antimotility agents.[4,62]

Kaolin-pectin suspension and attapulgite add bulk and produce firmer stools, but they do not reduce stool volume.[47] Additionally, although these agents are not absorbed and have few side effects, they may adsorb other substances or medications in the gastrointestinal tract if taken concomitantly. Bismuth subsalicylate (BSS) demonstrates antimicrobial activity against enteropathogens such as *E. coli*, *Salmonella*, *Shigella*, and *Campylobacter* and is effective in treating traveler's diarrhea.[63] Other potential mechanisms for its efficacy include antisecretory activity, enterotoxin inactivation, and prevention of bacterial attachment to intestinal mucosa.[61] The regimen for BSS is 30 mL every 30 minutes up to 8 doses. An alternative regimen is 2 tablets 4 times daily. The primary side effect of BSS is blackening of the tongue and the stool (which can be confused with melena). Tinnitus, encephalopathy, and salicylate toxicity have been reported with chronic use. Patients with hypersensitivity to aspirin or who are taking oral anticoagulants should not be treated with BSS.[61,63] Certain formulations of BSS also contain calcium carbonate, which should not be taken with selected antibiotics (i.e., tetracyclines, quinolones). Although BSS has been shown to be a safe and effective adjunct to ORT for infants and children, there still may be some concern, if only theoretical, over the potential development of Reye's syndrome.[54,64]

Antimicrobial Therapy

There are no effective antimicrobial agents for viral GE. The use of antibiotics to treat bacterial GE depends on the infecting organism, the severity and chronicity of the infectious process, and the effectiveness of the antibiotic in reducing the severity or carrier state of the illness. Because many of the GE infections experienced by ambulatory patients are self-limiting, antibiotic therapy is not routinely recommended unless the infection is severe or disseminated or the patient is chronically symptomatic, debilitated, or immunocompromised.

One of the important considerations in deciding whether to use antimicrobial therapy for GE, and then which one to use, is the development or presence of antimicrobial resistance. The indiscriminate use of antibiotics in humans and animals is clearly related to the development and prevalence of multiresistant strains of pathogenic organisms. Multiresistant *Salmonella*, *Shigella*, and ETEC have been associated with epidemics in developing countries.[65,66] Therefore, the choice to institute antimicrobial therapy in the face of a normally self-limiting disease such as GE should be made cautiously. Antimicrobial resistance varies widely; changes with time; and depends on the agent, organism strain, and the year or specific geographical location. When needed, antibiotics must be chosen carefully with knowledge of susceptibility patterns of the likely pathogen and area, prior therapy, and the patient's condition, in order to minimize the potential for side effects and the development of resistance. The Internet can provide up-to-date information and recommendations regarding prophylaxis and treatment of travel-related infections for patients and health care providers.[67]

The primary goals of antibiotic therapy in the management of infectious GE are to decrease the duration of symptomatic illness, prevent complications, and reduce the excretion of pathogenic organisms and further spread of disease.[68] The utility of such therapy depends on the specific organism involved and the timely institution of therapy. Antibiotics appear to be of most value in *Shigella*, ETEC, cholera, and *Campylobacter* infections and of least value in *Salmonella* and *Yersinia* GE. They may be of some value in noncholera *Vibrio*, *Aeromonas*, and *Plesiomonas* infections in certain patients. Table 71.6 lists the drug(s) of choice by causative agent and the conditions under which antibiotic therapy is considered most appropriate. Table 71.7 lists the usual drug, dose, side effect, and monitoring parameters by drug entity for agents used in the management of infectious GE.

Ampicillin and amoxicillin are effective agents for GE caused by ampicillin-sensitive strains of *Shigella* or *Salmonella*. Therapy for *Shigella* infections has been shown to be beneficial in decreasing the duration and severity of diarrhea and is generally recommended.[4] In contrast, treatment of *Salmonella* GE does not demonstrate these benefits but may be useful in systemic or disseminated infections.[4,69] Ampicillin and amoxicillin are available orally, are well tolerated, and can be given to both adults and children.

Tetracycline or doxycycline has been successfully used to treat GE caused by *Shigella*, ETEC, and *V. cholerae*. However, resistance of these organisms to tetracycline has been increasing, to the point that it can be used as an alternative agent or when susceptibility data are available.[24] Tetracycline should not be given to pregnant women or children under age 12 years because of the potential for unwanted, permanent staining of teeth. It is also associated with photosensitivity reactions, probably secondary to skin accumulation. Patients taking tetracycline should be advised to take appropriate precautions (e.g., sunscreen) when exposed to sunlight. Doxycycline may be preferred over tetracycline because it is better tolerated, is given less frequently, requires no adjustment for renal impairment, and is available in both oral and IV formulations.

Chloramphenicol has been used to treat systemic *Salmonella* and *Campylobacter* infections caused by susceptible strains, although it is not considered first-line therapy for either pathogen. Although rare, bone marrow suppression, both dose related and idiosyncratic, has been associated with chloramphenicol. If used, judicious monitoring of all hematopoietic cell lines is necessary to limit toxicity. Chloramphenicol serum concentrations should be less than 25 mg/L to reduce the probability of dose-related bone marrow suppression.

Trimethoprim/sulfamethoxazole (TMP/SMX) remains an important drug in the armamentarium used to treat bacterial GE. It is effective as either first- or second-line therapy in GE caused by ETEC, *Aeromonas*, *Plesiomonas*, *Shigella*, and ampicillin-resistant *Salmonella* infections.[4,63] TMP/SMX may cause rash, vomiting, fever, Stevens-Johnson syndrome, hemolytic anemia, nephrotoxicity, and bone marrow suppression. It is less likely than tetracycline to cause photosensitivity reactions when used

Table 71.6 ▪ Antibiotics of Choice for Bacterial Gastroenteritis

Organism	Indication	Drug(s) of Choice	Alternative Drugs
Salmonella spp.	Disseminated disease or high-risk patient	TMP/SMX, FQ	Amox, Amp, Chloro, TG ceph
Shigella spp.	Gastroenteritis (dysentery)	TMP/SMX, FQ	Amp, Tetra, Azithro
Campylobacter spp.	Gastroenteritis, bacteria	FQ, Norflox, Azithro	Chloro, Doxy
ETEC	Moderate to severe traveler's diarrhea	TMP/SMX, FQ	Norflox, Doxy
Vibrio cholerae	Gastroenteritis	FQ, Doxy	TMP/SMX, Chloro, Erythro
Yersinia spp.	Bacteremia	FQ, Norflox	Doxy, TMP/SMX, TG ceph, Chloro, Gent
Aeromonas spp.[a]	Persistent diarrhea	TMP/SMX	FQ, Norflox, Chloro, Tetra, Gent, TG ceph
Plesiomonas spp.[a]	GE	TMP/SMX	FQ, Chloro, Doxy

Source: References 72, 73.

Amox, amoxicillan; *Amp,* ampicillin; *Azithro,* azithromycin; *Chloro,* chloramphenicol; *Clinda,* clindamycin; *Doxy,* doxycycline; *Erythro,* erythromycin; *ETEC,* enterotoxigenic *Escherichia coli; FQ,* fluoroquinolone (ciprofloxacin, ofloxacin, etc., except norfloxacin); *Gent,* gentamicin; *Norflox,* norfloxacin; *Tetra,* tetracycline hydrochloride; *TG ceph,* third-generation cephalosporin; *TMP/SMX,* trimethoprim–sulfamethoxazole.

[a]Strain-specific susceptibility testing should be used to guide treatment.

Table 71.7 ▪ Antibiotic Dosing and Monitoring Data

Drug	Dosage	Adverse Effects	Monitoring Parameters
Ampicillin	Adult: 500 mg q6hr or 50–100 mg/kg/day Children: 50–200 mg/kg/day	Rash (3%), diarrhea, nausea (10%) Hypersensitivity, hematologic—less common	Skin changes (rash onset 4–5 days) GI: assess changes in symptoms despite cure of infection
Trimethoprim–sulfamethoxazole (TMP/SMX) Cotrimoxazole	Adult: TMP/SMX, 160 mg (TMP) q12h Children >6 weeks: TMP/SMX, 5 mg/kg TMP	Rash (5%), Stevens-Johnson syndrome (rare), bone marrow suppression (anemia, neutropenia), nephrotoxicity; increased incidence of adverse effects in patients with AIDS	Skin changes: progressive rash with periorbital or oral blisters may indicate Stevens-Johnson syndrome—discontinue drug Hematologic: CBC with differential platelet count Nephrotoxicity: serum creatinine, urine output
Tetracycline HCl	Adult: 250–500 mg QID Children >12 years: 25–30 mg/kg/day divided QID Do not give with drugs or food containing divalent or trivalent cations—Fe, Ca, Mg, Al	Nausea, vomiting, epigastric pain (common) Photosensitivity, antianabolic effect aggravates uremia	GI: assess changes in symptoms despite cure of infection Photosensitivity: apply sunscreen
Doxycycline	Adult: 100 mg QD or BID Children >12 years: 4–5 mg/kg/day in 2 doses on first day, followed by 2–2.5 mg/kg in 2 doses	Dental and bone effects (permanent staining of teeth least likely with doxycycline), hematologic reactions, hepatoxicity (rare, results in fatty infiltration of the liver)	Hematologic: CBC, platelet count
Erythromycin	Adult: 250–500 mg QID Children: 30–50 mg/kg/day divided QID	Nausea, vomiting, abdominal cramping (15–60%), hepatotoxicity (cholestatic jaundice; estolate most, ethyl succinate least), reversible ototoxicity with high IV doses; inhibitor of cP450 hepatic metabolism of theophylline, cyclosporine, warfarin; increases bioavailability of digoxin	GI: assess changes in symptoms despite cure of infection Hepatic: monitor liver transaminases, total bilirubin Drug interactions: monitor theophylline, cyclosporine and digoxin levels; monitor INR (or PT) to assess warfarin pharmacodynamics
Azithromycin	Adult: 500 mg × 1, 250 mg QD Children: 10 mg/kg × 1 loading dose, then 5 mg/kg QD Do not give with food—bioavailability reduced 50%	Nausea, vomiting, abdominal cramping (3–5%); hepatotoxicity and ototoxicity uncommon; inhibitor of cP450 hepatic metabolism	Same as erythromycin
Chloramphenicol	Adult: 500 mg QID Children: 25–100 mg/kg/day divided QID	Nausea, vomiting, diarrhea: aplastic anemia (1 in 500–100,000 patients treated, irreversible), gray syndrome (infants and children), bone marrow suppression (dose related); inhibits metabolism of tolbutamide, phenytoin, dicumarol	GI: assess changes in symptoms despite cure of infection Hematologic: CBC with differential, reticulocyte count Monitor serum levels with dosage adjustment Drug interactions: monitor phenytoin levels
Ciprofloxacin Norfloxacin Ofloxacin	Adult: 500–700 mg BID 400 mg BID 200–400 mg BID Children: not recommended Do not give orally with drugs or food containing divalent or trivalent cations—Fe, Ca, Mg, Al	Nausea, vomiting, diarrhea (5%), CNS (headache, dizziness, tremors, restlessness more common with elderly and renally impaired)	GI: assess changes in symptoms despite cure of infection CNS: evaluate changes in mental status, consider reduced dosage in elderly and renally impaired Drug interactions: monitor theophylline levels

AIDS, acquired immunodeficiency syndrome; *CBC*, complete blood cell count; *CNS*, central nervous system; *GI*, gastrointestinal; *INR*, international normalized ratio; *PT*, prothrombin time.

in the management of traveler's diarrhea. Because of its significant tubular secretion in the kidney, dosing adjustments for renal dysfunction are needed. Additionally, TMP/SMX may compete with creatinine for excretion by this pathway and cause a slight, but clinically insignificant, elevation in serum creatinine values.

Macrolides, such as erythromycin or azithromycin, are considered either first- or second-line therapy for treating infectious GE caused by *C. jejuni,* depending on the geographical susceptibility patterns of the organism. Erythromycin and azithromycin are available in both oral and IV forms. Intravenous therapy may be necessary in cases of disseminated disease. The major adverse effect associated with macrolides is gastrointestinal intolerance, typically manifested by nausea and abdominal cramping, which can be seen with both oral and IV formulations. Azithromycin has a more favorable pharmacokinetic profile, allowing once-daily dosing, and is generally better tolerated than erythromycin. Reversible cholestatic jaundice has been seen with erythromycin, primarily with the estolate salt of the drug. Liver transaminases should be monitored in patients receiving either erythromycin or azithromycin. Reversible hearing loss and phlebitis may be seen with the IV form of erythromycin as well.

The fluoroquinolones have become the drugs of choice for treatment of most bacterial organisms causing infectious GE.[4,63] Nalidixic acid was the first quinolone used to treat GE infections. Other, newer fluoroquinolones, such as ciprofloxacin, norfloxacin, and ofloxacin, have been shown to be effective in treating GE infections due to *Shigella, Salmonella, Campylobacter, E. coli, Yersinia,* and *Vibrio.* In general, these agents reduce the duration of the illness by 24 hours and may reduce associated complications and mortality rates as well.[70,71] The broad-spectrum activity of these agents and concern over resistance to other drugs has led to the widespread prophylactic and empiric use of fluoroquinolones for GE. The result has been the alarming increase in fluoroquinolone resistance of several important GE pathogens, such as *Salmonella, E. coli,* and *Campylobacter,* in several countries. Some have suggested a link between this increased resistance among human pathogens to the veterinary use of quinolones.[71] Given these concerns, the decision to use this important, and still very effective, class of antibiotics should be made carefully to preserve its value in the management of GE and other serious infectious diseases.

Regimens for the fluoroquinolones vary based on the organism and severity of the disease. Dosages of ciprofloxacin, norfloxacin, and ofloxacin range from 500 to 1000 mg, 400 mg, and 200 mg, respectively, with frequencies of a single dose, once or twice daily.[4,63,72] These agents are not approved for use in children or pregnant women because of concern over the development of arthropathy. Quinolones have been used safely in children and pregnancy for multiple indications when no alternative therapies were viable; however, their routine use for treatment of GE in these populations is not justified.[71] Other side effects reported with quinolones include gastrointestinal upset, rash, and dizziness.

Other antibiotics having activity against enteropathogens that can be used as alternative agents include some oral and IV cephalosporins, amoxicillin-clavulanic acid, aztreonam, and aminoglycosides.[21,31,72,73]

ALTERNATIVE THERAPIES

The use of biotherapeutic (or probiotic) agents, vitamin A, and zinc as treatments for diarrhea has been investigated. Probiotic therapy consists of administering organisms such as *Lactobacillus* or *Bifidobacterium* to favorably alter the intestinal flora and normalize intestinal function. The data are inconsistent regarding the efficacy of such therapy to date. Similarly, some studies of vitamin A and zinc treatment for diarrhea have demonstrated efficacy, whereas others have not. Further research is needed to determine the value of these therapies in the management of patients with infectious GE.[54,59,74,75]

FUTURE THERAPIES

Future directions for treatment of infectious GE will focus on prophylaxis through use and development of vaccines, investigation of new antidiarrheals (e.g., zaldaride, berberine derivatives, α_2-adrenergic agonists, prostaglandin and leukotriene antagonists, chloride channel blockers, calmodulin inhibitors, enkephalinase inhibitors, and newer somatostatin analogues), and further defining the roles of probiotics, vitamin A, and zinc as adjunct therapies.[54,62,76]

IMPROVING OUTCOMES

Given the continued prevalence and substantial morbidity and mortality associated with infectious GE, it is clear that improvements can be made in its prevention and treatment. One group of authors has eloquently reviewed and identified the areas of health care and outcomes that must be improved related to GE in the United States. Documented contributing factors to GE-related mortality in the United States include lack of parental knowledge of the signs and importance of dehydration, limited access to care, inadequate treatment by physicians, and poor community hygiene. Paradoxically, there are also data to suggest that some children are hospitalized unnecessarily and that IV therapy and medications are overused. One study cited by these authors estimated the average cost per GE case for children under age 3 years to be $289, which annualizes to between 0.6 and 1.0 billion dollars. Contributing factors to overutilization include overestimation of the degree of dehydration by physicians, inappropriate recommendations from physicians to delay feeding and ORT secondary to vomiting, and use of therapies by physicians (IV over ORT, antibiotics, antidiarrheals) in contrast to medical literature and expert opinion. Other reasons cited include financial constraints, office staff training, and reimbursement considerations. These factors related to underuse, overuse, and inappropriate use of therapies for GE affect all of the therapeutic goals for this disease. Further information must be obtained regarding the reasons for and influences on physician and parental practices and the impact on patient outcomes.[77] Such information should assist in the development of interventions targeted toward more cost-effective and appropriate management of GE in the United States. The Pediatric Gastroenteritis Patient Outcomes Research Project is conducting a study of the effectiveness and safety of home GE treatment in patients treated in a variety of settings.[56]

In most cases, educational efforts should be directed at the caregivers, not the patients, because many of the patients are children. Parents or adult patients should receive education regarding signs of dehydration or worsening condition, advice on use or avoidance of antibiotics or antidiarrheal medications, administering ORT (type, duration, amount), directions for refeeding, recommendations for appropriate (and inappropriate) foods or fluids, and instructions for skin care and good hygiene to prevent further transmission.[19] Several national and local medical associations (e.g., AAP) provide patient care instructions for parents on the Internet.

KEY POINTS

- Infectious GE remains a significant cause of morbidity and mortality worldwide. Most cases of GE are viral, are self-limiting in nature, and may be endemic or cause outbreaks related to contaminated water or food.
- GE-associated diarrhea results from impaired absorption or increased secretion of fluid, electrolytes, and nutrients in the intestine. GE pathogens cause diarrhea primarily by destruction of the intestinal surface villi and production of toxins.
- Diagnosis of GE involves careful history of travel, medications, underlying diseases, contacts, and recent food or water ingestion. Evaluation of the appearance, quantity, and duration of the diarrhea and a microscopic examination of the stool are often helpful. Stool cultures are usually of little benefit and can be costly.
- The primary goals for treatment of GE involve providing supportive care, appropriate oral fluid and electrolyte therapy, and nutritional management.
- Oral fluid therapy is the preferred method of rehydration. The indications for intravenous fluid therapy are limited, and the need for such therapy should be determined based on a careful evaluation of the patient's clinical status and degree of dehydration.
- Commercially available oral rehydration solutions are recommended for use in treating GE-induced diarrhea. "Clear liquids" such as cola, broth, fruit juices, or sports drinks should be avoided because they provide inadequate electrolyte replacement and contain excess sugars.
- Maintenance of breastfeeding and institution of early refeeding is recommended to assist in intestinal repair and prevent malnutrition. A mixed diet of complex carbohydrates, lean meats, yogurt, fruits, and vegetables is preferred. Restrictive diets, such as the BRAT diet, should be avoided.
- The use of antidiarrheal agents is infrequently useful or necessary. The appropriateness of such therapy should be based on the likely pathogen, expected duration of disease, clinical presentation (i.e., no fever or bloody stools), and potential side effects.
- The need for and choice of antibiotic therapy should be evaluated based on duration of disease, likely pathogen, potential side effects, and concern of presence or development of antimicrobial resistance. The most commonly used antibiotics for GE are trimethoprim/sulfamethoxazole and the fluoroquinolones.
- Future directions in the management of GE will include the development and use of vaccines and newer antidiarrheal agents and evaluation of probiotic agents, vitamin A, and zinc as adjunctive therapies.
- Research efforts should be directed at defining the reasons for the inappropriate physician and parental practices that result in overuse and underuse of health care resources to treat GE and the clinical and financial outcomes of these practices.

REFERENCES

1. Bern C, Martines J, de Zoysa I, et al. The magnitude of the global problem of diarrhoeal diseases: a ten year update. Bull World Health Organ 70:705–714, 1992.
2. Glass RI, Lew JF, Gangarosa RE, et al. Estimates of morbidity and mortality for diarrheal diseases in American children. J Pediatr 118:S27–S33, 1991.
3. Kilgore PE, Holman RC, Clarke MJ, et al. Trends of diarrheal disease-associated mortality in US children, 1968 through 1991. JAMA 274:1143–1148, 1995.
4. Dupont HL. Guidelines on acute infectious diarrhea in adults. Am J Gastroenterol 92:1962–1975, 1997.
5. Gangarosa RE, Glass RI, Lew JF, et al. Hospitalizations involving gastroenteritis in the Unites States, 1985: the special burden of the diseases among the elderly. Am J Epidemiol 135:281–290, 1992.
6. Mandell GL, Bennett JE, Dolin R. Principles and practice of infectious diseases. New York: Wiley, 1995;1:76, 77, 79–81.
7. Shewmake RA, Dillon B. Food poisoning. Causes, remedies, and prevention. Postgrad Med 103:125–129, 134, 136, 1998.
8. Mines D, Stahmer S, Shepherd SM. Poisonings: food, fish, shellfish. Emerg Med Clin North Am 15:157–177, 1997.
9. Lew EA, Poles MA, Dieterich DT. Diarrheal diseases associated with HIV infection. Gastroenterol Clin North Am 26:259–290, 1997.
10. Neild PJ, Nelson MR. Management of HIV-related diarrhoea. Int J STD AIDS 8:286–296, 1997.
11. Fekety R. Guidelines for the diagnosis and management of *Clostridium difficile*-associated diarrhea and colitis. American College of Gastroenterology, Practice Parameters Committee. Am J Gastroenterol 92:739–750, 1997.
12. Cleary RK. *Clostridium difficile*-associated diarrhea and colitis: clinical manifestations, diagnosis, and treatment. Dis Colon Rectum 41:1435–1449, 1998.
13. Wilcox MH. *Clostridium difficile* infection: appendix. J Antimicrob Chemother 41(Suppl C):71–72, 1998.
14. Green KY. The role of human caliciviruses in epidemic gastroenteritis. Arch Virol Suppl 13:153–165, 1997.
15. Blacklow NR, Greenberg HB. Viral gastroenteritis. N Engl J Med 325:252–264, 1991.
16. Northrup RS, Flanigan TP. Gastroenteritis. Pediatr Rev 15:461–471, 1994.
17. Bishop RF. Natural history of human rotavirus infection. Arch Virol Suppl 12:119–128, 1996.

18. Lieberman JM. Rotavirus and other viral causes of gastroenteritis. Pediatr Ann 23:529–535, 1994.
19. Harrison MS. Rotavirus: an overview–from discovery to vaccine. Pediatr Nurs 24:317–323, 1998.
20. Glass RI, Noel J, Mitchell D, et al. The changing epidemiology of astrovirus-associated gastroenteritis: a review. Arch Virol Suppl 12:287–300, 1996.
21. Stutman HR. *Salmonella*, *Shigella*, and *Campylobacter:* common bacterial causes of infectious diarrhea. Pediatr Ann 23:538–543, 1994.
22. Eliason BC, Lewan RB. Gastroenteritis in children: principles of diagnosis and treatment. Am Fam Physician 58:1769–1776, 1998.
23. Buchwald DS, Blaser MJ. A review of human salmonellosis II. Duration of excretion following infection with nontyphi *Salmonella*. Rev Infect Dis 6:345–356, 1984.
24. Farthing M, Feldman R, Finch R, et al. The management of infective gastroenteritis in adults. A consensus statement by an expert panel convened by the British Society for the Study of Infection. J Infect 33:143–152, 1996.
25. Altekruse SF, Swerdlow DL, Stern NJ. Microbial food borne pathogens. *Campylobacter jejuni*. Vet Clin North Am Food Anim Pract 14:31–40, 1998.
26. Qadri SM, Kayali S. Enterohemorrhagic *Escherichia coli*. A dangerous food-borne pathogen. Postgrad Med 103:179–180, 1998.
27. Hyams KC, Bourgeouis AL, Merrel BR, et al. Diarrheal disease during Operation Desert Shield. N Engl J Med 325:1423–1428, 1991.
28. Afghani B, Stutman HR. Toxin-related diarrheas. Pediatr Ann 23:549–555, 1994.
29. Bell BP, Goldoft M, Griffin PM, et al. A multistate outbreak of *Escherichia coli* O157:H7-associated bloody diarrhea and hemolytic uremic syndrome from hamburgers: the Washington experience. JAMA 272:1349–1353, 1994.
30. Slutsker L, Ries AA, Maloney K. A nationwide case-control study of *Escherichia coli* O157:H7 infection in the United States. J Infect Dis 177:962–966, 1998.
31. San Joaquin VH. *Aeromonas*, *Yersinia*, and miscellaneous bacterial enteropathogens. Pediatr Ann 23:544–548, 1994.
32. Bottone EJ. *Yersinia enterocolitica:* the charisma continues. Clin Microbiol Rev 10:257–276, 1997.
33. Sanchez JL, Taylor DN. Cholera. Lancet 349:1825–1830, 1997.
34. Holmberg SD. Vibrios and *Aeromonas*. Infect Dis Clin North Am 2:655–676, 1988.
35. Meng J, Doyle MP. Emerging issues in microbiological food safety. Annu Rev Nutr 17:255–275, 1997.
36. Soave R, Herwaldt BL, Relman DA. Cyclospora. Infect Dis Clin North Am 12:1–12, 1998.
37. Goodgame RW. Understanding intestinal spore-forming protozoa: cryptosporidia, microsporidia, isospora, and cyclospora. Ann Intern Med 124:429–441, 1996.
38. Bourke B, Chan VL, Sherman P. *Campylobacter upsaliensis:* waiting in the wings. Clin Microbiol Rev 11:440–449, 1998.
39. Jamieson FB, Wang EE, Bain C, et al. Human torovirus: a new nosocomial gastrointestinal pathogen. J Infect Dis 178:1263–1269, 1998.
40. Bennet RG, Greenough WB. Approach to acute diarrhea in the elderly. Gastroenterol Clin North Am 22:517–533, 1993.
41. Golding J, Emmett PM, Rogers IS. Gastroenteritis, diarrhoea and breast feeding. Early Hum Dev 49(Suppl):S83–S103, 1997.
42. Guarino A, Canani RB, Russo S, et al. Oral immunoglobulins for treatment of acute rotaviral gastroenteritis. Pediatrics 93:12–16, 1994.
43. Dellert SF, Cohen MB. Diarrheal disease: established pathogens, new pathogens, and progress in vaccine development. Gastroenterol Clin North Am 23:637–654, 1994.
44. Anonymous. Prevention of rotavirus disease: guidelines for use of rotavirus vaccine. American Academy of Pediatrics. Pediatrics 102:1483–1491, 1998.
45. Scott DA. Vaccines against *Campylobacter jejuni*. J Infect Dis 176(Suppl 2):S183–S188, 1997.
46. Chaturvedi S, Chaturvedi S. Oral vaccines for cholera control. Natl Med J India 10:17–18, 1997.
47. Park SI, Giannella RA. Approach to the adult patient with acute diarrhea. Gastroenterol Clin North Am 22:483–497, 1993.
48. Acra SA, Ghishan GK. Electrolyte fluxes in the gut and oral rehydration solutions. Pediatr Clin North Am 43:433–449, 1996.
49. Guerrant RL, Bobak DA. Bacterial and protozoal gastroenteritis. N Engl J Med 325:327–340, 1991.
50. Kroser JA, Metz DC. Evaluation of the adult patient with diarrhea. Prim Care 23:629–647, 1996.
51. Center for Disease Control and Prevention. The management of acute diarrhea in children: oral rehydration, maintenance, and nutritional therapy. MMWR 41:1–20, 1992.
52. Weinberg AK, Minaker KL. Dehydration–evaluation and management in older adults. JAMA 274:1552–1556, 1995.
53. Liebelt EL. Clinical and laboratory evaluation and management of children with vomiting, diarrhea, and dehydration. Curr Opin Pediatr 10:461–469, 1998.
54. American Academy of Pediatrics. Practice parameter: the management of acute gastroenteritis in young children. Pediatrics 97:424–433, 1996.
55. Snyder JD. Use and misuse of oral therapy for diarrhea: comparison of U.S. practices with the American Academy of Pediatrics recommendations. Pediatrics 87:28–33, 1991.
56. Gavin N, Merrick N, Davidson B. Efficacy of glucose-based oral rehydration therapy. Pediatrics 98:45–51, 1996.
57. Desjeux JF, Briend A, Butzner JD. Oral rehydration solution in the year 2000: pathophysiology, efficacy and effectiveness. Baillieres Clin Gastroenterol 11:509–527, 1997.
58. Khiri-Maung U, Greenough WB. Cereal-based oral rehydration therapy I. Clinical studies. J Pediatr 118:572–579, 1991.
59. Duggan C, Nurko S. "Feeding the gut": the scientific basis for continued enteral nutrition during acute diarrhea. J Pediatr 131:801–808, 1997.
60. Sullivan PB. Nutritional management of acute diarrhea. Nutrition 14:758–862, 1998.
61. Powell DW, Szauter KE. Nonantibiotic therapy and pharmacotherapy of acute infectious diarrhea. Gastroenterol Clin North Am 22:683–707, 1993.
62. Schiller LR. Review article: antidiarrhoeal pharmacology and therapeutics. Aliment Pharmacol Ther 9:87–106, 1995.
63. Ericsson CD. Travelers' diarrhea: epidemiology, prevention and self-treatment. Infect Dis Clin North Am 12:285–303, 1998.
64. Figueroa-Quintanila D, Salazar-Lindo E, Sack B, et al. A controlled trial of bismuth subsalicylate in infants with acute watery diarrheal disease. N Engl J Med 328:1653–1658, 1993.
65. Rowe B, Ward LR, Threlfall EJ. Multi-drug resistant *Salmonella typhi*: a worldwide epidemic. Clin Infect Dis 24(Suppl 1):S106–S109, 1997.
66. Sack RB, Rahman M, Yunus M, et al. Antimicrobial resistance in organisms causing diarrheal disease. Clin Infect Dis 24(Suppl 1):S102–S105, 1997.
67. Freedman DO. Keeping current: travel medicine resources available on the Internet. Infect Dis Clin North Am 12:543–547, 1998.
68. Askenazi S, Cleary TG. Antibiotic treatment of bacterial gastroenteritis. Pediatr Infect Dis J 10:140–148, 1991.
69. Grisant KA, Jaffe DM. Dehydration syndromes: oral rehydration and fluid replacement. Emerg Med Clin North Am 9:565–588, 1991.
70. Waiz A. The new quinolones in the treatment of diarrhoea and typhoid fever. Drugs 49(Suppl 2):32–135, 1995.
71. Moss PJ, Read RC. Empiric antibiotic therapy for acute infective diarrhoea in the developed world. J Antimicrob Chemother 35:903–913, 1995.
72. Gilbert DN, Moellering RC, Sande MA. The Sanford guide to antimicrobial therapy. 28th ed. Hyde Park, VT: Antimicrobial Therapy Inc., 1998:12–14.
73. Mandell GL, Bennett JE, Dolin R. Principles and practice of infectious diseases. New York: Wiley, 1995;2:194, 201, 205, 208, 214.
74. Lewis SJ, Freedman AR. Review article: the use of biotherapeutic agents in the prevention and treatment of gastrointestinal disease. Aliment Pharmacol Ther 12:807–822, 1998.
75. Bhan MK, Bhandari N. The role of zinc and vitamin A in persistent diarrhea among infants and young children. J Pediatr Gastroenterol Nutr 26:446–453, 1998.
76. Caeiro JP, DuPont HL. Management of travellers' diarrhoea. Drugs 56:73–81, 1998.
77. Merrick N, Davidson B, Fox S. Treatment of acute gastroenteritis: too much and too little care. Clin Pediatr 35:429–435, 1996.

CHAPTER 72

INFECTIVE ENDOCARDITIS

Shirley M. Palmer

DEFINITION

Endocarditis is an infection of the inner lining of the heart and the mucosa that underlies it. However, the term refers most commonly to an infection of a heart valve. The mural endocardium, papillary muscles, and chordae tendineae can be involved in the infection, but the complications and clinical manifestations usually arise from the involvement of the tricuspid, mitral, or aortic valves.[1,2]

Subacute disease is an indolent infection that may produce signs and symptoms over periods as long as several months before a diagnosis is made. Acute infection is of rapid onset, with fulminant symptoms. Commonly, patients with subacute disease have all of the "classical" manifestations of the disease. However, the diagnosis is now suspected in any febrile illness of unclear cause, so progression to chronicity is becoming less common.[2,3]

TREATMENT GOALS: INFECTIVE ENDOCARDITIS

- Eradicate infection through use of antimicrobial therapy to sterilize the infected valve and surrounding structures. Antimicrobials used in treatment of endocarditis should always be bactericidal.
- Administer antimicrobials in high doses to penetrate into the valvular vegetation at the site of infection.
- Prolong therapy (2 to 6 weeks or longer) to achieve complete sterilization.
- If necessary, use combination therapy for adequate bactericidal activity.
- Monitor for toxicity of antimicrobials and complications of endocarditis.
- Surgery may be indicated to excise infected tissue and repair or replace the affected valve and restore cardiac function.
- Prevent death from severe hemodynamic compromise or from complications arising from embolic phenomena.
- Prevent recurrent episodes through administering prophylactic antibiotics before procedures that result in transient bacteremic episodes.

EPIDEMIOLOGY

There are approximately 15,000 to 20,000 new cases of infective endocarditis (IE) each year in the United States.[4]

Etiology

The clinical spectrum of IE has changed significantly in the past few decades. Infection caused by viridans streptococci, which were responsible for 70 to 80% of all cases in the 1960s and 1970s, has declined; now only 30 to 40% of cases are caused by these organisms.[2,3] Enterococci are the causative pathogens in approximately 5 to 18% of cases, and other streptococci account for an additional 15 to 25% of cases.[2] Staphylococci account for 20 to 35% of all cases, and account for the majority of isolates among injection drug users (IDUs).[2,5] The incidence of methicillin-resistant isolates has increased significantly, accounting for 40% of isolates of *Staphylococcus aureus* in IDUs at one medical center, and 84 to 87% of coagulase-negative staphylococci isolates in cases of prosthetic valve endocarditis occurring in the first year after surgery.[6,7] Gram-negative bacteria account for up to 10% of cases, most frequently in patients with prosthetic valves or in IDUs.[2,6] Fungi, particularly *Candida albicans,* are seen in 5% of cases or less.[1,2] Anaerobic endocarditis is rare. Up to 20% of cases may be culture negative; this could result from incorrect diagnosis, prior administration of antibiotics, failure to isolate slow-growing fastidious organisms (e.g., HACEK group [*Haemophilus* spp., *Actinobacillus actinomycetemcomitans, Cardiobacterium hominis, Eikenella corrodens, Kingella kingae*], nutritionally variant streptococci, or anaerobes), or nonbacterial etiology.[2]

Risk Factors

Risk factors associated with the development of IE include intravenous (IV) drug use, presence of intravascular devices, some types of underlying valvular heart disease, or the presence of a prosthetic heart valve. IDUs develop endocarditis more frequently than the general population, probably because of frequent nonsterile IV injections. The most common valve affected is the tricuspid valve, although other valves also may be affected. The bacteriology of IE in this population is primarily composed of *S. aureus* (50 to 60%), streptococci (15%), and Gram-negative bacilli and fungi (25 to 35%).[6]

The incidence of intravascular device–related IE, once thought to be uncommon, is increasing. A recent review of all *S. aureus* IE cases occurring in Denmark over a 10-year period found that 33% of cases were nosocomially acquired, and 25% of these were associated with infected intravascular devices.[8] A group of investigators at Duke University Medical Center determined that 50.8% of *S. aureus* IE cases were associated with intravascular devices, and over half of these infections were community acquired.[9] In a previous study, the primary investigator found that the prevalence of endocarditis in patients with intravascular catheter–related *S. aureus* bacteremia was 23%, which has led to the suggestion that all such patients should routinely undergo transesophageal echocardiography (TEE) to assist in early detection of IE and permit prompt institution of appropriate antimicrobial therapy.[10,11]

Certain individuals with congenital or acquired valvular heart defects are predisposed to developing IE. These conditions include mitral valve prolapse, degenerative valvular lesions, rheumatic heart disease, ventricular septal defect, coarctation of the aorta, and congenital bicuspid aortic valve.[2] The risk of infection is greater with some conditions than others. For example, patients with mitral valve prolapse are approximately eight times more likely to develop IE than patients in the general population.[3] IE in patients with preexisting valvular damage usually results from transient bacteremia with organisms that colonize mucosal surfaces and are considered normal flora. The most common sites of infection are the mitral and aortic valves. Viridans streptococci, which are found in the mouth, are responsible for the majority of cases of native valve endocarditis in non-drug users.[12] The remainder of cases are due to enterococci, other streptococci, and Gram-negative bacilli.

The other group of patients who are at special risk for developing IE are those who have prosthetic cardiac valves. Prosthetic valve endocarditis (PVE) occurring within the first 2 months after surgery (i.e., early PVE) is caused by organisms introduced during or shortly after surgery while the patient is still in the hospital. The most frequently cultured organisms are coagulase-negative staphylococci (35%), followed *by S. aureus* (17%), Gram-negative bacilli (16%), and fungi (10%).[13] Infections occurring more than 2 months after surgery (i.e, late PVE) are usually caused by the same organisms that produce diseases on native valves (i.e., primarily streptococci); however, endocarditis caused by coagulase-negative staphylococci may not be detected until months after surgery because of its indolent course.[7] For this reason, some investigators have proposed changing the definition of "early" PVE to include infections occurring during the first year after valve replacement.[14,15] The rate of PVE ranges from 1 to 4% during the first year after surgery and is approximately 1% per year thereafter.[3] Endocarditis is especially devastating in patients with prosthetic valves because fatal complications can occur quickly. A recent study by the Department of Veterans Affairs found overall mortality rates of 46%, with no difference between early versus late PVE. However, the mortality rate was twice as high in patients with New York Heart Association Class III or IV congestive heart failure as compared with those in Classes I and II.[16] Other factors associated with poor prognosis include onset within 12 months of implantation; Gram-negative, fungal, or *S. aureus* etiology; and aortic valve involvement.[2,17]

There has been a significant trend in recent years toward an increase in the age of patients with IE.[2,3,18] This is at least partly due to marked decreases in the prevalence of rheumatic heart disease, the longevity of persons in modern society (leading to degenerative valvular lesions), and increasing numbers of older patients with prosthetic cardiac valves.[3,18] Although increased age was associated with a poorer prognosis in previous years, a recent study found the mortality rate in elderly patients to be similar to that of younger patients, which the authors attribute to improved diagnostic sensitivity of TEE, leading to earlier diagnosis.[18]

The overall mortality rate for all forms of IE is approximately 25 to 30%. However, the mortality rate ranges from 10 to 15% in penicillin-sensitive streptococcal endocarditis to 90% or more in fungal infection.[2,19] Factors associated with a poor prognosis include heart failure, renal failure, left-sided (aortic or mitral valve) involvement, infection of a prosthetic valve, cerebral embolism, and infection with Gram-negative bacilli or fungi.[2,20]

PATHOPHYSIOLOGY

As mentioned previously, the tissues involved in IE are primarily the tricuspid, mitral, and aortic valves; the valve of the pulmonary artery is rarely infected. The tricuspid valve is the most common site of infection in IDUs. The mitral and aortic valves are also involved in this group of patients, as well as in patients with underlying valve pathology. Damage to the mitral and aortic valves leads to more severe hemodynamic alterations than does tricuspid disease.[1,2] Lesions of the chordae, the atrial or ventricular walls, and the pulmonary artery or aorta are considered satellite infections to the primary valvular involvement.[1]

Four factors are necessary in the pathogenesis of the infection: (1) a previously damaged cardiac valve, (2) a platelet-fibrin thrombus, (3) bacteremia, and (4) bacterial adherence.[1] In published series of patients with fatal IE, autopsy revealed that the mitral valve was involved in 86%, the aortic valve in 55%, the tricuspid valve in 20%, and the pulmonic valve in only 1%.[2] Correlating the pressure gradient across these valves with the relative frequency of infection makes a strong argument for mechanical stress as an important factor in the pathogenesis of IE. Similarly, the hemodynamic alterations that occur across an incompetent valve result in abnormal "jets" of blood that may damage the endocardium and provide a locus for infection. This change in hemodynamics also creates a low-pressure "sink" that sets up an additional site for infection. Consequently, vegetations in IE are most commonly found on the low-pressure side of the valve: the atrial surfaces of the mitral and tricuspid valves and the ventricular surface of the aortic valve.[1,2]

Once the endothelial surface of the valve is damaged, collagen is exposed, and a sterile platelet-fibrin thrombus is formed. This is called nonbacterial thrombotic endocarditis (NBTE).[1,2] The next critical factor in the pathogenesis of the infection is the presence of bacteremia. Bacteremia or fungemia may arise from other foci of infection. In addition, transient bacteremias with the potential for producing endocarditis have been described following tooth extraction, periodontal surgery, liver biopsy, endoscopy or sigmoidoscopy, and manipulations of the genitourinary tract. The organisms causing IE in these cases can usually be traced to the site of the procedure. For example, viridans streptococci, nonenterococcal group D streptococci, and other facultative organisms are normal flora of the nasopharynx. Enterococci and Gram-negative bacilli usually arise from the urinary or gastrointestinal tracts. Staphylococci are found on the skin and may colonize the nasopharynx. Fungi may arise from the bowel, as can certain Gram-negative and anaerobic organisms. Bacteria and fungi may also colonize certain areas of skin and thus gain entrance to the circulation via intravenous catheters.[1,2]

The final step in the development of IE occurs when organisms adhere to the thrombus. The adherence properties of an organism correlate directly with the ability of that organism to produce endocarditis.[1,2] For instance, some strains of streptococci and staphylococci produce virulence factors such as dextran or fibrinonectin that promote adherence to traumatized endothelial cells.[1] Production of an extracellular polysaccharide matrix, or slime, allows coagulase-negative staphylococci to adhere to prosthetic materials and resist phagocytosis.[7] Once organisms adhere to the thrombus, they begin to multiply. Within 24 hours, the bacteria undergo a period of exponential growth, reach a very high inoculum (approximately 10^9 colony-forming units [cfu]/g), and enter a "resting" stage of low metabolic activity.[21] Additional platelet-fibrin deposition occurs, resulting in sequestration from leukocytes and enlargement of the infected thrombus, now termed a vegetation.[1,21] The vegetation is the source of prolonged and continuous bacteremia, the hallmark sign of IE.

COMPLICATIONS

Complications from IE may be classified as cardiac or extracardiac. The most common cardiac complication is congestive heart failure, which is the leading cause of death in patients with IE.[15,22,23] Less common complications include intracardiac abscesses, conduction defects, infection- or immune complex–mediated pericarditis, and myocardial infarction.[22,23]

Extracardiac complications are usually related to embolic events, which occur in at least one-third of patients with IE.[2] Persons with tricuspid valve IE commonly have pulmonary emboli, whereas those with left-sided IE are more likely to have systemic embolic events. Many patients develop renal insufficiency, which may be caused by several factors such as metastatic abscesses within the kidney from infected emboli (predominantly staphylococcal infection), infarction of the kidney from compromised blood flow caused by aseptic emboli, immune-complex nephritis caused by deposition of immunoglobulins and complement on the glomerular basement membrane, or even nephrotoxicity of antimicrobials used for treatment.[2] Splenic artery emboli may result in splenomegaly and abdominal pain in patients with subacute presentation.[2] Involvement of the central nervous system occurs in 20 to 40% of patients with IE, most commonly in those with left-sided involvement or *S. aureus* etiology.[24] The predominant manifestations are cerebral embolism and mycotic aneurysm, with meningitis, brain abscess, encephalopathy, or seizures occurring less frequently. Presenting symptoms differ depending on the type of manifestation or location of the emboli but almost always include headache. Various imaging techniques (e.g., computerized tomography, magnetic resonance imaging) may be useful for diagnosis of central nervous system involvement; neurosurgery may be indicated in cases of aneurysm or intracranial bleeds.[24]

CLINICAL PRESENTATION AND DIAGNOSIS

Signs and Symptoms

The classic signs and symptoms of IE, such as Osler's nodes, Janeway lesions, clubbing of the fingers, splinter hemorrhages, and retinal lesions, are now uncommon.[1,17] The primary reason for this is the high index of suspicion for the disease in a patient with fever of unknown origin, leading to an earlier diagnosis, before the development of these more chronic findings. The most common signs and symptoms are a heart murmur or a change in a previously noted murmur, fever, embolic episodes, splenomegaly, skin manifestations (primarily petechiae), weakness, dyspnea, night sweats, anorexia, weight loss, and malaise.[2,17] These are not present in all cases, but the most crucial

Table 72.1 ▪ DUKE Criteria for Diagnosis of Infective Endocarditis

Definite Infective Endocarditis	
Pathologic criteria	
	Microorganisms: demonstrated by culture or histology in a vegetation, *or* in a vegetation that has embolized, *or* in an intracardiac abscess, *or*
	Pathologic lesions: vegetation or intracardiac abscess present, confirmed by histology showing active endocarditis.
Clinical criteria (using definitions listed in Table 72.2)	
	2 major criteria, *or*
	1 major criterion plus 3 minor criteria, *or*
	5 minor criteria
Possible Infective Endocarditis	
Findings consistent with infective endocarditis that fall short of "Definitive" but not "Rejected."	
Rejected	
Firm alternative diagnosis explaining evidence of infective endocarditis, *or*	
Resolution of manifestations of endocarditis, with antibiotic therapy for 4 days or less, *or*	
No pathologic evidence of infective endocarditis at surgery or autopsy, after antibiotic therapy for 4 days or less.	

Source: Durack DT, Lukes AS, Bright DK, et al. New criteria for diagnosis of infective endocarditis: utilization of specific echocardiographic findings. Am J Med 96:200–209, 1994. Copyright 1994, with permission from Excerpta Medica Inc.

criterion for the diagnosis of the disease is positive blood cultures.

Diagnosis

Investigators from Duke University Medical Center have recently proposed new criteria for the diagnosis of IE (Tables 72.1 and 72.2).[25] The new Duke criteria incorporate echocardiographic findings into the classification schemes and have been found to be more sensitive than the older von Reyn criteria.[26]

Echocardiography is the technique of choice for identifying vegetations and is a very important tool for the diagnosis of IE.[17,27] The development of transesophageal imaging has facilitated higher-resolution imaging by moving the transducer from outside of the chest wall to immediately adjacent to the heart. In contrast to the standard transthoracic echocardiography (TTE), TEE is much more sensitive (greater than 86% detection of vegetations versus only 58% for TTE).[4,27] TEE is superior to TTE for identifying small vegetations, vegetations on either pulmonic or prosthetic valves, and intracardiac abscesses.[4,19] However, TEE is a more invasive procedure and is often reserved for cases in which TTE is nondiagnostic.[3]

The bacteremia in IE is usually continuous, but low grade.[2] In practice, three blood cultures taken over an extended time period in a patient who is not critically ill should produce a very high yield. In acutely ill patients, two or three blood cultures should be taken rapidly from different sites before starting antibiotic therapy. Other criteria that may support the diagnosis of endocarditis include fever, immunologic manifestations, and vascular phenomena (Table 72.2).

IE in IDUs is frequently heralded by neurologic dysfunction or pulmonary emboli.[2,6,17] This may misdirect

Table 72.2 ▪ Definitions of Terminology Used in DUKE Criteria

Major Criteria
Positive blood culture for infective endocarditis
Typical microorganism for infective endocarditis from 2 separate blood cultures:
Viridans streptococci, *Streptococcus bovis,* HACEK group, *or*
Community-acquired *S. aureus* or enterococci, in the absence of a primary focus, *or*
Persistently positive blood culture, defined as recovery of a microorganism consistent with infective endocarditis from
(i) Blood cultures drawn more than 12 hours apart, *or*
(ii) All of three or a majority of four or more separate blood cultures, with first and last drawn at least 1 hour apart
Evidence of endocardial involvement
Positive echocardiogram for infective endocarditis
(i) Oscillating intracardiac mass, on valve or supporting structures, or in the path of regurgitant jets, or on implanted material, in the absence of an alternative anatomic explanation, *or*
(ii) Abscess, *or*
(iii) New partial dehiscence of prosthetic valve, *or*
New valvular regurgitation (increase or change in preexisting murmur not sufficient)
Minor Criteria
Predisposition: predisposing heart condition or intravenous drug use
Fever: ≥38°C (100.4°F)
Vascular phenomena: major arterial emboli, septic pulmonary infarcts, mycotic aneurysm, intracranial hemorrhage, conjunctival hemorrhages, Janeway lesions
Immunologic phenomena: glomerulonephritis, Osler's nodes, Roth spots, rheumatoid factor
Microbiologic evidence: positive blood culture[a] but not meeting major criterion as noted previously, or serologic evidence of active infection with organism consistent with infective endocarditis
Echocardiogram: consistent with infective endocarditis but not meeting major criterion as noted previously

Source: Durack DT, Lukes AS, Bright DK, et al. New criteria for diagnosis of infective endocarditis: utilization of specific echocardiographic findings. Am J Med 96:200–209, 1994. Copyright 1994, with permission from Excerpta Medica Inc.

HACEK, Haemophilus spp., *Actinobacillus actinomycetemcomitans, Cardiobacterium hominis, Eikenella* spp., and *Kingella kingae.*

[a]Excluding single positive cultures for coagulase-negative staphylococci or organisms that do not cause endocarditis.

the efforts toward a diagnosis, which again points to the importance of obtaining sufficient blood cultures in the febrile patient with a history of symptoms consistent with IE.

TREATMENT

Pharmacotherapy

The cure of IE is difficult and requires sterilization of the vegetation. Sequestering the infecting organisms within an avascular vegetation provides protection from the circulating antibodies and white blood cells. In the absence of humoral or cellular immune mechanisms, antibiotics must be capable of bactericidal activity. This fact has been proven clinically by the failure of bacteriostatic antibiotics such as the tetracyclines, erythromycin, and chloramphenicol to cure endocarditis. In addition, organisms in a vegetation exhibit reduced metabolic activity and are less susceptible to antimicrobials, which are primarily effective against rapidly dividing cells. The high organism load within the vegetation may also result in decreased effectiveness of drug therapy. Thus, organisms that appear to be sensitive in vitro using standard inocula (10^5/mL) may exhibit "tolerance" to the antimicrobial at the high inocula encountered in vivo (10^9 to 10^{10}/g).[28] Combination therapy often is necessary to overcome this tolerance and to achieve effective bactericidal activity, such as when treating enterococcal infection, or is used to shorten total course of therapy (from 4 weeks to 2 weeks) for highly susceptible organisms. Failure of antibiotics to penetrate in sufficient concentrations to the core of the vegetation also contributes to treatment difficulty.[29] All of these factors combined necessitate the use of high-dose, bactericidal antimicrobial therapy for a prolonged duration in order to achieve sterilization. Anticoagulant therapy for the treatment of endocarditis (other than that necessary for the management of a prosthetic valve) is contraindicated because of the risk of hemorrhage. The theoretical benefit of decreasing vegetation size is unfounded in the clinical setting.

Empiric therapy is most often instituted before culture results are known, especially in patients who are acutely ill. The choice of empiric therapy should be based on the most likely infecting organism, as well as the institution's or community's resistance patterns. For example, an elderly man with a history of enterococcal urinary tract infections should be treated for enterococcal IE. Likewise, an IDU with acute disease should be treated for disease due to *S. aureus* until culture results are obtained; if in a community where a high incidence of IDUs are known to have methicillin-resistant *S. aureus*, empiric use of vancomycin may be warranted. Therapy should be revised as soon as culture and susceptibility results are available, even if patients are responding favorably to empiric therapy. Clinical improvement usually occurs within 4 to 10 days; however, it is not unusual for a patient to remain bacteremic for 5 to 7 days after therapy is instituted. Prolonged bacteremia (i.e., longer than 7 days) may indicate emergence of resistant subpopulations, inadequate antimicrobial therapy, or presence of abscesses or other foci of infection. The patient's antibiotic regimen should be reevaluated, and TEE may be conducted or repeated to assess the need for surgery. Table 72.3 lists the most recent recommendations of the American Heart Association (AHA) for treating common types of endocarditis.[12]

Streptococcal Infection (viridans streptococci, *S. bovis*)

Most streptococci (except enterococci) are usually highly susceptible to penicillin G (minimum inhibitory concentration [MIC] <0.1 μg/mL), and therapy with penicillin alone for 4 weeks is highly effective.[2,12] A 4-week regimen of ceftriaxone administered once daily has also been found to be as effective as penicillin and facilitates outpatient treatment.[30] Vancomycin is the drug of choice for patients with severe β-lactam allergy. A 2-week regimen of penicillin and an aminoglycoside is an appropriate alternative in patients with uncomplicated IE, but it may be more toxic because of the aminoglycoside.[12] A 2-week regimen of ceftriaxone and netilmicin dosed once daily has also been found to be effective for uncomplicated streptococcal IE.[31] Netilmicin is not commonly used in the United States; however, other aminoglycosides (e.g., gentamicin) may be substituted. When IE is caused by streptococci that are resistant to penicillin (MIC > 0.1 μg/mL and < 0.5 μg/mL), combination therapy with a penicillin (4 weeks) plus an aminoglycoside (2 weeks) is recommended. IE caused by nutritionally variant streptococci or viridans streptococci with penicillin (MICs > 0.5 μg/mL) should be treated with a 4- to 6-week course of penicillin or ampicillin plus an aminoglycoside for the entire course. The same regimen is also recommended for streptococcal PVE, but a full 6-week course is required.[12]

Enterococcal Infection

Enterococcal IE is difficult to treat because enterococci are resistant to penicillin (MIC ~ 4 μg/mL) and vancomycin (MIC ~ 2 μg/mL) and are not killed by these drugs when used alone. Enterococci also are resistant to standard concentrations of aminoglycosides; however, adding aminoglycosides to penicillin, ampicillin, or vancomycin may result in synergistic killing of most organisms. This situation requires a special aminoglycoside susceptibility study to predict whether synergy will be achieved. If the isolate is inhibited by less than 2000 μg/mL of streptomycin or less than 500 μg/mL of gentamicin, the organism exhibits only low-level resistance and adding the aminoglycoside to the β-lactam or vancomycin will probably result in synergy. An MIC greater than or equal to 2000 μg/mL of streptomycin and greater than or equal to 500 μg/mL of gentamicin is considered to be high-level resistance, indicating that synergy will not be obtained with penicillin or vancomycin.[12,32] High-level gentamicin resistance is common in some isolates of enterococci and is now being encountered in viridans streptococci.[2,32] In some centers, as many as

Table 72.3 ▪ Antimicrobial Therapy for Native Valve (NV) and Prosthetic Valve (PV) Endocarditis

Organism	Regimens (preferred regimen listed first)	Dosage and Route	Duration (weeks)
Streptococci, NV (penicillin MIC ≤0.1 μg/mL)	Penicillin G	12–18 MU/day IV	4
	Ceftriaxone	2 g IM/IV once daily	4
	"Short Course" Regimen[a]		
	Penicillin G	12–18 MU/day IV	2
	plus		
	gentamicin[b]	1 mg/kg q8hr IV[c]	2
	"Short Course" Regimen[a]		
	Ceftriaxone	2 g IM/IV once daily	2
	plus		
	gentamicin	4 mg/kg IV once daily	2
	Vancomycin	15 mg/kg q12hr IV[d]	4
Streptococci, NV (penicillin MIC >0.1 μg/mL but <0.5 μg/mL)	Penicillin G	18 MU/day IV	4
	plus		
	gentamicin[b]	1 mg/kg q8hr IV[c]	2
	Vancomycin	15 mg/kg q12hr IV[d]	4
Streptococci, NV (penicillin MIC >0.5 μg/mL	Penicillin G	18–30 MU/day	4–6
	plus		
	gentamicin[b]	1 mg/kg q8hr IV[c]	4–6
	Ampicillin	2 g IV q4hr	4–6
	plus		
	gentamicin[b]	1 mg/kg q8hr IV[c]	4–6
	Vancomycin	15 mg/kg q12hr IV[d]	4–6
Streptococci, PV	Penicillin G	12–18 MU/day IV	6
	plus		
	gentamicin[b]	1 mg/kg q8hr IV[c]	2
Enterococci, NV	Penicillin G	18–30 MU/day	4–6
	plus		
	gentamicin[b]	1 mg/kg q8hr IV[c]	4–6
	Ampicillin	2 g IV q4hr	4–6
	plus		
	gentamicin[b]	1 mg/kg q8hr IV[c]	4–6
	Vancomycin	15 mg/kg q12hr IV[d]	4–6
	plus		
	gentamicin[b]	1 mg/kg q8hr IV[c]	4–6
Enterococci, PV	Penicillin G	18–30 MU/day	≥6
	plus		
	gentamicin[b]	1 mg/kg q8hr IV[c]	≥6
	Ampicillin	2 g IV q4hr	≥6
	plus		
	gentamicin[b]	1 mg/kg q8hr IV[c]	≥6
	Vancomycin	15 mg/kg q12hr IV[d]	≥6
	plus		
	gentamicin[b]	1 mg/kg q8hr IV[c]	≥6
Methicillin-susceptible staphylococci, NV	Nafcillin or oxacillin	2 g IV q4hr	4–6
	+/−		
	gentamicin	1 mg/kg q8hr IV[c]	3–5 days
	Cefazolin	2 g IV q8hr	4–6
	+/−		
	gentamicin	1 mg/kg q8hr IV[c]	3–5 days
	"Short Course" Regimen[e]		
	Nafcillin *or* oxacillin	2 g IV q4hr	2
	plus		
	gentamicin	1 mg/kg q8hr IV[c]	2
	Vancomycin	15 mg/kg q12hr IV[d]	4–6
	+/−		
	gentamicin	1 mg/kg q8hr IV[c]	3–5 days

(continued)

Table 72.3 *(continued)*

Organism	Regimens (preferred regimen listed first)	Dosage and Route	Duration (weeks)
Methicillin-susceptible staphylococci, PV	Nafcillin or oxacillin	2 g IV q4hr	≥6
	plus		
	gentamicin	1 mg/kg q8hr IV[c]	2
	plus		
	rifampin	300 mg PO q8hr	≥6
Methicillin-resistant staphylococci, NV	Vancomycin	15 mg/kg q12hr IV[d]	4–6
	+/−		
	gentamicin	1 mg/kg q8hr IV[c]	3–5 days
Methicillin-resistant staphylococci, PV	Vancomycin	15 mg/kg q12hr IV[d]	≥6
	plus		
	gentamicin	1 mg/kg q8hr IV[c]	2
	plus		
	rifampin	300 mg PO q8hr	≥6
HACEK organisms	Ceftriaxone	2 g IM/IV once daily	4
	Ampicillin	2G IV q4hr	4
	plus		
	gentamicin	1 mg/kg q8hr IV[c]	4

Adapted from Wilson WR, Karchmer AW, Dajani AD, et al. Antibiotic treatment of adults with infective endocarditis due to streptococci, enterococci, staphylococci, and HACEK microorganisms. JAMA 274(21):1706–1713, 1995. Copyright 1995, American Medical Association.

[a]Short-course regimens indicated in uncomplicated streptococcal IE only.

[b]May substitute streptomycin (7.5 mg/kg q12hr) for strains exhibiting high-level resistance to gentamicin (>500 μg/mL) and sensitivity to streptomycin (MIC <2000 μg/mL).

[c]Dosage must be adjusted for renal dysfunction (target peak ~ 3 μg/mL, trough <0.5 μg/mL).

[d]Dosage must be adjusted for renal dysfunction (target peak ~ 30–45 μg/mL, trough ~ 10–15 μg/mL).

[e]Short-course regimen indicated only for uncomplicated, right-sided IE due to methicillin-sensitive strains of *S. aureus* in IDUs.

60% of *Enterococcus faecium* isolates are resistant to high levels of gentamicin.[2,17,32] Approximately 30 to 50% of these gentamicin-resistant strains are susceptible to streptomycin, and the penicillin–streptomycin combination will be bactericidal.[32] Because of intrinsic resistance of *E. faecium* to most other aminoglycosides, only gentamicin and streptomycin are routinely tested and used.[32]

The preferred regimen for treating enterococcal IE consists of penicillin or ampicillin plus an aminoglycoside for 6 weeks. Traditional dosing of aminoglycosides (i.e., every 8 hours for normal renal function) is recommended, because studies have shown that once-daily dosing regimens are suboptimal for enterococcal IE.[33–35]

Increasing numbers of enterococci are highly resistant to multiple antimicrobials, including aminoglycosides, penicillins, and glycopeptides (e.g., vancomycin). Treatment options for these situations are limited. In patients with ampicillin-sensitive, high-level aminoglycoside-resistant strains, the traditional penicillin–aminoglycoside combination is unlikely to be effective.[32,36] Therapy with high-dose penicillin G or ampicillin alone for 6 to 12 weeks may be effective, but adjunctive surgery may be required.[12,32,36] Experimental models of endocarditis suggest that continuous IV infusion of penicillin may be more effective than intermittent bolus administration of the same total daily dose.[32] However, experience with these regimens in humans is limited, and it is not known if continuous infusion regimens will achieve adequate concentrations in endocardial vegetations.

Some isolates of enterococcus (especially *E. faecium*) are found to be resistant to penicillins by virtue of the production of β-lactamase or by alteration of penicillin-binding proteins (PBPs). The β-lactamase–producing strains are effectively treated with a β-lactam/β-lactamase inhibitor combination (e.g., ampicillin and sulbactam) plus an aminoglycoside (if the isolate is aminoglycoside susceptible). The presence of penicillin resistance mediated by PBP alteration necessitates the use of vancomycin in combination with an aminoglycoside. This regimen is considered suboptimal therapy because glycopeptides are less rapidly bactericidal than β-lactams.[2,17]

Finally, vancomycin-resistant enterococci (VRE) have also emerged as pathogens. Most VRE isolates in the United States are *E. faecium* and are often resistant to all cell wall–active agents (e.g., penicillins, cephalosporins), aminoglycosides, and numerous other antibiotics.[37] Hence, therapy selection is extremely difficult. If the isolate is susceptible to ampicillin with an MIC of 32 mg/L or less, high-dose ampicillin therapy may be effective.[37] If resistant to ampicillin, additional susceptibility testing to other antimicrobial agents and possibly even time-kill curves with various combinations may help guide therapy. In vitro and animal studies suggest that some isolates may be inhibited synergistically by combinations of β-lactams, glycopeptides, and aminoglycosides.[36] Combination therapy with fluoroquinolones and β-lactams or aminoglycosides has also been reported to be effective in vitro; however, animal studies have had conflicting results.[36] There are anecdotal reports of the effectiveness of minocycline, doxycycline, chloramphenicol, and rifampin–gentamicin–ciprofloxacin in treating other systemic VRE infections, but these agents have not been studied prospectively in humans in a clinical trial.[37] One new combination agent with good in vitro activity against vancomycin-resistant *E. faecium* is quinupristin–dalfopristin (Synercid), a pristinamycin derivative. This agent has been used for treating VRE infections with some success; however, in vitro data suggest that it may not be bactericidal against enterococci, which is necessary for successful treatment of endocarditis. In addition, Synercid has little activity against *E. faecalis* isolates. Other experimental classes of antibiotics currently being investigated for treating VRE infections include oxazolidinones, glycylcyclines, everninomycins, lipopeptides, and newer fluoroquinolones.[37] The most reliable management for endocarditis caused by multiple resistant strains of enterococci appears to be surgical replacement of the valve accompanied by the best available medical therapy for very prolonged periods.[2,12]

Staphylococcal Infection

IE may be caused by coagulase-positive staphylococci *(S. aureus)* or coagulase-negative staphylococci *(S. epidermidis). Staphylococcus aureus* is an extremely virulent pathogen that is capable of infecting both native and prosthetic valves.

Almost all staphylococci produce β-lactamase (e.g., "penase"), which makes them resistant to penicillins. IE due to penicillin-sensitive strains (approximately 2%) may be treated with penicillin G. The drugs of choice for treatment of β-lactamase–producing, methicillin-sensitive strains of *S. aureus* (MSSA) are oxacillin and nafcillin. Adding an aminoglycoside for the initial 2 weeks of therapy was not shown in clinical trials to improve overall outcomes; therefore, use of gentamicin is advocated only during the first 3 to 5 days of therapy to potentially achieve more rapid clearance of bacteremia and to reduce the time during which patients are febrile.[3] First-generation cephalosporins such as cefazolin may be used in cases of mild penicillin allergy (i.e., mild rash), although experience with these agents is minimal and has been associated with reported failures. Thus, this may be a situation for penicillin (i.e, nafcillin) desensitization. Vancomycin may be substituted for nafcillin or oxacillin in patients with immediate hypersensitivity reactions to β-lactams. However, in numerous studies using time-kill curves, in animal models, and in clinical trials, vancomycin has been shown to be less rapidly bactericidal than β-lactam antibiotics and suboptimal outcomes have been documented.[3,12,38,39] Based on such data, vancomycin should be used only when absolutely indicated. The standard duration of therapy for native valve IE due to MSSA is 4 to 6 weeks. Shorter courses of therapy have been found to be effective only in IDUs with uncomplicated right-sided disease; these patients may be treated with nafcillin plus an aminoglycoside for a full 2 weeks.[40] IDUs with evidence of left-sided or metastatic disease should receive the standard course of therapy, as should patients with β-lactam allergy, because a short, 2-week course of vancomycin plus tobramycin has been shown to be ineffective.[12,40]

Patients who are infected with methicillin-resistant *S. aureus* (MRSA) should receive vancomycin for 4 to 6 weeks, and gentamicin may be added for at least the first 3 to 5 days. Few alternatives to vancomycin exist for MRSA. Studies have assessed the efficacy of IV and oral ciprofloxacin for treatment of *S. aureus* (particularly MRSA) endocarditis.[3,41] The addition of rifampin to the regimen appears to prevent the inevitable emergence of quinolone-resistant isolates in a particular patient. Unfortunately, widespread ciprofloxacin resistance in the community may render this combination ineffective. In in vitro studies, animal models, and small studies, imipenem has been found to be effective for treating IE due to MSSA or MRSA.[42–44] A large-scale clinical trial is ongoing. An additional treatment alternative may be trimethoprim–sulfamethoxazole with or without rifampin. This agent was effective in the treatment of some cases of right-sided IE due to MRSA, although failures occurred in some patients with MSSA.[45]

Patients with staphylococcal *(S. aureus* and *S. epidermidis)* PVE require at least 6 weeks of therapy. The use of oral rifampin in high doses (300 mg tid) has been shown to improve sterilization of infected prosthetic material and is recommended to be used in combination with nafcillin–oxacillin or vancomycin for the entire course.[12] Gentamicin should be added during the first 2 weeks of therapy, if the isolate is susceptible. If aminoglycoside resistant, substitution of a fluoroquinolone may be considered.[12]

A high incidence of coagulase-negative staphylococci are methicillin resistant. Endocarditis due to these organisms, usually found on prosthetic valves, should be treated with vancomycin plus rifampin for the entire 6 weeks, with an aminoglycoside added for the first 2 weeks of treatment.[12]

Gram-Negative Infection

Gram-negative bacillary endocarditis should be treated for at least 6 weeks with bactericidal antibiotics to which the infecting organisms are sensitive. The empiric treatment of Gram-negative endocarditis should include an aminoglycoside at maximum doses (5 to 8 mg/kg/day) in combination with a β-lactam compound.[2,4,17] Third-generation cephalosporins (e.g., cefotaxime, ceftizoxime, ceftriaxone), extended-spectrum penicillins (e.g., piperacillin, mezlocillin), fluoroquinolones, and imipenem may provide adequate therapy for endocarditis caused by aerobic Gram-negative bacilli.

IE due to *Pseudomonas aeruginosa* is most commonly seen in IDUs.[4,46] Combination therapy with high doses of an antipseudomonal β-lactam plus an aminoglycoside (5 to 8 mg/kg/day) is required, in conjunction with valve replacement in patients with left-sided disease, in order to achieve a cure.[4,6,46] In spite of "adequate" therapeutic regimens, morbidity and mortality from pseudomonal IE remains high.[4,6]

HACEK organisms occur in 5 to 10% of cases of native valve endocarditis. Treatment with a third-generation cephalosporin or ampicillin plus gentamicin for 3 to 4 weeks for native valve infection and 6 weeks for prosthetic valve infection is recommended. Alternative therapy for penicillin-allergic patients includes trimethoprim–sulfamethoxazole or fluoroquinolones, although clinical data with these drugs is lacking.[12]

Other Organisms

The treatment of other forms of endocarditis is less well established. Infections caused by anaerobes, although rare, are associated with a high mortality rate.[2] These infections tend to be very destructive and often require surgical intervention. Many anaerobic organisms such as those found in the oropharynx are highly susceptible to penicillin G. For penicillin-resistant organisms such as *Bacteroides fragilis* and related species, another bactericidal agent such as metronidazole should be chosen. β-Lactam/β-lactamase inhibitor combinations (e.g., ampicillin–sulbactam, piperacillin–tazobactam, ticarcillin–clavulanate) and imipenem are also active in vitro against *B. fragilis* and most other anaerobes, and may be considered. Clindamycin and chloramphenicol are bacteriostatic and should be avoided.[2]

Fungal endocarditis is virtually impossible to cure without surgery, and even with seemingly adequate fungicidal therapy, the mortality rate is very high. This is probably due to several reasons: the invasiveness of the organisms; the large friable vegetations produced on the valve, causing a high rate of major embolic complications; the lack of fungicidal activity with available antifungal agents; and the negligible penetration of the antifungal agent into the vegetation.[2,47,48] Patients at risk for fungal endocarditis include IDUs; recent prosthetic valve recipients; and patients recently hospitalized who had surgery, received broad-spectrum antibiotics, received hyperalimentation, or had long-term intravenous catheters.[48] Fungal species most frequently associated with IE are *Aspergillus* and *Candida*.[19,47,48] The mainstay of therapy is amphotericin B given for a prolonged period of time, along with early valve replacement.[47] Use of liposomal amphotericin B formulations may be better tolerated, but efficacy studies are needed. The addition of 5-flucytosine (5-FC) for treating *Candida* infections may be considered; however, toxicities include dose-related bone marrow suppression, which may be worsened by drug accumulation secondary to amphotericin-induced impaired renal function. Fluconazole and itraconazole have in vitro activity against many fungi, but these agents are fungistatic, and data to support use in fungal IE are lacking.[2,48]

Nonpharmacologic Therapy

Valve replacement is indicated for many intractable complications of endocarditis. Indications for surgery include severe hemodynamic compromise, valvular obstruction, evidence of intracardiac extension or abscess, persistent bacteremia, relapse following "adequate" therapy, an infecting organism that is resistant to available antimicrobials, fungal IE, left-sided pseudomonal IE, more than one major embolic event, and instability of an infected prosthetic valve.[4,46,49,50]

PREVENTION

Bacteremia from most sources usually is transient and nearly always inconsequential in the normal individual. However, in the patient with congenital or acquired heart disease or a prosthetic valve, any bacteremia may lead to endocarditis. In assessing the risk of a bacteremia to an individual patient, important considerations include the incidence of bacteremia with a given procedure, as well as the most likely organisms, the type of cardiac abnormality, and possibly the concentration of the bacteria in the bloodstream.[51]

Only indirect evidence from animal studies demonstrates the effect of prophylactic systemic antibiotics in bacteremia-producing procedures. There are no prospective controlled trials of endocarditis prophylaxis in humans, and the recommended regimens are derived from experiments in the rabbit model. The AHA recommends the use of prophylactic antimicrobials before, during, and after a procedure likely to produce a bacteremia.[52] These include all dental procedures likely to induce gingival bleeding, tonsillectomy–adenoidectomy, surgical procedures or biopsy involving respiratory mucosa, bronchoscopy, incision and drainage of infected tissue, and various genitourinary and gastrointestinal procedures. Table 72.4 lists cardiac conditions for which prophylaxis is recommended and those for which it is not believed to be necessary.[52] Table 72.5 lists dental and other procedures for which prophylaxis is or is not recommended.[52] Patients who have a history of rheumatic fever with residual valvular disease should receive a prophylactic regimen recommended by the AHA before specific surgical and dental procedures, because drug regimens used to prevent recurrence of acute rheumatic fever are not adequate for prevention of endocarditis.[53] If the patient is currently receiving a penicillin for secondary prevention of rheumatic fever, it is recommended that a non-penicillin regimen be used for endocarditis prophylaxis.[53] The AHA guidelines for prophylaxis are summarized in Tables 72.6 and 72.7.[52]

Table 72.4 ▪ Cardiac Conditions

Endocarditis Prophylaxis Recommended	Endocarditis Prophylaxis Not Recommended
High-risk category Prosthetic cardiac valves, including bioprosthetic and homograph valves Previous bacterial endocarditis Complex cyanotic congenital heart disease (e.g., single-ventricle states, transposition of the great arteries, tetralogy of Fallot) Surgically constructed systemic pulmonary shunts or conduits Moderate-risk category Most other congenital cardiac malformations Acquired valvular dysfunction (eg., rheumatic heart disease) Hypertrophic cardiomyopathy Mitral valve prolapse with valvular regurgitation, thickened leaflets, or both	Isolated secundum atrial septal defect Surgical repair of atrial septal defect, ventricular septal defect, or patent ductus arteriosis (without residua beyond 6 months) Previous coronary artery bypass graft surgery Mitral valve prolapse, without regurgitation Physiologic, functional, or innocent heart murmurs Previous Kawasaki disease without valvular dysfunction Previous rheumatic fever without valvular dysfunction Cardiac pacemakers and implanted defibrillators

Source: Adapted from Dajani AS, Taubert KA, Wilson W, et al. Prevention of bacterial endocarditis–recommendations by the American Heart Association. JAMA 277(22):1794–1801, 1997. Copyright 1997, American Medical Association.

Table 72.5 ▪ Dental or Surgical Procedures

Endocarditis Prophylaxis Recommended	Endocarditis Prophylaxis Not Recommended
Dental procedures Dental extractions Periodontal procedures including surgery, scaling and root planing, probing, and recall maintenance Dental implant placement and reimplantation of avulsed teeth Endodontic (root canal) instrumentation or surgery only beyond the apex Subgingival placement of antibiotic fibers or strips Initial placement of orthodontic bands but not brackets Intraligamentary local anesthetic injections Prophylactic cleaning of teeth or implants where bleeding is anticipated Respiratory tract procedures Tonsillectomy or adenoidectomy Surgical operations that involve respiratory mucosa Bronchoscopy with rigid bronchoscope Gastrointestinal tract procedures Sclerotherapy for esophageal varices Esophageal stricture dilation Endoscopic retrograde cholangiography with biliary obstruction Biliary tract surgery Surgical operations that involve intestinal mucosa Genitourinary tract procedures Prostatic surgery Cystoscopy Urethral dilation	Dental procedures Restorative dentistry (operative and prosthodontic) Local anesthetic injections Intracanal endodontic treatment; after placement and buildup Placement of rubber dams Postoperative suture removal Placement of removable prosthodontic or orthodontic appliances Taking of oral impressions Fluoride treatments Orthodontic appliance adjustment Shedding of primary teeth Respiratory tract procedures Endotracheal intubation Bronchoscopy with a flexible bronchoscope Tympanostomy tube insertion Gastrointestinal tract procedures Transesophageal echocardiography Endoscopy with/without gastrointestinal biopsy Genitourinary tract procedures Vaginal hysterectomy Vaginal delivery Cesarean section In uninfected tissue: Urethral catheterization, uterine dilation and curettage, therapeutic abortion, sterilization procedures, or insertion/removal of intrauterine devices Other procedures Cardiac catheterization, including balloon angioplasty Implanted cardiac pacemakers, implanted defibrillators, and coronary stents Incision or biopsy of surgically scrubbed skin Circumcision

Source: Adapted from Dajani AS, Taubert KA, Wilson W, et al. Prevention of bacterial endocarditis–recommendations by the American Heart Association. JAMA 277(22):1794–1801, 1997. Copyright 1997, American Medical Association.

Table 72.6 ▪ Prophylactic Regimens for Dental, Oral, Respiratory Tract, or Esophageal Procedures

Situation	Agent	Adult Regimen
Standard prophylaxis	Amoxicillin	2 g PO, 1 hr before procedure
Unable to take oral medications	Ampicillin	2 g IM/IV, within 30 min of procedure
Penicillin allergy	Clindamycin	600 mg PO, 1 hr before procedure
	or	
	cephalexin or cefadroxil	2 g PO, 1 hr before procedure
	or	
	Azithromycin or clarithromycin	500 mg PO, 1 hr before procedure
Penicillin allergy, unable to take oral medications	Clindamycin	600 mg IV within 30 min of procedure
	or	
	cefazolin	1 g IV within 30 min of procedure

Adapted from Dajani AS, Taubert KA, Wilson W, et al. Prevention of bacterial endocarditis—recommendations by the American Heart Association. JAMA 277(22):1794–1801, 1997. Copyright 1997, American Medical Association.

Table 72.7 ▪ Prophylactic Regimens for Genitourinary and Gastrointestinal (excluding esophageal) Procedures

Situation	Agent	Adult Regimen
High-risk patients	Ampicillin	Ampicillin 2 g IM/IV
	plus	*plus*
	gentamicin	gentamicin 1.5 mg/kg within 30 min of procedure,
		followed by
		ampicillin 1 g IM/IV
		or
		amoxicillin 1 g PO 6 hr later
High-risk patients, penicillin allergy	Vancomycin	Vancomycin 1 g IV over 1–2 hr
	plus	*plus*
	gentamicin	Gentamicin 1.5 mg/kg; infusions completed within 30 min of procedure
Moderate-risk patients	Amoxicillin	Amoxicillin 2 g PO 1 hr before procedure
	or	*or*
	ampicillin	ampicillin 2 g IM/IV within 30 min before procedure
Moderate-risk patients, penicillin allergy	Vancomycin	Vancomycin 1 g IV over 1–2 hr; infusion completed within 30 min of procedure

Source: Adapted from Dajani AS, Taubert KA, Wilson W, et al. Prevention of bacterial endocarditis—recommendations by the American Heart Association. JAMA 277(22):1794–1801, 1997. Copyright 1997, American Medical Association.

KEY POINTS

- IE is a potentially life-threatening infection that requires early recognition and aggressive and prolonged treatment for successful management.
- High-dose antimicrobial therapy is needed because IE is difficult to treat as a result of an absence of host defenses, poor penetration of antibiotics, high organism burden, and reduced metabolic state of organisms at the site of infection.
- Combination therapy is required for treatment of IE due to *Pseudomonas aeruginosa*, enterococcus species, or tolerant organisms.
- Combination therapy also may be useful to shorten the overall duration of therapy for susceptible organisms (e.g., *S. aureus*, streptococci) as long as a penicillin is part of the regimen.
- Infections due to multidrug-resistant pathogens such as enterococcus are increasing in prevalence, and combinations of antibiotics are commonly used to achieve synergistic bactericidal effects.
- Surgical removal of the infected valve is often necessary in patients with the following characteristics: severe hemodynamic compromise; intracardiac abscess; Gram-negative, fungal, or other nonbacterial etiology; infection caused by resistant organisms; PVE; relapse after "adequate" therapy; and multiple embolic events.
- Newer antimicrobials such as quinupristin–dalfopristin, lipopeptides, glycylcyclines, and fluoroquinolones may have a role in the treatment of IE.
- A minimum of 6 weeks of therapy is required for successful treatment of PVE, and replacement of the infected prosthesis may be necessary.
- Prevention of infection is best achieved by recognition of patients at risk, identification of clinical situations likely to produce bacteremia, and use of the recommended prophylactic regimens.

REFERENCES

1. Sullam PM, Drake TA, Sande MA. Pathogenesis of endocarditis. Am J Med 78(6B):110–115, 1985.

2. Scheld WM, Sande MA. Endocarditis and intravascular infections. In: Mandell GL, Bennett JE, Dolin R, eds. Principles and practice of infectious diseases. 4th ed. New York: Churchill Livingstone, 1995:740–783.
3. Bayer AS. Infective endocarditis. Clin Infect Dis 17:313–322, 1993.
4. Bayer AS, Bolger AF, Taubert KA, et al. Diagnosis and management of infective endocarditis and its complications. Circulation 98:2936–2948, 1998.
5. Chambers HF, Korzeniowski OM, Sande MA, et al. *Staphylococcus aureus* endocarditis: clinical manifestations in addicts and non-addicts. Medicine 62:170–177, 1983.
6. Levine DP, Crane LR, Zervos MJ. Bacteremia in narcotic addicts at the Detroit Medical Center. II. Infectious endocarditis: a prospective comparative study. Rev Infect Dis 8:374–396, 1986.
7. Whitener C, Caputo GM, Weitekamp MR, et al. Endocarditis due to coagulase-negative staphylococci. Infect Dis Clin North Am 7:81–96, 1993.
8. Roder BL, Wandall DA, Frimodt-Meller N, et al. Clinical features of *Staphylococcus aureus* endocarditis: a 10-year experience in Denmark. Arch Intern Med 159:462–469, 1999.
9. Fowler VG Jr, Sanders LL, Kong LK, et al. Infective endocarditis due to *Staphylococcus aureus*: 59 prospectively identified cases with follow-up. Clin Infect Dis 28:106–114, 1999.
10. Fowler VG Jr, Li J, Corey GR, et al. Role of echocardiography in evaluation of patients with *Staphylococcus aureus* bacteremia: experience in 103 patients. J Am Coll Cardiol 30:1072–1078, 1997.
11. Watanakunakorn C. Editorial response: increasing importance of intravascular device-associated *Staphylococcus aureus* endocarditis. Clin Infect Dis 28:115–116, 1999.
12. Wilson WR, Karchmer AW, Dajani AD, et al. Antibiotic treatment of adults with infective endocarditis due to streptococci, enterococci, staphylococci, and HACEK microorganisms. JAMA 274:1706–1713, 1995.
13. Threlkeld MB, Cobbs CG. Infectious disorders of prosthetic valves and intravascular devices. In: Mandell GL, Bennett JE, Dolin R, eds. Principles and practice of infectious diseases. 4th ed. New York: Churchill Livingstone, 1995:783–793.
14. Vlessis AA, Khaki A, Grunkemeier GL, et al. Risk, diagnosis and management of prosthetic valve endocarditis: a review. J Heart Valve Dis 6:443–465, 1997.
15. Caulderwood SB, Swinski LA, Karchmer AW, et al. Prosthetic valve endocarditis: analysis of factors affecting outcome of therapy. J Thorac Cardiovasc Surg 92:776–783, 1986.
16. Grover FL, Cohen DJ, Oprian C, et al. Determinants of the occurrence of and survival from prosthetic valve endocarditis. J Thorac Cardiovasc Surg 108:207–214, 1994.
17. Molavi A. Endocarditis: recognition, management, and prophylaxis. Cardiovasc Clin 23:139–174, 1993.
18. Werner GS, Schulz R, Fuchs JB, et al. Infective endocarditis in the elderly in the era of transesophageal echocardiography: clinical features and prognosis compared with younger patients. Am J Med 100:90–97, 1996.
19. Nassar RM, Melgar GR, Longworth DL, et al. Incidence and risk of developing fungal prosthetic valve endocarditis after nosocomial candidemia. Am J Med 103:25–32, 1997.
20. Siddiq S, Missri J, Silverman DI. Endocarditis in an urban hospital in the 1990s. Arch Intern Med 156:2454–2458, 1996.
21. Durack DT, Beeson PB. Experimental bacterial endocarditis I. Colonization of a sterile vegetation. Br J Exp Path 53:44–49, 1972.
22. Wilson WR, Giuliani ER, Danielson GK, et al. Management of complications of infective endocarditis. Mayo Clin Proc 47:162–170, 1982.
23. Weinstein L. Life-threatening complications of infective endocarditis and their management. Arch Intern Med 146:953–957, 1986.
24. Tunkel AR, Kaye D. Neurologic complications of infective endocarditis. Neurol Clin 11:419–440, 1993.
25. Durack DT, Lukes AS, Bright DK, et al. New criteria for diagnosis of infective endocarditis. Am J Med 96:200–209, 1994.
26. Von Reyn CF, Levy BS, Arbeit RD, et al. Infective endocarditis: analysis based on strict case definitions. Ann Intern Med 94:505–511, 1981.
27. Daniel WG, Mugge A. Transesophageal echocardiography. N Engl J Med 332:1268–1279, 1995.
28. Baldassarre JS, Kaye D. Principles and overview of antibiotic therapy. In: Kaye D, ed. Infective endocarditis. New York: Raven Press, 1992:169–190.
29. Carbon C, Cremieux AC, Fantin B. Pharmacokinetic and pharmacodynamic aspects of therapy of experimental endocarditis. Infect Dis Clin North Am 7:37–51, 1993.
30. Francioli P, Etienne J, Hoigne R, et al. Treatment of streptococcal endocarditis with a single daily dose of ceftriaxone sodium for 4 weeks. JAMA 267:264–267, 1992.
31. Francioli P, Ruch W, Stamboulian D, and the International Infective Endocarditis Study Group. Treatment of streptococcal endocarditis with a single daily dose of ceftriaxone and netilmicin for 14 days: a prospective multicenter study. Clin Infect Dis 21:1406–1410, 1995.
32. Eliopoulos GM. Aminoglycoside-resistant enterococcal endocarditis. Infect Dis Clin North Am 7:117–133, 1993.
33. Fantin B, Carbon C. Importance of the aminoglycoside dosing regimen in the penicillin-netilmicin combination for treatment of *Enterococcus faecalis*–induced experimental endocarditis. Antimicrob Agents Chemother 34:2387–2391, 1990.
34. Marangos MN, Nicolau DP, Quintiliani R, et al. Influence of gentamicin dosing interval on the efficacy of penicillin-containing regimens in experimental *Enterococcus faecalis* endocarditis. J Antimicrob Chemother 39:519–522, 1997.
35. Schwank S, Blaser J. Once versus thrice-daily netilmicin combined with amoxicillin, penicillin, or vancomycin against *Enterococcus faecalis* in a pharmacodynamic in vitro model. Antimicrob Agents Chemother 40:2258–2261, 1996.
36. Landman D, Quale JM. Management of infections due to resistant enterococci: a review of therapeutic options. J Antimicrob Chemother 40:161–170, 1997.
37. Murray BE. Vancomycin-resistant enterococci. Am J Med 101:284–293, 1997.
38. Small PM, Chambers HF. Vancomycin for *Staphylococcus aureus* endocarditis in intravenous drug abusers. Antimicrob Agents Chemother 34:1227–1231, 1990.
39. Levine DP, Fromm BS, Reddy BR. Slow response to vancomycin or vancomycin plus rifampin therapy among patients with methicillin-resistant *Staphylococcus aureus* endocarditis. Ann Intern Med 115:674–680, 1991.
40. Chambers HF. Short-course combination and oral therapies of *Staphylococcus aureus* endocarditis. Infect Dis Clin North Am 7:69–79, 1993.
41. Heldman AW, Hartert TV, Ray SC, et al. Oral antibiotic treatment of right-sided staphylococcal endocarditis in injection drug users: prospective randomized comparison with parenteral therapy. Am J Med 101:68–76, 1996.
42. Palmer SM, Rybak MJ. An evaluation of the bactericidal activity of ampicillin/sulbactam, piperacillin/tazobactam, imipenem, or nafcillin alone and in combination with vancomycin against methicillin-resistant *Staphylococcus aureus* (MRSA) in time-kill curves with infected fibrin clots. J Antimicrob Chemother 39:515–518, 1997.
43. Chandrasekar PH, Levine DP, Price S, et al. Comparative efficacies of imipenem-cilastatin and vancomycin in experimental aortic valve endocarditis due to methicillin resistant *Staphylococcus aureus*. J Antimicrob Chemother 21:461–469, 1988.
44. Dickinson G, Rodriguez K, Arcey S, et al. Efficacy of imipenem/cilastatin in endocarditis. Am J Med 78(6A):117–121, 1985.
45. Markowitz N, Quinn EL, Saravolatz LD. Trimethoprim-sulfamethoxazole compared to vancomycin for the treatment of *Staphylococcus aureus* infection. Ann Intern Med 117:390–398, 1992.
46. Komshian SV, Tablan OC, Palutke W, et al. Characteristics of left-sided endocarditis due to *Pseudomonas aeruginosa* in the Detroit Medical Center. Rev Infect Dis 12:693–702, 1990.
47. Gilbert HM, Peters ED, Lang SJ, et al. Successful treatment of fungal prosthetic valve endocarditis: case report and review. Clin Infect Dis 22:348–354, 1996.
48. Rubinstein E, Lang R. Fungal endocarditis. Eur Heart J 16(Suppl B):84–89, 1995.
49. Alsip SG, Blackstone EH, Kirklin JW, et al. Indications for cardiac surgery in patients with active infective endocarditis. Am J Med 78(6B):138–148, 1985.
50. Moon MR, Stinson EB, Miller DC. Surgical treatment of endocarditis. Prog Cardiovasc Dis 40:239–264, 1997.
51. Durack DT. Prevention of infective endocarditis. N Engl J Med 332:38–44, 1995.
52. Dajani AS, Taubert KA, Wilson W, et al. Prevention of bacterial endocarditis–recommendations by the American Heart Association. JAMA 277:1794–1801, 1997.
53. Dajani A, Taubert K, Ferrieri P, et al. Treatment of acute streptococcal pharyngitis and prevention of rheumatic fever: a statement for health professionals. Pediatrics 96:758–764, 1995.

CHAPTER 73

CENTRAL NERVOUS SYSTEM INFECTIONS

Constance M. Pfeiffer and Lisa M. Avery

The central nervous system (CNS) is composed of the brain and spinal cord. The brain is surrounded by membranes (the meninges) and is protected by the skull. CNS infections can occur in the membranes between the skull and the brain (meningitis) or within the brain itself (encephalitis or brain abscesses) or may be associated with an indwelling CNS device (i.e., shunt infections).

CNS infections are associated with significant morbidity and mortality. These infections are caused by a variety of pathogens, including bacteria, viruses, fungi, and parasites. Predisposing factors for the development of CNS infections include sinusitis, otitis media, head injury, and the presence of systemic infections.

TREATMENT GOALS: CENTRAL NERVOUS SYSTEM INFECTIONS

- Diagnose and initiate therapy promptly. A delay in therapy of a few hours may result in increased morbidity and mortality.
- Base treatment on the site or type of infection (i.e., meningitis, abscess versus shunt infection), the suspected pathogens and their anticipated susceptibilities, and individual patient characteristics.
- Use only antimicrobials that have a bactericidal mechanism of action, including all agents in a combination regimen.
- Select antimicrobials that have good penetration through the blood–brain barrier (BBB) and achieve adequate cerebrospinal fluid (CSF) drug concentrations.
- Ensure high-dose antimicrobial dosage regimens to ensure adequate CSF concentrations that should exceed the minimum bactericidal concentration (MBC) of the pathogen by at least 8 to 10 times.
- Note that because of the unidirectional flow of CSF, direct instillation of antibiotics into the CSF (via lumbar puncture or intraventricular) will only achieve therapeutic antibiotic concentrations *below* the point of instillation.

Meningitis

EPIDEMIOLOGY

A variety of factors influence the suspected etiology of meningitis. Age (Table 73.1), underlying risk factors (e.g., immunocompromise), and seasonal variations can be useful in directing empiric therapy. In adults, three organisms–*Neisseria meningitidis, Streptococcus pneumoniae,* and *Haemophilus influenzae*–are most commonly responsible for meningitis. Gram-negative meningitis is extremely rare in adults, except when postneurosurgical meningitis occurs. However, meningitis due to enteric organisms, most frequently *Escherichia coli,* is common in neonates. Geriatric patients are more likely to develop meningitis due to *Listeria monocytogenes,* although *S. pneumoniae* and *N. meningitidis* are still the most common pathogens in this age-group.[1,2]

Age alone cannot be used as the only criterion for empiric antibiotic therapy selection. Several other factors should influence the decision-making process. Nosocomial meningitis or status-post open head trauma increases the index of suspicion for gram-negative bacilli and staphylococcal infections. Specifically, patients with indwelling shunts may develop *Staphylococcus epidermidis* meningitis (frequently methicillin resistant). Other risk factors can also predispose patients to development of certain types of meningitis. Alcoholism, asplenia, bacterial pneumonia, sinusitis, head trauma, immunosuppression, and sickle cell disease increase the likelihood of *S. pneumoniae* meningitis. Lyme meningitis due to *Borrelia burgdorferi* (neuroborreliosis) is becoming more common in areas endemic for Lyme disease.

PATHOPHYSIOLOGY

Pathogens are thought to infect the meninges through three pathways: hematogenous seeding, direct inoculation (trauma, neurosurgery), or contiguous spread from a parameningeal focus (e.g., sinusitis, dental surgery). Virulence factors may also play a role for certain meningeal pathogens. Encapsulated organisms such as *S. pneumoniae* and *H. influenzae* type b are more easily able to cross the BBB into the CNS, and they are also more resistant to phagocytosis in the bloodstream; *N. meningitidis* use pili on their cell surface to breach and attach to the mucosal barrier.

Once pathogens have entered the CNS, a cascade of events occurs. The presence of bacterial cell wall products triggers the production of cytokines, including interleukin-1, tumor necrosis factor, and prostaglandin E_2, which initially lead to increased blood flow to the brain. These cytokines also increase BBB permeability by interfering with the integrity of capillary tight junctions, allowing cerebral edema to occur. Cytotoxins released from neutrophils, and possibly the bacteria itself, also contribute to the development of cerebral edema.

Intracranial pressure rises secondary to increased blood flow and edema, resulting in decreased cerebral perfusion. The inflammatory process can result in vasculitis and thrombotic events that contribute to the overall cerebral ischemia, which may ultimately result in significant neurologic sequelae.

CLINICAL PRESENTATION AND DIAGNOSIS

Signs and Symptoms

Symptoms of meningitis may occur acutely, within 24 hours, or insidiously, over 1 to 7 days. Acute meningitis is associated with a higher fatality rate (50%) and is most commonly caused by bacteria. Subacute meningitis may be caused by viral, mycobacterial, fungal, or bacteria infection and is generally associated with a lower mortality

Table 73.1 ▪ Common Pathogens That Cause Meningitis (Arranged by Patient Age-Group)

Age-Group	Common Pathogens	Empiric Treatment
Neonates	Group B streptococcus *Listeria monocytogenes* Gram-negative bacilli Gram-positive bacilli	Ampicillin + cefotaxime or an aminoglycoside
Infants (1–3 months)	*Streptococcus pneumoniae* *Neisseria meningitidis* Rarely, *Haemophilus influenzae* pathogens seen in neonates	Ampicillin + cefotaxime or ceftriaxone + dexamethasone
3 months to 50 years	*Streptococcus pneumoniae* *Neisseria meningitidis* Rarely, *Haemophilus influenzae*	Cefotaxime or ceftriaxone ± vancomycin
Older adults (>50 years)	*Streptococcus pneumoniae* *Listeria monocytogenes* Gram-negative bacilli	Ampicillin + cefotaxime or ceftriaxone ± dexamethasone

rate (less than 25%).[3] A patient with either acute or subacute meningitis may have symptoms of meningeal inflammation such as vomiting, headache, lethargy, confusion, or neck stiffness. Fever, rigors, myalgias, and photophobia are seen as well. Less commonly, patients experience focal symptoms such as seizures, cranial nerve palsies, or hemiparesis. The clinical presentation in neonates and in older adults is more insidious. Neonates and young infants lack the meningeal signs and symptoms but may display hypothermia or hyperthermia, listlessness, lethargy, high-pitched crying, nausea, vomiting, anorexia, poor eating habits, irritability, and seizures. Late clinical manifestations in infants include neck stiffness and a full fontanelle. Older adults may have only new-onset confusion and no other cardinal signs, such as fever or nuchal rigidity, so meningitis can easily be misdiagnosed.

On physical examination patients may have nuchal rigidity or meningismus, positive Kernig's or Brudzinski's sign, and papilledema. Kernig's sign is elicited by placing the patient in the supine position and then flexing the thigh perpendicular to the abdomen with the knee also in the flexed position. As the leg is extended, the patient with meningitis resists leg extension. Brudzinski's sign is evident when forward neck flexion results in the flexion of the hips and knees. A petechial or purpuric rash predominantly on the extremities is consistent with *N. meningitidis*, although it may also occur with streptococci or *H. influenzae* infections.

Diagnosis

It is imperative that a rapid diagnosis of meningitis be made to ensure prompt, appropriate therapy. A lumbar puncture (LP) is used to confirm the diagnosis and identify the pathogen. The goal is to obtain and evaluate the CSF within 30 minutes of presentation. However, first it must be determined whether it is safe to perform the LP (i.e., rule out contraindications to performing an LP, such as a mass lesion, brain abscess, or subdural empyema). This may be done by examining the patient for the presence of focal neurologic signs. The patient should also be evaluated for papilledema, hemiparesis, aphasia, ataxia, and visual field defects, which may suggest an extreme increase in intracranial pressure. If papilledema or neurologic signs are present, an LP is contraindicated because of the risk of brain herniation. Computerized tomography (CT) or magnetic resonance image (MRI) may be performed before an LP to help in the assessment process. There is some debate about whether CT should be performed before all LPs. Proponents believe that neurologic signs may be missed because of the patient's inability to participate in a complete neurologic examination. Papilledema or lack thereof is not a reliable marker of the presence or absence of increased ICP and therefore should not be used as the sole safety indicator.

In patients who have focal neurologic signs, blood cultures should be drawn and appropriate empiric antibiotics given before completion of imaging studies and LP. Sterilization of the spinal fluid may take several hours, and therefore CSF cultures may still be positive despite administration of antibiotics.

Before removing the CSF an opening pressure can be measured. In meningitis, pressures generally exceed 200 mm H_2O (normal: < 150 mm H_2O in supine position). Pressures greater than 600 mm H_2O may be consistent with intracranial masses. A repeat LP may be necessary if treatment response is inadequate.

The CSF is also evaluated for gross visual turbidity, cell analysis, glucose and protein concentrations, and Gram stain and culture. A normal CSF sample should be colorless and clear. In bacterial meningitis, the CSF may be cloudy; but in fungal and viral meningitis the fluid is generally clear. A pleocytosis (increased number of white blood cells) with a predominance of neutrophils is consistent with bacterial meningitis. A lymphocytic pleocytosis is consistent with fungal, mycobacterial, or viral infections, although viral meningitis may have an initial neutrophilic predominance. Characteristics of the CSF in adults with various types of meningitis are summarized in Table 73.2. In neonates, the total normal number of white blood cells in the CSF is higher than in adults (Table 73.3); by age 1 year, the normal values are the same as those in adults. The glucose concentration in normal CSF fluid is 50 to 60% (or 0.5:1 ratio) of the simultaneous serum glucose, generally 3 to 6.1 mmol/L (70 to 110 mg/dl). In bacterial, fungal, and mycobacterial infections, the CSF–blood glucose ratio is generally less than 0.5, whereas in viral meningitis the CSF–blood glucose ratio is normal. For an accurate assessment of CSF glucose a plasma glucose sample should be obtained before the LP. This is especially important in diabetic patients whose plasma glucose may be elevated; therefore, the relative glucose in the CSF may appear normal. Another issue that should be considered is whether the patient received dextrose 50% (D50) in the emergency room before the lumbar puncture. The time for glucose to reach equilibrium between the blood and CSF after D50 administration is a minimum of 30 minutes, and it may take up to 4 hours. Effects on CSF glucose will not be seen if the D50 injection was given less than 30 minutes before the LP.[1–5]

An elevated protein concentration is a sign of disruption of the BBB. In adults the normal protein concentrations range is 20 to 40 mg/dl. Although protein elevation is a nonspecific finding, in meningitis it is generally elevated (100 to 500 mg/dl), except in viral meningitis, where the concentrations are somewhat lower (50 to 100 mg/dl). In neonates the normal protein concentration is 20 to 150 mg/dl because of the immaturity of the BBB; by age 1 year, the upper limit of normal decreases to 45 mg/dl.[1–5]

Some clinicians advocate the use of measurement of lactate in the CSF to aid in the differential diagnosis of viral meningitis versus bacterial meningitis. If the concentration of lactate in the CSF is more than 6 mmol/L, the patient probably has bacterial meningitis; if the concentration is less than 3 mmol/L, the patient probably has viral meningitis.

Table 73.2 ▪ Cerebrospinal Fluid Characteristics in Meningitis

Pathogen	White Blood Cell Count (cells/m³)	Predominant Cell Type in Differential	Glucose Ratio (cerebrospinal fluid to blood)	Protein Concentration (mg/dL)
None (normal cerebrospinal fluid)	<5	Lymphocytes Monocytes	0.5–0.6	20–40
Bacterial	1000–100,000	Neutrophils	<0.5	100–500
Fungal	10–1000	Lymphocytic	<0.5	100–500
Mycobacteria	100–400	Lymphocytic	<0.5	100–500
Viral	10–1000	Lymphocytic (polymorphonuclear leukocytes early)	0.5–0.6	50–100

Table 73.3 ▪ Normal Values for Cerebrospinal Fluid in Pediatric Populations

	Full-Term Neonate	Infant	Child
White blood cell count	0–25 cells/mm³	0–8 cells/mm³	0–5 cells/mm³
Protein concentration	20–150 mg/dL	14–45 mg/dL	15–45 mg/dL
Glucose concentration	20–40 mg/dL	70–90 mg/dL	50–80 mg/dL

A Gram stain of the CSF provides another tool for rapid diagnosis of bacterial meningitis and can be used to guide empiric therapy.[6] A causative bacterial organism may be detected on Gram stain in up to 60 to 80% of untreated patients and in 40 to 60% of patients who have already received some antibiotic therapy.[5,6] The diagnostic accuracy of the Gram stain is related to the concentration of bacterial colonies and the particular microorganism involved. Greater than 10^5 colony-forming units (cfu) per milliliter of bacteria correlates with a positive Gram stain.[5] If tuberculous or cryptococcal meningitis is suspected, acid-fast stain or India ink stain, respectively, is used.

CSF cultures are positive in 70 to 80% of cases of bacterial meningitis and can help direct antibiotic therapy. Blood cultures are positive in 40 to 60% of patients with *H. influenzae,* meningococcal, and pneumococcal meningitis.

Other cultures may be of some use if systemic infections sources are identified as the potential etiology of meningitis, such as respiratory and urinary tract cultures. As in other types of infection, the patient may have a peripheral leukocytosis (white blood cell count >10,000/mm³). Other diagnostic tests include fungal cultures, cryptococcal antigen testing, and Venereal Disease Research Laboratory (VDRL) test to rule out neurosyphilis.

Rapid diagnostic tests play a role in identifying the causative organism, especially for patients who received antibiotics before LP or in patients with negative results from Gram stain or culture procedures. The latex agglutination test detects the polysaccharide antigen of *H. influenzae* type b, *S. pneumoniae*, *N. meningitidis*, *E. coli* K1, and group Bstreptococci from either CSF, serum, or urine. The results are generally available in 20 to 30 minutes. The overall sensitivity of the latex agglutination test ranges from 50 to 100%; however, the sensitivity is lower for *N. meningitidis.*[7] The limulus test detects endotoxins produced by gram-negative organisms. However, this test is not widely used because it lacks specificity and specimens are easily contaminated. Polymerase chain reaction (PCR) techniques are currently being investigated for utilization in rapid diagnosis of CNS infections, including herpesvirus infections.

TREATMENT

Pharmacokinetic and Pharmacodynamic Considerations

The presence of the BBB and the unidirectional flow of CSF complicate the treatment of CNS infections. The tightly joined endothelial cells of brain capillaries form the BBB, which acts as a semipermeable membrane, regulating drug concentrations entering and exiting the CSF. To ensure adequate CSF bactericidal activity, therapy must include only those antimicrobials that can penetrate the BBB and achieve adequate levels in the CSF. Factors influencing the ability of drugs to cross the BBB are lipophilicity, degree of ionization, molecular weight, and complexity of structure. Nonionized, lipophilic, low-molecular-weight molecules passively diffuse across the BBB more readily than large, complex, hydrophilic, or ionized molecules. Because only free drug is capable of traversing the BBB, agents that are highly protein bound are at a potential disadvantage.

Meningeal inflammation that occurs along with meningitis actually enhances the penetration of certain antibiotics through the BBB (Table 73.4). Although the exact mechanism is unknown, it may be related to the impairment of active transport pumps and the disruption of the tight junctions of the capillaries. For example, the penicillin class of drugs achieves low CSF concentrations when the meninges are normal, but in the presence of meningitis and inflamed meninges, much higher concentrations are achievable. Because the degree of inflammation correlates with the percentage of antibiotic penetration, when inflammation decreases, as occurs with the healing process, the percentage of antibiotic penetration also decreases. Additionally, concomitant corticosteroid use causes a decrease in inflammation, a decrease in BBB permeability, and thus a decrease in CSF antibiotic concentration. Adjuvant corticosteroid use has been advocated in several instances of bacterial meningitis treatment, so antibiotic dosages and CSF penetration must be assessed carefully.

To control the active secretion of substances, the BBB also has a series of transport pumps. These stereospecific carriers remove weak organic acids such as penicillin, ampicillin, nafcillin, and cefazolin from the CSF through the choroid plexus. These "exit pumps" are saturable and may be inhibited by weak organic acids such as probenecid.

To optimize antibiotic concentrations in the CNS and overcome the permeability and secretory problems of the BBB, the direct instillation of antibiotics into the CSF is also an option. CSF is produced at a rate of 0.5 ml per minute by the choroid plexus and flows unidirectionally from lateral ventricles to the third and fourth ventricles and then to the subarachnoid space. CSF then flows through the subarachnoid space into the spinal column.

Table 73.4 ▪ Cerebrospinal Fluid (CSF) Penetration–Drug Characteristics

Achieve Adequate CSF Concentration Without Meningeal Inflammation	Achieve Adequate CSF Concentration Only if Meningeal Inflammation Exists	Do Not Achieve Adequate CSF Concentrations
Sulfonamides	Penicillins	Aminoglycosides
Trimethoprim	Penicillin G	Vancomycin
Chloramphenicol	Ampicillin	Polymyxin
Isoniazid	Nafcillin	Amphotericin B
Metronidazole	Antipseudomonal penicillins	
Fluconazole	Imipenem	
Flucytosine	Meropenem	
Pyrazinamide	Aztreonam	
	Third-generation cephalosporins	
	Quinolones	
	Ciprofloxacin	
	Ofloxacin	
	Rifampin	

This unidirectional flow is important to remember when administering drugs directly into the CSF because therapeutic levels of antibiotic will be achieved below the site of injection, but not above.

Drugs can be introduced directly into the CSF at a variety of sites and routes. Intraventricular injection is the most invasive, consisting of placement of a subcutaneous reservoir with a catheter that is placed directly into one of the lateral ventricles. Intrathecal administration requires that a needle be inserted into the subarachnoid space. Intracisternal administration is the injection of drug at the base of the skull, and intralumbar administration is for injection via a lumbar puncture site. These administration methods are used as adjunctive therapy and never as a sole method of drug administration.

Once the issue of drug penetration into the CSF has been addressed, the pharmacodynamic properties of the antimicrobial must be considered. As in endocarditis and osteomyelitis, the antibiotic chosen for the treatment of CNS infections must be bactericidal. This is an important factor because, compared with blood, the CSF has decreased immunoglobulins, complement, and opsonic activity, which results in impaired phagocytic activity against encapsulated bacteria. Bactericidal antibiotics include agents such as penicillins, cephalosporins, vancomycin, quinolones, penems, and aminoglycosides. The concentrations of bactericidal agents must exceed the MBC of the organism by at least 8 to 10 times to achieve the maximum rate of bacteria kill.[1]

Agents such as erythromycin, clindamycin, and tetracycline are bacteriostatic and should not be used for treatment of meningitis. Although chloramphenicol is considered to be bacteriostatic for most organisms, it does have bactericidal activity against certain bacteria (e.g., *S. pneumoniae, H. influenzae,* and *N. meningitidis*), and, therefore, is an option for the treatment of meningitis due to these pathogens. Use of bacteriostatic agents in combination with bactericidal agents may result in antagonism and is thus not recommended.

Empiric treatment of suspected meningitis is guided by the age of the patient (Table 73.1), expected pathogens (Table 73.5), and results of the Gram stain of the CSF (Table 73.6), if available. Empiric therapy generally consists of a third-generation cephalosporin and sometimes one or more additional antibiotics as indicated by patient-specific characteristics. Common regimens are ceftriaxone 2 g every 12 hours or cefotaxime 2 g every 4 to 6 hours.[3,4] The addition of vancomycin or ampicillin may be indicated in certain patient populations. Pathogen-specific treatment is discussed in the following sections.

Pharmacotherapy

Streptococcus pneumoniae Meningitis

Streptococcus pneumoniae, commonly called pneumococcus, is a gram-positive coccus seen on Gram stain in pairs or short chains. It is an encapsulated organism with 85 different serotypes. In 40 to 50% of cases, the patient has

Table 73.5 ▪ Common Pathogens That Cause Meningitis and Empiric Antibiotic Therapy in Patient Populations

Patient Type	Common Pathogens	Empiric Therapy
Alcoholic or debilitated patient (chronic illness)	*Streptococcus pneumoniae* *Listeria monocytogenes* Gram-negative bacilli	Ampicillin + ceftriaxone Dexamethasone
Impaired cellular immunity (high-dose steroids, lymphoma, myeloma, etc.)	*Listeria monocytogenes* Gram-negative bacilli *(Pseudomonas aeruginosa)*	Ampicillin + ceftazidime
Postneurosurgery or head trauma	*Streptococcus pneumoniae* *Staphylococcus aureus* Gram-negative bacilli (enteric gram-negative bacilli and *Pseudomonas aeruginosa*)	Vancomycin + ceftazidime

Table 73.6 ▪ Empiric Antibiotic Therapy for Meningitis Using Cerebrospinal Fluid Gram Stain Morphological Information

Gram Stain Result	Likely Pathogen	Empiric Therapy
Gram-negative bacilli	*Haemophilus influenzae* Enteric organisms *Pseudomonas aeruginosa*	Ceftazidime and aminoglycoside (add dexamethasone if pediatric patient)
Gram-negative cocci	*Neisseria meningitidis*	Penicillin G or ceftriaxone or cefotaxime
Gram-positive bacilli	*Listeria monocytogenes*	Ampicillin and aminoglycoside IV
Gram-positive cocci	*Streptococcus pneumoniae*	Vancomycin and ceftriaxone or cefotaxime (consider dexamethasone)

a concomitant pneumococcal pneumonia or otitis media infection.[8]

Empiric therapy for *S. pneumoniae* in the past included penicillin or ampicillin. Although penicillin has been the first-line agent, there has recently been an increase in the rates of pneumococci resistance to penicillin therapy. Now antibiotic resistance rates are as high as 25% in some areas of the United States.[9] Resistance to β-lactam antimicrobials results from alterations in the penicillin-binding proteins of the bacterial cell wall.[10] The Centers for Disease Control and Prevention (CDC) has standardized the classification of penicillin resistance. *Streptococcus pneumoniae* is considered sensitive to penicillin if the minimum inhibitory concentration (MIC) is 0.6 μg/mL or less. If the MIC is 0.1 to 1.0 μg/mL, the isolate is classified as intermediate, and if the MIC is 2.0 μg/mL or greater, the strain is considered resistant, previously referred to as high-level resistance. Cephalosporins are not currently affected to the same degree as penicillins, possibly because cephalosporins bind to several different penicillin-binding proteins. Therefore, susceptibility testing should include ceftriaxone or cefotaxime even for known penicillin-resistant strains. Resistance to cephalosporins is defined as MIC greater than 0.5 μg/mL. Some data indicate that this MIC value may be too conservative.[6] Antibiotics that typically exhibit cross-resistance include chloramphenicol, erythromycin, trimethoprim–sulfamethoxazole, aminoglycosides, and tetracycline. Risk factors for the development of penicillin resistance include age less than 5 years, frequent antibiotic use, and the use of prophylactic antibiotics to prevent chronic infections, such as otitis media.[11]

Because of the high rate of penicillin resistance, empiric therapy for patients with proven or suspected pneumococcal meningitis should include vancomycin in addition to ceftriaxone or cefotaxime until sensitivity results are available. A less conservative approach would be to continue to use monotherapy with ceftriaxone or cefotaxime. However, the number of case reports of cephalosporin-resistant isolates has been increasing.[12]

A secondary complication arises from the revised empiric therapy for potential penicillin-resistant *S. pneumoniae* infection because empiric therapy may sometimes include the adjuvant dexamethasone. Dexamethasone, due to its antiinflammatory effect, decreases vancomycin penetration in adults and, therefore, is generally not recommended. If a steroid is used, the preferred regimen is ceftriaxone IV plus rifampin PO or IV. In children, dexamethasone has not been shown to decrease vancomycin penetration to a significant degree and should be included in the empiric regimen in combination with cefotaxime or ceftriaxone in children receiving steroids. It appears that timing of dexamethasone is important in pneumococcal meningitis, with administration before or concurrently with antibiotics having better outcome. Short courses (i.e., first 2 days of therapy) of corticosteroid administration may be optimal.[13]

Clinical studies evaluating these regimens are few, and recommendation changes will occur when the results of future clinical trials are available. Monotherapy with vancomycin or rifampin is not appropriate because of vancomycin's erratic CSF penetration and the rapid development of rifampin resistance during rifampin monotherapy. Empiric therapy for patients with severe penicillin allergies (i.e., anaphylaxis) should include vancomycin in addition to rifampin. Cephalosporins and penems (meropenem and imipenem) should not be used in these patients because they may cause life-threatening allergic cross-sensitivity reactions.

Once sensitivity results are available, empiric therapy can be modified to provide narrower coverage. The treatment of choice in patients with penicillin-sensitive strains (MIC ≤0.6 μg/mL or less) is high-dose penicillin or ampicillin. Treatment of intermediately sensitive strains of pneumococcus (MIC 0.1 to 1.0 μg/mL) includes either high-dose penicillin (500,000 U/kg/day) or, if the MIC for cephalosporins is less than 0.5 μg/mL, either ceftriaxone or cefotaxime. Vancomycin, the drug of choice for high-level penicillin resistance, is sometimes used in combination with rifampin and ceftriaxone. In experimental meningitis, the combination of vancomycin and ceftriaxone was synergistic even in cases in which the MIC was greater than 0.5 μg/ml for ceftriaxone.[14] In pediatric patients who are not responding after 24 to 48 hours of therapy with vancomycin plus cefotaxime or ceftriaxone, rifampin may be added or substituted for vancomycin.[15] The duration of therapy is 10 to 14 days.

Alternative therapies for treatment of penicillin-resistant strains include chloramphenicol, imipenem, meropenem, cefpirome, cefepime, trovafloxacin, clinafloxacin, and streptogranin antibiotics. Chloramphenicol has been used to treat meningitis in children with resistance to penicillin and cephalosporins. It has been associated with poor outcomes (death, serious neurologic deficits, and poor clinical response), despite the fact that MIC values suggested sensitivity to this drug.[6] Imipenem has been reported to be effective, both in intermediate and resistant strains; however, the risk of seizures is high and it is therefore not routinely recommended for meningitis or other CNS infections. Meropenem is a carbapenem that has activity similar to imipenem but differs in its stability against renal tubular dehydropeptidases; therefore, meropenem does not require the enzyme inhibitor cilastatin. Meropenem has also been shown to have a lower incidence of seizures. This may prove to be an option in cephalosporin-resistant strains, although there is currently a lack of clinical data. The fourth-generation cephalosporins, cefpirome and cefepime, have in vitro activity against *H. influenzae, Pseudomonas aeruginosa*, meningococcus, and strains of penicillin-resistant pneumococci. Trovafloxacin, clinafloxacin, and other newer-generation fluoroquinolones have excellent activity against resistant pneumococci and gram-negative pathogens and achieve excellent penetration into the CNS. The incidence of trovafloxacin-associated hepatic dysfunction must be considered when determining its role in the treatment of meningitis.

A 23-valent polysaccharide vaccine to prevent systemic pneumococcal infection has been available since 1983. Because 90% of all pneumococcal isolates are covered, the vaccine should be highly recommended to patients at risk of infection. Proper vaccination should decrease the incidence of pneumococcal infections, including resistance strains, because six of the seven serotypes commonly associated with resistance are contained in the vaccine.[16] As of this writing, recommendations for vaccination with pneumococcal vaccine are (1) immunocompetent adults 65 years of age or older; (2) immunocompetent adults and children (younger than 2 years of age) with chronic illnesses such as cardiovascular or pulmonary disease, diabetes mellitus, alcoholism, cirrhosis, or CSF leaks (patients who receive the vaccine before they are 65 years of age must be revaccinated 5 years after the first dose); (3) adults or children (older than 2 years of age) with functional or anatomic asplenia (e.g., sickle cell disease or splenectomy); and (4) immunocompromised adults and children (older than 2 years of age) with disease.[15,16] Immunocompromised patients include patients with the following diagnoses: congenital immunodeficiency; human immunodeficiency virus (HIV) infection; leukemia; Hodgkin's disease; non-Hodgkin's lymphoma; multiple myeloma; generalized malignancy; bone marrow or organ transplant; therapy with alkylating agents, antimetabolites, radiation, or systemic corticosteroids; chronic renal failure; or nephrotic syndrome.[16]

The vaccine is not recommended in children younger than 2 years of age, because they are unable to mount an adequate immune response. The usual dose of the vaccine is 0.5 mL given intramuscularly or subcutaneously. Side effects include local reactions at the injection site, low-grade fever, weakness, myalgias, and rash, although the incidence is low. Chemoprophylaxis is recommended in children with functional or anatomic asplenia in addition to vaccination. Prophylaxis with penicillin G or V may be given at a dose of 125 mg PO twice a day in children younger than age 5 years and 250 mg PO twice a day in children age 5 years or older.[15,16]

Neisseria meningitidis Meningitis

Neisseria meningitidis is a gram-negative organism that causes both endemic and epidemic disease. Due to the success of *H. influenzae* type b vaccination programs, *N. meningitidis* has become the leading cause of bacterial meningitis in the United States, with an estimated 2600 cases per year[2,17] and a fatality rate of approximately 10% despite antibiotic therapy to which strains remain clinically sensitive.[2,16,18] The incidence of endemic meningococcal disease increases in the late winter to early spring. Children 3 to 12 months of age, asplenic patients, and patients with C3 and C5–9 complement deficiencies have increased incidence of meningococcal disease. Previously, military recruits had high rates of serogroup C meningococcal disease; however, since the advent of routine meningococcal vaccination of recruits, incidence has decreased substantially. HIV-infected persons do not appear to be at increased risk for epidemic serogroup A meningococcal disease; however, they may be at increased risk for sporadic meningococcal disease or disease caused by other serogroups.[19,20] Asymptomatic colonization of the upper respiratory tract is common, and transmission from person to person occurs through inhalation of droplets of respiratory secretions. Close contacts of *N. meningitidis*-infected patients are at increased risk for development of disease.

Neisseria meningitidis has multiple serogroups known to cause invasive disease. In multistate surveillance during 1989–1991, serogroups B and C accounted for the majority of *N. meningitidis* meningitis cases (46 and 45%, respectively); serogroup W-135, serogroup Y, and strains unable to be typed accounted for most of the remaining cases.[2] Incidence of disease due to serogroup Y appears to be increasing.[21] Serogroup A, an uncommon cause of endemic disease in the United States, is the most common cause of epidemic disease elsewhere in the world.[18,20] Statewide epidemics and localized community outbreaks in the United States have been due to serogroups B and C.[22,23]

Clinical features of *N. meningitidis* infection include rapid onset with meningococcemia of fever, chills, malaise, and a rash. The rash may be maculopapular, petechial, or urticarial. In fulminant disease, the rash may become puerperal and is associated with a syndrome of disseminated intravascular coagulation, shock, coma, and death (Waterhouse-Friderichsen syndrome). This may occur within a few hours of presentation despite adequate antibiotic therapy. Other signs of meningococcal meningitis are common to infection with other pathogens.

When the CSF Gram stain reveals gram-negative cocci, meningococcal meningitis is assumed and empiric therapy can be directed toward that organism.[6] The drug of choice for the treatment of meningococcal meningitis is penicillin G administered as 4 million units every 4 hours for 7 days for adults with normal renal function.[7,15,24,25] Penicillin dose adjustment should be considered in patients with an estimated creatinine clearance of less than 30 mL/min. Rare strains of *N. meningitidis* are resistant or relatively resistant to penicillin. Cefotaxime (2 g every 4 to 6 hours) or ceftriaxone (2 g every 12 to 24 hours) are used as second-line agents for patients with penicillin allergy, although cross-sensitivity is sometimes seen. Chloramphenicol may be used in patients with allergy to both penicillin and cephalosporins. Other alternatives include sulfonamides and fluoroquinolones. No data support the use of corticosteroids in the treatment of meningococcal meningitis.[26] In fact, there is some concern that corticosteroids may adversely affect the ability of antibiotics to achieve adequate penetration of the CSF, leading to recrudescence and relapses.

Penicillin does not cure the carrier state and eradicate *N. meningitidis* from the nasopharynx; therefore, patients also must be treated with oral rifampin 10 mg/kg (maximum 600 mg) every 12 hours for 2 days.[24,27] Respiratory isolation should be instituted for 24 hours after therapy initiation to avoid transmission. Household, child care center, and nursery school contacts should be given antibiotic prophylaxis as soon as possible after exposure to the primary case is discovered. Prophylaxis of medical care workers is not recommended unless exposure to respiratory secretions from doing mouth-to-mouth resuscitation, intubation, or suctioning occurs before 24 hours of adequate antibiotics are administered. The drug of choice for prophylaxis is rifampin, administered in the same dosing regimen as that used for nasopharynx eradication.[15–17] A 4-day regimen of 20 mg/kg/day (maximum 600 mg) is also effective.[15] Ceftriaxone (250 mg adults, 125 mg children younger than age 12 years) given as a single intramuscular dose has been proven more effective than rifampin in eradicating serogroup A *N. meningitidis;* however, efficacy has not been confirmed for other strains.[28] Sulfisoxazole and ciprofloxacin (500 mg as a single dose) have also been used with some success.

A quadrivalent meningococcal vaccine is commercially available. The vaccine is active against serogroups A, C, Y, and W-135. Unfortunately, no vaccine is available with activity against serogroup B, the most common cause of meningococcal infection. The vaccine is given as a single 0.5 mL dose and consists of 50 μg of each of the purified bacterial capsular polysaccharides. Routine vaccination of children is not recommended, because infants are the highest-risk group and generally exhibit a poor response to all but the serogroup A component.[15,28] Vaccination should be considered in children older than 2 years of age in high-risk groups, including functional or anatomically asplenic patients and those with terminal complement component deficiency. The vaccine may be considered as an adjunct to antibiotic prophylaxis and may be useful in containing outbreaks of meningococcal disease due to the represented serogroups. Military recruits are routinely vaccinated, due to the frequency of serogroup C infection in this population.[15,16] Vaccination of college students residing in dormatories is now recommended by the American College Health Association and the Advisory Committee on Immunization Practices (ACIP).

Haemophilus influenzae type b Meningitis

Haemophilus influenzae type b is an encapsulated gram-negative pleomorphic coccobacillus. Approximately 30 to 50% of children carry *Haemophilus* asymptomatically in the nasopharynx, generally as the avirulent, nonencapsulated species. These nonencapsulated strains are a common cause of otitis media, sinusitis, and bronchitis, and up to 80% of adults are carriers.[1] Colonization by the type b conjugate ranges from 2 to 5%. Children younger than 2 years old are at the highest risk of developing infection with this organism, as are adults with predisposing factors such as sickle cell disease, asplenia, immunodeficiency states, malignancy, head trauma, neurosurgery, sinusitis, otitis media, or CSF leak. Alaskan Eskimo, Apache, and Navajo Native Americans also are at increased risk due to genetic factors. Patients commonly develop meningitis after an upper respiratory tract infection or otitis media. Complications of *H. influenzae* meningitis include deafness, blindness, seizure disorders, behavior disorders, and a decrease in school performance.

Previously, empiric therapy for this pathogen was ampicillin. However, this has recently been revised because of the increase in frequency of plasmid-mediated β-lactamase production, now seen in up to 12 to 40% of isolates. Presently, ceftriaxone and cefotaxime are the first-line empiric agents. They also have excellent in vitro activity against the other most commonly encountered meningeal pathogens, have few serious adverse reactions and drug interactions, and have been shown to rapidly sterilize CSF cultures. Disadvantages of chloramphenicol are the drug-drug interactions affecting the metabolism of other agents through cytochrome P-450, such as phenytoin, rifampin, carbamazepine, and phenobarbital, and the serum drug concentration monitoring that must be done to ensure adequate therapy. Cefuroxime was previously used in the treatment of bacterial meningitis, but clinical studies demonstrated an increase in hearing loss in cefuroxime-treated children compared with third-generation cephalosporins, possibly due to a delayed sterilization of CSF fluid.[29] Duration of therapy is 7 to 10 days in uncomplicated cases.

Chemoprophylaxis is recommended to stop contact spread, similar to meningococcus. Rifampin is used because it eradicates nasopharyngeal carriage of *H. influenzae* type b.[16] Minocycline is an alternative, although its CNS side effects discourage its use. Rifampin prophylaxis is recommended for all household contacts, children and adults, if there is one unvaccinated contact younger than 4 years of age. The only exclusion is pregnancy, due to the unknown risk of rifampin exposure to the fetus. A *household contact* is defined as an individual residing with the index patient or a nonresident who spent 4 or more hours with the index patient for at least 5 of the 7 days preceding the day of hospital admission of the index patient.[15] In households with a fully vaccinated, immunocompromised child, all members should receive rifampin prophylaxis due to the possibility of inadequate immune response to the vaccine. Because most secondary cases occur the first week after the patient has been hospitalized, prophylactic therapy should be administered promptly. Some benefit may be gained through therapy instituted up to 7 days after the index case. If the family does require prophylaxis and the index case was treated with ampicillin or chloramphenicol before hospital discharge, the index case should also receive rifampin prophylaxis.[16] Prophylaxis of the index case is not necessary if the patient received either cefotaxime or ceftriaxone, because these drugs eradicate *H. influenzae* from the nasopharynx.[15]

The recommendations are controversial for patients who attend a day care center or nursery school. Rifampin is indicated if one case of *H. influenzae* meningitis occurs at a day care facility that is attended by any unvaccinated child who is younger than 2 years of age and whose contact time is greater than 25 hours per week. Unvaccinated children should receive a dose of conjugate vaccine and should then complete the vaccination series. If the children are older than 2 years of age there is no need for rifampin. If two or more cases of invasive disease occur within 60 days and unvaccinated or incompletely vaccinated children are exposed, all children and supervisory personnel should promptly receive rifampin therapy.[15]

The dose of rifampin is 20 mg/kg (maximum 600 mg) PO every day for 4 doses.[15] Formal dosing guidelines are not available for children younger than 1 month of age, but some experts recommend 10 mg/kg (maximum 600 mg) daily for 4 days.[16] If children cannot swallow the capsules, rifampin powder may be mixed in applesauce before administration, or a 1% suspension in simple syrup may be compounded. Side effects include an orange-red discoloration of the urine and other body fluids, gastrointestinal disturbances, headache, drowsiness, dizziness, and elevated liver enzymes. Patients wearing soft contact lenses should be counseled regarding the possibility of permanent staining of their lenses during therapy. Rifampin is also a potent inducer of hepatic microsomal cytochrome P-450 enzymes and may lower the concentrations of multiple drugs, including oral contraceptives, glucocorticoids, and oral anticoagulants.

Since the development of the vaccine, the incidence of *H. influenzae* type b meningitis has dramatically declined by more than 90%.[30] *Haemophilus influenzae* type b conjugate vaccine contains antigenic capsular polysaccharide ribosylribitol phosphate –(PRP). It is coupled to carrier proteins such as diphtheria toxoid (PRP-D), *Neisseria meningitidis* protein (PRP-OMP), tetanus toxoid (PRP-T), or diphtheria CRM197 (mutant) protein (HbOC). Currently three doses of either HbOC or PRP-T are recommended at 2, 4, and 6 months or two doses given at 2 and 4 months for PRP-OMP. PRP-D is not recommended for children younger than 12 months. Booster doses of any of the four conjugate vaccines are given at 12 to 15 months. The vaccine does not affect nasopharyngeal carriage.

Listeria monocytogenes Meningitis

Listeria monocytogenes is a gram-positive aerobic bacillus that may be mistaken for the diphtheroids present in normal skin flora. Pregnant women, newborns, older adults, and immunocompromised persons are predisposed to *Listeria* infections. The incidence of *Listeria* infection is greatest in the summer and early fall. Contaminated coleslaw, milk, and cheeses have been the source of outbreaks associated with food poisoning.[4] Antibiotics that have activity against *Listeria* include penicillin G, ampicillin, erythromycin, trimethoprim–sulfamethoxazole, chloramphenicol, rifampin, tetracyclines, and aminoglycosides. In bacterial meningitis, when *Listeria* is one of the suspected pathogens (i.e., Gram stain reveals gram-positive bacilli or the patient is older than 50 years of age, debilitated, or an alcoholic), empiric therapy should consist of a third-generation cephalosporin combined with ampicillin, because cephalosporins have no activity against this organism. However, because only trimethoprim–sulfamethoxazole and aminoglycosides are bactericidal against *Listeria,* penicillin monotherapy of *Listeria* meningitis has led to mortality rates as high as 30%.[31] Therefore, the treatment of choice for documented *Listeria* meningitis includes ampicillin in combination with an aminoglycoside, either intravenously or intrathecally.[7,31] The aminoglycoside is added because of its documented in vitro synergy.[32–34] Trimethoprim–sulfamethoxazole is an alternative therapy for patients with penicillin allergy. Meropenem appears to have in vitro activity against *Listeria* and achieves adequate CSF drug concentrations.[35,36] Further study is necessary to evaluate the efficacy of meropenem in treating *Listeria* meningitis in humans.

Gram-Negative Bacillary Meningitis

Gram-negative bacilli are an uncommon cause of meningitis. Patients more likely to develop gram-negative meningitis include older adults, neonates, the immunocompromised, and patients with a history of recent trauma or neurosurgery. Although *S. pneumoniae* is the most common pathogen if a CSF leak is present, *S. aureus* and gram-negative infections are also common in this setting. *Enterobacteriaceae* (especially *E. coli* and *Klebsiella* species) and *Pseudomonas* species are the most commonly implicated gram-negative pathogens. Gram-negative meningitis in the older adult generally has a poor prognosis and involves a protracted clinical course.

Before the introduction of third-generation cephalosporins such as ceftazidime and cefotaxime, aminoglycoside therapy with or without chloramphenicol resulted in gram-negative meningitis mortality rates of 40 to 90%.[37] Treatment of gram-negative bacterial meningitis was revolutionized by the advent of third-generation cephalosporins, which result in cure rates of 78 to 94%.[7,38] These agents have excellent activity versus gram-negative organisms and achieve high levels in the CSF. The greatest experience in gram-negative infections is with cefotaxime[25,39,40] and ceftazidime.[41,42] Usual dosage of cefotaxime is 2 g every 4 hours. If *Pseudomonas* is implicated, ceftazidime 2 to 3 g every 6 to 8 hours plus intrathecal and systemic aminoglycoside therapy may be used empirically.[25] Once sensitivity to ceftazidime is established, the need for aminoglycoside may be reassessed. Although aminoglycosides cover a wide range of gram-negative pathogens, they do not penetrate well into the CSF. Therefore, when these antibiotics are used they are often delivered directly into the CSF through intrathecal administration. Preservative-free formulations of gentamicin or amikacin are used in doses of 8 mg and 20 to 30 mg daily, respectively.[25] However, even with intrathecal administration, therapeutic aminoglycoside levels are not obtained in the ventricles. Ventriculitis is commonly associated with gram-negative meningitis and may require intraventricular aminoglycoside administration through a reservoir. In resistant cases of coliform or *Pseudomonas* meningitis, direct instillation of gentamicin 4 mg every 12 hours into the lateral ventricles is sometimes used.

If initial therapy with cefotaxime or ceftazidime with or without an aminoglycoside fails or is contraindicated because of allergy, alternative agents with gram-negative activity may be used. Imipenem should be avoided because of its propensity to induce seizures (incidence of greater than 30% of treated patients in one series).[43,44] Meropenem may be a reasonable alternative.[45] Trimethoprim–sulfamethoxazole is occasionally used when β-lactam antibiotics cannot be tolerated; however, recurrences with this regimen are common. Fluoroquinolones and aztreonam are other possible alternatives.

Treatment of gram-negative bacterial meningitis should be guided by in vitro susceptibility patterns once a final identification of the organism is made, and therapy should be continued for 14 days after cultures become negative.

Fungal Meningitis

The two most common causes of fungal meningitis are *Cryptococcus neoformans* and coccidioidomycosis.[46] Bird droppings, rotten fruits and vegetables, wood rot, and soil contain cryptococcus. Infection occurs through inhalation of the aerosolized spores, which results in primary pulmonary disease that disseminates to the central nervous system. The onset of disease is gradual, generally over 4 or more weeks, and it is most prevalent in the immunosuppressed.[47] Patients most commonly experience headache along with alteration in mental status, nuchal rigidity, fever, and papilledema. Examination of the CSF reveals a pleocytosis. Diagnosis is made by India ink stain, culture, and latex agglutination test, which identifies the circulating capsular antigen, in serum of CSF. With these three methods the diagnosis can be made in 98 to 99% of cases.[47]

The preferred treatment regimen in individuals who do not have HIV infection is amphotericin 0.5 to 1 mg/kg/day and flucytosine 100 to 150 mg/kg/day for 6 weeks. A total of 1 to 2 g of amphotericin should be administered. The combination of flucytosine and amphotericin has been found to be superior to amphotericin alone in patients who do not have HIV infection, leading to successful outcomes in 75% of treated patients.[48] A recent study in HIV-infected patients with cryptococcal meningitis found that the addition of flucytosine 100 mg/kg/day during the first 2 weeks of amphotericin therapy did not improve clinical response.[49] Fluconazole achieves good CSF concentration, is available as an oral agent, and is better tolerated than amphotericin. Studies have shown efficacy with fluconazole as primary therapy in HIV-infected patients who have good prognostic signs. There is a high rate of relapse, so chronic suppressive therapy is often given. The usual regimen for cryptococcal meningitis in HIV-infected patients is amphotericin B 0.7 mg/kg/day for 2 weeks followed by fluconazole 800 mg/day orally for 2 days and then 400 mg/day for 8 weeks and 200 mg/day indefinitely.[48,49]

Therapy with amphotericin B may cause significant adverse drug reactions, including nephrotoxicity, electrolyte abnormalities, infusion-related toxicities, anemia, thrombocytopenia, and phlebitis. Not only is amphotericin toxic, it also achieves low CSF concentrations. Flucytosine (5-FC) is associated with bone marrow suppression, nausea and vomiting, and liver abnormalities.

Coccidioidomycosis is caused by *C. immitis*. This fungus is present in the soil of southwestern United States, Mexico, and Central America. Hyphal segment fragments release arthroconidia, the infectious particles, which are aerosolized and inhaled. Once inhaled, the infection disseminates within 3 to 6 months to the skin, musculoskeletal system, and meninges. In tissues, the spherules develop and form endosporins. People at increased risk of CNS infection include immunocompromised persons, infants, older adults, non-Caucasian persons (highest in black, Filipino, and Asian persons), males, and pregnant women. Headache is the most common symptom of fungal meningitis. Symptoms of meningeal irritation are usually absent. Approximately 90% of patients die within 12 months without active treatment.[50] Amphotericin either intrathecally, intracisternally, or intravenously is used. The azoles also have activity against coccidioidomycosis. Comparative trials with the azoles and amphotericin are not available, but because of the advantages of azoles, fluconazole, itraconazole, and ketoconazole may be used. Similar to cryptococcus, maintenance therapy is required because the relapse rate is high.

Viral Meningitis

Aseptic meningitis is defined as the presence of meningeal signs and symptoms, as well as CSF abnormalities consistent with meningitis, but stains and cultures are negative for bacteria or fungi. The most common causes of aseptic meningitis are viruses, particularly enterovirus, herpes, lymphocytic choriomeningitis, and mumps.[51,52] Drugs have also been implicated as a cause of aseptic meningitis (Table 73.7).[53]

Table 73.7 ▪ Aseptic Meningitis Syndrome–Drug-Related Causes

Ibuprofen
Trimethoprim–sulfamethoxazole
Sulindac
Naproxen
Tolmetin
Diclofenac
muromonab-CD3 (Orthoclone OKT3)
Carbamazepine
Immune globulin
Phenazopyridine
Vaccines–mumps and rubella

Enteroviruses are members of the picornavirus family and consist of poliovirus, coxsackievirus A and B, and echovirus. These agents are the most common causes of aseptic meningitis.[51] Transmission of these viruses occurs via fecal-oral and respiratory routes. Infants, children, and young adults (age less than 40 years) are at risk for development of enteroviral infections. Symptoms are either gradual or abrupt and are similar to bacterial meningitis. Focal neurologic symptoms are uncommon. An increased incidence of infections is usually seen in the late summer and early fall in temperate climates. Enteroviral infections are self-limited. Patients are given supportive care, including hydration and pain control.[53]

Herpes simplex virus types 1 and 2 have both been associated with CNS infections. Herpes simplex virus type 1 (HSV1) has been associated with meningoencephalitis, and herpes simplex virus type 2 (HSV2) is predominantly associated with meningitis. The diagnosis and treatment of herpes simplex CNS infections is reviewed during the discussion of encephalitis.

IMPROVING OUTCOMES

The use of corticosteroids as adjunctive therapy in meningitis remains controversial. The pathogenesis of meningitis, as reviewed earlier, consists of the release of cytokines that cause brain edema, increased intracranial pressure, and enhanced BBB permeability. Steroids inhibit the synthesis of these cytokines, thus blocking this cascade of events. CSF inflammation normalizes more rapidly with steroid therapy. Steroids may reduce the penetration of antibiotics into the CSF. A rabbit model of meningitis showed a decrease in CSF concentrations and a delay in CSF sterilization when either ceftriaxone or vancomycin was combined with dexamethasone. This may be detrimental in cases where the MIC of the pathogen is increased and the achievable concentration at the site of infection is decreased. Side effects of steroids are also a concern; there has been an increase in reports of secondary fevers and an increased risk of gastrointestinal bleeding with 4-day steroid regimens.[26,54,55] However, these effects are not seen with the 2-day regimen (0.4 mg/kg IV every 12 hours), which appears to have equal efficacy to the 4-day regimen.[13,26]

There is evidence of the beneficial effects of steroid therapy in meningitis. The addition of dexamethasone to cephalosporin therapy has resulted in a reduction of neurologic sequelae, especially hearing loss, in children. A meta-analysis of clinical trials since 1988 confirms the benefit of corticosteroid treatment in *H. influenzae* type b infection, and the Infectious Diseases Committee of the American Academy of Pediatrics advocates the use of dexamethasone for the treatment of meningitis caused by *H. influenzae*.[13,17]

Studies also suggest the utility of steroids in *S. pneumoniae* meningitis in children.[13] Evidence of benefit is strongest for the prevention of hearing loss. Significant adverse effects do not seem to be problematic with the 2-day steroid regimen, which should prove as effective as the 4-day regimen. When corticosteroid therapy is commenced with or before parenteral antibiotics, it may prevent the increased release of endotoxin due to the initiation of antibiotic therapy.

There is no evidence supporting the efficacy of corticosteroids in minimizing neurologic sequelae from *N. meningitidis*, fungal, or viral meningitis.

Encephalitis

EPIDEMIOLOGY

Encephalitis is a direct infection of the brain parenchyma. Viruses are by far the most common pathogen associated with encephalitis (although fungi, rickettsiae, and protozoans have also been implicated), and viral encephalitis will be the main focus of the discussion here. Viruses associated with encephalitis include arboviruses (most common), varicella-zoster virus, herpes simplex virus, measles, mumps, cytomegalovirus, HIV, and rabies.[56,57]

PATHOPHYSIOLOGY

The virus enters the CNS through hematogenous spread. The organism may enter the bloodstream through the respiratory or gastrointestinal tract or may be introduced through an insect or animal bite. Viral replication occurs at the site of entry, followed by spilling into the systemic circulation, and, finally, infection of distant sites, including the CNS. In the CNS, cell dysfunction due to viral invasion and inflammatory changes similar to those seen in meningitis occur.

CLINICAL PRESENTATION AND DIAGNOSIS

Signs and Symptoms

Clinical manifestations include a prodrome for several days that may consist of myalgia, fever, malaise, rash, or mild upper respiratory symptoms. Following the prodromal period, headache, drowsiness, change in mental status, and meningismus signify the development of encephalitis. As the infection progresses, drowsiness and confusion increase and may eventually lead to coma. Seizures are common, and focal signs associated with the area of the brain where the infection is concentrated may appear. Intracranial pressure may be increased.[54]

Diagnosis

The symptoms of viral encephalitis mimic a large range of other disease states, including bacterial meningitis, fungal or protozoan encephalitis, brain abscess, neoplasm, and drug overdose; these etiologies should be ruled out quickly. Peripheral blood smear should be examined for parasites and blood cultures obtained. Increased intracranial pressure should be ruled out before lumbar puncture is obtained. CT, electroencephalogram (EEG), or radionuclide brain scan should be performed to identify any focal lesions, masses, or cerebral edema. Focal infarctions in the temporal lobes may indicate herpes simplex infection. The CSF exhibits leukocytosis, usually predominantly lymphocytes, although polymorphonuclear neutrophil leukocytes (PMN) may be present in early stages. Red cells may be present if a necrotizing component is present, as is seen in herpes simplex encephalitis. Glucose content is normal, protein is raised, and organisms are not found on Gram stain. HSV2 can be cultured from the CSF, but HSV1 cannot. Rapid diagnosis of herpesvirus encephalitis using brain biopsy or PCR assay[56] is imperative, because a specific and effective therapy is available. The mortality rate of untreated herpes encephalitis is 60 to 80%.[57–61]

Symptoms are generally nonspecific for the different viruses; however, several organisms (e.g., herpes simplex, rabies) demonstrate tropism for certain areas of the brain and the resulting focal signs can increase the index of suspicion for a particular pathogen. Because of the commonality of symptoms of encephalitis, patient history can be an important consideration in determining the probable causative pathogen. Signs of infection outside the CNS may be helpful in diagnosing cases of encephalitis secondary to varicella, measles, mumps, or herpes simplex. Cytomegalovirus encephalitis is generally seen in infants and the immunocompromised, including organ transplant patients and HIV-infected patients. Travel history, season, or evidence or history of insect or animal bite may also provide clues to pathogen identity. Japanese encephalitis is the most common arbovirus infection worldwide and is endemic in Japan, Southeast Asia, China, India, and the Philippines. Eastern equine encephalitis occurs in the Atlantic and Gulf coasts of the United States and occurs mainly in summer and autumn. Evidence of a dog, cat, or raccoon bite increases suspicion for rabies infection, especially in endemic areas. Brain biopsy has been used when herpes simplex virus is suspected; however, there is no guarantee that the biopsy specimen contains virus, so its yield can be low. Despite efforts to determine the causative organism, in approximately one-third of cases no identification is made.

TREATMENT

Treatment of viral encephalitis is, with the exception of herpes simplex virus, primarily symptomatic. Anticonvulsants are used to control seizure activity; adequate nutrition, hydration, and oxygen are provided as needed; and cerebral edema is treated with intubation and hyperventilation, diuretics, or corticosteroids.[54] The use of dexamethasone in these patients is controversial because of the theoretical inhibition of interferon synthesis, which may impair host defense mechanisms against the virus.[57]

Comparative studies have found parenteral acyclovir to be superior to vidarabine for the treatment of herpes encephalitis.[58-61] Therefore, acyclovir is widely accepted as the drug of choice.[58-62] Herpes simplex virus should be treated with acyclovir 10 mg/kg IV infused over 1 hour every 8 hours for 14 to 21 days. Rapid institution of acyclovir treatment has been shown to decrease mortality rates to less than 30%.[62] Survival and recovery may be predicted by the patient's neurologic status at time of presentation. Acyclovir resistance has been reported, especially in patients with a history of prior or chronic acyclovir treatment.[63] In these cases vidarabine 15 mg/kg/day as a continuos infusion is given for 10 days, although clinical experience with HSV-resistant encephalitis is limited.

Brain Abscess

EPIDEMIOLOGY

Approximately 1 in 10,000 hospital admissions are due to a brain abscess, with males (2:1 versus females) less than 20 years of age having the highest incidence. Contiguous infection, hematogenous dissemination, or direct trauma may be the cause. Paranasal sinus, middle ear, mastoid, and dental infections result in contiguous spread either by direct extension or through vascular channels. The result is generally a single abscess. Concurrent sinusitis or dental infections commonly cause frontal lobe brain abscesses. Temporal lobe or cerebellar abscesses may be the result of otitis media.[64]

Multiple metastatic abscesses are caused by hematogenous spread from pulmonary infections, osteomyelitis, dental abscess, endocarditis, and skin pustules. Diverse pathogens may be involved in this clinical situation, and their identity depends on the original source of the bacteremia. Table 73.8 outlines common sources of brain abscesses and the associated pathogens. In approximately 25% of cases no apparent source of infection can be identified.[65]

Certain patient populations are at increased risk of brain abscesses. Children with cyanotic congenital cardiac anomalies, such as tetralogy of Fallot (i.e., right-to-left shunts), are at increased risk for development of hematogenously spread brain lesions. Infants and neonates develop brain abscess caused by gram-negative organisms. Immunocompromised patients are at increased risk of fungal abscesses caused by *Candida, Aspergillus, C. neoformans, Blastomyces, Histoplasma, Mucor,* and *Rhizopus. Listeria monocytogenes* and *Nocardia asteroides* also cause infections in immunocompromised persons. *Toxoplasma gondii* causes brain abscess in patients with acquired immunodeficiency syndrome (AIDS).

PATHOPHYSIOLOGY

A brain abscess is a potentially life-threatening infection precipitated by a focal suppurative process within the brain parenchyma. Brain abscesses result from bacterial, fungal, or parasitic infections that seed an area of necrosis in the brain. Bone fragments and debris caused by neurosurgery and cranial trauma may serve as a nidus of infection in some cases. The pathology of brain abscess formation can be divided into four stages.[66] Stage 1 is an early cerebritis that occurs on day 1 to day 3. Day 4 to day 9 marks the beginning of stage 2, or the late cerebritis phase. Fibroblasts produce the reticulin network that is the framework for the collagen capsule. At this stage there is maximal edema. From day 10 through day 13 (stage 3), the capsule becomes more developed around the necrotic center (early encapsulation stage). The capsule serves as a protective structure by controlling the spread of infection and limiting the destruction of brain parenchyma. Encapsulation is completed in stage 4, the late capsule stage.[66]

Table 73.8 ▪ Brain Abscess: Common Pathogens by Risk Factor

Cause	Pathogens	Recommended Therapy
Sinusitis	Streptococci Staphylococci Anaerobes *Haemophilus influenzae*	Third-generation cephalosporin and metronidazole
Otitis media/ mastoiditis	Streptococci *Bacteroides* Gram-negative organisms	Third-generation cephalosporin and metronidazole
Dental infections	*Fusobacterium* *Bacteroides* Streptococci	Penicillin and metronidazole
Cranial trauma and neurosurgery	*Staphylococcus aureus* Streptococci	Nafcillin or vancomycin (MRSA)

MRSA, methicillin-resistant *Staphylococcus aureus.*

CLINICAL PRESENTATION AND DIAGNOSIS

Signs and Symptoms

The clinical symptoms of patients with brain abscesses are nonspecific and depend on the size and location of the abscess, number of lesions, virulence of the organism, host response, and severity of cerebral edema that accompanies the abscess. Patients may either have abrupt symptoms or insidious onset over weeks. Most patients develop a constant, progressively worsening headache that is not relieved with analgesics. Nausea and vomiting occur as a sign of increasing intracranial pressure. Patients may have a low-grade fever (less than 101.5°F), focal neurologic deficits, and changes in mentation. The spectrum of consciousness can range from mild confusion to a coma. Obtunded or comatose individuals have a worse prognosis. In a study of 45 consecutive cases, the most common symptoms were headache (72%), fever (42%), seizure (35%), nausea and vomiting (35%), and confusion (26%).[67] Symptoms may also provide clues to the area of the brain infected. Parietal lobe abscesses are associated with the development of hemiparesis; ataxia and nystagmus are associated with cerebellar lesions. Symptoms common in infants include vomiting, irritability, seizures, poor feeding, enlarging head circumference, and bulging fontanelles.

Table 73.9 ▪ Antibiotics Used in Central Nervous System Infections

Drug	Dosing in Children	Dosing in Adults	Side Effects
Penicillin G	250,000–400,000 U/kg/day divided in 6 doses (q4hr)	3–4 million U q4hr (up to 24 million U/day)	Leukopenia Anemia Seizures in renal failure
Ampicillin	100–200 mg/kg/day divided in 4 doses	2 g q4hr	
Nafcillin/Oxacillin	100 mg/kg/day divided in 4 doses	2 g q4hr	Hepatotoxicity[b] Acute interstitial nephritis
Ceftriaxone	100 mg/kg/day divided q12–24hr[a]	1–2 g q12–24hr (up to 4 g/day)	Gastrointestinal upset Biliary sludging
Ceftazidime	225–300 mg/kg/day divided in 3 or 4 doses	2 g q6–8hr	
Cefotaxime	225–300 mg/kg/day divided in 3 or 4 doses	2 g q4hr	
Rifampin	20 mg/kg/day divided in 2 doses		
Aminoglycosides Gentamicin Tobramycin Amikacin		Gentamicin/tobramycin: IT: 8–10 mg QD IV: 2 mg/kg load Maintenance dosing to follow per drug target levels Amikacin: IT: 20–30 mg QD IV: 15 mg/kg load Maintenance dosing to follow per drug target levels	Nephrotoxicity Ototoxicity
Vancomycin	60 mg/kg/day divided in 4 doses	IV: 1–2 g q8–12hr Intraventricular: 10 mg/day Target peak serum concentration: 35–40 μg/mL Trough concentration: 10–15 μg/mL	Red-man (neck) syndrome Nephrotoxicity Ototoxicity Leukopenia
Chloramphenicol	75–100 mg/kg/day divided in 4 doses	IV: 75–100 mg/kg/day divided in 4 doses (up to 6 g/day)	Aplastic anemia Thrombocytopenia Leukopenia Gray baby syndrome
Amphotericin B	IV: 0.3–1.0 mg/kg/day	IT: 25–300 μg q48–72hr (max 500 μg–1 mg) IV: 0.3–1.0 mg/kg/day	Fever Chills Nephrotoxicity Hypokalemia Hypomagnesemia
Fluconazole		400 mg loading dose on day 1, then 200 mg QD	Gastrointestinal upset Elevated liver enzymes
Flucytosine		150 mg/kg/day divided q6hr	Myelosuppression Anemia Hepatitis Nausea Vomiting Diarrhea

IT, intrathecal.

[a]q24h dosing may be appropriate for penicillin-sensitive strains. Strains that are intermediate or resistant require q12h dosing.

[b]Oxacillin has higher incidence of hepatotoxicity.

Diagnosis

Unlike meningitis, diagnosis of brain abscesses does not depend on CSF findings. Lumbar punctures are contraindicated because the diagnostic utility is poor and the risks are high. Blood and urine cultures are also rarely helpful. The peripheral white blood cell count may be mildly elevated (<15,000/mL^3), as may the erythrocyte sedimentation rate (45 to 50 mm/hr). CT and MRI aid in making an early diagnosis and in monitoring therapy. The sensitivity of these procedures exceeds 95%, and they confirm the exact location of the lesion. To identify the causative organism, aspiration of the abscess is performed. This sample is then stained and cultured for potential pathogens, including both aerobic and anaerobic organisms.

TREATMENT

Once the diagnosis is confirmed, antibiotic therapy alone or combined with surgery is the cornerstone of treatment. Surgical procedures include excision or aspiration of the purulent material. These procedures not only remove the purulent material, but also decrease mass effect and intracranial pressure. Generally, if CT suggests cerebritis and the abscess is less than 2.5 cm, antibiotics can be initiated and the patient observed for response.[65,66] Otherwise, the abscess should be surgically drained.

Antibiotics used for the treatment of brain abscesses must be bactericidal and able to achieve high tissue concentrations in the brain. This does not always correlate with CSF concentrations. Antibiotics such as chloramphenicol, metronidazole, penicillin, nafcillin, vancomycin, trimethoprim–sulfamethoxazole, and third-generation cephalosporins achieve therapeutic concentrations (Table 73.9). Another consideration when choosing appropriate therapy is that agents should not be inactivated or rendered unstable by an acidic environment or purulent material, because both exist within the abscess. Organisms that are sensitive to aminoglycosides have reduced susceptibility when the pH is low (i.e., acidic environment). A third-generation cephalosporin (cefotaxime 2 g every 4 hours or ceftriaxone 2 g every 12 hours) plus metronidazole (7.5 mg/kg every 6 hours or 15 mg/kg every 12 hours) are commonly used.[65] High-dose penicillin G (20 to 24 million units per day) has also been used in combination with metronidazole with good results.[65] The duration of therapy ranges from 4 to 8 weeks but is dependent on the patient's response. Other appropriate empiric regimens, based on likely source of infection and common pathogens, are listed in Table 73.8.

Corticosteroids have been used as adjuvant therapy, although no significant benefit has been observed in survival. Steroids reduce cerebral edema and mass effect, but they also reduce the host defense mechanism and decrease antibiotic concentrations. This may cause a delay in killing of the organism.

Corticosteroids may be beneficial in patients with elevated intracranial pressure or significant mass effect causing neurologic deficits. In these cases, corticosteroids might prevent potentially life-threatening cerebral edema and herniation. High-dose corticosteroids (dexamethasone 10 mg every 6 hours) is usually given until the patient is stabilized and then tapered over 3 to 7 days.[65] In severe cases of elevated intracranial pressure, mannitol and intubation with hyperventilation may be necessary.

Long-term neurologic sequelae may result from brain abscesses. These include seizures, cognitive dysfunction, focal neurologic deficits, and epilepsy. Mortality rates associated with this entity ranged from 40 to 60% in the preantibiotic era.[68,69] Now, with availability of CT, diagnosis is made earlier and mortality rates range from 0 to 24%.[70] Recurrence rate ranges from 5 to 10%, and recurrence usually occurs within 6 weeks of treatment. This may be due to inadequate antibiotic therapy, incorrect antibiotic, failure to aspirate a large abscess, presence of a foreign body, or failure to eradicate underlying source of infection. Rupture of an intraventricular brain abscess is associated with an extremely high mortality rate (greater than 80%).[65] Craniotomy and debridement of the abscess site may be necessary.

Shunt Infections

EPIDEMIOLOGY

Hydrocephalus is an abnormal increase in the amount of CSF resulting in enlargement of the ventricles, which can result in brain atrophy. To relieve this pressure, ventriculoperitoneal (VP) and ventriculoatrial (VA) shunts are placed. A VP shunt relieves pressure by draining CSF into the peritoneal cavity; VA shunts drain into the right atrium. The shunts are composed of a proximal ventricular catheter, a one-way valve or subcutaneous reservoir, and a distal catheter inserted into the peritoneum or right atrium.[71] Because the CSF shunts interfere with the normal host defenses, they are associated with infections. Infection rates are between 2 and 40%.[72]

PATHOPHYSIOLOGY

Bacteria are introduced either retrograde from the distal end of the shunt, through wound or skin infections, hematogenously, or most commonly by colonization at the time of shunt placement surgery.

Organisms that make up the skin flora are the most common pathogens in shunt-related infections. *Staphylo-*

coccus epidermidis produces a "slime layer" composed of an exopolysaccharide substance that not only increases its adherence to the foreign body, but also decreases the activity of the antibiotic. Second to *S. epidermidis, S. aureus* is also isolated in the majority of cases. Gram-negative organisms, such as *E. coli, Klebsiella* species, *Proteus* species, and *Pseudomonas* species, may cause infections. *Haemophilus influenzae, S. pneumoniae, N. meningitidis,* and fungal infections occur less commonly.[71,72]

CLINICAL PRESENTATION AND DIAGNOSIS

Signs and Symptoms

The symptoms of shunt infections are nonspecific. The most common problems experienced are related to the malfunctioning of the shunt, such as headache, nausea, lethargy, and changes in mental status. Patients may have a low-grade fever (temperature greater than 100°F). If a VP shunt is in place, abdominal symptoms may be present. Infections of VA devices may result in chronic bacteremia and septic pulmonary emboli.[71]

Diagnosis

Diagnosis of a shunt infection is made based on blood cultures, CSF Gram stain, and cultures taken directly from the reservoir. In shunt infections, the CSF sample usually has increased protein and neutrophils, but the glucose concentration may be normal.

TREATMENT

Effective treatment consists of administrating antibiotics and removing the shunt, either by externalization of the distal ends of the catheter or by complete removal.

Antibiotics can be given either intraventricularly through the reservoir or intravenously. Treatment of *S. epidermidis* and methicillin-resistant *Staphylococcus aureus* (MRSA) includes vancomycin 2 g/day with the addition of rifampin 10 to 20 mg/kg/day. Vancomycin can also be given intraventricularly at a dose of 10 mg/day in adults. The goal is to maintain both serum and CSF vancomycin trough concentrations between 10 and 20 μg/mL. Elevated vancomycin concentrations may cause neurotoxicity; therefore, CSF levels are helpful in maintaining therapy within the therapeutic range.[71,72] An alternative therapy would be trimethoprim–sulfamethoxazole 10 to 20 mg/kg/day with or without rifampin. Methicillin-sensitive *S. aureus* is treated with penicillinase-resistant penicillins such as nafcillin at doses of at least 12 g/day.[72] Gram-negative enteric organisms other than *P. aeruginosa* respond to treatment with either ceftriaxone or cefotaxime. Ceftazidime 2 g IV every 8 hours, with the addition of an aminoglycoside in some cases, is used for treatment of *P. aeruginosa.*[72]

Pharmacoeconomics of Central Nervous System Infections

Pharmacoeconomic considerations of central nervous system infections primarily concern chemoprophylaxis of meningitis and vaccination programs. Unfortunately, there is a paucity of pharmacoeconomic analysis of these measures. Adherence to the criteria set forth for the use of chemoprophylaxis and vaccination against *N. meningitidis* and *H. influenzae* infections should reduce the cost of these interventions to society, and their appropriate application should ensure reduction of disease. Obviously, these measures can lead to the avoidance of epidemics and endemic outbreaks, as evidenced by the success of meningococcal vaccine in decreasing meningitis incidence in military recruits. Widespread vaccination against *H. influenzae* infection in children has caused a dramatic decline in the frequency of meningitis due to this organism. Quantification of the cost-effectiveness of widespread vaccination against *N. meningitidis* and the further refinement of the chemoprophylaxis guidelines may be necessary in the future.

KEY POINTS

- Initiate therapy promptly. A delay in therapy of a few hours may result in an increase in morbidity and mortality.
- Use antimicrobials that are bactericidal.
- Select antimicrobials that have good penetration into the CSF.
- Antimicrobials should be dosed appropriately to ensure adequate CSF penetration and should exceed the MBC by 8 to 10 times.
- When instilling antibiotics directly into the CSF, remember that therapeutic antibiotic levels are achieved *below* the point of instillation, but not above.

Meningitis

- Empiric antibiotic therapy should be directed by the Gram stain of CSF (if available) and the patient's age and underlying health status. Empiric regimens usually contain a third-generation cephalosporin (e.g., ceftriaxone) with or without additional antibiotics (ampicillin, vancomycin).

- Corticosteroids should be used in childhood *H. influenzae* meningitis and should be considered in *S. pneumoniae* meningitis (pediatric or adult) to decrease the incidence of long-term neurologic deficits, specifically hearing loss.
- Exposed contacts to meningitis index cases with *H. influenzae* and *N. meningitidis* may require chemoprophylaxis.
- Vaccines are available to decrease the incidence of disease, and, therefore, perhaps meningitis, due to *H. influenzae, N. meningitidis,* and *S. pneumoniae* in at-risk populations.

Encephalitis

- Treatment of most types of viral encephalitis is symptomatic (e.g., anticonvulsants, nutritional support, reduction of increased intracranial pressure).
- Rapid diagnosis to rule out herpes simplex infection is imperative, because directed therapy is available.
- Acyclovir is the drug of choice for herpes encephalitis and has been proven to significantly reduce morbidity and mortality.

Brain Abscess

- Antibiotic therapy may not be sufficient to cause resolution of brain abscesses larger than 2.5 cm; therefore, surgical drainage is often indicated.
- Antibiotic therapy is directed by the suspected source of infection (if identifiable) and the results of culture or Gram stain of the abscess aspirate. Empiric therapy should be broad spectrum and cover both aerobes and anaerobes.
- Duration of antibiotic therapy is generally 6 to 8 weeks, but it may be longer depending on clinical response.

Shunt Infections

- Removal of the shunt is most often recommended
- Empiric therapy is directed toward nosocomial pathogens, including methicillin-resistant staphylococci (*S. aureus* and *S. epidermidis*) and nosocomial gram-negative bacilli.

REFERENCES

1. Tunkel AR, Scheld WM. Acute meningitis. In: Mandell GL, Bennett JE, Dolin R, eds. Principles and practice of infectious diseases. 4th ed. New York: Churchill Livingstone, 1995;1:831–864.
2. Jackson LA, Wenger JD. Laboratory-based surveillance for meningococcal disease in selected areas–United States, 1989–1991. In: CDC surveillance summaries (June). MMWR 42(SS-2):21–30, 1993.
3. Durand ML, Calderwood SB, Weber DJ, et al. Acute bacterial meningitis in adults: a review of 493 episodes. N Engl J Med 328:21–28, 1993.
4. Wispelwey B, Tunkel AR, Scheld WM. Bacterial meningitis in adults. Infect Dis Clin North Am 4:645–659, 1990.
5. Greenlee JE. Approach to diagnosis of meningitis, cerebrospinal fluid evaluation. Infect Dis Clin North Am 4:583–599, 1993.
6. Quagliarello VJ, Scheld WM. Treatment of bacterial meningitis. N Engl J Med 336:708–716, 1997.
7. Tunkel AR, Wispelwey B, Scheld WM. Bacterial meningitis: recent advances in pathophysiology and treatment. Ann Intern Med 112:610–623, 1990.
8. Miller LG, Choi C. Meningitis in older patients: how to diagnose and treat a deadly infection. Geriatrics 52:43–55, 1997.
9. Hoffmann J, Cetron MS, Farley MM, et al. The prevalence of drug-resistant *Streptococcus pneumoniae* in Atlanta. N Engl J Med 333:481–486, 1995.
10. Coffey TJ, Daniels M, McDougal LK, et al. Genetic analysis of clinical isolates of *Streptococcus pneumoniae* with high-level resistance to expanded spectrum cephalosporins. Antimicrob Agents Chemother 39:1306–1313, 1995.
11. Breiman RF, Butler JC, Tenover FC, et al. Emergence of drug-resistant pneumococcal infections in the United States. JAMA 271:1831–1835, 1994.
12. Gold H, Moellering RC. Antimicrobial resistance. N Engl J Med 335:1445, 1996.
13. McIntyre PB, Berkey CS, King SM. Dexamethasone as adjunctive therapy in bacterial meningitis: A meta analysis of randomized clinical trials since 1988. JAMA 278:925–931, 1997.
14. Friedland IR, Shelton S, Paris M, et al. Dilemmas in diagnosis and management of cephalosporin-resistant *Streptococcus pneumoniae* meningitis. Pediatr Infect Dis J 12:196–200, 1993.
15. Committee on Infectious Diseases, American Academy of Pediatrics. In: Peter G, ed. 1997 red book: report of the committee on infectious diseases. 24th ed. Elk Grove Village, IL: American Academy of Pediatrics, 1997:222, 357–363, 410–418.
16. Lieberman JM, Greenberg DP, Ward JI. Prevention of bacterial meningitis, vaccines and chemoprophylaxis. Infect Dis Clin North Am 4, 1990: 703–729.
17. Control and prevention of meningococcal disease. Recommendations of the Advisory Committee on Immunization Practices (ACIP). MMWR 46(RR-5): 1–7, 1997.
18. Jackson LA, Tenover FC, Baker C, et al. Prevalence of *Neisseria meningitidis* relatively resistant to penicillin in the United States, 1991. J Infect Dis 169:438–441, 1994.
19. Pinner RW, Onyango F, Perkins BA, et al. Epidemic meningococcal disease in Nairobi, Kenya, 1989. J Infect Dis 166:359–364, 1992.
20. Stephens DS, Hajjeh RA, Baughman WS, et al. Sporadic meningococcal disease in adults: results of a 5-year population-based study. Ann Intern Med 123:937–940, 1995.
21. Serogroup Y meningococcal disease–Illinois, Connecticut, and selected areas, United States, 1989–1996. MMWR 45:1010–1013, 1996.
22. Jackson LA, Schuchat A, Reeves MW, Wenger JD. Serogroup C meningococcal outbreaks in the United States: an emerging threat. JAMA 273:383–389, 1995.
23. Serogroup B meningococcal disease–Oregon, 1994. MMWR 44:121–124, 1995.
24. Luby JP. Southwestern Internal Medicine Conference: Infections in the central nervous system. Am J Med Sci 304:379–391, 1992.
25. Kaplan SL. New aspects of prevention and therapy of meningitis. Infect Dis Clin North Am 6:197–213, 1992.
26. Schaad UB, Kaplan SL, McCracken GH. Steroid therapy for bacterial meningitis. Clin Infect Dis 20:685–690, 1995.
27. Schwartz B, Al-Ruwais A, A'Ashi J, et al. Comparative efficacy of ceftriaxone and rifampin in eradicating pharyngeal carriage of group A *Neisseria meningitidis*. Lancet 1:1239–1242, 1988.
28. Goldschneider I, Lepow ML, Gotschlich EG, et al. Immunogenicity of group A and group C meningococcal polysaccharides in human infants. J Infect Dis 128:769–772, 1973.
29. Schaad UB, Suter S, Gianella-Borradori A, et al. A comparison of ceftriaxone and cefuroxime for the treatment of bacterial meningitis in children. N Engl J Med 322:141–147, 1990.
30. Adams WG, Deaver KA, Cochi SL, et al. Decline of childhood *Haemophilus influnzae* type b (Hib) disease in the Hib vaccine era. JAMA 269:221–226, 1993.
31. Skogberg K, Syrjanen J, Jahkola M, et al. Clinical presentation and outcome of listerosis in patients with and without immunosuppressive therapy. Clin Infect Dis 14:815–821, 1992.
32. Trautmann M, Wagner J, Chahin M, Weinke T. *Listeria* meningitis: report of ten recent cases and review of current therapeutic recommendations. J Infect 10:107–114, 1985.
33. Hansen PB, Jensen TH, Lykkegaard S, Kristensen HS. *Listeria monocytogenes* meningitis in adults. Sixteen consecutive cases 1973–1982. Scand J Infect Dis 19:55–60, 1987.
34. Lorber B. Listeriosis. Clin Infect Dis 24:1, 1997.
35. Nairn K, Shepherd GL, Edwards JR. Efficacy of meropenem in experimental meningitis. J Antimicrob Chemother 36(Suppl A):73–84, 1995.

36. Dagan R, Velghe L, Rodda JL, et al. Penetration of meropenem into the cerebrospinal fluid of patients with inflamed meninges. J Antimicrob Chemother 34:175–179, 1994.
37. Cherubin CE, Marr JS, Sierra MF, et al. *Listeria* and gram negative bacillary meningitis in New York City 1972–1979. Am J Med 71:199–209, 1981.
38. Cherubin CE, Corrado ML, Nair SR, et al. Treatment of gram negative bacillary meningitis. Role of new cephalosporin antibiotics. Rev Infect Dis 4(Suppl): S453–464, 1982.
39. Jacobs RF. Cefotaxime treatment of gram negative enteric meningitis in infants and children. Drugs 35(Suppl2):185–189, 1988.
40. Kaplan SL, Patrick CC. Cefotaxime and aminoglycoside treatment of meningitis caused by gram-negative enteric organisms. Pediatr Infect Dis J 9:810–814, 1990.
41. Fong IW, Tomkins KB. Review of *Pseudomonas aeruginosa* meningitis with special emphasis on treatment with ceftazidime. Rev Infect Dis 7:604–612, 1985.
42. Rodriguez WJ, Khan WN, Cocchetti DM, et al. Treatment of *Pseudomonas aeruginosa* meningitis with or without concurrent therapy. Pediatr Infect Dis J 9:83–87, 1990.
43. Calandra GB, Brown KR, Grad LC, et al. The efficacy results and safety profile of imipenem/cilastatin from the clinical research trials. J Clin Pharmacol 28:120–127, 1988.
44. Wong VK, Wright HT Jr, Ross LA, et al. Imipenem/cilastatin treatment of bacterial meningitis in children. Pediatr Infect Dis J 10:122–125, 1991.
45. Donnelly JP, Horrevorts AM, Sauerwein RW, et al. High-dose meropenem in meningitis due to *Pseudomonas aeruginosa.* Lancet 339:1117, 1992.
46. Medoff G, Kobayashi GS. Systemic fungal infections: an overview. Hosp Pract 2:41–52, 1991.
47. Bennett JE, Dismukes W, Duma R. A comparison of amphotericin B alone and combined with flucytosine in the treatment of cryptococcal meningitis. N Engl J Med 301:126–131, 1979.
48. Van Der Horst CM, Saag MS, Cloud GA, et al. Treatment of cryptococcal meningitis associated with acquired immune deficiency syndrome. N Engl J Med 337:15, 1997.
49. Stevens DA. Coccidiomycosis. N Engl J Med 332:1077–1082, 1995.
50. Nelson S, Sealy DP, Schneider EF. The aseptic meningitis syndrome. Am Fam Physician 48:809–815, 1993.
51. Marinac JS. Drug and chemical-induced aseptic meningitis: a review of the literature. Ann Pharmacother 26:813–821, 1992.
52. Rubeiz H, Roos RP. Viral meningitis and encephalitis. Semin Neurol 12:165–177, 1992.
53. Lambert HP. Meningitis. J Neurol Neurosurg Psych 57:405–415, 1994.
54. Lebel MH, Frey BJ, Syrogrannopoulos GA. Dexamethasone therapy for bacterial meningitis. Results of two double-blind, placebo controlled trials. N Engl J Med 319:964–971, 1988.
55. Anderson M. Management of cerebral infection. J Neurol Neurosurg Psych 56:1243–1258, 1993.
56. Domingues RB, Tsanacles AM, Pannuti CS, et al. Evaluation of the range of clinical presentations of herpes simplex encephalitis by using polymerase chain reaction assay of cerebrospinal fluid samples. Clin Infect Dis 25:86–91, 1997.
57. Hirsch MS. Herpes simplex virus. In: Mandell GL, Bennett JE, Dolin R, eds. Principles and practice of infectious diseases, 4th ed. New York: Churchill Livingstone, 1995;2:1336–1345.
58. Whitley RJ, Alford CA, Hirsch MS, et al. Vidarabine versus acyclovir therapy of herpes simplex encephalitis. N Engl J Med 314:144–149, 1986.
59. Skoldenberg B, Forsgren M. Acyclovir versus vidarabine in herpes simplex encephalitis. Scand Infect Dis 47:89–96, 1985.
60. Skoldenberg B, Forsgren M, Alestig K, et al. Acyclovir versus vidarabine in herpes simplex encephalitis. Randomised multicenter study in consecutive Swedish patients. Lancet 2:707–711, 1984.
61. Peterslund NA. Herpes zoster associated encephalitis: clinical findings and acyclovir treatment. Scand J Infect Dis 20:583–592, 1988.
62. O'Brien JJ, Campoli-Richards DM. Acyclovir: an updated review of its antiviral activity, pharmacokinetic properties and therapeutic efficacy. Drugs 37:233–309, 1989.
63. Gately A, Gander R, Johnson P. Herpes simplex virus type 2 meningoencephalitis resistant to acyclovir in a patient with AIDS. J Infect Dis 161:711, 1990.
64. Britt RH, Enzmann DR. Clinical stages of human brain abscesses on serial CT scans after contrast infusion. Computerized tomographic, neuropathological and clinical correlations. J Neurosurg 59:972–989, 1983.
65. Mathisen GE, Johnson JP. Brain abscess. Clin Infect Dis 25:763–781, 1997.
66. Chun CH, Johnson JD, Hofstetter M, et al. Brain abscess, a study of 45 consecutive cases. Medicine 65:415–431, 1986.
67. Garfield J. Management of supratentorial intracranial abscess: a review of 200 cases. Br Med J 2:7, 1969.
68. Bellar AJ, Sahar A, Praiss I. Brain abscess. Review of 89 cases over 30 years. J Neurol Neurosurg Psychiatry 36:757, 1973.
69. Small M, Dale BAB. Intracranial suppuration 1969–1982–a 15 year review. Clin Otolaryngol 9:315, 1984.
70. Gorbach SL, Bartlett JG, Blacklow NR. Infectious diseases. 9th ed. Philadelphia: WB Saunders, 1992.
71. Luer MS, Halton J. Vancomycin administration into the cerebrospinal fluid: a review. Ann Pharmacother 27:912–921, 1993.
72. Kaufmann BA, Tunkel AR, Pryor JC, et al. Meningitis in the neurosurgical patient. Infect Dis Clin North Am 4:677–701, 1990.

CHAPTER 74

BONE AND JOINT INFECTIONS

Gregory V. Stajich and Sybelle A. Blakey

Osteomyelitis

DEFINITION

Osteomyelitis is a microbial infection of the bone associated with bacteria, fungi, and rarely mycobacteria. The result of this invasion is an inflammatory destructive process. Osteomyelitis can occur in any bone of the body. It begins as an acute infection and if left untreated may progress to a chronic disease. Factors such as the anatomic site of bone involved, the chronicity and extent of infection, the patient's age, the presence of prosthetic devices, the causative agent, and concomitant host diseases influence the clinical manifestations, therapy, and prognosis of the disease. Despite the advent of more potent antimicrobial therapy and enhanced diagnostic procedures and surgical techniques, the treatment of osteomyelitis continues to pose a diagnostic and therapeutic challenge. The discussion in this chapter is limited to infections of bacterial origin.

TREATMENT GOALS: OSTEOMYELITIS

- Arrest the infectious process.
- Prevent permanent bone damage and deformity.
- Reverse all signs and symptoms of disease.
- Prevent chronic infection.

EPIDEMIOLOGY

Depending on its pathogenesis, osteomyelitis can be categorized as either hematogenous or contiguous to a focus of infection. Contiguous osteomyelitis may be associated with vascular insufficiency (Table 74.1). Each type of osteomyelitis can be further categorized as either acute or chronic depending on the stage of illness (i.e., onset of symptoms and the duration of clinical manifestations).

Hematogenous osteomyelitis describes an infection whose source of bacteria is from the bloodstream. More than 85% of cases occur in children under 17 years of age. In this situation the long bones are usually affected; in adults the thoracic or lumbar vertebrae are involved. At any age, males are more likely to acquire hematogenous osteomyelitis.[1]

In contrast to hematogenous osteomyelitis, contiguous osteomyelitis has a biphasic age distribution. In younger individuals the source tends to be trauma and its associated surgery, whereas in older adults the risk factors of decubitus ulcers and infected joint prostheses are common.[2] Osteomyelitis can result from bacterial inoculation of the bone from an exogenous source or from extension of an adjacent soft tissue infection.

The last type of osteomyelitis, contiguous with vascular insufficiency, is usually seen in older individuals (between

Table 74.1 ▪ Categorization of Osteomyelitis

Type	Age Distribution	Bones Involved	Major Clinical Findings	Microbiology
Hematogenous	1–20 years >50 years	Long bones Vertebrae	Initial episode Fever Local tenderness Local swelling Decreased range of motion Recurrent episode Exudative drainage	Single pathogen
Contiguous	>50 years	Femur Tibia Skull Mandible	Initial episode Fever Erythema Swelling Sinus tract formation Recurrent episode Exudative drainage Sinus tract formation	Polymicrobial
Contiguous with vascular insufficiency	>50 years	Feet Toes	Initial and recurrent episode Pain[a] Swelling Erythema Exudative drainage Ulceration	Polymicrobial

Source: Reference 59.
[a]May be blunted by concurrent neuropathy.

50 and 70 years of age) with vascular insufficiency (e.g., diabetes mellitus, peripheral vascular disease). These infections develop as an extension of an existing localized infection and can affect the toes, metatarsals, tarsals, or hindfoot. This type of osteomyelitis is often polymicrobial and involves various bones; therefore, therapy generally differs from that of other types of osteomyelitis.

Acute osteomyelitis describes an infection with an onset of a few days to a week. It is usually a disease of children that is caused by a single pathogen, the predominant organism being *Staphylococcus aureus.* Alternatively, chronic osteomyelitis is predominantly seen in adults. A variety of factors have been used to define chronic osteomyelitis, including the chronicity of the disease, unresponsiveness to antibiotic therapy, and the presence of necrotic bone or a sinus tract.

Etiology

The most common bacterial causes of osteomyelitis are shown in Table 74.2. *Staphylococcus aureus* is the most common cause of infection in hematogenous osteomyelitis where it accounts for 60 to 90% of isolates in children.[3] One reason for this high rate is due to children's skeletal anatomy, which favors entrapment of organisms.[4] In the neonatal period, hematogenous osteomyelitis is caused by *Enterobacteriaceae* (especially *Escherichia coli*), group B streptococci, and *S. aureus.* In children older than 5 years of age, *Haemophilus influenzae* was once a prevalent pathogen, but its incidence has decreased due to the routine immunization of infants.[5] In children older than 5 years of age and in adolescents, the most commonly isolated pathogens are reported to include *S. aureus,* group A streptococci, and *Streptococcus pneumoniae.*[6] In adults, *S. aureus* is also the most common causative organism, where it has been isolated in up to 75% of cases.[7] In addition, gram-negative enteric bacilli may be isolated in up to one-third of cases and streptococci (including enterococci) in fewer than 10% of cases. Patients with sickle cell disease are often infected with *S. aureus* or *Salmonella* species, and *Pseudomonas aeruginosa* has been reported to cause infection in intravenous drug users. Polymicrobial infections are common in adult osteomyelitis and may include three or more pathogens. Anaerobes such as *Bacteroides fragilis,* other *Bacteroides* species, *Fusobacterium, Clostridium,* and microaerophilic cocci can also be significant pathogens in osteomyelitis.[8]

Risk Factors

Risk factors for the development of osteomyelitis are outlined in Table 74.3. The identification and knowledge of specific risk factors can aid in the early diagnosis of osteomyelitis in some patients and perhaps prevention of the infection in others.

Hematogenous dissemination of bacteria is one of the most important risk factors for the development of acute hematogenous osteomyelitis. This infection is predominantly a disease of children. Identification of septic foci that are associated with the promotion of bacteremia is important for overall treatment and pathogen recognition. For example, acute pharyngitis, minor lacerations, cellulitis, and cutaneous abscesses have been implicated as sources of bacteremia in children with acute osteomyelitis.[9] Another risk factor for bacteremia is the long-term use of indwelling vascular access catheters for hyperalimentation or for the administration of chemotherapeutic agents.

In older adults, gram-negative organisms and *Staphylococcus epidermidis* may cause osteomyelitis of the vertebral bodies. This infection may arise from primary sites in the gastrointestinal or urinary tract. A strong association has been documented between urinary tract infections and osteomyelitis of the vertebral bodies.[10] Intravenous drug use is the last predisposing factor as microorganisms are injected and cause various bacterial infections (i.e., endocarditis and osteomyelitis). Common infecting organisms include *P. aeruginosa, Serratia marcescens,* and *S. aureus.*[11]

Neonatal osteomyelitis also has associated risk factors. Placement of umbilical catheters following a complicated delivery or the use of frequent heel sticks for obtaining blood samples for laboratory tests have preceded the development of osteomyelitis in this age-group.

Osteomyelitis may also evolve from either direct bacterial inoculation (e.g., traumatic injury) or contiguous spread from an adjacent infectious focus. Direct inoculation can occur from a variety of sources such as penetrating trauma from open injuries to bone, reduction of fractures, orthopedic and diagnostic procedures, gunshot wounds, and animal bites.[12] In many cases, the sterile bone is directly penetrated and inoculated. The pathogen(s) may originate from the penetrating object or from the patient's skin. Osteomyelitis from a contiguous soft tissue infection is the most important pathogenesis in adults. The primary foci for these infections include soft tissue infections close to the bone, as in the case of osteomyelitis of the mastoid bone, which can originate from malignant otitis media or a paranasal sinus infection. Another example of contiguous osteomyelitis is mandibular osteomyelitis observed in patients with poor oral hygiene or chronic infections of the teeth. Postoperative wound infections following orthopedic correction of the skeleton, neurosurgery, median sternotomy, and oral surgery are also major sources of contiguous osteomyelitis.

Concurrent underlying diseases or conditions are recognized as predisposing risk factors to the development of osteomyelitis. Sickle cell anemia and related hemoglobinopathies are reported to predispose patients to the development of osteomyelitis due to *Salmonella* species.[13] Diabetes mellitus with vascular insufficiency often predisposes patients to chronic draining ulcers and cellulitis of the feet and toes, which promotes the development of contiguous osteomyelitis.[14] Decubitus ulcers, or pressure sores, in chronically debilitated bedridden patients also are a major risk factor. Chronic osteomyelitis may develop due to inadequate or delayed management of acute osteomyelitis, unrecognized bone infection, inappropriate antibiotic pharmacotherapy (choice, dose, duration), or inadequate surgical drainage.

PATHOPHYSIOLOGY

Animal models have long been used to explore the pathogenesis of osteomyelitis. In these studies, normal bone has been shown to be highly resistant to infection. The presence of a foreign body (e.g., a prosthetic device),

Table 74.2 ▪ Commonly Isolated Organisms in Monomicrobial Osteomyelitis

Neonate (<1 month)	Infants and Children (1 month–5 years)	Children and Adolescents (5–16 years)	Adults (>16 years)
S. aureus	*S. aureus*	*S. aureus*	*S. aureus*
Group B streptococci	*H. influenzae*	Group A streptococcus	Streptococci (including enterococci)
Enterobacteriaceae (especially *E. coli*)	Group A streptococci	*S. pneumoniae*	Gram-negative bacilli
	S. pneumoniae		Anaerobes

Table 74.3 ▪ Risk Factors Associated with the Development of Osteomyelitis

Hematogenous	Contiguous	Contiguous with Vascular Insufficiency
Bacteremic foci	Direct inoculation	Diabetes mellitus
Noninvasive	Penetrating trauma	Peripheral vascular disease
Acute pharyngitis	Open reduction of fracture	Pressure ulcer
Minor laceration	Gunshot wound	
Cellulitis	Orthopedic procedure	
Cutaneous abscess	Diagnostic procedure	
Sickle cell anemia	Animal bite	
Respiratory/urinary tract infection	Puncture wound	
Invasive	Adjacent foci	
Intravenous catheter	Surgery	
Intravenous drug user	Postoperative wound infection	
Hemodialysis	Soft tissue infection	
Heel stick	Poor oral hygiene	
Nonpenetrating trauma	Chronic tooth infection	

trauma, or a large inoculum of microorganisms lays the groundwork for the development of osteomyelitis.[15,16]

Acute hematogenous osteomyelitis in children usually involves the metaphysis of a long bone such as the femur. The pathogenesis is thought to involve the capillary ends of the nutrient artery, which make sharp turns under the epiphyseal growth plate and enter into large venous sinusoids where blood flow slows considerably (Fig. 74.1). Additionally, the capillary lining lacks phagocytic cells. These anatomic and physiologic features favor the growth of microorganisms. Following hematogenous seeding of the bone, the host's inflammatory response ensues. Vascular permeability is increased, resulting in edema and an influx of polymorphonuclear leukocytes. Cytokines, toxic oxygen radicals, and proteolytic enzymes generated by the inflammatory response destroy surrounding tissue, including bone. Prostaglandins, generated in response to bone disruption, decrease the threshold for bacterial infection of the bone.[17] Intraosseal pressure increases as pus collects and is confined within the rigid bone. In children, the cortical section of the bone and the metaphyses are much thinner than in adults. There is also less adherence of the periosteum to the underlying cortex. The culmination of these factors is extension of the suppurative process from the metaphysis through the cortex and into the subperiosteal space. The blood supply to the outer cortical bone may be further diminished due to the pressure leading to the development of dead bone or sequestra. In adults, the infectious process usually remains intramedullary due to the thicker cortex and tightly bound periosteum. Infecting microorganisms have attributes that aid in the development of osteomyelitis. *Staphylococcus aureus,* the most common etiologic agent, adheres to bone, cartilage, and prosthetic devices via adhesins that are specific for bone components (e.g., collagen, laminin, fibronectin).[18] The ability of *S. aureus* to survive within leukocytes after phagocytosis may explain some chronic bone infections.[19]

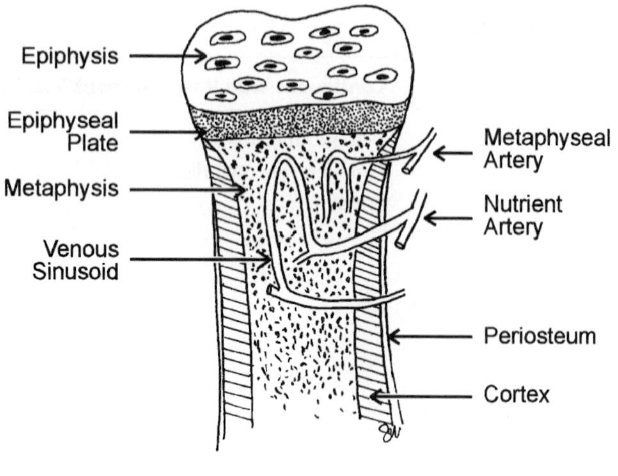

Figure 74.1. Cross section of a bone.

CLINICAL PRESENTATION AND DIAGNOSIS

Signs and Symptoms

Osteomyelitis secondary to hematogenous spread is often preceded by the signs and symptoms consistent with bacteremia: fever, malaise, chills, headache, nausea, vomiting, and myalgias (Table 74.1). Local symptoms include pain, swelling, tenderness, decreased range of motion in an adjacent joint, or suppuration at the involved site. In adults, osteomyelitis secondary to hematogenous spread usually affects the vertebrae. If diagnosis is delayed, the disease may progress to vertebral destruction and paralysis.[20]

With osteomyelitis secondary to a contiguous focus, infections are prevalent in the bones that are more prone to fracture or open reduction surgical procedures (e.g., femur, tibia). Fever may be present during the initial episode, but major symptoms are generally confined to the infected area and consist of pain, tenderness, swelling, and redness.

In patients with diabetes or vascular insufficiency osteomyelitis occurs almost exclusively in the feet.[21] This population may have claudication or extremity neuropathy, which blunts both perception of local injury and the inflammatory response. Local skin infection can progress insidiously to the bone. The clinical presentation of these patients is often dichotomous. If advanced neuropathy exists, the infection is often painless. However, if acute bony destruction occurs, excruciating pain may be elicited on physical examination.[22] Other symptoms include swelling, erythema, exudative drainage, and ulceration.

Acute osteomyelitis due to hematogenous spread or a contiguous focus can progress to a chronic infection. This recalcitrant disease is characterized by repeated therapeutic failures. This type of osteomyelitis cannot be cured until the nidus of infection has been removed. Antimicrobials often control the disease, but surgical debridement is usually necessary to eradicate the infection. The common characteristic for all types of chronic osteomyelitis is the presence of vascular thrombosis or sequestra. Sequestra provide a bacterial milieu for persistence of the infection and perpetuation of the inflammatory process. This results in eventual vascular thrombosis and further development of necrotic bone.[23] In addition, glycocalyx formation acts as a barrier to hormonal and cellular host defenses while enhancing the attachment of microorganisms to the bone or foreign bodies.[24]

Diagnosis

No single laboratory test is specific for the diagnosis of osteomyelitis. However, some tests are indicative of osteomyelitis. A definitive diagnosis can be made only with microbiological identification of the pathogen(s) from a bone specimen. In acute hematogenous osteomyelitis, the diagnosis rests with isolation of the pathogen from the bone lesion or blood culture. Bone biopsies or aspirates (83%) are superior to blood cultures (32%) in yielding organisms.[5,25]

Other tests that are of importance include a white blood cell count (WBC) and an erythrocyte sedimentation rate (ESR). A leukocytosis, with a left shift, may be consistent with an infectious process such as osteomyelitis. However, it has been reported that a normal WBC may occur in 40 to 75% of patients with acute osteomyelitis.[26] Although nonspecific, ESRs are frequently elevated in excess of 20 mm/hr in acute untreated osteomyelitis. An ESR that returns to normal during the course of therapy may be a favorable prognostic sign. The ESR is not a reliable laboratory test in many patients who have inflammatory diseases, collagen vascular illnesses, or sickle cell disease; in patients receiving corticosteroids; or in neonates.[27] In neonates and children, C-reactive protein, another nonspecific indicator of inflammation, typically begins to decline within 6 hours of initiation of appropriate therapy.[28]

A culture diagnosis of contiguous osteomyelitis may be more complex. Because osteomyelitis arises from a contiguous abscess, cellulitis, or penetration of the overlying skin, culture specimens obtained from subcutaneous or other surrounding tissues may also need evaluation. These may be obtained either by direct needle biopsy or at the time of surgical debridement. Caution should be exercised when evaluating culture specimens obtained from superficially draining sinus tracts because these areas may be heavily colonized. The results in this case may be misleading and not indicative of the actual pathogen of the site of infection. When vertebral osteomyelitis is suspected, blood cultures and needle biopsy guided by fluoroscopic or computed tomographic guidance have been successful.[29]

In chronic osteomyelitis, blood cultures and drainage from the sinus tract are often not reliable.[30] In the case where tissue and blood cultures are negative, direct subperiosteal or metaphyseal needle aspiration is required to make a definitive diagnosis. Bone biopsy specimens should be carefully cultured and stained for aerobes, anaerobes, mycobacteria, and fungi.

A variety of imaging methods can be used in the diagnosis of osteomyelitis. Early findings may be easily missed and may include adjacent soft tissue swelling, periosteal thickening or elevation, and focal osteopenia.[22] Radiography may be used at initial presentation and at follow-up; however, radiographic changes in the bone may lag 2 weeks behind the development of infection. With appropriate antimicrobial therapy, radiologic improvements may also lag behind clinical symptom improvement. Other imaging techniques, such as computed tomography (CT), nuclear imaging studies (e.g., technetium and gallium), magnetic resonance imaging (MRI), and positron emission tomography (PET) have improved disease detection and can reveal bony abnormalities even when plain radiographs are normal. These are more expensive techniques and are usually reserved for cases in which the diagnosis is equivocal.

Technetium 99m methylene diphosphonate is the current radiopharmaceutical of choice for nuclear imaging.[31] Following intravenous administration of the radionuclide, the skeletal system is imaged or scanned. Abnormal findings consistent with osteomyelitis are related to the Technetium 99m uptake ability of the inflamed tissues due to increased bone metabolic activity and blood flow. This radionuclide is highly sensitive but not specific, so scanning studies may also be positive in the presence of other inflammatory processes such as trauma, tumor, or arthritis.[27] Gallium 67 citrate is a more selective radionuclide that is taken up by polymorphonuclear leukocytes that have mobilized to the site of bacterial infection.

MRI and CT have excellent resolution and can detect edema, destruction of the medulla, cortical destruction, periosteal reaction, articular damage, and soft tissue involvement, even when plain radiographs are normal.[32] MRI has recently emerged as the preferred imaging technique for the diagnosis of osteomyelitis and soft tissue infections and is superior to CT in establishing the level of involvement of the infection. CT is preferred for establishing cortical bone destruction or sequestra or as a guide for drainage or biopsy.[33] PET is another noninvasive method that assesses perfusion and metabolic states of tissue. PET enables detection and demonstration of the extent of chronic osteomyelitis with a high degree of accuracy.[34]

TREATMENT

Pharmacotherapy

Because the treatment of osteomyelitis involves a protracted commitment to antibiotic therapy, careful evaluation and diagnosis are paramount. The keys to effective treatment are identifying the pathogen(s) and their antibiotic sensitivities, initiating appropriate empiric antimicrobial therapy before the culture and sensitivity results are known, and delivering adequate quantities of the antibiotic to the site of infection.

Parenteral Antibiotic Therapy

Empiric antimicrobial regimens should provide adequate antistaphylococcal coverage and take into consideration other probable organism(s) based on potential risk factors and patient history. After culture and sensitivity results are known, the therapy can be tailored to reflect the infecting organism(s) and their respective sensitivity profile. Initial empiric therapy usually consists of high-dose parenteral antibiotics because these regimens achieve high steady-state bone and serum concentrations more quickly than orally administered drugs. However, both parenteral and oral antibiotics are effective for the treatment of osteomyelitis, as long as serum and bone concentrations are adequate for eradication of the infecting organism(s). Most clinicians recommend initial parenteral therapy for a variable amount of time, followed by oral therapy for the remainder of treatment.[35,36] The duration of antibiotic therapy for treatment of osteomyelitis has not been fully elucidated. The best cure rates are obtained when parenteral therapy is administered for a minimum of 4 to

6 weeks.[37] However, the duration of therapy can vary depending on the etiology of the infection. For example, acute hematogenous osteomyelitis caused by *H. influenzae, Neisseria meningitidis,* and *S. pneumoniae* may be treated with shorter courses in a minimum of 14 days, whereas *S. aureus* and enteric gram-negative organisms usually require a minimum of 4 weeks.[38] Most clinicians prefer to use the amelioration of clinical signs, normalization of laboratory parameters (e.g., WBC and ESR), and improvement in radiographic findings in determining the patient-specific length of therapy for osteomyelitis from contiguous foci or for chronic osteomyelitis. The management of osteomyelitis in children and adults often includes surgery and immobilization in addition to antibiotic therapy.

In neonates, surgical intervention by debridement of necrotic tissue is controversial and less frequently desired.[3] A parenteral regimen is usually initiated and may be completed with oral antibiotics. The most commonly employed empiric antimicrobial regimens according to age-group and likely organisms are summarized in Table 74.4. Intravenous penicillinase-resistant penicillins (e.g., nafcillin, oxacillin) have the advantages of good bone penetration, bactericidal activity, and low cost. One disadvantage is the short half-life of these drugs, which results in a more frequent dose administration schedule. Additionally, the potential for penicillin-induced hypersensitivity or anaphylactic reactions exists. An alternative antibiotic is an intravenous first-generation cephalosporin, such as cefazolin. This drug can be used in some penicillin-allergic patients (e.g., in patients who have inconsequential rash from penicillin) and has the advantage of good activity against *S. aureus* and some gram-negative organisms, such as *E. coli.* If a patient has had a serious allergic reaction to β-lactam antibiotics, clindamycin or vancomycin can be used in the treatment of staphylococcal osteomyelitis.

Appropriate antimicrobial therapy for polymicrobial contiguous osteomyelitis, with or without vascular insufficiency, may include an aminoglycoside (e.g., gentamicin) added to the antistaphylococcal regimens described earlier. Patients receiving aminoglycosides must be carefully monitored because of the potential for ototoxicity and nephrotoxicity, especially in older adults or those with renal dysfunction. Alternatives include monotherapy with a broad-spectrum β-lactam antibiotic such as cefotaxime, ceftizoxime, or ceftriaxone. All three agents are highly active against *S. aureus* and common *Enterobacteriaceae* species. Ceftazidime is less active against *S. aureus,* but it is the most active cephalosporin against *P. aeruginosa.*[39,40] The current standard of care for the treatment of this infection, following surgical debridement, is a 4- to 6-week course of antibiotic therapy directed at organisms isolated from the culture.[41]

Anaerobic bacteria have been isolated in both acute hematogenous and contiguous osteomyelitis. Intraabdominal infections are often a source of anaerobic bacteremia. Anaerobic osteomyelitis of the mandible or the cranial and facial bones may result from the relatively high numbers of anaerobes present in the normal flora of the oral cavity. The most common form of chronic osteomyelitis due to anaerobes, however, is that related to underlying peripheral vascular disease. This syndrome is almost always associated with long-standing diabetes mellitus and, in nondiabetics, with severe peripheral vascular disease.

Special populations may require alternative therapy, such as those with nosocomial or prosthetic joint infections, intravenous drug users, or those with sickle cell disease. An empiric regimen for a patient with a hemoglobinopathy would be a penicillinase-resistant penicillin plus a third-generation cephalosporin or a fluoroquinolone (adults only). Intravenous drug users should begin therapy that is active against *P. aeruginosa,* such as a fluoroquinolone or the combination of a third-generation cephalosporin plus an aminoglycoside. Patients with prosthetic joint devices may develop infections with organisms such as *S. epidermidis* or *Propionibacterium* species and may require vancomycin.[42]

Oral Antibiotic Therapy

Characteristics such as improved bioavailability, good activity against the usual pathogens, and relatively nontoxic side effect profiles make oral antibiotics attractive for long-term treatment of osteomyelitis. Other factors include the realization that prolonged intravenous antibiotic therapy is associated with iatrogenic complications (e.g., phlebitis, local and vascular infection, excess fluid administration, patient discomfort) and economic pressures to provide optimal patient care for the lowest cost. A variety of oral agents have been used, including penicillins, cephalosporins, clindamycin, and fluoroquinolones.[43,44] In most instances, therapy is initiated with a parenteral antibiotic and then completed with an appropriate oral agent along with aggressive patient monitoring.

In children with hematogenous osteomyelitis, a brief course of intravenous antibiotics (typically 3 to 10 days) may be switched to oral therapy for several additional weeks of therapy.[45] The serum bactericidal titer (SBT) is reported to be a useful indicator of the potential adequacy of oral therapy in children with infections due to *S. aureus.*[46] The SBT assesses the ability of serial dilutions of the patient's serum to kill the patient's infecting organism. When these tests are used, a peak serum sample is drawn and a target SBT of 1:8 or greater and a trough titer of 1:2 or greater are recommended.[46,47]

In adults, the quinolones are promising agents for the treatment of gram-negative osteomyelitis, including that due to *P. aeruginosa.* Long term suppressive therapy with this class of drugs can attenuate the signs and symptoms of chronic refractory osteomyelitis.[48] The quinolones have demonstrated excellent efficacy versus *Enterobacteriaceae.* Further studies comparing the quinolones to traditional intravenous antibiotic regimens are needed before the quinolones supplant these agents in the treatment of

Table 74.4 ▪ Empiric Antibiotic Treatment of Osteomyelitis and Infectious Arthritis According to Age-Group and Probable Organisms

Age-Group	Probable Pathogens	Gram Stain	Antibiotic Regimens of Choice[a] (drug, dose, route, and frequency of administration)
Neonates (<1 month)	*S. aureus*	Gram-positive cocci in clusters	**One of the following:** (Frequency determined by postnatal age and weight) Nafcillin/oxacillin 100 mg/kg/day Cefazolin 50 mg/kg/day Vancomycin[b] 30 mg/kg/day **Plus one of the following:** (Frequency determined by postnatal age and weight) Gentamicin[b,c] 3 mg/kg/day Cefotaxime[d] 100 mg/kg/day
	Group B streptococci	Gram-positive cocci in pairs/chains	
	E. coli	Gram-negative bacilli	
Infants, children, and adolescents (1 month to 16 years)	*S. aureus*	Gram-positive cocci in clusters	**One of the following:** Nafcillin/oxacillin 50 mg/kg IV q6hr Cefazolin 25 mg/kg IV q6–8hr Clindamycin 10 mg/kg IV q6hr Vancomycin[b] 10 mg/kg IV q6–8hr (Cefotaxime[d,e] 50 mg/kg IV q6hr)
	Group A streptococci	Gram-positive cocci in pairs/chains	
	S. pneumoniae[f]		
	H. influenzae	Gram-negative bacilli	
	Enterobacteriaceae		
Adults (>16 years)	*S. aureus*	Gram-positive cocci in clusters	**One of the following:** Nafcillin/oxacillin 2 g IV q6hr Cefazolin 2 g IV q8hr Clindamycin 600 mg IV q8hr Vancomycin[b] 1 g IV q12hr (±Gentamicin[b–d] 5 mg/kg IV QD)
	Streptococci spp.	Gram-positive cocci in pairs/chains	
	N. gonorrhoeae (infectious arthritis only)	Gram-negative diplococci	Ceftriaxone 1 g IV QD
	Enterobacteriaceae *P. aeruginosa* *Salmonella*	Gram-negative bacilli	**One of the following:** Piperacillin 3–4 g IV q4–6hr + gentamicin[b–d] Ceftazidime[d] 2 g IV q8hr or ceftriaxone[d] 1 g IV QD Ciprofloxacin[d] 400 mg IV q12hr
	Anaerobes		**One of the following:** Clindamycin 600 mg IV q8hr Metronidazole 500 mg IV q6hr
	Mixed infections (aerobic and anaerobic)		**One of the following:** Imipenem/cilastatin 500 mg IV q6hr Ticarcillin/clavulanate 3.1 g IV q6hr Piperacillin/tazobactam 3.375–4.5 g IV q6hr Ampicillin/sulbactam 3 g IV q6hr Alatrofloxacin[g] 200 mg IV QD

[a] Doses based on normal renal function.
[b] Requires pharmacokinetic monitoring.
[c] Aminoglycosides may be given once a day or in multiple doses.
[d] Drug class representative.
[e] Add if Gram stain shows gram-negative bacilli.
[f] Great geographic variability in degree/prevalence of drug-resistant *S. pneumoniae*.
[g] Due to potential liver toxicity, use only in patients with life-threatening infections where benefits outweigh risks.

osteomyelitis due to other organisms such as *P. aeruginosa* and *S. aureus.* The indiscriminate use of quinolones is especially concerning given the ability of *S. aureus* to develop resistance during treatment. However, the quinolones may be used in combination with rifampin to help minimize resistance and improve outcomes even in patients with prostheses.[37] Quinolones are not approved for use in the pediatric population because of the potential for arthropathy or chondrodysplasia.[49]

Antibiotic Bone Concentrations

Debate continues over the relevance of antibiotic concentrations in infected bone. Clinical studies have failed to demonstrate that antibiotic bone concentrations considerably above the minimum inhibitory concentration (MIC) of the infecting organism are required for effective treatment of osteomyelitis.[50,51] There are several reasons for this controversy. A variety of sampling techniques and assay methods were used in these studies when bone samples were obtained from patients without bone infections who were undergoing orthopedic procedures. The vascular supply to infected bone may significantly affect antibiotic bone concentration. Infected tissue that is highly vascularized will achieve higher antibiotic bone concentrations than an area with compromised blood flow. Animal models of bone infection are being used to clarify the relationship between antibiotic bone concentrations and the treatment of osteomyelitis.[52]

Home Antibiotic Therapy

Administering parenteral antibiotics on an outpatient basis is an obvious alternative to hospitalization in patients who need long-term treatment of selected infectious diseases such as osteomyelitis and endocarditis. This method of treatment is a safe, efficacious, and cost-effective alternative to prolonged hospitalization.[53] A candidate for outpatient parenteral antibiotic therapy must meet three criteria: (1) the infection must require treatment beyond the expected duration of hospitalization, (2) the patient must be otherwise medically stable, and (3) there must be no equally effective and safe oral antibiotic regimen.[54] Therapy should be initiated in the hospital, where observation for untoward effects and overall tolerability of the regimen can be assessed. Once the patient is sent home, drugs are administered through a peripheral venous access site (e.g., intermittent needle therapy), a central catheter (e.g., peripheral intravenous central catheter), or directly through a Hickman-Broviac catheter. Intermittent needle therapy has a disadvantage in that the needle must be replaced every 3 days. Also, patients often complain of local pain and inflammation. Central catheters generally remain in place for the duration of therapy. Hickman-Broviac catheters have the disadvantage of requiring minor surgery for placement. To ensure the safety and efficacy of outpatient parenteral antibiotic therapy, the expertise of the physician and pharmacist must be combined.[55] Pharmacologic considerations include safety, efficacy, stability, and storage conditions. Patient factors include manual dexterity, ability of friends or family to assist, expense, proximity to a medical center for drug supplies and follow-up, and minimal interference with activities of daily living. Despite these considerations, outpatient parenteral therapy can be a cost-saving tool when compared with the expense of prolonged hospitalization.

Local Antibiotic Therapy: Antibiotic-Impregnated Beads

Antibiotic-impregnated beads may be used as an alternative treatment or in conjunction with systemic antibiotic therapy for the treatment of osteomyelitis. This form of local antibiotic therapy originated with the use of antibiotic-impregnated bone cement for the treatment of infected arthroplasties. From this concept evolved the use of antibiotic-impregnated cement beads, which are strung on surgical steel wire, for the treatment of local bone and soft tissue infections. Several antibiotics, including aminoglycosides, vancomycin, penicillins, cephalosporins, clindamycin, and erythromycin, have been incorporated into cement beads. In this system, polymethyl methacrylate (PMMA) acts as a carrier for the antibiotic. The release of antibiotic from the bead follows a bimodal pattern. Approximately 5% of the antibiotic is released within the first 24 hours, and the remainder is released over several weeks or months.[56]

Impregnated PMMA beads have a number of advantages over systemic antibiotic therapy. Parenteral antibiotic therapy and its associated high serum concentrations may lead to nephrotoxic, ototoxic, or allergic events. Additionally, due to poor vascularization in the area of infected bone, high doses of parenteral antibiotics are often required for adequate penetration into necrotic areas. Use of impregnated beads results in local antibiotic concentrations that are 5 to 10 times higher than concentrations achieved via systemic administration.[56] The PMMA used as a carrier for the antibiotic has not been shown to significantly alter the host's normal immune response but remains a concern.

A number of disadvantages also exist. Not all antibiotics are suitable candidates for incorporation into cement beads. Drug characteristics that must be taken into consideration include the following: (1) the drug must be heat stable up to 100°C due to the exothermic reaction generated when mixing the bone cement, (2) the antibiotic must be water soluble so that it can easily diffuse through the cement, (3) the antibiotic should have a low incidence of hypersensitivity reactions, and (4) the antibiotic should be bactericidal at low concentration. An additional surgical procedure is required to remove the beads.

Nonpharmacologic Therapy

Surgery

Infections in the bone have long been a formidable foe of orthopedic surgeons. Surgical intervention should be undertaken if pus is found on bone biopsy or aspiration or if a metaphyseal cavity is seen on the initial radiograph. The surgical approach consists of draining and irrigating the abscess and sinus tracts. This procedure is supplemented by preoperative and postoperative antibiotics given systemically or locally as antibiotic-impregnated beads. If no abscess is found, antibiotic therapy alone should be effective. If a patient does not show symptomatic improvement after 36 to 48 hours of empiric antibiotic therapy, the bone may need to be reaspirated and debrided. In adult osteomyelitis, any contiguous infectious processes should be evaluated for surgical drainage. Surgical debridement is required to excise avascular tissue and necrotic bone in patients with chronic infection.

Hyperbaric Oxygen

Hyperbaric oxygen (HBO) therapy has been used in the treatment of osteomyelitis.[57] HBO is administered by placing the patient in an enclosed chamber where oxygen pressures greater than sea level, usually 2 atmospheres, can be effected. Hypoxia at the site of infection results in poor wound healing. By attenuating the hypoxic environment in infected tissues, HBO promotes the formation of a collagen matrix and subsequent angiogenesis. Increasing the oxygen tension also revives and amplifies neutrophil-mediated killing of bacteria. Several studies have demonstrated beneficial effects of HBO when it is used in the treatment of chronic refractory osteomyelitis.[57] However, the scarcity of well-designed studies and the lack of randomized, well-controlled prospective studies make it difficult to support the routine use of HBO therapy. The cost-effective use of HBO as a standard regimen in the treatment of osteomyelitis is controversial. An average treatment regimen for osteomyelitis consists of 20 to 30 sessions lasting 90 minutes each with the cost for one session between $300 and $400.[57] Adverse effects of HBO include reversible myopia, mild to moderate pain secondary to barotrauma (rupture of the middle ear, cranial sinuses, teeth, or lungs), and, rarely, self-limiting seizures. HBO is adjunctive therapy and should always be used in conjunction with surgery and antibiotics. It should be reserved for cases of chronic refractory osteomyelitis that have not responded to standard surgical and antibiotic therapy.

IMPROVING OUTCOMES

The treatment of osteomyelitis involves prompt initiation of broad-spectrum antibiotics active against staphylococci, streptococci, and common enteric gram-negative rods as soon as possible after the onset of symptoms. This may minimize the number of patients who require extensive surgical debridement or those who may develop chronic osteomyelitis. Patients with acute osteomyelitis have the best prognosis, having an approximately 80% cure rate when parenteral antibiotics are maintained for more than 4 weeks and appropriate surgical intervention is employed.[46] Children with acute osteomyelitis can expect similar results if, after initial parenteral antibiotics, oral therapy compliance can be assured. Peak SBT values of 1:8 or greater are monitored to optimize therapy.

In the case of chronic osteomyelitis, the prognosis is substantially less favorable. Unsuccessful results have been attributed to several factors: short-term antibiotic treatment, poor bone penetration by antibiotics, existence of bone abscesses and sequestra, presence of foreign bodies, and the frequent nosocomial origin of pathogens that are often resistant to several antibiotics.[58] The combination of proper surgical debridement of dead bone and sequestra along with appropriate antibiotic treatment is critical and may increase follow-up success rates to 50%.[59] Patients for whom surgical debridement was unsuccessful or contraindicated may require long-term suppressive treatment with antibiotics to control their infections.

Outpatient intravenous antibiotic therapy represents a safe and cost-effective method for treating conditions such osteomyelitis and infectious arthritis.[55] Education of patients regarding compliance with the antibiotic regimen is extremely helpful in ensuring successful therapy. Outpatient intravenous antibiotic therapy requires selection of patients who are both medically and psychologically stable. Patients must learn to properly manage drugs and equipment, care for their intravenous access site, administer the medications, and recognize complications. Patients are trained by a pharmacist or nurse employed by the hospital or home care pharmacy. Administration of intravenous antibiotics in the home represents only one of several methods of administration outside of the hospital. For patients who are not candidates for home intravenous therapy, medications may be administered in physicians' offices, outpatient clinics, day-stay clinics, and emergency departments. Patient instructions for administration of intravenous antibiotics are listed in Table 74.5.

PHARMACOECONOMICS

The treatment of osteomyelitis often involves a protracted commitment to long-term parenteral antibiotics and surgical debridement, which can entail a major financial burden. In the era of prospective reimbursement of providers, it is not prudent to prolong hospitalization of an afebrile, stable patient for the sole purpose of administering 4 to 6 weeks of intravenous antibiotics. Outpatient

Table 74.5 ▪ Patient Instructions for Administering Intravenous Antibiotics

1. Remove antibiotic from refrigerator and thaw (if applicable).
2. Draw heparin solution into syringe and replace needle.
3. Hang intravenous bag above arm.
4. Establish fluid level in chamber and purge air.
5. Cleanse intravenous catheter stopper with alcohol.
6. Connect intravenous tubing to catheter.
7. Establish appropriate flow rate.
8. Complete infusion and use heparin flush.
9. Carefully dispose of used materials to prevent needle-stick injuries.

Source: Reference 55.

parenteral antibiotic therapy, via clinic visits, home health agencies, or self-administration, can substantially reduce hospital costs. Patient education, compliance, and follow-up visits are essential for successful eradication of the infection.

SUMMARY

Infection of bone remains difficult to treat, despite recent advances in antimicrobial therapy, diagnostic procedures and tests, and refinements in surgical techniques. When left untreated, osteomyelitis can result in significant systemic disease and bone deformity. The medical management involves accurate classification of the disease, identification of the offending pathogen via culture, surgical debridement, radiologic procedures, laboratory studies, and prompt high-dose antimicrobial therapy. Most β-lactam and aminoglycoside antibiotics penetrate normal and infected bone adequately but do not penetrate necrotic bone. Chronic osteomyelitis may require several months of treatment with intravenous and oral antibiotics and is associated with a less favorable prognosis. The majority of cases of acute osteomyelitis can be treated with monotherapy for a minimum of 4 weeks and are associated with a favorable prognosis. The oral fluoroquinolones are probably the most promising agents for the treatment of osteomyelitis caused by gram-negative bacilli. Hyperbaric oxygen may be useful as adjunctive therapy for chronic, refractory patients. Administering antibiotics at home has been shown to be a safe and cost-effective alternative in specific patients who would otherwise need prolonged hospitalization. Oral antibiotic therapy offers advantages in convenience and comfort for the patient and avoids iatrogenic disease and nosocomial superinfections, but it requires good patient compliance, careful follow-up, and laboratory monitoring.

Infectious Arthritis

DEFINITION

Infectious arthritis begins acutely in a single joint and is characterized by an inflammatory reaction of the joint space, synovium, synovial fluid, and articular cartilage. It is a closed-space infection with swelling, tenderness, and accumulation of pus in the joint. The yearly incidence varies from 2 to 10 per 100,000 in the general population to 30 to 70 per 100,000 in patients with rheumatoid arthritis and in patients with joint prostheses.[60,61] Prompt diagnosis and treatment are important to minimize damage to the joint or prevent spread of the infection to contiguous bone and soft tissue. Bacteria are the most common cause of joint infections, but fungi, viruses, and chlamydia have also been isolated. This discussion deals exclusively with bacterial arthritis.

TREATMENT GOALS: INFECTIOUS ARTHRITIS

- The treatment goals for infectious arthritis are essentially identical to those described in the osteomyelitis section. An additional goal is to prevent permanent joint damage leading to functional limitations and chronic pain.

EPIDEMIOLOGY

The pathogens that cause infectious arthritis vary considerably with the age of the patient. A few bacterial species cause the majority of cases, although given the right set of conditions any microorganism may infect a joint.

Etiology

The most common bacterial causes of infectious arthritis are listed in Table 74.6. *Staphylococcus aureus* is the most common organism isolated in newborns. Group B streptococci and *Enterobacteriaceae,* especially *E. coli,* have also been isolated and may be important pathogens.[62] In children under 2 years of age, *H. influenzae* type b is the predominant pathogen followed by *S. aureus* and *Streptococcus* species (e.g., group A, group B, and *S. pneumoniae*). Gram-negative enteric bacilli (e.g., *E. coli, Proteus* species, *Salmonella* species, and occasionally *Pseudomonas* species) also cause infectious arthritis in both infants and children. *Neisseria gonorrhoeae* is the most common cause of infectious arthritis in young, otherwise healthy, sexually active adults. *Staphylococcus aureus* is a major cause of infectious arthritis in older adults, and *S. epidermidis* is the leading cause in patients with prosthetic joints. Infections with gram-negative bacilli usually occur in patients age 60 years or older, often as a septic complication of a chronic joint disease. Anaerobic streptococci have been isolated as a complication of traumatic injuries, and *S. aureus* and *P. aeruginosa* cause infectious arthritis complicating intravenous drug use.

Risk Factors

An important risk factor for infectious arthritis is hematogenous seeding of a joint during either a transient or persistent bacteremia.[61] Because of the large number of total joint arthroplasties being done, joint prostheses have become the most important risk factor for infectious arthritis.[63] Joints may be inoculated during surgery, or, rarely, during aspiration or intraarticular steroid injection.[64] Puncture wounds (e.g., bites, stepping on a nail) represent other rare sources of bacterial joint inoculation. Host factors, such as age, preexisting joint disease, and immunosuppression, may also predispose a patient to

Table 74.6 ▪ Commonly Isolated Bacteria in Infectious Arthritis

Neonates (<1 month)	Infants and Children (1 month–5 years)	Children and Adolescents (5–16 years)	Adults (>16 years)
S. aureus Group B streptococci *Enterobacteriaceae*	*H. influenzae* *S. aureus* Group A, B streptococci *S. pneumoniae* Gram-negative bacilli	*S. aureus* Group A streptococci Gram-negative bacilli	*N. gonorrhoeae* *S. aureus* *S. epidermidis* *Enterobacteriaceae* *P. aeruginosa* Group A, B streptococci *S. pneumoniae*

infectious arthritis. Age greater than 80 years, diabetes mellitus, and rheumatoid arthritis are all reported independent risk factors for infectious arthritis.[61] Previous joint damage, such as that from rheumatoid arthritis, osteoarthritis, gout, and recent joint trauma, also appears to increase the risk of infectious arthritis.[61] Patients with impaired host defense systems, either through direct immunosuppressive therapy (e.g., systemic or intraarticular corticosteroid), or from primary malignancy (e.g., lymphoma) are also reported to be at greater risk.[65] Infections in these patients are usually associated with gram-negative bacilli. Intravenous drug users have a high rate of infection due to *P. aeruginosa* or *S. aureus*.[66] There is a rising incidence of infectious arthritis in patients who are infected with the human immunodeficiency virus.[67]

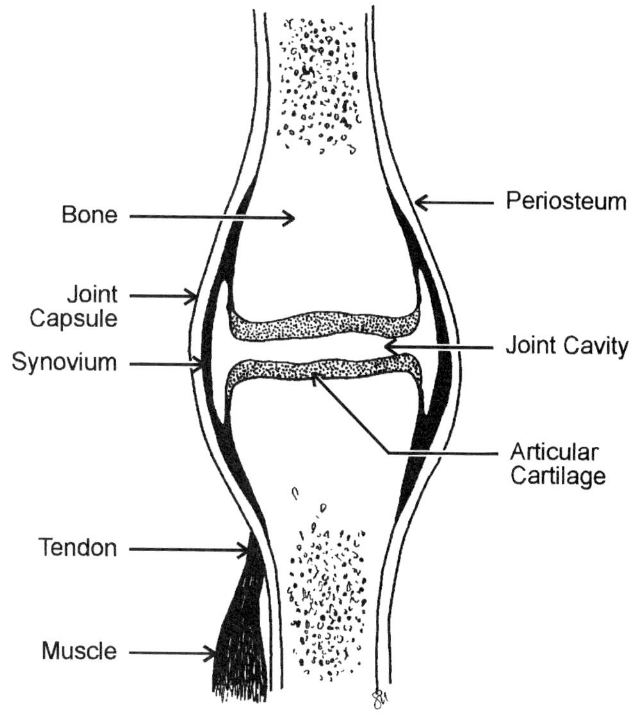

Figure 74.2. Major structures of a joint.

PATHOPHYSIOLOGY

The development of infectious arthritis is usually secondary to hematogenous spread of infection to a joint from a distant focus or may represent extension from infected bone. The latter is especially true in children younger than 1 year of age when the epiphyseal growth plate contains infection.

Once the organisms invade the joint space, the infection usually develops in the microvasculature of the synovial membrane (Fig. 74.2). At this site, the bacteria proliferate rapidly and trigger an acute inflammatory synovitis. This response is activated by bacteria engulfed by macrophages, synoviocytes, and migrating polymorphonuclear cells and is associated with the release of proteolytic enzymes, which can destroy intraarticular cartilage in as little as 3 days.[68] The infectious process induces a joint effusion, which increases intraarticular pressure, mechanically impeding blood and nutrient supply to the joint.[63] The continued inflammatory process may lead to destruction of the cartilage and invasion of the adjacent bone, causing osteomyelitis.[69]

CLINICAL PRESENTATION AND DIAGNOSIS

Signs and Symptoms

Nongonococcal infectious arthritis varies widely in manifestations. Usually it causes a painful monoarticular joint with swelling and redness that is sometimes associated with fever and chills. The patient has substantial limitation in the range of motion of the joint as a result of the swelling and tenderness. The knee is involved in the majority of cases (40 to 50%), followed by the hip (20 to 25%), ankle, elbow, shoulder, and joints of the hand,[70] although hip infections are more common in young children.[60] A hip or shoulder effusion is often difficult to detect on physical examination, and therefore the use of imaging studies is important in establishing the diagnosis of infectious arthritis.[71] Polyarticular infectious arthritis is most likely to occur in patients with rheumatoid arthritis or other collagen vascular diseases, in intravenous drug users, or in patients with overwhelming sepsis.[72]

Neisseria gonorrhoeae is the most common cause of infectious arthritis in young, otherwise healthy, sexually active adults and is a potentially serious complication of a urogenital infection. Unlike nongonococcal arthritis, gonococcal arthritis is usually polyarticular.[68] If left untreated, 1 to 3% of infections have been reported to disseminate to the synovial fluid and cause arthritis, which can cause various degrees of joint tissue damage.[63] Typical symptoms of gonococcal arthritis include inflammation, swelling, warmth, redness of the overlying skin, pain, and restriction of motion in the affected joints. This manifestation of disseminated gonococcal infection is three times more common in women, perhaps because their initial infection is asymptomatic compared with males and may go untreated for longer. Symptomatic bacteremia may or may not precede gonococcal arthritis.

Diagnosis

The definitive diagnosis of infectious arthritis requires isolation and identification of bacteria from the synovial fluid by Gram stain or culture. The synovial fluid culture is positive in 90% of nongonococcal cases.[73] In gonococcal infectious arthritis, *N. gonorrhoeae* is often not recovered early from the synovial fluid and blood cultures are positive in only approximately 20% of cases. If a patient has the clinical presentation of gonococcal infectious arthritis and negative synovial fluid cultures, the presumptive diagnosis is made if gonococci are isolated from another site (e.g., urogenital tract, blood, rectum, or throat).[74]

The presumptive diagnosis of infectious arthritis can be supported by the following laboratory data: (1) Gram stain of the joint fluid; (2) synovial fluid leukocytosis greater than 50,000/mm^3 with polymorphonuclear leukocytes greater than 75%; (3) decreased synovial fluid glucose relative to the patient's serum glucose; and (4) increased synovial fluid lactate dehydrogenase, protein, and lactic acid, although such increases are nonspecific and may be seen in inflammatory joint diseases.[68] The absence of uric acid or calcium pyrophosphate dihydrate crystals in the synovial fluid rules out gout and pseudogout, respectively. The ESR and C-reactive protein are elevated in the majority of patients and can be used to monitor therapy. Amplification of bacterial DNA by polymerase chain reaction (PCR) is a promising technique that may be more widely used in the future to allow a more rapid and accurate diagnosis of most bacterial infections. PCR has been shown to be 96% specific and 76% sensitive in detecting *N. gonorrhoeae* DNA in the synovial fluid.[75]

Early radiologic evaluation of the joint is generally nonspecific, showing only joint effusion or soft tissue swelling. Radionuclide imaging, CT, and MRI are far more sensitive than plain films in early septic arthritis.[63]

TREATMENT

Pharmacotherapy

The treatment of infectious arthritis involves microbiologic assessment, immediate antibiotic therapy, and joint aspiration. The empiric antibiotic regimen should be based on the Gram stain of aspirated fluid, as well as the patient's age and concomitant risk factors. Even if the Gram stain of aspirated fluid is negative, an empiric antibiotic regimen that covers *S. aureus* and streptococci species should be initiated.[76] In this case, infection is likely and prompt initiation of empiric antibiotics will decrease the potential for long-term sequelae. Table 74.4 outlines empiric antibiotic regimens for the most common causative organisms. Modifications of the empiric antibiotic regimen can be made once definitive culture and sensitivity results are known. Parenteral antibiotic therapy is usually administered for 2 to 4 weeks. Shorter courses of parenteral treatment with an early switch to oral antibiotics are often efficacious in treating children or in adults with gonococcal arthritis.[76]

Successful treatment of infectious arthritis is contingent on the antibiotic's ability to adequately penetrate the joint space and achieve sufficient synovial concentrations. Most antibiotics (e.g., penicillins, cephalosporins, aminoglycosides, and fluoroquinolones) achieve a maximal concentration in synovial fluid several times higher than the MIC for the most common infecting organisms. Intraarticular administration of antibiotics is usually unnecessary and not recommended because it may cause a secondary chemical synovitis.[63] Although aminoglycosides are reported to achieve adequate concentrations in the joint fluid, their activity is diminished in acidic environments (low pH). Drainage of purulent exudate, which has a low pH, is paramount when using this class of drugs.[77]

Nonpharmacologic Therapy

As with osteomyelitis, patients with suppurative arthritis are best managed with a combination of antibiotic therapy and debridement procedures. Methods of debridement for arthritis are done routinely with needle aspiration, but may include arthroscopy and open surgical drainage with drainage tube placement. Needle aspiration is used mostly on peripheral joints such as the elbow, wrist, knee, and ankle. Axial joints such as the shoulder, sternoclavicular joint, and hip undergo open drainage.[68] Intermittent or even daily needle aspiration may be needed during the first weeks of therapy with fluid laboratory results of the repeated aspiration serving as a clinical indicator. Parameters to be monitored are the volume of synovial fluid, total cell count, and percentage of polymorphonuclear leukocytes, which should decrease with each aspiration.

IMPROVING OUTCOMES

The overall prognosis for infectious arthritis is generally favorable and has not changed much over the past few decades despite more effective antibiotics and improved methods of joint drainage. Prompt use of therapeutic dosages of antibiotics administered within the first week of the infection can produce complete symptomatic recovery with little if any residual limitation of joint motion. Permanent joint damage develops in 50% of cases, and nongonococcal infectious arthritis has been associated with a mortality rate of 10%.[60,62] The majority of deaths occur in patients with underlying risk factors such as sepsis, rheumatoid arthritis, and malignancy.

A favorable prognosis is usually contingent on several host factors. In children the prognosis is correlated with several parameters, such as the particular joint involved, type of organism, adequate drainage, appropriate antibiotic coverage, and time of initiation of treatment relative to the onset of symptoms. Infections of the hip are associated with the highest rate of sequelae, and the morbidity in these cases may not be evident until months or years later. In adults the outcome of treatment is considerably poorer if the offending organism is not eradicated from the synovial fluid within 6 days of initiating therapy or if the patient is over 60 years old.[69] *Staphylococcus aureus* has the greatest propensity for causing chronic problems.[61]

SUMMARY

Infectious arthritis arises from hematogenous spread of organisms through the synovial membrane or from direct extension from a contiguous infection. The most common causative organism is *Staphylococcus aureus,* although other pathogens, such as streptococci species, *Enterobacteriaceae, Pseudomonas aeruginosa,* and *Neisseria gonorrhoeae,* have also been isolated. The initial presentation demonstrates a painful, erythematous, and swollen joint. The diagnosis rests on isolation of the pathogen from joint fluid obtained during needle aspiration or debridement. Optimal treatment includes the prompt and judicious use of β-lactam antimicrobial agents coupled with drainage of the affected joint. The duration of therapy can range from 2 to 4 weeks, depending on the offending pathogen. Infectious arthritis is associated with low mortality rates and few residual symptoms if recognized and treated properly and with alacrity.

KEY POINTS

- It is important to make the diagnosis of osteomyelitis or infectious arthritis early in the course of the disease because the prognosis depends on the rapidity and adequacy of treatment.
- Typical physical findings in a patient with acute hematogenous osteomyelitis include tenderness over the involved bone and decreased range of motion in adjacent joints.
- Except for culture results, no single laboratory test is diagnostic of osteomyelitis or infectious arthritis. Therefore, careful monitoring of the trends of the WBC with differential, ESR, and perhaps C-reactive protein are required.
- The diagnosis of infectious arthritis rests on the isolation of the pathogen(s) from joint fluid obtained by aspiration or from debridement.
- Children with acute bone pain and tenderness and signs of systemic sepsis should be considered to have osteomyelitis until proven otherwise.
- *Staphylococcus aureus* is the most common pathogen causing both osteomyelitis and infectious arthritis, although other microbes are often found depending on the age of the patient, concomitant disease states, and risk factors.
- Young, otherwise healthy, sexually active adults who have joint pain and stiffness should be evaluated and cultured for gonococcal infection.
- The basic principles for the treatment of osteomyelitis and infectious arthritis include adequate debridement procedures followed by identification of the organism, selection of the correct antibiotic, and delivery of adequate quantities of the antibiotic to the site of infection for an extended period of time.
- Surgical debridement and joint aspiration are important primary treatment modalities that should be used in conjunction with appropriate antibiotic therapy.
- There is little difference in effectiveness between oral and intravenous administration of antibiotics as long as both achieve serum concentrations sufficient to eradicate the pathogen(s).
- In the treatment of osteomyelitis, oral agents may be efficacious if used in the appropriate patient population and if compliance can be ensured.
- Long-term therapy with quinolones with or without rifampin may be needed in chronic refractory disease, especially in patients with prostheses.
- Outpatient parenteral antibiotic therapy may, in specific patients, be a cost-saving tool when compared with the expense of prolonged hospitalization for the sole purpose of administering intravenous antibiotics.
- The duration of antibiotic therapy for treatment of acute osteomyelitis has not been fully elucidated; however, the best cure rates are obtained when parenteral therapy is administered for a minimum of 4 to 6 weeks. More prolonged therapy (i.e., months) may be necessary for chronic osteomyelitis.

REFERENCES

1. David R, Barron BJ, Madewell JE. Osteomyelitis, acute and chronic. Radiol Clin North Am 25:1171–1201, 1987.
2. Mader JT, Shirtliff M, Calhoun JH. Staging and staging application in osteomyelitis. Clin Infect Dis 25:1303–1309, 1997.
3. Gentry LO. Antibiotic therapy for osteomyelitis. Infect Dis Clin North Am 4(3):485–499, 1990.
4. Nelson JD. Acute osteomyelitis in children. Infect Dis Clin North Am 4:513–522, 1990.
5. Karwowska A, Davies HD, Jadavji T. Epidemiology and outcome of osteomyelitis in the era of sequential intravenous-oral therapy. Pediatr Infect Dis J 17(11):1021–1026, 1998.
6. Faden H, Grossi M. Acute osteomyelitis in children: reassessment of etiologic agents and their clinical characteristics. Am J Dis Child 145:65–69, 1991.
7. Gentry LO. Approach to the patient with osteomyelitis. In: Kelley WN, ed. Textbook of internal medicine. 3rd ed. Philadelphia: Lippincott-Raven, 1997:1560–1565.
8. Dirschl DR, Almekinders LC. Osteomyelitis: common causes and treatment recommendations. Drugs 45(1):29–43, 1993.
9. Anderson JR, Scobie WG, Watt B. The treatment of acute osteomyelitis in children: a 10-year experience. J Antimicrob Chemother 7(Suppl A):43–50, 1981.
10. Wald ER. Risk factors for osteomyelitis. Am J Med 78(Suppl 6B):206–212, 1985.
11. Vibhagool A, Calhoun J, Mader JP, et al. Therapy of bone and joint infections. Hosp Formul 28:63–85, 1993.

12. Hass DW, McAndrew MP. Bacterial osteomyelitis in adults: evolving considerations in diagnosis and treatment. Am J Med 101:550–561, 1996.
13. Burnett MW, Bass JW, Cook BA. Etiology of osteomyelitis complicating sickle cell disease. Pediatr 101(2):296–297, 1998.
14. Lipsky BA. Osteomyelitis of the foot in diabetic patients. Clin Infect Dis 25:1318–1326, 1997.
15. Norden CW. Lessons learned from animal models of osteomyelitis. Rev Infect Dis 10:103–110, 1988.
16. Belmatoug N, Cremieux AC, Bleton R, et al. A new model of experimental prosthetic joint infection due to MRSA: a microbiologic, histopathologic, and MRI characterization. J Infect Dis 174:414–417, 1996.
17. Nair SP, Meghji S, Wilson M, et al. Bacterially induced bone destruction: mechanism and misconceptions. Infect Immun 64:2371–2380, 1996.
18. Hermann M, Vandaux PE, Pittet D, et al. Fibronectin, fibrinogen and laminin act as mediators of adherence of clinical staphylococcal isolates to foreign material. J Infect Dis 158:693–701, 1988.
19. Hudson MC, Ramp WK, Nicholson NC, et al. Internalization of *S. aureus* by cultured osteoblasts. Microbial Pathogenesis 19:409–419, 1995.
20. Bamberger DM. Osteomyelitis: a commonsense approach to antibiotic and surgical treatment. Postgrad Med 94(5):177–184, 1993.
21. Caputo GM, Cavanagh PR, Ulbrecht JS, et al. Assessment and management of foot disease in patients with diabetes. N Engl J Med 331:854–860, 1994.
22. Lew DP, Waldvogel FA. Current concepts: osteomyelitis. N Engl J Med 336(14):999–1007, 1997.
23. Gutman L. Acute, subacute, and chronic osteomyelitis and pyogenic arthritis in children. Curr Probl Pediatr 15(12):1–72, 1985.
24. Marrie TJ, Costerton JW. Mode of growth of bacterial pathogens in chronic polymicrobial human osteomyelitis. J Clin Microbiol 22:924–933, 1985.
25. Sonnen GM, Henry NK. Pediatric bone and joint infections. Diagnosis and antimicrobial management. Pediatr Clin North Am 43(4):933–947, 1996.
26. Waldvogel FA, Papageorgiou PS. Osteomyelitis: the past decade. N Engl J Med 303:360–370, 1980.
27. Stuart J, Whicker JT. Tests for detecting and monitoring the acute phase response. Arch Dis Child 63:115–117, 1988.
28. Unkila-Kallio L, Kallio MJT, Peltola H. The usefulness of C-reactive protein levels in the identification of concurrent septic arthritis in children who have acute hematogenous osteomyelitis. A comparison with the usefulness of the erythrocyte sedimentation rate and the white blood-cell count. J Bone Joint Surg Am 76-A(6):848–853, 1994.
29. Howard CB, Einhorn M, Dagan R, et al. Fine-needle bone biopsy to diagnose osteomyelitis. J Bone Joint Surg Br 76:311–314, 1994.
30. Patzakis MJ, Wilkins J, Kumar J, et al. Comparison of the results of bacterial cultures from multiple sites in chronic osteomyelitis of long bones. A prospective study. J Bone Joint Surg Am 76(5):664–666, 1994.
31. Tumeh SS, Tohmeh AG. Nuclear medicine techniques in septic arthritis and osteomyelitis. Rheum Dis Clin North Am 17:559–583, 1991.
32. Schauwecker DS. The scintigraphic diagnosis of osteomyelitis. Am J Rheum 158:9–18, 1992.
33. Magid D. Computed tomographic imaging of the musculoskeletal system. Radiol Clin North Am 32:255–273, 1994.
34. Guhlmann A, Brecht-Krauss D, Suger G, et al. Chronic osteomyelitis: detection with FDG PET and correlation with histopathologic findings. Radiology 206(3):749–754, 1998.
35. Mader JT, Calhoun JH. Osteomyelitis. In: Mandell GL, Douglas RG, Bennett JE Jr, eds. Principles and practice of infectious diseases. New York: Churchill Livingstone, 1995:1039–1051.
36. Cierny G, Mader JT. Adult chronic osteomyelitis. Orthopedics 7:1557–1564, 1984.
37. Rissing JP. Antimicrobial therapy for chronic osteomyelitis in adults: role of the quinolones. Clin Infect Dis 25:1327–1333, 1997.
38. Dagan R. Management of acute hematogenous osteomyelitis and septic arthritis in the pediatric patient. Pediatr Infect Dis J 12:88–93, 1993.
39. Gentry LD. Role for newer beta-lactam antibiotics in the treatment of osteomyelitis. Am J Med 78(Suppl 6A):134–139, 1985.
40. Tice AD. Osteomyelitis. Hosp Pract 28(Suppl 2):36–39, 1993.
41. Nelson JD, Norden C, Mader JT, et al. Evaluation of new antiinfective drugs for the treatment of acute hematogenous osteomyelitis in children. Clin Infect Dis 15(Suppl 1):S162–S166, 1992.
42. Lew DP, Pittet D, Waldvogel FA. Infections that complicate the insertion of prosthetic devices. In: Mayhall CG, ed. Hospital epidemiology and infection control. Baltimore: Williams & Wilkins, 1996:731–748.
43. MacGregor RR, Graziani AL. Oral administration of antibiotics: a rational alternative to the parenteral route. Clin Infect Dis 24:457–467, 1997.
44. Black J, Hunt TL, Godley PJ, et al. Oral antimicrobial therapy for adults with osteomyelitis or septic arthritis. J Infect Dis 155:967–972, 1987.
45. Syrogiannopoulos GA, Nelson JD. Duration of antimicrobial therapy for acute suppurative osteoarticular infections. Lancet 1:37–40, 1988.
46. Marshall GS, Mudido P, Rabalais GP, et al. Organism isolation and serum bactericidal titers in oral antibiotic therapy for pediatric osteomyelitis. South Med J 89:67–70, 1996.
47. Vosti K. Serum bactericidal test: past, present, and future use in the management of patients with infections. Curr Clin Top Infect Dis 10:43–55, 1989.
48. Waldvogel FA. Use of quinolones for the treatment of osteomyelitis and septic arthritis. Rev Infect Dis 11(Suppl 5):S1259–S1263, 1989.
49. Zabraniecki L, Negrier I, Vergne P, et al. Fluoroquinolone induced tendinopathy: report of six cases. J Rheum 23(3):516–520, 1996.
50. Fitzgerald RH. Antibiotic distribution in normal and osteomyelitic bone. Orthop Clin North Am 15:537–545, 1984.
51. LeFrock J, Smith BR. The penicillins and bone penetration of antibiotics. J Foot Surg 26(Suppl 1):S34–S41, 1987.
52. Cremieux A, Carbon C. Experimental models of bone and prosthetic joint infections. Clin Infect Dis 25:1295–1302, 1998.
53. Rich D. Physicians, pharmacists, and home infusion antibiotic therapy. Am J Med 97(2A):3–8, 1994.
54. Gilbert DN, Dworkin RJ, Raber SR, et al. Outpatient parenteral antimicrobial drug therapy. N Engl J Med 337(2):829–838, 1997.
55. Brown RB. Selection and training of patients for outpatient intravenous antibiotic therapy. Rev Infect Dis 13(Suppl 2):S147–S151, 1991.
56. Henry SL, Galloway KP. Local antibacterial therapy for the management of orthopaedic infections. Clin Pharmacokinet 29(1):36–45, 1995.
57. Tibbles PM, Edelsberg JS. Medical progress: hyperbaric-oxygen therapy. N Engl J Med 334(25):1642–1648, 1996.
58. Galankis N, Giamarellou H, Moussat T, et al. Chronic osteomyelitis caused by multi-resistant gram-negative bacteria; evolution of treatment with newer quinolones after prolonged follow-up. J Antimicrob Chemother 39:241–246, 1997.
59. Norden CW. Osteomyelitis. In: Mandell GL, Douglas RG, Bennett JE, eds. Principles and practice of infectious diseases. 3rd ed. New York: Wiley, 1990:922–930.
60. Morgan DS, Fisher D, Merianos A, et al. An 18 year clinical review of septic arthritis from tropical Australia. Epidemiol Infect 117:423–428, 1996.
61. Kaandorp CJE, vanSchaardenburg D, Krijnen P, et al. Risk factors for septic arthritis in patients with joint disease: a prospective study. Arthritis Rheum 38:1819–1825, 1995.
62. Ryan MJ, Kavanaugh R, Wall PG, et al. Bacterial joint infections in England and Wales: analysis of bacterial isolates over a four year period. Br J Rheumatol 36:370–373, 1997.
63. Goldenberg DL. Septic arthritis. Lancet 351:197–202, 1998.
64. LeDantec L, Maury F, Flipo RM, et al. Peripheral pyogenic arthritis. A study of one hundred seventy-nine cases. Revue Rheum 63:103–110, 1996.
65. Goldenberg DL. Septic arthritis and other infections of rheumatologic significance. Rheum Dis Clin North Am 17(1):49–56, 1991.
66. Brancos MA, Peris P, Miro JM, et al. Septic arthritis in heroin addicts. Semin Arthritis Rheum 21:81–87, 1991.
67. Saraux A, Taelman H, Blanche P, et al. HIV infections as a risk factor for septic arthritis. Br J Rheumatol 36:333–337, 1997.
68. Cimmino MA. Recognition and management of bacterial arthritis. Drugs 54(1):50–60, 1997.
69. Smith JW. Infectious arthritis. Infect Dis Clin North Am 4(3):523–538, 1990.
70. Brooks GF, Pons VG. Septic arthritis. In: Hoeprich PD, Jordan MC, Ronald AR, eds. Infectious diseases. 5th ed. Philadelphia: Lippincott, 1994:1382–1389.
71. Zimmerman B 3rd, Mikolich DJ, Lally EV. Septic sacroiliities. Semin Arthritis Rheum 26:592–604, 1996.
72. Dubost JJ, Fis I, Denis P, et al. Polyarticular septic arthritis. Medicine 72:296–310, 1993.
73. Goldenberg DL, Reed JI. Bacterial arthritis. N Engl J Med 312:764–771, 1985.
74. Wise CM, Morris CR, Wasilauskas BL, et al. Gonococcal arthritis in an era of increasing penicillin resistance: presentations and outcomes in 41 recent cases (1985–1991). Arch Intern Med 154:2690–2695, 1994.
75. Liebling MR, Arkfeld DG, Michelini G, et al. Identification of *Neisseria gonorrhoeae* in synovial fluid using the polymerase chain reaction. Arthritis Rheum 37:702–709, 1994.
76. Smith JM, Piercy EA. Infectious arthritis. Clin Infect Dis 20:225–231, 1995.
77. Hamed KA, Tam JY, Prober CG. Pharmacokinetic optimisation of the treatment of septic arthritis. Clin Pharmacokinet 21:156–163, 1996.

CHAPTER 75

SEXUALLY TRANSMITTED DISEASES

Vicky Dudas and Thomas C. Hardin

DEFINITION

Sexually transmitted diseases (STDs), which are occasionally referred to as venereal diseases, are infections that are caused by a variety of pathogenic microorganisms, as summarized in Table 75.1. It is generally accepted that patients with one sexually transmitted disease are at greater risk for the development of other sexually transmitted diseases, either concurrently or at some later point in time. Additionally, sexual partners of patients with diagnosed STDs are at high risk for the development of STDs. Age is an important risk factor given that the incidence of STDs is much higher in persons in their teens and twenties. Although rates of STDs are higher in men than in women, it is important to remember that the usual clinical manifestations are more obvious in men, leading to a larger percentage of men seeking treatment. Over the past decade, primarily because of concern about transmission of the human immunodeficiency virus (HIV), much effort

Table 75.1 ▪ Sexually Transmitted Pathogens and Associated Disease

Pathogens	Corresponding Clinical Syndrome/Disease
Bacteria	
Neisseria gonorrhoeae	Gonorrhea
Treponema pallidum	Syphilis
Haemophilus ducreyi	Chancroid
Calymmatobacterium granulomatis	Granuloma inguinale
Gardnerella vaginalis	Nonspecific vaginitis
Mycoplasma	
Ureaplasma urealyticum	Nongonococcal urethritis
Chlamydia	
Chlamydia trachomatis	Nongonococcal urethritis or lymphogranuloma venereum
Viruses	
Herpes simplex type II (or I)	Herpes genitalis
Human immunodeficiency virus	Acquired immunodeficiency syndrome (AIDS)
Hepatitis A, B, and C	Hepatitis
Human papillomavirus (HPV)	Condylomata acuminata
Poxvirus	Molluscum contagiosum
Parasites	
Trichomonas vaginalis	Trichomoniasis or nonspecific vaginitis
Giardia lamblia	Giardiasis
Entamoeba histolytica	Amebiasis
Phthirus pubis	Pediculosis
Sarcoptes scabiei	Scabies

has been directed toward changes in sexual practices to reduce the potential for transmission of disease by sexual contact.[1] In addition, because many STDs are asymptomatic, STD screening programs are a critical component in treatment and prevention of transmission.[2] Nevertheless, sexually transmitted diseases continue to be an important public health concern, with annual costs for treatment of non–acquired immunodeficiency syndrome (AIDS) STDs in the United States of over 5 billion dollars.[3]

This chapter is organized into three general sections: a review of common urethritis syndromes, discussion of infections associated with genital ulceration, and limited comments on less common STDs. Several diseases that are transmitted by sexual contact, such as hepatitis, HIV infection, AIDS, and parasitic infections, are discussed in other chapters of this text.

TREATMENT GOALS: SEXUALLY TRANSMITTED DISEASES

- Prevent disease transmission.
- Completely eradicate the infectious pathogen.
- Eliminate or alleviate clinical symptoms.
- Prevent associated long-term sequelae.

PREVENTION GUIDELINES

It is the responsibility of health care professionals to educate persons at risk for acquiring an STD. It is important to detect disease in asymptomatic patients and in those who are unlikely to seek treatment to reduce transmission rates. In addition, it is important to remember that for every patient with an STD requiring therapy, there are one or more infected sexual partners who should be identified and treated regardless of the appearance of symptoms.

The most effective method of preventing the transmission of STDs (including HIV) is the use of a latex condom used consistently and correctly, with or without spermicide with each act of sexual intercourse. Currently there is a female condom (Reality) available, which is a lubricated polyurethane sheath with a diaphragm-like ring at each end. Female condoms provide an alternative for women and should reduce the risk of STDs; however, to date they have been shown to prevent the transmission of only trichomoniasis. Vaginal spermicides can reduce the risk of cervical chlamydia and gonorrhea, but their effect on preventing transmission has not been evaluated.[4] Case-control studies have shown that the use of a diaphragm protects against cervical gonorrhea, chlamydia, and trichomoniasis.[4]

Urethritis Syndromes

The sexually transmitted disease that is most commonly seen is urethritis, or inflammation of the urethra, which usually presents clinically as a urethral discharge that may be accompanied by dysuria (painful or difficult urination). Clinically, urethritis is usually divided into either gonococcal or nongonococcal syndromes on the basis of the infecting pathogen. Nationwide, chlamydia (nongonococcal urethritis) is much more common than gonococcal urethritis (gonorrhea).[5] However, gonorrhea tends to be seen more frequently in STD clinics, possibly because of differences in socioeconomic factors and clinical presentation. In addition, gonorrhea is considered a reportable disease in all states whereas chlamydia is not. Although the usual clinical features of gonococcal and nongonococcal urethritis differ to some degree, there is sufficient overlap in presentation to make distinguishing between the two syndromes difficult.[6]

Gonorrhea

EPIDEMIOLOGY

Although the actual incidence of gonorrhea is unclear because of the large number of asymptomatic carriers and unreported cases, an estimated 600,000 new infections occur each year in the United States. It is caused by *Neisseria gonorrhoeae,* a Gram-negative aerobic coccus that usually grows in pairs (diplococci). Individuals between ages 15 and 24 years have the highest reported incidence of gonorrhea. The incidence of gonorrhea is reported to be 10 times greater in nonwhites than in whites. Other risk factors for gonorrhea include low socioeconomic status, urban residence, single marital status, and a previous history of gonococcal infections.[7]

PATHOPHYSIOLOGY

Gonorrhea primarily effects the epithelium and mucous membranes of the lower genital tract; however, it may also involve the eyes, oropharynx, and anus. Humans appear to be the only natural host for this intracellular pathogen. Transmission of gonorrhea is almost always by sexual intercourse, although perinatal transmission of the disease may occur. Once the gonococci are attached to the cell membranes by pili, one of the primary virulence factors, they are pinocytosed. Subsequently, polymorphonuclear leukocytes invade the tissue, leading to secretion of purulent exudates. The rate of male to female transmission of gonorrhea during sexual intercourse is reported to be higher than transmission from female to male, probably because the cervix is a more accessible target. The risk of transmission from an infected female to her male partner ranges from 20% to 40% per episode of unprotected vaginal intercourse; transmission risk from an infected male to his female partner has been reported to be closer to 50% and up to 90% per episode.[7,8]

CLINICAL PRESENTATION AND DIAGNOSIS

Signs and Symptoms

The clinical presentation of gonorrhea varies greatly in individuals. It may or may not be complicated and may or may not cause symptoms. In men, the incubation period for gonococcal urethritis is usually 2 to 7 days; the majority of patients develop symptoms within a week of the initial infection. The clinical presentation of gonorrhea is usually characterized by profuse, purulent urethral discharge that is associated with dysuria. Many cases of gonorrhea in men are asymptomatic and resolve spontaneously over the course of several weeks without specific treatment. However, up to 10% of untreated cases may be further complicated by the development of acute epididymitis, periurethral abscess, acute prostatitis, seminal vesiculitis, or urethral strictures.

In women, gonorrhea primarily involves the endocervix and the urethra. Most women develop acute symptoms within 10 days of infection, consisting of increased vaginal discharge and dysuria that are often overlooked because they tend to be nonspecific. Progression to salpingitis may occur in up to 15% of untreated women and usually is characterized by the development of acute abdominal or pelvic pain. In addition, 25 to 65% of women with gonorrhea are also coinfected with *Chlamydia trachomatis* or *Trichomonas vaginalis.*[4] Approximately 15% of women with untreated gonorrhea develop pelvic inflammatory disease, which may be associated with infertility and ectopic pregnancies if inadequately managed.

Infectious involvement of other body sites by *N. gonorrhoeae* can also be seen. Pharyngeal gonococcal infection, developed after orogenital sexual activity with an infected partner, is more common in females and homosexual males. The presentation is often asymptomatic, but symptoms resembling acute streptococcal pharyngitis may occur. Anal transmission of *N. gonorrhoeae* in women is generally by perianal contamination with vaginal discharge; in men it is usually through receptive anal intercourse with an infected partner. Most cases of anorectal gonorrhea are asymptomatic, but anal pruritus, constipation, tenesmus, and rectal bleeding have been observed in association with this condition.[7] Ocular gonococcal infection most commonly involves the conjunctiva and is often considered secondary to autoinoculation from fingers contaminated through sexual contact with an individual with urogenital gonorrhea. Gonococcal conjunctivitis may be serious and requires timely initiation of aggressive antibiotic therapy to prevent corneal ulceration. Disseminated gonococcal infection secondary to hematogenous spread is uncommon but is often considered the cause of septic arthritis in otherwise healthy young adults. Most patients with disseminated gonococcal infection do not have significant fevers or elevated white blood cell counts but commonly have monoarticular arthritic complaints in the wrist, knee, or ankle (any joint can be involved). In addition, a striking pustular, erythematous rash, located primarily on the extremities, is also common in patients with bacteremia secondary to *N. gonorrhoeae.*[4,7]

Newborns who are exposed to gonococci in utero or during delivery are at risk for the development of gonococcal ophthalmia neonatorum, a sight-threatening infection of the conjunctiva. Fortunately, this condition is rare today in the United States because of the use of aggressive ophthalmic prophylaxis after delivery.

Diagnosis

The diagnosis of gonorrhea is best made by identification of *N. gonorrhoeae* from a specimen taken from an involved site. In women, cultures taken from the cervix produce the highest yield, but urethral cultures are also acceptable. Men should have both urethral and anal cultures performed. Cultures can become positive within 24 to 48 hours.

Culturing and susceptibility testing of the organism is important for diagnosis in areas where drug-resistant *N. gonorrhoeae* is a concern in determining therapeutic options.[4,9] An alternative diagnostic technique that is commonly used in clinics to evaluate the collected specimen is Gram staining. If intracellular Gram-negative diplococci are observed, a presumptive diagnosis of gonorrhea is made, pending confirmation by subsequent culture. In males, Gram-stain evaluation of the urethral discharge is both highly sensitive and highly specific; therefore, culture confirmation is not considered necessary. However, the Gram stain is not considered acceptable as the sole method to diagnose gonococcal infection of the pharynx or rectum or in women with endocervical infection.[7] Rapid diagnostic tests based on detection of gonococcal antigens or cellular components do not have better sensitivity or specificity than Gram stain and culture and are therefore infrequently used, but they may have a role in asymptomatic individuals.

THERAPEUTIC PLAN

A number of treatment options for the management of gonococcal disease are available to the practicing clinician. Most cephalosporins and fluoroquinolones have potent in vitro and in vivo activity against *N. gonorrhoeae.* Historically, penicillins, tetracyclines, and sulfonamides were used widely as therapy for gonococcal infections, but widespread resistance now prevents their clinical use. Discovered in the 1970s, penicillinase-producing strains of *N. gonorrhoeae* make up a significant number of strains throughout the world. Table 75.2 summarizes the current Centers for Disease Control and Prevention (CDC) treatment recommendations for gonococcal infections.[10] Selection of a specific therapeutic regimen must be based

Table 75.2 ▪ CDC Recommendations for Treatment of Gonococcal Infections

Presentation	Drug Regimen	Cost[a]	Alternative Regimens/Comments
Uncomplicated gonorrhea of the cervix, urethra, rectum, and pharynx (see comments)[b]	Cefixime[c] 400 mg PO in single dose *or* Ceftriaxone 125 mg IM in single dose *or* Ciprofloxacin 500 mg PO in single dose *or* Ofloxacin 400 mg PO in single dose **PLUS (cotreatment of *Chlamydia* with any of the above)** Doxycycline 100 mg PO BID for 7 days *or* Azithromycin 1 g PO in single dose	$6.80 $25.00 $3.60 $4.30 $3.00 $18.60	Ceftizoxime 500 mg IM, cefotaxime 500 mg IM, cefotetan 1 g IM, cefoxitin 2 g IM with probenecid 1 g orally. Limited clinical experience. Other quinolones may be used but limited clinical data available. Quinolones and tetracyclines are contraindicated in pregnancy and children. If first-line therapy is contraindicated, spectinomycin 2 g IM in a single dose can be used.
Disseminated gonococcal infection[d,e]	Ceftriaxone 1g IV or IM q24hr *or* if β-lactam allergy: Ciprofloxacin 400 mg IV q12hr *or* Ofloxacin 400 mg IV q12hr *or* Spectinomycin 2 g IM q12hr Continue for 24–48 hr after improvement, then continue oral therapy for a total of 7 days: Cefixime 400 mg PO BID *or* Ciprofloxacin 500 mg PO BID *or* Ofloxacin 400 mg BID	$40.00 $30.00 $26.40 $21.18 Variable	Cefotaxime 1 g IV q8hr. Ceftizoxime 1 g IV q8hr.
Gonococcal conjunctivitis (adult)	Ceftriaxone 1 g IM as single dose	$40.00	Infected eye should be lavaged with saline solution one time.
Gonococcal ophthalmia neonatorum	Ceftriaxone 25–50 mg/kg IV or IM in a single dose, not to exceed 125 mg	Variable	Topical antibiotic therapy alone is inadequate and is unnecessary with systematic therapy.
Disseminated gonococcal infections in infants	Ceftriaxone 25–50 mg/kg IM or IV QD for 7 days or 10–14 days for documented meningitis	Variable	If meningitis is present, treat for 10–14 days.

[a]Based on 1998 Red Book AWP for daily drug costs or total drug costs for single-dose regimens.

[b]Patients should refer sex partners for evaluation and treatment. Patients should avoid sexual intercourse until therapy is completed and they are symptom free.

[c]NOTE: Pharyngeal infections are more difficult to treat. Cefixime should not be used.

[d]Gonococcal meningitis: ceftriaxone 2 g IV q12hr × 2 weeks.

[e]Gonococcal endocarditis: ceftriaxone 2 g IV q12–24hr × 4 weeks.

Table 75.3 ▪ Selected Pharmacokinetics of Antibiotics Active Against *Neisseria gonorrhoeae*

Antimicrobial Agent	Dose/Route	Peak Serum Concentration (mg/L)	$t_{1/2}$ (hr)	MIC_{90} (μg/mL)
Cefixime	400 mg PO	3.7	3–4	<0.03
Ceftriaxone	125 mg IM	12–15	7–8	<0.06
Ciprofloxacin	500 mg PO	2.4	4	<0.25
Ofloxacin	400 mg PO	2.9	4–5	<0.625

Source: Reference 9.

Table 75.4 ▪ CDC Recommendations for Treatment of Chlamydial Infections

Presentation	Initial Drug Regimen	Alternatives/Comments
Uncomplicated urethritis, endocervical or rectal infection	Azithromycin 1 g PO as a single dose *or* Doxycycline 100 mg PO BID for 7 days	Erythromycin base 500 mg QID *or* Erythromycin ethylsuccinate 800 mg PO QID *or* Ofloxacin 300 mg PO BID for 7 days
Urethritis during pregnancy	Erythromycin base 500 mg PO QID for 7 days *or* Amoxicillin 500 mg PO TID for 7 days	Erythromycin base 250 mg QID for 14 days Erythromycin ethylsuccinate 800 mg PO QID for 7 days Erythromycin ethylsuccinate 400 mg PO QID for 14 days *or* Azithromycin 1 g orally as single dose
Ophthalmia neonatorum	Erythromycin 50 mg/kg/day PO QID for 10–14 days	
Lymphogranuloma venereum	Doxycycline 100 mg PO BID for 21 days	Erythromycin base 500 mg PO QID for 21 days

Patients should refer sex partners for evaluation and treatment. Patients should avoid sexual intercourse until therapy is completed and they are symptom free.

on careful consideration of efficacy and safety, allergy history, age, pregnancy, patient preference, and costs.

TREATMENT

Many clinicians consider intramuscular ceftriaxone to be the treatment of choice for noncomplicated gonorrhea; this choice is based on extensive clinical evaluations demonstrating effective clearing of gonococcal infections from all sites.[4,9] Resistance to ceftriaxone has not been reported to date, so concern about potential treatment failure is reduced. Previous CDC treatment guidelines recommended an intramuscular ceftriaxone dose of 250 mg, but single doses as low as 62.5 mg have been reported to produce 100% cure rates in noncomplicated gonorrhea.[9] The currently recommended ceftriaxone regimen of 125 mg allows for a smaller volume for intramuscular injection and a lower drug cost. The serum levels of ceftriaxone are well above the minimum inhibitory concentration (MIC_{90}) of the organism, as shown in Table 75.3. There are limited data suggesting that intramuscular ceftriaxone provides adequate coverage for incubating syphilis as well, a therapeutic benefit that other treatment options do not have.[11] The most common adverse effects associated with IM ceftriaxone are pain at the injection site and gastrointestinal side effects such as nausea and diarrhea.

Cefixime is the only oral cephalosporin that is recommended by the CDC for the treatment of gonococcal infections. A cefixime dose of 400 mg is effective for urethral disease but has not been well studied for pharyngeal infection and does not provide activity against incubating syphilis.[12] The oral dose has been demonstrated to have cure rates of approximately 97%; however, it does not provide serum levels as high as those produced by ceftriaxone, as shown in Table 75.3. The main side effect associated with cefixime is gastrointestinal complaints such as nausea and diarrhea. Other oral agents approved by the Food and Drug Administration (FDA) for gonorrhea (e.g., cefuroxime axetil and cefpodoxime) are less well studied.

The preferred fluoroquinolones, ciprofloxacin and ofloxacin, are also highly effective oral alternatives for the treatment of uncomplicated gonorrhea but are contraindicated for use during pregnancy and for children under age 18. Ofloxacin is more active than ciprofloxacin against *C. trachomatis* but requires prolonged dosing (7 to 10 days) for successful treatment of chlamydial infections (Table 75.4). Other fluoroquinolones have been used, such as enoxacin 400 mg PO for one dose, lomefloxacin 400 mg PO for one dose, and norfloxacin 800 mg PO for one dose. Gonococcal resistance to the fluoroquinolones has been widely reported in Asia, Australia, and the United Kingdom, and there have been reports of decreasing susceptibility to fluoroquinolones in several regions of the United States.[13,14] The overall prevalence of gonorrhea with decreased susceptibility to fluoroquinolones was reported to be 0.4% in 1997. Fluoroquinolone-resistant gonorrhea demonstrates an MIC of 1.0 μg/mL or greater to ciprofloxacin and 2 μg/mL or greater to ofloxacin.[10] The fluoroquinolones provide no activity against *T. pallidum.*

A single 2000 mg oral dose of azithromycin provides a 95% cure rate for uncomplicated gonorrhea.[15] Unfortunately, at this dose azithromycin is expensive and causes considerable gastrointestinal intolerance such that it is not considered an option for routine treatment of gonorrhea. One benefit of a single dose of azithromycin for gonorrhea is that it also provides coverage for concomitant chlamydial infection that might be present.

Spectinomycin was once a commonly used alternative to β-lactam treatment of gonorrhea. Today it is useful only for patients with urogenital or anal infections who are unable to tolerate therapy with either a cephalosporin or fluoroquinolone.[4,9]

Disseminated gonococcal infections are best treated with a prolonged course of intravenous ceftriaxone, cefotaxime, or ceftizoxime. Therapy should be continued for 24 to 48 hours after significant clinical improvement (e.g., decrease in fever and white blood cell count), then followed with a suitable oral agent for another 7 days. Gonococcal endocarditis and meningitis require several weeks of intravenous antibiotic therapy.[7]

Topical therapy with either 1% silver nitrate, 1% tetracycline, or 0.5% erythromycin is recommended by the American Academy of Pediatrics for immediate postpartum administration to all newborns, but it is insufficient to treat gonococcal ophthalmia neonatorum in a baby born to a mother with active gonorrhea. A single intramuscular or intravenous dose of ceftriaxone 25 to 50 mg/kg (not to exceed 125 mg total) is thought to be adequate treatment for both gonococcal ophthalmia neonatorum and gonococcal conjunctivitis in adults.[4]

IMPROVING OUTCOMES

Routine follow-up is not necessary for patients who are treated with a regimen recommended in the CDC guidelines because of the very low treatment failure rates that have been reported. Patients who are treated with alternative regimens should be evaluated within 3 to 7 days to ensure resolution of symptoms. In most cases, persistence of clinical signs and symptoms indicates reinfection rather than treatment failure or may indicate coinfection with another infectious pathogen, such as *C. trachomatis.* In either case the patient needs another diagnostic workup along with aggressive identification and treatment of all recent sexual partners.[10]

Nongonococcal Urethritis

EPIDEMIOLOGY

Nongonococcal urethritis is more common than gonorrhea in the United States. The most common cause of nongonococcal urethritis, *Chlamydia trachomatis,* accounts for up to 55% of cases. An estimated 4 million Americans contract chlamydia each year. It is an obligate intracellular organism that has features of both bacteria and viruses.[16,17] *Chlamydia* species, like viruses, require host cellular material for replication, yet like bacteria maintain their cellular identity. There are 15 known serovars of *C. trachomatis.* The lymphogranuloma venerum strains produce invasive infections; the remaining strains produce superficial infections of epithelial cells. It is estimated that almost 50% of individuals with gonorrhea are coinfected with *C. trachomatis.*[18] Other pathogens that can also produce a urethritis syndrome include the bacterium *Ureaplasma urealyticum,* identified in approximately 20 to 40% of cases, and the parasite *T. vaginalis,* seen in fewer than 10% of patients.[16,17] However, approximately 20 to 30% of men with urethritis fail to demonstrate either gonococcal or common nongonococcal pathogens on evaluation. These cases of urethritis may be due to yeasts, viruses, and other bacteria that are difficult to culture or identify.[16] Risk factors associated with chlamydial infection include change in partner, sexually active adolescents, lower socioeconomic status, and African American race.[18]

CLINICAL PRESENTATION AND DIAGNOSIS

Signs and Symptoms

The clinical presentation of nongonococcal urethritis cannot be distinguished easily from the clinical features of gonococcal urethritis. Common symptoms of nongonococcal urethritis in men include dysuria, polyuria, and the presence of a mucoid urethral discharge within several weeks of exposure; however, approximately 25% of men are asymptomatic.[16] Unlike gonorrhea, the discharge seen in nongonococcal urethritis is typically mucoid or mucopurulent, and dysuria is present in fewer than 50% of cases. In addition, *C. trachomatis* is responsible for the majority of cases of acute epididymitis in men.

The majority of women with chlamydial urethral infections are clinically asymptomatic, making the identification of these individuals almost impossible.[18] Dysuria and urinary frequency are uncommon with urethral infections, but when symptoms occur, a mucopurulent discharge from the endocervicitis is most commonly seen. Symptoms associated with chlamydial infection are usually much less severe than those associated with gonorrhea. In one study, 70% of the chlamydial infections were detected during screening, at which time the women were asymptomatic.[19] Chlamydia is a major cause of pelvic inflammatory disease, which may subsequently lead to tubal infertility or ectopic pregnancy. In a manner similar to gonorrhea, chlamydia may be transmitted to an infant during vaginal delivery through an infected birth canal. The most common presentations in the neonate are conjunctivitis and nasopharyngeal infection.

Diagnosis

Identification of the infecting organism for most cases of nongonococcal urethritis is hampered because the two most common pathogens, *C. trachomatis* and *U. urealyticum,* cannot be cultured by routine laboratory procedures. Therefore, the diagnosis of nongonococcal urethritis usually depends on the presence of a characteristic urethral discharge (microscopically greater than four polymorphonuclear leukocytes per oil immersion field on a smear of an intraurethral swab specimen), the exclusion of gonorrhea, and a clinical response to therapy. Serologic tests that are specific for chlamydia and tissue-culturing techniques are thought to be unnecessary for the management of STDs in general clinical practice.[16] Rapid office tests using an enzyme immunoassay for the diagnosis of chlamydia infections are now available and are reported to offer excellent sensitivity and specificity.[20] Additional tests that allow rapid identification of chlamydial antigens in genital secretions are the enzyme-linked immunoabsorbent assay (ELISA) and the direct fluorescent antibody (DFA) test. Both tests are highly sensitive and specific.[21]

THERAPEUTIC PLAN

A number of antibiotic regimens have been evaluated for the clinical management of nongonococcal urethritis. The recent CDC treatment guidelines shown in Table 75.4 recommend a regimen of doxycycline 100 mg orally twice a day for 7 days.[10] Azithromycin orally as a single 1000 mg dose is equivalent to doxycycline in the treatment of nongonococcal urethritis.[22,23] Both doxycycline and azithromycin have cure rates greater than 95% in cases of nongonococcal urethritis.[24] Doxycycline is an inexpensive 7-day regimen that requires patient compliance because of multiple daily dosing. The toxicities of doxycycline include nausea and vomiting and the potential for phototoxicity. The bioavailability of doxycycline is reduced if taken concomitantly with multivalent ions such as iron; however, it can be administered without regard to meals or dairy products. Although azithromycin is an expensive alternative, it may be useful in patients with poor compliance with treatment or minimal follow-up. A single 1000 mg oral dose can be administered under direct patient observation to ensure compliance. Diarrhea, nausea, dizziness, and headache have been reported in fewer than 3% of treated patients. Alternative regimens that have been indicated by the CDC include erythromycin base 500 mg and erythromycin ethylsuccinate 800 mg orally four times a day for 7 days. These regimens are considered to be less efficacious than doxycycline or azithromycin.[10] Many patients cannot tolerate such high doses of erythromycin because of gastrointestinal side effects. If necessary, lower dosages of 250 mg for the base or 400 mg for the ethylsuccinate salt can be used, but the duration of treatment should be extended to 14 days.[16]

Ofloxacin has been evaluated for the treatment of nongonococcal urethritis. On the basis of the limited data available, ofloxacin appears to be similar to doxycycline in efficacy, with treatment success rates approaching 100%.[24,25] The dose of ofloxacin that has been used most often is 300 mg orally twice daily for 7 days. Larger doses (up to 400 mg twice daily) administered for shorter periods of time (5 days) have also been studied in a limited number of patients. Ofloxacin is more expensive than doxycycline, and, unlike azithromycin, it does not afford the opportunity for improved patient compliance. Ciprofloxacin has limited activity against *C. trachomatis* and should not be considered a therapeutic option for the treatment of nongonococcal urethritis.[26] Although the newer fluoroquinolones (e.g., levofloxacin) have FDA approval for the treatment of *C. trachomatis*, there are limited clinical data with these agents and neither agent is recommended by the CDC.

When considering therapy for pregnant women, erythromycin base should be used because doxycycline and ofloxacin are contraindicated. Doxycycline can cause permanent discoloration of the teeth during tooth development, and the quinolones have been shown to cause cartilage damage in juvenile animal species. Azithromycin is potentially an acceptable agent for use during pregnancy (pregnancy category B); however, clinical experience with this agent is not nearly as extensive as with erythromycin. See Table 75.4 for treatment of pediatric infections.

IMPROVING OUTCOMES

As with the treatment of gonorrhea, no specific patient follow-up is required unless symptoms persist after completion of therapy or recur shortly thereafter. Patients should be strongly encouraged to refer recent sexual partners for evaluation and treatment, regardless of the presence of clinical signs and symptoms of infection. Additionally, patients should be instructed to abstain from sexual intercourse until treatment has been completed and there is evidence that the infection has been cured. An alternative to abstinence would be careful use of a condom and contraceptive foam.

PHARMACOECONOMICS

Several pharmacoeconomic studies have been done evaluating the costs of azithromycin versus doxycycline. Although the acquisition cost of azithromycin therapy is considerably higher than that of doxycycline, it offers the advantage of single-dose treatment, thereby increasing compliance. Several studies have reported that when patient compliance is considered, azithromycin may be more cost-effective than doxycycline.[27,28]

Ulcerogenic Genital Infections

The development of genital ulcerations is associated with several sexually transmitted diseases, particularly syphilis, genital herpes simplex infections, and chancroid. Each of these diseases is discussed separately.

Syphilis

EPIDEMIOLOGY

Syphilis is an important contagious disease that can have many different manifestations.[29,30] The incidence of syphilis in the United States reached a peak during World War II and then declined after the introduction of penicillin in the late 1940s. In the 1960s the number of reported cases of syphilis rose slightly and then plateaued until the mid-1980s, when the incidence again began to rise. In 1990 over 50,000 cases were reported in the United States, up nearly 10% from 1989.[31] The reported incidence of 20 cases per 100,000 individuals is a 75% increase from 1985. However, syphilis rates have declined since 1991. The CDC reports that primary and secondary syphilis cases declined 84% from 1990 to 1997.[32] Syphilis continues to be more prevalent in non-Hispanic blacks, and infections are more concentrated in the southern region of the United States. The majority of new cases occur among individuals who are 15 to 30 years old, and many individuals have concurrent HIV infection. Various studies have shown the prevalence of syphilis in patients with HIV infection to be as high as 36%.[35] Although syphilis is most commonly transmitted through sexual intercourse, the organism can also be transmitted through placental transfer (congenital syphilis), by the administration of fresh human blood, by kissing or touching active lesions, or by accidental inoculation.[33]

The spirochete *Treponema pallidum* is the causal agent of syphilis. This unicellular organism is elongated and tightly coiled and divides approximately every 30 hours. The human is the only natural host. Unfortunately, the organism cannot be grown in vitro. The disease is usually transmitted by direct contact with an active infectious lesion, which teems with approximately 10^7 organisms per gram of tissue.[30] *Treponema pallidum* penetrates intact skin or mucous membranes and, within hours, invades regional lymphatics and blood vessels. Dissemination throughout the body is rapid. Any organ system can be infected, including the central nervous system.

CLINICAL PRESENTATION AND DIAGNOSIS

Signs and Symptoms

Syphilis can be divided clinically into five stages: incubating, primary, secondary, latent, and tertiary (late) syphilis.[30,31,34,35] The incubation period usually lasts about 3 weeks, appears to be directly related to the size of the inoculum, and may range from 3 days to 3 months. During this period the individual is asymptomatic and noninfectious, and serologic tests are usually negative. The hallmark of primary syphilis is the development of a painless chancre in as many as 60% of patients at the site of initial inoculation. The lesion consists of spirochetes, histiocytes, and plasma cells. Multiple chancres may occur; this feature is usually observed in HIV-infected individuals. Not all patients develop a chancre, and some chancres are atypical in appearance or so small and inconspicuous that they are undetected. Painless regional lymphadenopathy (bubo) can be present. Chancres quickly erode and ulcerate, developing a smooth base with raised borders that usually heals spontaneously within several weeks, accompanied by resolution of lymphadenopathy.

Secondary syphilis, or disseminated syphilis, is a generalized illness that develops approximately 2 to 8 weeks after contact and may begin before complete resolution of the chancre. Essentially all untreated patients progress to secondary syphilis. The presentation is most often characterized by classic lesions of the skin and mucous membranes.[35] The rash most often starts as reddish or copper-colored macular lesions appearing on the truncal extremities but may also appear maculopapular, papular, or pustular. The soles of the feet and palms of the hands are commonly involved. It is not uncommon to also detect similar nonpainful lesions on mucous membranes. These lesions usually persist for up to a week. Generalized lymphadenopathy is also often present. Constitutional symptoms are common and include headache, fever, sore throat, malaise, myalgias, arthralgias, anorexia, and weight loss. Condylomata lata are flat, hypertrophic lesions resembling warts that develop in moist areas and contain spirochetes. Involvement of other organ systems is possible and may include the development of immune-complex glomerulonephritis, syphilitic hepatitis, and synovitis. The central nervous system (CNS) is asymptomatically involved in nearly 30% of cases of secondary syphilis. Unless there is clinical evidence of CNS infection, evaluation of the cerebrospinal fluid (CSF) is not indicated. Serologic tests are positive in 65 to 85% of cases of secondary syphilis.[35]

Latent syphilis refers to a period of time during which there are no clinical manifestations of disease but the serologic tests for syphilis are positive. Early latent syphilis, generally considered to be the first 4 years, is the time when relapses of secondary syphilis may occur, and the patient is considered to be infectious. More than 90% of relapses, most often mucocutaneous in nature, occur in the first year, and it is widely believed that each relapse is clinically less florid than the previous episode. Late latent syphilis may continue for the balance of the patient's life or may progress to tertiary syphilis.[35] During late latent syphilis, relapses are rare, and the patient is not considered to be infectious. Nevertheless, in utero transmission of disease is possible during latent syphilis.

Approximately 30% of untreated patients progress to late (tertiary) syphilis, a slowly progressive disease that can affect any system in the body years after initial infection. Clinically, late syphilis is often classified as either neurosyphilis, cardiovascular syphilis, or gummatous syphilis (late benign syphilis), a condition that is characterized by the development of hyperimmune granulomas, known as gummas, that often involve the skin and the bones.

Approximately 10% of untreated patients progress to the development of neurosyphilis. As mentioned, CNS involvement is initially asymptomatic and can be detected only by evaluation of the CSF. Under ideal situations, all patients should have evaluation of the CSF at 1 year after diagnosis and treatment of syphilis to detect evidence of residual CNS disease, such as pleocytosis, increased protein, decreased glucose, or positive nontreponemal antigen test. Examination of the CSF is also indicated for all HIV-positive patients with syphilis. The clinical manifestations of symptomatic neurosyphilis may include focal or generalized seizures, visual disturbances, paresthesias, altered reflexes, speech disturbances, pupillary abnormalities, dementia, and stroke. Tabes dorsalis is a manifestation resulting from degeneration of the dorsal columns of the spinal cord; it is characterized by ataxia with a wide-based gait, impotence, urinary incontinence or retention, paroxysms of intense shooting pain (usually in the legs), and loss of reflexes.[33,35]

Congenital syphilis results from transplacental transmission of spirochetes to the fetus in utero. Babies who are born to mothers who acquire syphilis during pregnancy are at a higher risk of developing congenital syphilis than are those whose mothers acquired syphilis before pregnancy. Although nearly 75% of cases of congenital syphilis are diagnosed after age 10 years, some cases manifest very early after birth. Early cases often cause rhinitis and a diffuse maculopapular rash that may result in significant epithelial sloughing. Additionally, there may be generalized osteochondritis and perichondritis, eventually leading to bone destruction. Neonatal death from congenital syphilis is usually due to pneumonia, pulmonary hemorrhage, or hepatic failure. Patients with late congenital syphilis may have Hutchinson's triad, which includes Hutchinson's teeth (short, narrow, barrel-shaped incisors with a central notch), interstitial keratitis (photophobia, eye pain, tearing), and nerve deafness.

Diagnosis

Using dark-field microscopy, silver staining, or specific immunofluorescence or immunoperoxidase stains of transudate or tissue from the lesion can easily identify *T. pallidum* spirochetes.

The most direct method for establishing the diagnosis of syphilis is demonstration of *T. pallidum* on dark-field microscopic examination of fluid or tissue taken from a suspicious cutaneous lesion or lymph node.[29,30,36] Because *T. pallidum* is susceptible to environmental changes, it is recommended that any clinical specimen taken from a patient with suspected syphilis be examined immediately. Because of their highly characteristic spiral shape and motility, viable treponemes are easy to distinguish under microscopic examination. Dark-field microscopic examination of material from the oral cavity may not be useful in diagnosing syphilis because nonpathogenic spirochetes can be members of the normal oral flora. An alternative to dark-field microscopy that has been implemented in many clinical laboratories is the use of a direct fluorescence antibody test (DFA-TP), which has greater specificity for *T. pallidum* and does not require immediate examination.[37]

In the absence of suitable pathologic specimens to examine, the diagnosis of syphilis can be based on serologic testing.[30,38] The serologic tests that are used in the diagnosis of syphilis are classified as either nontreponemal or treponemal. Two commonly used nontreponemal antibody tests, Venereal Disease Research Laboratories (VDRL) and rapid plasma reagin (RPR), are quantitative measurements of antibodies against cardiolipin. These tests report serum titers that correlate with disease activity, with higher titers consistent with more active disease. These tests are inexpensive and easy to perform and are therefore often used for routine screening of patients. However, the test may remain reactive at low titers after treatment (serofast state) or become negative after 5 to 10 years, even without treatment (serorevert).[38] In some patients with secondary syphilis a prozone phenomenon may occur, leading to a false-negative VDRL test. This is due to an excess of antibody relative to antigen and may be corrected by dilution of the patient's serum before testing.[37] These tests can be used for patient monitoring and evaluation of therapy. Titers should fall and become nonreactive within 1 year after successful treatment of primary syphilis and within 2 years after effective treatment of secondary syphilis. Patients who are treated for late syphilis usually become nonreactive after a period of up to 5 years.[39] Other nontreponemal tests that have been used include the reagin screen test, the automated reagin test, and the unheated serum reagin test.[36]

Specific treponemal antibody tests, such as the fluorescent treponemal antibody-absorbed test (FTA-abs), are highly sensitive and specific. The positive predictive value of the FTA-abs test is 100% for the initial or any subsequent symptomatic case of syphilis. Unfortunately, because this specific treponemal test usually remains positive for life, despite treatment, it is much less reliable in the evaluation of asymptomatic patients with a previous history of treated syphilis.[31] Two additional treponemal antibody tests that are useful in the diagnosis of syphilis are the microhemagglutination assay for antibodies to *T. pallidum* (MHATP) and the hemagglutination treponemal test for syphilis (HATTS). These tests are less expensive and easier to perform than the FTS-abs test but are also somewhat less sensitive in diagnosing early syphilis.[40]

THERAPEUTIC PLAN

Four basic principles guide the current treatment strategy for syphilis: (1) the requirement of a minimum treponemicidal antibiotic concentration; (2) maintenance of continuous antibiotic concentration above this minimum inhibitory concentration; (3) adequate duration of therapy; and (4) the fact that the response to treatment is inversely related to the duration of the infection.[41] The specific CDC recommendations for the preparation, dosage, and duration of therapy are based on the stage and clinical manifestations of the disease at the time of treatment and are summarized in Table 75.5.[42]

TREATMENT

On the basis of more than 50 years of experience, the drug of choice for the treatment of all stages of syphilis is parenteral penicillin G.[42,43] *Treponema pallidum* is highly

Table 75.5 ▪ Recommended Treatment Regimens for All Stages of Syphilis in Patients Not Infected with Human Immunodeficiency Virus

Disease Stage	Adult Regimen	Child Regimen	Adult Penicillin Allergy
Sexual contact to infectious case of syphilis	Benzathine penicillin G, 2.4 million units IM as single-dose therapy		Doxycycline 100 mg PO BID for 14 days *or* Tetracycline, 500 mg PO QID for 14 days
Primary or secondary syphilis	Benzathine penicillin G, 2.4 million units IM as single-dose therapy	Benzathine penicillin G, 50,000 U/kg IM as single-dose therapy (max. 2.4 million units)	Doxycycline, 100 mg PO BID for 14 days *or* Tetracycline, 500 mg PO QID for 14 days
Early, latent syphilis (less than 1 yr duration)	Treat as primary or secondary syphilis		
Late, latent syphilis (greater than 1 yr duration)	Benzathine penicillin G, 2.4 million units IM weekly for 3 doses	Benzathine penicillin G, 50,000 U/kg IM weekly for 3 doses (max. 2.4 million units/dose)	Doxycycline, 100 mg PO BID for 28 days *or* Tetracycline, 500 mg PO QID for 28 days
Late syphilis (not neurosyphilis)	Treat as late, latent syphilis		
Neurosyphilis	Aqueous penicillin G, 12–24 million units/day IV (administered as 2–4 million units q4hr) for 10 to 14 days *or* Procaine penicillin G, 2.4 million units IM once daily PLUS probenecid 500 mg PO QID, both for 10–14 days (acceptable regimen only if compliance can be ensured)		Desensitize; then give IV aqueous penicillin G
Syphilis in pregnancy	Treat as appropriate with parenteral penicillin		Desensitize; then give parenteral penicillin
Congenital syphilis	N/A	Aqueous penicillin G, 100,000–150,000 U/kg/day (administered as 50,000 U/kg IV q12hr during the first 7 days of life, and q8hr thereafter, for 10–14 days) *or* Procaine penicillin G, 50,000 U/kg IM once daily as a single dose for 10–14 days	

Source: Reference 32.

Table 75.6 ▪ Oral Penicillin Desensitization Protocol[a]

Dose Number for Penicillin V Suspension[b]	Suspension Concentration (U/mL)	Dose (mL)	Dose (U)	Cumulative Dose (U)
1	1,000	0.1	100	100
2	1,000	0.2	200	300
3	1,000	0.4	400	700
4	1,000	0.8	800	1,500
5	1,000	1.6	1,600	3,100
6	1,000	3.2	3,200	6,300
7	1,000	6.4	6,400	12,700
8	10,000	1.2	12,000	24,700
9	10,000	2.4	24,000	48,700
10	10,000	4.8	48,000	96,700
11	80,000	1.0	80,000	176,700
12	80,000	2.0	160,000	336,700
13	80,000	4.0	320,000	656,700
14	80,000	8.0	640,000	1,296,700

Source: Reference 32.

[a] The penicillin dose should be diluted in 30–45 mL of water and administered orally.

[b] The interval between individual doses is 15 minutes; therefore elapsed time for desensitization is 3 hours 45 minutes.

sensitive to the effects of penicillin. Unfortunately, there have been no adequately controlled clinical trials to clearly define the optimal penicillin regimen for the treatment of various stages of syphilis. In addition, the data addressing nonpenicillin therapy are extremely limited. The current treatment guidelines for syphilis use benzathine penicillin G as first-line therapy for primary, secondary, and latent syphilis. Alternative therapeutic options for patients with significant penicillin allergy are limited. The use of doxycycline, 100 mg orally every 12 hours, or tetracycline, 500 mg orally every 6 hours, is considered an acceptable alternative treatment. There is less clinical experience with doxycycline, but compliance should be better. Erythromycin, 500 mg orally every 6 hours, has undergone limited evaluation but may be associated with high treatment failure rates, particularly in pregnancy.[29,42,43] The use of first-generation cephalosporins has shown limited efficacy but unacceptably high treatment failure rates. Also, ceftriaxone has undergone clinical studies in small numbers of patients with syphilis, and the results are promising.[11,38] Unfortunately, adequate data do not exist at this time to clearly define the appropriate use of ceftriaxone in the treatment of syphilis; however, a once-daily regimen may be considered if treponemicidal levels in the blood can be maintained for 8 to 10 days.[42]

Parenteral penicillin G is the only therapy that is documented to be effective in the management of syphilis during pregnancy and for neurosyphilis; therefore, patients who are allergic to penicillin should be treated with penicillin following desensitization. Patients who have positive skin tests to either the major or minor determinants of penicillin allergy can usually be safely desensitized over a 4- to 6-hour period using oral penicillin V suspension as outlined in Table 75.6.[44] Once desensitized,

Table 75.7 ▪ Recommended Treatment Regimens for Syphilis in Patients Infected with Human Immunodeficiency Virus

Disease Stage	Adult Regimen	Alternative Regimen
Primary and secondary	Benzathine penicillin G, 2.4 million units IM as single-dose therapy (some experts suggest multiple doses)	None; must desensitize and treat with penicillin
Latent	Benzathine penicillin G, 2.4 million units IM weekly for 3 doses	None; must desensitize and treat with penicillin

patients should be maintained on penicillin continuously until completion of the treatment course.

Many clinicians treat primary and secondary syphilis in HIV-infected patients more aggressively than in non–HIV-infected patients, using three intramuscular doses of benzathine penicillin G administered at weekly intervals (Table 75.7).

Occasionally, within the first 24 hours of treatment for early syphilis, the patient will experience a Jarisch-Herxheimer reaction, an acute, benign, febrile episode that is commonly accompanied by myalgias, transient adenopathy, and headache lasting for several hours. This reaction is thought to be caused by release of treponemal antigens due to rapid lysis of the organism by antibiotics. It is important that the clinician recognize this reaction as being independent of the drug regimen and not consider it to be an allergic reaction to the therapeutic agent used. If necessary for patient comfort, acetaminophen or aspirin can be used for symptomatic relief.

IMPROVING OUTCOMES

The CDC recommends serologic follow-up of patients who are treated for syphilis in order to evaluate the therapeutic outcome. Quantitative nontreponemal tests should be performed at 6, 12, and 24 months after completion of therapy for primary, secondary, and latent syphilis.[42] For patients with neurosyphilis, the CSF should be examined every 6 months until the cell count is normal. If the cell count remains abnormal at 24 months, re-treatment is suggested. A quantitative nontreponemal test every 2 to 3 months until it is nonreactive is recommended as a follow-up for congenital syphilis. The adequacy of treatment for syphilis during pregnancy should be evaluated with nontreponemal serologic testing on a monthly basis. HIV-infected patients should be evaluated clinically and serologically more frequently for treatment failure at 3, 6, 9, 12, and 24 months after therapy. Patients who fail to demonstrate a fourfold reduction in titer over a 3-month period or who show a fourfold increase in titer between tests should be re-treated.

Herpes Genitalis

Genital herpes, or herpes genitalis, is an acute inflammatory infection caused by the double-stranded DNA herpes simplex virus (HSV).[45]

EPIDEMIOLOGY

Genital herpes is the most commonly encountered cause of genital ulceration in the United States and can involve the male and female genital tracts with equal prevalence. Studies have shown that people with multiple sexual partners have an increased chance of acquiring herpes infection. Based on serologic data, it is reported that more than 40 million Americans are currently infected with genital herpes.[46] HSV type 2 (HSV-2) is the predominant viral type associated with herpes genitalis, and HSV type 1 (HSV-1) is most closely associated with oropharyngeal disease; however, each virus can cause infections in both anatomic areas. Humans are the only reservoir for transmission to other humans. Primary genital herpes develops after transmission of the virus by direct contact of the recipient's mucous membranes or skin with infected secretions or mucocutaneous surface of an infected sexual partner.[47] After inoculation there is an incubation period ranging from 2 to 20 days when the HSV replicates locally in epithelial cells, eventually causing a localized inflammatory response and ulceration. The virus also migrates via peripheral neurons to the sacral ganglia, where latency is established. After latency, a stimulus (physiologic, immunologic, or emotional factors) can produce periodic viral reactivation of symptomatic disease or asymptomatic viral shedding. The factors that contribute to this reactivation are poorly understood at present.[48] Transmission of HSV-2 often occurs in individuals who are unaware that they have the infection or are asymptomatic when transmission occurs.

CLINICAL PRESENTATION AND DIAGNOSIS

Signs and Symptoms

The clinical manifestations and recurrence rates of genital herpes are influenced by the viral type and numerous host-related factors, such as gender, immunocompetence, site of infection, and previous infection with HSV.[45] A significant number of HSV-2 infections are asymptomatic. First-episode infection (primary infection) occurs in individuals with HSV-1 or HSV-2 infections, in the absence of serum antibody to either type of HSV, and causes severe manifestations. Nonprimary first-episode infections tend to cause less severe manifestations because individuals already have serum antibodies to either of the herpes types; patients with serum antibodies to HSV-2 seldom develop genital HSV-1 infection[48]

A significant percentage of patients with primary HSV infection experience a prodromal flulike syndrome with fever, headache, malaise, and diffuse myalgias. After a brief incubation period of 2 to 20 days (average of 4 to 7 days), local symptoms develop, consisting of genital itching, tenderness, and dysuria. Typically, the lesions start as painful papules or vesicles that spread rapidly over the genital region, often clustering together to form large areas of shallow ulceration. The pain and irritation gradually increase over the first week, reaching maximum intensity between days 7 and 11 of infection, then slowly recede over the next week. Over the course of several weeks, the cutaneous ulcers crust over and eventually reepithelialize. Crusting does not occur with lesions on mucous membranes.[45,48] Viral shedding occurs during the period from development of the initial lesion until approximately the eleventh or twelfth day of illness. First-episode nonprimary genital herpes infections tend to be milder than primary infections. Patients experience lower incidence and shorter duration of prodromal flulike symptoms.

The symptoms of recurrent HSV infection are similar to those seen with primary episodes, without the systemic manifestations. The symptoms often appear to be more severe in women than men, possibly because of the extent of involved mucosal surface. In general, recurrent symptoms are milder than those seen with primary infection, are localized to the genital area, and usually last from 5 to 7 days.

Complications of genital herpes infection occur most commonly after primary episodes and usually result from the spread of genital disease or by autoinoculation of the virus. HSV infection of the rectum, pharynx, and eye are not unusual. Central nervous system involvement can include aseptic meningitis, transverse myelitis, or sacral radiculopathy. Blood-borne dissemination of HSV infection may accompany primary mucocutaneous infection in immunocompromised patients or during pregnancy. HSV infection of neonates who were exposed during pregnancy or delivery is associated with extremely high morbidity and mortality, with a case-fatality rate approaching 50%.[50] Herpes infections tend to be more prolonged and severe in immunocompromised patients (e.g., HIV, solid organ transplant).

Diagnosis

Because a number of other diseases are associated with genital ulceration, the diagnosis of herpes genitalis often requires laboratory testing. The easiest, but least sensitive and specific, technique is examination of cells scraped from the base of a typical lesion or ulcer (Tzanck smear) and stained by Giemsa or Papanicolaou stain.[45] Evidence of multinucleated giant cells with intranuclear inclusions is characteristic of HSV infection. Identification of HSV in tissue culture processed from a specimen taken from a symptomatic patient is the most sensitive and specific method for confirmation of primary HSV infection but is expensive and time-consuming to perform. Serologic demonstration of HSV infection is useful for confirming the diagnosis of primary HSV infection, for determining the HSV serotype (if a serotype-specific assay is used), and for distinguishing between primary and reactivated infections, because recurrent genital herpes rarely induces a significant increase in anti-HSV antibodies.[48,50] However, therapeutic decisions should not be postponed until the results are obtained.

THERAPEUTIC PLAN

The goals in treating herpes genitalis are to decrease the duration and severity of active infection, prevent associated complications, decrease the frequency of recurrence, and reduce the period of viral shedding and infectivity.[45] It is important to remember that these drugs do not eradicate latent virus or affect the risk or severity of recurrences after the drug is discontinued. To date, acyclovir, famciclovir, and valacyclovir have been shown to be effective in the clinical management of genital herpes. These antivirals are associated with reductions in viral shedding, decreases in the severity and duration of symptoms, and accelerated lesion healing of first-episode HSV genital infections. The use of 5% acyclovir topical ointment in cases of genital herpes should be discouraged because of lack of demonstrated efficacy.[50] The recommended regimens for management of primary herpes genitalis are summarized in Table 75.8. In first-episode cases, prompt initiation of antiviral therapy is associated with reduction in symptoms within 48 hours.[45,48] Acyclovir dosages should be reduced for patients with significant renal dysfunction. There is no advantage to using parenteral acyclovir instead of oral acyclovir except for patients with severe disease or complications who require hospitalization and cannot take acyclovir orally. In order to decrease the frequency of recurrent genital herpes, many patients with recurrent infection may benefit from chronic administration of antiviral therapy; therefore, treatment options (episodic treatment or daily suppressive therapy) should be discussed with patients as shown in Table 75.9.

To derive benefit, episodic antiviral therapy has to be started at the beginning of the prodrome or when lesions are first noted, because recurrent episodes of genital herpes in immunocompetent patients are self-limited.[45] In patients with more than six episodes per year, daily dosing of acyclovir for chronic suppressive therapy to prevent recurrences has been reported to reduce the frequency of recurrences by nearly 75%. If suppressive therapy is started, the current recommendation is to discontinue therapy after 12 months of continuous treatment in order to reassess the patient's rate of recurrence.[46] Although the potential for adverse effects from long-term acyclovir administration and the possibility of developing acyclovir-resistant strains of HSV are concerns, clinical data suggest few cumulative acyclovir toxicities and no significant changes in HSV susceptibility to acyclovir after prolonged acyclovir use for up to 6 years.[45,51] Safety and efficacy have been demonstrated among patients receiving daily therapy with valacyclovir and famciclovir for 1 year.[52,53] There

Table 75.8 ▪ Recommended Regimens for Treatment of Herpes Genitalis

Type of Infection	Recommended Regimen	Cost[a]	Alternative Regimen
First episode of genital herpes[b]	Acyclovir 400 mg PO TID for 7–10 days	$6.90	Acyclovir 5–10 mg/kg IV q8hr for 5–7 days or until clinical resolution (only for patients who require hospitalization)
	or		
	Acyclovir 200 mg PO 5 times daily for 7–10 days	$6.00	
	or		
	Famciclovir 250 mg PO TID for 7–10 days	$9.60	
	or		
	Valacyclovir 1 g PO BID for 7–10 days	$7.30	
First-episode of herpes proctitis	Acyclovir 400 mg PO 5 times daily for 10 days[c]	$11.45	As above

[a]Based on 1998 Red Book AWP for daily drug costs

[b]Treatment may be continued for >10 days until clinical resolution occurs.

[c]Clinical experience is lacking with famciclovir and valacyclovir, but they should be effective.

Table 75.9 ▪ Recommended Regimens for Recurrent Episodes of Herpes Genitalis

Type of Infection	Recommended Regimen	Type of Infection	Recommended Regimen
Recurrent infection	Acyclovir 400 mg PO TID for 5 days *or* Acyclovir 200 mg PO five times daily for 5 days *or* Acyclovir 800 mg PO BID for 5 days *or* Famciclovir 125 mg PO BID for 5 days *or* Valacyclovir 500 mg PO BID for 5 days	Daily suppressive therapy	Acyclovir 400 mg PO BID *or* Famciclovir 250 mg PO BID *or* Valacyclovir 250 mg PO BID *or* Valacyclovir 500 mg PO QD *or* Valacyclovir 1000 mg PO QD

have been limited reports of apparent acyclovir-resistant strains of HSV in patients with genital herpes. Foscarnet, 40 mg/kg intravenously every 8 hours (or 60 mg/kg every 12 hours) until clinical resolution, is the recommended treatment alternative in such cases.[46] Based on clinical experience, immunocompromised patients may benefit from higher doses of antivirals (acyclovir 400 mg tid five times daily, famciclovir 500 mg bid) for daily suppressive therapy because these patients may have more severe cases.

The safety of systemic acyclovir therapy during pregnancy has not been clearly established, although there is currently no evidence to suggest that acyclovir is teratogenic in humans.[46,49,50] Current recommendations are to avoid acyclovir therapy for HSV infections during pregnancy unless there is life-threatening infection as evidenced by encephalitis, hepatitis, or pneumonitis.[46]

TREATMENT

Acyclovir, a guanosine analog, is selectively taken up by HSV-infected cells and undergoes serial phosphorylation to the active form, acyclovir triphosphate. This triphosphorylated moiety acts to inhibit HSV DNA polymerase and viral replication. Both HSV-1 and HSV-2 are inhibited by concentrations of acyclovir that are achieved in serum and body tissues at the currently recommended dosages.[50] Unlike acyclovir, both famciclovir and valacyclovir are prodrugs. After oral administration, valacyclovir, the L-valyl ester (prodrug) of acyclovir, is hydrolyzed to acyclovir, and famciclovir is converted to its active form, penciclovir.[54,55] To exert an antiviral effect, all of these agents must become activated within the cell to a monophosphate form by thymidine kinase, an enzyme found predominantly in virally infected cells. The end result is inhibition of viral DNA synthesis. Of note, acyclovir-resistant strains of HSV and varicella-zoster virus are usually cross-resistant to penciclovir because the most common mechanism of resistance is a deficiency of thymidine kinase.

When compared with acyclovir, the pharmacokinetic profiles of the new analogs offer improved features. The oral bioavailability of acyclovir is poor, limited to only 15 to 30%; however, the bioavailability of acyclovir after valacyclovir administration is substantially increased to 54%.[54] Serum concentrations derived from 1 to 2 g of valacyclovir given orally four times daily are comparable to those achieved with administration of 5 to 10 mg/kg of intravenous acyclovir every 8 hours. Famciclovir, a prodrug, is converted to penciclovir, which has excellent oral bioavailability (77%).[55] Both acyclovir and penciclovir are predominantly cleared by the kidneys. In patients with renal insufficiency, accumulation can result; therefore, reduced doses are necessary. The antivirals are well tolerated in immunocompetent patients. When compared with placebo, adverse events were similar in patients taking either agent. No differences in incidence of adverse effects between famciclovir or valacyclovir compared with acyclovir were noted in comparative genital herpes trials. The most common adverse effects in clinical trials include gastrointestinal upset, diarrhea, headache, insomnia, dizziness, and fatigue. To date, there are essentially no clinically significant drug interactions with these drugs.[54,55]

Of concern, in comparative clinical trials involving immunocompromised patients given higher doses of valacyclovir (greater than 3 g/day), more cases of thrombotic thrombocytopenic purpura/hemolytic uremic syndrome (TTP/HUS) have been observed in patients receiving valacyclovir versus acyclovir.[56] The overall incidence of TTP/HUS in valacyclovir-treated patients is less than 3%, and the median time to occurrence of this complication is 53 days (range 8 to 100 days). To date, TTP/HUS has not been observed in immunocompetent patients or in immunocompromised patients given valacyclovir in doses of 3 g/day or less.[56] Therefore, valacyclovir has not been approved by the FDA for use in immunocompromised patients.

Patients with genital herpes should be advised to refrain from sexual activity while genital lesions are present. In addition, sexual partners of infected individuals should be evaluated and counseled about the lifelong nature of the disease. Successful management of genital HSV infection involves educating the patient about the natural history of the infection (i.e., the potential for recurrent episodes, asymptomatic viral shedding, and sexual transmission, especially because this often occurs during asymptomatic periods).

Chancroid

EPIDEMIOLOGY

Chancroid is a sexually transmitted disease caused by *Haemophilus ducreyi,* a small, Gram-negative, facultative anaerobic bacillus that is particularly hard to grow in culture. Most experts agree that genital herpes and primary syphilis are responsible for the majority of ulcerative genital lesions in developed countries, and chancroid accounts for most of the genital ulcers in developing societies.[57,58] Nevertheless, since the early 1980s, there have been several significant outbreaks of chancroid in the United States and Canada. Men, especially uncircumcised men, have a higher incidence of infection than women.[57]

For several years, the epidemiologic relationship between the presence of genital ulcers, such as chancroid, and heterosexual transmission of the human immunodeficiency virus has been recognized, particularly in Africa. It is believed that contact between the infectious ulcer of one sexual partner and mucous membranes of the other partner leads to this viral transmission. Therefore, identification and treatment of patients with chancroid, as well as other infections such as genital herpes that lead to the formation of genital ulcers, are important in limiting the spread of HIV.

CLINICAL PRESENTATION AND DIAGNOSIS

Signs and Symptoms

The incubation period for chancroid ranges from 3 to 10 days. The chancre starts as a tender, papule-like lesion with surrounding erythema and progresses over several days to an eroded, pustular ulcer that can be quite painful, particularly in men.[57] Many women with chancroid are asymptomatic. Over time, several of these small lesions can coalesce to form giant ulcers. The presence of painful inguinal lymphadenitis is seen concurrently in approximately 50% of cases and is often unilateral. Inflamed lymph nodes can progress to the development of formed buboes, which may rupture spontaneously in severe cases. Superinfection of the ulcerative lesions by enteric aerobic and anaerobic pathogens may further complicate the condition.[57]

Diagnosis

The definitive diagnosis of chancroid is dependent on the identification of *H. ducreyi* from culture on special media from samples collected from the ulcer or bubo. Because the proper media for culture is not widely available, the diagnosis is generally made by the exclusion of other diseases that produce inguinal ulceration, such as herpes genitalis, lymphogranuloma venereum, and syphilis.[57,58]

THERAPEUTIC PLAN

The CDC recommends systemic antibiotic therapy with any one of the following regimens: azithromycin 1000 mg orally as a single dose, ceftriaxone 250 mg intramuscularly as a single dose, ciprofloxacin 500 mg bid for 3 days, or erythromycin base 500 mg orally every 6 hours for 7 days.[58] Each of these regimens has proven to be highly effective in non–HIV-infected patients with chancroid. Most clinicians should not routinely recommend single-dose therapy for HIV-infected patients because of reported higher treatment failure rates.[59]

An alternative regimen that has not been as thoroughly evaluated is amoxicillin 500 mg plus clavulanic acid 125 mg orally three times daily for 7 days.[57,59] Cefotaxime is also an effective treatment option for chancroid, but multiple parenteral doses are required for optimal cure rates. Three successive daily intramuscular doses of 1 g cefotaxime produced a 95% cure rate; a single 1 g intramuscular dose cured only 53% of patients.[59] Other cephalosporins have not been studied as therapy for chancroid. Trimethoprim plus sulfamethoxazole (co-trimoxazole) is no longer a recommended treatment option for chancroid because of reports of *H. ducreyi* developing increased resistance to this combination.[59]

Patients should be reexamined several days after starting therapy to ensure that symptomatic improvement is observed. The time for complete healing may be several weeks, and significant scarring of tissues is common. Relapse after apparent healing has been reported in up to 5% of cases.[59] All known recent sexual contacts of the patient with chancroid should be evaluated and treated if possible.

Selected Other Sexually Transmitted Diseases

Trichomoniasis

EPIDEMIOLOGY

Trichomoniasis is a common condition caused by the flagellated, motile protozoan *Trichomonas vaginalis.*[60] In the United States, approximately 3 million females are treated for trichomoniasis annually; the incidence among males is unknown.[61] Individuals who have multiple sexual partners or are concurrently infected with another STD appear to be at increased risk for trichomoniasis. This supports the contention that trichomoniasis is an STD. Transmission between sexual partners is further confirmed by reports of recovery of *T. vaginalis* from 66 to 100% of female sexual partners of infected men and 30 to 40% of male partners of infected women.[62] For unclear reasons, trichomoniasis appears to be less common in women who use barrier contraception or oral contraceptives. Nonvenereal transmission can also occur from contact with colonized materials, such as towels and clothing. Neonates can acquire the organism during normal vaginal delivery.[63]

CLINICAL PRESENTATION AND DIAGNOSIS

Signs and Symptoms

Trichomoniasis is thought to be an asymptomatic and self-limited disease in most men and neonates, often requiring no specific therapy.[64,65] Up to 50% of women with vaginal trichomoniasis are asymptomatic. However, symptoms may develop after an incubation period ranging from 1 to 4 weeks. Common complaints include malodorous grayish or yellow-green vaginal discharge, dysuria, pruritus in the genital area, and vulvovaginal tenderness. Signs and symptoms may be exacerbated during menstruation, possibly because of increased vaginal pH facilitating an increase in organism growth.[65]

Diagnosis

Laboratory findings include an elevated vaginal pH (greater than 4.5) and large numbers of neutrophils seen on microscopic evaluation on the wet mount prep of the discharge. Evaluation of a wet mount prep from a vaginal swab remains the easiest, cheapest, and most widely used diagnostic technique employed.[60] Traditional stains, such as the Gram, Giemsa, and acridine orange stains, are not helpful in the diagnosis of trichomoniasis but should be done on all samples because of the high likelihood of concurrent disease in infected patients.[60] Culture of *T. vaginalis* from collected specimens is the most sensitive diagnostic technique available but requires up to 48 hours for necessary growth, reducing the clinical usefulness of culture for clinical diagnosis.[65]

THERAPEUTIC PLAN

The treatment of choice for trichomoniasis in both men and women is oral metronidazole.[60,66] With the recent availability of metronidazole gel as a treatment for bacterial vaginosis, topical metronidazole for trichomoniasis has been considered. Systemic therapy is superior to topical intravaginal treatment for women because organisms in the urinary tract are treated as well, thereby reducing the likelihood of relapse.[65] A single 2 g oral dose of metronidazole or 500 mg orally twice daily for 7 days for women has resulted in cure rates of 90% to 95%.[60,65,66] This probably holds true for men as well, although data are lacking to confirm this belief. A metronidazole regimen of 375 mg orally twice daily for 7 days has been recommended for approval as an alternative regimen by the FDA Anti-Infective Advisory Committee based on pharmacokinetic data.[66] As with any STD, it is important to treat all sexual partners as well to prevent reinfection. When sexual partners are treated simultaneously with metronidazole, the cure rate increases to greater than 95%.[60] Infants with symptomatic trichomoniasis or with prolonged (greater than 4 weeks) colonization after birth can be treated with parenteral metronidazole, 10 to 30 mg/kg/day for 7 days.[65] No specific follow-up is required unless signs and symptoms of infection continue.

TREATMENT

Metronidazole therapy is associated with some well-recognized side effects, particularly mild nausea, which are more common with large single doses. Peripheral neuropathy, manifesting as numbness and paresthesias, is also associated with metronidazole therapy, especially in patients who take large doses for prolonged periods of time. Metronidazole can interfere with alcohol metabolism by blocking alcohol dehydrogenase, producing an "Antabuse-like" or "disulfiram-like" reaction consisting of severe nausea, vomiting, and flushing when the two are taken concomitantly. The use of metronidazole during pregnancy is contraindicated, most importantly during the first trimester. Data suggest that metronidazole use during the second and third trimesters of pregnancy is safe; however, most clinicians do not consider specific therapy for trichomoniasis to be necessary during pregnancy unless the symptoms are severe.[65]

When the clinician is faced with an apparent failure of metronidazole, consideration must be given to the possibility of failure due to poor compliance, reinfection of the patient by an infected sexual partner, or the potential of infection by metronidazole-resistant organisms. Although *T. vaginalis* resistance to metronidazole appears to be increasing, alternative therapies are limited.[63] Current therapeutic options for infections caused by suspected or known metronidazole-resistant organisms include treatment for 7 to 10 days with daily oral doses of 2 g of metronidazole, with or without concurrent use of metronidazole 0.5% gel intravaginally.[65]

Lymphogranuloma Venereum

EPIDEMIOLOGY

Lymphogranuloma venereum (LGV) is caused by the invasive serotypes of *Chlamydia trachomatis,* the same pathogen that is associated with the development of nongonococcal urethritis in many patients.[67] LGV is a relatively rare disease in the United States and must be differentiated clinically from such other conditions as lymphoma, syphilis, chancroid, plague, tularemia, and genital herpes. Like other STDs, LGV is more common among individuals with multiple sexual contacts, in urban rather than rural areas, and in lower socioeconomic populations.[68]

CLINICAL PRESENTATION AND DIAGNOSIS

Signs and Symptoms

The most common clinical manifestation of LGV is tender inguinal lymphadenopathy, which is most commonly unilateral. This inguinal adenopathy appears 2 to 6 weeks after the development of an unremarkable herpetiform vesicle at the site of inoculation. The initial vesicle often goes unnoticed, particularly in women. Within 2 weeks, the inflamed inguinal node (bubo) may progress to fluctuance and rupture through the skin, forming sinus tracts that are slow to heal. This occurs in fewer than 30% of cases.[68] The remaining cases slowly form firm inguinal masses without suppuration. In females and homosexual males, LGV can cause perianal or perirectal inflammation that can progress to the formation of colonic fistulas or strictures. These patients may have rectal bleeding or rectal discharge of pus. In severe cases, patients may appear systemically ill. Laboratory findings are usually nonspecific and may consist of slightly elevated white blood cell counts, elevated erythrocyte sedimentation rate, and mild increases in hepatic transaminases.

Diagnosis

The diagnosis of LGV is based largely on the clinical presentation of significant inguinal adenopathy in the absence of another etiology. Isolation of *C. trachomatis* from an aspirated swollen bubo is possible in up to one-third of cases but requires special culture techniques that are not available in most laboratories. Serologic documentation of antichlamydial antibodies by microimmunofluorescence or ELISA is thought to be sensitive and more specific than complement fixation but can lead to false-positive results because of the widespread prevalence of other chlamydial infections in the at-risk population.

THERAPEUTIC PLAN

The recommended treatment of choice for LGV is doxycycline, 100 mg orally twice daily for 21 days, as shown in Table 75.4.[68,69] Alternative antibiotic regimens include erythromycin, 500 mg orally four times daily for 21 days, or sulfisoxazole, 500 mg orally four times daily for 21 days. Erythromycin is the treatment of choice for pregnant females. Although it is expected that azithromycin should offer similar efficacy to that of erythromycin as alternative therapy to doxycycline, insufficient clinical data are available to support its widespread use at this time. Swollen, inflamed lymph nodes may require surgical aspiration or incision and drainage for optimal care.

In general, appropriate antibiotic therapy and surgical intervention, if necessary, cure LGV and prevent further tissue damage and scarring. However, patients should be followed clinically until resolution of signs and symptoms of the disease. Sexual partners should be evaluated and treated appropriately if urethral or cervical chlamydial infection is detected.

Human Papillomavirus Infection—Condylomata Acuminata

EPIDEMIOLOGY

Condylomata acuminata, or genital warts, are venereal infections caused by human papillomavirus (HPV).[70] Genital HPV infection is the second most common venereal disease seen in STD clinics in the United States; it is responsible for more than 1 million office visits annually. Papillomaviruses are double-stranded DNA viruses that often produce squamous epithelial tumors. The virus has been shown to penetrate and infect the basal cell layer, the only site of actively dividing cells in the epithelium. More than 70 types of HPV have been identified; they contribute to a wide range of lesions, including plantar warts, laryngeal carcinoma, and cervical dysplasia. The HPV types that are considered to be primarily responsible for genital warts are HPV-6 and HPV-11.[70] These HPV types are easily transmitted during sexual intercourse. Genital warts are almost always the result of anal intercourse, particularly in homosexual men.

The natural history of untreated genital warts is variable. Some may grow larger, some regress, and many stay the same over time. Several years ago, it was commonly believed that, if left untreated, large genital warts would progress to malignancy. As techniques to identify particular types of HPV have become available, it has become clear that the risk of genital warts progressing to cancerous lesions is very small.[72] The HPV types that are most strongly associated with the development of cervical cancer are not the same types that are associated with genital warts. Additionally, the rates of noncervical genital cancers are extremely low in the United States, whereas the prevalence of genital HPV infections is very high.

CLINICAL PRESENTATION AND DIAGNOSIS

Signs and Symptoms

Condylomata acuminata may be asymptomatic, with only occasional anogenital pruritus and burning.[70] These lesions are usually known as flat condylomas and are identified as shiny white plaques after the application of dilute (3 to 5%) acetic acid solution to the site. The common locations for these flat warts are the penis, anus, vagina, vulva, and cervix. Large, hyperplastic, exophytic warts with raised, pinkish-colored papules are the classic condylomata acuminata.[73] These larger lesions may be associated with increased pain, bleeding, burning, and soiling of undergarments.

Diagnosis

Condylomata acuminata should be differentiated from other anogenital growths, such as molluscum contagiosum, moles, and skin tags. HPV cannot be grown in tissue culture; therefore, diagnosis is based on gross clinical appearance and confirmed by biopsy.[73] Histologic evidence of koilocytosis, the characteristic finding of HPV infection, can be observed with appropriate staining techniques, such as the Papanicolaou smear. Recently, newer techniques, such as DNA hybridization and polymerase chain reaction, have expanded the ability to identify specific HPV types, but these procedures are not currently useful for clinical screening.[72]

THERAPEUTIC PLAN

The treatment options for genital warts are frequently associated with significant pain and expense and with frustrating results because of poor responses or recurrences.[70,74] Many experts believe that recurrences of genital warts are much more commonly due to reactivation of subclinical infection than to reinfection by a sexual partner.[75] Eradication of genital HPV infection is not accomplished by any therapeutic option that is currently available. Although aggressive techniques for removal of the warts do produce cosmetic benefits, the surrounding tissues usually remain subclinically infected with HPV.

The plant resin podophyllin, applied as a 10 to 25% solution in compound tincture of benzoin, has traditionally been the most common initial treatment. Podophyllin has been shown to inhibit mitosis, leading to cell death. Topical applications of limited amounts (less than 0.5 mL per application) are made to the lesions and followed by thorough washing in 1 to 4 hours.[75] Applications can be repeated weekly as needed by health care providers to avoid the possibility of complications. In several clinical trials, podophyllin treatment was associated with initial clearance of warts in 32 to 79% of patients, with recurrence within 9 months seen in 27 to 65% of patients.[72] Systemic absorption of topically applied podophyllin can occur. The use of podophyllin is contraindicated during pregnancy.

The preferred self-treatment preparation is podofilox (podophyllotoxin), the most biologically active component of podophyllin as a 0.5% solution or gel.[76] Limited topical application of podofilox (less than 0.25 mL per application) is made to warts twice daily for 3 days, followed by a 4-day period of no treatment. Treatment cycles can be repeated as needed for up to four cycles. Complete clearance of warts has been described in 45 to 88% of patients, with recurrence within 3 months observed in 33 to 60% of these patients.[72] Local irritation associated with the use of podofilox is usually mild but does appear to be more frequent than that reported with podophyllin use. Podofilox has not been approved for the treatment of perianal, rectal, vaginal, or urethral warts.

An alternative treatment is imiquimod 5% cream applied once daily at bedtime, three times a week for as long as 16 weeks. Six to 10 hours after application the treatment area should be washed with mild soap. Like podophyllin, podofilox and imiquimod are contraindicated during pregnancy. These treatments are patient-applied therapies.

An alternative treatment option that is administered by the provider is trichloroacetic acid (80 to 90%) applied to the genital warts followed by powdering of the area with talc or baking soda to remove excess unreacted acid. Application can be made at weekly intervals as required.[70] Cryotherapy, performed by a health care provider using liquid nitrogen or a cryoprobe, produces results similar to those reported with podofilox and podophyllin.[72] In limited uncontrolled studies, topical 5% 5-fluorouracil has been reported to produce complete clearance of vulvovaginal warts in up to 68% of women, with 6- to 12-month recurrence rates of less than 10%. Intralesional injection of interferon-α 2b for external genital warts produced complete clearing in 44 to 60% of patients, and no recurrences were seen in these patients with limited short-term follow-up.[72] When intralesional interferon injection was combined with topical podophyllin, the response observed was superior to that seen with podophyllin alone, particularly in non–HIV-infected patients who had warts for less than 1 year. Systemic interferon administration in combination with other treatment options has not been associated with any improvement in response rates. The use of CO_2 laser therapy has produced disappointing results in limited clinical evaluations.[72]

KEY POINTS

- Health care professionals have a responsibility to contribute to the efforts to reduce the ever-expanding prevalence of sexually transmitted diseases.
- Infected patients and their sexual partners must be identified and treated appropriately, consistent with recently published CDC guidelines.
- Infected patients and their sexual partners must be counseled about the nature of their disease and methods that can be used to reduce the transmission of all STDs.
- Advances in drug therapy have led to safe and effective treatment regimens for most STDs that are also relatively inexpensive and easy to follow.
- Compliance has been enhanced for several diseases through the development of regimens requiring only a single dose of medication.

REFERENCES

1. Piot P, Islam MQ. Sexually transmitted diseases in the 1990s: global epidemiology and challenges for control. Sex Transm Dis 21(Suppl 2):S7–S13, 1994.
2. Gerbase A, Rowley J, Mertens T. Global epidemiology of sexually transmitted diseases. Lancet 351(S3):2–4, 1998.

3. Centers for Disease Control and Prevention. Addressing emerging infectious disease threats: a prevention strategy for the United States. Atlanta, GA: US Department of Health and Human Services, Public Health Service, 1994.
4. Adimora AA, Hamilton H, Holmes KK, et al. Sexually transmitted diseases: companion handbook. 2nd ed. New York: McGraw-Hill, 1994:25–40.
5. Centers for Disease Control and Prevention. Summary of notifiable diseases, United States, 1996. MMWR Morb Mortal Wkly Rep 45(53):1–81, 1997.
6. Rothenberg R, Judson FN. The clinical diagnosis of urethral discharge. Sex Transm Dis 10:24–28, 1983.
7. Handsfield HH, Sparling PF. *Neisseria gonorrhoeae.* In: Mandell GL, Bennet JE, Dolin R, eds. Principles and practice of infectious diseases. 4th ed. New York: Churchill Livingstone, 1995:1909–1926.
8. Judson F. Gonorrhea. Med Clin North Am 74:1353–1366, 1990.
9. Moran JS, Levine WC. Drugs of choice for the treatment of uncomplicated gonococcal infections. Clin Infect Dis 20(Suppl 1):S47–S65, 1995.
10. Centers for Disease Control and Prevention. 1998 Guidelines for treatment of sexually transmitted diseases. MMWR Morb Mortal Wkly Rep 47(RR-1):49–70, 1998.
11. Hook EW, Roddy RE, Handsfield HH. Ceftriaxone therapy for incubating and early syphilis. J Infect Dis 158:881–884, 1988.
12. Handsfield HH, McCormack WM, Hook EW, et al. A comparison of single dose cefixime with ceftriaxone as treatment for uncomplicated gonorrhea. N Engl J Med 325:1337–1341, 1991.
13. Centers for Disease Control and Prevention. Decreased susceptibility of *Neisseria gonorrhoeae* to fluoroquinolones: Ohio and Hawaii, 1992–1994. MMWR Morb Mortal Wkly Rep 43(18):325–327, 1994.
14. Centers for Disease Control and Prevention. Fluoroquinolone-resistant *Neisseria gonorrhoeae*–San Diego, CA, 1997. MMWR Morb Mortal Wkly Rep 47(20):405–408, 1998.
15. Handsfield HH, Dalu ZA, Martin DH, et al. Multicenter trial of single-dose azithromycin vs. ceftriaxone in the treatment of uncomplicated gonorrhea. Sex Transm Dis 21:107–111, 1994.
16. Adimora AA, Hamilton H, Holmes KK, et al. Sexually transmitted diseases: companion handbook. 2nd ed. New York: McGraw-Hill, 1994:271–280.
17. Bowie WR, Wang SP, Alexander ER, et al. Etiology of non-gonococcal urethritis: evidence for *Chlamydia trachomatis* and *Ureaplasma urealyticum.* J Clin Invest 59:735–742, 1977.
18. Martin DT. Chlamydial infections. Med Clin North Am 74:1367–1388, 1990.
19. Schacter J, Stoner E, Moncada JL, et al. Screening for chlamydial infection in women attending family planning clinics: evaluation of presumptive indicators for therapy. West J Med 138:375, 1983.
20. Coleman P, Varitek V, Muchahwar IK, et al. Testpack chlamydia: a new rapid assay for the detection of *Chlamydia trachomatis.* J Clin Microbiol 27:2811–2814, 1989.
21. Black CM. Current methods of laboratory diagnosis of *Chlamydia trachomatis* infections. Clin Microbiol Rev, 10:160–184, 1997.
22. Martin DH, Mroczkowski TF, Dalu ZA, et al. A controlled trial of a single dose of azithromycin for the treatment of chlamydial urethritis and cervicitis. N Engl J Med 327:921–925, 1992.
23. Whatley JD, Thin RN, Mumtaz G, et al. Azithromycin vs doxycycline in the treatment of non-gonococcal urethritis. Int J STD AIDS 2:248–251, 1991.
24. Weber JT, Johnson RE. New treatments for *Chlamydia trachomatis* genital infection. Clin Infect Dis 2(Suppl):S66–S71, 1995.
25. Augenbraun MH, Cummings M, McCormack WM. Management of chronic urethral symptoms in men. Clin Infect Dis 15:714–715, 1992.
26. Hooton TM, Rogers MR, Medina TG, et al. Ciprofloxacin compared with doxycycline for nongonococcal urethritis: ineffectiveness against *Chlamydia trachomatis* due to relapsing infection. JAMA 264:1418–1421, 1990.
27. Magid D, Douglas J, Schwartz S. Doxycycline compared with azithromycin for treating women with genital *Chlamydia trachomatis* infections: An incremental cost-effectiveness analysis. Ann Intern Med 124:389–399, 1996.
28. Lea A, Lamb HM. Azithromycin. A pharmacoeconomic review of its use as a single-dose regimen in the treatment of uncomplicated urogenital *Chlamydia trachomatis* infections in women. Pharmacoeconomics 12:596–611, 1997.
29. Adimora AA, Hamilton H, Holmes KK, et al. Sexually transmitted diseases: companion handbook. 2nd ed. New York: McGraw-Hill, 1994:63–86.
30. Tramont EC. *Treponema pallidum* (syphilis). In: Mandell GL, Bennet JE, Dolin R, eds. Principles and practice of infectious diseases. 4th ed. New York: Churchill Livingstone, 1995:2117–2133.
31. Centers for Disease Control. Primary and secondary syphilis: United States, 1981–1990. MMWR Morb Mortal Wkly Rep 40(19):314–323, 1991.
32. Centers for Disease Control. Primary and secondary syphilis: United States, 1997. MMWR Morb Mortal Wkly Rep 47(24):493–497, 1997.
33. Hook EW, Marra CM. Acquired syphilis in adults. N Engl J Med 326:1060–1069, 1992.
34. Chapel TA. The signs and symptoms of secondary syphilis. Sex Transm Dis 7:161–165, 1980.
35. Flores J. Syphilis–a tale of twisted treponemes. West J Med 163:552–559, 1995.
36. Fitzgerald TJ. Treponema. In: Balow A, Hausler WJ, Herrmann KL, et al., eds. Manual of clinical microbiology. 5th ed. Washington, DC: American Society for Microbiology, 1991:567–571.
37. Larsen SA. Syphilis. Clin Lab Med 9:545–557, 1989.
38. Quinn TC, Zenilman J, Rompalo A. Sexually transmitted diseases: advances in diagnosis and treatment. Adv Intern Med 39:149–196, 1994.
39. Romanowski B, Sutherland R, Fick GH, et al. Serologic response to treatment of infectious syphilis. Ann Intern Med 114:1005–1009, 1991.
40. Zenker PN, Rolfs RT. Treatment of syphilis, 1989. Rev Infect Dis 12(Suppl 6):S590–S609, 1990.
41. Wolters EC. Treatment of neurosyphilis. Clin Neuropharmacol 10:143–154, 1987.
42. Centers for Disease Control. 1998 guidelines for treatment of sexually transmitted diseases. MMWR Morb Mortal Wkly Rep 47(RR-1):29–49, 1998.
43. Rolfs RT. Treatment of syphilis, 1993. Clin Infect Dis 20(Suppl 1):S23–S38, 1995.
44. Wendel GD, Stark BJ, Jamison RB, et al. Penicillin allergy and desensitization in serious infections during pregnancy. N Engl J Med 312:1229–1232, 1985.
45. Adimora AA, Hamilton H, Holmes KK, et al. Sexually transmitted diseases: companion handbook. 2nd ed. New York: McGraw-Hill, 1994:135–154.
46. Centers for Disease Control. 1998 guidelines for treatment of sexually transmitted diseases. MMWR Morb Mortal Wkly Rep 47(RR-1):20–24, 1998.
47. Guinan ME, Wolinsky SN, Reichman RC. Epidemiology of genital herpes simplex virus infection. Epidemiol Rev 7:127–132, 1985.
48. Whitley R, Kimberlin D, Roizman B. Herpes simplex viruses. Clin Infect Dis 26:541–555, 1998.
49. Blanchier H, Huraux JM, Hurauz-Rendu C, et al. Genital herpes and pregnancy: preventive measures. Eur J Obstet Gynecol Reprod Biol 53:33–38, 1994.
50. de Ruiter A, Thin RN. Genital herpes: a guide to pharmacologic therapy. Drugs 47:297–304, 1994.
51. Fife KH, Crumpacker CS, Mertz GJ, et al. Recurrence and resistance patterns of herpes simplex virus following cessation of 6 years of chronic suppression with acyclovir. J Infect Dis 169:1338–1341, 1994.
52. Reitano M, Tyring S, Lang W, et al. Valaciclovir for the suppression of recurrent genital herpes simplex virus infection: a large scale dose range-finding study. J Infect Dis 178:603–610, 1998.
53. Diaz-Mitoma F, Sibbald G, Shafron S, et al. Oral famciclovir for the suppression of recurrent genital herpes. JAMA 280:887–892, 1998.
54. Perry CM, Faulds D. Valaciclovir. A review of its antiviral activity, pharmacokinetic properties and therapeutic efficacy in herpesvirus infections. Drugs 52:754–772, 1996.
55. Perry CM, Wagstaff AJ. Famciclovir: a review of its pharmacological properties and therapeutic efficacy in herpesvirus infections. Drugs 50:396–415, 1995.
56. Acyclovir product information (package insert). Data on file. Glaxo Wellcome Inc. 1996.
57. Adimora AA, Hamilton H, Holmes KK, et al. Sexually transmitted diseases: companion handbook. 2nd ed. New York: McGraw-Hill, 1994:87–92.
58. Centers for Disease Control and Prevention. 1998 guidelines for treatment of sexually transmitted diseases. MMWR Morb Mortal Wkly Rep 47(RR-1):18–20, 1998.
59. Schulte JM, Schmid GP. Recommendations for treatment of chancroid, 1993. Clin Infect Dis 20(Suppl 1):S39–S46, 1995.
60. Adimora AA, Hamilton H, Holmes KK, et al. Sexually transmitted diseases: companion handbook. 2nd ed. New York: McGraw-Hill, 1994:212–222.
61. Kent HL. Epidemiology of vaginitis. Am J Obstet Gynecol 165:1168–1176, 1991.
62. Muller M, Rein ME. *Trichomonas vaginalis.* In: Holmes KK, Mardh PA, Sparking PF, et al., eds. Sexually transmitted diseases. 2nd ed. New York: McGraw-Hill, 1990:481–492.
63. Grossman JH, Galash RP. Persistent vaginitis caused by metronidazole-resistant trichomoniasis. Obstet Gynecol 76:521–522, 1990.
64. Kriega JN, Jenny C, Verdon M, et al. Clinical manifestations of trichomoniasis in men. Ann Intern Med 118:844–949, 1993.
65. Rein MF. Trichomoniasis vaginalis. In: Mandell GL, Bennet JE, Dolin R, eds. Principles and practice of infectious diseases. 4th ed. New York: Churchill Livingstone, 1995:2493–2497.
66. Centers for Disease Control and Prevention. 1998 guidelines for treatment of sexually transmitted diseases. MMWR Morb Mortal Wkly Rep 47(RR-1):74–75, 1998.
67. Perine PL, Osoba AO. Lymphogranuloma venereum. In: Holmes KK, Mardh PA, Sparling PF, et al., eds. Sexually transmitted diseases. 2nd ed. New York: McGraw-Hill, 1990:195–204.

68. Adimora AA, Hamilton H, Holmes KK, et al. Sexually transmitted diseases: companion handbook. 2nd ed. New York: McGraw-Hill, 1994:56–62.
69. Centers for Disease Control. 1998 guidelines for treatment of sexually transmitted diseases. MMWR Morb Mortal Wkly Rep 47(RR-1):27–28, 1998.
70. Adimora AA, Hamilton H, Holmes KK, et al. Sexually transmitted diseases: companion handbook. 2nd ed. New York: McGraw-Hill, 1994: 162–174.
71. Reid R, Greenberg M, Jenson AB, et al. Sexually transmitted papilloma viral infections. I. The anatomic distribution and pathologic grade of neoplastic lesions associated with different viral types. Am J Obstet 156:212–218, 1987.
72. Stone KM. Human papillomavirus infection and genital warts: update on epidemiology and treatment. Clin Infect Dis 20(Suppl 1):S91–S97, 1995.
73. Howley PM, Schlegel R. The human papillomaviruses: an overview. Am J Med 85:155–172, 1988.
74. Kraus ST, Stone KM. Management of genital infection caused by human papillomavirus. Rev Infect Dis 12(Suppl 6):S620–S632, 1990.
75. Centers for Disease Control and Prevention. 1998 guidelines for treatment of sexually transmitted diseases. MMWR Morb Mortal Wkly Rep 47(RR-1):88–98, 1998.
76. Podofilox for genital warts. Med Lett Drugs Ther 33:117–118, 1991.

CHAPTER 76

HUMAN IMMUNODEFICIENCY VIRUS (HIV) INFECTION—ANTIRETROVIRAL THERAPY

Betty J. Dong

DEFINITION

Human immunodeficiency virus (HIV) is a retrovirus that can be divided into HIV-1 and HIV-2. HIV-1 is the predominant infection found in the United States and is the subtype addressed in this chapter. HIV-2 is found primarily in Africa. Both types of HIV infection deplete the helper T-lymphocytes (CD4 cell/mm^3), resulting in continued destruction of the immune system, and leading to the occurrence of opportunistic infections and malignancies. A person infected with HIV is defined by the Centers for Disease Control and Prevention (CDC) as having positive antibodies against HIV (positive HIV test), with 200 or more helper T-lymphocytes (CD4 cell/mm^3), and the absence of an acquired immunodeficiency syndrome (AIDS)-defining illness.[1] By definition then, an HIV-infected person with AIDS has fewer than 200 cells/mm^3 CD4 cells or the presence of an AIDS-defining illness (Table 76.1).

TREATMENT GOALS: HIV INFECTION

During the last decade, promising evidence of immune system reconstitution, and dramatic reductions in opportunistic infections, disease progression to AIDS, and death from the use of potent combinations of antiretroviral agents have led to widespread enthusiasm that HIV might be eradicated.[2–4] However, the discovery of latent, resting reservoirs of HIV that are inaccessible to current antiretroviral agents have dampened optimism for a "cure."[5–7] Eradication of HIV is highly unlikely and effective antiretroviral therapy is required chronically to maintain viral suppression and reduce disease progression. During the next decade, effective therapies aimed at continued suppression of HIV replication and targeted at resting HIV reservoirs will be critical to prolong survival and renew hopes for a "cure." The goals of antiretroviral therapy are to:

- Reduce symptoms from HIV infection and delay disease progression to AIDS.
- Minimize AIDS-related opportunistic infections and malignancies.
- Improve quality of life and prolong survival.
- Reduce viral load to undetectable levels or lowest levels possible for as long as possible.
- Maintain durability of viral suppression.
- Eliminate resting reservoirs of HIV.
- Increase CD4 lymphocyte count.
- Reduce viral resistance and drug failure.
- Reconstitute the immune system.

Table 76.1 ▪ 1993 AIDS-defining Illness from CDC

Candidiasis of esophagus, bronchi, trachea, or lungs
Cervical cancer, invasive
Coccidioidomycosis, disseminated or extrapulmonary
Cryptococcoses, extrapulmonary
Cryptosporidiosis, chronic intestinal (>1 month duration)
Cytomegalovirus disease other than liver, spleen, or nodes
Cytomegalovirus retinitis with vision loss
Encephalopathy, HIV-related
Herpes simplex: chronic ulcers (>1 month), bronchitis, pneumonitis, or esophagitis
Histoplasmosis, disseminated or extrapulmonary
Isosporiasis, chronic intestinal (>1 month)
Kaposi's sarcoma
Lymphoma Burkitt's (or equivalent term)
Lymphoma immunoblastic (or equivalent term)
Lymphoma, primary, of brain
Mycobacterium avium complex or *Mycobacterium kansasii*, disseminated or extrapulmonary
Pneumocystis carinii pneumonia (PCP)
Pneumonia, recurrent
Progressive multifocal leukoencephalopathy (PML)
Salmonella septicemia, recurrent
Toxoplasmosis of the brain
Tuberculosis
Wasting syndrome, HIV-related

Source: Reference 1.

- Prevent perinatal transmission from mother to fetus.
- Prevent HIV infection from high-risk occupational or nonoccupational exposures.
- Design effective therapeutic regimens that minimize drug adherence problems.
- Reduce total pill burden and minimize interference with quality of life.

EPIDEMIOLOGY

HIV infection is acquired by contact with infected blood or hazardous body fluids through unprotected sexual intercourse, contact with contaminated drug paraphernalia, transfusion of infected blood products, and vertical transmission from mother to infant. Although urine, tears, and saliva can contain HIV, transmission is rare. Protease-like inhibitor substances found in saliva can inhibit HIV's ability to enter the white blood cells.[8] One case of HIV infection, reported after deep kissing, is presumed related to contact with infected blood from poor dentition and gingivitis. Individuals who lack a coreceptor required for HIV cell entry do not acquire HIV infection despite repeated high-risk exposures.[9]

Experts estimate infection risks from a single unprotected sexual exposure with an infected sexual partner at 1/1000 to 1/10,000 depending on the type of the exposure.[10] The highest probability of HIV transmission is associated with unprotected receptive anal intercourse (0.8 to 3.2%) with a partner infected with HIV; lower risks are estimated with vaginal intercourse (0.05 to 0.15%). The risk of HIV infection after a percutaneous occupational exposure to a contaminated needle is estimated to be 0.3% or 1/300. The likelihood of infection is increased by a deep puncture, a device used in an artery or vein, a visibly bloody device, or exposure to a source patient who died of AIDS within 2 months. The risk from bloody mucocutaneous exposures (e.g., eye or mouth splashes) is estimated to be 1/3000. The estimated HIV probability after the use of contaminated injection drug paraphernalia (0.67%) is slightly higher than that associated with a puncture in an occupational setting, which may reflect the greater volume of blood transferred when sharing. In two large trials, the risks of perinatal HIV transmission to the infant was reported to be 19 and 23%.[11,12] The greatest risk for perinatal transmission likely occurs near to or during delivery. HIV can also be transmitted through breast milk; and breastfeeding should be avoided in mothers infected with HIV. Since 1985, surveillance of U.S. blood products have significantly reduced the chance of contaminated transfusions; the risk is estimated to be 1/450,000 to 1/660,000 transfusions or two cases per million.

Worldwide, the United Nations Joint Commission on AIDS (UNAIDS) estimates that 33.6 million adults and children are living with HIV/AIDS. In 1997, there were 5.8 million new cases of HIV infection globally; of which 2.1 million were in women. As of December 1997, there are 641,086 Americans living with AIDS. From January 1994 through June 1997, HIV was diagnosed in 72,905 persons residing in 25 states with HIV/AIDS surveillance programs.[13] Of these, AIDS was the initial diagnosis in 28% (20,215 persons). HIV infection was the initial diagnosis in 72% (52,690 persons); of whom 18% were infected through heterosexual contact. The groups at highest risk included African Americans (57%), men who have sex with men (32%), and women (28%). Substantial increased rates of infections were also noted in Hispanics (10%) and young adults aged 13 to 24 years of age. People aged 50 years or older represented approximately 10% of new AIDS cases diagnosed in 1995. Although the epidemic has disproportionately affected certain ethnic minorities, ethnicity is not considered a risk factor for HIV but a marker for other factors that might be predictive of increased risk for HIV infection (e.g., low income, history of injection drug use, high-risk sex, lack of education). Since the beginning of the epidemic, more than 11.7 million have died from AIDS. AIDS constitutes the fifth leading cause of death among Americans aged 25 to 44 years, and is the primary cause of death among African Americans in that age group. For the first time, the CDC recorded a 25% reduction in AIDS-related deaths between 1995 and 1996 that was primarily attributed to the introduction of highly active antiretroviral combinations, and effective prophylaxis against opportunistic infections.[2–4]

PATHOPHYSIOLOGY

The RNA-containing HIV virus requires the creation of proviral DNA within the host to complete its life cycle and infect other cells (Fig. 76.1). The envelope of the HIV virus contains a structure known as glycoprotein (gp 120) that binds to the CD4 receptor. Cell entry also requires the presence of a chemokine coreceptor, CCR5.[9] Viral RNA is uncoated before being transcribed by the reverse transcriptase (RT) enzyme into proviral DNA. The proviral DNA is integrated into the host nucleus by the integrase enzyme. The integrated viral genes may remain inactive or be transcribed back into genomic RNA and messenger RNA, which are then translated into viral proteins. Finally, the viral proteins are cleaved by the protease enzyme into new HIV particles, assembled, and new infectious virions are released to infect other cells.

Viral kinetics, replication, and clearance have been clarified. Viral replication is an ongoing and dynamic process that results in the progressive destruction of CD4 lymphocytes and continued immune depletion. Approximately 1 to 10 billion virions are produced daily to maintain a steady state of viral replication, even during a period of clinical latency. Using mathematical modeling, the half-life of free virus is estimated to be 6 hours. Infected memory CD4 lymphocytes serve as latent reservoirs of HIV infection, making eradication difficult.[5–7] It has been estimated that antiretroviral therapy would have to be maintained for a minimum of 5 to 7 years in order to eliminate these latent reservoirs; larger reservoirs would require durations of 10 years or more.[14]

After initial HIV infection, there is immediate widespread dissemination of the virus to other lymphatic systems and organs (e.g., brain). The majority of persons during primary infection exhibit some nonspecific symptoms of an acute viral infection. High plasma viremia (HIV RNA viral load or burden >10^7 copies/mL) is detected in blood and present in sexual organs and secretions. Infectivity is high during acute primary infection. During acute infection, the appearance of potent, cytotoxic CD8 T-lymphocytes from a highly activated immune system limits viral replication and reduces symptomology as plasma viremia declines.[15,16] In adults, a new steady-state plasma HIV RNA "viral setpoint" is established 6 months or longer after the initial infection that can remain stable for months or years before progression to AIDS. Because infected individuals have different steady-state levels of viral replication, it is important to identify their plasma HIV RNA level before starting therapy. In infants infected with HIV, the new viral "setpoint" is often not reached until more than a year after infection.

The time course of progression to AIDS can be quite variable in adults; however, average durations of 10 to 11 years are reported in the absence of antiretroviral therapy. Approximately 5 to 10% of persons infected with HIV

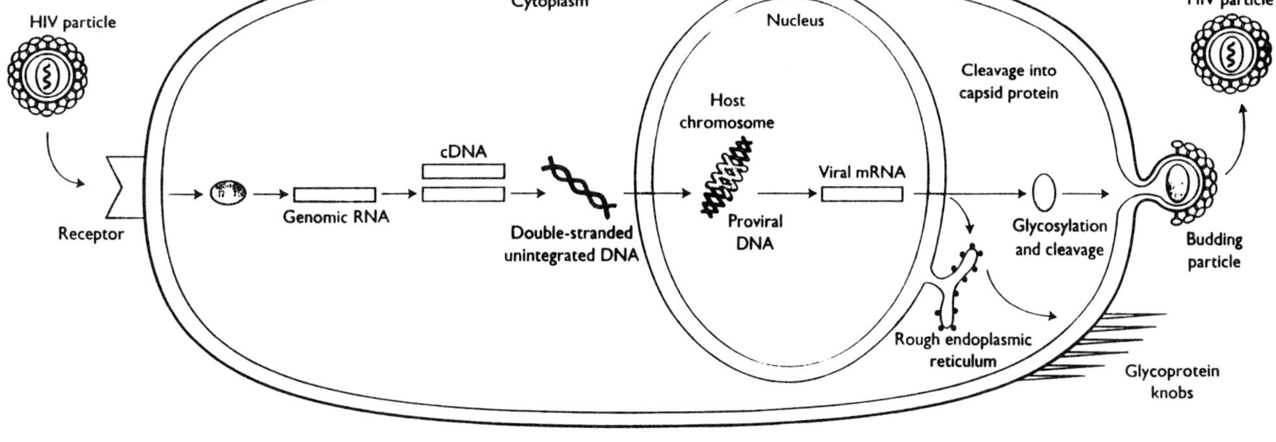

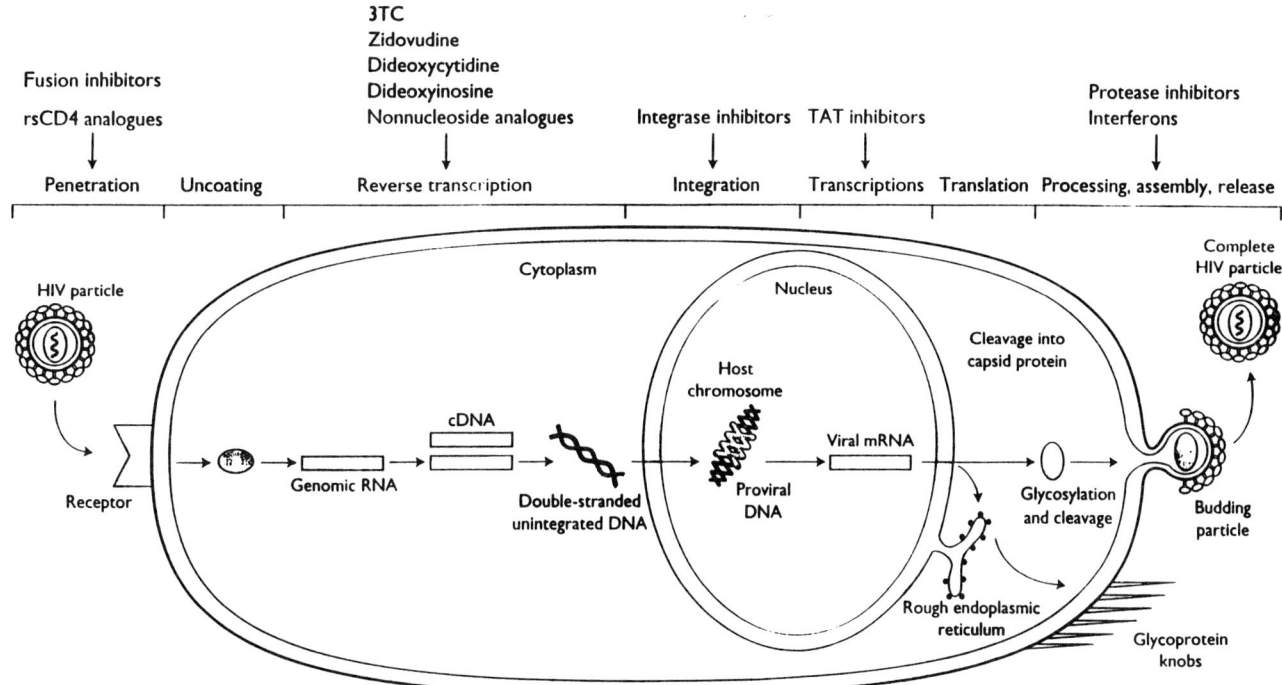

Figure 76.1. Life cycle of HIV-1 and sites of action for antiretroviral therapy. Adapted with permission from Mandell GL, Mildvan D. Atlas of infectious diseases. 2nd ed. Philadelphia: Current Medicine, 1997, vol I, ch 19.

have not been reported to progress to AIDS and are identified as long-term nonprogressors (LTNP). These HIV-infected LTNP remain asymptomatic with stable CD4 counts and low plasma viremia more than 15 years after their infection. It is believed that a strong humoral immune response from strong cytotoxic T-lymphocyte responses (e.g., enhanced CD8+ suppression) limits cell death (apoptosis) and disease progression.[17] Currently, there is no accurate commercial method to identify these long-term nonprogressors.

The CD4+ cell count has been used as an indicator of the extent of immune damage and risk of opportunistic infections rather than the plasma viral load tests. Persons with CD4 counts lower than 200 cells/mm^3 are predisposed to a variety of opportunistic infections, including *Pneumocystis carinii* pneumonia (Table 76.1). As the CD4 counts drop below 50 cells/mm^3, the prevalence of other infections, including *Mycobacterium avium-intracellulare* and *Cytomegalovirus* disease, increases. A landmark study showed that steady-state plasma HIV RNA levels are highly predictive of disease progression and can be elevated in persons with normal or low levels of CD4 counts. Persons with the highest viral loads depleted CD4+ counts quicker, had more rapid disease progression to AIDS, and died earlier than those with the lowest viral loads.[18] Although an inverse relationship is usually seen between viral load and CD4+ counts, a small percentage of persons may exhibit discordance between CD4+ and viral load. The significance of this discordance is unknown.

Treatment with highly active antiretroviral agents (HAART) has produced dramatic reductions in AIDS-related hospitalizations, opportunistic infections, and prolonged time of survival. Potent antiretroviral therapy can extend the time to development of AIDS and death in persons infected with HIV.[2–4] HAART is also the best treatment for HIV-related complications, including HIV-related nephropathy and progressive multifocal leukoencephalopathy (PML).[19,20] HAART may also allow modifications of primary and secondary antibiotic prophylaxis for multiple opportunistic infections.[21,22] In children with symptomatic HIV disease, HAART has produced improvements not only in immunologic and virologic measures but also in neurodevelopment and growth. Data on long-term outcome and efficacy in children are limited and clinical trials are needed.

CLINICAL PRESENTATION AND DIAGNOSIS

Signs and Symptoms

The clinical presentation of an acute primary HIV infection can be confused with a typical viral illness; however, it should be suspected in persons with a history of high-risk behaviors or presence of sexually transmitted disease. Common signs and symptoms are nonspecific, generally occur within days to weeks after the initial exposure, and include fever, fatigue, myalgias, arthralgias, headache, lymphadenopathy, pharyngitis, and oral lesions.[23] A maculopapular rash is present in 40 to 80% of persons during the acute illness. Symptoms last approximately 10 to 14 days but may continue for several weeks; prolonged symptoms are indicative of a poorer prognosis and more rapid disease progression.

Patients with established HIV infection can remain clinically asymptomatic for many years, or develop symptomatic disease (e.g., unexplained low-grade fevers, thrush, or symptoms of AIDS) (Table 76.1).

Diagnosis

Established HIV infection is diagnosed by finding antibodies to HIV in the plasma using various serological testing methods. The initial screening test for detection of anti-HIV antibodies is the ELISA (enzyme-linked immunosorbent assays). However, because a false-positive ELISA can occur in those with collagen vascular diseases, chronic hepatitis, and other conditions, all positive ELISA results must be confirmed by a Western blot before a diagnosis of HIV infection can be made. The accuracy of the Western blot is excellent, the specificity (likelihood that a person without infection will have a negative test) and sensitivity (likelihood that a person with infection will have a positive test) is greater than 99.9%. In neonates, the diagnosis of HIV infection is difficult because of the presence of passive maternal HIV antibodies, which can persist for many months.

A major disadvantage of serial HIV testing by ELISA, and then the Western blot, is that the 1- to 2-week delay for availability of test results can result in loss of infected persons for followup and treatment. In 1995, 25% of persons testing HIV positive and 33% of persons testing negative did not return for their results.[24] The only rapid HIV assay licensed by the FDA, SUDS (Single-Use Diagnostic System), can provide accurate results within 10 to 15 minutes of testing and may improve followup. Validation of these results in persons infected with HIV have demonstrated comparable sensitivity to standard tests but a lower specificity (91.8 to 99.5%); therefore, no further confirmatory testing is needed if the SUDS test is negative. However, to eliminate the possibility of a false-positive test, a positive SUDS test should be considered inconclusive until the results are confirmed by the Western blot.

Urine and saliva tests for HIV infection may be useful when collection of blood is not possible. OraSure HIV-1, an FDA-approved oral device for use by health care workers, uses a specially treated pad that is placed between the lower cheek and gum for 2 minutes. The pad creates an osmotic gradient that draws out HIV antibodies from the tissues of the oral mucosa transudate before the pad is sent for testing by HIV-1 enzyme immunoassay (EIA). All positive EIA are repeated and then confirmed by OraSure Western blot. Results are comparable to those obtained by serum testing, yielding a specificity of 99.9%. The Sentinel HIV-1 Urine EIA is a urine HIV-1 test approved by the FDA in August 1996 that is only available to health care professionals. The sensitivity and specificity of this test to detect HIV antibodies in urine (99.3%) are less than HIV tests for serum and saliva. A repeatedly positive urine EIA should be confirmed by a serum Western blot.

One home HIV-1 testing kit, Home Access HIV-1 Test System, is available in pharmacies and by mail. Confide, another home testing kit marketed in 1996, was withdrawn because of testing difficulties. The advantages of home testing are confidentiality and convenience if the $40 to $50 expenses are not prohibitive. Concerns about adequate pre- and post-test counseling and support for patients with positive results have not been documented. The user pricks a fingertip with the supplied lancet to collect the blood specimen, which is then sent to a central testing laboratory. The reported sensitivity and specificity is 100% provided that the specimens are collected properly. Once the specimens are received, EIA results are available by telephone within 3 to 7 days. All persons with positive or indeterminate results are referred immediately to a counselor. New home HIV tests that could provide results in less than 10 minutes are currently awaiting FDA approval and are expected on the market in the near future.

During primary HIV infection, the routine diagnostic HIV tests are not positive until 22 to 27 days after the acute infection.[23] In a high-risk patient with a negative Western blot test, elevated plasma viral RNA levels (e.g., >50,000 copies/mL) or the detection of the p24 antigen can establish the diagnosis of an acute HIV infection. Because false-positive results can occur, the diagnosis of HIV infection should not be made on the basis of low viral titers (<3000 RNA copies/mL). A positive Western blot is essential to confirm the existence of HIV infection.

Monitoring Viral Assays

The ability to measure the viral load (VL) or burden (amount of virus in the blood) has revolutionized HIV care. Plasma HIV RNA assays can assess the risk of disease progression and evaluate the efficacy of antiretroviral therapy.[18] The commercially available plasma HIV RNA assays differ in sensitivity so that it is critical to use the same assay to evaluate and monitor VL changes. The first generation RNA assays include the branched DNA (bDNA by Chiron), reverse transcriptase polymerase chain reaction (RT-PCR by Roche Amplicor), and nucleic acid sequence based amplification (NASBA by Organon). The NASBA and RT-PCR both amplify the viral RNA to detectable levels, whereas the bDNA technique amplifies the detection signal from the viral RNA. The lower limit of assay detection for the bDNA is 500 copies/mL, whereas the RT-PCR by Amplicor and NASBA is 400 copies/mL. Plasma HIV RNA levels obtained by the RT-PCR are approximately two times higher than those obtained by the bDNA assay. Compared to these first generation plasma HIV RNA assays, the newer ultrasensitive assay can detect levels of HIV RNA as low as 20 to 50 copies/mL.

Before starting antiretroviral therapy, establishment of a baseline VL is recommended to monitor the effectiveness of the antiretroviral regimen. The baseline is determined by averaging at least two viral loads taken a few weeks apart that do not differ by more than 0.5 $\log^{10}$. Within 2 to 8 weeks after starting an effective antiretroviral regimen that the virus is sensitive to, a 0.5 to 1 log (tenfold) reduction in plasma HIV RNA from baseline should be observed. Although the goal of therapy is an undetectable VL (e.g., below the current assay's limits of detection), it is important to note that the maximal reduction in VL may not occur until 4 to 6 months after starting therapy. Therefore, changes in therapy before this time are not recommended if there is a consistent downward trend in VL reduction, indicating a therapeutic response. Patients with advanced HIV disease or those with a history of multiple combination therapies may not ever attain complete viral suppression. Even patients with undetectable viral loads measured by the less sensitive viral assays often show detectable viral levels when measured by the ultrasensitive assays. Routine monitoring of VL is recommended every 8 to 12 weeks after starting therapy or after a change in the antiretroviral regimen. Treatment failure is suggested by a greater than 0.5 $\log^{10}$ increase in viral load when compared with the patient's most recent VL. Therefore, before establishing treatment failure, it is imperative to eliminate any factors that might elevate plasma HIV RNA levels transiently and alter interpretation of viral loads. For example, viral loads should not be determined within 1 month following immunizations or treatment of concurrent infections (e.g., herpes, tuberculosis, etc.).

THERAPEUTIC PLAN

National HIV disease guidelines on antiretroviral agents in adults have been published by the Department of Health and Human Services (DHHS) and the Henry J. Kaiser Family Foundation.[25] Similar recommendations for antiretroviral therapy in adults have also been developed by the International AIDS Society, USA panel.[26] Additional guidelines for using antiretroviral agents in pediatrics, pregnancy, for prophylaxis after occupational exposures, and a statement regarding prophylaxis after nonoccupational exposures have been developed by the Centers for Disease Control and Prevention (CDC).[27–30] Updates in these national guidelines can be obtained at the following websites: http://hivinsite.ucsf.edu; http://ucsf.itsa.edu/warmline; http://www.cdc.gov. The British HIV Association Guidelines recommend a more conservative approach to care of the adult infected with HIV.[31] Physicians with greater experience in the care of persons infected with HIV may be more knowledgeable about current treatment guidelines that may impact on the quality of care given.[32]

The major classes of antiretroviral agents include the nucleoside reverse transcriptase inhibitors (NRTI)

Table 76.2 ▪ Nucleoside Reverse Transcriptase Inhibitors

Drug	Dosage Forms	Usual Doses
Zidovudine (ZDV, AZT) (Retrovir) In combination with 3TC	100-mg caps, 300-mg tabs; 10 mg/mL syrup; 10 mg/mL IV Combivir (3TC 150 mg + ZDV 300 mg)	200 mg TID or 300 mg BID (500–600 mg/day); 100 mg TID if needed to decrease anemia; Renal dysfunction: CrCl <25 mL/min 100 mg TID
Didanosine (ddI) (Videx)	25-, 50-, 100-, 150-, 200-mg chewable tabs; 100-, 167-, 250-mg powder packets; reconstituted pediatric powder (dilute with antacid) 10 mg/ml	(>60 kg) 200 mg BID or 400 mg QD (>60 kg) 125 mg BID or 300 mg QD (>60 kg) PWD 250 mg BID (<60 kg) 167 mg BID Renal dysfunction: CrCl 26–49 mL/min <25 mL/min (>60 kg) 200 mg QD 100 mg QD (<60 kg) 125 mg QD 50 mg QD
Zalcitabine (ddC) (Hivid)	0.375-, 0.75-mg tablets; 0.1 mg/mL syrup (investigational)	(>60 kg) 0.75 mg TID (<60 kg) 0.375 mg TID Renal dysfunction: CrCl 10–40 mL/min 0.75 mg BID <10 mL/min 0.75 mg QD
Stavudine (d4T) (Zerit)	15-, 20-, 30-, 40-mg capsules; 1 mg/mL solution	(>60 kg) 20–40 mg BID (<60 kg) 15–30 mg BID Lower dosages decrease risk of peripheral neuropathy. Renal dysfunction: CrCl 26–49 mL/min <25 mL/min ≥60 kg 40 mg QD 20 mg QD ≤60 kg 30 mg QD 15 mg QD
Lamivudine (3TC) (Epivir) In combination with ZDV	150-mg tablets; 10 mg/mL syrup; Combivir (3TC 150 mg + ZDV 300 mg)	(>50 kg) 150 mg BID (<50 kg) 2 mg/kg BID Renal dysfunction: CrCl 26–49 mL/min 150 mg QD 10–25 150 mg LD 100 mg QD <10 150 mg LD 25–50 mg QD 300 mg BID
Abacavir (ABC, 1592) (Ziagen)	300-mg tablets; 20 mg/mL liquid	No dosage adjustment for renal dysfunction.

CrCl, creatinine clearance; *LD,* loading dose.

(Table 76.2), the protease inhibitors (PI) (Table 76.3), and the nonnucleoside reverse transcriptase inhibitors (NNRTI) (Table 76.4). Adjuncts include hydroxyurea.

TREATMENT

Initiating Antiretroviral Therapy

Before starting any antiretroviral therapy, it is essential that clinicians educate patients about the need for strict adherence to these complex regimens in order to minimize the potential for drug failure and drug resistance. Willingness of the patient to be responsible for therapy, as well as the prognosis for AIDS-free survival, should be established before starting therapy. There is general consensus that all persons infected with HIV with AIDS or symptomatic HIV disease should promptly receive aggressive antiretroviral therapy. In asymptomatic individuals infected with HIV, the optimal time to start antiretroviral therapy is controversial; however, it is generally accepted that treatment should be started before immunologic and clinical deterioration occurs. In asymptomatic persons, the benefits of early intervention are less clear; therefore, some experts recommend that HIV+ persons should receive aggressive therapy, whereas others advocate delaying therapy until absolutely necessary.[33–35] For asymptomatic persons with CD4+ cell counts higher than 400 cells/mm^3 and low viral RNA levels (<30,000 copies/mL), treatment may be deferred, given that the benefits of early treatment in this cohort are unknown and might actually reduce the protective CD8 antiviral response. Observation and a delay in starting therapy may be appropriate, given the complexities and toxicities of treatment and the possibility that such persons might be long-term nonprogressors. The DHHS guidelines offer therapy to all asymptomatic persons infected with HIV with a plasma HIV RNA greater than 10,000 (bDNA) to 20,000 (RT-PCR) copies/mL or CD4+ cells less than 500/mm^3.[25] The International AIDS Society is more aggressive and recommends starting therapy in all

Special Administration Instructions	Selected Adverse Effects	Potential for Drug Interactions (see Table 76.9)
Can be given with meals to reduce nausea.	Headaches, fatigue, nausea, insomnia, anemia, neutropenia, thrombocytopenia, hepatitis, increase LFT, myopathy with >6 mo use, lactic acidosis with hepatic steatosis (rare)	Avoid concurrent bone marrow suppressive agents (e.g., ganciclovir induction, trimethoprim-sulfamethoxazole treatment).
Administer on an empty stomach (1 hr before or 2 hr after a meal) and at least >2 hr from agents whose absorption is impaired by the buffer. Must chew or crush 2 tablets/dose for adequate buffer.	Nausea, vomiting, diarrhea, painful peripheral neuropathy, pancreatitis, hyperglycemia, hyperuricemia, hypertriglyceridemia, hyperamylasemia, increase LFT, lactic acidosis with hepatic steatosis (rare)	Avoid or limit alcohol or other pancreatic toxins (e.g., IV pentamidine). Avoid concurrent neurotoxic agents (e.g., ddC).
Can be given with/without meals.	Nausea, headache, malaise, painful peripheral neuropathy, aphthous oral ulcer, pancreatitis, esophageal ulcers, rash, lactic acidosis with hepatic steatosis (rare)	Avoid alcohol or other pancreatic toxins (e.g., IV pentamidine). Avoid concurrent neurotoxic agents (e.g., ddI).
Can be given with/without meals	Painful peripheral neuropathy, insomnia, anxiety, panic reactions, increase LFT, lactic acidosis with hepatic steatosis (rare)	Avoid concurrent neurotoxic agents (e.g., ddC). Avoid antagonistic combination of ZDV and d4T.
Can be given with/without meals	Headache, fatigue, nausea, peripheral neuropathy, increase LFT, lactic acidosis with hepatic steatosis (rare); pancreatitis in children	No significant DI
Can be given with/without meals	Nausea, headache, malaise, diarrhea, abdominal pain, lactic acidosis with hepatic steatosis (rare). 3–5% hypersensitivity reaction which can be life-threatening: *Do not rechallenge*	No significant DI

asymptomatic patients with plasma HIV RNA levels (>5,000 [bDNA] to 10,000 [RT-PCR] copies/mL) regardless of the CD4 cell counts.[26] Others advocate that therapy should be started in women infected with HIV earlier (e.g., at lower viral loads) since they may have a 60% higher risk of progressing to AIDS than men with the same viral load. A viral load of 5,000 copies/mL in women was considered equivalent to 10,000 copies in men.[36] Guidelines for starting antiretroviral therapy are summarized in Table 76.5.

Selecting Antiretroviral Therapy Regimens

The basic principles for successful antiretroviral therapy are summarized in Table 76.6. Because the first therapeutic regimen selected in an antiretroviral-naive person is often the most successful in achieving maximal and durable viral suppression, it is a very important therapeutic decision that should be thoroughly planned. Preparing and educating the patient about the complexities of the therapeutic regimen before initiating therapy are essential. Similarly, the ability of a regimen to achieve these goals declines as the number of failed regimens increases or as the HIV progresses. An undetectable viral load is also associated with a lower risk of de novo mutations developing during selective pressure of therapy. Because the virus is error prone during viral replication, the likelihood of drug resistance is minimized if viral replication is low or undetectable. HIV must develop several mutations to become resistant to combination therapy, and mutations can only arise as a consequence of de novo mutations in the presence of antiretroviral agents. Development of resistance can limit future treatment options, because resistance developing within a class of agents usually confers resistance to other agents within the same class.

The goal of treatment should be to achieve maximal suppression to an undetectable viral load and possibly,

Table 76.3 ▪ Protease Inhibitors*

Drug	Dosage Forms	Usual Doses	Special Administration Instructions	Common Adverse Effects	Potential for Drug Interactions (see Table 76.9)
Saquinavir (HG-SAQ) (Invirase)	200-mg hard gel capsules	600-mg TID Doses of 3200–7200 mg/day more effective but not FDA approved.	Take 3 capsules/dose TID within 2 hr of a large/high-fat meal.	Generally well tolerated. GI (diarrhea, nausea, abdominal pain), headache, elevated LFTs, hyperlipidemia, hyperglycemia, lipodystrophy	Least potent CYP3A4 enzyme inhibitor
Saquinavir (SG-SAQ) (Fortovase)	200-mg soft-gel capsules. Three times improved bioavailability over HG-SAQ.	1200 mg TID	Take 6 capsules/dose TID with large meal.		
Dual saquinavir/ ritonavir combination therapy		400 mg BID HG or SG SAQ (see Table 76.7)*	Grapefruit juice increases saquinavir absorption (variable)		
Ritonavir (RTV) (Norvir)	100-mg capsules or 80 mg/mL oral solution (contains 43% ETOH) Both contain significant amount of ETOH.	Titration schedule: 300 mg BID (days 1–2) 400 mg BID (days 3–5) 500 mg BID (days 6–13) to full therapeutic 600 mg BID on day 14. No titration needed if lower dosages of RTV used in combination with other PI.	Take 6 capsules/dose or 7.5 mL BID with meals to minimize GI symptoms; can mix oral solution with Advera, chocolate milk, or Ensure. Separate administration of RTV from antacids/ddI by more than 2 hr.	GI (nausea, diarrhea, vomiting, anorexia, abdominal pain), fatigue, weakness, numbness, circumoral paresthesia (tingling around the lips), change in taste, dizziness, headache, elevated LFTs, antabuse reaction, hyperlipidemia, hyperglycemia, lipodystrophy	Potent CYP3A4, CYP2D, and other isoenzyme inhibitor; induction of glucuronosyl transferases
Indinavir (IDV) (Crixivan)	200-, 300-, and 400-mg capsules	800 mg q8hr ATC Dosage adjustment in liver disease to 600 mg q8hr Avoid in renal failure See dual PI*	Take 2 capsules/dose q8hr on empty stomach (1 hr before or 2 hr after a meal) or with light meal (skim milk, juice, coffee, tea, dry toast, corn flakes). Avoid high-fat, high-calorie meal, and grapefruit juice that decreases absorption. Hydration (minimum of 6 glasses H_2O/day) to prevent kidney stones. Separate administration of IDV from antacids/ddI by more than 2 hr	Kidney stones GI (nausea, diarrhea, vomiting, abdominal pain) Neurologic: headache, insomnia, change in taste. Hyperlipidemia, hyperglycemia, lipodystrophy. Asymptomatic: hyperbilirubinemia, hepatitis	Moderate CYP3A4 enzyme inhibitor
Nelfinavir (NFV) (Viracept)	250-mg tablets 50-mg/g oral powder	750 mg TID or 1250 mg BID	Take 3 tablets/dose with meals TID *or* 5 tablets/dose with meals BID.	Diarrhea, nausea, hyperlipidemia, hyperglycemia, lipodystrophy	Moderate CYP3A4 enzyme inhibitor
Amprenavir (APV) (Agenerase)	50-, 150-mg tablets 15 mg/mL oral solution	1200 mg BID (contains 1744 IU of vitamin E)	Take 8 tablets/dose with or without meals BID.	Rash, diarrhea, headache	Moderate CYP3A4 enzyme inhibitor

Source: References 84, 85, 102, 104.

*See Table 76.7 for recommended dosages of dual PI regimens.

Table 76.4 ▪ Nonnucleoside Reverse Transcriptase Inhibitors

Drug	Dosage Forms	Usual Doses	Special Administration Instructions	Common Adverse Effects	Potential for Drug Interactions (see Table 76.9)
Nevirapine (NVP) (Viramune)	200 tablets; 10 mg/mL suspension	200 mg daily for the first 14 days, then if no rash increase 200 mg BID	Can be given with meals and with ddI/ antacids.	Skin rash (30–50%) can be severe, headache, diarrhea, nausea; increase LFT, hepatitis. Dose escalation can reduce the incidence of rash. Cross-reactivity of rash with other NNRTI unknown.	CYP3A4 enzyme inducer, including its own metabolism
Delavirdine (DLV) (Rescriptor)	100-mg tablets	400 mg TID (4 × 100 mg table in >3 oz of water to produce slurry)	Can be given with meals; separate administration by >1 hr from ddI/antacids.	Rash, headache; cross-reactivity of rash with other NNRTI unknown.	CYP3A4 enzyme inhibitor
Efavirenz (EFV) (Sustiva)	50-, 100-, 200-mg capsules	600 mg QD hs or 200 mg TID	Can be administered at bedtime with low-fat meal.	Headaches, dizziness, "disconnected" lightheadedness, nightmares, rash. Avoid in pregnancy owing to possible teratogenicity.	CYP3A4 inhibitor and inducer

Table 76.5 ▪ Prescribing Guidelines for Antiretroviral Agents: Initiation of Therapy

Clinical Category	CD4 T Cell Count and HIV Viral Load	Treatment Recommendations	Treatment Regimens (see Table 76.7)
Symptomatic (AIDS, thrush, unexplained fever)	Any value	Treat	2 NRTI Plus 1 PI 2 NRTI Plus 2 PI 2 NRTI plus 1 NNRTI 2 NRTI plus NNRTI + PI 3 NRTI
Asymptomatic	CD4 count <500/mm^3 *or* HIV RNA >5,000–10,000 (bDNA) *or* >10,000–20,000 (RT-PCR)	Offer therapy; willingness of patient to accept therapy is critical. Benefits outweigh risks of therapy.	Same as above
Asymptomatic	CD4 count <500/mm^3 *and* HIV RNA >5,000–10,000 (bDNA) *or* >10,000–20,000 (RT-PCR)	Delay therapy and observe *or* treat. Unknown benefits.	Same as above
Pregnancy	Any value	Treat mother and passively treat fetus.	Same as above, but ZDV should be included in the maternal regimen. Optimal dosage or time to start treatment unclear.
Newborn	Any value, treat if born to high risk or HIV+ mother	All neonates. All infants born to HIV-infected mothers will be HIV+ owing to transfer of maternal IgG antibodies through 18 mo of age.	For the neonate, 6 weeks of ZDV 2 mg/kg q6hr beginning within 1 to 8 hr of birth. A 1-week regimen after delivery might also be effective.
Primary HIV infection	Any value	Offer therapy; benefits may outweigh risks.	Same as above
Occupational and non-occupational exposure prophylaxis	N/A	Treat within 72 hr of risky exposure; benefits not documented for non-occupational exposures.	2NRTI ± PI (indinavir or nelfinavir). Add PI for higher risk exposures.

Source: References 25–30.

eradication; therefore, the most potent regimens should be used initially, if possible, in antiretroviral-naive persons. Monotherapy is no longer recommended, because incomplete viral suppression can encourage development of resistance. Similarly, the magnitude and durability of viral suppression is lower with dual antiretroviral combinations compared with combinations containing three or more agents.

The optimal combinations of antiretroviral agents are unknown; however, most guidelines recommend starting with a minimum of two nucleoside reverse transcriptase inhibitors (NRTI) plus either one or two PIs, or an NNRTI (Tables 76.5 and 76.7).[25,26] Others advocate a more aggressive regimen containing four or five agents for more rapid HIV suppression.[37] Protease-containing combinations appear to be more potent than NNRTI-containing combinations; therefore, they may be more appropriate for persons with symptomatic HIV disease or AIDS. Only one study to date (e.g., efavirenz) suggests that an NNRTI-containing regimen is comparable to a PI-containing regimen. NNRTI-containing combinations are attractive initial regimens because they spare the PI for future use and avoid bothersome PI toxicities and drug-drug interactions. Alternatively, a NRTI could be combined with a PI and a NNRTI. Other regimens under investigation include three drug combinations of NRTIs (e.g., zidovudine plus lamivudine plus abacavir). Virologic success rates of 60 to 90% have been reported using the preceding regimens in HIV-naive persons; results are less dramatic in antiretroviral-experienced

Table 76.6 ▪ Principles of Antiretroviral Therapy

- An undetectable viral load is the goal of therapy.
- Adherence is critical to maintain viral suppression and minimize the emergence of viral resistance.
- Avoid monotherapy to prevent the emergence of resistance and drug failure.
- Three or more antiretroviral agents are more effective than two agents.
- Your first regimen is your best chance for viral suppression.
- Treatment is most effective in antiretroviral-naive than in antiretroviral-experienced persons.
- Never add a single agent to a failing regimen.
- Resistance to one drug is likely to confer resistance to another drug in the same class.

Table 76.7 ▪ Possible Antiretroviral Treatment Options for Combination Therapy[a]

Class of ARV	Potential ARV Combinations (usual dosages unless specified)	Regimens/Combinations to Avoid	Comments
2 NRTI	ZDV + ddI ZDV + ddC ZDV + 3TC d4T + 3TC d4T + ddI ABC + ZDV ABC + ddI ABC + 3TC ABC + d4T ABC + ddC	d4T + ZDV (antagonistic) ddI + ddC (overlapping toxicity) ddC + d4T (overlapping toxicity) ddC + 3TC (weak viral suppression)	Avoid monotherapy. Optimal use of 3TC is in a 3-drug suppressive regimen to avoid the emergence of 3TC resistance.
3 NRTI	2 NRTI Plus ABC (see above)	See above	Data limited. Other regimens may be effective. Triple NRTI might be option in antiretroviral naïve subjects.
1 PI	Indinavir Nelfinavir Ritonavir SGC Saquinavir (Fortovase)	Avoid HG-SAQ as sole PI owing to poor bioavailability	Select PI based on patient's ability to adhere with special administration requirements, drug–drug interactions, and toxicity profile.
Dual protease inhibitor	RTV 400 mg BID + SAQ 400 mg BID RTV 400 mg BID + IDV 400 mg BID RTV 200 mg BID + IDV 800 mg BID RTV 400 mg BID + NFV 750 mg BID NFV 750 mg TID + SG SAQ 800 mg TID NFV 1250 mg BID + SG-SAQ 1000 mg BID NFV 750 mg or 1000 mg BID + IDV 1000 mg BID	IDV + SAQ (antagonistic in vitro)	RTV + SAQ dual PI regimen of choice. RTV + IDV eliminates need of administering IDV on an empty stomach.
1 NNRTI	Efavirenz Nevirapine	Dual NNRTI regimens	EFV-containing regimen compared favorably to a PI containing regimen. DLV might also be effective but data limited. No head-to-head comparisons among NNRTI.

[a]See Table 76.5 for treatment recommendations.

Source: References 25–30, 85.

persons, although long-term data are lacking. Clinical issues, including drug toxicity, laboratory abnormalities, medication adherence, and drug–drug interactions should be considered before selecting any antiretroviral regimen. These considerations are more complex when treating persons with more advanced illness on multiple drug therapies, or when there are concomitant issues such as dementia, substance abuse, psychiatric disorders, or homelessness.[38,39] Salvage regimens (e.g., for persons failing multiple regimens) include combinations containing hydroxyurea or investigational agents available by expanded access (e.g., ABT 378/Ritonavir) from pharmaceutical companies.

Certain combinations of antiretroviral agents should be avoided because of potential antiviral antagonism, lack of proven efficacy, or overlapping toxicity profiles (Table 76.7). Likewise, certain combinations of agents, such as dual protease inhibitor therapy, can increase effective PI levels and promote adherence by reducing the daily number of tablets taken. In an effort to take advantage of a particular PI drug–drug interaction, a standard combination is to use a potent PI inhibitor of the cytochrome P450 system to reduce the metabolism of the coadministered PI, thereby permitting lower doses of each PI to be given. A typical example is the combination of ritonavir increasing drug concentrations and therefore, the activity of concomitant saquinavir. Other examples of dual PI combination therapy are shown in Table 76.7.

Once maximal viral suppression has been achieved using an aggressive induction regimen, investigators have evaluated the feasibility of giving a less intensive antiretroviral regimen for maintaining viral suppression. After achieving viral suppression, three studies agree that less intensive maintenance regimens are not as successful in suppressing the virus as continuation of the induction regimen.[40–42] Therefore, once maximal viral suppression occurs, the initial antiretroviral regimen should be maintained to continue maximal viral suppression.

Changing Antiretroviral Therapy

Changes in antiretroviral regimens should be considered for documented treatment failures, unmanageable drug toxicity, patient intolerance leading to nonadherence, or use of a suboptimal regimen. If therapy has to be discontinued because of drug intolerance, all agents should be stopped simultaneously to minimize the emergence of drug resistance.[43,44] When selecting a new regimen, it is appropriate to substitute another agent from the same drug class responsible for causing the drug toxicity. However, if a regimen must be changed owing to treatment failure (i.e., increase in VL >0.5 $\log^{10}$ from last VL), or administration of a suboptimal regimen, it is preferable that the patient receive at least two to three new agents to minimize the development of resistance. Viral resistance can be detected in vitro using phenotypic and genotypic assays (Table 76.8). Commercially available genotypic assays can identify specific nucleic acid changes known to cause resistance; however, their results should be interpreted carefully.[45] Currently, genotypic assays may help identify resistance to various antiretroviral agents; therefore, those agents should be avoided. However, they do not identify which agents may be clinically effective. Long-term studies using genotypic assays are currently lacking and these assays are neither routinely recommended nor FDA approved. Phenotypic assays are more difficult to perform but might provide more accurate information about viral replication in the presence of the drug (e.g., concentrations of the drug required to inhibit 50% [IC_{50}] or 90% [IC_{90}] of viral replication).

Table 76.8 ▪ Mutations Associated with Antiretroviral Resistance

	Codon Mutations
Nucleoside Reverse Transcriptase Inhibitors (NRTI)	
Zidovudine (ZDV)	T215Y,[a] M41L
Didanosine (ddI)	L74V[a], K65R, M184V
Zalcitabine (ddC)	K65R,[a] M184V
Stavudine (d4T)	150T,[a] V75T[a]
Lamivudine (3TC)	M184V[a]
Abacavir (ABC)[b]	M184V, R65K, L74V, Y115F
Adefovir (ADF)	K65R,[a] T69D, K10E
Non-Nucleoside Reverse Transcriptase Inhibitors (NNRTI)	
Nevirapine (NVP)	K103N,[a] Y181C,[a] 188L V108I[a]
Delavirdine (DLV)	K103N/T,[a] Y181C[a]
Efavirenz (EFV)	K103N,[a] Y181C,[a] Y188L, V108I[a]
Protease Inhibitors (PI)	
Saquinavir (SAQ)	G48V,[a] L90M,[a] V82A
Ritonavir (RTV)	V82A/F,[a] I54V/L, A71V/L, M36I, 184V,[a] L90M[a]
Indinavir (IDV)	V82A/F,[a] M46I/L, 184V,[a] L90M[a]
Nelfinavir (NFV)	D30N,[a] A71V, 184V, L90M
Amprenavir (APV)	I50V,[a] M46I,[a] I47V, L10F

Source: References 44, 45.
[a]Critical mutations.
[b]Two to three concurrent mutations are necessary for significant mutation.

Pharmacotherapy in Pregnancy

HIV infection in pregnant women should be managed similarly to HIV infection in nonpregnant women (Table 76.5).[28] Combination antiretroviral therapy, similar to combinations described in the preceding for adults infected with HIV, is currently recommended (Table 76.7). Pregnancy should not preclude use of optimal therapeutic regimens because of possible teratogenicity issues. Two therapeutic issues need to be considered when using antiretroviral agents in pregnancy: effective antiretroviral therapy for the mother, and effective antiretroviral chemoprophylaxis to reduce the risk of vertical transmission and toxicity to the fetus. However, because the long-term impact of antiretroviral therapy on the fetus is unknown, the decision to institute antiretroviral therapy during pregnancy should include a discussion with the mother of the risks and benefits to her and her fetus. Women infected with HIV should be counseled not to breastfeed to avoid HIV transmission to the newborn through breast milk.

Several clinical trials support the use of zidovudine (ZDV) as part of any antiretroviral regimen to prevent perinatal transmission, although the optimal regimen, time of initiation, or duration of treatment is unclear. In 1994, a clinical trial (ACTG 076) found that ZDV monotherapy, orally starting at 14 to 34 weeks gestation, intravenously during delivery, and orally to the newborn for the first 6 weeks of life, reduced the risk of HIV transmission from mother to child by 66%.[11] The principal toxicity in the newborn was anemia that was reversible after drug discontinuation. Long-term followup (mean of 4.2 years) in these children who received zidovudine in utero and during the first 6 weeks of life revealed no significant adverse effects.[46] Another trial suggested comparable fetal protection when a short-term regimen of ZDV alone was given orally from 36 weeks of gestation, throughout labor and delivery, but without an infant component.[12] Interim data from 1357 subjects enrolled in the UNAIDS, United Nations Programme on HIV/AIDS Perinatal Transmission Trial (PETRA) found that ZDV and 3TC, started at delivery and administered for 1 week only to both the mother and child, reduced vertical transmission of HIV by 37%.[47] However, if antiretroviral therapy was started at 36 weeks gestation, continued through labor, and administered to both mother and child for 1 week only following delivery, perinatal HIV transmission was reduced by 50%. Last, an abbreviated ZDV regimen initiated intrapartum or in the first 48 hours of infant life was found to be effective, suggesting that postexposure prophylaxis may be responsible for ZDV's efficacy.[48] Based on these trials, all women should receive HIV counseling and treatment, and ZDV should be included in the maternal antiretroviral regimen. However, ZDV monotherapy is not recommended because incomplete viral suppression can lead to resistance and reduce the efficacy of future antiretroviral agents in the mother. If ZDV is not part of the initial regimen, addition or substitution of ZDV for other NRTIs is highly recommended.

The CDC guidelines give several possible treatment plans to reduce the risk of perinatal transmission depending on the clinical scenario.[28] For pregnant women infected with HIV who have not had prior antiretroviral therapy in their first trimester of pregnancy, decisions to delay therapy until at least after 10 to 12 weeks gestation should be entertained to reduce the possible risk of teratogenicity. For women infected with HIV already receiving antiretroviral therapy during the first trimester of pregnancy, the women should be counseled about the risks and benefits to themselves and their babies. Stopping therapy could lead to rebound in viral load in the mother, which could have adverse effects on both the mother and the fetus. If the decision is to stop therapy during the first trimester, all antiretroviral agents should be stopped and reintroduced simultaneously after the first trimester to avoid inducing resistance. For women in labor or for infants in whom no prior maternal antiretroviral therapy has been administered, administration of intrapartum intravenous zidovudine and the 6-week oral zidovudine to the newborn is highly recommended.

Postexposure Prophylaxis for Occupational and Nonoccupational Exposures

The benefits of postexposure prophylaxis (PEP) after an occupational percutaneous exposure have been established. A case-control study of health care workers found that the use of zidovudine alone within hours of the exposure reduced the risk of HIV transmission by 80%.[49] It is anticipated that exposure through high-risk sex or sharing of intravenous drug use paraphernalia is expected to be comparable to the risks associated with occupational exposure. The CDC recommends immediate initiation of two to three potent antiretroviral combinations after a high-risk occupational exposure.[29] The typical combinations are similar to those used in persons infected with HIV (Tables 76.5 and 76.7). The risks and benefits of PEP should be clearly explained before therapy is started. Side effects or concerns about potential side effects can limit initiation and completion of therapy. The CDC found that approximately one-third of health care workers who started PEP did not complete their therapy. CDC guidelines have also been provided for nonoccupational exposures after sexual exposures or injection drug use.[30] Benefits of PEP after a nonoccupational exposure have not been established.

Therapy for Acute Primary HIV Infection

Currently, there are no outcome data to support the use of antiretroviral agents in the treatment of acute HIV infection; data in support of early therapy are limited.[23] Nevertheless, most experts agree that early intervention with aggressive antiretroviral therapy appears valid. A discussion of the risks and benefits of antiretroviral therapy is appropriate before therapy is instituted. The theoretical benefits of early antiretroviral therapy include limiting systemic viral dissemination by suppressing the initial burst of viremia, decreasing the severity of the acute illness, changing the "viral setpoint" that may affect the rate of disease progression, and decreasing the emergence of resistant strains by suppressing viral replication. Acute antiretroviral prophylaxis is warranted only after a discussion of the risks and benefits of early intervention. The therapeutic regimens are similar to those used for the treatment of HIV infection (e.g., 2 NRTI and a PI). Although the duration of therapy is unknown, it is likely that chronic treatment will be required, because viral rebound has occurred after stopping treatment.

Antiretroviral Agents

Nucleoside Reverse Transcriptase Inhibitors

The nucleoside reverse transcriptase inhibitors were the first class of antiretroviral agents (ARV) approved for the treatment of HIV infection. There are currently six NRTI agents available (Table 76.2), with many others under investigation, including lobucavir. The NRTI continue to be essential agents in the treatment of HIV infection, especially when used in a combination of three or more highly active antiretroviral agents. Traditionally, two

NRTI have been used in combination with ARV agents from different classes, such as the NNRTI and PI. All the NRTI are prodrugs that need to be converted intracellularly to their active form before exerting their antiviral activity. Because the NRTI are not inducers or inhibitors of the cytochrome P450 system, drug interactions are not as problematic as with the PI or NNRTI. However, pharmacodynamic interactions should be monitored. Resistance has been described for all the NRTI and develops more rapidly in patients with advanced disease and high levels of viral replication. All toxicities with the NRTI have been attributed to mitochondrial toxicity.

Zidovudine (Retrovir)

Zidovudine (ZDV, Retrovir) was the first FDA-approved antiretroviral agent that was modestly effective in delaying disease progression to AIDS in those with asymptomatic HIV disease and CD4 counts lower than 500 cells/mm^3 (ACTG 019).[50] The time-limited and suboptimal benefits of ZDV monotherapy were first evident during The European Concorde Trial. No difference in clinical endpoints were observed at 3 years of followup in 1749 asymptomatic persons infected with HIV randomized to either immediate or delayed ZDV therapy (begun after the development of AIDS-related symptoms).[51] The durability of ZDV monotherapy in delaying disease progression has been estimated to be approximately 12 to 24 months. Although ZDV monotherapy is no longer recommended, its efficacy in preventing perinatal transmission from mother to child and as postexposure prophylaxis of health care workers following a high-risk occupational exposure is undisputed.[28,49] Several important trials, including AIDS Clinical Trials Group (ACTG) 175, Delta, and the Community Providers for Clinical Research in AIDS (CPCRA) have demonstrated the superiority of dual nucleoside analog therapy over ZDV monotherapy in delaying disease progression to AIDS or death. These results are particularly impressive in antiretroviral-naive patients.[52–54] The benefits of combination therapy in ZDV-experienced persons with advanced HIV infection were less evident. The combination of ZDV plus stavudine (d4T) should be avoided because antagonism has been demonstrated.[55] A preliminary analysis of ACTG 290 found that ZDV-experienced persons who received the combination of ZDV plus d4T had an unexpected rapid decline in their CD4 cells.[56]

ZDV is a thymidine analog that requires intracellular phosphorylation to its active moiety, ZDV-5N-triphosphate (ZDV-TP). Because of its structural similarity to thymidine triphosphate, the viral DNA copy incorporates the ZDV-TP, resulting in proviral DNA chain termination or competitive RT antagonism to block further viral replication (Fig. 76.1). Zidovudine is well absorbed; its bioavailability is approximately 60%. Plasma ZDV concentrations are highly variable; efficacy and toxicity plasma concentrations have not been established. Its penetration into the cerebrospinal fluid (CSF) is considered advantageous in the treatment of HIV-related dementia.[57] The optimal dosage and dosing frequency of zidovudine are unknown. Originally, based on an intracellular half-life of 3 to 4 hours, ZDV was administered at 200 mg five to six times daily. Subsequent studies have shown that ZDV 300 mg two times a day or 200 mg three times a day appear equally effective but may be less toxic. Dosage adjustment is required in severe renal insufficiency (Table 76.2).[58] However, higher dosages of ZDV (e.g., 1000 to 1200 mg daily) may be required for the management of HIV dementia or HIV-related thrombocytopenia.[59,60]

The toxicities of ZDV are well known (Table 76.2). During the first 6 weeks of therapy, complaints of nausea, vomiting, anorexia, bloating, headache, malaise, insomnia, confusion, or flulike symptoms should be expected; however, these tend to resolve with continued therapy or by dividing the dose (e.g., 200 mg t.i.d. instead of 300 mg b.i.d.). Hematological toxicities, including neutropenia and anemia, are less severe with the lower dosages used (e.g., <600 mg per day), but tend to predominate in those with advanced HIV infection or in those patients receiving concomitant marrow suppressive agents (e.g., induction doses of ganciclovir, TMP/SMX doses for treatment of PCP). Therefore, it is recommended that ZDV should be discontinued during induction doses of ganciclovir (Table 76.9). Higher serum concentrations of ZDV monophosphate (ZDV-MP) observed in those with low CD4 counts compared with seronegative volunteers may be responsible for the bone marrow suppression.[61] Anemia, which can be severe (e.g., hemoglobin <9 g/dL), usually occurs after 6 to 8 weeks of therapy, and responds to blood transfusions, erythropoietin, dosage reduction, or alternatively, changing to a less bone marrow suppressive antiretroviral agent. Macrocytosis, usually asymptomatic, develops in most patients after several weeks of ZDV and is a good indicator of adherence. The administration of granulocyte colony-stimulating factor (G-CSF) for ZDV-induced neutropenia (<500 cells/mm^3) may permit continued ZDV therapy; however, changing to an alternative antiretroviral agent when debilitating anemia occurs is easier and more cost effective. Myopathy, reported in 6 to 18% of patients, occurs after prolonged therapy (>6 months) and is reversible after stopping the drug.[62] An elevated creatinine kinase level (CPK) can confirm this idiosyncratic reaction in patients with symptoms of muscle pain and weakness. Hepatitis and hyperpigmentation of the nails and skin are infrequent. Although one case of cardiomyopathy and two retinal abnormalities were reported in children who received ZDV in utero, growth and development were considered to be normal.[46] Complete blood count (CBC), platelets, and liver function tests should be monitored at baseline, then every 2 to 4 weeks for 3 months, and then every 3 months or as necessary based on symptomology.

Resistance to ZDV is associated with a codon 215 mutation in the RT gene; codon 70, 41, 67, and/or 219 mutations may also be important (Table 76.8). Fortunately, little cross-resistance exists between these ZDV-inducing mutations and other NRTI resistance.

Table 76.9 ▪ Selected Pharmacodynamic and Pharmacokinetic Drug Interactions with Selected Antiretroviral Agents

Antiretroviral Agent	Interacting Drugs	Interaction	Recommendations
ZDV	Ganciclovir	Concomitant bone marrow suppression	Stop ZDV during ganciclovir induction therapy.
ddI	Isoniazid, ddC, vincristine, d4T	Increased risk of peripheral neuropathy	Use cautiously and if possible, avoid coadministration.
ddI	Quinolones, tetracyclines, ketoconazole, itraconazole, ritonavir, indinavir, delavirdine	Impaired absorption by ddI	Separate coadministration by at least 2 hr.
ddI	Alcohol, systemic pentamidine, ddC	Increased risk of pancreatitis	Use cautiously and if possible, avoid coadministration.
ddC	Isoniazid, ddI, vincristine, d4T	Increased risk of peripheral neuropathy	Use cautiously and if possible, avoid coadministration.
ddC	Alcohol, systemic pentamidine, ddI	Increased risk of pancreatitis	Use cautiously and if possible, avoid coadministration.
Protease inhibitors*	Terfenadine, cisapride, astemizole, ergot alkaloids, triazolam, midazolam	Potential for life-threatening arrhythmias owing to enzyme inhibition by PI	Avoid coadministration. Use nonsedating antihistamines (e.g., loratadine) or other sedative hypnotics (e.g., lorazepam, temazepam).
Protease inhibitors*	Rifabutin	Decreased PI efficacy due to enzyme induction by rifabutin. Increased rifabutin toxicity owing to 200% increased rifabutin level	Avoid coadministration with RTV and SAQ. Decrease rifabutin to 150 mg QD when combined with IDV, NFV, APV. Increase IDV to 1000 mg q8hr. Increase NFV to 1 gm TID.
Non-nucleoside RT†	Rifabutin	Decreased NNRTI/rifabutin efficacy owing to enzyme induction. Increased rifabutin toxicity with DLV	Avoid coadministration of DLV and rifabutin. Increase rifabutin dose to 450 mg QD with EFV.
PI and NNRTI*†	Rifampin	Decreased PI/NNRTI efficacy owing to enzyme induction by rifampin	Avoid coadministration, consider rifabutin.
Ritonavir	Amiodarone, bepridil, buproprion, clorazepate, piroxicam, propoxyphene, diazepam, estolazolam, flurazepam, clozapine, encainide, flecainide, propafenone, quinidine, merperidine, pimozide, zolpidem, terfenadine. Also see PI.	Potential for life-threatening arrhythmias and increased toxicity of drugs owing to CYP3A4 inhibition by ritonavir	Avoid coadministration. See comments under PI.
Saquinavir	Efavirenz	Decreased saquinavir levels 60% owing to enzyme induction by efavirenz.	Avoid coadministration. Dual PI therapy with RTV+ SAQ can prevent EFV interaction.
Indinavir	Efavirenz	Decreased IDV levels owing to enzyme induction by efavirenz	Increase IDV to 1 g q8hr.
Delavirdine	Terfenadine, astemizole, alprazolam, midazolam, triazolam, cisapride, ergot alkaloids	Potential for life-threatening arrhythmias and increased toxicity of drugs owing to enzyme inhibition by delavirdine	Avoid coadministration.
Delavirdine	Indinavir	Increased IDV levels 40% owing to enzyme inhibition	Decrease IDV to 600 mg q8hr.
Delavirdine ritonavir, indinavir	Buffered products, including antacids and ddI	Impaired absorption of ARV agents by buffered products	Separate coadministration by at least 2 hr.
Ritonavir	Disulfiram, metronidazole	Disulfiram reaction	Avoid coadministration.
Saquinavir, delavirdine	Phenytoin, phenobarbital, carbamazepine	Enzyme induction and potential reduction of effective PI and NNRTI levels	Use cautiously or avoid coadministration.
Ritonavir, nelfinavir, nevirapine	Oral contraceptives	Decreased efficacy of oral contraceptives	Use additional or alternative forms of contraception or change to another PI (e.g., indinavir) or NNRTI (e.g., efavirenz).

*PI = SAQ, RTV, IDV, NFV, APV+.

†NNRTI = EFV, NVP, DLV.

Source: References 84, 85, 102, 104.

Didanosine (Videx)

Didanosine (ddI, Videx) was the second NRTI approved in the United States and Canada for treatment of HIV infection in adults or children who failed or were intolerant to ZDV. Although ddI is less potent than ZDV in terms of its HIV inhibitory concentrations, ddI has improved activity within monocytes and macrophages, known reservoirs for HIV infection. Synergy of ddI with other NRTI, NNRTI, and hydroxyurea has been demonstrated. Initial phase I studies of ddI monotherapy have reported subjective improvements in symptoms and CD4 counts. The efficacy of ddI was compared with ZDV in a randomized, double-blind trial of ddI monotherapy versus ZDV monotherapy in ZDV-experienced persons with a mean CD4 count of 95 cells/mm^3. At a mean followup of 55 weeks, persons receiving ddI had a lower incidence of new AIDS-defining events or disease progression compared with those receiving ZDV, but there was no survival advantage.[63] Comparable results were reported with ddI in ZDV-experienced persons by the Community Program for Clinical Research on AIDS (CPCRA).[64] Several clinical trials involving dual nucleoside analogs have demonstrated the superiority of ddI monotherapy or ddI-containing combinations over ZDV in the treatment of ARV-naive and ZDV-experienced persons.

The active form of ddI, a purine nucleoside analog RT inhibitor, is dideoxyadenosine triphosphate (ddATP) whose long intracellular half-life of greater than 12 hours permits twice-daily dosing. Didanosine differs considerably from ZDV in its pharmacokinetic, pharmacodynamic, and tolerability profile. Penetration of ddI into the CSF is lower than ZDV, which might limit its usefulness in HIV dementia. The CSF to plasma concentration ratio for ddI is low, 0.2 compared with 0.6 for ZDV. Because ddI is highly acid labile, a buffered environment is required for adequate absorption. Food can also limit ddI absorption by 50%. Therefore, instructions to administer two chewable tablets per dose on an empty stomach (1 hour before or 2 hours after meals) are critical to enable sufficient buffer for proper absorption. The dosage of ddI is 200 mg (2 of the 100 mg tablets) two times a day for persons weighing more than 60 kg and 125 mg two times a day for those less than 60 kg. New data indicate that a once-daily regimen of ddI (400 mg if >60 kg) at bedtime may be equally efficacious and improve adherence.[65] Approximately 50% of ddI is excreted in the urine and dosage reductions are recommended in those with significant renal impairment (Table 76.2).[58]

Gastrointestinal side effects, including nausea and diarrhea, are most prominent and probably most likely owing to the buffer. Painful peripheral neuropathy is the most serious toxicity of ddI, affecting approximately 13 to 34% of those on therapy. Symptoms of tingling, burning, pain, numbness in distal extremities, and sensations of "walking on golf balls" are intermittent initially, but worsen with continued administration. Symptoms can be disabling but usually resolve slowly (e.g., several weeks) after drug discontinuation. Prompt recognition of peripheral neuropathy is required to prevent irreversible neurologic damage. Neuropathy is more frequent in those with a history of neuropathy or concurrent use of neurotoxins (e.g., isoniazid). Pancreatitis has been reported in 7% of persons receiving prolonged ddI therapy. This risk increases to 27% in those with a prior history of pancreatitis. Fatalities have occurred from ddI-associated pancreatitis. Patients should be educated about the signs and symptoms of pancreatitis (e.g., anorexia, nausea, vomiting, abdominal pain), informed about the dangers of concurrent alcohol intake, and instructed to contact their pharmacist or primary physician immediately if the preceding symptoms occur. An elevated amylase level can confirm the diagnosis of pancreatitis in persons presenting with the preceding complaints. Persons with a history of pancreatitis, renal impairment, and active alcohol intake are at greater risk for pancreatitis and should be considered poor candidates for ddI therapy. Both pancreatitis and peripheral neuropathy need to be distinguished from an HIV-related etiology. Rarely, elevated hepatic transaminases, rash, and hyperuricemia occur. Hematological toxicities to ddI are uncommon.

Several potential drug–drug interactions with ddI should be anticipated (Table 76.9). Because medications that require an acidic environment for absorption can be impaired by the buffer, this drug–drug interaction may be avoided by administering ddI at least 2 hours apart from delavirdine, ritonavir, indinavir, quinolones, tetracyclines, ketoconazole, and itraconazole. Also, one should avoid or use cautiously agents with overlapping ddI toxicities that can increase the risk of peripheral neuropathy (e.g., isoniazid, vincristine, ddC) or pancreatitis (e.g., ddC, intravenous pentamidine). A complete blood count, amylase, hepatic transaminases, and uric acid should be monitored at baseline and every 4 weeks initially during the first 3 months of therapy, and then as warranted based on symptomology.

Zalcitabine (Hivid)

Zalcitabine (ddC, Hivid) was FDA approved in 1992 for combination therapy with ZDV. Although ddC is extremely potent in vitro, zalcitabine monotherapy or combination therapy has been disappointing. No significant differences in disease progression or death were observed after a change from ZDV to the combination of ZDV plus ddC in ZDV-experienced persons with advanced HIV infection (ACTG 155). However, a larger increase in the CD4 count was noted in those with less severe HIV disease receiving the ddC-containing regimen.[66] In antiretroviral-naive patients, the combinations of ddC plus ZDV or ZDV plus ddI were equivalent and superior to ZDV monotherapy. In ZDV-experienced persons with less advanced HIV disease, the ddC-containing regimen was inferior to the combination of ddI plus ZDV. Based on the preceding data, ddC is widely regarded as the weakest of the available NRTI and is most effective when used in combination therapy for antiretroviral-naive patients. Didanosine is considered a superior agent compared with ddC for combination therapy.

Like other nucleoside analogs, ddC requires intracellular activation to the active triphosphate for antiviral activity. Zalcitabine is well absorbed, with approximately 90% oral bioavailability after oral dosing.[67] Similar to ddI, ddC has poor central nervous system (CNS) penetration; its CSF to plasma ratio is 0:2. The half-life is short, 2.6 hours, so that dosing three times a day is necessary. The dosage of ddC is 0.75 mg three times a day; no special administration instructions are necessary. However, because ddC is predominantly excreted renally (70%) as unchanged drug, dosage reduction in patients with severe renal impairment is recommended (Table 76.2).[58] Toxicity with ddC is similar to ddI; painful peripheral neuropathy and pancreatitis predominate. In an open label study, peripheral neuropathy was more frequent with ddC (44%) than ddI (22%), whereas pancreatitis occurred more often with ddI (29%). Generally, the same precautions and patient education identified in the preceding for ddI to reduce the risk of peripheral neuropathy and pancreatitis are germane for ddC administration. Oral aphthous ulcers and esophagus ulcerations are two unusual complications of ddC therapy. Complaints of pain with swallowing and mucocutaneous "canker sores" can be difficult to treat but usually resolve after stopping the drug. Other infrequent toxicities include hematological abnormalities, rash, fatigue, and gastrointestinal complaints of nausea, vomiting, and diarrhea. Hyperamylasemia without symptoms of pancreatitis can occur.

Drug interactions with ddC are infrequent (Table 76.9). Agents that can increase the risk of peripheral neuropathy (e.g., isoniazid, vincristine, ddI) or pancreatitis (ddI, intravenous pentamidine) should be avoided if possible or used cautiously with ddC. Patients receiving ddC should be monitored for symptoms of pancreatitis, peripheral neuropathy, and aphthous ulcers. Baseline evaluation of complete blood count, transaminases, and amylase are appropriate; repeat monitoring is dependent on symptomology and use of concurrent medications.

Stavudine (Zerit)

Stavudine (d4T, Zerit) is a thymidine-based nucleoside analog that received fast-track approval by the FDA in 1994 based on survival data from two clinical trials. The first trial, a phase III, multicenter, randomized, double-blind trial (BMS AI 455-019), compared d4T versus continued ZDV monotherapy in 822 ZDV-experienced persons with a median CD4 cell count of 235 cells/mm^3. A slightly reduced risk of developing a new AIDS-defining event or death was observed in the group receiving d4T-therapy compared with those receiving ZDV. A survival advantage was also apparent in a randomized, double-blind, parallel track trial in persons infected with HIV who failed or were intolerant of ZDV and ddI therapy. In this trial, survival between the d4T 20-mg two times a day and 40-mg two times a day dosage regimens were comparable. A synergistic effect of d4T and ddI has been demonstrated in vitro. The combination of d4T and ddI has produced potent and sustained virologic and immunologic benefits in antiretroviral-experienced persons.[68–70] Preliminary data reported a 0.7 to 1.8 log^{10} mean reduction in baseline viral load and changes in CD4 cell counts of −22 to +141 cells. This potent combination was well tolerated. The most common reason for drug discontinuation was peripheral neuropathy, particularly in persons with CD4 counts lower than 200 cells/mm^3. These data suggest that the combination of d4T and ddI may be a particularly potent NRTI combination in pretreated persons.

The combination of d4T and ZDV has shown antagonism in vitro and should be avoided. Clinically, a decline in CD4 counts was observed in patients receiving this combination (ACTG 290).[56] Preliminary results suggest that these negative effects might be attributed to competition for the same activating enzyme because both d4T and ZDV share the thymidine kinase enzyme for phosphorylation to the active TP moiety. In vitro data found that d4T-TP levels were reduced by more than 95% with ZDV, whereas d4T had no effect on the phosphorylation of ZDV owing to the higher affinity of ZDV than d4T for the enzyme. Preliminary data suggest that previous use of ZDV might also impair the future antiretroviral activity of d4T. In a small group of six persons infected with HIV, the intracellular phosphorylation of d4T to the active triphosphate was impaired for several weeks following ZDV use.[55] The effects of current d4T use affecting future use of ZDV are unknown.

Stavudine is rapidly absorbed with a bioavailability of approximately 86%. The intracellular half-life is about 4 hours. Significant levels of d4T were attained in CSF that exceeded the in vitro IC_{50} concentrations for most wild-type HIV-1 strains, causing reduction of CSF HIV RNA concentrations.[71] The FDA-approved dosage is 40 mg two times a day for patients weighing more than 60 kg and 30 mg two times a day for those weighing less than 60 kg. Lower dosages of 20 mg two times a day for those more than 60 kg and 15 mg two times a day for those less than 60 kg are appropriate for those at an increased risk of neuropathy. Dosage reduction is required in renal insufficiency because approximately 50% of d4T is excreted unchanged in the urine (Table 76.2).[58]

Stavudine is generally well tolerated. The major toxicity is a dose-related peripheral neuropathy; an incidence of 15 to 20% has been reported in clinical trials. The symptoms of neuropathy are similar to those seen with other neurotoxic agents (e.g., ddI). Symptoms usually resolve after drug discontinuation. Stavudine-induced neuropathy is dose-dependent. In a parallel track trial, efficacy was comparable but the incidence of neuropathy was lower in those receiving d4T 20 mg two times a day (15%) compared with those receiving d4T doses of 40 mg two times a day (21%). If neuropathy develops on full dosages of d4T (e.g., 40 mg b.i.d.), a dosage reduction to 20 mg two times a day should be attempted before therapy is discontinued. Other reported toxicities include pancreatitis, transaminase elevations, headache, nausea, and vomiting. Hematological toxicity is infrequent.

Lamivudine (Epivir)

Lamivudine (3TC, Epivir), a cytosine triphosphate analog, was approved in 1995 as the fourth NRTI for HIV infection. Lamivudine is also indicated for the treatment of hepatitis B infection.[72] The CAESAR (Canada, Australia, Europe, and South Africa) Trial was the first trial to demonstrate a survival benefit for a 3TC-containing regimen.[73] This trial randomized the addition of placebo, 3TC, or 3TC plus loviride to the underlying antiretroviral regimen of 1840 antiretroviral-experienced persons with median CD4+ cell counts of 126 cells/mm^3. A significant 54% reduction in the risk of disease progression occurred in those receiving 3TC, but the addition of loviride provided no additional benefits on outcome.

Lamivudine monotherapy should be avoided since resistance can develop rapidly from a mutation at the M184V codon (Table 76.8). Therefore, 3TC should be used only in a fully suppressive viral regimen (e.g., combination with two or more ARV) to prevent the emergence of resistance and the loss of antiviral activity. Several combinations of 3TC and NRTI have been studied and found to possess durable antiviral activity. The synergistic combination of 3TC and ZDV delayed the emergence of resistance to ZDV, and improved virologic and immunologic measures in four double-blind trials.[74–77] In the NUCA (United States) and the NUCB (Europe) trials, the combination of ZDV plus 3TC, compared with ZDV or 3TC alone, sustained a 1 log decline in viral load from baseline that persisted through week 52 in antiretroviral-naive patients. CD4 cell counts also improved by 60 to 80 cells/mm^3. In antiretroviral-experienced persons, the combination of ZDV plus 3TC was superior to ZDV alone or the combination of ZDV plus ddC; however, the effects on CD4 cell counts and viral load were less impressive. Preliminary results suggest that the commonly used combination of d4T and 3TC is a potent dual NRTI regimen.[78,79] The ALTIS study, an open label pilot trial in 83 persons infected with HIV who have a median CD4 cell count of 258 cells/mm^3 and a viral load of more than 15K copies/mL, showed that the combination of d4T plus 3TC was superior in antiretroviral-naive compared with experienced patients. At 24 weeks, a viral load reduction of 1.66 log^{10} copies/mL and a CD4 count increase of 108 cells occurred in the naive group compared with a 0.5 log^{10} reduction and a 46 CD4 cell count increase in the experienced group. A greater proportion of naive patients (21%) achieved an undetectable viral load compared with only 5% in the experienced group. The combination was safe and well tolerated.

The mean oral bioavailability of 3TC is 82% and is not affected by meals. It is phosphorylated intracellularly to 3TC-TP, which has a long intracellular half-life of 10 to 15 hours that permits twice daily dosing. Significant concentrations of 3TC are attained in the CSF. In one study, 3TC exceeded the in vitro IC_{50} concentrations for most wild-type HIV-1 strains, causing reduction of CSF HIV RNA concentrations.[71] The recommended dosage of 3TC is 150 mg two times a day. Dosage reduction is required in renal impairment because 79% of 3TC is eliminated unchanged in the urine (Table 76.2).[58] Lamivudine is very well tolerated. In clinical trials, the addition of 3TC to ZDV did not increase adverse effects or laboratory abnormalities. Headache, diarrhea, and occasionally, neutropenia have been reported. Lamivudine has been associated with paronychia.[80] No clinically significant drug–drug interactions have been reported.

Abacavir (Ziagen)

Abacavir (ABC, Ziagen), the newest NRTI approved in December 1998 by the FDA, is a promising addition to the current antiretroviral agents for adults and children.[81] Abacavir is intracellularly phosphorylated to its monophosphate form before subsequent conversion by cytosolic enzymes and cellular kinases to the active carbovir triphosphate moiety. In vitro, abacavir displays synergy when combined with zidovudine, nevirapine, and amprenavir; and additive effects with most NRTI (e.g., ddI, ddC, d4T, 3TC). The bioavailability of abacavir is excellent (≥75%) and its CNS penetration is similar to zidovudine. ABC is conveniently dosed 300 mg two times a day and can be administered without regard to meals. The majority of abacavir is metabolized; only 11 to 13% of the drug is excreted unchanged. Similar to other NRTI, no clinically significant drug–drug interactions have been identified. Resistance may develop less rapidly to ABC when compared with other agents. Multiple mutations are required before in vitro resistance to ABC develops (Table 76.8). For example, the 184 mutation confers high-level resistance to 3TC but only a tenfold increase in resistance to abacavir. The potential for cross-resistance is minimal between ABC and d4T or ZDV, whereas overlap in resistance is reported in vitro with ddI, ddC, and 3TC. Resistance to multiple NRTI reduced the effectiveness of ABC. Patients who have had extensive exposure to ZDV, 3TC, and other NRTs may have a minimal response to regimens containing abacavir.

The potency of ABC-containing combinations on viral suppression has been demonstrated in several clinical trials involving antiretroviral-naive and -experienced persons, including children. HIV RNA levels in the CSF have also declined with an ABC-containing regimen. The magnitude of viral suppression ranges from a median reduction of 1.48 to 1.84 log^{10} during monotherapy to mean reductions of greater than 2 log^{10} when used in ARV-containing combination. An ongoing, open-label, phase II trial (CNA2002) of 44 antiretroviral-naive subjects (baseline HIV RNA ≥30,000 copies/mL and CD4 ≥100 cells/mm^3) receiving the ABC/ZDV/3TC combination, provides evidence of a sustained virologic response.[82] By week 72, significant reductions in viral load were observed, 72% of the subjects had undetectable viral loads (<400 copies/mL), and 50% achieved fewer than 50 copies/mL. CD4 counts increased by a median of 150 cells from baseline. An open label prospective trial evaluated the double combination of ABC 300 mg two times a day and a PI, amprenavir 1200 mg orally two times a day in 41 treatment-naive patients with more than 400 CD4 cells/mm^3 and an HIV RNA of more than 5000 copies/mL. At the end of 48 weeks, all patients had undetectable viral loads, many as low as 5 copies/mL. Lymph node biopsies revealed normalization of percentage of CD4/CD8 cells. ABC also reduced viral load more than 1 log^{10} in nine of 15 ZDV, d4T, 3TC, and ddI-experienced persons who had ABC added to their existing ARV regimen. In all trials, CD4 cell counts continue to increase during therapy. ABC has been safely used in combination with ZDV, 3TC, NVP, and the PI.

FDA approval was based on virologic results from three phase III studies. Preliminary results at 16 weeks in antiretroviral-naive subjects receiving the triple NRTI combination of ABC/ZDV/3TC versus the "gold standard" protease inhibitor-containing regimen of IDV/ZDV/3TC showed no difference between the two regimens in achieving undetectable viral loads. A multicenter, double-blind, phase III trial randomized 173 HIV-infected ARV-naive subjects to the triple combination of ABC/3TC/ZDV or to placebo/3TC/ZDV. Subjects were stratified based on HIV RNA at study entry. Preliminary data at 16 weeks showed that viral suppression was comparable irrespective of baseline viral load in those receiving the triple combination. In the intent-to-treat analysis, 54% of those receiving the triple combination achieved HIV RNA levels less than 50 copies/mL compared with 15% in those on the dual combination.[83] In a phase III study of experienced children, 13% of those receiving the triple combination of ABC/3TC/ZDV achieved an undetectable viral load (<400 copies/mL) compared with only 2% of those on the dual combination of ZDV/3TC. The median increase in CD4 in those receiving the triple combination counts (i.e., 69 cells/mm^3) were superior to those given the two-drug regimens (9 cells/mm^3). Based on the potency and durability of viral suppression, a triple NRTI combination containing ABC appears to be an alternative initial treatment option in antiretroviral-naive persons.

Abacavir is well tolerated. Adverse effects reported from clinical trials include nausea, vomiting, malaise/fatigue, headache, muscle pain, abdominal pain, diarrhea, rash, and sleep disorders. Clinicians need to be aware of, and patients need to be alerted about, a potentially fatal hypersensitivity reaction that has been reported in about 3 to 5% of study subjects. Symptoms usually occur within the first 6 weeks of therapy and are heralded by the onset of fever; concomitant symptoms in about half of the subjects might include rash, nausea, oral lesions, conjunctivitis, and respiratory symptoms. Once stopped, the reaction subsides within a few days. Resuming abacavir is absolutely contraindicated because fatalities have been reported on rechallenge. Patients should be instructed to contact their pharmacist or doctor if these symptoms occur. A Medication Guide is issued to each patient by Glaxo Wellcome to alert patients about this potentially fatal reaction.

Adefovir dipivoxil (Preveon)

Adefovir dipivoxil (Preveon) belongs to a unique class of antiretroviral agents, the nucleotide analogs. Unlike other NRTIs, which must be activated by intracellular phosphorylation, adefovir contains its own phosphate group and requires no activation for its antiviral effects. Adefovir also exhibits activity against herpes virus, cytomegalovirus, and hepatitis B viruses, which may be advantageous in HIV+ persons coinfected with these viral pathogens. The mean oral bioavailability of adefovir is approximately 30%, but is increased to 40% with meals. The long intracellular half-life of 16 to 18 hours permits once-daily dosing. The majority of adefovir is renally excreted; unchanged drug and dosage adjustments are required in renal dysfunction. There are no known significant drug interactions. Common adverse effects include nausea, vomiting, malaise, and diarrhea. Elevations in hepatic transaminases and creatinine phosphokinases are reported. An unusual toxicity of adefovir is carnitine depletion, the clinical consequences of which are unclear in adults. Nevertheless, concurrent carnitine supplementation is necessary during adefovir therapy to normalize carnitine levels. The most serious toxicity is a dose-related nephrotoxicity. Proteinuria and elevations in serum creatinine are more common at the higher dosages of adefovir (120 mg). Fanconi's syndrome, a proximal tubular defect characterized by renal failure, wasting of electrolytes, glucose, protein, and renal tubular acidosis, is reported. The dosage in clinical trials ranged from daily doses of 40 to 120 mg, but it is expected that the approved dosage will be 60 mg, which might reduce the renal toxicity. Cross-resistance with other NRTIs appears limited. Moderate reductions in adefovir viral susceptibility occur in vitro with mutations at K65R, T69D, and K70E; similar results have not been shown in vivo (Table 76.8). Interestingly, the M184V mutation, usually associated with 3TC resistance, may enhance the activity of adefovir.

Information about the antiviral activity of adefovir is limited. In a double-blind phase II/III trial (GS 408), 442 patients with a mean baseline CD4 count of 355 cells/mm^3 and mean VL log^{10} 4.4 copies/mL, were randomized to add adefovir 120 mg daily or placebo to their preexisting antiretroviral regimen. About 39% of these patients were failing therapy with protease inhibitors (PIs). Preliminary results at 24 weeks showed a dismal mean decrease in VL of 0.39 log^{10}. Based on these observations, adefovir may not be an extremely potent antiviral agent.

Protease Inhibitors

The available PIs include soft gel saquinavir (SG-SAQ), hard-gel saquinavir (HG-SAQ), ritonavir (RTV), indinavir (IDV), nelfinavir (NFV), and amprenavir (APV).[84,85] All the PIs differ in their pharmacokinetics, tolerability, and drug interaction profile (Tables 76.3 and 76.9). The protease inhibitors are thought to act primarily at the end of the HIV life cycle to cause the formation of noninfectious immature virions (Fig. 76.1). Cleavage of these polyproteins is required for the formation of infectious virions; therefore, noninfectious mature virions are produced when PI are used.

The introduction of PIs in late 1995 revolutionized the care of persons infected with HIV and renewed hope for those affected by the HIV epidemic. These agents represent a major advance in the management of HIV disease and have dramatically altered disease progression to AIDS, reduced HIV-related hospitalizations owing to opportunistic infections, and prolonged survival.[2–4] Patients gained weight, felt stronger, and rejoined the work force. Significant improvements in CD4 cell counts and profound suppression of viral replication were observed, even in advanced HIV disease.[85] The inclusion of a PI within a dual NRTI regimen, or highly active antiretroviral therapy (HAART), is often recommended as initial therapy. Monotherapy with the PI should be avoided to prevent the emergence of resistance and subsequent drug failure. A comprehensive review of clinical trials, including dual PI trials, are summarized in Rana et al.[85]

Despite their undisputed effectiveness, several complex clinical issues are associated with the use of these agents. Adherence is critical, as loss of antiviral efficacy has been correlated with poor pill taking and loss of viral suppression.[86] The high pill burden and coordination with meals make these agents laborious to take; proper instructions are key to improve adherence.[87] The potential for life-threatening drug-drug interactions are significant because the PI are substrates of, and are metabolized by, the cytochrome P450 system (Table 76.9). The most potent P450 enzyme inhibitor is ritonavir. Indinavir, nelfinavir, and amprenavir are moderate inhibitors, whereas saquinavir is the least potent inhibitor. Drug resistance is shared among the class of PIs; therefore, development of resistance to one PI can confer resistance to another (Table 76.8). Last, new adverse effects have been identified (Table 76.10), a consequence of their rapid approval and limited knowledge about their long-term toxicity.

Lipodystrophy, diabetes, hyperlipidemia, and anecdotal reports of atherosclerotic complications have been described, causing concern about their long-term safety.[88–93] Lipodystrophy is characterized by central fat redistribution, including a "buffalo hump," augmented breast size in women, and increased abdominal girth (e.g., "crixbelly") associated with peripheral wasting of the buttocks, face, and extremities. Hypercholesterolemia, hypertriglyceridemia, and insulin resistance might also be present. The prevalence of lipodystrophy is unknown; however, incidences of 10 to 64% have been reported.[90] Usually, the lipodystrophy occurs after prolonged therapy and is associated with beneficial effects on well being, improved CD4 counts, and reductions in viral load. The etiology of this syndrome is unknown. Most experts believe that it is related to the use of protease inhibitors, although similar symptoms have also been reported in the absence of PI therapy. Diabetes is uncommon and occurs in those with risk factors for diabetes.[94–96] Treatment of hyperglycemia with diet, oral hypoglycemic agents, or insulin is effective, permitting continued use of the PI. Troglitazone, a cytochrome P450 enzyme inducer, should be used cautiously because it might reduce the efficacy of the PI. Hyperlipidemia can be managed with HGM-CoA reductase inhibitors, niacin, cholesterol binders, or fibric acid derivatives (e.g., gemfibrozil). Coadministration of simvastatin and lovastatin, whose metabolism is impaired by the PI, should be avoided because of the potential for rhabdomyolysis and acute renal failure. Pravastatin, atorvastatin, and possibly fluvastatin, are less likely to cause this toxic reaction and are recommended.[97] For isolated hypertriglyceridemia, the fibric acid derivatives (e.g., gemfibrozil) are indicated, but response may be poor. Ongoing studies are addressing the interaction of the statins with the PI. Creatinine phospokinase (CPK) levels should be routinely monitored, if

Table 76.10 ▪ Metabolic Adverse Effects Associated with the Protease Inhibitors

Adverse Effect	Potential Mechanism	Counseling	Treatment Recommendations
Hyperglycemia/diabetes	Related to insulin resistance	Signs and symptoms of diabetes: decrease wt if obese, decrease carbohydrate intake, increase exercise	Diet, oral hypoglycemics, insulin, metformin. Avoid troglitazone (P450 enzyme inducer).
Hyperlipidemia Hypercholesterolemia Hypertriglyceridemia	Unknown mechanism of action	Decrease cardiac risk factors: decrease wt if obese, increase exercise, stop smoking, BP control	Diet, niacin, fibric acid derivatives, HGMCo reductase inhibitors. Avoid simvastatin and lovastatin owing to risk of rhabdomyolysis and renal failure.
Abnormal fat distribution Increased abdominal girth, increased breast size, "buffalo hump," peripheral wasting	Unknown mechanism	Cosmetic; likely to reverse if stop PI	Stop PI if bothersome. Growth hormone may be effective.

Source: References 88–91.

warranted, for complaints of muscle weakness, muscle pain, or new renal dysfunction. Currently, there are no recommendations to stop PI therapy unless the lipodystrophy is of significant cosmetic concern to the patient, or if control of metabolic abnormalities is inadequate. Treatment of the lipodystrophy with growth hormone might be effective.[98,99] Changing to a less potent PI might reduce some of the effects on the lipid profile. For example, ritonavir appears to produce the most pronounced effect on triglyceride levels compared with other PI.

Hard-gel Saquinavir (Invirase)

The hard-gel formulation of saquinavir (HG-SAQ, Invirase) was approved by the FDA in December 1995 as the first member of this new antiretroviral class. It is the least potent of the currently approved PI; like all PI, it should not be used as monotherapy to prevent the emergence of resistance. FDA approval was based on favorable surrogate marker changes in three double-blind studies involving persons infected with HIV at different stages of their disease.[84,85] Modest increases in CD4 counts of 40 to 50 cells/mm^3 and declines in viral load of 0.5 log^{10} were found in ZDV-experienced patients who received the triple combination of HG-SAQ/ZDC/ddC compared with those receiving the dual combinations of ZDV/ddC and ZDV/HG-SAQ.[100] A beneficial effect on outcome endpoints has been observed with the combination of HG-SAQ/ddC. In 940 zidovudine-experienced, patients infected with HIV (NV 14256), a 66% reduction in deaths and a 50% decrease in the risk of disease progression to the first AIDS-defining event occurred in those receiving HG-SAQ 600 mg plus ddC 0.75 mg three times a day compared with those on ddC or saquinavir monotherapy.[101] Various ongoing studies will compare the safety and efficacy of the old and new SAQ formulations.

The mean absolute bioavailability of HG-SAQ is poor because of its large first-pass effect, about 4% being absorbed when taken with a high-fat meal. The soft-gel saquinavir (SG-SAQ, Fortovase) formulation was developed to overcome the poor bioavailability of the HG-SAQ.[102] Dissolving saquinavir in Capmul MCM90, a liquid of mono- and diglycerides medium-chain fatty acids, increases the bioavailability to 12%. The terminal elimination half-life of SAQ is approximately 13 hours and the drug is rapidly metabolized to inactive metabolites by the cytochrome P4503A4 isoenzyme. The FDA-approved dosage of HG-SAQ 600 mg three times a day should be administered with a high-fat meal to improve its bioavailability. However, data suggest that this FDA-approved dosage may be suboptimal. Doses of 3600 to 7200 mg per day of HG-SAQ monotherapy achieved a mean maximal viral load reduction of 1.1 to 1.5 log^{10}, respectively. At 24 weeks, these effects were sustained, producing a 0.5 log^{10} to 0.9 log^{10} reduction in viral load, respectively. Additionally, increases in CD4 counts of 100 cells above baseline were noted and resistance was also lower.[103] Unfortunately, the expense and tremendous pill burden make these high dosages of HG-SAQ impractical and cumbersome. However, the pill burden of the new soft gel formulation, at an approved dosage of 1200 mg three times a day or 18 capsules per day, is not much better. Medications or foods (e.g., ketoconazole, grapefruit juice, ritonavir) that inhibit the P4503A4 enzyme system have been observed to significantly increase plasma concentrations of HG-SAQ. Thus, purposely combining ritonavir plus either saquinavir formulation has improved compliance by reducing the pill burden and producing significant rises in CD4 cell counts and a drop in HIV-1 RNA levels.[103] Plasma levels of saquinavir in combination with RTV are 60-fold higher than when SAQ is given alone. A single-dose study of SAQ plus ranitidine increased the bioavailability of SAQ by 67% in 12 healthy subjects. Similarly, enzyme inducers (e.g., rifampin, rifabutin, nevirapine, efavirenz, anticonvulsants) that can significantly reduce SAQ levels should be completely avoided. An upward saquinavir dosage adjustment might be appropriate if coadministration is required with the aforementioned agents. Efavirenz reduced saquinavir levels by 60% and coadministration is not recommended. Rifabutin 300 mg per day reduces the steady-state AUC of saquinavir by 40%. Although SAQ is not a strong enzyme inhibitor, coadministration of SAQ with astemizole, cisapride, ergot alkaloids, triazolam, and midazolam should be avoided because of the increased risk of cardiac arrhythmia and excessive sedation (Table 76.9).

Saquinavir is very well tolerated. Gastrointestinal effects, including nausea, diarrhea, and abdominal pain are the most common. During high-dose saquinavir therapy or in combination with ritonavir, diarrhea, cough, rash, and elevated transaminases were more frequent. Laboratory abnormalities include increased levels of creatine phosphokinase, hyperglycemia, hypercholesterolemia, hypertriglyceridemia, and elevated transaminases.

Ritonavir (Norvir)

Ritonavir (RTV, Norvir) was approved by the FDA in March 1996 as the second licensed PI in the United States.[84,85,104] In March 1997, an FDA indication for treatment of children with HIV infection or AIDS was approved. Two phase I/II trials of ritonavir monotherapy (1000 to 1200 mg per day) demonstrated a potent reduction in VL of 1 to 2 log^{10} and significant increases in CD4 cell counts of 230 cells/mm^3. Sustained virologic benefits were not observed with lower doses.[105,106] Approval was based on ritonavir's striking clinical benefits, including beneficial changes in immunologic and virologic surrogate markers, improved quality of life, reductions in disease progression, and a survival advantage. Abbott's M94-247 was a double-blind, multicenter study that randomized 1090 persons infected with HIV with a mean CD4 count of 32 cells/mm^3 on at least two other antiretroviral agents, to either ritonavir 600 mg two times a day or placebo. After 6 months, 34% of those receiving a placebo developed an AIDS-defining event or died, compared with 17% for the ritonavir group.

The cumulative mortality was 10.1% on placebo compared with 5.8% in those receiving RTV.[107] Although ritonavir is an extremely potent PI, its poor tolerability and its extensive drug interaction profile are of concern.

Ritonavir is available as capsules, which require refrigeration, and as a liquid, which is stable at room temperature for 30 days. Availability of ritonavir capsules has been limited by problems of drug crystallization. Ritonavir is well absorbed and should be administered with food to minimize the gastrointestinal intolerance. Decreased absorption occurs when RTV is administered with antacids; therefore, patients should be instructed to separate RTV and antacids, including ddI, by at least 2 hours. Of the PI, ritonavir is the most potent inhibitor of the cytochrome (CYP) 4503A isoenzymes and the potential for fatal drug-drug interactions is significant (Table 76.9).[104] Coadministration of ritonavir with astemizole, terfenadine, cisapride, various antiarrhythmics, and several sedative-hypnotics (e.g., triazolam, midazolam) is contraindicated because of the potential for cardiac arrhythmias and oversedation. Caution is also required when ritonavir is coadministered with a wide variety of agents, including narcotics and psychotropics, whose metabolism is inhibited by ritonavir; a dosage adjustment might be required to prevent toxicity. Ritonavir can also induce glucuronosyl transferases, decreasing efficacy of oral contraceptives, thyroxine, and theophylline. Alternate forms of contraception are recommended and an upward dosage adjustment for thyroxine and theophylline might be necessary. Enzyme inducers, such as rifampin and rifabutin, can reduce the efficacy of ritonavir, and should be avoided. The significant alcohol content of ritonavir liquid and capsules can produce a disulfiram reaction in those receiving disulfiram or metronidazole. Because of the potential for significant drug–drug interactions with ritonavir, pharmacists should review the patient's medication profile before starting therapy. However, this potent enzyme inhibition has been advantageous in certain situations by increasing the amount of poorly bioavailable agents (e.g., saquinavir).

Ritonavir is the most problematic PI to administer because of its poor tolerability profile, leading to a high rate of drug discontinuation. Patients should be instructed that ritonavir can cause frequent gastrointestinal side effects, including nausea, vomiting, anorexia, abdominal pain, diarrhea, and taste disturbances, especially during the first 2 to 4 weeks of therapy. These symptoms are correlated with high plasma concentrations of ritonavir and can be minimized by slowly escalating the dose of ritonavir. Ritonavir induces its own metabolism, causing high, initial plasma levels to fall and reducing its side effects with continued dosing. It is recommended that ritonavir be started at 300 mg two times a day and increased over 1 to 2 weeks, in 100-mg increments as tolerated, to 600 mg two times a day (Table 76.3). The gastrointestinal symptoms are less problematic when lower dosages of 200 to 400 mg two times a day of ritonavir are used in combination with other PI (Table 76.7); dose escalation is not required. Proper instructions to administer ritonavir capsules or liquids with meals, juices, and so on are essential to increase palatability and improve adherence. Several suggestions, including coating the tongue with peanut butter and disguising the medication with ice cream, jelly, or chocolate syrup have been recommended to improve the palatability of the liquid. Circumoral paresthesia (25%), peripheral paresthesia (5 to 6%) asthenia, fatigue, and headaches are self-limiting and do not necessitate stopping the drug. Hematological toxicity is infrequent. Laboratory abnormalities include hypertriglyceridemia, hyperglycemia, hypercholesterolemia, and elevations in transaminases and creatine kinase. Triglyceride levels can exceed 1000 mg/dL (11 mmol/L); however, pancreatitis is uncommon. The adverse effects of ritonavir on the lipid profile have raised concerns about potential long-term complications from atherosclerotic disease. Anecdotal reports of vascular complications have been reported.[92,93] Ritonavir appears to be more likely than other PIs to cause lipid abnormalities, and changing to a less potent inhibitor might correct the hyperlipidemia. CPK should be routinely monitored, and if warranted, for complaints of muscle weakness, muscle pain, or new renal dysfunction. Abnormal fat accumulations (e.g., lipodystrophy) have also been reported.[88–91]

Indinavir (Crixivan)

Indinavir (IDV, Crixivan), the third PI approved, received accelerated FDA licensing in March 1996. Approval was based on impressive immunologic and virologic changes in surrogate markers during several phase II/III studies.[84,85] Merck 035, a randomized, double-blind trial conducted in 97 ZDV-experienced but 3TC-naive patients, compared IDV alone, the triple combination of IDV/ZDV/3TC, and the dual nucleoside combination of ZDV/3TC.[108] The baseline median CD4 count was 144 cells/mm^3 and the VL was 43,190 copies/mL. After 24 weeks, the greatest viral load reduction of 1.77 log^{10} occurred with the triple combination therapy compared with 1.24 log^{10} and 0.83 log^{10} in the monotherapy and dual combination arms, respectively. Mean CD4+ cell count increases at 24 weeks were 86, 100.6, and 46.3 cells/mm^3 for the three respective groups. At 24 weeks, 90% of those receiving the triple combination achieved undetectable viral loads that were sustained at 48 weeks, compared with 43% for IDV alone, and 0% for those in the dual NRTI arms. The Merck 020 study was an open-label trial comparing IDV monotherapy with ZDV-ddI and the combination of IDV/ZDV/ddI in 78 antiretroviral-naive patients with a median CD4+ cell count of 150 cells/mm^3 and a viral load of 117,000 copies/mL. After 24 weeks, patients receiving the triple combination arm were more likely to achieve undetectable viral loads (60%) compared with 15% for the other groups.[109] Merck 033, a phase III study, randomized 742 antiretroviral-naive patients with a mean CD4 count of 254 cells/mm^3 and mean viral load of 19,000 copies/mL, to ZDV alone, IDV alone, or ZDV/IDV. At 24 weeks, the groups receiving IDV alone or the IDV-containing combination achieved undetectable viral loads in 40 and 50% of patients, respectively, results that were not statistically different. However, the emergence of genotypic resistance to either drug was less in the IDV-combination arm, suggesting improved virologic activity over IDV monotherapy. Merck 039, a double-blind, phase II/III study, randomized 320 3TC and PI-naive patients with advanced HIV disease (CD4 count <50 cells/mm^3 and median VL of approximately 90,000 copies/mL) to ZDV/3TC, IDV monotherapy, or ZDV/3TC/IDV. Subjects receiving the triple combination had a median 2.2 $\log^{10}$ drop in viral load, a mean 86-cell increase in CD4 counts, and 65% achieved an undetectable viral load compared with only 4% on IDV alone and 0% on the dual NRTI arm.[110] These several trials demonstrate that triple combination therapy is associated with improved and sustained virologic and immunologic benefits compared with dual NRTI or IDV alone and delays the emergence of resistance. Treatment-naive subjects derive greater benefits than those with more advanced HIV disease.

In addition to impressive changes in surrogate markers, a beneficial effect on outcome has been demonstrated for an indinavir-containing combination. ACTG 320, a double-blind trial, randomized 1156 lamivudine and PI-naive subjects with mean CD4 of 86 cells/mm^3, to the dual combination of ZDV/3TC or triple combination of ZDV/3TC/IDV.[111] After 38 weeks, the study was prematurely terminated because of significant differences in clinical disease progression and mortality between the dual and triple combination arms. Approximately 50% fewer disease progression events occurred in those receiving ZDV/3TD/IDV compared with the ZDV/3TC group. Rates were 6 and 11% ($P = .001$), respectively; and for those with CD4 counts less than 50 cells/mm^3, 11 and 20%, respectively ($P = .005$). Eight subjects in the triple combination arm died compared with 18 receiving the dual combination ($P = .042$).

Indinavir is rapidly absorbed, but its bioavailability is reduced with meals. Patients should be reminded to administer IDV on an empty stomach (1 hour before meals or 2 hours after) for maximal benefit. If gastrointestinal symptoms are intolerable, IDV can also be ingested with a light, low-fat, low-protein meal. Indinavir has been detected in CSF, most likely related to its lower protein binding (60%) to α-$_1$acid glycoprotein compared with other PI.[112] Similar to ritonavir, drug interactions are of concern because indinavir is also metabolized by the CYP3A4 isoenzyme. About 20% of IDV is eliminated unchanged in the urine; no dosage adjustments are required in renal dysfunction.[58] The dosage of indinavir is 800 mg every 8 hours around the clock to maintain effective plasma levels. A study, evaluating an indinavir dosing interval of every 12 hours achieved suboptimal trough concentrations, and has been abandoned. However, a two times a day dosing regimen administered without regard to meals, may be effective when indinavir is combined with nelfinavir or ritonavir (Table 76.7).[113] In cirrhosis, the dosage of indinavir should be reduced to 600 mg every 8 hours. In patients receiving hemodialysis, no dosage modification is recommended if liver function is normal. Hemodialysis should be performed at the end of the indinavir dosing interval.[114] Coadministration of indinavir with agents whose metabolism will be inhibited, including terfenadine, astemizole, triazolam, midazolam, and ergots, should be avoided to prevent potentially fatal complications (Table 76.9). Coadministration of indinavir and rifampin also should be avoided to prevent loss of indinavir's antiretroviral activity. Coadministration of indinavir and rifabutin requires a dosage reduction of rifabutin to prevent rifabutin toxicity and uveitis. Decreased absorption occurs when IDV is administered with antacids; therefore, patients should be instructed to separate IDV and antacids, including ddI, by at least 2 hours.

Indinavir is better tolerated than ritonavir. The principal complication of indinavir is nephrolithiasis, caused by crystallization of the drug in the kidney. Kidney stones have been reported in 4 to 8% of patients.[115,116] Symptoms include nausea, flank pain (with or without hematuria), dysuria, urgency, renal colic, and renal obstruction leading to renal dysfunction. Oral hydration with 1.5 to 2 liters of noncaffeinated beverages daily is recommended to prevent stone formation; higher fluid intakes may be necessary in warmer climates. Patients unable (e.g., uncontrolled heart failure) or unwilling to comply with hydration should be considered poor candidates for IDV therapy. Stopping IDV therapy is not always necessary to reverse urologic symptoms or resolution of the stone. If aggressive hydration does not relieve symptoms, and renal obstruction persists, then discontinuing therapy is warranted. Asymptomatic indinavir crystalluria, reported in 20% of patients receiving indinavir, did not predict development of renal stones, and is not an indication for stopping therapy. Indinavir can cause mild gastrointestinal complaints of nausea (12 to 32 %), vomiting (4 to 12%), abdominal pain (8 to 9%), diarrhea (4.5%), and symptoms of gastroesophageal reflux (2%). Headache, fatigue, and weight gain can also occur. Lipodystrophy, a syndrome of abnormal central fat redistribution and peripheral wasting, sometimes referred to as "crixbelly," has been associated with all PI but is frequently reported with indinavir owing to its widespread use.[88,89] Laboratory abnormalities include hyperglycemia, lipid abnormalities, and mild to moderate asymptomatic hyperbilirubinemia (usually >2.5 mg/dL), which do not warrant drug discontinuation. However, symptoms of jaundice or hepatitis do necessitate stopping the drug to prevent further liver damage.[117]

Nelfinavir (Viracept)

Nelfinavir (NFV, Viracept) was the fourth PI approved by the FDA in March 1997 for adults and children infected with HIV. Clinical experience with this PI is the most limited and studies are ongoing.[84,85] Improvement of immunologic and virologic surrogate markers has been demonstrated but there are no data showing a delay in disease progression or a survival advantage.[118] The combination of

500 or 750 mg of NFV three times a day plus d4T versus d4T monotherapy was administered to 307 PI and d4T-naive subjects with a mean CD4 count of 279 cells/mm^3 and mean viral load of 141,000 copies/mL (Agouron 506). At 24 weeks, the NFV-containing regimens achieved approximately a 1-log viral load reduction compared with a 0.5-log^{10} decline in those receiving d4T monotherapy. Similarly, 19 to 20% of those receiving either nelfinavir regimen achieved an undetectable viral load compared with only 2% of those receiving d4T monotherapy. Protocol 511, a multicenter, double-blind study, randomized 297 antiretroviral-naive patients to ZDV/3TC plus nelfinavir (500 mg t.i.d. or 750 mg t.i.d.) or the combination of ZDV/3TC and placebo. The mean baseline CD4 was 288 cells/mm^3 and the mean baseline viral load was 153,044 copies/mL. At 24 weeks, both of the nelfinavir-containing regimens achieved superior results compared with the placebo group. However, 75% of those receiving the higher NFV dosing regimen had undetectable viral loads compared with 60% of those on the lower dose NFV regimen.[119] Increases in CD4 count were similar in the two nelfinavir groups. Both of these trials demonstrate that NFV is a potent protease inhibitor and that the higher dosing regimen is preferable.

Nelfinavir is well absorbed, and plasma levels are increased two to three times when NFV is administered with meals. The half-life is approximately 3.5 hours and NFV undergoes metabolism by hepatic CYP3A4 isoenzymes. The FDA recommended dosage is 750 mg three times a day; however, pharmacokinetic data indicate that a 1250-mg two times a day regimen is equally effective and more convenient.[120] Nelfinavir is most similar to indinavir in its drug interaction profile (Table 76.9). Like other PI, nelfinavir should not be administered with terfenadine, astemizole, cisapride, or ergots to avoid the potential for cardiac arrhythmias. Rifampin can significantly reduce NFV levels and coadministration is not recommended. The combination of nelfinavir and saquinavir increases the AUC of saquinavir by 392% and can be an effective treatment combination (Table 76.7). Because nelfinavir can reduce the efficacy of combination oral contraceptives by enzyme induction, an alternative or additional form of contraception (e.g., barrier contraceptives) is recommended.

Nelfinavir is the best tolerated of the available PI.[84] The major adverse effect of nelfinavir is mild to moderate diarrhea, which can be bothersome in 15 to 32% of those receiving nelfinavir. The diarrhea may be managed with over-the-counter antidiarrhea agents and was responsible for study discontinuation in less than 2% of subjects. Similar to other PI, nelfinavir is associated with lipodystrophy, lipid abnormalities, and hyperglycemia. Less common side effects include rash, headache, nausea, and flatulence.

Amprenavir (Agenerase)

Amprenavir (APV, Agenerase) is a "fast-track" PI FDA-approved in in April 1999.[121] Preliminary phase III data (ACTG 347) demonstrate significant virologic activity when APV is combined with 3TC and ZDV in PI and 3TC-naive subjects with a median baseline CD4 cell count of 305 cells/mm^3 and HIV-RNA of 37,889 copies/mL.[122] Undetectable viral loads were achieved in the majority of patients; and 63% of patients maintained durable viral suppression for 48 weeks. Clinical studies indicate that APV's antiviral activity is comparable to other PIs. A median VL reduction of 2.65 log^{10} from baseline is reported when APV is used in combination with other antiretroviral agents. Amprenavir has been safely given with ABC, ZDV, 3TC, and other PIs, including SAQ-SG, IDV, and NFV. In vitro, synergy was demonstrated when APV was combined with ZDV, ddI, ABC, or saquinavir; additive effects were seen with IDV or RTV. In vitro, the principal mutation producing a twofold reduction in susceptibility to APV occurs at codon 50, a mutation not found in other PIs, which may make cross-resistance to other PIs less likely (Table 76.8). Isolates resistant to APV showed limited cross-resistance to saquinavir or indinavir. Additional mutations at codons 46 and 47 produced a three- to 14-fold reduction in amprenavir susceptibility.

Amprenavir is 90% protein bound to α_1-acid glycoprotein. The half-life of APV is approximately 9 hours, permitting twice-daily dosing. The approved dosage is 1200 mg two times a day taken with or without food. Adherence might be difficult owing to the high pill burden of 8 tablets taken per dose, totaling 16 tablets daily. Amprenavir undergoes biliary excretion and is an inhibitor of the hepatic P450 CYP3A4 and CYP2C19 isoenzyme system. Its inhibitory potency is less than RTV, similar in potency to those of nelfinavir and indinavir, and greater than those of saquinavir. Its drug interaction profile requires further clarification, but is likely to be similar to other PIs (Table 76.9). Ritonavir and ketoconazole can significantly increase APV concentrations and dosage adjustments may be required. No dosage adjustments are recommended when APV is coadministered with IDV or NFV. EFV can decrease AMV levels and its coadministration is not recommended. Similar to other PIs, the coadministration of rifampin and APV should be avoided; and rifabutin doses need to be reduced when administered with APV to prevent rifabutin toxicity (e.g., uveitis). Amprenavir appears well tolerated. Adverse effects reported in more than 10% of patients receiving amprenavir monotherapy include rash, diarrhea, and headache. Rarely, Stevens-Johnson syndrome has been reported.

Non-Nucleoside Reverse Transcriptase Inhibitors

The non-nucleoside reverse transcriptase inhibitors (NNRTIs) include nevirapine, delavirdine, and efavirenz (Table 76.4). Unlike the NRTIs, the NNRTIs do not require activation by cellular phosphorylation for its antiretroviral activity. The NNRTIs do not have activity against HIV-2. The NNRTIs inactivate the HIV-1 RT by noncompetitively binding directly to the HIV-RT structure, likely at amino acid positions 100 and 103 (Fig. 76.1). Substitutions of the RT amino acids residues at these positions confer resistance to their antiviral activity. All the NNRTIs bind to the same RT enzyme pocket so that cross-resistance among the NNRTIs is likely despite their structural dissimilarities (Table 76.8). K103N was the predominant viral mutant, followed by Y188L or V108I mutations, that was observed among HIV+ persons experiencing viral rebound on efavirenz monotherapy. The NNRTIs should not be used as monotherapy but should be used only in combination with other antiretroviral agents to prevent the rapid emergence of resistance. Similar to the PIs, drug interactions are of concern, since the NNRTIs are metabolized by the hepatic CYP3A4 isoenzymes and can be either enzyme inducers or inhibitors (Table 76.9). Unlike most of the PIs, these agents are also attractive because they penetrate the blood-brain barrier. Although the NNRTIs are less potent agents than the PIs, there is considerable enthusiasm about the use of effective protease-sparing regimens as concerns about drug resistance and new adverse effects of the PIs (e.g., lipodystrophy, hyperlipidemia) increase.

Nevirapine (Viramune)

Nevirapine (NVP, Viramune) was the first NNRTI approved by the FDA in June of 1996. In December 1998, NVP received an FDA indication for the treatment of children infected with HIV. It is a dipyridodiazepinone analog with specific and potent inhibitory activity against the HIV-1 RT enzyme; it is also active against ZDV-sensitive and -resistant viruses. Early studies in treatment-experienced patients with advanced HIV disease only showed modest reductions in viral load and improvements in CD4 cell counts. However, more dramatic immunologic and virologic improvements were reported in treatment-naive patients when NVP was used in combination with 2 NRTI to sustain its antiretroviral activity and prevent the emergence of resistance. ACTG 241 was a placebo-controlled study of 398 ZDV-experienced patients with CD4 cell counts of 135 to 140 cell/mm^3, who were randomized to receive either NVP/ddI/ZDV or the ZDV/ddI/placebo combination. After 48 weeks, no difference was noted between the two groups in terms of clinical progression to AIDS or death, although a sustained 0.5 log^{10} reduction in viral load and a maximum 34 CD4 cells/mm^3 increase from baseline was achieved with the NVP-containing regimen. The best response was obtained in those with CD4 counts greater than 200 cells at baseline.[123] ACTG 193 randomized 1313 treatment-experienced patients with mean CD4 cell counts of 20 cells/mm^3 to ZDV alternating with ddI, or ZDV/ddC, or ZDV/ddI, or NVP/ddI/ZDV. Compared with the dual regimens, the triple combination group had the lowest mortality rate (36%) and the longest survival time (median 112 weeks).[124] This study suggest a favorable but modest clinical benefit of a NVP triple combination for patients with more advanced disease. The most impressive data for NVP is obtained from the INCAS (Italy, Netherlands, Canada, Australia) Trial, a double-blind, controlled study that randomized 151 treatment-naive patients with a mean CD4+ count of 376 cells/mm^3 to ZDV/NVP or ZDV/ddI or ZDV/NVP/ddI.[125] The NVP/ddI/ZDV triple combination produced a greater and sustained reduction in plasma viral load (2.18 log^{10}) than either of the dual regimens (1.55 log^{10} vs. 0.9 log^{10}). At week 52, the proportion of patients with HIV-1 RNA levels below 20 copies/mL were 51, 12, and 0% with ZDV/ddI/NVP, ZDV/ddI, and ZDV/NVP arms, respectively (P <.001). The greatest increase in CD4 cell counts of 120 cells/mm^3, and the greatest reduction from baseline viral load (1.7 log^{10}) also occurred in those receiving triple combination. Although disease progression or death were lower for those receiving the triple combination regimen (12%), it was not significantly different from both of the dual regimens (23%, 25%, P = .08). The INCAS trial suggests that a NVP triple combination might be an effective protease-sparing regimen.

The safety and pharmacokinetics of NVP has also been evaluated in seven HIV-1 infected pregnant women who received a single 200-mg oral dose at the onset of labor.[28] Their infants also received a single oral 2-mg/kg dose at 2 to 3 days of age. Although NVP elimination was impaired, the half-life of NVP was prolonged to 66 hours in the mother (compared with 45 hours in the nonpregnant female) and to 36.8 hours in the neonate (compared with 24.8 hours in children). No adverse effects were noted. A phase III perinatal transmission prevention clinical trial is under way to evaluate the efficacy of NVP in pregnancy and the newborn.

Nevirapine is well absorbed (bioavailability of 93%) and is not affected by food, antacids, or ddI. Approximately 60% of NVP is protein bound, permitting NVP to penetrate the CSF, attaining levels about 50% of those achieved in the plasma. The half-life ranges from 22 to 84 hours (mean 40 hours), suggesting that a daily dosing regimen may be effective. Similar to the PI, NVP is metabolized by the hepatic CYP3A4 isoenzymes. NVP is an enzyme inducer and has the potential to reduce blood levels of various medications (e.g., saquinavir), including inducing its own metabolism. Metabolic autoinduction of NVP results in an up to twofold increase in NVP systemic clearance after chronic administration of 200 to 400 mg daily for 1 to 2 weeks. Autoinduction also results in a reduction of its half-life from 45 hours to 25 to 30 hours after chronic administration. Therefore, a dose-escalation of NVP is recommended to minimize high drug concentrations and possibly, reduce adverse effects, primarily rash. Careful monitoring is required if NVP is coadministered with rifampin, rifabutin, oral contraceptives, triazolam, and midazolam (Table 76.9). The dosage of NVP is 200 mg every day for the first 2 weeks to reduce the incidence of rash, and then, if no rash, the dose should be increased to 200 mg two times a day. A once-daily 400-mg dosage is under investigation.

The dose-limiting side effect of NVP is a diffuse, erythematous, maculopapular rash that can occur in as many as 50% of subjects. The rash typically occurs within the first few weeks of administration and its occurrence is minimized by dose escalation. However, the rash may not always disappear with continued NVP administration and the dose should not be increased to twice-daily administration if the rash persists. Antihistamines can alleviate symptoms but NVP should be stopped if the rash is severe or if constitutional symptoms (e.g., fever, blister) are present. Drug discontinuation is required in 6% of cases. Patients should be instructed about the characteristics of the rash and to contact their pharmacist or physician if the rash persists. Rarely, life-threatening Stevens-Johnson syndrome has been reported (0.5%). Other adverse reactions reported include headache, dizziness, fever, fatigue, nausea, ulcerative stomatitis, abdominal pain, diarrhea, and elevated transaminases.

Delavirdine (Rescriptor)

Delavirdine (DLV, Rescriptor) is the second NNRTI approved for treatment of HIV-1 infection in adults. It is a bis(heteroaryl) piperazine and is chemically distinct from nevirapine. Although the approval package was sent to the FDA in November of 1996, delavirdine's approval was delayed until April 1997 because of the weakness of the data presented. Clinical data on DLV are very limited and there are no data confirming a survival advantage or delay in disease progression. Protocol 017 randomized treatment-experienced patients with mean CD4 cell counts of 135 cell/mm^3 to DLV 400 mg three times a day plus ddI or ddI monotherapy. The trial was stopped at 6 months because there was no statistical difference in mortality or disease progression between the two groups. Protocol 021 randomized less experienced patients with a mean CD4 cell counts of 325 cells/mm^3 to ZDV plus DLV at doses of 200, 300, or 400 mg three times a day.

The bioavailability of DLV is 85% and can be administered without regard to meals. The preferred method to administer DLV is to make a slurry of four (100-mg) tablets, dissolved in 3 to 4 oz of water, which improves its bioavailability by 20%. Absorption of DLV is decreased if administered with buffered products; therefore, patients should be instructed to separate DLV and antacids, including ddI by at least 2 hours (Table 76.9). The penetration of DLV into the CNS is more limited than NVP because of DLV's higher protein binding (98%). Delavirdine is also metabolized by the cytochrome P4503A4 system; however, unlike NVP, DLV is an enzyme inhibitor, and may inhibit its own metabolism. Coadministration of DLV with terfenadine, astemizole, cisapride, alprazolam, midazolam, triazolam, ergots, and amphetamines should be avoided because toxic blood levels of these drugs can produce cardiac arrhythmias and oversedation. Enzyme inducers, including rifampin, rifabutin, and the anticonvulsants (e.g., phenytoin, carbamazepine, and phenobarbital) can reduce DLV's efficacy and coadministration is not recommended.

Delavirdine's tolerability profile is very similar to NVP. A diffuse, erythematous, maculopapular, pruritic, skin rash is the most frequent complaint, occurring in 20 to 40% of study subjects. The rash usually occurs during the first few weeks of DLV dosing, and is self-limiting in 85% of patients despite drug continuation. Antihistamines can alleviate the pruritus and rash. In severe cases, the drug should be stopped to avoid progression to systemic symptoms of fever, facial swelling, mucosal involvement, or desquamation. Dose escalation of DLV is not helpful to reduce the occurrence of the rash. The cross-reactivity of rash from DLV or NVP is unknown but is expected to be low based on its different chemical structures. Other adverse effects include headache, nausea, diarrhea, and fatigue. Laboratory abnormalities include increased transaminases, and rarely, anemia and neutropenia.

Efavirenz (Sustiva)

Efavirenz (EFV, Sustiva) is the third NNRTI approved by the FDA in late September 1998 for the treatment of HIV-1 infection in adults and children.[126] Similar to all the NNRTI, its optimal use is in combination with at least two other antiretroviral agents to prevent the rapid emergence of resistance. Like other antiretroviral agents, viral suppression is more pronounced in antiretroviral-naive than in experienced patients. Efavirenz is unique among the NNRTIs because it is the initial NNRTI recommended by the DHHS Panel on Clinical Practices for Treatment of HIV Infection as an effective "protease-sparing" alternative.[25] The superiority of an EFV-containing combination was shown in a large, multicenter, open label, head-to-head trial (Dupont 006) that randomized 450 antiretroviral-naive or minimally pretreated patients to the triple combination of EFV/ZDV/3TC, the "gold standard" regimen of IDV/ZDV/3TC, or the dual combination of EFV/IDV.[127] This study was sufficiently powered to evaluate equivalence between the IDV/EFV combination and the triple combination of ZDV/3TC/IDV. Despite an open-label design and short followup of 48 weeks, using an "intent-to-treat" analysis, it was statistically significant that 64% of those receiving the EFV triple combination achieved an undetectable viral load compared with 44% on the IDV-containing regimen, and 43% on the dual EFV/IDV regimen. Adverse effects leading to discontinuation were higher in the IDV triple combination arm (37.8%) versus the EFV triple combination (20.8%) that may have biased the results favorably toward EFV. Nevertheless, the data are convincing enough that experts believe that EFV can be a comparable PI alternative.

Multiple trials of efavirenz-containing combinations have demonstrated significant immunologic and durable virologic activity, although currently there are no data demonstrating a survival advantage.[126] Efavirenz has been studied in combination with d4T, ZDV, 3TC, IDV, and NFV. A multicenter, double-blind, placebo-controlled, dose-ranging study evaluated the antiretroviral activity and safety of EFV 200 to 600 mg in combination with open-label ZDV and 3TC in 137 antiretroviral-naive patients. At 36 weeks of followup, 100% of patients receiving the highest EFV 600-mg dosage achieved an undetectable VL and an increase from baseline of 102 CD4 cells compared with 80 to 88% of those receiving the lower doses of EFV.[128] A multicenter, double-blind, phase II pilot study observed durable activity of an EFV/IDV combination on HIV-

RNA suppression and CD4 recovery for up to 72 weeks.[129] Protease inhibitor and NNRTI-naive persons infected with HIV ($n = 101$) were randomized to the combination of EFV/IDV or to IDV alone, with the addition of d4T and EFV after 12 weeks. At 72 weeks irrespective of the baseline plasma RNA level, 85% of those receiving the combination of EFV/IDV achieved an undetectable VL compared with 71% on the triple regimen of IDV/d4T/EFV. The EFV/IDV arm reported significant increases in CD4 count of 243 cells compared with 175 cells for the IDV arm. A 48-week multicenter, open label, nonrandomized study enrolled 30 antiretroviral-naive and 33 NNRTI and PI-naive persons infected with HIV on EFV 600 mg daily and nelfinavir (NFV) 750 mg every 8 hours with food.[130] Preliminary results at 16 weeks showed that 55.4% of patients achieved an undetectable VL by the ultrasensitive assay. No statistically significant differences were identified in antiretroviral-naive or experienced patients. A significant increase in CD4 count (61.9 cells) from baseline was observed in the experienced group. An ongoing study, comparing the addition of efavirenz, nelfinavir, or EFV/NFV to new NTRI in antiretroviral-experienced persons, showed that the VL was undetectable in 64% on NFV, 69% on EFV, and 81% on the combination of EFV plus NFV at 16 weeks. A double-blind, multicenter study (33 sites) randomized 237 patients on 2 NRTI to IDV/placebo or to EFV/IDV. At 24 weeks, 73.5% of those on EFV combination compared with 45.1% on the IDV combination achieved a plasma RNA less than 50 copies/mL by ultrasensitive assay.[131] Both combinations similarly elevated CD4 counts.

EFV can be taken with or without food; however, a high-fat meal should be avoided to limit increased absorption. Its long half-life of more than 40 hours permits daily dosing. Therapeutic CSF concentrations of EFV have been reported, similar to other NNRTIs.[126] Efavirenz is metabolized by the hepatic CYP3A4, and is both an inhibitor and inducer of the P450 system (Table 76.9). The administration of EFV with cisapride, astemizole, rifampin, and terfenadine is contraindicated. The combination of the soft-gel saquinavir formulation as the sole PI and efavirenz produced a clinically significant 60% decline in saquinavir concentrations, limiting use of this combination until further information is available. For persons receiving the combination of 400 mg two times a day of SAQ plus RTV 400 mg two times a day, it is not necessary to increase the dosage of SAQ when EFV is added. However, some clinicians have empirically increased the dosage of SAQ to 800 mg twice a day. Data from the manufacturer of RTV reported no increase in adverse effects in normal volunteers who took RTV 400 mg two times a day and SAQ 800 mg two times a day. The metabolism of IDV is increased about 35% by EFV, necessitating an IDV dosage increment to 1 g every 8 hours. No dosage adjustment of nelfinavir or ritonavir is required with EFV. It can be given at bedtime or divided into three daily doses if necessary to minimize the CNS adverse effects.

CNS side effects from efavirenz can be disabling in up to 50% of patients. Typical symptoms include fatigue, dizziness, headache, insomnia, "feelings of disconnection," and impaired concentration; however, confusion, stupor, agitation, hallucinations, abnormal dreaming, euphoria, paresthesias, nervousness, and somnolence are also reported. Patients should be educated that these CNS side effects are transient and should resolve within 1 month despite drug continuation. Instructions to take the efavirenz at bedtime can alleviate some of these CNS symptoms. Patients with a history of baseline altered mental status, psychiatric disturbances, or confusion may not be appropriate candidates for EFV therapy. Other side effects include nausea, headache, and a rash that usually do not require drug discontinuation; serious rash is less common than other marketed NNRTI. In a phase II trial, adverse effects were reported in 58% ($n = 54$) of patients and included grade II rash (10.7%), diarrhea (6%), abdominal pain (9%), nausea (6%), headache (5%), hematuria (8%), and elevations in transaminases (5%). EFV should be avoided in pregnant women until further data are available because congenital malformations have been reported in monkeys. Barrier contraceptives are recommended during EFV use in women of childbearing age.

ALTERNATIVE THERAPIES

Hydroxyurea (HU, Hydrea), a chemotherapeutic agent, is increasingly being used in persons who have failed multiple antiretroviral agents (e.g., salvage therapy).[132] It may also be beneficial in acute primary infection by reducing CD8-mediated killing of CD4 cells. In 11 patients treated with hydroxyurea, ddI, and IDV or NFV within 2 months of infection, CD4 cell counts increased and viral load remained undetectable throughout treatment. Additionally, there was no HIV RNA detected in the lymph nodes in two patients, and absence of viral rebound was noted in one patient after stopping therapy.[133] Hydroxyurea alone does not have any antiviral activity. However, hydroxyurea is often combined with ddI or d4T, and other antiretroviral agents, including a PI. A synergistic effect of hydroxyurea and ddI has been shown in vitro. Hydroxyurea depletes deoxynucleoside triphosphates, particularly dATP required for DNA synthesis, by inhibiting ribonucleoside reductase. Because ddI competes with dATP for DNA synthesis, HU facilitates the increased uptake of ddI or other NRTI for incorporation into the DNA. Although impressive reductions in viral load have been reported, outcome data are limited. The Swiss HIV Cohort Study randomized 144 antiretroviral-naive persons (mean VL 4.5 $\log^{10}$ and mean CD4 370 cells/mm^3) to ddI/d4T/HU 500 mg two times a day or ddI/d4T per placebo.[134] At 12 weeks, 54% ($n = 39/72$) of patients receiving HU achieved the primary endpoint (VL <200 copies/mL) compared with 28% ($n = 20/72$) in the placebo group. Using the ultrasensitive assay (<20 copies/mL), 19% of those receiving HU had undetectable VL compared with 8% in the placebo group. Although mean VL reduction was 2.3 $\log^{10}$ in the HU group versus 1.7 $\log^{10}$ in the placebo group, the increase in CD4 counts was lower in the HU group than the placebo group. The combination of ddI/d4T/HU was also reported to be superior to the combination of ddI/HU. Hydroxyurea is given in dosages of 500 mg to 1 g two times a day. Neutropenia, bone marrow toxicity, and reduced CD4 counts have been reported. Patients with pre-existing bone marrow suppression, especially those with a CD4 count less than 50 cells/mm^3 or an absolute neutrophil count less than 2000 cell/mm^3, may not be appropriate candidates for hydroxyurea. A complete blood count, including hematocrit, hemoglobin, platelets, white blood cell counts, and CD4 counts, should be routinely monitored in patients receiving hydroxyurea-containing combinations. Until further comparative or outcome data are available, HU should be reserved as salvage therapy for those failing or intolerant of conventional agents.

FUTURE THERAPIES

Several new agents within the existing antiretroviral classes are under investigation (Table 76.11). New NRTIs include 2′-3′-dideoxy-5-fluoro-3′thiacytidine (FTC), a fluorinated "me-too" 3TC agent with a similar resistance profile. Lodanosine, or FddA, is a fluorinated analog of ddI that is acid stable, eliminating the need for a buffer. The nucleotide analog, *bis*-POC-PMPA (tenofovir) is similar to adefovir but has greater potency and does not cause carnitine depletion. Several "second generation" PIs are in phase II and III trials, including ABT-378, tipranavir (PNU-140690), DMP-450, and AG 1776. ABT-378 is usually combined with ritonavir to significantly increase ABT's blood level, permitting once daily administration. Several "second-generation" NNRTIs under investigation, including S-1153, AG 1549, DMC 961, and DMC 963, possess potent antiviral activity against the K103N mutation that confers drug resistance to currently available NNRTIs.

Table 76.11 ▪ Future Therapies Under Investigation

Nucleoside reverse transcriptase inhibitors	FTC (2′-3′-dideoxy-5-fluro-3′ thiacytidine) Lodanosine (FddA) Bis-POC-PMPA (tenofovir) Lobucavir
Protease inhibitors	ABT-378 (Abbott) Tipranavir (PNU-140690) DMP-450 AG1776 (Agouron)
Non-nucleoside reverse transcriptase inhibitors	AG 1549 (Agouron) DMC 961, DMC 963 S-1153
Novel strategies	Peptide fusion inhibitor (T-20) Zinc fingers
Immunotherapy	Interleukin-2

Other NNRTIs under investigation include MKC-442, carboxanilide analogs with very long half-lives, and calanolide A.

Novel strategies will focus on an essential step in the life cycle of HIV, preventing HIV entry and infection of CD4 lymphocytes and other target cells. The peptide fusion inhibitor, T-20, inhibits HIV from entering the target cells by hindering the gp41 protein on the virus.[135] Preliminary results in four out of 16 infected persons receiving the highest doses of T-20 are promising. Intravenous administration of 100 mg of T-20 two times a day for 2 weeks produced 99% reductions of plasma HIV-RNA without significant toxicity. However, concerns about durability of its antiviral activity, resistance, poor oral bioavailability, and tissue penetration are additional issues that will need to be addressed before T-20 will be clinically feasible. Also under investigation are agents that inhibit cell entry by blocking interaction of the gp 120 with the CCR5 coreceptor.

Interleukin-2 (IL-2) is currently being studied in the treatment of HIV infection. In 44 patients already receiving HAART, 5-day cycles of 9 million units per day of IL-2 administered every 6 weeks or whenever the CD4 count fell below 1.25-fold of baseline, produced increases in CD4 counts and fewer opportunistic infections compared with 20 patients on HAART alone.[136] Three out of 14 persons infected with HIV were reported to have had virtually a "cure" following therapy with IL-2 and standard antiretrovirals. IL-2 is designed to flush HIV from latently infected cells in order to expose it to the antiretrovirals. HIV could not be cultured from 330 million immune cells taken from the three patients. Hopes of eradication may be premature until patients are taken off therapy to see if the virus rebounds. Adverse effects of IL-2 include flulike symptoms, including myalgias, fever, malaise, and fatigue. Elevations in viral load occur after IL-2 therapy so that adequate antiretroviral therapy must occur before receiving IL-2 therapy. Immunotherapeutic approaches that transfer protective cytotoxic lymphocyte cells using autologous HIV-1 *gag*-specific CD8+ cells clones appear promising.[137]

An effective and safe AIDS vaccine is not expected before the year 2003. The ability of the virus to rapidly mutate and evolve is a major obstacle and challenge to the development of a vaccine. Two ongoing phase III trials in the United States and Thailand are evaluating a gp 120-envelope vaccine; results will not be available until 2003.

IMPROVING OUTCOMES

Patient Education

Antiretroviral agents are extremely complex regimens that need to be properly administered and taken by the patient to maximize therapeutic efficacy. Therefore, patient education and an assessment of the patient's ability to comply with therapy are essential before therapy is started. Discussion should include proper administration of the regimen, the brand and generic names of the drugs, the number of pills taken per dose, the frequency of doses, total number of pills taken daily, coordination with meals, storage conditions, drug interactions, adverse effects, and availability of the pharmacist for consultation.[138] The relationship between adherence, viral load response, viral resistance, drug failure, and impact on future regimens need to be emphasized.[139] The pharmacist should ensure that the patient has a clear understanding of the information discussed. Counseling by pharmacists to increase medication adherence and knowledge about HIV disease has been effective in reducing viral load.[140]

Methods to Improve Patient Adherence to Drug Therapy

Reported rates of adherence to HIV therapy, defined as missed doses, incorrect dosages, or incorrect time of administration, range from 46 to 88%.[138] Using a Medication Event Monitoring System (MEMS), an ACTG study indicated that 82% of doses were taken but only 55 to 76% were taken at the right time, and 27% took the right dosage. In 10 ACTG clinics reporting nonadherence rates of 11 to 36%, the most common explanations given for missed dosages were forgetfulness and disruption of daily routine (e.g., being away from home, long clinic visits, and number of blood tests). Only 10% missed doses because of adverse events. Additional barriers to compliance include the patient's actual or perceived state of health (e.g., threat posed by the disease, perceived self-benefit), the complexity of the therapeutic regimen, the patient-provider relationship (e.g., mutual respect), and psychological barriers (e.g., mental disturbance; substance abuse, including alcohol; unstable living situations; lack of support system).[38,39]

Several strategies and devices can enhance medication adherence. Because forgetfulness is common, written instructions, individualized medication organizers, and reminder devices (e.g., programmable watch, beepers, electronic pillboxes) should supplement verbal medication instructions. Pharmacists have achieved undetectable viral load by educating patients about HIV disease, simplifying the medication regimen, and using medication reminders.[140] Simple instruction sheets identifying the time of pill administration can be helpful. Directly observed therapy has been recommended to improve medication adherence in persons infected with HIV.

PHARMACOECONOMICS

The use of new AIDS drugs, such as the PI, reduces nondrug costs. The database of California's Medi-Cal Program was used to assess mortality and health care costs in over 6000 persons infected with HIV receiving protease inhibitors.[141] Monthly mortality rates per 100 person years in July 1994 fell from 42.8 to 10.6 in December 1996 as the number of persons using PIs increased. Although direct pharmacy costs increased from $543 to $779, overall costs fell from $1959 to $1261 per patient per month during this same time period due to reduced hospitalization days. Hospitalization days dropped from 2.9 per 100 person days to 1.0 per 100 person days during the 2½ years, lowering monthly inpatient costs per person from $727 to $156. Clinical Partners, which conducted a study in conjunction with Merck, reported that monthly drug costs for patients in Texas and California enrolled in health care plans between January 1995 and December 1997, rose from $200 to $1100; however, monthly non-drug costs decreased from $1300 to $200. Over the last 14 months, the average monthly costs remained at $1300.

KEY POINTS

- Management of HIV infection with HAART have dramatically reduced the progression of HIV to AIDS, reduced hospitalizations for opportunistic infections, improved overall health and well being, and prolonged survival.
- Therapy with HAART may permit modification of antibiotics for primary and secondary prophylaxis of opportunistic infections.
- Therapy with a minimum of two nucleoside analogs and one to two PIs or an NNRTI is considered the standard of care.
- Therapy is most effective in antiretroviral-naive patients compared with experienced persons.
- The goals of therapy are to improve survival by reducing the viral load to undetectable levels for as long as possible to maintain durable viral suppression, prevent the emergence of resistance, and prevent drug failure.
- Patient adherence to these complicated regimens is essential to avoid the emergence of drug resistance and drug failure.
- Eradication of HIV is not yet achievable due to the presence of latent reservoirs that are inaccessible to current antiretroviral therapy.
- Reconstitution of the immune system appears promising if therapy is started during the initial primary infection.
- Antiretroviral therapy is protective against mother-to-child HIV transmission, against occupational exposures in health care workers, and possibly against nonoccupational exposures.
- Lipodystrophy, diabetes, hyperlipidemia, and vascular accidents are disturbing side effects of HAART.
- Significant drug–drug interactions with PIs and NNRTIs could be fatal and should be anticipated.
- Hydroxyurea is a popular alternative therapy used primarily in combination with other antiretrovirals for patient failing multiple antiretrovirals (salvage regimen).
- Promising future therapies include IL-2, T-20 fusion inhibitors, and vaccines.

REFERENCES

1. Centers for Disease Control and Prevention. 1993 revised classification system for HIV infection and expanded surveillance case definition for AIDS among adolescents and adults. MMWR 41(RR-17):1–19, 1992.
2. Detels R, Munoz A, McFarlane G, et al. Effectiveness of potent antiretroviral therapy on time to AIDS and death in men with known HIV infection duration. JAMA 280:1497–1503, 1998.
3. Palella FJ, Delaney KM, Moorman AC, et al. Declining morbidity and mortality among patients with advanced human immunodeficiency virus infection. N Engl J Med 338:853–860, 1998.
4. Hogg RS, Heath KV, Yip B, et al. Improved survival among HIV-infected individuals following initiation of antiretroviral therapy. JAMA 279:450–454, 1998.
5. Finzi D, Hermankova M, Pierson T, et al. Identification of a reservoir for HIV-1 in patients on highly active antiretroviral therapy. Science 278:1295–1300, 1997.
6. Chun TW, Stuyver L, Mizell SB, et al. Presence of an inducible HIV-1 latent reservoir during highly active antiretroviral therapy. Proc Natl Acad Sci USA 94:13193–13197, 1997.
7. Chun TW, Engel D, Berrey MM, et al. Early establishment of a pool of latently infected, resting CD4 (+) T cells during primary HIV-1 infection. Proc Natl Acad Sci USA 95:8869–8873, 1998.
8. Rothenberg RB, Scarlett M, delRio C, et al. Oral transmission of HIV. AIDS 12:2095–2105, 1998.
9. Moore JP. Co-receptors: implications for HIV pathogenesis and therapy. Science 276:51–52, 1997.
10. Katz M, Gerberding JL. The care of persons with recent sexual exposure to HIV. Ann Intern Med 128:306–312, 1998.
11. Connor EM, Sperling RS, Gelber R, et al. Reduction of maternal-infant transmission of human immunodeficiency virus type 1 with zidovudine treatment. N Engl J Med 331:1173–1180, 1994.
12. Centers for Disease Control and Prevention. Administration of zidovudine during late pregnancy and delivery to prevent perinatal HIV transmission: Thailand 1996–1998. MMWR 47(RR-8):151–153, 1998.
13. Centers for Disease Control and Prevention. Diagnosis and reporting of HIV and AIDS in states with integrated HIV and AIDS surveillance–United States, January 1994–June 1997. MMWR 47:309–314, 1998.
14. Ho DD. Toward HIV eradication or remission: the tasks ahead. Science 280:1866–1867, 1998.
15. Robbins PA, Roderiquez GL, Peden KW, et al. Human immunodeficiency virus type 1 infection of antigen-specific CD4 cytotoxic T lymphocytes. AIDS Res Hum Retroviruses 14:1397–1406, 1998.
16. Greenough TC, Brettler DB, Somasundaran M, et al. Human immunodeficiency virus type 1-specific cytotoxic T lymphocytes (CTL), virus load, and CD4 T cell loss: evidence supporting a protective role for CTL in vivo. J Infect Dis 176:118–125, 1997.
17. Liegler TJ, Yonemoto W, Elbeik T, et al. Diminished spontaneous apoptosis in lymphocytes from human immunodeficiency virus-infected long-term non-progressors. J Infect Dis 178:669–679, 1998.
18. Mellors JW, Munoz AM, Giorgi VJ, et al. Plasma viral load and CD4+ lymphocytes as prognostic markers of HIV-1 infection. Ann Intern Med 126:946–954, 1997.
19. Wali RK, Drachenberg CI, Papadimitriou JC, et al. HIV-1 associated nephropathy and response to highly-active antiretroviral therapy (letter) Lancet 352:783–784, 1998.
20. Albrecht H, Hoffmann C, Degen O, et al. Highly active antiretroviral therapy significantly improves the prognosis of patients with HIV-associated progressive multifocal leukoencephalopathy. AIDS 12:1149–1154, 1998.
21. Fisher M. Should we be stopping opportunistic infection prophylaxis in the era of HAART? J Infect 36:iv, 1998.
22. Lopez JC, Pena JM, Miro JM, et al. Discontinuation of PCP prophylaxis (PRO) is safe in HIV-infected patients (PTS) with immunological recovery with HAART. Preliminary results of an open, randomized, and multicentric clinical trial (GESIDA04/98). In Abstracts of the 6th Conference on Retroviruses and Opportunistic Infections. January 31–February 4, 1999, Chicago, IL. Abstract LB7.
23. Kahn JO, Walker BD. Acute human immunodeficiency virus type 1 infection. N Engl J Med 339:33–39, 1998.
24. Centers for Disease Control and Prevention. Update: HIV counseling and testing using RAPID tests–United States, 1995. MMWR 47:211–215, 1998.
25. Department of Health and Human Services and Henry J. Kaiser Family Foundation. Guidelines for the use of antiretroviral agents in HIV-infected adults and adolescents. MMWR 47(RR-5):43–82, 1998.
26. Carpenter CCJ, Cooper DA, Fischl MA, et al. Antiretroviral therapy in adults. Updated recommendations of the International AIDS Society–USA Panel. JAMA 283:381–390, 2000.
27. Centers for Disease Control and Prevention. Guidelines for the use of antiretroviral agents in pediatric HIV infection. MMWR 47(RR-4):1–43, 1998.
28. Centers for Disease Control and Prevention. Public Health Service Task Force recommendations for the use of antiretroviral drugs in pregnant women infected with HIV-1 for maternal health and for reducing perinatal HIV-1 transmission in the United States. MMWR 47(RR-2):1–30, 1998.
29. Center for Disease Control and Prevention. Public Health Service guidelines for management of health-care worker exposures to HIV and recommendations for postexposure prophylaxis. MMWR 47(RR-7):1–33, 1998.
30. Center for Disease Control and Prevention. Public Health Service statement for management of possible sexual, injecting-drug-use, or other nonoccupational exposure to HIV, including considerations related to antiretroviral therapy. MMWR 47(RR-17):1–15, 1998.
31. Gazzard B, Moyle G. 1998 revision to the British HIV Association Guidelines for antiretroviral treatment of HIV seropositive individuals. Lancet 352:314–316, 1998.
32. Brosgart CL, Mitchell TF, Coleman RL, et al. Clinical experience and choice of drug therapy for human immunodeficiency virus disease. Clin Infect Dis 28:14–22, 1999.
33. Walker BD, Basgoz N. Treat HIV-1 infection like other infections–treat it. JAMA 280:91–93, 1998.
34. Levy JA. Caution: should we be treating HIV infection early? Lancet 352:982–983, 1998.
35. Burman WJ, Reves RR. The case for conservative management of early HIV disease. JAMA 280:93–95, 1998.
36. Farzadegan H, Hoover DR, Astemborski J, et al. Sex differences in HIV-1 viral load and progression to AIDS. Lancet 352:1510–1514, 1998.
37. Weverling GJ, Lange JM, Juriaans S, et al. Alternative multidrug regimen provides improved suppression of HIV-1 replication over triple therapy. AIDS 12:F117–F122, 1998.
38. Bangsberg D, Tulsky JP, Hecht RM, et al. Protease inhibitors in the homeless. JAMA 278:63–65, 1997.
39. Strathdee SA, Palepu A, Cornelisse PG, et al. Barriers to use of free antiretroviral therapy in injection drug users. JAMA 280:547–549, 1998.
40. Havlir DV, Marschner IC, Hirsch MS, et al. Maintenance antiretroviral therapies in HIV infected subjects with undetectable plasma HIV RNA after triple drug therapy. N Engl J Med 339:1261–1268, 1998.
41. Pialoux G, Raffi F, Brun-Vezinet B, et al. A randomized trial of three maintenance regimens given after three months of induction therapy with zidovudine, lamivudine, and indinavir in previously untreated HIV-1 infected patients. N Engl J Med 339:1269–1276, 1998.
42. Reijers MH, Weverling GJ, Jurriaans S, et al. Maintenance therapy after quadruple induction therapy in HIV-1 infected individuals: Amsterdam Duration of Antiretroviral Medication (ADAM) study. Lancet 352:185–190, 1998.
43. Wainberg MA, Friedland G. Public health implications of antiretroviral therapy and HIV drug resistance. JAMA 279:1977–1983, 1998.
44. Boden D, Markowitz M. Resistance to human immunodeficiency virus type 1 protease inhibitors. Antimicrob Agents Chemother 42:2775–2783, 1998.
45. Hirsch MS, Conway B, D'Aquila RT, et al. Antiretroviral drug resistance testing in adults with HIV infection. Implications for clinical management. JAMA 279:1984–1991, 1998.
46. Culnane M, Fowler M, Lee SS, et al. Lack of long-term effects of in utero exposure to zidovudine among uninfected children born to HIV-infected women. JAMA 281:151–157, 1999.
47. Saba J, on behalf of the PETRA Trial Study Team. Interim analysis of early efficacy of three short ZDV/3TC combination regimens to prevent mother-to-child transmission of HIV-1: the PETRA trial. In Abstracts of the 6th Conference on Retroviruses and Opportunistic Infections. January 31–February 4, 1999, Chicago, IL. Abstract S7.
48. Wade NA, Birkhead GS, Warren BL, et al. Abbreviated regimens of zidovudine prophylaxis and perinatal transmission of the human immunodeficiency virus. N Engl J Med 339:1409–1414, 1998.
49. Centers for Disease Control and Prevention. Case-control study of HIV seroconversion in health-care workers after percutaneous exposure to HIV-infected blood–France, United Kingdom, and United States, January 1988–August 1994. MMWR 44:929–933, 1995.
50. Volberding PA, Lagakos SW, Grimes JA, et al. A comparison of immediate with deferred zidovudine therapy for asymptomatic HIV-infected adults with CD4 cell counts of 500 or more per cubic millimeter. N Engl J Med 333:408–413, 1995.

51. Concorde Coordinating Committee. Concorde: MRC/ANRS randomized double-blind controlled trial of immediate vs. deferred zidovudine in symptom-free HIV infection. Lancet 343:871–888, 1994.
52. Hammer SM, Katzenstein DA, Hughes MD, et al. A trial comparing nucleoside monotherapy with combination therapy in HIV-infected adults with CD4 cell counts from 200 to 500 per cubic millimeter. N Engl J Med 335:1081–1090, 1996.
53. Delta Coordinating Committee. Delta: a randomized double-blind controlled trial comparing combinations of zidovudine plus didanosine or zalcitabine with zidovudine alone in HIV-infected individuals. Lancet 348:283–291, 1996.
54. Saravolatz LD, Winslow DL, Collins G, et al. Zidovudine alone or in combination with didanosine or zalcitabine in HIV-infected patients with the acquired immunodeficiency syndrome or fewer than 200 CD4 cells per cubic millimeter. Investigators for the Terry Beirn Community Program for Clinical Research on AIDS. N Engl J Med 335:1099–1106, 1996.
55. Sommadossi JP, Zhou XJ, Moore J, et al. Impairment of stavudine (d4T) phosphorylation in patients receiving a combination of zidovudine (ZDV) and d4T (ACTG 290). In Abstracts of the 5th Conference on Retroviruses and Opportunistic Infections. February 1–5, 1998, Chicago, IL. Abstract 3.
56. Havlir DV, Friedland G, Pollard R, et al. Combination zidovudine (ZDV) and stavudine (d4T) therapy versus other nucleosides. Report of two randomized trials (ACTG 290 and 298). In Abstracts of the 5th Conference on Retroviruses and Opportunistic Infections. February 1–5, 1998, Chicago, IL. Abstract 2.
57. Burger DM, Kraaijeveld CL, Meenhorst PL, et al. Penetration of zidovudine into the cerebrospinal fluid of patients infected with HIV. AIDS 7:1581–1587, 1993.
58. Hilts AE, Fish DN. Dosage adjustments of antiretroviral agents in patients with organ dysfunction. Am J Health Syst Pharm 55:2528–2533, 1998.
59. Sidtis JJ, Gatsonis C, Price RW, et al. Zidovudine treatment of the AIDS dementia complex. Results of a placebo-controlled trial. Ann Neurol 33:343–349, 1993.
60. Landonio G, Cinque P, Nosari A, et al. Comparison of two dose regimens of zidovudine in an open, randomized, multicentre study for severe HIV-related thrombocytopenia. AIDS 7:209–212, 1993.
61. Barry M, Wild M, Veal G, et al. Zidovudine phosphorylation in HIV-infected patients and seronegative volunteers. AIDS 8:F1–F5, 1994.
62. Dalakas MC, Illa I, Pezeshkpour GH, et al. Mitochondrial myopathy caused by long-term zidovudine therapy. N Engl J Med 322:1098–1105, 1990.
63. Kahn JO, Laggakos SW, Richman DD, et al. A controlled trial comparing continued zidovudine with didanosine in human immunodeficiency virus infection. The NIAID AIDS Clinical Trials Group. N Engl J Med 327:581–587, 1992.
64. Abrahms DI, Goldman AI, Launer C, et al. A comparative trial of didanosine or zalcitabine after treatment with zidovudine in patients with the human immunodeficiency virus infection. N Engl J Med 330:657–662, 1994.
65. Hoetelmans RM, van Heeswijk RP, Profijt M, et al. Comparison of the plasma pharmacokinetics and renal clearance of didanosine during once and twice daily dosing in HIV-infected individuals. AIDS 12:F211–F216, 1998.
66. Fischl MA, Stanley K, Collier AC, et al. Combination and monotherapy with zidovudine and zalcitabine in patients with advanced HIV disease. The NIAID AIDS Clinical Trials Group. Ann Intern Med 122:24–32, 1995.
67. Gustavson LE , Fukuda EK, Rubio FA, et al. A pilot study of the bioavailability and pharmacokinetics of 2′,3′-dideoxycytidine in patients with AIDS or AIDS-related complex. J Acquir Immune Defic Syndr 3:28–31, 1990.
68. Pollard R, Peterson D, Hardy D, et al. Stavudine (d4T) and didanosine (ddI) combination therapy in HIV-infected subjects: antiviral effect and safety in an on-going pilot, randomized, double-blind trial. In Abstracts of the 11th International Conference on AIDS. July 7–12, 1996, Vancouver, Canada. Abstract Th. B293.
69. Raffi F, Reliquet V, Auger S, et al. Efficacy and safety of stavudine and didanosine combination therapy in antiretroviral experienced patients. AIDS 12:1999–2005, 1998.
70. Durant J, Rahelinirina V, Delmas B, et al. A pilot study of the combination of stavudine (d4T) and didanosine (ddI) in patients with <350 CD4/mm^3 and who are not eligible for a treatment with ZDV. In Abstracts of the 4th Conference on Retroviruses and Opportunistic Infections. January 22–26, 1997, Washington, DC. Abstract 553.
71. Foudraine NA, Hoeteimans RM, Lange JM, et al. Cerebrospinal-fluid HIV-1 RNA and drug concentrations after treatment with lamivudine plus zidovudine or stavudine. Lancet 351:1547–1551, 1998.
72. Dienstag JL, Perrillo RP, Schiff ER, et al. A preliminary trial of lamivudine for chronic hepatitis B infection. N Engl J Med 333:1657–1661, 1995.
73. CAESAR Coordinating Committee. Randomized trial of addition of lamivudine or lamivudine plus loviride to zidovudine-containing regimens for patients with HIV-1 infection: the CAESAR trial. Lancet 349:1413–1421, 1997.
74. Eron JJ, Benoit SL, Jemsek J, et al. Treatment with lamivudine, zidovudine, or both in HIV-positive patients with 200 to 500 CD4+ cells per cubic millimeter. North American HIV Working Party. N Engl J Med 333:1662–1669, 1995.
75. Katlama C, Ingrand D, Loveday C, et al. Safety and efficacy of lamivudine-zidovudine combination therapy in antiretroviral-naive patients. A randomized controlled comparison with zidovudine monotherapy. JAMA 276:118–125, 1996.
76. Staszewski S, Loveday C, Picazo JJ, et al. Safety and efficacy of lamivudine-zidovudine combination therapy in zidovudine-experienced patients: a randomized controlled comparison with zidovudine monotherapy. Lamivudine European HIV Working Group. JAMA 276:111–117, 1996.
77. Bartlett JA, Benoit SL, Johnson VA, et al. Lamivudine plus zidovudine compared with zalcitabine plus zidovudine in patients with HIV infection: a randomized, double-blind, placebo-controlled trial. North American HIV Working Party. Ann Intern Med 125:161–172, 1996.
78. Rouleau D, Conway B, Raboud J, et al. Stavudine plus lamivudine in advanced human immunodeficiency virus disease: a short-term pilot study. J Infect Dis 176:1156–1160, 1997.
79. Katlama C, Valantin MA, Calvez V, et al. ALTIS: a pilot study of D4T/3TC in antiretroviral naive and experienced patients. In Abstracts of the 4th Conference on Retroviruses and Opportunistic Infections. January 22–26, 1997, Washington, DC. Abstract LB4.
80. Zerboni R, Angius AG, Cusini M, et al. Lamivudine-induced paronychia (letter). Lancet 351:1256, 1998.
81. Foster RH, Faulds D. Abacavir. Drugs 55:729–736, 1998.
82. Staszewski S, Katlama C, Harrer T, et al. Abacavir (ABC, 1592) combination therapy in HIV-infected adults: durability to 72 weeks. In Abstracts of the 12th World AIDS Conference. June 28–July 3, 1998, Geneva, Switzerland. Abstract 12212.
83. Fischl M, Greenberg S, Clumeck N, et al. Safety and activity of abacavir (ABC, 1592) with 3TC/ZDV in antiretroviral-naive subjects. In Abstracts of the 12th World AIDS Conference. June 28–July 3, 1998, Geneva, Switzerland. Abstract 12230.
84. Flexner C. HIV-protease inhibitors. N Engl J Med 338:1281–1292, 1998.
85. Rana KZ, Dudley MN. Human immunodeficiency virus protease inhibitors. Pharmacotherapy 19:35–39, 1999.
86. Vanhove GR, Schapiro JM, Winter MA, et al. Patient compliance and drug failure in protease inhibitor monotherapy. JAMA 276:1955–1956, 1996.
87. Von Bargen J, Moorman A, Holmberg S. How many pills do patients with HIV infection take (letter). JAMA 280:29, 1998.
88. Lo JC, Mulligan K, Tai VW, et al. "Buffalo hump" in men with HIV-1 infection. Lancet 351:867–870, 1998.
89. Miller KD, Jones E, Yanovski JA, et al. Visceral abdominal-fat accumulation associated with use of indinavir. Lancet 351:871–875, 1998.
90. Carr A, Samaras K, Burton S, et al. A syndrome of peripheral lipodystrophy and insulin resistance in patients receiving HIV protease inhibitors. AIDS 12:F51–F58, 1998.
91. Carr A, Samaras K, Chisholm DJ, et al. Pathogenesis of HIV-1 protease inhibitor-associated peripheral lipodystrophy, hyperlipidemia, and insulin resistance. Lancet 351:1881–1883, 1998.
92. Henry K, Melroe H, Huebesch J, et al. Coronary artery disease associated with protease inhibitors. Lancet 351:1328, 1998.
93. Gallet B, Pulik M, Genet P, et al. Vascular complications associated with use of HIV protease inhibitors. Lancet 351:1958–1959, 1998.
94. Walli R, Herfort O, Michl GM, et al. Treatment with PI associated with peripheral insulin resistance and impaired oral glucose tolerance in HIV-infected patients. AIDS 12:F167–F173, 1998.
95. Dube MP, Johnson DL, Currier JS, et al. Protease inhibitor-associated hyperglycemia. Lancet 350:713–714, 1997.
96. Kaufman MB, Simionatto C. A review of protease inhibitor-induced hyperglycemia. Pharmacotherapy 19:114–117, 1999.
97. Henry K, Melroe H, Huebesch J, et al. Atorvastatin and gemfibrozil for protease-inhibitor related lipid abnormalities (letter). Lancet 352:1031–1032, 1998.
98. Mauss S, Wolf E, Moser-Juenemann C, et al. Successful treatment of PI-induced visceral abdominal fat accumulation with R-human growth hormone. Abstracts of the 4th International Congress on Drug Therapy in HIV Infection, Glasgow, Scotland. AIDS 12(Suppl 4):S53, 1998. Abstract P 145.
99. Torres R, Unger K. The effect of recombinant human growth hormone on protease-inhibitor-associated fat maldistribution. In Abstracts of the 6th

Conference on Retroviruses and Opportunistic Infections. January 31–February 4, 1999, Chicago, IL, Abstract 675.
100. Collier AC, Coombs R, Schoenfeld DA, et al. Treatment of human immunodeficiency virus infection with saquinavir, zidovudine, and zalcitabine. N Engl J Med 334:1011–1017, 1996.
101. Lalezari J, Haubrich R, Burger HU, et al. Improved survival and decreased progression of HIV in patients treated with saquinavir (Invirase, SQV) plus HIVID (zalcitabine, ddC). In Abstracts of the XI International Conference on AIDS. July 7–12, 1996, Vancouver, Canada. Abstract LB.B 6033.
102. Perry CM, Noble N. Saquinavir soft-gel capsule formulation. A review of its use in patients with HIV infection. Drugs 55:461–486, 1998.
103. Schapiro JM, Winters MA, Stewart F, et al. The effect of high dose saquinavir on viral load and CD4+ T cell counts in HIV-infected patients. Ann Intern Med 124:1039–1050, 1996.
104. Hsu A, Granneman GR, Bertz RJ. Ritonavir. Clinical pharmacokinetics and interactions with other anti-HIV agents. Clin Pharmacokinet 35:275–291, 1998.
105. Markowitz M, Saag M, Powderly WG, et al. A preliminary study of ritonavir, an inhibitor of HIV-1 protease, to treat HIV-1 infection. N Engl J Med 333:1534–1539, 1995.
106. Danner SA, Carr A, Leonard JM, et al. A short-term study of the safety, pharmacokinetics, and efficacy of ritonavir, an inhibitor of HIV-1 protease. N Engl J Med 333:1528–1533, 1995.
107. Cameron W, Health-Chiozzi M, Danner S, et al. Randomised placebo-controlled trial of ritonavir in advanced HIV-1 disease. The advanced HIV disease ritonavir study group. Lancet 351:543–549, 1998.
108. Gulick RM, Mellors JW, Havlir D, et al. Treatment with indinavir, zidovudine and lamivudine in adults with human immunodeficiency virus infection and prior antiretroviral therapy. N Engl J Med 337:734–739, 1997.
109. Massari R, Conant M, Mellors J, et al. A phase II open-label randomized study of the triple combination of indinavir, zidovudine (ZDV) and didanosine (ddI) versus indinavir alone and zidovudine/didanosine in antiretroviral-naive patients. In Abstracts of the 3rd Conference on Retroviruses and Opportunistic Infections. January 28–February 1, 1996, Washington, DC. Abstract 200.
110. Hirsch M, for the protocol 039 (indinavir) study group, Meibohm A, Rawlins S, et al. Indinavir (IDV) in combination with zidovudine (ZDV) and lamivudine (3TC) in ZDV-experienced patients with CD4 cell counts <50 cells/mm^3. In Abstracts of the IV Conference on Retroviruses and Opportunistic Infections. January 22–26, 1997, Washington, DC. Abstract LB7.
111. Hammer SM, Squires KE, Hughes MD, et al. A controlled trial of two nucleoside analogues plus indinavir in persons with human immunodeficiency virus infection and CD4 cell counts of 200 per cubic millimeter or less. N Engl J Med 337:725–733, 1997.
112. Stahle L, Martin C, Svensson JO, et al. Indinavir in cerebrospinal fluid of HIV-infected patients (letter). Lancet 350:1823, 1997.
113. Burger DM, Hugen PW, Prins J, et al. Pharmacokinetics of indinavir in a BID regimen with or without low-dose ritonavir. Abstracts of the 4th International Congress on Drug Therapy in HIV Infection, Glasgow, Scotland. AIDS 12(Suppl 4):S10, 1998. Abstract OP2.7.1.
114. Guardiola JM, Mangues MA, Domingo P, et al. Indinavir pharmacokinetics in haemodialysis-dependent end-stage renal failure (letter). AIDS 12:1395, 1998.
115. Daudon M, Estepa L, Viard JP, et al. Urinary stones in HIV-1 positive patients treated with indinavir. Lancet 349:1294–1295, 1997.
116. Kopp JB, Miller KD, Mican JM, et al. Crystalluria and urinary tract abnormalities associated with indinavir. Ann Intern Med 127:119–125, 1997.
117. Brau N, Leaf HI, Wieczorek RI, et al. Severe hepatitis in three AIDS patients treated with indinavir (letter) Lancet 349:924–925, 1997.
118. Moyle GJ, Youle M, Higgs C, et al. Safety, pharmacokinetics, and antiretroviral activity of the potent, specific human immunodeficiency virus protease inhibitor nelfinavir: results of a phase I/II trial and extended follow-up in patients infected with human immunodeficiency virus. J Clin Pharmacol 38:736–743, 1998.
119. Powderly W, Sension M, Conant M, et al. The efficacy of Viracept (nelfinavir mesylate, NLF) in pivotal phase II/III double-blind randomized controlled trials as monotherapy and in combination with d4T or AZT/3TC. In Abstracts of the IV Conference on Retroviruses and Opportunistic Infections. January 22–26, 1997. Washington, DC. Abstract 370.
120. Peterson A, Johnson M. Long term comparison of BID and TID dosing (Viracept) nelfinavir in combination with statuvudine (d4T) and lamivudine (3TC) in HIV patients. In Abstracts of the 12th World AIDS Conference. June 28–July 3, 1998, Geneva, Switzerland. Abstract 12224.
121. Adkins JC, Faulds D. Amprenavir. Drugs 56:837–842, 1998.
122. Murphy R, Degruttola V, Gulick R, et al. 141W94 with or without zidovudine/3TC in patients with no prior protease inhibitor or 3TC therapy–ACTG 347. In Abstracts of the 5th Conference on Retroviruses and Opportunistic Infections. February 1–5, 1998, Chicago, IL. Abstract 512.
123. D'Aquila RT, Hughes MD, Johnson VA, et al. Nevirapine, zidovudine, and didanosine compared with zidovudine and didanosine in patients with HIV-1 infection. A randomized, double-blind, placebo-controlled trial. National Institute of Allergy and Infectious Disease AIDS Clinical Trials Group Protocol 241 Investigators. Ann Intern Med 124:1019–1030, 1996.
124. Henry K, Thierny C, Kahn J, et al. A randomized, double-blind placebo-controlled study comparing combination nucleoside and triple therapy for the treatment of advanced HIV disease (CD4<50/mm^3). In Abstracts of the IV Conference on Retroviruses and Opportunistic Infections. January 22–26, 1997, Washington, DC. Abstract LB6.
125. Montaner JSG, Reiss P, Cooper D, et al. A randomized, double-blind trial comparing combinations of nevirapine, didanosine, and zidovudine for HIV-infected patients. The INCAS Trial. JAMA 279:930–937, 1998.
126. Adkins JC, Noble S. Efavirenz. Drugs 56:1055–1064, 1998.
127. Tashima K, Staszewski S, Morales-Ramirez J, et al. A phase III, multicenter, randomized, open label study to compare the antiretroviral activity and tolerability of efavirenz (EFV) + indinavir (IDV), versus EFV + zidovudine (ZDV) + lamivudine (3TC), versus IDV + ZDV + 3TC at 24 weeks (Study DMP 266-006). In Abstracts of the 6th Conference on Retroviruses and Opportunistic Infections. January 31–February 4, 1999, Chicago, IL. Abstract LB16.
128. Haas DW, Seekins D, Cooper R, et al. A phase II, double-blind, placebo-controlled, dose ranging study to assess the antiretroviral activity and safety of efavirenz (EFV, Sustiva, DMP 266) in combination with open-label zidovudine (ZDV) with lamivudine (3TC) at 36 weeks (DMP 266-005). In Abstracts of the 12th World AIDS Conference. June 28–July 3, 1998, Geneva, Switzerland. Abstract 22334.
129. Riddler S, Kahn J, Hicks C, et al. Durable clinical anti-HIV-1 activity (72 weeks) and tolerability for efavirenz (DMP 266) in combination with indinavir (IDV) (DMP 266-003, Cohort IV). In Abstracts of the 12th World AIDS Conference. June 28–July 3, 1998, Geneva, Switzerland. Abstract 12359.
130. Mildvan D, Martin G, Eyster M, et al. Initial effectiveness and tolerability of nelfinavir (NFV) in combination with efavirenz (EFV, Sustiva, DMP 266) in antiretroviral therapy naive or nucleoside analogue experienced HIV-1 infected patients: characterization in a phase II, open label, multicenter study at 16 weeks (DMP 266-024). In Abstracts of the 12th World AIDS Conference. June 28–July 3, 1998, Geneva, Switzerland. Abstract 22386.
131. Fessel WJ, Haas DW, Delapenha RA, et al. A phase III, double-blind, placebo-controlled, multicenter study to determine the effectiveness and tolerability of the combination of efavirenz (EFV, Sustiva, DMP 266) and indinavir (IDV) versus indinavir in HIV-1 infected patients receiving nucleoside analogue (NRTI) therapy at 24 weeks (DMP266-020). In Abstracts of the 12th World AIDS Conference. June 28–July 3, 1998, Geneva, Switzerland. Abstract 22343.
132. Romanelli F, Pomeroy C, Smith KM. Hydroxyurea to inhibit human immunodeficiency virus-1 replication. Pharmacotherapy 19:196–204, 1999.
133. Lisziewicz J, Jessen H, Finzi D, et al. HIV suppression by early treatment with hydroxyurea, didanosine, and a protease inhibitor (letter). Lancet 352:199–200, 1998.
134. Rutschmann OT, Opravil M, Iten A, et al. ddI + d4T +/-hydroxyurea for HIV-1 infection. In Abstracts of the 5th Conference on Retroviruses and Opportunistic Infections. February 1–5, 1998, Chicago, IL. Abstract 656.
135. Kilby MJ, Hopkins S, Venetta TM, et al. Potent suppression of HIV-1 replication in humans by T-20, a peptide inhibitor of Gp41-mediated virus entry. Nat Med 4:1302–1307, 1998.
136. Hengge UR, Goos M, Esser S, et al. Randomized, controlled phase II trial of subcutaneous interleukin-s in combination with highly active antiretroviral therapy (HAART) in HIV patients. AIDS 12:F225–F234, 1998.
137. Brodie SJ, Lewinsohm DA, Patterson BK, et al. In vivo migration and function of transferred HIV-1 specific cytotoxic T cells. Nat Med 1:34–41, 1999.
138. Tseng AL. Compliance issues in the treatment of HIV infection. Am J Health Syst Pharmacol 55:1817–1824, 1998.
139. Altice FL, Friedland GH. The era of adherence to HIV therapy. Ann Intern Med 129:503–505, 1998.
140. Graham KK, Beeler LH, Sension MG, et al. Interventions and patient outcome from a pharmacist-based HIV medication adherence referral clinic. In Abstracts of the 12th World AIDS Conference. June 28–July 3, 1998, Geneva, Switzerland. Abstract 32323.
141. Chen M, Rains J, Hiehle G, et al. Mortality and health care costs for 6,297 AIDS patients in California before and after protease inhibitors. In Abstracts of the 12th World AIDS Conference. June 28–July 3, 1998, Geneva, Switzerland. Abstract 12264.
142. Centers for Disease Control and Prevention. Prevention and treatment of tuberculosis among patients infected with human immunodeficiency virus: principles of therapy and revised recommendations. MMWR 47(RR-20):1–78, 1998.

CHAPTER 77

HUMAN IMMUNODEFICIENCY VIRUS INFECTION–ASSOCIATED OPPORTUNISTIC INFECTIONS

Robert C. Stevens

Opportunistic infections have a profound effect on the morbidity and mortality of individuals coinfected with the human immunodeficiency virus (HIV). By definition, when a person infected with HIV develops certain opportunistic infections, that individual is diagnosed with the acquired immunodeficiency syndrome (AIDS). The quality of life of patients with AIDS can be markedly affected after developing an opportunistic infection because of the need in most cases for lifelong therapies to prevent relapse of the clinical infection. This chapter discusses the pathophysiology, clinical presentation, and treatment of selected opportunistic infections in patients with AIDS including *Pneumocystis carinii* pneumonia (PCP), toxoplasmosis encephalitis (TE), disseminated *Mycobacterium avium* complex (MAC) infection, and cytomegalovirus (CMV) retinitis. Important opportunistic fungal infections for AIDS patients are discussed elsewhere in this volume.

Pneumocystis carinii Pneumonia

Pneumocystis carinii is an organism of low virulence in healthy persons; however, the ubiquitous organism causes pneumonia in immunocompromised subjects. Most people in the United States are infected with *P. carinii* by the age of 4 years but do not develop pneumonia because of an intact host defense system.[1] Significant knowledge about this pathogen has been acquired over the past 20 years since the AIDS epidemic was first uncovered. Most notable are improved measures for prevention, and alternatives for treatment, of acute *Pneumocystis carinii* pneumonia (PCP) infection.

TREATMENT GOALS: *PNEUMOCYSTIS CARINII* PNEUMONIA

- Ability to categorize patients who have mild to moderate or severe PCP, because therapy is somewhat dependent on disease severity.
- Selection of the most efficacious drug therapy that is least likely to cause adverse events in a patient infected with HIV. Most drugs used to treat PCP are associated with significant toxicity, which often results in therapy switches or early discontinuation.
- PCP prevention—the hallmark of treatment.
- Early identification of persons infected with HIV who would benefit from primary PCP prophylaxis.
- Counseling of patients about the need for secondary prophylaxis to prevent further episodes of PCP after successful completion of acute therapy.

EPIDEMIOLOGY

Early in the AIDS epidemic, PCP was the indicator disease in more than 60% of newly diagnosed AIDS cases. The widespread implementation of effective preventative measures (i.e., primary drug prophylaxis) has significantly decreased the percent of incidence of this infection. Adherence to drugs for PCP prophylaxis and potent antiretroviral regimens, coupled with a decrease in the number of individuals acquiring new HIV infection, have had pronounced effects on reducing the overall incidence of PCP.

PATHOPHYSIOLOGY

P. carinii is a slow-growing, unicellular eucaryote whose genetic sequence is linked to the fungal kingdom.[1] Its inability to grow on fungal media and its susceptibility to antiprotozoal agents, however, incline clinicians to view *P. carinii* as a parasite despite the molecular evidence that it is a fungus. Transmittal of the organism is likely to require inhalation of an infectious inoculum. Once inhaled, the organism resides in the alveoli generating large numbers of organisms in the setting of T-lymphocyte depletion caused by HIV. Significant production of *P. carinii* alters the alveolar capillary permeability resulting in impairment of gas exchange. Poor distribution of inspired air into alveoli that are obstructed with the organism, fluid, and inflammatory mediators leads to ventilation-perfusion mismatch. This clinical description is similar to the pathogenesis of the adult respiratory distress syndrome discussed in Chapter 82, Bacteremia and Sepsis.

CLINICAL PRESENTATION AND DIAGNOSIS

Signs and Symptoms

The primary target of infection is the lungs, with pneumonia accounting for more than 95% of *P. carinii* infections. More than 90% of patients have pulmonary complaints, primarily cough, shortness of breath, and tachypnea. Nonspecific constitutional symptoms such as fever, night sweats, fatigue, or weight loss also are observed. Since *P. carinii* is a much slower-growing organism than pyogenic bacteria, there is an indolent onset of pulmonary symptoms in persons infected with HIV. These patients may have fever and complain of lethargy and progressive onset of dyspnea on exertion over 2 to 4 weeks before seeking medical attention. The chest radiograph reveals the characteristic bilateral patchy infiltrates. Radiologic appearance lags behind clinical deterioration or improvement. Occasionally, fine basilar rales may be encountered on auscultation, but otherwise physical examination of the pulmonary system is often normal.

Patients with AIDS who develop PCP often have an elevation of serum lactate dehydrogenase (LDH). The sensitivity of an elevated LDH for PCP in this population is between 83 and 100%, with greater sensitivity in critically ill patients than ambulatory patients.[1] Although serum LDH is nonspecific for PCP, it is elevated less frequently with other types of pneumonia. The value of LDH is in evaluating prognosis and response to treatment. A strong correlation exists between degree of LDH elevation and survival. A high or rising LDH while on antipneumocystis therapy correlates with a worse prognosis, a failure of therapy, and increased mortality, whereas a low or a declining serum LDH value suggests the opposite trend.

Diagnosis

Individuals infected with HIV who present with pulmonary and nonspecific constitutional symptoms consistent with PCP, and with a chest radiograph revealing bilateral infiltrates, should have samples collected either by induced sputum or fiberoptic bronchoscopy with bronchoalveolar lavage to isolate the *P. carinii* cysts. Recovery of cysts from sputum or lungs is the definitive diagnosis.

PSYCHOSOCIAL ASPECTS

There are still occasions when the diagnosis of PCP, or another opportunistic infection, signifies the first moment that a patient learns of his or her possible or probable infection with HIV. As improbable as it may seem, there are individuals who participate in high-risk behavior relative to acquiring HIV (i.e., intravenous drug use), but do not know of their HIV status until they seek medical care for their ailing health caused by an opportunistic infection. The implications can be devastating, especially if the individual is seriously ill from the opportunistic infection. These patients require counseling about their newly diagnosed HIV status, as well as how to best resolve the acute episode of PCP.

It is imperative to provide the patient with support and candid information about AIDS so the person will not dwell in a state of denial and thus increase the likelihood of nonadherence to therapy. The more knowledge the person has about AIDS, the more likely he or she will cope well with this infection. Pertinent advice includes information on transmission of the virus, how to discuss his or her HIV status with family and loved ones, arrangement for follow-up care in HIV clinics, and financial resources to support medical and social care.

TREATMENT

Pharmacotherapy for Acute *Pneumocystis carinii* Pneumonia

The selection of appropriate antipneumocystis agents for patient-specific conditions requires an understanding of the subtleties in drug selection and monitoring. The first process in drug selection involves categorizing the pneumonia into mild to moderate PCP versus severe PCP. Mild to moderate PCP is defined by a patient's PaO_2 on room air greater than or equal to 70 mm Hg or an alveolar-arterial oxygen difference [(A-a) DO_2] less than 35 mm Hg. Severe PCP is defined as PaO_2 on room air less than 70 mm Hg or A-a gradient greater than or equal to 35 mm Hg. (The A-a gradient is the difference between the ideal alveolar partial pressure of oxygen [ideal PAO_2] less the measured arterial partial pressure of oxygen [measured PaO_2].) Table 77.1 lists the first-line and alternative treatment methods for PCP.

Mild to Moderate PCP

The schema for therapy of mild to moderate PCP is depicted on the left side of the algorithm in Figure 77.1. Trimethoprim-sulfamethoxazole (TMP-SMX) is widely considered the drug of choice.[2–4] No other drug or drug combination has been demonstrated to be superior to TMP-SMX in efficacy. However, TMP-SMX-induced adverse events are common; therefore, TMP-SMX dosage regimen modifications or drug therapy switches are often indicated.[5]

Commonly observed toxicities associated with TMP-SMX in persons infected with HIV include rash, gastrointestinal distress, neutropenia, thrombocytopenia, elevated liver transaminases, hyperkalemia (TMP acts akin to a potassium-sparing diuretic), hyponatremia, and renal dysfunction. Typically, these toxicities manifest within the first 1 to 2 weeks of therapy.

Morbilliform rash, the most frequent adverse event with TMP-SMX, is commonly self-limiting; rarely have patients infected with HIV developed severe skin reactions. There is no absolute contraindication to a person infected with HIV who has had a prior nonmucous membrane involving nondesquamating dermatological reaction to TMP-SMX to receive the drug in the future, should the individual present with acute PCP or need prophylaxis treatment. In patients with AIDS who develop a rash while on TMP-SMX, it is acceptable to continue treatment provided no mucous membranes are involved and no skin has vesiculated. The mild rash or pruritus can be alleviated with antihistamines if needed.

Neutropenia is a concentration-dependent toxicity of TMP-SMX and can be minimized with appropriate dose modification. Dosing TMP-SMX at 15 mg/kg/day instead of 20 mg/kg/day, or adjusting the dose to obtain TMP concentrations of 5 to 8 μg/mL 1.5 hours after intravenous infusion or oral ingestion, has been shown to lower the incidence of neutropenia.[6] Attempts to ameliorate the bone marrow suppression with folinic acid (analogous to the "leucovorin rescue" practiced with methotrexate in treatment of leukemia) was associated with higher rates of therapeutic failure and death compared with placebo in AIDS patients with PCP treated with TMP-SMX.[7]

Clinicians should also be aware of the nonspecific central nervous system (CNS) adverse effects associated with TMP-SMX, including fine tremors, headache, nervousness, light-headedness, insomnia, drowsiness, and acute psychosis. These toxicities can be concentration-dependent and appear to be more intense at daily doses of 20 mg/kg of the trimethoprim component.[8] Dosage reduction (12–15 mg/kg/day) is appropriate empirically and if CNS toxicity occurs. One may also reduce the risk of the potentiating CNS side effects by careful review and monitoring of concurrent medication use to avoid other drugs that may have a similar CNS toxicity profile.

Clearly, toxicities associated with TMP-SMX require the need for alternative therapies. The AIDS Clinical Trials Group (ACTG) 108 study compared oral TMP-SMX with oral TMP-dapsone and clindamycin-primaquine in 181 patients infected with HIV with PCP.[2] Survival and dose-limiting toxicity (36, 24, and 33% for each drug combination, respectively) did not differ among the three treatment arms. Elevation of serum aminotransferase levels to more than five times the baseline value was more frequent in the TMP-SMX group ($P = .003$), and one or more serious hematologic toxicities (neutropenia, anemia, thrombocytopenia, or methemoglobinemia) occurred more frequently in the clindamycin-primaquine group ($P = .01$). These findings provide clinicians with a better perspective on appropriate drug selection for individual patients (Fig. 77.1).

Table 77.1 ▪ Treatment of *Pneumocystis carinii* Pneumonia in Patients with HIV

Therapy Type	First-Line Therapy	Alternative Therapy	Comment
Acute infection	TMP (15 mg/kg/day) + SMX (75 mg/kg/day) divided in 3–4 daily doses PO/IV × 21 days	Pentamidine (4 mg/kg/day IV or IM) × 21 days	TMP-SMX is the preferred regimen
	TMP (15 mg/kg/day PO or IV) + dapsone (100 mg/day PO × 21 days)	Atovaquone/suspension (750 mg PO BID with food) × 21 days	See text and Figure 77.1 for appropriate selection of other regimens
	Clindamycin (600 mg every 6–8 hr PO or IV) + primaquine (30 mg base PO/day) × 21 days	Alternative considerations for refractory infections or side effects with standard agents: trimetrexate (45 mg/m²/day IV × 21 days + leucovorin (20 mg/m² IV or PO every 6 hr) × 24 days	Adverse events to sulfonamides (rash, fever, leukopenia, hepatitis, etc.) most common at 1–2 wk
			Patients with severe pneumonia PaO_2 <70 mm Hg) should receive corticosteroids (prednisone, 40 mg PO BID × 5 days, then 40 mg/day) × 5 days, then 20 mg/day until completion of treatment)
Prophylaxis	TMP-SMX (1 SS/day, 1 DS/day, or 1 DS 3 times/week)	Dapsone (50 mg BID or 100 mg/day)	Prophylaxis is indicated for any HIV-infected patient with a history of *Pneumocystis carinii* pneumonia, CD4+ count <200/mm³, unexplained fever (>100EF) for >2 weeks, or a history of oropharyngeal candidiasis
		Dapsone (50 mg/day) + pyrimethamine (50 mg/week) + leucovorin (25 mg/week)	
		Dapsone (200 mg/week) + pyrimethamine (75 mg/week) + leucovorin (25 mg/week)	Efficacy shown in controlled studies only for TMP-SMX, dapsone (± pyrimethamine), and aerosolized pentamidine
		Aerosolized pentamidine (300 mg) every month via Respirgard II nebulizer—pretreatment with β_2 agonist (albuterol, 2 Puffs)	Aerosolized pentamidine should not be used in patients with CD4 + counts <100/mm³ because of diminished efficacy
		Pentamidine (4 mg/kg) IM or IV q2wk	

Source: Reproduced with permission from Stevens RC. Opportunistic infections in AIDS due to protozoal and *Mycobacterium avium* complex. In Carter BL, Lake KD, Raebel MA, et al, eds. Pharmacotherapy self-assessment program. 3rd ed. Kansas City, MO: American College of Clinical Pharmacy, 1998:129–130.

TMP, trimethoprim; *SMX,* sulfamethoxazole; *SS,* single-strength TMP-SMX tablet; *DS,* double-strength TMP-SMX tablet.

TMP-dapsone can be used as an alternative in subjects infected with HIV who are intolerant to TMP-SMX. Patients who develop a mild rash from TMP-SMX and are subsequently changed to TMP-dapsone can also develop a rash from dapsone in up to 22% of cases.[9] Dapsone is a sulfonamide moiety and cross-sensitivity is observed. A TMP-SMX rash, presumably owing to the sulfa entity, however, does not preclude the use of dapsone.

Dapsone-induced methemoglobinemia can occur in up to two-thirds of persons infected with HIV; however, most individuals who are not deficient in the enzyme NADH-methemoglobin-reductase are asymptomatic. The manifestations of methemoglobinemia include cyanosis, headache, dizziness, drowsiness, stupor, fatigue, ataxia, dyspnea, tachycardia, nausea, and vomiting. Severe methemoglobinemia can lead to hemolysis owing to a change in iron oxidation state with impairment of oxygen transport. Dapsone and other potential hemolyzing agents should be discontinued, and methylene blue (1–2 mg/kg in a 1% saline solution given once intravenously over 10–15 minutes) should be administered as an antidote if methemoglobin concentrations exceed 20%, or at lower concentrations of methemoglobin if patients are severely symptomatic. Dapsone can also cause hemolysis, especially in patients who are deficient in the enzyme glucose-6-phosphate dehydrogenase (G6PD).

Rash, diarrhea, bone marrow suppression, hemolysis, and methemoglobinemia have been reported with clindamycin-primaquine.[2] It seems sensible to avoid this combination if possible in patients with underlying diarrhea due to HIV-gastroenteropathy or invasion of the gastrointestinal tract by some other diarrhea-causing opportunistic pathogen (e.g., CMV, *Cryptosporidium*, *Mycobacterium avium* complex [MAC]).

Atovaquone, an oral agent, has been shown to be better tolerated than TMP-SMX and pentamidine in patients

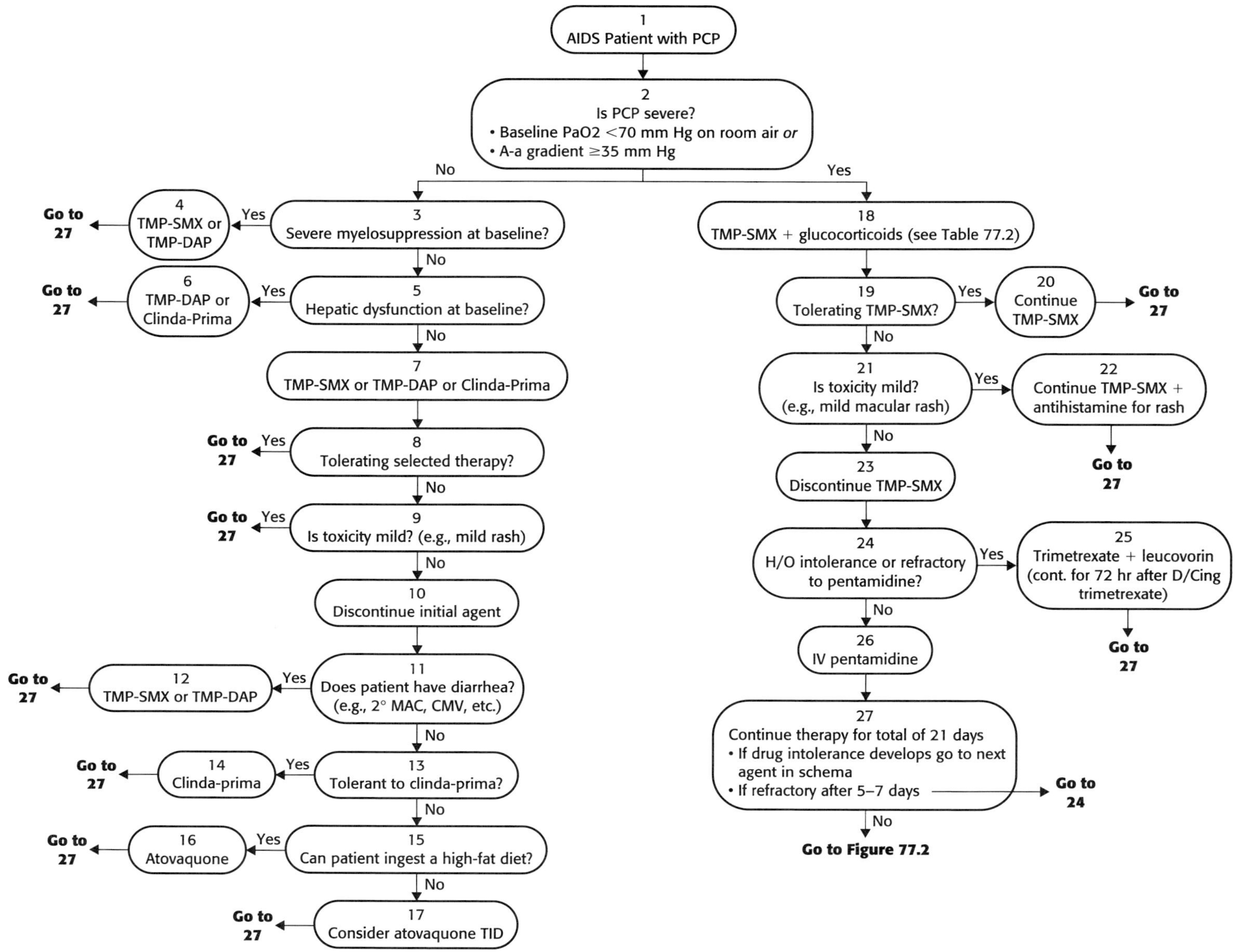

Figure 77.1. Algorithm for acute therapy of *Pneumocystis carinii* pneumonia (PCP). The schema is divided into therapies for mild to moderate pneumonia and severe pneumonia. Duration of therapy is 21 days, followed by lifelong secondary prophylaxis (Fig. 77.2). Doses are provided in Table 77.1. Atovaquone is the suspension formulation. *A-a gradient,* alveolar-arterial oxygen difference (refer to footnote in text for calculation of A-a gradient); *Clinda-Prima,* clindamycin-primaquine; *CMV,* cytomegalovirus; *MAC, Mycobacterium avium* complex; *PaO_2,* arterial partial pressure of oxygen; *TMP-DAP,* trimethoprim-dapsone; *TMP-SMX,* trimethoprim-sulfamethoxazole. (Reproduced with permission from Stevens RC. Opportunistic infections in AIDS due to protozoal and *Mycobacterium avium* complex. In: Carter BL, Lake KD, Raebel MA, et al., eds. Pharmacotherapy self-assessment program. 3rd ed. Kansas City, MO: American College of Clinical Pharmacy, 1998:131.)

with mild to moderate PCP; however, it is associated with a higher rate of therapeutic failure.[10,11] In some patients, this may be explained in part because of reduced bioavailability of the drug when the drug is not administered with a high-fat meal. Atovaquone absorption is enhanced with fatty foods. Persons infected with HIV should be instructed to take atovaquone with fatty foods because poor absorption is considered to be the most likely explanation for its inferior therapeutic response compared with TMP-SMX. Consumption of a high-fat diet can be problematic in this patient population because they can develop diarrhea secondary to the fatty foods, and diarrhea is linked to therapeutic failures and higher mortality in atovaquone-treated patients.[10,11] Macular rash is the most common adverse effect. Hematologic toxicity from atovaquone is rare. Atovaquone is perhaps the best tolerated antipneumocystis agent, but the lower therapeutic response necessitates restricting this agent to patients with mild to moderate PCP. Atovaquone is not indicated for initial treatment of severe PCP.

Severe PCP

Severe PCP requires parenteral antipneumocystis therapy, adjunctive glucocorticoids, and aggressive supportive care (e.g., supplemental oxygen, nutrition support–low albumin is a risk factor for a poor prognosis). A patient can be switched to oral therapy once he or she is clinically stable. TMP-SMX, the first-line parenteral therapy, followed by intravenous pentamidine, is an alternate for treatment of severe PCP.

Intravenous pentamidine is the most frequently prescribed alternative for TMP-SMX in patients with severe PCP who have significant intolerance to TMP-SMX, or who have not quickly responded to therapy (Fig. 77.1). In general, patients should not be labeled as TMP-SMX therapeutic failures until a minimum of 5 days of therapy are completed. Patients with severe infection often deteriorate during the first few days of therapy because of worsening oxygen desaturation. This is most likely because of release of cytokines from alveolar macrophages during the acute inflammatory process and lysis of *P. carinii* cysts after exposure to appropriate therapy. Thus, switching to alternative therapy would be premature during this transient decompensation period.

Commonly, parenteral pentamidine causes serious side effects including nephrotoxicity, hypotension, and hypoglycemia. Other serious complications include elevations in liver transaminases, hyperkalemia, hyperglycemia, leukopenia, thrombocytopenia, acute pancreatitis, and ventricular arrhythmias. A 5-year retrospective review of the incidence of parenteral pentamidine-associated adverse effects at San Francisco General Hospital in patients infected with HIV who received at least 5 days of pentamidine therapy found that 72% of the patients experienced an adverse effect.[12] Nephrotoxicity occurred in 45%, hypoglycemia in 24%, and pancreatitis in 9% of patients receiving pentamidine.

Nephrotoxicity caused by pentamidine is related to cumulative exposure, making renal damage unlikely in the first 5 to 7 days of therapy. Empiric dosage reduction (3 mg/kg/day) has been used in mild to moderate PCP, and especially after azotemia has developed, but the efficacy of this dosage has not been well established in severe PCP.[13] The concurrent use of other nephrotoxic drugs may increase the risk of renal injury.

Hypoglycemia caused by pentamidine, which occurs in 10 to 50% of patients with AIDS, is potentially the most dangerous toxicity because of its insidious onset. This side effect has been associated with use of higher doses, prolonged therapy, and repeated courses of intravenous pentamidine. A statistically significant relationship has been observed between hypoglycemia and nephrotoxicity.[12] Pentamidine exerts a lytic effect on pancreatic B cells, causing a sudden influx of insulin into the systemic circulation. No guidelines have been established for monitoring blood glucose, but daily assessment seems advisable. The optimal time for sample collection is unknown. It can be theorized that blood glucose should be ascertained within 4 hours post-pentamidine infusion based on the assumption that a temporal relationship exists between lysis of the B cells and the maximum tissue drug concentration. However, fatal hypoglycemia has occurred 2 weeks after the drug was stopped, presumably owing to pentamidine's high tissue affinity and subsequent drug accumulation. In hypoglycemic patients, it would be prudent to determine blood glucose Accu-checks every 4 to 6 hours for the first 24 to 48 hours, two to three times daily for the following 10 to 14 days, then daily for the remainder of therapy. Patient-specific monitoring programs would need to be structured dependent on the individual's baseline glucose control.

The role of adjunctive corticosteroids in patients with AIDS who have severe PCP is indisputable. Several well-controlled studies indicate that pulmonary failure (PaO_2 <75 mm Hg), the need for mechanical ventilation, and mortality rates were all significantly reduced in AIDS patients with PCP randomized to receive corticosteroids.[14,15] Negative outcomes from these studies revealed patients to experience mild, localized, mucocutaneous, herpetic lesions as the most significant complication in the steroid-treated patients. Subsequent investigations have shown that short-course steroid use has not enhanced the risk of developing active tuberculosis or relapses of other AIDS-related infections.

These trials collectively led to a consensus statement that recommended adjunctive corticosteroids be prescribed within 72 hours of initiating antipneumocystis therapy in AIDS patients with severe *P. carinii* pneumonia. Dosage guidelines for prednisone, including a tapering schedule, are listed in Table 77.1. Methylprednisolone, with appropriate dosage adjustment for potency differences, can be used when patients are unable to ingest oral prednisone.

Prophylaxis Pharmacotherapy

Chemoprophylaxis is either primary (directed against preventing the initial episode of clinical PCP) or secondary (directed against relapses or recurrences following treatment of an acute infection). The United States Public Health Service (USPHS) recommends that adults and adolescents with HIV infection should receive prophylaxis against PCP if they have a CD4 lymphocyte count of less than 200/mm^3, unexplained fever (>100°F [>38°C]) for more than 2 weeks, or a history of oropharyngeal candidiasis (Fig. 77.2).[16] Some clinicians may use a slightly higher CD4 lymphocyte count of 225 to 250 cells/mm^3, if the patient has had a downward trend pattern of CD4 cell count over the preceding months. Any patient who has recovered from an episode of acute PCP should receive secondary prophylaxis therapy.

A controversial aspect of PCP prophylaxis lies with the duration of prophylaxis endpoint. The potent effect of highly active antiretroviral treatment (HAART) that utilizes triple-drug combinations on suppressing the HIV RNA viral load has been impressive. Often RNA viral load drops below the limits of assay detection, and with it the subsequent restoration of CD4 cell counts above 200/mm^3. This result has led some clinicians to withdraw PCP prophylaxis. An early report in patients following initiation of HAART provides results from 78 patients ($n = 62$ primary, $n = 16$ secondary prophylaxis) who discontinued PCP prophylaxis when their CD4+ cell counts rose above 200/mm^3.[17] In this report, no episodes of PCP occurred during a mean follow-up of 12.7 months. These early findings appear promising; however, clinicians should wait until long-term follow-up data are available that establish the efficacy of this intervention before instituting widespread deviations from the USPHS prophylaxis guidelines.[16] This precaution is warranted because the repertoire of CD4 lymphocytes that increases secondary to HAART therapy may not restore all of the CD4 cell lines; therefore, there may be some qualitative difference in the functional capacity of these restored cells.

TMP-SMX, dapsone monotherapy, dapsone plus pyrimethamine, and aerosolized pentamidine are the more common agents used to prevent PCP (Fig. 77.2). No single agent or combination has been shown to be superior to TMP-SMX.[18,19]

ACTG 081 was a randomized trial to evaluate three regimens for primary PCP prophylaxis: TMP-SMX one double-strength tablet containing TMP 160 mg, and SMX 800 mg given twice daily (a high dose relative to current recommendations); dapsone 50 mg twice daily; and aerosolized pentamidine 300 mg once monthly.[18] Overall, the estimated 36-month risk of PCP was 18, 17, and 21%, for TMP-SMX, dapsone, and aerosolized pentamidine, respectively. These differences were not significant. However, for patients with a baseline CD4+ count less than 100/mm^3, the risk was 33% for aerosolized pentamidine compared to 19% for TMP-SMX and 22% for dapsone ($P = .04$). Although aerosolized pentamidine was better tolerated compared to the systemic agents, the inhaled product had two significant limitations (1) the aerosolized group had increased mortality among patients who entered the study with fewer than 100 CD4+ lymphocytes/mm^3 and (2) the group had greater numbers of patients with toxoplasmosis. Thus, this study demonstrates the advantage of systemic chemoprophylaxis, particularly TMP-SMX, over inhalation therapy in preventing PCP.

Use of aerosolized pentamidine for prophylaxis has some limitations, including the following: (1) less efficacy compared with TMP-SMX in controlled trials, especially in persons infected with HIV who have advanced immunodeficiency (CD4 <100 cells/mm^3); (2) increased rates of extrapulmonary foci of *P. carinii* infection and pneumothorax; (3) increased risk of PCP manifesting as an upper lobe disease owing to poor distribution of the aerosolized drug to this region; (4) lack of prophylaxis against toxoplasmosis and bacterial infections; and (5) high cost.

Aerosolized pentamidine's clear advantage, however, is its minor toxicity. Side effects (primarily cough, wheezing, and dyspnea during inhalation administration) are mild and infrequent causes of drug discontinuation. These bronchoconstrictive reactions can be diminished or prevented by administration of an inhaled β_2-agonist (e.g., albuterol, two 100-Fg puffs) before aerosolized pentamidine. Also, an inhaled β_2-agonist can be used as needed for bronchoconstriction during or after aerosolized pentamidine.

IMPROVING OUTCOMES

The most efficient, cost-effective method to organize treatment of PCP is not well defined, as evidenced by the geographic variation in the management and outcome of AIDS-related pneumocystis pneumonia. Geographic variations in mortality were accounted for by differences in severity of illness at admission, insurance status (private versus public versus no insurance), and in-hospital patient management. The latter may be prolonged because of inefficiencies in arranging home care coordination or outpatient follow-up. Independent of severity of illness, strategies to promote timely diagnostic tests and access to appropriate pharmaceuticals, including outpatient management if the subject is clinically stable, may reduce the variability observed in outcomes.

When the desired outcomes for either acute PCP therapy or PCP prophylaxis are not achieved, then a detailed review of the patient's entire medication regimen is needed. One must reassess whether the patient received optimal treatment, as well as what the new treatment options are. Specific questions that should be asked are presented algorithmically in Figure 77.1. Is the patient receiving his or her medication according to schedule? Have the dosages been adjusted for the patient's weight and renal function? (Refer to Table 77.1 for appropriate dosing regimens.) Is the patient receiving adjunctive corticosteroids if indicated for severe PCP? Does the patient have significant nausea and vomiting or diarrhea?

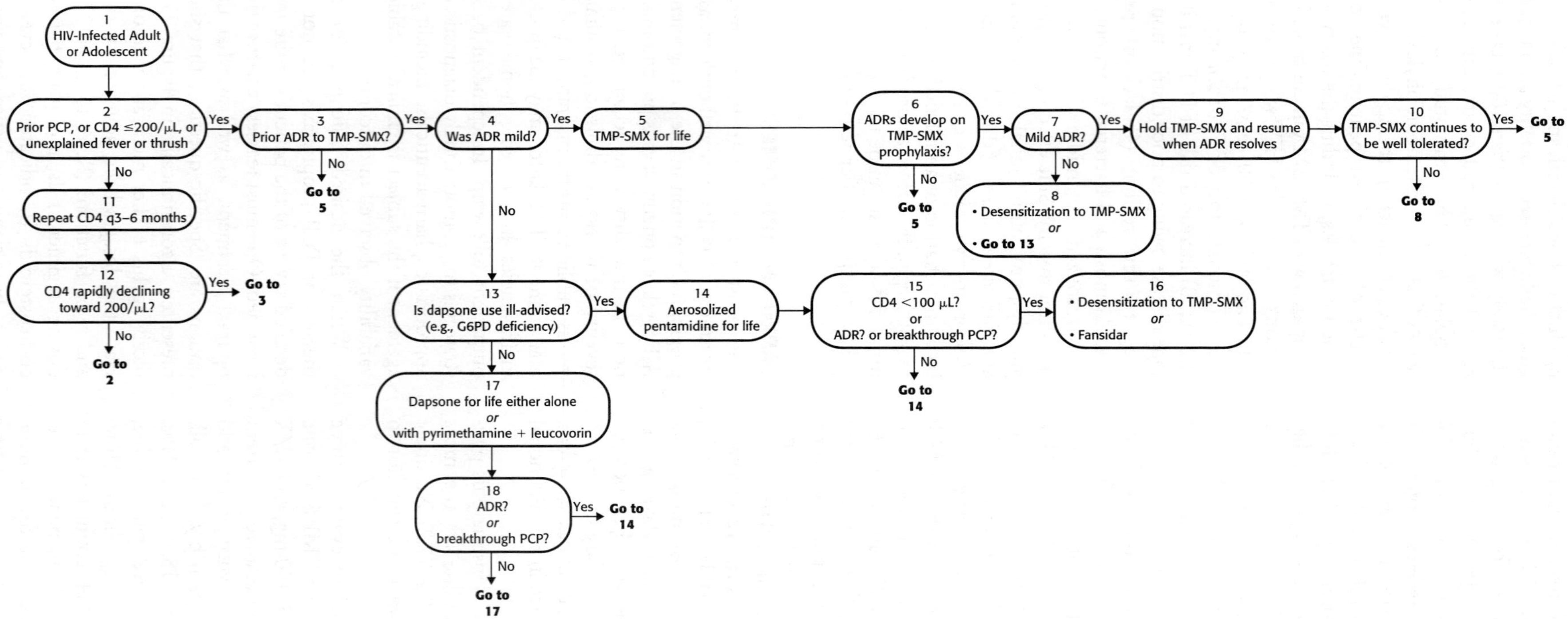

Figure 77.2. Algorithm for primary and secondary prophylaxis of *Pneumocystis carinii* pneumonia (PCP). Prophylaxis therapy is lifelong. Refer to Table 77.1 for recommended doses. *ADR,* adverse drug reaction; *CD4,* T-lymphocyte helper cells; *G6PD,* glucose-6-phosphate dehydrogenase; *TMP-SMX,* trimethoprim-sulfamethoxazole. (Reproduced with permission from Stevens RC. Opportunistic infections in AIDS due to protozoal and *Mycobacterium avium* complex. In: Carter BL, Lake KD, Raebel MA, et al., eds. Pharmacotherapy self-assessment program. 3rd ed. Kansas City, MO: American College of Clinical Pharmacy, 1998:136.)

If so, avoid clindamycin-primaquine and atovaquone or consider intravenous therapy. Has adequate time elapsed (minimum of 5 days) to enable an adequate assessment of the efficacy of the regimen in question?

Without question, widespread PCP prophylaxis has had a profound effect. The most obvious effect is that the percentage of new PCP cases categorized as the initial AIDS-defining illness has decreased. As health systems continue to be taxed and further constrain valuable resources, it is conceivable that patients may inadvertently lose access to care or pharmaceuticals. Pharmacists are in a unique position to remain at the forefront of ensuring that persons infected with HIV receive optimal prophylaxis for PCP. This is achieved through close monitoring of the patient's CD4+ lymphocytes, selection of chemoprophylaxis based on the individual's medication history, and, perhaps most important, constant support and motivation to enhance adherence. These activities probably do more to extend the quality of life than any other intervention short of behavioral modifications and strict adherence to antiretroviral therapy.

Toxoplasmosis Encephalitis

Toxoplasma gondii is a protozoal pathogen that is among the most prevalent causes of CNS infections in individuals infected with HIV. The primary disease associated with *T. gondii* infection is toxoplasmosis encephalitis (TE), but other sites may be affected, including the eye (retinochoroiditis), lung (pneumonitis), heart, skin, liver, or gut.

TREATMENT GOALS: TOXOPLASMOSIS ENCEPHALITIS

- Design a drug treatment for acute opportunistic infection and prophylaxis of TE (both primary and secondary), as with PCP.
- Design a treatment scheme that includes appropriate monitoring parameters to assess efficacy and tolerance in a person infected with HIV and TE.
- Develop an alternative treatment regimen in a patient with a history of intolerance to sulfonamides.
- Select the appropriate drug for secondary prophylaxis of *T. gondii* infection and counsel patients on how to minimize their risk to toxoplasmosis.
- Identify subjects infected with HIV who may benefit from primary prophylaxis of toxoplasmosis.

EPIDEMIOLOGY

The prevalence of *T. gondii* antibodies among adults infected with HIV is 8 to 16% in major urban areas of the United States.[20] The prevalence is higher (≥25%) in certain ethnic groups, especially Hispanics and Haitians. For example, TE is observed in 12 to 40% of patients with AIDS of Haitian origin who live in Florida.

Toxoplasmosis most often occurs in persons infected with HIV when the CD4+ lymphocyte count is less than 100 cells/mm^3. Ingestion of undercooked or raw meat containing tissue cysts and vegetables or other food products contaminated with oocysts, as well as direct contact with cat feces, are major modes of transmission of the parasite.

PATHOPHYSIOLOGY

Once *T. gondii* is ingested and reaches the systemic circulation, it has a high predilection for the CNS. The response of the brain to *T. gondii* infection can vary from a granulomatous reaction to a severe focal or generalized necrotizing encephalitis.[20] Perivascular inflammatory cell infiltrates can lead to fibrosis or necrosis, which can result in hemorrhage or thrombosis, accounting for neurologic signs and symptoms. Necrotizing lesions are not dependent on the host's inflammatory response because severe necrotizing processes may occur with minimal or no inflammation, suggesting that the parasite causes lysis of infected cells.[21]

CLINICAL PRESENTATION AND DIAGNOSIS

Signs and Symptoms

The clinical presentation of TE is typically a mixture of focal and generalized neurologic deficits. The presentation varies from a subacute course worsening over several weeks to a more acute fulminant process. The most frequent manifestations (usually in more than half of patients in published series) are fever, headache, disorientation, lethargy, and hemiparesis.[20] Seizures are the cause of patients seeking medical attention in one-third of patients with AIDS who have TE. Headache can be focal and generalized, and can be relentless in intensity, with marginal relief from nonsteroidal antiinflammatory agents or acetaminophen.

Diagnosis

Brain imaging studies (computed tomography [CT] or magnetic resonance imaging [MRI] scans) typically reveal multiple, bilateral, hypodense, enhancing mass lesions. So classic are these findings that the presence of multiple ring-enhancing lesions on CT or MRI scans in a patient with AIDS is assumed to be indicative of clinical TE, until proven otherwise. A single lesion is uncharacteristic of TE and more often associated with CNS lymphoma. The presumptive diagnosis of TE is thus made in persons infected with HIV with positive serology for *T. gondii* antibodies and who have CNS changes and imaging studies consistent with TE as described. A brain biopsy to confirm the diagnosis of TE is *not* typically completed unless the patient fails to improve clinically by 10 to 14 days of empiric TE therapy or actually clinically deteriorates over at least 3 days of therapy.[20]

TREATMENT

Pharmacologic intervention in the management of toxoplasmosis in individuals infected with HIV is divided into acute therapy, maintenance therapy (i.e., secondary prophylaxis), and primary prophylaxis (Table 77.2).

Table 77.2 ▪ Treatment of *Toxoplasma gondii* Encephalitis in Patients with AIDS

Therapy Type	First-Line Therapy	Alternative Therapy	Comment
Acute therapy	Pyrimetharnine (200 mg loading dose) then pyrimethamine (50–75 mg/day) PO × 3–6 weeks + leucovorin (10–25 mg/day) PO + sulfadiazine (1 g q6hr) × 3–6 weeks	Pyrimethamine (200 mg loading dose) then pyrimethamine (50–75 mg/day) PO × 3–6 weeks + *one* of the following: clarithromycin (1 g PO q12hr) or atovaquone suspension (750 mg PO q8hr) or azithromycin (1200–1500 mg/day PO) or dapsone (100 mg/day PO)	All HIV-infected persons who respond to acute therapy must receive lifelong maintenance therapy
	Pyrimethamine + leucovorin (above doses) + clindamycin (600 mg PO or IV q6hr) × 3–6 weeks	TMP (20 mg/kg/day) + SMX (100 mg/kg/day) divided in 3 to 4 doses	TMP-SMX is inferior against *T. gondii* compared to first-line therapies
			Leucovorin (10–25 mg/day) should be given along with and continued for 72 hr after stopping pyrimethamine Corticosteroids are indicated only for life-threatening cerebral edema/brain mass
Maintenance therapy	Pyrimethamine (25–75 mg/day) + leucovorin (10–25 mg/day) + sulfadiazine (500–1000 mg PO q6hr)	Pyrimethamine (50–100 mg/day) + leucovorin	Maintenance therapy with pyrimethamine-clindamycin does not provide effective prophylaxis against *P. carinii* pneumonia and alternatives are needed (e.g., TMP-SMX)
	Pyrimethamine (25–75 mg/day) + leucovorin (10–25 mg/day) + clindamycin (300–450 mg PO q6–8hr)	Pyrimethamine (50 mg/day) + leucovorin + *one* of the following: atovaquone suspension 750 mg every 8 hr or clarithromycin 1000 mg q12hr or azithromycin 1200–1500 mg/day Pyrimethamine (25 mg) + sulfadoxine (500 mg) PO 2 times/week (equal to Fansidar 1 tablet twice weekly) + leucovorin (10–25 mg/Fansidar dose)	
Primary prophylaxis	TMP-SMX (1 DS tablet/day)	TMP-SMX (1 SS tablet/day)	Strong support for primary prophylaxis in HIV-infected patients with positive *T. gondii* serology plus CD4+ count <200/mm³
		Pyrimethamine (50 mg/week) + leucovorin (25 mg/week) + dapsone (50 mg/day) Pyrimethamine (25–75 mg/week) + leucovorin (25 mg/week) + dapsone (100–200 mg/week)	

Source: Reproduced with permission from Stevens RC. Opportunistic infections in AIDS due to protozoal and *Mycobacterium avium* complex. In Carter BL, Lake KD, Raebel MA, et al, eds. Pharmacotherapy self-assessment program, 3rd ed. Kansas City, MO: American College of Clinical Pharmacy, 1998:129–130.

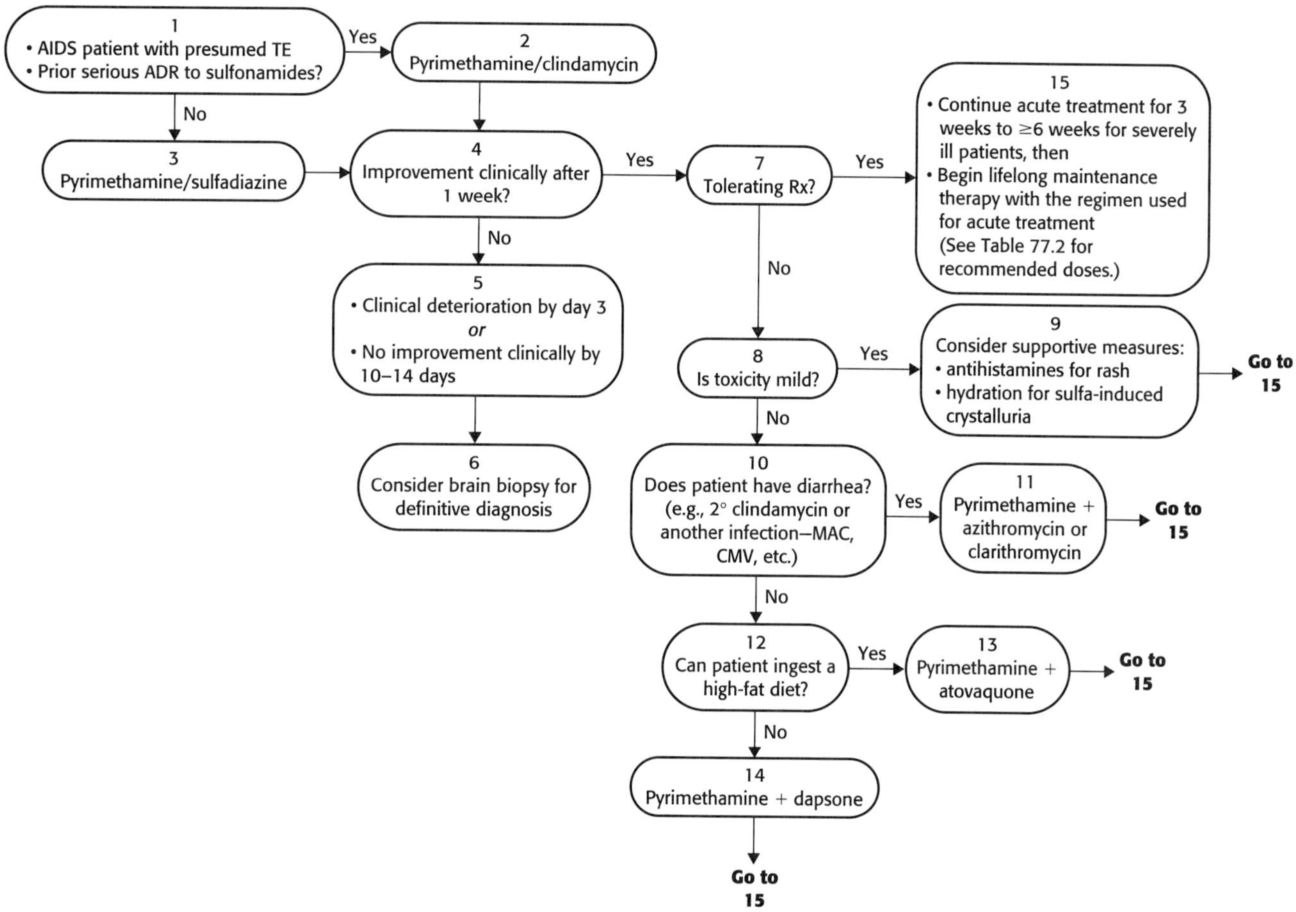

Figure 77.3. Algorithm for empiric treatment of toxoplasmic encephalitis (TE). Following acute therapy of TE, lifelong maintenance therapy is required to prevent relapse. Leucovorin (folinic acid) should be administered with pyrimethamine. Atovaquone is the suspension formulation. *ADR,* adverse drug reaction; *CMV,* cytomegalovirus; *MAC, Mycobacterium avium* complex. (Reproduced with permission from Stevens RC. Opportunistic infections in AIDS due to protozoal and *Mycobacterium avium* complex. In: Carter BL, Lake KD, Raebel MA, et al., eds. Pharmacotherapy self-assessment program. 3rd ed. Kansas City, MO: American College of Clinical Pharmacy, 1998:139.)

Acute Therapy

Empiric therapy is the combination of pyrimethamine and sulfadiazine or clindamycin, plus "leucovorin rescue" for the pyrimethamine-associated toxicities (Fig. 77.3). TE dosage regimens are listed in Table 77.2. Either therapy option has comparable clinical efficacy outcomes for acute TE therapy, but most experts prefer pyrimethamine-sulfadiazine because of its more established use and better outcome for secondary prophylaxis or maintenance therapy.[22,23] This regimen should be continued for at least 3 weeks, and 6 weeks or more in severe episodes or in patients responding slowly. Monotherapy, which may show initial benefits, is associated with high rates of relapse, even while the drug is continued. For this reason, it is recommended that all therapeutic regimens include two drugs for the entire duration of therapy. Similar treatment scenarios described for TE should also be applied to the management of extraneuronal toxoplasmosis.

Pyrimethamine is the cornerstone for current treatment of AIDS-related CNS toxoplasmosis. It is greater than 10 times more potent than TMP in interfering with dihydrofolate synthetase; this may explain why TMP-SMX is inferior to pyrimethamine-sulfadiazine.[24] TMP-SMX should not be considered therapeutically equivalent until a randomized comparative trial proves otherwise. In the rare event of a patient having concurrent PCP and TE, the combination of pyrimethamine-sulfadiazine should be prescribed. No additional drugs are needed for therapy of concurrent infections from these two protozoal pathogens.

Treatment-terminating adverse reactions may be experienced by up to 40% of patients.[20,21] The most notable toxicities of pyrimethamine are rash and dose-related bone marrow suppression that results in neutropenia, thrombocytopenia, and megaloblastic anemia. Hematologic suppression can be expected at pyrimethamine doses of 75 to 100 mg/day.

Leucovorin (folinic acid) is recommended to prevent pyrimethamine-induced "cytopenias." As noted in the PCP section, concurrent use of leucovorin with TMP-SMX for acute PCP is contraindicated; however, this is not true with pyrimethamine, where "leucovorin rescue" is recommended. It is important to note that folic acid must not be substituted for leucovorin because it is reported that folic acid will inhibit the activity of pyrimethamine against *T. gondii*.[20]

Adverse effects from sulfadiazine commonly include rash, nephrotoxicity with crystalluria, blood dyscrasias, and CNS effects. There have been few reports of life-threatening sulfadiazine-associated rashes, which should not preclude the use of sulfadiazine for patients who experience a macular rash. Crystalluria is reversed with hydration, alkalinization of the urine, and dose reduction.[25] Sulfadiazine can cause an encephalitislike syndrome that can be clinically indistinguishable from worsening TE to the clinician who is not suspicious of such toxicity.

Alternative therapies, including atovaquone, the extended-spectrum macrolide antibiotics (i.e., azithromycin), and dapsone, are being investigated for patients experiencing unmanageable toxicity to the mainstay regimens for TE. Relapse occurred in approximately 50% of patients in whom atovaquone was used alone for acute and subsequent maintenance therapy.[26] Currently the ACTG is conducting a multicenter trial to assess the efficacy of atovaquone in combination with pyrimethamine. Pending the outcome of this trial, it seems reasonable to use atovaquone with pyrimethamine or sulfadiazine.[20] Clarithromycin with pyrimethamine (plus leucovorin) had similar efficacy to standard regimens in a small noncomparative clinical trial.[27] Azithromycin has good in vitro activity and it is reasonable to substitute for clarithromycin. Dapsone-pyrimethamine has been used in limited cases, but appears to be an acceptable alternative. Appropriately conducted clinical trials are needed to assess the role of these alternative combinations in treating AIDS-related TE.

Adjunctive corticosteroid therapy with dexamethasone to relieve inflammation and cerebral edema frequently is required for management of patients with intracranial hypertension caused by the mass effect of *T. gondii* abscesses. The response rate, time to response, and mortality in patients who received corticosteroids was no different compared with those who did not receive steroids.[28] At present, patients with AIDS-related TE should receive corticosteroids only when it is absolutely necessary and for no more than 2 weeks if possible.[20] No quantifiable guidelines (e.g., extent of cerebral edema or elevation of intracranial pressure) exist to determine when to initiate dexamethasone. The dosage is dependent on clinical severity.

Maintenance Therapy (Secondary Prophylaxis)

The relapse rate after 12 months of TE in patients with AIDS who do not receive maintenance therapy is 50 to 80%.[20] Thus it is essential that patients with AIDS who successfully complete acute TE therapy be "maintained" on lifelong antitoxoplasma agents. Some patients even relapse while on maintenance therapy, and undoubtedly, poor adherence or drug intolerance contributes to this relapse rate. Maintenance doses are usually lower (as low as 25 mg/day) compared with those used for acute therapy (Table 77.2).

The regimen of pyrimethamine-sulfadiazine with leucovorin appears to have a lower relapse rate than other drug regimens and thus is recommended most often for maintenance therapy.[20] Unlike the efficacy of TMP-SMX given three times weekly for secondary PCP prophylaxis, pyrimethamine-sulfadiazine administered twice weekly had a high relapse rate of 30% by 12 months. Relapse rates for daily administration of pyrimethamine-sulfadiazine was only 6% by 12 months.[29] Thus, the latter regimen should be taken daily for secondary prophylaxis (maintenance therapy) of TE. However, administration twice weekly may be an option in those patients unable to continue daily use because of significant drug intolerance. Importantly, patients receiving pyrimethamine-sulfadiazine for TE maintenance therapy do not need further PCP prophylaxis because of activity against both pathogens with this regimen.[30]

Pyrimethamine-clindamycin is an alternative for maintenance therapy in patients with intolerance to sulfonamides because of a higher rate of relapse. Furthermore, this combination is less desirable because it does not prevent PCP. Pyrimethamine-sulfadoxine (Fansidar) is another alternative that offers the advantage of being dosed as one tablet orally twice weekly. Leucovorin (10 to 25 mg orally) should be added on the days of the week that the patient takes pyrimethamine-sulfadoxine. Side effects were relatively common (40%), with 7% of patients discontinuing therapy because of toxicity.[31] Pyrimethamine used alone at daily doses of 50 and 100 mg had relapse rates of 10 to 28% and 5%, respectively; thus suggesting that the higher dose may offer good protection in patients with AIDS who are unable to tolerate sulfonamides, clindamycin, or any of the other less-studied agents.

Primary Prophylaxis

Despite the availability of effective regimens, toxoplasmosis in patients with AIDS is associated with a mortality rate of 70% by 12 months after diagnosis.[20] This statistic alone strongly supports the use of primary prophylaxis in persons infected with HIV who are at the greatest risk of TE when their CD4 cell count is less than 200/mm^3 (as is the circumstance when 90% of TE cases occur). In addition, persons infected with HIV who are seronegative for *T. gondii* antibodies should receive instructions on how to protect themselves from initial inoculation or newly acquired infection. Such measures include: (1) eating meat that is well cooked (not pink or bloody); (2) avoiding touching mouth and eyes (i.e., mucous membranes) while handling raw meat; (3) washing hands thoroughly after handling raw meat; (4) washing all kitchen utensils, cutting boards, and surfaces that come in contact with raw meat with hot soapy water; (5) washing fresh fruit and vegetables before consumption; and (6) avoiding contact, if possible, with cat feces or cat litter boxes, or wearing gloves when disposing of cat litter.

In various reports, TMP-SMX, pyrimethamine-dapsone, and pyrimethamine-sulfadoxine were effective in preventing TE (Table 77.2). A randomized trial that compared TMP-SMX with pyrimethamine-dapsone indicated that both regimens are effective for toxoplasmosis.[32] However, the TMP-SMX regimen appeared to be more protective against PCP.[32,33] It must be emphasized that between these two regimens, up to 40 to 60% of patients will experience side effects and 2 to 12% will require discontinuation of therapy. Pyrimethamine alone is not considered a first-line agent for primary prophylaxis because of its less protective effect compared with TMP-SMX.[34,35]

Trimethoprim-sulfamethoxazole in low doses used intermittently for PCP prophylaxis prevents toxoplasmosis in patients with AIDS with positive *Toxoplasma* antibodies.[32,33] Thus, measures to enhance TMP-SMX adherence and minimize intolerance are critical. Until other preventive agents are identified, every effort (intermittent dose schedules, desensitization protocols, use of antihistamines) should be performed to maintain patients with AIDS whose CD4+ counts are less than 100/mm^3 on TMP-SMX for prophylaxis against *P. carinii* and *T. gondii*.

Mycobacterium avium Complex

Disseminated *Mycobacterium avium* complex (MAC) is an opportunistic infection observed in persons infected with HIV who have a more advanced stage of AIDS compared with PCP or TE, as represented by a lower CD4 count. Recently, significant advances have been made in the management and prevention of MAC infections. Although MAC is not yet curable in the HIV-infected host, these advances have resulted in fewer symptoms and prolonged survival. Preliminary findings suggest that implementation of HAART regimens appears to significantly decrease the occurrence of MAC initially, although the long-term effect on occurrence is not established.[36] These preliminary results underscore the importance of restoration of the immune system in persons with AIDS.

TREATMENT GOALS: *MYCOBACTERIUM AVIUM* COMPLEX

- Construct a treatment regimen that provides the most efficacious outcome while minimizing drug intolerance and the potential for the significant drug interactions that are associated with anti-MAC therapy.
- Identify subjects infected with HIV who may benefit from primary prophylaxis of MAC infections.
- Implement HAART regimens along with appropriate regimens against MAC as the most effective strategy for treating disseminated MAC infections.[37]
- Make certain that all anti-MAC regimens contain an extended-spectrum macrolide antibiotic (azithromycin or clarithromycin).
- Although the optimal regimen for treatment of MAC is not firmly established (i.e., two versus three drugs), the goals of therapy are well defined: Reduce or eradicate the number of *M. avium* organisms, ameliorate the symptoms of infection, and enhance the quality and duration of life.

EPIDEMIOLOGY

The state of immunodeficiency in persons infected with HIV is the single most important factor that predicts risk of MAC infection. Disseminated MAC has occurred almost exclusively in individuals with advanced HIV infection, especially in patients with CD4+ cell counts less than 50/mm^3.[16] There is an inverse relationship between risk of acquiring MAC and the CD4+ count; the risk is extremely high (approaches 80% by 12 months) when the CD4+ count is less than 10/mm^3. Hopefully, this will change as more patients are exposed to the potency of HAART regimens and MAC prophylaxis. In the absence of these chemotherapeutic interventions, the yearly rate of development of MAC is 20 to 25%, following an initial AIDS-defining illness and a CD4+ count less than 100/mm^3.

PATHOPHYSIOLOGY

Mycobacterium avium complex organisms are ubiquitous environmental saprophytes found in soil, water, animals, birds, food, and tobacco. The portal of entry for MAC into the body is presumed to be the gastrointestinal tract or the lungs. Macrophages in the small bowel can be found to be teeming with mycobacterial invasion and respiratory isolation of MAC frequently precedes disseminated disease. It is unknown whether MAC infection results primarily from acquisition of the organism from environmental exposure or reactivation of latent endogenous infection. Person-to-person transmission is unlikely, as suggested by the absence of an increased risk of developing the disease among individuals infected with HIV who are housemates or close contacts of those with MAC disease.

Nearly all patients infected with HIV with MAC have positive mycobacterial blood cultures. MAC has also been isolated from liver, spleen, lymph nodes, lung, adrenals, colon, kidney, and bone marrow. The organism can colonize the stool, urine, or respiratory secretions, which may or may not be associated with localized symptoms.

CLINICAL PRESENTATION AND DIAGNOSIS

Signs and Symptoms

The disabling complications associated with MAC include fever, malaise, night sweats, severe weight loss, anemia, neutropenia, diarrhea, abdominal pain, and malabsorption. These manifestations can result in profound fatigue, weakness, and emaciation that ultimately marginalize the quality of life for these patients.

Diagnosis

Special blood culture techniques for isolating mycobacteria with nearly 100% sensitivity are available. Time to culture positivity ranges from 5 to 51 days. It is uncommon for blood cultures to be negative when there is a positive histologic diagnosis from lymph node, liver, or bone marrow biopsies. In a prospective natural history study at San Francisco General Hospital among persons infected with HIV, the following were sensitive predictors of MAC bacteremia: (1) CD4+ cell count less than 50/mm^3, (2) history of fever for more than 30 days, (3) hemocrit less than 30%, or (4) a serum albumin level less than 3.0 g/dL.[38]

TREATMENT

Pharmacotherapy

Monotherapy of MAC in patients with AIDS is not effective.[39] Although patients may have an initial improvement, symptoms subsequently recur and the organisms proliferate. This suggests that monotherapy only provides a transient benefit, organisms can re-emerge, and resistance can develop. With one billion plus MAC organisms burdening the immunodeficient host, a relatively large number of resistant organisms will exist as wild-type strains. Under the selective pressure of single-drug therapy, resistant organisms will continue to proliferate in the infected tissue. Thus, the most appropriate therapy of MAC in persons infected with HIV is polypharmacy, which parallels the management of tuberculosis (Table 77.3).

Various treatment schemes for MAC have been studied to ascertain the most effective and best-tolerated regimens. The ideal regimen remains unclear. However, the USPHS Task Force recommended that disseminated MAC therapy be based on several principles that were constructed from the accumulated reported data: (1) treatment regimens should contain at least two drugs; (2) every regimen should contain a macrolide–either azithromycin or clarithromycin; (3) patients who develop MAC while receiving rifabutin prophylaxis should be managed the same as patients who were not taking rifabutin; and (4) therapy should be lifelong.[40]

A minimum of two drugs is essential for MAC therapy in the person infected with HIV (Table 77.3). Every regimen should contain a macrolide such as clarithromycin or azithromycin. Most experience with the macrolides is with clarithromycin.[39–43] Azithromycin is less active in vitro but attains higher intracellular concentrations. It offers the advantage of not being associated with as many significant drug interactions as clarithromycin. Ethambutol is preferred by most experts as the second drug because it has good in vitro activity, was superior to clofazimine when each was combined with a macrolide, is generally well tolerated in the doses used clinically, and does not have the potential drug interactions that are associated with rifabutin.[40–43]

Table 77.3 ▪ Treatment of *Mycobacterium avium* Complex in Patients with AIDS

Therapy Type	First-Line Therapy	Alternative Therapy	Comment
Acute therapy	Multidrug regimen of at least 2 drugs: clarithromycin (500 mg PO BID) or azithromycin (500 mg/day PO) + ethambutol (15 mg/kg/day PO)	None	Resistance develops with monotherapy
	Addition of a 3rd or 4th agent to the above regimens are equivocal but may include: rifabutin (450–600 mg/day PO) or ciprofloxacin (750 mg po 1–2 times daily) or clofazamine (100–200 mg/day PO)		Mortality is higher when clarithromycin dose exceeds 1000 mg/day
			Mortality was increased when clofazamine was added to clarithromycin + ethambutol. Its use must be carefully weighed
Prophylaxis	Clarithromycin (500 mg PO BID)	Rifabutin (300 mg/day PO)	Prophylaxis is recommended when CD4+ counts <50/mm^3
	Azithromycin (1200 mg/week PO)		

Source: Reproduced with permission from Stevens RC. Opportunistic infections in AIDS due to protozoal and *Mycobacterium avium* complex. In Carter BL, Lake KD, Raebel MA, et al, eds. Pharmacotherapy self-assessment program, 3rd ed. Kansas City, MO: American College of Clinical Pharmacy, 1998:129–130.

Approximately two-thirds of patients receiving the macrolide-ethambutol regimen can be anticipated to become culture negative.[41,42] Overall, MAC colony-forming units can be expected to decrease by about 1 to 2 logs from baseline with appropriate therapy.[40] The time course for clinical response to MAC therapy is variable. However, the majority of patients who defervesce and improve symptomatically do so after 2 weeks. The symptoms at 4 weeks should not continue at the same intensity as baseline if the patient is experiencing a beneficial response.

It is not clear if adding a third or even a fourth agent to the initial two-drug regimen (a macrolide and ethambutol) significantly increases the clinical response or degree of mycobacterial eradication. Additional agents that may be considered are rifabutin, clofazimine, ciprofloxacin, and, in some situations, amikacin. Selection of which agent to add is patient specific. With the administration of protease inhibitors and the potential for drug interactions with rifabutin, use of this antimycobacterial has become more complicated. If coadministration of rifabutin and a protease inhibitor is necessary, indinavir and nelfinavir are the preferred protease inhibitors, and the dose of rifabutin should be reduced by 50% with either of these drugs. Clofazimine has a slow onset of action and has the undesirable side effect of skin hyperpigmentation; however, it is rarely the cause of severe toxicity. However, clofazimine added to a regimen of clarithromycin and ethambutol for MAC bacteremia in patients with AIDS was shown not to contribute to clinical response and was associated with higher mortality.[42] This finding provides compelling evidence to question the continued use of clofazimine in the therapy of MAC infection. High doses of ciprofloxacin (750 mg 1–2 times per day) may cause intolerable gastrointestinal distress. Intravenous ciprofloxacin and intravenous or intramuscular amikacin should be considered in patients with severe symptomatic disease in whom gastrointestinal absorption of the oral medications may be marginal.

Adverse Effects of Anti-MAC Agents

Adverse effects associated with anti-MAC drugs are not as notorious for treatment-terminating events such as the drugs used for PCP or toxoplasmosis. The macrolides are well tolerated, with gastrointestinal disturbances (e.g., anorexia, diarrhea, abdominal pain) being the most common adverse effects, which can be alleviated by dividing the dose and administering it more frequently throughout the day. Taste perversion has been associated with clarithromycin.

Ethambutol can cause hyperuricemia or acute gout, but is an infrequent observation in the HIV-infected population. Retrobulbar neuritis is rarely seen with ethambutol at the dose recommended for MAC (15 mg/kg/day), but is possible when dosages are not adjusted in patients with renal impairment. A pink to brownish-black discoloration of the skin is a common adverse effect of clofazimine. Other sites affected by these color changes are conjunctiva, tears, sweat, urine, feces, and nasal secretions. The discolorations are not a source of any symptoms but can be a troubling cosmetic problem to the concerned patient. Peripheral neuropathies associated with clofazimine warrant further precaution and counseling (for patient understanding of the symptoms of peripheral neuropathy) in patients receiving antiretroviral therapy with didanosine, zalcitabine, or stavudine. These antiretrovirals can cause peripheral neuropathy. The high dose of ciprofloxacin recommended for MAC can result in headaches and restlessness.

Rifabutin, like rifampin, causes orange discoloration of bodily secretions, transaminase elevations, myalgias and arthralgias, rash, and hematologic toxicities. Uveitis is associated with rifabutin and appears to be a concentration-dependent toxicity.[44] Symptoms include acute onset of ocular pain, blurry vision, photophobia, and diminished visual acuity. Rifabutin should be discontinued when these symptoms occur. Ophthalmic corticosteroids or atropine drops cause rapid improvement in symptoms and clinical findings. In mild cases, rifabutin can be restarted with close monitoring for symptoms and careful review of the patient's medication profile to avoid drugs that may increase the rifabutin concentrations.

Drug Interactions Associated with Anti-MAC Agents

Drug interactions with agents used in MAC regimens are extensive and many are clinically significant. This is a primary area in which pharmacists can provide significant input into drug selection to avoid drug interactions that may affect efficacy or accentuate toxicity. Careful review of the patient's concurrent medications is essential to avoid drug interactions during therapy or prophylaxis of MAC.

Clarithromycin, an inhibitor of the cytochrome P450 metabolic pathway, can increase the serum concentrations of theophylline, carbamazepine, digoxin, warfarin, cisapride, or astemizole. Increased concentrations of the latter two drugs can be arrhythmogenic and lead to fatal ventricular arrhythmias. The product labeling for indinavir and ritonavir note that these protease inhibitors can increase clarithromycin concentrations by 53 and 77%, respectively.

A bidirectional drug interaction is observed between clarithromycin and rifabutin. Clarithromycin can inhibit the metabolism of rifabutin and its active metabolite. The area under the concentration-time curve (AUC) for rifabutin increased approximately twofold when coadministered with clarithromycin. The higher rifabutin concentrations may be associated with greater toxicity (e.g., uveitis). Conversely, rifabutin, an inducer of the cytochrome P450 pathway, can decrease the mean plasma concentration of clarithromycin by up to 30%. The impact of this bidirectional interaction on clinical efficacy is not known. No guidelines for dosage modifications exist. Thus, close patient monitoring for therapeutic response and toxicity is imperative. Azithromycin may be a more suitable macrolide when combined with rifabutin because the former is not typically associated with drug interactions via P450 inhibition (e.g., unlike clarithromycin, azithromycin does not cause a clinically significant interaction with theophylline).

Rifabutin, like rifampin but to a lesser extent, is an enzyme inducer and as such, can increase the hepatic metabolism of certain drugs (e.g., protease inhibitors, ketoconazole, and dapsone) used in the management of persons infected with HIV. It would seem prudent to avoid dapsone for PCP prophylaxis in patients requiring rifabutin for MAC therapy. Zidovudine AUC can be decreased by 30% when administered with rifabutin, but the clinical significance of this potential interaction is not known. Fluconazole can increase concentrations of rifabutin and its active metabolite by at least 80%.[45] Rifabutin, unlike rifampin, does not alter fluconazole metabolism.

Recommendations for the use of rifabutin with protease inhibitors have been suggested. The indinavir and nelfinavir product labeling recommends that the rifabutin dose be reduced by half when used concurrently. Rifabutin 300 mg per day may reduce indinavir concentrations by 32%, and indinavir may increase rifabutin concentrations by 204%. Ritonavir product labeling lists rifabutin as a contraindicated concomitant medication. Ritonavir can increase rifabutin concentrations fourfold.

Ciprofloxacin can increase serum concentrations of theophylline, caffeine, warfarin, and cyclosporine. Concurrent administration of cation-containing antacids will decrease ciprofloxacin absorption significantly. This can be avoided by giving the quinolone 2 hours before the antacid. Didanosine can also reduce the bioavailability of ciprofloxacin and doses should be spaced several hours apart.

Prophylaxis Pharmacotherapy

Up to 40% of individuals with advanced HIV infection are likely to develop MAC; thus, strategies for preventing this disease in patients at risk should be a high priority.[40] Because there are few clearly delineated risk factors for developing MAC other than a low CD4+ count, any prophylaxis has to be applied to the entire HIV-infected population at greatest risk (i.e., patients with CD4+ cells <50/mm^3).

Combined results from two randomized, placebo-controlled trials of rifabutin prophylaxis in more than 1100 patients infected with HIV with median CD4+ cell counts in the mid-50s/mm^3, demonstrated that rifabutin 300 mg per day reduced the incidence of MAC bacteremia by one-half.[46] This result was almost exclusively observed in those patients with CD4+ counts less than or equal to 75/mm^3 at study entry, and there was no benefit in patients with CD4+ counts greater than 100/mm^3. Overall survival did not differ between the two groups, but the trial was not designed to show such differences.

Lifelong rifabutin prophylaxis may not be feasible in selected patients. Adverse effects that may limit the use of rifabutin are neutropenia, thrombocytopenia, rash, nausea, flatulence, hepatitis, and arthralgias. A red-orange discoloration of urine, tears, sweat, or other body fluids can occur; soft contact lenses may be permanently stained. Patients receiving antiretroviral therapy with protease inhibitors generally, as a precaution, should not be administered rifabutin prophylaxis. As noted previously, if coadministration is necessary, the dose of rifabutin should be reduced by 50% when given with indinavir or nelfinavir, which are the preferred protease inhibitors in this setting because ritonavir is contraindicated with rifabutin.

Two randomized clinical trials have established clarithromycin or azithromycin as first-line agents for MAC prophylaxis.[47,48] In a placebo-controlled trial with patients having a median CD4+ count of 25 cells/mm^3, clarithromycin (500 mg twice daily) was well tolerated, reduced MAC infection by more than 60%, and reduced mortality.[47] Clarithromycin-treated patients had an increased incidence of taste perversion (11 versus 2%) compared with placebo. In the second trial conducted by the California Collaborative Treatment Group, weekly azithromycin was compared with daily rifabutin or the combination of both drugs in 693 persons infected with HIV who have CD4+ cell counts less than 100/mm^3.[3,48] The incidence of MAC infection at 1 year was 15.3% with rifabutin, 7.6% with weekly azithromycin, and 2.8% with both drugs. Dose-limiting toxicity was more common with the two-drug regimen. Survival was similar in all three groups.

As a result of these two trials, the USPHS recommends clarithromycin or azithromycin as the preferred prophylactic agents in persons infected with HIV with CD4+ counts less than 50 cells/mm^3.[16] Although the azithromycin-rifabutin combination is more effective than azithromycin alone, the additional cost, increased occurrence of adverse effects, added potential to incur drug interactions, and absence of a difference in survival when compared with azithromycin alone do not warrant a routine recommendation for this regimen.[48] Rifabutin is an alternative prophylactic agent in patients intolerant to macrolides (Table 77.3).

Azithromycin may be preferred because it is often easier for patients to take medication once weekly than twice daily as with clarithromycin, drug interactions are less problematic, and it is less costly. Patients unable to tolerate the two 600-mg tablets of azithromycin may split the regimen and take one tablet in the morning and one tablet in the evening until gastrointestinal tolerance develops. The two 600-mg tablets can be taken with or without food, unlike the capsules, which should be taken on an empty stomach. The tablets can simplify medication administration for patients receiving protease inhibitors because the latter drugs also require close attention to timing of meals.

IMPROVING OUTCOMES

Patient Education

The effectiveness of MAC therapy or prevention involves an understanding by the person infected with HIV of the opportunistic infection and the complexity of the medications used in its management. Other therapies (e.g., antiretrovirals, PCP prophylaxis) may confuse the patient and lead to poor adherence to the prescribed medications. Another caveat is that it may be necessary to coach the patient through the first 2 to 4 weeks to adhere to the MAC regimen, because a response usually is not immediate. Mycobacteria grow slowly, symptoms are insidious, and response to treatment is slow. Therefore, patients may need to be coaxed to adhere to treatment in the first few weeks, especially if they state that the drugs are not helping them to feel better.

Methods to Improve Patient Adherence to Drug Therapy

Without question, patient outcomes can be improved if the pharmacotherapist is able to simplify the anti-MAC drug regimen, whether it be for lifelong treatment of MAC or its prevention. Simplifying anti-MAC drug regimens so that dosing schemes are convenient (once-daily dosing of azithromycin and ethambutol), drug interactions are minimized (avert rifabutin if possible), and drugs whose bioavailability are affected by food are avoided (azithromycin capsules) are thought processes needed for effective disease management. Incorporation of these strategies in patient care will ultimately enhance adherence and improve outcomes in persons infected with HIV with MAC infection.

PHARMACOECONOMICS

Preliminary results have been reported on the cost effectiveness of drug regimens to prevent MAC infections in persons with AIDS.[49] The investigators developed a decision analytic simulation model of advanced HIV disease to project costs, life expectancy, and cost effectiveness in U.S. dollars per quality-adjusted life year saved. Azithromycin prophylaxis, begun after the CD4+ cell count declined to $50/mm^3$, was the most cost-effective MAC prophylaxis strategy compared with clarithromycin, rifabutin, combination therapies, and no MAC prophylaxis.

Cytomegalovirus

Infection with cytomegalovirus (CMV) is a common opportunistic infection in persons with AIDS that can result in significant morbidity and diminished quality of life if not treated properly. End-organ diseases affected by CMV are retinitis, colitis, and encephalitis. This section will limit the discussion to CMV retinitis because this accounts for 75 to 85% of CMV disease in patients with AIDS.

TREATMENT GOALS: CYTOMEGALOVIRUS

- Utilize new treatment modalities for CMV disease, which have enhanced the options for treatment and prevention of this opportunistic viral infection.
- Reverse or attenuate the retinitis, which ultimately can lead to blindness.Use ganciclovir or foscarnet as first-line therapy depending on the underlying clinical conditions in patients while limiting cidofovir to those subjects with refractory CMV disease.
- Discuss with the patient the role and potential complications associated with ganciclovir intraocular implant.
- Consider ganciclovir for prevention of CMV disease in persons with advanced AIDS who are CMV-seropositive and willing to commit to lifelong prevention.

EPIDEMIOLOGY

Retinitis is the most common manifestation of CMV infection in persons with AIDS. Clinical evidence of CMV retinitis occurs in as many as 40% of subjects infected with HIV, and autopsy series have revealed that CMV retinitis is present in up to 30% of patients.[50] Persons infected with HIV who are CMV-seropositive with a CD4+ cell count less than $50/mm^3$ are at greatest risk of CMV retinitis. Preliminary reports have shown the profound effect of HAART therapy on reducing the occurrence of CMV disease in patients with AIDS. In one center, the incidence of CMV disease was reduced by 80% because of combination antiretroviral therapy.[51]

PATHOPHYSIOLOGY

Ophthalmologic examination shows large creamy to yellowish-white granular areas of retinal necrosis and edema that follow a vascular distribution and can be hemorrhagic. This observation has been coined as a "cottage cheese and catsup" appearance. These pathophysiologic changes may be isolated early on at the periphery of the fundus; however, if left untreated the lesions progress within 2 to 3 weeks.[50] Ultimately, irreversible damage to the retina occurs, leading to diminished visual acuity and eventually blindness. Retinitis usually begins unilaterally, but can progress to contralateral involvement in patients with systemic CMV viremia.

CLINICAL PRESENTATION AND DIAGNOSIS

Signs and Symptoms

Decreased visual acuity, presence of floaters or light flashes, or unilateral loss of the central or peripheral visual field is the usual presenting complaint of patients with AIDS with CMV retinitis. (Floaters are spots in front of the eyes that "float" across a person's visual field.) Patients may be asymptomatic initially or may have poorly defined complaints about their vision. Photophobia or ocular pain are not associated with CMV retinitis.

Most patients with CMV retinitis have good vision at presentation, with 70 to 80% having a visual acuity of 20/40 or better.[52,53] Despite systemic therapy with ganciclovir or foscarnet, progressive visual loss occurs over time. In 287 patients with CMV retinitis, the median time to vision of 20/200 or worse in an eye with retinitis was 13.4 months and to bilateral vision of 20/200 or worse, 21.1 months.[52]

Diagnosis

The diagnosis of CMV retinitis is clinical. Virtually all patients infected with HIV with CMV retinitis have CD4+ cell counts less than 50/mm^3 and are seropositive for CMV. An ophthalmologist can establish the diagnosis with examination of both fundi by indirect ophthalmoscopy after pupillary dilation and finding the "cottage cheese and catsup" appearance.

PSYCHOSOCIAL ASPECTS

Irreversible vision loss as a result of retinitis can be devastating because it affects all aspects of one's daily activities. Suddenly, what once was routine becomes dependent on others–patients may be unable to drive a motor vehicle or complete simple errands. Reading books or watching television may no longer be possible. Obviously, it may be overwhelming to cope with the implications of such drastic alterations in lifestyle. Professional counseling can be offered, but perhaps more important is the provision of necessary support services to compensate for any lifestyle changes.

TREATMENT

The management of CMV retinitis involves three phases: (1) induction therapy for acute infection, (2) lifelong maintenance therapy following completion of the induction phase, and (3) prevention of CMV disease. More than one treatment regimen could be appropriate in most settings; thus, individual patient characteristics such as potential for overlapping drug toxicities and quality of life issues are considered in designing treatment schemes.

Pharmacotherapy—Induction and Maintenance Therapy

Daily intravenous (IV) infusions of ganciclovir or foscarnet, or weekly then biweekly IV infusions of cidofovir are each appropriate initial choices for induction and maintenance therapy for CMV retinitis.[54] Induction therapy is for 14 to 21 days followed by lifelong maintenance therapy (Table 77.4). Ganciclovir and foscarnet require lifelong daily intravenous infusions. The cost and inconvenience of these infusions and the risk of serious infections associated with central venous catheters are problematic.[55] The prolonged dosing interval for IV cidofovir may offset the need for a central line catheter and offer the patient greater flexibility in lifestyle; however, problems with nephrotoxicity may diminish the advantage of weekly dosing. The median time to the first progression of retinitis while on therapy with IV ganciclovir, IV foscarnet, or IV cidofovir ranges from 47 to 104 days, 53 to 93 days, and 64 to 120 days, respectively.[54] Oral ganciclovir should not be used as monotherapy for induction therapy because the limited bioavailability reduces its efficacy. Oral ganciclovir (4500 or 6000 mg/day) can be used for maintenance

Table 77.4 ▪ Treatment of Cytomegalovirus Retinitis in Patients with AIDS

Therapy Type	First-Line Therapy	Alternative Therapy	Comment
Induction therapy	Ganciclovir (5 mg/kg IV q12hr) for 14–21 days	Cidofovir (5 mg/kg IV once a week) for 2 weeks + probenecid pretreatment (2 g given 3 hr prior to infusion and 1 g at 2 hr and 8 hr postinfusion) with hydration before each dose	Monitor WBC with differential for ganciclovir-induced neutropenia
	Foscarnet (90 mg/kg IV q12 hr) for 14–21 days		Foscarnet IV infusion is over 2 hr and requires 500–1000 mL of 0.9% saline solution with each dose to minimize nephrotoxicity Cidofovir requires premedication with probenecid to minimize nephrotoxicity
Maintenance therapy	Ganciclovir (5 mg/kg IV once daily)	Ganciclovir (3–6 g PO daily in 3 divided doses with food)	Oral ganciclovir should *not* be used for maintenance therapy in patients with immediate sight-threatening disease
	Foscarnet (90–120 mg/kg IV once daily)	Cidofovir (5 mg/kg IV q2wk)	
Primary prophylaxis	Ganciclovir (1 g PO 3 times daily)		Prophylaxis may be considered for HIV-infected persons who are CMV seropositive and who have CD4+ cell counts <50/mm^3

therapy as long as the patient has no immediate sight-threatening disease.[54,56]

Preliminary results published in abstract have suggested that maintenance therapy of CMV retinitis may be stopped in patients infected with HIV responding to HAART regimens as evidenced by increasing CD4+ cell counts and undetectable HIV RNA viral loads.[54] Caution is advised in being overly optimistic in interpreting these results because the patient sample size was small and follow-up was short-term. Withdrawal of maintenance therapy requires validation from controlled studies prior to recommending this intervention.

Ganciclovir intraocular implant is a novel approach to drug delivery for CMV retinitis. The implant requires intraocular surgery and is subject to surgical complications. Many patients have immediate transient blurred vision with their current glasses that resolves within a few weeks. Approximately 10% of patients who received implants complain of a vision-compromising event. The benefit of this drug delivery device is that the median time to progression of disease (216–226 days) is significantly prolonged compared with the IV therapies.[57] The implant is depleted of ganciclovir after 5 to 8 months and must be replaced, which exposes the patient to subsequent risk (e.g., surgical complication, retinal detachment). The outcome of undergoing several reimplantation procedures is not known.[57] The major adverse event is retinal detachment, which can be a cause of substantial visual impairment. In addition, the local effect of the implant does not protect against disease that may develop in the contralateral eye.

Bone marrow suppression (neutropenia, thrombocytopenia) is the most significant adverse effect with systemic ganciclovir. Concentration-dependent neutropenia can be reversed with the use of granulocyte colony-stimulating factor, starting at a dose of 300 μg three times per week and then titrating the dose over time.[55] It is imperative to assess kidney function (estimate creatinine clearance) and adjust the dose accordingly because ganciclovir is primarily renally eliminated as the unchanged drug. The complete blood count (including white blood cells with differential) should be monitored at least weekly during induction therapy and weekly during the maintenance phase. Patients should be switched to foscarnet if neutropenia is severe (<500 to 1000 cells/mm^3).

Dose-limiting toxicities occur in approximately 30% of patients who receive IV foscarnet and include nephrotoxicity, electrolyte imbalances, nausea, malaise, genital ulcers, and neurologic symptoms.[54] Patients should be hydrated before and during the infusion to reduce the risk of nephrotoxicity, which can be augmented with concurrent administration of other nephrotoxic agents (e.g., amphotericin B, IV pentamidine, aminoglycosides). Supplementing potassium, magnesium, and calcium is often required during foscarnet therapy. An infusion pump should be used to control the rate of infusion (2 hours). The controlled infusion rate may ameliorate renal toxicity and the infusion-related malaise and neurotoxic effects. The serum creatinine and electrolytes should be monitored at least twice weekly during induction and weekly during maintenance therapy.

Nephrotoxicity is the most serious adverse effect of cidofovir therapy and can be prolonged and irreversible.[58,59] Concurrent probenecid and hydration with normal saline is required before each dose of cidofovir to minimize renal toxicity. The concomitant use of other nephrotoxic drugs, including nonsteroidal anti-inflammatory drugs (NSAIDs), should be discontinued 1 week before initiating cidofovir therapy.[54] The dose should be modified as listed in the product labeling for changes in renal function. Other adverse effects include neutropenia, metabolic acidosis, uveitis, and ocular hypotony. The serum creatinine, urinalysis (proteinuria), and white blood cell count (with differential) should be checked within 48 hours of each dose of cidofovir. Ocular examination should be performed monthly. Discontinue therapy for 3+ proteinuria if serum creatinine increases by 0.5 mg/dL above baseline, or if intraocular pressure decreases by 50% of baseline value.[54]

PHARMACOTHERAPY–PREVENTION THERAPY

Prophylaxis with oral ganciclovir may be considered for persons infected with HIV who are CMV seropositive and who have a CD4+ cell count of less than 50/mm^3.[16] This recommendation is based on results from a placebo-controlled trial of 725 patients in which the risk of developing CMV disease was reduced by one-half (26 to 14%).[60] These results were not supported in another clinical trial.[61] Current practice is to consider oral ganciclovir prevention on an individual case basis, explain the implications to the patient, and incorporate the patient's desires in the decision process.

IMPROVING OUTCOMES

Patient Education

Early recognition of CMV retinitis is most likely to occur when the patient has received information about the topic, and thus, is an important intervention for preventing severe CMV disease.[16] Patients should be made aware of the significance of increased floaters in the eye and should be advised to assess their visual acuity regularly by simple techniques such as reading newsprint. Patients should be instructed to seek medical attention should any visual changes occur.

Methods to Improve Patient Adherence to Drug Therapy

Daily IV infusions of ganciclovir or foscarnet requires major adjustments in the lifestyle of patients to accommodate drug administration. This can disrupt routine activities such as work or other obligations. Alternative maintenance therapies such as oral ganciclovir or IV cidofovir should be considered with the patient. As noted previously, oral ganciclovir is acceptable for maintenance therapy provided the patient has no immediate sight-threatening disease.

KEY POINTS

Pneumocystis carinii Pneumonia

- TMP-SMX is the drug regimen of choice for acute therapy and prophylaxis of PCP.
- Macular rash is a common adverse effect of sulfonamides in patients with AIDS, but should not necessarily preclude future use of these drugs.
- Adjunctive corticosteroids should be administered within 72 hours of starting antipneumocystis therapy for severe PCP, defined as a PaO_2 less than 70 mm Hg or A-a gradient greater than 35 mm Hg.
- Atovaquone is an alternative for treatment of mild to moderate PCP in patients who have no diarrhea and are able to ingest the oral suspension with fatty foods.
- Prophylaxis with systemic agents (TMP-SMX or dapsone) is recommended in persons infected with HIV with a CD4+ count of less than 200 cells/mm^3. Aerosolized pentamidine is an alternate in patients with CD4+ counts between 100 to 200 cells/mm^3.
- Importantly, patients receiving pyrimethamine-sulfadiazine for TE maintenance therapy do not need further PCP prophylaxis because of activity against both pathogens with this regimen.

Toxoplasmosis Encephalitis

- Pyrimethamine-sulfadiazine is the preferred regimen for treating acute toxoplasmic encephalitis and subsequent maintenance therapy (i.e., secondary prophylaxis). Patients should be well-hydrated to reduce the chances of sulfadiazine-induced crystalluria.
- Leucovorin (folinic acid) is recommended to prevent bone marrow suppression caused by pyrimethamine.
- Patients should receive instructions on how to protect themselves from infection of newly acquired *T. gondii* (e.g., eat meat that is well done, thoroughly wash fresh fruits and vegetables, wear latex gloves when handling cat litter boxes).

Mycobacterium avium Complex

- Treatment regimens should contain a macrolide (azithromycin or clarithromycin) and ethambutol.
- Drug interactions with anti-MAC agents are significant and require careful review of the medication profile to avoid complications especially with clarithromycin (cytochrome P450 inhibitor) and rifabutin (cytochrome P450 inducer).
- A macrolide (preferably azithromycin over clarithromycin) is the first-line agent for prophylaxis of MAC infection in persons infected with HIV with CD4+ cell counts less than 50/mm^3.

Cytomegalovirus Retinitis

- Intravenous ganciclovir or foscarnet are generally regarded as first-line drugs to treat CMV retinitis. Neutropenia and nephrotoxicity are frequent and serious adverse effects encountered with these drugs, respectively.
- Ganciclovir intraocular implant is a novel drug delivery system that significantly prolongs the time to progression of disease. The implant must be replaced when the drug supply is exhausted (about 5–8 months), and the long-term outcome of multiple reimplantation procedures is not known.
- Intravenous cidofovir should be used for refractory disease. Concurrent use of probenecid and hydration with normal saline is required before each dose to minimize renal toxicity.

REFERENCES

1. Stansell JD, Huang L. *Pneumocystis carinii* pneumonia. In: Sande MA, Volberding PA, eds. The medical management of AIDS. 5th ed. Philadelphia: Saunders, 1997:275–300.
2. Safrin S, Finkelstein DM, Feinberg J, et al. Comparison of three regimens for treatment of mild to moderate *Pneumocystis carinii* pneumonia in patients with AIDS. A double-blind, randomized trial of oral trimethoprim-sulfamethoxazole, dapsone-trimethoprim, and clindamycin-primaquine. ACTG 108 Study Group. Ann Intern Med 124:792–802, 1996.
3. Klein NC, Duncanson FP, Lenox TH, et al. Trimethoprim-sulfamethoxazole versus pentamidine for *Pneumocystis carinii* pneumonia in AIDS patients: results of a large prospective randomized treatment trial. AIDS 6:301–305, 1992.
4. Fishman JA. Treatment of infection due to *Pneumocystis carinii*. Antimicrob Agents Chemother 42:1309–1314, 1998.
5. Stein DS, Stevens RC. Treatment-associated toxicities: incidence and mechanisms. In: Sattler FR, Walzer PD, eds. *Pneumocystis carinii*. London: Bailliere Tindall, 1995:505–530.
6. Sattler FR, Cowan R, Nielsen DM, et al. Trimethoprim-sulfamethoxazole compared with pentamidine for treatment of *Pneumocystis carinii* pneumonia in the acquired immunodeficiency syndrome. A prospective, noncrossover study. Ann Intern Med 109:280–287, 1988.
7. Safrin S, Lee BL, Sande MA. Adjunctive folinic acid with trimethoprim-sulfamethoxazole for *Pneumocystis carinii* pneumonia in AIDS patients is associated with an increased risk of therapeutic failure and death. J Infect Dis 170:912–917, 1994.
8. Stevens RC, Laizure SC, Williams CL, et al. Pharmacokinetics and adverse effects of 20-mg/kg/day trimethoprim and 100-mg/kg/day sulfamethoxazole in healthy adult subjects. Antimicrob Agents Chemother 35:1884–1890, 1991.
9. Holtzer CD, Flaherty JF, Coleman RL. Cross-reactivity in HIV-infected patients switched from trimethoprim-sulfamethoxazole to dapsone. Pharmacotherapy 18:831–835, 1998.
10. Hughes W, Leoung G, Kramer F, et al. Comparison of atovaquone with trimethoprim-sulfamethoxazole for the treatment of *Pneumocystis carinii* pneumonia in patients with the acquired immunodeficiency syndrome (AIDS). N Engl J Med 328:1521–1527, 1993.
11. Dohn MN, Weinberg WG, Torres RA, et al. Oral atovaquone compared with intravenous pentamidine for *Pneumocystis carinii* pneumonia in patients with AIDS. Ann Intern Med 121:174–180, 1994.
12. O'Brien JG, Dong BJ, Coleman RL, et al. A 5-year retrospective review of adverse drug reactions and their risk factors in human immunodeficiency virus-infected patients who were receiving intravenous pentamidine therapy for *Pneumocystis carinii* pneumonia. Clin Infect Dis 24:854–859, 1997.
13. Conte J Jr, Chernoff D, Feigal D Jr, et al. Intravenous or inhaled pentamidine for treating *Pneumocystis carinii* pneumonia in AIDS. A randomized trial. Ann Intern Med 113:203–209, 1990.
14. Bozzette SA, Sattler FR, Chiu J, et al. A controlled trial of early adjunctive treatment with corticosteroids for *Pneumocystis carinii* pneumonia in the acquired immunodeficiency syndrome. California Collaborative Treatment Group. N Engl J Med 323:1451–1457, 1990.
15. Gagnon S, Boota AM, Fischl MA, et al. Corticosteroids as adjunctive therapy for severe *Pneumocystis carinii* pneumonia in the acquired immunodeficiency syndrome. A double-blind, placebo-controlled trial. N Engl J Med 323:1444–1450, 1990.

16. Centers for Disease Control and Prevention. 1997 USPHS/IDSA guidelines for the prevention of opportunistic infections in persons infected with human immunodeficiency virus. MMWR 46(RR-12):1–46, 1997.
17. Schneider MME, Borleffs JCC, Stolk RP, et al. Discontinuation of prophylaxis for *Pneumocystis carinii* pneumonia in HIV-1-infected patients treated with highly active antiretroviral therapy. Lancet 353:201–203, 1999.
18. Bozzette SA, Finkelstein DM, Spector SA, et al. A randomized trial of three antipneumocystis agents in patients with advanced human immunodeficiency virus infection. N Engl J Med 332:693–699, 1995.
19. Hardy WD, Feinberg J, Finkelstein DM, et al. A controlled trial of trimethoprim-sulfamethoxazole or aerosolized pentamidine for secondary prophylaxis of *Pneumocystis carinii* pneumonia in patients with the acquired immunodeficiency syndrome. ACTG Protocol 021. N Engl J Med 327:1842–1848, 1992.
20. Subauste CS, Wong SY, Remington JS. AIDS-associated toxoplasmosis. In: Sande MA, Volberding PA, eds. The medical management of AIDS. 5th ed. Philadelphia: Saunders, 1997:343–362.
21. Mariuz P, Bosler EM, Luft BJ. Toxoplasmosis in individuals with AIDS. Infect Dis Clin NA 8:365–381, 1994.
22. Katlama C, De Wit S, O'Doherty E, et al. Pyrimethamine-clindamycin vs. pyrimethamine-sulfadiazine as acute and long-term therapy for toxoplasmic encephalitis in patients with AIDS. Clin Infect Dis 22:268–275, 1996.
23. Dannemann BR, McCutchan JA, Israelski DM, et al. Treatment of toxoplasmic encephalitis in patients with AIDS: a randomized trial comparing pyrimethamine plus clindamycin to pyrimethamine plus sulfonamides. Ann Intern Med 116:33–43, 1992.
24. Canessa A, Del Bono V, De Leo P, et al. Cotrimoxazole therapy of *Toxoplasma gondii* encephalitis in AIDS patients. Eur J Clin Microbiol Infect Dis 11: 125–130, 1992.
25. Becker K, Jablonowski H, Haussinger D. Sulfadiazine-associated nephrotoxicity in patients with the acquired immunodeficiency syndrome. Medicine 75: 185–194, 1996.
26. Kovacs JA. Efficacy of atovaquone in treatment of toxoplasmosis in patients with AIDS. Lancet 340:637–638, 1992.
27. Fernandez-Martin J, Leport C, Morlat P, et al. Pyrimethamine-clarithromycin combination for therapy of acute *Toxoplasma* encephalitis in patients with AIDS. Antimicrob Agents Chemother 35:2049–2052, 1991.
28. Luft BJ, Hafner R, Korzun AH, et al. Toxoplasmic encephalitis in patients with the acquired immunodeficiency syndrome. N Engl J Med 329:995–1000, 1993.
29. Podzamczer D, Miro JM, Bolao F, et al. Twice-weekly maintenance therapy with sulfadiazine-pyrimethamine to prevent recurrent toxoplasmic encephalitis in patients with AIDS. Ann Intern Med 123:175–180, 1995.
30. Heald A, Flepp M, Chave JP, et al. Treatment of cerebral toxoplasmosis protects against *Pneumocystis carinii* pneumonia in patients with AIDS. Ann Intern Med 115:760–763, 1991.
31. Ruf B, Schurmann D, Bergmann F, et al. Efficacy of pyrimethamine/sulfadoxine in the prevention of toxoplasmic encephalitis relapses and *Pneumocystis carinii* pneumonia in HIV-infected patients. Eur J Clin Microbiol Infect Dis 12:325–329, 1993.
32. Podzamczer D, Salazar A, Jimenez J, et al. Intermittent trimethoprim-sulfamethoxazole compared with dapsone-pyrimethamine for simultaneous primary prophylaxis of pneumocystis pneumonia and toxoplasmosis in patients infected with HIV. Ann Intern Med 122:755–761, 1995.
33. Podzamczer D, Santin M, Jimenez J, et al. Thrice weekly cotrimoxazole is better than weekly dapsone-pyrimethamine for the primary prevention of *Pneumocystis carinii* pneumonia in HIV-infected patients. AIDS 7:501–506, 1993.
34. Leport C, Chêne G, Morlat P, et al. Pyrimethamine for primary prophylaxis of toxoplasmic encephalitis in patients with human immunodeficiency virus infection: a double-blind, randomized trial. J Infect Dis 173:91–97, 1996.
35. Jacobson MA, Besch CL, Child C, et al. Primary prophylaxis with pyrimethamine for toxoplasmic encephalitis in patients with advanced human immunodeficiency virus disease: results of a randomized trial. J Infect Dis 169:384–394, 1994.
36. Jouan M, Cambau E, Baril L, et al. Decreased incidence of disseminated MAC infection in 689 AIDS patients receiving antiretroviral treatment with protease inhibitors. Abstract I-30. 37th Interscience Conference on Antimicrobial Agents and Chemotherapy. Toronto, Ontario, Canada, September 28-October 1, 1997.
37. Wright J. Current strategies for the prevention and treatment of disseminated *Mycobacterium avium* complex infection in patients with AIDS. Pharmacotherapy 18:738–747, 1998.
38. Chin DP, Reingold AL, Horsburgh CR Jr, et al. Predicting *Mycobacterium avium* complex bacteremia in patients with the human immunodeficiency virus: a prospectively validated model. Clin Infect Dis 19:668–674, 1994.
39. Chaisson RE, Benson CA, Dubé MP, et al. Clarithromycin therapy for bacteremic *Mycobacterium avium* complex disease. A randomized, double-blind, dose-ranging study in patients with AIDS. Ann Intern Med 121:905–911, 1994.
40. Centers for Disease Control and Prevention. Recommendations on prophylaxis and therapy for disseminated *Mycobacterium avium* complex for adults and adolescents infected with human immunodeficiency virus. MMWR 42(RR-9): 17–20, 1993.
41. Dubé MP, Sattler FR, Torriani FJ, et al. A randomized evaluation of ethambutol for prevention of relapse and drug resistance during treatment of *Mycobacterium avium* complex bacteremia with clarithromycin-based combination therapy. J Infect Dis 176:1225–1232, 1997.
42. Chaisson RE, Keiser P, Pierce M, et al. Clarithromycin and ethambutol with or without clofazimine for the treatment of bacteremic *Mycobacterium avium* complex disease in patients with HIV infection. AIDS 11:311–317, 1997.
43. Shafran SD, Singer J, Zarowny DP, et al. A comparison of two regimens for the treatment of *Mycobacterium avium* complex bacteremia in AIDS: rifabutin, ethambutol, and clarithromycin versus rifampin, ethambutol, clofazimine, and ciprofloxacin. N Engl J Med 335:377–383, 1996.
44. Havlir D, Torriani F, Dubé M. Uveitis associated with rifabutin prophylaxis. Ann Intern Med 121:510–512, 1994.
45. Narang PK, Trapnell CB, Schoenfelder JR, et al. Fluconazole and enhanced effect of rifabutin prophylaxis. N Engl J Med 330:1316–1317, 1994.
46. Nightingale SD, Cameron W, Gordin FM, et al. Two controlled trials of rifabutin prophylaxis against *Mycobacterium avium* complex infection in AIDS. N Engl J Med 329:828–833, 1993.
47. Pierce M, Crampton S, Henry D, et al. A randomized trial of clarithromycin as prophylaxis against disseminated *Mycobacterium avium* complex infection in patients with advanced acquired immunodeficiency syndrome. N Engl J Med 335:384–391, 1996.
48. Havlir DV, Dubé MP, Sattler FR, et al. Prophylaxis against disseminated *Mycobacterium avium* complex with weekly azithromycin, daily rifabutin, or both. N Engl J Med 335:392–398, 1996.
49. Freedberg K, Scharfstein JA, Seage GR III. The cost-effectiveness of prophylaxis for *Mycobacterium avium* complex in AIDS. Abstract 44238. 12th World AIDS Conference. Geneva, Switzerland, June 28–July 3, 1998.
50. Drew WL, Stempien MJ, Erlich KS. Management of herpesvirus infections (CMV, HSV, VZV). In: Sande MA, Volberding PA, eds. The medical management of AIDS. 5th ed. Philadelphia: Saunders, 1997:381–388.
51. Moore R, Keruly JC, Gallant J, et al. Decline in mortality rates and opportunistic disease with combination antiretroviral therapy. Abstract 22374. 12th World AIDS Conference. Geneva, Switzerland, June 28–July 3, 1998.
52. Jabs DA. Ocular manifestations of HIV infection. Trans Am Ophthalmol Soc 93:623–683, 1995.
53. Studies of Ocular Complications of AIDS Research Group and the AIDS Clinical Trials Group. Foscarnet-ganciclovir cytomegalovirus retinitis trial 4: visual outcomes. Ophthalmology 101:1250–1261, 1994.
54. Whitley RJ, Jacobson MA, Friedberg DN, et al. Guidelines for the treatment of cytomegalovirus diseases in patients with AIDS in the era of potent antiretroviral therapy. Arch Intern Med 158:957–969, 1998.
55. Studies of Ocular Complications of AIDS Research Group and the AIDS Clinical Trials Group. Mortality in patients with the acquired immunodeficiency syndrome treated with either foscarnet or ganciclovir for cytomegalovirus retinitis. N Engl J Med 326:213–220, 1992.
56. Drew WL, Ives D, Lalezari JP, et al. Oral ganciclovir as maintenance treatment of cytomegalovirus retinitis in patients with AIDS. N Engl J Med 333:615–620, 1995.
57. Musch DC, Martin DF, Gordon JF, et al. Treatment of cytomegalovirus retinitis with a sustained-release ganciclovir implant. N Engl J Med 337:83–90, 1997.
58. Lalezari JP, Stagg RJ, Kuppermann BD, et al. Intravenous cidofovir for peripheral cytomegalovirus retinitis in patients with AIDS. A randomized, controlled trial. Ann Intern Med 126:257–263, 1997.
59. Studies of Ocular Complications of AIDS Research Group in Collaboration with the AIDS Clinical Trials Group. Parenteral cidofovir for cytomegalovirus retinitis in patients with AIDS: the HPMPC peripheral cytomegalovirus retinitis trial. A randomized, controlled trial. Ann Intern Med 126:264–274, 1997.
60. Spector SA, McKinley GF, Lalezari JP, et al. Oral ganciclovir for the prevention of cytomegalovirus disease in persons with AIDS. N Engl J Med 334:1491–1497, 1996.
61. Brosgart CL, Louis TA, Hillman DW, et al. A randomized, placebo-controlled trial of the safety and efficacy of oral ganciclovir for prophylaxis of cytomegalovirus disease in HIV-infected individuals. AIDS 12:269–277, 1998.

CHAPTER 78

MYCOTIC INFECTIONS

Annie Wong-Beringer

The incidence and spectrum of invasive fungal infections have increased dramatically over the past two decades.[1] Advances in medical technology and therapies such as bone marrow or solid-organ transplantation, use of invasive monitoring devices, mechanical ventilation, parenteral nutrition, broad-spectrum antimicrobial agents, intensive cancer chemotherapies, corticosteroids, and other immunosuppressives predispose patients to invasive fungal infections.[2,3] Adding to this growing population of susceptible hosts are individuals infected with HIV.

Medically important fungi causing systemic fungal infections can be classified as endemic versus opportunistic. Endemic pathogens are those capable of causing disease in otherwise healthy individuals as well as in immunocompromised hosts who reside in a specific geographic location; infections tend to be more disseminated and rapidly progressive in the latter population.[4] The three major pathogens that cause endemic mycoses in North America are *Coccidioides immitis*, *Histoplasma capsulatum*, and *Blastomyces dermatitidis*. In contrast, opportunistic pathogens such as *Candida* sp., *Aspergillus* sp., and *Cryptococcus neoformans* generally cause invasive disease in patients with overt immunosuppression.

The diagnosis of invasive fungal diseases is based on a combination of two or more of the following: careful evaluation of the clinical presentation of signs and symptoms, blood cultures, results of serologic testing, diagnostic imaging, and tissue biopsies for histopathology and cultures. Although associated mortality with invasive candidiasis and aspergillosis are extremely high in immunocompromised hosts, early diagnosis generally is difficult to establish with existing tests or studies.[5] Current research focuses on the development of newer methods using DNA and RNA gene probes, polymerase chain reactions (PCRs), and detection of fungal antigen and fungal metabolites in the early diagnosis and monitoring of therapeutic response of invasive fungal diseases.

TREATMENT GOALS: MYCOTIC INFECTIONS

- Determine the spectrum and severity of mycotic infections, which vary depending on the immune status of the host and pathogen.
- Understand the patient's risk factors for and etiology of immunosuppression, because the treatment goals may differ dramatically according to patient immune status and pathogen.
- Understand that immunocompetent patients usually do not require specific antifungal therapy for endemic mycoses.
- Use prolonged or lifelong secondary prophylaxis following acute initial treatment of primary fungal infections for some individuals (e.g., patients who are HIV-positive).
- Use aggressive therapy with high-dose amphotericin B in patients who experience prolonged and profound neutropenia secondary to cytotoxic chemotherapy, because they are at high risk for acute life-threatening systemic opportunistic mycoses such as disseminated candidiasis and invasive aspergillosis.
- Understand that primary antifungal prophylaxis administered during the period of prolonged and profound neutropenia may improve infectious morbidity and mortality in susceptible hosts.

Epidemiology and Clinical Presentation of Endemic Mycoses

Histoplasmosis

Histoplasmosis is an endemic mycosis caused by the pathogenic fungus, *Histoplasma capsulatum*. The organism was first described by Samuel Darling at the turn of the twentieth century. Histoplasmosis occurs throughout the world; however, the geographic distribution of this fungus in the United States prevails primarily along the Mississippi and Ohio river valleys and in other central, southeastern, and mid-Atlantic states. *H. capsulatum* is a dimorphic fungus that exists as a mold in soil or culture media at temperatures of less than 37°C (98.6°C) and as budding yeasts at 37°C or higher.[6] Infection is initiated following inhalation and distribution of the spores to the lungs. The spores convert promptly to the tissue-invasive yeast form on entering the mammalian hosts.[6]

T-cell immunity appears to be most critical in determining the outcome of infection. Individuals with impaired T-cell immunity, such as those with HIV infection, succumb to the severe and disseminated form of the disease. In fact, histoplasmosis has been recognized as an AIDS-defining illness since 1987; it is the most commonly diagnosed endemic mycosis in patients with HIV.[4]

EPIDEMIOLOGY

Factors accounting for the specific geographic distribution of *Histoplasma capsulatum* in the United States are not fully understood. However, humid environments along fertile river valleys appear to be favorable for growth of the organism. In addition, bird or bat droppings enhance the rate of sporulation, thereby increasing the number of infectious particles. Old buildings or urban parks inhabited by birds or bats, farms, bird roosts, and caves are sources of exposure to *H. capsulatum*. Exposure to spores may result from activities such as demolishing or remodeling old structures, clearing brush from urban parks, cleaning chicken coops, and repairing damaged chimneys. Spores can be spread by wind over large areas, and can be found even 10 years after birds have abandoned their roosts.[7]

CLINICAL PRESENTATION AND DIAGNOSIS

Host factors such as underlying immunosuppression and enhanced immunity from prior infection are important determinants of the outcome of infection. Environmental factors also play an important role in the severity of illness and attack rates. Exposure in enclosed areas rather than in the outdoors, for longer duration, or to high inoculum of spores usually results in more severe clinical disease.[7]

Signs and Symptoms

Pulmonary

The majority of symptomatic patients (80%) experience self-limiting acute disease that resembles an influenzalike illness.[7] Improvement of symptoms usually occurs within a few weeks. Inflammatory complications such as arthritis, severe arthralgia accompanied by erythema nodosum, and pericarditis may occur in up to 10% of patients. Management with anti-inflammatory agents is adequate without the need for antifungal therapy. In about 10% of symptomatic patients, histoplasmosis may present as cavitary disease resembling tuberculosis.[7] Chronic pulmonary symptoms (less severe than tuberculosis) and apical lung lesions that progress with inflammation, cavitation, and fibrosis are characteristic of this form of illness. Many such patients have underlying chronic obstructive pulmonary disease.

Disseminated

Disseminated histoplasmosis occurs rarely in patients without overt immunosuppression, at a rate of 1 in 2000 to 5000.[7] In contrast, disseminated disease occurs in 95% of cases in patients with AIDS.[4] The incidence of histoplasmosis in patients with HIV residing in endemic areas is 2 to 5% versus less than 1% in nonendemic areas. Most adults present with subacute illness characterized by low-grade fever, weight loss, and fatigue.[7] Untreated illness may last up to 20 years with asymptomatic periods interrupted by clinical illness. Central nervous system (CNS) involvement in the form of lymphocytic meningitis or cerebritis may complicate 10 to 20% of those with severe underlying immunosuppression. Focal organ involvement is uncommon. In patients with AIDS, 90% of disseminated disease occurs in those with CD4 counts below 200/μL.[4] The majority of patients present with low-grade fever, fatigue, weight loss of 1 to 3 months' duration, and respiratory symptoms such as cough and dyspnea. Approximately 10 to 20% of patients develop a syndrome resembling septicemia with shock, respiratory insufficiency, hepatic and renal failure, and intravascular coagulation with coagulopathy.

Diagnosis

A number of tests currently are available for the diagnosis of histoplasmosis, which include serologic tests for antibodies, antigen detection, fungal cultures, and fungal stains.[4,7] In general, serologic tests for antibodies are positive in 90% of otherwise healthy patients with active symptomatic disease.[7] As for patients with AIDS who have disseminated disease, antigen detection from urine and serum is the most sensitive method for diagnosis. Cultures of bone marrow, blood, urine, and sputum are recommended for all patients suspected to have disseminated histoplasmosis; bone marrow cultures provide the highest yield with positive results in more than 75% of cases.[7]

Blastomycosis

Blastomycosis is an endemic fungal infection caused by *Blastomyces dermatitidis.* Like *Histoplasma capsulatum*, this organism is a thermal dimorphic fungus that lives in the soil.[4] The geographic distribution of this organism overlaps that of *Histoplasma capsulatum* in much of the central and southeastern United States, and extends farther to the north and west, including Northern Wisconsin, northern Minnesota, and the adjacent areas of south-central Canada.[8] The United States appears to be the most heavily endemic area for *Blastomyces dermatitidis* in the world. Blastomycosis is an uncommon disease even among residents in endemic areas and is the least common opportunistic endemic mycosis in patients with AIDS.[4] The immunologic defense to *B. dermatitidis* in normal hosts is not fully understood. It is thought that both cellular and humoral immunity are important in controlling infection.[9] The disease is acquired through inhalation of conidia, with the lungs being the primary site of infection. Secondary spread to extrapulmonary sites may occur concurrent with the respiratory illness or after the respiratory illness has resolved.[8]

EPIDEMIOLOGY

The precise epidemiology of blastomycosis is less well understood than other endemic mycoses such as histoplasmosis and coccidioidomycosis.[8] The lack of a reliable skin test for large-scale surveys and the difficulty in isolating *B. dermatitidis* from soil do not allow for a precise determination of the endemic area and the ecologic niche of the fungus. Current evidence suggests that nitrogen-rich soil along rivers, streams, and lakes enhances growth of the fungus. Incidentally, many sporadic cases or outbreak cases occurred in close proximity to recreational water. Sporadic cases most commonly occur in males between 25 and 50 years of age who have heavy vocational or recreational exposure to woods and streams. Unlike histoplasmosis, where virtually every resident in endemic areas has acquired primary infection (as indicated by a positive skin test), exposure and infection with blastomycosis is less universal. Late reactivation of a primary infection may occur as long as 40 years after initial exposure.[10]

CLINICAL PRESENTATION AND DIAGNOSIS

Signs and Symptoms

Pulmonary blastomycosis occurs in up to 80% of all patients with a highly variable clinical presentation.[8] Five distinct symptomatology may be seen:

1. Asymptomatic illness detectable only as part of an outbreak
2. Brief flulike illness, usually with rapid resolution
3. Acute illness resembling bacterial pneumonia
4. Subacute or chronic illness with a symptomatic complex resembling tuberculosis or lung cancer
5. Fulminant infection with acute respiratory distress syndrome (ARDS)

The latter presentation, in which severe gas exchange abnormality and diffuse infiltrates are present, is associated with a mortality of more than 50%.[8] Most sporadic cases present with subacute or chronic pulmonary symptoms resembling tuberculosis or lung cancer. Approximately 25% of those patients have concurrent skin or bone involvement. Conversely, symptomatic cases that occur during point-source outbreaks tend to present with flulike illness or acute illness that resembles bacterial pneumonia.

Extrapulmonary manifestations most commonly involve the skin in the form of verrucous or ulcerative lesions, followed by bone (osteomyelitis), prostate (prostatitis), and CNS (cranial abscesses or meningitis) involvement. The CNS may be involved in 5 to 10% of disseminated cases.[8] In general, multiple visceral organ involvement and CNS disease are common among immunocompromised patients.[4,9]

Unlike other endemic mycoses, blastomycosis occurs rarely in patients with AIDS, and 90% of those affected have advanced disease with a CD4 count of less than 200/μL.[4] Fulminant respiratory failure and ARDS occur in 20 to 30% of patients, whereas disseminated cutaneous lesions may be present in one-third of patients. CNS involvement has been reported in up to 40% of patients with AIDS. Death owing to overwhelming pulmonary disease, with or without extrapulmonary manifestations, has been reported in up to 40% of patients with AIDS in contrast to a mortality rate of 2 to 3% in otherwise normal hosts. Most deaths occur within 4 weeks of diagnosis.

Diagnosis

Definitive diagnosis of blastomycosis is based on demonstration of the organism by culture or stain of body fluids or tissue specimen.[4,8] The easiest and most rapid method is by direct visualization of the organism in expectorated sputum or aspirated pus after 10% potassium hydroxide digestion. Cultures are positive in 90% of cases, but it may take several weeks to obtain the results. Serologic tests for antibodies are negative in most cases and a negative result does not exclude diagnosis. Reliable tests for antigen are not yet available for diagnostic purposes.

Coccidioidomycosis

Coccidioidomycosis is caused by *Coccidioides immitis*, a thermal dimorphic fungus like *H. capsulatum* and *B. dermatitidis*. In soil, it grows as a mold with arthroconidia but converts to a spherule containing 200 to 400 endospores each in host tissues. The number of multiplying coccidioidal organisms is significantly higher than *H. capsulatum* or *B. dermatitidis,* which may explain the higher incidence of clinical infection following exposure to *C. immitis*.[11] Primary pulmonary infection occurs in the susceptible host when airborne arthroconidia generated by dust storms or strong winds are inhaled.[12] T-cell immunity is critical for control of infection. Host immune response results in the production of immunoglobulin M (IgM) and immunoglobulin G (IgG) antibodies; although they do not confer specific protection to disease development, serologic tests measuring antibody levels have diagnostic and prognostic value.[12]

EPIDEMIOLOGY

The geographic distribution of *C. immitis* is along the warm and dry southwestern region of the United States; the southern San Joaquin Valley of California and southern Arizona are the most heavily endemic areas.[12] Hence, the popular terms "valley fever" and "desert rheumatism" are used to describe the common manifestations of coccidioidomycosis. Dusty conditions during late summer and fall, especially following rainy winters, predispose residents or travelers in endemic areas to the acquisition of airborne arthroconidia. Epidemiologic investigation of a recent large outbreak of coccidioidomycosis that occurred after the January 1994 Northridge earthquake in California confirms that dust cloud-generating events are significant risks for acquisition of infection.[13] Because T-cell immunity is a key defense to coccidioidal infection, patients with the following conditions are at risk for developing severe pulmonary and disseminated disease: HIV positive, AIDS, hematologic malignancies, organ transplantation, third trimester pregnancy, and recent postpartum. In the nonimmunocompromised population, disseminated disease is more likely to occur in the very old and very young. Interestingly, for unknown reason, patients belonging to certain ethnic groups (in order of descending risk) are predisposed to the development of disseminated disease: Filipino, African American, Native American, Hispanic, and Asian.[12]

CLINICAL PRESENTATION AND DIAGNOSIS

Signs and Symptoms

The majority (60%) of patients infected with coccidioidomycosis are asymptomatic. Approximately 40% develop symptoms with a spectrum of manifestations ranging from mild to moderate influenzalike illness, pneumonia, and disseminated disease.[14] The incubation period for the onset of symptoms following exposure is usually 1 to 4 weeks.

Acute respiratory illness often is misdiagnosed as viral bronchitis; respiratory symptoms usually last several days and are often accompanied by myalgia, malaise, and fatigue that may persist for several weeks.[11] In 15 to 20% of patients, a distinctive rash develops during the acute illness, either as erythema nodosum with raised painful nodules over the tibial or ankle areas or as a more diffuse erythema multiforme.[11] Arthritis of the ankle or other joints may be involved symmetrically. This is often called "desert rheumatism" and represents a self-limited immune complex reaction. A minority (5%) of acute coccidioidomycosis cases progress to complicated pulmonary disease with persistence of a pulmonary nodule or cavity.[14] Patients with diabetes mellitus are more likely to be affected. One-third of the cavities may close spontaneously within 2 years of its discovery, whereas the remainder may be complicated by secondary bacterial infections or persistent hemoptysis that require excision.[11] Diffuse pulmonary infiltrates accompanied by respiratory failure is noted more frequently in patients with AIDS compared with individuals without AIDS, and has an associated mortality of 70%.[4]

Disseminated disease develops in approximately 1% of symptomatic patients. In contrast to the general population, about 15% of patients with AIDS develop extrapulmonary manifestations.[4] Secondary spread to virtually all organs except the gastrointestinal tract has occurred.[12] The most frequent extrapulmonary manifestations is the development of granulomas or abscess on the skin, followed by synovitis and osteomyelitis. Meningitis is the most severe form of dissemination and is responsible for the majority of deaths owing to coccidioidomycosis, which may occur within 2 to 3 weeks of the onset of pulmonary symptoms or may follow an asymptomatic primary infection. The course of meningitis ranges from indolent to rapidly fatal within a few days.[12] Clinical presentation may be nonspecific and subtle with headache, weakness, mental status changes, weight loss, and occasional hydrocephalus. Cerebrospinal fluid (CSF) findings are marked by lymphocytic pleocytosis, elevated protein, and decreased glucose, with cultures often negative for the organism.

Diagnosis

Definitive diagnosis is made with fungal culture and stains of blood, tissue, and fluids.[11,12] However, blood cultures are frequently negative. Growth of the organism on appropriate media typically is apparent in 3 to 5 days. Histopathologic evidence of spherules with characteristic endosporulation also may confirm diagnosis. More than 50% of adult patients living in endemic areas have a positive reaction to the skin test, whereas a negative skin test does not rule out coccidioidomycosis.[14] A negative reaction in those with severe infection is a poor prognostic sign and may reflect an inability of the host to mount an adequate cell-mediated immunity.[11] Serologic tests measuring IgM and IgG antibodies to *C. immitis* are available commercially and are both sensitive and specific.[11] The diagnosis of coccidioidomycosis can be confirmed by positive serologic test results in the presence of acute illness. IgM is measured by an immunodiffusion method and is reported qualitatively as positive or negative. A positive result indicates acute disease activity, either initially or during a later exacerbation. On the other hand, complement-fixing (CF) IgG antibody in serum and CSF is measured quantitatively.[11] The quantity of antibody titers parallels the antigen (fungal) load to which the antibodies are developing. High-serum IgG titers (>1:64) predict the likelihood for dissemination of infection especially with the reversal of a previously positive skin test.[12] In addition, serial measurement of CF IgG titers at 3- to 4-week intervals during the period of illness is useful for monitoring disease progression. A positive CF IgG test of the CSF is the most useful test for confirming the diagnosis of coccidioidal meningitis.[11,12]

Epidemiology and Clinical Presentation of Opportunistic Mycoses

Cryptococcosis

Cryptococcus neoformans is an opportunistic fungal pathogen that causes invasive diseases primarily in patients with underlying immunodeficiency and rarely in hosts with normal defenses. It exists as an encapsulated yeast surrounded by a polysaccharide capsule and has a worldwide distribution.[15] Infection is acquired via inhalation of the spores of *C. neoformans* into the lungs. In patients with intact T-cell immunity, primary infection usually is contained within the lungs, whereas rapid dissemination to other sites, most notably the CNS, occurs in immunocompromised hosts.

EPIDEMIOLOGY

More than 20 species of *Cryptococcus* are known; however, *C. neoformans* is essentially the only human pathogen. The organism grows most abundantly in avian excreta, particularly pigeon droppings.[15] *C. neoformans* also has been isolated from nonavian sources such as fruits, vegetables, and dairy products. Four serotypes (A, B, C, and D) of *C. neoformans* are based on the antigenic determinants of the polysaccharide capsule.[15] The varieties of *C. neoformans* serotypes are *neoformans* and *gattii*. Epidemiologic evidence suggests differences in geographic distribution, host preference related to immune status, clinical course, and response to therapy between the two varieties.[16] Var. *neoformans* is ubiquitous, whereas var. *gattii* has geographic limitation to tropical and subtropical areas (e.g., southern California, Australia, Southeast Asia, Brazil, and Central America), particularly in the soil under eucalyptus trees. The majority (90%) of infections with *C. neoformans* var. *neoformans* occur in immunocompromised hosts, whereas var. *gattii* affects primarily immunocompetent hosts with a predilection for invasion of the CNS. Patients infected with the latter variety have more neurologic complications, such as altered mental status, papilledema, focal deficits, ataxia, and seizures. In addition, infections owing to var. *gattii* tend to have a protracted course and are less responsive to therapy.

In the pre-AIDS era, lymphoreticular malignancies, organ transplantation, diabetes, cirrhosis, malnutrition, and corticosteroid therapy were risk factors predisposed to cryptococcosis.[15] Since the beginning of the AIDS epidemic, cryptococcosis occurs primarily in patients with advanced HIV disease (CD4 count <100 cells/μL) and has become the fourth leading opportunistic infection in this population.[15] It is estimated that up to 10% of patients with AIDS in western countries will develop cryptococcal meningitis, whereas up to 30% of patients in sub-Saharan Africa are affected.[17] In a minority of patients (20 to 30%) infected with *C. neoformans*, no predisposing risk factors or underlying condition are apparent.[18]

CLINICAL PRESENTATION AND DIAGNOSIS

Signs and Symptoms

Pulmonary

Cryptococcal infection most often affects the lungs and CNS. Even though the lung is the portal of entry, pulmonary cryptococcosis is relatively uncommon.[15] In immunocompetent hosts, the infection is usually mild and localized with spontaneous resolution.[18] In contrast, the mortality rate associated with cryptococcal pneumonia in patients with AIDS exceeds 40%.[19] Most patients with AIDS and pulmonary cryptococcosis have disseminated disease; about 60 to 70% have concurrent meningeal involvement. In normal hosts, concurrent CNS involvement with pulmonary disease is more likely associated with infection owing to *C. neoformans* var. *gattii*.[15] Some have suggested that all patients with pneumonia or colonization be evaluated with a lumbar puncture to rule out CNS involvement despite the absence of obvious neurologic signs or symptoms.[15]

Central Nervous System

Cryptococcal meningitis is the most common manifestation of disseminated disease. Acute presentation with neurologic sequelae is much more common in immunocompetent hosts.[15] Conversely, 75 to 90% of patients with AIDS present with subacute meningitis or meningoencephalitis characterized by fever, malaise, and headache.[19] Approximately 30% may present with altered mental status, confusion, lethargy, personality change, and memory loss. Overt signs of meningismus such as neck stiffness and photophobia are uncommon among patients with AIDS. Also, response to infection in CSF is usually blunted with normal protein and sugar accompanied by a mild pleocytosis. CNS complications include hydrocephalus, visual or hearing loss, cranial nerve palsies, ataxia, seizures, and dementia. The mortality rate ranges between 10 and 30%, with most deaths occurring within the first few weeks of illness.[18] Various prognostic signs have been associated with poor outcomes of CNS disease in patients with AIDS (Table 78.1). Relapse rates of CNS disease in patients who do not have AIDS is 15 to 25% compared with more than 50% in those who do have AIDS.[19]

Other Sites

Cryptococcosis may involve other sites such as the skin, skeletal system, and prostate gland in decreased frequency.[18] Cutaneous disease may be present in 10% of the disseminated cases, appearing as papules, tumors, vesicles, abscesses, cellulitis, and lesions resembling molluscum contagiosum in patients with AIDS. More important, persistent but usually asymptomatic infection of the prostate gland may occur in as many as 29% of patients with AIDS, and serves as a source for subsequent relapse after completion of primary therapy.[18]

Diagnosis

Diagnosis of cryptococcosis is made by isolating the organism from a sterile body site, by histopathology, or by cryptococcal capsular antigen testing. Blood cultures are positive in 70% of patients with AIDS who are infected with *C. neoformans*.[19] India ink stain outlines the polysaccharide capsule of the yeast. Results from direct examina-

Table 78.1. ▪ Prognostic Signs Associated with Poor Treatment Outcomes of Cryptococcal Meningitis in AIDS

Prognostic Signs
Altered mental status at presentation
Elevated opening cerebrospinal pressure
Low CSF leukocyte count (<20 cells/mm^3)
High CSF cryptococcal antigen titers (≥1:8)
High serum cryptococcal antigen titers (≥1:32)

tion of the CSF are positive for India ink stain in more than 80% of patients with AIDS and approximately 50% of the time in normal hosts with meningeal involvement.[15] The latex agglutination test for cryptococcal polysaccharide antigen has a sensitivity and specificity exceeding 95%.[15] Testing for antigen in serum is a useful initial screening test in patients with AIDS who present with fever and headaches. A positive serum antigen test indicates the need for lumbar puncture; about 99% of patients with cryptococcal meningitis have positive serum antigen test.[15] Secondary infection with *Trichosporon beigelii* can cause false-positive results owing to cross-reactivity with the antigen. Serial measurement of antigen titers during therapy does not appear to be helpful in monitoring disease response or predicting relapse.[15]

Aspergillosis

Aspergillosis, the most common invasive mold infection worldwide, is caused by the ubiquitous fungus *Aspergillus* spp. Approximately 150 species have been identified thus far. Pathogenic species that commonly cause invasive diseases include *A. fumigatus, A. flavus, A. niger, A. terreus,* and *A. nidulans.*[20] *A. fumigatus* is the predominant species causing invasive aspergillosis; it accounts for approximately 90% of all cases. *A. fumigatus* is the most rapidly growing species and has very small spore size, allowing deep penetration into the lungs; both characteristics are likely to contribute to its pathogenicity. The growth rate of *A. fumigatus* and *A. flavus* may be accelerated by 30 to 40% in the presence of physiologic and pharmacologic concentrations of hydrocortisone.[20] The rate of progression of invasive diseases may be closely related to the growth rate of the organisms. Macrophage ingestion and killing of the spores and extracellular killing of hyphae by neutrophils are the primary host defenses against *Aspergillus* in the lungs.[20] Corticosteroids can substantially impair the functions of both macrophages and neutrophils. T-cell function is thought to be important in the more chronic forms of invasive aspergillosis.

EPIDEMIOLOGY

Aspergillus spp. are ubiquitous in the air and environment. They can be found in decomposing vegetable material, cellars, potted plants, pepper and spices, unfiltered marijuana smoke, and showerheads and hot water faucets. In addition, the release of large quantities of spores into the air is associated with local construction work, which represents a major risk factor for immunocompromised patients susceptible to the development of invasive aspergillosis.[21] Thus, the primary means of reducing the risk of acquiring the organisms for at-risk patients is the use of hepafiltration or laminar airflow to remove *Aspergillus* spores from the air. In addition, pharmaceutical agents are used to remove *Aspergillus* from surface areas.[21]

Although aspergillosis has been documented in immunocompetent patients, the occurrence is unusual. Those at highest risk for acquiring invasive diseases are patients in the following categories: bone marrow and solid organ transplant recipients, people with profound neutropenia, and those with severe burns. Other at-risk groups include individuals with underlying diseases such as late-stage AIDS, chronic granulomatous disease, and diabetes mellitus.[20]

CLINICAL PRESENTATION AND DIAGNOSIS

Signs and Symptoms

Clinical manifestations and the rate of disease progression vary among different patient groups.[20,21] Typically, individuals who are the least immunocompromised have prominent signs and symptoms with an indolent progression of disease over a 2- to 3-month period (from onset to diagnosis). In contrast, patients who are the most immunocompromised are least likely to have symptoms and may progress within 7 to 10 days from onset of disease to death. The respiratory tract is the primary portal of entry, accounting for 80 to 90% of invasive aspergillosis. Other possible sites of entry include damaged skin or operative wounds, the cornea, and the ear, which have resulted in burn-associated cutaneous aspergillosis, prosthetic valve endocarditis, keratitis, and catheter-site infection.

Aspergillosis can present as acute and chronic invasive pulmonary disease, tracheobronchitis, acute and chronic sinusitis, and disseminated disease in the form of cutaneous or cerebral infection.

Pulmonary

Acute invasive pulmonary aspergillosis occurs primarily in immunocompromised hosts. Prolonged neutropenia is a major risk factor for developing disease; as many as 70% of patients may be affected if the duration of neutropenia extends to or beyond 34 days.[22] Up to one-third of patients with acute invasive pulmonary disease are asymptomatic initially.[20] As the disease progresses, early symptoms may consist of dry cough with fever and nonspecific chest pain. Dyspnea and hypoxemia with normal white blood cell (WBC) count are characteristic of diffuse bilateral disease. Those with focal disease tend to progress slower and have a more favorable prognosis because surgical resection is a therapeutic option. Hemoptysis can occur with focal disease without warning and can be life threatening.[20] Plain chest radiographs are extremely heterogeneous but cavitated lesions or nodular shadows with and without cavitation are highly suspicious. As many as 30% of neutropenic bone marrow transplant patients with invasive aspergillosis have normal chest radiographs in the week preceding death.[21] More commonly, the clinical presentation of acute pulmonary aspergillosis in immunocompromised hosts is one of unremitting fever and the development of lung infiltrates despite broad-spectrum antibacterial therapy.

Chronic invasive aspergillosis occurs less frequently than acute aspergillosis.[20] Affected patients commonly have underlying conditions such as AIDS, chronic granulomatous disease, diabetes mellitus, alcoholism, and corticosteroid use. Presenting signs and symptoms are more prominent and tend to extend over weeks or months; they include chronic productive cough, mild to moderate hemoptysis, low-grade fever, malaise, and weight loss. Patients with chronic disease are usually strongly positive for antibodies to *Aspergillus*; this finding can be used to infer the diagnosis when bronchial biopsies are contraindicated or negative for *Aspergillus* hyphae.

Tracheobronchitis

Among immunocompromised patients, aspergillus tracheobronchitis occurs more commonly in patients with AIDS and lung transplant recipients.[20] Approximately 25% of the patients with tracheobronchitis have no apparent immunocompromise. Notably, in lung transplant recipients, it is difficult to differentiate *Aspergillus* colonization of the airways from infection. The majority of patients (80%) are symptomatic with cough, fever, dyspnea, chest pain, and hemoptysis. Airway disease ranges from excess mucous production and inflammation to ulceration and extensive pseudomembranous tracheobronchitis. Death usually results from respiratory insufficiency secondary to occlusion of airways or disseminated aspergillosis.

Sinusitis

Invasive aspergillus sinusitis can occur either as acute rhinosinusitis or chronic invasive sinusitis.[20] *A. flavus* is more commonly a cause of sinusitis. Acute rhinosinusitis is relatively common in neutropenic patients and bone marrow transplant recipients and rare in solid organ transplant recipients. Common signs and symptoms include fever, cough, epistaxis, and headache. Sinus pain, nasal discharge, and sore throat may occur. Local extension to palate, orbit, or brain is common and may occur relatively rapidly.[23] Relapse of disease during episodes of neutropenia and relapses of leukemia can be expected after initial response to treatment.[20]

Chronic invasive sinusitis occurs in healthy or somewhat immunocompromised patients; the latter typically are those with diabetes and alcoholism.[20] The disease usually progresses over months. Signs and symptoms are typical of chronic sinusitis, such as visual (e.g., diplopia, pain in the eye) and olfactory disturbances, and headaches with absence of fever. Complications such as bony destruction and osteomyelitis of the base of the skull may occur. Management requires surgical debridement with prolonged antifungal therapy.

Disseminated

In most patients who die of invasive aspergillosis, disseminated disease is often a postmortem diagnosis, unless cutaneous or cerebral aspergillosis is suspected and diagnosed before death. Cutaneous aspergillosis most commonly is associated with the intravenous–catheter site in neutropenic patients.[20] Premature neonates and children with AIDS also may develop invasive fungal dermatitis. Surgical wounds infected with *Aspergillus* may occur preoperatively or postoperatively; occurrence in liver transplant recipients are relatively common. Cutaneous disease in burn patients tends to occur over a rapidly progressive course, typically refractory to treatment.[24] The clinical appearance of cutaneous lesions is characterized by raised erythema that rapidly increase in size, with the center of the lesion changing from red to purple and finally to black with possible ulceration. The rate of progression is most rapid in those who are neutropenic. The lesions usually progress over several days in those with circulating neutrophils and are associated with pain and discomfort. In general, cutaneous aspergillosis is most responsive to antifungal therapy, with the exception of burn-associated aspergillosis.[20]

Cerebral aspergillosis accounts for 10 to 20% of the cases of invasive aspergillosis.[20,24] In patients who are profoundly neutropenic, altered mental status and seizures may be the presenting signs shortly before death. Individuals who are relatively less immunocompromised may have more focal features such as headaches and occasional fever. Radiologic evidence by computed tomography (CT) scans reveals either multiple hypodense lesions or ring-enhancing lesions with surrounding edema. CSF findings are abnormal but nonspecific. Definitive diagnosis is based on biopsy or aspiration of the lesion but is rarely performed because of the clinical status of the patient or coagulation problems.

Diagnosis

Once aspergillosis is suspected based on clinical grounds, radiologic evaluation should be performed immediately using CT or magnetic resonance imaging (MRI).[20] Plain radiographs of chest or sinuses early in the course of disease may be falsely negative or insensitive. Surgical resection or tissue biopsy should be performed on identification of a lesion. In those who are not surgical candidates or in whom surgical resection is not possible owing to diffuse pulmonary disease, bronchoscopy and bronchoalveolar lavage are recommended.

Laboratory diagnosis of invasive aspergillosis is based on a combination of approaches including detection of organism in tissue by direct microscopic examination, isolation, and identification of pathogen in culture, and detection of an immunologic response to the pathogen or some other marker of its presence, such as metabolic product.[20,21] Microscopy and culture should be performed on fluids obtained from bronchoalveolar lavage or on pus obtained from aspirated pulmonary lesions, infected sinuses, or abscesses. Typically, microscopy allows direct identification of *Aspergillus* from the preceding specimens based on the presence of hyphae; however, several other fungi may have similar microscopic and histologic appearances. Hence, further confirmation of the diagnosis should be made by culture of the preceding specimens. In addition, serologic methods used to detect the presence of galactomannan or antibodies to *Aspergillus* have been shown to be useful adjuncts in aiding clinicians in identifying invasive aspergillosis in hematology patients as well as in solid organ transplant recipients.[23] However, the sensitivity and specificity of the available assays are less than optimal to recommend routine use in the clinical setting.[20]

Given the rapid rate of progression of invasive aspergillosis from onset to death in those profoundly immunocompromised, delay in diagnosis and treatment is usually fatal. Frequently in clinical practice, aggressive empirical therapy for acute invasive aspergillosis is initiated based on a combination of clinical, radiologic, or microbiologic features before definitive proof of a diagnosis, which is based ideally on the histologic documentation of tissue invasion by hyphae and a positive culture of *Aspergillus*.

Candidiasis

Candida sp. are opportunistic pathogens that are a part of the normal human commensals. *Candida* as a cause of oral lesions was first identified in the 1840s. The appearance of all forms of *Candida* infections has arisen only following the introduction of antibiotics into clinical use in the 1940s.[25] Over the past decade, the incidence of infections owing to *Candida* sp. has increased dramatically. Data reported to the National Nosocomial Infections Surveillance (NNIS) system from participating hospitals in the United States between 1980 and 1989, reveal an increase in the rate of nosocomial candidemia by 500% in large teaching hospitals and by 219 and 370% in small teaching hospitals and large nonteaching hospitals, respectively.[26] Most recent data from the NNIS system (1990 to 1992) indicate that *Candida* sp. are now the sixth most common nosocomial pathogen overall and the fourth most common bloodstream pathogen.[27] Invasive candidiasis is associated with considerable morbidity and mortality. Based on a case-control study well matched for age, sex, service, underlying diagnosis, and duration of hospital stay, nosocomial candidemia was found to result in an excess mortality of 38% and those who survived spent an extra 30 days in the hospital.[28]

Candida organisms are yeasts that exist microscopically as small (4 to 6 μm), thin-walled, ovoid cells that reproduce by budding. Other morphologic forms such as pseudohyphae and hyphae also can be seen in clinical specimens for most *Candida* sp. except *C. glabrata*.[29] More than 150 *Candida* sp. have been identified previously; however, approximately 10 are considered important human pathogens. The pathogenic species include *C. albicans, C. tropicalis, C. parapsilosis, C. glabrata* (formerly classified as *Torulopsis glabrata*), *C. krusei, C. guilliermondii, C. lusitaniae, C. kefyr* (*C. pseudotropicalis*), *C. rugosa,* and *C. stellatoidea* (now considered *C. albicans*).[25] Speciation of the pathogens is important owing to the varied pathogenic potential and susceptibility to antifungal agents. A rapid presumptive identification of *Candida albicans* usually can be made by performing the specific germ tube test.[30] Hyphal outgrowths from the yeast cells occur only for *C. albicans* following incubation at 37°C (98.6°F) in horse serum for 2 to 3 hours, which allows it to be differentiated from other species. Identification of a germ tube negative *Candida* sp. (presumably *non-albicans*) relies on a combination of morphologic and biochemical testing. All pathogenic species are capable of causing similar spectrums of disease ranging from mucocutaneous to disseminated disease.[31] Breakdown of the normal host defense mechanisms is necessary for *Candida* organisms to become pathogens. An intact integument is required for protection against cutaneous invasion. Once invasion occurs, functioning neutrophils, macrophages, and lymphocytes are important host defenses against the development of systemic disease.[25]

EPIDEMIOLOGY

Candida sp. can be found in soil, inanimate objects, hospital environments, and food.[25] More important, the organisms are normal commensals of humans and are commonly found on diseased skin, along the entire gastrointestinal (GI) tract, in expectorated sputum, along the female genital tract, and in urine in patients with indwelling Foley catheters.[25] A majority of the infections arise from an endogenous source, with the GI tract or skin being the most likely portals of entry. However, exogenous acquisition of the organism is possible. For example, oral thrush in a newborn can result from the acquisition of *Candida* from the vagina of the mother during birth. In addition, *Candida* balanitis can be acquired through sexual contact with a partner who has *Candida* vaginitis.

Patients at risk for the development of invasive candidiasis include cancer patients, premature neonates, heroin addicts, burn patients, patients undergoing abdominal surgery, and organ transplantation recipients.[25,31]

Table 78.2. ▪ Susceptibility of Bloodstream Isolates of *Non-albicans Candida* spp. to Fluconazole

Candida spp. Isolated	MIC_{50} (μg/mL)
C. albicans	0.25
C. tropicalis	1.0
C. parapsilosis	1.0
C. glabrata	16
C. krusei	32

Source: Adapted from Pfaller MA. Nosocomial candidiasis: emerging species, reservoirs, and modes of transmission. Clin Infect Dis 22(Suppl 2):S89–S94, 1996. With permission.

Specifically, risk factors predisposed to the development of candidemia are prior treatment with multiple antibiotics, prolonged hospital stay, prior central venous catheterization, parenteral hyperalimentation, corticosteroid use, prior hemodialysis, and prior colonization at sites other than blood.[25,31,32] Antibiotics allow the proliferation of *Candida* sp. in the GI tract by suppressing normal bacterial flora, whereas instrumentation with catheters or other invasive monitoring devices provide a conduit for entry of *Candida* sp. into the bloodstream.

Candida albicans is the predominant cause of both focal and invasive infections. *C. albicans* has been reported to account for 50 to 70% or more of cases of invasive candidiasis, followed by *C. tropicalis, C. glabrata,* and *C. parapsilosis.*[33] Notably, recent data indicate an apparent shift to an increasing proportion of invasive infections caused by non-*albicans* species presumably related to the widespread use of antifungal agents such as fluconazole.[31] In general, *non-albicans Candida* sp. as a group are considered less susceptible than *C. albicans* to the azoles (Table 78.2).[33]

CLINICAL PRESENTATION AND DIAGNOSIS

Signs and Symptoms

Candidiasis can be broadly categorized as mucocutaneous or deep invasive infections.[31] The two categories of infection tend to have a distinct set of predisposing factors and diagnostic and treatment approaches. The more common forms of mucocutaneous candidiasis among susceptible patients are oropharyngeal (thrush), esophageal, and vulvovaginal candidiasis. Invasive syndromes are often hematogenous in origin ranging from catheter-related transient candidemia to acute disseminated candidiasis characterized by candidemia accompanied by simultaneous spread of the infection to one or more noncontiguous organs, and chronic disseminated candidiasis (previously known as hepatosplenic candidiasis). Focal organ involvement such as candidiasis involving the brain, heart, bone, and joint can occur and is presumably owing to hematogenous spread of the infection. Peritonitis may result from local processes and spread secondary to bowel injury.

Mucocutaneous Candidiasis

Thrush and Esophagitis

Oropharyngeal candidiasis (thrush) occurs generally among patients with disruption of local defenses or damage to the mucosal membranes resulting from radiation or cytotoxic chemotherapy and those receiving local or systemic antibiotics or corticosteroids.[25] In addition, the incidence of thrush is high among patients with malignancies or defects in cell-mediated immunity such as AIDS. Every year more than 60% of patients with HIV who have CD4 counts lower than 100/μL will develop disease complicated by frequent recurrences.[35] Oral thrush is characterized by creamy white, curdlike patches on the tongue and other mucosal surfaces that are removable by scraping.[25]

Esophageal involvement usually occurs by direct spread of oral disease, although a number of patients with *Candida* esophagitis have no associated oral disease.[25] Esophagitis most commonly occurs in patients receiving cytotoxic chemotherapy. In addition, approximately 10 to 20% of patients with AIDS have *Candida* esophagitis.[35] In esophagitis, white patches resembling thrush can be seen endoscopically along the esophagus. Symptoms consist of pain and difficulty swallowing, a feeling of obstruction on swallowing, and substernal chest pain. In extensive disease, bleeding and perforation may occur.[25]

Vulvovaginitis

Vulvovaginal candidiasis is estimated to occur at least once during reproductive years in 75% of women with no recognizable predisposing factors.[36] However, identifiable risk factors include broad-spectrum antibiotics, high estrogen-containing oral contraceptives, poorly controlled diabetes, and pregnancy. Among patients infected with HIV, one large cross-sectional study found similar incidence (9%) of vaginal candidiasis compared with patients who do not have HIV.[35] Clinical signs and symptoms include whitish cheesy discharge, vulvovaginal pruritus, irritation, soreness, dyspareunia, and burning on micturition.[36]

Deep Organ Involvement

Candidemia and Acute Disseminated Candidiasis

Candidemia is defined as the isolation of *Candida* sp. from at least one blood culture. The syndromes of candidemia can be subdivided into catheter-related candidemia limited to the bloodstream and acute disseminated candidiasis with hematogenous spread of the infection to one or more noncontiguous organs.[31] Catheter-related candidemia typically occurs in medical or surgical patients with an indwelling central venous catheter. Presenting signs often include an abrupt onset of fever and local signs of inflammation at the site of the catheter. Prognosis is usually good. Prompt response can be expected with antifungal therapy and removal of the infected catheter.

Acute disseminated candidiasis is a fulminant infection most often seen in neutropenic patients, burn patients, and postoperative patients.[25,31] In the latter group, those who have had organ transplantation, heart surgery, or GI tract surgery are at greatest risk.[25] Disseminated candidiasis typically presents as overwhelming sepsis with no distinct clinical features. Multiple organs usually are involved, with formation of microabscesses, most commonly in the kidney, brain, myocardium, and eye. Endophthalmitis and macular or erythematous cutaneous lesions are suggestive signs of disseminated disease but often are absent.[31] In the neutropenic patient, the most common manifestation is persistent fever despite broad-spectrum antibiotic therapy. Prognosis of disseminated candidiasis is heavily dependent on underlying disease, physiologic status of the patient (i.e., APACHE II score), degree of immunosuppression, and the extent of disease when antifungal therapy is instituted.[31]

Chronic Disseminated Candidiasis

Chronic disseminated candidiasis (also known previously as hepatosplenic candidiasis) is a distinct form of hematogenous candidiasis seen almost exclusively in patients with leukemia or bone marrow transplantation.[31] Infection of the liver or spleen presumably occurs during the period preceding chemotherapy-induced neutropenia. Candidemia may be detected occasionally during this period; however, the disease does not manifest itself until after neutrophil recovery. The typical patient will have persistent fever after neutrophil recovery and complain of abdominal pain. Multiple lesions are revealed on CT scans of the liver or spleen. Elevation of alkaline phosphatase and other liver function tests are usually present.[21]

Candiduria

Lower urinary tract infection is thought to occur via ascending route from the bladder. On the other hand, pyelonephritis can occur as a result of ascending or hematogenous spread.[25] Distinguishing infection versus colonization by the presence of *Candida* sp. in the urine is difficult.[37] Unlike bacterial urinary tract infection, in candiduria the quantity of organisms and the presence of pyuria do not significantly correlate with the presence of infection.[37] In patients with an indwelling Foley catheter, colonization of the urine with *Candida* sp. is common. In addition, candiduria may simply indicate the filtering of the organism during an episode of hematogenous spread in the critically ill patient and may be the only positive culture indicating disseminated disease.[31] In light of the relatively low sensitivity of blood cultures in diagnosing patients with disseminated candidiasis, a positive urine culture often poses a diagnostic and therapeutic dilemma for the clinician.

Diagnosis

Mucocutaneous Candidiasis

The diagnosis of oropharyngeal and esophageal candidiasis is based on the clinical appearance and the demonstration of hyphae, pseudohyphae, or yeast forms obtained from scraping the lesions using a 10% potassium hydroxide smear. Similarly, vulvovaginal candidiasis can be diagnosed by clinical presentation, direct microscopy using either saline solution or a 10% potassium hydroxide smear in addition to the presence of normal vaginal pH.

Deep Organ Involvement

Hematogenous spread is essential in disseminated candidiasis. Hence, prompt and accurate detection of *Candida* sp. in the bloodstream is tantamount to the diagnosis of disseminated disease. However, the diagnosis of hematogenous candidiasis remains elusive because of the low sensitivity of blood cultures. Several series have reported positive blood cultures in less than 50% of patients with autopsy-proven invasive candidiasis.[31] In addition, routine blood cultures may take several days to become positive. Serologic tests based on the detection of antibodies, antigen, or metabolites of the *Candida* sp. are not routinely recommended and few are commercially available.[21]

Owing to the lack of distinct clinical presentation and reliable diagnostic methods for disseminated candidiasis, some have suggested a clinical approach to aid clinicians in making the diagnosis.[31] Multiple risk factors have been shown to predict the likelihood of disseminated candidiasis in a given patient. Based on these risk factors, disseminated candidiasis should be considered for patients who have persistent, unexplained fever in conjunction with some combination of the following: neutropenia, prolonged duration of intensive care stay (>7 days), prolonged use of multiple antibacterial agents, prolonged use of intravascular catheters, and colonization with *Candida* at one or more body sites.

Treatment and Outcomes of Endemic Mycoses and Opportunistic Mycoses

Antifungal pharmacotherapy for systemic infections is limited to a few pharmacologic classes compared with antibacterial agents. An overview of the pharmacology of systemically available antifungal agents, which include amphotericin B, ketoconazole, itraconazole, fluconazole, 5-flucytosine, and terbinafine, is provided in the following sections. The current status and utility of antifungal susceptibility testing to guide therapy are also discussed. In addition, the role in therapy for each agent is detailed with respect to endemic and opportunistic mycoses.

GENERAL TREATMENT GUIDELINES

Pharmacotherapy

The three major classes of systemic antifungal agents in clinical use consist of the polyenes (amphotericin and nystatin), the azole derivatives, and the allylamines–thiocarbamates (terbinafine), all of which target fungal cell membranes either by interacting with or inhibiting ergosterol.

Amphotericin B

Amphotericin B has been available for more than 40 years and remains the gold standard for the treatment of systemic fungal infections. However, its use is associated with drug-related toxicities. The optimal dosage and duration of amphotericin B are largely empiric; total dosage generally has been determined by patient response and tolerance. Daily dosage varies from 0.5 to 1.5 mg/kg depending on the host's immune status, site, severity, and type of infection.[38–40] An initial 1-mg test dose of amphotericin is recommended traditionally in order to observe for anaphylactic reaction, which occurs on rare occasions; however, recent clinical experience suggests that this practice may not be necessary and may significantly delay therapy in those who are acutely ill.[38] In fact, for life-threatening infections, many clinicians advocate that a dose of 0.25 mg/kg be initiated on the first day of therapy followed by full-dose therapy on subsequent days of treatment. Adverse effects associated with systemic administration of amphotericin B are primarily acute infusion-related (e.g., fever, chills, rigors) and dose-limiting nephrotoxicity. Premedications with acetaminophen 10 mg/kg, diphenhydramine 50 mg, meperidine 25 to 60 mg administered one-half hour before amphotericin B infusions have been shown to reduce the incidence of fever and chills.[38] Hydrocortisone 25 mg added to the infusion also has reduced febrile reactions. Thrombophlebitis can also occur and can be minimized with the use of central venous line for administration, dilute solutions (<0.1 mg/mL), or the addition of heparin 500 to 1000 U/L of solution. The most significant adverse effect is nephrotoxicity. Reversible nephrotoxicity develops in approximately 80% of patients with receipt of at least 500 mg total dose of amphotericin B.[38] Irreversible renal damage occurs rarely and usually does not occur unless the total dose exceeds 4 to 5 g.[38] Efforts to minimize or reverse nephrotoxicity include the use of sodium loading, mannitol administration, and alternate-day administration. Infusion of 0.5 L of sodium chloride 0.9% over 30 minutes before and after completion of the amphotericin B infusion is advocated by some for patients at the first sign of rising serum creatinine (Scr) and blood urea nitrogen (BUN) concentrations.[41] However, caution must be exercised when liberalizing salt intake in patients with congestive heart failure (CHF), renal failure, or cirrhosis with ascites. The recently available lipid-formulated amphotericin B products (e.g., Abelcet, Amphotec, AmBisome) clearly are associated with a lower incidence of nephrotoxicity in comparison to the conventional formulation.[42] Clinical experience with the use of these products is limited to patients who are intolerant of or refractory to amphotericin B deoxycholate. Renal tolerance is usually defined as Scr greater than or equal to 2.5 mg/dL or doubling of baseline Scr in compassionate use studies and clinical trials. Thus far, no direct comparative data between lipid products has been published. Efficacy data from animal models of fungal infections suggest differential activity for the three commercially available lipid formulations. In addition, none of the lipid-based products demonstrates superior efficacy when prospectively compared with amphotericin B deoxycholate against invasive candidiasis and cryptococcal meningitis. At present, use of these expensive agents should be considered for salvage therapy.

Azoles

Ketoconazole, which was introduced in the 1980s, was the first systemically useful azole in the treatment of invasive mycoses. Ketoconazole offers a less toxic treatment alternative of endemic mycoses in the outpatient setting compared to amphotericin B. However, the high doses required (>800 mg/day) for treatment are associated with frequent toxicities.[43] Since the introduction of fluconazole and itraconazole in the 1990s, the use of ketoconazole has been replaced largely by the newer agents owing to their greater efficacy and tolerability. Fluconazole and itraconazole are available in oral and parenteral formulations. Both drugs are highly active against endemic mycoses; itraconazole is more effective than fluconazole against histoplasmosis and blastomycosis. In addition, they have variable activity against the yeasts and molds that cause invasive diseases. Non-*albicans Candida* species as a group are less susceptible to fluconazole and itraconazole, whereas *Aspergillus* spp. are susceptible only to itraconazole.[43] Despite the favorable adverse effect profile, itraconazole and fluconazole each has its unique limitations.[43,44] Oral absorption of itraconazole is poor and variable. A new oral solution has improved bioavailability over the capsule form. However, both formulations of itraconazole require an acidic medium for drug dissolution; thus, drug absorption is problematic in patients with HIV who have achlorhydria, or in those receiving concurrent antacids or H_2-antagonists. Serum levels should be measured to ensure adequate absorption. In contrast, fluconazole has excellent bioavailability and its absorption is not pH-dependent. All three azoles inhibit mammalian cytochrome P-450 enzyme families; ketoconazole is the most potent and fluconazole the least potent inhibitor.[96] In general, the magnitude of interaction increases when higher doses of azoles are employed. Clinically significant drug interactions have been documented when azoles are coadministered with terfenadine, astemizole, cisapride, cyclosporine, phenytoin, and rifampin. Simultaneous administration of the azoles with terfenadine, astemizole, and cisapride is contraindicated because of the potential occurrence of

Table 78.3. ▪ Dosage Adjustment in Renal and Hepatic Impairment

Drug	Renal Impairment CrCl (mL/min) >50–90	10–50	<10	Hepatic Impairment
Amphotericin	No change	No change	No change	No change
Fluconazole	No change	Decrease dosage 50%	Decrease dosage 75%	No change
Itraconazole	No change	No change	No change	Monitor carefully
Flucytosine	q6hr–normal daily dosing	q12–24hr Decrease 50–75% daily	q24hr Decrease 75% daily	No change
Terbinafine	No change	Decrease dosage 50%	Unknown	Unknown

life-threatening arrhythmias. Azole-induced inhibition of cyclosporine metabolism results in an increase in cyclosporine trough concentration and area under the curve; thus, close monitoring of cyclosporine serum concentrations and renal function is important in patients receiving both agents. In addition, rifampin and phenytoin may induce the metabolic clearance of ketoconazole and itraconazole (and, to a lesser extent, fluconazole), resulting in treatment failure of fungal infections. Phenytoin metabolism also can be inhibited by fluconazole; nystagmus and ataxia as a result of excessive phenytoin concentrations have been reported in a few patients in whom phenytoin and fluconazole were concomitantly administered.

Notably, owing to their relatively favorable safety profile compared with amphotericin, the azoles have assumed widespread use in the treatment of specific fungal infections as well as for prophylactic and suppressive therapy. However, the emergence of azole-resistant pathogens is being reported increasingly, particularly among oropharyngeal isolates of *Candida albicans* from patients infected with HIV. The clinical utility of these drugs may become limited in the near future with the continued use of these agents.[45,46,101]

Other Agents

5-Flucytosine is a nucleoside analog with limited utility owing to its narrow spectrum of activity, its toxicities, and the rapid emergence of resistance when used alone. Its role in therapy has been in combination with amphotericin B for treating cryptococcal meningitis and invasive aspergillosis. Maintaining a serum level of 5-flucytosine below 100 mg/mL is recommended to avoid dose-related bone-marrow toxicities. Dosage reduction is required in renal dysfunction.[47] Table 78.3 provides recommendations on dosage adjustment for selected antifungal agents in renal and hepatic impairment.[97,98] Terbinafine is an allylamine with a broad spectrum of in vitro activity, which includes *Aspergillus* sp. In addition, it has been demonstrated to act synergistically with the azoles against azole-resistant *Candida* sp.[44] The role of terbinafine in the treatment of invasive diseases currently is being evaluated. New antifungal drug targets are currently under investigation.[48] Agents that inhibit the biosynthesis of fungal cell wall components (chitin and glucan) have shown broad in vitro activity against pathogenic fungi; few have shown promise in animal models of invasive mycoses and are being evaluated in early clinical trials.

Antifungal Susceptibility Testing

The use of antifungal susceptibility testing to guide therapy may become the standard of care in the near future as the number and spectrum of fungal infections increases, reports of antifungal resistance continues, and new antifungal agents are developed. Studies correlating antifungal susceptibility testing results with in vivo outcome of fungal infections are ongoing. A reference method for in vitro susceptibility testing of yeasts has been standardized only recently.[93] A clear correlation between in vitro results and in vivo outcome has been demonstrated only for the use of azoles in the treatment of oropharyngeal candidiasis in patients infected with HIV.[94] In vitro results predicting in vivo outcomes for other clinical situations such as candidemia have not yet been shown.[95] A standardized method for in vitro testing of molds is still being developed. At present, the utility of antifungal susceptibility testing is limited to defining azole susceptibility in the oropharyngeal *Candida* isolates from patients with HIV and to reference laboratories involved in the surveillance of resistance or investigations of new compounds.

TREATMENT OF ENDEMIC MYCOSES

The majority of patients infected with endemic fungal pathogens (*H. capsulatum, B. dermatitidis,* and *C. immitis*) are asymptomatic or have self-limited acute pulmonary disease that does not require treatment with antifungal agents.[49] A minority of patients with the following clinical presentations may develop fulminant or chronic progressive disease requiring specific therapy: acute pulmonary disease accompanied by severe respiratory distress; chronic pulmonary cavitary disease; extrapulmonary dissemination involving skin, bone, CNS, and others.[7,8] Those who have underlying immunodeficiency also are candidates for antifungal therapy. Among the major endemic mycoses, coccidioidomycosis is most refractory to treatment, particularly the meningeal form of disease.[50] Lifelong maintenance therapy following acute treatment to prevent relapse is indicated in patients infected with HIV who have endemic mycoses and may be required in all patients with coccidioidal meningitis.[4,50] According to the 1997 U.S. Public Health Service Guidelines, primary prevention against histoplasmosis is recommended for residents living in endemic areas who have advanced HIV infection (CD4 count <100/μL) owing to the prevalence of disease and the severity of presentation in this patient population.[51] Routine prevention against primary infection with blastomycosis and coccidioidomycosis is not recommended currently for patients who are HIV positive.

Amphotericin B has been the mainstay of treatment of endemic mycoses. However, therapy often is complicated by acute infusion-related adverse effects and dose-limited nephrotoxicity. Recent introduction of the azoles provides less toxic treatment alternatives. Of note, patients who are immunocompromised or who have life-threatening or meningeal disease have been excluded from studies using the azoles. In addition, direct comparison between amphotericin B and the azole drugs has not been performed in controlled trials for endemic mycoses.[52] Nonetheless, response to treatment appears slower with the azoles by comparison with historical controls.[52] Hence, use of amphotericin B is currently indicated for treating patients with ARDS, sepsis syndrome, or other evidence of overwhelming infection with the endemic mycoses (including those with meningeal involvement, with the exception of coccidioidal meningitis).[53] A total dosage of 1.0 to 2.5 g of amphotericin B generally is recommended.[38] Daily dosage ranges from 0.7 to 1.5 mg/kg with administration of the drug until the disease is inactive or for a total of 2 to 3 months, depending on the host's response.[12,50,53] Therapy usually can be switched to itraconazole in patients who are clinically stable; thus, the total dosage or duration of amphotericin B may be shorter than that stated in the preceding.

Local administration via intra-articular injections of amphotericin B may be useful either as a primary therapy or as an adjunct to systemic therapy or surgery in coccidioidal synovitis or osteomyelitis.[12,50] Direct lumbar or cisternal injections or intraventricular administration via an Ommaya reservoir have been used to administer the drug along with parenteral administration for the treatment of coccidioidal meninigitis.[50] Because the drug is extremely irritating to the meninges, neurologic sequelae such as paraparesis, numbness, and severe headache have resulted. In addition, cisternal administration carries the potential risks of brain puncture or hemorrhage.[50] Treatment is initiated at an extremely low dosage (0.025 mg) and increased in a stepwise fashion until a maximum of 0.5 to 0.7 mg is reached.[50] Safer treatment with high-dose fluconazole and itraconazole for meningitis has been studied and now has largely replaced the use of this mode of administration.[54,55]

Itraconazole is considered the drug of choice for histoplasmosis and blastomycosis in nonimmunocompromised patients who do not have life-threatening or meningeal disease.[44] Itraconazole administered at dosages of 200 to 400 mg daily for a duration of 6 to 24 months has been associated with a response rate of 86 and 95% for histoplasmosis and blastomycosis, respectively.[56] Treatment is recommended for 6 months, or 3 months after all lesions have resolved. Patients with chronic cavitary pulmonary histoplasmosis are less responsive to itraconazole and may require therapy for at least 1 year or longer.[53]

Acute treatment with amphotericin B followed by lifelong maintenance therapy with itraconazole 200 to 400 mg per day is recommended to prevent relapse in patients who have HIV with histoplasmosis.[4,7] Itraconazole has been shown to be effective for induction therapy in patients who have HIV with mild to moderate disease, and as lifelong maintenance therapy. In an open-label, nonrandomized prospective trial, itraconazole therapy at 300 mg twice a day for 3 days followed by 200 mg twice a day for 12 weeks resulted in an 85% response (50/59) in patients with AIDS and disseminated histoplasmosis.[52] Patients with CNS involvement or severe clinical manifestations were excluded from the study. In a separate study involving a similar group of patients, fluconazole induction therapy at 800 mg per day for 12 weeks followed by maintenance therapy at 400 mg per day resulted in a 74% response.[57] However, the 1-year relapse rate with high-dose fluconazole therapy (800 mg/day) was substantially higher when compared with patients receiving itraconazole at 200 mg per day as maintenance therapy (47% versus <5%).[57,58] Ketoconazole is not an acceptable treatment option in patients with AIDS owing to the low response rate of less than 20%.[59]

Fluconazole is less active than itraconazole against blastomycosis and histoplasmosis, and is considered second-line therapy.[43,53] It is indicated for patients who cannot tolerate or adequately absorb itraconazole. A minimum dosage of 400 to 800 mg per day is required for treatment over a duration of at least 6 months.[57] However, for nonmeningeal coccidioidomycosis, response rates appear similar with fluconazole and itraconazole treatment at 400 mg per day.[56,57,60,61] A comparative trial evaluating the two azoles for the treatment of coccidioidomycosis is currently underway. Fluconazole is considered the drug of choice for most patients with coccidioidal meningitis, which obviates the need for intrathecal administration of amphotericin B. Fluconazole administered at 400 mg per day orally for up to 4 years resulted in a 79% (37/47) response rate.[54] Most improvement occurred within 4 to 8 months after starting therapy. Only two patients developed confusion during treatment, whereas alopecia was noted in three patients. Similarly, itraconazole treatment at 300 to 400 mg per day for a median of 10 months in eight evaluable patients with meningitis was associated with a favorable response.[55]

Despite these encouraging results with azole therapy for coccidioidal meningitis, a followup study on 18 patients in whom azole therapy had been discontinued because of a presumption of cure indicates that the relapse rate is unacceptably high.[62] Those patients were treated for a median duration of 37 months; 14 of 18 patients relapsed with disseminated disease, resulting in three deaths. Relapses occurred at 2 weeks to 30 months after treatment discontinued. Although the azoles appear to be safer alternatives to intrathecal administration of amphotericin, lifelong suppressive therapy is likely required for meningitis.

Specifically, for histoplasmosis, measurement of antigen levels in blood and urine samples is useful for monitoring treatment response and detection of early relapse.[7] When measured at 3- to 4-month intervals, a relative increase in antigen levels of more than two units compared with previously measured levels suggests recurrence of disease. Reinduction therapy may be instituted to control this recurrence. As for coccidioidomycosis, baseline evaluation of the skin test reactivity and CF antibody titers are recommended for all patients receiving therapy to help determine the duration as well as the response to treatment.[50] Persistently negative skin test reactivity in a patient with disseminated disease is associated with high likelihood of relapse when treatment is discontinued. A decreasing CF antibody titer during the treatment course is predictive of a positive response.

TREATMENT OF OPPORTUNISTIC MYCOSES

Cryptococcosis

Pulmonary disease in normal hosts resolves spontaneously and can be observed without antifungal therapy along with careful followup. The introduction of safe and effective oral agents such as fluconazole has prompted some to advocate therapy for all patients regardless of underlying immune status.[18]

Patients with progressive pulmonary disease, those with accompanying extrapulmonary involvement, and all immunocompromised patients should receive antifungal therapy. Amphotericin B with or without flucytosine is recommended for a total dosage of 1.0 to 1.5 g.[18] The optimal total dosage and duration is unknown; however, therapy should continue until there is clinical and radiographic resolution of disease with eradication of the organisms from sputum cultures or bronchoalveolar lavage. Fluconazole therapy at 200 to 400 mg per day for a duration of 3 to 6 months may be considered for those with mild to moderately severe pulmonary disease.[63]

All patients with cryptococcal meningitis require treatment (Table 78.4). In patients without AIDS, combination therapy of amphotericin B with flucytosine for 6 weeks has been established as the regimen of choice based on two early prospective randomized comparative trials.[64,65] It is notable that the incidence of adverse effects (e.g., bone

Table 78.4. ▪ Antifungal Therapy for Cryptococcal Meningitis

Patient Subgroups	Antifungal Regimen
Non-AIDS	Amphotericin B 0.3 mg/kg/day + 5-flucytosine 150 mg/kg/day in four divided doses × 6 weeks
AIDS	
Induction	Amphotericin B 0.7 mg/kg/day ± 5-flucytosine 100 mg/kg/day in two to three divided doses × 2 weeks, then fluconazole or itraconazole 400 mg/day × 8 weeks[a]
Maintenance (lifelong)	Fluconazole 200 mg every day
Prophylaxis	*Not* recommended routinely

[a]A switch to oral azole therapy after 2 weeks is appropriate only for patients who are clinically stable or who have improved.

marrow suppression and liver enzyme abnormalities) owing to flucytosine 150 mg/kg per day was high; 30 of 194 patients developed leukopenia, 22 of 194 developed thrombocytopenia, and 13 of 194 developed hepatitis.[65] The development of toxic effects was significantly correlated with the presence of flucytosine serum concentrations of greater than or equal to 100 μg/mL for 2 weeks or more. Approximately 50% of the toxic reactions occurred within the first 2 weeks and more than 90% within the first 4 weeks of therapy.

Antifungal therapy in patients with AIDS has been carefully evaluated in several large comparative trials over the past 10 years. Early studies have established the superior efficacy of amphotericin B with or without flucytosine over fluconazole for the acute treatment of cryptococcal meningitis in AIDS.[66,67] Fluconazole alone compared with the combined regimen was associated with higher mortality rates during the first 2 weeks of therapy (15 versus 8%) and a longer period to CSF sterilization (64 versus 42 days).[67] Similarly, more failures and relapses were observed for patients receiving itraconazole compared with combination therapy of amphotericin and flucytosine in another prospective randomized comparative trial.[68] The most recent trial evaluated a two-step treatment strategy consisting of amphotericin at higher dosages (0.7 mg/kg/day) for 2 weeks (step 1) followed by 8 weeks of either itraconazole or fluconazole 400 mg per day (step 2).[69] A total of 381 patients were randomized to receive amphotericin alone or in combination with flucytosine 100 mg/kg per day in step 1. The addition of flucytosine did not significantly improve survival at 2 weeks or shorten the time to negative CSF cultures. For the group receiving amphotericin B alone, mortality at 2 weeks was 6% with negative CSF cultures in 51% of the patients. When compared with regimens employed in previous studies, the short-term use of high dosage amphotericin with or without flucytosine during initial therapy was associated with lower mortality (6 versus 14 to 18%) and higher rates of CSF sterilization (50 versus 20%) at 2 weeks. The overall efficacy (complete resolution of symptoms) for this two-step regimen was 70% at 10 weeks. Of note, the strategy of changing therapy to an azole at 2 weeks cannot be recommended for patients who did not improve or who had clinical deterioration after 2 weeks of high-dose amphotericin therapy because those patients were excluded from enrollment onto step 2 of the study.

Alternative treatment strategies also have been evaluated in a limited number of patients. The combination of fluconazole 400 mg per day with flucytosine 150 mg/kg per day for 10 weeks resulted in negative CSF cultures after a median time of 23 days in 75% of study patients.[70] Based on the shorter time to CSF sterilization, flucytosine appears to enhance the efficacy of fluconazole; however, 30% of patients had dose-limiting adverse reactions to flucytosine requiring discontinuation of the drug. In addition, the safety and efficacy of a lipid formulation of amphotericin B (i.e., Abelcet) also has been compared prospectively with conventional formulation for the treatment of cryptococcal meningitis in patients with AIDS.[71] Comparable treatment success was observed for both formulations despite the use of lipid-formulated amphotericin B at five times the treatment dosage of conventional formulation (42 versus 50%, respectively). However, a higher number of recipients of the lipid formulation had persistent positive CSF cultures at the end of treatment despite symptom resolution. A disproportionate share of negative prognostic factors was present in the Abelcet group, suggesting that perhaps amphotericin B lipid complex may be less effective in that subgroup. In addition, the cost effectiveness of using the lipid formulations of amphotericin for this indication will need to be addressed considering the low rates of nephrotoxicity (4%) when amphotericin was given at high dosage for 2 weeks in the aforementioned trial.[69]

Similar to endemic mycoses, cryptococcosis in patients with AIDS is associated with a 50 to 60% relapse rate after completion of primary therapy.[19] Hence, lifelong maintenance therapy is recommended. Fluconazole has been established as the maintenance treatment of choice by two controlled trials.[72,73] At daily dosages of 200 mg per day, fluconazole therapy resulted in no relapse compared with 15% in placebo patients.[74] When compared to amphotericin B (1 mg/kg per week), recipients of fluconazole 200 mg per day had fewer relapses (2 versus 18%).[73] In addition, when administered at the same daily dosages, itraconazole was less effective than fluconazole as maintenance therapy in preventing relapses.[74]

Routine administration of fluconazole for primary prophylaxis is currently not recommended by the United States Public Health Service/Infectious Disease Society of America owing to the low incidence of disease, lack of survival benefit, concerns for development of both *Candida* and *Cryptococcus* resistance, and cost.[51] Prophylaxis may be administered selectively to those who have CD4 less than 50 cells/μL and may have a need for prophylaxis against other fungal infections.

Aspergillosis

Antifungal therapy for invasive aspergillosis is limited primarily to two agents with useful clinical activity against the organism; they are amphotericin B and itraconazole. However, therapy with either agent is limited by potential drug toxicities and significant drug interactions. Terbinafine, a systemically available oral allylamine recently approved for treating onychomycosis, demonstrates similar in vitro activity against *Aspergillus* compared with amphotericin B and itraconazole. Limited experience derived from compassionate use primarily in immunocompetent patients appears encouraging for the treatment of invasive bronchopulmonary aspergillosis.[75–77] More studies involving larger numbers of patients, particularly those who are immunocompromised, will have to be performed to determine the role of terbinafine in the treatment of invasive aspergillosis.

In general, treatment response for invasive aspergillosis has been disappointing with an overall response rate of 34% for amphotericin B.[78] Results from noncomparative open-label trials with itraconazole suggest similar response rates in immunocompromised patients.[79,80] The response rate and overall mortality vary substantially among different host groups in relation to underlying disease status, site of disease, and disease management. In one review on the therapeutic outcomes of more than 1200 cases of invasive aspergillosis involving the lungs, sinus, and brain in immunocompromised patients, the crude mortality rates (regardless of whether treatment was or was not given) were 86, 66, and 99%, respectively.[78] Among patients who lived long enough to receive at least 14 days of therapy for pulmonary aspergillosis, bone marrow transplant and liver transplant recipients had poorer responses compared with renal and heart transplant recipients (20 to 33% versus 83%). Virtually no patients with cerebral aspergillosis survived despite treatment; however, diagnosis was first made at autopsy for the majority of the patients.[24,78] Various factors other than the host group and site of infection have been suggested to predict poor response to treatment (Table 78.5).[78]

Early diagnosis and prompt initiation of aggressive antifungal therapy are extremely important. Amphotericin B is considered the first line of therapy for invasive aspergillosis in immunocompromised hosts. Itraconazole may be preferable for treating tracheobronchitis owing to its relative safety and effectiveness.[20] In neutropenic patients, rapid escalation (within 2 days) of the daily dosage of amphotericin to 1 mg/kg per day or higher is recommended.[24] Invasive aspergillosis has occurred in patients receiving amphotericin B at 0.5 mg/kg per day during empiric therapy for febrile neutropenia.[78] Of note, no prospective studies have been performed to correlate dosage with outcomes; the recommended dosage is based on the patient's ability to tolerate the drug. The optimal duration for amphotericin B therapy is unknown; cumulative dosages of 1.5 to 4 g or treatment duration of 4 to 6 weeks after complete hematologic recovery usually have

Table 78.5. ▪ Factors Predictive of Poor Response to Antifungal Therapy of Invasive Aspergillosis

Factors
Leukemic relapse
Persistent neutropenia
No reduction in immunosuppression
Diffuse pulmonary disease
Major hemoptysis
Delayed therapy
Low dosages of amphotericin B, especially during neutropenia
Undetectable or low serum itraconazole concentrations
Lack of secondary prophylaxis during another episode of neutropenia
Angioinvasion (histologically evident)

Source: Adapted from Denning DW. Therapeutic outcome in invasive aspergillosis. Clin Infect Dis 23:608–615, 1996. With permission.

been recommended. The median treatment duration in patients who received itraconazole therapy in open-label trials was 4 to 12 months.[79,80] A loading dose of itraconazole 200 mg three times a day for the first 3 days is used to achieve a steady state sooner because of the long half-life of the drug, followed by 200 mg two times a day. Consolidation therapy with itraconazole for prolonged periods may be appropriate for those who have achieved clinical improvement and have recovered from neutropenia. Limited experience suggests that higher dosages of itraconazole (800 mg/day) may have a role in the treatment of cerebral aspergillosis.[81] Serum levels of itraconazole should be obtained to ensure adequate absorption. Patients who failed treatment or developed disease during prophylactic therapy have low or undetectable serum concentrations, suggesting that a minimum effective concentration is required for therapeutic response; however, the optimal target concentration has not been determined.[24]

In the patient who achieved initial response to therapy, secondary prophylaxis may be important to administer to prevent relapse during further episodes of immunosuppression from cancer chemotherapy or bone marrow transplantation, or during treatment of acute allograft rejection.[20,24] Prophylactic administration of amphotericin B (1 mg/kg/day) should commence immediately before or at the same time as cytotoxic chemotherapy begins, and should continue until neutrophil recovery in those with prior documentation of invasive aspergillosis is achieved. Primary prophylaxis in neutropenic patients also has been employed with either low-dose amphotericin B or itraconazole with variable success. A subset of patients who failed to respond to initial treatment with amphotericin B have responded to subsequent treatment with itraconazole or lipid-formulated amphotericin B products (e.g., Abelcet, Amphotec, AmBisome).[42,79,80] Based on available animal and uncontrolled clinical data, at least five times the daily dosages of conventional amphotericin B formulation should be used when a lipid-formulated product is employed for the treatment of aspergillosis. No prospective comparative studies have been performed to address the relative efficacy among different formulations of amphotericin B thus far. It is clear that the lipid formulations of amphotericin B afford less nephrotoxicity than conventional forms, but at a much higher drug-acquisition cost. In addition, preliminary evidence from clinical trials of voriconazole (an investigational Triazole) in the treatment of invasive aspergillosis appears encouraging.[82]

Owing to the poor outcomes associated with existing agents, some have recommended the use of combination therapy with amphotericin B for the empirical treatment of invasive aspergillosis.[24] 5-Flucytosine and rifampin have been shown to be synergistic or additive with amphotericin B in experimental models of aspergillosis. Greater clinical success has been found with the combination of amphotericin B and 5-flucytosine in the treatment of cerebral and pulmonary aspergillosis, perhaps reflecting better tissue penetration with 5-flucytosine.[24] However, 5-flucytosine is not recommended for use in patients in whom serum concentrations cannot be monitored rapidly to maintain serum concentrations less than 100 μg/mL because of the potential of dose-related toxicities.[83] With respect to the addition of rifampin to amphotericin B, more favorable response was not shown for neutropenic patients treated with the combination for pulmonary aspergillosis.[24] In addition, the potent enzyme-inducing properties of rifampin pose significant drug interactions with cyclosporine and corticosteroid therapy in transplant recipients.

Candidiasis

Mucocutaneous Candidiasis

Oral thrush may be treated effectively with local antifungal therapy. In more extensive cases, systemic therapy may be used (Table 78.6). In esophagitis, systemic therapy usually is required because of the need for longer contact time. Among the azoles, fluconazole is proven superior to ketoconazole in patients with AIDS, which is likely owing to the presence of achlorhydria and the fact that absorption of fluconazole is not dependent on an acidic pH medium. In a randomized, double-blind comparative trial, itraconazole oral solution achieved similar clinical response rates as fluconazole (94 versus 91%).[85] Both were given at 100 to 200 mg per day for 3 to 8 weeks to patients infected with HIV. Recently, mucosal candidiasis refractory to fluconazole is an evolving problem in patients with advanced HIV disease.[35] Progressive immunosuppression and frequent exposure to antifungal agents are associated with the development of refractory disease. Some experts define fluconazole treatment failure as persistent or progressive disease after a 2-week course of fluconazole 200 mg daily. Treatment with oral solutions of itraconazole or amphotericin B in fluconazole-refractory patients

Table 78.6. ▪ Antifungal Therapy for Oropharyngeal and Esophageal Candidiasis

Forms of Candidiasis	Antifungal Regimen
Oropharyngeal and Esophageal	*Local therapy*[a]
	Nystatin suspension 100,000 U/mL, 4–6 mL four times a day
	Amphotericin B suspension 100 mg/mL, 5 mL four times a day
	Clotrimazole troches 10 mg four–five times a day
	Systemic therapy
	Ketoconazole 200–400 mg PO four times a day
	Fluconazole 100–200 mg PO four times a day
	Itraconazole 100–200 mg PO four times a day
Fluconazole-refractory disease in AIDS	Fluconazole 400–800 mg PO four times a day or two times a day
	Itraconazole solution 40 mg/mL, 2.5–5 mL PO two times a day
	or
	Amphotericin B 0.5–1.0 mg/kg per day IV four times a day

[a]Systemic therapy for esophageal candidiasis may be used for extensive cases of oropharyngeal disease.

has resulted in response rates of 60 and 44%, respectively.[35] Systemic amphotericin B therapy may be required for patients who do not respond to the above oral therapies or who have severe disease or esophageal involvement. Treatment duration is based on response, but is typically 7 to 10 days for oropharyngeal and at least 21 days for esophageal disease.

A number of topical and systemic antifungal agents are available for treating vulvovaginal candidiasis.[36] The different formulations of topical agents that are available include creams, vaginal tablets, and suppositories; the choice of treatment is a matter of patient preference rather than a difference in efficacy. All of the azole topical agents are highly effective, resulting in cure rates exceeding 80% with no clear difference in clinical efficacy for individual agents.[36] Single-dose oral fluconazole or itraconazole has shown comparable efficacy with multidose conventional topical azole therapy for uncomplicated vulvovaginal candidiasis. However, patients with severe disease respond better to 7-day topical azole therapy than single-dose fluconazole. Similarly, those with a history of recurrent infection (i.e., four or more episodes of proven infection during a 12-month period) are recommended to receive a longer course of therapy, 10 to 14 days rather than 5 to 7 days. More than one dose of fluconazole is noted to achieve clinical and mycologic remission in this subgroup. Topical azole therapy is associated with low incidence of local side effects and may be used in the first trimester of pregnancy.[36] Systemic azole therapy is not currently recommended for use during pregnancy. Single-dose fluconazole is infrequently associated with GI intolerance, headache, and rash.

Candiduria

Removal of an indwelling urinary catheter is essential in the eradication of *Candida* from the urine.[86] Local therapy with amphotericin B 50 mg in 1 L of sterile water as a continuous or intermittent irrigation of the bladder has been successful in greater than 90% of the cases.[37] Fluconazole (50 to 200 mg/day) offers the convenience of oral administration for ambulatory patients.[86,102] Response rates are comparable to amphotericin B bladder irrigation. However, infections owing to *non-albicans Candida* have reportedly persisted or failed fluconazole therapy. Treatment of upper tract infection requires the use of systemic therapy. Surgical intervention to correct the underlying obstructive abnormalities may be necessary to eliminate recurrent *Candida* colonization and subsequent infections of the urinary tract.[37]

Candidemia and Disseminated Candidiasis

Amphotericin B has been the mainstay of antifungal therapy for the treatment of invasive candidiasis. Fluconazole is an attractive alternative in light of the dose-limiting nephrotoxicity of amphotericin B. Until recently, efficacy data on fluconazole for the treatment of invasive candidiasis have largely been open-label and uncontrolled.

Fluconazole was compared to amphotericin B in a large, randomized controlled trial in nonimmunocompromised patients with candidemia.[87] Patients were administered either amphotericin B 0.5 to 0.6 mg/kg per day or fluconazole 400 mg per day intravenously then by mouth for 17 and 18 days, respectively. Treatment success was similar in both groups (79% amphotericin versus 70% fluconazole). Catheter-related candidemia was present in 72% of the patients with *C. albicans* as the predominant pathogen.

In another prospective comparative trial that included neutropenic patients, fluconazole 400 mg per day was compared with amphotericin B (25 to 50 mg/day up to 0.67 mg/kg/day) in the treatment of documented or presumed invasive candidiasis.[88] A total of 142 patients were evaluable; at least half in each group were neutropenic patients (<1000 cells/mm^3). Approximately 40% of the patients were treated for presumed invasive candidiasis; a presumed diagnosis was made only for neutropenic and postoperative patients. Overall response rates were not different between fluconazole- and amphotericin-treated patients (66 versus 64%). As in the previous study, fewer side effects were noted among fluconazole recipients compared with amphotericin B. Currently, combination therapy with fluconazole and amphotericin B for the treatment of invasive candidiasis is being evaluated.

The recent availability of lipid-formulated amphotericin B products has prompted investigation of the comparative efficacy of amphotericin B lipid complex (ABLC, e.g., Abelcet) versus conventional amphotericin B formulation in the treatment of invasive candidiasis.[89] Patients were prospectively randomized to receive either ABLC 5 mg/kg per day or amphotericin 0.6 to 1.0 mg/kg per day. The major underlying disorders were hematologic malignancy and solid tumors; approximately 15% of the patients in both groups were neutropenic at baseline. Candidemia was present in 85% of the patients, with *C. albicans* as the predominant pathogen. Comparable response rates were noted despite much higher dosages used (65% ABLC versus 61% amphotericin B). Nephrotoxicity was significantly less in the ABLC group. Comparative efficacy studies of prospective randomized design have not been performed for the other two commercially available lipid-formulated amphotericin B products (Amphotec, AmBisome) in the treatment of invasive candidiasis.

Based on findings from prospective comparative trials, fluconazole appears to be as efficacious as amphotericin B in the treatment of catheter-related candidemia owing to *C. albicans* in nonneutropenic patients. However, treatment experience of fluconazole in neutropenic hosts with proven invasive candidiasis remains limited. Amphotericin B should be considered a first-line therapy in the treatment of critically ill patients with candidemia or acute disseminated candidiasis in whom the portal of entry is non–catheter related and the causative pathogen is a *non-albicans Candida* species (such as *C. glabrata* or *C. krusei*). Amphotericin B lipid complex should be reserved for those who developed renal insufficiency secondary to conventional formulation. For those with chronic disseminated candidiasis, initial treatment with a brief course of amphotericin B (0.5 to 1.0 mg/kg/day) followed by a prolonged course of fluconazole is recommended.[31] Treatment experience with other invasive forms of candidiasis, such as endophthalmitis, peritonitis, and endocarditis are anecdotal and noncomparative.

IMPROVING OUTCOMES

Prolonged neutropenia is a significant risk factor for the development of invasive fungal infections, notably aspergillosis and candidiasis.[21] Associated mortality is high, whereas the diagnosis of invasive disease remains elusive. Thus, management strategies have included the use of antifungal prophylaxis and empiric therapy in those at high risk for developing invasive disease.[99,100]

Fluconazole prophylaxis at a high dosage (400 mg/day) during prolonged neutropenia following bone marrow transplantation has been shown to decrease the incidence of invasive candidiasis and mortality in a placebo-controlled trial. However, routine fluconazole prophylaxis has resulted in the selection of fluconazole-resistant *Candida* spp. (i.e., *C. krusei* and *C. glabrata*) in some centers and also *Aspergillus* as the cause of superinfections.[90,91] Thus, some advocate the use of fluconazole as prophylaxis only in those patients who are likely to have profound (<100 cells/mm^3) and protracted neutropenia (>10 days), and particularly those colonized with *Candida* or *Aspergillus*.[31]

In a large, prospective randomized trial of empirical treatment of febrile neutropenic patients who failed to respond to broad-spectrum antibacterial therapy, patients who were randomized to receive amphotericin B deoxycholate at 0.6 mg/kg per day developed proven fungal infections at an incidence of 8%.[92] Candidemia and invasive pulmonary aspergillosis accounted for the majority of infections. Although emergent infections were not prevented entirely, empirical therapy with amphotericin B, initiated at 96 hours after persistent fever despite antibacterial therapy, appears to be highly effective in controlling invasive fungal infections in neutropenic hosts.

KEY POINTS

- Advances in medical technology and therapies have attributed to a dramatic increase in the incidence and spectrum of invasive fungal infections over the past two decades.
- Medically important fungi causing systemic fungal infections can be classified as endemic versus opportunistic, with *Coccidioides immitis, Histoplasma capsulatum*, and *Blastomyces dermatitidis* being the major endemic pathogens, whereas *Candida* sp., *Aspergillus* sp., and *Cryptococcus* sp. are opportunistic pathogens causing invasive disease in patients with overt immunosuppression.
- The majority of patients infected with endemic fungal pathogens are asymptomatic or have self-limited acute pulmonary disease that does not require treatment with antifungal agents.
- Itraconazole is considered the drug of choice for histoplasmosis and blastomycosis in nonimmunocompromised patients who do not have life-threatening or meningeal disease, whereas amphotericin is the mainstay of treatment for critically ill patients with overwhelming infection.
- The risk for developing invasive candidiasis and aspergillosis is directly related to the duration and degree of neutropenia.
- Individuals who are the most immunocompromised are the least likely to have symptoms and have a rapidly fatal course with invasive aspergillosis.
- In clinical practice, aggressive empirical therapy for acute invasive aspergillosis is initiated based on a combination of clinical, radiologic, or microbiologic features before a diagnosis is proven definitively.
- *Candida* sp. is now the sixth leading nosocomial pathogen with an apparent shift to an increasing proportion of infections owing to *non-albicans Candida* sp.
- Speciation of *Candida* is important because of the varied pathogenic potential and susceptibility to anti-

fungal agents; *non-albicans Candida* sp. as a group are considered less susceptible than *C. albicans* to the azoles.

- Distinguishing infection versus colonization by the presence of *Candida* sp. in the urine is difficult, particularly in patients with indwelling urinary catheters.
- Disseminated candidiasis should be considered for patients who have persistent, unexplained fever in conjunction with some combination of the following: neutropenia, prolonged duration of intensive care stay (>7 days), prolonged use of multiple antibacterial agents, prolonged use of intravascular catheters, and colonization with *Candida* at one or more body sites.
- Lipid-formulated amphotericin B products clearly are associated with lower incidence of nephrotoxicity in comparison to conventional deoxycholate formulation. However, use of such expensive agents should be reserved for salvage therapy because superior efficacy has not been proven.
- Fluconazole appears to be as efficacious as amphotericin B in the treatment of catheter-related candidemia owing to *C. albicans* in non-neutropenic patients.
- Fluconazole prophylaxis in neutropenic hosts may result in the selection of fluconazole-resistant *Candida* sp. and also *Aspergillus* as the cause of superinfections.
- The emergence of azole-resistant *Candida* sp. is being reported increasingly, particularly among oropharyngeal isolates of *C. albicans* from patients with advanced HIV disease who have received repeated courses of azole treatment for oropharyngeal candidiasis.

REFERENCES

1. Beck-Sague CM, Jarvis WR. Secular trends in the epidemiology of nosocomial fungal infections in the U.S. 1980–1990. J Infect Dis 167:1247–1251, 1993.
2. Anaissie EJ. Opportunistic mycoses in the immunocompromised hosts: experience at a cancer center and review. Clin Infect Dis 14(1 Suppl):43–53, 1993.
3. Pfaller MA, Wenzel R. The impact of changing epidemiology of fungal infections in the 1990s. Eur J Clin Microbiol Infect Dis 11:287–291, 1992.
4. Wheat J. Endemic mycoses in AIDS: a clinical review. Clin Microbiol Rev 8:146–159, 1995.
5. Rinaldi MG. Problems in the diagnosis of invasive fungal disease. Rev Infect Dis 13:493–495, 1991.
6. Deepe GS Jr. Histoplasma capsulatum: darling of the river valleys. ASM News 63:599–604, 1997.
7. Wheat LJ. Diagnosis and management of histoplasmosis. Eur J Clin Microbiol Infect Dis 8:480–490, 1989.
8. Davies SF, Sarosi GA. Epidemiological and clinical features of pulmonary blastomycosis. Sem Respir Infect 12:206–218, 1997.
9. Pappas PG. Blastomycosis in the immunocompromised patients. Sem Respir Infect 12:243–251, 1997.
10. Bradsher RW. Therapy of blastomycosis. Sem Respir Infect 12:263–267, 1997.
11. Barbee RA. Coccidioidomycosis: now a national problem. J Respir Dis 14:785–796, 1993.
12. Einstein HE, Johnson RH. Coccidioidomycosis: new aspects of epidemiology and therapy. Clin Infect Dis 16:349–356, 1993.
13. Schneider E, Hajjeh RA, Spiegel RA, et al. A coccidioidomycosis outbreak following the Northridge, Calif, earthquake. JAMA 277:904–908, 1997.
14. Stevens DA. Coccidioidomycosis. N Engl J Med 332:1077–1082, 1995.
15. Denning DW. Invasive aspergillosis. Clin Infect Dis 26:781–805, 1998.
16. Aberg JA, Powderly WG. Cryptococcosis. Adv Pharmacol 37:215–251, 1997.
17. Peachey PR, Gubbins PO, Martin RE. The association between cryptococcal variety and immunocompetent and immunocompromised hosts. Pharmacotherapy 18:255–264, 1998.
18. Zeind CS, Cleveland KO, Menon M, et al. Cryptococcal meningitis in patients with acquired immunodeficiency syndrome. Pharmacotherapy 16: 547–561, 1996.
19. Dismukes WE. Management of cryptococcosis. Clin Infect Dis 17(Suppl 2):S507–S512, 1993.
20. Powderly WG. Cryptococcal meningitis and AIDS. Clin Infect Dis 17:837–842, 1993.
21. Warnock DW. Fungal complications of transplantation: diagnosis, treatment and prevention. J Antimicrob Chemother 36(Suppl B):73–90, 1995.
22. Gerson SL, Talbot GH, Hurwitz S, et al. Prolonged granulocytopenia: the major risk factor for invasive pulmonary aspergillosis in patients with acute leukemia. Ann Intern Med 100:345–351, 1984.
23. Tomee JF, Mannes GP, van der Bij W, et al. Serodiagnosis and monitoring of aspergillus infections after lung transplantation. Ann Intern Med 125:197–201, 1996.
24. Denning DW, Stevens DA. Antifungal and surgical treatment of invasive aspergillosis: review of 2,121 published cases. Rev Infect Dis 12:1147–1201, 1990.
25. Edwards JE Jr. Candida species. In: Mandell GL, Douglas RG, Bennett JE, eds. Principles and practice of infectious diseases. 4th ed. New York: Churchill Livingstone, 1995:2289.
26. Banerjee SN, Emori TG, Culver DH, et al. Secular trends in nosocomial primary bloodstream infections in the United States, 1980–1989. Am J Med 91(Suppl 3B):S86–S89, 1991.
27. Emori TG, Gaynes RP. An overview of nosocomial infections, including the role of the microbiology laboratory. Clin Microbiol Rev 6:428–442, 1993.
28. Wey SB, Mori M, Pfaller MA, et al. Hospital-acquired candidemia: the attributable mortality and excess length of stay. Arch Intern Med 148:2642–2645, 1988.
29. Odds FC. Pathogenesis of candidosis. In: *Candida* and candidosis. A review and bibliography. 2nd ed. London: Bailliere Tindall, 1988:236–278.
30. Taschdjian CL, Burchall JJ, Kozinn PJ. Rapid identification of *Candida albicans* by filamentation on serum and serum substitutes. Am J Dis Child 99:212–215, 1960.
31. Rodriguez LJ, Rex JH, Anaissie EJ. Update on invasive candidiasis. Adv Pharmacol 37:349–400, 1997.
32. Wenzel RP. Nosocomial candidemia: risk factors and attributable mortality. Clin Infect Dis 20:1531–1534, 1995.
33. Pfaller MA. Nosocomial candidiasis: emerging species, reservoirs, and modes of transmission. Clin Infect Dis 22(Suppl 2):S89–S94, 1996.
34. Rex JH, Pfaller MA, Barry AL, et al. Antifungal susceptibility testing of isolates from a random multicenter trial of fluconazole versus amphotericin B as treatment of nonneutropenic patients with candidemia. Antimicrob Agents Chemother 39:40–44, 1995.
35. Fichtenbaum CJ, Powderly WG. Refractory mucosal candidiasis in patients with human immunodeficiency virus infection. Clin Infect Dis 26:556–565, 1998.
36. Sobel JD, Faro S, Force RW, et al. Vulvovaginal candidiasis: epidemiologic, diagnostic, and therapeutic considerations. Am J Obstet Gynecol 178:203–211, 1998.
37. Wong-Beringer A. Treatment of funguria. JAMA 267:2780–2785, 1992.
38. Gallis HA, Drew RH, Pickard WW. Amphotericin B: 30 years of clinical experience. Rev Infect Dis 12:308–329, 1990.
39. Nagata MP, Gentry CA, Hampton EM. Is there a therapeutic or pharmacokinetic rationale for amphotericin B dosing in systemic *Candida* infections? Ann Pharmacother 30:811–818, 1996.
40. Drutz DJ, Spickard A, Rogers DE, et al. Treatment of disseminated mycotic infections: a new approach to amphotericin B therapy. Am J Med 45:405–418, 1968.
41. Gardner ML, Godley PJ, Wasan SM. Sodium loading treatment for amphotericin B-induced nephrotoxicity. Ann Pharmacother 24:940–946, 1990.
42. Wong-Beringer A, Jacobs RA, Guglielmo BJ. Lipid formulations of amphotericin B: clinical efficacy and toxicities. Clin Infect Dis 27:608–618, 1998.
43. Como JA, Dismukes WE. Oral azole drugs as systemic antifungal therapy. N Engl J Med 330:263–272, 1994.
44. Kauffman CA, Carver PL. Antifungal agents in the 1990s: current status and future developments. Drugs 53:539–549, 1997.
45. Denning DW, Baily GG, Hood SV. Azole resistance in Candida. Eur J Clin Microbiol Infect Dis 16:261–280, 1997.

46. White TC, Marr KA, Bowden RA. Clinical, cellular, and molecular factors that contribute to antifungal drug resistance. Clin Microbiol Rev 11:382–402, 1998.
47. Francis P, Walsh TJ. Evolving role of flucytosine in immunocompromised patients: new insights into safety, pharmacokinetics, and antifungal therapy. Clin Infect Dis 15:1003–1018, 1992.
48. Kurtz MB. New antifungal drug targets: a vision for the future. ASM News 64:31–39, 1998.
49. Ampel NM, Wieden MA, Galgiani JN. Coccidioidomycosis: clinical update. Rev Infect Dis 11:897–911, 1989.
50. Drutz DJ. Amphotericin B in the treatment of coccidioidomycosis. Drugs 26:337–346, 1983.
51. CDC. USPHS/IDSA guidelines for the prevention of opportunistic infections in persons infected with human immunodeficiency virus. MMWR 48(No. RR-10):1–59, 1999.
52. Wheat J, Hafner R, Korzun AH, et al. Itraconazole treatment of disseminated histoplasmosis in patients with the acquired immunodeficiency syndrome. Am J Med 98:336–342, 1995.
53. Kauffman CA. Role of azoles in antifungal therapy. Clin Infect Dis 22(Suppl 2):S148–S153, 1996.
54. Galgiani JN, Catanzaro A, Cloud GA, et al. Fluconazole therapy for coccidioidal meningitis. Ann Intern Med 119:28–35, 1993.
55. Tucker RM, Denning DW, Dupont B, et al. Itraconazole therapy for chronic coccidioidal meningitis. Ann Intern Med 112:108–112, 1990.
56. Dismukes WE, Bradsher RW Jr, Cloud GC, et al. Itraconazole therapy for blastomycosis and histoplasmosis. Am J Med 93:489–497, 1992.
57. Wheat J, MaWhinney S, Hafner R, et al. Treatment of histoplasmosis with fluconazole in patients with acquired immunodeficiency syndrome. Am J Med 103:223–232, 1997.
58. Hecht FM, Wheat J, Korzun AH, et al. Itraconazole maintenance therapy for histoplasmosis in AIDS: a prospective, multicenter trial. J AIDS Hum Retrovirol 16:100–107, 1997.
59. Wheat LJ, Connolly-Stringfield PA, Baker RL, et al. Disseminated histoplasmosis in the acquired immunodeficiency syndrome: clinical findings, diagnosis and treatment, and review of the literature. Medicine 69:361–373, 1990.
60. Graybill JR, Stevens DA, Galgiani JN, et al. Itraconazole treatment of coccidioidomycosis. Am J Med 89:282–290, 1990.
61. Catanzaro A, Fierer J, Friedman PJ. Fluconazole in the treatment of persistent coccidioidomycosis. Chest 97:666–669, 1990.
62. Dewsnup DH, Galgiani JN, Graybill JR., et al. Is it ever safe to stop azole therapy for *Coccidioides immitis* meningitis? Ann Intern Med 124:305–310, 1996.
63. Yamaguchi H, Ikemoto H, Watanabe K, et al. Fluconazole monotherapy for cryptococcosis in non-AIDS patients. Eur J Clin Microbiol Infect Dis 15:787–792, 1996.
64. Bennett JE, Dismukes WE, Duma RJ, et al. A comparison of amphotericin B alone and combined with flucytosine in the treatment of cryptococcal meningitis. N Engl J Med 301:126–131, 1979.
65. Dismukes WE, Cloud G, Gallis HA, et al. Treatment of cryptococcal meningitis with combination amphotericin B and flucytosine for four as compared with six weeks. N Engl J Med 317:334–341, 1987.
66. Larsen RA, Leal MAE, Chan LS. Fluconazole compared to amphotericin B plus flucytosine for cryptococcal meningitis in AIDS. Ann Intern Med 113:183–187, 1990.
67. Saag MS, Powderly WG, Cloud GA, et al. Comparison of amphotericin B and fluconazole in the treatment of acute AIDS-associated cryptococcal meningitis. N Engl J Med 326:83–89, 1992.
68. DeGans J, Portegeis P, Tiessens G, et al. Itraconazole compared with amphotericin B plus flucytosine in AIDS patients with cryptococcal meningitis. AIDS 6:185–190, 1992.
69. Van der Horst CM, Saag MS, Cloud GA, et al. Treatment of cryptococcal meningitis associated with the acquired immunodeficiency syndrome. N Engl J Med 337:15–21, 1997.
70. Larsen RA, Bozzette SA, Jones BE, et al. Fluconazole combined with flucytosine for treatment of cryptococcal meningitis in patients with AIDS. Clin Infect Dis 19:741–745, 1994.
71. Sharkey PK, Graybill JR, Johnson ES, et al. Amphotericin B lipid complex compared with amphotericin B in the treatment of cryptococcal meningitis in patients with AIDS. Clin Infect Dis 22:315–321, 1996.
72. Bozzette SA, Larsen RA, Chiu J, et al. A placebo-controlled trial of maintenance therapy with fluconazole after treatment of cryptococcal meningitis in the acquired immunodeficiency syndrome. N Engl J Med 324:580–584, 1991.
73. Powderly WG, Saag MS, Cloud GA, et al. A controlled trial of fluconazole or amphotericin B to prevent relapse of cryptococcal meningitis in patients with the acquired immunodeficiency syndrome. N Engl J Med 326:793–798, 1992.
74. Saag MS, Cloud GC, Graybill JR, et al. Comparison of fluconazole versus itraconazole as maintenance therapy of AIDS-associated cryptococcal meningitis. [Abstr No. I218]. In: Program and Abstracts of the 35th Interscience Conference on Antimicrobial Agents and Chemotherapy. San Francisco: American Society for Microbiology, 1995:244.
75. Schiraldi GF, Colombo MD, Harari S, et al. Terbinafine in the treatment of non-immunocompromised compassionate cases of bronchopulmonary aspergillosis. Mycoses 39:5–12, 1996.
76. Schiraldi GF, Cicero SL, Colombo MD, et al. Refractory pulmonary aspergillosis: compassionate trial with terbinafine. Br J Dermatol 134(Suppl 46):25–29, 39–40, 1996.
77. Harari S, Schiraldi GF, De Juli E, et al. Relapsing aspergillus bronchitis in a double lung transplant patient, successfully treated with a new oral antimycotic agent. Chest 111:835–836, 1997.
78. Denning DW. Therapeutic outcome in invasive aspergillosis. Clin Infect Dis 23:608–615, 1996.
79. Denning DW, Lee JY, Hostetler JS, et al. NIAID Mycoses Study Group multicenter trial of oral itraconazole therapy for invasive aspergillosis. Am J Med 97:135–144, 1994.
80. Stevens DA, Lee JY. Analysis of compassionate use itraconazole therapy for invasive aspergillosis by the NIAID Mycoses Study Group Criteria. Arch Intern Med 157:1857–1862, 1997.
81. Sanchez C, Mauri E, Dalmau D, et al. Treatment of cerebral aspergillosis with itraconazole: do high doses improve the prognosis? Clin Infect Dis 21:1485–1487, 1995.
82. Schwartz S, Milatovic D, Thiel E. Successful treatment of cerebral aspergillosis with a novel Triazole (voriconazole) in a patient with acute leukemia. Br J Haematol 97:663–665, 1997.
83. Summers KK, Hardin TC, Gore SJ, et al. Therapeutic monitoring of systemic antifungal therapy. J Antimicrob Chemother 40:753–764, 1997.
84. Laine L, Dretler RH, Conteas C, et al. Fluconazole compared with ketoconazole for the treatment of Candida esophagitis in AIDS: a randomized trial. Ann Intern Med 117:655–660, 1992.
85. Wilcox CM, Darouiche RO, Laine L, et al. A randomized, double-blind comparison of itraconazole oral solution and fluconazole tablets in the treatment of esophageal candidiasis. J Infect Dis 176:227–232, 1997.
86. Fisher JF, Newman CL, Sobel JD. Yeast in the urine: solutions for a budding problem. Clin Infect Dis 20:183–189, 1995.
87. Rex JH, Bennett JE, Sugar AM, et al. A randomized trial comparing fluconazole with amphotericin B for the treatment of candidemia in patients without neutropenia. N Engl J Med 331:1325–1330, 1994.
88. Anaissie EJ, Darouiche RO, Abi-Said D, et al. Management of invasive candidal infections: results of a prospective, randomized, multicenter study of fluconazole versus amphotericin B and review of the literature. Clin Infect Dis 23:964–972, 1996.
89. Anaissie EJ, White MH, Uzun O, et al. Amphotericin B lipid complex vs amphotericin B for treatment of invasive candidiasis: a prospective, randomized multicenter trial [abstract no. LM21]. In: Program and Abstracts of the 35th Interscience Conference on Antimicrobial Agents and Chemotherapy. San Francisco: American Society for Microbiology, 1995:330.
90. Wingard JR, Merz WG, Rinaldi MG, et al. Increase in Candida krusei infection among patients with bone marrow transplantation and neutropenia treated prophylactically with fluconazole. N Engl J Med 325:1274–1277, 1991.
91. Wingard JR, Merz WG, Rinaldi MG, et al. Association of Torulopsis glabrata infections with fluconazole prophylaxis in neutropenic bone marrow transplant patients. Antimicrob Agents Chemother 37:1847–1849, 1993.
92. Walsh TJ, Finberg RW, Arndt C, et al. Liposomal amphotericin B for empirical therapy in patients with persistent fever and neutropenia. National Institute of Allergy and Infectious Diseases Mycoses Study Group. N Eng J Med 340:764–771, 1999.
93. Pfaller MA, Rex JH, Rinaldi MG. Antifungal susceptibility testing: technical advances and potential clinical applications. Clin Infect Dis 24:776–784, 1997.
94. Rex JH, Pfaller MA, Galgiani JN, et al. Development of interpretive breakpoints for antifungal susceptibility testing: conceptual framework and analysis of in vitro-in vivo correlation data for fluconazole, itraconazole, and candida infections. Clin Infect Dis 24:235–247, 1997.
95. Rex JH, Pfaller MA, Barry AL, et al. Antifungal susceptibility testing of isolates from a randomized multicenter trial of fluconazole versus amphotericin B as treatment of nonneutropenic patients with candidemia. Antimicrob Agents Chemother 39:40–44, 1995.
96. Gillum JG, Israel DS, Polk RE. Pharmacokinetic drug interactions with antimicrobial agents. Clin Pharmacokinet 25:450–482, 1993.

97. Aweeka FT. Drug reference table. In: Handbook of drug therapy in liver and kidney disease. 1st ed. Boston: Little, Brown, 1991:291–322.
98. Terbinafine, Itraconazole. In: The use of antibiotics: a clinical review of antibacterial, antifungal and antiviral drugs. 5th ed. Oxford: Butterworth-Heinemann, 1997:1327, 1418.
99. Lortholary O, Dupont B. Antifungal prophylaxis during neutropenia and immunodeficiency. Clin Microbiol Rev 10:477–504, 1997.
100. Gubbins PO, Bowman JL, Penzak SR. Antifungal prophylaxis to prevent invasive mycoses among bone marrow transplantation recipients. Pharmacotherapy 18:549–564, 1998.
101. Ghannoum MA, Rice LB. Antifungal agents: mode of action, mechanisms of resistance, and correlation of these mechanisms with bacterial resistance. Clin Microbiol Rev 12:501–517, 1999.
102. Sobel JD, Kauffman CA, McKinsey D, et al. Candiduria: a randomized, double-blind study of treatment with fluconazole and placebo. Clin Infect Dis 30:19–24, 2000.

CHAPTER 79

PARASITIC INFECTIONS

R. Chris Rathbun

Parasitic diseases are a major cause of morbidity and mortality worldwide. Parasitism involves a relationship in which an animal host is injured as a result of close and prolonged contact by an infecting organism.[1] Knowledge of the parasite life cycle is critical to understanding the pathogenesis, treatment, and prevention of infection. The incidence of parasitic infections overall is increasing in the United States secondary to recent immigration trends, increased foreign travel to endemic areas, and immunosuppression secondary to HIV infection.

This chapter covers the major parasitic infections such as protozoal infections (e.g., malaria, cryptosporidiosis, giardiasis), helminthic infections (e.g., ascariasis, enterobiasis), and ectoparasites (e.g., lice, scabies). Special emphasis is placed on diseases that occur in the United States or represent a significant threat to international travelers. Parasitic infections such as American trypanosomiasis (Chagas' disease) caused by *Trypanosoma cruzi*, leishmaniasis, and amebiasis (*Entamoeba histolytica*) are not included. The reader is referred to recent reviews on these topics.[2–4]

TREATMENT GOALS: PARASITIC INFECTIONS

- Eliminate disease manifestations and prevent complications.
- Prevent the acquisition and spread of infection to other individuals.
- Use chemoprophylaxis to prevent clinical manifestations of malaria; eliminate parasitemia and hepatic reservoirs and prevent vascular complications secondary to *Plasmodium falciparum* infection.
- Alleviate diarrheal symptoms and reduce stool passage of infective spores in patients with intestinal protozoa (e.g., *cryptosporidia, Giardia*).
- Decrease or eliminate worm infestation and reduce passage of infective forms (e.g., eggs, larvae, cercariae) into the environment for patients with helminthic infections.
- Eliminate infestation and prevent spread to other individuals for patients with lice or scabies.

Protozoan Diseases

Malaria

EPIDEMIOLOGY

Plasmodium species responsible for human malaria include *P. falciparum*, *P. vivax*, *P. malariae*, and *P. ovale*. Each year, malaria afflicts approximately 500 million people and causes 2.7 million deaths worldwide.[5] Plasmodium species are spread by *Anopheles* mosquitoes, which are endemic in tropical areas such as sub-Saharan Africa, Asia, Central and South America, and portions of Turkey, Greece, and the Middle East. Other mechanisms of transmission include blood transfusions, needle sharing, and parturition. At the start of the twentieth century more than 500,000 cases of malaria occurred annually in the United States; approximately 1000 cases are now reported each year.[6,7]

PATHOPHYSIOLOGY

Infection is acquired from the female *Anopheles* mosquito when saliva containing sporozoites is injected during a blood meal. Sporozoites spread hematogenously to the liver, resulting in development of exoerythrocytic forms (tissue schizonts, hypnozoites) within hepatocytes. Merozoites are released from tissue schizonts into the circulation approximately 1 to 2 weeks later, leading to invasion of erythrocytes. *P. falciparum* merozoites proliferate within erythrocytes of all ages, whereas other malarial species are restricted to certain subpopulations. Within erythrocytes, merozoites consume hemoglobin and mature to ring, trophozoite, and schizont stage parasites or to sexual male and female gametocyte forms by asexual replication. Rupture of schizont-infected red cells occurs after 48 hours (72 hours with *P. malariae*), releasing merozoites that perpetuate erythrocytic invasion. Ingestion of gametocyte-infected red blood cells by *Anopheles* mosquitoes leads to fertilization of male and female forms within the mosquito gut and development of sporozoites that migrate to the mosquito's salivary glands, completing the infectious cycle. Relapse of disease does not occur with *P. falciparum* or *P. malariae* infection; however, *P. ovale* and *P. vivax* hypnozoites can become activated weeks to months following resolution of initial infection.[7]

CLINICAL PRESENTATION AND DIAGNOSIS

Signs and Symptoms

The presentation of malaria is typically nonspecific and includes fever, malaise, headache, rigors, and diaphoresis in more than 80% of patients. Symptom onset commonly occurs approximately 2 weeks after exposure. Anorexia, nausea, and vomiting occur in approximately 33% of patients and diarrhea, cough, and abdominal pain occur in approximately 16%. Tachypnea, tachycardia, hypotension, and altered consciousness also may occur. Splenomegaly (~25%) and hepatomegaly (~20%) can develop as the disease progresses. Cycling of fever every 48 to 72 hours (tertian or quartan pattern) because of synchronized schizont rupture may occur, especially with prolonged, untreated illness.[6,7]

Falciparum malaria can rapidly become life threatening because of adherence of parasitized cells to vascular endothelium, producing microvascular disease secondary to flow obstruction. Acute renal failure, symmetrical encephalopathy (i.e., cerebral malaria) manifesting as seizures and coma, and pulmonary edema may occur. Severe anemia secondary to hemolysis and decreased hematopoiesis along with thrombocytopenia and hypoglycemia are common. Hyperbilirubinemia due to hemolysis also may be prominent.[8] Parasitemia greater than 5% with concomitant end-organ disease or shock in nonimmune individuals is associated with a poor prognosis.[9]

Diagnosis

Microscopic evaluation of Giemsa-stained blood smears, ideally obtained at 12- to 24-hour intervals over 36 to 72 hours, is used most frequently for diagnosis.[7] Thick smears are used to optimize parasite detection. Thin smears viewed under oil immersion magnification are used to examine characteristic species morphology. Alternatively, diagnosis can be made by using a finger prick test strip containing monoclonal antibody to *Plasmodium* histidine-rich protein 2 (ParaSight-F test), buffy coat examination with acridine dye staining, DNA hybridization, or DNA or mRNA amplification by polymerase chain reaction (PCR).[6,8] Antibody testing for most species also is available from the Centers for Disease Control and Prevention (CDC), but the clinical value of these tests has not yet been fully defined.

TREATMENT

Pharmacotherapy

Uncomplicated *P. vivax*, *P. malariae*, *P. ovale*, and chloroquine-sensitive *P. falciparum* infections should be treated with chloroquine (Tables 79.1 and 79.2). Chloroquine dosage may be described as amounts of chloroquine phosphate or amounts of chloroquine base; careful note should be taken because the dosage varies significantly between the two. Dosage for children is often weight-based; however, doses for children should not exceed routine adult doses, which are composed of a loading dose of oral chloroquine base 600 mg (or chloroquine phosphate 1000 mg, or 10 mg/kg of chloroquine base for children) followed by chloroquine base 300 mg (5 mg

Table 79.1 ▪ Malaria Chemoprophylaxis[a]

Drug	Adult Dose	Pediatric Dose (per weight or age)	Side Effects	Comments
Chloroquine PO_4 (250 mg, 500 mg tablet)	500 mg (salt) PO once/ week beginning 1–2 wk before departure and continuing for 4 wk after leaving malarious area	8.3 mg/kg (salt) (maximum 500 mg)	Freguent: pruritus, nausea, headache Occasional: photophobia, reversible corneal opacities, partial alopecia Rare: nerve deafness, blood dyscrasia nail/ mucous membrane discoloration, retinopathy, myopathy, psychosis	▪ Take with food ▪ Safe for use in pregnancy ▪ May exacerbate psoriasis ▪ Children: tablets can be pulverized and placed in gelatin capsules
Hydroxychloroquine sulfate (200 mg tablet)	400 mg (salt) PO once/ week beginning 1–2 wk before departure and continuing for 4 wk after leaving malarious area	6.5 mg/kg (salt) (maximum 400 mg)	(Same as Chloroquine)	▪ Alternative to chloroquine ▪ Take with food ▪ Safe for use in pregnancy ▪ May exacerbate psoriasis
Mefloquine (250 mg tablet)	250 mg (salt) PO once/wk beginning at least 2 wk before departure and continuing for 4 wk after leaving malarious area	15–19 kg: ¼ tablet/wk 20–30 kg: ½ tablet/wk 31–45 kg: ¾ tablet/wk >45 kg: adult dose	Common: nausea, diarrhea, headache, dizziness, strange dreams, insomnia Rare: seizures, psychosis	▪ Pregnancy category C ▪ Contraindications: history of psychosis, epilepsy, cardiac conduction abnormalities
Doxycycline (100 mg tablet, capsule)	100 mg PO once daily beginning 1–2 days before departure and continuing for 4 wk after leaving malarious area	>8 yr: 2 mg/kg/day (maximum 100 mg)	Frequent: GI upset, photosensitivity, vaginal candidiasis Occasional: azotemia in renal disease Rare: allergic reactions blood dyscrasias	▪ Not for use in pregnancy
Primaquine (15 mg base tablet)	30 mg (base) PO once daily beginning 1 day before departure and continuing for 1 wk after leaving malarious area	0.5 mg/kg (base) (maximum 30 mg)	Frequent: hemolytic anemia (G6PD[b] deficiency) Occasional: abdominal pain, nausea, vomiting, methemoglobinemia Rare: leukopenia	▪ Alternative to doxycycline ▪ Not for use in pregnancy ▪ Rule out G6PD deficiency
Proguanil[c] (100 mg tablet)	200 mg PO once daily beginning 1 day before departure and continuing in combination with weekly chloroquine	<2 yr: 50 mg/day 2–6 yr: 100 mg/day 7–10 yr: 150 mg/day >10 yr: 200 mg/day	Frequent: anorexia, nausea, mouth ulcers Rare: hematuria	▪ Safe for use in pregnancy ▪ Less effective than mefloquine or doxycycline in chloroquine-resistant area

[a]Adapted with permission from Kain KC, Keystone JS. Malaria in travelers: epidemiology, disease, and prevention. Infect Dis Clin North Am 12:267–284, 1998; and Wyler DJ. Malaria: overview and update. Clin Infect Dis 16:449–458, 1993.

[b]*G6PD,* glucose-6-phosphate dehydrogenase.

[c]Not available in the United States.

base/kg) at 6, 24, and 48 hours.[9] A nonstandard regimen compressing dosage to 36 hours has also been described.[10] Pruritus is a common adverse effect in individuals with dark skin.

Hydroxychloroquine sulfate may be substituted using the necessary conversion (200 mg hydroxychloroquine sulfate salt = 155 mg chloroquine base) if chloroquine phosphate (250 mg salt = 156 mg base) is not available. A single oral dose of the combination product pyrimethamine-sulfadoxine (three tablets in adults or 1 mg pyrimethamine-20 mg sulfadoxine/kg in children) may be used by travelers for self-treatment. Defervescence and resolution of symptoms and parasitemia should occur within 72 hours of treatment initiation. To prevent infection relapses, patients with *P. vivax* and *P. ovale* infection living in nonendemic areas should also receive a 2-week course of primaquine base 15 mg daily for adults (0.25 mg base/kg/day for children) to eradicate hepatic hypnozoites.[9]

Patients with mild glucose-6-phosphate dehydrogenase (G6PD) deficiency, defined as 10 to 60% residual enzyme activity, should alternatively receive primaquine 45 mg once weekly (0.8 mg base/kg/week for children) for 8 weeks to minimize development of hemolytic anemia. Primaquine should not be used in patients with severe

Table 79.2 ▪ Pharmacokinetics of Antimalarials

Drug	Absorption	Protein Binding	$t_{1/2}$[a]	Distribution	Metabolism/Excretion
Chloroquine	89%	61%	41 d[a]	Eye, liver, spleen, kidneys, RBCs[a]	Hepatic; active desethyl metab.;[a] >50% renal
Mefloquine	High[b]	99%	20 d	RBCs	Hepatic; biliary
Doxycycline	>90%	90%	15–25 hr	Breast milk	30% feces; 40% renal
Quinine	>90%	80%	8–21 hr	Breast milk	Hepatic
Quinidine (IV)[a]	NA[a]	80%	6–13 hr	Breast milk	Hepatic; <25% renal
Primaquine	>90%	—[c]	4–10 hr	—[c]	Hepatic

[a]$t_{1/2}$, half-life; d, day; RBCs, red blood cells, metab., metabolite(s); IV, intravenous; NA, not applicable.
[b]Reports of >85% absorption represent relative difference between liquid and tablet formulations.
[c]Information not available.

G6PD deficiency (<10% residual enzyme activity) or in patients who are pregnant.[11]

Patients with suspected chloroquine-resistant falciparum malaria should receive oral quinine sulfate 650 mg every 8 hours (25 to 30 mg/kg/day for children) in conjunction with doxycycline 100 mg daily (2 to 3 mg/kg/day for children) or tetracycline 250 mg four times daily (20 mg/kg/day in divided doses for children) for 7 days.[9] Risk versus benefits assessment should be made when considering tetracyclines for children. Cinchonism (e.g., tinnitus, nausea, headache, blurred vision) and electrocardiogram (ECG) changes (i.e., QTc interval prolongation) can occur with quinine. For women who are pregnant or children younger than 8 years old, single-dose pyrimethamine-sulfadoxine should be used in place of a tetracycline. Clindamycin is also given with quinine, but is less preferred in this context because of resistance concerns and toxicity.[12] Single-dose mefloquine 15 mg base/kg followed by a second 10 mg base/kg dose 8 to 24 hours later in nonimmune patients is also effective for drug-resistant falciparum malaria; however, neurologic toxicities make it a less desirable first-line therapy.[9,12]

Patients (both children and adults) with severe malaria should be treated with intravenous quinidine gluconate. A loading dose of 10 mg base/kg (maximum 600 mg) in 250 mL of normal saline infused over 1 to 2 hours should be given, followed by a continuous infusion at 0.02 mg/kg per minute, until oral therapy can be started. If parenteral therapy is needed for more than 48 hours, then serum drug concentrations should be monitored and dose reduction may be necessary. Quinidine serum concentrations should be maintained between 3 and 7 mg/L and the dosage should be decreased if the QTc interval becomes prolonged by more than 25% from its baseline value.[9] Therapy can be continued with quinine sulfate to complete a 3-day course for chloroquine-resistant falciparum malaria and a 7-day course for multidrug-resistant falciparum malaria in combination with 7 days of a tetracycline.[12]

Chemoprophylaxis is indicated in all nonimmune individuals traveling to malarious areas where mosquito exposure is likely. Mefloquine is the drug of choice when traveling to chloroquine-resistant areas, especially for *P. falciparum*. In areas where mefloquine resistance is high or therapy is contraindicated, doxycycline should be used.[13,14] Daily doses of azithromycin 250 mg can be used in place of doxycycline for women who are pregnant and children younger than 8 years old; however, azithromycin is less effective.[15] Primaquine is an effective alternative to doxycycline for prevention of both falciparum and vivax malaria, but it is associated with significant gastrointestinal side effects.[16] Chloroquine is the drug of choice in geographic areas with low resistance. A summary of dosage guidelines and side effects for individual prophylactic agents is listed in Table 79.1.

Nonpharmacologic Therapy

Exchange transfusions are indicated in nonimmune patients with severe falciparum malaria where parasitemia exceeds 15%; they also should be considered in patients with 5 to 10% parasitemia or in those with altered mental status or renal or pulmonary complications.[9,17] Hemodialysis or peritoneal dialysis may be necessary in patients who develop renal failure.

FUTURE THERAPIES

Artemisinin and its derivatives, artesunate and artemether, are rapid-acting antimalarials that have been used widely in China for treatment of drug-resistant falciparum malaria.[18,19] These compounds are highly effective; however, pharmacokinetic studies are needed before approval can be considered in the United States. Malarial proteases are central to invasion of erythrocytes and subsequent release of merozoites. Synthetic peptide inhibitors of plasmodial cysteine and aspartic proteases are in the early stages of development.[20] Efforts to develop an effective malaria vaccine have been disappointing; however, preliminary results of a recombinant circumsporozoite protein vaccine are promising.[21] Atovaquone-proguanil (Malarone) has demonstrated effectiveness for prophylaxis and treatment of malaria and is expected to be licensed in the United States soon.[12,22]

Cryptosporidiosis, Isosporiasis, Microsporidiosis, and Cyclosporiasis

EPIDEMIOLOGY

The intestinal spore-forming protozoa include cryptosporidia, Isospora, microsporidia, and Cyclospora. Principal species infecting humans include *Cryptosporidium parvum*, *Isospora belli*, *Cyclospora cayetanensis*, and the microsporidia species *Enterocytozoon bieneusi* and *Encephalitozoon intestinalis* (formerly *Septata intestinalis*). Fecal–oral spread is the predominant route of transmission; however, ingestion of fecally contaminated water or food also has led to widespread community outbreaks.[23,24] In Milwaukee, an estimated 403,000 people developed symptomatic cryptosporidia infection in 1993 secondary to contamination of the municipal water supply.[25] Infection is more common in developing countries where sanitation is poor; however, predilection for serious, symptomatic infection in immunocompromised patients (AIDS, organ-transplant) has become apparent.[23,26]

PATHOPHYSIOLOGY

The life cycles of cryptosporidia, Isospora, microsporidia, and Cyclospora are similar in that infection occurs by ingestion of spores. Sporozoites are released from ingested spores by contact with bile salts and pancreatic enzymes. Invasion of intestinal epithelium in the small bowel follows, resulting in marked distortion of the villus architecture in some patients. Malabsorption of vitamin B_{12}, D-xylose, and fat may occur with more severe infection. Schizogony (asexual reproduction) leads to the formation of merozoites that reinfect the host's intestinal lining and perpetuate infection. Other merozoites develop into sexual forms, resulting in formation of oocysts (spores). Oocysts are excreted in the stool or may sporulate and release their sporozoites within the host, causing autoinfection.[23] *Encephalitozoon* spp. also infect macrophages, leading to secondary infections in the kidney, liver, brain, and sinuses.[26] Infection with *Isospora belli*, *Cyclospora cayetanensis*, and microsporidia species is limited to humans; however, *Cryptosporidium parvum* causes disease in both humans and animals.[23]

CLINICAL PRESENTATION AND DIAGNOSIS

Signs and Symptoms

Diarrhea, with or without abdominal cramping, is the primary clinical manifestation and may occasionally be accompanied by nausea, vomiting, and fever. Symptoms typically occur 7 to 10 days following ingestion of oocysts. Disease severity varies considerably among patients; stool frequency may be intermittent versus continuous, watery, and high volume (12 to 17 L/day). Immunocompetent patients typically have acute, self-limiting disease lasting 3 to 25 days; although, disease can last for months to years in some patients. Immunocompromised patients (e.g., those with AIDS, cancer, or IgA deficiency) are prone to chronic, life-threatening diarrhea, malabsorption, and dehydration. Biliary tract invasion has been described with cryptosporidia, microsporidia, and Isospora in patients with AIDS. Hepatitis, nephritis, peritonitis, pneumonia, keratoconjunctivitis, and encephalitis with seizures may develop with disseminated *Encephalitozoon intestinalis* infection.[23,26]

Diagnosis

Diagnosis is routinely established on the basis of stool smears for cysts. Oocyst size and shape are used to differentiate among organisms. Modified, acid-fast stains are effective for detecting cryptosporidia, Isospora, and Cyclospora. Sensitivity can be improved by stool-concentrating techniques or by using a cryptosporidial immunofluorescent stain. Microsporidia are best visualized in body fluids using a modified trichrome or fluorochrome stain; however, small bowel biopsy tends to be more sensitive for intestinal disease. Absence of fecal leukocytes and erythrocytes differentiates infection from other intestinal pathogens. Centrifugation enhances detection of microsporidia in respiratory secretions and urine.[23]

TREATMENT

Pharmacotherapy

Palliative therapy with antidiarrheal agents (e.g., bismuth subsalicylate, loperamide, kaolin and pectin, diphenoxylate) can be used to provide temporary relief of symptoms.[27] Infection with Cyclospora in immunocompetent patients should be treated with 160 mg of trimethoprim and 800 mg of sulfamethoxazole (one double-strength [DS] tablet) twice a day for 7 days.[28] For patients with Isospora, one DS tablet four times a day for 10 days followed by one DS tablet twice a day for 3 weeks should be used.[29] Patients with HIV infection should receive one DS tablet four times a day for 10 days for Cyclospora and Isospora; chronic suppressive therapy with one DS tablet three times a week is routinely necessary because relapses are common.[29,30] Pyrimethamine 50 to 75 mg with folinic acid 10 mg per day can be used to treat Isospora in persons infected with HIV with sulfonamide allergy, followed by pyrimethamine 25 mg and folinic acid 5 mg per day indefinitely.[31]

No uniformly effective therapy has been identified for patients with chronic cryptosporidial infection.[27] Paromomycin 500 mg three to four times a day for 2 to 4 weeks is effective in decreasing stool frequency in approximately 66% of patients and may reduce or eliminate oocyst shedding; however, it does not prevent biliary tract invasion in patients infected with HIV.[32] Relapse is common following discontinuation of therapy, necessitating suppressive therapy with 500 mg twice a day. Variable success has been observed with the macrolide antibiotics, spiramycin, azithromycin, and roxithromycin. Spiramycin 3 to 4 g per day in divided doses is associated with severe gastrointestinal irritation and showed no benefit in a placebo-controlled trial.[33] Roxithromycin 300 mg twice a day has produced clinical and parasitologic improvement in uncontrolled, open-label studies.[34,35] Azithromycin 900 mg per day demonstrated improvement in oocyst shedding and clinical endpoints (e.g., decreased stool frequency and weight loss) in a double-blind, placebo-controlled trial.[33] Azithromycin serum concentrations correlated with treatment response, suggesting that dosages greater than 900 mg per day may be necessary. A small, open-label trial evaluating combination therapy with paromomycin (1 g bid) and azithromycin (600 mg/day) for 4 weeks followed by paromomycin alone for 8 weeks has produced the best clinical results to date; however, it was not placebo-controlled.[36] A pilot study evaluating letrazuril, a congener of diclazuril, in patients infected with HIV with confirmed cryptosporidiosis demonstrated clinical improvement and eradication of oocyst shedding at dosages of 150 to 200 mg per day.[37] Double-blind, placebo-controlled trials with letrazuril are needed. Octreotide, a synthetic somatostatin analog, has been used (100 to 500 μg subcutaneously every 8 hours) to reduce diarrheal symptoms; however, it does not eliminate cyst passage in the stool and is an expensive alternative to traditional antidiarrheal therapies.[27,33]

Biological immunomodifiers may serve as promising alternatives to current treatment approaches. Hyperimmune bovine colostrum (HBC), given orally and by duodenal or biliary tract infusion, can produce dramatic symptomatic improvement but does not consistently eradicate oocyst shedding. Oral bovine transfer factor (BTF), a lymph node extract obtained from calves inoculated with cryptosporidia, produces similar results. Utility of these therapeutic methods is currently limited by routine availability, potency standardization, and lack of comparative studies.[27,33]

For *Encephalitozoon intestinalis*, albendazole 400 mg orally twice a day for 2 to 4 weeks produces clinical improvement and eradicates intestinal spore shedding.[38] Chronic suppressive therapy with 400 mg twice a day may be necessary to prevent relapse in patients infected with HIV. Albendazole displays in vivo activity against other microsporidia species, with the exception of *Enterocytozoon bieneusi*, for which no effective treatment currently exists. Fumagillin, an antibiotic produced by *Aspergillus fumigatus*, has been used topically for keratoconjunctivitis secondary to *Encephalitozoon* spp.[39] Fumagillin 20 mg three times a day by mouth for 2 to 3 weeks is effective for treating *Enterocytozoon bieneusi*-induced diarrhea in patients with AIDS, but is associated with thrombocytopenia.[40] Thalidomide has been associated with symptomatic relief of microsporidia infection in patients with AIDS but requires further study.[41]

Primary prophylaxis to prevent symptomatic infection with spore-forming protozoa is not currently recommended in patients infected with HIV; however, prophylaxis for *Mycobacterium avium* complex with either clarithromycin 500 mg twice a day or rifabutin 300 mg a day is associated with a lower incidence of symptomatic cryptosporidiosis.[42] In addition, initiation of antiretroviral therapy for HIV infection has been associated with symptom resolution, parasitologic cure, and disease prevention, presumably resulting from improvement in cell-mediated immunity.[26,33,43]

Nonpharmacologic Therapy

Fluid and electrolyte replacement is the mainstay of therapy in patients with severe dehydration.[27] Diets consisting of medium-chain triglycerides may help decrease the severity of diarrhea.[44] Parenteral nutrition may be necessary in patients with prolonged malabsorption. Cholecystectomy or sphincterotomy and stent placement may be necessary in patients with biliary tract disease.[32]

FUTURE THERAPIES

More than 100 known compounds have been screened for anticryptosporidial activity with limited success to date.[45] TNP-470 (AGM-1470) is an investigational semisynthetic fumagillin analog with in vivo activity against microsporidia that appears to be less toxic than fumagillin. TNP-470 is currently being evaluated in phase II studies for Kaposi's sarcoma and may also prove to be useful in treating microsporidia.[46]

Giardiasis

EPIDEMIOLOGY

Giardia lamblia (also known as *G. duodenalis* or *G. intestinalis*) is a flagellated, intestinal protozoan that is a common cause of diarrheal illness worldwide. Numerous waterborne outbreaks have been documented in mountainous regions throughout the United States. Infection occurs through ingestion of fecally contaminated food or water or by fecal–oral contact.[47]

PATHOPHYSIOLOGY

Exposure of ingested cysts to gastric acid and pancreatic enzymes releases pear-shaped trophozoites that colonize and replicate in the small bowel. Trophozoites attach to the intestine by means of an adhesive disk. Encystation by trophozoites follows within the ileum.[48] Disruption of the brush border membrane may occur; however, mucosal invasion is rare.

Table 79.3 ▪ Pharmacokinetics of Antiprotozoals

Drug	Absorption	Protein Binding	$t_{1/2}$[b]	Distribution	Metabolism/Excretion
Metronidazole	99%	11%	8.5 hr	CSF 16–100%, breast milk[b]	30–60% hepatic; 20–40% renal
Furazolidone	Poor	—[a]	—[a]	—[a]	33% renal
Paromomycin	Poor	N/A[b]	N/A	N/A	Feces

[a]Information not available.
[b]$t_{1/2}$, half-life; CSF, cerebrospinal fluid; N/A, not applicable.

CLINICAL PRESENTATION AND DIAGNOSIS

Signs and Symptoms

Acute, self-limiting diarrhea lasting 1 to 3 weeks occurs in 25 to 50% of infected patients. Symptoms begin 1 to 2 weeks following ingestion of cysts. Stools are typically greasy and foul-smelling but may be watery and profuse at symptom onset. Significant weight loss (≥10 lb) occurs in more than half of all patients. Malaise, nausea, abdominal cramping, bloating, and flatulence are also common. Gastric infection may develop in patients with achlorhydria. A subset of patients develop chronic diarrhea associated with protein, D-xylose, and vitamins A and B_{12} malabsorption. Steatorrhea also may be observed. Lactose intolerance lasting several weeks is commonly observed following resolution of infection. Children are frequently more symptomatic than adults.[45,47,48]

Diagnosis

Examination of fresh, iodine-stained stool or preserved (10% buffered formalin), trichrome or iron hematoxylin-stained stool for cysts is routinely used. Sensitivity approaches 90% with three stool samples. Occasionally, motile trophozoites can be visualized in feces by saline wet mount. Fecal leukocytes typically are absent. In difficult cases, proximal jejunal biopsy by endoscopy may be necessary. Small bowel biopsy may appear normal or reveal spruelike lesions.[47] Alternatively, the Enterotest (HDC Corporation) can be used, in which a gelatin capsule containing a nylon string is anchored in the mouth, ingested, and allowed to pass into the jejunum. After 4 to 6 hours, the string is removed and examined for presence of trophozoites within the adsorbed mucus.[47] Immunofluorescence (IFA) and enzyme-linked immunosorbent assays (ELISA) to detect stool antigen also are available and are 85 to 98% sensitive and 90 to 100% specific.[45]

TREATMENT

Oral metronidazole (Table 79.3) 250 mg three times a day for 5 to 7 days in adults or 5 mg/kg three times a day for 7 days in children is the treatment of choice for *Giardia* and is 80 to 95% effective.[28,47] Side effects include metallic taste, nausea, dizziness, headache, and a disulfiram reaction when taken with alcohol or alcohol-containing foods or drugs (i.e., elixirs). Reversible neutropenia may occur rarely. Furazolidone 100 mg four times a day for 7 to 10 days also has been used in adults and 2 mg/kg four times a day for 10 days in children (>1 month), but is less effective. However, a convenient oral suspension (50 mg/15 mL) is available for children. Side effects include nausea, vomiting, brown discoloration of the urine, and mild hemolysis in G6PD-deficient patients.[47] Albendazole 400 mg per day for 5 days or bacitracin 120,000 U (USP) for 10 days is also reportedly effective.[28] Treatment is typically deferred during pregnancy; however, if disease severity warrants, paromomycin 25 to 30 mg/kg per day in three divided doses for 5 to 10 days during the first trimester or metronidazole during the second or third trimester carries a low teratogenic risk.[28,47]

Helminthic Diseases

EPIDEMIOLOGY

Helminthic parasites consist of the nematodes (roundworms; e.g., *Ascaris*, *Enterobius*, *Trichuris*), trematodes (flukeworms; e.g., *Schistosoma*), and cestodes (tapeworms; e.g., *Taenia*). More than 25% of the world's population is infected with helminthic parasites. In the United States, *Enterobius* affects approximately 50 million people, *Ascaris* affects 4 million, and *Trichuris* affects 2.2 million people. Approximately 400,000 immigrants from endemic areas are infected with *Schistosoma* in the United States. Fecal–oral spread is the predominant means of transmission for intestinal nematodes and cestode larvae. Infection with adult cestodes (e.g., *Taenia*) and tissue nematodes (e.g., *Trichinella*) is acquired by eating raw or undercooked meat.[49] Trematode infection (e.g., *Schistosoma*) occurs by contact with fresh water inhabited by larval forms.

PATHOPHYSIOLOGY

Given the complex life cycle of helminths, most adult worms do not multiply within humans. Therefore, infestation with multiple worms is the result of separate infection events. Exceptions to this are seen when the organism life cycle is completed within the human host (e.g., *Strongyloides*) or when infection occurs during the organism's larval stage (e.g., larva migrans, cysticercosis, hydatidosis).[50]

Roundworm infection occurs through ingestion of parasite eggs (*Enterobius*, *Trichuris*, *Ascaris*) or from external skin penetration by larvae (hookworm, *Strongyloides*). Adult worms of *Trichuris* and *Enterobius* mature in the large intestine and cecum, respectively, from larvae released from ingested eggs. *Ascaris* larvae burrow through the small intestine and spread hematogenously to the lungs, where they penetrate the alveolar space, migrate up the trachea, are swallowed, and mature to adult worms within the small intestine. After skin penetration, hookworm and *Strongyloides* larvae reach the small intestine in a similar manner.[51]

Beef, pork, or fish tapeworm (*Taenia saginata*, *T. solium*, *Diphyllobothrium latum*) infection occurs from ingestion of cyst-infected tissue when excystation in the gut leads to development of a mature tapeworm in the intestine. Gravid proglottids are released into the intestinal lumen, depositing numerous eggs in the feces. Incidental ingestion of eggs by animal hosts or humans leads to larval tissue invasion and cyst formation (e.g., cysticercus [*T. solium*], hydatid cyst [*Echinococcus*]).[52]

Schistosoma infection occurs from fresh water exposure when cercariae penetrate the skin and migrate to the lungs and liver where they mature to adult worms. Adult worms ultimately descend to the urinary bladder or portal venous system and release eggs into the urine or feces. Miracidia hatch from eggs in fresh water and infect the species-specific snail host, leading to cercariae formation.[53]

CLINICAL PRESENTATION AND DIAGNOSIS

Signs and Symptoms

Disease severity is related to the intensity of infection within the affected tissue. Asymptomatic infection is common with low organism burdens. In patients who are symptomatic, nocturnal anal pruritus is characteristic of enterobiasis. Diarrhea, weight loss, and protein and iron malabsorption occur with hookworm. Heavy infection with *Trichuris* can result in bloody diarrhea, mild anemia, growth retardation, or rectal prolapse.[51] Abdominal cramping, vomiting, and diarrhea caused by intestinal or biliary obstruction can occur with heavy *Ascaris* or *T. saginata* infections.[51,52] Migration of hookworm, *Ascaris*, and *Strongyloides* larvae can cause pulmonary infiltration and eosinophilia ("Löeffler-like" syndrome), and localized skin erythema, rash, and pruritus at the site of larval skin entry. Strongyloidiasis in immunocompromised individuals can be life threatening because of larval dissemination throughout the body ("hyperinfection syndrome"), resulting in secondary Gram-negative sepsis.[51] Acute *Schistosoma* infection can cause a serum sickness-like illness (Katayama fever) owing to intravascular egg deposition. Long-term infection can result in species-specific, chronic granuloma formation in venules of the portal, genitourinary, and pulmonary systems, leading to obstructive manifestations such as portal hypertension.[53] Seizures, hydrocephalus, coma, and death can result from cysticerci in the brain (neurocysticercosis).[53,54]

Diagnosis

Definitive diagnosis is commonly made by microscopic examination of fecal specimens collected over several days for eggs or intact proglottids. Stool concentration techniques can increase the sensitivity of *Schistosoma* egg and *Strongyloides* larvae detection. Transparent adhesive tape applied to the perianal region in the morning is useful for detecting adult female pinworms (*Enterobius*). The Enterotest can be used to detect *Strongyloides* larvae in duodenal fluid. Computed tomography and magnetic resonance imaging are used to detect neurocysticerci and hydatid cysts. Eosinophilia is more commonly observed with ascariasis, hookworm, strongyloidiasis, and occasionally taeniasis. Serologic tests are of limited utility because of lack of standardization.[51–54]

TREATMENT

Treatment of helminthic infection is indicated in all patients, regardless of the degree of symptoms. Mebendazole 100 mg twice a day for 3 days or a single 500-mg dose (for mass treatment programs of both children and adults) is used for trichuriasis, ascariasis, and hookworm (Table 79.4). Expulsion of worms through the nose and mouth can occur with heavy *Ascaris* infections. Patients should be advised to drink fruit juices to minimize worm adherence to mucous membranes. A single dose of mebendazole (100 mg) or pyrantel pamoate (11 mg/kg [maximum 1 g]) repeated several times at 1- to 2-week intervals is typically necessary to cure *Enterobius*.[28,55] Asymptomatic close family members should be treated concurrently to minimize reinfection. Albendazole 400 mg a day for 3 days is 80% curative for trichuriasis.[55] A single 400-mg dose is as effective as mebendazole for ascariasis, is more effective against hookworm, and is better tolerated.[56] Alternatively, pyrantel pamoate 11 mg/kg as a single daily dose for 1 or 3 days can be used to treat *Ascaris* or hookworm, respectively.[28]

Single-dose ivermectin 150 to 200 mcg/kg in one dose for 1 to 2 days is the treatment of choice for uncomplicated strongyloidiasis (cure rate 83 to 100%).[28,57] Thiabendazole 25 mg/kg/dose given twice daily (maximum 3 g per day) for 2 days also can be used; however, gastrointestinal and central nervous system side effects are common.[55] Albendazole in dosages ranging from 400 to 800 mg per day for 3 days is less effective (cure rate 38 to 95%) but better tolerated than thiabendazole, making it an attractive alternative.[55] Thiabendazole remains the preferred agent

Table 79.4 ▪ Pharmacokinetics of Anthelmintics

Drug	Absorption	Protein Binding	$t_{1/2}$[a]	Distribution	Metabolism/Excretion
Albendazole	5–10%	70%	8–12 hr (metab.)[a]	CSF 25–50%[a]	Hepatic; active sulfoxide metabolite
Mebendazole	2–10%	95%	3–9 hr	—[b]	Feces; hepatic
Thiabendazole	>90%	—[b]	—[b]	—[b]	Hepatic; renal (metab.)
Pyrantel pamoate	Poor	—[b]	—[b]	—[b]	50% feces; <15% renal
Praziquantel	>80%	80%	0.8–1.5 hr	CSF 25%, breast milk	Hepatic; renal (metab.)
Ivermectin	—[b]	93%	27 hr	Liver, adipose	Hepatic; feces (metab.)

[a] $t_{1/2}$, half-life; CSF, cerebrospinal fluid; metab., metabolite(s).
[b] Information not available.

for disseminated strongyloidiasis; experience with ivermectin is currently limited.[50]

Praziquantel is highly effective for most tapeworm and flukeworm infections and is the drug of choice for schistosomiasis.[55] Single-dose therapy (5 to 10 mg/kg) for adults and children is effective for *Taenia saginata*, *Taenia solium*, and *Diphyllobothrium latum*. Flukeworm infections are treated with 25 mg/kg per dose given two or three times a day for 1 to 2 days. For schistosomiasis, 20 mg/kg two to three times a day for 1 day is used.[50] For treatment of neurocysticercosis, praziquantel 15 to 20 mg/kg per dose given three times a day for 15 days or albendazole 400 mg (or 7.5 mg/kg/dose for children) twice a day for 8 to 30 days is recommended.[28] Corticosteroid and antiepileptic drugs are frequently administered to reduce adverse reactions from cyst rupture. However, it has been reported that these drug combinations can cause significant drug interactions with praziquantel resulting in a decrease in its serum concentrations. These decreases may require serum drug concentration monitoring or empiric dose increases.[54] Albendazole is considered preferable for neurocysticercosis in cases where drug therapy is deemed necessary (for adults >60 kg administer 400 mg bid with meals; for <60 kg administer 15 mg/kg/day divided into two doses/day).[28,54,55] Duration of therapy may be as long as 1 month.

Side effects are uncommon with mebendazole and albendazole and include abdominal pain, nausea, vomiting, headache, dizziness, and rare allergic reactions. Liver function abnormalities, alopecia, and leukopenia can occur with prolonged therapy at high dosages. Both agents should be avoided during the first trimester of pregnancy and can be dosed the same in adults and children when treating intestinal nematodes. Albendazole's serum concentrations can be increased fivefold when taken with a fatty meal. Mebendazole and albendazole come in 100-mg and 200-mg chewable tablets, respectively. Tablets may be chewed, crushed and mixed with food, or swallowed whole.[55] Pyrantel pamoate is available over the counter in 180-mg capsules, 50-mg/mL and 144-mg/mL oral solutions, and a 50-mg/mL oral suspension. Side effects are mild owing to poor absorption and include nausea, vomiting, anorexia, and diarrhea. Praziquantel comes in 600-mg triscored tablets. Adverse effects are mild and include headache, dizziness, malaise, nausea, vomiting, and abdominal pain.[55] Ivermectin comes in 6-mg tablets and is associated with pruritus, dizziness, fever, edema, and postural hypotension.[55] Coadministration of cimetidine with mebendazole, albendazole, or praziquantel leads to higher serum concentrations and greater efficacy for extraintestinal helminth infections.[55]

Ectoparasites

EPIDEMIOLOGY

Lice infestation (pediculosis) is caused by *Pediculus humanus* var. *corporis* (human louse), var. *capitis* (head louse), and *Phthirus pubis* (pubic or crab louse). Head lice outbreaks are common among school age children. Human scabies is highly infectious and is caused by the itch mite, *Sarcoptes scabiei* var. *hominis*. Institutional outbreaks can occur in hospitals and nursing homes. Norwegian (crusted) scabies is a severe variant of scabies that typically occurs in immunocompromised or institutionalized individuals. Lice and scabies mites are distributed worldwide.[58,59]

PATHOPHYSIOLOGY

Adult female lice lay fertilized eggs (nits) on hair shafts or clothing fibers. Nymphs emerge 7 to 10 days later and proceed to obtain a blood meal. Saliva from lice nymphs, injected during the meal causes a localized hypersensitivity reaction within the skin. Adult female scabies mites lay two to three eggs daily for 4 to 6 weeks within narrow burrows in the stratum corneum layer of the epithelium. Larvae emerge in approximately 3 days. Localized hypersensitivity develops to dead mites, eggs, larvae, and their excrement. Infestation is generally limited to five to ten mites in immunocompetent hosts versus more than 10,000 in individuals with Norwegian scabies.[58,60]

CLINICAL PRESENTATION AND DIAGNOSIS

Pruritic, erythematous lesions are characteristic of lice infestation. Head lice are typically localized within the temporal and occipital areas but can involve the entire scalp. Body lice reside predominantly in the seams of clothing and produce small macules and papules on the trunk. Crab lice are found on pubic, axillary, or truncal hair, or eyelashes, and cause pruritus of affected areas and distinctive small bluish lesions (maculae ceruleae). Adult lice are difficult to see; however, nits are readily visible on hair shafts.[58] Scabies is characterized by intensely pruritic, erythematous papules. Classic linear burrows may be visible within interdigital web spaces or on wrists and ankles. Norwegian scabies produces generalized, crusted nodules and plaques, frequently involving the nails. Wet mount evaluation of skin scrapings can reveal the presence of organisms, eggs, or fecal pellets.[59] Secondary bacterial infections may develop with either pediculosis or scabies.

TREATMENT

Topical permethrin (1 to 5%) is the treatment of choice for lice and scabies.[28] Head and crab lice are treated with 1% permethrin. After shampooing and towel drying, the hair and scalp are saturated with permethrin 1%, wrapped in a towel for 10 minutes, and then rinsed thoroughly. Nits can be removed by applying a solution of equal parts vinegar and water to the hair and using a fine-toothed comb dipped in vinegar. One application is 97 to 99% effective but should be repeated after 1 week if lice and nits remain. For crab lice, permethrin 1% should be applied to affected areas in a similar fashion, except the eyelids where a thin layer of petrolatum should be placed. Sexual contacts should be treated concurrently. Body lice can be eliminated by laundering clothing in hot water and ironing seams.[58] Permethrin 5% cream is the preferred treatment for scabies. One application is massaged into the entire skin surface (except the face) and washed off after 8 to 14 hours. Household and sexual contacts should be treated at the same time. For Norwegian scabies, permethrin should be applied following a 10-minute lukewarm bath, applied again in 12 hours, and rinsed off after 12 more hours. Treatment should be repeated in 1 week. Clothing and bed linens should be cleaned in hot, soapy water and dried in the dryer's hot cycle.[59] Lindane 1% is also effective against lice and scabies but is associated with severe side effects (e.g., aplastic anemia, seizures) owing to systemic absorption and is less effective than permethrin. In addition, lindane-resistant lice and scabies have been reported.[61] Side effects associated with permethrin include pruritus, mild burning or stinging, tingling, numbness, and rash. Permethrin is contraindicated in patients with known hypersensitivity to chrysanthemums, pyrethrins, or pyrethrinoids. Other alternatives to permethrin include topical pyrethrins and piperonyl butoxide or single-dose oral ivermectin (200 mcg/kg). Systemic antihistamines and antibiotics are used to relieve pruritus and treat secondary bacterial infections.[28,62]

Psychosocial Aspects, Outcomes, and Pharmacoeconomics of Parasitic Infections

PSYCHOSOCIAL ASPECTS

Cultural beliefs regarding acquisition of parasitic infections influence the use of preventive strategies and appropriate therapy in developing countries. Herbal remedies and spiritualists are commonly used in endemic malarial areas.[63] Travelers' misconceptions about disease risk and severity can produce complacency about using chemoprophylaxis and seeking medical attention.[64] The common misconception that head lice infestation is related to poor personal hygiene can lead to poor self-image in affected children. Institutionalized individuals may refuse presumptive therapy during scabies outbreaks because of denial.

IMPROVING OUTCOMES

Patient Education

The most effective means of managing parasitic infections is disease prevention. Travelers in developing countries or wilderness areas can avoid infection by treating water with iodine, boiling for 1 minute, or drinking canned or bottled beverages. Chloride water treatment alone is ineffective against *G. lamblia* and *C. parvum*. Microfilters with pore sizes less than or equal to 2 μm also can be used to filter water for small volume use; however, the reliability of this method remains to be critically evaluated. When traveling in endemic malarial areas, preventive measures such as wearing pants and long-sleeved shirts, applying insect repellent containing DEET (N,N diethylmethyltoluamide), spraying aerosolized pyrethrins in living and sleeping areas, and sleeping in properly screened or enclosed areas should be used to minimize mosquito exposure. Travelers can obtain updated information from the CDC Web site (http://www.cdc.gov), from CDC's annual pamphlet entitled "Health Information for International Travel" (publication number CDC 95-8280), or from their local health department.[65]

Disease Management Strategies to Improve Patient Outcomes

Patient adherence is critical to maintaining the activity of antimalarial therapies and in preventing disease onset. Chemoprophylaxis regimens should be started before departure to endemic malarial areas so that side effects can be managed effectively, and therapeutic drug concentrations are achieved within the individual. Travelers should be informed of the importance of adhering to chemoprophylaxis regimens throughout their stay and to take precautionary measures to avoid mosquito exposure. Given the magnitude of helminthic infection worldwide, the World Health Organization has recommended that community-wide treatment be performed in endemic areas to prevent ongoing dissemination of infection. Improvement in growth and academic performance has been observed in treated children.[55] Simultaneous administration of anthelmintics also has been advocated to treat coinfection with multiple organisms.[55]

PHARMACOECONOMICS

Chemoprophylaxis is a cost-effective approach to decreasing the morbidity and mortality associated with malaria; however, in areas where attack rates are low, presumptive therapy may be preferred when the incidence of adverse effects with chemoprophylaxis exceeds the incidence of disease.[64] When chemoprophylaxis is indicated, once-weekly agents (mefloquine, chloroquine) are preferable to those administered daily (doxycycline). Annual mass treatment programs for geohelminths and schistosomiasis have been demonstrated to be cost effective in developing countries by decreasing disease manifestations and transmission. Despite its lower effectiveness for strongyloidiasis, albendazole is more cost effective than thiabendazole for mass treatment programs owing to better tolerance and improved patient adherence.[55] Similarly, mebendazole is less effective than albendazole for hookworm; however, generic mebendazole is significantly lower in cost, making it attractive for mass treatment programs targeting mixed helminthic infections.[56]

KEY POINTS

- The goals of antiparasitic therapy are to treat disease symptoms, eradicate responsible pathogens, minimize complications, and reduce disease transmission.
- Malaria is caused by *Plasmodium* spp. transmitted by *Anopheles* mosquito vectors.
- Selection of appropriate chemoprophylaxis, minimizing mosquito exposure, and patient adherence are critical to malaria prevention.
- Falciparum malaria can rapidly become life threatening; therefore, prompt institution of appropriate antiprotozoal therapy and supportive treatment is necessary.
- Poor sanitation and fecal–oral spread can lead to infection with intestinal protozoans (e.g., cryptosporidia, microsporidia, Isospora, Cyclospora, Giardia) and intestinal helminths.
- Asymptomatic infection or mild symptoms are common with intestinal protozoans and low-density helminthic infection.
- Individuals with HIV infection are more prone to developing chronic diarrhea and extraintestinal infection with intestinal protozoans.
- Intestinal infection with *Giardia lamblia* ranges from asymptomatic cyst passage to acute, self-limited diarrhea to chronic, severe diarrhea associated with significant weight loss, malabsorption, and lactose intolerance.
- Effective treatments for Cyclospora, Isospora, and microsporidia are available; however, no reliable therapy exists for chronic cryptosporidia infection.
- Treatment strategies for helminthic infections are directed at decreasing symptomatology, reducing worm burdens, and preventing spread of infection.
- Benzimidazoles and pyrantel pamoate are preferred agents for intestinal roundworms, whereas praziquantel is used for tapeworms, flukeworms, and schistosomes.
- Metronidazole is the drug of choice for *Giardia*; however, furazolidone is frequently used in children due to ease of administration and mild side effects.
- Lice and scabies infestations are characterized by development of pruritic, erythematous skin lesions secondary to localized skin hypersensitivity.
- Topical permethrin (1–5%) is the treatment of choice for lice and scabies.

REFERENCES

1. Markell EK, Voge M, John DT, eds. Medical parasitology. 7th ed. Philadelphia: Saunders, 1992:6.
2. Kirchhoff LV. American trypanosomiasis (Chagas' disease)–a tropical disease now in the United States. N Engl J Med 329:639–644, 1993.
3. Berman JD. Human leishmaniasis: clinical, diagnostic, and chemotherapeutic developments in the last 10 years. Clin Infect Dis 24:684–703, 1997.
4. Ravdin JI, Petri Jr WA. *Entamoeba histolytica* (amebiasis). In: Mandell GL, Douglas Jr RG, Bennett JE, eds. Principles and practice of infectious diseases. 4th ed. New York: Churchill Livingstone, 1995:2395–2408.
5. Nussenzweig RS, Zavala F. A malaria vaccine based on a sporozoite antigen (editorial). N Engl J Med 336:128–129, 1997.
6. Kain KC, Keystone JS. Malaria in travelers: epidemiology, disease, and prevention. Infect Dis Clin North Am 12:267–284, 1998.
7. Wyler DJ. Malaria: overview and update. Clin Infect Dis 16:449–458, 1993.
8. Krogstad KJ. Plasmodium species (malaria). In: Mandell GL, Douglas Jr RG, Bennett JE, eds. Principles and practice of infectious diseases. 4th ed. New York: Churchill Livingstone, 1995:2419, 2421, 2425.

9. White NJ. The treatment of malaria. N Engl J Med 335:800–806, 1996.
10. Pussard E, Leppers JP, Clavier F, et al. Efficacy of a loading dose of oral chloroquine in a 36-hour treatment schedule for uncomplicated *Plasmodium falciparum* malaria. Antimicrob Agents Chemother 35:406–409, 1991.
11. Lee LH, Caserta MT. Malaria: update on treatment. Pediatr Infect Dis J 17:342–343, 1998.
12. Barat LM, Bloland PB. Drug resistance among malaria and other parasites. Infect Dis Clin North Am 11:969–987, 1997.
13. Ohrt C, Richie TL, Widjaja H, et al. Mefloquine compared with doxycycline for the prophylaxis of malaria in Indonesian soldiers. A randomized, double-blind, placebo-controlled trial. Ann Intern Med 126:963–972, 1997.
14. Wolfe MS. Protection of travelers. Clin Infect Dis 25:177–184, 1997.
15. Andersen SL, Oloo AJ, Gordon DM, et al. Successful double-blinded, randomized, placebo-controlled field trial of azithromycin and doxycycline as prophylaxis for malaria in western Kenya. Clin Infect Dis 26:146–150, 1998.
16. Soto J, Toledo J, Rodriquez M, et al. Primaquine prophylaxis against malaria in nonimmune Colombian soldiers: efficacy and toxicity. A randomized, double-blind, placebo-controlled trial. Ann Intern Med 129:241–244, 1998.
17. Panosian CB. Editorial Response: exchange blood transfusion in severe falciparum malaria–the debate goes on. Clin Infect Dis 26:853–854, 1998.
18. Boele van Hensbrock M, Onyiorah E, Jaffar S, et al. A trial of artemether or quinine in children with cerebral malaria. N Engl J Med 335:69–75, 1996.
19. Hien TT, Day NPJ, Phu NH, et al. A controlled trial of artemether or quinine in Vietnamese adults with severe falciparum malaria. N Engl J Med 335:76–83, 1996.
20. Rosenthal PJ. Proteases of malaria parasites: new targets for chemotherapy. Emerg Infect Dis 4:49–57, 1998.
21. Stoute JA, Slaoui M, Heppner G, et al. A preliminary evaluation of a recombinant circumsporozoite protein vaccine against *Plasmodium falciparum* malaria. N Engl J Med 336:86–91, 1997.
22. Looareesuwan S, Viravan C, Webster HK, et al. Clinical studies of atovaquone, alone or in combination with other antimalarial drugs, for treatment of acute uncomplicated malaria in Thailand. Am J Trop Med Hyg 54:62–66, 1996.
23. Goodgame RW. Understanding intestinal spore-forming protozoa: cryptosporidia, microsporidia, Isospora, Cyclospora. Ann Intern Med 124:429–441, 1996.
24. Guerrant RL. Cryptosporidiosis: an emerging, highly infectious threat. Emerg Infect Dis 3:51–57, 1997.
25. MacKenzie WR, Hoxie NJ, Proctor ME, et al. A massive outbreak in Milwaukee of cryptosporidium infection transmitted through the public water supply. N Engl J Med 331:161–167, 1994.
26. Didier ES. Microsporidiosis. Clin Infect Dis 27:1–8, 1998.
27. Ungar BLP. Cryptosporidium. In: Mandell GL, Douglas Jr RG, Bennett JE, eds. Principles and practice of infectious diseases. 4th ed. New York: Churchill Livingstone, 1995:2507.
28. Anonymous. Drugs for parasitic infections. Med Lett Drugs Ther 40:1–12, Jan 2, 1998.
29. Pape JW, Verdier RI, Boney M, et al. Cyclospora infection in adults infected with HIV: clinical manifestations, treatment, and prophylaxis. Ann Intern Med 121:654–657, 1994.
30. Pape JW, Verdier RI, Johnson WD. Treatment and prophylaxis of *Isospora belli* infection in patients with the acquired immunodeficiency syndrome. N Engl J Med 320:1044–1047, 1989.
31. Ackers JP. Gut coccidia–Isospora, Cryptosporidium, Cyclospora, and sarcocystis. Semin Gastrointest Dis 8:33–44, 1997.
32. Hashmey R, Smith NH, Cron S, et al. Cryptosporidiosis in Houston, Texas. A report of 95 cases. Medicine (Baltimore) 76:118–139, 1997.
33. Ritchie DJ, Becker ES. Update on the management of intestinal cryptosporidiosis in AIDS. Ann Pharmacother 28:767–778, 1994.
34. Sprinz E, Mallman R, Barcellos S, et al. AIDS-related cryptosporidial diarrhea: an open study with roxithromycin. J Antimicrob Chemother 41(Suppl B):S85–S91, 1998.
35. Uip DE, Lima AL, Amato VS, et al. Roxithromycin in treatment for diarrhea caused by *Cryptosporidium* spp. in patients with AIDS. J Antimicrob Chemother 41(Suppl B):S93–S97, 1998.
36. Smith NH, Cron S, Valdez LM, et al. Combination therapy for cryptosporidiosis in AIDS. J Infect Dis 178:900–903, 1998.
37. Blanshard C, Shanson DC, Gazzard BG. Pilot studies of azithromycin, letrazuril and paromomycin in the treatment of cryptosporidiosis. Int J STD AIDS 8:124–129, 1997.
38. Molina JM, Chastang C, Goguel J, et al. Albendazole for treatment and prophylaxis of microsporidiosis due to *Encephalitozoon intestinalis* in patients with AIDS: a randomized double-blind controlled trial. J Infect Dis 177:1373–1377, 1998.
39. Diesenhouse MC, Wilson LA, Corrent GF, et al. Treatment of microsporidial keratoconjunctivitis with topical fumagillin. Am J Ophthalmol 115:293–298, 1993.
40. Molina JM, Goguel J, Sarfati C, et al. Potential efficacy of fumagillin in intestinal microsporidiosis due to *Enterocytozoon bieneusi* in patients with HIV infection: results of a drug screening study. The French Microsporidiosis Study Group. AIDS 11:1603–1610, 1997.
41. Sharpstone D, Rowbottom A, Francis N, et al. Thalidomide: a novel therapy for microsporidiosis. Gastroenterology 112:1823–1829, 1997.
42. Holmberg SD, Moorman AC, Von Bargen JC, et al. Possible effectiveness of clarithromycin and rifabutin for cryptosporidiosis chemoprophylaxis in HIV disease. JAMA 279:384–386, 1998.
43. Carr A, Marriott D, Field A, et al. Treatment of HIV-1-associated microsporidiosis and cryptosporidiosis with combination antiretroviral therapy. Lancet 351:256–261, 1998.
44. Wanke CA, Plesko D, DeGirolami PC, et al. A medium chain triglyceride-based diet in patients with HIV and chronic diarrhea reduces diarrhea and malabsorption: a prospective, controlled trial. Nutrition 12:766–771, 1996.
45. Thielman NM, Guerrant RL. Persistent diarrhea in the returned traveler. Infect Dis Clin North Am 12:489–501, 1998.
46. Coyle C, Kent M, Tanowitz HB, et al. TNP-470 is an effective antimicrosporidial agent. J Infect Dis 177:515–518, 1998.
47. Hill DR. *Giardia lamblia.* In: Mandell GL, Douglas Jr RG, Bennett JE, eds. Principles and practice of infectious diseases. 4th ed. New York: Churchill Livingstone, 1995:2487–2490.
48. Ortega YR, Adam RD. Giardia: overview and update. Clin Infect Dis 25:545–549, 1997.
49. VandeWaa EA, Henderson JD, White Jr GL, et al. Common helminth infections: battling wormlike parasites in primary care. Clin Rev 8:75–92, 1998.
50. Liu LX, Weller PF. Antiparasitic drugs. N Engl J Med 334:1178–1184, 1996.
51. Mahmoud AAF. Intestinal nematodes (roundworms). In: Mandell GL, Douglas Jr RG, Bennett JE, eds. Principles and practice of infectious diseases. 4th ed. New York: Churchill Livingstone, 1995:2526–2530.
52. King CH. Cestodes (tapeworms). In: Mandell GL, Douglas Jr RG, Bennett JE, eds. Principles and practice of infectious diseases. 4th ed. New York: Churchill Livingstone, 1995:2544–2548, 2550.
53. Mahmoud AAF. Trematodes (schistosomiasis) and other flukes. In: Mandell GL, Douglas Jr RG, Bennett JE, eds. Principles and practice of infectious diseases. 4th ed. New York: Churchill Livingstone, 1995:2538–2541.
54. White AC. Neurocysticercosis: a major cause of neurological disease worldwide. Clin Infect Dis 24:101–113, 1997.
55. de Silva N, Guyatt H, Bundy D. Anthelmintics: a comparative review of their clinical pharmacology. Drugs 53:769–788, 1997.
56. Albonico M, Smith PG, Hall A, et al. A randomized controlled trial comparing mebendazole and albendazole against *Ascaris, Trichuris,* and hookworm infections. Trans R Soc Trop Med Hyg 88:585–589, 1994.
57. Gann PH, Neva FA, Gam AA. A randomized trial of single- and two-dose ivermectin versus thiabendazole for treatment of strongyloidiasis. J Infect Dis 169:1076–1079, 1994.
58. Wilson BB. Lice (pediculosis). In: Mandell GL, Douglas Jr RG, Bennett JE, eds. Principles and practice of infectious diseases. 4th ed. New York: Churchill Livingstone, 1995:2558–2560.
59. Wilson BB. Scabies. In: Mandell GL, Douglas Jr RG, Bennett JE, eds. Principles and practice of infectious diseases. 4th ed. New York: Churchill Livingstone, 1995:2560–2562.
60. Mackey SL, Wagner KF. Dermatologic manifestations of parasitic diseases. Infect Dis Clin North Am 8:713–743, 1994.
61. Brown S, Becher J, Brady W. Treatment of ectoparasitic infections: review of the English-language literature, 1982–1992. Clin Infect Dis (20-suppl 1):S104–S109, 1995.
62. Meinking TL, Taplin D, Hermida JL, et al. Treatment of scabies with ivermectin. N Engl J Med 333:26–30, 1995.
63. Ahorlu CK, Dunyo SK, Afari EA, et al. Malaria-related beliefs and behavior in southern Ghana: implications for treatment, prevention and control. Trop Med Int Health 2:488–499, 1997.
64. Schlagenhauf P, Steffen R, Tschopp A, et al. Behavioral aspects of travelers in their use of malaria presumptive therapy. Bull WHO 73:215–221, 1995.
65. Centers for Disease Control and Prevention. Health information for international travel 1996–1997, Department of Health and Human Services, Atlanta, GA, 1997 (http://www.cdc.gov/travel/index.htm).

CHAPTER 80

SURGICAL ANTIBIOTIC PROPHYLAXIS

Ronald L. Braden

DEFINITION

Surgical antibiotic prophylaxis is the use of preoperative and postoperative antibiotics to decrease the incidence of postoperative infections.

TREATMENT GOALS: SURGICAL ANTIBIOTIC PROPHYLAXIS

- Decrease the incidence of postoperative infections.
- Minimize the adverse effects of these antibiotics on the microflora of the patient and the overall bacterial resistance in a particular institution.

EPIDEMIOLOGY OF POSTOPERATIVE INFECTIONS

Twenty-five percent of all nosocomial infections are postoperative wound infections.[1] Haley et al.[2] demonstrated that surgical wound infections can be responsible for an additional week of hospitalization and an increase by approximately 20% in the overall cost of care. This cost is estimated to exceed $1.5 billion per year in the United States. Administration of prophylactic antibiotics in certain surgical procedures can decrease postoperative infections, decrease length of hospital stay, and reduce the overall cost of care.

Inappropriate or indiscriminate use of prophylactic antibiotics can increase the cost of care by increasing drug cost, increasing drug toxicity, increasing microorganism resistance, and increasing laboratory costs. Prophylactic antibiotics can account for 30 to 40% of total antibiotic usage in some hospitals and inappropriate usage remains a significant problem. Pharmacy practitioners must become more astute in the development and implementation of cost-control measures in prevention of postoperative wound infections.[3]

PATHOPHYSIOLOGY OF POSTOPERATIVE INFECTIONS

Surgical wound infection does not necessarily follow bacterial contamination. The predominate organisms involved are the endogenous microflora at the surgical site. The development of a surgical wound infection is dependent upon a complex interaction between the patient's host-defense response, intrinsic bacterial factors, and local tissue factors.[4,5] Factors that increase the risk of surgical wound infection are as follows.

1. Host-defense response factors: Patients with an underlying host-defense deficit are at increased risk of surgical wound infection (e.g., extremes of age, malnutrition, diabetes, corticosteroid therapy, or other immunologic deficiency)
2. Bacterial factors
   a. Degree of wound contamination
   b. Bacterial virulence
   c. Microbial resistance to prophylactic antibiotics
3. Local tissue factors
   a. Blood supply and tissue hypoxia
   b. Necrotic material
   c. Presence of hematoma
   d. Presence of a foreign body

CLASSIFICATION OF SURGICAL WOUNDS

The Ad Hoc Committee of the Committee on Trauma of the National Research Council developed a standard classification of surgical wounds in 1964.[6] This classification identified four basic categories of wound contamination and the resultant postoperative infection rate expected within each category (Table 80.1).

RISK FACTORS FOR POSTOPERATIVE INFECTIONS

The risk of postoperative infection is dependent on patient factors, intraoperative factors, and perioperative management. Factors that have been identified as increasing the risk of postoperative infection are listed in Table 80.2. Regardless of the wound classification, emergency surgical procedures have a higher postoperative infection rate than the same elective operative procedure. Institutions in which a high volume of an operative procedure is performed have a lower postoperative infection rate than those institutions in which the operative procedure is performed less frequently.[7] Operative procedures that last longer have a higher postoperative infection rate regardless of their wound classification.

TREATMENT OF POSTOPERATIVE INFECTIONS

Principles of Antibiotic Prophylaxis

Prophylactic antibiotics are indicated when the risk of postoperative infection is high or when the consequence of infection is excessive morbidity or mortality.[8] Antibiotic selection should be based on the spectrum of antimicrobial activity, pharmacokinetic profile, drug toxicity, and positive results from well-controlled clinical trials. The benefit of the prophylactic antibiotic must always clearly outweigh its risks.

Antimicrobial Spectrum

The antimicrobial agent chosen for an individual patient should have activity against the most common pathogens that cause surgical wound infections (Table 80.3). The

Table 80.1 ▪ National Research Council Wound Classification Criteria

Classification	Criteria
Clean (<2%)[a]	Elective (not urgent or emergency), primarily closed; no acute inflammation or transection of gastrointestinal, oropharyngeal, genitourinary, biliary, or tracheobronchial tracts; no surgical technique break (e.g., elective inguinal herniorrhaphy)
Clean-contaminated (<10%)	Urgent or emergency procedure that is otherwise clean; elective gastrointestinal, oropharyngeal, biliary, or tracheobronchial tracts; minimal spillage and/or minor technique break; re-operation via clean incision within 7 days; blunt trauma, intact skin, negative exploration (e.g., vagotomy and pyloroplasty)
Contaminated (20%)	Acute, nonpurulent inflammation; major break in surgical technique or major spill from hollow organ; penetrating trauma <4 hr old; chronic open wounds to be grafted or covered (e.g., acute, nonperforated, nongangrenous appendicitis)
Dirty (40%)	Purulence or abscess; preoperative perforation of gastrointestinal, oropharyngeal, biliary, or tracheobronchial tracts; penetrating trauma >4 hr old (e.g., perforated appendicitis with abscess)

Source: Reference 8.
[a]Wound infection rates appear in parentheses.

Table 80.2 ▪ Factors Associated with Increased Risk of Postoperative Infection

Patient Factors	Perioperative Factors	Intraoperative Factors
Extremes of age	>48 hr preoperative hospitalization	Intraoperative contamination
Malnutrition	No preoperative shower	Lengthy operation
Obesity	Early shaving of site (>4 hr)	Excessive electrocautery
Associated problems	Hair removal	Prosthetic material
Diabetes	Prior antibiotic therapy	Wound drainage
Hypoxemia		Bloody wound fluid drainage
Previous infection		Epinephrine wound injection
Corticosteroid therapy		Intraoperative hypotension
Recent operation		Massive transfusion
Chronic inflammation		Skin preparation with alcohol/hexachlorophene
Prior site irradiation		

Source: Reference 8.

Table 80.3 ▪ Recommendations for Prophylactic Antibiotic Agents for Adults

Procedure	Bacteria	Antibiotic Agent	Dose
Cardiac: all with cardiopulmonary bypass	*Staphylococcus aureus, Staphylococcus epidermidis,* diphtheroids, Gram-negative enterics	Cefazolin[a] or cefuroxime	1–2 g pre-induction, 1 g every 8 hr for 48 hr
Noncardiac vascular: aortic resection prosthetic bypass	*S. aureus, S. epidermidis,* diphtheroids, Gram-negative enterics	Cefazolin[a]	1–2 g pre-induction, 1 g every 8 hr for 24 hr
Orthopedic: insertion of prosthetic joints, open operations	*S. aureus, S. epidermidis*	Cefazolin[a]	1 g pre-induction
Neurosurgery	*S. aureus, S. epidermidis*	Cefazolin[a]	1–2 g pre-induction
Head and neck: operations involving transection of the oropharyngeal mucosa (see text)	Oral aerobes and anaerobes, *S. aureus, S. epidermidis*	Cefazolin[a] + clindamycin	1–2 g pre-induction + 600 mg pre-induction
Gastroduodenal: ulcer patients treated with H_2 blockers, bleeding duodenal ulcer, gastric cancer	Oropharyngeal flora and Gram-negative enterics, *S. aureus*	Cefazolin[a]	1–2 g pre-induction
Biliary: all open and laparoscopic procedures	Gram-negative enterics, *S. aureus, Enterococcus faecalis,* clostridia	Cefazolin[a]	1–2 g pre-induction
Colorectal: operations that involve the colon and/or rectum	Enteric aerobes and anaerobes	Oral neomycin/ erythromycin	See below[c]
		Cefoxitin[b]	1 g pre-induction
Appendectomy: simple appendicitis	Enteric aerobes and anaerobes	Cefoxitin[b]	1 g pre-induction
Cesarean section	Enteric aerobes and anaerobes, *E. faecalis,* group B streptococci	Cefazolin[a]	1 g after umbilical cord is clamped
Hysterectomy	Enteric aerobes and anaerobes, *E. faecalis,* group B streptococci	Cefazolin[a]	1 g pre-induction

Source: References 8, 9.

[a]Vancomycin 1 g IV can be substituted for patients with severe type 1 β-lactam allergies.

[b]Cefoxitin, cefotetan, or cefmetazole.

[c]Oral neomycin 1g + erythromycin base 1g given orally the day before surgery at 1, 2, and 11 PM, + cefoxitin[b] 1g IV preinduction.

agent does not need to possess antibacterial activity against all of the endogenous microbial flora at the surgical site; use of agents with an excessively broad spectrum of activity increases the risk of microbial resistance and superinfection without an increase in effectiveness. Third-generation cephalosporins exemplify this point: despite their increased antimicrobial activity, these agents have not proven to be superior to first-generation cephalosporins in any operative procedure.[10]

Pharmacokinetics

The pharmacokinetic profile of the prophylactic agent is also an extremely important factor. Burke[11] demonstrated the importance of adequate serum concentrations of the prophylactic antibiotic at the time of surgical incision in an experimental animal model. Because most antibiotics distribute rapidly into tissue compartments after intravenous administration, total body clearance and volume of distribution become the most important pharmacokinetic variables. Intraoperative factors such as blood loss, fluid replacement, and alteration of blood flow to the liver and kidneys may cause significant alterations in the clearance and volume of distribution of prophylactic antibiotics.[12] Guglielmo et al.[13] demonstrated a significant increase in volume of distribution and elimination half-life of cefamandole in patients undergoing elective vascular surgery. The increased volume of distribution resulted in low serum concentrations of the antibiotic at the time of prosthetic graft placement, which would theoretically place the patient at increased risk of postoperative infection.

Timing of Antibiotic Administration

The most common error encountered in surgical prophylaxis is in the timing of antibiotic doses. As previously stated, Burke demonstrated the importance of adequate serum concentrations of the prophylactic antibiotic at the time of incision in experimental animals.[11] This finding was confirmed by Polk et al.[12] in a prospective clinical trial in which inappropriate time of drug administration was an independent risk factor for postoperative infection. Classen et al.[14] prospectively monitored the timing of antibiotic prophylaxis and studied the occurrence of surgical wound infections in patients undergoing elective clean or clean-contaminated surgical procedures. Patients receiving prophylactic antibiotics during the 2 hours before the initial surgical incision had the lowest overall surgical wound infection rate. "On call" dosing of prophylactic antibiotics may result in early drug administration because of an unforeseen delay in the beginning of the operative procedure and may result in inadequate tissue concentrations of the drug at the time of the initial surgical incision. Therefore, this practice should be strongly discouraged.

Duration of Prophylaxis

Antibiotic administration continued longer than 24 to 48 hours has been shown to decrease the risk of surgical wound infection after most operative procedures, but may increase toxicity, increase cost, alter the patient's microflora, and alter the microflora of the institution.[15] Single-dose prophylaxis for most operative procedures provides the optimal balance of reducing surgical wound infections while decreasing adverse drug effects.[16]

SUGGESTED ANTIBIOTIC REGIMENS FOR SELECTED SURGICAL PROCEDURES

Cardiac Operations

Cardiac operations are classified as clean surgical procedures and pose a low risk for surgical wound infection. Cardiac operative procedures such as pacemaker or defibrillator placement pose a low risk for postoperative infection and require single-dose antibiotic prophylaxis only. However, in cardiac operations that involve placement of prosthetic material, such as prosthetic valve replacement, the excessive morbidity and mortality of endocarditis and mediastinitis mandate the use of prophylactic antibiotics. The pathogens most commonly responsible for postoperative infection include *Staphylococcus aureus, Staphylococcus epidermidis,* and diphtheroid species. In most institutions, first-generation cephalosporins possess good activity against these pathogens and have remained the standard against which other antibiotics are compared. Cefazolin, a first-generation cephalosporin with a relatively long elimination half-life, has remained the most commonly prescribed prophylactic agent. Several investigations have compared newer cephalosporins with varying results. Slama et al.[17] compared cefamandole, cefazolin, and cefuroxime. Their results indicate that cefamandole and cefuroxime are both superior to cefazolin in overall wound infection rates; however, other investigators have been unable to reproduce these results and the choice of agent remains an area of controversy.[18,19] The choice of agent in this setting should be based on the individual institution's sensitivities; however the literature supports cefazolin as the prophylactic agent-of-choice in most cardiothoracic operations. Some practitioners recommend prolonged postoperative prophylactic antibiotics if the patient has been in the hospital awaiting surgery for >48 hours. This practice has not been shown to be more efficacious in altering postoperative infection rates and increases the risk of colonization of the patient with multidrug-resistant microorganisms.[20] This practice should be strongly discouraged.

Noncardiac Vascular Procedures

Like cardiac operations, noncardiac vascular procedures are classified as clean, and the most common pathogens are *S. aureus* and *S. epidermidis*. The incidence of postoperative infection is increased with insertion of vascular prosthesis or in procedures involving the groin.[21–23] Several authors have demonstrated the efficacy of three-dose cefazolin prophylaxis and cefazolin remains the prophylactic agent-of-choice in these procedures.[22,23] Prophylactic antibiotics have not been shown to improve outcomes for carotid endarterectomy or brachial artery repair when prosthetic material is not inserted. Therefore, prophylactic antibiotics are not indicated for these operative procedures.[24,25] In institutions with a significant incidence of methicillin-resistant *S. aureus* infection, vancomycin is an acceptable alternative agent but the Centers for Disease Control and Prevention criteria should be followed.[26]

Orthopedic Procedures

As with the previously described operative procedures, orthopedic procedures are clean and pose a low risk for infection; therefore, no antibiotic prophylaxis is necessary in most orthopedic procedures. However, the morbidity and mortality associated with prosthetic joint infections is extremely high and warrants the use of prophylactic antibiotics whenever prosthetic joints are placed. The most common pathogens are *S. aureus* and *S. epidermidis*. Cefazolin is the prophylactic agent of choice. It has significantly reduced postoperative infections and demonstrated adequate tissue and bone concentration and posses a low risk of toxicity.[27] The duration of antibiotic prophylaxis is somewhat controversial, but courses of longer than 48 hours after prosthetic device implantation offer no added benefit; therefore, single-dose or short-term antibiotic prophylaxis is indicated.[27,28]

Neurosurgical Procedures

The benefit of prophylactic antibiotics has not been well documented in clean neurosurgical operations without shunt placement, but the practice is common. *S. aureus* and *S. epidermidis* are the predominate pathogens, with Gram-negative aerobes being somewhat more common in cerebrospinal fluid (CSF) shunt infections. A review of the literature published by Haines[29] supports the use of prophylactic antibiotics, including cefazolin, cloxacillin, and vancomycin as monotherapy, and cefazolin plus gentamicin and gentamicin plus vancomycin as combination therapy.[29] These agents have been shown to reduce postoperative infection rates, but the choice of the most effective prophylactic agent remains difficult and should be based on the individual institution's antimicrobial sensitivities.[29–32] Limited data are available regarding CSF shunt procedures, but applying knowledge from other procedures involving prosthetic material would mandate the use of prophylactic antibiotics because of the extreme morbidity and mortality of postoperative infections associated with these procedures. From the available literature, cefazolin monotherapy appears effective in reducing the surgical wound infection rate in neurosurgical operations and should be considered the preferred prophylactic agent.

Head and Neck Procedures

Head and neck operations should be divided into two categories: clean procedures in which no transection of the oropharyngeal mucosa occurs and clean-contaminated procedures where transection of the oropharyngeal tract does occur. Clean procedures include parotidectomy, thyroidectomy, and submandibular gland excision. The infection rate for these procedures is low, and routine prophylactic antibiotics are not recommended.[33] Clean-contaminated procedures performed without prophylactic antibiotics have produced surgical wound infection rates of 24 to 87% and appropriate perioperative antibiotics have been shown to reduce the postoperative infection rate by approximately 50%.[34] The predominate pathogens in clean-contaminated head and neck procedures are the normal flora of the mouth and oropharynx. Multiple prophylactic antibiotic regimens have been proven effective in reducing surgical wound infection rates; however, the preferred regimens are cefazolin 1 to 2 g plus clindamycin or clindamycin plus gentamicin. Metronidazole appears to be as effective against anaerobic bacteria as clindamycin and may be substituted. Recently, ampicillin/sulbactam has been shown to be equal to standard regimens, although further study is required to identify the most optimal antibiotic prophylaxis in these operative procedures.[35] The duration of prophylactic antibiotic administration should not exceed 24 hours in these patients undergoing clean-contaminated procedures.[36]

Gastroduodenal Procedures

Surgical wound infection rates of the upper gastroduodenal tract (esophageal and gastroduodenal procedures) have been documented to be a function of gastric pH. Disease states or drugs that increase pH are well known to increase the incidence of postoperative infection.[37] The predominate pathogens in gastroduodenal operations are normal mouth flora, skin flora, and to a lesser extent, bowel flora. Several cephalosporins have been proven to be effective in reducing postoperative infection rates, and cefazolin has been studied in a single-dose regimen and appears to have equal efficacy to that of multidose regimens. The preferred regimen is cefazolin 1 to 2 g as a single dose at the induction of anesthesia.[38,39]

Biliary Tract Operations

The postoperative infection rate of biliary tract operations is directly related to the presence or absence of microorganisms in the bile. The infection rate of patients with positive bile cultures is reported to be approximately 36% while the infection rate of patients with sterile bile is <5%.[40,41] Risk factors for positive bile cultures include acute cholecystitis, biliary tract obstruction, and age older than 70.[42] The most common organisms found in biliary tract surgery are *Escherichia coli, Klebsiella* species, enterococci, streptococci, and staphylococci. Cephalosporins have shown good activity in biliary tract surgery and a meta-analysis by Meijer et al.[43] concluded that perioperative antibiotics should be used in all patients undergoing biliary tract surgery. Although patients with sterile biliary tracts appear to gain little or no benefit, preoperative identification of these patients is not possible. Cefazolin is the preferred agent and should be given as a single pre-induction dose.

Appendectomy

The incidence of surgical wound infections after appendectomy is highly variable and is dependent on the status of the appendix at the time of surgery. In uncomplicated appendicitis the infection rate is reported to be 4 to 9% without perioperative antibiotics and 1 to 5% with antibiotics.[44] The most common pathogens isolated after appendectomy are anaerobic organisms such as *Bacteroides fragilis* and aerobic Gram-negative organisms such as *E. coli,* streptococci, staphylococci, and enterococci are identified less frequently but may be associated with antibiotic treatment failure. Antibiotic regimens found to be effective in significantly reducing postoperative complications have included cefoxitin, cefotaxime, mezlocillin, and clindamycin.[44,45] The first-generation cephalosporins, cefazolin and cephalothin, have not been proven to be effective in reducing postoperative infections and do not appear to be appropriate prophylactic agents.[46,47] Cefoxitin, cefotetan, or cefmetazole given as a single-dose preinduction regimen appears to be the preferred regimen in uncomplicated appendicitis.[45] Antibiotic use in complicated appendicitis is classified as treatment, not prophylaxis, and is therefore not included in this discussion.

Colorectal Procedures

Surgical wound infections are responsible for excessive morbidity and mortality after elective colorectal surgery, which mandates the use of effective prophylactic antibiotics. Risk factors for postoperative infections include impaired host defenses, age older than 60, hypoalbuminemia, inadequate bowel preparation, and spillage of colonic contents with bacterial contamination of the surgical wound.[48] The goal of surgical prophylaxis in colorectal surgery is to reduce the risk of wound contamination by bacteria spilled from the colon and rectum during the surgical procedure. This is accomplished most effectively by use of mechanical bowel preparation, preoperative oral antibiotics, and parenteral perioperative antibiotics.[8] Mechanical bowel preparation reduces fecal bulk but does not significantly alter the concentration of microorganisms in the stool and does not decrease surgical wound infection rates.[49] Addition of oral antibiotics such as erythromycin and neomycin to mechanical bowel preparation decreases postoperative infections, and the addition of a perioperative parenteral cephalosporin such as cefoxitin, cefotetan, or cefmetazole can further decrease postoperative infection rate to <10% for elective colorectal procedures.[50] The preferred prophylactic regimen would include the following: (1) 4 L of a polyethylene glycol-electrolyte lavage solution given the day before surgery, plus (2) oral neomycin sulfate 1g and erythromycin base 1 g given after the bowel preparation is completed at 1, 2, and 11 PM the day before surgery, plus (3) cefoxitin, or a similar agent, at induction of anesthesia.

Cesarean Section

The risk of postoperative infection in cesarean section appears to be related to host factors and can be divided into high- and low-risk populations. High-risk patients are women who have not received prenatal care, are undernourished, undergo multiple vaginal examinations, have prolonged labor, and have undergone frequent invasive monitoring. The risk of postpartum endometritis is reported to be as high as 85% in the high-risk patient whereas it is 5 to 10% for the low-risk patient.[51] Appropriate prophylactic antibiotics can reduce the incidence of postoperative infection by 50 to 70% as documented by controlled clinical trials.[52] The preferred prophylactic regimen is cefazolin 1 g given after umbilical cord clamping. Administration of the drug after cord clamping is intended to minimize toxicity to the infant.

Hysterectomy

The incidence of postoperative infection after vaginal hysterectomy without prophylactic antibiotics is reported to be as high as 40%, whereas appropriate prophylactic antibiotics can reduce this incidence to <10%.[53] Risk factors for postoperative infection include low socioeconomic status, extremes of age, obesity, diabetes, and prior instrumentation of the genitourinary tract. Postoperative infections are caused by a variety of aerobic and anaerobic organisms, with *Bacteroides* species being the predominant anaerobe. However, single-dose cefazolin has proven as effective as extended spectrum cephalosporins and is the preferred prophylactic agent.[53]

FUTURE THERAPIES

Our understanding of the issues of surgical antibiotic prophylaxis have increased significantly over the past 30 years. Issues remaining to be resolved include development of a better risk stratification system to identify those patients at highest risk for postoperative infections and improved therapeutic plans for those patients.[53] The emergence of bacterial resistance also challenges the efforts to minimize postoperative would infections.

IMPROVING OUTCOMES

Prophylactic antibiotics play a significant role in the perioperative management of surgical patients. The resultant decrease in postoperative infections serves to decrease morbidity and mortality, which in turn can limit the length of the hospital stay and cut health care delivery costs in general. In using antibiotic prophylaxis, however, the pharmacist should consider the following criteria to extend its safety and efficacy. First, pharmacists should be actively involved in the process to ensure that the antibiotic's benefit outweighs the risk of treatment. Second, the pharmacist must be aware of the institution's microflora sensitivity patterns to base antibiotic selection on the appropriate spectrum of antimicrobial activity. Third, antibiotic dosing should be scheduled so that adequate tissue concentrations are achieved during the critical period and postoperative prophylaxis is limited to the shortest effective time. By being aware of the above considerations and being actively involved in the medication use process, the pharmacist is well positioned to improve surgical antibiotic prophylaxis and to help ensure that a successful surgical result is realized.

KEY POINTS

- Identification of patients at risk for postoperative infection should be based on the surgical wound classification and the patient-specific risk factors for infection.
- Antibiotics should be chosen that possess an antimicrobial spectrum of activity that adequately covers the microflora expected for each operative procedure.
- Antimicrobial agents should be chosen that achieve adequate tissue concentrations at the surgical site and are effective against the most common pathogens.
- Doses of antimicrobial agent should be given to maintain therapeutic tissue concentrations for the duration of the surgical procedure.
- The timing of antimicrobial prophylaxis administration is critical. Antimicrobial agents should not be given as "on call" doses, but should be administered when anesthesia is induced to provide effective concentrations during the procedure.
- Antimicrobial agents should be administered for the shortest period of time proven effective in decreasing the rate of postoperative infections.

REFERENCES

1. McGowan JE Jr. Cost and benefit of perioperative antimicrobial prophylaxis: methods for economic analysis. Rev Infect Dis 13(Suppl 10):S879–S889, 1991.
2. Haley RW, Schaberg DR, Crossley KB, et al. Extra charges and prolongation of stay attributable to nosocomial infections: a prospective interhospital comparison. Am J Med 70:51–58, 1981.
3. Haley RW. Measuring the costs of nosocomial infections: methods for estimating economic burden on the hospital. Am J Med 91(Suppl 3B):32S–38S, 1991.
4. Kernodle DS, Kaiser AB. Postoperative infections and antimicrobial prophylaxis. In: Mandell GL, Bennett JE, Dolin R, eds. Principles and practice of infectious disease. 4th ed. New York: Churchill Livingstone, 1995:2742–2756.
5. Nichols RL. Surgical infections and choice of antibiotics. In: Sabiston DC. Sabiston's essentials of surgery. 1st ed. Philadelphia: WB Saunders, 1997:141–168.

6. Ad Hoc Committee of the Committee on Trauma, Division of Medical Sciences, National Academy of Sciences-National Research Council. Postoperative wound infections: the influence of ultraviolet irradiation of the operating room and various other factors. Ann Surg 160(Suppl 2):23, 1964.
7. Farber BF, Kaiser DL, Wenzel RP. Relation between surgical volume and incidence of postoperative wound infection. N Engl J Med 305:200–204, 1981.
8. Page CP, Bohnen JM, Fletcher JR, et al. Antimicrobial prophylaxis for surgical wounds. Guidelines for clinical care. Arch Surg 128:79–88,1993.
9. Antimicrobial prophylaxis in surgery. Med Lett Drugs Ther 41(1060):75–80, 1999.
10. DiPiro JT, Bowden TA Jr, Hooks VH 3d. Prophylactic parenteral cephalosporins in surgery. Are the newer agents better? JAMA 252:3277–3279, 1984.
11. Burke JF. Effective period of preventive antibiotic action in experimental incisions and dermal lesions. Surgery 50:161, 1961.
12. Polk HC, Lopez-Mayor JF. Postoperative wound infection: a prospective study of determinant factors and prevention. Surgery 66:97–103, 1969.
13. Guglielmo BJ, Salazar TA, Rodondi LC, et al. Altered pharmacokinetics of antibiotics during vascular surgery. Am J Surg 157:410–412, 1989.
14. Classen DC, Evans RS, Pestotnik SL, et al. The timing of prophylactic administration of antibiotics and the risk of surgical-wound infection. N Engl J Med 326:281–286, 1992.
15. Guglielmo BJ, Hohn DC, Koo PJ, et al. Antibiotic prophylaxis in surgical procedures. A critical analysis of the literature. Arch Surg 118:943–955, 1983.
16. DiPiro JT, Cheung RP, Bowden TA Jr, et al. Single dose systemic antibiotic prophylaxis of surgical wound infections. Am J Surg 152:552–559, 1986.
17. Slama TG, Sklar SJ, Misinki J, et al. Randomized comparison of cefamandole, cefazolin, and cefuroxime prophylaxis in open-heart surgery. Antimicrob Agents Chemother 29:744–747, 1986.
18. Conklin CM, Gray RJ, Neilson D, et al. Determinants of wound infection incidence after isolated coronary artery bypass surgery in patients randomized to receive prophylactic cefuroxime or cefazolin. Ann Thorac Surg 46:172–177, 1988.
19. Gentry LO, Zeluff BJ, Cooley DA. Antibiotic prophylaxis in open-heart surgery: a comparison of cefamandole, cefuroxime, and cefazolin. Ann Thorac Surg 46:167–171, 1988.
20. Niederhauser U, Vogt M, Vogt P, et al. Cardiac surgery in a high-risk group of patients: is prolonged postoperative antibiotic prophylaxis effective? J Thorac Cardiovasc Surg 114:162–168, 1997.
21. Szilagyi DE, Smith RF, Elliott JP, et al. Infection in arterial reconstruction with synthetic grafts. Ann Surg 186:321–333, 1972.
22. Goldstone J, Moore WS. Infection in vascular prostheses: clinical manifestations and surgical management. Am J Surg 128:225–233, 1974.
23. Landreneau MD, Raju S. Infections after elective bypass surgery for lower limb ischemia: the influence of preoperative transcutaneous arteriography. Surgery 90:956–961, 1981.
24. Kaiser AB, Clayson KR, Mulherin JL Jr, et al. Antibiotic prophylaxis in vascular surgery. Ann Surg 188:283–289, 1978.
25. Pitt HA, Postier RG, MacGowan AW, et al. Prophylactic antibiotics in vascular surgery: topical, systemic, or both? Ann Surg 192:356–364, 1980.
26. Mangram AJ, Horan TC, Pearson ML, et al. Guidelines for prevention of surgical site infection, 1999. Infect Control Hosp Epidemiol 20(4):247–278, 1999.
27. Van Meirhaeghe J, Verdonk R, Verschraegen G, et al. Flucloxacillin compared with cefazolin in short-term prophylaxis for clean orthopedic surgery. Arch Orthop Trauma Surg 108:308–313, 1989.
28. Nelson CL. Prevention of sepsis. Clin Orthop 222:66–72, 1987.
29. Haines SJ. Efficacy of antibiotic prophylaxis in clean neurosurgical operations. Neurosurgery 24:401–405, 1989.
30. Geraghty J, Feely M. Antibiotic prophylaxis in neurosurgery. A randomized control trial. J Neurosurg 60:724–726, 1984.
31. Bullock R, van Dellen JR, Ketelbey W, et al. A double-blind placebo-controlled trial of perioperative prophylactic antibiotics for elective neurosurgery. J Neurosurg 69:687–691, 1988.
32. van Ek B, Dijkmans BA, van Dulken H, et al. Effect of cloxacillin prophylaxis on the bacterial flora of craniotomy wounds. Scand J Infect Dis 22:345–352, 1990.
33. Johnson JT, Wagner RL. Infection following uncontaminated head and neck surgery. Arch Otolaryngol Head Neck Surg 113:368–369, 1987.
34. Friberg D, Lundberg C. Antibiotic prophylaxis in major head and neck surgery when clean-contaminated wounds are established. Scand J Infect Dis Suppl 70:87–90, 1990.
35. Weber RS. Wound infection in head and neck surgery: implications for perioperative antibiotic treatment. Ear Nose Throat J 76:795–798, 1997.
36. Righi M, et al. Short-term versus long-term antimicrobial prophylaxis in oncologic head and neck surgery. Head Neck 18:399–404, 1996.
37. Gatehouse D, Dimock F, Burdon DW, et al. Prediction of wound sepsis following gastric operations. Br J Surg 65:551–554, 1978.
38. Pories WJ, Van RA, Burlingham BT, et al. Prophylactic cefazolin in gastric bypass surgery. Surgery 90:426–432, 1981.
39. Lewis RT, Goodall RG, Marien B, et al. Efficacy and distribution of single dose preoperative antibiotic prophylaxis in high-risk gastroduodenal surgery. Can J Surg 34:117–122, 1991.
40. Cainzos M, Potel J, Puente JL. Prospective randomized controlled study of prophylaxis with cefamandole in high risk patients undergoing operations upon the biliary tract. Surg Gynecol Obstet 160:27–32, 1985.
41. Stone HH, Hooper CA, Kolb LD et al. Antibiotic prophylaxis in gastric, biliary and colonic surgery. Ann Surg 184:443–452, 1976.
42. Chetlin SH, Elliot DW. Preoperative antibiotics in biliary surgery. Arch Surg 107:319–323, 1973.
43. Meijer WS, Schmitz PI, Jeekel J. Meta-analysis of randomized, controlled clinical trials of antibiotic prophylaxis in biliary tract surgery. Br J Surg 77:283–290, 1990.
44. Bauer T, Vennits B, Holm B, et al. Antibiotic prophylaxis in acute nonperforated appendicitis. The Danish Multi-Center Study Group III. Ann Surg 209:307–311, 1989.
45. Winslow RE, Dean RE, Harley JW. Acute nonperforating appendicitis. Efficacy of brief antibiotic prophylaxis. Arch Surg 118:651–655, 1983.
46. Donovan IA, Ellis D, Gatehouse D, et al. One-dose antibiotic prophylaxis against wound infection after appendicectomy: a randomized trial of clindamycin, cefazolin sodium and a placebo. Br J Surg 66:193–196, 1979.
47. Panichi G, Pantosti AL, Marsiglio F, et al. Cephalothin or cefoxitin in appendicectomy? J Antimicrob Chemother 6:801–804, 1980.
48. Nichols RL. Prophylaxis for elective bowel surgery. In: Wilson, SE, Williams RA, Finegold S. Intra-abdominal infections. New York: McGraw-Hill, 1982: 267–285.
49. Bartlett JG, Condon RE, Gorbach SL, et al. Veterans Administration Cooperative Study on bowel preparation for elective colorectal operations: impact of oral antibiotic regimen on colonic flora, wound irrigation cultures and bacteriology of septic complications. Ann Surg 188:249–254, 1978.
50. Stellato TA, Danziger LH, Gordon N, et al. Antibiotics in elective colon surgery: a randomized trial of oral, systemic, and oral/systemic antibiotics for prophylaxis. Am Surg 56:251–254, 1990.
51. Anstey JT, Sheldon GW, Blyth JG. Infectious morbidity after primary cesarean section in a private institution. Am J Obstet Gynecol 136:205–210, 1980.
52. Mugford M, Kingston J, Chalmers I. Reducing the incidence of infection after caesarean section: implications of prophylaxis with antibiotics for hospital resources. Br Med J 299:1003–1006, 1989.
53. Soper DE, Yarwood RL. Single-dose antibiotic prophylaxis in women undergoing vaginal hysterectomy. Obstet Gynecol 69:879–882, 1987.
54. Nichols RL. Surgical infections: prevention and treatment 1965 to 1995. Am J Surg 172:68–74, 1996.

CHAPTER 81

INFECTIONS IN THE IMMUNOSUPPRESSED PATIENT

William J. McIntyre

The human immune system serves many functions including homeostasis, surveillance, and defense. Defects in host defense can lead to a variety of infectious complications. This chapter reviews specific defects in the immune system and the infectious complications associated with those defects and discusses primarily the treatment of infection in neutropenic patients. However, many of the principles and treatments discussed in the section on neutropenia can also be applied to other immunocompromised patients. Acquired immune deficiency syndrome (AIDS) and its associated opportunistic infections are discussed in Chapter 77.

TREATMENT GOALS: INFECTIONS IN IMMUNOSUPPRESSED PATIENTS

- Identify inherited and acquired risk factors for infection in immunosuppressed patients.
- Identify the most common bacterial, fungal, and viral pathogens in immunosuppressed patients.
- Recommend appropriate empiric therapies for immunosuppressed patients based on patient-specific risk factors:
  - Identify forms of inherited immunocompromised states.
  - Define neutropenia.
  - Calculate an absolute neutrophil count.
  - Recommend an appropriate empiric regimen for a neutropenic patient.
  - List indications for the empiric use of antifungal agents in the immunosuppressed patient.
  - List indications for the empiric use of antiviral agents in the immunosuppressed patient.
  - Identify "low-risk" candidates for outpatient management of neutropenic fever.
  - Describe the indications for the use of prophylactic hematopoietic growth factors.

PATHOPHYSIOLOGY

An immunocompromised state is created by defects in the immune system. Immunodeficiency or immunosuppression occurs in patients as a result of either an inherited or an acquired defect. Inherited disorders are usually diagnosed shortly after birth and include diseases such as severe combined immune deficiency syndrome (SCIDS) and agammaglobulinemia. Acquired disorders can occur at any point in a patient's life and can be the result of chemotherapy, immunosuppressive agents (e.g., azathioprine, cyclosporine, and corticosteroids), radiation, or viruses (e.g., human immunodeficiency virus). The severity of the immunodeficiency varies in both inherited and acquired disorders. The types of infections seen in these patients are related to the specific defect and the severity of that defect. Defects can be seen in any component of the immune system. These defects can be generally classified into disorders of the mucocutaneous barriers, granulocytes, cellular immunity, complement synthesis, and antibody formation.[1,2]

The mucocutaneous barriers of the skin and respiratory, gastrointestinal (GI), and genitourinary tracts provide the body's initial and primary defense against pathogens. The loss of mucocutaneous barriers offers pathogens access to the host's internal organs. Breaches in mucocutaneous barriers are often iatrogenic, produced by a number of medical devices (central venous catheters, Foley catheters, and endotracheal tubes), procedures (surgery), and treatments (chemotherapy and radiation). Mechanical malfunctions may also occur, such as loss of the mucociliary mechanism of the lungs and decreased saliva production by salivary glands, resulting in a decreased ability to clear organisms from the bronchopulmonary tree and GI tract.[1]

Effects upon granulocytes can be quantitative or functional. A number of investigators have correlated the incidence of infection to the total granulocyte count, also called the absolute neutrophil count (ANC). A patient's ANC is determined by multiplying the total number of white blood cells (WBCs) by the percentage of circulating granulocytes (mature granulocytes plus band-immature white cell forms) that is obtained from a WBC differential count. In general, patients are said to be neutropenic or granulocytopenic if their total granulocyte count falls below 1000 cells/mm^3. However, some institutions use the stricter criterion of an ANC of ≤500 cells/mm^3 to define neutropenia. As the total granulocyte count falls below 1000 cells/mm^3, the rate of infection increases. When the total number of granulocytes falls below 100 cells/mm^3, the incidence of infection approaches 100%.[3] In some clinical practices the absolute phagocyte count (APC) is used. In addition to neutrophils the APC uses the number of circulating monocytes.

Granulocytopenic patients are particularly susceptible to infections by bacteria. The duration of granulocytopenia also has a profound effect on the rate of mortality from infections. The longer the patient is granulocytopenic, the greater the risk of infection by organisms. Granulocytes can also have functional abnormalities, which can be inherited or iatrogenic. Certain antineoplastic drugs, such as L-asparaginase and the vinca alkaloids, cause functional abnormalities that alter the granulocyte's ability to migrate and phagocytose bacteria, thus increasing the patient's susceptibility to infection.

The cellular immune system is primarily based on the interactions between macrophages and T lymphocytes. Cellular immunity provides protection against specific fungi, viruses, and protozoans. Impairment of cellular immunity is seen in patients who receive immunosuppressive agents (e.g., the corticosteroids or cyclosporine) and in patients with certain types of cancer (e.g., chronic lymphocytic leukemia, Hodgkin's disease, and non-Hodgkin's lymphoma).

Defects in complement synthesis, in antibody production, and in monocyte/macrophage systems can lead to recurrent pneumonia and sepsis by encapsulated organisms, such as *Streptococcus pneumoniae.* This increase in infection is caused by a loss of ability to opsonize bacteria. Opsonization describes the ability of antibodies and/or complement to attach to a pathogen, thereby enhancing its phagocytosis by monocytes and macrophages. Defects in opsonization and in the monocyte/macrophage system are seen in patients with complement deficiencies (angioedema), impaired antibody function (chronic lymphocytic leukemia), and decreased macrophage function (splenectomy).

Knowing the specific immune deficiency that a patient is experiencing helps predict likely pathogens and aid in choosing the appropriate initial therapies. However, patients rarely have just one specific deficiency. In immunocompromised hosts, a number of the components of the immune system are usually affected. This point is well illustrated in patients undergoing cancer treatment. In many patients with cancer, the disease itself predisposes the patient to infection. Tumors can invade normal tissues leading to tissue destruction, necrosis, and loss of normal barriers. Tumor invasion of the bone marrow can lead to "crowding out," a decreased production of normal hematopoietic cells, thus resulting in leukopenia. In addition, hematologic tumors, such as lymphoma, leukemia, and myeloma, may directly impair cell-mediated and antibody-mediated immunity.

Cancer treatment modalities affect host defenses. For the delivery of chemotherapy and supportive care, patients often require central venous catheters and Foley catheters. These devices provide a site for pathogenic invasion and colonization, particularly by Gram-positive bacteria and fungi. Mucocutaneous barriers may be further compromised by radiation- and chemotherapy-induced mucositis. Patients with mucositis have a predilection for developing infections by Gram-negative bacteria and *Candida* species. In addition to producing bone marrow suppression and neutropenia, individual antineoplastic agents may affect specific functions of the immune system as illustrated in Table 81.1.[4] Prolonged treatment with antineoplastic drugs has an impact on cellular immunity, as well as on granulocyte function. Compromised cellular immunity increases the risk of developing an opportunistic fungal or viral infection.

Among the most immunocompromised patients are children with SCIDS. SCIDS is an autosomal disorder characterized by a lack of cellular and humoral immunity. Patients with SCIDS fail to produce antibodies upon exposure to an antigen and fail to respond to cutaneous skin testing (anergy). During the first year of life, patients frequently present with opportunistic infections caused by *Candida, Pneumocystis carinii,* and viruses.

In the past, SCIDS was fatal unless the patient received a bone marrow transplant or was maintained in a protective environment–"bubble children." Recently, new approaches have been attempted. Forty percent of patients with SCIDS have a deficiency in adenosine deaminase (ADA).[5] ADA is responsible for preventing the toxic accumulation of deoxyadenosine in lymphocytes. Replace-

Table 81.1 ▪ Examples of the Effects of Chemotherapy Agents on the Immune System

Effect	Sample Agent
Myelosuppression	Alkylating agents Antimetabolites
Impaired cellular immunity	Cyclophosphamide Corticosteroids
Impaired antibody dysfunction	Cyclophosphamide Corticosteroids Alkylating agents Antimetabolites
Impaired chemotaxis	Vincristine
Phagocyte dysfunction	Corticosteroids

Table 81.2 ▪ Causes of Death in Neutropenic Patients

Complication	% Patients with Findings
Infection	35
Hemorrhage	27
Progression of cancer	18
Miscellaneous	20
Renal insufficiency	
Myocardial infarction	
Carcinoma meningitis	
Acute pulmonary edema	

ment therapy using pegademase bovine (polyethylene glycol-modified ADA bovine, [Adagen]) at 15 IU/kg IM weekly has benefited some patients. Gene therapy is currently being evaluated as a possible means to incorporate the ADA gene into the patients' lymphocytes.[6]

Among the most severe of the iatrogenic immunocompromised states is found in patients undergoing bone marrow transplantation (BMT). The myelotoxic conditioning regimens for BMT consist of high-dose chemotherapy and/or radiation that produces severe and prolonged neutropenia. To prevent graft-versus-host disease and graft rejection in patients receiving donor bone marrow (allogenic BMT), T-cell function must be suppressed. This is achieved either through purging the donor marrow of T cells or through the use of immunosuppressive agents, such as cyclosporine, methotrexate, and corticosteroids. Deficiencies in both antibody function and cellular immunity have been found to exist for up to 2 years after BMT.

The largest group of immunosuppressed patients are those receiving antineoplastic agents. Once neutropenia develops, these patients are highly susceptible to infection. Fever in a neutropenic patient is treated as a medical emergency; death due to sepsis may occur within 48 to 72 hours, if the appropriate antibiotic treatment is not initiated immediately. The rest of this chapter focuses on the treatment of the neutropenic patient.

CLINICAL PRESENTATION AND DIAGNOSIS

Over the past 20 years, great strides have been made in the treatment of infections in the neutropenic patient.[7] Even though the initial morbidity and mortality from infection have diminished substantially as a result of improvements in antibiotic therapy, infection is still the leading cause of death in patients with cancer (Table 81.2).[7,8] The reasons for this are not completely clear. In one retrospective review of 410 neutropenic patients with fever, 49 died during or after the neutropenic episode.[8] Nineteen died from bacterial or fungal infection. The remainder of the deaths were caused by noninfectious complications including disease progression.

The treatment of cancer has been refined, and chemotherapeutic regimens are becoming much more aggressive. Therefore, more patients are developing neutropenia for a longer period of time, and consequently have a greater risk of developing a life-threatening infection. Investigators have also shown that the more advanced the cancer, the greater the chance the patient will die of an infection.[9] Fungal organisms are becoming increasingly implicated as the cause of infections and death in the neutropenic patient. In one study, up to 58% of autopsies performed on patients who died of cancer showed pathologic signs of an invasive fungal infection.[10] Infections due to fungi are often more difficult to eradicate than bacterial infections. The Infectious Diseases Society of America has published guidelines for treatment of febrile neutropenic patients.[11]

Signs and Symptoms

The classic signs of infection (e.g., redness, swelling, tenderness, and heat) are absent owing to the lack of granulocytes. Often, the only sign of infection is fever, and fever is not always caused by infection. Fever can be induced by the administration of blood products and medications, further complicating the diagnosis. In actuality, infection is only documented in approximately 60% of neutropenic patients presenting with fever (Table 81.3).[1] Therefore, most often antibiotic treatment is initiated without any documented of the infective organism (empiric).

Diagnosis

Diagnosing an infection in a granulocytopenic patient can be difficult. Because the treatment must be initiated empirically, the clinician must know what organism to suspect. In 80% of the culture-documented infections in neutropenic patients, the infecting organism is either a Gram-negative or Gram-positive bacterium. The most common organisms are *Pseudomonas aeruginosa, Escherichia coli, Klebsiella pneumoniae, Staphylococcus aureus, and Staphylococcus epidermidis.* The other 20% of the documented infections are caused by fungi, viruses, or protozoans. Before the release of methicillin, the majority of the infections were caused by Gram-positive bacteria. Subsequently, Gram-negative bacteria became the primary cause

Table 81.3 ▪ Outcome of Infection in the Febrile Neutropenic Patient

Evidence of Infection	% Patients with Findings
Documented infection	60
Microbiologically documented (infection with bacteremia)	20
Microbiologically documented (infection without bacteremia)	20
Clinically documented infection	20
Fever of undetermined origin	20
Fever of noninfectious origin (e.g., blood product, medication)	20

of infection in neutropenic patients. In general, the pattern appears to be changing again; infections caused by *P. aeruginosa* are decreasing, and infections caused by Gram-positive organisms are increasing. *S. epidermidis* has become a major pathogen because of use of central venous catheters (e.g., Hickman catheters) in patients with cancer.[12,13] The increased incidence of infection by *S. epidermidis* is important because this organism is often (i.e., >60 to 80%) methicillin-resistant. The main point that needs to be emphasized is that the primary group of organisms causing infections in this patient population is always changing. Therefore, it is important for the clinician to know the primary pathogens cultured from neutropenic patients at their setting or institution.[14]

The sources of infection in neutropenic patients are primarily the GI tract (i.e., normal flora from the mouth and alimentary canal) and the respiratory tract (Table 81.4). Pizzo et al.[15] demonstrated that 80% of infections arise from organisms that colonize the patient. However, 50% of these organisms were acquired by the patient in the hospital and may be resistant to standard antibiotics. It would appear from the above data that surveillance cultures (cultures used to monitor colonization) would supply beneficial information. However, investigation has shown that routine use of surveillance cultures is not cost-effective.[16] Surveillance cultures were of limited value because (1) no one site of colonization consistently predicted the offending pathogen; (2) other potential pathogens were usually cultured at the same time; (3) if a useful culture was obtained it was usually after initiation of antibiotic therapy; and (4) the current practice of using broad-spectrum antibiotics covers the vast majority of potential pathogens in the neutropenic host.[16] Therefore, surveillance cultures should not be used routinely to monitor colonization of patients.

When granulocytopenic patients develop a fever, a careful physical examination should be performed to locate any possible source of infection. The patient's medication and transfusion records should be checked to ensure that the fever is not related to either of these potential causes. Before antibiotic therapy is initiated, culture specimens should be obtained from the following fluids or sites: sputum, urine, throat, and blood. Duplicate sets of blood cultures should be obtained if a patient has a central venous catheter (i.e., one set from the central venous catheter and one set from a peripheral venipuncture). Duplicate cultures may help determine if the central venous catheter site is infected. In the case of an infected catheter site, blood cultures from the catheter may be positive, whereas peripheral blood cultures are negative. Specimens for culture should also be taken from area that appears infected, such as a venipuncture site or bone marrow aspiration site. After the appropriate cultures have been collected, empiric antibiotic therapy should be initiated immediately to prevent early mortality.

Table 81.4 ▪ Source of Infection in a Neutropenic Patient

Oral cavity	Nose and sinuses
Trachea, bronchi, or lungs	Intravenous catheter sites
Intestine and esophagus	

TREATMENT

Pharmacotherapy

Antibacterial Therapy

Antibiotic therapy will be empiric and chosen to be effective against the most common pathogens seen at the institution. Antibiotic therapy in the febrile neutropenic patient has traditionally been combination therapy with either two or three drug regimens. However, with the introduction of the broad-spectrum antipseudomonal cephalosporins (e.g., cefoperazone, ceftazidime, and cefepime) and the carbapenems (imipenem/cilastatin and meropenem), single-agent therapy is a consideration. In selecting empiric therapy three principles should always be followed. First, antibiotics must be administered at the maximum prescribed dose. Next, broad-spectrum therapy should be selected whether the clinician decides to administer single-agent or combination therapy. Finally, the choice of antibiotic(s) must take into account the resistance patterns of the institution.[12]

Many antibiotic combinations have been investigated in the treatment of infections in the neutropenic patient. Antibiotic combinations fall into four categories:

1. An antipseudomonal β-lactam plus an aminoglycoside.
2. A semisynthetic penicillin plus a third-generation cephalosporin (double β-lactam).
3. A third-generation anti-pseudomonal cephalosporin or carbapenem (monotherapy).
4. Vancomycin plus any of the above regimens, depending on various factors.

With the emergence of vancomycin-resistant enterococci (VRE), there is an increased need to limit the use of empiric vancomycin. One approach may be to include vancomycin in the initial regimen, but to discontinue the vancomycin if cultures for Gram-positive organisms are negative. A second approach in stable patients is to restrict the use of empiric vancomycin and to add vancomycin if cultures are positive for methicillin-resistant organisms,

Other factors important in the selection of antibiotics include rapidity of bactericidal activity, efficacy in the neutropenic patient, pharmacokinetics of the antibiotics, potential for synergy between the antibiotics, and toxic effects.[12] Table 81.5 lists a number of studies that investigated the treatment of infections in the granulocytopenic patient. In general, early morbidity and mortality are seen from infection with Gram-negative organisms. Therefore, the majority of regimens initially protect against Gram-negative bacteria.[10] Recently however, group A streptococci have been associated with fulminant

Table 81.5 ▪ Antibiotic Combinations Studied in the Neutropenic Patient

Drugs	Overall % Responses	Reference
Semisynthetic penicillins and aminoglycosides		
Carbenicillin-gentamicin	83	17
Ticarcillin-amikacin	80	18
Ticarcillin-gentamicin	97	19
Third-generation cephalosporin-aminoglycoside		
Moxalactam-amikacin	83	18
Ceftazidime-tobramycin	71	20
Cefoperazone-amikacin	88	21
Semisynthetic penicillins and third-generation cephalosporins		
Piperacillin-moxalactam	77	22
Ticarcillin-moxalactam	65	23
Miscellaneous combinations		
Piperacillin-vancomycin	72	24
Trimethoprim/sulfamethoxazole plus ticarcillin	7	25

infections. When the literature is reviewed, it becomes obvious that the majority of antibiotic studies show a 65 to 97% overall response rate when appropriate antibiotic combinations are used. Therefore, Table 81.5 is not a list of the "ideal" combinations, but it provides a reference point when comparing antibiotic combinations.

When combination antibiotic regimens are used, the antibiotics included in the combination should be synergistic. The organism should be susceptible to at least two of the antibiotics for the patient to receive the maximum benefit from the combination regimen. In neutropenic patients, Klastersky et al.[26] showed that if two synergistic antibiotics (against the cultured organism) were used the cure rate of infection was 80%. If the antibiotics used were not synergistic, the cure rate was only 49%. Even if the antibiotics used do not demonstrate true synergy, studies have shown as long as the agents are active against the cultured organism the response rate is improved when compared to regimens in which only one of the antibiotics shows activity.[27,28] In addition, the bactericidal activity of the antibiotics is important to consider. Bactericidal activity can be measured by drawing peak or trough serum samples to measure the activity of the antibiotics administered by performing serial dilutions of the serum, which are then cultured with the patient's infecting organism. A peak serum bactericidal titer of 1:16 or greater correlated with a favorable clinical response in 87% of infected neutropenic patients.[28] Trough serum bacteria titers are reported to provide no additional information.

Some investigators have challenged the need for an aminoglycoside in empiric regimens. It is important to note that aminoglycosides have been found to be less effective in neutropenia patients.[29] In one study, the addition of an aminoglycoside to an antipseudomonal penicillin had no advantage over the antipseudomonal penicillin alone.[30] If aminoglycosides are used in an antibacterial regimen, peak and trough levels of the aminoglycoside should be monitored regularly. Concentrations of gentamicin or tobramycin that should be attained in this patient population are between 6 and 8 μg/mL for the peak level and between 1 and 2 μ/mL for the trough level.[31]

With the introduction of the third-generation cephalosporins, there has been renewed interest in monotherapy (single-agent therapy) for the treatment of infections in neutropenic patients. Good results have been obtained in trials with monotherapy. The benefits of single-agent therapy in the neutropenic patient include the following: nephrotoxicity can be avoided because aminoglycosides are not being used; patients receive less intravenous fluid, and single-agent therapy is less expense therapy than traditional combination therapy. However, single-agent therapy does have some drawbacks. With single-agent therapy, the antibiotic being used must be effective against the infecting organism. If not, the patient basically has no antibiotic protection. The third-generation cephalosporins have gaps in their protective effects (i.e., Gram-positive organisms). Also, the beneficial effects of synergism will not be utilized. The third-generation cephalosporins have theoretical advantages because they provide broad protection against Gram-negative bacteria, they attain high bactericidal concentrations in the serum, and many have long plasma half-lives. Imipenem/cilastatin has also been shown to be effective as a single agent. Ceftazidine and imipenem/cilastin have been compared in a randomized trial. Both regimens were equally effective for the management of fever in neutropenic patients.[32] However, the addition of an agent for protection against anaerobic bacteria (metronidazole and clindamycin) was more frequent in patients treated with ceftazidine, whereas patients treated with imipenem/cilastatin experienced more episodes of nausea. More than half of the patients in the trial required modification of the initial monotherapy. Table 81.6 lists some studies that have investigated single-agent therapy. In all of these studies, the investigators recommended either close monitoring of the patient for treatment failures or the addition of a second agent

Table 81.6 ▪ Monotherapy–Single-Agent Antibiotic Studies in Febrile Neutropenic Patients

Drug	Average Dose	Overall % Response	Reference
Ceftazidime	2 g q8hr	95	31
Ceftazidime	2 g q8hr	60	20
Cefoperazone	6 g q12hr	77	21
Moxalactam	1.5 g q8hr	80	33
Imipenem	500 mg q6hr	74	34

initially to protect against Gram-positive organisms. Therefore, at the present time, single-agent therapy is not recommended without close observation of the patient. These regimens may require early modification. It is recommend that monotherapy be limited to patients with an ANC of 500 to 1000 cells/mm^3 who are experiencing short periods of neutropenia.[35]

Antifungal Therapy

If febrile neutropenic patients do not respond to antibacterial agents within 4 to 7 days and no evidence of bacterial infection is documented, antifungal therapy should be initiated.[36] After bacteria, fungi are the next most likely cause of infection in the neutropenic patient. The incidence of fungal infection increases dramatically in patients with prolonged granulocytopenia.[1,3,7,10] A major obstacle in the treatment of fungal infections is making the diagnosis. Fungal cultures can be negative in the presence of a true fungal infection.[10] In addition, no good serologic tests for the diagnosis of fungal infections currently exist.[36] On the other hand, fungal organisms can be cultured from a number of different sites and fluids including those from nares, throat, sputum, and stool.[37] Often, fungal organisms cultured from these sites represent only colonization; yet, in the febrile neutropenic patient, the risk is too great and treatment should be initiated. A true diagnosis of fungal infection can only be made when the culture is obtained from a sterile site or by histologic examination.[3]

The majority of these infections are caused by *Candida albicans*. However, other *Candida* species such as *Candida glabrata, Candida krusei,* and *Candida tropicalis* must be considered. *Candida* species tend to infect the mucous membranes of the GI and urinary tracts, but can cause cutaneous or disseminated infections. Other common fungal pathogens include *Aspergillus*, *Fusarium*, and *Trichosporon* species.

Aspergillus infections occur rarely in immunocompetent patients. In an immunosuppressed patient, the organism is pathogenic, and infection is often fatal. In most cases, patients acquire the organism by inhalation of *Aspergillus* spores dispersed in the air. Because *Aspergillus* organisms are normally present in the soil, fungal spores may seed the air in areas near excavation or construction. Outbreaks of *Aspergillus* infections during periods of construction support this. *Aspergillus* infections occur primarily in two sites of the body: the sinuses and the lungs. Risk factors for infection include prolonged granulocytopenia (>30 days), severe neutropenia (ANC <100 cells/mm^3 for >7days), and graft versus host disease. Although prolonged granulocytopenia is the major risk factor for the development of fungal infection, broad-spectrum antibiotic and corticosteroid therapy can influence the development of fungal infection.[38]

Aspergillosis actually is a rare disease, but it is extremely difficult to treat.[39] Treatment of the infection must be extremely aggressive with resection of the infected area if possible followed by administration of amphotericin B. The *Aspergillus* organism is only moderately sensitive to amphotericin B. Rifampin or flucytosine have been used in combination with amphotericin B to increase efficacy.[40] Amphotericin B as single-drug therapy remains the "gold standard " for fungal infections. However, the possibility of severe side effects makes many clinicians somewhat reluctant to initiate amphotericin B as empiric therapy. Fluconazole, although it is a fungistatic drug, has gained some acceptance as empiric therapy.

Amphotericin B has activity against *C. albicans* but limited efficacy against *Aspergillus* and *Cryptococcus*. The dose of amphotericin B is 0.5 to 1.0 mg/kg of body weight per day. The manufacturer of amphotericin B recommends that a test dose of 1 mg be administered and followed by slow titration up to the calculated maintenance dose to limit adverse reactions. However, in neutropenic patients with a documented fungal infection, the dose should be escalated rapidly to the maintenance dose. Early initiation of amphotericin B therapy may decrease the risk of invasive fungal disease.[14] The duration of amphotericin B therapy depends on whether a positive diagnosis of a fungal infection has been made. The patient with a verified fungal infection should receive a total of 500 to 3000 mg of amphotericin B. If no positive diagnosis of a fungal infection has been made, the drug may be stopped when the total neutrophil count is greater than 500 cells/mm^3.[36]

Amphotericin B side effects can fall into two categories: immediate and dose related. Immediate side effects include fever, chills, and rigor. Patients receiving amphotericin B can be pretreated with acetaminophen, diphenhydramine, and hydrocortisone in an attempt to eliminate the immediate symptoms. Often, pretreatment is not effective, and the patient must endure the side effects. Long-term adverse effects from amphotericin B include renal toxicity and, rarely, bone marrow suppression. If patients develop renal toxicity due to amphotericin B, they will lose large amounts of potassium and magnesium. If renal failure does develop, it is usually reversible once the drug has been discontinued. Lipid-complex amphotericin B products are associated with decreased renal toxicity compared to amphotericin B. Data for the use of lipid-complex amphotericin B products are still limited in neutropenic patients.[41]

Ketoconazole is an oral antifungal agent with good activity against *C. albicans*.[39] An imidazole derivative, ketoconazole is only effective against fungal organisms in a growth phase. This medication is only indicated for superficial *Candida* infection and should never be prescribed when an invasive process is suspected or diagnosed. Side effects include adrenal suppression and hepatotoxicity. The usual dose of ketoconazole is 200 to 400 mg/day. Ketoconazole requires an acidic environment for absorption from the GI tract.

Fluconazole is the first of a new class of broad-spectrum bis-triazole antifungal agents. The fungistatic activity of fluconazole is related to the inhibition of fungal cytochrome P-450 sterol ^{14}C α-demethylation, resulting in an accumulation of ^{14}C α-methyl sterols in the fungus. Fluconazole is currently approved for use in oropharyngeal candidiasis, systemic candidal infections, and cryptococcal meningitis. Its role in treatment of neutropenic patients remains to be defined.[40] It is promising because of its lack of toxicity compared to amphotericin B. The usual oral dose for systemic candidiasis is 400 mg the first day, followed by 200 mg every day for 4 weeks. For esophageal candidiasis, the dose is 200 mg the first day followed by 100 mg every day for 2 weeks. Because fluconazole is eliminated by the kidneys, the dose must be adjusted in patients with renal insufficiency. The use of fluconazole in patients with cryptococcal meningitis is discussed in Chapter 77. Itraconazole, an oral triazole, has excellent activity against *Aspergillus* species, but its role in the treatment of granulocytopenia is yet to be clearly defined.[42]

Antiviral Therapy

Viral infections can be seen in patients with acute leukemia who are neutropenic as a result of aggressive chemotherapy, but the infections occur more frequently in patients receiving organ transplants (i.e., kidney, heart, liver, and bone marrow).[43] Patients receiving organ transplants may be severely immunosuppressed to prevent rejection of the transplanted organ. Viruses are responsible for up to 33% of deaths in the population with transplants.[44] The mortality from viral infection (particularly from cytomegalovirus [CMV] infection) is extremely high in patients with bone marrow transplants.[45,46] Viral infection can either be a primary infection in which the host is infected for the first time or a reactivated infection where the virus has been harbored in a nerve root ganglion (e.g., herpes viruses) or within WBCs (e.g., CMV). The main goal in the treatment of viral infections is to prevent the spread of the virus systemically (i.e., to the brain, lungs, or GI tract). At no time should an immunosuppressed patient receive live or attenuated viral vaccines, because these vaccines may result in viral infection.

Herpes simplex virus (HSV) infections can be caused by either type I or type II viruses. In the immunocompromised host, approximately 85% of the infections affect the oral cavity with the other 15% involving the genital area.[47] An oral herpes infection is usually diffuse and can be extremely painful, preventing the patient from taking in adequate oral nutrition. The herpetic lesion can also serve as a focus for secondary bacterial infections.[47] Herpes infections frequently occur within the first 17 days after the initiation of chemotherapy for patients with bone marrow transplants.[46]

The treatment of choice for HSV infections is acyclovir.[48,49] Acyclovir is a prodrug, which is metabolized by viral thymidine kinase. The metabolized drug is a potent inhibitor of herpes simplex and varicella zoster DNA polymerases. Acyclovir has been shown to be highly effective in the treatment of herpes infections in various types of immunosuppressed patient populations.[47,49] It has significantly reduced morality related to HSV in patients with bone marrow transplants.[46] The intravenous dose used in the treatment of herpes simplex is 5 mg/kg of body weight every 8 hours (or 250 mg/m^2 every 8 hours). There are relatively few side effects from this acyclovir regimen, except for thrombophlebitis in peripheral veins owing to the alkaline nature of the drug. Also, normal urine output should be maintained during therapy to prevent crystallization of the drug in the renal tubules. The dose of acyclovir should be adjusted in patients with significant renal failure because it, and its metabolites are eliminated renally. Topical acyclovir alone should not be prescribed in patients with widespread disease because of an increased risk of disseminated viral disease.[44]

Varicella-zoster virus (VZV), in its initial infection, is a communicable virus of the herpes family. It usually causes chickenpox in childhood upon initial exposure (primary disease) and then becomes latent. In immunosuppressed patients, the virus may reactivate, usually visible along a dermatomal pattern. VZV can also cause disseminated infection with pneumonia, encephalitis, hepatitis, and pancreatitis, but rarely in immunocompetent patients. In an investigation of children receiving chemotherapy for malignancies who subsequently developed VZV infection, 32% developed disseminated disease and 7% died of the infection.[50] The greatest risk of developing disseminated VZV occurred in patients whose total granulocyte count was below 500 cells/mm^3. Therefore, children with malignancies, immunosuppressed patients, and patients with bone marrow transplants who are exposed to someone with primary VZV (e.g., chickenpox) whose respiratory secretions are infectious, should receive passive immunization with varicella-zoster immune globulin (VZIG). The dose of VZIG is based on the patient's body weight and the varicella serum titer. VZV infection can be treated successfully with either vidarabine or acyclovir. Vidarabine has been shown to be effective in the treatment of varicella-zoster if it is initiated within 72 hours from the onset of the symptoms.[50] The intravenous dose of vidarabine is 10 mg/kg of body weight per day given as a continuous 12-hour infusion. However, the side effects of vidarabine such as GI distress, fluid overload, megaloblastic anemia, hallucinations, and seizures have limited its clinical usefulness. The treatment of choice for VZV is acyclovir.[51] The best clinical results with resolution of symptoms are seen when the acyclovir is administered early in the course of the disease.[50] The intravenous dose of acyclovir for the treatment of a VZV infection is higher than that for HSV infection (10 mg/kg of body weight every 8 hours or 500 mg/m^2 every 8 hours). Again, dosage adjustment of acyclovir is needed in patients with significant renal impairment.

CMV is an opportunistic virus from the herpes family, which causes few symptoms in an immunocompetent patient,[51] but becomes a serious pathogen in immunosuppressed patients. CMV infection in the population with bone marrow transplants is responsible for 15 to 20% of all deaths. Infection from CMV can cause pneumonia, retinitis, hepatitis, and bone marrow suppression, as just some of its disseminated manifestations.[45] CMV disease can originate from a primary infection or can be caused by reactivation of the latent virus, as with VZV. CMV can also be transmitted by a blood transfusion or organ transplantation as CMV is sequestered in WBCs.[45,52] Infection in the lungs is usually the most severe form. Patients with CMV pneumonia present with fever, dyspnea, and a nonproductive cough. On chest x-ray, the infection appears as an interstitial pneumonia with bilateral infiltrates. Respiratory function deteriorates rapidly, with patients often dying of respiratory failure.

A number of antiviral medications have been tried in the past for treatment of CMV disease including vidarabine, acyclovir, and interferon, but none of these drugs has effectively controlled the infection.[51–53] On the other hand, ganciclovir, foscarnet, and intravenous immunoglobulin (IVIG) have demonstrated some efficacy. Studies with ganciclovir have been conducted in patients with bone marrow transplants who have documented CMV pneumonia.[53] Despite good in vitro activity against CMV, ganciclovir alone did not change the outcome of the disease. Similarly, in limited trials in patients with bone marrow transplants, foscarnet was of limited value. The combination of ganciclovir and IVIG has been the most effective treatment of CMV infection and has been reported to increase survival, although mortality was still high.[54] Single-agent therapy with ganciclovir and foscarnet may be more useful in the treatment of disseminated CMV infection in other immunosuppressed patient populations (e.g., patients with AIDS and patients with renal transplants)[55] and in patients who have CMV infections in organs other than the lung (e.g., retina, liver, or GI tract).

Epstein-Barr virus (EBV), another herpes virus (notably causing mononucleosis), has been associated with pneumonia and leukopenia in the immunosuppressed patient population. EBV-associated lymphoma has also been described in patients receiving transplants with bone marrow that was T-cell depleted.[56] High-dose acyclovir and α-interferon have been used to treat the infection.[57]

Antibacterial Decontamination Therapy and Other Prophylaxis Regimens

Patients in protective isolation also receive total microbial suppression that includes both antibacterial and antifungal prophylaxis. Topical cleaners are applied to decontaminate the skin, and oral nonabsorbable antibiotics are given to clean the GI tract. Examples of nonabsorbable antibiotics that have been used include oral vancomycin (500 mg) and oral gentamicin (160 mg) given three to four times a day.[58] Although in the era of VRE, widespread use of oral vancomycin is not routinely recommended. The nonabsorbable antibiotic regimens that are used are not very palatable and compliance after several weeks is poor. In addition, if patients stop taking the oral antibiotic, they can be colonized with organisms that are resistant to many antibiotics and ultimately they become infected with these resistant organisms.[15]

An alternative method of microbial prophylaxis is called selective decontamination, which involves the use of antimicrobial agents to selectively suppress Gram-negative organisms. Selective decontamination involves a concept of colonization resistance. The concept of colonization resistance states that anaerobic bacteria provide protection in the GI tract from colonization with pathogenic bacteria and if the anaerobic bacteria are killed off, colonization with pathogenic organisms will occur. Therefore, if antibacterial agents that suppress Gram-negative organisms but leave anaerobic flora intact are given orally, colonization with a more virulent organism should not be seen. The two antimicrobial agents that have been administered as selective decontaminates are trimethoprim/sulfamethoxazole and nalidixic acid. The drug that has been most studied for this effect is the former. Results from the various studies have been somewhat contradictory. The dose of trimethoprim/sulfamethoxazole in studies investigating selective decontamination ranged from one single-strength tablet to one double-strength tablet orally two to three times a day. From these studies, trimethoprim/sulfamethoxazole appears to decrease the rate of infection in patients who are neutropenic for a prolonged period of time (longer than 7 days).[59–63] Patients with short-term neutropenia, however, have not had significant benefits from trimethoprim/sulfamethoxazole prophylaxis.[63] Trimethoprim/sulfamethoxazole has been compared directly to nalidixic acid for decontamination antibacterial prophylaxis.[64] Both of the therapies were efficacious, but the investigator stated that both regimens had disadvantages. The GI tracts of patients in both study groups became colonized with resistant organisms, which could have lead to superinfection. The primary disadvantage of trimethoprim/sulfamethoxazole is its myelosuppressive side effects, which in turn could prolong the neutropenia. In several studies, the period of neutropenia for patients receiving trimethoprim/sulfamethoxazole was longer than that of the control group.[64] Ciprofloxacin has been shown to be an effective alternative to trimethoprim/sulfamethoxazole.[65] However, because quinolones are so broad-spectrum, there is the concern of increased fungal overgrowth. In summary, it appears that both total microbial decontamination and selective decontamination are effective in decreasing the incidence of infections when used appropriately, but should only be used for patients who are expected to have an extremely prolonged neutropenic episode.[15,64,66]

Antifungal agents are also administered prophylactically to decrease the incidence of superficial fungal infections and fungal colonization caused by *C. albicans*, which may eventually lead to serious systemic infection. The agents used include nystatin suspension (15 mL orally four times a day), clotrimazole troches (10 mg orally five times a day), ketoconazole (200 to 400 mg orally once a day), and fluconazole (200 to 400 mg daily). One of these medications is usually combined with an antibacterial prophylactic regimen to give broad-spectrum coverage for both fungal and bacterial organisms. In patients undergoing BMT, prophylactic fluconazole has been shown to effectively decrease systematic candidiasis. All of these drugs are efficacious in the treatment of superficial fungal infection and suppression of *Candida* in the GI tract, but both nystatin suspension and clotrimazole troches can cause nausea and vomiting. Ketoconazole may be more effective than nystatin, but in a comparison study, there was an increase in colonization of torulopsis.[67] Therefore, the selection of an antifungal prophylactic agent should be made according to the patient's preference.

Antiviral prophylaxis is aimed primarily at HSV and CMV. In both cases antiviral prophylaxis should only be administered to patients who are going to be severely immunosuppressed (i.e., patients with acute leukemia undergoing induction therapy, and patients with bone marrow transplants).[68] Again the prophylactic antiviral agent of choice for HSV is acyclovir.[6,69] Acyclovir 5 mg/kg every 8 hours is given at the same dose used for treatment. The use of prophylactic medication for the prevention of CMV infection appears to be effective. In several studies, intravenous immunoglobulins have been administered to patients with bone marrow transplants to prevent CMV pneumonitis.[70,71] These include CMV-selected immunoglobulins (CMV-IVIG) and IVIG. Cost must be a consideration because IVIG therapy is expensive. Therefore, the administration of IVIG for viral prophylaxis is limited to high-risk populations (e.g., patients with bone marrow transplants).[72]

P. carinii is another opportunistic organism causing pneumonia (PCP) in immunosuppressed patients. Patients who are infected with *P. carinii* develop pneumonia and respiratory failure. Studies have demonstrated that a double-strength trimethoprim/sulfamethoxazole tablet given twice a day or three times per week is adequate to treat PCP in severely immunosuppressed patients.[73–75]

Adjunctive Therapy

The hematopoietic growth factors, granulocyte-macrophage colony-stimulating factor (GM-CSF) and granulocyte colony-stimulating factor (G-CSF), have both been used in the treatment of and prophylaxis for neutropenia. GM-CSF produces an increase in granulocytes, monocytes, and eosinophils. G-CSF affects the precursors of the neutrophil lineage. In addition, the administration of these agents may cause the release of other stimulating factors, which may directly or indirectly affect other cell lines, such as erythrocytes and platelets. Through stimulating monocyte and myeloid precursors, these agents have been shown to decrease the duration of neutropenia and thereby decrease the risk of infection.[76,77] The American Society of Clinical Oncology recommended the guidelines shown in Table 81.7 for use of hematopoietic growth factors.

Table 81.7 ▪ ASCO Guidelines for Colony-Stimulating Factor Use

Generally recommended
1. Myelosuppressive regimens with an incidence of neutropenia >40%
2. In patients experiencing febrile neutropenia in prior episodes of chemotherapy, where chemotherapy dose reduction is not indicated
3. After autologous bone marrow transplantation
4. Mobilization for collection of peripheral blood progenitor cells

Special uses
1. In patient with prolonged neutropenia or at high risk of sepsis
2. In neutropenic patients with myelodysplasia
3. With caution, in patients with acute myeloid leukemia after initial therapy

Not generally recommended
1. In afebrile neutropenic patients
2. After allogeneic bone marrow transplantation

Not generally recommended
1. Concurrently with chemotherapy
2. To support chemotherapy dose intensity outside of a clinical trial
3. For acute myeloid leukemia priming, outside a clinical trial

Recommended dosages
- Neutropenia
  - G-CSF 5 μg/kg/day SC started 24 to 72 hr postchemotherapy until ANC >10,000 cells/mm^3
  - GM-CSF 250 μg/kg/day IV over 2 hr or SC started 24 to 72 hr postchemotherapy until ANC >10,000 cells/mm^3
- Bone marrow transplantation
  - G-CSF 10 to 20 μg/kg/day SC started 24 to 72 hr postchemotherapy until ANC >10,000 cells/mm^3
  - GM-CSF 250 μg/kg/day IV over 2 hr or SC started 24 to 72 hr postchemotherapy until ANC >10,000 cells/mm^3

G-CSF, granulocyte colony-stimulating factor; *GM-CSF*, granulocyte-macrophage colony-stimulating factor.

At standard doses, both GM-CSF and G-CSF are well tolerated; side effects are usually limited to fever, chills, rash, fluid retention, and bone pain. Higher doses have been associated with more serious adverse effects, such as pulmonary edema and effusions. The frequency of bone pain increases in proportion to the dose. Nonsteroidal anti-inflammatory drugs have been reported to relieve this pain.

The efficacy and safety of administering granulocyte transfusions therapeutically and prophylactically in neutropenic patients have been investigated. Granulocyte transfusions have some benefit in neutropenic patients with documented infection.[78] Conversely, studies looking at the potential benefits of administering prophylactic granulocytes have shown no advantage in the groups receiving these transfusions,[79,80] and in one study the granulocyte prophylaxis group did slightly worse.[80] Adverse reactions seen from the GM-CSF and G-CSF transfusions, such as pulmonary infiltrates, increased incidence of activated CMV infections, and cross-matching problems, also limit the utility of this therapy.

Therefore, at the present time, granulocyte transfusion should only be administered to patients with a documented infection that is not responding to appropriate antibiotic therapy.[78]

Nonpharmacologic Therapy

Prophylactic antibiotics and protective environment procedures have been beneficial in certain neutropenic patient populations. Theoretically, the number of infections in all neutropenic patients could be reduced because 80% of the documented infections arise from endogenous bacterial and fungal flora.[15] Therefore, if the number of organisms colonizing a patient are decreased or completely eliminated, the infection rate in these patients could be reduced. If a prophylactic regimen used to decrease colonization were effective, morbidity and mortality would also be reduced. In addition, complications from systemic antibiotic administration would be decreased because patients would not require antibiotics as often. There are four strategies that can be used to decrease the rate of infection. They include (1) bolstering the host defense mechanisms; (2) reducing damage to natural body barriers; (3) reducing the acquisition of new organisms from the environment; and (4) suppressing the potential pathogenic organisms that currently colonize the patient.[15] The benefits of these strategies, however, have only been shown in patients with prolonged neutropenia.

The first three strategies are measures used in the general care of the patient. Procedures to enhance host defenses include proper nutrition, use of immunostimulants, and resolution of neutropenia as rapidly as possible. The most important aspect of bolstering the host defense is proper nutrition. If the patient has good nutritional intake, his or her response to stress and infection will be improved.

Protection of natural host barriers helps limit access of potential pathogens to the systemic circulation. Limiting the number of venipunctures and bone marrow aspirations will decrease the number of breaks in the skin. Rectal administration of drugs should be avoided to avert the induction of enteric bacteria into the blood. Invasive procedures such as urinary catheterization should be avoided to prevent colonization. Health care personnel and visitors should wash their hands thoroughly each time they enter a patient's room to help prevent the transfer of organisms from patient to patient. Attention to these general aspects of infection control can help reduce infectious complications in the neutropenic patient.

A strategy that can decrease the rate of infection by more than 50% is protected environment isolation.[81] Protective isolation involves the use of laminar airflow rooms and total microbial suppression. Laminar airflow rooms use high-efficiency particulate air filters (e.g., HEPA filters) to remove bacteria, fungi, mycobacteria, and spores from the air. Laminar flow combined with "good housekeeping" methods and reduced microbial content of food and beverages (cooked meats and no fresh fruits or vegetable) does decrease exposure to pathogens. Protective environment isolation does decrease the rate of infection in neutropenic patients; however, it also has some major drawbacks. The first is patient compliance; patients in this protected environment are not allowed to leave their room during the period of neutropenia (which can last 2 months or longer in some patients). Thus, these isolation techniques place a great deal of psychologic stress on the patient and decrease compliance. Finally, facilities for protective isolation are expensive, and many hospitals cannot afford these techniques.

IMPROVING OUTCOMES

Traditionally, neutropenic patients with fever have been hospitalized and treated with IV antibiotics until the neutropenia resolved. However, the availability of effective oral agents and IV antibiotics with longer half-lives has made outpatient treatment of select neutropenic patients with fever possible.[82] Outpatient treatment of neutropenic patients with fever should be limited to those patient who are "low risk." Although what factors truly identify low-risk patients remain controversial, in general, a low risk patient is medically stable (stable vital signs and no metabolic or electrolyte disorders), is expected to have a short duration of neutropenia, has ANC >100 cells/μL, and has a solid tumor.[83] Patients with cancer that is unresponsive to therapy are at risk for complications during neutropenic episodes and are classified as "high risk."[83] In addition, patients should live within close proximity to a medical facility, have good oral intake, have good family or caregiver support, and be reliable. In most trials using outpatient approaches to the treatment of fever in neutropenic patients, patients are seen at the medical facility, given a dose of IV antibiotics, and monitored for a period of time. Stable patients are discharged with an IV or oral regimen. Oral regimens consist of fluoroquinolones or third-generation oral cephalosporins; IV regimens use once or twice daily dosing regimen, such as ceftriaxone plus amikacin. Further research is needed to determine which empiric regimens are best for ambulatory neutropenic patients.[83]

Patients must be carefully monitored. Up to 21% of patients in a prospective trial required hospitalization. Although the indications for hospitalizing a patient being treated on an outpatient regimen have not been clearly delineated, potential indications include persistent fever (>5 days), a deterioration in medical condition, or positive cultures. However, many patients with positive cultures have been successfully treated as outpatients without hospitalization.

The duration of antibiotic therapy in a neutropenic patient is a topic of debate in the literature. If a patient's neutropenia and fever resolve during treatment with antibiotic(s), the antibiotic(s) can be discontinued 7 days after the febrile episode. The controversy involves patients who are still neutropenic 7 days after the fever resolves. A study performed by Pizzo et al.[84] investigated the duration of antibiotic therapy in this patient population. Neutropenic patients in this study were randomly assigned either to continue antibiotics after being afebrile for 7 days or to have their antibiotics discontinued. The patients in the group who continued to receive antibiotic therapy developed no further infectious complications. However, in the group in which the antibiotics were discontinued, for 41% of the patients antibiotic therapy was restarted within 2 days because of recurrence of fever and/or clinical signs of infection. No superinfection occurred in the group who continued to receive antibiotics. Some clinicians still feel that antibiotics should be discontinued after the patient has been afebrile for several days to reduce the possibility of superinfection.[12] Factors that must be considered in the decision to stop antibiotics in a patient who is still neutropenic include the degree of neutropenia, existing sources of infection (mucositis), and the overall stability of the patient's condition.[32]

Patients in whom fever persists for longer than 3 days should be reevaluated.[32] Possible considerations include resistance to current drug regimens, inadequate doses of antibiotics, and nonbacterial causes. Evidence of progressive disease suggests the need to reassess the current antibiotic regimen; if vancomycin was not a part of the initial regimen, it should be added. Persistent fever after 1 week of therapy usually dictates the addition of antifungal therapy. Antifungal therapy should be continued for 2 weeks. If no locus for a fungal infection is found, antifungal therapy may be stopped. Empiric use of antiviral therapy is usually only recommended if evidence of viral disease exists. Should fever persist despite the addition of amphotericin B, coverage for anaerobic bacteria should be considered.

If patients have persistent fever and pulmonary infiltrates while receiving broad-spectrum antibiotics, other opportunistic infections must be considered.[78,84] In addition to *Aspergillus*, pulmonary infiltrates may be caused by other fungal organisms, such as *Zygomycetes*, *Cryptococcus*, and *Histoplasma*.[85] Other potential pathogens include mycobacteria, *Chlamydia*, *Nocardia*, *Legionella*, and *Pneumocystis*. Bronchoalveolar lavage may be helpful in delineating the causative organism, although open lung biopsy may still be necessary.

In patients with positive culture results, antibiotic therapy may be targeted to the cultured organism. However, broad-spectrum coverage should be maintained owing to the possibility of a mixed infection. Patients with positive culture results should receive a 10- to 14-day course of appropriate antibiotic therapy.

In monitoring a neutropenic patient, the clinician should focus on two areas. First and of primary importance is to establish the status of the patient's neutropenia and identity the infecting organism. The second task is to monitor the patient for drug side effects and toxicities and to make appropriate adjustments in therapy.

Once the initial workup is complete and empiric therapy is started, the attention of the clinician should be focused on delineating the causative organism and monitoring the status of the patient for signs of a worsening condition, sepsis, and drug toxicity. As stated earlier, granulocytopenic patients may not have the typical symptoms of infection. The patient must be carefully watched for subtle changes. Complaints of fatigue, changes in mood, or changes in mental status may be the only signals of a deteriorating condition. Vital signs must be carefully monitored for signs of sepsis, such as increased heart rate, increased respiratory rate, and decreased blood pressure. The state of the neutropenia should be assessed daily by obtaining complete blood counts with differential. Identification of the causative organism must be rigorously pursued. Obtaining of daily blood specimens for culture has been advocated.

The side effects from antibiotic therapy depend on the antibiotic(s) chosen. Close monitoring is indicated in this population, because many of the patients are receiving multiple agents. Concurrent or prior exposure to one agent may predispose the patient to the toxicities of other agents. There are certain side effects that are very common in the neutropenic patient. Nephrotoxicity can result from aminoglycosides. Studies investigating the incidence of nephrotoxicity from aminoglycosides show a range between 0 and 15%.[31,33,34] The incidence of nephrotoxicity may be higher when the aminoglycosides are combined with other nephrotoxic drugs such as cephalothin,[34] amphotericin B, or vancomycin. Ototoxicity may also occur with aminoglycosides, with an incidence ranging from 6.2% to 17%.[31,32]

Fluid and electrolyte problems may also occur with antibiotics. Patients receiving semisynthetic penicillins often lose large amounts of potassium in their urine during therapy because of the potassium-wasting effect of the penicillin. Additional amounts of potassium and magnesium can also be lost if the patient is receiving amphotericin B. Thus, serum potassium and magnesium levels should be monitored closely in patients prone to potassium wasting. Finally, combination antibiotic therapy along with the administration of amphotericin B and acyclovir can substantially increase the amount of fluid a patient is receiving. This increase in fluid comes from the additional diluent required to administer the drug intravenously. The result may be volume overload and edema.

KEY POINTS

- The prognosis for immunosuppressed patients without correction of their underlying disease or removal of the causative agent is poor. In the majority of cases, the patient will remain immunocompromised and have recurrent bouts of infection.
- The treatment of infections in the immunocompromised host is difficult and requires diligence.
- Immunosuppressed patients require close monitoring for any signs or symptoms of infection.
- Patients must be treated aggressively and promptly to prevent morbidity and mortality.

- Gram-negative infections are still the most frequently encountered. However, the incidence of Gram-positive infections is on the rise once again.
- The importance of knowing the etiologic trends of pathogens at the individual institution cannot be overemphasized.
- Initial treatment in most immunosuppressed patients remains empiric.
- Monotherapy with antibacterial agents is becoming increasingly popular, but combination therapy still remains the standard of practice.
- In patients who remain febrile, the additional use of antifungal therapy is indicated.
- Use of colony-stimulating factors may be indicated in limited situations.

REFERENCES

1. Schimpff SC. Overview of empiric antibiotic therapy for the febrile neutropenic patient. Rev Infect Dis 7:5734–5740, 1985.
2. Cone LA, Woodard D, Heim NA. Clinical experience in the diagnosis and treatment of infection in the compromised host. Clin Ther 4(Suppl):45–53, 1981.
3. Pizzo PA. Granulocytopenia and cancer therapy. Cancer 54:2649–2661, 1984.
4. Haskell CM, ed. Cancer treatment Philadelphia: WB Saunders, 1990.
5. Hirschlorn R. Overview of biochemical abnormalities and molecular genetics of adenosine deaminase deficiency. Pediatr Res 33(1 Suppl):S35–S41, 1993.
6. Blaese R. Development of gene therapy for immunodeficiency: adenosine deaminase deficiency. Pediatr Res 33(1 Suppl);S49–S53, 1993.
7. Bodey GP. The treatment of febrile neutropenia: from the Dark Ages to the present [Historical article]. Support Care Cancer 5:351–357, 1997.
8. Rossi C, Klastersky J. Initial empirical antibiotic therapy for neutropenic fever: analysis of the causes of death. Support Care Cancer 4:207–212, 1996.
9. Schlier JP, Weerts D, Klastersky J. Causes of death in febrile granulocytopenic cancer patients receiving empiric antibiotic therapy. Eur J Cancer Clin Oncol 20:55–60, 1984.
10. Armstrong D, Young LS, Meyer JD, et al. Infectious complications of neoplastic disease. Med Clin North Am 55:729–745, 1971.
11. Hughes WT, Armstrong D, Bodey GP, et al. 1997 guidelines for the use of antimicrobial agents in neutropenic patients with unexplained fever. Infectious Diseases Society of America. Clin Infect Dis 25:551–573, 1997.
12. Bodey GP. Antibiotics in patients with neutropenic. Arch Intern Med 144:1845–1851, 1984.
13. Wade JC, Schimpff SC, Newman KA, et al. *Staphylococcus epidermidis*: an increasing cause of infection in patients with granulocytopenia. Ann Intern Med 97:503–508, 1982.
14. Klastersky J. Management of infection in granulocytopenic patients. J Antimicrob Chemother 12:102–104, 1983.
15. Pizzo PA, Schimpff SC. Strategies for the prevention of infection in the myelosuppressed or immunosuppressed cancer patients. Cancer Treat Rep 67:223–233, 1983.
16. Kramer BS, Pizzo PA, Robichaud KJ. Role of serial microbiologic surveillance and clinical evaluation in the management of cancer patients with fever and granulocytopenia. Am J Med 72:561–568, 1982.
17. Lau WK, Young LS, Black RE, et al. Comparative efficacy and toxicity of amikacin/carbenicillin versus gentamicin/carbenicillin in leukopenic patients: a randomized prospective trial. Am J Med 62:959–966, 1977.
18. DeJongh CA, Wade JC, Schimpff SC, et al. Empiric antibiotic therapy for suspected infection in granulocytopenic cancer patients. A comparison between the combination of moxalactam plus amikacin and ticarcillin plus amikacin. Am J Med 73:89–96, 1982.
19. Love LJ, Schimpff SC, Hahan DM, et al. Randomized trial of empiric antibiotic therapy with ticarcillin in combination with gentamicin, amikacin or netilmicin in febrile patients with granulocytopenia and cancer. Am J Med 66:603–610, 1979.
20. Fainstein V, Bodey GP, Bolivar ER, et al. A randomized study of ceftazidime compared to ceftazidime and tobramycin for the treatment of infection in cancer patients. J Antimicrob Chemother 12(Suppl A):101–110, 1983.
21. Piccart M, Klastersky J, Lagast MH, et al. Single-drug versus combination empirical therapy for gram-negative bacillary infections in febrile cancer patients with and without granulocytopenia. Antimicrob Agents Chemother 26:870–875, 1984.
22. Wintson DJ, Baines RC, Ho WC, et al. Moxalactam plus piperacillin versus moxalactam plus amkacin in febrile granulocytopenic patients. Am J Med 77:442–450, 1984.
23. Fainstein V, Bodey GP, Bolivar R, et al. Moxalactam plus ticarcillin or tobramycin for treatment of febrile episodes in neutropenic cancer patients. Arch Intern Med 144:1766–1770, 1984.
24. Jade AL, Bolivar R, Fainstein V, et al. Piperacillin plus vancomycin in the therapy of febrile episodes in cancer patients. Antimicrob Agents Chemother 26:295–299, 1984.
25. Keating MJ, Lawson R, Grose W, et al. Combination therapy with ticarcillin and sulfamethoxazole-trimethoprim for infection in patients with cancer. Arch Intern Med 141:926–930, 1981.
26. Klastersky J. Treatment of severe infections in patients with cancer. The role of new acyl-penicillins. Arch Intern Med 142:1984–1987, 1982.
27. Young LS. Use of aminoglycoside in immunocompromised patients. Am J Med 79(Suppl A):21–27, 1985.
28. Sculier JP, Klastersky J. Significance of serum bactericidal activity in gram negative bacillary bacteremia in patients with and without granulocytopenia. Am J Med 76:429–435, 1984.
29. Bodey GP. Aminoglycoside use in the compromised host. In: Whelton A, Neu HC, eds. The aminoglycosides. New York: Marcel Dekker, 1982:557–583.
30. Rolston KV, Berkey P, Bodey GP, et al. A comparison of imipenem to ceftazidime with or without amikacin as empiric therapy in febrile neutropenic patients Arch Intern Med 152:283–291, 1992.
31. Pizzo PA, Hathorn JW, Hiemenz J, et al. A randomized trial comparing ceftazidime alone combination antibiotic therapy in cancer patients with fever and neutropenic. N Engl J Med 315:552–558, 1986.
32. Freifeld AG, Walsh T, Marshall D, et al. Monotherapy for fever and neutropenia in cancer patients; a randomized comparison of ceftazidine versus imipenem. J Clin Oncol 13:165–176, 1995.
33. Stambaugh JE, McAdams J. The efficacy and safety of moxalactam in the treatment of acute bacterial infections in immunosuppressed patient with cancer. Curr Ther Res 31:864–871, 1982.
34. Mortimer J, Miller S, Black D, et al. Comparison of cefoperazone and mezlocillin with imipenem as empiric therapy in febrile neutropenic cancer patients. Am J Med 85(Suppl):21–30, 1988.
35. Hughes WT, Armstrong D, Bodey GB, et al. Guidelines for the use of antimicrobial agents in neutropenic patients with unexplained fever. J Infect Dis 161:381–396, 1990.
36. Cohen J. Empirical antifungal therapy in neutropenic patients. J Antimicrob Chemother 13:409–411, 1984.
37. Schubert MM, Peterson DE, Meyers JD, et al. Head and neck aspergillosis in patients undergoing bone marrow transplantation. Cancer 57:1092–1096, 1986.
38. Gerson SL, Talbot GH, Hurwitz S, et al. Prolonged granulocytopenia: the major risk factor for invasive pulmonary aspergillosis in patient with acute leukemia. Ann Intern Med 100:345–351, 1984.
39. Meunier-Carpentier F. Treatment of mycoses in cancer patients. Am J Med 74(Suppl):74–78, 1983.
40. Preston SL, Briceland LL. Fluconazole for antifungal prophylaxis in chemotherapy-induced neutropenia. Am J Health-Syst Pharm 52:164–173, 1995.
41. Prentice HG, Hann IM, Herbrecht R, et al. A randomized comparison of liposomal versus conventional amphotericin B for the treatment of pyrexia of unknown origin in neutropenic patients. Br J Haematol 98:711–718, 1997.
42. Jennings TS, Hardin TC. Treatment of aspergillosis with itraconazole. Ann Pharmacother 27:1206–1211, 1993.
43. Prentice HG, Hann IM. Antiviral therapy in the immunocompromised patient. Br Med Bull 41:367–373, 1985.
44. Burns WH, Saral R. Opportunistic viral infections. Brit Med Bull 41:46–49, 1985.
45. Wong KK, Hirsch MS. Herpes virus infections in patients with neoplastic disease, diagnosis and therapy. Am J Med 76:464–478, 1984.
46. Straus SE, Smith HA, Brickman C, et al. Acyclovir for chronic mucocutaneous herpes simplex virus infection in immunosuppressed patients. Ann Intern Med 96:270–277, 1982.
47. Wade JC, Newton B, McLaren C, et al. Intravenous acyclovir to treat mucocutaneous herpes simplex virus infection after bone marrow transplantation. Ann Intern Med 96:265–269, 1982.
48. Whitley RJ, Soong SJ, Dolin R, et al. Early vidarabine therapy to control the complications of herpes zoster in immunosuppressed patients. N Engl J Med 307:971–975, 1982.

49. Balfour HH, Bean B, Laskin OL, et al. Acyclovir halts progression of herpes zoster in immunocompromised patients. N Engl J Med 308:1448–1453, 1983.
50. Balfour HH, McMonigal KA, Bean B. Acyclovir therapy of varicella-zoster virus infections in immunocompromised patients. J Antimicrob Chemother 12(Suppl B):169–179, 1983.
51. Skinhj P, Anderson HK, Moller J, et al. Cytomegalovirus infection after bone marrow transplantation: relation of pneumonia to postgrafting immunosuppressive treatment. J Med Virol 14:91–99, 1984.
52. Meyer JD, Wade JC, McGuffin RW, et al. The use of acyclovir for cytomegalovirus infections in the immunocompromised host. J Antimicrob Chemother 12(Suppl B):181–193, 1983.
53. Shepp DH, Dandliker PS, Miranda P, et al. Activity of 9-[2-hydroxy-1-(hydroxymethyl)ethoxymethyl] guanine in the treatment of cytomegalovirus pneumonia. Ann Intern Med 103:368–373, 1985.
54. Emamuel D, Cunningham I, Jules-Elysee K, et al. Cytomegalovirus pneumonia after bone marrow transplantation successfully treated with the combination of ganciclovir and high dose intravenous immune globulin. Ann Intern Med 109:777–782, 1988.
55. Bach MC, Bagwell SP, Knapp NP, et al. 9(1,3-Dihydroxy-2-propoxymethyl) guanine for cytomegalovirus infection in patients with the acquired immunodeficiency syndrome. Ann Intern Med 103:381–382, 1985.
56. Papadopoulos EB, Ladanyi M, Emanuel D, et al. Infusions of donor leukocytes to treat Epstein-Barr virus-associated lymphoproliferative disorders after allogeneic bone marrow transplantation. N Engl J Med 330:1231–1233, 1994.
57. Taguchi Y, Purtilo DT, Okano M. The effect of intravenous immunoglobulin and interferon-alpha on Epstein-Barr virus-induced lymphoproliferative disorder in a liver transplant recipient. 57:1813–1815, 1994.
58. Malarme M, Meunier-Carpentier F, Klastersky J. Vancomycin plus gentamicin and co-trimoxazole for prevention of infections in neutropenic cancer patients (a comparative, placebo-controlled pilot study). Eur J Cancer Clin Oncol 17:1315–1322, 1981.
59. Kauffman CA, Liepman MK, Bergman AG. Trimethoprim/sulfamethoxazole prophylaxis in neutropenic patients. Am J Med 74:599–607, 1983.
60. Riben PD, Louie TJ, Lank BA, et al. Reduction in mortality from gram negative sepsis in neutropenic patients receiving trimethoprim/sulfamethoxazole therapy. Cancer 51:1587–1592, 1983.
61. Wade JC, Schimpff SC, Hargadon MT, et al. A comparison of trimethoprim/sulfamethoxazole plus nystatin with gentamicin plus nystatin in the prevention of infections in acute leukemia. N Engl J Med 304:1057–1062, 1981.
62. Martino P, Venditti M, Concetta M, et al. Co-trimoxazole prophylaxis in patients with leukemia and prolonged granulocytopenia. Am J Med Sci 287:7–9, 1984.
63. Weiser B, Lange M, Fialk MA, et al. Prophylactic trimethoprim-sulfamethoxazole during consolidation chemotherapy for acute leukemia: a controlled trial. Ann Intern Med 95:436–438, 1981.
64. Wade JC, deJongh CA, Newman KA, et al. Selective antimicrobial modulation as prophylaxis against infection during granulocytopenia: trimethoprim-sulfamethoxazole vs. nalidixic acid. J Infect Dis 147:624–633, 1983.
65. Dekker A, Rozenberg-Arska M, Verhoef J. Infection prophylaxis in acute leukemia: a comparison of ciprofloxacin with trimethoprim-sulfamethoxaozole and colistin. Ann Intern Med 106:7–12, 1987.
66. Denning D, Flulle HH, Hellriegel KP. Chemoprophylaxis of bacterial infection in granulocytopenic patients. Okolologie 19:57–58, 1987.
67. Shepp DH, Klosterman A, Siegel MS, et al. Comparative trial of ketoconazole and nystatin for prevention of fungal infection in neutropenic patients treated in a protective environment. J Infect Dis 152:1257–1263, 1985.
68. Hann IM, Prentice HG, Blacklock HA, et al. Acyclovir prophylaxis against herpes virus infections in severely immunocompromised patients: randomized double blind trial. Br Med J 287:384–388, 1983.
69. Prentice HG. Use of acyclovir for prophylaxis of herpes infections in severely immunocompromised patients. J Antimicrob Chemother 12(Suppl B):153–159, 1983.
70. Condie RM, O'Reilly RJ. Prevention of cytomegalovirus pneumonia with high-dose intravenous, hyperimmune; native, unmodified cytomegalovirus globulin. Am J Med 76(Suppl):134–141, 1984.
71. Winton DJ, Ho WG, Lin CH, et al. Intravenous immunoglobulin for modification of cytomegalovirus infection associated with bone marrow transplantation. Am J Med 76(Suppl):128–133, 1984.
72. Purdy BD, Plaisance KI. Infection with the human immunodeficiency virus: epidemiology, pathogenesis, transmission, diagnosis, and manifestations. Am J Hosp Pharm 46:1185–1209, 1989.
73. Gualtieri RJ, Donowitz GR, Kaiser DL, et al. Double-blind randomized study of prophylactic trimethoprim/sulfamethoxazole in granulocytopenic patients with hematologic malignancies. Am J Med 74:934–940, 1983.
74. Gordin FM, Simon GL, Wafsy CB, et al. Adverse reactions to trimethoprim-sulfamethoxazole in patients with the acquired immunodeficiency syndrome. Ann Intern Med 100:495–499, 1984.
75. Small CB, Harris CA, Friedland GH, et al. The treatment of *Pneumocystis carinii* pneumonia in acquired immunodeficiency syndrome. Arch Intern Med 145:837–840, 1985.
76. Nemunaitis J, Singer JW, Buckner D, et al. Use of recombinant human granulocyte-macrophage colony-stimulating factor in graft failure after bone marrow transplantation. Blood 76:245–253, 1990.
77. Glaspy JA, Golde DW. Granulocyte colony-stimulating factor: preclinical and clinical studies. Semin Oncol 19:386–394, 1992.
78. American Society of Clinical Oncology. American Society of Clinical Oncology recommendations for the use of hematopoietic colony-stimulating factors: evidence-based, clinical practice guidelines. J Clin Oncol 12:2471–2508, 1994.
79. Strauss RG, Connett JE, Gale RP, et al. A controlled trial of prophylactic granulocyte transfusions during initial induction chemotherapy for acute myelogenous leukemia. N Engl J Med 305:597–603, 1981.
80. Young LS. Prophylactic granulocytes in the neutropenic host. Ann Intern Med 96:240–241, 1982.
81. Schimpff SC. Infection prevention during profound granulocytopenia. New approaches to alimentary canal microbial suppression. Ann Intern Med 93:358–361, 1980.
82. Escalante CP, Rubenstein EB, Rolston KV. Outpatient antibiotic therapy for febrile episodes in low-risk neutropenic patients with cancer. Cancer Invest 15:237–242, 1997.
83. Davis DD, Raebel MA. Ambulatory management of chemotherapy-induced fever and neutropenia in adult cancer patients. Ann Pharmacother 32:1317–1323, 1998.
84. Pizzo PA, Robichaud KJ, Gill FA, et al. Duration of empiric antibiotic therapy in granulocytopenic patients with cancer. Am J Med 67:194–200, 1979.
85. Winston DJ, Ho WG, Gale RP. Therapeutic granulocyte transfusion for documented infections. Ann Intern Med 97:509–519, 1982.

CHAPTER 82

BACTEREMIA AND SEPSIS

Alan H. Mutnick, Elizabeth A. Beltz, and Dena M. Behm Dillon

DEFINITION

Bacteremia refers to the presence of viable bacteria in the bloodstream. The presence of fungi, parasites, viruses, and other pathogens in the blood is described in a similar fashion (i.e., fungemia, parasitemia, viremia, etc.).[1] Sepsis is a term used to describe the physiologic events that take place in the body in response to an infection.[2,3] These events are triggered either by the bacteria themselves or by their toxic byproducts, which are released into the circulation.

Bacteremia is defined as bacteria in the blood confirmed by blood cultures. Bacteremia may be low grade and transient (e.g., dental cleaning/manipulations) or may be constant and high grade (e.g., bacterial endocarditis). It may be associated with primary or secondary infectious processes. Nosocomial bacteremia may be associated with peripheral and central intravenous devices, intravascular hemodynamic monitoring devices, hemodialysis catheters, and total parenteral nutrition solutions.

Appropriately drawn blood samples for cultures are crucial to the correct diagnosis and/or confirmation of bacteremia (as discussed later in this chapter). The choice of antimicrobial agents should be based on the clinical presentation, the Gram stain results, the suspected infectious source, and a variety of patient factors. Antimicrobial therapy may then be modified based on results of confirmatory blood cultures and susceptibility patterns. In addition to rapid initiation of antibiotic therapy, another crucial step is the correction of predisposing or contributing factors (i.e., correction of neutropenia, removal of foreign bodies such as catheters or surgical hardware, and drainage of an abscess). The duration of antibiotic therapy is determined by the primary site of infection; the causative organism(s), concurrent medical problems, the degree of immunocompetence, and the continued presence or removal of infected foreign bodies.

The American College of Chest Physicians/Society of Critical Care has attempted to more accurately define the term "sepsis" to standardize the terminology used and to eliminate confusion among clinicians and researchers.[4] Because of the consensus that other noninfectious events can trigger a clinical response within the body, a recommendation was made to use the phrase, "systemic inflammatory response syndrome" (SIRS) as a general description for an inflammatory process, independent of its cause.[4] Consequently, sepsis becomes a subset of SIRS and would include SIRS that is the result of an infectious process (Fig. 82.1).

As can be seen from Figure 82.1, patients within circle A develop an infection. The etiology of the infection could include bacteria, fungi, parasites, or viruses. Many of these organisms are able to exist within the bloodstream and result in bacteremias, fungemias, parasitemias, or viremias. All of these bloodstream pathogens are able to induce physiologic changes, such as (1) body temperature greater than 38°C or less than 36°C, (2) heart rate greater than 90 bpm, (3) respiratory rate greater than 20 breaths/min or $PaCO_2 < 32$ torr, and (4) alterations in white blood cell count such as a white blood cell count greater than 12,000/mm^3, a count less than 4,000/mm^3, or the presence of more than 10% immature white blood cells (bands), and result in sepsis as shown in area B. However, those infectious processes resulting in sepsis as well as those noninfectious processes (e.g., burns, pancreatitis, or trauma) able to induce physiologic changes such as those listed above are considered to make up circle C–SIRS.[1]

According to this newly proposed classification, all patients with sepsis suffer from SIRS, but the converse is not always true, because other etiologic events besides

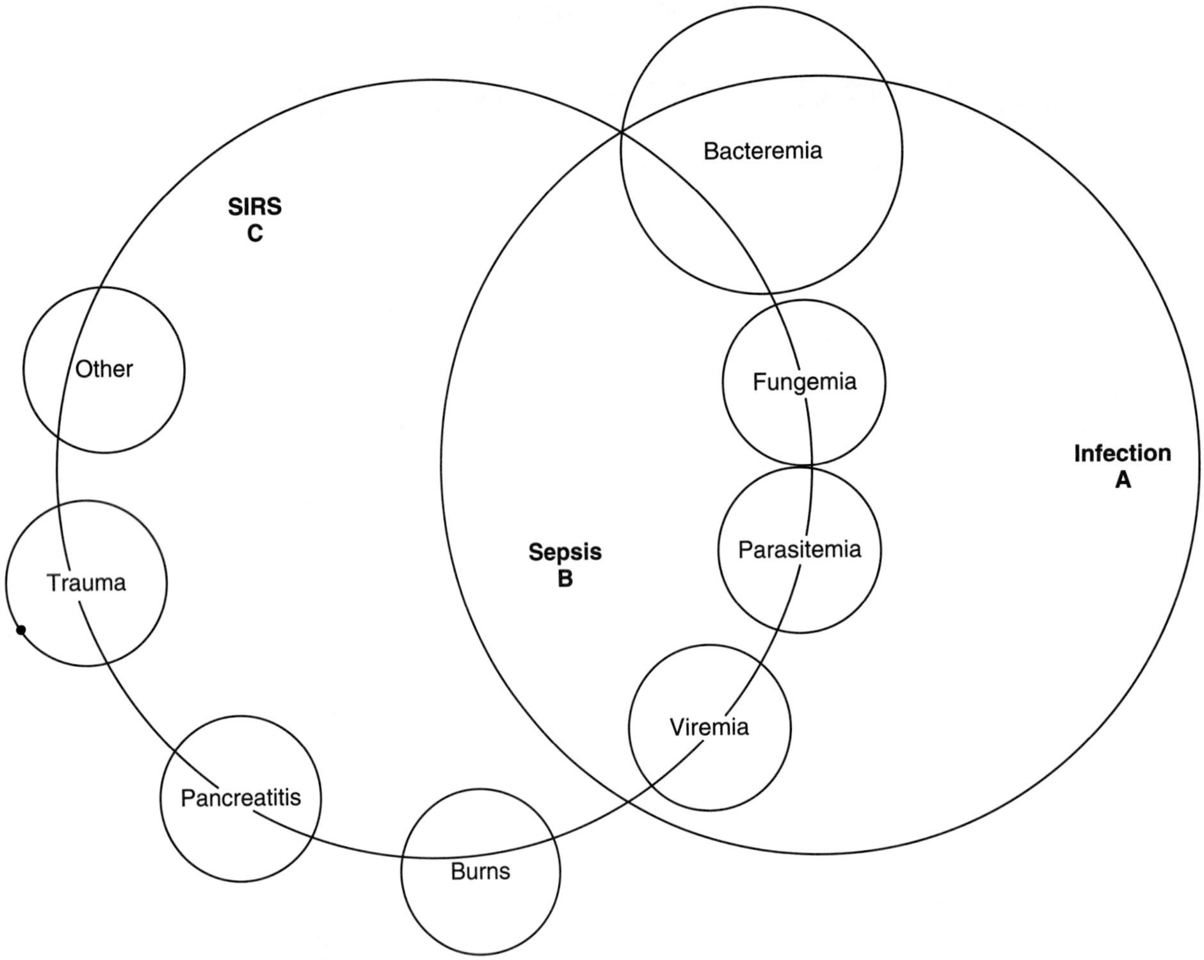

Figure 82.1. The relationship between systemic inflammatory response syndrome (SIRS) sepsis, infection, and bacteremia. (Adapted with permission from Bone RC, Balk RA, Cerra FB, et al. The ACCP/SCCM Consensus Conference Committee: definitions for sepsis and organ failure and guidelines for the use of innovative therapies in sepsis. Chest 101:1644–1655, 1992.)

sepsis contribute to the development of SIRS. As will be seen later in this chapter, confusion and the inability to have consistent definitions for the various clinical entities that encompass sepsis have made it difficult to compare therapeutic modalities, develop consistency among clinical trials, and identify the incidence of this clinical entity in patient populations.

TREATMENT GOALS: BACTEREMIA AND SEPSIS

- In general, deter the long-term consequences that can result from the disease process. These consequences include adult respiratory distress syndrome (ARDS) and disseminated intravascular coagulation (DIC), which can result in increased morbidity and mortality.
- Eradicate the source of infection through the use of antibiotics and correct neutropenia, remove foreign bodies, and perform surgical drainage when appropriate.
- Ensure resolution of ARDS by maximizing oxygenation while minimizing compromise of cardiac output and lung injury.
- Provide supportive care for patients with ARDS and prevent complications such as nosocomial pneumonia, stress ulcers, and deep vein thromboses.
- Use anticoagulation to prevent DIC, treat underlying causes, and support the patient while healing occurs.
- Stabilize respiratory and hemodynamic parameters.
- Correct hypotension while maintaining adequate organ perfusion.

EPIDEMIOLOGY

As mentioned earlier, the lack of consistency in defining the clinical entities of sepsis has made it difficult to determine the true incidence of this potentially life-threatening condition. The purpose of the Consensus Conference was to develop a working definition for the various clinical entities and provide a framework for future clinical research, epidemiologic evaluation, and therapeutic modalities.[1]

Reports from national publications reveal a significant increase of 139% in the incidence of septicemia during the years between 1979 and 1987, from 73.6 to 175.9 cases per 100,000 persons.[5] In this report, septicemia was considered a disease associated with the presence and persistence of pathogenic microorganisms or their toxins in the blood. Although the above-mentioned incidence was based on a working definition which is in close agreement to that developed by the Consensus Conference, the reporting of incidences of septic shock developing in patients with septicemia shows a large variability. An epidemiologic study involving eight academic medical centers was conducted using a random sample of all patients in intensive care units (ICUs), all patients not in ICUs who had blood drawn for cultures, all patients who died in an emergency department or ICU, and all patients who received a novel therapy for sepsis syndrome.[6] The authors concluded that sepsis occurred in a mean of 2.0 patients per 100 hospital admissions, a much higher incidence than reported in previous investigations.[7] This higher incidence could be the result of sicker patients, more nosocomial infections, and the fact that patients not in ICUs were included in this surveillance. Reports in the literature have suggested that septic shock develops in 17% of patients seen initially with coagulase-negative staphylococcal infections,[8] in 47% of patients with bacteremia,[7] and in 30% of patients without bacteremia.[7]

What has become clear in the literature is that patients who develop septic shock have a poor prognosis, with mortality rates reported to be as high as 90% and as low as 10%.[7–14] Once again, the disparity in the incidence reported may be a reflection of differences in defining the various clinical entities as sepsis.

PATHOPHYSIOLOGY

The initial event believed to be responsible for activating the "sepsis cascade" involves the release of a toxin into the circulation.[15] The form of toxin released into the circulation depends on the invading pathogen. Endotoxins are released into the circulation from select Gram-negative bacteria whereas Gram-positive bacteria or yeast cell wall products and viral or fungal antigens are believed to be capable of activating the sepsis cascade as well.[16,17]

After the toxin gains access to the circulation, it is able to stimulate the release of numerous mediators, which results in endothelial damage and activation of the coagulation cascade and complement system (Fig. 82.2). As described in Table 82.1, each mediator released is capable of inducing various physiologic changes dependent on the specific mediator. If the body becomes unable to restore normal physiologic function, the generalized inflammatory response produces the clinical syndrome of sepsis. As endothelial damage continues in a specific site, sepsis evolves into severe sepsis (previously called septic syndrome). If severe sepsis is associated with systolic blood pressure less than 90 mm Hg, it becomes sepsis-induced hypotension, which, if allowed to persist despite fluid resuscitation along with the presence of hypoperfusion abnormalities or organ dysfunction, results in septic shock.[4]

We have attempted to oversimplify the important triggering events for the reader to gain an appreciation for the changes occurring during the sepsis cascade. However, it would be inappropriate to assume that the process is as straightforward as our oversimplified description may lead one to believe. In fact, the chemical mediators may have different effects on various organ systems and may stimulate as well as inhibit various events within the sepsis cascade. Additionally, different chemical mediators may or may not be present in significant concentrations with different septic events. Many unanswered questions still exist about the exact pathophysiologic events that take place during the sepsis process.

COMPLICATIONS

Complications observed in the sepsis syndrome secondary to bacterial etiologies include hypotension, ARDS, bleeding, DIC, leukopenia, thrombocytopenia, and organ failure, including lung (acidosis or cyanosis), kidney (oliguria, anuria, or acidosis), liver (jaundice), and heart (congestive heart failure). The appearance and progression of these complications/symptoms are variable and may be influenced by underlying disease processes.[12] The appropriate management of these complications is critical to a positive clinical outcome and will be discussed in a subsequent section of this chapter.

Adult Respiratory Syndrome

ARDS, also called acute respiratory distress syndrome, is defined as acute respiratory failure characterized by increased microvascular and epithelial permeability pulmonary edema, with a major oxygenation defect, and relatively normal cardiac function.[18] ARDS was first described during World War I as a syndrome associated with thoracic trauma, but the first description involving nontraumatic etiologies appeared in 1967.

ARDS is always seen in the face of recognized clinical predispositions and usually occurs within the first 72 hours of insult.[18,19] These predisposing conditions may be direct insults to the lungs such as pneumonia, aspiration of gastric contents, or toxic inhalations, or they may be indirect insults, which include sepsis, trauma, and pancreatitis.[18–20] Sepsis is a leading cause of ARDS. It is estimated that 30 to 40% of patients with bacterial sepsis will develop ARDS.[18,20,21] The mortality from ARDS is reported to be 40 to 60%.[19,21,22]

Disseminated Intravascular Coagulation

DIC is a common complication of sepsis. This occurs when the normal balance between fibrin formation and the fibrinolytic system is disrupted and results in the stimulation of the coagulation process and fibrin formation.[23] DIC is associated with many clinical entities including infections, trauma, and malignancy.[23]

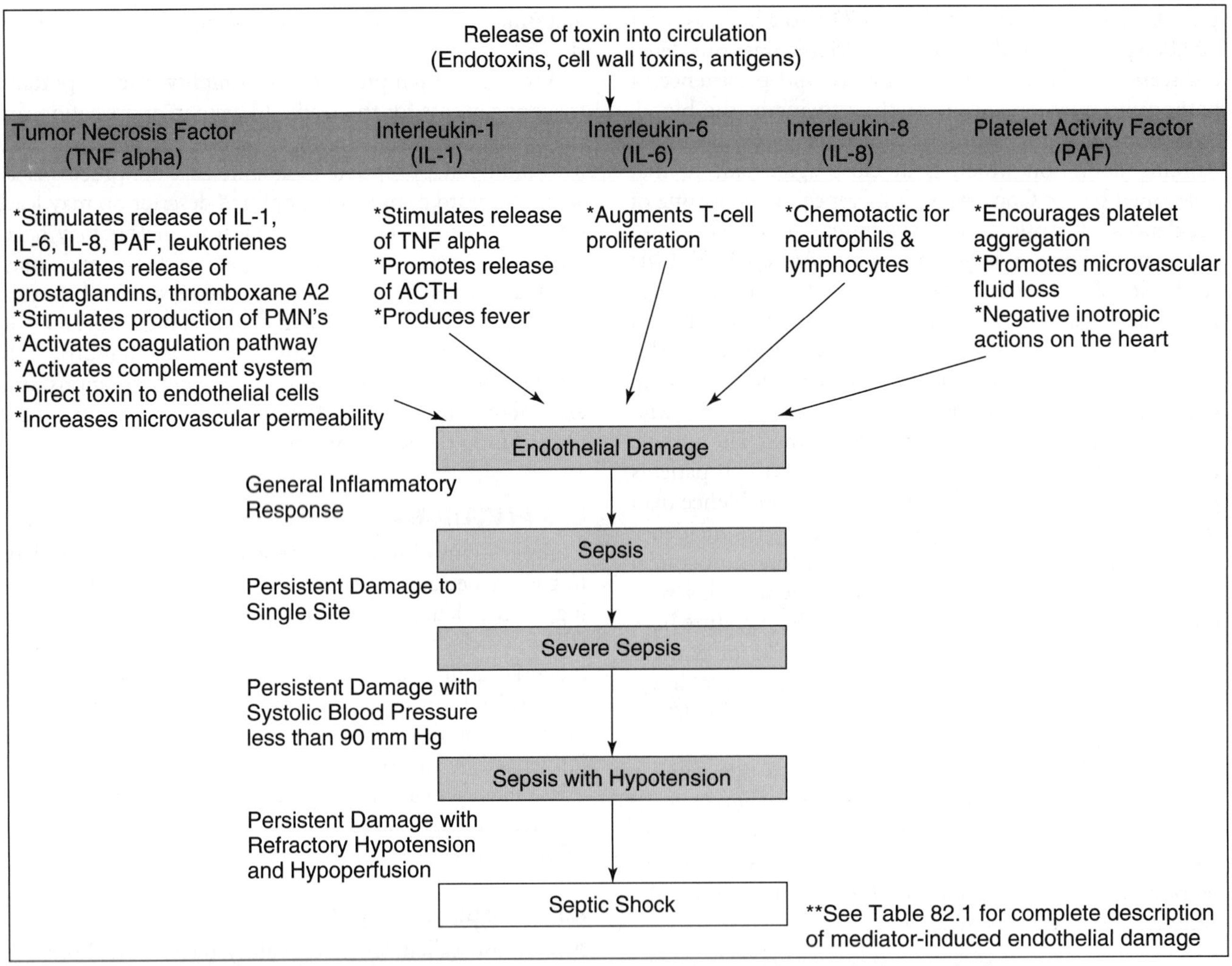

Figure 82.2. Sepsis-cascade pathway. *ACTH,* adrenocorticotropin; *IL,* interleukin; *PAF,* platelet-activating factor; *PNM, TNF-α,* tumor necrosis factor-α

CLINICAL PRESENTATION AND DIAGNOSIS

Signs and Symptoms

As should be evident to the reader at this time, the clinical presentation of sepsis is not easily defined because of the numerous biologic mediators that are released in response to sepsis and their respective impacts on the patient. Additionally, the duration of illness, degree of endotoxin release, and underlying comorbidities may present with differing degrees of organ dysfunction.

The clinical presentation of the sepsis syndrome can be variable as a result of the patient's underlying condition(s), particularly the presence of leukopenia. The sepsis syndrome is a dynamic process with symptoms that may progress rapidly in a given patient. The primary physical symptoms associated with bacterial etiologies of sepsis syndrome as described by Young[12] include fever, chills, hyperventilation, hypothermia, skin lesions, and/or changes in mental status. Hyperventilation may precede the onset of fever and chills in many patients. The presence of skin lesions may be useful in identifying a potential pathogen. Ecthyma gangrenosum lesions have been commonly associated with *Pseudomonas aeruginosa* bacteremia. Erythroderma is often seen with staphylococcal or streptococcal infections. Mental status changes could be seen in central nervous system infections and may be complicated by concomitant drug therapy.

The presence of predisposing factors such as surgery, organ transplantation, chemotherapy, other immunocompromise, or recent trauma may assist in the diagnosis and provide clues to potential pathogens. Data on previous and/or current antimicrobial therapy as well as Gram stain and culture results are important in defining the possible etiologic agent. Two sets of blood specimens for culture should be drawn from different peripheral sites at the time of first clinical suspicion of bacteremia or sepsis.[24] Ideally, these cultures should be performed before the initiation of antimicrobial therapy. Also, specimens from urine, sputum, and other obvious sources of infection should be taken and sent expeditiously to the microbiology laboratory for culture. Gram stain results for collected specimens should be available within hours of specimen collection and are valuable in the selection of the initial antimicrobial therapy. It must be noted, however, that bacteremia is only present in about 45% of patients with sepsis. Therefore, negative blood culture results should not lessen the importance of proper clinical diagnosis and initiation of appropriate supportive therapies.

Because of the dynamic changes that occur in the patient with sepsis, the patient may present with routine findings such as fever, tachycardia, tachypnea, leukocytosis with a left shift (indicating the presence of more immature

Table 82.1 ▪ Select Mediators of Endothelial Damage in Sepsis and Their Selected Actions[a]

Mediator	Major Effects
Tumor necrosis factor α (TNF-α)	• Stimulates release of interleukin-1, interleukin-6, interleukin-8, platelet-activating factor, leukotrienes, thromboxane A_2, and prostaglandins; may be able to stimulate macrophages directly to promote its own release • Has only a weak effect on T cells • Stimulates production of polymorphonuclear (PMN) cells by bone marrow; enhances phagocytic activity of PMN cells • Promotes adhesion of endothelial cells, PMN cells, eosinophils, basophils, monocytes, and occasionally, lymphocytes • Activates common pathway of coagulation and complement system • Direct toxin to vascular endothelial cells; increases microvascular permeability • Acts directly on hypothalamus to cause fever
Interleukin-1 (IL-1)	• Stimulates release of TNF-α, interleukin-6, interleukin-8, platelet-activating factor, leukotrienes, thromboxane A_2, and prostaglandins; may also be capable of stimulating its own production • Activates resting T cells to produce lymphocytes and other products; supports B-cell proliferation and antibody production; is cytotoxic for insulin-producing B cells • Promotes adhesion of endothelial cells, PMN cells, eosinophils, basophils, monocytes, and occasionally lymphocytes • Promotes PMN cell activation and accumulation • Increases endothelial precoagulant activity and endothelial release of plasminogen activator inhibitor • Acts synergistically with TNF-α; enhances tissue cell sensitivity to TNF-α • Promotes release of adrenocorticotropic hormone • Acts directly on hypothalamus to produce fever
Interleukin-6 (IL-6)	• Acts as a helper cell for T- and B-cell activation; interacts synergistically with IL-1 to affect thymocyte proliferation; in combination with TNF-α, augments T-cell proliferation • Promotes PMN cell activation and accumulation
Interleukin-8 (IL-8)	• Is chemotactic for both neutrophils and lymphocytes; induces tissue infiltration of both • Inhibits endothelial-leukocyte adhesion and decreases the hyperadhesion induced by them
Platelet-activating factor (PAF)	• Stimulates release of TNF-α, leukotrienes, and thromboxane A_2 • Promotes leukocyte activation and subsequent free radical formation • Encourages platelet aggregation, leading to thrombosis • Markedly alters microvascular permeability, thereby promoting microvascular fluid loss • Stimulates calcium influx-efflux in endothelial cells; causes cells to retract and lose reciprocal contact and promotes albumin diffusion in endothelial cells • Exerts a negative inotropic effect on the heart; lowers arterial blood pressure • May attenuate effects of endotoxin on hyperglycemia and hyperlactacidemia • May cause gastrointestinal ulceration, specifically in the duodenum and jejunum • Induces blood-brain damage and vasoconstriction; may be neurotoxic
Thromboxane A_2	• Promotes release of endothelium-derived relaxing factor; may stimulate prostacyclin production • Causes platelet aggregation and neutrophil accumulation • Increases vascular permeability • Produces vasoconstricton of vascular beds and pulmonary bronchoconstriction
Leukotriene B_4	• Promotes neutrophil chemotaxis and adhesion of neutrophils to endothelium • Is weakly chemotactic for eosinophils • Increases vascular permeability
Leukotriene C_4, D_4, E_4	• Stimulate release of prostacyclin • Decrease coronary blood flow and myocardial contractility; increase pulmonary vascular resistance • Have mild vasoconstrictive effects and enhance vasoconstrictive effects of epinephrine and norepinephrine
Prostacyclin	• Inhibits platelet aggregation and adhesion • Inhibits thrombus formation; may have fibrinolytic activity • Acts synergistically with prostaglandin E_2 to increase the effects of serotonin and bradykinin on vascular permeability • Causes vasodilation and increased blood flow • Exerts beneficial effects on tissue perfusion during the early stages of sepsis • Produces smooth muscle relaxation

[a]For a more comprehensive listing of all mediators, see reference 15.

white blood cells), findings similar to those for many other infectious as well as noninfectious processes. However, under the right conditions (poor nutritional status, debilitated or compromised host state, virulent organisms, and release of significant toxins), the patient may quickly develop other findings suggestive of the various sequelae associated with sepsis.

Diagnosis

The recommendations from the American College of Chest Physicians/Society of Critical Care Medicine Consensus conference[4] require that two or more of the following conditions must exist as a result of infection for a patient to be considered to have sepsis:

1. Temperature >38°C or <36°C;
2. Heart rate >90 bpm;
3. Respiratory rate >20 breaths/min or $PaCO_2$ <32 torr; or
4. White blood cell count >12,000/mm^3, <4,000/mm^3, or >10% immature (band) forms.

Additionally, the conference provided the following guidelines to differentiate the varying dynamic changes that may be associated with sepsis and its comparison to severe sepsis, septic shock, and multiple organ dysfunction syndrome:

- *Severe Sepsis*–Sepsis associated with organ dysfunction, hypoperfusion, or hypotension; clinical manifestations could include lactic acidosis, oliguria, or an alteration in mental status.
- *Septic Shock*–Sepsis with hypotension, despite adequate fluid resuscitation, along with abnormalities of inadequate perfusion; clinical manifestations could include lactic acidosis, oliguria, or an acute alteration in mental status.
- *Multiple Organ Dysfunction Syndrome*–Presence of altered organ status in an acutely ill patient so that normal homeostasis cannot be maintained.

The diagnostic workup for ARDS includes a chest radiograph, which shows a progression to diffuse, alveolar infiltrates.[25] Arterial blood gas results show hypoxemia with a ratio of PaO_2 to percentage oxygen inspired ≤ 200.[18]

Invasive hemodynamic monitoring is usually necessary to distinguish ARDS from congestive heart failure (cardiogenic pulmonary edema) because the chest radiograph is similar in appearance in both circumstances.[25] Because ARDS is from a pulmonary edema of a noncardiogenic origin, readings from a pulmonary artery catheter would be expected to show a relatively normal cardiac output with a relatively normal pulmonary capillary wedge pressure (estimating left ventricular end-diastolic pressures).[19,26]

Pathologic changes, usually only seen on autopsy, include virtually airless lungs, heavy with fluid on gross examination.[21] Microscopic findings vary depending on the phase of ARDS.[21] Initially, alveolar spaces are filled with proteinaceous fluid and inflammatory cells (acute phase) progressing through a subacute or organizing phase with a final fibrotic phase.[21]

DIC is best diagnosed with a combination of coagulation tests.[23] Because fibrinogen is converted to fibrin in DIC, fibrinogen levels are usually low and fibrinogen degradation products are elevated.[23] Plasmin generation and subsequent lysis of factors V and IX causes an increase in prothrombin time and thrombin time.[23] Partial thromboplastin time is prolonged because of consumption and degradation of factors V, VIII, IX, and XI. The platelet count is also typically low.[23]

Clinically, the patient with DIC typically is bleeding (often profuse) accompanied by thrombotic disorders. For example, the patient may have necrosis of the skin secondary to thromboses at the same time they are bleeding profusely from puncture sites and into organs. Microvascular thrombi may lead to organ damage.[23]

In the remaining sections of this chapter, the reader will be introduced to the various clinical strategies used to reduce the morbidity and mortality associated with sepsis. However, as will become apparent during the discussion, the release of multiple chemical mediators along with their varying effects on different organ systems requires multiple treatment modalities to combat the aggressive nature of the various clinical entities associated with sepsis.

THERAPEUTIC PLAN

At this time, national guidelines do not exist for the management of the patient with bacteremia or sepsis. Because of the varied etiologies associated with the development of the sepsis syndrome and its many sequelae, therapeutic regimens have been developed with the intention of aggressively treating infection as well as protecting and treating affected organ systems. In this section, the various therapeutic strategies will be described as they relate to the acute infective process as well as to its associated complications.

TREATMENT

Pharmacotherapy

The initial choice of antibiotic therapy in a patient with presumed sepsis or bacteremia will be empiric in most instances. Antibiotics should be targeted to the known infections as much as possible, although empiric broad-spectrum coverage is appropriate in sepsis when the etiologic agent(s) have not yet been identified. Prophylactic antibiotics have not been shown to be useful. Additionally, their use may promote antibiotic resistance.[19] Selection of therapy should be based on

1. Suspected source of infection and likely bacterial pathogen;
2. Community- or hospital-acquired organism;
3. Bacterial susceptibility or resistance patterns in a given hospital or community; and
4. Patient factors such as allergy history and/or the presence of organ dysfunction and/or immunocompromise.

Antibiograms based on hospital- or patient care unit-specific antibiotic susceptibilities are very useful in the initial selection of antibiotic(s). In a prospective surveillance study of 1754 patients with sepsis syndrome in 80 U.S. hospitals, 389 Gram-negative blood isolates were identified.[27] Table 82.2 summarizes the identities of these isolates. A more recent prospective surveillance study of 12,759 patients in eight tertiary care centers reported that 31% of the septic episodes involved Gram-positive organisms, 39.8% involved Gram-negative organisms, 6.1% involved fungi, 2% involved intra-abdominal organisms, and 16.3% were polymicrobial.[6] Based on this information and on other published data, it would seem that the initial empiric antibiotic therapy in patients with suspected sepsis syndrome should include a combination of antibiotics to cover a wide spectrum of Gram-negative as well as Gram-positive organisms, including streptococci and staphylococci (methicillin-resistant *Staphylococcus aureus* and coagulase-negative species). Combination antibiotic therapy further (1) affords coverage for "polymicrobial" bacteremia, (2) prevents the development of bacterial resistance by eradicating subpopulations of bacteria resistant to one of the drugs of the combination, and (3) provides additive or synergistic bactericidal effects over that achieved with single-drug therapy.

Given the environmental and patient factors described previously, the initial empiric antibiotic therapy combination might include

1. An extended spectrum penicillin (piperacillin or mezlocillin) or a third- or fourth-generation cephalosporin combined with an aminoglycoside.
2. If anaerobes are suspected (genitourinary source, trauma, or gastrointestinal source), metronidazole can be added to the above combination or a penicillinase inhibitor-β-lactam combination such as piperacillin-tazobactam; ticarcillin clavulanate can be substituted and combined with an aminoglycoside. Imipenem can also be combined with an aminoglycoside.
3. If an indwelling intravascular catheter is a possible source, and methicillin resistance is common with the *S. aureus* at the institution, add vancomycin to either 1 or 2 above.[12,28]

Table 82.2 ▪ Frequency of Gram-Negative Isolates from 1754 Patients with Sepsis Syndrome in 80 U.S. Hospitals

Organism	No. of Isolates (%) (*N* = 389)
Escherichia coli	155 (39.85)
Klebsiella species	49 (12.6)
Enterobacter species	29 (7.46)
Pseudomonas species	46 (11.83)
Bacteroides species	11 (2.83)
Proteus species	15 (3.86)
Mixed	30 (7.71)
Miscellaneous	54 (13.88)

Source: Reference 27.

4. If the patient is immunocompromised, see Chapter 81, Infections in the Immunosuppressed Patient.

Antibiotics administered to treat the sepsis syndrome should always be given initially by parenteral routes. As the patient's clinical condition improves, oral antibiotics may be considered after cessation of fever if the pathogen is susceptible to an oral alternative and only if the patient is clinically stable and able to take oral medications.

There is a potential advantage to having consistent blood levels of antibiotics that exhibit concentration-independent killing. With concentration-independent drugs such as the penicillins and cephalosporins, efficacy is associated with the amount of time that the serum drug concentration is greater than the minimum inhibitory concentration (MIC). Investigators are therefore researching the possibility of using continuous administration of certain antibiotics. Continuous infusion has been associated with reduced bacteremia compared with intermittent antibiotic therapy.[29] A study in healthy humans found that continuous infusion resulted in serum drug concentrations exceeding the drug's MIC for 100% of the 24-hour period versus 52 to 82% with intermittent dosing.[30] Unfortunately, most of the data supporting the use of continuous administration are in vitro and animal data.[31,32] Because of the lack of controlled studies in humans, whether intermittent or continuous intravenous administration of antibiotics is optimal is still not resolved.

Doses of antibiotics must be modified based on the degree of hepatic and/or renal dysfunction. Initial regimens may require frequent modification owing to the dynamic nature of the sepsis syndrome. Individualization of drug therapy using pharmacokinetic models is particularly important with the aminoglycoside-type antibiotics. Peak aminoglycoside serum concentrations of 8 to 12 times the MIC of the bacteria have been associated with a positive clinical outcome.[33] Extended interval aminoglycoside therapy may offer promise in the therapy of serious Gram-negative infections.[34,35] The role of aminoglycosides in the therapy of the sepsis syndrome has not been clearly defined at this time, as no trials published to date have researched the use of extended-interval dosing specifically for sepsis.

Modification of the initial antibiotic regimen may be required. After culture and susceptibility data from initial blood, urine, sputum, and/or wound specimens become available, the initial antibiotic regimen must be evaluated for appropriateness and modification may be required.

The clinical condition of the patient may deteriorate somewhat after antibiotic therapy is initiated. It is thought that this may be caused by the release of bacterial endotoxins as a result of the bactericidal effects of the antimicrobials.

The optimal duration of antibiotic therapy in the sepsis syndrome is difficult to define. It is dependent on a number of factors such as the site of infection, bacterial organism(s), the continued presence and/or removal of infected foreign bodies, concomitant medical problems, and the degree of immunocompetence. Typically, the duration of therapy should be 10 to 14 days or longer if infection persists at the primary site.[12] If the patient is immunocompromised, the treatment may need to be even longer. The antibiotics should not be stopped until the patient is afebrile for at least 4 to 7 days, has a resolving infection, and has a neutrophil count of at least $500/mm^3$ and increasing.[12]

Immunotherapy of Sepsis

Ziegler et al.[36] conducted a study using human antiserum to endotoxin produced by *Escherichia coli* J5 (J5 antiserum) in bacteremic patients. Deaths due to sepsis were reduced 22% compared to the control group (39%). In patients with profound shock, mortality was reduced 44% compared to control subjects (77%).[36] This study provided the first clinical evidence that reduction of the endotoxin effect might improve patient outcome in Gram-negative bacteremia and shock. Prophylactic administration of J5 antiserum in high-risk surgical patients improved outcome in infected patients in a later study.[37] Although these early results were promising, widespread use of antiendotoxin antiserum is not feasible because of the large number of volunteers needed to generate the antiserum. Additionally, the risks of disease transmission as well as the lack of predictable consistent interlot potency militate against common clinical application. The application of monoclonal antibody (mAb) technology avoids some of the above problems and has led to the development of mAbs directed against endotoxin and tumor necrosis factor α(TNF-α).[38–42]

Two large randomized controlled trials were conducted to evaluate the use of human monoclonal antiendotoxin antibody (HA1A) and murine monoclonal antiendotoxin antibody (E5) in the treatment of Gram-negative sepsis and shock. Ziegler et al.[43] conducted a randomized double-blind trial involving 543 patients with sepsis. Patients were randomly assigned to be treated with HA1A or placebo. Two hundred (37%) patients had Gram-negative bacteremia proven by blood cultures. Forty-nine percent of patients with Gram-negative bacteremia receiving placebo died. Thirty percent of patients receiving HA1A died. In the 196 patients with Gram-negative bacteremia who were followed to hospital discharge or death, 45 of 93 (48%) given placebo were alive and discharged compared to 65 of 103 (63%) of patients treated with HA1A.[43]

Greenman et al.[44] conducted a prospective, randomized, double-blind, placebo-controlled trial of E5 in 486 patients with Gram-negative sepsis. A total of 316 patients had confirmed Gram-negative sepsis. Administration of E5 resulted in significantly greater survival in patients with Gram-negative sepsis without shock. Resolution of organ failure was seen more frequently in these patients: in 19 of 35 (54%) receiving E5 compared to 8 of 27 (30%) in the placebo group.[44] Critical review and analysis of these studies by the scientific community produced much controversy and debate.[45] Trials of HA1A and E5 have shown that these agents have no effect on patient mortality.[46,47] Nebacumab (HA1A) was removed from all European markets in 1994. It was withdrawn from further research in the United States because of lack of efficacy.[48]

TNF-α appears to have a central role in the release of cytokines that cause the pathophysiologic changes associated with the sepsis syndrome and other inflammatory conditions.[49,50] Its nomenclature is based on its early use in oncologic studies. Injection of endotoxin induces a rise in TNF-α concentrations, which is associated with onset of chills, headache, fever, and tachycardia. Elevated TNF-α levels have been associated with adverse outcomes in sepsis.[51] Antibodies to TNF-α might, therefore, provide an effective treatment modality for the sepsis syndrome.[52]

A large multicenter prospective trial of mAb to human TNF-α versus placebo in 994 patients was performed. Patients with septic shock (N=478) demonstrated a trend toward a reduction in all-cause mortality at 3 days after infusion. There was no significant difference in all-cause mortality for all patients who received TNF-α mAb compared to placebo. Serious adverse effects were reported in 4.6% of treated patients.[53] Further studies focused on the subset of patients with sepsis syndrome and shock due to the results of the above study, which showed a greater benefit in that population. For example, the International Sepsis Trial (INTERSEPT II), randomly assigned 1879 patients with septic shock to receive TNF-α mAb or placebo.[54] Neither a decrease in organ failure nor an improvement in survival was found.

Further clinical studies need to be performed to evaluate the role of specific mAbs in the treatment of sepsis. Soluble interleukin-1 receptors and receptor antagonists showed promise early in animals and in human phase II trials.[50] However, a more recent trial showed no overall significant increase in survival, and another study was stopped because no effect was detected.

Many reasons for the failure of immunotherapy for sepsis have been proposed. Cytokines are thought to have both advantageous and damaging effects during sepsis, so inhibiting them may lead to advantageous or damaging results. Studies conducted in the future may help to better determine particular cases in which these therapies may prove to be beneficial.[55] Researchers continue to impart additional aspects of the immunologic response and to search for possible novel treatments.[56]

Supportive Pharmacotherapy

Aside from antibiotics, a patient with sepsis or septic shock requires prompt stabilization of respiratory and hemodynamic parameters. Stabilization of respiratory function is achieved with supplemental oxygen, close monitoring of arterial blood gases, and, if necessary, mechanical ventilation.[57]

Hypotension is commonly present and should be initially treated with rapid fluid administration to raise the blood pressure and achieve adequate tissue perfusion.[57] It should be noted that the use of positive pressure mechanical ventilation transiently decreases the patient's blood pressure. This transient hypotension usually responds to fluids. If fluid administration does not achieve the desired effects or if the patient develops signs of fluid overload, a sympathomimetic agent should be used.[57] Dopamine is the agent used initially in most cases. At low doses (2 to 5 μg/kg/min), dopamine acts on the dopaminergic receptors, increasing renal blood flow.[58] At higher doses (5 to 10 μg/kg/min), β-receptors are stimulated to a greater degree than α-receptors, while at doses greater than 10 μg/kg/min, the effect is primarily on α-receptors, causing an increased systemic vascular resistance.[58] At this point, dopamine has essentially the same effects as norepinephrine. When either agent is used, it should be titrated to achieve an adequate blood pressure to maintain tissue perfusion. Other agents (Table 82.3) may also be used to increase blood pressure.

It is important to keep in mind that as the vasoconstrictor effects increase, blood flow is decreased to many organs, including the kidneys, liver, and gastrointestinal tract. Therefore, the minimal dose necessary to maintain an adequate blood pressure should be used. In some cases, dobutamine may be used to increase myocardial contractility and cardiac output.

Hemodynamic parameters are usually monitored by invasive means in the critically ill septic patient. This may involve the placement of an arterial line to provide continuous blood pressure monitoring and placement of a pulmonary artery catheter to monitor fluid status and cardiac output.[57]

The use of corticosteroids as adjunctive therapy in sepsis has been well studied. Two placebo-controlled trials demonstrated no reduction in mortality.[59,60] In fact, a higher mortality rate was seen in the corticosteroid group, which was attributed to secondary infections. Therefore, the use of corticosteroids is not recommended as adjunctive therapy for sepsis.

Therapy of ARDS is primarily supportive, aimed at maintaining homeostasis (gas exchange, organ perfusion, and aerobic metabolism) while the acute lung injury resolves. The mainstay of supportive therapy is mechanical ventilation, which is closely monitored and customized to the individual patient.[19,61] The goal is to maximize oxygenation with minimal compromise of cardiac output and minimizing lung injury secondary to barotrauma and/or delivery of toxic concentrations of oxygen (>50%).[61]

Table 82.3 ▪ Vasoactive Drugs Used in Sepsis

Drug	Dose	Receptor Activity
Dopamine	2–20 μg/kg/min	Dopaminergic, α, β
Norepinephrine	2 μg/min and titrate	α, β
Epinephrine	0.05–0.2 μg/kg/min	α, β
Phenylephrine	20–200 μg/min	α_1
Dobutamine	2–15 μ/kg/min	β_1

[a]Dosage guidelines only; must be titrated to the desired effect.

Although ARDS is caused by increased permeability of pulmonary vasculature rather than volume overload, most physicians prefer to minimize patients' pulmonary capillary wedge pressures as much as possible while still maintaining an adequate cardiac output and blood pressure with adequate perfusion of end-organs.[19,62] Diuretics are useful, but volume status must be carefully monitored.[62]

Few pharmacologic interventions have been shown to clearly offer benefit in ARDS. Large studies are lacking in the literature, but agents that have been studied and found to offer no benefit include exogenous lung surfactant, acetylcysteine (an antioxidant), ibuprofen, and alprostadil.[19] Clinical trials involving ketoconazole and pentoxifylline require larger study groups to evaluate their role in sepsis; however, neither treatment looks promising.[19]

The use of corticosteroids in ARDS has been a subject of great controversy. Whereas studies have not found corticosteroids to be useful in the early or later phases of ARDS[59,60,63] and in fact may predispose the patient to infections, these agents may be useful during the fibroproliferative stage.[64,65] Some authors recommend initiating a 1- to 2-week trial of corticosteroids 1 to 2 weeks after the onset of ARDS in patients with severe disease who show no sign of improvement.[19]

Recovery from ARDS may take several weeks. Supportive care and measures to prevent complications such as nosocomial pneumonia, stress ulcers, and deep vein thromboses continue to be the mainstay of therapy for patients with ARDS.[19]

For DIC treat the underlying cause and give the patient support while healing occurs.[23] Fresh frozen plasma is commonly given when necessary.[23] Although controversial, heparin (which inhibits thrombin formation) may be used in patients for whom supportive measures are inadequate. When used for DIC, heparin is given as a continuous infusion at a low dose (300 to 500 U/hr).[23] Other anticoagulants, such as warfarin, have been used unsuccessfully.[23]

Nonpharmacologic Therapy

Hemofiltration (an established method for treatment of acute renal failure) may remove harmful substances, such as circulating mediators and cytokines, thus reducing their damaging effects. Continuous hemofiltration has been shown to improve hemodynamics, pulmonary function, and survival rates in animal models; however, the data in humans to date have not been as promising. A study by Heering et al.[66] determined that continuous venovenous hemofiltration can remove TNF-α and cytokines; however, a reduction in the blood levels of cytokines was not evident. Another study by Matamis et al.[67] failed to demonstrate beneficial hemodynamic effects. The correlation between a change in the concentration of inflammatory mediators and a change in hemodynamic parameters has not yet been established. Large randomized studies are needed to determine the utility of renal replacement therapy for the treatment of sepsis, but such studies are difficult to conduct because of the variability of technique between institutions. Therefore, this treatment remains controversial and still unproven.[68]

FUTURE THERAPIES

Even with appropriate antibiotic therapy and other adjunctive therapies, sepsis may progress to shock, cellular damage, and the death of the patient. The core endotoxin components of the cell wall of Gram-negative bacteria act as messengers or signals for macrophages to release biologically active "triggers" such as TNF-α and other cytokines as detailed earlier in this chapter. These cytokines produce many of the manifestations of sepsis syndrome including hypothermia, tachypnea, tachycardia, and organ dysfunction. Blocking or modification of the actions of endotoxin and/or these cytokines may confer the ability to augment or blunt the physiologic and pathologic manifestations of sepsis and its sequelae. It has been hypothesized that early clinical interventions with these treatment modalities might save lives in patients with sepsis.

A promising agent in the treatment of ARDS is inhaled nitric oxide. Nitric oxide acts as a selective pulmonary vasodilator. Its use in neonatal pulmonary hypertension is well described. Although its use in ARDS is still under investigation, it may prove useful for patients in whom conventional maneuvers have not optimized the oxygenation.[19]

PHARMACOECONOMICS

The literature on the pharmacoeconomics specifically pertaining to the treatment of bacteremia and sepsis is lacking. A study by Dasta and Armstrong[69] designed to evaluate the economic impact of patients in ICUs reported that patients who had a primary diagnosis of sepsis had more drugs administered per day (10.8 ± 2.5) than the mean for all patients in surgical ICUs (8.6 ± 3.0), they had the largest revenue loss ($54,738 per patient versus the average of $17,803), and they had the highest percentage of pharmacy to total hospital charges (18.8 ± 8.5% versus the average of 13.6 ± 7.7%).

Although as previously stated, there have been no trials researching the use of extended-interval dosing specifically for sepsis, an article published in *Pharmacoeconomics* pertains to the use of once-daily aminoglycoside administration in patients with Gram-negative sepsis.[70] It reviews the theoretical benefit of this dosing regimen based on literature from the 1970s pointing to the need for "adequate" serum concentrations early in the course of treatment because of the high mortality rate. Cost benefits of using this dosing regimen can result from decreased preparation/administration costs, decreased wastage associated with decreased frequency of daily administration, decreased monitoring costs due to a reduced number of samples needing to be taken, decreased costs associated with toxicity, and decreased costs of treatment failure.

KEY POINTS

- The successful management of sepsis with its attendant high mortality relies on early clinical suspicion, rapid diagnosis, and appropriate choice of antimicrobial agents based on clinical presentation, suspected source of infection, and a variety of underlying patient-specific factors.
- Use of traditional treatment modalities such as prompt fluid resuscitation and ventilatory and blood pressure support is fundamental to the clinical management of this syndrome.
- Because of the direct or indirect release of numerous chemical mediators by endotoxins as well as bacteria, yeast, viruses, or fungal antigens, there can be rapid progression of the syndrome.
- Rapidly evolving manifestations include decline in organ functions, and the development of life-threatening conditions such as ARDS and DIC.
- These rapid changes require prompt modification of drug dosing, application of therapeutic drug monitoring, and close monitoring in a patient's hemodynamic status to adjust primary therapy as well as supportive therapy.
- The optimal cost-effective application of newer technology such as the use of monoclonal antibodies and hemofiltration is awaiting further results of ongoing clinical trials.
- Only through continued research and the proper application of the results to the management of the patient with sepsis can the overall outcome of this syndrome be improved.

REFERENCES

1. Bone RC, Balk RA, Cerra FB, et al. The ACCP/SCCM Consensus Conference Committee: definitions for sepsis and organ failure and guidelines for the use of innovative therapies in sepsis. Chest 101:1644–1655, 1992.
2. Balk RA, Bone RC. The septic syndrome: definition and clinical implications. Crit Care Clin 5:1–8, 1989.
3. Ayres SM. SCCM's new horizons conference on sepsis and septic shock. Crit Care Med 13:864–866, 1985.
4. Members of the American College of Chest Physicians/Society of Critical Care Medicine Consensus Conference Committee. Definitions for sepsis and organ failure and guidelines for the use of innovative therapies in sepsis. Crit Care Med 20:864–874, 1992.
5. Increase in National Hospital Discharge Survey rates for septicemia–United States. 1979–1987. MMWR Morb Mortal Wkly Rep 39:31–34, 1990.
6. Sands KE, Bates DW, Lanken PN, et al. Epidemiology of sepsis syndrome in 8 academic medical centers. JAMA 278:234–240, 1997.
7. Bone RC, Fisher CJ Jr, Clemmer TP, et al. Sepsis syndrome: a valid clinical entity. Crit Care Med 17:389–393, 1989.
8. Martin MA, Pfaller MA, Wenzel RP. Coagulase-negative staphylococcal bacteremia. Ann Intern Med 110:9–16, 1989.
9. Tran DD, Groeneveld AB, van der Meulen J, et al. Age, chronic disease, sepsis, organ system failure, and mortality in a medical intensive care unit. Crit Care Med 18:474–479, 1990.
10. Dunn DL. Immunotherapeutic advances in the treatment of gram-negative bacterial sepsis. World J Surg 11:233–240, 1987.
11. The Veteran's Administration Systemic Sepsis Comparative Study Group. Effect of high-dose glucocorticoid therapy on mortality in patients with clinical signs of systemic sepsis. N Engl J Med 317:659–665, 1987.
12. Young LS. Sepsis syndrome. In: Mandell GL, Douglas RG, Bennett JE, et al.

Principles and practice of infectious diseases. 4th ed. Philadelphia: Churchill Livingstone, 1995:690–705.
13. Sprung CL, Caralis PV, Marcial EH, et al. The effects of high-dose corticosteroids in patients with septic shock. A prospective, controlled study. N Engl J Med 311:1137–1143, 1984.
14. Parker MM, Parillo JE. Septic shock: hemodynamics and pathogenesis. JAMA 250:3324–3327, 1983.
15. Bone RC. The pathogenesis of sepsis. Ann Intern Med 115:457–469, 1991.
16. Tracey KJ, Lowry SF, Cerami A. Cachectin/TNF-alpha in septic shock and septic adult respiratory distress syndrome [Editorial]. Am Rev Respir Dis 138:1377–1379, 1988.
17. Fong Y, Lowry SF, Cerami A. Cachectin/TNF: a macrophage protein that induces cachexia and shock. JPEN J Parenter Enteral Nutr 12:72S–77S, 1988.
18. Hyers TM. Prediction of survival and mortality in patients with adult respiratory distress syndrome. New Horiz 1:466–470, 1993.
19. Kollef MH, Shuster DP. The acute respiratory distress syndrome. N Engl J Med 332:27–37, 1995.
20. Fowler AA, Hamman RF, Good JT Jr, et al. Adult respiratory distress syndrome: risk with common predispositions. Ann Intern Med 98:593–597, 1983.
21. Goldsberry DT, Hurst JM. Adult respiratory distress syndrome and sepsis. New Horiz 1:342–347, 1993.
22. Suchyta MR, Clemmer TP, Elliott CO, et al. The adult respiratory distress syndrome: a report of survival and modifying factors. Chest 101:1074–1079, 1992.
23. ten Cate H, Brandjes DPM, Wolters HJ, et al. Disseminated intravascular coagulation: pathophysiology, diagnosis, and treatment. New Horiz 1:312–323, 1993.
24. Chandrasekar PH, Brown WJ. Clinical issues of blood cultures. Arch Intern Med 154:841–849, 1994.
25. Wheeler AP, Carroll FE, Bernard GR. Radiographic issues in adult respiratory distress syndrome. New Horiz 1:471–477, 1993.
26. Parrillo JE, Parker NM, Natanson C, et al. Septic shock in humans: advances in the understanding of pathogenesis, cardiovascular dysfunction, and therapy. Ann Intern Med 113:227–242, 1990.
27. Conboy K, Welage LS, Walawander CA, et al. Sepsis syndrome and associated sequelae in patients at high risk for gram-negative sepsis. Pharmacotherapy 15:66–77, 1995.
28. Conte JE Jr. Empiric antibiotic therapy. In: Manual of antibiotics and infectious diseases. 8th ed. Baltimore: Williams & Wilkins, 1995:54–61.
29. Mercer-Jones MA, Jadjiminas DJ, Heinzelmann M, et al. Continuous antibiotic treatment of experimental abdominal sepsis: effects on organ inflammatory cytokine expression and neutrophil sequestration. Br J Surg 85:385–389, 1998.
30. Nicolau DP, Nightingale CH, Banevicius MA , et al. Serum bactericidal activity of ceftazidime: continuous infusion versus intermittent injections. Antimicrob Agents Chemother 40:61–64, 1996.
31. Mouton JW, Vinks AA. Is continuous infusion of beta-lactam antibiotics worthwhile? Efficacy and pharmacokinetic considerations. J Antimicrob Chemother 38:5–15, 1996.
32. Vondracek TG. Beta-lactam antibiotics: is continuous infusion the preferred method of administration? Ann Pharmacother 29:415–424, 1995.
33. Moore RD, Lietman PS, Smith CR. Clinical response to aminoglycoside therapy: importance of the ratio of peak concentration to minimal inhibitory concentration. J Infect Dis 155:98–99, 1987.
34. Marik PE, Lipman J, Kobillski S, et al. A prospective randomized study comparing once versus twice-daily amikacin dosing in critically ill adult and pediatric patients. J Antimicrob Chemother 28:753–764, 1991.
35. Nicolau DP, Freeman CD, Belliveau PP, et.al. Experience with a once-daily aminoglycoside program administered to 2,184 adult patients. Antimicrob Agents Chemother 39:650–655, 1995.
36. Ziegler EJ, McCutchan JA, Fierer J, et al. Treatment of gram-negative bacteremia and shock with human antiserum to a mutant *Escherichia coli*. N Engl J Med 307:1225–1230, 1982.
37. Baumgartner J-D, Glauser MP, McCutchan JA, et al. Prevention of gram-negative shock and death in surgical patients by antibody to endotoxin core glycolipid. Lancet 2:59–63, 1985.
38. Chmel H. Role of monoclonal antibody therapy in the treatment of infectious disease. Am J Hosp Pharm 47(Suppl 3):S11–S15, 1990.
39. Wenzel RP. Anti-endotoxin monoclonal antibodies–a second look. N Engl J Med 326:1151–1152, 1992.
40. Zarowitz BJ. Human monoclonal antibody against endotoxin. Ann Pharmacother 25:778–783, 1991.
41. Olsen KM, Campbell GD. E5 monoclonal immunoglobulin M antibody for the treatment of gram-negative sepsis. Ann Pharmacother 25:784–790, 1991.
42. Pennington JE. Therapy with antibody to tumor necrosis factor in sepsis. Clin Infect Dis 17(Suppl 2):S515–S519, 1993.
43. Ziegler EJ, Fisher CJ, Sprung CL, et al. Treatment of gram-negative bacteremia and septic shock with HA-1A human monoclonal antibody against endotoxin. N Engl J Med 324:428–436, 1991.
44. Greenman RL, Schein RMH, Martin MA, et al. A controlled clinical trial of E5 murine monoclonal IgM antibody to endotoxin in the treatment of gram-negative sepsis. JAMA 266:1097–1102, 1991.
45. Warren HS, Danner RL, Munford RS. Antiendotoxin monoclonal antibodies. N Engl J Med 326:1153–1156, 1992.
46. Bone RC, Balk RA, Fein AM, et al. A second large controlled clinical study of E5, a monoclonal antibody to endotoxin: results of a prospective, multicenter, randomized, controlled trial. Crit Care Med 23:994–1005, 1995.
47. McCloskey RV, Straube RC, Sanders C, et al. Treatment of septic shock with human monoclonal antibody HA-1A. Ann Intern Med 121:1–5, 1994.
48. Rybacki JJ. Nebacumab (Drug Evaluation Monograph). In: Gelman CR, Rumack BH, Hutchison TA, eds. DRUGDEX System.
49. Beutler B, Cerami A. Cachectin: more than a tumor necrosis factor. N Engl J Med 316:379–384, 1987.
50. Michie HR, Spriggs DR, Manoque KR, et al. Tumor necrosis factor and endotoxin induce similar metabolic responses in human beings. Surgery 104:280–286, 1988.
51. Casey LC, Balk RA, Bone RC. Plasma cytokine and endotoxin levels correlate with survival in patients with the sepsis syndrome. Ann Intern Med 119:771–778, 1993.
52. Dinarello CA, Gelfand JA, Wolff SM. Anticytokine strategies in the treatment of the systemic inflammatory response syndrome. JAMA 269:1829–1835, 1993.
53. Abraham E, Wunderink R, Silverman H, et al. Efficacy and safety of monoclonal antibody to human tumor necrosis factor alpha in patients with sepsis syndrome. JAMA 273:934–941, 1995.
54. Abraham E, Anzueto A, Gutierrez G, et al. Double-blind randomised controlled trial of monoclonal antibody to human tumour necrosis factor in treatment of septic shock. NORASEPT II Study Group. Lancet 351:929–933, 1998.
55. Reinhart K, Karzai W. Treatment of sepsis: what has changed during the last decades? Acta Anaesth Scand 111(Suppl):174–176, 1997.
56. Vincent JL. Search for effective immunomodulating strategies against sepsis. Lancet 351:922–923, 1998.
57. Light RB. Septic shock. In: Principles of critical care. 1st ed. New York: McGraw-Hill, 1992:1172–1185.
58. Complete prescribing information. Intropin (dopamine HCl injection). Puerto Rico: DuPont Pharmaceuticals, August 1992.
59. Luce JM, Montgomery AM, Marks JD, et al. Ineffectiveness of high-dose methylprednisolone in preventing parenchymal lung injury and improving mortality in patients with septic shock. Am Rev Respir Dis 138:62–68, 1988.
60. Bone RC, Fisher CJ Jr, Clanner TP, et al. Early methylprednisolone treatment for septic syndrome and the adult respiratory distress syndrome. Chest 92:1032–1036, 1987.
61. Marini JJ. New options for the ventilatory management of acute lung injury. New Horiz 1:489–503, 1993.
62. Shuster DP. The case for and against fluid restriction and occlusion pressure reduction in adult respiratory distress syndrome. New Horiz 1:478–488, 1993.
63. Bernard GR, Luce JM, Sprung CL, et al. High-dose corticosteroids in patients with the adult respiratory distress syndrome. N Engl J Med 317:1565–1570, 1987.
64. Hooper RG, Kearl RA. Established ARDS treated with a sustained course of adrenocorticosteroids. Chest 97:138–143, 1990.
65. Meduri GU, Belenchia JM, Estes RJ, et al. Fibroproliferative phase of ARDS: clinical findings and effects of corticosteroids. Chest 100:943–952, 1991.
66. Heering P, Morgera S, Schmitz FJ, et al. Cytokine removal and cardiovascular hemodynamics in septic patients with continuous venovenous hemofiltration. Intensive Care Med 23:288–296, 1997.
67. Matamis D, Tsagourias M, Koletsos K, et al. Influence of continuous hemofiltration-related hypothermia on hemodynamic variables and gas exchange in septic patients. Intensive Care Med 20:431–436, 1994.
68. De Vriese AS, Vanholder RC, De Sutter JH, et al. Continuous renal replacement therapies in sepsis: where are the data? Nephrol Dial Transplant 13:1362–1364, 1998.
69. Dasta JF, Armstrong DK. Pharmacoeconomic impact of critically ill surgical patients. DICP 22: 994–998, 1988.
70. Parker SE, Davey PG. Once-daily aminoglycoside administration in gram-negative sepsis. Pharmacoeconomics 7:393–402, 1995.

CHAPTER 83

SKIN AND SOFT TISSUE INFECTIONS

Jeanne Hawkins Van Tyle and Neeta Bahal O'Mara

Bacteria normally colonize the skin without causing infection. Normal skin flora include a variety of aerobic and anaerobic bacteria and fungi (Table 83.1). The body's best defense against bacterial infection is an intact skin barrier. A variety of bacterial infections of the skin may occur (Table 83.2). Infections may be primary or secondary. The common etiologic agents and empiric treatment options vary depending on the infection, as summarized in Table 83.2. This chapter describes several of the more common skin infections, including cellulitis, impetigo, erysipelas, periorbital cellulitis, decubitus ulcers, and diabetic foot ulcers.

Cellulitis

DEFINITION

Cellulitis is defined as an acute, spreading infection of the skin and subcutaneous tissue.[1]

EPIDEMIOLOGY

Although cellulitis may affect patients of all ages, more than one-half of patients who develop cellulitis have an underlying condition such as drug or alcohol abuse, obesity, diabetes mellitus, peripheral vascular disease, or preexisting edema.[2] The presence of a foreign body, such as an intravenous catheter, also increases the risk of developing cellulitis.

Table 83.1 ▪ Normal Skin Flora

Bacteria	
	Staphylococcus epidermidis[a]
	Diphtheroids
	Corynebacterium spp.[a]
	Propionibacterium acnes[a]
	Staphylococcus aureus
	Streptococcus spp.
	Streptococcus pyogenes
	Peptococcus
	Mycobacterium spp.
	Bacillus spp.
Fungi	
	Malassezia furfur[a]
	Candida spp.

[a]Most common organisms.

PATHOPHYSIOLOGY

Cellulitis may occur when the skin barrier is broken, as in a cut, bite, or abrasion. Other causes of cellulitis include infection from a contiguous site (e.g., osteomyelitis) or due to hematogenous spread.

Although any organism may cause cellulitis, the most common bacterial causes are group A streptococci and *Staphylococcus* species.[1] In addition, in certain populations, other organisms are prevalent (Table 83.3). For example, patients with diabetes may develop cellulitis caused by multiple organisms, including Gram-negative organisms and anaerobic organisms (see Diabetic Foot Infections later in this chapter). *Haemophilus influenzae* was considered a common pathogen in children before the *H. influenzae* vaccine was introduced.

CLINICAL PRESENTATION AND DIAGNOSIS

Cellulitis most commonly affects the head, neck, and upper and lower extremities.

Signs and Symptoms

The most common signs and symptoms associated with cellulitis include pain, tenderness, erythema, swelling, and warmth at the site of infection.[2] Less often, patients have

Table 83.2 ▪ Common Bacterial Infections of the Skin

Lesion	Common Etiologic Agents	Treatment Options
Primary infections		
Cellulitis	Group A *Streptococcus* *S. aureus*	PRSP; 1st-generation cephalosporin, azithromycin,[a] clarithromycin,[b] AM/CL
Impetigo	Group A *Streptococcus* *S. aureus*	Oral 1st- or 2nd-generation cephalosporin, erythromycin, AM/CL, azithromycin,[a] clarithromycin, mupirocin
Erysipelas	Group A *Streptococcus*	PRSP, cefazolin, AM/CL
Periorbital cellulitis	Group A *Streptococcus* *S. aureus* Enterobacteriaceae	Parenteral 1st-generation cephalosporin, PRSP, TC/CL, AM/SB, 2nd- or 3rd-generation parenteral cephalosporin
Secondary infections		
Chronic ulcers (decubitus)	Polymicrobic; can include coliform bacteria, peptostreptococci, enterococci, *Bacteroides* spp., *Proteus* spp., *C. perfringens, P. aeruginosa*	CephFrag + APAG, imipenem + cilastatin, TC/CL, PIP/TZ, CIP + clindamycin
Diabetic foot ulcers	Polymicrobic; can include *S. aureus, B. fragilis, C. perfringens, P. aeruginosa,* peptostreptococci, enterococci, *Proteus* spp.	CephFrag + APAG, imipenem + cilastatin, TC/CL, PIP/TZ, CIP + clindamycin

PRSP, penicillinase-resistant synthetic penicillin (e.g., nafcillin or dicloxacillin); *AM/CL,* amoxicillin + clavulanate; *TC/CL,* ticarcillin + clavulanate; *AM/SB,* ampicillin + sulbactam; *CephFrag,* cephalosporins with significant *B. fragilis* activity (i.e., cefoxitin or cefotetan); *APAG,* antipseudomonal aminoglycoside; *PIP/TZ,* piperacillin + tazobactam; *CIP,* ciprofloxacin.

[a]Indication approved by the U.S. Food and Drug Administration.

[b]Unlabeled use.

lymphangitis (streaks of erythema spreading from the area of cellulitis) and enlarged and tender lymph nodes. Some patients may experience a prodrome, which may include chills, malaise, anorexia, nausea, and vomiting.[2] Fever and white blood cell count elevation may occur in some patients but are not present in all.

Diagnosis

Needle aspiration of the infected area may identify the pathogenic organism in up to 60% of patients,[3] but other investigators report lower yields.[4,5] In general, needle aspiration and cultures of the infected area are unnecessary in uncomplicated cases because empiric therapy is effective in the majority of cases.[6] Obtaining cultures should be considered if the infection is complex; if there is an increased risk of complications, as in very young patients or older adults and in patients with diabetes, peripheral vascular disease, or immunosuppression; and if a standard course of antibiotics has failed.[7,8]

Table 83.3 ▪ Common Microorganisms Causing Cellulitis in Specific Patient Populations

Normal healthy population	Group A streptococci *S. aureus*
Children	Group A streptococci *Staphylococcus* spp. *H. influenzae*
Diabetic patients	*Staphylococcus* spp. *Streptococcus* spp. Gram-negative organisms Anaerobic organisms
Hospitalized patients[10]	*Staphylococcus* spp. (including coagulase-negative staphylococci) *Streptococcus* spp., Gram-negative organisms (*Hemophilus spp., E. coli, Klebsiella, Pseudomonas* spp.)

TREATMENT

Pharmacotherapy

Optimal cellulitis treatment is based on a number of factors, including the most likely causative organisms, penetration of the antibiotic to the site of infection, concurrent medications, medication allergies, patient compliance issues, and cost. The most likely organism may vary depending on patient age and concomitant diseases such as diabetes mellitus or human immunodeficiency virus (HIV) infection (Table 83.3). Commonly used outpatient antibiotic regimens for uncomplicated cellulitis are listed in Table 83.4.

Empiric therapy of uncomplicated cellulitis should be effective against *Streptococcus* species and *Staphylococcus aureus.* Table 83.4 summarizes commonly used outpatient antibiotic regimens for uncomplicated cellulitis treatment. Although penicillin and erythromycin are effective against streptococci, they do not treat penicillinase-producing staphylococci, which are the majority of all staphylococcal organisms. Therefore, oral therapy with a penicillinase-resistant synthetic penicillin (PRSP) such as dicloxacillin or a first-generation cephalosporin such as cephalexin is preferred. If intravenous therapy is indicated, empiric therapy with a β-lactamase–stable penicillin such as nafcillin or a first-generation cephalosporin such as cefazolin may be used. For patients who live in a nursing home or who have been recently or are currently hospitalized, methicillin-resistant *S. aureus* (MRSA) may be a causative organism. Therefore, vancomycin therapy may be necessary until culture and sensitivity results are known.

Once the causative organisms and sensitivities are known, therapy may be changed to provide the most appropriate antibiotic for the organisms that are identified. If streptococci are identified as the causative organism, oral penicillin VK (250 to 500 mg four times a day) or intravenous penicillin G (1 to 2 million U every 4 to 6 hours) can be used. Oral erythromycin (250 to 500 mg four times a day) and intravenous erythromycin (500 mg every 6 hours) are suitable alternatives in a patient who is allergic to penicillins and cephalosporins. If MRSA is identified, intravenous vancomycin should be used.

A variety of the newer intravenous antibiotics have been evaluated in cellulitis treatment. Several investigators have evaluated the use of ceftriaxone in children and adults with cellulitis.[9] Advantages cited include activity against the most common pathogens associated with cellulitis and the ability to administer once daily while maintaining sustained tissue concentrations above the mean inhibitory concentration (MIC) for the common pathogens. Ampicillin–sulbactam[10] and ticarcillin–clavulanate[11] have also been used successfully to treat cellulitis infections. Although many of the newer agents have demonstrated efficacy equivalent to that of traditional therapies of cellulitis, cost generally is higher and should be considered when selecting these newer agents. In addition, the antibiotic that is most active against the causative agent and has the narrowest spectrum should be chosen to avoid promoting antimicrobial resistance.

In patients who may have Gram-negative organisms (i.e., in diabetic patients, prolonged hospitalization, immunocompromised patients), empiric therapy should be broadened to include the likely pathogens. Typically, an aminoglycoside such as gentamicin or tobramycin may be added to a penicillin or cephalosporin. If anaerobic organisms are suspected, the antibiotic regimen should include clindamycin or metronidazole. Another alternative is the use of a penicillin (ampicillin–sulbactam, ticarcillin–clavulanate, piperacillin–tazobactam) or a cephalosporin (cefoxitin or cefotetan) that has activity against anaerobic organisms including *Bacteroides fragilis.*[11]

Nonpharmacologic Therapy

Nonpharmacologic therapy of cellulitis consists of resting and elevating the affected area and applying moist heat.

Table 83.4 ▪ Commonly Used Outpatient Antibiotic Regimens for Treating Uncomplicated Cellulitis

Generic Name	Brand Name	Adult Dosage	Pediatric Dosage
Penicillin antibiotics			
Penicillin V	Pen-Vee K, V-Cillin K, others	250–500 mg q6–8h	15–62.5 mg/kg/day divided q6–8h
Dicloxacillin	Dynapen, Pathocil, others	125–250 mg q6h	12–25 mg/kg/day divided q6h
Amoxicillin–clavulanate	Augmentin	250 mg (of amoxicillin) q8h or 500–875 mg q12h	20–45 mg/kg/day (of amoxicillin) divided q12h
First-generation cephalosporin antibiotics			
Cephalexin	Keflex, Keftabs, others	250–500 mg q6–12h	25–50 mg/kg/day divided q6–12h
Cefadroxil	Duricef, Ultracef	1 g as single dose or divided q12h	30 mg/kg/day divided q12h
Cephradine	Velosef	250–500 mg q6–12h	25–50 mg/kg/day divided q6–12h
Macrolide antibiotics			
Erythromycin	ERYC, Ery-Tab, EES, others	250–500 mg q6h	30–50 mg/kg/day divided q6h
Clarithromycin	Biaxin	250 mg q12h	15 mg/kg/day divided q12h
Azithromycin	Zithromax	500 mg/day × 1 day, then 250 mg/day on days 2–5	10 mg/kg on day 1 5 mg/kg q24h on days 2–5
Others			
Clindamycin	Cleocin, others	150–450 mg q6h	20–30 mg/kg/day divided q6h

Moist heat is preferred to minimize edema around the infected site[8] and to promote suppuration and drainage.[12] Surgery may be necessary if an abscess is present. Depending on the severity, extent, and location of the infection, the patient can be treated with oral antibiotics as an outpatient or as an inpatient using intravenous antibiotics. Patients with deep infections of the hand, orbital or facial cellulitis, or deep human or animal bites, and patients who are seriously ill or immunocompromised are often hospitalized and treated initially with parenteral antibiotics. After improvement, patients may complete therapy with oral antibiotics.

Impetigo

DEFINITION

Impetigo is one of the most common, contagious, superficial bacterial skin infections and occurs predominantly in children. Initially, impetigo presents as vesicles, which become pustules that rupture and form honey-crusted lesions. The vesicles usually occur on exposed areas of the skin such as the face and extremities after trauma.

PATHOPHYSIOLOGY

The most common causative organism is group A streptococci, although *S. aureus* may also be present. It is unclear whether *S. aureus* is a primary cause or a secondary invader of the infected site.

CLINICAL PRESENTATION AND DIAGNOSIS

Conditions in which there is a break in the skin, such as chickenpox, abrasions, and burns, are predisposing factors to the development of impetigo. Diagnosis can be made by history and examination, but a culture must be obtained from the base of a lesion that has had the crust removed for definitive diagnosis.

TREATMENT

Pharmacotherapy

The most effective therapy of impetigo is controversial.[13] Although some investigators claim that systemic therapy is necessary, others argue that topical therapy is sufficient. Penicillin has long been considered the drug of choice.[1] However, this is being questioned.[13–15] In one study, only 53% of patients responded to oral penicillin V therapy, whereas cloxacillin therapy was effective in 100%.[15] Consequently, a 7-day course of therapy with a penicillinase-resistant antibiotic (cloxacillin, cephalexin, cefaclor, cefadroxil, amoxicillin–clavulanic acid, erythromycin, azithromycin, or clarithromycin) aimed at both group A streptococci and *S. aureus* may be preferred.[15–20] Erythromycin therapy should be avoided in geographic areas where there is a high rate of erythromycin-resistant *S. aureus*.

Mupirocin ointment (Bactroban), a topical antibiotic, has activity against Gram-positive organisms including group A streptococci and *S. aureus*. It is applied as a 2% ointment to the affected area two or three times daily. A number of studies[16,19–22] comparing oral erythromycin with topical mupirocin have supported the efficacy of topical mupirocin. Consequently, topical mupirocin may be the treatment of choice in patients whose lesions are not widespread.[23] Regardless of the agent used, impetigo should respond to treatment within 7 days. If no improvement is seen, antimicrobial resistance or noncompliance with the prescribed regimen should be considered.

Erysipelas

DEFINITION

Erysipelas is a superficial skin infection that presents with the abrupt onset of a fiery red rash, hence the nickname *St. Anthony's fire.*

PATHOPHYSIOLOGY

The most common cause of erysipelas is group A streptococci, but other *Streptococcus* species, *H. influenzae,* and staphylococci have also been implicated. Bacteria enter through a break in the skin such as a scratch, cut, or lesion such as chickenpox lesions.[12] Facial erysipelas may occur after a streptococcal upper respiratory tract infection.[18] Patients often develop blisters, and malaise, myalgia, chills, fever, nausea, and vomiting may be present.

CLINICAL PRESENTATION AND DIAGNOSIS

The rash typically occurs in the lower extremities but may also occur on the face, ears, or arms.[24] It affects people of all ages but appears to be more common in neonates, infants, and older adults. It occurs more commonly in patients with underlying diseases but can occur in previously healthy people.[25] Diagnosis is made by examination of the rash and on clinical appearance.

TREATMENT

Pharmacotherapy

Penicillin is the drug of choice for erysipelas. It may be administered orally or intravenously, depending on the severity of the infection. Other agents that may be used include ampicillin, amoxicillin, nafcillin, oxacillin, dicloxacillin, erythromycin, clindamycin, and cephalosporins such as cefazolin, cephalexin, cefadroxil, cefuroxime axetil, and cefaclor.[12,26] Empiric therapy with a second-generation cephalosporin such as cefaclor or cefuroxime axetil may be needed to ensure adequate treatment for *H. influenzae* in nonimmunized children.[12] Oral antibiotics should be continued for 10 to 14 days or until the rash has resolved.[27,28] Recurrence of erysipelas may occur and is more common in immunocompromised patients and patients with a history of venous insufficiency. Although it is unknown why recurrences occur, there may be an association with pharyngeal carriage of group A streptococci. Therefore, prophylactic antibiotics (penicillin V orally or benzathine penicillin intramuscular) have been used to reduce the rate of recurrences in high-risk patients.[29,30]

Nonpharmacologic Therapy

Although nonpharmacologic therapy (bed rest, elevation of the affected area, and cool, moist dressings) is helpful, antibiotic therapy is the mainstay of therapy. Without antibiotics, the mortality rate has been to reported to be as high as 80% in neonates.[25]

Periorbital Cellulitis

DEFINITION

Periorbital cellulitis involves the superficial area around the eye and may represent a medical emergency.

EPIDEMIOLOGY

Periorbital cellulitis is an infection that most commonly affects infants and children. An upper respiratory tract infection, sinusitis, or conjunctivitis often precedes periorbital cellulitis. At other times, it may follow trauma such as a scratch, abrasion, or insect bite.[31] The most common causative organisms include *Staphylococcus* species, *Streptococcus* species, and *H. influenzae.* The incidence of *H. influenzae* periorbital cellulitis has dramatically declined in recent years after the routine administration of *H. influenzae* type B vaccine to all children 2 months and older.

CLINICAL PRESENTATION AND DIAGNOSIS

The eyelid and orbit is edematous, erythematous, warm, painful, and tender. Progression may occur with vision changes and increased intraocular pressure. In addition, fever and leukocytosis are present.[32]

TREATMENT

Pharmacotherapy

Empiric antibiotic therapy with parenteral antibiotics should be initiated immediately. Therapy should be targeted to cover streptococci and staphylococci in all infants and children, and *H. influenzae* may be an important pathogen in nonimmunized children. Intravenous penicillinase-resistant penicillins such as nafcillin, oxacillin, ampicillin–sulbactam or a first-generation cephalosporin such as cefazolin is effective against streptococci and *S. aureus* (not methicillin-resistant staphylococci). Second-generation cephalosporins such as cefuroxime are effective against *H. influenzae* in addition to streptococci and staphylococci. A clinical response such as fever reduction and symptom resolution typically occurs within 24 to 72 hours. After such a response, oral antibiotic therapy with amoxicillin–clavulanic acid, trimethoprim–sulfamethoxazole, or cefadroxil or other cephalosporin should be continued for 7 to 10 days.[31,32] Cefixime, a third-generation agent, may not be active against *S. aureus*.

Nonpharmacologic Therapy

Topical wet compresses may provide some symptomatic relief.

Pressure Sores (Decubitus Ulcers, Bed Sores)

DEFINITION

Pressure sores[33–40] result from ischemic necrosis and ulceration of tissues overlying a bony prominence that has been subjected to prolonged pressure against an external object such as a bed, wheelchair, cast, or splint. This pressure may be sufficient to occlude small vessels and result in irreversible ischemic changes. These lesions often develop into infected ulcers.

TREATMENT GOALS: PRESSURE SORES

- Relieve pressure and pain.
- Provide adequate nutritional support.
- Remove devitalized tissues.
- Promote granulation and reepithelization of tissue.
- Eliminate sources of moisture such as fluids of incontinence, perspiration, or wound drainage.

EPIDEMIOLOGY

Pressure ulcers are a serious problem that affects approximately 9% of all hospitalized patients and 23% of all patients in nursing homes according to the Agency for Health Care Policy and Research (AHCPR).[33]

PATHOPHYSIOLOGY

Immobility is the most important risk factor. Four factors critical to formation of pressure sores are pressure, shear, friction, and moisture. Shearing is produced by the sliding of parallel surfaces of tissue in unequal fashion, as when the head of the bed is raised and the patient slides toward the foot of the bed. Friction generated by pulling a patient across a bedsheet may result in tissue trauma and ulcer development. Moisture from perspiration or incontinence may lead to maceration and skin irritation that weaken the epidermal barrier. These lesions are most often seen in patients who have diminished or absent sensation, patients with spinal cord injury[41] or degenerative neurologic disease, or those who are debilitated, demented, emaciated, or paralyzed.[42] Other risk factors for pressure sores include advanced age,[43] poor nutrition, and low arteriolar pressure.

CLINICAL PRESENTATION AND DIAGNOSIS

Signs and Symptoms

Pressure sores most commonly occur in tissues over the sacrum and the heels and may involve skin, muscle, and bone. More than 95% of pressure sores are located on the lower body.

Classification

Clinical staging[33] or grading helps to guide management (Table 83.5). Stage I lesions involve only the epidermis, stage II ulcers extend into the dermis, stage III ulcers are deep lesions that extend into the subcutaneous tissues, and stage IV lesions extend into muscle and bone. Deep lesions often take months to heal, and extensive surgical treatments are needed. Figure 83.1 illustrates the classification of lesions based on lesion depth and tissue involvement.

Diagnosis

Accurate identification of risk factors is essential to preventing pressure sores. Several authors have proposed risk assessment scales.[44–47] One such scale, the Braden Scale,[45–47] includes six subscales that reflect sensory perception, skin moisture, activity level, mobility, nutritional

Table 83.5 ▪ Classification of Pressure Sores

Stage	Description	Treatment
I	Lesion involves only the epidermis; nonblanchable erythema of the intact skin.	Pressure relief and local wound care
II	Partial-thickness loss; ulcer extends into the dermis.	Pressure relief and local wound care
III	Full-thickness loss; deep ulcer extends into the subcutaneous tissue and fascia.	Pressure relief, surgery, and systemic antibiotics if needed
IV	Ulcer extends into muscle, bone, or joint.	Radical surgery and systemic antibiotics to treat osteomyelitis if present

Source: The National Pressure Advisory Panel.

status, and friction and shear. A score of 16 or less out of a possible 23 points predicts ulcer development. The Braden Scale has shown high reliability with different assessors, including nurse aides, licensed practical nurses, and registered nurses. The size, number, and location of pressure ulcers must be documented to allow evaluation of the effectiveness of the treatments. The key to prevention is early recognition of predisposing factors and measures to prevent pressure on sensitive areas, frequent position changes, frequent visual skin inspection, and keeping the predisposed skin areas clean and dry. Durable medical goods and special supplies are useful in these patients. The use of sheepskin or egg-crate mattresses has been suggested, but objective data suggest that they do not lower pressures sufficiently to prevent pressure sores. Many institutions have nursing policies that combine air mattresses with frequent repositioning.

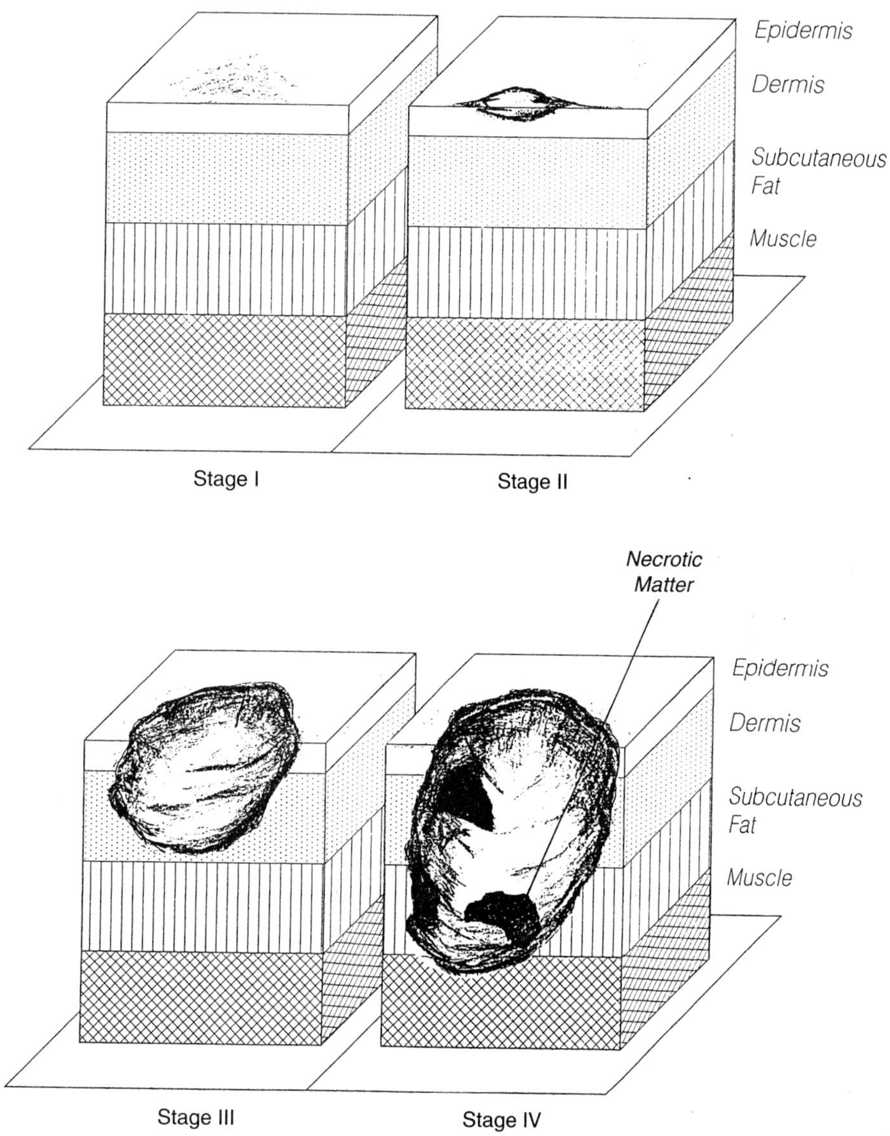

Figure 83.1. Classification of pressure sores.

PSYCHOSOCIAL ASPECTS

All patients being treated for pressure ulcers should undergo a psychosocial assessment to determine the patient's ability to comprehend information and motivation to adhere to the treatment program. At minimum, the assessment should include mental status, learning ability, and signs of depression.

THERAPEUTIC PLAN

Ulcer treatment must be planned with the understanding that it is like an iceberg, with only a small visible surface and an extensive unknown base. Many treatments for pressure ulcers have been recommended without adequate evidence to support their use. The treatment of stage I and stage II lesions is primarily local. If the patient cannot adequately oxygenate the tissue, systemic antibiotics are unlikely to have high penetration into the area. Figure 83.2 is an AHCPR algorithm for pressure ulcer treatment.[33]

TREATMENT

Pharmacotherapy

Local Therapy

The role of pharmaceutical debriding agents is less well defined. Many products that are used as debriding agents are applied to the wound on gauze. Mechanical debridement through the use of gauze dressings may allow earlier development of granulation tissue. Mechanical debridement with wet-to-dry dressings is painful and may traumatize the wound.[48] Wet-to-moist or wet-to-wet debridement may accomplish the same result while causing less discom-

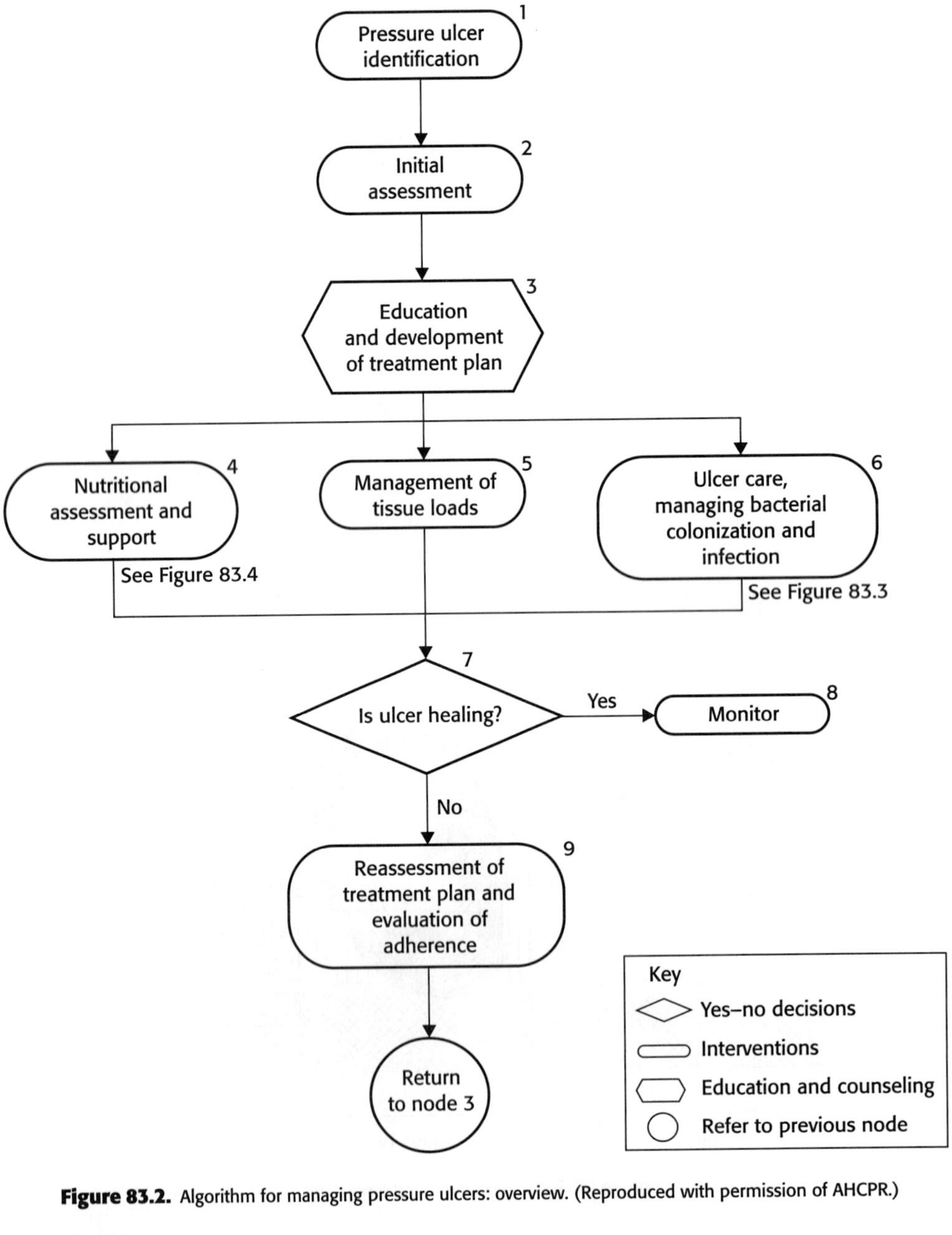

Figure 83.2. Algorithm for managing pressure ulcers: overview. (Reproduced with permission of AHCPR.)

fort. Gauze interacts physically with the wound surface and can cause dry-to-dry debridement, wet-to-dry debridement, or wet-to-wet debridement.

Absorbent materials such as dextranomer (Debrisan) microbeads have been used on moist ulcers. Dextranomer is a sterile, chemically inert, hydrophilic substance that removes exudate from the wound surface via an osmotic pressure mechanism. It is available as a paste or bead preparation. When sprinkled onto open wounds, these products are thought to act through the formation of a gel that removes fluids, microbes, and debris from the wound through capillary forces.

Enzymatic debridement has been used to clean pressure sores that are covered with eschar. Eschar is the scab or slough produced by the wound. Travase (casein in mineral oil and polyethylene glycol) is a sutilain that acts to selectively digest necrotic soft tissue by proteolytic actions. A moist environment is necessary for optimal enzymatic activity. The wound is cleaned and irrigated with normal saline. A thin layer of Travase ointment is applied to the site and covered with a moist dressing. The site should be cleansed and redressed three or four times a day for best results. The action of the casein is impaired by certain agents such as benzalkonium chloride, hexachlorophene, nitrofurazone, and thimerosal that may be used as preservatives in other products. Antibiotics such as penicillin, neomycin, and streptomycin do not affect the enzyme activity. Santyl is collagenase in white petrolatum. Collagenase is able to dissolve undenatured collagen fibers that retard healing. Collagenase is effective within a narrow pH range of 6 to 8. Collagenase ointment is applied directly to deep wounds with a tongue depressor or onto a sterile gauze. In the presence of an infection, the topical antibiotic should be applied first. It is used once daily and is compatible with neomycin–polymyxin B–bacitracin ointment. Elase is fibrinolysin and desoxyribonuclease in petrolatum. The enzyme activity probably is exhausted at the end of 24 hours. Desoxyribonuclease is isolated from bovine pancreas. It acts to depolymerize desoxyribonucleic acids and DNA in necrotic tissue. The wound should be cleaned with saline and then gently dried before the ointment is used. The dressing is changed two or three times a day with warm saline flushes at dressing change.

It is doubtful whether antiseptics (Table 83.6) have any beneficial effects on open ulcers. The contact time between antiseptic and microbe is too brief for bactericidal effects, and antiseptics may inhibit wound healing. The clinical practice guidelines published by AHCPR specifically state that antiseptics should not be used to treat pressure sores. Normal saline is the recommended cleansing solution for most pressure ulcers.

The topical antibiotics (Table 83.7) do not penetrate deeper tissues. Antibiotic dressings may not enhance healing and may induce microbial resistance. Neomycin-based products may produce allergic reactions. Infected pressure sores warrant culture and sensitivity testing with appropriate parenteral antibiotics if bacterial infection is documented.[49] Figure 83.3 from AHCPR guides the clinician through a preferred pathway for managing bacterial colonization and local and systemic infection. A 2-week trial of topical antibiotics (e.g., an agent such as silver sulfadiazine) for clean pressure ulcers that are not healing should be considered. Silver sulfadiazine is a broad-spectrum agent with activity against Gram-positive and Gram-negative bacteria. It has been used in pressure ulcers and infected leg ulcers.[50] Topical metronidazole may be effective on infected ulcers that produce a characteristic foul odor. A number of studies[51–53] have used once- or twice-daily application of topical metronidazole with promising results. This indication is not approved by the U.S. Food and Drug Administration (FDA). In a study by Pierleoni,[53] topical metronidazole 1% was applied to sterile gauze in infected decubitus ulcers every 8 hours. Microbiologic efficacy was documented. It may be combined with oral therapy in suspected or documented susceptible anaerobic infections. A commercially available gel contains metronidazole 0.75% in a water-soluble gel (MetroGel Curatek).

Table 83.6 ▪ Topical Antiseptic Agents

Generic Name	Trade Name	Note or Caution
Chlorhexidine	Hibiclens	Associated with corneal opacification
Povidone–iodine	Betadine	Associated with hypothyroidism
Hydrogen peroxide	Various	Cytotoxic; may impair healing; no longer recommended
Acetic acid	Various	Cytotoxic; may impair healing; no longer recommended
Sodium hypochlorite	Dakin's solution	Cytotoxic; may impair healing; no longer recommended

Chemicals used as antiseptics may kill the microflora in a wound but may also damage delicate, newly forming skin. The Agency for Health Care Policy Research Clinical Practice Guidelines do not recommend any topical antiseptic.

Table 83.7 ▪ Topical Antibiotic Agents

Suggested role in pressure ulcers with purulent drainage and/or foul odor:
- Silver sulfadiazine
- Gentamicin
- Bacitracin
- Mupirocin (Bactroban)
- Metronidazole gel (MetroGel; not approved by the U.S. Food and Drug Administration)

Systemic Therapy

Systemic antibiotics[54] are indicated only when there is evidence of advancing cellulitis, sepsis, bacteremia, or osteomyelitis. Because ulcer debridement may result in tran-

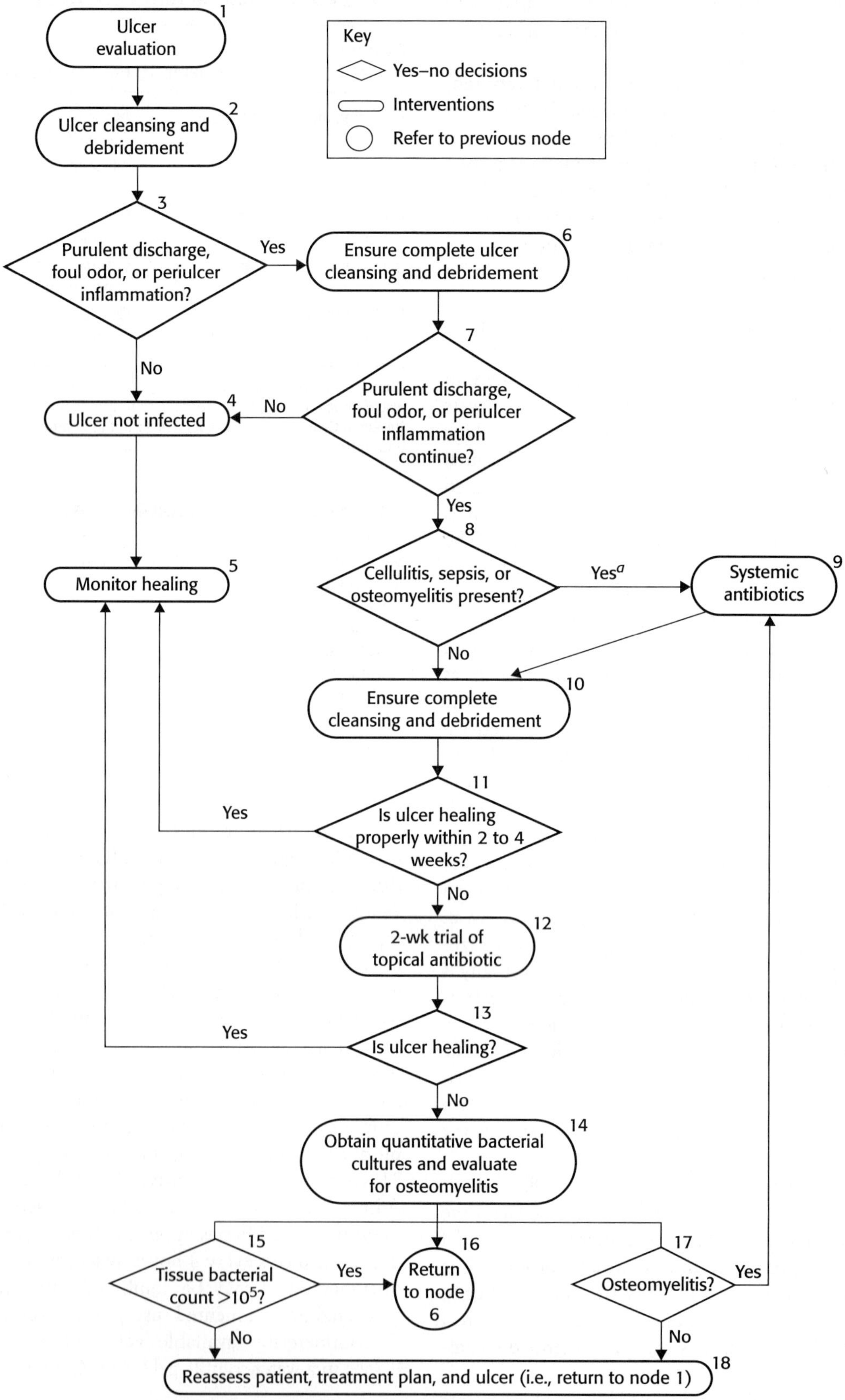

[a]Suspicion of sepsis warrants urgent medical evaluation and treatment. Sepsis treatment is not discussed in this guideline.

Figure 83.3. Algorithm for managing bacterial colonization and infection. (Reproduced with permission of AHCPR.)

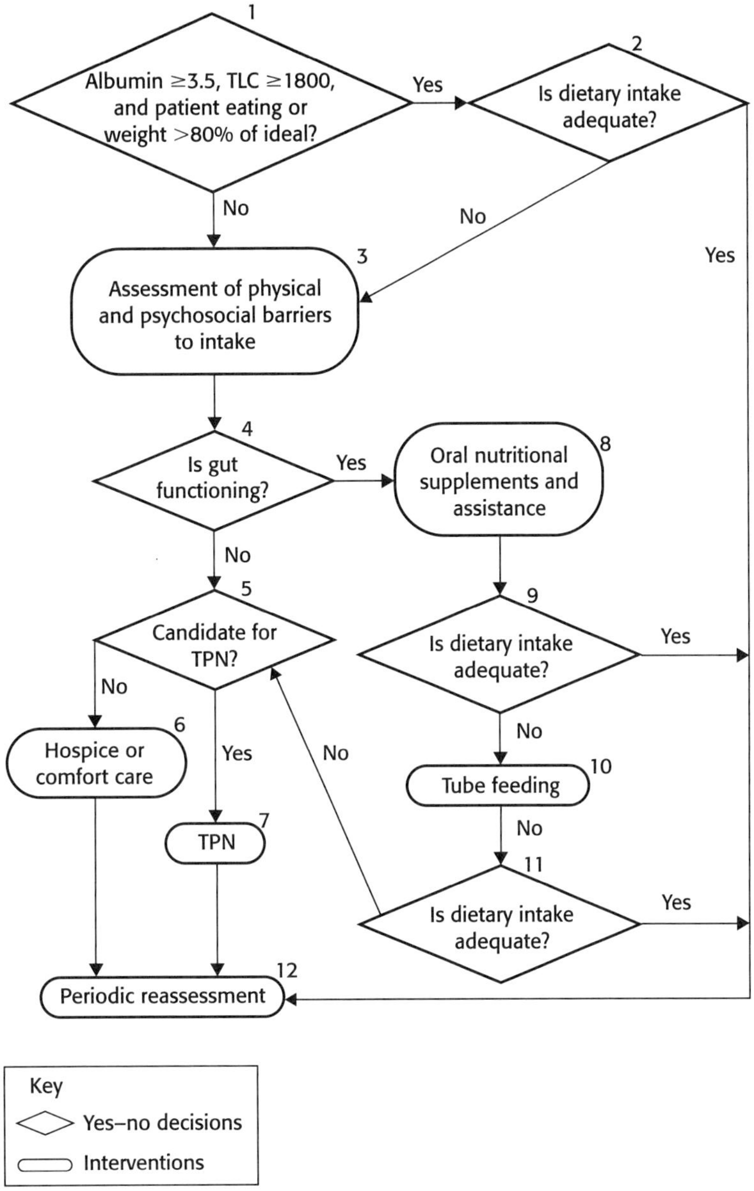

Figure 83.4. Algorithm for nutritional assessment and support of patients with pressure sores. *TLC*, total lymphocyte count; *TPN*, total parenteral nutrition. (Reproduced with permission of AHCPR.)

sient bacteremia in about 50% of patients, prophylaxis for bacterial endocarditis seems prudent in patients with artificial valves or other risk factors who need debridement.

Nonpharmacologic Therapy

Nutrition

Attention to nutritional status is essential in managing pressure ulcers at all stages.[55] Figure 83.4 is an algorithm to help clinicians ensure that the diet of the patient with a pressure ulcer contains nutrients that are adequate to support healing.[33] Hypoalbuminemic patients have been shown to be at higher risk for developing pressure sores and exhibit slower rates of healing. Nutritional monitoring with attention to dietary protein is essential. In addition, ascorbic acid supplementation (500 mg twice daily) and zinc sulfate have been suggested, but study flaws make interpreting this treatment difficult.

Local Care

The mainstay of therapy is local care.[56] Managing an established ulcer involves treating underlying medical conditions, providing proper nutrition and hydration, and using dressings or procedures that facilitate tissue repair. The goal of therapy is to produce a local wound environment that enhances wound healing. Table 83.8 summarizes local wound therapies for pressure ulcers. The environment to promote wound healing is warm, moist, and clean and has an adequate blood supply. This promotes wound healing by permitting the formation of healthy granulation tissue. Polyurethane films such as Tegaderm and OpSite may help

Table 83.8 ▪ Local Wound Therapy for Pressure Ulcers

Therapy	Examples	Notes
Cleanse with normal saline or lactated Ringer's		Avoid antiseptic solutions.
Moist environment dressings	Granuflex, Cutinova hydro	
Enzymatic debridement	Elase, Travase	May also damage healing tissue.
Skin barrier products (used primarily for stages I and II)	Polyurethane: OpSite, Tegaderm, Bioclusive, Ensure-It	
	Hydrogel: Vigilon, Geliperm, IntraSite	Dressings interact with wound exudate, producing a soft, moist gel that enables removal of the dressings with little damage to the newly formed tissue. Dressings stay in place for 1–7 days.
	Hydrocolloid: DuoDerm, Comfeel, Restore	Opaque and impermeable to oxygen and water.

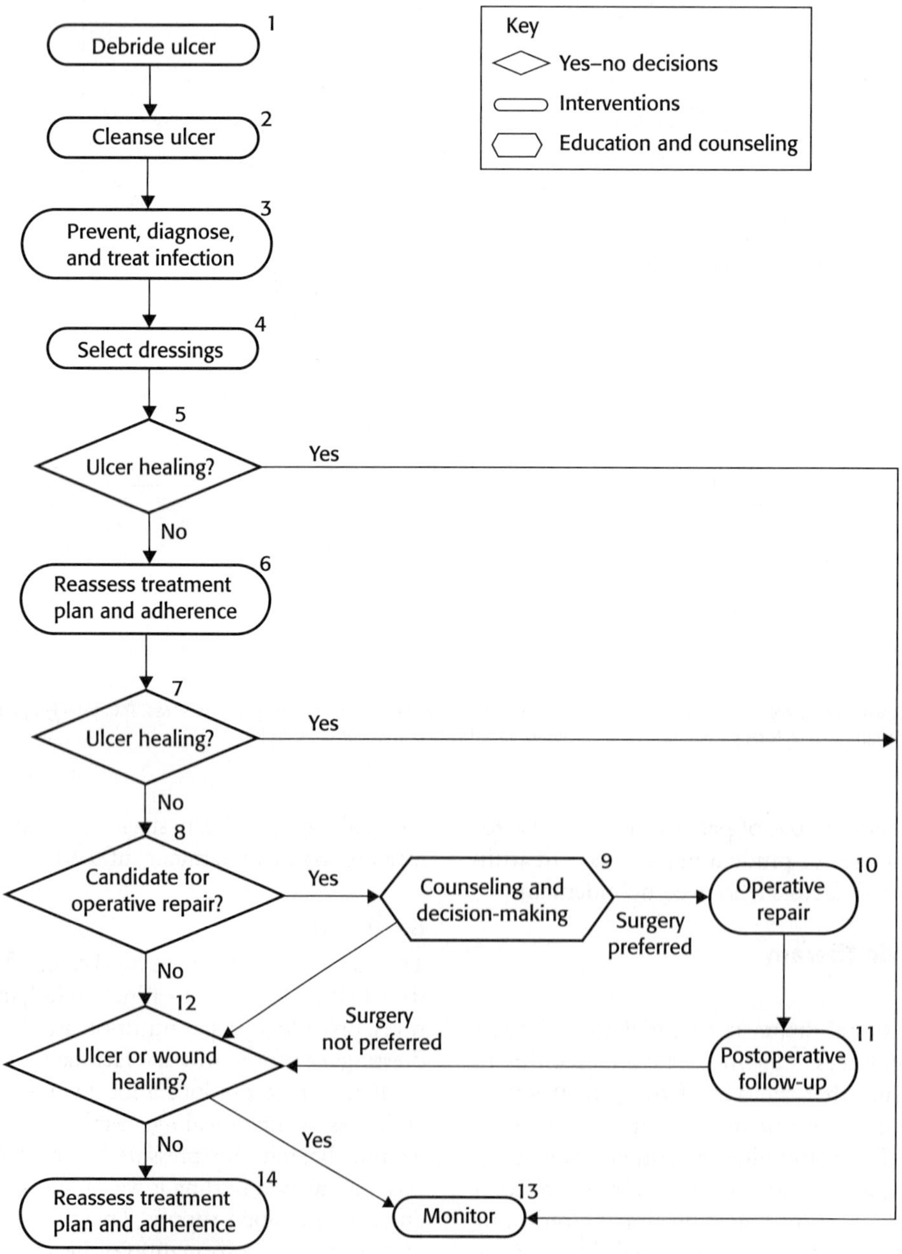

Figure 83.5. Algorithm for pressure ulcer care. (Reproduced with permission of AHCPR.)

to reduce friction between skin and bedsheets and may prevent further skin maceration. OpSite is a semipermeable, gas-permeable, transparent polyurethane film that permits perspiration evaporation but is impermeable to bacterial entry. DuoDerm is an impermeable, opaque, hydrocolloid dressing that forms a gellike wound covering on absorption of wound exudate. This is helpful to prevent and treat stage I lesions.

Surgery

Debridement is the process of cleaning an open wound by removing foreign material and dead tissue so that healing can occur. Removing dead tissue is necessary to prevent the dead tissue from promoting infection and to start reepithelialization of the area. Figure 83.5 outlines initial care of the pressure ulcer, including debridement and wound care.[33] Extensive necrotic material can be removed rapidly and effectively by surgical debridement. Most clinicians prefer irrigation after surgical debridement.

IMPROVING OUTCOMES

Educational programs for preventing pressure ulcers should include information on risk factors, assessment of common areas, and the importance of reducing pressure, friction, and shear. Because many patients are older adults, it is important to assess mental status and cognitive abilities. The family or the caregiver should attend educational programs as well.

Bacterial Diabetic Foot Infections

DEFINITION

Foot ulcers are among the most common causes of hospitalization for patients with diabetes mellitus.[57–59] Diabetic foot ulcers are caused by prolonged pressure over bony prominences of the foot. The pressure results in a loss of substance on the cutaneous surface. This causes a gradual disintegration and necrosis of the tissues. These lesions may be unnoticed in patients with peripheral neuropathies associated with a loss of sensation to the area.

TREATMENT GOALS: BACTERIAL DIABETIC FOOT INFECTIONS

- Control infection promptly.
- Retard progression of neuropathy through glycemic control.
- Eliminate pressure or shear forces.
- Educate the patient about prevention and follow-up care.

EPIDEMIOLOGY

The foot of the diabetic patient is susceptible to all forms of trauma. Common results of trauma are infection and gangrene. Foot infection is the most common complication of diabetes that warrants hospitalization. This complication accounts for more than 20% of all hospitalizations and is the most common cause of foot amputation in diabetic patients.[60] The amputation rate is approximately 60 per 10,000 people with diabetes per year. The U.S. Department of Health's goal for the year 2000 is a 40% reduction in the amputation rate in patients with diabetes.

PATHOPHYSIOLOGY

Many factors are involved in diabetic foot ulcer development;[61,62] three major factors are neuropathy, vascular insufficiency, and immunologic defects. Neuropathy, which includes sensory disturbances and autonomic neuropathy with anhidrosis, vasodilation, edema, and erythema, causes structural and functional changes in the foot that alter weight bearing, muscle function, and support and normal pain sensations. Classic neuropathic ulcers occur most often on the plantar surfaces of the foot. Vascular insufficiency and angiopathy are risk factors for foot infections and for the prognosis of these infections. Finally, diabetic patients are impaired hosts. Granulocytes from poorly controlled diabetic patients exhibit defects in phagocytosis. Because of these and other factors, the diabetic foot ulcer and infection present unique management problems. These ulcers may involve only superficial tissues or may involve deeper tissues and structures. A grading system using a six-point scale (0 to 5) has been proposed by Wagner.[63]

CLINICAL PRESENTATION AND DIAGNOSIS

Signs and Symptoms

Typical signs and symptoms of infection may not be present because the neuropathy renders infection and gangrene painless in the diabetic patient. For this reason, prophylactic foot care is essential. If an ulcer is detected, all weight bearing should be eliminated. Early incision, drainage, and identification of the organisms may obviate further surgery.

Diagnosis

Deep tissue cultures for both anaerobic and aerobic organisms provide the most reliable microbiologic information. It must be determined whether the infection is mild or life-threatening. Bacteriologic investigations reveal a polymicrobic spectrum (average of three to six organisms) in most diabetic infections. Gram-negative and Gram-positive aerobes and anaerobes are common. *S. aureus, S. epidermidis, Corynebacterium,* group D streptococci, *Pseudomonas, Klebsiella* species, *Enterobacter* species, and anaerobic Gram-positive cocci are most common.[64–67]

PSYCHOSOCIAL ASPECTS

A properly educated patient can make informed decisions about his or her daily care. A full psychosocial assessment should be performed to determine the patient's ability to comprehend information. A minimum assessment of mental status, learning ability, and psychological well-being can help practitioners understand patient education needs. Diabetic patients need many medications and medical supplies. Issues such as cost and transportation can play an important role in the therapeutic success. Visual changes and sensory changes have a major impact on prevention, recognition, and treatment.

TREATMENT

Pharmacotherapy

Objective data about the efficacy of various antibiotic treatments are lacking. Oral antimicrobial therapy is acceptable for treating mild, superficial lesions if the infection is in the early stages and has minimal drainage but gangrene and systemic symptoms are absent. If there is no improvement after 48 to 72 hours of treatment, intravenous therapy should be initiated.[68] Antibiotic selection depends on assumptions made from available studies,[64,65] many of which are inappropriately designed. A prospective study of outpatient oral treatment of mild diabetic foot infections compared 2-week courses of cephalexin (500 mg four times daily) and clindamycin (300 mg four times daily). Researchers found that both agents were effective and produced comparable rates of cure or improvement (96% clindamycin versus 86% cephalexin). Systemic antibiotic treatment is clearly indicated when there is evidence of cellulitis, septicemia, or osteomyelitis.[69,70]

Some general therapeutic concepts can be suggested. Because diabetic patients are impaired hosts and have granulocyte defects, bactericidal antibiotics are preferred, and prolonged courses of treatment may be needed. The prevalence of vascular insufficiency suggests the need for higher dosages and longer courses to obtain adequate tissue penetration. The recommended length of therapy for soft tissue infection is 2 to 3 weeks. The appropriate time to switch from intravenous to oral antimicrobial therapy is variable. These infections are presumed to be polymicrobic with aerobes and anaerobes. Empiric therapy should provide broad coverage until culture results are available. The higher incidence of renal insufficiency in diabetic patients necessitates cautious use and careful monitoring of nephrotoxic agents such as the aminolycosides. Ampicillin–sulbactam, ticarcillin–clavulanate, piperacillin–tazobactam, and cefoxitin or cefotetan are reasonable agents because of their broad spectrum of activity against most anticipated organisms. Table 83.9 lists agents that may be useful in treating diabetic foot infections. Even with careful treatment and monitoring, amputation may be necessary under certain conditions.

Nonpharmacologic Therapy

Other considerations in diabetic foot ulcer care should recognize that ulcer healing might take a long time because

Table 83.9 ▪ Antibiotic Regimens for Infected Diabetic Ulcers

Appearance	Infection	Possible Treatment Regimen
Limited in extent	Aerobic Gram-positive cocci	PO: clindamycin × 14 days PO: 1st-generation cephalosporin cephalexin × 14 days PO: amoxicillin + clavulanate IV: cefazolin PO: ciprofloxacin + clindamycin PO: trimethoprim–sulfamethoxazole
Chronic, recurrent, limb-threatening	Polymicrobic (both aerobes and anaerobes)	Cefoxitin Oral ciprofloxacin + clindamycin
	If septic	Imipenem + cilastatin Ticarcillin–clavulanate Piperacillin–tazobactam PRSP–APAG–clindamycin Vancomycin–metronidazole–azetreonam Ampicillin–sulbactam Ceftizoxime Ampicillin–APAG–clindamycin

PRSP, penicillinase-resistant synthetic penicillin; *APAG,* antipseudomonal aminoglycoside.

of the underlying poor circulation and tissue oxygenation. Nutritional monitoring and support are essential. Anemia should be corrected to enhance tissue oxygenation. Although it is usually more difficult to control blood glucose in diabetic patients with active infections, adequate glucose control is essential to enhance treatment success. During the acute infection, diabetic patients may need higher dosages of oral sulfonylurea agents or insulin. Major complications include sepsis syndrome, contiguous osteomyelitis, and transient bacteremia during ulcer manipulation. Because ulcer debridement may result in transient bacteremia, prophylaxis for bacterial endocarditis seems prudent in patients with artificial valves or other indications who need debridement.

FUTURE THERAPIES

Investigations on the pharmacologic application of growth factors and cytokines to wounds has increased our knowledge of normal and impaired wound healing, but clinical benefit in controlled studies has not been seen.[71]

IMPROVING OUTCOMES

The patient and all caregivers need to learn the basics of foot care. In patients with reduced vision secondary to retinopathy, the role of the family and caregivers becomes very important. The patient should be instructed to follow a program of proper footwear, education, and regular foot care. Diabetic education programs can be an important source of information, resulting in better glycemic control and fewer lower-extremity infections.

KEY POINTS

- Skin and soft tissue infections are common. Treatment demands knowledge of the anticipated skin pathogens and the status of the host's defense mechanisms.
- Acute skin and soft tissue infections usually are treated successfully if appropriate debridement is performed.
- Periorbital cellulitis is a very serious infection and may be a medical emergency.
- Decubitus ulcers and diabetic foot ulcers result from an interplay of complex host factors and tissue microorganism invasion. Often these infections are not curable and necessitate chronic care.

REFERENCES

1. Swartz MN. Cellulitis and superficial infections. In: Mandell GL, Douglas RG Jr, Bennett JE, eds. Principles and practices of infectious diseases. 4th ed. New York: Churchill Livingstone, 1995:909–929.
2. Ginsberg MB. Cellulitis: analysis of 101 cases and review of the literature. South Med J 74:530–533, 1981.
3. Fleisher G, Ludwig S, Campos J. Cellulitis: bacterial etiology, clinical features and laboratory findings. J Pediatr 97:591–593, 1980.
4. Hook EW III, Hooton TM, Horton CA, et al. Microbiologic evaluation of cutaneous cellulitis in adults. Arch Intern Med 146:295–297, 1986.
5. Sigurdsson AF, Gudmundsson S. The etiology of bacterial cellulitis as determined by fine-needle aspiration. Scand J Infect Dis 21:537–542, 1989.
6. Powers RD. Soft tissue infections in the emergency department: the case for the use of "simple" antibiotics. South Med J 84:1313–1315, 1991.
7. Sachs MK. The optimum use of needle aspiration in the bacteriologic diagnosis of cellulitis in adults. Arch Intern Med 150:1907–1912, 1990.
8. Lindbeck G, Powers R. Cellulitis. Hosp Pract (Off Ed) 28(Suppl 2):10–14, 1993.
9. Gainer RB. Ceftriaxone in the treatment of serious infections. Skin and soft tissue infections. Hosp Pract (Off Ed) 26(Suppl 5):24–30, 1991.
10. Campoli-Richards DM, Brogden RN. Sulbactam/ampicillin. A review of its antibacterial activity, pharmacokinetic properties, and therapeutic uses. Drugs 33:577–609, 1987.
11. Tan JS, Wishnow RM, Talan DA, et al. The piperacillin/tazobactam skin and skin structure study group. Treatment of hospitalized patients with complicated skin and skin structure infections: double-blind, randomized, multicenter study of piperacillin–tazobactam versus ticarcillin–clavulanate. Antimicrob Agents Chemother 37:1580–1586, 1993.
12. Ben-Amitai D, Ashkenazi S. Common bacterial skin infections in childhood. Pediatr Ann 22:225–233, 1993.
13. Dagan R. Impetigo in childhood. Changing epidemiology and new treatments. Pediatr Ann 22:235–240, 1993.
14. Demidovich CW, Wittler RR, Ruff ME, et al. Impetigo: current etiology and comparison of penicillin, erythromycin and cephalexin therapies. Am J Dis Child 144:1313–1315, 1990.
15. Dagan R, Bar-David Y. A double blind study comparing erythromycin and mupirocin for treatment of impetigo in children: implication of a high prevalence of erythromycin-resistant Staphylococcus aureus strain. Antimicrob Agents Chemother 36:287–290, 1992.
16. Jacob RF, Brown WD, Chartrand S, et al. Evaluation of cefuroxime axetil and cefadroxil suspension for the treatment of pediatric skin infections. Antimicrob Agents Chemother 36:1614–1618, 1992.
17. Blumer JL, Lemon E, O'Horo J, et al. Changing therapy for skin and soft tissue infections in children: have we come full circle? Pediatr Infect Dis J 6:117–122, 1987.
18. Bisno AL, Stevens DL. Streptococcal infections of skin and soft tissues. N Engl J Med 334:240–245, 1996.
19. Sadick NS. Current aspects of bacterial infections of the skin. Dermatol Clin 15:341–349, 1997.
20. Goldfarb J, Crenshaw D, O'Hord J, et al. Randomized clinical trial of topical mupirocin versus oral erythromycin for impetigo. Antimicrob Agents Chemother 32:1780–1783, 1988.
21. Britton JW, Fajardo JE, Krafte-Jacos B. Comparison of mupirocin and erythromycin in the treatment of impetigo. J Pediatr 117:827–829, 1990.
22. McLinn S. Topical mupirocin vs systemic erythromycin treatment for pyoderma. Pediatr Infect Dis J 7:785–790, 1988.
23. Barton LL, Friedman AD, Sharky AM, et al. Impetigo contagiosa, III: comparative efficacy of oral erythromycin and topical mupirocin. Pediatr Dermatol 6:134–138, 1989.
24. Canoso JJ, Barza M. Soft tissue infections. Rheum Dis Clin North Am 19:293–307, 1993.
25. Fekety FR Jr. Erysipelas. In: Demis DJ, ed. Clinical dermatology. Philadelphia: JB Lippincott, 1992;3(16):1–4.
26. Kahn RM, Goldstein EJC. Common bacterial skin infections. Postgrad Med 93:175–182, 1993.
27. Bratton RL, Nesse RE. St. Anthony's fire: diagnosis and management of erysipelas. Am Fam Physician 51:401–404, 1995.
28. Eriksson B, Jorup-Rönström C, Karkkonen K, et al. Erysipelas: clinical and bacteriologic spectrum and serological aspects. Clin Infect Dis 23:1091–1098, 1996.
29. Sjöblom AC, Eriksson B, Jorup-Rönström C, et al. Antibiotic prophylaxis in recurrent erysipelas. Infection 21:390–393, 1993.
30. Kremer M, Zuckerman R, Avraham Z, et al. Long-term antimicrobial therapy in the prevention of recurrent soft-tissue infections. J Infect 22:37–40, 1991.
31. Siddens JD, Gladstone GJ. Periorbital and orbital infections in children. J Am Osteopath Assoc 92:226–230, 1992.
32. Malinow I, Powell KR. Periorbital cellulitis. Pediatr Ann 22:241–246, 1993.
33. Bergstrom N, Bennett MA, Carlson CE, et al. Pressure ulcer treatment. Clinical practice guideline. Quick reference guide for clinicians, No. 15. Rockville, MD: US Department of Health and Human Services, Public Health Service, Agency for Health Care Policy and Research. AHCPR pub. no. 95-0653, Dec. 1994.
34. National Pressure Ulcer Advisory Panel. Pressure ulcer prevalence, cost and risk assessment: consensus development conference statement. Decubitus 2:24–28, 1989.
35. Brandeis GH, Morris JN, Nash DJ, et al. The epidemiology and natural history of pressure ulcers in elderly nursing home residents. JAMA 264:2905–2909, 1990.

36. Young JB, Dobrzanski S. Pressure sores: epidemiology and current management concepts. Drugs Aging 2:42–57, 1992.
37. Goode PS, Allman RM. The prevention and management of pressure ulcers. Med Clin North Am 73:1511–1524, 1989.
38. Leigh IH, Bennett G. Pressure ulcers: prevalence, etiology, and treatment modalities. Am J Surg 167:(Suppl 1A) 25S–30S, 1994.
39. Longe RL. Current concepts in clinical therapeutics: pressure sores. Clin Pharm 5:669–681, 1986.
40. Spoelhof GD, Ide K. Pressure ulcers in nursing home patients. Am Fam Physician 47:1207–1215, 1993.
41. Ditunno JF Jr, Formal CS. Chronic spinal cord injury. N Engl J Med 330:550–556, 1994.
42. Hunter SM, Cathcart-Silberberg T, Langemo DK, et al. Pressure ulcer prevalence and incidence in a rehabilitation hospital. Rehab Nurs 17:239–242, 1992.
43. Allman RM. Pressure ulcers among the elderly. N Engl J Med 320:850–853, 1989.
44. Gosnell DJ. Assessment and evaluation of pressure sores. Nurs Clin North Am 22:339–415, 1987.
45. Bergstrom N, Braden BJ, Laguzza A, et al. The Braden scale for predicting pressure sore risk. Nurs Res 36:205–210, 1987.
46. Bergstrom N, Demuth PJ, Braden BJ. A clinical trial of the Braden scale for predicting pressure sore risk. Nurs Clin North Am 22:417–428, 1987.
47. Bergstrom N, Braden B. A prospective study of pressure sore risk among institutionalized elderly. J Am Geriatr Soc 40:747–758, 1992.
48. Stuzin J, Engrav L, Buehler P. Care of open wounds. Compr Ther 8:32–34, 1982.
49. Rogers KG. The rational use of antimicrobial agents in simple wounds. Emerg Med Clin North Am 10:753–766, 1992.
50. Payne CM, Bladin C, Colchester AC, et al. Argyria from excessive use of topical silver sulfadiazine [letter]. Lancet 340:126, 1992.
51. Jones PH, Willis AT, Ferguson IR. Treatment of anaerobically infected pressure sores with topical metronidazole. Lancet 1:214, 1978.
52. Baker PG, Haig G. Metronidazole in the treatment of chronic pressure sores and ulcers. Practitioner 225:569–573, 1981.
53. Pierleoni EE. Topical metronidazole therapy for infected decubitus ulcers. J Am Geriatr Soc 32:775–781, 1984.
54. Leaper DJ. Prophylactic and therapeutic role of antibiotics in wound care. Am J Surg 167:(Suppl 1A):15S–19S, 1994.
55. Telfer NR, Moy RL. Drug and nutrient aspects of wound healing. Dermatol Clin 11:729–737, 1993.
56. Howell JM. Current and future trends in wound healing. Emerg Med Clin North Am 10:655–663, 1992.
57. Burton CS III. Management of chronic and problem lower extremity wounds. Dermatol Clin 11:767–773, 1993.
58. Kertesz D, Chow AW. Infected pressure and diabetic ulcers. Clin Geriatr Med 8:835–852, 1992.
59. Laing P. Diabetic foot ulcers. Am J Surg 167(Suppl 1A):31S–36S, 1994.
60. Newman LG, Waller J, Palestro CJ, et al. Unsuspected osteomyelitis in diabetic foot ulcers. JAMA 266:1246–1251, 1991.
61. Caputo GM, Cavanagh PR, Ulbrecht JS, et al. Assessment and management of foot disease in patients with diabetes. N Engl J Med 331:854–860, 1994.
62. Caputo GM, Joshi N, Weitekamp MR. Foot infections in patients with diabetes. Am Fam Physician 56:195–202, 1997.
63. Wagner FW. The dysvascular foot: a system for diagnosis and treatment. Foot Ankle 2:64–122, 1981.
64. Peterson LR, Lissack LM, Canter K, et al. Therapy of lower extremity infections with ciprofloxacin in patients with diabetes mellitus, peripheral vascular disease, or both. Am J Surg 86:801–808, 1989.
65. Lipsky BA, Pecoraro RE, Larson SA, et al. Outpatient management of uncomplicated lower-extremity infections in diabetic patients. Arch Intern Med 150:790–797, 1990.
66. Wheat LJ, Allen SD, Henry M, et al. Diabetic foot infections. Arch Intern Med 146:1935–1940, 1986.
67. Mertz PM, Ovington LG. Wound healing microbiology. Dermatol Clin 11:739–747, 1993.
68. West NJ. Systemic antimicrobial treatment of foot infections in diabetic patients. Am J Health Syst Pharm 52:1198–1207, 1995.
69. Gentry LO. Therapy with newer oral β-lactam and quinolone agents for infections of the skin and skin structures: a review. Clin Infect Dis 14:285–297, 1992.
70. Leichter SB, Schaefer JC, O'Brian JT. New concepts in managing diabetic foot infections. Geriatrics 46:24–30, 1991.
71. Pierce GF, Mustoe TA. Pharmacologic enhancement of wound healing. Annu Rev Med 46:467–481, 1995.

CHAPTER 84

SUPPORTIVE CARE THERAPIES FOR PATIENTS WITH CANCER

Kirsten M. Duncan, Gary Ogawa, and Unamarie Clibon

Supportive care therapies are critical to the physical and emotional well-being of the patient with cancer. Supportive care agents increase the chance that chemotherapy and radiation can be administered at the optimal dose and on schedule. They also are crucial in minimizing the serious side effects that may diminish the patient's quality of life and compliance with future cancer treatment. The use of supportive care therapy for patients with cancer has become even more important with recent advances in the treatment of cancer. Supportive care therapies have allowed increases in the dose intensity of cancer therapies, for example, high-dose chemotherapy for bone marrow transplantation, new chemotherapy combinations that previously were associated with intolerable side effects, or high-dose radiation. Increased dose intensity is associated with an improved survival rate for patients with certain cancers.

Supportive care agents are used to prevent and manage chemotherapy and radiation-related toxicities from diagnosis to ultimate outcome. This chapter discusses agents used to prevent oral complications such as mucositis, xerostomia, constipation and diarrhea, and nausea and vomiting and hematologic complications such as anemia, neutropenia, and thrombocytopenia and cytoprotective agents to prevent specific chemotherapy-induced toxicities. Additional therapeutic modalities covered in other chapters that are important to consider in the overall management of a patient with cancer include nutritional support, management of fever and infection in immunocompromised patients, and pain management.

Oral Complications

Mucositis

Annually there are approximately 400,000 cases of treatment-induced damage to the oral cavity.[1] Oral complications that arise as a result of cancer therapy, particularly chemotherapy and localized radiation therapy, include mucositis, xerostomia (dry mouth), bacterial, fungal, or viral infection, dental caries, loss of taste, trismus, and osteoradionecrosis.[2] As severe oral damage may occasionally result in life-threatening complications, effective supportive therapies for prevention and treatment are vital to the positive clinical outcome for a cancer patient.

Mucositis, also referred to as stomatitis, is generalized inflammation of the oral mucosal membranes. This is an important complication to address as it can be a dose-limiting toxicity for both chemotherapy and radiotherapy.

TREATMENT GOALS: MUCOSITIS

- Avoid the complications associated with mucositis, provide pain relief, promote healing, and prevent local and systemic infection.[3]
- By avoiding these complications and maintaining a good quality of life, help patients complete their scheduled cancer therapy and improve therapeutic outcome.

EPIDEMIOLOGY

The incidence and severity of mucositis vary from patient to patient. The probability of developing mucositis is dependent upon the treatment modality. Approximately 40% of patients treated with standard chemotherapy develop mucositis compared to 76% of patients who receive high-dose chemotherapy and undergo bone marrow transplantation. Between 30 and 60% of patients receiving radiation therapy for cancer of the head and neck develop mucositis, and greater than 90% of patients receiving concomitant chemotherapy and localized radiation therapy will be affected.[1,4] There are patient-related and treatment-related risk factors that may predict which patients are more likely to develop mucositis (Table 84.1).[4] Patients with risk factors need to be followed closely and preventive measures should be used to diminish the incidence and severity of mucositis.

PATHOPHYSIOLOGY

The development of mucositis occurs through two mechanisms. First is the direct effect of the chemotherapy or radiation on the oral mucosa, termed direct stomatotoxicity. Second is the indirect result of myelosuppression or indirect stomatotoxicity.

Direct Stomatotoxicity

The mucosal epithelial cells undergo rapid turnover, usually every 7 to 14 days, which makes these cells susceptible to the effects of cytotoxic therapy.[4] Both chemotherapy and localized radiation therapy can cause direct stomatotoxicity by interfering with cellular growth and maturation such that the ability of the oral mucosa to regenerate is compromised.[4] The incidence and severity of chemotherapy-induced mucositis depend upon the specific agent, the dose, and the method of administration (i.e., IV bolus versus IV infusion). The severity of radiation-induced mucositis depends upon the type of radiation, the volume of irradiated tissue, the daily fraction, and the cumulative dose.[4] The onset of mucositis can also vary. Patients who receive standard-dose chemotherapy develop mucositis within 5 to 7 days after the administration of chemotherapy.[6] Patients undergoing bone marrow transplantation often exhibit oral complications approximately 10 days after the treatment regimen has started,[7] while radiation-induced mucositis usually appears during the third to the fifth week of radiation therapy.[6] Mucositis is generally self-limiting, and in nonmyelosuppressed patients whose oral lesions are not complicated by fungal, bacterial, or viral infection, healing occurs within 2 to 3 weeks.[4,8] The sites most often affected include the lips, cheeks, soft palate, floor of the mouth, and the ventral surface of the tongue.[1,4]

Table 84.1 ▪ Risk Factors for the Development of Mucositis

Factor	Comments
Patient-related	
Hematologic malignancy	Oral complications may be associated with the underlying hematologic malignancy, particularly if the patient has severe neutropenia.[5]
Younger age	There is a higher incidence of hematologic malignancy in younger patients. Additionally, younger patients have a higher mucosal turnover rate than do elderly patients.
Poor oral hygiene (dental caries, gingival disease, chronic oral infection)	If these patients receive aggressive mouth care, they can diminish their chances of oral complications.
Poor nutritional status	Malnutrition interferes with tissue repair thus impairs the mucosal healing.
Seropositive for herpes simplex virus or history of flare	Prophylactic acyclovir should be considered for patients at high risk for reactivation.
Treatment-related	
Stomatotoxic chemotherapy (alkylating agents, antimetabolites, hydroxyurea, procarbazine)	Drugs differ in their ability to cause mucositis; furthermore, stomatotoxicity can be dose-related. Methotrexate and 5-fluorouracil are among the most stomatotoxic agents.
Radiation therapy	Radiation therapy to the head and neck region (>4000–5000 cGy) and total body irradiation increase the risk for developing mucositis.
Concomitant chemotherapy and radiotherapy	Combined modality therapy may accelerate the onset and increase the incidence and severity of oral complications.

Indirect Stomatotoxicity

Gram-negative bacteria and fungal infections may result in direct invasion of the oral mucosa and indirectly cause mucositis.[9] Patients are at increased risk for oral infections when they are neutropenic, and this is usually when indirect stomatotoxicity appears. The onset of mucositis secondary to myelosuppression varies depending upon the timing of the neutrophil nadir associated with the chemotherapy agent administered, but typically develops anywhere from 10 to 21 days after chemotherapy administration.[6]

CLINICAL PRESENTATION AND DIAGNOSIS

Before cancer therapy is initiated, all patients should undergo a comprehensive dental evaluation to document baseline parameters, to identify risk factors, and to develop strategies to diminish oral complications.

Patients with mucositis can have many symptoms. Mucositis usually begins with swelling, redness, and erythema of the mucosal membranes followed by the development of white elevated desquamative areas that progress into painful pseudomembranous lesions.[4] Once the mucosal surface is damaged, patients are more susceptible to both local secondary infection and systemic infection; therefore, the lesions of patients with febrile neutropenia should be cultured to rule out bacterial, fungal, or viral infection.

Patients may complain of pain, dry mouth, and burning and/or tingling of the lips.[10] The pain associated with mucositis is often intense and can be exacerbated by attempts to eat, drink, swallow, or speak. The pain may be so severe that it limits adequate nutritional and liquid intake, thus putting patients at increased risk for dehydration and malnutrition.

In assessing mucositis, a complete history of the patient's complaints and risk factors should be obtained, with particular attention paid to the onset and duration of the lesions, the presence of pain or fever, aggravating or relieving factors, and the patient's ability to eat, drink, and talk. A thorough oral examination to evaluate the appearance of the mucositis is also important. A number of laboratory parameters should be obtained to rule out infection or dehydration (i.e., complete blood count, platelet count, electrolyte panel, blood urea nitrogen, and serum creatinine).

PSYCHOSOCIAL ASPECTS

Mucositis adversely affects the patient's quality of life. Patients may be frustrated or embarrassed by the difficulty associated with performing the most basic functions, such as speaking, eating, and controlling saliva. In some cases, the symptoms may be so unbearable that patients may not comply with the remainder of their cancer therapy.

PREVENTION

One of the most important measures to prevent mucositis is strict adherence to a meticulous oral care regimen. Patients and their family members should be thoroughly counseled on the importance of maintaining good oral hygiene (Table 84.2).

The prophylactic measures most commonly used include rinses to remove debris and soothe tissues, chlorhexidine gluconate oral rinse to diminish plaque accumulation, and oral cryotherapy before 5-fluorouracil (5-FU) administration (Table 84.3). Cryotherapy (ice chips) temporarily vasoconstricts the mucosal vasculature, thus decreasing the direct toxic effects of 5-FU. Patients should avoid commercial rinses containing alcohol or phenol because they can be drying to the mucosal tissue and result in further irritation. There are numerous other prophylactic approaches including sucralfate suspension, allopurinol mouthwash to lessen the severity of 5-FU-induced mucositis, chamomile mouthwash, and antimicrobial agents (i.e.,

Table 84.2 ▪ Oral Maintenance to Prevent Mucositis

Refer patient to a dentist for a comprehensive examination to identify and correct any potential complications *before* cancer therapy is initiated (the identification of infection requires prompt therapy with the appropriate antimicrobial agent to prevent systemic infection).

Encourage patients to seek professional dental care throughout cancer therapy as necessary.

Instruct patients to brush teeth with a soft bristle toothbrush and fluoridated toothpaste after every meal and before bedtime (patients may use a sponge dipped in chlorhexidine gluconate 0.12% oral rinse if unable to brush); the toothbrush should be changed monthly.

Recommend that patients floss teeth daily (contraindicated in the presence of thrombocytopenia or severe pain).

Encourage good nutrition with adequate protein and fluid intake (2 L of fluid daily) and recommend avoidance of spicy, acidic, hot, or irritating foods.

PTA lozenges consisting of polymixin B, tobramycin, and amphotericin B) to prevent infection. The data supporting the use of these agents are either inconclusive or lacking and they cannot be recommended as a standard of care. To lessen the impact of radiation therapy, patients should have protective radiation stents to protect normal dentition or appropriate radiation shields to protect dental implants. Furthermore, patients should be discouraged from wearing dentures once radiation therapy begins, especially at night.

TREATMENT

Presently, there are no proven effective therapeutic strategies that either prevent mucositis or reduce the severity or duration once it develops. Consequently, there are very few well-conducted randomized, placebo-controlled trials evaluating various modalities to manage mucositis. Difficulties associated with evaluating published studies include different patient populations, variable cancer treatments, and lack of a universally accepted grading system to document the severity of mucositis. Much of the available treatment information is anecdotal, and the efficacy and safety of the majority of the mucositis treatment regimens have not yet been established.

The treatment of mucositis is primarily palliative and focused on symptom management. For mild to moderate mucositis, ice chips or popsicles may provide adequate pain relief for some patients.[3] The mainstays of therapy for mucositis are oral rinses or mouthwashes that cleanse the mucosa and provide pain relief. Rinses can be those used for prophylaxis of mucositis or those containing a coating agent or local anesthetic (Table 84.4). Sucralfate has also been evaluated with mixed results. Sucralfate forms an ionic bond with tissue proteins, creating a protective barrier and may also stimulate the production of prostaglandin E_2, which increases blood flow to the oral mucosa.[4] Oral rinses can be a single agent or a combination of several agents from different categories and may include an antifungal or corticosteroid; however, there are no controlled trials documenting the efficacy of combination rinses. Patients should be instructed to use rinses as needed for pain and before eating to diminish the pain associated with swallowing. Oral rinses used to treat mucositis are generally not associated with significant side effects; however, there are several important points of

Table 84.3 ▪ Prevention of Mucositis

Measure	Administration
Saline rinse	Dissolve 1/2 tsp sodium chloride in 8 oz of water; swish in oral cavity for at least 2–3 min and expectorate at least 4 times daily
Sodium bicarbonate rinse	Dissolve 1 tsp sodium bicarbonate (baking soda) in 1 pint of warm water; swish in oral cavity for at least 2–3 min and expectorate at least 4 times daily
Sodium chloride and sodium bicarbonate combination rinse	1 tsp baking soda in 8 oz of sterile saline; swish in oral cavity for at least 2–3 min and expectorate at least 4 times daily
Cold water rinse	Swish in oral cavity for at least 2–3 minutes at least 4 times daily
Chlorhexidine gluconate 0.12% oral rinse	Swish in oral cavity for 30 sec and expectorate 2–4 times daily (for patients undergoing treatment for leukemia or bone marrow transplantation)
Cryotherapy	Beginning 5 min before 5-flourouracil administration, continuously swish ice chips in the mouth for 30 min[11,12a]

[a]*Note:* A trial comparing the efficacy of 30 versus 60 min of cryotherapy demonstrated no significant difference in outcome.[12]

Table 84.4 ▪ Pharmacologic Management of Mucositis

Agent	Dosing Recommendation
Coating agents	
Magnesium and aluminum based antacids (e.g., Maalox, Mylanta), Kaopectate	Used in various amounts in combination mouthwashes to provide a soothing effect
Sucralfate slurry	1 g swished for 2 min 4–6 times daily
Local anesthetics	
Lidocaine viscous 2%	5–15 mL swished and expectorated q2–3 hr PRN
Dyclonine HCl 0.5 or 1%	5–15 mL swished and expectorated q2–3 hr PRN
Diphenhydramine	12.5 mg swished and expectorated QID (dissolve 25 mg in approximately 45 mL warm water)[3]
Benzocaine 20% spray	1–2 sprays PRN
Benzocaine in orabase	Apply to affected (localized) lesions q2–3 hr PRN

caution. Xylocaine viscous 2% and dyclonine hydrochloride 0.5 to 1% may cause numbing of the oral cavity, which can make swallowing difficult and put some patients at risk for aspiration.[13] Although diphenhydramine does not cause numbing of the oral cavity, it can cause sedation if it is ingested.[3] For pain associated with severe mucositis, oral or parenteral narcotics may be required (refer to Chapter 54 for pain management strategies).[14] If mucositis interferes with nutritional intake or has a negative impact on the patient's quality of life, the dosage of chemotherapy may need to be decreased in future cycles or the schedule of radiotherapy may need to be delayed until adequate healing has occurred. This is undesirable as decreasing the intensity of cancer therapy may have a negative impact on the patient's ultimate outcome, namely response rate and survival. Furthermore, should patients experience severe fluid or weight loss, oral supplementation or even intravenous hydration may be necessary.

Other agents have been studied for the management of mucositis; however, owing to a lack of convincing data, they are not currently considered the standard of care and in some cases are experimental. Examples include hematologic growth factors (granulocyte-macrophage colony-stimulating factor [GM-CSF] and granulocyte colony-stimulating factor [G-CSF]), allopurinol mouthwash, leucovorin, glutamine, uridine, propantheline, vitamin E, vitamin C and glutathione, azelastine hydrochloride, β-carotene, kamillosan liquid (chamomile; not available in the United States), aspirin, silver nitrate, prostaglandins, indomethacin, benzydamine (not available in the United States), corticosteroids, Oratect gel, and sodium alginate.

FUTURE THERAPIES

Clinicians are beginning to understand more about mucositis on a molecular level, and new approaches to the prevention and treatment of mucositis are being explored. The following agents are in the early stages of development or in clinical trials, and more information is needed to prove their safety and efficacy. New approaches include biologically active factors that inhibit cellular regeneration such as tumor growth factor β and epidermal growth factor. Other treatment modalities that may show promise in the management of mucositis include amifostine, capsaicin, and laser therapy.

Table 84.5 ▪ Patient Education

Strict compliance with oral care maintenance using gentle techniques
Keep oral tissues, including lips, moist
Maintain a bland diet and avoid spicy or acidic foods
Avoid or diminish alcohol and smoking consumption
Use ice chips and popsicles to provide relief from pain and discomfort
Maintain compliance with the cancer therapy regimen

IMPROVING OUTCOMES

Patient understanding and compliance with proper mouth care regimens are critical to minimize the morbidity associated with mucositis (Table 84.5). By effectively managing mucositis and its associated complications, clinicians are more likely to deliver the cancer regimen as scheduled, which could improve response rate and survival. Effectively managing the adverse effects of cancer therapy decreases the costs associated with caring for the patient with cancer. Furthermore, if mucositis can ultimately be prevented, clinicians may be able to increase the dose intensity of chemotherapy and radiotherapy regimens to improve patient outcome.

Xerostomia

Xerostomia, or dryness of the mouth, is commonly associated with radiation therapy for head and neck cancer. Because xerostomia can be uncomfortable for the patient with cancer as well as increase the risk for additional oral complications, is it important that it be diagnosed and appropriately managed.

TREATMENT GOALS: XEROSTOMIA

- Stimulate salivary flow.
- Replace lost secretions.
- Protect the dentition.
- Prevent complications associated with xerostomia such as mucositis.[4]

PATHOPHYSIOLOGY

Healthy adults secrete up to 1.5 L of saliva daily.[7] Saliva is important in maintaining mucosal health: it moistens the oral cavity and clears it of debris and oral flora, it is an integral component of digestion, and it is important for speaking and swallowing.[4,7] Radiation therapy damages the salivary glands such that saliva production is decreased. One study found that the average salivary flow rate decreased 57% after 1 week of radiation, 67% after 6 weeks of radiation therapy, and 95% 3 years after treatment was completed.[1] There exists a relationship between the dose and location of radiation, the volume of irradiated tissue, and the extent of damage to the salivary glands. Generally, damage is reversible in patients who receive less than 6000 cGy, while changes may be permanent in patients who receive greater than 6000 cGy.[4] There may be additional causes that exacerbate the radiation-induced xerostomia such as concomitant medications (tricyclic antidepressants, antipsychotics, antihistamines, antihypertensives, and diuretics), concurrent illnesses (diabetes mellitus and interstitial nephritis), and vitamin A and nicotinic acid deficiencies.[4] It is important to thoroughly investigate and eliminate, if possible, all potential causes of xerostomia as they predispose the patient with cancer to more serious oral complications such as mucositis, oral infection, dental caries and decalcification, periodontitis, gingival erosion, and abscesses.[4]

Table 84.6 ▪ Management of Xerostomia

Maintain good oral hygiene
Debride the tongue using a soft toothbrush
Use saliva substitutes or water rinses 4–6 times daily to keep the mouth moist and aid in swallowing
Drink liquids frequently (avoid caffeinated beverages)
Eat moistened or pureed foods
Use sugar-free candy (i.e., lemon candy) or gum PRN
Apply lubrication to the lips (e.g., Blistex or Aquaphor)
Discontinue or decrease smoking or alcohol consumption

CLINICAL PRESENTATION AND DIAGNOSIS

There are no standardized grading scales to document the severity of xerostomia. It is important to document all patient-reported signs and symptoms. Patients primarily complain of dryness in the mouth. As eating and swallowing become more difficult, patients may experience loss of appetite and weight loss.

TREATMENT

Keeping the mouth moist is the most important aspect of managing xerostomia. This can be achieved using pharmacologic and nonpharmacologic interventions (Table 84.6). Oral pilocarpine 5 mg PO TID has been shown to stimulate salivary secretion and relieve symptoms in patients who have residual salivary function.[15–17] The major side effect associated with pilocarpine is sweating. There are also several saliva substitutes that are commercially available; however, most patients find these substitutes do not work well and can be costly.[7] Water rinses may be more acceptable to patients and should be used before and during meals and additionally as needed. Other measures that patients may try include sugarless gum and candy, sucking on ice chips, or use of a humidifier.[1]

The Food and Drug Administration (FDA) recently approved amifostine for the reduction of moderate to severe xerostomia in patients receiving radiation therapy postoperatively for head and neck cancers.

Constipation and Diarrhea

Lower gastrointestinal toxicity, including constipation and diarrhea, is common in patients with cancer. Approximately 4 to 10% of patients with cancer develop diarrhea (this increases to 43% after bone marrow transplantation), and greater than 50% of patients referred to a palliative care setting, or hospice, suffer from constipation.[18,19]

TREATMENT GOALS: CONSTIPATION AND DIARRHEA

- Prevent the development of constipation and diarrhea.
- If the patient has either constipation or diarrhea, help bring about prompt resolution to prevent associated complications.

PATHOPHYSIOLOGY

Although there are numerous etiologies that may contribute to the development of diarrhea and constipation in the patient with cancer, there are several causes that are specific to the population with cancer (Tables 84.7 and 84.8). The cells of the gastrointestinal tract (as with the oral mucosa) proliferate rapidly, and they are at increased risk of damage from chemotherapy or radiation therapy.

Irinotecan (CPT-11), an agent used to treat advanced colon and rectal cancers, is commonly associated with severe diarrhea. There are two types of diarrhea associated with irinotecan: early onset (within 24 hours of administra-

Table 84.7 ▪ Possible Causes of Diarrhea in the Patient with Cancer

Endocrine tumors
Vipoma
Malignant carcinoid tumor
Gastrinoma
Medullary carcinoma of the thyroid
Partial bowel obstruction by tumor
Graft versus host disease
Cancer therapy
Chemotherapy (particularly irinotecan, 5-fluorouracil +/− leucovorin or interferon alfa)
Radiation therapy
Supportive therapy
Enteral nutrition
Laxatives
Antacids

Sources: References 18, 19.

Table 84.8 ▪ Possible Causes of Constipation in the Patient with Cancer

Bowel obstruction by tumor	Patient-related
Cancer therapy	Decreased mobility
Vinca alkaloids	Malnutrition
Supportive therapies	
Opioid therapy	
Nonsteroidal anti-inflammatory drugs	

Sources: References 19, 20.

tion) and late onset (more than 24 hours after administration). Early diarrhea is due to cholinergic causes and is generally self-limiting. Late diarrhea can be prolonged and may be associated with significant morbidity.

TREATMENT

In general, the approach to the management of diarrhea and constipation is no different from that of patients without cancer. For a detailed treatment plan, refer to Chapter 27. Irinotecan-induced diarrhea is so prevalent that drugs to treat and prevent it have been standardized and should be administered to all patients. Because the early-onset diarrhea is cholinergic in nature, atropine 1 mg IV should be administered (after ruling out a history of cardiac disease) immediately. Patients should receive prophylaxis with atropine in all subsequent cycles of irinotecan therapy. At the first sign of late-onset diarrhea, patients should be given loperamide 4 mg to be followed by loperamide 2 mg PO every 2 hours (not to exceed 16 mg/24 hr) until the patient has not had a bowel movement for at least 12 hours.[21]

Chemotherapy-Induced Nausea and Vomiting

According to data collected in 1983,[22] patients with cancer expressed significant concerns regarding the adverse side effects of chemotherapy-induced nausea and vomiting. In 1983, vomiting was the number one concern of patients undergoing chemotherapy while nausea was second. In 1993,[23] after the development of newer antiemetic strategies, vomiting fell to fifth yet nausea continued to be their number one fear.

It is extremely distressing and debilitating for patients with cancer to experience severe nausea and vomiting secondary to antineoplastic treatment, especially with the current use of combination chemotherapy and dose-intensified regimens. Known complications of protracted emesis include dehydration, electrolyte and acid-base imbalance, possible esophageal tearing or rib fracture, aspiration pneumonitis, a decreased nutritional state, and potential inability to continue curative therapy.[24] Family, friends and co-workers often also share this level of discomfort. It is therefore essential that effective antiemetic therapy be used to provide positive outcomes for everyone.

TREATMENT GOALS: CHEMOTHERAPY-INDUCED NAUSEA AND VOMITING

- Use antiemetic agents with proven effectiveness, in the correct dose or combinations, properly timed, to eliminate difficulties with nausea and/or vomiting and allow continuation of chemotherapy as planned.
- Because chemotherapeutic agents induce nausea and/or vomiting with widely varying potentials and via a variety of mechanisms, match the antineoplastic drug and dose being used to the appropriate antiemetic agent, combination, and dose.
- Use aggressive antiemetic therapy to eliminate the cost of treating any complication secondary to protracted nausea or vomiting.
- Provide total symptom management to ensure the comfort of the patient.

EPIDEMIOLOGY

The incidence and severity of nausea and/or vomiting depend on a variety of factors related to both the antineoplastic drug and patient. Hesketh et al.[25] have tabulated the emetogenic potential of single antineoplastic agents and/or combinations in a comprehensive manner and ranked them according to their emetogenic potential.

Table 84.9 similarly ranks the emetogenic potential of various antineoplastic agents from acute I (most severe) to acute IV (where the use of an antiemetic is optional). Note that in contrast to the five emetogenic levels proposed by Hesketh et al.,[25] this table has only four categories (emetogenic potential IV and V have been combined, as treatment is similar). The ranking found in Table 84.9 also integrates data from several studies and adds specific mg/m^2 doses as published elsewhere.[26–29]

One must also not fail to recognize important patient-related risk factors for postchemotherapy nausea and vomiting (Table 84.10). In providing optimal care for patients with cancer, it is essential that risk factors be carefully reviewed and evaluated before any treatment is begun. This provides a means to deliver effective symptom management while maintaining the highest quality of life possible.[30]

Table 84.9 ▪ Emetogenic Potential[a]

- Acute I agents (includes BMT doses of ANY chemotherapeutic agent, regardless of category or route)
  - Emetogenic potential >90%
    - Carmustine >250 mg/m^2
    - Cisplatin ≥50 mg/m^2
    - Cyclophosphamide >1500 mg/m^2
    - Dacarbazine ≥500 mg/m^2
    - Mechlorethamine
    - Pentostatin
    - Streptozocin
  - Emetogenic potential 60–90%
    - Amifostine 740–910 mg/m^2
    - Carboplatin ≥1000 mg/m^2
    - Carmustine ≤250 mg/m^2
    - Cisplatin <50 mg/m^2
    - Cyclophosphamide >750 mg/m^2 but ≤1500 mg/m^2
    - Cytarabine >1000 mg/m^2
    - Dactinomycin >1500 mg/m^2
    - Doxorubicin >60 mg/m^2
    - Ifosfamide >2000 mg/m^2
    - Methotrexate >1000 mg/m^2
    - Plicamycin (for testicular cancer, not hypercalcemia)
- Acute II agents
  - Emetogenic potential 30–60%
    - 5-Azacytadine
    - Carboplatin <1000 mg/m^2
    - Cyclophosphamide ≤750 mg/m^2
    - Daunorubicin
    - Doxorubicin 20–60 mg/m^2
    - Epirubicin ≤90 mg/m^2
    - Fluorouracil ≥1000 mg/m^2
    - Idarubicin
    - Ifosfamide ≤2000 mg/m^2
    - Irinotecan
    - Melphalan (IV)
    - Methotrexate 250–1000 mg/m^2
    - Mitoxantrone <15 mg/m^2
- Acute III agents
  - Emetogenic potential 10–30%
    - Amifostine 200–340 mg/m^2
    - L-Asparaginase
    - Cytarabine <250 mg/m^2
    - Docetaxel
    - Doxorubicin ≤20 mg/m^2
    - Liposomal doxorubicin
    - Etoposide <200 mg/m^2
    - Fluorouracil <1000 mg/m^2
    - Gemcitabine
    - Interferons
    - Methotrexate >50 mg/m^2, but <250 mg/m^2
    - Mitomycin-C
    - Paclitaxal
    - Teniposide
    - Thiotepa
    - Topotecan
- Acute IV agents (antiemetics are not generally required with these agents)
  - Emetogenic potential <10%
    - Bleomycin
    - Cladribine
    - Fludarabine
    - Methotrexate ≤50 mg/m^2
    - Rituximab
    - Vincristine
    - Vinblastine
    - Vinorelbine
- Oral agents (carefully evaluate need for antiemetic therapy based on patient symptoms)
  - Acute I: procarbazine, lomustine
  - Acute II: cyclophosphamide, altretamine
  - Acute III: melphalan, 6-mercaptopurine
  - Acute IV: busulfan, chlorambucil, hydroxyurea, 6-thioguanine, L-phenylalanine mustard

[a]Rule with combination agent regimens (except for acute IV agents):
When more than one agent is administered the emetogenic potential of the combination is generally increased by one category, based on the highest category of the individual agents.
If the patient has a history of migraine headaches, move up one category and avoid ondansetron.

PATHOPHYSIOLOGY

Previously the path for drug-induced emesis was believed to be a simple one wherein blood-borne agents acted directly on the chemoreceptor trigger zone (CTZ) located in the area postrema of the fourth ventricle of the brain.[31] The CTZ then stimulated the vomiting center (VC) found on the dorsal lateral reticular formation of the medulla. Once triggered, the VC then initiates the body's act of emesis by integrating the actions of several body organs and systems (Fig. 84.1). Because dopamine is a major neurotransmitter between the CTZ and the VC, most antiemetic agents used have traditionally been antagonists of the dopamine type 2 receptor (D_2) such as the phenothiazines (prochlorperazine) or the butyrophenones (haloperidol or droperidol). Prochlorperazine is still considered by most to be an effective general antiemetic agent.

From work performed in animals, it is known that stimulation of the VC is a very complex process that

Table 84.10 ▪ Risk Factors for Postchemotherapy Nausea and Vomiting

- Highly emetogenic, high-dose, or combination chemotherapy
- Multiple cycles of chemotherapy
- Longer infusion time for chemotherapy
- Concurrent radiation therapy
- Prechemotherapy nausea or vomiting
- History of nausea and/or vomiting with chemotherapy
- Increased level of apprehension and/or anxiety
- Sensitivity to motion sickness or morning sickness
- Generally a patient of younger age (younger greater risk than older)
- Generally a patient of the female sex (female greater risk than male)

Note: A history of chronic ethanol consumption protects against nausea and/or vomiting.

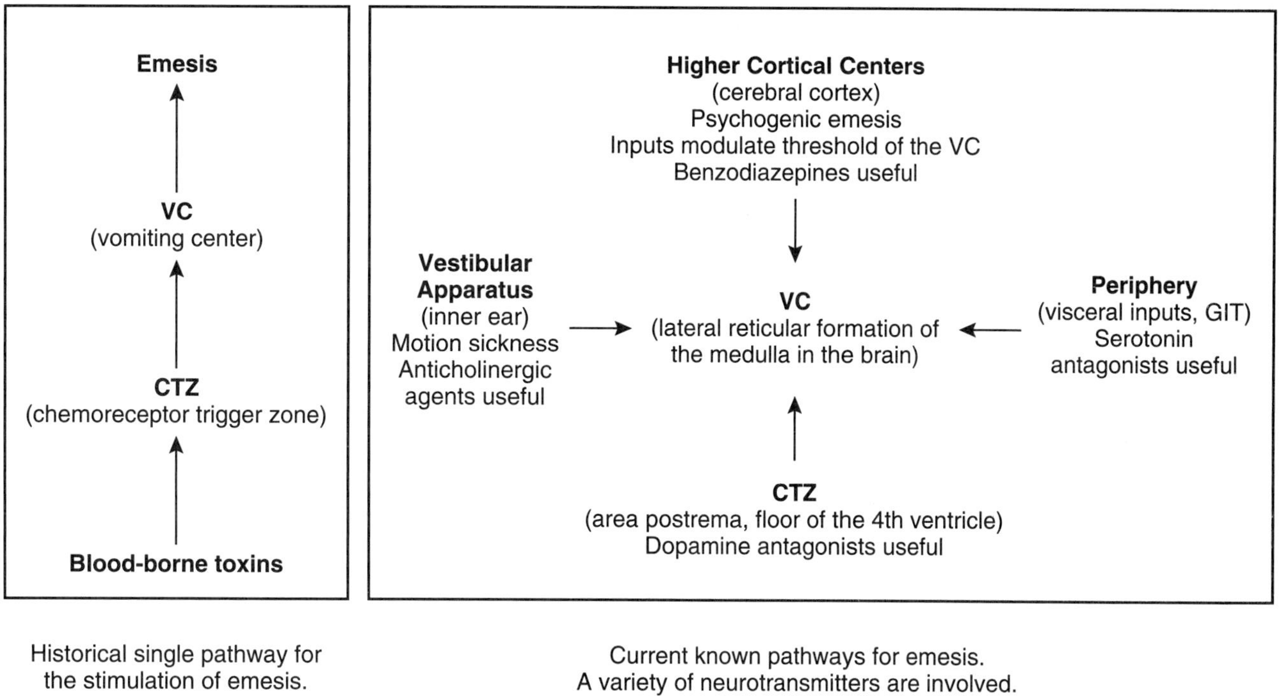

Figure 84.1. Emetogenic pathways. *CTZ*, chemoreceptor trigger zone; *GIT, gastrointestinal tract; VC*, vomiting center.

derives inputs from several areas: the CTZ, vestibular apparatus, periphery, and higher cortical centers.[32] Although it can aggravate nausea and vomiting secondary to chemotherapy when the patient is driving home after treatment, input from the vestibular apparatus is not believed to play a primary role in chemotherapy-induced emesis.

The introduction of cisplatin also allowed further discovery of new stimulatory pathways to the VC, as it induced a different type of severe emesis. Acute cisplatin-induced emesis was refractory to even the most aggressive use of standard dopamine antagonists, and thus it currently serves as a standard to test the efficacy of new antiemetic agents and treatment strategies.[33] Metoclopramide when administered intravenously every 2 hours in very high doses (1 to 3 mg/kg) was able to demonstrate a degree of effectiveness against cisplatin emesis.

Studies in animals indicated that complete surgical ablation of the CTZ failed to block emesis due to cisplatin. This understanding initiated the search for other inputs (ones from the periphery) that fed into the VC and could stimulate emesis after antineoplastic therapy. This led to an understanding of the role that serotonin plays in emesis and how metoclopramide in high doses acts as a weak serotonin antagonist.[33,34]

The role of serotonin is not fully understood, but it is currently felt that chemotherapeutic agents such as cisplatin cause enterochromaffin cells within the gastrointestinal tract to secrete serotonin. This neurotransmitter then stimulates emesis via multiple pathways both peripherally and centrally (either via vagal afferents or via direct action on the CTZ and VC). The serotonin type 3 receptor blocking agents (5-HT-3 antagonists) are our most effective class of agents against chemotherapy-induced emesis to date, as they not only block the action of serotonin but also inhibit further release of serotonin from the enterochromaffin cells.

These blocking agents do not have a linear response curve but actually exhibit a saturation or plateau phenomena.[35] Thus, higher doses of 5-HT-3 antagonists do not necessarily provide an enhanced antiemetic response. Recent studies have been able to show that significantly decreased doses of these agents can be used without affecting desired patient outcomes and overall antiemetic response. The synergistic effect demonstrated with combining 5-HT-3 antagonists and dexamethasone and the use of higher dexamethasone doses allows an even further reduction of the 5-HT-3 antagonist dose[36] and the overall cost of treatment.

Additional reductions in treatment cost can also be realized with use of oral 5-HT-3 antagonists and oral dexamethasone, all of which possess good oral bioavailability and efficacy. With enterochromaffin cells located within the gastrointestinal tract, oral 5-HT-3 agents offer the additional effect of blocking local serotonin receptors and thus reducing serotonin secretion.[37]

CLINICAL PRESENTATION AND DIAGNOSIS

It is extremely important to determine the exact etiology of nausea and vomiting in a patient with cancer before using an antiemetic agent for symptom management

(Table 84.11). Often obstruction of the gastrointestinal tract secondary to tumor invasion or heavy use of opiates or increased intracranial pressure from metastatic processes to the brain may be the true cause of nausea and protracted vomiting.[38] In these cases the use of an antiemetic agent is of limited benefit to the patient compared to correction of the primary problem.

Chemotherapy-related nausea and vomiting can present in three different ways: acute, delayed, and anticipatory. Nausea and vomiting are normally acute and take place within the first 24 hours after the administration of antineoplastic agent(s). Some agents can also produce a phenomena of delayed nausea, classically observed with cisplatin or high-dose cyclophosphamide chemotherapy, which begins after the first 24 hours and can last for several days.[33] Anticipatory nausea and vomiting are a conditioned or learned response that usually follows after one or more courses of emetogenic chemotherapy.[32] The nausea and vomiting experienced in this case have no relation to chemotherapy administration and can be triggered by a variety of associated sights or smells.[38]

Acute Emesis

Defined as emesis within the first 24 hours postchemotherapy, acute emesis is best controlled with prophylactic combinations of oral and/or intravenous antiemetics. Usually a 5-HT-3 antagonist combined with a steroid such as dexamethasone works well. The use of oral or intravenous dexamethasone has been documented to greatly enhance the efficacy of any antiemetic agent.[33] Because of its relatively low cost (compared to the 5-HT-3 antagonists) and low potential for side effects, the current recommendation is to use a 20-mg oral or intravenous dose for maximum protection. The dose of 5-HT-3 agent administered should be stratified according to the particular chemotherapeutic agent and dose used. This will minimize treatment cost, while providing optimal patient coverage. Refer to Table 84.12 for dosing recommendations.

Table 84.11 ▪ Initial Workup and Diagnosis

Risk factors for postchemotherapy nausea and vomiting
Other nonchemotherapy etiologies (e.g., acute abdominal emergencies, central nervous system disorders, acute systemic infections, fluid/electrolyte imbalances, etc.)
Fluid status (check hydration: skin turgor, weight, creatinine, blood urea nitrogen)
Comprehensive metabolic panel
Serum magnesium
Hepatic function panel (rule out electrolyte imbalance, electrolyte depletion, and renal/hepatic dysfunction
Vital signs (rule out fever, dehydration)
Orientation/mentation (rule out central nervous system disorder)
Evaluation of medications (opioids, digoxin, theophylline, oral antibiotics, etc.)
Active prechemotherapy nausea/vomiting: may need to move up one treatment class

Source: OnCare Treatment Guideline for Antiemetic Therapy, updated 1998.

Delayed Nausea and Vomiting

Studies indicate that this is frequently seen with the intravenous administration of high doses of cisplatin and cyclophosphamide.[34,38–40] The nausea and vomiting begin 1 or 2 days after treatment and can last for several days. The exact cause for delayed nausea and vomiting is poorly understood, and this syndrome is rather difficult to treat. We currently do not have highly effective antiemetics to combat this problem. It is hoped that the new class of oral neurokinin-1 (NK-1) receptor antagonists will prove helpful in this area.[41,42] Currently oral agents such as metoclopramide or ondansetron along with dexamethasone are used, although they have limited effectiveness.[33,43–45]

Anticipatory Nausea and Vomiting

This is a conditioned response that is learned after one or more courses of emetogenic chemotherapy during which the patient has had a difficult time.[32] The stimulus in this case comes from the higher or cortical centers of the brain transmitting impulses directly into the vomiting center, thereby greatly lowering the normal threshold for emesis. Triggers for this can be numerous, from the mere smell of isopropyl alcohol, to the reddish color of doxorubicin, to the sight of a chemotherapy nurse in public. All can elicit profound nausea and possibly immediate emesis.[39]

Anticipatory nausea and vomiting can be approached in two ways. The first is to aggressively treat the patient with adequate antiemetics to prevent a distressing experience from ever happening. The second is to use agents such as benzodiazepines to calm the patient and induce antegrade amnesia. Benzodiazepines act not only to calm and relax the patient but also to elevate the emesis threshold back to normal. With the antegrade amnesia induced by the benzodiazepines the patient may not remember enough to form a conditioned response.[46] Lorazepam is commonly administered sublingually at a dose of 1 or 2 mg to prevent anticipatory nausea and vomiting.

Benzodiazepines are also useful in reducing the level of fear and anticipation when the patient receives treatment. Fear can also cause significant stress for the patient and decrease the threshold for nausea and vomiting. Use of benzodiazepines the night before to induce sleep not only serves to provide a good night's rest but also calms the patient before treatment.

PSYCHOSOCIAL ASPECTS

It is extremely difficult for patients to deal with both a diagnosis of cancer and its many treatments. Surgery, radiation therapy, and chemotherapy are all associated with a wide variety of feared complications and side effects. The situation can be made more distressing if those involved also suffer from severe nausea and/or vomiting secondary to chemotherapy.

Table 84.12 ▪ Antiemetic Treatment Guideline[a]

Acute I Emetogenic Agents (Emetogenic Potential from 60 to >90%)

For each day of chemotherapy (start before chemotherapy)

- Granisetron 10 μg/kg IVP × 1 dose, or 2 mg PO × 1 dose, or 1 mg PO BID × 2 doses

or

- Ondansetron 16 to 20 mg IV × 1 dose (over 15 min), or 8 mg PO q8hr × 3 doses

or

- Dolasetron 100 mg IVP or 1.8mg/kg IVP × 1 dose, or 100mg PO × 1 dose

with

- Dexamethasone 8 to 20 mg IVP/PO × 1 dose
- (Optional) Additional dexamethasone 8 mg IVP/PO q6hr × 3 doses, to begin 6 hr after initial dose

If continued emesis in first 24 hr, treatment options include

- Prochlorperazine 10 mg IVP q6hr and/or
- Lorazepam 1 to 2 mg IVP/SL q6hr (useful if anticipatory vomiting is suspected)

or

- Metoclopramide 1 mg/kg IV q3hr × 2 doses with
- Diphenhydramine 25–50 mg IVP q3hr × 2 doses

or

- Another first-line agent from the list above

(Optional) At bedtime, the evening before chemotherapy

- Prochlorperazine 10 mg regular or 15 mg long-acting PO × 1 dose

or

- Promethazine 12.5–25 mg PO × 1 dose

and/or

- Lorazepam 1–2 mg PO/SL × 1 dose

Patients may repeat dose(s) the next day upon arrival for treatment.

If continued emesis after 24 hr

- Prochlorperazine 10 mg regular or 15 mg long-acting PO or 25 mg PR q6hr × 24 hr

or

- Promethazine 12.5–25 mg PO or 25 mg PR q6hr × 24 hr

or

- Haloperidol 1 mg PO q6hr × 24 hr

or

- Metoclopramide 20 mg PO q6hr, with

Diphenhydramine 25–50 mg PO q6hr

For cisplatin- and cyclophosphamide-containing regimens, refer to prophylactic regimen for delayed emesis.

Acute II Emetogenic Agents (Emetogenic Potential from 30 to 60%)

For each day of chemotherapy (start before chemotherapy)

- See treatment recommendations for acute I emetogenic agents, except:
- Ondansetron 8–10 mg IV × 1 dose (over 15 min) or 8 mg PO BID × 2 doses

(Optional) At bedtime, the evening before chemotherapy

See treatment recommendations for acute I emetogenic agents

If continued emesis during or after the first 24 hr

- See treatment recommendations for acute I emetogenic agents

Acute III Emetogenic Agents (Emetogenic Potential from 10 to 30%)

For each day of chemotherapy (start before chemotherapy)

- Dexamethasone 20 mg IVP/PO × 1 dose, then 8 mg IVP/PO q6hr × 3 doses

and/or

- Prochlorperazine 10 mg IVP, 10 mg regular, or 15 mg long-acting PO q6hr × 4 doses
- Metoclopramide 20 mg IVP/PO q6hr × 4 doses
- For some Acute III agents, use of any antiemetic is totally optional

If continued emesis within the first 24 hr

- Add another first-line agent from the list above

with

- Lorazepam 1–2 mg IVP/SL q6hr × 3 doses

(Optional) At bedtime, the evening before chemotherapy

- Prochlorperazine 10 mg regular or 15 mg long-acting PO × 1 dose

with

- Lorazepam 1–2 mg PO/SL × 1 dose

(continued)

Both nausea and vomiting have a direct impact on patients and their sense of well-being and control. They also have a detrimental impact and toll on family, friends, and co-workers. Severe nausea or vomiting may prevent the patient from participating in family activities and continuing to play a vital role in the workplace or community. There is also a significant impact on the physical, psychological, social, and spiritual dimensions of patients' quality of life.[47]

Dietary or behavioral interventions can assist with minimizing nausea or vomiting. Avoidance of spicy, greasy, or smelly foods and eating smaller more frequent meals can help. The timing of chemotherapy may also be important, as treatment first thing in the morning after a good night's sleep on an empty stomach is favored by some. Acupressure (sea sickness bands), herbal remedies (ginger), distraction (watching videos, playing video games, or imagery), or self-hypnosis can also assist in minimizing nausea and vomiting without the requirement for prescription medications.[48,49]

TREATMENT

Refer to Table 84.12 for evidence-based recommendations for the treatment of acute, anticipatory, delayed, and radiation-induced emesis. Recommendations are broken into those to be used as initial treatment for symptom management within the first 24 hours and those used for subsequent treatment for periods beyond 24 hours.

Table 84.12 *(continued)*

Patients may repeat dose(s) the next day upon arrival for treatment.

If continued emesis after 24 hr

- Haloperidol 1 mg IVP/PO q6hr × 24 hr
- If inadequate response, next cycle treat patient as Acute II

Acute IV Emetogenic Agents (Emetogenic Potential <10%)

- Antiemetic therapy is generally not necessary nor required with agents in this class

Anticipatory Nausea and Vomiting

Physician/nurse to evaluate need (in addition to standard antiemetics) the night before treatment

- Lorazepam 1–2 mg PO/SL at bedtime, with a repeat dose upon arrival for treatment

Behavioral interventions (use volunteer cancer support services)

- Relaxation (sleep, nap, or watch videotapes)
- Guided imagery
- Hypnosis (self-hypnosis)
- Distraction (music, books on tape, video games)

Delayed Nausea and Vomiting

Use as prophylactic treatment with high-dose cisplatin or cyclophosphamide (Acute I); administer the following after the initial 24 hr of acute antiemetics

(Evaluate need for intravenous hydration if delayed nausea and vomiting are severe.)

This combination can be used for the active treatment of delayed nausea/vomiting

- Metoclopramide 0.5 mg/kg/dose IV or PO QID (rounded to nearest 10 mg) × 4 days, with
- Dexamethasone 8 mg IVP or PO BID × 2 days, then 4 mg IVP or PO BID × 2 days

This combination should be used for prophylaxis only

- Ondansetron 8 mg IVP or PO BID × 3 days, with
- Dexamethasone 8 mg IVP or PO BID × 3 days

If inadequate response, then with the next cycle add (for 3 to 4 days)

- Prochlorperazine 10 mg IVP, or 10 mg regular or 15 mg long-acting PO, or 25 mg PR q6hr

with

- Lorazepam 1 mg PO/SL q6hr

Radiation-Induced Nausea and Vomiting

(For radiation to the extremities only, no antiemetics are normally needed.)

If a patient develops a problem with nausea and vomiting

- Prochlorperazine 10 mg IVP before each radiation treatment,
- then 10 mg IVP/PO q6hr daily for the 2 days after treatment is completed

with

- Dexamethasone 10 mg IVP before each treatment,
- then 4 mg IVP/PO q6hr daily also for the 2 days after treatment is completed

or

- Ondansetron 8 mg PO q8hr on each treatment day,

then continue for 2 more days post completion

or

- Granisetron 2 mg PO × 1dose or 1 mg PO BID × 2 doses on each treatment day, then continue for 2 more days after completion

If continued emesis in the first 24 hr

- Metoclopramide 20 mg IVP/PO q4–6hr, with
- Diphenhydramine 25–50 mg IVP/PO q4–6hr

Source: OnCare Treatment Guideline for Antiemetic Therapy, updated 1998.

[a]Extensive prechemotherapy education and alleviation of patient fears are critical to minimize or eliminate potential difficulties with nausea and/or vomiting.

Options are also offered for additional treatment within the first 24 hours and medications to be taken at bedtime the evening before chemotherapy.

Studies such as those conducted by Seynaeve et al.[50] demonstrated how both the dose and cost of 5-HT-3 antagonists could be reduced significantly without compromising overall patient outcome. A total of 535 chemotherapy-naive patients who received cisplatin (50 to 120 mg/m^2)-containing regimens participated in a randomized, double-blind, parallel study and were given single doses of ondansetron 8 or 32 mg intravenously or a bolus dose of 8 mg followed by continuous infusion of 1 mg/hr for 24 hours (total 32 mg). Complete and major control (≤2 emetic episodes) of acute emesis was achieved by 78% in the 32-mg group, 74% in the 8-mg group, and 74% in the bolus plus infusion group. The investigators thus concluded that a single intravenous dose of ondansetron 8 mg given before chemotherapy was as effective as a 32-mg daily dose in the prophylaxis of acute cisplatin-induced emesis.

MONITORING AND FOLLOW-UP

To determine and track the outcome of antiemetic therapy it is important to use standardized measurement tools. Table 84.13 identifies the National Cancer Institute criteria to assess the degree of nausea and/or vomiting. These measurements should be taken from patient interviews and documented after each cycle of treatment to determine whether antiemetic therapy was successful or whether a change in drug selection or dose is required. Patient-reported symptoms should also include an assessment of potential antiemetic drug-related toxicity, the most common being dystonic reactions. Appropriate medications can be prescribed if these side effects persist.

If symptoms of nausea and vomiting persist despite the use of proper antiemetics, it would be wise to determine the true reason for continued nausea and/or vomiting. These include acute abdominal emergencies, various infections, disorders of the central nervous system, and possibly toxicity due to other medications being taken by

Table 84.13 ▪ Monitoring and Follow-Up

Document Degree of Nausea (NCI grading)

- Grade 0 None
- Grade 1 Able to eat, reasonable intake
- Grade 2 Intake significantly decreased, but can eat
- Grade 3 No significant intake

Document Degree of Vomiting (NCI/WHO grading)

- Grade 0 None
- Grade 1 1 episode in 24 hr
- Grade 2 2–5 episodes in 24 hr
- Grade 3 6–10 episodes in 24 hr
- Grade 4 >10 episodes in 24 hr, or requiring parenteral support

If Persistent Nausea and/or Vomiting, Rule Out Other Causes

- Acute abdominal emergencies (acute appendicitis, acute cholecystitis, intestinal obstruction, or acute peritonitis)
- Infections (bacterial, fungal, or viral) (acute systemic infections, infections of the GI tract [rule/out parasitic], or inner ear infections)
- Central nervous system disorders (Increased intracranial pressure due to neoplasms, meningitis, bleeding, etc.)
- Medication related (opioid side effects, oral antibiotic side effects, digoxin toxicity, or theophylline toxicity)

For Persistent Nausea and Vomiting Monitor

- Fluid status
- Blood pressure
- Orientation/mentation
- Blood chemistry
- Vital signs

Medication Toxicity Monitoring

- Signs and symptoms of dystonic reactions: check for pseudoparkinsonism (mask-like faces, drooling, tremors, cogwheel rigidity, shuffling gate, akathesia, muscle rigidity, and dystonia)
- Management of dystonic reaction: diphenhydramine 25 to 50 mg PO/IM/IVP QID, or benztropine 1 to 2 mg PO/IM/IVP BID

Source: OnCare Treatment Guideline for Antiemetic Therapy, updated 1998.
NCI, National Cancer Institute; *WHO,* World Health Organization.

the patient. For these causes the use of antiemetics may not only be useless but also inappropriate.

As nausea and vomiting continue, one needs to carefully monitor the patient to prevent potential dehydration and serum electrolyte abnormalities.

FUTURE THERAPIES

New research is providing exciting information on the future of antiemetic therapy. Animal studies targeting blockers of substance P (a neurokinin neuropeptide) demonstrate significant activity against a wide range of nausea and vomiting syndromes.[42,47] It appears that substance P is involved in numerous pathways that stimulate both nausea and vomiting. Thus, an inhibitor of substance P at the NK-1 receptor may provide significant relief from these symptoms. Current studies are underway to determine the effectiveness of NK-1 receptor antagonists for the treatment of delayed nausea and vomiting. We have scant knowledge of the syndrome of delayed nausea and vomiting and little to offer patients in terms of effective therapy.[42]

IMPROVING OUTCOMES

The aggressive use of potent and effective antiemetics improves overall outcome for the patient by allowing treatment to proceed as planned with the doses of antineoplastic agents necessary to achieve a desired response.[51] Patients can quickly return to normal family, work, and community activities and the need for prolonged hospitalization because of the complications of nausea and vomiting is avoided.

With the advent of 5-HT-3 antagonists and their enhanced efficacy combined with dexamethasone, chemotherapy-induced nausea and vomiting can easily be prevented or greatly minimized. Today we are fortunate to have a better understanding of emetic pathways and also have many more antiemetic agents to select from. Optimal use of these agents has made the treatment of cancer tolerable and the completion of therapy more likely. With the future use of NK-1 receptor antagonists, both acute and delayed emesis may rapidly become a thing of the past.

Complications Treated with Stimulatory Cytokines

Several proteins have been developed that stimulate various steps of hematopoiesis and are designated as growth factors or stimulatory cytokines. These proteins are produced in vivo and bind to specific cell receptors to stimulate stem cell proliferation and differentiation.

Hematopoiesis proceeds from a stem cell in an orderly, timed fashion to mature cells (Fig. 84.2). Presently, G-CSF (filgrastim), GM-CSF (sargramostim), oprelvekin (IL-11), and recombinant human erythropoietin (rhuEPO) are available in the United States. In the future, recombinant human thrombopoietin will also be available.

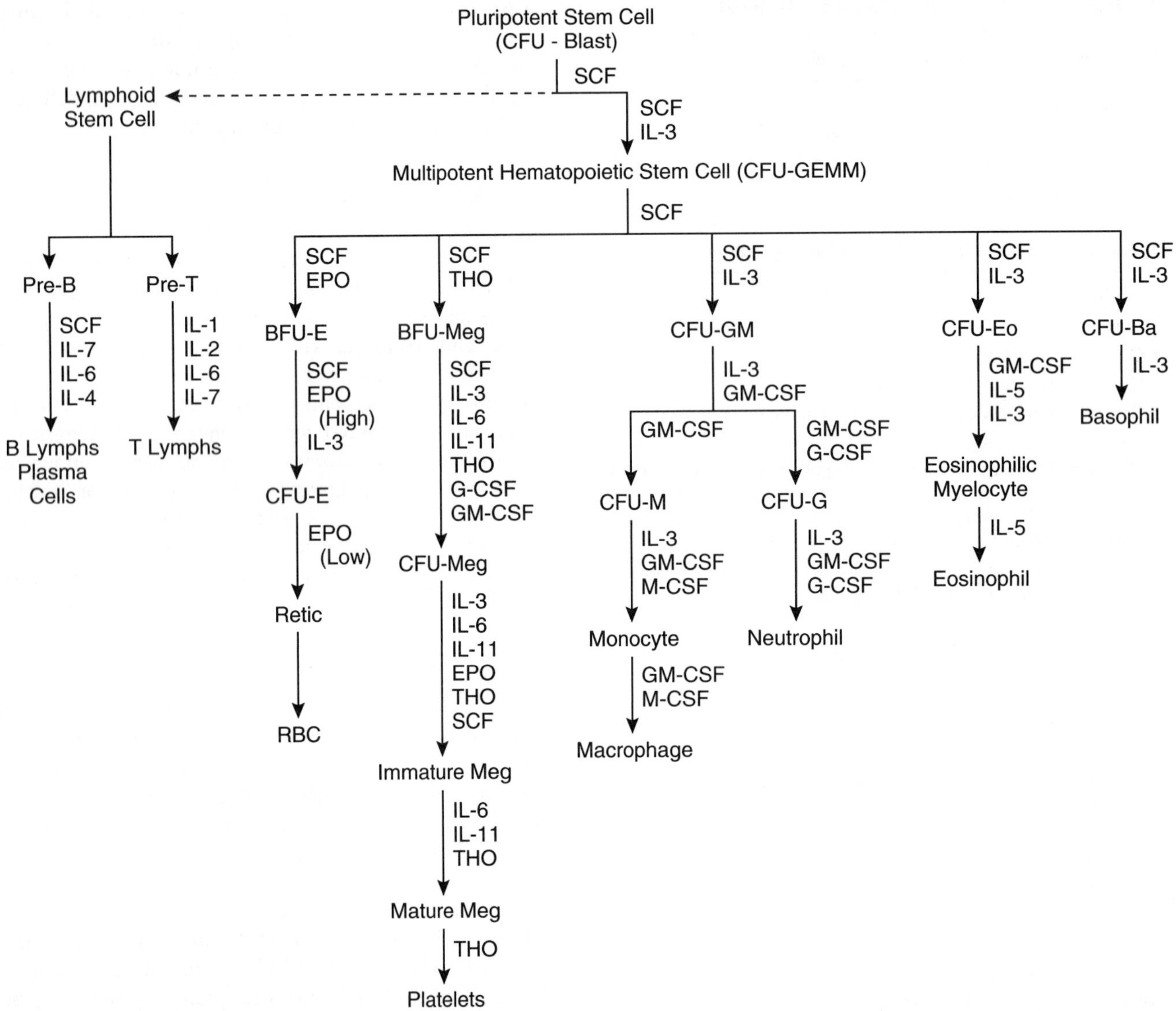

Figure 84.2. Hematopoiesis. *Ba,* basophil; *BFU,* blast-forming unit; *CFU,* colony-forming unit; *CSF,* colony-stimulating factor; *E,* erythroid; *Eo,* eosinophil; *EPO,* erythropoietin; *G,* granulocyte; *GEMM,* granulocyte, erythroid, macrophage, megakaryocyte; *GM,* granulocyte-macrophage; *IL,* interleukin; *Lymphs,* lymphocytes; *M,* macrophage; *Meg,* megakaryocyte; *Retic,* reticulocyte; *SCF,* stem cell factor/steel factor; *THO,* thrombopoietin.

Chemotherapy-Induced Neutropenia: Myelopoiesis Cytokines

Chemotherapy can have numerous toxic effects on the bone marrow. Of concern is chemotherapy-induced neutropenia (CIN). Patients experience CIN when the absolute neutrophil count (ANC) falls below 500/μL. At this time, patients are most vulnerable to bacterial, fungal, and viral infections.

TREATMENT GOALS: CHEMOTHERAPY-INDUCED NEUTROPENIA

- Prevent CIN and its associated infection risk by primary and secondary uses of myelopoiesis cytokines with standard-dose chemotherapy as well as use after high-dose cytotoxic therapy with bone marrow transplantation (BMT).
- Mobilize peripheral blood progenitor cells.

PATHOPHYSIOLOGY

Chemotherapy-induced neutropenic infections are the primary life-threatening event of any chemotherapy course. The duration and severity of CIN are the most important predictors of infection risk. Myelopoiesis growth factors decrease the time that granulocyte counts remain below 500/μL, decrease the incidence of febrile neutropenia, and decrease the number of infectious complications in patients with high-dose autologous BMT or allogeneic BMT. CSFs are also effective for mobilizing progenitor cells into peripheral blood to harvest for autologous or allogeneic transplantation.

TREATMENT

Recombinant (r) GM-CSF is a 127-amino acid glycosylated protein derived from yeast cultures. Original clinical trials used a nonglycosylated form from *Escherichia coli* cultures (molgramostim); however, this is no longer available due to its higher toxicity profile.[52] rGM-CSF stimulates granulopoiesis at the colony-forming unit (CFU)-GM level (Fig. 84.2). G-CSF is a 175-amino acid nonglycosylated protein derived from *E. coli* cultures. It stimulates granulopoiesis at the CFU-G level. There are no comparative trials testing the efficacy of G-CSF versus GM-CSF. There are small, varied differences reported depending upon which indication was investigated. The American Society of Clinical Oncology (ASCO) guidelines appropriately consider both agents equally effective for the prevention of CIN.[53]

ASCO guidelines recommend primary (or prophylactic, with the first course of chemotherapy) use of CSF if the expected incidence of febrile neutropenia with a chemotherapy regimen is 40% or greater. Special circumstances that support CSF usage with chemotherapy regimens for which the incidence of febrile CIN is less than 40% are: poor performance status, advanced cancer, preexisting neutropenia secondary to disease, extensive prior chemotherapy, previous radiation to the pelvis (as this area contains a large amount of bone marrow), open wounds, or concomitant active infections.

Secondary use of CSF is defined as use after a previous febrile CIN episode or previous CIN when dose reduction or delay is not appropriate, e.g., adjuvant chemotherapy in breast cancer. Silber et al.[54] correlated first-cycle ANC nadirs with a predicted need for CSF in subsequent chemotherapy courses. Presently, their mathematical model is complex but soon guidelines using first-cycle nadir counts may be used to select patients who should receive CSF with subsequent cycles for dose maintenance.

The use of CSFs in patients who are already neutropenic and febrile is recommended only if serious prognostic comorbidities are present. Studies have not yet supported a decrease in the number of neutropenic days or duration of hospitalization. Serious concomitant illnesses include pneumonia, hypotension, and multiorgan dysfunction.

CSFs are not routinely recommended for dose escalation outside of clinical trials. Filgrastim (G-CSF) absorption and distribution follow first-order pharmacokinetics. The volume of distribution is 150 mL/kg and the serum half-life is approximately 3.5 hours after either subcutaneous or intravenous administration. Sargramostim (GM-CSF) absorption and distribution also follow first-order pharmacokinetics. The half-life after intravenous administration is 60 minutes and after subcutaneous administration is 162 minutes. Thus, daily administration is recommended. The ANC after G-CSF use is discontinued falls rapidly for 1 to 3 days before a new, lower baseline level is maintained. The time to reach a desired neutrophil count with GM-CSF may be 1 day longer, but the ANC levels are more sustained with little or no decrease after discontinuation. CSF doses (Table 84.14) should begin 24 to 72 hours after chemotherapy and continue past the neutrophil nadir. The original recommendations were to treat to until an ANC of 10,000/μL was reached, but most clinicians now treat until ANC is greater than 1500 to 2500/μL for 2 consecutive days or for a maximum of 14 days. CSFs should be discontinued at least 24 hours before the next chemotherapy course. Discontinuation of CSFs 48 hours before the next cycle of chemotherapy has also been shown to decrease the chance of worsening CIN with subsequent cycles.[55] Theoretically, cytotoxic chemother-

Table 84.14 ▪ Myelopoiesis Cytokines

	GM-CSF	G-CSF
Dose	BSA 1.0 = 250 μg; 0.5 mL[a] BSA 1.2 = 300 μg; 0.6 mL BSA 1.4 = 350 μg; 0.7 mL BSA 1.6 = 400 μg; 0.8 mL BSA 1.8 = 450 μg; 0.9 mL BSA 2.0 = 500 μg; 1.0 mL	≤70 kg = 300 μg vial >70 kg = 480 μg vial or 5μg/kg/day
Route	SC IV	SC IV
Side effects		
More common	Arthralgia Myalgia Medullary bone pain Headache Skin rash Itching	Arthralgia Myalgia Medullary bone pain Headache Skin rash Itching
Less frequent or rare	Fever Excessive leukocytosis Redness or pain at injection site Shortness of breath Anaphylactic reaction Transient supraventricular arrhythmia Capillary leak syndrome Vasculitis Weakness	Excessive leukocytosis Redness or pain at injection site Anaphylactic reaction Transient supraventricular arrhythmia Splenomegaly Fever Sores on skin Vasculitis Weakness

GM-CSF, granulocyte-macrophage colony-stimulating factor; *G-CSF*, granulocyte colony-stimulating factor.

[a]Based on standard 250 μg/m² BSA; doses in 50 μg increments.

apy could result in greater CIN if given when the bone marrow is being stimulated by CSFs.

Refer to Table 84.14 for side effects associated with CSF administration. Particular side effects that should be managed appropriately include temperature elevation, site reactions, and bony pain or arthralgias. Temperature elevation can occur 30 minutes to 4 hours after injection and usually maximizes at 38°C or less. Patients can take acetaminophen or ibuprofen before injection to prevent this reaction. If temperature rises above 38.2°C or does not respond to antipyretics, an underlying infection must be considered. Site reactions are typically localized and caused by the injection technique. The injection sites need to be rotated, and the CSF should be injected at room temperature. It is often helpful to cool the skin with ice for a few minutes before injection. Bony medullary pain or arthralgias are common reactions and can be treated with analgesics typically used for mild to moderate pain. Rarely, the pain can be severe but usually resolves 1 to 3 days after CSF use is discontinued. Capillary leak syndrome previously reported with molgramostim is rarely associated with the yeast-derived GM-CSF product that is currently available.[56]

There are several precautions with CSF use. Administration with combined chemotherapy and radiotherapy has not been studied, and the use of CSF with daily radiation therapy may worsen neutropenia or damage the bone marrow. Lithium results in rapid release of neutrophils as they develop; thus close monitoring is warranted in patients receiving concomitant lithium and CSF therapy. Lower CSF doses and/or a shorter duration of therapy may be required when concomitant lithium therapy is being administered. Sargramostim is contraindicated in patients sensitive to yeast-derived products while filgrastim is contraindicated in patients sensitive to *E. coli*-derived products.

Chemotherapy-Induced Anemia: Erythropoiesis Cytokines

Anemia in patients with cancer may have several potential causes.[57] The causes must be differentiated to assure that all treatable causes are identified. Cancer may cause anemia directly by the following: acute or chronic blood loss, intratumor bleeding, erythrophagocytosis, hypersplenism, splenomegaly, and bone marrow replacement. Anemia also results from inhibitory cytokines produced by the cancer or physiologic effects of the cancer. This anemia may, in part, be similar to the anemia of chronic disease. Mechanisms involve abnormalities of iron usage and/or blunted erythropoietic bone marrow response by inhibitory cytokines. A few such cytokines are tumor necrosis factor α, interleukin (IL)-6, IL-1, and interferon-γ. Immune hemolytic anemias, microangiopathic hemolysis, primary bone marrow failure and nutritional deficiencies also must be considered before labeling anemia in a patient with cancer as a cancer- or chemotherapy-induced anemia.

TREATMENT GOALS: CHEMOTHERAPY-INDUCED ANEMIA

- Maintain hemoglobin level during chemotherapy and/or radiation therapy.
- Maintaining an appropriate hemoglobin level will decrease fatigue and improve quality of life while avoiding the risk of red blood cell transfusions.

PATHOPHYSIOLOGY

The most common cause of anemia in a patient with cancer is chemotherapy or radiotherapy. Therapy-induced anemia is caused by stem cell death, committed progenitor cell death, blockage or delay in hematopoiesis cell cycling, or damage to mature cells. Patients at highest risk for therapy-induced anemia are those who are anemic before therapy or undergo combined modality treatment.

TREATMENT

Erythropoietin acts similarly to a hormone in erythropoiesis. It is secreted by the kidney in response to low oxygen tension. It stimulates a narrow range of erythropoiesis at early burst-forming unit, erythroid (BFUe) but primarily at colony-forming unit, erythroid (CFUe), and its presence at subsequent levels of development appears to stop apoptosis (Fig. 84.2). The common clinical indications for therapeutic use are chemotherapy-induced anemia, radiation-induced anemia, anemia associated with renal failure, human immunodeficiency virus-associated anemia, and anemia due to myelodysplastic syndromes.

rhuEPO administration in patients undergoing cancer chemotherapy and radiotherapy results in a 40 to 70% response rate with at least a 2 g/dL increase in hemoglobin level and a decrease in the need for red blood cell transfusions by 30 to 80%.[58,59] An increased hemoglobin level has also been associated with improved quality of life.[60,61]

rhuEPO is a 165-amino acid glycoprotein derived from mammalian cells and is identical to isolated natural erythropoietin. rhuEPO demonstrates first-order pharmacokinetics after intravenous administration. Subcutaneous administration results in peak serum concentrations in 12 to 24 hours that decline slowly thereafter with a half-life of 7 to 18 hours.[62] Patients with normal renal function have a half-life that is 20% shorter after IV administration. The half-life in patients with chronic renal failure is 4 to 13 hours and is not affected by dialysis. In patients undergoing dialysis, decreased doses (by 32%) can be administered subcutaneously to maintain hematocrit levels of 30 to 33%.

Doses of 150 to 300 U/kg should be administered three times per week. Initiate therapy at 150 U/kg three times per week and increase if no or little response occurs within 2 to 4 weeks. Hemoglobin level and reticulocyte counts are monitored at 2-week intervals and iron, transferrin, and ferritin at 4-week intervals. Before rhuEPO is started, adequate levels of vitamin B_{12}, folate, and iron should be confirmed by laboratory tests. Several investigators have tried to determine predictive factors for cancer-induced anemia that is responsive to rhuEPO. There are no reliable predictive factors; even pre-erythropoietin levels of several hundred (normal 10 to 20 U/L) do not predict unresponsiveness. Some investigators do not use rhuEPO if endogenous erythropoietin levels are 1000 U/L or greater, while other investigators use cutoff levels of 500 U/L or greater; more information is needed in this area. Presently, a therapeutic trial is the only way to determine responsiveness.

The etiology of failures, if all other causes of anemia are eliminated, is generally unknown. A small group of failures, though, may be related to functional iron deficiency.[63] This is caused by impaired bone marrow utilization of iron stores. Early evidence shows that administration of iron (IV), when transferrin saturation is 15% or less or ferritin is 100 ng/mL or less, improves the response to rhuEPO response and allows decreased doses of rhuEPO to be administered in patients with renal failure.[64–66]

The side effects of rhuEPO are minimal. Medullary bone pain is reported most commonly. The hypertension from increased red blood cell mass seen in patients with renal failure is rare in patients with cancer.

Chemotherapy-Induced Thrombocytopenia: Thrombopoiesis Cytokines

Chemotherapy-induced thrombocytopenia is a significant and increasing problem in patients with cancer. Of patients with solid tumors who are undergoing chemotherapy, 25% develop thrombocytopenia with platelet counts less than 50×10^9/L, whereas 10 to 15% have platelet counts less than 20×10^9/L.[67] The depth and duration of thrombocytopenia are correlated with serious bleeding. Patients with a platelet count less than 20×10^9/L for 7 days have a 10% risk of bleeding whereas patients with similar low counts for 14 days have a 60% risk.[68] With the availability of G-CSF and GM-CSF to prevent neutropenia, thrombocytopenia is now often the dose-limiting toxicity related to chemotherapy administration.

TREATMENT GOALS: CHEMOTHERAPY-INDUCED THROMBOCYTOPENIA

- Prevent chemotherapy-induced thrombocytopenia through use of thrombopoiesis cytokines.
- In so doing, decrease the risk of serious bleeding complications and the need for platelet transfusions and allow chemotherapy administration to proceed on schedule.

PATHOPHYSIOLOGY

Several growth factors/cytokines are involved in thrombopoiesis: IL-1, IL-3, IL-6, IL-11, and Mpl ligand, known as thrombopoietin (THO) (Fig. 84.2). Mpl ligand increases platelet production by inducing early marrow precursors in a dose-dependent manner. Its presence contributes to proliferation, but it is not required in the final stages of platelet development. rTHO is under development by Genentech. This product showed promise for chemotherapy-induced thrombocytopenia in early phase I/II trials.[69]

TREATMENT

The only product currently approved by the FDA is oprelvekin (IL-11). IL-11 primarily has maturational effects on megakaryocytes but with IL-3 and stem cell factor (SCF) enhances proliferation of early progenitors as well (Fig. 84.2).[70] Oprelvekin is a nonglycosylated, 177-amino acid protein, produced in *E. coli.* The terminal half-life is approximately 7 hours. There is no accumulation with daily administration at either the 25 or 50 μg/kg recommended doses.

Oprelvekin has been shown to increase platelet counts at the chemotherapy nadir and decrease the need for platelet transfusions when used in patients with severe thrombocytopenia from a previous chemotherapy course.[71] It has also been shown (compared with placebo) to decrease platelet transfusions and speed platelet recovery with initial dose-intense chemotherapy.[72] In clinical studies, oprelvekin's clinical benefit was definite and statistically significant, but 30% of the oprelvekin-treated group still required at least one platelet transfusion.

Oprelvekin is given at 50 μg/kg/day subcutaneously starting the day after chemotherapy and is continued for 10 to 21 days. Platelet counts increase within 5 to 9 days and can continue to increase for up to 7 days after injections are discontinued.

Side effects of oprelvekin are minimal. Plasma volume expansion can occur and cause dyspnea, peripheral edema, and transient atrial arrhythmias. These side effects are usually self-limiting and are reversible after discontinuation. Transient atrial arrhythmias have occurred at the

50 μg/kg/day dose and greater, and they have been characterized as brief without sequelae. Oprelvekin is not directly arrhythmogenic and the atrial arrhythmias are probably associated with increased plasma volume. Thiazide diuretics can be used to decrease plasma volume expansion. Minor arthralgias, skin rash, conjunctival redness, and fatigue can also occur. Oprelvekin has been used with G-CSF and GM-CSF without any evidence of adverse reactions, pharmacokinetic profile change, or altered therapeutic benefit of either drug.

Cytokine support of thrombopoiesis is evolving. As other products become available, their use alone or with oprelvekin will develop. Severe chemotherapy-induced thrombocytopenia and use of a limited supply blood product (platelet transfusions) may soon be preventable in most patients. Oprelvekin is the first step in that direction.

Complications Treated with Cytoprotective Agents

Chemotherapy-Induced Organ Toxicity: Cytoprotective Agents

There are now three established drugs used in conjunction with chemotherapy to reduce the severity and/or prevent a specific organ toxicity or toxicity profile. Two of these agents allow dose-intense chemotherapy for the malignancy while protecting an organ from the toxic effects of therapy. Mesna and dexrazoxane protect against specific side effects: ifosfamide-induced hemorrhagic cystitis and doxorubicin-induced cardiotoxicity, respectively. The third agent, amifostine, is a general cytoprotectant. It is approved for cisplatin-induced renal toxicity and bone marrow toxicity but is useful in many situations.

TREATMENT GOALS: CHEMOTHERAPY-INDUCED ORGAN TOXICITY

- Administer cytoprotective agents with chemotherapy to reduce or prevent specific chemotherapy-induced organ toxicities.
- Enable continuation of scheduled chemotherapy.

TREATMENT

Mesna

Cyclophosphamide and ifosfamide can cause hemorrhagic cystitis and fibrosis due to the metabolite acrolein. Mesna (sodium-2-mercaptoethanesulfonate) protects the uroepithelium by binding acrolein to its free sulfhydryl groups, thus forming a nontoxic, stable compound. Mesna can also bind other metabolites of ifosfamide such as 4-hydroxy-ifosfamide and chloracetaldehyde. It has been shown to be superior to hydration and urinary alkalinization in preventing hemorrhagic cystitis.[73]

Mesna is oxidized to dimesna in the circulation. Approximately 50% is glomerularly filtered and converted back to mesna by renal tubular glutathione reductase and is available in urine as intact mesna with free sulfhydryl groups. Mesna has a short plasma half-life compared to ifosfamide and is water soluble with little tissue penetration. The efficacy of ifosfamide is not altered by mesna.

Mesna is currently available only in an intravenous form, but there are data for oral administration as well.[74] Intravenous dosing results in urinary concentrations twice those with oral administration. Urinary excretion of an intravenous dose is complete in 4 hours but orally administered doses result in urinary levels for at least 8 hours. Intravenous mesna must be given frequently (every 4 hours) to protect the uroepithelium after ifosfamide dosing. Mesna is given at 60% of the ifosfamide dose in three equal doses: just before chemotherapy and then 4 hours and 8 hours after chemotherapy. An alternative method of administration uses a mesna 200 mg loading dose followed by a constant infusion of mesna with ifosfamide over 24 hours. During the constant infusion, the mesna dose is equivalent to the ifosfamide dose. Adverse reactions to mesna are minor and include nausea, diarrhea, headache, and fatigue.

Dexrazoxone

Dexrazoxane is a dioxopiperazine analog of EDTA that is hydrolyzed intracellularly to its active form. It then binds iron and prevents iron-mediated free radical formation responsible for doxorubicin-induced cardiotoxicity.[75]

Doxorubicin is a highly active chemotherapy agent in many malignancies and is included in first-line regimens for breast cancer, many lymphomas, sarcomas, and small cell lung cancer. Doxorubicin use is limited by dose-related cardiotoxicity. Use of dexrazoxane has been shown to allow higher cumulative doses of doxorubicin with 90%

less cardiotoxicity up to cumulative doxorubicin doses of 750 mg/m^2.[76]

Dexrazoxane administration must be completed 30 minutes before doxorubicin administration at a dose ratio of 10:1. Slow intravenous push or rapid infusion is recommended. Adverse reactions include enhanced myelosuppression and pain at the injection site. Several other side effects reported in studies are most likely caused by doxorubicin: alopecia, nausea, vomiting, fatigue, and anorexia. The myelosuppression appears to be dose-related and is more common at doses of 600 mg/m^2 and higher. Extensive pharmacokinetic studies have demonstrated that doxorubicin's pharmacokinetics are not altered by concurrent administration with dexrazoxane and that dexrazoxane, itself, is myelosuppressive. There are no reported cumulative toxicities with dexrazoxane.[77]

Doxorubicin is an important chemotherapy agent and amelioration of its dose-limiting toxicity is an important advance. It is unknown how useful dexrazoxane will be with other anthracyclines, idarubicin and daunorubicin or the anthracenedione, mitoxantrone.

Amifostine

Amifostine was initially developed by Walter Reed Medical Center as a cell protector from radiation associated with nuclear war. It has been investigated more recently as a cytoprotector for the effects of certain chemotherapy agents and radiotherapy.

Amifostine is a phosphorylated aminothiol drug metabolized to free thiol by alkaline phosphatase enzyme in the cell membrane of normal tissue. This allows selective action on normal tissue versus malignant tissue, which has lower activity of this cell membrane-associated enzyme. The increased free thiol concentration intracellularly binds free radicals generated by certain chemotherapy agents or radiation therapy and protects the cell.

Amifostine is a broad range cytoprotectant. Clinical studies in ovarian cancer and non-small cell lung cancer have consistently shown decreases in mucositis, renal toxicity, bone marrow suppression, and neurologic toxicity with platinum-based chemotherapy regimens.[78] Decreased effectiveness against tumors has not been seen in those cancer types. In head and neck cancer, decreased incidence of mucositis and xerostomia due to radiation therapy has also been documented.[79] Amifostine, recently, has been shown to protect the bone marrow better than G-CSF after carboplatin therapy.[80] In early studies, amifostine has shown beneficial effects in myelodysplastic syndromes.[81] Three- and 5-day regimens at 200 mg/m^2 have improved platelet counts, ANCs, and hemoglobin levels. This effect could be important in a disease with few therapeutic options.

Amifostine has a short half-life (α half-life less than 1 minute and β half-life of 8 minutes) and is 90% cleared from the plasma in 6 minutes. It is given intravenously over less than 10 minutes, 30 minutes before chemotherapy. It is not effective if given after chemotherapy. The dosage was originally 910 mg/m^2, but current recommendations are 740 mg/m^2 before cisplatin or carboplatin. In patients undergoing radiation therapy, 200 mg/m^2/day given over 3 minutes has been shown to protect against xerostomia and mucositis.

Amifostine has several side effects, which may limit its use. During intravenous administration, hypotension can be significant (a 20 mm Hg drop in systolic blood pressure is average). This effect can be reduced by having the patient well hydrated and by limiting the infusion time to 10 minutes or less. Prehydrating the patient with 1 L of intravenous fluids 2 hours before amifostine and having the patient remain supine for 30 minutes after the infusion has decreased the incidence of this side effect. If hypotension occurs, discontinue the amifostine infusion. The baseline blood pressure usually returns to normal in 5 minutes, and then amifostine administration can be resumed. The guidelines for quantitative blood pressure changes and altered infusion rates are detailed in the prescribing information.

Nausea with or without vomiting is also a common side effect, which can be successfully prevented with premedications: dexamethasone and a 5-HT-3 receptor antagonist. These antiemetics should be administered at least 1 hour before amifostine, and the patient should be instructed to take oral antiemetics in addition 3 to 6 hours before amifostine. Other adverse reactions reported include allergic reactions and decreased calcium levels.

Amifostine is an effective cytoprotectant and can be used in many chemotherapy and/or radiotherapy protocols. The side effects of hypotension and nausea/vomiting limited its use initially. The new lower dosing recommendation, combined with hydration, antiemetics, and limited infusion time have controlled these side effects. Amifostine is an effective protectant of hematopoiesis, peripheral nerves, and oral/esophageal mucosa and also protects against the nephrotoxic effects of platinum drugs as well.

FUTURE THERAPIES

Several cytoprotectant compounds are currently under investigation. IL-15 has been used to prevent diarrhea induced by irinotecan. Myeloid progenitor inhibitory factor-1 has been investigated in phase I studies as a bone marrow protector of neutrophils and platelets. Keratinocyte growth factor shows promise as a protector against mucositis in radiation and chemotherapy regimens and high-dose chemotherapy with stem cell support.

KEY POINTS

- When used appropriately, supportive care therapies for the patient with cancer diminish some of the complications associated with chemotherapy and radiation; this has many important implications. It increases the chances that cancer therapy will be delivered at the optimal dosage intensity and on schedule, it improves quality of life, both physically and emotionally, and in some cases it allows for increased dosage intensity which may improve survival for patients with some cancers.

- Recently, great strides have been made in the development of supportive care strategies in terms of identifying, preventing, and treating the complications associated with the delivery of chemotherapy and radiation.
- While we are still searching for effective therapies for some complications, we have found pharmacologic therapies that have vastly improved the treatment of others. For example, although there is currently no effective treatment for mucositis and management is primarily preventive, new compounds are being investigated. The discovery of the 5-HT-3 antagonists has dramatically decreased the incidence and severity of nausea and vomiting. Furthermore, the hematologic support agents have improved the outcomes in patients receiving cancer therapy that may cause neutropenia (CSFs), anemia (rhuEPO), and thrombocytopenia (oprelvekin). There are also a number of cytoprotective agents that can be used to diminish the incidence of particular side effects: mesna for ifosfamide-induced hemorrhagic cystitis, dexrazoxane for doxorubicin-induced cardiotoxicity, and amifostine for a broad range of toxicities.
- There is intensive ongoing research devoted to the identification of supportive care therapies that will improve the outcomes, in terms of improved quality of life and increased survival rates, for patients with cancer. It is an area that will continue to grow with our quest to improve cancer therapies.

REFERENCES

1. Dose AM. The symptom experience of mucositis, stomatitis, and xerostomia. Semin Oncol Nurs 11:248–255, 1995.
2. Zlotolow IM. General considerations in prevention and treatment of oral manifestations of cancer therapies. In: Berger A, Portenoy RK, Weissman DE, eds. Principles and practice of supportive oncology. Philadelphia: Lippincott-Raven, 1998:237.
3. Kinzie BJ. Treatment of stomatitis associated with antineoplastic-drug therapy. Clin Pharm 7:14–17, 1988.
4. Berger AM, Kilroy TJ. Oral complications. In: DeVita VT Jr, Hellman S, Rosenberg SA, eds. Principles and practice of oncology 5th ed. Philadelphia: Lippincott-Raven, 1997:2714.
5. National Institutes of Health. Oral complications of cancer therapies: diagnosis, prevention, and treatment. NIH Consens Statement 7:1–11, 1989.
6. Verdi CJ. Cancer therapy and oral mucositis. Drug Saf 9:185–195, 1993.
7. Carl W. Oral complications of local and systemic cancer treatment. Curr Opin Oncol 7:320–324, 1995.
8. Haskell CM. Principles of cancer chemotherapy. In: Haskell CM, ed: Cancer treatment. 4th ed. Philadelphia: WB Saunders, 1995:42.
9. Loprinzi CL, Foote RL, Michalak J. Alleviation of cytotoxic therapy-induced normal tissue damage. Semin Oncol 22(2, Suppl 3):95–97, 1995.
10. Solomon MA. Oral sucralfate suspension for mucositis. N Engl J Med 315:459–460, 1986.
11. Mahood DJ, Dose AM, Loprinzi CL, et al. Inhibition of fluorouracil-induced stomatitis by oral cryotherapy. J Clin Oncol 9:449–452, 1991.
12. Rocke LK, Loprinzi CL, Lee JK, et al. A randomized clinical trial of two different durations of oral cryotherapy for the prevention of 5-fluorouracil-related stomatitis. Cancer 72:2234–2238, 1993.
13. Epstein JB. The painful mouth. Infect Dis Clin North Am 2:103–202, 1988.
14. Berger AM, Kilroy TJ. Oral complications of cancer therapy. In: Berger A, Portenoy RK, Weissman DE, eds. Principles and practice of supportive oncology. Philadelphia: Lippincott-Raven, 1998:223.
15. Fox PC, Atkinson JC, Macynski AA, et al. Pilocarpine treatment of salivary gland hypofunction and dry mouth (xerostomia). Arch Intern Med 151:1149–1152, 1991.
16. Greenspan D, Daniels TE. Effectiveness of pilocarpine in postradiation xerostoma. Cancer 59:1123–1125, 1987.
17. Johnson JT, Ferretti FA, Nethery J, et al. Oral pilocarpine for postirradiation xerostomia in patients with head and neck cancer. N Engl J Med 329:390–395, 1993.
18. Cox GJ, Matsui SM, Lo RS, et al. Etiology and outcome of diarrhea after bone marrow transplantation: a prospective study. Gastroenterology 107:1398–1407, 1994.
19. Mercadante S. Diarrhea, malabsorption, and constipation. In: Berger A, Portenoy RK, Weissman DE, eds. Principles and practice of supportive oncology. Philadelphia: Lippincott-Raven, 1998:191.
20. Bruera E, Suarez-Almazor M, Velasco A, et al. The assessment of constipation in terminal cancer patients admitted to a palliative care unit: a retrospective review. J Pain Symptom Manage 9:515–519, 1994.
21. Rothenberg ML, Eckardt JR, Kuhn JG, et al. Phase II trial of irinotecan in patients with progressive or rapidly recurrent colorectal cancer. J Clin Oncol 14:1128–1135, 1996.
22. Coates A, Abraham S, Kaye SB, et al. On the receiving end: patient perception of the side effects of cancer chemotherapy. Eur J Cancer 19:203–208, 1983.
23. Griffin AM, Butow PN, Coates AS, et al. On the receiving end. V: patient perceptions on the side effects of cancer chemotherapy in 1993. Ann Oncol 7:189–195, 1996.
24. Graves T. Emesis as a complication of cancer chemotherapy: pathophysiology, importance, and treatment. Pharmacotherapy 12:337–345, 1992.
25. Hesketh PH, Kris MG, Grunberg SM, et al. Proposal for classifying the acute emetogenicity of cancer chemotherapy. J Clin Oncol 15:103–109, 1997.
26. Aapro M. Methodological issues in antiemetic studies. Invest New Drugs 11:243–253, 1993.
27. Tortorice PV, O'Connell MB. Management of chemotherapy-induced nausea and vomiting. Pharmacotherapy 10:129–145, 1990.
28. Foot ABM, Hayes C. Audit of guidelines for effective control of chemotherapy and radiotherapy induced emesis. Arch Dis Child 71:475–480, 1994.
29. Currow DC, Noble PD, Stuart-Harris R. The clinical use of ondansetron. Med J Aust 162:145–149, 1995.
30. Osaba D, Zee B, Pater J, et al. Determinants of postchemotherapy nausea and vomiting in patients with cancer. J Clin Oncol 15:116–123, 1997.
31. Borrison HL, Wang SC. Physiology and pharmacology of vomiting. Pharmacol Rev 5:193–230, 1953.
32. Grunberg SM, Hesketh PJ. Control of chemotherapy-induced emesis. N Engl J Med 329:1790–1796, 1993.
33. Gralla RJ, Rittenberg C, Peralta M, et al. Cisplatin and emesis: aspects of treatment and a new trial for delayed emesis using oral dexamethasone plus ondansetron beginning at 16 hours after cisplatin. Oncology 53:86-91, 1996.
34. Del Favero A, Roila F, Tonato M. Reducing chemotherapy-induced nausea and vomiting: current perspectives and future possibilities. Drug Saf 9:410–428, 1993.
35. Grunberg SM. Antiemetic drugs: essential pharmacology. In: Tonato M, ed. Antiemetics in the supportive care of cancer patients. Berlin: Springer Verlag, 1996:25–33.
36. Pectasides D, Mylonakis A, Varthalitis J, et al. Comparison of two different doses of ondansetron plus dexamethasone in the prophylaxis of cisplatin-induced emesis. Oncology 54:1–6, 1997.
37. Blaver P. A pharmacological profile of oral granisetron (Kytril tablets). Semin Oncol 22(Suppl 10):3–5, 1995.
38. Lichter I. Nausea and vomiting in patients with cancer. Hematol Oncol Clin North Am 10:207–220, 1966.
39. Stewart A. Optimal control of cyclophosphamide-induced emesis. Oncology 53(Suppl 1):32–38, 1996.
40. Martin M. The severity and pattern of emesis following different cytotoxic agents. Oncol 53(Suppl 1):26–31, 1996.
41. Bountra C, Gale JD, Gardner CJ, et al. Towards understanding the etiology and pathophysiology of the emetic reflex: novel approaches to antiemetic drugs. Oncology 53(Suppl 1):102–109, 1996.
42. Lakhbir S, Field MJ, Hughes J, et al. The tachykinin NK1 receptor antagonists PD 154075 blocks cisplatin-induced delayed emesis in the ferret. Eur J Pharmacol 321:209–216, 1997.
43. Hesketh P. Management of cisplatin-induced delayed emesis. Oncology 53(Suppl 1):73–77, 1996.

44. Tavorath R, Hesketh PJ. Drug treatment of chemotherapy-induced delayed emesis. Drugs 52:639–648, 1996.
45. Kris MG, Roila F, De Mulder PHM, et al. Delayed emesis following anticancer chemotherapy. Support Care Cancer 6:228–232, 1998.
46. Laszlo J, Clark RA, Hanson DC, et al. Lorazepam in cancer patients treated with cisplatin: a drug having antiemetic, amnesic and anxiolytic effects. J Clin Oncol 3:864–869, 1985.
47. Grant M. Introduction: nausea and vomiting, quality of life, and the oncology nurse. Oncol Nurs Forum 24:5–7, 1997.
48. King CR. Nonpharmacologic management of chemotherapy-induced nausea and vomiting. Oncol Nurs Forum 24:41–47, 1997.
49. Suekawa M, Ishige A, et al. Pharmacological studies on ginger. I. Pharmacological actions of pungent constituents, (6)-gingerol and (6)-shogaol. J Pharmacobiodyn 7:836–848, 1984.
50. Seynaeve C, Schuller J, Buser K, et al. Comparison of the anti-emetic efficacy of different doses of ondansetron, given as either a continuous infusion or a single intravenous dose, in acute cisplatin-induced emesis. A multicentre, double-blind, randomised, parallel group study. Br J Cancer 66:192–197, 1992.
51. Marty M. Future trends in cancer treatment and emesis control. Oncology 50:159–162, 1993.
52. Rowe JM, Anderson JW, Mazza JJ, et al. A randomized placebo-controlled phase III study of granulocyte-macrophage colony-stimulating factor in adult patients: a study of the Eastern Cooperative Oncology Group (E1490). Blood 86:457–462, 1995.
53. American Society Clinical Oncology. Update of recommendations for the use of hematopoietic colony stimulating factors: evidence-based, clinical practice guidelines. J Clin Oncol 14:1957–1960, 1996.
54. Silber JH, Fridman M, DiPaola, RS, et al. First-cycle blood counts and subsequent neutropenia, dose reduction, or delay in early stage breast cancer therapy. J Clin Oncol 16:2392–2400, 1998.
55. Vivianne CG, Tijan-Heijnen, Biesma B, et al. Enhanced myelotoxicity due to granulocyte colony stimulating factor administration until 48 hours before the next chemotherapy course in patients with small cell lung carcinoma. J Clin Oncol 16:2708–2714, 1998.
56. Bunn PA, Crowley J, Kelly, K, et al. Chemoradiotherapy with or without granulocyte-macrophage colony stimulating factor in the treatment of limited-stage small-cell lung cancer: a prospective phase III randomized study of the Southwest Oncology Group. J Clin Oncol 13:1632–1641, 1995.
57. Ludwig H, Fritz E: Anemia in cancer patients. Semin Oncol 25(Suppl):2–6, 1998.
58. Glaspy J, Bukowski R, Steinberg D, et al. Impact of therapy with epoetin alpha or clinical outcomes in patients with nonmyeloid malignancies during cancer chemotherapy in community oncology practice. J Clin Oncol 15:1218–1234, 1997.
59. Cascinu S, Fedeli A, Del Ferro E, et al. Recombinant human erythropoietin treatment in cisplatin-associated anemia: a randomized, double-blind trial with placebo. J Clin Oncol 12:1058–1062, 1994.
60. Cella D. Factors influencing quality of life in cancer patients: anemia and fatigue. Semin Oncol 25(Suppl 7):43–46, 1998.
61. Leitgeb C, Pecherstorfer M, Fritz E, et al. Quality of life in chronic anemia of cancer during treatment with recombinant human erythropoietin. Cancer 73:2535–2542, 1994.
62. Kaufman JS, Reda DJ, Fye CL, et al. Subcutaneous compared with intravenous epoetin in patients receiving hemodialysis. N Engl J Med 339:578–583, 1998.
63. Weinberh ED. The role of iron in cancer. Eur J Cancer Prev 5:19–36, 1996.
64. Henry D, Mason B, Staddon A, et al. Efficacy of Infed plus recombinant human erythropoietin (rhuEPO) in treating anemia in cancer patients with suboptimal response to rhuEPO: a pilot study [Abstract 230]. Proc Am Soc Clin Oncol 17:59a, 1998.
65. Adamson JW. The relationship of erythropoietin and iron metabolism to red blood cell production in humans. Semin Oncol 21(Suppl 13):9–15, 1994.
66. Fishbane S, Frei GL, Maesaka J. Reduction in recombinant human erythropoietin doses by the use of chronic intravenous iron supplementation. Am J Kidney Dis 26:41–46, 1995.
67. Dutcher J, Schiffer C, Aisner J, et al. Incidence of thrombocytopenia and serious hemorrhage among patients with solid tumors. Cancer 53:557–562, 1984.
68. Rebulla P, Finazzi G, Marangoni F, et al. The threshold for prophylactic platelet transfusions in adults with acute myeloid leukemia. N Engl J Med 337:1870–1875, 1997.
69. Kaushansky K. Thrombopoietin. N Engl J Med 339:746–754, 1998.
70. Du X, Williams DA. Interleukin II: review of molecular, cell biology and clinical use. Blood 89:3897–3908, 1997.
71. Tepler I, Elias L, Smith JW, et al. A randomized placebo-controlled, trial of recombinant human interleukin-11 in cancer patients with severe thrombocytopenia due to chemotherapy. Blood 87:3607–3614, 1996.
72. Issacs C, Robert N J, Bailey A, et al. Randomized placebo-controlled study of recombinant human interleukin-II to prevent chemotherapy induced thrombocytopenia in patients with breast cancer receiving dose-intensive cyclophosphamide and doxorubicin. J Clin Oncol 15:3368–3377, 1997.
73. Schoenike SE, Dana WJ. Ifosfamide and mesna. Clin Pharm 9:179–191, 1990.
74. Goren MP. Oral administration of mesna with ifosfamide. Semin Oncol 23(Suppl 16):91–96, 1996.
75. Seifert CF, Nesser ME, Thompson DF. Dexrazoxane in the prevention of doxorubicin-induced cardiotoxicity. Ann Pharmacother 28:1063–1072, 1994.
76. Speyer JL, Green, MD, Felerluch-Jacquotte A, et al. ICRF-187 permits longer treatment with doxorubicin in women with breast cancer. J Clin Oncol 10:117–127, 1992.
77. Hellman K. Cardioprotection by dexrazoxane (Cardioxane; ICRF-187): progress in supportive care. Support Care Cancer 4:305–307, 1996.
78. Capizzi RL. Amifostine: the preclinical basis for broad-spectrum selective cytoprotection of normal tissues from cytotoxic therapies. Semin Oncol 23:2, 1996.
79. Buntzel J, Schuth J, Kuttner K, et al. Radiochemotherapy with amifostine cytoprotection for head and neck cancer. Support Care Cancer 6:155–160, 1998.
80. Anderson H, Mercer V, Thatcher N. A phase III randomized trial of carboplatin and amifostine versus carboplatin and G-CSF in patients with inoperable non-small cell lung cancer (NSCLC) [Abstract 1787]. Proc Am Soc Clin Oncol 17:465a, 1998.
81. List AF, Farah B, Heaton R, et al. Stimulation of hematopoiesis by amifostine in patients with myelodysplastic syndrome. Blood 90:3364–3369, 1997.

CHAPTER 85

CHRONIC LEUKEMIAS

Betsy Althaus

Chronic myelogenous leukemia (CML) and chronic lymphocytic leukemia (CLL) are hematologic malignancies that occur primarily in older adults. Patients usually survive several years beyond the diagnosis of leukemia, even in the absence of treatment. Over time, the chronic leukemias become more aggressive and less responsive to treatment. CML is curable only with an allogeneic bone marrow transplant (BMT), which is available to about 20 to 30% of patients. CLL is incurable at this time.

New therapies are emerging that contribute to prolonged survival and may possibly lead to a cure for patients with chronic leukemia. Patients with chronic leukemia are benefiting from the knowledge and application of new therapeutic approaches, including the use of biologic agents, advances in hematopoietic stem cell transplants, new effective chemotherapy, and improved supportive care. As these advances in treatment are made available for patients, care must be taken to safeguard patient quality of life. The new approaches under development will warrant evaluations of cost:benefit ratios.

Chronic Myelogenous Leukemia

CML is a hematologic malignancy originating from a leukemic transformation in a clonal pluripotent stem cell. Ninety-five percent of patients display a characteristic (9; 22) chromosome translocation, the Philadelphia chromosome. The disease progresses through two or three stages, eventually culminating in a leukemic blast crisis.[1] The first stage is an early chronic phase in which the patient is minimally symptomatic that may last 3 to 5 years. In this early phase of the disease, the leukemic cells retain the ability to differentiate and mature into granulocytes. The leukemia may then go through a transition phase or accelerated phase of several months' duration, in which the symptoms are more pronounced and more refractory to medication. CML invariably causes a fatal leukemic blast crisis, unless the leukemic clone has been eradicated, and normal hematopoiesis is restored. At this time, the only potential cure for CML is an allogeneic hematopoietic stem cell transplant or BMT.

TREATMENT GOALS: CHRONIC MYELOGENOUS LEUKEMIA

- Provide curative therapy by eradicating the leukemic cells and restoring normal hematopoiesis. A cure for CML is currently available only through allogeneic bone marrow (or hematopoietic stem cell) grafts, which are available for about 20 to 30% of patients with CML.

- For patients who are not candidates for allogeneic stem cell grafting, prolong the chronic phase of the disease as long as possible to provide for prolonged survival with minimal symptoms.

EPIDEMIOLOGY

CML accounts for approximately 20% of all cases of leukemia, with an incidence of 1 to 1.5 cases per 100,000 population. The median age at diagnosis is 67 years, although patients may be diagnosed at any age.[2] There is a slight male to female predominance in a ratio of about 1.5:1.[3]

The etiology of the leukemogenic transformation is unclear. There appears to be no hereditary component. Chemical leukemogens are not distinctly identified, but may include benzene and chemotherapy. No role for viral involvement has been observed. Exposure to ionizing radiation appears to have an etiologic role in some cases. Survivors of atomic bomb explosions, radiologists, and patients exposed to large amounts of radiation have an increased incidence of CML.[4]

PATHOPHYSIOLOGY

The key event in the evolution of CML appears to be the translocation of proto-oncogene *c*-ABL located on the long arm of chromosome 9 to the *BCR* gene on the long arm of chromosome 22. A reciprocal translocation occurs, and the *BCR* gene on chromosome 22 is translocated to chromosome 9. A *BCR-ABL* gene is formed on chromosome 22, and an *ABL-BCR* gene is formed on chromosome 9. The role of the *ABL-BCR* product is unknown. The *BCR-ABL* gene is transcribed into an 8.5-kb mRNA, which is translated into a 210-kD protein. The expression of the *BCR-ABL* gene to the p210BCR/ABL tyrosine kinase protein is linked to the oncogenic transformation to CML. The mechanism through which this transformation occurs is unclear.[5] The resultant t(9;22) chromosomal translocation is named the Philadelphia (Ph) chromosome.

Further chromosomal abnormalities occur as the disease progresses to the accelerated and blastic phase. Examples of these acquired abnormalities include trisomy 8, an additional Ph chromosome, and isochromosome 17q.[6]

CLINICAL PRESENTATION AND DIAGNOSIS

Signs and Symptoms

Chronic Phase

The onset of symptoms is usually gradual. Common presenting symptoms are fatigue, weight loss, anorexia, abdominal fullness, early satiety, and sweating. Physical findings commonly include splenomegaly, hepatomegaly, sternal tenderness, pallor, and palpable lymph nodes. Laboratory findings include an elevated white blood cell (WBC) count, often greater than 100×10^9/L. Basophilia, eosinophilia, and monocytosis are typical. Most patients have normochromic, normocytic anemia. Many patients have thrombocytosis. The lactic acid dehydrogenase (LDH), uric acid, and serum vitamin B_{12} levels are usually above normal. The leukocyte alkaline phosphatase level is nearly always low. The bone marrow is hypercellular.[3,4,6]

Progression to Accelerated and Blast Phase

The disease may progress from the chronic phase to the accelerated phase and then to blast crisis or may move directly from the chronic phase to the blast phase. The transition may occur at any time in the course of the disease. Although the chronic phase usually lasts several years, there is no guarantee that the CML will not rapidly advance to blast crisis. As the disease moves into the accelerated phase, medication is no longer as effective as in the chronic stage and laboratory test results and clinical findings will worsen. New cytogenetic abnormalities will appear. Patients entering the accelerated phase may report fever, night sweats, weight loss, myalgias, and arthralgias.

Patients in the blastic phase of CML have signs and symptoms of acute leukemia. CML will evolve to acute myeloid leukemia (AML) in about two-thirds of patients and to acute lymphocytic leukemia (ALL) in about one-third. The acute leukemic phase of CML is more refractory to therapy than is de novo acute leukemia. CML that transforms into ALL is more responsive to therapy than CML that transforms into AML.[3,4,6]

Diagnosis

CML is commonly diagnosed incidentally after the detection of a high WBC count on routine screening. The patient with symptoms most frequently reports asthenia, abdominal discomfort, weight loss, and fever. On physical examination, the majority of patients have splenomegaly. Hepatomegaly is also common. The WBC count is elevated in more than 90% of patients, with many having a WBC count greater than 100×10^9/L. Anemia and thrombocytosis are usually present. The bone marrow shows hyperplasia of myeloid cells. Analysis generally shows less than 5% blasts. Cytogenetic analysis, an examination of the chromosomes in metaphase in the leukemic cells, is necessary to confirm the presence of the Ph chromosome.[3,4,6]

PSYCHOSOCIAL ASPECTS

CML is usually diagnosed when patients have few symptoms. They will be told that they have leukemia that is incurable without an allogeneic BMT and that the chance of a successful BMT is greatest if it is performed during the chronic phase and within the first year of diagnosis. Therefore, at a time in their disease when they are feeling well, patients have to choose between the possibility of their CML remaining in the chronic phase for 3 to 5 years with a decreased chance of cure or undergoing an early BMT with its attendant risk of early death but with the chance of cure. If the patient chooses to wait for disease progression before undergoing BMT, the likelihood of cure with BMT is reduced. Family members may feel guilty if they are not eligible as bone marrow donors. If the patient undergoes a BMT and dies from transplant-related complications, the related donor may feel that he or she contributed to patient harm. Patients who are too old for transplant or without suitable donors will be faced with the knowledge that the leukemia is incurable.

THERAPEUTIC PLAN

The only curative therapy available for a patient with CML is allogeneic bone marrow or stem cell transplant. This approach is available only to patients who have a suitable donor and who are young enough to tolerate the procedure and the subsequent toxic effects of allogeneic transplant. All patients with chronic-phase CML who are younger than 40 years of age with a matched sibling donor should undergo BMT. Although the upper age limit at which a BMT is too dangerous is controversial, it has been advancing over the years because supportive care has led to improved survival even in older patients. The decision to perform a BMT in patients older than 50 years of age may be based on the patient's functional status and overall health and not on age alone. The timing of the transplant is also controversial. Survival is markedly improved if the transplant is performed during the chronic phase of CML and in the first year from diagnosis. However, the patient is often asymptomatic or minimally symptomatic during this time, and it may be difficult for the patient to decide to undergo a life-threatening procedure when he or she feels well.[3–6]

The patient variables considered in treatment decisions include patient age, patient functional status, phase of disease (chronic versus blast crisis), and donor availability. Treatment options include chemotherapy and/or interferon (INF)-α, allogeneic BMT with matched sibling donor, allogeneic BMT with unrelated donor, or experimental autologous BMT.

TREATMENT

Treatment by Phase

Chronic Phase

If CML is in the chronic phase and an allogeneic BMT is unavailable or inappropriate because of the patient's age or Karnofsky performance status, the standard treatment options are busulfan, hydroxyurea, or IFN-α alone or in combination with chemotherapy. The goal of therapy for CML in the chronic phase is to prolong survival and minimize symptoms by achieving a complete hematologic response and a complete cytogenetic response. Complete hematologic response is generally defined as the return to normal hematologic laboratory values and the absence of any signs or symptoms of CML. A complete cytogenetic response is the disappearance of the Ph chromosome, also described as the absence of all Ph-positive metaphases. A partial cytogenetic response has been variously defined. A useful definition is the presence of the Ph chromosome in less than 35% of the metaphases.[4] Busulfan, hydroxyurea, and INF-α usually provide a complete hematologic response. A cytogenetic response is rarely if ever achieved with busulfan or hydroxyurea. Interferon can provide a complete cytogenetic response in 9 to 26% of patients, and a partial cytogenetic response in about the same percentage.

Busulfan

Busulfan was at one time the most effective agent available for the chronic phase of CML, but its use has been supplanted by agents with less toxicity and more efficacy. Busulfan is an alkylsulfonate alkylating agent, which is not cell cycle specific. It is well absorbed orally. The half-life in adults is 2.1 to 2.6 hours. Busulfan is metabolized in the liver, and the metabolites are renally cleared. The primary effect at low doses is to suppress granulocytopoiesis. Busulfan use may lead to a delayed, prolonged, and profound myelosuppression. This effect requires that patients receiving busulfan be carefully monitored, so that the dose can be decreased or the drug stopped before the target WBC count is reached. Because blood counts continue to drop after busulfan is discontinued, the drug must be stopped at about double the desired WBC count to prevent dangerously low WBC counts. Pancytopenia from busulfan is frequently fatal. Patients must be monitored closely to avoid this complication. Skin hyperpigmentation is common. An infrequent but serious complication of chronic busulfan therapy is pulmonary fibrosis. The initial symptoms include fever, dry cough, and dyspnea. Busulfan should be discontinued while other possible causes of pulmonary symptoms, such as infection, are ruled out. If the patient is thought to have busulfan-induced pulmonary dysplasia, further therapy with busulfan is absolutely contraindicated. No effective treatment for the pulmonary complications of busulfan is known. The patient may develop pulmonary failure, which usually results in death within 6 months of the onset of pulmonary symptoms. An Addison-like syndrome can rarely develop with chronic busulfan therapy, with symptoms of anorexia, weakness, hypotension, and fatigue.[7–10]

Busulfan is commercially available as 2-mg tablets. It may be given either daily or intermittently. On the intermittent schedule the usual dose is 0.1 mg/kg/day orally.[4] Once the WBC count decreases by half, the dose should be reduced by half. When the WBC count falls below 20×10^9/L, busulfan should be stopped and restarted when the WBC rises to 50×10^9/L. Alternatively, busulfan can be given as a 4 mg/day dose, holding the dose when the WBC falls below 10×10^9/L.[3] Advantages to the use of busulfan in chronic-phase CML are that it is effective in most patients in achieving a hematologic remission, it is given orally, it is inexpensive, and it is generally well tolerated. Busulfan's role in treatment of chronic-phase CML has been largely replaced by hydroxyurea, which has fewer side effects, has a dose that is easier to titrate, and may provide improved survival.

Hydroxyurea

Hydroxyurea is a ribonucleotide diphosphate reductase inhibitor. Ribonucleotide reductases catalyze the conversion of ribonucleotides to deoxyribonucleotides. Hydroxyurea may have other mechanisms of action as well. Hydroxyurea is cell cycle specific for the S phase, causing cell arrest at G_1 to S.[7–11] Its oral bioavailability is 73 to 127%.[12,13] The half-life is about 3.5 to 4.5 hours. Hydroxyurea is both hepatically metabolized and renally excreted. The usual dose is 20 to 30 mg/kg/day or 1.5 to 2 g/day. The drug is commercially available in 500-mg tablets. The dose should be adjusted downward for patients with leukopenia or thrombocytopenia. The primary adverse effect is bone marrow suppression. Gastrointestinal effects are uncommon at usual doses.[7–11]

An unusual and infrequent complication of chronic hydroxyurea use is the development of cutaneous leg ulcers. The ulcers are usually painful and may be multiple. The ulcers heal or markedly improve after hydroxyurea is discontinued.[14]

Hydroxyurea is used in chronic-phase CML to control blood counts. It does not delay or prevent the transition to blast crisis. It has few side effects, and the dose is easily titrated. It is preferred over busulfan because of its greater tolerability with fewer side effects and no severe adverse effects, because of its ease of dose adjustment, and because it appears to provide a survival advantage compared to busulfan.[15] It may be used as a single agent or combined with INF-α or other agents.

Interferon-α

INF-α has been found to be useful in patients with CML for inducing both a complete hematologic remission and a major or complete cytogenetic response.[16,17] Questions being explored about the use of INF-α include which patients are most likely to benefit, what is the most effective dose, what is the most effective duration of use, when is it appropriate to discontinue INF-α, and how best to combine chemotherapy with INF-α. Because INF-α does not benefit all patients, is expensive, and has side effects that may make it difficult for patients to continue therapy, careful attention to patient selection and monitoring is important to achieve the best response with the least toxicity.

The side effects of INF-α may decrease the patient's sense of well-being. These side effects include flu-like symptoms of malaise, fever, chills, and aching. The symptoms are sometimes relieved by acetaminophen. Tachyphylaxis to these side effects usually develops within weeks. Anorexia, nausea, and diarrhea are common. Fatigue and depression may be significant. INF-α should be avoided in patients with clinical depression (Table 85.1).[17,18]

In general, the recommended dose of INF-α is 5 million U/m²/day, adjusted to the patient's tolerance of side effects. In at least one study a dose lower than 5 million U/m²/day subcutaneously was used and equal efficacy was reported[19]; however, other studies have observed a dose-response effect, suggesting a better response with the standard dose.[17,18]

Table 85.1 ▪ Recommendations for Interferon-α Administration

In general, the recommended dose of INF-α is 5 million U/m²/day, adjusted to the patient's tolerance of side effects.
Try to give full dose of INF-α if possible, adjusting to patient tolerance to side effects and effect on quality of life.
Begin the INF-α at a low dose for several days to allow the patient time to adjust to the side effects. A reasonable beginning dose is 3 million U SC daily. Then increase the dose toward the intended dose.
Add hydroxyurea 0.5–2 g orally daily to decrease the WBC count to $\leq$10–20 × 10^9/L. It is reasonable to continue both agents. If one drug needs to be stopped because of a low WBC count, discontinue the hydroxyurea before altering the INF-α.
Give INF-α at bedtime.
Instruct the patient to take acetaminophen with each dose to decrease fever and myalgias.

Source: References 17, 18.

INF-α, interferon alpha; *WBC*, white blood cell.

The best time to begin therapy for optimal response is in the early chronic phase, when the patient has more Ph-negative polyclonal hematopoiesis. Most patients achieving a hematologic response will have it within the first 3 months of therapy. Most patients who achieve a cytogenetic response will have it within the first 12 months of treatment, but it may take as long as 18 months.[20]

For patients with chronic-phase CML, there is an improved 5-year survival rate when INF-α is used, compared to chemotherapy.[20] A comparison of INF-α to busulfan in the early chronic phase found a 54% predicted survival rate at 5 years for patients receiving INF-α and a 32% predicted 5-year survival rate for those receiving busulfan.[21]

The UK Medical Research Council[22] found a survival advantage for patients treated with INF-α over those treated with conventional chemotherapy, hydroxyurea, or busulfan. The comparison was made by combining results from all patients who did not receive INF-α therapy and comparing them to the INF-α group. The hydroxyurea group showed a 5-year survival similar to that for the INF-α group (46% compared to 52%). It is not clear if this is a statistically different response. The survival advantage existed even for patients who did not show evidence of a cytogenetic response.

In a meta-analysis of seven randomized trials, the 5-year survival rate with INF-α was 57%, compared to 42% with chemotherapy.[20] However, in some studies, no survival advantage of INF-α over hydroxyurea was seen. The Benelux Study Group found no advantage in survival for the combination of INF-α and hydroxyurea compared to hydroxyurea alone.[23] Low-dose INF-α (3 × 10^6 U 5 days/week) was used. The survival of the INF-α group was similar to that seen in other studies. The hydroxyurea group showed better survival than that seen in other studies. The German CML Study Group also found no difference in survival between hydroxyurea and INF-α groups,[24] while the Italian Cooperative Study Group found a significant survival advantage with the use of INF-α.[25] A comparison of the German and Italian studies suggested that the different findings are based on differences of study design and that the combination of INF-α and hydroxyurea is more effective than each agent used alone.[26] The potential benefits of the combination of INF-α and hydroxyurea include possible additive effects that may provide a survival advantage and earlier hematologic remission, and therefore earlier relief of disease symptoms for the patient. A long-term follow-up of the Italian Cooperative Study Group reported that the significant improvement in survival seen in the INF-α study arm compared to the chemotherapy arm was maintained over time. Of 218 patients, 26% achieved either a complete or major cytogenetic response. In nine patients (4%), the complete cytogenetic response has continued for more than 8 years.[27] The German CML Study Group is conducting a randomized trial comparing INF-α 5 million U/m^2/day and hydroxyurea 40 mg/kg/day to hydroxyurea alone in patients with chronic phase CML who had no prior therapy.[28]

In one study, the combination of low-dose cytarabine and INF-α appeared to increase survival in patients with chronic-phase CML compared to treatment with INF-α alone.[29] The dose of INF-α used was 5 million U/m^2/day, and the dose of cytarabine was 20 mg/m^2/day for 10 days out of every month. Patients also were given hydroxyurea 50 mg/kg/day until complete hematologic remission was obtained. There was an increase in hematologic and cytogenetic remissions. However, there were more side effects in the combination treatment group. Cytarabine contributed thrombocytopenia, nausea, vomiting, diarrhea, mucositis, weight loss, asthenia, and skin rashes to the usual side effects of INF-α therapy. About one-half of the patients in the study receiving the combination therapy discontinued treatment because of side effects compared to one-third of patients treated with INF-α alone. Patient quality of life or functional status between combination therapy and INF-α alone was not compared. Because of the observed increase in cytogenetic response and improved survival, it is reasonable to provide combination therapy with low-dose cytarabine and INF-α, despite the increase in side effects.

It appears that INF-α probably prolongs the survival of patients who achieve a major cytogenetic response. However, it may take more than 12 months for the cytogenetic response to occur, and it would be useful to be able to make an early prediction about which patients are likely to eventually respond to continued INF-α therapy. Some investigators have attempted this. Preliminary guidelines based on a large single-institution study have been developed[30] (Table 85.2). The authors recommend that INF-α therapy should be continued in patients who have more than a 10% chance of achieving a major cytogenetic response, if an allogeneic transplant is not available to them. They found that pretreatment risk factors for a low chance of response are spleen size more than 5 cm below the costal margin, and platelet count greater than 700 × 10^9/L. The decision algorithm appears to be fairly complex. At 3 months, interferon should be discontinued in patients who achieve no better than a partial hematologic response and have pretreatment risk factors (splenomegaly or thrombocytosis). At 6 months, patients with a complete hematologic response and a minor cytogenetic response have a 60% chance of achieving a major cytogenetic response. Patients with a complete hematologic response and no cytogenetic response and no pretreatment risk factors have a 38 to 45% chance of achieving a major cytogenetic

Table 85.2 ▪ Treatment Continuation/Discontinuation Algorithm for Interferon-α in Patients with CML

Evaluation Time from Start of IFN-α	Patient Characteristics	IFN-α Therapy Decision
3 mo	Less than or equal to a partial hematologic response and poor pretreatment risk factors (splenomegaly ≥5 cm below the costal margin or pretreatment platelet count ≥700 × 10^9/L)	Discontinue IFN-α
6 mo	Less than or equal to a partial hematologic response and poor pretreatment risk factors Complete hematologic response, no cytogenetic response, and no pretreatment risk factors or	Discontinue IFN-α
	Complete hematologic response, no cytogenetic response, and poor pretreatment risk factors (splenomegaly ≥5 cm below the costal margin or pretreatment platelet count ≥700 × 10^9/L)	Continue IFN-α
12 mo	Less than or equal to a partial hematologic response or Complete hematologic response, no cytogenetic response, and poor pretreatment risk factors (splenomegaly ≥5 cm below the costal margin or pretreatment platelet count ≥700 × 10^9/L)	Discontinue IFN-α
	Complete hematologic response, no cytogenetic response, and no poor pretreatment risk factors	May offer to continue IFN-α for 6 mo

INF-α, interferon alpha.

response. Both of these groups should continue INF-α therapy. Patients with no cytogenetic response at 6 months, and pretreatment risk factors of thrombocytosis or splenomegaly have a less than 10% chance of achieving a major cytogenetic response. INF-α should be stopped and other treatment options offered. At 12 months, if patients with pretreatment risk factors have no cytogenetic response, INF-α therapy should be stopped. However, patients with no cytogenetic response at 12 months, but with a complete hematologic response and no pretreatment risk factors, have a 16 to 26% chance of achieving a major cytogenetic response and can be offered INF-α therapy for another 6 months. It is assumed that achieving a major cytogenetic response confers a survival advantage.[17]

These findings have been supported by a single institution trial reporting that failure to have a hematologic response at 3 months predicted a low probability of a cytogenetic response to INF-α and that a major or complete cytogenetic response to INF-α is associated with prolonged survival.[31]

It is not known if patients with a long-term complete cytogenetic response from INF-α can be considered cured. Patients may have no detectable Ph chromosome, yet still have residual *BCR-ABL* transcript. The absence of the *BCR-ABL* transcript is a molecular complete remission. Molecular complete remissions have been observed in recipients of BMTs. There are some patients with a long-term complete cytogenetic response from INF-α who also have been observed to have nondetectable *BCR-ABL*.[28,32] It is possible that these patients have been cured of CML without a BMT, but further follow-up is required.

The cost-effectiveness of INF-α has been calculated by two investigators.[33,34] For a therapy to be considered worthwhile, the marginal cost-effectiveness should be less than $50,000 per quality-adjusted life year (QALY). One trial found the marginal cost-effectiveness to be $34,800 per QALY saved.[33] The model used $1,500 as the estimated drug cost for INF-α for 1 month at a dose of 5 million U/m^2/day. A second trial estimated the marginal cost-effectiveness to be $89,500 or $63,000 per QALY saved, depending on the scenario.[34] The authors estimated the monthly cost of INF-α to be $2,750 for a mean dose of 8 million U/m^2/day. In the second analysis, therefore, INF-α was not found to be a cost-effective therapy. Both groups of authors reported that the models are most sensitive to manipulation of drug cost.

STI-571

STI-571 is a new investigational agent that is showing promise in CML.[35] The BCR-ABL transcript of CML has tyrosine kinase activity, which is necessary for its ability to cause leukemic transformation. STI-571 is an ABL protein tyrosine kinase inhibitor. In phase I testing in CML patients who have failed INF-α therapy, the drug has produced exciting results. Patients have rapidly achieved a hematologic complete response in 96% (23/24) of patients, and some patients have achieved a cytogenetic response. STI-571 is given orally on a daily schedule and has minimal side effects.

Homoharringtonine

Homoharringtonine is an investigational agent presently in phase II clinical trials that may show usefulness in CML. It is a plant alkaloid derived from the *Cephalotaxus fortuneii* tree. In a group of patients with late chronic-phase CML, most of whom had received previous treatment with INF-α, homoharringtonine was able to produce a complete hematologic remission in 72% and a complete cytogenetic remission in 9% of those with active disease.[36] The dose used in the study was 2.5 mg/m^2/day as a continuous intravenous infusion given on an outpatient basis for 14 days, followed by maintenance therapy of 2.5 mg/m^2/day for 7 days per month. Toxic effects were mild and included mild diarrhea, nausea, vague chest pain, tachycardia, headache, and fatigue. Fever or infection occurred with 25% of induction courses. Neutropenia and thrombocytopenia were common.

Accelerated Phase

Patients with CML in the accelerated phase have a 6- to 18-month survival. There is no standard therapy for accelerated-phase CML. The treatment goal is to provide symptom palliation and a return to chronic-phase CML. Generally, each patient must be assessed and treated with an individualized treatment plan, modified for disease response and patient tolerance. A patient with accelerated-phase CML has circulating blasts, and these blasts can be immunophenotyped to determine if the CML is transforming into a myeloid or lymphoid blast crisis phase. The patient may then receive treatment appropriate for the associated acute leukemia. Patients receiving a BMT during the accelerated phase have a much lower survival rate than during the chronic phase.

Blast Phase

Patients with blast-phase CML have an expected survival of 2 to 3 months. The goal of treatment is to provide symptom palliation and a return to chronic-phase CML. Patients should be managed with therapy for acute leukemia. Many patients have disease resistant to this therapy. Patients with a lymphoid blast crisis are more likely to respond than patients with a myeloid blast crisis. BMT during a blast crisis provides a 0 to 20% chance for long-term survival. For some patients with blast-phase CML a second chronic phase may be achieved, in which case a BMT should be performed, if there is an available donor. Patients in blast crisis may benefit from the investigational agent STI-571.[37]

Bone Marrow Transplant

Allogeneic Bone Marrow Transplant

Allogeneic BMT has the potential to cure CML and is the treatment of choice for young patients with chronic-phase

CML. A human leukocyte antigen (HLA)-matched sibling donor is available for only 20 to 25% of patients with CML. The probability of long-term survival for patients receiving a BMT in the chronic phase is 60 to 80% and less than 20% for patients in blast crisis. Survival outcomes appear to be more favorable if the patient receives a BMT within 1 year of diagnosis. Younger patients have better outcomes, but the upper age limit is controversial and is advancing as supportive care improves.[2]

A retrospective study compared survival after HLA-identical allogeneic BMT versus treatment with INF-α or hydroxyurea. The group included patients from 15 to 55 years of age. The study described better survival with INF-α or hydroxyurea in the first 18 months from diagnosis. Survival figures for the BMT group did not surpass those of the hydroxyurea/INF-α group until 5.5 years from the initial diagnosis. If BMT was delayed for more than 1 year after diagnosis, the survival advantage from BMT decreased. At 7 years, the survival probability in the transplant group was 58% and in the hydroxyurea/INF-α group the survival probability was 32%.[38]

The usual preparative regimens for BMT in patients with CML are cyclophosphamide and total body irradiation or cyclophosphamide and busulfan. Modified preparative regimens with less toxic effects and equal efficacy continue to show promise in reducing the mortality from BMT, making it available to an older age group.[39]

Unrelated Donor Bone Marrow Transplant

The use of unrelated donors for BMT carries increased risk for the patient. More failure to engraft the new marrow is seen, and graft-versus-host disease (GVHD) occurs more frequently and is more severe. Because of the increased risk with unrelated donor BMTs, the decision to perform this type of transplant in a patient with CML who is feeling well can be difficult.[40,41]

Most recommendations for unrelated donor transplants for CML have included an upper age limit for patients of 35 to 45 years. It is possible that this age limit may be raised. A review of unrelated donor transplants for CML showed a 74% 5-year survival rate for patients younger than 50 years who received matched unrelated donor transplants within the first year of diagnosis.[41] This high survival may reflect improved supportive care, including antiviral and antifungal prophylaxis.

A decision analysis for unrelated donor BMT compared transplant within the first year from diagnosis (early transplant), delayed transplant, and no transplant.[40] The study concluded that unrelated donor transplant performed within the first year was superior in quality-adjusted expected survival to no transplant, but that it takes 4 years before survival for patients receiving an early transplant is improved over that for patients with no transplant. Delayed transplant (i.e., transplant later than 1 year from diagnosis) also showed increased quality-adjusted expected survival compared to no transplant, although it took 6 years to realize this difference.

A model of the cost-effectiveness of unrelated donor BMT compared to therapy with INF-α or hydroxyurea has been developed.[42] Compared to INF-α therapy, the cost-effectiveness ratio for an unrelated donor BMT is $51,800 for each QALY gained and compared to hydroxyurea it is $55,000. When the model parameter estimates were manipulated to simulate changes in clinical scenarios, the cost-effectiveness ratio ranged from $32,600 to $126,800 QALY. The authors conclude that while unrelated donor BMT is very expensive, it is cost-effective for a carefully selected patient population in whom it can significantly prolong life.

A patient with chronic-phase CML who is younger than 50 years old and who lacks a matched sibling donor should be offered a matched, unrelated donor transplant, if a donor is available, and the institution is experienced in performing unrelated donor marrow transplants. Older patients in the same situation should be given a trial of INF-α.[2]

Relapse After Bone Marrow Transplant

Relapse after BMT may be hematologic or cytogenetic. It is common for the Ph chromosome to be detectable for several months after the transplant. This does not necessarily herald relapse. The persistence of the Ph chromosome for more than 6 months after transplant, the reappearance of the Ph chromosome after it has disappeared, or a rising proportion of Ph-positive metaphases are triggers to begin therapy for relapse. Two approaches that have been successful for treating CML relapse after BMT are donor lymphocyte infusion (DLI) and the use of INF-α. DLI appears to be more effective in eradicating the Ph chromosome; however, there is significant toxicity in the form of loss of engraftment or severe GVHD, with as much as 20% mortality. INF-α appears to provide cytogenetic remission in a significant number of patients with cytogenetic relapse, without causing life-threatening toxic effects.[43,44] A reasonable strategy may be to offer INF-α therapy to patients with cytogenetic relapse, and if they do not have remission within 1 year, to offer DLI. Patients with hematologic relapse may receive either INF-α or DLI. There may be a role for combination therapy using a modified dose of DLI and INF-α.[43]

Autologous Bone Marrow Transplant

It may be possible to obtain long-term survival in patients through an infusion of Ph chromosome-negative autologous peripheral blood progenitor cells.[45] Some investigators have reported that treatment in the early chronic phase, before initiation of INF-α therapy, may allow for collection of more Ph-negative stem cells. In one study, patients received a course of intensive conventional chemotherapy, followed by granulocyte colony-stimulating factor. Peripheral blood progenitor cells were pheresed when blood count results were beginning to improve. These patients then received preparative regimens of high-dose chemotherapy with or without total body irradiation, followed by infusion of the previously mobilized stem cells. Half of the patients achieved Ph-negative marrow, but follow-up has been short.[46] With allogeneic BMT, the duration of remission seems to depend on the graft-versus-leukemia (GVL) effect. With the GVL effect, the donor hematopoietic cells recognize persistent leukemia cells as foreign and act to eradicate them. This effect is absent in autograft recipients. It may be necessary to provide post-transplant maintenance therapy such as INF-α to patients receiving autografts. Autografting may prove useful for patients without matched donors or who are outside the age limit to tolerate allogeneic grafting. This procedure is investigational and should be performed in the context of a clinical trial.

Chronic Lymphocytic Leukemia

CLL is a slowly progressing leukemia that may be quiescent for years and occurs primarily in older adults. It is not curable, but in many patients does not decrease survival compared to the normal population. Therefore, CLL is usually not treated unless the patient is symptomatic, or the rate of disease progression increases.

CLL is a malignancy of monoclonal small mature lymphocytes, which have prolonged survival and which proliferate and accumulate in the blood, bone marrow, lymph nodes, spleen, and liver. Ninety-five percent of patients have B-cell CLL; 5% have T-cell CLL.

TREATMENT GOALS: CHRONIC LYMPHOCYTIC LEUKEMIA

- Prolong survival and palliate disease symptoms, while maintaining good quality of life.[47] There is no known curative therapy for CLL. Aggressive therapy with BMT may be an appropriate consideration in younger patients with risk factors for poor survival, but this approach is investigational.

EPIDEMIOLOGY

The cause of CLL is unknown. Radiation and drug exposure do not seem to be risk factors. There may be an increased risk with industrial exposure for agricultural and asbestos workers.[48] CLL is primarily a disease of older adults, and its incidence increases with age. The median age at diagnosis is 65 years.[40] More men than women are affected, by a ratio of about 2:1. CLL is the most commonly occurring leukemia in Western Europe and North America, but is uncommon in Japan and China. Immigrants from Japan to the West do not acquire an increased risk for the disease.[48]

PATHOPHYSIOLOGY

CLL may result from a mutational change that prevents normal programmed cell death (apoptosis), rather than from increased cell proliferation.[49] It is speculated that a normal CD5-positive lymphocyte is transformed via multiple mutational steps into a monoclonal leukemic cell line that lacks normal apoptotic mechanisms, which then accumulates.[47] Most CLL cells (about 95%) are in the quiescent G_0 stage of the cell cycle. Symptoms of CLL arise from accumulation of leukemic lymphocytes in organs and tissues and from immune dysfunction.

CLINICAL PRESENTATION AND DIAGNOSIS

Signs and Symptoms

Patients are often asymptomatic at diagnosis, with the diagnosis being made when a routine complete blood count is done. Patients with symptoms may report typical "B" symptoms of weight loss, fever, fatigue, and night sweats. They may experience early satiety or a feeling of abdominal fullness from splenomegaly or hepatomegaly. They may notice enlarged lymph nodes and may report frequent infections.

Diagnosis

The diagnosis of CLL is based on an absolute lymphocyte count in the blood of 5×10^9/L. The leukemic cells are normal-appearing small mature lymphocytes. They have monoclonal expression of either κ or λ light chains. There is a smaller than normal amount of surface immunoglobulin.[50] B lymphocytes in CLL express surface antigens CD5, CD19, CD20, and CD23. If a bone marrow aspirate and biopsy are performed, more than 30% of nucleated cells must be lymphoid for a diagnosis of CLL.

There are two staging systems for CLL: the Rai system[51] and the Binet system.[52] The Rai system is used primarily in the United States and the Binet system is used mostly in Europe. Both systems are useful and either can be applied. The two systems stage CLL based on evidence of lymphocyte infiltration into tissue and organs and on evidence of impaired bone marrow function, as seen by anemia or thrombocytopenia. Patients with low-risk disease exhibit lymphocytosis only, and have a median survival of longer than 10 years. Patients with high-risk disease have lymphocytosis with anemia or thrombocytopenia and have a median survival of 2 years (Table 85.3).[53] One useful prognos-

Table 85.3 ▪ Staging Systems Used for Chronic Lymphocytic Leukemia

System and Risk	Stage	Definition	Percentage of Patients with CLL in Stage	Survival Median (yr)	Survival 10-Year (%)
Rai staging system					
Low	0	Lymphocytosis only	31	>10	59
Intermediate	I	Lymphocytosis and lymphadenopathy	35	9	
	II	Lymphocytosis and splenomegaly with or without lymphadenopathy or hepatomegaly	26	5	
High	III	Lymphocytosis and anemia, with or without organomegaly	6	2	
	IV	Lymphocytosis, anemia, and thrombocytopenia, with or without organomegaly	2	2	
Binet staging system					
Low	A	Lymphocytosis, with enlargement of <3 lymphoid areas[a]	63	>10	51
	A′	Stage A with lymphocyte count of ≤30,000/mm³ and hemoglobin concentration of ≥120 g/L	49	>10	56
	A″	Stage A with lymphocyte count of >30,000/mm³, hemoglobin concentration of <120 g/L, or both	14	7	38
Intermediate	B	Lymphocytosis, with enlargement of ≥3 lymphoid areas	30	5	
High	C	Lymphocytosis and either anemia or thrombocytopenia, or both	7	2	

Source: Reprinted with permission from Dighiero G, Maloun K, Desablens B, et al. Chlorambucil in indolent chronic lymphocytic leukemia. N Engl J Med 338: 1506–1514, 1998. Data from references 51, 52, and 60.

[a]The following lymphoid areas are included: cervical, axillary, and inguinal (whether unilateral or bilateral), spleen, and liver.

tic indicator is lymphocyte doubling time. Lymphocyte doubling time of less than 1 year is associated with a much worse prognosis. The typical patient with CLL usually develops a higher stage of disease slowly over several years. The patient then requires more treatment, and the treatment gradually needs to be more aggressive to control symptoms, bringing with it more side effects of therapy.

In a small percentage of patients, CLL may transform abruptly into a large-cell non-Hodgkin's lymphoma that is resistant to treatment. This is called Richter's transformation or Richter's syndrome. The patient will have fever, increased lymphadenopathy, a rising LDH level, and widespread tissue infiltration of lymphoma cells. It occurs in 3 to 15% of patients with CLL. Few patients with Richter's transformation survive longer than 6 to 8 months. There is controversy over whether the lymphoma arises from the original malignant clone or is from a separate, distinct clone. It appears that the lymphoma arises from the original clone in at least two-thirds of patients.[48,54]

Patients with CLL may develop autoimmune reactions against hematopoietic cells. Autoimmune hemolytic anemia is estimated to occur in 5 to 37% of patients with CLL.[55] Pure red cell aplasia may be present in 6% of patients. Idiopathic thrombocytopenia occurs in 2 to 3% of patients. The cause of the autoimmune dysfunction is not well understood.

The immune dysfunction seen in patients with CLL contributes significantly to the morbidity of the disease. The mechanism for the immune dysfunction is multifaceted and includes impairment in both humoral and cell-mediated immune function.[56] The malignant CLL B cell functions poorly as an antigen-presenting cell. The B cell to T cell interaction is weakened. There are a decreased number of normal B cells, and their immune function may be downregulated by cytokine production from the malignant B-cell clone. This may contribute to the low levels of immunoglobulin usually seen in patients with CLL. T cells in patients with CLL may be anergic. Natural killer (NK) cells have a decreased ability to become activated and to lyse target cells. NK cell mediation of antibody-dependent cell-mediated cytotoxicity is decreased. There is a proposed mechanism in which the dysfunction of the NK cells and T cells in patients with CLL may lengthen the survival of the malignant B-cell clone and so contribute to the progression of the disease.

Infectious complications are a major manifestation of the immune dysfunction seen in CLL. The majority of deaths in patients with CLL that are actually due to CLL are from bacterial infections. The usual infecting organisms are *Staphylococcus aureus, Streptococcus pneumoniae, Haemophilus influenzae, Escherichia coli, Klebsiella pneumoniae,* and *Pseudomonas aeruginosa.* With the recent increased use of purine analogs such as fludarabine, cladribine, and pentostatin, a new group of infecting organisms has been observed.[57] These include *Listeria, Pneumocystis, Mycobacterium tuberculosis, Nocardia, Candida, Aspergillus,* and herpes viruses. The risk for these infections increases if the patient receives corticosteroids concurrently or before purine analog therapy.[58]

PSYCHOSOCIAL ASPECTS

Patients may be told that they have incurable leukemia and that they do not need treatment. This confuses most patients. Patients with low-stage disease may have no symptoms or have symptoms that are controlled with an oral medication taken once or twice a month. The change to a more aggressive disease will develop gradually, usually over several years. The patient is usually elderly and may have other medical problems, some of which may be more life threatening or may affect the person's quality of life more distinctly than does CLL. If the patient is young with high-risk disease, he or she may be faced with a choice between a BMT with its multiple risks, which has not yet been shown to improve survival but may ultimately control the leukemia, or standard therapy, which is usually well tolerated but does not prolong survival.

TREATMENT

Patients with CLL are usually only treated if they develop uncomfortable symptoms, such as increasing adenopathy, or constitutional symptoms, such as fatigue and weight loss, develop significant anemia or thrombocytopenia, or show evidence of more rapid disease progression, such as a lymphocyte doubling time of less than 1 year.

Pharmacotherapy

Alkylating Agents

When the decision is made to treat a patient with CLL, the initial therapy is usually chlorambucil, an oral alkylating agent. It may be given at 0.1 mg/kg daily, or at 4 mg/kg every 2 to 4 weeks, or as a 0.7 mg/kg total dose over 4 days every month. It is available as a 2-mg tablet and is well absorbed orally. Chlorambucil is hepatically metabolized, with hepatic and renal clearance of the metabolites. The half life is 2 to 8 hours. The dose is adjusted for disease response and myelosuppression. Chlorambucil is well tolerated and has mild side effects other than myelosuppression. The use of chlorambucil in patients with CLL does not prolong survival but does control disease symptoms. It has been shown to be as effective as more aggressive and more toxic combinations of chemotherapy such as cyclophosphamide, vincristine, and prednisone (CVP) or cyclophosphamide, melphalan, and prednisone.[59–61] No advantage has been found for starting chlorambucil therapy in patients in the early stage of disease.[53] Prednisone may be added to chlorambucil in an oral dose of 40 mg/m^2/day for 5 days every month. Other schedules have also been used. The addition of prednisone to chlorambucil does not prolong survival, but may increase symptom improvement in lymphadenopathy and splenomegaly. It appears to have particular value in patients who have immune-mediated anemia or thrombocytopenia. Because of emerging evidence suggesting that prior steroid therapy may contribute to the risk of opportunistic infection in patients who eventually receive one of the purine analogs such as fludarabine, an attempt should be made to limit the use of prednisone to those patients who show response of CLL-related anemia or thrombocytopenia to steroid therapy.

Cyclophosphamide, another alkylating agent, appears to have efficacy equal to that of chlorambucil. The usual dose is 1 to 2 mg/kg/day. When cyclophosphamide in combination with other chemotherapy agents is compared to single-agent chlorambucil, no clear advantage has been seen.

The alkylating agent (either chlorambucil or cyclophosphamide) is usually continued until the patient's symptoms have responded and no additional improvement is seen, or until the patient experiences myelotoxicity.[62] The drug can then be stopped. If the patient's disease symptoms recur or worsen after therapy is discontinued, it is reasonable to renew treatment with the same agent. If the disease progresses while the patient is receiving therapy, the alkylating agent should be discontinued, and another agent such as a purine analog should be started.

Purine Analogs

The three purine analogs that have shown efficacy in CLL are fludarabine, cladribine, and pentostatin. The most experience is with fludarabine. It has been approved for use in the treatment of CLL refractory to alkylating agents. Cladribine has also been shown to be effective for this indication. Pentostatin has not been used as extensively and may show less efficacy than fludarabine and cladribine in the treatment of CLL. There appears to be cross-resistance between fludarabine and cladribine, and a patient whose disease is refractory to one of these agents is unlikely to respond to the other.

Fludarabine phosphate is a water-soluble analog of adenosine and is a fluorinated analog of the antiviral drug vidarabine. It is resistant to adenosine deaminase. Fludarabine is first dephosphorylated to 2-fluoro-ara-adenine and is then converted intracellularly to 2-fluoro-ara-adenosine triphosphate (ATP), which is the active form. It inhibits DNA polymerase, and ribonucleotide reductase. Fludarabine is also effective against the nonproliferating cells of CLL, possibly by inducing apoptosis. The half-life of 2-fluoro-ara-adenine is about 10 hours, with a clearance of 8.9 L/hr/m^2 and a volume of distribution of 98 L/m^2. Fludarabine is primarily cleared renally, and the dose should be adjusted for renal impairment, although exact guidelines are not available. The usual dose for the treatment of B-cell CLL is 25 mg/m^2/day IV over 30 minutes daily for 5 days every 4 weeks. The drug should be continued for three cycles after the maximal response has been achieved.[8,9,63] It should be discontinued for disease progression or for the development of hemolytic anemia. The usual and expected side effect is myelosuppression, which may be cumulative. It is possible that colony-stimulating factors after fludarabine may be useful in reducing the myelosuppression, allowing for the administration of fludarabine therapy on the planned schedule. The use of colony-stimulating factors may also decrease infections.[64] At high doses of fludarabine, severe irreversible neurotoxicity has been observed, but these doses are no longer in use.[65] Rarely patients may develop interstitial pneumonitis. Opportunistic infections are common, especially in patients who have had extensive prior therapy or have received steroids. Patients may even develop infections after the first dose of fludarabine without a history of steroid use.[66] Patients should be carefully monitored for infection, and care must be taken not to miss infections such as *Pneumocystis carinii* pneumonia (PCP), listeriosis, tuberculosis, herpes infections, and *Candida* or *Aspergillus* infections.[67,68] Consideration should be given to the use of PCP prophylaxis for all patients receiving fludarabine. It should be required in patients with CLL who have a current or previous history of corticosteroid use. The role for prophylaxis against herpes and fungal infections is yet to be determined.

There may be an increased risk of hematologic immune manifestations such as hemolytic anemia in fludarabine-treated patients. Although hemolytic anemia is common in patients with CLL, the purine analogs appear to further promote its occurrence. A causal relationship has not been firmly established. Most patients with fludarabine-associated hemolytic anemia have a recurrence if the drug is given again, which carries a high risk of mortality. Patients who develop hemolytic anemia with any of the purine analogs should not receive further therapy with any drug in this class.[68,69]

In previously treated patients with high Rai stage disease, the response rate to fludarabine is 31 to 36%.[70] The response rate is improved in patients who receive fludarabine as first-line therapy and has been reported to be as high as 78% in one series.[71] Although fludarabine is effective in achieving a response, there is no evidence that its use as first-line therapy instead of chlorambucil improves overall survival. It is also unknown whether there are quality of life differences between treatment with chlorambucil and fludarabine regimens.

Cladribine is a chlorinated analog of adenosine. It is resistant to adenosine deaminase. Deoxycytidine kinase phosphorylates cladribine intracellularly to 2-Cd-adenosine monophosphatase (AMP), which is then converted to 2-Cd-ATP. 2-Cd-AMP is incorporated into DNA. 2-Cd-ATP inhibits ribonucleotide reductase. Cladribine also shows activity in resting cells by depleting nicotinamide adenine dinucleotide levels. Ultimately, the activity of cladribine results in apoptosis, even in quiescent lymphocytes.[8,9] The half-life is 5 to 6 hours; plasma clearance is about 980 mL/hr/kg, with a large amount of variability. The volume of distribution is about 9 L/kg. It is not known how cladribine is cleared from the body, but there is some renal clearance. Although approved for use in hairy cell leukemia where it is the drug of choice, it has also shown substantial activity in CLL.[72,73] The usual dose is 0.1 mg/kg/day as a continuous IV infusion daily for 7 days every 4 weeks. Other similar schedules have been used in clinical studies, with a usual maximum dose of 0.7 mg/kg per cycle (e.g., 0.12 mg/kg/day IV over 2 hours daily for 5 days).[74] Bone marrow suppression is the usual and expected side effect. As with fludarabine, infections are a common occurrence, and patients should be monitored closely. Fever, even without infection, is common. Nausea may occur, but it is usually mild. High doses of cladribine, which are not in clinical use, have produced neurotoxicity. Immune hematologic effects have occurred with the use of cladribine in patients with CLL. Cladribine has been associated with an increased risk of hemolytic anemia, which may be fatal.[75] If hemolytic anemia develops while the patient is receiving therapy, the drug should be discontinued, and the patient should not be given additional therapy with cladribine or another purine analog. If the patient has a history of disease (CLL)-related autoimmune hemolytic anemia, it is appropriate to attempt therapy with a purine analog, as some patients have shown resolution of disease-related autoimmune hemolytic anemia when treated with fludarabine or cladribine. At this time, pentostatin for CLL should be reserved for use in the context of a clinical trial.

Therapy for patients with CLL for whom treatment is indicated should begin with chlorambucil. If the patient has a good performance status and is young, the use of fludarabine as first-line therapy may be considered because it may provide a higher response rate and a longer remission. However, it has more severe and dangerous side effects, requires IV administration, and is expensive compared to chlorambucil. It is not known whether fludarabine improves survival compared to chlorambucil. If a patient receiving chlorambucil either fails to respond or has disease progression, the patient should be treated with either fludarabine or cladribine, because these agents are less toxic than combination therapy such as COP (cyclophosphamide, vincristine [Oncovin], and prednisone) or CHOP (cyclophosphamide, hydroxydaunorubicin, vincristine [Oncovin], and prednisone) and may be more effective.[76] At this time, fludarabine should probably be chosen over cladribine for CLL, as their efficacy and safety profile are similar, but fludarabine is approved for the indication, is easier to administer, and is less expensive. If a patient fails to respond to a purine analog or shows disease progression while receiving therapy, combination therapy such as CHOP may be considered. Careful consideration must be given to the patient's quality of life and performance status before initiating therapy that will not prolong survival and that has significant toxic effects in elderly, heavily pretreated patients.

Intravenous Immunoglobulin

Hypogammaglobulinemia is a frequent finding in patients with CLL and may contribute to the incidence of bacterial infections. The administration of IV immunoglobulin was found to reduce the incidence of bacterial infections but not to prolong survival. The study used immunoglobulin 400 mg/kg IV every 3 weeks. A lower dose may also provide a similar benefit. In general, intravenous immunoglobulin is not recommended as standard therapy for patients with CLL. It may be appropriate in a patient with advanced disease and low immunoglobulin levels who has frequent bacterial infections requiring hospitalization.[77] Intravenous immunoglobulin may be useful in the management of autoimmune hemolytic anemia. One recommended dosing schedule is 400 mg/kg/day IV for 5 days, repeated as needed.[78]

CAMPATH-1H

CAMPATH-1H, an investigational agent in phase II clinical trials, is a human anti-CD52 monoclonal antibody. CD52 antigen is expressed on the surface of more than 95% of human B and T lymphocytes. There appears to be some activity of CAMPATH-1H even in heavily pretreated patients with CLL, including patients who have received purine analogs.[79,80] Some patients have achieved a complete response. The primary toxic effect is immune suppression and a high frequency of infections is seen. CAMPATH-1H may prove to be a useful agent in the management of CLL. Its place in therapy is yet to be determined.

Bone Marrow Transplant

The role of BMT in the management of CLL is controversial. The age of most patients with CLL is above the limit for allogeneic BMT. The value of autologous BMT in a disease in which the bone marrow is heavily infiltrated with disease may be limited. Patients with low-stage disease often have the same life expectancy as age-matched control subjects. No survival advantage has yet been demonstrated using BMT in patients with CLL. Nevertheless, in patients younger than 55 years of age with good performance status and Rai stage III or IV disease, allogeneic BMT may be considered.[81,82] In patients between 55 and 65 years old with good performance status and high Rai stage disease, an autologous BMT may be appropriate. Several investigators have reported the feasibility of transplant under these conditions, reporting a high percentage of patients achieving a complete response, and in some studies, low transplant-related mortality.[83–85] One study reported that prior treatment with fludarabine might reduce the incidence of GVHD, owing to its immunosuppressive effects.[86] Patients undergoing either autologous or allogeneic BMT for CLL should be treated within the framework of a clinical study.

An exciting new development is the use of nonablative and less-toxic preparative regimens for allogeneic BMT. This approach harnesses the GVL effect to provide the antileukemic response, instead of relying on the intensity of the chemotherapy and radiation therapy to eradicate the leukemic cells. The milder preparative regimen decreases the toxic risks of transplantation, making it more tolerable for older patients.[87]

Nonpharmacologic Therapy

Patients may sometimes benefit from the removal of their spleen. In particular, patients with refractory anemia or thrombocytopenia often show improvement after splenectomy.[88] Splenic radiation has also been of value for patients with symptomatic splenomegaly that does not respond to drug therapy.

IMPROVING OUTCOMES

Infection is the leading cause of death in patients with CLL. Many of the infections are common bacterial infections that can be treated with standard antibiotics. Patients need to be educated about the signs and symptoms of infections and instructed to seek medical evaluation when these signs and symptoms occur.

KEY POINTS

Chronic Myelogenous Leukemia

- The earlier an allogeneic transplant is performed in the course of CML, the better the chance for long-term disease-free survival.
- Patients with chronic-phase CML who are younger than 50 years old with a matched sibling donor should undergo an allogeneic BMT within the first year from diagnosis.
- Patients without a donor for a BMT and patients who are older and in poor health are not candidates for BMT.
- There are many patients with CML who do not fit into the above categories. Making decisions about treatment of these patients is difficult and should be done on a case-by-case basis.
- Patients without a matched sibling donor or patients who are older than 50 years of age should be given a trial of INF-α. Patients may receive combination therapy with INF-α and hydroxyurea and/or cytarabine. In the absence of a complete cytogenetic response, allogeneic BMT should be offered, if age and functional status allow and a donor is available.

Chronic Lymphocytic Leukemia

- CLL is incurable at this time
- Many patients with CLL do not require treatment. Patients with low-stage disease do not benefit from the addition of drug therapy.
- Patients are at high risk for infection both from the disease and from drug therapy and therefore require careful monitoring.
- Autoimmune hematologic disease is common.
- Aggressive therapy such as BMT should be reserved for patients with good performance status and progressive disease.

REFERENCES

1. Sokal JE, Baccarani M, Russo D, et al. Staging and prognosis in chronic myelogenous leukemia. Semin Hematol 25:49–61, 1988.
2. Lee SJ, Anasetti C, Horowitz MM, et al. Initial therapy for chronic myelogenous leukemia: playing the odds [Editorial]. J Clin Oncol 16:2897–2903, 1998.

3. Athens JW. Chronic myeloid leukemia. In: Lee GR, Bithell TG, Foerster J, et al. Wintrobe's clinical hematology. 9th ed. Philadelphia: Lea & Febiger, 1993: 1969–1998.
4. Cortes JE, Talpaz M, Kantarjian H. Chronic myelogenous leukemia: a review. Am J Med 100:555–570, 1996.
5. Goldman, J. Chronic myeloid leukemia: new strategies for cure [Ham-Wasserman lecture]. Education Program, American Society of Hematology, 1997:1–7.
6. Ferrajoli A, Fizzotti M, Liberati AM, et al. Chronic myelogenous leukemia: an update on the biological findings and therapeutic approaches. Crit Rev Oncol Hematol 22:151–174, 1996.
7. Hardman JG, Limbird LE, Molinoff PB, et al., eds. Goodman & Gilman's the pharmacological basis of therapeutics. 9th ed. New York: McGraw-Hill, 1996.
8. Dorr RT, Von Hoff DD. Cancer chemotherapy handbook. 2nd ed. Norwalk, CT: Appleton & Lange, 1994.
9. Chabner BA, Longo DL. Cancer chemotherapy and biotherapy. 2nd ed. Philadelphia: Lippincott-Raven, 1996.
10. Package labeling. Busulfan. Research Triangle Park, NC: GlaxoWellcome, 1996.
11. Package labeling. Hydroxyurea. New Jersey: Bristol Laboratories, 1996.
12. Gwilt PR, Tracewell WG. Pharmacokinetics and pharmacodynamics of hydroxyurea. Clin Pharmacokinet 34:347–358, 1998.
13. Rodriguez GI, Kuhn JG, Weiss GR, et al. A bioavailability and pharmacokinetic study of oral and intravenous hydroxyurea. Blood 91:1533–1541, 1998.
14. Best PJ, Daoud MS, Pittelkow MR, et al. Hydroxyurea-induced leg ulceration in 14 patients. Ann Intern Med 128:29–32, 1998.
15. Hehlmann R, Heimpel H, Hasford J, et al. Randomized comparison of busulfan and hydroxyurea in chronic myelogenous leukemia: prolongation of survival by hydroxyurea. Blood 82:398–407, 1993.
16. Wetzler M, Kantarjian H, Kurzrock R, et al. Interferon-α therapy for chronic myelogenous leukemia. Am J Med 99:402–410, 1995.
17. Kantarjian HM, Smith TL, O'Brien S, et al. Prolonged survival in chronic myelogenous leukemia after cytogenetic response to interferon-α therapy. Ann Intern Med 122:254–261, 1995.
18. Deisseroth AB, Kantarjian H, Andreef M, et al. Chronic leukemias. In: DeVita VT, Hellman S, Rosenberg SA, eds. Cancer: principles and practice of oncology. 5th ed. Philadelphia: Lippincott-Raven, 1997.
19. Schofield JR, Robinson WA, Murphy JR, et al. Low doses of interferon-α are as effective as higher doses in inducing remissions and prolonging survival in chronic myeloid leukemia. Ann Intern Med 121:736–744, 1994.
20. Chronic Myeloid Leukemia Trialists' Collaborative Group. Interferon alfa versus chemotherapy for chronic myeloid leukemia: a meta-analysis of seven randomized trials. J Natl Cancer Inst 89:1616–1620, 1997.
21. Ohnishi K, Ohno R, Tomonaga M, et al. A randomized trial comparing interferon-α with busulfan for newly diagnosed chronic myelogenous leukemia in chronic phase. Blood 86:906–916, 1995.
22. Allan NC, Richards SM, Shepherd PCA. UK Medical Research Council randomized, multicentre trial of interferon-α n1 for chronic myeloid leukaemia: improved survival irrespective of cytogenetic response. Lancet 345:1392–1397, 1995.
23. The Benelux CML Study Group. Randomized study on hydroxyurea alone versus hydroxyurea combined with low-dose interferon-α 2b for chronic myeloid leukemia. Blood 91:2713–2721, 1998.
24. Hehlmann R, Heimpel H, Hossfield DK, et al. Randomized study of the combination of hydroxyurea and interferon alpha versus hydroxyurea monotherapy during the chronic phase of chronic myelogenous leukemia (CML Study II). Bone Marrow Transplant 17(Suppl 3):S21–S24, 1996.
25. The Italian Cooperative Study Group on Chronic Myeloid Leukemia. Interferon alfa-2a as compared with conventional chemotherapy for the treatment of chronic myeloid leukemia. N Engl J Med 330:820–825, 1994.
26. Hasford J, Baccarani M, Hehlmann R, et al. Interferon-α and hydroxyurea in early chronic myeloid leukemia: a comparative analysis of the Italian and German chronic myeloid leukemia trials with interferon-α. Blood 87:5384–5391, 1996.
27. The Italian Cooperative Study Group on Chronic Myeloid Leukemia. Long-term follow-up of the Italian trial of interferon-α versus conventional chemotherapy in chronic myeloid leukemia. Blood 92:1541–1548, 1998.
28. Hehlmann R, Heimpel H, Hasford J, et al. Randomized comparison of interferon-α with busulfan and hydroxyurea in chronic myelogenous leukemia. Blood 134:4064–4077, 1994.
29. Guilhot F, Chastang C, Michallet M, et al. Interferon alfa-2b combined with cytarabine versus interferon alone in chronic myelogenous leukemia. N Engl J Med 337:223–229, 1997.
30. Sacchi S, Kantarjian HM, Smith TI, et al. Early treatment decisions with interferon-alfa therapy in early chronic-phase chronic myelogenous leukemia. J Clin Oncol 16:882–889, 1998.
31. Mahob FX, Fabres C, Pueyo S, et al. Response at three months is a good predictive factor for newly diagnosed chronic myeloid leukemia patients treated by recombinant interferon-α. Blood 92:4059–4065, 1998.
32. Kurzrock R, Estrov Z, Kantarjian H, et al. Conversion of interferon-induced, long-term cytogenetic remissions in chronic myelogenous leukemia to polymerase chain reaction negativity. J Clin Oncol 16:1526–1531, 1998.
33. Kattan MW, Inoue Y, Giles FJ, et al. Cost-effectiveness of interferon-α and conventional chemotherapy in chronic myelogenous leukemia. Ann Intern Med 125:541–548, 1996.
34. Liberato NL, Quaglini S, Barosi G. Cost-effectiveness of interferon alfa in chronic myelogenous leukemia. J Clin Oncol 15:2673–2682, 1997.
35. Druker BJ, Talpaz M, Resta D, et al. Clinical efficacy and safety of an ABL specific tyrosine kinase inhibitor as targeted therapy for chronic myelogenous leukemia. American Society of Hematology Annual Meeting, December 1999, Abstract 1639.
36. O'Brien S, Kantarjian H, Keating M, et al. Homoharringtonine therapy induces responses in patients with chronic myelogenous leukemia in late chronic phase. Blood 3322–3326, 1995.
37. Druker BJ, Kantarjian H, Sawyers CL, et al. Activity of an ABL specific tyrosine kinase inhibitor in patients with BCR-ABL positive acute leukemias, including chronic myelogenous leukemia in blast crisis. American Society of Hematology Annual Meeting, December 1999, Abstract 3082.
38. Gale RP, Hehlmann R, Zhang M, et al. Survival with bone marrow transplantation versus hydroxyurea or interferon for chronic myelogenous leukemia. Blood 91:1810–1819, 1998.
39. Keleman E, Masszi, Renenyi P, et al. Reduction in the frequency of transplant-related complications in patients with chronic myeloid leukemia undergoing BMT preconditioned with a new, non-myeloablative drug combination. Bone Marrow Transplant 21:747–749, 1998.
40. Lee SJ, Kuntz KM, Horowitz MM, et al. Unrelated donor bone marrow transplantation for chronic myelogenous leukemia: a decision analysis. Ann Intern Med 127:1080–1088, 1997.
41. Hansen JA, Gooley TA, Martin PJ, et al. Bone marrow transplants from unrelated donors for patients with chronic myeloid leukemia. N Engl J Med 338:962–968, 1998.
42. Lee SJ, Anasetti C, Kuntz KM, et al. The costs and cost-effectiveness of unrelated donor bone marrow transplantation for chronic phase chronic myelogenous leukemia. Blood 92:4047–4052, 1998.
43. Higano CS, Chielens D, Raskind W, et al. Use of α-2a-interferon to treat cytogenetic relapse of chronic myeloid leukemia after bone marrow transplantation. Blood 90:2549–2554, 1997.
44. Steegman JL, Casado F, Granados E, et al. Treatment of chronic myeloid leukemia relapsing after allogeneic bone marrow transplantation: the case for giving interferon [Correspondence]. Blood 91:2617–2618, 1998.
45. McGlave PH, De Fabritiis P, Deisseroth A, et al. Autologous transplants for chronic myelogenous leukemia: results from eight transplant groups. Lancet 343:1486–1491, 1994.
46. Carella AM, Cunningham I, Lerma E, et al. Mobilization and transplantation of Philadelphia-negative peripheral-blood progenitor cells early in chronic myelogenous leukemia. J Clin Oncol 15:1575–1582, 1997.
47. Rozman C, Montserrat E. Chronic lymphocytic leukemia. N Engl J Med 333:1052–1057, 1995.
48. Flinn IW, Grever M. Chronic lymphocytic leukemia. Cancer Treat Rev 22:1–13, 1996.
49. Reed JC. Molecular biology of chronic lymphocytic leukemia. Semin Oncol 25:11–18, 1998.
50. Cheson BD, Bennett JM, Grever M, et al. National Cancer Institute-sponsored working group guidelines for chronic lymphocytic leukemia: revised guidelines for diagnosis and treatment. Blood 87:4990–4997, 1996.
51. Rai KR, Sawitsky A, Cronkite EP, et al. Clinical staging of chronic lymphocytic leukemia. Blood 46:219–234, 1975.
52. Binet JL, Auquier A, Dighiero G, et al. A new prognostic classification of chronic lymphocytic leukemia derived from a multivariate survival analysis. Cancer 48:198–206, 1981.
53. Dighiero G, Maloum K, Desablens B, et al. Chlorambucil in indolent chronic lymphocytic leukemia. N Engl J Med 338:1506–1514, 1998.
54. Giles FJ, O'Brien SM, Keating MJ. Chronic lymphocytic leukemia in (Richter's) transformation. Semin Oncol 25:117–125, 1998.
55. Diehl LF, Ketchum LH. Autoimmune disease and chronic lymphocytic leukemia: autoimmune hemolytic anemia, pure red cell aplasia, and autoimmune thrombocytopenia. Semin Oncol 25:80–97, 1998.
56. Bartik MM, Welker D, Kay NE. Impairments in immune cell function in B cell chronic lymphocytic leukemia. Semin Oncol 25:27–33, 1998.
57. Morrison VA. The infectious complications of chronic lymphocytic leukemia. Semin Oncol 25:98–106, 1998.

58. Anaissie EJ, Kontoyiannis DP, O'Brien S, et al. Infections in patients with chronic lymphocytic leukemia treated with fludarabine. Ann Intern Med 129:559–566, 1998.
59. Raphael B, Anderson JW, Silber R, et al. Comparison of chlorambucil and prednisone versus cyclophosphamide, vincristine, and prednisone as initial treatment of chronic lymphocytic leukemia: long-term follow-up of an Eastern Cooperative Oncology Group randomized clinical trial. J Clin Oncol 9:770–776, 1991.
60. French Cooperative Group on chronic lymphocytic leukemia: a randomized clinical trial of chlorambucil vs COP in stage B chronic lymphocytic leukemia. Blood 75:1422–1425, 1990.
61. Montserrat E, Alcala A, Alonso C, et al. A randomized trial comparing chlorambucil plus prednisone versus cyclophosphamide, melphalan, and prednisone in the treatment of chronic lymphocytic leukemia stages B and C. Nouv Rev Fr Hematol 30:429–432, 1998.
62. Faguet GB. Chronic lymphocytic leukemia: an updated review. J Clin Oncol 12:1974–1990, 1994.
63. Package labeling. Fludarabine. Richmond, CA: Berlex Laboratories, 1996.
64. O'Brien S, Kantarjian H, Beran M, et al. Fludarabine and granulocyte colony-stimulating factor (G-CSF) in patients with chronic lymphocytic leukemia. Leukemia 11:1631–1635, 1997.
65. Cheson BD, Vena DA, Foss FM, et al. Neurotoxicity of purine analogs: a review. J Clin Oncol 12:2216–2228, 1994.
66. Hequet O, de Jaureguiberry JP, Jaubert D, et al. Listeriosis after fludarabine treatment of chronic lymphocytic leukemia. Hematol Cell Ther 39:89–91, 1997.
67. Byrd JC, Hargis JB, Kester KE, et al. Opportunistic pulmonary infections with fludarabine in previously treated patients with low-grade lymphoid malignancies: a role of *Pneumocystis carinii* pneumonia prophylaxis. Am J Hematol 49:135–142, 1995.
68. Cheson BD. Infectious and immunospuppressive complications of purine analog therapy. J Clin Oncol 13:2431–2448, 1995.
69. Weiss R, Freiman J, Kweder SL, et al.. Hemolytic anemia after fludarabine therapy for chronic lymphocytic leukemia. J Clin Oncol 16:1885–1889, 1998.
70. Sorenson MJ, Vena DA, Fallavollita A, et al.. Treatment of refractory chronic lymphocytic leukemia with fludarabine phosphate via the group C protocol mechanism of the National Cancer Institute: five-year follow-up report. J Clin Oncol 15:458–465, 1997.
71. Keating MJ, O'Brien S, Lerner S, et al. Long-term follow-up of patients with chronic lymphocytic leukemia (CLL) receiving fludarabine regimens as initial therapy. Blood 92:1165–1171, 1998.
72. Tallman MS, Hakiman D, Zanzig C, et al. Cladribine in the treatment of relapsed or refractory chronic lymphocytic leukemia. J Clin Oncol 13:983–998, 1995.
73. Juliusson G, Liliemark J. Long-term survival following cladribine (2-chlorodeoxyadenosine) therapy in previously treated patients with chronic lymphocytic leukemia. Ann Oncol 7:373–379, 1996.
74. Robak T, Blasinska-Morawiec M, Krykowski E, et al. Intermittent 2-hour intravenous infusions of 2-chlorodeoxyadenosine in the treatment of 110 patients with refractory or previously untreated B-cell chronic lymphocytic leukemia. Leuk Lymphoma 22:509–514, 1996.
75. Robak T, Blasinska-Morawiec M, Krykowski E, et al. Autoimmune haemolytic anaemia in patients with chronic lymphocytic leukaemia treated with 2-chlorodeoxyadenosine (cladribine). Eur J Haematol 58:109–113, 1997.
76. The French Cooperative Group on CLL, Johnson S, Smith AG, et al. Multicentre prospective randomised trial of fludarabine versus cyclophosphamide, doxorubicin, and prednisone (CAP) for treatment of advanced-stage chronic lymphocytic leukaemia. Lancet 347:1432–1438, 1996.
77. Cooperative group for the study of immunoglobulin in chronic lymphocytic leukemia. N Engl J Med 319:902–907, 1988.
78. Flores G, Cunningham-Rundles C, Newland AC, et al. Efficacy of intravenous immunoglobulin in the treatment of autoimmune hemolytic anemia: results in 73 patients. Am J Hematol 44:237–242, 1993.
79. Osterberg A, Dyer MJS, Bunjes D, et al. Phase II multicenter study of human CD52 antibody in previously treated chronic lymphocytic leukemia. J Clin Oncol 54:1567–1574, 1997.
80. Dyer MJ, Kelsey SM, Mackay HJ, et al. In vivo 'purging' of residual disease in CLL with Campath-1H. Br J Haematol 97:669–672, 1997.
81. Flinn IW, Vogelsang G. Bone marrow transplant for chronic lymphocytic leukemia. Semin Oncol 25:60–64, 1998.
82. Michallet M, Archimbaud E, Bandini G, et al. HLA-identical sibling bone marrow transplantation in younger patients with chronic lymphocytic leukemia. Ann Intern Med 124:311–315, 1996.
83. Rabinowe SN, Soiffer RJ, Gribben JG, et al. Autologous and allogeneic bone marrow transplantation for poor prognosis patients with B-cell chronic lymphocytic leukemia. Blood 82:1366–1376, 1993.
84. Khouri IF, Keating MJ, Vriesendorp HM, et al. Autologous and allogeneic bone marrow transplantation for chronic lymphocytic leukemia: preliminary results. J Clin Oncol 12:748–758, 1994.
85. Dreger P, von Neuhoff N, Kuse R, et al. Early stem cell transplantation of chronic lymphocytic leukaemia: a chance for cure? Br J Cancer 77:2291–2297, 1998.
86. Khouri IF, Przepiorka D, van Besien, et al. Allogeneic blood or marrow transplantation for chronic lymphocytic leukaemia: timing of transplantation and potential effect of fludarabine on acute graft-versus-host disease. Br J Hematol 97:466–473, 1997.
87. Khouri IF, Keating M, Korbling M, et al. Transplant-lite: induction of graft-versus-malignancy using fludarabine-based nonablative chemotherapy and allogeneic blood progenitor-cell transplantation as treatment for lymphoid malignancies. J Clin Oncol 16:2817–2824, 1998.
88. Cusack JC Jr, Seymour JF, Lerner S, et al. Role of splenectomy in chronic lymphocytic leukemia. J Am Coll Surg 185:237–243, 1997.

CHAPTER 86

ACUTE LEUKEMIAS

John N. McCormick and R. Michelle Sanders

Overview

The leukemias are a group of neoplastic diseases of the blood-forming cells of the bone marrow, which result in the proliferation and accumulation of immature and generally defective blood cells in both the bloodstream and the bone marrow.[1] This may result in anemia, thrombocytopenia, and granulocytopenia as well as infiltration of other sites such as lymph nodes, kidney, spleen, testes, and the central nervous system (CNS). The cells involved are usually leukocytes, but several different forms of the disease may be manifested, according to which leukocyte cell line is involved (Fig. 86.1). The leukemias are universally fatal if untreated, generally due to complications resulting from the leukemic infiltration of the bone marrow and replacement of normal hematopoietic precursor cells. These fatal complications are usually hemorrhage and infection.[1] The natural history of untreated leukemia has led to the classifications of "acute" and "chronic" leukemia, referring to the rapidity of death, with average survival for untreated acute leukemia of about 3 months. Patients with chronic leukemia generally have more differentiated types of malignant cells and survive somewhat longer without treatment.

Acute leukemias are classified according to the predominant cell type involved. Because of significant differences in age distribution, responses to treatment, and prognosis, the acute leukemias are divided into acute lymphocytic leukemia (ALL) and acute myelogenous leukemia (AML). AML can be further divided into additional subtypes, depending on the cell line involved (Figs. 86.1 and 86.2): myelocytic, myelomonocytic, monocytic, promyelocytic, erythrocytic, and several other very rare types. However, because the response to treatment is similar for all these relatively uncommon types of leukemia, they are generally treated in the same fashion and referred to collectively as AML. In this chapter, ALL and AML will be discussed separately with regard to pathophysiology, treatment, and prognosis.

TREATMENT GOALS: ACUTE LEUKEMIAS

- The basis for therapy depends on a number of factors that include morphology, biologic markers, immunology, genetic alterations, and other known risk factors of the leukemia.
- Rapidly achieve a complete clinical and hematologic remission with the use of multidrug combination chemotherapy.
- Maintain complete remission by eradicating any residual, undetectable disease with the use of radiation, central nervous system therapy, and adjuvant multidrug chemotherapy, considering maximum effect and reduction of late toxic effects.
- Provide excellent supportive care that will continue to treat toxic effects of therapy and provide a good quality of life during and after leukemia therapy.

EPIDEMIOLOGY

Approximately 25,700 new cases of acute leukemia are identified each year in the United States, according to the National Cancer Institute's Surveillance, Epidemiology, and End Results program.[2] About 20,400 Americans die of leukemia each year. Overall, leukemias account for about 2% of all new cancer cases and about 4% of cancer deaths. Despite the overall low incidence rate in children younger than 15 years of age, the acute leukemias are the most common malignancy and rank second only to accidents in mortality for this age group.[2]

The causes of acute leukemias are generally not known. Viruses have been shown to produce some types of leukemia in animals (e.g., feline leukemia), and the Epstein-Barr virus has been implicated as the causative agent of Burkitt's lymphoma in Africans and of some types of nasopharyngeal carcinoma.[3] Currently, attention is being focused on the isolation of the human T-cell leukemia virus from a human lymphoma. Persons who have previously been exposed to radiation, with or without antineoplastic drugs, are also at greater risk of developing leukemia. In addition, numerous genetic derangements (particularly Down's syndrome), exposure to benzene, pesticides, and smoking have been associated with a higher incidence of acute leukemia.[4] However, in most children and adults, the cause of leukemia cannot be identified, and probably numerous factors interact to result in the malignant condition.

Despite differences in appearance and clinical behavior, all hematologic neoplasms have in common the fact that they are clonal; that is, all cells composing the malignant population in a given patient are derived from a single mutant precursor cell.[5] The neoplastic clones have two important features compared to normal cells. First, they appear to possess an advantage over normal hematopoietic clones that results in growth of the malignant population at the expense of normal cells. Second, there is an imbalance between proliferation and differentiation. Most malignant populations are made up of poorly differentiated cell types that ordinarily would not proliferate or be found in the bloodstream in large numbers. However, the malignant transformation of these cells results in immature cell types that proliferate but do not further differentiate.

It is useful to review the process of normal production of cellular blood elements. As shown in Figure 86.1, pluripotent stem cells differentiate, mature, and proliferate to form mature cells that exist in the peripheral circulation. These stem cells have virtually unlimited potential for self-renewal. They are capable of responding to physiologic needs by inducing production of progenitor cells committed to mature separately into lymphoid cells or myeloid cells. The myeloid cells differentiate to form erythrocytes, megakaryocytes, granulocytes, and monocytes, whereas the lymphoid cells form circulating B and T lymphocytes. As maturation proceeds in the various cellular lineages, the proliferative capacity becomes progressively restricted until eventually it is lost completely. Therefore, mature cells must be continually replaced as they complete their life cycle. Various stimulatory factors, such as erythropoietin, thrombopoietin, and colony-stimulating factors, regulate the proliferation and differentiation of committed precursor cells, derived from the

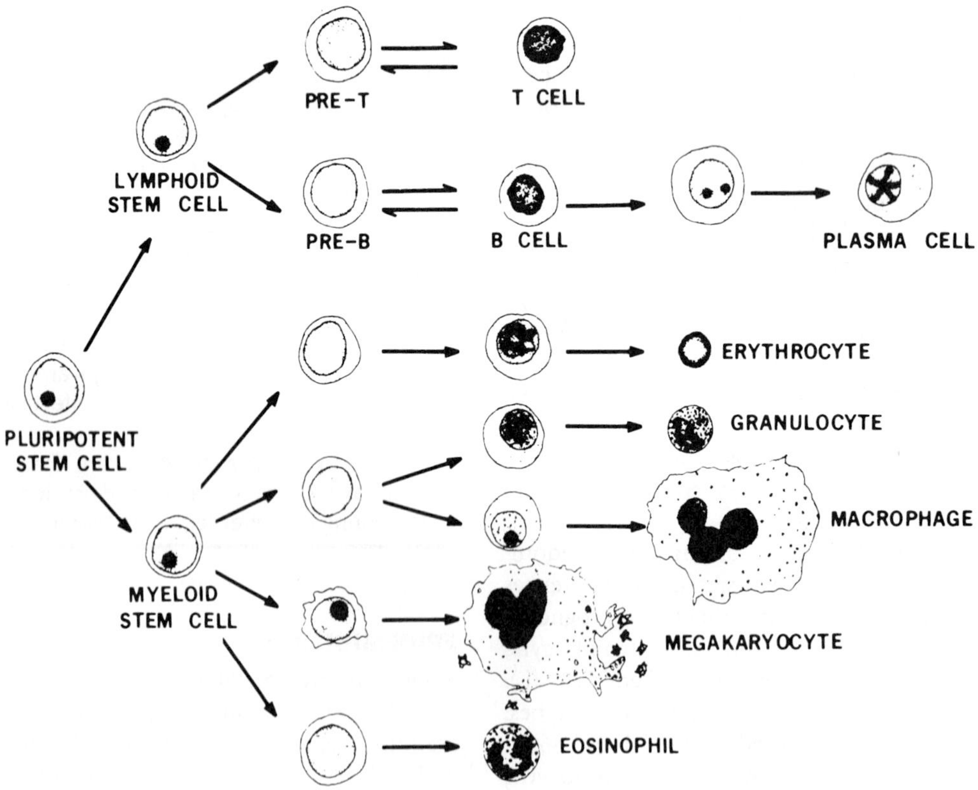

Figure 86.1. A schematic model of hematopoiesis showing clonal derivation of mature lymphoid and hemic cells from a pluripotent stem cell. (Reprinted with permission from Altman AJ, Schwartz AD. Malignant diseases of infancy, childhood and adolescence. Philadelphia: WB Saunders, 1983:187–238.)

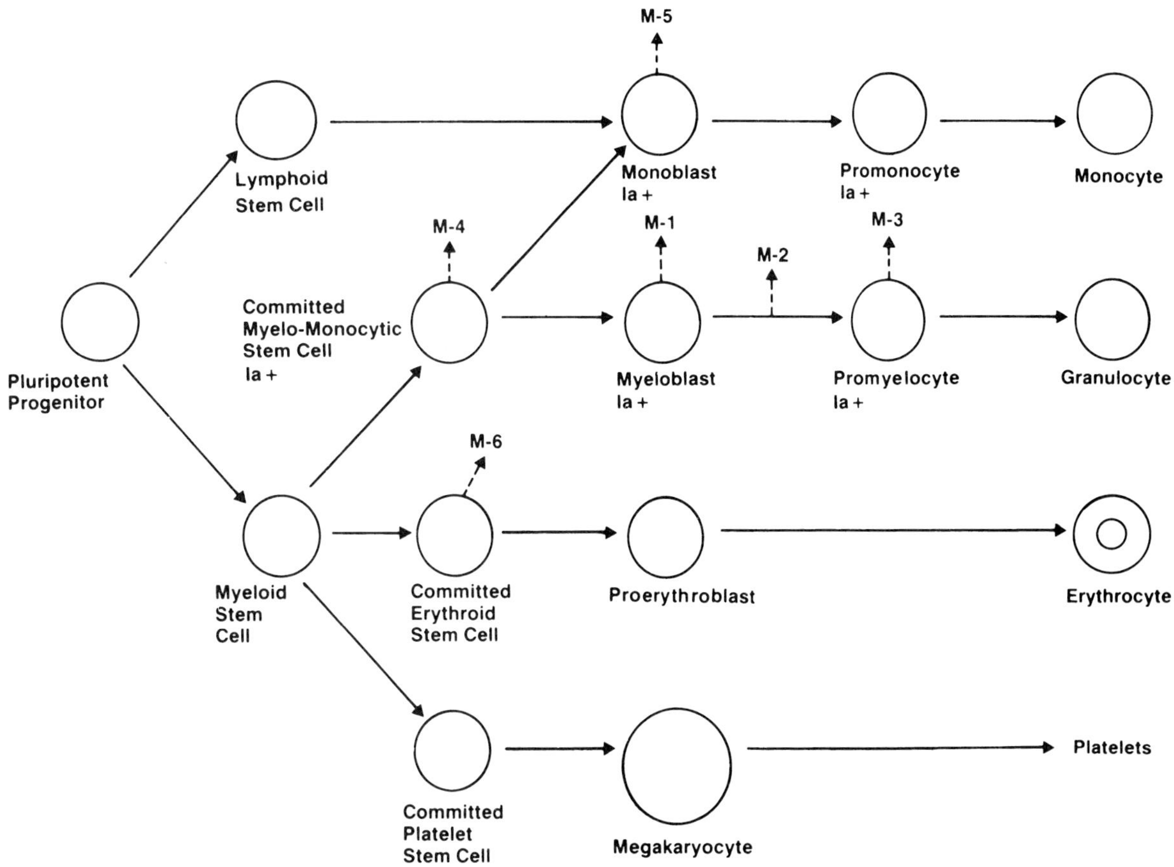

Figure 86.2. Myeloid differentiation and relationship to French-American-British (FAB) classification of acute myelogenous leukemia. *M1,* undifferentiated myeloid; *M2,* early (?) differentiated myeloid; *M3,* promyelocytic; *M4,* myelomonocytic; *M5,* monocytic; *M6,* erythroleukemia. (Reprinted with permission from Fernbach DJ. Natural history of acute leukemia. In: Sutow WW, Fernbach DJ, Vietti TJ, eds. Clinical Pediatric Oncology. 3rd ed. St Louis, MO: CV Mosby, 1984:332–377.)

pluripotent stem cells. Leukemia cells do not undergo terminal differentiation and thus do not lose their proliferative potential. The leukemic cell population continues to expand, and normal bone marrow elements may be "crowded out," resulting in the characteristic signs of bone marrow failure, which generally bring patients to medical attention.

CLASSIFICATIONS OF ACUTE LEUKEMIAS

Acute leukemias are classified depending on the cell of origin. However, additional classifications of leukemia have been developed to further identify differences in the clinical course, response to treatment, and prognosis of various types of acute leukemia. An important development introduced in the 1970s is the French-American-British (FAB) system of nomenclature that is now widely used to classify the morphologic subgroups of acute leukemias.[6] The FAB system is summarized in Table 86.1.

In addition to the FAB system, immunologic and biochemical markers, and specific genetic abnormalities are used to classify and identify subtypes of leukemia cells. Immunologic "markers" refer to the surface immunoglobulin (SIg) found on the cell membrane of malignant leukocytes or to their cytoplasmic immunoglobulins (CIg). As normal cells undergo differentiation, these markers change and may be used to determine the degree of differentiation achieved by the malignant cell line. This permits identification of the type of cell involved and leads to further classification. Genetic alterations (e.g., chromosomal gains or losses, resulting in hyperdiploidy or hypodiploidy, respectively; chromosomal translocations, and deletion or inactivation of tumor-suppressor genes) are found in most patients with lymphoid leukemia.[7]

The development of hybridoma techniques and unlimited quantities of specific monoclonal antibodies has led to more precise identification of specific immunologic markers in the classification of ALL and to a revised immunologic classification system (Table 86.2). Because leukemic lymphoblasts lack specific morphologic or cytochemical features, immunophenotyping is necessary for diagnosis. Although monoclonal antibodies against 166 different clusters of differentiation (CD) molecules on human leukocytes exist, only a few are truly lineage specific.[8] T-lineage ALL is documented based on a positive reaction with the highly sensitive monoclonal antibody CD7 plus

Table 86.1 ▪ The French-American-British (FAB) Cooperative Group Classification of Acute Leukemias

FAB Designation	Common Terms (Abbreviations) for Leukemic Subgroups	Predominating Cell Type	Unique Clinical or Laboratory Features
L1	Acute lymphocytic leukemia, childhood (ALL)	Microlymphoblasts	
L2	Acute lymphocytic leukemia, adult (ALL)	Mixed lymphoblasts, prolymphoblasts	
L3	Burkitt's-type leukemia	Lymphocytes	
M0	Minimal myeloid differentiation	Undifferentiated	Blasts often express CE34 and terminal deoxynucleotidyl transferase
M1	Acute myelocytic leukemia, undifferentiated; acute myelogenous, acute granulocytic	Myeloblasts	
M2	Acute myelocytic leukemia, differentiated	Mixed myeloblasts, promyelocytes	Myeloblastomas (especially orbital)
M3	Acute progranulocytic leukemia	Hypergranular promyelocytes	Disseminated intravascular coagulation
M4	Acute myelomonocytic leukemia (AMML)	Mixed myelocytes, monocytes	Infants, extramedullary leukemia
M5	Acute monocytic leukemia (AMOL)	Monocytes	Infants, extramedullary leukemia, second leukemia after epipodophyllotoxins
M6	Erythroleukemia	Mixed erythroblasts, erythrocytes, myelocytes	
M7	Megakaryoblastic leukemia	Megakaryoblasts	Down's syndrome

Table 86.2 ▪ Classification of Acute Lymphocytic Leukemia by Morphologic Characteristics, Immunophenotype, and Chromosome Number[a]

Category	Frequency (%)
FAB morphologic classification system	
L1	80
L2	17
L3	3
Immunophenotype	
Early pre-B	57
Pre-B	25
Transitional pre-B	1
B-cell	2
T-cell	15
Ploidy	
Hypodiploid (<45 chromosomes)	7
Diploid (normal 46 chromosomes)	8
Pseudodiploid (46 chromosomes, with abnormalities)	42
Hyperdiploid (47–50 chromosomes)	15
Hyperdiploid (>50 chromosomes)	27
Triploid/tetraploid	1

FAB, French-American-British.

[a]On the basis of 500 consecutive patients with newly diagnosed disease (ages ≤18 years) treated at St. Jude Children's Research Hospital (from references 6 and 7).

the highly specific monoclonal antibody CD3. B-lineage ALL can be confirmed based on positive reactions with antibodies CD19 and CD79a, respectively.[9] B-lineage classification includes three major subtypes: B-cell (expression of surface immunoglobulin heavy chains and either κ or λ light chains), pre-B (presence of cytoplasmic immunoglobulin), and early pre-B (no surface and cytoplasmic immunoglobulins). Transitional B cells, which express cytoplasmic and surface immunoglobulin chains and surrogate light-chain proteins, appear to define a clinically distinct form of ALL. T cells may also be classified according to the degree of differentiation (early, intermediate, or late), but this classification of T-cell ALL has limited clinical significance.[10] The prognosis associated with these various subgroups of ALL will be discussed later.

Biochemical markers refer to altered concentrations of intracellular enzymes, which may be found in various forms of leukemia. Terminal deoxynucleotidyl transferase is an intracellular enzyme that is generally not detected in mature lymphocytes but is found in most patients with ALL, excluding those with the B-cell subtype. It may also be found in up to 5% of patients with AML. Reactions with myeloperoxidase and Sudan black stain, on the other hand, are positive predominantly in AML. The periodic acid-Schiff reaction is positive in ALL and is useful in differentiating it from AML.[11]

In actual practice, the classification of acute leukemia in a particular patient is based on the combination of morphology and immunologic and biochemical studies. These studies generally correlate with one another and are used to confirm the suspected classification in a patient. Figure 86.2 shows the correlation between FAB classification, immunologic markers, and biochemical markers for subgroups of ALL and AML, respectively.

Genetic abnormalities in patients with acute leukemia have contributed greatly to the understanding of the pathogenesis of the disease. Alterations in the *p53* suppressor gene are found in acute leukemia. Normal *p53* allows cells to stop in the G_1 phase of the cell cycle. Inactivation of *p53* allows cells to proliferate unregulated, which occurs in acute leukemia.[12] Mutations of the *ras* gene may lead to unregulated proliferation and differentiation, a characteristic of acute leukemia.[13] Several chromosomal translocations are well documented in acute leukemia and provide information on risk and prognosis of disease. *MLL* gene rearrangements located on chromosome 11q23, positive Philadelphia chromosome translocation on chromosome 9;22, and alterations in chromosome 4;11 confer a poor prognosis. However, an excellent outcome is expected in patients who have the *TEL-AML1* fusion on chromosome 12;21.[14]

CLINICAL PRESENTATION AND DIAGNOSIS

The initial presenting symptoms of acute leukemia differ very little for ALL and AML. The complaints that most often bring patients to medical attention are fatigue, weight loss, fever, pallor, purpura, and pain.[15] These symptoms result from bone marrow failure. Anemia occurs because of inadequate erythrocyte production, infections are caused by inadequate neutrophil production, and bleeding is the result of inadequate platelet production. In addition, infiltration of leukemia cells into the liver, spleen, or lymph nodes may result in hepatosplenomegaly, lymphadenopathy, and bone and joint pain. Table 86.3 lists the frequency of presenting complaints among patients with ALL. These complaints may be present for a few days or even a few weeks; rarely, there may be a history of these symptoms for several months before diagnosis. The most common symptom at diagnosis is the presence of fever, occurring in about 60% of patients. Although patients may be neutropenic at diagnosis, fever appears to be due to the leukemia itself because 70% of these patients become afebrile within 72 hours of beginning induction therapy without antibiotics.[16] Nevertheless, empiric antibiotic therapy is usually begun in febrile, neutropenic patients at diagnosis of leukemia because the risk of serious systemic infections in such patients cannot be ignored.

Table 86.3 ▪ Frequency of the More Common Presenting Complaints Among Children with Acute Lymphocytic Leukemia

Finding	Percent
Fever	61
Pallor	55
Hemorrhage	52
Anorexia	33
Fatigue	30
Bone pain	23
Abdominal pain	19
Joint pain	15
Lymphadenopathy	15
Weight loss	13

Patients with newly diagnosed leukemia may have a total white blood cell (WBC) count that is markedly elevated, normal, or markedly depressed. A very high circulating WBC count (hyperleukocytosis) is associated with a poorer prognosis. This condition can also be life threatening because blasts can occlude small vessels in vital organs. Additionally, most of the white cells in the circulation are immature blast forms; therefore, they are incapable of mounting a response to bacterial infections. Thus, most patients with leukemia have an increased risk of opportunistic infections at diagnosis.

The diagnosis of acute leukemia is not usually difficult to establish. A bone marrow aspirate is performed to allow examination of the cellular elements of the bone marrow. It is often hypercellular, with 60 to 100% blast cells. A minimum of 25% blast cells is considered adequate to establish the diagnosis of acute leukemia, but most commonly this is an all-or-none diagnosis, and the pattern is obvious. Abnormal cells found in the peripheral blood may be suggestive of acute leukemia but usually are not considered diagnostic, because bizarre mononuclear cells may be seen in the blood of patients with viral illnesses. If blasts or other unidentified cells are seen in the peripheral blood, the diagnosis must be confirmed by a bone marrow examination.

THERAPEUTIC PLAN

The modern cure-oriented approach to the treatment of any malignant condition usually involves some combination of surgery, radiation, and chemotherapy. Although surgery is important in the treatment of solid tumors, it is impossible to surgically remove tumor tissue in leukemia, and therefore surgery has a minor supportive role.

Radiation therapy has a larger role in leukemia, but it is not used alone as a curative modality. It is important in the treatment of either occult or overt leukemia in the CNS. High-dose radiotherapy is also used to obliterate functional bone marrow as part of the preparation for bone marrow transplants. It may also be used in individual patients to reduce the size of an infiltrative leukemic mass, particularly when functional impairment of an organ or joint is involved.

Drug Therapy

Drug therapy remains the primary modality for the treatment of acute leukemias with the goal of treatment for both AML and ALL being the complete eradication of any detectable disease. Beginning with the use of aminopterin in childhood ALL in 1948,[17] additional effective agents have been identified and introduced into routine clinical use. The clinical indications and common toxic effects of the drugs routinely used to treat acute leukemia today are summarized in Table 86.4.

For all phases of leukemia, it has been clearly demonstrated that drugs used in combination are superior to

Table 86.4 ▪ Principal Toxic Effects and Clinical Indications for Drugs Used to Treat Leukemia

Drug	Acute Delayed Indications	Delayed	Indications
Plant alkaloids			
Etoposide	Nausea and vomiting; hypotension with rapid administration; hypersensitivity reactions (2–20%); vesicant with extravasation	Bone marrow depression; alopecia, oral ulceration	AML (induction 200 mg/m^2 CI for 3 days) ALL (150–300 mg/m^2 weekly pairs)
Vincristine	Vesicant reaction with extravasation; mild emetogenicity	Neurotoxicity; peripheral neuropathy, jaw pain, paralytic ileus, foot drop, decreased reflexes, constipation; alopecia; bone marrow depression	ALL (remission induction and continuation: 1–1.5 mg/m^2 weekly pairs)
Antimetabolites			
Cladribine (2-CDA)	Mild nausea and vomiting; rash	Bone marrow depression; immunosuppression	AML 8.9 mg/m^2/day × 5 days CI
Cytarabine	Nausea, vomiting, diarrhea, rash	Bone marrow depression; CNS toxicity; interstitial pneumonitis; pulmonary capillary leak (high dose)	ALL (200–300 mg/m^2 weekly or alternating pairs) If intrathecally: 28–36 mg AML (100 mg/m^2 CI days 1–7 or 250 mg/m^2 CI days 1–5) AML high dose: 2–3 g/m^2 IV q12hr days 1, 3, and 5 or 6
Fludarabine	Nausea and vomiting	Bone marrow depression; megaloblastosis; oral ulceration; fever and arthralgias; diarrhea; alopecia; rash on soles and palms	AML 50–150 mg/m^2/day × 5 days over 30 min IV
Mercaptopurine	Occasional nausea and vomiting	Bone marrow depression; liver damage	ALL (continuation therapy: 75–100 mg/m^2/day)
Methotrexate	Dose-related nausea and vomiting; diarrhea (usually mild); rash	Bone marrow depression; oral and gastrointestinal ulceration; nephrotoxicity (high doses); hepatic cirrhosis (low dose) and elevated liver transaminases; pulmonary infiltration (fibrosis/pneumonitis); CNS toxicity (high dose and intrathecal therapy)	ALL (intrathecal 6–12 mg, low doses orally or IV 40 mg/m^2 dose, high doses IV 1500–5000 mg/m^2 over 2–24 hr)
Thioguanine	Occasional nausea and vomiting 1 or 2 days after administration	Bone marrow depression	AML (100 mg/m^2 daily to twice daily days 1–7)
Antibiotics			
Daunorubicin	Nausea and vomiting; diarrhea; vesicant—local reactions at infiltration site; red urine, 1 or 2 days after administration	Bone marrow depression; cardiotoxicity; stomatitis; alopecia; potentiation of radiation	AML (45 mg/m^2 CI over 3 days) Doses may be decreased to 30 mg/m^2 in older adults ALL (25 mg/m^2 IV once a week for 2–3 wk)
Doxorubicin	Nausea and vomiting; diarrhea; local reactions at infiltration site; red urine, 1 or 2 days after administration	Bone marrow depression; cardiotoxicity; stomatitis; alopecia; potentiation of radiation	AML (30 mg/m^2 CI over 3 days)
Idarubicin	Nausea and vomiting; diarrhea; local reactions at infiltration site; red urine, 1 or 2 days after administration	Bone marrow depression; cardiotoxicity; stomatitis; alopecia; potentiation of radiation	AML 12 mg/m^2 for 2–3 days
Mitoxantrone	Nausea and vomiting; diarrhea; local reactions at infiltration site; blueish-green urine, 1 or 2 days after administration	Bone marrow depression; cardiotoxicity; stomatitis; alopecia; potentiation of radiation	AML 12 mg/m^2 for 2–3 days
Alkylating agents			
Cyclophosphamide	Nausea and vomiting (sometimes delayed)	Bone marrow depression; immunosuppression; alopecia; hemorrhagic cystitis; sterility; secondary malignancies; SIADH	ALL (150–300 mg/m^2 IV alternating weekly pairs)

(continued)

Table 86.4 *(continued)*

Drug	Acute Delayed Indications	Delayed	Indications
Miscellaneous			
Asparaginase	Nausea and vomiting; fever; anaphylaxis; local reaction	Hepatotoxicity; hyperglycemia; pancreatitis; abdominal pain; coagulation defects; CNS depression	ALL induction (10,000 U/m^2/day IM QOD to weekly for 6–9 doses)
All-*trans* retinoic acid[21]	Fever; progressive increase in WBC without symptoms ATRA syndrome: increased WBC count with symptoms of fever, respiratory distress, weight gain, lower extremity edema, pleural effusions, hypotension, and sometimes renal failure[18–20]	Increase in transaminases; increase in triglycerides; bone pain; headaches; increased calcium; dry lips and mucosa; pseudotumor cerebri	AML (M3)-APL (45 mg/m^2/day) To reduce side effects doses of 25 mg/m^2/day have been effective

ATRA, all-*trans* retinoic acid; *AML,* acute myelogenic leukemia; *ALL,* acute lymphocytic leukemia; *APL,* acute promyelocytic leukemia; *CNS,* central nervous system; *SIADH,* syndrome of inappropriate secretion of diuretic hormone; *WBC,* white blood cell.

single agents. The rationale for combination therapy is that several effective agents with different mechanisms of action are more likely to destroy different subpopulations of leukemia cells and reduce the potential for development of drug resistance. The practical problem in the design of clinical treatment programs is to use the optimal number of agents in the most effective dosages and sequence. Several principles guide the use of combination chemotherapy for malignant diseases: (1) each of the drugs used should have demonstrated single-agent activity against the tumor; (2) the drugs should have different mechanisms of action; (3) the drugs used should have minimally overlapping toxicities; and (4) the maximal optimal doses should be used, scheduled with respect to specific tumor cell kinetics.

The optimal use of anticancer drugs is limited by our incomplete understanding of their mechanisms of action, mechanisms of resistance to them, and their interactions. In addition, our understanding of the biology of tumors and the factors that control their growth is incomplete. Current research directed at elucidating the cellular mechanisms that govern both the reproduction of malignant cells and their response to anticancer drugs is expected to improve our use of the drugs currently available as well as to lead to the development of new agents.

Bone Marrow Transplantation

Bone marrow transplantation (BMT) is a treatment modality that has an important role in the treatment of AML, particularly during the first remission. BMT has also been useful in producing cures in patients with ALL who have had a relapse and receive a transplant during their second remission and in patients with ALL with a poor prognosis, such as infants and those with Philadelphia chromosome, who receive a transplant during their first remission. This procedure typically includes total body irradiation, with or without high-dose chemotherapy (cyclophosphamide, cytarabine, busulfan, and etoposide have all been used), to kill residual leukemia cells and produce irreversible bone marrow suppression. Bone marrow is obtained from either a human leukocyte antigen-matched donor (allogeneic), an identical twin (syngeneic), or a patient in remission (autologous). Bone marrow is harvested from the iliac crest of the donor and then intravenously infused into the patient. Engraftment usually occurs in about 2 to 3 weeks. BMT has a number of hazards. First, there is the complication of graft-versus-host disease (GVHD), which results from the T lymphocytes in the donor marrow reacting against host tissue. GVHD primarily occurs after allogeneic transplantation. Second, there is the risk of infection as a result of immunosuppression. Viral and fungal infections are especially common and difficult to treat. A third common complication is veno-occlusive disease of the liver, a fibrous obliteration (either partial or complete) of small hepatic venules leading to thrombosis, endophlebitis, fibrosis, and portal hypertension with ascites. Finally, there is the risk of relapse of leukemia despite the intensive therapy.

Acute Lymphocytic Leukemia

Childhood ALL represents one of the cancer treatment success stories of recent years. Long-term survival in children receiving modern therapy is now about 73%. In adults, however, the survival rate remains approximately 30%.[22] Several distinct phases of therapy, each with a specific rationale, have been developed, and current efforts to improve the cure rate of ALL have focused on refining and optimizing therapy for each of these phases.

TREATMENT

Induction Therapy

Complete remission (CR), defined as the complete eradication of all detectable disease, may be produced in at least 95% of patients with ALL with induction therapy. Patients in CR have no evidence of leukemia and may lead relatively normal lives while in remission. However, patients in remission may have as many as 10^8 leukemia cells in their bodies, but this mass of cells remains clinically undetectable. Remission induction therapy is capable of eradicating up to 99.9% of the total body burden of malignant cells, but since patients may have 10^{10} to 10^{12} leukemia cells at diagnosis, a substantial number of cells remain to be eliminated after patients achieve a clinical CR.

The objectives of initial remission induction are to (1) eradicate as many leukemia cells as possible, within the limits of biologic tolerance, and (2) reestablish normal hematopoiesis and general good health. "Standard" remission induction therapy generally consists of two or more drugs. Prednisone and vincristine are almost always used, and this combination produces a CR in more than 90% of patients. However, the intensity of the initial treatment influences the duration of remission, and addition of a third agent, either asparaginase or an anthracycline (daunorubicin or doxorubicin), appears to increase the fraction of patients who remain in continuous complete remission (CCR) and are eventually cured.[23-25] Therefore, induction regimens generally include at least three drugs: prednisone, vincristine, and either asparaginase or an anthracycline.

Consolidation Therapy

Consolidation therapy refers to a period of intensive therapy administered after achievement of CR. The purpose of consolidation therapy is to secure the CR by eradicating as many of the remaining leukemic cells as possible, within the limits of biologic tolerance. Consolidation therapy may consist of different combinations of agents or repeated courses of the regimen used to achieve the initial clinical remission.

Central Nervous System Therapy

An important site of initial relapse in patients who achieve a CR is the CNS. After conventional induction therapy alone, up to 60% of patients may have their initial reappearance of malignant blast cells in the CNS,[26] probably because of poor penetration across the blood–brain barrier by the drugs used to induce remission. The precise definition of CNS disease has been somewhat controversial. The two most commonly accepted definitions of CNS disease are as follows: (1) a total cerebrospinal fluid (CSF) WBC count greater than 5 cells/μL and the presence of blast cells in the CSF or with cranial nerve palsy and (2) the presence of any number of blasts regardless of cell counts in the CSF.

The presence of the CNS as a "pharmacologic sanctuary" for ALL led to the recognition that specific CNS therapy is an essential component of treatment for this disease. Proposed by George and Pinkel in the 1960s,[27] CNS therapy has reduced the CNS relapse rate to less than 10%.[28] The mainstay of CNS therapy has been cranial irradiation, either with spinal irradiation or intrathecal administration of methotrexate. The dose originally used was 2400 cGy delivered over 2 to 3 weeks, but more recently, it has been shown that 1800 cGy provides adequate treatment, with less toxicity and morbidity.[29] Intrathecal methotrexate has been used with success in place of spinal irradiation, resulting in less myelosuppression and growth abnormalities.[30] The usual dose for patients older than 3 years of age is 12 mg/m^2.[31] Cytarabine or hydrocortisone, or both, may be added to methotrexate to further improve the effectiveness of CNS therapy. Recent data have suggested that the treatment for CNS disease should be intensified based on prognostic factors as well as on the CNS disease at diagnosis, reserving cranial irradiation and multiple intrathecal doses for those at greater risk for relapse. Therefore, patients with non-T-cell, non-B-cell ALL who have less than 5 cells/μL in the CSF, regardless of blasts, would receive less CNS prophylaxis and no irradiation in the context of highly effective chemotherapy.[26,32]

Another approach to CNS treatment is the use of high-dose methotrexate intravenously, without irradiation.[33] This therapy consists of methotrexate in doses of 500 mg/m^2 or more, infused over 24 hours. The long infusion time is intended to improve penetration of methotrexate across the blood–brain barrier. Although CSF methotrexate concentrations are typically only 1% or less of the concurrent plasma concentrations,[34] use of high-dose methotrexate allows prolonged high plasma concentrations to achieve cytocidal methotrexate concentrations in the CSF. Leucovorin "rescue" is then administered to prevent excessive and intolerable toxicity to normal tissues. High-dose intravenous methotrexate may be combined with intrathecal methotrexate to further boost CSF concentrations. Doses as high as 33.6 g/m^2 have been used[35] to achieve CSF concentrations of 10 μM from intravenous methotrexate alone. However, no improvement in overall survival has been shown as a result of using this approach. In general, high-dose methotrexate may result in a slightly higher CNS relapse rate than cranial irradiation with intrathecal methotrexate,[36] but overall disease-free survival does not appear to be different. This suggests that high-dose methotrexate may improve control of disease in the bone marrow as well. In addition, cranial irradiation results in more significant CNS toxicities than does high-dose methotrexate.

The optimal dose of high-dose methotrexate in the treatment of ALL has not been defined. One study[37] identified a relationship between plasma methotrexate concentration and the probability of relapse. Patients received 15 courses of methotrexate 1000 mg/m^2, given as a 200 mg/m^2 loading dose, followed by 800 mg/m^2 over

24 hours. This therapy was delivered as CNS therapy during the first 75 weeks of continuation therapy. Patients who achieved steady-state plasma concentrations greater than 16 μM for at least half their courses were more likely to remain in CCR than patients whose plasma concentrations were lower. The variability in plasma concentrations was due solely to interpatient differences in drug elimination since all patients were treated with identical methotrexate doss. This study provides insight into how best to use methotrexate for ALL and offers guidance in selecting a dose of methotrexate that will yield optimal cytotoxic exposure and the best results. A potential role for prospective pharmacokinetic monitoring of high-dose methotrexate to improve its therapeutic benefit in ALL patients is also discussed.

Monitoring methotrexate serum concentrations in all patients receiving high doses is warranted. The leucovorin rescue dose should be adjusted based on the clearance of the methotrexate and the measured serum levels. Aggressive hydration with alkalinization improves clearance of methotrexate while leucovorin should prevent many of the unwarranted side effects of methotrexate. The amounts of fluid, alkalinization, and leucovorin are increased with delayed clearance as defined by the elevated methotrexate level.

The preceding data for the use of CNS prophylaxis and high-dose methotrexate for control or prevention of CNS disease and/or relapse is in the context of intense systemic therapy. Recent data suggest that the addition of epipodophyllotoxins to the systemic therapy may result in better CNS cytotoxicity because of documented CNS penetration.[38] Another approach to improving control of CNS disease is the use of dexamethasone instead of prednisone during maintenance therapy.[39]

Maintenance Therapy

Of patients who have a achieved a CR, only a small proportion (perhaps 15%) will be long-term survivors if no additional therapy is administered.[40] Continuation, or maintenance, therapy appears to be necessary to eradicate the remaining leukemia cells that are undetectable during remission. The growth fraction of leukemia cells is relatively small, and the cell cycle time is fairly long. Therefore, only a small fraction of the total number of leukemia cells is susceptible at any given time to the effects of most anticancer drugs that are cell cycle phase-specific agents. Hence, a prolonged period of exposure to anticancer drugs is necessary to further reduce the malignant population. The most common maintenance therapy has consisted of a two-drug combination of mercaptopurine and methotrexate.[40] Mercaptopurine is given orally in doses of 50 to 90 mg/m^2/day, and methotrexate is given either orally, intravenously, or intramuscularly at doses of 15 to 30 mg/m^2/wk.

The optimal duration of maintenance therapy is not known, and current guidelines are based on empiric trial-and-error approaches. Most treatment programs use 2 to 6 years of maintenance therapy. In determining the length of maintenance therapy, the risk of off-therapy relapses must be considered in comparison to the risks of undesirable toxic effects of the therapy. Therapy may be stopped after 30 months of CCR or at least 12 months of continuous remission after an isolated nonmedullary relapse (CNS or testes). Results of several large long-term studies indicate that 70% of patients who elect to have therapy stopped in this fashion will remain disease-free and be long-term survivors.[40]

Although maintenance therapy is well tolerated, a significant problem is relapse while the patient is receiving therapy. A substantial fraction (perhaps 40%) of patients have a relapse during the maintenance phase of therapy, presumably as a result of the development of resistant disease. In addition, maintenance therapy is immunosuppressive and associated with the risk of opportunistic infections. Therefore, alternative strategies have been used to overcome both the development of resistance and to reduce the risk of infections and other complications.

Approaches to prevent bone marrow relapse during remission have included increasing the number of drugs administered during remission, periodic repetition of the agents used to induce the initial remission (referred to as "reinforcement" pulses), and intermittent rather than continuous chemotherapy. Use of more than two agents simultaneously does not appear to improve the rate of disease-free survival but does increase the toxicity of the therapy.[41] A recent approach to improving event-free survival includes a delayed reintensification phase, or reinduction.[26]

One approach to the maintenance therapy of ALL is rotational use of non-cross-resistant anticancer drugs early in therapy. This concept is based on the somatic mutation theory of Luria and Delbrück[42] and its further development by Goldie and Coldman.[43,44] This hypothesis states that intense early therapy and sequential or rotational use of multiple non-cross-resistant agents during maintenance therapy will reduce the likelihood of the emergence of a drug-resistant subpopulation of leukemia cells. Patients who have bone marrow relapses during this phase of therapy account for the largest fraction of patients who die of ALL, undoubtedly because of development of resistance, either by mutation or by selection, to the methotrexate-mercaptopurine combination usually administered during this phase of therapy. The rationale for administering additional non-cross-resistant agents during maintenance therapy is to reduce the opportunity for resistance to be manifested to the primary drug combination. Therefore, other effective agents such as etoposide, cyclophosphamide, cytarabine, teniposide, or additional anthracyclines may be administered during the maintenance phase of therapy in addition to the more customary methotrexate and mercaptopurine. However, the negative aspect is the increase in toxicity that may be encountered with some of these other agents. Because up to 50% of patients may be cured with the relatively well-tolerated methotrexate-mercaptopurine combination, the addition of more toxic drugs during continuation therapy may

Table 86.5 ▪ Adverse Prognostic Factors at Diagnosis of Acute Lymphocytic Leukemia

Age	Hematologic findings
<2 years	Elevated WBC count
>10 years	Elevated hemoglobin
Sex	Decreased platelet count
Male	FAB morphology
Race	L2, L3
Nonwhite	Immunologic markers
Physical findings	T-cell or B-cell leukemia
Hepatosplenomegaly	Cytogenetics
Lymphadenopathy	DNA index <1.16
Mediastinal mass (on chest roentgenogram)	Translocations
Lymphoblasts in CNS	Philadelphia chromosome

CNS, central nervous system; *WBC*, white blood cell; *FAB*, French-American-British.

result only in more morbidity for patients who may be cured with less aggressive therapy. This dilemma points out the need to develop a better understanding of the various subtypes of ALL and significant prognostic factors to more readily identify those patients who would be expected to do well with less intense therapy.

PROGNOSIS

Numerous variables are associated with the likely prognosis for patients with ALL. Table 86.5 lists some of the most widely recognized factors. Age at diagnosis is important, with children younger than 2 years of age and those older than 10 years of age having a higher mortality rate with current standard therapy. Several studies have shown that males have a slightly greater risk of relapse than females, even after accounting for nonmedullary relapses in the testes, which apparently act as a pharmacologic sanctuary from systemic anticancer drugs. WBC count at diagnosis is universally recognized as an important prognostic factor since higher WBC counts represent a greater tumor burden and are associated with a poorer outcome. T-cell and mature B-cell leukemias are associated with a poorer prognosis than leukemia expressing other SIgs. Many series have shown that nonwhite patients may have a poorer prognosis although there has been speculation that this may be due, at least in part, to socioeconomic factors that may cause delays in diagnosis and treatment. A thymic or mediastinal mass on chest roentgenograms is a feature of high-risk disease, although this is often associated with T-cell disease. Patients with lymphoblasts detectable in the CSF at diagnosis have a poorer prognosis.

Genetic characteristics, in addition to clinical factors, also have prognostic significance. Ploidy, defined as the number of chromosomes present in leukemic clones, is an established prognostic factor. The types and frequency of various ploidies are summarized in Table 86.2. Leukemic cell clones with more than 53 chromosomes or a ratio of DNA content greater than 1.15 times normal (sometimes referred to as the "DNA index") are more responsive to treatment and this type of disease has a better prognosis.[45] Cytogenetic studies have shown that leukemic clones that exhibit various types of translocations are associated with a poorer prognosis. For example, in children younger than 1 year of age, 70 to 80% have rearrangement of the *MLL* gene, indicative of poor prognosis.[46] In adolescent and adult patients, poor prognostic factors include the frequency of *MLL* rearrangements and the presence of the Philadelphia chromosome.[9]

These risk factors often cosegregate; patients with T-cell leukemia often have a high WBC count, for example. Therefore, none of these factors should be regarded as having completely independent prognostic value, and any treatment plan that uses these factors to individualize therapy should consider how these factors interact and correlate with one another. It appears likely that as our understanding of the molecular biology of leukemia improves, the genetically oriented prognostic factors will gradually replace the more traditional clinical factors in assigning risk categories and designing treatment regimens. On the other hand, any prognostic factor is important relative only to the treatment currently used. If a major new treatment advance is found, all currently used prognostic factors could lose their predictive value.

Acute Myelogenous Leukemia

AML differs in many respects from ALL, particularly with regard to its age distribution and prognosis. Whereas ALL is primarily a childhood disease, AML is primarily a disease of adults. In addition, in both children and adults, it has proved much more resistant to treatment, and to achieve a cure, most patients require much more intense, toxic, and myelosuppressive therapy than that required for ALL. The most successful treatment programs available today result in cure rates of no more than about 40% of all patients with AML. In addition, the more intense therapy results in greater morbidity and mortality, particularly in older patients, and may limit the amount of effective therapy that can be administered. BMT has a more well-established role in the treatment of AML for those patients who have an acceptably matched donor.

TREATMENT

Remission Induction Therapy

Although early attempts to treat AML used the same drugs that had been found to be successful in ALL, the two groups of diseases are quite different in their biologic characteristics and their responses to therapy. The two most effective agents in the treatment of AML are cytarabine and daunorubicin. Almost all current treatment protocols administer 5 to 10 days of cytarabine by continuous infusion. Daunorubicin is administered daily for 2 or 3 days, either before cytarabine or simultaneously at the beginning of the cytarabine continuous infusion. This standard induction combination known as 7+3 will result in CRs in 64 to 75% of patients.[47–50] However, the challenge in the treatment of AML is to maintain remission. Relapses are usually due to resistant disease in the bone marrow; isolated extramedullary relapses are uncommon. In addition, relapses occur earlier than with ALL, generally during the first year after diagnosis. Therefore, most current treatment regimens have emphasized early intense therapy, but use a shorter duration of therapy, relative to that for ALL. Other drugs that may be used in the treatment of AML are etoposide, fludarabine, cladribine, thioguanine, amsacrine, mitoxantrone, and idarubicin.[51,52] In recent research the replacement of daunorubicin with idarubicin has resulted in not only a higher CR rate but also longer remission and survival.[53–55] Suppression of the WBCs and platelets appears to be greater in the idarubicin and cytarabine combination.[53] The Children's Cancer Group and the Australian Leukemia Study Group recently reported that intensification of induction chemotherapy prolongs remissions in both children and adults with AML. These data are consistent with the concept that early leukemia cell kill prevents the emergence of drug-resistant leukemia clones.[56] Recent data also suggest that high doses of cytarabine at 3 g/m^2 administered on alternate days for 8 doses compared with conventional doses of cytarabine will significantly prolong remission and disease-free survival. However, there is clear evidence that intensified induction therapy will result in significantly more myelosuppression during postremission therapy.[57] Current treatment approaches for both adults[58] and children[59] with AML have recently been reviewed.

Central Nervous System Therapy

Treatment of the CNS is of lesser importance in AML since the primary reason for treatment failure is bone marrow relapse. Although lymphoblasts are found in the CSF more frequently in AML than in ALL, treatment of the CNS is often limited to intrathecal drugs, with irradiation administered at the end of therapy to patients with CNS disease at diagnosis. CNS treatment delivered earlier has no effect on disease-free survival because of the inadequacy of systemic therapy and bone marrow relapses. Intrathecal therapy usually consists of methotrexate, cytarabine, and hydrocortisone.

Postremission Therapy

Chemotherapy

Postremission consolidation therapy is an integral component of virtually all contemporary clinical trials for AML. Without continued intensification therapy or BMT, survival rates are less than 30% at 5 years. Because of these results, intensification therapy or the "ultimate intensification" of BMT has been explored with a suggested benefit on survival. In those patients with M3 AML, all-*trans* retinoic acid (ATRA) has been combined with cytarabine and daunorubicin, demonstrating a significant improvement in leukemia-free survival. Early results using ATRA alone revealed a CR rate of 85 to 90%, but relapse occurred within 1 year in most patients. Also what is known as the "ATRA syndrome" occurred in one-third to one-half of the patients and was fatal for some. This syndrome, which is characterized by a rapid increase in WBC counts, appears to be minimized with the combination of intensive chemotherapy. Disease-free survival rates as high as 75 to 81% with CR rates of 90% have been achieved with ATRA and chemotherapy.[60–65]

Bone Marrow Transplantation

Allogeneic BMT from a fully histocompatible family donor was evaluated in children and young adults with AML in first remission as an alternative to continued chemotherapy.[66–68] The early results were quite favorable compared with chemotherapy with leukemia-free survival rates of 50 to 65% at 5 years. However, with increasing age and the presence of unfavorable cytogenetic abnormalities these rates decrease.[69] Cassileth et al.[70] reviewed patients between 16 and 55 years of age and compared high-dose cytarabine, allogeneic transplantation, and autologous transplantation as postremission therapy. Each group received one course of chemotherapy postremission, consisting of idarubicin and cytarabine, and then was given either of the three modalities. The results revealed better survival for those patients receiving chemotherapy than those receiving autologous transplantation. A marginal advantage was seen in those receiving chemotherapy compared with those receiving allogeneic transplantation. The use of matched, unrelated or mismatched family donors should be reserved for the patient in a second or subsequent remission. BMT is complicated by the occurrence of both acute and chronic GVHD, and only a limited number of patients with AML (25 to 40%) have compatible bone marrow donors. Therefore, bone marrow transplants do not offer a universal cure for this disease. Several large prospective randomized studies of AML in pediatric patients have concluded that autologous BMT is not superior to intensive chemotherapy in the first remission.[71–74]

PROGNOSIS

Prognostic factors for AML are less well defined than for ALL, primarily because the overall survival is much poorer. Nevertheless, a number of variables have been identified

Table 86.6 ▪ Adverse and Favorable Prognostic Factors at Diagnosis of Acute Myelocytic Leukemia

Adverse	FAB morphology
Age	M4 or M5 (with high WBC, <2 yr old and extramedullary disease)
>60 years	Cytogenetics
<2 years	All abnormal karyotypes (approximately 55–85% are abnormal)
Sex	Monosomy 7
Male	*Favorable*
Secondary AML or prior myelodysplastic syndrome	Down's syndrome with AML
Hematologic findings	FAB M1 with Auer rods
Elevated WBC count (>100,000/μL)	t(8;21) (adult only)
Extramedullary leukemia (non-CNS)	inv16/M4Eo subtype
	t(15;17)

AML, acute myelocytic leukemia; *WBC,* white blood cell; *CNS,* central nervous system; *FAB,* French-American-British.

that are associated either with a poor likelihood of achieving a clinical remission or with a short remission. These factors are summarized in Table 86.6. Variables associated with a poor prognosis are advancing age, a high WBC count, and a high degree of bone marrow involvement. Cytogenetic studies are becoming increasingly important for prognosis as well as treatment selection. A normal karyotype is associated with a favorable prognosis, as well as a number of specific chromosomal abnormalities such as t8;21 in adults with AML.[75,76]

Supportive Therapy for Acute Leukemias

The improving prognosis for the acute leukemias is due in large part to the advancements in supportive care that have occurred over the past 10 years. Deaths during induction therapy due to hemorrhage, infections, and metabolic derangements have been reduced as a consequence of the improved ability to manage these complications. In addition, deaths during remission due to opportunistic infections are less frequent today, and certain types of lethal infections, notably *Pneumocystis carinii* pneumonia, have been virtually eradicated from the population of leukemia patients. Use of central venous catheters has also simplified the delivery of complicated chemotherapy regimens although these devices are associated with significant complications of their own. The use of enteral and parenteral nutritional support has also been important in the management of these patients. All of these factors have permitted the routine use of more intense therapies in an attempt to develop effective, curative therapy for acute leukemia.

Infection in the immunosuppressed, granulocytopenic patient with cancer remains a significant cause of morbidity and mortality. The risk of life-threatening septicemia or pneumonia increases dramatically as the patient's granulocyte count decreases and as the duration of the granulocytopenia increases.[77] Since immunosuppressed patients are unable to mount a response to infectious organisms, the common clinical signs of infection (leukocytosis and purulence) may be absent. Therefore, fever is of supreme importance in diagnosing infections in the granulocytopenic patient, and the presence of fever in such patients should be regarded as a medical emergency. Infections that are not promptly treated progress rapidly, and death from septicemia or pneumonia may occur in a few hours. Prompt institution of empiric broad-spectrum antibiotic coverage will prevent mortality in most cases.

A potentially lethal opportunistic infection for immunosuppressed patients is pneumonia caused by *P. carinii.* This organism is ordinarily innocuous and is found virtually everywhere in the environment. However, in immunosuppressed patients with cancer, who are not necessarily granulocytopenic, it can produce a potentially fatal infection, and in the past has been a major cause of death during remission for patients with ALL. Low daily doses of trimethoprim/sulfamethoxazole (TMP/SMX) administered prophylactically during remission prevented this infection in virtually all immunosuppressed patients with ALL.[78] Equally effective protection can be achieved by administering TMP/SMX for only 3 consecutive days each week.[79] This reduced exposure has the advantage of fewer adverse effects, primarily, the occurrence of systemic mycoses. Although neutropenia has been reported as an unwanted consequence of prophylaxis with TMP/SMX in some studies, no increase in neutropenia was detected in this study. For those few patients who cannot tolerate TMP/SMX, dapsone and inhaled pentamidine are viable alternatives and have been found to be safe and effective.[80]

Tumor lysis syndrome (TLS) is a complication of the initial antileukemic therapy in some patients, particularly those with a very high initial WBC count. These metabolic derangements are more often seen in those with ALL, especially the T- and B-cell types, than in those with AML.[81] TLS refers to the metabolic disturbances found with a very brisk response to induction therapy that results in significant cell death and the release of intracellular nucleoproteins into the circulation. The purine byproducts of these nucleoproteins are metabolized by xanthine oxidase to uric acid, which in high concentrations can produce obstructive urate nephropathy. The metabolic disturbances include hyperuricemia, hyperphosphatemia, hyperkalemia, and hypocalcemia. Patients may also experience acute renal failure. There is a clear association with hyperuricemia and acute renal failure.[82,83] Other factors that influence the risk of acute renal failure in those with TLS include hyperphosphatemia, low glomerular filtration rate before therapy, xanthinuria, intravascular volume depletion, and infiltration of renal parenchyma by malignant cells.[82–84] Therefore, the goals of treatment of TLS are to prevent renal failure and the worsening of metabolic disturbances. This is primarily done through increasing the excretion of the aforementioned metabolic contents. Vigorous hydration and urinary alkalinization (to increase the solubility of uric acid in the urine) should be initiated in patients with an initial high WBC count. However, alkalinization of the urine may lead to massive phosphate crystalluria because phosphate precipitates at alkaline pH so the goal of alkalinization should be to maintain urine pH between 6.5 and 7.0.[85]

Administration of allopurinol, a xanthine oxidase inhibitor, prevents the production of uric acid and the development of nephropathy. However, xanthine nephropathy must be considered during allopurinol therapy, especially if impaired renal function decreases the elimination of allopurinol. This would require a decrease in the dose of allopurinol. Currently, an agent, the enzyme urate oxidase, which converts uric acid to the water-soluble metabolite allantoin, thereby lowering plasma uric acid concentrations as well as urinary uric acid excretion is being investigated.[86]

Because of the bone marrow suppressive effects of both the disease and its therapy, most patients need extensive support with blood products, including platelet, erythrocyte, and occasionally, granulocyte transfusions. Hemorrhages are a cause of significant morbidity and mortality in patients with leukemia, and the ability to collect platelets either from whole blood or by plasmapheresis is essential in the modern therapy of leukemia. The hematocrit may be decreased as a result of decreased erythrocyte production, and packed red blood cells may be required to maintain the hematocrit at adequate levels. Granulocyte transfusions have no apparent role in the prevention of infection but, along with antibiotic therapy, may be effective in treating documented sepsis. However, because of the cost of preparing granulocyte transfusions, the very short life span of transfused granulocytes in the patient, and the serious side effects of granulocyte transfusions, this procedure is usually reserved for only the most gravely ill patients.

Cytokines (granulocyte colony-stimulating factor [G-CSF] and granulocyte-macrophage colony-stimulating factor [GM-CSF]) have been widely used in the treatment of patients with solid tumors and lymphomas to shorten the length and severity of neutropenia after treatment with antineoplastic drugs. The use of cytokines in acute leukemias has been less widespread. Although occasional patients may benefit from cytokine support during treatment for ALL, in general, the treatment does not produce prolonged neutropenia, and the benefit of cytokine use has not been established. In a pediatric study of 164 patients with ALL, aged 2 months to 17 years, patients received either G-CSF 10 mg/kg/day or placebo after remission induction therapy. The results found no benefit in infection site, neutropenia hospitalizations, or disease-free survival.[86a] In AML, cytokine use was initially avoided because of concern that cytokines, which stimulate the growth and release of cells from the myelocytic lineage, could potentially stimulate growth of leukemia cells as well. However, two recent double-blind, placebo-controlled studies[87,88] have evaluated the use of GM-CSF to reduce the length and severity of neutropenia in elderly patients being treated for primary acute myelocytic leukemia. The results of these studies were somewhat different. In the larger study,[87] 388 patients older than 60 years of age were evaluated, and no significant benefit of cytokine treatment was identified. The authors conclude that GM-CSF use cannot be recommended in such patients. However, in the smaller study,[88] 124 patients between 55 and 70 years of age were evaluated, and GM-CSF treatment was associated with shorter time to neutrophil recovery, a reduction in overall treatment-related toxicity, a reduction in infectious toxicity, and longer survival time. This article concluded that GM-CSF treatment was safe and efficacious in this group of patients. GM-CSF is generally considered a useful supportive measure in the elderly patient with AML. The G-CSF treatment, when used in the elderly patients with AML, has not demonstrated an equivalent effect.[89]

Disseminated intravascular coagulation is an occasional but life-threatening complication of AML, particularly for patients with progranulocytic leukemia (M3 AML), and results in severe hemorrhages. It is characterized by thrombocytopenia, hypofibrinogenemia, decreased factor V levels, and increased levels of fibrin split products. It is treated with low-dose heparin.

KEY POINTS

- Tremendous advances have been made in the treatment of the acute leukemias over the past 10 years, and the successes that have been achieved in the treatment of childhood ALL serve as a model for treatment of other human malignancies.
- Today, acute leukemias are potentially curable diseases in many patients, and considerable prolongation of a

useful and productive life can be achieved for many others.

- Current research efforts in immunology and molecular biology are likely to lead to powerful new treatments.
- AML is typically a disease of adults while ALL is a disease of childhood.
- AML is generally more resistant to treatment than ALL.
- Initial presenting symptoms result from bone marrow failure and include fatigue, weight loss, fever, pallor, purpura, and pain.
- A diagnosis of acute leukemia is made by performing a bone marrow aspirate, which contains a minimum of 25% blast cells.
- The primary treatment modality is chemotherapy for both AML and ALL.
- BMT plays an important role in the treatment of AML.
- Childhood ALL represents one of the success stories of cancer treatment.
- The treatment phases involved in ALL therapy include induction, consolidation, CNS, and maintenance treatment.
- The treatment phases for AML include remission induction and postremission therapy with either chemotherapy or BMT.
- ALL induction therapy involves the use of prednisone, vincristine, and either asparaginase or an anthracycline.
- The 7+3 regimen (cytarabine + daunorubicin) is the standard of care in AML for remission induction.
- Fever in a granulocytopenic patient should always be considered a medical emergency and requires immediate empiric antibiotic therapy.
- TLS is common in those with an initially high WBC count and consists of hyperphosphatemia, hyperuricemia, hyperkalemia, and hypocalcemia.
- Disseminated intravascular coagulation is a life-threatening complication primarily associated with M3 AML (promyelocytic leukemia).

REFERENCES

1. Clarkson B. The acute leukemias. In: Thorn GW, Adams RD, Braunwald E, et al., eds. Harrison's principles of internal medicine. 8th ed. New York: McGraw-Hill, 1977:1767–1777.
2. Wingo PA, Tong T, Bolden S. Cancer statistics. CA Cancer J Clin 45:8–30, 1995.
3. Gallo RD, Wong-Staal F. Retroviruses as etiologic agents of some animal and human leukemias and lymphomas and as tools for elucidating the molecular mechanism of leukemogenesis. Blood 60:545–556, 1982.
4. Sandler DP, Ross JA. Epidemiology of acute leukemia in children and adults. Semin Oncol 24:3–16, 1997.
5. Altman AJ, Schwartz AD. Malignant diseases of infancy, childhood and adolescence. Philadelphia: WB Saunders, 1983:187–238.
6. Bennett JM, Catovsky D, Daniel M-T, et al. Proposals for the classifications of the acute leukemias; French-American-British (FAB) co-operative group. Br J Haematol 33:451–458, 1976.
7. Pui C-H. Acute lymphoblastic leukemia. Pediatr Clin North Am 44:831–846, 1997.
8. Kishimoto T, Goyert S, Kikutani H, et al. CD antigens 1996. Blood 89:3502, 1997.
9. Pui C-H, Evans W. Acute lymphoblastic leukemia. N Engl J Med 339:605–615, 1998.
10. Pui C-H. Childhood leukemias (medical progress). N Engl J Med 332:1618–1630, 1995.
11. Pui C-H, Behm FG, Crist WM. Clinical and biologic relevance of immunologic marker studies in childhood acute lymphoblastic leukemia. Blood 82:343–362, 1993.
12. Marks DI, Kurz BW, Link MP, et al. High incidence of potential p53 inactivation in poor outcome childhood acute lymphoblastic leukemia at diagnosis. Blood 87:1155–1161, 1996.
13. Cline MJ. The molecular basis of leukemia. N Engl J Med 330:328–336, 1994.
14. Rubnitz JE, Downing JR, Pui C-H, et al. TEL gene rearrangement in acute lymphoblastic leukemia: a new genetic marker with prognostic significance. J Clin Oncol 15:1150–1157, 1997.
15. Fernbach DJ. Natural history of acute leukemia. In: Sutow WW, Fernbach DJ, Vietti TJ. Clinical pediatric oncology. 3rd ed. St Louis: CV Mosby, 1984:332–377.
16. Freeman AI, Pantazopoulos N, DeCastro L, et al. Infections in children with acute leukemia. Med Pediatr Oncol 1:67–73, 1975.
17. Farber S, Diamond LK, Mercer RD, et al. Temporary remissions in acute leukemia in children produced by folic antagonist 4-ametho-pteroylglutamic acid (aminopterin). N Engl J Med 238:787–793, 1948.
18. Fenaux P, Castaigne S, Chomienne C, et al. All trans retinoic acid treatment for patients with acute promyelocytic leukemia. Leukemia 6:64–72, 1992.
19. Gratas C, Menot ML, Dresch C, et al. Retinoic acid supports granulocytic but not erythroid differentiation of myeloid progenitors in normal bone marrow cells. Leukemia 7:1156–1162, 1993.
20. Castaigne S, Chomienne C, Daniel MT, et al. All trans retinoic acid as a differentiating therapy for acute promyelocytic leukemias. I, Clinical results. Blood 76:1704–1709, 1990.
21. Lazzarino M, Regazzi MB, et al. Clinical relevance of all-trans retinoic acid pharmacokinetics and its modulation in acute promyelocytic leukemia. Leuk Lymphoma 23:539–543, 1996.
22. Lapart G, Larson R. Treatment of adult acute lymphoblastic leukemia. Semin Oncol 24:70–82, 1997.
23. Jacquillat C, Weil M, Gemon MF, et al. Combination therapy in 130 patients with acute lymphoblastic leukemia (protocol 06 LA 66-Paris). Cancer Res 33:3278–3284, 1973.
24. Ortega JA, Nesbit ME Jr, Donaldson MH, et al. L-Asparaginase, vincristine and prednisone for induction of first remission in acute lymphocytic leukemia. Cancer Res 37:535–540, 1977.
25. Sackman JF, Pavlovsky S, Penalver JA, et al. Evaluation of induction of remission, intensification and central nervous system prophylactic treatment in acute lymphoblastic leukemia. Cancer 34:418, 1974.
26. Tubergen DG, Gilchrist GS, O'Brien RT, et al. Improved outcome with delayed intensification for children with acute lymphoblastic leukemia and intermediate presenting features: a Children's Cancer Group phase III trial. J Clin Oncol 11:527–537, 1993.
27. George P, Pinkel D. CNS radiation in children with acute lymphocytic leukemia in remission [Abstract]. Proc Amer Assoc Cancer Res 6:22, 1965.
28. Aur RJA, Simone JV, Hustu HO, et al. A comparative study of central nervous system irradiation and intensive chemotherapy early in remission of childhood acute lymphocytic leukemia. Cancer 29:381, 1972.
29. Nesbit ME, Robison LL, Littman PS, et al. Presymptomatic central nervous system therapy in previously untreated childhood acute lymphoblastic leukaemia: comparison of 1800 rad and 2400 rad. A report for Children's Cancer Study Group. Lancet 1:461, 1981.
30. Aur RJA, Hustu HO, Verzosa MS, et al. Comparison of two methods of preventing central nervous system leukemia. Blood 42:349–357, 1973.
31. Bleyer WA. Clinical pharmacology of intrathecal methotrexate. II. An improved dosage regimen derived from age-related pharmacokinetics. Cancer Treat Rep 61:1419–1425, 1977.
32. Gilchrist GS, Tubergen DG, Sather HN, et al. Low numbers of CSF blasts at diagnosis do not predict for the development of CNS leukemia in children with intermediate-risk acute lymphoblastic leukemia: a Children's Cancer Group report. J Clin Oncol 12:2594–2600, 1994.
33. Freeman AI, Weinberg V, Brecher ML, et al. Comparison of intermediate-dose methotrexate with cranial irradiation for the post-induction treatment of acute lymphocytic leukemia in children. N Engl J Med 308:477–484, 1983.
34. Evans WE, Crom WR, Yalowich JC. Methotrexate. In: Evans WE, Schentag JJ, Jusko WJ, eds. Applied pharmacokinetics; principles of therapeutic drug monitoring. 2nd ed. Spokane: Applied Therapeutics, 1986:1009–1056.
35. Balis FM, Savitch JL, Bleyer WA, et al. Remission induction of meningeal leukemia with high-dose intravenous methotrexate. J Clin Oncol 3:485–489, 1985.
36. Freeman AI, Weinberg VE, Brecher ML, et al. Comparison of intermediate-dose methotrexate with cranial irradiation for the post-induction treatment of acute lymphocytic leukemia in children. N Engl J Med 308:477–484, 1983.
37. Evans WE, Crom WR, Abromowitch M, et al. Clinical pharmacodynamics of

high-dose methotrexate in acute lymphocytic leukemia; identification of a relation between concentration and effect. N Engl J Med 314:471–477, 1986.
38. Relling MV, Mahmoud H, Pui C-H, et al. Intravenous etoposide therapy achieves potentially cytotoxic concentrations in cerebrospinal fluid of children with acute lymphoblastic leukemia [Abstract]. Proc Annu Meet Am Assoc Cancer Res 35:A1438, 1994.
39. Jones B, Freeman AI, Shuster JJ, et al. Lower incidence of meningeal leukemia when prednisone is replaced by dexamethasone in the treatment of acute lymphocytic leukemia. Med Pediatr Oncol 19:269–275, 1991.
40. Simone JV, Rivera G. Management of acute leukemia. In: Sutow WW, Fernbach DJ, Vietti TJ, eds. Clinical pediatric oncology. 3rd ed. St Louis: CV Mosby, 1984:378–402.
41. Aur RJA, Simone JV, Verzosa JS, et al. Childhood acute lymphocytic leukemia: study VIII. Cancer 42:2123–2134, 1978.
42. Luria SE, Delbrück M. Genetics 28:491–511, 1943.
43. Goldie JH, Coldman AJ. A mathematical model for relating the drug sensitivity of tumors to their spontaneous mutation rate. Cancer Treat Rep 63:1727–1733, 1979.
44. Goldie JH, Coldman AJ, Gudauskas GA. Rationale for the use of alternating non-cross-resistant chemotherapy. Cancer Treat Rep 66:439–449, 1982.
45. Williams DL, Tsiatis A, Brodeur GM, et al. Prognostic importance of chromosome number in 136 untreated children with acute lymphoblastic leukemia. Blood 60:864–871, 1982.
46. Pui C-H, Kane JR, Crist WM. Biology and treatment of infant leukemia. Leukemia 9:762–769, 1995.
47. Lister TA, Rohatiner AZS. The treatment of acute myelogenous leukemia in adults. Semin Hematol 19:172–192, 1982.
48. Gale RP. Advances in the treatment of acute myelogenous leukemia. N Engl J Med 300:1189–1199, 1979.
49. Gale RP, Foon KA, Cline M, et al. Intensive chemotherapy for acute myelogenous leukemia. Ann Intern Med 94:753–757, 1981.
50. Mayer RJ, Davis RB, Schiffer CA, et al. Intensive post-remission chemotherapy in adults with acute myeloid leukemia. N Engl J Med 3331:896–903, 1994.
51. Santana VM, Hurwitz CA, Blakley RL, et al. Complete hematologic remissions induced by 2-chlorodeoxyadenosine in children with newly diagnosed acute myeloid leukemia. Blood 84:1237–1242, 1994.
52. Gandhi V. Fludarabine for treatment of adult acute myelogenous leukemia. Leuk Lymphoma 11(Suppl 2):7–13, 1993.
53. Wiernik PH, Banks PC, Case DC, et al. Cytarabine plus idarubicin or daunorubicin as induction and consolidation therapy for previously untreated adults with acute myeloid leukemia. Blood 79:313–319, 1992.
54. Berman E, Heller G, Santorsa J, et al. Results of a randomized trial comparing idarubicin and cytosine arabinoside with daunorubicin and cytosine arabinoside in adult patients with newly diagnosed acute myelogenous leukemia. Blood 77:1666–1674, 1991.
55. Vogler WR, Velez-Garcia E, Omura G, et al. A phase 3 trial comparing daunorubicin or idarubicin combined with cytosine arabinoside in acute myelogenous leukemia. J Clin Oncol 10:1103–1111, 1992.
56. Woods W, Kobrinsky N, Buckley J, et al. Timed-sequential induction therapy improves post-remission outcome in acute myeloid leukemia: a report from the Children's Cancer Group. Blood 87:4979–4989, 1996.
57. Bishop JF, Matthews JP, Youg GA, et al. A randomized study of high dose cytarabine in induction in acute myeloid leukemia. Blood 87:1710–1717, 1996.
58. Stone RM, Mayer RJ. Treatment of the newly diagnosed adult with de novo acute myeloid leukemia. Hematol Oncol Clin North Am 7:47–64, 1993.
59. Hurwitz CA, Mounce KG, Grier HE. Treatment of patients with acute myelogenous leukemia: review of clinical trials of the past decade. J Pediatr Hematol Oncol 17:185–197, 1995.
60. Chessells JM, O'Callaghan U, Hardisty RM: Acute myeloid leukemia in childhood: clinical features and prognosis. Br J Haematol 6:555–564, 1986.
61. Creutzig U, Ritter J, Schellong G: Identification of two risk groups in childhood acute myelogenous leukemia after therapy intensification in study AML-BFM-83 as compared with study AML-BFM-78. Blood 75:1932–1940, 1990.
62. Ravindranath Y, Steuber CP, Krischer H, et al. High dose cytarabine for intensification of early therapy of childhood acute myeloid leukemia: a Pediatric Oncology Group study. J Clin Oncol 9:572–580, 1991.
63. Tallman M, Anderson J, Schiffer C, et al. Phase III randomized study of all-trans-retionic acid (ATRA) vs. daunorubicin and cytosine arabinoside as induction therapy and ATRA vs observation as maintenance therapy for patients with previously untreated acute promyelocytic leukemia [Abstract]. Blood 86:125, 1995.
64. Wells R, Woods W, Lamphin B, et al. Impact of high dose cytarabine and asparaginase intensification on childhood acute myeloid leukemia: a report from the Children's Cancer Group. J Clin Oncol 11:538–545, 1993.
65. Kanamaru A, Takemoto Y, Tanimoto M, et al. All-trans retionic acid for the treatment of newly diagnosed acute promyelocytic leukemia. Blood 85:1202–1206, 1995.
66. Sanders JE, Thomas ED, Buckner CE, et al. Marrow transplantation of children in first remission of acute nonlymphoblastic leukemia: an update. Blood 66:460–462, 1985.
67. Woods W, Kobrinsky N, Neudorf S, et al. Intensively timed induction therapy followed by autologous or allogeneic bone marrow transplantation for children with acute myeloid leukemia or myelodysplastic syndrome: A Children's Cancer Group pilot study. J Clin Oncol 11:1448–1457, 1993.
68. McGlave PB, Haake RJ, Bostrom BC, et al. Allogeneic bone marrow transplantation for acute nonlymphocytic leukemia in first remission. Blood 72:1512–1517, 1988.
69. Leith CP, Kopecky KJ, Godwin J, et al. Acute myeloid leukemia in the elderly: assessment of multidrug resistance (MDR1) and cytogenetics distinguishes biologic subgroups with remarkably distinct responses for standard chemotherapy: a Southwest Oncology Group study. Blood 89:3323–3329, 1997.
70. Cassileth PA, Harrington DP, Appelbaum FR, et al. Chemotherapy compared with autologous or allogeneic bone marrow transplantation in the management of acute myeloid leukemia in first remission. N Engl J Med 339:1649–1656, 1998.
71. Ravindranath Y, Yeager A, Chang M, et al. Autologous bone marrow transplantation versus intensive consolidation chemotherapy for acute myeloid leukemia in childhood. N Engl J Med 334:1428–1434, 1996.
72. Amadori S, Testi AM, Arico M, et al. Prospective comparative study of bone marrow transplantation and postremission chemotherapy for childhood acute myelogenous leukemia. J Clin Oncol 11:1046–1954, 1993.
73. Lowenberg B, Verdonck LJ, Dekker AW, et al. Autologous bone marrow transplantation in acute myeloid leukemia in first remission: results of Dutch prospective study. J Clin Oncol 8:287–294, 1990.
74. Harousseau JL, Cahn JY, Pignon B, et al. Comparison of autologous bone marrow transplantation and intensive chemotherapy as postremission therapy in adult myeloid leukemia. Blood 90:2978–2986, 1997.
75. Arthur DC, Berger R, Golomb HM, et al. The clinical significance of karyotype in acute myelogenous leukemia. Cancer Genet Cytogenet 40:203–216, 1989.
76. Fourth International Workshop on Chromosomes in Leukemia, 1982. Clinical significance of chromosomal abnormalities in acute nonlymphoblastic leukemia. Cancer Genet Cytogenet 11:332–350, 1984.
77. Schimpff SC. Therapy of infection in patients with granulocytopenia. Med Clin North Am 61:1101–1118, 1977.
78. Hughes WT, Kuhn S, Chaudhary S, et al. Successful chemoprophylaxis for *Pneumocystis carinii* pneumonitis. N Engl J Med 297:1419–1426, 1977.
79. Hughes WT, Rivera GK, Schell MJ, et al. Successful intermittent chemoprophylaxis for *Pneumocystis carinii* pneumonitis. N Engl J Med 316:1627–1632, 1987.
80. Slavin MA, Hoy JF, Stewart K, et al. Oral dapsone versus nebulized pentamidine for *Pneumocystic carinii* pneumonia prophylaxis: an open randomized prospective trial to assess efficacy and haematological toxicity. AIDS 6:1169–1174, 1992.
81. Bunin NJ, Pui CH: Differing complications of hyperleukocytosis in children with acute lymphoblastic or acute nonlymphoblastic leukemia. J Clin Oncol 3:1590–1595, 1985.
82. Kjellstrand CM, Cambell DC II, von Hartitzsch B, et al. Hyperuricemic acute renal failure. Arch Intern Med 133:349–359, 1974.
83. Jones DP, Stapleton FB, Kalwinsky D, et al. Renal dysfunction and hyperuricemia at presentation and relapse of acute lymphoblastic leukemia. Med Pediatr Oncol 18:283–286, 1990.
84. Band PR, Silverberg DS, Henderson JE, et al. Xanthine nephropathy in a patient with lymphosarcoma treated with allopurinol. N Engl J Med 283:354–357, 1970.
85. Jones DP, Mahmoud H, Chesney RW. Tumor lysis syndrome: pathogenesis and management. Pediatr Nephrol 9:206–212, 1995.
86. Pui C-H, Relling MV, et.al. Urate oxidase in prevention and treatment of hyperuricemia associated with lymphoid malignancies. Leukemia 11:1813–1816, 1997.
86a. Pui CH, Boyett JM, Hubes WT, et al. Human granulocyte colony-stimulating factor after induction chemotherapy in children with acute lymphoblastic leukemia. N Engl J Med 336:1781–1787, 1997.
87. Stone RM, Berg DT, George SL, et al. Granulocyte-macrophage colony-stimulating factor after initial chemotherapy for elderly patients with acute myelogenous leukemia. N Engl J Med 332:1671–1677, 1995.
88. Rowe JM, Anderson JW, Mazza JJ, et al. A randomized placebo-controlled phase III study of granulocyte-macrophage colony-stimulating factor in adult patients (< 55 to 70 years of age) with acute myelogenous leukemia: a study of the Eastern Cooperative Oncology Group (E1490). Blood 86:457–462, 1995.
89. Godwin JE, Kopecky KJ, Head DR, et al. A double-blind placebo-controlled trial of granulocyte colony-stimulating factor in elderly patients with previously untreated acute myeloid leukemia. A Southwest Oncology Group study. Blood 91:3607-3615, 1998.

CHAPTER 87

LYMPHOMAS

Rebecca S. Finley and Clarence L. Fortner

DEFINITION

Lymphoid malignancies may manifest in either the bone marrow and peripheral blood or in any other tissue where lymphocytes may aggregate. When they present as extramedullary tumors arising primarily in the lymph nodes or other sites, these tumors are called lymphomas; when the bone marrow is the predominant site of the disease, they are classified as leukemias. Lymphomas are generally separated into Hodgkin's disease (HD) and non-Hodgkin's lymphomas (NHLs). The term "non-Hodgkin's lymphomas" represents multiple diseases with diverse morphologic, immunophenotypic, chromosomal, and clinical features.

TREATMENT GOALS: LYMPHOMAS

- Attempt cure of disease with combination chemotherapy regimens
- Produce significant, long-term remission of disease
- Minimize side effects of therapy

PATHOPHYSIOLOGY

Anatomy and Physiology of the Lymphoreticular System

The lymphoreticular system constitutes the anatomic basis of both cellular and humoral immunity. Lymphocytes are the principal cellular component of the lymphoreticular system and are widely distributed in the body both singly and in aggregated centers (most commonly the lymph nodes). Reticulum cells and cells of the monocyte-macrophage series are also included in this system. Lymphoid cells originate in the bone marrow, undergo differentiation, and migrate by way of the blood and lymphatic vessels to populate the other lymphoreticular tissues (Fig. 87.1). As lymphocytes differentiate, their morphologic appearance changes, and they sequentially express different cell surface antigens. T lymphocytes are processed through the thymus gland and are responsible for cell-mediated immunity. T lymphocytes are the predominant lymphocytes in peripheral blood and occupy the deep cortex of the lymph nodes. B lymphocytes are derived from the bone marrow and confer humoral immunity. B lymphocytes constitute only 10 to 15% of circulating lymphocytes and predominate in the follicles of the lymph nodes.

Malignant Transformation

Most lymphomas can be classified by their cellular origin; however, the precise cellular origin of HD has been difficult to establish. In recent years, newly identified immunologic characteristics suggest that the characteristic cells of HD, the Reed-Sternberg (R-S) cells may be some type of altered B cell.[1] Also, because HD is predominantly a disease of lymph nodes, it has been suggested that R-S cells might also come from some type of rare cell that resides only in lymphoid tissue.[2]

NHLs result from the malignant transformation of normal lymphoid cells at specific stages of differentiation. Like other malignancies, cytogenetic abnormalities have been identified that are associated with NHLs. In contrast to many other types of malignancies, however, most NHLs have only one or a very few cytogenetic changes. The most common type of changes are oncogenes activated by chromosomal translocations or tumor suppressor genes inactivated by chromosomal deletions or mutations.[3] After the malignant transformation, there is a clonal expansion of the malignant cells. Although some NHL cells may morphologically resemble the normal lymphocyte or lympho-

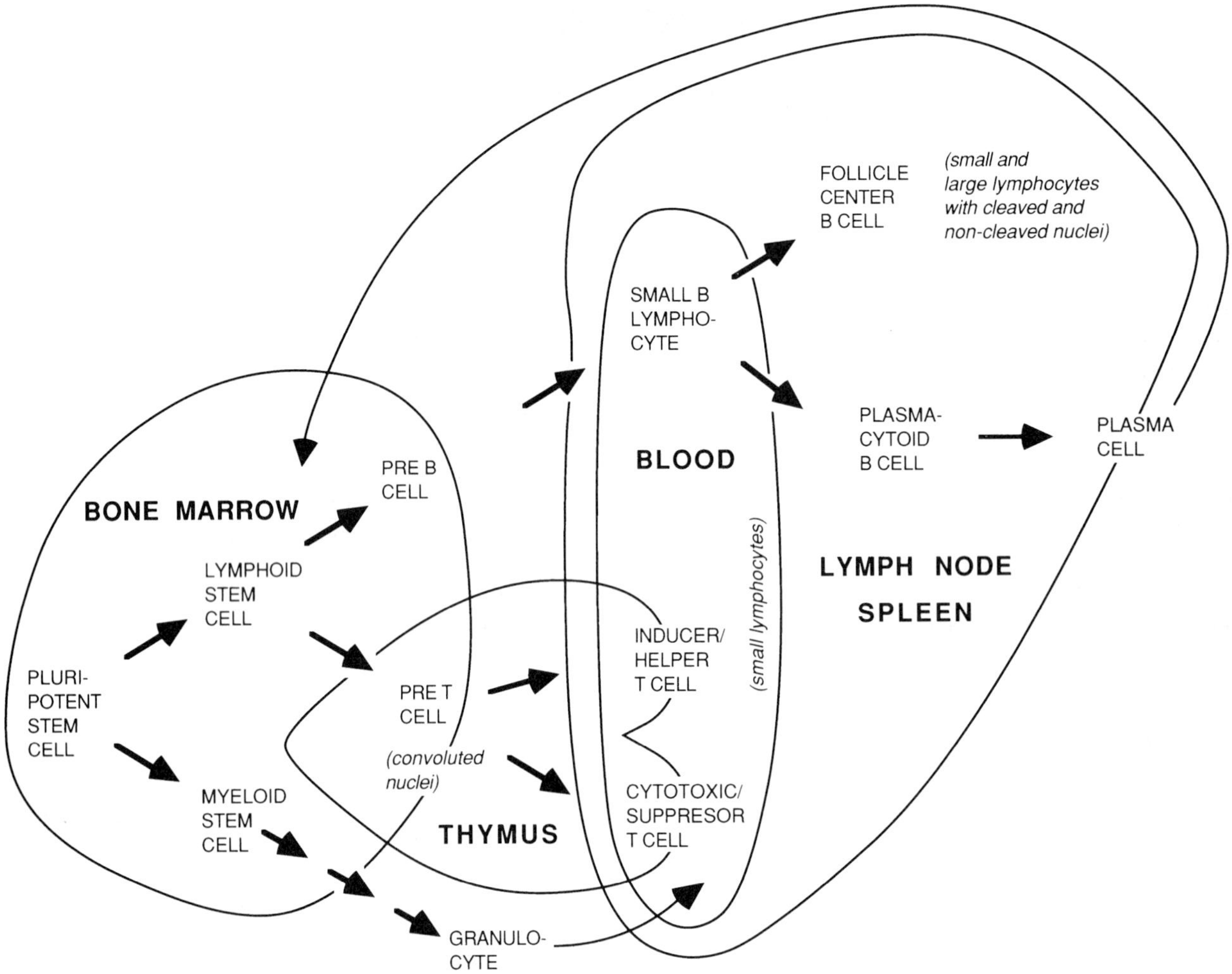

Figure 87.1. Tissue distribution of lymphocytes. (Reprinted with permission from Aisenber AC. Cell lineage in lymphoproliferative disease. Am J Med 74:680, 1983.)

cyte precursor at the stage when the transformation occurred, others may appear quite different. Lymphoma cells, however, tend to retain the same immunophenotype as their normal counterparts, and thus assessment of the cell surface antigens may be used to determine the exact type of NHL. The clinical course of the NHL is influenced by the stage at which the malignant transformation occurs. If the transformation occurs in a stage where rapid proliferation normally occurs, the lymphoma is likely to be a rapidly progressive disease. If the transformation occurs in more mature cells or progenitor resting stages, the lymphoma is likely to progress more slowly. In developed countries such as the United States, most adult NHLs are derived from B lymphocytes (85%), whereas only about 15% are of T-cell origin.

EPIDEMIOLOGY

Incidence

The incidence of lymphomas in the United States appears to be rising. The incidence of NHL has been reported to have increased 50% over the past 15 years while the incidence of HD has decreased slightly, probably owing to more accurate diagnoses. The American Cancer Society estimated that during 1999 there will be 7,200 new cases of HD and 56,800 new cases of NHL, with 1,300 and 25,700 deaths attributed to each disease, respectively.[4] Although the precise reason for the increase in lymphomas is unknown, both the aging of the U.S. population and the increased number of persons with severe immunosuppression are believed to be at least partially responsible.[5] The incidence of NHL increases steadily from childhood to age 80, and it is more common in males than in females.[6] HD exhibits a bimodal incidence curve, with the first peak occurring in the late 20s, after which there is a decline in incidence until about age 45. After age 45, the incidence increases steadily with age. HD is also more common in males than females[7] and more common in Whites than Blacks. Interestingly, an increased risk of HD correlates with an increasing level of education.[8]

Etiology

Although the etiology of most lymphomas is unknown, a number of factors have been associated with an increased risk. Patients with immunodeficiency disorders, either acquired (e.g., acquired immunodeficiency syndrome [AIDS] or caused by immunosuppressive therapies) or congenital (e.g., Wiskott-Aldrich syndrome, ataxia-telangiectasia), appear to have an increased risk of NHL.[5,9,10] Patients receiving chronic immunosuppressive therapy after organ transplantation to prevent graft rejection have a substantial risk. It has been estimated that 2% of patients with renal transplants and 5% of patients with heart transplants ultimately develop a NHL.[11] Patients who undergo allogeneic bone marrow or peripheral blood stem cell transplants are also at increased risk.[11] In each of these situations, it appears that the risk correlates with the severity of immunosuppression.[12] Chronic inflammation associated with autoimmune disorders such as Hashimoto's thyroiditis or Sjögren's syndrome[5] promotes the development of mucosa-associated lymphoid tissue (MALT), which can ultimately progress to lymphoma. Patients with autoimmune disorders such as rheumatoid arthritis or systemic lupus erythematosus frequently receive chronic immunosuppressive therapy; however, it is not clear whether it is the underlying autoimmune disorder or the immunosuppression that increases their risk of NHL.[11,13]

Infectious etiologies have been suggested for both NHL and HD. The Epstein-Barr virus (EBV) has been the most extensively studied viral pathogen. EBV is the cause of infectious mononucleosis and when it infects B lymphocytes in vitro, it can transform them into immortal lymphoblastoid cell lines.[11,14,15] EBV has been linked with the development of Burkitt's lymphoma in African children[16,17] and with HD.

There has been a small (3-fold), but consistent, increased risk of HD among persons who have had infectious mononucleosis.[18–20] Also, in some series, the proportion of patients with HD who have elevated titers of antibody against EBV is larger than expected and enhanced activation of EBV may precede the development of HD.[21–25] An important finding is that DNAs of EBV and EBV-encoded genes[26] have been detected in some R-S cells[27–33]; however at least 50% of patients with HD show no evidence of EBV. It is not clear whether EBV has a direct role in the development of HD or whether EBV infection is a result of a decreased immune competency that is linked to the pathogenesis of HD.[23] Also, because of the high prevalence of EBV in the general population, coincidence cannot be entirely ruled out. Epidemiologic studies reported clustering of patients with HD in a high school.[34,35] Familial studies also suggested an increased risk in first-degree relatives, especially siblings of young adult patients,[36] and there is an association of HD with certain leukocyte antigens.[37] Overall, there is no evidence to support the hypothesis that HD is transmitted by person-to-person contact.[24]

Two other viruses have also been associated with the development of lymphomas. Human T-cell leukemia virus type 1 is transmitted through sexual contact and infected blood products and has been isolated from adult T-cell lymphoma/leukemias.[38] The Kaposi's sarcoma-associated herpes virus has also been isolated from some patients with AIDS-related lymphomas.[39]

In recent years, gastric infection with *Helicobacter pylori* has been implicated in the pathogenesis of primary gastric lymphomas. The chronic gastritis that results from the infection leads to MALT, which may progress to lymphoma.[40–42]

Other environmental, occupational, and therapeutic exposures associated with an increased risk of NHL include pesticides, solvents, woodworking, and some cancer chemotherapy drugs.[43] Ionizing radiation may also induce lymphomas, as evidenced by the increased incidence in survivors of Hiroshima and patients irradiated for ankylosing spondylitis.[1,44] Chronic phenytoin use may lead to a condition known as lymphoid hyperplasia or pseudolymphoma. In most cases, this condition regresses when the phenytoin is discontinued.[45]

Pathology

The diagnosis and classification of malignant lymphoma can be made by biopsy and histopathologic examination under a light microscope. In recent years, immunophenotypic and cytogenetic assessment of lymphoma cells have also aided in differentiating the various subtypes of lymphomas.

A biopsy specimen of HD reveals a heterogeneous cellular population of normal-appearing lymphocytes (predominantly helper T cells), eosinophils, plasma cells, and R-S cells. These R-S cells, the characteristic malignant cells of HD, are multinucleated giant cells that are usually required to make a pathologic diagnosis. The normal appearing host inflammatory cells that surround the R-S cells are the body's response to the tumor. Although 35 to 40% of patients with HD have cytogenetic abnormalities, no specific chromosomal marker has been identified. Several classifications have been used to categorize HD into various subtypes. The Rye classification (based on morphology) was widely used in the past, but the availability of more immunologic and molecular information has resulted in a new classification by the International Lymphoma Study Group. This system makes an important distinction between nodular lymphocyte predominance HD and the other subtypes, which are often called classic HD (Table 87.1).[46]

Nodular lymphocyte predominance Hodgkin's disease (NLPHD) represents about 5% of all HD cases. It differs both morphologically and immunologically from classic HD in that the R-S cells have vesicular, polylobulated nuclei resembling popcorn. As the name implies, a nodular pattern is almost always present and the background (infiltrate surrounding the R-S cells) is predominantly lymphocytes. The immunophenotype of NLPHD lacks the HD-associated antigens, CD15 and CD30, but expresses CD45 and B-cell associated antigens (CD19, CD20, CD22, and CD79a). NLPHD is often diagnosed while in the early stages (I or II), and most patients have a complete response (CR)to therapy with 90% of patients

Table 87.1 ▪ Comparison of REAL and Rye Classifications of Histologic Subtypes Found in Hodgkin's Disease

REAL Classification	Rye Classification
Lymphocyte predominance, nodular (with or without diffuse	Lymphocyte predominance, nodular (most cases)
Classic Hodgkin's Disease	
Lymphocyte-rich classic disease	Lymphocyte predominance, diffuse (most cases) Lymphocyte predominance, nodular (some cases)
Nodular sclerosis	Nodular sclerosis
Mixed cellularity	Mixed cellularity (most cases)
Lymphocyte depletion	Lymphocyte depletion

surviving >10 years.[1] However, patients with NLPHD have a higher risk of development of NHL than those with other types of HD.[47]

Classic HD is defined by the presence of R-S cells with a background of either nodular sclerosis, mixed cellularity, or lymphocyte depletion. A lymphocyte-rich subtype has also been recently described. Immunologically, cells are CD15- and CD30-positive and lack T- and B-cell antigens. Although most patients show cytogenetic abnormalities, no specific abnormality is characteristic for the disease.

The mixed-cellularity subtype contains an infiltrate of lymphocytes, epithelioid histiocytes, eosinophils, neutrophils, and plasma cells.[1] It represents 15 to 30% of all cases and may be seen at any age. Patients may be seen at any clinical stage and abdominal lymph node and splenic involvement are relatively common.

Lymphocyte-depleted HD is characterized by a predominance of variant R-S cells, with a hypocellular background. This subtype is the least common, accounting for <1% of cases and is most commonly seen in older patients and human immunodeficiency virus (HIV)-positive patients. Patients with the lymphocyte-depleted subtype often have symptomatic and disseminated disease.

Nodular-sclerosing HD is characterized by a nodular pattern with fibrous bands separating the nodules. The background contains lymphocytes, histiocytes, plasma cells, neutrophils, and eosinophils. Necrosis is frequently seen. This is the most common type of HD, accounting for 60 to 80% of all cases. It most frequently occurs in adolescents and young adults but can occur at any age. It is associated with a good prognosis, especially in localized disease.

HD cells release various cytokines that produce local and systemic reactions. These cytokines include interleukin (IL)-1, IL-2, IL-5, IL-6, tumor necrosis factor, interferon-γ, granulocyte-macrophage colony-stimulating factor, granulocyte colony-stimulating factor, macrophage colony-stimulating factor, and tumor growth factor-β. It is believed that release of these cytokines contributes to the "B" symptoms (i.e., fever, night sweats, and weight loss) and tumor growth factor-β may play a role in the fibrosis of nodular sclerosing HD.[48]

Unlike HD, the cellular origin of the various NHLs is well established. The classification of NHLs is based on their cellular origin (and at what point during lymphocyte differentiation the malignant transformation occurred), morphologic, cytogenetic, and immunologic characteristics of the malignant cells. Many different histologic classification systems have been used over the years. In the past, the Rappaport system, based solely on morphology, has been the most commonly used.[49]

Many attempts have been made to develop a classification system that will integrate morphologic and prognostic information with the evolving knowledge of the functional classification of lymphocytes. From 1976 until 1980 the National Cancer Institute (NCI) sponsored a multi-institutional study in which the consensus of 12 notable pathologists (Working Formulation of Non-Hodgkin's Lymphomas) grouped lymphomas according to biologic aggressiveness or grade.[50] The major groups (low-, intermediate-, and high-grade) of the Working Formulation were based primarily upon differences in survival. More recently, 19 renowned international hematopathologists (The International Lymphoma Study Group) have advocated the Revised European-American Lymphoma (REAL) classification in a further attempt to resolve international discrepancies in nomenclature[51] (Table 87.2). This system uses genetic, molecular, and immunologic information as well as morphology to define specific disease entities. Since its initial description, clinicians and pathologists have suggested a clinical grouping schema for the REAL classification that separates both the B- and T-cell lineage lymphomas according to the clinical course of the disease into (1) indolent (low-risk), (2) aggressive (intermediate-risk), and (3) highly aggressive (high-risk). Many of the indolent lymphomas have a follicular or nodular histologic pattern where bands of connective tissue create a nodular pattern throughout the involved lymph nodes. Commonly, indolent lymphomas are not diagnosed until they are stage III or IV because patients may be relatively asymptomatic until that time. They are characterized by a slow clinical progression with only moderate sensitivity to chemotherapy, and patients are rarely cured, although some survive for many years with active disease. Pathologically, many of the aggressive and highly aggressive lymphomas have a diffuse pattern where the disease completely replaces the normal architecture of the lymph node. The aggressive lymphomas have a more rapid clinical course and if untreated, patients usually die within 3 to 6 months. These lymphomas are much more sensitive to chemotherapy; many patients experience prolonged disease-free intervals and approximately 35 to 40% are cured. Patients with highly aggressive lymphomas will die within several weeks if effective treatment is not initiated. With aggressive therapy many of these patients may also respond very well.[52] Although controversial, the

Table 87.2 ▪ Comparison of the Rappaport, Working Formulation, and REAL Classifications for Non-Hodgkin's Lymphomas

Rappaport[49]	Working Formulation[50]	REAL B-Cell[51]	REAL T-Cell[51]
	Low grade		
Lymphocytic, well-differentiated	A. Malignant lymphoma: small lymphocytic consistent with chronic leukemia; plasmacytoid	B-cell CLL/PLL/SLL Marginal zone/MALT Mantle cell Lymphoplasmacytic immunocytoma	T-cell CLL/PLL LGL ATL/L (chronic and smoldering types)
Nodular (follicular) lymphocytic, poorly differentiated	B. Malignant lymphoma: follicular, predominantly small cleaved by diffuse areas; sclerosis	Follicle center, follicular, grade 1 Mantle cell Marginal zone/MALT	
Nodular (follicular) mixed lymphocytic and histiocytic	C. Malignant lymphoma: follicular mixed, small cleaved and large cell sclerosis	Follicle center, follicular, grade II Marginal zone/MALT	
	Intermediate grade		
Nodular (follicular) histiocytic	D. Malignant lymphoma: follicular, predominantly large-cell diffuse areas slcerosis	Follicle center, follicular, grade III	
Diffuse lymphocytic, poorly differentiated	E. Malignant lymphoma: diffuse small cleaved cell sclerosis	Mantle cell Follicle center, diffuse small cell Marginal zone/MALT	T-cell CLL/PLL LGL ATL/L Angioimmunoblastic Angiocentric
Diffuse mixed, lymphocytic and histiocytic	F. Malignant lymphoma: diffuse mixed, small and large cell sclerosis, epithelioid cell component	Large B-cell lymphoma (rich in T cells) Follicle center, diffuse small cell Lymphoplasmacytoid Marginal zone/MALT Mantle cell	Peripheral T-cell, unspecified ATL/L Angioimmunoblastic Angiocentric Intestinal T-cell lymphoma
Diffuse histiocytic (with or without sclerosis)	G. Malignant lymphoma: diffuse large cell cleaved cell, noncleaved cell sclerosis	Diffuse large B-cell lymphoma	Peripheral T-cell, unspecified ATL/L Angioimmunoblastic Angiocentric Intestinal T-cell lymphoma
	High grade		
Diffuse histiocytic (with or without sclerosis)	H. Malignant lymphoma: large cell, immunoblastic plasmacytoid clear cell polymorphous epithelioid cell component	Diffuse large B-cell lymphoma	Peripheral T-cell, unspecified ATL/L Angioimmunoblastic Angiocentric Intestinal T-cell Anaplastic large cell
Lymphoblastic (with or without convoluted cells)	I. Malignant lymphoma: lymphoblastic convoluted cell, nonconvoluted cell	Precursor B-lymphoblastic	Precursor T-lymphoblastic
Diffuse, undifferentiated (Burkitt's and non-Burkitt's type)	J. Malignant lymphoma: small cleaved, Burkitt's tumor; follicular areas	Burkitt's High grade B-cell, Burkitt-like diffuse large B-cell	Peripheral T-cell unspecified

CLL, chronic lymphocytic leukemia; *PLL,* prolymphocytic leukemia; *SLL,* small lymphocytic lymphoma; *MALT,* mucosa-associated lymphoid tissue; *LGL,* large granular lymphocyte leukemia; *ATL/L,* adult T-cell leukemia/lymphoma.

Table 87.3 ▪ Morphologic and Clinical Characteristics of Selected Non-Hodgkin's Lymphomas

REAL Classification	Morphology	Clinical Characteristics
Indolent		
Follicle center lymphoma, follicular	Cleaved and large noncleaved follicle center cells; pattern of growth is at least partially follicular and diffuse areas may be present; 40–60% progress to diffuse large B-cell lymphoma	Most common adult lymphoma in US, comprising 35–40% of all NHL and 75–80% of indolent B-cell lymphomas; affects mostly older adults; spleen and bone marrow frequently involved along with many lymph nodes
Mantle cell lymphoma	Small to medium sized lymphoid cells with slightly irregular or "cleaved" nuclei	About 5% of adult NHL in US: affects mostly older adults; patients usually have widespread disease
Aggressive		
Diffuse large B-cell lymphoma	Large cells that resemble centroblasts or immunoblasts; some may be rich in small T lymphocytes or histiocytes	Accounts for 30–40% of adult NHL; may be seen in any age group, but primarily adults; often presents with single or multiple rapidly enlarging masses; up to 40% occur extranodally (e.g., stomach, CNS, bone, kidney)
Peripheral T-cell lymphomas, unspecified	Mixture of small and large atypical cells; diffuse or occasionally interfollicular proliferation that ranges from atypical small cells to medium size or large cells	Less than 15% of lymphomas in US; most frequently affects adults; may be accompanied by eosinophilia, pruritis, or hemophagocytic syndromes; may involved lymph nodes, skin, liver, spleen, and other viscera
Highly aggressive/acute lymphomas/leukemias		
Precursor T-lymphoblastic lymphoma, leukemia	Lymphoblasts slightly larger than small lymphocytes but smaller than cells or large B-cell lymphoma	40% of childhood lymphomas and 15% of acute lymphoblastic leukemia; patients predominantly adolescent and young adult males; mediastinal masses and peripheral lymphadenopathy common. CNS involvement also common
Burkitt's lymphoma	Medium-sized cells with round nuclei, multiple nucleoli, and basophilic cytoplasm; extremely high rate of cell proliferation	Most common in children; rare in adults and often associated with AIDS; most present in abdomen, ovaries, or kidneys, rarely seen as acute leukemia with circulating tumor cells

NHL, non-Hodgkin's lymphoma; *CNS*, central nervous system; *AIDS*, acquired immunodeficiency syndrome.

prognosis associated with T cell-derived NHL is probably worse than that for B-cell tumors.[53] The morphologic, histologic, and clinical features of some of the NHLs are presented in Table 87.3.

As mentioned previously, specific cytogenetic changes are frequently associated with some types of lymphomas (Table 87.4), and lymphoma cells typically have the immunologic characteristics of their normal cell of origin (Table 87.5). Identification of these factors has become increasingly important in establishing a precise diagnosis, defining a treatment plan, and predicting overall prognosis. Burkitt's lymphoma, which is composed of noncleaved small cells, carries a poor prognosis. Burkitt's lymphoma is of B-lymphocyte origin and has been recognized as a clinicopathologic entity for many years. In the United States, Burkitt's lymphoma occurs primarily in adults and accounts for less than 5% of NHL. Although a definite association of Burkitt's lymphoma in African children with EBV has been established, EBV-positive tumors are rare in Americans.

T-cell lymphomas are far less common than B-cell lymphomas, especially in adults. Tumors of differentiated T cells frequently arise in the lymph nodes and skin (e.g., mycosis fungoides and Sézary syndrome) or may be widespread (i.e., T-cell leukemia). The cellular appearance of T-cell malignancies varies and may include cytologic types ranging from small, atypical lymphoid cells to large and often convoluted lymphoid cells. Mycosis fungoides, a cutaneous T-cell lymphoma, is characterized by proliferation of mature T cells (helper or inducer cells). Its prognosis

Table 87.4 ▪ Examples of Cytogenetic Lesions Associated with Specific Lymphomas

Lymphomas	Chromosomal Translocation	Proto-Oncogene	Tumor Suppressor Gene
Diffuse large cell lymphoma	t(14;18)(q32;q11) t(2;18)(p11;q11) t(18;22)(q11;q11) t(3;?)(q27;?)	*BCL-2* *BCL-6*	*p53*
Burkitt's lymphoma	t(8;14)(q24;q32) t(2;8)(p11;q24) t(8;22)(q24;q11)	*c-MYC*	*p53*
Mantle cell lymphoma	t(11;14)(q13;q32)	*BCL-1/ CCND1*	
Cutaneous T-cell lymphoma	der(10)(q24)	*LYT-10*	

Source: Reference 3.

Table 87.5 ▪ Examples of Immunophenotypic Characteristics of Non-Hodgkin's Lymphoma

Lymphoma	CD5	CD10	CD23	CD43	CD103	Pan-T (CD2, CD3)	NK (CD16, CD56)
Indolent							
Lymphoplasmacytoid	–	–	–	–/+	–/+	–	–
MALT	–	–	–/+	–/+	–/+	–	–
Follicular	–	+/–	–/+	–	–/+	–	–
Mantle cell	+	–	–	+	–	–	–

Lymphoma	CD45	CD19	CD20	CD3	CD5	CD7	CD10
Aggressive							
Diffuse large B-cell	+	+	+	–	–/+	–	–/+
Anaplastic large B-cell	+/–	–	–	+/–	+/–	NA	–
Peripheral T-cell	+	–	–	+/–	+/–	+/–	–
Highly aggressive							
Burkitt's	+	+	+	–	–	–	+

Source: Reference 5.
NK, natural killer; *MALT,* mucosa-associated lymphoid tissue.

is related to the stage of the disease, with most patients having a chronic course. The Sézary syndrome is closely related to mycosis fungoides and generally represents a leukemic phase.

Precursor lymphoblastic lymphoma/leukemia represents less than 10% of NHLs and is closely related to T-cell acute lymphoblastic leukemia. It is more common in adolescents and young adults and, without very aggressive treatment, confers a poor prognosis. About one-half of lymphoblastic lymphomas are characterized morphologically by convoluted nuclear configurations.

CLINICAL PRESENTATION AND DIAGNOSIS

Signs and Symptoms

General

Most patients with lymphomas have superficial lymphadenopathy. Although superficial lymphadenopathy in adults is most frequently related to an acute infectious process, biopsy should be performed on discrete hard lymph nodes, particularly if they are fixed or matted. The cervical nodes are the most common site of presentation in HD (65 to 80%), but this presentation is less common in NHL (30 to 40%). HD is believed to be unifocal in origin, probably beginning with a single lymph node. Spread occurs to adjacent nodes via lymph channels and either by direct extension into adjacent organs or by blood vessel invasion with dissemination to the spleen, bone marrow, liver, bone, and other organs.[11] Supraclavicular and mediastinal lymphadenopathy are also common in HD.

In NHL, with disease initially confined to the lymph nodes, there is a tendency for spread to contiguous lymphatic sites or occasionally, to adjacent extranodal sites. In contrast to HD, NHL spreads more rapidly to distant nodal and extranodal sites via the bloodstream, similar to the metastatic dissemination of many other tumors. The presentation of NHL depends on the histology of the disease. Indolent NHL may initially present with slowly progressive, nontender peripheral lymphadenopathy that may wax and wane spontaneously, whereas aggressive and highly aggressive NHLs generally progress steadily. The natural history of some indolent (follicular) lymphomas is progression to a diffuse pattern as well as a shift from the small, relatively slowly proliferating cells to large, more rapidly proliferating cells.

Twenty to 35% of patients with NHL have disease only outside the lymph nodes. The majority of the extranodal lymphomas exhibit a diffuse pattern. The most commonly involved extranodal site is the head and neck area, followed by the gastrointestinal tract. Other primary extranodal sites include the skin, central nervous system (CNS), liver, lung, testes, and bone marrow. When bone marrow involvement occurs, half of the patients show some evidence of disease dissemination in the blood.[54]

In rare patients, HD may present with massive mediastinal adenopathy causing superior vena cava obstruction accompanied by headache; congestion of the face; subcutaneous edema involving the face, neck, and thorax; and cough and dyspnea (see "Complications" below). Lymphoblastic lymphoma may also present with mediastinal adenopathy, which may also produce vena cava obstruction. NHL, and less commonly HD, may present with massive retroperitoneal adenopathy that may obstruct the ureters or the inferior vena cava, giving rise to ascites and edema in the lower extremities.

At initial presentation 20% of patients with NHL and 30 to 40% of patients with HD experience systemic or constitutional symptoms (fever, night sweats, weight loss, and pruritus).[1,5] These symptoms may develop about the same time as the lymph node enlargement or may occasionally precede the detection of adenopathy. They generally subside rapidly with treatment, and their reappearance at any time in the course of the disease represents an unfavorable prognostic sign. In patients with HD, the frequency of systemic symptoms increases with the stage of disease, age of the patient, and unfavorable histologic subtype.

Lymphomas Associated with Human Immunodeficiency Virus Infection

Since the AIDS epidemic began in 1981, the number of reports of lymphoma in patients with AIDS and HIV infection has steadily increased. In 1985 the Centers for Disease Control and Prevention (CDC) amended its case definition of AIDS to include patients with high-grade, B-cell NHL and documented HIV infection.[55] HIV infection is not believed to be directly responsible for the malignant transformation from normal lymphocyte to lymphoma. Rather, the effect of EBV on infected B cells, proto-oncogene activation by EBV, overexpression of IL-6 and IL-10, oncogene activation, and tumor suppressor gene loss have been implicated.[56]

The incidence of lymphoma associated with HIV infection is not unexpected because various other immunodeficiency disorders have also been associated with an increased incidence of lymphomas.[5,9,10] Currently the CDC predicts that 40% of patients who survive longer than 36 months with a diagnosis of AIDS will develop NHL. The risk correlates with the degree of immunosuppression (i.e., CD4 count).[56] NHLs of several histologic types,[57–60] as well as HD,[61,62] have been reported in patients with AIDS; however, the most frequent types have been large cell immunoblastic, small noncleaved cell (Burkitt's and Burkitt's-like) and diffuse large cell.[63] Although the incidence of HD is higher in HIV-infected men, it is not listed as an AIDS-defining illness. Most lymphomas in this population present at advanced stages, with unusual clinical features including prodromal manifestations, a high frequency of extranodal and CNS involvement, and usually a poor prognosis with respect to the histologic subtypes.[64] Although the disease may appear at any site, gastrointestinal, bone marrow, central nervous system, and hepatic involvement are far more common than in non-HIV-infected patients with NHL.[56,60] It is estimated that up to 25% of HIV-associated NHLs are confined to only the CNS.

Diagnosis and Staging

Decisions regarding appropriate therapy for a patient with a lymphoma depend upon the correct morphologic diagnosis and accurate assessment of the extent of disease. Diagnosis of lymphoma requires histopathologic confirmation of lymph node biopsy. When lymphadenopathy is present, one or more complete nodes must be excised. Needle biopsies are generally not adequate. When primary extranodal lymphoma presents with regional or distant adenopathy, both sites should be examined histologically to ensure a correct diagnosis. Extranodal disease is sometimes mistaken for solid tumors in certain sites (e.g., stomach, breast, or testicle), and it is not until surgical removal and pathologic examination that the tumor is discovered to be a NHL.

Hodgkin's Disease

Staging systems have been developed to facilitate therapeutic planning and communication of data concerning the natural history of the disease and treatment outcomes. The Ann Arbor staging system (Table 87.6) was developed in 1971 for use in HD and was revised in 1989.[65] It also is widely used for staging of NHL. In HD this system has been reproducible and predictive of response to therapy. The Ann Arbor Classification is divided into four stages, and each stage is further subdivided into A (asymptomatic) and B (symptomatic) groups. As the disease progresses from stage I to stage IV, the prognosis becomes worse. The presence of symptoms (designated B) also confers a worse prognosis. The clinical symptoms associated with HD are general rather than specific and include unexplained weight loss of more than 10% of the body weight, unexplained fever with temperature above 38°C (100.4°F), and night sweats. A patient may experience additional symptoms such as pruritus or alcohol-induced pain, but they generally do not correlate with the severity of disease and are not considered in the staging evaluation.

When localized extranodal disease is contiguous to involved lymph nodes (often in the lungs or vertebrae adjacent to involved lymph nodes), staging is based on the

Table 87.6 ▪ Ann Arbor (Cotswold) Classification for the Staging of Hodgkin's Disease

Stage I	Disease involvement of a single lymph node region (I) or lymphoid structure (e.g., spleen, thymus) or a single localized extrnodal organ or site (I_E)
Stage II	Disease involvement of two or more lymph node regions on the same side of the diaphragm (II); localized contiguous involvement of one extranodal organ or site and lymph node region on the same side of the diaphragm (II_E); the number of anatomic sites is indicated by a subscript (e.g., II_3)
Stage III	Disease involvement of lymph node regions on both sides of the diaphragm (III); may also be accompanied by localized involvement of an extralymphatic organ or site (III_E) or by involvement of the spleen (III_S), or both (III_{SE}) III_1 indicates with or without involvement of splenic, hilar, celiac, or portal nodes III_2 indicates involvement of para-aortic, iliac, or mesenteric nodes
Stage IV	Diffuse or disseminated disease involvement of one or more extranodal organs or tissues, with or without associated lymph node enlargement

Designations applicable to any stage of disease

A	Asymptomatic
B	Symptomatic: weight loss 10% of body weight, unexplained fever with temperature above 38°C (100.4°F), and night sweats
X	Designates bulky disease as >1/3 widening of the mediastinum or >10 cm maximum dimension of nodal mass
E	Involvement of a single extranodal site that is contiguous or proximal to the known nodal site

Staging should be identified as clinical stage (CS) or pathologic stage (PS)

Table 87.7 ▪ Recommended Staging Procedures for Hodgkin's Disease and Non-Hodgkin's Lymphomas

Required procedures
1. Detailed history with special attention to the presence (and duration) or absence of systemic symptoms (i.e., fever, unexplained sweating, unexplained weight loss)
2. Careful physical examination with special attention to all lymph node areas; size of liver and spleen
3. Adequate surgical biopsy reviewed by an experienced hemopathologist
4. Routine laboratory tests including complete blood count, erythrocyte sedimentation rate, liver and renal function tests, serum uric acid
5. Radiologic examination of the chest, gastrointestinal tract, and skeletal system or any areas of bone tenderness
6. Computed tomography (CT) scan or magnetic resonance imaging (MRI) of the chest
7. Abdominal and pelvic CT scan

Procedures necessary under certain circumstances
1. Bilateral lower extremity lymphography in patients who present with inguinal or iliac Hodgkin's disease (HD)
2. Exploratory laparotomy and splenectomy in patients with clinical stage I-II HD
3. Bilateral bone marrow biopsy in patients with clinical stage III HD

appropriate lymph node involvement followed by the subscript "E," which denotes direct extension. This type of disease confers a more favorable prognosis than clearly disseminated (stage IV) disease. In general, the "E" designation is used in patients with extranodal disease that is so limited in extent and location that it can be easily irradiated.

The diaphragm has key significance in the staging of HD. It is the reference point from which the extent (or stage) of HD is measured. If the disease is confined to lymph nodes on only one side (above or below) of the diaphragm, the disease is considered to be localized, and the prognosis is generally better than if the disease were more disseminated and present on both sides of the diaphragm.

Procedures necessary for accurate clinical staging of HD are listed in Table 87.7. A detailed patient history is obtained, making note of the presence or absence of symptoms, and a thorough physical examination must be performed, giving particular attention to areas of bone tenderness and the size of the liver and spleen. Laboratory tests and procedures are used to detect clinical abnormalities that may implicate a specific organ or organ system invaded by HD. Further pathologic staging is then necessary to definitively diagnose HD in tissues that have been implicated by the clinical staging procedures. Pathologic staging involves biopsy and microscopic examination of the suggestive tissue. More aggressive staging techniques have included exploratory laparotomy and splenectomy. In the past, these procedures have made tremendous contributions in staging accuracy and knowledge of the natural history of HD; however, current recommendations specify that laparotomy should be performed only if management decisions depend upon the identification of abdominal disease, and in some of these situations, laparoscopy combined with needle biopsies of marrow may substitute for this procedure. Laparotomy is of most value in identifying those patients with clinical stages I and II disease who might be eligible for treatment with radiation therapy alone (i.e., patients with negative laparotomy results verifying pathologic stage I or II disease).[66] If systemic chemotherapy is already considered essential to the patient's management, based on noninvasive studies such as computed tomography (CT) or magnetic resonance imaging (MRI), then staging laparotomy becomes inconsequential. Although the overall morbidity is low, laparotomy plus splenectomy increases the risk of sepsis from encapsulated organisms (i.e., *Streptococcus pneumoniae, Haemophilus influenzae*), varicella zoster infection, and bowel obstruction resulting from adhesions among the intestinal loops. Therefore, the decision to perform such a staging procedure must be carefully weighed, especially because a CT or MRI scan is easy to administer and noninvasive.

Non-Hodgkin's Lymphoma

NHLs are not as predictable in their patterns of involvement, nor do they reflect discrete changes in their prognosis with changes in stages, as seen with HD. In spite of these limitations, the Ann Arbor staging system has been widely used for defining patient groups in clinical trials. However, much effort has been spent on identifying other factors that have prognostic significance for patients with NHL. Such factors relate to the extent of the lymphoma (lactate dehydrogenase, β_2-microglobulin, stage, number of disease sites, extent of extranodal disease, and bone marrow involvement), the patient's response to the disease (Karnofsky performance status and B symptoms), and the patient's ability to tolerate therapy (age, performance status, and bone marrow involvement).[5,67] Other disease-related variables such as the rate of proliferation of tumor cells, the immunophenotype, and cytogenetic abnormalities also have been reported to correlate with survival, and it is likely that they will soon be widely used to establish prognosis.

In contrast to those with HD, patients with NHL are more likely to have disseminated disease, so local therapeutic options such as surgery and radiation therapy are less commonly used. Therapeutic options in NHL are also more likely to be limited because of the advanced age or concomitant illnesses of the patient. Because of the divergent clinical features of patients with NHL, no rigid or routine staging plan is appropriate for all patients. Many of the staging procedures used in HD (Table 87.7) are used for the NHLs, although they are less applicable because of the high prevalence of extranodal disease. These staging procedures should be carefully considered with regard to the histologic subtype, the individual patient, and the anticipated and available therapy. Extensive staging procedures should be reserved for clinical trials or for patients in whom a specific therapeutic alternative, such as radiation therapy, is available.

As in HD, a thorough physical examination and routine laboratory tests are aimed at the detection of potential sites of involvement, the rate of lymph node enlargement, and the presence of B symptoms. Renal and hepatic function should also be evaluated to assess for signs of organ involvement and to ascertain the patient's ability to tolerate aggressive therapy. Although the bone marrow is frequently involved in NHL, peripheral blood abnormalities are uncommon. Bilateral bone marrow aspirations and biopsies are generally indicated for patients with indolent follicular lymphomas or clinically advanced aggressive and highly aggressive histologic subtypes. The frequency of bone marrow involvement ranges from 5 to 15% in patients with diffuse large B-cell lymphoma to 55 to 85% of patients with follicular lymphoma. Although relatively uncommon in diffuse large B-cell lymphoma, bone marrow involvement may predict CNS involvement, and patients with this finding should receive a lumbar puncture with examination of the cerebrospinal fluid.

Gastrointestinal studies are indicated in patients with abdominal symptoms or masses and in patients with nasopharyngeal lymphomas, to obtain prognostic information, to plan therapy, and to establish involvement or impending obstruction of the gastrointestinal or genitourinary tract. A chest x-ray or chest CT scan is usually done to identify hilar and mediastinal lymphadenopathy and effusions. ^{67}Ga scans are also done to identify sites of disease. Abdominal CT scans are used for assessment of retroperitoneal and intra-abdominal disease, As in HD, there is no justification for routine staging laparotomy, and this procedure should be used only when it will influence management decisions.

TREATMENT

The treatment of lymphomas primarily includes radiation therapy and chemotherapy. Surgery, although useful in the management of many other malignancies, does not play a major role. Today the only roles for surgery in lymphomas are (1) initial staging and diagnostic procedures; (2) relief of obstruction related to a localized lymph node enlargement not responding to therapy; (3) management of a gastrointestinal lymphoma, to reduce the rate of perforation or hemorrhage; and (4) management of complications of lymphomas such as hypersplenism.

Lymphomas were recognized early on as being very responsive to radiation therapy, and until the end of the 1960s radiation therapy was the only successful modality that could, under appropriate circumstances, achieve cure for some lymphomas. Although radiation therapy has been used since the early 1900s, it was not until the 1950s, the era of megavolt radiation (using ^{60}Co and linear accelerators), that the use of large fields, exposing entire lymph node chains to radiation in the range of 3500 to 4000 cGy was possible. With these advances in technique, the therapeutic results of patients with all types of lymphomas have improved progressively.

Radiation therapy essentially has the same effect on cellular biochemistry as do the alkylating agents used in chemotherapy. DNA replication is prevented by interference with the cross-links necessary to maintain the double-helix DNA molecule. Proliferating tissue, characteristic of malignancies, is especially radiosensitive because of its constant DNA production necessary for cell division. The epithelial lining of the gastrointestinal tract is also rapidly dividing tissue and frequently encountered side effects with radiation therapy are radiation-induced pharyngitis, esophagitis, and gastroenteritis. The rapid production of cells in the bone marrow makes this site very susceptible to radiation-induced bone marrow suppression. It is therefore important that vital, uninvolved organs and viscera be shielded during radiation therapy to minimize radiation-induced toxicities. Possible radiation fields used for the treatment of lymphomas are described in Table 87.8.

The use of drugs in the management of neoplastic diseases was developed after the end of World War II, and lymphomas and leukemias were among the first tumors to respond to such chemotherapy. In general, with single-agent chemotherapy, the CR rate has rarely exceeded 20 to 30%, so the treatment of lymphomas requires the use of drug combinations. Combination chemotherapy uses drugs with different mechanisms of action that attack proliferating cells at different stages of cell replication.

Although the great majority of cytotoxic drugs can produce objective responses in lymphomas, it was in 1970 with the four-drug regimen known as MOPP (*m*echlorethamine or Mustargen, vincristine or *O*ncovin, *p*rednisone, and *p*rocarbazine) that DeVita et al.[68] showed that chemotherapy could induce a high rate of complete remission in patients with advanced HD. Later, the ability

Table 87.8 ▪ Radiation Therapy Fields Used in the Management of Lymphomas

Mantle: Encompasses mediastinal, hilar, and bilateral supraclavicular, infraclavicular, cervical, and auxillary node chains, with lead shields shaped to lungs, heart, and spinal cord

Inverted-Y: Encompasses splenic or splenic pedicle, para-aortic, iliac, inguinal, and femoral node chains, with lead shields for rectum and bladder, iliac and upper femoral bone marrow, and "gap" at junction with mantle fields

Para-aortic/hepatic: Encompasses splenic hilar and para-aortic node chains and entire right lobe of liver, usually joined across another "gap" by a separate pelvic field

Waldeyer: Encompasses preauricular nodes and lymphatic tissues of Waldeyer's ring when clinically involved or when adenopathy is present in high cervical nodes

Total nodal: Encompasses all lymph node regions above the diaphragm (cervical, supra- and infraclavicular, axillary, mediastinal) and all lymph node regions below the diaphragm (periaortic, retroperitoneal, inguinal, and splenic regions)

Subtotal nodal: Encompasses the mantle plus para-aortic, spleen and pedicle fields

Involved field: Encompasses only the known involved sites

Extended field: Encompasses known involved sites plus contiguous uninvolved regions

Table 87.9 ▪ Criteria for Treatment Response

Complete response (CR): Disappearance of all signs and symptoms of the disease; this includes the return to normal of all previously abnormal parameters and a negative second biopsy of known involved extranodal sites
Partial response (PR): A reduction of 50% in the product of the longest perpendicular diameters of all measurable lesions
Minimal response (MR) or no change: A reduction of <50% in the product of the longest perpendicular diameters of all measurable lesions
Treatment failure (TF): Increase in size of any lesion and/or appearance of new lesion(s)

of chemotherapy to produce long-term remissions (i.e., cure) in patients with HD and certain NHL histologic subtypes was confirmed.

After radiation therapy or chemotherapy has been administered to a patient with lymphoma, the patient's response to treatment must be assessed. Standard criteria are generally used for the objective evaluation of treatment response (Table 87.9) so that various therapies may be compared in a consistent manner. Objective reduction of the disease manifestations usually begins within the first month after the start of treatment. However, this depends on the histologic type of lymphoma and is usually more rapid in HD than in NHL.

Selection of the appropriate type of therapy depends upon confirmation of the histologic subtype and the extent of the disease, as well as any patient-specific factors (e.g. age or concomitant illness) that may influence the patient's ability to withstand treatment. With few exceptions, the initial approach to management of malignant lymphomas must have curative intent, regardless of disease extent and histologic type.

Hodgkin's Disease

Early-Stage (I, II, and III_A) Hodgkin's Disease

Stages I and II HD are very amenable to radical external beam radiation therapy (i.e., high doses of radiation with curative intent), because in these stages the disease is present in a few well-defined, focal areas.[69] Treatment may be limited to the known involved sites (i.e., involved field, IF), given to only the known involved sites plus contiguous uninvolved regions (i.e., extended field, EF), or delivered to all major lymphoid regions (i.e., total nodal irradiation, TNI). It is generally recommended that local tumor masses receive "boost therapy" to a minimum dose of 4000 to 4400 cGy, whereas apparently uninvolved areas treated for subclinical disease appear to be controlled adequately with doses of about 3600 cGy. The usual dose is 150 to 220 cGy/day administered 5 days each week, so the total duration of treatment is 4 to 6 weeks.

With either TNI or subtotal nodal irradiation (sTNI), the 10-year relapse-free survival rate (which is often equated to cure) in patients with pathologic (confirmed by laparotomy) stages I and II HD is 75 to 80%.[70–72] If only the IF is irradiated, the response rate has been poorer (38%) than with TNI, although overall survival was comparable at 5 years (90%) because most patients who have a relapse after radiation will respond to chemotherapy.[73] The use of chemotherapy with radiation (combined modality therapy) appears to reduce the relapse rate but it does not improve the overall survival.[1,74] sTNI is not associated with significantly more toxicity than that experienced with IF, although it dramatically improves relapse-free survival; therefore, this technique is generally considered the standard approach for stages I and II disease. About 50% of patients with a large (greater than one-third of the largest transverse chest diameter) mediastinal mass have a relapse when treated with radiation therapy alone[75]; therefore, most investigators advocate the use of chemotherapy plus irradiation. Likewise, patients with bulky axillary disease or significant involvement of the pleura, lung, or pericardium should also receive combined modality therapy.[76,77] Fever, weight loss, age older than 40 years, mixed cellularity or lymphocyte depleted histology, or male sex may predict an increased likelihood of occult abdominal disease in patients with clinically staged disease (without laparotomy), and most experts recommend either a staging laparotomy to rule out occult disease or combined modality therapy. A regimen of four cycles of ABVD chemotherapy (see below) with limited radiation therapy is recommended.[78]

Some evidence indicates that treatment of early-stage disease with chemotherapy alone is at least as effective as radiation therapy. When patients with stages I_B, II_A, or III_A disease were randomly assigned to receive either radiation or MOPP chemotherapy, Longo et al.[79] reported a CR rate of 96% in each arm of the study. At a median follow-up of 7.5 years, 35% of patients in the radiation group and 13% of patients who received MOPP therapy had a relapse. The projected 10-year disease-free survival for patients receiving radiation therapy is 60% versus 86% for MOPP-treated patients ($P = .009$), although overall survival was not significantly different. Systemic chemotherapy eliminates the need for the patient to undergo a laparotomy or splenectomy with the associated morbidity. However, the acute toxic reactions associated with chemotherapy may be worse than those associated with radiation. Further follow-up of this and other similar trials is necessary to assess late and chronic treatment-related side effects.

For patients with stage III_A disease the 5-year relapse-free survival when treated with radiation alone is only 35 to 66%, although overall survival ranges from 80 to 92% at 5 years, emphasizing the effectiveness of salvage treatment.[80] Currently, it is believed that radiation therapy alone is inadequate in stage III_A disease and that combination chemotherapy is the treatment of choice for patients with III_A disease who do not have mediastinal involvement.[81] Several clinical studies have reported improved relapse-free survival with the use of chemotherapy plus radiation.[82–84] Other studies suggest that combined modality therapy does not increase the long-term disease-free survival rate compared to chemotherapy alone[85,86]; however, it is superior in patients with bulky mediastinal disease. In addition, combined modality therapy is associated with more toxicity.[87]

Stages III_B and IV Hodgkin's Disease

Chemotherapy with or without radiation therapy is the treatment of choice for patients with stage III_B or IV HD. Stage IV disease is not well suited for radiation therapy, because sites of the disease in this stage may be so numerous and diffuse that localized radiation cannot be effectively administered. Parenchymal organs cannot tolerate curative doses of radiation, and the presence of HD in these areas precludes the use of radical radiation. Stage IV disease is therefore treated primarily with systemic chemotherapy, which can reach all sites of disease. "Spot" radiation is also used in stage IV disease for palliative treatment to anatomical areas of disease involvement not responding to chemotherapy and causing pain, tenderness, or obstruction.

The drug combination that was first successful in producing long-term remissions in HD is MOPP. Pioneered by DeVita et al.,[68] MOPP therapy has endured and is still considered by many to be a valuable front-line chemotherapy for HD[88,89] (Table 87.10). After 20 years of experience with this regimen at the NCI, 159 of 198 patients (80%) achieved a complete remission, with 54% of these patients remaining disease free at 20 years. MOPP therapy is given in cycles that repeat every 28 days. Over 1000 patients have been treated with the MOPP regimen in reported clinical trials. The average CR rate has been 67% (44 to 87%) with a long-term disease-free survival of at least 50% in all studies.[1] Patients should receive a minimum of six complete cycles of therapy (or two cycles after documentation of CR) at maximally tolerated doses. When doses have been attenuated, lower remission and survival rates have been reported.[1,90] Although it appears that full-dose chemotherapy predicts the best response, it is possible that patients with poorer prognosis disease are unable to tolerate full-dose treatment. When patients are considered to be in complete remission, which must be determined by appropriate restaging, two more cycles of chemotherapy should be given. Once complete remission has been achieved, there is no real advantage in prolonging treatment or administering any type of maintenance therapy. Similar chemotherapy regimens have yielded comparative results and toxicities (Table 87.10). In addition to MOPP and MOPP derivatives, other novel combination chemotherapy regimens have shown excellent results when used as first-line therapy. Bonadonna et al.[91] first described the ABVD regimen (doxorubicin or *A*driamycin, *b*leomycin, *v*inblastine, and *d*acarbazine) (Table 87.10) in patients who

Table 87.10 ▪ Combination Chemotherapy Regimens Used in Hodgkin's Disease

Acronym	Agents	Dose (mg/m²)	Treatment Days	Frequency of Cycles
MOPP	Mechlorethamine	6 IV	1, 8	Every 28 days
	Vincristine (Oncovin)	1.4 IV	1,8	
	Procarbazine	100 PO	1 through 14	
	Prednisone	40 PO	1 through 14, cycles 1 and 4	
ABVD	Doxorubicin	25	1,15	Every 28 days
	Bleomycin	10	1,15	
	Vinblastine	6	1,15	
	Dacarbazine	375	1,15	
MVPP	Mechlorethamine	6	1,8	Every 28 days
	Vinblastine	10	1,8,15	
	Procarbazine	100	1–15	
	Prednisolone	40	1–15	
MOPP/ABV	Mechlorethamine	6	1	Every 28 days
	Vincristine	1.4 (max 2 mg)	1	
	Prednisone	40	1–14	
	Procarbazine	100	1–7	
	Doxorubicin	35	8	
	Bleomycin	10	8	
	Vinblastine	6	8	
EVA	Etoposide	100	1–3	Every 28 days
	Vinblastine	6	1	
	Doxorubicin	50	1	
EPOCH	Etoposide	200 CIV	1 thru 4	Every 29 days
	Vincristine	1.6 CIV	1 thru 4	
	Doxorubicin	40 CIV	1 thru 4	
	Cyclophosphamide	750 IV	6	
	Prednisone	60 PO	1 thru 6	
CEP	Lomustine	80 PO	1	
	Etoposide	100 PO	1 thru 5	
	Prednimustine	60 PO	1 thru 5	

Source: Reference 1.

had a relapse after MOPP therapy.[91] After their very positive results, they undertook a prospective study to evaluate MOPP versus MOPP alternating with ABVD.

Goldie and Coldman[92] proposed that during treatment, malignant cells may mutate and become resistant to therapy. The use of alternating, non-cross-resistant chemotherapy regimens has been suggested as a possible means of improving the CR rate and lengthening the median duration of disease-free survival by exposing tumor cells to an increased number of cytotoxic drugs. This strategy offers the possibility of reducing treatment failures caused by overgrowth of singly, doubly, or even multidrug-resistant phenotypes. The ABVD regimen consists of drugs that are individually non-cross-resistant with the agents in the MOPP regimen. This combination has demonstrated a CR rate as high as that for the MOPP regimen and has been proven to be effective in patients with disease resistant to MOPP therapy. In a randomized study of patients with advanced HD, alternating monthly cycles of MOPP and ABVD (MOPP/ABVD) were compared to MOPP therapy alone. The rates of CR (89 versus 74%) and 8-year relapse-free survival for patients achieving a CR were superior (73 versus 45%) for the MOPP/ABVD regimen, with a similar incidence of serious toxic reactions.[93,94]

Klimo and Connors[95] reported the results of a similar hybrid regimen (MOPP/ABV) (Table 87.10), in which seven drugs were administered in single monthly cycles. This regimen omitted dacarbazine and increased the dose of doxorubicin from 25 to 35 mg/m^2; 13% of the patients also received some local radiation therapy. The CR rate was 97.5%, and at a median follow-up of 3.5 years, the overall survival rate was 93.5% and the relapse-free survival was 90.5%. Glick et al.[96] also reported a CR rate of 81% and a 22-month relapse-free survival of 80% using this hybrid regimen. However, another large randomized trial reported equivalent outcomes for ABVD alone versus the alternating regimen.[97] Today, ABVD alone is the most common first-line therapy in use, largely because patients are generally able to tolerate full doses better than they do with MOPP.

Over the past 25 years, it has become apparent that several factors influence the overall long-term response to HD therapies. Factors that have a negative impact on potential cure include age (>40 years), stage of disease, number of extranodal sites, and constitutional symptoms.[98–100] After chemotherapy is initiated, the rate of tumor regression and the dose intensity (i.e., amount of drug administered per unit of time) also appear to influence the duration of response and survival.[89,101] Review of outcome data has shown that the best overall results are seen in subsets of patient who received chemotherapy at closest to the intended dose and schedule (without dose attenuation or delay between cycles).[5] The dose intensity of the mechlorethamine, procarbazine, and vincristine has each been suggested to correlate with outcome in MOPP or MOPP-derivative regimens.[89,94,101–105] For example, although the original MOPP regimen includes 1.4 mg/m^2 of vincristine, many clinicians have limited each dose to a maximum of 2 mg. The use of full doses is associated with significant neurotoxicity, but no patient was permanently disabled if a sliding-scale dose, taking into account the patient's symptoms, was used. Conversely, no study using the 2-mg dose maximum has shown results as good as the original regimen, and retrospective analyses have shown that the dose of vincristine does have an impact on treatment results.[81]

The most common dose-limiting toxic reaction of many of the other drugs used in HD regimens is myelosuppression. Therefore, the use of colony-stimulating factors in combination with chemotherapy regimens may allow for a higher dose intensity to be tolerated.

Despite the success of first-line therapies (both radiation and chemotherapy) for HD, 20 to 50% of patients either will have disease that is initially refractory to primary treatment or will have a relapse after primary treatment.[106] Chemotherapy such as the MOPP or ABVD regimens is also appropriate therapy for patients who have a disease relapses after radiation therapy.[88,107] DeVita et al.[88] reported that 94% of patients whose disease recurred after local irradiation achieved a complete remission with MOPP therapy.[88]

The optimal management for patients who have a relapse after primary chemotherapy (e.g., MOPP) or for those in whom initial chemotherapy failed is not clearly established. At the NCI, 59% of 32 patients who had a relapse after MOPP therapy achieved a complete remission when retreated with MOPP. Patients whose first complete remission was longer than 1 year were more likely to achieve a second complete remission. The duration of the second remission was also longer in patients whose initial remission was longer than 1 year.[108] Overall, about 35% of patients who have a relapse after an initial chemotherapy-induced complete remission have a long-term disease-free survival.[5]

A number of other antineoplastic agents, including doxorubicin, carmustine, lomustine, etoposide, vinblastine, dacarbazine, and bleomycin, have demonstrated significant activity in HD. These agents have been assembled in various combinations (Table 87.10). If the initial CR was longer than 1 year, patients may be retreated with the same therapy or a non-cross-resistant regimen. For relapses in patients who initially received ABVD, retreatment with ABVD may be difficult because of the risks of cumulative doxorubicin cardiotoxicity and bleomycin pulmonary toxicity. Useful salvage regimens include etoposide, vinblastine or vincristine, and doxorubicin (EVA) and lomustine, etoposide, and prednimustine (CEP).[109–111] In patients who previously had a relapse after MOPP or whose disease was resistant to MOPP, a 40% CR rate was reported and 31% of these patients remained disease-free at a median follow-up of 42 months after treatment with EVA.[109] This regimen incorporated another active agent, etoposide,[112] into the treatment of HD and has the potential advantage of less emetogenic complications and pulmonary toxicity than many of the other second-line regimens.

Patients in whom first-line therapy fails are much less likely to respond to other conventional therapies.[113] Even if such patients do achieve a complete remission with second-line therapy, it is likely to be brief. Prognosis is influenced by the stage of the disease at initial diagnosis and at relapse, the status of B symptoms at relapse, the patient's performance status, whether it is a first or later relapse, the number of failed chemotherapy regimens, whether it is relapsed or refractory disease, and the duration of the prior remission.[114]

The use of high-dose chemotherapy with allogeneic or autologous bone marrow transplant may offer better chances for long-term survival.[115–117] With this treatment approach, the CR rates have ranged from 40 to 70%, and 20 to 49% of patients appear to have a long remission (>2 years).[118–126] A recent report by the Autologous Blood and Marrow Transplant Registry on 122 HD patients who failed to achieve a CR after one or more conventional regimens reported that 50% achieved a CR after high-dose therapy.[127] The best treatment results are seen in patients with low tumor volumes, good performance status, and chemotherapy-sensitive disease (i.e., showing some indication of tumor response before bone marrow transplant). Rappaport et al.[128] reported a projected 3-year event (relapse)-free survival for patients with minimal disease (all areas ≤2 cm) of 70% versus 15% for patients with bulky disease. In one series, human leukocyte antigen-identical allogeneic marrow recipients had a statistically lower relapse rate than recipients of autologous marrow, although survival, event-free survival, and nonrelapse-related mortality were not different.[117] Clinical trials have reported 8 to 20% treatment-related deaths. Many of these deaths and other treatment morbidities are associated with the profound myelosuppression before bone marrow engraftment. Numerous trials using colony-stimulating factors have now reported accelerated myeloid recovery, fewer febrile days, and shorter hospitalizations.[129,130]

Non-Hodgkin's Lymphoma

The management for NHLs depends upon many factors, including the age of the patient, presence of concomitant disease, and the stage and histologic subgroup of the primary disease.

Indolent Non-Hodgkin's Lymphoma

Stage I and II Indolent Non-Hodgkin's Lymphoma

Fewer than 10% of patients with indolent NHL (Table 87.2) have localized disease (i.e., stage I or II) at the time of diagnosis. Local or regional radiation therapy is generally very effective in achieving disease control in the irradiated areas.[131] However, although many patients experience long disease-free intervals, at least 40 to 50% will have a recurrence of the disease within 10 years.[52] Chemotherapy, either alone or in combination with radiation therapy, does not appear to improve the disease-free survival in patients with early-stage disease. If patients have a relapse after an initial response to radiation therapy, it is usually at a different anatomical site.

Stage III and IV Indolent Non-Hodgkin's Lymphoma

More than 50 to 75% of patients with low-grade lymphomas have stage III or IV disease at initial diagnosis.[132,133] Few of these patients can be cured. Treatment options for patients with favorable histologic subtype disease and advanced disease include total nodal irradiation, total body irradiation, single-agent chemotherapy, and combination chemotherapy.

A number of agents, including mechlorethamine, melphalan, chlorambucil, cyclophosphamide, vincristine, vinblastine, doxorubicin, carmustine, fludarabine, and etoposide have activity against the follicular (low-grade) lymphomas. Although CR rates as high as 65% have been reported with several of these agents and the duration of relapse-free survival may be up to several years, this type of therapy is not considered to be curative. With the use of molecular biology techniques, it appears that many patients with follicular NHL in apparent complete remission still have cells containing cytogenetic evidence of the disease.[134] In an attempt to improve results observed with single-agent therapy, a number of combination chemotherapy regimens have been developed. Initially, one of the most widely used regimens was the CVP (cyclophosphamide, vincristine, and prednisone) regimen. Although studies with this regimen suggested higher CR rates than with single-agent therapy, the overall disease-free survival and survival were not significantly altered. In response to this information, a number of more aggressive regimens (e.g., CHOP [cyclophosphamide, hydroxydaunomycin, vincristine (Oncovin), and prednisone]-bleomycin, C-MOPP [cyclophosphamide plus MOPP], m-BACOD [methotrexate, bleomycin, doxorubicin (Adriamycin), cyclophosphamide, vincristine (Oncovin) and dexamethasone], and COPP [cyclophosphamide, vincristine (Oncovin), procarbazine and prednisone]) with and without radiation therapy have been investigated; however, overall survival was not improved.

The nucleoside analogs, pentostatin, cladribine, and fludarabine have all shown activity in the treatment of the follicular lymphomas in patients for whom other conventional therapy as well as first-line therapy has failed. The impressive results with them as single-agents have led investigators to incorporate these agents in combination regimens.[135–139] Interferon alfa-2b has recently been approved for the treatment of clinically aggressive follicular NHL in conjunction with anthracycline-containing combination chemotherapy. In an NCI-sponsored trial, 13 (4 CRs, 9 partial responses) of 24 patients responded to a regimen of 50 million units/m^2 given three times weekly. The responses were seen in patients with both lymph node and extranodal disease. The median duration of response was 8 months.[140] Several studies have subsequently demonstrated that the addition of interferon alfa to combination chemotherapy regimens prolongs the duration of remission and, in some studies, it has also prolonged the overall survival compared to chemotherapy alone.[141–143]

The newest approach to treating indolent lymphomas has been the use of monoclonal antibodies targeted at cell surface antigens. The CD20 antigen is expressed on the surface of more than 90% of the B-cell lymphomas. Because this antigen does not shed, modulate, or internalize, it is an ideal target for antibody therapy. If the antigen was shed from the surface the monoclonal antibody would bind to it in the serum and never reach the tumor cell. Likewise, if the antigen was altered or internalized within the cell the antibody would not recognize or could not reach its target. Initial trials with the chimeric human-mouse anti-CD20 monoclonal antibody, rituximab (Rituxan) demonstrated biological efficacy in producing transient depletion of B-cells and a good safety profile.[144] After binding to the CD20 antigen, rituximab induces lysis of the cell. A multicenter, single-arm trial reported a 48% response rate in 166 patients with low-grade or follicular lymphomas who had progressive disease that had relapsed or failed to respond to previous conventional therapy. Although most of the responses were partial, the median duration of response was projected to be 10 to 12 months.[145] After the marketing of this product in 1998, the manufacturer did report that several deaths had been reported in patients with bulky disease that were presumably related to a massive cell lysis and metabolic complications within several hours after the initial dose. Therefore, it has been recommended that patients with high tumor burdens be closely monitored during and after therapy until the risk of such a reaction has passed. Recently, rituximab has been combined with cytotoxic chemotherapy. Czuczman et al.[146] reported an overall response rate of 95% (55% CR) in 40 patients who received six infusions of rituximab (375 mg/m^2) in combination with six courses of CHOP chemotherapy. Thirty-one of these patients had not received any prior therapy. The combination of chemotherapy plus rituximab did not appear to cause any additional toxicity over what would be anticipated with the individual regimens.

Because of the indolent nature of this disease, some clinicians have suggested that asymptomatic patients may not require immediate therapy after the initial diagnosis. Clinicians who have advocated this alternative strategy emphasize that close monitoring and follow-up of patients is always necessary and that therapy can be delayed until the disease progresses and the patient becomes symptomatic. This approach is appealing, especially in older patients who are less likely to tolerate the side effects of chemotherapy. Several randomized trials have evaluated whether immediate therapy is superior to this "watch and wait approach," and the results have not established a clear-cut superiority for either approach. French investigators and researchers at Stanford University both reported comparable survival rates with both initial treatment strategies.[147–149] Conversely, clinicians at the Memorial Sloan-Kettering Cancer Center in New York observed that the median survival for patients treated with the watch and wait approach was only 4 years versus the 5 to 9 years frequently reported for patients who receive initial aggressive therapy.[150] All experts do seem to agree that patients with bulky disease (very large lymph nodes or masses) or systemic symptoms should receive immediate treatment after diagnosis.

Patients who do not achieve a CR after initial therapy often receive various palliative therapies for many years. High-dose chemotherapy with autologous bone marrow or peripheral stem cell transplantation has also been used for patients who fail to achieve a CR or for other high-risk patients. A monoclonal antibody or a cytotoxic agent is used to purge the patient's marrow of malignant cells before reinfusion. Although CRs are often reported and several groups have observed event-free survivals of longer than 3 to 4 years, it is uncertain if the cure rate is increased.[151,152] A longer disease-free survival is almost certainly associated with a better quality of life for the patient and probably fewer treatment-related side effects. Unfortunately, most patients with indolent lymphomas still cannot be cured, usually receive multiple different treatment regimens throughout the course of their disease, and inevitably have a relapse after varying durations of response. Patients eventually die of unrelated causes, toxicity of the therapy, progressive disease, or transition to a more aggressive type of lymphoma.

Aggressive Non-Hodgkin's Lymphoma

Localized (Stage I and II) Aggressive Non-Hodgkin's Lymphoma

Although in the past, patients with stage I and II aggressive histologic subtypes were often managed with radiation therapy, randomized studies have confirmed that combination chemotherapy with radiation therapy produces superior 5-year disease-free survival rates (76 to 88%) versus radiation alone (32 to 45%).[153,154] Chemotherapy alone may be sufficient for some patients; however some studies have shown that patients with bulky tumor masses or extranodal disease clearly benefit from radiation therapy in addition to the chemotherapy.[155] Often three cycles of a regimen such as CHOP (Table 87.11) followed by irradiation of the involved area are recommended.

Advanced Stage (III and IV) Aggressive Non-Hodgkin's Lymphoma

Combination chemotherapy is clearly the most beneficial therapy for patients with advanced stage aggressive NHL. Unlike the indolent nature of the follicular histologic subtypes, patients with these more aggressive histologic subtypes may succumb to their disease rapidly, unless they receive and respond to appropriate therapy. For more than 20 years it has been recognized that many patients with aggressive histologic subtype lymphomas can be cured with chemotherapy; however, the optimal regimen has been widely debated.

CHOP is a first-generation regimen that has been widely used over the past 2 decades. It has consistently produced complete remissions in 45 to 55% of patients and cure in approximately 30 to 35%. With the intent of increasing the percentage of long-term, disease-free survivors, many other regimens have been investigated (Table 87.11). These regimens have used other active agents such as bleomycin, etoposide, cytarabine, and methotrexate as well as the agents used in the CHOP regimen. In addition to combining active drugs, many regimens have also used innovative approaches to scheduling in an attempt to maximize the response while maintaining acceptable degrees of toxicity. Examples of such regimens include the M-BACOD and

Table 87.11 ▪ Combination Chemotherapy Regimens for the Treatment of Aggressive Non-Hodgkin's Lymphoma

Acronym	Agents	Dose (mg/m²)	Treatment Days	Frequency of Cycles
CHOP	Cyclophosphamide	750	1	Every 21 days
	Doxorubicin	50	1	
	Vincristine	1.4 (max 2 mg)	1	
	Prednisone	100	1–5	
M-BACOD	Methotrexate (MTX)	3000	14	Every 21 days
	Bleomycin	4	1	
	Doxorubicin	45	1	
	Cyclophosphamide	600	1	
	Vincristine	1	1	
	Dexamethasone	6	1–5	
	Leucovorin	Dose determined per MTX levels		
MACOP-B	Methotrexate	400	8, 36, 64	Every 28 days
	Doxorubicin	50	1, 15, 29, 43, 57, 71	
	Cyclophosphamide	350	1, 15, 29, 43, 57, 71	
	Vincristine	1.4	8, 22, 36, 50, 64, 78	
	Bleomycin	10	22, 50, 78	
	Prednisone	75 (total)	1–63, taper 64–78	
ProMACE-CytaBOM	Cyclophosphamide	650	1	Every 21 days
	Doxorubicin	25	1	
	Etoposide	120	1	
	Prednisone	60	1–15	
	Cytarabine	300	8	
	Bleomycin	5	8	
	Vincristine	1.4	8	
	Methotrexate	120	8	
	Leucovorin	25 q6	9	

Source: References 5, 156.

the ProMACE (prednisone, methotrexate, cyclophosphamide, doxorubicin [Adriamycin], and etoposide) combinations, in which the relatively nonmyelosuppressive high-dose methotrexate with leucovorin rescue is given between the myelosuppressive agents to prevent regrowth of the lymphoma between cycles of the treatment. A 75% CR rate was reported for M-BACOD, and initial projections predicted that 55 to 60% of patients would be cured.[157] The MACOP-B (methotrexate, doxorubicin [Adriamycin], cyclophosphamide, vincristine [Oncovin], prednisone, and bleomycin) regimen includes weekly administration of active agents for 12 weeks, with myelosuppressive and nonmyelosuppressive intravenous agents given on alternating weeks. The reported CR rate with this regimen is 84%, with a predicted median duration of response of greater than 2 years. This initial evidence suggested that this regimen was as effective as other regimens, although it can be administered in one-half the time or less.[158]

Although many such trials reported complete remission rates and overall survival durations that appeared to be superior to those with the original CHOP regimen, it quickly became apparent that these outcome measures were also influenced by the histologic subtype and other prognostic factors. In addition, most of these trials were single-arm studies that were conducted in single institutions. Often, the results could not be replicated at other sites. Subsequently, a large (899 eligible patients), multi-institutional, randomized trial reported that remission rates and overall survival at 3 years did not differ significantly whether CHOP, MACOP-B, m-BACOD, or ProMACE-CytaBOM (cytarabine, bleomycin, vincristine, and methotrexate) was used (Table 87.12). Because there were fewer severe toxicities and fatalities in the CHOP group, these investigators concluded that it remains the best available treatment.[156] Several other randomized trials have also failed to show any advantage for the newer generation regimens over CHOP and most of the newer regimens have caused more severe toxicities.[159] Thus, in 1999 CHOP remains the most widely used regimen for aggressive NHL. It is important to note, however, that with CHOP or any of the other regimens evaluated in the

Table 87.12 ▪ Comparison of a Standard Regimen (CHOP) with Three Intensive Chemotherapy Regimens for Advanced Non-Hodgkin's Lymphoma

Regimen[a]	6-Yr Overall Survival (%)	Fatal Toxicities (%)
CHOP	33	1
m-BACOD	36	5
ProMACE-CytaBOM	34	3
MACOP-B	32	6

Source: Intergroup Trial of 899 patients with Stage III and IV aggressive NHL.[156]

[a]See Table 87.11 for drugs included in regimens.

randomized trial, the overall long-term survival (i.e., cure) rates remain at less than 40%, demonstrating the need for continued research for more effective treatment strategies.

Over the years the importance of dose-intensity has been emphasized in the treatment of aggressive NHL. Although the treatment regimens are effective, they also produce serious side effects. In patients experiencing toxic reactions it is often tempting to prolong the interval between courses of therapy to allow more recovery time. However, the specified schedule must be adhered to, whenever possible, to produce the best results. In many cases, prolongation by even 1 week may be associated with rapid tumor regrowth. Few clinical trials have directly addressed the significance of maintaining dose intensity in treatment of the aggressive lymphomas. The National Cancer Institute of Canada clinical trials group compared standard BACOP with BACOP that included escalated doses of doxorubicin in patients with previously untreated, advanced intermediate- and high-grade (Working Group Classification) NHL. The standard dose doxorubicin group received 25 mg/m^2 on days 1 and 8 of each cycle and the escalated dose group received 40 mg/m^2. There were no differences in response rate, disease-free survival, and survival during a median 65 months follow-up; however, because of granulocytopenia (no colony-stimulating factor was given) only 47% of patients were able to tolerate the escalated dose of doxorubicin beyond the first cycle.[160] A meta-analysis of 22 studies, however, suggested that dose intensity may correlate with remission rate in advanced-stage intermediate-grade lymphoma.[161] The availability of colony-stimulating factors has somewhat reduced morbidity related to neutropenia when the high-dose regimens are used.

For patients with aggressive NHL, only those who achieve a CR will have a long, disease-free survival. Factors that appear to adversely affect the ability to attain a CR include advanced-stage disease, the presence of systemic symptoms, bone marrow or liver involvement, gastrointestinal masses greater than 10 cm in diameter, a hemoglobin level less than 12 g/dL, and a lactate dehydrogenase level greater than 250 U.[162] Other factors that may also adversely affect the prognosis include more than three sites of disease involvement, advanced age, or a slow response to initial therapy.[163] Variability in response rates to similar regimens in different clinical trials may be a result of a different mix of prognostic factors in the patient population. If patients with poor prognostic factors do attain a complete remission, then overall survival does not appear to be compromised.

Because major prognostic factors have been identified, it has been suggested that patients with more favorable prognostic factors may be safely managed with less aggressive treatment. This strategy has been termed *risk-related therapy*. Although it is recommended that patients without high-risk prognostic factors receive a minimum of six courses of CHOP therapy, more aggressive therapies have been evaluated for patients with high-risk disease if they initially show evidence of response to the conventional regimen.

If the disease responds favorably to a conventional regimen (e.g., CHOP), it is deemed to be chemotherapy-sensitive. Because the dose-response relationship for the sensitive aggressive lymphomas is typically quite steep, the use of high-dose chemotherapy (with bone marrow or peripheral stem cell rescue) has been postulated to offer a greater chance of cure for these high-risk patients. At least one randomized trial in high-risk patients who initially achieved a CR with conventional therapy reported that the 5-year disease-free survival was superior for those who received high-dose chemotherapy than for those who received additional conventional-dose chemotherapy.[164] Other investigators have advocated initial high-dose therapy without assessing for chemosensitivity.[165,166] A potential advantage of this approach is that tumor cells are not exposed to initial chemotherapy and therefore have no opportunity to develop acquired resistance. A potential disadvantage is that patients with de novo resistant disease would receive very toxic and expensive high-dose therapy with little chance of meaningful response.

Maintenance chemotherapy after achievement of a CR does not appear to prolong survival in patients with most types of NHL. Patients whose disease does not respond to initial chemotherapy or who have a relapse in less than 1 year should be given non-cross-resistant regimens. However, the results of salvage treatments for NHLs are far less encouraging than those described for HD. Patients whose initial remission exceeds 1 year may benefit from retreatment with the original regimen, but only 5 to 10% of patients who have a relapse after chemotherapy-induced CR have a long-term disease-free survival (i.e., cure) with conventional chemotherapy regimens.[167]

High dose chemotherapy with or without total body irradiation combined with autologous or allogeneic bone marrow transplant is also widely used as salvage therapy for patients with NHL.[117,128,168,169] The patients who are most likely to benefit from this type of therapy are those who achieve a CR after conventional salvage chemotherapy and those who only achieve a partial response after initial chemotherapy.[170] When used as salvage therapy in patients who have had a relapsed or had disease that was refractory to first-line therapy, CR rates of 40 to 60% have been reported, with 15 to 20% long-term survivors.[171–174] Higher cure rates (35 to 40%) have been reported for subgroups of patients who underwent this treatment approach when their tumors remained sensitive to chemotherapy (i.e., after a first relapse).

Highly Aggressive Non-Hodgkin's Lymphoma

Precursor lymphoblastic lymphoma/leukemia (T-cell type) generally occurs in adolescents and young adults. These patients are more likely to have bone marrow, mediastinal, and CNS involvement than those with other lymphomas. Encouraging results have been reported with regimens similar to those used to treat acute lymphoblastic leukemia with CNS prophylaxis and maintenance chemotherapy.

Systemic chemotherapy is the treatment of choice for Burkitt's lymphoma. Although aggressive chemotherapy regimens have achieved durable systemic remissions, many patients have relapses in the CNS. Therefore, such regimens should be augmented with intermittent intrathecal methotrexate or cytarabine prophylaxis. The initial chemotherapy regimen must contain high doses of cyclophosphamide, and commonly used regimens also include vincristine, doxorubicin, prednisone, and high-dose methotrexate. Regimens such as these are producing 2- to 3-year disease-free survival rates in the range of 50 to 70%.[175–177]

Other Lymphomas

There are five well-established treatment modalities for mycosis fungoides and Sézary syndrome: (1) topical therapy with mechlorethamine, (2) photochemotherapy with psoralen and ultraviolet light, (2) electron beam therapy to the whole body, (4) systemic chemotherapy, and (5) interferon-α.[5,178] Patients with disease limited to plaque lesions (without erythroderma or other tissue involvement) generally respond well to topical mechlorethamine or photochemotherapy, but most patients experience have a relapse within a few years. Electron beam irradiation also produces CRs in most patients with only plaque lesions and in some patients with more extensive disease, although relapse generally occurs within 3 years. Systemic chemotherapy is reserved for patients with disease that has spread to other organs. Combination chemotherapy regimens used in mycosis fungoides are similar to those used in other NHLs. Although these regimens produce CRs in about 25% of patients, the duration of response is usually brief.[5]

Recently denileukin diftitox (Ontak) was approved by the Food and Drug Administration for treatment of persistent or recurrent cutaneous T-cell lymphoma (including mycosis fungoides or the Sézary syndrome) when malignant cells express the CD25 subunit of the IL-2 receptor. Denileukin diftitox is a fusion protein containing part of the diphtheria toxin and IL-2. It is designed to direct the cytocidal action of diphtheria toxin to cells that express the IL-2 receptor. After binding with the receptor on the cell surface, cellular protein synthesis is inhibited, resulting in cell death within hours. Subunits of the IL-2 receptor are found on many cutaneous T- cell lymphoma cells; however, before denileukin diftitox therapy malignant cells must be tested for CD25 expression. The recommended treatment regimen is 9 or 18 μg/kg/day via intravenous infusion over at least 15 minutes for 5 consecutive days every 21 days. A randomized, double-blind study reported overall response rates of 23 and 36% with these doses, respectively.[179]

Human Immunodeficiency Virus-Associated Lymphomas

For patients with AIDS-related lymphomas the prognosis is much poorer than for patients with similar histologic subtypes who are not infected with HIV. Within the AIDS-associated lymphoma group, patients with a Karnofsky performance status less than 70%, a history of AIDS before diagnosis of lymphoma, a history of opportunistic infections, bone marrow involvement, other extranodal involvement, or a CD4 cell count of less than 100/dL have all been reported to have a shorter survival.[180,181] Obviously most of these prognostic factors are related to the underlying severity of the HIV infection or AIDS and it is uncertain at this time how improved antiretroviral therapies and supportive care will influence the prognosis associated with lymphoma in this group.

Because of the aggressiveness and extent of these lymphomas, intensive chemotherapy regimens similar to those used for aggressive non-HIV lymphomas have been used. CR rates have been somewhat less than those reported for those regimens in the non-HIV population, but several in vestigators have reported significant CR rates (>50%).[182–185] CR rates have been highest in patients without the poor prognostic factors mentioned above. Despite these encouraging responses, many investigators have reported median survivals of less than 1 year[182–185] with patients either dying of AIDS-related complications (e.g., opportunistic infections), treatment toxicity, or recurrent disease.

The high incidence of treatment-related complications and mortality has led to the use of less intensive regimens. The AIDS Clinical Trials Groups reported the results of a low-dose M-BACOD (50% dose of doxorubicin and cyclophosphamide) regimen with CNS and *Pneumocystis carinii* prophylaxis followed by zidovudine. Forty-six percent of 42 patients achieved a CR, with a median duration of 14 months.[186]

Evidence suggests that patients without poor prognostic signs who are able to tolerate combination chemotherapy and achieve a CR may experience a 1- to 2-year disease-free survival. Concomitant administration of hematopoietic growth factors and antiretroviral therapy has been reported by some to ameliorate some chemotherapy-related toxicities. Sparano et al.[187] reported that the concomitant use of didanosine and filgrastim with a 96-hour infusion regimen of cyclophosphamide, doxorubicin, and etoposide significantly reduced neutropenia and red blood cell transfusion requirements; however, the incidence of chemotherapy-induced CD4 or CD8 lymphopenia was not reduced. Fewer opportunistic infections were noted when dideoxycytidine was added to the M-BACOD regimen[188]; however, a high incidence of opportunistic infections and additive hematologic toxicities were also reported when zidovudine was added to a low-dose chemotherapy regimen.[189] The role of protease inhibitors is currently being evaluated. One group of investigators also reported a 243% increase in the p24 antigen in patients receiving concomitant sargramostim (GM-CSF), which they attributed to the expansion of macrophages.[190]

Unfortunately, with currently available therapeutic options, few patients attain a long-term disease-free survival. Therefore, less intensive (lower-dose) regimens that are associated with fewer complications and comparable response and survival outcomes are reasonable at this time.[191]

Methyl-glyoxal-bis guanylhydrazone (MGBG), an investigational agent, may be considered in patients with AIDS-related lymphoma who have a relapse or refractory disease.[192] MGBG provides another mechanism of action in that it interferes with polyamine biosynthesis. It also crosses the blood–brain barrier and has no significant myelotoxicity. Another investigational agent, a monoclonal antibody (anti-B4) conjugated with ricin, has been used in patients with AIDS-related lymphoma who have a relapse or refractory disease.[193] This agent was administered at a low dose over 28 days and may be associated with tumor responses with acceptable toxicity. Other trials have shown that relatively low doses of aldesleukin (IL-2) has increased CD4 counts, natural killer cells, and interferon-γ gene expression. It is currently being studied in HIV-related lymphomas.[194,195] Results from ongoing clinical trials such as these and additional new therapies are in great demand.

COMPLICATIONS

Patients with malignant lymphomas may experience a wide variety of complications, which may be secondary to either the disease or the therapy (Table 87.13). Although many of the disease-related complications have been reduced or eliminated through the use of more effective therapies, the use of more aggressive treatment regimens has resulted in more treatment-related complications. Additionally, the increased cure rate for HD and many of the NHLs has stimulated concern of late and long-term treatment-associated toxic reactions.

Many disease-related complications result from infiltration or obstruction of organs, tissues, or blood vessels by the lymphoma. Rapidly growing lymphomas (e.g., nodular sclerosing HD, and lymphoblastic lymphoma) may produce obstruction of the superior vena cava. Patients with this complication frequently exhibit shortness of breath; swelling of the face, neck and upper extremities; headache; and sensations of choking. The occurrence of superior vena cava syndrome should be considered an oncologic emergency. Therapy must often be initiated before a tissue diagnosis is made (if this is the initial presentation of the lymphoma) and includes immediate radiation therapy to the mass, diuretics, and combination chemotherapy.

Table 87.13 ▪ Serious Complications Associated with Lymphomas (and the Treatment of Lymphomas)

- Disease-related
  - Superior vena cava obstruction
  - Spinal cord compression
  - Central nervous system infiltration
  - Renal failure
  - Immunologic abnormalities
  - Pleural effusion
  - Hemolytic anemia
- Treatment-related
  - Chemotherapy-related
    - Granulocytopenia and infection
    - Tumor lysis syndrome
    - Gonadal injury/sterility
    - Secondary leukemia
    - Organ damage (e.g., renal, hepatic, cardiac) secondary to specific agents
  - Radiation therapy-related
    - Tumor lysis syndrome
    - Pneumonitis
    - Pericarditis
    - Hypothyroidism

Lymphoma masses may occasionally cause compression of the spinal cord. At initial diagnosis, this is generally more common with HD than NHL; however, it is more common overall in patients with relapses or refractory NHL and HIV-associated lymphomas. The most common presenting symptom is central back pain. As the degree of compression progresses, other neurologic symptoms develop (e.g., motor dysfunction, paresthesias, and incontinence) and paraplegia may result if no treatment is given. Appropriate therapy depends upon the extent of compression. If detected early enough, chemotherapy and/or radiation therapy may elicit a rapid improvement. In some patients with more advanced spinal cord compressions, emergency surgery (laminectomy) followed by radiation therapy may be required. Corticosteroids are also used to prevent edema or promote its resolution. These agents may also have a direct oncolytic effect as well.

Some lymphomas may infiltrate the CNS and develop meningeal seeding (leptomeningeal involvement). Signs of this complication include headache, nausea and vomiting, and lethargy. Confirmation of meningeal involvement is made by examination of the cerebrospinal fluid, and treatment includes corticosteroids and intrathecal chemotherapy agents (e.g., methotrexate and cytarabine) and radiation therapy. Intracerebral lymphomas may also occur, but these are generally primary tumors (now most commonly seen in patients with HIV) and not complications of other systemic disease.

Renal failure in patients with lymphoma may be caused by infiltration of the kidneys or obstruction of the ureters by the lymphoma. Infiltration of the kidneys is usually treated with systemic therapy (although low-dose, local radiation therapy may occasionally be used), and urethral obstruction may be treated with local radiation therapy combined with systemic chemotherapy.

As would be anticipated from the nature of the disease, immunologic abnormalities commonly occur in patients with malignant lymphomas. Abnormalities in delayed hypersensitivity, particularly cutaneous anergy, develop with extensive involvement of lymphatic tissues or severe lymphocytopenia. Depressed cell-mediated immunity (T lymphocyte) is associated with a high risk of opportunistic infections, including tuberculosis, salmonellosis, toxoplasmosis, and herpes zoster. This is particularly true in patients with HD. In some cases, infection may precede diagnosis of the disease.[196] Furthermore, patients may continue to have an underlying T-cell function deficit that persists after their disease is in remission.[197] Radiation and chemotherapy also contribute to the decreased immunologic functions and subsequent infectious complication.

Granulocytopenia secondary to myelosuppressive chemotherapy also predisposes patients to serious infections. Gram-negative bacilli (i.e., *Escherichia coli, Klebsiella pneumoniae, Pseudomonas aeruginosa*) and Gram-positive cocci (*Staphylococcus aureus* and *Staphylococcus epidermidis*) are the pathogens most commonly responsible for infections during granulocytopenia. As chemotherapy regimens have become more aggressive, especially those used in NHL, the degree and duration of granulocytopenia have increased, placing more patients at risk for infectious complications. Fortunately, the availability of colony-stimulating factors (filgrastim and sargramostim) has ameliorated this risk substantially.Acute and chronic toxic reactions associated with the administration of combination chemotherapy are determined by the individual agents included in the treatment regimen. In addition to myelosuppression, these may include nausea and vomiting, mucositis, neurotoxicity, cardiotoxicity, skin changes, and pulmonary toxicity. Many of these toxic reactions are avoidable or reversible if the clinician(s) managing the patient is familiar with the agents being used and their associated risks. The major long-term complications of chemotherapy of lymphomas are sterility and the risk of second malignancies.

Testicular function in adult men is particularly susceptible to injury by many chemotherapeutic agents. The MOPP regimen has been reported to cause azoospermia and germinal aplasia in more than 80% of men receiving this regimen.[198] Although chemotherapy-associated azoospermia is generally persistent, recovery may be observed in a small portion of patients several years after the cessation of therapy. A comparison of the MOPP and ABVD regimens revealed that azoospermia occurred in 100% of MOPP-treated men but in only 15 to 35% of those receiving ABVD therapy. In addition, spermatogenesis almost always reappeared in the ABVD-treated men.[199,200] This information may be important in planning treatment for young men with HD who are concerned about preservation of fertility after treatment.

Gonadal injury also occurs in women after combination chemotherapy. Ovarian failure is associated with arrest of follicular maturation or frank destruction of ova and follicles. Unlike the profound effects of the MOPP regimen on testicular function, it appears to produce ovarian dysfunction and amenorrhea in only 40 to 50% of women.[108,201] Ovarian injury from MOPP therapy is correlated with age at treatment, with older patients (older than age 35) much more likely to experience persistent amenorrhea.[202] Persistent amenorrhea also appears to be less common after ABVD therapy than after MOPP therapy.[199]

The potential of myelodysplasia and second malignancies, particularly acute nonlymphocytic leukemia, is a well-documented complication associated with HD and/or its therapy. Several studies have provided convincing evidence that the risk of leukemia varies markedly with the form of therapy for HD. Secondary leukemias occur in 2 to 3% of patients who have received MOPP with or without radiotherapy and the 10-year cumulative risk of such patients is between 5 and 10%.[203–205] Leukemia has usually developed between 3 and 10 years after initiation of treatment for HD, and in most patients HD has been in complete remission when the leukemia develops. The risk of acute leukemia after ABVD therapy appears to be negligible. Patients with HD are also at increased risk of developing NHL. NHLs apparently occur more frequently after combined radiation and chemotherapy.[206] Patients with HD may also have a slight increased risk of developing solid tumors.[205] In particular, an excess risk for lung cancer has been observed in patients who received radiation therapy (in the irradiated field).[205] Patients treated for NHL also have an increased risk of developing acute nonlymphocytic leukemia and the intensity of therapy appears to be correlated with the likelihood of developing a secondary leukemia.

Complications after radiation therapy are largely related to the field that has been irradiated, although fatigue generally occurs in most patients. Nausea, vomiting, mucositis/esophagitis, diarrhea, and anorexia commonly occur after abdominal radiation, while dryness of the mouth and throat, dysphagia, alteration in taste, and increased dental caries may occur after irradiation of the head and neck regions. Bone marrow depression may occur during the abdominal-pelvic irradiation and may require interruption of treatment. In addition to these acute side effects, long-term complications may pose more serious problems. Long-term effects are usually related to the volume of normal tissue that has been irradiated, the total dose given, and the size of the daily dose administered. They include radiation pneumonitis, pericarditis, nephritis, hepatitis, growth retardation (in children), and hypothyroidism.

CONCLUSION

Most lymphomas are sensitive to radiation therapy and to many chemotherapeutic agents. Combination chemotherapy regimens can now successfully cure HD and aggressive NHLs in many patients. In addition, many other patients experience a significant prolongation of disease-free survival after chemotherapy. It is likely that high-dose chemotherapy with bone marrow transplantation, monoclonal antibodies, and other biologic response modifiers (e.g., interferon) will assume a much more prominent role in the management of lymphomas in the future.

Management of patients with lymphomas requires not only an understanding of the disease process and its appropriate therapy but also an understanding of the variety of complications that may arise secondary to the disease or its therapy. These complications include opportunistic infections, obstruction by the tumor, secondary malignancies, and chemotherapy- and radiation-associated toxicities. Anticipation and appropriate management of these complications can greatly reduce the overall morbidity experienced by the patient.

KEY POINTS

- Lymphoid malignancies that present as extramedullary tumors arising primarily in the lymph nodes are called lymphomas, whereas lymphoid malignancies occurring predominantly in the bone marrow are leukemias.

- Lymphomas are broadly divided into HD and NHLs. Each of these groups includes various subtypes distinguished by morphologic, immunophenotypic, chromosomal, and clinical features.
- Treatment is determined by the classification and stage of the lymphoma at diagnosis as well as patient-specific factors that influence a patient's ability to tolerate therapy.
- Early-stage HD may be successfully treated with radiation therapy; however, advanced stages should be treated with combination chemotherapy. Chemotherapy regimens such as ABVD or MOPP produce long-term disease-free remissions in more than 50% of patients.
- Early-stage NHL may also be treated with radiation therapy. Advanced-stage indolent (follicular or low-grade) lymphomas may be treated with CVP, CHOP, or interferon in combination with cytotoxic chemotherapy.
- CHOP is the most widely recommended regimen for first-line treatment of advanced aggressive NHL.
- High-dose chemotherapy with peripheral blood or bone marrow stem cell rescue is a widely used strategy to treat patients with HD and NHL that are refractory to standard therapies.

REFERENCES

1. DeVita VT, Mauch PM, Harris NL. Hodgkin's disease. In: DeVita VT, Hellman S, Rosenberg SA, eds. Cancer. Principles and practice of oncology. 5th ed. Philadelphia: Lippincott-Raven, 1997:2242–2283.
2. Delsol G, Meggetto F, Brousett P, et al. Relation of follicular dendritic reticulum cells to Reed-Sternberg cells of Hodgkin's disease with emphasis on the expression of CD21q antigen. Am J Pathol 142:1729–1738, 1993.
3. Gaidano G, Dalla-Favera R. Molecular biology of lymphomas. In: DeVita VT, Hellman S, Rosenberg SA, eds. Cancer. Principles and practice of oncology. 5th ed. Philadelphia: Lippincott-Raven, 1997:2231–2245.
4. American Cancer Society. Cancer statistic 1999. New York: American Cancer Society, 1999.
5. Shipp MA, Mauch PM, Harris NL. Non-Hodgkin's lymphomas. In: DeVita VT, Hellman S, Rosenberg SA, eds. Cancer: Principles and practice of oncology. 5th ed. Philadelphia: Lippincott-Raven, 1997:2165–2219.
6. Cantor KP, Fraumeni JF. Distribution of non-Hodgkin's lymphoma in the United States between 1950 and 1975. Cancer Res 40:2645–2652, 1980.
7. MacMahon B. Epidemiological evidence of the nature of Hodgkin's disease. Cancer 10:1045–1054, 1957.
8. Mueller NE. Hodgkin's disease. In: Schnottenfeld D, Fraumani J, eds. Cancer epidemiology and prevention. 2nd ed. New York: Oxford University Press, 1992
9. Penn I. The incidence of malignancies in transplant recipients. Transplant Proc 7:323, 1975.
10. Matas AJ, Hertel BF, Rosai J, et al. Post-transplant malignant lymphoma. Distinctive morphologic features related to its pathogenesis. Am J Med 61:716, 1976.
11. Levine AM. Lymphoma complicating immunodeficiency disorders. Ann Oncol 5(Suppl 2):29–35, 1994.
12. Morrison VA, Dunn DL, Manivel CJ, et al. Clinical characteristics of post-transplant lymphoproliferative disorders. Am J Med 97:14–24, 1994.
13. Kamel OW, van de Rijn M, Hanasono MM, et al. Immunosuppression-associated lymphoproliferative disorders in rheumatic patients. Leuk Lymphoma 16:363–368, 1995.
14. Aisenberg AC. Coherent view of non-Hodgkin's lymphoma. J Clin Oncol 13:2656–2675, 1995.
15. McKnight H, Cen H, Riddler SA, et al. EBV gene expression, EBNA antibody responses and EBV+ peripheral blood lymphocytes in post-transplant lymphoproliferative disease. Leuk Lymphoma 15:9–16, 1994.
16. Reedman BM, Klein G. Cellular localization of an Epstein-Barr virus (EBV)-associated complement fixing antigen in producer and nonproducer lymphoblastoid cell lines. Int J Cancer 11:499–520, 1973.
17. Blattner WA, Gibbs WN, Saxinger C, et al. Human T-cell leukaemia/lymphoma virus-lymphomareticular neoplasia in Jamaica. Lancet 2:61–64, 1983.
18. Miller RW, Beebe GW. Infectious mononucleosis and the empirical risk of cancer. J Natl Cancer Inst 50:315–321, 1973.
19. Connolly RR, Chistene BW. A cohort study of cancer following infectious mononucleosis. Cancer Res 34:1172–1178, 1974.
20. Rosdahl N, Larsen SO, Clemmensen J. Hodgkin's disease in patients with previous mononucleosis, 30 years experience. Br Med J 2:253–256, 1974.
21. Gottlieb-Stematsky T, Vonsover A, Ramot B, et al. Antibodies to Epstein-Barr virus in patients with Hodgkin's disease and leukemia. Cancer 36:1640–1645, 1975.
22. Evans AS, Gutensohn NM. A population-based case-control study of EBV and other viral antibodies among persons with Hodgkin's disease and their siblings. Int J Cancer 34:149–157, 1984.
23. Mueller N, Evans A, Harris NL, et al. Hodgkin's disease and Epstein-Barr virus. Altered antibody pattern before diagnosis. N Engl J Med 320:689–695, 1989.
24. MacMahon B. Epidemiological evidence of the nature of Hodgkin's disease. Cancer 10:1045–1052, 1957.
25. Mueller NA, Evans A, Harris NL, et al. Hodgkin's disease and Epstein-Barr virus. Altered antibody patterns before diagnosis. N Engl J Med 320:689–695, 1989.
26. Pallesen G, Hamilton-Dutoit SJ, Rowe M, et al. Expression of Epstein-Barr virus latent gene products in tumour cells of Hodgkin's disease. Lancet 337:320–322, 1991.
27. Weiss LM, Strickler JG, Warnke RA, et al. Epstein-Barr viral DNA in tissues of Hodgkin's disease. Am J Pathol 129:86–91, 1987.
28. Weiss LM. Gene analysis and Epstein-Barr viral genome studies of Hodgkin's disease. Int Rev Exp Pathol 33:165–184, 1992.
29. Weiss LM, Movahed LA, Warnke RA, et al. Detection of Epstein-Barr viral genomes in Reed-Sternberg cells of Hodgkin's disease. N Engl J Med 320:502–506, 1989.
30. Boiocchi M, Carbone A, DeRe V, et al. Is the Epstein-Barr virus involved in Hodgkin's disease. Tumori 75:345–350, 1989.
31. Bignon YJ, Bernard D, Cure H, et al. Detection of Epstein-Barr viral genomes in lymph nodes of Hodgkin's disease patients. Mol Carcinog 3:9–11, 1990.
32. Uhara H, Sato Y, Mukai K, et al. Detection of Epstein-Barr DNA in Reed-Sternberg cells of Hodgkin's disease using the polymerase chain reaction and in situ hybridization. Jpn J Cancer Res 81:272–278, 1990.
33. Anagnostopoulos I, Hummel M, Stein H. Epstein-Barr virus and Hodgkin's disease. Forum 6:36–42, 1996.
34. Vianna NJ, Greenwald P, Davies JNP. Extended epidemic of Hodgkin's disease in patients with previous mononucleosis, 30 years experience. Br Med J 2:253–256, 1974.
35. Vianna JH, Dolan AK. Epidemiological evidence for transmission of Hodgkin's disease. N Engl J Med 289:499–502, 1973.
36. Grufferman S, Cole P, Smith PG, et al. Hodgkin's disease in siblings. N Engl J Med 296:248–250, 1977.
37. Prazak J, Hermanska Z. Study of HLA antigens in patients with Hodgkin's disease. Eur J Haematol 43:50–53, 1989.
38. Reitz M. Human T-cell leukemia virus, type 1, and human leukemia and lymphoma. In: Cossman J, ed. Molecular genetics in cancer diagnosis. New York: Elsevier, 1990:163.
39. Cesarman E, Chang Y, Moore PS, et al. Kaposi's sarcoma-associated herpesvirus-like DNA sequences in AIDS-related body-cavity-based lymphomas. N Engl J Med 332:1186–1191, 1995.
40. Parsonnet J, Hansen S, Rodriguez L, et al. *Helicobacter pylori* infection and gastric lymphoma. N Engl J Med 330:1267–1271, 1994.
41. Wotherspoon AC, Ortiz-Hidalgo C, Falzon MR, et al. *Helicobacter pylori*-associated gastritis and primary B-cell lymphoma. Lancet 338:1175–1176, 1991.
42. Eidt S, Stolte M, Fischer R. *Helicobacter pylori* gastritis and primary gastric non-Hodgkin's lymphomas. J Clin Pathol 47:436–439, 1994.
43. Rabkin CS, Devesa SS, Zahm SH, et al. Increasing incidence of non-Hodgkin's lymphoma. Semin Hematol 30:286–296, 1993.
44. Anderson RE, Nishiyama H, Yohei I, et al. Pathogenesis of radiation related leukemia and lymphoma. Speculations based primarily on experience of Hiroshima and Nagasaki. Lancet 1:1060–1062, 1972.
45. Olsen JH, Boice JD, Jensen JP, et al. Cancer among epileptic patients exposed to anticonvulsant drugs. J Natl Cancer Inst 81:803–808, 1989.
46. Harris NL, Jaffe ES, Stein H, et al. A revised European-American classification of lymphoid neoplasms: a proposal from the International Lymphoma Study Group. Blood 84:1361–1392, 1994.
47. Bennett M, MacLennan K, Vaughan Hudson G, et al. Non-Hodgkin's lymphoma arising in patients treated for Hodgkin's disease in the BNLI: a 20-year experience. British National Lymphoma Investigation. Ann Oncol 2(Suppl 2):83–92, 1991.

48. Kradin ME, Agnarsson BA, Ellingsworth LR, et al. Immunohistochemical evidence of a role for transforming growth factor beta in the pathogenesis of nodular sclerosing Hodgkin's disease. Am J Pathol 136:1209–1214, 1990.
49. Rappaport H. Tumors of the hematopoietic system. In: Atlas of Tumor Pathology. Section III, Fascicle 8. Washington DC: Armed Forces Institute of Pathology, 1966.
50. National Cancer Institute sponsored study of classification of non-Hodgkin's lymphomas. Summary and description of a working formulation for clinical usage. Cancer 49:2112–2135, 1982.
51. Harris NL, Jaffe ES, Stein H, et al. A revised European-American Classification of lymphoid neoplasms: A proposal from the International Lymphoma Study Group. Blood 84:1361–1392, 1994.
52. Mac Manus MP, Hoppe R. Is radiotherapy curative for stage I and II low-grade follicular lymphoma? Results of a long-term follow-up study of patients treated at Stanford University. J Clin Oncol 14:1282–1298, 1996.
53. Armitage JO: Treatment of Non-Hodgkin's lymphoma. N Engl J Med 328:1023–1030, 1993.
54. Foucar K. Incidence and patterns of bone marrow and blood involvement by lymphoma in relationship to the Lukes-Collins classification. Blood 54:1417–1422, 1979.
55. Centers for Disease Control. Revision of the case definition of acquired immunodeficiency syndrome for national reporting–United States. MMWR Morb Mortal Wkly Rep 34:373–375, 1985.
56. DeMario MD, Liebowitz DN. Lymphomas in the immunocompromised patient. Semin Oncol 25:492–502, 1998.
57. Ziegler JL, Drew WL, Miner RC, et al. Outbreak of Burkitt's-like lymphoma in homosexual men. Lancet 2:631–633, 1982.
58. Snider WD, Simpson DM, Aronyk KE, et al. Primary lymphoma of the nervous system associated with acquired immunodeficiency syndrome [Letter]. N Engl J Med 308:45, 1983.
59. Ciobanu N, Adreeff M, Safai B, et al. Lymphoblastic neoplasia in a homosexual patient with Kaposi's sarcoma. Ann Intern Med 98:151–155, 1983.
60. Ioachim HL, Cooper MC, Hellman GC. Lymphomas in men at high risk for acquired immune deficiency syndrome. Cancer 56:2831–2842, 1985.
61. Biggar RJ, Horm J, Goedert JJ, et al. Cancer in a group at risk of acquired immunodeficiency syndrome (AIDS) through 1984. Am J Epidemiol 126:578–586, 1987.
62. Rabkin CS, Biggar RJ, Horm JW. Increasing incidence of cancers associated with the human immunodeficiency virus epidemic. Int J Cancer 47:692–696, 1991.
63. Kaplan L, Straus D, Testa M, et al. Randomized trial of standard dose mBACOD with GM-CSF vs. reduced dose mBACOD for systemic HIV-associated lymphoma: ACTG 142 [Abstract]. Proc Am Soc Clin Oncol 14:288, 1995.
64. Ziegler JL, Beckstead JA, Volberding PA, et al. Non-Hodgkins lymphoma in 90 homosexual men. Relation to generalized lymphadenopathy and the acquired immunodeficiency syndrome. N Engl J Med 311:565–570, 1984.
65. Lister TA, Crowther D, Sutcliffe SB, et al. Report of a committee convened to discuss the evaluation and staging of patients with Hodgkin's disease: Cotswolds Meeting. J Clin Oncol 7:1630–1636, 1989.
66. Ng AK, Weeks JC, Mauch PM, et al. Laparotomy versus no laparotomy in the management of early-stage, favorable-prognosis Hodgkin's disease: a decision analysis. J Clin Oncol 17:241–252, 1999.
67. Shipp MA. Prognostic factors in aggressive non-Hodgkin's lymphoma: who has "high-risk" disease? Blood 83:1165–1173, 1994.
68. DeVita VT, Serpick A, Carbone P: Combination chemotherapy in the treatment of advanced Hodgkin's disease. Ann Intern Med 73:881–895, 1970.
69. Hoppe RT. Radiation therapy in the management of Hodgkin's disease. Semin Oncol 17:704–715, 1990.
70. Leslie NT, Mauch PM, Hellman S. Stage IA to IIB supradiaphragmatic Hodgkin's disease: Long-term survival and relapse frequency. Cancer 55: 2072–2078, 1985.
71. Lee CK, Aeppli DM, Bloomfield CD, et al. Curative radiotherapy for laparotomy-staged IA, IIA, IIIA Hodgkin's disease: an evaluation of the gains achieved with radical radiotherapy. Int J Radiat Oncol Biol Phys 19:547–549, 1990.
72. Farah R, Ultmann J, Griem M, et al. Extended mantle radiation therapy for pathologic stage I and II Hodgkin's disease. J Clin Oncol 6:1047–1058, 1988.
73. Gladstein E. Radiation in Hodgkin's disease: past achievements and future progress. Cancer 39:837–842, 1977.
74. Koziner B, Myers J, Cirrincione C, et al. Treatment of stages I and II Hodgkin's disease with three different therapeutic modalities. Am J Med 80:1067–1078, 1986.
75. Mauch P, Goodman R, Hellman S. The significance of mediastinal involvement in early stage Hodgkin's disease. Cancer 42:1039–1045, 1978.
76. Leopold KA, Canellos GP, Rosenthal D, et al. Stage IA-IIB Hodgkin's disease: staging and treatment with large mediastinal adenopathy. J Clin Oncol 7:1059–1065, 1989.
77. Zittoun R, Audebert A, Hoemi B, et al. Extended versus involved fields irradiation combined with MOPP chemotherapy in early clinical stages of Hodgkin's disease. J Clin Oncol 3:207–214, 1985.
78. Bonadonna G. Modern treatment of malignant lymphomas: a multidisciplinary approach? The Kaplan Memorial Lecture. Ann Oncol 5(Suppl 2):5–16, 1994.
79. Longo DL, Glatstein E, Duffy PL, et al. Radiation therapy versus combination chemotherapy in the treatment of early-stage Hodgkin's disease: seven year results of a prospective randomized trial. J Clin Oncol 9:906–917, 1991.
80. Portlock CS. Hodgkin's disease. Med Clin North Am 68:629–740, 1984.
81. Longo DL. The use of chemotherapy in the treatment of Hodgkin's disease. Semin Oncol 17:716–735, 1990.
82. Stein RS, Golomb HS, Wiernik PH, et al. Anatomic substages of stage IIIA Hodgkin's disease: followup of a collaborative study. Cancer Treat Rep 66:733–741, 1982.
83. Hoppe RT, Cox RS, Rosenberg SA, et al. Prognostic factors in pathologic stage III Hodgkin's disease. Cancer Treat Rep 66:743–749, 1982.
84. Mouch PM, Rosenthal DS, Canellos GP, et al. Improved survival for stage IIIA and IIIB Hodgkin's disease patients treated with combined radiation therapy (RT) and chemotherapy. Proc Am Soc Clin Oncol 2:213, 1983.
85. Lister TA, Dorreen MS, Faux M, et al. Treatment of stage III_A Hodgkin's disease. J Clin Oncol 1:745–749, 1983.
86. Crowther D, Wagstaff J, Deaken D, et al. A randomized study comparing chemotherapy alone and chemotherapy followed by radiotherapy in patients with pathologically staged III_A Hodgkin's disease. J Clin Oncol 2:892–897, 1984.
87. Brookman MA, Longo DL. Concomitant illness in patients treated for Hodgkin's disease. Cancer Treat Rev 13:77–111, 1986.
88. DeVita VT, Simon RM, Hubbard SM, et al. Curability of advanced Hodgkin's disease with chemotherapy: long-term follow up of MOPP treated patients at the National Cancer Institute. Ann Intern Med 92:587–595, 1980.
89. Longo DL, Young RC, Wesley M, et al. Twenty years of MOPP therapy for Hodgkin's disease. J Clin Oncol 4:1295–1306, 1986.
90. van Rijswijk RE, Haanen C, Dekker AW, et al. Dose intensity of MOPP chemotherapy and survival in Hodgkin's disease. J Clin Oncol 7:1776–1782, 1989.
91. Straus DJ, Myers J, Lee BJ, et al. Treatment of advanced Hodgkin's disease with chemotherapy and irradiation. Controlled trial of two versus three alternating potentially non-cross resistant drug combinations. Am J Med 76:270–278, 1984.
92. Goldie JH, Coldman AJ. A mathematical model for relating the drug sensitivity of tumors to their spontaneous mutation rate. Cancer Treat Rep 63:1727–1733, 1979.
93. Santoro A, Bonadonna G, Bonfante V, et al. Alternating drug combinations in the treatment of advanced Hodgkin's disease. N Engl J Med 306:770–775, 1982.
94. Bonadonna G, Valgussa P, Santoro A. Alternating non-cross-resistant combination chemotherapy or MOPP in stage IV Hodgkin's disease. Ann Intern Med 104:739–746, 1986.
95. Klimo P, Connors JM. An update on the Vancouver experience in the management of advanced Hodgkin's disease treated with the MOPP/ABV hybrid program. Semin Hematol 25:34–40, 1988.
96. Glick J, Young ML, Harrington D, et al. MOPP/ABV hybrid chemotherapy for advanced Hodgkin's disease significantly improves failure-free and overall survival: the 8-year results of the intergroup trial. J Clin Oncol 16:19–26, 1998.
97. Canellos GP, Anderson JR, Propert KJ, et al. Chemotherapy of advanced Hodgkin's disease with MOPP, ABVD, or MOPP alternating with ABVD. N Engl J Med 327:1478–1484, 1992.
98. Oliver IN, Wolf MM, Cruickshank D, et al. Nitrogen mustard, vincristine, procarbazine, and prednisolone for relapse after radiation in Hodgkin's disease. Cancer 62:233–239, 1988.
99. Pillai GN, Hagemeister RB, Valasquez WS, et al. Prognostic factors for stage IV Hodgkin's disease treated with MOPP, with or without bleomycin. Cancer 55:691–697, 1985.
100. Wagstaff J, Gregory WM, Swindell R, et al. Prognostic factors for survival in stage III_B and IV Hodgkin's disease: a multivariate analysis comparing two specialist treatment centres. Br J Cancer 58:487–492, 1988.
101. Carde P, MacKintosh FR, Rosenberg SA. A dose and time response analysis of the treatment of Hodgkin's disease with MOPP chemotherapy. J Clin Oncol 1:146–153, 1983.
102. Canellos GP. Can MOPP be replaced in the treatment of advanced Hodgkin's disease? Semin Oncol 17(Suppl 2):2–6, 1990.
103. Levis A, Vitolo U, CioccaVasina MA, et al. Predictive value of the early response to chemotherapy in high-risk stages II and III Hodgkin's disease. Cancer 60:1713–1719, 1987.

104. Green JA, Dawson AA, Fell LF, et al. Measurement of drug dosage intensity in MVPP therapy in Hodgkin's disease. Br J Clin Pharmacol 9:511–514, 1980.
105. Van Rijswijk RE, Haanen C, Dekker AW, et al. Dose intensity of MOPP chemotherapy and survival in Hodgkin's disease. J Clin Oncol 7:1776–1782, 1989.
106. Gibbs GE, Peterson BA, Kennedy BJ, et al. Long-term survival of patients with Hodgkin's disease: treatment with cyclophosphamide, vinblastine, procarbazine, and prednisone. Arch Intern Med 141:897–900, 1981.
107. Santoro A, Viviana S, Villarreal CJ, et al. Salvage chemotherapy in Hodgkin's disease irradiation failures: superiority of doxorubicin-containing regimens over MOPP. Cancer Treat Rep 70:343–348, 1986.
108. Fisher RI, DeVita VT, Hubbard SM, et al. Prolonged disease-free survival in Hodgkin's disease with MOPP reinduction after first relapse. Ann Intern Med 90:761–763, 1979.
109. Canellos GP, Petroni GR, Barcos M, et al. Etoposide, vinblastine, and doxorubicin: an active regimen for the treatment of Hodgkin's disease in relapse following MOPP. Cancer and Leukemia Group B. J Clin Oncol 13:2005–2011, 1995.
110. Bonadonna G, Viviani S, Valagussa P, et al. Third-line salvage chemotherapy in Hodgkin's disease. Semin Oncol 12(Suppl 2):23–25, 1985.
111. Santoro A, Viviani SS, Valagussa P, et al. CCNU, etoposide and prednimustine (CEP) in refractory Hodgkin's disease. Semin Oncol 13(Suppl 1):23–26, 1986.
112. Taylor RE, McElwin TJ, Barrett A, et al. Etoposide as a single agent in relapsed advanced lymphoma–a phase II study. Cancer Chemother Pharmacol 7:175–177, 1982.
113. Harker WG, Kushlan P, Rosenberg SA. Combination chemotherapy for advanced Hodgkin's disease after failure of MOPP: ABVD and B-CAVe. Ann Intern Med 101:440–446, 1984.
114. Canellos GP. Is there an effective salvage therapy for advanced Hodgkin's disease? Ann Oncol 2(Suppl 1):1–7, 1991.
115. Vose JM, Bierman PJ, Armitage JO. Hodgkin's disease: the role of bone marrow transplantation. Semin Oncol 17:749–757, 1990.
116. Williams SF, Bitran JD. The role of high-dose therapy and autologous bone marrow reinfusion in the treatment of Hodgkin's disease. Hematol Oncol Clin North Am 3:319–329, 1989.
117. Anderson JE, Litzow MR, Appelbaum FR, et al. Allogeneic, syngeneic, and autologous marrow transplantation for Hodgkin's disease: the 21-year Seattle experience. J Clin Oncol 11:2342–2350, 1993.
118. Jagannath S, Armitage JO, Dicke KA, et al. Prognostic factors for response and survival after high-dose cyclophosphamide, carmustine, and etoposide with autologous bone marrow transplantation. J Clin Oncol 7:179–185, 1989.
119. Carella AM, Congiu AM, Gaozza E, et al. High-dose chemotherapy with autologous bone marrow transplantation in 50 advanced resistant Hodgkin's disease patients: an Italian Study Group report. J Clin Oncol 6:1411–1416, 1988.
120. Gribben JG, Linch DC, Singer CRJ, et al. Successful treatment of refractory Hodgkin's disease by high-dose combination chemotherapy and autologous bone marrow transplantation. Blood 73:340–344, 1989.
121. Goldstone AH. EBMT experience of autologous BMT (ABMT) in non-Hodgkin's lymphoma and Hodgkin's disease. Bone Marrow Transplant 1(Suppl):289–292, 1986.
122. Phillips GL, Solff SN, Herzig RH, et al. Treatment of progressive Hodgkin's disease with intensive chemoradiotherapy and autologous bone marrow transplantation. Blood 73:2086–2092, 1989.
123. Vose JM, Bierman PJ, Armitage JO. Hodgkin's disease: the role of bone marrow transplantation. Semin Oncol 17:749–757, 1990.
124. Jones RJ, Piantadosi S, Mann RB, et al. High-dose cytotoxic therapy and bone marrow transplantation for relapsed Hodgkin's disease. J Clin Oncol 8:527–537, 1990.
125. Reese DE, Barnett MJ, Conners JM, et al. Intensive chemotherapy with cyclophosphamide, carmustine, and etoposide followed by autologous bone marrow transplantation for relapsed Hodgkin's disease. J Clin Oncol 9:1871–1879, 1991.
126. Desch CE, Lasala MR, Smith TJ, et al. The optimal timing of autologous bone marrow transplantation in Hodgkin's disease patients after a chemotherapy relapse. J Clin Oncol 10:200–209, 1992.
127. Lazarus HM, Rowlings PA, Zhang M-J, et al. Autotransplants for Hodgkin's disease in patients never achieving remission: a report from the Autologous Blood and Marrow Transplant Registry. J Clin Oncol 17:534–545, 1999.
128. Rappaport AP, Rowe JM, Kouides PA, et al. One hundred autotransplants for relapsed or refractory Hodgkin's disease and lymphoma: value of pretransplant disease status for predicting outcome. J Clin Oncol 11:2351–2361, 1993.
129. Taylor K Mc, Jagannath S, Spinolo JA, et al. Recombinant human granulocyte colony-stimulating factor hastens recovery after high-dose chemotherapy and autologous bone marrow transplantation in Hodgkin's disease. J Clin Oncol 7:791–799, 1989.
130. Nemunaitis J, Singer JW, Buchner CD, et al. Use of recombinant human granulocyte-macrophage colony-stimulating factor in autologous marrow transplantation for lymphoid malignancies. Blood 72:834–836, 1988.
131. Portlock CS. Management of the low-grade non-Hodgkin's lymphomas. Semin Oncol 17:51–59, 1990.
132. Chabner BA, Johnson RE, Young R, et al. Sequential non-surgical and surgical staging of non-Hodgkin's lymphomas. Ann Intern Med 85:149–154, 1976.
133. Rosenberg SA. Validity of Ann Arbor staging of the non-Hodgkin's lymphomas. Cancer Treat Rep 61:1023–1027, 1977.
134. Gribben JG, Freedman AS, Woo SD, et al. All advanced stage non-Hodgkin's lymphomas with polymerase chain reaction amplifiable breakpoint of bcl-2 have residual cells containing the bcl-2 re-arrangement at evaluation and after treatment. Blood 78:3275–3280, 1991.
135. Redman JR, Cabanillas F, Velasquez WS, et al. Phase II trial of fludarabine phosphate in lymphoma: an effective new agent in low-grade lymphoma. J Clin Oncol 10:790–794, 1992.
136. Tefferi A, Witzig T, Reid J, et al. Phase I study of combined 2-chlorodeoxyadenosine and chlorambucil in chronic lymphocytic leukemia and low-grade lymphoma. J Clin Oncol 12:569–574, 1994.
137. Saven A, Emanuele S, Kosty M, et al. 2-Chlorodeoxyadenosine activity in patients with untreated, indolent non-Hodgkin's lymphoma. Blood 86:1710–1716, 1995.
138. Solal-Celigny P, Brice P, Brousse N, et al. Phase II trial of fludarabine monophosphate as first-line treatment in patients with advanced follicular lymphoma: a multicenter study by the Groupe d'Etude des Lymphomes de l'Adulte. J Clin Oncol 14:514–519, 1996.
139. Hochster H, Oken H, Bennett I, et al. Efficacy of cyclophosphamide (CYC) and fludarabine (FAMP) as first line therapy of low-grade non-Hodgkin's lymphoma (NHL)-ECOG 1491 [Abstract]. Blood 84:383a, 1994.
140. Foon KA, Sherwin SA, Abrams PG. Treatment of advanced non-Hodgkin's lymphoma with recombinant leukocyte A interferon. N Engl J Med 311: 1148–1152, 1984.
141. Andersen JW, Smalley RV. Inteferon alfa plus chemotherapy for non-Hodgkin's lymphoma: five-year follow-up [Letter]. N Engl J Med 329:1821–1822, 1993.
142. Solal-Celigny P, Lepage E, Brousse N, et al. Doxorubicin-containing regimen with or without interferon alfa-2b for advanced follicular lymphomas: final analysis of survival and toxicity in the Groupe d'Etude des Lymphomes Folliculaires 86 Trial. J Clin Oncol 16:2332–2338, 1998.
143. Cole BF, Solal-Celigny P, Gelber RD, et al. Quality-of-life adjusted survival analysis of interferon alfa-2b treatment for advanced follicular lymphoma: an aid to clinical decision making. J Clin Oncol 16:2339–2344, 1998.
144. Maloney DG, Liles TM, Czerwinski DK, et al. Phase I clinical trial using escalating single-dose infusion of chimeric anti-CD20 monoclonal antibody (IDEC-C2B8) in patients with recurrent B-cell lymphoma. Blood 84:2457–2466, 1994.
145. McLaughlin P, Grillo-Lopez AJ, Link BK, et al. Rituximab chimeric anti-CD20 monoclonal antibody therapy for relapsed indolent lymphoma: half of patients respond to a four-dose treatment program. J Clin Oncol 16:2825–2833, 1998.
146. Czuczman MS, Grillo-Lopez AJ, White CA, et al. Treatment of patients with low-grade B-cell lymphoma with the combination of chimeric anti-CD20 monoclonal antibody and CHOP chemotherapy. J Clin Oncol 17:268–276, 1999.
147. Brice P, Bastion Y, Lepage E, et al. Comparison in low-tumor-burden follicular lymphomas between an initial no-treatment policy, prednimustine, or interferon alfa: a randomized study from the Groupe d'Etude des Lymphomes Folliculaires. Groupe d'Etude des Lymphomes de l'Adulte. J Clin Oncol 15:1110–1117, 1997.
148. Horning S, Rosenberg S. The natural history of initially untreated low-grade non-Hodgkin's lymphomas. N Engl J Med 311:1471–1475, 1984.
149. Rosenberg SA. The Karnofsky Memorial Lecture. The low-grade non-Hodgkin's lymphoma: challenges and opportunities. J Clin Oncol 3:299–310, 1985.
150. Straus D, Gaynor JJ, Lieberman PH, et al. Non-Hodgkin's lymphomas: characteristics of long-term survivors following conservative treatment. Am J Med 82:847–856, 1987.
151. Freedman A, Neuberg D, Gribben J, et al. Autologous bone marrow transplantation in relapsed low grade non-Hodgkin's lymphoma [Abstract]. Bone Marrow Transplant 203, 1995.
152. Rohatiner A, Johnson P, Price C, et al. Myeloblative therapy with autologous bone marrow transplantation as consolidation therapy for recurrent follicular lymphoma. J Clin Oncol 12:1177–1184, 1994.
153. Monfardini S, Banfi A, Bonadonna G, et al. Improved five year survival after combined radiotherapy-chemotherapy for stage I-II non-Hodgkin's lymphoma. Int J Radiat Oncol Biol Phys 6:125–134, 1980.

154. Nissen NI, Ersboll J, Hansen HS, et al. A randomized study of radiotherapy versus radiotherapy plus chemotherapy in stage I-II non-Hodgkin's lymphomas. Cancer 52:1–7, 1983.
155. Glick J, Kim K, Earle J, et al. An ECOG randomized phase III trial of CHOP vs CHOP + radiotherapy for intermediate grade early stage non-Hodgkin's lymphoma [Abstract]. Proc Am Soc Clin Oncol 14:391, 1995.
156. Fisher RI, Gaynor ER, Dahlberg S, et al. Comparison of a standard regimen (CHOP) with three intensive chemotherapy regimens for advanced non-Hodgkin's lymphoma. N Engl J Med 328:1002–1006, 1993.
157. Skarin AT, Canellos GP, Rosenthal DS, et al. Improved prognosis of diffuse histiocytic and undifferentiated lymphoma by use of high dose methotrexate alternating with standard agents (M-BACOD). J Clin Oncol 1:91–98, 1983.
158. Klimo P, Connors JM. MACOP-B chemotherapy for the treatment of diffuse large-cell lymphoma. Ann Intern Med 102:596–602, 1985.
159. Gordon L, Harrington D, Anderson J, et al. Comparison of a second-generation combination chemotherapeutic regimen (m-BACOD) with a standard regimen (CHOP) for advanced diffuse non-Hodgkin's lymphoma. N Engl J Med 327:1342–1349, 1992.
160. Meyer RM, Quirt IC, Skillings JR, et al. Escalated as compared with standard doses doxorubicin in BACOP therapy for patients with non-Hodgkin's lymphoma. N Engl J Med 329:1770–1776, 1993.
161. Meyer RM, Hryniuk WM, Goodyear MDE. The role of dose intensity in determining outcome in intermediate-grade non-Hodgkin's lymphoma. J Clin Oncol 9:339–347, 1991.
162. Fisher RI, Hubbard SM, DeVita VT, et al. Factors predicting long-term survival in diffuse mixed, histiocytic, or undifferentiated lymphoma. Blood 58:45–50, 1981.
163. Vose JM, Armitage JO, Weisenburger DD, et al. The importance of age in survival of patients treated with chemotherapy for diffuse large-cell lymphoma–rapidly responding patients have more durable remissions. J Clin Oncol 4:160–164, 1986.
164. Haioun C, Lepage E, Gisselbrecht C, et al. Autologous bone marrow transplantation (ABMT) versus sequential chemotherapy for aggressive non Hodgkin's lymphoma (NHL) in first complete remission (CR): a study of 542 patients (LNH87-2 Protocol) [Abstract]. Blood 86:457a, 1995.
165. Shipp M, Neuberg D, Janicek M, et al. High-dose CHOP as initial therapy for patients with poor prognosis aggressive non-Hodgkin's lymphoma: a dose-finding pilot study. J Clin Oncol 13:2916–2923, 1995.
166. Gianni AM, Bregni M, Siena S, et al. High-dose chemotherapy and autologous bone marrow transplantation compared with MACOP-B in aggressive B-cell lymphoma. N Engl J Med 336:1290–1297, 1997.
167. Cabanillas F. Experience with salvage regimens at M.D. Anderson Hospital. Ann Oncol 2(Suppl 1):31–32, 1991.
168. Kessinger A, Nademanee A, Forman SJ, et al. Autologous bone marrow transplantation for Hodgkin's and non-Hodgkin's lymphoma. Hematol Oncol Clin North Am 4:577–587, 1990.
169. Williams SF. The role of bone marrow transplantation in the non-Hodgkin's lymphomas. Semin Oncol 17:88–95, 1990.
170. Haq R, Sawka CA, Franssen E, et al. Significance of a partial or slow response to front-line chemotherapy in the management of intermediate-grade or high-grade non-Hodgkin's lymphoma: a literature review. J Clin Oncol 12:1074–1084, 1994.
171. Phillips GL, Herzig RH, Lazarus HM, et al. Treatment of resistant malignant lymphoma with cyclophosphamide, total body irradiation, and transplantation of cryopreserved autologous marrow. N Engl J Med 310:1557–1561, 1984.
172. Armitage JO, Gingrich RD, Klassen LW, et al. Trial of high-dose cytarabine, cyclophosphamide, total-body irradiation, and autologous marrow transplantation for refractory lymphoma. Cancer Treat Rep 70:871–875 1986.
173. Takvorian T, Canellos GP, Ritz J, et al. Prolonged disease free survival after autologous bone marrow transplantation in patients with non-Hodgkin's lymphoma with a poor prognosis. N Engl J Med 316;1499–1505, 1987.
174. Armitage JO. Treatment of non-Hodgkin's lymphoma. N Engl J Med 328:1023–1030, 1993.
175. Schwenn MR, Blattner SR, Lynch E, et al. HiC-COM: a 2-month intensive chemotherapy regimen for children with stage III and IV Burkitt's lymphoma and B-cell acute lymphoblastic leukemia. J Clin Oncol 9:133–138, 1991.
176. Soussain C, Patte C, Ostronoff M, et al. Small noncleaved cell lymphoma and leukemia in adults: a retrospective study of 65 adults treated with the LMB pediatric protocols. Blood 85:664–674, 1995.
177. Magrath I, Adde M, Shad A, et al. Adults and children with small non-cleaved-cell lymphoma have a similar excellent outcome when treated with the same chemotherapy regimen. J Clin Oncol 14:925–934, 1996.
178. Cutaneous T-cell lymphoma (mycosis fungoides). Lancet 347:871–876, 1996.
179. Package insert. ONTAK. San Diego, CA: Ligand Pharmaceuticals, 1999.
180. Levine AM, Sullivan-Halley J, Pike MC, et al. Human immunodeficiency virus-related lymphoma: Prognostic factors predictive of survival. Cancer 68:2466–2472, 1991.
181. Kaplan LD, Abrams DI, Feigel E, et al. AIDS-associated NHL in San Francisco. JAMA 261:719–724, 1991.
182. Gill PS, Levine AM, Krailo M, et al. AIDS-related malignant lymphoma: results of prospective treatment trials. J Clin Oncol 5:1322–1328, 1987.
183. Bermudez MA, Grant KM, Rodvien R, et al. Non-Hodgkin's lymphoma in a population with or at risk for acquired immunodeficiency syndrome: indications for intensive chemotherapy. Am J Med 86:71–76, 1989.
184. Knowles DM, Chamulak GA, Subar M, et al. Lymphoid neoplasia associated with the acquired immunodeficiency syndrome (AIDS). Ann Intern Med 108:744–753, 1988.
185. Lowenthal DA, Straus DJ, Campbell SW, et al. AIDS-related lymphoid neoplasia. Cancer 61:2325–2337, 1988.
186. Levine AM, Wernz JC, Kaplan L, et al. Low-dose chemotherapy with central nervous system prophylaxis and zidovudine maintenance in AIDS-related lymphoma: a prospective multi-institutional trial. JAMA 266:84–88, 1991.
187. Sparano JA, Wiernik P, Hu X, et al. Pilot trial of infusional cyclophosphamide, doxorubicin, and etoposide plus didanosine and filgrastim in patients with human immunodeficiency virus-associated non-Hodgkin's lymphoma. J Clin Oncol 14:3026–3035, 1996.
188. Levine AM, Espina B, Tulpule A, et al. Low dose m-BACOD with concomitant dideoxycytidine: an effective regimen in AIDS-related lymphomas [Abstract]. Blood 82:387, 1993.
189. Tirelli U, Errante D, Oksenhendler E, et al. Prospective study with combined low-dose chemotherapy and zidovudine in 37 patients with poor-prognosis AIDS-related non-Hodgkin's lymphoma. Ann Oncol 3:843–847, 1992.
190. Kaplan LD, Kahn JO, Crowe S, et al. Clinical and virologic effects of recombinant human granulocyte-macrophage colony stimulating factor in patients receiving chemotherapy for immunodeficiency virus-related non-Hodgkin's lymphoma: results of a randomized trial. J Clin Oncol 9:929–940, 1991.
191. Kaplan LD, Straus DJ, Testa MA, et al. Low-dose compared with standard-dose M-BACOD chemotherapy for non-Hodgkin's lymphoma associated with human immunodeficiency virus infection. N Engl J Med 336:1641–1648, 1997.
192. Levine AM, Tulpule A, Tessman D, et al. Mitoguazone therapy in patients with refractory or relapsed AIDS-related lymphoma: results from a multicenter phase II trial. J Clin Oncol 15:1094–1103, 1997.
193. Tulpule A, Anderson LJ, Levine AM, et al. Anti-B4 (CD 19) monoclonal antibody, conjugated with ricin (B4 blocked ricin:B4BR) in refractory AIDS-lymphoma [Abstract]. Proc Am Soc Clin Oncol 13:10, 1994.
194. Kovacs JA, Baseler M, Dewar RJ, et al. Increases in CD4 T lymphocytes with intermittent courses of IL-2 in patients with human immunodeficiency virus infection. N Engl J Med 332:567–575, 1995.
195. Bernstein ZP, Porter MM, Gould M, et al. Prolonged administration of low-dose IL-2 in human immunodeficiency virus-associated malignancy results in selective expansion of innate immune effectors without significant clinical toxicity. Blood 85:3287–3297, 1995.
196. Hohl RJ, Schilsky RL. Nonmalignant complications of therapy for Hodgkin's disease. Hematol Oncol Clin North Am 3:331–343, 1989.
197. Vanhaelan CPJ, Fisher RI. Increased sensitivity of T cells to regulation by normal suppressor cells persists in long-term survivors with Hodgkin's disease. Am J Med 72:385–390, 1982.
198. Schilsky RL, Sherins RJ. Adverse effects of treatment: gonadal dysfunction. In: DeVita VT, Hellman S, Rosenberg SA, eds. Cancer. Principles and practice of oncology. 2nd ed. Philadelphia: JB Lippincott, 1985: 2032.
199. Santoro A, Viviani S, Zucali R, et al. Comparative results and toxicity of MOPP vs ABVD combined with radiotherapy in PS IIB, III Hodgkin's disease [Abstract]. Proc Am Soc Clin Oncol 2:223, 1983.
200. Bonadonna G, Santoro A. ABVD chemotherapy in the treatment of Hodgkin's disease. Cancer Treat Rev 9:21–35, 1982.
201. Chapman RM, Sutcliffe SB, Malpas JS. Cytotoxic-induced ovarian failure in women with Hodgkin's disease. I. Hormone function. JAMA 242:1877–1881, 1979.
202. Schilsky RL, Serins RJ, Hubbard SM, et al. Long term follow up of ovarian function in women treated with MOPP chemotherapy for Hodgkin's disease. Am J Med 71:552–556, 1981.
203. Pedersen-Bjergaard J, Larsen SO. Incidence of acute nonlymphocytic leukemia, preleukemia, and acute myeloproliferative syndrome up to 10 years after treatment of Hodgkin's disease. N Engl J Med 307:965–971, 1982.
204. Coltman CA, Dixon DO. Second malignancies complicating Hodgkin's disease: A Southwest Oncology Group 10-year follow-up. Cancer Treat Rep 66:1023–1033, 1982.
205. VanLeeuwen FE, Somers R, Taal BG, et al. Increased risk of lung cancer, non-Hodgkin's lymphoma and leukemia following Hodgkin's disease. J Clin Oncol 7:1046–1058, 1989.
206. Krikorian JG, Burke JS, Rosenberg SA, et al. Occurrence of non-Hodgkin's lymphoma after therapy for Hodgkin's disease. N Engl J Med 300:452–458, 1979.

CHAPTER 88

BREAST CANCER

Suzanne Fields Jones and Howard A. Burris III

TREATMENT GOALS: BREAST CANCER

- Treatment of breast cancer varies by disease stage at diagnosis and patient-specific prognosis factors.
- The goal of treatment of early-stage disease is cure. A combination of surgery, radiation, hormonal therapy, or chemotherapy is used to achieve this goal.
- The combination of surgery, radiation, and chemotherapy is also used for locally advanced disease and may result in disease cure or palliation.
- The goals of treatment of metastatic disease are symptom palliation and possibly prolonged survival. Chemotherapy, hormonal therapy, and/or radiation therapy are used in this setting.

EPIDEMIOLOGY

Incidence and Mortality

Breast cancer is the most common malignancy diagnosed in women in the United States and is the second most common cause of cancer death in women, surpassed only by lung cancer. Approximately 182,800 new cases of breast cancer are expected to be diagnosed in the United States during 2000, and an estimated 41,200 people are expected to die with breast cancer this year.[1] The incidence of breast cancer, which had increased steadily over the last two decades due to improved awareness and earlier detection of the disease through screening, has more recently remained relatively stable. The mortality rate from breast cancer also appears to be beginning to decline, which may be due to detection of disease at an earlier stage and improvements in adjuvant treatment.

ETIOLOGY

The etiology of breast cancer is unknown, but several predisposing risk factors for the disease have been determined. These factors can be divided into three major categories: genetic or familial, endocrine, and environmental factors (Table 88.1).

Women who have a first-degree relative (mother or sister) with breast cancer have a twofold to threefold increased risk of developing breast cancer.[2,3] This risk may be increased further if more than one first-degree relative is diagnosed with the disease, the relative is of a young age at the time of diagnosis, or the relative has bilateral breast cancer.[4] Women who have a personal history of breast cancer have a higher probability than the average woman of developing primary breast cancer in the contralateral breast.[3]

A small percentage of breast cancers can be classified as hereditary cancers. The majority of these hereditary cancers are caused by mutations in the BRCA1 and BRCA2 genes, and a small percentage are associated with other rare cancer syndromes such as Li-Fraumeni syndrome or Cowden disease.[5] It is estimated that the risk of developing breast cancer in women who carry BRCA1 and BRCA2 mutations is 33% by age 50 and 56% by age 70.[6] As a result, many women may want to undergo genetic testing for breast cancer. However, the interpretation of the genetic test results and management of patients with positive results is a controversial issue. Although women who test positive for BRCA1 and BRCA2 are at increased risk for development of breast cancer, the appropriate management of these patients remains a challenge for physicians. Women who test positive for BRCA1 and

Table 88.1 ▪ Risk Factors for Breast Cancer Development

Personal history of breast cancer
Family history of breast cancer in first-degree relatives
Proliferative benign breast disease
Early menarche, late menopause
Nulliparity
First pregnancy after age 35
Exogenous estrogens (postmenopausal hormone replacement therapy, oral contraceptives)
Obesity (menopausal weight gain, fat distribution)
Dietary factors—alcohol, high-fat diet
Radiation

BRCA2 should be encouraged to practice intensified early detection methods for breast cancer via monthly breast self-examinations, clinician breast examination every 6 to 12 months, and annual mammography beginning between ages 25 and 35 years.[5] Prophylactic mastectomy and chemoprevention with tamoxifen remain controversial in this patient population. Furthermore, a negative BRCA1 and BRCA2 genetic test should not be misinterpreted. When women with a personal or family history of breast cancer were tested for BRCA1 mutations, only 16% tested positive.[7] Based on their history, these women are still at greater risk for developing breast cancer than the general population and should be encouraged to practice routine screening for breast cancer detection despite the negative genetic test results. Further education and research in the area of genetic testing for breast cancer are warranted.

Patients with benign breast disease have an increased risk of developing breast cancer if they have proliferative lesions with atypical hyperplasia.[2,3] Their risk is increased further if there is also a positive family history for breast cancer. Patients in these higher-risk groups may warrant close monitoring for breast cancer development, but other patients with benign breast disease (e.g., fibrocystic or "lumpy" breast) should be treated similar to the general population.

Both endogenous and exogenous hormones have also been associated with an increased risk for breast cancer. The incidence of breast cancer is thought to correlate with prolonged high levels of estrogen in the bloodstream, which would occur in women with long menstrual histories. As a result, women with early menarche (age less than 12) or late menopause (age greater than 55) are at higher risk for the development of breast cancer.[8,9] Women who have never been pregnant are also at a greater risk for breast cancer than women who have given birth. However, the age at which a woman experiences her first full-term pregnancy also influences her risk of developing breast cancer. A first full-term pregnancy after age 35 increases the risk for breast cancer because of hormonal changes and latent breast tissue differentiation that occur during pregnancy, particularly the first pregnancy.[3,8] Theoretically, increasing the number of menstrual cycles with either oral contraceptive use or postmenopausal hormone-replacement therapy could be associated with an increased risk of breast cancer. However, the studies that have been published in this area to date show conflicting results. Most studies have been conducted retrospectively with numerous hormone preparations and have shown no relation between oral contraceptives and breast cancer. In a meta-analysis of the case-control studies available in the literature through 1989, a positive trend in the risk of breast cancer was noted among premenopausal women who used oral contraceptives for an extended period before their first term pregnancy.[10] Several studies have also suggested an increased risk of breast cancer in women taking oral contraceptives during the perimenopausal period.[8] Decreased exposure of breast cells to estrogens and progestins could be obtained by using the combination of a gonadotropin-releasing hormone agonist and very low dose hormone replacement for contraception. This type of contraception could possibly be beneficial in reducing the lifetime risk of breast cancer and should be explored further because of the large number of women using combination-type oral contraceptives.

Prolonged duration of postmenopausal hormone-replacement therapy (HRT) has also been associated with an increased risk of breast cancer in studies conducted in both Europe and the United States, but additional large prospective studies will be required to determine the true association between exogenous estrogen administration and the risk of breast cancer.[11] The relief of menopausal symptoms and protection from the morbidity and mortality of cardiovascular disease and osteoporosis experienced with postmenopausal estrogen replacement must be considered when weighing the risks and benefits of exogenous hormone therapy.

The use of HRT in postmenopausal women or younger women with premature menopause with a prior history of breast cancer is controversial, because no randomized clinical trials have been conducted to date in this population. Many breast tumors are positive for estrogen receptors and are thought to grow in the presence of estrogen. Therefore, physicians are reluctant to prescribe HRT in women with a history of breast cancer. Estrogen HRT in postmenopausal women decreases the symptoms associated with menopause, reduces the risk of cardiovascular disease, and minimizes the development of osteoporosis. Raloxifene, an estrogen receptor modulator approved by the Food and Drug Administration (FDA) for the treatment of osteoporosis, produces favorable effects on bone and lipids and may reduce the risk of breast and endometrial cancer. The use of tamoxifen in postmenopausal women with a history of breast cancer decreases the risk of contralateral breast cancer, cardiovascular disease, and osteoporosis, but it does not improve menopausal symptoms. Some postmenopausal patients with a history of breast cancer choose to take estrogen replacement therapy and should be followed very closely with regular breast examinations and mammograms. Randomized clinical trials in postmenopausal women or younger women with therapy-induced premature menopause and a prior history of breast cancer are warranted to determine the appropriateness of HRT in this population.

Based on the incidence rates of breast cancer in various countries, it is thought that environmental factors contribute to the development of breast cancer in women. Western countries such as the United States have high breast cancer rates, whereas Eastern countries such as Japan have a low incidence of the disease. Furthermore, when people migrate from Japan to the United States, they gradually acquire the higher incidence rates of their new environment.[12] The difference in breast cancer rates is thought to be partially due to dietary differences between the two populations, specifically the amount of fat that is consumed in the diet. Data obtained from several large prospective studies have failed to show a direct correlation between high-fat diets and the risk of breast cancer.[13] Obesity has also been associated with increased estrogen levels, but it has been directly associated only with an increased risk of breast cancer in postmenopausal women.[2,12] More recent research indicates that the weight gain and increases in central body fat that occur during menopause are associated with an increased risk of postmenopausal breast cancer, possibly due to the concomitant alterations in ovarian hormones, glucose metabolism, and breast cancer growth factors that occur.[14] Women who are physically active during adolescence and young adulthood may also have a decreased risk of developing breast cancer possibly due to infrequent or irregular menstrual cycles and maintaining a lean body weight.[15] Although several logical explanations support the protective effect of exercise in protecting against breast cancer development, no studies have conclusively demonstrated this relationship.[16] The combination of all or several of these factors probably contributes to the development of breast cancer in many women.

Several prospective and case-control studies have consistently demonstrated a positive correlation between alcohol consumption and the risk of breast cancer. These studies are somewhat difficult to compare because the amount and type of alcohol consumed has varied with each study. However, a meta-analysis of 16 studies uncovered a dose-response relationship between alcohol consumption and breast cancer risk.[17] The combined data indicate that women who consume two drinks per day have a 40 to 70% increased risk for breast cancer compared with women who did not drink at all. Furthermore, a study conducted in premenopausal women also demonstrated that ingestion of approximately two alcoholic drinks per day increases sex steroid hormone levels, further strengthening the relationship between alcohol ingestion and breast cancer risk.[18]

Survivors of the atomic bomb blasts during World War II have experienced an increased incidence of breast cancer due to radiation exposure.[19] Similar breast cancer incidence rates have also been reported in women treated with radiation for mastitis, women receiving multiple fluoroscopies for the treatment of tuberculosis, and women receiving mantle radiation for the treatment of Hodgkin's disease. There is a 10- to 15-year latency period between radiation exposure and tumor development, and women over 40 years of age at the time of exposure are believed to experience little or no increased risk for breast cancer. It is thought that prepubertal and pubertal girls who receive radiation therapy have the highest risk for radiation-induced breast cancer because of the sensitivity of the breast tissue to the effects of radiation. This tissue sensitivity decreases with increasing age. Some physicians have expressed concern about the use of repeated screening mammographies in women, due to the link between radiation exposure and breast cancer. However, the amount of radiation a woman is exposed to during a mammogram is extremely low, most women undergoing mammography are greater than 40 years of age, and there have been no case reports to date of breast cancer development secondary to mammography screening.

PATHOPHYSIOLOGY

Breast Anatomy and Tumor Development

Human breast tissue is composed primarily of connective tissue and fat. There is also an elaborate duct system within the breasts that is used during lactation. Breast tissue has an abundant blood supply and an extensive lymphatic network. Lymphatic drainage of the mammary tissues flows into the axillary, interpectoral, and internal mammary lymph nodes. This is important because breast cancer commonly spreads via the lymphatic system, and metastatic disease is often discovered in the regional lymph nodes at the time of diagnosis (Fig. 88.1).

A woman's breast tissue and glands begin to develop around the time of puberty, due to the influence and interaction of sex hormones. However, the amount of breast development occurring at puberty is limited and the majority occurs during the first pregnancy. The large amounts of estrogen and progesterone produced by the ovaries during pregnancy stimulate rapid growth and terminal differentiation of immature breast tissue. A delay in the terminal differentiation of breast tissue until a later age may help explain why women who become pregnant for the first time after age 35 have an increased risk for breast cancer development, because immature cells are more susceptible to cycling estrogen effects and estrogens are known to initiate tumor growth.[20]

Pathogenesis of Breast Cancer

The development of breast cancer occurs when breast cells lose their normal differentiation and proliferation controls. The proliferation of these abnormal cells, or tumor cells, is influenced by various hormones, oncogenes, and growth factors. There is strong evidence to suggest that estrogen directly and indirectly stimulates the growth of tumor cells.[21] Furthermore, numerous growth factors that also play a role in tumor development are secreted by the breast cancer cells themselves. These factors can be classified as either autocrine (if they stimulate their own growth) or paracrine (if they have an effect on other cells). Examples of the autocrine growth factors include transforming growth factor alpha (TGF-α) and insulin-like growth factors

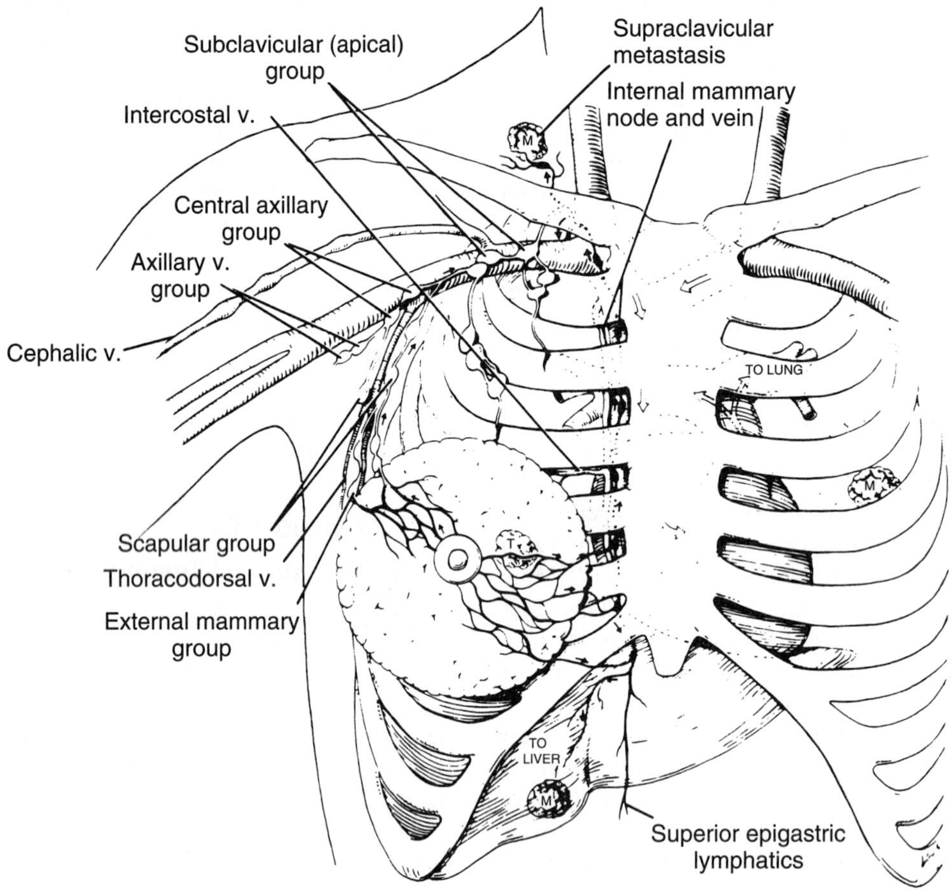

Figure 88.1. Breast tissue drainage and its relationship to tumor metastases. (From Copeland EM III, Bland KI. The breast. In: Sabiston DC Jr, ed. Essentials of surgery. Philadelphia: WB Saunders, 1987, with permission.)

I and II (IGF-I and IGF-II). Transforming growth factor beta (TGF-β), platelet-derived growth factor (PDGF), and procathepsin D (52K protein) are all paracrine growth factors. The exact mechanism of tumor development is not completely understood, but tremendous progress has been made in this area with the discovery of the autocrine and paracrine growth factors. The mechanism of action of several of the hormonal agents used for the treatment of breast cancer involves the alteration of the growth factors involved in tumor development. Trastuzumab, a monoclonal antibody that binds specifically to growth factor receptors on the malignant cell surface, has been approved by the FDA for use in metastatic disease.

CLINICAL PRESENTATION AND DIAGNOSIS

Signs and Symptoms

Breast cancer masses tend to be painless, solitary, unilateral, hard, irregular, and nonmobile. Patients may also have skin changes, nipple discharge, or axillary lymphadenopathy. On presentation, any woman with suspected benign or malignant breast disease should have a mammography. Furthermore, any breast mass that is suggestive of malignancy by mammography or on physical examination should be biopsied by either fine needle aspiration, core needle biopsy, incisional biopsy, or excisional biopsy. Although needle aspirations and core biopsies provide enough evidence for a histologic diagnosis of breast cancer, they do not delineate the size of the tumor or allow for estrogen receptor determination of the tumor.[22]

Detection and Diagnosis

Early detection of breast cancer is critical because patients with limited-stage disease have a better prognosis. Three complementary screening techniques have been shown to be effective for breast cancer detection: breast self-examination (BSE), physical examination by a physician, and mammography.

A large number of breast cancers are discovered by patients themselves during regular BSEs. Breast self-examination is a simple procedure that should be performed by all women over age 20 on a monthly basis. In a meta-analysis of 12 studies evaluating BSE, it was determined that women who performed monthly examinations were more likely to have smaller tumors with negative axillary lymph nodes at diagnosis as compared with those who did not perform monthly examinations.[23] In a small prospective study, BSE resulted in more limited disease at diagnosis and a small improvement in 5-year survival for patients performing monthly BSEs.[24] Currently, the American Cancer Society recommends that all women perform monthly BSEs, and numerous educational brochures and breast models are available to aid women in this procedure. However, in order for BSE to be an effective screening tool, women must be compliant with their examinations.

A physical examination conducted by a trained physician is also an important screening technique for breast cancer detection. The American Cancer Society recommends that women over age 40 have a yearly physical examination by their physician. Women between ages 20 and 40 should have a physical examination conducted by their physician every 3 years. Although mammography is more sensitive for detecting small breast tumors than physical examination, approximately 10% of palpable masses are missed by mammography.[25] Therefore, it is critical that both physical examinations and screening mammography be performed. When the two procedures are used together, it is estimated that greater than 90% of diagnosed breast cancers are detected.[22]

The importance of physical examination and mammography as screening tools to detect breast cancer has been confirmed with two large, randomized prospective clinical trials–the Health Insurance Plan of Greater New York (HIP) and the Breast Cancer Detection Demonstration Project (BCDDP). The HIP study randomized 31,000 women between ages 40 and 64 to receive an initial screening examination plus mammography with three annual follow-up screenings.[26] The matched control group for the study consisted of 31,000 additional women who received only routine medical care. At the 5-year analysis, a 38% reduction in the breast cancer mortality rate was noted in the patients receiving annual physical examinations and mammography compared with the control group. Furthermore, the reduction in mortality rate has persisted throughout 18 years of follow-up and remains at 23%.[27] The BCDDP enrolled 280,000 women between ages 35 and 72 at centers throughout the United States who were screened with physical examination and mammography between 1973 and 1980.[28] The women were also instructed about BSE and were encouraged to perform monthly examinations. There were 4275 breast cancers diagnosed during the study period, and approximately one-third of these were less than 1 cm in size at the time of diagnosis. The BCDDP further supported the utilization of screening mammography because 40% of the tumors were detected by mammography alone. In the 20-year analysis of the study, the data indicate that women diagnosed with noninvasive breast cancers have a low breast cancer mortality rate (97.2% adjusted cancer survival rate, 78.5% observed rate). In women with invasive cancers, survival was related to the size of the tumor and lymph node status at diagnosis. These results were consistent across all age-groups enrolled on the study and underline the importance of screening mammography.

A great deal of controversy regarding the benefit of mammography screening in women between ages 40 and 49 has surfaced in the recent oncology literature. The reason for this controversy is that the set of clinical trial data from the individual trials was subsequently analyzed in subsets determined by patient age, although the original design of the trials did not allow for this stratification.[29] When analyzed by subgroup, the studies lose their statistical power because sufficient numbers of women ages 40 to 49 were not enrolled in the trials. However, when all of the randomized controlled trials are analyzed in a meta-analysis, a mortality reduction of 25 to 30% is achieved in women who begin mammography screening by age 40. As a result of this controversy, The National Cancer Institute convened a panel of experts to obtain a consensus on the data in the literature. The panel concluded that the data currently available do not warrant a recommendation for screening mammography for all women 40 years of age or older. The panel also recommended that the decision to undergo mammography in women ages 40 to 49 should be left up to the individual patient and that it is the responsibility of health care professionals to educate the patient regarding the risks and benefits of screening mammography so that she can make an informed decision. The panel also stated that third-party payors should reimburse the cost of the mammogram for women who choose to have the study performed so that financial issues will not influence a woman's individual decision. Despite these statements, the American Cancer Society continues to recommend that all women begin annual or biannual mammography screening at age 40. The current American Cancer Society guidelines for breast cancer detection are listed in Table 88.2.

The benefits of early detection by mammography have only recently begun to be realized. Since 1980, the number of women over 40 years of age who have ever had a mammogram has increased by more than 200%.[30] At the same time, the incidence of breast cancer detection has increased by approximately 32%, with the majority of the tumors being diagnosed at an early stage. It is hoped that this increase in early detection and treatment will subsequently result in a decrease in breast cancer mortality rates.

Table 88.2 ▪ American Cancer Society Guidelines for Breast Cancer Detection

Age Group	Screening Recommendation
20–39	Monthly breast self-examination Breast physical examination every 3 years Baseline mammogram at age 35–39
40–49	Monthly breast self-examination Yearly breast physical examination Mammogram every 1–2 years
>50	Monthly breast self-examination Yearly breast/physical examination and mammogram

Breast Cancer Staging

The TNM classification system is the most commonly accepted staging system for breast cancer. Tumor size (T) is described on a scale of 0 to 4 based on characteristics of the primary tumor. Extent of lymph node involvement (N), based on location and palpability, and the presence or absence of distant metastases (M), are also included in the system. In the management of breast cancer, the ipsilateral axillary, internal mammary, and pectoral nodes are all considered regional spread of the disease. Involvement of any other lymph nodes, including the supraclavicular, cervical, or contralateral internal mammary lymph nodes, is considered distant metastases. Table 88.3 describes the TNM staging system used for breast cancer.

PSYCHOSOCIAL ASPECTS

In addition to the physical changes that occur in a woman's life as a result of breast cancer treatment, the patient must also cope with many psychosocial issues. The changes in appearance that occur due to surgery (breast removal) or chemotherapy (alopecia) may create problems with self-image or perceived acceptance by family and friends. It may also be difficult for healthy women diagnosed with breast cancer to make the transition from the role of caregiver in the family to the role of "care receiver." The possible inability to continue working plus the costs of treatment may place additional financial burdens on families during this time. Many women may find it difficult to deal with the numerous added stresses associated with a cancer diagnosis and should be encouraged to participate in support groups that exist to address these and many other issues.

THERAPEUTIC PLAN

The goal of treatment in breast cancer varies by the stage of disease at diagnosis and patient-specific prognostic factors. Most breast cancer disease (excluding metastatic disease) is treated for cure. Some patients with isolated metastases that can be resected may also be treated for cure. Most often, if the disease recurs it is nonresectable, making the goal of cure nearly impossible. When cure is not possible, the goals of treatment are to prolong survival and palliate symptoms.

Noninvasive Breast Cancer

The increased use of mammography and subsequent increase in suspicious breast masses has led to more frequent diagnosis of lobular carcinoma in situ (LCIS). LCIS is confined to the lobules and terminal ducts, is nonpalpable, and is not detected radiographically by mammography.[3] It is most often diagnosed incidentally in premenopausal women and is not considered a malignancy in and of itself, but its presence may predispose women to the development of breast cancer in the future. Standard treatment for LCIS consists of close observation of the patient following the excisional biopsy with regular physical examinations and mammograms for the development of breast cancer.

The increased use of mammography has also led to an increase in the diagnosis of ductal carcinoma in situ (DCIS).[31] In contrast to LCIS, DCIS occurs more commonly in postmenopausal women, is visible on radiologic evaluation, and is often palpable. Patients with DCIS are managed with mastectomy or lumpectomy with or without radiation. No studies directly comparing the two procedures have been conducted. However, the National Surgical Adjuvant Breast and Bowel Project (NSABP) has conducted a trial comparing lumpectomy and lumpectomy plus radiation in patients with DCIS.[32] At 8-year follow-up, patients who received lumpectomy plus radiation had a decreased incidence of both invasive and noninvasive ipsilateral breast cancers compared with patients who received lumpectomy alone. In patients who received lumpectomy plus radiation therapy, the cumulative incidence of invasive ipsilateral breast cancer was only 3.9%, suggesting that lumpectomy plus radiation is sufficient treatment for patients with DCIS and that mastectomy is not warranted.

Early-Stage Breast Cancer

Approximately 75 to 80% of women diagnosed with breast cancer have stage I or II disease at the time of diagnosis. In the early days of breast cancer management, the primary mode of treatment was a radical mastectomy. The goal of this treatment was to remove the breast, underlying tissues, and regional lymph nodes. However, as surgical skills and patient management improved, the modified radical mastectomy, which spares the pectoralis muscles and some high axillary lymph nodes, became acceptable for the treatment of primary disease and patients were spared the sequelae associated with a radical mastectomy. *Breast conservation treatment* is defined as lumpectomy or partial mastectomy accompanied by axillary node dissection and followed by radiation therapy. A large randomized trial conducted by NSABP demonstrated that overall survival and disease-free survival were equivalent in patients who underwent total mastectomy, lumpectomy alone, or lumpectomy plus breast radiation.[33] Furthermore, in patients who were treated with lumpectomy plus radiation, the incidence of recurrence of a tumor in the ipsilateral breast was 10% versus 35% for patients treated with lumpectomy alone. Although the addition of radiation to surgery does not improve survival as compared with surgery alone, the rate of local recurrence is reduced threefold in patients who receive combination surgery and radiation.[34] These findings suggest that the combination of lumpectomy and radiation is appropriate therapy for patients with early-stage breast cancer.

The necessity of axillary node dissection in patients with early-stage breast cancer is currently a controversial issue. With the increased use of mammography, the number of tumors ≤1 centimeter in diameter at diagnosis has increased dramatically.[35] The majority of these small tumors also do not have nodal involvement at the time of

Table 88.3 ▪ TNM Staging System for Breast Cancer

Primary Tumor (T)

TX	Primary tumor cannot be assessed
T0	No evidence of primary tumor
Tis	Carcinoma in situ: intraductal carcinoma, LCIS, or Paget's disease of the nipple with no tumor
T1	Tumor 2 cm or less in greatest dimension
T1mic	Microinvasion 0.1 cm or less in greatest dimension
T1a	Tumor more than 0.1 cm but not more than 0.5 in greatest dimension
T1b	Tumor more than 0.5 cm but not more than 1 cm in greatest dimension
T1c	Tumor more than 1 cm but not more than 2 cm in greatest dimension
T2	Tumor more than 2 cm but not more than 5 cm in greatest dimension
T3	Tumor more than 5 cm in greatest dimension
T4	Tumor of any size with direct extension to (a) chest wall or (b) skin, only as described below:
T4a	Extension to chest wall
T4b	Edema (including peau d'orange) or ulceration of the skin of the breast or satellite skin nodules confined to the same breast
T4c	Both (T4a and T4b)
T4d	Inflammatory carcinoma

NOTE: Paget's disease associated with a tumor is classified according to the size of the tumor.

Regional Lymph Nodes (N)

NX	Regional lymph nodes cannot be assessed (e.g., previously removed)
N0	No regional lymph node metastasis
N1	Metastasis to movable ipsilateral axillary lymph node(s)
N2	Metastasis to ipsilateral axillary lymph node(s) fixed to one another or to other structures
N3	Metastasis to ipsilateral internal mammary lymph node(s)

Pathologic Classification (pN)

pNX	Regional lymph nodes cannot be assessed (e.g., previously removed, or not removed for pathologic study)
pN0	No regional lymph node metastasis
pN1	Metastasis to movable ipsilateral axillary lymph node(s)
pN1a	Only micrometastasis (none larger than 0.2 cm)
pN1b	Metastasis to lymph node(s), any larger than 0.2 cm
pN1bi	Metastasis in 1 to 3 lymph nodes, any more than 0.2 cm and all less than 2 cm in greatest dimension
pN1bii	Metastasis to 4 or more lymph nodes, any more than 0.2 cm and all less than 2 cm in greatest dimension
pN1biii	Extension of tumor beyond the capsule of a lymph node metastasis less than 2 cm in greatest dimension
pN1biv	Metastasis to a lymph node 2 cm or more in greatest dimension
pN2	Metastasis to ipsilateral axillary lymph nodes that are fixed to one another or to other structures
pN3	Metastasis to ipsilateral internal mammary lymph node(s)

Distant Metastasis (M)

MX	Distant metastasis cannot be assessed
M0	No distant metastasis
M1	Distant metastasis (includes metastasis to ipsilateral supraclavicular lymph nodes[s])

STAGE GROUPING

Stage 0	Tis	N0	M0	Stage IIIA	T0	N2	M0
Stage I	T1[a]	N0	M0		T1[a]	N2	M0
Stage IIA	T0	N1	M0		T2	N2	M0
	T1[a]	N1[b]	M0		T3	N1	M0
	T2	N0	M0		T3	N2	M0
Stage IIB	T2	N1	M0	Stage IIIB	T4	Any N	M0
	T3	N0	M0		Any T	N3	M0
				Stage IV	Any T	Any N	M1

Source: Reprinted with permission from American Joint Committee on Cancer (AJCC) cancer staging manual. 5th ed. Philadelphia: Lippincott-Raven, 1997.

[a] T1 includes T1mic.

[b] The prognosis of patients with N1a is similar to that of patients with pN0.

diagnosis. Furthermore, the use of adjuvant systemic therapy in node-negative patients, as well as node-positive patients, shifts the purpose of axillary node dissection at diagnosis to a prognostic indicator only. Finally, the elimination of the lymph node dissection from breast conservation treatment would significantly decrease the morbidity of the surgical procedure (specifically the lymphedema and limitation of arm motion and strength).[36] As a result, researchers are investigating the use of sentinel lymph node detection as a possible alternative to lymph node dissection for detecting lymph node metastases.[37,38] The sentinel lymph node is the first node that receives lymphatic drainage from a tumor. It can be detected by injecting a blue dye or radioactive colloid around the primary tumor and following the drainage pathway of the dye or colloid. The sentinel node can then be biopsied to determine the presence or absence of lymphatic metastases. Using the blue dye injection technique, sentinel node dissection was 100% predictive of the axillary nodal status in 100 patients.[37] Additionally, 67% of patients had disease involvement in the sentinel lymph node only. Radioisotope lymphoscintigraphy has also been used in breast cancer patients to identify the sentinel lymph node, but this technique has proven more difficult. Nonetheless, the preliminary results of sentinel lymph node dissection are believed to be positive, and this may lead to the avoidance of axillary node dissection, particularly in patients with a negative sentinel lymph node.

Adjuvant therapy is chemotherapy or hormonal therapy that is administered in an attempt to treat the residual micrometastatic disease that remains after surgery. In May 1988, the National Cancer Institute issued a clinical alert to physicians concerning the use of adjuvant hormonal or cytotoxic chemotherapy in the treatment of women with node-negative breast cancer (stage I).[39] This alert was issued due to the results of four randomized clinical trials utilizing adjuvant therapy in node-negative breast cancer patients.[40–43] Although the treatment regimens used in the four trials were different, all demonstrated a statistically significant increase in disease-free survival in patients with node-negative disease (Table 88.4). However, overall survival was not prolonged significantly in any of these studies.

Since the clinical alert was issued regarding adjuvant therapy in node-negative patients, a new series of clinical trials has been conducted in this patient population in an attempt to determine the most appropriate treatment regimen. In a large study conducted by NSABP, patients with node-negative, estrogen-receptor–positive breast cancer were randomized to receive tamoxifen alone versus tamoxifen plus cyclophosphamide, methotrexate, and fluorouracil (CMF).[44] At 5-year follow-up, disease-free survival was significantly prolonged in patients receiving CMF plus tamoxifen versus those receiving tamoxifen alone. The Southwest Oncology Group (SWOG) conducted a similar study in which node-negative patients were stratified as high risk or low risk based on tumor size and S-phase fraction.[45] The high-risk patients were randomized to receive CMF with or without tamoxifen or cyclophosphamide, doxorubicin, and fluorouracil (CAF) with or without tamoxifen, and the low-risk patients were followed without adjuvant therapy. The addition of tamoxifen to the chemotherapy regimens was beneficial only in patients who were estrogen-receptor positive, and the CAF regimen appeared to be marginally superior to CMF. The low-risk patients did as well as or better than the high-risk patients with observation only and no adjuvant therapy.

Because the disease-free survival rate in node-negative patients receiving no adjuvant therapy is 70 to 90%, many physicians question whether all patients with node-negative disease should receive adjuvant therapy, particularly patients with tumors less than 1 centimeter in diameter. Furthermore, the acute and delayed toxicities, as well as the direct cost and cost-effectiveness of the therapy, must be considered. Indirect costs in the form of drug toxicities and decreased quality of life during therapy are difficult to quantitate, but they should be included when weighing the risks and benefits of adjuvant therapy. Acute toxicities, such as nausea, vomiting, mucositis, and myelosuppression, resulted in patient death in a small percentage of patients in the randomized clinical trials. Long-term toxicities in the form of secondary malignancies (leukemia following alkylating agents and endometrial cancers following tamoxifen therapy), venous and arterial thrombosis, and congestive heart failure secondary to anthracycline admin-

Table 88.4 ▪ Clinical Trials of Adjuvant Therapy for Node-Negative Breast Cancer

			Disease-Free Survival		
Trial	**No. Patients**	**Treatment Regimen**	**Treated**	**Control**	***P* Value**
Ludwig V[40]	1275	CMF × 1 month[a]	77%	73%	0.04
Intergroup[41]	406	CMFP × 6 months[b]	84%	69%	0.0001
NSABP B13[42]	679	MF × 12 months[c]	80%	71%	0.003
NSABP B14[43]	2644	TAM × 5 years[d]	83%	77%	<0.00001

[a]Cyclophosphamide 400 mg/m² IV D 1 and 8; methotrexate 40 mg/m² IV D 1 and 8; fluorouracil 600 mg/m² D 1 and 8. (Leucovorin 15 mg IV/PO D 1 and 8 was also given to 69% of patients.)

[b]Cyclophosphamide 100 mg/m² PO D 1–14; methotrexate 40 mg/m² IV D 1 and 8; fluorouracil 600 mg/m² IV D 1 and 8; prednisone 40 mg/m² PO D 1–14.

[c]Methotrexate 100 mg/m² IV D 1 and 8; fluorouracil 600 mg/m² IV D 1 and 8 (leucovorin 10 mg/m² PO q6hr × 6 doses).

[d]Tamoxifen 10 mg PO BID.

istration were not addressed due to the relatively short follow-up period. These delayed toxicities, however, are increasingly important when the survival benefits associated with adjuvant therapy are minimal or nonexistent, as in patients with tumors smaller than 1 centimeter.

A recent study evaluated quality of life in women with early-stage breast cancer who received adjuvant treatment 2 to 5 years previously.[46] The self-rated quality of life was generally favorable, with less than one-third of patients reporting moderate to severe symptoms. However, sexual function did appear to be compromised following adjuvant therapy. Another interesting finding from the study was that 65% of patients stated that they were willing to undergo 6 months of chemotherapy for a 5% increase in likelihood of cancer cure. Another survey of breast cancer survivors found a similar willingness to receive chemotherapy for a low degree of benefit.[47] The women surveyed would have undergone chemotherapy for a median life expectancy improvement of 3 to 6 months or an improvement of less than 1% in the risk of recurrence. However, this survey also revealed that many women are incompletely informed about their prognosis and the impact of adjuvant therapy. Women appear to overestimate the risk of early relapse and the effectiveness of adjuvant therapy.

Continued research in the area of adjuvant therapy for node-negative breast cancer is clearly warranted. Due to the discrepancies in the data collected to date, physicians are encouraged to enroll their newly diagnosed patients in large, prospective randomized clinical trials. Outside the clinical trial setting, the decision to treat node-negative breast cancer with chemotherapy or hormonal therapy must be made on an individual basis. The presence or absence of prognostic factors and the patient's desire to receive treatment should influence the physician's final judgment concerning adjuvant therapy. It is also imperative that physicians try to improve the education of patients regarding the risk of disease relapse, as well as the potential benefits of adjuvant therapy. Clinicians are currently working to develop a computer-based tool to provide individualized estimates of the risk of relapse and mortality for patients with early-stage breast cancer to aid physicians and patients in the adjuvant therapy decision.[48]

The management of stage II breast cancer (tumor smaller than 5 cm with positive nodal involvement) is more straightforward based on the results of more than 100 randomized trials using systemic adjuvant therapy. Although the results of the individual trials are often contradictory, a meta-analysis conducted by the Early Breast Cancer Trialists' Collaborative Group indicates that systemic adjuvant therapy can prolong disease-free and overall survival in stage II breast cancer.[49] This analysis involved 133 randomized trials in which 75,000 women were enrolled.

There were 44 trials in which systemic adjuvant chemotherapy (both single agent and combination regimens) were compared with no-adjuvant therapy.[50] An overall reduction in the odds of recurrence as a result of treatment in patients receiving adjuvant chemotherapy was 21%, regardless of patient age and treatment regimen. When analyzed by patient age, the reduction in the annual odds of recurrence was significantly greater in women under age 50 (28%) than in older patients (17%). A concomitant decrease in the odds of death with treatment was 11% for all patients (17% for patients less than 50 years of age, 9% for patients 50 years of age or older). Furthermore, the use of combination chemotherapy regimens appeared to be more effective than single-agent regimens, and prolonged treatment with chemotherapy (longer than 6 months) had no survival advantage over short-term therapy. A large individual study conducted by the Cancer and Leukemia Group B in women with node-positive disease receiving adjuvant chemotherapy also suggests that disease-free and overall survival are significantly longer in patients who receive full doses of scheduled therapy.[51] As a result, clinicians should try to avoid chemotherapy dose reductions in the adjuvant setting, so that the maximal benefit of therapy may be achieved. The availability of the hematopoietic growth factors may make this more feasible.

Although combination chemotherapy regimens have proven to be more effective than single-agent therapy, the optimal combination regimen has not been determined and the choice of an adjuvant combination chemotherapy regimen may be a difficult one. Table 88.5 describes some of the combination regimens used in the treatment of breast cancer. Numerous drug combinations were used in

Table 88.5 ▪ Combination Chemotherapy Regimens Used in the Treatment of Breast Cancer

Regimen	Drug	Dose
CMF (28 day)	Cyclophosphamide	100 mg/m²/day PO days 1–14 or 600 mg/m²/day IV D 1
	Methotrexate	40 mg/m²/day IV D 1 and 8
	Fluorouracil	600 mg/m²/day IV D 1 and 8
Repeat every 28 days		
CMF (21 day)	Cyclophosphamide	600 mg/m²/day IV D 1
	Methotrexate	40 mg/m²/day IV D 1
	Fluorouracil	600 mg/m²/day IV D 1
Repeat every 21 days		
AC	Doxorubicin	60 mg/m²/day IV D 1
	Cyclophosphamide	600 mg/m²/day IV D 1
Repeat every 21 days		
FAC or CAF	Fluorouracil	500 mg/m²/day IV D 1 and 8
	Doxorubicin	50 mg/m²/day IV D 1
	Cyclophosphamide	600 mg/m²/day IV D 1
Repeat every 21–28 days		
CFM (CNF, FNC)	Cyclophosphamide	500–600 mg/m²/day IV D1
	Fluorouracil	500–600 mg/m²/day IV D 1
	Mitoxantrone	10–12 mg/m²/day IV D 1
Repeat every 21 days		

the various clinical trials, but the combination of cyclophosphamide, methotrexate, and fluorouracil has been studied most extensively. Doxorubicin has demonstrated significant activity as single-agent therapy in phase II clinical trials in breast cancer patients and has produced increased response rates when used in combination chemotherapy regimens.[52,53] Although conducted in patients with node-negative disease, a recent study comparing CAF and CMF was completed by SWOG.[45] As stated previously, CAF appeared to be marginally superior to CMF, but the toxicities were also increased with CAF. Some clinicians may choose to restrict the doxorubicin-containing regimens to the metastatic disease setting because doxorubicin-refractory patients have historically been very difficult to treat. However, the approval of new chemotherapeutic agents, such as the taxanes and capecitabine, for the refractory disease setting may change this practice. The taxanes have demonstrated the best single-agent activity of any drug tested to date in the refractory disease setting. As a result, researchers are currently conducting studies to determine whether the incorporation of the taxanes into combination regimens used for early-stage disease (i.e., adjuvant therapy) will improve disease-free or overall survival in patients with breast cancer.

The meta-analysis of randomized trials of adjuvant tamoxifen therapy in early breast cancer has been updated.[54] Fifty-five trials enrolling 37,000 women were included in the analysis. The primary benefit of adjuvant tamoxifen therapy was seen in patients with estrogen-receptor–positive tumors or for whom no receptor measurement was available. This patient population experienced a 20% decrease in mortality rate and a 34% decrease in the annual odds of recurrence with adjuvant tamoxifen therapy. In contrast to the previous analysis, the beneficial effects of adjuvant tamoxifen therapy did not appear to be related to age, because both premenopausal and postmenopausal patients demonstrated benefit. In women with estrogen-receptor–negative tumors, no statistical benefit in decreased recurrence or mortality was noted. The data also suggest that about 5 years of adjuvant tamoxifen produces a substantially greater delay in disease recurrence as compared with 1 or 2 years of tamoxifen administration. The potential benefit of greater than 5 years of tamoxifen therapy has not been evaluated fully to date and awaits maturation of current clinical data. However, preliminary data suggest no added benefit of prolonged administration (i.e., greater than 5 years).[55] The meta-analysis also indicated that the addition of 5 years of tamoxifen to chemotherapy was substantially better than the administration of chemotherapy alone. The recommended order of administration of tamoxifen and chemotherapy (concurrent versus consecutive administration) remains to be determined in large randomized clinical trials; a preliminary trial suggests that the initiation of tamoxifen before combination chemotherapy might be detrimental, particularly in patients with estrogen-receptor–negative tumors.[56]

In summary, the management of stage II breast cancer depends primarily on patient age and estrogen-receptor status. All premenopausal women should be treated with 6 months of adjuvant systemic chemotherapy, regardless of their estrogen-receptor status. The most commonly used adjuvant regimen is CMF. Preliminary data suggest that the addition of 5 years of tamoxifen to chemotherapy increases the benefit of adjuvant therapy, but the data from clinical trials exploring chemoendocrine combinations must be further analyzed. In postmenopausal estrogen-receptor–positive patients, adjuvant endocrine therapy in the form of oral tamoxifen for a duration of 5 years is the treatment of choice. The addition of adjuvant chemotherapy may prove beneficial in this patient subset as well. Adjuvant therapy for postmenopausal patients with estrogen-receptor–negative disease is somewhat less straightforward. Adjuvant systemic chemotherapy alone or in combination with endocrine therapy has proven beneficial in this patient subset. Numerous trials designed to answer clinical questions about the management of patients with early (stages I and II) breast cancer are currently underway. In order to determine optimal adjuvant therapy regimens and treatment durations, all physicians should encourage patients receiving adjuvant therapy to participate in clinical trials when they are available. Physicians also must monitor patients closely for the development of recurrent breast cancer after their initial breast cancer diagnosis. The American Society of Clinical Oncology (ASCO) has issued recommended breast cancer surveillance guidelines.[57] Generally, women with a history of breast cancer should perform monthly BSE and undergo annual mammography of both the preserved and contralateral breast. The patient should also have a complete history and physical examination every 3 to 6 months for the first 3 years after diagnosis, then every 6 to 12 months for 2 years, and then annually. ASCO does not recommend bone scans, chest radiographs, hematologic blood counts, tumor markers, liver ultrasonograms, or computed tomography as part of routine follow-up.

Locally Advanced Breast Cancer

Patients diagnosed with locally advanced breast cancer (stage III disease) have tumors larger than 5 cm or direct tumor involvement of the skin or underlying chest wall. These patients also have extensive lymph node involvement. Because of the bulk of disease at the time of diagnosis, surgical management is generally not feasible. Furthermore, standard treatment modalities are minimally effective, resulting in poor survival rates in these patients. In an attempt to improve the overall survival rates in women with locally advanced disease, researchers began to use combined modality therapy.[58] Radiation therapy, systemic chemotherapy, and surgery have all been used in various regimens in randomized clinical trials. Neoadjuvant therapy involves the use of chemotherapy before surgery to decrease the size of the tumor and improve resectability. Other advantages of neoadjuvant chemotherapy include earlier treatment of micrometastatic disease, intact tumor vasculature resulting in improved drug delivery, the ability to determine tumor responsiveness to chemotherapy in vivo, and the ability to customize postsurgical systemic therapy based on this response. After neoadjuvant chemotherapy, patients may receive radiation therapy, surgery alone, or a combination of the two modalities. However, the local control rates achieved in studies using the combination of surgery and radiation therapy after chemotherapy are greater than the control rates obtained with either modality alone.[59] When all three modalities are combined, more than 90% of patients with locally advanced breast cancer are disease free after treatment, and many remain disease free for up to 3 to 5 years.

Because of the success of neoadjuvant therapy in the treatment of locally advanced disease, investigators are beginning to explore the use of neoadjuvant therapy in earlier-stage disease. The results from a preliminary study conducted by NSABP indicate that preoperative doxorubicin and cyclophosphamide reduced the size of most tumors and decreased the incidence of positive nodes at the time of surgery. As a result, more patients were able to undergo breast conservation surgery instead of mastectomy, which may lead to improved quality of life for breast cancer patients.[60] Many questions remain to be answered about the use of combined modality therapy in patients with stage III disease at diagnosis: Which combined treatment regimen is the most effective? How many courses of neoadjuvant therapy should be administered before surgery? Which drugs should be used for neoadjuvant therapy? Should patients also receive systemic adjuvant therapy (either chemotherapy or endocrine therapy) postoperatively? Randomized clinical trials designed to answer some of these questions are currently being conducted, and results remain to be determined.

Metastatic Breast Cancer

Radiation therapy, hormonal therapy, and chemotherapy have all been used in the treatment of metastatic breast cancer to palliate the patient and possibly prolong survival. Because "cure" is not the primary goal of therapy at this point, the easiest, least toxic treatment that can provide the best possible response is generally preferred. Breast cancer can metastasize to virtually any site, but the most common sites include bone, lung, pleura, liver, soft tissue, and the central nervous system. The choice of therapy for metastatic disease is based on the site of disease involvement and the presence or absence of certain patient characteristics.[2,61] For example, patients who experience a longer disease-free survival (2 years or longer), have disease that is primarily located in bone or soft tissue, have responded to primary endocrine therapy, and are late premenopausal or postmenopausal will most likely respond to endocrine therapy. The most important factor predicting response to hormonal therapy, however, is the presence of estrogen receptors (ER) and progesterone receptors (PR) on tumor tissues. From 50 to 60% of ER-positive patients and 75 to 85% of ER- and PR-positive patients have a chance of responding to hormonal therapy, whereas those with no hormone receptors have a 90% chance of failure with hormone therapy.[2] Chemotherapeutic drugs are most commonly used as palliative therapy in patients who would not be expected to respond to hormonal therapy (i.e., patients with rapidly progressive lung, liver, or bone marrow disease) or patients who have failed to respond to initial treatment with endocrine therapy.[61] Radiation therapy is primarily used to control symptomatic disease such as bone metastases, metastatic brain lesions, and spinal cord compressions. Both brain and spinal cord metastases seldom respond to chemotherapy and hormonal manipulations, but they do respond somewhat to irradiation.

The most common endocrine therapies used in the management of metastatic breast cancer are listed in Table 88.6. The response rates to all types of endocrine therapy are equivalent, so it is prudent to begin therapy with the least toxic agent. Furthermore, there does not appear to be any advantage to combining hormonal treatments rather than administering the single agents sequentially. If a patient fails to respond to initial hormonal therapy or progresses during therapy after an initial response, an alternative hormonal manipulation should be attempted, because multiple responses may occur. The median duration of response to the first attempt at hormonal manipulation is usually in the range of 9 to 12 months, and the duration of any subsequent responses is generally shorter.[62] First-line hormonal therapy should be administered for at least 6 to 8 weeks before disease response is assessed. After initiation of therapy, some patients may experience a flare (or worsening) of their disease that may or may not be accompanied by hypercalcemia. Therapy may need to be withheld or decreased during this initial period, but treatment can usually continue. Furthermore, 5 to 10% of patients may actually experience regression of their tumor when therapy is withdrawn.[62] If a patient becomes refractory to hormonal therapy at any time, combination chemotherapy should be employed.

Ovarian ablation (oophorectomy) via surgery or radiation has been used as first-line therapy in the treatment of premenopausal women with metastatic breast cancer in the past, and produced response rates of 30 to 45%.[63] However, the development of pharmacologic agents that block estrogen binding or produce medical castration has resulted in drug therapy as first-line treatment and the avoidance of the morbidity and mortality associated with surgery or radiation. Administration of luteinizing hormone–releasing hormone (LHRH) analogs suppresses ovarian estrogen production in premenopausal women.[64] After an initial stimulation of ovarian hormone production, the LHRH analogs downregulate the luteinizing hormone–releasing factor receptors, resulting in ablation of ovarian hormone production that is reversible after drug discontinuation. In postmenopausal women, tamoxifen therapy is the first-line treatment of choice because of ease of administration and lack of serious side effects. Compara-

Table 88.6 ▪ Endocrine Therapies Used for Metastatic Breast Cancer

Class	Drug	Dose	Side Effects
Antiestrogen	Tamoxifen Toremifene	20 mg PO QD 60 mg PO QD	Disease flare, hot flashes, nausea, vomiting, edema, vaginal discharge; rare: thrombophlebitis, ocular abnormalities, and endometrial cancer
LHRH analogs (equivalent to surgical oophorectomy)	Leuprolide Goserelin	7.5 mg SQ q28d 3.6 mg SQ q28d	Ammenorrhea, hot flushes, occasional nausea
Progestins	Medroxyprogesterone acetate Megestrol acetate	400–1000 mg IM Q week 40 g PO QID	Weight gain, hot flashes, vaginal bleeding
Aromatase inhibitors	Aminoglutethimide with hydrocortisone 40 mg/day Anastrozole (selective inhibitor)	250 mg PO BID × 2 weeks then QID 1 mg PO QD	Lethargy, skin rash, ataxia, nystagmus, postural dizziness, diarrhea, asthenia, nausea, headache, hot flashes
Estrogens	Diethylstilbestrol Ethinylestradiol Conjugated estrogens	5 mg PO TID 1 mg PO TID 2.5 mg PO TID	Nausea/vomiting, fluid retention, hot flashes, anorexia, hepatic dysfunction, thromboembolism
Androgens	Fluoxymesterone	10 mg PO BID	Deepening voice, alopecia, hirsutism, facial/truncal acne, fluid retention, menstrual irregularities, cholestatic jaundice

Table 88.7 ▪ Toxicities of Commonly Used Antineoplastic Agents

Drug	Toxicity
Cyclophosphamide	Myelosuppression, nausea/vomiting, alopecia, hemorrhagic cystitis, stomatitis
Methotrexate	Myelosuppression, mucositis, diarrhea, nausea/vomiting, hepatic dysfunction, nephrotoxicity
Fluorouracil (FU)/capecitabine	Myelosuppression, mucositis, alopecia, nausea/vomiting, diarrhea, skin hyperpigmentation/photosensitivity, cerebellar ataxia (FU only), hand-foot syndrome
Vinblastine/vinorelbine	Neurotoxicity, constipation, alopecia, myelosuppression, injection site reactions, skin necrosis after extravasation
Doxorubicin	Myelosuppression, nausea/vomiting, alopecia, stomatitis, radiation recall, skin necrosis after extravasation, cardiotoxicity (occurs more frequently with cumulative doses 550 mg/m^2)
Mitoxantrone	Myelosuppression, nausea/vomiting, alopecia, mucositis, urine discoloration, cardiotoxicity
Paclitaxel/docetaxel	Myelosuppression, hypersensitivity reactions (require premedications), paresthesia/neuropathy, myalgias and arthralgias (greater with paclitaxel), nausea, vomiting, diarrhea, alopecia, fluid retention (docetaxel), cutaneous reactions (docetaxel)
Trastuzumab	Fever, chills, diarrhea, cardiac dysfunction

tive trials between tamoxifen and other forms of endocrine therapy (e.g., estrogen, progestins, aromatase inhibitors, androgens) have not demonstrated superiority of tamoxifen based on clinical response, but the toxicity profiles do support the use of tamoxifen initially over other therapies. However, this may change with the increased use of tamoxifen in the adjuvant disease setting.

Approximately 35 to 50% of patients who respond initially to tamoxifen therapy experience a response to second-line hormonal therapy.[64] Progestins, aromatase inhibitors, and androgens are second-line hormonal choices. The choice of second- and third-line endocrine therapy is currently based on toxicity, cost, and ease of administration, rather than response, due to the comparable response rates between agents. The recommended doses, routes of administration, and side effects reported with the endocrine therapies used for metastatic breast cancer are listed in Table 88.6.

Patients with rapidly progressive disease or who do not fulfill the criteria for treatment with endocrine therapy should receive chemotherapy initially. Patients who fail to respond to endocrine therapy should also be treated with chemotherapy. The chemotherapeutic agents that have demonstrated activity in the treatment of breast cancer include doxorubicin, cyclophosphamide, fluorouracil, methotrexate, mitoxantrone, vinblastine, vinorelbine, mitomycin C, thiotepa, melphalan, paclitaxel, docetaxel, trastuzumab, and capecitabine. The objective response rates reported with these drugs as single-agent therapy range from 20 to 68%.[61,65–69] Table 88.7 describes some of the toxicities associated with the commonly used antineoplastic agents. Historically, the combination regimens listed in Table 88.5, as well as numerous ad hoc combination regimens, have been used in the metastatic disease setting because of the presumed increase in activity with combination therapy. However, some of the newer single chemotherapeutic agents have produced responses equivalent to those obtained with combination regimens, particularly in the anthracycline-refractory disease setting.

Single-agent paclitaxel was approved for the treatment of breast cancer after failure of combination chemotherapy for metastatic disease or relapse within 6 months of adjuvant therapy.[70] The recommended dose of paclitaxel for metastatic breast cancer is 175 mg/m^2 intravenously over 3 hours every 3 weeks. Clinical trials exploring alternative schedules, such as weekly dosing, are currently ongoing. Similarly, docetaxel was approved for the treatment of patients with locally advanced or metastatic breast cancer who have progressed during prior chemotherapy or have relapsed during anthracycline-based adjuvant therapy.[71] In phase II trials conducted in patients who had documented disease resistant to anthracycline-based therapy, docetaxel produced an overall response rate of 41% at doses of 100 mg/m^2. This is the highest response rate that has been reported with single-agent therapy in anthracycline-resistant disease. In a randomized phase III study comparing single-agent docetaxel and single-agent doxorubicin in patients with metastatic breast cancer who had failed prior alkylating chemotherapy, docetaxel produced a significantly higher response rate (47% versus 32%), prolonged time to disease progression (26 weeks versus 21 weeks), and prolonged overall survival (15 versus 14 months).[72] In another randomized phase III trial comparing single-agent docetaxel with the combination of mitomycin C and vinblastine in patients with metastatic breast cancer who had previously failed an anthracycline-containing regimen, docetaxel again produced an increased response rate (30% versus 11.6%) and prolonged time to disease progression (19 weeks versus 11 weeks).[73] However, most important, survival was increased with docetaxel as compared with the mitomycin C plus vinblastine combination (12-month survival: 49% versus 33%; 18-month survival: 33% versus 21%). Docetaxel is administered at a dose of 60 to 100 mg/m^2 intravenously over 1 hour with doses repeated every 21 days. Patients with hepatic impairment experienced increased hematologic toxicity in the clinical trials, so the drug should be used with caution in patients with elevated liver function tests. Both paclitaxel and docetaxel are attractive agents for patients with metastatic disease who have failed prior anthracycline therapy or for whom further anthracycline therapy is not indicated. Further study of these drugs as single agents or in combination regimens is currently underway, and the optimal dose and schedule of both agents remain to be determined.

Capecitabine is a prodrug that is converted to fluorouracil after oral administration. The drug has been approved by the FDA for the treatment of patients with metastatic breast cancer resistant to both paclitaxel and an anthracycline-containing chemotherapy regimen or resistant to paclitaxel and for whom further anthracycline therapy is not indicated (e.g., patients who have received cumulative doses of 400 mg/m^2 of doxorubicin or doxorubicin equivalents).[74] The recommended starting dose of capecitabine is 2500 mg/m^2/day administered orally twice daily with food for 2 consecutive weeks followed by 1 week of rest (21-day cycles). Subsequent doses should be adjusted based on toxicities encountered during treatment. The most common toxicities associated with therapy include diarrhea, nausea, vomiting, stomatitis, and hand-foot syndrome. In women enrolled in the clinical trials who had failed both paclitaxel and an anthracycline, capecitabine produced an overall response rate of 26%.[74] The convenience of oral administration also makes capecitabine an attractive agent for the metastatic disease setting because the primary goal of treatment is palliation.

Researchers have recently developed a humanized monoclonal antibody, trastuzumab, which binds to the HER2 receptor and is the perfect example of translational research from the laboratory to clinical practice. Trastuzumab was recently approved by the FDA for the treatment of patients with metastatic breast cancer whose tumors overexpress the HER2 protein and who have received one or more chemotherapy regimens for their metastatic disease. HER2 overexpression has been correlated with decreased disease-free and overall survival in breast cancer patients, and approximately 25 to 30% of breast cancers overexpress HER2.[75] In the initial phase II trial in patients with metastatic breast cancer who had received extensive prior therapy and overexpressed HER2, weekly intravenous administration of single-agent trastuzumab produced an overall response rate of 12%.[76] This response rate was also confirmed in a large open-label trial conducted in 222 women who had received one or two prior cytotoxic regimens for metastatic disease.[77] In this population, trastuzumab produced an overall response rate of 16% with a median duration of 9.1 months. The addition of trastuzumab to front-line chemotherapy for metastatic disease has also recently been evaluated. A total of 469 patients were randomized to receive paclitaxel, doxorubicin, and cyclophosphamide (PAC) or doxorubicin and cyclophosphamide (AC) with or without weekly trastuzumab.[78] The median time to progression was longer in patients receiving chemotherapy plus trastuzumab versus patients receiving chemotherapy alone (7.6 months versus 4.6 months). Furthermore, the overall response rate in patients receiving chemotherapy plus trastuzumab was 48% versus 32% in patients receiving chemotherapy alone. Based on these data, trastuzumab is also indicated in combination with paclitaxel for the treatment of patients with metastatic breast cancer whose tumors overexpress HER2 and who have not received chemotherapy for their metastatic disease. Trastuzumab appears to be well tolerated overall, with fever and chills being the most commonly reported side effects. However, patients who received trastuzumab plus AC appeared to have a higher incidence of cardiac dysfunction. The etiology of the increased cardiac dysfunction remains to be determined.

Doxorubicin has demonstrated significant activity in the adjuvant treatment of breast cancer and in the treatment of metastatic disease. Unfortunately, however, doxorubicin dosing is limited by the development of cardiomyopathy, which occurs with cumulative lifetime doses of greater than 400 mg/m^2. As a result, patients commonly cannot be re-treated with doxorubicin when they develop metastatic disease because of the doses they received in the adjuvant setting. Dexrazoxane is an intracellular chelating agent that interferes with the generation of iron-mediated free radicals, which are thought to be responsible for anthracycline-induced cardiotoxicity. The drug is approved for the reduction of the incidence and severity of cardiomyopathy associated with doxorubicin administration in women with metastatic breast cancer who have received a cumulative doxorubicin dose of 300 mg/m^2 and who, in their physician's opinion, would benefit from continuing therapy with doxorubicin.[79] Dexrazoxane is administered at a dexrazoxane:doxorubicin ratio of 10:1 and is given by IV push or infusion 30 minutes before doxorubicin administration. Although the approval of dexrazoxane would allow patients to receive higher cumulative lifetime doses of doxorubicin, many clinicians choose to use alternative agents such as the taxanes or capecitabine in the metastatic disease setting because of their significant antitumor activity, lack of cross-resistance with doxorubicin, and ease of administration.

The approval of pamidronate, a bone resorption inhibitor, for the treatment of osteolytic bone metastases is another advancement in the management of patients with metastatic breast cancer. The administration of 90 mg of pamidronate intravenously over 2 hours every 3 to 4 weeks in conjunction with standard chemotherapy or hormonal therapy resulted in a decrease in the number of skeletal complications in women with metastatic disease as compared with placebo.[80] The median time to onset of the first skeletal complication was also significantly prolonged in patients receiving pamidronate. A recent update of this study indicated that the decrease in osteolytic bone lesions was sustained when dosing was extended to 2 years, and no unexpected adverse events occurred with prolonged pamidronate administration.[81]

In summary, the goal of treatment of metastatic disease is palliation. As a result, patient quality of life should play a role in treatment decisions. The new agents approved for metastatic breast cancer, such as the taxanes, trastuzumab, and capecitabine, offer promising alternatives for patients with anthracycline-resistant disease. However, the data on the use of these new drugs as single agents or in combination regimens are limited, so additional clinical trials are warranted. Furthermore, the optimal duration of treatment in women with metastatic disease remains to be determined.

PROGNOSIS

The natural history of breast cancer varies greatly among patients. Some patients have extremely aggressive disease that progresses rapidly; others are diagnosed with disease that follows a more indolent course. Because of these variations, the ability to predict which patients will experience a better disease prognosis is extremely important. Table 88.8 lists some of the prognostic factors that have been determined in breast cancer patients to date. The most commonly assessed prognostic factors include nodal status, tumor size, hormone receptor status, histologic grade, and cell proliferation indices. The remaining prognostic factors are still considered investigational until there are sufficient data to support their clinical utility.

Table 88.8 ▪ Prognostic Factors in Breast Cancer

Prognostic Factor	Favorable	Unfavorable
Nodal involvement	Absent	Present
Tumor size	Small	Large
Histologic grade	Well differentiated	Poorly differentiated
Estrogen receptor	Positive	Negative
Progesterone receptor	Positive	Negative
S-phase fraction	Low	High
Mitotic index	Low	High
Ploidy	Diploid	Aneuploid
Thymidine labeling index	Low	High
HER2/neu (c-erbB-2)	Absent	Present
p53	Absent	Present
Microvessel density (angiogenesis)	Low	High

The single most important prognostic factor at the time of diagnosis is the extent of axillary lymph node involvement. Numerous studies have confirmed the significance of nodal involvement for predicting disease recurrence and survival. The number of affected nodes is directly related to disease recurrence and indirectly related to survival. In patients with no nodal involvement at diagnosis, the 10-year survival rate is approximately 75%. As nodal involvement increases to 1 to 3 nodes and 4 to 9 nodes, the 10-year survival rate decreases to 62% and 42%, respectively.[82] When 10 or more nodes are involved, the 10-year survival rate decreases dramatically to only 20%. Tumor size at the time of diagnosis is also an important prognostic factor for breast cancer.[83] Although large tumors have a greater tendency to metastasize to axillary lymph nodes, tumor size is also an independent predictor for breast cancer recurrence. Patients with well-differentiated tumors also have a better prognosis than patients with poorly differentiated tumors, making histologic grade an important prognostic factor as well.

Another important prognostic factor is estrogen- and progesterone-receptor status. A tumor is considered estrogen-receptor positive if the cytosol protein concentration is ≥10 fmol/mg. Laboratory assays for the determination of estrogen receptor content in tumors were originally developed to predict tumor response to hormonal therapy. However, in 1977 Knight and colleagues recognized the prognostic importance of estrogen-receptor status by demonstrating a higher rate of disease recurrence in patients with estrogen-receptor–negative tumors.[83,84] Furthermore, in patients with node-positive disease, the presence of progesterone receptors in tumor tissue indicates improved disease-free survival compared with patients without progesterone receptors.

The rate of tumor cell proliferation has also demonstrated prognostic significance in breast cancer recurrence.

Rate of cell proliferation can be determined using either the tritiated thymidine labeling index or DNA flow cytometry, which determines the percentage of tumor cells actively dividing in the S-phase of the cell cycle. Both techniques indicate that patients with rapidly proliferating tumors (high S-phase fraction, high mitotic index) have a decreased disease-free survival compared with patients with slowly proliferating tumors.[85,86] Additionally, flow cytometry can detect the presence of abnormal DNA content, or aneuploidy, in breast cancer cells. Patients with aneuploid tumors also appear to have a decreased disease-free survival.[86]

Tumor concentrations of breast cancer growth factors and their receptors have also been measured to determine prognostic significance. Increased levels of the HER-2/neu (c-erbB-2) oncogene, a protein that promotes tumor cell development, have been correlated with decreased disease-free and overall survival in patients with node-positive disease.[75] Cathepsin D is a protease that promotes tumor cell growth and possibly disease metastasis. In the original analysis conducted by researchers at the University of Texas Health Science Center at San Antonio in women with node-negative disease, high levels of cathepsin D were associated with a decreased disease-free and overall survival rate.[87] However, a subsequent larger analysis failed to confirm this original data. As a result, the role of cathepsin-D as a prognostic factor remains unclear. Expression of the tumor suppressor gene p53 may also predict prognosis. Patients with node-negative breast cancer who express p53 appear to have a decreased disease-free and overall survival rate when compared with patients who do not express the p53 gene.[82] Other prognostic factors for breast cancer are the vascular growth factors, such as vascular endothelial growth factor, platelet-derived endothelial cell growth factor, and fibroblast growth factors.[88,89] Early laboratory studies suggest that tumor angiogenesis (blood vessel growth) is an independent and highly significant prognostic factor for lymph node involvement and predicts survival. Tumors that have high microvessel density are more likely to metastasize and bode a worse prognosis as well.

Predicting disease recurrence in patients with breast cancer is a difficult task, especially in patients with negative nodal involvement at the time of diagnosis. The ability to determine prognostic factors for disease recurrence would be extremely useful clinically, because patients with a poor prognosis could be treated more aggressively initially in an attempt to prolong survival, and patients with a very low risk of recurrence could avoid unnecessary adjuvant systemic therapy.

FUTURE THERAPIES

Although progress has been made in the treatment of breast cancer, further improvements in therapy are necessary. Current avenues of research include new methods of administration for commercially available drugs and the development of new drugs. Continuous infusion therapy, sequential or alternating therapy with other agents, and the use of liposome-encapsulated doxorubicin are ways in which researchers are attempting to decrease the toxicities and increase the efficacy of doxorubicin administration.[90,91] The search for synergistic drug combinations using conventional agents and new therapeutic agents such as the taxanes, vinorelbine, trastuzumab, and capecitabine is also underway. It is hoped that new combination regimens will increase response rates and overall survival. The use of the newer chemotherapeutic agents in both the adjuvant and the metastatic settings is also being explored. Several oral antineoplastic agents that have activity in breast cancer and could be added to the drug armamentarium are also currently being studied in clinical trials.

The epidermal growth factor receptor has an established role as an oncogene in the development and progression of breast cancer. The development of monoclonal antibodies directed against the EGF receptor is also being investigated as therapy for breast cancer.[89,92] Several novel agents that inhibit angiogenesis are also entering clinical trials to determine their activity in the treatment of breast cancer, because angiogenesis plays such an important role in tumor progression.[88,89,93] Other antineoplastic agents, such as farnesyl-protein transferase inhibitors, metalloproteinase inhibitors, and telomerase inhibitors, are also being investigated in preclinical and early clinical trials.[94]

For many antineoplastic agents there is a linear relationship between dose and tumor response, but the toxic effects of the drug on the marrow limit the dose that can be administered. High-dose chemotherapy intensification with or without autologous bone marrow support or peripheral blood stem cell transplantation is actively being investigated for the treatment of breast cancer.[95,96] Currently, approximately 50% of transplants for breast cancer are conducted in patients with local disease and 50% are conducted in patients with metastatic disease, with more than half of patients being transplanted within 1 year of their diagnosis. The 3-year survival rate after transplant in patients in the transplant registry by stage was as follows: stage 2, 74%; stage 3, 70%; inflammatory disease, 52%; and metastatic disease, 30%. When the results for early breast cancer are compared with data recorded in the American Surveillance, Epidemiology, and End Results Registry (SEER), there does not appear to be an improvement in overall survival with high-dose therapy (SEER 3-year survival data: stage 2, 73%; stage 3, 56%; and inflammatory disease, 50%).[97] There also does not appear to be a survival advantage in metastatic disease when the data are compared with historical data from M. D. Anderson. Currently, large cooperative group prospective randomized studies are underway to determine the effectiveness of high-dose therapy in the treatment of breast cancer. Unfortunately, of the patients enrolled in the Autologous Blood and Marrow Transplant Registry, only 11% with early high-risk breast cancer and 1% with metastatic disease were enrolled in clinical trials. Therefore, accrual to these protocols has been relatively slow. In a preliminary study evaluating high-dose therapy in patients with metastatic disease, all patients received two to four cycles of induction therapy and were then randomized to receive observation alone with high-dose therapy at relapse or immediate high-dose therapy. Surprisingly, overall survival was better in the group that received high-dose therapy at relapse (3.2 years versus 1.7 years).[98] As a result, clinicians, breast cancer patients, and third-party payors all anxiously await the data from the randomized cooperative group studies. The benefits of treatment must outweigh the increased cost and toxicities of high-dose therapy for this to become standard treatment.

PREVENTION

Tamoxifen has been shown to decrease the risk of developing a second primary carcinoma in the contralateral breast in women diagnosed with breast cancer.[54] Additionally, tamoxifen significantly decreased total cholesterol and low-density lipoprotein cholesterol levels in postmenopausal women receiving 2 years of adjuvant therapy for node-negative breast cancer.[99] Plasma high-density lipoprotein levels were also increased, resulting in lipoprotein profiles that are favorable for the prevention of coronary heart disease and atherosclerosis. Another positive effect of tamoxifen is a decrease in bone density loss due to retarded bone resorption.[100] However, the estrogenic effects of tamoxifen may cause venous thrombosis and endometrial cancer with prolonged administration.[101,102] Therefore, in order to use tamoxifen in a chemopreventive setting, the benefits of therapy must outweigh the risks. Using a relative risk model, Ragaz and Coldman[103] predicted that the decrease in death secondary to contralateral breast cancer and cardiovascular events as a result of tamoxifen would outweigh the slight increase in mortality from endometrial cancer and thromboembolic episodes in breast cancer survivors.

The preliminary data from the Breast Cancer Prevention Trial conducted by NSABP and the National Cancer Institute also support this finding and resulted in the FDA approval of tamoxifen for reducing the incidence of breast cancer in women at high risk for developing the disease.[104] A total of 13,388 women who were considered at increased risk for developing breast cancer (based on personal or family history) were enrolled in the study and randomized to receive tamoxifen 20 mg daily or placebo daily for 5 years. At a median follow-up of 3.6 years, there were 85 cases of invasive breast cancer diagnosed in women taking tamoxifen versus 154 cases in women on placebo (45% reduction in the rate of breast cancer). The rate of diagnosis of noninvasive breast cancer was also lower in women taking tamoxifen. Women receiving tamoxifen had fewer hip, wrist, and spine fractures (47 versus 71), but there was no difference in cardiovascular events between the two groups. As expected, the number of cases of endometrial cancer (33 versus 14), pulmonary embolism (17 versus 6), and deep vein thrombosis (30 versus 19) was higher in the tamoxifen group than in the placebo group and appeared to occur most often in women greater than 50 years of age at enrollment. Similar preliminary results have also been reported with raloxifene in postmenopausal women with osteoporosis, except the risk of endometrial cancer was decreased.[105] Raloxifene is a selective estrogen-receptor modulator approved for the treatment of osteoporosis that has estrogenic effects on bone and lipids and anti-estrogenic effects on the endometrium (in contrast to tamoxifen). As a result of these studies, a large randomized clinical trial is planned that will directly compare tamoxifen and raloxifene. Although these data would support the use of tamoxifen in patients similar to those enrolled in the aforementioned protocol, they cannot be extrapolated to the general population. However, longer follow-up of the current studies and data obtained from additional studies may support generalized chemoprevention in the future with tamoxifen or another agent. The use of synthetic retinoids as chemoprevention is also being explored.[94]

CONCLUSION

Advances in the areas of early detection methods, genetic testing, primary surgical treatment, radiation therapy, and chemotherapy or hormonal therapy for adjuvant and metastatic disease have occurred due to the willingness of both physicians and patients to participate in randomized, controlled clinical trials and the long-term analysis of these trial results. However, many unanswered questions remain regarding the etiology, detection, treatment, and prevention of breast cancer, so continued intensive research is warranted.

KEY POINTS

- Noninvasive breast cancer (LCIS and DCIS) is generally easily controlled with surgery alone or surgery plus radiation.
- Early-stage breast cancer (stages I and II) is most often managed with breast-conserving surgery and radiation. Adjuvant hormonal therapy or chemotherapy is indicated in stage II patients, and the treatment approach depends on estrogen-receptor status and age.
- Locally advanced breast cancer (stage III) is most effectively managed with combined-modality therapy. When all three modalities are combined, more than 90% of patients are disease free after treatment and may remain disease free for up to 3 to 5 years.
- The goals of treatment for metastatic breast cancer are to prolong survival and palliate symptoms. The choice of therapy depends on the site of disease involvement and patient-specific characteristics. Although patients with metastatic breast cancer will most likely die of their disease, many patients can achieve durable responses to treatment that allow them to lead prolonged lives with good quality.

- Many new therapies, including monoclonal antibodies and the taxanes, have helped prolong survival in patients with metastatic disease and may also be beneficial in the treatment of earlier-stage disease.

REFERENCES

1. Greenlee RT, Murray T, Bolden S, et al. Cancer statistics, 2000. CA Cancer J Clin 50:7–33, 2000.
2. Hutchins L, Broadwater R Jr, Lang NP, et al. Breast cancer. Dis Mon 36: 63–125, 1990.
3. Abeloff MD, Lichter AS, Niederhuber JE, et al. Breast. In: Abeloff MD, Armitage JO, Lichter AS, Niederhuber JE, eds. Clinical oncology. New York: Churchill Livingstone, 1995:1617–1714.
4. Anderson DE. A genetic study of human breast cancer. J Natl Cancer Inst 48:1029–1034, 1972.
5. Matloff ET, Peshkin BN. Complexities in cancer genetic counseling: breast and ovarian cancer. PPO Updates Principles and Practice of Oncology 12:1–11, 1998.
6. Struewing JP, Hartge P, Wacholder S, et al. The risk of cancer associated with specific mutations of BRCA1 and BRCA2 among Ashkenazi Jews. N Engl J Med 336:1401–1408, 1997.
7. Couch FJ, DeShano ML, Blackwood MA, et al. BRCA1 mutations in women attending clinics that evaluate the risk of breast cancer. N Engl J Med 336:1409–1415, 1997.
8. Henderson DE. Endogenous and exogenous endocrine factors. Hematol Oncol Clin North Am 3:577–598, 1989.
9. Jawed Iqbal M, Taylor W. Hormonal and reproductive factors–new evidence. In: Stoll BA, ed. Women at high risk to breast cancer. Dordrecht: Kluwer Academic, 1989:41–46.
10. Romieu I, Berlin JA, Colditz G. Oral contraceptives and breast cancer. Review and meta-analysis. Cancer 66:2253–2263, 1990.
11. Roy JA, Sawka CA, Pritchard KI. Hormone replacement therapy in women with breast cancer: do the risks outweigh the benefits? J Clin Oncol 14:997–1006, 1996.
12. London S, Willett W. Diet and the risk of breast cancer. Hematol Oncol Clin North Am 3:559–576, 1989.
13. Hunter DJ, Spiegelman D, Adami HO, et al. Cohort studies of fat intake and the risk of breast cancer–a pooled analysis. N Engl J Med 334:356–361, 1996.
14. Ballard-Barbash R. Anthropometry and breast cancer. Body size–a moving target. Cancer 74(Suppl 3):1090–1100, 1994.
15. Frisch RE, Wyshak G, Albright NL, et al. Lower prevalence of breast cancer and other cancers of the reproductive system among former college athletes compared to nonathletes. Br J Med 52:885–891, 1985.
16. Hoffman-Goetz L, Husted J. Exercise and breast cancer: review and critical analysis of the literature. Can J Appl Physiol 19:237–252, 1994.
17. Longnecker MP, Berlin JA, Orza MJ, et al. A meta-analysis of alcohol consumption in relation to risk of breast cancer. JAMA 260:652–656, 1988.
18. Reichman ME, Judd JT, Longcope C, et al. Effects of alcohol consumption on plasma and urinary hormone concentrations in premenopausal women. J Natl Cancer Inst 85:722–727, 1993.
19. Goss PE, Sierra S. Current perspectives on radiation-induced breast cancer. J Clin Oncol 16:338–347, 1998.
20. Pike MC, Krailo MD, Henderson DE, et al. Hormonal risk factors, breast tissue age and age-incidence of breast cancer. Nature 303:676–770, 1983.
21. Osborne CK, Arteaga CL. Autocrine and paracrine growth regulation of breast cancer: clinical implications. Breast Cancer Res Treat 15:3–11, 1990.
22. Stockdale FE. Breast cancer. In: Rubenstein E, Federman DD, eds. Scientific American medicine. New York: Scientific American, 1990:1–16.
23. Hill D, White V, Jolley D, et al. Self examination of the breast: is it beneficial? Meta-analysis of studies investigating breast self examination and extent of disease in patients with breast cancer. Br Med J 297:271–275, 1988.
24. Huguley CM, Brown RL, Greenberg RS, et al. Breast self-examination and survival from breast cancer. Cancer 62:1389–1396, 1988.
25. Kopans DB. Breast cancer detection, diagnosis, and radiation therapy. In: Rich MA, Hager JC, Keydar I, eds. Breast cancer: progress in biology, clinical management, and prevention. Boston: Kluwer Academic, 1989:71–84.
26. Shapiro S, Strax P, Venet L. Periodic breast cancer screening in reducing mortality from breast cancer. JAMA 215:1777–1785, 1971.
27. Shapiro S, Venet W, Strax P, et al. Current results of the breast cancer screening randomized trial: The Health Insurance Plan of Greater New York study. In: Day NE, Miller AB, eds. Screening for breast cancer. Toronto: Hans Huber, 1988:3–15.
28. Smart CR, Byrne C, Smith RA, et al. Twenty-year follow-up of the breast cancers diagnosed during the Breast Cancer Detection Demonstration Project. CA Cancer J Clin 47:134–149, 1997.
29. Kopans DB. Breast cancer screening: women 40–49 years of age. PPO Updates Principles and Practice of Oncology 8:1–11, 1994.
30. Newcomb PA, Lantz PM. Recent trends in breast cancer incidence, mortality, and mammography. Breast Cancer Res Treat 28:97–106, 1993.
31. Winchester DP, Strom EA. Standards for diagnosis and management of ductal carcinoma in situ (DCIS) of the breast. CA Cancer J Clin 48:108–128, 1998.
32. Fisher B, Dignam J, Wolmark N, et al. Lumpectomy and radiation therapy for the treatment of intraductal breast cancer: findings from National Surgical Adjuvant Breast and Bowel Project B-17. J Clin Oncol 16:441–452, 1998.
33. Fisher B, Anderson S, Redmond CK, et al. Re-analysis and results after 12 years of follow-up in a randomized clinical trial comparing total mastectomy with lumpectomy with or without irradiation in the treatment of breast cancer. N Engl J Med 333:1456–1461, 1995.
34. Early Breast Cancer Trialists' Collaborative Group. Effects of radiotherapy and surgery in early breast cancer. An overview of the randomized trials. N Engl J Med 333:1444–1455, 1995.
35. Cady B, Stone MD, Schuler JG, et al. The new era in breast cancer: invasion, size, and nodal involvement dramatically decreasing as a result of mammographic screening. Arch Surg 131:301–308, 1996.
36. Haffty BG, Ward B, Pathare P, et al. Reappraisal of the role of axillary lymph node dissection in the conservative treatment of breast cancer. J Clin Oncol 15:691–700, 1997.
37. Giuliano AE, Jones RC, Brennan M, et al. Sentinel lymphadenectomy in breast cancer. J Clin Oncol 15:2345–2350, 1997.
38. Leong SPL. The role of sentinel lymph nodes in human solid cancer. PPO Updates Principles and Practice of Oncology 12:1–12, 1998.
39. Clinical Alert from the National Cancer Institute. Breast Cancer Res Treat 12:3–5, 1988.
40. Ludwig Breast Cancer Study Group. Prolonged disease-free survival after one course of perioperative adjuvant chemotherapy for node-negative breast cancer. N Engl J Med 320:491–496, 1989.
41. Mansour EG, Gray R, Shatila AH, et al. Efficacy of adjuvant chemotherapy in high-risk node-negative breast cancer. An intergroup study. N Engl J Med 320:485–490, 1989.
42. Fisher B, Redmond C, Dimitrov NV, et al. A randomized clinical trial evaluating sequential methotrexate and fluorouracil in the treatment of patients with node-negative breast cancer who have estrogen-receptor-negative tumors. N Engl J Med 320:473–478, 1989.
43. Fisher B, Costantino J, Redmond C, et al. A randomized clinical trial evaluating tamoxifen in the treatment of patients with node-negative breast cancer who have estrogen-receptor-positive tumors. N Engl J Med 320:479–484, 1989.
44. Fisher B, Dignam J, Wolmark N, et al. Tamoxifen and chemotherapy for lymph node-negative, estrogen receptor-positive breast cancer. J Natl Cancer Inst 89:1673–1682, 1997.
45. Hutchins L, Green S, Ravdin P, et al. CMF versus CAF with and without tamoxifen in high-risk node-negative breast cancer patients and a natural history follow-up study in low-risk node-negative patients: first results of intergroup trial INT 0102. Proc Am Soc Clin Oncol 17:1a, 1998.
46. Lindley C, Vasa S, Sawyer WT, et al. Quality of life and preferences for treatment following adjuvant therapy for early-stage breast cancer. J Clin Oncol 16:1380–1387, 1998.
47. Ravdin PM, Siminoff LA, Harvey JA. Survey of breast cancer patients concerning their knowledge and expectations of adjuvant therapy. J Clin Oncol 16:515–521, 1998.
48. Siminoff LA, Ravdin PM, Gerson N, et al. Impact of a personal computer based tool for providing individualized estimates of outcomes for patients with early breast cancer. Proc Am Soc Clin Oncol 17:105a, 1998.
49. Systemic treatment of early breast cancer by hormonal, cytotoxic, or immune therapy. 133 randomized trials involving 31,000 recurrences and 24,000 deaths among 75,000 women. Early Breast Cancer Trialists' Collaborative Group [2 parts]. Lancet 339:1–15, 71–85, 1992.
50. Early Breast Cancer Trialists' Collaborative Group. Polychemotherapy for early breast cancer: an overview of the randomised trials. Lancet 352:930–942, 1998.
51. Wood WC, Budman DR, Korzun AH, et al. Dose and dose intensity of adjuvant chemotherapy for stage II, node-positive breast carcinoma. N Engl J Med 330:1253–1259, 1994.
52. Namer M. Anthracyclines in the adjuvant treatment of breast cancer. Drugs 45(Suppl 2):4–9, 1993.
53. Hortobagyi GN, Buzdar AU. Present status of anthracyclines in the adjuvant treatment of breast cancer. Drugs 45(Suppl 2):10–19, 1993.

54. Early Breast Cancer Trialists' Collaborative Group. Tamoxifen for early breast cancer: an overview of the randomized trials. Lancet 351:1451–1467, 1998.
55. Fisher B, Dignam J, Bryant J, et al. The worth of five versus more than five years of tamoxifen therapy for breast cancer patients with negative lymph nodes and estrogen receptor-positive tumors. J Natl Cancer Inst 88:1529–1542, 1996.
56. International Breast Cancer Study Group. Effectiveness of adjuvant chemotherapy in combination with tamoxifen for node-positive postmenopausal breast cancer patients. J Clin Oncol 15:1385–1394, 1997.
57. American Society of Clinical Oncology. Recommended breast cancer surveillance guidelines. J Clin Oncol 15:2149–2156, 1997.
58. Hortobagyi GN. Multidisciplinary management of advanced primary and metastatic breast cancer. Cancer 74(Suppl 1):416–423, 1994.
59. Hortobagyi GN. Comprehensive management of locally advanced breast cancer. Cancer 66:1387–1391, 1990.
60. Fisher B, Brown A, Mamounas E, et al. Effect of preoperative chemotherapy on local-regional disease in women with operable breast cancer: findings from National Surgical Adjuvant Breast and Bowel Project B-18. J Clin Oncol 15:2483–2493, 1997.
61. Wong K, Henderson IC. Management of metastatic breast cancer. World J Surg 18:98–111, 1994.
62. Buzdar AU. Current status of endocrine treatment of carcinoma of the breast. Semin Surg Oncol 6:77–82, 1990.
63. Davidson NE. Ovarian ablation as treatment for young women with breast cancer. Monogr Natl Cancer Inst 16:95–99, 1994.
64. Santen RJ, Manni I, Harvey H, Redmond C. Endocrine treatment of breast cancer in women. Endocrine Reviews 11:221–265, 1990.
65. Garber JE, Henderson IC. The use of chemotherapy in metastatic breast cancer. Hematol Oncol Clin North Am 3:807–821, 1989.
66. Norton L. Salvage chemotherapy of breast cancer. Semin Oncol 21(4 Suppl 7):19–24, 1994.
67. Arbuck SG, Dorr A, Friedman MA. Paclitaxel (Taxol) in breast cancer. Hematol Oncol Clin North Am 8:121–140, 1994.
68. Chevallier B, Fumoleau P, Kerbrat P, et al. Docetaxel is a major cytotoxic drug for the treatment of advanced breast cancer: a phase II trial of the Clinical Screening Cooperative Group of the European Organization for Research and Treatment of Cancer. J Clin Oncol 13:314–322, 1995.
69. Jones AL, Smith IE. Navelbine and the anthrapyrazoles. Hematol Oncol Clin North Am 8:141–152, 1994.
70. Taxol (paclitaxel) package insert. Bristol-Myers Squibb Company, Princeton, 1997.
71. Taxotere (docetaxel) package insert. Rhone-Poulenc Rorer, Collegeville, 1998.
72. Chan S, Friedrichs K, Noel D, et al. A phase III study of Taxotere (T) vs doxorubicin (D) in patients (pts) with metastatic breast cancer (MBC) who have failed an alkylating containing regimen. Breast Cancer Res Treat 46:23, 1997.
73. Nabholtz JM, Thuerlimann B, Beswoda WR, et al. Taxotere improves survival over mitomycin C vinblastine in patients with metastatic breast cancer who have failed an anthracycline containing regimen: final results of a phase III randomized trial. Proc Am Soc Clin Oncol 17:101a, 1998.
74. Xeloda (capecitabine) package insert. Roche Laboratories, Nutley, 1998.
75. Tandon AK, Clark GM, Chamness GC, et al. HER-2/neu oncogene protein and prognosis in breast cancer. J Clin Oncol 7:1120–1128, 1989.
76. Baselga J, Tripathy D, Mendelsohn J, et al. Phase II study of weekly intravenous recombinant humanized anti-p185HER2 monoclonal antibody in patients with HER2/neu-overexpressing metastatic breast cancer. J Clin Oncol 14:737–744, 1996.
77. Cobleigh MA, Vogel CL, Tripathy D, et al. Efficacy and safety of Herceptin (humanized anti-her2 antibody) as a single-agent in 222 women with HER2 overexpression who relapsed following chemotherapy for metastatic breast cancer. Proc Am Soc Clin Oncol 17:97a, 1998.
78. Slamon D, Leyland-Jones B, Shak S, et al. Addition of Herceptin (humanized anti-HER2 antibody) to first line chemotherapy for HER2 overexpressing metastatic breast cancer (HER2+/MBC) markedly increases anticancer activity: a randomized multinational controlled phase III trial. Proc Am Soc Clin Oncol 17:98a, 1998.
79. Zinecard (dexrazoxane) package insert. Pharmacia Upjohn, Kalamazoo, 1996.
80. Hortobagyi GN, Theriault RL, Porter L, et al. Efficacy of pamidronate in reducing skeletal complications in patients with breast cancer and lytic lesions. N Engl J Med 335:1785–1791, 1996.
81. Hortobagyi GN, Theriault RL, Lipton A, et al. Long-term prevention of skeletal complications of metastatic breast cancer with pamidronate. J Clin Oncol 16:2038–2044, 1998.
82. Fisher ER, Anderson S, Redmond C, et al. Pathologic findings from the National Surgical Adjuvant Breast Project Protocol B-06: 10-year pathologic and clinical prognostic discriminants. Cancer 71:2507–2514, 1993.
83. Donegan WL. Tumor-related prognostic factors for breast cancer. CA Cancer J Clin 47:28–51, 1997.
84. Clark GM, McGuire WL. Steroid receptors and other prognostic factors in primary breast cancer. Semin Oncol 15(Suppl 1):20–25, 1988.
85. Silvestrini R, Daidone MG, Valagussa P, et al. 3H-thymidine labeling index as a prognostic indicator in node-positive breast cancer. J Clin Oncol 8:1321–1326, 1990.
86. Clark GM, Dressler LG, Owens MA. Prediction of relapse or survival in patients with node-negative breast cancer by DNA flow cytometry. N Engl J Med 320:627–633, 1989.
87. Ravdin PM, Tandon AK, Allred DC, et al. Cathepsin D by Western blotting and immunohistochemistry: failure to confirm correlations with prognosis in node-negative breast cancer. J Clin Oncol 12:467–474, 1994.
88. Harris AL, Fox S, Bicknell R, et al. Gene therapy through signal transduction pathways and angiogenic growth factors as therapeutic targets in breast cancer. Cancer 74(Suppl 3):1021–1025, 1994.
89. Gasparini G, Harris AL. Clinical importance of the determination of tumor angiogenesis in breast carcinoma: much more than a new prognostic tool. J Clin Oncol 13:765–782, 1995.
90. Valagussa P, Brambilla C, Bonnadonna G. Chemotherapy of advanced disease. In: Hoogstraten B, Burn I, Bloom JHG, eds. UICC current treatment of cancer: breast cancer. Berlin: Springer-Verlag, 1989:233–256.
91. Treat J, Greenspan A, Forst D, et al. Antitumor activity of liposome-encapsulated doxorubicin in advanced breast cancer: Phase II study. J Natl Cancer Inst 82:1706–1710, 1990.
92. Baselga J, Mendelsohn J. The epidermal growth factor receptor as a target for therapy in breast carcinoma. Breast Cancer Res Treat 29:127–138, 1994.
93. Fan T-PD, Jaggar R, Bicknell R. Controlling the vasculature: angiogenesis, antiangiogenesis, and vascular targeting of gene therapy. Trends Pharmacol Sci 16:57–66, 1995.
94. Piccart MJ, Hortobagyi GN. Conclusions: future strategies in the treatment of breast cancer. Semin Oncol 24(Suppl 3):S3-34–S3-40, 1997.
95. Antman KH, Rowlings PA, Vaughan WP, et al. High-dose chemotherapy with autologous hematopoietic stem-cell support for breast cancer in North America. J Clin Oncol 15:1870–1879, 1995.
96. Lazarus HM. Hematopoietic progenitor cell transplantation in breast cancer: current status and future directions. Cancer Investigation 16:102–126, 1998.
97. Ravdin PM, Callander NS, Hortobagyi GN. Registry results and high-dose therapy. J Clin Oncol 16:387–388, 1998.
98. Peters WP, Jones RB, Vredenburgh J, et al. A large prospective, randomized trial of high-dose combination alkylating agents (CPB) with autologous cellular support (ABMS) as consolidation for patients with metastatic breast cancer achieving complete remission after intensive doxorubicin-based induction therapy. Proc Am Soc Clin Oncol 15:121, 1996.
99. Love RR, Newcomb PA, Wiebe DA, et al. Effects of tamoxifen therapy on lipid and lipoprotein levels in post-menopausal patients with node-negative breast cancer. J Natl Cancer Inst 82:1327–1332, 1990.
100. Fornander T, Rutgrist LE, Siöberg HE, et al. Long-term adjuvant tamoxifen in early breast cancer: effect on bone mineral density in post-menopausal women. J Clin Oncol 8:1019–1034, 1990.
101. Love RR. Tamoxifen therapy in primary breast cancer: biology, efficacy, and side effects. J Clin Oncol 7:803–815, 1989.
102. Stearns V, Gelmann EP. Does tamoxifen cause cancer in humans? J Clin Oncol 16:779–792, 1998.
103. Ragaz J, Coldman A. Survival impact of adjuvant tamoxifen on competing causes of mortality in breast cancer survivors, with analysis of mortality from contralateral breast cancer, cardiovascular events, endometrial cancer, and thromboembolic episodes. J Clin Oncol 16:2018–2024, 1998.
104. Fisher B, Costantino JP, Wickerham DL, et al. Tamoxifen for prevention of breast cancer: report of the National Surgical Adjuvant Breast and Bowel Project P-1 Study. J Natl Cancer Inst 90:1371–1388, 1998.
105. Cummings SR, Norton L, Eckert S, et al. Raloxifene reduces the risk of breast cancer and may decrease the risk of endometrial cancer in post-menopausal women. Two-year findings from the multiple outcomes of raloxifene evaluation (MORE) trial. Proc Am Soc Clin Oncol 17:2a, 1998.

CHAPTER 89

LIVER TUMORS

Robert J. Stagg and Jennie T. Chang

Liver tumors are classified as primary tumors, those arising from the hepatobiliary system, or secondary tumors, those metastasizing to the liver from a primary tumor of extrahepatic origin, and as being either benign or malignant. Liver tumors, as a group, are one of the most common malignancies in the world. In Europe and North America, metastatic adenocarcinomas are the most frequently occurring liver tumors, and in Africa and Southeast Asia, primary hepatocellular carcinoma is the most prevalent hepatic malignancy. Primary and metastatic liver tumors account for approximately 20% of cancer-related deaths in the United States. Because of the liver's vital physiologic role, hepatic tumors often govern patient survival, even in the presence of any extrahepatic tumor. Primary and metastatic liver tumors will be discussed separately because they have distinct biologic and clinical features.

Anatomy and Physiology of the Liver

The liver is a wedge-shaped organ that is suspended from the diaphragm and lies in the right upper quadrant of the abdomen (Fig. 89.1). The liver consists of three lobes: the right lobe, which is the largest; the left lobe; and the caudate lobe, which is the smallest and is located on the dorsal aspect of the liver. The right lobe is further subdivided into the anterior and posterior segments, and the left lobe is subdivided into the medial and lateral segments.

The liver has a dual blood supply, coming from both the portal vein and the hepatic artery. Normal hepatic parenchyma receives the majority of its blood supply from the portal vein, whereas hepatic tumors receive the majority of their blood supply from the hepatic artery.[1] Several of the modalities employed in the treatment of hepatic tumors exploit this unique finding. The blood from both the portal vein and the hepatic artery is drained from the liver by the hepatic vein, which returns it to the inferior vena cava, immediately below the right atrium. The vena cava lies in a groove on the dorsal aspect of the liver. Each segment of the liver has its own biliary system; these systems join intrahepatically to form the right and left hepatic ducts and then unite as they exit the liver to form the common bile duct. The hepatic artery enters and the portal vein and bile duct exit the liver at the hilum in a region known as the porta hepatis.

The liver performs a number of critical physiologic functions, including producing and excreting bile (including bilirubin), synthesizing proteins (including albumin, gamma globulins, and several clotting factors), and metabolizing foodstuffs, drugs, and toxins. Hepatic tumors may interfere with these physiologic functions.

After damage by surgical resection, disease, or toxic insult, an otherwise healthy liver is capable of regenerating to its original size. However, an impaired liver, such as a cirrhotic liver, may not be able to regenerate after such an insult. Liver regeneration occurs through hypertrophy of the remaining liver parenchyma. The liver's ability to regenerate enables it to tolerate treatment modalities, such as surgical resection, cryosurgery, and chemoembolization, that are employed in the treatment of liver tumors. Patients with cirrhotic livers may not tolerate these therapies as well. Liver regeneration appears to be regulated by a variety of

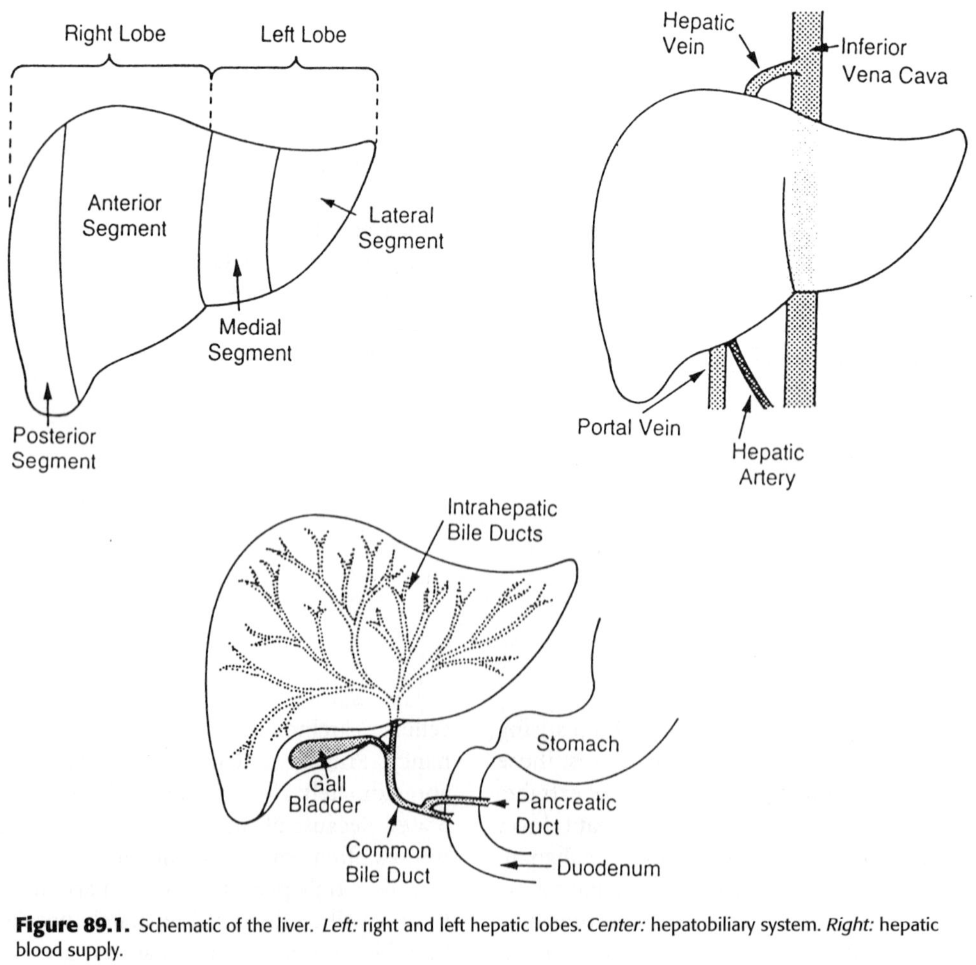

Figure 89.1. Schematic of the liver. *Left:* right and left hepatic lobes. *Center:* hepatobiliary system. *Right:* hepatic blood supply.

growth factors, including epidermal growth factor (EGF), hepatocyte growth factor (HGF), transforming growth factor α and β (TGF-α and TGF-β), fibroblast growth factor (FGF), interleukin 1-α (IL-1), and hepatopoietin-B. The precise interactive role of each of these growth factors in initiating and subsequently terminating liver regeneration has not been fully elucidated. Liver regeneration is essentially complete within a few months of initiation.

Primary Liver Tumors

Table 89.1 lists the various types of benign and malignant primary liver tumors.

Benign Primary Liver Tumors

INFANTILE HEMANGIOENDOTHELIOMA

Infantile hemangioendothelioma is a benign tumor of vasculoendothelial origin that occurs in the first 6 months of life. Because of the vascular nature of this tumor, a bruit can sometimes be heard over the liver. Approximately one-half of the patients also have a cutaneous hemangioma. In addition, patients may have hepatomegaly, congestive heart failure secondary to arteriovenous shunting, thrombocytopenia, or microangiopathic hemolytic anemia, and up to one-third of patients have hemolytic jaundice.[2] Asymptomatic patients can be followed without treatment because spontaneous regression of the tumor may occur within 1 year. However, patients with symptomatic congestive heart failure should be managed medically with diuretics and inotropic agents. If medical management is unsuccessful, symptoms may be controlled with steroids, radiotherapy, or hepatic arterial ligation. Surgical resection may also be used in patients with intractable cardiac failure or refractory consumptive coagulopathy.[3]

CAVERNOUS HEMANGIOMA

Cavernous hemangioma is the most common benign tumor of the liver, occurring in up to 7% of the population. It is hypervascular and most commonly occurs in women in the fourth, fifth, or sixth decade of life. It increases in size during pregnancy or estrogen administration. Hemangiomas are usually asymptomatic and are most often found incidentally at autopsy. Occasionally, patients develop symptoms, including right upper quadrant pain, fever, early satiety, or vomiting. Only severely symptomatic patients and those having lesions larger than 10 cm who are at risk for intraperitoneal hemorrhage should be treated. For such patients, surgical resection is the treatment of choice.[4] Additional therapeutic modalities that have been employed include steroids, radiation, hepatic arterial ligation, and embolization.[5]

Table 89.1 ▪ Primary Liver Cancers

Benign	Malignant
Infantile hemangioendothelioma	Hepatocellular carcinoma
Cavernous hemangioma	Hepatoblastoma
Hepatic cell adenoma	Intrahepatic cholangiocarcinoma
Focal nodular hyperplasia	Angiosarcoma
	Epithelioid hemangioendothelioma
	Undifferentiated sarcoma

HEPATIC CELL ADENOMA

Hepatic adenoma occurs primarily in young women of childbearing age and usually manifests as a large solitary mass in the liver. Oral contraceptives, anabolic steroids, and type 1 glycogen storage disease have been implicated in the etiology of hepatic adenoma.[6] It is not known whether the development of hepatic adenoma in women taking oral contraceptives is due to the estrogen or progesterone component and whether the reduction in the estrogen content of many oral contraceptives will decrease the incidence of this tumor. Complete spontaneous regression, as well as progression, has been noted in women after discontinuation of an oral contraceptive. Rare cases of malignant transformation of hepatic adenoma to hepatocellular carcinoma have been reported.[7] Surgical resection of a persistent hepatic adenoma is the preferred treatment because of its propensity to rupture and the possibility of malignant transformation. There is no role for radiation or chemotherapy in the management of this disease. Oral contraceptives and anabolic steroids should be strictly avoided in all patients with a history of resected or unresected hepatic adenoma.

FOCAL NODULAR HYPERPLASIA

Focal nodular hyperplasia is a hypervascular tumor that occurs most often in females and manifests as an asymptomatic hepatic mass. It can occur at any age, including childhood, and is usually asymptomatic. The etiology of focal nodular hyperplasia is largely unknown, but oral contraceptives have been reported to be a possible cause.[6] Patients with focal nodular hyperplasia often have coexisting congenital heart disease or other tumors, including cavernous hemangiomas, glioblastomas, astrocytomas, pheochromocytomas, and multiple endocrine neoplasias.[8] Treatment is generally not indicated because this tumor is rarely symptomatic and is not premalignant, but surgical resection has been successfully employed in symptomatic patients.[9] The long-term prognosis of this tumor is excellent.

Malignant Primary Liver Tumors

Hepatocellular carcinoma is the most prevalent malignant tumor of the liver and will be the major focus of this section. Other primary malignant tumors rarely occur, but warrant mention.

HEPATOBLASTOMA

Hepatoblastoma is the most common primary malignant liver tumor in young children, affecting approximately 1 child per 100,000. It is usually diagnosed before age 5 but has been rarely reported in adults. It may be familial and occurs twice as frequently in males as in females. It may occur in conjunction with congenital anomalies such as tetralogy of Fallot, persistent ductus arteriosis, or extrahepatic biliary atresia. Hepatoblastoma usually manifests as a solitary mass that may be encapsulated. The most common presenting symptom is abdominal swelling. Serum α-fetoprotein is elevated in the majority of cases. If untreated, hepatoblastoma is uniformly fatal. Approximately 30 to 50% of patients with hepatoblastoma are cured by surgical resection, which is the treatment of choice whenever feasible. Preoperative chemotherapy, chemoembolization, or radiation may reduce tumor bulk, allowing removal of an originally unresectable tumor.[10] Postoperative adjuvant chemotherapy has also been administered to patients with hepatoblastoma, but its utility remains unclear.[11] Encouraging results have been obtained in patients with unresectable hepatoblastoma confined to the liver who have undergone liver transplantation, although further study is needed to determine its role.[12] Systemic chemotherapy, typically with a cisplatin- or doxorubicin-based regimen, can be employed for patients with unresectable hepatic tumor or extrahepatic disease, but it is generally not curative.

INTRAHEPATIC CHOLANGIOCARCINOMA

Intrahepatic cholangiocarcinoma is a tumor arising from the intrahepatic bile ducts and is the second most common malignant primary tumor of the liver. Occasionally, tumors contain a mixture of cholangiocarcinoma and hepatocellular carcinoma. Intrahepatic cholangiocarcinoma may arise from a peripheral bile duct or a major intrahepatic duct and has a low tendency to metastasize. Cholangiocarcinomas arising from the intrahepatic bile ducts in the hilum of the liver are known as Klatskin tumors. Patients with Crohn's disease, sclerosing cholangitis, biliary atresia, ulcerative colitis, and hepatolithiasis are at increased risk for developing cholangiocarcinoma. The median survival of untreated patients is approximately 6.5 months, although patients who have small peripheral tumors may survive much longer. Surgical resection is occasionally curative and should be performed whenever possible. Liver transplant may also have a role in the management of locally confined cholangiocarcinoma. Penn[13] reported the results in 109 patients with intrahepatic or hilar cholangiocarcinoma, from liver transplant centers throughout the world, who underwent orthotopic liver transplantation. The 2- and 5-year actuarial survival rates were 30 and 17%, respectively.[13] Systemic chemotherapy is employed for patients with unresectable or metastatic tumor. A partial response rate of 31% was reported with intravenous 5-fluorouracil, mitomycin, and doxorubicin.[14] Responses have also been observed with intraarterial chemotherapy.[15]

ANGIOSARCOMA

Angiosarcoma, though uncommon, is the most frequently occurring sarcoma of the liver. It grows rapidly and is often accompanied by thrombocytopenia. Approximately 40% of cases are associated with exposure to a carcinogen, specifically thorium oxide (Thorotrast), vinyl chloride, arsenic, or radium.[16] There can be a latency period of up to 40 years from the carcinogen exposure to the development of the angiosarcoma.[17] It is a rapidly progressive tumor, metastasizing to the lungs, porta hepatis, lymph nodes, or spleen. Angiosarcomas occasionally rupture, leading to hemoperitoneum. Resection offers the only potential for cure and is the treatment of choice whenever feasible. Radiation or chemotherapy may produce partial responses in unresectable lesions, although the experience with these modalities is limited.[16] Patients with unresectable angiosarcoma usually survive less than 1 year.

EPITHELIOID HEMANGIOENDOTHELIOMA

Epithelioid hemangioendothelioma is a rare vascular tumor of the liver.[18] It occurs primarily in middle age and more frequently in women than in men. In some patients, the development of epithelioid hemangioendothelioma appears to be causally related to the use of oral contraceptives. Epithelioid hemangioendothelioma causes hepatic fibrosis and frequently infiltrates the hepatic and portal veins. Clinically, it often manifests in a manner similar to that of Budd-Chiari syndrome. Various treatments have been employed, including liver transplantation, partial hepatectomy, chemotherapy, and radiation. It can be very slow growing, with 25% of patients with an unresectable tumor surviving longer than 5 years from diagnosis.

UNDIFFERENTIATED SARCOMA

Undifferentiated (embryonal) sarcoma of the liver is a term used to describe a group of very rare pediatric sarcomas of the liver that defy categorization since they lack cellular differentiation.[19] The tumor rarely metastasizes but spreads by direct invasion into adjacent organs. It is usually rapidly fatal, although cures have been reported with surgical resection. Radiation and chemotherapy have been used in the treatment of unresectable lesions and metastatic disease, but their utility is unclear.

Hepatocellular Carcinoma

DEFINITION

Hepatocellular carcinoma (HCC), also known as hepatoma, accounts for 40% of childhood and 90% of adult malignant primary tumors of the liver. It is more common in males than in females. HCC rarely occurs in adults before age 40 and increases in frequency thereafter, with the peak incidence occurring in the sixth decade of life. HCC is uncommon in the United States, with approximately 3000 to 4000 cases diagnosed annually.[20] However, it is one the most prevalent cancers in Asia, sub-Saharan Africa, and the South Pacific Islands and is estimated to cause 1.25 million deaths worldwide each year.

TREATMENT GOALS: HEPATOCELLULAR CARCINOMA

- Whenever feasible, concentrate treatment on curing the patient through surgical removal of the HCC or use a treatment modality that causes local tumor necrosis, such as cryotherapy.
- When cure is not feasible, either because of extensive hepatic involvement or the presence of extrahepatic metastases, treat those patients desiring therapy with a modality that has a reasonable chance of producing a response while maintaining the patient's quality of life.

EPIDEMIOLOGY

HCC is frequently associated with preexisting liver disease. In the United States, approximately 50% of patients with HCC have underlying cirrhosis secondary to alcohol, postnecrotic cirrhosis, or hemochromatosis.[21] Primary biliary cirrhosis and the cirrhosis associated with Wilson's disease do not appear to significantly predispose patients to developing HCC. It is estimated that approximately 5% of all patients with cirrhosis will eventually develop HCC.

Chronic active hepatitis B infection is the most important predisposing factor worldwide.[22] Epidemiologic studies reveal a high incidence of HCC in patients residing in those regions where hepatitis B is endemic. Patients chronically infected with hepatitis B have a 10- to 390-fold increased risk of developing HCC. The method by which chronic hepatitis B infection causes hepatic oncogenesis is not completely understood, but three possible mechanisms have been proposed. The first postulates that viral infection results in chronic inflammation and hepatocyte regeneration, leading to random mutations in the host genome and malignant transformation. The second theory postulates that there is targeted integration of hepatitis B regulatory genes adjacent to specific sites in the host genome, resulting in activation of host proto-oncogenes or inactivation of tumor suppressor genes and subsequent malignant transformation. The final theory postulates that random integration of the hepatitis B genome into the host genome occurs and that malignant transformation is a direct result of the oncogenic action of the integrated viral genes or viral gene products. Whatever the mechanism, approximately 80% of HCC worldwide is thought to be the result of prior hepatitis B infection. Thus the hepatitis B virus appears to rank in importance with tobacco as a human carcinogen.

Hepatitis C infection also predisposes patients to developing HCC.[23] Hepatitis C infection is present in about 15% of HCC patients in the United States and 76% of patients in Japan.[24,25] Little is known about the exact mechanism by which hepatitis C produces hepatic oncogenesis.

Aflatoxin B1, a toxin produced by *Aspergillus flavus*, has also been implicated as a possible cause of HCC.[26] It appears to cause HCC by producing distinct point mutations in the p53 tumor suppressor gene. Aflatoxins are present on several foodstuffs consumed in large quantities in those parts of the world having a high incidence of HCC. These include rice, peanuts, soybeans, corn, wheat, bread, milk, and cheese, especially when they are stored in unrefrigerated conditions.

Case reports in the literature suggest an association between hormone exposure and the development of HCC. Women and men have developed HCC after exposure to oral contraceptives and androgens, respectively.[27,28] However, it remains to be determined whether the ingestion of hormones is causally related to the development of HCC.

Finally, certain inherited metabolic disorders, including hemochromatosis, glycogen storage disease, α_1-antitrypsin deficiency, and tyrosinemia, predispose patients to develop HCC.

PATHOPHYSIOLOGY

HCC is a grayish white to bright yellow tumor that is usually not encapsulated. Occasionally, however, encapsulated HCC is found in older patients and is a slower-growing and less invasive tumor than typical HCC.[29] Three major categories of HCC have been described based on its macroscopic appearance. The most common type is the nodular form in which the liver is studded with tumor. The second is the massive type, which manifests as a large mass and is sometimes associated with small satellite lesions. The last type is the diffuse form, which is the rarest and manifests as scattered tumor throughout the liver. The diffuse form always occurs in association with cirrhosis.

Eight different histologic subtypes of HCC have been identified based on the microscopic appearance of the tumor (Table 89.2). The hepatic variant, also known as the trabecular variant, is the most common. The fibrolamellar variant is noteworthy because it is usually solitary and has a better prognosis than the other types of HCC.[30] It occurs primarily in women between ages 15 and 30 and is not associated with cirrhosis. The clear cell variant may also be associated with a better prognosis.

HCC often infiltrates the diaphragm and invades the intrahepatic portal veins. Less often the tumor invades the hepatic vein or bile duct. Frequently, regional lymph nodes are involved with tumor, but unless this occurs in the porta hepatis, such involvement usually does not alter the patient's clinical course. At autopsy, 40 to 50% of patients with HCC are found to have distant metastases. The lung is the most common site of metastases, although almost any organ can be involved. The presence of metastatic disease rarely alters the patient's outcome because the tumor burden in the liver usually determines the duration of survival.

CLINICAL PRESENTATION AND DIAGNOSIS

Signs and Symptoms

Unfortunately, HCC is not typically symptomatic until there is advanced disease. The most common symptoms are abdominal pain, abdominal distension, fatigue, anorexia, weight loss, and fevers. On examination, most patients have hepatomegaly. Less often, patients have ascites, edema, or jaundice. Rarely, patients have hemorrhage secondary to esophageal varices. Although uncommon in North American patients, patients in Asia and Africa frequently (10 to 20%) have spontaneous rupture of their HCC with intraperitoneal hemorrhage.

Many laboratory abnormalities may be present in a patient with HCC. The hepatic transaminases and alkaline phosphatase are usually elevated, and the bilirubin is elevated in up to 50% of patients. Because of the decreased synthetic ability of the liver and the cachectic state of patients, the albumin level is often decreased, and the prothrombin time (PT) and partial thromboplastin time (PTT) may be elevated. A mild anemia and a reactive leukocytosis frequently occur. Rarely, erythrocytosis is present in patients having HCC with underlying cirrhosis. Hypoglycemia occurs in two distinct subpopulations of patients with HCC. The first group consists of patients with good performance status who have an acquired form of glycogen storage disease, secondary to their tumor, with reduced hepatocellular levels of glucose 6-phosphatase and a phosphorylase required for the breakdown of glycogen. The second group consists of terminal patients in whom hepatic gluconeogenesis is impaired. Approximately one-third of patients have high serum cholesterol levels. Finally, some patients have hypercalcemia due to either bone metastases or a parathormone-like substance produced by the tumor.

Diagnosis

The diagnostic workup of a patient suspected of having HCC generally proceeds from the physician's clinical suspicion based on the patient's presenting signs and symptoms, to laboratory tests, to noninvasive radiologic studies, and then to tissue biopsy. The clinician usually first suspects the possibility of a hepatic malignancy when the patient complains of right upper quadrant pain or an enlarged liver is detected on physical examination. When these signs and symptoms occur in a patient with a prior history of hepatitis B or cirrhosis, a diagnosis of HCC must be considered.

Laboratory tests may be helpful in the diagnosis, but most are nonspecific. The most useful laboratory test is the α-fetoprotein (AFP). AFP is a glycoprotein synthesized by fetal liver, fetal intestine, and yolk sac cells. Levels are very high before birth and fall to normal adult levels of less than 10 ng/mL after delivery. AFP is elevated (greater than 100 ng/mL) in about 75 to 90% of patients who have HCC.[31] Although levels are elevated in a few other malignant conditions, the frequency of elevated levels in patients with HCC makes this a useful initial test. When elevated, the AFP level can also be used to follow a patient's clinical course because it usually falls with response to therapy and rises with progressive disease. Ferritin levels are elevated in patients with HCC. However, it is also

Table 89.2 • Histologic Variants of Hepatocellular Carcinoma

Hepatic or trabecular	Giant cell
Pleomorphic	Clear cell
Adenoid or acinar	Fibrolamellar
Sclerosing	Mixed

elevated in most patients with uncomplicated cirrhosis and thus lacks specificity.[32] In addition, ferritin levels do not correlate with therapeutic response, as does AFP.

Several radiologic tests may be used to confirm the presence of a hepatic mass and to subsequently follow the course of the disease. Arteriography may be used to assist in the diagnosis of HCC when other radiographic techniques fail. On arteriographic examination, HCC typically has a dilated feeding artery with a hypervascular tumor bed. Radionuclide liver-spleen scanning with technetium sulfur colloid is simple to perform, inexpensive, and not associated with morbidity, but it is rarely used because of its inability to image the rest of the abdomen. Ultrasound is similarly inexpensive and is not associated with morbidity, but it is incapable of detecting hepatic lesions less than 1 cm in size and has limited utility in determining the presence of extrahepatic tumor. Although they are more expensive, computed tomography (CT) and magnetic resonance imaging (MRI) are the most frequently employed methods for imaging a hepatic malignancy. These techniques are more sensitive than ultrasound and allow visualization of the entire abdomen. However, the most sensitive radiographic technique for detecting a hepatic lesion is intraoperative ultrasound. This procedure should be performed whenever hepatic resection is contemplated because it is more sensitive for detecting lesions than even the surgeon's visual and tactile inspection of the liver.[33]

These radiographic techniques are useful for documenting the presence of a hepatic mass and following the course of disease once the diagnosis has been confirmed and therapy has been instituted, but by themselves, they do not provide a definitive diagnosis of HCC. This requires pathologic examination of a tissue specimen. Tissue specimens may be obtained by percutaneous biopsy, peritoneoscopy with directed needle biopsy, or open biopsy at laparotomy.

Screening

Theoretically, screening patients who are at high risk for developing HCC should result in the detection of the malignancy earlier, thus allowing potentially curative surgery to be performed in a larger number of patients. However, although some early HCCs are detected by screening high-risk patients with AFP levels or ultrasound, no definitive outcome advantage has been observed.[34–39]

PSYCHOSOCIAL ASPECTS

The diagnosis of HCC has a major impact on patients and their family members. Patients have to cope with the diagnosis of a potentially rapidly fatal illness, as well as the anxiety of contemplating the aggressive surgical and medical treatments used in this disease. Thus patients and their family members must be educated about HCC and its treatment options, as well as assisted with the emotional impact of the diagnosis itself.

Because HCC occurs most frequently in Asia, many HCC patients in the United States are immigrants. As a result, patients and their family members often do not speak fluent English. In such cases, it is essential that translators assist with the education of the patient and their family members. In addition, in some Asian countries, patients are typically not informed that they have terminal cancer. As a result, it is not uncommon to have family members request that the patient not be fully informed regarding their diagnosis and prognosis. This situation requires discussion with the family, so that an approach can be agreed on that allows the patient to be appropriately informed of his or her treatment options.

TREATMENT

Surgical resection and orthotopic liver transplantation of HCC are potentially curative modalities and should be employed whenever feasible. Cryosurgery, intratumoral alcohol injection, and radiofrequency ablation are three modalities that may be useful in patients with potentially resectable HCCs who are not candidates for surgical resection because of underlying liver disease or other comorbid illnesses. Patients with unresectable but liver-predominant disease are most frequently treated with systemic chemotherapy, intraarterial chemotherapy (with or without Lipiodol; see Intraarterial Lipiodol Chemotherapy later in this chapter), or chemoembolization. Other alternatives for these patients include hepatic artery ligation, embolization, and radiation (external beam radiation or radioimmunotherapy). Systemic chemotherapy is the only alternative for patients who have significant extrahepatic tumor.

Surgical Resection

Surgical resection of HCC is the most widely employed modality that offers a potential for cure. Partial hepatectomy is associated with significant morbidity and mortality (3 to 15%), especially in patients with underlying liver disease, and therefore should only be attempted with curative intent.[40–58] Unfortunately, the majority of patients are not candidates for surgical resection because their intrahepatic tumor is too extensive, their underlying liver disease limits their ability to withstand the surgical procedure, or they have extrahepatic disease. Approximately one-third of patients are considered candidates for resection following preoperative staging of their tumor, and of those, approximately two-thirds are found to be unresectable at surgery because of the presence of extrahepatic tumor or previously undiagnosed intrahepatic tumor. Thus only about 10 to 15% of patients with HCC have resectable disease. Occasionally, unresectable HCC may be rendered resectable with chemotherapy, radiation, or both.[59]

Table 89.3 summarizes the results of surgical resection for HCC. The 5-year survival rates for patients having undergone a potentially curative resection ranged from 15

Table 89.3 ▪ Results of Surgical Resection for Hepatocellular Carcinoma

Author/Year	Number of Patients	Perioperative Mortality (%)	5-Year Survival (%)	Reference
Lin/1987	225	8	18	40
Chen/1989	120	4	32[a]	41
Toshihara/1990	119	15	33	42
Choi/1990	174	13	15	43
Yamanaka/1990	128	6	54	44
Kobayashi/1990	180	3	49	45
Tsuzuki/1990	119	15	39	46
Iwatsuki/1991	76	6	33	47
Gozzetti/1993	168	8	36	48
Kawarada/1994	149	4	39	49
Tani/1997	90	4	38	50
Yamasaki/1991	427	3	41	51
Nagashima/1996	50	12	53	52
Takenaka/1996	280	2	50	53
Chen/1997	382	4	46	54
Makuuchi/1998	352	1	47	55
Takayama/1998	163	1	51	56
Lise/1998	100	11	38	57
Philosphe/1998	67	4	38	58

[a]Four-year survival.

to 54%. Approximately 20% of the 5-year survivors ultimately die of recurrent disease; thus approximately 25% of the resected patients are cured of HCC. Factors associated with an increased likelihood of cure include having adequate hepatic function to withstand the surgery, a tumor smaller than 5 cm, negative resection margins, a well-differentiated tumor, an encapsulated tumor, lack of vascular invasion, or having the fibrolamellar variant of HCC.[32,41] In addition, patients without viral hepatitis are at a decreased risk for recurrence of HCC.

The role of adjuvant chemotherapy following resection has not been fully elucidated. Data from a small study in Asia suggest that adjuvant intraarterial chemotherapy may improve disease-free and overall survival of patients with HCC.[60] However, a recent randomized study comparing surgical resection with or without adjuvant chemotherapy reported a higher incidence of overall recurrence, extrahepatic recurrence, and a shorter disease-free survival for the group that received adjuvant intraarterial chemotherapy.[61]

Orthotopic Liver Transplantation

Orthotopic liver transplantation (OLT) has been performed in patients who have locally confined but unresectable HCC. Unfortunately, the results with OLT have been somewhat disappointing, with 3-year survival rates of approximately 50% and long-term survival rates of only 20%.[62–70] A retrospective review of OLT in HCC conducted at the University of Pittsburgh reported no difference in 3-year survival rates between HCC patients who underwent hepatectomy and those who underwent OLT.[45] However, patients who had underlying cirrhosis had a 3-year survival rate of only 5.9% with hepatectomy compared with a 42.9% survival rate with OLT. These results, which have been confirmed in a retrospective review reported by Bismuth and colleagues,[71] may be explained by the elimination of the cirrhotic liver. A prospective randomized trial of cirrhotic patients with HCC comparing surgical resection to OLT has not been conducted and thus a definitive benefit of OLT in cirrhotic patients has not been proved. Three tumor characteristics are thought to negatively affect patient survival after transplantation: a tumor greater than 5 cm, vascular invasion, and a poorly differentiated tumor.[72]

Two small subpopulations of HCC patients appear to benefit significantly from OLT. Patients with fibrolamellar HCC have a 50% disease-free survival after OLT,[73,74] and patients with a small HCC discovered incidentally at the time of OLT for end-stage liver disease have an 80% likelihood of long-term survival.[65]

In an attempt to improve on the results with OLT for HCC, recent studies have combined OLT with perioperative chemotherapy. In one study, doxorubicin was administered preoperatively to 20 HCC patients who subsequently underwent OLT and resulted in an estimated 3-year survival of 59%.[75] In another trial, 10 patients were treated with perioperative cisplatin and α-interferon followed by OLT, and 9 of 10 patients were alive 1 year after OLT.[76] Venook and colleagues[77] treated 11 patients with preoperative chemoembolization, and 10 were alive without recurrence at a median follow-up of 40 months. In another trial, 25 patients treated with 6 months of postoperative intravenous 5-fluorouracil, doxorubicin, and cisplatin had a 46% 3-year survival rate compared with 5.8% in a historical control patient population.[78] These pilot studies suggest that perioperative chemotherapy may increase the cure rate of OLT, but a prospective randomized trial must be performed before definitive conclusions can be drawn.

Cryosurgery

Cryosurgery utilizes a probe circulating liquid nitrogen through its tip, which is inserted into a tumor under intraoperative ultrasound guidance to induce freezing temperatures within a tumor, resulting in necrosis. The use of multiple freeze-thaw cycles increases the percentage of tumor cells killed.[79] Cryosurgery is relatively well tolerated. However, in the largest published experience to date, only 12 of 60 (20%) patients were alive 3 years after cryosurgery.[80] It may be most useful in patients with resectable disease who are not candidates for partial hepatectomy due to underlying liver disease, such as cirrhosis.

Radiofrequency Ablation

Radiofrequency ablation, like cryosurgery, is a technique used to produce necrosis of individual tumors.[81] Under ultrasound or magnetic resonance guidance, radiofrequency energy is transmitted to the tumor via electrode needles, resulting in tumor necrosis. Like cryosurgery, radiofrequency ablation appears to be most useful in treating small tumors in patients with underlying liver disease who are not good surgical candidates.

Percutaneous Alcohol Injection

Percutaneous injection of absolute ethyl alcohol directly into a tumor under ultrasound guidance is capable of producing histologically confirmed complete responses in small HCCs by inducing dehydration and intracellular coagulation, leading to necrosis, vascular occlusion, and fibrosis. The volume of ethyl alcohol injected depends on the size of the tumor and its vascularity, but it is generally 2 to 8 mL. The distribution of alcohol within the tumor during the injection is evaluated by ultrasound. In various studies, percutaneous alcohol injection for small, typically solitary, HCCs resulted in a 3-year survival of 55 to 70%.[82–84] Castells and colleagues[82] compared the outcome of 30 patients treated with percutaneous alcohol injection with 33 patients treated with surgical resection. Two years after the procedure, 66% of the percutaneous alcohol–treated group compared with 45% of the surgical resection group had recurrence of their tumor, although the survival rates were similar for the two groups.[82] As with cryosurgery and radiofrequency ablation, percutaneous alcohol injection appears to be most useful in the rare patient who has potentially resectable HCC, but it is not a good candidate for surgical resection because of underlying liver disease.

Radiotherapy

Standard external beam radiation is of limited benefit in the management of HCC because of the inherent intolerance of normal liver parenchyma to radiation. Doses to the liver in excess of 3000 rads produce radiation hepatitis in a significant number of patients.[85] Patients with underlying liver disease develop radiation hepatitis at even lower doses. Some partial responses to external beam radiation at doses of 2000 to 3000 rads fractionated over 7 days have been reported, although survival does not appear to be extended.[86] Three-dimensional radiation treatment can minimize the radiation dose to liver and allow a higher dose of radiation to be delivered to the HCC than conventional external beam radiation.[87,88] Whether this approach will improve on the results obtained with standard external beam radiation remains to be determined.

Other approaches of delivering radiotherapy to the tumor while minimizing exposure to the normal liver tissue are under investigation. One such approach is the administration of radioimmunoglobulin targeted to a tumor antigen. Initial studies of iodine-131 polyclonal antiferritin antibody plus chemotherapy and external beam radiation produced encouraging results, but a subsequent randomized trial comparing this approach to chemotherapy alone failed to produce a survival advantage.[89] In addition, significant myelosuppression was observed. Two alternative methods of delivering regional radiotherapy are the administration of intraarterial iodine-131 radiolabeled Lipiodol and neutron-activated yttrium-90 containing glass microspheres.[90,91] In a study comparing epirubicin Lipiodol versus iodine-131 radiolabeled Lipiodol, similar results were observed for the two treatments.[92] In a study investigating the use of intraarterial yttrium-90 microspheres, significant antitumor activity was observed at tumor doses exceeding 120 Gy.[93]

Hormonal Therapy

Hormonal agents such as megestrol acetate and tamoxifen citrate have been investigated for the treatment of HCC because some HCCs are estrogen-receptor positive, as are some breast cancers.[94] Based on this finding, patients with HCC have been treated with megestrol acetate or tamoxifen citrate.[94–96] Although occasional responses were observed in these early studies, two well-designed, multicenter studies have found that tamoxifen citrate is comparable to placebo for the treatment of HCC.[97,98] In a recent study, megestrol acetate failed to produce any responses in 32 patients with HCC.[99]

Intravenous Chemotherapy

Intravenous chemotherapy is of limited benefit in altering the natural history of HCC. However, it is the only therapeutic option for the majority of patients who have widely metastatic disease. The experience with single-agent chemotherapy is summarized in Table 89.4. Doxorubicin is the agent with the most reproducible activity, producing responses in approximately 20% of patients. It is usually administered intravenously in doses of 20 to 75 mg/m^2 every 21 days.[100–108] 4′-Epirubicin and mitoxantrone also appear to have activity against HCC.[109–113]

5-Fluorouracil has been administered both orally[102,114,115] and intravenously[115–118] to patients with HCC. By both routes, the response rates have been low. Amsacrine, dichloromethotrexate, etoposide, cisplatin, and α-interferon have all produced occasional responses, but the overall response rates with these agents have been low.[104,119–129] Various combination regimens have been studied, but none have improved on the results obtained with single-agent therapy.

Intraarterial Chemotherapy

Because of the discouraging results obtained with intravenous chemotherapy, administration directly into the hepatic artery has been used to increase the drug exposure (concentration versus time) to the tumor and thus enhance efficacy.[130,131] The drug exposure is most dramatically increased when the agent being administered has a rapid total body clearance because intraarterial infusion enables the drug to be delivered in a high concentration to the tumor before its elimination from the body. An additional benefit is derived from intraarterial administration when the agent has a high first-pass hepatic extraction. The high first-pass hepatic extraction of the drug leads to a lower

Table 89.4 ▪ Results of Single-Agent Intravenous Chemotherapy for Hepatocellular Carcinoma

Drug	Number of Patients	Responses	Response Rate (%)	Reference
Doxorubicin	41	6/41	15	100
	44	14/44	32	101
	57	9/57	16	102
	74	22/74	30	103
	28	8/28	29	104
	35	3/35	9	105
	52	6/52	11	106
	45	11/45	24	107
	109	11/109	10	108
	485	**91/485**	**19**	
Mitoxantrone	22	6/22	27	109
	20	0/20	0	110
	42	**6/42**	**14**	
4′-Epidoxorubicin	18	3/18	17	111
	13	3/13	23	112
	33	3/33	9	113
	64	**9/64**	**14**	
5-Fluorouracil	12	6/12	50	114
	48	0/48	0	102
	21	0/21	0	115
	10	1/10	10	116
	8	0/8	0	117
	15	1/15	7	118
	114	**8/114**	**7**	
Amsacrine	23	3/23	13	119
	16	0/16	0	120
	20	1/20	5	121
	35	1/35	3	122
	94	**5/95**	**5**	
Dichloro-methotrexate	14	0/14	0	123
	7	3/7	43	124
	21	**3/21**	**14**	
Etoposide	24	3/24	13	125
	38	7/38	18	104
	62	**10/62**	**16**	
Cisplatin	13	1/13	8	126
	26	4/26	15	127
	39	**5/39**	**13**	
Interferon	28	2/28	7	128
	25	2/25	8	129
	53	**4/53**	**8**	

systemic drug exposure than with intravenous administration and thus fewer adverse effects. Table 89.5 lists the total body clearance rates and hepatic extraction ratios of chemotherapeutic agents commonly used to treat hepatic malignancies.[132–137] Floxuridine, 5-fluorouracil, and doxorubicin have rapid total body clearance and high hepatic extraction ratios. Therefore, the intraarterial administration of these agents results in a substantial increase in drug exposure at the tumor site and a decrease in systemic exposure. In contrast, cisplatin and mitomycin C have relatively slow total body clearance and low hepatic extraction ratios. Thus intraarterial administration of these agents produces fewer changes in the tumor and less systemic drug exposure.

In the past, hepatic intraarterial chemotherapy was most commonly administered via a radiographically placed transcutaneous catheter inserted into the hepatic artery via the femoral or brachial artery. This can be successfully accomplished in approximately 80% of patients but is associated with several complications, including catheter migration, drug misperfusion, infection, catheter thrombosis, hepatic arterial thrombosis, and arterial emboli. To avoid catheter migration, transcutaneous catheters may be surgically placed and secured in the hepatic artery. Although this approach prevents catheter migration, the other difficulties of a transcutaneous catheter remain.

The advent of totally implantable ports and pumps in the early 1980s made the administration of long-term hepatic intraarterial chemotherapy feasible. Implanted ports are surgically placed into a subcutaneous pocket, and the catheter is inserted in a ligated gastroduodenal artery, with the tip at the hepatic artery. Implanted ports are most useful for the administration of bolus chemotherapy. Continuous-infusion chemotherapy via implanted ports requires the use of an external infusion device and is therefore technically cumbersome. Totally implantable pumps have made it feasible to administer infusional hepatic intraarterial chemotherapy in the outpatient setting (Fig. 89.2). Table 89.6 lists the characteristics of the various constant-flow and programmable implantable pumps. The pumps, like the ports, are placed into a subcutaneous pocket, and the catheter is inserted in a ligated gastroduodenal artery with the tip at the hepatic artery. All the devices have a drug chamber that is filled by percutaneously passing a needle into the inlet septum and injecting the next course of therapy. In addition, the pumps have a side port that may be used for bolus administration of chemotherapy.

Table 89.7 summarizes the clinical results with single-agent hepatic arterial chemotherapy in the treatment of HCC. Although the clinical trials are few and have small patient populations, the response rates are higher than those reported with intravenous chemotherapy. Single-agent intraarterial floxuridine produces a response in approximately 55% of patients.[117,138] Because of the high first-pass hepatic extraction of floxuridine, intraarterial infusions do not produce systemic toxicity. However, hepatobiliary toxicity may occur, including biliary sclerosis and cholecystitis. Biliary sclerosis is a potentially serious toxicity that results from floxuridine-induced inflammation and subsequent thrombosis of the peribiliary vascular plexus, which causes ischemic damage to the bile duct.[139] Serious biliary toxicity can usually be prevented with careful monitoring and appropriate dosage adjustments.

Table 89.5 ▪ Total Body Clearances and Hepatic Extractions of Drugs Administered by Hepatic Intraarterial Infusion

Drug	Total Body Clearance (mL/min)	Hepatic Extraction Ratio (%)	Reference
Floxuridine	4800	95	132
Doxorubicin	2000	50	133
5-Fluorouracil	1000	80	134,135
Cisplatin	600	24	136
Mitomycin C	575	10	137

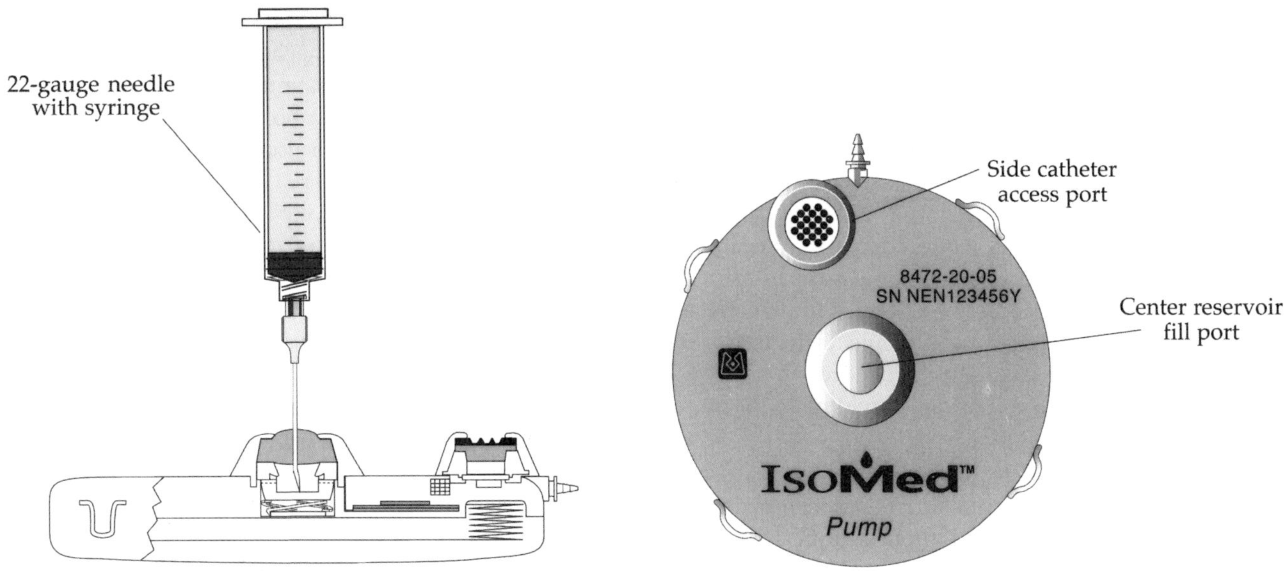

Figure 89.2. Medtronics (Minneapolis, Minn.) Isomed implantable pump *(left)* and cross section of implantable pump *(right)*.

Table 89.6 ▪ Implantable Pumps

Device	Diameter	Weight	Volume	Flow Rate	Side Port	Battery	Alarms	Cost
Constant Flow								
Arrow (Model 3000)	78 mm	137 g	30 mL	0.37–1.2 mL/day	No[a]	No	No	$4995
Arrow (Model 3000-16)	61 mm	98 g	16 mL	0.37–1.3 mL/day	No	No	No	$4995
Medtronic (IsoMed)	77 mm	113–120 g	20, 35, 60 mL	0.5–4.0 mL/day	Yes	No	No	–
Programmable								
Medtronic (SynchroMed)	7.0 cm	165–185 g	10, 18 mL	0.1–21.6 mL/day	Optional	Yes	Low volume Low Battery	$7485–8285

[a]Access into pump and hepatic intraarterial catheter achieved via the same central port using different needles.

Prophylactic cholecystectomy is recommended if repeated courses of hepatic intraarterial floxuridine are to be administered. Additionally, gastritis and gastroduodenal ulceration have occurred as a result of misperfusion of floxuridine into the stomach and duodenum. This can be prevented by surgically ligating the arterial feeders to the stomach arising from the hepatic artery. Although 5-fluorouracil has not been tested as a single agent in the United States, results from Japan indicate that it may have activity similar to floxuridine when administered intraarterially for HCC.[140] Doxorubicin also appears to have enhanced activity when infused intraarterially, with response rates of 40 to 50%.[103,140–144] Mitomycin C has also been reported to have significant efficacy when administered intraarterially.[32] However, detailed response data are not available. Finally, hepatic intraarterial cisplatin, mitoxantrone, epirubicin, and ifosfamide have produced some responses in patients with HCC.[145–151]

High response rates have also been reported with combination intraarterial chemotherapy. Responses were observed in 8 of 15 (53%) patients receiving intraarterial mitomycin C, 5-fluorouracil, vinblastine, vincristine, and doxorubicin;[152] 8 of 12 (67%) patients receiving floxuridine, doxorubicin, and mitomycin C;[153] and 8 of 13 (61%) patients receiving floxuridine, leucovorin, doxorubicin, and cisplatin.[154] It remains unclear whether combination intraarterial chemotherapy is superior to single-agent intraarterial chemotherapy.

Intraarterial Lipiodol Chemotherapy

Lipiodol is an ethyl ester of the fatty acid of poppyseed oil, containing 38% iodine by weight; it is used as lymphangiogram dye. After intraarterial injection, Lipiodol concentrates in HCC. As a result of this finding, lipophilic chemotherapeutic agents have been administered intraarterially in conjunction with Lipiodol in an attempt to facilitate the delivery of the chemotherapeutic agent into the tumor cell. The drugs most commonly combined with Lipiodol are doxorubicin and styrene-maleic acid–neocarzinostatin (SMANCS). SMANCS is a conjugation of neocarzinostatin, a proteinaceous antitumor antibiotic, and copolystyrene-maleic acid, a drug used to treat hepatic malignancies in Asia. Studies with intraarterial Lipiodol and doxorubicin or SMANCS have reported responses in 30 to 40% of patients.[155] In a recent study, intraarterial Lipiodol and SMANCS produced an overall response rate of 40% (27% complete response rate) in 30 HCC patients.[156] A randomized study comparing hepatic intraarterial cisplatin and doxorubicin to hepatic intraarterial cisplatin, doxorubicin, and Lipiodol failed to demonstrate an advantage for the Lipiodol-containing regimen.[157] Thus further comparative studies are needed to ascertain whether Lipiodol has a role in the management of HCC.

Hepatic Artery Ligation

Surgical ligation of the hepatic artery has been performed in patients who have HCC without significant extrahepatic involvement in an attempt to produce tumor necrosis secondary to ischemia. This approach has been used as a single modality and in combination with chemotherapy.[158,159] Responses with hepatic arterial ligation are often transient because extrahepatic collateral arteries develop rapidly, reperfusing the tumor.[160] The procedure is generally well tolerated, with hepatic pain, fever, and elevated hepatic enzymes being the most prevalent adverse events. Rarely, hepatic artery ligation causes hepatic necrosis, resulting in death. Patients with severely compromised hepatic function or portal vein thrombosis should not undergo this procedure. Although frequently employed in the past, hepatic artery ligation is rarely used today because occlusion of the hepatic artery can be accomplished radiographically (i.e., embolization), and permanent loss of the hepatic artery precludes its use for other liver-directed treatments, such as intraarterial chemotherapy or chemoembolization. Ligation of the hepatic artery has also been used to stop intraabdominal bleeding from a ruptured HCC,[161] but this can also be accomplished angiographically with coiling or embolization;[162] thus it is rarely employed for this purpose.

Table 89.7 ▪ Results of Single-Agent Intraarterial Chemotherapy for Hepatocellular Carcinoma

Drug	Number of Patients	Responses	Response Rates (%)	Reference
Floxuridine	16	9	56	117
	28	15	54	138
	44	**24**	**55**	
Fluorouracil	9	2	22	140
Doxorubicin	10	4	40	113
	13	6	46	141
	2	1	50	142
	6	3	50	143
	19	8	42	144
	19	8	42	140
	69	**30**	**44**	
Cisplatin	16	3	19	145
	33	18	55	146
	10	4	40	147
	59	**25**	**42**	
Mitoxantrone	22	6	27	148
	23	6	26	149
	45	**12**	**27**	
Epirubicin	53	8	15	150
Ifosfamide	16	6	38	151

Embolization and Chemoembolization

Two related modalities, embolization and chemoembolization, are frequently used to treat unresectable but liver-predominant HCC. Embolization of HCC involves radiographic placement of a percutaneous catheter into the hepatic artery and injection of an embolizing substance that occludes the arterial blood flow at the tumor capillary level, thus producing tumor ischemia. Embolizing substances that have been administered include Angiostat (5 to 75 U) (Target Therapeutics, Los Angeles, CA); Ethibloc (Ethicon, Hamburg, West Germany); Gelfoam cubes (1 to 3 mm) (Pharmacia and Upjohn, Kalamazoo, MI); Ivalon particles (150 to 500 U) (Unipoint Lab, High Point, NC); and autologous blood clot. Gelfoam powder (40 to 60 U) (Pharmacia and Upjohn, Kalamazoo, MI) has also been used, but this substance is no longer commercially available in the United States. The various embolizing substances achieve different levels and durations of arterial blockade; the optimal embolizing substance is yet to be determined. Embolization is preferred over hepatic artery ligation because it is nonsurgical and associated with fewer collateral arteries. In one study of HCC patients who had failed hepatic arterial chemotherapy, 6 of 9 patients responded to embolization.[163] In Japan, 120 patients with HCC were treated with Gelfoam embolization, and 90% responded with 1-, 2-, and 3-year survival rates of 44, 29, and 15%, respectively.[164]

Chemoembolization combines the tumor ischemia produced by embolization with prolonged high intratumoral concentrations of chemotherapy. This is accomplished by infusing embolizing microspheres that contain chemotherapeutic agents or a mixture of concentrated chemotherapy with an embolizing substance into the hepatic artery. In two studies, biodegradable albumin microspheres containing mitomycin C were used to embolize patients with HCC, and responses were observed in 7 of 7 (100%) patients and 15 of 20 (75%) patients.[165,166] In another study, chemoembolization with Gelfoam and doxorubicin, mitomycin C, and cisplatin produced responses in 12 of 50 (24%) patients and liquefaction necrosis in 70% of patients.[167] Additional studies employing mitoxantrone, epirubicin, doxorubicin, and Lipiodol chemoembolization have obtained similar response rates.[168,169] In a study comparing cisplatin chemoembolization to supportive care, chemoembolization reduced tumor size and α-fetoprotein levels but did not affect overall survival.[170]

Both embolization and chemoembolization are generally well tolerated, with liver pain, fever, and elevated liver function enzymes being the most prevalent adverse events.

Table 89.8 ▪ Prognostic Variables in Patients with Hepatocellular Carcinoma

Factor	Favorable	Unfavorable
Resectability	Yes	No
Liver function	Normal LFTs Bilirubin ≤36 μmol/L Normal albumin Normal PT, PTT No ascites No portal hypertension	Abnormal LFTs Bilirubin >36 μmol/L Hypoalbuminemia Abnormal PT, PTT Ascites Portal hypertension
Metastases	No	Yes
Performance status	Ambulatory	Bedridden
Age	≤45 years	>45 years
Sex	Female	Male
Country	North American	African, Asian
Histology	Fribrolamellar variant Clear cell variant	Remaining histologies
Tumor encapsulation	Encapsulated tumor	Nonencapsulated tumor
Cirrhosis	No	Yes

Rare cases of acute renal failure, necrosis of the bile ducts or gallbladder, and hemoperitoneum have been reported. Additionally, if the embolizing substance is inadvertently injected into an area other than the tumor capillary bed, necrosis of that region may result.

PROGNOSIS

HCC is an aggressive malignancy that usually carries a grave prognosis. The reported median survival in untreated patients from the time of diagnosis varies from 1 to 6 months. Several factors are of prognostic importance (Table 89.8).[171] The most important of these is the resectability of the tumor. Surgical removal offers the only potential cure for HCC.

A patient's performance status is of prognostic significance, with ambulatory patients surviving longer than those who are bedridden. The percentage of liver involved with tumor at the time of presentation is inversely related to the duration of survival. Additionally, the location of tumors within the liver can alter outcome. Patients with tumor near the porta hepatis may deteriorate rapidly because a small increase in tumor volume may cause compression of the inferior vena cava, portal vein, hepatic artery, and bile duct leading to subsequent ascites, edema, and jaundice.

The patient's baseline liver function is also important, with those patients having normal liver function tests, bilirubin, albumin, and PT and PTT having the best prognosis. Patients with ascites, edema, or esophageal varices have a poorer prognosis. Patients having the fibrolamellar or clear cell variants of HCC and those with encapsulated tumors generally survive longer. Although metastatic disease itself rarely determines outcome, its presence suggests a more aggressive tumor and is associated with a shorter survival.

Other important prognostic factors include the patient's age, sex, country of origin, and the presence or absence of cirrhosis. Patients 45 years of age or younger have a better prognosis than those over 45, and female patients survive longer than their male counterparts. Patients with otherwise normal livers survive longer and respond better to chemotherapy than those with cirrhosis.

PREVENTION

Because very few patients with HCC are cured, prevention of HCC is the most appealing approach to decrease the incidence of HCC.[172] As previously discussed, hepatitis B appears to be a major etiologic cause of HCC. Vertical transmission from mother to infant is the most common method of hepatitis B transmission in endemic areas. Vaccination of newborns with a hepatitis B vaccine can prevent vertical transmission and thus eliminate the predisposition for subsequently developing HCC.[173] Pilot data from Shanghai and Gambia have demonstrated that such a strategy is effective in preventing transmission of hepatitis B in endemic areas.[174,175] In addition, a universal hepatitis B vaccination program in Taiwan demonstrated a significant decline in the incidence of HCC.[176] A cost-benefit analysis of newborn vaccination has shown that it is justifiable even in areas of intermediate endemicity.[177] It is estimated that worldwide vaccination against hepatitis B could reduce the incidence of HCC by up to 60%.[172] In addition, the risk of patients with chronic active hepatitis B developing hepatocellular carcinoma may be reduced by the administration of α-interferon.[178] Other factors that may reduce the incidence of HCC include reducing alcohol intake, reducing exposure to aflatoxin B1, and decreasing the incidence of hepatitis C infection.[179]

Secondary Malignant Liver Tumors

Metastases to the liver may occur from virtually any malignancy. Of all organs in the body, the liver is the most common site of blood-borne metastases. In an autopsy series of 9497 cancer patients, 8055 (84.8%) had metastatic disease, and 4444 (46.8%) had liver metastases.[180] Liver metastases may be the only site of metastatic disease or part of a more widely metastatic process. Hepatic metastases occur most frequently in patients with primary tumors originating in organs drained by the portal vein, including tumors of the stomach, small intestine, colon, pancreas, gallbladder, and extrahepatic biliary tract. However, some malignancies such as breast cancer, lymphomas, testicular cancer, and ocular melanoma, which arise in organs having nonportal sources of venous drainage, are also associated with a high incidence of liver metastases.

The factors contributing to the high incidence of liver metastases in cancer patients are complex and not fully understood. On an ultrastructural level, the sinusoidal fenestrations of the liver may be more permeable to metastatic cells than the capillary endothelium of other organs. Further, the liver has relatively little connective tissue, which in other organs may act as a physical barrier to metastatic cells. From a physiologic standpoint, the liver, as the organ that filters the blood, may inherently be more efficient than other organs at removing metastatic cells from the blood. Last, in patients with tumors originating in organs drained by the portal circulation, the liver is the first organ encountered by the metastatic cells after their release into the bloodstream and thus is the organ presented with the highest burden of metastatic cells. The remainder of the discussion on liver metastases will focus on colorectal cancer because it is the most common tumor that metastasizes to the liver.

Colorectal Cancer Metastatic to the Liver

DEFINITION

Colorectal cancer affects about 1 person out of every 20 in the United States and most Westernized countries. If diagnosed early, colorectal cancer has a high cure rate. However, many patients have metastatic disease at diagnosis or subsequently develop metastatic disease. The most common site of metastases from colorectal cancer is liver.

TREATMENT GOALS: COLORECTAL CANCER METASTATIC TO THE LIVER

- For patients with resectable disease confined to the liver, attempt to cure patients by surgical removal.
- For patients with incurable extensive hepatic involvement and extrahepatic involvement, try to produce a response; this is intended to result in improved survival without significantly impairing the patient's quality of life.
- Treat patients with unresectable disease confined to the liver with hepatic intraarterial chemotherapy or systemic chemotherapy.
- Limit treatment to systemic chemotherapy for patients with significant extrahepatic involvement.

EPIDEMIOLOGY

Approximately 129,400 new cases were diagnosed in 1999, and approximately 40% of all patients diagnosed with colorectal cancer die of metastatic disease to their liver.[20] At the time of diagnosis, approximately 15 to 25% of these patients have metastatic disease in the liver, and another 25% of patients develop metastasis later during the course of disease. The liver is the most common site of metastatic involvement, followed by the lung.

CLINICAL PRESENTATION AND DIAGNOSIS

Signs and Symptoms

Often liver metastases are diagnosed incidentally during surgery in patients without antecedent signs or symptoms suggestive of hepatic involvement or during routine follow-up. The most common complaints in patients with symptomatic liver metastases include abdominal pain, abdominal distension, anorexia, weight loss, fatigue, jaundice, and unexplained fever.

Diagnosis

The diagnosis of a patient suspected of having liver metastases generally proceeds from the physical examination, to laboratory tests, to radiographic imaging, and then to tissue biopsy. The most common finding on physical examination is hepatomegaly. In patients with advanced hepatic metastases, the tumor may occlude the bile duct, portal vein, or inferior vena cava, resulting in jaundice, portal hypertension (ascites, esophageal varices), or lower extremity edema, respectively. In some cases, patients with primary colorectal cancer may have synchronous liver metastases; in other cases, the liver metastases may appear months to years after the initial diagnosis of the primary tumor.

Approximately 60% of patients with hepatic metastases have elevated levels of alanine aminotransferase (ALT), aspartate aminotransferase (AST), lactic dehydrogenase (LDH), or alkaline phosphatase (AP).[181] In addition, serum bilirubin levels are often elevated in patients with advanced hepatic metastases. The greater the extent of liver involvement, the more likely these tests will be elevated. No single liver enzyme test is superior to the others for detecting liver metastases. Although hepatic enzyme elevations are somewhat useful in identifying patients who may have liver metastases, elevations can occur in patients without liver metastases, and thus these tests lack specificity.

Another laboratory test that is helpful in diagnosing colorectal cancer is the carcinoembryonic antigen (CEA) level. CEA is a glycoprotein that is produced in small amounts by normal columnar epithelial cells (normal value less than 4 ng/mL). CEA is elevated in 60 to 80% of patients with colorectal cancer. The CEA level tends to fall with tumor regression and to rise with disease progression.

Although colorectal cancer at any site may produce CEA, levels greater than 20 ng/mL are most frequently associated with liver metastases.[182,183] Approximately 70% of patients with colorectal cancer metastatic to the liver have elevated CEA levels. However, because CEA is elevated in a variety of other malignant and nonmalignant conditions, it lacks diagnostic specificity. Thus its major role lies in screening patients for recurrent disease and monitoring patients known to have metastases who are receiving treatment.

Several radiographic techniques are helpful in diagnosing liver metastases.[184,185] Computed tomography and magnetic resonance imaging are the two preferred radiographic techniques for detecting liver metastases. These methods are more expensive than others, but they are more able to accurately detect small lesions, are more reproducible, and allow for simultaneous imaging of the remainder of the abdomen. Ultrasound is inexpensive and does not expose patients to radiation, but intestinal gas, excessive fat, and overlying ribs can interfere with imaging. Thus small lesions may go undetected. Radionuclide liver-spleen scanning using technetium sulfur colloid is simple to perform but is associated with high false-positive and false-negative results, is unable to image extrahepatic tumor, and often does not detect lesions smaller than 2 cm. Gamma camera imaging following the administration of indium-111 satumomab pendetide can be used in addition to other radiographic techniques to assist in the detection of colorectal cancer metastatic to the liver.[186]

When liver-associated laboratory tests and radiographic techniques are used together, the combined sensitivity in diagnosing liver metastases increases to 90%, whereas alone, the sensitivities are 60 and 80%, respectively.[187]

Tissue biopsy in order to confirm the presence of liver metastases is usually unnecessary in colorectal cancer patients because data from the patient's history, physical examination, laboratory tests, and radiographic studies are usually sufficient to make the diagnosis. If a tissue specimen is required to confirm the diagnosis, it may be obtained by percutaneous biopsy, peritoneoscopy with needle-directed biopsy, or open biopsy at laparotomy.

PSYCHOSOCIAL ASPECTS

Patients with synchronous liver metastases must cope with the diagnosis and treatment of their primary colorectal cancer, as well as their liver metastases. Typically, treatment of the primary tumor involves surgical resection of the tumor in the colon or rectum. If a colostomy is performed, this represents an additional psychologic issue for the patient. The liver metastases may be treated with surgery, chemotherapy, or both. After surgery, patients must cope with their prognosis. The prognosis can range from a high likelihood of cure to a projected survival of only a few months.

Patients who develop metachronous liver metastases must cope with the recurrence of their disease. In addition, as with patients who have synchronous metastases, they must cope with the surgical or medical treatment being undertaken, as well as their prognosis.

TREATMENT

Several modalities have been employed either alone or in combination in the treatment of colorectal cancer metastatic to the liver, including surgical resection, radiotherapy, hepatic arterial ligation, intravenous chemotherapy, hepatic intraarterial chemotherapy, cryotherapy, and gene therapy. The following is a discussion of the results obtained with these treatments.

Surgical Resection

Surgical resection offers a potential cure for patients with colorectal cancer metastatic to the liver, and thus should be performed whenever removal of all the apparent metastatic disease can be safely accomplished. Evidence of extrahepatic disease and more than four hepatic lesions are contraindications to resection; thus resection is feasible in only approximately 20% of patients. The results with surgical resection are summarized in Table 89.9.[188–208] The operative mortality rate in these studies ranged from 0 to 8%. The operative mortality rate is highest in patients who undergo extensive resections and those with a significant comorbid illness. The 5-year survival rate ranged between 18 and 45%. Patients with solitary metastases, those without extrahepatic disease, those who are female, those with synchronous metastases (compared with those who develop metachronous metastases), those with clear margins of resection, and those whose primary originated in the colon (compared with the rectum) survive longer after resection.

Intraoperative ultrasound with palpation is commonly used in an attempt to identify and resect any disease that was not apparent on preoperative radiographic imaging. In one study, detection of hepatic lesions by intraoperative ultrasound had a 97% accuracy rate compared with a 78% accuracy rate when preoperative radiographic imaging, surgical inspection, and palpation were used.[187] Additionally, radioimmunoguided surgery has been employed in an attempt to identify and resect inapparent hepatic tumor. The impact of intraoperative ultrasound and radioimmunoguided surgery on survival after resection is yet to be determined. Adjuvant chemotherapy is not routinely used after the surgical removal of hepatic metastases from colorectal cancer, but results from a pilot study suggest that it may be beneficial.[209]

Radiotherapy

External beam radiation plays a limited role in the management of liver metastases from colorectal cancer because of the liver's inherent radiosensitivity. As mentioned earlier, lifetime doses of greater than 3000 rads are associated with a high incidence of radiation hepatitis.[85] Fractionated doses of 1800 to 2400 rads can provide pain

Table 89.9 ▪ Results of Surgical Resection for Colorectal Cancer Metastatic to the Liver

Author/Year	Number of Patients	Operative Mortality (%)	Survival 3 year	Survival 5 year	Reference
Hughes/1989	800	–	–	32	188
Adloff/1990	55	2	–	20	189
Doci/1991	100	5.0	–	30	190
Petrelli/1991	62	8	–	28	191
Nakamura/1992	31	3	–	45	192
Rosen/1992	280	4.0	47	25	193
van Ooijen/1992	118	7.6	–	21	194
Gayowski/1994	204		43	32	195
Fuhrman/1995	107	2.8	–	44	196
Jatzko/1995	66	4.5	–	30	197
Scheele/1995	434	4.4	45	33	198
Scott/1995	49	4	58	18	199
Nordlinger/1996	1568	2	44	28	200
Marmorale/1996	73	1.4	–	27	201
Fong/1997	456	2.8	59	38	202
Jenkins/1997	131	3.8	42	25	203
Rees/1997	107	0.7	47	30	204
Shirabe/1997	31		42	39	205
Taylor/1997	123	0	–	34	206
Elias/1998	136	1.5	–	28	207
Ohlsson/1998	111	3.6	37	25	208

relief for patients with symptomatic metastases. However, external beam radiotherapy does not prolong survival.[210] Radiotherapy has been used in combination with chemotherapy, although it is unclear whether the outcome is superior to that obtained with chemotherapy alone.[211]

Cryotherapy

Cryotherapy is another treatment option for patients with colorectal cancer metastatic to the liver. In various studies, 20 to 51% of patients were alive without evidence of disease at median follow-ups of 14 to 26 months after cryotherapy.[212] In one study, 136 patients with unresectable disease who underwent cryosurgery had a median survival of 30 months.[213] In a trial in which cryotherapy plus postoperative regional chemotherapy was used to treat residual disease after resection in 20 patients, the median survival was 32 months.[214]

Hepatic Arterial Ligation

As with HCC, ligation of the hepatic artery has been performed in patients with liver metastases from colorectal cancer in an attempt to produce tumor necrosis secondary to ischemia.[215] Symptomatic improvement is observed in some patients after hepatic arterial ligation, but it is usually transient. In addition, ligation of the hepatic artery prevents its future use for other liver-directed therapies, such as intraarterial chemotherapy.

Intravenous Chemotherapy

Systemic chemotherapy is of limited benefit in the treatment of patients with colorectal cancer metastatic to the liver.[216] The agents possessing activity include 5-fluorouracil, irinotecan, mitomycin C, and lomustine (CCNU). Intravenous 5-fluorouracil produces partial responses in approximately 15 to 20% of patients. Several dosage schedules have been employed, but none is significantly superior to the others.[217] The most common side effects of intravenous 5-fluorouracil are nausea, vomiting, stomatitis, and myelosuppression. The cytotoxicity of 5-fluorouracil may be biochemically enhanced by the administration of leucovorin. Seven prospective randomized studies comparing 5-fluorouracil to 5-fluorouracil plus leucovorin have been conducted.[218–224] Six of the studies demonstrated a higher response rate, and two of the studies showed a survival advantage for 5-fluorouracil plus leucovorin. As a result, 5-fluorouracil plus leucovorin has become the standard first-line systemic chemotherapy regimen. Other agents, such as phosphonoacetyl-L-aspartic acid (PALA) and α-interferon, have also been given with 5-fluorouracil in an attempt to enhance its activity, but none has improved on the results achieved with 5-fluorouracil and leucovorin.

Irinotecan, a camptothecin analog, has produced response rates of 19 to 32% in patients with previously untreated colorectal cancer and 13 to 25% in patients with previously treated disease.[225–230] In a phase III trial comparing irinotecan to infusional 5-fluorouracil, irinotecan produced an overall survival that was 1.4 times greater than 5-fluorouracil.[231] The principal side effect of this agent is diarrhea; thus patients receiving this agent must adhere to a strict antidiarrheal regimen. Mitomycin C administered in doses of 10 to 15 mg/m^2 every 6 to 8 weeks also produces partial responses in approximately 15 to 20% of patients. However, cumulative myelosuppression and fatigue make continued administration difficult;[216] thus mitomycin C is usually reserved for patients who have failed 5-fluorouracil and irinotecan. Oral CCNU has limited activity against colorectal cancer and is typically reserved as the last treatment option. Its primary toxicity is delayed myelosuppression.

Other agents with promising activity that are undergoing investigation for the treatment of colorectal cancer include oxaliplatin, capecitabine, and raltitrexed. Single-agent oxaliplatin, a third-generation platinum derivative, has demonstrated activity against 5-fluorouracil refractory colorectal cancer.[232] In addition, in a randomized study, oxaliplatin, 5-fluorouracil, and leucovorin resulted in a higher response rate than 5-fluorouracil and leucovorin (57 versus 26%).[233] In phase II studies, capecitabine, an orally administered prodrug of 5-fluorouracil, has produced response rates comparable to 5-fluororuracil alone.[234–238] In three phase III studies, raltitrexed, a novel thymidylate synthase inhibitor, dosed once every 3 weeks, produced response rates comparable to 5-fluorouracil.[239–241]

Table 89.10 ▪ Results of Single-Agent Intraarterial Chemotherapy for Colorectal Cancer Metastatic to the Liver

Drug	Number of Patients	Response Rates (%)	Median Survival (months)	Reference
Floxuridine	81	88	26	242
	93	80	20	243
	77	83	13	244
	17	29	13	245
	24	73	22	246
	41	37	–	247
	14	36	–	248
	25	40	15	249
5-Fluorouracil	52	67	–	252
	369	55	–	253
	24	50	9	254
	30	34	10	255
	30	57	11.9	256

Hepatic Intraarterial Chemotherapy

Hepatic intraarterial chemotherapy has been widely used in the treatment of colorectal cancer metastatic to the liver. (For a complete discussion of the rationale of intraarterial chemotherapy, see Intraarterial Chemotherapy earlier in this chapter.) Table 89.10 summarizes the phase II results with single-agent hepatic intraarterial chemotherapy. The most commonly administered agent is floxuridine, in part because it is available in a convenient formulation for usage in the implantable pump. It has produced partial responses ranging from 29 to 88% and median survivals ranging from 13 to 26 months.[242–249] In an attempt to further augment the activity of intraarterial floxuridine, the addition of intraarterial leucovorin was studied, but the regimen produced prohibitive hepatobiliary toxicity.[250] A phase II study of intraarterial floxuridine, leucovorin, and dexamethasone demonstrated that the addition of dexamethasone reduced the biliary sclerosis.[251] 5-Fluorouracil has also been administered by hepatic intraarterial infusion with response rates ranging from 34 to 67% and median survival of 9 to 12 months.[252–256] The lower solubility of 5-fluorouracil (relative to floxuridine) prevents its use in the implantable pump, thus an external pump and a radiographically placed percutaneous catheter are required to administer the drug by continuous infusion.

To improve on the results obtained with single-agent intraarterial chemotherapy, various combination regimens have been investigated (Table 89.11). Unfortunately, the results have been similar to those obtained with single-agent intraarterial therapy, with the response rates ranging from 20 to 83% and the median survival times ranging from 8 to 22 months.[257–268] However, one combination regimen using alternating floxuridine and 5-fluorouracil may offer an advantage over other regimens since it appears to be associated with fewer side effects.[259]

Six randomized trials have been conducted comparing hepatic intraarterial floxuridine with systemic chemotherapy or no treatment (Table 89.12).[269–274] All studies reported a significantly higher response rate in the patients treated with intraarterial therapy, and two of the studies reported a survival benefit with intraarterial chemotherapy.[273,274] The two largest studies,[269,270] neither of which demonstrated a survival advantage for intraarterial therapy, allowed patients on the intravenous arm to receive intraarterial therapy at the time of hepatic tumor progression, thus confounding the survival analyses. A meta-analysis of the data from these six trials revealed that hepatic intraarterial chemotherapy produced a modest survival advantage when compared with intravenous chemotherapy.[275]

Gene Therapy

Recently, hepatic intraarterial p53 gene therapy has been investigated for the treatment of colorectal cancer metastatic to the liver. Venook and colleagues[276] administered a single dose of recombinant adenovirus encoding the human wild-type p53 gene by hepatic intraarterial infusion to 16 patients with colorectal cancer metastatic to the liver whose tumor had a mutant p53 gene. Although the single-dose treatment was well tolerated, with fevers being the principal toxicity, no responses were observed. The results of future studies will determine whether gene

Table 89.11 ▪ Results of Combination Intraarterial Chemotherapy for Colorectal Cancer Metastatic to the Liver

Drug	Number of Patients	Response Rates (%)	Median Survival (months)	Reference
Floxuridine and 5-fluorouracil	52	81	—	257
	48	54	—	258
	64	50	22	259
Floxuridine and mitomycin C	12	83	15	260
	40	20	14	261
Floxuridine and dichloromethotrexate	13	69	20	261
5-Fluorouracil and mitomycin C	20	55	8	262
	30	50	11	263
Floxuridine and mitomycin C	24	42	11	264
Floxuridine and mitomycin C and carmustine	29	52	12	265
Floxuridine and cisplatin and mitomycin C	36	70	12	266
5-Fluorouracil and doxorubicin and mitomycin C	23	35	22	267
Floxuridine and mitomycin C and carmustine	46	47	19	268

Table 89.12 ▪ Results of Randomized Trials Comparing Intravenous to Hepatic Intraarterial Chemotherapy for Colorectal Cancer Metastatic to the Liver

Author/Year	Number of Patients	Response Rate (%)		Survival (months)		Reference
		IV	IA	IV	IA	
Kemeny/1986	99	20	50	12	17	269
Hohn/1989	143	10	42	16	16.5	270
Chang/1987	64	17	62	11	16	271
Martin/1990	69	21	48	10.5	12.6	272
Rougier/1992	166	9	43	11	15	273
Allen-Mersh/1994	100	—	—	6.6	13.5	274

therapy will ultimately play a role in the treatment of colorectal cancer metastatic to the liver.

PROGNOSIS

In general, colorectal cancer metastatic to the liver portends a poor prognosis. Because of this, studies have been done to identify prognostic factors that may further define indications for resection. Although data remain inconclusive, regional lymph node involvement, CEA level, tumor size and location, and positive liver resection margins are consistent with poor outcome.[277–280] The most important prognostic factor by far is the resectability of the hepatic metastases. Surgical resection is the only potentially curative modality for liver metastases and should be performed whenever possible. The most important prognostic factor in patients with unresectable tumor is the extent of hepatic involvement.[281] The survival in untreated patients ranges from 2 to 22 months (median of 8 to 10 months); those patients who have the smallest amount of tumor survive the longest. Another important factor is the degree of histologic differentiation. Patients with well-differentiated tumors survive longer than those with poorly differentiated tumors.[282] In addition, patients with a poor performance status, significant weight loss, low albumin level, ascites, elevated hepatic enzymes, or bilirubin level have a shortened survival.

KEY POINTS

- Liver tumors are a diverse group of benign and malignant tumors comprising primary tumors, which arise from the hepatobiliary system, and secondary tumors, which metastasize to the liver from neoplasms elsewhere in the body.
- The most prevalent primary malignancy of the liver is hepatocellular carcinoma, also referred to as hepatoma, and the most common cause of hepatic metastases is colorectal cancer.
- Complete surgical removal by resection or, for primary malignant tumors, liver transplantation offers a potential for cure of malignant liver tumors and should be performed whenever feasible.

- Unfortunately, surgical removal is feasible in only approximately 10 to 15% of patients, and of those patients, only approximately 30% are cured.
- Cryosurgery, radiofrequency ablation, and percutaneous alcohol injection are three modalities that are useful in patients with potentially resectable disease who are not candidates for surgical removal because of underlying liver disease, such as cirrhosis.
- Several therapies have been used to treat patients with unresectable malignant liver tumors. Radiotherapy has been used, but it is of limited benefit because of the inherent intolerance of the normal hepatic parenchyma to radiation. Systemic chemotherapy has been used, but it produces responses in only 15 to 35% of patients.
- In patients who have liver-predominant disease, more encouraging results have been obtained with liver-directed therapies such as hepatic intraarterial chemotherapy with or without Lipiodol and chemoembolization.
- Further research is required to develop more efficacious therapies for liver tumors.

Hepatocellular Carcinoma

- HCC is the most common primary malignant tumor of the liver in adults.
- It is relatively uncommon in the United States, but is very prevalent in Asia, sub-Saharan Africa, and the South Pacific Islands.
- HCC is frequently associated with preexisting liver disease. Chronic active hepatitis B infection is the most important predisposing factor worldwide. In addition, hepatitis C infection, exposure to aflatoxin B1 or sex hormones, and certain inherited metabolic disorders predispose patients to developing HCC.
- Whenever feasible, the goal of therapy should be to cure the patient by surgical removal or a treatment modality that causes local tumor necrosis, such as cryotherapy.
- When cure is not feasible, either because of extensive hepatic involvement or the presence of extrahepatic metastases, the goal of treatment should be to treat those patients desiring therapy with a modality that has a reasonable chance of producing a response while maintaining the patient's quality of life. Patients with disease confined to the liver may be treated with either liver-directed therapies, such as chemoembolization or hepatic intraarterial chemotherapy, or systemic chemotherapy. Patients with significant extrahepatic disease may be treated with systemic chemotherapy.

Colorectal Cancer Metastatic to the Liver

- Colorectal cancer is the most common tumor that metastasizes to the liver.
- Whenever feasible, the goal of therapy should be to cure the patient by surgical removal or a treatment modality that causes local tumor necrosis, such as cryotherapy.
- When cure is not feasible, either because of extensive hepatic involvement or the presence of extrahepatic metastases, the goal of treatment should be to treat those patients desiring therapy with a modality that has a reasonable chance of producing a response while maintaining the patient's quality of life. Patients with disease confined to the liver may be treated with hepatic intraarterial chemotherapy or systemic chemotherapy. Patients with significant extrahepatic disease may be treated with systemic chemotherapy.

REFERENCES

1. Bierman HR, Byron RL Jr, Kelly LH, et al. Studies on the blood supply of tumors in man: III. Vascular patterns of the liver by hepatic arteriography in vivo. JNCI 12:107–227, 1951.
2. Yohannan MD, Abdulla AM, Patel PJ. Neonatal hepatic hemangioendothelioma: presentation with jaundice and microangiopathic hemolytic anemia. Eur J Pediatr 149:804–805, 1990.
3. Samuel M, Spitz L. Infantile hepatic hemangioendothelioma: the role of surgery. J Pediatr Surg 30:1425–1429, 1995.
4. Hobbs KE. Hepatic hemangiomas. World J Surg 14:468–471, 1990.
5. Lise M, Feltrin G, Da Pian PP, et al. Giant cavernous hemangiomas: diagnosis and surgical strategies. World J Surg 16(3):516–520, 1992.
6. Nichols FC, van Heerden JA, Weiland LH. Benign liver tumors. Surg Clin North Am 69:297–314, 1989.
7. Gordon SC, Reddy KR, Livingstone AS, et al. Resolution of a contraceptive steroid-induced hepatic adenoma with subsequent evolution into hepatocellular carcinoma. Ann Intern Med 105:547–549, 1986.
8. Wanless JR, Mawdsley C, Adams R. On the pathogenesis of focal nodular hyperplasia of the liver. Hepatology, 5:1194–1200, 1985.
9. Landen S, Siriser F, Bardoxoglou E, et al. Focal nodular hyperplasia of the liver. A retrospective review of 20 patients managed surgically. Acta Chir Belg 93(3):94–97, 1993.
10. Seo T, Ando H, Watonabe Y, et al. Treatment of hepatoblastoma: less extensive hepatic resection after effective preoperative chemotherapy with cisplatin and adriamycin. Surgery 123:407–414, 1998.
11. Evans AE, Land VJ, Newton WA, et al. Combination chemotherapy (vincristine, Adriamycin, cyclophosphamide, 5-fluorouracil) in the treatment of children with hepatoblastoma. Cancer 50:821–826, 1982.
12. Superina R, Bilik R. Results of liver transplantation in children with unresectable liver tumors. J Pediatr Surg 31:835–839, 1996.
13. Penn I. Hepatic transplantation for primary and metastatic cancer of the liver. Surgery 110:726–735, 1991.
14. Harvey JH, Smith FP, Schein PS. 5-Fluorouracil, mitomycin, and doxorubicin (FAM) in carcinoma of the biliary tract. J Clin Oncol 2:1245–1248, 1984.
15. Smith GW, Bukowski RM, Hewlett JS, et al. Hepatic artery infusion of 5-fluorouracil and mitomycin C in cholangiocarcinoma and gallbladder carcinoma. Cancer 54:1513–1516, 1984.
16. Locker GY, Doroshow JG, Zwelling LA, et al. The clinical features of hepatic angiosarcoma: a report of four cases and a review of the English literature. Medicine 58:48–64, 1979.
17. Azodo MV, Gutierrez OH, Greer T. Thorotrast-induced ruptured hepatic angiosarcoma. Abdom Imaging 18:78–81, 1993.
18. Dean PJ, Haggett RC, O'Hara CJ. Malignant epithelioid hemangioendothelioma of the liver in young women. Relationship to oral contraceptive use. Am J Surg Pathol 9:695–704, 1985.
19. Walker NI, Horn MJ, Strong RW, et al. Undifferentiated (embryonal) sarcoma of the liver. Pathologic findings and long-term survival after complete surgical resection. Cancer 69:52–59, 1992.
20. Landis Sh, Murray T, Bolden S, et al. Cancer statistics: 1999. CA Cancer J Clin 49:8–33, 1999.
21. Moertel CG. The liver. In: Holland JF, Frei E III, eds. Cancer medicine. Philadelphia: Lea & Febiger, 1973:1541–1547.
22. Popper G, Gerber MA, Thung SN. The relation of hepatocellular carcinoma to infection with hepatitis B and related viruses in man and animals. Hepatology 2:1S–9S, 1982.
23. Zala G, Havelka J, Altorfer J, et al. Hepatitis C and hepatoma. Schweiz Med Wochenschr 122:194–197, 1992.

24. Hassan F, Jeffers LJ, De Medina M, et al. Hepatitis C–associated hepatocellular carcinoma. Hepatology 12:589–591, 1990.
25. Kiyosawa K, Sodeyama T, Tanaka E, et al. Interrelationship of blood transfusion, non-A non-B hepatitis and hepatocellular carcinoma: analysis by detection of antibody to hepatitis C virus. Hepatology 12:671–675, 1990.
26. Gerbes AL, Caselmann WH. Point mutations of the p53 gene, human hepatocellular carcinoma and aflatoxins. J Hepatol 19:312–315, 1993.
27. Palmer JR, Rosenberg L, Kaufmann DW, et al. Oral contraceptive use and liver cancer. Am J Epidemiol 130:878–882, 1989.
28. Farrell GC, Uren RF, Perkins RW, et al. Androgen induced hepatoma. Lancet 1:430–431, 1975.
29. Okuda K, Musha H, Nakajima Y, et al. Clinicopathologic features of encapsulated hepatocellular carcinoma: a study of 26 cases. Cancer 40:1240–1245, 1977.
30. Ruffin MT. Fibrolamellar hepatoma. Am J Gastroenterol 85:577–581, 1990.
31. Waldmann TA, McIntire KR. The use of radioimmunoassay for alpha-fetoprotein in the diagnosis of malignancy. Cancer 34:1510–1515, 1974.
32. Okuda K, Ohtsuki T, Obata H. Natural history of hepatocellular carcinoma and prognosis in relation to treatment. Study of 850 patients. Cancer 56:918–928, 1985.
33. Salminen PM, Hockerstedt K, Edgren J, et al. Intraoperative ultrasound as an aid to surgical strategy in liver tumors. Acta Chir Scand 156:329–332, 1990.
34. Lok ASF, Lai CL. Alpha-fetoprotein monitoring in Chinese patients with chronic hepatitis B virus infection: role in the early detection of hepatocellular carcinoma. Hepatology 9:110–115, 1989.
35. Tremolda F, Benevegnu L, Drago C, et al. Early detection of hepatocellular carcinoma in patients with cirrhosis by alpha-fetoprotein, ultrasound, and fine-needle biopsy. Hepatogastroenterology 36:519–521, 1989.
36. Colombo M, De Franchis R, Del Ninno E, et al. Hepatocellular carcinoma in Italian patients with cirrhosis. N Engl J Med 325:675–680, 1991.
37. Regan LS. Screening for hepatocellular carcinoma in high risk individuals. Arch Intern Med 149:1741–1744, 1989.
38. McMahon BJ, London T. Workshop on screening for hepatocellular carcinoma. J Natl Cancer Inst 83:916–919, 1991.
39. Dodd GD, Miller WJ, Baron RL, et al. Detection of malignant tumors in end-stage cirrhotic livers: efficacy of sonography as a screening technique. Am J Roentgenol 159:727–733, 1992.
40. Lin TY, Lee CS, Chen KM, et al. Role of surgery in the treatment of primary carcinoma of the liver: a 31 year experience. Br J Surg 74:839–842, 1987.
41. Chen MF, Hwang TL, Jeng CB, et al. Hepatic resection in 120 patients with hepatocellular carcinoma. Arch Surg 124:1025–1028, 1989.
42. Toshihara T, Sugioka A, Veda M, et al. Hepatic resection for hepatocellular carcinoma. Surgery 107:551–560, 1990.
43. Choi TK, Edward CS, Fan ST, et al. Results of surgical resection for hepatocellular carcinoma. Hepatogastroenterology 37:172–173, 1990.
44. Yamanaka N, Okamoto, E, Toyosaka A, et al. Prognostic factors after hepatectomy for hepatocellular carcinoma. Hepatogastroenterology 37:172–173, 1990.
45. Kobayashi N, Kumada K, Yamaoka Y, et al. The outcomes of the operated hepatocellular carcinoma patients. Nippon Geka Hokan 59:369–376, 1990.
46. Tsuzuki T, Sugioka A, Ueda M, et al. Hepatic resection for hepatocellular carcinoma. Surgery 107:511–520, 1990.
47. Iwatsuki S, Starzl TW, Sheahan DG, et al. Hepatic resection versus transplantation for hepatocellular carcinoma. Ann Surg 214:221–229, 1991.
48. Gozzetti G, Mazziotti A, Grazi GL, et al. Surgical experience with 168 primary liver cell carcinomas treated with hepatic resection. J Surg Oncol 3(Suppl):59–61, 1993.
49. Kawarada Y, Ito F, Sakurai H, et al. Surgical treatment of hepatocellular carcinoma. Cancer Chemother Pharmacol 33:S7–S12, 1994.
50. Tani M, Edamoto Y, Kawai S, et al. Results of 90 consecutive hepatectomies for hepatocellular carcinoma: a multivariate analysis of survival. Semin Oncol 24:S6–S16, 1997.
51. Yamasaki S, Makuuchi M, Hasegawa H. Results of hepatectomy for hepatocellular carcinoma at the National Cancer Center Hospital. HPB Surg 3:235–249, 1991.
52. Nagashima I, Hamada C, Naruse K, et al. Surgical resection for small hepatocellular carcinoma. Surgery 119:40–45, 1996.
53. Takenaka K, Kawahara N, Yamamoto K, et al. Results of 280 liver resections for hepatocellular carcinoma. Arch Surg 131:71–76, 1996.
54. Chen MF, Jeng LB. Partial hepatic resection for hepatocellular carcinoma. J Gastroenterol Hepatol 12:S329–S334, 1997.
55. Makuuchi M, Takayama T, Kubota K, et al. Hepatic resection for hepatocellular carcinoma: Japanese experience. Hepatogastroenterology 45: 1267–1274, 1998.
56. Takayama T, Makuuchi M, Yamasaki S, et al. Systemic resection for hepatocellular carcinoma. Nippon Geka Gakkai Zasshi 99:241–244, 1998.
57. Lise M, Bacchetti S, Da Pian PD, et al. Prognostic factors affecting long term outcome after liver resection for hepatocellular carcinoma. Cancer 82:1028–1036, 1998.
58. Philosophe B, Greig PD, Hemming AW, et al. Surgical management of hepatocellular carcinoma: resection or transplantation? J Gastrointest Surg 2:21–27, 1998.
59. Sitzmann JV, Abrams R. Improved survival for hepatocellular cancer with combination surgery and multimodality treatment. Ann Surg 217:149–154, 1993.
60. Nakashima K, Kim Y, Okada K, et al. Prophylactic chemotherapy by regional arterial infusion in resected hepatoma patients. Gan To Kagaku Ryoho 19(Suppl):1489–1492, 1992.
61. Lai EC, Lo CM, Fan ST, et al. Post-operative adjuvant chemotherapy after curative resection of hepatocellular carcinoma: a randomized controlled trial. Arch Surg 133:183–188, 1998.
62. Hang CE, Jenkins RL, Rohrer RJ, et al. Liver transplantation for hepatic primary hepatic cancer. Transplantation 53:376–382, 1992.
63. Venook AP. Liver transplantation for primary hepatobiliary malignancy. Semin Gastrointest Dis 4:178–183, 1993.
64. Bismuth H, Ericzon BG, Rolles K, et al. Hepatic transplantation in Europe. Lancet 2:674–676, 1987.
65. Iwatsuki S, Gorden RD, Shaw BW, et al. Role of liver transplantation in cancer therapy. Ann Surg 202:401–407, 1985.
66. Jenkins RL, Pinson CW, Stone MD. Experience with transplantation in the treatment of liver cancer. Cancer Chemother Pharmacol 23(Suppl):S104–S109, 1989.
67. O'Grady JG, Polson RJ, Rolles K, et al. Liver transplantation for malignant disease. Ann Surg 207:373–379, 1988.
68. Ringe B, Wittekind C, Bechstein WO, et al. The role of liver transplantation in hepatobiliary malignancy. Ann Surg 209:88–98, 1989.
69. Olthoff KM, Millis JM, Rosove MH, et al. Is liver transplantation justified for the treatment of hepatic malignancies? Arch Surg 125:1261–1268, 1990.
70. Pichlmayr R. Can liver transplantation be applied for the treatment of liver cancer? Jpn J Surg 22:187–190, 1992.
71. Bismuth H, Chiche L, Adam R, et al. Liver resection versus transplantation for hepatocellular carcinoma in cirrhotic patients. Ann Surg 218:145–151, 1993.
72. Klintmalm GB. Liver transplantation for hepatocellular carcinoma: a registry report of the impact of tumor characteristics on outcome. Ann Surg 228:479–490, 1998.
73. Starzl TE, Iwatsuki S, Shaw BW, et al. Treatment of fibrolamellar hepatoma with partial or total hepatectomy and transplantation of the liver. Surg Gynecol Obstet 162:145–148, 1986.
74. Ringe B, Wittekind C, Weimann A, et al. Results of hepatic resection and transplantation for fibrolamellar carcinoma. Surg Gynecol Obstet 175:299–305, 1992.
75. Stone MJ, Klintmalm GBG, Polter D, et al. Neoadjuvant chemotherapy and liver transplantation for hepatocellular carcinoma: a pilot study in 20 patients. Gastroenterology 104:196–202, 1993.
76. Carr BI, Selby R, Madariaga J, et al. Prolonged survival after liver transplantation and cancer chemotherapy for advanced stage hepatocellular carcinoma. Transplant Proc 25:1128–1129, 1993.
77. Venook AP, Ferrell LD, Roberts JP, et al. Liver transplantation for hepatocellular carcinoma: results with preoperative chemoembolization. Liver Transpl Surg 1:242–248, 1995.
78. Olthoff KM, Rosove MH, Shackleton CR, et al. Adjuvant chemotherapy improves survival after liver transplant for hepatocellular carcinoma. Ann Surg 221:734–741, 1995.
79. Ravikumar TS, Steele GS. Hepatic cryosurgery. Surg Clin North Am 69:433–440, 1989.
80. Zhou XD, Tang ZY, Yu YQ, et al. Clinical evaluation of cryosurgery in the treatment of primary liver cancer. Cancer 61:1889–1892, 1988.
81. Lewin JS, Connell CF, Duerk JL, et al. Interactive MRI-guided radiofrequency interstitial thermal ablation of abdominal tumors: clinical trial for evaluation of safety and feasibility. J Magn Reson Imaging 8:40–47,1998.
82. Castells A, Bruix J, Bru C, et al. Treatment of small hepatocellular carcinoma in cirrhotic patients: a cohort study comparing surgical resection and percutaneous ethanol injection. Hepatology 18:1121–1126, 1993.
83. Ebara M, Kita K, Nagato Y, et al. Percutaneous ethanol injection for small hepatocellular carcinoma. Gan To Kagaku Ryoho 20:884–888, 1993.
84. Isobe H, Sakai H, Imari Y, et al. Intratumor ethanol injection therapy for solitary minute hepatocellular carcinoma. A study of 37 patients. J Clin Gastroenterol 18:122–126, 1994.
85. Ingold JA, Reed GB, Kaplan HS, et al. Radiation hepatitis. Am J Roentgenol 93:200–208, 1965.
86. Phillips R, Murikama K. Primary neoplasms of the liver. Results of radiation therapy. Cancer 4:714–720, 1960.

87. Lawrence TS, Tesser RJ, Ten Haken RK. An application of dose volume histograms to the treatment of intrahepatic malignancies with radiation therapy. Int J Radiat Oncol Biol Phys 20:555–561, 1991.
88. Robertson JM, Lawrence TS, Dworzanin LM, et al. Treatment of primary hepatobiliary cancers with conformal radiation therapy and regional chemotherapy. J Clin Oncol 11:1286–1293, 1993.
89. Order S, Pajak T, Leibel S, et al. A randomized prospective trial comparing full dose chemotherapy to 131 I antiferritin: an RTOG study. Int J Radiat Oncol Biol Phys 20:953–963, 1991.
90. Wollner I, Knutsen C, Smith P, et al. Effects of hepatic arterial yttrium 90 glass microspheres in dogs. Cancer 61:1336–1344, 1988.
91. Leung WT, Lau WY, HO S, et al. Selective internal radiation therapy with intra-arterial 131-iodine-Lipiodol in inoperable hepatocellular carcinoma. Proc Am Soc Clin Oncol 13:202, 1994.
92. Bhattacharya S, Novell JR, Dusheiko GM, et al. Epirubicin-Lipiodol chemotherapy versus 131-iodine-Lipiodol radiotherapy in the treatment of unresectable hepatocellular carcinoma. Cancer 76:2202–2210, 1995.
93. Lau WY, Leung WT, Ho S, et al. Treatment of inoperable hepatocellular carcinoma with intrahepatic arterial yttrium-90 microspheres: a phase I and II study. Br J Cancer 70:994–999, 1994.
94. Friedman MA, Demanes DJ, Hoffman PG. Hepatomas: hormone receptors and therapy. Am J Med 73:362–366, 1982.
95. Paliard P, Clement G, Saez S, et al. Treatment of hepatocellular carcinoma with tamoxifen [letter]. Gastroenterol Clin Biol 8:680–681, 1984.
96. Chao Y, Wu M, Liu Y, et al. Treatment of hepatocellular carcinoma with Megace. Proc Am Soc Clin Oncol 12:205, 1993.
97. Riestra S, Rodriquez M, Delgado M, et al. Tamoxifen does not improve survival of patients with advanced hepatocellular carcinoma. J Clin Gastroenterol 26:200–203, 1998.
98. Castells A, Bruix J, Bru C, et al. Treatment of small hepatocellular carcinoma in cirrhotic patients: a cohort study comparing surgical resection and percutaneous ethanol injection. Hepatology 18:1121–1126, 1993.
99. Chao Y, Chan WK, Wang SS, et al. Phase II study of megestrol acetate in the treatment of hepatocellular carcinoma. J Gastroenterol Hepatol 12:277–281, 1997.
100. Vogel CL, Bayley AC, Brockes RJ. A phase II study of adriamycin in patients with hepatocellular carcinoma from Zambia and the United States. Cancer 39:1923–1929, 1977.
101. Johnson PJ, Williams R, Thomas H, et al. Induction of remission in hepatocellular carcinoma with doxorubicin. Lancet 1:1006–1009, 1978.
102. Falkson G, Lavin P, Moertel CG, et al. Chemotherapy studies in primary liver cancer: A prospective randomized clinical trial. Cancer 42:2149–2156, 1978.
103. Olweny CLM, Katongole-Mbidde E, Bahendeka S, et al. Further experience in treating patients with hepatocellular carcinoma in Uganda. Cancer 46:2717–2722, 1980.
104. Melia WM, Johnson PJ, Williams R. Induction remission in hepatocellular carcinoma: a comparison of VP-16 with adriamycin. Cancer 51:206–210, 1983.
105. Yang P, Sheu J, Chen D, et al. Systemic chemotherapy of hepatocellular carcinoma with adriamycin alone and FAM regimen. In: Chemotherapy of hepatic tumors. Tokyo: Excerpta Medica, 1984:41–47.
106. Chlebowski RT, Brezechwa-Asjukiewicz A, Cowdon A, et al. Doxorubicin for hepatocellular carcinoma: clinical and pharmacokinetic results. Cancer Treat Rep 68:487–491, 1984.
107. Choi TK, Lee NW, Wong J, et al. Chemotherapy for advanced hepatocellular carcinoma: clinical and pharmacokinetic results. Cancer Treat Rep 68:487–491, 1984.
108. Sciarrino E, Simonetti RG, Moli SL, et al. Adriamycin treatment for hepatocellular carcinoma: experience with 109 patients. Cancer 56:2751–2755, 1985.
109. Dunk AA, Scott SC, Johnson PJ, et al. Mitoxantrone as single agent therapy in hepatocellular carcinoma: a phase II study. J Hepatol 1:395–404, 1985.
110. Lai KH, Tsai YT, Lee SD, et al. Phase II study of mitoxantrone in unresectable primary hepatocellular carcinoma following hepatitis B infection. Cancer Chemother Pharmacol 23:54–56, 1989.
111. Hochester HS, Green MD, Speyer J, et al. 4′-Epidoxorubicin (epirubicin) activity in hepatocellular carcinoma. J Clin Oncol 3:1525–1540, 1985.
112. Tan YO, Lim F. 4′-Epidoxorubicin as a single agent in advanced primary hepatocellular carcinoma: a preliminary experience. Ann Acad Med Singapore 15:169–171, 1986.
113. Shiu W, Leung N, Li M, et al. The efficacy of high dose 4′-epidoxorubicin in hepatocellular carcinoma. Jpn J Clin Oncol 18:235–237, 1988.
114. Kennedy PS, Lehane DE, Smith FE, et al. Oral fluorouracil therapy of hepatoma. Cancer 39:1930–1935, 1977.
115. Link JS, Bateman JR, Paroly WS, et al. 5-Fluorouracil in hepatocellular carcinoma: report of 21 cases. Cancer 39:1936–1939, 1977.
116. Davis HL, Ramirez H, Ansfield FJ. Adenocarcinomas of the stomach, pancreas, liver, and biliary tracts: survival of 328 patients treated with fluoropyrimidine therapy. Cancer 33:193–197, 1974.
117. Al-Sarraf M, Go TS, Kithier K, et al. Primary liver cancer: a review of the clinical features, blood groups, serum enzymes, therapy and survival of 65 cases. Cancer 33:574–582, 1974.
118. Tetef M, Doroshow J, Akman S, et al. 5-Fluorouracil and high-dose calcium leucovorin for hepatocellular carcinoma: a phase II trial. Cancer Invest 13:460–463, 1995.
119. Bukowski RM, Legna S, Saidi J, et al. Phase II trial of M-AMSA in hepatocellular carcinoma: a Southwest Oncology Group Study. Cancer Treat Rep 66:1651–1652, 1982.
120. Cheng E, Lightdale C, Young C, et al. Phase II trial of (m-AMSA) 4′-9 (acridinylamino)-methane-sulfon-m-aniside in primary liver cancer. Am Clin Oncol 6:211–213, 1983.
121. Amrein PC, Richards F, Coleman M, et al. Phase II trial of Amsacrine in patients with hepatoma: a Cancer and Leukemia Group B study. Cancer Treat Rep 68:923–924, 1984.
122. Falkson G, Coetzer B, Klaasen DJ. A phase II study of m-AMSA in patients with primary liver cancer. Cancer Chemother Pharmacol 8:305–310, 1982.
123. Vogel CL, Adamson RH, DeVita VT, et al. Preliminary clinical trials of dichloromethotrexate (NSC-29630) in hepatocellular carcinoma. Cancer Chemother Rep 56:249–258, 1972.
124. Tester WJ, Donehower RS, Eddy JL, et al. Evaluation of weekly escalating doses of dichloromethotrexate in patients with hepatocellular carcinoma and other solid tumors. Cancer Chemother Pharmacol 8:305–310, 1982.
125. Cavalli F, Rosenzweig M, Renard J, et al. A phase II study of oral VP-16-213 in patients with hepatocellular carcinoma. Proc Am Soc Clin Oncol 22:457, 1981.
126. Melia WM, Westaby D, Williams R. Diaminodichloride platinum (cisplatinum) in treatment of hepatocellular carcinoma. Clin Oncol 7:275–280, 1981.
127. Okada S, Okazaki N, Nose H, et al. A phase 2 study of cisplatin in patients with hepatocellular carcinoma. Oncology 50:22–26, 1993.
128. Gastrointestinal Tumor Study Group. A prospective trial of recombinant human interferon 2B in previously untreated patients with hepatocellular carcinoma. Cancer 66:135–139, 1990.
129. Lai LL, Wu PL, Lok AS, et al. Recombinant alpha-2-interferon is superior to doxorubicin for inoperable hepatocellular carcinoma: a prospective randomized trial. J Pharmacokinet Biopharm 2:257–285, 1974.
130. Eckman WW, Patlak CS, Fenstermacher JD. A critical evaluation of the principles governing the advantages of intra-arterial infusions. J Pharmacokinet Biopharm 2:257–285, 1974.
131. Chen HG, Gross JF. Intra-arterial infusion of anticancer drugs: theoretical aspects of drug delivery and review of responses. Cancer Treat Rep 64:31–40, 1980.
132. Ensminger WS, Rosowsky A, Raso V, et al. A clinical pharmacologic evaluation of hepatic arterial infusions of 5-fluoro-2′-deoxyuridine and 5-fluorouracil. Cancer Res 38:3784–3792, 1978.
133. Garnick MB, Ensminger WD, Israel M. A clinical pharmacologic evaluation of hepatic arterial infusion of adriamycin. Cancer Res 39:4105–4110, 1979.
134. Fraile RJ, Baker LH, Buroker TR, et al. Pharmacokinetics of 5-fluorouracil administered orally, by rapid intravenous and by slow infusion. Cancer Res 40:2223–2228, 1980.
135. Ensminger W, Stetson P, Gyves J, et al. Dependence of hepatic arterial fluorouracil pharmacokinetics on dose, route and duration of infusion. Proc Am Soc Clin Oncol 2:25, 1983.
136. Campbell TN, Howell SB, Pfeifle CE, et al. Clinical pharmacokinetics of intraarterial cisplatin in humans. J Clin Oncol 12:755–762, 1983.
137. Gyves JL, Ensminger W, Stetson P, et al. Clinical pharmacology of mitomycin C by hepatic arterial infusion. Proc Am Soc Clin Oncol 2:25, 1983.
138. Wellwood JM, Cady B, Oberfield RA. Treatment of primary liver cancer: response on regional chemotherapy. Clin Oncol 5:25–31, 1979.
139. Ludwig J, Kim CH, Wiesner RH, et al. Floxuridine-induced sclerosing cholangitis: an ischemic cholangiopathy. Hepatology 9(2):215–219, 1989.
140. Doci R, Bignami P, Bozzetti F, et al. Intrahepatic chemotherapy for unresectable hepatocellular carcinoma. Cancer 61:1983–1987, 1988.
141. Bern MM, McDermott W, Cady B. Intraarterial hepatic infusion and intravenous adriamycin for treatment of hepatocellular carcinoma: A clinical and pharmacology report. Cancer 42:399–406, 1978.
142. Urist MM, Balch CM. Intra-arterial chemotherapy for hepatoma using adriamycin administered via an implantable infusion pump. Proc Am Soc Clin Oncol 3:146, 1983.
143. Shepherd FA, Evans WK, Fine S, et al. Hepatic arterial infusion of mitoxantrone and adriamycin in the treatment of primary hepatocellular carcinoma. Proc Am Soc Clin Oncol 4:95, 1985.

144. Ukeda H, Kuroda S, Ohnoshi T, et al. Intra-arterial adriamycin for patients with hepatocellular carcinoma and metastatic carcinoma. Gan To Kagaka Ryoho 11:2579–2584, 1984.
145. Cheng E, Watson RC, Fortner J, et al. Regional intraarterial infusion of cisplatin in primary liver cancer. Proc Am Soc Clin Oncol 1:179, 1982.
146. Onohara S, Kobayashi H, Itoh Y, et al. Intra-arterial cis-platinum infusion with sodium thiosulfate protection and angiotensin II induced hypertension for treatment of hepatocellular carcinoma. Acta Radiol 29:197–202, 1988.
147. Kajanti M, Riassanen P, Kirkkunen P, et al. Regional intra-arterial infusion of cisplatin in primary hepatocellular carcinoma. A phase II study. Cancer 58:2386–2388, 1986.
148. Shepherd FA, Evan WK, Blackstein ME, et al. Hepatic artery infusion of mitoxantrone in the treatment of primary hepatocellular carcinoma. J Clin Oncol 5:635–640, 1987.
149. Shepherd FA, Evans WK, Blackstein ME, et al. Hepatic arterial infusion of mitoxantrone in the treatment of primary hepatocellular carcinoma. J Clin Oncol 5:635–640, 1987.
150. Ando K, Kirai K, Kubo Y, et al. Intra-arterial administration of epirubicin in the treatment of nonresectable hepatocellular carcinoma. Epirubicin Study Group for Hepatocellular carcinoma. Cancer Chemother Pharmacol 19:183–189, 1987.
151. Malik IA, Khan WA, Haq S, et al. A prospective phase II trial to evaluate the efficacy and toxicity of hepatic arterial infusion of ifosfamide in patients with inoperable localized hepatocellular carcinoma. Am J Clin Oncol 20:289–292, 1997.
152. Douglas CC. Prolongation of survival with periodic percutaneous multidrug arterial infusions in patients with primary and metastatic gastrointestinal carcinoma to the liver. Proc Am Soc Clin Oncol 21:416, 1980.
153. Patt YZ, Chuang VP, Wallace S, et al. Hepatic artery chemotherapy and occlusion for palliation of primary hepatocellular and unknown primary neoplasms in the liver. Cancer 51:1359–1363, 1983.
154. Patt YZ, Charnsangavej C, Lawrence D, et al. Hepatic arterial infusion for FUDR, leucovorin, adriamycin, and platinol: effective palliation for nonresectable hepatocellular carcinoma. Proc Am Soc Clin Oncol 11:165, 1992.
155. Kanematsu T, Matsumata T, Furuta T, et al. Lipiodol drug targeting in the treatment of primary hepatocellular carcinoma. Hepatogastroenterology 37:442–444, 1990.
156. Okusaka T, Okada S, Ishii H, et al. Transarterial chemotherapy with zinostatin stimalamer for hepatocellular carcinoma. Oncology 55:276–283, 1998.
157. Carr B, Iwatsuki S, Baron R. Intrahepatic arterial cisplatinum and doxorubicin with or without Lipiodol for advanced hepatocellular carcinoma: a prospective randomized study. Proc Am Soc Clin Oncol 12:219, 1993.
158. Lee YT, Irwin L. Hepatic artery ligation and adriamycin infusion chemotherapy for hepatoma. Cancer 41:12459–12555, 1978.
159. Nagasue N, Inokuchi K, Kobayashi M, et al. Serum alpha-fetoprotein levels after hepatic artery ligation and post-operative chemotherapy: Correlation with clinical status in patients with hepatocellular carcinoma. Cancer 40:615–618, 1977.
160. Charnsangavej C, Chuang VP, Wallace S, et al. Angiographic classification of hepatic arterial collaterals. Radiology 144:485–494, 1982.
161. Chearanai O, Plengvanit U, Asavanich C, et al. Spontaneous rupture of primary hepatoma: report of 63 cases with particular reference to the pathogenesis and rationale treatment by hepatic artery ligation. Cancer 51:1532–1536, 1983.
162. Soyer P, Levesque M, Zeittoun G, et al. Hemoperitoneum caused spontaneous rupture of hepatocellular carcinoma. Role of hepatic artery embolization in the therapeutic procedure. J Radiol 72:287–290, 1991.
163. Wallace S, Charnsangavej C, Carrasco H, et al. Infusion-embolization. Cancer 54:2751–2765, 1984.
164. Yamada R, Sato M, Kawabata M, et al. Hepatic artery embolization in 120 patients with unresectable hepatoma. Radiology 148:397–401, 1983.
165. Fujimoto S, Miyazaki M, Endoh F, et al. Biodegradable mitomycin C microspheres given intra-arterially for operable hepatic cancer. Cancer 56:2404–2410, 1985.
166. Ohnishi K, Tsuchiya S, Nakayama T, et al. Arterial chemoembolization of hepatocellular carcinoma with mitomycin C microcapsules. Radiology 152:51–55, 1984.
167. Venook A, Stagg R, Lewis B, et al. Chemoembolization for hepatocellular carcinoma. J Clin Oncol 8:1108–1114, 1990.
168. Civalleri D, Pellicci R, Decaro G, et al. Palliative chemoembolization of hepatocellular carcinoma with mitoxantrone, Lipiodol, and Gelfoam. A phase II study. Anticancer Res 16:937–941, 1996.
169. Kawai S, Tani M, Okamura J, et al. Prospective and randomized trial of Lipiodol-transcatheter arterial chemoembolization for treatment of hepatocellular carcinoma: a comparison of epirubicin and doxorubicin (second cooperative study). The Cooperative Study Group for Liver Cancer Treatment of Japan. Semin Oncol 24:S6-38–S6-45, 1997.
170. Groupe d'Etude et de Traitement du Carcinome Hepatocellulaire. A comparison of Lipiodol chemoembolization and conservative treatment for unresectable hepatocellular carcinoma. N Engl J Med 332:1256–1261, 1995.
171. Okuda K and the Liver Tumor Study Group of Japan. Primary liver cancers in Japan. Cancer 45:2663–2669, 1980.
172. Stuver SO. Toward global control of liver cancer? Semin Cancer Biol 8:299–306, 1998.
173. Xu ZY, Liu CB, Francis DP, et al. Prevention of perinatal acquisition of hepatitis B virus carriage using vaccine: preliminary report of a randomized, double-blind placebo-controlled and comparative trial. Pediatrics 76:713–718, 1985.
174. Sun ZT, Zhu Y, Stjernsward, et al. Design and compliance of HBV vaccination trial on newborns to prevent hepatocellular carcinoma and 5-year results of its pilot study. Cancer Detect Prev 15:313–318, 1991.
175. Fortuin M, Chotard J, Jack AD, et al. Efficacy of hepatitis B vaccine in the Gambian expanded programme on immunization. Lancet 341:1129–1131, 1993.
176. Chang MH, Chen CK, Lai MS, et al. Universal hepatitis B vaccination in Taiwan and the incidence of hepatocellular carcinoma in children. Taiwan Childhood Hepatoma Study Group. N Engl J Med 336:1855–1859, 1997.
177. Ginsburg GM, Shouval D. Cost benefit analysis of a nation-wide neonatal inoculation programme against hepatitis B in an area of intermediate endemicity. J Epidemiol Commun Health 46:587–594, 1992.
178. Ikeda K, Saitoh S, Suzuki Y, et al. Interferon decreases hepatocellular carcinogenesis in patients with cirrhosis caused by the hepatitis B virus: a pilot study. Cancer 82:827–835, 1998.
179. Recommendations for prevention and control of hepatitis C virus (HCV) infection and HCV-related chronic disease. Centers for Disease Control and Prevention. MMWR Morb Mortal Wkly Rep 47:1–39, 1998.
180. Weiss L, Gilbert HA, eds. Liver metastases. Boston: GK Hall, 1982.
181. Beck PR, Belfield A, Spooner RJ, et al. Serum enzyme elevations in colorectal cancer. Cancer 43:1772–1776, 1979.
182. Kemeny MM, Sugarbaker PH, Smith TJ, et al. A prospective analysis of laboratory tests and imaging studies to detect hepatic lesions. Ann Surg 195:163–167, 1982.
183. Szymendera JJ, Nowacki MP, Szawlowski AW, et al. Predictive value of plasma CEA levels: preoperative and postoperative monitoring of patients with colorectal carcinoma. Dis Colon Rectum 25:46–52, 1982.
184. Funven P, Makuuchi M, Takayasu K, et al. Preoperative imaging of liver metastases. Comparison of angiography, CT scan, and ultrasound. Ann Surg 202:573–579, 1985.
185. Schreve RH, Terpstra OT, Ausema L, et al. Detection liver metastases. A prospective study comparing liver enzymes, scintigraphy, ultrasonography, and computed tomography. Br J Surg 71:947–949, 1984.
186. Domingues JM, Wolff BG, Nelson H, et al. 111In-CYT-103 scanning in recurrent colorectal cancer: does it affect standard management? Dis Colon Rectum 39:514–519, 1996.
187. Knol JA, Marn CS, Francis IR, et al. Comparisons of dynamic infusion and delayed computed tomography, intraoperative ultrasound, and palpation in the diagnosis of liver metastases. Am J Surg 165(1):81–87, 1993.
188. Hughes K, Schilel J, Sugerbaker P, et al. Surgery for colorectal cancer metastatic to the liver. Surg Clin North Am 69:339–359, 1989.
189. Adloff M, Arnaud JP, Thebault Y, et al. Hepatic metastases of colorectal cancer. Should it be treated surgically? Report of 55 cases. Chirurgie 116:144–149, 1990.
190. Doci R, Genarri L, Bignami P, et al. One hundred patients with hepatic metastases from colorectal cancer treated by resection: analysis of prognostic determinants. Br J Surg 78:797–801, 1991.
191. Pettrelli N, Gupta B, Piedmonte M, et al. Morbidity and survival of liver resection for colorectal adenocarcinoma. Dis Colon Rectum 34:899–904, 1992.
192. Nakamura S, Yokoi Y, Suzuki S, et al. Results of extensive surgery for liver metastases in colorectal carcinoma. Br J Surg 79:35–38, 1992.
193. Rosen CB, Nagorney DM, Taswell HF, et al. Perioperative blood transfusions and determinants of survival after liver resection for metastatic colorectal carcinoma. Ann Surg 216:493–505, 1992.
194. van Ooijen B, Wiggers T, Meijer S, et al. Hepatic resections for colorectal metastases in The Netherlands. A multiinstitutional 10-year study. Cancer 70:28–34, 1992.
195. Gayowski TJ, Iwatsuki S, Madariaga JR, et al. Experience in hepatic resection for metastatic colorectal cancer: analysis of clinical and pathologic risk factors. Surgery 116:703–710, 1994.
196. Fuhrman GM, Curley SA, Hohn DC, et al. Improved survival after resection of colorectal liver metastases. Am Surg Oncol 2:537–541, 1995.
197. Jatzko GR, Lisborg, PH, Stettner HM, et al. Hepatic resection for metastases from colorectal carcinoma: a survival analysis. Eur J Cancer 31A(1):41–46, 1995.

198. Scheele J, Stang R, Altendorf-Hofmann A, et al. Resection of colorectal liver metastases. World J Surg 19:59–71, 1995.
199. Scott S, Carty N, Anderson L, et al. Liver resection for colorectal liver metastases. Eur J Surg Oncol 21:33–35, 1995.
200. Nordlinger B, Guiguet M, Vaillant JC, et al. Surgical resection of colorectal carcinoma metastasized to the liver. A prognostic scoring system to improve case selection, based on 1568 patients. Cancer 77:1254–1262, 1996.
201. Fong Y, Cohen AM, Fortner JG, et al. Liver resection for colorectal metastases. J Clin Oncol 15:938–946, 1997.
202. Marmorale C, Miconi G, De Luca S, et al. Surgical treatment of hepatic metastatic colorectal cancer. Ann Ital Chir 67:245–249, 1996.
203. Jenkins LT, Millikan KW, Bines SD, et al. Hepatic resection for metastatic colorectal cancer. Am Surg 63:605–610, 1997.
204. Rees M, Plant G, Bygrave S. Late results justify resection for multiple hepatic metastases from colorectal cancer. Br J Surg 84:1136–1140, 1997.
205. Shirabe K, Takenaka K, Gion T, et al. Analysis of prognostic risk factors in hepatic resection for metastatic colorectal carcinoma with special reference to the surgical margin. Br J Surg 84:1077–1080, 1997.
206. Taylor M, Forster J, Langer B, et al. A study of prognostic factors for hepatic resection for colorectal metastases. Am J Surg 173:467–471, 1997.
207. Elias D, Cavalcanti A, Sabourin JC, et al. Results of 136 curative hepatectomies with a safety margin of less than 10 mm for colorectal metastases. J Surg Oncol 69:88–93, 1998.
208. Ohlsson B, Stenram U, Tranberg KG. Resection of colorectal liver metastases: 25-year experience. World J Surg 22:268–277, 1998.
209. Curley SA, Roh MS, Chase JL, et al. Adjuvant hepatic arterial infusion chemotherapy after curative resection of colorectal liver metastases. Am J Surg 166:743–746, 1993.
210. Borgelt BB, Gelber R, Brady LW, et al. The palliation of hepatic metastases: results of Radiation Therapy Oncology Group pilot study. Int J Radiat Oncol Biol Phys 7:587–591, 1981.
211. Barone RM, Byfield JE, Goldfarb PB, et al. Intra-arterial chemotherapy using an implantable infusion pump and liver irradiation for the treatment of hepatic metastases. Cancer 50:850–862, 1982.
212. Seifert JK, Junginger T, Morris DL. A collective review of the world literature on hepatic cryotherapy. J R Coll Surg Edinb 43:141–154, 1998.
213. Weaver ML, Ashton JG, Zemel R. Treatment of colorectal liver metastases by cryotherapy. Semin Surg Oncol 14:163–170, 1998.
214. Hewitt PM, Dwerryhouse SJ, Zhao J, et al. Multiple bilobar liver metastases: cryotherapy for residual lesions after liver resection. J Surg Oncol 67:112–116, 1998.
215. Evans JT. Hepatic artery ligation in hepatic metastases from colon and rectal malignancies. Dis Colon Rectum 22:370, 1979.
216. Moertel CG. Chemotherapy of gastrointestinal cancer. N Engl J Med 299:1049–1052, 1978.
217. Ansfield R, Klotz J, Nealson T, et al. A phase II study comparing the utility of four regimens of 5-fluorouracil. Cancer 39:34–40, 1977.
218. Dorosow JH, Multhauf P, Leung L, et al. Prospective randomized comparison of fluorouracil versus fluorouracil and high-dose continuous infusion leucovorin calcium for the treatment of advanced measurable colorectal cancer in patients previously unexposed to chemotherapy. J Clin Oncol 8:491–501, 1990.
219. Erlichman C, Fine S, Wong A, et al. A randomized trial of fluorouracil and folinic acid in patients with metastatic colorectal carcinoma. J Clin Oncol 6:469–475, 1988.
220. Petrelli N, Douglas HO, Herra L, et al. The modulation of fluorouracil with leucovorin in metastatic colorectal carcinoma: a prospective randomized phase III trial. J Clin Oncol 7:1419–1426, 1989.
221. Poon MA, O'Connell MJ, Moertel CG, et al. Biochemical modulation fluorouracil: evidence of significant improvement of survival and quality of life in patients with advanced colorectal carcinoma. J Clin Oncol 7:1407–1418, 1989.
222. Valone FH, Friedman MA, Wittlinger PS, et al. Treatment of patients with advanced colorectal carcinomas with fluorouracil alone, high-dose leucovorin plus fluorouracil, or sequential methotrexate, fluorouracil, and leucovorin. A randomized trial of the Northern California Oncology Group. J Clin Oncol 7:1427–1436, 1989.
223. Petrelli N, Herrera L, Rustum Y, et al. A prospective randomized trial of 5-fluorouracil verus 5-fluorouracil and high dose leucovorin versus 5-fluorouracil and methotrexate in previously untreated patients with advanced colorectal carcinoma. J Clin Oncol 5:1559–1565, 1987.
224. Labianca R, Pancera G, Aitini E, et al. Folinic acid plus 5-fluorouracil versus equidose 5FU in advanced colorectal cancer. Phase III study of "GISCAD" (Italian Group for the Study of Digestive Tract Cancer). Ann Oncol 2:673–679, 1991.
225. Shimada Y, Yoshino M, Wakii A, et al. Phase II study of CPT-11, a new camptothecin derivative in metastatic colorectal cancer. J Clin Oncol 11:909–913, 1993.
226. Conti JA, Kemeny NE, Saltz LB, et al. Irinotecan is an active agent in untreated patients with metastatic colorectal cancer. J Clin Oncol 14:709–715, 1996.
227. Pitot HC, Wender DB, O'Connell MJ, et al. Phase II trial of irinotecan in patients with metastatic colorectal carcinoma. J Clin Oncol 15:2910–2919, 1997.
228. Rougier P, Bugat R, Douillard JY, et al. Phase II study of irinotecan in the treatment of advanced colorectal cancer in chemotherapy-naive patients and patients pretreated with fluorouracil-based chemotherapy. J Clin Oncol 15:251–260, 1997.
229. Shimada Y, Yoshino M, Wakui A, et al. Phase II study of CPT-11, a new camtothecin derivative, in metastatic colorectal cancer. CPT-11 gastrointestinal cancer study group. J Clin Oncol 11:909–913, 1993.
230. Von Hoff DD, Rothenberg ML, Pitot HC, et al. Irinotecan (CPT-11) therapy for patients with previously treated metastatic colorectal cancer: overall results of FDA-reviewed pivotal US clinical trials [abstract]. Proc Am Soc Clin Oncol 16:803, 1997.
231. Van Cutsem E, Bajetta E, Niederle N, et al. A phase III multicenter randomized trial comparing CPT-11 to infusional 5FU regimen in patients with advanced colorectal cancer after 5FU failure [abstract]. Proc Am Soc Clin Oncol 17:984, 1998.
232. Machover D, Diaz-Rubio E, de Gramont A, et al. Two consecutive phase II studies of oxaliplatin (L-OHP) for treatment of patients with advanced colorectal carcinoma who were resistant to previous treatment with fluoropyrimidines. Ann Oncol 7:95–98, 1996.
233. de Gramont A, Figer A, Seymour M, et al. A randomized trial of leucovorin and 5-fluorouracil with or without oxaliplatin in advanced colorectal cancer [abstract]. Proc Am Soc Clin Oncol 17:985, 1998.
234. Meropol NG, Budman DR, Creaven PK, et al. A phase I study of continuous twice daily treatment with capecitabine in patients with advanced and/or metastatic solid tumors [abstract]. Ann Oncol 7:298, 1996.
235. Taguchi T, Ishitani K, Saitoh K, et al. A Japanese phase I study of continuous twice daily treatment with capecitabine in patients with advanced and/or metastatic solid tumors [abstract]. Ann Oncol 7:299, 1996.
236. Hughes M, Planting A, Twelves C, et al. A phase I study of intermittent twice daily oral therapy with capecitabine in patients with advanced and/or metastatic solid cancer [abstract]. Ann Oncol 7:297, 1996.
237. Dirix LY, Bissett D, Van Oosterom AT, et al. A phase I study of capecitabine in combination with oral leucovorin in patients with advanced and/or metastatic tumours [abstract]. Ann Oncol 7:5980, 1996.
238. Findlay M, Van Cutsem E, Kocha W, et al. A randomized phase II study of Xeloda (capecitabine) in patients with advanced colorectal cancer [abstract]. Proc Am Soc Clin Oncol 16:798, 1997.
239. Pazdur R. Vincent M. Raltitrexed (Tomudex) versus 5-fluorouracil and leucovorin in patients with advanced colorectal cancer: results of a randomized, multicenter, North American trial [abstract]. Proc Am Soc Clin Oncol 16:801, 1997.
240. Harper P. Advanced colorectal cancer: results from the latest Tomudex (raltitrexed) comparative study [abstract]. Proc Am Soc Clin Oncol 16:802, 1997.
241. Cunningham D, Zalcerg JR, Rath U, et al. Final results of a randomized trial comparing Tomudex (raltitrexed) with 5-fluorouracil plus leucovorin in advanced colorectal cancer. Ann Oncol 7:961–965, 1996.
242. Balch CM, Urist MM, Soong SJ, et al. A prospective phase II clinical trial of continuous FUDR regional chemotherapy for colorectal metastases to the liver using a totally implantable pump. Ann Surg 198:567–573, 1983.
243. Niederhuber JE, Ensminger W, Gyves J, et al. Regional chemotherapy of colorectal cancer metastatic to the liver. Cancer 53:1336–1343, 1984.
244. Reed ML, Vaitkevicius VK, Al-Sarraf M, et al. The practicality of chronic hepatic artery infusion therapy of primary and metastatic hepatic malignancies: ten-year results in 124 patients in a prospective protocol. Cancer 47:402–409, 1981.
245. Weiss GR, Garnick MB, Osteen RT, et al. Long-term hepatic arterial infusion of 5-fluorodeoxyuridine for liver metastases using an implanted infusion pump. J Clin Oncol 1:337–344, 1983.
246. Kemeny MM, Goldberg DA, Browning S, et al. Experience with continuous regional chemotherapy and hepatic resection as treatment of hepatic metastases from colorectal primaries. A prospective randomized study. Cancer 55:1265–1270, 1985.
247. Kemeny N, Daly J, Oderman P, et al. Hepatic artery pump infusion: toxicity and results in patients with metastatic colorectal carcinoma. J Clin Oncol 2:595–600, 1984.

248. Riether RD, Khubchandani IT, Sheets JA, et al. A prospective study of continuous hepatic perfusion with implantable pump. Dis Colon Rectum 28:24–26, 1985.
249. Kemeny N, Seiter K, Niedzwiecki D, et al. A randomized trial of intrahepatic infusion of fluorodeoxyuridine with dexamethasone versus fluorodeoxyuridine alone in the treatment of metastatic colorectal cancer. Cancer 69:327–333, 1991.
250. Hohn DC, Roh M, Chase J, et al. Prohibitive toxicity with hepatic arterial infusion of low-dose floxuridine and folinic acid for colorectal liver metastases. Proc Am Soc Clin Oncol 10:459, 1991.
251. Kemeny N, Conti JA, Cohen A, et al. Phase II study of hepatic arterial floxuridine, leucovorin, and dexamethasone for unresectable liver metastases from colorectal carcinoma. J Clin Oncol 12:2288–2295, 1994.
252. Tandon RN, Bunnell IL, Cooper RG. The treatment of metastatic carcinoma of the liver by the percutaneous selective hepatic artery infusion of 5-fluorouracil. Surgery 73:118–121, 1973.
253. Ansfield FJ, Ramirez G. The clinical results of 5-fluorouracil intra-hepatic arterial infusion in 528 patients with metastatic cancer to the liver. Prog Clin Cancer 7:201–206, 1978.
254. Petrek JA, Minton JP. Treatment of hepatic metastases by percutaneous hepatic arterial infusion. Cancer 43:2182–2188, 1979.
255. Grage TB, Vassilopoulos PP, Shingleton WW, et al. Results of a prospective randomized study of hepatic arterial infusion with 5-fluorouracil versus intravenous 5-fluorouracil in patients with hepatic metastases from colorectal origin. Surgery 86:550–555, 1979.
256. Berger M. Hepatic infusion for metastatic colorectal cancer in a community hospital setting [abstract]. Proc Am Soc Clin Oncol 22:456, 1981.
257. Adson MA, van Heerden JA, Adson MH, et al. Resection of hepatic metastases from colorectal cancer. Arch Surg 119:647–651, 1984.
258. Oberfield RA, McCafferey JA, Polio J, et al. Prolonged and continuous percutaneous intra-arterial hepatic infusion chemotherapy in advanced metastatic liver adenocarcinoma from colorectal primary. Cancer 44:414–423, 1979.
259. Stagg RJ, Venook AP, Chase JL, et al. Alternating hepatic intra-arterial floxuridine and fluorouracil: a less toxic regimen for treatment of liver metastases from colorectal cancer. J Natl Cancer Inst 83:423–428, 1991.
260. Patt Y, Mavligit GM, Chaung VP, et al. Percutaneous hepatic arterial infusion of mitomycin C and floxuridine: an effective treatment for metastatic colorectal cancer to the liver. Cancer 46:261–265, 1980.
261. Shepard KV, Levin B, Karl RC, et al. Therapy for metastatic colorectal cancer with hepatic artery infusion chemotherapy using a subcutaneous implanted pump. J Clin Oncol 3:161–169, 1985.
262. Hatfield AK, Kammer BA, Danley RA, et al. Intermittent hepatic artery perfusions for symptomatic metastatic colon carcinoma [abstract]. Proc Am Soc Clin Oncol 1:102, 1982.
263. Theodors A, Bukowski RM, Lavery I, et al. Hepatic artery infusion with 5-fluorouracil and mitomycin-C in metastatic colorectal carcinoma phase II study. Med Pediatr Oncol 10:463–470, 1982.
264. Isenberg J, Fischbach R, Kruger I, et al. Treatment of liver metastases from colorectal cancer. Anticancer Res 16:1291–1295, 1996.
265. Patt YZ, Boddie AW Jr, Charnsangavej C, et al. Hepatic arterial infusion with floxuridine and cisplatin: overriding importance of antitumor effect versus degree of tumor burden as determinants of survival among patients with colorectal cancer. J Clin Oncol 4:1356–1364, 1986.
266. Cohen AM, Schaeffer N, Higgins J. Treatment of metastatic colorectal cancer with hepatic arterial combination chemotherapy. Cancer 57:1115–1117, 1986.
267. Wils J, Schlangen J, Naus A. Phase II study of hepatic artery infusion with 5-fluorouracil, adriamycin, and mitomycin C in liver metastases from colorectal carcinoma. Cancer Chemother Pharmacol 13:215–217, 1984.
268. Kemeny N, Cohen A, Seiter K, et al. Randomized trial of hepatic arterial floxuridine, mitomycin, and carmustine versus floxuridine alone in previously treated patients with liver metastases from colorectal cancer. J Clin Oncol 11:330–335, 1993.
269. Kemeny N, Reichman B, Oderman P, et al. Update of randomized study of intrahepatic vs systemic infusion of fluorodeoxyuridine in patients with liver metastases from colorectal carcinoma. Proc Am Soc Clin Oncol 5:89, 1986.
270. Hohn DC, Stagg RJ, Fridman MA, et al. A randomized trial of continuous intravenous versus hepatic intra-arterial fluorodeoxyuridine in patients with colorectal cancer metastatic to the liver: the Northern California Oncology Group Trial. J Clin Oncol 7:1646–1654, 1989.
271. Chang AE, Schneider PD, Sugarbaker PH, et al. A prospective randomized trial of regional versus systemic continuous 5-fluorodeoxyuridine chemotherapy in the treatment of colorectal liver metastases. Ann Surg 206:685–693, 1987.
272. Martin JK, O'Connell MJ, Wieand HS, et al. Intra-arterial floxuridine vs systemic fluorouracil for hepatic metastases from colorectal cancer. Arch Surg 125:1022–1027, 1990.
273. Rougier P, LaPlanche A, Huguier M, et al. Hepatic arterial infusion of floxuridine in patients with liver metastases from colorectal carcinoma: long-term results of a prospective randomized trial. J Clin Oncol 10:1112–1118, 1992.
274. Allen-Mersh TG, Earlam S, Fordy C, et al. Continuous hepatic artery floxuridine infusion prolongs overall and normal-quality survival in colorectal liver metastases patients. Proc Am Soc Clin Oncol 13:202, 1994.
275. Harmantas A, Rotstein LE, Langer B. Regional versus systemic chemotherapy in the treatment of colorectal carcinoma metastatic to the liver. Is there a survival difference? Meta-analysis of the published literature. Cancer 78:1639–1645, 1969.
276. Venook AP, Bergsland EK, Ring E, et al. Gene therapy of colorectal liver metastases using a recombinant adenovirus encoding WT P53 (SCH 58500) via hepatic artery infusion: a phase I study [abstract]. Proc Am Soc Clin Oncol 17:1661, 1998.
277. Rosen CB, Nagorney DM, Taswell HF, et al. Perioperative blood transfusions and determinants of survival after liver resection for metastatic colorectal carcinoma. Ann Surg 216:493–505, 1992.
278. Cady B, Stone MD, McDermott WV, et al. Technical and biological factors in disease-free survival after hepatic resection for colorectal cancer metastases. Arch Surg 127:561–569, 1992.
279. Hughes KS. Resection of the liver for colorectal carcinoma metastases: a multi-institutional study of indications for resection. Surgery 103:278–288, 1988.
280. Scheele J, Stangl R, Altendorf-Hofmann A, et al. Indicators of prognosis after hepatic resection for colorectal secondaries. Surgery 110:13–29, 1991.
281. Pettavel J, Morgenthaler F. Protracted arterial chemotherapy of liver tumors: an experience of 107 cases over a 12-year period. Prog Clin Cancer 7:217–233, 1978.
282. Goslin R, Steele G, Zamcheck N, et al. Factors influencing survival in patients with hepatic metastases from adenocarcinoma of the colon or rectum. Dis Colon Rectum 25:749–754, 1982.

CHAPTER 90

GASTROINTESTINAL CANCERS

Judy L. Chase, Dina K. Patel, VanAnh Trinh, and Richard D. Lozano

The gastrointestinal system is one of the most common sites of cancer in humans. This chapter will focus on colorectal, pancreatic, and gastric cancer. Hepatocellular (primary liver cancer) is discussed in detail in Chapter 89, Liver Tumors. Other gastrointestinal cancers that occur less frequently and that are not covered in this chapter include esophageal, biliary, small intestine, gallbladder, and appendiceal neoplasms.

TREATMENT GOALS: GASTROINTESTINAL CANCERS

- In general, surgery is the primary treatment and usually the only curative modality currently available. Early-stage disease can be treated with curative intent.
- Advanced, surgically unresectable disease is treated with palliative chemotherapy, radiation, or both. Response rates and survival of patients with advanced disease remain poor.

Colorectal Cancer

EPIDEMIOLOGY

Incidence

In the United States, more than 130,000 new cases of colorectal cancer are diagnosed yearly, representing approximately 15% of all cancer diagnoses.[1] Incidence rates for colorectal cancer have declined in recent years from a high of 53 per 100,000 in 1985 to 44 per 100,000 in 1994.[1] Overall, in the United States it is estimated that approximately 1 in 17 people will develop colorectal cancer in

Table 90.1 ▪ Risk Factors for Colorectal Cancer

Dietary	**Preexisting disease**
High animal fats and meat	Inflammatory bowel disease
Low fiber	Colorectal cancer
Genetic	Pelvic irradiation for cancer
Familial adenomatous polysis syndrome	Neoplastic colorectal polyps
Gardner's, Oldfield's, or Turcot's syndrome	**General**
Familial	All men and women over age 40
Familial colorectal cancer syndrome	Previous cholecystectomy
Hereditary adenocarcinomatosis syndrome	Previous ureterosigmoidostomy
Family history of colorectal cancer	

their lifetime. North America, Australia, New Zealand, and portions of Europe have the highest incidence of the disease. Africa and other underdeveloped countries tend to have a low incidence of colorectal cancer. In the United States, the median age at diagnosis is 70 for men and 73 for women, with the age-specific incidence rising steadily from the second to the ninth decade. Approximately 50,000 deaths per year are attributed to colorectal cancer in the United States, accounting for about 10% of cancer deaths.[1] The incidence appears to be relatively equally distributed between the sexes, with a slight male predominance. Colorectal cancer rates, unlike those for cancers of the lung, cervix, and prostate, show little socioeconomic correlation in the United States and other developed countries.

In the United States, the Seventh Day Adventists and Mormon religious groups have a diminished risk for colorectal cancer. The 20 to 50% reduction in risk is probably attributed to religious practices prohibiting alcohol and tobacco use and promoting some form of dietary moderation.[2,3]

Etiology

A specific cause of colorectal cancer has not been identified. Clinical risk factors include dietary practices, genetic factors, familial syndromes, other preexisting diseases, and advancing age (Table 90.1). Epidemiology and animal studies have determined that diets rich in animal fats and poor in fiber are associated with an increase in the risk of the disease.[4] Dietary fat may enhance colorectal carcinogenesis by a number of mechanisms. Dietary fat increases the production of secondary bile acids, which promote tumorigenesis and increase the proliferative activity of intestinal crypt cells.[5] Dietary fat may also enhance the damaging activity of intraluminal free fatty acids to the intestinal epithelium.[6]

Another correlate of dietary fat intake and the risk of colorectal cancer is meat consumption. In industrialized countries, including the United States, meat is the major source of dietary fat, and high-fat diets tend to be high in meat intake. It is still unclear whether the association of meat with colorectal cancer reflects the effect of fat, meat in general, or certain types of meat.

A number of animal, case control human, and epidemiologic studies have assessed the influence of dietary fiber on risk of colorectal cancer. The majority have found dietary fiber to be protective. The most widely accepted mechanism reflects the stool-bulking characteristics of dietary fiber. By increasing stool bulk, the concentration of potentially carcinogenic or epithelium-damaging agents are diluted out in the bowel lumen.[7] A second explanation involves dietary fiber enhancing fermentation by gut bacteria. This fermentation produces short-chain fatty acids that decrease the intraluminal pH, which may decrease the solubility and ionization of both free bile acids and free fatty acids, thus reducing the risk of colorectal cancer.[8] Third, some dietary fiber metabolites, such as butyrate, may have antineoplastic properties of their own.[9] However, a recent prospective study of 88,757 women by Fuchs and colleagues[10] concluded that their data did not support the existence of an important protective effect of dietary fiber against colorectal cancer. Other dietary factors, such as alcohol intake, have been studied and have produced conflicting data. Several epidemiologic studies have reported a direct association between alcohol ingestion and colorectal cancer, whereas other studies have found minimal or no association. A meta-analysis concluded that alcohol consumption and the increased risk of colorectal cancer was at best small, and no clear causative role could be established.[11]

Multiple genetic factors have been implicated in the development of colorectal cancer. First-degree relatives of persons with colorectal cancer have a threefold increased risk of developing the disease, thereby conferring a genetic etiology. Familial adenomatous polyposis is a rare inherited condition characterized by hundreds of large intestinal polyps. The majority of patients with this disease develop colorectal cancer by age 30. The extent to which other genetic factors, either in isolation or combined with environmental factors, contribute to the development of colorectal cancer requires continued research.

PATHOPHYSIOLOGY

Approximately 70% of all colorectal cancers occur in the sigmoid colon and rectum. The remainder occur in decreasing frequency in the ascending colon (16%), the transverse colon and splenic flexure (8%), and the descending colon (6%). Histologically, adenocarcinoma accounts for 90 to 95% of colorectal tumors. The remaining 5 to 10% of large bowel tumors are squamous cell carcinomas, undifferentiated carcinomas, rectal carcinoid, or, very rarely, sarcomas. The adenocarcinomas are further classified by grade. The grade is based on the degree of tumor differentiation, reflected by structural and cytologic features of the specimen. Grade 1 is the most differentiated, with well-formed tubules and the least nuclear polymorphism and mitoses. Grade 3 is the least differentiated, with only occasional glandular structures, and grade 2 is intermediate between grades 1 and 3. Poorly differentiated tumors are associated with a poor prognosis. Two histologic subtypes of colorectal adenocarcinoma, colloid or mucinous adenocarcinoma and signet ring cell carcinoma, are both associated with a more aggressive clinical course. They tend to occur more frequently in individuals less than 40 years of age. They also tend to be poorly differentiated and associated with a poor prognosis.

Colorectal adenocarcinomas tend to remain superficial for a long period of time, growing first into the lumen of the bowel, then slowly invading the deeper layers of the intestinal wall. The extent of tumor invasion into the bowel wall correlates both with the presence of lymph node metastases and, ultimately, patient survival. Colorectal cancer may spread by direct invasion of adjacent tissues and metastasize via lymphatic and hematogenous routes. The liver is the most common site of hematogenous metastases, followed by the lung. Involvement of other sites in the absence of liver or lung metastases is rare.

CLINICAL PRESENTATION AND DIAGNOSIS

Signs and Symptoms

The signs and symptoms of colorectal cancer are often subtle and nonspecific. Many patients may be completely asymptomatic and have colorectal cancer detected via routine screening procedures. The symptoms that are most commonly associated with colorectal cancer are the passage of blood around the stool or on the toilet paper; abdominal pain, which is frequently crampy and intermittent; and a change in bowel habits. The passage of bright red blood is most often seen with cancers of the rectum or sigmoid colon. Melena may result from right-sided colon tumors or obstructing tumors that retard the passage of fecal contents. Unexplained iron deficiency anemia may be the first sign in otherwise asymptomatic patients, especially in tumors located in the proximal colon. Any persistent change in bowel habits should be considered suspicious and deserves further evaluation. Such a change may be newly developed diarrhea, constipation, rectal pressure, or a change in stool caliber. These symptoms may mimic those of other bowel disorders such as diverticular disease, irritable bowel disease, or inflammatory bowel disease. More advanced colorectal cancer may produce unexplained weight loss. When compared with proximal colon cancers, left-sided tumors typically cause obstructive symptoms earlier in the disease course because stool in the distal colon is more solid and therefore less likely to pass easily through a narrowed lumen. Conversely, right-sided tumors can grow larger and into advanced disease and remain virtually asymptomatic.

Physical examination is usually unrevealing in early colorectal cancer. In advanced disease, a palpable abdominal mass, signs of bowel obstruction or perforation, hepatomegaly, or ascites may be present.

Screening

The natural history of colorectal cancer often involves a prolonged period of growth whereby many patients remain asymptomatic until advanced disease is present. Colorectal cancer presents a major health risk to the population, and routine screening of asymptomatic patients with the hope of early detection is recommended. The primary care physician should develop a colorectal screening strategy for adult patients as part of an annual physical examination. The screening program should include stool guaiac testing, digital rectal examination, and a flexible sigmoidoscopy. The routine screening procedures are listed in Table 90.2. Stool guaiac for occult blood may be useful as a means of early detection. Stool guaiac testing is not without problems. A negative test does not assure the absence of large bowel cancer and therefore should not be relied on as the sole screening test. Colonoscopy should be used for screening purposes in high-risk patients. Routine screening of individuals at average risk should begin at age 50. Individuals with high-risk factors (personal past history of colorectal cancer or adenomas, a family history of colorectal cancer or adenomas, inflammatory bowel disease) should begin screening at an earlier age. Patients with signs or symptoms of colorectal cancer are not candidates for screening but should be referred for a definitive examination and evaluation of their entire large bowel.

Diagnosis

Patients with any symptoms suggestive of colorectal cancer or a history of polyps should proceed with specific studies to establish a definitive diagnosis. The most widely used diagnostic tests are double-contrast barium enema and colonoscopy.[12] Colonoscopy is somewhat more sensitive than barium enema and offers the advantages of direct visualization of the tumor and the ability to biopsy lesions for immediate tissue diagnosis. However, colonoscopy tends be more expensive than barium enema. The double-contrast barium enema involves the rectal administration of barium combined with distension of the bowel lumen with air. The barium outlines the colonic wall and may reveal lesions as small as 1 to 2 cm. However, barium enema often cannot differentiate an early colon cancer from a benign polyp. Barium enema may be helpful in assessing the remainder of the bowel in patients in whom the colonoscope cannot be passed beyond the tumor

Table 90.2 ▪ Recommendations for Colorectal Cancer for the General Population

Procedure	Frequency
Digital rectal examination	Annual
Fecal occult blood tests	Annual
Flexible sigmoidoscopy/colonoscopy	Every 3–5 years

Table 90.3 ▪ TNM Staging Classification for Colorectal Cancer

Primary Tumor (T)

TX	Primary tumor cannot be assessed
T0	No evidence of primary tumor
T_{is}	Carcinoma in situ
T1	Tumor invades submucosa
T2	Tumor invades muscularis propria
T3	Tumor invades through muscularis propria into subserosa or into nonperitonealized pericolic or perirectal tissues
T4	Tumor directly invades other organs or structures or perforates visceral peritoneum

Regional Lymph Nodes (N)

NX	Regional lymph nodes cannot be assessed
N0	No regional metastasis
N1	Metastasis in 1 to 3 regional lymph nodes
N2	Metastasis in 4 or more regional lymph nodes

Distant Metastasis (M)

MX	Distant metastasis cannot be assessed
M0	No distant metastasis
M1	Distant metastasis

Stage Grouping

AJCC/UICC				Dukes
Stage 0	T_{is}	N0	M0	–
Stage I	T1	N0	M0	A
	T2	N0	M0	–
Stage II	T3	N0	M0	B
	T4	N0	M0	–
Stage III	Any T	N1	M0	C
	Any T	N2	M0	–
Stage IV	Any T	Any N	M1	

because of a narrowed bowel lumen. Therefore, barium enema and colonoscopy are often used together.

No blood tests are effective in identifying colorectal cancer. Carcinoembryonic antigen (CEA) is a tumor marker that can be measured in the blood and may be elevated in colorectal cancer. It is not specific to colorectal cancer, because it may be elevated in other gastrointestinal and nongastrointestinal malignancies. A marked elevation in CEA may indicate metastatic disease, especially to the liver, and may warrant further workup.[13] A normal or low preoperative level does not guarantee a small or localized primary lesion. CEA may be useful in screening after curative resection and in monitoring response to treatment; however, it should not be used as the sole screening or monitoring method. Other laboratory tests that should be included in the diagnostic workup are not specific to colorectal cancer and include the usual preoperative evaluations such as complete blood count, differential, platelets, serum chemistry, liver panel, electrolytes, and coagulation profile. Chest x-ray is often requested as a part of the standard preoperative workup but is not required for diagnosis. It may be used to rule out metastatic disease to the lung in patients with an already confirmed diagnosis of colorectal cancer. Patients with a recently diagnosed advanced colorectal cancer may also undergo computed tomography (CT) or ultrasound of the abdomen to assess the presence or absence of liver metastases. However, this is not required as part of the standard diagnostic workup and is used in selected patients with symptoms or laboratory test suggestive of liver metastases. CT of the pelvis is recommended for large, palpable abdominal masses or rectal tumors that may be associated with genitourinary involvement. Endorectal ultrasound is a relatively new procedure that may provide more accurate assessment of the depth of invasion into the bowel wall and the nodal status of patients with rectal tumors. Thus endorectal ultrasound may be able to determine the stage of rectal tumors before surgery.

Staging and Prognosis

The staging of colorectal cancer has been complicated by the development of multiple staging systems, many of which use the same descriptors to represent different stages. The TNM and the Dukes' staging systems are the most widely used and are presented in Tables 90.3 and 90.4, respectively; however, the TNM system is used more commonly now. Most investigators agree that the single most important prognostic factor for survival or recurrence after curative surgical resection is stage of the cancer. The 5-year survival rate for stage I is 80 to 90%, stage II 70 to 80%, stage III 30 to 50%, and stage IV less than 10%.[14] Stage is determined by the depth of penetration through the bowel wall, the presence and number of positive lymph nodes, and the presence of distant metastatic disease. Other factors that have a negative influence on prognosis include lymphatic vessel invasion, blood vessel invasion, mucinous or signet cell tumor type, colonic obstruction or perforation, lack of rectal bleeding, age under 40, male sex, symptomatic at diagnosis, high-grade tumors, tumors located in the rectosigmoid area, and elevated preoperative CEA levels.[15]

TREATMENT

Stage I, II, or III Colorectal Cancer

Surgery

Surgery with curative intent is the primary treatment modality for stage I, II, or III (Dukes' A, B, or C) colorectal cancers. Cancers of the colon are removed by a wide resection of the primary lesion together with all surround-

Table 90.4 ▪ Dukes' System for Staging of Colorectal Cancer (Astler-Collier Modification)

A	Lesions limited to the mucosa, nodes negative
B1	Extension through the mucosa but within the bowel wall, nodes negative
B2	Extension through the bowel wall, nodes negative
B3	Tumors adhere to or invade adjacent structures, nodes negative
C1	B1 with positive nodes
C2	B2 with positive nodes
C3	B3 with positive nodes
D	Distant metastatic disease

ing tissue that contains lymph nodes to which the tumor is likely to spread.[16] The specific surgical procedure used depends on the location of the primary tumor and its corresponding lymphatic drainage. A standard procedure for tumors of the right colon (cecum, ascending colon) is a right hemicolectomy, for left-sided tumors (transverse and descending colon) a left hemicolectomy, and for sigmoid tumors a sigmoid colectomy. Tumors in the upper portion of the rectum are usually treated with a low anterior resection with reanastomosis. Low rectal tumors often require an anteroposterior resection and colostomy. If the tumor involves adjacent organs such as the small bowel, bladder, uterus, or ovaries, an en bloc resection of the entire area is indicated.

Resection of the primary tumor is often warranted in patients with incurable metastatic disease found operatively or postoperatively. Resection of the primary tumor is intended to avoid local complications of cancer growth such as bleeding/hemorrhage, obstruction/perforation, and pain. Resection of the primary tumor in this setting has no impact on survival but may be associated with an improved quality of life. Patients with rectal cancer and distant metastatic disease at the time of diagnosis may receive palliative radiotherapy to the primary lesion instead of surgical resection.

Adjuvant Therapy

Rationale

The administration of treatments aimed at occult microscopic disease that may remain after complete surgical resection of all gross disease is termed *adjuvant therapy*. The goal of treatment when no disease is present is to decrease the risk of recurrences and ultimately prolong survival. Adjuvant therapy may involve systemic therapy with chemotherapy, local-regional therapy with radiation, or both, depending on the natural history of the primary neoplastic disease being treated. It is indicated when there is a high likelihood of recurrence and the potential benefit outweighs the risk of morbidity and costs. To obtain maximal benefit, the adjuvant therapy should be administered when the potential tumor burden is minimal (i.e., as soon as feasible after the primary surgical treatment), and it must be administered in maximally tolerated doses.[17] For adjuvant chemotherapy, the availability of agents with proven efficacy against measurable disease is required, because there is no way to evaluate efficacy in the adjuvant setting (no measurable disease) until failure occurs.

As discussed, surgical excision is the primary treatment of colorectal cancer, with approximately 80% of patients diagnosed at a stage when all gross tumor can be surgically removed. However, nearly 50% of patients develop recurrent disease and die from metastatic disease. Therefore, treatment directed at occult disease after complete surgical resection of the primary disease is warranted in an attempt to decrease recurrence. The risk of recurrence and ultimately survival is highly dependent on stage. The range of recurrence rates for a stage I lesion is 0 to 13%; the range of rates for stage II lesions is 11 to 61%; and the range of rates for stage III lesions is 32 to 88%.[18] Approximately 60 to 84% of recurrences become apparent within 2 years, and treatment depends on location, size, patient performance status, and prior therapy. Because the risk of recurrence after resection of a stage I colorectal tumor is low, the cost-benefit ratio does not warrant adjuvant therapy for these patients. Adjuvant therapy for stage II and III lesions is discussed in the following section. Because there are anatomic, natural history, and therapeutic differences between colon and rectal tumors, adjuvant therapy for each is addressed separately.

Adjuvant Therapy for Colon Cancer

Initially, adjuvant therapy after potentially curative surgical resection for large bowel cancer was attempted using alkylating agents, nitrogen mustard and thiotepa. These drugs have not been shown to have activity in advanced colorectal cancer, and it is therefore not surprising that they were ineffective in the adjuvant treatment of colorectal cancer. Subsequent trials focused on the use of 5-fluorouracil (5-FU) and fluorodeoxyuridine because these drugs had produced some responses in patients with metastatic disease. These drugs were first used alone and then in combinations with other agents, including semustine, vincristine, and bacillus Calmette–Guérin (BCG). None of the single-agent or combination trials resulted in decreased recurrence rates or improved survival compared with untreated controls.[19]

Levamisole, an anthelmintic agent, attracted interest for cancer therapy because of its presumed immunomodulatory activity. In the early 1980s a small nonrandomized trial reported levamisole to have activity in the adjuvant setting for colon cancer.[20] Subsequent trials investigated levamisole alone and in combination with 5-FU in the hope of achieving additive activity. Levamisole combined with 5-FU has been found to significantly reduce the recurrence rate. In stage III disease levamisole plus 5-FU reduced the recurrence rate by 40% and death rate by 33% compared with no adjuvant therapy.[21] On the basis of these results, a Consensus Panel convened by the National Institutes of Health recommended levamisole plus 5-FU as standard adjuvant treatment for patients with stage III colon cancer.[22] The dosing regimen is presented in Table 90.5. Any trials investigating the adjuvant treatment of stage III patients should incorporate levamisole plus 5-FU as the control arm. In stage II disease, no clear benefit of adjuvant therapy has been established. Levamisole plus 5-FU produced some reduction in recurrence rates and slight improvement in survival; however, these results are not statistically significant. It is suggested that patients with stage II colon cancer and high risk of recurrence factors, such as tumor perforation, adherence to or invasion of adjacent organs, or unfavorable cellular kinetic pattern (ploidy), be offered adjuvant treatment with levamisole plus 5-FU.[19] The Israel Cooperative Oncology Group reported findings from their randomized trial comparing 5-FU plus leucovorin to 5-FU plus levamisole

Table 90.5 ▪ Adjuvant Therapy for Stage III Colon Cancer

Agents	Dosage
Levamisole plus 5-FU	50 mg orally three times daily × 3 days repeated every 2 weeks × 1 year 450 mg/m^2 IV daily × 5 days, then beginning on day 28 450 mg/m^2 IV once a week × 48 weeks
Leucovorin plus 5-FU	500 mg/m^2 weekly × 6 weeks for 6 cycles 500 mg/m^2 weekly × 6 weeks for 6 cycles
Leucovorin plus 5-FU	20 mg/m^2 IV daily × 5 days every 28 days for 6 months 425 mg/m^2 IV daily × 5 days every 28 days for 6 months
Levamisole plus leucovorin plus 5-FU	50 mg orally three times daily × 3 days repeated every 2 weeks × 1 year 500 mg/m^2 weekly × 6 weeks for 6 cycles 500 mg/m^2 weekly × 6 weeks for 6 cycles

in the adjuvant setting. The results showed that there was equal efficacy between the two treatment arms and less toxicity associated with the 5-FU plus leucovorin group.[23]

The toxicity associated with levamisole includes nausea, vomiting, diarrhea, and dermatitis. These side effects are uncommon and usually mild. The toxicity associated with the levamisole plus 5-FU combination are those anticipated with 5-FU alone and include nausea, vomiting, diarrhea, stomatitis, dermatitis, and leukopenia. Again, the toxicity is usually mild and of short duration. Overall, the levamisole plus 5-FU combination is generally well tolerated.

5-Fluorouracil and leucovorin have been extensively studied in the treatment of metastatic colorectal cancer. As will be discussed later, the addition of leucovorin to 5-FU increases the response rates seen in metastatic disease compared with 5-FU alone. This has prompted the extensive investigation into the role of leucovorin plus 5-FU and the combination of leucovorin plus levamisole plus 5-FU in colon cancer adjuvant trials. A recent trial compared 5-FU plus leucovorin, 5-FU plus levamisole, and the combination of all three agents in approximately 2000 patients with stage II or III colorectal cancer. No significant differences were found among the three treatment arms with respect to disease-free or overall survival.[24]

Adjuvant Therapy for Rectal Cancer

Rectal cancer, which should be distinguished from colon cancer, is characterized by an increased risk of local recurrence and a comparable risk for distant metastases compared with colon cancer. The risk of local recurrence after surgical resection of a rectal tumor depends on disease extension beyond the rectal wall and the presence of lymph node involvement. Patients with tumor confined to the rectal wall and nodal involvement have a local recurrence rate of 20 to 40%. In patients with tumor extending beyond the rectal wall and negative lymph nodes, the recurrence rate is approximately the same, 20 to 35%. Patients with both tumor extending beyond the rectal wall and positive lymph nodes have a recurrence rate that is almost double, 40 to 70%.[25] Because of an increased risk of local recurrence with rectal cancer compared with colon cancer, adjuvant therapy has been approached with an increased emphasis on local-regional treatment with radiation therapy.

Postoperative radiation without chemotherapy has been shown to improve local control but has no effect on systemic recurrence or survival.[26–28] Adjuvant chemotherapy without radiation has been shown to decrease the incidence of systemic failure but has had no impact on local recurrence rates or survival. Adjuvant therapy using the combined modality approach of postoperative irradiation and chemotherapy has been shown to improve both local control and survival of resected high-risk rectal cancer patients.[28–30] The National Institutes of Health (NIH) Consensus Conference (1990) on adjuvant treatment of colon and rectal cancers recommends postoperative radiation and chemotherapy as standard adjuvant therapy for stage II and III rectal tumors.[22] The external beam pelvic radiation is usually delivered in doses of 50 to 55 Gy, combined with a 5-FU–based chemotherapy regimen. In the initial combined modality adjuvant trials, the chemotherapy consisted of 5-FU plus or minus methyl-CCNU. Current data suggest that in the adjuvant rectal setting, 5-FU alone affords equal efficacy and less toxicity than 5-FU plus methyl-CCNU when combined with radiation.[29,30] The best chemotherapy regimen is yet to be determined. Due to the positive results observed in colon cancer with continuous 5-FU, 5-FU plus levamisole, and 5-FU plus leucovorin, these chemotherapy regimens have recently been combined with radiation for the adjuvant treatment of rectal cancer. Tepper and colleagues[31] examined various combinations of 5-FU–based chemotherapy regimens (5-FU plus levamisole, 5-FU plus leucovorin, or 5-FU plus leucovorin and levamisole) combined with pelvic radiation in the adjuvant setting for rectal carcinoma. The initial results show no significant advantage with the addition of levamisole or with the three-drug combination.[31] Phase I and II trials are in progress to determine the role of oral UFT (uracil/tegafur), which is discussed in greater detail later in this chapter, with radiation therapy. UFT may provide an alternative for patients requiring continuous infusional 5-FU as a part of their combined-modality regimen.[32] Outside of a clinical trial, patients with stage II or III rectal cancer should receive adjuvant chemoradiation treatment with 50 to 55 Gy pelvic irradiation plus 5-FU or a 5-FU–based chemotherapy regimen.

There is some controversy regarding the sequencing of surgery and chemoradiation, because preoperative treatment appears to be equally beneficial and perhaps less toxic.[33] A theoretic advantage of preoperative irradiation is the potential damage to cells that may be spread locally or distantly at the time of resection. The major advantage of postoperative irradiation is the ability to avoid treatment of patients at low risk for local recurrence and those who have metastatic disease that was not diagnosed before surgery. Currently, it is suggested that any patient with rectal cancer in which the tumor penetrates through the bowel wall or has positive lymph nodes should receive adjuvant chemoradiation. Whether this therapy is administered preoperatively or postoperatively requires further clinical trials. Increased availability and expertise with endorectal ultrasound is required to determine the extent of bowel penetration and preoperative staging.

Advanced Colorectal Cancer (Stage IV)

Single-Agent Chemotherapy

Chemotherapy is usually the only feasible approach to controlling advanced (stage IV) colorectal cancer. The liver and lung are the most common sites of metastatic disease. Median survival of patients with advanced disease is usually only 6 to 10 months. For the most part, the treatment of advanced colorectal cancer is considered palliative. A few patients with small isolated liver metastases may undergo surgical resection, cryotherapy, or radiofrequency ablation, but this results in cure or long-term disease-free survival in only a small percentage of patients. The majority of patients with advanced or metastatic colorectal cancer may receive systemic chemotherapy that has no curative potential in an attempt to decrease symptoms and ultimately prolong survival. A number of single agents have been investigated, but the fluoropyrimidines are considered the mainstay of therapy for colorectal cancer.

5-FU is an antimetabolite that inhibits the formation of the DNA-specific nucleoside base thymidine. The main mechanism of action is believed to be inhibition of thymidylate synthase by FdUMP, the active metabolite of 5-FU. 5-FU exerts its major cytotoxicity during the S phase of the cell cycle. The plasma half-life of 5-FU is only 10 to 20 minutes, and the inhibition of thymidylate synthase after a bolus dose is also short.[34,35] Thus only a small fraction of cancer cells are susceptible to the toxic effects of 5-FU after bolus administration. This may theoretically limit the efficacy of 5-FU when administered by intravenous bolus. Infusional schedules have been investigated as a mechanism to overcome this limitation. 5-FU infusion durations ranging from 24 hours to greater than 10 weeks have been explored in clinical trials. Response rates for infusional 5-FU are generally 30 to 40%; however, no statistically significant survival advantage has been documented.[36] The commonly used dosage schedules for infusional 5-FU are presented in Table 90.6.[37–39] The dose-limiting toxicity of infusional 5-FU is usually mucositis, but may also include diarrhea or dermatitis; the dose-limiting toxicity of bolus 5-FU is usually myelosuppression, but may include mucositis and diarrhea. A distinct type of dermal toxicity, termed *palmar-plantar erythrodysesthesia* or *hand-foot syndrome,* may be seen in up to 30% of patients treated with prolonged infusions of 5-FU. This syndrome causes painful swelling and erythema of the hands and feet and may progress to painful desquamation. It is managed by prompt discontinuation of the 5-FU infusion at the onset of symptoms and reinstitution of treatment at reduced dosage after complete recovery from toxicity.

Combination Chemotherapy

Numerous combinations of chemotherapeutic agents have been explored in colorectal cancer. Most of these have combined one or more agents with 5-FU in an attempt to improve response rates. Drugs used in the combination regimens include 5-FU, cisplatin, semustine, mitomycin C, cyclophosphamide, DTIC, hydroxyurea, methotrexate, vincristine, and doxorubicin.[36] Thus far, no combination chemotherapy regimen has been shown to be superior to 5-FU alone and therefore cannot be recommended for use in colorectal cancer.

Biochemical Modulation of 5-FU

With the exception of the fluoropyrimidines, the virtual lack of available agents with activity against colorectal cancer has stimulated the search for methods to improve response rates with 5-FU. One method of overcoming the schedule dependence of 5-FU is to prolong the inhibition of thymidylate synthase by the coadministration of a reduced folate. Leucovorin (folinic acid, LCV) has been successfully used for this purpose. Leucovorin stabilizes the covalent bond between thymidylate synthase and FdUMP and thus increases the cytotoxicity of 5-FU.[40] Numerous studies have been completed using a variety of doses of leucovorin in combination with 5-FU. The response rates to 5-FU/leucovorin are 30 to 44%, a statistically significant improvement compared with 5-FU alone.[41–46] There also appears to be a trend toward improved survival with 5-FU/leucovorin, but this has reached statistical significance in only two studies thus far. Despite the lack of a clear-cut survival advantage, 5-FU plus leucovorin is considered standard therapy for ad-

Table 90.6 ▪ Infusional 5-FU Schedules for Advanced Colorectal Cancer

Infusion Duration	5-FU Dose	Frequency	Major Toxicity
24 hours	2.6 g/m²/day	Weekly	Myelosuppression Ataxia Mucositis
4–5 days	1.0 g/m²/day	Every 3–4 weeks	Mucositis
3–10 weeks	300 mg/m²/day	Continuous	Mucositis

vanced colorectal cancer by most oncologists at the present time. Doses for leucovorin have ranged from 15 to 500 mg/m^2/day, but data demonstrate that leucovorin doses of 20 mg/m^2/day effectively enhance 5-FU efficacy and are associated with less toxicity compared with high-dose leucovorin regimens.[43] Currently, the most commonly accepted dosage schedule of 5-FU/leucovorin incorporates the lower dosages of leucovorin. Some of the commonly used dosage schedules for the 5-FU plus leucovorin combination are presented in Table 90.7. It should be noted that, because of its mechanism of modulation, leucovorin should always be administered before or concomitantly with the 5-FU. The toxicity of the 5-FU and leucovorin combinations is qualitatively different from either the bolus or infusional 5-FU alone. In general, myelosuppression is not increased over what would be expected with 5-FU alone. However, lower doses of 5-FU are usually used when combined with leucovorin. Gastrointestinal toxicity in the form of diarrhea and mucositis is significantly increased with the addition of leucovorin and can produce life-threatening dehydration if not treated promptly. Hand-foot syndrome, which is rarely seen with bolus 5-FU, has been reported to occur frequently with the leucovorin plus 5-FU combination, even with bolus dosing.[46] A variety of other agents have been used to modulate the activity of 5-FU, including, but not limited to, methotrexate, interferon-α, dipyridamole, *N*-phosphonoacetyl-L-aspartate (PALA), and uridine.[47–50] However, more clinical research is required to determine the exact role of modulating agents in the treatment of colorectal cancer with 5-FU.

Regional Chemotherapy

Regional chemotherapy for the treatment of colorectal cancer usually refers to hepatic arterial infusion of chemotherapy for the treatment of liver metastases. This approach offers the advantage of substantially increasing the intensity of drug delivery to the liver while minimizing the systemic side effects. It is indicated in patients who have liver-only metastases and a good performance status. Hepatic arterial infusion for colorectal liver metastases is discussed in more detail in Chapter 89, Liver Tumors.

Table 90.7 ▪ Selected Dosage Schedules for 5-FU Plus Leucovorin in the Treatment of Advanced Colorectal Cancer

Drug	Dose, Route and Administration	Frequency
Leucovorin	20 mg/m^2 IV push, followed by	Times 5 days, repeated
5-FU	425 mg/m^2 IV push	Every 4–5 weeks
Leucovorin	500 mg/m^2 IV over 2–3 hours	Weekly
5-FU	600 mg/m^2 IV bolus during leucovorin	Weekly
Leucovorin	20 mg/m^2 IV push once weekly	Repeat every 5 weeks
5-FU	200 mg/m^2 IV continuous infusion × 28 days	
Leucovorin	200 mg/m^2 IV push	Times 5 days, repeated every 4–5 weeks
5-FU	370 mg/m^2 IV push	

FUTURE THERAPIES

New Agents

Irinotecan (CPT-11,Camptosar), a semisynthetic derivative of camptothecin, is a potent inhibitor of topoisomerase I, thereby causing DNA strand breaks and cell death. Phase II trials with irinotecan as first-line therapy for colorectal cancer revealed response rates of 19 to 32%. Irinotecan as second-line treatment of 5-FU–resistant colorectal carcinoma resulted in response rates of 13 to 25%.[51] A phase III multicenter randomized trial comparing irinotecan to infusional 5-FU in patients with metastatic colorectal cancer refractory to 5-FU showed significant improvement in overall survival in patients who received irinotecan.[52] Irinotecan has recently been approved by the Food and Drug Administration (FDA) as the standard second-line treatment for patients with advanced colorectal carcinoma. The recommended dose is 125 mg/m^2 IV weekly times 4 every 6 weeks. In vitro data suggest synergy between irinotecan and 5-FU; therefore, a variety of combinations of irinotecan and 5-FU are currently under investigation. The main toxicities associated with irinotecan are diarrhea (acute and delayed), myelosuppression, and nausea.[53,54] Recently, an alternative irinotecan dosing schedule of 350 mg/m^2 IV every 3 weeks has been approved for use in the United States. Toxicity with this regimen is similar to the weekly schedule.

Promising Investigational Agents

Oxaliplatin is a new third-generation platinum complex that exhibits increased therapeutic activity with reduced toxicity compared to cisplatin.

Oxaliplatin and 5-FU work synergistically. Phase II trials investigating different schedules of oxaliplatin plus 5-FU and leucovorin produced response rates of 46 to 58%.[55] The addition of oxaliplatin to the 5-FU and leucovorin combination increased the incidence and severity of toxicities. Oxaliplatin lacks nephrotoxicity, which is commonly associated with cisplatin and carboplatin. It has limited hematologic toxicity. The most common acute side effect seen with oxaliplatin is a transient peripheral neuropathy that is enhanced by exposure to cold.[55] Clinical trials have shown oxaliplatin to be active as a single agent and more effective in combination with 5-FU and leucovorin. There are still ongoing phase III trials expecting to confirm the role of oxaliplatin in treating colorectal cancer.

Raltitrexed (Tomudex) is a potent and specific thymidylate synthase inhibitor with activity in colorectal cancer. A 26% objective response rate has been reported in patients with advanced colorectal cancer.[56] In addition, in vitro studies have revealed synergistic activity with 5-FU. What makes raltitrexed an important agent in colorectal cancer is its lack of myelosuppression. The major toxicities associated with raltitrexed are asthenia, diarrhea, nausea, and vomiting. Raltitrexed is usually administered intravenously once every 21 days.

Capecitabine (Xeloda) is an orally administered prodrug of 5-FU. Capecitabine passes through the intestinal mucosa as an intact molecule and is then activated by a cascade of three enzymes that results in the intracellular release of 5-FU. Capecitabine is currently being investigated in patients who have failed 5-FU plus leucovorin, irinotecan, or both. The response rate is approximately 28% in patients with previously untreated metastatic colorectal carcinoma receiving 2500 mg/m^2/day PO on an intermittent schedule.[57] Side effects and toxicities are similar to those seen with infusional 5-FU such as hand-foot syndrome, diarrhea, nausea and vomiting, mucositis, and neutropenia.

Tegafur (ftorafur) is another 5-FU prodrug that has been combined with uracil to form a compound called UFT. Uracil inhibits the activity of hepatic dihydropyrimidine dehydrogenase (DPD), which is responsible for the elimination of greater than 80% of the administered 5-FU dose. UFT is administered orally and recently has been combined with oral leucovorin for the treatment of colorectal cancer. A 42% response rate has been reported in patients with advanced colorectal cancer.[58] The dose-limiting toxicity of this regimen is diarrhea. The oral dosing, initial response rates, and a favorable toxicity profile make UFT plus leucovorin an attractive alternative for the treatment of advanced colorectal cancer. Use of tegafur in the adjuvant setting also deserves further investigation.

There are a number of other oral products in addition to capecitabine and UFT, such as S-1 and 5-ethynyluracil, that are currently being studied for the treatment of colorectal cancer. These agents may best be used in the adjuvant setting due to their ease of administration and limited toxicity profile. They may also play a role as radiosensitizing agents for rectal cancer.

17-1a monoclonal antibody is a new agent that is being studied in the adjuvant setting. This antibody binds to a cell surface glycoprotein that is expressed preferentially on adenocarcinomas but also found on normal epithelial cells. Preclinical studies indicate that 17-1a monoclonal antibody induces antibody-dependent cell death. One clinical study in patients with stage III (Dukes' stage C) colorectal carcinoma revealed a 32% reduction in death rate and a 23% overall reduction in recurrence with 17-1a monoclonal antibody. Toxic effects were infrequent, with the most common effects being mild gastrointestinal symptoms.[59]

Table 90.8 ▪ Toxicities of Agents Used in Colorectal Cancer

Agent	Toxicities
5-fluorouracil (5-FU)	Nausea, vomiting, diarrhea, stomatitis, dermatitis, myelosuppression, palmar-plantar erythrodysesthesia
Leucovorin	Increased diarrhea and mucositis when administered with 5-FU
Levamisole	Nausea, vomiting, diarrhea, dermatitis
Irinotecan (CPT-11)	Diarrhea (acute and delayed), myelosuppression, nausea
Oxaliplatin	Peripheral neuropathy, mild myelosuppression, nausea, vomiting
Raltitrexed	Asthenia, diarrhea, nausea, vomiting
Capecitabine	Similar to those seen with infusional 5-FU
UFT	Diarrhea
17-1a monoclonal antibody	Mild gastrointestinal symptoms

Irinotecan, oxaliplatin, raltitrexed, capecitabine, and UFT plus leucovorin are important advances in the treatment of advanced colorectal cancer. The most efficacious dose and dosing schedule, reproducible response rates, and toxicity profiles, as well as the exact role of each of these agents in the treatment of colorectal cancer, require further investigation. In addition, continued research evaluating new agents, modulating agents, combination chemotherapy, and combined modality therapies is needed. Table 90.8 summarizes the toxicities associated with the agents used in the treatment of colorectal cancer.

CONCLUSION

Colorectal cancer is one of the most common malignancies and is a major health problem in the United States. Prevention and early detection programs have received attention in recent years as the incidence continues to rise, with a large proportion of patients diagnosed with already advanced disease. Prognosis has been directly associated with the depth of tumor invasion into or through the bowel wall. The initial treatment for colorectal cancer is surgery to remove the primary lesion and surrounding tissue. Adjuvant therapy for patients with localized disease has been shown to decrease recurrence rates and prolong survival. Treatment of advanced disease with chemotherapy remains palliative, and the results are limited by the availability of active agents. The fluoropyrimidines continue to be the most active and most commonly used agents in the treatment of colorectal cancer. Ongoing research evaluating biochemical modulation of 5-FU and identification of new agents will, it is hoped, yield increased response rates and improved survival in the future.

Pancreatic Cancer

EPIDEMIOLOGY

Incidence

Pancreatic cancer is a relatively rare malignancy, with approximately 29,000 new cases diagnosed in the United States in 1998.[1] The incidence has decreased slightly over the last two decades, primarily due to a steady decline in the rate for white males.[60–62] Carcinoma of the pancreas is mainly a disease of the elderly. More than 80% of cases occur between ages 60 and 80, and cases below age 40 are very rare.[60,62] There had been a slight male preponderance in the incidence, with male to female ratio being 1.7:1.0 in older epidemiologic studies.[61] This ratio gradually equalizes because the incidence rate has declined significantly in males since 1974.[60] Racial differences in incidence and mortality rates from pancreatic cancer have also been noticed. Incidence and mortality rates in blacks of both sexes are higher than in whites and other ethnic groups.[60] The incidence is higher in urban than in rural areas and higher in industrialized nations, implying that environmental factors play a role in the etiology.[63] Countries with a high incidence include Denmark, Sweden, Finland, Ireland, Austria, Czechoslovakia, Hungary, and certain areas of Canada.[63–65]

In the United States, approximately 28,900 deaths in 1998 are attributed to pancreatic cancer, making it the fourth most common cause of cancer death in both men and women.[1] Prognosis is dismal for patients diagnosed with pancreatic cancer, with median survival from the time of diagnosis being only 6 months.[61] Less than 5% of patients survive 5 years.[1,60] Carcinoma of the pancreas is one of the most aggressive solid tumors, representing a major public health problem and a significant clinical challenge.

Etiology

Many dietary and environmental factors have been implicated as possible etiologic factors in the development of pancreatic cancer, but definite causal relationships have not been established in the majority of cases. Strongest evidence points to cigarette smoking as a risk factor associated with pancreatic cancer. Results from animal studies suggest that nitrosamines in tobacco smoke are carcinogenic to the pancreas. Several case-control studies found a twofold to threefold increase in risk in smokers compared with nonsmokers.[66–70] Occupational exposure to certain chemicals has also been linked to an excess of pancreatic carcinoma. Employees of petroleum and chemical industries appear to be at especially high risk. Workers exposed to industrial solvents or petroleum products for more than 10 years have up to a fivefold increase in incidence of pancreatic cancer.[71] Stone miners, cement workers, gardeners, textile workers, and leather tanners are also among the high-risk group.[62,72] Numerous studies have examined the causative role of nutrition in the development of pancreatic cancer, with inconsistent results. Some found a positive correlation with total energy intake, carbohydrate ingestion, or meat consumption.[62,67,69] Others suggested a protective effect of diets high in fiber, fruits, and vegetables.[62] An increased risk for pancreatic cancer has also been attributed to alcohol or coffee consumption;[65,66] however, evidence is weak and inconsistent.

A connection between pancreatic malignancy and a number of medical conditions, such as diabetes mellitus and chronic pancreatitis, has long been suspected. Approximately 15% of patients diagnosed with pancreatic cancer have a history of diabetes mellitus, implying a causal relationship between diabetes mellitus and the development of pancreatic cancer.[73] However, in more than half of these patients, the onset of clinical diabetes preceded the diagnosis of pancreatic cancer by only a few months. This suggests that the cancer may cause insulin insufficiency, and diabetes manifesting many years before the diagnosis of pancreatic cancer would be better evidence for an etiologic correlation.[74] However, this line of reasoning has been counterbalanced by the argument that although the clinical diagnosis of diabetes was made very recent to the diagnosis of pancreatic cancer, undiagnosed diabetes may well have preceded the cancer by many years.[75] With regard to chronic inflammation of the pancreas, the issue remains controversial as well. Some studies have proposed a causal relationship between chronic pancreatitis and the development of pancreatic cancer.[76,77] However, others suggest that the long-term risk of pancreatic cancer in patients with chronic pancreatitis may actually be related to alcohol consumption, smoking, and selection bias.[78]

Recent advances in the understanding of human genetics have brought about an increasing appreciation for the hereditary influence on the etiology of pancreatic cancer. Abnormal changes in K-*ras*, an oncogene, or p53, p16, DPC4, and BRCA2, the tumor suppressor genes, have been linked with carcinoma of the pancreas.[79,80] Several genetic syndromes associated with pancreatic cancer, including hereditary pancreatitis, ataxia-telangiectasia, hereditary nonpolyposis colorectal cancer, familial atypical multiple mole-melanoma, Peutz-Jeghers, and familial breast cancer, have been described.[79,81,82] Identification of familial clusters of pancreatic cancer also facilitates genetic study of the disease. Although the overall percentage of pancreatic carcinoma that shows familial clustering remains uncertain, a crude estimate suggests that as many as 3 to 5% of all pancreatic cancers have a hereditary origin.[83]

PATHOPHYSIOLOGY

The pancreas lies transversely in the posterior part of the upper abdomen. The head of the pancreas is on the right side of the abdomen and rests against the curve of the duodenum. The body of the pancreas lies beneath the stomach, and the tail of the pancreas extends across the abdomen to the left side. The pancreas is virtually surrounded by other organs in the upper abdomen. However, unlike other organs, it cannot be palpated because of its posterior location. Because of its position and large functional reserve, symptoms of pancreatic disease, including cancer, often do not appear until the disorder is far advanced.

The pancreas is both an endocrine and an exocrine organ. Most tumors (95%) occur in the exocrine portion. Tumors of the endocrine portion are usually benign, whereas only 2% of tumors arising in the exocrine portion of the pancreas are benign. Malignant tumors may arise from pancreatic ductal epithelial cells, acinar cells, connective tissue, or lymphatic tissue. Histologically, ductal adenocarcinoma accounts for more than 80% of all pancreatic malignancies. The head of the pancreas is the site for approximately 60% of all pancreatic tumors, with 15% occurring in the body and tail, and 20% diffusely involving the gland.[84]

On gross examination, tumors of the pancreas usually appear hard, gritty, and whitish. The surrounding tissue often displays evidence of chronic pancreatitis. Tumors in the head of the pancreas are usually less than 5 cm in diameter at diagnosis and are often associated with pancreatic and common bile duct obstruction, adjacent duodenum invasion, and portal vein or superior mesentery artery occlusion. Tumors occurring in the tail of the pancreas are usually larger (5 to 10 cm) at the time of diagnosis and associated with splenic vein obstruction. Early subclinical metastases are characteristic of pancreatic cancer. Less than 20% of patients have disease confined to the pancreas at the time of diagnosis. Forty percent of patients have locally advanced (regional lymph nodes, adjacent organs) disease, and more than 40% have distant metastases at diagnosis.[60] The most commonly involved distant organ is the liver, followed by lung, bone, and brain.

CLINICAL PRESENTATION AND DIAGNOSIS

Signs and Symptoms

The early symptoms of pancreatic cancer tend to be very nonspecific and insidious in nature, thus delaying diagnosis in 80 to 90% of patients. Pain is the single most common presenting symptom and is usually the reason why patients seek medical attention. Pain, described as dull, constant, and radiating to the middle and upper back, is attributed to tumor invasion of the celiac and mesenteric plexus.[85–87] Because most tumors arise in the ductal system, biliary obstruction is common. Obstructive jaundice occurs in approximately 50% of all patients with pancreatic cancer and in up to 90% of patients with tumors in the head of the pancreas.[88] Obstructive jaundice is generally associated with less advanced disease because it forces patients to seek medical attention when the tumor is still localized and potentially resectable. Nausea, anorexia, weight loss, and fatigue are among the common complaints at presentation and can be attributed to both obstructive jaundice and gastrointestinal obstruction.[85,88] Pancreatic endocrine and exocrine insufficiency have also been reported, causing glucose intolerance, malabsorption, and steatorrhea.

Pancreatic cancer may spread by invading surrounding tissues or by metastasizing to distant sites. Direct invasion into the abdominal lymph nodes, liver, and gastroduodenum is often present at diagnosis. The liver and peritoneum are the most common sites of distant metastases and may be present in up to 40% of patients at the time of diagnosis. Less common sites of metastases include the lung, bone, and brain. The natural history of pancreatic cancer is highlighted by the early development of widespread metastatic disease, and death is often secondary to liver failure and malnutrition.[61]

Diagnosis

Because the symptoms of pancreatic cancer tend to be nonspecific and are often attributed to other medical conditions, a high index of suspicion is necessary to make an accurate and timely diagnosis. Pancreatic cancer should be included in the differential diagnosis of any patient with unexplained jaundice, pancreatitis, weight loss, and nonspecific upper abdominal or back pain. The goal of medical evaluation in a patient with suspected pancreatic cancer is to establish the presence or absence of a primary tumor, and if one is present to determine the extent of local and metastatic disease. The diagnostic evaluation usually begins with a physical examination to establish clinical correlation such as jaundice, weight loss, palpable mass, ascites, or metastatic disease. Blood tests are obtained to help evaluate jaundice, liver function, and pancreatic function. Serum amylase, lipase, alkaline phosphatase, and leucine aminopeptidase may increase in patients with pancreatic cancer. If the tumor involves the liver, levels of lactic dehydrogenase and the transaminases may be also be elevated.

The diagnostic workup continues with noninvasive radiologic studies and then, if necessary, proceeds to more invasive radiologic and endoscopic procedures, and eventually to tissue biopsy. Currently, contrast-enhancing helical CT is considered the mainstay imaging modality for both diagnostic and staging workup of pancreatic cancer.[89] Primary goals of CT are to detect the suspected pancreatic mass and to determine the resectability of the identified tumor. Many studies have confirmed the accuracy of helical CT in predicting resectability, with the resectability rate approaching 80%.[90] Although helical CT remains the preferred imaging test for diagnosis and staging of pancreatic cancer, it has its limitation in detecting small metastases to lymph nodes, liver, and peritoneum.[91]

More invasive procedures to aid in the diagnosis of pancreatic cancer include angiography, endoscopic retrograde cholangiopancreatography (ERCP), endoscopic ultrasonography (EUS), and laparoscopy. In the past, angiography was performed preoperatively to define vascular anomalies and to determine the anatomic relationship between the tumor and the major surrounding vessels. Currently, it has no place in the routine workup of pancreatic malignancy because helical CT can provide the same information.[91] ERCP does not provide additional diagnostic information if a pancreatic mass has been identified on CT. However, it still maintains an important role in the differential diagnosis of those patients who have a typical history of pancreatic cancer but do not have a pancreatic mass on CT.[61,91] In the absence of choledocholithiasis or a history of pancreatitis, obstructive lesions of the intrapancreatic portion of the common bile duct are almost always secondary to malignancy. Another role of ERCP is to place a stent to relieve obstructive jaundice in highly symptomatic patients who are not to be bypassed or resected shortly. EUS is a relatively new diagnostic tool developed for staging workup of pancreatic cancer. Using the wall of the stomach and duodenum as an acoustic window, EUS produces detailed images of the pancreas and can be helpful in detecting small intrapancreatic masses missed by CT. Its role in assessing vascular involvement is still controversial. EUS may also be used as a means of obtaining tissue biopsy and instituting celiac plexus neurolysis for pain management.[92] The role of EUS in the management of patients with pancreatic cancer has not yet been established. Some authors have advocated laparoscopy with peritoneal washing for cytology to further increase the resectability rate predicted by helical CT.[91,93] The peritoneum is the second most common site for pancreatic metastases; however, peritoneal seeding, typically a few millimeters in diameter, most likely fails to be detected by CT. Direct laparoscopic visualization of the peritoneum, omentum, and liver surface for tumor implants can potentially spare patients from an unnecessary laparotomy. However, more data are required to support the cost-effectiveness of the routine use of this procedure.

Once a suspected pancreatic mass is considered unresectable or if metastatic disease is present, histologic diagnosis should be obtained by direct fine-needle biopsy of the pancreas or percutaneous biopsy of a liver metastasis. If the tumor is considered resectable, the patient should be evaluated for surgery.

A variety of biologic substances identified in the serum of patients with pancreatic cancer may be considered tumor markers. At the current time, a number of potential markers have been identified, including CEA, tumor-associated carbohydrate antigen (CA 19-9), CA 125 antigen, and monoclonal antibody products (DUPAN-2, SPAN-1).[94] CEA is elevated in approximately 50% of patients with pancreatic cancer, but it is also increased in many other benign and malignant gastrointestinal diseases.[94] CA 19-9 is elevated in approximately 80% of patients with pancreatic cancer. Although there are some limitations to the clinical application of CA 19-9, reasonable data from worldwide studies support its promising role in the management of pancreatic cancer as a diagnostic adjunct, a prognostic indicator, and a monitoring tool.[95,96] CA 125 is elevated in less than 50% of patients with pancreatic cancer and is not clinically useful.[94] DUPAN-2 appears to be highly specific for identifying and following patients with pancreatic cancer, but it may also be elevated in patients with other gastrointestinal malignancies or diseases.[97] Further investigation into the development of more specific and sensitive tumor markers in pancreatic cancer is required before they will be considered to be consistently clinically useful.

Staging and Prognosis

The American Joint Committee on Cancer (AJCC) has developed staging criteria for adenocarcinoma of the pancreas. This system, also known as the TNM staging system, is based on the extent of the primary tumor, regional lymph nodes, and metastatic disease.[98] The TNM staging system is presented in Table 90.9. Unfortunately, this staging system is not clinically useful. It is difficult to apply because the lymph node status is difficult to assess without surgery. Moreover, the TNM stage does not correlate well with treatment or prognosis. Instead, for prognosis prediction and therapy decision, most centers

Table 90.9 ▪ TNM Staging System for Pancreatic Cancer

TX	Primary tumor cannot be assessed		
T0	No evidence of primary tumor		
T_{is}	Carcinoma in situ		
T1	Tumor limited to the pancreas ≤2 cm in greatest dimension		
T2	Tumor limited to pancreas >2 cm in greatest dimension		
T3	Tumor extends directly into any of the following: duodenum, bile duct, peripancreatic tissues		
T4	Tumor extends directly into any of the following: stomach, spleen, colon, adjacent large vessels		
NX	Regional lymph nodes cannot be assessed		
N0	Regional lymph nodes not involved		
N1	Regional lymph nodes involved		
pN1a	Metastasis in a single regional lymph node		
pN1b	Metastasis in multiple regional lymph nodes		
MX	Distant metastases cannot be assessed		
M0	No known distant metastases		
M1	Distant metastases present		
Stage 0	T_{is}	N0	M0
Stage I	T1–2	N0	M0
Stage II	T3	N0	M0
Stage III	T1–3	N1	M0
Stage IVA	T4	Any N	M0
Stage IVB	Any T	Any N	M1

Table 90.10 ▪ Clinical or Radiographic Staging System

Stage I	Resectable No local arterial or venous involvement No extrapancreatic disease
Stage II	Locally Advanced Local arterial or venous involvement No extrapancreatic disease
Stage III	Metastatic Distant metastases, typically to liver, peritoneum

rely on the clinical or radiographic staging system[61] (Table 90.10). It classifies pancreatic cancer into three groups: stage I disease is localized to the pancreas and is surgically resectable; stage II disease is locally advanced and not surgically resectable; stage III disease has metastatic spread. Obviously, patients with stage I disease have the best prognosis and are the only patients in whom the disease is curable. Unfortunately, less than 15% of patients are in stage I at the time of presentation. Most patients present with advanced disease–stage II or III–and are considered unresectable and incurable. These patients have a very poor prognosis, with less than 10% of them surviving 1 year after diagnosis.

TREATMENT

Surgery, radiation therapy, and chemotherapy are treatment options for patients with pancreatic cancer. Primary treatment goals vary with stage. For those patients with stage I disease, therapy is aimed toward a cure. With more advanced disease, the objectives of medical management are to prolong survival, palliate symptoms, and improve quality of life. Unfortunately, the available treatment options for this patient population have not significantly altered the natural history of the disease.

Localized, Resectable Pancreatic Cancer (Stage I)

Cancer of the pancreas usually manifests in advanced stages with local invasion into vital structures, making curative surgery an option for only a small number of patients. Before modern imaging technologies became available, laparotomy often revealed that the pancreatic malignancy was actually more advanced than what had been apparent on preoperative studies. Therefore, many patients ended up with incomplete tumor removal or palliative surgery. Unfortunately, data have shown that positive-margin resection does not provide additional survival benefit beyond what can be achieved with palliative chemoradiation alone.[99,100] Moreover, laparotomy carries with it a significant morbidity rate of 20 to 30% and a mean hospital stay of 3 to 4 weeks.[61]

Recently, high-quality helical CT has significantly increased the resectability rate, presuming strict observation of resectability criteria. For a resectable mass located in the head of the pancreas, a pancreaticoduodenectomy (Whipple procedure) is considered standard of care.[101] This operation involves the en bloc removal of the distal stomach and duodenum, the first portion of the jejunum, and the head and part of the body of the pancreas. Despite successful surgery with curative intent, the prognosis remains unfavorable even in this selected group of patients, with only 10 to 30% 5-year survival rates.[99] Long-term postoperative morbidity further reduces quality of life, with hemorrhage, infection, pancreatic fistula, and nutritional problems being the commonly encountered complications. Therefore, surgical procedures continue to be modified with an effort to improve cure rate and reduce morbidity. Currently, about one-third of all pancreatic surgeons in the United States advocate the pylorus-preserving Whipple procedure, in which the stomach and the pylorus are retained.[102] The potential advantage of this modification is that the nutritional sequelae of the standard pancreaticoduodenectomy, such as food dumping syndrome and diarrhea, can be avoided. So far, there is no evidence suggesting a survival disadvantage associated with this new surgical technique. Another surgical alternative is a total pancreatectomy,[103,104] which may have the advantage of preventing local recurrence. However, long-term survival rate after total pancreatectomy was not different from the Whipple procedure. Moreover, there are disadvantages associated with complete removal of the pancreas, such as pancreatic exocrine insufficiency and permanent diabetes mellitus requiring lifelong replacement therapy.

Incidence of local tumor recurrence status after curative resection is 50 to 80%. Patients who undergo pancreaticoduodenectomy alone have a median survival of 12 months. It is currently recommended that patients receive adjuvant treatment with chemoradiation to improve local-regional control. External-beam radiation therapy and concomitant 5-FU have been demonstrated to improve survival after curative resection by the Gastrointestinal Tumor Study Group (GITSG). The standard of care at the present is the delivery of 40 Gy in a split-course fashion plus 5-FU at 500 mg/m^2/day IV bolus for 3 days concurrently with each 20 Gy segment of radiation therapy. The 5-FU regimen is then continued weekly, beginning 1 month after completion of radiation, for a full 2 years. Median survival was 20 months with the multimodality approach compared with 11 to 12 months with surgery alone.[105,106]

Despite the clinical benefit of adjuvant chemoradiation, the delivery of multimodality therapy is delayed or omitted in 25% of patients due to prolonged recovery after pancreaticoduodenectomy.[107] This stems the interest in neoadjuvant chemoradiation. Preoperative chemoradiation offers several potential advantages. First, radiation appears to be more effective on well-oxygenated cells that have not been devascularized by surgery. Second, peritoneal tumor cell implantation due to surgical manipulation may be prevented by preoperative chemoradiation. Third, patients with disseminated disease evident on restaging after chemoradiation will not be subjected to laparotomy. Fourth, because chemoradiation is given first, delayed postoperative recovery will have no effect on the delivery of multimodality therapy.[61,108] Spitz and colleagues[107] have compared the neoadjuvant approach to the standard adjuvant chemoradiation. Preoperative radiotherapy was delivered at either 50.4 Gy in standard split course over 5.5 weeks or 30 Gy as rapid fractionation over 2 weeks. Postoperative irradiation was given to a total dose of 50.4 Gy in standard fractionation. Both preoperative and postoperative radiotherapy were carried out concomitantly with continuous-infusion 5-FU at 300 mg/m^2/day for 5 days weekly. At a median follow-up of 19 months, it was found that the delivery of preoperative and postoperative chemoradiation in patients who underwent potentially curative surgery for pancreatic adenocarcinoma led to similar treatment toxicity, patterns of tumor recurrence, and survival. This represents an approach to maximize the proportion of patients who receive all components of multimodality therapy and avoids the toxicity of pancreaticoduodenectomy in patients found to have metastatic disease at the time of restaging.

A novel approach of delivering chemoradiation involves the use of gemcitabine, a new pyrimidine antimetabolite, as a radiosensitizer. Recent evidence supporting gemcitabine's efficacy in the treatment of advanced pancreatic cancer, as well as its activity as a radiosensitizing agent, provides the rationale for the ongoing multi-institutional phase II study of preoperative external-beam radiation therapy and concomitant gemcitabine for patients with resectable adenocarcinoma of the pancreas.[108–111]

Another alternative to postoperative adjuvant chemoradiation is the use of electron-beam intraoperative radiation therapy (EB-IORT). EB-IORT is delivered after resection of the specimen but before initiating gastrointestinal reconstruction. Of note, EB-IORT prolongs the surgical procedure only an additional 30 to 40 minutes. The dose of EB-IORT ranges from 10 to 15 Gy. Initial results support the safety of adjuvant EB-IORT and suggest improved rates of local-regional control.[112,113] EB-IORT has also been added to preoperative chemoradiation and pancreaticoduodenectomy with good result. Pisters and colleagues[114] reported a median survival of 25 months at a median 37-month follow-up in the group of patients treated with preoperative chemoradiation, pancreaticoduodenectomy, and EB-IORT.

With better local-regional control with neoadjuvant or adjuvant chemoradiation, disease recurrence is primarily secondary to distant metastases. Prognosis remains dismal. The major barrier to progress in the treatment of pancreatic cancer lies in the absence of effective systemic therapies. Innovative therapeutic approaches continue to be developed and investigated in clinical trials, which will hopefully result in newer and more efficacious strategies to alter the natural history of the disease.

Localized, Unresectable Pancreatic Cancer (Stage II)

Patients who are found to have locally advanced unresectable disease at the time of operation can undergo palliative surgical bypass to correct impending biliary or gastrointestinal obstruction. These operations do not prolong survival, but they usually improve the quality of life for these patients. For treatment, patients with stage II disease can receive either 5-FU–based chemoradiation or gemcitabine.

Based on the results of a GITSG trial completed in 1981, patients with locally advanced pancreatic cancer who receive 5-FU–based chemoradiation have a median survival of about 10 months compared with 6 months in those who receive radiation alone.[115] Of note, the clinical benefit of chemoradiation is primarily limited to patients with good performance status. The optimal chemoradiation regimen is yet to be determined. In the GITSG trial, a split-course radiotherapy was delivered to a total dose of 40 to 60 Gy in combination with 5-FU at 500 mg/m^2/day IV bolus for the first 3 days of each 20 Gy course. Weekly maintenance 5-FU then followed at 500 mg/m^2 IV bolus for 2 years or until tumor progression. Several other combinations have also been used. With concurrent radiation, combination chemotherapy has not been proved to be superior to 5-FU alone[116,117]; therefore, it cannot be recommended. Many investigational radiotherapy techniques are currently being tested, including EB-IORT, high-energy particle-beam irradiation, and interstitial implantation of iodine-125.[112,113,118] Radiosensitizers other than 5-FU, such as bromodeoxyuridine, paclitaxel, cisplatin, and gemcitabine, have been looked at as well.[109–111,119,120] However, no randomized trials have been conducted to confirm the superiority of any of these modifications over the original regimen reported by the GITSG.

Gemcitabine, a pyrimidine antimetabolite, has been approved by the FDA as first-line therapy for both locally advanced and metastatic adenocarcinoma of the pancreas.[121–124] Gemcitabine is dosed at 1000 mg/m^2 weekly for 7 weeks followed by 1-week rest; each subsequent cycle is dosed at 1000 mg/m^2 weekly for 3 weeks followed by 1-week rest.[121] The advantage of gemcitabine in treating advanced pancreatic cancer lies in the clinical benefits it offers to patients with significant symptomatology. A randomized single-blinded phase III trial was conducted to compare the clinical benefit of 5-FU and gemcitabine in treating patients with advanced disease. The primary endpoint in this trial was the clinical benefit response measured by pain control, functional improvement, and weight gain.[125–127] Other secondary endpoints included time to tumor progression, median survival, and 1-year survival rate. At the conclusion of the trial, a significantly higher percentage of patients receiving gemcitabine experienced clinical benefit compared with those treated with 5-FU. Patients in the gemcitabine arm also had longer median survival and higher probability to survive 1 year than patients in the 5-FU arm. Toxicity was generally tolerable in both arms, with myelosuppression being the dose-limiting side effect for gemcitabine.[127] Because the major advantage of gemcitabine is symptomatic relief, it is reasonable to use gemcitabine in patients with poor performance status or with significant pain as an alternative to chemoradiation.

Metastatic Pancreatic Cancer (Stage III)

For patients with metastatic pancreatic cancer, systemic chemotherapy is the only treatment option. Until recently, the mainstay of therapy has been 5-FU, with modest response rate and little clinical benefit.[128] Several 5-FU doses and schedules have been used to treat metastatic carcinoma of the pancreas. To date, there is no consensus regarding the optimal dosing regimen for 5-FU in this clinical setting. Refer to Table 90.11 for commonly used dosing schedules, side effects, and monitoring parameters of 5-FU.

Attempts to modulate 5-FU activity with leucovorin, methotrexate, and interferon-α have failed to demonstrate additional therapeutic advantage.[129] To improve the disappointing results obtained with single-agent chemotherapy, combination chemotherapy has also been tried. Response rates with these combination regimens have ranged from 2 to 40%, with a median response rate of 20%.[130] This is not substantially different from the results seen with single-agent 5-FU.

Gemcitabine has provided some hope for patients with metastatic pancreatic cancer (Table 90.11). Despite its modest impact on survival, gemcitabine has been shown to significantly palliate pain and improve performance status. Due to its clinical benefit on symptomatology, gemcitabine has evolved to become the standard of care for patients with metastatic pancreatic cancer.[127]

FUTURE THERAPIES

With better local-regional control with chemoradiation, treatment failure and disease recurrence in patients with stage I or II disease are primarily secondary to distant metastases. Unfortunately, the available systemic chemotherapy has not significantly modified the natural history of the disease, necessitating the development of newer and more efficacious agents.

Marimastat represents a brand new class of chemotherapeutic agents, the matrix metalloproteinase inhibitors (MMPIs). Preclinical studies have shown that MMPIs can restrict the growth and regional spread of solid tumors, inhibit metastatic spread, and block neoplastic neovascularization. Marimastat is an oral MMPI with minimal

Table 90.11 ▪ Commonly Used Chemotherapeutic Agents in Pancreatic Cancer

Agent and Commonly Used Schedules	Side Effects	Monitoring Parameters	Comments
5-FU (bolus) 400–500 mg/m²/day × 5 days, repeated monthly	Nausea/vomiting	Control of nausea/vomiting	Level II emetogen Premedicate with phenothiazine antiemetic; have antiemetic available as needed
	Myelosuppression (primarily neutropenia)	CBC with differential and platelet Signs and symptoms (S/S) of infection or bleeding	
	Mucositis	S/S of mucositis Pain level Nutrition	Ensure good mouth care
	Diarrhea	Fluid and electrolytes Bowel habit S/S of dehydration	Instruct patients to report if three or more loose stools per day
	Photosensitivity		Instruct patients about photosensitivity
	Hair loss, nailbed changes		Usually partial hair loss
	Inflammation of tear ducts and lacrimal glands (dacryocystitis)		Instruct patients to report if eye problems occur Topical steroid may be useful for dacryocystitis
	Neurotoxicity	S/S such as headache, ataxia, confusion, nystagmus	Rare Discontinue 5-FU
Gemcitabine 1000 mg/m² weekly × 7 weeks followed by 1 week rest, then 1000 mg/m² weekly × 3 weeks, repeated monthly	Nausea/vomiting	Control of nausea/vomiting	Level II emetogen Premedicate with phenothiazine antiemetic; have antiemetic available as needed
	Acute infusion-related reactions (flushing, dyspnea, facial swelling, hypotension)		Slowing of infusion rate may be helpful
	Rash		Systemic steroid may be helpful
	Hair loss		Usually partial hair loss
	Myelosuppression (primarily neutropenia)	CBC with differential and platelet Signs and symptoms (S/S) of infection or bleeding	Dosing adjustment based on severity of neutropenia is required
	Proteinuria and hematuria	Urinalysis S/S of hematuria	Instruct patients to report change in color of urine or difficulty passing urine

toxicities. A multi-institutional, randomized, double-blind phase III trial comparing marimastat to placebo as adjuvant therapy in patients with resectable pancreatic cancer is ongoing.[131]

The multitargeted antifolate antimetabolites (MTAs) are another new class of antineoplastics. These agents can inhibit several enzymes intimately involved with folate metabolism, such as thymidylate synthase, dihydrofolate reductase, and glycinamide ribonucleotide formyl transferase. The MTAs possess broad-spectrum antitumor activity and have demonstrated response in patients with pancreatic cancer in phase I trials. The dose-limiting toxicity of these agents is myelosuppression. Phase II studies with these agents are being initiated.[132]

Dolastatin 10 is a potent antimitotic that binds to tubulin and inhibits the polymerization of purified tubulin, thus disrupting microtubule assembly. The exact binding site of the drug on tubulin has not been identified, but it is probably located near the vinca alkaloid binding sites. In vitro studies have demonstrated potent antiproliferative activity in a number of leukemias, lymphomas, and solid tumor cell lines. Phase I trials to define the maximal tolerated dose have been completed, with myelosuppression found to be the dose-limiting toxicity. Phase II studies with dolastatin are currently being conducted in patients with metastatic pancreatic cancer.[133,134]

The potential of combining gemcitabine with 5-FU has also been explored. A phase I study of gemcitabine with 5-FU and leucovorin has shown that the combination was tolerable.[111] Several phase II trials are being carried out using this combination in patients with advanced pancreatic cancer. These results should be available in the near future.[135]

Novel treatment strategies that utilize gene transfer technology open up a new frontier in cancer therapy. A number of genetic abnormalities have been detected in pancreatic tumor cells, and gene therapy may be a promising alternative to conventional approaches in treating pancreatic cancer. Approximately 60% of pancreatic cancer specimens have abnormalities in the p53 tumor suppressor gene,[79,136,137] and gene therapy targeting this genetic lesion is currently being investigated. Intratumoral injection with adenovirus ONYX-015, alone and in combination with gemcitabine, is under phase I study in patients with unresectable pancreatic tumors. ONYX-015 is an attenuated adenovirus that efficiently replicates in and lyses tumor cells deficient in p53 gene.[132,138,139] Also, K-*ras* mutation resulting in deregulated cell proliferation is found in 90% of pancreatic cancer.[79,136,137] Farnesyl transferase inhibitors, which inhibit the enzymatic activation required for *ras* function and transforming ability, have just entered phase I testing.[132,140]

IMPROVING OUTCOMES

The clinical course of pancreatic cancer is characterized by significant symptomatology, with survival usually measured in weeks to months. To date, the available treatment options have not significantly improved survival. Given this scenario, supportive care of the patient with pancreatic cancer often becomes more important than treatment of the primary disease. Supportive care for this patient population includes, but is not limited to, pain control, amelioration of psychosocial issues, nutritional support, relief of obstructive jaundice, and control of gastrointestinal symptoms (nausea, vomiting, constipation, gastrointestinal obstruction, etc.).[88,141,142]

Both obstructive jaundice and gastrointestinal obstruction can be managed by invasive measures. Biliary decompression can be achieved with nonoperative percutaneous or endoscopic stenting with low complication rates. However, in the long run, recurrent jaundice due to stent collapse can be a problem.[141] Development of self-expanding metallic stents may prolong the duration of stent patency.[143] Because of the higher complication rate, surgical biliary bypass, such as choledochoenterostomy or cholecystoenterostomy, is usually reserved for patients who also require bypass surgery to palliate impending gastrointestinal obstruction.[141] To manage gastrointestinal obstruction, a palliative gastrojejunostomy can be done.[141] Postoperative use of an H_2-antagonist is required to reduce the risk of stomal ulceration. Again, due to higher mortality and morbidity of major surgery in this patient population, nonoperative duodenal stenting is currently under investigation.

Pain is another supportive care issue that demands appropriate attention and management.[85,86] Effective pain control measures should be comprehensive, including pharmacologic approach, invasive techniques, and support group. For pharmacologic management of pain, the World Health Organization three-step analgesic ladder and the guidelines from the Agency for Health Care Policy and Research represent good community practice standards.[141,142,144–147] Invasive measures, such as chemical or surgical splanchnicectomy or percutaneous celiac plexus block, can be performed to complement opioid-based treatment.[148,149]

Psychosocial issues, typically described as depression, anxiety, and a feeling of doom, are commonly observed in patients with pancreatic cancer.[142] Psychologic and behavioral studies suggest higher rates of depression in this patient population than in those with other neoplasms.[150,151] Etiology of such depressive and anxiety symptoms is comprehensive, including the chemical imbalance secondary to the disease itself and the contribution of pain, terminal illness, and other life stressors. If such psychosocial issues are present, they must be taken seriously and treatment should be considered. The use of psychotherapy, cognitive-behavioral techniques, and psychotropic medications concomitant with proper management of other symptomatology can significantly abate depression and anxiety to enhance quality of life.[142]

CONCLUSION

Pancreatic cancer is a relatively rare but highly lethal disease, resulting in the death of more than 95% of patients within 5 years of diagnosis. The symptoms of this disease are vague and often attributed to more benign conditions, allowing the disease to progress to advanced stages before diagnosis. Only patients with very early disease are potentially curable, and the treatment of choice is surgical resection plus neoadjuvant or adjuvant radiation and chemotherapy. Effective treatments for advanced disease are still being sought. Because there is no consistently effective treatment for advanced disease, these patients should be entered into clinical trials whenever possible. Most patients experience progressive deterioration, and supportive care often becomes the mainstay of therapy. Patients often require supportive care that includes control of gastrointestinal symptoms (nausea, vomiting, diarrhea, constipation, and obstruction), pain control, and nutritional support.

Gastric Cancer

EPIDEMIOLOGY

Incidence

Gastric cancer was the leading cause of cancer deaths worldwide until the late 1980s.[152] In the United States the estimated total number of new gastric cancer cases in 1998 was approximately 22,600 (14,300 men and 8,300 women).[1] Over the last 60 years the incidence of gastric cancer in the United States has been declining. Worldwide the most prevalent areas for gastric cancer are Japan, South America (particularly Chile and Costa Rica), and Eastern Europe. Japan has the highest incidence by far, and it is the number one cause of death in that country.[153]

Etiology

The risk factors for the development of gastric cancer are believed to be associated with the environment. Diet is probably the most commonly postulated environmental factor studied in relation to gastric cancer. Diets including high concentrations of nitrates/nitrites, high salt intake, inappropriate food storage, food spoilage/fermentation, and other factors fostering nitrosamine formation have been related to increasing the risk of developing gastric cancer.[154] Diets that are rich in vitamin A and vitamin C lower the risk of gastric cancer.[155] Therefore, one proposed chemopreventive agent is ascorbic acid, or vitamin C. The mechanism of action of ascorbic acid is thought to be through this vitamin's ability to prevent the reduction of nitrous acid to N-nitroso compounds. These N-nitroso compounds are carcinogenic in the stomach.[156,157]

Another factor that may increase the risk of gastric cancer is chronic infection with *Helicobacter pylori. Helicobacter pylori* is commonly present in patients with severe gastritis and chronic atrophic gastritis. It is a common infection, with approximately 50% of adults over age 50 in North America and virtually 100% of adults in some developing or newly industrialized countries infected.[154] It is estimated that the incidence of gastric cancer is six times higher in a 100%-infected population when compared with a noninfected population.[158] Still, only a small percentage of the total number of patients infected with *H. pylori* develop gastric cancer.[159] Infection with *H. pylori* indirectly causes gastric cancer. The chronic gastritis secondary to *H. pylori* leads to an increase in cell turnover and intestinal metaplasia development.[160] Other risk factors increasing the occurrence of gastric cancer include family history, individuals from blood group A, and individuals with pernicious anemia, atrophic gastritis, prior gastric surgery, gastric polyps, or achlorhydria.[161] Individuals from lower socioeconomic classes tend to be at increased risk for the development of gastric cancer. This increased risk is thought to be secondary to dietary and environmental factors common in this population. Smoking has also been associated with increased risk of gastric cancer. However, alcohol consumption has not been shown to increase the risk of gastric cancer.

PATHOPHYSIOLOGY

The majority of malignant gastric cancers are adenocarcinomas, accounting for approximately 84% of all gastric neoplasms. The incidence of other less common histologic classifications include signet ring cell tumors (8%); mucinous adenocarcinomas (3%); and diffuse type adenocarcinoma, intestinal type adenocarcinoma, papillary adenocarcinoma, undifferentiated carcinoma, adenosquamous carcinoma, and tubular adenocarcinoma, each identified in less than 2% of patients.[162]

Approximately 30% of primary gastric cancers occur in the upper third of the stomach, 14% in the middle third, and 26% in the lower third. The incidence of proximal (upper third) gastric cancer has been increasing over the last 15 years.[163] The entire stomach may be involved in up to 10% of patients.[162] Gastric cancer has four major patterns of spread: direct extension into the surrounding tissues and organs such as the liver, diaphragm, pancreas, spleen, biliary tract, and transverse colon; nodal metastases, both local (perigastric, celiac axis, porta hepatis, retroperitoneal) and distant (Virchow's node, left axillary nodes); hematogenous spread to liver, lung, bone, and brain; and intraperitoneal dissemination in the pelvis.[161] Intraperitoneal spread may be evidenced by the presence of peritoneal implants or ascites.

CLINICAL PRESENTATION AND DIAGNOSIS

Signs and Symptoms

Patients with early gastric cancer are typically men (male to female ratio 1.5:1 to 2:1) who are 44 to 70 years of age. By the time gastric cancer is diagnosed in the United States, it is usually advanced. This is primarily because the signs and symptoms of early gastric cancer are vague and nonspecific and similar to those of peptic ulcer disease. The first signs and symptoms that patients may have are mild epigastric pain and dyspepsia. Approximately 40% of patients experience nausea and vomiting. Persistent vomiting may be associated with a distal cancer obstructing the pylorus. Patients with proximal lesions or lesions involving the gastroesophageal junction may have dysphagia as their primary symptom. When gastric cancer is still in the early stages, weight loss is minimal, in spite of anorexia. Only one-fourth of patients with early gastric cancer demonstrate signs and symptoms of upper gastrointestinal bleeding, with associated anemia. Once the disease has advanced, patients complain of significant weight loss (more than 10 pounds), abdominal pain, anorexia, hematemesis, guaiac-positive stools, and anemia. Other physical changes that might suggest advanced gastric cancer when observed in conjunction with the previous signs include palpable lymph nodes, palpable ovarian mass (Krukenberg tumor), hepatomegaly, palpable abdominal mass, ascites, jaundice, and cachexia.[164]

Many patients report experiencing the symptoms of mild epigastric pain for 21 to 36 months. Patients with advanced gastric cancer often relate having experienced symptoms for at least the previous 6 to 8 months. In general, the abdominal pain and discomfort experienced with either early or advanced gastric cancer is not relieved by food or antacids.[164]

A study to better understand gastric cancer was undertaken in the late 1980s by the American College of Surgeons and involved 18,365 patients.[162] Men outnumbered women in this study (63% and 37%, respectively). The median age of men was 68.4 years, and the median age of women was 71.9 years. The presenting features of these patients were evaluated and are listed in Table 90.12. The most common symptoms observed in more than 50% of the patients were weight loss and abdominal pain. Other frequently encountered symptoms included nausea, anorexia, dysphagia, and melena.

Table 90.12 ▪ Common Presenting Signs/Symptoms of Gastric Cancer

Weight loss	Dysphagia
Abdominal pain	Melena
Nausea	Early satiety
Anorexia	Ulcer-type pain

Diagnosis

The differential diagnosis between peptic ulcer disease and gastric cancer must be made in these patients, because the presenting signs and symptoms are so similar. Currently, no blood test that can be used in the definitive diagnosis of gastric cancer is available. Blood tests that may be useful in determining the extent of disease include complete blood count, liver function tests (bilirubin, alkaline phosphatase, LDH, ALT, AST), and CEA. CEA is not used as a diagnostic tool, because it is elevated in only 15 to 30% of patients with advanced disease.[165] CEA may be useful in assessment of response to treatment or evaluating recurrence after potentially curative surgical resection.

Historically, the diagnostic procedure performed on patients with upper gastrointestinal (GI) complaints has been the upper GI roentgenogram. However, over the last 10 to 15 years there has been a decrease in the use of upper GI roentgenogram and an increased use of upper GI endoscopy for the diagnosis of gastric symptomatology. The increase in the use of endoscopy demonstrates the usefulness of direct visualization of the stomach with an additional advantage of obtaining biopsy specimens. Thus esophagogastroduodenoscopy has become the diagnostic procedure of choice.[162]

Endoscopic ultrasonography (EUS) can also be performed to diagnose gastric cancer and the extent of disease. The main utility of EUS is in preoperative staging by enabling evaluation of the depth of cancer invasion into the gastric wall. EUS has a 91% accuracy rate in evaluating depth of invasion and may also be useful in diagnosing perigastric metastatic lymph nodes.[166]

Screening for early gastric cancer is currently being conducted in areas associated with a high risk of gastric cancer, primarily Japan, South America, and Eastern Europe. Again, esophagogastroduodenoscopy is the diagnostic procedure used in these areas.[164] Screening programs in Japan have increased the number of patients diagnosed with an early-stage gastric cancer by up to 40%.[167] Another diagnostic test often ordered for patients with suspected advanced gastric cancer is CT of the abdomen. This test is performed to evaluate the presence or absence of distant metastases.[161]

Staging and Prognosis

The staging of gastric cancer depends on the extent of the disease. This information is obtained during the diagnostic period for the patient (endoscopic procedures, radiology examinations). The TNM classification is used to describe the stage of gastric cancer as recommended by the AJCC (Table 90.13).[161] The percentage of patients presenting at the various stages are stage I (less than 5%), stage II (10 to 15%), stage III (17 to 20%), and stage IV (72%).[167]

Table 90.13 ▪ TNM Staging Classification for Gastric Cancer

Primary Tumor (+)	
T_{is}	Limited to mucosa; does not penetrate the basement membrane
T1	Mucosa or submucosa
T2	To or into but not through serosa
T3	Through serosa without invasion of adjacent tissue
T4a	Involves immediately adjacent structures or extends into esophagus or duodenum
T4b	Direct extension to liver, diaphragm, pancreas, abdominal wall, adrenals, kidney, retroperitoneum, or small bowel, or extraluminal extension to esophagus or duodenum
Regional Lymph Nodes (N)	
N0	No nodal involvement
N1	Perigastric nodes along lesser or greater curvature, within 3 cm of tumor
N2	Other regional lymph nodes—resectable
N3	Other intraabdominal nodes
Distant Metastases (N)	
N0	No distant metastases
N1	Distant metastases present
Stage 0	T_{is} N0 M0
Stage I	T1 N0 M0
Stage II	T2–3 N0 M0
Stage III	T1–3 N1–2 N0
	T4a N02
Stage IV	T1–4a N3 M0
	T4b Nany M0
	Tany Nany M1

The prognostic factors found to be most significant in predicting poor prognosis are depth of invasion and presence of lymph node metastasis.[168,169] The 5-year survival of patients with tumors invading only the mucosa is 91%; in comparison, the 5-year survival of patients with tumors invading adjacent organs is 6.6%. In patients with more than three positive lymph nodes, the 5-year survival is approximately 20%. Other factors that may have some role in predicting outcome include favorable histology (mucinous adenocarcinoma 5-year survival 38.6%) and location of the tumor (whole stomach 5-year survival 20%, upper third of stomach 5-year survival 29.1%). Overall the prognosis for patients diagnosed with gastric cancer is poor, mainly because only a few patients are diagnosed with early-stage disease. The overall survival is strongly correlated with stage at diagnosis. The 5-year survival rate for stage I gastric cancer is 90%; stage II, 70%; stage III, 45%; and stage IV, less than 10%.[168]

TREATMENT

Surgery

Surgery is the only therapeutic option that offers a potential cure for the gastric cancer patient. The amount of stomach removed should be enough to allow ample tumor-free margins, with the regional lymph nodes also being removed. Extension of the surgical margins into the adjacent organs should be done only if necessary, and a controversy surrounds the prophylactic removal of other lymph nodes (i.e., those not directly involved regionally).[170–175] In order to ensure tumor-free margins, either a subtotal or total gastrectomy will be performed, based on the location of the tumor in the stomach and on the pattern of spread of the tumor within the stomach. In general, tumors in the distal portion of the stomach can be best treated with a radical subtotal gastrectomy. Tumors in the middle third of the stomach often require a total gastrectomy. Tumors located in the proximal portion of the stomach and the cardia require a total gastrectomy, with the margins often extending into the distal esophagus.[176,177] However, complete resection of all gross disease with negative margins is still associated with a high rate of recurrent disease.

If a patient has locally advanced (invading other organs) or metastatic gastric cancer, surgery would only be considered with a palliative intent. The symptoms most commonly palliated include pain, hemorrhage, nausea, dysphasia, and obstruction. Again, this could be either a subtotal or total gastrectomy, depending on the location of the obstruction. Currently, palliation from symptom-producing gastric obstruction may also be achieved with endoscopic laser surgery. This often provides recanalization with minimal morbidity and mortality.[177]

Radiation

Radiation therapy has a limited role in the treatment of gastric cancer. This is primarily due to the difficulty in delivering the required dose to the stomach area. Many normal tissues in this area are highly radiosensitive: the spinal cord, kidneys, liver, and small intestines. The use of intraoperative radiation therapy (IORT) is one appealing route of radiation delivery in this patient population. This method allows delivery of the required doses of radiation directly to the tumor and does not exceed the tolerance level of the normal tissues. IORT has been used in combination with external beam radiation and with chemotherapy in the adjuvant setting. Rarely, radiation therapy may be used in advanced gastric cancer for palliation of pain.[178–181]

Chemotherapy

Neoadjuvant Chemotherapy

The goal of neoadjuvant chemotherapy is to improve resectability of tumors in patients with locally advanced disease by decreasing the tumor burden and, therefore, increasing the survival time. Gastric cancer patients who are candidates for neoadjuvant chemotherapy are those patients who have locoregional extension of disease (stage II and III) and are considered unresectable at diagnosis or those patients who are potentially resectable, but have bulky disease or other poor prognostic factors (cardial location or enlarged lymph nodes). The advantages of giving chemotherapy to these groups of patients before surgery are to (1) promote tumor regression, (2) increase local control rate, (3) allow for more conservative surgical procedures, and (4) define postoperative chemotherapy regimens for patients who have responded to chemotherapy preoperatively. Problems with neoadjuvant chemotherapy include (1) development of resistant clones to chemotherapy, (2) delay of local control measures (i.e., surgery), and (3) increased risk of metastatic spread.[182]

Many of the combinations of drugs used in the treatment of advanced disease have been used in the neoadjuvant setting in both patient types. Currently two randomized trials have compared neoadjuvant chemotherapy versus surgery alone. In the first trial, from Korea, patients with locally advanced gastric cancer were randomized to preoperative chemotherapy with cisplatin, etoposide, and 5-fluorouracil (PEF) followed by surgery versus surgery alone. The curative resection rate was 79% for treated patients versus 61% for the surgery alone patients.[183] In the second trial, from Japan, patients with advanced gastric cancer (stage IV) were randomized to preoperative chemotherapy with cisplatin, etoposide, mitomycin C, and UFT (tegafur plus uracil, 1:4 molar ratio) followed by surgery versus surgery alone. The curative resection rate was 38% for treated patients and 15% for the surgery alone patients. The median survival was 17 months and 8 months, respectively.[184] However, larger comparative Western trials between preoperative and postoperative chemotherapy must be completed to determine the true value of this therapy.[182,185–187]

Adjuvant Chemotherapy

Many trials with adjuvant chemotherapy regimens have been investigated in an effort to improve survival rates in resected gastric cancer patients. These adjuvant regimens have been compared with surgery alone. Single agents that have been used as adjuvant chemotherapy in separate trials are thiotepa, floxuridine, and high-dose mitomycin C.[188] Only mitomycin C demonstrated an increase in survival when compared with surgery alone.[189]

With the advent of combination chemotherapy regimens for the treatment of unresectable gastric cancer, combination regimens in the adjuvant chemotherapy setting have increased in use. The GITSG reported a survival benefit in the group of patients receiving adjuvant chemotherapy with 5-FU and methyl-CCNU.[190] These results, however, were not able to be duplicated in two separate confirmatory trials.[191,192] 5-FU, doxorubicin, and mitomycin C (FAM) is a regimen that has been tested extensively in the treatment of advanced disease. Two separate trials have evaluated FAM in the adjuvant setting, compared with surgery alone. Neither study demonstrated a survival advantage for adjuvant therapy over surgery alone. Other variations of the FAM regimen, as well as other combination chemotherapy regimens, have been studied in the adjuvant setting, again without affecting survival.[193]

In Japan, adjuvant chemotherapy is administered earlier in the patient's course of treatment. Often, at the time of surgery, intraperitoneal mitomycin C is administered, followed by intravenous mitomycin C administration the following day. Initially a significant survival benefit was reported for patients treated in this fashion. However, a more recent, larger study failed to show a survival advantage.[194] Additional studies have added intravenous 5-FU, which again demonstrated an improved survival advantage. Early administration of adjuvant chemotherapy, plus screening programs leading to early detection of gastric cancer, may be responsible for the improved survival of gastric cancer patients in Japan.[188,193,195,196] Additional trials are needed to further define the role of adjuvant chemotherapy in gastric cancer. Due to the lack of consistent clinical data, neoadjuvant and adjuvant therapies are not currently considered standard of practice in the United States and should be practiced only within the confines of clinical trials.

Chemotherapy of Advanced Disease

Numerous single agents have been tested in the treatment of advanced gastric cancer.[197] Of these agents tested, 5-FU, doxorubicin, mitomycin C, cisplatin, and more recently paclitaxel and docetaxel have demonstrate activity as single agents. Because of this single-agent activity, investigators have combined these agents in a number of varying regimens.[198–200] One of the first combinations used in advanced gastric cancer was 5-FU, doxorubicin, and mitomycin, also known as the FAM regimen (Table 90.14). In the initial study of the FAM regimen, a 42% partial response (PR) rate was reported with no complete responses (CRs) observed. The median survival of responding patients was 12.5 months, compared with 5.5 months for all patients.[201] Experience with the combination has since increased, and approximately 650 patients in various studies have received treatment with an FAM regimen. The overall response rate in these studies is approximately 30% (2% CR), and the median survival time is 6.9 months.[197]

Table 90.14 ▪ Combination Chemotherapy Regimens for the Treatment of Advanced Gastric Cancer

FAM[(201)]	5-FU	600 mg/m^2 days, 1, 8, 29, 36
	Doxorubicin	30 mg/m^2 days, 1, 29
	Mitomycin C	10 mg/m^2 day 1
FAMTX[(206)]	Methotrexate[a]	1500 mg/m^2 day 1
	5-FU	1500 mg/m^2 1 hour after MTX on day 1
	Doxorubicin	30 mg/m^2 day 15
ELF[(214)]	Etoposide	120 mg/m^2 days, 1, 2, 3
	Leucovorin	300 mg/m^2 days 1, 2, 3
	5-FU	500 mg/m^2 days 1, 2, 3
EAP[(218)]	Etoposide	120 mg/m^2 days 4, 5, 6
	Doxorubicin	20 mg/m^2 days 1, 7
	Cisplatin	40 mg/m^2 days 2, 8

[a]Leucovorin rescue started 24 hours after MTX.

Numerous other combination regimens have been compared with FAM. All regimens produced a response rate that was comparable to FAM with no difference in survival. The North Central Cancer Treatment Group (NCCTG) concluded after studying FAM versus single-agent 5-FU that 5-FU should be considered the standard treatment for advanced gastric cancer, because less expense and toxicities were observed with comparable response rates.[202] Other studies could not document statistically a survival advantage of one treatment over another.[203,204]

A four-arm study by the NCCTG compared 5-FU, doxorubicin, and methyl-CCNU (FAMe); 5-FU, doxorubicin, and cisplatin (FAP); and FAMe alternating with triazinate to single-agent 5-FU. Once again, single-agent 5-FU was less toxic than any of the combination regimens and the combination regimens did not demonstrate a survival advantage over the single agent.[205]

The combination of high-dose methotrexate, 5-FU, and doxorubicin (FAMTX, Table 90.14) produced a promising initial response rate of 63%. Other trials have resulted in lower response rates of 33 to 59%, with some severe toxicities (grade 4 neutropenia, grade 3 mucositis). FAMTX has been compared to FAM in an attempt to better define the toxicity of FAMTX in comparison to FAM, then considered standard treatment. The response rate for FAMTX in this trial was 41%; for FAM the response rate was lower than expected at 9%. Mucositis was more often observed in the FAMTX arm; thrombocytopenia was a cumulative toxicity of FAM. Overall, the toxicities of the two arms were comparable.[206] Multiple modifications of the FAMTX regimen have been reported; some of these modifications have included altering drug doses, substituting drugs, or adjusting the dosing schedule. None of these modification has provided survival or response advantages over other combination chemotherapy regimens.[207–209]

Because single-agent 5-FU is active in the treatment of advanced gastric cancer, biochemical modulation of 5-FU has been studied in this population. Studies have reported activity in 5-FU combinations with leucovorin, interferon-α, and methotrexate. Overall response rates of these biochemically modulated regimens are in the range of 8 to 50%. A higher complete and overall response rate has been observed with 5-FU and leucovorin when compared with single-agent 5-FU.[210–213]

ELF chemotherapy is a combination of leucovorin, 5-FU, and etoposide (Table 90.14). The original ELF regimen produced a 48% overall response rate (12% CR).[214] Modifications (l-leucovorin for d,l-leucovorin; oral etoposide for intravenous etoposide) of the ELF regimen have not affected the overall response rate.[215–216] PELF chemotherapy (cisplatin, epirubicin, leucovorin, 5-FU) has been compared to an FAM regimen. Patients receiving PELF demonstrated a higher overall response rate (43%) than the patients in the FAM arm. However, more grade 3 and 4 toxicities were reported in the PELF arm, and there was no survival advantage with PELF.[217]

The final combination chemotherapy regimen studied extensively in advanced gastric cancer has been etoposide, doxorubicin, and cisplatin (EAP) (Table 90.14). Response rates using this combination of agents have ranged from 20 to 72%.[218–221] Toxicities observed with EAP chemotherapy were leukopenia, thrombocytopenia, and mucositis.[219] In a comparison trial of EAP versus FAMTX, both regimens produced similar response rates and toxicities; however, the toxicities associated with EAP therapy were more severe and required longer hospitalizations.[220]

A more recent trial combining docetaxel and cisplatin conducted by the Swiss Group for Clinical Cancer Research achieved a 58% response rate.[222] Another trial combining paclitaxel and 5-FU reported a 63% response rate and median survival of 12 months.[223] These newer agents (paclitaxel, docetaxel), along with irinotecan and the oral 5-FU prodrugs (S-1, UFT, capecitabine), are currently being studied in various combinations.

Another route of drug administration that has been used in advanced gastric cancer patients is intraperitoneal. This procedure is used primarily for patients with peritoneal seeding. Hyperthermic perfusion with mitomycin C[224] and intraperitoneal cisplatin[225,226] has been reported as a safe method of direct chemotherapy administration for patients with peritoneal seeding only. Overall, the use of combination chemotherapy has improved the response rate in advanced gastric cancer patients; however, patient survival has demonstrated little improvement. Thus new agents are continuously being screened for the treatment of advanced gastric cancer. Outside of a clinical trial, the least expensive and least toxic chemotherapy regimens should be used in the treatment of advanced gastric cancer. See Table 90.15 for a summary of chemotherapy agents and toxicities currently used in the treatment of gastric cancer.

CONCLUSION

Because the signs and symptoms of early gastric cancer are so similar to those of peptic ulcer disease, gastric cancer is usually diagnosed in advanced stages. The treatment of gastric cancer depends on the stage of disease. As with other cancers of the gastrointestinal tract, surgery is the only means to achieve a cure. Patients who are able to undergo surgery for curative purposes are those with early-stage disease (stages I and II). In patients with locally advanced or metastatic disease, surgery is performed only as a palliative therapy. The role of neoadjuvant or adjuvant chemotherapy with or without radiation therapy must be explored further, because conflicting reports currently exist. Multiple combination chemotherapy regimens have been used in the treatment of unresectable gastric cancer, each providing the patient with varying response rates and toxicities. Unfortunately, none of the regimens provides the patient with an improved survival. Because of this, new agents and combinations continue to be studied in the treatment of gastric cancer.

Table 90.15 ▪ Toxicities of Chemotherapeutic Agents Used in Gastric Cancer

Agent	Toxicities
Cisplatin	Nausea, vomiting, diarrhea, nephrotoxicity, myelosuppression, peripheral neuropathy, ototoxicity
5-Fluorouracil	Nausea, vomiting, stomatitis, diarrhea, dermatitis, myelosuppression, palmar-plantar erythrodysesthesia, photosensitivity
Leucovorin	Increased diarrhea and stomatitis when used with 5-fluorouracil
Etoposide	Myelosuppression, nausea, vomiting, alopecia, hypotension
Doxorubicin	Myelosuppression, nausea, vomiting, alopecia, cardiotoxicity, mucositis
Mitomycin C	Myelosuppression (delayed), nausea, vomiting, pulmonary toxicity, hemolytic uremic syndrome
Methotrexate	Myelosuppression, nausea, vomiting, diarrhea, stomatitis, malaise, fatigue, alopecia
Paclitaxel	Myelosuppression, peripheral neuropathy, nausea, vomiting, alopecia, hypersensitivity reaction
Docetaxel	Myelosuppression, paresthesia, nausea, vomiting, hypersensitivity reaction, alopecia, fluid retention, rash, stomatitis, diarrhea
Irinotecan	Diarrhea, myelosuppression, nausea, vomiting
Capecitabine	Palmar-plantar erythrodysesthesia, diarrhea, photosensitivity, mucositis
UFT	Diarrhea, nausea, abdominal cramping, photosensitivity
S-1	Diarrhea, myelosuppression

KEY POINTS

- Of the GI tumors, those arising from the colon and rectum are most common.
- The prognosis for colorectal cancer is completely dependent on the depth of tumor invasion into or through the bowel wall.
- Early-stage disease can be cured with surgical resection, but advanced disease treatment remains palliative.
- Pancreatic cancer, although relatively rare in the United States, is one of the most lethal malignancies, resulting in death of more than 95% of patients within 5 years of diagnosis.
- Most patients with pancreatic disease have advanced disease at diagnosis, leading to poor outcomes.
- Because there is no truly effective treatment for advanced pancreatic cancer, patients should be encouraged to participate in clinical trials.
- Gastric cancer, like pancreatic cancer, is often diagnosed late in the course of the disease.
- With all of the GI tumors, surgery is the only modality that is currently curative.
- New agents and combinations are needed before significant progress can be made in curing advanced gastrointestinal tumors.

REFERENCES

1. Landis SH, Murry T, Bolden, et al. Cancer statistics. CA Cancer J Clin 48:6–29, 1998.
2. Phillips RL, Kuzma JW, Lotz TM. Cancer mortality among comparable members vs non-members of the Seventh Day Adventist Church. In: Cairns J, Lyon JL, Skolnick M, eds. Cancer incidence in defined populations. Cold Spring Harbor, NY: Cold Spring Laboratory, 1980:83–102.
3. Enstrom JE. Health and dietary practices and cancer mortality among California Mormons. In: Cairns J, Lyon JL, Skolnick M, eds. Cancer incidence in defined populations. Cold Spring Harbor, NY: Cold Spring Laboratory, 1980:69–90.
4. Ziegler RG, Devesa SS, Fraumeni JF, et al. Epidemiology pattern of colorectal cancer. In: DeVita VT, Hellman S, Rosenberg SA, eds. Important advances in oncology. Philadelphia: JB Lippincott, 1986:209–232.
5. Deschner EE, Cohen BI, Raicht RF. Acute and chronic effect of dietary cholic acid on colonic epithelial cell proliferation. Digestion 21:290–296, 1981.
6. Newmark HL, Wargovich MJ, Bruce WR. Colon cancer and dietary fat, phosphate, and calcium: a hypothesis. J Natl Cancer Inst 72:1323–1325, 1984.
7. Kritchevsky D. Dietary fiber and cancer. Nutr Cancer 6:213–219, 1985.
8. Yang CS, Newmark HL. The role of micronutrient deficiency in carcinogenesis. CRC Crit Rev Oncol Hematol 7:267–287, 1987.
9. Eastwoood M. Dietary fiber and risk of cancer. Nutr Rev 45:193–198, 1977.
10. Fuchs CS, Giovannucci EL, Colditz GA, et al. Dietary fiber and the risk of colorectal cancer and adenoma in women. N Engl J Med 340:169–171, 1999.
11. Longnecker MP, Orza MJ, Adams ME, et al. A metaanalysis of alcoholic beverage consumption in relation to risk of colorectal cancer. Cancer Causes Control 1:59–68, 1990.
12. Margulis AR, Thoeni RF. The present status of the radiologic examination of the colon. Radiology 167:1–5, 1988.
13. O'Dwyer PT, Mojzcski C, McCabe DP. Reoperation directed by carcinoembryonic antigen level: the importance of a thorough preoperative evaluation. Am J Surg 155:227–231, 1988.
14. Cohen AM, Mindky BD, Schilsky RL. Colon cancer. In: DeVita VT, Hellman S, Rosenberg SA, eds. Cancer: principles and practice of oncology. 4th ed. Philadelphia: JB Lippincott, 1993:929–977.
15. Bond JH. Screening and early detection. In: Wanebo HJ, ed. Colorectal cancer. St. Louis: Mosby, 1993:149–157.
16. Enker WE, Loffer UT, Block GE. Enhanced survival of patients with colon and rectal cancer is based upon wide anatomic resection. Ann Surg 190:350–360, 1979.
17. Steele G, Posner MR. Adjuvant treatment of colorectal adenocarcinoma. Curr Probl Cancer 17:223–269, 1993.
18. Devasa JM, Morales V, Enriques JM. Colorectal cancer: the basis for a comprehensive follow-up. Dis Colon Rectum 31:636–652, 1988.
19. Moertel CG. Accomplishment in surgical adjuvant therapy for large bowel cancer. Cancer 70:1364–1371, 1992.
20. Verhaegen H, DeCree J, DeCock W, et al. Levamisole therapy in patients with colorectal cancer. In: Terry WD, Rosenberg SA, eds. Immunotherapy of human cancer. New York: Excerpta Medica, 1982:225–229.
21. Moertel CG, Fleming TR, Macdonald JS, et al. Fluorouracil plus levamisole as effective adjuvant therapy after resection of stage III colon carcinoma: a final report. Ann Intern Med 122:321–326, 1995.
22. NIH Consensus Conference. Adjuvant therapy for patients with colon and rectal cancer. JAMA 264:1444–1450, 1990.
23. Peretz T, Figer A, Borovik R, et al. 5-FU + leucovorin as active and less toxic regimen than 5-FU + levamisole in the adjuvant therapy of colorectal cancer: Israel Cooperative Oncology Group. Proc ASCO 16:941, 1997.
24. Wolmark N, Rockette H, Mamounas EP. The relative efficacy of 5-FU + leucovorin + levamisole and 5-FU + leucovorin + levamisole in patients with Dukes' B and C carcinoma of the colon: first report of NSABP C-04 [abstract]. Proc Am Soc Clin Oncol 15:205, 460, 1996.
25. Gunderson LL, Martenson JA. Colorectal cancer: radiotherapy. In: Brain MC, Carbone PC, eds. Current therapy in hematology–oncology. 5th ed. St Louis: Mosby, 1995:371–384.
26. Gastrointestinal Study Group. Prolongation of the disease-free interval in surgically treated rectal cancer. N Engl J Med 312:1465–1472, 1985.
27. Douglass HO, Mayer RJ, Thomas PRM, et al. Survival after postoperative combination treatment of rectal cancer [letter]. N Engl J Med 315:1294, 1986.

28. Krook J, Moertel C, Gunderson LL, et al. Effective surgical adjuvant therapy for high-risk rectal carcinoma. N Engl J Med 324:709–714, 1991.
29. Weaver D, Lindblad AS. Gastrointesinal Tumor Study Group: radiation therapy and 5-fluorouracil with or without MeCCNU for the treatment of patients with surgically adjuvant adenocarcinoma of the rectum. Proc ASCO 9:106, 1990.
30. O'Connell M, Wieand HS, Krook J, et al. Lack of value for methyl-CCNU as a component of effective rectal cancer surgical adjuvant therapy: interim analysis of intergroup protocol 86-47-51. Proc ASCO 10:134, 1991.
31. Tepper JE, O'Connell MJ, Petroni GR, et al. Adjuvant postoperative fluorouracil-modulated chemotherapy combined with pelvic radiation therapy for rectal cancer: initial results of intergroup 0114. J Clin Oncol 15:2030–2039, 1997.
32. Minsky BD. Current and future directions in adjuvant combined-modality therapy of rectal cancer. Oncology 119(Suppl 10):61–68, 1997.
33. Rougier P, Nordlinger B. Larger scale trial for adjuvant treatment in high risk resected colorectal cancers. Rationale to test the combination of loco-regional and systemic chemotherapy and to compare l-leucovorin + 5-FU to levamisole + 5-FU. Ann Oncol 2:21–28, 1993.
34. Macmillan WE, Wolberg WH, Welling PG. Pharmacokinetics of fluorouracil in humans. Cancer Res 38:3479–3482, 1978.
35. Washtien WL, Santi DV. Intracellular free and macromolecular-bound metabolites of 5-fluorodeoxyuridine and 5-fluorouracil. Cancer Res 39:3397–3404, 1979.
36. Ahlgren JD. Colorectal cancer: chemotherapy. In: Ahlgren JD, Macdonald JS, eds. Gastrointestinal oncology. Philadelphia: JB Lippincott, 1992:339–357.
37. Seifert P, Baker LH, Reed MD, et al. Comparison of continuously infused 5-fluorouracil with bolus injection in patients with colorectal adenocarcinoma. Cancer 36:123–128, 1975.
38. Lokich JJ, Bothe A, Fine A, et al. Phase I study of protracted venous infusion of 5-fluorouracil. Cancer 48:2565–2568, 1981.
39. Ardalan B, Singh G, Silberman H. A randomized phase I and II study of short-term infusion of high-dose fluorouracil with and without *N*-(phosphonacetyl)-L-aspartic acid in patients with advanced pancreatic and colorectal cancers. J Clin Oncol 6:1053–1058, 1988.
40. Evans RM, Laskin JD, Hakala MT. Effect of excess folates and deoxyinosine on the activity and site of action of 5-fluorouracil. Cancer Res 41:3283–3295, 1981.
41. Petrelli N, Herrera L, Rustum Y, et al. A prospective randomized trial of 5-fluorouracil and high dose leucovorin versus 5-FU and methotrexate in previously untreated patients with advanced colorectal carcinoma. J Clin Oncol 5:1559–1565, 1987.
42. Petrelli N, Douglass HO, Herrera L, et al. The modulation of fluorouracil with leucovorin in metastatic colorectal carcinoma: a prospective phase III trial. J Clin Oncol 7:1419–1426, 1989.
43. Poon MA, O'Connell MJ, Moertel CG, et al. Biochemical modulation of fluorouracil: evidence of significant improvement of survival and quality of life in patients with advanced colorectal carcinoma. J Clin Oncol 7:1407–1408, 1989.
44. Doroshaw JH, Multhauf P, Leong L, et al. Prospective randomized comparison of fluorouracil versus fluorouracil and high dose continuous infusion leucovorin calcium for the treatment of advanced measurable colorectal cancer in patients previously unexposed to chemotherapy. J Clin Oncol 8:491–501, 1990.
45. Erlichman C, Fine S, Wong A, et al. A randomized trial of fluorouracil and folinic acid in patients with metastatic colorectal carcinoma. J Clin Oncol 6:469–475, 1988.
46. Poon MA, O'Connell MJ, Wieland HS, et al. Biochemical modulation of fluorouracil with leucovorin: confirmatory evidence of improved therapeutic efficacy in advanced colorectal cancer. J Clin Oncol 9:1967–1972, 1991.
47. Wadler SW, Schwartz EL, Goldman M, et al. Fluorouracil and recombinant alfa-2a-interferon: an active regimen against advanced colorectal carcinoma. J Clin Oncol 7:1769–1775, 1989.
48. Ardalan B, Singh G, Silberman H. A randomized phase I and II study of short-term infusion of high-dose fluorouracil with or without *N*-(phosphonacetyl)-L-aspartic acid in patients with advanced pancreatic and colorectal cancer. J Clin Oncol 7:1053–1058, 1988.
49. Grem JL, Fischer PH. Enhancement of 5-fluorouracil's anticancer activity by dipyridamole. Pharmacol Ther 40:349–371, 1989.
50. Klubes P, Leyland-Jones B. Enhancement of the antitumor activity of 5-fluorouracil by uridine rescue. Pharmacol Ther 41:289–302, 1989.
51. Punt CJA. New drugs in the treatment of colorectal carcinoma. Cancer 83:679–689, 1998.
52. Van Custem E, Bajetta E, Niederle K, et al. A phase III multicenter randomized trial comparing CPT-11 to infusional 5FU regimen in patients with advanced colorectal cancer after 5FU failure. Proc ASCO 17:984, 1998.
53. Bugat R, Rougier P, Douillard JY, et al. Efficacy of irinotecan HCl (CPT 11) in patients with metastatic colorectal cancer after progression while receiving a 5-FU based chemotherapy. Proc ASCO 14:567, 1995.
54. Abigerges D, Chabot GG, Armand JP, et al. Phase I and pharmacologic studies of the camptothecin analog irinotecan administered every 3 weeks in cancer patients. J Clin Oncol 13:210–221, 1995.
55. Missel JL. Oxaliplatin in practice. Br J Cancer 77(Suppl 4):4–7, 1998.
56. Zalcberg J, Cunningham D, Green M, et al. The final results of a large scale phase II study of the potent thymidylate synthase inhibitor tomudex (ZD1694) in advanced colorectal cancer. Proc ASCO 14:494, 1995.
57. Findlay M, Van Custem E, Kocha W, et al. A randomised phase II study of xeloda (capecitabine) in patients with advanced colorectal cancer [abstract]. Proc Am Soc Clin Oncol 16:227a, 798, 1997.
58. Pazdur R, Rhodes V, Lassere Y, et al. UFT plus leucovorin: a potentially effective oral regimen in colorectal carcinoma. Proc ASCO 13:590, 1994.
59. Riethmuller G, Schneider-Gadicke E, Schlimok G, et al. Randomised trial of monoclonal antibody for adjuvant therapy of Dukes' C colorectal carcinoma. Lancet 343:1177–1183, 1994.
60. Ries LAG, Kosary CL, Hankey BF, et al. SEER cancer statistics review, 1973–1995. Bethesda, MD: National Cancer Institute, 1998.
61. Evans DB, Abbruzzese JL, Rich TA. Cancer of the pancreas. In: DeVita Jr VT, Hellman S, Rosenberg SA, eds. Cancer: principles and practices of oncology. 5th ed. Philadelphia: Lippincott-Raven, 1997.
62. Gold EB, Goldin SB. Epidemiology of and risk factors for pancreatic cancer. Surg Oncol Clin North Am 7:67–88, 1998.
63. Parkin DM, Pisani P, Ferlay J. Global cancer statistics. CA Cancer J Clin 49:33–64, 1999.
64. Tominaga S, Kuroishi T. Epidemiology of pancreatic cancer. Semin Surg Oncol 15:3–7, 1998.
65. Ahlgren JD. Epidemiology of and risk factors in pancreatic cancer. Semin Oncol 23:241–250, 1996.
66. Silverman DT, Dunn JA, Hoover RN, et al. Cigarette smoking and pancreas cancer: a case-control study based on direct interviews. J Natl Cancer Inst 86:1510–1516, 1994.
67. La Vecchia C, Boyle P, Franceschi S, et al. Smoking and cancer with emphasis on Europe. Eur J Cancer 27:94–104, 1991.
68. Mack TM, Yu MC, Hanisch R, et al. Pancreas cancer and smoking, beverage consumption, and past medical history. J Natl Cancer Inst 76:49–60, 1986.
69. Zheng W, McLaughlin JK, Gridley G, et al. A cohort of smoking, alcohol consumption, and dietary factors for pancreatic cancer (United States). Cancer Causes Control 4:477–482, 1993.
70. Olsen GW, Mandel JS, Gibson RW, et al. A case-control study of pancreatic cancer and cigarettes, alcohol, coffee and diet. Am J Public Health 79:1016–1019, 1989.
71. Mancuso TF, El-Attar AA. Cohort study of workers exposed to betanaphthylamine and benzidine. J Occup Med 9:277–285, 1967.
72. Pietri F, Clavel F. Occupational exposure and cancer of the pancreas: a review. Br J Ind Med 48:583–587, 1991.
73. Karmody A, Kyle J. The association between carcinoma of the pancreas and diabetes mellitus. Br J Surg 56:362–364, 1969.
74. Gullo L, Pezzilli R, Morselli-Labate AM. Diabetes and the risk of pancreatic cancer. N Engl J Med 331:81–84, 1994.
75. Jones SC. Pancreatic cancer and diabetes [letter]. N Engl J Med 331:1526–1528, 1994.
76. Lowenfels AB, Maisonneuve P, Cavallini G, et al. Pancreatitis and the risk of pancreatic cancer. N Engl J Med 328:1433–1437, 1993.
77. Ekbom A, McLaughlin JK, Karlsson BM, et al. Pancreatitis and pancreatic cancer: a population-based study. J Natl Cancer Inst 86:625–627, 1994.
78. Karlson BM, Ekbom A, Josefsson S, et al. The risk of pancreatic cancer following pancreatitis: an association due to confounding? Gastroenterology 113:587–592, 1997.
79. Hruban RH, Petersen GM, Ha PK, et al. Genetics of pancreatic cancer: from genes to families. Surg Oncol Clin North Am 7:1–23, 1998.
80. Nomoto S, Nakao A, Ando N, et al. Clinical application of K-ras oncogene mutations in pancreatic carcinoma: detection of micrometastases. Semin Surg Oncol 15:40–46, 1998.
81. Goldstein AM, Fraser M, Struewing JP, et al. Increased risk of pancreatic cancer in melanoma-prone kindreds with $p16^{INK4}$ mutations. N Engl J Med 333:970–974, 1995.
82. Whelan AJ, Bartsch D, Goodfellow PJ. Brief report: a familial syndrome of pancreatic cancer and melanoma with a mutation in the CDKN2 tumor-suppressor gene. N Engl J Med 333:975–977, 1995.
83. Lynch HT, Smyrk T, Kern SE, et al. Familial pancreatic cancer: a review. Semin Oncol 23:251–275, 1996.
84. Wilentz RE, Hruban RH. Pathology of cancer of the pancreas. Surg Oncol Clin North Am 7:43–63, 1998.

85. Krech RL, Walsh D. Symptoms of pancreatic cancer. J Pain Symptom Manage 6:360–367, 1991.
86. Kelsen DP, Portenoy RK, Thaler HT, et al. Pain and depression in patients with newly diagnosed pancreas cancer. J Clin Oncol 13:748–755, 1995.
87. Passik SD, Breitbart WS. Depression in patients with pancreatic carcinoma: diagnostic and treatment issues. Cancer 78:625–626, 1996.
88. Lillemoe KD, Pitt HA. Palliation. Cancer 78:605–614, 1996.
89. Bluemke DA, Fishman EK. CT and MR evaluation of pancreatic cancer. Surg Oncol Clin North Am 7:103–124, 1998.
90. Furhman GM, Charnsangavej C, Abbruzzese JL, et al. Thin-section contrast enhanced computed tomography accurately predicts resectability of malignant pancreatic neoplasms. Am J Surg 167:104–113, 1994.
91. Steinberg WM, Barkin J, Bradley III EL, et al. Controversies in clinical pancreatology. Pancreas 17:24–30, 1998.
92. Stevens PD, Lightdale CJ. The role of endosonography in the diagnosis and management of pancreatic cancer. Surg Clin North Am 7:125–133, 1998.
93. Fernandez-del Castillo, Warshaw AL. Laparoscopic staging and peritoneal cytology. Surg Oncol Clin North Am 7:135–142, 1998.
94. Posner MR, Mayer RJ. The use of serologic tumor markers in gastrointestinal malignancies. Hematol Oncol Clin North Am 8:533–552, 1994.
95. Ritts RE, Pitt HA. CA 19-9 in pancreatic cancer. Surg Oncol Clin North Am 7:93–101, 1998.
96. Nakao A, Oshima K, Nomoto S, et al. Clinical usefulness of CA 19-9 in pancreatic carcinoma. Semin Surg Oncol 15:15–22, 1998.
97. Kiriyama E, Hayakawa T, Kondo T, et al. Usefulness of a new tumor marker, span-1, for the diagnosis of pancreatic cancer. Cancer 65:1557–1561, 1990.
98. American Joint Committee on Cancer. Exocrine pancreas. In: Fleming ID, Cooper JS, Henson DE, et al., eds. AJCC cancer staging manual. 5th ed. Philadelphia: Lippincott-Raven, 1997.
99. Nitecki SS, Sarr MG, Colby TV, et al. Long-term survival after resection for ductal adenocarcinoma of the pancreas. Is it really improving? Ann Surg 221:59–66, 1995.
100. Whittington R, Bryer MP, Haller DG, et al. Adjuvant therapy of resected adenocarcinoma of the pancreas. Int J Radiat Oncol Biol Phys 21:1137–1143, 1991.
101. Reber HA. Pancreas. In: Schwartz SI, Shires GT, Spencer FC, et al., eds. Principles of surgery. 7th ed. New York: McGraw-Hill, 1999.
102. Yeo CJ. Pylorus-preserving pancreaticoduodenectomy. Surg Oncol Clin North Am 7:143–156, 1998.
103. Brooks JR, Brooks DC, Levine JD. Total pancreatectomy for ductal cell carcinoma of the pancreas. Ann Surg 209:405–410, 1989.
104. Van Heerden JA, McIlrath DC, Ilstrup DM, et al. Total pancreatectomy for ductal cell carcinoma of the pancreas: an update. World J Surg 12:658–662, 1988.
105. Gastrointestinal Tumor Study Group. Further evidence of effective adjuvant combined radiation and chemotherapy following curative resection of pancreatic cancer. Cancer 59:2006–2010, 1987.
106. Kalser MH, Ellenberg SS. Pancreatic cancer: adjuvant combined radiation and chemotherapy following curative resection. Arch Surg 120:899–903, 1985.
107. Spitz FR, Abbruzzese JL, Lee JE, et al. Preoperative and postoperative chemoradiation strategies in patients treated with pancreaticoduodenectomy for adenocarcinoma of the pancreas. JCO 15:928–937, 1997.
108. Miller AR, Robinson EK, Lee JE, et al. Neoadjuvant chemoradiation for adenocarcinoma of the pancreas. Surg Oncol Clin North Am 7:183–197, 1998.
109. Lawrence T, Chang E, Hahn T, et al. Radiosensitization of pancreatic cancer cells by 2′,2′-difluoro-2′-deoxycytidine. Int J Radiol Oncol Biol Phys 34:867–872, 1996.
110. Robertson JM, Shewach DS, Lawrence TS. Preclinical studies of chemotherapy and radiation therapy for pancreatic carcinoma. Cancer 78:674–679, 1996.
111. Hidalgo M, Castellano D, Paz-Ares L, et al. Phase I–II study of gemcitabine and fluorouracil as a continuous infusion in patients with pancreatic cancer. JCO 17:585–592, 1999.
112. Roldan GE, Gunderson LL, Nagorney DM, et al. External beam versus intraoperative and external beam irradiation for locally advanced pancreatic cancer. Cancer 61:1110–1116, 1988.
113. Shibamoto Y, Manabe T, Baba N, et al. High dose, external beam and intraoperative radiotherapy in the treatment of resectable and unresectable pancreatic cancer. Int J Radiol Oncol Biol Phys 19:605–611, 1990.
114. Pisters PWT, Abbruzzese JL, Janjan NA, et al. Rapid-fractionation preoperative chemoradiation, pancreaticoduodenectomy, and intraoperative radiation therapy for resectable pancreatic adenocarcinoma. JCO 16: 3843–3850, 1998.
115. Moertel CG, Frytak S, Hahn RG, et al. Therapy of locally unresectable pancreatic carcinoma: a randomized comparison of high dose (6000 rads) radiation alone, moderate dose radiation (4000 rads) plus 5-FU, and high dose radiation plus 5-FU: the gastrointestinal tumor study group. Cancer 48:1705–1710, 1981.
116. Gastrointestinal Tumor Study Group. Treatment of locally unresectable carcinoma of the pancreas: comparison of combined-modality therapy (chemotherapy plus radiotherapy) to chemotherapy alone. J Natl Cancer Inst 80:751–755, 1988.
117. Boz G, De Paoli A, Roncandin M, et al. Radiation therapy combined with chemotherapy for inoperable pancreatic carcinoma. Tumori 77:61–64, 1991.
118. Dobelbower RR Jr, Merrick H, Ahuja R, et al. I-125 interstitial implant, precision high-dose external beam therapy, and 5-FU for unresectable adenocarcinoma of pancreas and extrahepatic biliary tree. Cancer 58:2185–2195, 1986.
119. Safran H, King TP, Choy H, et al. Paclitaxel and concurrent radiation for locally advanced pancreatic and gastric cancer: a phase I study. JCO 15:901–907, 1997.
120. Robertson JM, Ensminger WD, Walker S, et al. A phase I trial of intravenous bromodeoxyuridine and radiation therapy for pancreatic cancer. Int J Radiol Oncol Biol Phys 37:331–335, 1997.
121. Eli Lilly and Company. Gemzar (Gemcitabine HCl) injection, package insert. Indianapolis, 1996.
122. Noble S, Goa KL. Gemcitabine: a review of its pharmacology and clinical potential in non–small cell lung cancer and pancreatic cancer. Drugs 54:447–472, 1997.
123. Moore M. Activity of gemcitabine in patients with advanced pancreatic carcinoma. Cancer 78: 633–638, 1996.
124. Casper ES, Green MR, Kelsen DP, et al. Phase II trial of gemcitabine (2,2′-difluorodeoxycytidine) in patients with adenocarcinoma of the pancreas. Invest New Drug 12:29–34, 1994.
125. Burris III HA. Objective outcome measure of quality of life. Oncology 11:131–135, 1996.
126. Rothenberg ML, Abbruzzese JL, Moore M, et al. A rationale for expanding the endpoints for clinical trials in advanced pancreatic carcinoma. Cancer 78: 627–632, 1996.
127. Burris III HA. Improvements in survival and clinical benefit with gemcitabine as first-line therapy for patients with advanced pancreas cancer: a randomized trial. JCO 15:2403–2413, 1997.
128. Schnall SF, McDonald JS. Chemotherapy of adenocarcinoma of the pancreas. Semin Oncol 23:220–228, 1996.
129. DeCaprio, JA, Mayer RJ, Gonin R, et al. Fluorouracil and high dose leucovorin in previously untreated patients with advanced adenocarcinoma of the pancreas: results of a phase II trial. JCO9:2128–2133, 1991.
130. The Gastrointestinal Tumor Study Group. Phase II studies of drug combinations in advanced pancreatic carcinoma: fluorouracil plus doxorubicin plus mitomycin C and two regimens of streptozocin plus mitomycin C plus fluorouracil. JCO 4:1794–1798, 1986.
131. Rasmussen HS, McCann PP. Matrix metalloproteinase inhibition as a novel anticancer strategy: a review with special focus on batimastat and marimastat. Pharmacol Ther 75:69–75, 1997.
132. Von Hoff DD, Goodwin AL, Garcia L, et al. Advances in the treatment of patients with pancreatic cancer: improvement in symptoms and survival time. Br J Cancer78:9–13, 1998.
133. Bai R, Pettit GR, Hamel E, et al. Binding of dolastatin 10 to tubulin at a distinct site for peptide antimitotic agents near the exchangeable nucleotide and vinca alkaloid sites. Biochem Pharmacol 39:1941–1949, 1990.
134. Bagniewski PG, Pitot HC. Pharmacokinetics of dolastatin 10 in adult patients with solid tumors [abstract]. Proc Ann Am Assoc Cancer Res 38:A1492, 1997.
135. Cascinu S, Silva RR, Barni S, et al. Gemcitabine and 5-FU in advanced pancreatic cancer: a GISCAD phase II study [abstract]. Proc Am Soc Clin Oncol 17:264a, 1998.
136. Clary BM, Lyerly HK. Gene therapy and pancreatic cancer. Surg Oncol Clin North Am 7:217–237, 1998.
137. Takeda S, Nakao A, Miyoshi K, et al. Gene therapy for pancreatic cancer. Semin Surg Oncol 15:57–61, 1998.
138. Ganly I, Kirn D, Rodriguez GI, et al. Phase I trial of intratumoral injection with an E1B-attenuated adenovirus, ONYX-015, in patients with recurrent p53(–) head and neck cancer [abstract]. Proc Am Soc Clin Oncol 16:382, 1997.
139. Heise C, Sampson-Johannes A, Williams A, et al. ONYX-015, an E1B-attenuated adenovirus, causes tumor-specific cytolysis and antitumoral efficacy that can be augmented by standard chemotherapeutic agents. Nat Med 3:639–645, 1997.
140. Kohl NE, Omer CA, Conner MW, et al. Inhibition of farnesyl transferase induces regression of mammary and salivary carcinomas in ras transgenic mice. Nat Med 1:792–797, 1995.

141. Lillemoe KD. Palliative therapy for pancreatic cancer. Surg Oncol Clin North Am 7:199–217, 1998.
142. Alter CL. Palliative and supportive care of patients with pancreatic cancer. Semin Oncol 23:229–240, 1996.
143. Davids PH, Groen AK, Rauws EA, et al. Randomized trial of self-expanding metal stents versus polyethylene stents for distal malignant biliary obstruction. Lancet 340:1488–1492, 1992.
144. Caraceni A, Portenoy RK. Pain management in patients with pancreatic carcinoma. Cancer 78:639–653, 1996.
145. Lebovitz AH, Lefkowitz M. Pain management of pancreatic carcinoma: a review. Pain 36:1–11, 1989.
146. World Health Organization. Cancer pain relief and palliative care. Geneva: World Health Organization, 1990.
147. Agency for Health Care Policy and Research. Management of cancer pain: clinical practice guideline, number 9. Washington, DC: US Department of Health and Human Services, Agency for Health Care Policy and Research, 1994.
148. Lillemoe KD, Cameron JL, Kaufman HS, et al. Chemical splanchnicectomy in patients with unresectable pancreatic cancer: a prospective randomized trial. Ann Surg 217:447–457, 1993.
149. Kawamata M, Ishitani K, Ishikawa K, et al. Comparison between celiac plexus block and morphine treatment on quality of life in patients with pancreatic cancer pain. Pain 64:597–602, 1996.
150. Holland JC, Korzun AH, Tross S, et al. Comparative psychological disturbance in patients with pancreatic and gastric cancer. Am J Psychiatry 143:982–986, 1996.
151. Fras I, Litin EM, Pearson JS. Comparison of psychiatric symptoms in carcinoma of the pancreas with those in some other intra-abdominal neoplasm. Am J Psychiatry 123:1553–1562, 1967.
152. Boring C, Squires T, Ton J. Cancer statistics 1991. CA Cancer J Clin 41:28, 1991.
153. Mishima Y, Hirayama R. The role of lymph node surgery in gastric cancer. World J Surg 11:406, 1987.
154. Hwang H, Swyer J, Russell RM. Diet, *Helicobacter pylori* infection, food preservation and gastric cancer risk: are these new roles for preventive factors. Nutr Rev 52:75–83, 1994.
155. Hotz J, Goebell H. Epidemiology and pathogenesis of gastric carcinoma. In: Meyer HJ, Schnoll HJ, Hotz J, eds. Gastric carcinoma. New York: Springer-Verlag, 1989:3.
156. Tannenbaum SR, Wishnok JS, Leaf CD. Inhibition of nitrosamine formation by ascorbic acid. Am J Clin Nutr 53(Suppl):247S–250S, 1991.
157. Schorah CJ, Sobala GM, Sanderson M, et al. Gastric juice ascorbic acid: effects of disease and implications for gastric carcinogenesis. Am J Clin Nutr 53:287S–293S, 1991.
158. Eurogast. An international association between *Helicobacter pylori* infection and gastric cancer. Lancet 341:1359–1362, 1993.
159. Parsonnett J, Friedman GD, Vandersteen DP, et al. *Helicobacter pylori* infection and the risk of gastric carcinoma. N Engl J Med 325:1127–1131, 1991.
160. Graham DY. Benefits from elimination of *Helicobacter pylori* infection include major reduction in the incidence of peptic ulcer disease, gastric cancer, and primary gastric lymphoma. Prev Med 32:712–716, 1994.
161. Macdonald JS, Hill MC, Roberts IM. Gastric cancer: epidemiology, pathology, detection, and staging. In: Ahlgren J, Macdonald J, eds. Gastrointestinal oncology. Philadelphia: JB Lippincott, 1992:151–158.
162. Wanebo HJ, Kennedy BJ, Chmiel J, et al. Cancer of the stomach: a patient care study by the American College of Surgeons. Ann Surg 218:583–592, 1993.
163. Salvon-Harman JC, Nikulasson S, Stone MD, et al. Shifting proportions of gastric adenocarcinomas. Arch Surg 129:381, 1994.
164. Farley DR, Donohue JH. Early gastric cancer. Surg Clin North Am 72:401–421, 1992.
165. Ellis DJ, Spevis C, Kingston RD, et al. Carcinoembryonic antigen levels in advanced gastric carcinoma. Cancer 42:623–625, 1978.
166. Caletti G, Ferrari A, Brocchi E, et al. Accuracy of endoscopic ultrasonography in the diagnosis and staging of gastric cancer and lymphoma. Surgery 113:14–27, 1993.
167. Kaneko E, Nakamura T, Umeda N, et al. Outcome of gastric carcinoma detected by gastric mass survey in Japan. Gut 18:626, 1977.
168. Kim JP, Kim YW, Yang HK, et al. Significant prognostic factors by multivariate analysis of 3926 gastric cancer patients. World J Surg 18:872–878, 1994.
169. Lee WJ, Lee Ph, Yue SC, et al. Lymph node metastases in gastric cancer: significance of positive number. Oncology 52:45–50, 1995.
170. Boddie AW Jr. The role of lymphadenectomy in cancer, with particular reference to gastric cancer. Int Surg 79:6–10, 1994.
171. Behrns KE, Dalton RR, van Heerden JA, et al. Extended lymph node dissection for gastric cancer: is it of value? Surg Clin North Am 72:433–443, 1992.
172. Bonenkamp JJ, Van de Velde CJH, Sasako M, et al. R2 compared with R1 resection for gastric cancer: morbidity and mortality in a prospective, randomized trial. Eur J Surg 158:413–418, 1992.
173. Robertson CS, Chung SCS, Woods SDS, et al. A prospective randomized trial comparing R1 subtotal gastrectomy with R3 total gastrectomy for antral cancer. Ann Surg 220:176–182, 1994.
174. Bunt AMG, Hermans J, Boon MC, et al. Evaluation of the extent of lymphadenectomy in a randomized trial of Western- versus Japanese-type surgery in gastric cancer. J Clin Oncol 12:417–422, 1994.
175. Pacelli F, Doglietto GB, Ballantone R, et al. Extensive versus limited lymph node dissection for gastric cancer: a comparative study of 320 patients. Br J Surg 80:1153–1156, 1993.
176. Smith JW, Brennan MF. Surgical treatment of gastric cancer: proximal, mid and distal stomach. Surg Clin North Am 72:381–399, 1992.
177. Vezeridis MP. Wanebo HJ. Gastric cancer: surgical approach. In: Ahlgren J, Macdonald J, eds. Gastrointestinal oncology. Philadelphia: JB Lippincott, 1992:159–170.
178. Budach VGF. The role of radiation therapy in the management of gastric cancer. Ann Oncol 5(Suppl 3):S37–S48, 1994.
179. Tepper JE. Combined radiotherapy and chemotherapy in the treatment of gastrointestinal malignancies. Semin Oncol 19(Suppl 11):96–101, 1992.
180. Hallissey MT, Dunn JA, Ward LC, et al. The second British Stomach Cancer Group trial of adjuvant radiotherapy or chemotherapy in resectable gastric cancer: five-year follow-up. Lancet 343:1309–1312, 1994.
181. Calvo FA, Aristu JJ, Azinovic I, et al. Intraoperative and external radiotherapy in resected gastric cancer: updated report of a phase II trial. Int J Radiation Oncol Biol Phys 24:729–736, 1992.
182. Rougier P. Lasser P, Ducreux M, et al. Preoperative chemotherapy of locally advanced gastric cancer. Ann Oncol 5(Suppl 3):S59–S68, 1994.
183. Kang YK, Choi DW, Im YH, et al. A phase III randomized comparison of neoadjuvant chemotherapy followed by surgery for locally advanced stomach cancer [abstract]. Proc Am Soc Clin Oncol 15:215, 1996.
184. Yonemura Y, Sawa T, Kinoshita K, et al. Neoadjuvant chemotherapy for high-grade advanced gastric cancer. World J Surg 17:256–262, 1993.
185. Alexander HR, Grem JL, Pass HI, et al. Neoadjuvant chemotherapy of locally advanced gastric cancer. Oncology 7:37–41, 1993.
186. Kelsen D. Neoadjuvant therapy for gastrointestinal cancers. Oncology 7:25–31, 1993.
187. Leichman L, Silberman H, Leichman CG, et al. Preoperative systemic chemotherapy followed by adjuvant postoperative intraperitoneal therapy for gastric cancer: a University of Southern California pilot program. J Clin Oncol 10:1933–1942, 1992.
188. Agboola O. Adjuvant treatment in gastric cancer. Cancer Treat Rev 20:217–240, 1994.
189. Grau JJ, Estape J, Alcobendas F, et al. Positive results of adjuvant mitomycin C in resected gastric cancer: a randomized trial on 134 patients. Eur J Cancer 29A:340–342, 1993.
190. Gastrointestinal Tumor Study Group. Controlled trial of adjuvant chemotherapy following curative resection for gastric cancer. Cancer 49:1116–1122, 1982.
191. Engstrom PF, Lavin PT, Douglass HO Jr, et al. Postoperative adjuvant 5-fluorouracil plus methyl-CCNU for gastric cancer patients: Eastern Cooperative Oncology Group Study (EST 3275). Cancer 55:1868–1873, 1985.
192. Higgins GA, Amadeo JH, Smith DE, et al. Efficacy of prolonged intermittent therapy with combined 5-FU and methyl-CCNU following resection for gastric carcinoma. A Veterans Administration Surgical Oncology Group report. Cancer 52:1105–112, 1983.
193. Douglass HO Jr. Gastric cancer: current status of adjuvant therapy. Oncology 3:61–66, 1989.
194. Kelsen D. Adjuvant and neoadjuvant therapy for gastric cancer. Semin Oncol 23:379–389, 1996.
195. Bleiberg H, Gerard B, Deguiral P. Adjuvant therapy in resectable gastric cancer. Br J Cancer 66:987–991, 1992.
196. Lise M, Nitti D, Marchet A, et al. Adjuvant treatment for gastric cancer. Anticancer Drugs 2:433–445, 1991.
197. Kelsen D. The use of chemotherapy in the treatment of advanced gastric and pancreas cancer. Semin Oncol 21(Suppl 7):58–66, 1994.
198. Macdonald JS, Gastric cancer: chemotherapy of advanced disease. Hematol Oncol 10:37–42, 1992.
199. Ajani JA, Fairweather J, Dumas P, et al. A phase II study of Taxol in patients with advanced untreated gastric carcinoma [abstract]. Proc Annu Meet Am Soc Clin Oncol 16:A933, 1997.
200. Taguchi T. A late phase II study of docetaxel in patients with gastric cancer [abstract]. Proc Annu Meet Am Soc Clin Oncol 16:A934, 1997.

201. Macdonald JS, Schein PS, Woolley PV, et al. 5-fluorouracil, doxorubicin, and mitomycin (FAM) combination chemotherapy for advanced gastric cancer. Ann Intern Med 93:533–536, 1980.
202. Cullinan SA, Moertel CG, Fleming TR, et al. A comparison of three chemotherapeutic regimens in the treatment of advanced pancreatic and gastric carcinoma. Fluorouracil vs. fluorouracil and doxorubicin vs. fluorouracil, doxorubicin and mitomycin. JAMA 253:2061–2067, 1985.
203. Figoli F. Galligioni E, Crivellari D, et al. Evaluation of two consecutive regimens in advanced gastric cancer. Cancer Invest 93:257–262, 1991.
204. Kim NY, Park YS, Heo DS, et al. A phase III randomized study of 5-fluorouracil, doxorubicin, and mitomycin C versus 5-fluorouracil alone in the treatment of advanced gastric cancer. Cancer 71:3813–3818, 1993.
205. Cullinan SA, Moertel CG, Wieand HS, et al. Controlled evaluation of three drug combination regimens versus fluorouracil alone for the therapy of advanced gastric cancer. J Clin Oncol 12:412–416, 1994.
206. Wils JA, Klein HO, Wagener DJT, et al. Sequential high-dose methotrexate and fluorouracil combined with doxorubicin a step ahead in the treatment of advanced gastric cancer: a trial of the European Organization for Research and Treatment of Cancer Gastrointestinal Tract Cooperative Group. J Clin Oncol 9:827–831, 1991.
207. Murad AM, Santiago FF, Petroianu A, et al. Modified therapy with 5-fluorouracil, doxorubicin, and methotrexate in advanced gastric cancer. Cancer 72:37–41, 1993.
208. Pyrhonen S, Kuitunen T, Nyandoto P, et al. Randomized comparison of fluorouracil, epidoxorubicin and methotrexate plus supportive care with supportive care alone in patients with non-resectable gastric cancer. Br J Cancer 71:587–591, 1995.
209. Roelofs EMJ, Wagener DJY, Conroy T, et al. Phase II study of sequential high-dose methotrexate and 5-fluorouracil alternated with epirubicin and cisplatin in advanced gastric cancer. Ann Oncol 4:426–428, 1993.
210. Wilke H, Stahl M, Schmoll HJ, et al. Biochemical modulation of 5-fluorouracil by folinic acid or alpha-interferon with and without other cytostatic drugs in gastric, esophageal, and pancreatic cancer. Semin Oncol 19(Suppl 3):215–219, 1992.
211. Konishi T, Hiraishi M, Mafune K, et al. Therapeutic efficacy and toxicity of sequential methotrexate and 5-fluorouracil in gastric cancer. Anticancer Res 14:1277–1280, 1998.
212. Louvet C, deGramont A, Demuynck B, et al. High-dose folinic acid, 5-fluorouracil bolus and continuous infusion in poor-prognosis patients with advanced measurable gastric cancer. Ann Oncol 2:229–230, 1991.
213. Vanhoefer U, Wilke H, Weh HJ, et al. Weekly high-dose 5-fluorouracil and folinic acid as salvage treatment in advanced gastric cancer. Ann Oncol 5:850–851, 1994.
214. Wilke H, Preusser P, Fink U, et al. High dose folinic acid, etoposide and 5-fluouracil in advanced gastric cancer. A phase II study in elderly patients or patients with cardiac risk. Invest New Drugs 8:65–70, 1990.
215. DiBartolomeo M, Bajetta E, deBraud F, et al. Phase II study of the etoposide, leucovorin and fluorouracil combination for patients with advanced gastric cancer unsuitable for aggressive chemotherapy. Oncology 52:41–44, 1995.
216. Taal BG, Teller FGM, ten Bokkel Huinink WW, et al. Etoposide, leucovorin, 5-fluorouracil combination chemotherapy for advanced gastric cancer: experience with two treatment schedules incorporating intravenous or oral etoposide. Ann Oncol 5:90–92, 1994. 227.
217. Cocconi G, Bella M, Zironi S, et al. Fluorouracil, doxorubicin, and mitomycin combination versus PELF chemotherapy in advanced gastric cancer: a prospective randomized trial of the Italian Oncology Group for Clinical Research. J Clin Oncol 12:2687–2693, 1994.
218. Preusser P, Wilke H, Achterrath W, et al. Phase II study with the combination of etoposide, doxorubicin, and cisplatin in advanced measurable gastric cancer. J Clin Oncol 7:1310–1317, 1989.
219. Bajetta E, diBartolomeo M, deBraud F, et al. Etoposide, doxorubicin, and cisplatin treatment in advanced gastric cancer: a multicentre study of the Italian Trials in Medical Oncology (ITMO) Group. Eur J Cancer 30A:596–600, 1994.
220. Kelsen D, Atiq OT, Saltz L, et al. FAMTX versus etoposide, doxorubicin and cisplatin: a random assignment trial in gastric cancer. J Clin Oncol 10:541–548, 1992.
221. Haim M, Tsalik M, Robinson E. Treatment of gastric adenocarcinoma with the combination of etoposide, adriamycin and cisplatin: comparison between two schedules. Oncology 51:102–107, 1994.
222. Roth AD, Maibach R, Martinelli G, et al. Taxotere-cisplatin in advanced gastric carcinoma: a promising drug combination [abstract]. Eur J Cancer 33(Suppl 8):S275, 1997.
223. Murad AM, Guimaraes RC, Aragao BC, et al. Paclitaxel plus fluorouracil: a novel and very active regimen for advanced gastric cancer. A phase II trial [abstract]. Eur J Cancer 33(Suppl 8):S277, 1997.
224. Fujimoto S, Takahashi M, Kobayashi K, et al. Relation between clinical and histologic outcome of intraperitoneal hyperthermic perfusion for patients with gastric cancer and peritoneal metastasis. Oncology 50:338–343, 1993.
225. Tsujitani D, Okuyama T, Watanabe A, et al. Intraperitoneal cisplatin during surgery for gastric cancer and peritoneal seeding. Anticancer Res 13:1831–1834, 1993.
226. Jones AI, Trott P, Cunningham D, et al. A pilot study of intraperitoneal cisplatin in the management of gastric cancer. Ann Oncol 5:123–125, 1994.

CHAPTER 91

LUNG CANCER

Kristan M. Augustin

Lung cancer is the leading cause of cancer death in both men and women in the United States. It is estimated that in 2000 164,100 new cases will be diagnosed and 156,900 deaths will be related to this disease.[1] Lung cancer is divided into two distinct classes that have important prognostic and therapeutic implications. Approximately 80% of new cases diagnosed are non–small cell lung cancer (NSCLC), whereas only a minority of cases are small cell lung cancer (SCLC). Although vast improvements in diagnosis, treatment, and prevention of lung cancer have been made over the past few years, prognosis is poor, with less than 20% of patients alive 5 years after diagnosis. This disease costs an estimated $8 billion annually and makes up approximately 20% of all cancer costs in the United States.[2]

EPIDEMIOLOGY

Lung cancer was once a disease that affected primarily men. However, with the changing trends in women's smoking habits over the past decades, the number of lung cancer deaths in women surpasses that caused by breast cancer and is estimated to represent 25% of all cancer deaths in 1998. Although there appears to be a higher mortality rate in African American men than in Caucasian men, the rates are comparable between African American and Caucasian women. The incidence of lung cancer increases with age, with the diagnosis of most patients occurring between ages 55 and 65 years. Finally, people living in developed countries are more likely to develop lung cancer, with the highest rates of lung cancer deaths observed in the United States, Hungary, and Denmark.

Most epidemiologic studies conclude that lung cancer may be preventable. More than 80% of patients with lung cancer have a history of smoking cigarettes. This risk factor is further supported by the epidemiologic correlation between smoking trends and the incidence and mortality of patients with lung cancer. In the 1930s, it was noted that the number of men who smoked was increasing, with women following this trend nearly 20 years later. What was once thought to be a disease that affected primarily men now includes a significant number of women.[3]

The risk of developing lung cancer appears to be related to the number, duration, and type of tobacco products smoked. Compared to a nonsmoker, people who smoke 20 cigarettes a day have a 20-fold higher risk of developing lung cancer. Additionally, the duration of smoking increases risk, with adults who start smoking during adolescence and continue throughout their lifetime at greatest risk. Cigarettes are the most significant risk factor, but pipes and cigars are also risk factors. Finally, the amount of tar and nicotine found in cigarettes may play a role in lung cancer development. Adding filters and reducing tar from 35 mg to approximately 13 mg appears to reduce the risk but does not eliminate it.

Smoking is the largest modifiable risk factor for lung cancer. Cessation of cigarette smoking is known to significantly decrease the risk of developing lung cancer. This benefit is not observed for at least 5 years and increases with each subsequent year of abstinence. Therefore, much support exists for smoking cessation and prevention programs, particularly in adolescents and young adults, to reduce the incidence of new cases of lung cancer.

Environmental tobacco smoke, also known as secondhand or passive smoking, has long been of concern as a potential cause of lung disease. Known carcinogens present in environmental tobacco smoke may cause lung cancer in nonsmokers. Those who live with a smoker or are exposed to at least 20 cigarettes a day are at a 30% higher risk of developing lung cancer than those who do not.[4] A report published by the U.S. Surgeon General confirmed this finding in 1986. Since then, laws have been passed and reforms initiated to prevent smoking in many public areas.[5]

Asbestos and radon are two occupational risk factors correlated with lung cancer. Lung cancer was first noted in mine, mill, insulation, textile, and shipyard workers exposed to asbestos. Those exposed had a relative risk eight times that of nonexposed workers. In workers who are exposed to both asbestos and cigarette smoke, the risk increases to 45 times that of a nonexposed worker.[6]

Radon has been known to cause respiratory problems and death in silver miners since the sixteenth century. It may leak indoors through the soil, basements, and crawl spaces. This inert gas decomposes and emits α-particles, which damage cells in the lung. Uranium miners exposed to the gas and particles are believed to be at increased risk, but the cases are complicated by exposure to other substances, including arsenic, silica, and tobacco. In combination with tobacco smoke, radon poses an even greater risk of lung cancer.

Other substances postulated to increase the risk of lung cancer include arsenic, formaldehyde, ether, chromium, polycyclic aromatic hydrocarbons, nickel, and silica. Additionally, case reports suggest that lung cancer may develop secondary to interstitial fibrosis caused by tuberculosis, chronic fibrosis, and chronic obstructive pulmonary disease.

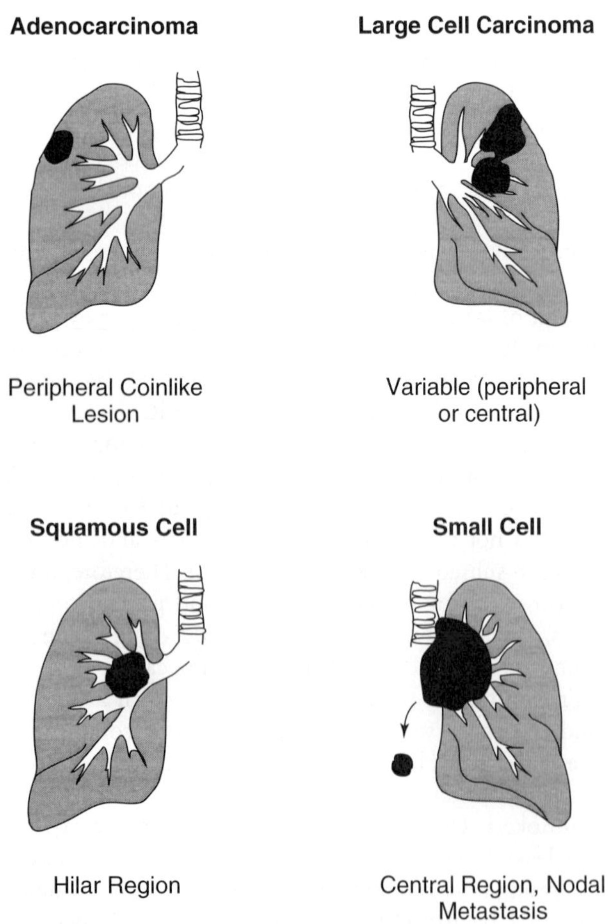

Figure 91.1. Size and location of each cellular type of lung cancer. (*Source:* Harvey JC, Beattie EJ. Lung cancer. Clinical Symposia 45:2–34.)

PATHOPHYSIOLOGY

Lung malignancies are categorized as NSCLC or SCLC (Fig. 91.1). By classifying the type of lung cancer, one can better determine treatment strategies and prognosis. NSCLC accounts for more than 80% of cases diagnosed each year. NSCLCs do not proliferate as rapidly as SCLCs and are characterized as one or more histologic types that include adenocarcinoma, squamous cell, and large cell carcinoma. Adenocarcinoma is the most common histologic type of NSCLC and typically presents as a small peripheral coinlike lesion (less than 4 cm), with metastases occurring early, often before diagnosis. This type of NSCLC is more likely to occur in nonsmokers and women than the other types of lung cancer. Squamous cell carcinoma is most often observed in men and smokers. It is a rapidly growing tumor that presents in the central or hilar regions of the lung. It may remain localized and cavitate, or it may spread to regional lymph nodes. Large cell carcinoma is an anaplastic tumor that generally presents as a large and bulky peripheral lesion. It is known to rapidly proliferate and metastasize to both local and distant sites. Small cell carcinoma is a rapidly growing and aggressive tumor. It typically arises from the central region of the lung but occasionally appears in the periphery. Early metastases are common, with a majority occurring outside the hemithorax. A lung cancer that presents as multiple nodules in different lobes or the contralateral lung is called a synchronous tumor. Each nodule may be of the same or different cell type, and the prognosis in these patients generally is poor.

CLINICAL PRESENTATION AND DIAGNOSIS

Signs and Symptoms

The anatomic location of the lesion and the extent of disease usually determine how this carcinoma presents. Tumors in the periphery typically are asymptomatic and are discovered on a chest radiograph obtained for some other medical condition. Centrally located tumors usually present earlier, with nonspecific symptoms that often are mistaken for other respiratory disorders, including pneumonia. Cough is the most common symptom in patients with lung cancer. However, this symptom may be present for years before diagnosis because many of these patients have a history of smoking. The patient must be questioned about a change in frequency and severity of coughing because it usually worsens as the tumor progresses. Dyspnea is also a nonspecific symptom that may worsen with obstruction. Hemoptysis may present as one of the first new symptoms, but it is also nonspecific and often confused with other respiratory conditions including tuberculosis, bronchitis, and aspergillosis. The invasion of the left recurrent laryngeal nerve may cause compression and vocal cord paralysis, resulting in hoarseness. Postobstructive pneumonia, fatigue, and anorexia with weight loss may also be present.

Pancoast's, Horner's, and superior vena cava syndromes

sometimes are present at diagnosis. Compression of the brachial plexus causing shoulder and arm pain is called Pancoast's syndrome. Facial swelling often is a sign that the tumor is compressing or invading the superior vena cava and is characterized as superior vena cava syndrome. Horner's syndrome may be present secondary to the invasion of the sympathetic ganglia resulting in ptosis, myosis, and ipsilateral anhydrosis.

Paraneoplastic syndromes often are present in patients with SCLC. These syndromes can produce signs and symptoms at a site distant from the primary lesion and its metastases. Syndrome of inappropriate antidiuretic hormone (SIADH) may present in up to 50% of patients with SCLC. Severe dilutional hyponatremia may cause disorientation, seizures, and coma if not promptly treated. Other endocrinologic abnormalities include atrial natriuretic peptide and ectopic adrenocorticotropic hormone secretion. Lambert–Eaton Myasthenic Syndrome is a rare but damaging neurologic paraneoplastic syndrome that may produce profound muscular weakness. Paraneoplastic cerebellar degeneration and paraneoplastic encephalomyelitis may also occur, resulting in various neuromuscular and neurologic sequelae.

Metastases may be present at diagnosis in both NSCLC and SCLC. Common sites of metastasis include the liver, bone, brain, contralateral lung, and adrenal glands. Often patients present with different signs and symptoms, including pain, headaches, seizures, and elevated liver function tests. These are often a result of extrathoracic disease and must be evaluated to determine the exact stage of the disease and appropriate treatment.

Diagnosis

Careful evaluation of the symptoms is important. A complete physical examination and medical history provide valuable information. Additionally, blood chemistries and complete blood count should be obtained to evaluate for abnormalities. Patients thought to be at high risk for lung cancer should get a chest radiograph to evaluate pulmonary nodules, mediastinal widening, pleural effusions, and potential osseous metastases. A computed tomographic (CT) scan should be performed for patients with probable or definite lung cancer to further define the tumor, determine the extent of mediastinal involvement, detect pericardial involvement or chest wall invasion, and identify additional lung masses. Histologic or cytologic diagnosis should be performed using at least one of five methods. Sputum collection for cytology may be performed, but typically a bronchoscopy is performed in all patients with central lesions. Alternatively, a transthoracic needle aspiration of peripheral lesions may be performed. In patients with mediastinal lymph nodes larger than 1 cm, mediastinoscopy should be performed for histologic diagnosis and for additional staging information (Fig. 91.2). Patients with pleural effusions should undergo thoracentesis or thoracoscopy to better visualize and biopsy the pleural nodules, pleural surface, and ipsilateral lymph nodes. Finally, intraoperative staging involving the removal of the primary lesion and the ipsilateral mediastinal lymph nodes also confirms the diagnosis. Evaluation of distant metastasis usually is performed only in symptomatic patients or those with advanced disease.

For patients in whom surgical resection is a treatment option, pulmonary function tests should be obtained to identify those at risk for postoperative complications. The most common procedure is the forced expiratory volume in 1 second (FEV_1) technique. Patients with an FEV_1 less than 800 mL are at greatest risk for postoperative morbidity and mortality and generally are considered poor surgical candidates. Other pulmonary function tests that may be performed to determine risk include a split function perfusion scan, arterial blood gases, diffusing capacity of lung for carbon monoxide (DLCO), and maximum voluntary ventilation.

Staging

Lung cancer is staged both clinically at the time of diagnosis with noninvasive tools and pathologically after the surgically resected specimen is evaluated. The TNM classification schema is used for staging lung cancer (Tables 91.1 and 91.2).[7,8] *T* refers to the size and extent of the tumor, *N* represents the involvement of regional lymph nodes, and *M* denotes distant metastatic disease. It is a universally accepted system that groups patients with similar extent of disease and facilitates treatment and prognosis decisions. Additionally, it groups patients with similar characteristics together for analysis in clinical trials. Although the TNM system is used for all histologies, it is more applicable to NSCLC. SCLC can be staged according to this system, but very few patients are candidates for surgical staging at the time of diagnosis. Thus, patients with SCLC usually are classified as having limited or extensive disease using the Veterans Administration Lung Cancer Therapy Group (VALG) system.[9,10] Limited disease is defined as a tumor that may be treated within a single, tolerable radiotherapy port. It was suggested that this definition be clarified to include tumors limited to one hemithorax with regional lymph node metastases, including hilar, ipsilateral, and contralateral mediastinal; ipsilateral and contralateral supraclavicular nodes; and with ipsilateral pleural effusion independent of whether the cytology findings are positive or negative.[11] Approximately two-thirds of patients diagnosed with SCLC have extensive disease that refers to all tumor burden that exceeds limited disease.

PSYCHOSOCIAL ASPECTS

Upon learning of the diagnosis of lung cancer, patients exhibit a wide variety of emotions and behaviors. Anger, shock, fear, and sadness are common feelings at diagnosis. Guilt is often present because patients feel that lung cancer was brought on by their lifestyle. Some patients may become depressed, whereas others exhibit signs of denial.

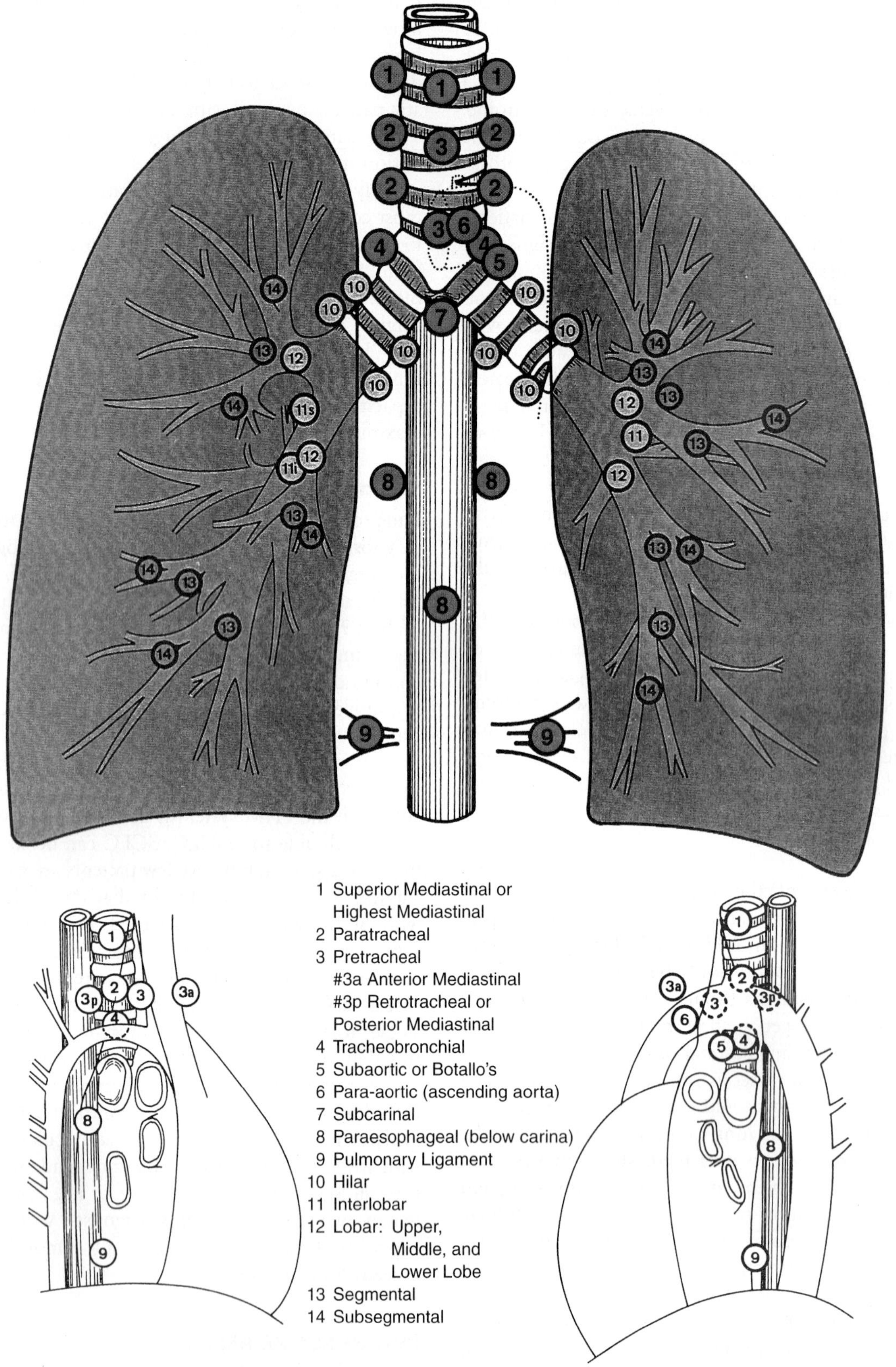

Figure 91.2. Thoracic lymph node map. (*Source:* Naruke T, Suemasu K, Ishikawa S. Surgical treatment for lung cancer with metastasis to mediastinal lymph nodes. J Thorac Cardiovasc Surg 71[2]:279–285, 1976.)

Additionally, the quality of life of these patients is greatly affected by their illness and may ultimately play a role in their psychological well-being. The patients' symptoms may affect their ability to complete daily activities by interfering with physical and psychological functions, as well as their social, sexual, occupational, and spiritual interactions. The psychological, emotional, and social concerns of these patients must be addressed and treated accordingly. Support groups, counseling, medications, and religion often play a role in comforting patients with lung cancer and improving their quality of life.

Table 91.1 ▪ TNM Classification of Lung Cancer

Primary tumor (T)	
TX	Primary tumor cannot be assessed or tumor proven by malignant cells present in sputum or bronchial washings but not visualized by imaging or bronchoscopy.
T0	No evidence of primary tumor.
T_{is}	Carcinoma in situ.
T1	Tumor ≤3 cm in greatest dimension, surrounded by lung or visceral pleura, without bronchoscopic evidence of invasion more proximal than the lobar bronchus[a] (i.e., not the main bronchus).
T2	Tumor with any of the following features of size or extent: >3 cm in greatest dimension Involves the main bronchus, ≥2 cm distal carina Invades the visceral pleura Associated with atelectasis or obstructive pneumonitis that extends to the hilar region but does not involve the entire lung.
T3	Tumor of any size that directly invades the chest wall (including superior sulcus tumors), diaphragm, mediastinal pleura, or parietal pericardium; tumor in the main bronchus <2 cm distal the carina but without involvement of the carina; or associated atelectasis or obstructive pneumonitis of the entire lung.
T4	Tumor of any size that invades the mediastinum, heart, great vessels, esophagus, vertebral body, carina, or tumor with a malignant pleural effusion.[b]
Regional lymph nodes (N)	
NX	Regional lymph nodes cannot be assessed.
N0	No regional lymph node metastasis.
N1	Metastasis to ipsilateral peribronchial or ipsilateral hilar lymph nodes and intrapulmonary nodes involved by direct extension of the primary tumor.
N2	Metastasis to ipsilateral mediastinal or subcarinal lymph node(s).
N3	Metastasis to contralateral mediastinal, contralateral hilar, ipsilateral or contralateral scalene, or supraclavicular lymph node(s).
Distant metastasis (M)	
MX	Presence of distant metastasis cannot be assessed.
M0	No distant metastasis.
M1	Distant metastasis present.[c]

Source: Reference 8.

[a]The uncommon superficial tumor of any size with its invasive component limited to the bronchial wall, which may extend proximal to the main bronchus, is also classified T1.

[b]Most pleural effusions associated with lung cancer are caused by tumor. However, in a few patients multiple cytopathologic examinations of pleural fluid show no tumor. In these cases, the fluid is nonbloody and is not an exudate. When these elements and the clinical judgment dictate that the effusion is not related to the tumor, the effusion should be excluded as a staging element and the patient's disease should be staged T1, T2, or T3. Pericardial effusion is classified according to the same rules.

[c]Separate metastatic tumor nodule(s) in the ipsilateral nonprimary lobe(s) of the lung are classified as M1.

Table 91.2 ▪ Stage Grouping (TNM) of Lung Cancer

Stage	T	N	M	5-yr Survival Rate After Treatment (%)
0	T_{is}	N0	M0	Not available
IA	T1	N0	M0	67
IB	T2	N0	M0	57
IIA	T1	N1	M0	55
IIB	T2	N1	M0	39
	T3	N0	M0	38
IIIA	T3	N1	M0	25
	T1	N2	M0	23
	T2	N2	M0	23
	T3	N2	M0	23
IIIB	T4	N0	M0	7
	T4	N1	M0	7
	T4	N2	M0	7
	T1	N3	M0	3
	T2	N3	M0	3
	T3	N3	M0	3
	T4	N3	M0	3
IV	Any T	Any N	M1	1

Source: Reference 7.
TNM, tumor, node, and metastasis.

TREATMENT

Non–Small Cell Lung Cancer

NSCLC accounts for the majority of lung cancer cases. Male patients and those with a poor performance status, weight loss greater than 5%, and advanced stage have a poorer prognosis. The treatment goals for early-stage NSCLC are to cure the patient of the disease and prolong survival in those who cannot be cured.

Surgery is considered the cornerstone of therapy and offers the only true potential for cure. Radiation therapy, with or without chemotherapy, often is added to the treatment regimen. The treatment goals for late-stage NSCLC are to prolong survival and palliate symptoms. Untreated, most patients die within 1 year of diagnosis.

Stage I

Surgical resection is considered standard of care for treating stage I patients. The preferred surgical procedure for patients who are in good physical condition is a lobectomy with hilar and mediastinal lymph node dissection. Any lesser surgical procedure, such as a wedge resection or segmentectomy, may compromise the prognosis of these patients. Although there is no difference in operative morbidity or mortality, there appears to be an increase in local recurrence and decreased survival after limited resection.[12,13] Currently, there is no proven role for adjuvant chemotherapy or radiation after a lobectomy in stage I NSCLC. Therefore, the addition of adjuvant chemotherapy and/or radiation to surgery should be limited to clinical trials.

Complete resection often is contraindicated in patients with compromised pulmonary function, those older than 70 years, those with a medical condition that prohibits surgery, and those who refuse surgery. In these patients a segmentectomy or wedge resection may be performed in an attempt to prolong survival. Radiation therapy is an alternative modality used in an attempt to improve local control of the tumor and possibly prolong survival in medically inoperable stage I lung cancer. Radiation dosages of at least 60 Gy typically are administered with minimal complications and result in a 13 to 17% overall survival rate.[14,15] Patients who are younger, have tumors less than 4 cm in size, with squamous cell histology, and are asymptomatic upon diagnosis have a better prognosis after radiotherapy than other patients with unresectable NSCLC.

Stage II

As in stage I NSCLC, surgical resection is the treatment of choice for stage II tumors. Postoperative radiotherapy may reduce the incidence of local recurrences but has no impact on overall survival, generally because distant metastases occur.[16,17] Therefore, adjuvant thoracic irradiation should be limited to investigational protocols. Adjuvant chemotherapy after complete resection has been evaluated in several clinical trials that produced conflicting results. However, the chemotherapy regimens administered may not have been optimal, and further studies evaluating neoadjuvant and adjuvant therapy are needed.[18–24] Therefore, chemotherapy is also not recommended in medically operable stage II NSCLC outside of a clinical trial setting because its benefit has not been defined clearly. Patients with unresectable or incompletely resected stage II lung cancer may benefit from adjuvant chemotherapy and/or radiotherapy, but the exact role of chemotherapy and/or radiotherapy in this setting is still under investigation.

Stage IIIA

T3 Disease

Surgery is the treatment of choice for patients with T3N0-1 disease. Postoperative radiation therapy often is used in patients with positive margins, but no compelling evidence supports its use. Additionally, combined adjuvant chemotherapy and radiotherapy has not been clearly proven and therefore is not recommended unless used in the setting of a clinical trial.

N2 Disease

Treatment of patients with N2 disease is very controversial. Patients with ipsilateral or subcarinal mediastinal lymph nodes have a poor prognosis. Although complete resection provides good local control, most patients die from systemic metastases, with less than 20% alive at 5 years.[25–27] Radiotherapy as monotherapy may be an option in patients with inoperable N2 disease, but very few patients are alive at 5 years without tumor recurrence. Therefore, it seems logical that postoperative radiation and/or chemotherapy would prevent disseminated recurrences and prolong survival. However, several clinical trials evaluating adjuvant therapy produced negative results, with no difference in disease-free or overall survival in completely resected patients with N2 disease compared to surgery alone.[17,19,28] Additional trials comparing chemoradiotherapy to radiotherapy alone, after complete resection, in patients with N2 disease also failed to prolong survival or time to recurrence.[29,30]

Postoperative radiation therapy is indicated for patients who had complete resection with positive lymph nodes or resection with margins positive for disease and those who develop recurrent disease, and are unable to undergo surgery. It reduces local recurrence, but there is no supporting evidence of a survival benefit, most likely because of distant metastasis.

Complete resection is needed to improve the chance of long-term survival. In an attempt to improve resectability and survival, several studies have evaluated neoadjuvant chemotherapy alone or in combination with radiotherapy. The goal of preoperative therapy is to reduce the size of the tumor, improve the chance for a complete resection, potentially downstage the tumor, decrease the chance of local relapse, and treat potential micrometastatic disease that may be present in locally advanced but potentially resectable disease. In a nonrandomized trial, Martini et al.[31] evaluated mitomycin C, vindesine or vinblastine, and high-dose cisplatin (MVP) administration before surgery. Overall survival at 5 years was 17%, with a median survival of 19 months. Survival was improved in patients who were completely resected, with a 5-year survival rate of 26%. These results were confirmed in a similar nonrandomized study conducted by Burkes et al.[32] that enabled several patients with unresectable disease to undergo thoracotomy and prolong survival after MVP administration. Kirn et al.[33] conducted a nonrandomized study in which 60 patients received platinum-containing regimens followed by surgical resection. Patients with complete resections appear to benefit from neoadjuvant chemotherapy, with a 2-year survival rate of 67%. In two small randomized trials, chemotherapy administered before surgical resection was compared with surgery alone. Roth et al.[34] randomized 60 patients to receive either three courses of preoperative cyclophosphamide, etoposide, and cisplatin (CEP) or resection alone. Patients who responded to neoadjuvant chemotherapy and had a complete resection were given three additional courses of chemotherapy. A survival advantage in patients receiving preoperative chemotherapy was observed, with 56% of patients alive at 3 years. Rosell et al.[35] compared the combination of mitomycin, ifosfamide, and cisplatin (MIP) as neoadjuvant therapy and surgery as monotherapy in 60 patients. Survival and disease-free survival were significantly higher in the chemotherapy group than in those treated with surgery alone. Although the sample size was small for the randomized trials, the data are significant and must be confirmed in larger clinical trials.

The addition of radiotherapy to chemotherapy before surgery may provide some benefit to patients with potentially resectable stage IIIA disease. Three nonrandomized clinical studies evaluated a cisplatin-based regimen and radiation therapy before and after resection. These studies found a potential benefit in the patients' survival, but treatment-related morbidity and mortality were common.[36–38] Future randomized clinical trials must be conducted to further define the role of combination neoadjuvant therapy in this setting.

Patients with unresectable disease have a poor prognosis. Primary chemoradiotherapy may be an option for this group of patients. Although it does not have a profound impact on overall survival and the rate of local failure is great, it is superior to thoracic irradiation as monotherapy.[39–41]

Although the optimal induction regimen has not been found, there are several options to offer these patients. Currently, preoperative regimens using chemotherapy, chemoradiotherapy, and radiotherapy alone appear promising. Until treatment for stage IIIA lung cancer is clearly delineated, these patients should be treated in a clinical trial setting.

Superior Sulcus Tumor

This tumor is located in the apex of the lung, invades the first rib, and involves the stellate ganglion and brachial plexus. Shoulder pain, rib erosion, and Horner's syndrome often are present and are called Pancoast's syndrome. Preoperative radiotherapy may reduce tumor size, facilitating en bloc resection of the involved lung, chest wall, and T1 nerve root. Adjuvant radiotherapy may be of benefit in patients with residual disease. Currently there is no proven role for chemotherapy with this type of tumor.

Stage IIIB and IV

Stage IIIB NSCLC is more locally advanced than stage IIIA lung cancer and generally is considered unresectable. Prognosis is poor, with a 5-year survival rate of less than 7%. Patients with T4 disease have tumors that invade the heart, trachea, esophagus, vertebral body, or the carina, and treatment consists of radiotherapy alone or in combination with chemotherapy. Patients with contralateral mediastinal or hilar lymph nodes or supraclavicular or scalene lymph nodes have N3 disease, and radiation therapy alone yields poor results. These patients should receive chemotherapy in addition to radiotherapy.

Palliative therapy, also called best supportive care, is the standard treatment for patients with metastatic NSCLC (stage IV) unless they are enrolled in a clinical trial. Surgical excision of a solitary brain metastasis followed by radiation is indicated in patients with responsive disease in an attempt to prolong survival. In patients with single metastatic lesions in other areas of the body, surgical excision is the standard of care. Furthermore, radiotherapy often is administered to palliate symptoms from the primary tumor and metastatic sites. Often these patients are admitted to the hospital for intensive supportive care. Several studies have evaluated the effectiveness, both clinically and financially, of administering best supportive care compared to chemotherapy in chemotherapy-naive patients with advanced NSCLC.[42–44] Not only was a modest survival advantage observed in patients receiving chemotherapy, but the patients' quality of life was improved, with a reduction in symptoms and the ability to continue normal daily activities. Additionally, chemotherapy was found to be cost-effective in these patients because it reduced the symptoms, number and duration of hospital admissions, and number of palliative radiotherapy treatments administered. Although these studies demonstrate a benefit of delivering chemotherapy rather than best supportive care, it is important to note that the eligibility criteria and chemotherapy administered varied between the studies. The differences include a wide variety of chemotherapy regimens administered with different durations of treatment, delivery of minimally active drugs in certain regimens, and the study population included patients with either stage IIIB and IV NSCLC or just stage IV in the analysis. Despite these differences, chemotherapy appears to be cost-effective and confers a survival advantage to patients with unresectable advanced NSCLC.

Only a few chemotherapeutic agents produce response rates of at least 15% in NSCLC, and none improve survival as single agents (Table 91.3). Cisplatin is regarded as the most active and important agent in treating NSCLC. Carboplatin has marginal activity by itself in treating NSCLC, but when it is used in combination with etoposide, the response rates are similar to that observed with cisplatin–etoposide regimens, without the toxicity.

Multimodality therapy has been evaluated in the setting of advanced NSCLC, with regimens including cisplatin producing better responses. Regimens commonly used to treat NSCLC are listed in Table 91.4. Furthermore, regimens that add radiotherapy produce results that trend toward a survival advantage. Sause et al.[41] evaluated patients with nonresectable NSCLC who were randomized to receive either standard radiotherapy, twice-daily radiotherapy, or cisplatin plus vinblastine in addition to radiotherapy. Approximately 50% of the patients in each arm had stage IIIB disease. Although the results were not statistically significant, there was a trend toward prolonged survival in the combination therapy arm. Kreisman et al.[45] compared these two agents plus radiotherapy with radiation monotherapy. This study also found a trend toward increased survival in patients with stage IIIB disease. The combination of cisplatin and etoposide with radiation was evaluated in patients with stage IIIA and IIIB NSCLC in a randomized trial performed by the Southwest Oncology Group.[46] In this trial, resection was attempted in patients who responded to treatment or had stable disease. Seventy-eight percent of the patients with stage IIIB disease were eligible for resection after receiving chemo-

Table 91.3 ▪ Chemotherapeutic Agents Active in Non–Small Cell Lung Cancer

Chemotherapy Agent	Common Adverse Drug Events	Monitoring Parameters[a]
Carboplatin	Thrombocytopenia, neutropenia, anemia, nausea and vomiting, mucositis, stomatitis, alopecia, peripheral neuropathy, hypomagnesemia, hypokalemia, hypocalcemia, hypophosphatemia, and liver function test elevations	Complete blood count with differential, magnesium, potassium, calcium, inorganic phosphorus, total bilirubin, alkaline phosphatase, SGPT, LDH, urine output, and weight
Cisplatin	Nephrotoxicity (renal tubular damage), acute and delayed nausea and vomiting (may be severe), high-frequency hearing loss, myelosuppression, peripheral neuropathy, hypomagnesemia, hypokalemia, hyponatremia, hypocalcemia, hypophosphatemia, and mild alopecia	BUN, creatinine, complete blood count with differential, magnesium, potassium, sodium, calcium, inorganic phosphorus, urine output, and weight
Docetaxel	Myelosuppression, nausea and vomiting, stomatitis, diarrhea, fluid retention, rash, alopecia, myalgia, and arthralgia	Complete blood count with differential, urine output, and weight
Etoposide	Myelosuppression, nausea and vomiting, hypotension, mucositis, alopecia, and diarrhea	Complete blood count with differential and blood pressure
Gemcitabine	Myelosuppression, nausea and vomiting, diarrhea, stomatitis, pain, alopecia, and elevated liver enzymes	Complete blood count with differential, total bilirubin, LDH, SGPT, and alkaline phosphatase
Ifosfamide	Myelosuppression, nausea and vomiting (may be severe), hemorrhagic cystitis, dysuria, nephrotoxicity, neurotoxicity (including lethargy, ataxia, mental status changes, disorientation, seizures, and coma), and alopecia	Complete blood count with differential, urinalysis as indicated, BUN, creatinine
Irinotecan	Myelosuppression, diarrhea, nausea and vomiting, vasodilation, headache, and dizziness	Complete blood count with differential
Mitomycin C	Delayed myelosuppression, mild nausea and vomiting, stomatitis, diarrhea, hemolytic uremic syndrome, creatinine elevation, dyspnea, alopecia, and interstitial pneumonia	Complete blood count with differential, chest radiograph as indicated, and creatinine
Paclitaxel	Hypersensitivity reactions (especially without premedication), myelosuppression, mucositis, nausea and vomiting, peripheral neuropathy, alopecia, myalgia, and arthralgia	Complete blood count with differential
Vinblastine	Myelosuppression, constipation, mild nausea and vomiting, paraesthesia, alopecia, and muscle pain	Complete blood count with differential
Vinorelbine	Myelosuppression, mild nausea and vomiting, constipation, transient liver function test elevations, peripheral neuropathy, myalgia, arthralgia, and alopecia	Complete blood count with differential, total bilirubin, alkaline phosphatase, LDH, and SGPT

[a]Patient should be monitored clinically for symptomatic toxicities.
SGPT, serum glutamic–pyruvic transaminase; *LDH*, lactate dehydrogenase; *BUN*, blood urea nitrogen.

therapy and radiotherapy. The results of this study are encouraging because the pattern of relapse and 3-year survival rate is similar to that in patients with stage IIIA disease. Further studies must be conducted to evaluate the risk and benefit potential of adding surgery to treat this group of patients.

Newer agents with activity against NSCLC as monotherapy include paclitaxel, docetaxel, vinorelbine, gemcitabine, and irinotecan. The taxane, paclitaxel, is an antimicrotubule agent that has excellent activity against advanced NSCLC. When it is used a single agent in patients with stage IIIB or IV disease, overall response rates range from 21 to 25%.[47–49] In combination with cisplatin or carboplatin, response rates increase to greater than 35%.[50–55] Based on the results of these studies, the combination of paclitaxel with either cisplatin or carboplatin is now incorporated into many treatment plans and clinical trials for treating this advanced disease. Docetaxel is similar to paclitaxel and produces response rates greater than 20% in untreated patients with advanced NSCLC.[56–58] Although grade 4 neutropenia is often observed, response rates improve when docetaxel is administered in combination with cisplatin in clinical trials.[59–61] The camptothecin analog irinotecan produces response rates greater than 30% as monotherapy in previously untreated advanced NSCLC.[62,63] Myelosuppression and diarrhea are the common side effects observed with this chemotherapeutic agent. In combination with cisplatin, response rates improved to 48 to 54% with tolerable toxicities.[64] Gemcitabine is a new antimetabolite with single-agent activity in NSCLC. In several clinical trials, this pyrimidine analog produced objective response rates of approximately 20%, with weekly dosages ranging from 800 to 2800 mg/m^2 and tolerable toxicity.[65–68] The mild toxicity profile of gemcitabine makes it an ideal agent to use in combination with cisplatin, which results in objective response rates greater than 30%.[69–71] Vinorelbine, the semisynthetic analog of vinblastine, is approved by the Food and Drug Administration for first-line treatment of patients with advanced NSCLC. This agent interferes with microtubule assembly, which results in mitosis inhibition. In patients with inoperable NSCLC, vinorelbine produces an objective response rate of 29% and median survival of 33 weeks when intravenous dosages of 30 mg/m^2 are administered weekly.[72] Not only is the combination of vinorelbine and cisplatin superior to vinorelbine alone, but it results in improved objective response rate and survival than cisplatin as monotherapy or the combination of cisplatin and vindesine.[73,74]

Compared with the combination regimen containing etoposide and cisplatin, both gemcitabine and vinorelbine as monotherapy are more cost-effective, with parallel efficacy in relation to duration of survival.[75,76] The cost savings probably result from the reduction in the number of hospital days needed to administer the agents and treatment of drug-related toxicities observed with gemcitabine and vinorelbine. Additionally, the ability to administer these two medications on an outpatient basis further contributes to a cost savings. The clinical and financial effectiveness observed with these two agents make them excellent treatment options in this patient population. Further pharmacoeconomic analyses of the other new agents are needed.

Recurrent or Refractory Disease

Second-line therapy for patients who do not respond to an initial platinum-based regimen is undefined. However, several options are available and may benefit the patient by prolonging survival, palliating symptoms, and improving quality of life. Newer agents, including docetaxel, paclitaxel, vinorelbine, or irinotecan, may offer a survival advantage to patients with a good performance status.[77] An alternative to the newer agents with documented activity in NSCLC is participation in studies involving investigational agents with unknown activity. Finally, best

Table 91.4 ▪ Common Chemotherapy Regimens for Treating Non–Small Cell Lung Cancer

Drug	Dosage	Schedule
EP		Repeat course every 3–4 wk.
Etoposide	60–120 mg/m^2 IV on days 1–3	
Cisplatin	50–120 mg/m^2 IV on day 1	
CEP		Repeat course every 4 wk.
Cyclophosphamide	500 mg/m^2 IV on day 1	
Etoposide	100 mg/m^2 IV on days 1–3	
Cisplatin	100 mg/m^2 IV on day 1	
CAP		Repeat course every 4 wk.
Cyclophosphamide	400 mg/m^2 IV on day 1	
Doxorubicin	40 mg/m^2 IV on day 1	
Cisplatin	50–60 mg/m^2 IV on day 1	
MVP		Repeat course every 6 wk.
Mitomycin	8 mg/m^2 IV on days 1 and 29	
Vinblastine	3–4.5 mg/m^2 IV on days 1, 8, 29, then every 2 wk	
Cisplatin	80-120 mg/m^2 IV on days 1 and 29	
ICE		Repeat course every 4 wk.
Ifosfamide	1–1.2 g/m^2 IV on days 1 and 2	
Cisplatin	100 mg/m^2 IV on days 1 and 8	
Etoposide	60–75 mg/m^2 IV on days 1–3	
Vinorelbine	30 mg/m^2 IV on day 1	Repeat weekly until disease progression.
Cis-Vinorelbine		Repeat cycle every 3 wk.
Cisplatin	80-120 mg/m^2 IV on day 1	
Vinorelbine	30 mg/m^2 IV on days 1, 8, and 15	
Cis-Tax		Repeat cycle every 3–4 wk.
Cisplatin	60–90 mg/m^2 IV on day 1	
Paclitaxel	135–215 mg/m^2 IV on day 1	
Carbo-Vinorelbine		Repeat cycle every 4 wk.
Carboplatin	AUC 7 IV on day 1	
Vinorelbine	25 mg/m^2 IV on days 1, 8, and 14	
Carbo-Tax		Repeat cycle every 3 wk.
Carboplatin	AUC 5–7.5 IV on day 1	
Paclitaxel	135 mg/m^2 IV on day 1	

AUC, area under the curve. Dosage based on creatinine clearance using the Calvert equation: AUC(Creatinine clearance + 25).

supportive care measures, as defined previously, may be administered to patients with a poor performance status or those who do not want to continue receiving potential curative therapy.

Despite the advancements recognized with the novel chemotherapeutic agents, prolonged survival in patients with advanced NSCLC has not significantly improved over the past few years. Further clinical trials evaluating the new chemotherapeutic agents in combination are warranted. Additional studies assessing the efficacy and toxicity of newer agents are needed. Finally, newer selective approaches including monoclonal antibodies, gene therapy involving intralesional injection of adenovirus p53, and antisense oligodeoxynucleotides are being investigated in an attempt to improve the survival rate of patients with NSCLC.

Small Cell Lung Cancer

SCLC differs from NSCLC in its histology, great propensity for early widespread metastatic dissemination, and sensitivity to chemotherapeutic agents. SCLC is an aggressive tumor, with most patients presenting with locally bulky disease, mediastinal nodes, and either subclinical or detectable metastases at diagnosis. Often these patients develop this malignancy later in life, between the ages of 50 and 70 years, thus making aggressive treatment regimens difficult to tolerate. Additionally, those presenting with extensive disease, a weight loss of more than 5%, and male gender have a poorer prognosis, once again limiting the usefulness of aggressive regimens. The treatment goals for patients with SCLC are to cure the few patients who present with limited stage disease through a combination of radiation, surgery, and chemotherapy and to prolong life and palliate symptoms in the majority of patients who present with extensive stage disease. Untreated, these patients live less than 12 weeks.

Limited Disease

Chemotherapy is the cornerstone of treatment for SCLC. Several chemotherapeutic agents have significant activity against SCLC as monotherapy (Table 91.5). Aggressive regimens including combination chemotherapy appear to produce higher response rates and are needed for treating limited disease (Table 91.6). The most common regimens used include cyclophosphamide, doxorubicin, and vincristine (CAV) and etoposide and platinum (EP). Although CAV and EP produce similar response and survival rates, EP has become the regimen of choice in treating limited disease SCLC secondary to the neurologic and cardiac toxicities observed with CAV.[78,79] In patients with untreated limited disease, the combination of carboplatin and etoposide appears to minimize toxicity without diminishing efficacy.[80–82] Thus, this regimen may be a suitable alternative to EP in older adults or medically compromised patients. Adding paclitaxel to carboplatin and oral etoposide may be an option. Although severe myelosuppression is common, this regimen shows promising results, and comparison trials with carboplatin and etoposide alone are being conducted.[83,84] Maintenance chemotherapy does not appear to prolong survival, but it does prolong time to recurrence. Although SCLC is very chemosensitive, approximately 50% of the patients relapse locally with chemotherapy alone.

SCLC is sensitive to radiotherapy but cures a only small number of patients with limited disease. Additionally, local recurrence occurs in a majority of patients when chemotherapy is administered alone. Therefore, thoracic irradiation added to combination chemotherapy was evaluated in patients with limited disease and found to provide better local control and improve overall survival. Perry et al.[85] compared the efficacy of chemotherapy alone, chemotherapy plus concurrent radiotherapy, and three cycles of sequential chemotherapy followed by radiation therapy in 426 patients with limited SCLC. All patients received cyclophosphamide, etoposide, and vincristine. Etoposide was replaced with doxorubicin after the completion of radiotherapy. Patients who received chemotherapy alone had higher rates of chest failures and lower rates of response and survival than patients receiving thoracic irradiation. There was no difference in local relapse or survival in either group receiving radiotherapy. Doxorubicin is a radiosensitizer, but it also produces significant cardiotoxicity when administered concurrently with radiation therapy. Therefore, avoiding regimens containing doxorubicin during thoracic irradiation is common practice, making EP with radiotherapy the preferred regimen. Several studies evaluating the concurrent thoracic radiotherapy and EP administration have produced overall response rates greater than 80% and projected 2-year survival rates of 42 to 83%.[86–88] Incorporation of concurrent radiotherapy during the first or second course of the chemotherapy regimen results in enhanced survival. Although the combination of EP and thoracic irradiation is the cornerstone of treatment in limited disease SCLC, it confers significant toxicity, including weight loss, esophagitis, and pulmonary dysfunction compared with either modality alone.

Surgery in patients with SCLC is controversial. Several years ago surgery was considered the treatment of choice, but a study conducted by the British Medical Research Council concluded that surgery was inferior to radiotherapy in promoting long-term survival.[89] This resulted in the abandonment of surgery as the primary treatment modality in SCLC. However, a few years later in a retrospective trial conducted by the Veterans Administration Surgical Oncology Group, patients with very limited disease (T1N0M0 and possibly T1N1M0 or T2N0M0) benefited from potentially curative resection, with a reduction in local recurrences observed.[90] Adding postoperative chemotherapy further enhances the overall survival observed in these patients.[91,92] Thus, complete surgical resection is indicated in patients with limited disease who are good surgical candidates, followed by intensive chemotherapy with or without chest irradiation.

Table 91.5 ▪ Chemotherapeutic Agents Active in Small Cell Lung Cancer

Chemotherapy Agent	Common Adverse Drug Events	Monitoring Parameters[a]
Carboplatin	Thrombocytopenia, neutropenia, anemia, nausea and vomiting, mucositis, stomatitis, alopecia, peripheral neuropathy, hypomagnesemia, hypokalemia, hypocalcemia, hypophosphatemia, and liver function test elevations	Complete blood count with differential, magnesium, potassium, calcium, inorganic phosphorus, total bilirubin, alkaline phosphatase, SGPT, LDH, urine output, and weight
Carmustine	Nausea and vomiting, myelosuppression (delayed), alopecia, lethargy, hepatotoxicity, and nephrotoxicity	Complete blood count with differential, total bilirubin, LDH, alkaline phosphatase, SGPT, BUN, and creatinine
Cisplatin	Nephrotoxicity (renal tubular damage), acute and delayed nausea and vomiting (may be severe), high-frequency hearing loss, myelosuppression, peripheral neuropathy, hypomagnesemia, hypokalemia, hyponatremia, hypocalcemia, hypophosphatemia, and mild alopecia	BUN, creatinine, complete blood count with differential, magnesium, potassium, sodium, calcium, inorganic phosphorus, urine output, weight
Cyclophosphamide	Myelosuppression, cardiotoxicity (including congestive heart failure), alopecia, nausea and vomiting (may be severe), anorexia, diarrhea, stomatitis, and hemorrhagic cystitis	Complete blood count with differential, urine output, weight, urinalysis as indicated
Docetaxel	Myelosuppression, nausea and vomiting, stomatitis, diarrhea, fluid retention, rash, alopecia, myalgia, and arthralgia	Complete blood count with differential, urine output, and weight
Doxorubicin	Cardiotoxicity (including cardiomyopathy and congestive heart failure), nausea and vomiting, myelosuppression, anorexia, mucositis, diarrhea, alopecia, palmar plantar erythrodysesthesia, and radiation recall	Urine output, weight, and complete blood count with differential
Etoposide	Myelosuppression, hypotension, nausea and vomiting, mucositis, alopecia, and diarrhea	Complete blood count with differential and blood pressure
Gemcitabine	Myelosuppression, nausea and vomiting, diarrhea, stomatitis, pain, alopecia, and elevated liver enzymes	Complete blood count with differential, total bilirubin, LDH, SGPT, and alkaline phosphatase
Ifosfamide	Myelosuppression, nausea and vomiting (may be severe), hemorrhagic cystitis, dysuria, nephrotoxicity, neurotoxicity (including lethargy, ataxia, mental status changes, disorientation, seizures, and coma), and alopecia	Complete blood count with differential, urinalysis as indicated, BUN, creatinine
Irinotecan	Myelosuppression, diarrhea, nausea and vomiting, vasodilation, headache, and dizziness	Complete blood count with differential
Lomustine	Myelosuppression (delayed), nausea and vomiting, hepatotoxicity, nephrotoxicity, and pulmonary fibrosis	Complete blood count with differential, total bilirubin, alkaline phosphatase, LDH, SGPT, BUN, creatinine, and chest radiograph as indicated
Methotrexate	Myelosuppression, nausea and vomiting, stomatitis, malaise, fatigue, dizziness, fever, alopecia, and radiation recall	Complete blood count with differential
Paclitaxel	Hypersensitivity reactions (especially without premedication), myelosuppression, mucositis, nausea and vomiting, peripheral neuropathy, alopecia, myalgia, and arthralgia	Complete blood count with differential
Topotecan	Myelosuppression, diarrhea, abdominal pain, nausea and vomiting, dyspnea, asthenia, pain, and alopecia	Complete blood count with differential
Vincristine	Myelosuppression, constipation, alopecia, neurotoxicity (including peripheral neuropathy, SIADH, paralytic ileus, and neuromuscular difficulties), myalgias, and alopecia	Complete blood count with differential
Vinorelbine	Myelosuppression, mild nausea and vomiting, constipation, transient liver function tests elevations, peripheral neuropathy, myalgia, arthralgia, and alopecia	Complete blood count with differential, total bilirubin, alkaline phosphatase, LDH, and SGPT

[a]Patient should be monitored clinically for symptomatic toxicities.

SGPT, serum glutamic–pyruvic transaminase; *LDH,* lactate dehydrogenase; *BUN,* blood urea nitrogen; *SIADH,* syndrome of inappropriate secretion of antidiuretic hormone.

Table 91.6 ▪ Common Chemotherapy Regimens for Treating Small Cell Lung Cancer

Drug	Dosage	Schedule
EP		Repeat every 3 wk.
Etoposide	80–120 mg/m² IV on days 1–3	
Cisplatin	75–100 mg/m² IV on day 1	
CAV		Repeat every 3 wk.
Cyclophosphamide	750–1000 mg/m² IV on day 1	
Doxorubicin	40–50 mg/m² IV on day 1	
Vincristine	1.4 mg/m² IV on day 1 (maximum dosage 2 mg)	
CEV		Repeat every 3–4 wk.
Cyclophosphamide	1000 mg/m² IV on day 1	
Etoposide	50 mg/m² IV on day 1, then 100 mg/m² PO on days 2–5	
Vincristine	1.4 mg/m² IV on day 1 (maximum dosage 2 mg)	
CAE		Repeat every 3 wk.
Cyclophosphamide	1000 mg/m² IV on day 1	
Doxorubicin	45 mg/m² IV on day 1	
Etoposide	50 mg/m² IV on days 1–5	
ICE		Repeat every 4 wk.
Ifosfamide	2 g/m² IV on days 1–3	
Carboplatin	300–600 mg/m² IV on day 1 or 3	
Etoposide	60–100 mg/m² IV on days 1–3	
CODE		
Cisplatin	25 mg/m² IV every wk for 9 wk	
Vincristine	1 mg/m² IV (maximum dosage 2 mg) IV on wk 1, 2, 4, 6, and 8	
Doxorubicin	25 mg/m² IV on wk 1, 3, 5, 7, and 9	
Etoposide	80 mg/m² IV on wk 1, 3, 5, 7, and 9	
VIP		Repeat cycle every 4 wk.
Ifosfamide	1.2 g/m² IV on day 1	
Cisplatin	20 mg/m² IV on days 1 and 8	
Etoposide	37.5 mg/m²/day PO on days 1–3	
EC		Repeat every 3–4 wk.
Etoposide	60–100 mg/m² IV on days 1–3	
Carboplatin	300–400 mg/m² IV on day 1	
Etoposide	100 mg/m²/day PO on days 1–5	Repeat every 3–4 wk.
Topotecan	1.5 mg/m² IV on days 1–5	Repeat every 3 wk.

Prophylactic Cranial Irradiation

There is a higher incidence of brain metastases in patients with SCLC than in those with other histologic types. It is reported that up to 50% of patients have brain involvement at autopsy despite treatment. Additionally, the probability of developing brain metastases increases as survival is prolonged with multimodality treatment. Central nervous system metastases are present in 50 to 80% of patients surviving 2 years.[93,94] Once metastases of the brain occur, the symptoms can be devastating and often result in death. Treatment with cranial irradiation and corticosteroids often improves neurologic symptoms and may result in a partial or complete response, but long-term survival is rare.

Preventing central nervous system metastases is ideal but difficult to achieve. Prophylactic cranial irradiation (PCI) has been widely studied in both retrospective and prospective clinical trials. However, putting this treatment modality into practice is highly controversial. Early studies concluded that the development of brain metastases was significantly reduced in patients receiving PCI, but no significant survival advantage was observed. Furthermore, some patients develop brain metastases despite PCI. However, in patients with limited disease who achieve a complete remission after initial therapy, a survival benefit is suggested, supporting the addition of this treatment modality to the treatment plan in this select group of patients.[95]

PCI is not without complications. Acute toxicities often are mild and include alopecia, headaches, fatigue, skin erythema, and disturbances in taste, appetite, and hearing. In long-term survivors, delayed complications are the most devastating and a reason for controversy. Gradual intellectual decline, short-term memory loss, optic atrophy, fine motor skill impairment, gait difficulty, and speech impairment often are reported. Additionally, diffuse cerebral atrophy, white matter abnormalities, and ventricular enlargement often are noted on CT and magnetic resonance imaging scans.

There are a few alternatives to prophylactic cranial irradiation. For patients who do not achieve a complete remission with initial therapy, have extensive disease, are older, or have a poor performance status, a watch and wait policy is recommended. Combination chemotherapy regimens including agents that penetrate the blood–brain barrier, resection of an isolated lesion, and whole brain or stereotatic radiation are potential therapies that may be implemented when brain metastases occur in an attempt to provide symptomatic relief and prolong survival.

Extensive Disease

A majority of patients with SCLC present with extensive disease. Chemotherapy is the treatment of choice, and regimens similar to those administered in limited disease are used. Chemotherapy produces objective responses in a majority of patients, but less than 5% of patients are alive at 5 years. Clinical trials involving gemcitabine, irinotecan, paclitaxel, topotecan, and vinorelbine have produced promising results.[96–99] Future trials with these agents in combination with other chemotherapeutic agents may result in new regimens that improve the outcome of patients with extensive disease. Thoracic irradiation reduces the rate of local recurrence but has no impact on response or survival and should not be administered with a curative intent. Nonetheless, radiotherapy plays a role in palliating symptoms of the primary tumor and its metastases.

Refractory or Recurrent Disease

Successful treatment with salvage regimens in patients who do not respond to chemotherapy or whose disease recurs is rare and brief. Patients treated initially with a regimen not containing etoposide or cisplatin may achieve a brief response to these two agents lasting 3 to 36 weeks.[100,101] Administering oral etoposide daily is an alternative therapy that minimally prolongs survival with tolerable toxicities.[102] The newer agents, including docetaxel, irinotecan, topotecan, and vinorelbine, have produced objective response rates but have had little impact on survival.[103–108]

Treatment for Older Adults

Nearly one-fourth of all patients diagnosed with SCLC are older than 65 years. These patients generally cannot tolerate aggressive treatment regimens because of poor performance status or concomitant illnesses. Thus, most prefer to treat these patients with regimens not associated with life-threatening toxicities but realize the survival benefit for these patients may be compromised. Oral etoposide is an effective agent in SCLC that has acceptable toxicities, including myelosuppression and alopecia. When it is given to patients as palliative treatment, overall response rates exceed 50% and overall survival is greater than with supportive care alone. Thus, this agent is an acceptable option for older or medically compromised patients with SCLC.

Complications

Many complications may occur during chemotherapy administration (Tables 91.3 and 91.5). Often the regimen-related toxicities are tolerable and self-limiting, but occasionally long-term effects occur that may compromise the patient's health and quality of life. Often the gastrointestinal tract is affected by the drugs administered. Nausea and vomiting commonly occur, vary in intensity, and may warrant antiemetics. The emesis may occur acutely or be delayed, as is often observed with agents such as cisplatin and cyclophosphamide. Additionally, diarrhea, stomatitis, and anorexia complicate the patient's health. Supplemental nutrition and hydration may be necessary, as well as good oral hygiene to avoid infections. Myelosuppression including neutropenia, thrombocytopenia, and anemia may result but usually does not warrant using a colony-stimulating growth factor. With chemotherapeutic agents such as carmustine and lomustine, the myelosuppression may be delayed up to 8 weeks. Cardiotoxicity appears as congestive heart failure or as a cardiomyopathy warranting symptomatic treatment. Laboratory abnormalities may occur, including electrolyte disturbances warranting supplementation. Additionally, laboratory results may indicate hepatic dysfunction or renal failure. Cisplatin often causes hypomagnesemia and other electrolyte alterations. Additionally, renal tubular damage, peripheral neuropathy, and ototoxicity are potential side effects of cisplatin that may not be reversible. Although carboplatin may cause these toxicities to a lesser extent, it reduces the platelet count sharply. Other treatment-related toxicities include pulmonary toxicity and neurotoxicity.

Radiation therapy produces several acute and delayed side effects (Table 91.7).[109,110] Side effects that occur within 90 days of completing radiotherapy are considered acute and reflect local tissue damage. Fatigue and myelosuppression are common after treatment, and rarely adult respiratory distress syndrome may occur. Erythema and desquamation may present acutely, whereas fibrosis and telangiectasia occur months and even years after radiotherapy. Mucositis is common during and after radiotherapy. It is generally self-limiting and may be treated with analgesics and good oral hygiene. Late esophageal strictures may warrant repeated endoscopic dilation. Rarely, fistulas and perforation may occur. Pericarditis may occur within the first 90 days after treatment. It is generally self-limiting and is treated with analgesics, antipyretics, and occasionally antiarrhythmic agents. Heart failure and coronary stenosis may occur months after treatment. Radiation pneumonitis occurs in 5 to 15% of patients within 1 to 4 months after therapy. It typically presents with dyspnea, cough, low-grade fever, and pleuritic chest pain. Usually only supportive care is needed, but in severe cases steroids should be administered. Pulmonary fibrosis

Table 91.7 ▪ Complications Associated with Radiotherapy

Fatigue	Skin erythema and desquamation
Myelosuppression	Skin fibrosis and telangiectasia
Adult respiratory distress syndrome	Pericarditis
Mucositis	Heart failure and coronary stenosis
Esophageal strictures, fistulas, and perforation	Pneumonitis
	Pulmonary fibrosis

generally presents 3 to 18 months after radiotherapy completion. Patients may be asymptomatic, and treatment is supportive care only.

As previously discussed, chemotherapy and radiotherapy often are combined in multimodality regimens. These combinations may potentiate the toxicities observed with chemotherapy or radiation alone increasing the morbidity associated with the treatment plan. Care should be taken to minimize these effects in patients receiving aggressive therapy.

IMPROVING OUTCOMES

Upon diagnosis, patients should be counseled on means of treating their disease, relieving the symptoms, and preventing recurrence. Reviewing treatment options and the toxicities of each therapy helps the patient to understand the expectations associated with each modality chosen. Smoking cessation should be strongly encouraged in patients who smoke. Not only will it assist in relieving symptoms, but it may prevent additional primary tumors. Nicotine patches, nicotine gum, and bupropion often are used. Enrollment in programs that offer counseling and support, in addition to medication, may further benefit a patient's effort to stop smoking.

Published reports postulate that diets high in fruits and vegetables may protect against lung cancer. This is based on the concept that these foods include antioxidants, which may reduce the concentration or prevent the formation of free radicals and excited oxygen species, which may play a role in lung cancer development. However, in chemoprevention trials to date, the vitamins most likely to work in this regard, vitamin A or β-carotene, do not appear to protect against lung cancer.[111,112] Additionally, trials looking at the effects of cis-retinoic acid and green tea on lung cancer are currently being conducted. Enrollment in studies similar to these may be beneficial to patients with lung cancer.

KEY POINTS

- Lung cancer continues to be the leading cause of cancer death among men and women worldwide.
- This disease affects primarily patients with a history of cigarette smoking and therefore may be preventable.
- Accurate histologic and staging classification is important in determining treatment options and prognosis.
- NSCLC is not as aggressive as SCLC and is classified into adenocarcinoma, squamous cell, and large cell carcinoma.
- SCLC is an aggressive and rapidly proliferating tumor with metastases often detectable at diagnosis.
- Current treatment of patients with lung cancer is controversial and summarized as follows:
  - Complete surgical resection alone is the cornerstone of treatment for patients with stage I and II NSCLC.
  - Patients with stage IIIA NSCLC should receive chemotherapy, chemoradiotherapy, or radiotherapy before surgical resection.
  - Prognosis is poor in patients with stage IIIB and IV NSCLC, with less than 7% of these patients alive at 5 years.
  - Stage IIIB and IV NSCLC is considered unresectable, and chemotherapy and/or radiotherapy in a clinical setting generally is offered as palliative therapy.
  - Chemotherapy plus radiotherapy is the standard of care for patients with limited disease SCLC.
  - Etoposide and cisplatin or cyclophosphamide, doxorubicin, and vincristine are the regimens most often administered to patients with limited disease SCLC.
  - Surgery is indicated in patients with limited disease SCLC who are in good health.
  - Prophylactic cranial irradiation is indicated in patients with limited disease SCLC who achieve a complete remission after primary therapy.
  - Prognosis is poor in patients with extensive disease SCLC, with less than 5% of patients alive at 5 years.
  - Chemotherapy is the treatment of choice in patients with extensive disease SCLC.
  - Despite the many diagnostic and therapeutic improvements developed over the past few years, prognosis for patients with lung cancer is still poor.
  - New agents, combination regimens, and newer selective approaches must be investigated further to improve response rates and prolong survival.
  - Until further therapeutic breakthroughs occur, prevention is the only means of controlling this disease.

REFERENCES

1. Greenlee RT, Murray T, Bolden S, et al. Cancer Statistics, 2000. CA Cancer J Clin 50:7–33, 2000.
2. Deist CE, Hailer BE, Smith TJ. Economic considerations in the care of lung cancer patients. Curr Opin Oncol 8:126–132, 1996.
3. US Department of Health, Education, and Welfare. Smoking and Health. Report of the Advisory Committee to the Surgeon General of the Public Health Service. Rockville, MD: US Department of Health, Education, and Welfare, Public Health Service, PHS pub no. 1103, 1964.
4. Garfinkel L, Auerbach O, Joubert L. Involuntary smoking and lung cancer: a case-control study. J Natl Cancer Inst 75:463–469, 1985.
5. US Department of Health and Human Services. The health consequences of involuntary smoking: a report of the Surgeon General. Washington, DC: USHS Publication no. CDC 87-8398, 1986.
6. Selikoff IJ, Hammond EC, Chung J. Asbestos exposure, smoking and neoplasia. JAMA 204:106–112, 1968.
7. Mountain CF. Revisions in the international system for staging lung cancer. Chest 111:1710–1717, 1997.
8. Anonymous. Lung. In: AJCC cancer staging manual. 5th ed. Philadelphia: Lippincott-Raven, 1997:127–137.
9. Hide L, Yee J, Wilson R, et al. Cell type and the natural history of lung cancer. JAMA 193:140–142, 1965.
10. Stitik FP. The new staging of lung cancer. Adv Chest Radiol 32:635–647, 1994.
11. Stahel RA, Ginsberg R, Havemann K, et al. Staging and prognostic factors in small cell lung cancer: a consensus report. Lung Cancer 5:119–126, 1989.
12. Harpole DH, Herndon JE, Young WG, et al. Stage I non-small cell lung cancer. Cancer 76:787–796, 1995.
13. Ginsberg RJ, Rubinstein LV. Randomized trial of lobectomy versus limited

resection for T1 N0 non-small cell lung cancer. Ann Thorac Surg 60:615–623, 1995.
14. Graham PH, Gebski VJ, Stat M, et al. Radical radiotherapy for early non-small cell lung cancer. Int J Radiat Oncol Biol Phys 31:261–266, 1995.
15. Sandler HM, Curran WJ, Turrisi AT. The influence of tumor size and pre-treatment staging on outcome following radiation therapy alone for stage I non-small cell lung cancer. Int J Radiat Oncol Biol Phys 19:9–13, 1990.
16. Weisenburger TH, Gail M. Effects of postoperative mediastinal radiation on completely resected stage II and stage III epidermoid cancer of the lung. N Engl J Med 315:1377–1381, 1986.
17. Stephens RJ, Girling DJ, Bleefen NM, et al. The role of post-operative radiotherapy in non-small-cell lung cancer: a multicentre randomised trial in patients with pathologically staged T1-2, N1-2, and M0 disease. Br J Cancer 74:632–639, 1996.
18. Holmes EC. Surgical adjuvant therapy for stage II and stage III adenocarcinoma and large cell undifferentiated carcinoma. Chest 106(Suppl 6):293S–296S, 1994.
19. Figlin RA, Piantodosi S. A phase 3 randomized trial of immediate combination chemotherapy vs delayed combination chemotherapy in patients with completely resected stage II and III non-small cell carcinoma of the lung. Chest 106(Suppl 6):310S–312S, 1994.
20. Feld R, Rubinstein L, Thomas PA. Adjuvant chemotherapy with cyclophosphamide, doxorubicin, and cisplatin in patients with completely resected stage I non-small-cell lung cancer. J Natl Cancer Inst 85:299–306, 1993.
21. Shields TW, Humphrey EW, Eastridge CE, et al. Adjuvant cancer chemotherapy after resection of carcinoma of the lung. Cancer 40:2057–2062, 1977.
22. Niiranen A, Niitamo-Korhonen S, Kouri M, et al. Adjuvant chemotherapy after radical surgery for non-small-cell lung cancer: a randomized study. J Clin Oncol 10:1927–1932, 1992.
23. Shields TW, Higgins GA, Humphrey EW, et al. Prolonged intermittent adjuvant chemotherapy with CCNU and hydroxyurea after resection of carcinoma of the lung. Cancer 50:1713–1721, 1982.
24. Girling DJ, Stott H, Stephens RJ, et al. Fifteen-year follow-up of all patients in a study of post-operative chemotherapy for bronchial carcinoma. Br J Cancer 52:867–873, 1985.
25. Van Klaveren RJ, Festen J, Otten HJ, et al. Prognosis of unsuspected but completely resectable N2 non-small cell lung cancer. Ann Thorac Surg 56:300–304, 1993.
26. Goldstraw P, Mannam GC, Kaplan DK, et al. Surgical management of non-small-cell lung cancer with ipsilateral mediastinal node metastasis (N2 disease). J Thorac Cardiovasc Surg 107:19–28, 1994.
27. Watanabe Y, Shimizu J, Oda M, et al. Aggressive surgical intervention in N2 non-small cell cancer of the lung. Ann Thorac Surg 51:253–261, 1991.
28. Ohta M, Tsuchiya R, Shimoyama M, et al. Adjuvant chemotherapy for completely resected stage III non-small-cell lung cancer. J Thorac Cardiovasc Surg 106:703–708, 1993.
29. Pisters KMW, Kris MG, Gralla RJ, et al. Randomized trial comparing postoperative chemotherapy with vindesine and cisplatin plus thoracic irradiation with irradiation alone in stage III (N2) non-small cell lung cancer. J Surg Oncol 56:236–241, 1994.
30. Lad T. The comparison of CAP chemotherapy and radiotherapy to radiotherapy alone for resected lung cancer with positive margin or involved highest sampled paratracheal node (stage IIIA). Chest 106(Suppl 6):302S–306S, 1994.
31. Martini N, Kris MG, Flehinger BJ, et al. Preoperative chemotherapy for stage IIIa (N2) lung cancer: the Sloan-Kettering experience with 136 patients. Ann Thorac Surg 55:1365–1374, 1993.
32. Burkes RL, Ginsberg RJ, Shepherd FA, et al. Induction chemotherapy with mitomycin, vindesine, and cisplatin for stage III unresectable non-small-cell lung cancer: results of the Toronto phase II trial. J Clin Oncol 10:580–586, 1992.
33. Kirn DH, Lynch TJ, Mentzer SJ, et al. Multimodality therapy of patients with stage IIIA, N2 non-small-cell lung cancer. J Thorac Cardiovasc Surg 106:696–702, 1993.
34. Roth JA, Fossella F, Komaki R, et al. A randomized trial comparing perioperative chemotherapy and surgery with surgery alone in resectable stage IIIA non-small-cell lung cancer. J Natl Cancer Inst 86:673–680, 1994.
35. Rosell R, Gomez-Codina J, Camps C, et al. A randomized trial comparing preoperative chemotherapy plus surgery with surgery alone in patients with non-small cell lung cancer. N Engl J Med 330:153–158, 1994.
36. Elais AD, Skarin A, Gonin R, et al. Neoadjuvant treatment of stage IIIA non-small cell lung cancer: long-term results. Am J Clin Oncol 17:26–36, 1994.
37. Strauss GM, Herndon JE, Sherman DD, et al. Neoadjuvant chemotherapy and radiotherapy followed by surgery in stage IIIA non-small-cell carcinoma of the lung: report of a Cancer and Leukemia Group B phase II study. J Clin Oncol 10:1237–1244, 1992.
38. Rusch VW, Albain KS, Crowley JJ, et al. Surgical resection of stage IIIA and stage IIIB non-small-cell lung cancer after concurrent induction chemoradiotherapy. J Thorac Cardiovasc Surg 105:97–106, 1993.
39. Dillman RO, Seagren SL, Propert KJ, et al. A randomized trial of induction chemotherapy plus high-dose radiation versus radiation alone in stage III non-small cell lung cancer. N Engl J Med 323:940–945, 1990.
40. LeChevalier T, Arrigada R, Quoix E, et al. Radiotherapy alone versus combined chemotherapy and radiotherapy in nonresectable non-small-cell lung cancer: first analysis of a randomized trial in 353 patients. J Natl Cancer Inst 83:417–423, 1991.
41. Sause WT, Scott C, Taylor S, et al. Radiation therapy oncology group (RTOG) 88-08 and Eastern Cooperative Oncology Group (ECOG) 4588: preliminary results of a phase III trial in regionally advanced, unresectable non-small-cell lung cancer. J Natl Cancer Inst 87:198–205, 1995.
42. Jaakkimainen L, Goodwin PJ, Pater J, et al. Counting the costs of chemotherapy in a National Cancer Institute of Canada randomized trial in non-small-cell lung cancer. J Clin Oncol 8:1301–1309, 1990.
43. Souquet PJ, Chauvin F, Boissel JP, et al. Meta-analysis of randomised trials of systemic chemotherapy versus supportive treatment in non-resectable non-small cell lung cancer. Lung Cancer 12(Suppl 1):S147–S154, 1995.
44. Evans WK. Cost-effectiveness of gemcitabine in stage IV non-small cell lung cancer: an estimate using the Population Health Model Lung Cancer Module. Semin Oncol 24(Suppl 7):S7-56–S7-63, 1997.
45. Kreisman H, Lisbona A, Olson L, et al. Effect of radiologic stage III substage on nonsurgical therapy of non-small cell lung cancer. Cancer 72:1588–1596, 1993.
46. Albain KS, Rusch VW, Crowley JJ, et al. Concurrent cisplatin/etoposide plus chest radiotherapy followed by surgery for stages IIIA (N2) and IIIB non-small-cell lung cancer: mature results of Southwest Oncology Group phase II study 8805. J Clin Oncol 13:1880–1892, 1995.
47. Chang AY, Kim K, Glick J, et al. Phase II study of Taxol, merbarone, and piroxantrone in stage IV non-small-cell lung cancer: the Eastern Cooperative Oncology Group Results. J Natl Cancer Inst 85:388–394, 1993.
48. Murphy WK, Fossella FV, Winn RJ, et al. Phase II study of Taxol in patients with untreated advanced non-small-cell lung cancer. J Natl Cancer Inst 85:384–388, 1993.
49. Hainsworth JD, Thompson DS, Greco A. Paclitaxel by 1-hour infusion: an active drug in metastatic non-small-cell lung cancer. J Clin Oncol 13:1609–1614, 1995.
50. Belli L, LeChevalier T, Gottfried M, et al. Phase I/II trial of paclitaxel plus cisplatin as first-line chemotherapy for advanced non-small cell lung cancer: preliminary results. Semin Oncol 22:29–33, 1995.
51. Pirker R, Krajnik G, Zochbauer S, et al. Paclitaxel/cisplatin in advanced non-small-cell lung cancer (NSCLC). Ann Oncol 6:833–835, 1995.
52. Klastersky J, Sculier JP. Dose-finding study of paclitaxel (Taxol) plus cisplatin in patients with non-small cell lung cancer. Lung Cancer 12(Suppl 2):S117–S125, 1995.
53. Langer CJ, Leighton JC, Comis RL, et al. Paclitaxel and carboplatin in combination in the treatment of advanced non-small-cell lung cancer: a phase II toxicity, response, and survival analysis. J Clin Oncol 13:1860–1870, 1995.
54. Muggia FM, Vafai D, Natale R, et al. Paclitaxel 3-hour infusion given alone and combined with carboplatin: preliminary results of dose-escalation trials. Semin Oncol 22(Suppl 9):63–66, 1995.
55. Schutte W, Bork I, Sucker S. Phase II trial of paclitaxel and carboplatin as first-line treatment in advanced non-small cell lung-cancer (NSCLC) [abstract]. Proc Am Soc Clin Oncol 15:1208, 1996.
56. Cerny T, Kaplan S, Pavlidis N, et al. Docetaxel (Taxotere) is active in non-small-cell lung cancer: a phase II trial of the EORTC early clinical trials group (ECTG). Br J Cancer 70:384–387, 1994.
57. Francis PA, Rigas JR, Kris MG, et al. Phase II trial of docetaxel in patients with stage III and IV non-small-cell lung cancer. J Clin Oncol 12:1232–1237, 1994.
58. Fosella FV, Lee JS, Murphy WK, et al. Phase II study of docetaxel for recurrent or metastatic non-small-cell lung cancer. J Clin Oncol 12:1238–1244, 1994.
59. Le Chevalier T, Belli L, Monnier A, et al. Phase II trial of docetaxel (Taxotere) and cisplatin in advanced non-small cell lung cancer (NSCLC): an interim analysis [abstract]. Proc Am Soc Clin Oncol 14:1059, 1995.
60. Cole JT, Gralla RJ, Marques CB, et al. Phase I-II study of cisplatin + docetaxel (Taxotere) in non-small cell lung cancer (NSCLC) [abstract]. Proc Am Soc Clin Oncol 14:1087, 1995.
61. Zalcberg J, Millward M, McKeage M, et al. Phase II trial of docetaxel and cisplatin in advanced non-small-cell lung cancer. J Clin Oncol 16:1948–1953, 1988.
62. Douillard JY, Ibrahim N, Riviere A, et al. Phase II study of CPT-11 in

non-small cell lung cancer (NSCLC) [abstract]. Proc Am Soc Clin Oncol 14:1118, 1995.
63. Fukuoka M, Niitani H, Suzuki A, et al. A phase II study of CPT-11, a new derivative of camptothecin, for previously untreated non-small-cell lung cancer. J Clin Oncol 10:16–20, 1992.
64. Masuda N, Fukuoka M, Takada M, et al. CPT-11 in combination with cisplatin for advanced non-small-cell lung cancer. J Clin Oncol 10:1775–1780, 1992.
65. Abratt RP, Bezwoda WR, Falkson G, et al. Efficacy and safety profile of gemcitabine in non-small-cell lung cancer: a phase II study. J Clin Oncol 12:1535–1540, 1994.
66. Anderson H, Lund B, Bach F, et al. Single-agent activity of weekly gemcitabine in advanced non-small-cell lung cancer: a phase II study. J Clin Oncol 12:1821–1826, 1994.
67. Fossella FV, Lippman SM, Shin DM, et al. Maximum tolerated dose defined for single-agent gemcitabine: a phase I dose-escalation study in chemotherapy-naïve patients with advanced non-small-cell lung cancer. J Clin Oncol 15:310–316, 1997.
68. Gatzemeier U, Shepherd FA, Le Chevalier T, et al. Activity of gemcitabine in patients with non-small cell lung cancer: a multicentre, extended phase II study. Eur J Cancer 32A:243–248, 1996.
69. Shepherd FA, Burkes R, Cormier Y, et al. Phase I dose-escalation trial of gemcitabine and cisplatin for advanced non-small-cell lung cancer: usefulness of mathematic modeling to determine maximum tolerable dose. J Clin Oncol 14:1656–1662, 1996.
70. Sandler AB, Ansari R, McClean J, et al. A Hoosier Oncology Group phase II study of gemcitabine plus cisplatin in non-small cell lung cancer (NSCLC) [abstract]. Proc Am Soc Clin Oncol 14:1089, 1995.
71. Steward WP, Dunlop DJ, Dabouis G, et al. Phase I/II study of gemcitabine and cisplatin in the treatment of advanced non-small cell lung cancer: preliminary results. Semin Oncol 23:43–47, 1996.
72. Depierre A, Lemarie E, Dabouis G, et al. A phase II study of Navelbine (vinorelbine) in the treatment of non-small-cell lung cancer. Am J Clin Oncol 14:115–119, 1991.
73. Le Chevalier T, Brisgand D, Douillard JY, et al. Randomized study of vinorelbine and cisplatin versus vindesine and cisplatin versus vinorelbine alone in advanced non-small-cell lung cancer: results of a European multicenter trial including 612 patients. J Clin Oncol 12:360–367, 1994.
74. Wozniak AJ, Crowley JJ, Balcerzak SP, et al. Randomized trial comparing cisplatin with cisplatin plus vinorelbine in the treatment of advanced non-small-cell lung cancer: a Southwest Oncology Group study. J Clin Oncol 16:2459–2465, 1998.
75. Copley-Merriman C, Martin C, Johnson N, et al. Economic value of gemcitabine in non-small cell lung cancer. Semin Oncol 23(Suppl 10):90–98, 1996.
76. Evans WK, Le Chevalier T. The cost-effectiveness of Navelbine alone or in combination with cisplatin in comparison to other chemotherapy regimens and best supportive care in stage IV non-small cell lung cancer. Eur J Cancer 32A:2249–2255, 1996.
77. Fossella FV, Lee JS, Hong WK. Management strategies for recurrent non-small cell lung cancer. Semin Oncol 24:455–462, 1997.
78. Evans WK, Shepherd FA, Feld R, et al. VP-16 and cisplatin as first-line therapy for small-cell lung cancer. J Clin Oncol 3:1471–1477, 1985.
79. Einhorn LH. Cisplatin and VP-16 in small-cell lung cancer. Semin Oncol 13(Suppl 3):3–4, 1986.
80. Bishop JF, Raghavan D, Stuart-Harris R, et al. Carboplatin (CBDCA, JM-8) and VP-16-213 in previously untreated patients with small-cell lung cancer. J Clin Oncol 5:1574–1578, 1987.
81. Kosmidis PA, Samantas E, Fountzilas G, et al. Cisplatin/etoposide versus carboplatin/etoposide chemotherapy and irradiation in small-cell lung cancer: a randomized phase III study. Semin Oncol 21(Suppl 6):23–30, 1994.
82. Ellis PA, Talbot DC, Priest K, et al. Dose intensification of carboplatin and etoposide as first-line combination chemotherapy in small-cell lung cancer. Eur J Cancer 31A:1888–1889, 1995.
83. Gatzemeier U, Jagos U, Kaukel E, et al. Paclitaxel, carboplatin, and oral etoposide: a phase II trial in limited-stage small cell lung cancer. Semin Oncol 24(Suppl 12):S12-149–S12-152, 1997.
84. Hainsworth JD, Gray JR, Stroup SL, et al. Paclitaxel, carboplatin, and extended-schedule etoposide in the treatment of small-cell lung cancer: comparison of sequential phase II trials using different dose-intensities. J Clin Oncol 15:3464–3470, 1997.
85. Perry MC, Eaton WL, Propert KJ, et al. Chemotherapy with or without radiation therapy in limited small-cell carcinoma of the lung. N Engl J Med 316:912–918, 1987.
86. Johnson BE, Grayson J, Woods E, et al. Limited stage small cell lung cancer treated with concurrent etoposide/cisplatin plus BID chest radiotherapy [abstract]. Proc Am Soc Clin Oncol 8:888, 1989.
87. Johnson DH, Kim K, Turrisi AT, et al. Cisplatin & etoposide + concurrent thoracic radiotherapy administered once versus twice daily for limited-stage small cell lung cancer: preliminary results of an intergroup trial [abstract]. Proc Am Soc Clin Oncol 13:1105, 1994.
88. Turrisi AT, Glover DJ, Mason BA. A preliminary report: concurrent twice-daily radiotherapy plus platinum-etoposide chemotherapy for limited small cell lung cancer. Int J Radiat Oncol Biol Phys 15:183–187, 1988.
89. Fox W, Scadding JC. Medical Research Counsel comparative trial of surgery and radiotherapy for primary treatment of small celled or oat celled carcinoma of the bronchus. Lancet 2:63–65, 1973.
90. Shields TW, Higgins GA, Matthews MJ, et al. Surgical resection in the management of small cell carcinoma of the lung. J Thorac Cardiovasc Surg 84:481–488, 1982.
91. Meyer JA. Five-year survival in treated stage I and II small cell carcinoma of the lung. Ann Thorac Surg 42:668–669, 1986.
92. Karrer K, Shields TW, Denck H, et al. The importance of surgical and multimodality treatment for small cell bronchial carcinoma. J Thorac Cardiovasc Surg 97:168–176, 1989.
93. Komaki R, Cox JD, Whitson W. Risk of brain metastasis from small cell carcinoma of the lung related to length of survival and prophylactic irradiation. Cancer Treat Rep 65:811–814, 1981.
94. Nugent JL, Bunn PA, Matthews MJ, et al. CNS metastases in small cell bronchogenic carcinoma. Cancer 44:1885–1893, 1979.
95. Arriagada R, Le Chevalier T, Borie F, et al. Prophylactic cranial irradiation for patients with small-cell lung cancer in complete remission. J Natl Cancer Inst 87:183–190, 1995.
96. Cormier Y, Eisenhauer E, Muldal A, et al. Gemcitabine is an active new agent in previously untreated extensive small cell lung cancer. Ann Oncol 5:283–285, 1994.
97. Kudoh S, Fujiwara Y, Takada Y, et al. Phase II study of irinotecan combined with cisplatin in patients with previously untreated small-cell lung cancer. J Clin Oncol 16:1068–1074, 1998.
98. Schiller JH, Kyung-Mann K, Hutson P, et al. Phase II study of topotecan in patients with extensive-stage small-cell carcinoma of the lung: an Eastern Cooperative Oncology Group Trial. J Clin Oncol 14:2345–2352, 1996.
99. Iaffaioli RV, Facchini G, Tortoriello A, et al. Phase I study of vinorelbine and paclitaxel in small-cell lung cancer. Cancer Chemother Pharmacol 41:86–90, 1997.
100. Porter LL, Johnson DH, Hainsworth JD, et al. Cisplatin and etoposide chemotherapy for refractory small cell carcinoma of the lung. Cancer Treat Rep 69:479–481, 1985.
101. Evans WK, Osoba D, Feld R, et al. Etoposide (VP-16) and cisplatin: an effective treatment for relapse in small-cell lung cancer. J Clin Oncol 3:65–71, 1985.
102. Johnson DH, Greco FA, Strupp J, et al. Prolonged administration of oral etoposide in patients with relapsed or refractory small-cell lung cancer: a phase II trial. J Clin Oncol 8:1613–1617, 1990.
103. Smyth JF, Smith IE, Sessa C, et al. Activity of docetaxel (Taxotere) in small cell lung cancer. Eur J Cancer 30A:1058–1060, 1994.
104. Masuda N, Fukuoka M, Kusunoki Y, et al. CPT-11: a new derivative of camptothecin for the treatment of refractory or relapsed small-cell lung cancer. J Clin Oncol 10:1225–1229, 1992.
105. Perez-Soler R, Glisson BS, Lee JS, et al. Treatment of patients with small-cell lung cancer refractory to etoposide and cisplatin with the topoisomerase I poison topotecan. J Clin Oncol 14:2785–2790, 1996.
106. Furuse K, Kubota K, Kawahara M, et al. Phase II study of vinorelbine in heavily previously treated small cell lung cancer. Oncology 53:169–172, 1996.
107. Jassem J, Karnicka-Mlodkowska H, van Pottelsberghe C, et al. Phase II study of vinorelbine (Navelbine) in previously treated small cell lung cancer patients. Eur J Cancer 29A:1720–1722, 1993.
108. Ardizzoni A, Hansen H, Dombernowsky P, et al. Topotecan, a new active drug in the second-line treatment of small-cell lung cancer: a phase II study in patients with refractory and sensitive disease. J Clin Oncol 15:2090–2096, 1997.
109. Machtay M, Friedberg JS. The role of radiation therapy in the management of non-small cell lung cancer. Semin Thorac Cardiovasc Surg 9:80–89, 1997.
110. Van Houtte P, Danhier S, Mornex F. Toxicity of combined radiation and chemotherapy in non-small cell lung cancer. Lung Cancer 10(Suppl 1):S271–S280, 1994.
111. Omenn GS, Goodman GE, Thornquist MD, et al. Effects of a combination of beta carotene and vitamin A on lung cancer and cardiovascular disease. N Engl J Med 334:1150–1155, 1996.
112. Hennekens CH, Buring JE, Manson JE, et al. Lack of effect of long-term supplementation with beta carotene on the incidence of malignant neoplasms and cardiovascular disease. N Engl J Med 334:1145–1149, 1996.

CHAPTER 92

PROSTATE CANCER

Carol Balmer

DEFINITION

Carcinoma of the prostate gland is a malignancy of the male genitourinary tract and the most common cancer in men in the United States.

TREATMENT CONSIDERATIONS

Prostate cancer is a disorder of older men. It usually is a slowly growing cancer, and in many men it never becomes clinically evident. Because of the age of patients at diagnosis and the characteristic slow growth of prostate cancer, it is more common to die with a diagnosis of prostate cancer than to die of this disease. This has led some clinicians to question whether it should be treated at all. Treatment decisions in prostate cancer, more than any other cancer, depend on the patient's age and medical condition. These factors combine to determine the treatment goals for patients with prostate cancer.

TREATMENT GOALS: PROSTATE CANCER

- Attempt curative interventions for patients with localized disease who have symptoms of prostate cancer or are likely to live for more than 10 years after diagnosis.
- Avoid treatment interventions that increase morbidity without a corresponding increase in length or quality of life.
- Preserve sexual, bladder, and bowel function and quality of life.
- Relieve symptoms of localized and metastatic disease.
- Minimize the side effects of treatment.

EPIDEMIOLOGY

Incidence

The estimated incidence of prostate cancer is 1999 was 179,500 men in the United States. This figure represents 29% of new cancers in men and 15% of new invasive cancers. About 37,000 deaths from prostate cancer occur, accounting for 13% of cancer deaths in men.[1] Only lung cancer is responsible for more cancer deaths.

It is important to note that the 1999 incidence figures show a dramatic decline from peak estimates in 1997 of 334,500 new cases per year (Table 92.1).[2] The incidence of prostate cancer appeared to increase very rapidly during the late 1980s and early 1990s, more than doubling within a few years. Because prostate cancer is a cancer of older men, some of the statistical increase resulted from aging of the U.S. population. However, the most important factor in the increase was significant improvement in methods of detection. During the late 1980s and early 1990s, prostate-specific antigen (PSA) blood testing became widely used as a screening test for prostate cancer. Its use was implemented in widely publicized

Table 92.1 ▪ Incidence of Prostate Cancer and Prostate Cancer Deaths, Based on Annual Predictions

Year	Incidence	Deaths
1984	76,000	25,000
1989	103,000	28,500
1993	165,000	35,000
1994	200,000	38,000
1995	244,000	40,400
1996	317,000	41,400
1997	334,500	41,800
Adjustment	209,900	–
1998	184,500	39,200
1999	179,300	37,000

Source: References 1, 3, 4.

"Prostate Awareness Weeks" in which inexpensive prostate screening was made available.[3] This resulted in the diagnosis of thousands of men with prostate cancer, most at an earlier stage of disease than previously had been possible. It is likely that without PSA testing, many of these men would have remained undiagnosed for years or might never have been diagnosed. This phenomenon resulted in what appeared to be a very rapid rate of growth over a brief period. Statistical estimates extrapolated from the slope of the steeply rising incidence rate curve were used to project the number of new cases of prostate cancer in future years. Once the pool of early-diagnosed prostate cancer cases was depleted, however, the incidence rate of prostate cancer began to decline and adjustments to the earlier estimates were made.[2,5] Current estimates remain much higher than the pre-PSA figures, but it was also evident that clinically detectable prostate cancer was increasing even before PSA measurements became available. The real increase in prostate cancer remains to be established.[4]

Despite the great changes in the incidence estimates for prostate cancer, the predicted number of deaths has remained fairly stable for the last several years. This wide discrepancy between incidence and mortality has raised questions about the clinical significance of early-stage prostate cancer and fueled the controversies about the need for widespread screening and the need to treat patients with early-stage disease.[4,6]

Etiology

The causes of prostate cancer remain unknown, although recent studies have contributed to the understanding of prostate cancer etiology. Some facts and associations are well established.

Prostate cancer is a disease of older men, with the mean age at presentation about 70 years. The incidence of prostate cancer increases more quickly with age than does any other malignancy.[7] During 1993–1995, the last period for which data are available, the probability of developing prostate cancer was about 1 in 10,000 for men less than 39 years of age, 1 in 55 for men aged 40 to 59, and 1 in 7 for those aged 60 to 79. The lifetime risk is estimated at 1 in every 6 men.[1]

African American men have the highest incidence of prostate cancer in the world. In the United States, the incidence of prostate cancer in African American men is approximately twice the prostate cancer rate of Whites. Prostate cancer is also more deadly in African Americans than in Whites; 5-year survival rates are about 15% lower for black men than white men in the United States.[8] In contrast, Asian American men develop prostate cancer at only half of the rate of Whites.

Androgens are essential for prostate cancer development. The primary circulating androgen is testosterone, which is converted by the enzyme 5-α reductase to dihydrotestosterone (DHT), the form that controls cell division in prostate cells.

There is evidence that differences in androgen levels or their regulation account for some of the racial differences in prostate cancer incidence. Testosterone levels in young African American men are about 15% higher than in age-matched Whites, a difference that may account for some of the higher risks of prostate cancer in this population. Testosterone levels are not correspondingly lower in Japanese men, but 5-α reductase activity is markedly less, which could result in lower levels of DHT.[9]

Family history is strongly associated with prostate cancer incidence. The magnitude of familial risk increases when the affected relative is diagnosed with prostate cancer at an early age and when more than one first-degree relative is affected.

Several chromosomal alterations are associated with an inherited predisposition to prostate cancer. Some chromosomal alterations are the presence of the PRCA1 (prostate cancer 1) gene and the HPC1 (hereditary prostate cancer 1) gene. Prostate cancers developing in families with linkage to the HPC1 allele characteristically occur at a younger age, and are higher grade and more clinically advanced at diagnosis, than cancers in families that do not carry this gene. Prostate cancer risk also is tripled or quadrupled in carriers of mutations in BRCA1 and BRCA2, the genes associated with hereditary breast or ovarian cancer.[10] Other chromosomal alterations may be important in prostate carcinogenesis, particularly loss or inactivation of tumor suppressor genes, which normally prevent cancerous growth.

Dietary factors also are associated with prostate cancer, perhaps because circulating androgen levels are altered by diet. The strongest dietary association is with increased animal fat intake. A diet high in saturated fats has also been correlated with a more rapid progression of disease in men with previously diagnosed prostate cancer.[11] Recently, prostate cancer risk has been inversely associated with selenium levels as measured in toenails[12] and with high levels of vitamin E intake.[13]

Insulin-like growth factor–I (IGF-I) is made by the liver in response to growth hormone and promotes carcinogenesis in prostate cancer cells in vitro. High levels of IGF-I have recently been shown to be a strong predictor of prostate cancer risk.[14]

Epidemiologic evidence suggests a slightly higher risk for developing prostate cancer in men who have undergone vasectomy. The increase in risk begins about 20 years after the vasectomy. A biologic mechanism to explain the association has not been established, and it is not yet certain that the association is causal.[7,15]

Negative associations also are important in mapping etiologic and epidemiologic factors. Prostate cancer is not associated with tobacco smoking. No occupational exposures have been convincingly linked with prostate cancer, nor has presence of benign prostatic hypertrophy (BPH), the normal overgrowth of the prostate that occurs with age. Sexual activity and sexually transmitted infections are not associated with prostate cancer.[7]

PATHOPHYSIOLOGY

Normal Anatomy

The prostate is a small, heart-shaped gland about an inch and a half in diameter. It is located at the base of the urinary bladder and completely surrounds the first inch of the urethra. It lies slightly above the rectum (Fig. 92.1). The prostate gland is surrounded by a fibrous capsule and is composed primarily of acinar or glandular tissue. The neurovascular bundles that control penile erection lie in grooves along the prostate gland, just outside the fibrous capsule. The normal function of the prostate is the production of a milky secretion called prostatic fluid, which adds to the volume of the ejaculate during sexual intercourse. Normal growth and the growth of malignant prostate tissues are controlled by androgens. Although testosterone has some effect on prostate tissue, DHT formed from testosterone is the primary androgen that controls prostate cell growth and differentiation.

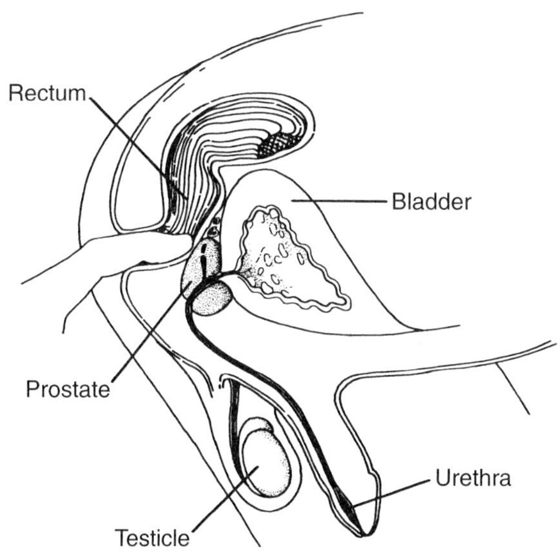

Figure 92.1. Male anatomy and digital rectal exam.

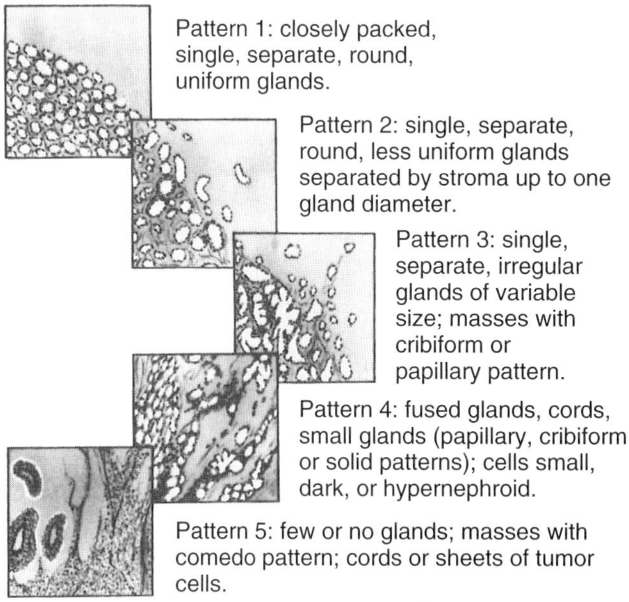

Pattern 1: closely packed, single, separate, round, uniform glands.
Pattern 2: single, separate, round, less uniform glands separated by stroma up to one gland diameter.
Pattern 3: single, separate, irregular glands of variable size; masses with cribiform or papillary pattern.
Pattern 4: fused glands, cords, small glands (papillary, cribiform or solid patterns); cells small, dark, or hypernephroid.
Pattern 5: few or no glands; masses with comedo pattern; cords or sheets of tumor cells.

Figure 92.2. Gleason pathologic scoring system for prostate cancer. (Reprinted with permission from Trump DL, Shipley WU, Dillioglugil O, et al. Neoplasms of the prostate. In: Holland JF, Frei E III, Past RC Jr, et al., eds. Cancer medicine. 4th ed. Baltimore: Williams & Wilkins, 1997:2129.)

Anatomically, the prostate gland is divided into three zones: transitional (surrounding the urethra), central, and peripheral. Most prostate cancers arise in the peripheral zone of the prostate, in the posterior lobe.[16,17]

Pathology

About 98% of prostate cancers arise from glandular tissues and are pathologically classified as adenocarcinomas. Prostate cancers are graded pathologically by their degree of differentiation, or how much (well differentiated) or how little (poorly differentiated) they resemble normal prostate tissue. This grading has prognostic value because well-differentiated tumors tend to grow more slowly and behave less aggressively than poorly differentiated tumors. The most widely used system is the Gleason grading system. In this system, cancers are assigned two scores, each from 1 to 5, that are added to make a total score from 2 (very well differentiated) to 10, which indicates a very poorly differentiated carcinoma (Fig. 92.2).

DNA ploidy status of tumors also is assessed for prognostic purposes. Tumors that are primarily diploid, demonstrating 46 chromosomes like normal human somatic cells, tend to behave less aggressively than those with a high proportion of aneuploid cells, which have an irregular number of chromosomes.[17]

Both normal and malignant prostate tissues produce PSA, a glycoprotein with serine protease activity. Because PSA is produced exclusively by prostatic tissue and circulates in the blood, it has become an important tumor marker for prostate tissue growth. However, PSA is produced by normal and hypertrophied prostate tissue (BPH) as well as malignant tissue, so it is not a specific

Table 92.2 ▪ Clinical Uses of Prostate-Specific Antigen Measurements

Screening asymptomatic populations, in combination with digital rectal exam
Assessing clinical importance of biopsy-detected cancers
Assessing disease prognosis
Staging prostate cancer as a guideline to appropriate initial treatment
Assessing efficacy of radical prostatectomy or radiation therapy
Monitoring patients for disease recurrence after surgery or radiation
Evaluating objective response to hormone therapy or chemotherapy
Evaluating efficacy of new agents in prostate cancer management

marker for prostate cancer. It is somewhat quantitative. Both the absolute level and the rate of increase (PSA velocity) reflect the activity of the prostate tissue growth process. PSA has many roles in prostate cancer screening, diagnosis, monitoring, and management (Table 92.2).[16,18]

CLINICAL PRESENTATION AND DIAGNOSIS

Prostate cancer usually is a slow-growing cancer, with a long doubling time that may exceed 2 years. Although prostate cancer grows slowly, if it does become clinically active, it will progress relentlessly in the absence of treatment and eventually will threaten the patient's life.

Prostate cancer always begins in the prostate gland, then spreads in one or more of three ways. It can spread locally by direct extension, penetrating the fibrous prostate capsule to invade adjacent structures such as the seminal vesicles and bladder wall. The most serious sequelae of local spread is urinary obstruction, which can result from compression of the urethra or the bladder neck. Prostate cancer may also spread through the lymphatic system or through the blood. Blood-borne metastatic spread carries prostate cancer cells to the bones, overwhelmingly the most common site of metastases. The bones that are located physically near the prostate, that is, those of the lower spine, pelvis, and proximal femurs, are the most common early sites of bony spread, although prostate cancer typically affects many bones in its advanced stages. Bone metastases are typically either osteoblastic (tumor that builds onto bone) or a combination of osteoblastic and osteolytic (bone dissolving) lesions. Osteoblastic tumor masses growing on the spine may compress the spinal cord and produce paralysis or loss of bowel or bladder control. Other metastatic sites of spread are lungs, liver, and soft tissue, especially lymph nodes.[6,16,19]

Signs and Symptoms

The anatomy and natural history of prostate cancer account for its presenting signs and symptoms. Prostate cancer usually is asymptomatic in its early stages because the growth in the prostate is small at first and is usually near the periphery of the gland. Larger tumor masses may produce urinary obstructive symptoms. Because the prostate physically surrounds the urethra, overgrowth of the prostate can compress the urethra and compromise urine flow. Because most prostate cancers grow in the outer areas of the prostate, these urinary symptoms are much less commonly caused by prostate cancer than by noncancerous overgrowth of prostate tissue, or BPH, in which the tissue overgrowth typically is in the central area of the prostate gland. However, when obstructive symptoms occur secondary to prostate cancer, they are indistinguishable from those produced by BPH. These include difficulty in initiating the urine stream, urgency, frequency, nocturia, dribbling, and incomplete bladder emptying.[16,20]

Too often, prostate cancer spreads before it produces serious local symptoms that bring patients to medical care. The presenting symptoms usually are attributable to metastatic spread to the bones, particularly low back pain. Prostate cancer is so common that evaluating unexplained low back pain in men older than 50 should include a PSA measurement to screen for prostate cancer. In patients with advanced metastatic disease at the time of diagnosis, the presenting symptoms may be those of spinal cord compression: lower extremity weakness or paralysis or loss of bowel or bladder control. Prostate cancer in these patients must be treated as a medical emergency. Anemia, weakness, or weight loss may also be presenting signs of advanced disease.[16,20]

Screening

Cancer screening refers to testing asymptomatic people who are at risk for a specific cancer. Because prostate cancer usually is asymptomatic in its early and most curable stages, increasing public health efforts have been devoted to widespread screening of populations at risk. The American Cancer Society recommends yearly screening with a PSA and digital rectal exam (DRE) beginning at age 50 for men with a life expectancy of at least 10 years. Annual screening should start at a younger age (often specified as 40 or 45 years of age) for men at high risk, such as African Americans and patients with a strong family history.[21]

Despite the potentially life-saving benefits of these prostate cancer screening programs, their value remains controversial. Some of the controversy can be explained by the natural history of prostate cancer. One of the most unusual features of prostate cancer, and one that still confounds understanding, is that the histologic prevalence of prostate cancer is much greater than its clinical incidence. Autopsy series evaluating prostates from men who died of unrelated causes have demonstrated cancer in about 30% of men over 50 and in 67% of men in their 80s. These figures represent more than 10 million men in the United States who have cancer foci physically present in their prostate glands. In contrast, the 179,300 new patients diagnosed in 1999 represent less than 2% of these men. Most histologically detectable cancers do not progress within the lifetime of the host and are called latent or clinically unimportant cancers. Those that threaten the life or well-being of the host are called clinically important.

One of the most important challenges in effective prostate cancer control and screening is to find objective criteria to distinguish between these two forms of prostate cancer.[22]

The argument against widespread screening programs for asymptomatic men is that most prostate cancers that are detected are likely to remain latent and will never cause clinical symptoms during that person's lifetime. Because of the advanced age of patients with prostate cancer, even those in whom the disease becomes clinically evident are statistically more likely to die of causes other than prostate cancer. The argument continues that diagnosing a patient with prostate cancer may lead to costly treatments that may be unnecessary in that patient but produce well-defined morbidity. Opponents of screening say that this violates the medical principle to "do no harm."[18]

Supporters of screening programs argue that the screening tests used (PSA and DRE) have limited utility in detecting latent cancers. The majority of cancers detected by these programs have proved to be clinically important in follow-up and probably would have progressed if left untreated. In this context, widespread screening, particularly of younger patients with a greater than 10-year life expectancy, is seen as an ethical and economical public health initiative because treating early-stage disease is less costly than treating advanced disease. To reduce prostate cancer mortality, men who are most likely to suffer with and die from prostate cancer must be diagnosed and treated.[6,18,23] Very recently, the first evidence of objective benefit of screening on survival was found by Labrie et al.,[24] who compared prostate cancer death rates in a large cohort of screened and unscreened men in Quebec City. Annual death rates from prostate cancer were 2.7 times greater in unscreened men than in men who were screened for prostate cancer.

Newer refinements of PSA measurements continue to add to the specificity and clinical utility of PSA testing. Examples are PSA velocity, which indicates the rate of rise of PSA from year to year, PSA density, which compensates for the size of the prostate gland, use of age-specific values (Table 92.3), comparisons of free and total forms of PSA, and measurement of membrane-bound forms of PSA.[18,25]

Table 92.3 ▪ Guide to Interpreting Prostate-Specific Antigen Values

Value (ng/mL)[a]	SI Units (pmol/L)[b]	Interpretation
0–4	0–118	Normal range, age nonspecific
0–2.5	0–74	Age-specific normal range, ages 40–49
0–3.5	0–103	Age-specific normal range, ages 50–59
0–4.5	0–132	Age-specific normal range, ages 60–69
0–6.5	0–191	Age-specific normal range, ages 70–79
4–10	118–294	Overlap area of benign prostatic hypertrophy and prostate cancer
>10	>294	High likelihood of prostate cancer
<0.2	<6	Expected level after radical prostatectomy

Source: Reference 3.

[a]Hybritech Tandem assay.

[b]SI units are not used in the prostate cancer literature and are provided here for reference only (conversion factor 29.412).

Diagnosis

The tests most widely used in screening, PSA and DRE, are also cornerstones of prostate cancer diagnosis. Although PSA testing is not specific for prostate cancer, it is the single most accurate method for prostate cancer detection. Patients with PSA levels greater than 4 ng/mL, or greater than age-specific values listed in Table 92.3, should be evaluated with DRE. Because most prostate cancers arise in the posterior lobe of the prostate, which can be palpated through the rectal wall (Fig. 92.1), DRE has long been a clinically useful diagnostic tool. Prostate cancers are felt as hard nodules in the otherwise rubbery glandular tissue. DRE may also detect extension of cancerous growth into tissues adjacent to the prostate. Suspicious or equivocal results after PSA and DRE are evaluated further using transrectal ultrasound (TRUS), which can visualize prostate size, nodules, and invasion of periprostatic tissues.

TRUS is also used to guide prostate biopsy, the definitive diagnostic test. Current standards of practice for prostate biopsy use high speed spring-loaded gunlike biopsy devices to take needle biopsy samples of the prostate through the rectal wall. At least six needle cores of tissue, distributed throughout the gland, usually are taken. Gunlike biopsy devices have made this an outpatient procedure of little discomfort and very low morbidity and have increased the reliability of tissue sampling.[26]

Staging

Once prostate cancer has been detected, the histologic grade or degree of cell differentiation (Gleason stage) and DNA ploidy status are assessed as indicators of prognosis. These tests are discussed in the Pathophysiology section of this chapter. Limited metastatic workup, including a bone scan, chest radiograph, liver function tests, and serum phosphatases, is also performed to assess extent and stage of disease. Pelvic imaging studies to evaluate lymph node involvement may be performed but do not reliably detect small lymph nodes.

Two staging systems for prostate cancer are in widespread use and have important prognostic significance. They are outlined in Table 92.4. The American Urologic Association Whitemore–Jewett staging system, which uses an A, B, C, D classification, remains the most commonly used. Although most solid tumors are staged in a four-stage system, there are some important differences in the classification pattern for prostate cancers. Stage A represents microscopic disease, which is not a stage category for other solid tumors. Stage B indicates one or more palpable nodules (similar to stage A or I in most other solid tumor classifications). Stage C refers to bulky local disease with extension outside of the prostate capsule but specifically excludes cancers with lymph node involvement. Prostate cancer is the only solid tumor in which stage D (IV) indicates lymph node involvement. The patient's disease is classified as D_1 disease when pelvic lymph nodes are the only detected site of metastases. Metastatic spread to bones or other distant sites is D_2 prostate cancer. An additional but unofficial designation of D_3 sometimes is used for hormone-refractory prostate cancer (HRPC), discussed later in this chapter. The other staging system in common use is the TNM classification, which stages prostate cancer based on the primary tumor (T), lymph node involvement (N), and presence or absence of distant metastases (M) (Table 92.4).[27] Survival of patients with prostate cancer is closely tied to stage of disease (Table 92.5).

Table 92.4 ▪ Staging Classification Systems for Prostate Cancer

AUA	Description	TNM	Description
		TX	Primary tumor cannot be assessed.
		T_0	No evidence of primary tumor.
A	No palpable tumor.	T_1	Clinically inapparent tumor, not palpable or visible by imaging.
A_1	Focal.	T_{1a}	5% or less of tissue.
A_2	Diffuse.	T_{1b}	More than 5% of tissue.
		T_{1c}	Tumor identified by needle biopsy because of elevated prostate-specific antigen.
B	Confined to prostate.	T_2	Tumor confined within the prostate but detectable clinically.
B_1	Small, discrete nodule.	T_{2a}	Tumor involves half of a lobe or less.
B_2	Large or multiple nodules.	T_{2b}	Tumor involves more than half of a lobe but not both lobes.
		T_{2c}	Tumor involves both lobes.
C	Localized to periprostatic area.	T_3	Tumor extends through capsule.
C_1	No involvement of seminal vesicles.	T_{3a}	Extracapsular extension on one side.
		T_{3b}	Extracapsular extension on both sides.
C_2	Involvement of seminal vesicles.	T_{3c}	Tumor invades seminal vesicles.
		T_4	Tumor fixed or invades adjacent structures other than those listed in T_3.
D	Metastatic disease.	N_1	Metastasis in a single lymph node, 2 cm or less.
D_1	Pelvic lymph node metastases.	N_2	Metastasis in single lymph node, >2 cm but <5 cm, or multiple lymph nodes none >5 cm.
		N_3	Metastasis in lymph node >5 cm.
D_2	Metastases to bone or distant lymph nodes or other organs.	M_1	Distant metastases.

Source: Reference 27.
AUA, American Urologic Association; *TNM,* tumor, node, and metastasis.

Table 92.5 ▪ Risk of Death and Cure Rates by Prostate Cancer Stage

Stage[a]	Percentage of Patients	10-yr Survival (%)[b]	Estimated Cure Rate (%)	Prognosis
All stages	100	51	32	
Stage A	10	95	85	Treatment may be unnecessary.
Stage B	30	80	65	Often curable.
Stage C	10	60	25	Occasionally curable.
Stage D_1	20	40	<5	Rarely curable.
Stage D_2	30	10	<1	Incurable.

Source: Adapted from Scardino PT, Weaver R, Hudson MA. Early detection of prostate cancer. Hum Pathol 23:211–222, 1992.
[a]Stage is based on clinical stage, pelvic lymph node dissection, bone scan, and acid phosphatase.
[b]Cancer-specific survival rates.

PSYCHOSOCIAL ASPECTS

Psychosocial issues are important in prostate cancer screening and treatment decisions. Until the mid-1980s, prostate cancer was poorly addressed in the United States. Perhaps because of the close association of prostate function and male sexual performance, many men were unwilling to discuss prostate function or to undergo the rectal examinations needed for screening. As a result of focussed public education and public awareness efforts, the willingness of men to undergo prostate cancer testing and treatment has increased.

There are other important psychosocial considerations. Prostate cancer significantly shortens life. Men with clinically localized prostate cancer, the most favorable form, lose an estimated 33% of their remaining life expectancy.[6] The life expectancy of men with advanced prostate cancer is even more severely compromised. Most of this time sacrificed to prostate cancer occurs during the typical retirement years, the time during which most men plan to enjoy life. Treatments for prostate cancer commonly produce impotence, incontinence, feminization, and weakness, and can discourage men from selecting potentially curative treatment. It is important that public education issues be continued, targeted at populations at highest risk for prostate cancer and those most likely to benefit from early treatment.

THERAPEUTIC PLAN

Prostate cancer treatment has been outlined by health care organizations. Two algorithms are presented: treating patients with clinically localized disease (Fig. 92.3) and treating patients with advanced disease (Fig. 92.4).

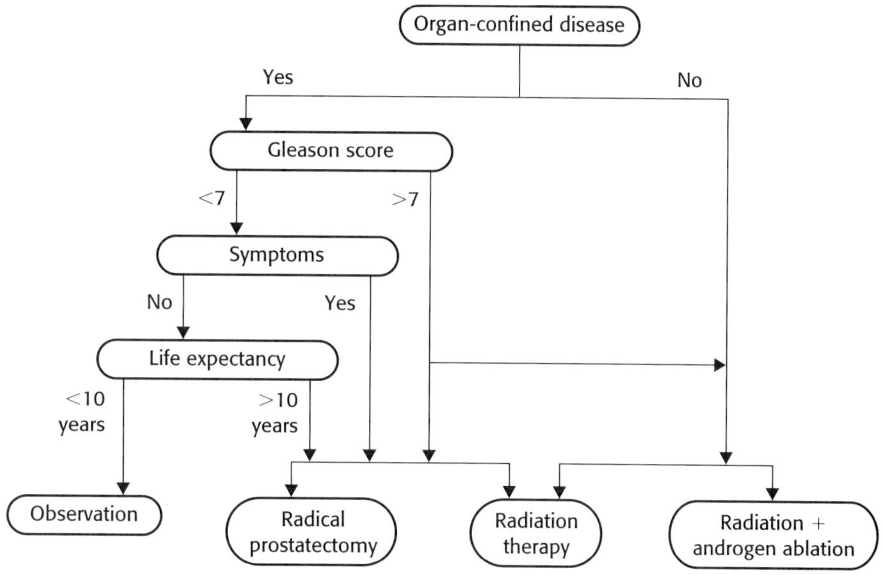

Figure 92.3. Treatment algorithm for localized prostate cancer. (*Source:* References 18, 29, 30.)

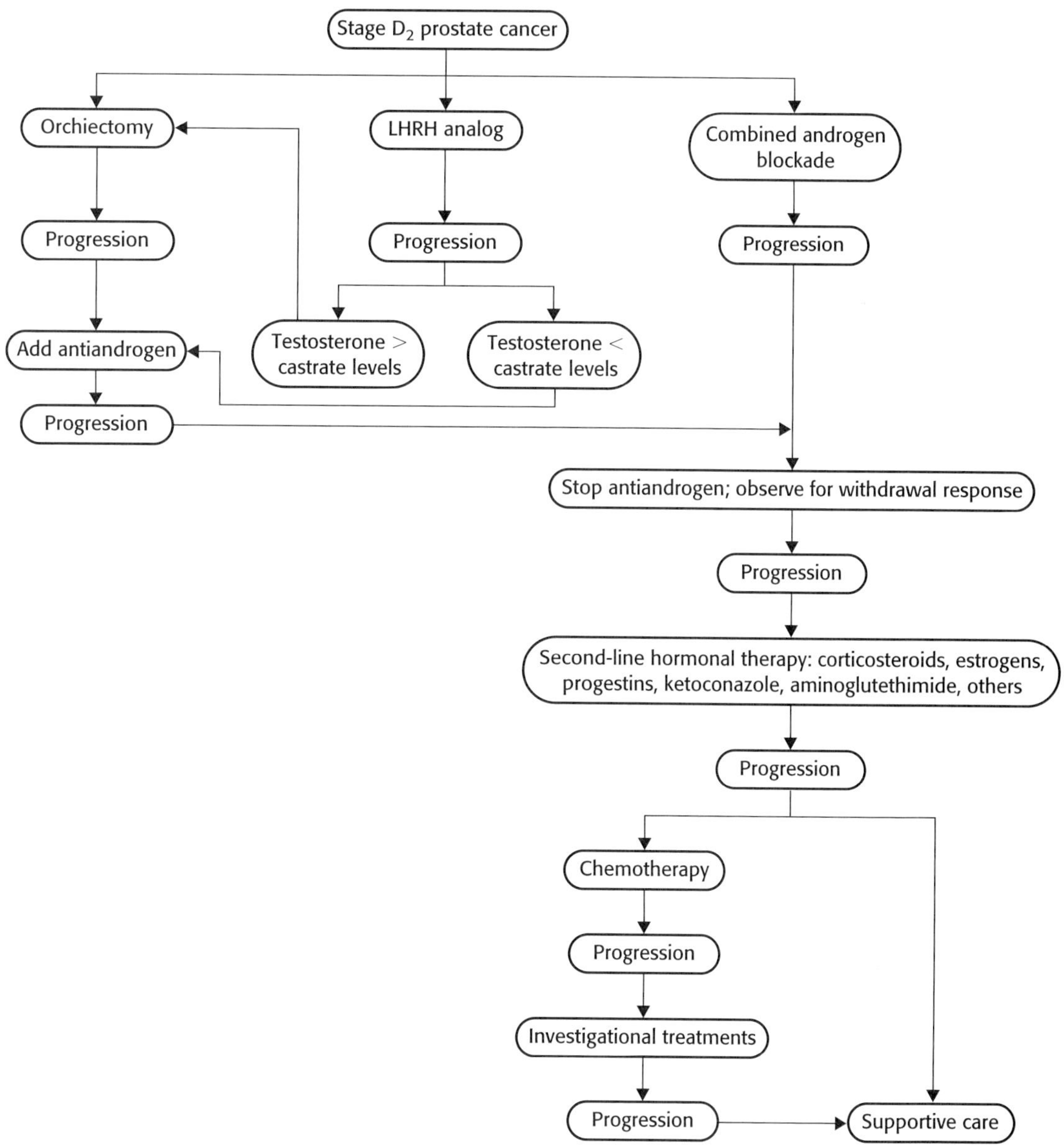

Figure 92.4. Treatment algorithm for advanced disease. *LHRH,* luteinizing hormone–releasing hormone.

TREATMENT

Clinically Localized Disease

There are several primary treatment options for cancer that is clinically localized to the prostate gland (stages A and B): surgery, radiation therapy, cryotherapy, or close observation without treatment.

Surgery

The standard of treatment is radical prostatectomy, or surgical removal of the prostate gland, plus pelvic lymph node dissection. This procedure offers the best chance to eradicate cancer that is confined to the prostate. PSA levels decline to levels equal to those in women (less than 0.2 ng/mL) after successful removal of all prostatic tissue with this surgery. Survival at 15 years is approximately 90%. Radical prostatectomy has been technically improved in recent years but still entails significant risks of morbidity, and related mortality up to 2%. The most common complications are impotence, with an incidence of 30 to 60%, and urinary incontinence (5 to 15%).[16,30,31]

Impotence was nearly universal with earlier radical prostatectomy techniques. The cavernous neurovascular bundles that carry the enervation for erectile control run in channels along each side of the prostate gland and traditionally were removed with the prostate. Nerve-sparing surgical techniques can preserve one or both neurovascular bundles in men with localized cancer that does not involve these structures. Return of erections sufficient for penetration and intercourse depends on the patient's age, extent of tumor, and erectile capacity before surgery. Best success is achieved when both neurovascular bundles are preserved in younger men with good erectile function before surgery.[30,31] Potency lost from the effects of surgery may be restored nonpharmacologically with vacuum erection devices or penile prostheses. Pharmacologic methods include transurethral alprostadil (prostaglandin E_1)[32] or oral sildenafil.[33]

Urinary incontinence is a less common but also very troublesome consequence of radical prostatectomy. Eighty to 95% of men recover normal urinary continence or report only stress-induced spotting within 18 months after surgery in large controlled series. The remainder need pads to keep their outer garments dry or are totally incontinent. Urinary incontinence can be treated with pelvic floor muscle exercises, anticholinergic or α-adrenergic agonists, anti-incontinence clamps, or implantation of inflatable urinary sphincters. Other surgical complications include blood loss, urethral stricture, rectal injury, thromboembolism, and wound infection. Surgery-related death occurs in 0.1 to 2% of patients.[30,31,34]

Radiation

Destruction of the prostate with radiation therapy is a satisfactory alternative to surgery for men with localized prostate cancer who are not good surgical candidates because of advanced age or concomitant health problems. Local radiation may be accomplished by external beam irradiation, which uses high-energy photon beams produced from linear accelerators, or by implantation of seeds of radioactive substances (iodine-125 or palladium-103). Use of implanted sources of radiation is called interstitial radiation or brachytherapy.

External beam radiation is the most commonly used and best evaluated method of radiation therapy. This generally entails radiation therapy sessions 5 days a week for 7 to 8 weeks. PSA levels drop much more slowly after radiation therapy than after surgery, often taking many months to reach nadir. Levels are also less likely to become undetectable after external beam radiation therapy than after radical prostatectomy, suggesting that eradication of cancerous tissue is not always complete. Radiation is most likely to produce satisfactory results in patients with pretreatment PSA levels less than 15 ng/mL. External beam radiation and radical prostatectomy are considered comparably efficacious if the PSA is reduced to zero. Although overall long-term survival rates are lower than with surgery, the differences may not be clinically important in older men. Administering androgen ablative hormone therapy (discussed later) before and during external beam radiation therapy has recently been shown to result in higher disease-free survival than radiation alone in patients with bulky stage B prostate cancers.[35–38]

Rectal or bladder irritation and bleeding are the most common acute complications of radiation therapy. Bladder irritation may respond to anticholinergic drugs; rectal irritation may be relieved with rectal corticosteroids. Proctitis or cystitis persist for many years in 3 to 8% of patients. Newer radiation techniques use three-dimensional conformational methods to plan the radiation dosage to the prostate, producing less damage to nearby organs such as the bladder and rectum. Although impotence develops much more slowly with radiation therapy than with surgery, the eventual risk of impotence from external beam radiation is approximately the same as with nerve-sparing surgical techniques. Chronic urinary incontinence is uncommon.[16,39]

Brachytherapy, or interstitial radiation therapy, delivers a high dosage of radiation to the prostate, with relative sparing of nearby normal tissue. The greatest advantage of implants over external beam radiation techniques is that the radiation procedure is accomplished as a 1-day outpatient procedure rather than with weeks of daily radiation therapy visits. Interstitial radiation is less toxic than external beam radiation and is comparably effective for low-risk patients (PSA levels of 10 ng/mL or lower and low Gleason scores). It is inferior to external beam radiation for higher-risk patients.[40,41]

Cryoablation

Cryoablative therapy entails destroying tissues by freezing. Freezing produces cell injury and cell death through a combination of direct mechanical shock (such as rupture of cell membranes from ice crystal formation), osmotic shock resulting from cell dehydration as water is transferred from intracellular to extracellular spaces, and cellular hypoxia. In cryotherapy of the prostate, the prostate tissue is frozen by means of perineally inserted cryoprobes. Cryotherapy destruction of the prostate can be used to treat localized tumors in low-risk patients and to treat patients with local tumor recurrence. It has not yet been compared with other methods in prospective randomized trials.[42]

Observation

The fourth modality for treating localized disease is observation, also called watchful waiting or expectant management. This is a much-debated issue in prostate cancer management. Prostate cancer usually is slow-growing and occurs late in life, so that many men diagnosed with prostate cancer die of unrelated causes, whether or not the cancer is treated. Treating localized disease is costly and can result in long-term complications such as impotence, incontinence, and rectal pain that compromise quality of life. Yet 37,000 men still die of this painful, debilitating disease each year, so clearly the difficulty lies in patient selection. Observation with careful follow-up is an appropriate decision choice for men with a life-expectancy of less than 10 years who have low-grade, localized prostate cancers. Younger men with a longer projected period of risk should be offered potentially curative treatment. A large randomized trial, the Prostate Intervention Versus Observation Trial (PIVOT) is currently under way to compare mortality and cost-effectiveness of radical prostatectomy or observation without treatment in patients with localized prostate cancer and should conclusively resolve this controversy.[16,43]

In summary, patients with localized prostate cancer have several treatment options:

- Radical prostatectomy is the most effective local therapy but carries significant risks of impotence and incontinence.
- External beam radiation is a good treatment alternative for patients unable or unwilling to undergo radical prostatectomy. Radiation produces slower PSA responses, is less effective in eradicating local tumor, and entails 6 to 8 weeks of daily treatment.
- Combinations of external beam radiation therapy and hormone therapy may improve outcome.
- Interstitial radiation with implanted radioisotope seeds produces results comparable to those of external beam radiation in men with low-risk prostate cancer. The implantation is a 1-day outpatient procedure.
- Prostate cryotherapy has not been tested in prospective randomized trials but appears to produce results comparable to those of radiation in men with low-risk disease.
- Observation may be a feasible option in men with low-grade, well-localized tumors who have a life expectancy of less than 10 years. Careful follow-up is needed.

Locally Advanced Disease

It is unlikely that patients with prostate cancer that has penetrated the prostate capsule and spread locally (stage C) will be cured by either radical prostatectomy or radiation therapy. Most of these patients have clinically undetectable micrometastases at the time of diagnosis, which eventually cause disease recurrence.

Radical prostatectomy can be used to treat small tumors that have penetrated the prostate capsule but is rarely curative. Attempts to improve the effectiveness of surgery by shrinking the size of the tumor mass preoperatively with hormonal agents (neoadjuvant therapy) have not been proven to decrease relapse. Administering androgen ablative hormone therapy in this manner is called downstaging because the intent is to convert the tumor from clinical stage C, in which the tumor extends beyond the prostate, to stage B disease.[44]

External beam radiation therapy is the most commonly used treatment for patients with stage C prostate cancer. As a single therapy, however, it is limited in its ability to provide long-term control of locally extensive prostate cancer. Neoadjuvant hormone therapy has also been studied in combination with radiation. The rationale is similar to that of its use in combination with surgical resection of the prostate: androgen ablative hormone therapy decreases the volume of tumor to be radiated, which may permit lower dosages of radiation to be administered. Randomized trials have proven that neoadjuvant hormone therapy decreases the local prostate cancer recurrence rate and results in disease-free survival longer than that of radiation therapy alone.[45,46]

One trial in which hormone therapy was administered during radiation therapy and for 3 years after completion of radiation treatments demonstrated for the first time that combined hormone therapy and radiation also results in higher overall survival rates than radiation alone.[47] The long duration of hormone administration in this trial makes it difficult to compare its results with those of true neoadjuvant trials in which hormone therapy was administered on a short-term basis before and during radiation therapy. Long-term administration after completion of radiation therapy may be more accurately considered adjuvant rather than neoadjuvant therapy.

Metastatic Disease

Hormonal therapy is the cornerstone of metastatic prostate cancer treatment. Prostate tissue growth is known to be fed by androgens, the male sex hormones. This applies to normal prostate tissue, to BPH, and to prostate cancers, although the sensitivity of individual cells or clones within a tumor mass may vary. Prostate cancer masses are heterogeneous; that is, all of the cells are not identical. Some are called hormone dependent. These cells die when androgenic hormones are withdrawn. Hormone-sensitive cells stop growing until resupplied with androgen. Some prostate cancer cells are believed to be hormone independent and are unaffected by the presence or absence of androgen.[48,49]

The goal of all hormonal interventions for prostate cancer management is androgen ablation, removing the

Table 92.6 ▪ Hormonal Agents for Managing Prostate Cancer

Drug Name	Usual Dosing	Monitoring Parameters
Aminoglutethimide (inhibits adrenal steroid synthesis)	250 mg PO 4 × daily	Self-limited rash; sedation, somnolence or lethargy; steroid replacement with dexamethasone needed; drug interactions.
Bicalutamide (nonsteroidal antiandrogen)	50 mg PO/day	Same as flutamide.
Flutamide (nonsteroidal antiandrogen)	250 mg PO q8h	Monitor LFTs (especially first 2 mo of therapy); diarrhea; gynecomastia.
Goserelin acetate (LHRH analog)	3.6 mg SC q4wk (or 10.8 mg SC q12wk)	Same as leuprolide acetate.
Ketoconazole (inhibits adrenal and testicular steroid synthesis)	400 mg PO q8h	Nausea and vomiting; monitor LFTs; gynecomastia; may need corticosteroid replacement therapy. Do not administer with terfenadine or astemizole.
Leuprolide acetate (LHRH analog)	7.5 mg IM/mo (or 22.5 mg IM q3mo or 30 mg q4mo)	Flare reaction first 4 wk (increased bone pain; risk of spinal cord compression; urinary obstruction); hot flashes; anemia with prolonged use.
Megestrol acetate (progestin; steroidal antiandrogen)	160 PO mg/day in 2–4 divided doses	Weight gain; impaired glucose control; fluid retention.
Nilutamide (nonsteroidal antiandrogen)	300 mg/day × 30 days, then 150 mg/day	Same as flutamide; monitor for new exertional dyspnea or worsening of preexisting dyspnea; delayed adaptation to dark.
Prednisone (corticosteroid)	5–10 mg/day	Fluid retention; impaired glucose control; mood changes; gastrointestinal bleeding; opportunistic infections.

Disease response is monitored in all patients by prostate-specific antigen measurements, pain symptoms, bone scan, and radiographic studies of soft tissue masses, if present. Impotence is common from androgen ablative therapies. Usual dosages and specific monitoring parameters are noted in table.

LFTs, liver function tests; *LHRH,* luteinizing hormone–releasing hormone.

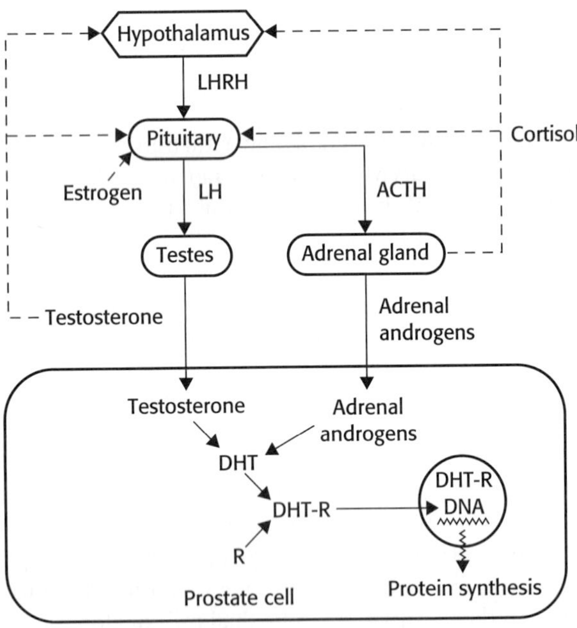

Figure 92.5. Influence of endocrine system on prostate cell growth. *ACTH,* adrenocorticotropic hormone; *DHT,* dihydrotestosterone; *LH,* luteinizing hormone; *LHRH,* luteinizing hormone–releasing hormone; *R,* receptor.

stimulatory effects of male hormones from prostate cancer cells. There are many ways to accomplish this goal. To put the different hormonal interventions (Table 92.6) in context, it is necessary to review the normal regulation of male hormone secretion.[48–50] These relationships are diagrammed in Figure 92.5.

Testosterone is the primary androgen. About 90% of circulating androgens are produced by the testes; the balance is produced by the adrenal glands. This proportion varies from patient to patient, and in some patients the adrenal gland is a very important source of androgens. Androgen production is regulated by a negative feedback system that includes the hypothalamus and the pituitary, in addition to the testes and adrenal glands.

Secretion of testosterone by the testes is regulated in the brain. The hypothalamus acts as a sensor that registers changes in circulating levels of hormones. When it detects low levels of testosterone, the hypothalamus secretes luteinizing hormone–releasing hormone (LHRH). This is also called gonadotropin-releasing hormone (GnRH). Under the stimulation of LHRH, the pituitary gland secretes luteinizing hormone (LH), a gonadotropin. LH stimulates the Leydig cells of the testes to secrete testosterone. A similar feedback loop controls steroid hormone production in the adrenal glands. The adrenals cannot produce testosterone directly but produce androgenic precursors that can be enzymatically converted to testosterone in many peripheral tissues.[48,50]

Testosterone is the main circulating androgen, but within the prostate it is transformed into DHT by 5-α reductase. Although both testosterone and DHT can stimulate the same androgen receptors in the prostate, DHT has more than twice the affinity of testosterone for these receptors. DHT's actions within prostate cells are believed to be similar to those of other steroid hormones: DHT binds to specific receptors in the cytoplasm and is transferred to the nucleus, where the hormone-induced effects on gene transcription ultimately result in the synthesis of proteins that produce the hormone's biologic effects.

Guidelines for Hormonal Therapy

Hormonal interventions for prostate cancer control are possible at every site in the hypothalamic–pituitary–gonadal–adrenal axis, at the point of conversion of testosterone to DHT, and at the hormone receptor level. Possible hormonal interventions differ in their mechanisms, advantages, and disadvantages, but some general guidelines apply broadly to their application in the treatment of prostate cancer[48–50]:

- The goal of all hormone therapy for prostate cancer is androgen ablation.
- About 85% of patients with prostate cancer have an objective or subjective response (relief of symptoms) to first-line hormonal therapy.
- With few exceptions, all of these hormonal interventions are effective and have comparable response rates.
- Choice of treatment depends on patient and physician preference, cost considerations, concomitant medical conditions, and rapidity of response needed.
- Hormone therapy is palliative. It does not cure patients with prostate cancer and in general does not prolong overall survival, although disease-free survival may be lengthened.
- The average duration of response to first-line hormone therapy is 1 to 2 years.
- Second-line hormone interventions have a much lower likelihood and shorter duration of response.
- Most hormone ablative therapies produce impotence and loss of libido (sexual desire). Hot flashes and feminizing effects such as gynecomastia (breast enlargement) and loss of male-distributed body hair are common.

First-Line Hormonal Interventions

Surgical Castration

Huggins et al.[51] were the first investigators to recognize the hormonal dependence of prostate cancer in the early 1940s and to treat it with a hormone therapy. They noted dramatic improvement in their patients with prostate cancer after surgical castration. Nearly 5 decades later, surgical removal of the testes (orchiectomy) remains the standard against which other hormone therapies are evaluated. It is still a widely used first-line treatment for metastatic prostate cancer. The external location of the testes makes orchiectomy an outpatient surgical procedure with very low physical morbidity. Castration may relieve prostate cancer symptoms very rapidly; patients may report relief of pain from bone metastases within hours of the procedure. This makes it the hormone intervention of choice in emergent situations such as impending paralysis from spinal cord metastases. Other advantages are its cost-effectiveness and lack of compliance problems. Subcapsular orchiectomy, in which the testes are excised but the scrotal sac remains, helps overcome the cosmetic disadvantages of this surgery, but it remains unacceptable to many patients. Orchiectomy carries negative psychologic and gender-related associations and is not reversible. It produces impotence and loss of libido in nearly 100% of patients. Hot flashes and weight gain are also common.[49,50]

Medical Castration

The availability of medical alternatives to surgical castration made prostate cancer therapy more acceptable to many patients. Estrogens were the first form of medical castration and were widely used in patients with prostate cancer in the 1960s and 1970s. Estrogens have many hormonal effects but primarily interfere with the release of LHRH from the hypothalamus, with subsequent decreases in LH production, and eliminate the hormonal signal for testosterone production by the testes.[49]

Diethylstilbestrol (DES) has been the most widely used estrogen. Its use and dosing were studied in a series of Veterans Administration Urological Research Group (VACURG) trials.[52] The first VACURG trial proved that 5 mg DES per day was as effective as orchiectomy in treating metastatic prostate cancer but more toxic, causing an excess of cardiovascular deaths. The next VACURG trial compared DES dosages of 0.2, 1, and 5 mg. The 0.2-mg dosage was not effective. The 1-mg dosage produced fewer cardiovascular complications and similar response rates to 5 mg, although castration levels of testosterone were not achieved consistently. Without strong objective data, an empiric 3-mg dosage became the standard of practice. At these dosages, the incidence of edema (15 to 20%), thrombophlebitis or embolus (5 to 10%), and myocardial infarction, angina, or congestive heart failure (about 5%) were still significant. Gynecomastia and breast tenderness, nausea, loss of libido, and impotence were also common. Use of estrogens as a means of medical castration went out of favor with the advent of the LHRH (or GnRH) analogs leuprolide and goserelin. Manufacture of oral DES has been discontinued in the United States. Other estrogens probably would produce similar clinical and toxic effects but have not been widely studied in patients with prostate cancer.[49,50]

The use of LHRH analogs (Table 92.6) to treat an androgen-dependent disorder such as metastatic prostate cancer seems counter to the logic of androgen ablation because it is LHRH that begins the cascade of signals that results in testosterone production. An LHRH analog should theoretically increase testosterone and stimulate the growth of prostate cancer. This is exactly what happens during the first several days of leuprolide or goserelin administration. Symptoms of prostate cancer such as bone pain and urinary obstruction may increase. This is called the flare phenomenon. However, chronic administration disrupts the normal pulsatile release of LHRH and inhibits LHRH receptors in the pituitary. This suppresses LH production and, ultimately, testosterone production. Castrate levels of testosterone are achieved within 4 weeks.

LHRH analogs are as effective as orchiectomy or DES in treating metastatic prostate cancer and avoid the cardiovascular complications and some of the feminization that estrogens produce. Disadvantages are the high cost, lack of oral formulations, high incidence of hot flashes, and risk of tumor flare. Flare symptoms occur in up to 10% of patients. Although they are usually manifest as a manageable increase in bone pain, flares can be very serious in patients with tumor masses near the spinal cord or obstructing urine flow. Special caution is needed during initiation of leuprolide or goserelin therapy in these patients. Tumor flare can be prevented by concomitant antiandrogen administration (discussed later). The main advantage of LHRH analogs over orchiectomy is reversibility of their effects, although it may take several months for testosterone levels to return to normal after LHRH analog therapy is stopped.[48–50]

Combined Androgen Blockade

Both orchiectomy and LHRH analogs very effectively eliminate testicular androgens. Neither intervention affects adrenal androgens, which normally account for 5 to 10% of male androgen production. Even this low level of androgens can stimulate prostate cancer growth. Combined androgen blockade (CAB), also called total or maximal androgen blockade, refers to combination therapies designed to eliminate the effects of testicular and adrenal androgens. Orchiectomy or an LHRH analog is combined with an androgen receptor antagonist (antiandrogen) to prevent any physiologic effects from adrenally produced androgens. Three nonsteroidal antiandrogens are available in the United States: flutamide, bicalutamide, and nilutamide (Table 92.6). All inhibit the uptake and binding of testosterone and DHT to nuclear receptors in a competitive manner. Testosterone production is not affected and may increase when antiandrogens are given without testicular suppression. These high serum testosterone levels may override the competitive androgen blockade, and for that reason antiandrogens are not approved or recommended as single-agent therapy. However, monotherapy with antiandrogens offers some quality of life benefits, including preservation of libido and sexual potency, and is sometimes administered to patients who refuse other hormones to avoid compromising sexual functioning.[53]

Adding antiandrogens to testicular suppressive therapies substantially increases costs and moderately increases toxicity. All commercially available nonsteroidal antiandrogens can cause gynecomastia, diarrhea, and increases in liver function tests. Diarrhea is greatest with flutamide, and rare fatal hepatotoxicity has been attributed to its use. Bicalutamide and flutamide can produce hematuria. Nilutamide produces delayed adaptation to dark, alcohol intolerance, and rare interstitial lung disease.[49]

The clinical benefit of total androgen blockade remains controversial. Small, nonrandomized studies in the early 1980s suggested better survival rates in patients with prostate cancer who received total androgen blockade than in historical controls treated with monotherapy. A landmark controlled trial (Southwest Oncology Group Intergroup Study 0036), which randomized patients to leuprolide plus either flutamide or placebo, was published in 1989.[54] This study demonstrated a 7-month survival advantage for patients on the combination therapy arm. Analysis of a small subset of patients with minimal metastatic disease and good performance status showed greater benefit, with a 20-month survival advantage at 5 years. This was the first time that hormone therapy had been proven to prolong survival in patients with metastatic prostate cancer. The survival benefit was accomplished with a modest increase in overall toxicity. Combination regimens quickly became the standard of care for initial treatment of patients with stage D_2 prostate cancer.[49]

Since that study was published, many randomized trials have sought to confirm or refute its findings. No study has shown a dramatic difference in favor of CAB or testicular suppression alone, nor have they shown differential responses for patients with good performance status and minimal disease. Two large, randomized trials demonstrated results very similar to those of the Intergroup study described earlier, with an overall survival advantage of about 7 months in patients on CAB in one study and similar progression-free survival advantage in patients on CAB in the other study. Many more individual trials have not shown a statistically significant difference in overall survival or progression-free survival.[49] Meta-analyses of controlled studies using nonsteroidal antiandrogens, but not steroidal antiandrogens such as cyproterone acetate, suggest a small benefit in progression-free survival and overall survival for patients receiving combined therapy.[55,56] Balanced with these benefits are substantial increases in costs and the added toxicity of the antiandrogen. One analysis of quality of life found that patients treated with CAB (orchiectomy plus flutamide) had worse emotional functioning and overall poorer quality of life.[57] For these reasons, many practitioners question whether the modest improvements in survival that seem possible with total androgen blockade are clinically meaningful.[58] Complete androgen blockade is not supported by current data for all patients with metastatic prostate cancer but may be appropriate for carefully selected patients.

Other important considerations in hormonal prostate cancer management are the questions of intermittent compared with continuous androgen suppression and that of immediate versus deferred treatment for advanced prostate cancer.

The goal of intermittent androgen suppression is to help maintain the hormonal responsiveness of prostate cancers by treating patients with cycles of treatment and treatment cessation followed by tumor regrowth. Treatment is continued until the PSA level nadirs, then treatment is stopped until the PSA begins to increase again. After a hormonal treatment cycle, patients are able to stay off hormonal treatment for an average of 9 months. During these off-treatment periods, quality of life improves significantly because toxicity decreases. Costs of treatment may be reduced, and the time to development of hormone resistance and tumor progression may be delayed. The impact of intermittent androgen therapy on disease progression and survival remains to be determined.[49,59]

The question of immediate versus deferred treatment of advanced prostate cancer is based on the general principle in advanced cancer that treatment is palliative rather than curative. Palliation traditionally is viewed as relief of symptoms, so from this perspective it is not reasonable to treat unless the patient has symptoms that can be improved. Palliation must be viewed in a broader scope of lengthening symptom-free intervals to improve quality of life. However, increasing data support the immediate treatment of asymptomatic patients with locally advanced or metastatic prostate cancer rather than deferring treatment until patients are symptomatic. Immediate treatment slows disease progression and the development of metastatic pain and complications.[60]

Second-Line Hormonal Interventions

Treatment options for patients who do not respond to hormone therapy (hormone-resistant, about 15% of patients) or who eventually become refractory to treatment (all other patients) are limited. Second-line hormone interventions have lower response rates, shorter durations of effect, and greater toxicity than the first-line therapies outlined earlier.

Manipulation of Antiandrogens

About one-third of patients whose prostate cancer progresses during combination therapy that includes an antiandrogen will benefit from stopping the antiandrogen (antiandrogen withdrawal syndrome). First recognized with flutamide, this phenomenon has now been documented on withdrawal of other antiandrogens as well. The mechanism of this effect is unknown, but evidence suggests that the antiandrogen begins to act as an androgen rather than an antiandrogen during prolonged therapy, perhaps because of mutations in androgen receptors. Antiandrogen withdrawal is the least toxic and most cost-effective second-line hormonal intervention for patients who have previously been controlled on CAB.[61,62]

Adding antiandrogens can be considered in patients who have not previously received them, followed by withdrawal of the antiandrogen upon further progression to assess a withdrawal response.[48] Anecdotally, patients may also respond to a change in antiandrogens after progression on one drug in that class.

As fewer patients are treated with CAB as first-line therapy, more patients are coming to care after failure of LHRH analogs or orchiectomy alone. Although the value of specific interventions has not been well documented in this setting, it has been recommended that testosterone levels be measured in patients who have been treated with LHRH analogs. Patients who do not have castrate testosterone levels may benefit from orchiectomy.

Estrogens

Estrogen therapy, discussed earlier, remains a second-line option for patients with progressive prostatic cancer who do not have elevated risk factors for thromboembolic complications such as a history of stroke. Manufacture of oral DES was stopped in 1997, but other estrogens are expected to have similar therapeutic and toxic effects. It is important that patients be counseled about the cardiovascular risks and other side effects before deciding to begin estrogen treatment.[63]

Aminoglutethimide or Ketoconazole

Adrenal androgens can be suppressed with aminoglutethimide or ketoconazole, an antifungal agent (Table 92.6). Both agents block adrenal steroid production by blocking cytochrome P-450; ketoconazole also interferes with testicular steroid production. Glucocorticoid replacement is necessary with aminoglutethimide treatment and sometimes with ketoconazole. Aminoglutethimide is used primarily as a second-line treatment in patients who have progressed after other agents. Ketoconazole lowers serum testosterone levels very rapidly and can be used as short-term treatment in patients with impending spinal cord compression when orchiectomy is not possible. High dosages are needed and may produce severe hepatitis.[50]

Miscellaneous Agents

Corticosteroids decrease PSA by more than 50% in about one-third of patients with hormone-refractory progressive prostate cancer. They may act in part by suppressing adrenal androgen production through feedback effects on adrenocorticotropic hormone (ACTH) production, although other mechanisms appear to be involved as well. Only low dosages (10 to 20 mg prednisone daily) are needed.[64] Megestrol acetate is a progestin that inhibits pituitary LH secretion and is also weakly antiandrogenic. Side effects associated with its use include fluid retention, impaired glucose control, and weight gain.[64] Finasteride, a 5-α reductase inhibitor, prevents the conversion of testosterone to DHT. It has very modest effects in advanced prostate cancer but is appealing in its ability to preserve potency.[65]

Cytotoxic Chemotherapy

Cytotoxic chemotherapy produces only low rates of objective responses (defined as disappearance of or more than 50% decrease in size of all detected tumor masses) and has not been widely accepted as therapy for patients with HRPC. No single agent or combination chemotherapy regimen has yet been proven to prolong survival.[68] Prostate cancer cells are inherently resistant to most conventional cytotoxic agents. Another consideration is that cytotoxic chemotherapy has its greatest effects against rapidly dividing cells; the very slow doubling time of prostate cancer cells may partially account for this low level of efficacy.

HRPC management with cytotoxic chemotherapy has increased in use and credibility in the past decade. Some of this change can be attributed to changes in how efficacy is measured. Most patients with HRPC have bone metastases as their major or only metastatic site, but no methods satisfactorily measure bone disease. Only 10% of patients with HRPC have measurable soft tissue disease, and objective response rates in these patient subsets cannot accurately be extrapolated to patients with bone metastases. Decrease in PSA levels often is used as a surrogate indicator of response but does not uniformly correlate with tumor response. For these reasons, quality of life indicators of response such as pain relief, decreased use of analgesics, and improvements in performance status are accepted by the U.S. Food and Drug Administration (FDA) as evidence of efficacy in patients with advanced prostate cancer. When drug efficacy is measured by these parameters, clinical benefit as defined by symptom relief is possible in a significant number of patients.[48,67]

Only one chemotherapy regimen has received FDA approval for treating symptomatic patients with HRPC based on these parameters. Mitoxantrone plus prednisone was demonstrated to be more effective than prednisone alone in palliating symptoms of HRPC in a carefully controlled trial.[68] Twenty-nine percent of patients on the combination regimen experienced significant pain relief, compared with 12% of patients on prednisone ($P = .01$). Duration of palliative response was also significantly longer, 43 weeks versus 18 weeks ($P < .0001$), although there was no difference in overall survival.

Other single agents with objective efficacy include cyclophosphamide, doxorubicin, cisplatin, estramustine, vinblastine, vinorelbine, etoposide, paclitaxel, and docetaxel. Single-agent objective response rates rarely exceed 10%. Combining these agents (Table 92.7) can increase response rates, although objective response rates for patients with measurable disease remain low.

The most consistent results have been obtained with combination regimens that contain estramustine. This is an unusual oral agent that combines an alkylating agent with an estrogen. It was originally designed as a means of targeting the alkylator to hormone-sensitive cells. More recent studies indicate that its mechanism of action is distinct from that of either of the two components. It is now recognized to work as an antimitotic agent with antimicrotubule effects. Estramustine is minimally effective as a single agent in patients with HRPC. In combination with other agents with antimicrotubular activity such as the vincas or taxanes, however, estramustine can produce palliative or PSA responses in up to 75% of patients with HRPC in small phase II nonrandomized trials. Palliative or PSA response rates of 25 to 40% are more representative. Encouraging results have also been achieved with combinations of estramustine and etoposide. No regimen has yet emerged as superior, and no true standard of care exists for cytotoxic chemotherapy for patients with HRPC.[16,69,70]

Table 92.7 ▪ Examples of Combination Chemotherapy Regimens with Palliative Activity in Patients with Hormone-Refractory Prostate Cancer

Mitoxantrone plus prednisone
Cyclophosphamide plus dexamethasone
Cyclophosphamide plus etoposide
Doxorubicin plus cyclophosphamide
Estramustine plus vinblastine
Estramustine plus vinorelbine
Estramustine plus docetaxel
Estramustine plus doxorubicin
Estramustine plus paclitaxel
Estramustine plus etoposide
Estramustine plus etoposide plus paclitaxel
Estramustine plus etoposide plus vinorelbine
Estramustine plus etoposide plus cisplatin or carboplatin
Estramustine plus doxorubicin plus vinblastine

Nonpharmacologic Therapy for Advanced Prostate Cancer

The major form of nonpharmacologic therapy for patients with advanced prostate cancer is orchiectomy, discussed earlier as a first-line androgen ablative therapy. Radiation therapy plays an important role in managing pain secondary to bone metastases in patients with advanced disease. It is administered by external beam techniques to palliate isolated painful bone sites. Multiple painful sites may be radiated systemically with bone-targeting radioisotopes. Two products are currently available: strontium-89 and samarium-153. These agents accumulate in bone at sites of increased turnover, such as metastatic tumor sites, and release low levels of radiation to nearby tissues. Onset of pain relief is gradual but lasts for several months, with little toxicity except bone marrow suppression.[71]

There is mounting evidence that diet affects not only the development of prostate cancer but also the progression of disease. Low-fat diets were shown to slow the progression of human prostate cancer xenografts (transplanted tissue) in nude mice. Human studies to evaluate the impact of similar diets in men with prostate cancer are under way.[72]

ALTERNATIVE THERAPIES

Probably the most widely used alternative therapies in prostate cancer management are herbal estrogens. The best studied product is PC-SPES, a combination of eight different herbs. Although promoted as a nonhormonal treatment for prostate cancer, it has recently been proven to have estrogenic activities. In a small trial, six of eight men with stage D_2 prostate cancer responded to PC-SPES treatment, achieving castrate testosterone levels, and PSA decreased in all eight patients, similar to responses produced by pharmacologic dosages of estrogens such as DES. Treatment with PC-SPES is also believed to carry the thromboembolic risks of estrogen therapy.[73] Other popular alternative therapies include modified citrus pectin, a fruit derivative that is promoted as decreasing the risk of metastatic spread by decreasing adhesion of cancer cells; vitamin supplementation; and selenium supplementation.

Several agents are used for symptom management. Saw palmetto is widely used for managing urinary obstructive symptoms. It is an herbal product with pharmacologic effects similar to those of finasteride and with established efficacy in relieving symptoms of BPH. It is not known to affect prostate cancer growth but may improve obstructive symptoms in patients with prostate cancer by reducing coexisting BPH. Hot flashes (vasomotor flushes) are a common side effect of many androgen ablative therapies. They may respond to vitamin E supplementation, herbal estrogens, or the phytoestrogens in soy products.

FUTURE THERAPIES

Despite the availability of many palliative treatments for prostate cancer, more than 37,000 men die of prostate cancer each year, enduring disease courses that are often relentless, painful, and debilitating. Truly effective treatments for HRPC have not yet been discovered. These unsatisfactory options for disease management have stimulated research for new treatments for patients with prostate cancer. Several avenues of research are being investigated.

Suramin is an investigational polysulfonated napthylurea used to treat African sleeping sickness. Its antitumor activity may depend on tumor growth factors inhibition or apoptosis induction (programmed cell death). The palliative superiority of suramin over placebo when combined with replacement dosages of hydrocortisone has been established in patients with HRPC. Pain and analgesic use decreased and disease progression was delayed in a large double-blind trial.[74]

Liarozole is a retinoic acid metabolism–blocking agent that promotes differentiation in cancer cells by increasing retinoic acid levels within the tumor cells. It can produce objective responses and decrease PSA in men with HRPC.[75]

Many investigative therapies target apoptosis, programmed cell death. Prostate cancers are believed to be mixtures of androgen-dependent and androgen-independent cells. Androgen-dependent cells undergo rapid apoptosis when androgens are withdrawn. Prostate cancer regrowth is attributable to takeover by androgen-independent tumor cells, which give rise to apoptosis-resistant clones. Some of the methods being explored to increase apoptosis of prostate cancer cells include using novel chemicals and natural products to induce apoptotic effects in slow-growing cells, interfering with molecules that regulate apoptosis, or modifying signal transduction pathways involved in apoptosis.[76]

Immunologic approaches to prostate cancer focus on vaccine therapies, often based on synthetic forms of prostate-associated antigens or genetically modified immune cells such as dendritic cells, the most potent antigen-presenting cells of the immune system. Dendritic cells capture proteins, digest them, and present the antigenic peptides to other cells of the immune system.[77] Gene therapies are used to augment normal immune response approaches against prostate cancer cells, to restore or increase tumor levels of tumor suppressor genes such as p53, or to counteract oncogenes, such as those that interfere with apoptosis or disrupt normal cell function.[78]

IMPROVING OUTCOMES

Outcome evaluation in prostate cancer is complicated by the advanced age of most patients and the slow growth of the disease. It is one of the few cancers in which treatment may not be necessary for all patients. In some cases, the best outcomes are achieved with no treatment.

Patient Education

It is only in recent years that prostate cancer has been openly discussed in the lay press. It is still common for men to be confused about precisely what the prostate is, where it is located, or how it functions. Significant changes in public awareness have taken place in a short time. Celebrities with prostate cancer have made their conditions public to encourage other men to be screened for prostate cancer and to educate the public about prostate cancer symptoms. Prostate Awareness Weeks have educated and screened thousands of men at risk for prostate cancer. Excellent patient education brochures are available through the American Cancer Society and the National Cancer Institute.

Methods to Improve Patient Adherence to Drug Therapy

LHRH analogs are the most commonly used drugs for prostate cancer treatment. Unfortunately, the two most commonly used products, leuprolide and goserelin, must be administered parenterally. Initially, only immediate-release formulations were available, necessitating daily subcutaneous injections. Depot forms soon were developed that permitted monthly injections, to improve patient adherence to drug therapy. In the late 1990s, extended-depot formulations that released drug over 3- or 4-month periods were marketed, further simplifying dosing. Once-yearly and every-2-year formulations are under investigation. Once-daily antiandrogens (bicalutamide and nilutamide) may result in better compliance than the every-8-hour dosing regimens necessitated by the pharmacokinetics of flutamide.

Treatment adherence also is improved by preventing or managing undesirable side effects of treatment. Most surgical, radiation, and hormonal interventions for prostate cancer produce impotence. Loss of sexual functioning can have a serious negative impact on quality of life and treatment satisfaction and can adversely affect patient willingness to initiate or continue therapy. Mechanical aids to produce penile erections, such as vacuum devices, have limited acceptance, as do intercavernous injections of pharmacologic vasodilators. Recent availability of effective and less intrusive methods to produce erections (intraurethrally administered alprostadil and oral sildenafil) have been welcomed by men with prostate cancer and are likely to improve acceptance of prostate cancer treatments.[32,33]

Hot flashes are a common and troublesome side effect of surgical castration and LHRH analogs. These vasoactive flushes are centrally mediated and produce sensations of heat and sweating that persist for several minutes. They can occur as often as 30 or 40 times a day and often awaken patients from sleep. Hot flashes can be controlled in about 75% of patients with low dosages of megestrol acetate, 20 mg twice daily.[79] The antidepressant agent venlafaxine hydrochloride has recently been shown to decrease the frequency and severity of hot flashes in men who have undergone androgen deprivation treatments.[80]

Disease Management Strategies to Improve Patient Outcomes

Several disease management interventions for prostate cancer in the last few years have been shown to improve outcome. Examples of strategies that have improved outcomes in patients with localized disease are nerve-sparing surgical techniques for radical prostatectomy, development of cryosurgery and brachytherapy techniques, more widespread use of three-dimensional conformal radiation therapy techniques, and combinations of androgen ablative therapy with radiation treatment. Outcomes in patients with advanced disease have been most affected by liberalization of criteria for drug approval for patients with HRPC that have permitted drug approval based on decreases in pain and improved well-being.

PHARMACOECONOMICS

Much of the economic debate in prostate cancer management centers on the cost-effectiveness of screening. One comprehensive analysis was based on 20-year literature review and estimated cost-effectiveness of projected outcomes after one DRE and PSA measurement. Using favorable assumptions, screening appears cost-effective in men less than 69 years old.[81]

Another economic analysis compared the costs of palliative chemotherapy with mitoxantrone and prednisone with those of prednisone alone in symptomatic men with HRPC in whom quality of life outcomes were measured. Comparisons included hospital admissions, outpatient visits, diagnostic tests, chemotherapy, radiation, and palliative care. The mean total cost of care was slightly less in men who received the combination regimen. Cost–utility analysis favored mitoxantrone plus prednisone and led the authors to conclude that treatments that reduce symptoms and improve quality of life can reduce overall costs of care.[82]

PREVENTION

Improved understanding of factors that affect prostate cancer growth has important implications for prostate cancer prevention. A large chemoprevention trial, the Prostate Cancer Prevention Trial (PCPT), is currently under way in men at high risk of prostate cancer. A total of 18,000 men have been randomized to long-term treatment with the 5-α reductase inhibitor finasteride or to placebo. It is proposed that androgen reduction by finasteride will prevent prostate cancer development. Results of the PCPT will be available in the year 2004.[83]

Potential dietary interventions to decrease the risk of prostate cancer include vitamin E or selenium supplementation and reduced consumption of red meat and dairy products.[7,12,13]

Limited evidence suggests that growth hormone injections should be avoided because growth hormone may increase levels of insulin-like growth factor.[14]

KEY POINTS

- Prostate cancer is a disease of older men and is the most common cancer in men.
- The apparent incidence of prostate cancer increased dramatically in the past decade because of the availability of PSA testing; incidence predictions have recently been revised downward.
- The cause of prostate cancer is unknown, although race, family history, and genetic changes are known to increase risk.
- Early diagnosis offers the best opportunity for cure, but the value of screening programs remains controversial because many prostate cancers are biologically latent and would not produce symptoms within the lifetime of the patient.
- Prognosis is determined by Gleason pathologic score and stage of disease.
- Treatment options for patients with localized prostate cancer include radical prostatectomy, radiation therapy, and cryotherapy. Observation is a treatment option in patients with low-grade tumors and a life expectancy of less than 10 years.
- Combinations of hormonal therapies with radiation therapy increase duration of response and progression-free survival.
- Androgen ablation is the cornerstone of treatment for metastatic prostate cancer. It is palliative rather than curative.
- First-line hormonal treatments for metastatic prostate cancer include orchiectomy, an LHRH analog, or CAB. The choice of hormonal therapy depends on patient preference, costs, and other medical conditions.
- Options for second-line hormonal therapy include antiandrogen addition or withdrawal, estrogens, progestins, corticosteroids, aminoglutethimide, and ketoconazole.
- The role of cytotoxic chemotherapy in HRPC management is increasing, based on symptom relief and improved quality of life. Mitoxantrone plus prednisone is the only approved regimen; combinations of antimicrotubule agents are also promising.

- Alternative therapies include herbal estrogenic products, modified citrus pectin, and products for symptom management.
- Economic evaluations have demonstrated the value of widespread screening and the value of palliative chemotherapy.
- Future directions include development of prostate cancer vaccines, apoptosis-inducing agents, and gene therapy.

REFERENCES

1. Landis SH, Murray T, Bolden S, et al. Cancer statistics, 1999. CA Cancer J Clin 49:8–31, 1999.
2. Parker SL, Tong T, Bolden S, et al. Cancer statistics, 1997. CA Cancer J Clin 47:5–27, 1997.
3. Crawford ED. Prostate cancer awareness week: September 22 to 28, 1997. CA Cancer J Clin 47:288–296, 1997.
4. Garnick MB, Fair WR. Prostate cancer: emerging concepts, Part II. Ann Intern Med 125:205–212, 1996.
5. Wingo PA, Landis S, Ries LAG. An adjustment to the 1997 estimate for new prostate cancer cases. CA Cancer J Clin 47:239–242, 1997.
6. Abbas F, Scardino PT. The natural history of clinical prostate cancer [editorial]. Cancer 80:827–833, 1997.
7. Haas GP, Sakr WA. Epidemiology of prostate cancer. CA Cancer J Clin 47:273–287, 1997.
8. Robbins AS, Whittemore AS, VanDen Eeden SK. Race, prostate cancer survival, and membership in a large health maintenance organization. J Natl Cancer Inst 90:986–990, 1998.
9. Ross RK, Coetzee GA, Reichardt J, et al. Does the racial–ethnic variation in prostate cancer risk have a hormonal basis? Cancer 75:1778–1782, 1995.
10. Lindor NM, Greene MH, Mayo Familial Cancer Program. The concise handbook of family cancer syndromes. J Natl Cancer Inst 90:1039–1072, 1998.
11. Bairati I, Meyer F, Fradet Y, et al. Dietary fat and advanced prostate cancer. J Urol 159:1271–1275, 1998.
12. Yoshizawa K, Willett WC, Morris SJ, et al. Study of prediagnostic selenium level in toenails and the risk of advanced prostate cancer. J Natl Cancer Inst 90:1219–1224, 1998.
13. Heinonen OP, Albanes D, Virtamo J, et al. Prostate cancer and supplementation with alpha-tocopherol and beta-carotene: incidence and mortality in a controlled trial. J Natl Cancer Inst 90:440–446, 1998.
14. Chan JM, Giovannucci E, Andersson SO, et al. Plasma insulin-like growth factor-I and prostate cancer risk: a prospective study. Science 279:563–566, 1998.
15. John EM, Whittemore AS, Wu AH, et al. Vasectomy and prostate cancer: results from a multiethnic case-control study. J Natl Cancer Inst 87:662–669, 1995.
16. Trump DL, Shipley WU, Dillioglugil O, et al. Neoplasms of the prostate. In: Holland J. Cancer medicine. 4th ed. Baltimore: Williams & Wilkins, 1997:2125–2164.
17. Bostwick DG. Pathology of prostate cancer. In: Ernstoff MS, Heaney JA, Peschel RE, eds. Prostate cancer. Malden, MA: Blackwell, 1998:15–47.
18. Woolf SH. Screening for prostate cancer with prostate-specific antigen: an examination of the evidence. N Engl J Med 303:1401–1405, 1995.
19. Adolfsson J, Rutqvist LE, Steineck G. Prostate carcinoma and long-term survival. Cancer 80:748–752, 1997.
20. Cersosimo RJ, Carr RJ. Prostate cancer: current and evolving strategies. Am J Health Syst Pharm 53:381–396, 1996.
21. von Eschenbach A, Ho R, Murphy GP, et al. American Cancer Society guidelines for the early detection of prostate cancer: update 1997. CA Cancer J Clin 47:261–264, 1997.
22. Hanks GE, Myers CE, Scardino PT. Cancer of the prostate. In: Devita VT, Hellman S, Rosenberg SA, eds. Cancer: principles and practice of oncology. Philadelphia: JB Lippincott, 1997:1322–1385.
23. Gomella LG. The Will Rogers phenomenon in prostate cancer: a good thing. Cancer J Sci Am 4:19–21, 1998.
24. Labrie F, Dupont A, Candas B, et al. Decrease of prostate cancer death by screening: first data from the Quebec prospective and randomized study [abstract]. Proc Am Soc Clin Oncol Annual Meeting 17:1, 1998.
25. Beduschi C, Oesterling JE. Percent free prostate-specific antigen: the next frontier in prostate-specific antigen testing. Urology 51(Suppl 5A):98–109, 1998.
26. Foster HE Jr, Lytton B. Diagnostic evaluation of prostate cancer. In: Ernstoff MS, Heaney JA, Peschel RE, eds. Prostate cancer. Malden, MA: Blackwell, 1998:48–61.
27. Anonymous. Genitourinary sites. In: Fleming ID, Cooper JS, Henson DE, et al., eds. AJCC cancer staging manual. 5th ed. Philadelphia: Lippincott-Raven, 1997:219–224.
28. Millikan R, Logothetis C. Update of the NCCN guidelines for treatment of prostate cancer. Oncology 11:180–193, 1997.
29. LaRocca RV. Prostate cancer. In: Djulbigovic B, Sullivan DM, eds. Decision making in oncology: evidence-based management. New York: Churchill-Livingstone, 1997:317–323.
30. Catalona WJ. Surgical management of prostate cancer. Cancer 75:1903–1908, 1994.
31. Lepor H, Guerena M. Surgical management of prostate cancer. In: Ernstoff MS, Heane JA, Peschel RE, eds. Prostate cancer. Malden, MA: Blackwell, 1998:91–106.
32. Padma-Nathan H, Hellstrom WJG, Kaiser FE, et al. Treatment of men with erectile dysfunction with transurethral alprostadil. N Engl J Med 336:1–7, 1997.
33. Goldstein I, Lue TF, Padma-Nathan H, et al. Oral sildenafil in the treatment of erectile dysfunction. N Engl J Med 338:1397–1404, 1998.
34. Zincke H, Bergstralh EJ, Blute ML, et al. Radical prostatectomy for clinically localized prostate cancer: long-term results of 1,143 patients from a single institution. J Clin Oncol 12:2254–2263, 1994.
35. Lawton C, Winter K, Murray K, et al. Updated results of the Phase III Radiation Oncology Group Trial 85-31 evaluating the potential benefit of androgen deprivation following standard radiation therapy for unfavorable prognosis carcinoma of the prostate [abstract]. Proc Am Soc Clin Oncol Annual Meeting 18:1195, 1999.
36. Lee WR, Hanks GE, Schultheiss TE, et al. Localized prostate cancer treated by external-beam radiotherapy alone: serum prostate-specific antigen–driven outcome analysis. J Clin Oncol 13:464–469, 1995.
37. Crook JM, Bahadur YA, Bociek RG, et al. Radiotherapy for localized prostate cancer. Cancer 79:328–336, 1997.
38. Reni M, Bolognesi A. Prognostic value of prostate specific antigen before, during, and after radiotherapy. Cancer Treat Rev 24:91–99, 1998.
39. Nguyen LN, Pollack A, Zagars GK. Late effects after radiotherapy for prostate cancer in a randomized dose–response study: results of a self-assessment questionnaire. Urology 51:991–997, 1998.
40. D'Amico AV, Whittington R, Malkowicz SB, et al. Biochemical outcome after radical prostatectomy, external beam radiation therapy, or interstitial radiation therapy for clinically localized prostate cancer. JAMA 280:975–980, 1998.
41. Sharkey J, Chovnick SD, Behar RJ, et al. Outpatient ultrasound-guided palladium 103 brachytherapy for localized adenocarcinoma of the prostate: a preliminary report of 434 patients. Urology 51:796–803, 1998.
42. Schmidt JD, Doyle J, Larison S. Prostate cryoablation: update 1998. CA Cancer J Clin 48:239–253, 1998.
43. Chodak GW, Thisted RA, Gerger GS, et al. Results of conservative management of clinically localized prostate cancer. N Engl J Med 330:242–248, 1994.
44. Gibbons RP. Prostate carcinoma: surgical management of regional disease. Cancer 78:2455–2460, 1996.
45. Pilepich MV, Krall JM, Al-Sarraf M, et al. Androgen deprivation with radiation therapy compared with radiation therapy alone for locally advanced prostatic carcinoma: a randomized comparative trial of the Radiation Therapy Oncology Group. Urology 45:616–623, 1995.
46. Leverdiere J, Gomez JL, Cusan L, et al. Beneficial effect of combination hormonal therapy administered prior to and following external beam radiation therapy in localized prostate cancer. Int J Radiat Oncol Biol Phys 37:247–252, 1997.
47. Bolla M, Gonzalez D, Warde P, et al. Improved survival in patients with locally advanced prostate cancer treated with radiotherapy and goserelin. N Engl J Med 337:295–300, 1997.
48. Downing AJ, Tannock IF. Systemic treatment for prostate cancer. Cancer Treat Rev 24:283–301, 1998.
49. Goktas S, Crawford ED. Optimal hormonal therapy for advanced prostatic carcinoma. Semin Oncol 26:162–173, 1999.
50. Brufsky A, Kantoff PW. Hormonal therapy for prostate cancer. In: Ernstoff MS, Heaney JA, Peschel RE, eds. Prostate cancer. Malden, MA: Blackwell, 1998:160–180.
51. Huggins C, Stevens R, Hodges C. The effect of castration on advanced carcinoma of the prostate gland. Arch Surg 43:209–223, 1941.
52. Blackard CE. The Veterans' Administration cooperative urological research group studies of carcinoma of the prostate: a review. Cancer Chemother Rep 59:225–227, 1975.

53. Boccon-Gibod L. Are non-steroidal anti-androgens appropriate as monotherapy in advanced prostate cancer? Eur Urol 33:159–164, 1998.
54. Crawford ED, Eisenberger MA, McLeod DG, et al. A controlled trial of leuprolide with and without flutamide in prostatic carcinoma. N Engl J Med 321:419–424, 1989.
55. Caubet J, Tosteson TD, Dong EW, et al. Maximum androgen blockade in advanced prostate cancer: a meta-analysis of published randomized controlled trials using nonsteroidal antiandrogens. Urology 4971–4978, 1997.
56. Bennett L, Tosteson TD, Schmitt BP, et al. Maximum androgen-blockade with medical or surgical castration in advanced prostate cancer: a meta-analysis of 9 published randomized controlled trials and 4,128 patients using flutamide. Prostate Cancer Prostatic Dis 2:4–8, 1999.
57. Moinpour CM, Savage MJ, Troxel A, et al. Quality of life in advanced prostate cancer: results of a randomized therapeutic trial. J Natl Cancer Inst 90:1537–1544, 1998.
58. Eisenberger MA, Blumenstein BA, Crawford ED, et al. Bilateral orchiectomy with or without flutamide for metastatic prostate cancer. N Engl J Med 339:1036–1042, 1998.
59. Theyer G, Hamilton G. Current status of intermittent androgen suppression in the treatment of prostate cancer. Urology 52:353–359, 1998.
60. Medical Research Council Prostate Cancer Working Party Investigators Group. Immediate versus deferred treatment for advanced prostatic cancer: initial results of the Medical Research Council trial. Br J Urol 79:235–246, 1997.
61. Scher HI, Kelly WK. Flutamide withdrawal syndrome: its impact on clinical trials in hormone-refractory prostate cancer. J Clin Oncol 11:1566–1572, 1993.
62. Huan SD, Gerridzen RG, Yau JC, et al. Antiandrogen withdrawal syndrome with nilutamide. Urology 49:632–634, 1997.
63. Smith DC, Redman BG, Flaherty LE, et al. A phase II trial of oral diethylstilbestrol as a second-line hormonal agent in advanced prostate cancer. Urology 52:257–260, 1998.
64. Sartor O, Weinberger M, Moore A, et al. Effect of prednisone on prostate-specific antigen in patients with hormone-refractory prostate cancer. Urology 52:252–256, 1998.
65. Osborn JL, Smith DC, Trump DL. Megestrol acetate in the treatment of hormone refractory prostate cancer. Am J Clin Oncol 20:308–310, 1997.
66. Tannock IF. Is there evidence that chemotherapy is of benefit to patients with carcinoma of the prostate? J Clin Oncol 3: 1013–1021, 1985.
67. Dowling AJ, Panzarella T, Tannock IF. Relationship between changes in serum prostatic specific antigen and palliative response following treatment of symptomatic hormone-refractory prostate cancer. Abst Proc Am Soc Clin Oncol 17:1248, 1998.
68. Tannock IF, Osaba D, Stockler MR, et al. Chemotherapy with mitoxantrone plus prednisone or prednisone alone for symptomatic hormone-resistant prostate cancer: a Canadian randomized trial with palliative end points. J Clin Oncol 14:1756–1764, 1996.
69. Upadhyaya H, Vogelzang NJ. Chemotherapy for prostate cancer. In: Ernstoff MS, Heaney JA, Peschel RE, eds. Prostate cancer. Malden, MA: Blackwell, 1998:181–202.
70. Raghavan D, Koczwara B, Javle M. Evolving strategies of cytotoxic chemotherapy for advanced prostate cancer. Eur J Cancer 33:566–574, 1997.
71. Mertens WC, Filipczak LA, Ben-Josef E, et al. Systemic bone-seeking radionuclides for palliation of painful osseous metastases: current concepts. CA Cancer J Clin 48:361–374, 1998.
72. Wynder EL, Fair WR. Prostate cancer nutrition adjunct therapy [editorial]. J Urol 156:1364–1365, 1996.
73. DiPaola RS, Zhang H, Lambert GH, et al. Clinical and biologic activity of an estrogenic herbal combination [PC-SPES] in prostate cancer. N Engl J Med 339:785–791, 1998.
74. Small EJ, Marshall ME, Reyno L, et al. Superiority of suramin + hydrocortisone over placebo + hydrocortisone: results of a multi-center double-blind phase III study in patients with hormone refractory prostate cancer [abstract]. Proc Am Soc Clin Oncol Annual Meeting 17:1187, 1998.
75. Debruyne FJM, Murray R, Fradet Y, et al. Liarozole, a novel treatment approach for advanced prostate cancer: results of a large randomized trial versus cyproterone acetate. Urology 52:72–81, 1998.
76. Tang DG, Porter AT. Target to apoptosis: a hopeful weapon for prostate cancer. Prostate 32:284–293, 1997.
77. Tjoa BA, Lodge PA, Salgaller ML, et al. Dendritic cell-based immunotherapy for prostate cancer. CA Cancer J Clin 49:117–128, 1999.
78. Malkowicz SB, Johnson JO. Gene therapy for prostate cancer. Hematol Oncol Clin North Am 12:649–663, 1998.
79. Loprinzi CL, Michalak JC, Quella SK, et al. Megestrol acetate for the prevention of hot flashes. N Engl J Med 331:347–352, 1994.
80. Loprinzi CL, Pisansky TM, Fonseca R, et al. Pilot evaluation of venlafaxine hydrochloride for the therapy of hot flashes in cancer survivors. J Clin Oncol 16:2377–2381, 1998.
81. Coley CM, Barry MJ, Fleming C, et al. Early detection of prostate cancer. Part II: estimating the risks, benefits, and costs. Ann Intern Med 126:468–479, 1997.
82. Bloomfield DJ, Krahn MD, Neogi T, et al. Economic evaluation of chemotherapy with mitoxantrone plus prednisone for symptomatic hormone-resistant prostate cancer: based on a Canadian randomized trial with palliative end points. J Clin Oncol 16:2272–2279, 1998.
83. Thompson IM, Coltman CA Jr, Crowley J. Chemoprevention of prostate cancer: the Prostate Cancer Prevention Trial. Prostate 33:217–221, 1997.

CHAPTER 93

PEDIATRIC SOLID TUMORS

Martha G. Danielson and Susannah E. Koontz

The annual incidence of cancer in children is approximately 140 per million.[1] Despite this low incidence, cancer is second only to accidents as the cause of death in children ages 1 to 14 years, making it the leading cause of death attributed to disease in this population.[2] The incidence of all cancers in this age-group is slightly greater in males than females (1.13:1).[3] Slight upward trends in the incidence of cancer in the pediatric population have been identified recently, especially in infants.[4,5] However, survival from childhood cancer continues to improve (Tables 93.1 and 93.2).[2,4] These increases in survival rates are attributed to the use of more effective combination chemotherapy given as adjuvant therapy; dose-intensified chemotherapy regimens; and refined diagnostic, surgical, and radiotherapy techniques to treat tumors.[6] In all, approximately 65% of children diagnosed with cancer achieve a cure.[7]

Solid tumors account for more than 40% of all pediatric malignancies (Fig 93.1),[8] and peak incidence varies with tumor type. For example, neuroblastoma, retinoblastoma, rhabdomyosarcoma, and Wilms' tumor are more common in infants and toddlers, whereas osteosarcoma and Ewing's sarcoma have their peak incidence during adolescence.[3] Solid tumors, unlike hematologic malignancies, require one or more of the following: surgery, radiation, multiagent chemotherapy, and immunotherapy. Thus the organization of efforts from the pediatric oncologist, pathologist, radiologist, surgeon, and other health care professionals such as nurses, pharmacists, dieticians, psychologists, and social workers is vital to achieving the stated treatment goals.

Table 93.1 ▪ Incidence of Solid Tumors in U.S. Infants 1979–1981 Compared with 1989–1991

Type	1979–1981 Rate[a]	1989–1991 Rate[a]
Neuroblastoma	51	60
Central nervous system tumor	24	33
Retinoblastoma	22	29
Sarcoma	10	11
Renal	26	24
All cancers[b]	189	220

Source: Reference 4.

[a]Per million U.S. children age less than 1 year.

[b]Includes all tumor histologies.

Table 93.2 ▪ Five-Year Relative Survival Rates for Children Under Age 15

	Five-Year Relative Survival Rates (%)		
	Year of Diagnosis		
Site	1960–1963	1974–1976	1986–1993[a]
Bones and joints	20	54	64
Central nervous system	35	54	61
Neuroblastoma	25	52	65
Soft tissue	38	60	73
Wilms' tumor	33	74	92
All cancers[b]	28	56	72

Source: Reference 2.

[a]The difference in 1974–1976 rate and 1986–1993 rate is statistically significant ($P < 0.05$).

[b]Excluding basal and squamous cell skin cancers and in situ carcinomas except urinary bladder.

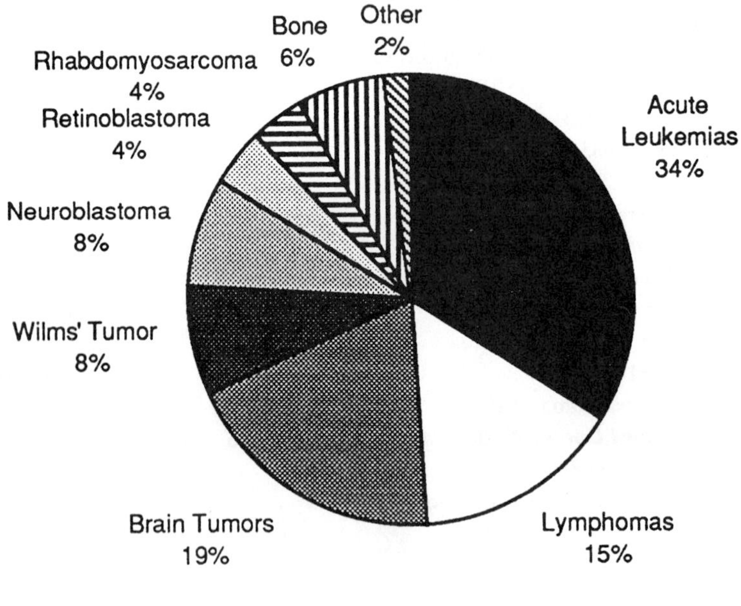

Figure 93.1. Relative incidence of pediatric malignancies. (*Source:* Gurney JG, Severson RK, Davis S, et al. Incidence of cancer in children in the United States: sex-, race-, and 1-year age-specific rates by histology type. Cancer 75:2168–2195, 1995.)

This chapter introduces the reader to the more common pediatric solid tumors. An overview of epidemiology, clinical presentation and diagnosis, and prognosis is given for each tumor type. Treatment modalities and supportive care issues relating to pharmaceutical care encountered in clinical practice are emphasized. Where appropriate, the reader is referred to primary literature for more detailed information.

TREATMENT GOALS: PEDIATRIC TUMORS

- Eradicate the primary tumor and systemic disease.
- Minimize and treat toxicities relating to therapy.
- Identify and manage long-term sequelae of therapy.
- Use a multidisciplinary approach incorporating multimodal therapy to achieve treatment goals.

Overview

TREATMENT MODALITIES

The four major modalities used in patients with solid tumors are surgery, radiation therapy, chemotherapy, and immunotherapy. Surgery remains the primary treatment for most solid tumors and serves three functions:

1. Diagnosis and staging
2. Treatment
3. Prevention

Visual inspections and tissue samplings for pathologic evaluations can provide the basis for staging, which in turn can facilitate the determination of subsequent therapy. Total resection, debulking, metastatic resection, palliation, and reconstruction procedures are examples of the role of surgery in treatment algorithms. Prophylactic surgical procedures in certain patients have reduced the likelihood of developing malignancies. The goal of surgery is maximal tumor resection while minimizing the chance of deformities.

Maximizing the local control of a tumor is the goal of radiation therapy. Radiotherapy is usually administered in a series of small exposures (fractions) for a period of a few minutes. Typically, radiotherapy is scheduled to last 1 to 7 weeks with administration occurring once or twice a day for 5 days per week. Radiation works by damaging cellular DNA (by causing ionization of atoms and the formation of free radicals), and cell death occurs when irradiated cells attempt to replicate. The effects of radiation therapy are most pronounced on rapidly dividing cells, making malignancies an excellent target for this treatment modality. However, rapidly dividing healthy cells (namely bone marrow stem cells and gastrointestinal cells) are often damaged by radiation therapy, and significant toxicities (neutropenia, thrombocytopenia, nausea, vomiting, diarrhea, mucositis, etc.) are the result.[6] Fractionated radiation and dose reductions used in combination with chemotherapy have decreased radiation-related toxicities.[9] Long-term toxicities from radiation therapy include cardiac toxicity; learning disabilities; and impaired development of soft tissues, teeth, and visual structures, which results in decreased muscle mass and cosmetic deformities.[10]

The majority of pediatric malignancies are chemosensitive. Chemotherapy can be administered before surgery or radiation (neoadjuvant therapy) or can be given as adjuvant therapy following other treatment modalities. It is also used as the primary modality to treat unresectable metastatic disease. Regimens used in pediatric solid tumors consist of multiple agents. The rationale of combination chemotherapy is that using numerous agents with different mechanisms of action allows for synergistic or additive effects while minimizing the likelihood of drug resistance.[11] Additionally, studies using dose-intensive therapies, regimens in which agents are given at higher doses over shorter intervals, have demonstrated promising results.[12] Multidrug resistance (MDR) is beginning to surface in pediatric patients with solid malignancies. The identification of p-glycoprotein-mediated MDR is currently a controversial topic with conflicting reports validating the need for additional research.[13] Agents most commonly used in solid tumors are summarized in Table 93.3 and are discussed in more detail, where appropriate, throughout the chapter.

The fourth treatment modality in pediatric solid malignancies is immunotherapy. Immunotherapy, which includes growth-differentiating agents, gene therapy, and biologic therapy, is used to augment a patient's own immune system or can be used to directly transfer immunity through the incorporation of physiologic proteins in the defense of cancer. Interferons, interleukins, monoclonal antibodies, and retinoids are examples of such agents. This area of therapy continues to be one of great interest, and the exact role of these agents in solid tumors has yet to be defined.

SUPPORTIVE CARE

With the introduction of dose-intensive chemotherapy regimens, the incidence and frequency of side effects have increased. Some of these adverse reactions include severe myelosuppression, mucositis, nausea, and vomiting. Delays in subsequent cycles of chemotherapy are common because hospitalization for febrile neutropenia and dehydration is the primary mechanism to manage such toxicities. Resultant delays in subsequent chemotherapy, as well as reductions in the doses of the agents, can have a negative impact on tumor response and survival.[14]

Recent advances in supportive care therapies have allowed more patients to remain on their therapy schedules with fewer side effects. Granulocyte colony-stimulating

Table 93.3 ▪ Commonly Used Chemotherapeutic Agents in Pediatric Solid Malignancies

Drug	Class	Spectrum of Use	Route	Common Toxicities	Key Monitoring Parameters
Methotrexate (MTX)	Antimetabolite	Osteosarcoma Medulloblastoma	IV, PO	Myelosuppression, mucositis, nausea, vomiting, diarrhea, rash, alopecia, hepatotoxicity, renal (high doses)	CBC, lytes, liver enzymes, SCr, BUN, UOP
Cyclophosphamide (Cytoxan) (CTX)	Alkylator	Rhabdomyosarcoma Ewing's sarcoma Neuroblastoma Wilms' tumor	IV, PO	Myelosuppression, nausea, vomiting, diarrhea, hemorrhagic cystitis, alopecia, SIADH, cardiac toxicity (high doses)	CBC, lytes, Scr, BUN, UOP
Ifosfamide (Ifex) (IFOS)	Alkylator	Rhabdomyosarcoma Osteosarcoma Ewing's sarcoma Neuroblastoma	IV	Myelosuppression, nausea, vomiting, diarrhea, hemorrhagic cystitis, neurotoxicity, alopecia, renal tubular acidosis, electrolyte disturbances	CBC, lytes, SCr, BUN, UOP
Cisplatin (Platinol) (CDDP)	Alkylator	Brain tumors Osteosarcoma Neuroblastoma Germ cell tumors	IV	Myelosuppression, nausea, vomiting, renal toxicity, electrolyte disturbances, ototoxicity, anaphylaxis, neurotoxicity	CBC, lytes, SCr, BUN, uric acid, UOP
Carboplatin (Paraplatin) (CBDCA)	Alkylator	Brain tumors Osteosarcoma Neuroblastoma	IV	Myelosuppression, nausea, vomiting, hepatotoxicity, electrolyte abnormalities	CBC, liver enzymes, lytes
Doxorubicin (Adriamycin) (DOX, ADR)	Antitumor antibiotic	Most solid tumors	IV	Myelosuppression, nausea, vomiting, diarrhea, alopecia, radiation recall reaction, cardiotoxicity	CBC, lytes, bilirubin (for dose adjustments)
Dactinomycin (Cosmegen)	Antitumor antibiotic	Wilms' tumor Ewing's sarcoma Rhabdomyosarcoma	IV	Myelosuppression, nausea, vomiting, diarrhea, alopecia, radiation recall reaction, photosensitizer, hepatotoxicity	CBC, lytes, liver panel
Mechlorethamine (Mustargen)	Alkylator	Brain tumors	IV	Myelosuppression, nausea, vomiting, hyperuricemia, anaphylaxis	CBC, lytes, uric acid
Lomustine (CeeNU) (CCNU)	Alkylator	Brain tumors	PO	Myelosuppression, nausea, vomiting, hepatotoxicity, neurotoxicity, alopecia	CBC, lytes, liver panel
Procarbazine (Matulane)	Alkylator	Brain tumors	PO	Myelosuppression, nausea, vomiting, diarrhea, alopecia, neurotoxicity	CBC, lytes
Dacarbazine (DTIC-Dome) (DIC)	Alkylator	Brain tumors	IV	Myelosuppression, nausea, vomiting, flulike symptoms, photosensitizer	CBC, lytes
Vincristine (Oncovin) (VCR)	Vinca alkaloid	Most solid tumors	IV	Neurotoxicity, peripheral neuropathy, constipation, alopecia, SIADH, hypotension	Lytes, blood pressure
Etoposide (VePesid) (VP-16)	Topoisomerase inhibitor	Brain tumors Neuroblastoma Ewing's sarcoma Rhabdomyosarcoma	IV, PO	Myelosuppression, nausea, vomiting, mucositis, alopecia, hypotension (IV formulation), anaphylaxis	CBC, lytes, blood pressure

BUN, blood urea nitrogen; *CBC,* complete blood cell count with differential; *lytes,* electrolyte panel; *SCr,* serum creatinine; *SIADH,* syndrome of inappropriate antidiuretic hormone; *UOP,* urine output.

factor (G-CSF, filgrastim) and granulocyte–macrophage colony-stimulating factor (GM-CSF, sargramostim) are growth factors that stimulate the production of white blood cells. These agents have demonstrated their benefit in oncology by shortening the period and degree of neutropenia in some patients. Newer antiemetics have a defined role in pediatrics as well. When compared with traditional antiemetics (prochlorperazine, chlorpromazine, and metoclopramide administered in high doses), the nonsedating serotonin ($5\text{-}HT_3$) receptor antagonists (ondansetron, granisetron, dolasetron) have provided patients with effective control of nausea and vomiting with fewer side effects.[15] Other supportive measures in the pediatric population include blood products (red blood cells and platelets), hyperalimentation, broad-spectrum antibiotics, pain management, and fluid and electrolyte replacement.

Autologous hematopoietic stem-cell rescue following myeloablative chemotherapy (with or without radiotherapy) continues to be a subject of investigation. This process involves the collection of hematopoietic stem cells from a patient before the administration of lethal doses of chemotherapy or radiation, which produces profound myelosuppression. After the administration of the chemotherapy regimen that is intended to ablate residual tumor, the collected stem cells are reinfused to restore the patient's bone marrow. This technique has been studied in patients in whom survival is estimated to be less than 30%, and, although mixed results have been reported, some patients have shown great benefit.[16–18] This therapy may gain a more defined role in the future after additional studies are performed.

CLINICAL TRIALS AND RESEARCH

The importance of research in pediatric oncology is almost immeasurable and is vital to perpetuate the advances seen in past decades. As previously mentioned, the approach to the pediatric cancer patient is multidisciplinary. The collaboration of research efforts from several institutions can facilitate this process. The two national collaborative groups in the United States are the Childrens Cancer Group (CCG) (which also has affiliations in Canada and Australia) and the Pediatric Oncology Group (POG). In the future, these groups will merge into one organization. Another important institution to pediatric oncology research is the Surveillance, Epidemiology and End Results (SEER) program, a tumor registry of the National Cancer Institute (NCI) that facilitates the assimilation of data relating to cancer.

In the United States, approximately 20% of patients enrolled in clinical studies are children, and 80 to 90% of all children treated for cancer receive treatment at institutions that are affiliated with CCG or POG.[1] Members of these organizations meet periodically within their groups to review current data, revise treatment standards based on their data, and discuss future therapy plans. Conducting studies at several institutions allows for greater patient accrual, which can expedite the research process and validate results more quickly. Thus the most effective therapy for pediatric malignancies can be ascertained sooner. Additionally, these patients are more likely to receive follow-up care that is meticulously documented, allowing for the observation of delayed effects following treatments and determination of appropriate interventions and treatments for these long-term sequelae. Therefore, enrollment of children in clinical studies should be strongly encouraged.

LONG-TERM SEQUELAE AND SECONDARY MALIGNANCIES

Because the majority of children treated for a childhood malignancy become long-term survivors, late effects and secondary malignancies are a concern for the clinician. Secondary malignancies are estimated to occur in 3 to 12% of patients within 20 years of diagnosis and are most frequently associated with alkylating agents, nitrosoureas, and epipodophyllotoxins.[19–21] The actual manifestations of delayed toxicities following chemotherapy or radiotherapy and their appropriate management should remain an integral part of the therapeutic plan for each patient. Common complications following treatment are summarized in Table 93.4.[7,20,22,23]

Table 93.4 ▪ Long-Term Effects After Treatment for Childhood Malignancies

Organ System	Offending Agent(s)	Manifestations	Monitoring Parameters
Endocrine	Radiation therapy to the head, neck, or central nervous system or chemotherapy to the central nervous system	Impaired growth Abnormal pubertal progression Hypothyroidism	Height, weight, growth velocity, scoliosis examination Growth velocity and development Thyroid-stimulating hormone and T4 measurements, size of thyroid
Reproductive	Males: radiation to the testes or central nervous system, nitrosoureas, procarbazine	Azoospermia, oligospermia, decreased testicular size	Testosterone, follicle-stimulating hormone, luteinizing hormone, testicular volume, semen analysis
	Females: radiation to the pelvis, nitrosoureas, procarbazine	Amenorrhea, oligomenorrhea, precocious puberty, ovarian dysfunction	Estrogen, follicle-stimulating hormone, luteinizing hormone, menstrual history
Renal	Nephrectomy (Wilms' tumor), cisplatin, cyclophosphamide, ifosfamide	Decreased glomerular filtration rate, chronic cystitis, tubular necrosis, Fanconi's syndrome, vesicouretal reflux	Serum creatinine, blood urea nitrogen, yearly urinalysis, blood pressure, possible renal ultrasound
Cardiac	Radiation to the thorax, doxorubicin, mitoxantrone, high-dose cyclophosphamide	Left ventricular dysfunction, coronary artery disease, congestive heart failure, arrhythmias	Chest X-ray, electrocardiogram, echocardiogram, lipid profile, consider exercise testing or radionuclide angiocardiogram if total anthracycline dose exceeds 550 mg/m^2 or in high-risk patients
Pulmonary	Whole lung irradiation, bleomycin, nitrosoureas, busulfan, methotrexate, cyclophosphamide	Decreased lung volume, restrictive airway disease, decreased cardiac output diffusion, decreased exercise tolerance	Chest X-ray, pulmonary function tests
Liver	Radiation to the abdomen, methotrexate, 6-mercaptopurine	Elevation of bilirubin and liver enzymes, liver fibrosis, hepatitis, cirrhosis	Liver enzyme panel, serologies for hepatitis, imaging studies
Central nervous system	Cranial irradiation and central nervous system chemotherapy	Decreased attention span, memory loss, leukoencephalopathy, brain necrosis, cerebrovascular accident	Cognitive learning tests, computed tomography

Source: References 7, 20, 22, 23.

Brain Tumors

Neoplasms of the brain are second only to leukemia in their frequency during childhood and are the most common solid tumors in children under 15 years of age. A multidisciplinary approach has allowed for improvements in diagnostic, surgical, and radiation techniques and in chemotherapeutic regimens, influencing a change in overall 5-year survival rates from 35% in the early 1960s to better than 60% in the early 1990s.[2] Brain tumors are a heterogeneous group of neoplasms with tissue type and site of tumor incidences varying with the patient's age.

TREATMENT GOALS: PEDIATRIC BRAIN TUMORS

- Management of the child with a brain tumor is highly individualized. Site and type of tumor are two of the most important variables that dictate therapy.
- The health professional's role in the care of children with brain tumors involves monitoring not only chemotherapeutic regimens and antiemetic therapy, but also supportive care drugs used for cerebral edema, seizure control, endocrine abnormalities, infections, pain management, and conscious sedation.

EPIDEMIOLOGY

All central nervous system (CNS) tumors account for approximately 20% of cancers in children under age 15 years. The incidence of brain tumors in males is slightly greater than in females (1.13:1), and Caucasians have a higher incidence than African Americans (1.25:1).[3] The exact etiology of brain tumors remains unclear, and there is no universally accepted nomenclature system because the classification of primary brain tumors remains controversial. Epidemiologic studies have failed to specifically identify causative agents responsible for the development of brain tumors.

CLINICAL PRESENTATION AND DIAGNOSIS

Signs and Symptoms

Clinical manifestations of brain neoplasms depend on tumor location, age, and development level of the child and are often vague. Generalized symptoms include nausea; vomiting; and diffuse, frequent headaches habitually occurring in the morning on awakening. These symptoms, commonly mistaken for evidence of an infectious illness, migraine, or tension headache, may indicate the presence of increased intracranial pressure (ICP) and hydrocephalus, which is often associated with infratentorial tumors that obstruct flow of the cerebrospinal fluid (CSF) through the cerebral ventricles. Localizing symptoms may include gait disturbances and ataxia, seizures, visual field defects, neuroendocrine abnormalities, facial and extraocular muscle palsies, and hemiparesis. Diagnosis may be difficult in children less than 2 years of age because of nonspecific, nonlocalizing signs and symptoms such as irritability, listlessness, failure to thrive, vomiting, developmental delay, and progressive macrocephaly.[24]

Diagnosis

Magnetic resonance imaging (MRI) or computed tomography (CT) is used to diagnose and determine size, location, and tumor density of CNS neoplasms and are also performed postoperatively to assess the volume of a residual tumor. For tumors with a high propensity for metastasis into the CSF, such as medulloblastoma, posterior-fossa ependymoma, and germ-cell tumors, spinal

Table 93.5 ▪ Distribution of Common Brain Tumors in Children, According to Location and Histologic Appearance

Location and Type of Tumor	Percentage of All Brain Tumors
Infrantentorial	
Primitive neuroectodermal tumor (medulloblastoma)	20–25
Low-grade astrocytoma, cerebellar	12–18
Ependymoma	4–8
Malignant glioma, brainstem	3–9
Low-grade astrocytoma, brainstem	3–6
Other	2–5
Total	45–60
Supratentorial hemispheric	
Low-grade astrocytoma	8–20
Malignant glioma	6–12
Ependymoma	2–5
Mixed glioma	1–5
Ganglioglioma	1–5
Oligodendroglioma	1–2
Choroid-plexus tumor	1–2
Primitive neuroectodermal tumor	1–2
Meningioma	0.5–2
Other	1–3
Total	25–40
Supratentorial midline	
Suprasellar	
Craniopharyngioma	6–9
Low-grade glioma, chiasmatic-hypothalamic	4–8
Germ-cell tumor	1–2
Pituitary adenoma	.05–2.5
Pineal region	
Low-grade glioma	1–2
Germ-cell tumor	.05–2
Pineal parenchymal tumor	.05–2
Total	15–20

Source: Reference 24.

Table 93.6 ▪ Common Perioperative Problems of Childhood Brain Tumors with Pharmacologic or Surgical Solutions

Perioperative Problem	Type of Tumors Involved	Preoperative and Intraoperative Management	Postoperative Management
Peritumoral edema	Large tumors; smaller tumors in critical areas such as the brainstem	Corticosteroids (e.g., dexamethasone [Decadron] at a dose of 0.05–0.1 mg/kg or body weight 4 times daily) are administered.	Corticosteroids are tapered within several days of surgery, particularly if tumor resection is extensive.
Obstructive hydrocephalus	Intraventricular or periventricular tumors	An external ventricular drain is placed before tumor resection is begun.	If the tumor resection opens the cerebrospinal fluid pathways, drainage established by ventriculostomy can often be discontinued within several days of surgery. Patients in whom progressive ventriculomegaly develops or who have an enlarging pseudomeningocele require definitive diversion of cerebrospinal fluid. Although a shunt poses a theoretical risk of peritoneal seeding of the tumor, this has not been confirmed in studies.[a]
Seizures	Tumors of the cerebral hemispheres; tumors that will require cerebral retraction during their removal	An anticonvulsant agent, such as phenytoin (Dilantin), is started preoperatively and continued during surgery.	In children without prior seizures, anticonvulsant drugs can generally be stopped within several months of surgery. In patients with a history of preoperative seizures who undergo complete tumor removal and are rendered seizure free, anticonvulsant agents can often be discontinued within several months of surgery.
Hypothalamic-pituitary hormonal insufficiency	Tumors arising in and around the hypothalamus	An evaluation of endocrine function is useful if the child is clinically stable. "Stress" doses (doses several times the normal maintenance dose) of a corticosteroid, such as hydrocortisone, are administered before and during surgery. Because diabetes insipidus may develop during surgery, fluid balance must be monitored closely.	Doses of corticosteroids can be decreased to maintenance levels during the first postoperative week. Fluid balance and electrolyte levels are monitored closely and controlled by administration of appropriate fluids and, if indicated, vasopressin. Detailed postoperative and, often, follow-up endocrine testing is required to determine long-term needs for hormonal replacement.

Source: Reference 24.
[a]See reference 24.

MRI and a cytologic examination of CSF are performed for staging purposes. To achieve sharp images, movement during MRI and CT must be kept to a minimum; thus children are often immobilized and heavily sedated before the examination.

Tumors are commonly classified by their location and are broadly divided into two categories: (1) supratentorial neoplasms, including cerebral hemispheric and midline tumors; and (2) infratentorial neoplasms, including brain stem and cerebellar tumors (Table 93.5).[24] Unlike adults, in whom most brain tumors are located supratentorially near the cerebral hemispheres, 50 to 60% of CNS tumors in children older than 1 year arise infratentorially in the posterior fossa. The most prevalent histology is glial in origin and includes a broad variety of tumor types, most commonly low-grade astrocytoma. The medulloblastoma, of primitive neuroectodermal origin, is a malignant cerebellar tumor that has a marked propensity to invade the meninges and parenchymal tissue and is the most common distinct tumor type of childhood brain neoplasms. Midline tumors, such as craniopharyngiomas and pineal tumors, occur near the optic chiasm and often cause visual field defects, hydrocephalus, and extraocular muscle palsies.[25]

TREATMENT

Surgery

The specific management of brain malignancies depends on tumor type and location. To make a histologic diagnosis and reduce tumor burden, surgery is often the first task of a series of interventions. Surgical cure, however, is not often an obtainable goal because the anatomic location of many tumors does not allow for total resection. Maximal tumor removal must be balanced against the risk of causing severe neurologic damage to the patient. Short-term external ventricular drains or long-term internal ventriculoperitoneal shunts are often placed to drain CSF in patients with obstructive hydrocephalus. Table 93.6 summarizes the perioperative supportive care issues often seen in clinical practice when treating patients with brain tumors.[24]

Radiotherapy

Brain tumors have customarily been treated with maximum tolerated doses of 5000 to 6000 cGy administered in once-daily fractions of 180 to 200 cGy over 5 to 6 weeks. Radiation hyperfractionation, the administration of larger numbers (twice-daily doses) of smaller fractions of radiotherapy over an equivalent period, may allow for higher total doses with less morbidity and intensified tumor kill.[26] Results of studies in brain stem gliomas have been mixed.[27] Other advances include sophisticated approaches that allow more restricted administration of radiation to the tumor while minimizing exposure of surrounding tissue. Brain stem tumors are often surgically inaccessible; therefore, primary treatment is radiotherapy with or without combination chemotherapy.[24] For neoplasms that have a propensity to metastasize throughout the neuraxis, craniospinal irradiation may be indicated.[25]

Acute adverse effects of brain irradiation include transient exacerbation of local neurologic signs; radiation sickness with symptoms of nausea, vomiting, loss of appetite, drowsiness, and irritability; xerostomia and sialadenitis; hair loss; bone marrow suppression in those receiving craniospinal irradiation; skin erythema, breakdown, and hyperpigmentation; and the somnolence syndrome, a period of extreme drowsiness that may occur 4 to 8 weeks after the completion of a course of treatment with recovery in 1 to 2 weeks. Late side effects include significant learning disabilities, personality changes, bone and soft tissue malformations, cerebral necrosis, and retardation of linear growth due to decreased release of hormones from the hypothalamic-pituitary axis such as growth hormone and thyroid-stimulating hormone.[28]

Chemotherapy

Achieving therapeutic antineoplastic drug concentrations in the brain is problematic because of poor penetration of the blood-brain barrier (BBB) by most agents. Determinants of BBB penetration embody physiochemical and pharmacokinetic drug properties and pathophysiology of the tumor itself. Chemotherapeutic agents of low molecular weight, of high lipid solubility, and that unionize at physiologic pH have the highest chance of crossing the BBB. Pharmacokinetic properties such as low serum protein binding and long elimination half-life may also improve drug entrance. The pathophysiology of large CNS masses creates a paradoxical situation in which permeability of the BBB is enhanced at the necrotic center, but reduced around the viable periphery of the tumor where antineoplastic effects are desired. However, clinical trials have demonstrated that some water-soluble agents (platinum analogs and classical alkylators) have significant activity in certain brain tumors that may be a result of increased BBB permeability induced by the malignancy. The efficacy of chemotherapy agents also depends on tumor growth kinetics.

Chemotherapy has been studied mostly in poor-risk patients in the following situations: primary therapy for recurrent brain tumors in older studies; as adjuvant therapy after surgery or radiation therapy in newly diagnosed patients; and as postoperative neoadjuvant (preirradiation) therapy. Early studies demonstrated that chemotherapy could produce regression of recurrent tumors but rarely produced cures. As adjuvant therapy to radiotherapy and surgery, chemotherapy regimens have significantly increased 5-year survival rates in children with at least partially resected supratentorial or cerebellar malignant astrocytomas[29] and in children with high-risk medulloblastoma.[30,31] Preirradiation chemotherapy regimens were conceptualized to assess drug-induced tumor responses before radiotherapy and to improve survival results over conventional postirradiation therapy. Further, this schedule may help avoid additive toxicity, such as prolonged myelosuppression and enhanced cisplatin ototoxicity that may result when radiation is followed by chemotherapy. These methods may improve drug entry into the tumor before radiotherapy-induced vascular changes occur, and certain agents may act as radiation sensitizers. Children less than 3 years of age are at an increased risk of developing severe long-term neurologic deficits from irradiation because myelinization of the brain is usually not complete before this age. For this reason, in these children, preirradiation chemotherapy is often preferred as initial postoperative treatment over radiation, allowing radiotherapy to be delayed or deferred for a few years until the brain is more mature.[32]

Lomustine (CCNU) and vincristine are the prototypic agents used in malignant gliomas. Lomustine is a low-molecular-weight, lipid-soluble, oral agent that easily crosses the BBB. Vincristine, although it penetrates the BBB poorly, has been shown to be active in the treatment of brain tumors since the 1960s. In the latter 1970s and early 1980s, methotrexate, cyclophosphamide, and cisplatin were found to have significant activity in recurrent tumors, especially medulloblastoma. Unfortunately, the use of methotrexate and cisplatin in previously irradiated patients is constrained by a high occurrence rate of severe leukoencephalopathy and ototoxicity, respectively.[33,34] The more recent use of the analog carboplatin may reduce the neurotoxic, nephrotoxic, and ototoxic effects of cisplatin, but it may increase the incidence of myelosuppression. Corticosteroids are often added to the chemotherapy regimen to minimize cerebral edema secondary to the drug therapy. Table 93.7 summarizes common chemotherapy combinations (and their acronyms) that have been used in brain tumors.[35]

FUTURE THERAPIES

Brainstem gliomas are usually unresectable, relatively unresponsive to current chemotherapeutic regimens, and

Table 93.7 ▪ Chemotherapy Combinations for Pediatric Brain Tumors

Regimen	Dosage/Route	Comments
"PCV"		
CCNU	100 mg/m² PO, day 1 or day 2	Every 6 weeks × 8 cycles (1 year)
Vincristine[a]	1.5 mg/m² IV (max 2 mg), days 1, 8, ±15	
Prednisone	40 mg/m² PO, days 1–14	
OR		
Procarbazine	100 mg/m² PO days 1–14	
"MOPP"		
Nitrogen Mustard	6 mg/m² IV, days 1, 8	Every 4 weeks × 12 cycles (1 year)
Vincristine[a]	1.4–1.5 mg/m² IV (max 2 mg), days 1, 8	
Procarbazine	100 mg/m² PO, days 1–14	
Prednisone	40 mg/m² PO, days 1–14	
"8-in-1"		
Vincristine[a]	1.5 mg/m² IV, hour 0	Every 4–6 weeks × 10–24 cycles
CCNU	100 mg/m² PO, hour 0	
Procarbazine	75 mg/m² PO, hour 1	
Hydroyurea	1500–3000 mg/m² PO, hour 2	
Cisplatin	60–90 mg/m² IV, hours 3–9	
Ara-C	300 mg/m² IV, hour 9	
Cyclophosphamide	300 mg/m² IV, hour 12	
OR		
Dacarbazine	150 mg/m² IV, hour 12	
Methylprednisolone	300 mg/m² IV, hours 0, 6, 12	
Cisplatin Combinations		
Cisplatin+	90–100 mg/m² IV, day 1	Every 3–4 weeks
Vincristine[a]	1.5 mg/m² IV, day 1	Various combinations with cisplatin, which is a very active agent in medulloblastoma and ependymoma
OR		
Etoposide	150 mg/m² IV, day 3 and 4	
OR		
Cyclophosphamide	1000 mg/m² IV, day 1	

Source: Reference 35.
[a]Maximum dose 2.0 mg.

generally have a median survival of less than 1 year after radiotherapy.[24] Recurrent tumors are also associated with a poor prognosis. Preliminary studies of dose-intensified, marrow-ablative chemotherapy regimens, along with autologous transplantation or peripheral stem-cell rescue for recurrent malignant gliomas and medulloblastoma, have shown promise. Newer studies will evaluate this strategy for newly diagnosed aggressive brain tumors, including brain stem gliomas.[36]

PROGNOSIS

The 5-year survival rate is best in children with cerebellar astrocytomas (91%) and worst for those with brain stem gliomas (18%).[37] Less than one-third of patients in poor-risk categories (high-grade astrocytomas, including glioblastoma multiforme, unresectable medulloblastomas, anaplastic ependymomas, unresectable brain stem tumors, and in children less than 4 years of age) become long-term survivors.

Neuroblastoma

Neuroblastoma is the most common extracranial solid tumor in children and the fourth most common pediatric malignancy. It is the most common malignant neoplasm in the newborn and in children between 1 and 12 months of age.[3] Neuroblastoma is thought to be derived from the embryonic neural crest that forms the adrenal medulla and sympathetic nervous system. A small, blue, round-cell tumor, neuroblastoma consists of dense nests of cells separated by fibrovascular bundles. It is important for the pathologist to differentiate between neuroblastoma and other small, round-cell tumors such as Ewing's sarcoma, lymphoma, rhabdomyosarcoma, and Askin's tumor.

EPIDEMIOLOGY

Fifty percent of all malignancies diagnosed in the first month of life are neuroblastoma.[38,39] The median age at diagnosis is approximately 2 years, and neuroblastoma rarely occurs after age 10 years. There is little difference in the incidence between males and females. Caucasians are more likely to develop neuroblastoma than African Americans (1.31 : 1), and racial differences are most pronounced during the first year of life.[3] Genetic abnormalities associated with neuroblastoma include deletions on the short arm of chromosome 1 and N-*myc* oncogene (also known as *MYCN*) amplification.[40]

Urinary catecholamine metabolites, namely homovanillic acid (HVA) and vanillylmandelic acid (VMA), are elevated in more than 85% of children with neuroblastoma.[41] Mass screening for these substances has been performed in Japan since 1972. The evidence suggests that 65% of all childhood neuroblastomas can be detected clinically or by screening at or before 12 months of age. It further suggests that many of the cases detected by screening are not in the poor prognostic category.[39] The application of mass screening is currently being evaluated to determine whether it is beneficial or harmful and at what individual and societal costs, although previous trials suggest that mass screening does not reduce mortality rates.[41]

CLINICAL PRESENTATION AND DIAGNOSIS

Signs and Symptoms

Neuroblastoma can occur anywhere along the sympathetic nervous system. The most common site of the primary tumor is in the abdomen (adrenal gland [40%] or a retroperitoneal paraspinal ganglion [25%]), thoracic cavity (15%), or pelvis (5%). Thoracic primaries are more common in children less than 1 year of age. Metastatic disease is identified in 50% of infants and two-thirds of older children at diagnosis. The most common sites of metastasis are lymph node, bone marrow, bone, liver, and subcutaneous tissue. Spontaneous regression of neuroblastoma is occasionally observed in young infants; it occurs extremely rarely in older children. Further, the tumor may undergo differentiation to a more mature and benign tumor type classified as a ganglioneuroma. Tumors with mixed pathologic characteristics (benign and malignant cells) are termed *ganglioneuroblastoma*.[38,42]

Signs and symptoms at presentation depend on the location of the primary and metastatic sites. The most common presentation is that of an abdominal or flank mass that is firm and irregular and crosses the midline. Thoracic neuroblastoma presents as a posterior mediastinal mass and is usually found coincidentally on a routine chest radiograph. High thoracic and cervical masses can be associated with Horner's syndrome, which consists of unilateral ptosis, myosis, and anhydrosis. Paraspinal tumors may extend into neuronal foramina of the vertebral bodies and result in symptoms related to compression of nerve roots and spinal cord. The range of symptoms includes radicular pain, subacute paraplegia, and bowel and bladder dysfunction. Constitutional symptoms include weight loss, anorexia, intermittent fever, hypertension (due to compression of the renal vasculature), secretory diarrhea (due to increased vasoactive intestinal peptide), and irritability.[42]

Diagnosis

Physical examination should include a check for spinal cord compression and hypertension. Laboratory workup should include a complete blood cell count, liver and renal function tests, and urine analysis for urinary catecholamines. Chest radiograph, CT or MRI, skeletal survey, abdominal ultrasound, and bone marrow aspirate and biopsy should be done to determine location, size, extent, and possible metastatic disease. Cytogenetic evaluation including N-*myc* oncogene copy number and DNA index should be performed to assist in assessing the patient's prognosis. A definitive diagnosis is made under one of the following circumstances: (1) an unequivocal pathologic diagnosis made from tumor tissue by light microscopy with or without immunohistology, electron microscopy, or increased serum or urine catecholamines or metabolites; or (2) bone marrow aspirate or trephine biopsy containing tumor cells and increased serum or urine catecholamines or metabolites.[42]

In 1987, the International Neuroblastoma Staging System (INSS) was proposed that would lead to uniformity in staging patients with neuroblastoma for clinical trials and biologic studies worldwide. The INSS combines features from two other widely used staging systems used by CCG (Evans' staging system) and POG, which are detailed elsewhere.[42] Table 93.8 summarizes the INSS along with treatment and prognosis for each stage of disease.[43] Clinical, radiographic, and surgical evaluation of the child with neuroblastoma forms the foundation for the INSS.

TREATMENT

The treatment of neuroblastoma is a combination of surgery, radiotherapy, and chemotherapy. The stage of the tumor, age of the patient, and biologic features of the tumor determine the role of each treatment modality. Infants less than 1 year of age commonly have a small primary tumor and metastases to the skin, liver, or bone marrow (stage IVS). Their disease often regresses spontaneously, and only supportive care is necessary.[38] Chemotherapy remains the backbone of the multimodality treatment plan.

Surgery

Surgery is an important treatment modality and is usually the first in a series of treatments for neuroblastoma. Primary surgical procedures are vital in providing an initial diagnosis, in providing tissue samples for pathologic evaluation, and for appropriately staging the patient. Another goal of the surgeon is to excise as much tumor as possible. Those patients with localized disease (stages I and II) require no additional treatment after surgery. In some

Table 93.8 ▪ International Neuroblastoma Staging System and Treatment Summary

Stage	Staging Criteria	Incidence	Treatment	Survival at 5 Years
1	Localized tumor confined to the area of origin, complete gross excision with or without microscopic residual disease; identifiable ipsilateral and contralateral lymph nodes negative microscopically	5%	Surgery alone, chemotherapy with recurrence	90% or greater
2a	Unilateral tumor with incomplete, gross excision; identifiable ipsilateral and contralateral lymph nodes negative microscopically	10%	Surgery plus postoperative chemotherapy with 5 courses of cyclophosphamide plus doxorubicin	70–80%
2b	Unilateral tumor with complete or incomplete gross excision; with positive ipsilateral regional lymph nodes: identifiable contralateral lymph nodes negative microscopically	10%	Surgery plus postoperative chemotherapy with 5 courses of cyclophosphamide plus doxorubicin	70–80%
3	Tumor infiltrating across the midline with or without regional lymph node involvement; or, midline tumor with bilateral regional lymph node involvement	25%	Surgery plus postoperative chemotherapy with 5 courses of cyclophosphamide plus doxorubicin	40–70% (depending on completeness of surgical resection)
4	Dissemination of the tumor to distant lymph nodes, bone, bone marrow, liver, or other organs (except as defined in stage 4s)	60%	Aggressive chemotherapy with cyclophosphamide plus doxorubicin then cisplatin plus teniposide plus radiotherapy; consider dose intensification with ABMT for older children	More than 60% if age at diagnosis is younger than 1 year; 20% if age at diagnosis is older than 1 year and under 2 years; 10% if age at diagnosis is over 2 years
4s	Localized primary tumor as defined for stage 1 or 2 with dissemination limited to liver, skin, or bone marrow.	5%	Individualized therapy, not standardized	More than 80%

Source: Reference 43.

cases, surgery is delayed until chemotherapy is administered (neoadjuvant chemotherapy), which may convert a partial response to a complete one. Complications from surgical procedures are relatively uncommon (5 to 25%) and occur most frequently in abdominal tumors.[42]

Radiotherapy

Neuroblastoma is considered a radiosensitive tumor. Tumoricidal doses of 15 to 30 cGy are generally used to treat residual tumor after surgery or chemotherapy.[42] Radiotherapy is also used in palliation of symptoms for end-stage disease. Radioactive-labeled meta-iodobenzylguanidine (MIBG) has been used in Europe for diagnostic and therapeutic purposes. MIBG is known to be taken up by catecholamine-secreting tumors, such as pheochromocytomas and immature neuroblastoma cells. Using this specificity, MIBG radiolabeled with ^{125}I and ^{131}I has been used for detection of neuroblastoma and evaluated for antitumor activity in small phase I and II studies, but currently it is not widely available in the United States. MIBG may be ultimately useful for the treatment of residual tumor following surgery in stage III patients or palliation of bone pain. Use of this therapy may advantageously decrease the patient's overall exposure to radiation while increasing the total dose of radiation delivered to the tumor. The myelosuppressive effects of MIBG on tumor-infiltrated bone marrow have been problematic. Future studies will better define its role in the diagnosis and therapy of neuroblastoma.[44]

Chemotherapy

The primary treatment modality in neuroblastoma is chemotherapy. A number of agents have demonstrated activity in neuroblastoma in several single-agent phase II trials. Examples of these agents, which have yielded response rates of 34 to 45%, include cyclophosphamide, cisplatin, doxorubicin, vincristine, etoposide, and teniposide.[42] Combination chemotherapy has been shown to be more effective than single-agent therapy. Dose-intensified regimens have produced excellent local responses, but the duration of response has been limiting. High-dose chemotherapy followed by purged autologous stem-cell rescue, after initial induction chemotherapy, has produced promising results in patients with advanced disease.[45] This modality will probably be incorporated into future treatment protocols.

Biologic Therapy

Because neuroblastoma cells are known at times to undergo spontaneous regression or maturation to benign tumors, indicating that these cells may be regulated by natural defense mechanisms, newer research strategies are focusing on biologic manipulation of minimal residual disease. These strategies include exploitation of the body's own defense system with interleukin-2-stimulated natural killer cells and attempts to achieve tumor maturation with the use of vitamin B_{12} and retinoic acid.[43,46] In a recent CCG randomized trial, isotretinoin (13-*cis*-retinoic acid) was found to significantly improve event-free survival in high-risk neuroblastoma patients when administered after either intensive chemotherapy alone or after intensive chemoradiotherapy supported by purged autologous bone marrow transplantation. Based on these results, the author recommends utilization of isotretinoin as part of standard therapy for minimal residual disease after consolidation therapy is complete. The dose used in this study was 160 mg/m^2/day for 14 consecutive days each month for 6 months.[47] Another area of exploration is eradication of disease via monoclonal antibodies against the cell surface disganglioside antigen, G_{D2}, specifically located on neuroblastoma cells. Radioactive ^{131}I-coupled G_{D2} antibodies have been administered as therapy for neuroblastoma.[42] Responses have been seen in patients with disseminated disease, but those with large tumor masses were resistant to this therapy. Monoclonal antibodies may also be useful in purging tumor cells from bone marrow ex vivo before reinfusion of autologous marrow after dose-intensive therapy.

IMPROVING OUTCOMES

Two commonly used agents in the treatment of neuroblastoma are cisplatin and etoposide, both of which require specific and careful monitoring. Cisplatin, a platinum analog, can cause profound renal dysfunction that is dose related, as well as related to cumulative dose. Nephrotoxicity from cisplatin, which can be reversible, exhibits as an increase in serum creatinine and blood urea nitrogen (BUN) as a result of renal tubular damage. Adequate hydration is vital in reducing the likelihood of nephrotoxicity. Many protocols require that hydration begin before the administration of cisplatin and continue for at least 24 hours after the completion of cisplatin administration. Hydration is usually given as 3000 to 3600 mL/m^2/day (twice maintenance fluids) in an effort to maintain urine output at a rate of 2 to 3 ml/kg/hr. In addition to urine output, BUN, and serum creatinine, daily weights and serum electrolytes, particularly potassium and magnesium, are closely monitored as well.

Table 93.9 ▪ Factors Associated with a Poor Prognosis in Neuroblastoma

Age >1 year
Advanced disease (stage 3 or 4)
Urinary catecholamine ratio of VMA/HVA ≤1
Serum ferritin >143 ng/mL
Lactate dehydrogenase >1500 U/mL
Neuron-specific enolase >100 ng/mL
N-*myc* oncogene amplification
Diploid karyotype (DNA index = 1)
Allelic loss or deletion associated with chromosome 1

Source: References 40, 42, 48, 49.

Etoposide can cause hypotension, especially if the drug is administered rapidly. Although this phenomenon can occur in both adults and children, and monitoring parameters for both populations are blood pressure and pulse, significant differences exist in normal mean values between these two groups. In general, children have lower blood pressures and higher pulse rates than adults. Monitoring for etoposide-related hypotension and tachycardia should include a baseline blood pressure and pulse rate followed by serial measurements until the completion of the infusion.

PROGNOSIS

The most important prognostic factors for neuroblastoma are the age of the patient at the time of diagnosis, the stage at diagnosis, and the site of the primary tumor. Patients with primary tumors of the adrenal gland appear to have a poorer prognosis than patients with tumors originating at other sites, particularly the thorax. The survival of patients with a localized, surgically resected tumor without distant metastasis is 75 to 90%; however, patients greater than 1 year old with distant metastasis at presentation have only a 10 to 30% 2-year disease-free survival rate.[38,48] Infants tend to have a better prognosis than do older children. The presence of the N-*myc* oncogene is found predominantly in patients with advanced disease and is associated with a rapid tumor progression and a poor prognosis.[49] Indicators associated with a poor prognosis in neuroblastoma are listed in Table 93.9.[40,42,48,49]

Wilms' Tumor

Wilms' tumor (WT), also known as nephroblastoma or renal embryoma, is the most common renal neoplasm in children. This tumor, which was first extensively described by Max Wilms more than 100 years ago, has a peak incidence during the second and third year of life and rarely occurs after age 6. Recent research has demonstrated the genetics of WT to be complex, and several genetic anomalies have been identified in patients with WT, including germline mutations within the WT1 gene. However, the precise etiology of WT remains unclear.

TREATMENT GOALS: WILMS' TUMOR

- The treatment of WT relies on the coordination of multidisciplinary efforts from the surgeon, radiation oncologist, and medical oncologist.
- A complete surgical excision of the tumor is the primary goal of treatment.
- Adjuvant radiation and chemotherapy are added to some treatment courses in patients in whom benefit has been previously demonstrated; thus the therapeutic approach to the child with WT depends on several factors.

EPIDEMIOLOGY

The incidence of WT, which accounts for approximately 6.1% of all childhood cancers, is greater in girls than boys (0.78:1), and African American children are more likely to develop WT than Caucasian children (0.88 : 1).[3] Boys are more likely than girls to develop WT at a younger age; and bilateral disease, which accounts for approximately 4 to 8% of cases, more frequently occurs in the younger child. Several carcinogens during the prenatal period have been implicated in the development of WT, although definitive correlation is lacking. Examples of these exposures include cigarette smoking, alcohol, coffee, pesticides, oral contraception use, hair dyes, and industrial hydrocarbons.[50]

When WT occurs in the child with no genetic predisposition or family history, it is termed *sporadic*. *Familial* WT is reserved for those patients with a genetic predisposition to the development of WT or when WT occurs as a feature of a specific genetic disorder. One syndrome associated with an increased incidence of WT is the WAGR syndrome (WT, aniridia, genitourinary anomalies, and mental retardation). The WAGR syndrome is associated with abnormalities of the WT1 gene on chromosome 11. Other syndromes in which WT is a feature are the Beckwith-Weidemann syndrome and the Denys-Drash syndrome.[51]

CLINICAL PRESENTATION AND DIAGNOSIS

Signs and Symptoms

Most children are found to have abdominal swelling or an asymptomatic palpable mass when they are examined by their physician. Other symptoms, which occur in 20 to 30% of patients, are fever, malaise, abdominal pain, and gross or microscopic hematuria. Approximately 25% of patients have hypertension as a result of increased renin activity. Metastatic disease at the time of presentation is rare (15% of patients) and usually occurs in the lung (85%), the liver (7%), or both sites (8%).[51,52]

Diagnosis

Diagnostic techniques are directed toward the primary goal of verifying the presence of WT and differentiating it from neuroblastoma. WT arises intrarenally and distorts the calyceal region of the kidney. Neuroblastoma occurs extrarenally and displaces rather than distorts cells in the kidney. In general, an abdominal ultrasound is sufficient for providing proper evaluation of the kidney in determining whether the mass is cystic or solid. Extrarenal involvement of other abdominal organs can be verified by CT; however, the benefit of this diagnostic technique in the child with WT is lacking because the decision to perform a laparotomy is usually supported by results from the ultrasound.[53] A chest x-ray can verify the presence of metastasis.

The physical examination should include a careful exploration to locate and size the tumor. Any movement during respiration should be carefully noted. These findings assist the physician in distinguishing WT from neuroblastoma or splenomegaly. Laboratory evaluation should include a complete blood cell count with differential, liver function tests, serum calcium, BUN, serum creatinine, and urinalysis. When the diagnosis of WT is confirmed, the child is staged accordingly (Table 93.10),[54] and a therapeutic plan is outlined.

TREATMENT

Research in the area of WT has been facilitated through the formation of the National Wilms' Tumor Study Group (NWTSG). Increased survival rates have been achieved primarily through the multidisciplinary efforts of several institutions in four separate collaborations from 1969 (NWTS-1) to 1994 (NWTS-4). Each study yielded impor-

Table 93.10 ▪ Staging of Wilms' Tumor (NWTS-4)

I. Tumor limited to the kidney and completely excised. The surface of the renal capsule is intact. The tumor was not ruptured before or during removal. There is no residual tumor apparent beyond the margins of excision.

II. Tumor extends beyond the kidney, but is completely excised. There is regional extension of the tumor (i.e., penetration through the outer surface of the renal capsule into the perirenal soft tissues). Vessels outside the kidney substance are infiltrated or contain tumor thrombus. The tumor may have been biopsied or there has been local spillage of tumor confined to the flank. There is no residual tumor apparent at or beyond the margins of excision.

III. Residual nonhematogenous tumor confined to the abdomen. Any of the following may occur:
   a. Lymph nodes on biopsy are found to be involved in the hilus, the periaortic chains, or beyond.
   b. There has been diffuse peritoneal contamination by the tumor such as by spillage of tumor beyond the flank before or during surgery, or by tumor growth that has penetrated through the peritoneal surface.
   c. Implants are found on the peritoneal surface.
   d. The tumor is not completely resectable because of local infiltration into vital structures.

IV. Hematogenous metastases. Deposits beyond stage III (e.g., lung, liver, bone, and brain).

V. Bilateral renal involvement at diagnosis. An attempt should be made to stage each side according to the above criteria on the basis of extent of disease before therapy.

Source: Reference 54.

Table 93.11 ▪ Summary of Significant Findings in the NWTS Collaborations

Study (Registration Dates)	Significant Conclusions
NWTS-1 (1969–1973)	1. In children less than 2 years old with stage I favorable histology, postoperative radiation had no benefit. 2. The combination of vincristine and dactinomycin was more effective than either drug alone in stage II or III disease.
NWTS-2 (1974–1978)	1. For children with stage I favorable histology, 15 months of vincristine and dactinomycin was no more effective than 6 months of therapy. 2. The addition of doxorubicin to vincristine and dactinomycin improved relapse-free survival rates in stage II–IV disease.
NWTS-3 (1979–1986)	1. For stage I disease, 11 weeks of vincristine and dactinomycin without radiation is effective therapy. 2. For stage II favorable histology disease, vincristine and dactinomycin without radiation for 15 months was equivalent to vincristine and dactinomycin with radiation or with doxorubicin. 3. For patients with stage II favorable histology, the addition of abdominal radiation did not improve survival. 4. 1000 cGy abdominal radiation was equivalent to 2000 cGy in stage III favorable histology. 5. For stage III favorable histology, the addition of doxorubicin to vincristine and dactinomycin was more beneficial than vincristine and dactinomycin together. 6. The addition of cyclophosphamide to vincristine, dactinomycin, and doxorubicin did not improve survival in stage IV favorable histology, but the addition of cyclophosphamide to the three-drug regimen may benefit those patients with stage II–IV anaplastic histology.
NWTS-4 (1986–1994)	1. Pulse-intensive chemotherapy regimens are as effective as standard regimens. 2. For stage II–IV favorable histology, 6 months of therapy is as effective as 15 months.

Source: References 52, 55–59.

tant findings that have molded current therapeutic practices to provide the most effective and economical treatment to the WT patient while reducing treatment-related morbidity and mortality. A summary of significant findings from each collaboration appears in Table 93.11.[52,55–59]

Surgery

Surgery is an essential component of treatment in WT. Complete excision of the tumor without spillage is the surgeon's goal. Surgery facilitates proper staging and provides an opportunity to assess tumor location and spread. Inspection of the contralateral kidney for WT, which may have been missed on diagnostic evaluation, is imperative during surgery. The surgeon also looks for invasion or thrombosis of the renal artery and vein. After the tumor is excised, the surgeon inspects the liver to determine if there is any tumor involvement. Finally, lymph node sampling is performed to determine the possibility of hematogenous seeding.[52]

Radiotherapy

WT is a radiosensitive tumor; however, not every patient will benefit from radiotherapy, as demonstrated by the NWTS-1, NWTS-2, and NWTS-3.[53–57] For patients who are diagnosed with stage I or II WT with favorable histology, radiation therapy is not indicated if vincristine and dactinomycin are administered. For those patients with stage III WT with favorable histology, a dose of 1000 cGy is effective if given in combination with vincristine, dactinomycin, and doxorubicin. If tumor spillage occurs during surgery and is confined to the flank, radiation is not advocated. However, if spillage occurs throughout the abdomen, radiation therapy is given. For patients with pulmonary metastases visible on plain chest radiographs, whole-lung irradiation (dose of 1200 cGy) is recommended.[52]

Chemotherapy

The first pediatric solid tumor found to be responsive to chemotherapy (dactinomycin) was WT. Other single agents with activity in WT are vincristine, doxorubicin, and cyclophosphamide. The NWTS-1, NWTS-2, and NWTS-3 demonstrated that combination chemotherapy was superior to single-agent therapy. The NWTS-4 determined that "pulse-intensive" therapy was as effective as standard chemotherapy regimens and patients with stage II, III, or IV WT with favorable histology do not achieve a greater benefit with 15 months of therapy than with 6 months of therapy. Pulse-intensive therapy regimens allow for dactinomycin and doxorubicin to be given as a single dose rather than smaller, divided doses. This form of chemotherapy also has proven to be of economical benefit. The regimens studied in the NWTS are detailed elsewhere.[52,54,60] In general, chemotherapy is initiated soon after surgery. Preoperative chemotherapy is reserved for those patients with very large tumors requiring debulking before surgery.

FUTURE THERAPIES

The NWTS-5 opened in 1995 as a single-arm trial to examine biologic features of WT in an effort to predict outcome. Several other questions will be examined in this trial as well. The issue of management with surgery alone will be examined in those patients under age 2 with stage I WT with favorable histology and tumors weighing less than 550 g. For older patients and patients with larger tumors, as well as those patients with stage I anaplastic disease and stage II WT with favorable histology, treatment will not change from current recommendations, which is an 18-week regimen of pulse-intensive dactinomycin and vincristine. Patients with stage III or IV WT with favorable histology and focal anaplasia stage II, III, or IV will receive radiation therapy in addition to 24 weeks of pulse-intensive dactinomycin, vincristine, and doxorubicin. New chemotherapy regimens involving etoposide and carboplatin in addition to radiation will be analyzed for those patients designated as high risk.[59]

IMPROVING OUTCOMES

Therapeutic interventions in patients with WT often involve the pharmacist. For patients who receive radiation therapy during their treatment, dose reductions of chemotherapeutic agents are necessary. Dactinomycin and doxorubicin are known to have two types of interactions with radiotherapy–enhancement of radiation effects and a "radiation recall" reaction.[61–63] Radiation recall, or reactivation, is a recurrence of the effects of radiation, especially in mucous membranes and the skin, for up to several weeks after radiation following the administration of chemotherapy. To decrease the likelihood of occurrence in patients requiring radiation, doses of dactinomycin and doxorubicin should be decreased by 50% during and for up to 6 weeks after radiotherapy.

Pulse-intensive therapy has shown great benefit in patients with WT. The NWTS-4 provided evidence that patients experienced less hematologic toxicity than previously reported despite the administration of myelosuppressive chemotherapy in higher doses.[60] However, the regimens studied in the NWTS-4 were not absent of side effects. Dactinomycin is associated with hepatotoxicity causing transient elevations in liver function tests. The NWTS-4 demonstrated an increase in the incidence of hepatotoxicity (as well as the observation of acute veno-occlusive disease) when compared with the NWTS-3. The initial pulse-intensive dose of 60 μg/kg was thought to be excessive and was reduced to the 45 μg/kg dose. However, follow-up analysis has found the current pulse-intensive regimen, as well as the standard dose of 15 μg/kg/day for 5 days, to have more hepatotoxicity than that reported in the NWTS-3. The pathogenesis of these observations remains unknown.[64,65] It is important for health care professionals to recognize this condition, which usually occurs within the first 3 months after diagnosis, and not confuse it with other causes for liver dysfunction. Liver enzymes usually return to baseline values within 2 weeks of discontinuing therapy. A reduction in dactinomycin dose should be made if a patient's liver function tests are elevated. If laboratory values are greater or continue to rise, dactinomycin should be held until values return to a range that is more appropriate for its use.

The dose of dactinomycin used in patients with WT illustrates an important concept in pediatric oncology. The dose of this chemotherapeutic agent is expressed as an amount (μg) per amount of body weight (kg) rather than amount per body surface area (m^2) that is usually seen with other protocols. After analysis of data from NWTS-2, it was noted that an unusually large number of infants died from regimen-related toxicities.[66] Doses in the NWTS-4 for this same age-group were reduced by 50%. Results were more favorable with fewer toxicities without compromise in therapeutic efficacy.[67] These findings illustrate the need for alternative dosing methods in infants, which is most likely due to the fact that infants, when compared with children and adults, have a larger body surface area to weight ratio. An approximate conversion of a dose/m^2 to a dose/kg can be made by dividing the dose/m^2 by 30, which is based on the assumption that the average 30 kg child has a body surface area of 1 m^2.

PROGNOSIS

Children diagnosed with WT have an excellent overall survival rate, and more than 90% of these patients achieve a cure. Through the collaborative research efforts of several institutions in the NWTS, tumor histology has emerged as the most important prognostic indicator. Based on the appearance of the tumor tissue, patients are broadly classified as favorable histology or unfavorable histology. Approximately 85% of patients with WT are classified as favorable histology, and 4-year overall survival rates for these patients, as demonstrated in the NWTS-3, are significant: stage I (95.6%), stage II (91.1%), stage III (90.9%), and stage IV (80.9%).[53] Additional factors linked to prognosis are lymph node involvement and distant metastasis.

Sarcomas

A sarcoma is a malignant neoplasm formed by proliferation of embryonic mesenchymal cells, which normally give rise to connective tissue, including blood, bone, cartilage, and muscle tissue. Sarcomas in children can be divided into two principle categories, bone sarcomas and soft tissue sarcomas, which are further subdivided into various tumor types. Bone sarcomas occur with a peak incidence in adolescents and most commonly include osteosarcoma and Ewing's sarcoma. Soft tissue sarcomas are made up of a multitude of histologic types, of which the subtype rhabdomyosarcoma makes up at least one-half of all cases. A more detailed pathologic description of pediatric soft tissue tumors is described elsewhere.[68]

Rhabdomyosarcoma

Rhabdomyosarcoma (RMS), a very aggressive tumor first described by Weber in 1854,[69] is thought to arise from primitive mesenchymal tissue that mimics immature striated muscle. The two major histologic subtypes of RMS, which may or may not have prognostic significance, are embryonal (53%) and alveolar (21%). Embryonal cells, which resemble striated muscle, are more commonly found in younger children with involvement in the head and neck or genitourinary tract. Alveolar cells, which resemble lung parenchymal cells, occur more frequently in adolescents and usually involve the trunk or extremities.[70]

TREATMENT GOALS: RHABDOMYOSARCOMA

- Treatment strategies for RMS encompass several therapeutic modalities.
- Surgery, if feasible, is directed at removing as much tumor as possible.
- Surgery is usually followed by radiation, which is given to reduce residual tumor and local microscopic disease.
- Chemotherapy is administered to eradicate micrometastases.

EPIDEMIOLOGY

The incidence of RMS in males exceeds that of females (1.44 : 1), and there is a slight preponderance in Caucasians when compared with African Americans (1.15 : 1) with racial differences being more pronounced in females.[3,70] The majority of RMS is seen in children under age 6; however, a second peak in incidence occurs in late adolescence (15 to 19 years). Rhabdomyosarcoma has been associated with an increased incidence of maternal breast cancer and an increased number of cancers in siblings.[71] This familial manifestation is referred to as the Li-Fraumeni cancer family syndrome and may be associated with alterations in the p53 tumor suppressor gene.[72] Additionally, a strong correlation exists between alveolar RMS and translocations on chromosomes 2 and 13.[73]

CLINICAL PRESENTATION AND DIAGNOSIS

Signs and Symptoms

Presenting symptoms of RMS are widely variable because this tumor can arise anywhere in the body. The most common sites for occurrence are the head and neck region, the genitourinary tract, and the extremities. Common signs and symptoms depending on location are summarized in Table 93.12.[70]

The natural progression of RMS involves local invasion of adjacent organs or structures and distant metastases by lymphatic and hematogenous spread. The most common sites of metastases include the lungs, liver, bone and bone marrow, and CNS.

Table 93.12 ▪ Signs and Symptoms of Rhabdomyosarcoma Based on Tumor Location

Tumor Location	Signs and Symptoms
Head and neck region	Nausea, vomiting, headache, cranial nerve palsies, hypertension, proptosis, ophthalmoplegia, epistaxis, sinus obstruction with or without nasal discharge
Genitourinary tract	Hematuria, urinary obstruction, constipation, vaginal discharge, painless scrotal or inguinal enlargement
Extremities	Swelling of the affected site, possibly accompanied by pain, tenderness, and redness

Source: Reference 70.

Diagnosis

Diagnostic techniques commonly employed in the diagnosis of RMS include biopsies, radiographic studies, CT, and MRI. Biopsies are essential for histologic diagnosis, and radiographic evaluation assists in determining the location of lesions and the extent of metastasis, if applicable. Preoperative CT with or without contrast, which historically has been considered the imaging modality of choice, enables the radiation therapist to ascertain the extent of tumor involvement and thus plan treatment fields accordingly. More recently, MRI has become more popular because of the ability to provide superior soft tissue contrast when compared with CT imagery. Bone marrow involvement can be confirmed with bone marrow aspirates and biopsies. Lumbar puncture is necessary for all cases of parameningeal involvement and in some primary tumors involving sites in the head and neck.[70]

Precise determination of the location and amount of disease is critical in treating a patient with RMS because staging can direct therapy and predict prognosis. Today, there are two classification systems employed in clinical practice to stage patients with RMS. The more widely accepted staging system is the surgicopathologic clinical group (CG) system developed by members of the Intergroup Rhabdomyosarcoma Studies (IRS). The other staging system is the site-based tumor-node-metastasis (TNM) system, which, historically, has been used in adult patients with RMS. The CG system is based on the amount of tumor following surgery and the degree of tumor dissemination. Because surgery techniques vary among surgeons, the CG system is often criticized for its lack of consistency. Additionally, important prognostic factors such as tumor size and site location are not incorporated in the CG system. Therefore, the IRS committee adopted a modified TNM classification system, which is not dependent on subjective factors such as the surgeon's skill and incorporates the tumor's size, location, and biologic properties.[69,70] Currently, the IRS-IV study is comparing the utility of the two staging systems. The reader is referred elsewhere for the details of these classification systems.[70]

TREATMENT

Surgery

Although patients with completely resected tumors have the best prognosis, most patients with RMS do not have tumors that are completely resectable either because of their location or their extensive invasion into surrounding tissues. Thus surgery is followed by other treatment modalities. In some circumstances, incisional biopsies may be preferred to surgery, such as in cases where surgery may create cosmetic disfigurements or the tumor is in close proximity to vital blood vessels and nerves. Secondary excision may be feasible after tumor debulking with chemotherapy with or without radiotherapy. Occasionally, second-look procedures after chemotherapy alone may spare a patient from radiation treatments if no residual tumor is present.

Radiotherapy

Radiation therapy in doses of 4000 to 5000 cGy is indicated when there is either local or metastatic macroscopic or microscopic residual disease that is unresectable. It may also be indicated for tumors with unfavorable histology or primary lesions of the extremity in any stage. Chemotherapy in patients with bulky disease may allow tumor reduction, permitting the use of better-defined radiation fields. Patients with parameningeal lesions with extension into the brain parenchyma, meninges, or CSF receive intrathecal chemotherapy (methotrexate, cytarabine, and hydrocortisone) plus craniospinal irradiation.[74] Hyperfractionated irradiation to the primary site is being studied to determine if this method can decrease toxicity, especially the retardation of growing bone. A pilot study comparing standard radiation doses (5040 cGy) to hyperfractionated doses (5940 cGy) in combination with chemotherapy in children with localized but nonresectable RMS and metastatic RMS suggested that acute toxicities with hyperfractionated radiation may be less than conventional, once-daily radiotherapy protocols.[75] Additional studies are ongoing to confirm these findings. Brachytherapy, the delivery of radiation to a carefully restricted volume via an implanted radioactive device, may be indicated for critically located, incompletely resected tumors. This internal radiation strategy may lower the radiation fibrosis in adjacent normal structures associated with external radiotherapy that inherently allows more radiation scatter.[70]

Chemotherapy

Chemotherapy is an integral part of treatment for RMS in that all patients receive chemotherapy regardless of stage because of the high risk of disseminated disease. Chemotherapy also decreases the need for radiation in some patients. Treatment length varies with stage; patients with stage I disease usually require 1 year of therapy, whereas patients with stage II, III, or IV disease require at least 2 years of therapy because the majority of relapses occur within 2 years of starting therapy. The prototypic chemotherapy regimen employed in RMS is vincristine, actinomycin D, and cyclophosphamide (VAC). Doxorubicin was used in early trials (RMS-I and RMS-II) in combination with VAC; however, its use has declined because its addition to VAC did not improve overall survival and it was found to be associated with serious delayed cardiotoxicity in approximately 2% of patients.[76,77]

Newer combinations of agents, including etoposide, ifosfamide, cisplatin, and melphalan, have been compared with VAC therapy in more recent studies (IRS-III and IRS-IV).[78,79] These studies also explored giving dose-intensive chemotherapy (involving dose escalations of cyclophosphamide and ifosfamide) early in therapy to improve outcome while sparing patients surgical procedures and excessive radiation treatments. Melphalan was found to be an active agent in previously untreated patients but was highly myelosuppressive. Ifosfamide and etoposide have demonstrated favorable activity in pilot studies. Therapy complications following chemotherapy have included hemorrhagic cystitis, Fanconi's syndrome, and secondary neoplasms.

FUTURE THERAPIES

Currently the IRS-V, a study that is assigning patients to one of four histologic subgroups and is exploring risk-directed therapy, is using G-CSF with combination chemotherapy to reduce the duration of neutropenia after highly myelosuppressive regimens. Another agent, topotecan, is currently being evaluated for utility in RMS.[80]

IMPROVING OUTCOMES

Patient Monitoring

Ifosfamide is commonly employed in the treatment of RMS. This is an alkylating agent with significant renal and neurologic toxicities. After the administration of ifosfamide, myelosuppression ensues and granulocytes reach their nadir in 10 to 14 days with recovery occurring in 3 weeks. Thrombocytopenia is more commonly associated with higher doses. Hemorrhagic cystitis is common and requires judicious hydration of the patient before and for up to 72 hours after ifosfamide infusions. Mesna administration, which serves as a uroprotectant, should accompany the infusion of ifosfamide and continue for 24 hours after its completion. The total dose of mesna is generally 60 to 120% of the ifosfamide dose on a weight-per-weight basis.

Fanconi's syndrome, or proximal renal tubular acidosis, which is characterized by tubular wasting of glucose, protein, sodium, potassium, calcium, phosphate, and bicarbonate, is a significant dose-dependent nephrotoxicity after the administration of ifosfamide. An increase in serum creatinine is also characteristic of renal damage from ifosfamide. Other predisposing factors to developing Fanconi's syndrome are young age, unilateral nephrectomy, cumulative dose of ifosfamide, and concomitant administration of platinum chemotherapy.[81,82] The total dose of ifosfamide is also a risk factor in the development of Fanconi's syndrome. Once a cumulative dose of 72 g/m^2 is achieved, a change in therapy (to cyclophosphamide) should be considered to decrease the likelihood of adverse reactions.

Neurologic toxicities are common at higher doses of ifosfamide and generally manifest as somnolence, confusion, and disorientation. Nausea and vomiting can be a significant problem after the administration of ifosfamide but generally is well controlled with the use of antiemetics. Because ifosfamide undergoes hepatic activation, mild, transient increases in liver enzymes have been reported. Notable monitoring parameters in patients receiving ifosfamide are serum creatinine, BUN, complete blood cell count with differential, electrolytes, calcium, phosphorus, liver enzymes, urine analysis, and urine output.

Patient Education

The importance of hydration and adequate urine output should be enforced. Oral hydration to ensure continued diuresis at home should be encouraged. The patient should be made aware of manifestations of hemorrhagic cystitis, and any blood or clots in the urine should be reported immediately. Drugs that are inducers of P-450 enzymes have the potential to interact with ifosfamide, and their use should be carefully monitored.

Trimethoprim–sulfamethoxazole (TMP/SMX, Bactrim) administration is strongly suggested to prevent *Pneumocystis carinii* infections. Regimens studied in the IRS studies can be profoundly myelosuppressive and warrant prophylactic antibiotic administration. Several dosage regimens for TMP/SMX are employed in clinical practice; a widely accepted regimen is 5 mg/kg/day (based on the trimethoprim component) divided two times per day given on Monday, Wednesday, and Friday. Patients and their caregivers should be counseled to maintain adequate fluid intake and avoid prolonged sun exposure while on therapy. A rash that develops during therapy should be reported to a health care professional immediately.

PROGNOSIS

Several prognostic indicators have been elucidated in RMS.[70,83] The extent of tumor at the time of diagnosis appears to be the most important and the strongest predictor of outcome. Patients with metastasis have a poorer prognosis than patients with localized disease. Total surgical resection of tumor confers a better prognosis than residual disease. The tumor's histopathologic subtype is a useful prognostic indicator (embryonal has a better prognosis than alveolar); however, research suggests that tumor location is the more important tumor characteristic in predicting outcome. The tumor's primary site is important because it affects the length of time before a diagnosis is made, the feasibility of surgical resection, and the likelihood of metastasis. Sites with a favorable prognosis are orbit, paratesticular, gastrointestinal, prostate, and genitourinary tract; sites with an unfavorable prognosis are the extremities, retroperitoneum, intrathoracic, head and neck, trunk, perineal, ear, and sinuses.[84] Younger age and early response to chemotherapy are additional favorable prognostic indicators. Overall, 70% of children diagnosed with RMS can be expected to survive 5 or more years.[69]

Osteosarcoma

Osteosarcoma (OS), the most common bone neoplasm occurring in children, is a primary malignant tumor of mesenchymal origin characterized by the production of osteoid tissue (immature bone) by the malignant proliferating spindle cell stroma.[85] The past three decades have produced more favorable treatment outcomes; however, up to one-half of all patients diagnosed with OS do not realize a cure. Despite a more detailed understanding of the pathophysiology of OS, questions revolving around therapy remain, and, as research continues, determination of these answers is anticipated in the near future.[85,86]

TREATMENT GOALS: OSTEOSARCOMA

- The goals of therapy for OS are local control of the primary tumor and eradication of distant microscopic disease, which is always assumed to be present at diagnosis.
- Because radiation is ineffective, surgery and chemotherapy are the two treatment modalities used to manage patients.

EPIDEMIOLOGY

Osteosarcoma is primarily a cancer of adolescence, and peak incidence occurs during the second decade of life (age 14 years for males and age 13 years for females). The current overall incidence of OS in children less than 15 years old is slightly greater in females than in males (0.97 : 1); however, historically, more males develop OS than females. Racial differences in OS are not varied, with the rate of OS in African American children slightly exceeding the rate in Caucasian children (0.87 : 1).[3] The exact incidence and gender and racial differences of OS are debated because SEER data are restricted to persons less than 15 years old.[87]

The growth spurt seen during puberty is probably the basis for peak incidence during adolescence, suggesting a relation of the development of malignancy to rapid bone proliferation. In fact, the most likely sites of tumor are the distal femur, proximal tibia, and proximal humerus, all of which are the metaphyseal portions of bones, which undergo the most rapid growth during adolescence. Predisposing factors to OS have not been identified in children, although previous ionizing radiation and Paget's disease have been implicated in older patients. Children with hereditary retinoblastoma have a significantly greater chance of later developing OS, suggesting a genetic predisposition in some patients. Deregulation of the p53 tumor suppressor gene also appears to be important in the development of OS.[85,86]

CLINICAL PRESENTATION AND DIAGNOSIS

Signs and Symptoms

OS can occur in any bone, but approximately one-half of tumors arise in the knee.[87] The majority of patients have a chief complaint of pain over the site of disease. A soft tissue mass is not present in all cases. Symptoms usually occur a few weeks to several months before medical evaluation is conducted. If symptomatology is thought to be secondary to injury, evaluation can be furthered delayed. Fever, weight loss, and adenopathy, all of which are more suggestive of advanced disease, may also be present. At the time of diagnosis, most patients have micrometastatic disease and up to 20% of patients have visible signs of distant metastasis, usually appearing as tumors in the lung. Lymph node spread in OS is rare because bones lack a lymphatic system.[85,87]

Diagnosis

Radiographic evaluation plays a pivotal role in OS; it not only makes the determination of the presence of disease, but it can be helpful, although not definitive, in assisting the clinician in assessing tumor response to chemotherapy. Plain film radiographs are part of the initial series of studies ordered and allow the clinician to determine the extent of bone involvement and the presence of any pathologic fractures. The exact location of tumor is best made with the aid of MRI and CT. CT can also detect pulmonary metastasis. Radionuclide bone scans are used to identify the extent of the primary tumor and are instrumental in determining the presence of metastatic disease.

Laboratory evaluation in the patient with OS is limited. Serum alkaline phosphatase can be elevated in up to 40% of patients. Although it is a poor indicator of the extent of tumor, it can be used as a prognostic indicator. Serum lactate dehydrogenase (LDH) is another laboratory marker that can be elevated in patients.

A universal staging system is not employed in the diagnosis of OS because most tumors are considered high grade. The only delineation made in patients with OS is local disease versus metastatic disease.[85]

TREATMENT

Surgery

Because radiation therapy is not active in OS, surgery is the only means of local control of tumor. Past surgical techniques were limited to limb amputation, and outcomes were poor despite these radical procedures. Fewer than 25% of patients lived several years beyond surgery. Today surgical techniques have been refined to include limb-sparing techniques. These procedures are made possible with the use of neoadjuvant chemotherapy and incorporate CT and MRI diagnostic procedures early in the treatment process. Other surgical procedures include resection of pulmonary nodules in patients with limited lung disease, which may provide long-term survival results in some patients.[85,87]

Chemotherapy

The importance of chemotherapy in OS is evident–less than 20% of patients survive with surgery alone. Administration of chemotherapy can occur before or after surgery. Adjuvant chemotherapy is generally administered for 6 to 9 months after surgery and has increased disease-free survival rates and overall survival rates significantly to more than 65% and approximately 50%, respectively, in patients with nonmetastatic disease.[88–90] Neoadjuvant chemotherapy has gained popularity in the past decade and offers several advantages. It allows the surgeon more time to develop a plan and to construct prosthetic devices for the patient, facilitating limb-salvage techniques. Metastatic disease is treated earlier in the disease course, and, by administering chemotherapy as first-line therapy, tumor response can be assessed, which can then be correlated with outcome.

Because OS is a relatively drug-resistant tumor, patients require intensive doses of active agents given over a specified time (dose-intensive chemotherapy). Agents with demonstrated activity in OS include cisplatin,[88–90] doxorubicin,[12,88–90] ifosfamide,[91] and methotrexate with leucovorin rescue.[92] Ifosfamide has demonstrated its most beneficial effects in patients with very large tumor burdens.[93] High-dose methotrexate (HDMTX) regimens involve the administration of methotrexate in doses of up to 12 g/m^2 over 4 to 6 hours followed by the administration of leucovorin 24 hours after methotrexate until a desired concentration of methotrexate is achieved (less than 0.1 $\mu M/L$). Because methotrexate is renally eliminated, measures are employed by the clinician to enhance its excretion and decrease the likelihood of toxicities. These methods include adequate hydration (2 to 3.5 $L/m^2/day$) to ensure diuresis and administering sodium bicarbonate (PO or IV) or acetate (IV) to alkalinize the urine, which promotes excretion of methotrexate metabolites. When these prophylactic measures are instituted, side effects from methotrexate, which include nausea, vomiting, mucositis, stomatitis, rash, and myelosuppression, are minimized. Certain drugs are avoided in these patients during methotrexate therapy to minimize methotrexate accumulation and direct insult to the kidney. Examples of other nephrotoxic drugs include cisplatin, amphotericin B, aminoglycosides, and cyclosporine. Nonsteroidal anti-inflammatory drugs and TMP/SMX administration is avoided because these agents compete with methotrexate for renal tubular excretion and can lead to prolonged elevations in methotrexate serum concentrations.[94]

FUTURE THERAPIES

Muramyl-tripeptide conjugated with phosphatidyl ethanolamine (MTP-PE) may have a role in the future treatment of OS. A derivative of bacillus Calmette-Guérin vaccine, MTP-PE is encapsulated into liposomes, which facilitates its delivery, and promotes the in vitro activation of monocytes. These activated monocytes have a tumoricidal effect against OS. Preliminary data show that it is safe for administration to humans, but in vivo efficacy data are currently lacking.[85]

IMPROVING OUTCOMES

Patient Monitoring

With respect to HDMTX therapy, monitoring serum methotrexate levels is the pharmacist's primary concern. Serial methotrexate levels should be obtained at designated times after the infusion of the dose. Based on the concentration at a designated time period, leucovorin dosing may need modification to reach the desired endpoint. Recommendations for leucovorin adjustments are described in more detail elsewhere.[94,95] Renal function should be monitored as well. Serum creatinine and BUN should be followed to assess renal function. Urine output should be noted as well to determine if diuresis is adequate (usually a goal of 2 to 3 ml/kg/hr). Monitoring urine pH (to maintain above 6.5 to 7) is also advisable to ensure alkalinization of the urine. Although mild myelosuppression is common, it can be monitored by serial complete blood cell counts with differentials. Significant but reversible elevations in liver transaminases and increases in bilirubin and prothrombin time are not uncommon, and the monitoring of liver chemistries is warranted. Nausea, vomiting, mucositis, and stomatitis should be noted for two reasons. First, electrolyte disturbances can occur with vomiting, and replacement therapy via adequate hydration is common. Second, if oral intake is limited or impaired, oral medications may need to be switched to intravenous administration to prevent a compromise in patient care.

Patient Education

It is important to educate patients and their families with regard to adequate hydration while on an HDMTX protocol. Vigorous intravenous hydration is given before and in the hours after the methotrexate infusion. Patients should be encouraged to drink plenty of fluids as well to ensure adequate hydration and diuresis. Patients should report nausea and vomiting that interferes with their ability to take oral medications, particularly if they are receiving leucovorin as tablets. Because methotrexate can cause a rash, patients should be advised to remain out of the sun for prolonged periods of time, and they should be educated on protective methods to avoid sunburn. Key drug-drug interactions should be explained to patients and their temporary avoidance should be stressed.

PROGNOSIS

Prognostic indicators in OS have been reported in the literature with varied implications and interpretations. Some indicators that confer a poorer prognosis are male gender; large tumor burden; a shorter time interval from disease to treatment; tumors located at the proximal femur, humerus, and axial skeleton; and elevated alkaline phosphatase and LDH.[96,97] Age was once considered a prognostic indicator (with young age having a poorer outcome) but must be further evaluated because many trials exclude older children and young adults.[86] Tumor necrosis of greater than 90% after neoadjuvant chemotherapy appears to be the most important characteristic in children with a favorable clinical outcome.[87] Despite the identification of these prognostic factors, patients are not stratified to receive a particular treatment regimen based on their presence or absence.[97]

Ewing's Sarcoma

First described in 1921 by James Ewing, Ewing's sarcoma (ES) is the second most common primary bone cancer diagnosed in children. Ewing's sarcoma is a small round-cell neoplasm belonging to a family of tumors of neural histogenesis. Although it usually arises in the bone, ES may originate in soft tissue. Treatment of ES more closely parallels RMS than that of OS. Also included in this family, but excluded from this discussion, is peripheral primitive neuroectodermal tumor.

TREATMENT GOALS: EWING'S SARCOMA

- The treatment goals of ES are similar to those of OS—local control of tumor and management of micrometastatic disease.
- Surgery and chemotherapy are used to achieve these goals. Radiation therapy is an effective tool for the treatment of ES.

EPIDEMIOLOGY

The peak incidence of ES occurs in the second decade of life and rarely occurs before age 5 or after age 30.[3,98] In children less than age 15 years, the incidence in males is similar to that in females (1.08 : 1) and both sexes have a peak incidence at age 13 years. There are, however, striking differences in the high incidence in Caucasian children when compared with African American children of the same age (11.0 : 1). In fact, ES is the childhood malignancy with the most remarkable difference in racial incidence.[3]

The exact cause of ES has yet to be determined. Ewing's sarcoma is not associated with familial cancer syndromes and does not appear to be inherited or associated with other congenital diseases of childhood. Radiation exposure does not appear to attribute to the development of ES. Cytogenetic studies in children with ES have produced valid associations with certain genetic rearrangements. The most common genetic anomalies in ES include the t(11;22) translocation and the t(21;22) translocation. As a result, molecular assays are being used to aid the clinician in diagnosing ES.[99]

CLINICAL PRESENTATION AND DIAGNOSIS

Signs and Symptoms

More than 90% of children have pain and swelling at the site of tumor. The pain may be intermittent at first, which may delay medical evaluation, but usually progresses to being persistent and severe. A palpable mass is not always present at diagnosis, and patients rarely have paraplegia. Fever is present in approximately 20% of patients. When fever is accompanied by leukocytosis, an infectious etiology is usually suspected, and an incorrect diagnosis, such as osteomyelitis, may be made. Other presenting findings that have been reported are weight loss and an increase in sedimentation rate.[98–100]

Diagnosis

A variety of diagnostic tests are performed on the patient with suspected ES in order to define the exact location of the tumor, estimate the size of the tumor, and determine the presence of metastasis. Ewing's sarcoma primarily affects long tubular bones of the lower extremities, especially the femur. The most common axial site of involvement is the pelvis. Unlike OS, which primarily damages the ends of bones, ES causes damage to bones in more central locations between the diaphysis and metaphysis. Plain radiographs can easily demonstrate the damage caused by ES, which is referred to as "onion skinning." CT and MRI are used to complement one other. MRI is more sensitive than CT for detecting abnormalities but can overestimate tumor involvement, which necessitates confirmatory studies by CT.[98–100]

Clinically detectable metastatic disease is present in approximately 20% of patients at the time of diagnosis. The most common site of metastasis is the lung (50% of patients). Other locations for metastatic ES are bone (25% of patients), bone marrow (10 to 20% of patients), and rarely the liver and lymph nodes. Because there is a high rate of metastatic disease at the time of presentation, diagnostic procedures including CT of the chest, bone scan, and bone marrow aspirate and biopsy should be performed. There is no definitive tumor marker in ES; however, one-half of all patients with ES have an elevated erythrocyte sedimentation rate. An elevated LDH is a common finding as well. There is no universal staging schemata for ES; the only delineation made at the time of diagnosis is local disease versus metastatic disease.[98–100]

TREATMENT

Ewing's sarcoma is a radiosensitive tumor. Local control is achieved through surgery or radiation, and chemotherapy is always given adjuvantly to treat microscopic metastatic disease either before or after local control measures.

Local Control

Radiation therapy is reserved for those patients with small tumor. Doses of radiation used to control ES are fairly high (5500 to 6000 cGy), and, until recently, radiation was given over the entire affected bone. However, improved techniques are being employed to deliver radiation over more refined fields, which can decrease the toxicity of this therapy. Radiation is advantageous in ES because it can significantly decrease the soft tissue component before chemotherapy or surgery. Surgery is reserved for larger tumors because it has been demonstrated that applying radiation to these tumors is associated with higher local failure rates. Surgery may be a better option for local control in cases which radiation would cause significant morbidity. Another indication for surgery is cases in which radiation would have an increased likelihood of morbidity. Such cases include the presence of small rib lesions; cases in which the primary tumor occurs in expendable bones, such as the clavicle, body of the scapula, and proximal tibia, and in small well-confined lesions of the ileum; and cases in which the tumor involves weight-bearing bones or major growth sites.[98]

Chemotherapy

Vincristine, dactinomycin, and cyclophosphamide have been recognized as single agents with activity in ES since the early 1960s. As a result, their use in combination (VAC) was one of the first therapeutic regimens used in patients with ES. Doxorubicin was found to have activity in ES in the 1970s, and several institutions added it to the VAC regimen (VACAdr).[100] The benefit of the addition of doxorubicin was investigated by a collaborative study, the Intergroup Ewing's Sarcoma Study I (IESS-I), in the United States. This study compared the VAC regimen with the VACAdr regimen and found the latter regimen superior. The study also demonstrated the importance of dose-intensive chemotherapy in ES, in that the administration of VACAdr at 3-week intervals versus 6-week intervals was associated with less incidence of relapse.[101] A recent study examining these regimens in extraosseous ES showed no difference in response rates between these regimens; however, these results must be interpreted with caution because identification of patients with extraosseous ES has become more precise.[99,102] A second study (IESS-II) employing the VACAdr regimen confirmed the importance of dose intensity by demonstrating the superiority of high-dose intermittent cyclophosphamide over moderate-dose continuous cyclophosphamide.[103]

More recently, the roles of ifosfamide and etoposide in the treatment of ES have been investigated. Ifosfamide has been substituted for cyclophosphamide in the VACAdr regimen with mixed results.[104,105] The addition of both ifosfamide and etoposide alternating with the VACAdr regimen has been shown to produce higher response rates when compared with VACAdr alone, particularly for those patients with localized tumors and good prognostic indicators at the time of diagnosis.[106–108] The 5-year event-free survival rate for patients with nonmetastatic disease at diagnosis treated on the standard VACAdr regimen was 52% compared with 68% for patients who received the addition of ifosfamide and etoposide to their chemotherapy, a statistically significant difference. However, the addition of ifosfamide or etoposide is associated with more adverse effects and significantly more morbidity than the VACAdr regimen.

FUTURE THERAPIES

Collaborative research continues in determining the most appropriate chemotherapy regimen for ES. A combined CCG and POG trial that examines the utility of dose intensification of alkylating agents used in previous studies is currently being conducted. Another promising treatment modality in ES is the use of autologous stem-cell transplantation. This process allows the administration of large doses of chemotherapy to patients followed by the reinfusion of previously collected stem cells as "rescue" therapy. Patients with high-risk ES have been successfully treated with stem-cell transplantation after the failure of conventional therapy.[16,109] Additional studies involving larger patient cohorts are necessary before the exact role of stem-cell transplantation can be determined.

IMPROVING OUTCOMES

Doxorubicin is known to cause congestive heart failure, and effects may be delayed by as much as 20 years. Recognized risk factors to anthracycline-induced cardiac toxicity, which can involve a decrease in diastolic function and a decrease in left ventricular free wall thickness, are mediastinal radiation and cumulative doxorubicin dose. Patients should be monitored accordingly for several years after therapy.[110–114]

PROGNOSIS

Several prognostic indicators have been identified for patients with ES. The following are suggestive of a poor prognosis at the time of diagnosis: increase in LDH, large tumor size (larger than 8 cm), the presence of constitutional symptoms, metastatic disease, older age, and a primary tumor site that is axial (pelvic).[99,100] Other poor prognostic indicators that have been recently identified and warrant additional investigation for their confirmation are an increased albumin and the presence of tumor cells in the bone marrow but not in the blood.[115,116] Almost 70% of patients who present with local disease will achieve a cure. In contrast, of the approximately 20% of patients who are diagnosed with metastatic disease, only a third will achieve a cure.[117]

Retinoblastoma

Although it accounts for a small percentage of pediatric malignancies, retinoblastoma (RB) is the most common intraocular tumor in children. It also serves as the prototype and model for understanding the heredity and genetics in childhood cancer. It is a tumor of the embryonic neural retina consisting of closely packed, round, undifferentiated small cells with darkly stained nuclei and scant cytoplasm.[118] The chance of survival is excellent overall; however, the chance of a secondary neoplasm in children with the hereditary form of RB is extremely high.

TREATMENT GOALS: RETINOBLASTOMA

- The treatment of RB is highly individualized and is determined based on several factors, including the stage at diagnosis.
- The primary goal of treatment is management of the local tumor and the preservation of vision, if feasible.
- A secondary treatment goal is the monitoring of patients with RB for secondary neoplasms, most notably osteosarcoma, for several years after treatment.

EPIDEMIOLOGY

Retinoblastoma represents less than 3% of pediatric malignancies and rarely occurs after age 5. There is a slight preponderance of RB in females (0.86 : 1) and in African Americans (0.87 : 1).[3] The incidence of RB is 1 in 18,000 live births, which translates to approximately 200 new cases of RB being diagnosed in the United States each year.[119] Genetic abnormalities associated with RB are numerous, the most notable being deletions on chromosome 13 involving the two RB alleles localized to the 13q14 region.[118]

Delineation among types of RB is made based on the presence of disease in one or both eyes and if the disease is inherited. The incidence of bilateral involvement ranges from 20 to 30%.[119] More specifically, of all cases of RB, 60% are nonhereditary and unilateral, 25% are hereditary and bilateral, and 15% are hereditary and unilateral.[120] Thus bilateral disease is always inherited. Because there is a strong correlation of disease development with the presence of genetic anomalies, patients with a strong family history of RB often undergo frequent, meticulous eye examinations during the first 3 to 4 years of life.

CLINICAL PRESENTATION AND DIAGNOSIS

Most cases of RB in the United States are diagnosed while the tumor is confined to the intraocular space. Bilateral RB, which usually is multifocal involving numerous tumors in both eyes, is diagnosed earlier than unilateral disease. The most common sites of metastases are the CNS and the bone and bone marrow via hematogenous seeding. Lymphatic extension is less common because the eye does not have significant lymphatic drainage.[118]

Signs and Symptoms

The most common presenting symptom (56 to 62%) is leukocoria (also called cat's eye reflex or white eye), which is the result of retinal detachment. Strabismus (20 to 24%) occurs secondary to pressure from the tumor. Less common signs and symptoms are eye pain, ocular cellulitis, vitreous hemorrhage, glaucoma, and poor vision.[121] Metastatic disease, which occurs when the tumor spreads along the optic nerve and invades the subarachnoid space of the CNS or involves lymphatic or hematologic seeding, is associated with anorexia, nausea, vomiting, weight loss, and headache.[118]

Diagnosis

Ophthalmoscopic examination can suffice to make the clinical diagnosis of RB. However, retinal detachment and vitreous hemorrhage can make examination difficult; thus pupillary dilation and examination under anesthesia is necessary to fully evaluate the patient's retina. Metastatic workup includes CT and MRI of the globe, orbits, and CNS; lumbar puncture for CSF evaluation; and a bone marrow biopsy and aspirate to confirm the presence of bone marrow involvement.[122] After diagnosis, the patient is staged accordingly. The Reese-Ellsworth staging system, introduced in 1963, is the widely accepted classification schemata employed in clinical practice today (Table 93.13).[123]

Table 93.13 ▪ Reese-Ellsworth Staging Classification of Retinoblastoma

Group 1 (very favorable)
A. Solitary tumor, smaller than 4 disk diameters[a] at or behind the equator.
B. Multiple tumors, none larger than 4 disk diameters, all at or behind the equator.

Group 2 (favorable)
A. Solitary tumor, 4–10 disk diameters in size, at or behind the equator.
B. Multiple tumors, 4–10 disk diameters in size, behind the equator.

Group 3 (doubtful)
A. Any lesion anterior to the equator.
B. Solitary tumors larger than 10 disk diameters behind the equator.

Group 4 (unfavorable)
A. Multiple tumors, some larger than 10 disk diameters.
B. Any lesion extending anteriorly to the ora serrata.

Group 5 (very unfavorable)
A. Tumors involving more than half the retina.
B. Vitreous seeding.

Source: Reference 123.
[a]1 disk diameter = 1.5 mm.

TREATMENT

Treatment is highly individualized in the child with RB. Several factors are considered when determining treatment options. The size of the tumor, the number of lesions, disease location, and the feasibility of vision preservation determine therapy. Historically, enucleation and external beam radiation have been the only viable therapeutic options. Advances in surgical techniques have expanded therapeutic options in those with limited disease. Chemotherapy does not have a significant role in RB and is reserved for patients with extraocular disease. Optimally, therapy is directed at eradicating the tumor while preserving vision.

Surgery

Surgical techniques have extended beyond enucleation to include cryotherapy and photocoagulation. Enucleation remains the therapeutic option when the potential for vision preservation does not exist or when conservative therapy fails to control the tumor. It is most commonly performed in children with unilateral advanced disease. Removal of the globe should be accompanied by resection of an adequate length of the optic nerve to ensure a free margin. Children can be fitted with an artificial eye as early as 6 weeks after this generally painless procedure. Enucleation has no significant morbidity and mortality except in younger children (less than 3 years), who experience cessation of orbital development after surgery, which leads to a sunken orbit as the face continues to grow.

Cryotherapy and photocoagulation are techniques used to manage small tumors (usually less than 4 disc diameters) or tumors that appear after radiotherapy. Cryotherapy is most advantageous when used to control tumors in the anterior part of the retina. This technique employs a small probe placed directly on the conjunctiva or sclera that ultimately interrupts the microvascularization of the tumor when intracellular ice crystals are produced. Photocoagulation, used in managing tumors located in the posterior retina, involves an argon laser that encircles the tumor, causing its ischemic necrosis after occlusion of the blood vessels that supply the tumor.[118]

Radiotherapy

Retinoblastoma is a radiosensitive tumor. Radiation therapy is the preferred treatment option when the tumor is confined to the globe and the chance for vision preservation exists. It is preferred over photocoagulation and cryotherapy when tumors are large. Delivery of 4500 to 5400 cGy over 4.5 to 6 weeks, given as 180 to 200 cGy daily 5 days per week, is the dose widely used in practice, although the optimum fractionation and total dose warrants further investigation. The experiences from St. Jude Children's Research Hospital suggest that a total dose of 4000 cGy may provide the maximal benefit because doses beyond this do not confer greater benefit and are associated with an increase in morbidity.[124] Patients with brain metastases receive full cranial or craniospinal radiation as well. Complications of therapy are atrophy of the orbital bone, vasculitis, vitreous hemorrhage, optic neuropathy, retinopathy, glaucoma, and cataracts.[125] Another complication seen in patients with the hereditary form of RB is an acceleration in the interval until a second malignancy results. Methods to decrease complications from radiation therapy are delivery of localized therapy, using smaller fractions of radiation per dose, and using radioactive plaques. Radioactive plaques deliver radioactive isotopes (e.g., cobalt 60) directly to small tumors located in the posterior retina.[118]

Chemotherapy

The role of chemotherapy in the treatment of RB has been minor and is generally reserved for patients with extraocular or recurrent disease. Intraocular penetration of chemotherapy agents is poor, and chemotherapy has failed to demonstrate an increase in survival or an increase in vision preservation.[126] Although RB is a fast-growing tumor, which, logically, would make it an excellent target for chemotherapy, this tumor type commonly expresses the multidrug-resistant glycoprotein p170, a factor that contributes to the poor activity of many chemotherapeutic agents.

Single agents found to be active in RB are cyclophosphamide (47% response rate), doxorubicin (33%), and vincristine (16%). Combination chemotherapy has produced mixed results, and duration of response has ranged from 1 to 5 months. Combination regimens have included vincristine, cyclophosphamide, and dactinomycin; cyclophosphamide and doxorubicin; and cisplatin and teniposide. Intrathecal methotrexate has been used in patients with cerebral spinal fluid involvement with minimal response.[127]

More recently, chemotherapy given as chemoreduction in the initial management of RB confined intraocularly has been examined in a prospective pilot study.[128] Vincristine, etoposide, and carboplatin given in combination for two cycles followed by ocular examination under anesthesia was studied in 20 patients with 54 tumors in 31 eyes. Although the results were not indicative of a curative modality, tumor regression was seen in all cases. Eleven eyes were spared from radiation therapy, and enucleation was avoided in all cases where indicated.

FUTURE THERAPIES

Studies such as those mentioned previously will be continued in the future to determine the precise role of chemoreduction in the management of patients with RB. Cyclosporine given in combination with chemotherapy to reverse the effects of the MDR gene is another area of ongoing research in patients with RB. Refined radiation techniques and the use of heavy-particle radiation are also newer treatment modalities. High-dose chemotherapy followed by autologous stem-cell rescue remains an experimental therapeutic approach in patients with advanced disease and has shown promise in patients with bone or bone marrow involvement.[129] Gene therapy directed at the RB1gene is a distant but probable treatment modality.

IMPROVING OUTCOMES

Continued monitoring and long-term follow-up are crucial in the patient with RB, particularly those patients with the hereditary form of the disease. The risk of developing osteosarcoma or a soft tissue sarcoma as a secondary malignancy is greatly enhanced in those patients who receive radiation. In fact, a dose-response relationship is evident.[130] Frequent eye examinations under anesthesia should be performed until age 5. Additional eye examinations and physicals should continue indefinitely at the discretion of the physician.

PROGNOSIS

When RB is detected early, the prognosis for complete recovery is excellent. Survival exceeds 90% in those patients with limited disease confined to the globe. Extension beyond the orbit or metastases to the brain or bone marrow confers a poor prognosis. The survival rate in these patients is reported to range from 35 to 80%.[118]

KEY POINTS

- Although childhood cancer is rare, mortality from this disease is second only to accidents as a cause of death in children under age 15 years.
- Survival outcomes for children with solid tumors have been greatly improved over the last three decades by a multimodal approach and intensive combination chemotherapy, and for many patients there is now hope for long-term survival. More than 60% of children diagnosed with cancer achieve a cure.
- Intense treatment regimens to invoke cure, however, are more toxic than past therapies, and management of patients requires extensive supportive care by a team of dedicated health care professionals. With children often surviving into adulthood, long-term follow-up of these patients is crucial to assess and ultimately prevent chronic toxicities of therapy.
- Solid tumors account for approximately 40% of pediatric malignancies.
- Enrollment of children in clinical trials is strongly encouraged to allow for greater patient accrual, more rapid reporting of research results, and an increased likelihood of long-term monitoring of patients.

- Secondary malignancies and late side effects following chemotherapy are a concern in pediatric patients, and appropriate monitoring should be part of routine physicals.
- Pediatric brain tumors are a heterogeneous group of neoplasms, and treatment is highly individualized based on patient age and tumor type and location.
- The management of neuroblastoma, the most common extracranial solid tumor in children, involves a combination of surgery, radiotherapy, chemotherapy, and immunotherapy.
- Several recent advances have been made in the treatment of Wilms' tumor, the most common renal neoplasm occurring in children, conferring an overall survival rate of more than 90%.
- In children, sarcomas, which are characterized by proliferation of embryonic mesenchymal cells, can be divided into two broad categories (bone and soft tissue), although treatment of each type is highly specific.
- Retinoblastoma serves as the prototype and model for understanding genetics in childhood cancer, because many patients survive the initial diagnosis of retinoblastoma but are at an increased risk of developing a second neoplasm, most notably osteosarcoma.

REFERENCES

1. Bleyer WA. The impact of childhood cancer on the United States and the world. CA Cancer J Clin 40:355–367, 1990.
2. Landis SH, Murray T, Bolden S, et al. Cancer statistics, 1998. CA Cancer J Clin 48:6–29, 1998.
3. Gurney JG, Severson RK, Davis S, et al. Incidence of cancer in children in the United States: sex-, race-, and 1-year age-specific rates by histology type. Cancer 75:2168–2195, 1995.
4. Kenney LB, Miller BA, Gloeckler Reis LA, et al. Increased incidence of cancer in infants in the US: 1980–1990. Cancer 82:1396–1400, 1998.
5. Gurney JG, Davis S, Severson RK, et al. Trends in cancer incidence among children in the US. Cancer 78:532–541, 1996.
6. Berg SL, Grisell DL, DeLaney TF, et al. Principles of treatment of pediatric solid tumors. Pediatr Clin North Am 38:249–267, 1991.
7. DeLaat CA, Lampkin BC. Long-term survivors of childhood cancer: evaluation and identification of sequelae of treatment. CA Cancer J Clin 42:263–282, 1992.
8. Novakovic B. US childhood cancer survival, 1973–1987. Med Pediatr Oncol 23:480–486, 1994.
9. Trott KR. Chronic damage after radiation therapy: challenge to radiation biology. Int J Radiat Oncol Biol Phys 10:907–913, 1984.
10. Kun LE. General principles of radiation therapy. In: Pizzo PA, Poplack DG, eds. Principles and practices of pediatric oncology. 3rd ed. Philadelphia: Lippincott-Raven, 1997:289–321.
11. Goldie JH, Coldman AJ. The genetic origin of drug resistance in neoplasms: implications for systemic therapy. Cancer Res 44:3643–3653, 1984.
12. Kawai A, Sugihara S, Kunisada T, et al. The importance of doxorubicin and methotrexate dose intensity in the chemotherapy of osteosarcoma. Arch Orthop Trauma Surg 115:68–70, 1996.
13. Kuttesch JF Jr. Multidrug resistance in pediatric oncology. Invest New Drugs 14:55–67, 1996.
14. Lepage E, Gisselbrecht C, Haioun C, et al. Prognostic significance of received relative dose intensity in non-Hodgkin's lymphoma patients: application of LNH-87 protocol. Ann Oncol 4:651–656, 1993.
15. Jacobson SJ, Shore RW, Greenberg M, et al. The efficacy and safety of granisetron in pediatric cancer patients who had failed standard antiemetic therapy during anticancer chemotherapy. Am J Pediatr Hematol Oncol 16:231–235, 1994.
16. Burdach S, Jurgens H, Peters C, et al. Myeloablative radiochemotherapy and hematopoietic stem-cell rescue in poor-prognosis Ewing's sarcoma. J Clin Oncol 11:1482–1488, 1993.
17. Atra A, Pinkerton R. Autologous stem cell transplantation in solid tumours of childhood. Ann Med 28:159–164, 1996.
18. Graham-Pole J, Gee A, Emerson S, et al. Myeloablative chemoradiotherapy and autologous bone marrow infusions for treatment of neuroblastoma: factors influencing engraftment. Blood 78:1607–1614, 1991.
19. Mike V, Meadows AT, Zimmerman LE. Incidence of second malignant neoplasms in children: results of an international study. Lancet 2:1326–1331, 1982.
20. Marina N. Long-term survivors of childhood cancer: the medical consequences of cure. Pediatr Clin North Am 44:1021–1042, 1997.
21. Smith MB, Xue H, Strong L, et al. Forty-year experience with second malignancies after treatment of childhood cancer: analysis of outcome following the development of the second malignancy. J Pediatr Surg 28:1342–1349, 1993.
22. Dennis M, Hetherington CR, Spiegler BJ. Memory and attention after childhood brain tumors. Med Pediatr Oncol 26(Suppl 1):25–33, 1998.
23. Hopewell JW. Radiation injury to the central nervous system. Med Pediatr Oncol 26(Suppl 1):1–9, 1998.
24. Pollack IF. Brain tumors in children. N Engl J Med 331:1500–1510, 1994.
25. Albright AL. Pediatric brain tumors. CA Cancer J Clin 43:272–288, 1993.
26. Lassoff SJ, Allen J, Epstein F, et al. Advances in surgery: brain stem and spinal cord tumors in children. In: Bleyer A, Packer R, eds. Pediatric neuro-oncology: new trends in clinical research. New York: Hardwood Academic, 1992:278–297.
27. Packer RJ, Boyett JM, Zimmerman RA, et al. Hyperfractionated radiation therapy (72 Gy) for children with brain stem gliomas. a Childrens Cancer Group phase I/II trial. Cancer 72:1414–1421, 1993.
28. Heideman RL, Packer RJ, Albright LA, et al. Tumors of the central nervous system. In: Pizzo PA, Poplack DG, eds. Principles and practice of pediatric oncology. 3rd ed. Philadelphia: Lippincott-Raven, 1997:633–697.
29. Sposto R, Ertel IJ, Jenkin RD, et al. The effectiveness of chemotherapy for treatment of high grade astrocytoma in children: results of a randomized trial. A report from the Childrens Cancer Study Group. J Neurooncol 7:165–177, 1989.
30. Evans AE, Jenkin DT, Sposto R, et al. The treatment of medulloblastoma. Results of a prospective randomized trial of radiation therapy with and without CCNU, vincristine, and prednisone. J Neurosurg 72:572–582, 1990.
31. Packer RJ, Sutton LN, Goldwein JW, et al. Improved survival with the use of adjuvant chemotherapy in the treatment of medulloblastoma. J Neurosurg 74:433–440, 1991.
32. Duffner PK, Horowitz ME, Krischer JP, et al. Postoperative chemotherapy and delayed radiation in children less than three years of age with malignant brain tumors. N Engl J Med 328:1725–1731, 1993.
33. Friedman HS, Oakes JW. The chemotherapy of posterior fossa tumors in childhood. J Neurooncol 5:217–229, 1987.
34. Schell MJ, McHaney VA, Green AA, et al. Hearing loss in children and young adults receiving cisplatin with and without prior cranial radiation. J Clin Oncol 7:754–760, 1989.
35. Lanzkowsky P. Central nervous system malignancies. In: Lanzkowsky P, ed. Manual of Pediatric Hematology and Oncology. 2nd ed. New York: Churchill Livingstone, 1995:397–417.
36. Finlay JL. High-dose chemotherapy followed by bone marrow "rescue" for recurrent brain tumors. In: Bleyer A, Packer R, eds. Pediatric neuro-oncology: new trends in clinical research. New York: Hardwood Academic, 1992:278–297.
37. Duffner PK, Cohen ME, Myers MH, et al. Survival of children with brain tumors: SEER program, 1973–1980. Neurology 36:597–601, 1986.
38. Carlsen NLT. Neuroblastoma: epidemiology and pattern of regression. Am J Pediatr Hematol Oncol 14:103–110, 1992.
39. Goodman SN. Neuroblastoma screening data. Am J Dis Child 145: 1415–1422, 1991.
40. Matthay KK. Neuroblastoma: a clinical challenge and biologic puzzle. CA Cancer J Clin 45:179–194, 1995.
41. Craft AW, Parker L. Screening for neuroblastoma: 20 years and still no answer. Eur J Cancer 32A:1540–1543, 1996.
42. Brodeur GM, Castleberry RP. Neuroblastoma. In: Pizzo PA, Poplack DG, eds. Principles and practice of pediatric oncology. 3rd ed. Philadelphia: Lippincott-Raven, 1997:761–797.
43. Philip T. Overview of current treatment of neuroblastoma. Am J Pediatr Hematol Oncol 14:97–102, 1992.
44. Niethammer D, Handgretinger R. Clinical strategies for the treatment of neuroblastoma. Eur J Cancer 31A:568–571, 1995.

45. Matthay KK, Harris R, Reynolds CP, et al. Improved event-free survival (EFS) for autologous bone marrow transplantation (ABMT) vs. chemotherapy in neuroblastoma: a phase III randomized Childrens Cancer Group (CCG) study [abstract 2018]. Proc Am Soc Clin Oncol 17:525a, 1998.
46. Israel MA. Disordered differentiation as a target for novel approaches to the treatment of neuroblastoma. Cancer 71:3310–3313, 1993.
47. Reynolds CP, Villablanca JG, Stram DO, et al. 13-*cis*-retinoic acid after intensive consolidation therapy for neuroblastoma improves event-free survival: a randomized Childrens Cancer Group (CCG) study [plenary session 5]. Proc Am Soc Clin Oncol 17:2a, 1998.
48. Evans AE, D'Angio GJ, Propert K, et al. Prognostic factors in neuroblastoma. Cancer 59:1853–1859, 1987.
49. Look AT, Hayes FA, Shuster JJ, et al. Clinical relevance of tumor cell ploidy and N-myc amplification in childhood neuroblastoma. A Pediatric Oncology Group study. J Clin Oncol 9:581–591, 1991.
50. Olshan AF, Breslow NE, Falletta JM, et al. Risk factors for Wilms' tumor. Report from the National Wilms' Tumor Study. Cancer 72:938–944, 1993.
51. Petruzzi MJ, Green DM. Wilms' tumor. Pediatr Clin North Am 44:939–952, 1997.
52. Green DM, Coppes MJ, Breslow NE, et al. Wilms' tumor. In: Pizzo PA, Poplack DG, eds. Principles and practice of pediatric oncology. 3rd ed. Philadelphia: Lippincott-Raven, 1997:733–759.
53. Green DM, D'Angio GJ, Beckwith JB, et al. Wilms' tumor. CA Cancer J Clin 46:46–63, 1996.
54. Mehta MP, Bastin KT, Wiersma SR. Treatment of Wilms' tumor. Current recommendations. Drugs 42:766–780, 1991.
55. D'Angio GJ, Evans AE, Breslow N, et al. The treatment of Wilms' tumor. Results of the National Wilms' Tumor Study. Cancer 38:633–646, 1976.
56. D'Angio GJ, Evans A, Breslow N, et al. The treatment of Wilms' tumor. Results of the Second National Wilms' Tumor Study. Cancer 47:2302–2311, 1981.
57. D'Angio GJ, Breslow N, Beckwith JB, et al. Treatment of Wilms' tumor. Results of the Third National Wilms' Tumor Study. Cancer 64:349–360, 1989.
58. Green D, Breslow N, Beckwith J, et al. A comparison between single dose and divided dose administration of dactinomycin and doxorubicin. A report from the National Wilms' Tumor Study Group [abstract]. Proc ASCO 15:460, 1996.
59. Wiener JS, Coppes MJ, Ritchey ML. Current concepts in the biology and management of Wilms' tumor. J Urol 159:1316–1325, 1998.
60. Green DM, Breslow NE, Evans I, et al. The effect of chemotherapy dose intensity on the hematological toxicity of the treatment of Wilms' tumor. A report from the National Wilms' Tumor Study. Am J Pediatr Hematol Oncol 16:207–212, 1994.
61. D'Angio GJ, Farber S, Maddock CL. Potentiation of x-ray effects by actinomycin D. Radiology 73:175–177, 1959.
62. Donaldson SS, Glick GM, Wilbur JR. Adriamycin activating a recall phenomenon after radiation therapy. Ann Intern Med 81:407–408, 1974.
63. Greco FA, Bereton HD, Kent H, et al. Adriamycin and enhanced radiation reaction in normal esophagus and skin. Ann Intern Med 85:294–298, 1976.
64. Green DM, Finklestein J, Norkool P, et al. Severe hepatic toxicity after treatment with single-dose dactinomycin and vincristine. A report of the National Wilms' Tumor Study. Cancer 62:270–273, 1988.
65. Green DM, Norkool P, Breslow NE, et al. Severe hepatic toxicity after treatment with vincristine and dactinomycin using single-dose or divided dose schedules. A report from the National Wilms' Tumor Study. J Clin Oncol 8:1525–1530, 1990.
66. Jones B, Breslow N, Takashima J, et al. Toxic deaths in the Second National Wilms' Tumor Study. J Clin Oncol 2:1028–1033, 1984.
67. Morgan E, Baum E, Breslow N, et al. Chemotherapy-related toxicity in infants treated according to the Second National Wilms' Tumor Study. J Clin Oncol 6:51–55, 1988.
68. Coffin CM, Dehner LP. Pathologic evaluation of pediatric soft tissue tumors. Am J Clin Pathol 109(Suppl 1):S38–S52, 1998.
69. Pappo AS, Shapiro DN, Crist WM. Rhabdomyosarcoma. Biology and treatment. Pediatr Clin North Am 44:953–972, 1997.
70. Wexler LH, Helman LJ. Rhabdomyosarcoma and the undifferentiated sarcomas. In: Pizzo PA, Poplack DG, eds. Principles and practice of pediatric oncology. 2nd ed. Philadelphia: Lippincott-Raven, 1997:799–829.
71. Hartley AL, Birch JM, Blair V, et al. Patterns of cancer in the families of children with soft tissue sarcoma. Cancer 72:923–930, 1993.
72. Malkin D, Li FP, Strong LC, et al. Germ line p53 mutations in a familial syndrome of breast cancer, sarcomas, and other neoplasms. Science 250:1233–1238, 1990.
73. Pappo AS, Shapiro DN, Crist WM, et al. Biology and therapy of pediatric rhabdomyosarcoma. J Clin Oncol 13:2123–2139.
74. Wexler LH, Helman LJ. Pediatric soft tissue sarcomas. CA Cancer J Clin 44:211–247, 1994.
75. Donaldson SS, Asmar L, Breneman J, et al. Hyperfractionated radiation in children with rhabdomyosarcoma–results of an Intergroup Rhabdomyosarcoma pilot study. Int J Radiat Oncol Biol Phys 32:903–911, 1995.
76. Maurer HM, Beltangady M, Gehan EA, et al. The Intergroup Rhabdomyosarcoma Study–I. A final report. Cancer 61:209–220, 1988.
77. Maurer HM, Gehan EA, Beltangady M, et al. The Intergroup Rhabdomyosarcoma Study–II. Cancer 71:1904–1922, 1993.
78. Crist W, Gehan EA, Ragab AH, et al. The Third Intergroup Rhabdomyosarcoma Study. J Clin Oncol 13:610–630, 1995.
79. Ruymann F, Crist W, Wiener E, et al. Comparison of two doublet chemotherapy regimens and conventional radiotherapy in metastatic rhabdomyosarcoma: improved overall survival using ifosfamide/etoposide compared to vincristine/melphalan in IRSG-IV [abstract 1874]. Proc Am Soc Clin Oncol 16:521a, 1997.
80. Vietti T, Crist W, Ruby E, et al. Topotecan window in patients with rhabdomyosarcoma: an IRSG study [abstract 1837]. Proc Am Soc Clin Oncol 16:510, 1997.
81. Skinner R, Sharkey IM, Pearson ADJ, et al. Ifosfamide, mesna, and nephrotoxicity in children. J Clin Oncol 11:173–190, 1993.
82. Loebstein R, Koren G. Ifosfamide-induced nephrotoxicity in children: critical review of pediatric risk factors. Pediatrics 101:E8, 1998.
83. Rodary C, Gehan EA, Flamant F, et al. Prognostic factors in 951 nonmetastatic rhabdomyosarcoma in children: a report from the International Rhabdomyosarcoma Workshop. Med Pediatr Oncol 19:89–95, 1991.
84. Tsokos M, Webber B, Parham DM, et al. Rhabdomyosarcoma. A new classification scheme related to prognosis. Arch Pathol Lab Med 116:847–855, 1992.
85. Link MP, Eilber F. Osteosarcoma. In: Pizzo PA, Poplack DG, eds. Principles and practice of pediatric oncology. 3rd ed. Philadelphia: Lippincott-Raven, 1997:889–920.
86. Whelan JS. Osteosarcoma. Eur J Cancer 33:1611–1619, 1997.
87. Meyers PA, Gorlick R. Osteosarcoma. Pediatr Clin North Am 44:973–989, 1997.
88. Eilber F, Giuliano A, Eckardt J, et al. Adjuvant chemotherapy for osteosarcoma: a randomized prospective trial. J Clin Oncol 5:21–26, 1987.
89. Winkler K, Beron G, Delling G, et al. Neoadjuvant chemotherapy of osteosarcoma: results of a randomized cooperative trial (COSS-82) with salvage chemotherapy based on histological tumor response. J Clin Oncol 6:329–337, 1988.
90. Link MP, Goorin AM, Miser AW, et al. The effect of adjuvant chemotherapy on relapse-free survival in patients with osteosarcoma of the extremity. N Engl J Med 314:1600–1606, 1986.
91. Harris MB, Cantor AB, Goorin AM, et al. Treatment of osteosarcoma with ifosfamide: comparison of response in pediatric patients with recurrent disease versus patients previously untreated: a pediatric oncology group study. Med Pediatr Oncol 24:87–92, 1995.
92. Goorin A, Strother D, Poplack D, et al. Safety and efficacy of l-leucovorin rescue following high-dose methotrexate for osteosarcoma. Med Pediatr Oncol 24:362–367, 1995.
93. Voute PA, van den Berg H, Behrendt H. Ifosfamide in the treatment of pediatric malignancies. Semin Oncol 23(Suppl 7):8–11, 1996.
94. Chu E, Allegra C. Antifolates. In: Chabner BA, Longo DL, eds. Cancer chemotherapy and biotherapy. 2nd ed. Philadelphia: Lippincott-Raven, 1996:109–148.
95. Ackland SP, Schilsky RL. High-dose methotrexate: a critical reappraisal. J Clin Oncol 5:2017–2031, 1987.
96. Hudson M, Jaffe MR, Jaffe N, et al. Pediatric osteosarcoma: therapeutic strategies, results, and prognostic factors derived from a 10-year experience. J Clin Oncol 8:1988–1997, 1990.
97. Davis AM, Bell RS, Goodwin PJ. Prognostic factors in osteosarcoma: a critical review. J Clin Oncol 12:423–431, 1994.
98. Horowitz ME, Tsokos MG, DeLaney TF. Ewing's sarcoma. CA Cancer J Clin 42:300–332, 1992.
99. Grier HE. The Ewing family of tumors. Ewing's sarcoma and primitive neuroectodermal tumors. Pediatr Clin North Am 44:991–1004, 1997.
100. Horowitz ME, Malawer MM, Woo SY, et al. Ewing's sarcoma family of tumors: Ewing's sarcoma of the bone and soft tissue and the peripheral primitive neuroectodermal tumors. In: Pizzo PA, Poplack DG, eds. Principles and practice of pediatric oncology. 3rd ed. Philadelphia: Lippincott-Raven, 1997:831–863.
101. Nesbit ME, Gehan EA, Burgert EO Jr, et al. Multimodal therapy for the management of primary, nonmetastatic Ewing's sarcoma of bone: a long-term follow-up of the first intergroup study. J Clin Oncol 8:1664–1674, 1990.
102. Raney RB, Asmar L, Newton WA Jr, et al. Ewing's sarcoma of soft tissues in childhood: a report from the Intergroup Rhabdomyosarcoma Study, 1972 to 1991. J Clin Oncol 15:574–582, 1997.

103. Burgert EO Jr, Nesbit ME, Garnsey LA, et al. Multimodal therapy for the management of nonpelvic, localized Ewing's sarcoma of bone: Intergroup Study IESS-II. J Clin Oncol 8:1514–1524, 1990.
104. Jurgens H, Exner U, Kuhl J, et al. High-dose ifosfamide with mesna uroprotection in Ewing's sarcoma. Cancer Chemother Pharmacol 24(Suppl 1):S40–S44, 1989.
105. Oberlin O, Habrand JL, Zucker JM, et al. No benefit of ifosfamide in Ewing's sarcoma: a nonrandomized study of the French Society of Pediatric Oncology. J Clin Oncol 10:1407–1412, 1992.
106. Grier H, Krailo M, Link M, et al. Improved outcome in non-metastatic Ewing's sarcoma and PNET of bone with the addition of ifosfamide and etoposide to vincristine, cyclophosphamide, adriamycin, and actinomycin: a Childrens Cancer Group and Pediatric Oncology Group report [abstract 1443]. Proc Am Soc Clin Oncol 13:421, 1994.
107. Grier H, Krailo M, Tarbell N, et al. Adding ifosfamide and etoposide to vincristine, cyclophosphamide, adriamycin, and actinomycin improves outcome in non-metastatic Ewing's and PNET: update of CCG/POG study. Med Pediatr Oncol 27:259–265, 1996.
108. Wexler LH, DeLaney TF, Tsokos M, et al. Ifosfamide and etoposide plus vincristine, doxorubicin, and cyclophosphamide for newly diagnosed Ewing's sarcoma family of tumors. Cancer 78:901–911, 1996.
109. Atra A, Whelan JS, Calvagna V, et al. High-dose busulphan/melphalan with autologous stem cell rescue in Ewing's sarcoma. Bone Marrow Transplant 20:843–846, 1997.
110. Von Hoff DD, Layard MW, Basa P, et al. Risk factors for doxorubicin-induced congestive heart failure. Ann Intern Med 91:710–717, 1979.
111. Goorin AM, Borrow RW, Goldman A, et al. Congestive heart failure due to adriamycin cardiotoxicity: its natural history in children. Cancer 47:2810–2816, 1981.
112. Steinherz LJ, Steinherz PJ, Tan CTC, et al. Cardiac toxicity 4 to 20 years after completing anthracycline therapy. JAMA 266:1672–1677, 1991.
113. Hausdorf G, Morf G, Beron G, et al. Long term doxorubicin cardiotoxicity in childhood: non-invasive evaluation of the contractile state and diastolic filling. Br Heart J 60:309–315, 1988.
114. Steinherz LJ, Graham T, Hurwitz R, et al. Guidelines for cardiac monitoring of children during and after anthracycline therapy: report of the cardiology committee of the Childrens Cancer Study Group. Pediatrics 89:942–949, 1992.
115. Aparicio J, Munarriz B, Pastor M, et al. Long-term follow-up and prognostic factors in Ewing's sarcoma. A multivariate analysis of 116 patients from a single institution. Oncology 55:20–26, 1998.
116. Fagnou C, Michan J, Peter M, et al. Presence of tumor cells in bone marrow but not blood is associated with adverse prognosis in patients with Ewing's tumor. J Clin Oncol 16:1707–1711, 1998.
117. Sandoval C, Meyer WH, Parham DM, et al. Outcome in 43 children presenting with metastatic Ewing sarcoma: the St. Jude Children's Research Hospital experience, 1962 to 1992. Med Pediatr Oncol 26:180–185, 1996.
118. Donaldson SS, Egbert PR, Newsham I, et al. Retinoblastoma. In: Pizzo PA, Poplack DG, eds. Principles and practice of pediatric oncology. 3rd ed. Philadelphia: Lippincott-Raven, 1997:699–715.
119. Devesa SS. The incidence of retinoblastoma. Am J Ophthalmol 80:263–265, 1975.
120. Knudson AG Jr. Mutation and cancer: statistical study of retinoblastoma. Proc Natl Acad Sci USA 68:820, 1971.
121. Abramson DH, Frank CM, Susman M, et al. Presenting signs of retinoblastoma. J Pediatr 132:505–508, 1998.
122. Arrigg PG, Hedges TR III, Char DH. Computed tomography in the diagnosis of retinoblastoma. Br J Ophthalmol 67:588–591, 1983.
123. Reese AB, Ellsworth RM. The evaluation and current concept of retinoblastoma treatment. Trans Am Acad Ophthalmol Otolarygol 65:169–172, 1963.
124. Fontanesi J, Pratt CB, Hustu HO, et al. Use of irradiation for therapy of retinoblastoma in children more than 1 year old: the St. Jude Shildren's Research Hospital experience and review of literature. Med Pediatr Oncol 24:321–326, 1995.
125. Pradhan DG, Sandridge AL, Mullaney P, et al. Radiation therapy for retinoblastoma: a retrospective review of 120 patients. Int J Radiat Oncol Biol Phys 39:3–13, 1997.
126. Schvartzman E, Chantada G, Fandino A, et al. Results of a stage-based protocol for the treatment of retinoblastoma. J Clin Oncol 14:1532–1536, 1996.
127. White L. Chemotherapy for retinoblastoma: where do we go from here? Ophthalmic Paediatr Genet 12:115–130, 1991.
128. Shields CL, De Potter P, Himelstein BP, et al. Chemoreduction in the initial management of intraocular retinoblastoma. Arch Ophthalmol 114:1330–1338, 1996.
129. Namouni F, Doz F, Tanguy ML, et al. High-dose chemotherapy with carboplatin, etoposide and cyclophosphamide followed by a haematopoietic stem cell rescue in patients with high-risk retinoblastoma: a SFOP and SFGM study. Eur J Cancer 33:2368–2375, 1997.
130. Wong FL, Boice JD Jr, Abramson DH, et al. Cancer incidence after retinoblastoma. Radiation dose and sarcoma risk. JAMA 278:1262–1267, 1997.

CHAPTER 94

GYNECOLOGIC CANCERS

Janet A. Lyle

In 1998 there were approximately 80,400 new cases of gynecologic cancer and 27,100 gynecologic cancer deaths in the United States. Together, they are the fourth most common cause of cancer death in women, preceded by lung, breast, and colorectal cancers.[1] This chapter focuses on the three most common gynecologic cancers: ovarian, endometrial, and cervical. The other gynecologic cancers (vulvar, vaginal, and gestational trophoblastic diseases) are less common.

TREATMENT GOALS: GYNECOLOGICAL CANCERS

- Prevent gynecologic cancer by recognizing and avoiding any identified risk factors.
- Detect early; many cancers, especially cervical and endometrial cancers, may be curable if detected early, and cancers usually are more responsive to therapy when disease is limited.
- Cure the patient.
- Prolong survival.
- Maintain the patient's functional status and quality of life.
- Relieve disease symptoms.

Ovarian Cancer

Ovarian cancer is the second most common gynecologic cancer and the leading cause of gynecologic cancer death in the United States. In 1998 there were an estimated 25,400 new cases of ovarian cancer, with 14,500 deaths attributed to the disease.[1] The lifetime risk of developing ovarian cancer in the United States is approximately 1.5%, and 1 woman in 100 die of this disease.[2]

EPIDEMIOLOGY

Etiology

Although the cause of ovarian cancer is unknown, several risk factors have been identified. The most identifiable risk factors are nulliparity or low parity and unsuppressed ovulation. Women who have had at least two children have a 30% lower ovarian cancer risk. Each additional pregnancy decreases the risk by another 10 to 15%. Using oral contraceptives also protects against ovarian cancer and may reduce the risk by up to 30 to 60% depending on the duration of use.[2,3] Use of the infertility drug clomiphene for more than 1 year has been shown to increase the risk of borderline and invasive ovarian tumors twofold to threefold.[4]

Incidence

The highest incidence of ovarian cancer occurs in industrialized countries, particularly northern and western Europe and North America. The exception is Japan, which has one of the lowest rates of ovarian cancer in the world. Environmental factors appear to play a role because Japanese women who have migrated to the United States have a risk of ovarian cancer that by the second generation approaches the rate of white women born in the United States. Asbestos and talc are the two main industrial chemicals associated with an increased risk. Until recently, most talc powders contained asbestos. When applied on the perineum, talc can be absorbed through the vagina or cervix, reaching the ovaries by retrograde flow. A diet that is high in meat and animal fat has also been implicated as a causative factor in some studies.[2,3]

Risk Factors

The most important risk factor for ovarian cancer is a family history of ovarian cancer. A small subset of ovarian cancer cases have a genetic link and appear to be inherited as an autosomal dominant trait. Although hereditary ovarian cancer constitutes only 5 to 10% of the total ovarian cancer cases, women with two or more first-degree relatives with ovarian cancer may have up to a 50% chance of developing the disease. In contrast, a woman with no family member with ovarian cancer has only a 4 to 5% chance of developing the disease.[2] Three hereditary patterns of ovarian cancer have been identified: site-specific ovarian cancer, breast and ovarian cancer, and ovarian cancer associated with colorectal cancer. In patients with the breast and ovarian cancer syndrome, there is a 50% higher risk of ovarian cancer among women who have a history of breast cancer and vice versa. The gene responsible for most cases of this syndrome has been identified as BRCA1, located on chromosome 17q.[2,5]

PATHOPHYSIOLOGY

Histology

The most common malignant ovarian tumor is epithelial ovarian cancer, representing more than 90% of cases; the remainder are stromal tumors (less than 10%) and germ cell tumors (2 to 3%). Epithelial ovarian cancer occurs most often in postmenopausal women, with a peak incidence in the 50- to 70-year range. Black women in the United States have a lower incidence than white women. Stromal tumors tend to be detected at earlier stages and have a more benign course. The mean age of women developing these tumors is 40 years. Usually they are treated with surgery because the response to radiation or chemotherapy is poor. Although germ cell tumors are uncommon, they are important because they occur in young women of childbearing potential and are highly curable. The peak incidence occurs in the early 20s, with a higher incidence in Asian and black women. Many tend to be highly aggressive, but most present at an early stage and are very responsive to treatment with surgery and chemotherapy.[2] Only epithelial cell ovarian cancer is addressed in this chapter.

Pathogenesis

Tumor dissemination occurs primarily by contiguous growth, surface shedding, and lymphatic spread. Hematogenous spread of ovarian cancer is rare. The tumor originates and grows in the ovary and invades the ovarian capsule. Pelvic structures become involved by direct contact with the tumor. The tumor can shed cells into the peritoneal cavity, whether or not the capsule is disrupted. These cells are carried by the peritoneal fluid to sites on the peritoneal surfaces, where they form micrometastases. Free-floating tumor cells are removed from the peritoneal cavity by lymphatic channels in the diaphragm. Tumor spread also occurs via the lymphatics from the ovary. Therefore, common sites of tumor spread include the peritoneum, diaphragm, omentum, bowel surfaces, and retroperitoneal lymph nodes. Distant organs at risk include the liver, lungs, pleura, kidneys, bone, adrenal glands, bladder, and spleen in decreasing order of frequency.[2,6] Impaired pleural lymphatic drainage may result in malignant pleural effusions, which can be the first extraperitoneal sign of ovarian cancer.[6]

CLINICAL PRESENTATION AND DIAGNOSIS

Signs and Symptoms

Ovarian cancer usually is asymptomatic in its early stages, and only 15 to 25% of cases are confined to the ovaries at the time of diagnosis. Because the ovaries are in a spacious pelvic cavity, the tumor can grow considerably before producing symptoms. When symptoms do develop, they usually are a sign of advanced disease and may include nausea, dyspepsia, vaginal bleeding, abdominal distension, or lower abdominal discomfort, usually nonspecific and intermittent.[2] Unfortunately, these symptoms often are confused with gastrointestinal disease and treated symptomatically. It is therefore essential that women with lower abdominal symptoms have a thorough physical and pelvic exam, especially perimenopausal or postmenopausal women who have other risk factors for ovarian cancer.

Diagnosis

If an ovarian mass is detected on pelvic exam, the diagnostic workup usually includes an ultrasound to characterize ovarian enlargement. Transvaginal ultrasound is a useful, noninvasive procedure that can define disease in the pelvis and differentiate ascites from an ovarian cyst. A computed tomography (CT) scan may be helpful in obtaining additional diagnosis and staging information when combined with oral and intravenous contrast. Peritoneal cytology, whereby ascitic fluid is aspirated to identify malignant cells, is another technique that may be useful in diagnosing ovarian cancer, but it is not used routinely in the United States.[2] Efforts to develop a screening test for ovarian cancer have focused on imaging methods such as transvaginal ultrasound, but cost and a high rate of false-positive results have limited its usefulness as a screening tool. Color flow Doppler imaging is being used to differentiate benign from malignant ovarian tumors based on differences in vascularity between normal and malignant tissue.[7]

Tumor markers that can detect disease are a helpful monitoring tool. CA-125 is the most useful marker for ovarian cancer. This antigen, identified by a monoclonal antibody to human ovarian cancer, is common to most epithelial ovarian cancers. It is elevated (more than 35 U/mL) in more than 80% of patients with this type of ovarian cancer but in only 1% of the normal population. Unfortunately, it is a nonspecific indicator, and elevated levels can be seen in patients with other gynecologic cancers and in patients with benign conditions such as pancreatitis, endometriosis, pelvic inflammatory disease, and cirrhosis.[7] It is also associated with a significant number of false negatives in early disease. For this reason it is not a useful screening tool alone for the diagnosis of ovarian cancer. CA-125 does correlate with the stage and extent of disease and is useful in monitoring the response to therapy in patients who have elevated levels at the time of diagnosis. Patients with CA-125 levels that remain elevated after a course of chemotherapy are likely to have a residual tumor. Conversely, a fall in CA-125 after chemotherapy has been associated with increased patient survival.[8] Other tumor markers that may be useful in ovarian cancer are listed in Table 94.1. Macrophage colony-stimulating factor (M-CSF) and the OVX1 antigen, which is present on high–molecular-weight mucin, have been found to be complementary with CA-125.[9] The hope is that a combination of tumor markers, especially OVX1 and CA-125, will improve the sensitivity of early detection and prove to be effective in ovarian cancer screening. Because no current screening tool is effective in diagnosing early stage ovarian cancer, prophylactic oophorectomies should be considered after age 35, if childbearing is complete, for women in high-risk groups.[5]

Table 94.1 ▪ Clinically Useful Tumor Markers in Ovarian Cancer

Marker	Types of Tumor Identified
CA-125	Nonmucinous epithelial ovarian cancer
CA 19-9	Mucinous epithelial ovarian cancer
Carcinoembryonic antigen	Mucinous epithelial ovarian cancer
NB70K	Mucinous epithelial ovarian cancer
Lipid-associated sialic acid	Advanced stage epithelial ovarian cancer
Interleukin 6	Advanced stage epithelial ovarian cancer
Interleukin 10	Advanced stage epithelial ovarian cancer
Macrophage colony-stimulating factor	Nonmucinous epithelial ovarian cancer
OVX1 antigen	Nonmucinous epithelial ovarian cancer
α-Fetoprotein	Endodermal sinus tumor Embryonal cell carcinoma
Human chorionic gonadotropin	Ovarian choriocarcinoma Embryonal cell carcinoma Mixed germ cell tumors
Lactate dehydrogenase	Dysgerminoma

Source: Deppe G. Ovarian cancer: advances in management. Surg Clin North Am 71:1285–1302, 1991.

TREATMENT

Pharmacotherapy

Initial Therapy

Chemotherapy has become the most common form of therapy for patients with advanced ovarian cancer. Numerous chemotherapeutic agents (Table 94.2) from a variety of classes are effective, but the alkylating agents such as cyclophosphamide, melphalan, and chlorambucil were the first agents with documented activity, producing objective response rates of approximately 40% when used as single agents. However, 5-year survival was poor (less than 10%) for patients with advanced disease.

In the late 1970s, cisplatin was considered the most active agent in treating ovarian cancer, with overall response rates of 60% and complete response rates of 20 to 40% when used as a single agent.[10] Significant side effects include nausea and vomiting, nephrotoxicity, ototoxicity, peripheral neuropathy, and bone marrow suppression. A meta-analysis of 45 clinical trials of chemotherapy in ovarian cancer demonstrated better response and survival rates with cisplatin-based regimens than with chemotherapy regimens not containing cisplatin.[11] There was also a modest survival benefit when cisplatin combination regimens were compared with cisplatin monotherapy. The standard chemotherapeutic regimen for advanced ovarian cancer became six cycles of the two-drug combination of cisplatin and another alkylating agent, cyclophosphamide. Response rates ranged from 60 to 80%, with complete remission rates of 20 to 25%.

Many studies have concluded that carboplatin can be substituted for cisplatin as first-line therapy with no difference in response rates, disease-free progression, or

Table 94.2 ▪ Commonly Used Chemotherapeutic Agents in Gynecologic Cancers

Drug	Dosage	Dosage Adjustment	Side Effects	Comments
Cisplatin	50–100 mg/m^2	Reduce if CrCl <50 mL/min.	Severe nausea and vomiting, myelosuppression, peripheral neuropathy, ototoxicity, nephrotoxicity	Vigorous hydration decreases risk of nephrotoxicity.
Carboplatin	Area under the curve of 6–7	Reduce if CrCl <60 mL/min, avoid if <15 mL/min.	Neutropenia, thrombocytopenia	400 mg/m^2 is equivalent to cisplatin 100 mg/m^2.
Cyclophosphamide	500–750 mg/m^2	Reduce if CrCl <50 mL/min.	Myelosuppression, hemorrhagic cystitis	Hydration decreases the risk of hemorrhagic cystitis.
Ifosfamide	1000–1500 mg/m^2/day for 5 days		Myelosuppression, hemorrhagic cystitis, CNS toxicity	Must be administered with MESNA to avoid hemorrhagic cystitis.
Doxorubicin	40–60 mg/m^2	Reduce if bilirubin >1.5 mg/dl; avoid if bilirubin >5 mg/dl	Myelosuppression, mucositis, cardiotoxicity	Vesicant; cardiac toxicity is cumulative; dosage should not exceed 550 mg/m^2.
Paclitaxel	135–175 mg/m^2		Myelosuppression, flulike symptoms, alopecia, flushing	Hypersensitivity reactions are caused by the cremophor vehicle and are reduced with premedications.
Altretamine	260 mg/m^2/day PO, 14–21 days every 28 days		Nausea, vomiting, peripheral neuropathy, CNS toxicity	Gastrointestinal toxicity can be reduced by giving the dose after meals.
Topotecan	1.5 mg/m^2/day × 5		Myelosuppression	

CrCl, creatinine clearance; *MESNA,* 2-mercaptoethanesulfonate; *CNS,* central nervous system.

survival rates.[10,11] Carboplatin is a second-generation platinum compound that is less nephrotoxic, ototoxic, neurotoxic, and emetogenic than cisplatin and is therefore easier to administer and tolerate. The combination of carboplatin and cyclophosphamide was compared with cisplatin and cyclophosphamide in two large North American trials.[12,13] Both studies demonstrated a better therapeutic index with the carboplatin-containing regimen and no difference in survival. The combination of carboplatin and cyclophosphamide became an accepted first-line therapy for advanced ovarian cancer. Carboplatin is more myelosuppressive than cisplatin, however, and can cause significant thrombocytopenia. Consideration should be given to switching to cisplatin rather than compromising the carboplatin dosage if severe myelosuppression occurs because the colony-stimulating factors (e.g., granulocyte CSF, granulocyte–macrophage CSF) are not useful in preventing or treating thrombocytopenia. Although a carboplatin dosage of 400 mg/m^2 is therapeutically equivalent to 100 mg/m^2 cisplatin, many investigators now use the Calvert formula[14] to calculate a carboplatin dosage based on a target area under the curve (AUC) as follows:

$$\text{Dosage (mg)} = \text{Target AUC (Glomerular filtration rate } + 25)$$

Unlike cisplatin, approximately 70% of the carboplatin is excreted in the urine, primarily by glomerular filtration. Thus, pretreatment renal function has a direct effect on efficacy and toxicity of carboplatin. The glomerular filtration rate can be measured directly or can be estimated by using creatinine clearance. A target AUC of 6 to 7 is used to maximize the dosage of carboplatin without causing excessive toxicity.

Doxorubicin has a response rate of approximately 30% as a first-line single agent in ovarian cancer and has also been extensively studied in combination chemotherapy regimens. Four major randomized trials have compared cisplatin plus cyclophosphamide with or without doxorubicin in advanced ovarian cancer. Individually, there were no significant differences in complete remission, disease-free progression, or overall survival.[10] However, a meta-analysis of these trials documented a 7% survival advantage for patients receiving the doxorubicin-containing regimens.[15] It is unclear whether this occurred because doxorubicin was added or because the dosages of cisplatin and cyclophosphamide in the three-drug regimen were greater than those in the two-drug regimens in three of the trials. Because there is only a modest survival benefit and doxorubicin greatly increases the toxicity of the regimen (e.g., myelosuppression, cardiotoxicity, mucositis), the combination of a platinum compound and cyclophosphamide remained first-line therapy for advanced ovarian cancer.

More recently, paclitaxel has been shown to have significant activity in advanced ovarian cancer. Its unique mechanism of action involves binding to and stabilizing cellular microtubules, thereby inhibiting mitosis. Very high response rates have been documented in heavily pretreated patients. Significant side effects include bone marrow suppression, alopecia, myalgias, and peripheral neuropathy. Pretreatment with dexamethasone 10 to 20 mg, diphenhydramine 25 to 50 mg, and cimetidine 300 mg can reduce the incidence of hypersensitivity reactions, which are thought to be secondary to the cremophor vehicle or a rapid infusion rate. Given the high activity of paclitaxel in recurrent disease, it was evaluated as first-line therapy in advanced ovarian cancer treatment. A pivotal trial compared cisplatin and cyclophosphamide with cisplatin and a 24-hour infusion of paclitaxel.[16] The overall response rates were 73% versus 60%, progression-free survival 18 months versus 13 months, and overall survival 38 months versus 24 months, respectively, favoring the paclitaxel arm. This trial established a new standard regimen for patients with advanced ovarian cancer. Paclitaxel followed by cisplatin results in less neutropenia and equal efficacy and is therefore the preferred sequence of administration.[17] Another study, conducted in women previously treated with a platinum-containing regimen, concluded that a 3-hour paclitaxel infusion was as effective as a 24-hour infusion with reduced myelosuppression.[18] This mode of administration is more convenient for outpatient administration and has not been associated with an increased incidence of hypersensitivity reactions. The incidence of neurotoxicity and ototoxicity is similar in patients who receive either cisplatin and cyclophosphamide or cisplatin and paclitaxel.[17,19] These side effects do not appear to be a function of infusion rate. Two recent studies have demonstrated the safety and effectiveness of combined paclitaxel and carboplatin in patients with recurrent ovarian cancer and in chemotherapy-naive stage III and IV ovarian cancer.[20,21] The overall response rates were 75 and 78%, with complete response rates of 67 and 61%, respectively. Because the combination of paclitaxel and carboplatin is highly effective, easy to administer, and well tolerated, it is now considered first-line therapy in advanced ovarian cancer. Questions remain about the proper infusion rate and dosage of paclitaxel, however. Combination chemotherapy regimens used to treat ovarian cancer are described in Table 94.3.

Salvage Therapy

Although the majority of patients achieve a complete remission after induction chemotherapy, 40 to 50% of patients with advanced disease relapse within 2 years after platinum-based chemotherapy.[10] Patients who relapse after initial platinum-based chemotherapy or have bulky residual disease after therapy are candidates for salvage chemotherapy. The likelihood of a response to salvage chemotherapy in ovarian cancer is influenced by the initial response to chemotherapy and the time interval to recurrence. The longer the treatment-free interval, the greater the response rate. Retreatment with platinum-based chemotherapy has an established role for patients who initially responded to this therapy and have had a disease-free interval of at least 6 months. Patients who did not respond to platinum-based chemotherapy or who have a short disease-free interval should be treated with paclitaxel. Overall response rates of 30 to 40% have been documented with paclitaxel monotherapy in heavily pretreated patients with recurrent disease.[10] Responses are seen in patients who have platinum-sensitive and platinum-resistant disease. An overall response rate of 53% has been demonstrated in patients with recurrent ovarian cancer treated with the combination of paclitaxel and cisplatin and a median survival of more than 23 months for responders.[22] Patients who do not respond to platinum- or paclitaxel-based chemotherapy can be treated with single-agent salvage therapy or are encouraged to enter a clinical trial.

Table 94.3 ▪ Selected Regimens for Epithelial Ovarian Cancer

CP	Cyclophosphamide 750 mg/m² IV day 1 Cisplatin 75 mg/m² IV day 1 Repeat cycle every 28 days
CC	Cyclophosphamide 600 mg/m² IV day 1 Carboplatin AUC 6–7 IV day 1 Repeat cycle every 28 days
CT	Cisplatin 75 mg/m² IV day 1 Paclitaxel 135 mg/m² IV over 24 hr day 1 or Paclitaxel 175 mg/m² IV over 3 hr day 1 Repeat cycle every 21 days
Carbo-Taxol	Carboplatin AUC 6–7 IV day 1 Paclitaxel 135 mg/m² IV over 24 hr day 1 or Paclitaxel 175 mg/m² IV over 3 hr day 1 Repeat cycle every 21 days
CAP	Cyclophosphamide 500 mg/m² IV day 1 Doxorubicin 50 mg/m² IV day 1 Cisplatin 50 mg/m² IV day 1 Repeat cycle every 21 days

AUC, area under the curve.

Other agents that have documented activity as salvage therapy include altretamine (hexamethylmelamine), ifosfamide, etoposide, and tamoxifen. Oral etoposide as second-line therapy produced a 26.8% response rate (7.3% complete response) in platinum-resistant patients and a 34.1% response rate (14.6% complete response) in platinum-sensitive patients.[23] It is administered daily for 3 out of every 4 weeks and is tolerated fairly well. Myelosuppression is the dose-limiting side effect. The overall response rate for the other agents generally is less than 20%, with a median duration of response of approximately 8 months.[2,10] Of these, altretamine (hexamethylmelamine) is the only drug approved for this indication. It is administered orally in four divided doses but gastrointestinal (nausea, vomiting, diarrhea) and central nervous system (peripheral neuropathy, agitation, confusion) side effects may be dose limiting. Several new agents have been evaluated in advanced ovarian cancer. Topotecan is a new topoisomerase I inhibitor that inhibits relaxation of supercoiled DNA, resulting in single- and double-stranded DNA breaks. The dose-limiting toxicity is myelosuppression, especially neutropenia and thrombocytopenia, but the nonhematologic side effects are mild. It was recently approved as second-line therapy in advanced ovarian cancer. Response rates of 13.8 to 20.5% were documented in three large clinical trials in women who either did not respond to or relapsed after platinum-based chemotherapy. Response to topotecan was higher in platinum-sensitive patients.[24] Another trial showed no statistically significant difference in efficacy between topotecan and paclitaxel in patients who did not respond to or relapsed after platinum-based chemotherapy, but there was a trend in favor of topotecan for overall response rate, time to disease progression, and survival.[25] Gemcitabine is a pyrimidine analog that resembles cytarabine (ARA-C) and works by competing with the natural nucleotide deoxycytidine triphosphate for incorporation into DNA. It is approved for treating pancreatic cancer, but a 19% response rate was seen in a phase II study in platinum-resistant patients with ovarian cancer.[26] It has a mild side effect profile that includes myelosuppression (dose limiting), flulike symptoms, peripheral edema, rash, and elevated liver function tests. Another taxane, docetaxel, has shown similar activity to paclitaxel, but with considerably more toxicity.[10] The drug can cause peripheral edema, pleural effusions, skin toxicity, peripheral neuropathy, and severe lethargy. The prophylactic use of dexamethasone can reduce the incidence of fluid retention and skin toxicity with this agent.

Intraperitoneal Chemotherapy

Intraperitoneal chemotherapy was selected as a potential treatment for ovarian cancer because the disease spreads primarily within the peritoneal cavity, and direct intraperitoneal instillation of chemotherapy achieves extremely high concentrations at the site of the tumor while minimizing systemic toxicity of the drug. Optimal agents for intraperitoneal therapy have a high molecular weight and low lipid solubility, are slowly cleared from the peritoneal cavity, and are minimally toxic to the peritoneum. Cisplatin appears to be the drug of choice for intraperitoneal administration, achieving a peritoneal cavity to plasma concentration ratio of 10 to 20. A study comparing intraperitoneal and intravenous cisplatin, in addition to intravenous cyclophosphamide, in optimally debulked stage III ovarian cancer showed a higher response rate in the intraperitoneal arm (47% versus 36%) and an 8-month survival advantage.[27] In addition, there were significantly fewer toxic effects in the patients receiving intraperitoneal therapy. However, this study was initiated before paclitaxel became available. The peritoneal route of paclitaxel has also been studied, achieving levels in the peritoneal cavity approximately 1000 times greater than those in the plasma. Early results with intraperitoneal use show promising results (61% complete response) in patients with microscopic residual disease.[28]

Intraperitoneal therapy involves instilling chemotherapeutic agents directly into the peritoneal cavity through a specialized catheter or a surgically placed subcutaneous port. The drug usually is diluted into 1.5 to 2 L normal saline to ensure adequate distribution throughout the cavity. It is then instilled over 30 to 60 minutes and the remainder usually is removed after a dwell time of approximately 6 hours. The most common complications are catheter failure, abdominal pain, and peritonitis. Limitations of intraperitoneal therapy include variability of drug distribution throughout the peritoneal cavity, limited ability of agents to penetrate into tumor nodules, adequacy of drug delivery to tumor after regional drug delivery, and limited ability of high concentrations of chemotherapy within the peritoneal cavity to overcome drug resistance.[29] Potential candidates for intraperitoneal therapy include patients with early stage, high-grade lesions, patients with very small residual disease after systemic chemotherapy, or patients with negative findings at second-look surgery, but it remains an investigational procedure. There is no evidence of substantial activity in patients with bulky residual disease.

High-Dose Therapy

A significant dose–response relationship exists for cisplatin used to treat ovarian cancer over a dosage range of 25 to 100 mg/m^2. Dose-limiting side effects, especially peripheral neuropathy, limit dosages to 100 mg/m^2, and there is no evidence that a cisplatin dosage greater than 75 mg/m^2 per cycle should be used in combination chemotherapy regimens.[2] Consequently, most clinical trials of high-dose chemotherapy focus on carboplatin, the dose-limiting effect of which is bone marrow suppression. Carboplatin is an ideal candidate for high-dose chemotherapy regimens with hematopoietic growth factors (granulocyte CSF, granulocyte–macrophage CSF) and peripheral stem cell rescue. It has been used in combination with other alkylating agents, such as cyclophosphamide, melphalan, or thiotepa, in various high-dose regimens for ovarian cancer. The overall response of high-dose chemotherapy regimens is 71%, with a 43% complete response rate. Although the response rates are high, the median time to progression is 6 months, with only 14% of patients disease free at 1 year.[30] Progression-free survival and overall survival were 7 and 13 months, respectively, for patients with advanced ovarian cancer treated with high-dose carboplatin, mitoxantrone, and cyclophosphamide followed by autologous stem cell transplant.[31] Both values were higher in patients with a low tumor burden and platinum-sensitive disease. These patients seem to be the best candidates for high-dose therapy with hematologic support, but additional randomized clinical trials are needed to evaluate this therapy before it can be used in routine practice.

Nonpharmacologic Therapy

Surgery

Early Disease Surgery

Surgery is sufficient for treating well-differentiated stage IA and IB ovarian tumors. These tumors are associated with an excellent patient survival, and additional therapy is not needed. After a thorough staging laparotomy, patients undergo a total abdominal hysterectomy, bilateral salpingo-oophorectomy, omentectomy, and any tumor debulking that can be accomplished. The uterus and contralateral ovary can be preserved in selected patients with early disease who want to preserve fertility if optimal staging was achieved.[32] Patients with poorly differentiated tumors (grade 3), dense adhesions, or stage IC or II disease have a higher risk of relapse and need additional therapy with systemic chemotherapy. Intra-abdominal radiation and radioactive phosphorus have also been used as adjuvants to surgery in early ovarian cancer but with much less enthusiasm in the United States.[6,33]

Advanced Disease Surgery

Patients with advanced disease at the time of the staging laparotomy should undergo surgery to remove as much of the primary tumor and metastatic disease as possible (cytoreductive surgery). Because complete disease removal usually is not possible, the goal is to reduce the tumor size to less than 2 cm in diameter, which can improve patient comfort and leave fewer cancer cells to be eradicated by chemotherapy. Cytoreduction improves blood supply to the tumor and causes a higher percentage of resting tumor cells to become actively dividing cells, which increases sensitivity to subsequent chemotherapy or radiation therapy.[6] It may also remove any existing resistant tumor clones.[32] Optimal debulking surgery is feasible in 70 to 90% of patients when performed by a specialist in gynecologic oncology. This is important because the volume of disease left after cytoreductive surgery has a significant impact on patient survival.[34] When optimal debulking at presentation cannot be performed, surgery may be done after a brief course of chemotherapy to make the disease operable. A large, randomized trial demonstrated a 6-month improvement in progression-free and overall survival in patients who underwent optimal debulking after three cycles of chemotherapy.[35]

A second-look operation may be helpful in evaluating the peritoneal cavity for evidence of disease. This procedure is a surgical laparotomy in a patient with no clinical evidence of disease after primary surgery and subsequent chemotherapy and is intended to determine the response to therapy. Less invasive assessments of patient response such as a CT scan and CA-125 determination are not reliable in detecting residual tumor. Patients with residual disease at the time of surgery may benefit from further cytoreductive surgery, which can improve disease status before salvage chemotherapy. A negative second look can also identify patients with chemotherapy-sensitive tumors who may be candidates for further consolidation therapy.[2,32] However, the direct benefit of second-look operations remains controversial. Ovarian cancer recurs in 30 to 50% of patients regardless of whether a pathologic complete response is achieved on second look. The procedure may also miss microscopic disease or cancer that has spread beyond the abdominal cavity. The operation is a major surgical procedure with inherent complications, and traditional second-line therapies have not demonstrated a significant effect on overall survival.[32,36] The recent development of more effective second-line and salvage therapies may add to the potential value of second-look operations in ovarian cancer management, but at this time there is little justification for a second-look laparotomy outside a clinical trial setting. A framework for using second-look laparotomy to manage ovarian cancer is outlined in Figure 94.1.

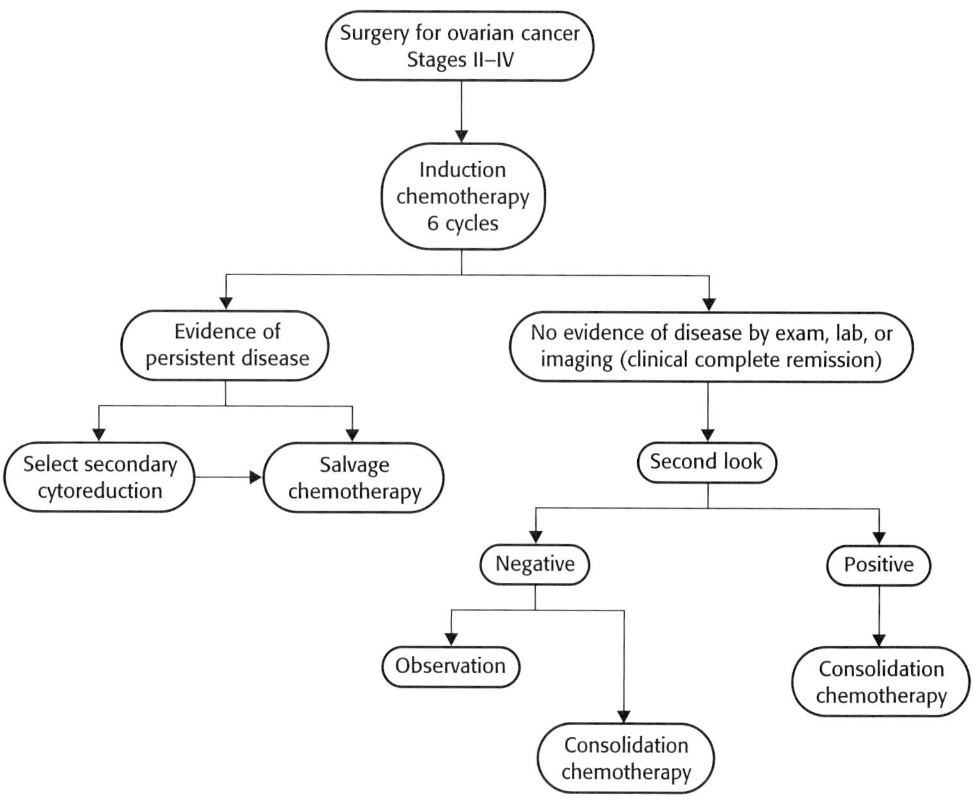

Figure 94.1. Algorithm for using second-look laparotomy to manage ovarian cancer.

Radiation Therapy

Radiation may be used as primary adjuvant therapy (additional therapy administered after the primary tumor mass has been eliminated by the initial treatment modality) after surgery in patients with stage I or early stage II ovarian cancer or in a study setting after a negative second look in advanced disease. Radiation must be directed to both the pelvis and the upper abdomen to prevent relapses throughout the peritoneal cavity. Many normal tissues such as the kidney and the liver are also radiosensitive, a situation that limits the dosage of radiation that can be administered safely. The dosage of radiation depends on the size of the tumor and is fractionated into multiple doses delivered over several weeks. For whole-abdomen radiation, the standard dosage is 2500 to 3000 cGy to the abdomen and 4500 cGy to the pelvis, areas of macroscopic disease and areas at higher risk of relapse. The overall toxicity and complexity of whole-abdomen radiation and the effectiveness of chemotherapy have limited its usefulness for early stage ovarian cancer, and its role has declined in the United States in recent years. In advanced disease, radiation usually is reserved for inoperable tumors that are unresponsive to chemotherapy or as salvage therapy for persistent or symptomatic disease. It is also being explored in combination with chemotherapy in advanced and optimally debulked disease.[2,37]

The most common side effect of radiation therapy for ovarian cancer is radiation enteritis. This syndrome is dose-related and may include diarrhea, nausea, vomiting, and weight loss. These gastrointestinal symptoms usually subside a few weeks after therapy completion. Radiation-induced hepatitis and nephritis can occur with dosages greater than 2500 cGy, especially if precautions have not been taken to minimize organ exposure during treatment. The most serious complication is small bowel obstruction, which usually warrants surgical correction. Radiation may also cause bone marrow suppression with a subsequent reduction in peripheral blood counts, which return to normal after therapy cessation. However, irradiated bone marrow can remain impaired for extended periods, and this should be considered for patients who may later receive myelosuppressive chemotherapy.[2]

Radioactive phosphorus (^{32}P) or chromic phosphate is a radioisotope that emits β-particles with a tissue penetration range of 1 to 2 mm. It has a half-life of 14.3 days. Intraperitoneal ^{32}P instillation can sterilize microscopic peritoneal tumor but cannot effectively treat larger tumors.[2] Unfortunately, distribution may be quite variable within the peritoneal cavity because of adhesions or loculations that are secondary to surgery. The usual ^{32}P dosage is 10 to 20 mCi, diluted in 1 to 1.5 L saline, which is instilled into the peritoneal cavity. This delivers approximately 6000 cGy of radiation to the peritoneum and approximately 7000 cGy to the omentum.[33] Side effects include abdominal pain (15 to 20%), peritonitis (2 to 3%), and small bowel obstruction (5 to 10%). Because of its low toxicity, it can be useful as adjuvant therapy in patients with negative second-look operations. The difficulty in administering ^{32}P, the maldistribution of radioisotopes, and the incidence of late bowel complications have reduced enthusiasm for this therapy in early stage ovarian cancer. In addition, ^{32}P therapy does not have a survival advantage over cisplatin-based chemotherapy.[33,37]

Table 94.4 ▪ Comprehensive Staging Laparotomy for Suspected Early Ovarian Carcinoma

Vertical incision that allows adequate visualization and palpation of structures in the upper abdomen and retroperitoneum
Peritoneal washings (pelvis, paracolic gutters, hemidiaphragms)
Inspection and palpation of all peritoneal and mesenteric surfaces
Biopsy of any lesions or adhesions
Total abdominal hysterectomy and bilateral salpingo-oophorectomy
Infracolic omentectomy
Random peritoneal biopsies (bladder, cul de sac, bilateral pelvic peritoneum, paracolic gutters, hemidiaphragms)
Pelvic and para-aortic lymphadenectomy (inspection and palpation only are inadequate)
Appendectomy (optional)

Source: Reference 32.

Table 94.5 ▪ International Federation of Gynecology and Obstetrics Staging for Carcinoma of the Ovary

Stage I	Tumor limited to the ovaries.
Stage IA	Tumor limited to one ovary; capsule intact, no tumor on ovarian surface. No malignant cells in ascites or peritoneal washings.
Stage IB	Tumor limited to both ovaries; capsules intact, no tumor on ovarian surface. No malignant cells in ascites or peritoneal washings.
Stage IC	Tumor limited to one or both ovaries with ruptured capsule, tumor on ovarian surface, or malignant cells in ascites or peritoneal washings.
Stage II	Tumor involving one or both ovaries with pelvic extension.
Stage IIA	Extension or metastases on the uterus or tubes. No malignant cells in ascites or peritoneal washings.
Stage IIB	Extension to other pelvic tissues. No malignant cells in ascites or peritoneal washings.
Stage IIC	Tumor is either stage IIA or IIB with malignant cells in ascites or peritoneal washings.
Stage III	Tumor involving one or both ovaries with microscopically confirmed peritoneal metastasis outside the pelvis or regional lymph node metastasis. Any liver capsule metastasis.
Stage IIIA	Microscopic peritoneal metastasis beyond the pelvis.
Stage IIIB	Macroscopic peritoneal metastasis beyond the pelvis 2 cm or less in the greatest dimension.
Stage IIIC	Peritoneal metastasis beyond the pelvis more than 2 cm in the greatest dimension or regional lymph node metastasis.
Stage IV	Distant metastasis (excludes peritoneal metastasis). Any liver parenchymal metastasis. If pleural effusion is present, it must have positive cytology.

PROGNOSIS

The most significant prognostic indicators for ovarian cancer are the disease stage at the time of surgery, the amount of residual disease after initial surgical resection, and the histologic type and grade of the tumor.[2,34] Ovarian cancer warrants careful surgical exploration for proper disease staging (Table 94.4). Patients need to undergo a thorough exploratory laparotomy, which determines the location and extent of macroscopic disease. If macroscopic disease is not found, a careful search for microscopic disease is undertaken, which includes abdominal washings and multiple biopsies. The most commonly used staging classification is the International Federation of Gynecology and Obstetrics (FIGO) system, outlined in Table 95.5. Because ovarian cancer often is asymptomatic in its early stages, most patients are in FIGO stages III or IV at the time of diagnosis. If surgical exploration reveals bulky abdominal disease, then cytoreductive surgery becomes the goal rather than a staging procedure.[6] Accurate staging is critical for proper ovarian cancer management, but unfortunately inadequate staging or understaging is common. The 5-year survival rate is 60 to 90% for patients with stage I disease and 40 to 60% for patients with stage II disease. This is significantly lower in patients with stage III disease (15 to 20%) and stage IV disease (less than 5%).[2,34]

The histologic subtype also plays a role in determining patient prognosis, especially in early stage ovarian cancer. Clear cell and mucinous cell types appear to be associated with a poorer prognosis. Approximately 10 to 20% of ovarian tumors have a histologic appearance between benign cysts and malignant carcinomas and are called borderline tumors. These are associated with an 80 to 90% 5-year survival rate, regardless of the stage of the disease, and the majority of these patients are cured with surgery alone. The value of histologic grade as an independent prognostic variable is not clearly established. Tumor grade may be the most important prognostic factor in stage I disease, but its value seems to decrease in patients with advanced disease. Patients with a well-differentiated tumor (grade 1) or a moderately well-differentiated tumor (grade 2) have significantly higher 5-year survival rates than do patients with poorly differentiated tumors (grade 3).

There is an inverse relationship between the size of residual tumor after surgery and patient survival, emphasizing the importance of optimal debulking surgery. Aggressive surgical removal is also beneficial in terms of response to subsequent chemotherapy and quality of life.[34] Although there does not seem to be a correlation between the CA-125 value before the primary operation and survival, a high correlation has been demonstrated when measured 1 month after the third course of chemotherapy in patients with stage III or IV ovarian cancer.[9] Younger age and good performance status also have been identified as favorable prognostic factors.[34]

Cervical Cancer

Cancer of the cervix is the third most common female genital cancer in the United States, with an estimated 13,700 new cases of invasive cervical cancer in 1998 and 4900 deaths attributed to the disease.[1] It is one of the few types of cancers that can be prevented by an inexpensive mass screening program for detecting preinvasive lesions. Most deaths from this disease can be prevented by routine screening and early detection. Cervical cancer usually occurs in the fifth or sixth decade, but preinvasive lesions often occur in women less than 40 years of age.[38]

EPIDEMIOLOGY

Cervical cancer is more common in women of low socioeconomic status and with a smoking history. In the United States, the incidence is greatest in Native American, African American, and Hispanic American women. It is associated with sexual intercourse at a younger age, multiple sexual partners or partners who have had multiple sexual partners, pregnancy at a younger age, and multiple pregnancies.[38] Because cervical cancer has many characteristics of a sexually transmitted disease, many infectious agents have been implicated. The strongest association is with the human papillomavirus (HPV), which is now considered the biggest risk factor for cervical cancer. It has been identified in more than 90% of invasive cervical cancers. Of the more than 20 different HPV types of identified in the human genital tract, types 16 and 18 are the most common.[39]

PATHOPHYSIOLOGY

Histology

Squamous cell carcinoma makes up 80 to 90% of all cervical cancers. These are further differentiated into large cell keratinizing, large cell nonkeratinizing, and small cell nonkeratinizing cell types. Adenocarcinomas make up approximately 10% of cases, with most subtypes containing glandular features. Adenosquamous cell and small cell carcinomas are rare.[40] Invasive tumors usually are defined as exophytic or endophytic (endocervical) lesions. Exophytic lesions protrude from the cervix into the vagina, are friable, and bleed easily. They may be less extensive than they appear on first examination. Endophytic lesions are located in the endocervical canal of a normal-appearing cervix and can be more extensive than they appear. These lesions may become large enough to distend the cervix and create barrel-shaped lesions.[41]

Pathogenesis

Cervical carcinoma begins at the squamous–columnar junction between the endocervical canal and cervix, a site of continuous metaplastic change. The precursor lesion is called dysplasia or cervical intraepithelial neoplasia (CIN), which precedes the development of invasive cervical cancer. CIN is characterized by cellular immaturity and disorganization and increased mitotic change. Progression from CIN to invasive disease can be quite long, with 66% of all patients developing invasive carcinoma within 10 years. The tumor becomes invasive when it breaks through the basement membrane into the underlying tissue. Cervical cancer usually progresses in a predictable manner, and tumor dissemination generally is a function of the extent of local tumor invasion. The disease can spread by direct extension into the vagina or endometrium, then to the walls of the pelvis, the bladder, and the rectum. In addition to local invasion, tumor spread can occur through the rich lymphatic network of the cervix, which anastomoses with those of the lower uterus. It spreads initially to lymph nodes in the pelvis, then to the para-aortic lymph nodes and distant sites. The most common sites of distant spread are the lung, extrapelvic nodes, liver, and bone.[41]

CLINICAL PRESENTATION AND DIAGNOSIS

Signs and Symptoms

Patients with preinvasive cervical cancer usually are asymptomatic, and the disease is detected by a Papanicolaou (Pap) smear performed during a routine pelvic examination. Patients with early invasive disease can have symptoms of vaginal discharge or intermittent vaginal bleeding, often after coitus. As the lesion progresses, the vaginal discharge becomes more pronounced. In advanced disease, symptoms may include lower extremity edema, flank or leg pain, urinary incontinence, hematuria, and constipation, which are indicative of pelvic invasion.[41]

Diagnosis

Current recommendations are that annual pelvic examinations and Pap smear screening begin when a woman has become sexually active or reaches age. If three or more consecutive exams are normal, the Pap smear may be performed less often, at the physician's discretion, in women who are at low risk for cervical cancer. The accuracy of the Pap smear test largely depends on the quality of the specimen. Although false-negative results range from 15 to 25%, the long interval between the appearance of dysplasia and the development of invasive disease allows multiple opportunities to detect preinvasive lesions in most patients.[38] As Pap smear screening has become more prevalent, CIN is now more common than invasive cervical cancer, particularly in women younger than 50 years, and the mortality rate from cervical cancer has dropped significantly.[1]

If abnormal findings are discovered on the Pap smear, colposcopy should be performed to identify abnormal areas that warrant biopsy and to determine the extent of the lesion. The colposcope is a low-power magnification device that allows visualization of mucosal abnormalities. All visible lesions should be biopsied. Cervical conization or cone biopsy (removal of a cone-shaped portion of tissue from the cervix) is indicated when colposcopy is inadequate or when no gross lesions are visible.[38] Further evaluation may include a chest radiograph to rule out lung metastases and a pyelogram to rule out ureteral obstruction, cystoscopy, and proctoscopy. CT scan and magnetic resonance imaging (MRI) are helpful in assessing local disease but not as accurate in determining nodal involvement.[41]

TREATMENT

Pharmacotherapy

Most women with cervical cancer are cured with surgery, radiation therapy, or a combination of the two. Until recently, only patients with advanced disease or recurrent disease after surgery and radiation were candidates for chemotherapy. The goal in recurrent disease is primarily palliation. Unfortunately, response rates have remained low, partly because drug delivery is impaired by vascular damage and poor bone marrow reserve from prior pelvic radiation. Patients who have not received prior surgery or radiation have much higher response rates to chemotherapy. In addition, extrapelvic disease tends to be more responsive than disease confined to the pelvis.[42] The only statistically significant factors determining response to chemotherapy in a recent study were age and site of recurrence. Patients who were older were more likely to respond, and the response rate was almost 20% higher for patients in whom disease recurred outside the irradiated field.[43]

Single agents that have activity in cervical cancer treatment are listed in Table 94.6. Overall response rates are consistently less than 25%, and most responses are partial and of short duration. Cisplatin is regarded as the most active agent in cervical cancer, with overall response rates ranging from 18 to 31%. Doubling the dosage from 50 to 100 mg/m^2 resulted in a higher response rate, but toxicity was also higher and it had no effect on response duration or overall survival.[42] Because cisplatin is nephrotoxic, it must be given with caution to patients with advanced disease, who often have obstruction of one or more ureters and impaired renal function. Results with carboplatin as a single agent have been disappointing. Ifosfamide may be one of the most active single agents in cervical cancer, with response rates ranging from 16 to 50% in chemotherapy-naive patients. Trials evaluating the combination of ifosfamide and a platinum compound reported response rates of 50 to 62%, but ifosfamide must

Table 94.6 ▪ Single-Agent Chemotherapy for Cervical Cancer

Drug	Overall Response (%)
Alkylating agents	
Cyclophosphamide	15
Chlorambucil	25
Ifosfamide	29
Platinum compounds	
Cisplatin	22
Carboplatin	15
Antimetabolites	
Fluorouracil	20
Methotrexate	18
Plant alkaloids	
Vincristine	18
Vinorelbine	18
Paclitaxel	18
Antitumor antibiotics	
Doxorubicin	17
Bleomycin	10
Topoisomerase-1 inhibitors	
Irinotecan	21
Topotecan	18

be administered and monitored carefully to prevent the incidence of hemorrhagic cystitis. The three-drug combination of bleomycin, ifosfamide, and a platinum compound produced even higher response rates of 65 to 100% in patients without prior radiation.[44] The results from these small phase II trials prompted a large, randomized trial that compared cisplatin alone with cisplatin plus ifosfamide and cisplatin plus an investigational agent, dibromodulcitol, in advanced or recurrent squamous cell carcinoma of the cervix. Adding ifosfamide to cisplatin improved the response rate from 19 to 33% but caused significantly more toxicity (neutropenia, peripheral neuropathy, nephrotoxicity, and encephalopathy). There was also no improvement in progression-free and overall survival in any group.[45]

Among the newer chemotherapeutic agents, paclitaxel, irinotecan, and vinorelbine have significant activity in refractory cervical cancer. Although paclitaxel has demonstrated significant activity in other gynecologic malignancies, it has only moderate activity (18% response rate) in cervical cancer.[44,46] Both irinotecan and topotecan have demonstrated activity in this disease, but irinotecan has produced more favorable results. Like topotecan, it inhibits the enzyme topoisomerase I but its dose-limiting toxicity is a combination of neutropenia and diarrhea. The drug also causes significant nausea and vomiting, skin rash, and fatigue. Response rates of 15 to 24% have been documented in relapsed disease.[46] Vinorelbine is a new vinca alkaloid derived from vinblastine. An overall response rate of 18% was documented in patients with advanced or recurrent cervical cancer who had never received chemotherapy. Significant side effects included neutropenia, nausea, vomiting, stomatitis, and rarely, neurotoxicity.[47] Unfortunately, even for these newer agents, duration of response usually is only a few months, and there has been no impact on overall survival.

Despite the lack of a survival benefit with currently available chemotherapy regimens in advanced cervical cancer, several recent studies have demonstrated a significant improvement in overall survival with the combination of chemotherapy and radiation therapy for patients with locally advanced disease. Concurrent chemotherapy can inhibit the repair of sublethal damage from radiation. In addition, the cytotoxic effect may reduce the tumor bulk and lead to reoxygenation of the tumor, thereby making it more radiation sensitive. In one study, patients with bulky stage IB cervical cancer were treated with radiation therapy alone or in combination with weekly cisplatin, followed in all patients by adjuvant hysterectomy. Cervical cancer recurrence at 3 years was 21% in the cisplatin group and 37% in the radiation-only group. Overall survival was also significantly higher in the cisplatin group (83% versus 74%). The size of the tumor and the histologic grade were significant prognostic factors.[48] In another study, patients with stage IIB through IVA (or high-risk stage IB or IIA) cervical cancer were treated with either radiation therapy to the pelvis and para-aortic lymph nodes or pelvic radiation alone plus two cycles of cisplatin and fluorouracil (days 1 to 5 and 22 to 26 of radiation therapy). Disease-free survival at 5 years was 40% in the radiation-alone group and 67% in the combined therapy group. Overall survival rates were 58 and 73%, respectively.[49] The last study compared radiation therapy in combination with concurrent chemotherapy, which consisted of either cisplatin alone, cisplatin, fluorouracil, and hydroxyurea, or hydroxyurea alone in patients with stage IIB through IVA disease without para-aortic lymph node involvement. Both groups that received cisplatin had a higher rate of progression-free survival and overall survival.[50] Although moderate and severe side effects occurred more often with combined modality treatment in all of these studies (primarily hematologic and gastrointestinal), these effects were self-limiting. The results of these trials provide compelling evidence to support cisplatin-based chemotherapy in combination with radiation therapy as a new standard of care for women with locally advanced cervical cancer.

Nonpharmacologic Therapy

Superficial Ablative Therapy

Patients with CIN or stage 0 disease can be treated with superficial ablative therapy consisting of cryotherapy, laser vaporization, or a loop excision procedure. Each can be done in an outpatient setting under local anesthesia, and each is well tolerated. Overall cure rates are in the 80 to 90% range. Loop electrosurgical excision is a procedure in which a charged electrode (fine wire loop) is used to excise the lesion. It is becoming the preferred treatment because it is easily learned and inexpensive and preserves the excised lesion for histopathologic evaluation. The diagnosis and treatment can therefore be completed in one visit in most cases.[51] Patients with mild dysplasia need no further therapy because most lesions resolve spontaneously. Conization is performed when the entire lesion cannot be visualized by colposcopy, there is evidence of endocervical involvement, the biopsy is not consistent with the Pap smear results, and there is no evidence of invasive disease. Surgery and radiation are the primary treatment modalities for invasive cervical cancer and are equally effective in early disease.[41] The use of adjuvant chemotherapy in advanced disease has not been established clearly, and most chemotherapeutic agents have limited activity in cervical cancer. The treatment modalities for cervical cancer are outlined in Table 94.7.

Surgery

Surgery is the therapy of choice in early invasive cervical cancer. Patients with stage IA1 tumors (less than 3 mm depth of invasion) have a low risk of lymph node metastases and a recurrence rate of only 4.2%. A total abdominal hysterectomy without lymph node resection is recommended for these patients with what is now called microinvasive carcinoma of the cervix. Patients with stage IA2 (3 to 5 mm depth of invasion), IB1, and IIA disease have a higher incidence of lymph node metastasis, and a radical hysterectomy with pelvic lymph node dissection is recommended.[52] A 5-year survival rate of more than 90% in stage IA disease and 80 to 90% in stage IB or IIA disease can be achieved after surgery or radiation alone. Survival drops to approximately 45% for patients with stage IB or IIA disease who have pelvic lymph node involvement. Although results with surgery and radiation therapy are equivalent in this patient population, surgery usually is preferred over radiation for young and medically fit patients. Reproductive function can be preserved and vaginal atrophy and stenosis can be avoided with a surgical approach. Complications from radical hysterectomy include urinary fistula, bladder dysfunction, pulmonary embolism, small bowel obstruction, lymphocyst formation, and infection.[38]

Radiation Therapy

Radiation therapy is appropriate in all stages of cervical cancer. For early stage disease (stage IA, IB, and IIA), the choice of radiation or surgery depends on patient factors and local expertise. Appropriate indications for radiation therapy in this patient population include older women, patients who are medically inoperable, and tumors that are larger than 4 cm in diameter. Larger tumors usually have deep stromal invasion and are at high risk for lymph node involvement. Radiation also is used after surgery in early stage disease if the tumor has metastasized to pelvic or para-aortic lymph nodes. The goal in this setting is to prevent a local recurrence, but it is uncertain whether this affects overall patient survival. For all other stages of cervical cancer, radiation is the treatment of choice. The 5-year survival rate is 65 to 75% for stage IIB disease, 35 to 50% for stage IIIB disease, and 15 to 20% for stage IVA disease.[38]

Intracavitary radiation or brachytherapy may be used as a single modality to treat stage IA disease if surgery is not an option. Brachytherapy is delivered by applicators that are inserted in the vagina and uterus and arranged next to the cervix. These applicators are loaded with radioactive cesium or iridium and deliver high dosages of radiation to the primary tumor and paracervical tissues while minimizing radiation effects to the rectum and bladder. Complications of intracavitary therapy include uterine perforation and infection.[41,53] The treatment of choice for stage IB, II, or III disease is external beam irradiation combined with two or more intracavitary applications. The local failure rate was significantly reduced and the 4-year survival improved when two or more intracavitary applications were compared with one application in patients with stage IIB disease.[54] External beam irradiation treats the primary cervical tumor and the potential sites of regional spread. It is delivered to a field that includes the pelvic lymph nodes at a dosage of 150 to 200 cGy/day. The para-aortic lymph nodes are included in the radiation field if they are involved or in high-risk patients.[55] The pelvis receives a total dosage of 4000 to 5000 cGy and the tumor itself a total dosage of 7500 to 9000 cGy with the combination of external beam radiation and brachytherapy. Patients with locally advanced disease usually begin with a course of external beam therapy to shrink bulky disease before brachytherapy is initiated.

The most common side effects during external beam irradiation are acute reactions such as fatigue, diarrhea, and mild bladder irritation. Late tissue reactions may occur months or years after therapy and can include vaginal stenosis and vaginal adhesions. Visceral perforation, rectal bleeding or fistula, hematuria, ureteral stricture, and very rarely, small bowel obstruction are more serious reactions and occur in fewer than 10% of treated patients. Late tissue reactions are dose-related and may warrant hospitalization or surgery.[38,52] They are more common in patients who have had prior abdominal or pelvic surgery or chemotherapy. In an effort to decrease the incidence of late complications, hyperfractionated radiotherapy schedules were developed. Hyperfractionation consists of dosages of 110 to 160 cGy per fraction two times a day, which allows

Table 94.7 ▪ Treatment Modalities for Cervical Cancer

Stage	Treatment
IA1	Total hysterectomy or brachytherapy
IA2, IB1, IIA	Radical hysterectomy or external beam RT and brachytherapy
IB2, IIB	External beam RT +/– brachytherapy and cisplatin-based chemotherapy
III, IVA	External beam RT +/– brachytherapy and cisplatin-based chemotherapy
IVB	Chemotherapy with or without RT

RT, radiation therapy.

delivery of therapeutic dosages with less toxicity. This method of administration allows the slowly proliferating tissues in which late complications occur to repair the damaged DNA before the next dose of radiation. Their repair capacity is excellent when very small dosages of radiation are used but is lost when dosages exceed 200 cGy per dose. The principle of hyperfractionation also applies to brachytherapy.[55]

PROGNOSIS

The most significant prognostic variables in early stage cervical cancer appear to be tumor size, depth of tumor invasion, vascular invasion, and lymph node involvement.[56] Other prognostic variables include stage, tumor volume, grade, and histologic type. Unlike for ovarian cancer, the staging of cervical cancer is based on clinical assessment of the patient, not on a surgical procedure, and is described in Table 94.8. Prognosis is worse with advancing stage, but the predictive value of the staging system may result from the correlation of stage and tumor volume.[41] Tumor size can be useful in predicting behavior; larger tumors generally are associated with greater spread and a worse prognosis even in stage I disease. Positive lymph nodes indicate a larger tumor, deep invasion of the tumor, and lymphatic spread. Patients with adenocarcinoma and adenosquamous carcinoma tend to have higher rates of lymph node metastases and a less favorable prognosis than do patients with squamous-cell carcinoma of the same stage. Small cell carcinoma had a very poor prognosis. A correlation between the tumor grade and survival is stronger for adenocarcinomas than for squamous cell carcinomas, with poorly differentiated tumors associated with a worse outcome.[40] The prognosis for invasive cancers also depends on the associated HPV type. The 5-year disease-free survival was 100% for patients with intermediate-risk tumors (HPV 31, 33, 35, 52, 58), 58% for patients with HPV16-positive tumors, and 38% for patients with HPV18-positive tumors. In addition,

Table 94.8 ▪ International Federation of Gynecology and Obstetrics Staging for Carcinoma of the Cervix

Stage I	Tumor confined to the uterus (extension to corpus should be disregarded).
Stage IA	Invasive carcinoma diagnosed only by microscopy.
Stage IA1	Tumors with stromal invasion 3 mm or less in depth taken from the base of the epithelium and 7 mm or less in horizontal spread.
Stage IA2	Tumors with stromal invasion more than 3 mm and not more than 5 mm with a horizontal spread 7 mm or less.
Stage IB	Clinically visible lesion confined to the cervix or microscopic lesion greater than a stage IA2.
Stage IB1	Clinically visible lesion 4 cm or less in greatest dimension.
Stage IB2	Clinically visible lesion more than 4 cm in greatest dimension.
Stage II	Tumor invades beyond the uterus but not to the pelvic wall or to the lower third of the vagina.
Stage IIA	Tumor without parametrial invasion.
Stage IIB	Tumor with parametrial invasion.
Stage III	Tumor extends to the pelvic wall, involves the lower third of the vagina, or causes hydronephrosis or a nonfunctioning kidney.
Stage IIIA	Tumor involves the lower third of the vagina, no extension to the pelvic wall.
Stage IIIB	Tumor extends to the pelvic wall or causes hydronephrosis or nonfunctioning kidney.
Stage IV	Tumor extension beyond the true pelvis.
Stage IVA	Tumor invades the mucosa of the bladder or rectum.
Stage IVB	Distant metastasis.

HPV-negative patients tend to have a poorer prognosis than those who are HPV positive.[39] Women who are infected with the human immunodeficiency virus are a unique subset of patients who are at risk for cervical carcinoma. These patients present with more advanced disease, have a poorer response to treatment, and overall have a poorer prognosis.[57]

Endometrial Cancer

Endometrial cancer is the most common gynecologic malignancy in the United States, representing almost half of all new cases diagnosed annually. Although approximately 36,100 cases were diagnosed in 1998, only 6300 deaths were attributed to the disease (2.3% of all cancer deaths in women), primarily the result of early diagnosis.[1] The incidence and mortality rates have been fairly constant since 1989. Endometrial cancer generally occurs in white postmenopausal women with an average age at diagnosis of 60 years. The incidence is lower in black and Asian women.[58]

EPIDEMIOLOGY

The endometrium is a complex tissue that is responsive to endogenous and exogenous hormone fluctuations. Prolonged unopposed estrogen exposure results in hyperstimulation of the endometrium and is the major risk factor for endometrial cancer. Estrogen replacement therapy used to control symptoms in postmenopausal women without concomitant progesterone therapy is associated with a 4- to 14-fold increase in risk.[59] Other risk factors related to estrogen exposure include estrogen-secreting tumors, nulliparity or low parity, early menarche, and late menopause. The use of a combination oral contraceptive appears to be protective. Medical disorders such as hypertension, diabetes mellitus, gallbladder disease, and obesity also increase the risk of endometrial cancer. Adipose tissue can convert androstenedione from the adrenals to the weak estrogen estrone. In a small subset of patients, there is a genetic predisposition, and the risk of developing endometrial cancer in these families is as high as 50%.[58] Finally, there is a relationship between tamoxifen, which is used extensively to treat and prevent breast cancer, and the development of endometrial cancer. Although the drug is primarily an antiestrogen, it may also exhibit mild estrogenic effects. This risk does not outweigh the significant benefits of tamoxifen in patients with breast cancer, but these women must be monitored carefully to detect premalignant endometrial lesions.[59,60]

PATHOPHYSIOLOGY

Histology

The most common endometrial cancer cell type is adenocarcinoma, which accounts for approximately 75 to 80% of all cases. Grade 1 tumors have identifiable endometrial glands and are well differentiated, and grade 3 tumors are predominantly solid and entirely undifferentiated. Major subtypes include papillary, secretory, ciliated, and adenocarcinoma with squamous differentiation (formerly adenosquamous carcinoma). Less common and more aggressive cell types include papillary serous (5 to 10%), mucinous (1%), clear cell (4 to 5%), squamous cell (less than 1%), mixed (10%), and undifferentiated.[61]

Pathogenesis

Endometrial cancer arises in the glandular component of the uterine lining and can be small and focal or diffusely involve the uterine cavity. The tumor usually is friable, with focal areas of ulceration or hemorrhage. Local extension accounts for disease in the ovary, vagina, or cervix. Invasion into the myometrium can also occur, resulting in spread to adjacent tissues such as the bladder or fallopian tubes. Because of the rich lymphatic network of the uterus, nodal metastases can occur in the pelvic, para-aortic, and superficial inguinal nodes. Hematogenous spread is uncommon, and sites of distant spread can include lung, liver, bone, and brain.[58]

CLINICAL PRESENTATION AND DIAGNOSIS

Signs and Symptoms

Abnormal vaginal bleeding is reported by the majority of women with endometrial cancer and allows early detection. Because it is a disease of postmenopausal women, this is usually recognizable, but the diagnosis should be considered in premenopausal women with heavy or prolonged bleeding. Pain can also be reported, but this usually signifies advanced disease. Occasionally, asymptomatic women with endometrial cancer have abnormalities detected by cervical cytology, but less than 50% of women have an abnormal Pap smear.

Diagnosis

Endometrial cancer is diagnosed by dilation and curettage or by endometrial biopsy. The latter has become more popular because it is an outpatient procedure and, if adequately performed, has a diagnostic accuracy equivalent to that of surgical curettage under anesthesia.[58] Once the diagnosis is made, further testing includes a thorough physical examination, laboratory studies, and a chest radiograph. For advanced disease, ultrasound, CT scan, and pyelography may be useful in determining tumor spread to the pelvic lymph nodes, para-aortic area, and possibly the liver. MRI and ultrasound are ineffective in defining primary tumor invasion in the myometrium.[62]

There are no specific tumor markers for endometrial cancer, but serum CA-125 may be elevated in more than one-half of patients with the disease. A baseline level can be beneficial because if it is elevated, the level can be followed during and after treatment to evaluate the response to therapy and to help predict recurrence of the disease.[63] Although there are no adequate screening tests for endometrial cancer, women 40 years and older should have an annual pelvic exam. Endometrial biopsy is recommended at menopause and periodically thereafter for women at high risk of developing the disease.[1] The Pap smear is an unreliable screening tool. MRI and ultrasound are highly accurate in detecting early endometrial proliferation but are not cost-effective as screening modalities. In addition, ultrasound interpretation of endometrial thickening often is erroneous in tamoxifen-treated patients.[59]

TREATMENT

Pharmacotherapy

Hormonal Therapy

The normal endometrium contains receptors to both estrogen and progesterone and is very sensitive to both. Progesterone exerts a maturational effect, and progestins have been used to treat advanced or recurrent endometrial cancer because of their systemic activity and low-grade toxicity. Response to these agents is correlated with the presence and level of progesterone receptors. Higher response rates can be achieved in patients with a low tumor burden, a low-grade tumor, and disease outside a prior radiation field. Many different progestins have been studied, but the most widely used are medroxyprogesterone acetate and megestrol. The response rates are similar at 15 to 30%, but almost all patients eventually experience disease progression. Medroxyprogesterone may take 12 weeks to produce a response, and daily oral therapy achieves better results than weekly intramuscular injections. The side effects of fluid retention and weight gain may be problematic for patients who already have hypertension or obesity. Tamoxifen can induce progesterone receptors in some patients with endometrial cancer and has been successful as a single agent in advanced disease. The overall response rate is equivalent to that of the progestins in patients who have never received hormonal therapy, but it has no effect in patients who have become resistant to earlier hormonal therapy. The use of tamoxifen is controversial because of its association with endometrial cancer in patients taking the drug for breast cancer. Gonadotropin-releasing hormones also appear to have similar activity to the progestational agents but are more difficult to administer.[59,64]

Chemotherapy

Chemotherapy is reserved for women with advanced disease (which is fairly uncommon) or extrapelvic recurrent disease. Experience with adjuvant chemotherapy after surgery in patients with high-risk early stage disease is limited, and it has not improved patient survival. The chemotherapy agents that have the best activity in endometrial cancer include doxorubicin, cisplatin, and carboplatin, with an overall response rate of 25 to 30%. Other single agents with significant activity are listed in Table 94.9. Most responses are partial, however, and the duration of response averages only 3 to 5 months.[59,65] Paclitaxel produced an impressive response rate of 36% in a recent clinical trial and shows promise in this disease.[66] In an effort to improve the results of single-agent chemotherapy, various combination regimens have been evaluated, most of them containing doxorubicin. These regimens have produced response rates of up to 60% in patients with advanced or recurrent disease, but the average duration of response is only 6 to 8 months.[65] The best results have been documented with the combination of cisplatin and doxorubicin, which produced an overall response rate of 45% in a large, randomized trial comparing it with doxorubicin alone.[67] Therefore, doxorubicin alone or in combination with cisplatin is considered the standard chemotherapy regimen for women with recurrent endometrial cancer. Few patients obtain long-term survival, however, and the toxicity can be significant in this patient population. About 50% of treated patients develop grade 3 or 4 hematologic toxicity, and nephrotoxicity, neurotoxicity, and cardiotoxicity are other potential side effects. Paclitaxel is being evaluated in combination chemotherapy regimens and may show promise in this disease. Adding hormonal therapy to chemotherapy regimens has not improved response rates.[65]

Table 94.9 ▪ Single-Agent Chemotherapy in Endometrial Cancer

Drug	Overall Response (%)
Platinum compounds	
Cisplatin	25
Carboplatin	30
Antimetabolites	
Fluorouracil	21
Plant alkaloids	
Vincristine	18
Paclitaxel	36
Antitumor antibiotics	
Doxorubicin	28
Epirubicin	26

Nonpharmacologic Therapy

Surgery

Surgery is the treatment of choice for patients with early stage endometrial cancer. Patients with stage I disease that is well differentiated should undergo a total abdominal hysterectomy and bilateral salpingo-oophorectomy with peritoneal cytology. Selected pelvic lymph nodes may be removed. If lymph nodes are negative in stage IA and IB disease, no postoperative treatment is indicated. Pelvic and para-aortic lymph nodes are sampled if there is deep invasion of the myometrium, for grade 2 and 3 tumors, and for rare histologic types. If there is intraperitoneal spread of the tumor, an omentectomy, multiple peritoneal biopsies, and debulking are recommended.[62] Surgery may also be indicated for women who present with advanced primary cancers, followed by adjuvant therapy. It is not recommended for patients with recurrent disease because of the lack of effective regional and systemic therapy.[58]

Radiation Therapy

Patients with stage I disease who are not candidates for surgery because of severe medical problems or who refuse surgery can be treated with radiation alone, but there have been reports of inferior cure rates. Radiation may be indicated after surgery for patients with stage I disease who have deeply invasive (stage IC) or high-grade tumors and in patients with stage II disease because of the high risk of extrauterine spread. Although adjuvant radiation therapy may prevent pelvic recurrence, it has not been proven to influence overall survival in these patients.[58] Radiation is commonly delivered by external beam to the pelvis at a dosage of 4000 to 4500 cGy over a period of 5 to 7 weeks. The para-aortic lymph nodes are also radiated if they are positive. External beam radiation can effectively treat the pelvic lymph nodes and areas of bulky disease, but high dosages can result in unacceptable bowel and rectal toxicity. Brachytherapy is commonly used in conjunction with external beam radiation to increase the total dosage delivered to the primary tumor to approximately 5000 to 7000 cGy. The brachytherapy sources may be placed adjacent to the tumor inside a cavity, such as the vagina, or directly within the tumor itself.

Radiation therapy has been given preoperatively and postoperatively, with comparable results. Advantages of preoperative radiation include radiating while the uterus has an intact blood supply and is well oxygenated, reducing the tumor mass that will be removed surgically, and a possible lower complication rate. However, postoperative radiation allows prior surgical staging to determine prognosis and determine which patients are candidates for additional therapy, and most institutions in the United States advocate this approach.[68] The majority of patients with stage III disease are not candidates for initial surgery and are treated with external pelvic irradiation and brachytherapy, with subsequent surgery for persistent disease. Radiation therapy can also be used to treat recurrent endometrial cancer that is confined to the vagina or a specific region in the pelvis. Its use in bulky pelvic disease in stage IV patients is primarily palliative.

PROGNOSIS

Endometrial cancer is highly curable when it is diagnosed early, and the stage of the disease at diagnosis has a direct influence on survival. The FIGO staging system is based on a surgical staging procedure and is described in Table 94.10.Patients with stage I disease have a 90% disease-free survival. Survival decreases as the cancer spreads outside the endometrium. The 5-year disease-free survival is 83% for stage II and 43% for stage III.[69] The prognostic factors can be divided into two groups that are incorporated into the staging system. The first group consists of uterine risk factors and includes histologic type and grade, depth of myometrial invasion, cervical extension, and vascular space invasion. All of the uncommon endometrial cell types such as papillary serous, clear cell, and squamous cell carcinomas are associated with a greater risk for extrauterine metastases and a poorer prognosis. Patients with well-differentiated tumors (grade 1) tend to have disease that is limited to the surface of the endometrium. Those with less differentiated tumors (grade 2 and 3) are more likely to have myometrial invasion, which is associated with lymph node involvement and distant metastases, and therefore decreased survival. Cervical involvement also increases the probability of lymph node metastases. The second group consists of extrauterine risk factors and includes pelvic lymph node metastases, aortic lymph node metastases, adnexal metastases, positive peritoneal cytology, and distant organ metastases, which are all associated with a poorer prognosis.[62,69] One report found progesterone receptor levels to be the single most important prognostic indicator in early stage endometrial cancer. Patients with progesterone receptor levels of 100 or more had a 3-year disease-free survival of 93%, compared with 36% for patients with progesterone levels less than 100.[70] Most progesterone receptor–positive tumors are well differentiated and are easily treated by initial therapy. In addition, positive progesterone receptors can predict responsiveness to progestational therapy. More recent studies have found that molecular markers such as DNA ploidy, proliferative activity (S-phase fraction), the P-53 tumor suppressor gene, and oncogene overexpression (e.g., Her-2/neu, K-ras) may be helpful in determining which patients are at high risk for extrauterine metastases.[69]

Table 94.10 ▪ International Federation of Gynecology and Obstetrics Staging for Endometrial Carcinoma

Stage I	Tumor confined to the corpus uteri.
Stage IA	Tumor limited to the endometrium.
Stage IB	Tumor invades one-half of the myometrium or less.
Stage IC	Tumor invades more than one-half of the myometrium.
Stage II	Tumor invades the cervix but does not extend beyond the uterus.
Stage IIA	Endocervical glandular involvement only.
Stage IIB	Cervical stromal invasion.
Stage III	Local or regional spread.
Stage IIIA	Tumor involves the serosa or adnexa (direct extension or metastasis) or cancer cells in ascites or peritoneal washings.
Stage IIIB	Vaginal involvement (direct extension or metastasis).
Stage IIIC	Metastasis to the pelvic or para-aortic lymph nodes.
Stage IV	Extension beyond the true pelvis.
Stage IVA	Tumor invades the bladder or bowel mucosa.
Stage IVB	Distant metastasis, including metastasis to intra-abdominal lymph nodes other than para-aortic or inguinal lymph nodes.

KEY POINTS

- There is no effective screening tool to date for ovarian cancer.
- The most identifiable risk factors for ovarian cancer are a family history, nulliparity or low parity, and unsuppressed ovulation.
- Chemotherapy is the most common form of therapy for patients with ovarian cancer, and the first-line regimen consists of a platinum compound and paclitaxel.
- Cervical cancer can be curable if detected early by a Pap smear performed during routine pelvic examinations.
- The biggest risk factor for cervical cancer is HPV, and the disease occurs most often in women who experience sexual intercourse at a younger age, multiple sexual partners, pregnancy at a younger age, and multiple pregnancies.
- Most patients with cervical cancer are treated with surgery or radiation therapy, although recent studies have demonstrated a significant improvement in overall survival with the combination of chemotherapy and radiation therapy for patients with locally advanced disease.

- Endometrial cancer usually is curable because vaginal bleeding allows early detection.
- Major risk factors for endometrial cancer include unopposed estrogen exposure, nulliparity or low parity, early menarche, and late menopause.
- Surgery is the treatment of choice for patients with endometrial cancer; chemotherapy is reserved for women with advanced disease, and responses usually are partial and of short duration.
- New chemotherapeutic agents and multimodality therapy are improving the outcome for patients with advanced gynecologic cancer.

REFERENCES

1. Cancer Facts & Figures. Atlanta, GA: American Cancer Society, 1998.
2. Ozols RF, Schwartz PE, Eifel PJ. Ovarian cancer, fallopian tube carcinomas and peritoneal carcinoma. In: Devita VT, Hellman S, Rosenberg SA. Cancer: principles and practice of oncology. 5th ed. Philadelphia: Lippincott-Raven, 1997:1502–1539.
3. Daly M, Obrams GI. Epidemiology and risk assessment for ovarian cancer. Semin Oncol 25:255–264, 1998.
4. Rossing MA, Daling JR, Weiss NS, et al. Ovarian tumors in a cohort of infertile women. N Engl J Med 331:771–776, 1994.
5. Claus EB, Schwartz PE. Familial ovarian cancer. Cancer 76:1998–2003, 1995.
6. Hoskins WJ. Surgical staging and cytoreductive surgery of epithelial ovarian cancer. Cancer 71:1534–1540, 1993.
7. Van Nagell JR, Gallion HH, Pavlik EJ, et al. Ovarian cancer screening. Cancer 76:2086–2091, 1995.
8. Mogensen O. Prognostic value of CA 125 in advanced ovarian cancer. Gynecol Oncol 44:207–212, 1992.
9. Berek JS, Bast RC. Ovarian cancer screening. The use of serial complementary tumor markers to improve sensitivity and specificity for early detection. Cancer 76:2092–2096, 1995.
10. Lorigan PC, Crosby T, Coleman RE. Current drug treatment guidelines for epithelial ovarian cancer. Drugs 51:571–584, 1996.
11. Advanced Ovarian Cancer Trialists Group. Chemotherapy in advanced ovarian cancer: an overview of randomized clinical trials. BMJ 303:884–890, 1991.
12. Alberts DS, Green S, Hannigan EV, et al. Improved therapeutic index of carboplatin plus cyclophosphamide versus cisplatin plus cyclophosphamide. Final report by the Southwest Oncology Group of a phase III randomized trial in stages III and IV ovarian cancer. J Clin Oncol 10:706–717, 1992.
13. Swenerton K, Jeffrey J, Stuart G. Cisplatin-cyclophosphamide versus carboplatin-cyclophosphamide in advanced ovarian cancer: a randomized phase III study of the National Cancer Institute of Canada Clinical Trials Group. J Clin Oncol 10:718–726, 1992.
14. Calvert AH, Newell DR, Gumbrell LA, et al. Carboplatin dosage: prospective evaluation of a simple formula based on renal function. J Clin Oncol 7:1748–1756, 1989.
15. The Ovarian Cancer Meta-Analysis Project. Cyclophosphamide plus cisplatin versus cyclophosphamide, doxorubicin, and cisplatin chemotherapy of ovarian carcinoma: a meta-analysis. J Clin Oncol 9:1668–1674, 1991.
16. McGuire WP, Hoskins WJ, Brady MF, et al. Cyclophosphamide and cisplatin compared with paclitaxel and cisplatin in patients with stage III and stage IV ovarian cancer. N Engl J Med 334:1–6, 1996.
17. Rowinsky EK, Gilbert MR, McGuire WP, et al. Sequences of taxol and cisplatin: a phase I and pharmacologic study. J Clin Oncol 9:1692–1703, 1991.
18. Eisenhauer EA, ten Bokkel Huinink WW, Swenerton KD, et al. European-Canadian randomized trial of paclitaxel in relapsed ovarian cancer: high-dose versus low-dose and long versus short infusion. J Clin Oncol 12:2654–2666, 1994.
19. Cavaletti G, Graziella B, Crespi V, et al. Neurotoxicity and ototoxicity of cisplatin plus paclitaxel in comparison to cisplatin plus cyclophosphamide in patients with epithelial ovarian cancer. J Clin Oncol 15:199–206, 1997.
20. Bookman MA, McGuire WP, Kilpatrick D, et al. A phase I study of the Gynecologic Oncology Group. J Clin Oncol 14:1895–1902, 1996.
21. Huizing MT, van Warmerdam LJC, Rosing H, et al. Phase I and pharmacologic study of the combination paclitaxel and carboplatin as first line chemotherapy in stage III and IV ovarian cancer. J Clin Oncol 15:1953–1964, 1997.
22. Goldberg JM, Piver MS, Hempling RE, et al. Paclitaxel and cisplatin combination chemotherapy in recurrent epithelial ovarian cancer. Gynecol Oncol 63:312–317, 1996.
23. Rose PG, Blessing JA, Mayer AR, et al. Prolonged oral etoposide as second-line therapy for platinum-resistant and platinum-sensitive ovarian carcinoma: a Gynecologic Oncology Group study. J Clin Oncol 16:405–410, 1998.
24. Brogden RN, Wiseman LR. Topotecan: a review of its potential in advanced ovarian cancer. Drugs 56:709–723, 1998.
25. ten Bokkel W, Gore M, Carmichael J. Topotecan versus paclitaxel for the treatment of recurrent epithelial ovarian cancer. J Clin Oncol 15:2183–2193, 1997.
26. Lund B, Neijt JP. Gemcitabine in cisplatin-resistant ovarian cancer. Semin Oncol 23:72–76, 1996.
27. Alberts DS, Liu PY, Hannigan EV, et al. Intraperitoneal cisplatin plus intravenous cyclophosphamide versus intravenous cisplatin plus intravenous cyclophosphamide for stage III ovarian cancer. N Engl J Med 335:1950–1955, 1996.
28. Markman M, Brady MF, Spirtos, NM, et al. Phase II trial of intraperitoneal paclitaxel in carcinoma of the ovary, tube, and peritoneum: a Gynecologic Oncology Group study. J Clin Oncol 16:2620–2624, 1998.
29. Markman M. Intraperitoneal therapy of ovarian cancer. Semin Oncol 25: 356–360, 1998.
30. Fennelly D. The role of high-dose chemotherapy in the management of advanced ovarian cancer. Curr Opin Oncol 8:415–425, 1996.
31. Stiff PJ, Bayer R, Kerger C, et al. High-dose chemotherapy with autologous transplantation for persistent/relapsed ovarian cancer: a multivariate analysis of survival for 100 consecutively treated patients. J Clin Oncol 15:1309–1317, 1997.
32. Boente MP, Chi DS, Hoskins WJ. The role of surgery in the management of ovarian cancer: primary and interval cytoreductive surgery. Semin Oncol 25:326–334, 1998.
33. Young RC, Pecorelli S. Management of early ovarian cancer. Semin Oncol 25:335–339, 1998.
34. Friedlander ML. Prognostic factors in ovarian cancer. Semin Oncol 25:305–315, 1998.
35. van der Burg MEL, van Lent M, Buyse M, et al. The effect of debulking surgery after induction chemotherapy on the prognosis in advanced epithelial ovarian cancer. N Engl J Med 332:629–634, 1995.
36. Muderspach L, Muggia FM, Conti PS. Second-look laparotomy for stage III epithelial ovarian cancer: rationale and current issues. Cancer Treat Rev 21:499–511, 1995.
37. Lanciano R, Reddy S. Update on the role of radiotherapy in ovarian cancer. Semin Oncol 25:361–371, 1998.
38. Cannista SA, Niloff JM. Cancer of the uterine cervix. N Engl J Med 334:1030–1038, 1996.
39. Lombard I, Vincent-Salomon A, Validire P, et al. Human papillomavirus genotype as a major determinant of the course of cervical cancer. J Clin Oncol 16:2613–2619, 1998.
40. Benda JA. Pathology of cervical carcinoma and its prognostic implications. Semin Oncol 21:3–11, 1994.
41. Eifel PJ, Berek JS, Thigpen JT. Cancer of the cervix, vagina and vulva. In: Devita VT, Hellman S, Rosenberg SA. Cancer: principles and practice of oncology. 5th ed. Philadelphia: Lippincott-Raven, 1998:1502–1539.
42. Omura GA. Chemotherapy for cervix cancer. Semin Oncol 21:54–62, 1994.
43. Brader KR, Morris M, Levenback C, et al. Chemotherapy for cervical carcinoma: factors determining response and implications for clinical trial design. J Clin Oncol 16:1879–1884, 1998.
44. Thigpen T, Vance R, Khansur T, et al. The role of paclitaxel in the management of patients with carcinoma of the cervix. Semin Oncol 24(Suppl 2):S2-41–S2-46, 1997.
45. Omura G, Blessing J, Vaccarello L, et al. A randomized trial of cisplatin versus cisplatin plus mitolactol versus cisplatin plus ifosfamide in advanced squamous carcinoma of the cervix by the Gynecologic Oncology Group [abstract]. Gynecol Oncol 60:120–121, 1996.
46. Eisenhauer EA, Vermorken JB. New drugs in gynecologic oncology. Curr Opin Oncol 8:408–414, 1996.
47. Morris M, Brader KR, Levenback C, et al. Phase II study of vinorelbine in advanced and recurrent squamous cell carcinoma of the cervix. J Clin Oncol 16:1094–1098, 1998.
48. Keys HM, Bundy BN, Stehman FB, et al. Cisplatin, radiation, and adjuvant hysterectomy compared with radiation and adjuvant hysterectomy for bulky stage Ib cervical carcinoma. N Engl J Med 340:1154–1161, 1999.
49. Morris M, Eifel PJ, Lu J, et al. Pelvic radiation with concurrent chemotherapy compared with pelvic and para-aortic radiation for high risk cervical cancer. N Engl J Med 340:1137–1143, 1999.
50. Rose, PG, Bundy BM, Watkins EB, et al. Concurrent cisplatin-based

radiotherapy and chemotherapy for locally advanced cervical cancer. N Engl J Med 340:1144–1153, 1999.
51. Bloss JD. The use of electrosurgical techniques in the management of premalignant diseases of the vulva, vagina, and cervix: an excisional rather than an ablative approach. Am J Obstet Gynecol 169:1081–1085, 1993.
52. Sevin BU, Nadji M, Averette HE, et al. Microinvasive carcinoma of the cervix. Cancer 70:2121–2128, 1992.
53. Marcial VA, Marcial LV. Radiation therapy of cervical cancer. Cancer 71:1438–1445, 1993.
54. Coia L, Won M, Lanciano R, et al. The patterns of care outcome study for cancer of the uterine cervix. Cancer 66:2451–2456, 1990.
55. Rotman M, Pajak TF, Choi K, et al. Prophylactic extended-field irradiation of para-aortic lymph nodes in stages IIB and bulky IB and IIA cervical carcinomas. JAMA 274:387–393, 1995.
56. Sevin BU, Nadji M, Lampe B, et al. Prognostic factors of early stage cervical cancer treated by radical hysterectomy. Cancer 76:1978–1986, 1995.
57. Maiman M, Fruchter RG, Guy L, et al. Human immunodeficiency virus infection and invasive cervical carcinoma. Cancer 71:402–406, 1993.
58. Burke TW, Eifel PJ, Muggia FM. Cancer of the uterine body. In: Devita VT, Hellman S, Rosenberg SA. Cancer: principles and practice of oncology. 5th ed. Philadelphia: Lippincott-Raven, 1997:1478–1499.
59. Cohen CJ, Rahaman J. Endometrial cancer: management of high risk and recurrence including the tamoxifen controversy. Cancer 76:2044–2052, 1995.
60. Barakat BR. Tamoxifen and endometrial neoplasia. Clin Obstet Gynecol 39:629–640, 1996.
61. Gordon MD, Ireland K. Pathology of hyperplasia and carcinoma of the endometrium. Semin Oncol 21:64–70, 1994.
62. Mikuta JJ. Preoperative evaluation and staging of endometrial cancer. Cancer 76:2041–2043, 1995.
63. Rose PG, Sommers RM, Reale FR, et al. Serial serum CA 125 measurements for evaluation of recurrence in patients with endometrial carcinoma. Obstet Gynecol 84:12–16, 1994.
64. Lentz SS. Advanced and recurrent endometrial carcinoma: hormonal therapy. Semin Oncol 21:100–106, 1994.
65. Burke TW, Gershenson DM. Chemotherapy as adjuvant and salvage treatment in women with endometrial carcinoma. Clin Obstet Gynecol 39:716–727, 1996.
66. Ball HC, Blessing JA, Lentz SS, et al. A phase II trial of taxol in advanced and recurrent adenocarcinoma of the endometrium: a Gynecologic Oncology Group study [abstract]. Gynecol Oncol 56:120, 1995.
67. Thigpen J, Blessing H, Homesley J, et al. Phase III trial of doxorubicin +/– cisplatin in advanced or recurrent endometrial carcinoma. Proc Am Soc Clin Oncol 12:261, 1993.
68. Nag S. Modern techniques of radiation therapy for endometrial cancer. Clin Obstet Gynecol 39:728–744, 1996.
69. Homesley HD, Zaino R. Endometrial cancer: prognostic factors. Semin Oncol 21:71–78, 1994.
70. Ingram SS, Rosenman J, Heath R, et al. The predictive value of progesterone receptor levels in endometrial cancer. Int J Radiat Oncol Biol Phys 17:21–27, 1989.

CHAPTER 95

SKIN CANCERS AND MELANOMAS

Laura Boehnke Michaud

The skin is the largest organ in the human body. It comprises the epidermis, dermis, and subcutaneous tissues. Skin performs many functions, including protection from the environment, synthesis of vitamin D, thermoregulation, and sensations of touch and temperature. Several different cell and tissue types make up the skin and its appendages (hair follicles and apocrine, eccrine and sebaceous glands). These components can transform to produce many different benign and malignant tumors.[1] This chapter focuses on the most common skin neoplasms (basal cell and squamous cell carcinoma) and the most life-threatening skin cancer, cutaneous melanoma. Tumor registries divide skin cancers into two broad categories: nonmelanoma skin cancer and melanoma.

TREATMENT GOALS: SKIN CANCERS AND MELANOMAS

- The treatment goal for the vast majority of patients with nonmelanoma skin cancer is curative.
- Of the nonmelanoma skin cancers, basal cell carcinoma is generally less aggressive than squamous cell carcinoma.
- Melanoma is highly curable in its early stages (stages I and II), but it is associated with a much worse prognosis in the later stages and is nearly uniformly fatal after metastases have occurred.
- In patients with metastatic melanoma, the focus is on palliation of symptoms, improvement in quality of life, and prolongation of life.

Nonmelanoma Skin Cancer

EPIDEMIOLOGY

Incidence

Nonmelanoma skin cancer (NMSC) is the most common cancer in the United States and many other countries (e.g., Australia, New Zealand, United Kingdom). In the United States, basal cell carcinoma (BCC) and squamous cell carcinoma (SCC) are estimated to account for more than 1 million new cases and 1900 deaths annually.[2] These numbers are believed to be grossly underestimated due to the fact that most cases of skin cancer are managed in a private clinic setting and are subsequently not recorded with tumor registries. Studies designed to investigate underreporting have been performed in Australia and the United Kingdom and indicate that the incidence of NMSC is significantly underestimated in these countries.[3,4,5]

Table 95.1 ▪ Risk Factors Associated with Nonmelanoma Skin Cancer

Ultraviolet radiation	Immunosuppression
Chemicals[a]	Viruses[a]
Chronic inflammation	Genetic factors

[a]Questionable etiologic relationship with nonmelanoma skin cancer (see text).

Etiology

Ultraviolet Radiation and Skin Type

Several factors have been determined to influence the incidence of skin cancer (Table 95.1). Two major factors are ultraviolet (UV) radiation exposure and skin type. UV light is subdivided by wavelength into UV-A, UV-B, and UV-C. These divisions and the wavelengths involved are shown in Figure 95.1. This figure also depicts the depth of penetration by each type of UV light and the protective role of the ozone layer. UV-A and UV-B light are considered harmful to humans, but their effects on biologic systems are still being characterized. UV-B radiation consists of short wavelengths, absorbed by the skin and responsible for sun-induced erythema, photoaging, and photocarcinogenesis. UV-A light is not absorbed by the ozone layer, and it penetrates deep into the dermal layer of the skin, producing erythema, immediate pigment

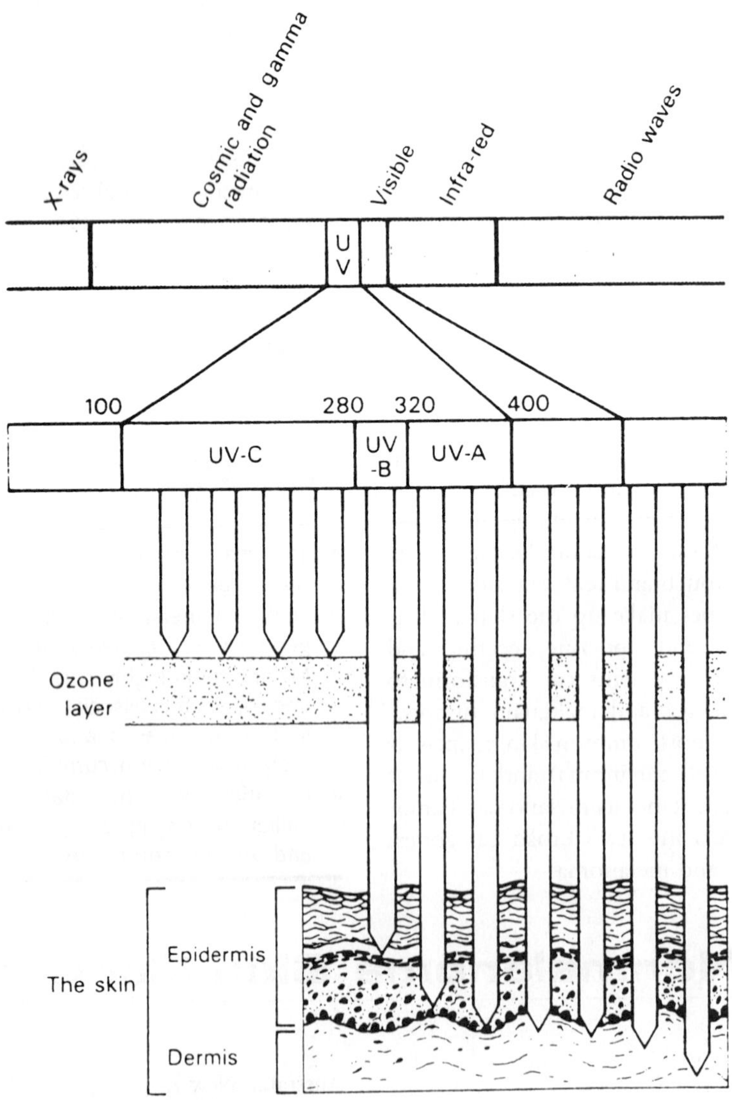

Figure 95.1. Solar electromagnetic spectrum showing depth of penetration of radiation into the skin. (Reprinted with permission from Emmett AJJ, ORourke MGE, eds. Malignant skin tumours. New York: Churchill Livingstone, 1991:24.)

Table 95.2 ▪ Factors Influencing Ultraviolet Radiation Exposure

Amount of ozone	Season of the year
Latitude	Occupation
Altitude	Recreational activities
Reflective surfaces	Clothing requirements (styles)
Time of day	

darkening, delayed melanogenesis, and elastosis and other dermal connective tissue damage.

UV-B energy can be absorbed by many cellular components, including DNA, lipids, and proteins.[6] DNA absorbs strongly in the UV-B spectrum, partially governing the nature of damage produced by sunlight. UV-A radiation exerts its genotoxic effects indirectly, possibly through production of reactive oxygen species.[6] Effects of UV radiation on other cellular components, including the immune system and DNA-repair mechanisms, may also play a major role in skin carcinogenesis.[7] Tumor cell initiation, represented by DNA damage, may be induced by UV radiation, as well as other compounds and exposures.[1] Effects on surrounding normal cells allow for clonal expansion of the initiated cells, a process termed *tumor cell promotion.* Both initiation and promotion are required for carcinogenesis to occur. UV radiation may also act as a promoter in skin, inducing apoptosis in surrounding normal cells and allowing space for expansion of tumor cells.[1]

The amount of UV light reaching the earth's surface at any given place depends on several factors (Table 95.2). The ozone layer determines the amount of UV-B light that penetrates the atmosphere. Many theories attribute the rise in skin cancer incidence over the past two decades to the depletion of the ozone layer and the change in lifestyle seen in modern society (i.e., increased recreational sun exposure and decreased clothing requirements).[3] However, these assumptions have never been proven in any study to date. Geographic location, age at time of exposure, and the amount and type of UV exposure appear to play an important role in the epidemiology of skin cancer. There are numerous studies in the literature investigating this topic, most of which are retrospective reviews. Although there is consensus that UV exposure is an important factor in determining risk, there is little consensus regarding age at time of exposure and amount and type of exposure in relation to predisposition.[8]

Skin type influences the effects of UV radiation in humans. Skin types are divided into six types based on sunburning and suntanning history (Table 95.3).[1] Types I and II are at highest risk for skin cancers. Skin cancers are rare in African Americans, with SCCs being more prevalent than BCCs in this population.[9] There is evidence to support an increased risk of both BCC and SCC in people of older age, with freckling skin, and with blue eyes.[3] SCC and BCC are most common on sun-exposed areas of the body (e.g., head, neck, and dorsum of the hands).[1] Although older age is associated with an increased risk of NMSC, as chronic sun exposure has shifted from occupational to recreational, the incidence of skin cancer in younger patients is increasing. For SCC, total cumulative exposure to UV light is the primary risk factor.[10] For BCC, risk is better correlated with the tendency to sunburn (i.e., skin type).[1] Increases in recreational UV radiation exposure are believed to contribute to the rising incidence of skin cancer in the United States, but decreased clothing requirements and a societal focus on tanning have also influenced the incidence of skin cancer in most countries.

Chemical Carcinogenesis

Carcinogenesis is a process generally occurring over a span of 10 to 50 years and progressing from initiation through promotion and ultimately to carcinogenesis. Basic changes in DNA configuration take place in cells during initiation (i.e., purine and pyrimidine substitutions, dimers, deletions). At this point, cells may progress to malignancy (if promoted effectively) or remain unchanged for life. Cells must be completely initiated for promotion to occur. Promoters cause reversible inflammation and hyperplasia, allowing for clonal expansion of initiated cells, which lead to carcinogenesis in cells that have been completely initiated.[1] Chemical carcinogenesis was first reported in chimney sweeps of the 1700s who acquired scrotal SCC secondary to arsenic present in the soot of chimneys.[11] Most chemical carcinogenesis data since this time have been established in laboratory animals and cannot be directly applied to humans. Several chemicals act as initiators and promoters that may influence the risk of cancer. Tar, a compound containing polycyclic aromatic hydrocarbons and used to treat psoriasis, acts as an initiator. Benzoyl peroxide, used to treat acne, is a known promoter. Many other agents used to treat skin disorders are initiators and promoters, but long-term use of these agents has never been associated with an increased incidence of malignancy.[1] The two-hit theory of carcinogenesis, requiring both initiation and promotion, is an accepted hypothesis by scientists worldwide and seems to explain why these products are not always associated with an increased incidence of cancer.

Table 95.3 ▪ Skin Types

Skin Type	Suntanning and Sunburning History	Skin Color
I	Always burns, never tans	White
II	Always burns, minimal tan	White
III	Burns often, tans gradually	Light brown
IV	Burns minimally, tans well	Moderate brown
V	Burns rarely, tans profusely	Dark brown
VI	Never burns, deeply pigmented	Black

Source: Reference 1.

Chronic Inflammation and Irritation

Chronic inflammation and irritation can predispose a patient to skin cancer in the affected area. For example, cancers can develop in an area of chronic ulcers and scars of burns. Betel nuts and chewing tobacco cause chronic irritation of the mucosal surface of the mouth and can lead to SCC of the oral cavity and lip.[1]

Immunosuppression

Chronic UV-B exposure produces changes in host immunity by producing generalized defects in antigen-presenting cells and inducing the formation of suppressor T cells. UV radiation also produces changes in both the number and type of Langerhans cells present in human skin.[1] These alterations in the immune system allow development and progression of skin cancers. Clinical examples of this phenomenon are found in renal transplant recipients, in whom the most common cancers are NMSCs.[12] In these patients, the incidence of SCC has been shown to be significantly higher than the general population, with lesions developing about 3 to 5 years after transplantation. The ratio of SCC to BCC in the general population is 0.2:1. In a study of 523 renal transplant recipients reported out of Toronto, the ratio of SCC to BCC was 2.3:1.[13] These data lead us to believe that immunosuppression plays a role in the development of skin cancers, but details relating to this relationship are not well understood.

Viral Oncogenesis

Data demonstrate that the presence of human papillomavirus (HPV) may be associated with an increased risk of cutaneous malignancies. HPV types 5, 8, 14, 16, 17, and 33 have been associated with various epidermal carcinomas and carcinoma of the cervix.[1] These viruses appear to be oncogenic, but conclusive evidence of causation is not available.

Genetic Factors

Many genetic syndromes are associated with an increased incidence of skin neoplasms. These genodermatoses are listed in Table 95.4. Patients with xeroderma pigmentosum (XP) are known to be extremely susceptible to UV radiation–induced cancers secondary to a defect in the DNA-excision repair mechanism. This supports the theory that photodamage to DNA plays a major role in UV radiation–induced carcinogenesis.[1]

Table 95.4 ▪ Genodermatoses Associated with Cancers of the Skin

Genodermatoses	Associated Skin Cancers
Xeroderma pigmentosum	Basal cell and squamous cell carcinomas Malignant melanoma
Basal cell nevus syndrome	Basal cell carcinomas
Familial atypical mole and melanoma syndrome	Malignant melanoma
Multiple self-healing epithelioma of Ferguson-Smith	Squamous cell carcinoma
Torre's syndrome	Sebaceous adenomas
Cowden's syndrome	Hair follicle tumors
Gardner's syndrome	Cutaneous cysts (may progress to carcinoma)
Carney's syndrome	Myxomas (benign connective tissue tumor)
Oculocutaneous albinism	Basal cell and squamous cell carcinoma Malignant melanoma

The tumor suppressor gene, p53, has been shown to be mutated in 90% of SCCs of the skin and 50% of BCCs.[7] Mutations in p53 found in SCCs and actinic keratoses (AKs) are nearly uniformly secondary to UV radiation exposure and generally occur in only one allele, requiring a second insult to result in carcinogenesis. BCCs are associated with lesions on both p53 alleles, and both mutations are usually related to UV exposure.[7] The ras oncogene is mutated in 10 to 40% of NMSCs,[14] and many other chromosomal regions are lost in SCCs and AKs, including, but not limited to, 9q, 13q, 17p, 17q, and 3p.[7]

Basal Cell Carcinoma

Basal cell carcinoma represents 75 to 80% of all reported cases of nonmelanoma skin cancer in the United States.[1] It is three times more common than all other cancers combined in Australia.[15] BCC is generally less invasive than SCC and rarely metastasizes, with a mortality rate of 0.03%.[15] The morbidity from BCC may profoundly affect the lives of patients with disfiguring lesions and scars from treatment. Most commonly associated with chronic sun (UV light) exposure in fair-skinned older adults, BCC rarely occurs under age 40. BCC occurs more frequently in men than in women.[1]

CLINICAL PRESENTATION AND DIAGNOSIS

Signs and Symptoms

BCC arises from the basal layer of cells in the epidermis and its appendages. Malignant basal cells are not able to mature into keratinocytes and retain their ability to divide beyond the basal layer, becoming a bulky neoplasm. BCC generally begins as a slow-growing, shiny, skin-colored to pink, firm, well-circumscribed, raised, dome-shaped papule. As the nodule increases in size, its center may become ulcerated, surrounded by a pearly, rolled border. Telangiectasias are often seen on the surface of the lesion. Classification of these lesions is a complex process that lacks uniformity and clear definition. The World Health Organization (WHO) classification contains 10 variations and is based on histopathologic features. A simplified schema has been suggested by a number of authors, basing the classification of lesions on generally recognized forms of growth pattern: (1) nodular, including micronodular; (2) infiltrative, including morphea; (3) superficial, apparently multicentric; and (4) mixed, including a combination of any two or all of these types.[15] Utilization of this classification system allows for appropriate decisions to be made regarding prognosis and treatment. Also, it is reproducible and fairly easy to use. However, because of the lack of uniformity across studies and reports, discrepancies still exist.

Nodular BCC represents approximately 50% of all BCCs.[15] Peripheral palisading of nuclei, a phenomenon characteristic of BCC, is prominent in the nodular type and produces an effect on the surrounding stroma that is required to allow for expansion of malignant cells.[1,15] These lesions have a nodular clinical appearance and may have central necrosis with cyst or microcyst formation. The size of the nodules in the dermis may determine prognosis. Micronodular BCC (15%), consisting of small nodules less than 0.15 mm in diameter, is a subgroup that is more likely to recur.[16] The most common site of nodular BCC is the head and neck area.[1] Multiple lesions may appear simultaneously on any part of the body.[1,9] Figure 95.2 is an illustration of this type of BCC.

Infiltrative BCC represents approximately 10 to 20% of all BCCs. The important feature in its presentation appears to be the shape of the cells in the dermis. Groups of cells vary in size and have irregular spiky projections, and palisading is poorly developed or absent. Larger groups are located centrally and superficially, with smaller groups in the periphery of the dermis where they infiltrate between collagen. In a subvariant termed *morphea* type (5%), all cell groups are small, the stroma is densely sclerotic and fibrous, and irregular islands and cords of cells infiltrate the stroma in a configuration that appears parallel to the skin surface.[15] In other classification schemes, this is often referred to as the sclerosing or morphea-type lesion.[1] They usually manifest as a yellow, sclerotic, scarlike patch with indistinct margins. These typically appear on the face and neck areas and may go undetected for a long period of time.[1]

Superficial, apparently multifocal lesions represent approximately 15% of all BCCs.[15] They are termed this because of the small buds of cells that grow down from the dermis into the superficial dermis, while remaining attached to the base of the epidermis. This often occurs over a wide area of skin and is intermittently separated by normal epidermis. Although the downgrowths appear to be separated by normal epidermis, this is in fact one lesion with the groups of cells being interconnected at the epidermal basal layer.[15] This type of growth is often referred to as multifocal and may be associated with more deeply invasive growth. Clinically, these appear as a flat, erythematous, scaly patch surrounded by a fine, threadlike

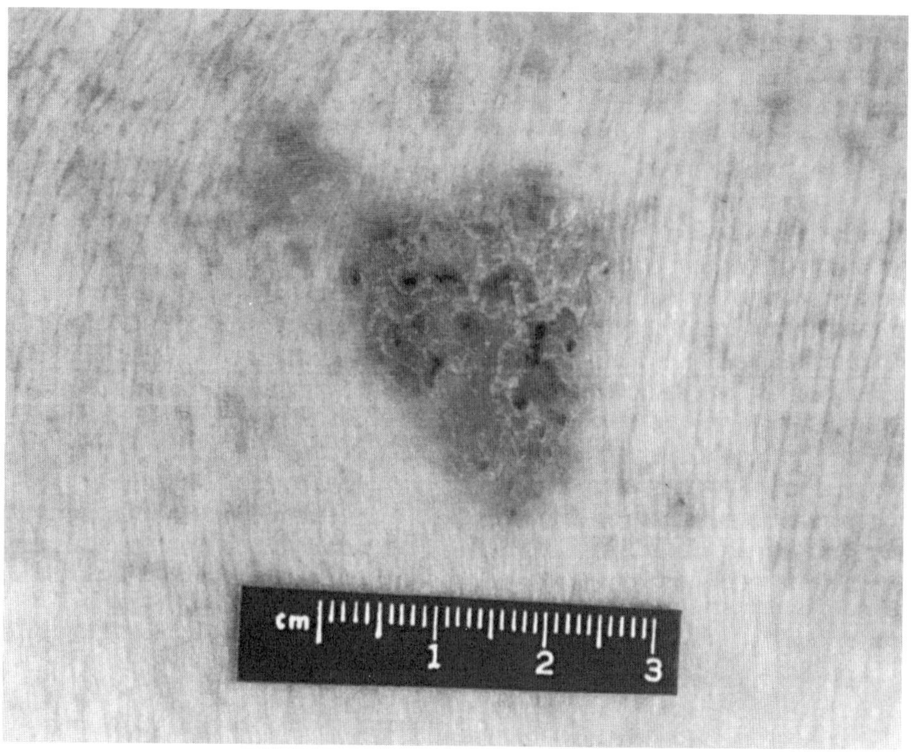

Figure 95.2. Nodular basal cell carcinoma.

pearly border.[1] These lesions most commonly occur on the trunk and, to a lesser degree, on the extemities.[15]

Mixed lesions represent approximately 10 to 15% of all BCCs. Superficial and infiltrative patterns of growth often occur in combination and are seen at the lateral or deep margins and may contribute to an incomplete removal of the lesion.

The appearance of a pigment in any of these lesions can occur and may facilitate removal of the lesion, secondary to the obvious appearance of the resected specimen margins.[17] This occurs most commonly in the nodular or superficial types of lesions. Only 2% of all lesions are pigmented in the White population, but this incidence is much higher in Black[18] and Japanese[19] populations.

Basosquamous cell carcinomas appear to have a biologic behavior and pathologic features that represent both BCC and SCC.[1,15] Consensus is lacking regarding what constitutes this definition. If a lesion within this category exhibits a prominent squamous component it may be more likely to recur and metastasize. It would be beneficial to avoid this terminology and instead record the growth pattern and differentiation in unequivocal terms. However, if a lesion exhibits a considerable area of squamous carcinoma, the prognosis may be more like that of pure squamous carcinoma.

Staging

Staging for NMSCs is based on the tumor-node-metastasis (TNM) staging system adopted by the American Joint Committee on Cancer (AJCC). Because BCC so rarely metastasizes even to local lymph nodes, size has been the most important factor for prognosis and treatment planning (Table 95.5).[20] Most BCCs manifest as T1 lesions (2 cm or less). Secondary to neglect, some lesions grow to be very large (T3, greater than 5 cm) and may invade underlying structures (T4). On entering the bone or blood circulation, BCCs metastasize. There have been approximately 300 reported cases of metastatic BCC in the world literature to date.[1]

Table 95.5 ▪ American Joint Committee on Cancer Staging for Basal Cell Carcinoma and Squamous Cell Carcinoma

Stage	Tumor (T)[a]	Nodes (N)[b]	Metastases (M)[c]
0	T_{is}	N0	M0
I	T1	N0	M0
II	T2	N0	M0
	T3	N0	M0
III	T4	N0	M0
	Any T	N1	M0
IV	Any T	Any N	M1

Note: If multiple simultaneous tumors are identified, the tumor with the highest T category is classified and the number of separate tumors are indicated in parentheses—for example, T2(5).

Source: Reference 20.

[a] T_{is} = carcinoma in situ; T1 = ≤2 cm; T2 = >2 cm and ≤5 cm; T3 = >5 cm; T4 = invades deep extradermal structures (cartilage, skeletal muscle, or bone).

[b] N0 = no regional lymph node metastases; N1 = regional lymph node metastases.

[c] M0 = no distant metastases; M1 = distant metastases.

PROGNOSIS

The incidence of recurrent lesions is dependent on the size of the lesion and the length of follow-up. Large BCCs (greater than 2 cm) have a higher recurrence rate than smaller tumors. One study reported that 33% of BCC recurrences occurred within 1 year after treatment, 66% within 3 years, and 82% within 5 years.[21] Of these recurrences, 18% did not become apparent until 5 to 10 years later, emphasizing the need for long-term follow-up. Up to 70% of metastases occur in regional lymph nodes that can be surgically removed; however, distant metastases may occur in lungs, bones, liver, and other viscera.[1] The median survival of patients with distant metastases is approximately 10 to 14 months.[1] Primary tumor size and resistance of the primary tumor to surgery and radiation increase the propensity for metastases.

The histologic type of lesion and ability to completely resect the lesion are thought to be important factors in determining prognosis. Infiltrative and micronodular tumors are more likely to be incompletely excised.[15] Superficial, apparently multifocal tumors may be incompletely excised without demonstrating tumor cells at the surgical margins. Complete resection is key in determining the likelihood of recurrence. Incompletely excised tumors demonstrate a recurrence rate of 33 to 39% compared with a recurrence rate of 1% for tumors that are thought to be completely excised.[22,23]

Squamous Cell Carcinoma

Squamous cell carcinoma is the second most common skin cancer and represents approximately 20% of all reported cases.[1] SCC is more invasive and has a greater propensity for metastases than BCC. One literature review noted a weighted average metastatic rate of 2.3 or 5.2%, dependent on follow-up of less than or greater than 5 years, respectively.[24] SCCs are most common in Whites, with the incidence being higher in males than females.[10] UV radiation is a predisposing factor for SCC with cumulative sun exposure leading to an increased incidence with increasing age.[10] UV-A alone may play a role in the development of SCC, as may PUVA treatments (psoralen plus UV-A for the treatment of psoriasis).[1,10] Long-term PUVA treatments have been associated with a risk up to

30 times that of the general population.[25] This issue is controversial, with studies also showing no increased risk of SCC with PUVA treatments. However, the follow-up and treatment duration of most negative studies are short.[26] Long-term risks associated with PUVA treatments also appear to be related to the presence of other exposures, including ionizing radiation, arsenic, and methotrexate. There is a strong dose-response relationship between PUVA and development of SCC, and patients continue to have an increased risk after discontinuation of therapy.[26]

The presence of actinic keratoses is a risk factor for SCC. AKs are the most common premalignant skin lesions and have histologic similarities to SCC in situ (see pathophysiology section). Untreated AK can spontaneously remit, remain stable, or progress to SCC. Studies have estimated that 1 to 10.2% of AK lesions eventually develop into SCC.[10] There is a great deal of controversy regarding the rate of malignant transformation, and as many as 25% of lesions may spontaneously remit. However, 60% of newly diagnosed SCCs occur at the site of a previous AK.[27,28] These studies controlled for as many risk factors as possible; however, the number of known risk factors makes trial design complex and difficult to analyze.

SCC lesions occurring on mucous membranes are most common in persons with a history of heavy smoking and alcohol use. Chewing tobacco and betel nuts are associated with development of SCC of the oral cavity.

PATHOPHYSIOLOGY

SCC is a tumor of keratinizing cells, arising from stratified squamous epithelium and growing to invade the dermis. Confined to the epidermal layer, these tumors are defined as SCC in situ, referred to as Bowen's disease. Once they have invaded the dermis, they can track along tissue planes, perichondrium, or periosteum. SCC grows more rapidly than BCC but has similar invasive characteristics, causing tissue destruction. In contrast to BCC, SCC has a much greater potential for regional and distant metastases.[1]

CLINICAL PRESENTATION AND DIAGNOSIS

Signs and Symptoms

SCC appears as a flesh-colored or erythematous raised, firm papule.[10] It may be crusted with keratin products and may ulcerate and bleed in later stages. SCC in the area of AK has somewhat different characteristics from those that appear on normal skin (de novo SCC). With an SCC that arises from an AK, the lesion appears as a plaque or a nodule with a warty scale covering. These lesions bleed easily with minor trauma and may have telangiectasias on their surface.[1] De novo SCC may have a slightly raised, indurated border (Fig. 95.3). Invasion can occur and manifests as a firm, erythematous nodule with a center core that may be ulcerated. The surface may be smooth or warty and papillomatous and may contain telangiectasias.[1] Infiltrative lesions are often attached to underlying tissues and cartilage. This is a sign of aggressive tumor growth. SCC occurs most commonly on the face, head, and neck, followed by the upper extremities and trunk.[10] SCC may also occur on mucous membranes. These lesions may appear in the oral cavity and lip, can invade other structures of the face, and are more likely to metastasize.

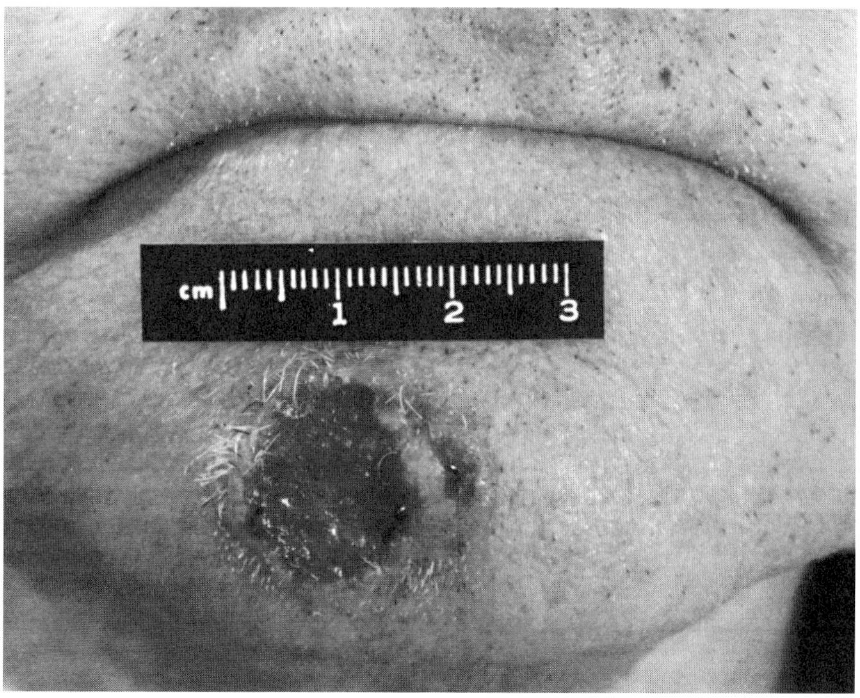

Figure 95.3. De novo squamous cell carcinoma (arising from normal tissue).

Staging

The AJCC has identified the TNM staging system as the system to be used for all skin cancers (Table 95.5).[20] For SCC this is inadequate because of the lack of inclusion of key prognostic variables. The TNM system takes into account the diameter and depth of invasion, as well as the involvement of cartilage, muscle, or bone, but fails to consider anatomic site, etiology, and host immunosuppression, among other prognostic factors.

PROGNOSIS

The frequency of metastases is dependent on anatomic site, histologic features, etiology, host immunosuppression, diameter, depth of invasion, neurotropism, and prior treatment. Some factors have more prognostic significance than others. Mucosal SCC is more aggressive than cutaneous SCC and metastasizes more frequently.[29] SCC of the lip has a worse prognosis than cutaneous SCC but a better prognosis than SCC of the penis, scrotum, or anus.[29] Histologic features that determine levels of differentiation have been shown to be of prognostic significance. Tumors with a greater percentage of well-differentiated cells have a better prognosis than those with a greater percentage of poorly differentiated cells.[10,29]

The etiology of SCC also determines prognosis. Lesions that occur secondary to immunosuppressive disorders are more likely to metastasize than lesions appearing secondary to UV light exposure.[10] SCCs that arise from chronic lesions, such as scars or ulcers, are associated with higher rates of metastases than lesions found on normal skin.[10]

Generally, larger and deeper primary lesions are more likely to metastasize. According to some reports, lesions greater than 2 cm in diameter make up the majority of metastatic cases, and lesions larger than 1 cm in diameter make up the majority of recurring SCCs.[29] A report based on the size and depth of invasion demonstrated a risk of metastasis of 1.4% with T1 lesions, 9.2% with T2 lesions, and greater than 13% with T3 or T4 lesions.[30] In this study, SCCs with a depth of less than 2 mm never metastasized. Those with a depth between 2 and 6 mm had a metastatic rate of 4.5%, and those with a depth greater than 6 mm had a 15% metastatic rate.[30] Depth of invasion of skin cancers can be classified by skin level of deepest invasion. Clark's levels (I through V), which were initially developed for cutaneous melanomas, have been used to study SCC.[29] Penetration to Clark's level IV (the reticular dermis) has been associated with a greater potential for metastases.

Perichondrial, periosteal, and perineural invasion correlate with poor prognoses.[29] Lesions exhibiting perineural invasion typically have higher recurrence rates. However, with the acceptance of Mohs' surgery, this rate has decreased significantly but is still higher than lesions lacking this characteristic.[10] Recurrent lesions are historically more difficult to treat than primary lesions, demonstrating the importance of aggressive first-line treatment when the opportunity for cure is optimal. Metastases most commonly occur to the parotid lymph nodes from primary lesions on the temple or ear.[10] If treated aggressively and early, multimodality therapy including surgery, chemotherapy, or radiation therapy can produce cure rates of more than 50%.[10] If the nodal metastases measure less than 3 cm or are confined to the superficial parotid nodes, cure rates can reach 85 to 95%.[10] The 5-year disease-free survival (DFS) rates for SCC are listed in Table 95.6.

Treatment of Nonmelanoma Skin Cancers

Once the diagnosis of NMSC is confirmed with a biopsy, the treatment planning begins. Planning requires consideration of the type of skin cancer; anatomic location; size; general health and age of the patient; and whether the lesion is primary, recurrent, or metastatic. SCCs require that a wide margin be removed or treated because of their aggressive nature.[1,10] Smaller BCC lesions can be treated with curettage and electrodesiccation.[1] The anatomic location of the lesion also influences the rate of recurrence. Lesions located along the embryonal fusion planes (the midface under the eyes; periauricular and postauricular areas; the paranasal, nasolabial, and inner canthal areas) have the potential for deep invasion and higher recurrence rates.[1] Cosmetic results of treatment are also considered during planning. A lesion located on the eyelids or the tip of the nose requires a tissue-sparing approach (i.e., radiation therapy or Mohs' micrographic surgery).[1] Cryotherapy and topical fluorouracil treatments are also effective for BCC but generally are associated with lower cure rates.[1] Mohs' micrographic surgery is generally used for BCC lesions that have poorly defined margins or for recurrent lesions.

The general health of the patient is key in treatment planning. Unless the disorder can be corrected before surgery, patients with coagulopathies require a less invasive procedure to decrease the risk of bleeding. If travel is a problem (e.g., older adults, debilitated patients or those without transportation), procedures requiring one or two office visits are better than those requiring 10 to 15 office visits. The chance of infection is higher in immunosuppressed patients and should be considered if compliance and cleanliness are of concern.[1]

Treatment choices include curettage with electrodesiccation, cryotherapy, surgical excision (including Mohs' micrographic surgery), radiation therapy, and chemotherapy (topical and systemic). These are listed in Table 95.6.

Table 95.6 ▪ Management of Nonmelanoma Skin Cancer

Method	Indications	5-Year Disease-Free Survival	Comments
Curettage and electrodesiccation	Nodular BCC Anatomic areas with low recurrence rates	77–97% (BCC)	Skilled, experienced practitioners' cure rates are 95–97%.
Cryotherapy	Best for nodular and recurrent BCC Best anatomic locations are eyelid, nose, ear, chest, back, or tip of the nose	95–99% (BCC) 90% (AK)	Lack specimen for pathologic review to check margins. Best results with very small tumors (<0.5 cm).
Surgical excision	Best for aggressive or large lesions Wider margins required for SCC, morphea-type, and recurrent BCC	96% (all nonmelanoma skin cancers)	Skin grafts may be required for wound closure.
Mohs' micrographic surgery	Lesions that do not have well-defined border Recurrent or morphea-type tumors Large tumors (>2 cm) Incompletely excised tumors Tumors within radiation dermatitis Anatomic areas with high recurrence rates	98% (BCC) 96.5% (recurrent BCC) 93% (SCC)	Very complex, time-consuming procedure. Only done at a few institutions. Highest disease-free survival.
Radiation	Reserved for treatment of lesions not amenable to other treatment modalities Lesions along the embryonal fusion plane Good for lesions on eyelids, periorbital region, medial triangle of cheek, earlobe, and nose	96.4% (BCC) 91.9% (SCC)	Areas of radiation are at higher risk of developing other cutaneous malignancies.
Photodynamic therapy	Not a treatment of choice yet Investigational treatment	CR 88–100% (Photophrin)	Persistent photosensitivity for 8–10 weeks.
Chemotherapy			
Topical	5-FU only approved agent Treatment of choice for multiple AK Very small superficial BCC (not amenable to other treatment modalities) Older adult patients not eligible for other treatments	79% (superficial BCC)	If used after curettage, recurrence rate is decreased. Not generally used as single-modality therapy.
Systemic	Neoadjuvant combination chemotherapy has been investigated	CR 26% PR 54% (SCC skin or lip)	Not commonly used for nonmelanoma skin cancer; less effective. Used in conjunction with other treatments (e.g., radiation therapy).

AK, actinic keratosis; *BCC,* basal cell carcinoma; *CR,* complete response; *PR,* partial response; *SCC,* squamous cell carcinoma.

Curettage and Electrodesiccation

Curettage is performed with a curet, a pencil-like instrument with a round or oval tip, sharpened on one side. The tumor is debulked down to the normal tissue, using sound and texture differences to distinguish between normal tissue and tumor. The tumor is removed with a 2 to 3 mm margin of normal tissue. Electrodesiccation may follow curettage, destroying any tumor cells remaining at the base and periphery of the excision site and producing hemostasis. This procedure uses an electrical current to produce sufficient heat, causing tissue damage at the point of contact. Increasing the amperage (current) causes more heat, deeper penetration, and more tissue damage and scarring.[1]

The overall DFS rate with this procedure is 77 to 97%.[1] The rate of recurrence depends on patient selection and practitioner skill in performing the procedure. Skilled, experienced practitioners produce DFS rates as high as 95 to 97%; less experienced dermatology residents perform less adequately, with higher recurrence rates.[1] Lesions with more aggressive histology, larger size, longer history, or locations in high-risk anatomic areas are not candidates for this procedure as primary treatment. Use of this procedure is reserved for minimally invasive BCCs and SCC in situ lesions. The disadvantage to this procedure is the lack of margin control. Many clinicians believe that the cure rates published in the literature (as high as 99%) are actually much lower, due to careful patient selection and a high degree of skilled practitioners used in the published studies.[10]

Cryotherapy

Cryotherapy uses liquid nitrogen (–195.5°C) to freeze viable tissue. Freezing causes formation of extracellular and intracellular ice, abnormal concentration and crystallization of electrolytes, and denaturation of lipoprotein complexes that are lethal to the cells.[1] A 3 to 5 mm margin is required to maximize cure rates.[1] The temperature of the tissue is measured with a thermocoupler inserted underneath the tumor. A temperature sufficient for cell death is at least –50°C.[1] The tissue is allowed to thaw, and then the procedure is repeated for best results.[1]

This technique is best suited for patients who have pacemakers or are poor surgical candidates. Cryotherapy is most effective in lesions that are less than 2 cm and are located on the eyelid, nose, ear, chest, back, or tip of the nose.[1] This is the recommended procedure for recurrent BCCs and tumors with well-defined margins.[1,10] Studies with cryotherapy of SCC are limited, and cryotherapy is not routinely used for invasive lesions of this type.[10] Cryotherapy is contraindicated in morphea-type BCCs, patients with cold intolerance (e.g., cryoglobulinemia, Raynaud's disease), lesions in certain anatomic locations (free margin of eyelid, vermilion border of the lip, ala nasi, anterior and posterior ear, or scalp), or tumors larger than 3 cm.[1] The adverse reactions related to cryotherapy include edema, oozing, erosions, hemorrhaging, and secondary infections. Re-epithelialization may take as long as 10 weeks.[31] The cosmetic results obtained with cryotherapy are very good, with the exception of hypopigmentation and hyperpigmentation. Hyperpigmentation usually fades within a few months after the procedure.[1]

The DFS rates achieved with cryotherapy are very high. One study reported a 99% 5-year DFS rate using cryotherapy in extremely small BCCs (most tumors were 0.5 cm or smaller).[32] Most studies report a recurrence rate of less than 5% with skilled, experienced practitioners performing the procedure.[9] One disadvantage is the lack of pathologic evidence of tumor-free margins. The margins are determined by sight only. Tumor cells could be left behind, predisposing the patient to recurrence; therefore, only very superficial lesions should be treated with this technique.[1,9,29] Use of cryotherapy for actinic keratoses is effective with a few individual lesions and has a very low recurrence rate (10%), but it is not recommended for patients with multiple AKs.[33]

Surgery

Surgical excisions use a scalpel to make an elliptical incision, removing the entire tumor with a 3 to 5 mm margin for BCC and a margin of several centimeters for SCC.[1,10] The optimal tumor-free margin required for SCC has not been determined, but it is well accepted that wider margins than for BCCs are needed. For recurrent or morphea-type BCC, a wide margin is required (e.g., 1 cm).[1] Large tumors with deep invasion also require wider surgical margins. Regional lymph node dissection is required only when lymph nodes are clinically palpable. Skin grafts are occasionally required for wound closure. These grafts take 5 to 7 days to be accepted and 2 to 3 months to become mature and cosmetically acceptable.[1] A skin flap is a piece of tissue that is attached on one side to the donor area and carries its own blood supply and is another option for wound closure.[1] The decision to perform a surgical excision is made after evaluating all other treatment options. DFS rates with surgery alone for NMSC have been reported to be 96%.[9,29] Surgical excisions are contraindicated in patients with coagulation disorders, unless corrected before surgery.

Mohs' Micrographic Surgery

Frederick Moh first described this technique for tumor removal in 1930.[1,31] The procedure is depicted in Figure 95.4. A scalpel is used to make a saucer-shaped excision with a 45-degree angle to provide a specimen with a beveled edge. A map is drawn to correspond to the specimen removed. The specimen is then divided, numbered, and color coded on the edges. Corresponding numbers and color codes are marked on the map. Serial frozen sections are performed. The saucer shape and the angled edge allow for viewing of all surfaces. Any remaining tumor is marked on the map, and excision is repeated until the tumor is completely excised. With this procedure, minimal normal skin is sacrificed and cosmetic results are usually very good, depending on the size of the area excised and the anatomic location of the tumor. Occasionally skin grafts or flaps are required for coverage of very large lesions, but these are not needed as often as with surgical excisions.[1,10]

Mohs' micrographic surgery is indicated if the tumor recurrence rate is high (embryonal fusion planes of the midface, nasal area, or periauricular areas), if the tumor borders are not well-defined, if the tumors are recurrent, in morphea-type BCC, for incompletely excised or large tumors (larger than 2 cm), and for tumors within radiation dermatitis. Infiltrative, micronodular and multifocal BCCs are most appropriately managed with Mohs' micrographic surgery if possible.[15] Five-year DFS rates with Mohs' micrographic surgery are higher than with any other treatment modality (98% for primary BCC, 96.5% for recurrent BCC, and 93% for SCC).[34,35] This treatment approach is now recognized as the standard method of excision for primary and recurrent NMSCs.

Radiation

BCCs and SCCs are radiosensitive tumors. Because of the lack of pathologic confirmation of clear margins and radiation-related morbidity, this method is reserved for lesions that are not amenable to other treatment modalities. Patients with tumors located on the eyelids; periorbital region; and medial triangle of the cheek, earlobe, and nose are good candidates for radiotherapy. Skin cancers along the embryonal fusion plane can be successfully treated with radiation. This method of treatment is not recommended for use in tumors located on the trunk, extremities, dorsum of the hands, or scalp or those arising in sweat and sebaceous glands. It is also not recommended for tumors greater than 8 cm in diameter, morphea-type

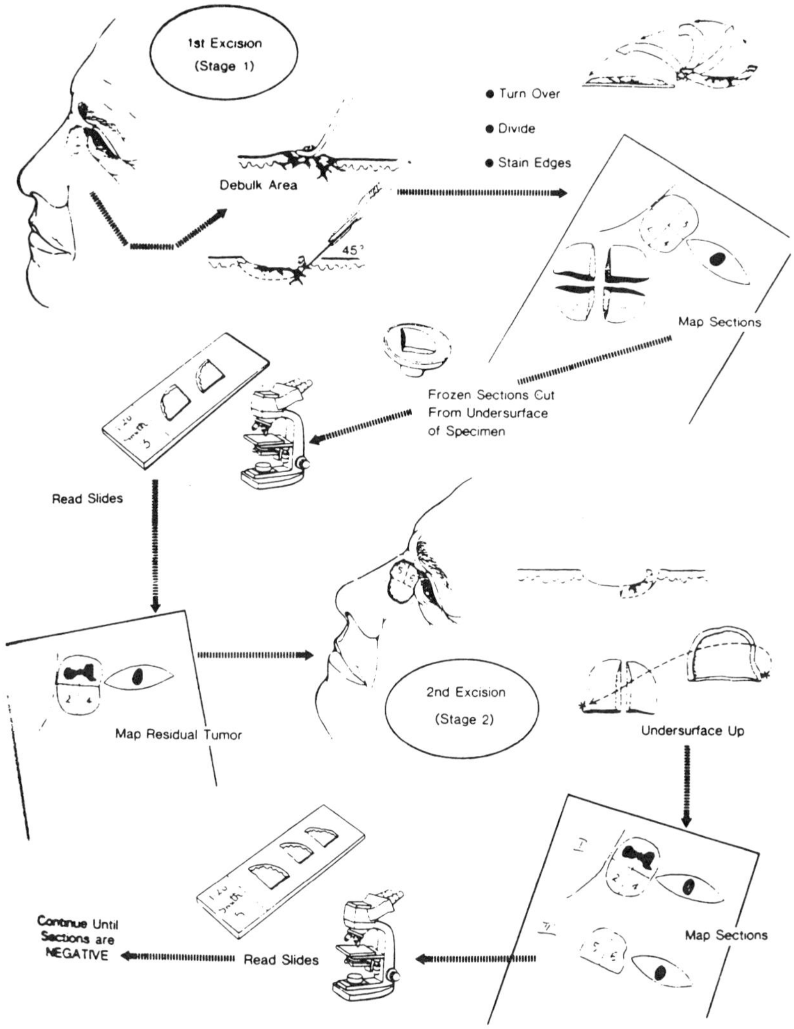

Figure 95.4. Schematic representation of the techniques of Mohs' micrographic surgery. (Reprinted with permission from Safai B. Cancers of the skin. In: DeVita VT, Hellman S, Rosenberg SA, eds. Cancer: principles and practice of oncology. 4th ed. Philadelphia: Lippincott, 1993:1602.)

BCC, intraoral lesions, or tumors that occur on the upper lip growing into a nostril. Radiation is a good choice for patients who are poor surgical risks and for palliation of very large tumors in older adults.[35] DFS rates with this treatment modality are 96.4% for BCC and 91.9% for SCC.[1] Immediate sequelae are erythema, loss of eyelashes when treating the eyelids, and mucositis when treating the nose. Long-term sequelae include radiation dermatitis, which may manifest as atrophy, telangiectasias, hyperpigmentation or hypopigmentation, and precancerous lesions.[1] Radiated areas have a higher risk for the development of other skin neoplasms.[1,31] These reasons contribute to the decision to reserve radiation for lesions not amenable to other treatment modalities.

Photodynamic Therapy

Photodynamic therapy is a new technique for treatment of superficial BCCs. This technique uses tumor-sensitizing drugs to selectively target tumor cells in the skin. A light is required to activate the drugs to produce free radical formation and tissue damage. Many agents are under investigation, including porphyrin-, chlorine-, and phthalocyanine-containing substances that produce free radicals when subjected to certain wavelengths of light. The first compound to be approved by the Food and Drug Administration (FDA), a hematoporphyrin derivative (HPD, Photophrin), is given intravenously and is preferentially taken up by tumor cells. When exposed to laser light, the drug is activated and the tumor is killed. Photophrin is approved for treatment of esophageal cancer only. One study reported a complete response rate of 88 to 100% when treating primary and recurrent BCCs, depending on the dose received by the tumor bed and the nature of the lesion.[36] Re-treatment of recurrences resulted in a 100% complete response rate. SCC lesions appear to respond to PDT, but at a lower rate than BCC, requiring higher doses to achieve acceptable results.[37] Complete response rates with skin metastases have been reported to be 74% with lesions from a variety of primary sites.[38] Patients with multiple lesions or large areas that are affected are particularly suited for PDT.[37] Generalized photosensitivity for 8 to 10 weeks after administration of this agent is a major problem.[36] Newer agents have been developed to circumvent these problems. One agent, 5-aminolevulinic acid (ALA), has been applied topically to skin cancer lesions and illuminated with different types of light sources.[37,39] Photodynamic therapy is not yet the treatment of choice for any cancer, and the higher recurrence rates make it inferior to other proven modalities of treatment. However, future investigations may target difficult to treat or recurrent lesions, as well as patients with multiple or large affected areas. Further clinical studies must be done to identify the role of photodynamic therapy in the treatment of primary and secondary skin cancers.

Chemotherapy

Topical chemotherapy is useful for treatment of precancers and cancers of the skin, but cure rates are generally higher with surgical procedures. The efficacy of topical agents depends on their ability to penetrate the lesion and be absorbed by the target cells. Fluorouracil (5-FU) is the only topical chemotherapy agent to date that has shown efficacy against NMSC and precancerous lesions (e.g., actinic keratoses). This agent is believed to preferentially penetrate sun-damaged skin, where the protective layer is deficient. Because of its selectivity for rapidly dividing cells, 5-FU has a greater effect on premalignant and malignant cells than on normal cells. 5-FU is an antimetabolite that inhibits the action of thymidylate synthetase. Thymidylate synthetase is the enzyme responsible for the methylation of 2-deoxyuridylic acid to thymidylic acid, which is a key step in the synthesis of DNA and cellular reproduction.

Topical 5-FU is the treatment of choice for multiple AK. It must be applied to an entire area of skin and should not be used to "spot treat" small areas of AK.[40] A patient with AK on the face must have the entire face treated, not just the visible lesions. This ensures treatment of occult lesions in the affected area. Under special circumstances, superficial BCC can be treated with topical 5-FU. This is not the treatment of choice for these lesions, but it can be useful in patients who refuse surgery or are not good surgical candidates.[1] Older adults with multiple other medical problems are candidates for topical 5-FU. One disadvantage of this treatment choice is the lack of penetration into deep tissues of the dermis. The reported 5-year cumulative recurrence rate for superficial BCC treated with 5-FU topical therapy alone is 21%.[41] This can be improved if curettage is used as primary treatment before 5-FU to debulk the tumor, resulting in a 5-year cumulative recurrence rate of 6%.[41] Topical 5-FU is contraindicated for nodular BCC and for all SCC, due to their more invasive characteristics. Use of 5-FU for treatment of these lesions should be reserved for patients who are not candidates for other therapies. Optimal areas for use of 5-FU are the facial areas, the dorsum of the hand, and the lower extremities. Biopsy should be performed after treatment is complete to ensure that there are no hidden cells that will put the patient at risk for recurrence. Long-term close follow-up is required for all patients with precancers and cancers of the skin, but, most important, for patients with more aggressive lesions.

Fluorouracil is available topically in a cream or solution (Effudex) in 1%, 2%, and 5% concentrations. Inflammation is a clinical indicator of efficacy and is expected in the cancerous or precancerous area (not in normal skin). Mild to moderate inflammation is sufficient to obtain results. An increase in potency of the agent is required if there is insufficient inflammation at the treatment site. There are no clinical data demonstrating a difference between these available concentrations if adequate erythema is achieved. 5-FU should be administered once or twice a day for several weeks (2 to 10 weeks).[40] Duration of therapy is determined by the location and type of lesion being treated. Lesions on the dorsum of the hands and the forearms tend to be thicker, requiring longer treatment periods. Certain types of precancerous skin disorders are more aggressive, have a higher rate of recurrence, and require longer treatment periods.

5-FU solution is applied with a soft brush and the cream with a fingertip. Using a plastic occlusive dressing can increase the time of contact of 5-FU with the lesion, theoretically increasing the response.[40] This method is useful in treating more aggressive lesions. Concomitant use of topical 13-all-*trans*-retinoic acid (tretinoin, Retin-A) enhances the effect of 5-FU.[40] Steroid cream can be used to alleviate inflammation after treatment is complete without affecting overall response of the tumor.[40] Patients experience photosensitivity while using 5-FU, and this reaction is more severe when combined with tretinoin cream. Patients should be instructed to use a sunscreen and to cover with clothing when exposed to the sun in order to prevent severe sunburns. Contact hypersensitivity to the vehicle and the 5-FU has been reported.[40] This reaction differs from the expected erythema in that vesicles are seen in the area of contact and itching is reported. The usual manifestations associated with the expected erythema produced by 5-FU are described as burning or stinging and *not* itching.[40] Extemporaneous compounding of 5-FU with a different vehicle may prevent recurrence of this problem. 5-FU can cause severe irritation of the conjunctiva or nares if allowed to enter the eyes or nose, respectively.[42] Therefore, contact with these areas should be avoided. Patients should wash their hands carefully after applying 5-FU, with instructions not to touch the eyes or nasal membranes while the fingers are still contaminated with 5-FU.

Systemic administration of 5-FU alone or with cisplatin has not been effective in the treatment of BCC. *Neoadjuvant therapy* is defined as any treatment used before definitive local therapy, in hopes of (1) determining sensitivity of the lesion and (2) decreasing the size of the lesion allowing for tissue-sparing procedures. Large SCCs (greater than 5 cm) have been treated neoadjuvantly with combination chemotherapy. A study using CFB (cisplatin

100 mg/m^2 on day 1, 5-FU 650 mg/m^2/day continuous infusion for 5 days, and bleomycin 15 mg IV bolus on day 1 followed by continuous-infusion bleomycin [16 mg/m^2/day] for 5 days) demonstrated complete response rates of 26% and partial response rates of 54% in patients with SCC of the skin or lip greater than 5 cm in diameter.[43] This strategy, when combined with surgical excision, may be useful in down-staging lesions, improving cosmetic results, and limiting the need for reconstruction. Systemic chemotherapy has also been used to treat SCC of the mucous membranes. Topical nitrogen mustard and BCNU have been used to successfully treat cutaneous T-cell lymphoma (mycoses fungoides), but they are not effective against BCC or SCC.

Immune therapy with intralesional interferon-α (IFN-α) or interleukin-2 (IL-2) has been reported to be effective in BCC, SCC, AK, and metastatic lesions of the skin from a variety of cancers.[29,44] The administration of these drugs is required for several weeks in order to see a response, and the optimal doses required have yet to be determined. Many patients receiving interferon-α experience a flulike syndrome associated with systemic absorption of the drug. These agents may offer an alternative to surgery, but further data are needed to determine their role in the treatment of NMSCs and precancerous lesions.

Retinoids are still under clinical investigation both topically and systemically for prevention and treatment of skin cancer. In some malignant cell lines, retinoids induce cell differentiation, inhibit tumor promotion and induction, and may interfere with tumor initiation.[45] Treatment of AK and BCC with retinoids alone is thought to be less effective than standard treatment modalities.[45] Robinson and Kligman[46] evaluated topical 5-FU in conjunction with topical tretinoin for treatment of AK. Response rates on the forearms were 25% for 5-FU alone and 100% for combination treatment, and response rates on the hands were 0% for 5-FU alone and 90% for combination treatment. Differences in side effects and relapse rates were not commented on in this report and these data have not been substantiated, but this does represent promising results.

Cutaneous Melanoma

EPIDEMIOLOGY AND RISK FACTORS

Incidence

Melanoma is estimated to be the seventh most frequently diagnosed cancer in 1999, with approximately 44,000 new cases (3.6% of all cancers in the United States) and 7300 deaths in 1999, accounting for 1.3% of all cancer deaths in the United States.[47] Melanoma has increased at a rate faster than that of any other cancer over the past 30 years. In 1935, the estimated lifetime risk of developing melanoma was 1 in 1500. In 1980, the incidence increased to 1 in 250 and in 1985 to 1 in 135; this trend continues into the 1990s. It is estimated that by the year 2000 the lifetime risk will be 1 in 90 (Fig. 95.5).[48] This increase in incidence is exponential, whereas the increase in mortality has been linear (Fig. 95.6).[49] This is thought to be due to early detection secondary to screening programs, which have led to an increase in the percentage of earlier-stage lesions. These patients are highly curable and positively influence overall survival. In a study done in Alabama looking at incidence and mortality of melanoma between 1955 and 1982, an increase in thinner, more curable lesions in the latter years was reported.[50]

The median age at diagnosis of melanoma is approximately 45 years, much younger than most other cancers.[51] Melanoma is rare in childhood (less than 15 years old). The peak incidence for most forms of melanoma is reached at approximately 50 years of age and then declines. This distributive pattern of incidence may be related to recreational sun exposure in early adult life, which corresponds to an increased incidence of melanoma in early middle age. This pattern holds true for superficial spreading and nodular melanomas but not for lentigo maligna melanomas (LMMs). LMM is related to cumulative sun exposure, causing the incidence to increase with age and become most common in the latter years of life.[52] Melanoma incidence does not differ substantially among the sexes. Males have a greater incidence of melanoma on the trunk and females on the lower extremities, but the overall incidence is similar.[52,53] Table 95.7 lists the risk factors associated with cutaneous malignant melanoma.

Risk Factors

Skin, hair, and eye color have long been recognized as determinates of risk for melanoma. In a review of the literature, Armstrong and English found a relative risk of developing melanoma ranging from one to three for persons with "light" skin color.[52] In this same review, they found that red hair, compared with dark brown to black hair, infers a twofold to fourfold increase in risk and fair hair infers less than a twofold increase in risk.[52] The skin's reaction to sunlight is also important in determining risk. People who burn easily rather than tanning, after relatively short exposures to UV light, are at increased risk (types I and II, Table 95.3). With the exception of LMM, people with outdoor occupations do not appear to have an increased risk of melanoma. The only form of melanoma associated with cumulative (chronic) sun exposure has been LMM.[53] All other forms of melanoma have been better associated with intermittent sun exposure, especially during childhood. Blistering sunburns during childhood

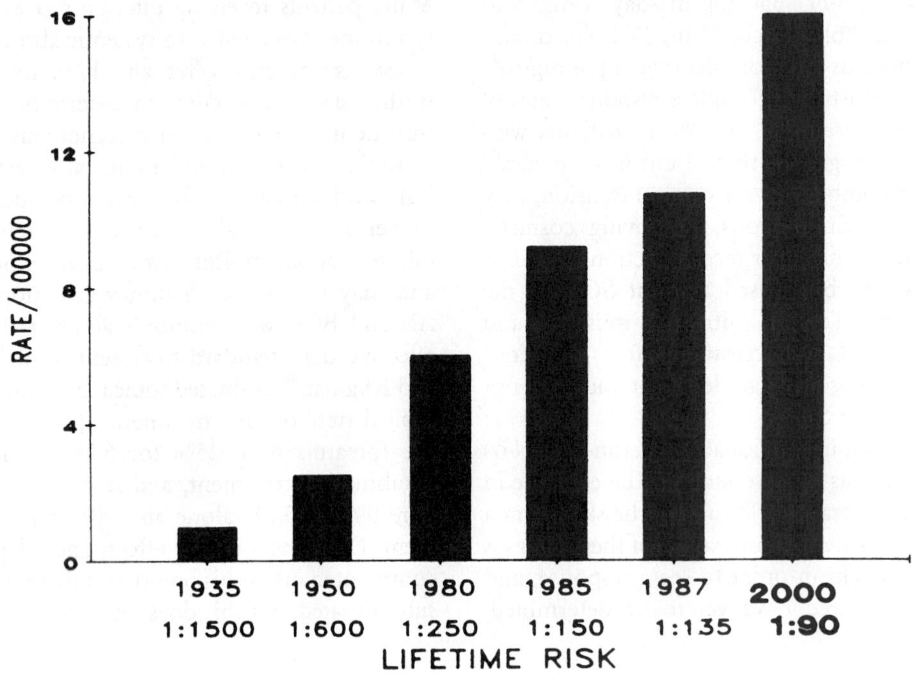

Figure 95.5. Past, current, and projected lifetime risk of a person in the United States developing malignant melanoma. (Reprinted with permission from Rigel DS, Kopf AW, Friedman RJ. The rate of malignant melanoma in the US: are we making an impact? J Am Acad Dermatol 17:1050, 1987.)

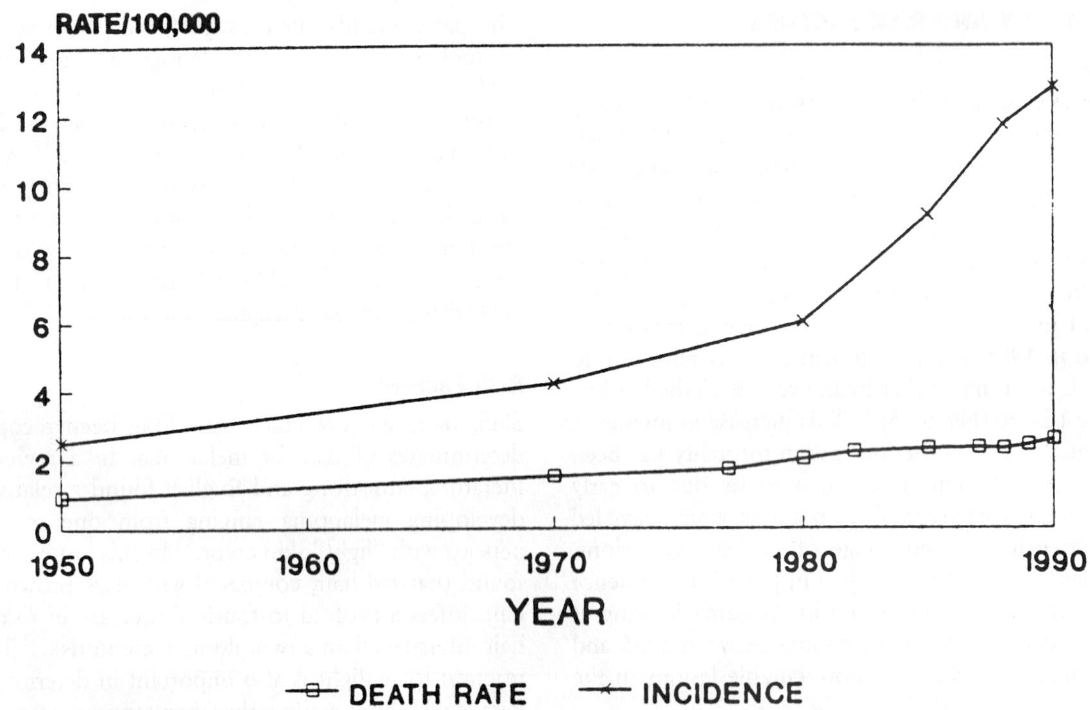

Figure 95.6. Comparison of melanoma incidence and mortality rates in the United States (1990 figures estimated). (Reprinted with permission from Grin-Jorgensen CM, Rigel DS, Friedman RJ. The worldwide incidence of malignant melanoma. In: Balch CM, Houghton AN, Milton GW, et al. Cutaneous melanoma. 2nd ed. Philadelphia: Lippincott, 1992:29.)

or adolescence have been associated with increased risk of developing melanoma.[53] Excessive intermittent (recreational) UV radiation exposure, in conjunction with light coloring and easy burning from sunlight, seems to be the most important risk factor for developing melanoma. Although these facts appear to be straightforward, there is a great deal of controversy regarding the role of UV radiation in the etiology of melanoma.

Freckling, whether in adulthood or childhood, is a risk factor for developing melanoma.[54] Benign melanocytic nevi (moles) are no longer believed to be premalignant lesions. However, the number, size, and type of nevi play an important role in risk assessment.[54] The data are controversial as to the number of benign melanocytic nevi associated with increased incidence of melanoma. Different measures and combinations of number and size of lesions have been applied, and no consensus has been developed to assist in analyzing risk. One study demonstrated a significantly increased risk of nonfamilial melanoma developing in persons with more than 120 small (less than 5 mm in diameter) nevi, more than five large (5 to 10 mm in diameter) nevi, and at least one atypical-appearing nevus.[55] All nevi should be closely monitored for changes that may indicate increased growth or malignant potential. Atypical (dysplastic) nevi are characteristically different from benign melanocytic nevi and are thought to be associated with a much higher incidence of melanoma than persons without these lesions (see etiology section).[54]

People who have a previous melanoma are at increased risk of developing a second primary melanoma.[53] Patients with familial melanoma are at greater risk of developing multiple primary melanomas. However, only 4 to 10% of melanoma patients describe a history of melanoma in a first-degree relative, demonstrating that familial melanoma is uncommon.[51,53] Atypical mole syndrome (AMS) is now used to describe dysplastic nevus syndrome. This is an inherited disorder in which family members have atypical moles and are at increased risk for developing melanoma.[56] Recently, debate has evolved over the nature of this genetic trait and association with melanoma risk. Linkage analysis studies appear to correlate melanoma and the AMS to the short-arm region of chromosome 1.[54] Debate surrounds the actual penetrance, incidence, and significance of a genetic lesion in this location.[54] Familial atypical mole and melanoma syndrome (FAMMS) occurs when two or more family members have melanoma within a family of individuals with atypical mole syndrome.[56] Atypical moles may be premalignant lesions or a marker of increased risk of developing melanoma. The actual rate of malignant conversion of an atypical mole to melanoma is small and varies among kindreds.[56] Xeroderma pigmentosum, a rare autosomal recessive disorder characterized by deficient repair of DNA damage caused by UV-B light, is associated with more than a 1000-fold increase in incidence of skin cancer, including melanoma.[52] These observations lead us to believe that a relationship exists between the immune system and genetics that determines reactions to melanoma antigens (see etiology section).

Table 95.7 ▪ Risk Factors for Melanoma

Fair skin/hair coloring
Freckling
Sunburns easily/tans poorly
Blistering sunburns in childhood or adolescence
Indoor occupation/intermittent sun exposure
Personal/family history of melanoma
Benign melanocytic nevi
>120 small nevi (<5 mm diameter)
>5 large nevi (5–10 mm diameter)
Atypical (dysplastic) nevi (one or more)

Etiology

Ultraviolet Radiation

The precise cause of melanoma is unknown, but host factors and environmental exposures have been most extensively studied. Ultraviolet radiation is proposed to be the most important etiologic agent responsible for the development of cutaneous melanoma. The exact role UV radiation plays in the etiology of melanoma is of great debate, and although discoveries surrounding this relationship have been numerous, there are still many questions left to answer. People with light coloring (skin, hair, eyes) are at increased risk of developing melanoma, indicating that pigmentation may play a role in protecting the skin from the effects of UV radiation. Also, there is a correlation between childhood exposure to UV radiation and increasing incidence of melanoma. In contrast to these data, the lack of predisposition in those with outdoor occupations tends to weaken the association of UV exposure to developing melanoma.[54] Many studies attempting to induce melanomas in animals with UV radiation have failed.[53] Aside from lentigo maligna melanoma, melanomas do not occur most frequently on the face, the most sun-exposed area of the body.[53] These facts further complicate the association between sun exposure and melanoma. Many investigators now believe that the intermittent, recreational UV radiation exposure that has become more frequent in the 1980s and 1990s has substantially contributed to the rise in incidence of this cancer and is the most important environmental risk factor for development of melanoma.[53,54]

Although most clinicians accept the role of UV radiation in the etiology of melanoma and other neoplasms of the skin, the data to support this relationship are not consistent. In an update, Elwood[8] reviews the epidemiologic data regarding UV radiation and its relationship with cutaneous melanoma. The varied results from the available studies indicate the complexity of the issue. The clearly positive associations appear to be found in measures of potential sun exposure (e.g., residence in more sunny rather than less sunny places).[8] Case control studies indicate that geographic location is a determinate of risk, most powerfully seen in migratory studies. UV radiation, although a single factor, is complex in terms of measuring exposure.[8] Hours of exposure are usually measured. However, actual exposure depends on many other factors, such as geographic location (latitude, altitude), skin type of the population being measured, type of exposure (intermittent, chronic, natural sun, tanning lamps), amount of skin exposed, and many other factors. In summary, there is little consensus as to the most appropriate methods for assessing risk secondary to UV exposure.

As mentioned in the NMSC section, UV-B radiation has been most commonly linked to skin cancers and is responsible for the erythematous reaction of the skin after excessive sun exposure. UV-A radiation is believed to have effects on the immune system that may play a role in the development of skin cancers.[57] The extent of involvement of UV-A radiation in the development of melanomas has not been fully elucidated. There has been speculation as to the risk of fluorescent lights, sun lamps, and tanning beds in the development of melanomas. The data are controversial, with studies showing an increased relative risk[58–60] and no difference in relative risk[61–63] in those exposed to these types of light sources compared with the general population.

Factors that determine the extent of UV radiation exposure were discussed earlier. The closer to the equator one lives, the greater the risk of developing melanoma. This is a generally well accepted rule; however, there are exceptions. For example, Norway and Sweden (northern Europe) have higher incidences of melanoma than Italy and France (southern Europe).[52] These anomalies may be due to the fact that ethnic skin coloring darkens with increasing proximity to the equator. Also, there are other environmental factors that determine the amount of UV radiation exposure that are not accounted for by latitude alone (e.g., altitude, reflective surfaces, time of day of exposure, season of the year).

Genetics

Genetics play a major role in certain types of melanoma, especially the familial form mentioned earlier. Also, individuals with a personal history of melanoma are at increased risk of developing a second lesion. This indicates the presence of a genetic predisposition. Data indicate a linkage to chromosome 1p, and other data have indicated that chromosome 9p21 may also be an important locus in developing melanoma.[64] This region appears to be similar to the CDKN2 gene, which encodes for a cell cycle regulator p16. CDKN2 binds to cyclin-dependent kinases (CDKs) in vitro and is a principal negative regulator of cell replication. Mutation of this gene appears to be present in some melanoma kindreds, but is not related to the development of atypical nevi.[64] Conclusive data relating genetic predispositions to melanoma incidence are still awaited, and ongoing studies are addressing these issues. If the linkage to CDKN2 is confirmed, new agents targeting this pathway (CDK inhibitors) may provide a novel therapeutic alternative for melanoma. Many other genes have been implicated in the etiology of melanoma. More than likely multiple genetic lesions, in conjunction with other host and environmental factors, are responsible for the biologic progression of a normal melanocyte to a malignant melanoma.

Other Etiologic Factors

The effects of hormonal manipulations on the incidence of melanoma have been studied. These studies stem from the observation that nevi often undergo changes in appearance during pregnancy and puberty. This observation was attributed to changes in hormone levels in the body, especially increases in circulating estrogen. Oral contraceptives have been associated with increased incidence of melanoma in only a few studies, and in all of these the increase could be attributable to chance due to the small number of cases and the lack of control for other, well-documented risk factors (e.g., sun exposure).[65,66] The same situation exists for exogenous estrogen replacement therapy.[67–69]

Other factors have been studied, including the effects of alcohol, tobacco, coffee, tea, dietary fat, parity, age at first pregnancy, hair dyes, surgery, prior skin problems, and viruses. None of these factors has been proven to have a consistent relationship with the risk of developing melanoma.[52]

PATHOPHYSIOLOGY

Melanomas arise from melanocytes that are located in the epidermal-dermal junction of the skin and the choroid of the eye. Melanocytes can also be found in the meninges, mucosa of the alimentary and respiratory tracts, and lymph node capsules. Melanocytes are dendritic pigmented cells that produce melanin. These cells arise from the neural crest early in fetal development. It usually takes 4 to 6 weeks for the melanocytes to migrate to their final destinations.

Melanin is produced in melanosomes, organelles located in the cytoplasm of melanocytes, and is synthesized from tyrosine. Many of the compounds produced along this pathway are cytotoxic and have been targets for potential therapeutic interventions. There are several types of melanin, ranging from black (eumelanin) to red-yellow (pheomelanin). Skin color is dependent on the type of melanin and melanosomes produced and their interactions with neighboring keratinocytes, not the density of melanocytes in the skin.[70] The differences in genetics that determine skin color, and, therefore, the type of melanosomes and melanin produced, are not entirely identified to date. However, it is generally accepted that many different genes collaborate to determine skin color, texture, and anomalies.

The most important proteins used to identify melanomas are S-100 and HMB-45. S-100 is expressed by nearly all melanomas, but it is also expressed by sarcomas, nerve sheath tumors, and a subset of carcinomas. HMB-45 is more specific for melanoma cells but is not always present in metastatic melanomas.[54] These proteins are used most effectively when applied together with a panel of markers specialized to identify and differentiate melanomas.

Several types of pigmented lesions must be differentiated from melanoma lesions. These lesions are listed in Table 95.8. Normal epidermal melanocytes accumulate to develop common acquired nevi. This occurrence is thought be related to sun exposure. Common acquired nevi are benign in nature and in small numbers do not impose an increased risk of melanoma. These lesions mature through characteristic phases of growth and development, beginning as flat, focal proliferations of melanocytes within the epidermis, and occasionally progress to include the dermis.[70] Atypical (dysplastic) nevi do not go through these predictable developmental stages. They manifest as asymmetric, irregularly shaped, hazy-bordered, irregularly pigmented lesions and may range in diameter from 2 mm to greater than 6 mm.[71] It has been reported that most primary cutaneous melanomas arise from an atypical nevus. However, the vast majority of atypical nevi do not progress to melanoma.[72] Histopathologic confirmation must be obtained for any lesion with the aforementioned characteristics.

Melanoma cells differ from normal epidermal melanocytes in their ability to grow independent of exogenous growth factors, invade into tissues, and metastasize.[70] Melanoma cells usually have marked chromosomal anomalies with two general phases of growth. The radial growth phase is the early phase of horizontal growth with little invasion into surrounding tissue. This phase of growth is characteristically slow, but it is most notable by the examiner's eye. In contrast, the vertical growth phase is not recognized by examination, due to changes taking place beneath the epidermal layer of skin. Vertical growth is expressed in later phases of melanoma progression, being required for extension into the dermal or subcutaneous layers of the skin or metastases to other organs. Clark and colleagues[73] proposed a model for tumor progression from normal melanocyte to melanoma (Fig. 95.7). This theory begins with a benign nevus undergoing atypical (dysplastic) changes (distortion of the cell architecture). Most of these atypical lesions spontaneously regress over time, as is typical for most precancerous lesions, but occasionally undergo transformation into an upregulated proliferation of melanocytes confined solely to the epidermal layer of the skin (melanoma in situ). During the radial growth phase, primary melanomas may develop the characteristics to invade the basement membrane of the epidermis, but they usually do not have the capacity to survive in the new dermal environment. These thin lesions, when removed surgically, have a very high cure rate. If left intact, these lesions may develop the capacity to survive in the dermal layer and potentially metastasize and survive in other tissues. Nodular melanomas do not exhibit a radial growth phase and have a greater potential for metastases from their onset. These lesions are the only exceptions to the progression theory.[74]

Normal melanocytes require growth factors from other cells (paracrine growth factors) for proliferation. Some of these substances have been identified and include basic fibroblast growth factor (bFGF), insulin, insulin-like growth factor (IGF-1), hepatocyte growth factor (HGF), and c-kit ligand.[74] Melanoma cells can proliferate without the need for exogenous growth factors. This led to the discovery that melanomas can produce autocrine growth factors that would otherwise be supplied by the cellular environment. Several autocrine growth factors have been identified in cell culture systems of melanoma cells. The production of bFGF by melanoma cell lines in vitro has been well characterized and seems to be an early event in progression of melanoma cells.[70] Melanocyte growth-stimulating activity (MGSA), platelet-derived growth factor (PDGF), transforming growth factor alpha (TGF-α), interleukin-6 (IL-6), and interleukin-8 (IL-8) are also thought to be autocrine growth factors produced by melanoma cells, but are less well characterized.[70,74] Expression of only one of these factors is not sufficient to cause malignant transformation to melanoma. Transforming growth factor beta (TGF-β) and possibly interleukin-1 (IL-1) are believed to prevent the growth of melanoma cell lines in vitro.[70,74] The relatively quiescent nature of normal melanocytes leads to the assumption that numerous negative control mechanisms are working in concert to control growth. These mechanisms would need to be turned off for transformation into a highly invasive

Table 95.8 ▪ Differential Diagnosis of Pigmented Cutaneous Lesions

Common Lesions	Uncommon Lesions
Seborrheic keratosis	Hemangioma
Subungual hematoma	Pigmented basal cell carcinoma
Compound nevus	Blue nevus
Junctional nevus	Pigmented dermatofibroma
Lentigo	Kaposi's sarcoma
	Cutaneous T-cell lymphoma
	Tattoo

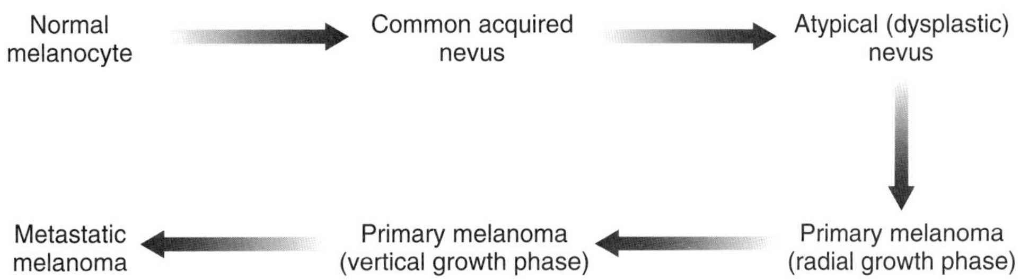

Figure 95.7. Clark's model of tumor progression from normal melanocyte to melanoma. (Adapted from Balch CM, Houghton AN, Peters LJ. Cutaneous melanoma. In: DeVita VT, Hellman S, Rosenberg SA, eds. Cancer: principles and practice of oncology. 4th ed. Philadelphia: Lippincott, 1993:1615.)

melanoma.[74] Paracrine factors seem to play a role in melanoma growth and differentiation, including insulin-like growth factor and epidermal growth factor, which have been shown to stimulate growth of melanoma cells.[70,74] Inhibitory factors (TGF-β, IL-6) may play a role in confining early melanomas to the epidermal layer.[72] Resistance to these factors emphasizes an important aspect of melanoma progression in that later stages of the disease are biologically and genetically different from earlier-stage lesions.[72] Adhesion molecules and angiogenesis factors are being investigated to define their role in the evolution of melanoma cells, enabling them to exist in foreign environments (e.g., other tissue sites) and metastasize.[74] It is rapidly becoming evident that there are complex cellular systems involved in the growth and progression of melanoma, and these interactions are being investigated for development of prognostic indicators, therapeutic interventions, and predictors of response.

Many suppressor genes and oncogenes have been investigated in relation to growth stimulation and inhibition. Chromosomes 1, 6, and 9 are most often found to contain abnormalities in melanomas.[74] Melanoma cells have been found to abnormally express common tumor suppressor genes identified for other cancers, including p53, NF1 (neurofibromatosis-1 tumor suppressor gene), nm 23 (metastasis suppresser gene), and c-kit (oncogene expression is diminished in melanomas). Familial melanoma (atypical mole syndrome) has been studied extensively to reveal the genetic link that increases these patients' susceptibility to melanoma, implicating both chromosome 1 and 9 as possible loci for genes involved in susceptibility to familial melanoma.[74,75]

CLINICAL PRESENTATION AND DIAGNOSIS

Signs and Symptoms

Melanomas can occur anywhere on the body, but are most commonly found on the lower extremities in women and the trunk in men. Typical features of cutaneous melanoma are variegation, irregular raised surface, irregular border with indentations, and ulceration of the surface. The American Cancer Society (ACS) has developed the ABCD rules for identification of suspected lesions.[76] These rules incorporate the aforementioned features into an easily remembered acronym:

Asymmetry
Border irregularity
Color variegations
Diameter greater than 6 mm (the size of a pencil tip eraser)

The key in diagnosing melanoma is recognizing that *any change* in a pigmented lesion is significant. Any pigmented lesion that undergoes a change in size, shape, color, texture, or sensation should be biopsied to rule out melanoma. This includes lesions that lose color and become amelanotic. Itching, burning, or pain in a pigmented lesion should always arouse suspicion of melanoma. However, most patients have none of these symptoms.[54,77]

Four major histologic classifications exist for melanomas: superficial spreading, nodular, lentigo maligna, and acral lentiginous (Table 95.9, Fig. 95.8). Superficial spreading melanomas (SSMs) are the most common variety, making up 70% of all melanomas.[54] These lesions usually arise from a preexisting nevus and evolve slowly over 1 to 5 years, but they also can manifest after only a few months. The majority of existence for these lesions is spent in the radial growth phase, eventually progressing to the vertical phase of growth, invading the dermis and other underlying tissues and acquiring the capacity to metastasize.[54] Some lesions never progress to the vertical growth phase; however, determining which lesions will progress is not currently possible. These lesions occur at any age after puberty and are more common in women than men.[54] The ABCD rules apply most appropriately to SSMs.[76]

Nodular melanoma (NM) is the second most common subset of melanomas, accounting for 15 to 30% of all melanomas.[54] These lesions are more aggressive, lacking a radial growth phase and growing undetected, vertically into the underlying structures. The undetected growth of these lesions predisposes them to late diagnosis with regional spread more likely evident at presentation.[54]

Table 95.9 ▪ Classification of Cutaneous Malignant Melanoma

Subtype	Percent of All Melanomas	Characteristics
Superficial spreading	70	1. Initial phase of radial growth 2. Progresses to predominantly vertical growth
Nodular	15–30	1. Rapid growth (over weeks to months) 2. Uniformly blue-black, dome-shaped nodule (amelanotic variants exist) 3. No discernible phase of radial growth
Lentigo maligna	4–10	1. Primarily on sun-exposed skin of older adults, most often on face 2. Closely linked to cumulative sun exposure 3. Arise from lentigo ("age spots") 4. After decades of radial growth develop nodular areas
Acral-lentiginous	2–8 (in Whites)	1. Most often found on palms, soles, nail beds, and mucous membranes 2. Sunlight not a factor 3. More common in African Americans, Asians, and Hispanics

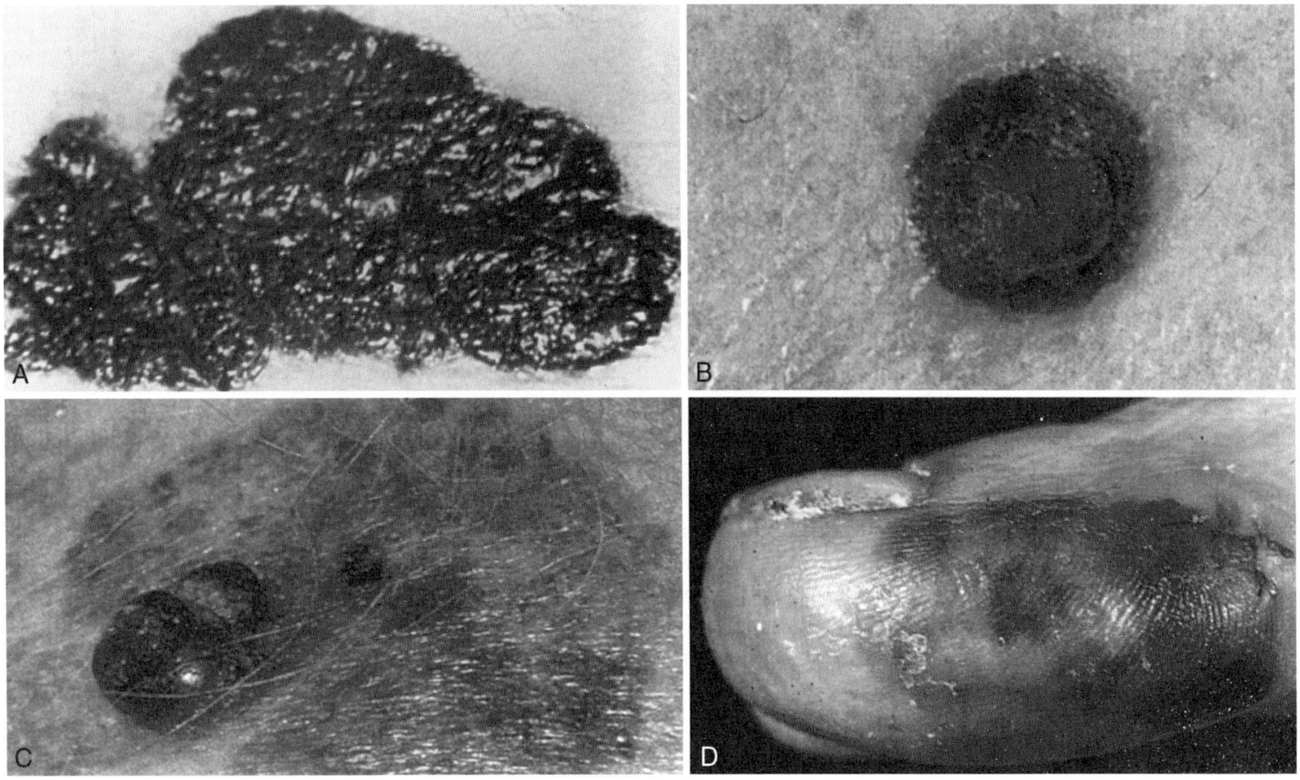

Figure 95.8. Four major histologic classifications for melanomas. **A.** Superficial spreading melanoma. **B.** Nodular melanoma. **C.** Lentigo maligna melanoma. **D.** Acral lentiginous melanoma. (Reprinted with permission from Balch CM, Houghton AN, Peters LJ. Cutaneous melanoma. In: DeVita VT, Hellman S, Rosenberg SA, eds. Cancer: principles and practice of oncology. 4th ed. Philadelphia: Lippincott, 1993:1614.)

These lesions tend to arise from normal skin rather than preexisting nevi and can occur anywhere on the body. The most common areas are the trunk, head, and neck and are true to their name, having a dome shape with sharply demarcated borders.[54] NMs are typically diagnosed between 40 and 50 years of age, but they can occur at any age and are more common in men than women.[54] NMs are usually 1 to 2 cm in diameter but can be much larger. They are characteristically dark brown to black, can have shades of blue color, but are amelanotic (lacking pigment) in approximately 5% of cases.[54] The ABCD rules do not apply to these characteristic lesions.[76]

LMM arises from the precursor or in situ lesion (lentigo maligna), which is light brown and flat with markedly irregular borders, usually appearing on sun-exposed areas of skin in older adults.[54] If invasion is documented within a lentigo maligna, the lesion is considered to be LMM.[54] These lesions are closely related to cumulative lifetime UV radiation exposure. The radial growth phase can last for as long as 5 to 15 years or more, converting to the vertical growth phase, which manifests as a nodule or papule within the lentigo maligna lesion. This form of melanoma is less common than SSM or NM and has less propensity to metastasize. LMM represents only 4 to 10% of all cutaneous melanomas.[54] These lesions are usually located on the face, with the nose and cheeks most commonly affected. The average age at diagnosis is 70 years; it is very uncommon in those younger than 50 years of age.[54] Lentigo malignas tend to be large (greater than 3 cm), and changes within the lesion are often overlooked because of their slow-growing nature. If neglected, LMM have the potential to spread and become aggressive. The diagnosis requires that sun-related changes be evident in the dermis and epidermis.[54]

Acral lentiginous melanomas (ALMs) are the most common melanomas in dark-skinned people such as African Americans, Asians, and Hispanics, representing 35 to 60% of melanomas diagnosed but making up only 2 to 8% of melanomas in Whites.[54] These lesions arise on the palms, soles, beneath the nail plate, or in the mucous membranes, and they are large, with the average diameter at diagnosis being 3 cm.[54] These lesions appear to have little correlation with exposure to UV radiation. They occur most commonly in older people (average age in the sixties).[54] ALM is present an average of 2.5 months before diagnosis, demonstrating its more aggressive nature. These lesions often are confused with LMM because of their light brown, flat appearance. The growth can be deceptive, growing undetected vertically with little evidence of change from the surface. These lesions are more aggressive than SMM or LMM and therefore have a poorer prognosis.[54] Subungual melanoma is one particular type of ALM. The median age at diagnosis is 55 to 65 years, and it is equally common in males and females.[54]

Melanoma can metastasize anywhere in the body, with the most common sites of metastases at first relapse being skin, subcutaneous tissue, and distant lymph nodes.[54] Lung, liver, brain, and the gastrointestinal tract are the next most common sites. In-transit metastases are defined as lesions located between the primary site of the lesion and the first major regional lymph node basin.[54] These lesions are thought to originate from cells trapped in the lymphatics. They are usually observed in the subcutaneous or intracutaneous layer of the skin (i.e., satellitosis). Local recurrences are defined as any tumor that occurs within 5 cm of the scar of a previously excised melanoma.[54]

Patients with stage I, II, or III melanoma rarely have changes in radiographic evaluations if micrometastases are present, but instead have symptoms.[54] Particular attention should be paid to signs or symptoms of central nervous system involvement. Also, blood in the stool and gastrointestinal symptoms can be possible indicators of metastatic disease. Although some patients remain stable for months, others have rapid progression of disease with clinical deterioration within weeks. The clinical course of any individual patient is difficult to predict and should be followed carefully by close monitoring of symptoms and signs relevant to the most common sites of metastases, as well as any other change in symptoms experienced.

Staging and Prognosis

If melanoma is suspected, biopsy is required for diagnosis. Several characteristics must be considered when determining biopsy technique. Microstaging, to determine the full thickness of the lesion, is essential and must be performed with the initial biopsy. Therefore, excisional biopsy (removing the entire lesion) is the optimal biopsy procedure for lesions suspected of melanoma.[53] Other characteristics that must be considered are the location of the lesion (amount of tissue coverage) and the size of the lesion. It is difficult to completely excise a large lesion on the face with acceptable cosmetic results. In these cases, a punch biopsy can be done in the most raised, deeply pigmented portion of the lesion, reaching its full depth. Another alternative is an incisional biopsy. Shave, needle, curettage, and saucerization biopsies are contraindicated for any primary pigmented lesion suspected of melanoma. These procedures may compromise the integrity of the histologic confirmation. The needle biopsy technique may be useful to document nodal metastases of melanoma.[53]

Microstaging, an integral part of staging and management of melanoma (Fig. 95.9), currently is accomplished using two methods. Breslow's method uses an ocular micrometer to measure the total height (not just depth) of the lesion from the granular layer to the area of deepest

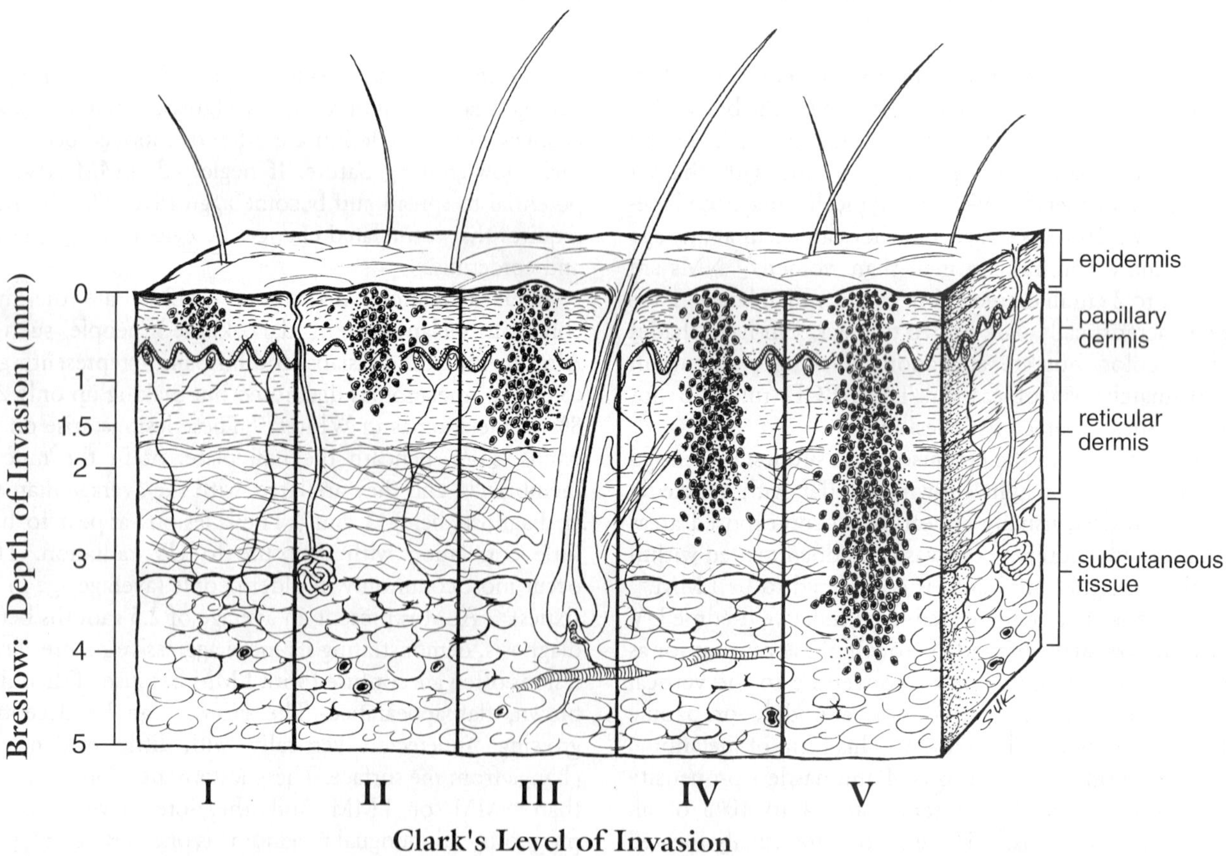

Figure 95.9. Pathologic microstaging of melanoma. Breslow's levels measure tumor thickness in millimeters (mm) and are shown on the left-hand side of the figure. Clark's levels measure the depth of invasion by tissue level of deepest penetration and are depicted across the bottom of the figure.

Table 95.10 ▪ Pathologic Microstaging for Cutaneous Malignant Melanoma

Breslow's Levels[a]	Clark's Levels	
≤0.75 mm	I	Confined to the epidermis
0.76–1.49 mm	II	Extends into the papillary dermis
1.50–2.49 mm	III	Up to but not extending into the reticular dermis
2.50–3.99 mm	IV	Extending into the reticular dermis
≥4.00 mm	V	Extending into the subcutaneous tissue

[a]Uses an ocular micrometer to measure the total height of the lesion from the granular layer to the area of deepest penetration.

Table 95.11 ▪ Traditional Three-Stage System for Cutaneous Malignant Melanoma

Stage		Criteria	5-Year Survival Rate (%)
I	(thickness in mm)	Skin only	79
	≤0.75		96
	0.76–1.49		87
	1.50–2.49		75
	2.50–3.99		66
	≥4.00		47
II	Any thickness	Nodal metastases	36
III	Any thickness	Distant metastases	5

penetration.[78] If the lesion is ulcerated, measurements are made from the base of the ulcer to the deepest portion of the lesion; if it is raised above the normal surface of the skin, the measurements are taken from the highest point to the deepest point of the lesion. Breslow's levels are listed in Table 95.10. Clark and colleagues[79] developed microstaging levels based on the depth of invasion into the skin rather than thickness of the lesion (Table 95.10). In several studies looking at the prognostic significance of these two methods of microstaging, Breslow's measures of tumor thickness demonstrated more accurate and reproducible ability to predict the risk for metastases.[78,80]

The original three-stage system for melanoma incorporated local, regional, and distant spread of the disease into three simple stages. This staging system categorized approximately 85% of patients in stage I, preventing detection of discernible differences in risk for metastases and death (Table 95.11).[50] With the observations of the prognostic significance of tumor thickness and level of invasion, the AJCC developed a new staging system incorporating these prognostic factors into the classic TNM staging system used for most solid tumors. The most current acceptable staging system is presented in Table 95.12.[20] Figure 95.10 illustrates the overall survival rates of patients using the new staging system, demonstrating that stage is now a better predictor of survival.[20]

Many prognostic factors have been identified to assist in treatment planning and determination of risk with melanoma.[81] Tumor thickness, as measured in millimeters, is the single most important prognostic factor for patients with stage I and II melanomas. There are not thought to be any natural breakpoints for categories of thickness, but rather a continuous correlation of survival to tumor thickness exists.[81] The categories made by Breslow were arbitrary cutoff points, but they have been accepted for staging purposes and are thought to impart some separation in terms of risk of recurrence and overall survival. Clark's levels of invasion are also of prognostic significance, with an inverse correlation between increasing level of invasion and survival. Ulceration of the primary lesion is a strong indicator of poor prognosis for stage I, II, and III melanoma. Ulceration and tumor thickness are thought to be closely correlated, with ulcerated lesions manifesting as thicker lesions than those without ulceration.[81] For stage I and II lesions, patients with lesions on the extremities have a better survival rate than those with lesions on the trunk or head and neck. Of these extremity lesions, those on the upper extremities have a slightly better survival rate than those on the lower extremities.[81] Gender was of prognostic significance for stage I and II lesions, with women having a better survival rate than men. A primary reason for this survival advantage is the fact that lesions in women tend to occur more commonly on the extremities and are less often ulcerated.[81] Older patients tend to have thicker lesions and tend to have a worse prognosis than younger patients, using 50 years of age as an arbitrary cutoff point.[81] When matched thickness for thickness, all of the different types of melanoma have similar prognosis except for LMM. LMM has the best prognosis, regardless of thickness of the lesion or age of the patient.[81]

Many powerful prognostic variables have been identified since this staging system was adopted. Clinicians around the world are calling for needed revisions in the current system to incorporate some of these important factors. The questionable significance of Clark's levels has been heavily debated in the literature. In a critical analysis by Buzaid and colleagues,[82] reanalysis of the combined melanoma database from the University of Alabama at

Table 95.12 ▪ American Joint Committee on Cancer Staging System for Cutaneous Malignant Melanoma

T	Breslow's (mm)	Clark's	N	
1	≤0.75	II	1	Nodal metastasis ≤3 cm
2	0.76–1.50	III	2	Nodal metastasis >3 cm
3	1.51–4.00	IV	M	
4	>4.00	V	1	Distant metastasis

Stage	Criteria
I	T1 or T2, N0, M0
II	T3 or T4, N0, M0
III	Any T, N1 or N2, M0
IV	Any T, Any N, M1

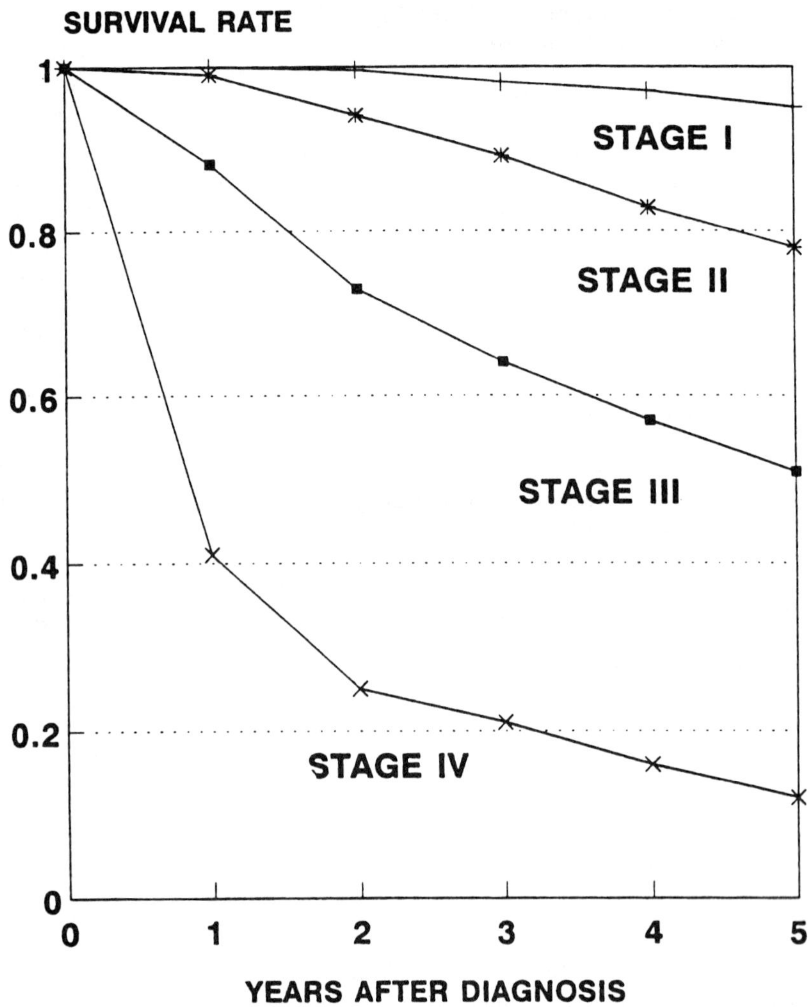

Figure 95.10. Relative survival rates according to the stage of disease. Data taken from 8479 patients who were diagnosed between 1977 and 1982. Patients are listed in the Surveillance, Epidemiology, and End Results Program of the National Cancer Institute. Stage I represents 4286 patients; stage II, 3328; stage III, 649; and stage IV, 216. (Reprinted with permission from American Joint Committee on Cancer. Manual for staging of cancer. 4th ed. Philadelphia: Lippincott, 1995:144.)

Birmingham and the Sydney Melanoma Unit revealed that Clark's level of invasion had little prognostic significance beyond that of tumor thickness for melanomas thicker than 1 mm. Also in this report, cutoffs for tumor thickness were reanalyzed for best statistical fit, and it was found that ranges of less than 1 mm, 1 to 2 mm, 2 to 4 mm, and greater than 4 mm appear to be the best cutoffs for tumor thickness. Other factors such as tumor ulceration and the presence of tumor-infiltrating lymphocytes are thought to be important prognostic indicators.[83] Many models incorporating several different prognostic factors have been developed and evaluated to better predict outcomes. These models have not been confirmed in large prospective trials, but they may prove to be more effective than single prognostic factors. See reference 83 for more details regarding proposed changes in the staging of melanoma.

The presence of microscopic lymph node metastases may assist is identifying higher-risk subsets of patients within specific tumor thickness categories. Methods of lymphatic mapping and sentinel node biopsy are being investigated as a relatively noninvasive means of staging the nodal basin. Coupling this technique with serial sectioning, advances in immunohistochemistry and new molecular markers (e.g., polymerase chain reaction for tyrosinase) may enhance the ability to determine prognosis for stage I and II patients.[83]

For patients with stage III melanoma, clinically involving regional lymph nodes, the number of metastatic lymph nodes involved was the best predictor of survival. Patients with only one lymph node involved had significantly better 10-year survival rates than those with two to four nodes and five or more nodes (40%, 18%, and 9%, respectively).[81] Currently the staging system separates nodal status by size (less than 3 cm or greater than 3 cm). However, there are few data in the literature to substantiate this designation.[83]

The single most important prognostic variable for patients with stage IV (distant metastases) disease is the number of metastatic sites involved. Patients with one site of metastases have a median survival of 7 months, compared with 4 months for those with two sites and 2 months for those with three or more sites. Patients with metastases to skin, subcutaneous tissues, and distant lymph nodes, the most common sites of first relapse, have a median survival of 7 months, and 25% remain alive at 1 year. The next most common site of first relapse is the lung, having the best median survival of 11 months if isolated. Metastases to brain, liver, and bone impart a median duration of survival of 2 to 6 months, with a 1-year survival rate of only 8 to 10%.[81] The length of disease-free interval also appears to be of importance for metastatic patients, depicting the growth rate of the tumor.[83] The dismal prognosis evident with metastatic disease, compared with local disease (stage I and II), is powerful information to advocate screening programs worldwide. These efforts are discussed later.

TREATMENT

For melanoma, surgical excision is, generally, the most effective treatment modality. Even in selected cases of metastatic disease, the optimal palliative treatment includes surgical resection of the lesion(s). Metastatic lesions are generally not responsive to other treatment modalities and should be considered relatively radiotherapy and chemotherapy resistant. Although this is true, much of the research with melanoma lies in the arena of systemic therapy for metastatic melanoma and adjuvant treatment of patients after removal of involved lymph nodes by several different modalities. Patients with advanced disease have a poor prognosis; therefore, any treatment modality recommendation must emphasize the importance of an acceptable quality of life. Recent promising results with immunotherapy brings hope for a future of novel treatment modalities with vaccines and gene-targeting therapies. Table 95.13 outlines treatment strategies for cutaneous malignant melanoma by stage of disease.

Surgery

Excision of Primary Melanoma

For stage I and II melanomas, the treatment of choice is surgical excision of the primary lesion, down into the subcutaneous tissue, plus a radius of normal-appearing tissue.[84] This can often be performed in the office using local anesthesia, depending on the location of the lesion and margins required. With excision alone, the overall risk of local recurrence is about 3% for stages I and II.[84] The prognostic significance of tumor thickness obtained from microstaging enticed investigators to challenge the standard use of radical excisions (at least 5 cm of tumor-free margin) for *all* melanoma lesions. Many investigators set out to prove that thinner margins are appropriate for thinner lesions, without compromising overall survival, rate of metastases, or incidence of local recurrence. Lesions less than 1 mm thick are thought to be safely excised with a 1 cm margin. Based on data from the WHO Melanoma Programme[85] and the Intergroup Melanoma Study,[86] the recommended margin of excision for lesions between 1 and 2 mm should be based on the anatomic location of the lesion and the need for a skin graft for closure versus primary closure. Those 1 to 2 mm lesions that would require a skin graft with a 2 cm excision should employ the 1 cm margin. This would lessen the risk for complications from skin grafting while maintaining a very low risk of local recurrence. Lesions between 2 and 4 mm thick should use the 2 cm margin for optimal local control. Excisional requirements for thicker lesions (larger than 4 mm) have not been studied in a randomized, controlled manner, but the current recommendations are to excise these lesions with a 2 to 3 cm margin.[87] Melanoma in situ lesions (contained in the epidermis) have a minimal risk of recurring locally and do not have the capability to metastasize. The recommended tumor-free margin for these lesions is at least 0.5 to 1 cm.[88] Table 95.13 outlines treatment recommendations for melanoma.

For primary cutaneous melanomas on the fingers or toes, digital amputation is required. It is important to

Table 95.13 ▪ Treatment Strategies for Cutaneous Malignant Melanoma by Stage of Disease

Stage	Treatment of Choice	5-Year Disease-Free Survival[a]	Comments
I and II[a]	Surgical excision	47–97%	LMMs have the best prognosis and can often be treated with thinner margins or radiotherapy.
<1 mm	1 cm margin		CMMs on fingers and toes require digital amputation.
1–2 mm	1–2 cm margin (see text)		ERLND and lymph node mapping are controversial (see text).
2–4 mm	2 cm margin		Consider adjuvant interferon for T4 lesions (see text).
>4mm	2–3 cm margin		
III	Surgical excision of primary and involved regional lymph nodes	20–40%	Removal of the entire nodal basin is usually performed. Adjuvant interferon is indicated for these patients. Isolated limb perfusion has response rates of up to 100% (see text). Intralesional bCG may be used to treat satellite lesions (see text).
IV	Biochemotherapy (chemotherapy plus biologic therapy; see text), surgical excision, or both	<5%	Selected lesions in the lung, brain, subcutaneous tissues can be resected for palliation of symptoms. Chemoimmunotherapy has been shown to prolong survival in patients with stage IV disease. Resection of isolated lung or subcutaneous metastases may prolong survival in 15–30% of patients (see text).

bCG, bacillus Calmette-Guérin; *CMM,* cutaneous malignant melanoma; *ERLND,* elective regional lymph node dissection; *LMM,* lentigo maligna melanoma.

[a]Information on stage I and II CMM is divided into these categories in the studies available to date. These are not the same divisions seen in the staging system shown in Table 95.12.

preserve enough of the digit to ensure adequate functioning. These procedures require at least a 1 cm margin of skin be removed at the time of amputation.[84] The ear can usually be partially amputated or wedge resected, reserving complete amputation for recurrent lesions or widespread disease. Ear prostheses are available for patients requiring this type of surgery.[84]

Elective Lymph Node Dissection

Removal of normal-appearing regional lymph nodes in hopes of decreasing the incidence of distant failure is termed *elective lymph node dissection* (ELND). ELND is a controversial procedure and may or may not be associated with improved survival. This procedure is based on the belief that melanoma metastasizes sequentially, first spreading to the regional lymph nodes and then to distant sites. Opponents of the procedure note the successes with surgical excision of the primary alone for stage I and II patients as reasons not to inflict this type of morbidity on patients who may not have microscopic disease in the lymph nodes.[89] The hypothesis that earlier removal of lymph nodes positively affects survival has not been consistently supported in clinical trials evaluating ELND versus wide local excision of the primary alone. Proponents for ELND state that for those patients with microscopic nodal metastases, early diagnosis and removal may bring good survival odds, potentially preventing further distant metastases from occurring.[90] Two recently completed randomized prospective trials are expected to report their long-term results, which may help resolve this issue.[90] These contemporary studies also take into account the influence of now recognized prognostic variables that may identify a high-risk subset of patients.

One resolution to this controversy lies in a new procedure that can stage the suspected lymph node basin without requiring full dissection. This procedure is termed *intraoperative lymphatic mapping and sentinel node biopsy.*[91] A vital blue dye is injected into the dermis just adjacent to the primary melanoma lesion. The first node to collect the dye is biopsied, the so-called sentinel node. If this node is positive for microscopic disease, lymphadenectomy can be done. However, if this node is negative, the procedure can be halted and the patient is spared an unnecessary surgery. The identification rate with this procedure is reported to be 85 to 90% with low false-negative rates.[90] Many cutaneous sites have ambiguous lymph drainage, making it more difficult to identify the sentinel node. Lymphoscintigraphy has been used to better identify sentinel nodes in areas with ambiguous lymph drainage. In this procedure, ^{99m}Tc-labeled colloid combined with vital blue dye is injected and a g-counter is used in the operating room to locate the sentinel node. This procedure is reported to have a false-negative rate of less than 1%.[90] This technique of lymphatic mapping with biopsy may be useful for staging purposes and to more effectively choose those patients who would benefit from adjuvant therapy.

The issue of ELND remains one of the most controversial topics concerning patients with melanoma. Ongoing studies investigating lymph node mapping with sentinel node biopsy and selective lymph node dissection (if indicated) may prove this to be the treatment of choice for regional lymph node basins.[90] Results of these studies are anxiously awaited.

Therapeutic Lymph Node Dissection

Lymphadenectomy performed when clinically apparent nodes are found is termed *therapeutic dissection.* Clinically evident regional lymph node involvement (stage III) is managed primarily with surgical resection. Long-term disease-free survival after lymphadenectomy is predicted to be 20 to 40% for stage III melanoma patients. The adverse effects of lymphadenectomy depend on the site of resection. The ilioinguinal lymph node basins drain the lower extremities. After resection of these basins, there is noticeable edema in approximately 26% of patients at long-term follow-up, but only 5% and 3% of patients, respectively, report pain or functional deficit.[54] Leg exercises, elastic stockings, diuretics, and perioperative antibiotics have been shown to prevent edema in these patients. Complications with axillary node dissection are infections (7%), seroma (27%), hemorrhage (1%), and arm edema (1%).[54] Cervical and parotid lymph nodes can also be removed with similar complications. Nerve damage occurring in the location of these lymph nodes (close proximity to the cranial nerves) is rarely seen but is always a possibility.[54]

Surgical Management of Metastases

Patients with distant metastases have a poor prognosis, with a median survival of 5 to 8 months and a 5-year survival rate of less than 5%. Resections of metastatic lesions can offer palliation of symptoms but rarely affect survival rates. Resection of isolated pulmonary or subcutaneous metastases is associated with prolonged survival in up to 15 to 30% of patients.[55] At this point in the disease process, emphasis is placed on quality of life rather than quantity.

Radiation

Radiotherapy for Primary Melanomas

The use of radiation for treatment of melanoma is controversial. Initial reports of complete radioresistance among all melanomas have been challenged. With early stages of melanoma, surgery alone is the standard of care with very high cure rates (greater than 95%). Treatment of primary melanomas with conventional radiation is limited to LMM lesions. Many of these lesions occur on the face in older adults and may require extensive reconstruction if surgery is performed. Radiotherapy can be useful for these patients with little morbidity and very good clinical and cosmetic results. In one series, using fractionated doses of radiation to treat 28 patients with LMM, only 2 patients recurred, but some lesions took as long as 24 months to fully regress after radiation.[92] The long-term adverse effects with radiation are skin pallor, telangiectasias, and atrophy in the area of treatment (approximately 10%).[92]

Adjuvant Radiotherapy

The use of radiotherapy after surgery has been studied in cases where optimal resection would be disfiguring and where the risk of local relapse is high. Ang and colleagues,[93] in an investigation of 174 patients with cutaneous melanoma of the head and neck who were at high risk for local recurrence, concluded that adjuvant radiation can decrease local recurrence rates but has little effect on survival. Survival is at least equal to that seen with conventional approaches. The role for adjuvant radiation is small, but it can be instrumental if a disfiguring surgical procedure can be avoided. Radiation, in place of dissection, of the lymph node basins is possible and may be associated with less morbidity than that with dissection. Randomized, controlled studies must be done in order to better identify the role for adjuvant radiotherapy, either to the primary sites or to the nodal basins.

Radiotherapy for Distant Metastases

Distant sites of metastases may be treated with radiation. The most common indications for radiotherapy are treatment of subcutaneous, dermal, lymph node, brain, or bone metastases. Palliation of symptoms can often be accomplished with radiotherapy directed toward the specific site of involvement. Spinal cord compression or other lesions not amenable to surgery can also be radiated for palliation. If a patient is not a surgical candidate, based on other medical criteria, radiotherapy is a reasonable option for treatment of metastatic melanoma.[54] Radiation fractions greater than 4 Gy are usually required to achieve a response.[94] This dose of radiation may predispose patients to more acute and chronic sequelae resulting from the radiation effects on normal tissues. Therefore, the decision to radiate should include a detailed examination of other treatment modalities, carefully assessing the risks and benefits of each type of therapy in relation to potential efficacy and adverse events, as well as patient and tumor characteristics.

Hyperthermia and Isolated Limb Perfusion

Hyperthermia

Hyperthermia, or warming the body, has been studied both alone and in conjunction with radiotherapy and chemotherapy as a treatment modality for a number of cancers. Warming is accomplished with the use of a water-circulating mattress that has adjustable heating components. Hyperthermia in the range of 40 to 45°C is cytotoxic against melanoma cells when used alone.[94] One rationale behind the combination of hyperthermia and radiotherapy (thermoradiotherapy) is that hyperthermia will potentially bring radioresistant cells out of their dormant state, thereby making them more susceptible to the effects of radiotherapy. Also, resistance mechanisms differ between hyperthermia and radiation. Therefore, the combination increases the chance that cells resistant to one modality may be susceptible to the other.[94] Thermoradiotherapy is thought to be an active treatment modality. A randomized trial of patients with recurrent or metastatic melanoma was conducted; patients were assigned to receive radiotherapy alone or with hyperthermia. In a univariate analysis of tumor control rates, a significant advantage was demonstrated with the addition of hyperthermia (46% versus 28%, respectively; $p = 0.008$).[95] Effects on normal tissue did not appear to be significantly worse with the addition of hyperthermia. These effects have been verified by other investigators.[94] The logistics of this treatment approach may limit making this the standard method of radiotherapy for melanoma.

Isolated Limb Perfusion

Isolated limb perfusion with and without hyperthermia has been studied, particularly in patients with multiple lesions on an isolated extremity (Fig. 95.11). The goal of limb perfusion is to maximize the concentration of drug in the affected limb while minimizing the systemic side effects of chemotherapy. This procedure has been used adjuvantly for subclinical micrometastases and therapeutically for local recurrences, as well as in-transit or satellite metastases.[96] Many agents have been used either alone or in combination and include melphalan, actinomycin D, mechlorethamine, dacarbazine, cisplatin, carboplatin, tumor necrosis factor (TNF), and IFN-β and IFN-γ. The drug most studied and most effective is melphalan, which has complete response rates of about 54% (range 26 to 81%).[96] In the presence of hyperthermia (40 to 41.5°C), one study demonstrated an increase in complete response rates from 32 to 76%.[97] Survival data have not yet determined whether adjuvant isolated limb perfusion is superior to surgery alone for melanomas thicker than 1.5 mm. There are currently two studies underway to investigate this question. For treatment of bulky in-transit metastases, this technique is very encouraging and should be considered standard of care, especially as an alternative to amputation. Combination of melphalan, TNF-α, and IFN-γ has shown promising results in the treatment of bulky, in-transit metastases. This combination has reported overall response rates of 100%, complete responses of 90%, and acceptable regional and systemic toxicity.[98] Although these data were substantiated in a phase II trial for recurrent melanomas,[99] subsequent data have failed to demonstrate a significant improvement in the duration of response or recurrence rate.[96] The National Cancer Institutes (NCI) is currently conducting a study randomizing patients to receive isolated limb perfusion with melphalan alone or in combination with TNF-α, to substantiate the response rates previously described and to determine their durability. It must be emphasized that any remaining nodules after isolated limb perfusion require resection to avoid local recur-

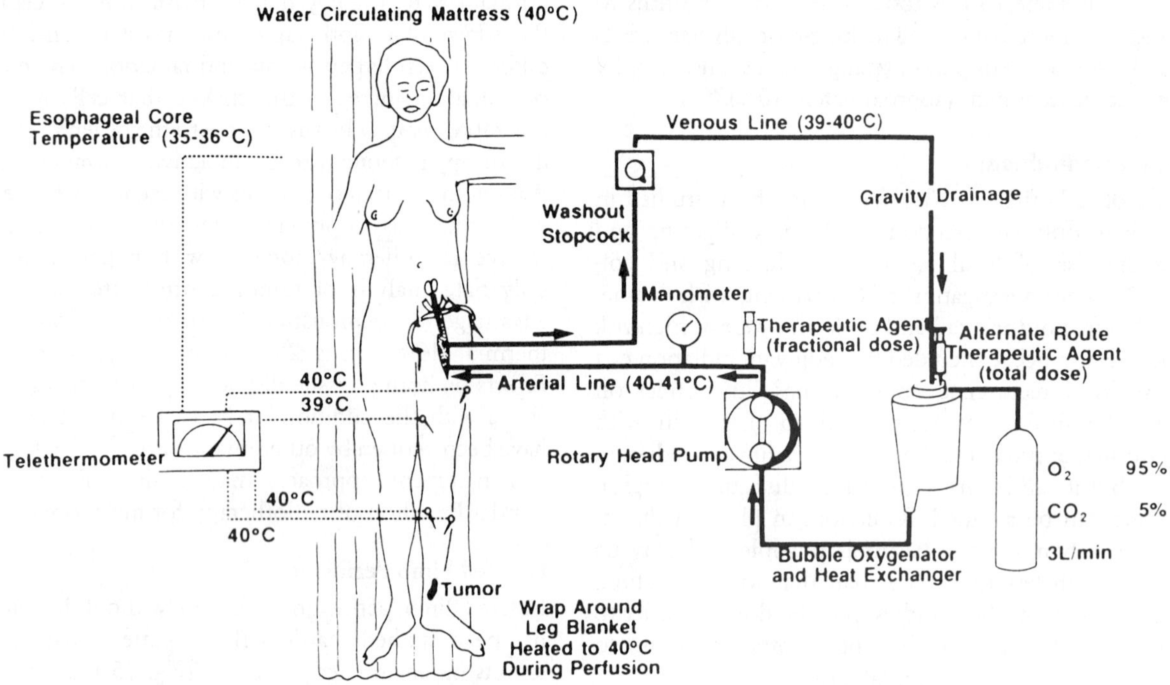

Figure 95.11. Isolated limb perfusion with hyperthermia for lower limb melanoma. (Reprinted with permission from Krementz ET, Ryan RF, Muchmore JH, et al. Hyperthermic regional perfusion for melanoma of the limbs. In: Balch CM, Houghton AN, Milton GW, et al, eds. Cutaneous melanoma. 2nd ed. Philadelphia: Lippincott, 1992:405.)

rences.[96] This treatment modality does appear to have a role in the management of melanoma, but an experienced team of experts is required to maximize benefits and minimize toxicity associated with the procedure.

Intralesional Therapy

Metastatic skin lesions have been treated with a number of different agents given by intralesional injection. The most common agent used is bacillus Calmette-Guérin (bCG). This treatment has been associated with regression of lesions, sometimes with durable remissions of several months to years.[100] Occasionally, satellite lesions adjacent to the lesion injected will also respond, demonstrating a local immune response. This type of treatment is useful only if the lesions are confined to a very small area and is not superior to surgery (the treatment of choice).

Systemic Therapy

Adjuvant Therapy

Historically, adjuvant therapy for stage I, II, and III melanoma demonstrated no survival advantage over surgery alone. Agents such as bCG, *Corynebacterium parvum,* and levamisole were not successful in treating these patients, and chemotherapy agents produced similar results, including high-dose chemotherapy with autologous bone marrow transplantation.[101] Trials with immunotherapy were surprisingly positive and represent the only data available significantly affecting the survival of melanoma patients. The Eastern Cooperative Oncology Group (ECOG), North Central Cancer Treatment Group (NCCTG), and WHO have all reported trials investigating the role of adjuvant IFN-α (Table 95.14). All of the trials employed different dosing schedules, route of administration, duration of therapy, and type of IFN. The risk groups enrolled in the trials were slightly different, and this may have affected the overall results.

The ECOG trial (E1684) and NCCTG both used high-dose regimens of IFN. In the ECOG trial patients received a loading dose of IFN-α-2b 20 MU/m^2/day IV 5 days a week for 4 weeks, then 10 MU/m^2/day SC three days a week for the next 48 weeks to complete a full year's therapy.[102] This trial is the only trial to date to demonstrate a survival benefit when used in the adjuvant setting for melanoma and was the primary study used by the FDA Oncologic Drug Advisory Committee (ODAC) for approval of IFN-α-2b (Intron-A). Therapy was initiated after primary resection of disease in patients with deep primary lesions (T4, AJCC stage IIB) or regional lymph node metastases (N1, AJCC stage III). All patients underwent regional lymphadenectomy and wide local excision. Prolongation of median survival (2.8 to 3.8 years, $p = 0.02$) and relapse-free survival (1.0 to 1.7 years, $p = 0.002$) were both statistically significant for the overall trial.[102] Stage III patients made up 89% of the population studied and demonstrated the greatest benefit in terms of prolonged overall and relapse-free survival.[103] A small subset of stage IIB patients failed to show benefit, but imbalance in the treatment groups was found in terms of the presence of primary ulceration. Because of the small numbers of patients in this group, further subset analysis, controlling for ulceration, could not be completed. Early in the trial,

Table 95.14 ▪ Randomized Clinical Trials of Adjuvant Interferon for High-Risk Melanoma

Study Group	Type of Interferon	Dose and Schedule	Median Survival (years)	Patient Population (*n*)
ECOG (E1684)[102]	IFN-α-2b	20 MU/m²/day IV × 5 days per week × 4 weeks, then 10 MU/m²/day SC three times per week × 48 weeks	2.8 vs 3.8 ($p = 0.02$)	T4 (stage IIB) or N1 (stage III); completely resected; major benefit in the stage III group only ($n = 287$)
NCCTG[106]	IFN-α-2a	20 MU/m²/day IM three times per week × 12 weeks	6.0 vs 4.4 ($p = 0.53$)	Stage IIA/B (T <1.69 mm thick) or stage III ($n = 262$)
WHO Trial 16[107]	IFN-α-2a	3 MU SC three times per week × 3 years	No difference	Recurrent nodal metastases fully resected ($n = 426$)

ECOG, Eastern Cooperative Oncology Group; *IFN,* interferon; *IM,* intramuscular; *IV,* intravenous; *MU,* million units; *NCCTG,* North Central Cancer Treatment Group; *SC,* subcutaneous; *WHO,* World Health Organization.

this treatment regimen had substantial toxicity, and more than 50% of patients discontinued therapy before completion. A dose-adjustment scheme was developed to improve the safety of administration with this regimen. See Table 95.15 for details of IFN dose adjustments used in this and subsequent trials. With this adjustment scheme, discontinuation rates of 26% were seen in the overall analysis. Long-term durable results are seen, with 37% of patients in the treatment arm disease free at 5 years of follow-up, compared with only 26% in the observation arm. Concerns regarding quality of life and cost issues have been addressed in two subsequent analyses of these data for quality-of-life–adjusted survival time and cost of quality-adjusted life-year gained. In the Q-TWIST study, investigators compared the time patients gained without relapse and overall survival between the treatment and observation groups.[104] The IFN group gained a median of 8.9 months without relapse and 7 months of overall survival time. The treated group experienced severe treatment-related side effects for an average of 5.8 months. The net result was that patients in the IFN-treated group had more quality-adjusted survival time than the observation group. This analysis was retrospective and relied on the clinicians' reporting of side effects experienced when determining time with symptoms. Cost analysis of the data also determined that benefits of IFN over a lifetime yield incremental cost per life-year or quality-adjusted life-year of less than $16,000 for both.[105] This compares favorably with the Canadian benchmark of $20,000 per quality of life-year gained, identifying a meaningful intervention.

The NCCTG study used a high-dose IFN-α-2a regimen, consisting of 20 MU/m²/day IM three times a week for 12 weeks.[106] Patients with resected stage IIA/B melanoma of greater than 1.69 mm depth or stage III disease were studied. No significant impact on overall survival or relapse-free interval was noted when the entire study population was analyzed, but a trend toward benefit was noted among patients with stage III disease. Differences in duration of treatment, type of IFN, method of administration, and patient characteristics compared with the ECOG regimen may have affected these results, but these factors cannot be further analyzed.

Table 95.15 ▪ Adjuvant Interferon Dose Adjustment Recommendations[a]

Parameters	Dose Recommended
Starting dose	20 MU/m²/day IV × 5 days per week × 4 weeks, then 10 MU/m²/day SC three times per week × 48 weeks
If ANC < 500/mm³ or SGPT/SGOT >5 × ULN	1. Hold therapy until labs return to normal 2. Restart therapy at 50% dose level
If ANC <250/mm³ or SGPT/SGOT >10 × ULN; or, at 50% dose level, patient still having problems	Discontinue therapy

ANC, absolute neutrophil count; MU, million units; SC, subcutaneous; SGOT, serum glutamic-oxaloacetic transaminase (aspartate aminotransferase); SGPT, serum glutamate pyruvate transaminase (alanine aminotransferase); ULN, upper limit of normal.

[a]Per Food and Drug Administration recommendations in Intron product information, Schering Corporation, March 1997.

The WHO Melanoma Programme Trial randomized 426 patients with resected recurrent nodal disease to receive IFN-α 3 MU SC three times a week for 3 years or observation.[107] Initial results indicated a relapse-free survival benefit, but on further follow-up, relapse-free and overall survival were no different between the treatment and observation arms. Ongoing trials have been designed to answer many of the questions now raised regarding adjuvant therapy for melanoma. Currently, the standard regimen for adjuvant IFN therapy is that utilized in the ECOG 1684 trial mentioned previously and approved by the FDA (Table 95.15).

Toxicities occurring in more than 20% of patients receiving high-dose IFN according to the ECOG regimen consist of fatigue (96%), neutropenia (92%), fever (81%), myalgia (75%), anorexia (69%), vomiting/nausea (66%), increased serum glutamic-oxaloacetic transaminase (SGOT) (63%), headache (62%), chills (54%), depression (40%), diarrhea (35%), alopecia (29%), altered taste sensation (24%), dizziness/vertigo (23%), and anemia (22%).[102] Severe, life-threatening toxicities (ECOG grade 3 or 4) occurring in greater than 10% of patients include neutropenia/leukopenia (26%), fatigue (23%), fever (18%), myalgia (17%), headache (17%), chills (16%), and increased SGOT (14%).[102] Management of these side effects is crucial in maintaining quality of life for the patient and requires an intimate knowledge of the characteristics and treatment of events that can positively affect quality of life. Low-dose IFN regimens have fewer adverse events and are tolerated by most patients. Adverse events occurring most frequently with low-dose IFN are mild to moderate in severity and include flulike symptoms (fever, headache, chills, myalgia) and fatigue. Premedication with acetaminophen may help with these symptoms. Many aspects of adjuvant IFN therapy, such as optimal dose and duration of therapy, are unknown. It does appear that high doses and long durations of therapy are required to achieve a survival benefit. The choice of IFN subtype (2a or 2b) may be important. In other disease states, a difference between the two agents has been suspected but never proven, and many clinicians consider these agents therapeutically equivalent. The trials to date support the use of IFN-α-2b only in the adjuvant setting, but ongoing trials are attempting to clarify this issue.

Metastatic Melanoma

Chemotherapy

Currently, the only role for systemic chemotherapy in melanoma is for treatment of metastatic disease. Conventional chemotherapy has little activity against melanoma. Many agents show minimal activity with response rates of 10 to 20% (Table 95.16). Dacarbazine (DTIC) is the most active single-agent chemotherapy for melanoma, with responses seen in 20% of patients.[108] Median duration of response is approximately 1 year. Although prolongation of survival is questionable with chemotherapy, palliation of symptoms can be accomplished in some patients, improving their quality of life if the chemotherapy is tolerable.

DTIC is a severe emetogen, with up to 90% of patients vomiting in the absence of premedication with strong antiemetics before treatment. Serotonin antagonists have improved this toxicity, and the addition of dexamethasone to the antiemetic regimen decreases nausea and emesis further. A flulike syndrome can occur with large single doses of dacarbazine, manifesting as fever, myalgia, and malaise. The onset is within 7 days and can last as long as 3 weeks.[109] Other acute reactions with high-dose therapy include a severe photoreaction with exposure to sunlight, and hypotension has been observed during the infusion. Myelosuppression is mild to moderate, is dose related, and predominantly affects the granulocytes and platelets. Alopecia, facial flushing, facial paresthesias, and hepatic toxicity are rarely reported.[109] With the introduction of new antiemetics to control nausea and vomiting, dacarbazine is tolerated fairly well when given as a single agent.

DTIC may be given in a number of different schedules and dosages. Daily schedules lasting 10, 5, or 2 days have been described, as have single bolus injections. The most common regimens are (1) 800 to 1000 mg/m^2 as a bolus injection given once, (2) 250 mg/m^2/day for 5 days as daily bolus injections, and (3) 4.5 mg/kg/day for 10 days as daily bolus injections. These treatment regimens are repeated every 3 to 4 weeks. There is no difference in response rates with these schedules, but there is less nausea and vomiting with lower, daily doses. Doses up to 2000 mg/m^2 as single injections are associated with dose-limiting flulike reactions and hypotension. Doses up to 2500 mg/m^2 given as a continuous infusion over 24 hours have been investigated with hemibody radiation in patients with metastatic melanoma, but no improvement in responses was seen compared with standard doses and toxicity was much worse with continuous infusions.[109] Patients with liver metastases from melanoma have been treated with intraarterial DTIC at similar doses as described for intravenous administration, with overall responses of 41% and less intense systemic toxicity.[110] There have been a few case studies of intrathecal or intraventricular DTIC administration for leptomeningeal melanoma, with questionable safety and efficacy.[111,112] An oral derivative of dacarbazine, temozolomide, has recently shown activity against metastatic melanoma with a response rate of 21% in 56 patients, with the major toxicity being myelosuppression.[113] Temozolomide remains investigational, but further studies are ongoing.

Nitrosoureas are less active than DTIC but are widely used in combination regimens. Carmustine (BCNU), lomustine (CCNU), and semustine (methyl-CCNU) are most extensively studied in melanoma. These agents are lipid soluble and cross the blood-brain barrier, but they usually lack significant activity against melanoma brain metastases.[108] In contrast, fotemustine, a new nitrosourea, has induced some measurable responses in melanoma brain lesions. In two phase II trials, 184 patients were treated with fotemustine; 40 (22%) responses were noted, including 4 complete responses, and eleven of the responses were in brain metastases.[114,115] Fotemustine has also been used intra-arterially for isolated hepatic metastases. In a small study of 13 patients receiving intra-arterial fotemustine, response rates reached 60%, but quick relapses were seen in other visceral organs.[116] Vinca

Table 95.16 ▪ Chemotherapy Agents with Significant Activity Against Cutaneous Malignant Melanoma

Carboplatin	Lomustin (CCNU)
Carmustine (BCNU)	Paclitaxel
Cisplatin (CDDP)	Semustine (MeCCNU)
Dacarbazine (DTIC)	Vinblastine (VBL)
Docetaxel	Vincristine
Fotemustine	Vindesine

alkaloids have been shown to have some activity against melanoma and are often employed in combination regimens. Vindesine is used largely in Europe, where it is commercially available, and vinblastine is more commonly used in the United States.[108]

Cisplatin, in standard doses (50 to 100 mg/m^2), has demonstrated only minimal responses, but in higher doses (60 to 150 mg/m^2) with amifostine (WR2721, Ethyol) response rates of 53% were seen.[117] Median duration of response was 4 months, and no complete responses were demonstrated. Amifostine is a renal protectant being studied with cisplatin and is thought to potentiate the antitumor effects of cisplatin in this particular study. The dose-limiting toxicity with this combination was peripheral neuropathy. Intrahepatic chemoembolization with cisplatin and polyvinyl sponge has been investigated for liver metastases from melanoma. Responses of 25 to 50% have been reported, with durations of 2 to 19 months.[118] Carboplatin, a derivative of cisplatin, has shown minimal activity (11% response rate) against melanoma as a single agent,[119] but it may be beneficial in high-dose regimens and other standard-dose combination regimens in the adjuvant or metastatic setting.

Paclitaxel appears to have fairly promising activity against melanoma. In a review of clinical phase II studies of paclitaxel in metastatic melanoma, 73 patients were evaluable, with overall response rates of 16% and stable disease in 14%.[120] Median duration of response was approximately 5 months (range 1 to 17 months), no different from historic controls. These data warrant further investigation of paclitaxel in combination regimens. Docetaxel, a derivative of paclitaxel, has been evaluated in a phase II trial and demonstrated a 17% response rate (5 partial responses out of 30 patients).[121]

Betulinic acid is a pentacyclic triterpene extract from the stem bark of white birch trees. This novel compound appears to be selectively cytotoxic for human melanoma cells in vitro and in athymic nude mice.[122] The mechanism of antitumor activity is believed to be through induction of apoptosis. The agent appears to have minimal toxicity and is under preclinical development for the treatment and prevention of melanoma.

Combination Chemotherapy

In response to the less than optimal results seen with single-agent chemotherapy, clinicians naturally investigated combination regimens in hopes of improving responses. Because DTIC has minimal toxicity, adding another agent must clearly show a survival advantage to warrant the added toxicity. Many two-drug regimens have been investigated, but they have failed to show such a survival advantage. Three-drug regimens have been investigated, but little comparative data to single-agent DTIC are available. Some common regimens that show activity are listed in Table 95.17. The BOLD regimen has come under some scrutiny due to the inclusion of bleomycin, an agent without activity against melanoma and an agent with pulmonary toxicity after lifetime cumulative doses of 300 to 400 mg/m^2. Regimens used most frequently combine DTIC, cisplatin, carmustine (BCNU), vinblastine, or vindesine. In Europe, the combination of DTIC, cisplatin, and vindesine has demonstrated response rates of 30 to 40%.[123] A similar regimen has been used in the United States at MD Anderson Cancer Center, substituting vinblastine for vindesine (CVD regimen). This regimen has produced response rates of up to 40%.[124] Unfortunately, these regimens do not represent synergistic activity and may not warrant the added toxicity in metastatic patients in whom quality of life is most meaningful.

Table 95.17 ▪ Combination Chemotherapy Regimens Used to Treat Metastatic Malignant Melanoma

Regimen Name	Chemotherapy Agents	Dose and Schedule of Administration
BOLD	Bleomycin	15 U D1,4 q3–4wk
	Vincristine	1 mg/m^2 D1,4 q3–4wk
	Lomustine (CCNU)	80 mg/m^2 D1 q3–4wk
	Dacarbazine (DTIC)	200 mg/m^2/day D1–5 q3–4wk
DTIC/CDDP/ Vindesine	Dacarbazine	250 mg/m^2/day D1–5 q3–4wk
	Cisplatin (CDDP)	100 mg/m^2 D1 q3–4wk
	Vindesine	3 mg/m^2 D1 q3–4wk
CVD	Cisplatin	20 mg/m^2/day D2–q3–4wk
	Vinblastine (VBL)	1.6 mg/m^2/day D1–5 q3–4wk
	Dacarbazine	800 mg/m^2 D1 q3–4wk
Dartmouth	Cisplatin	25 mg/m^2/day D1–3 q3wk
	Carmustine (BCNU)	150 mg/m^2 D1 q6wk
	Dacarbazine	220 mg/m^2/day D1–3 q3wk
	Tamoxifen	20 mg PO QD

The four-drug regimen of DTIC, cisplatin, carmustine, and tamoxifen has shown response rates of up to 53% in treated patients. This regimen, developed by Del Prete and colleagues,[125] is often referred to as the Dartmouth regimen and has been extensively studied by McClay and colleagues.[126] The crucial component is thought to be the addition of tamoxifen to the regimen. When tamoxifen was not given, response rates fell to 10%, and rose again to 52% when tamoxifen was added back to the regimen.[126] Tamoxifen does, however, impart more significant toxicity to the regimen with increased incidence of thromboembolic disorders and hot flashes. Historically, the Dartmouth regimen has not been able to improve overall survival compared with DTIC alone, but a preliminary analysis of a randomized study directly comparing these two regimens demonstrated an advantage with the combination regimen. Response rates (22% versus 6%) and median survival (36 weeks versus 28 weeks) were greater with the Dartmouth regimen than with single-agent

DTIC.[127] ECOG is attempting to confirm this difference in a similar study currently underway in the United States, but results will not be available for some time.

The mechanism of tamoxifen in this regimen is not clear, and as a single agent, tamoxifen has *no* activity against melanoma. The presence of estrogen receptors in melanoma cells has not been confirmed since the advent of more accurate methods of detection for these receptors. Estrogen may play a role in melanoma cell growth that has yet to be elucidated, but it may not be related to the effects seen with tamoxifen. Synergy with tamoxifen has been demonstrated with cisplatin, carboplatin, nitrogen mustard, doxorubicin, and vinblastine in vitro.[128] Carmustine has also been suggested to have a synergistic interaction with tamoxifen. Tamoxifen is known to bind to the p170 glycoprotein responsible for multidrug resistance, potentially preventing efflux of the cytotoxic drug from the cytoplasm and overcoming drug resistance. Data from McClay and colleagues[129] did not show this to be the mechanism of synergy with cisplatin or carboplatin, but these agents are not generally associated with this mechanism of resistance. Other proposed mechanisms of action include tamoxifen acting directly on melanoma cells, interacting with the cellular autocrine or paracrine factors involved in melanoma growth and proliferation.

High doses of chemotherapy with autologous bone marrow support have been investigated for metastatic melanoma. Overall responses have ranged from 40 to 65%, with complete response rates as high as 15%.[100] Unfortunately, this approach has demonstrated no survival advantage. The toxicity of these regimens makes the risk-to-benefit ratio unacceptable at this time, preventing the endorsement of such treatment outside the context of a clinical trial.

Immunotherapy

Melanomas are the single most frequent tumor type to undergo spontaneous regression (up to 3 to 4% of lesions),[128] leading to the belief that the body has an antitumor defense mechanism that is functional in some melanomas. This has directed researchers to investigate the immune system as a potential target for therapy and modulation of the natural history of this disease.

IFN-α was one of the first immunotherapies developed to augment the body's immune system. IFN-α augments tumor cell expression of histocompatibility antigens necessary for immune recognition and destruction of tumor cells.[130] Initial results with natural purified IFN-α showed infrequent responses, but responses with recombinant human IFN-α have been much better (average 20%).[128] The best results are seen with daily or three times a week doses in the range of 10 MU/m^2, given intravenously, intramuscularly, or subcutaneously.[130] Investigators in one trial started patients on IFN-α-2a at a dose of 50 MU/m^2 IM three times a week, but had to reduce the dose to 12 MU/m^2 three times a week due to adverse events. At the reduced dose level, the overall response rate was 20%, but most responses were short lived and there was no significant impact on survival.[131] Another trial demonstrated significant responses (44%) when IFN-α-2b was given to patients who failed to respond to multiple injections of a melanoma vaccine (Melacine). The median duration of response was 11 months, and responders had a median survival of 32 months.[132] These results suggest an interaction between active specific immunotherapy and IFN-α, which may be related to effects of IFN on major histocompatibility complex (MHC) class I expression and cytotoxic T-lymphocyte activity. Many different regimens of IFN-α are used for the treatment of metastatic melanoma, and the optimal dose, schedule of administration, and duration of therapy are controversial. Combinations of vaccines with IFN are discussed later in this chapter.

The most common adverse effects associated with IFN-α are a flulike syndrome, consisting of myalgias, fever, headache, chills, and anorexia. With continued treatment, patients generally experience a decrease in these symptoms. Premedication with acetaminophen has proven to be helpful in tolerating standard doses (3 to 6 MU/m^2). With high doses (greater than 6 MU/m^2), these effects are intensified and prolonged, leading to less symptom relief with acetaminophen premedication. Neutropenia and increases in serum transaminases occur infrequently but may require discontinuation of therapy. In contrast to the adjuvant data discussed earlier, the different types of IFN-α (2a, 2b, 2c) seem to have similar activity against metastatic melanoma.

IFN-β binds to the same cell-surface receptor as IFN-α, but it is unclear whether the subsequent actions on melanoma cells are similar. The side effects of IFN-β are similar to those of IFN-α. IFN-γ binds to a specific receptor on the cell surface and has biologic properties that are very different from those of IFN-α. Systemic administration of single-agent IFN-γ has little activity against melanoma.

Interleukin-2 (IL-2), initially referred to as T-cell growth factor, is produced by lymphocytes and is responsible for many immunoregulatory functions. IL-2 can amplify immune responses by promoting growth of activated T cells, resulting in enhancement of both specific and nonspecific antitumor cytotoxicity. Specific antitumor cytotoxicity is T-cell mediated, whereas nonspecific antitumor cytotoxicity is mediated by natural killer cells. Also related to the amplification of the immune response is the induction of other cytokines, including TNF-α and IFN-γ. IL-2 does not have any direct antitumor activity, but rather acts through immunologic enhancement to kill cancer cells. This was the first agent to demonstrate that an immunologic intervention can induce significant anticancer effects.[130]

IL-2 as a single agent generates response rates of 15 to 20% in metastatic melanoma.[130] When incubated with lymphatic cells in vitro, IL-2 activates the lymphoid cells to become cytotoxic to tumor cells. These lymphocytes, called lymphokine-activated killer (LAK) cells, can be administered systemically to patients in conjunction with IL-2 administration. In vitro studies of metastatic melanoma cells incubated with IL-2 have shown an increase in tumor-infiltrating lymphocytes (TIL cells). TIL cells can

Table 95.18 ▪ Selected Interleukin-2 Regimens for Metastatic Melanoma

Administration	Interleukin-2 Source	*N*	Dose	Schedule	Overall Response (%)
Bolus	Cetus	134	7.2×10^5 IU/kg	TID × 5 days, q15d	17
	Cetus	46	6.0×10^5 IU/kg	TID × 5 days, q15d	22
	HLR	44	6.0×10^6 IU/m^2 [a]	TID × 5 days, q15d	5
	Cetus	42	$36–60 \times 10^6$ IU/m^2 [b]	D1,3,5, qwk	10
Continuous	Russel	37	$16–24 \times 10^6$ IU/m^2	Per day	22
	Cetus	33	18×10^6 IU/m^2 [c]	Per day, days 1–5, 10–15, q2wk	12
	HLR	33	3×10^6 IU/m^2 [d]	Per day, days 1–5, 13–17, 21–24, 28–31	9
	Cetus	33	$18–22.5 \times 10^6$ IU/m^2	Per day, max 4.5 days, then days 11–15	3

Source: Reference 135.

Cetus, Cetus-Oncology division, owned by Chiron Corporation, Emeryville, CA; *HLR,* Hoffman LaRoche; *IU,* international units; *TID,* three times a day.

[a]Dose expressed in Biological Response Modification Program (BRMP) units corresponding to 16×10^6 IU.

[b]Originally given as outpatient, but later modified because of toxicity and dose reduced from 60 to 36×10^6 IU/m^2.

[c]Interleukin-2 given with a median duration of treatment of 8 weeks. A second cycle was given after a free interval of 9 to 16 days.

[d]Dose expressed in BRMP units corresponding to 7.8×10^6 IU.

also be administered to patients in conjunction with IL-2. Studies of these combinations (LAK or TIL cells with IL-2) have shown results similar to those of IL-2 alone, and most centers no longer use these complicated regimens. Responses with IL-2 may be delayed, with initial increases in tumor volume secondary to inflammation. Of these responses, a greater proportion (usually one-third) are complete compared with conventional chemotherapy.

Although no direct comparisons have been performed, in general, response rates, quality, and duration of responses are superior with high-dose IL-2 compared with lower doses of IL-2 or IFN-α. In a report of the experience of the NCI Surgery Branch with the use of high-dose IFN-α, tumor response appeared to correlate with the amount of IL-2 delivered.[133] Different doses and schedules of IL-2 have been investigated to try to maximize the antitumor response while minimizing toxicity. The largest single institution experience has been with the NCI bolus regimen of interleukin 7.2×10^5 IU/kg intravenously three times a week for 5 days given every 15 days.[134] Continuous infusion regimens with lower cumulative doses have been given over several days with similar response rates and toxicity. However, response duration appears to be shorter, and fewer complete responses are seen with continuous infusion regimens.[135] One possible mechanism for this difference may be that T cells are activated only after short-term treatment with high-doses of IL-2. See Table 95.18 for selected bolus and continuous infusion IL-2 single-agent regimens.

Multiorgan system toxicity is commonly associated with high-dose IL-2, requiring specialized units capable of providing intensive care and management of these toxicities. Table 95.19 contains a partial list of the most common toxicities associated with high-dose IL-2 and their management. The cardiovascular events and capillary-leak syndrome are the most life-threatening adverse events associated with high-dose IL-2 and lead to solid organ toxicities, such as pulmonary edema and hypotension.[130] The capillary-leak syndrome is believed to be largely mediated by TNF-α, which is associated with a similar situation seen in septic shock. Although steroids can ameliorate this reaction, they may also diminish the antitumor effects of IL-2.[130] An intimate knowledge of the details of administration and toxicity management are required to adequately care for patients receiving these regimens. Many patients are unable to tolerate the toxicity and prefer to discontinue therapy, and some patients develop severe, life-threatening toxicity that mandates discontinuation. With a better understanding of the incidence and management of IL-2–associated adverse events, these regimens can now be safely administered by experienced clinicians.[136]

Combining IL-2 and IFN has been largely unsuccessful, resulting in short responses in 8 to 15% of patients. An exception to this has been the regimen developed by Keilholz and colleagues,[137] consisting of "decrescendo" interleukin-2 and interferon. This regimen begins with IL-2 at 1 mg/m^2/day and tapers over 5 days with a fixed dose of IFN-α (10 MU/m^2/day SC for 5 days). A 41% response rate was demonstrated with the "decrescendo" schedule compared with a fixed dose of IL-2 at 1 mg/m^2/day for 5 days of 18%. Although this was not a randomized comparison, these results are intriguing. In a prospective randomized trial comparing IL-2 alone versus IL-2 plus IFN-α-2a, no significant improvement in responses was demonstrated with the addition of IFN.[138]

Monoclonal antibodies (mAbs) targeting specific antigens present on the melanoma cell surface are also being explored for the treatment of melanoma. With the technology advancements of the last several years, humanized mAbs are now available and are thought to be active against certain targeted cancers. Two such agents have recently gained FDA approval and are now commercially available in the United States (rituximab and trastuzumab). Several different cell-surface antigens have been targeted

Table 95.19 ▪ Adverse Events Associated with High-Dose Interleukin-2

Adverse Event	Associated Symptoms	Management
Capillary leak syndrome	Fluid retention, weight gain, pulmonary edema, hypotension	Administer vasopressors (pure α-sympathomimetic agent) and fluid support for hypotension
Cardiac	Arrhythmias, decreased myocardial contractility, angina, myocardial infarction	Manage capillary leak and treat any arrhythmias appropriately
Neurologic	Parasthesias, constipation, confusion, agitation, hallucinations, lethargy, somnolence, seizures, coma	May have to discontinue therapy; may take a few days to reverse after discontinuation, but are fully reversible
Renal dysfunction	Oliguria, azotemia	Renal-dose dopamine to enhance renal blood flow
Gastrointestinal	Nausea, vomiting, diarrhea, stomatitis	Prophylactic antiemetics (nausea/vomiting), diphenoxylate+atropine (diarrhea), and histamine-2 blockers (gastrointestinal ulceration/bleeding)
Elevations in liver function tests	Transient increases in aminotransferases, alkaline phosphatases, and total bilirubin	May require discontinuation of therapy; usually return to normal a few days after discontinuation
Hematologic	Anemia, thrombocytopenia, leukopenia in first few days (secondary to demargination); then rebound leukocytosis	Monitor for signs/symptoms of infections, especially related to central venous access devices; erythropoietin may be beneficial for anemia.
Constitutional symptoms	Fever, chills, myalgias, arthralgias, fatigue	Premedicate with acetaminophen or indomethacin[a]
Other	Hypothyroidism, rash	May require discontinuation of therapy; rash seen with subcutaneous administration at injection site

[a]Indomethacin may exacerbate the renal dysfunction associated with interleukin-2 and may be detrimental to the patient.

for this type of therapy with two main strategies in mind. MAbs can be given alone to activate the host immune system or can be conjugated to cytotoxic agents, such as radioisotopes or plant toxins (e.g., ricin A chain). Unconjugated mAbs have most commonly targeted the gangliosides GD2 and GD3. The most extensively studied mAb has been R24, which targets GD3. Toxicity seen with R24 administration is mild to moderate with a maximum tolerated dose (MTD) of 1200 mg/m^2 cumulative dose given over 5 to 7 days.[139] When administered in this manner the dose-limiting toxicity (DLT) is malignant hypertension secondary to the increased serum levels of catecholamines. This most likely occurs due to reactivity of the mAb R24 with the adrenal medulla, an organ with similar developmental origin to the melanocyte. No other end-organ toxicity has been noted, even in relation to reactivity of the mAb with the skin or eye. Responses have been seen at a dose of 30 mg/m^2 daily, with a small number of durable responses (some lasting more than 2 years).[140] The optimal immunologic or antitumor dose is not known at this time. Many ongoing trials are addressing these issues. The use of mAbs against GD2 are limited in their effects on peripheral nerves, causing severe neuropathic pain in some patients.[141] This is believed to occur secondarily to the reactivity of the mAb with peripheral nerve fibers.

Conjugated mAbs have also reached the clinical trial arena and have demonstrated some responses in melanoma patients. An mAb to the glycoprotein p97 antigen conjugated to iodine 131 has been shown to deliver 500 mCi of radiation to the tumor site.[142] This conjugated mAb has a DLT of thrombocytopenia and neutropenia, indicating the effects of marrow irradiation. Ricin A chain, a highly potent inhibitor of protein synthesis, has been conjugated to a number of different antibodies with mild toxicity, including flulike symptoms and hepatic enzyme elevations.[143] In a phase II trial with 46 melanoma patients, this type of conjugate (xomasyme-mel) produced one complete response and three partial responses for an overall response rate of 9%.[144] All of these antibodies are mouse derived and carry with them the potential for host IgG (human antimouse antibody), which will inactivate the delivered agent. New technology has allowed mouse antibodies to be humanized to avoid this reaction. Many humanized antibodies against melanoma have been developed and are entering clinical trials.

The principles involved in melanoma mAbs have also been used to develop melanoma vaccines. The goal of a vaccine is to stimulate the host immunity to reject the targeted diseased cell, in this case melanoma cells (specific immunotherapy). Nonspecific immunotherapy uses agents such as intact microorganisms, haptens, or protein products to stimulate the immune system without targeting specific tumor antigens (termed an *adjuvant*). Specific and nonspecific immunotherapeutics are often given together to maximize immune response.[145] The number and type of potential antigen targets present on the melanoma cell surface varies between patients and between cells within the same tumor nodule.[145] This fact makes the development of a specific vaccine that would be generally applicable a very difficult task. The identification of several cell-surface melanoma antigens has allowed for expansion of this technology.

Vaccines range from complex mixtures of antigens, such as whole-cell vaccines, to purified single antigens. Whole-cell vaccines may be derived from autologous or allogeneic (pooled) tumor cells. Autologous vaccines are not very immunogenic and require a potent adjuvant to elicit an immune response. Trials are ongoing to improve the immunogenicity of these types of vaccines. Another avenue taken by researchers to develop a vaccine has been to use cell-surface antigens that have been shed from several different cell lines and combine these into one vaccine, potentially increasing the chances of eliciting an immune response in the patient.[145] The polyvalent whole-cell melanoma vaccine (PMCV) has been compared with non-PMCV therapies in the adjuvant therapy of metastases that have been excised in a historical, case-controlled analysis.[146] Median survival for the PMCV arm was 36 months; the non-PMCV arm was 19 months. Prospective, randomized trials comparing PMCV with observation are currently underway in the adjuvant therapy of both primary and metastatic melanomas.

Viruses can also be used to elicit tumoricidal immune responses. In ongoing studies, the vaccinia virus is being used to target melanoma cells by infecting a melanoma cell line with the virus and collecting the nucleus-free cell lysate to produce a vaccine. One such product, vaccinia melanoma cell lysate (VMCL) vaccine, in a phase II trial of patients with AJCC stage III melanoma, demonstrated 5-year survival rates of 50% for vaccine recipients compared with 34% for historical controls.[147] Mechanical lysates are formed when cell lines are disrupted to create a lysate vaccine without associated viral antigens. Melacine is an example of such a lysate vaccine and is administered with the adjuvants detox and cyclophosphamide to enhance immunogenicity.[145] As mentioned previously, this vaccine may act with IFN-α to enhance cytotoxicity,[132] and this combination is being tested in a randomized, phase III trial currently underway. Vaccines containing ganglioside antigens, specifically GM2, are formed from cells that are incubated with Tice bCG and then collected and administered to the patient with adjuvant cyclophosphamide. When conjugated to keyhole limpet hemocyanin (KLH), which acts as a carrier protein, and administered with the adjuvant QS-21, this vaccine becomes superior in terms of generating cytotoxic antibodies.[145] This preparation (GM2-KLH/QS-21) is currently being compared with IFN-α for the postsurgical adjuvant therapy of patients with AJCC stage III melanoma who have undergone complete resection (ECOG E-1694). While the results of ongoing trials are awaited, new technology improving these molecules advances to better understand and take advantage of the biology of melanoma, the host immune system, and their interactions.

Combination Biochemotherapy

Single-agent chemotherapy is minimally effective against metastatic melanoma, and combination chemotherapy regimens have not proven better than single-agent dacarbazine. The potential advantage in combining chemotherapy with immunotherapy lies in the hope that different mechanisms of action will enhance the rate and duration of responses. Combination chemotherapy with the CVD regimen described previously has been investigated with the addition of IL-2 and IFN-α.[148] This combination is thought to be sequence dependent. Alternating CVD with IL-2/IFN-α (biotherapy) every 6 weeks has shown similar responses to those obtained with CVD alone. Biotherapy administered after CVD followed by a sandwich of biotherapy/chemotherapy/biotherapy appears to be superior to CVD alone (response rates 73% versus 40%, respectively).[148] Table 95.20 outlines this regimen of CVD/biotherapy sequential chemoimmunotherapy. Simultaneous administration of biotherapy and CVD also appears to be superior to CVD alone (response rates 63% versus 40%, respectively). However, only the sequential therapy with CVD/biotherapy has shown a significant increase in progression-free survival (8 versus 4 months, $p = 0.005$) and overall survival (12 versus 9 months, $p = 0.006$) compared with CVD alone (historical controls).[149] A prospective, randomized trial comparing CVD alone with CVD/biotherapy described in Table 95.20 is underway at MD Anderson Cancer Center. It is important to mention that this regimen is extremely toxic, requiring hospitalization for both the chemotherapy and biotherapy portions of the regimen. Renal-dose dopamine is given as a standard for all patients during the biotherapy portion of the regimen, in order to maintain renal perfusion during the IL-2 infusion. This regimen has been important for developing the sequencing aspects of chemoimmuno-

Table 95.20 ▪ Legha Biochemotherapy Sequential Regimen

CVD		Biotherapy	
Cisplatin	20 mg/m²/day IV × 4 days	IFN-α	5 MU/m² SC × 5 days
Vinblastine	1.6 mg/m²/day IV × 5 days	IL-2	3 MU/m² IV CI over 24 hr × 4 days
Dacarbazine	800 mg/m² IV × 1 day		

DAY:	1–5	6–11	12–16	17–22	23–26	27–32	33–42	43–48
	CVD Course 1	BIO	Break	BIO	CVD	BIO	Break	CVD Course 2

Only sequential therapy (CVD followed by BIO), shown here, has been superior to CVD alone.

BIO, biotherapy; *CI,* continuous infusion; *IFN-α,* interferon-α; *IL-2,* interleukin-2; *IV,* intravenous; *MU,* million units; *SC,* subcutaneous.

therapy and confirming that combining chemotherapy and biotherapy does increase survival, but more feasible outpatient regimens must be developed to improve the quality of life of these patients.

Richards[150] used a different chemotherapy regimen in conjunction with IL-2, IFN-α, and tamoxifen. Carmustine (150 mg/m^2), dacarbazine (220 mg/m^2), and cisplatin (25 mg/m^2) were combined on days 1 through 3 and 22 through 24. IL-2 (1.5×10^6 IU/m^2 IV every 8 hours) and IFN-α (6×10^6 IU/m^2 subcutaneously once daily) were given on days 4 through 8 and 17 through 21. Tamoxifen (10 mg) was given twice daily for 6 weeks. Of the 34 patients who were evaluable, 20 (59%) had objective responses and 8 (24%) of those were complete. This is impressive in comparison to other combination trials. The sites of metastases in this trial were not reported, but one patient with hepatic metastases had a complete response. This is a small, noncomparative trial warranting further investigation.

Many different combinations of chemotherapy and immunotherapy are being investigated around the world. Many of these show greater responses than those of conventional therapy with either modality alone. These regimens have not been compared with each other, nor have they been compared with standard therapy with either chemotherapy or immunotherapy alone. Acceptance of any of these combination regimens as standards of therapy will have to wait until further evidence of a survival benefit or an increase in palliative efficacy is shown.

No Treatment

Dismal responses to conventional treatment regimens and short survival spans bring to light the question of risks versus benefits. The treatment regimens currently being investigated have a considerable amount of toxicity associated with their administration, especially regimens including high-dose IL-2. If the benefits of these regimens do not include increased overall survival with good quality of life, the benefits may not be worth the risks. In fact, many clinicians would consider no treatment a reasonable option for patients with metastatic melanoma. Treatment with an investigational regimen in a controlled clinical trial is the only way to ensure that the options these patients have continue to expand.

SCREENING AND PREVENTION

A key factor in increasing overall survival with all types of skin cancer is early diagnosis, improving the odds of the patient evading subclinical metastases at the time of diagnosis. This is particularly true for melanoma, which, if detected early in its radial phase, is curable, but in its later stages is deadly. Key issues that make screening for a disease successful are (1) a sensitive and specific screening tool; (2) disease prevalence that is high enough to warrant screening; (3) potential outcomes that are serious enough to warrant the expense and effort of screening; (4) a disease that is relatively slow growing and not immediately life threatening; (5) a screening tool that is simple, inexpensive, and acceptable to the population being screened; (6) early diagnoses that result in better overall survival rates and improved prognoses; and (7) the screening should lead to more effective treatment at an earlier stage.[151] Skin cancer is one disease that meets these criteria.

Screening for skin cancer consists of visual inspection of the skin and subsequent referral for biopsy and histologic evaluation of any suspicious lesion. This is a simple and inexpensive process, but it poses some challenges. Visual inspection is defined differently by different investigators. Several studies to date have demonstrated the impact of a trained practitioner in recognizing significant cutaneous diseases. Successful skin cancer screening programs must include the participation of such practitioners. After attending a screening program, most people are able to learn the procedure for visual self-inspection. For average-risk patients, the use of self-examinations is adequate with self-referral to a physician if any suspicious lesion is found. For high-risk patients, a professional examination with mole mapping, documenting, and following of all skin lesions is key for early detection and a positive impact on mortality. This method is both sensitive and specific, as well as economically sound. For example, the National Melanoma/Skin Cancer Prevention Program in the United States relies on volunteers to provide the screenings and facilities. The prevalence of skin cancer is obviously high enough to warrant mass screening. The serious potential outcome of melanoma is also apparent, as evidenced by the extremely high mortality rate of metastatic melanoma. However, melanoma, in its radial growth phase, is slow growing, highly curable, and not immediately life threatening. With new treatment options such as monoclonal antibodies, vaccines, and other new agents, earlier treatment will be more effective and lead to better overall survival rates with improved prognoses.

The most reliable method for determining the success of a screening program is a reduction in mortality rate from the cancer. The efficacy of screening or early detection programs has not been tested in randomized trials. Many countries around the world have shown increases in the numbers of melanomas detected and decreases in the thickness of the melanomas found. These statistical trends theoretically equate into reduced mortality rates, but this has not been proven.

In conjunction with disease screening, public education efforts lead, not only to more effective screening programs, but also to more effective prevention. UV radiation exposure has been associated with skin cancer of all kinds. Limiting exposure to UV radiation through the use of sunscreens and protective clothing has never been shown to decrease the incidence of skin cancer in humans. However, in animal studies it is evident that sunscreens effectively decrease the amount of UV radiation penetrating the dermis. Theoretically, this action will decrease the physiologic effects of UV radiation. Recently under debate, the use of sunscreens may actually lead to an increase in the amount of UV radiation a person is exposed to. A false sense of security may be present when sunscreens are used. Unfortunately, until the complex mechanism of action of UV radiation is outlined and the efficacy of sunscreens is determined, these actions of prevention must be coupled with decreased time spent outdoors during periods of intense sunlight and avoidance of artificial UV sources such as tanning beds. These actions are most critical for prevention of NMSC. The association of melanoma with UV radiation is less well defined, but cutaneous melanoma may be somewhat preventable with these same measures.

Preventive medicine is based on the premise that the natural history of disease can be interrupted at three major points, preventing progression to the more severe stages of disease.[152] Primary prevention focuses on improving overall health and risk reduction. This can be related to skin cancer and melanoma in the efforts made to educate the public about the dangers of UV radiation exposure and the importance of avoiding such exposure. Secondary prevention in relation to cancer includes tools for screening and early diagnosis, leading to treatment of early, more curable stages of cancer. This applies to skin cancers and melanomas, as discussed earlier. Tertiary prevention refers to treatment of cancer patients to avoid complications and recurrences. In reference to skin cancer and melanoma, the efforts described previously are tertiary approaches to the prevention of recurrences and complications from cancer. Earlier interventions theoretically offer better outcomes, but these approaches are often more difficult to execute.

Primary prevention associated with skin cancer and melanoma can be accomplished through behavior modification (e.g., covering up when in the sun) or through administration of agents that interfere with the carcinogenic process (chemoprevention). Chemoprevention has been studied with both systemic and topical retinoids. Prevention of new skin cancer lesions has been reported with oral isotretinoin, oral etretinate, and topical tretinoin in people with genetic dermatoses such as xeroderma pigmentosum and nevoid basal cell carcinoma syndrome.[45] The doses required to maintain prevention are high, and withdrawal of therapy leads to regression and loss of preventive activity, requiring high-dose, chronic maintenance therapy.[45] A large, randomized, placebo-controlled trial of chemoprevention with retinol has been reported to decrease the incidence of SCC, but not BCC, in a moderate-risk population of 2297 participants.[153] Oral retinol was given for 3 to 5 years at a dose of 20,000 IU daily. Patients enrolled had at least 10 AKs within the past year or no more than two prior SCCs or BCCs, resided in Arizona for at least 5 years, had a daily dietary intake of vitamin A of 10,000 IU or less, and did not have a diagnosis of xeroderma pigmentosum or basal cell nevus syndrome. The total number of new diagnoses of SCC were 113 in the retinol group and 136 in the placebo group (hazard ratio [HR] = 0.74; 95% confidence intervals [CI] = 0.56 to 0.99; $p = 0.04$).[153] Differences in the number of new diagnoses of BCC did not reach statistical significance between the retinol and placebo arms (HR = 1.06; 95% CI = 0.86 to 1.32; $p = 0.36$).[153] The incidence of adverse events was not clearly outlined in this trial. The authors state that the drug was well tolerated. This trial provides intriguing results to consider for patients who meet these risk requirements. The general, widespread acceptance of retinol as a preventive agent for skin cancer requires further study to determine which populations will stand to benefit from such interventions. Also, the long-term safety of agents such as this is of considerable importance when use is primarily confined to healthy participants who may be unnecessarily exposed to adverse events without much hope for substantial benefit. Determination of the optimal retinoid compound, dosages, and utility of combinations with other preventive agents is currently being investigated and may assist in the development of preventive strategies that are meaningful. Vaccines are also being investigated for prevention of melanoma in high-risk populations such as patients with atypical mole (dysplastic nevus) syndrome. These trials are ongoing, but will provide vital information concerning the pathophysiology of these diseases.

KEY POINTS

- Skin cancer is often a forgotten cancer because of its generally benign nature. However, the incidence and importance of this set of diseases is profound.
- NMSC is not extremely threatening in terms of mortality, but it is highly detrimental in terms of morbidity and number of patients affected.
- Melanoma is extremely life threatening, especially in its later stages, and poses a great threat to the general population secondary to its rapidly increasing incidence.
- The management of patients with NMSC is summarized in the following key points:
  - Treatment planning should consist of consideration of the type of skin cancer; anatomic location; size; general health and age of the patient; and whether the lesion is primary, recurrent, or metastatic.
  - SCCs generally require that a wider margin of normal tissue be removed to ensure optimal treatment.
  - Smaller BCC lesions may be removed with curettage followed by electrodesiccation.
  - Other treatment modalities are also used in some circumstances, including cryotherapy, Mohs' micrographic surgery, radiation, and chemotherapy (topical or systemic).
- Therapy for melanoma is more controversial, aggressive, and multidisciplinary in nature. Key points regarding the management of melanoma are as follows:
  - Surgical excision is the mainstay of therapy for all stages of melanoma.
  - Wide surgical margins are required for most lesions, with 1 to 2 cm margins being adequate for most primary lesions.

- Elective lymphadenectomy is a controversial procedure and may not be associated with improved survival.
- Lymphatic mapping with sentinel lymph node biopsy and selective lymphadenectomy is often used to determine the nodal status of the area surrounding the tumor bed.
- In addition to appropriate systemic therapy, surgical resection of involved lymph nodes and solitary visceral metastases is indicated in most cases.
- Adjuvant therapy with IFN-α is indicated for patients with clinically positive lymph nodes after complete surgical resection of the primary lesion and any involved lymph nodes.
- The approved dose of IFN-α for adjuvant therapy of melanoma consists of a prolonged regimen with high doses that are associated with significant toxicity.
- The most active single chemotherapy agent for the treatment of melanoma is dacarbazine.
- Combination chemotherapy has not demonstrated superior efficacy compared with single-agent chemotherapy.
- Combination biochemotherapy has demonstrated significantly greater activity compared with historical data for other types of treatment regimens.
- Many different regimens exist for biochemotherapy of melanoma; they are extremely toxic and often require hospitalization for administration.

- The detrimental outcome seen with lesions not amenable to surgery provides the impetus for development of many new treatment modalities. These include new immunotherapies, chemotherapies, monoclonal antibodies, and vaccines.
- Using new and currently available therapeutic agents in different combinations and with different modalities of treatment is leading the search for better therapeutic outcomes. With the development of gene therapy on the horizon, new hopes for better survival rates are strengthened.
- In conjunction with all of these treatment hopes, the emphasis on prevention and screening is imperative. These tools may someday obviate the need for more effective therapeutic modalities.

REFERENCES

1. Safai B. Management of skin cancer. In: DeVita VT, Hellman S, Rosenberg SA, eds. Cancer: principles and practice of oncology. 5th ed. Philadelphia: Lippincott-Raven, 1997:1883–1933.
2. American Cancer Society. Cancer facts and figures 1998: selected cancers. Available from http://www.cancer.org/statistics/cff98/selectedcancers.html.
3. Osterlind A. Etiology and epidemiology of melanoma and skin neoplasms. Curr Opin Oncol 3:355–359, 1991.
4. Roberts DL. Incidence of nonmelanoma skin cancer in West Giamorgan, South Wales. Br J Dermatol 122:399–404, 1990.
5. Emmett AJJ, O'Rourke MGE, eds. Malignant skin tumours. New York: Churchill Livingstone, 1991:24.
6. Griffiths HR, Mistry P, Herbert KE, et al. Molecular and cellular effects of ultraviolet light-induced genotoxicity. Crit Rev Clin Lab Sci 35(3):189–237, 1998.
7. Brash DE. Molecular biology of skin cancer. In: DeVita VT, Hellman S, Rosenberg SA, eds. Cancer: principles and practice of oncology. 5th ed. Philadelphia: Lippincott-Raven, 1997:1879–1883.
8. Elwood JM. Melanoma and sun exposure. Semin Oncol 23(6):650–666, 1996.
9. Hacker SM, Browder JF, Ramos-Caro FA. Basal cell carcinoma: choosing the best method of treatment for a particular lesion. Postgrad Med 93(8):101–104, 106, 108, 111, 1993.
10. Goldman GD. Squamous cell cancer: a practical approach. Semin Cutaneous Med Surg 17(2):80–95, 1998.
11. Potter M. Percival Pott's contribution to cancer research. Natl Cancer Inst Monogr 10:1, 1963.
12. Dreno B, Mansat E, Legoux B, Litoux P. Skin cancers in transplant patients. Nephrol Dial Transplant 13:1374–1379, 1998.
13. Gupta AK, Cardella CJ, Haberman HF. Cutaneous malignant neoplasms in patients with renal transplants. Arch Dermatol 122:1288–1293, 1986.
14. Ananthaswamy HN, Pierceall WE. Molecular mechanisms of ultraviolet radiation carcinogenesis. Photochem Photobiol 52:1119, 1990.
15. Rippey JJ. Why classify basal cell carcinomas? Histopathology 32:393–398, 1998.
16. Hendrix JD Jr, Parlette HL. Micronodular basal cell carcinoma. Arch Dermatol 132:295–298, 1996.
17. Maloney ME, Jones DB, Sexton FM. Pigmented basal cell carcinoma: investigation of 70 cases. J Am Acad Dermatol 27:74–78, 1992.
18. Abreo F, Sanusi ID. Basal cell carcinoma in North American blacks: Clinical and histopathologic study of 26 patients. J Am Acad Dermatol 25:1005–1011, 1991.
19. Kikuchi A, Shimizu H, Nishikawa R. Clinical and histopathological characteristics of basal cell carcinoma in Japanese patients. Arch Dermatol 132:320–324, 1996.
20. American Joint Committee on Cancer. Manual for staging of cancer. 5th ed. Philadelphia: Lippincott-Raven, 1997:157–161.
21. Rowe DE, Carroll RJ, Day CL. Long-term recurrence rates in previously untreated (primary) basal cell carcinoma: implications for patient follow-up. J Dermatol Surg Oncol 15:315–328, 1989.
22. Pascal RR, Hobby LW, Lattes R, et al. Prognosis of "incompletely excised" versus "completely excised" basal cell carcinoma. Plast Reconstr Surg 41:328–332, 1968.
23. Gooding CA, White G, Yatsuhashi M. Significance of marginal extension in excised basal cell carcinoma. N Engl J Med 273:923–924, 1965.
24. Rowe DE, Carroll RJ, Day CL. Prognostic factors for local recurrence, metastasis, and survival rates in squamous cell carcinoma of the skin, ear, and lip: implications for treatment modality selection. J Am Acad Dermatol 26:976–990, 1992.
25. Stern RS, Laird N for the Photochemotherapy Follow-up Study. The carcinogenic risk of treatments for severe psoriasis. Cancer 73:2759–2764, 2994.
26. Morison WL, Baughman RD, Day RM, et al. Consensus workshop on the toxic effects of long-term PUVA therapy. Arch Dermatol 134:595–598, 1998.
27. Marks R, Foley P, Goodman G, et al. Spontaneous remission of solar keratoses: The case for conservative management. Br J Dermatol 115:649–655, 1986.
28. Marks R, Rennie G, Selwood T. Malignant transformation of solar keratoses to squamous cell carcinoma. Lancet 1:795–797, 1988.
29. Kwa RE, Campana K, Moy RL. Biology of cutaneous squamous cell carcinoma. J Am Acad Dermatol 26:1–26, 1992.
30. Breuninger H, Black B, Rassner G. Microstaging of squamous cell carcinomas. Am J Clin Pathol 94:624–627, 1990.
31. Vargo NL. Basal and squamous cell carcinomas: An overview. Semin Oncol Nurs 7(1):13–25, 1991.
32. Kuflik EG, Gage AA. The five-year cure rate achieved by cryosurgery for skin cancer. J Am Acad Dermatol 24:1002–1004, 1991.
33. Hacker SM, Flowers FP. Squamous cell carcinoma of the skin: will heightened awareness of risk factors slow its increase? Postgraduate Med 93(8):115–118, 120–121, 125–126, 1993.
34. Lawrence CM. Mohs surgery of basal cell carcinoma–a critical review. Br J Plast Surg 46:599–606, 1993.
35. Albright SD. Treatment of skin cancer using multiple modalities. J Am Acad Dermatol 7:143–171, 1982.
36. Wilson BD, Mang TS, Stoll H, et al. Photodynamic therapy for the treatment of basal cell carcinoma. Arch Dermatol 128:1597–1601, 1992.
37. Allison RR, Mang TS, Wilson BD. Photodynamic therapy for the treatment of nonmelanomatous cutaneous malignancies. Semin Cutaneous Med Surg 17(2):153–163, 1998.
38. Cairnduff F, Stringer MR, Hudson EJ, et al. Superficial photodynamic therapy with topical 5-aminolevulinic acid for superficial primary and secondary skin cancer. Br J Cancer 69(3):605–608, 1994.
39. Svanberg K, Andersson T, Killander D, et al. Photodynamic therapy of non-melanoma malignant tumours of the skin using topical amino levulinic acid sensitization and laser irradiation. Br J Dermatol 130:743–751, 1994.

40. Cullen SI. Topical fluorouracil therapy for precancers and cancers of the skin. J Am Geriatr Soc 12:529–535, 1979.
41. Epstein E. Fluorouracil paste treatment of thin basal cell carcinomas. Arch Dermatol 121:207–213, 1985.
42. Dillaha CJ, Jansen GT, Honeycutt WM, et al. Selective cytotoxic effect of topical 5-fluorouracil. Arch Dermatol 88:247–256, 1963.
43. Sadek H, Azli N, Wendling JL, et al. Treatment of advanced squamous cell carcinoma of the skin with cisplatin, 5-fluorouracil, and bleomycin. Cancer 66:1692–1696, 1990.
44. Tahery DP, Moy RL. Immunotherapy and skin cancer. J Dermatol Surg Oncol 18:584–586, 1992.
45. Peck GL. Topical tretinoin in actinic keratosis and basal cell carcinoma. J Am Acad Dermatol 15:829–835, 1986.
46. Robinson TA, Kligman AM. Treatment of solar keratoses of the extremities with retinoic acid and 5-fluorouracil. Br J Dermatol 92(6):703–706, 1975.
47. Landis SH, Murray T, Bolden S, et al. Cancer statistics, 1999. CA Cancer J Clin 49:8–31, 1999.
48. Rigel DS, Kopf AW, Friedman RJ. The rate of malignant melanoma in the US: are we making an impact? J Am Acad Dermatol 17:1050, 1987.
49. Grin-Jorgensen CM, Rigel DS, Friedman RJ. The worldwide incidence of malignant melanoma. In: Balch CM, Houghton AN, Milton GW, et al, eds. Cutaneous melanoma. 2nd ed. Philadelphia: Lippincott, 1992:27–39.
50. Balch CM, Soong SJ, Milton GW, et al. Changing trends in cutaneous melanoma over a quarter century in Alabama, USA, and New South Wales, Australia. Cancer 52:1748–1753, 1983.
51. Dreiling L, Hoffman S, Robinson WA. Melanoma: epidemiology, pathogenesis, and new modes of treatment. Adv Intern Med 41:553–604, 1996.
52. Armstrong BK, English DR. Epidemiologic studies. In Balch CM, Houghton AN, Milton GW, et al, eds. Cutaneous melanoma. 2nd ed. Philadelphia: Lippincott, 1992:12–26.
53. Koh HK. Cutaneous melanoma. N Engl J Med 325(3):171–182, 1991.
54. Balch CM, Reintgen DS, Kirkwood JM, et al. Cutaneous melanoma. In: DeVita VT, Hellman S, Rosenberg SA, eds. Cancer: principles and practice of oncology. 5th ed. Philadelphia: Lippincott-Raven, 1997:1947–1994.
55. Grob JJ, Gouvernet J, Aymar D, et al. Count of benign melanocytic nevi as a major indicator of risk for non-familial nodular and superficial spreading melanoma. Cancer 66:387–395, 1990.
56. Lee JE. Factors associated with melanoma incidence and prognosis. Semin Surg Oncol 12:379–385, 1996.
57. Drolet BA, Connor MJ. Sunscreens and the prevention of ultraviolet radiation–induced skin cancer. J Dermatol Surg Oncol 18:571–576, 1992.
58. Swerdlow AJ, English JSC, MacKie RM, et al. Fluorescent lights, ultraviolet lamps, and risk of cutaneous melanoma. Br Med J 297:647–650, 1988.
59. Walter SD, Marrett LD, From L, et al. The association of cutaneous melanoma with the use of sunbeds and sunlamps. Am J Epidemiol 131:232–243, 1990.
60. MacKie RM, Freudenberger R, Aitchison TC. Personal risk-factor chart for cutaneous melanoma. Lancet ii:487–490, 1989.
61. Elwood JM, Williamson C, Stapleton PJ. Malignant melanoma in relation to moles, pigmentation, and exposure to fluorescent and other lighting sources. Br J Cancer 52:65–74, 1986.
62. Gallagher RP, Elwood JM, Hill GP. Risk factors for cutaneous malignant melanoma–the Western Canada Melanoma Study. Recent Results Cancer Res 102:38–55, 1986.
63. Osterlind A, Tucker MA, Stone BJ, et al. The Danish case-control study of cutaneous malignant melanoma: II. Importance of UV-light exposure. Int J Cancer 42:319–324, 1988.
64. Cannon-Albright LA, Kamb A, Skolnick M. A review of inherited predisposition to melanoma. Semin Oncol 23(6):667–672, 1996.
65. Ramcharan S, Pellegrin FA, Ray R, et al. The Walnut Creek Contraceptive Drug Study. Vol III. An interim report. NIH pub no 81-564. Washington, DC: US Government Printing Office, 1981.
66. Holly EA, Weiss NS, Liff JM. Cutaneous melanoma in relation to exogenous hormones and reproductive factors. J Natl Cancer Inst 70:827–831, 1983.
67. Holman CDJ, Armstrong BK, Heenan PJ. Cutaneous malignant melanoma in women: exogenous sex hormones and reproductive factors. Br J Cancer 50:673–680, 1984.
68. Beral V, Evans S, Shaw H. Oral contraceptive use and malignant melanoma in Australia. Br J Cancer 50:681–685, 1984.
69. Beral V, Ramcharan S, Faris R. Malignant melanoma and oral contraceptive use among women in California. Br J Cancer 36:804–809, 1977.
70. Herlyn M, Houghton AN. Biology of melanocytes and melanoma. In: Balch CM, Houghton AN, Milton GW, et al, eds. Cutaneous melanoma. 2nd ed. Philadelphia: Lippincott, 1992:82–92.
71. Crutcher WA, Cohen PJ. Dysplastic nevi and malignant melanoma. Am Fam Physician 42(2):372–385, 1990.
72. Albino AP, Reed JA, McNutt NS. Molecular biology of cutaneous malignant melanoma. In: DeVita VT, Hellman S, Rosenberg SA, eds. Cancer: principles and practice of oncology. 5th ed. Philadelphia: Lippincott-Raven, 1997:1935–1946.
73. Clark WH Jr, Elder ED, Guerry D IV, et al. The precursor lesions of superficial spreading and nodular melanoma. Hum Pathol 15:1147–1165, 1984.
74. Lu C, Kerbel RS. Cytokines, growth factors and the loss of negative growth controls in the progression of human cutaneous malignant melanoma. Curr Opin Oncol 6:212–220, 1994.
75. Gruis NA, Bergnam W, Frants RR. Locus for susceptibility to melanoma on chromosome 1p. N Engl J Med 322(12):853–854, 1990.
76. Friedman RJ, Rigel DS, Kopf AW. Early detection of malignant melanoma: the role of physician examination and self-examination of the skin. CA Cancer J Clin 35:130–151, 1985.
77. Fitzpatrick TB, Milton GW, Balch CM, et al. Clinical characteristics. In: Balch CM, Houghton AN, Milton GW, et al, eds. Cutaneous melanoma. 2nd ed. Philadelphia: Lippincott, 1992:223–233.
78. Breslow A. Thickness, cross-sectional areas and depth of invasion in the prognosis of cutaneous melanoma. Ann Surg 172:902–908, 1970.
79. Clark WH Jr, Ainsworth AM, Bernardino EA, et al. The developmental biology of primary human malignant melanomas. Semin Oncol 2:83–103, 1975.
80. Balch CM, Murad TM, Soong SJ, et al. A multifactorial analysis of melanoma: Prognostic histopathological features comparing Clark's and Breslow's staging methods. Ann Surg 188:732–742, 1978.
81. Balch CM, Soong SJ, Shaw HM, et al. An analysis of prognostic factors in 8500 patients with cutaneous melanoma. In: Balch CM, Houghton AN, Milton GW, et al, eds. Cutaneous melanoma. 2nd ed. Philadelphia: Lippincott, 1992:165–187.
82. Buzaid AC, Ross MI, Balch CM, et al. Critical analysis of the American Joint Committee on Cancer staging system for cutaneous melanoma and proposal of a new staging system. J Clin Oncol 15:1039–1051, 1997.
83. Ross M. Modifying the criteria of the American Joint Commission on Cancer staging system in melanoma. Curr Opin Oncol 10:153–161, 1998.
84. Singletary SE, Balch CM, Urist MM, et al. Surgical treatment of primary melanoma. In: Balch CM, Houghton AN, Milton GW, et al, eds. Cutaneous melanoma. 2nd ed. Philadelphia: Lippincott, 1992:269–274.
85. Veronesi U, Cascinelli N. Narrow excision (1 cm margin), a safe procedure for thin cutaneous melanoma. Arch Surg 126:438–441, 1991.
86. Balch CM, Urist MM, Karkousis CP, et al. Efficacy of 2 cm surgical margins for intermediate-thickness melanomas (1 to 4 mm): results of a multi-institutional randomized surgical trial. Ann Surg 218:262–269, 1993.
87. Timmons MJ. Malignant melanoma excision margins: making a choice. Lancet 340:1393–1395, 1992.
88. Goldsmith LA, Askin FB, Chang AE, et al. Diagnosis and treatment of early melanoma. JAMA 268:1314–1319, 1992.
89. Crowley NJ. The case against elective lymphadenectomy. Surg Oncol Clin North Am 1:223–243, 1992.
90. Ross MI. Surgical management of stage I and II melanoma patients: approach to the regional lymph node basin. Semin Surg Oncol 12:394–401, 1996.
91. Morton DL, Wen DR, Wong JM. Technical details of intra-operative lymphatic mapping for early stage melanoma. Arch Surg 127:392–399, 1992.
92. Harwood AR. Conventional fractionated radiotherapy for 51 patients with lentigo maligna and lentigo maligna melanoma. Int J Radiat Oncol Biol Phys 9:1019–1021, 1983.
93. Ang KK, Byers RM, Peters LJ, et al. Regional radiotherapy as adjuvant treatment for head and neck malignancy melanoma. Arch Otolaryngol Head Neck Surg 116:169–172, 1990.
94. Schmidt-Ullrich RK, Johnson CR. Role of radiotherapy and hyperthermia in the management of malignant melanoma. Semin Surg Oncol 12:407–415, 1996.
95. Overgaard J, Gonzales D, Hulshof MC, et al. Randomized trial of hyperthermia as adjuvant to radiotherapy for recurrent or metastatic melanoma: European Society for Hyperthermia Oncology. Lancet 345:540–543, 1995.
96. Hohenberger P, Kettelhack C. Clinical management and current research in isolated limb perfusion for sarcoma and melanoma. Oncology 55:89–102, 1998.
97. Cavaliere R, Cavaliere F, Deraco M, et al. Hyperthermic antiblastic perfusion in the treatment of stage IIIA-IIIAB melanoma patients: comparison of two experiences. Melanoma Res 4(Suppl 1):5–11, 1994.
98. LeJeune FJ, Liereard D, Leyvraz A, et al. Regional therapy of melanoma. Eur J Cancer 29A:606–612, 1993.
99. Lienard D, Eggermont AM, Schraffordt Koops H, et al. Isolated perfusion of the limb with high-dose TNF-alpha, interferon-gamma and melphalan for melanoma stage III. Melanoma Res 4(Suppl 1):21–26, 1994.
100. Ho RCS. Medical management of stage IV malignant melanoma. Cancer 75(2):735–741, 1995.

101. Agarwala SS, Kirkwood JM. Adjuvant therapy of melanoma. Semin Surg Oncol 14:302–310, 1998.
102. Kirkwood JM, Strawderman MH, Ernstoff MS, et al. Interferon alfa-2b adjuvant therapy of high-risk resected cutaneous melanoma: the Eastern Cooperative Oncology Group Trial EST 1684. J Clin Oncol 14:7–17.
103. Kirkwood JM, Strawderman MH, Ernstoff MS, et al. Adjuvant therapy of high risk melanoma: the role of high-dose interferon alfa-2b. In: Salmon S, ed. Adjuvant therapies of cancer, VIII. Philadelphia: Lippincott-Raven, 1997: 251–257.
104. Cole BF, Gelber RD, Kirkwood JM, et al. A quality-of-life-adjusted survival analysis of interferon alfa-2b adjuvant treatment for high-risk resected cutaneous melanoma: an Eastern Cooperative Oncology Group Study (E1684). J Clin Oncol 14:2666–2673, 1996.
105. Hillner BE, Kirkwood JM, Atkins MB, et al. Economic analysis of adjuvant interferon alfa-2b in high-risk melanoma based on projections from Eastern Cooperative Oncology Group 1684. J Clin Oncol 15:2351–2358, 1997.
106. Creagan ET, Dalton RJ, Ahmann DL, et al. Randomized, surgical adjuvant clinical trial of recombinant interferon alfa-2a in selected patients with malignant melanoma. J Clin Oncol 13:2776–2783, 1995.
107. Cascinelli N. Evaluation of efficacy of adjuvant rIFNa 2A in melanoma patients with regional node metastases (Meeting Abstract #1296). Proc Annu Meet Am Soc Clin Oncol 14: , 1995.
108. Nathan FE, Mastrangelo MJ. Systemic therapy in melanoma. 14:319–327, 1998.
109. Dorr RT, Von Hoff DD. Cancer chemotherapy handbook. 2nd ed. CT: Appleton & Lange, 1994:343–349.
110. Einhorn LH, McBride CM, Luce JK, et al. Intraarterial infusion therapy with 5-(3,3-dimethyl-1-triazeno)imidazole-4-carboxamide (NSC-45388) for malignant melanoma. Cancer 32(4):749–755, 1973.
111. Yamasaki T, Kikuchi H, Yamashita J, et al. Primary spinal intramedullary malignant melanoma: case report. Neurosurgery 25:117–121, 1989.
112. Champagne MA, Silver HKB. Intrathecal dacarbazine treatment of leptomeningeal malignant melanoma. J Natl Cancer Inst 84:1203–1204, 1992.
113. Bleehen NM, Newlands ES, Lee SM, et al. Cancer research campaign phase II trial of temozolomide in metastatic melanoma. J Clin Oncol 13:910–913, 1995.
114. Jacquillat C, Khayat D, Banzet P, et al. Final report of the French multicenter phase II study of the nitrosourea fotemustine in 153 evaluable patients with disseminated malignant melanoma including patients with brain metastases. Cancer 66:1873–1878, 1990.
115. Falkson CI, Falkson G, Falkson HC. Phase II trial of fotemustine in patients with metastatic malignant melanoma. Invest New Drugs 12:251–254, 1994.
116. Khayat D, Cour V, Bizzari JP, et al. Fotemustine (S 10036) in the intra-arterial treatment of liver metastasis from malignant melanoma: a phase II study. Am J Clin Oncol 14(5):400–404, 1991.
117. Glover D, Glick JH, Weiler C, et al. WR 2721 and high-dose cisplatin: an active combination in the treatment of metastatic melanoma. J Clin Oncol 5:574–578, 1987.
118. Mavligit G, Charnsangavej C, Carrasco CH, et al. Regression of ocular melanoma metastatic to the liver after hepatic arterial chemoembolization with cisplatin and polyvinyl sponge. J Am Med Assoc 260:974–976, 1988.
119. Chang A, Hunt M, Parkinson DR, et al. Phase II trial of carboplatin in patients with metastatic malignant melanoma: a report from the Eastern Cooperative Oncology Group. Am J Clin Oncol 16(2):152–155, 1993.
120. Wiernik PH, Einzig AI. Taxol in malignant melanoma. Monogr Natl Cancer Inst 15:185–187, 1993.
121. Aamdal S, Wolff I, Kaplan S, et al. Docetaxel (Taxotere) in advanced malignant melanoma: a phase II study of the EORTC Early Clinical Trials Group. Eur J Cancer 30A:1061–1064, 1994.
122. Pisha E, Chai H, Lee IS, et al. Discovery of betulinic acid as a selective inhibitor of human melanoma that functions by induction of apoptosis. Nature Med 1:1046–1051, 1995.
123. Gundersen S. Dacarbazin, vindesine, and cisplatin combination chemotherapy in advanced malignant melanoma: a phase II study. Cancer Treat Rep 71:997–999, 1987.
124. Legha SS, Ring S, Papadopoulos N, et al. A prospective evaluation of a triple-drug regimen containing cisplatin, vinblastine, and dacarbazine (CVD) for metastatic melanoma. Cancer 64:2024–2029, 1989.
125. Del Prete SA, Maurer LH, O'Donnell J. Combination chemotherapy with cisplatin, carmustine, dacarbazine, and tamoxifen in metastatic melanoma. Cancer Treat Rep 68:1403–1405, 1984.
126. McClay EF, Mastrangelo MJ, Berd D, et al. Effective combination chemo/hormonal therapy for malignant melanoma: experience with three consecutive trials. Int J Cancer 50:553–556, 1992.
127. Sileni VC, Nortilli R, Medici M, et al. BCNU (B), cisplatin (C), dacarbazine (D) and tamoxifen (T) (BCDT) in metastatic melanoma (MM): results of a randomized phase II study (Meeting Abstract). Proc Ann Meet Am Soc Clin Oncol 16:495, 1997.
128. Kirkwood JM. Systemic therapy of melanoma. Curr Opin Oncol 6:204–211, 1994.
129. McClay EF, Albright K, Jones J, et al. Modulation of cisplatin (DDP) sensitivity by tamoxifen (TAM) in human malignant melanoma. Proc Am Soc Clin Oncol 10:291, 1991.
130. Bear HD, Hamad GG, Kostuchenko PJ. Biologic therapy of melanoma with cytokines and lymphocytes. Semin Surg Oncol 12:436–445, 1996.
131. Creagan ET, Ahmann DL, Frytak S, et al. Three consecutive phase II studies of recombinant interferon alfa-2a in advanced malignant melanoma. Cancer 59(3 Suppl):638–646, 1987.
132. Mitchell MS, Jakowatz J, Harel W, et al. Increased effectiveness of interferon alfa-2b following active specific immunotherapy for melanoma. J Clin Oncol 12:402–411, 1994.
133. Royal RE, Steinberg SM, White D, et al. Correlates of response of IL-2 therapy in patients treated for metastatic renal cancer and melanoma. Cancer J Sci Am 6:91–98, 1996.
134. Rosenberg SA, Yang JC, Topalian SL, et al. Treatment of 283 consecutive patients with metastatic melanoma or renal cell cancer using high-dose bolus interleukin-2. JAMA 271:907–913, 1994.
135. Philip PA, Flaherty L. Treatment of malignant melanoma with interleukin-2. Semin Oncol 24(1 Suppl 4):S4-32–S4-38.
136. Kammula US, White DE, Rosenberg SA. Trends in the safety of administration of high dose interleukin-2 in patients with metastatic cancer (Meeting Abstract #1684). Proc Annu Meet Am Soc Clin Oncol 17:437a, 1997.
137. Keilholz U, Scheibenbogen C, Brossart P, et al. Interleukin-2–based immunotherapy and chemoimmunotherapy in metastatic melanoma. Recent Results Cancer Res 139:383–390, 1995.
138. Sparano JA, Fisher RI, Sunderland M, et al. Randomized phase III trial of treatment with high-dose interleukin-2 either alone or in combination with interferon alfa-2a in patients with advanced melanoma. J Clin Oncol 11:1969–1977, 1993.
139. Bajorin DB, Chapman PB, Wong G, et al. A phase I trial of high-dose R24 mouse monoclonal antibody in patients with metastatic melanoma (Meeting Abstract). Proc Am Assoc Cancer Res 32:265, 1991.
140. Lichtin A, Illiopoulos D, Guerry D, et al. Therapy of melanoma with an anti-melanoma ganglioside monoclonal antibody. A possible mechanism of a complete response (Meeting Abstract). Proc Annu Meet Am Soc Clin Oncol 7:247, 1988.
141. Goodman GE, Beaumier P, Hellstrom I, et al. Pilot trial of murine monoclonal antibodies in patients with advanced melanoma. J Clin Oncol 3:340, 1985.
142. Larson SM, Carrasquillo JA, Krohn KA, et al. Localization of 131-I labeled p97-specific Fab fragments in human melanoma as a basis for radiotherapy. J Clin Invest 72:2101, 1983.
143. Vitteta ES, Fulton RJ, May RD, et al. Redesigning nature's poisons to create anti-tumor reagents. Science 238:1098, 1987.
144. Selvaggi K, Saria EA, Schwartz R, et al. Phase I/II study of murine monoclonal antibody-ricin a chain (xomasyme-mel) immunoconjugate plus cyclosporine a in patients with metastatic melanoma. J Immunother 13:210, 1993.
145. Ollila DW, Kelley MC, Gammon G, et al. Overview of melanoma vaccines: active specific immunotherapy for melanoma patients. Semin Surg Oncol 14:328–336, 1998.
146. Hsueh EC, Nizze A, Essner R, et al. Adjuvant immunotherapy with polyvalent melanoma cell vaccine (PMCV) prolongs survival after complete resection of distant melanoma metastases (Meeting Abstract). Proc Am Soc Clin Oncol 16:492, 1997.
147. Hershey P. Active immunotherapy with viral lysates of micrometastases following surgical removal of high-risk melanoma. World J Surg 16:251–260, 1992.
148. Buzaid AC, Legha SS. Combination of chemotherapy with interleukin-2 and interferon-alfa for the treatment of advanced melanoma. Semin Oncol 21(6):23–28, 1994.
149. Legha S, Buzaid AC, Ring S, et al. Improved results of treatment of metastatic melanoma with combined use of biotherapy and chemotherapy (biochemo) (Abstract). Proc Am Soc Clin Oncol 13:394, 1994.
150. Richards JM. Sequential chemoimmunotherapy for metastatic melanoma. Semin Oncol 18(5):91–95, 1991.
151. Cole P, Morrison AS. Issues in population screening for cancer. J Natl Cancer Inst 64:1263–1272, 1980.
152. Bal DG, Nixon DW, Foerster SB, Brownson RC. Cancer prevention. In: Murphy GP, Lawrence W, Lenhard RE, eds. American Cancer Society textbook of clinical oncology. 2nd ed. Atlanta: American Cancer Society, 1995: 40–63.
153. Moon TE, Levine N, Cartmel B, et al. Effect of retinol in preventing squamous cell skin cancer in moderate-risk subjects: a randomized, double-blind, controlled trial. Cancer Epidemiol Biomark Prev 6(11):949–956, 1997.

CHAPTER 96

PEDIATRIC AND NEONATAL THERAPY

Robert H. Levin

Pediatric Pharmacology

Pediatrics is a branch of medicine that deals with the care and treatment of the diseases of humans from birth through adolescence, with specific terminology defined for different age groups (Table 96.1). Within pediatrics, which became a specialty in the twentieth century, there are as many medical specialties as there are in adult internal medicine.

Neonates, infants, and children require unique considerations since age-related differences in physiology alter the pharmacokinetics of many drugs. In infants, particularly in neonates, differences in drug absorption, distribution, excretion, metabolism, and sensitivity affect the use and dosing of drugs. Pediatric dosing also involves various methods of calculating doses and consideration of appropriate drug formulations. The child's family or caretakers must be included in any discussion of medical treatment that involves the administration of drugs to the child. The issue of compliance or adherence with therapeutic regimens rests on the willingness of others to assist in the child's medical care.

TREATMENT GOALS: PEDIATRIC PHARMACOLOGY

- Know the differences between absorption of drugs in infants and children compared to adults.
- Appreciate the differences in drug distribution, metabolism, and excretion in infants and children.
- See how infants and children may be more sensitive to drug effects than adults.
- Know the techniques for successful administration of drugs to children in order to achieve the highest level of adherence to medication regimens.
- Know about the new FDA regulations concerning children.
- Appreciate the unique adverse drug effects that can occur in children.

DEVELOPMENTAL PHARMACOLOGY

Drug Absorption

Drugs are most frequently administered to children orally. Neonates have potentially altered drug absorption as a

Table 96.1 ▪ Pediatric Definitions

Category	Age
Premature	<38 wk gestation
Newborn, neonate	Birth to 1 mo old
Infant, baby	1–24 mo
Young child	2–5 yr
Older child	6–12 yr
Adolescent	13–18 yr

result of decreased production of gastric acid that also reduced gastric emptying time. Neonates have a relative achlorhydria. Those drugs that are absorbed in the stomach, by remaining in the stomach for an additional 6 to 8 hours, may have enhanced effects as a result of increased absorption. Although gastric acid production increases and the pH decreases rapidly over the first 24 hours of life, levels of gastric acid equivalent to those of an adult are not reached until the child is about 1 year old. This causes a decreased absorption of acidic drugs such as aspirin. As the neonate matures into infancy, the gastrointestinal transit time increases so that a sustained-release drug formulation passes through the intestine very quickly. For example, in case of Theo-Dur Sprinkles only about 50% of the drug is absorbed in children less than 5 years old. The hydrolytic enzyme system of the newborn or infant may not be sufficient for absorption of certain drugs. Oral phenytoin is inadequately absorbed in infants under 6 months old, necessitating doses greater than usual (15 to 20 mg/kg/day) to produce therapeutic serum levels.[1] Finally, conditions such as diarrhea markedly decrease the absorption of orally administered drugs.

The rectal route is employed more frequently in young children than in adults, since children frequently have difficulty swallowing medications. No specific physiologic differences influence rectal absorption of medication in children; however, problems have been documented with certain suppository dosage forms. Outdated suppositories or those exposed to air may have erratic melting characteristics that cause decreased and unpredictable drug absorption, which have been reported with those containing aminophylline. Appropriate therapeutic responses occur with suppositories of aspirin, acetaminophen, prochlorperazine, promethazine, glycerin, and others.

Ointments, lotions, and creams are commonly used for topical treatment of localized skin lesions that usually occur in the diaper area in infants and on the trunk, limbs, and face in children. A number of factors should be considered before selecting a topical agent. Infants, in contrast to older children, have a proportionally larger skin surface area that is capable of absorbing more topical drugs, especially if the drugs are applied to the perineum and face. Inflammation increases the amount of drug absorbed, as does the occlusion that occurs with plastic-coated diapers. An infant's skin is very sensitive so that a number of chemicals frequently cause local irritation (e.g., parabens, methyl salicylate).

The parenteral route, frequently used in hospitalized children, is seldom needed for medication administration in ambulatory children except for immunizations or insulin administration to diabetics. Infants have a small muscle mass, and intramuscular injections must be given in the lateral thigh rather than the arm or buttock. Absorption from intramuscular sites in neonates is slower and more erratic because of the smaller muscle mass and blood supply. Therefore, in neonates, the intravenous route is preferred because this route ensures that most drugs are 100% absorbed.

Drug Distribution

Most drugs are primarily distributed into the aqueous portion of the body. The body weight of neonates is about 75% water; therefore, the volume of distribution of many drugs is increased. For example, the volume of distribution of theophylline in a neonate is approximately 1 L/kg compared to 0.48 L/kg in a 6-year-old. In addition, the total body water of neonates is 56% extracellular fluid and many drugs are primarily distributed in total body water. Body water composition gradually falls to 40% extracellular and 60% intracellular water and 60% total body water by 1 year of age (Table 96.2).[2] Many drugs are less avidly bound to plasma proteins in neonates and plasma protein concentrations are also lower in neonates. This produces a higher unbound fraction of drugs such as phenytoin and sulfasoxazole, leading to an increased clearance and decreased half-life. A higher unbound fraction can also lead to increased toxicity. Thus phenytoin, which is normally 90% protein-bound, may be only 70% bound in neonates or premature infants. Serum levels of phenytoin are reported as total phenytoin levels, so that a level of 10 mg/L (90% protein bound) really means that the unbound active level of the drug is 1 mg/L. Therefore, toxic effects could occur when there is a low serum albumin level causing a 70% binding of phenytoin where the unbound level is 3 mg/L.

Table 96.2 ▪ Percentages of Body Water[a]

Age (Weight)	Extracellular Water (%)	Intracellular Water (%)	Total Body Water (%)
Premature baby (1.5 kg)	60	40	83
Full-term baby (3.5 kg)	56	44	74
5 mo old (7.0 kg)	50	50	60
1 yr old (10.0 kg)	40	60	59
Adult male	40	60	60

Source: Reference 2.

[a]Developmental changes from birth to adulthood. The extracellular and intracellular water are each expressed as a percentage of total body weight. Total body water is expressed as a percentage of body weight.

Drug Metabolism

Liver metabolism is the predominant method for drug transformation. Liver enzymes are present at birth and are stimulated to proliferate by the buildup of endogenous substrate. Each of the enzyme systems matures at a different rate but there are sufficient enzymes at 3 days postpartum, in a full-term infant, to adequately metabolize endogenous substrates. Bilirubin requires metabolism through the glucuronyl transferase pathway. This pathway matures slowly so that by 1 to 2 weeks of neonatal age, it is capable of also glucuronidating exogenous substances. It is at this time that drugs dependent on this pathway can be safely used. If chloramphenicol were to be given IV to an infant less than 1 week old, at the usual dose for children of 100 mg/kg/day, the drug would accumulate and cause cardiovascular collapse and cyanosis, which is known as "gray baby syndrome."[3] If required, though a rare occurrence these days, chloramphenicol in a dose of 25 mg/kg/day can be used in the first week of neonatal life.[3]

Bilirubin itself can be toxic to the newborn. The unconjugated, protein-bound fraction of bilirubin crosses into the brain very readily. When serum bilirubin levels reach 12 to 20 mg/dL, bilirubin will cross the blood-brain barrier and cause a yellow staining of the brain called kernicterus. Kernicterus may progress to irreversible brain damage and death when bilirubin levels are greater than 21 mg/dL. Irreversible brain damage can also occur at lower bilirubin serum levels of 12 to 20 mg/dL, if drugs such as sulfasoxazole, aspirin, or caffeine are given to the neonate. These drugs displace bilirubin from albumin and allow it to pass into the brain. Placing the infant under fluorescent lights usually treats bilirubin levels over 12 mg/dL. The light metabolizes the bilirubin in the skin to harmless metabolites, which are then excreted by the kidney. Other forms of treatment are phenobarbital, which induces liver enzymes, or exchange blood transfusions.

Drug Excretion

The kidneys excrete both metabolized and unmetabolized drugs. Drugs are also excreted through the gastrointestinal tract, lungs, and sweat glands. With most drugs, these latter pathways are of only limited importance. Neonatal kidney function matures rapidly. At birth, a full-term newborn has approximately 33% of the glomerular filtration rate and renal tubular excretion capacity of an adult. This capacity is about 15% or less in premature infants. The capacity to excrete a solute load quickly increases in the first few weeks of life to about 50% of adult levels at 1 month of age. This change is reflected in the decreasing half-lives of penicillin and carbenicillin in neonates (Table 96.3).[4,5] Doses of drugs that depend to a large degree on renal excretion (e.g., aminoglycosides and penicillins) must therefore be adjusted for the neonate. For example, gentamicin is given every 12 hours in the 1-week-old and every 8 hours in the 2- to 4-week-old neonate. Because of the rapidly changing characteristics of the newborn, drug level monitoring should be employed for aminoglycosides. Doses should be based on the neonate's age and weight. Drugs for normal infants and older children are administered in the usual therapeutic doses with no adjustment needed for renal function. At about 9 to 12 months of age, the infant kidney is functioning at adult levels.

Table 96.3 ▪ Age-Dependent Half-Life of Antibiotics in Serum

	Carbenicillin		Penicillin	
Age Group (Days Old)	Number Patients	Average Half-Life (hr)	Number of Patients (Average Age in Days)	Average Half-Life (hr)
1–3	13	5.7	–	–
4–7	23	4.2	7 (3.7)	3.21
8–14	13	3.4	13 (9.5)	1.74
15–21	2	2.2	6 (18.5)	1.4
22–45	4	1.5	–	–

Source: References 4, 5.

Drug Sensitivity

Neonates and infants are more sensitive to the effects of many drugs because of the immaturity of their organs. The central nervous system matures slowly and reaches adult levels at about 8 years of age. Because of this and the increased permeability of the blood-brain barrier, the neonate appears to be especially sensitive to the depressant effects of drugs such as phenobarbital, morphine sulfate, chloral hydrate, and chlorpromazine. Codeine and meperidine, however, do not produce this exaggerated effect in neonates.

The cardiovascular system usually functions adequately in the neonate and infant except in times of stress, when exaggerated responses may occur. General anesthetics may cause cardiovascular depression. Diuretics or antihypertensives in normal doses may induce severe hypotension.

The temperature regulating system is unstable and immature in the neonate and infant. Many drugs cause wide fluctuations in temperature and have exaggerated responses in neonates and infants. Drugs in therapeutic doses that normally lower temperature, such as aspirin and acetaminophen, can also raise the temperature when taken in toxic doses (Tables 96.4 and 96.5).[6] The skin, in addition to its immature thermal regulatory ability, increased permeability, and large surface area, is also more sensitive to drugs. This drug sensitivity may be either allergic or toxic and may occur throughout infancy and childhood. Allergic reactions are the most common and may be the immediate-onset type such as urticaria, angioneurotic edema, and anaphylaxis, or the delayed-onset types such as erythema multiforme or a fixed drug eruption. These drug-induced reactions mimic skin eruption caused by other processes. The most common drugs leading to skin reactions in pediatrics are sulfonamides, tetracycline, penicillins, isoniazid, cephalosporins, barbiturates, phen-

Table 96.4 ▪ Drugs Causing Hyperthermia

Drug	Comment
Salicylates[a] Aspirin Sodium salicylate Methyl salicylate (oil of wintergreen) Diflunisal	Increase temperature with toxicity and cause sweating and dehydration
Nonsteroidal anti-inflammatory agents[a] Ibuprofen, naproxen Indomethacin Mefenamic acid Piroxicam	Increase temperature with toxic doses
Dinitrophenols Herbicides, fungicides Nitrophenols Miscellaneous pesticides Insecticides	Increase temperature up to 2 days after heavy exposure, whether inhaled, ingested, or by skin contact
Anticholinergics Atropine Scopolamine Belladonna Benztropine Propantheline, etc.	High temperature can result from large doses or repeated therapeutic doses
Sympathomimetics Amphetamine and congeners Ephedrine Epinephrine Propylhexedrine inhalers, etc. Cocaine	Large doses cause chills and fever
Para-aminophenols[a] Acetaminophen	Large doses cause sweating and chills and probably fever
Antihistamines Diphenhydramine Hydroxyzine, etc.	Large doses cause fever
Boric acid	Large doses cause fever
Thyroid preparations Levothyroxine	Large doses cause fever
Alcohol[a]	Large doses cause fever
Antipsychotics[a] Phenothiazines Chlorpromazine Tricyclic antidepressants Amitriptyline Others MAO inhibitors Haloperidol	Overdoses cause fever
Phencyclidine (PCP)	Overdoses cause fever

Source: Reference 6.
[a]Also causes hypothermia (see Table 96.5).

ytoin, chloral hydrate, phenothiazines, narcotics, aspirin, indomethacin, iodides, griseofulvin, and topical antihistamines. There are a number of other adverse drug effects that occur in children: (a) growth suppression with tetracycline and corticosteroids; (b) sexual precocity with androgens; (c) neurotoxicity with hexachlorophene; (d) prepubertal effects with levodopa; (e) intracranial hypertension with corticosteroids, nalidixic acid, vitamins A and D, and nitrofurantoin; (f) jaundice with novobiocin, sulfonamides, and vitamin K; and (g) a bulging fontanel and tooth-staining with tetracycline.[7]

Drug Administration

Dosing

Children are not small adults. Doses for neonates must be tailored for their age, weight, and decreased liver and kidney function. Doses given on a milligram-per-kilogram basis that have established efficacy in neonates, infants, and children can be found in a number of sources.[8,9] Drugs that are very toxic, such as cancer chemotherapeutic agents, should be, for better accuracy, dosed on a milligram-per-square-meter basis. Body surface area takes into account the child's height and weight and is especially

Table 96.5 ▪ Drugs Causing Hypothermia

Drug	Comment
Salicylates[a] Aspirin Sodium salicylate Methyl salicylate (oil of wintergreen) Diflunisal	Lower fever in therapeutic doses
Nonsteroidal anti-inflammatory agents[a] Ibuprofen, naproxen Indomethacin Mefenamic acid Piroxicam	Decrease temperature with therapeutic doses
Para-aminophenol[a] Acetaminophen	Therapeutic doses will lower fever
Phenylbutazone Indomethacin Colchicine	Usually used for arthritis and gout but can be used to lower temperature
Chlorpromazine[a] Other phenothiazine also	Lower fever
Cholinergic agents Physostigmine Pilocarpine Neostigmine	Large dose or repeated small doses cause profuse sweating and cold extremities
Topical agents Water Alcohol[a] Volatile oils Menthol, etc.	Local cooling causes lower temperature
Sedative hypnotics Barbiturates Alcohol Benzodiazepines Diazepam	Overdoses decrease fever, causes sympatholytic syndrome
Opiates	Overdoses decrease fever by causing sympatholytic syndrome
Clonidine	Overdoses decrease fever by causing sympatholytic syndrome
Hypoglycemic agents Tolbutamide	Overdoses decrease fever

Source: Reference 6.
[a]Also causes hyperthermia (see Table 96.4).

useful for children who are not normal for their age in either height or weight. If necessary, the body surface area can be calculated from a child's height and weight, or a suitable nomogram can be used (Fig. 96.1). If a dose for a drug cannot be found in appropriate texts or current publications, the drug may not be suitable for pediatric use. This factor should be evaluated carefully before any dose is calculated. There are many formulas to calculate doses by the child's weight, age, body surface area, or height; however, all are inaccurate and should not be used.

In neonates, infants, and young children, the accurate and timely administration of oral or parenteral doses is particularly important. This requires precise dose calculation, measurement, and delivery, especially for parenteral medications. Microinfusion devices for intravenous infusion of drugs must deliver small volumes of fluids and medications accurately and safely. These neonatal microinfusion devices deliver intravenous fluid or medication in increments of tenths of a milliliter and have safeguards against uncontrolled free flow of fluid.[10,11] The syringe pump is the most accurate device available because there is absolute control of the volume delivered. A retrograde system is another system employed, especially in neonates, to keep fluid administration to a minimum. Here the drug is administered in tubing between two three-way stopcocks in a direction away from the patient, hence retrograde, while an equal volume of maintenance solution is injected into an empty syringe so that the volume to the patient remains constant. Also, one needs to take care when using standard syringes with "dead space" in the needle hubs so that the drug contained in these dead spaces is not injected into the neonate. In order to avoid injecting the "dead space overdose," use only syringes with permanently affixed needles and no dead space.

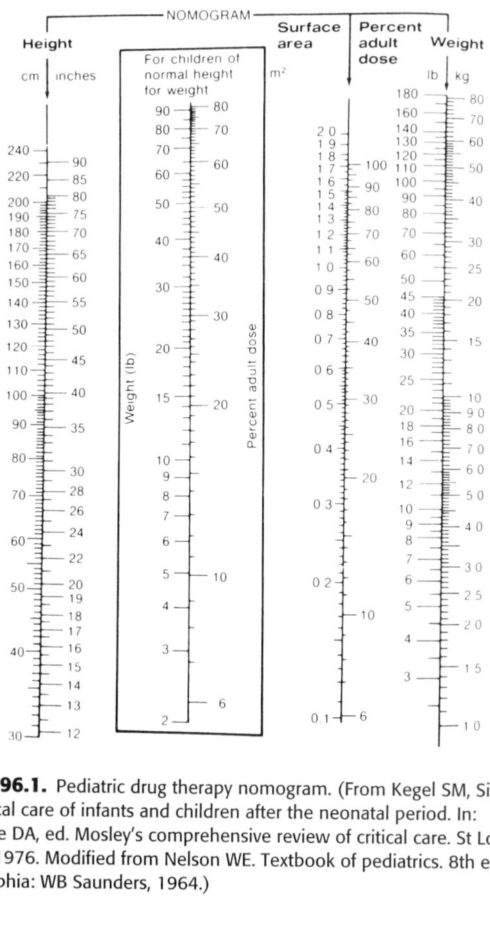

Figure 96.1. Pediatric drug therapy nomogram. (From Kegel SM, Singer MI. Critical care of infants and children after the neonatal period. In: Zschoche DA, ed. Mosley's comprehensive review of critical care. St Louis: Mosby, 1976. Modified from Nelson WE. Textbook of pediatrics. 8th ed. Philadelphia: WB Saunders, 1964.)

Compliance

Compliance is the term most health care providers use and write about when describing a patient's successful completion of their drug therapy regimen. However, when counseling a patient about their medications, would you rather they are compliant or adherent to their drug therapy? It seems we should want our patients to be adherent rather than compliant to their regimens according to the definitions below.

> *Compliance* is defined by Webster as
>
> 1. a. The act of complying with a wish, request, or demand; acquiescence. b. *Medicine.* Willingness to follow a prescribed course of treatment.
> 2. A disposition or tendency to yield to the will of others.
>
> Adherence is defined by Webster as
>
> 1. The process or condition of adhering.
> 2. Faithful attachment; devotion: *"Adherence to the rule of law . . . is a very important principle."*
>
> (William H. Webster)*

Most adherence studies of adult ambulatory patients reveal that 50 to 70% of patients fail to complete a course of therapy. In addition, 90% of patients make at least some error in taking their medication, such as a missed dose or a dose taken at the incorrect time. In pediatrics similar adherence problems occur. Very ill children are often unwilling to take medications. Becker et al.[12] studied mothers whose children had otitis media and were treated with oral penicillin. Mothers who were the most diligent in completing drug therapy had the following traits: (a) they were concerned about the child's health and current illness; (b) they felt that the illness was a major threat to the child's health and welfare; (c) they had confidence in the child's physician and the prescribed medication; (d) they had a more satisfactory experience with their pediatric clinic; (e) they actively endeavored to keep the child healthy and prevent future illness; and (f) they were better able to manage the problems of everyday life. In contrast, those mothers who complied less well with the medication regiment had opposite attitudes to the above. Additionally, these latter mothers thought their health was bad and were more concerned with their own health problems than with the health problems of their child. To achieve maximum success with medication regimens, therefore, health care personnel should emphasize and reinforce those traits that lead to increased adherence. Mattar et al.[13]

**The American Heritage Dictionary of the English Language, Third Edition,* © 1992 by Houghton Mifflin Company. Electronic version licensed from InfoSoft International, Inc. All rights reserved.

reported that by emphasizing verbal and written patient instructions and providing calibrated measuring devices and calendars, pharmacists were able to achieve adherence levels of 51% in a cohort of 33 patients being treated with antibiotics for otitis media. In comparison, only 8.5% of 200 control patients were compliant.

Drugs that are taken only once or twice a day, are easy to swallow and palatable, and are easy to use, carry, and store should increase adherence. The person giving medications should approach the child firmly but gently. A provocative, angry, or punishing attitude will increase the child's hostility and defensive medication-avoidance behavior. This adversary behavior affects adherence and interferes with good relationships even in adolescents. The adolescent has all the adherence considerations of the child plus those of the adult; therefore, adolescents need to be knowledgeable about and in control of their medications.

FEDERAL REGULATORY CHANGES

Since the enactment of the 1938 Food, Drug, and Cosmetic Act, as amended in 1962, the Food and Drug Administration (FDA) has had the responsibility of approving drugs for infants, children, and adults. The FDA requires that all drugs be tested for efficacy and safety only in adults prior to their approval for licensing in the United States. Information about drug use for infants, children, and adolescents is only included in the package insert if the newly-licensed drug is specifically tested and indicated for treatment of children. Since 1979, the FDA has required that all drugs to be used for children must have adequate, well-controlled clinical studies in children before any pediatric use information could be included in the package insert or label. Therefore, most new drugs approved in the U.S. have no pediatric information in the product insert, even if they have been successfully used in children.

About 80% of prescription drugs licensed in the U.S. never receive formal approval from the FDA for use in children because pharmaceutical companies do not want to spend large sums of money required for the needed extensive research. This realistically leaves the provider taking care of children with no guidance from the FDA or manufacturer about the drug's use and leaves the child as a "therapeutic orphan." Alternate publications and textbooks must be used as they serve as the only repository of information on the use of these drugs in children. However, the FDA had finally changed its regulations, and was accepting and actively soliciting labeling supplement applications as of January 1995, in order to increase the information included on labels and package inserts about drug use in children.

Manufacturers had until December 13, 1996, to submit these labeling supplement applications for a marketed drug if available information, e.g., clinical trials or experience, literature reports, or other information supports pediatric-use labeling. That new regulation allowed manufacturers to extrapolate adult clinical trial efficacy data to children if the course of the disease and effects of the drug are similar in both populations. The data included must be accompanied by pediatric-specific information on dosing, safety, indications, pharmacokinetics, and pharmacological considerations. In addition, the FDA requires manufacturers to submit pediatric-use information as part of their first application for a new drug. For the first time, children would no longer be "therapeutic orphans" and would be considered as a special population in the drug development process. Unfortunately, this voluntary regulation did not achieve its goal, and the FDA was forced to elaborate new regulations.

The FDA proposed additional regulations in August 1997, which were finalized in December 1998.[14] The new pediatric guidelines are part of the FDA Modernization Act of 1997 (21 U.S.C. 355a[b], and Public Law 105-115, subsection 505A) which amended the Federal Food, Drug, and Cosmetic Act and the Public Health Service Act. The effective date of this rule is April 1, 1999. Manufacturers have 20 months after this date to submit their data on pediatric safety and effectiveness. The important highlights of this Modernization Act are as follows:

- New drugs and biological products have pediatric labeling for approved uses when they are approved, or shortly thereafter.
- A presumption that all new products will be studied in children, unless the manufacturer receives an exemption because the drug will not be used in a substantial number (>50,000) of pediatric patients.
- Require pediatric studies in already marketed drugs and biological products where pediatric labeling is needed for effective use in children, that are used in a substantial number (>50,000) of pediatric patients, and would provide a therapeutic advantage over existing treatments.

This means that any new approved chemical entity or biologic products must contain safety and effectiveness information for any relevant pediatric age group for which it is indicated. It also means that pediatric indications will be needed for all marketed drugs when there is a change in indications, new dosage forms, new dosage regimens, new active ingredients, or new routes of administration. A manufacturer does not have to do additional controlled trials in children if the course of the disease being studied and the effects of the drug are similar in adults and children. However, additional data would have to be provided on dosing, pharmacokinetics, and safety in children.

The FDA can grant a waiver for this requirement of pediatric studies only under certain conditions. The product must meet both of the following conditions: (a) It does not represent a therapeutic pediatric benefit over existing products; and (b) it would not be used in >50,000 pediatric patients. The following list of proposed diseases where pediatric indications will probably be waived is: Alzheimer's disease, age-related macular degeneration, prostate cancer, breast cancer, non-germ cell ovarian cancer, renal cell cancer, hairy cell leukemia, uterine cancer, lung cancer, squamous cell cancers of the oropharynx, pancreatic cancer, colorectal cancer, basal cell and squamous cell cancer, endometrial cancer, osteoarthritis, Parkinson's disease, amyotrophic lateral sclerosis, arteriosclerosis, infertility, and symptoms of menopause. The FDA can also grant a waiver for additional pediatric studies in drugs that are commonly used or are of therapeutic importance in children if:

- The product is likely to be ineffective or unsafe in children.
- Pediatric studies are either impossible or impractical to do because the population is too geographically dispersed or small.
- Needed pediatric formulations cannot be developed using reasonable efforts.

This act requires the FDA, after consultation with pediatric research experts, to produce a list from already approved drugs with adult indications that includes those drugs for which additional information about pediatric use is needed. The FDA, after consultation with and recommendations from pediatric experts, released its Pediatric Priority List on May 20, 1998, after reviewing all currently adult approved medications.[15] The criteria for inclusion on the priority list are any of the following:

- The product is a significant improvement over other products for an approved pediatric indication for use in the treatment, diagnosis or prevention of a disease; or
- The drug will be used in >50,000 pediatric patients; or
- The drug is in a class or for an indication where additional pediatric data are needed.
- The list not only lists the individual medications, but also indicates the appropriate pediatric age groups for each drug, and will be revised as needed. This list can be viewed at the following Web site: http://www.fda.gov/cder/pediatric.

In addition to these new pediatric regulations, several professional organizations are also in the process of developing pediatric categories of use. The American Society of Health-System Pharmacists (ASHP), the American Academy of Pediatrics (AAP), and the FDA are discussing a system of categorizing the use of drugs in pediatrics analogous to the FDA pregnancy categories of A, B, C, D, and X. The proposed categories, as discussed in an article by K. Zenk,[16] are reproduced below:

- Category A: Adequate studies have not demonstrated any risk specific to pediatric patients.
- Category B: Adequate studies have not been done, but no data indicating risk specific to pediatric patients have been reported.
- Category C: Risks specific to pediatric patients exist with agents in the same or related therapeutic classes.
- Category D: Adequate studies have not been done and no data indicating risk specific to pediatric patients have been reported; however, because of the toxicity of the drug, less toxic alternatives should be considered.
- Category X: Adequate studies have demonstrated risk specific to pediatric patients.

There will be additional information accompanying these designations, e.g., specific age of children if applicable, specific problems occurring in children, and specific therapeutic indications.

ADVERSE EFFECTS IN PEDIATRIC DRUG THERAPY

Physicians and other health care providers can also minimize costly prescription errors by being more careful when writing or filling prescriptions according to a medication error study done by Physician Insurers of America.[17] Four types of medication errors accounted for 37.4% of the total liability claims in this study: (a) incorrect or inappropriate dosage; (b) inappropriate medication for the medical condition being treated; (c) failure to monitor for drug side effects; and (d) communication failure between physician and patient. The other medication errors that occurred in this study were caused by illegible handwriting and related mistakes in writing prescriptions (inappropriate length of treatment, method, site, route of administration of drugs), failure to take an adequate medical history, failure to monitor drug levels, side effects, drug effects, drug allergies, prescribing inappropriate or contraindicated medications, or pharmacist errors when filling the prescription. Antibiotics, glucocorticoids, and analgesics (narcotic, non-narcotic, narcotic antagonists) accounted for 34.9% of the patient's claims to the insurance company. Errors in pediatric patients were most likely to be caused by drugs used for respiratory problems and from intravenous fluid use.

This study recommended a number of risk management steps quoted below that physicians (also appropriate for other health care professionals) might use to reduce medication errors.

- Chart all prescriptions and refills on a medication flow sheet.
- Post medication allergies on the chart in a consistent and conspicuous manner.
- Obtain and document medication histories from patients and update as necessary.
- Read the medical record for contraindications to medications, allergies, and excessive number of refills.
- Review authoritative references before prescribing unfamiliar medications for the correct dosage, contraindications, and side effects.
- Educate patients about their medications, using such resources as the AMA's "Patient Medication Instructions" or "United States Pharmacopoeia" leaflet program.
- Obtain and document informed consent for the prescription of medications with potentially significant drug complications and side effects.
- Closely monitor patients for drug side effects.
- Closely monitor drug usage, particularly with controlled substances.
- Periodically re-evaluate patients on chronic analgesic or psychotropic therapy for the indications for, and efficacy of continued therapy.
- Obtain specific drug allergy information for antibiotics (penicillin and sulfa), NSAIDs, anticonvulsants, and diuretics.

There is also a federally mandated program to report serious adverse drug reactions, "The FDA Medical Products Reporting Program" called MedWatch. Any adverse event should be reported that produces any serious undesirable experience associated with the use of a medical product in a patient. A serious event in a patient is one that is either life-threatening, prolongs or causes a hospital admission, causes a disability or congenital anomaly, or requires intervention to prevent permanent impairment or damage. Complete information and reporting forms can be found on the FDA web site, http://www.fda.gov/medwatch/report. Complete information for pharmacists has also been published by ASHP.[18]

The Pediatric Pharmacy Advocacy Group, Inc. (PPAG) is a non-profit voluntary organization composed of health care providers interested in promoting safe and effective medication use in children. It also has a Pediatric Adverse Drug Event and Reaction Reporting System (PADR). The purpose of this system is to serve as a uniform way of collecting and reporting adverse drug events in children. Forms can be filled via the Internet at http://www.ppag.org/padr.htm, and subsequently sent to the MedWatch program.

PSYCHOSOCIAL ASPECTS

Mothers who were the most diligent in completing drug therapy had the following traits: (a) they were concerned about the child's health and current illness; (b) they felt that the illness was a major threat to the child's health and welfare; (c) they had confidence in the child's physician and the prescribed medication; (d) they had a more satisfactory experience with their pediatric clinic; (e) they actively endeavored to keep the child healthy and prevent future illness; and (f) they were better able to manage the problems of everyday life. The person giving medications should approach the child firmly but gently.

Infant Nutrition

Healthy growth and development of children are the major focuses for "Well Baby" clinics. During visits to the clinics, the parents are informed about proper nutrition, breastfeeding, maternal diet, and drugs to be avoided. Synthetic infant formulas, baby foods, and table foods are also discussed. Proper nutrition and the use of prophylactic agents such as immunizations prevent diseases. The advantages and possible adverse effects of each immunization are thoroughly discussed with the parents prior to their administration to the child, and are thoroughly reviewed in this book in Chapter 65.

TREATMENT GOALS: INFANT NUTRITION

- Parents are informed about proper nutrition, breastfeeding, maternal diet, and drugs to be avoided.
- The feeding of synthetic infant formulas, baby foods, and table foods are also discussed with parents.

BREASTFEEDING

Human breast milk is the most healthy and complete food for the full-term infant. It should be the only source of nutrition for infants up to 6 months of age.[19,20] Breastfeeding is usually supplemented with food in the child over 6 months old. In the United States, of those infants who are breast-fed, over 50% are breast-fed until at least 3 months of age. This decreases to 25% of 6-month-old infants, and less than 5% of 9- to 12-month-old infants are still breastfeeding. In some cultures, however, children at 4 to 6 years of age are still breastfeeding to gain needed protein. There are advantages to breastfeeding; it is less expensive than infant formula, the breast is an antiseptic environment, and breast milk has proteins of better biologic value, curds that are easier to digest, more easily absorbed fat, immunoglobulins, lysozymes, antistreptococcal enzymes, complement, lactoferrin, and macrophages that decrease infections.

Infants in the United States who breast-feed have a lower incidence of gastrointestinal disease, respiratory disease, otitis media, and allergies.[21] There is also mounting evidence that breastfeeding is somewhat protective against developing obesity, allergy, arteriosclerosis, cystic fibrosis, celiac disease, early onset diabetes, and other metabolic disorders in adulthood.[22] There are also advantages for the mother; breastfeeding enhances postpartum recovery, returns women to their prepartum weight quicker, and enhances maternal-infant bonding.[16]

There are disadvantages to breastfeeding. The mother must want to nurse in order for it to be satisfactory and rewarding for her and the infant. The breasts must be prepared for nursing during the last trimester of pregnancy. Sometimes pain, inconvenience, engorgement, minor infections, and inflammation are associated with breastfeeding. The mother should have an adequate diet and must be careful about taking drugs that are excreted into breast milk. The mother should not breast-feed if she has active, untreated tuberculosis, breast cancer, breast reduction surgery, or a serious infection. In many cases, active support and encouragement by health care personnel overcome most, if not all, of the maternal apprehension about breastfeeding. The maternal use of medications can be carefully planned in order to least affect the breastfeeding infant. See Chapter 100 on pregnancy and lactation.

Normal Breast Physiology

The breast is composed of glandular, fibrous, and adipose tissue and rests on a bed of connective tissue. The glandular tissue is composed of 15 to 20 lobes arranged radially around the nipple. Strands of fibrous tissue connect the lobes, and adipose tissue occupies the space between and around the lobes. Each lobe is divided into several lobules and connected by alveolar tissue, blood vessels, and ducts (Fig. 96.2a).[23] Each lobule contains a small lactiferous duct. Eventually these lactiferous ducts unite and form a single main canal for each lobe. These 15 to 20 main canals each become dilated and form a reservoir (sinus lactiferous) for milk storage and finally merge and pass through the nipple.

The functioning part of the breast is the alveoli or acini (sacs) in the lobule (Fig. 96.2b). It is in the acini that milk is produced and secreted into the lactiferous ducts. Drugs cross from the blood in the capillary beds through the acini epithelium and into the lactiferous ducts. See Chapter 100.

Normal Composition of Milk

The composition of milk is determined by the mammary gland with little or no external control.[24,25] The milk occurs in three forms: colostrum, transitional, and mature milk. Colostrum, which serves as a precursor of milk, may be expressed from the breasts as early as the fourth month of pregnancy, but it usually appears after parturition. It is scanty the first few days after birth, becomes well established on the third or fourth day, and usually continues for no more than five days. It has, however, been known to continue for as long as 10 days. Colostrum is a transudate consisting primarily of serum albumin (3 to 5%) and cast-off epithelium (colostrum corpuscles) that has undergone fatty degeneration. It has a higher specific gravity than mature milk (1.030–1.060 compared with 1.026–1.036) and also a higher average pH (7.7 compared with 6.8). It is richer in vitamin A, sodium, potassium, and other minerals but lower in sugar and fat. Colostrum is quickly modified by the mammary gland into transitional milk.

Transitional milk is produced within the first week of breastfeeding. It usually lasts for a few weeks, during which time a moderate increase in fat and sugar and gradual decrease in proteins and minerals occurs. Milk finally matures near the end of the first month of lactation.

Mature milk has between 0.9 and 1.6% protein, 2 to 6% fat, and 6.5 to 8% lactose. The composition of milk at the beginning of a feeding is highest in protein and lowest in fat. This is reversed toward the end of the feeding. The effect of this on the excretion of drugs is unknown.

Once established, mature milk varies little in composition.[2,23] If the mother has adequate nutritional intake, her diet can be quite varied without affecting milk composition or volume. A deficiency in maternal diet will

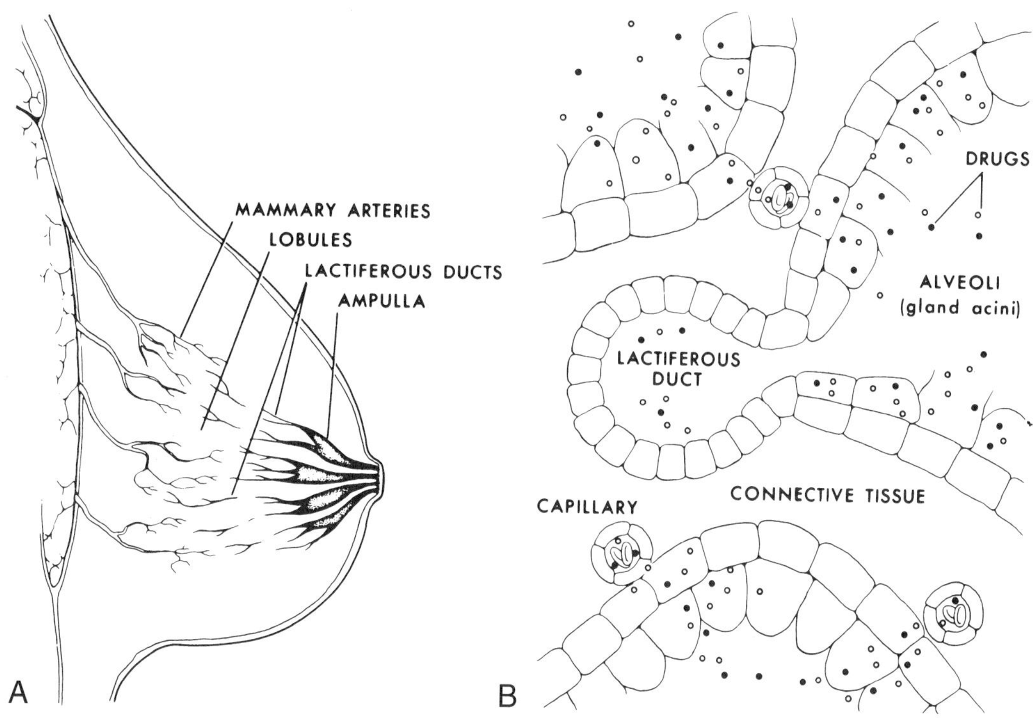

Figure 96.2. **A,** Cross-section of the breast; **B,** Magnified cross-section of lobule capillaries. (*Source:* Reference 21.)

first cause a decrease in the quantity of milk but will not affect milk composition unless the mother's tissue stores are depleted. A decreased water intake will cause maternal thirst before it affects milk production.

Control of Milk Production

The initiation and maintenance of milk production has not been adequately studied; however, the evidence regarding physiologic and endocrine factors in lactation is better understood now.[24] Lactation usually begins at birth or shortly thereafter. The inhibition of lactation during pregnancy is assumed to be the result of the high estrogen or progesterone levels. The effects of estrogen on milk secretion are dose dependent. At low endogenous levels occurring post partum, milk secretion occurs, whereas lactation is inhibited by high doses of estrogen (diethylstilbestrol given postpartum). In most women, low-dose oral contraceptives do not decrease lactation even when given immediately postpartum.[25] Estrogen may work partly by affecting prolactin (lactogenic factor), which is secreted from the anterior pituitary.

Prolactin is presently under extensive investigation in an effort to delineate its true role during pregnancy and lactation.[26] During pregnancy, prolactin, estrogen, progesterone, and human growth hormone stimulate breast development. There are high concentrations of prolactin during pregnancy and breastfeeding, but low concentrations after birth in the absence of breastfeeding. If breastfeeding is successful and unrestricted, the high levels of prolactin have been reported to be contraceptive.[27] This contraceptive effect is seen only in certain societies and has not been observed in the U.S., where formula supplements are frequently given.

The posterior pituitary, in addition to the anterior pituitary, is involved in and stimulated when an infant breast-feeds. The release of oxytocin by the posterior pituitary initiates the "letdown" reflex. Oxytocin stimulates the expression or ejection of milk from the breast, the letdown reflex, whereas prolactin stimulates milk production. The letdown reflex is responsive to other internal and external factors. The actions and sounds associated with nursing can initiate this reflex. In contrast, distractions such as fright, pain, and emotional distress can inhibit milk expression. It is hypothesized that the high levels of the catecholamines, adrenaline, and norepinephrine produced in such circumstances cause vasoconstriction in the mammary circulation that prevents oxytocin from reaching the contractile cells.[19] Excessive doses of medications that also release endogenous catecholamines (e.g., amphetamines and most decongestants) may interfere with milk secretion.

Quantity of Milk Produced

The quantity of milk produced depends upon the demands of the infant. If the infant's demand is increasing, milk supply will adjust accordingly within two days and vice versa. The actual secretion of milk is a discontinuous process. During feeding there is increased milk secretion as a result of the depletion of milk stores. In all probability, drugs are excreted into milk in larger amounts when the milk is being actively secreted. To derive the total quantity of drug ingested (measured as milligrams per deciliter), it is necessary to know the quantity of milk ingested by the infant. This depends on the age and weight of the infant (Table 96.6). See Chapter 100 for a discussion of drugs excreted in breast milk. If women cannot breastfeed, prepared infant formulas are the best substitute and are covered in Chapter 97, Pediatric and Neonatal Nutrition.

Table 96.6 ▪ Quantities of Milk Ingested

Amount at Each Feeding[a] (mL)	Age (weeks)
20–45	1
30–90	2
40–140	4
60–150	6
75–165	12
90–175	16
120–225	24

[a]Feedings are usually every 3–4 hours; quantity consumed depends on infant's weight.

Infants who are 6 to 12 months old usually do not require infant formulas; cow's milk alone plus baby food provides adequate nutrition for this age group. If cow's milk is used, the daily intake should be kept to one quart or less. Greater than 1 quart/day can lead to milk intolerance, diarrhea, and iron-deficiency anemia secondary to the large intake of protein, which may cause an enteropathy. Reducing the intake of milk to less than a quart and supplementing with iron-rich infant food resolve the enteropathy and its sequelae. The infant foods used should be those with the least possible added salt, sugar, and monosodium glutamate (MSG). These substances are added to improve the taste for increased adult acceptability. The added sodium and MSG have been causally implicated in predisposing susceptible infants to developing hypertension as adult.[28] The inclusion of MSG in infant food seems unwarranted. The added sugar may predispose infants to obesity by increasing the total number of fat cells.

The use of infant foods usually starts at 6 months of age with cereals and then the addition of vegetables, fruits, and meats as tolerated to avoid colic. The daily intake of infant foods for the 8- to 12-month-old should consist of two or more servings of meat, four or more servings of vegetables, one or more servings of citrus fruits, and four or more servings of bread or cereal. The size of each serving should increase as the child grows. Junior foods that contain small chunks of solid food are usually begun at 8 to 12 months of age. Adult table food is usually begun at 1 year of age. If the child receives a normal, varied diet that contains the required nutrients, no added supplements are needed. Giving a normal child additional vitamins and minerals adds nothing to health and is an unneeded expense. Vitamins and minerals should only be used if nutritional deficiencies have been documented.

PSYCHOSOCIAL ASPECTS

Breastfeeding should be the only source of nutrition for infants up to 6 months of age because it is more healthy for the infant, and more personally satisfying for the successful mother. There are also advantages for the mother for breastfeeding; it enhances postpartum recovery, it returns women to their prepartum weight quicker, and it enhances maternal-infant bonding.

Fevers in Children

One of the most common symptoms of illness is fever, which is a mechanism for fighting off infection. It is one of the most common childhood complaints. It is important to separate mild febrile disease from a serious infection.

TREATMENT GOALS: FEVERS IN CHILDREN

- Learn when to be concerned about a fever, and what its causes are.
- Know which drugs cause fevers, and which ones are used to treat fevers.

EPIDEMIOLOGY

The causes of mild fevers in children are usually upper respiratory infections and lower respiratory infections caused by assorted viruses, including influenza. Bacterial infections that cause otitis media, sore throat, urinary tract infections, or respiratory infections also quite commonly cause fever.

COMPLICATIONS

Children who are at the greatest risk for complications from a febrile illness, and who must be watched carefully if they develop a sudden fever, are those that are: (a) less than 2 months old with a rectal temperature over 38°C; (b) those 6 to 24 months old with a rectal temperature over 39°C; or (c) any child with a rectal temperature over 40°C. Children less than 2 months old do not manifest the usual signs and symptoms of systemic disease, for example, fever or inflammation, and it is therefore very difficult to diagnose serious disease in these infants before it becomes life threatening. Children between 6 and 24 months with a fever are at high risk of having an infection caused by either *Streptococcus pneumoniae*, or if unimmunized, *H. influenzae*. Children at any age with high fevers (more than 40°C rectally) are at great risk of having bacterial sepsis or meningitis.

Children who have prolonged undiagnosed fevers (>38°C rectally) for more than 2 weeks in duration are classified as having a fever of unknown origin (FUO). There are a number of causes of FUOs, as depicted in Table 96.7. These unexplained fevers require an extensive workup and are generally serious.

Table 96.7 ▪ Causes of Fever of Unknown Origin

Causes	Age <6 yr (%)	Age 6–14 yr (%)	Age >14 yr (%)
Infections	65	38	36
Neoplastic diseases	8	4	19
Autoimmune diseases	8	23	13
Miscellaneous	13	17	25
Undiagnosed (FUOs)	6	18	7

TREATMENT

Fever does not have to be pharmacologically treated unless it is causing morbidity or is debilitating for the patient. Fevers should be treated if the patient is irritable, very sick, delirious, or has shaking chills or seizures. In bacterial infections, the fever decreases as the child recovers and provides a convenient monitoring parameter for the efficacy of antibiotics.

The two most commonly used antipyretic analgesics for treating fevers in children are ibuprofen and acetaminophen. Aspirin can also be used; however, because of its association with Reye's syndrome, it is seldom used for treating fevers. The analgesic/antipyretic dose is the same on a milligram-for-milligram basis for both agents. The usual oral dose is 5 to 10 mg/kg/dose (about 65 mg/kg/day for acetaminophen and 40 mg/kg/day for ibuprofen) given every 4 to 6 hours for acetaminophen and every 6 to 8 hours for ibuprofen. If one agent at the maximum dose is not effective for lowering temperature, both agents can be used, alternating doses every 2 hours. An alternate strategy to employ is to give both agents at the same time every 6 to 8 hours. This avoids doubling the dose of either agent and causing toxicity. This approach can be used because the toxicities of these agents are different. Ibuprofen, due to direct mucosal irritation, causes gastrointestinal toxicity in children, and in overdoses usually leads to nausea, vomiting, abdominal pain, and metabolic acidosis. Acetaminophen, generally thought to be less toxic, may cause hepatic toxicity[29,30] when used in excessive doses. The hepatic toxicity is due to a buildup of a toxic metabolite, which binds to hepatocytes and causes their lysis. The buildup of this metabolite occurs when there is a depletion of its converting enzyme, glutathione, caused by large ingestions of acetaminophen.

Caution is needed when treating fevers or pain with analgesics in children or adolescents less than 19 years old with flu or varicella infections. Acetaminophen is the analgesic of choice because of the risk of developing Reye's syndrome. The syndrome usually starts in a patient recovering from varicella, who suddenly starts vomiting and deteriorates rapidly. Some patients may slowly get better but many go on to develop symptoms that consist of metabolic encephalopathy associated with hepatic failure. Although it is a rare disease, 204 cases were reported in 1984 which decreased to none as of 1989 in the United States.[31] Warnings about use of aspirin and Reye's syndrome began to appear on aspirin labels in 1984. The FDA required a warning on all aspirin-containing products: "Children and teenagers should not use this medicine (aspirin) for chickenpox or flu symptoms before a doctor is consulted about Reye's syndrome, a rare but serious illness." Patients and parents should be alerted to this warning. It is believed that this decrease in incidence of Reye's syndrome is due to the decreased use of aspirin for flu and varicella. The majority of cases of Reye's syndrome occur in children between 6 and 18 years old. Reye's syndrome may occur in children whether or not they have taken aspirin during their antecedent illness, but aspirin seems to increase the chances for developing this syndrome, possibly by altering the immune system of susceptible children and therefore increasing the virulence of the infection. It may also predispose the child to metabolic complications by acting as an additional insult.[32–36] The treatment for Reye's syndrome consists of fluid and electrolyte therapy for the patient's metabolic requirements and mannitol and other agents to reduce cerebral edema. Vitamin K, barbiturates, hypothermia, or corticosteroids may also be employed. The mortality rate is between 20 and 40%; permanent brain damage may occur in those who survive.[37]

PSYCHOSOCIAL ASPECTS

Fever does not have to be pharmacologically treated unless it is causing morbidity or is debilitating for the patient. Fevers should be treated if the patient is irritable, very sick, delirious, or has shaking chills or seizures.

KEY POINTS

- Health maintenance and disease prevention, including proper nutrition and an immunization program, are important aspects of the practice of pediatrics.
- Certain illnesses such as upper respiratory viral infections, otitis media, infantile diarrhea, and other febrile diseases are so common that every child can be expected to suffer several episodes before they are 6 years old.
- Proper therapy instituted quickly can prevent these minor diseases from becoming more serious. Although many of these pediatric diseases are treated in the same way as they are in adults, neonates, infants, and children have unique characteristics that call for additional knowledge of drug therapy.
- Considerations in drug therapy in pediatrics include the influence of normal growth and development on drug absorption, distribution, and elimination, as well as dosage formulation to facilitate adherence.

Pediatric Pharmacology

- There is decreased absorption of acidic drugs, phenytoin, sustained release theophylline in neonates and infants.
- The volume of distribution is increased for most drugs in neonates.
- Drugs should be adjusted for decreased hepatic clearance until a full-term newborn reaches the age of 2 weeks old.
- Drugs should be adjusted for decreased renal function until a full-term newborn reaches the age of 1 month.
- The neonate appears to be especially sensitive to the depressant effects of drugs such as phenobarbital, morphine sulfate, chloral hydrate, and chlorpromazine.
- Doses given on a milligram per kilogram basis that have established efficacy in neonates, infants, and children can be found in a number of sources.
- There are special parenteral delivery forms available for neonates to deliver very small amounts of fluid.
- To achieve maximum success with medication regimens, therefore, pharmacists should emphasize verbal and written patient instructions and provide calibrated measuring devices and calendars.
- The new FDA regulation for children means that any new approved chemical entity or biologic products contain safety and effectiveness information for any relevant pediatric age group for which it is indicated.
- The new FDA regulation also means that pediatric indications will be needed for all marketed drugs when there is a change in indications, new dosage forms, new dosage regimens, new active ingredients, or new routes of administration.
- Physicians and other health care providers can also minimize costly prescription errors by being more careful when writing or filling prescriptions.

Infant Nutrition

- Human breast milk is the most healthy and complete food for the full-term infant.
- Infants in the United States who breastfeed have a lower incidence of gastrointestinal disease, respiratory disease, otitis media, and allergies.
- The use of infant foods usually starts at 6 months of age with cereals, followed with the addition of vegetables, fruits, and meats as tolerated to avoid colic.

Fevers in Children

- Children who are at the greatest risk for complications from a febrile illness, and who must be watched carefully if they develop a sudden fever, are those that are: (a) less than two months of age with a rectal temperature over 38°C; (b) those 6 to 24 months old with a rectal temperature over 39°C; or (c) any child with a rectal temperature over 40°C.
- Children at any age with high fevers (more than 40°C rectally) are at great risk of having bacterial sepsis or meningitis.
- The two most commonly used antipyretic analgesics for treating fevers in children are ibuprofen and acetaminophen.
- Do not use aspirin when treating fevers or pain in children or adolescents less than 19 years old with flu or varicella infections because of the risk of causing Reye's syndrome.

REFERENCES

1. Watson PD, Powell JR, Mimaki T. Anticonvulsant usage. In: Jaffe ST, ed. Pediatric pharmacology and therapeutics: principles in practice. New York: Grune & Stratton, 1980:195–212.
2. Friis-Hansen B. Body composition during growth. Pediatrics 47:264, 1971.
3. Nelson JD. Antimicrobial drugs. In: Jaffe SJ, ed. Pediatric pharmacology and therapeutics: principles in practice. New York: Grune & Stratton, 1980: 187–198.
4. Nelson JD, McCracken GM. Clinical pharmacology of carbencillin and gentamicin in the neonate and comparative efficacy with ampicillin and gentamicin. Pediatrics 52:801, 1973.
5. McCracken GH, Ginsberg C, et al. Clinical pharmacology of penicillin in newborn infants. J Pediatr 82:692, 1973.
6. Levin RH, Maltz HE. Fluid balance in drug therapy. In: Waechter EH, Blake JB, eds. Nursing care of children. 9th ed. Philadelphia: JB Lippincott, 1976:102.
7. Facts and Comparisons Staff. Facts and comparisons. St Louis: Facts and Comparisons, 1998.
8. Zenk KE. Neonatal and pediatric dosing. In: Pagliaro LA, Levin RH, eds. Problems in pediatric drug therapy. Hamilton, IL: Drug Intelligence Publications, 1979.
9. Levin RH, Zenk KE. Medication table. In: Rudolph AM, ed. Pediatrics. 18th ed. Norwalk, CT: Appleton-Century-Crofts, 1987.
10. Zenk KE. Drug use in neonates. U.S. Pharmacist 11:H2–H20, 1986.
11. Zenk KE. Special delivery: delivering IV antibiotics to children. Nursing86 16:50–52, 1986.
12. Becker MH, Drachman RH, Kirscht JP. Predicting mothers' compliance with pediatric medical regimens. J Pediatr 81:843, 1972.
13. Mattar ME, Markello J, Jaffe SJ. Pharmaceutical factors affecting pediatric compliance. Pediatrics 55:101, 1975.
14. Federal Register 63(231), December 2, 1998.
15. FDA Docket No. 98N-0056, May 20, 1998.
16. Zenk KE. Challenges in providing pharmaceutical care to pediatric patients. Am J Hosp Pharm 51:688, 1994.
17. Reinso D. Pediatricians and the law: physicians can minimize costly prescription errors. American Academy of Pediatrics News 10:17, 1994.
18. ASHP. ASHP guidelines on adverse drug reaction monitoring and reporting. Am J Health Syst Pharm 52:417, 1995.
19. Lawrence RA. Breastfeeding: a guide for the medical profession. 4th ed. St Louis: Mosby, 1996:12–24.
20. Barness LA. Bases of weaning recommendations. J Pediatr 117(Suppl):S84–85, 1990.
21. Chen Y, Yu S, Li WX. Artifical feeding and hospitalization in the first 18 months of life. Pediatrics 81:52, 1988.
22. Lawrence RA. Breastfeeding and medical disease. Med Clin North Am 73:583–603, 1989.
23. Arena J. Contamination of the ideal food. Nutr Today 5:2, 1970.
24. Holt LE. Feeding techniques and diets. In: Barnett HL, ed. Pediatrics. 15th ed. New York: Meredith Corporation, 1972:148.
25. Jelliffe DB, Jelliffe EFP. The volume and composition of human milk in poorly nourished communities: a review. Am J Clin Nutr 31:492, 1978.
26. Gambrell R. Immediate postpartum oral contraception. Obstet Gynecol 36:101, 1970.
27. Jelliffe DB, Jelliffe EFP. Lactation, conception and the nutrition of the nursing mother and child. J Pediatr 81:829, 1972.
28. Committee on Nutrition. Sodium intake by infants in the United States. Evanston, IL: American Academy of Pediatrics, 1979.
29. APHA Project Staff. Handbook of non-prescription drugs. 7th ed. Washington, DC: American Pharmaceutical Association, 1982:123.
30. Anonymous. Aspirin or paracetamol. Lancet 2:287, 1981.
31. Centers for Disease Control. Summary of notifiable diseases, United States 1989. MMWR 38(54), 1990.
32. Anonymous. Salicylate labeling may change because of Reye's syndrome. FDA Drug Bull 12:9, 1982.
33. Waldman RJ, et al. Aspirin as a risk factor in Reye's syndrome. JAMA 247:3089, 1982.
34. Halpin TJ, Holtzhauer FJ, Campbell RJ, et al. Reye's syndrome and medication use. JAMA 248:687, 1982.
35. Starko KM, Ray CGJ, Dominguez LB, et al. Reye's syndrome and salicylate use. Pediatrics 66:859, 1980.
36. Hurwitz ES, Barrett MJ, Bregman D, et al. Public health service study on Reye's syndrome and medications. N Engl J Med 313:849, 1985.
37. Rudolph AM. Pediatrics. 18th ed. Norwalk, CT: Appleton-Century-Crofts, 1987.

CHAPTER 97

PEDIATRIC AND NEONATAL NUTRITION

Emily B. Hak and Richard A. Helms

In addition to basal requirements, pediatric patients require nutrients to meet the demands of growth and development. Failure to provide essential nutrients can result in growth retardation, immune system impairment, and neurologic deficits. The premature neonate presents a unique nutritional challenge to the clinician because transition to the extrauterine environment is a period of rapid lean body mass accretion and organ development. Thus preterm neonates require early nutritional intervention and consideration of developmental issues.

The most significant advance in the nutritional care of the high-risk neonate was the development of parenteral nutrition. The first report of the successful use of total parenteral nutrition in an infant occurred more than 50 years ago, but only in the last 30 years has parenteral nutrition been routinely used in children with a variety of surgical or medical conditions. Understanding of macronutrient and micronutrient metabolism and substrate requirements has grown over time and practitioners are now able to individualize nutrients based on age, weight, nutritional status, and disease. Enteral formulas have been developed to meet the specialized nutrient needs of preterm and term infants who are not fed human milk. Likewise, commercially available enteral formulas have been designed to meet the nutritional requirements of older children who cannot or should not eat. Standards have been developed to assist the clinician with appropriate nutrition therapies in hospitalized children.[1]

TREATMENT GOALS: PEDIATRIC AND NEONATAL NUTRITION

- Provide nutrients for basal requirements, growth and development, wound healing, and recovery from acute illness.
- Use the gastrointestinal tract whenever possible.
- Provide nutrients in a safe and effective manner.
- Continually evaluate response and adjust nutrient intake according to growth and age, with consideration of underlying conditions.
- Engage patient and parents or caregivers, whenever possible, in nutrition management.

NUTRITIONAL ASSESSMENT AND MONITORING

Similar nutritional assessment techniques are used clinically in both children and adults; however, children require special consideration for almost all parameters assessed.[2–5] Body composition in infants can be evaluated using dual-energy x-ray absorptiometry (DEXA), total body electrical conductivity (TOBEC), and magnetic resonance imaging (MRI) techniques.[6–8] However, because of the equipment and personnel expense and the need for patients to remain motionless during the study, these procedures will not likely be used in routine clinical pediatric practice.

Weight

Weight is the most important assessment tool used to evaluate nutritional outcome in children. All infants who are receiving parenteral nutrition should have their weight measured daily, unless medically prohibited. In these patients, the addition or deletion of clothing, diapers, wound dressings, or arm boards used to stabilize an intravenous line can alter the apparent weight, making interpretation of daily fluctuations difficult. Furthermore, significant variation in weight can be seen when different scales are used or when different caregivers perform the measurement. Because daily weight changes may relate to factors other than lean body mass accretion, an average should be made over several days. The younger the infant, the greater the gain per unit of body weight. Older children and adolescents may require less frequent weighing because growth is slower and detectable changes are fewer.

Intake and Output

Accurate assessment of intake and output is important in evaluating weight gain. Intake consists of substances delivered both enterally and parenterally, and should include fluid used in the delivery of medications and flushes as well as maintenance fluid infusion. Output includes urine, stool, nasogastric or gastrostomy tube drainage, chest tube outputs, emesis, blood loss, ventriculostomy drainage, and wound drainage. In an uncatheterized infant, urine and stool losses can be approximated by weighing diapers before and after elimination. If possible, urine and stool volumes should be recorded separately. Daily evaluation of weight in conjunction with assessment of total intake and output will aid in the evaluation of fluid balance and the source of weight gain.

Growth Charts

Growth charts derived from large populations of pediatric patients in the United States allow comparison of an individual child to an age-related population for length or height, weight, and head circumference.[9] In addition, estimates of appropriate average daily weight gains can be extrapolated from growth charts to better evaluate changes over a relatively short period. This is most useful in younger, smaller infants whose weight increases in g/kg/day are greater. Preterm infants should be plotted on an intrauterine growth curve or a growth curve developed for use in preterm neonates. Alternatively, a standard growth curve can be used and the postnatal age adjusted for length of gestation. Information determined from growth charts can be used to assess current nutritional status, to help identify nutritional deficits, and to differentiate between acute and chronic malnutrition.[10] In general, weight below the population standard indicates acute malnutrition, while both weight and height below the population standard suggests a more chronic problem.[11] Periodic plotting of weight and height allows evaluation of interindividual response to nutrition.[12]

Anthropometric Measurements

As with weight, age-related nomograms have been developed for arm circumference and triceps skinfold.[13] Using this nomogram, Frisancho calculated age-related percentiles for arm muscle area, arm muscle diameter, and arm muscle circumference.[14] Subscapular skinfold standards also have been developed.[15] To minimize variability between measurements, the same trained individual and same caliper type should be used to assess a given patient. As with weight, these assessments are valuable in evaluating interindividual progress.

Visceral Proteins

Serum albumin, transferrin, transthyretin (also known as prealbumin), and retinol-binding protein are the primary visceral protein markers used in nutritional assessment.[16–20] While the half-lives of visceral proteins in children are similar to adult values, age-related normal serum concentrations usually are lower in children. In healthy preterm infants and unhealthy term infants, transthyretin concentrations of 10.8 ± 3.9 and 9.7 ± 3.7 mg/dL, respectively, are reported,[20] whereas concentrations in adults are 23 to 41 mg/dL.[18] Transthyretin and retinol-binding protein concentrations increase following the provision of appropriate nutrients in otherwise healthy, appropriate-for-gestational-age infants[21] and premature infants.[22] Likewise, concentrations of these proteins increase in critically ill, malnourished infants receiving nutrition support.[23] Visceral protein markers are subject to concentration changes unrelated to nutrition status, including renal failure, iron status, liver function, and acute illness.[24]

Urine Studies

A nitrogen balance calculation measures the difference between total nitrogen output and intake (enteral and parenteral protein) during a 24-hour period. Although this is a relatively easy, noninvasive, reliable assessment of adequacy of intake in adults, problems exist with conducting these studies in neonates and infants.[25] One of the most common approaches used to collect urine in an uncatheterized pediatric patient requires a urine collection bag to be placed around the genital area with an adhesive and remain affixed securely for the collection period. Complications such as collection bags that do not fit adequately, adhesives that do not stick properly, skin breakdown under the adhesive, or stool contamination of the collected urine occur frequently. As an alternative means of estimating nitrogen losses for nitrogen-balance calculation, it has been proposed that urine be collected every 6 hours.[26] A newer method of urine and stool collection simply requires that all wet or soiled diapers be placed in a cooler after removal from the infant and collected over a 24-hour period. Soaking the diapers in a citrate buffer allows recovery of 90 to 95% of the nitrogen.[27] In addition, the total urine nitrogen (TUN) concentration relationship with urinary urea nitrogen is less predictable in neonates and critically ill children.[28] Despite these difficulties, skilled nursing care and accurate recording of intake and output enable the clinician to make a reasonable estimate of urinary nitrogen excretion.

Table 97.1 ▪ Daily Maintenance Fluid Requirement for Term Infants and Children

Weight	Fluid
Up to 10 kg	100 mL/kg[a]
>10–20 kg	1000 mL + 50 mL/kg for every kg >10 kg
>20 kg	1500 mL + 20 mL/kg for every kg >20 kg

[a]Preterm infants may require 120–150 mL/kg.

Adapted from Holliday MA, Segar WE. The maintenance need for water in parenteral fluid therapy. Pediatrics 19:823–832, 1957.

TUN is measured using pyrochemiluminescence, a method that is not available in many hospital clinical laboratories. Other measures of protein catabolism that have been used in pediatric patients include urinary 3-methylhistidine concentration to creatinine ratio.[29,30]

Immune Function

Assessments of immune function may not be helpful in assessing the nutritional status of infants and young children. The lack of an immunologic response to a specific challenge may not indicate malnutrition but may be secondary to immaturity or a lack of antigenic experience.[31,32] On the other hand, improved lymphocyte function and enhanced expression of T-cell populations has been reported in malnourished infants receiving short-term parenteral nutrition.[11,33] As with visceral proteins, underlying disease can affect response to immunologic stimulation.

FLUID REQUIREMENTS

Fluid needs are based on water losses from skin and respiration, urine and stool output, water accumulation in newly formed tissues, and water produced from carbohydrate oxidation.[34,35] Evaporative skin losses are related directly to body surface area and the quality of the skin as a barrier. Because the body surface area per unit weight is greater in children than in adults, evaporative losses are increased, which results in greater fluid requirements per unit weight in children. Fluid requirements are 90 to 100 mL per 100 kilocalories in children,[36,37] decreasing to 45 mL per 100 calories in adults. Maintenance fluid requirements for everyone except preterm neonates can be calculated from the equations described by Holliday and Segar (Table 97.1).[37]

Fluid requirements may be altered by immaturity, activity, environment, or pathology.[34,38,39] Soon after birth, the extracellular fluid volume contracts, and a diuresis resulting in weight loss occurs.[34,40] The percentage of extracellular fluid increases with increasing prematurity; the percentage of total body weight loss after birth is increased in premature neonates.[38] Organ immaturity (primarily kidney and skin) in the preterm neonate results in increased sensible and insensible water losses. In preterm neonates, the skin and subcutaneous tissue are thinner and more permeable, and the body surface area to body weight ratio is increased, resulting in increased evaporative losses.[41] In addition, infants may be under radiant warmers or require ultraviolet light therapy for treatment of neonatal jaundice, thereby further increasing evaporative water losses.[42] Renal immaturity may result in an inability to excrete a concentrated urine, which will increase the fluid volume that preterm neonates require.[43] Renal function matures with increasing postconceptional age; thus, the ability of neonates to regulate water and electrolyte metabolism improves with increasing age.[44] Certain diseases common in preterm neonates have been associated with excessive fluid intake, including bronchopulmonary dysplasia,[45] necrotizing enterocolitis,[46] intraventricular hemorrhage,[47] and patent ductus arteriosus.[48]

Like adults, children with congenital cardiac or renal anomalies, increased intracranial pressure, syndrome of inappropriate antidiuretic hormone (SIADH) secretion, or pulmonary edema may require varying degrees of fluid restriction. Conversely, patients with excessive fluid losses (e.g., gastric drainage, diarrhea or increased stool or ostomy output, vomiting, chest tube drainage, burn or wound exudate, fistula drainage, or patients under radiant warmers, ultraviolet lights, or with fever) may require additional fluids to compensate for these losses. These outputs should be replaced with fluids that are similar in volume and electrolyte composition (Table 97.2). In addition to electrolyte replacement, the albumin concentration can be measured in fluids that are expected to contain significant amounts of albumin, such as chest tube drainage or wound exudate. The addition of albumin to a replacement fluid may be the appropriate method to compensate for the estimated deficit.

PARENTERAL NUTRITION

Administration

Peripheral infusion of parenteral nutrition solutions is an alternative for patients who require short-term therapy, which is no more than 7 to 10 days in our experience. In small infants and children, peripheral access sites are limited. Unlike in adults, veins in the dorsum of the foot or hand or scalp veins often are used to establish venous

Table 97.2 ▪ Range of Electrolyte Composition (mEq/L) of Gastrointestinal Secretions

Secretion	Na^+	K^+	Cl^-	HCO_3^-
Saliva	35–60	10–20	15–35	50
Gastric	10–115	5–35	10–150	0
Pancreatic	115–155	5–10	55–110	70–90
Bile	130–165	5–15	80–120	35–50
Midjejunum	70–125	5–30	70–135	10–20
Ileostomy	90–140	5–30	60–135	15–50
Diarrhea	25–50	35–60	0–40	35–45

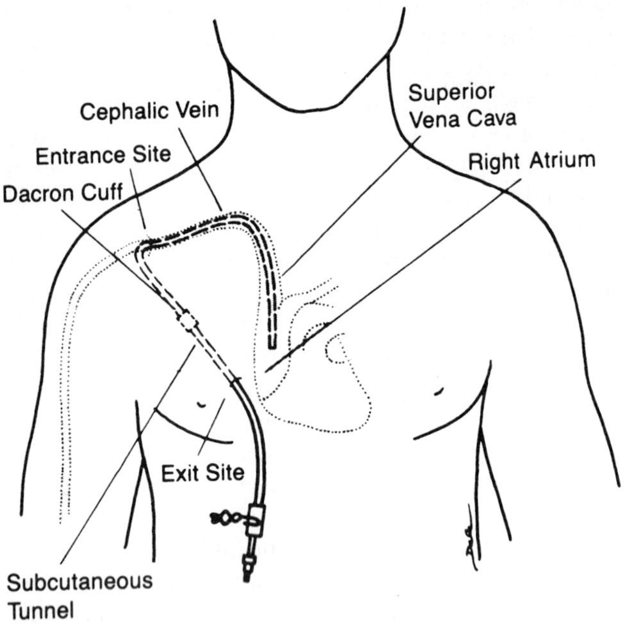

Figure 97.1. Placement of central venous catheter. The subclavian route as shown here is more commonly used in older children.

access. With peripheral access, the parenteral nutrition solution composition is limited because as osmolality increases, the risk for complications such as phlebitis and infiltration increases.[49] (This is discussed in more detail in the Parenteral Nutrition Complications section.)

In practice, the final osmolality for peripherally infused solutions (approximately 850 mOsm/L) is similar to that used in adults; however, the dextrose concentration is usually higher (10–12.5%) and amino acid concentration lower (2–3%). Compared with plasma (295 mOsm/L), these solutions are very hypertonic and may result in tissue irritation leading to injury if infiltration occurs. Concentrations of calcium and potassium, two known tissue irritants, should be limited in peripherally infused solutions. Although each patient's needs should be considered individually, limits of 10 mEq calcium per liter and 40 mEq potassium per liter may be prudent for most patients.

Peripheral parenteral nutrition can be used successfully in pediatric patients who are relatively well nourished and require parenteral nutrition for no more than 7 to 10 days. Between 50 to 75 kcal/kg/day and 2 to 3 g/kg/day of protein can be provided peripherally to infants, if fluids are not restricted and fat is well tolerated.

Percutaneous intravenous central (PIC) catheters have been used in very small neonates and in infants who require parenteral nutrition but who have poor peripheral venous access. Using sterile technique at the bedside, these catheters can be inserted into a peripheral vein and advanced into the central circulation. PIC catheters have remained in place for an average of 24 days, which is significantly longer than the usual 2 to 3 days that a peripheral Teflon or steel catheter remains in place. For PIC catheters that are centrally placed, solutions that contain more concentrated nutrients and, therefore, are more hypertonic can be infused. The risks associated with surgical central venous catheter placement are avoided as well.[50]

Children that require parenteral nutrition for an extended length of time should have a catheter placed surgically. The most frequently used central venous catheters for long-term access are the Broviac and Hickman catheters. The most common and convenient site for placement is the superior vena cava, with the catheter tip lying at the superior vena cava–right atrial junction (Fig. 97.1). Femoral insertion sites also are used, and the catheter is advanced to the inferior vena cava. The Dacron cuff is positioned subcutaneously near the exit site and stimulates the formation of a fibrous adhesion that anchors the catheter and prevents migration of pathogenic organisms from the skin surface to the catheter tip. The location of the exit site should be made with cosmetic considerations because scars may remain after catheter removal. If placement is not performed using fluoroscopy, a chest radiograph should be obtained immediately after insertion to verify appropriate catheter placement.

Totally implantable vascular-access devices can be used in larger pediatric patients who require long-term central venous access; they are best suited for intermittent therapies most likely in the home. Compared with external catheters, implanted catheters require less maintenance, are

Table 97.3 ▪ Typical Peripheral and Central Line Solutions Used in Infants and Children (per L)

	Dextrose 10% Solutions for Peripheral Use		Dextrose 25% Solutions for Central Use	
Solution name	CPF 3%	IPF 2.4%	CCF 3%	ICF 2.4%
Amino acid (g)	30[a]	24[b]	30[a]	24[b]
Dextrose (g)	100	100	250	250
Electrolytes				
Sodium	51 mEq	38.5 mEq	51 mEq	38.5 mEq
Potassium	20 mEq	20 mEq	20 mEq	20 mEq
Chloride	51 mEq	38.5 mEq	51 mEq	38.5 mEq
Acetate	12 mEq	8.2 mEq	12 mEq	8.2 mEq
Phosphate	5.5 mmol	8 mmol	5.5 mmol	8 mmol
Calcium	6 mEq	10 mEq	8 mEq	25 mEq
Magnesium	3 mEq	4 mEq	3 mEq	4 mEq
PTE[c]	NR	2 mL	2 mL	2 mL
Zinc	1 mg	1 mg	1 mg	1 mg
Multivitamin[d]				

CPF, child (>12 kg) peripheral formula; IPF, infant (<12 kg) peripheral formula; CCF, child central formula; ICF, infant central formula; NR, none required for short-term administration.

[a]Standard crystalline amino acid formulation.

[b]Pediatric crystalline amino acid formulation (L-cysteine HCl at 40 mg/g protein admixed at dispensing).

[c]Pediatric trace element solution, per mL: 1 mg Zn, 100 µg Cu, 25 µg Mn, 1 µg Cr, 15 µg Se.

[d]Pediatric multivitamin (Dosing recommendations can be found in Vitamins section.)

less noticeable, impose fewer restrictions on patient activity, and have a lower infection rate.[51,52] In most cases, a Huber needle that is bent at a 90° angle is required for insertion through the skin into the port, thus a needle stick occurs each time the catheter is used. According to product literature, the central silicone port can be punctured 1000 to 2000 times, depending on the brand. Extra care of the skin over the site is essential if infectious complications related to needle insertion are to be avoided.

Composition of Parenteral Nutrition Solutions

Typically, parenteral nutrition solutions for infants contain 2.5% amino acids, 10 to 25% dextrose, and electrolytes, vitamins, and minerals in amounts sufficient to meet the patient's estimated daily requirements (Table 97.3). The proportion of calories from each of the major nutrients should approach the percentages in the average enteral diet: 50 to 60% carbohydrate, 30 to 40% fat (higher percentage of fat is necessary in neonatal and infant diets), and 10 to 15% protein. Providing a balanced formula reduces the risk of toxicities or complications associated with excessive or inadequate administration of any single nutrient. Older children and adolescents may require a more concentrated amino acid solution (up to 5%) and lower dextrose concentrations depending on the fluid volume available for infusion. Intravenous fat emulsions (10 and 20%) offer a concentrated source of calories and provide essential fatty acids. In some institutions, the fat emulsion is added directly to the parenteral nutrition solution; this is referred to as a total nutrient admixture (TNA) or three-in-one mixture.[53] The use of TNAs in patients receiving pediatric amino acid products is subject to several compositional limitations including pH changes that alter calcium and phosphorus solubility and lipid particle instability resulting from a high–divalent-cation (primarily calcium) concentration. In addition, the ability to visualize particulates is lost, and a 0.2-micron filter cannot be used with TNAs because lipid particles range in size from 0.3 to 0.5 micron.

Protein Requirements

Initially, the nitrogen source in parenteral nutrition solutions was protein hydrolysates that were associated with hyperammonemia, compositional variability, occasional allergic reactions, and poor nitrogen usage in infants.[54] Because of these factors, common practice was to institute parenteral protein at a low dosage, typically 0.5 g/kg/day, in preterm neonates and to gradually increase dosage, based on tolerance, to the desired level. The introduction of crystalline amino acid products eliminated some of the original problems; however, the incorporation of hydrochloride salt forms of several amino acids resulted in acidosis in young infants. Inadequate arginine in at least one formulation resulted in hyperammonemia. Today, many amino acid mixtures are formulated using the freebase form of crystalline amino acids when possible, and the few that are unstable as a freebase, such as lysine, usually are added as the acetate salt, thereby decreasing the risk for metabolic acidosis. The amino acid source varies according to manufacturer; therefore, the electrolyte content of amino acid solutions is variable (Table 97.4). With these crystalline amino acid products, early introduction of protein at 1 to 2 g/kg in the preterm infant is well tolerated and is associated with increased growth, improved nitrogen balance, and improved catch-up growth,[55,56] and graduating amino acid dosages in parenteral nutrition is rarely indicated.

Table 97.4 ▪ Electrolyte Content and pH of Commercially Available Amino Acid Products (mEq/L)

	g/100 mL	OAc	Cl	Na	Phos[a]	pH
TrophAmine	6	56	<3	5		5–6
	10	97	<3	5		5–6
Aminosyn-PF	7	32.5		3.4		5–6.5
	10	46		3.4		5–6.5
Aminosyn	7	105		5.4		4.5–6
	10	148		5.4		4.5–6
Aminosyn II	7	50.3		31.3		5–6.5
	10	71.8		45.3		5–6.5
Novamine	15	151				5.2–6
FreAmine III	8.5	72	<3	10	10	6–7
	10	89	<3	10	10	6–7
Travasol	8.5	73	34			6–8
	10	87	40			6–8
Cysteine HCl	5		5.7			1.5–2

[a]Units are mmol/L.

Table 97.5 ▪ Parenteral Protein Requirements (g/kg/day)

Preterm	2.5–3.0
Infant/neonate	2.0–2.5
Infant	1.5–2.0
Preschool/school-age	1.0–1.5
Adolescent	0.8–1.5

Because of increased tissue anabolism, parenteral protein requirements in children are greater on a per kilogram basis than those in adults. Guidelines for protein dosages are presented in Table 97.5. Because of immaturity, the preterm infant and neonate also require qualitatively different amino acids for optimal growth and development.[57–59] Enzyme immaturity in the transsulfuration pathway prevents conversion of methionine to cysteine and cysteine to taurine, thereby rendering those two amino acids essential (Fig. 97.2). Similarly, phenylalanine hydroxylase insufficiency may limit the conversion of phenylalanine to tyrosine. Thus cysteine, taurine, tyrosine, and histidine are conditionally essential amino acids for preterm infants and neonates.

The reference or target ranges for individual plasma amino acid concentrations were determined 2 to 3 hours after a human milk feeding.[60] The distribution of amino acids present in a particular product is important because this directly affects plasma amino acid concentrations that are in active equilibrium with metabolically active cells,[54] thus, it was not surprising that plasma amino acid patterns in neonates and infants infused with standard amino acid products designed for use in adults differed from the target range.[57] Two pediatric-specific formulations (Aminosyn-PF; Abbott Laboratories, Chicago, IL and TrophAmine; McGaw, Inc., Irvine, CA) were developed to address these metabolic differences (Table 97.6). Both products require the addition of L-cysteine hydrochloride before infusion. These products contain less methionine and glycine, include the dicarboxylic amino acids (aspartate and glutamate) and taurine, and differ from each other in the amounts of methionine, tyrosine (lower in Aminosyn-PF), and taurine (lower in TrophAmine) that are added. Because of solubility difficulty, tyrosine is added in the form of *N*-acetyl L-tyrosine (NAT) to TrophAmine. NAT is not as efficiently converted to tyrosine in preterm neonates as it is in older infants and children; the clinical implications of this are not known.

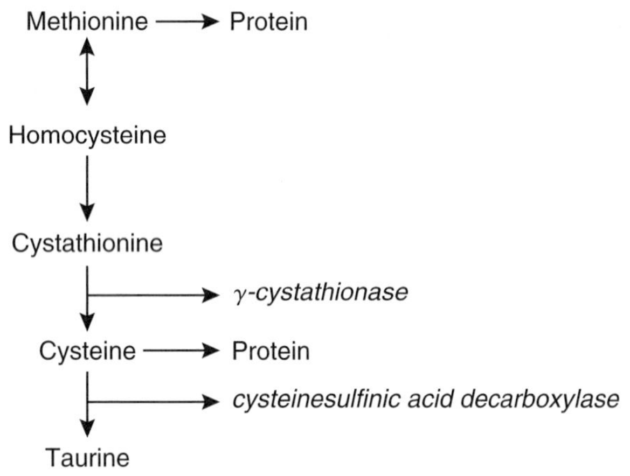

Figure 97.2. Metabolic pathway for the conversion of methionine to cysteine and taurine.

The proposed benefits of using pediatric amino acid solutions with added L-cysteine include enhanced growth, improved nitrogen retention, better calcium and phosphorus solubility, and, importantly, reduced risk for metabolic bone disease and cholestasis. Pediatric-specific amino acid formulations used in preterm post-surgical infants resulted in nitrogen balance and weight gain similar to that occurring during intrauterine growth.[57,58] Term neonates and older infants who received TrophAmine with L-cysteine supplementation also had age-appropriate weight gain and nitrogen retention.[59] Infants given peripheral parenteral nutrition with lower dosages of protein (as pediatric-specific amino acids), and more notably, calorie intakes that were below previously described requirements,

Table 97.6 ▪ Comparison of Parenteral Amino Acid Products

	Composition (mole %)			
Amino Acid	**Aminosyn-PF**	**TrophAmine**	**Aminosyn**	**FreAmine III**
L-Isoleucine	7.4	8.2	6.4	6.3
L-Leucine	11.6	14.1	8.4	8.4
L-Lysine	5.9	7.3	5.7	6.0
L-Methionine	1.5	2.9	3.1	4.3
L-Phenylalanine	3.3	3.9	3.1	4.1
L-Tryptophan	1.1	1.3	0.9	0.9
L-Threonine	5.5	4.6	5.1	4.0
L-Valine	7.1	8.8	8.0	6.8
L-Arginine	9.1	9.2	6.6	6.6
L-Histidine	2.6	4.1	2.3	2.2
L-Alanine	10.1	7.9	16.8	9.6
L-Proline	9.1	7.8	8.7	11.7
Glycine	6.6	6.4	19.9	22.5
L-Serine	6.1	4.8	4.7	6.8
L-Tyrosine	0.4	0.5	0.3	0
N-Acetyl-L-tyrosine[a]	0	1.2	0	0
L-Glutamic acid	7.2	4.5	0	0
L-Aspartic acid	5.1	3.1	0	0
L-Cysteine[b]	0	0.4	0	0
Taurine	0.7	0.3	0	0
Total	100.4	101.3	100.0	100.2

[a]As tyrosine equivalents.
[b]Admixed to Aminosyn-PF, TrophAmine.

had weight gain and positive nitrogen balance.[61] This is likely the result of optimal plasma availability of amino acids for anabolism. As reported by Beck et al.,[62] the lower incidence of cholestasis in very low–birth-weight neonates who received a pediatric amino acid formulation may be due in part to enhanced amino acid utilization. In addition, the lower solution pH allows more optimal dosing of calcium and phosphorus and anecdotally appears to decrease the incidence of metabolic bone disease.

Pediatric amino acid products are formulated to be supplemented with L-cysteine hydrochloride; however, this is not always done in practice because of the cost. The clinical implications of omitting L-cysteine are not known and only limited work has been published. The effect of cysteine supplementation was evaluated in postsurgical adults who received a pediatric amino acid product.[63] Those who received cysteine tended to have more positive nitrogen balances than those who received the pediatric amino acid product alone.[63] Interestingly, in a study in older children who received a pediatric amino acid with different L-cysteine dosages, plasma taurine–not cysteine–concentrations were directly related to the dose of L-cysteine given.[64]

Protein requirements of the older child and adolescent can be met parenterally using a standard crystalline amino acid formulation. Some incremental increases in protein intake, over those found in Table 97.5, may be required for the severely catabolic patient.

Caloric Requirements

Unlike adults who require nonprotein calories for basal metabolic demands, activity, and maintenance of body temperature, children require additional calories for growth and development. The most elegant work describing global and compartmental energy needs in preterm infants used indirect calorimetry.[65] Enterally fed low–birth-weight infants had global energy requirements of 150 kcal/kg/day. Approximately 18 kcal/kg/day were lost in stool; thus, 132 kcal/kg/day were required for metabolization to energy. Of these 132 kcal/kg/day, basal metabolism required 63 kcal/kg/day, activity required 4 kcal/kg/day, and the remaining 65 kcal/kg/day were required for growth.

Parenteral caloric requirements for optimal growth of the preterm infant and neonate range from 85 to 135 kcal/kg/day[5,65,66] and are similar to fluid requirements. However, short-term provision of lower calorie (60 to 70 kcal/kg) and pediatric amino acid intakes of 2.2 g/kg/day have been associated with a positive nitrogen balance and modest weight gain.[61] Caloric requirements (per kilogram body weight) decrease during the first year of life and continue to decrease until adult needs are approached (Table 97.7). As with protein, recommendations for caloric intake are merely guidelines for the practitioner. Assessment of clinical outcome, including weight gain, height or length, nitrogen balance, visceral and somatic protein measurements, and achievement of developmental milestones, should be used to determine the adequacy of delivered substrate.

Table 97.7 ▪ Parenteral Calorie Requirements (kcal/kg/day)

Preterm infant/neonate	85–130
Infant	90–120
1–6 yr	75–90
7–12 yr	50–75
13–18 yr	30–50

Carbohydrate

Dextrose is used almost exclusively as the carbohydrate calorie source. Neonates, particularly premature neonates, are less glucose-tolerant and are at risk for developing hyperglycemic-induced hyperosmolar coma and intraventricular hemorrhage.[67] Thus initial parenteral nutrition solutions should be limited to 5 g/kg/day of dextrose and should be advanced slowly by about 3 g/kg/day with close monitoring of serum glucose. Usually, older infants and children can be started on 10 g/kg/day (7 mg/kg/min) of dextrose, with dosages increasing by 5 g/kg every 12 to 24 hours, to a maximum of 30 to 35 g/kg/day, if the patient has a central venous catheter and is glucose-tolerant. Usually, dosages of 25 g/kg/day (17 mg/kg/min) when used with concomitant fat emulsion infusion are sufficient to achieve adequate weight gain in infants. With increasing age, maximum exogenous glucose oxidation rates decrease from approximately 12.5 mg/kg/min in infants to about 5 mg/kg/min in adults. Dextrose concentrations should be advanced slowly in all individuals under severe stress or those who are receiving corticosteroids, because hyperglycemia may develop even when dextrose intake is low.

Although higher dosages may not result in hyperglycemia, the maximum glucose oxidation rate may be exceeded and fat may accumulate, which can be desirable in an infant, particularly if he or she is undernourished. However, producing fat from carbohydrate is not energy efficient, results in increased CO_2 production, and may cause fatty infiltrations in the liver, all of which are undesirable. Glucose oxidation rates in children generally are higher than in adults; however, a study in burned children ages 1 to 11 years old who received parenteral nutrition during perioperative periods found that the maximum glucose oxidation rate was 5 mg/kg/min, similar to adults.[68] Even when glucose oxidation rates were exceeded, these patients were euglycemic, suggesting that the excess glucose entered nonoxidative pathways.[68]

Insulin may be used to facilitate glucose metabolism for patients who are carbohydrate intolerant. Very low–birth-weight infants are started on 0.05 units/kg/hr while older infants and children usually are started on dosages of 0.1 units/kg/hr of insulin with the dosage titrated to serum glucose concentration.[69] A concomitant insulin infusion will accomplish this better than adding insulin to the parenteral nutrition solution. The insulin dosage should be titrated to frequent (every 2 hours) assessments of blood glucose.

Fat

As in adults, infusion of fat emulsion prevents or reverses essential fatty acid deficiency (EFAD), provides a concentrated and isotonic source of calories, provides a more physiologic "diet," and prolongs survival time of peripheral intravenous lines in patients receiving parenteral nutrition. Fat emulsion products are compared in Table 97.8. Unlike adults, biochemical evidence of EFAD (a triene [5,8,11-eicosatrienoic acid with 3 double bonds] to tetraene [arachidonic acid with 4 double bonds] ratio above 0.4)[70,71] may be evident after a few days of no fat intake in preterm neonates (Fig. 97.3). Although linolenic acid does not reverse EFAD like linoleic acid does, evidence suggests that linolenic acid also may be essential.[72,73]

Table 97.8 ▪ Composition of 20% Fat Emulsions[a]

Ingredient or Characteristic	Liposyn III Abbott Laboratories	Intralipid Clintec Nutrition
Source		
Soybean oil (%)	20	20
Safflower oil (%)	–	–
Fatty acid distribution		
Linoleic acid (%)	54.5	50
Oleic acid (%)	22.4	26
Palmitic acid (%)	10.5	10
Linolenic acid (%)	8.3	9
Stearic acid (%)	4.2	3.5
Egg yolk phospholipids (%)	1.2	1.2
Glycerin (%)	2.5	2.25
Calories (per mL)	2	2

[a]In 10% fat emulsions, the oil sources are the same for each product but the amounts are halved, resulting in a higher phospholipid to triglyceride ratio and a 1.1 kcal/mL concentration.

The transport of free fatty acids across the mitochondria for beta oxidation and energy production is dependent on carnitine acyltransferase. Neonates and infants may have a relative insufficiency of the hydroxylase enzyme required in the final step of the in vivo synthesis of carnitine. Consistent with this finding, plasma carnitine concentrations are low in preterm neonates[74] and older infants receiving carnitine-free nutrition for more than a month since birth,[75] resulting in a limited capacity for fat oxidation. Supplementation of 10 to 20 mg/kg/day of carnitine for 7 days in older infants resulted in increased fat usage and plasma carnitine concentrations.[75] Decreased carnitine concentrations have been associated with gastroesophageal reflux disease and apnea in low-birth-weight infants, which has resolved with carnitine supplementation.[76]

Fat emulsion should be initiated at 0.5 g/kg/day in premature neonates. Term infants and infants older than one month can usually be started at 1 g/kg/day. If serum triglyceride or free fatty acid concentrations are within acceptable limits, the fat emulsion dosage can be increased by 0.25 to 0.5 g/kg/day up to 3 g/kg/day in preterm neonates and by 0.5 to 1 g/kg/day up to a maximum of 4 g/kg/day in term and older infants, as recommended by the American Academy of Pediatrics (AAP).[72] Ideally, fat emulsion is given continuously over 24 hours to promote clearance from the circulation.

Neonates, particularly those who are premature, frequently develop physiologic jaundice or unconjugated (indirect) hyperbilirubinemia because of their inability to conjugate bilirubin. Because the blood–brain barrier is immature in neonates, indirect bilirubin can cross into the brain and cause a yellow staining known as kernicterus that is associated with neurologic sequelae. Fatty acids and unconjugated bilirubin bind competitively to albumin; thus, unconjugated bilirubin can be displaced from

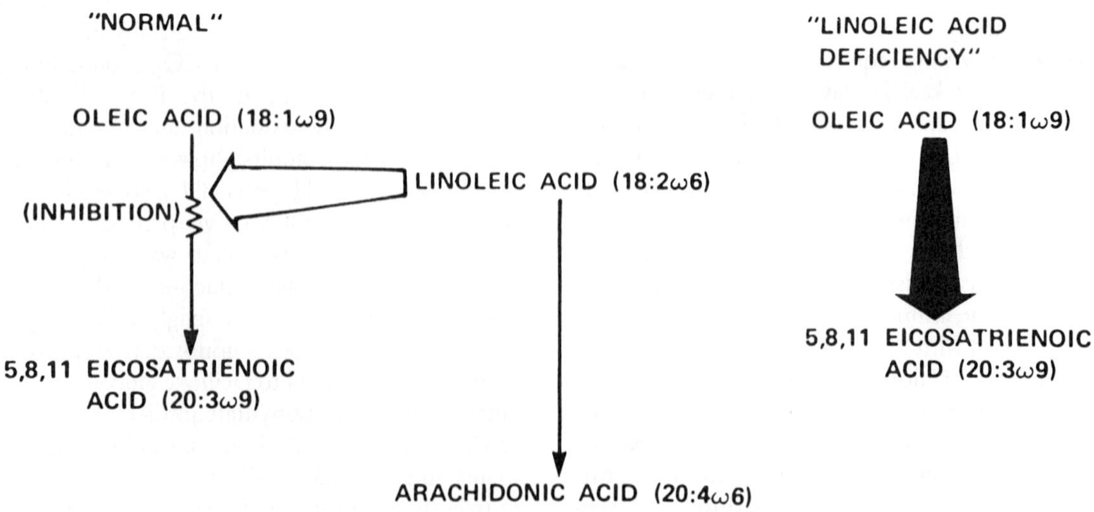

Figure 97.3. Essential fatty acid deficiency. Under "normal" conditions the large open arrow indicates linoleic acid's inhibition of the oleic acid conversion to 5,8,11-eicosatrienoic acid. During linoleic acid deficiency the solid arrow depicts enzymatic elongation and desaturation of oleic acid to form abnormal 5,8,11-eicosatrienoic acid, resulting in a greater triene to tetraene ratio. (Reprinted with permission from Pelham LD. Rational use of intravenous fat emulsions. Am J Hosp Pharm 38:198–208, 1981. American Society of Health-System Pharmacists, Inc. All rights reserved.)

high-affinity albumin-binding sites by free fatty acids. Andrew et al.[77] found that the molar ratio of serum-free fatty acids to albumin must exceed six for bilirubin to be displaced from high-affinity binding sites on albumin. Conversely, an in vitro study found that both Intralipid and Liposyn enhanced the reserve capacity for indirect bilirubin binding to albumin.[78] Therefore hyperbilirubinemia alone should not be an absolute contraindication to the use of intravenous fat emulsion, and provision of 2 to 4% of the total daily caloric requirement as fat emulsion to prevent EFAD should not present a problem.

The effects of fat emulsion on immune function are controversial and inconsistent. Both in vitro incubation of white blood cells with fat emulsion and in vivo infusion of fat emulsion inhibit leukocyte chemotaxis, phagocytosis, bactericidal capacity, and lymphoproliferation.[79–81] On the other hand, others report that fat either has no effect or that it restores and augments immune function.[31,82–84] These conflicting findings are probably secondary to the complexities (e.g., duration of exposure, lipid concentration and composition, responding cell type) of fatty acid and fatty acid metabolite interactions with immunoreactive cells. In practice, parenteral lipids are used conservatively in patients who are immunocompromised or who have sepsis, and serum triglycerides are monitored to assess tolerance.

The use of fat emulsion in neonates with pulmonary compromise also is controversial. Because fat emboli were found in pulmonary capillaries during postmortem examinations of neonates who received Intralipid, the infusion of fat emulsion in neonates with respiratory compromise was postulated to alter pulmonary function. These findings were subsequently attributed to artifact, which occurred secondary to a delay in the fixation of the lung after death.[85] Neonates less than one week of age with respiratory distress syndrome who received 1 g/kg of Intralipid over 4 hours had lower Po_2 values than age-related neonates who received no Intralipid.[86] However, the changes in Po_2 did not correlate with elevations in serum triglyceride concentration.[86] Oxygen diffusion in the lungs of premature neonates was not affected by infusion of Intralipid up to 4 g/kg/day over 24 hours.[87] Following the AAP recommendations to infuse the daily fat dosage over 24 hours whenever possible will help avoid excessive fat concentrations in the circulation and minimize potential changes in pulmonary microcirculation that may result in a lowering of Po_2.

The 10 and 20% concentrations of fat emulsion contain the same amount of phospholipid, resulting in a higher phospholipid to triglyceride ratio in the 10% (0.12) products compared with the 20% (0.06) products. Infants who were randomized to 7 days of continuous infusion 10% had higher plasma concentrations of phospholipid and cholesterol than those who received 20% fat emulsion.[88] In addition, the LDL cholesterol had greater total cholesterol and phospholipid concentrations in those who received 10% fat. Two-thirds of the phospholipid in 10% fat is in the form of liposomes, which may store cholesterol and apoproteins and potentially alter cholesterol regulation and triglyceride metabolism. Thus the 20% product should be used whenever possible.

Table 97.9 ▪ Daily Electrolyte Dosages (mEq/kg/day)

	Preterm Infants	Children and Term Infants
Sodium	2–8	2–5
Potassium[a]	1.4–10	2–3
Chloride	1.1–5	2–3
Magnesium	0.25–0.6	0.25–0.5
Calcium	2.5–3.5	1–2
Phosphate[b]	1.3–2	0.5–1

[a]Reflects patients receiving diuretics.
[b]Units are mmol/kg/day.

Electrolyte and Mineral Requirements

The reader is referred to Chapter 9 for a discussion of electrolytes and minerals. As with adults, factors such as hydration, cardiovascular status, renal function, and concurrent medications should be considered when determining electrolyte requirements in children.[89] In addition, age and organ maturity, in particular the kidney, should be considered in premature infants.

The daily maintenance electrolyte requirements for neonates, infants, and children are listed in Table 97.9.[25,34,37–39,89,90] As with adults, children with excessive gastrointestinal tract fluid losses should receive replacement with a solution composed of comparable electrolytes (Table 97.2). Replacement fluids are delivered most efficiently using a separate intravenous infusion.

Amino acid solutions also contain various amounts of anions (usually acetate) and cations, which should be considered when determining anion distribution (Table 97.4). L-Cysteine HCl provides additional chloride (5.7 mEq Cl/g L-cysteine) to parenteral nutrition solutions.

Sodium

Premature infants have functionally immature kidneys that may promote excessive urinary sodium losses.[91] Sodium requirements in these infants may be as high as 8 mEq/kg/day. When determining sodium needs, other sources of sodium such as flushes, continuous infusion of normal saline through arterial lines, or antibiotics as sodium salts should be considered.

Frequent causes of abnormal serum sodium concentrations in the pediatric population are vomiting and diarrhea. Patients receiving diuretics or those with certain renal disorders (e.g., renal tubular acidosis) have increased urinary sodium losses and often require additional sodium. Parenteral nutrition solutions high in sodium may be desirable in patients with closed head injury to increase serum osmolality and ultimately decrease intracranial pressure. Specific types of malignancies, pulmonary diseases, central nervous system disorders, and drugs (e.g., vincristine, carbamazepine, cyclophosphamide, barbiturates) may result in hyponatremia secondary to SIADH.

Potassium

Usual potassium dosages range from 2 to 4 mEq/kg/day; however, depending on organ maturity, presence of disease, and medications, much larger dosages may be needed in extreme cases. Preterm infants may have increased potassium requirements secondary to increased urinary losses resulting from immature renal function. Several factors affect potassium homeostasis including acid-base status, insulin, glucocorticoids, aldosterone, catecholamines, and renal potassium excretion. Vomiting, diarrhea, and draining fistulas are the primary causes of extrarenal potassium loss. In addition, metabolic alkalosis secondary to hydrogen ion losses, perhaps via the gastrointestinal tract, also may result in hypokalemia because potassium shifts intracellularly as hydrogen ions are shifted out of the cell. Diuretics, amphotericin, and cisplatin are frequent causes of drug-associated hypokalemia. Other drugs such as the aminoglycosides and penicillins[92] promote renal potassium excretion. Hypokalemia refractory to potassium supplementation may indicate a concurrent hypomagnesemia, which must be addressed before serum potassium concentrations can be maintained. Because potassium is the principal intracellular cation, the extent of potassium depletion by extracellular serum concentrations is difficult to estimate; therefore, frequent serum concentration monitoring is necessary.

Peripheral infusion of potassium is irritating to vessels, may be painful to the patient, and should be limited to about 40 mEq/L for peripherally infused solutions. Patients with central venous access can receive more concentrated solutions, but the maximum rate of potassium delivery should not exceed 0.5 to 1 mEq/kg/hr considering all sources. Patients receiving more than 0.5 mEq/kg/hr should be monitored by electrocardiogram because cardiac dysrhythmias may develop when potassium is infused rapidly.[93] Potassium is most efficiently replaced using continuous infusions because the transient increase in potassium serum concentration with a 1 mEq/kg dose infused over 2 hours may stimulate aldosterone and promote potassium renal elimination.

Infant serum samples often are hemolyzed because they are obtained by heel puncture, which may require considerable squeezing to obtain an adequate blood volume. Hemolysis releases intracellular potassium, causing an apparent elevation in serum potassium concentration. When hyperkalemia is noted in an asymptomatic patient, the phlebotomy method should be determined and the serum evaluated for visual evidence of hemolysis. Validation of the serum concentration by venipuncture may be desirable before aggressive treatment is undertaken.

Calcium

Calcium, the most abundant mineral in the body, is important to maintain the functional integrity of cellular membranes, neuromuscular activity, regulation of various endocrine and exocrine secretory activities, blood coagulation, and bone metabolism. In newborns, 98% of total body calcium is present in bone. Approximately 40% of total serum calcium is bound to serum proteins, and 80 to 90% of this calcium is bound to albumin. Variations in the serum protein concentration and serum pH proportionately alter protein-bound and total serum calcium concentrations.

Calcium homeostasis is regulated by parathyroid hormone (PTH), calcitonin, and vitamin D.[94] PTH and calcitonin respond reciprocally to acute changes in calcium and magnesium serum concentrations. Acute increases in these cations decrease PTH and increase calcitonin production. Likewise, an acute decrease in calcium concentration causes an increase in PTH concentration and a decrease in calcitonin, resulting in the mobilization of calcium from bone. Therefore, serum calcium concentration is neither a sensitive nor a specific measure of the adequacy of intake.

Calcium and phosphorus requirements are inversely related to postconceptional age. In utero calcium accretion rates at 36 weeks gestation are 5 to 7.5 mEq/kg/day of elemental calcium. Because of limitations in calcium and phosphorus solubility, it is impossible to provide an equivalent calcium dose and an appropriate phosphate dose either enterally or parenterally. Interestingly, adequate bone mineralization occurs with significantly less calcium than is accreted in utero as long as the appropriate amount of phosphate is also provided. A physiologic ratio of calcium and phosphate (1.7 mg:1 mg) promotes retention of these minerals in premature infants and minimizes parenteral-nutrition–related bone disease.[95,96] In addition to the inherently greater calcium requirements for normal bone mineralization, premature infants often have concurrent diseases that require aggressive diuretic therapy, which increases calcium urinary excretion,[97] or requires fluid restriction, which limits the amount of substrate that can be solubilized. Thus these infants are at increased risk for metabolic bone disease. Calcium and phosphorus solubility is enhanced with lower calcium and phosphorus concentrations, a lower pH, and colder temperature. The pediatric amino acid products have a lower pH and the addition of L-cysteine decreases the pH, thereby increasing calcium and phosphate solubility.[98–100] Therefore the number of calcium and phosphate dosages provided in pediatric amino acid-based formulations can be increased to more adequately address needs.

Calcium may react with phosphate to form monobasic or dibasic calcium phosphate, depending on pH. At low solution pH, the predominant form of calcium phosphate is monobasic, which is quite soluble. As the pH increases, more dibasic phosphate becomes available to bind with calcium, and precipitation occurs more easily.[98] Solutions compounded from amino acid products with a relatively high pH, such as FreAmine III (McGaw), have relatively low calcium phosphate solubility. In certain circumstances, L-cysteine HCl has been added to standard amino acid

Table 97.10 ▪ Chemical Characteristics of Phosphorus

Salt	Formula	Molecular Weight	Solubility with Calcium
Monobasic	$Ca(H_2PO_4)_2$	234.06	Moderate
Dibasic	$CaHPO_4$	136.06	Insoluble
Tribasic	$Ca_3(PO_4)_2$	310.20	Insoluble

products to decrease solution pH and enhance calcium phosphate solubility. Increased temperatures increase calcium ionization and thereby increase the likelihood of calcium phosphate precipitation. It is common for temperatures in the nursery or near the infant to be increased. For example, infants in isolettes or those receiving ultraviolet-light therapy have warmer environments that may cause solutions that are near the limit of calcium and phosphate solubility to precipitate near the infant, perhaps in the intravenous line. In some cases, precipitation has occurred within the catheter as the infusing solution was warmed by the patient's body temperature.

Because the calcium gluconate is less ionized in solution than the chloride salt, less precipitation occurs with the gluconate than with the chloride salt; thus, calcium supplementation in parenteral nutrition solutions is generally done with calcium gluconate.[101] Approximately 100 mg of calcium gluconate is equivalent to 0.46 mEq or 9.2 mg of elemental calcium, and 100 mg of calcium chloride is equivalent to 1.36 mEq or 27.2 mg of elemental calcium.

When compounding the solution, phosphate is added early in the process because it is concentrated (3 mmol/mL) and consumes a small volume compared to calcium and, therefore, is more likely to remain in the injection port. The addition of other additives helps clear the injection port of phosphate. Calcium is more dilute (0.456 mEq/mL) than phosphate salts and is added last.[102]

Phosphorus

Phosphate functions as a cofactor in multiple enzyme systems necessary for the metabolism of protein, carbohydrate, and fat, and is required for production of the high-energy adenosine triphosphate (ATP) bonds. Refeeding of a severely malnourished patient without adequate provision of phosphate has been associated with severe hypophosphatemia caused by total body phosphate depletion and increased intracellular shifting of phosphate during refeeding[103] and may result in death. Hypophosphatemia may also occur secondary to hyperparathyroidism (i.e., increased urinary phosphate excretion) or respiratory alkalosis (i.e., intracellular phosphate shifting). As with calcium, phosphorus is particularly important in bone growth, an important concern in pediatric patients. Phosphorus content, as the phosphate ion, in parenteral nutrition solutions is limited by solubility factors (for a more detailed discussion, see the previous section entitled Calcium).

Phosphate dosages provided to neonates and infants range from 1 to 2 mmol/kg. This amount can be provided to most patients who are not fluid restricted. Dosage requirements decrease to approximately 1 mmol/kg in older children and to 0.5 to 0.75 mmol/kg in adolescents and young adults. Because phosphate exists in three valence states that fluctuate with changing pH, phosphate requirements usually are described in millimoles (mmol) or milligrams (mg), not milliequivalents (mEq). The use of milliequivalents does not reflect the concentration of phosphorus in solution and may lead to dosing errors. For example, 1 mmol phosphate is equal to 31 mg elemental phosphorus and 3 mmol of phosphate is contained in either 4 mEq of sodium phosphate or 4.4 mEq of potassium phosphate. The different chemical states of phosphorus are listed in Table 97.10 and the dissociation constants of hydrogen phosphate are shown in Table 97.11.

Magnesium

Magnesium, the second most common intracellular cation, is necessary for numerous enzymatic reactions involving energy storage and use. Extracellular magnesium is used during neuromuscular transmission and is required for cardiovascular tone. Approximately 2% of the body's total magnesium is present in the extracellular compartment, whereas 98% is found intracellularly, primarily in bone.

Magnesium balance and serum magnesium concentration are largely determined by renal magnesium excretion, which is regulated primarily by the glomerular filtration rate, tubular reabsorption, and PTH. When necessary, the kidney can conserve or increase urinary magnesium excretion, depending on body stores.[94]

As with hypocalcemia, hypomagnesemia often is present in infants with DiGeorge's syndrome and those born to diabetic mothers. Neonatal hepatitis and congenital biliary atresia are commonly associated with hypomagnesemia.[104] Because magnesium is absorbed in the proximal jejunum, patients that undergo intestinal resection are at risk for developing hypomagnesemia. Similarly, patients with extensive diarrheal or ileostomy fluid losses may have increased magnesium losses. Diuretics, amphotericin, cyclosporine, and cisplatin increase urinary magnesium losses and may contribute to hypomagnesemia. Magnesium depletion may precipitate refractory hypokalemia or hypocalcemia.[105] Because magnesium is an intracellular cation that equilibrates rather slowly, increases in magnesium content in parenteral nutrition solutions may not

Table 97.11 ▪ Dissociation of Hydrogen Phosphate

pKa_1	pH 2.12	$H_3PO_4 \leftrightharpoons H^+ + H_2PO_4^-$
pKa_2	pH 7.21	$H_2PO_4^- \leftrightharpoons H^+ + HPO_4^{=}$
pKa_3	pH 12.67	$HPO_4^{--} \leftrightharpoons H^+ + PO_4^{\equiv}$

Table 97.12 ▪ Vitamin Content of Various Parenteral Vitamin Products

Vitamin	MVI-Pediatric[a]	MVI-12[b]	MULTI-12[c]	Cernevit[d]	MVC[e]
Usual dose	5 mL	10 mL	5 mL	5 mL	1 mL
Manufacturer	Astra	Astra	Sabex, Inc.	Baxter	Fujisawa
A (Retinol equivalents)	2300 IU	3300 IU	3300 IU	3500 IU	2000 IU
D (Ergocalciferol)	400 IU	200 IU	200 IU	220 IU	200 IU
E (d, l g Tocopherol acetate)	7 IU	10 IU	10 IU	11.2 IU	1 IU
K (Phytonadione)	200 μg	0	0	0	0
C (Ascorbic acid)	80 mg	100 mg	100 mg	125 mg	100 mg
B_1 (Thiamine)	1.2 mg	3 mg	3 mg	3.51 mg	10 mg
B_2 (Riboflavin)	1.4 mg	3.6 mg	3.6 mg	4.14 mg	2 mg
B_6 (Pyridoxine)	1 mg	4 mg	4 mg	4.53 mg	3 mg
Niacinamide	17 mg	40 mg	40 mg	48 mg	20 mg
Dexpanthenol	5 mg	15 mg	15 mg	17.25 mg	5 mg
Biotin	20 μg	60 μg	60 μg	69 μg	0
Folic acid	140 μg	400 μg	400 μg	414 μg	0
B_{12} (Cyanocobalamin)	1 μg	5 μg	5 μg	6 μg	0

[a]Contains 375 mg mannitol, sodium hydroxide, 50 mg polysorbate 80, 0.8 mg polysorbate 20, 58 mg butylated hydroxytoluene, and 14 mg butylated hydroxyanisole.

[b]Contains propylene glycol (30%), sodium citrate, citric acid, sodium hydroxide, polysorbate 20 (4.8%), butylated hydroxyanisole (0.0004%), butylated hydroxytoluene (0.0018%), and ethanolamine (2%).

[c]Vial 1 contains vegetable oil (0.0045%), polysorbate 80 (1.4%), and sodium hydroxide or hydrochloric acid to adjust pH. Vial 2 contains propylene glycol (30%) and citric acid or sodium citrate to adjust pH.

[d]Contains 250 mg glycine, 140 mg glycocholic acid, and 112.5 mg soybean phosphatides in one vial of lyophilized powder.

[e]Contains 56 mg polysorbate 80 and 75 mg mannitol packaged in 2 vials. Vial 1 is 4 mL, vial 2 is 1 mL.

restore intracellular magnesium concentrations for days. Infusion of bolus doses of magnesium results in increased amounts of magnesium urinary concentrations, and as with potassium, infusion of estimated deficits should be performed with continuously.

Vitamins

A parenteral multivitamin product based on Recommended Dietary Allowances (RDAs) for oral vitamins was formulated according to recommendations of the Nutrition Advisory Group (NAG) of the American Medical Association (AMA) in the 1980s. Twice during the 1990s parenteral vitamin manufacturing was suspended, and at least two significant parenteral vitamin shortages resulted. To prevent the potential morbidity and mortality from vitamin deficiencies, the Food and Drug Administration (FDA) allowed the distribution of vitamin products used in other countries in the United States. In the recommended dosages, the amounts of vitamins in most of these products are similar to the products manufactured in the United States; however, Cernevit is a completely different type of formulation that consists of soybean phosphatide micelles. Importantly, MVC does not contain biotin, folic acid, or B_{12}. The contents of these products are compared in Table 97.12.

Parenteral multivitamin preparations are sensitive to pH, light, and temperature. In addition, vitamins may interact with one another or adsorb to the plastic matrix of administration sets, decreasing bioavailability.[90] MVI pediatric contains retinol, which adsorbs to plastic tubing, significantly reducing the amount delivered. MVI pediatric also contains vitamin K, which is not in adult parenteral vitamins, and it contains twice the amount of vitamin D as the adult products.

Infants and children weighing 3 kg or more, up to 11 years of age, should receive the full single-dose vial (5 mL) daily. Medically stable infants and children receiving parenteral nutrition with this dosage maintain acceptable vitamin serum concentrations.[90] The FDA recommends that infants weighing 1 to 3 kg receive daily 65% (3.25 mL) of a single full dose and infants weighing less than 1 kg receive daily 30% (1.5 mL) of a single full dose. In the AMA/NAG consensus meeting in 1987, it was reported that using these dosages in preterm infants results in increased plasma concentrations of most water-soluble vitamins and low concentrations of vitamin A. These clinicians recommended that preterm infants be dosed at 2 mL/kg/day, with the maximum of 5 mL/day to address the problem with the water-soluble vitamins.[90] This decrease in dosage would also decrease the amount of vitamin A that is delivered, thereby compounding the problem with retinol adsorption to the tubing. Of further concern in premature neonates is the possible decreased metabolism of the polysorbate emulsifiers due to immature hepatic metabolic pathways. Because of these altered vitamin requirements and potential toxicity of the emulsifier, it was proposed that a separate intravenous multivitamin product be developed specifically for preterm infants.[90]

Children more than 11 years old should receive the adult multivitamin product at the recommended adult dosage. These preparations do not contain vitamin K, and, in general, they provide half the vitamin D dosage that is in the pediatric product. The remaining vitamins are present in greater amounts to address the RDA for adults. (For further discussion on this topic, see Chapter 12.)

Trace Elements

The trace elements constitute less than 0.01% of human body weight. Despite their low body content, trace elements have essential roles in biochemical processes including growth and development. Pediatric trace-element requirements have not been well defined, hence RDAs and reports of deficiency currently guide the intravenous dosage recommendations. Current recommendations for trace element dosing are shown in Table 97.13.

Because trace elements are stored during the last trimester of pregnancy, premature neonates have insufficient body stores that put them at increased risk of developing deficiencies. Patients with persistent diarrhea or excessive ostomy outputs have increased zinc losses in these body fluids and thus may require additional supplementation. Copper and manganese are excreted through the biliary system, and patients with severe liver disease, including cholestasis, should not receive these trace elements.[90] Conversely, patients with exterior biliary drainage or jejunostomies may have increased copper losses, resulting in increased requirements. Selenium deficiency may result in cardiomyopathy and skeletal muscle myopathy.[90] Selenium, chromium, and molybdenum are excreted primarily by the kidneys; thus doses should be adjusted in patients with renal insufficiency. Each trace element is available as a single-entity product for patients requiring an individualized approach to supplementation.

To complicate trace element supplementation, parenteral products are contaminated with a variety of elements, most notably aluminum and chromium, and concerns about potential toxicity have been expressed.[106] Children on long-term parenteral nutrition who received recommended dosages of chromium have plasma chromium concentrations from 5 to 10 times higher than normal.[107,108] This is likely due to significant amounts of chromium present as a contaminant in amino acid and electrolyte products that are not taken into consideration.[107,108] As research in this area progresses, trace element dosing in pediatric patients will change.

Parenteral Nutrition Complications

Technical

With parenteral nutrition, the most basic forms of nutrients are delivered directly into the bloodstream, bypassing normal digestive and absorptive processes. Frequently, intravenous access can be achieved by cannulating a peripheral vein or the inferior or superior vena cava with a surgically placed catheter (Fig. 97.1). Because of the nature of the solutions and catheters and the direct link to the bloodstream, a variety of technical and infectious complications are associated with parenteral nutrition.

The osmolality of parenteral nutrition solutions designed to infuse via peripheral veins usually ranges from 800 to 950, thus phlebitis can occur. Infiltration or extravasation of the catheter is an expected and usually benign event that results in infusion of fluid into the interstitial tissue. However, infants and small children who have limited extravascular tissue space and who may not be able to communicate pain adequately are at risk for developing complications, including localized swelling and edema, which may progress to necrosis.[109] The infiltrated site can be treated with hyaluronidase injections to increase the rate of solution absorption and decrease potential tissue damage. The addition of 1 to 2 units of heparin per mL of dextrose amino acid solution[110] and the concomitant infusion of fat emulsion with the dextrose and amino acid solution[111] increases the length of time to infiltration in infants receiving peripherally infused parenteral nutrition.

Patients who require parenteral nutrition for relatively long periods of time generally have central venous catheters placed for this purpose. In small infants and children with limited or difficult peripheral vascular access, a central venous catheter may be required, even if parenteral nutrition is required for a relatively short time.[112] Complications that occur at the time of catheter placement include pneumothorax, vein or cardiac perforation, chylothorax,[113] and bleeding. Following catheter placement, the catheter hub or line may be punctured, crack, or break. Damages to the hub or proximal (exposed) portion of the catheter can be repaired in many cases, but catheter removal may be necessary.

The infusate may extravasate or infiltrate into the thoracic or pericardial cavity. These fluids will be resorbed, in time, after the infusion is discontinued, but significant tissue injury may result. Furthermore, the abrupt discontinuation of a concentrated dextrose solution infusing into

Table 97.13 ▪ Trace Element Daily Requirements

Trace Element	Preterm[86] Neonates	Term[86] Neonates	<5 Years Old	Older[86] Children	Adults[87]
Zinc	400 μg/kg	300 μg/kg	100 μg/kg	5 mg	2.5–4 mg
Copper	20 μg/kg	20 μg/kg	0 μg/kg	200 μg	300–500 μg
Manganese	1 μg/kg	1 μg/kg	2–10 μg/kg	50 μg	150–800 μg
Chromium	0.2 μg/kg	0.2 μg/kg	0.14–0.2 μg/kg	5 μg	10–20 μg
Selenium	2–3 μg/kg	2–3 μg/kg	2–3 μg/kg	40 μg	40–80 μg
Iodide	1 μg/kg	1 μg/kg	1 μg/kg		

the central circulation may result in hypoglycemia. Extravasated or infiltrated solutions may accumulate in the pleural or pericardial region, resulting in respiratory or cardiac decompensation, and require chest tube placement.

Catheters may migrate out of position or be accidentally removed.[114] This problem is more common with percutaneously placed catheters than with the Broviac or Hickman silastic catheters that are tunneled and anchored by a Dacron cuff (Fig. 97.1).[115]

Catheters located in the right atrium may stimulate dysrhythmias by coming in contact with nodal tissue. These dysrhythmias may be resolved by pulling the catheter away from sensitive tissue.

Catheters may become occluded due to fibrin deposition,[116] precipitates,[117] or saponified material that accumulates within the lumen. In many instances, the catheter that is not completely occluded can be recannulated pharmacologically.[118–120] Fibrinolytic agents such as urokinase, streptokinase, or tissue plasminogen activator are useful in dissolving fibrin that partially occludes a catheter. Precipitates, such as calcium phosphate, may be dissolved by decreasing the pH inside the catheter with the instillation of 0.1 N HCl into the catheter.[118] Other agents such as ethanol may be used to dissolve saponified material.[119] Depending on the catheter volume, the appropriate agent is drawn into a 10 mL syringe and instilled in the lumen of the partially occluded catheter. After a defined period of time, usually 2 to 4 hours, the agent is withdrawn along with an additional 5 mL of blood, and the catheter is flushed. This ensures that any loosened debris from the catheter lumen is removed and not infused into the patient.

Metabolic

Metabolic complications include electrolyte and mineral abnormalities, aberrant plasma amino acid patterns (see section entitled Protein Requirements), metabolic bone disease, micronutrient deficiencies, cholestasis, hypersensitivity reactions, acid-base abnormalities, and alterations in pulmonary and immunologic function.[121]

Most electrolyte and mineral abnormalities and acid-base complications can be avoided with adequate monitoring and appropriate forethought when formulating solutions. Cholestasis and metabolic bone disease are two problems that are especially worrisome in pediatric patients; these will be discussed in more detail in the following sections.

Cholestasis

The etiology of cholestasis is multifactorial and complex, and it occurs most commonly in premature infants who are enterally fasted and receive long-term parenteral nutrition.[122] These infants are also at risk for infection, including hepatitis, and frequently receive medications, such as furosemide, that are associated with cholestasis; thus it remains a diagnosis of exclusion. In parenteral nutrition-associated cholestasis, proposed mechanisms include amino acid competition with bile salts for hepatocyte uptake, enhanced production of secondary bile salts,[123] and the provision of excessive calories and protein.[124] Increases in γ-glutamyltransferase (GGT) and direct bilirubin[125] are early indicators of cholestasis, but are not seen until after at least 10 days of parenteral nutrition. Initiation of small-volume enteral (trophic) feeding for gut stimulation is probably the most important intervention that should be initiated as soon as the patient is able to tolerate even minimal enteral feeding. Offering the patient a protein- and calorie-free period by cycling the parenteral nutrition solution off for a period of time during the day also may be beneficial. Phenobarbital, a choleretic agent, is not effective treatment for parenteral nutrition-associated cholestasis.[126] Cholecystokinin has been proposed as a useful agent to promote bile flow and potentially treat cholestasis, but there is insufficient experience to recommend its use for this purpose.[127] Finally, the use of a pediatric-specific amino acid formulation should be considered. These solutions normalize plasma amino acid patterns and should result in optimal substrate metabolism and minimize potential toxicity associated with amino acids. Cholestasis generally resolves when the parenteral nutrition is discontinued.

Bone Disease

As with cholestasis, the etiology of metabolic bone disease is multifactorial and may be related to inadequate calcium and phosphorus intake, end-organ resistance to vitamin D, increased calcium losses in the urine due to medications (in particular loop diuretics), and aluminum intake as a contaminant. Adequate calcium and phosphorus dosing significantly decreases the occurrence of metabolic bone disease in infants. Because the pediatric amino acid products inherently have a lower pH, more appropriate amounts of calcium and phosphorus can be given and, anecdotally, the occurrence of metabolic bone disease can be decreased. Aluminum is a significant contaminant in many parenteral fluids; therefore, those who receive large volume parenteral fluids may be at risk for aluminum accumulation not only in soft tissues such as the brain but also in bone, thereby resulting in osteomalacia.[128,129] Amino acid manufacturers set limits for aluminum content in the individual amino acids included in their products; therefore, contaminant aluminum in these products is minimal. Patients suspected of having osteopenia and rachitic changes should be evaluated by roentgenograms or radiographic densitometry.[130]

Other

Hypersensitivity reactions have been reported in patients receiving parenteral nutrition.[131–137] Anaphylaxis has been attributed to the amino acid solutions,[131] vitamin preparations,[132,133] magnesium sulfate,[131] fat emulsion,[134] iron, and soybean oil.[135] In addition, bradycardia[136] and diarrhea[137] have been associated with fat emulsion infusions.

A variety of hematologic abnormalities have been reported in patients receiving parenteral nutrition. Thrombocytopenia has been related to fat emulsion infusions and appears to be dose-related.[138] In contrast, an increased peripheral platelet count has also been described in preterm neonates on parenteral nutrition.[139] Parenteral nutrition-associated eosinophilia[139] occurs with greater frequency in premature neonates and appears to be self-limiting. Hemolysis due to lipid peroxidation of red blood cell membranes may be associated with failure to provide sufficient antioxidant (vitamin E) or antioxidant cofactors such as selenium.[140] Intravascular hemolysis has been reported with rapid infusion of fat emulsion in adults.[141,142]

Impairment of immune function has been described with deficiency or insufficiency of a variety of micronutrients including zinc;[143] selenium; pyridoxine and pantothenic acid;[144,145] vitamins E,[146,147] A, and D;[146] arginine;[148] and glutamine.[149]

Infection

Infection is a serious complication associated with central venous catheters and may be a blood-borne, exit-site, or tunnel-tract infection. Mechanisms include introduction of organisms into the bloodstream through the catheter, hematogenous spread, and potentially, bacterial translocation, a process in which normal bacteria present in the bowel crosses the intestinal lumen and enters the bloodstream. Because of problems with venous access in small children, central venous catheters are used for multiple purposes, increasing the risk for infection. Young children often play with their catheters or infusion sets and may chew on lines or disconnect their infusion, which further increases the risk for contamination. Infants who require parenteral nutrition often have bowel disease that results in frequent, loose stools that are difficult to contain; it is not uncommon for fecal material to come in contact with tubing, also increasing the risk for accidental contamination of catheters or solutions. Furthermore, premature neonates have a greater risk for infection because of immune system immaturity. In some cases, infections are polymicrobial. The incidence of central venous line infections is inversely related to age and in pediatric patients ranges from 42 to 57%.[150] Organisms that commonly result in infection in pediatric patients on long-term parenteral nutrition are listed in Table 97.14.[151]

Table 97.14 ▪ Microorganisms Cultured from Central Venous Catheters in Children on Home Parenteral Nutrition[151]

Staphylococcus epidermidis	25%
Klebsiella	12%
Staphylococcus aureus	10%
E. coli	6%
C. parapsilosis	5%
Gram-positive organisms	43%
Gram-negative organisms	36%
Fungi	13%
Polymicrobial	11%

Solution contamination is often suspected to be the source of the infection. Dextrose amino acid solutions are very hypertonic and poorly support bacterial growth; however, yeast will grow in these solutions. On the other hand, lipid products facilitate bacterial growth; thus, repackaging of lipid products is discouraged. Malassezia furfur is a fungal infection that is predominantly found in children, and it is almost exclusively associated with lipid infusion. Routine fungal cultures will not detect this organism.

Ideally, infected catheters are removed. However, in children who require long-term central access removal of infected catheters and placement of a new catheter in a different site after the infection is cleared may not be feasible. Once a vein has been cannulated, collateral veins develop around the site so that blood flow to an area is not compromised. Collateral vessels are tortuous and narrow and can rarely be cannulated. In addition, cannulated veins may become thrombosed or scarred, rendering them unsuitable for subsequent catheterization. Therefore the decision to remove a central line in a child who depends on this route for hydration and nutrition must be made judiciously. Placement of a catheter directly into the right atrium has been performed in children without an alternative catheterization site. In patients with catheter-related infection who continued to require central venous access, 55 to 89% of catheter-related infections were successfully treated in situ by administering appropriate antibiotics.[152,153] The appropriate dosage of the antimicrobial agent(s) should be infused through the infected catheter. In addition, antibiotics or antifungals can be instilled and allowed to reside in the catheter for varying lengths of time. Daily blood cultures are obtained through the catheter lumen(s) and from a peripheral site to ensure that the microorganism is being eradicated.[152,153] Multiple lumen catheters require careful evaluation because only one of the lumens may be infected. It is important that the infected lumen be effectively treated.

The body recognizes indwelling central venous catheters as foreign; fibrin can accumulate outside and inside the lumen of the catheter, particularly if the line is used for blood withdrawal.[116] Microorganisms may be harbored within the fibrin, providing a nidus for infection. Even appropriate microbial therapy may not penetrate through the fibrin web and eradicate microorganisms residing inside. Although urokinase, streptokinase, tissue plasminogen activator, and possibly HCl can dissolve the fibrin within the catheter lumen, it is less likely that fibrin around the outside of the catheter will be affected. Monthly treatment of central lines with a fibrinolytic has been suggested to decrease the number of central-line infections. However, dissolution of a fibrin sheath that is harboring a large number of microorganisms has the potential to release the microorganisms into the bloodstream. The resultant bacteremia may result in an acute septic event or seed distant sites.

The catheter exit site or tunnel tract may also become infected. Local antibiotic therapy may be used to treat certain exit-site infections; however, both exit-site and

Table 97.15 ▪ Recommended Dietary Allowances for Energy and Protein Intake

	Kilocalories/kg	g Protein/kg
Infants		
Birth–6 mo	108	2.2
>6–12 mo	98	1.6
>1–3 yr	102	1.2
4–6 yr	90	1.1
7–10 yr	70	1
Males		
11–14 yr	55	1
Females		
11–14 yr	47	1

Adapted from National Research Council. Recommended Dietary Allowances. 10th ed. Washington, DC: National Academy of Sciences, 1989.

tunnel-tract infections may require systemic antimicrobial therapy. In addition, more frequent central line dressing changes may be required.

ENTERAL NUTRITION

The AAP recommends that infants be breast fed whenever possible. (Chapter 96 discusses this in more detail.) However, many mothers elect to totally or partially bottle-feed for a variety of reasons. Special feeding nipples for bottles are available to avoid nipple confusion for breast-fed infants who receive some bottles. Infants who cannot be orally fed due to illness or disease may refuse the breast or bottle as they recover. Speech therapists or occupational therapists can work with infants and caregivers to facilitate the transition back to oral breastfeedings.

Table 97.16 ▪ Recommended Dietary Allowances for Vitamins and Minerals

	0–6 mo	>6–12 mo	>1–3 yr	4–6 yr	7–10 yr	Males 11–14 yr	Females 11–14 yr
Vitamins							
Fat soluble							
A (μg)	375	375	400	500	700	1000	800
D (μg)	7.5	10	10	10	10	10	10
E (mg)	3	4	6	7	7	10	8
K (μg)	5	10	15	20	30	45	45
Water soluble							
C (mg)	30	35	40	45	45	50	50
Thiamine (mg)	0.3	0.4	0.7	0.9	1	1.3	1.1
Riboflavin (mg)	0.4	0.5	0.8	1.1	1.2	1.5	1.3
Niacin (mg)	5	6	9	12	13	17	15
B_6 (mg)	0.3	0.6	1	1.1	1.4	1.7	1.4
Folate (μg)	25	35	50	75	100	150	150
B_{12} (μg)	0.3	0.5	0.7	1	1.4	2	2
Minerals							
Calcium (mg)	400	600	800	800	800	1200	1200
Phosphorus (mg)	300	500	800	800	800	1200	1200
Magnesium (mg)	40	60	80	120	170	270	280
Iron (mg)	6	10	10	10	10	12	15
Zinc (mg)	5	5	10	10	10	15	12
Selenium (μg)	10	15	20	20	30	40	45

Adapted from National Research Council. Recommended Dietary Allowances. 10th ed. Washington, DC: National Academy of Sciences, 1989.

Table 97.17 ▪ Infant Formulas[a]

	kcal/oz	Carbohydrate Source	Protein Source
Standard infant			
Enfamil with iron	20	Lactose	Nonfat milk solids
Similac with iron	20	Lactose	Nonfat milk
Concentrated, premature			
Similac Special Care with iron	24	Lactose, hydrolyzed corn starch	Nonfat milk, whey protein concentrate
Enfamil PM 24 with iron	24	Corn syrup solids, lactose	Whey, nonfat milk solids
Preemie SMA	24	Maltodextrins	Nonfat milk, whey
Transitional, premature			
NeoCare	22	Corn syrup solids, lactose	Nonfat milk, whey

[a]Formula content changes are possible. The authors suggest referring to the most recent publication of product literature or consulting clinical dietetics for product information.

[b]Contents of CHO, PRO, fat, Na, K, Ca, P, and Fe are per 100 mL.

MCT, medium-chain triglycerides.

This process may require a time commitment on the part of the primary caregiver, but most infants learn or relearn this skill quickly. Mothers who want to breastfeed but whose infants cannot be enterally fed initially may pump milk from their breasts and freeze their milk for later use.

Infant Formulas

The RDA is defined as the level of intake of essential nutrients that is judged by the Food and Nutrition Board, on the basis of scientific knowledge, to be adequate to meet known nutrient needs of healthy persons.[154] The RDA estimates generally exceed the nutrient requirements of most healthy infants and children but they provide guidelines for development of enteral formulas. They do not provide guidelines for premature infants and may not provide adequate allowances for infants and children with disease or during drug therapy. The RDA requirements of energy and protein for healthy infants and children are listed in Table 97.15. Energy required for growth is greatest during the newborn period. As infants grow, the total caloric requirement increases, but because of the increasing body size, the amount of kilocalories required per kilogram decreases. From infancy to childhood, protein requirements decrease more rapidly than energy requirements. This reflects an increase in activity (requiring energy) and a decrease in growth rates (requiring protein).

The RDAs for vitamin and minerals in infants and children are listed in Table 97.16. Although infant formulas contain vitamins and minerals, it is important to determine whether their total daily intake delivers the recommended amounts. Most infant formulas contain adequate amounts of iron. Premature infants may require additional vitamin supplementation.[155]

Concentrated premature infant formulas are available to meet the needs of infants with immature gastrointestinal tracts (Table 97.17).[155] The kilocalorie content of these formulas is 24 per ounce compared with 20 per ounce in standard infant formulas. Protein, carbohydrate, and fat components of these products require less complex digestive processes. These formulas contain primarily whey protein, which forms smaller curds that are more easily digested than casein. In addition, whey protein has an amino acid composition high in cysteine and low in tyrosine, making it more desirable for the premature infant with immature enzymatic pathways (the Protein Requirements section provides a more detailed discussion). Lactose, a reducing sugar, is the carbohydrate found in human milk; however, low-lactase activity is found in the intestinal mucosa of premature infants. Thus the lactose content of preterm formulas has been limited to 40 to 50% of the available carbohydrate. The remaining carbohydrate is provided in the form of maltodextrins or "corn syrup," which is a mixture of monosaccharides, oligosaccharides, and polysaccharides that relies on multiple digestive and absorptive pathways and results in enhanced utilization.

Premature infants frequently have a decreased ability to digest long-chain triglycerides (LCT) because of reduced bile-acid pool size and decreased pancreatic lipase activity. Thus 13 to 50% of fat in these formulas is provided as medium-chain triglycerides (MCTs) that are more easily absorbed because they do not require bile acids for solubilization nor do they require carnitine for transport into the mitochondria where beta oxidation occurs. However, MCTs do not provide essential fatty acids, thus a portion of fat must be supplied as LCT.

The nutrient distribution in standard infant formulas available for infants less than one year old reflects their distribution in human milk. The composition of these products is similar (Table 97.18) and, when reconstituted according to the standard formula, they contain 20 kilocalories per ounce. Infant formulas should have an osmotic load similar to that of human milk (277 to 303 mOsm/kg), to avoid diarrhea induced by a high osmotic load.

The protein in the specialized infant formulas Nutramigen, Pregestimil, and Alimentum is in the form of free amino acids and peptides that result from partial acid hydrolysis of cow's milk (Table 97.18). The protein in these formulas is easily digestible; thus they may be appropriate for infants with intestinal resection, cow's milk allergy, or other protein allergies. The fat content of Pregestimil and Alimentum is similar, containing about 50% MCTs, while Nutramigen contains 100% of its fat as

Fat Source	CHO[b] g	PRO g	Fat g	Na mEq	K mEq	mg Ca/mg P	Fe mg	mOsm kg H_2O
Coconut and soybean oils	6.9	1.5	3.8	0.9	1.9	52/35	1.3	300
Soybean and coconut oils	7.1	1.4	3.6	0.8	1.8	49/37	1.3	290
Coconut, soybean, and coconut oils	8.5	2.2	4.3	1.5	2.6	144/72	1.2	300
40% MCT; coconut and soybean oils	8.9	2.4	4.1	1.3	2.1	132/67	1.2	310
Coconut, safflower, and soybean oils	8.4	1.9	4.3	1.3	1.9	72/40	0.3	280
25% MCT; soy, coconut	7.7	1.9	4.1	1.1	2.7	32/14	1.3	250

Table 97.18 ▪ Specialized Infant Formulas[a]

	kcal/oz	Carbohydrate Source	Protein Source
Hypoallergenic			
Nutramigen	20	Corn syrup solids, modified corn starch	Casein hydrolysate
Pregestimil	20	Corn syrup solids, modified corn starch	Casein hydrolysate
Alimentum	20	Sucrose and modified tapioca starch	Casein hydrolysate
Other			
Portagen	20	Corn syrup solids, sucrose, 0.75 mg/qt lactose	Sodium caseinate
Isomil	20	Corn syrup and sucrose	Soy protein isolate
Neocate	20	Corn syrup solids	L-amino acids
Nursoy	20	Sucrose	Soy protein isolate
Prosobee	20	Corn syrup solids, glucose polymers	Soy protein isolate
SMA with iron	20	Lactose	Nonfat milk
Similac PM 60/40	20	Lactose	Whey protein, sodium caseinate
Lactofree	20	Corn syrup solids	Milk protein

[a]Formula content changes are possible. The authors suggest referring to the most recent publication of product literature or consulting clinical dietetics for product information.

[b]Contents of CHO, PRO, fat, Na, K, Ca, P, and Fe are per 100 mL.

MCT, medium-chain triglycerides.

Table 97.19 ▪ Formulas for Children From 1–10 Years[a]

	kcal/oz	Carbohydrate Source	Protein Source
Pediasure	30	Cornstarch, sucrose	Sodium caseinate, whey
Kindercal	30	Maltodextrin, sucrose	Calcium caseinate, sodium caseinate, milk protein concentrate
Peptamen Jr.	30	Maltodextrin	Whey protein
Vivonex Pediatric	24	Maltodextrin, modified starch	Free amino acids

[a]Formula content changes are possible. The authors suggest referring to the most recent publication of product literature or consulting clinical dietetics for product information.

[b]Contents of CHO, PRO, fat, Na, K, Ca, P, and Fe are per 100 mL.

MCT, medium-chain triglycerides.

LCTs. Portagen, a formula with 86% of its fat as MCTs and no lactose, is available for infants with significant steatorrhea that may occur with cystic fibrosis, pancreatic insufficiency, or intestinal resection. MCTs are not transported through the lymphatic system; therefore, Portagen has been used in patients with chylothorax because chyle production is minimized with this formula.

Lactose- and sucrose-free formulas (i.e., Isomil, Isomil SF, Nursoy, Prosobee; Table 97.18) are also available for infants with disaccharidase deficiency or specific types of carbohydrate intolerance. Because all of these formulas contain hypoallergenic soy protein, they may be indicated if cow's milk allergy is suspected. Low renal-solute formulas (e.g., PM 60/40, SMA) contain less sodium than other specialized formulas and are indicated when low-sodium intake is desirable (Table 97.18). Although these formulas have a whey-to-casein protein concentration of approximately 60 to 40% (more like human milk), the carbohydrate content is exclusively lactose.

Formulas have been developed and marketed for children between 1 and 10 years of age (Table 97.19). The protein concentration in these products is equal to or greater than that found in infant formulas and the percentage of carbohydrate is usually greater and fat is usually less than that found in infant formulas. Calcium and phosphorus is approximately equimolar in children's formulas, whereas in infant formulas there is a greater amount of calcium than phosphorus. In children's formulas the renal solute load is greater than that found in infant formulas. Pediasure and Kindercal are standard children's formulas, and Vivonex Pediatric is designed for children who require a more elemental feeding solution.

Formulas are available as ready-to-feed unit-of-use or multiple-use containers, concentrated liquids, or dry powders. Before feeding, formula should be stored in a cool, dry place because temperature extremes can cause irreversible physical and chemical changes. The ready-to-feed solutions should not be diluted before feeding unless the physician prescribes a dilute formula. The concentrated liquid and dry powder formulas require dilution or reconstitution before feeding. Instructions for the amount of water to be added are provided on each container. Failure to dilute concentrated formulas can result in hyperosmolality and dehydration. Regular tap water that meets federal drinking water standards is acceptable for reconstituting infant formula. However, in certain situations the physician may suggest sterilization of tap water before reconstitution, such as in the case of well water. Because salts are

Fat Source	CHO[b] g	PRO g	Fat g	Na mEq	K mEq	mg Ca/mg P	Fe mg	mOsm kg H_2O
Corn and soybean oils	8.9	1.9	2.6	1.4	1.9	63/42	1.3	320
55% MCT; coconut, safflower, and corn oils	6.9	1.9	3.7	1.4	1.9	63/42	1.3	320
50% MCT; coconut, safflower, and soybean oils	6.8	1.8	3.7	1.3	2	70/50	1.2	370
83% MCT; coconut, corn, and soybean oils	7.7	2.3	3.2	1.6	2.1	63/47	1.3	236
Coconut and soybean oils	6.7	1.8	3.6	1.3	1.8	70/50	1.2	250
Safflower oil, coconut and soy	7.1	1.9	2.8	0.9	2.4	75/56		342
Coconut, oleo, safflower, and soybean oils	6.9	2.1	3.6	0.8	1.9	63/44	1.3	296
Coconut, soybean, and corn oils	6.7	2.0	3.5	1	2.1	63/49	1.3	200
Coconut and soybean oils	7.1	1.5	3.6	0.6	2	42/28	1.2	300
Coconut and soybean oils	6.8	1.6	3.7	0.7	1.5	37/19	0.15	260
Palm olein, soy, coconut, and sunflower oils	7.0	1.5	3.7	1.0	1.9	55/37	1.2	

Fat Source	CHO[b] g	PRO g	Fat g	Na mEq	K mEq	mg Ca/mg P	Fe mg	mOsm kg H_2O
20% MCT; coconut, safflower, and soybean	11	3	5	1.7	3.4	97/80	1.4	310
20% MCT; coconut, corn, canola, and sunflower oils	13.5	3.4	4.4	1.6	3.4	85/85	1.1	310
60% MCT; coconut, soybean, and canola oils	13.7	3	3.8	2	3.4	100/80	1.4	260
68% MCT; coconut and soybean oils	13	2.4	2.4	1.7	3.1	97/80	1	360

added to chemically softened water, it should not be used to reconstitute infant formula. Commercially prepared sterile water is not necessary for formula preparation at home. Most city water supplies are fluoridated; however, sterile water and well water are not fluoridate, and supplementation may be required in infants who have formulas prepared using water from these sources.

Formula preparation should take place in a clean area, using clean utensils. The individual preparing the formula should have clean hands and use good technique, to avoid contaminating the formula during reconstitution. Immediately after reconstituting concentrated formula or opening a ready-to-feed multiple-use container, the portion required for an individual feeding should be put in an appropriate bottle for feeding and the remainder should be stored in a clean container in the refrigerator. After the infant has begun feeding, any formula left in the bottle after 2 hours should be discarded. Reconstituted formula can be stored in the refrigerator for up to 24 hours.

Smaller infants should be fed formula that is not cooler than room temperature and some infants may prefer warmed formula. Older infants do not require warmed formula but may prefer it. The bottle with the required amount of formula for a single feeding can be warmed with warm, running tap water. If a bottle warmer is used, electric warmers are preferred over water-containing warmers because of the potential for bacterial contamination of the water contained in the warmer. Microwaves should never be used to warm infant formula because hot spots can develop throughout the formula and may burn the infant. In addition, the excessive heat can physically alter the formula and degrade nutrients.

Concentrated liquids and dry powder formulas can be reconstituted to provide increased amounts of all substrates included in the formula. Standard reconstitution provides 20 kcal/oz; however, some infants require more concentrated formula due to fluid considerations. These products can be mixed with less water so that they contain 24, 27, or 30 kcal/oz. When formulas are concentrated in this manner, the protein, electrolyte, and mineral concentrations are also increased and should be considered. In lieu of concentrating formulas, other additives such as carbohydrate (e.g., polycose) or fat (e.g., medium chain triglycerides) can be admixed to enhance calorie content. The manufacturers recommend that medications not be added to infant formula because of potential drug–nutrient interactions.

After the initial opening, formula powder can be covered and stored in a cool, dry place for up to 4 weeks in the original container. Refrigeration is not necessary. However, opened liquid formula (ready-to-feed or concentrate) should be stored in the original container in the refrigerator and may be used for up to 48 hours after opening. Reconstituted formula no longer in the original container should be discarded if not used within 24 hours.

Oral electrolyte solutions, such as Pedialyte, Resol, and Rice-Lyte, are available for maintenance of fluid and electrolyte balance during mild-to-moderate diarrhea (Table 97.20). Rehydralyte contains more sodium and is better suited for use in infants with moderate-to-severe diarrhea than products containing less sodium. The World Health Organization (WHO) developed a rehydration solution formula that contains 3.5 g sodium chloride, 2.5 g sodium bicarbonate, 1.5 g potassium chloride, and 20 g glucose with distilled water added to make one liter of solution. The sodium concentration in the WHO solution is about 90 mEq/L. Other liquids such as Gatorade contain less sodium and are less suitable for fluid replacement in diarrhea.

Administration

The significance of the gastrointestinal tract in immune function has been recognized, and early enteral feedings are encouraged whenever possible, even in critically ill patients. Feeding tubes are placed soon after injury in patients with burns or after trauma and, as with premature infants, low-volume continuous enteral feedings are started and advanced as tolerated. In many of these patients, parenteral nutrition can be avoided entirely. In those who cannot tolerate formula advancement, low-volume continuous trophic feeds should be continued if possible.

Maturation of the gastrointestinal tract is directly related to postconceptional age, and premature neonates may be unable to be fed enterally immediately after birth. In addition, the suck and swallow reflex develops at 34 to 36 weeks of gestation; therefore, even with functional maturity of the gastrointestinal tract, these neonates may not be able to be fed orally. In these cases, a combination of parenteral and enteral feeding is used during the transition to full enteral, hopefully oral, feedings. To begin the transition to enteral feedings, a low volume of premature formula (or human milk that is provided in most cases by the infant's mother) is infused continuously through an orogastric or nasogastric tube. Volumes are advanced very gradually if the infant tolerates the formula. Regularly during this process, gastric residuals are aspirated through the tube and the volumes are measured to be sure the formula is progressing through the gastrointestinal tract. Abdominal distension and vomiting are indicative of too rapid an advancement in feedings, or either outlet or intestinal obstruction. Stool consistency, volume, and frequency are monitored. During this rather slow process, parenteral nutrition is used as the primary source of substrate; however, the infant is encouraged to suck a pacifier. As feedings progress, the parenteral nutrition solution is decreased and the infant may be offered a small volume of formula (or human milk) by bottle. Infants should be weighed daily and adequate calorie intake, considering both parenteral and enteral calories, should be maintained. Preterm neonates who develop abdominal distension and have evidence of intraluminal gas (pneumatosis intestinalis) on abdominal radiograph should have enteral feedings discontinued until they are evaluated for necrotizing enterocolitis. Initial therapy for this disease includes maintaining the patient's "nothing-by-mouth" status and providing parenteral nutrition and antibiotic therapy. Surgery is required for perforation.

Table 97.20 ▪ Infant Electrolyte Solutions (per L)

	kcal mEq	Na^+ mEq	K^+ mEq	Cl^- mEq	Citrate	mOsm
Rehydralyte	100	75	20	65	30	305
Pedialyte	100	45	20	35	30	250
Resol[a] *80*	50	20	50	34		269
Rice-Lyte	126	50	25	45	34	
Infalyte 77	50	20	40	30		251
WHO solution	80	90	30	80	30	330

[a]Each liter contains Ca^{2+} 4 mEq; phosphate 5 mmol; and Mg^{2+} 4 mEq.

Feeding routes in sick neonates, infants, and children are similar to those for adults and include orogastric, nasogastric, and transpyloric jejunal feeding routes and gastrostomy. The type of illness and length of time the patient has continued without oral feedings should be considered when reinstituting enteral feedings. Continuous low-volume feedings are often used initially; however, patients who are being fed into the stomach can be given an appropriate formula and volume for age as a bolus. When choosing the formula to be delivered, the feeding route should be considered.

Potential problems associated with enteral feedings include aspiration, formula intolerance, and malposition of the tube. Aspiration is a greater risk in patients with gastroesophageal reflux or intractable vomiting. Reflux precautions, including elevating the head of the bed and using low-volume, more-frequent or continuous feedings, are helpful. Medications that promote gastrointestinal motility including prokinetic agents (e.g., metoclopramide, bethanechol, cisapride) and those that decrease gastric secretions (e.g., histamine 2 antagonists, proton pump inhibitors) may be beneficial. The primary manifestation of formula intolerance is diarrhea. Changing to an age-appropriate elemental formula or fiber-containing formula (e.g., Pediasure with fiber in those more than one year old), or short-term therapy with an antiperistaltic agent such as loperamide may be indicated. Patients who develop abdominal distention may have an ileus or a malpositioned feeding tube and enteral feedings may be contraindicated. In this case, intestinal perforation may occur with continued feeding.

Gastrostomy-tube (G-tube) placement is indicated in patients with upper gastrointestinal tract anomalies (e.g., cleft palate, esophageal atresia), esophageal injury, or tracheoesophageal fistula. G-tubes can be placed percutaneously in older infants and children. Button type G-tubes are available and are aesthetically more pleasing than the standard G-tubes. Infants and children requiring prolonged tube feeding, such as patients with long-term coma or severe cardiac, neurologic, or respiratory disease, should be considered for G-tube placement. This route of administration facilitates intermittent bolus feeding.

Transpyloric jejunal feeding tubes may be used in infants and children with gastrointestinal anomalies or delayed gastric motility or after upper gastrointestinal surgery. The use of jejunostomy feeding tubes is increasing in children with the improved pediatric jejunal feeding tubes and refinement of surgical placement techniques. With jejunal feedings, continuous feedings are preferred because the small bowel cannot accommodate large volumes of fluid. Complications with jejunal feeding include malabsorption and bowel perforation.[156] In addition, the formula used in patients fed via jejunostomy may need to consist of less complex substrate, depending on the location of the feeding tube.

CONCLUSION

In this chapter the reader has been apprised of the uniqueness of pediatric nutritional needs and the limitations of assessment techniques used in children. It is important to remember that children are not small adults and therefore, should not be treated as such. Children (particularly neonates and infants) require quantitatively and qualitatively different nutrients than adults. Failure to address these unique substrate requirements can result in abnormal physical and neurologic growth and development. However, with an understanding of the unique needs of children, the appropriate nutrients can be provided, normal growth can be achieved, and developmental milestones can be met.

KEY POINTS

- In general, fluid requirements (mL/kg) and calorie requirements (kcal/kg) are inversely related to patient age and weight.
- Parenteral amino acids have been designed to result in plasma amino acid patterns similar to neonates and infants fed human milk.
- Many metabolic complications associated with parenteral nutrition in neonates and infants can be avoided with an understanding of micronutrient needs and appropriate monitoring.
- Fat requirements are higher in pediatric patients to provide for normal growth and development.
- Normal growth and development can be achieved with parenteral nutrition.
- Whenever possible, the enteral route of feeding should be used; the ideal infant enteral feeding is human milk.
- Infant formulas have been designed using human milk as a template for nutrient composition.

REFERENCES

1. ASPEN Board of Directors. Standards for hospitalized pediatric patients. Nutr Clin Pract 11:217–228, 1996.
2. Costa G. Determination of nutritional needs. Cancer Res 37:2419–2424, 1977.
3. Merritt RJ, Blackburn GL. Nutritional assessment and metabolic response to illness of the hospitalized child. In: Suskind RM, ed. Textbook of pediatric nutrition. New York: Raven Press, 1981:285.
4. Grant JP, Custer PG, Thurlow J. Current techniques of nutritional assessment. Surg Clin North Am 61:437–463, 1981.
5. Kerner JA, Sunshine P. Parenteral alimentation. Semin Perinatol 3:417–434, 1979.
6. Ponder SW. Clinical uses of bone densitometry in children: are we ready yet? Clin Pediatr 34:237, 1995.
7. Fiorotto ML, de Bruin NC, Brans YW, et al. Total body electrical conductivity measurements: an evaluation of current instrumentation for infants. Pediatr Res 37:94–100, 1995.
8. Olhager E, Thomas K, Wigstrom L, et al. Description and evaluation of a method based on magnetic resonance imaging to estimate adipose tissue volume and total body fat in infants. Pediatr Res 44:572–577, 1998.
9. Hamill PVV, Drizd TA, Johnson CL, et al. Physical growth: National Center for Health statistics percentiles. Am J Clin Nutr 32:607–629, 1979.
10. Waterlow JC. Some aspects of childhood malnutrition as a public health problem. BMJ 4:88–90, 1974.
11. Helms RA, Miller JL, Burckart FJ, et al. Clinical outcome as assessed by anthropometric parameters, albumin and cellular immune function in high-risk infants receiving total parenteral nutrition. J Pediatr Surg 18:564–569, 1983.
12. Gurney JM, Jelliffe DB. Arm anthropometry in nutritional assessment: nomogram for rapid calculation of muscle circumference and cross-sectional muscle and fat areas. Am J Clin Nutr 26:912–915, 1973.
13. Frisancho AR. Triceps skin fold and upper arm muscle size norms for assessment of nutritional status. Am J Clin Nutr 27:1052–1058, 1974.
14. Tanner JM, Whitehouse RH. Revised standards for triceps and subscapular skinfolds in British children. Arch Dis Child 50:142–145, 1975.
15. Ingenbleek Y, van den Schrieck H, de Nayer P, et al. Albumin, transferrin, and the thyroxine-binding prealbumin/retinol binding protein (TBPA-RBP) complex in assessment of malnutrition. Clin Chim Acta 63:61–67, 1975.
16. Rothschild MA, Oratz M, Schreiber SS. Albumin synthesis. N Engl J Med 286:748–757, 1972.
17. Awai M, Brown EB. Studies of the metabolism of I131-labeled human transferrin. J Lab Clin Med 61:363–396, 1963.
18. Oppenheimer JH, Surks MI, Bernstein G, et al. Metabolism of I-131 labeled thyroxine binding prealbumin in man. Science 149:748–751, 1965.
19. Peterson PA. Demonstration in serum of two physiological forms of the human retinol-binding protein. Eur J Clin Invest 1:437–444, 1971.
20. Thomas RM, Massoudi M, Byrne J, et al. Evaluation of transthyretin as a monitor of protein-energy intake in preterm and sick neonatal infants. JPEN J Parenter Enteral Nutr 12:162–166, 1988.
21. Giacoia GP, Watson S, West K. Rapid turnover transport proteins, plasma albumin, and growth in low birth weight infants. JPEN J Parenter Enteral Nutr 8:367–370, 1984.
22. Moskowitz SR, Pereira G, Spitzer A, et al. Prealbumin as a biochemical marker of nutritional adequacy in premature infants. Pediatr 102:749–753, 1983.
23. Helms RA, Dickerson RN, Ebbert ML, et al. Retinol-binding protein and prealbumin: useful measures of protein repletion in critically ill, malnourished infants. J Pediatr Gastroenterol Nutr 5:586–592, 1986.
24. Vehe KL, Brown RO, Kuhl DA, et al. The prognostic inflammatory and nutritional index in traumatized patients receiving enteral nutrition support. J Am Coll Nutr 10:355–363, 1991.
25. Heird WC, Winters RW. Total parenteral nutrition. J Pediatr 86:2–16, 1975.

26. Lopez AM, Wolfsdorf J, Razynski A, et al. Estimation of nitrogen balance based on a six-hour urine collection in infants. JPEN J Parenter Enteral Nutr 10:517–518, 1986.
27. van Goudoever JB, Wattimena JDL, Carnielli VP, et al. Effect of dexamethasone on protein metabolism in infants with bronchopulmonary dysplasia. J Pediatr 124:112–118, 1994.
28. Boehm KA, Helms RA, Storm MC. Assessing the validity of adjusted urinary urea nitrogen as an estimate of total urinary nitrogen in three pediatric populations. JPEN J Parenter Enteral Nutr 18:172–176, 1994.
29. Seashore JH, Huszar GB, Davis EM. Urinary 3-methylhistidine excretion and nitrogen balance in healthy and stressed premature infants. J Pediatr Surg 15:400–404, 1980.
30. Forbes GB, Bruining GJ. Urinary creatinine excretion and lean body mass. Am J Clin Nutr 29:1359–1366, 1976.
31. Lawton AR, Cooper MD. Ontogeny of immunity. In: Stiehm ER, Bulginiti VA, eds. Immunologic Disorders in Infants and Children. Philadelphia: WB Saunders, 1980:36.
32. Shannon DC, Johnson G, Rosen FS, et al. Cellular reactivity to Candida albicans antigen. N Engl J Med 275:690–693, 1966.
33. Helms RA, Herrod HG, Burckart GJ, et al. E-Rosette formation, total T-cells and lymphocyte transformation in infants receiving intravenous safflower oil emulsion. JPEN J Parenter Enteral Nutr 7:541–545, 1983.
34. Costarino A, Baumgart S. Modern fluid and electrolyte management of the critically ill premature infant. Pediatr Clin North Am 33:153–178, 1986.
35. Heely AM, Talbot NB. Insensible water losses per day by hospitalized infants and children. Am J Dis Child 90:251–256, 1955.
36. Levine SZ, Wheatlye MA. Respiratory metabolism in infancy and in childhood: daily heat production in infants, predictions based on insensible loss of weight compared with direct measurements. Am J Dis Child 51:1300–1323, 1936.
37. Holliday MA, Segar WE. The maintenance need for water in parenteral fluid therapy. Pediatrics 19:823–832, 1957.
38. Bell EF, Oh W. Fluid and electrolyte balance in very low birth weight infants. Clin Perinatol 6:139–150, 1979.
39. Perkin RM, Levin DL. Common fluid and electrolyte problems in the pediatric intensive care unit. Pediatr Clin North Am 27:567–586, 1980.
40. Friis-Hansen B. Body water compartments in children: changes during growth and related changes in body composition. Pediatrics 28:169–181, 1961.
41. Stuart HC, Sobel EH. The thickness of the skin and subcutaneous tissue by age and sex in childhood. J Pediatr 28:637–647, 1946.
42. Williams PR, Oh W. Effects of radiant warmer on insensible water loss in newborn infants. Am J Dis Child 128:511–514, 1974.
43. Leake RD, Zakuddin S, Trygstad CW, et al. The effects of large volume intravenous fluid infusion on neonatal renal function. J Pediatr 89:968–972, 1976.
44. Arant BS Jr. Developmental patterns of renal functional maturation compared in the human neonate. J Pediatr 92:705–712, 1978.
45. Van Marter LJ, Leviton A, Allred EN, et al. Hydration during the first days of life and the risk of bronchopulmonary dysplasia in low birth weight infants. J Pediatr 116:942–949, 1990.
46. Goldman HI. Feeding and necrotizing enterocolitis. Am J Dis Child 134:553–555, 1980.
47. Goldberg RN, Chung D, Goldman SL, et al. The association of rapid volume expansion and intraventricular hemorrhage in the preterm infant. J Pediatr 96:1060–1063, 1980.
48. Bell EF, Warburton D, Stonestreet BS, et al. Effect of fluid administration on the development of symptomatic patent ductus arteriosus and congestive heart failure in premature infants. N Engl J Med 302:598–604, 1980.
49. Phelps SJ, Helms RA. Risk factors affecting infiltration of peripheral venous lines in infants. J Pediatr 111:384–389, 1987.
50. Oellrich RG, Murphy MR, Goldberg LA, et al. The percutaneous central venous catheter for small or ill infants. Maternal Child Nursing 16:92–96, 1991.
51. Wurzel CL, Halom K, Feldman JG, et al. Infection rates of Broviac-Hickman catheters and implantable venous devices. Am J Dis Child 142:536–540, 1988.
52. Mirro J, Rao B, Kuman M, et al. A comparison of placement techniques and complications of externalized catheters and implantable port use in children with cancer. J Pediatr Surg 25:120–124, 1990.
53. Rollins CJ, Elsberry VA, Pollack KA, et al. Three-in-one parenteral nutrition: a safe and economical method of nutritional support for infants. JPEN J Parenter Enteral Nutr 14:290–294, 1990.
54. Stegink LD, Baker GL. Infusion of protein hydrolysates in the newborn infant: plasma amino acid concentrations. J Pediatr 78:595–602, 1971.
55. Thureen PJ, Anderson AH, Baron KA, et al. Protein balance in the first week of life in ventilated neonates receiving parenteral nutrition. Am J Clin Nutr 68:1128–1135, 1998.
56. Van Goudoever JB, Colen T, Wattimena JLD, et al. Immediate commencement of amino acid supplementation in preterm infants: effect on serum amino acid concentrations and protein kinetics on the first day of life. J Pediatr 127:458–465, 1995.
57. Helms RA, Christensen ML, Mauer EC, et al. Comparison of pediatric versus standard amino acid formulation in preterm neonates requiring parenteral nutrition. J Pediatr 110:466–470, 1987.
58. Adamkin DH, McClead RE, Desai NS, et al. Comparison of two neonatal intravenous amino acid formulations in preterm infants: a multicenter study. J Perinatol 11:375–382, 1991.
59. Heird WC, Dell RB, Helms RA, et al. Amino acid mixture designed to maintain normal plasma amino acid patterns in infants and children requiring parenteral nutrition. Pediatrics 80:401–408, 1987.
60. Polberger SK, Axelsson IE, Raiha NCR. Amino acid concentrations in plasma and urine in very low birth weight infants fed protein-unenriched human milk or protein-enriched human milk. Pediatrics 86:909–915, 1990.
61. Chessman K, Johnson M, Fernandes E, et al. Changing parenteral substrate requirements in neonates receiving a pediatric amino acid formulation. JPEN J Parenter Enteral Nutr 12:105, 1988. (abstract)
62. Beck R. Use of a pediatric parenteral amino acid mixture in a population of extremely low birth weight neonates: frequency and spectrum of direct bilirubinemia. Am J Perinatol 7:84–86, 1990.
63. Gazzaniga AB, Waxman K, Day AT, et al. Nitrogen balance in adult hospitalized patients with the use of a pediatric amino acid model. Arch Surg 123:1275–1279, 1988.
64. Helms RA, Storm MC, Christensen ML, et al. Cysteine supplementation results in normalization of plasma taurine concentrations in children receiving home parenteral nutrition. J Pediatr 134:358–361, 1999.
65. Reichman BL, Chessex P, Putet G, et al. Partition of energy metabolism and energy cost of growth in the very low-birth-weight infant. Pediatrics 69:446–451, 1982.
66. Zlotkin SH, Bryan MH, Anderson GH. Intravenous nitrogen and energy intakes required to duplicate in utero nitrogen accretion in prematurely born human infants. J Pediatr 99:115–120, 1981.
67. Thomas DB. Hyperosmolality and intraventricular haemorrhage in premature babies. Acta Paediatr Scand 65:429–432, 1976.
68. Sheridan RL, Yu Y, Prelack K, et al. Maximal parenteral glucose oxidation in hypermetabolic young children: a stable isotope study. JPEN J Parent Enter Nutr 22:212–216, 1998.
69. Collins JW Jr, Hoppe M, Brown K, et al. A controlled trial of insulin infusion and parenteral nutrition in extremely low birth weight infants with glucose intolerance. J Pediatr 118:921–927, 1991.
70. Press M, Kikuchi H, Shimoyana J, et al. Diagnosis and treatment of essential fatty acid deficiency in man. BMJ 2:247–250, 1974.
71. Pelham LD. Rational use of intravenous fat emulsions. Am J Hosp Pharm 38:198–208, 1981.
72. Committee on Nutrition, American Academy of Pediatrics. Commentary on parenteral nutrition. Pediatrics 71:547–552, 1983.
73. Bivins BA, Bell RM, Rapp RP, et al. Linoleic acid versus linolenic acid: what is essential. JPEN J Parenter Enteral Nutr 7:473–478, 1983.
74. Schiff D, Chan G, Seccombe D, et al. Plasma carnitine levels during intravenous feeding of the neonate. J Pediatr 95:1043–1046, 1979.
75. Helms RA, Whitington PF, Mauer EC, et al. Enhanced lipid utilization in infants receiving oral L-carnitine during long-term parenteral nutrition. J Pediatr 109:984–988, 1986.
76. Iofalla AK, Roe CR. Carnitine deficiency in apnea of prematurity. Pediatr Research 2:309A, 1995.
77. Andrew G, Chan G, Schiff D. Lipid metabolism in the neonate: II. The effect of Intralipid on bilirubin binding in vitro and in vivo. J Pediatr 88:279–284, 1976.
78. Burckart GJ, Whitington RF, Helms RA. The effect of two intravenous fat emulsions and their components on bilirubin to albumin. Am J Clin Nutr 36:521–526, 1982.
79. Nordenstrom J, Jarstrand C, Wienick A. Decreased chemotactic and random migration of leukocytes during Intralipid infusion. Am J Clin Nutr 32:2416–2422, 1979.
80. Jarstrand C, Berghem L, Lahnborg G. Human granulocyte and reticuloendothelial system function during Intralipid infusion. JPEN J Parenter Enteral Nutr 2:663–670, 1978.
81. Ladisch S, Poplark DG, Blaese RM. Inhibition of human lymphoproliferation by intravenous lipid emulsion. Clin Immunol Immunopathol 25:196–202, 1982.

82. Palmbald J, Brostrom O, Lahnborg G, et al. Neutrophil functions during total parenteral nutrition and Intralipid infusion. Am J Clin Nutr 35:1430–1436, 1982.
83. Strunk RC, Murrow BW, Thilo E, et al. Normal macrophage function in infants receiving Intralipid by low-dose intermittent administration. J Pediatr 106:640–645, 1985.
84. Escudier EF, Escudier BJ, Henry-Amar MC, et al. Effects of infused Intralipids on neutrophil chemotaxis during total parenteral nutrition. JPEN J Parenter Enteral Nutr 10:596–598, 1986.
85. Schroder H, Paust H, Schmidt R. Pulmonary fat embolism after Intralipid therapy-a postmortem artefact? Acta Paediatr Scand 73:461–464, 1984.
86. Pereira GR, Fox WW, Stanley CA, et al. Decreased oxygenation and hyperlipemia during intravenous fat infusions in premature infants. Pediatrics 66:26–30, 1980.
87. Brans YW, Dutton EB, Andrew DS, et al. Fat emulsion tolerance in very low birth weight neonates: effect on diffusion of oxygen in the lungs and on blood pH. Pediatrics 78:79–84, 1986.
88. Haumont D, Deckelbaum RJ, Richelle M, et al. Plasma lipid concentrations in low birth weight infants given parenteral nutrition with twenty or ten percent lipid emulsion. J Pediatr 115:787–793, 1989.
89. Arnold WC. Parenteral nutrition, and fluid and electrolyte therapy. Pediatr Clin North Am 37:449–461, 1990.
90. Greene HL, Hambidge KM, Schanler R, et al. Guidelines for the use of vitamins, trace elements, calcium, magnesium, and phosphorus in infants and children receiving total parenteral nutrition: report of the Subcommittee on Pediatric Parenteral Nutrient Requirements from the Committee on Clinical Practice Issues of The American Society for Clinical Nutrition. Am J Clin Nutr 48:1324–1342, 1988.
91. Sulyok E, Varga F, Gyory E, et al. Postnatal development of renal sodium handling in premature infants. J Pediatr 95:787–792, 1979.
92. Stapleton FB, Nelson B, Vats TS, et al. Hypokalemia associated with antibiotic treatment. Am J Dis Child 130:1104–1108, 1976.
93. Schaber DE, Uden DL, Stone FM, et al. Intravenous KCl supplementation in pediatric cardiac surgical patients. Pediatr Cardiol 6:25–28, 1985.
94. Popovtzer MM, Knochel JP, Kunnar R. Disorders of calcium, phosphorus, vitamin D, and parathyroid hormone activity. In: Schrier RQ, ed. Renal and Electrolyte Disorders. Boston: Little, Brown & Co., 1997:241–319.
95. Pelegano JF, Rowe JC, Carey DE, et al. Simultaneous infusion of calcium and phosphorus in parenteral nutrition for premature infants: use of physiologic calcium/phosphorus ratio. J Pediatr 114:115–119, 1989.
96. Koo WWK. Parenteral nutrition related bone disease. JPEN J Parenter Enteral Nutr 16:386–394, 1992.
97. Vileisis RA. Furosemide effect on mineral status of parenterally nourished premature neonates with chronic lung disease. Pediatrics 85:316–322, 1990.
98. Eggert LD, Rusho WJ, MacKay MW, et al. Calcium and phosphorus compatibility in parenteral nutrition solutions for neonates. Am J Hosp Pharm 39:49–53, 1982.
99. Lenz GT, Mikrut BA. Calcium and phosphate solubility in neonatal parenteral nutrient solutions containing Aminosyn-PF or TrophAmine. Am J Hosp Pharm 45:2367–2371, 1988.
100. Schmidt GL, Baumgartner TG, Fischlschweiger W, et al. Cost containment using cysteine HCl acidification to increase calcium/phosphate solubility in hyperalimentation solutions. JPEN J Parenter Enteral Nutr 10:203–207, 1986.
101. Henry RS, Jurgens RW Jr, Sturgeon R, et al. Compatibility of calcium chloride and calcium gluconate with sodium phosphate in a mixed TPN solution. Am J Hosp Pharm 37:673–674, 1980.
102. Niemiec PW Jr, Vanderveen TW. Compatibility considerations in parenteral nutrient solutions. Am J Hosp Pharm 41:893–911, 1984.
103. Solomon SM, Kirby DF. The refeeding syndrome: a review. JPEN J Parenter Enteral Nutr 14:90–97, 1990.
104. Tsang RC. Neonatal magnesium disturbances. Am J Dis Child 124:282–293, 1972.
105. Whang R, Aikawa JK. Magnesium deficiency and refractoriness to potassium repletion. J Chron Dis 30:65–68, 1977.
106. Hak EB, Storm MC, Helms RA. Chromium and zinc contaminant in components of parenteral nutrition solutions commonly used in infants and children. Am J Health-Syst Pharm 55:150–154, 1998.
107. Moukarzel AA, Song MK, Buchman AL, et al. Excessive chromium intake in children receiving total parenteral nutrition. Lancet 339:385–388, 1992.
108. Mouser J, Cochran EB, Helms RA, et al. Chromium concentrations in children on home TPN and the relationship to intake. JPEN J Parenter Enteral Nutr 18(Suppl):33S, 1994.
109. Brown AS, Hoelzer DJ, Piercy SA. Skin necrosis from extravasation of intravenous fluids in children. Plastic Reconstruct Surg 64:145–150, 1979.
110. Alpan G, Eyal F, Springer C, et al. Heparinization of alimentation solutions administered through peripheral veins in premature infants: a controlled study. Pediatrics 74:375–378, 1984.
111. Phelps SJ, Cochran EB. Effect of the continuous administration of fat emulsion on the infiltration of intravenous lines in infants receiving peripheral parenteral nutrition solutions. JPEN J Parenter Enteral Nutr 13:628–632, 1989.
112. Eichelberger MR, Rous PG, Hoelzer D, et al. Percutaneous subclavian venous catheters in neonates and children. J Pediatr Surg 16:547–552, 1981.
113. Ruggiero RP, Caruso G. Chylothorax–a complication of subclavian vein catheterization. JPEN J Parenter Enteral Nutr 9:750–753, 1985.
114. Gutcher G, Cutz E. Complications of parenteral nutrition. Semin Perinatol 10:196–207, 1986.
115. Welch GW, McKell DW, Silverstein P, et al. The role of catheter composition in the development of thrombophlebitis. Surg Gynecol Obstet 138:421–424, 1974.
116. Hoshal VL, Ause RG, Hoskins PA. Fibrin sleeve formation on indwelling subclavian central venous catheters. Arch Surg 102:353–358, 1971.
117. Breaux CW Jr, Duke D, Georgeson KE, et al. Calcium phosphate crystal occlusion of central venous catheters used for total parenteral nutrition in infants and children: prevention and treatment. J Pediatr Surg 22:829–832, 1987.
118. Duffy LF, Kerzner B, Gebus V, et al. Treatment of central venous catheter occlusions with hydrochloric acid. J Pediatr 114:102–104, 1989.
119. Pennington CR, Pithie AD. Ethanol lock in the management of catheter occulusion. JPEN J Parenteral Enteral Nutr 11:507–508, 1987.
120. Holcombe BJ, Forloines-Lynn S, Garmhausen LW. Restoring patency of long-term central venous access devices. J Intravenous Nursing 15:36–41, 1992.
121. Baker SS, Dwyer E, Queen P. Metabolic derangements in children requiring parenteral nutrition. JPEN J Parenter Enteral Nutr 10:279–281, 1986.
122. Black DD, Suttle EA, Whitington PF, et al. The effect of short-term total parenteral nutrition on hepatic function in the human neonate: a prospective randomized study demonstrating alteration of the hepatic canalicular function. J Pediatr 99:445–449, 1981.
123. Farrell MK, Balistren WF, Sucky FY. Serum-sulfated lithocholate as an indicator of cholestasis during parenteral nutrition in infants and children. JPEN J Parenter Enteral Nutr 6:30–33, 1982.
124. Whitington PF. Cholestasis associated with total parenteral nutrition in infants. Hepatology 5:693–696, 1985.
125. Beale EF, Nelson RM, Bucciarelli RL, et al. Intrahepatic cholestasis associated with parenteral nutrition in premature infants. Pediatrics 64:342–347, 1979.
126. Gleghorn EE, Merritt RJ, Subramanian N, et al. Phenobarbital does not prevent total parenteral-associated cholestasis in noninfected infants. JPEN J Parenter Enteral Nutr 10:282–283, 1986.
127. Doty JE, Pitt HA, Porter-Fink V, et al. Cholecystokinin prophylaxis of parenteral nutrition-induced gallbladder disease. Ann Surg 201:76–80, 1985.
128. Koo WWK, Kaplan LA, Horn J, et al. Aluminum in parenteral nutrition solution–sources and possible alternatives. JPEN J Parenter Enteral Nutr 10:591–595, 1986.
129. Klein GL, Alfey AC, Shike N, et al. Parenteral drug products containing aluminum as an ingredient or a contaminant; response to FDA notice of intent. Am J Clin Nutr 53:399–402, 1991.
130. Lyon AJ, Hawkes DJ, Doran M, et al. Bone mineralization in preterm infants measured by dual energy radiographic densitometry. Arch Dis Child 64:919–923, 1989.
131. Pomeranz S, Gimmon Z, Zvi AB, et al. Parenteral-nutrition-induced anaphylaxis. JPEN J Parenter Enteral Nutr 11:314–315, 1987.
132. Bullock L, Etchason E, Fitzgerald JF, et al. Case report of an allergic reaction to parenteral nutrition in a pediatric patient. JPEN J Parenter Enteral Nutr 14:98–100, 1990.
133. Market AD, Lew DB, Schropp KP, Hak EB. Anaphylactoid reaction associated with parenteral nutrition in a 4 year old. J Pediatr Gastroenterol Nutr 26:229–231, 1998.
134. Kamath KR, Berry A, Commins G. Acute hypersensitivity reaction to Intralipid. N Engl J Med 304:360, 1981.
135. Hiyama DT, Griggs B, Mittman RF, et al. Hypersensitivity following lipid emulsion infusion in an adult patient. JPEN J Parenter Enteral Nutr 13:318–320, 1989.
136. Sternberg A, Gruenevald T, Duetsch AA, et al. Intralipid-induced transient sinus bradycardia. N Engl J Med 304:422–423, 1981.
137. Connon JJ. Diarrhea possibly caused by total parenteral nutrition. N Engl J Med 301:273–274, 1979.
138. Campbell AN, Freedman MH, Pendarz PI, et al. Bleeding disorder from the "fat overload" syndrome. JPEN J Parenter Enteral Nutr 8:447–449, 1984.
139. Bhat AM Scanlon JW. The pattern of eosinophilia in premature infants. J Pediatr 98:612–616, 1981.

140. Rotruck JT, Pope AL, Banther HE, et al. Selenium: biochemical role as a component of glutathione peroxidase. Science 179:588–590, 1973.
141. Marks LM, Patel N, Kurtides ES. Hematologic abnormalities associated with intravenous lipid therapy. Am J Gastroenterol 73:490–495, 1980.
142. McGrath KM, Zalcberg JR, Slonim J. Intralipid induced haemolysis. Br J Haematol 50:376–378, 1982.
143. Golden MHN, Harland PAEG, Golden BE, et al. Zinc and immunocompetence in protein-energy malnutrition. Lancet 1:1226–1227, 1978.
144. Hodges RE, Bean WB, Ohlson MA, et al. Factors affecting human antibody response V. Combined deficiencies of pantothenic acid and pyridoxine. Am J Clin Nutr 11:187–199, 1962.
145. Axelrod AE. Immune process in vitamin deficiency states. Am J Clin Nutr 24:265–271, 1971.
146. Kinsella JE, Lokesh B, Broughton S, et al. Dietary polyunsaturated fatty acids and eicosanoids: potential effects on the modulation of inflammatory and immune cells: an overview. Nutrition 6:24–44, 1990.
147. Meydani SN, Yogeeswaran G, Liu S, et al. Fish oil and tocopherol-induced changes in natural killer cell-mediated cytotoxicity and PGE_2 synthesis in young and old mice. J Nutr 118:1245–1252, 1988.
148. Barbul A, Sisto DA, Waserkurg HL, et al. Arginine stimulates lymphocyte immune response in healthy human beings. Surgery 90:244–251, 1981.
149. Burke DJ, Alverdy JC, Aoys E, et al. Glutamine-supplemented total parenteral nutrition improves gut immune function. Arch Surg 124:1396–1399, 1989.
150. Vargas JH, Ament ME, Berquist WE. Long-term home parenteral nutrition in pediatrics. Ten years of experience in 102 patients. J Pediatr Gastroenterol Nutr 6:24–37, 1987.
151. Buchman AL, Moukarzel A, Goodson B, et al. Catheter-related infections associated with home parenteral nutrition and predictive factors for the need for catheter removal in their treatment. JPEN J Parenter Enteral Nutr 18:297–302, 1994.
152. Flynn PM, Shenep JL, Stokes DC, et al. In situ management of confirmed central venous catheter-related bacteremia. Pediatr Infect Dis J 6:729–734, 1987.
153. Hartman GE, Shochat SJ. Management of septic complications associated with Silastic catheters in malignancy. Pediatr Infect Dis J 6:1042–1047, 1987.
154. National Research Council. Recommended Dietary Allowances. 10th ed. Washington DC: National Academy Press, 1989: ch. 3–9.
155. Kennedy-Caldwell C, Caldwell MD, Zitarelli ME. Pediatric enteral nutrition. In: Rombeau JL, Caldwell MD, eds. Clinical Nutrition–Enteral and Tube Feeding. Philadelphia: WB Saunders, 1990:325–360.
156. American Academy of Pediatrics, Committee on Nutrition. Nutritional needs of low-birth-weight infants. Pediatrics 75:976–986, 1985.

CHAPTER 98

GYNECOLOGIC DISORDERS

Ronald J. Ruggiero

Disorders of the female reproductive tract are the reason for many gynecologic complaints and problems. Dysmenorrhea, the premenstrual syndrome, endometriosis, vaginitis, venereal warts, and estrogen replacement therapy for hot flushes, atrophic vaginitis, and the prevention of estrogen deficiency-induced osteoporosis require rational drug management. Observational studies indicate that estrogen replacement therapy alone (ERT) or estrogen replacement with progestational opposition for women with an intact uterus (HRT) probably help prevent coronary heart disease (CHD) and may help prevent colon cancer, cognitive decline, and Alzheimer's disease (AD). The recent introduction of the first in a series of selective estrogen receptor modulators (SERMs), raloxifene, developed as an alternative to ERT/HRT, has ushered in new challenges, choices, and concerns for the menopausal woman and her health care providers. The popular alternative medicine movement is luring a significant number of women into taking phytoestrogen-containing regimens rather than traditional, better studied ERT/HRT regimens, along with many other "natural" preparations that are in general poorly studied and regulated.

Teratogenicity should be considered when treating a woman with childbearing potential, and women who are taking potentially teratogenic drugs must use an effective method of contraception.

Dysmenorrhea

TREATMENT GOALS: DYSMENORRHEA

- Avoid lower abdominal spasmodic pains and other prostaglandin-induced effects.
- Efficacy monitoring of therapy is dependent solely upon the subjective responses of the patient.

EPIDEMIOLOGY

It is estimated that 30 to 50% of the 35 million women of childbearing age in the United States are affected by painful menstrual periods or dysmenorrhea, and 10 to 15% of those women are incapacitated for 1 to 3 days each month. Dysmenorrhea is the greatest single cause of absenteeism from school and work among young women.[1] The cost for the estimated 600 million work hours lost annually in the United States is approximately $2 billion.[2]

PATHOPHYSIOLOGY

Primary dysmenorrhea occurs during ovulatory cycles and, unlike secondary dysmenorrhea, has no detectable pelvic pathologic conditions, such as adhesions on the reproductive organs.

CLINICAL PRESENTATION AND DIAGNOSIS

The most common symptom that women experience is spasmodic pain of the lower abdomen that can radiate to the back and along the thighs. The pain is accompanied by one or more of the following systemic symptoms in more than 50% of patients: nausea and vomiting (89%), fatigue (85%), diarrhea (60%), lower backache (60%), and headache (45%). The duration is usually 48 to 72 hours, with the pain starting a few hours before or just after the onset of menstrual flow.[3]

The etiology of these symptoms has been determined to be related to the pharmacologic actions of prostaglandin (PG) E_2 (PGE_2) and $PGF_{2\alpha}$, which are formed from the phospholipids of dead cell membranes in the menstruating uterus. PGE_2 causes disaggregation of platelets and is a vasodilator, whereas $PGF_{2\alpha}$ mediates or potentiates pain sensations and stimulates smooth muscle contraction.[1] Additionally, estrogens can stimulate synthesis and/or release of $PGF_{2\alpha}$ and vasopressin that cause uterine hyperactivity, and for this reason, progestin-dominant combination oral contraceptives are often used to alleviate dysmenorrhea.[4]

TREATMENT

Table 98.1 lists drug therapy regimens currently used for primary dysmenorrhea, including nonsteroidal anti-inflammatory drugs (NSAIDs) and combination oral contraceptives (COCs).

Clinically, there is no way to predict whether a certain NSAID will give maximal benefit to any given patient based on current data in the literature. Few direct comparisons of one NSAID to another have been done. Even though most studies show superiority of the active drug over placebo, no single NSAID has been found to be superior, although some studies give mefenamic acid a slight edge. The initial selection should be tried for at least two to four cycles. If therapy is unsuccessful, some patients may still respond to another NSAID class, and NSAIDs are successful in 77 to 80% of patients with dysmenorrhea. Ibuprofen, naproxen, or naproxen sodium is the usual initial choice, with flurbiprofen and mefenamic acid being reserved for more difficult cases.

Patients should be told that NSAIDs need not be taken until the onset of symptoms because the half-life of prostaglandins is only minutes. With the short-term use of NSAIDs for dysmenorrhea, side effects are infrequent and usually mild. Gastrointestinal irritation is best avoided by taking the NSAIDs with food or milk. Other NSAIDs such

Table 98.1 ▪ Drug Therapy of Primary Dysmenorrhea

Drug	Usual Dose
NSAIDs	
Acetic acids	
Diclofenac[a] (CDOC)[b]	100 mg PO stat, then 50 mg TID
Indomethacin	25 mg PO TID
Tolmetin	400 mg PO TID
Sulindac	200 mg PO q4–6hr
Fenamates	
Mefenamic acid[a] (CDOC)	500 mg PO stat, then 250 mg q6hr
Meclofenamate	100 mg PO stat, then 50–100 mg q6hr
Oxicams	
Piroxicam	20 mg PO daily
Proprionic acids	
Flurbiprofen	50 mg PO QID
Ibuprofen[a] (CDOC)	400 mg PO q4hr
Naproxen[a] (CDOC)	500 mg PO stat, then 250 mg q6–8hr
Naproxen sodium[a] (CDOC)	550 mg PO stat, then 275 mg q6–8hr
Ketoprofen[a] (CDOC)	50 mg PO TID
Salicylic acids	
Diflunisal	1000 mg PO stat, then 500 mg q12hr
Combination oral contraceptives (28-day cycle pack, progestin dominant)	1 daily
Cyclooxygenase-2 inhibitor	
Refecoxib	50 mg daily for 5 days maximum with or without food
α-Adrenergic agonists[c]	
Clonidine	0.1 mg PO TID

NSAIDs, nonsteroidal anti-inflammatory drugs.

[a]FDA approved for primary dysmenorrhea.

[b]CDOC, clinical drug of choice: (a) No single NSAID has proven superiority—proprionic acids often used initially; (b) NSAIDs may be ineffective in 20 to 30% of patients; (c) combination oral contraceptives may be ineffective in 10% of patients.

[c]Only preliminary data available; therefore last therapeutic choice.

as aspirin should be avoided with the use of NSAIDs listed in Table 98.1 because they may greatly enhance side effects and toxic effects such as peptic ulceration, liver damage, and renal damage. Patients having allergies to aspirin, especially anaphylactic reactions, should be cautioned never to take NSAIDs in prescription or over-the-counter preparations.

Recently, the cyclooxygenase-2 (COX-2) inhibitor, rofecoxib, which has the potential benefit of fewer gastrointestinal side effects, was approved for the treatment of primary dysmenorrhea.

COCs relieve dysmenorrhea in 90% of patients, probably by a reduction in the amount of endometrium formed and consequently the amount of prostaglandins formed. Compliance with the COC regimen is essential for maintenance of anovulatory cycles.

Because NSAIDs do not relieve pain in 20 to 30% of patients with dysmenorrhea and COCs do not relieve pain in 10% of patients, another cause of dysmenorrhea has been proposed that includes excessive stimulation of the uterus by the adrenergic nervous system. In a recent report of four patients in whom therapy with NSAIDs and COCs failed, the α-adrenergic agonist clonidine in a dose of 0.1 mg three times daily worked very well.[5] Clonidine may therefore be useful as the last-alternative therapy although large, well-controlled studies are needed to confirm its efficacy in primary dysmenorrhea.

PHARMACOECONOMICS

The pharmacoeconomics of the management of primary dysmenorrhea is self-evident. The use of a generic NSAID would be most cost effective, followed by brand name NSAIDs, oral contraceptives (in patients who are not using oral contraception), and a COX-2 inhibitor.

Premenstrual Syndrome

DEFINITION

Unlike primary dysmenorrhea, there is no consensus on the definition of premenstrual syndrome (PMS). The most widely accepted definition states that the following criteria be met to document PMS[6]:

1. The signs and/or symptoms must occur cyclically, recur to some degree in the luteal phase (i.e., after ovulation) of the menstrual cycle, and are usually present to some degree each cycle.
2. During the follicular phase (i.e., before ovulation), the patient should be free of symptoms. There must be at least 7 symptom-free days in each cycle. Most patients do not have symptoms for several days after the onset of menses until near ovulation.
3. The combination of distressing physical, psychologic, or behavioral changes are sufficiently severe to result in deterioration of interpersonal relationships and/or interfere with normal activities.

TREATMENT GOALS: PREMENSTRUAL SYNDROME

- Alleviate the symptoms of PMS.
- Efficacy monitoring of therapy depends largely on the subjective responses of the patient and on the observations of persons close to her and the patient's health care providers.

EPIDEMIOLOGY

It is estimated that 30 to 80% of menstruating women experience symptoms of PMS, with 20 to 30% reporting moderate to severe symptoms. Absenteeism due to PMS is costly because 60% of women are in the workforce today.

CLINICAL PRESENTATION AND DIAGNOSIS

Table 98.2 lists many of the commonly reported chief symptoms of PMS. The etiology of PMS remains as elusive as the definition and the myriad of symptoms attributed to this disorder.

A new disorder category, premenstrual dysphoric disorder (PMDD), which occurs in 2 to 9% of menstruating women, was recently added to the "Depressive Disorders Not Otherwise Specified" section of the American Psychiatric Association's *Diagnostic and Statistical Manual of Mental Disorders, Fourth Edition* (DSM-IV). As found with PMS patients, PMDD patients experience symptoms for several days to 2 weeks during the luteal phase of the cycle. The most common symptoms of PMDD are low mood, tension, anger, irritability, mood swings, headache, bloating, and changes in appetite and sleep.[7] DSM-IV requires a minimum of five clinical symptoms, one of which must be related to mood (low mood, mood swings, tension, or irritability). These symptoms must be prospectively confirmed with some method of daily rating. The syndrome meets criteria only if it leads to functional impairment in either work or interpersonal areas.[8]

Table 98.3 lists the proposed DSM-IV criteria for PMDD.

TREATMENT

Pharmacotherapy

Table 98.4 lists the drug therapy regimens for PMS. Lack of consistent definition and paucity of carefully designed drug studies have led to less than satisfactory treatment of PMS.[12] Complicating the study results is the fact that placebo responses have been as high as 60 to 80% in many studies. No one drug has been shown to be superior or satisfactory for the long-term treatment of PMS. Many of the early studies available were not very helpful in choosing appropriate therapy. Numerous case reports and uncontrolled clinical trials describe beneficial effects for the agent being studied. However, the same agent's therapeutic benefit is often lacking when a placebo-controlled clinical trial is performed, as is the case with various forms of progesterone.[9] Because of this, most clinicians use stress reduction classes, counseling, and exercise programs along with drug therapy.

Patients must understand the empirical nature of the various therapies and realize that some patients have responded very well to any given drug, ancillary treatment, or combination of treatments.

In a recent double blind, placebo-controlled, 6-month crossover study using the gonadotropin-releasing hormone (GnRH) agonist leuprolide acetate, 3.75 mg intramuscularly monthly, or saline, both behavioral and physical symptoms of PMS were reduced and the GnRH agonist was well tolerated. Patients with moderate premenstrual depression improved but remained clinically symptomatic, and those with severe premenstrual depression showed no improvement by any efficacy measurement. The differential response to leuprolide suggests that it may be of value in diagnosing distinct subtypes of PMS.[11] This lends support to the theory that cyclic fluctuations in ovarian steroids are involved in the regulation of neuropeptides, which in turn modulate mood and behavior.[13]

Some authors believe that 80% of patients with PMS can be treated without drugs using education, stress reduction, and dietary modifications.[9,14] Some researchers are also studying alprazolam because of its anxiolytic and

Table 98.2 ▪ Symptoms of PMS

Psychological[a]	Somatic[a]
Anxiety	Abdominal bloating
Depression	Edema
Irritability	Weight gain
Wide mood swings	Constipation
Increased appetite	Hot flashes
Aggression	Breast pain
Lethargy or fatigue	Headache
Forgetfullness and reduced concentration	Acne
Sleep disorders	Rhinitis
Phobias	Palpitations

Source: Reference 6.

[a]In approximate order of frequency of occurrence.

Table 98.3 ▪ DSM-IV Proposed Criteria for Premenstrual Dysphoric Disorder

1. At least five symptoms in most cycles during the last year, including a minimum of one mood symptom, present in the last week of the luteal phase and absent in the week postmenses:
   - Depressed mood, feelings of hopelessness
   - Anxiety, tension, feeling "keyed up"
   - Affective lability
   - Lack of energy, lethargy
   - Persistent and marked anger or irritability
   - Decreased interest in usual activities
   - Difficulty concentrating
   - Changes in appetite
   - Changes in sleep
   - A subjective sense of being overwhelmed
   - Physical symptoms such as breast tenderness, bloating, or muscle pain
2. Symptoms must markedly interfere with work or interpersonal relationships.
3. Disturbance is not merely an exacerbation of another disorder.
4. Criteria 1, 2, and 3 are confirmed by daily ratings for two cycles.

Source: References 7, 8.

antidepressant effects during the symptomatic premenstrual days but its addiction liability must be noted. A recent study used 300 mg of micronized oral progesterone and 0.25 mg of alprazolam or placebo taken four times daily from day 18 of the menstrual cycle through day 2 of the next cycle. Oral micronized progesterone therapy was no better than placebo. In contrast, 37% of the alprazolam group experienced a 50% reduction in mental function, pain, and mood.[10]

Progesterone, in various forms, has been the most commonly prescribed therapy for PMS for several decades and yet is the most controversial. Uncontrolled clinical trials have consistently demonstrated that progesterone suppositories are an effective treatment for PMS, and they are the basis for the widespread use of progesterone therapy in the United States. Unfortunately, progesterone deficiency has never been proven to be a cause for PMS, and most controlled clinical trials have failed to demonstrate the superiority of progesterone therapy over placebo.[15] Advocates of progesterone therapy were unwilling to accept unfavorable clinical trial data because of the dilemma of having very few alternative agents to offer their patients with PMS.

The most recently studied and, oftentimes, most effective class of agents to treat the generalized symptoms of PMS are the selective serotonin reuptake inhibitors (SSRIs). Fluoxetine 20 mg daily has shown remarkable results.[16] Women with dysphoric PMS who also met DSM-IV criteria for PMDD entered a single-blind treatment with sertraline 100 mg/day for one full menstrual cycle. Responders were randomly assigned to a four-cycle double-blind placebo-controlled crossover study in which sertraline 100 mg/day or placebo was each given only during luteal phases of two consecutive menstrual cycles. The 11 patients who received both regimens responded well to continuous and luteal phase treatment. The authors concluded that because their patients started sertraline about a week before anticipated symptoms, the beneficial effect of the SSRI may be manifested much faster in patients with dysphoric PMS than in patients with major depressive or anxiety disorders in whom it usually takes 2 to 3 weeks to see relief. This might suggest a difference in the sensitivity of serotonergic systems in these patients.[17]

A recent thorough risk-benefit appraisal of drugs used in the management of PMS indicates that fluoxetine, alprazolam, and leuprolide in that order (or other members of their pharmacologic classes) currently provide the best relief of generalized PMS symptoms. Despite the success of these treatments, knowledge of the potential adverse effects of these agents and their management is essential and modulates their use in some patients.[16]

Nonpharmacologic Therapy

Finally, a recent study concluded that dietary supplementation with 1200 mg of elemental calcium from calcium

Table 98.4 ▪ Effectiveness of the Current Drug Therapy for Premenstrual Syndrome (PMS)[a]

Drug	Average Dose/Regimen	Average Patient Improvement[b] (%)
Spironolactone (CDOC)[c]	25 mg PO QID days 14–28	0–80
Various COCs (28's) (CDOC)	One PO daily days 1–28	0–29
Pyridoxine (CDOC)	50–500 mg PO days 1–28	0–76
Lithium	200 mg PO QID days 1–28	0–60
Mefenamic acid	500 mg PO TID days 14–28	0–92
Oil of evening primrose	3 g PO day 15 to menses	0–60
Progesterone suppositories[9] (CDOC)	200–400 mg PV days 14–28	0–60
Bromocriptine	1.25–2.5 mg PO BID day 14 to menses	0–80
Alprazolam[10d]	0.25–5.0 mg PO BID	37–75
Fluoxetine[16]	20 mg PO QID	0–100
Clonidine	17 μg/kg/day PO	100
GnRH agonist leuprolide acetate[11e]	3.75 mg IM q30days	0–100[f]

Sources: References 13, 14, 15.

[a]Three classes of agents have proven efficacy: benzodiazepines (especially alprazolam), gonadotropin-releasing hormone agonists (especially leuprolide), and selective serotonin uptake inhibitors (especially fluoxetine).[16]

[b]Study results vary greatly.

[c]CDOC, clinical drug of choice. In the treatment of PMS, the CDOCs are most often tried although none are satisfactory for long-term resolution of symptoms, and the studies available are not helpful in choosing therapy.

[d]The addictive quality of alprazolam is a main drawback, and many patients with PMS have a history of substance dependence, depression, and other psychiatric disorders.[10]

[e]Effective for the short term. Whether prolonged therapy would be safe and effective, or even necessary, remains to be determined. The only worrisome side effect is a substantial decrease in estradiol that could, with long-term use, lead to osteoporosis. The cost of gonadotropin-releasing hormone (GnRH) agonists such as leuprolide and nafarelin is prohibitive unless they are used as a last resort.

[f]Less effective in moderately depressed and ineffective in severely depressed. Caution—more than 75% of patients have worsening depression.

carbonate is a simple and effective treatment in PMS, resulting in a major reduction in overall luteal phase symptoms. By the third treatment cycle there was an overall 48% reduction in total symptom scores from baseline compared with a 30% reduction in the placebo group. Furthermore, all four symptom factors (negative affect, water retention, food cravings and pain) were significantly reduced.[18]

ALTERNATIVE THERAPY

Alternative therapies for mastodynia (breast pain) include caffeine restriction, vitamin E 200 to 600 IU/day, or oil of evening primrose 0.5 to 1.5 g twice daily. Mild PMS has been treated with 1.0 g of elemental calcium daily, pyridoxine 50 to 100 mg once or twice daily, magnesium 50 to 100 mg twice daily, or multivitamin with mineral supplements. Herbal products such as dong quai, red raspberry leaves, blue and black cohosh, and gingerroot are suggested by alternative health care providers.[19] Unfortunately there is little clinical evidence of the efficacy of these alternative therapies.

PHARMACOECONOMICS

Pharmacoeconomics would dictate a 3-month trial of elemental calcium and other less costly therapies before using SSRIs or leuprolide.

Endometriosis

TREATMENT GOALS

- Ameliorate pain.
- Correct menstrual irregularities and infertility by the suppression of ectopic endometrial implants.

EPIDEMIOLOGY

Possibly 5 to 15% of all premenopausal women have endometriosis to some degree. This disorder is a common abnormal pelvic finding in women older than 25 years of age and may be found in 40 to 50% of women who undergo surgery for the diagnosis and treatment of infertility. The average age at diagnosis is 28 years, and 75% of women with endometriosis are between 24 and 50 years old.[20]

The most widely accepted etiology of endometriosis involves retrograde menstruation. This is supported by findings that (1) retrograde menstruation is a common (90%) event in menstruating women with patent fallopian tubes, and (2) the anatomic distribution of endometriosis found at laparoscopy is consistent with retrograde menstruation. It has also been suggested that endometrial cells may successfully implant only in women with alterations in cell-mediated immunity and that such translocated cells may receive a stimulus for ectopic implantation and growth from activated macrophages.[21] There are at least four other possible etiologies of endometriosis: (1) ectopic functioning endometrium developing as a result of atypical development of germinal epithelium because various parts of the pelvic peritoneum are embryologically derived from totipotential coelomic epithelial cell elements; (2) metastases of normal endometrium spreading via uterine lymphatic vessels; (3) hematogenous spreading via blood vessels to distant sites; or (4) cell rests of Müllerian epithelium developing into functioning ectopic endometrial implants.

PATHOPHYSIOLOGY

Endometriosis is a disorder in which there is a presence of islands of endometrium in extrauterine locations, which exhibit the histologic and hormonal responsiveness of native endometrium. Cyclic change in these islands of endometrium is associated with menstrual-like bleeding and resultant localized inflammation.[20]

Endometriosis most commonly occurs within the pelvis, on or within the ovaries, on the peritoneum, or beneath the serosa of pelvic viscera. Extrapelvic endometriosis, which occurs less often, involves locations outside the genital tract, such as the bowel, rectum, appendix, umbilicus, scars, pleura, lung, kidney, ureter, bladder, and nerves.[22]

CLINICAL PRESENTATION AND DIAGNOSIS

The most frequent symptoms of genital tract endometriosis are secondary dysmenorrhea and pelvic pain, dyspareunia, menstrual irregularities, and infertility. Depending on the location of the extrapelvic endometriosis, the symptoms and signs vary. Interestingly, the severity of the disease does not directly correlate with the severity of the symptoms.[23]

TREATMENT

Danazol (Table 98.5) was the first hormonal agent approved by the Food and Drug Administration (FDA) for the treatment of endometriosis. Although considered an "antigonadotropin," its mechanism of action is much more complex in that it inhibits gonadotropin surge,

Table 98.5 ▪ Danazol Therapy for Endometriosis[a]

Dose[b]: Moderate-to-Severe Symptoms		400 mg PO BID	
Mild Symptoms		100–200 mg PO BID	
Side Effect	**Percent**	**Side Effect**	**Percent**
Weight gain	85	Decreased libido	20
Muscle cramps	52	Nausea	17
Decreased breast size	48	Headache	17
Flushing	42	Dizziness	10
Mood changes	38	Insomnia	10
Seborrhea	37	Rash	8
Depression	32	Increased libido	8
Sweating	32	Deepening voice	7
Edema	28	Increased low-density lipoprotein	<5
Change in appetite	28	Decreased high-density lipoprotein	<5
Acne	27	Increased hepatic enzymes	<5
Fatigue	25	Fetal masculinization	<5
Hirsuti	21		

Source: Reference 24.

[a]Although approved for the treatment of endometriosis, the considerable side effect profile and availability of newer, less troublesome therapies may have displaced danazol in this disorder.

[b]It is essential that therapy continue uninterrupted for 3 to 6 months but may be extended to 9 months if necessary. The dose may be adjusted to patient response.

NOTE: Cost to patient: 200 mg/day = $104 per month.
400 mg/day = $203 per month.
800 mg/day = $403 per month.

inhibits the action of steroidogenic enzymes, and interacts with androgen and progesterone receptors.[24]

Amenorrhea occurs with doses of 200 to 800 mg/day without significantly decreasing circulating levels of gonadotropins or estrogens. The manufacturer recommends use of a nonhormonal method of contraception because ovulation may occur and further warns that use of danazol during pregnancy could result in androgenic effects on the fetus that to date has been limited to clitoral hypertrophy and labial fusion of the external genitalia in the female fetus. The manufacturer further recommends that therapy begin during menstruation or after a negative result with a reliable pregnancy test.

Continuous oral progestational therapy with medroxyprogesterone acetate (MPA) is becoming popular because of its low cost and generally well-tolerated side effects compared to danazol. Although depot medroxyprogesterone acetate (DMPA) is available, oral administration may be preferable in the patient desiring to get pregnant because of the well-documented prolonged anovulatory effect of DMPA. At a daily oral dose of 50 mg for 4 months, MPA did not adversely alter serum concentrations of lipids or lipoproteins.[24] Table 98.6 lists average dose, duration, and side effects of MPA.

The inability of danazol to cause complete ovarian suppression and the high frequency of side effects associated with its use led to efforts to develop more effective agents. Long-acting GnRH agonists create a temporary and readily reversible "medical oophorectomy" and are currently the best therapy next to actual oophorectomy for the treatment of endometriosis. Endogenous GnRH is normally released in a circadian pattern every 60 to 90 minutes in the follicular phase. Downregulation of the pituitary gland occurs if the peptide is given continuously or as a long-acting synthetic agonist analog. Although GnRH agonists can be administered intravenously, intramuscularly, subcutaneously, intranasally, intravaginally, or rectally, only subcutaneous 28-day implants or once-daily doses, intramuscular monthly doses of depot forms, or twice-daily nasal sprays are currently used in the United States. Goserelin acetate subcutaneous implants, depot leuprolide acetate, and intranasal nafarelin acetate have been approved for the treatment of endometriosis by the FDA at this time. Table 98.7 lists average dosages, routes, duration and side effects for GnRH agonist preparations.

After 6 months of therapy, it has been shown that nafarelin decreased total vertebral bone mass by a mean of 5.9% at the end of treatment. Six months after completion of treatment, the total vertebral mass was still 1.4% below pretreatment levels. For this reason and because safety data for retreatment are not available, the manufacturer suggests performing bone density studies before retreating.

It is not clear which of these hormonal therapies is the most efficacious for symptomatic endometriosis.[24] Depot leuprolide, available in monthly or every 3 month dosage forms and the goserelin implant, that lasts for 28 days, have the advantage of avoiding the compliance problems that occur with daily injections or twice-daily nasal spraying.

Table 98.6 ▪ Medroxyprogesterone Acetate Therapy for Endometriosis

Dose: 30–50 mg PO daily[a]	
Side Effect	**Percent**
Amenorrhea	70
Weight gain	60
Edema, bloating	60
Dysfunctional bleeding	20
Anxiety, irritability	20
Cyclic bleeding	10
Depression	5

Source: Reference 24.

[a]Cost to patient: 30 mg daily = $46 per month.
50 mg daily = $74 per month.

Table 98.7 ▪ Gonadotropin-Releasing Hormone (GnRH) Agonists Therapy for Endometriosis

GnRH Agonist	Dosage Regimen/Route	Duration (mo)
Nafarelin (CDOC)[a]	200 μg in one nostril in the morning, 200 μg in the other nostril in the evening[b]	6
Buserlin	300 μg intranasally 3 times daily	6
Goserelin (CDOC)	3.6 mg subcutaneous biodegradable implant	6
Leuprolide	0.5 mg subcutaneously daily	6
Leuprolide (CDOC)	3.75 mg (depot) monthly	6

GnRH Agonist Side Effects

Hot flashes	Decreases libido
Vaginal dryness	Decreased bone mineral content

Source: References 24, 25.

[a]CDOC, clinical drug of choice.

[b]If amenorrhea does not occur after 2 months of treatment, use 1 spray (200 μg) into both nostrils in the morning and evening (total = 800 μg daily). Treatment should begin between days 2 and 4 of menses and not last for more than 6 months since safety data for retreatment are not available. Do not use topical nasal decongestants until 30 minutes after dosing. The manufacturer suggests use of a nonhormonal (barrier) method of contraception since the drug is pregnancy category X, having induced major malformations in 4 of 80 rat fetuses at 7 times the maximum human dose.

NOTE: Cost to patient: 400 μg/day = $45 per month.
800 μg/day = $86 per month.

[c]Clinical drug of choice. Depot leuprolide and the goserelin implant have the advantage of avoidance of compliance with daily injections or twice daily nasal sprays. With the goserelin implant, use of the required 16-gauge needle often requires a local anesthetic before insertion.

NOTE: Cost to patient: goserelin implant 3.6 mg/mo = $443 per month.
SC leuprolide 0.5 mg/day = $342 per month.
depot leuprolide 3.75 mg = $445 per month.

Although these hormonal therapies have proved effective in relieving pain and combating the histologic manifestations of endometriosis, currently no clear evidence validates the efficacy of any medical approach in treating infertility.[24]

Surgery is not necessarily a last approach in the treatment of endometriosis. Surgical techniques such as thermal ablation (destruction by heat) and cryoablation (destruction by freezing) are often used during the diagnostic laparoscopic evaluation of symptomatic patients.

Finally, the role of low-dose COCs in preventing endometriosis, in limiting progression of established disease, or in minimizing the risk of recurrence after hormonal and/or surgical therapy has not been clarified.[25] Only the lowest possible dose of estrogen should be used.[25] The cost to the patient is $15.00 to $30.00 per month.

PHARMACOECONOMICS

From a pharmacoeconomic standpoint, 80% of women who are seen with chronic pelvic pain have endometriosis. The annual cost of chronic pelvic pain in the United States is estimated to be $2.8 billion, with another $600 million for indirect costs. These costs do not include the cost of diagnostic procedures such as ultrasonography or laparoscopy or costs associated with complications of laparoscopy. Chronic pelvic pain accounts for approximately 10% of all gynecologic outpatient visits. Therefore, there may be clinical and economic benefits when GnRH agonists are used to treat endometriosis without a surgical diagnosis.[26]

Vaginitis (Vulvovaginitis)

EPIDEMIOLOGY

At least one-third of all women of childbearing age currently have one or more vulvovaginal infections. The chief symptoms are varying degrees of vaginal discharge, itching, and burning. The fear, shame, physical discomfort, esthetic revulsion, psychosexual problems, and embarrassment experienced as a result of vulvovaginal infections cause more unhappiness than any other gynecologic disorder, and the cost of treatment is substantial.[27]

PATHOPHYSIOLOGY

Normally, women of childbearing age have a thick, protective epithelium that is maintained by estrogen. A pH of 4.5 to 5.5 is maintained by the normal flora, which consists of a mixture of aerobic and anaerobic bacteria that break down epithelial cell carbohydrates, particularly glycogen, to lactic acid. The flora often includes clostridia, anaerobic streptococci (Peptostreptococcus), aerobic group D and B hemolytic streptococci, coliforms, and sometimes *Listeria*, in addition to the normally present Döderlein's bacilli (*Lactobacillus* species). If lactobacilli are suppressed by the administration of antibiotic drugs, yeasts or various bacteria normally present may become pathogenic by increasing in numbers and causing irritation and inflammation. After menopause, lactobacilli diminish, and a mixed flora predominates; the pH changes from acid to neutral or alkaline, which along with a thinning of the vaginal epithelium and a reduction of cervical mucus, leads to increased vaginal infections and atrophic vaginitis. Normally, cervical mucus has antibacterial activity and contains lysozyme. In some women, the vaginal introitus (vaginal entrance) contains a heavy flora similar to that of the perineum and perianal area, which may predispose them to recurrent urinary tract infections. Table 98.8 includes the vulvovaginitides. Herpes genitalis is discussed in Chapter 75.

Table 98.8 ▪ Prevalence of Various Vulvovaginitides in 1000 Consecutive Patients with Lower Genital Tract Infections (Gonorrhea and Syphilis Excluded)

Disorder	Incidence Number	Percentage	Percentage with One or More Other Pathogens[a]
Bacterial vaginosis	425	42.5	23.3
Vulvovaginal candidiasis	373	37.3	17.7
Trichomoniasis	142	14.2	37.7
Herpes genitalis	94	9.4	16.4
Condylomata acuminata	72	7.2	55.6

Source: Reference 27.

[a]One patient had five infections simultaneously, 2 had four, and 126 had two. Incidences and numbers of simultaneous infections depend on the patient population studied.

Bacterial Vaginosis

TREATMENT GOALS: BACTERIAL VAGINOSIS

- Restore the normal vaginal flora and alleviate the minimal vulvar itching and burning, the gray homogeneous discharge, and the fishy odor.
- Efficacy monitoring of the drug therapy does not require reexamination of the patient unless symptoms persist.

A taxonomic controversy is responsible for the many etiologies and names proposed for bacterial vaginosis (BV). The names formerly given to the disease, "*Haemophilus* vaginitis," "*Corynebacterium* vaginitis," and "*Gardnerella* vaginitis," reflected the suspected bacterial cause. Now, however, bacterial vaginosis is the preferred name, pointing to the vagina as one of the body sites in which normally colonizing bacteria may become pathogenic.

Normally, lactobacilli, the predominant vaginal organisms, control the growth of anaerobes and other bacteria by the production of hydrogen peroxide. If hydrogen peroxide is produced in very low levels, the mixed anaerobic and aerobic vaginal flora become free to proliferate 10- to 10,000-fold and grow *Gardnerella vaginalis*, which is normally present in 40 to 60% of women. *G. vaginalis* produces amino acids. Anaerobes produce enzymes that cleave these amino acids and form amines that increase vaginal pH, causing epithelial shedding that produces a discharge. Thus, a vicious cycle starts in which an elevated pH decreases lactobacilli, anaerobes predominate, and extremely high quantities of *G. vaginalis* are present.[28]

CLINICAL PRESENTATION AND DIAGNOSIS

Signs and Symptoms

The chief symptom of BV is vaginal discharge that has a characteristic foul "fish" odor that worsens after intercourse because of a shift to an alkaline pH in the vagina. This discharge is gray and homogeneous and often coats the labia. Minimal vulvovaginal itching and burning may occur.

In addition, BV has recently been associated with endometritis, pelvic inflammatory disease (PID), and vaginal cuff cellulitis after invasive procedures such as endometrial biopsy, hysterectomy, hysterosalpingography (x-ray film of the uterus and oviducts after the injection of radiopaque material), placement of intrauterine devices, cesarean section, and uterine curettage. The bacterial flora that characterizes BV has been found in the endometria and salpinges (fallopian tubes) of women who have PID. Treatment with metronidazole substantially reduces postabortion PID and is recommended for both symptomatic and asymptomatic women who have BV. More information is needed before recommending that asymptomatic women with BV be treated before other invasive procedures are performed.[29]

Diagnosis

There are four criteria used to diagnose bacterial vaginosis: (1) homogeneous vaginal discharge; (2) pH greater than 4.5; the presence of "clue cells" (a squamous epithelial cell whose border contains adherent *G. vaginalis*); and a positive "sniff" test (10% potassium hydroxide added to the discharge releases the rotten fish odor of amines).

TREATMENT

Clearly, metronidazole is the clinical drug of choice (CDOC) and therefore is the initial choice for treatment of BV in nonpregnant women. The use of metronidazole in pregnancy is controversial because although it was given a Pregnancy Category B rating , mutagenicity in bacteria, carcinogenicity in animal models, and potentiation of the fetotoxicity and teratogenicity of alcohol in mice have been observed. Recent studies suggest that BV in pregnant women is a factor in premature rupture of membranes, preterm labor, and premature delivery. Furthermore, BV organisms are often found in postpartum or postcesarean endometritis. The 1998 Guidelines for Treatment of Sexually Transmitted Diseases (1998 STD Guidelines) recommend that high-risk women (i.e., those who have previously delivered a premature infant) be screened and treated in the earliest part of the second trimester.

Metronidazole 250 mg orally three times daily for 7 days is the CDOC despite the theoretical and unproven concerns about its possible teratogenicity in humans. Metronidazole 2 g in a single dose or clindamycin 300 mg orally twice daily for 7 days are alternative regimens.[29]

Low-risk pregnant women (i.e., women who have not had a previous premature delivery) who have symptoms of BV may be treated with metronidazole 250 mg orally three times a day for 7 days or alternatively (1) metronidazole 2 g orally in a single dose, (2) clindamycin 300 mg orally twice a day for 7 days, or (3) metronidazole gel 0.75% one full applicator vaginally at bedtime daily for 5 days (NOTE: new dose since publication of the 1998 STD Guidelines that state twice daily). It is important to note that the 1998 STD Guidelines state that data are limited for the use of metronidazole vaginal gel during pregnancy. Also, the use of clindamycin vaginal cream during pregnancy is not recommended because the results of two randomized trials indicated an increase in the number of preterm deliveries in users.[29] Confusion arises because the FDA still allows the manufacturer of clindamycin vaginal cream to retain the pregnancy indication and promote its use in the second trimester of pregnancy based on safety and efficacy data pertaining to the microbiologic cure.

No clinical counterpart of BV is recognized in the male, and treatment of the male sex partner has not been shown to be beneficial for a woman's response to therapy or the likelihood of recurrence.[29]

Patients should be instructed to abstain from intercourse while taking the oral or vaginal form of the drug or to use condoms to obtain a good outcome. It is absolutely essential to complete the full course of therapy because symptoms may disappear before there is bacteriologic cure.

The current drug therapies for BV are summarized in Table 98.9.

Table 98.9 ▪ Drug Treatment of Bacterial Vaginosis[a]

Drug	Dose/Regimen
Recommended regimens for nonpregnant women	
Metronidazole (CDOC)[b]	500 mg PO BID for 7 days (95% overall cure rate)[29]
OR	
Metronidazole (CDOC)	2 g PO in a single dose (84% overall cure rate)[29]
OR	
Clindamycin vaginal cream (CDOC)	2%[c,d] app 1 p.v. h.s. for 7 days[29]
Metronidazole vaginal gel (CDOC)[f]	0.75%[e] app 1 p.v. h.s. for 5 days[29]
Alternative regimens for nonpregnant women	
Metronidazole (CDOC)	2 g PO in a single dose (84% overall cure rate)[29]
Metronidazole vaginal gel	0.75%[e] app 1 p.v. h.s. BID for 5 days[29]
Clindamycin (CDOC)	300 mg PO BID for 7 days[29]
Ampicillin	500 mg PO QID for 7 days[27]
Amoxicillin	500 mg PO TID for 7 days[27]
Cephradine	250 mg PO QID for 7 days[27]
Tetracycline	500 mg PO QID for 7 days[27]
Recommended regimen for high-risk pregnant women (previous preterm birth; treat if symptomatic or asymptomatic)	
Metronidazole (CDOC)	250 mg PO TID for 7 days[29]
Alternative regimens for high-risk pregnant women	
Metronidazole (CDOC)	2 g PO in single dose
Clindamycin (CDOC)	300 mg PO BID for 7 days[29]
Recommended regimen for low-risk pregnant women (no previous preterm birth and symptomatic)	
Metronidazole (CDOC)	250 mg PO TID for 7 days[29]
Alternative regimens for low-risk pregnant women	
Metronidazole (CDOC)	2 g PO in single dose[29]
Clindamycin (CDOC)	300 mg BID for 7 days[29]
Metronidazole vaginal gel	0.75[e,f] app 1 p.v. h.s. for 5 days[29]

[a]The principal goal of therapy is to relieve vaginal symptoms and signs. Many authorities do not recommend treatment of asymptomatic infection. Treatment of the male sex partner, who is always asymptomatic, has not been shown to be beneficial for the patient.

[b]CDOC, clinical drug of choice; oral metronidazole is clearly the best treatment.

[c]Recommended in pregnancy and as an alternative to metronidazole.

[d]Mean bioavailability is about 4%; contains mineral oil and may weaken latex condoms and diaphragms.

[e]Preferred by some health care providers because of lack of certain systemic side effects such as mild-to-moderate gastrointestinal upset and unpleasant taste, and mean peak serum concentration is <2% that of the standard 500 mg PO dose.

[f]New approved dose since the publication of the 1998 STD Guidelines that still recommend BID for 5 days.

Vulvovaginal Candidiasis

TREATMENT GOALS: VULVOVAGINAL CANDIDIASIS

- Restore normal vaginal flora and thereby alleviate the vulvar erythema; the fungal patches; the severe itching and burning of the vagina, vulva, or both; and the white, dry, curdlike vaginal discharge.
- Alleviation of symptoms is evidence of efficacy, and reexamination of the patient is unnecessary unless symptoms persist.
- Of all the drug therapies for vulvovaginal candidiasis (VVC), only nystatin is fungistatic and is therefore no longer recommended.[29] *Candida glabrata* is best treated with gentian violet.

EPIDEMIOLOGY

The female genital tract and bowel are colonized by *Candida albicans* in 90 to 95% of patients and *C. glabrata* in the other 5 to 10% and are asymptomatic. Because of this, the terms for symptomatic candidiasis or moniliasis have been replaced with the term *vaginal candidosis* by some authors. Approximately 75% of women will have one episode of VVC and 40 to 45% will have two or more episodes. Less than 5% will experience recurrent VVC (RVVC).[29]

Factors predisposing to VVC include:[27]

1. Pregnancy and "pseudopregnancy" from oral contraceptives by vaginal thinning from progestins, altered sexual habits (i.e., anal followed by vaginal intercourse), increased *Candida* colonization (but not infection).
2. Antibiotic therapy, by increasing candidal colonization as a result of suppression of bacterial competition from the genital tract and bowel, reduced phagocytosis of Candida, and direct growth stimulation of *Candida.*
3. Diabetes mellitus, if poorly controlled, by increased glucose secretions, or alterations in the immune system.

CLINICAL PRESENTATION AND DIAGNOSIS

The chief symptoms of VVC are severe itching of the vulva, vagina, or both and meatal (urethral external opening) dysuria. The vulvitis symptoms are often aggravated by tight clothing.

There are three criteria for the diagnosis of VVC: (1) thick, white, curdlike secretions; (2) pH ≤4.5; and (3) long threadlike fibers of mycelia with tiny buds of conidia attached that are apparent when 1 or 2 drops of 10% potassium hydroxide are added to a vaginal exudate slide (KOH preparation).

Nickerson's media is infrequently used to confirm the diagnosis before the treatments summarized in Table 98.10 are instituted.

TREATMENT

Patient compliance improves as the duration of therapy decreases. Fortunately, the 3-day therapies listed in Table 98.10 are approximately as effective as the 7-day therapies.[30,31] Single-day therapies, other than oral fluconazole, should only be used for uncomplicated mild or early VVC.

Patients should understand that strict compliance to the treatment is necessary, that creams are usually preferable to tablets or suppositories because some cream can be applied to the perineum, and that treatment should always be continued through menses, if it occurs, and when vaginal contraceptives are used. The patient should also be instructed to report any new vaginal irritation because vaginal irritation in 0 to 6.6% of users has been reported with miconazole >tioconazole >butoconazole >clotrimazole >nystatin. Irritation may necessitate changing the drug therapy. Terconazole use has been reported to cause headaches in 26% of the patients. When gentian violet is used, the patient should be advised of its permanent purple staining characteristics. If a patient uses gentian violet applied to tampons, she must be warned of the possible increased risk of toxic shock syndrome (TSS) and should be told that TSS is a rare illness that can be fatal and that is characterized by high fever (102°F or greater), hypotension, a sunburnlike rash with desquamation 1 to 2 weeks after onset, vomiting, or diarrhea. If TSS symptoms occur, the patient should discontinue tampon use and contact her physician immediately.

Recurrent Vulvovaginal Candidiasis

DEFINITION

RVVC is usually defined as four or more episodes of symptomatic VVC occurring annually and affects less than 5% of women. It may be due to:

1. Intestinal reservoir: Up to 100% correlation has been found between simultaneous infestations of *C. albicans* in the vaginal and fecal material. A persistent intestinal reservoir may recolonize the perianal area and lead to recurrent infection.[32]
2. Sexual transmission: Unequivocal proof that a colonized penis may transmit *C. albicans* is lacking even though circumstantial evidence shows that 5 to 25% of male partners of infected females may asymptomatically carry yeast, usually in the coronal sulcus. Some clinicians advocate treatment of the male for 7 days with a cream (Table 98.10).[32]

Table 98.10 ▪ Drug Treatment of Vaginal Candidiasis

Drug/Dose	Regimen (days)
Seven-day therapy	
Clotrimazole 1% Vag Cr (CDOC)[a,b,c]	App 1 p.v. h.s. × 7
Clotrimazole 100 mg Vag tabs[b,c]	Tab 1 p.v. h.s. × 7
Miconazole nitrate 2% Vag Cr[b,c]	App 1 p.v. h.s. × 7
Miconazole nitrate 100 mg Vag Supp[b,c]	Supp[b,c] 1 p.v. h.s. × 7
Terconazole 0.4% Vag Cr[b]	App 1 p.v. h.s. × 7
Tioconazole 80 mg Supp[b]	Supp 1 p.v. h.s. × 7
Three-day therapy[d]	
Butoconazole nitrate 2% Vag Cr[b,c]	App 1 p.v. h.s. × 3
Clotrimazole 1% Vag Cr[b,c]	App 1 p.v. BID × 3
Clotrimazole 100 mg Vag Tabs[b,c]	Tab 2 p.v. h.s. × 3
Miconazole nitrate 2% Vag Cr[b,c]	App 1 p.v. BID × 3
Miconazole nitrate 200 mg Vag Supp[b,c]	Supp[b] 1 p.v. h.s. × 3
Terconazole 80 mg Vag Supp[b]	Supp 1 p.v. h.s. × 3
Terconazole 0.8% Vag Cr[b]	App 1 p.v. h.s. × 3
One-day therapy[e]	
Clotrimazole 500 mg Vag Tab[b,f]	Tab 1 p.v. h.s. × 1
Fluconazole 150 mg PO tablet[g]	Tab 1 PO × 1
Tioconazole 6.5% Vag Oint[b,c]	App 1 p.v. h.s. × 1
Miscellaneous therapies	
Itraconazole 200 mg oral	Cap 1 PO BID × 3
Ketoconazole 200 mg Oral Tab[h]	Tab 1 PO BID × 3
Gentian violet tampons 5 mg[i]	Tampon 1 p.v. 1–2 times daily for 3–4 hr for 12 days
Miconazole Tampons 100 mg[j]	Tampon 1 p.v. h.s. × 5

Vag, vaginal; *cr*, cream; *App*, applicator; *Tab*, tablet; *supp*, suppository; *oint*, ointment; *cap*, capsules.

[a]CDOC, clinical drug of choice would be any of the 7-day therapies.

[b]NOTE: These creams and suppositories are oil based and may weaken latex condoms and diaphragms.

[c]Over-the-counter preparations. If symptoms persist after use or if there is a recurrence of symptoms within 2 months, medical care should be sought.[27]

[d]Three-day therapies are as effective as 7-day therapies except for pregnant, diabetic, or corticosteroid-using women. For these conditions, use only 7-day therapy.

[e]One-day therapy is approximately as effective as 2- or 3-day therapies for mild-to-moderate, sporadic, nonrecurrent VVC in a normal woman. Severe local or recurrent VVC in a woman with diabetes or other immune dysfunction caused by a less susceptible pathogen such as *Candida glabrata* may require 10–14 days of therapy. Any woman when symptoms persist after using an over-the-counter preparation or who has a recurrence within 2 months should seek medical care.[29]

[f]Single dose serves as a vaginal depot for at least 3 days.[30]

[g]Superior to 3 days of vaginal clotrimazole 200 mg, and symptoms were relieved more rapidly.[31]

[h]Should be the last treatment of choice for recurrent or persistent cases since the drug is hepatotoxic and is contraindicated in pregnancy because of its known teratogenic effects in rats manifested as limb deformities; clinically significant drug interactions may occur with astemizole, calcium channel antagonists, cisapride, coumadin, cyclosporin A, oral hypoglycemic agents, phenytoin, protease inhibitors, tacrolimus, terfenadine, theophylline, trimetrexate, and rifampin.

[i]Best treatment for *C. glabrata*. Caution: purple staining.

[j]Data on file for 123 patients, Advanced Care Products, claims 5 days to be as effective as 7 days of miconazole nitrate cream with similar side effects; the manufacturer claims that the therapeutic effect is not affected by menstruation. The use of nonmedicated tampons has been associated with an increased risk of toxic shock syndrome; this product is available only in California at the time of writing.

NOTE: If any first course fails, reconfirm diagnosis with microscopic examination and treat with an alternative drug.

NOTE: Any of the above medications[29] except ketoconazole, can be used for pregnant patients.

NOTE: Nystatin Vag Tabs 100,000 U are intentionally left off this table because they are only fungistatic, whereas all the other therapies are fungicidal.[29]

3. Therapy failure: *Candida* blastospores invade intact epithelial cells in the superficial layers of the vaginal mucosa to a depth of several layers and may reemerge weeks or months later when the epithelial cells are normally shed. Approximately 20 to 50% of women clinically responding by culture to standard antifungal therapy have positive culture results within 30 days.[32]

TREATMENT

For RVVC, the following regimens may be used. For nonpregnant women give ketoconazole 200 mg oral tablets, one twice daily for 3 days[33] or fluconazole 150 mg oral tablet once. Only male partners who experience symptomatic balanitis or penile dermatitis should be treated with a topical cream (Table 98.10) for 7 days. For pregnant women give nystatin 500,000-U oral tablets, one three times daily for 14 days, plus clotrimazole 1% vaginal cream applied once vaginally at bedtime for 14 days. Only male partners who experience symptomatic balanitis or penile dermatitis should be treated with topical antifungal creams (Table 98.10) for 14 days.

The 1998 STD Guidelines, however, state that the optimal treatment has not been established and that after confirmation by culture, maintenance therapy with ketoconazole 100 mg orally once daily can be used for up to 6 months. As part of the evaluation for predisposing conditions, human immunodeficiency virus (HIV) testing should only be done in women with predisposing factors for HIV infection. Women who have acute VVC and are HIV positive can have the same response to conventional antifungal therapy as HIV-negative women, and there is insufficient evidence to determine optimal treatment for RVVC in HIV-positive women at this time.[29]

Trichomonas Vaginitis

DEFINITION

Trichomoniasis is a disease of the vagina that also occurs in the lower urinary tract of men and women.

TREATMENT GOALS: TRICHOMONAS VAGINITIS

- Restore the normal vaginal flora and thereby alleviate the vaginal itching, burning, and the malodorous yellow-green or gray discharge.
- Reexamination is necessary only when symptoms persist.

EPIDEMIOLOGY

Sexual transmission is well recognized although transmission by communal fomites (substances capable of absorbing and transmitting the contagium of disease), such as toilet splash, gloves, and instruments, may occur rarely. Transmission to newborns from untreated mothers also occurs, and the child will require treatment. Male partners should be treated simultaneously because 80% may be culture positive.[27]

CLINICAL PRESENTATION AND DIAGNOSIS

Signs and Symptoms

The chief symptoms of *Trichomonas vaginitis* infection are variable, ranging from a mild yellow-green or gray vaginal discharge, to a moderate malodorous discharge, to itching, burning discharge with odor, to intermenstrual or postcoital bleeding. Dysuria is present in at least 10% of patients.

Diagnosis

There are four diagnostic parameters: (1) thick or thin white, yellow, green, or gray malodorous discharge; (2) pH 5.0 to 7.5; (3) highly motile, pear-shaped, unicellular *T. vaginalis* seen with saline mount microscopy (a flagellated protozoan about twice the size of a white blood cell); and (4) "strawberry" vagina or cervix, seen only in about 10% of patients, due to swollen papillae projecting through vaginal secretions

TREATMENT

Table 98.11 summarizes the current treatment of *T. vaginitis* in primary and recurrent cases. Unfortunately, metronidazole is the only adequately effective treatment and is therefore the CDOC. Because 80% of male partners may be culture positive, they must be treated simultaneously.

IMPROVING OUTCOMES

Patient education should include discussion of the necessity of strict compliance with the simultaneous treatment for both partners and the use of condoms until the regimen is completed. A metallic taste in the mouth and brown urine may occur. Patients taking metronidazole should avoid the consumption of alcohol because of the possibility of a disulfiram-type reaction.

Table 98.11 ▪ Drug Treatment of *Trichomonas* Vaginitis

Recommended regimen
  Metronidazole CDOC 500 mg tabs: 4 PO in a single dose
Alternate regimen
  Metronidazole 500 mg BID for 7 days

1. Male sex partners of infected women should be treated with regimen A or B.
2. Asymptomatic women should be treated with regimen A or B.
3. If failure occurs with either regimen, the patient should be treated with metronidazole 500 mg twice daily for 7 days.
4. If repeated failure occurs, the patient should be treated with a single 2-g dose of metronidazole daily for 3 to 5 days.
5. Patients for whom there are additional culture-documented treatment failures in which reinfection has been excluded should be managed in consultation with an expert who can determine the susceptibility of *Trichomonas vaginalis* to metronidazole.
6. Pregnant patients can be treated with 2 g of metronidazole in a single dose.
7. For lactating women, use regimen A, interrupting breast feeding for at least 24 hours after therapy.

Source: Reference 29.

The author recently comanaged a patient with culture susceptabilities by and recommendations from the Centers for Disease Control and Prevention, using furazolidione 100 mg per 5 g of 2% nonoxynol-9 contraceptive jelly, 5 g vaginally twice daily along with metronidazole 1 g orally twice daily for 14 days. Tinidazole, which generally has increased activity against *T. vaginalis,* is only available from a Canadian investigator and was ineffective against this patient's strain. A recent article reported the use of 6.25% (250 mg per 4 g applicatorful) paromomycin cream vaginally nightly for 14 days for patients with metronidazole resistance and 5 with allergy. Six of the 9 were cured.[34]

[a]Although the FDA has approved Flagyl 375 mg twice daily for 7 days on the basis of pharmacokinetic equivalency to metronidazole 250 mg three times daily for 7 days, there are no clinical data available and 1998 STD guidelines do not recommend its use.

Genital and Anal Warts (Condylomata Acuminata)

TREATMENT GOALS: GENITAL AND ANAL WARTS

- Destroy the human papillomavirus (HPV)-infected tissue, prevent recurrence and sexual transmission, and possibly prevent the sequelae of squamous cell genital cancer.
- Unfortunately, no therapy has been shown to eradicate HPV. HPV has been demonstrated in adjacent tissue after laser treatment of HPV-associated cervical intraepithelial neoplasia and after attempts to eliminate subclinical HPV by extensive laser vaporization of the anogenital area. Therefore, the goal of treatment is not the eradication of HPV.[29]
- Sex partners should be examined for evidence of warts and treated as needed.

EPIDEMIOLOGY

Approximately 60% of sexual partners of persons infected with condylomata acuminata develop genital or anal warts, with an average incubation period of 2 to 3 months. The typical lesions in women are most often found in the fourchette (the fold connecting the two labia minora posteriorly) and on the labia and less commonly found on other parts of the vulva, perineum, and anus. In addition, cervical warts are common. During pregnancy, genital warts tend to enlarge and grow more rapidly, taking on a cauliflower appearance. They may involve the labia and vagina rather than the perianal area and may render vaginal delivery difficult. The causative agent is the HPV. A decade ago, genital and anal warts were thought to be trivial lesions of little importance. However, today, as a result of a 460% increase in 15 years in the United States, they are recognized as one of the most important of the sexually transmitted diseases. There is an estimated 2% incidence of flat condyloma of the cervix of all women of childbearing age. These data suggest that genital and anal warts are being encountered as often as herpes genitalis and gonorrhea.[35]

Recently, many investigators have found that under certain circumstances some types of HPV (most commonly types 16, 18, 31, 33, 35, 45, and 56) are strongly associated with genital dysplasia and carcinoma.[36] Fortunately, most exophytic genital warts are most often caused by HPV types 6 and 11. However, a biopsy is needed in all instances of atypical, pigmented, or persistent warts. All women with anogenital warts should have a regular Pap smear.[29]

CLINICAL PRESENTATION AND DIAGNOSIS

The chief symptom reported by patients is an occasional itching of the lesions. Diagnosis is made by the presence of verrucose growths, usually on the vulva or genital area, and a positive sexual history.

TREATMENT

Treatment of genital warts should be guided by the preference of the patient, the available resources, and the experience of the health care provider. None of the available treatments is superior to other treatments, and no single treatment is ideal for all warts.[29] Patient-applied and provider-administered treatments of external genital warts, cervical warts, vaginal warts, urethral meatus warts, anal warts, and oral warts are summarized in Table 98.12. Treatments include cytotoxic, destructive, immunologic, and surgical methods. The cytotoxic treatment regimens with podophyllin, podofilox, or 5-fluorouracil and the destructive treatment with trichloroacetic acid are covered in Table 98.12.

Cryotherapy with liquid nitrogen or dry ice, electrosurgery, and carbon dioxide lasers[37] are other useful destructive treatments. Shave and scissor excision of larger lesions is an acceptable surgical method.

Imiquimod is the newest in a class of drugs called immune response modifiers. It induces the production five subtypes of the cytokine interferon-α, enhances cell-mediated cytolytic activity against viral targets, and thereby mimics the body's natural response to viral infections. New warts have been known to develop during treatmen.[29,38] Imiquimod cream may weaken latex diaphragms and condoms.

Estrogen Replacement Therapy

The female climacteric (a period of female life, preceding termination of the reproductive period, characterized by endocrine, somatic, and psychic changes, and ultimately menopause) is a clinical epoch secondary to the physiologic depletion of ovarian follicles. Menopause refers to the cessation of menses. A patient is postmenopausal after 1 year of amenorrhea secondary to ovarian failure secondary to lack of functional ovarian follicles. Surprisingly, this occurs in approximately 5% of women before reaching 40 years of age. It is estimated that more than

Table 98.12 ▪ Drug Treatment of Genital or Anal Warts (Condylomata Accuminata)[a]

External genital warts, recommended treatment[27]

Provider-administered

Trichloroacetic acid (TCA) or bichloroacetic acid (BCA) 80–90% (CDOC)[b]

1. Apply skin protectant[d] to surrounding tissues.
2. Treatment is adequate if a white color develops 30–60 seconds later.
3. Patient will experience a sharp, burning pain for 15–30 minutes.
4. Repeat weekly if necessary.

Podophyllin resin 10–25% in compound tincture of benzoin

1. Apply skin protectant[d] to surrounding tissues.
2. Apply <0.5 mL per treatment; treat <10 cm.^{2}
3. Wash off thoroughly in 1–4 hours.
4. If four applications fail, other treatments are indicated.
5. Not for extensive lesions or during pregnancy because podophyllin is absorbed and is toxic.

Patient-applied

Podofilox 0.5% topical solution

1. Apply skin protectant[c] to surrounding tissues.
2. Apply with a cotton-tipped applicator twice daily morning and evening (every 12 hours), for 3 consecutive days, then withhold use for 4 consecutive days. This 1-week cycle of treatment may be repeated up to four times until there is no visible wart tissue. If there is incomplete response after 4 treatment weeks, alternative treatment should be considered since the safety and effectiveness of more than 4 treatment weeks have not been established.
3. Treatment should be limited to less than 10 cm^2 of wart tissue and to no more than 0.5 mL of the solution per day.
4. Systemic absorption studies did not result in detectable serum levels. However, it should be used in pregnancy only if TCA or BCA therapy fails.

Imiquimod 5% cream (CDOC)

1. Apply with a finger at bedtime, three times a week for as long as 16 weeks.
2. The treatment area should be washed with mild soap and water 6–10 hours after application.
3. Warts may disappear by 8–10 weeks or sooner in many patients.
4. The safety of imiquimod during pregnancy has not been established.

5-Fluorouracil cream 5%[37] (CDOC)

1. Only for vaginal/cervical/penile warts.
2. Female: Insert ½ vaginal applicator (2.5 g) p.v. h.s. for 5 days.
   Male: Apply 1–2 nights weekly to entire penis; avoid the urethra; therapy is for 3 months; apply a tissue between underside of penis and scrotum, and wear a jockstrap to keep penis in place.
3. Female to apply a skin protectant[c] to vulva and urethra h.s. and a.m. after washing external genitalia.
4. Avoid during pregnancy because it may be teratogenic.

Cervical warts

High-grade squamous intraepithelial lesions (SIL) must be ruled out by an expert before treatment is begun.

Vaginal warts

Cryotherapy with liquid nitrogen, TCA or BCA 80–90%, or podophyllin 10–25%, as above.

Urethral meatus warts

Cryotherapy with liquid nitrogen or podophyllin 10–25%, as above.

Anal warts

Cryotherapy with liquid nitrogen or TCA or BCA 80–90%, as above.

Oral warts

Cryotherapy with liquid nitrogen or surgical removal.

Source: References 29, 35.

[a]Condoms should be used until warts disappear.

[b]CDOC, clinical drug of choice.

[c]Zinc oxide ointment 20%, silicone cream, or silver sulfadiazine 1% cream.

36 million women in the United States will become menopausal during the next decade.[39] By age 51.1, the average age of menopause, a woman can expect to live another 28 years. Therefore, more than 32 million women in the United States 51.1 years of age and older can expect to live 40% of their lives in a state of relative estrogen deficiency. The consequences of this estrogen deficiency include vasomotor instability, atrophic vaginitis, and osteoporosis.

TREATMENT GOALS: ESTROGEN REPLACEMENT

- Prevent menopausal symptoms, vaginal atrophy, dysuria secondary to estrogen deficiency, osteoporosis, and cardiovascular disease.
- Instruct all patients to perform monthly breast self-examinations and report any lumps or retractions discovered.

Table 98.13 ▪ Treatment of Hot Flushes and Equivalent Estrogen Replacement Therapy (ERT) Regimens[a]

Generic Name	Equivalent Regimen
Conjugated estrogens (CDOC)[b]	0.625 mg PO × 25 days/mo[c]
Esterified estrogens	0.625 mg PO × 25 days/mo[c]
Esterified estrogens with methyltestosterone 1.25 mg	0.625 mg one PO × 25 days/mo[c,d]
Estropipate	0.625 mg PO × 25 days/mo[c]
Ethinyl estradiol	0.2 mg PO × 25 days/mo[c]
17β-estradiol	0.5 mg × 25 days/mo[c]
17β-estradiol (transdermal)	0.05 mg patch to skin BIW[e]
Medroxyprogesterone acetate	20 mg PO daily[f]
Clonidine	0.2 mg PO BID[g]

[a]With all ERT regimens, add medroxyprogesterone acetate 5 mg for 10–14 days/month or 2.5 mg daily to prevent endometrial hyperplasia and possible malignancy in all women who have not had their uterus removed. Micronized progesterone 100 mg BID × 14d or 100 mg daily may also be used.

[b]CDOC, clinical drug of choice; conjugated estrogens are the initial choice because of the extensive literature on their use.

[c]Over 80% of ERT patients in the United States are given conjugated estrogens. Little in the literature supports the advantage of one preparation over another if equivalent doses are used.

[d]Only indicated for the treatment of moderate-to-severe vasomotor symptoms not improved by estrogens alone.

[e]75% effective similar to oral ERT; up to 20% minor skin irritation.[39] Least skin irritation if applied to buttocks. Recently also available as a once-weekly patch.

[f]Mechanism unknown; >70% effective; not an approved use; may be used when estrogens are contraindicated; about one-third of women with intact uteri may have vaginal bleeding. Progestins will not prevent vaginal atrophy and may not prevent osteoporosis.[40]

[g]α-Adrenergic agonist; <50% effective; dry mouth and sedation limit usefulness; not approved use; more studies needed; last choice.[41]

- Instruct patients to report any signs of jaundice such as yellowing of the skin or sclera.
- Instruct patients to report any irregular noncyclic bleeding because it may indicate neoplastic changes in the genital tract. Tell postmenopausal patients that they may have withdrawal bleeding when receiving cyclic regimens of estrogen and progestin (Table 98.13), as long as they have intact uteri.

Vasomotor Symptoms

Approximately 80% of women within the first year of ovarian failure or castration experience hot flushes that are caused by a decrease in the tone of arterioles, resulting in an increased blood flow to the skin and resultant rise in skin temperature. Hot flushes appear to be synchronous with increased hypothalamic release of GnRH. Because GnRH neurons are close to the centers that regulate temperature in the intact hypothalamus, it is likely that α-adrenergic stimulation of GnRH release concomitantly stimulates these centers. Although the symptoms may last for at least 5 years for 70% of this group, homeostatic adjustments eventually occur. The most likely explanation of why all women do not experience hot flushes seems to be varying amounts of endogenous estradiol (5 to 20 μg/day versus 50 to 300 μg/day before menopause) produced in the liver and adipose tissue. Obese women may produce twice as much estradiol as slender women. Some of these obese women may still experience symptoms.

TREATMENT GOALS: VASOMOTOR SYMPTOMS

- The treatment goals of ERT for women with hot flashes are not only to control temperature regulation but also to correct resultant sleep deprivation, which is thought to contribute to cognitive dysfunction in these patients.

CLINICAL PRESENTATION AND DIAGNOSIS

Signs and Symptoms

The chief vasomotor symptoms reported by patients are described as hot flushes or hot flashes occurring over the anterior part of the body, especially the chest, neck, and face. An episode lasts usually only a few minutes and is commonly precipitated by anxiety or excitement. The vasomotor symptoms vary considerably in duration, frequency, and severity. One variation, night sweats, is experienced by some patients who usually describe awakening at night, covered in perspiration, and throwing off the bed covers.

It is estimated that following physiologic menopause, 15% of patients seek treatment for vasomotor symptoms; 50% of reproductive-age women undergoing castration request treatment. The vasomotor symptoms themselves are not thought to be harmful, but they indicate an estrogen deficiency state and are usually treated on request. The lowest dosage of estrogen to reduce the vasomotor symptoms to a tolerable level should be used with reevaluation every 6 months. Reduced symptoms during the drug-free evaluation period are found within 2 to 5 years of menopause. Clinically, there is no reasonable means to follow the response to treatment other than subjective symptomatic improvement.

Diagnosis

All potential patients for estrogen therapy should undergo a baseline evaluation, including pelvic examination, cytology, breast examination, blood pressure, and a thorough history, to rule out the following absolute and relative contraindications:

- Absolute
  - Undiagnosed vaginal bleeding
  - Suspected breast cancer
  - Suspected endometrial cancer
  - Active venous thrombosis
- Possibly absolute (under debate)
  - History of breast cancer
  - History of endometrial cancer
  - Malignant melanoma
- Relative
  - Uterine fibroids
  - Endometriosis
  - History of cholelithiasis
  - History of migraine
  - Hypertriglyceridemia
  - Liver disease

TREATMENT

Recommended therapies for vasomotor symptoms and equivalent ERT doses and regimens[39–41] appear in Table 98.14.

Table 98.14 ▪ Currently Recommended Treatments for Vaginal Atrophy and Dysuria[a,b]

Generic Name	Regimen
Conjugated estrogen cream 0.625 mg/g (CDOC)[c]	0.2–1 g p.v. daily × 10, then BIW–TIW
Estropipate cream 1.25 mg/g	0.2–1 g p.v. daily × 10, then BIW–TIW
17-β-estradiol cream 0.1 mg/g	0.2–1 g p.v. daily × 10, then BIW–TIW
Dienestrol cream 0.01%	0.2–1 full applicator daily × 10, then BIW–TIW
Estradiol vaginal ring	p.v. for 90 days releases 7.5 μg/24 hr (0.6 μg absorbed)[d]

[a]Most experts recommend cyclic addition of 10–13 days of progestin monthly if the uterus is present to prevent endometrial hyperplasia and possible malignancy.

[b]These regimens are extrapolated from Dyer and Townsend[42] and differ from the manufacturer's recommendations.

[c]CDOC, clinical drug of choice.

[d]May become clinical drug of choice for patients with breast cancer.

IMPROVING OUTCOMES

Continuation of therapy is a major problem with patients receiving ERT/HRT. Many patients require additional interventions between visits to assure patient satisfaction and compliance. The role of the pharmacist as a proactive comanager of perimenopausal and menopausal women is currently being studied by the author and his specialty resident in women's health within the University of California, San Francisco National Center of Excellence in Women's Health. This is an area where the pharmacist can make a huge impact on the health care system and one that is sure to lead to reimbursement for cognitive services. Patient education should include the potential disease preventative effects as well as the symptomatic relief provided by ERT/HRT. The major adverse effects of estrogen therapy as well as instructions about the importance of yearly physical examinations, repeating the baseline tests should be stressed. Patients should also be warned taking estrogens combined with the adverse cardiovascular and neoplastic effects of smoking may contribute to these disorders although this has not been established in the literature.

Vaginal Atrophy, Atrophic Vaginitis, and Dysuria

Postmenopausal estrogen deficiency leads to a thinning of the vaginal epithelium, a decreased blood supply, dryness, and a change to a neutral or alkaline pH that predisposes to infection.

TREATMENT GOALS: VAGINAL ATROPHY, ATROPHIC VAGINITIS, DYSURIA

- Eliminate the atrophy, dysuria, and predisposition to vaginal infections caused by estrogen deficiency.

CLINICAL PRESENTATION AND DIAGNOSIS

The chief symptoms are vaginal discharge secondary to infection, complaints of painful intercourse (dyspareunia) due to dryness, and dysuria. Estrogens increase the vascularity and epithelial proliferation of the vagina, allowing greater lubrication, increased protection from vaginitis, and reduced vaginal trauma from coitus. The increased vascularity resulting from estrogen therapy is associated with increased blood flow through the periurethral venous plexus, leading to small increases in periurethral pressure occasionally sufficient to correct urinary stress incontinence.

TREATMENT

The atrophy and dysuria can be treated with equal effectiveness by either systemic or vaginally applied estrogen. However, the response to conjugated locally applied estrogen cream may be lost after 14 days because of tissue cornification or downregulation of the estrogen receptors. For this reason, the systemic effects and topical response may be erratic. This can be overcome by stopping treatment for 7 to 14 days and restarting using 0.1 mg daily rather than the 1.25- to 2.5-mg dose recommended by the manufacturer.[42] Conjugated estrogens, estropipate, and estradiol vaginal creams contain 0.625, 1.25, and 0.1 mg/g, respectively, and include applicators graduated from 1 to 4 g. One gram is roughly equivalent to a full applicator of dienestrol cream 0.01%.

A vaginal ring is available, which is therapeutically equivalent to the estrogen vaginal creams. It contains a total of 2 mg of estradiol and releases approximately 7.5 μg/24 hr for 3 months. Because approximately only 8% of the estradiol (0.6 μg) is systemically absorbed daily, serum levels of estradiol at steady state are within the range observed in untreated postmenopausal women (<50 pmol/L).[43] Because of the limited absorption, researchers are planning to test this product in women having a history of breast cancer for relief of the signs and symptoms of urogenital atrophy.

Conjugated estrogen vaginal cream and its equivalents have four times the activity of oral estrogens on local tissues. Patient instructions and warnings are basically the same as with oral estrogens because systemic estrogen levels may be reached. Most experts recommend the addition of 10 to 14 days of MPA 5 mg daily, 2.5 mg daily, or micronized progesterone 100 mg BID for 10 to 14 days or 100 mg daily in women with intact uteri to prevent endometrial hyperplasia and possible malignancy. Current recommended treatments for vaginal atrophy and dysuria are listed in Table 98.14.

Osteoporosis Secondary to Estrogen Deficiency

TREATMENT GOALS: OSTEOPOROSIS SECONDARY TO ESTROGEN DEFICIENCY

- Prevent and/or treat bone loss secondary to estrogen deficiency.

EPIDEMIOLOGY

Conservatively, osteoporosis secondary to estrogen deficiency may be responsible for 100,000 wrist fractures and 250,000 hip fractures annually in the United States. The cost of acute care may total $3 billion after hip fractures, and the mortality may be as high as 15 to 30%, or 27,000 to 60,000 deaths per year, for the year after a hip fracture, usually because of complications such as pneumonia, pulmonary embolism, or congestive heart failure. An additional 40,000 patients will require prolonged institutionalization,[45] and this helps bring the annual total of direct and indirect costs to $14 billion.[46]

In women, maximal mineral content in cortical bone of the radius occurs in the mid-30s and declines 3% per decade until menopause, at which time it declines 9% per decade until age 75 and thereafter returns to a 3% decline per decade, with as much as 66% skeletal loss by age 80. Of women older than age 60, 25% have spinal compression fractures, causing much pain and debilitation; by age 75, this figure reaches 50%.[45]

TREATMENT

Because which patients will be prone to osteoporosis cannot be predicted, all women who are postmenopausal or lack ovarian function or ovaries should receive ERT, when not contraindicated, soon after the diagnosis of estrogen deficiency. An exception to this may be African-American women, who have a greater bone mass and higher calcitonin levels than non-African-American women, leading to a low risk for osteoporosis. Some African-American women may need ERT only for premature surgical menopause, hot flushes, atrophic vaginitis, or estrogen-deficiency dysuria.

A decline in circulating estrogens enhances calcium efflux from bone mineral stores and increases the serum concentration of ionized calcium. This suppresses secretion of parathyroid hormone (PTH), which, in turn, reduces the synthesis of 1,25-dihydroxyvitamin D_3 by the renal tubular cells. The lowered concentration of 1,25-dihydroxyvitamin D_3 causes a decrease in the intestinal absorption of calcium. Studies of PTH and vitamin D have not demonstrated a consistent relationship between their levels and osteoporosis. However, calcitonin secretion progressively declines with age and estrogen deficiency. Calcitonin inhibits bone resorption and is known to be increased with ERT. Therefore, there may be beneficial effects on bone due to estrogens at nonestrogen or estrogen receptor sites.

Osteoporosis Prevention

TREATMENT GOALS: OSTEOPOROSIS PREVENTION

- ERT and HRT are approved for the prevention and treatment of osteoporosis.
- In some patients, the risks associated with hormonal therapy and the need for lifelong ERT/HRT to prevent osteoporosis have made both patients and practitioners hesitant to use ERT/HRT.

EPIDEMIOLOGY

The association of endometrial cancer with unopposed ERT exists. It is well known that estrogens stimulate the growth of the endometrium and that the resultant proliferation can potentially progress to atypical hyperplasia and adenocarcinoma. The highest incidence of endometrial cancer occurs in users of estrogens not opposed by progestins, the lowest incidence is seen in users of estrogen and progestin combination therapy, and intermediate incidence is seen in women not taking estrogens or progestins. Progestins decrease estrogen receptors in endometrial cells and induce estradiol dehydrogenase and isocitrate activity, which are the mechanisms whereby these cells metabolize estrogens.[42]

Although some studies have found that ERT/HRT increases the risk of breast cancer in postmenopausal women,[47,48] other studies have shown little or no relationship.[49,50] A reanalysis of epidemiologic data on more than 160,000 women from 51 investigation centers has shown a 2.3% increase in breast cancer risk per year, with women who have ever used estrogen having a statistically significant relative risk (RR) of 1.14, current users having a RR of 1.35, and with former users having a RR of 1.07 (not statistically different).[51] A recent study from Finland of 988 current users of ERT and 757 former users found that breast cancer morbidity did not increase in current users (RR 0.57 [95% confidence interval (CI) 0.27 to 1.20]) compared to former users (RR 0.94 [0.47 to 1.90]) and that the RR for breast cancer did not rise significantly (former users 0.96 [0.48 to 1.95]; current users 0.63 [0.30 to 1.35]).[52] Women taking ERT/HRT should be encouraged to perform monthly breast self-examinations, have regular physical examinations, and have mammography every 1 to 2 years after age 40 and annually after age 50.[39]

In general, epidemiologic data from case-control and cohort studies have suggested that postmenopausal estrogen confers a moderate degree of protection from coronary artery disease, with reductions in overall mortality rates for acute myocardial infarction in comparison with nonestrogen users.[53]

The Postmenopausal Estrogen/Progestin Interventions (PEPI) Trial has shown that estrogen alone, or in combination with a progestin, improves lipoproteins and lowers fibrinogen levels without detectable effects on postchallenge insulin or blood pressure. It further showed that conjugated equine estrogens 0.625 mg daily plus 200 mg of micronized oral progesterone for 12 days of the month had the most favorable effect on high-density lipoprotein cholesterol (HDL-C) with no excess risk of endometrial hyperplasia.[54]

The Heart and Estrogen/Progestin Replacement Study (HERS) was a 4.1 year randomized, double blind, placebo-controlled secondary prevention trial of 2,763 women using conjugated equine estrogen 0.625 mg plus MPA 2.5 mg daily as a treatment to protect against recurrent CHD. Additional patient risk factors for CHD included 18% of patients who had diabetes, 55% of patients who were overweight, and 13% who were smokers. HRT in these postmenopausal women did not reduce the overall incidence of recurrent myocardial infarction and CHD death compared with placebo (RR 1.52, 95% CI 1.01 to 2.29) in the first year. However, HRT resulted in fewer second events reducing linearly by the fourth and fifth years of treatment from 4.25 per 100 patients per year in the first year to 2.30 (RR 0.67, 95% CI 0.43 to 1.04). The rate of nonfatal heart attacks also reduced linearly from 3.13 during the first year to 1.39 by the fourth and fifth years. The study was not designed to evaluate primary prevention in a population of healthy women, which represents the most typical use of HRT. It looked at a subset of women with an average age of 67 years who had established CHD.[55] The results do suggest that there may be no cardiovascular benefit to beginning HRT in a woman with CHD at the age of 65 or older. Interestingly, 13 venous thromboembolic events (VTEs) occurred in the first year compared to 6 in the fourth and fifth year.[55] Five recently conducted studies in 1996 to 1997 consistently showed that between 1 and 2 additional VTEs per 10,000 healthy postmenopausal women can be attributed to current use of HRT.[56]

Gallbladder disease was significantly greater (RR 1.38, CI 1.00 to 1.92) among those on active treatment.[55]

TREATMENT

Current Drug Therapies to Prevent Estrogen-Deficiency Osteoporosis

The minimum effective dose of estrogen to prevent bone loss is conjugated estrogens 0.625 mg or the equivalent.[57] Combining elemental calcium 1500 mg/day and conjugated estrogen 0.3 mg produced an actual increase in vertebral trabecular mass over 2 years in one study.[58] In a recent 2-year study, women taking esterified estrogens 0.3, 0.625, or 1.25 mg daily had increases in spine bone mineral density of approximately 2, 3, and 5%.[59]

For those unable to tolerate estrogens, progestins alone

may be used because there is some evidence that they decrease bone turnover. Giving 150 mg of DMPA intramuscularly monthly has been suggested, although this has not been clearly established.[60] (NOTE: The original article incorrectly states that 150 mg was given on days 1 through 25 monthly: erratum published in Obstet Gynecol 63:4, 1984). The 21 patients given 150 mg of DMPA intramuscularly once monthly had significantly lowered urinary calcium/creatinine and hydroxyproline/creatinine ratios, which were similar to those of the 22 patients who received oral conjugated estrogens 0.625 mg on days 1 through 25 of each month. Unfortunately, the number of study patients was small and the study duration was only 3 months; therefore, the study needs to be verified with larger numbers of patients participating for a much longer time.

In a 3-year prospective study of 200 perimenopausal women suffering from various menopausal symptoms, these symptoms resolved in 6 months in the 100 women who were given a triphasic oral contraceptive containing levonorgestrel and ethinyl estradiol, with no adverse effects on liver function tests, blood glucose, blood pressure, or coagulation factors and with marked improvement in plasma lipid levels. At 3 years, the control subjects showed a loss of about 6% of bone mass compared to pretreatment levels, whereas the drug group did not lose bone mass, even though both groups averaged daily elemental calcium intake of 1000 mg.[61] However, with the triphasic contraceptive, the average daily intake of ethinyl estradiol is 32 μg compared to the 20-μcg normal ERT dose and actually is six times higher than the 5 μg dose that is approximately equivalent to conjugated equine estrogens (CEE) 0.625 mg.

Although not approved for this use, intermittent cyclic therapy with oral etidronate is effective in reversing the progressive loss of vertebral bone that occurs in postmenopausal osteoporosis.[62] Continuous high doses of etidronate may lead to the impairment of bone mineralization and the cessation of bone remodeling.

Therefore, to reduce bone resorption through the inhibition of osteoclastic activity, 400 mg of oral etidronate per day was given, after a 4-hour fast in the afternoon, with water for 2 weeks, because the average oral absorption is only 3% of the dose when fasting, followed by a 13-week period in which no drugs were taken. While the patients were taking etidronate, 500 mg of elemental calcium and 400 U of vitamin D supplements were taken in the morning. The 15-week cycles were repeated 10 times for a total of 150 weeks, resulting in small but significant increases in the bone mineral content of vertebrae and, after approximately 1 year of treatment, a stabilization in the progression of spinal deformity and a significant decrease in the rate of new vertebral fractures. Because of the long remodeling cycle in osteoporosis, the effects of antiresorptive agents such as etidronate are not likely to be fully apparent during the first year of therapy. Oral etidronate is well tolerated, and no significant side effects were noted during the study. A 4-year, prospective, randomized study in 15 postmenopausal women showed an additive effect of intermittent cyclical etidronate 400 mg daily for 14 days every 12 weeks and conjugated equine estrogens 0.625 mg daily plus DL-norgestrel 150 μg for 12 days each month over 4 years. Bone mineral density (BMD) increases in the lumbar spine were +10.4% in the combined treatment group versus +7.3% in the cyclic etidronate group and +7% versus +0.9%.[63] A recent study followed BMD in 425 postmenopausal women who had undergone hysterectomy taking alendronate (ALN) 10 mg/day, CEE 0.625 mg/day or both over 2 years compared to placebo. Lumbar spine BMD changes were +6%, +6%, +8.3%, and −0.6%, respectively, total hip BMD changes were +4%, +3.4%, +4.7%, and +0.3%, and femoral neck BMD changes were +2.9%, +2.6%, 4.2%, and −0.6%. Therefore, the combination increased spine and hip BMD more than either drug alone.[64] Whether or not combination therapy is cost-effective needs to be studied, and it should be reserved for patients at highest risk for bone loss and subsequent fracture.

ALN was the first drug in the bisphosphonate class to be approved for the prevention and treatment of osteoporosis in postmenopausal women. The Fracture Intervention Trial (FIT) found that 3 years of ALN therapy reduces the risk of vertebral, hip, and wrist fractures by about 50% in women with low BMD.[65] In a recent study, 55.8% of participants did not comply with one or more instructions for taking the drug by 3.1 months of use: 13.5% failed to comply with at least one of the recommended safety rules, and 51.7% disregarded rules relating to avoiding all foods for 30 minutes after taking the drug on an empty stomach and not taking liquids other than water. The most common reason for discontinuation in 28.6% of participants discontinued was the gastrointestinal problems that were reported by 32.7% of all users.[66]

Nasal salmon calcitonin 100 IU in the morning and 100 IU in the evening has been studied for the treatment of established osteoporosis in a 1-year double-blind, placebo-controlled study.[67] Further bone loss was prevented with no side effects. The patients also received 500 mg of elemental calcium daily. The FDA has approved this product for the treatment of osteoporosis after the manufacturer agreed to conduct additional studies of long-term effectiveness in preventing fractures because two clinical randomized trials demonstrated that daily use increased bone mass in the spine but not in the forearm or hip. Recently, the PROOF (Prevent Recurrence of Osteoporotic Fracture) study of 1255 women with osteoporosis reported a 39% reduction in new and/or worsening vertebral fractures per 1000 patient-years of with the use of 200 IU of nasal calcitonin daily through 5 years.[68]

A 2-year prospective study of 20 women using an estradiol transdermal system releasing 0.05 mg of estradiol per day for 3 weeks with the addition of a variety of progestins for the last 10 days of the hormonal cycle validated transdermal use of estradiol (i.e., the prevention of osteoporosis). The study was conducted for 24 months with 24 patients as control subjects. The vertebral mass of the control patients, measured by dual photon absorptiometry, decreased significantly (–4.3%) (P <.001), whereas treated women had a net gain of 5.4% (P <.001).[69]

Long-term studies evaluating the effect of transdermal 17β-estradiol on serum lipids are yet to be completed. One 24-week study found a significant increase in HDL-C and reductions in both total serum cholesterol and low-density lipoprotein (LDL) levels in 10 patients using a patch that released 0.1 mg of estradiol per day every day of the month.[70] A more recent, small study showed that both conjugated estrogens 0.625 mg and transdermal estradiol 0.05 mg used without a progestin did not produce significant changes in lipoproteins over the course of 12 months.[71] Larger numbers of patients using this therapy for a much longer duration are needed to verify this study and also the use of much more sophisticated methods for lipoprotein determinations.

The onset of symptoms of osteoporosis are insidious, and the condition leads to wrist fractures and painful spinal vertebral fractures in patients in their 60s, and hip fractures in patients in their 70s.

The Comparative Effect on Bone Density, Endometrium, and Lipids of Continuous Hormones as Replacement Therapy (CHART) study recently demonstrated that continuous low doses of ethinyl estradiol (5 or 10 μg daily with 1 mg of norethindrone acetate prevent endometrial proliferation, minimize vaginal bleeding, maintain a beneficial lipid profile, and provide an increase in BMC.[72]

Role of Calcium and Vitamin D Intake

Healthy postmenopausal women whose usual daily elemental calcium dietary intake is less than 400 mg lose mineral from the spine at a greater rate than those women whose intake is higher. In a recent study, in women who had undergone menopause 5 or fewer years earlier, bone loss from the spine was rapid and was not affected by supplementation with 500 mg of elemental calcium daily in addition to their normal daily intake with was lower than 400-mg or 400 to 650 mg. In women who had been postmenopausal for 6 years or more given placebo, bone loss was less rapid in those normally taking 400 to 650 mg of calcium. None of the women had used estrogen, glucocorticoids, or other medications known to affect calcium or bone metabolism within the past year in this double-blind, placebo-controlled, randomized trial to determine the effect of calcium on bone loss from the spine, femoral neck, and radius. During the 2-year study, those with the lower calcium intake maintained bone density at the femoral neck and radius but not the spine when treated with calcium carbonate. Although it has not been a consistent finding, increased rates of bone loss have been reported to occur for 2 to 5 years after menopause. The median daily intake of calcium in women over 44 years of age in the United States is known to be 475 mg.[73]

The 1999 Adequate Intake (AI) of the National Institute of Medicine is 1000 mg/day for women between 19 and 50 years of age and 1200 mg/day for women 51 years of age or more, whether or not the woman is taking ERT or HRT. These guidelines are based on calcium from the diet plus supplemental calcium.[74]

Vitamin D is necessary to absorb calcium. The 1999 AI of the National Institute of Medicine for vitamin D is 200 IU/day for women between the ages of 19 and 50, 400 IU/day for women between the ages of 51 and 70, and 600 IU/day for women older than 70 years of age.[74]

Although calcium citrate malate was more bioavailable and shown to be more effective than calcium carbonate in the study cited, it is not available commercially at this time.[73] For those requiring calcium supplementation, calcium carbonate is usually the easiest to take calcium source because it contains the most elemental calcium per tablet. It should be taken with meals to assure adequate stomach acid secretion to facilitate absorption.[44]

The main adverse effects of calcium supplementation are constipation in older adults and possible kidney stone formation in those predisposed persons who take at least 2000 mg of elemental calcium daily.

Dairy products are the best food source of calcium, with 8 oz of skim or whole milk containing roughly 300 mg of elemental calcium, 8 oz of yogurt having roughly 345 mg, 1 oz of cheese having 211 mg, and 8 oz of ice cream having 200 mg.[55] Dietary sources may be supplemented with oral calcium salts (Table 98.15).

Role of Progestins

There are two reasons for adding progestin to ERT therapy: (1) to reduce the risk of estrogen-induced irregular

Table 98.15 ▪ Oral Calcium Supplementation

Generic Preparation	% Ca^{2+}	Tablet Size (mg Ca^{2+}/Tab)	No./Day to Supply 1 g	Cost/Day ($)[a]
Calcium carbonate (CDOC)[c]	40	650 (260)	4	0.36
Dibasic calcium PO4	23	500 (115)	9	0.90
Calcium lactate	13	650 (84.5)	12	0.60
Calcium gluconate	9	650 (58.5)	17	0.85

Source: Reference 44.

[a]Based on average wholesale price, 1999 *Redbook*.

[b]CDOC, clinical drug of choice.

Table 98.16 ▪ Current Hormonal Replacement Therapy Regimen

Drug	Regimen	Reference
A. Cyclic sequential (estrogen days 1–25 + progestin days 13–16 through 25)		
1. Conjugated estrogens or equivalent[a] (CDOC)[b]	0.625 mg daily days 1–25 per month	57 (Table 98.13)
PLUS		
Medroxyprogesterone acetate or equivalent[c] (CDOC)	2.5–10 mg days 13–16 through 25 each month	76, 77
2. Conjugated estrogens or equivalent[a]	0.3 mg days 1 through 25 each month	58
PLUS		
Medroxyprogesterone acetate or equivalent[c]	2.5–10 mg days 13–16 through 25 each month	76, 77
AND		
daily elemental calcium intake	1500 mg daily	58
B. Cyclic combined (estrogen days 1–25 + progestin days 1–25)		
C. Continuous sequential (estrogen taken daily + progestin taken days 1–12)		
D. Continuous combined (estrogen daily + progestin daily)		
3. Conjugated estrogens or equivalent[a,d]	0.625 mg daily	75
PLUS		
Medroxyprogesterone acetate or equivalent[c,d]	2.5–5.0 mg daily	75
4. Depot medroxyprogesterone acetate[e]	150 mg intramuscularly monthly	60
5. Levonorgestrel plus ethinyl estradiol triphasic oral contraceptive[f]	Daily days 1 through 21 each month	61
6. Ethinyl estradiol	5 mcg daily	72
PLUS		
Norethindrone acetate	1 mg daily	
E. Constant estrogen/intermittent progestin		
1. 17β-estradiol	1 mg daily	
PLUS		
Norgestimate	0.09 mg days 4, 5, 6, 10, 11, 12, 16, 17, 18, 22, 23, 24, 28, 29, 30	99

[a]97% of women with intact uteri will experience withdrawal bleeding with this regimen until age 60, and 60% of those age 60–65 will experience withdrawal bleeding.[75]

[b]CDOC, clinical drug of choice.

[c]Norethindrone or norethindrone acetate 0.7–1 mg; DL-norgestrel 150 μg; micronized oral progesterone 150 mg twice daily.[75] Further studies are ongoing to find optimal doses of all progestins.[76,77]

[d]There is no convincing proof that continuous/combined therapy reduces progestin-induced problems as compared with sequential regimens.[75]

[e]Depot medroxyprogesterone acetate usually may be used where estrogens are contraindicated. Etidronate,[62] nasal salmon calcitonin,[67,68] and calcium carbonate alone[73] may also be of benefit for patients who cannot use estrogens.

[f]Needs further study and should be last choice.

bleeding, endometrial hyperplasia, and carcinoma; and (2) to enhance the effect on bone conservation. Unequivocal data showing that progestins favorably modify the response of the skeleton to estrogens are lacking, and endometrial protection remains the only well substantiated reason for adding progestin to estrogen regimens.[75]

When used sequentially for 10 to 13 days/mo, endometrial protection should occur for most patients with MPA 10 mg, or norethindrone or norethindrone acetate 0.7 to 1.0 mg, or DL-norgestrel 150 μg, or micronized progesterone 300 mg.[75] The PEPI trial found that micronized progesterone 200 mg for 14 days monthly was sufficient to prevent endometrial hyperplasia.[54]

Many patients experience some unwanted progestational effects: breast tenderness, bloating, edema, abdominal cramping, anxiety, irritability, and depression. The C-19-nortestosterone derivatives such as norgestrel, norethindrone, or norethindrone acetate possess some androgenic activity and thus tend to be associated with acne and greasy skin and hair. The first combination transdermal patches are now available. They release estradiol 0.05 mg/day plus either norethindrone acetate 0.14 or 0.25 mg/day. This preparation appears to minimize the unwanted androgenic side effects. The C-21 derivatives such as MPA are less androgenic and are more likely to be associated with depression and anxiety.[75]

Oral micronized progesterone, although an attractive alternative, has a significant first-pass hepatic metabolism and therefore requires large doses and in some patients twice-daily administration. Progesterone 200 to 300 mg/day causes drowsiness in approximately 30% of patients.[75] One study used 21 days of percutaneous 17β-estradiol gel in a dose of 1.5 mg (low dose) for the first 6 months and 3.0 mg (high dose) for 25 days if needed to control menopausal symptoms with two different doses of natural micronized progesterone. Maximal reduction of mitoses was noted on biopsies taken after 11 days of progesterone. No hyperplasia was observed after 5 to 7 years of 11 days of either 200 or 300 mg of natural micronized progesterone.[78] Micronized progesterone in peanut oil 100 mg capsules are currently used once daily continuously or twice daily for 14 days in HRT owing to the favorable results of the PEPI Trial.[54]

In an effort to reduce patient's exposure to MPA and

reduce side effects, cyclic hormone replacement using quarterly progestin was tried in 199 women given conjugated estrogen 0.625 mg daily and quarterly MPA 10 mg daily for 14 days over 1 year after having taken conjugated estrogens 0.625 mg/day with monthly cyclic MPA 5 or 10 mg for 1 to 5.4 years (mean 5.4 ± 4.5 years). Endometrial hyperplasia at baseline was 0.9% and after 1 year was 1.5%. Quarterly MPA resulted in longer menses (7.7 ± 2.9 versus 5.4 ± 2.0 days) and more reports of heavier menses (31.1 versus 8.0%). Of interest, despite these problems, women preferred the quarterly regimen by nearly 4:1.[79]

Unfortunately, when the same researchers tried biannual MPA, the incidence of endometrial hyperplasia was higher than acceptable (Bruce Ettinger, personal communication, unpublished data, 1994). As a matter of fact, they now prefer using MPA every other month rather than quarterly and are currently studying low-dose esterified estrogens 0.3 mg daily and MPA 10 mg daily for 14 days every 6 months.[80] Women who use these low doses of estrogens are less likely to have irregular bleeding, heavy bleeding, or breast tenderness.[81]

Probably the greatest benefit of HRT is reduction of the risk of death from cardiovascular disease, especially in women normally considered to be at high risk because of obesity, previous angina, or hypertension.[82] It is feared that the addition of a progestin may negate the beneficial estrogen effects and possibly increase the risk of cardiovascular disease. Therefore, the minimum dose of progestin for endometrial protection should be prescribed.[76]

There is also no proof that continuous, combined therapy of estrogen with progestin on a daily basis reduces the progestin-induced problems compared with sequential regimens. Additionally, there is a high incidence of unexpected vaginal bleeding in 18 to 58% of patients in 12 studies reported so far. With unopposed estrogen regimens, approximately 25% of patients experience regular withdrawal bleeding during each cycle. With sequential therapies, regular bleeding occurs in about 85% of patients, appearing as a light, predictable bleeding lasting 4 to 5 days. Over time, this bleeding often becomes lighter and shorter, and in some patients amenorrhea develops.[77] Table 98.17 summarizes the bleeding patterns from a double-blind, randomized study done with 1724 postmenopausal women over 1 year.[83]

Table 98.18 summarizes the incidences of endometrial hyperplasia from various HRT regimens versus continuous ERT at 6 and 12 months of treatment.[84] Table 98.13 summarizes current HRT regimens to prevent osteoporosis.

Table 98.17 ▪ Bleeding Patterns with Continuous Combined or Sequential Regimens of Conjugated Estrogens with Medroxyprogesterone Acetate

Regimen (Estrogen/Progestin)	% Amenorrhea	% Spot-BTB
1. Continuous combined 0.625 mg/2.5 mg	61.4	22.3
2. Continuous combined 0.625 mg/5.0 mg	72.8	12.7
3. Continuous sequential 0.625 mg daily/5.0 mg days 15–28	16.1	8.1
4. Continuous sequential 0.625 mg daily/10.0 mg days 15–28	18.8	8.3
5. Continuous 0.625 mg and placebo	75.5	14.6

Source: Reference 83.

Table 98.18 ▪ Incidence of Endometrial Hyperplasia in Continuous Combined, Continuous Sequential Conjugated Estrogens with Medroxyprogesterone Acetate and Conjugated Estrogen Alone Regimens

Regimen (Estrogen/Progestin)	Percent at 6 Months	12 Months
1. Continuous combined 0.625 mg/2.5 mg	<1	<1
2. Continuous combined 0.625 mg/5.0 mg	<1	<1
3. Continuous sequential 0.625 mg daily 5.0 mg days 15–28	<1	<1
4. Continuous sequential 0.625 mg daily 10.0 mg days 15–28	<1	<1
5. Continuous 0.625 mg and placebo	7	20

Source: Reference 84.

Selective Estrogen Receptor Modulators

With the approval of raloxifene as the first SERM, a new alternative to traditional ERT/HRT osteoporosis prophylaxis became available. At 60 mg/day, women in one study had an increase in spine and hip BMD of 1.6% while those taking placebo lost 0.8% in both areas.[85] Raloxifene has recently been shown to reduce vertebral fracture risk by 30% in a 3-year randomized clinical trial. Although raloxifene increased femoral neck bone density by 2.1%, there was no decrease in hip fractures.[86] A study comparing raloxifene 60 mg to CEE 0.625 mg plus MPA 2.5 mg daily showed similar effects on LDL-C with a 12 vs 14% reduction, respectively, no effect on total HDL-C and favorable effects on other factors such as HDL_2, which may lead to cardioprotection.[87] The incidence of breast cancer was 1.5/1000 patient-years in raloxifene patients versus 3.9/1000 patient-years in patients taking placebo,[88] which might be expected from a close relative of tamoxifen. Results from the recently completed MORE Randomized Trial showed that among postmenopausal women with osteoporosis, the risk of invasive breast cancer decreased by 76% over 3 years of treatment with raloxifene.[89] Endometrial thickening and endometrial cancer do not occur with raloxifene use.[85] The main side effects are hot flashes, leg cramps, and an increase in deep vein thrombosis similar to that seen in ERT/HRT and combination oral contraceptive users. Unfortunately, there is no estrogen deficiency syndrome benefit from raloxifene.

Effect of ERT/HRT on Alzheimer's Disease

The Leisure World Cohort of more than 8000 women demonstrated a reduction in the estimated risk of AD that was dependent on the dose of CEE used and the duration of use. The odds ratio for getting AD for women using CEE up to 0.625 mg was 0.78 and with CEE up to 1.25 mg and greater was 0.54. The odds ratios of getting AD were 0.83, 0.5, and 0.4 corresponding to up to 3, 4 to 14, or 15 or more years of use of estrogen.[90] More studies are underway with estrogens and AD. Although raloxifene has not been shown to be of benefit in prevention of AD, other SERMs are being studied for this indication.

Estrogen and Colon Cancer

Current as well as former users of estrogen have been shown to have reduced mortality from colon cancer by duration of use. Although there is a suggestion that women who use HRT represent a group that works to reduce colon cancer risk factors by controlling their diet, exercise, and smoking and by participating in regular colorectal screening, there is no evidence to support this suggestion. Although the precise mechanism of how estrogen might reduce colon cancer is unknown, it may affect bile acid metabolism or promote tumor suppressor activity through estrogen receptors.[91]

ALTERNATIVE THERAPY

Pharmaceutical-quality ipriflavone, a phytoestrogen isoflavone, slows bone reabsorption and stimulates collagen synthesis and has been approved in Europe and Japan for the treatment of osteoporosis. Supplementation with 600 mg/day increases bone mass in postmenopausal women.[92] Preliminary results of the beneficial effect of phytoestrogens on bone and in the prevention of endometrial and breast cancer are discussed in three recent reviews of alternative medicine as it pertains to the perimenopausal and menopausal woman.[93–95]

PHARMACOECONOMICS

When a postmenopausal woman takes 10 to 15 years of ERT or HRT, net life expectancy is increased, and there is a substantial impact on quality of life. The cost per quality-adjusted year of life saved over 15 years in a patient with no symptoms and no side effects is estimated to be $11,100 for ERT and $17,900 for HRT and for patients with side effects is $11,100 and $26,300, respectively. (NOTE: If side effects occur more utilization of health care services occurs and costs increase.) If breast cancer occurred, the cost would be $32,000 and $72,000, respectively. Most costs per year of life saved ranged from $15,000 to $25,000, which compares favorably to those that have been estimated for other commonly accepted medical practices such as mild-to-moderate diastolic hypertension, which has a range of $15,800 to $89,800.[96] This study did not estimate the savings that would be associated with HRT as a result of decreasing the incidence of coronary heart disease. It also did not take into consideration the cost of using bone densitometry. In the 1997 *Osteoporosis Pocket Guide to Prevention and Treatment of Osteoporosis,* the National Osteoporosis Foundation recommends that all postmenopausal women younger than age of 65 who have one or more risk factors for osteoporosis, all women aged 65 and older, postmenopausal women who are seen with fractures, women in whom bone mineral testing may facilitate the decision to take needed therapy, and women who have been receiving hormone replacement therapy for prolonged periods should be tested for BMD.[97] This screening is sure to add to up-front costs but in the long run should lead to a reduced number of fractures and lesser costs.

Many pharmacoeconomic models assume that there is 100% compliance with ERT/HRT. Unfortunately, a recent nationwide estimate using a large prescription claim database found that after 1 year 54.4% of the study subjects were noncompliant with HRT. Noncompliance was defined as taking less than 21/28 days of medication averaged over 1 year.[98]

KEY POINTS

The pharmacotherapies of gynecologic disorders have varying degrees of clinical efficacy. For example, prostaglandin inhibitors are very successful in the treatment of primary dysmenorrhea. At the other end of the spectrum is the marginal success of pharmacotherapy for PMS. Somewhere in between lies the success of the pharmacotherapies for endometriosis, the vulvovaginitides, and the disorders resulting from estrogen deficiency.

Three major clinical dilemmas result from these pharmacotherapies. First, the adequate treatment of the PMS remains elusive. Second, the validity and safety of long-term ERT/HRT for the prevention of osteoporosis and cardiovascular disease need further study. Noncompliance with ERT/HRT and other important pharmacotherapies should be limited by the initiation of proactive interventions by pharmacists. Finally, although not unique to gynecology, the dilemma of the teratogenic potential of all pharmacotherapies must be continually evaluated and reevaluated in women in their reproductive years.

Dysmenorrhea

- Dysmenorrhea is the single greatest cause of women's absenteeism for work.
- The etiology of dysmenorrhea is the pharmacologic actions of PGE_2 and $PGF_{2\alpha}$.

Endometriosis

- Endometriosis is a common abnormal pelvic finding in women older than 25 years of age.
- It is characterized by islands of endometrium that are associated with menstrual like bleeding and resultant localized inflammation.
- The use of a GnRH agonist without the surgical diagnosis of endometriosis has pharmacoeconomic benefits.

Vaginitis (Vulvovaginitis)

- At least one-third of all women of childbearing age currently have one or more vulvovaginal infections versus the normal vaginal flora.

Genital and Anal Warts (Condylomata Acuminata)

- Epidemiologically, genital and anal warts are among the most important sexually transmitted diseases.
- Certain stypes of HPV are strongly associated with genital dysplasia and carcinoma.

Estrogen Replacement Therapy

- ERT is used for symptomatic relief of vasomotor instability, vaginal atrophy, atrophic vaginitis, and dysuria.
- Estrogen replacement therapy can help in preventing and treating osteoporosis. ERT/HRT and the risk of breast cancer is controversial.
- The comparative roles of ERT/HRT, bisphosphonates, nasal calcitonin, and SERMs in the prevention of osteoporosis must be considered.
- The role of progestins in HRT.
- ERT/HRT in the prevention of CAD, AD, and colon cancer are of great importance and need further study.

REFERENCES

1. Smith RP. Drug therapy for dysmenorrhea. IMJ Ill Med J 169:22–25, 1986.
2. Dawood MY. Dysmenorrhea. Clin Obstet Gynecol 33:168–178, 1990.
3. Dysmenorrhea. ACOG Tech Bull 68:1–5, 1983.
4. Ekstrom P, Juchnicka E, Laudanski T, et al. Effect of an oral contraceptive in primary dysmenorrhea–changes in uterine activity and reactivity to agonists. Contraception 40:39–47, 1989.
5. Kleber HD, Kosten TR. Use of clonidine for dysmenorrhea in four patients. Psychosomatics 26:539–546, 1985.
6. Chihal HJ. Premenstrual syndrome: an update for the clinician. Obstet Gynecol Clin North Am 17:457–479, 1990.
7. Yonkers KA. Antidepressants in the treatment of premenstrual dysphoric disorder. J Clin Psychiatry 58(Suppl 14):4–10, 1997.
8. American Psychiatric Association. Diagnostic and statistical manual of mental disorders (DSM IV). 4th ed. Washington, DC: American Psychiatric Association, 1994.
9. Maddocks S, Hahn P, Moller F, et al. A double-blind placebo controlled trial of progesterone vaginal suppositories in the treatment of premenstrual syndrome. Am J Obstet Gynecol 154: 573–581, 1986.
10. Freeman EW, Rickels K, Sondheimer SJ, et al. A double-blind trial of oral progesterone, alprazolam and placebo in treatment of severe premenstrual syndrome. JAMA 274:51–57, 1995.
11. Brown CS, Ling FW, Andersen RN, et al. Efficacy of depot leuprolide in premenstrual syndrome: effect of symptom severity and type in a controlled trial. Obstet Gynecol 84:779–786, 1994.
12. Smith MA, Youngkin EQ. Managing the premenstrual syndrome. Clin Pharm 5:788–797, 1986.
13. True BL, Goodner SM, Burns EA. Review of the etiology and treatment of premenstrual syndrome. Drug Intell Clin Pharm 19:714–722, 1985.
14. Harrison W, Sharpe L, Endicott J. Treatment of premenstrual symptoms. Gen Hosp Psychiatry 7:54–65, 1985.
15. Smith S, Schiff I. The premenstrual syndrome-diagnosis and management. Fertil Steril 52:527–543, 1989.
16. Mortola JF. A risk-benefit appraisal of drugs used in the management of premenstrual syndrome. Drug Saf 10:160–169, 1994.
17. Halbreich U, Smoller JW. Intermittent luteal phase sertraline treatment of dysphoric premenstrual syndrome. J Clin Pyschiatry 58:399–402, 1997.
18. Thys-Jacobs S, Starkey P, Bernstein D, et al. Calcium carbonate and the premenstrual syndrome: effects on premenstrual and menstrual symptoms. Am J Obstet Gynecol 179:444–452, 1998.
19. Fankhauser MP. Psychiatric disorders in women: psychopharmacologic treatments. J Am Pharm Assoc (Wash) NS37:667–678, 1997.
20. Endometriosis. ACOG Tech Bull 184:1–6, 1993.
21. Guzick DS. Clinical epidemiology of endometriosis and infertility. Obstet Gynecol Clin North Am 16:43–59, 1989.
22. Markham SM, Carpenter SE, Rock JA. Extrapelvic endometriosis. Obstet Gynecol Clin North Am 16:193–219, 1989.
23. Galle PC. Clinical presentation and diagnosis of endometriosis. Obstet Gynecol Clin North Am 16:29–41, 1989.
24. Metzger DA, Luciano, AA. Hormonal Therapy of Endometriosis. Obstet Gynecol Clin North Am 16:105–121, 1989.
25. Erickson LD, Ory SJ. GnRH analogues in the treatment of endometriosis. Obstet Gynecol Clin North Am 16:123–145, 1989.
26. Glasser M. The clinical and economic benefits of GnRH agonist in treating endometriosis. Am J Manag Care 5(Suppl):S316–S325, 1999.
27. Gardner HL. Infectious vulvovaginitis. In: Monif GR, ed. Infectious diseases in obstetrics and gynecology. 2nd ed. Philadelphia: Harper and Row, 1982:515.
28. Sweet RL. Importance of differential diagnosis in acute vaginitis. Am J Obstet Gynecol 152:945–947, 1985.
29. 1998 guidelines for the treatment of sexually transmitted diseases. MMWR Morb Mortal Wkly Rep 47(RR-1):1–116, 1998.
30. Ritter W. Pharmacokinetic fundamentals of vaginal treatment with clotrimazole. Am J Obstet Gynecol 152:945–947, 1985.
31. Anderson GM, Barrat J, Bergan T, et al. A comparison of single-dose oral fluconazole with 3-day intravaginal clotrimazole in the treatment of vaginal candidiasis. Report of an international multicentre trial. Br J Obstet Gynecol 96:226–232, 1989.
32. Sobel JD. Epidemiology and pathogenesis of recurrent vulvovaginal candidiasis. Am J Obstet Gynecol 152:924–934, 1985.
33. Fregoso-Duenas F. Ketoconazole in vulvovaginal candidosis. Rev Infect Dis 2:620–624, 1980.
34. Nyirjesy P, Sobel JD, Weitz MV, et al. Difficult-to-treat trichomoniasis: results with paromomycin cream. Clin Infect Dis. 26:986–988, 1998.
35. Lynch PJ. Condylomata acuminata (anogenital warts). Clin Obstet Gynecol 28:142–151, 1985.
36. Genital human papillomavirus infections. ACOG Tech Bull 193:1–7, 1994.
37. Ferenczy A. Comparison of 5-fluorouracil and CO_2 laser for treatment of vaginal condylomata. Obstet Gynecol 64:773–778, 1984.
38. Beutner KR, Ferenczy A. Therapeutic approaches to genital warts. Am J Med 102(5A):28–37,1997.
39. Hormone replacement therapy. ACOG Educ Bull 247:1–10, 1998.
40. Schiff I, Tulchinsky D, Cramer D, et al. Oral medroxyprogesterone in the treatment of postmenopausal symptoms. JAMA 244:1443–1445, 1980.
41. Laufer LR, Erlik Y, Meldrum DR, et al. Effect of clonidine on hot flashes in postmenopausal women. Obstet Gynecol 60:583–586, 1982.
42. Dyer GI, Townsend PT. Dose related changes in vaginal cytology after topical conjugated equine oestrogens. Br Med J 284:789, 1982.
43. Schmidt G, Andersson S, Nordle O, et al. Release of 17-beta-oestradiol from a vaginal ring in postmenopausal women: pharmacokinetic evaluation. Gynecol Obstet Invest 38:253–260, 1994.
44. Bauwens SF, Drinka PJ, Boh L. Pathogenesis and management of primary osteoporosis. Clin Pharm 5:639–659, 1986.
45. DeFazio J, Speroff L. Estrogen replacement therapy: current thinking and practice. Geriatrics 40:32–48, 1985.
46. Osteoporosis. ACOG Educ Bull 246:1–9, 1998.
47. Colditz GA, Hankinson SE, Hunter DJ, et al. The use of estrogens and progestins and the risk of breast cancer in postmenopausal women. N Engl J Med 332:1589–1593, 1995.
48. Steiberg KK, Thacker SB, Smith SJ, et al. A meta-analysis of the effect of estrogen replacement therapy on the risk of breast cancer. JAMA 265:1985–1990, 1991.
49. Dupont WD, Page DL. Menopausal estrogen replacement therapy and breast cancer. Arch Intern Med 151:67–72, 1991.

50. Henrich JB. The postmenopausal estrogen/breast cancer controversy. JAMA 268:1900–1902, 1992.
51. Collaborative Group on Hormonal Factors in Breast Cancer. Breast cancer and hormone replacement therapy: collaborative reanalysis of data from 51 epidemiological studies of 52,705 women with breast cancer and 108,411 women without breast cancer. Lancet 350:1047–1059, 1997.
52. Sourander L, Rajala T, Rajala I, et al. Cardiovascular and cancer morbidity and mortality and sudden cardiac death in postmenopausal women on oestrogen replacement therapy (ERT). Lancet 352:1965–1969, 1998.
53. Henderson BE, Ross RK, Paganini-Hill A, et al. Estrogen use and cardiovascular disease. Am J Obstet Gynecol 154:1181–1186, 1986.
54. The Writing Group for the PEPI Trial. Effects of estrogen or estrogen/progestin regimens on heart disease risk factors in postmenopausal women. JAMA 273:199–208, 1995.
55. Hulley S, Grady D, Bush T, et al. Randomized trial of estrogen plus progestin for secondary prevention of coronary heart disease in postmenopausal women: the heart and estrogen/progestin replacement study (HERS). JAMA 280:605–613, 1998.
56. Castellsague J, Gutthann SP, Rodriguez LAG. Recent epidemiological studies of the association between hormone replacement therapy and venous thromboembolism. Drug Saf 18:117–123, 1998.
57. Lindsay R, Hart M, Clark DM. The minimum effective dose of estrogen for the prevention of postmenopausal bone loss. Obstet Gynecol 63:759–763, 1984.
58. Gordan GS, Gennant, HK. The aging skeleton. Clin Geriatr Med 1:95–118, 1985.
59. Genant H, Lucas J, Weiss S, et al. Low dose esterified estrogen therapy. Arch Intern Med 1577:2609–2615, 1997.
60. Lobo RA, McCormick W, Singer F, et al. Depo-medroxyprogesterone acetate compared with conjugated estrogens for the treatment of postmenopausal women. Obstet Gynecol 63:1–5, 1984.
61. Shargil AA. Hormone replacement therapy in perimenopausal women on a triphasic contraceptive compound: a three year prospective study. Int J Fertil 30:15–28, 1985.
62. Harris ST, Watts NB, Jackson RD, et al. Four-year study of intermittent cyclic etidronate treatment of postmenopausal osteoporosis: three years of blinded therapy followed by one year of open therapy. Am J Med 95:557–567, 1993.
63. Wimalawansa SJ. A four-year randomized controlled trial of hormone replacement therapy and bisphosphonate, alone or in combination, in women with postmenopausal osteoporosis. Am J Med 104:219–226, 1998.
64. Greenspan S, Bankhurst A, Bell N, et al. Effects of alendronate and estrogen, alone or in combination on bone mass turnover in postmenopausal osteoporosis. Bone 23:S174, 1998.
65. Black DM, Cummings SR, Karpf DB, et al. Randomised trial of effect of alendronate on risk of fracture in women with existing vertebral fractures. Lancet 348:1535–1541, 1996.
66. Ettinger B, Pressman A, Schein J, et al. Alendronate use among 812 women: Prevalence of gastrointestinal complaints, noncompliance with patient instructions, and discontinuation. J Manag Care Pharm 4:488–492, 1998.
67. Overgaard K, Riis BJ, Christiansen C, et al. Nasal calcitonin for the treatment of established osteoporosis. Clin Endocrin 30:435–442, 1989.
68. Silverman SL, Chestnut C, Andriano K, et al. Salmon calcitonin nasal spray (NS-CT) reduces risk of vertebral fracture(s) (VF) in established osteoporosis and has continuous efficacy with prolonged treatment: accrued 5 year worldwide data of the PROOF Study. Bone 23:S174, 1998.
69. Ribot C, Tremollieres JM, Louvet JP, et al. Preventive effects of transdermal administration of 17-beta-estradiol on postmenopausal bone loss: a 2-year prospective study. Obstet Gynecol 75(Suppl):42–55, 1990.
70. Stanczyk FZ, Shoupe D, Nunez V, et al. A randomized comparison of nonoral estradiol delivery in postmenopausal women. Am J Obstet Gynecol 159:1540–1546, 1988.
71. Erenus M, Kutlay K, Kutlay L, et al. Comparison of the impact of oral versus transdermal estrogen on serum lipoproteins. Fertil Steril 61:300–302, 1994.
72. Speroff L, Rowan J, Symons J, et al. The comparative effect on bone density, endometrium, and lipids of continuous hormones as replacement therapy (CHART study). JAMA 276:1397–1403, 1996.
73. Dawson-Hughes B, Dallal GE, Krall EA, et al. A controlled trial of the effect of calcium supplementation on bone density in postmenopausal women. N Engl J Med 323:878–883, 1990.
74. Standing Committee on the Scientific Evaluation of Dietary Reference Intakes, Food and Nutrition Board, Institute of Medicine: Calcium (Chapter 4); Vitamin D (Chaper 7). In: Dietary reference intakes for calcium, phosphorous, magnesium, vitamin D, and fluoride. Washington, DC: National Academy Press, 1999:71–145, 250–287.
75. Whitehead MI, Hillard TC, Crook D. The role and use of progestogens. Obstet Gynecol 75(Suppl):59–76, 1990.
76. Gambrell RD. Clinical use of progestins in the menopausal patient. J Reprod Med 27:531–538, 1982.
77. Lane G, Siddle NC, Ryder TA, et al. Is Provera the ideal progestogen for addition to postmenopausal estrogen therapy? Fertil Steril 45:345–352, 1986.
78. Moyer DL, de Lignieres B, Driguez P, et al. Prevention of endometrial hyperplasia by progesterone during long-term estradiol replacement: influence of bleeding pattern and secretory changes. Fertil Steril 59:992–997, 1993.
79. Ettinger B, Seby J, Citron JT, et al. Cyclic hormone replacement therapy using quarterly progestin. Obstet Gynecol 83:693–700, 1994.
80. Ettinger B, Pressman A, Vangessel A. Efficacy and safety of low-dosage esterified estrogens combined with 6-monthly progestin [Abstract 99.020]. Presented at the 10th Annual Meeting of the North American Menopause Society, New York, 1999.
81. Ettinger B. Personal perspective on low-dosage estrogen therapy for postmenopausal women. Menopause 6:273–276, 1999.
82. Henderson BE, Ross RK, Paganini-Hill A. Estrogen use and cardiovascular disease. J Reprod Med 30(Suppl):814–820, 1985.
83. Archer DF, Pickar JH, Bottiglioni F. Bleeding patterns in postmenopausal women taking continuous combined or sequential regimens of conjugated estrogens with medroxyprogesterone acetate. Obstet Gynecol 83:686–692, 1994.
84. Woodruff JD, Pickar JH. Incidence of endometrial hyperplasia in postmenopausal women taking conjugated estrogens (Premarin) with medroxyprogesterone acetate or conjugated estrogens alone. Am J Obstet Gynecol 170:1213–1223, 1994.
85. Delmas P, Bjarnason N, Mitlak B, et al. Effects of raloxifene on bone mineral density, serum cholesterol concentrations, and uterine endometrium in postmenopausal women. N Engl J Med 337:1641–1647, 1997.
86. Ettinger B, Black DM, Mitlak BH, et al. Reduction of vertebral fracture risk in postmenopausal women with osteoporosis treated with raloxifene. Results from a 3-year randomized clinical trial. JAMA 282:637–645, 1999.
87. Walsh BW, Kuller LH, Wild RA, et al. Effects of raloxifene on serum lipids and coagulation factors in healthy postmenopausal women. JAMA 279:1445–1451, 1998.
88. Jordan VC, Glusman JE, Eckert S, et al. Incident primary breast cancers are reduced by raloxifene: integrated data from multicenter, double blind, randomized trials in 12,000 postmenopausal women [Abstract]. Proc ASCO 17:122a, 1998.
89. Cummings SR, Eckert S, Krueger KA, et al. The effect of raloxifene on risk of breast cancer in postmenopausal women. Results from the MORE Randomized Trial. JAMA 281:2189–2197, 1999.
90. Paganini-Hill A. Alzheimer's disease in women–Can estrogen play a preventive role? Female Patient 23:10–20, 1998.
91. Calle EE. Hormone replacement therapy and colorectal cancer: interpreting the evidence. Cancer Causes Control 8:127–129, 1997.
92. Valente M, Bufalino L, Castignole GN, et al. Effects of 1-year treatment with ipriflavone on bone in postmenopausal women with low bone mass. Calcif Tissue Int 54:377–380, 1994.
93. Taylor M. Alternatives to conventional hormone replacement therapy. Comp Ther 23:514–532, 1997.
94. Israel D, Youngkin EQ. Herbal therapies for perimenopausal and menopausal complaints. Pharmacotherapy 17:970–984, 1997.
95. Aldercreutz H, Mazur W. Phyto-oestrogens and Western diseases. Ann Med 29:95–120, 1997.
96. Tosteson NA, Weinstein M, Schiff I. Cost-effectiveness analysis of hormone replacement therapy. In: Lobo RA: Treatment of the postmenopausal woman: basic and clinical aspects. New York, Raven Press, 1994:405.
97. Pocket guide to prevention and treatment of osteoporosis. Washington, DC: National Osteoporosis Foundation (NOF), 1997.
98. Faulkner DL, Young C, Hutchins D, et al. Patient noncompliance with hormone replacement therapy: a nationwide estimate using a large prescription claims database. Menopause 5:226–229, 1998.
99. Corson SL, Richart RM, Caubel P, et al. Effect of a unique constant-estrogen, pulsed progestin hormone replacement therapy containing 17β-estradiol and norgestimate on endometrial histology. Int J Fertil 44:279–285, 1999.

CHAPTER 99

CONTRACEPTION

Debbie Scholtz and Jannet M. Carmichael

DEFINITION

Contraception is literally the prevention of conception, but generally is taken to mean the prevention of pregnancy.

TREATMENT GOALS: CONTRACEPTION

- Help patient choose an acceptable method that will reliably prevent pregnancy.
- Teach patient to use the method effectively and consistently.
- Avoid or manage annoying or potentially dangerous adverse effects.

EPIDEMIOLOGY

The control of fertility is a frequent concern of women and health care providers the world over. In the United States alone, nearly half of all pregnancies each year are unintended.[1] The decisions of whether or not to use contraception and which method to use are not always easy to make. Significant advancements in contraception have been made in the last several years, resulting in methods that are much safer than in previous years, while maintaining high efficacy rates when used properly. Unfortunately there is still no 100% safe and effective contraceptive method besides complete abstinence. Health care providers, including pharmacists, can play a critical role in helping women and their partners choose and use the available methods as safely and effectively as possible.

PHYSIOLOGY

To understand the evolution of contraceptive methods, it is first necessary to review the physiology of the normal menstrual cycle.

The average menstrual cycle (Fig. 99.1) lasts 28 days with a range of 23 to 35 days. Several organ systems are involved in this cycle including the hypothalamus, pituitary gland, uterus, and ovaries. The changes that occur in the ovaries during this 28-day cycle can be divided into three phases: the follicular phase, ovulation, and the luteal phase.

The follicular phase lasts for approximately the first 14 days of the cycle. At the beginning of this phase, several follicles, each containing an oocyte, begin to enlarge, first independently and then in response to pituitary follicle-stimulating hormone (FSH). After 5 or 6 days one of the follicles begins to develop more rapidly. The granulosa cells of this follicle multiply, and under the influence of FSH and pituitary luteinizing hormone (LH), synthesize and release estrogens from the ovary at an increasing rate. Peripheral levels of estradiol begin to rise significantly by cycle day 7. The estrogens appear to inhibit FSH before midcycle (a negative feedback inhibition system); however, the high level and rate of increase of estrogen stimulates a surge of FSH and LH at the end of this phase, which in turn causes final-stage growth and rupture of the ovum (ovulation).

Ovulation ordinarily occurs at midcycle, on day 14 or 15. As estrogen levels peak, a surge of LH occurs, leading to follicular maturation and ovulation. The onset of the LH surge appears to be the most reliable indicator of impending ovulation, occurring 34 to 36 hours before follicle rupture. At the time of ovulation, the granulosa cells of the follicle begin to secrete progesterone.

The luteal phase follows, which is dominated by progesterone effects. Under the influence of LH, the ruptured follicle fills with blood and the surrounding theca and granulosa cells proliferate and replace the blood to form the corpus luteum. The cells of this structure produce estrogens and progesterone for the remainder of the cycle

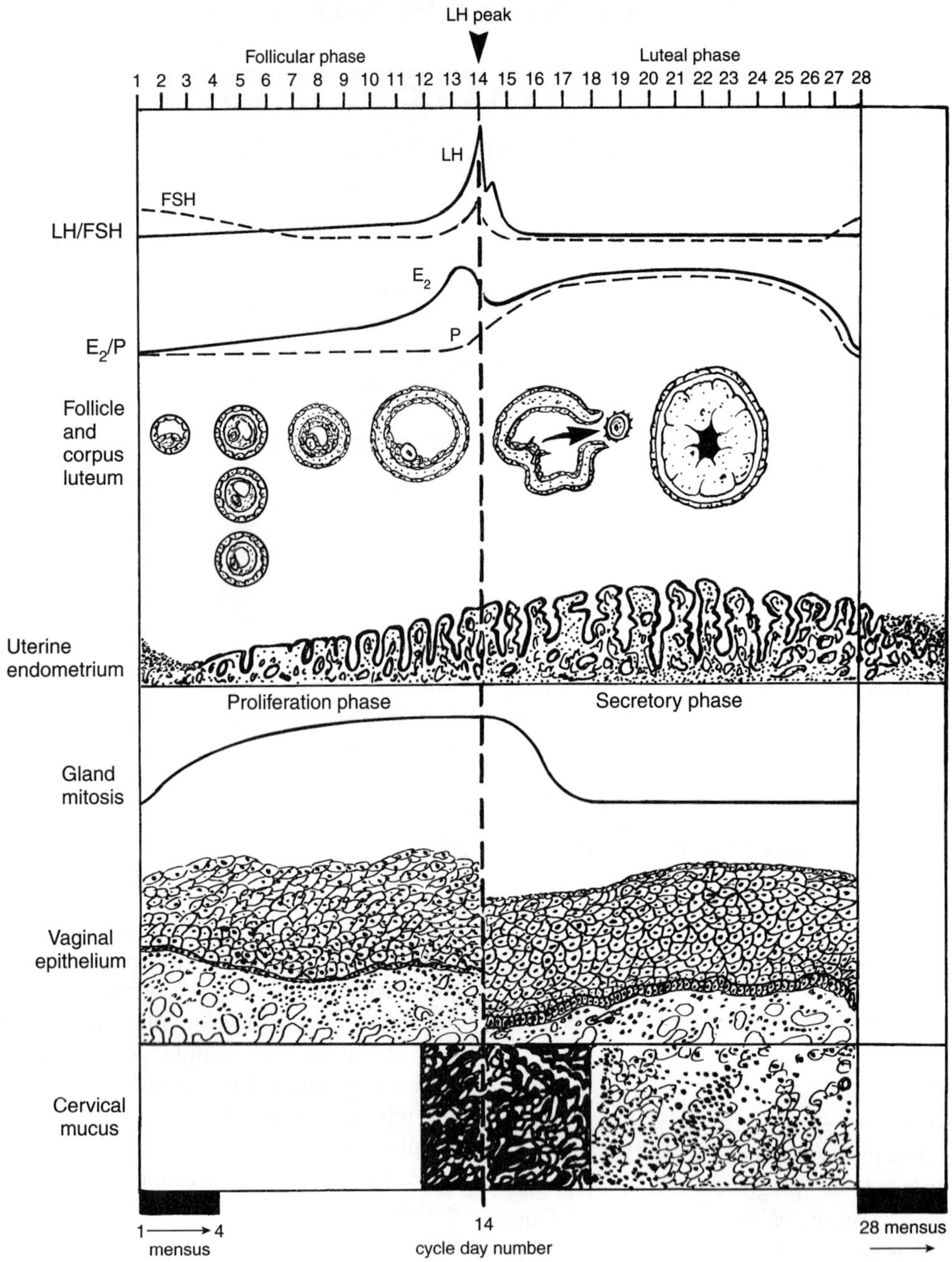

Figure 99.1. Composite changes in tissues and hormones during the reproductive cycle. E_2, estradiol; *FSH,* follicle-stimulating hormone; *LH,* luteinizing hormone; *P,* progesterone. (Reprinted with permission from Beckmann CRB, Ling FW, Herbert WNP, et al. Obstetrics and gynecology. 3rd ed. Baltimore, MD: Williams & Wilkins, 1998.)

unless pregnancy occurs. If pregnancy does not occur during this cycle, the corpus luteum begins to degenerate and ceases hormone production. This drop in serum levels of estrogen and progesterone results in endometrial shedding (menstruation) and the beginning of a new cycle. If pregnancy does occur, the corpus luteum remains active because it is stimulated by human chorionic gonadotropin derived from the developing placenta, thus maintaining the high levels of progesterone and estrogen necessary for pregnancy.

The changes that occur in the uterus over the 28-day cycle can also be divided into three phases: the menstrual phase, the proliferative phase, and the secretory phase. The menstrual phase starts on day 1 of the menstrual cycle with the sloughing of the old endometrium and the onset of vaginal bleeding. This phase lasts 3 to 6 days. The proliferative phase is a period of growth of the endometrial lining lasting from day 6 to day 14. Estrogen from the developing follicles is responsible for this growth as well as for the growth of uterine glands and the proliferation of uterine vessels. The secretory phase, which coincides with the luteal phase in the ovaries, is primarily under the influence of progesterone. During this phase, the endometrium becomes thicker and is held in place, the uterine glands branch, and the secretory function of these glands begins, thus preparing the endometrium for implantation should fertilization of the ovum occur.

THERAPEUTIC PLAN

There are many methods of contraception available, including surgical, pharmacologic, and nonpharmacologic methods. Surgical options include tubal ligation for women and vasectomy for men. These are generally considered permanent options, although they may be reversible under certain rare circumstances. Other options that involve men include condoms and natural family planning. All other options at this time are used by women. Figure 99.2 indicates the various methods available in a decision tree format. Table 99.1 compares the failure rates of these methods, both under "typical use" conditions and "perfect use" conditions. The decision to use a particular method is dependent on individual factors including the safety and efficacy of the method, the person's ability to use the method correctly, concurrent conditions, and the particular needs and desires of the couple.

METHODS OF CONTRACEPTION

Hormonal Contraception

Combination Oral Contraceptives

The use of female sex hormones to prevent the development of the ovum was suggested as early as 1931, but it was not until 1956, after the discovery of norethynodrel, that field trials were begun on what we now know as birth control pills.[2] In 1960, the U.S. Food and Drug Administration (FDA) first approved the use of Enovid 10, a combination pill containing 150 μg of mestranol and 9.85 mg of norethynodrel. Other products soon followed, containing varying amounts of estrogens and progestins.

Components: Estrogens and Progestins

All combination oral contraceptives (COCs) contain both an estrogenic compound and a progestin. Over the years, the amounts and types of these components have changed in attempts to lower side effects and improve efficacy.

The major natural estrogens produced by women are estradiol, estrone, and estriol. Estradiol is the major secretory product of the ovaries. Some estrone is also produced in the ovaries, although most estrone and estriol is formed in the liver from estradiol or converted in the peripheral tissues. To improve absorption and potency, synthetic estrogens were produced. Mestranol and ethinyl estradiol are the estrogens that have been used in the

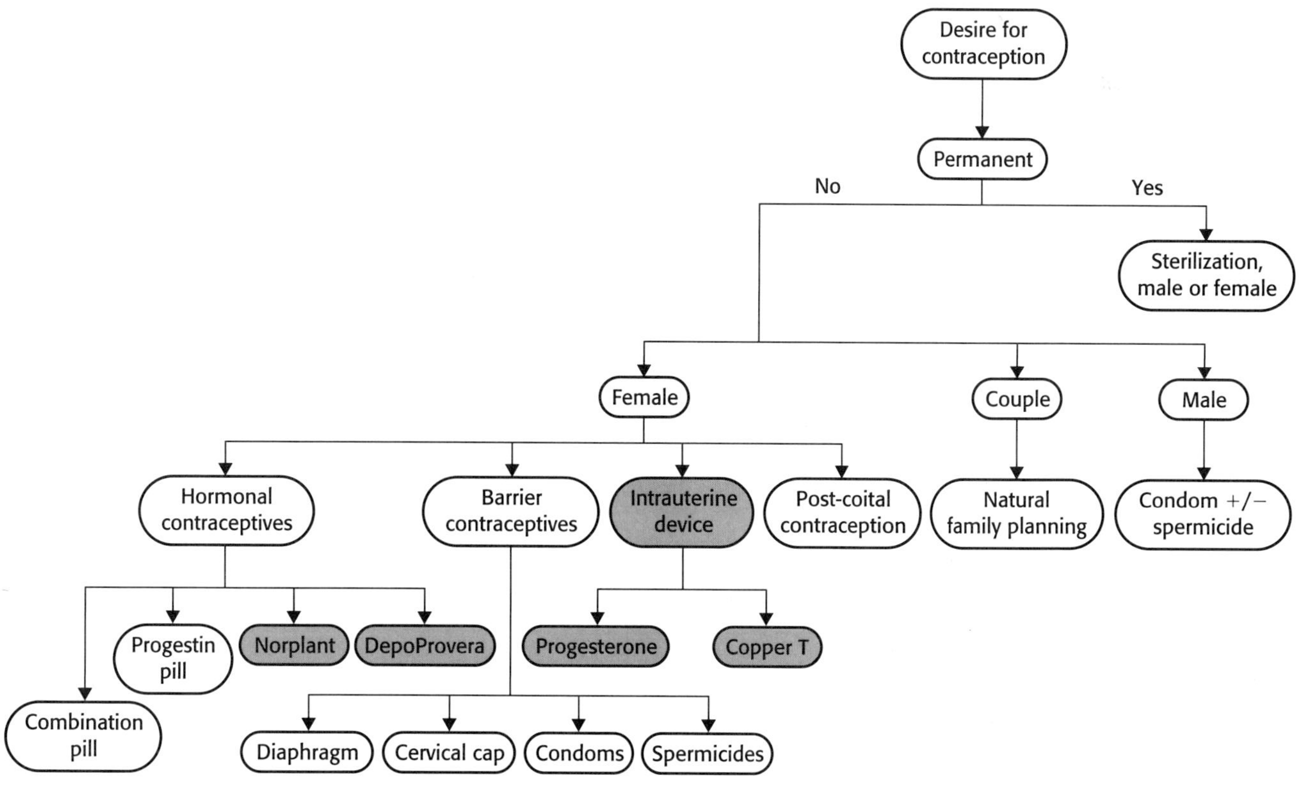

Figure 99.2. One of several possible algorithms to contraceptive choice. Shaded choices are less "use oriented," that is, require minimal action on the part of the couple to be effective. (Reprinted with permission from Beckmann CRB, Ling FW, Herbert WNP, et al. Obstetrics and gynecology. 3rd ed. Baltimore, MD: Williams & Wilkins, 1998.)

Table 99.1 ▪ Percentage of Women Experiencing an Unintended Pregnancy during the First Year of Typical Use and the First Year of Perfect Use of Contraception and the Percentage Continuing Use at the End of the First Year: United States

	% of Women Experiencing an Unintended Pregnancy within the First Year of Use		% of Women Continuing Use at One Year[c]
Method (1)	**Typical Use[a] (2)**	**Perfect Use[b] (3)**	**(4)**
Chance[d]	85	85	
Spermicides[e]	26	6	40
Periodic abstinence	25		63
Calendar		9	
Ovulation Method		3	
Symptothermal[f]		2	
Postovulation		1	
Cap[g]			
Parous women	40	26	42
Nulliparous women	20	9	56
Sponge			
Parous women	40	20	42
Nulliparous women	20	9	56
Diaphragm[g]	20	6	56
Withdrawal	19	4	
Condom[h]			
Female (reality)	21	5	56
Male	14	3	61
Pill			
Progestin only		0.5	
Combined		0.1	
IUD			
Progesterone T	2.0	1.5	81
Copper T 380A	0.8	0.6	78
LNg 20	0.1	0.1	81
Depo-Provera	0.3	0.3	70
Norplant and Norplant-2	0.05	0.05	88
Female sterilization	0.5	0.5	100
Male sterilization	0.15	0.10	100

Emergency contraceptive pills: treatment initiated within 72 hours after unprotected intercourse reduces risk of pregnancy by at least 75%[i]
Lactational amenorrhea method: a highly effective, *temporary* method of contraception[j]

Source: Reprinted with permission from Hatcher RA, Trussell J, Stewart F, et al. Contraceptive technology. 17th ed. New York: Ardent Media Inc., 1998.

[a]Among *typical* couples who initiate use of a method (not necessarily for the first time), the percentage who experience an accidental pregnancy during the first year if they do not stop use for any other reason.

[b]Among couples who initiate use of a method (not necessarily for the first time) and who use it *perfectly* (both consistently and correctly), the percentage who experience an accidental pregnancy during the first year if they do not stop use for any other reason.

[c]Among couples attempting to avoid pregnancy, the percentage who continue to use a method for 1 year.

[d]The percentages becoming pregnant in columns (2) and (3) are based on data from populations where contraception is not used and from women who cease using contraception to become pregnant. Among such populations, about 89% become pregnant within 1 year. This estimate was lowered slightly (to 85%) to represent the percentages who would become pregnant within 1 year among women now relying on reversible methods of contraception if they abandoned contraception altogether.

[e]Foams, creams, gels, vaginal suppositories, and vaginal film.

[f]Cervical mucus (ovulation) method supplemented by calendar in the *preovulatory* and basal body temperature in the postovulatory phases.

[g]With spermicidal cream or jelly.

[h]Without spermicides.

[i]The treatment schedule is one dose within 72 hours after unprotected intercourse, and a second dose 12 hours after the first dose. The Food and Drug Administration has declared the following brands of oral contraceptives to be safe and effective for emergency contraception: Ovral (1 dose is 2 white pills), Alesse (1 dose is 5 pink pills), Nordette or Levlen (1 dose is 4 light-orange pills), Lo/Ovral (1 dose is 4 white pills), Triphasil or Tri-Levlen (1 dose is 4 yellow pills).

[j]However, to maintain effective protection against pregnancy, another method of contraception must be used as soon as menstruation resumes, the frequency or duration of breastfeeds is reduced, bottle feeds are introduced, or the baby reaches 6 months of age.

United States. Mestranol is an inactive synthetic estrogen that is demethylated in the liver to form the active ethinyl estradiol. Only one current COC contains mestranol in a dose of 50 μg, which is roughly equivalent to 35 μg ethinyl estradiol. All other COCs contain 50 μg or less of ethinyl estradiol. Pills containing 50 μg or greater ethinyl estradiol are considered "high-dose."

Ethinyl estradiol undergoes extensive first-pass hepatic

metabolism, which can result in considerable patient-to-patient variation in plasma and urine steroid concentrations. Circulating ethinyl estradiol is highly bound to albumin. It is metabolized primarily by the hepatic cytochrome P-450 3A4 isoenzyme. Ethinyl estradiol also undergoes enterohepatic circulation and is excreted into the bile, deconjugated in the gastrointestinal (GI) system and reabsorbed into the bloodstream. This may result in a rebound of blood levels of estrogen 10 to 14 hours after administration.

The role of estrogen in preventing pregnancy occurs through several mechanisms.[3,4] First, negative feedback inhibition by estrogen on the hypothalamus and pituitary gland suppresses the release of FSH and LH, preventing the selection of a dominant follicle and subsequent ovulation. Estrogen also may contribute by altering the endometrial lining, allowing changes in secretions, which results in alternating areas of edema and dense cellularity. In larger doses, estrogen stimulates the degeneration of the corpus luteum (luteolysis).

Progestin use in COCs has changed considerably. Progesterone itself is the most important natural progestin and also serves as a precursor to the estrogens, androgens, and adrenocortical steroids. Progesterone is rapidly absorbed after parenteral administration, but is poorly absorbed when given orally. To overcome problems with absorption and high first-pass metabolism, synthetic progestins were developed. There are now eight different synthetic compounds in use in the United States, including the older norethindrone, norethindrone acetate, ethynodiol diacetate, norgestrel, levonorgestrel, and norethynodrel, and the newer desogestrel and norgestimate. All synthetic progestins used in COCs are 19-nortestosterones derived from testosterone and differ from each other in terms of their biologic activities. Unlike the estrogens, progestins can exhibit not only progestin effects, but also estrogenic and androgenic effects. This may result in subtle differences in side effects, but not in the ability to suppress ovulation. As a group, these agents exert their contraceptive effects by suppressing the release of LH (inhibiting ovulation), thickening the cervical mucus to hinder sperm transport, and producing an atrophic endometrial lining, which is inhospitable to implantation.

Progestins, like ethinyl estradiol, undergo first-pass metabolism.[3,4] Metabolism occurs in varying degrees in the intestinal wall and in the liver. Some of the older compounds (norethindrone acetate and ethynodrel diacetate) are converted to norethindrone, which exerts its activity and is then converted and excreted as sulfates and glucuronide. As first introduced, norgestrel was a mixture of D- and L-isomers. It has since been recognized that activity rests entirely with the levo form. Original products still contain the racemic norgestrel, but newer products contain half of the amount of levonorgestrel. There is enhanced potency of levonorgestrel and its derivatives of about 5-fold to 10-fold compared with norethindrone. Three derivatives of levonorgestrel represent the newest generation of orally active progestins: desogestrel, norgestimate, and gestodene (not currently available in the United States). It appears that neither desogestrel nor gestodene is converted to levonorgestrel, but norgestimate may undergo this transformation. However, one metabolite of norgestimate, 17-deacetylnorgestimate, is likely to also contribute to the pharmacologic response. Desogestrel is rapidly converted to 3-ketodesogestrel and is present in high circulating concentrations.

Together ethinyl estradiol and the progestin component work synergistically to produce very effective contraceptive effects. Compared to other methods of birth control, COCs remain one of the most effective forms. With perfect use (consistent and correct), only 1 of 1000 women using COCs may accidentally become pregnant during the first year. With typical use (not always consistent and correct), at least 30 of 1000 women (with some estimating the number to be closer to 50)[3] may become pregnant. Clearly, encouraging patients to strive for perfection with pill use will prevent many unintended pregnancies.

Risks

One reason why some women may be reluctant to take COCs consistently and correctly is a fear of possible adverse effects. It is important to discuss these fears and the potential risks as well as benefits before choosing this particular method. As stated earlier, older products contained higher doses of hormones and were associated with significant side effects. This reputation continues to linger despite evidence to the contrary with more modern products. Also, with extensive study, many benefits from the use of COCs have been identified.

Cardiovascular Disease. Historically, COCs have been associated with increased risks for myocardial infarction (MI) and stroke. Much debate continues on the exact relationship of COC use and the risk of MI and stroke. Early data showed that dangers during therapy seem to increase substantially with age and the presence of risk factors such as smoking greater than 15 cigarettes daily, preexisting hypercholesterolemia, diabetes mellitus, or hypertension.[5,6] Overall, oral contraceptives were found to multiply the effects of age and other risk factors for MI and stroke, rather than just add to them.[6] Because cigarette smoking is far more prevalent among women of reproductive age than any of these other risk factors, it becomes by far the most important factor.

Whereas early epidemiologic studies of high-dose oral contraceptives found significantly increased risks of developing cardiovascular disease among users of COCs, several trends have led to a reassessment of that risk. First, studies have become more sophisticated and now take into account the potentially confounding effects of cigarette smoking. Second, in recent years women have been evaluated more carefully before they begin to take oral contraceptives, and those women who have serious underlying medical problems and older women who smoke have been less likely to use oral contraceptives. Third, the formulations have changed dramatically; current formulations have a 3- to 4-fold decrease in estrogen dose and a 1-fold decrease in progestin dose compared with the formulations initially prescribed and studied. Hence the findings of early epidemiologic studies are probably less important with today's products.[7]

Use of oral contraceptives by healthy women who do not smoke does not appear to be associated with an increased risk of either MI or stroke.[8–11] Data from the United States and the United Kingdom have documented no increase in the risk of death from cardiovascular disease among contemporary users of oral contraceptives. Data from the Oxford Family Planning Association study[12] also support the hypothesis that oral contraceptives that contain less than 50 μg of estrogen are safer than high-dose formulations.

Some evidence suggests that the pathophysiology of MI among women who used oral contraceptives in earlier studies was thrombosis and not atherosclerosis.[2] First, most studies, including the large Nurses' Health Study[13,14] from the United States, have found no increased risk of MI among former users of COCs. If atherosclerosis were the cause, then the risk should remain elevated after women discontinued COCs. Corroborating evidence comes from autopsy studies of women who died of MI. Second, there does not appear to be a duration-related effect between length of oral contraceptive use and risk of infarction. This also argues against deposition of plaque as the pathophysiologic mechanism.

Hypertension. As with the increased risks for MI and stroke, older formulations of COCs have been associated with significant elevations of blood pressure as well. The risk of hypertension appears to be much lower when estrogen and progestin doses are lowered. Although some studies have shown no clinically significant changes in blood pressure in low-dose COC users versus nonusers,[15,16] others have shown mildly increased systolic and diastolic blood pressures,[17] and rarely, individual patients have experienced idiosyncratic reactions and have developed hypertension after they begin taking the pill. A recent large epidemiologic study[18] reported a relative risk of 1.8 in current users versus never-users, after adjustment for other risk factors for hypertension. This relative risk appeared to decrease in past users. The mechanism for contraceptive-induced changes in blood pressure is still unclear, with alterations in plasma angiotensinogen and increases in sodium and water retention being noted. Although these are primarily estrogenic effects, progestins may have a synergistic effect, as significant elevations in blood pressure have only been apparent in the combination products and not with either hormone alone.

Hypertension associated with COCs is reversible on discontinuation of the pills, but it may take up to 3 to 4 months to return to normal. It is prudent to monitor patients at the initiation of oral contraception and periodically (e.g., 3 months later) thereafter. If the blood pressure rises significantly, the method may have to be discontinued, although some women may tolerate a lower dose product with careful monitoring.

Thrombosis. The impact of COCs on the blood coagulation system has been less clear. Historically, users of high-dose COCs have had significantly increased risks of developing superficial thrombophlebitis and venous thrombosis versus nonusers. Fatalities as a result are exceedingly rare. As doses of estrogen were lowered to less than 50 μg, a marked drop in the incidence of fatal and nonfatal pulmonary embolism was noted, thus implying an estrogen dose-related effect.[2] A large number of changes in the blood coagulation process have been attributed to estrogen, including an increase in platelet aggregation, increases in several clotting factors and a decrease in antithrombin III activity.[19–21] Which of these changes plays the major role is not known at this time. The role of progestins is also unclear. It was generally accepted that the progestin component did not have a significant impact on clotting parameters, but several observational studies released in 1995 and 1996[22–25] seemed to refute this belief. In these reports, women using low-dose COCs containing either gestodene or desogestrel seemed to have an increased risk of thromboembolism compared to users of low-dose pills with the older progestins. This caused a great amount of concern about the safety of the newer agents. Further review and reanalysis of the data did not confirm the findings, but instead showed possible confounding and bias in the original studies.[26] Part of the problem may have been with patient selection, in that physicians may have prescribed these newer agents preferentially in patients who already had a higher risk for thromboembolism.[27] Also, duration of use may have been a confounding factor, in that it appears the risk for venous thromboembolism is greatest in the first year of use regardless of the formulation used.[28] Several recent studies have not been able to show significant differences between the older and newer progestins, but questions remain.[29,30] An explanation may involve differential effects of the different progestins on sensitivity to activated protein C, which acts as an endogenous anticoagulant.[31] Also, some women may have a newly identified genetic mutation called factor V Leiden, which also causes resistance to activated protein C and increases risk for deep vein thrombosis. The combination of the genetic mutation and a progestin that increases resistance to activated Protein C may help explain the epidemiologic observations, but more study is needed.

As with the other concerns for MI, stroke, and hypertension, patient selection remains the most important method of reducing the incidence of these adverse effects. Women who are already at high risk for cardiovascular problems (hypertension, smoking and older than 35 years, or diabetes with vascular complications) or have already had a cardiovascular or thromboembolic event should not use combination oral contraceptives.

Cancer. The data supporting the protective effects of COCs on the development of uterine and ovarian cancers are clear-cut; the effect of COCs on the risk of breast cancer is more complicated. Previous studies have found increased, decreased, or no change in risk in COC users.

More recent studies have shed some light on the risk in various subgroups of women. The Collaborative Group on Hormonal Factors in Breast Cancer published an extensive study in 1996, which reanalyzed the results of 54 studies.[32] This report indicated a small increase in relative risk of breast cancer in current users, which continues (although at an increasingly lower rate) in previous users up to 10 years after discontinuation. Thereafter, there was no increased risk in ever-users versus never-users. Also, it appeared that if breast cancer was diagnosed in a current or former user of COCs, the cancer was more likely to be less advanced, which possibly may impact survival rates. It still remains to be proven if estrogen use initiates the cancer or merely promotes its growth. Because breast neoplasms are relatively slow growing and usage patterns have changed considerably over the last 25 years, it will still be several years before the complete facts are known. Women may be reassured that the use of hormonal contraception does not increase the risk of breast cancer diagnosed in later life (after age 45), and overall the risk of developing any type of reproductive cancer is reduced.

Even more conflicting than the data on breast cancer are the studies evaluating the risk of cervical cancer. Several studies[33,34] have shown a slightly increased risk but it has been difficult to sort out the confounding risk factors such as multiple partners, coitus at an early age, and the role of human papilloma virus. Also, women using COCs are more likely to have regular cervical cancer screening as a prerequisite for renewal of prescriptions, which may partially explain an increase in diagnosis. It is reasonable to require yearly Pap smears in sexually active women taking COCs, with more frequent screening in those women deemed to be at high risk.

Hepatomas may occur in women taking oral contraceptives. A wide array of benign liver tumors has been reported, the most common of which are focal nodular hyperplasias and liver cell adenomas. Even though these tumors may rupture and bleed, since the advent of low-dose contraceptives, this complication has been quite rare. Hepatocellular cancer was also felt to be associated with COC use, but interestingly enough, there has not been an increase in death rates from liver cancer in the time since this method was introduced.[2]

Gallbladder Disease. Use of oral contraceptives was originally thought to increase the incidence of gallstones and cholecystitis by at least 2-fold. Estrogens alter the composition of bile, possibly by increasing cholesterol saturation of bile. With the decrease in estrogen content, this effect may be less common. One large prospective study showed the relative risk for symptomatic gallstones in ever-users of COCs to be 1.2, in long-term users 1.5, and in current users 1.6.[35] Overall, the incidence is quite low.

Benefits

Using controlled, cyclic doses of hormones, a woman's menstrual cycle can be more regulated and predictable. For most women, with continued use of COCs, the endometrial lining becomes thinner, resulting in less menstrual blood loss and reduced anemia, as well as reduced menstrual cramping or dysmenorrhea. Premenstrual symptoms such as depression, anxiety, and fluid retention may be lessened by the use of COCs,[36] but in some women these symptoms worsen.

Besides these benefits on the menstrual cycle itself, COCs offer other advantages. Perhaps most importantly, women who use COCs have a significantly lower risk than nonusers of COCs of developing either endometrial or ovarian cancer. In both cases, it appears that this protection increases the longer the woman takes COCs and continues for many years after they are discontinued.[37] Also, because of the inhibition of FSH and LH, ovarian stimulation is suppressed, and the incidence of functional ovarian cysts is reduced.[38] This appears to be somewhat dependent on dose, with older, higher-potency COCs offering the most benefit. Benign breast diseases such as fibroadenomas and cysts are also less likely to develop in COC users.[39] With the inhibition of ovulation, the chances for an ectopic pregnancy are markedly reduced.[40]

Acne and hirsutism may be either adversely affected or markedly improved by COCs, depending on the particular product. Combinations that are "estrogen-dominant" in their activity profile are useful in suppressing sebum production and reducing the production of androgenic hormones by the ovaries. Estrogens also increase sex hormone binding globulin levels by 3- to 4-fold, allowing increased binding of testosterone and a decrease in free testosterone. These effects result in reduced androgenic activity and improvement in acne and hirsutism. Progestins may have the opposite effects on sebum production and testosterone levels. If acne or hirsutism is a problem, it is advantageous to choose a COC which is estrogen dominant and/or contains a progestin with low androgenic activity (e.g., desogestrel or norgestimate).[2,41]

Precautions

Table 99.2 indicates which women should not receive combination oral contraceptives.

Types of Combination Oral Contraceptives

Table 99.3 lists the various formulations of COCs currently available on the U.S. market, and their relative activities. Although products containing 50 μg ethinyl estradiol are still available, the grand majority of women use products containing less than 35 μg. All come in either 21- or 28-day pill packs, with active pills being taken for the first 21 days of each cycle, and either no pills or inactive pills for the last 7 days. Menstruation usually occurs 1 to 4 days after the last active pill, and a new pack must always be started 7 days after the last active pill. Monophasic pills contain the same amount of ethinyl estradiol and progestin in each pill. Biphasic formulations, which are seldom used, vary the amount of progestin between the first 10 days and last 11 days. Triphasic pills came about as an attempt to further lower total progestin doses over the 21-day cycle and to more closely mimic physiologic

Table 99.2 ▪ Precautions in the Provision of Combined Oral Contraceptives (COCs)

Refrain from providing COCs for women with the following diagnoses (World Health Organization category 4):

Precautions	Rationale/Discussion
Deep vein thrombosis or pulmonary embolism, or a history thereof	Estrogens promote blood clotting. Thromboembolic events related to known trauma or an intravenous needle are not necessarily a reason to avoid use of pills.
Cerebrovascular accident (stroke), coronary artery or ischemic heart disease, or a history thereof	Estrogens promote blood clotting.
Structural heart disease, complicated by pulmonary hypertension, atrial fibrillation, or history of subacute bacterial endocarditis	Estrogens promote blood clotting.
Diabetes with nephropathy, retinopathy, neuropathy or other vascular disease; diabetes of more than 20 years duration	Estrogens promote blood clotting.
Breast cancer	Breast cancer is a hormonally sensitive tumor. In theory, the hormones in COCs might cause some masses to grow.
Pregnancy	Current data do *not* show that hormonal contraceptives taken during pregnancy cause any significant risk of birth defects. However, hormonal contraceptives should not be given to pregnant women.
Lactation (<6 weeks postpartum)	There is some theoretical concern that the neonate may be at risk due to exposure to steroid hormones during the first 6 weeks postpartum. COCs can diminish the volume of breast milk.
Liver problems: benign hepatic adenoma or liver cancer, or a history thereof; active viral hepatitis; severe cirrhosis	COCs are metabolized by the liver and their use may adversely affect prognosis of existing disease.
Headaches, including migraine, with focal neurologic symptoms	Focal neurologic symptoms such as blurred vision, seeing flashing lights or zigzag lines, or trouble speaking or moving may be an indication of an increased risk of stroke.
Major surgery with prolonged immobilization or any surgery on the legs	Increased risk for deep vein thrombosis and pulmonary embolism is seen.
Older than 35 years and currently a heavy smoker (20 or more cigarettes a day)	Smoking increases the risk for cardiovascular disease.
Hypertension, 160+/100+ or with vascular disease	Hypertension is an important risk factor for cardiovascular disease.

Source: Reprinted with permission from Hatcher RA, Trussell J, Stewart F, et al. Contraceptive technology. 17th ed. New York: Ardent Media Inc., 1998.

changes in hormonal levels. In these formulations, both the estrogen and progestin doses may change throughout the cycle. Two new formulations are of note. Estrostep is the only multiphasic COC in which the progestin dose is fixed and the estrogen dose is gradually increased from 20 μg to 35 μg. Mircette (not shown in Table 99.3) was approved in 1998 and is a monophasic pill containing low doses of estrogen (20 μg) and desogestrel (0.15 mg) and a shortened pill-free interval. After 21 active pills, 2 days of inactive pills are followed by 5 days of pills containing 10 μg ethinyl estradiol.

Initiation, Selection, and Monitoring

As evidenced by Table 99.3, there are many products from which to choose. Providing there are no reasons not to prescribe COCs and after obtaining a medical history, weight, blood pressure, and a Pap smear, any product containing 35 μg or less ethinyl estradiol may be recommended for the majority of women. Individual considerations will be discussed in the following sections.

All COCs can be initiated in one of three ways: (1) the first pill is taken on the first day of the menstrual period ("Day One start"), (2) the first pill is taken on the Sunday after the onset of menses ("Sunday start"), or (3) anytime, if the woman is definitely not pregnant. The Sunday start will result in future periods occurring during the week instead of the weekend, which may be preferable for some women. The Day One start provides immediate protection, so backup contraception is probably not necessary with this method.[3] With the other two methods, a backup method is recommended until seven consecutive pills have been taken.[3] Some clinicians recommend backup protection for the entire first month if patients may be inexperienced with daily pill taking and may miss pills. Patients should be advised to take the pill consistently every day at roughly the same time. Patients should also be informed what to do in the event of a missed pill. This is somewhat dependent on the type of pill being taken and at what point in the cycle the pill is missed. With low-dose pills, especially those containing 20 to 30 μg ethinyl estradiol, one missed pill could be enough to allow ovulation. Modest fluctuations in the levels of FSH and LH among pill users have been observed. This might indicate that follicular development may proceed to a greater extent in some women, resulting in more breakthrough ovulation. Because women who have taken oral contraceptives for a long period of time have ovaries in a semidormant state, they are less likely to experience breakthrough ovulation as a result of a missed pill. On the other hand, women who have not been taking oral contraceptives for long are more likely to have mature follicles ready for ovulation; they may be more affected by a missed pill. Contrary to popular belief, missing pills at midcycle is not the greatest risk period. A high level of hormones early in the cycle is necessary at the level of the hypothalamus for suppression of FSH and LH. Therefore, missing one pill on day 2, for example, would be more likely to result in pregnancy than missing a pill on day 20.

If one pill in the first 3 weeks is missed, it should be taken as soon as possible. If the missed pill is not remembered until the next day, the two pills should be taken together. Backup protection or abstinence may be recommended for the next 7 days. If two consecutive pills are missed during the first 2 weeks, then two should be taken daily for 2 days, followed by resumption of the regular dosing. Backup contraception should be used for the remainder of the cycle. If two pills are missed during the third week, it is recommended that the woman finish taking one active pill daily to the end of the pill pack and then immediately start using a new pack without a pill-free interval in between. If three pills are missed anytime, then the patient should stop the old pack and start over with a new pack. Again, when pills are missed, backup contraception should be used until seven pills have been taken. Manufacturers of individual products may suggest different approaches; it is prudent to consult the package insert

Table 99.3 ▪ Contraceptive Pill Activity[a] (Ranked According to Estrogen Content and Endometrial Potency)

Drug	Endometrial Activity (%)[b]	Estrogenic Activity (μg)[c]	Progestational Activity (mg)[d]	Androgenic Activity (mg)[e]
50 μg estrogen				
Ovral	4.5	42	1.3	0.80
Genora/Necon/Nelova/Norethin/Norinyl/Ortho-Novum 1/50	10.6	32	1.0	0.34
Ovcon 50	11.9	50	1.0	0.34
Norlestrin 1/50	13.6	39	1.2	0.53
Demulen 50/Zovia 1/50	13.9	26	1.4	0.21
Sub-50 μg estrogen monophasic				
Lo-Ovral	9.6	25	0.8	0.46
Ovcon 35	11.0	40	0.4	0.15
Desogen/Ortho-Cept	13.1	30	1.5	0.17
Levlen/Levora/Nordette	14.0	25	0.8	0.46
Ortho-Cyclen	14.3	35	0.3	0.18
Genora/Necon/Nelova/Norinyl/Norethin/Ortho-Novum 1/35	14.7	38	1.0	0.34
Brevicon/Modicon/Necon/Nelova 0.5/35	24.6	42	0.5	0.17
Loestrin 1.5/30	25.2	14	1.7	0.80
Alesse	26.5	17	0.5	0.31
Loestrin 1/20	29.7	13	1.2	0.53
Demulen/Zovia 1/35	37.4	19	1.4	0.21
Sub-50 μg estrogen multiphasic				
Ortho-Novum 7/7/7	14.5	48	0.8	0.25
Tri-Levlen/Triphasil/Trivora	15.1	28	0.5	0.29
Jenest	17.3	39	0.8	0.28
Necon/Nelova/Ortho-Novum 10/11	17.6	40	0.8	0.25
Ortho Tri-Cyclen	17.7	35	0.3	0.15
Tri-Norinyl	25.5	40	0.7	0.23
Estrostep	26.2	16	1.2	0.53
Progestin-only				
Ovrette	34.9	0	0.08	0.13
Micronor/Nor-QD	42.3	1	0.12	0.13

Source: Reprinted with permission from Dickey RP. Managing contraceptive pill patients. 9th ed. Durant, OK: Essential Medical Information Systems, 1998.

Information submitted to the US Food and Drug Administration by the manufacturer. These rates are derived from separate studies conducted by different investigators in several population groups, and, therefore, a precise comparison cannot be made, except when randomized comparative studies are used. Randomized comparative studies used are: NDA 18-985 (Ortho 7/7/7 and Jenest vs. Ortho 1 + 35); NDA 19-653 (Ortho-Cyclen vs. Lo-Ovral); Syntex laboratories study 17-6288 (Tri-Norinyl and Ortho 10/11 vs. Norinyl 1 + 35).

[a]Ranked according to estrogen content and endometrial potency.

[b]Women showing spotting and bleeding in third cycle of use.

[c]Estrogenic activity of entire tablet (mouse uterine assay) as ethinyl estradiol equivalents per day.

[d]Induction of glycogen vacucles in human endometrium as norethindrone equivalents per day.

[e]Methyltestosterone per 28 days by the rat ventral prostate assay.

as well. Patients should also be advised about the availability of emergency contraception (see subsequent section).

Side Effects. In the first one or two cycles, as the body adjusts to new hormone levels, some women experience side effects such as nausea and irregular bleeding or spotting. "Breakthrough bleeding" is a term used to describe this type of bleeding, which occurs between periods and has been difficult to quantify. For most women these problems tend to decrease substantially by the third cycle of pills, although for some women it may continue. If spotting or breakthrough bleeding continues after three cycles, the dose of estrogen or progestin can be adjusted (e.g., increasing the estrogenic potency or endometrial activity of the pill). Another option is to add additional estrogen, either estradiol 2 mg/day or conjugated equine estrogens 1.25 mg/day, taken along with the pill when bleeding occurs.[2]

Many side effects can be attributed to the estrogen or progestin component, either because of an excess effect or a deficiency. Table 99.4 lists various hormone-related effects. With the wide variety of products available with differing hormonal activities, it is possible to manipulate the levels in an attempt to reduce a particular effect. For example, if a woman complains of continued acne, one could suggest switching to a product with less androgens. Several guides are available that give detailed information on the evaluation of side effects and their management.[2,3,42] Clearly, it is important to first rule out the possibility of serious adverse effects before continuing or changing the pill. Patients should be counseled to watch for warning signs that may indicate a serious problem and to report them immediately (Table 99.5).

Table 99.4 ▪ Relation of Side Effects to Hormone Content

Estrogen Excess	Progestin Excess	Androgen Excess
Breast cystic changes	Cervicitis	Acne
Dysmenorrhea	Flow length decrease	Cholestatic jaundice
Heavy flow	Moniliasis	Hirsutism
Cervical extrophy	Increased appetite	Libido increase
Uterine fibroid growth	Depression	Oily skin and scalp
Chloasma	Fatigue	Rash/pruritus
Telangiectasias	Noncyclic weight gain	Edema
	Libido decrease	
Estrogen Deficiency	**Progestin Deficiency**	**Estrogen Excess or Progestin Deficiency**
Absence of withdrawal bleeding	Breakthrough bleeding days 10–21	Bloating
Breakthrough bleeding days 1–9	Delayed withdrawal bleeding	Dizziness
Continuous bleeding and spotting	Dysmenorrhea	Edema
Flow decrease	Heavy flow	Cyclic headache
Atrophic vaginitis		Irritability
Vasomotor symptoms		Leg cramps
		Nausea/vomiting
		Cyclic visual changes
		Cyclic weight gain

Source: Adapted with permission from Dickey RP. Managing contraceptive pill patients. 9th ed. Durant, OK: Essential Medical Information Systems, Inc., 1998.

Table 99.5 ▪ Combination Oral Contraceptive Warning Signs

Symptom	Possible Significance
A: Abdominal pain	Hepatic tumor, gallbladder disease, thrombosis
C: Chest pain (severe cough or shortness of breath)	Myocardial infarction or pulmonary embolism
H: Headache (severe dizziness or weakness)	Hypertension, migraines, or stroke
E: Eye problems (loss or blurring, speech problems)	Stroke or hypertension
S: Severe leg pain (calf or thigh)	Thrombosis

An increase in the frequency of headache (both tension and migraine) has been noted to occur. Approximately half of the women who develop vascular headaches with COCs report preexisting migraine attacks. There is evidence that falling estrogen levels may incite the cerebrovascular system to respond by producing cyclic migraine headaches.[43] Formulations that shorten the pill-free interval and provide very low doses of estrogen for the last several days may be useful for those women who suffer these menstruation-related migraines. Patients with new-onset migraines or worsening headaches after initiation of a COC should discontinue this method.

Increased corneal sensitivity, particularly contact lens discomfort, has been noted in about one of five women who take oral contraceptives.[44] Changes in corneal curvature and decreased tear secretion have been blamed for this side effect in oral contraceptive users and pregnant patients. A variety of ocular changes have been attributed to the pill, ranging from retinal vascular accidents to decreases in visual acuity and color changes.[45] Repeated prospective and retrospective studies failed to find a correlation between the use of birth control pills and many of these abnormalities, which are found normally in a population of women of reproductive age. However, caution should be exercised in prescribing oral contraceptives to women with known ophthalmologic disorders.

Depression has been noted occasionally in COC users. Because of the lack of well-controlled trials and underlying prevalence of depression in this patient population, much controversy exists as to the cause. Depending on the severity and whether there is a temporal relationship, one could try altering the hormonal potency by switching to a lower dose pill. Some women also seem to develop low pyridoxine levels while taking COCs and may respond to supplementation with 50 mg of vitamin B_6.[46] Careful monitoring of the depressed patient is recommended.

Drug Interactions. Evidence indicates that certain drugs may interfere with the efficacy of COCs. The converse is also true; COCs may modify the action of other drugs. Mechanisms thought to be responsible for these interactions include: (1) interference with steroid absorption or reabsorption through enterohepatic circulation; (2) stimulation or inhibition of hepatic metabolism; (3) displacement of steroids from their receptor sites; and (4) opposing steroid action by some physiologic effect.

Gastroenteritis has long been associated with decreased GI transit time and steroid absorption. Because ethinyl estradiol conjugates are excreted in the bile, broken down by gut bacteria to active hormone, and then reabsorbed, anything that increases GI motility (e.g., diarrhea or stimulant laxatives) could reduce circulating concentrations of oral contraceptives and lead to contraceptive failure. Likewise, broad-spectrum antibiotics such as ampicillin or tetracycline may eliminate the gut microflora that is necessary for this enterohepatic circulation. Numerous well-documented clinical reports have appeared of pregnancies in women who have not missed COC doses but were also taking an antibiotic. However, no well-designed clinical studies have been able to prove an increased failure rate or even lower plasma hormone levels in patients taking antibiotics.[47] Unfortunately, a definitive answer to this dilemma is unlikely to be provided from a prospective study for ethical reasons. The most conservative approach, recommended by the International Planned Parenthood Federation, is to use a back-up method of contraception for 2 weeks if a woman is taking a short course of a broad-spectrum antibiotic. They also suggest that after 2 weeks of antibiotic use, the intestinal flora recovers due to acquired resistance, so the risk of failure would be reduced, even with continued antibiotic use.[48]

The most clinically significant drug interactions occur with drugs that affect the hepatic metabolic enzymes through either induction or inhibition. Induction of microsomal enzymes results in increased clearance of the substrate, which in this case could lead to contraceptive failure and unintended pregnancy. Estrogens, including ethinyl estradiol, are substrates for the cytochrome P-450 3A4 isoenzyme and thus may be affected primarily by drugs that induce this particular enzyme. These include: rifampin, rifabutin, carbamazepine, felbamate, phenobarbital, phenytoin, primidone, and troglitazone.[49] Topiramate has also been reported to decrease estrogen levels through an unknown mechanism.[50] Options for patients requiring these medications include increasing the estrogenic strength of the pill to 50 μg (which may increase side effects) or, when possible, choosing another medication. Of the class of antiepileptic drugs, valproic acid, ethosuximide, vigabatrin, and lamotrigine do not appear to interfere with the metabolism of estrogen. Another proposed option is to "tricycle," which means to take active pills for 63 days in a row before having a pill-free week.[3] This method has not been thoroughly studied, but may be an appropriate choice in some circumstances. Griseofulvin use has also been reported to result in reduced serum hormone levels in several case reports.

Benzodiazepines, which undergo oxidation, appear to compete with COCs for these enzymes; this could result in reduced effectiveness of the contraceptive or increased effects of the benzodiazepine.[3] Reduced clearance has also been suggested for corticosteroids, theophylline, aspirin and acetaminophen.[3] Monitoring of a patient taking these drugs is recommended with possible dose reduction if increased effects are seen.

Special Patient Groups

Patients with Diabetes. Historically, patients with established diabetes taking older, high-dose COCs showed a worsening of carbohydrate intolerance. It appears that these changes are caused by the progestin component because estrogens do not affect carbohydrate metabolism.[51] The newer progestins (desogestrel, gestodene, and norgestimate) as well as low doses of COCs containing norethindrone, appear to have negligible effects on glucose tolerance.[52,53] Monophasic pills containing levonorgestrel have caused glucose intolerance in women who previously had gestational diabetes, but triphasic pills with levonorgestrel have not. A study in 1998[54] evaluating the risk for development of type II diabetes in Latino women who previously had gestational diabetes found no increased risk for those using a low-dose COC containing ethinyl estradiol and norethindrone. Risk was significantly increased for those women using a contraceptive containing a progestin only.

Generally, young women with a family history of diabetes or a personal history of gestational diabetes and some women with diabetes who do not have vascular complications can safely take low-dose COCs.

Women Older Than 35. Older women who are healthy and free of any contraindications can safely use low-dose COCs until menopause. The risk for MI seems to be increased primarily in those women who are older than 35 years of age and who also smoke. Estrogen-containing contraceptives are not recommended in this population.

Breastfeeding Patients. Estrogen in COCs appears to inhibit the action of prolactin in breast tissue receptors in a dose-related manner. This results in a decrease in milk production. Some constituents of COCs are found in breast milk as well, although adverse effects on infants have not been noted with the use of low-dose pills. Whereas some experts state that low-dose COCs can be used successfully in lactating women, others suggest that progestin-only pills are preferred. If estrogen-containing pills are used, they should be delayed at least until 6 weeks postpartum, with 8 to 12 weeks being suggested by some, to allow milk production to be fully established.[3]

Progestin-Only Contraceptives

Oral Forms

The second type of oral contraceptive is sometimes called the "mini-pill." This form does not contain estrogen and provides low doses of either norethindrone or norgestrel taken daily without a pill-free interval. Progestins prevent pregnancy by inhibiting ovulation, thickening the cervical mucus, and causing a thin atrophic endometrium. In this case though, ovulation is not inhibited with any predictability. Some women will continue to ovulate regularly, some will not, and others will ovulate sporadically.[3] The effectiveness of this method is thus less than that provided by the COC. Approximately 5% of women will become pregnant in the first year of typical use.

Even though this method of birth control is slightly less effective, it does offer some advantages, particularly in those women who should avoid estrogen. This includes those with estrogen-related adverse effects, smokers, and women who are breastfeeding, as well as those with a history of deep vein thrombosis or cardiovascular complications. The effectiveness in lactating women is nearly 100% because breastfeeding itself provides a contraceptive effect.[55] Progestin does not affect the quantity or quality of milk produced, making this an ideal form for this patient population, although many recommend initiating this method after 6 weeks postpartum.[3] Other benefits include reduced menstrual blood loss and anemia, decreased dysmenorrhea, less risk of endometrial cancer, and possibly a lower risk for pelvic inflammatory disease.

Because ovulation is not blocked consistently, and changes in cervical mucus can be affected by late pills, this is a method that requires absolute compliance with pill taking every 24 hours. Other than the higher failure rate, risks are few with the mini-pill. As with all other forms of hormonal birth control, it should not be used if a woman has unexplained vaginal bleeding, breast cancer, or active liver disease. Women with cardiovascular conditions or diabetes who choose this method should be carefully monitored.

Mini-pills can have unpredictable effects on the menstrual cycle. Women who continue to ovulate will have regular periods, but others will experience irregular periods and spotting. Some will develop amenorrhea. Women considering the mini-pill should be informed about these effects and should accept the high probability of unpredictable bleeding. In some women, symptoms of depression, premenstrual syndrome, or breast tenderness worsen, rather than decrease, while taking progestin-only pills.

Missed pills with this method are more of a concern. Some experts recommend that a backup method of birth control be used at all times or at least for the first cycle while the routine is being established. If a pill is delayed for more than 3 hours, it should be taken as soon as possible and backup contraception should be used for the following 48 hours. Women who miss two pills should take two pills for 2 days, use backup contraception, or consider emergency contraception if intercourse has already occurred.[3] Concurrent use with drugs that induce hepatic microsomal enzymes may result in unacceptable low levels of the progestin and contraceptive failure and thus should be avoided.

Injectable Medroxyprogesterone Acetate

Depot medroxyprogesterone acetate (DMPA) has been used for many years in other countries as an injectable contraceptive and was approved for use in the United States in 1992. The drug suppresses the preovulatory surge of LH and reduces levels of LH and FSH, thus inhibiting ovulation; it also produces the cervical mucus changes and endometrial growth changes discussed earlier.[2] It provides effective contraception, resulting in a 0.3% pregnancy rate in the first year of use. DMPA is given as a deep intramuscular injection in a dose of 150 mg every 12 weeks. Plasma levels of contraceptive are reached within 24 hours with peak concentrations in 20 days. The optimal time to initiate DMPA is within 5 days of the onset of menses. This ensures that the patient is not pregnant and prevents ovulation during the first month of use.

Along with providing the same benefits as the progestin-only pills, DMPA is also advantageous for women who have difficulty with daily compliance. Significant drug interactions are unlikely. Patients with sickle cell disease may experience improvements in their condition while receiving DMPA, possibly due to increased red blood cell stability and reduced painful crises.[56] Patients with seizures may experience a reduction in the frequency of seizures, which may be due to sedative effects of the hormone.[57,58]

Besides the general precautions with hormonal contraceptives, women considering DMPA should be aware that this is not a quickly reversible method. Because of the slow clearance of the drug from the body, it may take 6 to 12 months before fertility returns, which is a significant difference from other methods. Also allergic reactions are possible, although they are rare.

The most common side effect of DMPA is irregular bleeding. Rarely is the bleeding heavy; in most cases it results in prolonged light bleeding or spotting. Amenorrhea develops in at least 50% of women after 1 year of use, which may be seen as a benefit by some women. Weight gain, headaches, abdominal discomfort, breast tenderness, and depression also may occur and if significant may require discontinuation of the injections. Reduced bone density and reductions in high-density lipoprotein cholesterol levels have also been noted in DMPA users. Detailed guidelines on the management of adverse effects and delayed injections can be found in several references.[2,3,59]

Subdermal Implants

Another method of delivering progestin is by subdermal implants. Norplant contains levonorgestrel (216 mg total) in six flexible silicone rods, each about 3.4 cm long. Under local anesthesia, a small incision is made in the upper arm, and the implants are inserted subdermally in a fan-like distribution. The hormone is released at a fairly constant rate, which slowly declines over time, but provides very effective contraception for 5 years. The relatively low circulating levels of levonorgestrel are not sufficient to suppress the secretion of FSH and LH completely, but ovulation is suppressed at least 50% of the time.[3] Also, levonorgestrel in this form has the same impact on the endometrium and cervical mucus as with other forms. These effects and the lack of required compliance contribute to a low pregnancy rate of 0.05% in the first year and a cumulative rate of 3.9% after 5 years. It appears that heavier women have a slightly higher failure rate. If the implants are placed within 7 days of the onset of menses, backup contraception is only necessary for the first 3 days.[3]

Subdermal implants are an ideal choice for a woman who has difficulty complying with daily pill taking or regular injections and does not wish to become pregnant for several years. Should the woman decide to discontinue the method, fertility promptly returns on removal of the implants.

Pain on insertion or removal is possible, although the risk of infection is quite low. Removal of the implants can be difficult if they were not placed properly. Also, because of the low levels of hormones present, enzyme induction by drugs such as phenytoin or carbamazepine may lead to unacceptably low levels and contraceptive failure.

Irregular bleeding is a strong possibility with subdermal implants, and women should be prepared for this. Periods can be irregular, and bleeding can be heavy at times, although this tends to decrease with time. About 7 to 10% of women discontinue use in the first year because of irregular bleeding.[42] Most women return to regular cycles by 1 year. Some recommend the addition of nonsteroidal anti-inflammatory drugs or short courses of estrogen to control bleeding although this has not been systematically studied. Other reported side effects include headaches, nervousness, weight gain, acne, breast tenderness, and ovarian cysts.

Nonhormonal Contraception

A variety of nonhormonal contraceptive devices are available, including spermicidal agents, condoms, intrauterine devices, diaphragms, and cervical caps. The efficacy of these products in theory and in use is shown in Table 99.1.

Spermicidal Agents

Spermicidal agents are available without a prescription in a wide variety of forms, including film, foam, jelly, cream, suppositories, or tablets and may be used alone or in combination with other methods. Estimates of efficacy vary widely, because of the difficulty in controlling all the variables with a method that is quite user-dependent. Pregnancy rates may range from as low as 5 to 6% to more than 50%. These rates are improved when spermicides are combined with other methods.

The primary active ingredient used in the United States in nonoxynol-9, which kills sperm by disrupting the sperm cell membrane. For it to work properly, it must be applied on or near the cervix before intercourse. Products such as films, tablets, or suppositories must be inserted at least 15 minutes before intercourse to allow dissolution and dispersal of the product. When used alone, spermicides are effective for approximately 1 hour. More spermicide must be inserted for additional acts of intercourse.

Benefits of using spermicidal agents include their wide availability in pharmacies and grocery stores, low cost, and reduced risk of some sexually transmitted diseases such as gonorrhea, chlamydia, and trichomoniasis.[3] Unfortunately, it does not appear that nonoxynol-9 provides adequate protection against human immunodeficiency virus (HIV).[3]

Skin irritation or allergy may develop in either partner due to the spermicide or other ingredients. Switching to another form may be useful. Women with abnormal vaginal anatomy may have difficulty using these products properly. Serious adverse effects have not been reported. Also, several well-designed recent studies have shown no increased risk of congenital malformations in newborns[60] or spontaneous abortuses[61] of women who conceived while using spermicides.

With proper selection and appropriate use, these products can be used successfully. Careful attention to details such as timing and insertion techniques are important to emphasize.

Condoms

Due to their ability to prevent sexually transmitted diseases (STDs) and pregnancy, when used consistently and correctly, condoms are one of the most popular contraceptives. They are also accessible, inexpensive, and readily usable. During the 1980s, there was a dramatic increase in condom sales in the United States. Currently, condoms are made to be worn not only by men, but by women as well. Condoms for men are latex rubber sheaths that are worn over an erect penis during coitus. This mechanical barrier prevents transmission of the semen into the vagina. Although pregnancy rates are higher than for users of COCs, barrier methods are effective in preventing the transmission of STDs, including HIV, from either partner. Several in vitro and in vivo studies have demonstrated that latex condoms prevent the transmission of viruses, specifically herpes virus and HIV, when used for vaginal, orogenital, and anogenital intercourse.[62–64] In addition, *Chlamydia trachomatis* and gonorrheal infections can be prevented. There are also "natural membrane" condoms that are made of processed collagenous tissue from the intestinal caecum of lambs. This type of condom is more porous and does not block the transmission of infectious organisms, but may be used to prevent pregnancy in those with a sensitivity to latex. Currently numerous synthetic products are in development that would provide protection from STDs, as well as unintended pregnancy, for people with a sensitivity to latex.

More than 100 brands of condoms are available in different shapes, sizes, colors, and thicknesses. Some condoms have a small amount of spermicide applied to the inside and/or outside of the condom. Condoms are marketed rolled or unrolled, lubricated or unlubricated, and ribbed and may have reservoir ends to collect the semen. When the condom is put on, half an inch of empty space should be left at the tip if the condom does not have a reservoir end. To prevent spillage during withdrawal, the rim of the condom should be held against the base of the penis during withdrawal, promptly after ejaculation. A condom should be used only once.

Oil-based products (e.g., petroleum jelly, hand lotion, or vegetable oil) should never be used to lubricate a condom because they cause deterioration of the latex.

K-Y jelly, contraceptive foam, and saliva are acceptable lubricants. Trying to test a condom for holes by filling it up with water, as well as unrolling it and then sliding it over the penis, increases the probability of breakage.

There is a condom for females called the Reality condom, which has been available over the counter since 1993. It is a polyurethane sheath or pouch that is closed at one end and has two flexible polyurethane rings, one at each end. Polyurethane is stronger than latex and less likely to break or tear. The female condom is approximately 17 cm in length and 7.8 cm in diameter. As with male condoms, the female condom will help prevent pregnancy and is believed to prevent the transmission of STDs, although this has not been proven.[3] The pouch is prelubricated on the inside with a silicone-based lubricant, with an additional bottle of lubricant included.

The open end with the outer ring remains outside the vagina to cover the perineum. The inner ring is needed for insertion and to hold the pouch in place. When inserting the pouch, the inner ring is held between the thumb and middle finger while the index finger is placed on the pouch between the other two fingers. While squeezing the inner ring, the pouch is inserted as far as possible into the vagina to cover the cervix. The pouch should not be twisted. Removal of the pouch should occur before standing up by squeezing and twisting the outer ring and gently pulling. If the penis does not move freely in and out, if the outer ring is pushed inside, or if there is noise during intercourse, more lubricant can be applied. A new condom should be inserted before each additional act of intercourse.

There have been some problems with the acceptability of the female condom. The visibility of the outer ring, unpleasant noises during intercourse and problems with the initial insertion are common complaints. However, with careful training and practice, it is a useful method of contraception and probably protects against STDs.

Intrauterine Devices

The idea of inserting a foreign body into the uterus to prevent pregnancy is not new. The use of intrauterine stones dates back to ancient times. Natural fibers such as silkworm gut were investigated in the early 1900s. After World War II, artificial fibers and various types of polyethylene became available and were molded in many ways to produce intrauterine devices (IUDs). The copper-containing IUD gained popularity in the 1960s, and an IUD that slowly releases progesterone was an innovative development of the 1970s. Currently, IUDs are commonly used by women worldwide, but less than 1% of women in the United States choose them. Litigation concerning IUDs was responsible for many manufacturers voluntarily withdrawing their products, although at this point, litigation has significantly dropped off with an increased emphasis on patient selection, informed consent, and improved documentation.[3] There are two products available now in the United States. The copper T 380A (ParaGard by Ortho) is a copper-containing IUD that can be left in place for up to 10 years. The progesterone T (Progestasert System by Alza) is a T-shaped unit containing a reservoir of 38 mg of progesterone, which is designed to release 65 μg/day. It provides contraceptive action for 1 year. A third IUD, the levonorgestrel-20 IUD (by Leiras) may be approved in the United States soon. This one releases levonorgestrel at a constant rate of 20 μg/day for up to 5 years and may result in less menstrual blood loss.

The mechanism of action of the IUD depends on the type. Copper-containing IUDs appear to cause changes in uterine and tubal fluids, which alter sperm and ova transport and prevent fertilization.[65] Those IUDs containing hormones have the same types of effects on the uterus as other forms of progestin: thickening of cervical mucus, impairment of motility, and disruption of ovulation. Whether they also prevent fertilization has not been determined definitively.

As long as the IUD is inserted correctly and remains in place, it is a highly effective method (Table 99.1). Users should be taught to check for the string extruding from the cervix to ensure that the IUD has not been expelled.

The IUD is a reasonable option for women who need reliable, reversible long-term contraception, who cannot take hormones (for the Copper T 380A), and for whom compliance is a problem with other methods. Women in a mutually monogamous relationship who have already delivered at least one child may be better suited for this method, although with careful counseling, others may consider it as well.[3]

There is an increased risk of pelvic inflammatory disease (PID) in women with IUDs who are subsequently exposed to STDs. The risk appears to be greatest in the first few weeks after insertion and could have ramifications for the woman's future fertility.[66] Also, should a pregnancy occur while the IUD is in place, there is a significantly increased chance of spontaneous abortion occurring, even if the IUD is removed early. Other problems with the IUD include dysmenorrhea and abnormal bleeding or spotting. The IUDs containing hormones appear to decrease these types of side effects. Also, rarely the IUD may gradually work its way through the uterine wall and may need to be removed from the abdominal cavity by laparoscopic procedures. In the first year, up to 10% of women may spontaneously expel the IUD.

Women should be informed about warning signs when an IUD is inserted. Those warning signs requiring medical attention are reflected in this mnemonic[3]:

P: period late (pregnancy); abnormal spotting or bleeding
A: abdominal pain or pain with intercourse
I: infection exposure (any STD) or abnormal discharge
N: not feeling well, fever, chills
S: string missing, shorter or longer

The Diaphragm

The diaphragm is a flexible dome-shaped rubber cap that is available in several styles and diameters (50 to 95 mm). It is inserted into the vagina by the woman before intercourse and blocks the opening to the uterus by covering the cervix. The diaphragm must be fitted by a clinician and should be refitted at each annual examination or if the woman delivers a baby, aborts, or has a significant change in weight.

The most effective use of the diaphragm is in combination with spermicidal agents. The mechanical barrier is useful for holding the spermicide near the cervical os. Spermicides also aid insertion because of their lubricating properties. At least a teaspoonful of spermicidal jelly or cream should be placed into the dome and spread around the inside of the rim before insertion. The diaphragm must remain in place for at least 6 hours after intercourse. Oil-based products (e.g., petroleum jelly or lotions) may cause deterioration of the diaphragm and are not recommended. If additional lubrication is needed, more spermicide or a water-soluble lubricant may be used. Another full applicator of spermicide should be inserted into the vagina, leaving the diaphragm in place, before each subsequent coitus or if more than 6 hours has elapsed since the insertion. There may be a risk of toxic shock syndrome if the diaphragm is left in place for more than 24 hours. After it has been removed, the diaphragm should be washed and stored carefully. The diaphragm may be used during menses.

The key to successful diaphragm use is motivation. Many clinicians fail to recognize the diaphragm as a viable contraceptive option. However, because of its mechanical action, it represents a method of contraception practically devoid of side effects. The diaphragm is not advised for use in patients who have recurrent urinary tract infections or a history of toxic shock syndrome. Also, if there is a lack of trained personnel to fit the device or properly counsel the patient, it should not be used.

The Cervical Cap

There has been a resurgence of interest in a barrier method smaller than a diaphragm that fits over the cervix, called the cervical cap. A cap available in the United States is the Prentif Cavity-Rim Cervical Cap (manufactured by Lamberts Ltd.). The Prentif cap is made of natural rubber (latex) and is thimble-shaped. Spermicide is placed inside the dome before insertion. The cervical cap must be left in place for 6 hours after intercourse but can be left in for a maximum of 48 hours without adding more spermicide, even if intercourse is repeated. If additional lubrication is needed, a water-soluble lubricant or more spermicide may be used. The cervical cap should not be left in for more than 48 hours because of increased risk of toxic shock syndrome. As with the diaphragm, the cervical cap needs to be washed after use and stored carefully. The Prentif cap is manufactured in four sizes and should be fitted by a professional. Pregnancy rates are similar to those with other barrier methods; however in parous women the cap is slightly less effective than in nulliparous women. Because of concern over possible adverse effects on cervical tissue, caps should only be used in women with normal Pap smears. Smears should be checked after the first 3 months of use and annually thereafter. Use of the cap should be discontinued if the Pap smear becomes abnormal although studies have not shown an increase in cervical abnormalities in cap users.[67] The cap should also not be used in women with a history of toxic shock syndrome or repeated urinary tract infections or during any vaginal bleeding. It is important that both the clinician and the patient be comfortable inserting this device.

The Sponge

Another form of vaginal contraception is a nonprescription, disposable polyurethane foam sponge called the Today sponge. It is much smaller and thicker than a diaphragm, with a ribbon loop for removal. The sponge is impregnated with nonoxynol-9, which is activated by adding water shortly before insertion, and it can be left in place over the cervix for up to 24 hours. Contraceptive protection is provided for up to 24 hours regardless of the frequency of intercourse. It should be left in for at least 6 hours after intercourse. Its effectiveness is similar to that of the cervical cap, and it is most effective in nulliparous women. Production of the sponge was voluntarily halted by the manufacturer in 1995 because of an inability to comply with more stringent government-directed mandates at its manufacturing facility, but in 1999 Allendale Pharmaceuticals announced it had bought the sponge and intended to begin manufacturing it again.

Emergency Contraception

Emergency contraception is the use of a method after intercourse to prevent pregnancy. Many women and many health professionals do not know of the availability of emergency contraception, which is unfortunate given the high rate of unintended pregnancies. It has been known for years that a combination of high doses of estrogen and progestin is effective, but it was not until 1997 that the FDA published an opinion supporting the use of the products as safe and effective postcoital contraception.[68]

High doses of estrogen and progestin prevent pregnancy primarily by disrupting follicular development and inhibiting ovulation.[3] Sperm and ova transport may also be affected. If ovulation has already occurred, then pregnancy may not be prevented. True effectiveness rates are difficult to measure given all the underlying variables, but it has been estimated that approximately 74% of pregnancies are avoided that would otherwise have occurred.[3]

Emergency contraception may be advisable anytime unprotected intercourse has occurred, or when a known failure of another method has occurred (e.g., missed pills, broken condom, etc.). It is most effective when started within 24 hours of intercourse, but may be used up to 72 hours afterward. Recommended products and doses are listed in Table 99.6. Generally one dose is taken as soon as possible, with the second dose following 12 hours later. A commercial kit containing 4 pills, a urine pregnancy test, and patient information, became available in late 1998. Up to 50% of women will experience nausea, with vomiting occurring in 15 to 25%. Antinausea drugs such as meclizine or diphenhydramine can be taken before the hormones are taken. Women may also experience breast tenderness, headaches, abdominal pain, and dizziness.

Menstrual changes may also occur, and the next period may be earlier or delayed. If the period has not occurred within 3 weeks of using the emergency contraception, a pregnancy test should be performed. Reassurance can be given that should a pregnancy have occurred, there is little risk of adverse fetal effects as a result of using this method. Information about use of a regular form of birth control should also be provided. Women already taking oral contraceptives should resume their dosing the day after taking the second dose of the emergency contraceptive.

Table 99.6 ▪ Oral Contraceptives Used for Emergency Contraception in the United States

Brand	Pills per Dose	Ethinyl Estradiol per Dose (μg)	Levonorgestrel per Dose (mg)[a]
Nordette	4 light-orange pills[b]	120	0.60
Levlen	4 light-orange pills[b]	120	0.60
Lo/Ovral	4 white pills[b]	120	0.60
Triphasil	4 yellow pills[b]	120	0.50
Tri-Levlen	4 yellow pills[b]	120	0.50
Ovral	2 white pills[b]	100	0.50
Alesse	5 pink pills[b]	100	0.50
Ovrette	20 yellow pills[c]	0	0.75

Source: Reprinted with permission from Hatcher RA, Trussell J, Stewart F, et al. Contraceptive technology. 17th ed. New York: Ardent Media Inc., 1998.

[a]The progestin in Ovral, Lo/Ovral, and Ovrette is norgestrel, which contains two isomers, only one of which (levonorgestrel) is bioactive; the amount of norgestrel in each dose is twice the amount of levonorgestrel.

[b]The treatment schedule is one dose within 72 hours after unprotected intercourse and another dose 12 hours later.

[c]The treatment schedule in the only published prospective study of levonorgestrel was one 0.75 mg tablet (equivalent to 20 Ovrette pills) within 48 hours after unprotected intercourse and another tablet 12 hours later. However, interim data from a large World Health Organization study indicate that the regimen is effective when initiated up to 72 hours after unprotected intercourse.

PREGNANCY TERMINATION

Despite the availability and effectiveness of contraceptive methods, unintended pregnancies still occur at a high rate. Women choosing to end a pregnancy are faced with several difficult decisions. Currently, women may opt for either surgical or medical methods for pregnancy termination. Surgical methods are reviewed elsewhere.[3]

Medical options have not commonly been used in the United States, but this may change with the development of more effective methods. Mifepristone has been available in a few European countries for several years and has been recommended for approval by the FDA. Mifepristone is a competitive progesterone antagonist and acts by causing decidual breakdown and detachment of the embryo. It also may increase responsiveness to uterine prostaglandins, resulting in increased uterine contractions and expulsion. It appears to be most effective when given in early pregnancy, i.e., before 7 weeks or less.[69] It is given orally, often followed by oral or vaginal misoprostol, a prostaglandin E_1 analog, which improves efficacy.[70] Most women will experience cramping and bleeding, although it is very rarely severe.

Misoprostol is also sometimes used with methotrexate, which acts by blocking folic acid in fetal cells, disrupting their division. This combination also appears to be highly effective but has not been extensively studied.[71,72] Most protocols use an intramuscular injection of methotrexate, followed several days later with misoprostol tablets inserted vaginally.

All medical options require close monitoring, follow-up, and support. Also it is important to note that women can quickly become pregnant again after abortion, and options for contraception should be thoroughly discussed.

FUTURE METHODS

In addition to subdermal implants using fewer rods, studies are also progressing with vaginal rings that may contain a progestin alone or in combination with estrogen. These could be inserted by the woman and be left in place for up to 1 year. Long-acting injectables that include estrogen are being developed, which may improve the bleeding irregularities seen with DMPA. Other delivery methods being evaluated are topical gels and transdermal patches.

Hormonal contraception for men is also undergoing study. Options may include a long-acting shot, subdermal implants, or daily pills, all of which work by suppressing sperm production. Current research with nonhormonal methods is focusing on improvements of methods already available, such as male condoms that do not use latex, IUDs that do not cause uterine cramping, and vaginal barriers that are easy to insert and remove. Another avenue is the use of vaccines directed against sperm production in the male, but this method is several years away from being approved.[3,42]

IMPROVING OUTCOMES

Assisting patients in choosing an appropriate contraceptive method and teaching them to use it consistently and correctly should help reduce the rate of unintended pregnancies. For women who choose oral contraceptives it is important to stress the correct day to start the pills and how to avoid missing pills, such as choosing a time of day they will most likely remember or connecting the pill taking with another daily routine such as teeth brushing before bedtime. Patients should know what to do in event of a missed pill and should be encouraged to refill their prescriptions before they finish a pack. Many failures occur because the next cycle of pills is not started on time.

With barrier methods, the appropriate techniques for insertions and removal should be reviewed. It should also be recommended that patients keep adequate supplies on hand to encourage their consistent use.

Regardless of the method chosen, patients should also choose a backup method to have on hand if their primary method fails or if doses are missed. Patients should also be aware of the availability of emergency contraception and that only condoms provide protection against STDs. Finally, every sexually active woman should be reminded of the need for regular physical examinations and screening for cervical cancer.

KEY POINTS

- The choice of a particular method is dependent on individual factors, including the safety and efficacy of the method, the person's ability to use the method correctly, concurrent conditions, and the particular needs and desires of the couple.
- COCs can be used safely and effectively by many women, if properly selected, counseled, and monitored.
- COCs provide many contraceptive and noncontraceptive benefits, including significant reductions in ovarian and endometrial cancers.
- Risks of COC use increase in women who are already at risk for cardiovascular disease including smokers, patients with hypertension or moderate to severe diabetes, and those who have already suffered a vascular event such as a MI, cerebrovascular accident, or deep vein thrombosis.
- Many side effects of COCs may be managed by patient counseling and careful manipulation of the hormonal content.
- Progestin-only pills are not as effective as COCs but are good choices for women who are breastfeeding or who cannot take estrogen.
- DMPA and subdermal implants are highly effective forms of contraception and are good choices for those who have difficulty with compliance with other methods or who have significant problems with estrogen. Women who choose this method should be adequately counseled on the likelihood of irregular bleeding.
- Barrier methods can be effective contraceptives with proper counseling in motivated users. Condoms provide the greatest protection from sexually transmitted infections.
- IUDs and diaphragms can be used safely and effectively in properly selected patients.
- Patients should be aware of the availability of emergency contraception.

REFERENCES

1. Brown SS, Eisenberg L, eds. The best intentions: unintended pregnancy and the well-being of children and families. Washington, DC: National Academy Press, 1995.
2. Speroff L, Darney PD. A clinical guide to contraception. 2nd ed. Baltimore: Lippincott Williams & Wilkins, 1997.
3. Hatcher RA, Trussell J, Stewart F, et al. Contraceptive technology. 17th ed. New York: Ardent Media, 1998.
4. Guillebaud J. The pill and other hormones for contraception. 5th ed. Oxford, UK: Oxford University Press, 1997.
5. Mann JI, Doll R, Thorogood M, et al. Risk factors for myocardial infarction in young women. Br J Prev Soc Med 30:94–100, 1976.
6. Collaborative Group for the Study of Stroke in Young Women. Oral contraceptives and stroke in young women: associated risk factors. JAMA 231:718–722, 1975.
7. Grimes DA. The safety of oral contraceptives: epidemiologic insights from the first 30 years. Am J Obstet Gynecol 166:1950–1954, 1992.
8. Mischell DR. Contraception. N Engl J Med 320:777–787, 1989.
9. Sidney S, Siscovick DS, Petitti DB, et al. Myocardial infarction and use of low-dose oral contraceptives: a pooled analysis of 2 U.S. studies. Circulation 98:1058–1063, 1998.
10. Lewis MA. Myocardial infarction and stroke in young women: what is the impact of oral contraceptives? Am J Obstet Gynecol 179:S68–S77, 1998.
11. Schwartz SM et al. Stroke and use of low-dose oral contraceptives in young women: a pooled analysis of two U.S. studies. Stroke 29:2277–2284, 1998.
12. Mant D, Villard-Mackintosh L, Vessey MP, et al. Myocardial infarction and angina pectoris in young women. J Epidemiol Community Health 41:215–219, 1987.
13. Stampfer MJ, Willett WC, Colditz GA, et al. A prospective study of past use of oral contraceptive agents and risk of cardiovascular disease. N Engl J Med 319:1313–1317, 1998.
14. Colditz GA. Oral contraceptive use and mortality during 12 year follow up: The Nurses' Health Study. Ann Intern Med 120:821–826, 1994.
15. Blumenstein BA, Douglas MB, Hall WD. Blood pressure changes and oral contraceptive use: a study of 2676 black women in the southeastern United States. Am J Epidemiol 112:539–552, 1980.
16. Tsai CC, Williamson HD, Kirkland BH, et al. Low-dose oral contraception and blood pressure in women with a past history of elevated blood pressure. Am J Obstet Gynecol 151:28–32, 1985.
17. Wilson ES, Cruickshank J, McMaster M, et al. A prospective controlled study of the effect on blood pressure of contraceptive preparations containing different types and dosages of progestogen. Br J Obstet Gynecol 91:1254–1260, 1984.
18. Chasen-Taber L, Willett WC, Manson JE, et al. Prospective study of oral contraceptives and hypertension among women in the United States. Circulation 94:483–489, 1996.
19. Dugdale M, Masi AT. Hormonal contraception and thromboembolic disease, effects of oral contraceptives on hemostatic mechanisms. J Chron Dis 23:775-790, 1971.

20. Petersen C, Kelly R, Minard B, et al. Antithrombin III: a comparison of functional and immunologic assay. Am J Clin Pathol 69:500–504, 1978.
21. Howie PW, Mallinson AC, Prentice CRM, et al. Effect of combined estrogen-progestin oral contraceptives on antiplasmin and antithrombin activity. Lancet 2:1329–1332, 1970.
22. WHO Collaborative Study of Cardiovascular Disease and Steroid Hormone Contraception. Venous thromboembolic disease and combined oral contraceptives: results of international case-control study. Lancet 346:1575–1582, 1995.
23. WHO Collaborative Study of Cardiovascular Disease and Steroid Hormone Contraception. Effect of different progestogens in low estrogen oral contraceptives on venous thromboembolic disease. Lancet 346:1582–1588, 1995.
24. Jick H, Jick SS, Gurewich V, et al. Risk of idiopathic cardiovascular death and non fatal venous thromboembolism in women using oral contraceptives with differing progestogen components. Lancet 346:1589–1593, 1995.
25. Spitzer WO, Lewis MA, Heineman LA, et al. Third generation oral contraceptives and risk of venous thromboembolic disorders: an international case-control study. Transnational Research Group on Oral Contraceptives and the Health of Young Women. BMJ 312:83–88, 1996.
26. Lewis MA, Heineman LA, MacRae KD, et al. The increased risk of venous thromboembolism and the use of third generation progestogens: role of bias in observational research. The Transnational Research Group on Oral Contraceptives and the Health of Young Women. Contraception 54:5–13, 1996.
27. Westhoff CL. Oral contraceptives and venous thromboembolism: should epidemiologic associations drive clinical decision making? Contraception 54:1–3, 1996.
28. Lewis MA. The epidemiology of oral contraceptive use: a critical review of the studies on oral contraceptives and the health of young women. Am J Obstet Gynecol 179:1086–1097, 1998.
29. Farmer RD, Lawrenson RA, Thompson CR, et al. Population-based study of risk of venous thromboembolism associated with various oral contraceptives. Lancet 349:83–88, 1997.
30. Farmer RD, Todd JC, Lewis MA, et al. The risks of venous thromboembolic disease among German women using oral contraceptives: a database study. Contraception 57:67–70, 1998.
31. Rosing J, Tans G, Nicolaes GA, et al. Oral contraceptives and venous thrombosis: different sensitivities to activated protein C in women using second- and third-generation oral contraceptives. Br J Haematol 97:233–238, 1997.
32. Collaborative Group on Hormonal Factors in Breast Cancer. Breast cancer and hormonal contraceptives: collaborative reanalysis of individual data on 53,297 women with breast cancer and 100,239 women without breast cancer from 54 epidemiological studies. Lancet 347:1713–1727, 1996.
33. Thomas DB, Ray RM, World Health Organization Collaborative Study of Neoplasia and Steroid Contraceptives. Oral contraceptives and invasive adenocarcinomas and adenosquamous carcinomas of the uterine cervix. Am J Epidemiol 144:281–289, 1996.
34. Zondervan KT, Carpenter LM, Painter R, et al. Oral contraceptives and cervical cancer–further findings from the Oxford Family Planning Association Contraceptive Study. Br J Cancer 73:1291–1297, 1996.
35. Grodstein F, Colditz GA, Hunter DJ, et al. A prospective study of symptomatic gallstones in women: relation with oral contraceptives and other factors. Obstet Gynecol 84:207–214, 1994.
36. Mortola JF. A Risk-benefit appraisal of drugs used in the management of premenstrual syndrome. Drug Saf 10:160–169, 1994.
37. Harlap S, Kost K, Forrest JD. Preventing pregnancy, protesting health: a new look at birth control choices in the United States. New York The Alan Guttmacher Institute, 1991.
38. Broome M, Clayton J, Fotherby K. Enlarged follicles in women using oral contraceptives. Contraception 52:13–16, 1995.
39. WHO Scientific Group. Oral contraceptives and neoplasia. Technical Report Series No. 187. Geneva: WHO, 1992.
40. Franks AL, Beral V, Cates W, et al. Contraception and ectopic pregnancy risk. Am J Obstet Gynecol 163:1120–1123, 1990.
41. Redmond GP, Olson WH, Lippman JS, et al. Norgestimate and ethinyl estradiol in the treatment of acne vulgaris: a randomized, placebo-controlled trial. Obstet Gynecol 89:615–622, 1997.
42. Dickey RP. Managing contraceptive pill patients. 9th ed. Durant, OK: Essential Medical Information Systems, 1998.
43. Mattson RH, Rebar RW. Contraceptive methods for women with neurological disorders. Am J Obstet Gynecol 168:2027–2032, 1993.
44. Smith MB. A quantitative estimate of ocular iatrogenic disease in humans. J Am Optom Assoc 45:751–755, 1974.
45. Wood JR. Ocular complications of oral contraceptives. Opthalmic Semin 2:371–402, 1977.
46. Adams PW, Wynn V, Rose DP, et al. Effect of pyridoxine hydrochloride (vitamin B-6) upon depression associated with oral contraception. Lancet 1:897–901, 1973.
47. Helms SE, Bredle DL, Zajic J, et al. Oral contraceptive failure rates and oral antibiotics. J Am Acad Dermatol 36:705–710, 1997.
48. Kubba A. Drug interactions with hormonal contraceptives. IPPF Medical Bull 30:3–4, 1996.
49. Michalets EL. Update: clinically significant cytochrome p450 drug interactions. Pharmacotherapy 18:84–112, 1998.
50. Rosenfield W, Doose D, Walker S, et al. Effect of topiramate on the pharmacokinetics of an oral contraceptive containing norethindrone and ethinyl estradiol in patients with epilepsy. Epilepsia 38:317–323, 1997.
51. Spellacy WN. Carbohydrate metabolism during treatment with progestogen and low-dose oral contraceptives. Am J Obstet Gynecol 142:732–734, 1982.
52. Mestman JH, Schmidt-Sarosi C. Diabetes mellitus and fertility control: contraception management issues. Am J Obstet Gynecol 168:2012–2020, 1993.
53. Baird DT, Glasier AF. Hormonal contraception. N Engl J Med 328:1543–1549, 1993.
54. Kjos SL, Peters RK, Xiang A, et al. Contraception and the risk of type 2 diabetes mellitus in Latina women with prior gestational diabetes mellitus. JAMA 280:533–538, 1998.
55. Moggia AV, Harris GS, Dunson TR, et al. A comparative study of a progestin-only contraceptive versus nonhormonal methods in lactating women in Buenos Aires, Argentina. Contraception 44:31–43, 1991.
56. De Ceulaer K, Gruber C, Hayes R, et al. Medroxyprogesterone acetate and homozygous sickle-cell disease. Lancet 2:229–231, 1982.
57. Mattson RH, Cramer JA, Caldwell BV, et al. Treatment of seizures with medroxyprogesterone acetate: preliminary report. Neurology 34:1255–1258, 1984.
58. Mattson RH, Rebar RN. Contraceptive methods for women with neurologic disorders. Am J Obstet Gynecol 168:2027–2032, 1993.
59. Nelson AL. Counseling issues and management of side effects for women using depot medroxyprogesterone acetate contraception. J Reprod Med (Suppl) 41:391–400, 1996.
60. Louik C, Mitchell AA, Werle MM, et al. Maternal exposure to spermicides in relation to certain birth defects. N Engl J Med 317:474–478, 1987.
61. Strobino B, Kline J, Lai A, et al. Vaginal spermicides and spontaneous abortion of known karyotype. Am J Epidemiol 123:431–443, 1986.
62. Carey RF, Herman WA, Retta SM, et al. Effectiveness of latex condoms as a barrier to human immunodeficiency virus–sized particles under conditions of simulated use. Sex Transm Dis 16:230–234, 1992.
63. Centers for Disease Control and Prevention. Update: barrier protection against HIV infection and other sexually transmitted diseases. MMWR Morb Mortal Wkly Rep 42:589–591, 1993.
64. Weller S. A meta-analysis of condom effectiveness in reducing sexually transmitted HIV. Soc Sci Med 36:1635–1644, 1993.
65. Ortiz ME, Croxatto HB. The mode of action of IUDs. Contraception 36:37–53, 1987.
66. Farley TM, Rosenberg MS, Rowe PJ, et al. Intrauterine devices and pelvic inflammatory disease: an international perspective. Lancet 339:785–788, 1992.
67. Richwald GA, Greenland S, Gerber MM, et al. Effectiveness of the cavity-rim cervical cap: results of a large clinical study. Obstet Gynecol 74:143–148, 1989.
68. Food and Drug Administration. Prescription drug products; certain combined oral contraceptives for use as postcoital emergency contraception. Fed Regist 62:8610–8612, 1997.
69. Urquhart DR, Templeton AA, Shinewi F, et al. The efficacy and tolerability of mifepristone and prostaglandin in termination of pregnancy of less than 63 days gestation: UK multicentre study–final results. Contraception 55:1–5, 1997.
70. El-Refaey H, Rajasekar D, Abdalla M, et al. Induction of abortion with mifepristone and oral or vaginal misoprostil. N Engl J Med 332:983–987, 1995.
71. Hausknecht RU. Methotrexate and misoprostil to terminate early pregnancy. N Engl J Med 333:537–540, 1995.
72. Wiebe ER. Abortion induced with methotrexate and misoprostol. Can Med Assoc J. 154:165–170, 1996.

CHAPTER 100

DRUGS IN PREGNANCY AND LACTATION

Beth Logsdon Pangle

A pregnant woman takes an average of 3 medications and may take up to 15 medications during her pregnancy.[1–4] Symptoms commonly treated include pain, nausea and vomiting, gastrointestinal upset, edema, and the common cold. Concurrent diseases such as diabetes mellitus, infections, or hypertension may also require treatment.[5] At least 35% of pregnant women have taken some sort of medication during pregnancy, and 40% of pregnant women have taken medications during their first trimester.[6–8] These figures are impressive when you consider that many medications are taken without medical supervision and without a clear indication and may be taken immediately after conception before pregnancy is known. Although many pregnant women may be unnecessarily exposed to drugs, heightened public awareness of medication use and concern for the fetus has reduced drug use in pregnancy. Compared to women in the mid-1960s, women in the 1980s took less medication throughout pregnancy and during the first trimester.[9] However, the World Health Organization (WHO) completed an international survey of drug use in pregnancy involving nearly 15,000 pregnant women from 22 countries. Eighty-six percent of these women took a medication during pregnancy, receiving an average of 2.9 (range 1 to 15) prescriptions per pregnancy.[4] This survey did not take into account over-the-counter medications purchased without the advice of a physician. This extremely high drug utilization rate during pregnancy is then elevated by an increase in drug administration during the intrapartum period, when 79% of women in the WHO study received an average of 3.3 drugs. Little is known about the characteristics of the pregnant women who take medication, but one study identified nonwhite, unmarried, less educated women as less likely to use medication than other groups. This may be a result of less prenatal care within this population, and medical care may be associated with increased use of medications.[3] Also, surveys in Western countries indicate that 90 to 99% of women who are breastfeeding receive a medication during their first week postpartum, 17 to 25% at 4 months postpartum, and 5% of mothers receive chronic medications during breastfeeding.[10,11] With increasing information on the benefits of breast milk, which has nutritional and immunologic properties superior to those of infant formulas, the American Academy of Pediatrics (AAP) recommends breastfeeding for optimal nutrition during the first 6 months of life.[12] This increase in breastfeeding to more than 60% of American mothers today has led to questions regarding the safety and potential toxicity to neonates of drugs and chemicals that may be excreted in the breast milk.

The number of prescription and over-the-counter drugs available for human use is escalating each year. Attention should be paid to drugs that cause harm to the developing fetus. Out of nearly 1000 drugs evaluated for teratogenic potential, only about 30 are proven teratogens. A teratogen is an agent that is present during critical periods of development and is able to produce a congenital defect. The term "congenital defect" refers to major and minor malformations as well as functional abnormalities. Structural abnormalities that require major surgery or that are incompatible with life occur at an incidence of 2 to 4% in the United States. Approximately 10% of children have abnormal physical or mental development. Only 2 to 3% of all abnormalities are believed to be chemical or drug-induced.[13] However, this figure may be underestimated because many cases are not reported. Although the number of infants with defects due to drug exposure is relatively small, the use of drugs during pregnancy should be avoided unless absolutely necessary. However, as will be discussed, medication may be used during breastfeeding in many cases when necessary. Drugs with known or suspected teratogenic effects or nonteratogenic adverse effects, drugs contraindicated or to be used with caution during breastfeeding, and those drugs of choice in pregnancy and lactation are listed in Tables 100.1 through 100.6.

It is the responsibility of the clinician to counsel all patients with complete, accurate, and current information on the risks and benefits of using medications while pregnant or breastfeeding. The fetus or neonate must always be kept in mind as a potential recipient of the drug. Significant harm may come to the fetus or neonate if exposed to an agent. However, drugs are a welcome addition to managing the obstetric patient with chronic medical disorders, which could potentially harm the fetus if left untreated. An example is the use of insulin in pregnant women with diabetes. Compared with previous data, diabetic women today have fewer complications during pregnancy with close monitoring of glucose and the use of insulin. Mothers with a chronic disease, such as hypertension, who wish to breastfeed often are able to because their physicians can select drugs that are minimally excreted in breast milk, such as an angiotensin-converting enzyme inhibitor (ACEI) or a calcium channel blocker (CCB). Each patient should receive careful evaluation and counseling regarding her medical condition and the risks and benefits of the appropriate therapy.

In reviewing the literature, the clinician should keep in mind that data on drugs in pregnancy and lactation are constantly being updated and may appear to be contradictory. Much of the data arises from case reports that may not be generalized to all women. Sound professional judgment based on clinical assessment of the patient and an understanding of the literature must be combined with direct patient counseling before medication is taken during pregnancy or lactation. Patient involvement in the decision-making process is important. This chapter provides a general review of common issues relating to drug use in pregnancy and lactation. Other references should be consulted because this chapter is not meant to include all issues necessary to making patient-specific therapeutic decisions.

Table 100.1 ▪ Known Teratogens

Angiotensin-converting enzyme inhibitors
Alcohol
Androgens (i.e., danazol)
Anticonvulsants (i.e., carbamazepine, phenytoin, valproic acid)
Antineoplastics (i.e., cylophosphamide, methotrexate)
Cocaine
Diethylstilbestrol
Iodides
Isotretinoin
Lithium
Live vaccines
Tetracycline (especially weeks 24–26)
Thalidomide
Warfarin

Sources: References 14–16.

Table 100.2 ▪ Suspected Teratogens

Benzodiazepines (e.g., diazepam)	Oral hypoglycemics
Estrogens	Progestins
Methimazole	Tricyclic antidepressants
Quinolones	

Sources: References 14–16.

Table 100.3 ▪ Drugs with Nonteratogenic Adverse Effects

Antithyroid agents	Diuretics
Aminoglycosides	Isoniazid
Aspirin	Narcotics
Barbiturates	Nicotine
β-Blockers	Nonsteroidal anti-inflammatory drugs
Benzodiazepines	Oral hypoglycemics
Caffeine	Propylthiouracil
Chloramphenicol	Sulfonamides
Cocaine	

Sources: References 14–16.

Table 100.4 ▪ Drugs Contraindicated During Breastfeeding

Amiodarone	Heroin[b]
Amphetamines[a,b]	Isotretinoin
Bromocriptine[a,b]	Lithium[b]
Cocaine[b]	Marijuana[b]
Cyclophosphamide[b]	Methotrexate[b]
Cyclosporine[b]	Nicotine (smoking)[b]
Doxorubicin[a,b]	Phencyclidine (PCP)[b]
Ergotamine[b]	

Source: Reference 17.

[a]Drug is concentrated in human milk.

[b]Included in American Academy of Pediatrics statement.

LIMITATIONS IN THE LITERATURE

Since the early 1960s and the tragedy of the defects caused by thalidomide, the U.S. Food and Drug Administration (FDA) has required that all medications be shown to be safe and effective for the population intended for treatment before becoming commercially available. Unfortunately, because teratogenicity differences and pharmacokinetic drug properties exist between species, animal studies may not be extrapolated to humans.

Most human data regarding drugs during pregnancy or lactation are anecdotal. Although this type of information is not optimal, the importance of it should not be underestimated. In fact, every known teratogen has been identified by astute clinicians who recognized possible associations between drugs used by pregnant women and resulting malformations. Thalidomide and isotretinoin were first reported as teratogenic in case reports. Most case reports await further studies to verify associations. Unfortunately, few epidemiologic studies have been done. The well-known Collaborative Perinatal Project, performed from 1959 to 1965, collected data on a cohort of 50,282 mother-child pairs to investigate the teratogenic role of drugs. The rates of various birth defects in infants of drug-exposed women were compared to those of infants in nondrug-exposed women. These published results are a useful reference for drugs often used during pregnancy.[18]

Yet, even among well-controlled studies, collecting teratologic information is complicated and the data must be carefully evaluated.[19] For many studies and reports there is a lack of uniform definitions of malformations and diagnostic criteria, with most concentrating on major anatomical abnormalities detected at birth. Minor abnormalities are often omitted, and follow-up studies to detect abnormalities later in life are rare. Also, surveys of pregnant women can be limiting because maternal reporting of drugs taken during pregnancy is generally not accurate. Drugs taken, such as over-the-counter medications, may not be accounted for by the mother, and the correct dose or timing of ingestion may be inaccurate. Mothers of infants with birth defects tend to report more accurately than those with normal infants. Interviews with indication-oriented and drug-oriented questions may produce better recall. In summary, understanding that the data regarding drug use in pregnancy is influenced by multiple confounding factors is key in assessing the relative risk of exposure to the infant.

Table 100.5 ▪ Drugs to Be Used with Caution or That May Be of Concern during Breastfeeding

Acebutolol	Indomethacin
Alcohol (large amounts)[b]	Mesalamine (5-aminosalicylic acid)[b]
Aluminum antacids	Methadone (>20 mg/day)
Amantadine	Metoclopramide[a,b]
Antidepressants (amitriptyline, amoxapine, desipramine, clomipramine, doxepin, fluoxetine, fluvoxamine, imipramine, trazodone)[b]	Methimazole
Antipsychotics (chlorpromazine, haloperidol, mesoridazine, perphenazine)[b]	Metronidazole[b]
Atenolol	Nalidixic acid
Benzodiazepines (diazepam, lorazepam, midazolam, prazepam,[a] quazepam, temazepam)[b]	Nitrofurantoin
Chloramphenicol[b]	Phenobarbital[b]
Clemastine[b]	Primidone[b]
Gold salts	Phenytoin
	Salicylates (aspirin)[b]
	Sulfonamides[b]
	Sulfasalazine[b]

Source: Reference 17.
[a]Drug is concentrated in human milk.
[b]Included in AAP statement.

Table 100.6 ▪ Drugs of Choice

Drug Class	During Pregnancy	During Lactation
Analgesics	Acetaminophen	Acetaminophen
Anticoagulants	Heparin, preferably LMWH	Heparin or warfarin
Anticonvulsants	Phenobarbital	Carbamazepine, Ethosuximide, or valproic acid
Antidiabetics	Insulin	Insulin, tolbutamide
Antihypertensives	Methyldopa	ACE inhibitor or CCB
Anti-infectives	Penicillin or cephalosporin	Penicillin or cephalosporin
Corticosteroids	Prednisone	Prednisolone
Decongestants	Oxymetolazine drops/spray	Oxymetolazine drops/spray
GI protectants	Magnesium hydroxide, aluminum hydroxide, calcium carbonate, ranitidine, or sucralfate	Sucralfate or famotidine
Laxatives/stool softeners	Psyllium or docusate	Psyllium or docusate

Source: References 14, 17.
LMWH, low-molecular-weight heparin; *ACE,* angiotensin-converting enzyme inhibitor; *CCB,* calcium channel blocker; *GI,* gastrointestinal.

RESOURCES FOR INFORMATION

When risk to the fetus or infant is determined, there are several sources of information available. TERIS is a computer database that evaluates the potential for harm that could occur to the fetus if a mother takes a medication; this information is summarized in *Teratogenic Effects of Drugs: A Resource for Clinicians.*[20] This system relies primarily on human data and is designed to assess risk by rating agents from none to high in its potential for harm.

In 1979 the FDA devised a system that determines the teratogenic risk of drugs by considering the quality of data from animal and human studies (Table 100.7).[21] Benefits and risks of therapy are included for most drugs, providing therapeutic guidance for the clinician. Although category A is considered the safest category, some drugs with a B, C, or D rating are commonly used in pregnancy. Only category X denotes that a drug is contraindicated and there is no reason to risk using the drug during pregnancy.

Drugs in Pregnancy and Lactation, along with its quarterly updates, is an exhaustive reference that provides an up-to-date summary of available data on specific drugs.[15] Other potential sources for information include the drug manufacturer as well as medical journals. Most important,

Table 100.7 ▪ Food and Drug Administration Categories for Drug Use in Pregnancy

Category A: Controlled studies in women fail to demonstrate a risk to the fetus in the first trimester, and the possibility of fetal harm appears remote.

Category B: Either animal studies do not indicate a risk to the fetus and there are no controlled studies in pregnant women or animal studies have indicated fetal risk, but controlled studies in pregnant women failed to demonstrate a risk.

Category C: Either animal studies indicate a fetal risk and there are no controlled studies in women or there are no available studies in women or animals.

Category D: There is positive evidence of fetal risk but there may be certain situations where the benefit may outweigh the risk.

Category X: There is a definite fetal risk based on studies in animals or humans or based on human experience and the risk clearly outweighs any benefit to pregnant women.

Source: Reference 21.

the data should be carefully evaluated before inferring results to an individual patient. Regarding breastfeeding, most assessments were made with the assumption of a full-term, exclusively breastfed infant. Greater caution should be taken with preterm infants, whereas greater leniency may be used with older, partially breastfed infants. Also, maternal dose was based on standard dosing; therefore, high dosage regimens present higher risk to the infant. Because taking any medication while pregnant or lactating has some degree of risk, conservative use of all medications is warranted. The indications for the drug and the benefit of therapy should be clear, and every safeguard should be taken to decrease the risk of fetal or neonatal harm. Once the decision to use a medication is made, the lowest effective dose should be prescribed for the shortest possible duration. Also, a systematic approach has been proposed by the Drug Information Service of the University of California San Diego Medical Center to minimize infant exposure to drugs in breast milk with minimal disruption of nursing (Table 100.8).

CHOOSING A DRUG FOR A PREGNANT OR NURSING MOTHER

Many drug and nondrug factors should be considered before prescribing medications to a pregnant or nursing mother. Principles of teratology have been identified and timing of exposure during fetal development is the most important factor to consider. Knowing the developmental stage when insult is applied can aid in predicting the possible defect. Exposure around the time of conception and implantation may kill the fetus, possibly without the woman knowing she was pregnant. However, if exposure occurs during the first 14 days after conception when the cells are still totipotential (i.e., if one cell is damaged, another can assume its function), the fetus may not be damaged.[19,20,23] The most sensitive period is from implantation to the end of organogenesis, days 18 to 60, during which damage to the developing organs may occur.[18] From 8 weeks of gestation until birth, morphologic changes may occur as the developmental and growth phases continue, including brain maturation. Drugs administered during labor and delivery may also reach the infant and produce physiologic effects and fetal compromise after delivery. Drugs such as alcohol, however, may cause abnormalities throughout gestation.

Factors that influence teratogenicity of a drug include genotypes of the mother and the fetus, the embryonic stage at exposure, dose, duration of exposure, nature of the agent and the mechanism by which it causes a defect, simultaneous exposure to other drugs or environmental agents that may affect potential abnormalities, the maternal and fetal metabolism of the drug, and the extent to

Table 100.8 ▪ Stepwise Approach to Minimizing Infant Exposure

1. *Withhold the drug.* Some medications such as headache or cold-symptom medication is not essential and can be avoided with the mother's cooperation.
2. *Delay drug therapy.* If a mother is close to weaning her infant from breastfeeding, elective drug use or surgery can be postponed.
3. *Choose drugs that pass poorly into breast milk.* Within a class of drugs (i.e., β-blockers), there are large differences in the amount of drug distribution into milk among the different medications.
4. *Choose an alternative route of administration.* Minimizing maternal serum concentrations through use of locally applied drugs will also minimize drug concentrations in milk and the infant's dose of medication. These include inhaled or topical corticosteroids, inhaled bronchodilators or decongestants, for example.
5. *Avoid nursing at times of peak drug concentrations in milk.* A general rule is that peak concentrations occur in milk approximately 1–3 hours after an oral dose. Nursing just before a dose may help avoid this peak effect on the infant. However, this may not always be successful, particularly in neonates who nurse irregularly and often. This strategy work best for medications with short half-lives in nonextended-release dosage forms.
6. *Take medication before the infant's longest sleep period.* This is useful for long-acting drugs that may be given only once daily.
7. *Temporarily withhold breastfeeding when drug therapy is temporary.* If a dental or surgical procedure is undertaken with a short-course of postoperative medication, mothers may be able to pump extra milk before the procedure to use while not nursing or formula may be substituted. Pumping the breasts during the time of nursing abstinence is necessary to maintain milk flow and relieve engorgement. Breastfeeding may be resumed as early as one to two maternal half-lives (50–75% elimination) after the last dose in drugs where the concern is that particularly toxic serum concentrations will accumulate in the infant with repeated dosing. For drugs with a high potential of toxicity that even a small dose may be harmful, a delay of four to five half-lives (94–97% elimination) or longer may be advised.
8. *Discontinue nursing.* A small number of medications that may be necessary for the mother's health (i.e., cancer chemotherapy) are too toxic to allow nursing. In these cases, it is in the best interest of the child and mother to discontinue breastfeeding.

Source: Reference 22.

which the drug crosses the placenta.[24] Nonionizable drugs with molecular weights less than 600, high lipid solubility, and low protein binding readily cross the placenta. Fetal drug concentrations may be as low as 50% of maternal levels in some cases or may exceed maternal levels in others. Excretion of medication by the fetus occurs primarily via the fetal liver and the placenta. If a patient has already taken a medication before she seeks professional advice about the teratogenic risk, she should be given all information including an opinion of actual risk; however, the decision to continue the pregnancy should ultimately be made by the patient.

Human milk is a suspension of fat and protein in a carbohydrate and mineral solution. A nursing mother can produce 600 ml of breast milk per day containing 6 g of protein, 22 g of fat, and 42 g of lactose. Milk proteins, particularly casein and lactalbumin, and lactose are synthesized entirely from the mammary gland. The role of these proteins in drug binding has yet to be completely elucidated. Drug excretion into milk may be accomplished by binding to the proteins or the protein and/or fat components of the milk fat globule. It is also possible that lipid-soluble drugs may be sequestered in the milk fat globule. All of the nutrients achieve a concentration in the milk that provides ideal nutrients though 6 months of life.[15]

During breastfeeding, the amount of drug available to the nursing infant is influenced by maternal, drug, and infant factors (Table 100.9). Passive drug diffusion into breast milk occurs across a concentration gradient with the mammary epithelium serving as a semipermeable membrane. The concentration achieved depends on the concentration gradient, the molecular weight, the lipid solubility, the degree of drug ionization, and protein binding. Drugs with molecular weights less than 200 can cross from plasma to milk and weak bases can concentrate in milk because of the lower pH compared to plasma. Milk proteins, however, bind drugs much less efficiently than albumin. In addition, because neonates do not absorb and eliminate drugs as well as adults, drug administration to breastfeeding mothers may lead to prolonged elimination in neonates, allowing accumulation with repeated dosing. This may be exaggerated in preterm neonates.

Table 100.9 ▪ Factors Influencing Drug Concentration in Breastfed Infants

Maternal	Milk composition and pH Mammary blood flow Maternal drug metabolism
Drug	Molecular weight (<200) pKa Protein binding Lipid solubility Dose and dosing interval Formulation (i.e., immediate vs. sustained release)
Infant	Amount of breast milk consumed (i.e., fully vs. partially breastfed) Higher GI pH Altered GI flora Prolonged GI transit time Reduced amounts of bile salts and pancreatic enzymes Decreased affinity of neonatal proteins for drugs Greater percentage of body water and extracellular fluid volume Decreased hepatic and renal elimination

Source: Reference 22.
GI, gastrointestinal.

TREATMENT OF PREGNANCY-INDUCED DISEASES

Asthma

Asthma complicates up to 4% of pregnancies.[25,26] The effect pregnancy has on asthma is variable: it may improve, go unaltered, or worsen. Women with severe asthma before pregnancy are more likely to have difficulty with the disease during pregnancy. Maternal and fetal morbidity and mortality increases when asthma is not adequately treated. Neonatal or perinatal mortality, low birth weight, increased risk of transient tachypnea of the newborn, and increased risk of prematurity may be seen more often in pregnant asthmatic women than in normal control subjects. If asthma is controlled, infants are born with no greater risk for congenital abnormalities than the general population.[25–27] Complications may arise as a result of the disease or the drug therapy.

The improved outcome of mother and child associated with treating pregnant asthmatic women supports administration of medications to these women.[28,29] Inhaled β_2-agonists, such as albuterol, have been used successfully in treating mild and infrequent asthmatic episodes. Systemic effects are lessened by using aerosolized therapy, the preferred route of administration for pregnant women. These agents may cause maternal tachycardia, hyperglycemia or hypotension, or neonatal hypoglycemia. Based on results of one surveillance study of 1090 infants who were exposed in the first trimester, polydactyly may be associated with use in the first trimester.[15] Use of albuterol in the first trimester is limited, but use in the second and third trimester has not been linked to congenital defects. Terbutaline is another β-agonist that is commonly used as a tocolytic. There are no reports of adverse effects of albuterol use during lactation, and the β-agonists are considered compatible with breastfeeding.[15]

Theophylline in conjunction with inhalation therapy is considered safe in pregnancy and preferred in patients requiring long-term control.[30] Theophylline should be monitored throughout pregnancy to maintain nontoxic serum concentrations, particularly in the third trimester when a possible decrease in theophylline clearance and/or increase in volume of distribution takes place.[31] Theophylline crosses the placenta, and fetal concentrations are about equal to maternal concentrations. Adverse fetal or neonatal effects include jitteriness, cardiac arrhythmias, hypoglycemia, vomiting, tachycardia, and feeding difficulties. Theophylline does not appear to be associated with congenital defects. Theophylline is excreted in breast milk and may cause irritability and fretful sleep in infants.[22] Neonates may be more likely to be affected because of their slow elimination compared with older infants; therefore, extended-release preparations may be preferable.[15] This drug is considered compatible with lactation by the AAP with maternal plasma concentrations kept as low as therapeutically possible and infant concentrations obtained if adverse effects occur.[22,32]

If steroids are indicated, they should not be withheld.[27] Oral, IV, or inhaled therapy may be used as necessary to control acute attacks. Two reports of infants exposed to prednisone throughout gestation resulted in one with congenital cataracts and the other immunosuppressed. Any association between these abnormalities and steroid therapy has not been supported by other studies, however. No evidence has confirmed that prednisone increases fetal morbidity and mortality and the risk to the newborn is considered to be low.[27] However, spontaneous abortion, prematurity, and cardiac malformations have been documented from experience with 40 women treated with inhaled beclomethasone.[33] Flunisolide or triamcinolone have been suggested as alternative anti-inflammatory agents for inhalation, but documentation on their use is sparse. Corticosteroids occur in small quantities in breast milk; therefore, at standard doses (<20 mg/day of prednisone) or with single oral doses an infant is unlikely to receive significant amounts. With doses <20 mg/day or long-term therapy, prednisolone is preferred (it avoids a double peak concentration in milk from the prodrug effect), with nursing delayed until 3 to 4 hours after a dose.[15,22] Depot injections and inhaled corticosteroids present little or no risk to the nursing infant.[22]

Cromolyn sodium by inhalation is indicated for the prevention of asthmatic attacks. Cromolyn does not have significant systemic absorption, it is unknown whether it crosses the placenta. Currently, there is no evidence of an association between cromolyn and fetal malformations. It has been used without maternal or fetal harm.[29,34]

Coagulation Disorders

Despite pregnancy being a "hypercoagulable state" with increased risk of thromboembolism, the incidence is still low at 0.2 to 0.4%.[23,35] Pregnant women with thromboembolic disease or a history of thromboembolic disease or who are at an increased risk (i.e., antithrombin II or protein C or S deficiency) should receive anticoagulant therapy. Although such therapy has risks, the reduction of antepartum mortality rates from 13 to 1% in women with thromboembolic disease receiving anticoagulants supports treatment of the pregnant patient.[23]

The anticoagulant drug of choice in the pregnant patient is heparin. Heparin does not cross the placenta and has not been associated with congenital defects. Heparin has been used at doses of 5,000 U SC every 12 hours with little risk to the mother or fetus. However, 5,000 U every 12 hours may be inadequate prophylaxis during the second and third trimesters because of increasing heparin requirements in pregnancy. Doses more than 10,000 U every 12 hours may be needed.[36] Perinatal mortality rates are comparatively better for heparin therapy (3.6%) recipients than coumarin therapy recipients (26.1%).[37] Exposure to warfarin during the sixth to ninth week of gestation may result in fetal warfarin syndrome; defects of the central nervous system and skeletal system and facial defects may be seen with exposure throughout pregnancy. Stillbirths, spontaneous abortion, mental retardation, and impairment in physical growth may also occur. Although advantageous in many respects over other anticoagulants, the use of heparin has risks for the mother. Bleeding, particularly during delivery, and thrombocytopenia (incidence up to 15%) may occur. Use of heparin for protracted period of time (3 to 6 months) is associated with a reversible osteopenia and is more likely with doses more than 20,000 U/day.[35] Periodic monitoring of prothrombin time, activated partial thromboplastin time, hematocrit, and platelet count is useful. If bleeding occurs, heparin may be rapidly reversed with protamine sulfate. A general rule is 0.5 mg of protamine for every 100 U of heparin. Heparin does not pass into breast milk because of its high molecular weight.[15] Warfarin therapy does not appear to cause significant risk to the breastfeeding neonate with little or no drug diffusing into the breast milk and is considered compatible with nursing by the AAP.[32] Also, because of the oral route of administration with warfarin and the significant risk of osteoporosis associated with protracted heparin therapy, warfarin is the ideal anticoagulant for use during the postpartum period for maintenance therapy.

It appears that low-molecular-weight heparin (LMWH) may be at least as safe and effective as unfractionated heparin, without the need for laboratory monitoring and less risk of bleeding because of minimal effects on platelets and vascular permeability. LMWH also does not cross into the fetal circulation, but it is unknown whether LMWH causes less heparin-induced osteoporosis. In addition to animal studies, human studies involving more than 180 pregnancies in which LMWHs were used showed no increase in adverse fetal effects.[38] Despite lack of documentation, LMWHs still have a relatively high molecular weight and, as such, should not be expected to be excreted into human milk.[15]

Common Cold

The common cold often affects pregnant women whose resistance is weakened. The viruses causing the common cold have not been found to be teratogenic. However, determining the risk associated with most cold medications is difficult because of confounding variables such as the underlying illness and polypharmacy. The short-lived symptoms often include watery eyes and nose, coughing, sneezing, and congestion. If at all possible, medication therapy should be avoided. If medication must be used, combination products should be avoided and single agents be used to limit drug exposure.

If the patient's symptoms require an antihistamine, both chlorpheniramine and triprolidine have been commonly used in pregnancy. A significant increased risk of birth defects has been reported with brompheniramine use in the first trimester; therefore this drug is not recommended. Antihistamine use in the last 2 weeks of pregnancy was found to increase the risk of retrolental fibroplasia in exposed premature infants. Antihistamines are excreted into breast milk and the AAP recommends the use of clemastine with caution during breastfeeding.[32] Nasal cromolyn, beclomethasone, or flunisolide are useful alternatives.[22]

Minor malformations, including club foot and inguinal hernia, have been documented with first trimester use of decongestants. Of the decongestants, pseudoephedrine has not been associated with adverse outcomes. Phenylpropanolamine should be avoided because of possible significant physical deformations associated with early use.[13] Phenylephrine and oxymetazoline may be used as topical nasal decongestants, which advantageously limits systemic absorption. Pseudoephedrine is excreted in breast milk, but the AAP considers the drug to be compatible with breastfeeding.[32]

Antitussives and/or expectorants, such as dextromethorphan and guaifenesin, have been used in pregnant women despite little documentation of their use. Pregnant women should avoid those products containing alcohol, because of the risk of fetal alcohol syndrome, which has been documented in a woman who abused cough medication. The addition of alcohol in cough preparations should also discourage use in breastfeeding.

Constipation

Pregnant patients commonly complain of symptoms of constipation. Possible causes include increased pressure on colon and rectum, decreased peristalsis, increased progesterone, decreased motilin, or increased colonic absorption of water.[39] Patients experiencing constipation should add fiber to the diet and increase water intake. Moderate exercise helps maintain regularity.

Bulk-forming laxatives appear to be safe in pregnancy and lactation and are the agents of choice. Because these agents are not absorbed systemically, they do not pose a threat to the fetus or neonate. Adequate fluid intake needs to be stressed when taking bulk laxatives to prevent intestinal obstruction. Surfactants, such as docusate sodium, may be effective but limited information is available regarding use in pregnancy. Mineral oil should be avoided because of the risk of decreased absorption of fat-soluble vitamins. Use of senna in moderate doses is acceptable according to the AAP and it may be used as a second-line drug during lactation.[32]

Diabetes Mellitus

The risk of congenital abnormalities is three times greater in pregnant overt diabetics than in nondiabetic population.[40] Congenital anomalies result in 3 to 22% of infants born to diabetic mothers and are associated with poor glucose control compared to 2% incidence in the normal population.[41] Blood glucose control is elemental in decreasing the incidence of perinatal morbidity and mortality. When possible, pregnancy in the diabetic woman should be planned to prevent complications. It is important that the patient be normoglycemic before conception and during the first trimester because the congenital effects associated with diabetes are related to poor glucose control in the first eight weeks of gestation.[42]

Patients at highest risk of complications during pregnancy include those with vasculopathy, poor glucose control, a previous stillbirth, and medication noncompliance. Diabetes during pregnancy is commonly categorized according to the White classification.[43] This system classifies patients based on presence of vascular disease, age of onset, and duration of diabetes mellitus in the patient. The potential effects on the infant include macrosomia, polyhydramnios, malformations, respiratory distress syndrome, and fetal behavior and intellectual impairment. With good prenatal management, diabetic patients now have a 96% chance of delivering a healthy child.

During pregnancy, diabetic patients have an increased risk of ketoacidosis, which may occur at lower glucose concentrations than in the nonpregnant diabetic woman. Ketoacidosis is associated with a 50% perinatal mortality rate and can be prevented with close monitoring at home by the patient. Glycosylated hemoglobin monitoring once each trimester is helpful in assessing control. Most women should be able to maintain glucose levels between 60 and 120 mg/dL.[44] About 70% of pregnant diabetic women have increased insulin requirements after the 24th week, and requirements usually double by the end of pregnancy. Insulin has a large molecular weight and crosses the placenta minimally with indirect effects on the fetus, making insulin the treatment of choice by the American College of Obstetrics and Gynecologists for patients with type I and II diabetes as well as gestational diabetes if diet alone fails. The use of insulin provides the best glucose control.[45] Breastfeeding significantly reduces blood sugars, allowing a reduced dose of insulin.[22] Diabetic mothers may breastfeed without insulin passing into breast milk.[15]

Oral hypoglycemic agents are contraindicated during pregnancy because they cross the placenta and stimulate the fetal pancreas and potentiate fetal and neonatal hypoglycemia. They may also be associated with teratogenicity with no advantage over insulin in the pregnant patient, except the avoidance of an injection.[15] These agents should be discontinued before conception or as soon as possible after pregnancy is determined. Little information is available about the use of oral hypoglycemic agents during breastfeeding. Tolbutamide and chlorpropamide are excreted in breast milk in small quantities, and tolbutamide is the recommended agent during nursing.[22] No reports describe the use of glipizide or glyburide during lactation, but an excretion pattern similar to that of chlorpropamide or tolbutamide should be expected.[15]

Gestational diabetes develops during the second half of pregnancy in 2 to 3% of patients.[41] Women with gestational diabetes have a lessened risk of congenital abnormalities compared to women with overt diabetes because gestational diabetes generally does not occur until the 24th week of gestation, after organogenesis is complete. The patient with gestational diabetes is initially given a diabetic diet and home glucose monitoring. If glucose control is not achieved with diet alone, insulin should be started.

Tight glucose control should be maintained during labor and delivery to reduce the risk of neonatal hypoglycemia. During delivery, the mother should receive 5% dextrose with 10 Units of regular insulin per liter at a rate of 100 mL/hr. Glucose should be monitored every 1 to 2 hours with additional glucose or insulin given to maintain a glucose level of 100 mg/dL. Immediately after delivery, insulin requirements drop and remain low for 24 to 72 hours. The patient should be monitored closely to prevent hypoglycemic shock. If the mother chooses to breastfeed, lower insulin requirements are expected as well.

Epilepsy

Despite nearly one million American women of childbearing age having epilepsy, less than 1% of pregnancies are complicated by seizure disorders.[46] The primary goal in managing these patients is prevention of seizures with the fewest adverse effects on the fetus. Pregnancy has unpredictable effects on the frequency and severity of seizures. Overall, most women experience no change in the frequency of seizures during pregnancy, and some patients note a decrease in seizure frequency. One third of patients reportedly have an increase in frequency of seizures; however, with increased attention to management of anticonvulsant therapy during pregnancy, it is more likely that only 25% actually have an increase in seizure frequency.[47] Patients with epilepsy, both those taking medication and those not taking medication, have a higher incidence of delivering an infant with congential malformations and mental retardation.[46,48] Although it is difficult to separate the effects of medication from the effects of disease, literature reviews indicate that anticonvulsants are associated with an increase in congenital defects. Although teratogenicity does occur with anticonvulsants, the benefits of treatment in preventing maternal seizures outweigh the risk to the infant.

The AAP recommends that a patient who is seizure free for at least 2 years undergo a trial of medication withdrawal before becoming pregnant. Patient counseling should begin as soon as pregnancy is considered. The risk of delivering an infant with birth defects in healthy women is 2 to 4% and increases to 4 to 6% in pregnant epileptic women receiving monotherapy. Pregnant epileptic women have a greater than 90% chance of having a normal child.[49]

Further research is needed to determine which, if any, anticonvulsant is safest for mother and child. Serious risks are inherent with each agent. Monotherapy is preferred using the lowest effective dose possible to minimize risk. The clinician should be aware of the changes in anticonvulsant pharmacokinetics that occur during pregnancy, resulting in lower serum concentrations. These pharmacokinetic changes include increased renal and hepatic clearance, decreased protein-binding capacity, and increased volume of distribution. Despite lower serum concentrations, seizure frequency may not increase because free drug concentrations do not decline proportionately with total drug concentration. Anticonvulsant serum concentrations should be monitored throughout pregnancy and dose adjustments made based on serum concentration, frequency of seizures, and adverse effects.

Serious and sometimes fatal hemorrhagic disease of the newborn may occur and be seen within 24 hours after delivery in infants exposed to anticonvulsants. This is caused by a deficiency in vitamin K-dependent clotting factors, and all infants should be treated prophylactically with vitamin K 2 mg IM at birth.[48] Some physicians recommend administering oral vitamin K prophylactically to the mother during the last 2 to 4 weeks before expected delivery.[46] Prophylaxis is necessary because treatment may not be successful once there is clinical evidence of bleeding. Because folate deficiency occurs during anticonvulsant therapy, prophylactic administration of folic acid throughout gestation is recommended to prevent megaloblastic anemia and neural defects.[50]

Phenytoin causes fetal hydantoin syndrome, and effects may be evident in childhood. This syndrome includes school and learning problems, developmental problems, and physical abnormalities such as craniofacial abnormalities, growth retardation, limb defects, cardiac lesions, hernias, and distal digital and nail hypoplasias.[51] Many congenital malformations are surgically correctable. There is about a 10% risk for a fetus exposed to phenytoin to develop the full syndrome and about 30% risk for partial expression of the syndrome.[52] The teratogenic potential of phenytoin may be more closely related to the metabolites than to the parent drug. Genetic variations may help explain why some infants are affected and others are not affected after exposure to phenytoin.

Phenobarbital is the drug of choice in pregnant epileptic women because it appears to be less teratogenic than phenytoin.[48] During pregnancy, higher dosages are usually needed to maintain therapeutic serum levels. Similar to phenytoin, coagulopathy and folate deficiency may occur with phenobarbital use. Unlike phenytoin, phenobarbital may cause neonatal addiction and withdrawal symptoms, such as hyperactivity, feeding disturbances, tremulousness, or diarrhea. Withdrawal symptoms usually occur within 7 days of delivery, and symptoms may develop after discharge to home. Parents should be advised to monitor for symptoms at home and to be aware that the infant may require treatment with phenobarbital. Phenobarbital appears in milk in relatively large amounts, with drowsiness, potential feeding difficulties, infantile spasms after weaning, and one case of methemoglobinemia reported.[15,22,32] Phenobarbital may be used cautiously in low doses with close monitoring of infant behavior, weight gain, and periodic infant serum concentrations.[32]

Carbamazepine has been used in pregnancy and was previously thought to be less teratogenic than other anticonvulsants. However, reports indicate that carbamazepine is teratogenic and has been associated with defects such as spina bifida (1%), craniofacial defects, nail hypoplasia, and developmental delay.[53,54] According to the AAP, carbamazepine may be used during lactation, but occasional monitoring of infant serum drug levels may be indicated.[32]

The fetal valproate syndrome has been described in case reports with associations of cleft palate, renal defects, and neural tube defects (1 to 2%).[55,56] Minor and major cardiovascular and craniofacial malformations, mental and physical developmental deficiencies, and meningomyelocele have also occurred with its use in pregnancy. It appears that valproate, rather than its metabolite, is teratogenic and therefore valproate should be avoided during pregnancy.[57] However, low valproate concentrations are found in milk, and no adverse effects have been reported in breastfed infants.[15]

Data on use of the newer anticonvulsants, felbamate, gabapentin, lamotrigine, and topiramate, during pregnancy are limited, and they have been assigned a pregnancy risk category of C.[58] An international lamotrigine-exposure registry and follow-up study of 53 pregnant epileptic women showed no difference from birth outcomes in the general population.[59] The manufacturer of felbamate suggests that it be used with caution in breast-feeding mothers. Women receiving gabapentin, topiramate, or tiagabine should breastfeed only if the benefits outweigh the risks. Breastfeeding is not recommended while the mother is taking lamotrigine.[60]

Heartburn

Nearly 30 to 50% of pregnant women complain of heartburn, particularly during the third trimester.[61] This results from relaxation of the lower esophageal sphincter and increased pressure from the uterus onto the stomach, allowing regurgitation of stomach contents into the lower esophagus. Nonpharmacologic management should be tried initially and a low-fat diet is recommended. Patients should also avoid caffeine, spicy foods, orange juice, tomato juice, or peppermint. Small, frequent meals and avoiding meals just before bedtime often helps alleviate the symptoms. Elevating the head of the bed is sometimes effective as well. Antacids such as magnesium and/or aluminum hydroxides are usually effective and appear to be safe. Although sucralfate is an aluminum salt and aluminum has been associated with neurobehavioral and skeletal toxicity in animals, there is no evidence of absorption from the gastrointestinal tract and no reports of associated congenital defects when it is taken during pregnancy or adverse effects on breastfed infants.[61]

Drugs used in the nonpregnant patient to manipulate lower esophageal sphincter tone are not currently recommended during pregnancy. Antacids should be used rather than histamine-2 antagonists, bethanechol, cisapride, and metoclopramide. Despite the antiandrogenic effects of cimetidine, this effect is not present with ranitidine in animals or humans. Data indicate no association of ranitidine and fetal or neonatal effects when used throughout pregnancy, and it would be the preferred agent if a histamine-2 antagonist is needed. Because famotidine has less excretion in breast milk, it is the histamine-2 antagonist of choice during lactation.[22] The use of metoclopramide is classified by the AAP as a potential concern because of the possibility of defects in neural tube development in newborn animals. However, the AAP considers the use of cisapride as acceptable during breast feeding.[32]

Hemorrhoids

Hemorrhoids often develop or worsen during pregnancy owing to increased venous pressure below the uterus and constipation. Treating the constipation along with sitz baths are useful in reducing discomfort from hemorrhoids. External medications are preferred over those inserted into the rectum because of possible systemic absorption across the rectal mucosa.

Hypertension

Pregnancy-induced hypertension can be a serious and life-threatening obstetric complication. Gestational hypertension is diagnosed when the blood pressure exceeds 140/90 mm Hg in the absence of proteinuria or pathologic edema. Preeclampsia is divided into two forms, mild and severe. Mild preeclampsia is hypertension accompanied by proteinuria (>300mg/24 hr or 100 mg/dL in two random samples 6 hours apart) and/or pathologic edema. Preeclampsia is considered severe when proteinuria exceeds 4 g/24 hr or persistent values of 2+ are present by dipstick, blood pressure is 160/110 mm Hg, and/or severe headache, visual disturbances, or epigastric pain is noted. Eclampsia is the development of generalized seizures in a patient with pregnancy-induced hypertension. Pregnancy-aggravated hypertension is diagnosed in a patient with preexisting essential hypertension with diastolic increases of 15 mm Hg or systolic increases of 30 mm Hg after the 24th week of gestation. Preeclampsia is superimposed if proteinuria or pathologic edema is present.[6]

The incidence of preeclampsia is 5 to 8% in the United States.[6] Risk factors include first pregnancy (up to 85%), young or older maternal age, multiple gestation, family history, diabetes mellitus, essential hypertension, and molar pregnancies (i.e., tumor-like mass of cysts instead of embryo that grows from tissue of fertilized egg). Complications include intrauterine growth retardation (IUGR), placental insufficiency or abruption, and preterm labor and delivery. The incidence of complications increases in direct proportion to increased blood pressure.

Prevention of preeclampsia with low-dose aspirin has been suggested for patients are high risk of developing preeclampsia. Because of the potential imbalance of prostaglandins as a causative factor for preeclampsia, prophylactic aspirin has been studied. Low-dose aspirin has been shown to decrease thromboxane A_2 synthesis to a greater degree than the decrease in prostacyclin synthesis, which would theoretically normalize the ratio of thromboxane A_2 and prostacyclin. Aspirin 60 mg/day is started at 24 to 28 weeks of gestation and continued until onset of labor.[62,63] The usefulness of low-dose aspirin in preventing preeclampsia has been verified by several studies, but investigation continues to determine which patients are at highest risk for preeclampsia and might benefit from prophylaxis.[62–64] Although there have been no adverse effects noted in mothers or infants exposed to low-dose aspirin during pregnancy, unnecessary exposure to medication should be avoided if the risk of preeclampsia is low.[64] Low-dose aspirin has not been shown to be effective in preexisting preeclampsia/eclampsia.

The goal of treatment of preeclampsia is to decrease blood pressure, prevent or control seizures, and deliver a viable infant. Treatment for mild preeclampsia includes bed rest, daily urine protein measurements, and twice daily blood pressure monitoring. Diuresis usually begins within 48 hours with symptom regression within 5 days. Patients unable or unwilling to comply with these restrictions should be hospitalized. Antihypertensive medications have not been shown to be useful in prolonging gestation in pregnancies complicated by pregnancy-induced hypertension.[6] Women with severe preeclampsia must be hospitalized, IV or IM magnesium sulfate given to prevent seizures, and plans for induction of labor or cesarean delivery made. Magnesium sulfate is administered with a 4-g loading dose IV or IM followed by 1 to 3g/hr IV continuous infusion or 10 g (5 g in each buttock) plus 5 g every 4 hours IM. Intravenous administration may be preferred owing to the feasibility of rapid discontinuation if toxicity occurs as well as lack of pain that is associated with multiple large-volume IM injections. Convulsions not controlled by adequate serum concentrations of magnesium may respond to IV diazepam or phenytoin. Monitoring for signs of toxicity is extremely important with maintenance of serum concentrations at 4 to 7 mEq/L. Patient patellar reflexes, respiratory rate greater than 10/min, and urine output greater than 25 mL/hr should also be maintained. Neonates should be monitored for respiratory depression and hyporeflexia if exposed to magnesium sulfate for an extended period of time. Treatment of mild maternal magnesium toxicity includes 1 g of calcium gluconate, but calcium treatment may not be effective for hypermagnesemia of the neonate.

Treatment of severe hypertension (i.e., systolic greater than 160 mm Hg or diastolic at least 110 mm Hg) requires drug treatment to decrease the risk of maternal cerebrovascular accidents. Intravenous hydralazine is most commonly used at doses of 5 to 10 mg, followed by 10 mg every 20 minutes as needed to decrease diastolic pressure below 100 mm Hg. Hydralazine has not been clearly associated with congenital defects; however, three cases of neonatal thrombocytopenia and bleeding have been documented with its use. Patients may experience tachycardia, headache, flushing, tremors, and palpitations, and propranolol may be useful for combating the cardiac effects but should not be used alone for treatment of hypertension. Diazoxide is not recommended for control of blood pressure in patients with preeclampsia or eclampsia because of multiple serious adverse effects including maternal and neonatal hyperglycemia, maternal hypotension, and inhibition of labor. Labetalol, an α- and β-adrenergic blocker, is an acceptable alternative to hydralazine for the acute treatment of hypertension in preeclampsia/eclampsia. The recommended initial dose is 10 to 20 mg IV, and then the dose is doubled every 10 to 30 minutes until blood pressure is controlled or to a maximum of 300 mg. Continuous infusion of labetalol at 1 to 2 mg/min has also been used to achieve control, with reduction of the dose to 0.5 mg/min to maintain blood pressure. Labetalol has a faster onset with less tachycardia than hydralazine, but IV hydralazine tends to be more effective.[6,65] Neonatal bradycardia and mild transient hypotension have been reported rarely with labetalol. Nitroprusside has been used for life-threatening hypertensive emergencies, but should be avoided if possible because of the potential for neonatal cyanide toxicity.

If therapy is initiated during gestation for patients with hypertension without preeclampsia, methyldopa 250 mg two to three times daily has been used most often and remains the drug of choice.[66] Data regarding long-term effects fail to document physical or mental abnormalities caused by the drug. Using methyldopa reportedly increases fetal survival rates and decreases midtrimester fetal loss. Clonidine is an alternative agent that has been shown to be effective for severe hypertension in late pregnancy with no associated reports of congenital abnormalities.[67] However, because clonidine offers no advantage over methyldopa and there is more experience with methyldopa, methyldopa is generally the preferred agent. Hydralazine 10 to 25 mg two to three times daily has also been used as in conjunction with methyldopa when needed for chronic hypertension.

β-Blockers have been used in pregnancy for various indications. Effects on the mother and fetus vary among these agents because of their differences in pharmacokinetic and pharmacodynamic profiles. These drugs cross the placenta readily, producing fetal steady-state serum levels that approach maternal levels. Because of the potential for decreased fetal heart rate reactivity, the neonate exposed to these agents near delivery should be monitored for 24 to 72 hours after birth. Experience with atenolol, labetalol, and metoprolol in the first trimester is limited and additional study is needed to assess their effects. In the second and third trimesters, these agents have not been found to induce premature labor or produce congential malformations. Unlike methyldopa, no long-term follow-up studies past 1 year have been conducted for metoprolol, propranolol, or labetalol. Propranolol has been effective in doses of 80 to 140 mg/day, but IUGR, bradycardia, hypoglycemia, and neonatal respiratory distress syndrome may occur in newborns.[68] Metoprolol has been found to be safe at doses of 100 mg/day with decreased perinatal mortality when compared to hydralazine.[69] Atenolol has been used mainly in late pregnancy at doses of 50 to 100 mg/day. IUGR has been shown to be associated with atenolol therapy, especially when it is initiated early in pregnancy. However, one-year follow-up studies have found normal growth and development in children exposed in utero during the third trimester.[70] Labetalol may have fewer cardiac effects on the fetus because of its α- and β-blocking effects. Newborns should be observed for 24 to 48 hours because of the potential for transient hypotension or bradycardia, but the majority of infants do not appear to be adversely affected.[71] Sibai et al.[72] showed the association of growth retardation with labetalol use in the third trimester. Because of the lower excretion of drug in milk, labetalol, metoprolol, and propranolol would be preferred for use in breastfeeding mothers and is supported by the AAP.[15,22,32]

Despite widespread use of CCBs in the treatment of hypertension in the nonpregnant population, there is limited information available on the use of calcium channel blockers in pregnancy.[73,74] However, Magee et al.[75] completed a prospective, multicenter trial in 78 women with first-trimester exposure to CCBs blockers. They found no increased risk of congenital malformations compared to that of control subjects. CCBs have been shown to be effective in treating acute hypertension in a small number of patients near term, yet animal studies associated nifedipine use with fetal hypoxia, acidosis, and decreased uterine blood flow. Nifedipine may increase the neuromuscular blockade properties of magnesium sulfate and the combination should be avoided.[76] Although limited information is available, the AAP considers these agents safe for use in nursing mothers.[32]

ACEIs are contraindicated in pregnancy because they cause fetal and neonatal anuria, oligohydramnios, congentital malformations, and fetal death.[65,77] Mothers with exposure to ACEIs should receive counseling regarding potential adverse outcomes, and infants who were exposed should be monitored closely for renal failure and hypotension.[78] Captopril and enalapril are both found in small quantities in breast milk with no adverse effects in infants.[22] These agents are considered compatible with breastfeeding according to the AAP.[32]

The use of diuretics in pregnancy is controversial. The main concern regarding diuretic use is their effect on the volume status of the patient by decreasing plasma and extracellular volume, decreasing cardiac output, and decreasing placental and uterine perfusion. This may accentuate problems in women with previously contracted fluid volumes and preeclampsia. Thiazides and loop diuretics have been used in late gestation for refractory hypertension. Adverse effects of thiazide diuretics include neonatal hypoglycemia resulting from maternal hyperglycemia, electrolyte imbalances, thrombocytopenia, decreased weight gain, and increased perinatal mortality. Therefore, these agents are not first-line therapy for treatment of hypertension in pregnancy. The AAP considers thiazide diuretics compatible with nursing, but thrombocytopenia, lactation suppression, and allergic reactions are potential adverse effects of sulfonamide diuretics.[22,32] Loop diuretics may suppress the volume of milk produced and should be avoided.[22] Acetazolamide and spironolactone appear in negligible concentrations in milk and are compatible with breastfeeding.[22,32]

Although fetal loss is about 16% in women with mild hypertension and may reach 40% in women with severe hypertension, the primary goal of blood pressure management is to prevent maternal complications.

Nausea and Vomiting

The nausea and vomiting of pregnancy are usually mild and often referred to as "morning sickness." Up to 80% of pregnant women experience nausea and vomiting during pregnancy, most commonly during the first trimester.[58,79] Nausea and vomiting of pregnancy is distinguished from hyperemesis gravidarum, which is intractable vomiting leading to electrolyte imbalance, maternal weight loss, altered nutritional status, and at times, end-organ or neurologic damage. Hyperemesis gravidarum occurs in 1 in 1000 births and generally requires hospitalization and treatment with intravenous fluids, electrolytes, antiemetics, and sedation.[79] In very severe cases, peripheral or central parenteral nutrition may be necessary. Treatment with parenteral nutrition has been shown to be effective in providing the mother and fetus with adequate nutrition.

Symptoms usually begin within a few weeks of conception and continue through the first 4 months. Nausea is often apparent on arising but abates as the day progresses. Some women report nausea and vomiting throughout the day and in some patients it persists throughout the pregnancy.[80,81] Although symptoms are self-limiting, nearly 83% of women experiencing nausea and vomiting report taking medication for relief.[80]

The etiology of nausea and vomiting in pregnancy is unknown, but several possibilities are proposed, including increased concentrations of hormones during pregnancy and emotional and psychologic factors. Because the cause is unknown, treatment is focused on the symptoms. The goal of therapy is to eliminate the symptoms, improve the patient's quality of life, do no harm to the fetus, and prevent hyperemesis gravidarum from occurring. Conservative nonpharmacologic measures should be tried first. Mild to moderate nausea and vomiting may be managed by efforts such as instructing the patient to eat small, frequent meals. High-carbohydrate meals, crackers, or high-protein snacks may also be helpful. Spicy foods and noxious odors should be avoided, and many patients find relief by lying down. When nondrug measures fail or if the nutritional and metabolic health of the mother is at risk, drug therapy may be required. Although teratogenic risk cannot be ruled out for any drug, the risk involved with the current agents used for nausea and vomiting in pregnancy appears to be minimal. Meclizine is commonly used as the drug of choice; use in the first trimester has been associated with low teratogenic risk.[18] Dimenhydrinate has been used as an alternative with an apparently low risk of adverse outcomes.[82] When symptoms are not controlled and the health of the mother and fetus calls for drug therapy, phenothiazines (i.e., promethazine or prochlorperazine) may be used. Conflicting results have been reported regarding the safety of phenothiazines, so routine use is not recommended. Other agents that appear safe in pregnancy include metoclopramide, droperidol, or ondansetron.[83]

Pyridoxine deficiency has been hypothesized to cause nausea and vomiting of pregnancy. The demand for pyridoxine is increased during pregnancy, and women may develop a deficiency of this vitamin if supplementation is not given. However, the deficiency does not develop until the second or third trimester. Thus, this may not explain symptoms of nausea and vomiting that occur with normal pyridoxine levels or in the first trimester. Studies have been conducted on the efficacy of pyridoxine in eliminating symptoms, but this is yet to be proven.[84]

OTHER COMMONLY USED DRUGS OF ABUSE

In addition to counseling pregnant women regarding various prescription and nonprescription medications during pregnancy and lactation, other substances that are commonly used should not be overlooked. Pregnant women should be informed of the risks of using any of the following substances.

Alcohol

The worldwide incidence of fetal alcohol syndrome (FAS) is estimated to be between 1:300 and 1:2000 live births.[85,86] The syndrome is characterized by defects of the central nervous system, craniofacial abnormalities, and growth and mental difficulties. Affected infants can display a wide range of other abnormalities. Mental retardation is the most significant consequence. Nearly 30 to 40% of infants born to alcoholic women (i.e., ≥4 drinks/day) have complete FAS, and up to 70% may have partial expression of the syndrome, referred to as fetal alcohol effects (FAE). Additional maternal factors that may contribute to expression of the syndrome are poor nutrition, smoking, drug abuse, inadequate prenatal care, genetic disposition, and low socioeconomic status.

The effects are dose related, but the amount of ethanol that may be ingested without causing abnormalities is unknown. Two drinks per day has been related to decreased birth weight while binge drinking or drinking ≥6 drinks per day are associated with adverse physical and intellectual outcomes and possibly stillbirth.[87,88] Pregnant women should be informed that a safe level of consumption and the phase of development most susceptible are not known. Women should thus avoid alcohol throughout pregnancy and even when trying to conceive.

Although alcohol passes freely into breast milk, reaching concentrations of approximately maternal serum levels, the effects on infants have been considered insignificant except in rare cases or at very high concentrations. Potentiation of hypothrombinemic bleeding, a pseudo-Cushing's syndrome, has been reported in nursing infants of alcoholic mothers.[15] Alcohol ingestion of 1 g/kg daily decreases the milk ejection reflex. Alcohol should be used in moderation during lactation and nursing should be withheld temporarily after alcohol consumption (i.e., 1 to 2 hours per drink).[22] Despite potential effects in infants such as drowsiness, diaphoresis, deep sleep, weakness, decrease in linear growth, and abnormal weight gain, the AAP considers maternal ethanol use compatible with breastfeeding.[32]

Caffeine

Caffeine is found in various quantities in many beverages, analgesics, diet aids, and stimulants. On average, 1 cup of coffee can have up to 180 mg of caffeine, 1 can of soda up to 90 mg, and 1 oz of milk chocolate has 6 mg. Diet aids and stimulants contain 100 to 200 mg per dose. This makes caffeine the number one drug ingested by pregnant women. This potent central nervous system stimulant crosses the placenta, with fetal levels similar to maternal levels, but caffeine has not been shown to be a major teratogen in humans.[89] Numerous studies have been done to assess effects on the fetus, with results ranging from no effect to demonstration of complications.[18] These studies are difficult to interpret because of confounding factors, such as cigarette and alcohol use. Long-term data through age 7 have shown no effects of perinatal caffeine exposure on intelligence, attention, or physical growth.[90] A positive correlation exists between heavy caffeine use and cigarette smoking. High doses of caffeine may cause fetal breathing movements and cardiac arrhythmias. Currently studies are looking at the risk of spontaneous abortion and IUGR because of conflicting results in prior studies.[91] Conflicting results also have been published regarding difficulty to conceive and caffeine intake.[92,93] However, if a woman is having difficulty conceiving, it is reasonable to eliminate or decrease caffeine intake.

In summary, current studies document conflicting results, and the limitations of present studies make positive associations difficult. In 1980 the FDA advised all women, based on animal toxicity data, to avoid caffeine use during pregnancy. Although, when used in moderation, no association with congenital malformations, spontaneous abortions, preterm birth, and low birth weight has been proven.[15]

In breastfeeding, the concentrations of caffeine in breast milk after maternal ingestion is probably too small to be clinically important, and the AAP considers usual amounts of caffeine to be compatible with breast-feeding.[15,32] However, reports exist of infant jitteriness and difficulty sleeping with high maternal intake of caffeine (≥ 6 caffeinated drinks per day).[22]

Nicotine

Maternal smoking is one of the few known preventable causes of perinatal morbidity and mortality. Despite documentation and information regarding the adverse effects on the fetus and the mother, young women continue to be a large consumer group of smokers.[94] Fetal, neonatal, and infant mortality is increased, birth weight and length are decreased, gestation is shortened, and the frequency of fetal breathing movements is reduced. Complications of pregnancy such as abruptio placentae, premature rupture of membranes, amnionitis, and placenta previa may also occur. Changes in uterine and placental oxygenation or blood flow may be the cause of infant death, prematurity, or spontaneous abortions. Complications in infancy and childhood may evolve into deficits in long-term physical growth or intellectual and behavioral performance.[23,88,95]

The effect of smoking is dose related. Light smoking (less than 1 pack/day) was found to increase fetal death by 20% and heavy smoking (1 or more packs/day) increases the risk by 35%. Similarly, birth weight is lower with heavier smoking. According to the Surgeon General's report in 1990 on smoking cessation, women who quit smoking within the first trimester of pregnancy or before conception reduce the risk of having a low-birth-weight baby compared to those of women who never smoked.[96] Smoking cessation during pregnancy may also decrease the potential for death or preterm delivery. Birth weight may not be improved if the woman simply reduces the number of cigarettes smoked per day. All women should be informed of the risk of smoking on the fetus and encouraged to quit during pregnancy.

Both nicotine and its metabolite, cotinine, are concentrated in milk and excreted in amounts proportional to the number of cigarettes smoked by the mother.[22] Smoking is associated with infantile colic.[97] Nicotine shortens the period of breastfeeding by lowering maternal serum prolactin concentrations.[22] The AAP considers smoking to be contraindicated during breastfeeding.[32] Anderson[22] advises lactating women to stop or decrease smoking as much as possible, not to smoke before nursing, and not to smoke in the same room with the infant.

KEY POINTS

- Medication use in pregnancy and lactation is a complex issue, and efforts must be made to provide the patient, as well as the fetus or neonate, with the most safe and effective medication.
- Most medications taken by the mother reach the fetus to some extent.
- Patient education is imperative to ensure maternal involvement in the decision process regarding medication risk and benefit.

REFERENCES

1. Doering PL, Stewart RB. The extent and character of drug consumption during pregnancy. JAMA 239:843–846, 1978.
2. Rudd CC, Brazy GE. Drugs in the perinatal period: implications for the preterm infant. Pediatrics 14:30–37, 1988.
3. Buitendijk S, Bracjen MB. Medication in early pregnancy: prevalence of use and relationship to maternal characteristics. Am J Obstet Gynecol 165:33–40, 1991.
4. Collaberative Group on Drug Use in Pregnancy. An international survey on drug utilization during pregnancy. Int J Risk Saf Med 1:1,1991.
5. Bologa-Campeanu M, Koren G, Rider M, et al. Med Toxicol 3:307–323, 1988.
6. Cunningham FG, MacDonald PC, Grant NF, et al: Williams Obstetrics. 19th ed. Norwalk: Appleton & Lange, 1993.
7. Bodendorfer TW, Briggs GG, Gunning JE. Obtaining drug exposure histories during pregnancy. Am J Obstet Gynecol 135:490–494, 1979.
8. Bonati M, Bortolus R, Marchetti F, et al. Drug use in pregnancy: an overview of epidemiological (drug utilization) studies. Eur J Clin Pharmacol 38:325–328, 1990.
9. Rubin PC, Craig GF, Gavin K, et al. Br Med J 292:81–83, 1986.
10. Bennett PN, Matheson I, Dukes NMG, et al: Drugs and human lactation. Amsterdam: Elsevier, 1988.
11. Matheson I, Kristensen K, Lunde PKM. Drug utilization in breast feeding women. A survey in Oslo. Eur J Clin Pharmacol 38:453–459, 1990.
12. American Academy of Pediatrics. Policy statement based on task force report: the promotion of breast feeding. Pediatrics 69:654–661, 1982.
13. Oakley GP. Frequency of human congenital malformations. Clin Perinatol 13:545–554, 1986.
14. Koren G, Pastuszak A, Ito S. Drugs in pregnancy. N Engl J Med 338:1128–1137, 1998.
15. Briggs GG, Freeman RK, Yaffe SJ. Drugs in pregnancy and lactation. 5th ed. Baltimore: Williams & Wilkins, 1998.
16. McCombs J. Therapeutic considerations in pregnancy and lactation. In: Dipiro JT, Talbert RL, Yee GC, et al. Pharmacotherapy a pathophysiologic approach. Stanford: Appleton & Lange, 1997.
17. Logsdon BA. Drugs in lactation. J Am Pharm Assoc 37:407–418, 1997.
18. Heinonen OP, Slone D, Shappiro S. Birth defects and drugs in pregnancy. Littleton, CO: PSG Publishing, 1977.
19. Werler MM, Pober BR, Nelson K, et al. Reporting accuracy among mothers of malformed and nonmalformed infants. Am J Epidemiol 129:415–421, 1989.
20. Friedman JM. Teratogenic effects of drugs: a resource for clinicians. Baltimore: Johns Hopkins University Press, 1994.
21. Fed Regist 44:37434–37467, 1980.
22. Anderson PO. Drug use during breast-feeding. Clin Pharm 10:594–624, 1991.
23. Niebyl JR. Drug use in pregnancy. 2nd ed. Philadelphia: Lea & Febiger, 1988.
24. Dicke JM. Teratology: principles and practice. Med Clin North Am 73:567–582, 1989.
25. Perlow JH, Montgomery D, Morgan MA, et al. Severity of asthma and perinatal outcome. Am J Obstet Gynecol 167:963–967, 1992.
26. Clark SL. Asthma in pregnancy. Obstet Gynecol 82:1036–1040, 1993.
27. Demissie K, Marcella SW, Breckenridgee MB, et al. Maternal asthma and transient tachypnea of the newborn. Pediatrics 102:84–90, 1998.
28. Schwartz DB. Medical disorders in pregnancy. Emerg Med Clin North Am 5:509–528, 1987.
29. Stenius-Aarniala B, Piirila P, Teramo K. Asthma and pregnancy: a prospective study of 198 pregnancies. Thorax 43:12–18, 1988.
30. Carter BL, Driscoll CE, Smith GD. Theophylline clearance during pregnancy. Obstet Gynecol 68:555–559, 1986.
31. Greenberger PA. Asthma in pregnancy. Clin Perinatol 12:571–584, 1985.
32. American Academy of Pediatrics Committee on Drugs. The transfer of drugs and other chemicals into human breast milk. Pediatrics 93:137–150, 1994.
33. Greenberger PA, Patterson R. Beclomethasone dipropionate for severe asthma during pregnancy. Ann Intern Med 98:478–480, 1983.
34. Wilson J. Use of sodium cromoglycate during pregnancy: results on 296 asthmatic women. J Pharm Med 8:45–51, 1982.
35. Rutherford SE, Phelan JP. Clinical management of thromboembolic disorders in pregnancy. Crit Care Clin 7:809–828, 1991.
36. Dahlman TC, Hellgreen MS, Blomback M. Thrombosis prophylaxis in pregnancy with use of subcutaneous heparin adjusted by monitoring heparin concentrations. Am J Obstet Gynecol 161:420–425, 1989.

37. Ginsberg JS, Hirsh J, Turner DC, et al. Risks to the fetus of anticoagulant therapy during pregnancy. Thromb Haemost 61:197–203, 1989.
38. Wahlberg TB, Kher A. Low molecular weight heparin as thromboprophylaxis in pregnancy. Haemostasis 24:55–56, 1994.
39. West L, Warren J, Cutis T. Diagnosis and management of irritable bowel syndrome, constipation, and diarrhea during pregnancy. Gastroenterol Clin N Am 21:793–802, 1992.
40. Reece EA, Hobbins JC. Diabetic embryopathy: pathogenesis, prenatal diagnosis, and prevention. Obstet Gynecol Surv 41;325–335, 1986.
41. Barss VA. Diabetes and pregnancy. Med Clin North Am 73:685–700, 1989.
42. Gabbe SG. Management of diabetes mellitus in pregnancy. Am J Obstet Gynecol 153:824–828, 1985.
43. White P. Classification of obstetric diabetes. Am J Obstet Gynecol 149:171–173, 1984.
44. Landon MB, Gabbe SG. Diabetes mellitus and pregnancy. Obstet Gynecol Clin North Am 19:633–654, 1992.
45. Committee on Technical Bulletins of the American College of Obstetricians and Gynecologists. ACOG Technical Bulletin, No. 200, December 1994.
46. Yerby MS, Devinsky O. Epilepsy and pregnancy. Adv Neurol 64:53–63, 1994.
47. Devinsky O, Yerby MS. Women with epilepsy: reproduction and effects of pregnancy on epilepsy. Neurol Clin 12:479–495, 1994.
48. Dalessio DJ. Seizures and pregnancy. N Engl J Med 312:559–563, 1985.
49. American Academy of Pediatrics Committee on Drugs. Anticonvulsants and pregnancy. Pediatrics 63:331–333, 1979.
50. Delgado-Escueta AV, Janz D. Consensus guidelines: preconception counseling, management, and care of the pregnant woman with epilepsy. Neurology 42:149–160, 1992.
51. Buehler BA, Delimont D, Van Waes M, et al. Prenatal prediction of risk of the fetal hydantoin syndrome. N Engl J Med 322:1567–1572, 1990.
52. Lewis DP, VanDyke DC, Shimbo PJ, et al. Drug and environmental factors associated with adverse pregnancy outcomes. Part I: Antiepileptic drugs, contraceptives, smoking, and folate. Ann Pharmacother 32:802–817, 1998.
53. Jones KL, Lacro RV, Johnson KA, et al. Pattern of malformations in the children of women treated with carbamazepine during pregnancy. N Engl J Med 320:1661–1666, 1989.
54. Roza FW. Spina bifida in infants of women treated with carbamazepine during pregnancy. N Engl J Med 324:674–675, 1991.
55. DiLiberti JH, Farndon PA, Dennis NR, et al. The fetal valproate syndrome. Am J Med Genet 19:473–481, 1984.
56. Omtzigt JG, Los FJ, Grobbee DE, et al. The risk of spina bifida after first trimester valproate exposure in a prenatal cohort. Neurology 42:119–125, 1992.
57. Nau H, Tzimas G, Mondry M, et al. Antiepileptic drugs after endogenous retinoid concentrations: a possible mechanism of teratogenesis of anticonvulsant therapy. Life Sci 57:53–60, 1995.
58. Malone FD, D'Alton ME. Drugs in pregnancy: anticonvulsants. Semin Perinatol 21:114–123, 1997.
59. Eldridgge RR, Tennis P. Monitoring birth outcomes in the lamotrigine pregnancy registry [Abstract]. Epilepsia 36:90, 1995.
60. Chang SI, McAuley JW. Pharmacotherapeutic issues for women of childbearing age with epilepsy. Ann Pharmacother 32:794–801, 1998.
61. Baron TH, Ramirez B, Richter JE. Gastrointestinal motility disorders during pregnancy. Ann Intern Med 118:366–375, 1993.
62. Sibai BM, Caritis SN, Thom E, et al: Prevention of preeclampsia with low-dose aspirin in healthy, nulliparous pregnant women. N Engl J Med 329:1213–1218, 1993.
63. Hauth JC, Goldenberg RL, Parker CR, et al. Low-dose aspirin therapy to prevent preeclampsia. Am J Obstet Gynecol 168:1083–1093, 1993.
64. Imperiale TF, Petrulis AS. A meta-analysis of low-dose aspirin for the prevention of pregnancy-induced hypertensive disease. JAMA 266:261–265, 1991.
65. Kyle PM, Redman CWG. Comparative risk-benefit assessment of drugs used in the management of hypertension in pregnancy. Drug Saf 7:223–234, 1992.
66. National High Blood Pressure Education Working Group. Report on high blood pressure in pregnancy. Am J Obstet Gynecol 163:1691–1712, 1990.
67. Horvath JS, Phippard A, Korda A. Clonidine hydrochloride–a safe and effective antihypertensive agent in pregnancy. Obstet Gynecol 66:634–638, 1985.
68. Redmond GP. Propranolol and fetal growth retardation. Semin Perinatol 6:142–147, 1982.
69. Remuzzi G, Ruggenenti P. Prevention and treatment of pregnancy-associated hypertension: What have we learned in the last 10 years? Am J Kidney Dis 18:285–305, 1991.
70. Reynolds B, Butters L, Evans J, et al. First year of life after the use of atenolol in pregnancy associated hypertension. Arch Dis Child 59:1061–1063, 1984.
71. Pickles CJ, Symonds EM, Pipkin FB. The fetal outcome in a randomized trial of labetalol versus placebo in pregnancy-induced hypertension. Br J Obstet Gynecol 96:38–43, 1989.
72. Sibai BM, Gonzalez AR, Mabie WC, et al. A comparison of labetalol plus hospitalization versus hospitalization alone in the management of preeclampsia remote from term. Obstet Gynecol 70:323–327, 1987.
73. Goldberg CA, Schrier RW. Hypertension and pregnancy. Semin Nephrol 11:576–593, 1991.
74. Probst BD. Hypertensive disorders of pregnancy. Emerg Med Clin North Am 12:73–89, 1994.
75. Magee LA, Schick B, Donnenfeld AE, et al: The safety of calcium channel blockers in human pregnancy: a prospective, multicenter cohort study. Am J Obstet Gynecol 174:823–828, 1996.
76. Snyder SW, Cardwell MS. Neuromuscular blockade with magnesium sulfate and nifedipine. Am J Obstet Gynecol 161:35–36, 1989.
77. Shotan A, Wilderhorn J, Hurst A, et al. Risks of angiotensin-converting enzyme inhibition during pregnancy: experimental and clinical evidence, potential mechanisms, and recommendations for use. Am J Med 96:451–456, 1994.
78. Rosa FW, Bosco LA, Graham CF, et al. Neonatal anuria with maternal angiotensin-converting enzyme inhibition. Obstet Gynecol 74:371–374, 1989.
79. Walters WAW. The management of nausea and vomiting during pregnancy. Med J Aust 147:290–291, 1987.
80. Vellacott ID, Cooke EJA, James CE. Nausea and vomiting in early pregnancy. Int J Gynecol Obstet 27:57–62, 1988.
81. Gadsby R, Barnie-Adshead AM, Jagger C. A prospective study of nausea and vomiting during pregnancy. Br J Gen Pract 43:245–248, 1993.
82. Leathem AM. Safety and efficacy of antiemetics used to treat nausea and vomiting in pregnancy. Clin Pharm 5:660–668, 1986.
83. World MJ. Ondansetron and hyperemesis gravidarum. Lancet 341:185, 1993.
84. Sahakian V, Rouse D, Sipes S, et al. Vitamin B6 is effective therapy for nausea and vomiting: a randomized, double-blind, placebo-controlled study. Obstet Gynecol 78:33–36, 1991.
85. Council on Scientific Affairs American Medical Association. Fetal effects of maternal alcohol use. JAMA 249:2517–2521, 1983.
86. Committee on substance abuse and committee on children with disabilities. Fetal alcohol syndrome and fetal alcohol effects. Pediatrics 91:1004–1006, 1993.
87. Frequent alcohol consumption among women of childbearing age-behavioral risk factor surveillance system, 1991. MMWR Morb Mortal Wkly Rep 42:328–335, 1994.
88. Streissguth AP, Barr HM, Sampson PD. Moderate prenatal alcohol exposure: effects on child IQ and learning problems at age 7½ years. Alcohol Clin Exp Res 14:662–669, 1990.
89. Hill LM, Kleinberg F. Effects of drugs and chemicals on the fetus and newborn, part I. Mayo Clin Proc 59:707–716, 1984.
90. Barr HM, Streissguth AP. Caffeine use during pregnancy and child outcome: a 7-year prospective study. Neurotoxicol Teratol 13:441–448, 1991.
91. Mills JL, Holmes LB, Aarons JH, et al. JAMA 269:593–597, 1993.
92. Wilcox A, Weinberg C, Baird D. Caffeinated beverages and decreased fertility. Lancet 2:1453–1456, 1988.
93. Joesoef MR, Beral V, Rolfs RT, et al. Are caffeinated beverages risk factors for delayed conception? Lancet 1:136–137, 1990.
94. Cigarette smoking among women of reproductive age–United States, 1987–1992. MMWR-Morb Mortal Wkly Rep 43:789–797, 1994.
95. Olsen J, Pereira A, Olsen SF. Does maternal tobacco smoking modify the effect of alcohol on fetal growth? Am J Public Health 181:69–73, 1991.
96. Centers for Disease Control. The Surgeon General's 1990 Report on the Health Benefits of Smoking Cessation [Executive Summary]. MMWR Morb Mortal Wkly Rep 39:RR12, 1990.
97. Matheson I, Rivrud GN. The effect of smoking on lactation and infantile colic. JAMA 261:42–43, 1989.

CHAPTER 101

ALZHEIMER'S DISEASE

Darlene Fujimoto and Nathan Rawls

DEFINITION

In 1907 Alois Alzheimer, a neuropsychiatrist, first described a syndrome of clinical features characterized by a decline of memory and other cognitive functions in comparison with the patient's previous level of function.[1] This disease has an insidious onset, is progressive, and is differentiated by the exclusion of other diseases that would account for the cognitive deterioration and personality changes. This most common cause of dementia is called Alzheimer's disease (AD) or primary degenerative dementia of the Alzheimer's type (DAT). Disturbances in memory are the hallmark of this disease, but other cognitive functions such as language use, visual-spatial perception, and the ability to learn, solve problems, perform mathematical calculations, think abstractly, and make appropriate judgments are also affected.[2]

TREATMENT GOALS: ALZHEIMER'S DISEASE

- Accurately diagnose the cause of dementia in order to provide appropriate treatment. For example, in dementia due to stroke, medications such as aspirin may prevent further stroke and impairment.
- Recognize that some depressed patients may present with symptoms similar to Alzheimer's disease and require careful diagnosis and a therapeutic trial of an antidepressant, which may resolve the cognitive symptoms.
- Use medications to prevent progression of the disease. In Alzheimer's disease, new medications may slow the disease process and maintain the patient's function while sustaining the best quality of life.
- Treat other causes of dementia symptoms.
- Manage psychiatric symptoms if necessary.
- Provide a safe environment for the patient.
- Provide health maintenance and optimize sensory input (such as glasses for sight, hearing aids, walkers for ambulation).
- Maintain function: activities of daily living (ADLs) are self-maintenance skills such as dressing, bathing, eating, toileting, and ambulating; and instrumental activities of daily living (IADLs) are higher-order skills such as managing finances, driving a car, adhering to medication schedule, and using the telephone.
- Plan for future medical, financial, and legal decisions.
- Provide caregiver education and support.

EPIDEMIOLOGY

Alzheimer's disease primarily affects the elderly and is the cause of a majority of dementia cases. It affects more than 4 million people in the United States. More than 100,000 people die of Alzheimer's disease each year.[3] The prevalence of dementia doubles every 5 years from the ages of 60 to 90. A community-based study of elderly people found that 5 to 10% of the U.S. population over age 65 has Alzheimer's disease. The prevalence increases with age and may reach nearly 30 to 50% in those more than 85 years old.[4] Although the dementia syndrome may be caused by more than 70 disorders (Table 101.1), more than 50% of the cases are attributed to Alzheimer's disease; this is followed by dementia associated with stroke, or a combination of the two. Other significant causes of dementia

Table 101.1 ▪ Causes of Dementia Syndrome[a]

- Psychiatric Disorders
  - Depression
  - Delirium
  - Paranoid states
  - Schizophrenia
- Trauma
  - Subdural hematoma
  - Dementia pugilistica
- Drugs and Toxins
  - Anticholinergics
  - Antidepressants
  - Anticonvulsants
  - Alcohol
  - Benzodiazepines
  - Barbiturates
  - Propranolol
  - Methyldopa
  - Reserpine
  - Heavy metal poisoning
  - Organophosphates
- Metabolic
  - Renal failure
  - Fluid/electrolyte imbalances
  - Hypoglycemia/hyperglycemia
  - Hypothyroidism/hyperthyroidism
- Hepatic failure
  - Addison's disease
  - Cushing's syndrome
  - Hypopituitarism
  - Severe anemia
  - Hypoxia/anoxia
- Infections
  - AIDS
  - Neurosyphilis
  - Meningitis
  - Tuberculosis
  - Pneumonia
  - Creutzfeldt-Jakob (slow virus)
- Intracranial conditions
  - Hydrocephalus
  - Neoplasms
  - Strokes
- Degenerative neurological disorders
  - Alzheimer's disease
  - Pick's disease
  - Huntington's chorea
  - Parkinson's disease
  - Lewy body disease
- Cardiovascular
  - Congestive heart failure
  - Arrhythmia
  - Vascular occlusion
- Nutritional disorders
  - Vitamin B_{12} deficiency
  - Folate deficiency
  - Thiamine deficiency
- Collagen vascular disorders
  - Systemic lupus erythematosus
  - Temporal arteritis

[a]Table represents a partial list.

include Parkinson's disease, other neurodegenerative disorders such as Lewy body disease, toxins, and metabolic disorders. The putative risk factors for Alzheimer's disease include advancing age, a history of dementia, and Down's syndrome in a first-degree relative.[5] Other possible risk factors are previous head trauma, a family history of Down's syndrome, and thyroid disease.

Currently four genes are thought to be involved in the development of Alzheimer's disease. One genetic risk factor on chromosome 19, apolipoprotein E-4 (ApoE), is associated with late-onset (after age 60 to 65) Alzheimer's disease.[6] At least three autosomal-dominant genes have been identified and account for about one-half of early-onset symptoms (before age 60). These genes are presenilin 1 on chromosome 14,[7] rare ones such as presenilin 2 on chromosome 1, and amyloid precursor protein (APP) on chromosome 21.[8]

The etiology of Alzheimer's disease is unknown, but the effect of the disease process leads to neuronal injury. Evidence suggests that a chronic inflammatory process may contribute to neuron pathogenesis. The major biochemical abnormality observed in AD is a 40 to 90% reduction in the enzyme choline acetyltransferase in the cerebral cortex and hippocampus. The deficiency of this enzyme causes decreased synthesis of acetylcholine in the brain. The loss of acetyltransferase in the brain appears to begin before the onset of clinical symptoms. There seems to be a strong correlation between the degree of enzyme reduction, the amount of acetylcholine and the decline of mental status scores, and abnormal symptoms.

Although acetylcholine is the primary neurotransmitter deficit associated with Alzheimer's disease, other neurotransmitters have been implicated. The neuropeptide somatostatin often is deficient in patients with Alzheimer's disease, as is the number of somatostatin receptors. Variable losses in the amount of norepinephrine and the biosynthetic enzyme dopamine β-hydroxylase and decreases of serotonin may account for noncognitive symptoms of depression and aggression. Clinical symptoms exhibited may be the result of a combination of neurotransmitter deficiencies in different individuals.

PATHOPHYSIOLOGY

From brain autopsy studies, patients with Alzheimer's disease have been found to have cortical atrophy and a significant loss of neurons. Two hallmark histopathologic features linked to Alzheimer's are an increase in neuritic plaques and a high density of neurofibrillary tangles.[9] Neurofibrillary tangles are abnormal neurons containing bundles of paired helical filamentous structures wound around each other in the cytoplasm. Certain abnormally phosphorylated proteins, tau proteins, are components of the paired helical filaments. These abnormal proteins may interfere with the stability of microtubules and nerve cell functioning.

Neuritic plaques are small spheres containing β-amyloid protein, an insoluble protein deposit, which is a fragment from abnormally phosphorylated proteins (APP). APP overproduction may contribute to the buildup of β-amyloid protein and is thought to be toxic to neurons. In autopsy studies, the degree of plaque formation has been highly correlated with the degree of clinical impairment observed when the patient was alive.

Mutations of APP gene on chromosomes 21 and 14 have been linked to familial Alzheimer's disease.[10] Current research has shown a possible role for ApoE in the pathogenesis of Alzheimer's disease. ApoE is a protein that binds to the β-amyloid and is present in neuritic plaques and tangles. Because it makes amyloid deposition in plaques more likely it is considered a risk factor for developing late-onset Alzheimer's disease.[11] The identification of ApoE4 allele may eventually be used as a diagnostic aid or presymptomatic or risk testing for Alzheimer's disease.

CLINICAL PRESENTATION AND DIAGNOSIS

Signs and Symptoms

The pathophysiology of AD may begin long before clinical symptoms are apparent. There is an extended time course, with risk factors from genetic predisposition and environment in the clinical expression of the disease (Fig. 101.1). Alzheimer's disease causes a progressive deterioration in intellectual abilities such that it interferes with the person's ability to function in occupational or social situations. Several cognitive changes may occur, including: (a) progressive deterioration of short-term memory or the ability to learn and retain small amounts of information; (b) language dysfunction (aphasia) such as difficulty finding words and loss of auditory comprehension leading to inability to understand questions and follow directions; and (c) inability to draw and recognize two- and three-dimensional figures. In addition, patients may have difficulty balancing a checkbook, driving, using a telephone, and taking medications as prescribed. They may forget to turn off the stove while cooking, may become disoriented or lost, and may not be able to dress and feed themselves.

Eventually the patient loses the ability to care for himself or herself. Behavioral disturbances are prevalent and may increase as the disease progresses.

The onset of symptoms often is overlooked or dismissed as a natural progression of aging. In early or mild dementia, the most common symptoms include signs of depression, personality changes, and misidentifications. As the disease progresses, there may be increases in agitation, psychiatric symptoms such as mood disturbances, and psychotic symptoms such as delusions, hallucinations, and paranoia. The average duration of illness from clinical onset of symptoms to death is 8 to 11 years.

Medications may cause delirium or exacerbate an existing organic dementia. Patients with dementia are more sensitive to the central nervous system effects of all medications. Although delirium tends to have an abrupt onset and fluctuating course, its presentation may mimic the dementia syndrome. Many medications may cause memory impairment and confusion. Any medication the patient is taking should be evaluated for possible misadventures such as intoxication, drug interactions, and medication misuse.

The elderly use many medicines that are high in anticholinergic side effects; these effects are additive; therefore, more anticholinergic medications increase the likelihood that clinical symptoms will develop. It is critical to obtain an accurate list of medications and dosages the patient is taking, including nonprescription drugs and supplements. Discontinuing unnecessary medications, tapering to geriatric dosages, or changing the selection of medication to decrease side effects is an important process and may be a vital therapeutic intervention.

Diagnosis

In 1993, the U.S. Department of Health and Human Services convened an expert panel in order to set standards for education about the recognition and assessment of AD and related disorders.[12] Accurate and early diagnosis and appropriate treatment need to be improved in order to optimize the care of these persons. The main clinical findings include:

- Cognitive Impairment–memory, language, visual-spatial
- Functional Impairment–ADLs, IADLs
- Behavioral Symptoms–depression, agitation, aggression

The diagnosis of Alzheimer's disease should include a detailed medical history and evaluation using diagnostic criteria such as in DSM-IV (Table 101.2),[13] laboratories

Genetic predisposition	Amyloid deposition	Cell Damage	Inflammatory Response	Neuritic plaques, tangles, neuron/synapse loss
Age 0	20	40	60	80
	(Long Preclinical Phase)		(Age-related changes)	

Initiation Factors	Promoting Factors	Clinical Symptoms Appear	Clinical Diagnosis	Loss of Independence	Death
• Down's syndrome • Head Trauma • Genetic Factors ApoE-4 APP Presenillin I Presenillin II	Age Depression Stress Toxins Illness Hypothyroidism Illiteracy	Forgetfulness Changes in mood	Impairment of occupation or social function	Behavior Problems Incontinence Nursing home placement	

Long Preclinical Period
Genetic Risk
Age-related Changes
Promoting Factors
Appearance of Symptoms
Other Factors Modulate Course

Figure 101.1. Continuum of Alzheimer's disease progression.

Table 101.2 ▪ Diagnostic Criteria for Dementia of the Alzheimer's Type (DSM-IV)

A. The development of multiple cognitive deficits manifested by both
   (1) Memory impairment (impaired ability to learn new information or to recall previously learned information)
   (2) One (or more) of the following cognitive disturbances:
      (a) aphasia (language)
      (b) apraxia (impaired motor activities)
      (c) agnosia (failure to recognize or identify objects)
      (d) disturbance in executive functioning (i.e., planning, organizing, abstracting, sequencing)
B. The cognitive deficits in Criteria A1 and A2 each cause significant impairment in social or occupational functioning and represent a significant decline from a previous level of functioning.
C. The course is characterized by gradual onset and continuing cognitive decline.
D. The cognitive deficits in Criteria A1 and A2 are not due to any of the following:
   (1) Other central nervous system conditions that cause progressive deficits in memory and cognition (e.g., strokes, Parkinson's disease, subdural hematoma)
   (2) Systemic conditions that are known to cause dementia (eg., hypothyroidism, vitamin B_{12} or folic acid deficiency, neurosyphilis, HIV, infection)
   (3) Substance-induced conditions
E. The deficits do not occur exclusively during the course of a delirium.
F. The disturbance is not better accounted for by another Axis 1 disorder (e.g., major depressive disorder, schizophrenia).

Source: Reference 13.

(Table 101.3), and physical examination along with an assessment of functional performance and a mental status examination.[14] The Mini-Mental State Examination (MMSE) is the most frequently used brief mental status examination in the United States.[15]

Confirmation of the diagnosis of Alzheimer's disease requires postmortem examination or brain biopsy to identify characteristic neurofibrillary tangles and amyloid plaques. Computed tomography (CT), magnetic resonance imaging (MRI), and other neuroimaging technologies have proven useful in the diagnosis of other potential causes of dementia but do not confirm the diagnosis. Therefore the diagnosis of Alzheimer's disease is based on clinical assessment. It is estimated that experienced clinicians can correctly diagnose Alzheimer's disease in more than 80% of cases.[16]

PSYCHOSOCIAL

The diagnosis of Alzheimer's disease can have a profound effect on both the patient and the patient's family. During the early stages of the disease, while some memory remains intact, patients may experience anxiety, depression, and become hostile. Restrictions in activities such as driving, hobbies, and work can cause frustration and anger. As the dementia progresses, patients may be less upset by their losses while the caregiver's burden increases. The stress associated with caregiving for a patient with Alzheimer's disease may lead to anxiety, depression, and physical illness. Caregivers report social isolation, with fewer visits from friends and fewer opportunities to participate in normal daily activities. Caregivers often report poor sleep patterns and may neglect their own health needs due to the restrictions imposed by the continuous attention necessary to provide care for a patient with Alzheimer's disease.

The progression of Alzheimer's disease causes increased demands on caregivers and the health care system. Severe Alzheimer's disease has a profound impact on family members, particularly those involved in caring for the affected individual. Patients will develop dependence on others for total care and will often develop medical problems associated with decreased mobility. Psychotic symptoms and agitation may become significant concerns and cause stress to family members. Issues involving institutionalization, resuscitative measures, and life-support measures require family members to make difficult and often traumatic decisions. Family support services are particularly important in helping family caregivers cope with the emotional and social consequences of Alzheimer's disease.

THERAPEUTIC PLAN

Guidelines are available to assist in the early and accurate identification of Alzheimer's disease. The Agency for Health Care Policy Research (AHCPR) has published early assessment guidelines for this disease because early recognition may allow for better care planning by the patient and family.[17] Early identification will allow the use of new therapies, which may slow or halt the progression of this progressive dementia.

Guidelines for the pharmacologic management of cognitive changes caused by Alzheimer's disease have been developed by the Department of Veterans Affairs.[18] These guidelines provide a systematic approach to using donepezil and other drugs that enhance cholinergic function. These guidelines are dynamic, with periodic revisions, and can be located on the Internet at http://www.dppm.med.va.gov.

Table 101.3 ▪ Diagnostic Tests for Alzheimer's Disease

Mini-Mental State Examination (MMSE)
Neurologic history and examination
Laboratory tests (CBC, electrolytes, calcium, T4, TSH, B_{12}, syphilis serology)
CT scan
Lumbar puncture
Neuropsychologic testing (when indicated)
EEG
SPECT, PET
ApoE (not yet indicated)

Table 101.4 ▪ Guidelines for Treating Patients with Alzheimer's Disease

1. The differential diagnosis of cognitive impairment is imperative.
2. Before treatment, rigorously pursue the diagnosis of any treatable states that may cause dementia symptoms, especially evaluate for depression.
3. Avoid any unnecessary use of medications. Many medications cause symptoms that may be mistaken for dementia. The elderly have little reserve capacity against side effects and are therefore more prone to additive, adverse effects.
4. Individualize therapy. Each patient exhibits different behavioral and cognitive manifestations. Optimum dosages of medications used in treating Alzheimer's disease have not been established. Dosage must be individualized, monitored, and titrated frequently.
5. Because of the progressive nature of the disease, medications used to treat some symptoms may need to be adjusted and may be discontinued.
6. Carefully monitor patients on medications. Goals of therapy and evaluation for efficacy for drug therapy should be ongoing.
7. Discontinue ineffective or unnecessary medications.

TREATMENT

Historically, a wide variety of medications have been proposed to treat AD; however, most early trials were undertaken without an understanding of the pathophysiology of the disease. While the current armamentarium does not offer unequivocally effective treatment, medications are palliative and may delay symptom progression. Furthermore, several medications have been correlated with a decreased prevalence of AD. General guidelines for treating Alzheimer's patients are outlined in Table 101.4. Health care professionals should be informed about current modalities in order to guide treatments, therapy (Table 101.6), and assessment to discontinue ineffective medications.

There are two basic categories of Alzheimer's drug treatment. The most frequently used medications are symptomatic and help to control unwanted behaviors and maintain patient function. They do not affect the outcome of the disease process, and patients continue to decline. The other category is therapeutic or primary medications to treat Alzheimer's. These agents are used to slow disease progression or reverse the process; the majority are experimental. Currently, two cholinesterase inhibitors have been approved to treat mild to moderate AD. They have demonstrated cognitive improvement, some stabilization of behaviors and mood, and may slow the progression of the disease. In addition, some medications that may be protective against the development of Alzheimer's are being evaluated.[19]

Pharmacotherapy: Symptomatic Treatment

During the course of Alzheimer's disease, patients experience memory dysfunction, progressive loss of cognitive ability, difficulties in the use of language, disorientation, confusion, disruption of the sleep-wake cycle, personality changes, and a lack of emotional control that often results in anxiety, agitation, and aggression. Pharmacotherapy is often used to alleviate some of these symptoms. All psychotropics should be used with caution; those that are low in anticholinergic side effects are usually preferred. They should be started at low dosages and titrated according to therapeutic response and side effects.[20]

Antidepressants

Early stages of Alzheimer's disease are often accompanied by depressive symptoms that may respond to drug therapy. Depressive symptoms such as agitation, memory loss, and insomnia can be confused as dementia. Resolution of depression results in improvement of mood, functional abilities, and possibly cognitive abilities.[21] A therapeutic trial of antidepressants, preferably low in anticholinergic side effects, can be effective in treating "pseudodementia" or depressive symptoms. In general, antidepressants are encouraged and should be chosen for these patients as for any other depressed patient, by side-effect profiles and response to medication. Low dosages given once or twice a day are often beneficial. Sedating antidepressants such as trazodone and nefazodone can also be used for their calming effects, and to help decrease excessive excitation and agitation. A bedtime dose may alleviate insomnia. The select serotonin reuptake inhibitor (SSRIs) antidepressants are effective for depression and offer a preferable side effect profile, although they do have the potential for increasing anxiety symptoms, agitation, and insomnia.

Hypnotics

Insomnia is a common complaint of the elderly, and sleep disturbances are frequent with patients who have dementia. Sleep disturbance may be manifested by night awakening, pacing, trying to leave the environment, or searching for lost items. Sleep irregularities should be addressed initially with social interventions; regulating schedules, keeping patients active during the day, and preventing daytime napping all help to decrease nighttime insomnia. Sleep difficulties often distress patients and caregivers and can lead to exhaustion of caregivers. Sedating antidepressants such as trazodone, nefazodone, or nortriptyline given at bedtime may be beneficial.

When a hypnotic is absolutely necessary, the lowest dosage for the shortest duration should be used. The short-acting agents such as zolpidem (5 to 10 mg) and temazepam (7.5 mg) may be helpful. Longer half-life benzodiazepines should be avoided because of their tendency to accumulate and cause oversedation and an increased risk for falling. Diphenhydramine and other antihistamines have been used for sleep because of moderate sedating properties. However, the anticholinergic effects may increase confusion and psychotic symptoms and make them undesirable in this population.

Alcohol intake should be discontinued or kept to a minimum because of its effects on cognition, disruption of

Table 101.5 ▪ Drug Therapies in the Treatment of Alzheimer's Disease

Drug	Mode of Action	Evaluation/Comments
Precursors to acetylcholine (ACh): Choline, lecithin	Increase amount of ACh	Most clinical trials conclude not effective alone.
Acetylcholinesterase inhibitors: Tacrine, donepezil, physostigmine, Experimental drugs: Metrifonate, galanthamine, rivastigmine, velnacrine	Prevent the breakdown of ACh	Clinical modest effects on selected cognitive measures. May decrease negative behaviors. Currently several more drug trials in progress.
Cholinergic agonists: Bethanecol Experimental: Xanomeline	Muscarinic agonists	Some subjective improvement.
Other Therapeutic Agents:		
Ergoloid mesylates	Metabolic enhancer	Modest clinical effect, possibly due to mood elevation.
Estrogen	Increase blood flow to brain, alter amyloid protein metabolism, affect nerve growth factor	Mechanism for effect in Alzheimer's not known.
Nonsteroidal anti-inflammatory agents (NSAIDs)	May prevent degeneration if immune/inflammatory effects cause plaque and tangle formation	Reduced prevalence of Alzheimer's disease in rheumatoid groups vs. controls and some groups taking anti-inflammatory medication.
Nerve growth factors	May attenuate rate of degeneration of remaining ACh neurons	Based on animal studies, NIA workgroup concluded strong rationale for clinical trials.
Nimodipine	Inhibits calcium influx that occurs with cellular changes, may slow progression of disease	Less deterioration on some memory tests, minimal cognitive benefits.
Selegiline (l-Deprenyl)	Irreversible MAO-B inhibitor, acts as an antioxidant and increases adrenergic stimulation	Improvements in some cognitive testing, was comparable to vitamin E in delaying disease progression.
Vitamin E	Antioxidant, traps free radicals, may inhibit lipid peroxidation	Delayed Alzheimer's progression.
Acetyl-l-carnitine	Neuroprotective/promotes ACh synthesis	Some minimal benefits on cognitive tests.
Nootropic agents: piracetam, oxiracetam, aniracetam	Enhances brain metabolism/possibly neuroprotective	Many studies show increases cognitive tests and some symptoms, minimal benefits.

sleep pattern, and other side effects; furthermore, drug interactions and excessive intake can cause delirium or dementia.

All hypnotics should be used sparingly because of their widespread central nervous system depressant effects. They can increase confusion and memory impairment, worsen depressive symptoms, and aggravate most of the cognitive symptoms occurring in Alzheimer's disease. The efficacy of long-term, routine use of hypnotics has not been proven. Maintaining daytime activity and nocturnal sleep, and giving other sedating medications at bedtime and hypnotics "as needed" can sufficiently control insomnia.

Anxiolytics

Anxiety frequently affects patients who are experiencing memory loss. The elderly may manifest their anxiety in somatic forms such as agitation, motor restlessness, and insomnia. Buspirone is sometimes effective for the anxiety and agitation in Alzheimer's disease and has minimal side effects. Starting dosages such as 5 mg three times a day or 10 mg twice a day may be beneficial for anxiety and may benefit the patient with agitated symptoms occurring with dementia.[22] The effective dosage range is usually 15 to 30 mg/day with mild side effects of dizziness, drowsiness, and nausea. Buspirone should not be used "as needed" and takes several weeks for maximal effect.

The use of benzodiazepines for anxiety is limited by their side effects and possibility of worsening dementia symptoms. Short–half-life benzodiazepines in low dosages (e.g., lorazepam 0.5 to 1.0 mg) given once or twice a day may be useful. Because they act on the central nervous system, they may produce confusion, drowsiness, and amnesia, features that mimic and confound Alzheimer's disease. They can also cause gait instability and have been correlated with an increased frequency of falls.

Antipsychotics

Antipsychotics are indicated for the treatment of specific psychotic symptoms. Delusions are common, especially with suspiciousness or persecution (e.g., false claims that people are stealing misplaced items, or feeling that someone is trying to harm them); visual hallucinations are more common than auditory hallucinations in this population. Paranoia and severe agitation, which may be distressful to the patient or interfere with the caregiver's ability to provide care, may need treatment with medication.

No single agent is always superior. Antipsychotics do not affect higher cortical functions such as memory, judgment, and problem solving. The high-potency antipsychotics (haloperidol, fluphenazine) leave the patient more prone to extrapyramidal side effects such as pseudoparkinsonism and tardive dyskinesia. Low-potency agents (chlorpromazine, thioridazine) are anticholinergic and have cardiovascular side effects that make them undesirable in this population. The adverse effects may further impair the remaining physical and cognitive functions of patients with Alzheimer's disease. Movement may be decreased, hypotension may cause more falls, and sedation may exacerbate confusion. Low dosages of high-potency antipsychotics (haloperidol or risperidone 0.5 to 1 mg) given daily or divided twice a day are usually sufficient. The newer atypical antipsychotic agents (risperidone, olanzapine, 2.5 to 10 mg), which effect dopamine and serotonin, may be beneficial and have a more desirable extrapyramidal side effect profile. A late afternoon or early evening dose may lessen daytime sedation and decrease "sundowning" (a phenomenon of agitation and confusion worsening in the late afternoon and evening). It should be emphasized that antipsychotics should only be used for distressful, incapacitating symptoms. Brief hallucinations such as seeing children in their room or misperceptions that do not create distress to the patient are better left unmedicated. Caregivers should be educated about the temporary, benign nature of these episodes.

Agitation is a term that refers to a range of behavior disturbances that include verbal and physical aggression, combativeness, and disinhibition. Newly developed agitation may be a sign of a medical problem such as discomfort, pain, depression, delirium, constipation, lack of sleep, loneliness, and acute illness such as urinary tract infections. When these medical problems are controlled, the symptoms often resolve.

The efficacy of antipsychotics in controlling agitation is modest. Antipsychotic use should be minimized and is indicated only for symptoms that are harmful and distressing to the patient that cannot be controlled through all other means. They have potentially severe and possibly permanent side effects, including tardive dyskinesia and pseudoparkinsonism. Strict monitoring is imperative to prevent more harm than benefit from the use of these medications.

Mood Stabilizers

Agitation often occurs in nursing home residents and includes physically aggressive (striking out, grabbing), nonaggressive (wandering, restlessness), and verbally aggressive (cursing, constant screaming) behaviors. The frequency of agitated behavior increases with the progression of Alzheimer's disease.[23] Developing literature has suggested alternative drugs such as carbamazepine,[24,25] trazodone,[26] and β-blockers[27,28] for controlling significant and possibly dangerous behavior. Benefits have been shown, but studies are preliminary and include small sample populations of patients.[29] Caution should be taken with the use of β-blockers in this population. These patients frequently suffer from concurrent problems such as diabetes, chronic obstructive pulmonary disease, and heart block, which are contraindications to their use.

Valproic acid, an anticonvulsant used for mood stabilization, has shown some efficacy in treating nonpsychotic agitation. Relatively low dosages may improve symptoms of restlessness, vegetative signs, and striking behaviors with minimal side effects. The primary side effect is gastrointestinal disturbance, which is minimized by using the coated formulation, starting at a low dosage (125 mg BID to TID) and titrating slowly.[30]

Benefits of psychotropic medications are variable, and responses to agents are highly individual and limited by adverse effects. Psychotropics are useful and can improve behavior and function, easing patients' distress, and lessening the burden of care. Because Alzheimer's disease is progressive, therapy should be evaluated at least every 6 months to ensure that the fewest medications are being used in the lowest effective dosages. Tapering psychotropic medications in stabilized patients at regular intervals is an effective tool to assess the need for continued therapy.

Families and caregivers should be counseled. They must understand that psychotropic medications may improve some symptoms but they will not prevent further deterioration of function or progression of the disease. The caregivers' understanding of the disease process and the effects of drug therapy will often lessen the need to use these types of medications.

Pharmacotherapy: Therapeutic Treatments

Therapeutic drugs that slow progression of brain failure or reverse or alleviate disease symptoms are being evaluated. When Alzheimer's disease is further characterized, treatment will likely consist of a combination of medications. Drug therapy will probably affect the balance of cholinergic and other neurotransmitter systems because of the multiple neurochemical abnormalities and brain functions affected. Eventually, when more specific causes are known, therapies can be directed at reversing pathologic damage and disease progression. In addition, several medications are being studied for the possibility that they can prevent or slow the appearance of the clinical symptoms of Alzheimer's disease.

Cholinergic Agents

At present the cholinergic deficit hypothesis provides the most viable and consistent explanation of the memory impairment that occurs in Alzheimer's disease, but it does not account for all the clinical deficits. Neurochemical studies of patients with Alzheimer's disease consistently show a deficiency of the neurotransmitter, acetylcholine, and choline acetyltransferase, the enzyme that is responsible for synthesis of acetylcholine. A positive correlation has been reported between the degree of cognitive impairment of Alzheimer's disease patients and decreases in choline acetyltransferase and acetylcholine.[31] Comparisons between patients with Alzheimer's disease and age-matched controls have demonstrated neuron losses in the nucleus basalis of Meynert, an area that is thought to provide cholinergic input to the cortex and a major cholinergic pathway leading from the septum to the hippocampus, a structure that is critical to normal memory (and learning) functions.[32] Several pharmacologic efforts to augment cholinergic activity have focused on (a) increasing acetylcholine synthesis and release, (b) limiting acetylcholine breakdown by inhibiting acetylcholinesterase, and (c) directly stimulating acetylcholine receptors.[33,34]

Agents such as choline and lecithin (phosphatidylcholine) serve as precursors to acetylcholine, and large amounts have been shown to increase acetylcholine concentrations in the brain. Clinical trials of choline and lecithin have not shown convincing evidence that these substances improve cognition in patients with Alzheimer's disease. This is probably because the enzyme choline acetyltransferase, which is required for these precursors to be synthesized to acetylcholine, is depleted in Alzheimer's disease.

Two enzymes are responsible for the hydrolysis of acetylcholine (ACh): acetylcholinesterase (AChE) and butyrylcholinesterase (BChE). AChE is primarily responsible for ACh metabolism in the brain, and BChE has predominant activity in the periphery. A selective AChE agent without BChE effect is desirable and may decrease the side-effect profile such as gastrointestinal distress and hepatic effects.

Cholinesterase inhibitors (physostigmine, tacrine, donepezil) block AChE and increase the amount of available ACh in the synaptic cleft by limiting the breakdown of ACh. AChE inhibitors are currently the most extensively used and studied class of medications for the treatment of Alzheimer's disease. They show mild benefits and slight improvements in mental status, slowing of progression, and minimizing of behaviors.

Intravenous doses of physostigmine have shown statistically significant and transient improvement in visual recognition memory tests.[35] Although several studies corroborate improvements,[36,37] physostigmine use is limited by the short duration of action and adverse effects such as nausea, vomiting, diarrhea, dizziness, and headache.

Although several AChE inhibitors are under investigation, only two have been approved by the Food and Drug Administration. Tacrine was approved in 1993 and was the first drug indicated to treat mild to moderate Alzheimer's disease. Tacrine (tetrahydroaminoacridine, or THA) is a reversible cholinesterase inhibitor with a longer duration of action than physostigmine. Tacrine elevates ACh levels in the cerebral cortex and is a palliative treatment for Alzheimer's disease when used in therapeutic dosages.[38] Tacrine has shown dose-related benefits in cognitive function and attention tasks and improved measures of quality of life.[39,40] Tacrine does not alter the course of the progress of dementia, and a slow decline in function will continue.

A high prevalence (30%) of abnormal liver function tests (elevated transaminase), which usually return to normal with decreases in dosage or discontinuance of drug therapy, has been observed in patients treated with tacrine. A few occurrences of liver necrosis and jaundice also have been reported.[41] Tacrine should be used with caution by patients with gastrointestinal disease because it may increase gastric acid secretion and cardiovascular conditions. It has a vagotonic effect on pulse rate and can worsen bradycardia with sick sinus syndrome. Tacrine is metabolized by the cytochrome P-450 system, and most drug interactions are generally related to this. It should be used with caution for patients taking phenytoin, theophylline, and cimetidine.

Tacrine has a long titration schedule and is initiated at 10 mg four times a day for 6 weeks. If the patient tolerates the medication, it should be increased by 40 mg/day at 4- to 6-week intervals until a dosage of 120 to 160 mg/day is reached. Because of its short half-life (1.5 to 3.5 hours), tacrine is given four times a day and should be taken on an empty stomach because food decreases absorption.

Baseline liver function tests including bilirubin, aspartate transaminase (AST), and alanine aminotransferase serum enzyme activity (ALT,SGPT) are recommended. After each dosage increase, transaminase levels should be measured every other week from weeks 4 through 16; then monitoring may be performed every 3 months. If a patient develops ALT/SGPT elevations greater than three but less than five times normal, the dosage should be reduced by 40 mg/day and monitoring performed weekly. If the ALT/SGPT is greater than 5 times normal, the tacrine should be stopped and labs should be monitored until they are normal; a rechallenge may be considered.[42]

Adverse effects such as nausea, vomiting, loose stools, dizziness, and headache are common dose-related side effects and often limit tacrine use. Patients generally become tolerant to the peripheral cholinergic effects. This is the reason that medications such as tacrine have to be titrated to an effective, therapeutic dosage.

The newer agents in this class do not seem to have the same effects on liver function and have shown favorable side effect profiles and easier titration schedules.

Donepezil was the second AChE inhibitor approved to treat Alzheimer's disease in 1996. Donepezil is a reversible inhibitor of AChE indicated for the treatment of mild to moderate Alzheimer's disease. It is well absorbed and is metabolized by cytochrome P-450 with renal excretion of unchanged drug. It has a long elimination half-life of approximately 72 hours, which is not altered in the elderly or in patients with renal or hepatic dysfunction. Both 5-mg and 10-mg daily doses have shown patient improvement in a variety of clinical trials. The benefit of the 10-mg dose is not always clinically significant, but may provide additional benefit for some patients. The treatment course usually results in mild increases in cognitive testing using the Alzheimer's Disease Assessment Scale (ADAS-cog) and in caregiver impression scale, as well as a slowing of decline when compared to a placebo. Studies with a placebo washout period showed a decline in function within weeks until function declined to near baseline.[43]

Adverse effects are usually mild. The most common are

gastrointestinal, such as nausea and diarrhea, insomnia, fatigue, and muscle cramps. There is an increase in side effects from the 5-mg to the 10-mg dose, but over a 6-week titration period most side effects resolve and begin to approach the occurrence found in the 5-mg dose. Because of the relative ease of titration, starting at the 5-mg dose for 4 to 6 weeks and then increasing to 10 mg to evaluate for maximal benefit is recommended. If there are no side effects or mild effects, the patient should be left on the 10-mg dose given daily.

Although evidence supports the cholinergic hypothesis of memory and cognitive function, it is highly unlikely that this impairment is the sole disorder occurring in Alzheimer's disease. Alzheimer's disease represents multiple disorders and subtypes that share certain features and probably results from a combination of neuronal changes (such as a decrease in protein synthesis, production of abnormal proteins, and impaired energy production) and neurotransmitter deficits in the brain. With advancing knowledge of the causes of Alzheimer's disease, new therapies can be developed. The pharmacologic efforts to treat Alzheimer's disease have been based on various theories, and the list of therapies continues to grow.[44] Table 101.5 lists current treatments and several possible therapeutic agents being evaluated. Ultimately, therapy will probably consist of a combination of medications used to prevent clinical symptoms in those with a genetic predisposition and medications based on cause and specific symptoms. The optimal therapy will prevent or reverse the disease process itself.

Metabolic Enhancers

Discussed more for its historic than clinical importance in the treatment of Alzheimer's, Hydergine (ergoloid mesylates) has an FDA-approved indication for use in the cognitive decline of the elderly. Originally thought to act as a cerebral vasodilator, ergoloid mesylates are now classified as metabolic enhancers. Their proposed mechanisms in dementia treatment are to increase certain enzymes, alter glucose and oxygen use, and act as α-adrenoreceptor blockers, and as serotonin and dopamine agonists. How the pharmacologic effects are related to clinical efficacy is uncertain.[45]

The efficacy and dosage of ergoloid mesylates are questionable. Despite a preponderance of studies showing positive effects, the favorable results are variable from one study to another and tend to be more statistically significant than medically important.[46] Studies show some improvement in behavioral variables, including mood, attention, and performance of specific tasks, when ergoloid mesylates are given early in the course of dementia. This improvement may be related to a mild improvement

Table 101.6 ▪ Pharmacologic Therapy for Psychiatric Manifestations in the Demented Elderly

Drug	Usual Dose Range	Symptoms Treated	Comments/Side Effects
Antidepressants			
Fluoxetine	5–10 mg/AM	Depression	Agitation, anxiety, insomnia, drug interactions
Sertraline	25–100 mg/day	Agitation	Diarrhea, nausea
Nefazodone	50–200 mg/day	Depression	Constipation
Trazodone	25–200 mg/day		Sedation hypotension
Venlafaxine	25–75 mg/day		Hypertension with increased dose
Antipsychotics			
Haloperidol	0.25–2 mg/day	Psychosis, extreme aggression	Parkinsonism, akathisia, tardive dyskinesia, NMS
Olanzapine	2.5–10 mg/day		Sedation, minimal extrapyramidal symptoms (EPS)/Parkinsonism
Risperidone	0.5–2 mg/day		Minimal EPS
Quetiapine	25 mg BID to 400 mg/day		
Anticonvulsants			
Carbamazepine	100–400 mg/day	Agitation or aggression	Leukopenia, rash, hepatotoxicity
Divalproex sodium	500–1500 mg/day		Ataxia, cardiac and thyroid effect.
			Sedation, emesis, hepatotoxicity, hyperammonemia, bone marrow suppression
Anxiolytics			
Lorazepam	0.5–2 mg/day	Anxiety, agitation, aggression	Sedation, confusion, falls, rebound, dependence
Oxazepam	7.5–30 mg/day		Long-acting, falls
Clonazepam	0.5–1.5 mg/day		Dizziness, effect takes 2–6 wk
Buspirone	10–60 mg/day		
β-Adrenergics			
Propranolol	10–300 mg/day	Aggression, agitation, anxiety	Hypotension, caution in COPD, DM, asthma
Pindolol	5–40 mg/day		
Hypnotics			
Temazepam	7.5 mg/HS	Insomnia as needed	Sedation, ataxia, falls, confusion
Zolpidem	5–10 mg/HS		

Ranges based on published reports, prescribing information, and clinical experience.

in mood.[47] Once the disease has progressed, little effect is expected.

Optimal dosages for patients with Alzheimer's disease have not been established. However, some studies have used 6 to 12 mg/day; which is above the FDA-recommended dosage of 3 mg/day. Ergoloid mesylates can usually be safely administered with mild and occasionally adverse effects of gastrointestinal upset and bradycardia.

Nonpharmacologic Therapy

Managing the environment of the patient with Alzheimer's disease is an important treatment consideration. A safe, stable, comfortable environment will minimize the strain of decreasing mental capacities and lessen confusion and agitation. Patients should be stimulated and helped to function, but choices that may overwhelm and confuse them should be limited. Labeling items with names and laying out one change of clothes will help maintain the patient's ability to perform the activities of daily living. Alterations in surroundings such as room changes should be minimized; they may cause an increase in confusion and disorientation. Physical and psychosocial stressors such as minor surgery, bereavement, or institutionalization can and often will aggravate intellectual deficits in a demented patient. Within reason, familiar furnishings, diet, and routines should be maintained.

Caregiver training is important. Caregivers must understand the limitations of the patient's cognition and how that affects his or her behaviors and functioning. Patients are often confused and cannot process what is going on around them. Many of the interactions between patients and caregivers can be modified to best suit the patient and to prevent or minimize incidents that might lead to agitation and difficulty in caring for the individual.

A therapeutic approach should provide adequate emotional support for family members and those who provide daily patient care. Referring the family to the local branch of the Alzheimer's Association and to books such as *The Thirty-Six-Hour Day*[48] are often as valuable as current drug therapy. Relatives of Alzheimer's disease patients who are experiencing changes in the patient's cognitive abilities and personality and their relationship with the Alzheimer's disease patient grieve for their own losses.[49] Families must be educated about the disease process and expectations of therapy. There are no medical cures, and the disease waxes and wanes but is progressive. Often a rational presentation of the course will minimize fears, allow rational expectations, and enhance the family's ability to provide support to the patient without dependence on excessive medication. It must be remembered that all medications have toxicities, and many may exacerbate the symptoms they are supposed to relieve. Medications are often used to maintain patients in the home. Caregivers must understand the dangers of overmedicating and the need to administer medications only as directed. Families and the caregivers closest to the patients should be included in therapeutic decisions and often provide the best monitoring information.

ALTERNATIVE THERAPIES

Extracts of the ginkgo biloba (EGb) leaf are widely available as nonprescription supplements and are used by many people for their cognitive effects. The extracts contain many constituents such as flavonoids and terpenoids. Neuroprotective effects of EGb may be caused by reduced capillary fragility, antioxidant effects, and inhibition of platelet aggregation. In Germany, EGb 761 has been approved for treating dementia and cerebral circulatory disturbances. EGb 761 studies in the United States have shown benefits in short-term memory and caregiver behavior assessment. The adverse effects are usually mild gastrointestinal symptoms, headache, dizziness, and vertigo.[50] A variety of extracts are available in the United States; however, studies evaluating ginkgo biloba have been conducted using EGb 761 almost exclusively and knowledge of all the potential toxicities of ginkgo biloba treatment is limited. Although there is some evidence of mild efficacy using EGb 761, it is not proven effective. Because there is little control over the contents in preparation from company to company, ginkgo biloba should not be recommended at this time.

If patients with the disease do take this supplement, they should ensure that the main ingredient is EGb 761.

FUTURE THERAPIES

Following the lead of tacrine, and more recently donepezil, other cholinesterase inhibitors are under investigation. Metrifonate is an irreversible inhibitor of brain cholinesterase that has long-lasting effects.[51] Metrifonate is converted, in vivo, to 2,2-dichlorovinyl dimethyl phosphate (DDVP), which is the active metabolite of acetylcholinesterase. Metrifonate has been used for more than 30 years as a treatment for schistosomiasis and has only recently been studied in Alzheimer's disease. Preliminary clinical trials indicate benefits similar to other currently available cholinesterase inhibitors, with reports of low toxicity and once daily dosing. Another cholinesterase inhibitor is rivastigmine, which is reported to have regional selectivity for the hippocampus and cortex. Limited data indicate that rivastigmine is superior to placebo in treating Alzheimer's disease at 12 weeks of treatment. Effective dosages were greater than 6 mg daily, with nausea and vomiting the most frequent adverse effects. Preliminary data indicate that rivastigmine is effective in improving cognitive symptoms in patients with mild to moderate Alzheimer's disease.[52]

It has been hypothesized that the pathology of Alzheimer's may involve oxidative stress and the accumulation of free radicals, which lead to degeneration in the brain. Antioxidants and anti-inflammatory medications may also have neuroprotective effects by stimulating the production of nerve growth factor. Agents in this category may affect the processing of amyloid. They could be involved in disease modification and prevention of the occurrence of this disease.

Vitamin E (alpha-tocopherol) interacts with cell membranes, traps free radicals, and inhibits lipid peroxidation that damages cells. Selegiline, a monoamine oxidase-B inhibitor, may act as an antioxidant and reduce neuronal damage in AD progression. A study compared 341 patients with moderate AD who received vitamin E 2000 IU/day, selegiline 10 mg/day, both, or placebo showed benefit from either vitamin E or selegiline, but less with both combined.[53] Possible side effects from selegiline are insomnia, hallucinations, nausea, and dizziness. Vitamin E may interfere with vitamin K absorption and could reduce clotting. With current knowledge of the two agents, vitamin E is a preferable choice for most patients because it has fewer side effects and potential drug interactions than selegiline.

Recent evidence has supported a role for estrogens in both normal neural development and neuronal maintenance. It may delay the onset or slow the progression of AD by a variety of means including effects on nerve growth factor, increasing blood flow to the brain, and altering amyloid protein metabolism.[54] Estrogen may also be protective in AD with a possible 60% decrease in the risk of developing AD.[55] Because of the possible beneficial effect for AD and many other benefits of estrogen including decreasing osteoporosis and preventing cardiovascular disease, it should be recommended to women unless clinically contraindicated.

A few studies postulate a possible role of nonsteroidal anti-inflammatory drugs (NSAIDs) in the prevention or slowing of decline due to Alzheimer's. They may affect an inflammatory component in the formation of neuritic plaques. An evaluation of 1686 participants found the risk of AD was reduced by 50% in people who reported taking NSAIDs, with reduction to 60% with two or more years of NSAID use.[56] Although the evidence is encouraging, the frequent occurrence of side effects such as ulcers, GI distress, and nephrotoxicity with these agents make the prescribing of NSAIDs not recommended for elderly patients solely to prevent AD.

IMPROVING OUTCOMES

With the approval of more medications to treat Alzheimer's disease, compliance with medications becomes more important. Patients in early stages may be able to manage a limited number of medications given once or twice a day. But reminder systems and adherence evaluation should be performed periodically. Besides pharmacotherapy, a comprehensive plan should include adequate nutrition, correction of sensory deficits (e.g., glasses, hearing aid), and attention to the social environment.

Because of the lack of nursing home beds and their high costs, alternative care will become even more important in the future. Patients who are in early stages of Alzheimer's disease need education and counseling. When family members become involved in care, their understanding of drug therapy and the ability to comply with regimens should be evaluated. Care for the caregivers is often as important as care of the patient. Remember that an aging spouse may be on the borderline of competency and function, and the added burden of caring for a demented mate may be too much for the person to handle properly. When the caregiver gives out, the care system suffers. Day care and home care services are offered by various local agencies and provide different levels of supervision and activities for patients with Alzheimer's. Day care is especially important in providing much needed respite for the caregivers at home.

PHARMACOECONOMICS

The economic impact of Alzheimer's disease on health care is enormous and will be increasing as more people live longer. Costs to Medicaid in 1991 for Alzheimer's disease totaled $5.7 billion.[57] In understanding the total cost of care, both direct and indirect costs must be considered. Direct health care costs include clinic visits, medications, hospitalizations, and nursing home care. Nonmedical costs include social services, day care, home health services, and the cost of equipment for home care. Caregivers also have increased medical costs for the treatment of medical illness, depression, and increased hospitalizations associated with the stress of caregiving. Indirect costs include loss of productivity for both the patient and caregiver.[58] Using 1991 data, the annual national direct and total costs were estimated to be $20.6 billion and $67.3 billion, respectively.[57]

The cost of care for patients with Alzheimer's disease increases with the severity of the disease. Patients with advanced, severe dementia will usually require nursing home care, often for extended periods of time. Patients with Alzheimer's disease have a median length of nursing home stay that is more than 10 times the national average for all other diagnoses.[59] Efforts to slow the progression of the dementia and use assisted living or home care programs should have a positive impact on the future cost of care for patients with Alzheimer's disease. Drug therapies directed at stopping or slowing the progression of Alzheimer's disease will allow patients to remain in a less restrictive and less costly environment.

KEY POINTS

- Alzheimer's disease is a complex, progressive, degenerative disorder with no known cure.
- All potentially reversible dementias should be identified and treated before a diagnosis of Alzheimer's disease can be made.
- Patients with Alzheimer's disease may require pharmacologic treatment for depression, anxiety, and behavioral manifestations.
- A safe environment is essential for providing care for patients with Alzheimer's disease.
- Caregiver education and support are necessary to assist in maintaining Alzheimer patients in the least restrictive environment.
- New drug therapies may prevent the progression of Alzheimer's disease.

- When antipsychotics are used to control psychoses or disruptive behavior, the lowest dosage for the shortest period of time is recommended.
- Maintain the most appropriate level of care and to keep the patient as functional and comfortable for as long as possible.

REFERENCES

1. Huppert FA, Tym E. Clinical and neuropsychological assessment of dementia. Br Med Bull 42:11–18, 1986.
2. Katzman R. Alzheimer's disease. N Engl J Med 31:964–973, 1986.
3. Advisory Panel on Alzheimer's Disease. Alzheimer's Disease and Related Dementias: Acute and Long-term Care Services. Washington, DC: U.S. Dept. of Health and Human Services, 1996, NIH publication 96-4136.
4. Evans DA, Funkenstein HH, Albert MS, et al. Prevalence of Alzheimer's disease in a community population of older persons higher than previously reported. JAMA 262:2551–2556, 1989.
5. Fox JH, Heston LL, Terry RD. Zeroing in on Alzheimer's disease. Patient Care 20:68–91, 1986.
6. Saunders AM, Schmader K, et al. Apolipoprotein E4 allele distribution in late-onset Alzheimer's disease and in other amyloid-forming diseases. Lancet 342:710–711, 1993.
7. Schellenberg GD, Bird TD, et al. Genetic linkage evidence for a familial Alzheimer's disease locus on chromosome 14. Science 258:667–668, 1992.
8. Levy-Lahad E, Wijsman EM, et al. A familial Alzheimer's disease locus on chromosome 1. Science 269:970–972, 1995.
9. Caputo CB, Salama AI. The amyloid proteins of Alzheimer's disease as potential targets for drug therapy. Neurobiol Aging 10(5):451–461, 1989.
10. Liddell M, Williams J, Bayer A, et al. Confirmation of association between the e4 allele of apolipoprotein E and Alzheimer's disease. J Med Genet 31:197–200, 1994.
11. Mayeux R, Stern Y, Ottman R, et al. The apolipoprotein e4 allele in patients with Alzheimer's disease. Ann Neurol 34:752–754, 1993.
12. Anonymous. Recognition and Initial Assessment of Alzheimer's Disease and Related Dementias, Clinical Practice Guidelines: 19, AHCPR, Nov. 1996.
13. American Psychiatric Association. Diagnostic and Statistical Manual of Mental Disorders. 4th ed. Washington, DC: American Psychiatric Association, 1994: 142–143.
14. McKhann G, Drachman D, Folstein M, et al. Clinical diagnosis of Alzheimer's disease. Neurology 34:939–944, 1984.
15. Folstein MF, Folstein SE, McHugh PR. Mini-Mental State: A practical method for grading the cognitive state of patients for the clinician. Kidlington, UK: Elsevier Science, Ltd., 1974:196–198.
16. Becker JT, Boller F, Lopez OL, et al. Alzheimer research program. The natural history of Alzheimer's disease: description of study cohort and accuracy of diagnosis. Arch Neurol 51:585–594, 1994.
17. Early identification of Alzheimer's disease-type dementias. Clinical Guideline 19, Rockville, MD: Agency for Health Care Policy and Research, USHHS No. 96-0703, Sept. 1996.
18. Pharmacy benefits management–medical advisory panel. The Management of Cognitive Changes in Alzheimer's Disease. VHA PBM-SHG Publication No. 99-0013. Hines, IL: Pharmacy Benefits Management Strategic Healthcare Group, Veterans Health Administration, Department of Veterans Affairs, August 1999.
19. Van Reekum R, Black S, et al. Cognition enhancing drugs in dementia: A guide to the near future. Can J Psych 42(Suppl 1):35s–50s, 1997.
20. American Psychiatric Association. Practice guideline for the treatment of patients with Alzheimer's disease and other dementias of late life. Am J Psychiatr 154(Suppl 5):1–30, 1997.
21. Reifler BS, Larson E, Teri L, et al. Dementia of the Alzheimer's type and depression. J Am Geriatr Soc 34:855–859, 1986.
22. Sakauye DM, Camp CJ, et al. Effects of buspirone on agitation associated with dementia. Am J Geriatr Psychiatr 1:82–84, 1988.
23. Reisberg B, Franssen E, et al. Stage specific incidence of potentially remediable behavioral symptoms in aging and Alzheimer disease. Bull Clin Neurosci 54:95–112, 1989.
24. Lemke MR. Effect of carbamazepine on agitation in Alzheimer's inpatients refractory to neuroleptics. J Clin Psychiatry 56:354–357, 1995.
25. Tariot PN, Erb R, et al. Efficacy and tolerability of carbamazepine for agitation and aggression in dementia. Am J Psych 155:54–61, 1998.
26. Lebert F, Pasquier F, et al. Behavioral effects of trazodone in Alzheimer's disease. J Clin Psych 55:536–538, 1994.
27. Weiler PG, Mungas D, et al. Propranolol for the control of disruptive behavior in senile dementia. J Geriatr Psychiatry Neurol 1:226–230, 1988.
28. Greendyke RM, Kanter DR. Therapeutic effects of pindolol on behavioral disturbances associated with organic brain disease: a double-blind study. J Clin Psychiatry 47(8):423–426, 1986.
29. Schneider LS, Sobin PB. Non-neuroleptic treatment of behavior symptoms and agitation in Alzheimer's disease and other dementias. Psychopharmacol Bull 28:71–79, 1992.
30. Lott AD, McElroy SL, et al. Valproate in the treatment of behavioral agitation in elderly patients with dementia. J Neuropsychiatry Clin Neurosci 7:314–319, 1995.
31. Bartus RT, Dean RL, Beer B, et al. The cholinergic hypothesis of geriatric memory dysfunction. Science 217:408–414, 1982.
32. Davis BM, Mohs RC, Greenwald BS, et al. Clinical studies of the cholinergic deficit in Alzheimer's disease. 1: neurochemical and neuroendocrine studies. J Am Ger Soc 33:741–748, 1985.
33. Hollander E, Mohs RC, Davis KL. Cholinergic approaches to the treatment of Alzheimer's disease. Br Med Bull 42:97–100, 1986.
34. Kumar V, Calache M. Treatment of Alzheimer's disease with cholinergic drugs. Int J Clin Pharmacol Ther Toxicol 29:23–37, 1993.
35. Davis KL, Mohs RC. Enhancement of memory processes in Alzheimer's disease with multiple dose intravenous physostigmine. Am J Psychol 139:1421–1424, 1982.
36. Christie JE, Shering A, Ferguson J, et al. Physostigmine and arecoline effects of intravenous infusions in Alzheimer presenile dementia. Br J Psychol 138:46–50, 1982.
37. Thal LJ, Masur DM, Blau AD, et al. Chronic oral physostigmine without lecithin improves memory in Alzheimer's disease. J Am Geriatr Soc 37:42–48, 1989.
38. Summer WK, Majovski LV, Marsh GM, et al. Oral tetrahydroaminoacridine in long-term treatment of senile dementia, Alzheimer type. N Engl J Med 315:1241–1245, 1986.
39. Knapp MJ, Knopman DS, Soloman PR, et al. A 30-week randomized controlled trial of high-dose tacrine in patients with Alzheimer's disease. JAMA 271:985–991, 1994.
40. Davis KL, Thal LJ, Ganzu ER, et al. A double blind, placebo controlled multicenter study of tacrine for Alzheimer's disease. N Engl J Med 327:1253–1259, 1992.
41. Gamzu ER, Thal LJ, Davis KL. Therapeutic trials using tacrine and other cholinesterase inhibitors. Adv Neurol 51:241–245, 1990.
42. Cognex (tacrine) package insert, prescribing and use information.
43. Aricept (donepezil) package insert, prescribing and use information.
44. Schneider LS, Tariot PN. Emerging drugs for Alzheimer's disease: mechanisms of action and prospects for cognitive enhancing medications. Med Clin North Am 78:911–934, 1994.
45. Hollister LE, Yesavage J. Ergoloid. Mesylates for senile dementias: unanswered questions. Ann Intern Med 100:894–898, 1984.
46. Schneider LS, Olin JT. Overview of clinical trials of Hydergine in dementia. Arch Neurol 51:787–798, 1994.
47. Thompson TL, Filey CM, Mitchell WD, et al. Lack of efficiency of Hydergine in patients with Alzheimer's disease. N Engl J Med 323:445–448, 1990.
48. Mace NL, Rabins PV. The thirty-six-hour day: a family guide to caring for persons with Alzheimer's disease, related dementing illness, and memory loss in later life. 2nd ed. New York: Warner Books, 1992.
49. Howell M. Caretakers' views on responsibilities for the care of the demented elderly. J Am Geriatr Soc 32:657–660, 1984.
50. LeBars PL, Katz MM, et al. A placebo-controlled, double-blind, randomized trial of an extract of ginkgo biloba for dementia. JAMA 278:1327–1332, 1997.
51. Williams BR. Metrifonate: a new agent for the treatment of Alzheimer's disease. Am J Health Syst Pharm 56:427–431, 1999.
52. Spencer CM, Noble S. Rivastigmine: a review of its use in Alzheimer's disease. Drugs Aging 13:391–411, 1998.
53. Sano M, Ernesto C, et al. A controlled trial of selegiline, alpha-tocopherol, or both as treatment for Alzheimer's disease. N Engl J Med 336:1216–1222, 1997.
54. Birge SJ. The role of estrogen in the treatment of Alzheimer's disease. Neurol 48(Suppl 7):S36–S41, 1997.
55. Kawas C, Resnick S, et al. A prospective study of estrogen replacement therapy and the risk of developing Alzheimer's disease: The Baltimore Longitudinal Study of Aging. Neurology 48:1517–1521, 1997.
56. Steward WF, Kawas C, et al. Risk of Alzheimer's disease and duration of NSAID use. Neurology 48:626–632, 1997.
57. Ernst RL, Hay JW. The U.S. economic and social costs of Alzheimer's disease revisited. Am J Public Health 84:1261–1264, 1994.
58. Hamdy RC, Turnbull RM, Clar W, et al. Alzheimer's disease–a handbook for caregivers. St. Louis: Mosby, 1994.
59. Welch HG, Walsh JS, Larson EB. The cost of institutional care in Alzheimer's disease: nursing home and hospital care in a prospective cohort. J Am Geriatr Soc 40:221–224, 1992.

CHAPTER 102

GERIATRIC DRUG THERAPY

Susan W. Miller

TREATMENT GOALS: GERIATRIC DRUG THERAPY

- Resolve the symptoms of a specific condition and slow progression of the negative outcomes of the condition.
- Avoid medication related problems.
- Set an actual target clinical parameter for the problem being treated such as a specific blood pressure, glucose level, or reduction in incidences of problematic behaviors.
- Set an appropriate duration of therapy and consider dosage reductions or discontinue drugs at that time.
- Select the most appropriate pharmacologic alternative based on the patient's clinical status and comorbid conditions.
- Initiate therapy with a low dose (one-fourth to one-third the usual recommended dose) and increase slowly to account for prolonged drug half-life.
- Use the fewest number of medications possible.
- Minimize the number and dose of medications with effects on the central nervous system.
- Consider the effect of the selected medication on the functional ability and quality of life of the patient.

DEMOGRAPHICS AND DRUG-USAGE PATTERNS

Over 31 million people or 12.6% of the population in the United States are older than 65 years of age. By the year 2050, it is projected that this percentage will increase to about 22%, with the largest increases in the 75- to 84-year-old age group and the frail or 85 and older age group.[1] People reaching age 65 have an average life expectancy of an additional 17.2 years (18.2 years for women and 15.2 years for men).[2] Factors contributing to the growing numbers of older adults include the increased birth rate before 1920 and after World War II, the decrease in mortality associated with the development of antibiotics and vaccines, improvements in sanitation and technology, and a decline in midlife mortality from coronary artery disease.[3] The past 20 years have seen a revolution in our knowledge of how the processes of aging affect drug therapy. With this knowledge has come progress in caring for patients older than age 65. Advances in medical technology have enhanced studies of the physiologic changes of aging, and there is now a broader understanding of how physiologic changes affect the treatment of disease and the use of medications in older patients.[4]

Because older adults experience a higher rate of chronic conditions compared to the population at large, they are more likely to use health care services. They account for about 31% of all hospital discharges and 42% of all acute care hospital days. Older patients are admitted to hospitals more than three times as often as younger patients, are hospitalized 50% longer, and use twice as many prescription medications as the general population. Although only 5% of the total elderly population reside in a nursing home at any one time, about 20% spend some time in a nursing home during their lifetime. One of the fastest growing areas of health care delivery is that of personal care or assisted-living facilities, which offer room, board, and limited supervision and provision of care for older residents. These demographic changes will continue to have a major impact on health care manpower, practice, and expenditures.

Medication use among older adults is common, with national surveys of medication-use patterns indicating that elderly patients account for 30% of all medications prescribed in the United States, but also consume substantial quantities of over-the-counter medications.[5] Landmark studies have established the rates of medication use among various groups of older patients and include:

1. The Dunedin Study, a longitudinal, epidemiologic study starting in 1978 examining the drug usage patterns of an ambulatory, elderly population, showed the number of prescribed and nonprescribed drugs to increase from an average of 2.9 to 4.08 over a 10-year increase in age.[6]
2. The Boston Collaborative Drug Surveillance Program reported on drug use patterns in several hospitals and found the average number of drug exposures increased with age, from 6.3 per patient in the 16- to 25-year-old category to 9.7 in patients older than 65 years of age.[7]
3. Medication use in long-term care facilities has been reported to be high and the most recent investigations report an average of 5.85 routine medications and 3.03 as-needed medications per patient.[8] These numbers are affected by attention to compliance to regulations regarding medication use in these facilities and the role of the consultant pharmacist in the long-term care facility setting.[9]

PSYCHOSOCIAL ASPECTS

Geriatric patients use more medications compared to younger patients because they have more symptoms of disease. A second contributing factor to drug use in older patients is the psychosocial aspect of drug use. These psychosocial issues can cause either an increase or a decrease in medication use. Included in these psychosocial aspects is the attitude that medications are available that can cure most any disease or alleviate any symptom; therefore, a medication to manage any disease or symptom should be prescribed. Many older patients equate drugs (medications) with narcotics (dope) and therefore view them as something to be avoided. Research has shown an inverse correlation between the number of medications people take and their satisfaction with life and health. Increased consumption of medications has been reported in women who are not satisfied with their lives. Other opinions regarding medication use by geriatric patients include the beliefs that

- Physicians would not prescribe any medication that could be harmful.
- The Food and Drug Administration makes sure that all drugs are safe.
- Over-the-counter drugs are completely safe and are not really drugs.
- All drugs can be addicting.
- If a little dose of a drug is good then more would be better.
- Vitamins and herbal products are harmless because they are natural products.

It is important for pharmacists and other health care professionals to listen to older patients' opinions regarding drug therapy and respond to these with the best interest of the patient in mind.

MEDICATION-RELATED PROBLEMS IN GERIATRIC PATIENTS

Problems with medication therapy in geriatric patients can be described in different ways. Several terms that often appear in the literature are polypharmacy, adverse drug reactions (ADRs), appropriateness of therapy, and compliance.

Polypharmacy, or the use of multiple prescription and over-the counter medications, especially by older people with chronic health problems, has been identified as the principal drug safety issue of the future.[10] Patient acuity may be the most important determinant of medication usage in older adults. A review of studies on drug usage among geriatric patients has shown a wide variation in the number of drugs used among older people based on their relative independence or level of care.[11] Other major factors influencing medication use in older patients, especially medication usage in long-term care facilities are (1) the initiation of diagnosis-related groups (DRGs) emphasizing shorter hospital stays and therefore discharging patients who are not ready to go home (potentially on more medications) to nursing facilities[12] and (2) the effects of the Health Care Financing Administration (HCFA) regulations on stressing rational drug usage in nursing facilities and subsequent monitoring of drug therapy by pharmacists.[13,14]

The inability of older patients to manage their medications has been attributed to one-fourth of nursing home

Table 102.1 ▪ Potential Risk Factors for Identification of Elderly Nursing Facility Residents at High Risk for Drug-Related Problems

Specific medication	Class of medication
Digoxin	Anticonvulsants
Warfarin	Antiarrhythmics
Lithium	Antipsychotics
Theophylline	Antidepressants
Chlorpropamide	Sedative/hypnotics
Glyburide	Benzodiazepines
Patient characteristics	Histamine H_2 antagonists
Number of active chronic medical diagnoses (>6)	Nonsteroidal anti-inflammatory agents
Number of medication doses per day (>12)	Anticholinergics
Recent transfer from hospital	Angiotensin-converting enzyme inhibitors
Advanced age (>85 years)	Diuretics
Prior adverse drug reaction	New prescription for antibiotic
Cancer	Narcotic analgesics
Depression	
Low body weight or body mass index (<22 kg·m²)	
Six or more medications	
Cognitive impairment (including dementia)	
Decreased renal function (estimated creatinine clearance <50 mL/min)	

Source: Reference 21.

Table 102.2 ▪ Medications That Can Cause Mental Status Changes

Amantadine	Morphine
Anticholinergics and atropine	Narcotics
Barbiturates	Nonsteroidal anti-inflammatory agents
Benzodiazepines	Penicillin G procaine
Bromocriptine	Phenytoin
Buspirone	Pilocarpine
Caffeine	Propoxyphene
Calcium channel blockers	Propranolol
Captopril	Quinidine
Carbamazepine	Salicylates
Cephalosporins	Selective serotonin reuptake inhibitors
Corticosteroids	Selegiline
Digoxin	Sulfonamides
Estrogens	Theophylline
Fluoroquinolones	Trycyclic antidepressants
Histamine H_2 receptor antagonists	Valproic acid
Hydroxymethylglutaryl coenzyme A reductase inhibitors	Vinblastine
Levodopa	Vincristine
Meperidine	Zolpidem
Methyldopa	
Monoamine oxidase inhibitors	

Source: Reference 22.

admissions,[15] and up to 17% of hospital admissions of patients older than age 65 are attributable to ADRs.[16,17] Much of the ADR reporting in elderly patients was documented primarily in the nursing facility setting,[18,19] but elderly patients living in the community have also been shown to be at risk for drug-related problems.[20]

Among other factors, the use of multiple prescription medications for the management of chronic diseases in the aging population increases the risk for medication-related problems. Other risk factors for medication related problems have been identified and are included in Table 102.1.[21] Older patients are at increased risk for ADRs compared to younger patients and often have an atypical presentation of the ADR that may be confused with aging or disease progression. Cognitive impairment and behavioral changes frequently are the result of drug therapy; therefore, the medical evaluation of the older patient should include a thorough review of drug therapy to screen for possible drug-induced effects[22] (Table 102.2). In older patients, classic digoxin toxicity commonly presents as anorexia and weight loss instead of nausea and vomiting; further, instead of haloes and color vision changes, the older patient may complain of hazy or muddy vision. Suspected digoxin toxicity should be confirmed by electrocardiograms and digoxin serum levels from appropriately drawn blood samples. Additional factors contributing specifically to ADRs in geriatric patients are listed in Table 102.3.

More than one in six elderly Americans are taking prescription drugs that are not suited for geriatric patients and may lead to physical or mental deterioration and possibly death.[23] Recently, strategies have been developed in attempts to foster appropriate prescribing of medications in the geriatric population overall. The explicit criteria for determining potentially inappropriate medication use by elderly patients are listed in Table 102.4. These criteria were developed through a consensus panel of experts in geriatric care, geriatric pharmacology, geriatric

Table 102.3 ▪ Reasons for High Frequencies of Adverse Drug Reactions in Elderly Patients

Multiple chronic diseases requiring treatment with potent medications
Several physicians prescribing therapy independently
Inappropriate identification of altered presentation of adverse drug reactions
Patient noncompliance with prescribed medications
Inappropriate self-medication
Inadequate patient education about prescribed or over-the-counter medications
Age-related physiologic changes that alter drug kinetics and pharmacologic response to drugs

Table 102.4 ▪ Explicit Criteria for Inappropriate Medication Orders

Medications that should be avoided
- Sedative or hypnotic agents
  - Long-acting benzodiazepines
  - Meprobamate
  - Short-acting barbiturates
- Antidepressants
  - Amitriptyline
  - Combination antidepressants-antipsychotics
- Antihypertensive agents
  - Methyldopa
  - Propranolol
  - Reserpine
- Nonsteroidal anti-inflammatory drugs
  - Indomethacin
  - Phenylbutazone
- Oral hypoglycemic agents
  - Chlorpropamide
- Analgesic agents
  - Propoxyphene
  - Pentazocine
- Dementia treatments
  - Cyclandelate
  - Isoxsuprine
- Platelet inhibitors
  - Dipyridamole
- Muscle relaxants or antispasmodic agents
  - Cyclobenzaprine
  - Orphenidrate
  - Methocarbamol
  - Carisoprodol

Medications that should be avoided *(continued)*
- Gastrointestinal antispasmodic agents
  - Clidinium
  - Hyoscyamine
  - Dicyclomine
  - Belladonna

Medications with dosage limits
- Antipsychotic agents
  - Haloperidol
  - Thioridazine
- Digoxin
- Histamine blockers
  - Cimetidine
  - Ranitidine
- Iron supplements
- Short-acting benzodiazepines
  - Oxazepam
  - Thiazides
- Antihypertensive agents
  - Hydrochlorothiazide

Medications with duration limits
- Decongestants
  - Oxymetazoline
  - Phenylephrine
  - Pseudoephedrine
- Histamine blockers
- Short-acting benzodiazepines
  - Oxazepam
  - Triazolam
  - Alprazolam

Source: References 24, 25.

psychopharmacology, and nursing home care. These experts reached agreement on criteria defining inappropriate drug use in nursing home residents. The criteria relate to certain drugs that should not be used and doses and durations of therapy of some drugs that should not be exceeded in the older patient in a nursing facility.[24,25]

The Medication Appropriateness Index (MAI) is a rating scale that provides parameters for the evaluation of 10 key elements of medication prescribing.[26] For each parameter, the index has operational definitions, explicit instructions, and an assigned weight. The evaluator rates the medication as appropriate, marginally appropriate, or inappropriate, based on the operational definitions and then a medication appropriateness score is calculated. Higher scores indicate less appropriate prescribing. These parameters are listed in Table 102.5. Both the explicit criteria and MAI methods of prescribing and monitoring drug therapy stress the importance of considering the individual patient, his or her clinical and health status, and concomitant medications he or she is receiving, before prescribing additional medications. Despite these strategies for improving the prescribing of medications for geriatric patients, drug-related morbidity and mortality within nursing facilities still exist. It has been estimated that for every $1.00 spent on drugs in nursing facilities, $1.33 in health care resources are consumed in the treatment of drug-related problems in this patient population.[27]

Compliance is defined as the extent to which a patient's behavior coincides with a prescriber's planned medical regimen. Noncompliance or nonadherence with drug therapy occurs in one-half to one-third of elderly patients,[28] and most often too little medication is consumed.[29] Poor communication between health care professionals, coupled with declining cognitive function and complicated drug regimens are major reasons for noncompliance in older patients. Pharmacists should make a special effort to counsel these high-risk patients by providing both verbal reinforcement and written instructions to assure an understanding of why the drug was prescribed, its correct use, the proper administration time consistent with lifestyle and activities, and the common side effects. Upon refill visits to the pharmacy, the pharmacist should ask the patient and caregiver subtle and open-ended questions related to side effects and potentially serious ADRs. Eliminating unnecessary or duplicative therapy in addition to simplifying the drug regimen will help minimize ADRs and maximize compliance. Pharmacists should be aware of the major risk factors for noncompliance and assess each patient for the presence of possible risk factors (Table 102.6).

Table 102.5 ▪ Criteria of Medication Appropriateness Index

1. Is there an indication for the drug?
2. Is the medication effective for the condition?
3. Is the dosage correct?
4. Are the directions correct?
5. Are the directions practical?
6. Are there clinically significant drug-drug interactions?
7. Are there clinically significant drug-disease interactions?
8. Is there unnecessary duplication with other drug(s)?
9. Is the duration of therapy acceptable?
10. Is this drug the least expensive alternative compared to others of equal utility?

Source: Reference 26.

Table 102.6 ▪ Major Risk Factors for Noncompliance

Chronic disease or long-term therapy	Multiple medications
Use of multiple pharmacies	Multiple or complicated dosing schemes
Psychiatric illness	Ineffective communication with health care professionals
Cognitive impairment	
Multiple physicians	

EFFECTS OF AGING ON DRUG ACTIONS

It has been estimated that many of the ADRs encountered in elderly patients are the result of dose-related pharmacokinetic changes and thus may be prevented if these changes are considered when prescribing drug therapy.[30] The aging process alone can influence drug response by interfering in varying degrees with the fraction of drug absorbed (f), the plasma drug half-life ($t_{1/2}$), the volume of drug distribution in the body (V_d), and the metabolic and renal clearance from the body (Cl). By predicting which drugs are potentially affected by age-related changes, the correct dose and dosing interval can be better estimated. In addition to alterations in drug kinetics, age can also influence the pharmacologic response of drugs.

Absorption

Product formulation, inherent drug properties, and patient variables can influence the rate, and in some cases the extent of drug absorption in elderly patients. In terms of product formulation, it is common for a geriatric patient to have difficulty swallowing a tablet or capsule, and it is frequently necessary to use a liquid dosage form or to crush the tablet for administration with food or via a nasogastric tube. In general, extended-release, enteric-coated, and sublingual products should not be crushed because of adverse effects on absorption half-life and toxicity.

Age-related physiologic changes in the gastrointestinal tract include elevated gastric pH, delayed gastric emptying time, and decreases in both gastrointestinal motility and intestinal blood flow. These age-related physiologic changes alone do not seem to influence the passive transport mechanisms by which most drugs are absorbed.

Medications that undergo first-pass metabolism are absorbed more completely in the older patient. This requires both smaller initial and maintenance doses of these medications when used to manage chronic diseases (Table 102.7). The age-related delay in gastric emptying allows more contact time in the stomach for potentially ulcerogenic drugs such as the nonsteroidal anti-inflammatory drugs (NSAIDs), increases the frequency of drug interactions with antacids, provides more chance for binding, may increase absorption of poorly soluble drugs, and may delay the onset of action of the weakly basic drugs.

Age does reduce the active transport mechanisms involved in the absorption of sugars (galactose), vitamins (thiamine and folic acid), and minerals (calcium and iron). Because of these changes in absorption, as well as the fact that elderly patients often do not consume a balanced diet because of food preferences or economic reasons, the use of a multivitamin and mineral supplement should be considered.

Problems with bioavailability and bioequivalence have been reported with many medications, and the issue of generic substitution is especially important to the geriatric patient because medication costs are so vital to this population.[31] Studies have demonstrated wide bioavailability and bioequivalence differences when various brands of generic tolbutamide, phenytoin, prednisone, furosemide, digoxin, and levothyroxine are compared.[32] Indiscriminate switching among products should be avoided, especially for drugs in critical therapeutic categories such as cardiovascular or hormone replacement agents, and for medications prescribed for debilitated or frail patients.

Physiologic changes and diseases, such as acute congestive heart failure (CHF), often necessitate the use of the intravenous route of administration because of incomplete absorption via the oral and intramuscular routes. There is also a decrease in absorption of intramuscularly administered drugs in bedridden elderly patients, probably due to changes in regional blood flow and reduced muscle mass.

In conclusion, although the potential for problems with absorption of medications exists in geriatric patients, practice has shown these changes to be of little clinical significance. Changes in gastric motility and blood flow can affect the extent of absorption (peak concentration) and the rate of absorption (time to peak concentration), but completeness of absorption of drugs in geriatric patients is similar to that in younger patients; however, delays in onset of activity may occur.

Table 102.7 ▪ Medications Affected by Extensive First-Pass Hepatic Metabolism

Amitriptyline	Methylphenidate
Desipramine	Metoprolol
Dextropropoxyphene	Morphine
Dihydroergotamine	Nifedipine
Diltiazem	Nitroglycerin
5-Fluorouracil	Pentazocine
Hydralazine	Propranolol
Labetalol	Salicylamide
Lidocaine	Verapamil
6-Mercaptopurine	

Distribution

Increasing age can alter the distribution of a medication to the target organ. Although total protein is unaffected by aging, the plasma albumin portion often decreases in elderly, debilitated patients. Albumin acts as a drug carrier, binding the drug until it is needed. If albumin is decreased, there will be a resultant increase in active, unbound drug (free fraction). The importance of the increased free fraction is questionable because, while more free drug is available for receptor binding, more free drug is also available for metabolism and elimination.[33] In addition to age and diet, disease states such as cirrhosis, renal failure, and malnutrition can reduce albumin levels. Reduced protein binding is seen with phenytoin, but the drug is cleared from the plasma more rapidly as described above. Initial doses of most highly protein-bound drugs (greater than 90% protein bound) should be reduced and titrated slowly if there is evidence of decreased albumin. For extensively protein-bound drugs whose binding is reduced as a result of hypoproteinemia, practitioners should expect both therapeutic and toxic events at lower total serum concentrations.[34] If several highly protein-bound drugs are used together, the chance of the patient having a drug interaction increases. In the case of meperidine, there is a decrease in the binding to red blood cells with increasing age,[35] thus increasing the amount of free drug available systemically. This may result in an increased incidence of respiratory depression, or with meperidine's active metabolite, normeperidine, central nervous system (CNS) stimulation to the point of seizures. α_1-Acid glycoprotein (AAG) is a protein which also binds to some medications. AAG is described as an acute-phase reactant and can increase with age, especially in acutely ill patients and those with inflammation. The release of AAG may increase the protein binding of basic drugs, such as lidocaine and propranolol, decreasing the amount of unbound or active drug and thus decreasing the pharmacologic effect.[36,37]

Changes in the ratio of lean body weight to fat can also alter medication distribution and thus pharmacologic response. With aging, total body water is decreased, and total body fat is increased. These changes influence the onset and duration of action of highly tissue-bound drugs, such as digoxin and water-soluble drugs such as alcohol, lithium, or morphine. The dosages of most water-soluble drugs are based on an estimation of lean body weight[38]:

$$\text{Men} = 50 \text{ kg} + 2.3 \text{ (inches in height} > 5 \text{ ft)}$$

$$\text{Women} = 45 \text{ kg} + 2.3 \text{ (inches in height} > 5 \text{ ft)}$$

If actual weight is less than estimated body weight, the actual weight should be used in dosage calculations.

Between the ages of 18 and 85 years, there is an increase in total body fat in both women and men; lean body mass will eventually decrease in both groups as well. With increasing age, the volume of distribution of lipophilic drugs increases as a result of an increase in the fat:lean muscle ratio, diminished protein binding, and a decrease in total body weight. Fat-soluble drugs, including many CNS-active drugs, may have a delayed onset of action and subsequently accumulate in adipose tissue, prolonging their duration of action, sometimes with adverse effects on the patient.

Elimination

Drugs are primarily cleared from the body by metabolism in the liver, excretion by the kidneys, or some combination of the two processes. With increasing age, a decrease in total body clearance results in higher average plasma drug concentrations and an enhanced pharmacologic response, both of which could lead to drug toxicity. Age-related physiologic changes in the kidney influence drug elimination and response in the geriatric patient to a greater extent than age-related physiologic changes that occur in the liver.

Hepatic Metabolism

Age-related physiologic changes, such as reductions in liver mass, hepatic metabolizing enzyme activity, and liver blood flow may account for the decreased elimination of some hepatically metabolized medications in the elderly patient. Medications that are biotransformed in the liver may be affected by these changes. Drug metabolism can also be affected at all ages by gender, genetics, smoking, diet, concomitant drugs, and diseases. Hepatic metabolism is highly dependent on blood flow. From 25 years of age and up, there is a continual reduction in hepatic blood flow, and in the presence of CHF, hepatic blood flow is further compromised. With drugs that are highly dependent on hepatic metabolism, such as most β-blockers, lidocaine, theophylline, and the narcotic analgesics, the decrease in hepatic clearance could increase the plasma concentrations of these drugs to toxic levels.

In addition to alterations of hepatic blood flow, age influences the rate of hepatic clearance of drugs by causing changes in the intrinsic activity of some liver enzymes. Hepatic metabolism occurs by two mechanisms: the microsomal enzyme mixed-function oxidase system (phase I), which includes the cytochrome P-450 systems; and conjugation of the drug molecule with a glucuronide, a sulfa, or an acetyl moiety (phase II). Phase I metabolism may produce compounds with pharmacologic activity, while phase II metabolism usually produces inactive metabolites. Reductions in phase I metabolism are often noted in the geriatric patient, and several enzymatic reactions of the cytochrome P-450 systems are slowed dramatically with advancing age. Of the more than 30 cytochrome P-450 isoenzymes identified, the major ones responsible for drug metabolism include CYP3A4, CYP2D6, CYP1A2, and the CYP2C subfamily.[38] Vigilant monitoring of drug therapy is necessary to avoid life-threatening drug interactions among commonly prescribed medications (Table 102.8).

Table 102.8 ▪ Problematic Drugs Involving the Cytochrome P-450 Enzyme System

Antihistamines (selected nonsedating agents)	Macrolide antibiotics
Antipsychotic agents (selected agents)	Narcotic analgesics
Azole antifungal agents	Phenobarbital
β-Blockers (selected agents)	Phenytoin
Benzodiazepines (short- and intermediate-acting)	Quinolones (selected agents)
Carbamazepine	Tricyclic antidepressants (selected agents)
Cimetidine	Selective serotonin reuptake inhibitors (selected agents)
Cisapride	Warfarin
Hydroxymethyl glutaryl-coenzyme A reductase inhibitors	

Source: Reference 39.

Phase II metabolism is usually unaffected by aging. The clinical effect of these changes results in slowed metabolism and prolonged duration of action for those medications using phase I metabolic pathways, but not for those using phase II metabolic pathways.[38,39] Studies seem to suggest that in elderly patients initial doses of hepatically metabolized drugs should be reduced by one-third to one-half the usual recommended starting dose and then adjusted based on the clinical response.

Renal Elimination

The glomerular filtration rate (GFR) may decrease as much as 50% with increasing age, and this can directly affect the renal elimination of drugs or their active metabolites. Serum creatinine is frequently used to monitor renal function, but this test has limited usefulness for monitoring the GFR in the older patient. Significant elevations of serum creatinine do not occur unless a majority of the kidney function has deteriorated. The production of creatinine, which depends on muscle mass, is decreased in elderly patients; therefore an apparently normal serum creatinine in an older patient may not be a valid predictor of drug elimination. Blood urea nitrogen is also not a useful indicator of renal function because it can be affected by hydration status, diet, and blood loss.

The GFR is reduced owing to age-related decreases in renal mass, loss of functional nephrons, and diminished renal artery perfusion. A commonly used estimation of GFR in the geriatric population is the creatinine clearance (Cl_{Cr}) which correlates well with both GFR and tubular secretion. Creatinine clearance can be estimated by a standard equation developed by Cockroft and Gault[41] that takes into consideration age, body weight, and serum creatinine in patients with stable renal function:

$$Cl_{Cr}\,(\text{male}) = \frac{\text{lean body weight (kg)} \times (140 - \text{age in years})}{\text{serum creatinine} \times 72}$$

$$Cl_{Cr}\,(\text{female}) = 0.85 \times Cl_{Cr}\,(\text{male})$$

This, as well as other creatinine clearance-estimating equations in common clinical use, has been reported to provide unacceptable predictions of creatinine clearance in a representative sample of healthy older adults.[42] An evaluation of several methods of calculations and nomograms used to estimate creatinine clearance in older patients determined that the use of published equations and rounding low serum creatinine values up to 1.0 mg/dL caused a significant underestimation of actual creatinine clearance in older patients. This study suggested that the practice of rounding-up serum creatinine concentrations could potentially lead to underdosing of certain medications such as aminoglycosides.[43] It is important to remember that mathematical equations and nomograms are simply estimates of an individual's actual renal function, and although the estimates appear to be less accurate in the geriatric population, the difficulty in collecting 24-hour urine samples may preclude more accurate creatinine clearance determinations.

To avoid drug toxicity, dosages of renally excreted drugs (or active metabolites) must be adjusted if the creatinine clearance is less than 30 mL/min (Table 102.9). Many drug monographs now contain dosing guidelines based on declining renal function, and practitioners should refer to these or similar references for dosing guidelines for renally excreted drugs in the presence of varying degrees of renal failure. Dosage and/or interval adjustments are necessary to prevent drug related problems. (A summation of pharmacokinetic changes with aging is found in Table 102.10.)

Table 102.9 ▪ Examples of Medications Primarily Excreted by the Kidney

Acetazolamide	Histamine H_2 receptor antagonists
Allopurinol	Lithium
Amiloride	Methotrexate
Angiotensin-converting enzyme inhibitors	Metoclopramide
	Nadolol
Amantadine	Norfloxacin
Aminoglycosides	Penicillins
Atenolol	Probenecid
Cephalosporins	Procainamide
Chlorpropamide	Quinidine
Ciprofloxacin	Spironolactone
Digoxin	Sulfamethoxazole
Disopyramide	Sulfinpyrazone
Ethambutol	Thiazides
Fluconazole	Trimethoprim
Furosemide	Vancomycin

Table 102.10 ▪ Age-Related Physiologic Changes Affecting Pharmacokinetic Parameters

Parameter	Direction of Change
Absorption	
Gastric pH	Increase
Absorptive surface	Decrease
Splanchnic blood flow	Decrease
Gastrointestinal motility	Decrease
Gastric emptying rate	Decrease
Distribution	
Cardiac output	Decrease
Total body weight	Decrease
Lean body mass	Decrease
Serum albumin	Decrease
α-Acid glycoprotein	Increase
Body fat	Increase
Relative tissue perfusion	Decrease
Metabolism	
Hepatic mass	Decrease
Hepatic blood flow	Decrease
Hepatic function	Decrease
Hepatic enzyme activity	Decrease
Phase 1 reactions	Decrease
Phase 2 reactions	No change
Excretion	
Renal mass	Decrease
Renal blood flow	Decrease
Glomerular filtration rate	Decrease
Tubular secretion	Decrease

EFFECTS OF AGING ON DRUG RESPONSE

With increasing age, there is an increased intolerance to drugs as a result of altered pharmacodynamic response at the target organs. Altered response may be due to a reduction in receptor number and sensitivity, depletion of neurotransmitters, the presence of disease, or physiologic changes. With aging, there is evidence of a depletion in the neurotransmitters acetylcholine, dopamine, and serotonin; a depletion in several hormones; a decrease in the enzymatic degradation of monoamine oxidase; an impaired baroreceptor response to blood pressure changes; a decreased responsiveness to β-adrenergic receptors, and increased pain tolerance.[44] Each of these changes can affect the older patient's response to medications.

Many drugs routinely prescribed for geriatric patients have adverse effects on the CNS, such as cognitive impairment and memory loss. Careful monitoring of these agents is necessary to differentiate among drug effectiveness, adverse effects, or progression of a disease process. Altered end-organ sensitivity may result in exaggerated pharmacologic response, as seen with the barbiturates and benzodiazepines. Other drug classes affected include the narcotic analgesics, antihypertensive agents, anticholinergic agents, phenothiazines, and tricyclic antidepressants. It appears that geriatric patients are more sensitive to both the therapeutic and adverse effects of many of these agents; therefore, lower initial and maintenance doses are recommended. A diminished pharmacologic response is also possible and occurs with β-blockers, β-agonists, and some calcium channel blockers (CCBs).

Increased sensitivity to warfarin in the geriatric patient has been demonstrated and recommendations for warfarin prescribing are to reduce the average daily dosage by 30 to 40% and monitor carefully, keeping the international normalized ratio within the therapeutic range.[45] Elderly women have been reported to be more susceptible to the bleeding complications of heparin,[46] and hematuria has been shown to be a useful and sensitive clinical parameter to monitor for potential heparin or warfarin toxicity.

Dose adjustments of medications are often necessary because many of these same drugs are also influenced by age-related physiologic changes, especially drug distribution and elimination. The net effect in an individual patient is often difficult to predict. For example, in elderly patients, there is an increased bioavailability of β-blockers, but a decreased responsiveness at the receptor site level. Another example is that the inotropic effect of theophylline is increased with age, but the bronchodilator effect is decreased. The homeostatic reserves in geriatric patients are less efficient and result in unpredictable drug effects and an impaired ability to recover from drug induced problems (Fig. 102.1). Numerous drug therapies require special attention when prescribed for geriatric patients, and dosage titration should always be based on a balance between optimal clinical response and minimal adverse effects.

TREATMENT

Diabetes

Aging changes related to glucose metabolism include impaired pancreatic secretion of insulin, changes in the renal threshold for glucose, and impaired glucose tolerance. Goals of management for older patients include the following.

- To avoid associated problems or diabetes complications and have a reasonable life expectancy (10 years or more) strive for the best possible glycemic control without causing hypoglycemia: fasting blood glucose level of 100 to 120 mg/dL and post-prandial (pp) glucose of ≤180 mg/dL with hemoglobin $A1_c$ within 1% of upper limits of normal (4.0 to 6.0%).
- Less aggressive management is acceptable in patients with advanced diabetes complications or impaired cognitive function, who are unable to comply with regimen or have neuropsychiatric disorders: fasting blood glucose level >140 mg/dL and pp glucose of >200 to 220 mg/dL with hemoglobulin $A1_c$ of 8%.[47] (Patients maintained with hemoglobulin $A1_c$ >7% for any length of time have been shown to have an increase in complications associated with diabetes.)
- Selection of treatment modalities for the elderly diabetic patient should take into consideration comorbid conditions, concomitant drug therapy, side effect profile(s) of the drug therapy, route(s) of drug elimination, and ease of monitoring. Blood glucose monitoring provides the best index of control for the elderly diabetic patient because urine glucose monitoring has been shown to be unreliable due to age-related increases in the renal threshold.

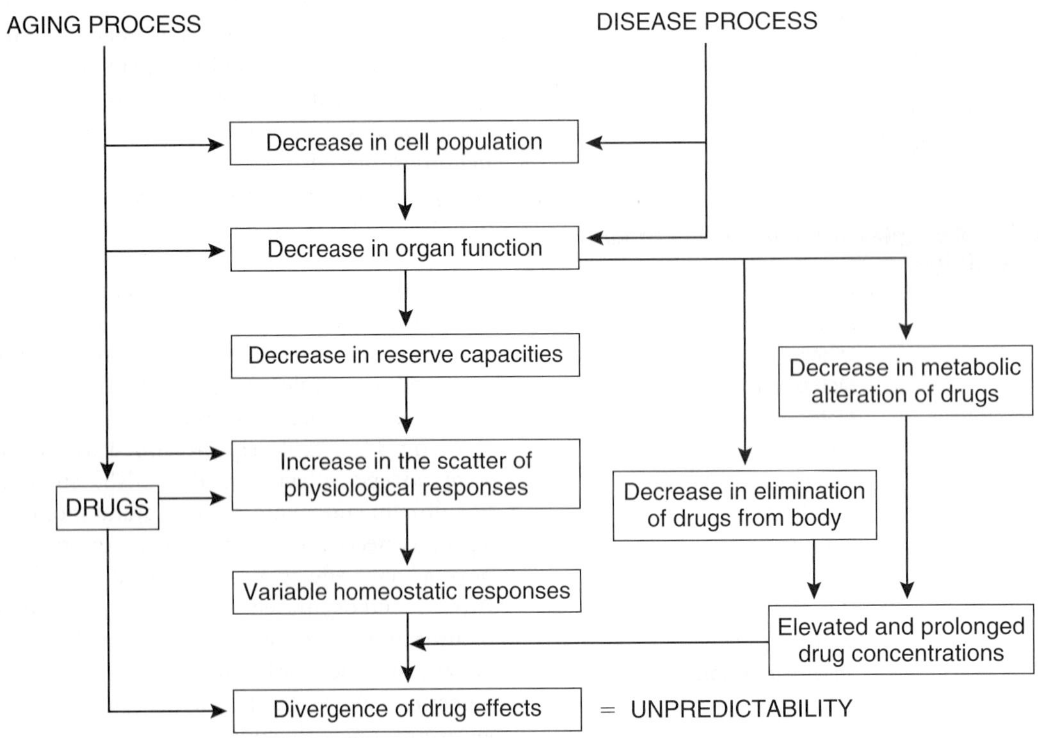

Figure 102.1. Unpredictability of drug effects in older adults. (Reprinted with permission from Henney HH. Altered drug effects in the elderly. U.S. Pharmacist 45[10]:41-50, 1985.)

Cardiovascular Disease

Aging produces several hemodynamic changes that may influence the choice of cardiovascular agents, such as an increase in peripheral vascular resistance and decreases in renal blood flow, plasma volume, plasma renin, aldosterone, and cardiac output. With an increase in peripheral vascular resistance, elderly patients may exhibit an enhanced response to vasodilators, especially diuretics, CCBs, and angiotensin-converting enzyme inhibitors (ACEIs).

Hypertension is very common among older patients. It has been shown that an elevated pulse pressure (systolic blood pressure [SBP] minus diastolic blood pressure [DBP]), which indicates reduced vascular compliance in large arteries, may be a better marker of increased cardiovascular risk than either SBP or DBP alone.[48] In practice, pulse pressures greater than 50 mmHg are considered to be elevated. This is particularly important to older patients who often have an isolated elevation of SBP (140 mm Hg or greater with a DBP less than 90 mm Hg). Although primary hypertension is the most common form of hypertension in older patients, practitioners must recognize that identifiable causes of hypertension such as atherosclerotic renovascular hypertension or primary aldosteronism may occur more frequently in older persons, especially in those whose hypertension was first seen after age 60 or is resistant to treatment.[49]

Large trials have shown that treatment of hypertension in older persons has major benefits in the form of fewer strokes, reduced incidence of coronary heart disease, cardiovascular disease, and heart failure, and longer life.[50–52] The Sixth Report of the Joint National Committee on Prevention, Detection, Evaluation, and Treatment of High Blood Pressure (JNC VI)[53] recommends that the goal of treatment of hypertension in older patients should be the same as that in younger patients (less than 140/90 mm Hg, if possible), although an interim goal of SBP less than 160 mm Hg may be necessary in those patients with significant systolic hypertension.

Initial therapy should address lifestyle modifications to include modest reduction in the use of salt and weight loss. Drug treatment should be initiated if lifestyle modifications are not successful in decreasing the blood pressure. Antihypertensive drug therapy should be implemented cautiously in older patients because they may be more sensitive to volume depletion and sympathetic inhibition than younger patients. Although all classes of antihypertensive medications have been shown to be effective in lowering blood pressure, thiazide diuretics or β-blockers in combination with thiazide diuretics are recommended because they have been shown to be effective in reducing mortality and morbidity as well.[54] Other initial therapy choices include the CCBs, ACEIs, and α-blockers, and studies are underway to determine the effect of these classes of drugs on the mortality and morbidity of hypertension. The JNC VI gives guidelines on drug therapy selection for hypertension in the presence of comorbid conditions and concomitant drug therapy.

With the age-related decline in renal function, the choice and dosage of a diuretic is important. Because older patients have a decreased plasma volume and lower levels of aldosterone, aggressive diuretic therapy to reduce blood pressure is generally not indicated. The recommendation is to initiate therapy with a small dose of hydrochlorothiazide (12.5 mg) or its equivalent, increasing to a maximum dose of 25 mg twice a day. For patients with a creatinine clearance of less than 30 mL/min, a loop diuretic such as furosemide, bumetanide, or metolazone is recommended because thiazide agents will be ineffective. Diuretic combinations with a potassium-sparing agent can be useful, but hyperkalemia may develop from reduced potassium excretion, the concurrent use of potassium supplements, or concurrent use of ACEIs.

Older patients often exhibit an impaired baroreceptor reflex response that makes them more susceptible to hypotension. Aggressive treatment of hypertension will often result in severe orthostasis, leading to falls and subsequent injuries. There is evidence of a 20 mm Hg or greater drop in blood pressure in one-fourth of healthy elderly patients undergoing positional changes. Drugs that interfere with the baroreceptor reflex, such as adrenergic-blocking agents, should be used cautiously because of the increased risk of falls and fractures.

Blood pressure should be measured in the standing as well as the sitting position, and antihypertensive treatments should be initiated with smaller dosages and in longer intervals than usual. Additional complications of aggressive antihypertensive therapy are cognitive dysfunction resulting from hypoperfusion to the brain and exaggerated side effects of the medications. In general, initial doses of antihypertensive agents for geriatric patients are reduced by one-third to one-half with slow titration until the desired response is achieved.

The Agency for Health Care Policy and Research Clinical Practice Guidelines[55] for the management of CHF reflect increased use of ACEIs because they have been shown to not only provide symptomatic relief with fewer side effects, but also to prolong survival in patients with mild, moderate, or severe CHF. The guidelines suggest that diuretics are indicated in patients with evidence of fluid overload, and the use of cardiac glycosides is restricted to those patients with severe systolic dysfunction or who are intolerant of or unresponsive to diuretic and/or ACEI therapy. Studies have shown that digoxin can be safely withdrawn in a majority of older patients if there is no evidence of heart failure and if the heart is in normal sinus rhythm, especially in the presence of subtherapeutic plasma levels of digoxin (<0.8 ng/mL).[56] Patients should be monitored for signs and symptoms of atrial fibrillation and CHF if withdrawal from digoxin is attempted.

Anxiety and Insomnia

As many as half of patients older than age 50 report experiencing insomnia, and it has been shown that hypnotic drug use increases with increasing age. Due to age-related changes in the CNS, a general guideline for doses of anxiolytics-sedative-hypnotics is to start with one-third to one-half the usual recommended initial dose or to extend the time interval between doses. Geriatric patients are more sensitive to the cortical depressant effects of the benzodiazepines (BZDs) and can appear to be cognitively impaired, depressed, or both as a result of chronic intoxication. In the older patient, BZDs are effective in reducing sleep latency, but chronic or repeated use can lead to overmedication, additive side effects, or hypersomnolence. When used regularly in the elderly, BZDs can cause significant toxicity, including dependence, hangover effect, dysphoria, and withdrawal symptoms on discontinuation. An increased risk of hip fracture has been correlated directly with the use of long-acting BZDs; users of short half-life BZDs had no significantly increased risk compared to control subjects.[57]

When selecting a BZD for use in geriatric patients, considerations should include specific symptoms and needs of the patient (i.e., sleep latency, sleep maintenance, and/or early morning wakening anxiety) and the metabolic pathway of the drug. Shorter-acting agents such as oxazepam, lorazepam, temazepam, and triazolam may be preferable. Nonbenzodiazepine agents such as buspirone and zolpidem are useful therapeutic alternatives, which lack the adverse effects of the BZDs. Chloral hydrate is a cost-effective hypnotic agent for use in the older patient; however, tolerance quickly develops in as little time as 1 week if the drug is used daily. Diphenhydramine is useful for occasional insomnia or anxiety in the geriatric patient, but the risk of anticholinergic delirium or worsening of the patient's cognitive state can occur if it is used too frequently, in excessive doses, or with other drugs that have anticholinergic properties. Recommended dosing information for anxiolytics and sedative/hypnotics is listed in Table 102.11.

Table 102.11 ▪ Recommended Maximum Doses of Anxiolytics, Sedatives, and Hypnotics

	Usual Daily Dose	
Medication	**Adult: Age <65 (mg/day)**	**Geriatric: Age ≥65 (mg/day)**
Benzodiazepine Anxiolytics		
Alprazolam	0.75–4	0.25–0.75
Chlordiazepoxide[a]	15–100	10–20
Clorazepate[a]	15–60	7.5–15
Diazepam[a]	6–40	1–5
Halazepam	60–100	20–40
Lorazepam	2–6	0.5–2
Oxazepam	30–120	10–30
Prazepam[a]	20–60	10–15
Benzodiazepine sedative/hypnotics		
Estazolam	1–2	0.5–1
Flurazepam[a]	15–30	15
Quazepam[a]	7.5–15	7.5
Temazepam	15–30	15
Triazolam	0.125–0.5	0.0625–0.125
Clonazepam	1.5–20	0.5–1.5
Other Anxiolytics and Sedatives		
Buspirone	15–60	10–60
Chloral hydrate	250–1000	250–500
Diphenhydramine	25–200	25–50
Hydroxyzine	25–600	10–50
Zolpidem	5–20	5–10

[a]Not recommended for use in geriatric patients.

Psychosis and Behavioral Problems

In the geriatric population, antipsychotic agents are useful for treatment of psychoses and severe behavioral manifestations associated with dementia. Behavioral symptoms occurring with dementia include anxiety, agitation, aggression, paranoia, hallucinations, and combativeness. When these symptoms occur, they are disturbing to both the patient and the care-giver. Guidelines that are a part of the Omnibus Budget Reconciliation Act (OBRA) require that before prescribing an antipsychotic agent for the management of a patient with dementia within a nursing facility, the clinical record must contain (in addition to the diagnosis of dementia), both quantitative and qualitative documentation of associated psychotic and/or agitated behaviors that present a danger to the patient or to others. Inappropriate indications for antipsychotic agents in patients with dementia include wandering, poor self-care, restlessness, impaired memory, anxiety, depression, insomnia, unsociability, indifference to surroundings, fidgeting, nervousness, uncooperativeness, or agitated behaviors that do not represent a danger to the resident or others. OBRA guidelines also require periodic (every 6 months) trial dosage reductions to determine the lowest effective dose for a particular patient.[58]

The phenothiazine antipsychotics (low-potency agents) have prominent sedative, cardiovascular, anticholinergic, and neurologic side effects that are often manifested in the elderly patient, most likely as a result of a deceased ability of the hepatic enzymes to metabolize the drugs to inactive metabolites and/or to altered receptor sensitivity. Nonphenothiazine antipsychotics (high-potency agents) are less sedating and cause less anticholinergic toxicity, but can cause more adverse neurologic effects such as tardive dyskinesia. The initial dose of either class of antipsychotic should be small and gradually increased according to the clinical response of the patient. Drugs may be given in divided doses or as a single daily dose, with small doses of "as-needed orders" for repeating the dose to determine the lowest effective dose and to minimize size effects. Maximum daily doses should be approximately one-fourth of those recommended in younger patients (Table 102.12).

The newer atypical antipsychotic agents such as clozapine, risperidone, olanzapine, and quetiapine are frequently prescribed to manage disruptive behaviors such as agitation, combativeness, or aggression, which occur in patients with dementia. Smaller dosages (compared to those useful for managing psychosis) are usually prescribed to manage the associated behaviors of patients with dementia, and currently clinical studies assessing specific maximum and minimum doses are being conducted.

Extrapyramidal symptoms have been shown to occur in up to 50% of all patients taking antipsychotic agents and between the ages of 60 and 80 years. Almost 90% of these reactions occur within the first 10 weeks of therapy. These side effects can be minimized by using the lowest effective dose of the antipsychotic agent or with an anticholinergic agent, such as benztropine or diphenhydramine. After 3 months of continuous therapy, the anticholinergic agent can be withdrawn without a recurrence of the extrapyramidal symptoms for most patients. Anticholinergic agents should not be used prophylactically because this exposes the patient to additional anticholinergic effects such as confusion and hallucinations. The incidence of tardive dyskinesia can be minimized by the proper use of anticholinergic drugs (attempting to maintain the balance between dopamine and acetylcholine), limiting the use of antipsychotic medications, and adjusting maintenance doses to the lowest effective levels. Alternative therapies for problem behaviors associated with dementia include lithium and selected anticonvulsants such as carbamazepine and valproic acid.[59]

Table 102.12 ▪ Recommended Maximum Doses of Oral Antipsychotics

Medication	Adult: Age <65 (mg/day)	Geriatric: Age ≥65 (mg/day)	Geriatric/ Dementia: Age ≥65 (mg/day)
Acetophenazine	300	150	20
Chlorpromazine	1600	800	75
Chlorprothixene	1600	800	75
Clozapine	450	25	50
Fluphenazine	40	20	4
Haloperidol	100	50	4
Loxapine	250	125	10
Mesoridazine	500	250	25
Molindone	225	112	10
Olanzapine	20	10	7.5[a]
Perphenazine	64	32	8
Promazine	500	50	150
Quetiapine	750	150	—[a]
Risperidone	16	4	2
Thioridazine	800	400	75
Thiothixene	60	30	7
Trifluoperazine	80	40	8
Trifluopromazine	100	20	

[a]—, limited clinical experience in this population.

Table 102.13 ▪ Recommended Dosage Ranges of Antidepressants

Medication	Adult: Age <65 (mg/day)	Geriatric: Age ≥65 (mg/day)
Amitriptyline[a]	75–300	25–150
Amoxapine[a]	150–600	25–300
Bupropion	225–450	50–100
Desipramine[b]	75–300	10–100
Doxepin	75–300	10–75
Fluoxetine	20–80	10–40
Fluvoxamine	50–300	—[c]
Imipramine	75–300	10–150
Maprotiline	75–300	25–75
Mirtazapine	15	—[c]
Nefazodone	300–600	—[c]
Nortriptyline[b]	75–300	10–75
Paroxetine[b]	20–50	10–30
Protriptyline	15–60	15–20
Sertraline [b]	75–200	25–200
Trazodone	150–600	25–150
Trimipramine	75–300	25–100
Venlafaxine	75–375	—[c]

[a]Not recommended for use in geriatric patients.
[b]Preferred agents in geriatric patients.
[c]—, limited clinical experience in this population.

Depression

Clinical depression is common among geriatric patients and is often underdiagnosed and therefore undertreated in the nursing facility population (and geriatric population in general).[60] The presentation of depression in an older patient can be atypical and dismissed as cognitive impairment, reaction to chronic illness, or an understandable response to institutionalizaion.[61] The older, tertiary amine antidepressants such as amitriptyline and imipramine are usually not recommended for most depressed geriatric patients because of their sedative and highly anticholinergic properties. The secondary amines such as desipramine and nortriptyline are preferable because of their lower incidence of and less severe side effects. The newer agents such as selective serotonin reuptake inhibitors are promoted to be better tolerated in the geriatric patient, despite limited clinical studies to support this claim.[62] Trazodone lacks anticholinergic side effects, but it is extremely sedating and can cause hypotension. It is recommended as an alternative antidepressant when others have failed. (The most common use of trazodone in current geriatric practice is as a sedative-hypnotic, owing to its strong sedative properties.) Recommended dosing information for antidepressants is listed in Table 102.13.

Mild-to-Moderate Pain

Many older patients suffer from some degree of chronic pain related most often to degenerative joint disease. NSAIDs are very commonly prescribed for this condition, but their use is problematic. NSAIDs have been shown to be hazardous in the older population because of their ability to cause renal insufficiency, gastrointestinal hemorrhage, and blood pressure elevations. Many of the adverse effects of NSAIDs result from the ability of these agents to inhibit the biosynthesis of prostaglandins. Prostaglandins function to maintain renal blood flow and GFR in the presence of reduced effective or actual circulatory volume, they mediate effects that protect the gastric and duodenal mucosa, and they play a role in the modulation of blood pressure. To limit the occurrence of these adverse effects, NSAID use should be limited to those situations in which it is absolutely necessary and NSAID use should be accompanied by monitoring of hemoglobin, hematocrit, renal function, and electrolytes. Inflammation is a rare cause of pain in chronic osteoarthritis, and an analgesic with few or no anti-inflammatory properties such as acetaminophen or nonacetylated salicylates may be more appropriate than an NSAID.[63]

Geriatric patients are significantly more sensitive to the pain-relieving effect of narcotics because of changes in receptor number and function, alterations in protein binding, and prolonged clearance of these agents. These changes allow narcotics to be more effective in smaller doses when used in geriatric patients compared to younger patients. The elderly, as a group, are more likely to develop narcotic side effects of constipation, respiratory depression, cough suppression, and cognitive impairment compared to younger patients.[64] No evidence yet allows the preference of one narcotic over another on the basis of age alone. The dosing of narcotic analgesics in the older patient should be done cautiously by increasing the dose until the patient obtains pain relief for at least 4 hours. The dose should be administered before the pain occurs to avoid anticipatory anxiety and behavioral reinforcement of drug use, especially in terminally ill patients with chronic pain. Adjuvant analgesic relief may be provided by the use of tricyclic antidepressants or NSAIDs.

PREVENTIVE CARE

Mortality and morbidity from pneumococcal pneumonia, influenza, and tetanus infections are very high in the geriatric population. Older patients show a response to antibody formation from the polyvalent pneumococcal vaccine comparable to that of a younger population.[65] All persons 65 years of age and older should receive the pneumococcal vaccine, including previously unvaccinated persons and persons who have not received vaccine within 5 years (and were less than 65 years of age at the time of vaccination). All persons who have unknown vaccination status should receive one dose of pneumococcal vaccine.[66] A favorable antibody response is likewise elicited from an annual influenza vaccine administered to a geriatric patient, with an efficacy rate of 70 to 80% against the influenza strains of the season. It usually takes 4 to 8 weeks to elicit a full antibody response, so vaccinations must be made in advance of the anticipated flu season. Although cases of tetanus have decreased dramatically as a result of mandatory pediatric vaccination programs, elderly individuals are a major at-risk population for this disease owing to declining titers with increasing age. Adults who have completed a primary series of tetanus immunization should receive booster doses every 10 years. The majority of elderly patients, particularly those with chronic diseases, should be immunized with a documented dose of polyvalent pneumococcal vaccine, an annual influenza vaccine, and a tetanus booster every 10 years.

CONCLUSION

Because of the many possibilities for age-related changes and medication actions and adverse effects, designing therapeutic regimens for geriatric patients can be complicated and unpredictable. When providing care for geriatric patients, it is necessary to continually reevaluate the need for existing and/or new medications. Proper medication use by geriatric patients should include optimization of drug therapy to meet the patient's medical needs, yet avoid drug-induced adverse effects; patient education to maximize patient adherence to drug therapy regimens; and regular review of the patient's drug therapy to screen for the following:

1. Is each medication necessary?
2. Are nonpharmacologic alternatives available?
3. Is the lowest effective dose being used?
4. Are there any unaddressed medical or drug-related problems?

Above all, communication among the pharmacist, the physician, the nurse, the patient, and the patient's caregiver is of utmost importance in meeting the goals(s) of therapy.

KEY POINTS

- Elderly patients account for 30% of all medications prescribed in the United States, but also consume substantial quantities of over-the-counter medications.
- Polypharmacy, or the use of multiple prescription and over-the-counter medications, especially by older people with chronic health problems, has been identified as the principal drug safety issue of the future.
- Older patients are at risk for ADRs compared to younger patients and often have an atypical presentation of the ADR that may be confused with aging or disease progression.
- More than one in six elderly Americans are taking prescription drugs that are not suited for geriatric

patients and may lead to physical or mental deterioration and possibly death.

- In both prescribing and monitoring medication therapy in geriatric patients, it is extremely important to consider the individual patient, his or her clinical and health status, and concomitant medications he or she is receiving.
- By predicting which drugs are potentially affected by age-related physiologic and pharmacokinetic changes, the correct dose and dosing interval can be more accurately estimated.
- Changes in gastric motility and blood flow can affect the extent of absorption and the rate of absorption, but completeness of absorption of medications in geriatric patients is similar to that in younger patients; however, a delay in the onset of activity may occur.
- The importance of increased free fraction of a medication (due to a decrease in binding to albumin) is questionable because while additional free drug is available for receptor binding, more free drug is also available for metabolism and elimination.
- Age-related physiologic changes in the kidney influence drug elimination and response in the geriatric patient to a greater extent than age-related physiologic changes that occur in the liver.
- To avoid drug toxicity, the dosages of renally excreted drugs (or active metabolites) must be adjusted if the creatinine clearance is less than 30 mL/min.
- With increasing age, there is an increased intolerance to medications as a result of altered pharmacodynamic response at the target organs.
- Because of the many possibilities for age-related change and medication actions and adverse effects, designing therapeutic regimens for geriatric patients can be complicated and unpredictable.
- When providing care for geriatric patients, it is important to continually reevaluate the need for existing and/or new medications.
- Regular review of the drug regimen of a geriatric patient should include asking the following questions: Is each medication necessary? Are nonpharmacologic alternatives available? Is the lowest effective dose being used? Are there any unaddressed medical or drug related problems?

REFERENCES

1. Monthly Vital Statistics Report. Hyattsville, MD: National Center for Health Statistics, 1996:43:6.
2. Fowles DG: A profile of older Americans: 1991. USDHHSAoA/AARP Publication No. PF3049(1291)D996, Washington DC, 1991.
3. Abrams WB, Berkow R: The Merck manual of geriatrics. Rahway, NJ: MSD Research Laboratories, 1995:1115–1123.
4. Steiner JF. Pharmacotherapy problems in the elderly. J Am Pharm Assoc NS36(7):431–467, 1996.
5. Koch K, Knapp DA: Highlights of drug utilization in office practice. National ambulatory medical care survey, 1985. Vital and health statistics, no. 143. DHHS Publication No. (PHS) 87-1250. Hyattsville, MD: National Center for Health Statistics, 1987.
6. Stewart RB, Moore MT, May FE, et al. Age Aging 20:182–188, 1991.
7. Miller DR: Drug surveillance utilizing epidemiologic methods. Am J Hosp Pharm 30:584–592, 1973.
8. Tobias DE, Pulliam CC. General and psychotherapeutic medication use in 878 nursing facilities: a 1997 national survey. Consult Pharm 12:1401–1408, 1997.
9. Kidder SW. Cost-benefit of pharmacist-conducted drug-regimen reviews. Consult Pharm 2: 394–398, 1987.
10. Healthy People 2000: national health promotion and disease prevention objectives. Washington, DC: U.S. Department of Health and Human Services, 1990.
11. Tobias DE, Pulliam CC. General and psychotherapeutic medication use in 372 nursing facilities: a national survey. Consult Pharm 9:449–461, 1994.
12. Tresch DD, Duthie EH, Newton M: Coping with diagnosis related groups. Arch Intern Med 148:1393–1396.
13. Simonson W. Consultant pharmacy practice. 2nd ed. Alexandria, VA: American Society of Consultant Pharmacists, 1991:13–26.
14. Health Care Financing Administration. State operations manual–provider certification transmittal no. 250. 1992(Apr): P139–P150.
15. Green LW, Mullen PD, Stainbrook GL. Programs to reduce drug errors in the elderly: direct and indirect evidence from patient education. J Geriatr Drug Ther 1:3–18, 1986.
16. Gurwitz JH, Avorn J. The ambiguous relation between aging and adverse drug reactions. Ann Intern Med 114:956–966, 1991.
17. Colley CA, Lucas LM. Polypharmacy: the cure becomes the disease. J Gen Intern Med 8:278–283, 1993.
18. Gurwitz JH, Soumerai SB, Avorn J. Improving medication prescribing and utilization in the nursing home. J Am Geriatr Soc 38:542–552, 1990.
19. Avorn J, Gurwitz JH. Drug use in the nursing home. Ann Intern Med 123:195–204, 1995.
20. Wilcox SM, Himmelstein DU, Woolhandler S. Inappropriate drug prescribing for the community-dwelling elderly. JAMA 272:292–296, 1994.
21. Fouts M, Hanlon J, Pieper C, et al. Identification of elderly nursing facility residents at high risk for drug-related problems. Consult Pharm 12:1103–1111, 1997.
22. Drugs that cause psychiatric symptoms. Med Lett Drugs Ther 40(1020):21–24, 1998.
23. Stover KA. GAO reports elderly not taking drugs properly. Pharmacy Today 1(14):8, 1995.
24. Beers MH, Ouslander JG, Fingold SF, et al. Inappropriate medication prescribing in skilled-nursing facilities. Ann Intern Med 117:684–689, 1992.
25. Beers MH. Explicit criteria for determining potentially inappropriate medication use by the elderly, an update. Arch Intern Med 157:1531–1536, 1997.
26. Hanlon JT, Schmader KE, Samsa GP, et al. A method for assessing drug therapy appropriateness. J Clin Epidemiol 45:1045–1051, 1992.
27. Bootman JL, Harrison DL, Cox E. The health care cost of drug-related morbidity and mortality in nursing facilities. Arch Intern Med 157:2089–2096, 1997.
28. Morrow D, Leirer V, Sheikh J. Adherence and medication instructions: review and recommendations. J Am Geriatr Soc 36:1147–1160, 1988.
29. Cooper JK, Love DW, Raffoul PR. Intentional prescription nonadherence (noncompliance) by the elderly. J Am Geriatr Soc 30:329–333, 1982.
30. Greenblatt DG, Sellers EM, Shader RI. Drug disposition in old age. N Engl J Med 306:1081–1088, 1982.
31. Miller SW, Strom JG. Drug-product selection: implications for the geriatric patient. Consult Pharm 5:30–37, 1990.
32. Riley TN, Ravis WS. Key concepts in drug bioequivalence. U.S. Pharm 12(2):40–53, 1987.
33. Hayes MJ, Langman MJS, Short AH. Changes in drug metabolism with increasing age. Br J Clin Pharmacol 2:73–79, 1975.
34. Greenblatt DJ, Sellers EM, Koch-Weser J. Importance of protein binding for the interpretation of serum or plasma drug concentrations. J Clin Pharmacol 22:259–263, 1982.
35. Mather LE, Tucker GT, Pflug AE, et al. Meperidine kinetics in man. Clin Pharmacol Ther 17:21–30, 1975.
36. Lalonde RL, Tenero DM, Burlew BS, et al. Effects of age on protein binding and disposition of propranolol stereoisomer. Clin Pharmacol Ther 47:447–455, 1990.
37. Davis D, Grossman SH, Kitchell BB, et al. Age related changes in the plasma protein binding of lidocaine and diazepam. Clin Res 28:234A, 1980.
38. Devine B. Gantamicin therapy. Drug Intel Clin Pharm 8:650–655, 1974.
39. Michalets EL. Update; clinically significant cytochrome P-450 drug interactions. Pharmacotherapy 18:84–112, 1998.
40. Vestal RE, Norris AH, Tobin JD, et al. Antipyrine metabolism in man:

influence of age, alcohol, caffeine, and smoking. Clin Pharmacol Ther 18:425–432, 1975.
41. Greenblatt DJ, Divoll M, Harmatz JS, et al. Oxazepam kinetics: Influence and effects of age and sex. J Pharmacol Exp Ther 215:86–91, 1980.
42. Cockroft DW, Gault MH. Prediction of creatinine clearance from serum creatinine. Nephron 16:31–41, 1976.
43. Malmrose LC, Gray SL, Peiper CF, et al. Measured versus estimated creatinine clearance in a high-functioning elderly sample: Mac Arthur foundation study of successful aging. J Am Geriatr Soc 41:715–721, 1993.
44. Smythe M, Hoffman J, Kizy K, et al. Estimating creatinine clearance in elderly patient with low serum creatinine concentrations. Am J Hosp Pharm 51:198–204, 1994.
45. Feely J, Cloakley D. Altered pharmacodynamics in the elderly. Clin Geriatr Med 6:269–283, 1990.
46. Gurwitz JH, Avorn J. Ross-Degnan D, et al. Aging and the anticoagulant response to warfarin therapy. Ann Intern Med 116:901–904, 1992.
47. Jick H, Slone D, Borda IT, et al. Efficacy and toxicity of heparin in relation to age and sex. N Engl J Med 279:284–286, 1968.
48. Standards of medical care for patients with diabetes mellitus. Diabetes Care 21(Suppl 1):S23–S31, 1998.
49. Madhaven S, Ooi WL, Cohen H, et al. Relation of pulse pressure and blood pressure reduction to the incidence of myocardial infarction. Hypertension 23:395–401, 1994.
50. Setaro JF, Black HR. Refractory hypertension N Engl J Med 69:997–999, 1994.
51. Staessen JA, Fagard R, Thijs L, et al. For the systolic hypertension (Syst-Eur) trial investigators. Morbidity and mortality in the placebo-controlled European trial on isolated systolic hypertension in the elderly. Lancet 350:757–764, 1997.
52. SHEP Cooperative Research Group. Prevention of stroke by antihypertensive drug treatment in older persons with isolated systolic hypertension: final results of the Systolic Hypertension in the Elderly Program (SHEP). JAMA 265:3255–3264, 1991.
53. National High Blood Pressure Education Program Working Group. National High Blood Pressure Education Program Working Group Report on Hypertension in the Elderly. Hypertension 23:275–285, 1994.
54. Joint National Committee on Detection, Evaluation, and Treatment of High Blood Pressure. The Sixth Report of the Joint National Committee on Prevention, Detection, Evaluation, and Treatment of High Blood Pressure (JNC VI). Arch Intern Med 157:2413–2446, 1997.
55. MacMahon S, Rodgers A. The effects of blood pressure reduction in older patients: an overview of five randomized controlled trials in elderly hypertensives. Clin Exp Hypertens 15:967–978, 1993.
56. Heart failure: evaluation and care of patients with left ventricular dysfunction. Clinical Practice Guideline No. 11. AHCPR Publication No. 94-0612. Rockville, MD: Agency for Health Care Policy and Research, Public Health Service U.S. Department of Health and Human Services, June 1994.
57. Gheorghiade M, Beller GA. Effects of discontinuing maintenance digoxin therapy in patients with ischemic heart disease and congestive heart failure in sinus rhythm. Am J Cardiol 51:1243–1250, 1983.
58. Ray WA, Griffin MR, Downey W. Benzodiazepines of long and short elimination half-life and the risk of hip fracture. JAMA 262:3303–3307, 1989.
59. Fed Regist 56(187):483, 1991.
60. Yeager BR, Farnett LE, Ruzicka SA. Management of the behavioral manifestations of dementia. Arch Intern Med 155:250–260, 1995.
61. Rovner BW, German PS, Brant IJ, et al. Depression and mortality in nursing home elderly. JAMA 265;993–996, 1991.
62. Board of Directors of the American Association for Geriatric Psychiatry, Clinical Practice Committee of the American Geriatrics Society and Committee on Long-Term Care and Treatment for the Elderly, American Psychiatric Association. Psychotherapeutic medications in the nursing home. J Am Geriatr Soc 40:946–949, 1992.
63. Song F, Freemantle N, Sheldon TA, et al. Selective serotonin reuptake inhibitors: meta-analysis of efficacy and acceptability. Br Med J 306:683–687, 1993.
64. Bradley JD, Brandt KD, Katz BP, et al. Comparison of an antiinflammatory dose of ibuprofen, and acetaminophen in the treatment of patients with osteoarthritis of the knee. N Engl J Med 325:87–91, 1991.
65. Kaiko RF, Wallenstein SL, Rogers AG, et al. Narcotics in the elderly. In: Reidenberg MM, ed. Med Clin North Am 66:1079–1089, 1982.
66. Ammann AJ, Schiffman G, Ausrian R. The antibody response to pneumococcal capsular polysaccharides in the aged individuals. Proc Soc Exp Biol Med 164:312–316, 1980.
67. Centers for Disease Control and Prevention. Prevention of pneumococcal disease: recommendations of the Advisory Committee on Immunization Practices (ACIP). MMWR Morb Mortal Wkly Rep 46(No. RR-8):1–10, 1997.

CHAPTER 103

CRITICAL CARE THERAPY

Bradley A. Boucher, G. Dennis Clifton, and Scott D. Hanes

Critical care medicine is a multidisciplinary subspecialty that has realized remarkable growth over the last three decades, paralleling advances in life support technologies. Individuals requiring intensive care unit (ICU) management include postoperative general surgical, cardiothoracic, and neurosurgical patients; victims of major trauma and burns; medical patients with acute respiratory failure and exacerbations of chronic diseases; and obstetric and neonatal patients. Common features among many of these patients are their complex pathophysiologic states and the use of a large number of pharmacologic agents in their management, many having a narrow therapeutic index. On average, these patients have 8 to 12 medications prescribed while being cared for in the ICU.[1] Table 103.1 lists categories of agents commonly administered to medical and surgical ICU patients. Recognition of the pharmacologic monitoring demands in the ICU by pioneering clinical pharmacists in the 1970s spawned the development of critical care as a specialty within the pharmacy profession.[1,2] Since that time, this focus area within pharmacology has grown immensely, with thousands of pharmacists providing care to ICU patients on a full- or part-time basis in virtually all types of ICU settings (e.g., medical ICUs, coronary care units, surgical ICUs, trauma and burn centers, neonatal ICUs, neurology/neurosurgical ICUs). In addition, scores of aspiring practitioners and researchers continue to receive postgraduate critical care pharmacy training annually. This chapter introduces the practice of critical care pharmacology by outlining several general principles relevant to the care of ICU patients and highlighting the management of medical problems frequently encountered in the critically ill patient population.

USE OF THE PROBLEM-ORIENTED METHOD

Developing a pharmacist-oriented problem list is an essential initial step in the process of formulating a monitoring and treatment plan for patients in general. Use of the problem-oriented approach is particularly important in the care of critically ill patients considering the relative complexities of their medical problems. Because these patients commonly have multi–organ system involvement, it is strongly recommended that the critical care pharmacy practitioner reflect on each respective organ system (e.g., central nervous system, pulmonary system, cardiovascular system) to determine whether a problem or potential problem amenable to pharmacologic therapy exists. In so doing, the formidable challenge of evaluating critically ill patients is significantly simplified by breaking down their medical problems into more manageable pieces. Furthermore, the task of identifying appropriate monitoring parameters for treatment success or failure, including drug toxicity, is much more easily accomplished. This latter task is aided substantially by the relative wealth of clinical and laboratory data available in critically ill patients for this purpose, compared to other hospitalized patients and the ambulatory patient care environment. A more thorough discussion and examples of the problem-oriented method can be found in the companion workbook for this text.

Table 103.1 ▪ Medications Commonly Administered in Medical and Surgical Intensive Care Units

Analgesics	Anxiolytics/antipsychotics
Antianginals	Bronchodilators
Antiarrhythmics	Catecholamines
Antimicrobials	Corticosteroids
Anticoagulants	Diuretics
Anticonvulsants	Inotropes
Antiemetics	Insulin
Antihypertensives/vasodilators	Neuromuscular blocking agents
Antipyretics (acetaminophen/ aspirin)	Stress ulcer prophylaxis (H_2-blockers/antacids/sucralfate)

TREATMENT GOALS: CRITICAL CARE THERAPY

- Minimize patient mortality and morbidity through the use of invasive and noninvasive monitoring, extensive observation, and intensive care by health care providers specialized in critical care medicine.
- Restore curable patients to an independent state following acute injury or illness.
- Restore or improve the baseline state of chronically ill patients following an acute exacerbation or deterioration of their illness.
- Use pharmacologic and supportive therapies (e.g., mechanical ventilation) to resuscitate unstable patients and restore them to physiologic stability.
- Use all pharmacotherapy in a rational and cost-effective manner.
- Individualize pharmacotherapy in patients with organ dysfunction through the application of relevant pharmacokinetic and pharmacodymanic principles.
- Maximize utilization of limited health care resources by appropriate selection and optional management of patients receiving expensive or technically sophisticated therapies.
- Provide emotional and psychological support to patients and family members thrust into the typically overwhelming and unknown environment of the ICU.

PHARMACOKINETIC AND PHARMACODYNAMIC CONSIDERATIONS

Critically ill patients undergo a number of physiologic changes during their acute stress that have the potential to dramatically affect drug disposition or response in these patients relative to more stable patients or healthy volunteers. Among these changes is a surge in catecholamines commonly observed in critically ill patients that can have significant effects on cardiac output (CO) and systemic vascular resistance (SVR). These effects in turn may result in increases or decreases in drug delivery to the kidneys and liver by altering renal and hepatic blood flow, respectively. Mechanical ventilation (MV) settings, especially very high positive end-expiratory pressure (PEEP), may also reduce hepatic blood flow. Another important hemodynamic alteration often observed in critically ill patients is hypotension accompanying various shock states (e.g., cardiogenic, hemorrhagic, septic, neurogenic). Prolonged hypotension may not only result in acute pharmacokinetic alterations, but in end-organ damage as well (e.g., acute renal failure [ARF], hepatic dysfunction, bowel ischemia). In severe ARF cases, patients may require hemodialysis or other forms of renal replacement therapy in order to sustain homeostasis. Drug removal by the particular type of renal replacement therapy is yet another important factor to consider relative to design of dosing regimens.

A number of other factors may affect drug disposition in critically ill patients. One of these factors is the release of cytokines during the acute phase response. Several in vitro and animal studies have provided evidence that many of the pro-inflammatory cytokines (e.g., interleukin-1 [IL-1], interleukin-6 [IL-6], and tumor necrosis factor [TNF]) decrease cytochrome P-450 enzyme concentrations or activity, which could affect many drugs used in the critical care setting that undergo hepatic oxidative metabolism.[3] Critically ill patients are also susceptible to protein binding changes as an indirect consequence of acute stress. For example, during the acute-phase response, patients typically become very catabolic, which can result in profound hypoalbuminemia. This may cause significant reductions in the protein binding of acidic drugs. Other patients receiving highly protein bound, basic drugs (e.g., lidocaine) may have significant increases in protein binding accompanying dramatic rises in α_1-acid glycoprotein (AAG) concentrations. The pharmacokinetic implications of these protein binding changes on the total and unbound drug concentrations are largely determined by the clearance properties of the drug in question (i.e., high extraction versus low extraction).[4] Finally, considering the large number of medications administered to critically ill patients, the potential for pharmacokinetic and pharmacodynamic drug interactions increases substantially. Although these interactions may be well tolerated in other patient populations, critically ill patients may be particularly susceptible to any associated adverse effects due to their unstable physiologic state.

Figure 103.1 summarizes the wide array of variables that may potentially affect drug disposition and response in critically ill patients. Superimposed on these many variables is the dynamic nature of the critically ill patient. For example, pharmacokinetic parameter estimates at one point in time may be dramatically different from those obtained only a short time later in the patient's hospital course. Thus critical care pharmacy practitioners facing the daunting task of designing treatment regimens and monitoring therapy in these individuals need to have a keen appreciation of these many factors. In addition, surveillance of the primary literature for pharmacokinetic and pharmacodynamic investigations of specific drugs in various critically ill patient subsets is of utmost importance. Despite the difficulty in conducting these investigations because of numerous confounding variables, increasing numbers of studies are being published each year. Readers are directed to the textbook entitled *The Pharmacologic Approach to the Critically Ill Patient*, third edition, focusing on drug use in the critically ill for a more comprehensive treatment of this topic.[5]

DRUG ADMINISTRATION IN THE INTENSIVE CARE UNIT

Individual patient care plans in critically ill patients should always include assessment of the most appropriate and cost-effective route of drug administration. All routes of drug administration, including intravenous (IV), intramuscular (IM), intraarterial, epidural, intraventricular, intrathecal, subcutaneous (SC), oral, sublingual, rectal, inhalation, and topical, are used in the ICU setting. The route of drug administration depends on available dosage forms, intended use of the agent, functionality and availability of the gut, duration of action, urgency of treatment, and the hemodynamic stability of the patient. The duration of action of cardiovascular acting agents is especially important when dealing with hemodynamically unstable patients. In these patients, IV administration of short-acting cardiovascular agents is generally preferred. The rapidity by which the desired effect takes place is also an important variable in deciding the type and route of drug administration. For example, the pharmacologic management of hyperkalemia may be performed over a period of hours by oral administration of sodium polystyrene sulfonate or more rapidly with the IV administration of insulin or sodium bicarbonate.

Intravascular

Antimicrobials, inotropes, vasopressors, vasodilators, and analgesics administered to critically ill patients are most commonly administered intravenously. Additionally, the IV route is often used to administer nutrition, blood products, fluids, and electrolytes. Unfortunately, IV drug therapy in the ICU is often complicated by large numbers of concurrent drugs, limited sites of access, fluid restriction, and drug incompatibilities. These factors require critical care practitioners to be knowledgeable about many facets of IV therapy.

The number of IV medications that must be administered simultaneously often exceeds the available number of IV access sites. Consequently, it is essential that the chemical compatibility of agents mixed or infused together be known. In addition, a fluid-restricted patient may require that drugs be mixed in the minimum amount of fluid possible. Manufacturers' package inserts, along with a variety of published references and charts, are available to assist clinicians in determining the compatibility and stability of various drugs.[6] These publications provide useful guidelines but do not cover all possible combinations of specific drugs, their concentrations, routes, or conditions of administration. Pharmacists must be cautious, and generally should avoid mixing drugs together when no compatibility or stability data exist. The absence of visual changes when two drugs are admixed or when a single drug is highly concentrated does not ensure compatibility or stability. An additional consideration is the ability of the infusion device to be used to accurately deliver a highly concentrated solution.

Most IV solutions are administered to critically ill patients through peripheral veins. Central venous administration of agents is used when pharmacologic agents or electrolytes may be damaging to peripheral veins or when peripheral venous access is limited or nonexistent. Vasopressor agents (e.g., norepinephrine, dopamine) should always be administered via a central vein. Peripheral venous administration of these agents is associated with the risk of ischemic necrosis and sloughing of superficial

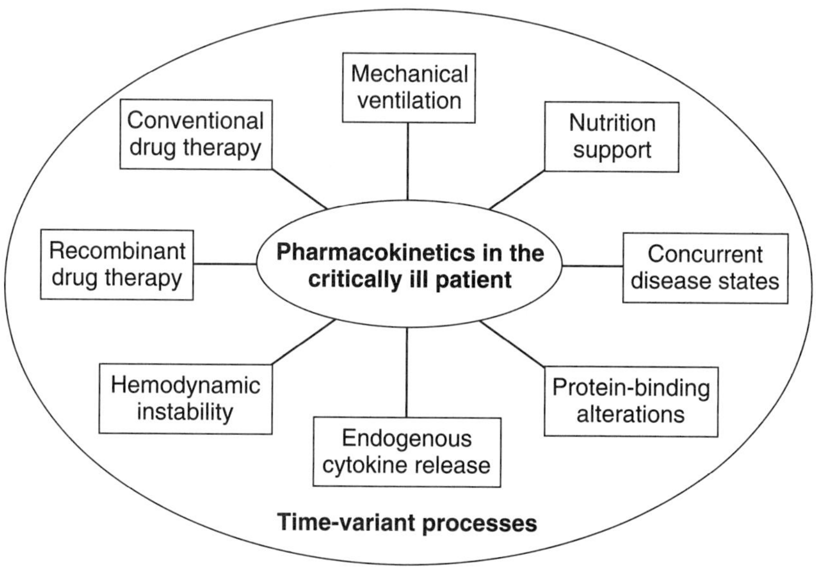

Figure 103.1. Potential factors affecting drug disposition in critically ill patients. The possibility of temporal changes in these factors must also be considered secondary to the dynamic nature of this patient subset.

tissues if extravasation occurs (i.e., infiltration of the catheter and solution out of the vein and into the surrounding tissues). If extravasation occurs, the medication should be discontinued and the tubing disconnected from the catheter. Highly concentrated solutions of certain agents (e.g., potassium chloride) may also be very irritating and damaging to the peripheral vein. A major concern for central venous catheters used for drug administration is the development of infection at the puncture site. This may lead to thrombophlebitis, venous thrombosis, embolism, or septicemia. Meticulous aseptic technique is essential for inserting and caring for the catheter. Other complications of central catheter placement include pneumothorax, systemic infection, arrhythmias (pulmonary artery catheter), pulmonary infarction, and air embolism.

Occasionally, drugs may be administered directly into an artery. The most common indication for this route is for local administration of a drug. For example, thrombolytic agents may be infused through a catheter whose tip is placed near an arterial thrombus. The high pressures encountered in the arterial circulation necessitate administration of such agents via an infusion pump capable of operating under these conditions. A catheter for monitoring arterial blood pressure and obtaining arterial blood gases is often placed in the radial or ulnar artery of critically ill patients. The patency of this catheter, or so called art line, is generally maintained with a slow-flowing heparinized solution.[7] These lines should not be used for drug administration.

Epidural

Epidural administration of narcotics, particularly morphine, fentanyl, sufentanil, alfentanil, and hydromorphone alone or in combination with local anesthetics such as bupivacaine, are very effective for the relief of acute pain.[8] The analgesic agent(s) may be administered by continuous infusion with or without intermittent bolus doses, or intermittent doses alone. Respiratory depression, however, is less common with continuous-infusion regimens. The incidence of pruritus, urinary retention, hypotension, vomiting, and sedation may be higher with this route of narcotic administration. Epidural analgesia is generally contraindicated in patients who have systemic infections, are receiving anticoagulant therapy, or have a coagulopathy. Only preservative-free medications should be administered directly into the epidural space. Epidural doses range from 1 to 10 mg for morphine, 50 to 100 μg for fentanyl, 25 to 50 μg for sufentanil, 0.7 to 1.0 mg for alfentanil, and 0.5 to 3 mg for hydromorphone.

Inhalational

The pulmonary route for local and systemic drug administration is frequently used in critically ill patients. Inhalation of β-adrenergic and muscarinic bronchodilators, corticosteroids, mucolytics, and antibiotics is used to achieve local effects in the lung. These agents, if commercially available, may be administered via metered-dose inhalers (MDIs) or by ultrasonic or jet nebulization. The choice of technique also depends on the ability of the patient to cooperate or assist with treatment. Nebulization treatments are generally more time consuming, require the use of specialized equipment and personnel, and are more expensive.[9] Nebulization treatments and MDIs can also be used in patients who are intubated and mechanically ventilated. When MDIs are used to administer agents through the ventilator circuit, the deposition of drug in the lung is highly variable, depending on whether a spacer is used, the type of spacer, and the length of the endotracheal tube. Lung deposition is generally less than that with spontaneously breathing patients. When using MDIs to administer drugs in mechanically ventilated patients, the normal dose should be doubled.[10] Actuation of the MDI should occur at the beginning of the inspiratory phase. Holding chambers that attach to the ventilatory circuit may increase the amount of aerosol delivered to the lungs. If an in-line holding chamber is used, the inhaler should be actuated 1 to 2 seconds before the mechanical breath.

Systemic administration of selective cardiovascular-acting agents via the endotracheal tube may be performed in emergency situations in which venous access has not yet been established. Agents in which endotracheal administration has proven to be effective include epinephrine, atropine, and lidocaine.[11] When administered by this route, a catheter for drug administration should be advanced beyond the tip of the endotracheal tube. Two to 2.5 times the normal dose should be administered followed by delivery of several quick breaths.[11]

Other Administration Routes

Although the intramuscular, subcutaneous, and oral routes of drug administration are frequently used in the intensive care unit, they cannot be used in every patient. Intramuscular, subcutaneous, and oral routes of administration require adequate blood flow to the site of administration for systemic absorption to occur. In patients with shock, the circulatory system redistributes blood flow away from the skeletal muscle, skin, and gastrointestinal system in order to preserve blood flow to vital organs. Thus both the extent and rate of systemic absorption may be severely affected in such conditions. Additionally, patients with thrombocytopenia, a coagulopathy, or those receiving anticoagulant medications should not receive intramuscular injections due to the increased risk of bleeding and hematoma formation. Many drugs cannot be given intramuscularly due to limited solubility, pH of the solution, or the injection volume. For example, intramuscular phenytoin is extremely painful due to the high pH required to manufacture a soluble formulation. When administering medications orally, the pharmacist should carefully monitor the gastrointestinal function of the patient. Significant changes in the extent or rate of absorption may occur in patients with gastroparesis, ileus, or diarrhea. Knowledge of food-drug interactions is also essential. For example, enteral feeds may significantly reduce the absorption of phenytoin, placing the patient at increased risk for seizure activity.[12]

SPECIAL PROBLEMS IN THE CRITICALLY ILL PATIENT

Central Nervous System

Pain and Anxiety

The most common central nervous system (CNS) problems encountered in critically ill patients are acute pain, anxiety, and agitation. Pain may be a consequence of direct trauma or medical and surgical procedures, or it may accompany underlying medical problems. Anxiety is the psychophysiologic response to the anticipation of real or imagined danger sensed by critically ill patients. Agitation (i.e., excitement accompanied by motor restlessness) may be present secondary to sleep deprivation and unfamiliarity with the ICU environment, in addition to pain. In extreme cases, these untoward feelings can progress to a state of delirium characterized by disorganized thinking, decreased level of consciousness, altered sensory perception, disorientation, or altered psychomotor activity.[13] Withdrawal symptoms in patients with a history of alcoholism are another common problem in critically ill patients, especially trauma victims. In order to minimize suffering and emotional stress in ICU patients, it is imperative that adequate attention be given to pain relief, sedation, and management of anxiety.

In general, the goal of analgesic therapy in these patients is to provide short-term symptomatic pain relief during the period of tissue healing. The tendency to undertreat acute pain has been highlighted in recent years.[14] The most commonly used analgesics for acute pain within the ICU setting are parenteral opiate analgesics, most notably morphine, fentanyl, and hydromorphone.[13] The use of meperidine in this setting is not recommended.[13] In addition to a short duration of action, meperidine also has an active metabolite that can accumulate and result in CNS excitation.[13] Effective analgesic dosage requirements of these agents can vary tremendously, emphasizing the need for individualization of therapy while monitoring closely for adverse effects. *Adverse effect* is a relative term, however, because sedation associated with the use of opiates is often an added benefit in the ICU setting. Alternatives to systemic analgesic therapy include regional nerve blocks and epidural infusions. Advantages of these techniques are decreased risk of respiratory depression, sedation, nausea, and hypomotility of the gastrointestinal tract.[15] Less potent analgesics such as acetaminophen and nonsteroidal anti-inflammatory drugs (e.g., ketorolac) should also be considered as the acute pain being experienced by the critically ill patient begins to subside. In the latter case, ketorolac use should be limited to 5 days or less to minimize adverse effects (e.g., gastrointestinal bleeding, acute renal failure).[16,17] The benzodiazepines, lorazepam, and midazolam are the most commonly used anxiolytics/sedatives in ICU patients. These agents are also considered first-line therapy in the management of alcohol withdrawal.[18] Antihistamines such as diphenhydramine are also used occasionally as a sedative in the ICU.[19] Parenteral haloperidol is the preferred agent used to manage delirium in the critically ill patient because of pharmacologic inhibition of dopaminergic activity in the CNS.[20] Propofol is the newest addition to those agents routinely used for sedation in critically ill patients. It is recommended as an alternative to benzodiazepines for short-term (less than 24 hours) sedation in the critically ill patient.[13] Use of individual treatment goals and objective assessment scales (Table 103.2) is recommended in managing these patients.[21,22] Neuromuscular blocking agents such as pancuronium and vecuronium are important adjunctive agents in agitated patients requiring mechanical ventilation. These agents

Table 103.2 ▪ Sedation and Agitation Scales

Ramsay Scale

Awake levels:
1. Patient anxious and agitated or restless or both
2. Patient cooperative, oriented, and tranquil
3. Patient responds to commands only

Asleep levels, depends on response to a light glabellar tap or loud auditory stimulus:
4. Patient responds briskly
5. Patient responds sluggishly
6. Patient does not respond

Riker Sedation-Agitation Scale

Score	Description	Example
+3	Immediate threat to safety	Pulling at endotracheal tube or catheters, trying to climb over bed rail, striking at staff
+2	Dangerously agitated	Requiring physical restraints and frequent verbal reminding of limits, biting endotracheal tube, thrashing side-to-side
+1	Agitated	Physically agitated, attempting to sit up, calms down to verbal instructions
0	Calm and cooperative	Calm, arousable, follows commands
−1	Oversedated	Difficult to arouse or unable to attend to conversation or commands
−2	Very oversedated	Awakens to noxious stimuli only
−3	Unarousable	Does not awaken to any stimuli

Source: References 21, 22.

should be administered with sedative agents to prevent further anxiety and emotional distress during the paralysis period. The anxiety accompanying paralytic use relates to the feeling of helplessness and fear with loss of voluntary muscle control. Use of peripheral nerve stimulators for monitoring neuromuscular blockers is relatively commonplace in ICUs using continuous paralytic therapy. Specifically, response to either train-of-four or a double-burst muscle twitch on stimulation by the peripheral nerve stimulator is the most frequently employed technique for monitoring neuromuscular blocking drugs. See reference 15 for a more detailed discussion regarding the use of peripheral nerve stimulators. Persistent paralysis after discontinuation is now appreciated as a significant risk associated with the use of neuromuscular blocking agents in ICU patients.[23] Hence, dosages and duration of therapy should be minimized as much as possible, with cessation of the paralytic therapy at least once daily to assess the need for continued paralysis.[24] Table 103.3 summarizes dosing regimens, typical onset of action, and duration of activity for the most commonly used analgesics, sedatives, and paralytics in the ICU setting.

Neurotrauma

In contrast to the symptomatic problems of pain and anxiety frequently encountered in critically ill patients, CNS disorders that may result in ICU admission include traumatic brain injury and spinal cord injury (SCI). Although not all patients with acute neurotrauma are admitted to an ICU, those with the most severe insults typically require supportive care and intensive monitoring. Patients suspected of having a head injury or SCI should undergo a thorough physical and neurologic examination along with computed tomography. The Glasgow Coma Scale (GCS) is the most widely used system to grade the arousal and functional capacity of the cerebral cortex in these patients.[25] A GCS of 3–8, 9–12, and 13–14 is consistent with severe, moderate, and minor head injury, respectively (Table 103.4). The possibility that ethanol or drug intoxication, hypoglycemia, severe electrolyte disturbances, infection, hypoxia, hypotension, or spinal cord injury may alter the initial neurologic examination should always be considered. Thus initial laboratory tests for all patients with suspected neurologic injury should include a urine drug screen, blood ethanol concentration, complete blood count, electrolytes, glucose, blood urea nitrogen, and serum creatinine.

The initial management goal in these patients is to establish an adequate airway and maintain breathing and circulation during the initial period of evaluation (ABCs of resuscitation). Control of increased intracranial pressure (ICP) is also a priority in head injury patients, considering its potential to decrease cerebral blood flow (CBF) and thus cerebral delivery of oxygen (CDO_2). Nonpharmacologic and pharmacologic approaches in managing increased ICP (i.e., greater than 20 mm Hg) include mild hyperventilation ($PaCO_2$ 35 mm HG or greater); elevating the patient's head to 30 degrees; moderate, controlled hypothermia (32° to 34°C); osmotic and loop diuretics; and barbiturate coma in refractory patients.[26] See reference 27 for a more extensive discussion of this topic. In addition to close monitoring of ICP, cerebral perfusion pressure (CPP), which is the difference between MAP and ICP (i.e., CPP = MAP – ICP), should also be monitored.

Table 103.3 ▪ Clinical Use of Selected Analgesics, Sedatives, and Paralytics Commonly Used in Critically Ill Patients

Agent	Dose	Onset of Action	Duration of Activity
Analgesics			
Morphine	2–10 mg q 1–2hr IV	<1 min	4–5 hr
	5–15 mg/hr IV infusion		
	5–10 mg q 4hr IM/SC	10–30 min	4–7 hr
Fentanyl	50–200 μg/hr IV infusion	30 sec	30–60 min
Hydromorphone	0.3–1.5 mg q1–2hr IV	5 min	3–4 hr
	0.45–1.5 mg/hr IV infusion		
Ketorolac	30 mg q 6hr IV	10 min	6 hr
Sedatives			
Lorazepam	1–4 mg q1–4hr IV	5–15 min	4 hr
Midazolam	1–5 mg q 1–2 hr IV	1–5 min	15 min–6 hr
	0.025–0.3 mg/kg/hr IV infusion		
Haloperidol	2–5 mg q 1–4hr IV	1 min	>24 hr
Propofol	1–8 mg/kg/hr IV infusion	<1 min	8–10 min
Skeletal muscle relaxants			
Pancuronium	0.01 mg/kg prn	2–5 min	75–90 min
	0.06–0.1 mg/kg/hr IV	3–6 min	
Vecuronium	0.05–0.1 mg/kg IV prn	3–5 min	25–40 min
	0.1–0.2 mg/kg/hr IV infusion		

Source: References 13, 15, 20, 24.

Table 103.4 ▪ Glasgow Coma Scale

	Response	Score
Eyes		
	Open spontaneously	4
	To verbal command	3
	To pain	2
	No response	1
Best Motor Response		
To verbal command	Obeys	6
To painful stimulus (pressure to nailbeds)	Localizes pain	5
	Flexion-withdrawal	4
	Flexion-abnormal (decorticate rigidity)	3
	Extension (decerebrate rigidity)	2
	No response	1
Best Verbal Response		
(Arouse patient with painful stimulus if necessary)	Oriented and converses	5
	Disoriented and converses	4
	Inappropriate words	3
	Incomprehensible sounds	2
	No response	1
	Total	3–15

Source: Reference 25.

The CPP is essentially the pressure gradient driving CBF. It is recommended that the CCP be maintained greater than 70 mm Hg in patients with severe head injury.[26]

Neurotrauma patients should generally be kept euvolemic, with systemic blood pressure maintained in a normotensive range in an attempt to sustain CBF without exacerbating elevations in ICP. Patients with systemic hypertension should receive α-blockers, β-blockers, or angiotensin converting enzyme inhibitors because they do not typically affect ICP. Use of sedatives (e.g., benzodiazepines, barbiturates) and opiate analgesics may also be effective in lowering transiently increased blood pressure. Use of the venodilators, nitroprusside and nitroglycerin, and selected calcium channel blockers (e.g., nicardipine, diltiazem) should be avoided because they may have the undesirable effect of increasing cerebral blood volume, thereby increasing ICP.

By maintaining ventilation and CDO_2, further cerebral ischemia may be prevented or attenuated. This is of utmost importance because ischemia is thought to trigger extension of the primary insult into uninjured tissue (i.e., secondary neuronal injury) following acute head injury and SCI. In essence, cerebral ischemia results in cellular hypoxia and loss of cell membrane integrity. This in turn can lead to major intracellular and extracellular ionic shifts, resulting in cytotoxic edema (with or without concurrent increased intracranial pressure), intracellular acidosis, electrical failure, and eventual generation of reactive oxygen species (e.g., oxygen free radicals). The importance of understanding the pathophysiology of secondary neuronal injury is readily apparent in light of the many promising pharmacologic strategies available or under investigation that attempt to modulate this destructive cascade of events. These strategies include calcium channel blockers, glutamate antagonists, opiate antagonists, and nonsteroidal anti-inflammatory drugs.[28]

Despite several unsuccessful attempts at attenuating secondary neuronal injury, the results of two landmark investigations provide optimism for further breakthroughs in this arena. The first investigation was the second National Acute Spinal Cord Injury Study (NASCIS 2).[29] In this multicenter study, SCI patients randomized to receive methylprednisolone 30 mg/kg IV over 15 minutes followed by a 5.4 mg/kg/hr infusion for 23 hours had a significant increase in motor and sensory function at 6 weeks and 6 months compared to placebo patients in those patients receiving therapy within *8 hours* after injury. Thus *all* future SCI patients should receive methylprednisolone within this 8-hour treatment window because there is no alternative therapy of proven benefit at present to offer these patients. Results of the follow-up trial referred to as NASCIS 3 corroborated the findings of NASCIS 2 and suggested that patients receiving therapy between 3 and 8 hours after injury have improved outcomes when treated with methylprednisolone for 48 hours versus 24 hours (i.e., 5.4 mg/kg/hr).[30] Unfortunately, patients receiving the longer duration of therapy also had more severe sepsis and pneumonia compared with those receiving 24 hours of methylprednisolone.[30]

Seizure Treatment and Prophylaxis

Seizures are caused by variety of conditions in ICU patients, including mechanical brain injury, cerebral hypoxia/ischemia, CNS infections, metabolic disorders, and chronic alcohol abuse.[31] Of these conditions, seizures in patients with moderate to severe head injury are of particular concern because the seizure activity can greatly increase cerebral metabolism. Thus head injury patients experiencing one or more seizures should receive initial therapy consisting of incremental IV doses of diazepam (5 to 40 mg) or lorazepam (2 to 8 mg) to terminate any active seizure activity, followed by IV phenytoin or fosphenytoin to prevent seizure recurrence. In addition, prophylactic phenytoin or fosphenytoin should be considered in patients with mild to moderate injury based on a landmark study by Temkin and colleagues in 1990.[32] Data from this study do not support the use of phenytoin beyond 7 days unless seizures are observed. Aggressive phenytoin therapy is recommended during the treatment period to maintain total concentrations in the range of 40 to 80 mmol/L (10 to 20 mg/L). This can generally be achieved using an adult IV loading dose of 18 to 20 mg/kg followed by an initial adult daily maintenance dose of

2.5 to 3.0 mg/kg every 12 hours. The potential for phenytoin's metabolism to increase as a function of time should also be considered in these patients. See Chapter 52 for a thorough discussion of managing non–trauma related seizures. The treatment of status epilepticus was reviewed by Lowenstein and Alldredge.[33]

Pulmonary System

Mechanical Ventilation

A high percentage of critically ill patients are mechanically ventilated for all or a portion of their intensive care unit stay. The objectives of mechanical ventilation (MV) include improvement of pulmonary gas exchange, relief of respiratory distress, alteration of pressure-volume relationships (e.g., atelectasis, decreased compliance), and allowance of lung and airway healing. Basic MV settings include the fraction of inspired oxygen (FiO_2) (i.e., the percent of oxygen contained in the inhaled gas), tidal volume (usually 5 to 15 mL/kg), and ventilation rate. Because of the toxic effects of oxygen to the lung, the lowest FiO_2 that will achieve satisfactory arterial oxygenation (arterial oxygen pressure [PaO_2] exceeding 60 mm Hg or arterial hemoglobin saturation [SaO_2] exceeding 90%) is used. PEEP is often used to prevent alveolar collapse at the end of expiration. The principal therapeutic effect of PEEP is to improve or maintain PaO_2 or SaO_2 while allowing a decrease in FiO_2. Mechanical ventilation, particularly when high levels of PEEP are used, may lower cardiac output. Increased transmural pressure causes a decrease in ventricular distensibility and increases in peripheral vascular resistance. Consequently, cardiac output is decreased secondary to decreased venous return and impaired contractility. See recent review articles for a more thorough discussion of MV therapy.[34]

Several important factors and variables should be considered and monitored by pharmacists caring for patients who receive MV (Table 103.5). Nosocomial pneumonia is a common complication of MV, occurring in approximately 30% of patients. Nosocomial pneumonia in these patients is associated with a greater than twofold risk of death.[35] If signs and symptoms of pneumonia appear, empiric antibiotic treatment aimed at the most likely pathogens (e.g., *Pseudomonas aeruginosa, Enterobacteriaceae*) should be promptly initiated. Infectious sinusitis also occurs frequently in mechanically ventilated patients, particularly those patients who have nasotracheal or nasogastric tubes.[36] The presence of infectious sinusitis also increases the likelihood of developing nosocomial pneumonia. Infectious sinusitis is most commonly caused by Gram-negative bacteria followed by Gram-positive bacteria and yeast. Other studies have suggested that MV may be an independent risk factor for the development of stress ulcers in critically ill patients.[37] Mechanical ventilation can also be an uncomfortable and frightening experience. Although use of proper ventilatory settings and reassurance of the patient are the primary treatments for distress and agitation, analgesics, sedatives, and neuromuscular blocking agents are also frequently used for patient comfort and optimal delivery of ventilation. Finally, MV can have significant hemodynamic effects, particularly decreased cardiac output and hypotension. These effects are a result of increased intrathoracic pressure generated by positive pressure breathing.

Table 103.5 ▪ Mechanical Ventilation Complications

Cardiovascular
• Hypotension • Decreased cardiac output • Decreased renal blood flow • Decreased hepatic blood flow • Decreased cerebral blood flow
Respiratory
• Pneumonia • Sinusitis • Pneumothorax
Gastrointestinal
• Ileus • Gastrointestinal distension • Stress ulceration/gastrointestinal hemorrhage

When weaning the patient from MV, a number of other factors should be considered to improve the patient's likelihood for successful extubation. These include adequate nutrition supplementation and correction of electrolyte disturbances, especially hypophosphatemia, which could impair oxygen delivery and respiratory muscle function.[38] Sedatives and narcotic analgesics should be used sparingly if at all when trying to wean patients from the ventilator. Optimization of bronchodilator therapy in patients with underlying obstructive or bronchospastic pulmonary disease may also aid in successful extubation of patients.

Acute Respiratory Distress Syndrome

The acute (formerly adult) respiratory distress syndrome (ARDS) is a condition involving impaired oxygenation associated with bilateral pulmonary infiltrates on frontal chest radiograph and a pulmonary artery capillary wedge pressure (PCWP) of 18 mm Hg or less. Injury is characterized by diffuse alveolar damage, increased vascular permeability, and the development of noncardiogenic pulmonary edema. When damage is severe, the air spaces fill with fluid, resulting in deterioration in gas exchange and mechanical properties of the lung.[39] ARDS may result from direct lung injury such aspiration of gastric contents or inhalation of toxins, or indirectly from conditions such as bacterial sepsis or pancreatitis. The mortality rate associated with ARDS approaches 50%, with most patients dying from the underlying predisposing illness, severe sepsis, or multiple organ dysfunction syndrome (MODS). The current clinical management of ARDS involves primarily supportive measures aimed at maintaining gas exchange and oxygen delivery. No specific measures currently exist to correct the abnormalities associated with ARDS. Mechanical ventilation with PEEP is typically required for at least 10 to 14 days in most patients. Extracorporeal membrane oxygenation (ECMO) may be used when ventilation is ineffective in providing adequate blood oxygenation. Fluid management is also important because intravascular hydrostatic pressures may contribute to pulmonary edema. Therapy should be aimed at achieving the lowest PCWP while maintaining an adequate CO. If sepsis is presumed to be the cause of ARDS, empiric antibiotic therapy should be instituted early. The use of high-dose corticosteroids is controversial and probably should not be used early in treatment unless a significant number of eosinophils are found in the blood or bronchoalveolar lavage fluid. Evidence suggests that a trial of methylprednisolone, 2 mg/kg/day for 32 days, beginning 1 to 2 weeks following the onset of ARDS in patients with severe disease may attenuate the fibroproliferative phase of the disorder.[40] A variety of other anti-inflammatory and vasodilatory agents have been investigated. These include cyclooxygenase inhibitors, proinflammatory cytokine inhibitors, pentoxifylline, prostaglandins E_1 and E_2, antioxidants, antiproteases, inhaled nitric oxide, and surfactant replacement therapy.[41] Unfortunately, none of these promising strategies has been demonstrated to conclusively alter the clinical course of ARDS.

Cardiovascular System

Principles of Oxygen Delivery and Consumption

The primary goal of life-support techniques used in modern critical care units is to achieve and maintain optimal tissue oxygenation. Although traditional hemodynamic monitoring of pressures and flow is important for providing measures of tissue perfusion, this monitoring does not allow assessment of oxygenation. Earlier studies have shown that oxygen transport monitoring is superior to hemodynamic monitoring alone, particularly in high-risk, critically ill patients.[42,43] However, interventions designed to achieve supraphysiologic indices (cardiac index, oxygen delivery, oxygen consumption) are not universal, secondary to equivocal evidence of efficacy[44] and possibly increased mortality rates.[45] A recent meta-analysis suggested that significantly decreased mortality rates may only occur in those who achieve supraphysiologic goals preoperatively or preventively.[46] Nonetheless, ensuring adequate tissue oxygenation is still the cornerstone of medical therapy in the critically ill patient.

Oxygen demand is dependent on the overall rate of tissue metabolism rate and the intrinsic ability of tissues to extract oxygen. Generally, little can be done to alter oxygen demand. However, interventions aimed at reducing metabolic rate such as lowering body temperature, skeletal muscle paralysis, or sedation may modestly lower overall oxygen demand. Hence, most interventions are directed at improving the transportation of oxygen to tissues. The delivery of oxygen (DO_2) to tissues is the product of cardiac index (CI) and arterial oxygen content (CaO_2). The actual amount of oxygen consumed at the tissue level (VO_2) may be calculated as the product of CI and the difference between CaO_2 and mixed venous oxygen content (CvO_2). Arterial and venous oxygen content are dependent on the hemoglobin concentration, the percent oxygen saturation of arterial or mixed venous hemoglobin (SaO_2 or SvO_2) and, to a minor extent, the amount of oxygen dissolved in plasma. The percentage of oxygen extracted by the tissues (O_2 ER) is calculated as $(CaO_2 - CvO_2)/CaO_2$. Oxygen transport variables, their calculation, and normal values are listed in Table 103.6. In

Table 103.6 ▪ Oxygen Transport Variables, Normal and Goal Values

Parameter	Abbreviation	Calculation	Normal Value	Goal
Arterial Hgb saturation	SaO_2	Measured	95–99	>95
Mixed venous oxygen saturation	SvO_2	Measured[a]	65–75%	>60
Arterial oxygen content	CaO_2	$(Hgb \times SaO_2 \times 1.34^b) + (PaO_2 \times 0.0031^c)$	17–20 mL O_2/dL	
Venous oxygen content	CvO_2	$(Hgb \times SvO_2 \times 1.34) + (PvO_2 \times 0.0031)$	12–15 mL O_2/dL	
Oxygen delivery	DO_2	$CI \times CaO_2 \times 10$	529–720 mL/min/m^2	>550
Oxygen consumption	VO_2	$(CaO_2 - CvO_2) \times CI \times 10$	100–150 mL/min/m^2	>167
Oxygen extraction ratio	O_2 ER	$(CaO_2 - CvO_2)/CaO_2$	22–30%	<31

CI, cardiac index (L/min/m^2); *Hgb*, hemoglobin (g/dL); *PaO_2*, arterial pressure of oxygen in blood (mm Hg); *PvO_2*, venous pressure of oxygen in blood (mm Hg).

[a]Obtained from pulmonary artery blood.

[b]Milliliters of O_2/1 g Hgb.

[c]Solubility coefficient of O_2 in plasma.

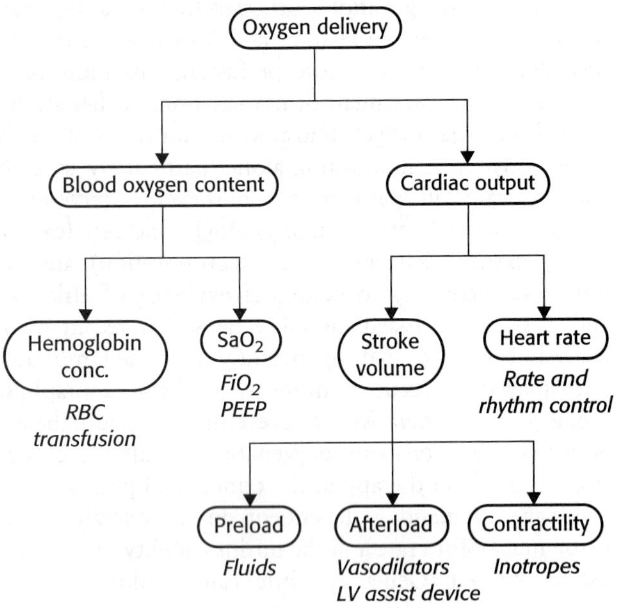

Figure 103.2. Factors influencing oxygen delivery to tissues. Means of altering each factor for improved oxygen delivery are provided in *italics*.

addition to SaO_2, SvO_2, CaO_2, CvO_2, DO_2, and VO_2, other clinical and laboratory parameters commonly used to monitor the adequacy of tissue oxygenation include arterial pH, total CO_2 content, lactic acid levels, blood pressure, heart rate, temperature, respiratory rate, urine output, and mental status.

In order to improve tissue oxygenation, oxygen delivery may be increased by altering CI, CaO_2, or both. One approach to improving tissue oxygenation is outlined in Figure 103.2. Patients who are anemic, and subsequently have a low hemoglobin concentration, may benefit from transfusion of red blood cells. Commonly used methods to improve SaO_2 include increases in FiO_2 and PEEP. Improvements in CO can be achieved by ensuring appropriate heart rate and stroke volume. Stroke volume is dependent on preload, afterload, and contractility. Pharmacologic therapies aimed at correcting these hemodynamic variables are addressed in other chapters of this textbook and include the use of fluids, vasodilators (e.g., nitroprusside), inotropes (e.g., dobutamine), and antiarrhythmics (including atropine, beta blockers, and digoxin). The maneuver that yields the greatest improvement in DO_2 as determined by calculating its effect on oxygen transport variables is generally the one that should be used. This is usually determined by assessing the clinical status of the patient in conjunction with hemodynamic measurements obtained from the pulmonary artery catheter. For instance, the volume status of the patient is estimated by analyzing the left-ventricular end-diastolic pressure (LVEDP). Unfortunately, many factors, particularly increasing PEEP, can significantly affect the accuracy of correlating LVEDP with left-ventricular end-diastolic volume. Recently, right-ventricular end-diastolic volume has proven to be a more reliable indicator of volume status than LVEDP.[47] Thus DO_2 may be more reliably optimized by assessing right rather than left ventricular function.

The drawback of oxygen transport monitoring as described is that it provides only an indication of global tissue oxygenation and may not detect regional or organ-specific mismatching of oxygen delivery and utilization. Tissue-specific markers of oxygen utilization such as gastric intramucosal pH have recently been developed and increasingly are being used to obtain evidence of regional adequacy of tissue oxygenation.[48]

Acute Myocardial Infarction

The medical management of uncomplicated acute myocardial infarction (AMI) is well established (see Chapter 43) as outlined in recently published practice guidelines.[49] In the absence of contraindications, treatment with thrombolytics and aspirin should be initiated within 30 minutes of patient presentation to the hospital. To achieve the greatest benefit, thrombolytics should be administered within 12 hours from the onset of symptoms. Intravenous or SC heparin should be initiated during alteplase therapy and immediately following streptokinase therapy. In those patients not receiving thrombolytic therapy, standard heparin or low-molecular-weight heparin should be initiated. Intravenous β-adrenergic blocking agents should be administered as early as possible in the course of therapy (i.e., within 12 hours), as should nitroglycerin. Chronic therapy with β-adrenergic blocking agents is also indicated unless the patient is at low risk for reinfarction. Oral angiotensin converting enzyme inhibitors are indicated in patients with anterior myocardial infarctions, particularly those with ejection fractions below 40%. Therapy should be initiated within 24 hours after the infarction and continued indefinitely to reduce left ventricular remodeling and development of congestive heart failure. In those patients without ST-segment elevation or an ejection fraction greater than 40%, therapy should be continued for at least 6 weeks. Additional consideration should be given as to providing adequate analgesia and correcting electrolyte disorders, particularly magnesium, because it may have cardioprotective effects. The role of glycoprotein IIb/IIIa receptor inhibitors, such as abciximab and tirofiban, can also be used in the treatment in AMI.

Cardiogenic Shock

Cardiogenic shock can occur as a complication of AMI in 6 to 20% of survivors. However, the incidence and related mortality of cardiogenic shock after an AMI is decreasing because of advances in medical and invasive therapy. A variety of other conditions such as acute myocarditis, sustained arrhythmia, and decompensation in patients with end-stage heart failure may also result in cardiogenic shock. Clinically, cardiogenic shock is defined as reduced cardiac index (less than 2.2 $L/min/m^2$) and evidence of tissue hypoxia (i.e., O_2 ER greater than 31%, oliguria, cyanosis, cool extremities, altered mentation) in the presence of adequate intravascular volume.

Specific treatment of cardiogenic shock is preceded by correcting problems of hypoxia, electrolyte abnormalities, acidosis, and restoring sinus rhythm.[50] Restoration of adequate DO_2 to tissues occurs primarily through improving myocardial systolic function (Fig. 103.2). Inotropic agents such as dobutamine, amrinone, milrinone, and vasodilators such as sodium nitroprusside work to improve forward blood flow and reduce pulmonary edema. Dobutamine is preferred to dopamine and norepinephrine in cardiogenic shock; however, the latter two agents are useful in patients who are profoundly hypotensive. The phosphodiesterase inhibitors, amrinone and milrinone, have both positive inotropic activity and vasodilatory action. The phosphodiesterase inhibitors can be used in conjunction with or substituted for dobutamine in cardiogenic shock because their mechanisms of action are different and thus additive. Sodium nitroprusside is particularly useful in reducing systemic vascular resistance (afterload), improving CI, and reducing myocardial VO_2. Sodium nitroprusside and nitroglycerin also lower left ventricular filling pressures (preload), which helps reduce oxygen consumption. These agents may also improve DO_2 by reducing pulmonary edema, improving gas exchange, and subsequently increasing blood oxygen content. Intra-aortic balloon counterpulsation, which increases diastolic coronary filling and decreases afterload, is used in cardiogenic shock, especially in patients with high systemic vascular resistance but low blood pressures (i.e., systolic less than 90 mm Hg.).

Cardiogenic shock secondary to right ventricular failure occurs less frequently and is a challenge to manage. Adequate filling pressures must be maintained because these patients are particularly sensitive to volume depletion. Dobutamine is used to increase right ventricular contractility and reduce pulmonary vascular resistance.

Acute Cardiac Arrhythmias

Ventricular and supraventricular cardiac arrhythmias are frequently encountered in critically ill patients. The specific management of acute cardiac arrhythmias is covered in Chapter 41. When cardiac arrhythmias occur in critically ill patients, they are often precipitated by some other event or abnormality. Correctable causes of cardiac arrhythmias such as electrolyte abnormalities, hypoxia, acid-base disturbances, and drug toxicity should always be assessed and managed if present. Pharmacologic management of cardiac arrhythmias can generally be discontinued once the underlying abnormality is corrected or the precipitating factor removed. If the arrhythmia persists, the goals of therapy are to control the ventricular rate (atrial arrhythmias), convert to sinus rhythm, maintain sinus rhythm, and prevent complications (e.g. ischemic stroke).

Hypertensive Emergencies and Urgencies

Hypertensive crisis is a term used to refer to hypertensive emergencies and hypertensive urgencies. A hypertensive emergency is severe hypertension (i.e., systolic blood pressure 180 mm Hg or greater, diastolic blood pressure 110 mm Hg or greater) associated with symptoms of end-organ damage. Included in this definition are patients with hypertension associated with complications such as acute congestive heart failure, AMI, unstable angina, hypertensive encephalopathy, intracranial hemorrhage, dissecting aortic aneurysm, or eclampsia. These patients should be hospitalized with immediate lowering of their blood pressure. The initial goal of therapy is to reduce MAP by no more than 25% (within minutes to 2 hours) and then toward 160/100 mm Hg within 2 to 6 hours.[51]

Hypertensive urgency is a term used to describe asymptomatic patients with severe hypertension where lowering of the blood pressure over a period of hours is desirable. Examples include patients with optic disc edema, progressive target organ complications, and severe perioperative hypertension.[51]

A variety of IV medications are available to treat hypertensive emergencies and urgencies. Sodium nitroprusside and labetalol have proven to be especially effective and safe for lowering blood pressure in these situations. Alternative agents include nicardipine and fenoldopam.[51] Use of the once popular maneuver of administering sublingual nifedipine should be avoided, due to serious adverse effects associated with its use and the inability to effectively control the fall in blood pressure. When hypertension is complicated by dissecting aortic aneurysm, sodium nitroprusside should be avoided and IV β-adrenergic blockers (esmolol), calcium antagonists (verapamil or diltiazem), or trimethaphan camsylate used. Oral medications agents used to treat hypertensive urgencies include loop diuretics, angiotensin converting enzyme inhibitors, α_2-agonists, and calcium channel blockers.[51]

Renal System

Acute renal failure (ARF), defined as an abrupt decrease in the glomerular filtration rate (GFR), is a relatively common problem observed in critically ill patients. This is not surprising considering that shock, sepsis, and trauma are among the leading causes of ARF.[52] A smaller number of patients have exacerbation of their chronic renal failure (CRF) as the problem precipitating ICU admission or as a concurrent disease state accompanying an independent acute problem. Regardless of the circumstances, it is essential that the critical care practitioner be aware of the potential for renal insufficiency to be present or to develop in ICU patients and be adept at evaluating their level of renal impairment. In essence, not only may specific treatment be warranted for reversing the ARF or managing the complications of CRF, but major adjustments in drug-dosing regimens and fluid and electrolyte management may be necessary. In addition, because critically ill patients are particularly susceptible to developing ARF, drugs that may induce renal failure should be identified and used cautiously. The most noteworthy of these agents are the aminoglycosides, amphotericin B, radiocontrast dye, cyclosporine, and nonsteroidal anti-inflammatory drugs (e.g., ketorolac).

Key laboratory tests and monitoring parameters in patients diagnosed or suspected of having acute renal insufficiency include serum creatinine, blood urea nitrogen, urine sodium, urine osmolality, urinalysis, urine creatinine, serum electrolytes, and urine output. After ruling out prerenal causes of ARF (e.g., dehydration, hemorrhage) and urinary obstruction, the primary goal of therapy should be to increase urinary output in oliguric patients, because nonoliguric patients have fewer complications and improved survival.[53] Drugs used for this purpose include mannitol 12.5 to 25 g IV repeated in 1 hour if no response, furosemide 100 mg IV followed by 240 mg IV in 1 hour if no response, and low-dose dopamine 1 to 5 μg/kg/min IV.[54] Despite ongoing use of these agents, clinical trials of diuretics in the treatment of ARF have failed to demonstrate improvements in mortality rates.[55] Restriction of fluids, dietary protein, and electrolytes, especially potassium, magnesium, and phosphorus, is also important in oliguric patients to maintain homeostasis. Treating the underlying cause of ARF, such as the use of antibiotics for infected patients and discontinuation of nephrotoxic drugs when feasible, is an additional consideration. General guidelines for dosage adjustments for renally eliminated drugs and active drug metabolites, including reference tables, can be found in reference texts.[56] A caveat to consider in applying these guidelines is that most equations used to estimate creatinine clearance (e.g., Cockroft and Gault) assume that the serum creatinine is at steady state. However, in patients with ARF, serum creatinine may be rising rapidly. Thus either special formulas that take this problem into account must be used,[57] or an acknowledgment must be made that the estimates obtained using the conventional formulas may be significantly overestimating the creatinine clearance.

In contrast to the diagnosis of ARF, the presence of CRF can usually be identified from the patient's history. When possible and appropriate, medications that the patient was receiving before admission should be continued as previously prescribed. Dosage adjustments for newly instituted medications should be made in a manner similar to adjustments in ARF patients, although in this instance, the problem of rapidly changing serum creatinine values is usually irrelevant. In both ARF and CRF patients, renal replacement therapy (i.e., hemodialysis, peritoneal dialysis, continuous arteriovenous hemodialysis) may be needed to maintain a homeostatic state. The effects of intermittent hemodialysis and continuous renal replacement therapies on drug dosing regimens and fluid and electrolyte supplementation is another important area for the critical care practitioner to understand in order to optimize care in these patients. A thorough discussion of this topic can be found in Chapter 23.

Gastrointestinal System

Colonization of the Gastrointestinal Tract and Nosocomial Infections

It has been recognized since the early 1970s that critically ill patients are at risk to develop superficial gastroduodenal lesions that can result in major gastric bleeding if untreated. Major risk factors for developing stress-induced gastrointestinal bleeding are presence of a coagulopathy and respiratory failure for greater than 48 hours.[37] A thorough discussion of the pathophysiology and treatment alternatives can be found in Chapter 24. Because of the significant morbidity and mortality associated with major gastric hemorrhage, critically ill patients typically receive stress ulcer prophylaxis consisting of one of the following agents: antacids, H_2-antagonists, or sucralfate. In the late 1980s, however, the practice of arbitrarily choosing among these equally efficacious alternatives was called into question by a study by Driks and colleagues.[58] They concluded that drugs raising the gastric pH (i.e., antacids and H_2-antagonists) were associated with a higher incidence of nosocomial pneumonia than sucralfate, a drug demonstrated to be effective for this indication without affecting gastric pH.[58] The explanation most frequently offered for this phenomenon is that when the gastric pH is raised, colonization of the stomach with Gram-negative bacteria will occur, with subsequent retrograde migration of the bacteria to the lungs. Since that time, numerous other studies have been conducted to settle the ensuing controversy. Although meta-analyses of these studies have reached varying conclusions, the evidence generally suggests a higher incidence of associated nosocomial pneumonia with antacids and H_2-antagonists compared to sucralfate.[37,59–61] In addition, sucralfate may also be the most cost-effective alternative.[62] Nonetheless, both H_2-antagonists and sucralfate continue to be used extensively in critically ill patients for the prophylaxis of stress ulcers. More recently, this practice has also been questioned by some investigators arguing that many, if not the majority, of patients receive no benefit from these drugs.[37] More studies are needed in specific ICU patient subsets to discern which critically ill patients are at greatest risk for major gastrointestinal bleeding before the practice of no treatment can be advocated.

Liver Dysfunction

Liver dysfunction is a relatively common finding in critically ill patients. Some patients may have a history of severe chronic liver disease (e.g., alcoholic cirrhosis), whereas others may develop acute hepatic dysfunction secondary to direct trauma, infectious hepatitis, or following an ischemic insult (e.g., hemorrhagic shock). From a therapeutic standpoint, one of the most important considerations in evaluating these patients is the potential for alterations in drug metabolism. Alterations in the synthetic functions of the liver can also affect drug dosing and monitoring in these patients. For example, protein binding can be dramatically decreased for acidic, highly protein-bound drugs secondary to hypoalbuminemia. Hyperbilirubinemia can result in protein-binding displacement as well. The pharmacodynamic profile of certain drugs such as anticoagulants may also be altered secondary to diminished clotting factor production and an increased sensitivity to CNS-active drugs.

Acknowledging the potential for pharmacokinetic and pharmacodynamic alterations in critically ill patients with suspected liver disease, several challenges face critical care practitioners in designing therapeutic drug regimens for an individual patient. One issue is that few, if any, hepatic processes are performed at 100% capacity. Therefore, even though liver dysfunction may be present, the effects of this impairment on drug metabolism may be insignificant. The liver also has reparative properties allowing function to return after an acute insult. Finally, unlike creatinine clearance, which is a good estimate of the glomerular filtration rate in patients with renal dysfunction, no analogous predictor of hepatic function is available for clinical use in patients with liver disease. Laboratory tests that are useful in identifying liver disease but not necessarily the extent of damage are: serum albumin, prothrombin time, bilirubin, and the liver enzymes, aspartate aminotransferase (AST), alanine aminotransferase (ALT), and alkaline phosphatase.[63] Thus careful attention to signs and symptoms of severe liver impairment (e.g., hepatic encephalopathy, hepatomegaly, splenomegaly), in conjunction with these laboratory tests, remains the most viable approach for assessing the level of residual hepatic function in a given patient. After making this assessment, tables summarizing the pharmacokinetic literature relative to the normal disposition pathway for a particular drug or citing specific clinical drug trial findings from patients with liver disease can be used as general guides for drug usage in those individuals deemed to have significant impairment.[63] The possibility of induction or inhibition of hepatic enzymatic function is yet another consideration in these patients. The use of potentially hepatotoxic drugs should also be carefully evaluated in those critically ill patients with evidence of hepatic dysfunction to avoid exacerbation of the condition.

Hematologic System

Coagulation and hematologic disorders are common in the ICU population. Routine laboratory monitoring should include a daily complete blood count with platelets, activated partial thromboplastin time (APTT), and prothrombin time (PT). Commonly encountered hematologic problems include anemia, thrombocytopenia, and neutropenia. The recognition of anemia and its treatment is covered Chapters 13 and 14. In the critical care setting, it is imperative that an adequate hematocrit and hemoglobin be maintained to ensure adequate tissue oxygenation. Transfusion of red blood cells in the form of whole blood or packed red blood cells may be necessary to maintain sufficient oxygen-carrying capacity.

Platelet Disorders

Thrombocytopenia is perhaps one of the most commonly encountered hematologic abnormalities in critically ill patients. As discussed in Chapter 14, a variety of factors may be responsible for the reduction in platelets seen in this population. Heparin-induced thrombocytopenia should be considered, particularly if platelet counts begin to fall precipitously following several days of therapy. If suspected, heparin administration should be discontinued and removed from all flush solutions (e.g., arterial and pulmonary artery catheters). Low-molecular-weight heparins and lepirudin may be alternatives in patients suffering from thrombocytopenia due to unfractionated heparin products.[64] Thrombocytopenia, secondary to sequestration, may also occur during extracorporeal circulation with procedures such as cardiopulmonary bypass or charcoal hemoperfusion.

Platelet dysfunction (secondary to drugs and organ abnormalities such as renal failure), splenomegaly, and cirrhosis are also encountered in the critically ill. Prolonged bleeding times caused by renal failure have empirically been treated with conjugated estrogens 0.6 mg/kg/day and IV desmopressin at a dose of 0.3 μg/kg. Cirrhosis-induced platelet dysfunction has also been treated with desmopressin.[65]

Disseminated Intravascular Coagulopathy

Disseminated intravascular coagulopathy (DIC), as discussed in Chapter 15, is a common occurrence in critically ill patients, especially those with viral, fungal, or bacterial sepsis, severe tissue injury or ischemia, and ARDS. Microvascular thrombosis associated with DIC may lead to further end-organ damage, including focal skin necrosis, ARF, seizures, and stroke. The management of DIC includes the treatment of the underlying disease while providing supportive measures to maintain circulation and oxygenation. Transfusion of blood products and coagulation factors is frequently administered in patients who demonstrate clinical manifestations of DIC.

Deep Venous Thrombosis

Critically ill patients, particularly those suffering major trauma, are at significant risk for the development of deep venous thrombosis (DVT) and the catastrophic occurrence of pulmonary embolism.[66] Risk factors for the development of DVT include tissue injury secondary to trauma and surgery, immobilization, venous stasis, and cardiac dysfunction. Unless specific contraindications exist, all critically ill patients should receive DVT prophylaxis. Prophylaxis generally consists of SC heparin 5000 to 10,000 U every 8 to 12 hours. Compression stockings and intermittent compression boots are alternatives for DVT prophylaxis in patients with contraindications to heparin treatment.

Fluid and Electrolyte Disturbances

The homeostatic mechanisms that maintain normal electrolyte concentrations are often impaired in critically ill patients. In many instances, these abnormalities are a direct result of the patient's primary illness (e.g., hyperkalemia with diabetic ketoacidosis), whereas in others the disturbance may be the result of secondary disorders or a consequence of therapy (e.g., diuretics). Proper correction of the electrolyte disorder is dependent on identification of its cause, estimation of the degree of abnormality, and selection of the appropriate replacement source. Electrolyte abnormalities most commonly observed in critically ill patients include hypokalemia, hypophosphatemia, hypomagnesemia, hypocalcemia, and hyperkalemia. The etiology and manifestations of these electrolyte disorders and their treatment are discussed in Chapter 9.

Nutritional Support

Appropriate nutritional support enhances immune function, reduces length of ICU stay, and increases survival. Nutritional support of hospitalized patients is covered in Chapter 12. Enteral nutrition, particularly when administered distal to the pylorus, can be initiated early in most critically ill patients and should be considered as first-line therapy for those requiring nutritional support. Advantages of enteral nutrition in this population include a decreased rate of complications and mortality, lower cost, improved gastrointestinal protection, and a lower infectious risk profile. The latter advantages may largely be explained by attenuation of bacterial translocation from the gut by maintaining function integrity of the gastrointestinal tract with enteral nutrition.

The selection of the specific route and formulation of the nutritional product depends on the goals of nutritional support, caloric requirements, and the specific nutrients to be delivered. The determination and administration of caloric needs is paramount in critically ill patients. Underfeeding may result in impaired host defenses, delayed wound healing, muscle wasting, and prolonged weaning from MV. Overfeeding is associated with hepatic dysfunction, elevated blood urea nitrogen, hyperglycemia, fluid overload, and excessive carbon dioxide production. The commonly used Harris-Benedict equation is often inaccurate in critically ill patients, resulting in both underprediction and overprediction of caloric needs. The measurement of resting energy expenditure by indirect calorimetry can be performed accurately in many critically ill patients and allows individualization of nutritional support. The use of a metabolic cart to measure resting energy expenditure may be particularly valuable in patients with multiple risk and stress factors that may make estimates by the Harris-Benedict equation highly inaccurate. Patients who fail to respond adequately to estimated nutritional needs may also benefit from the use of indirect calorimetry.

SIRS, CARS, and MODS

During periods of acute stress induced by sepsis, trauma, pancreatitis, and so on, critically ill patients undergo a number of metabolic changes secondary to activation of the sympathetic nervous system and the hypothalamic-pituitary-adrenal axis. Specific mediators involved in the acute-phase response include epinephrine, norepinephrine, cortisol, glucagon, pro-inflammatory cytokines such as IL-1, IL-2 , IL-6, IL-8 , and TNF.[67] The effect of this response is generally an acceleration of whole body metabolism proportional to the intensity of the initiating event or injury.[68] This can manifest itself as depletion of body stores of protein, fat, and carbohydrates or defects in intracellular energy metabolism that can ultimately contribute significantly to major organ dysfunction (e.g., lungs, heart, kidneys, gastrointestinal tract, CNS). Balancing the acute-phase response is an anti-inflammatory response mediated by substances such as IL-4, IL-10, IL-11, and IL-13, colony-stimulating factors, and soluble receptors to the pro-inflammatory mediators such as TNF and IL-1.[69] If the pro-inflammatory and anti-inflammatory mediators are balanced, homeostasis can be restored. When pro-inflammatory mediators dominate over anti-inflammatory mediators, an intense inflammatory response known as the systemic inflammatory response syndrome (SIRS) can occur.[69,70] Activation of polymorphonuclear neutrophils (PMNs), macrophages, the complement kinin, and coagulation pathways are key secondary events in this process. Relative tissue hypoxia and generation of reactive oxygen metabolites may be key events in the pathogenesis of organ failure in these patients. When these pathophysiologic processes affect two or more major organs it is referred to as the multiorgan dysfunction syndrome (MODS).[70] Regardless of the initiating event, MODS is a condition associated with significant morbidity and mortality in critically ill patients. If anti-inflammatory mediators dominate over pro-inflammatory mediators, a condition referred to as the compensatory anti-inflammatory response syndrome (CARS) can occur (Fig. 103.3).[69] This condition is characterized by anergy, an increased susceptibility to infection, or both.

Many different investigational therapeutic strategies have been employed that attempt to modulate SIRS in critically ill patients. One such strategy is early and aggressive nutritional support. The goal of nutritional supplementation in this setting is to meet the increased energy and protein requirements typically present in these patients and thus diminish catabolism of body tissue. Attempts have been made to augment anabolic processes. One example was administration of recombinant human growth hormone. However, S.D. Hellmann, MD, of Genentech, Inc., recommended in a letter in 1998 that this strategy be abandoned after an increased mortality rate was documented in patients receiving recombinant somatro-

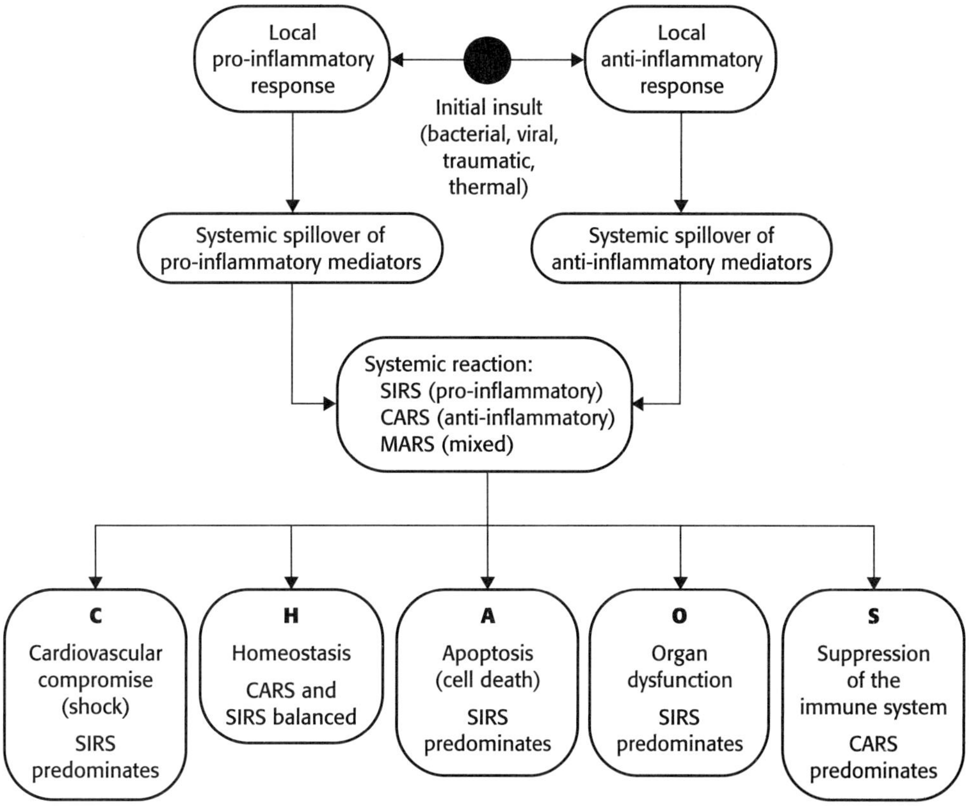

Figure 103.3. Clinical sequelae of the systemic inflammatory response syndrome (SIRS) and the compensatory anti-inflammatory response syndrome (CARS). MARS is the mixed antagonistic response syndrome. (Reprinted with permission from Bone RC: Sir Isaac Newton, sepsis, SIRS, and CARS. Crit Care Med 24:1125–1128, 1996.)

pin versus placebo in two major clinical investigations. Monoclonal antibodies directed against several of the pro-inflammatory cytokines or their receptors (e.g., anti-TNF antibody, IL-1 receptor antagonist) have also undergone clinical trials.[69] Unfortunately, all of these trials to date have failed to produce any beneficial effects. Another approach has been to develop antibodies to molecules responsible for binding PMNs to the endothelial cells during their migration following an inflammatory stimulus.[71] Other approaches include use of antioxidants, prostaglandin inhibitors, and mechanical removal of cytokines.[72] Despite these intense research efforts, it is clear that no single strategy will likely be successful in modulating SIRS and CARS in critically ill patients due to the overwhelming complexity of these syndromes. Nonetheless, improved understanding of the pathophysiology underlying SIRS and CARS and more sophisticated identification of patient subsets manifesting one or both of these syndromes offer some promise for affecting the devastating clinical course for these individuals in the future.

PHARMACOECONOMICS

Technologic advances in medical science, coupled with economic incentives, over the past three decades have led to a tremendous increase in the quantity and quality of critical care therapy provided to severely ill patients. This type of care is very expensive. An estimated $62 billion of the approximately $809 billion the United States spent on health care during 1992 was allocated to reimburse charges incurred in the ICU. Intensive therapy has been reported to be 3.8 times more expensive than general ward care and to account for 20% of total hospital charges. Because of the high cost of ICU treatment, national debates over rising health care costs, and mechanisms for reimbursement, the cost-effectiveness of health care provided in this setting is under increasing scrutiny.[73]

The introduction of new pharmacologic agents and an increased understanding of the properties and benefits of older agents have contributed significantly to the decrease in morbidity and mortality associated with critical illness. Considerable study has been devoted to determining the clinical benefit of various and competing pharmacologic therapies. Unfortunately, efficacy can no longer be the sole criterion that determines the use of a particular pharmacologic agent in caring for patients. This is particularly true in the critical care setting, where a patient's medication costs per day may reach into the thousands of dollars. A major question regarding the use of new and expensive agents, therefore, aside from their clinical efficacy, concerns their economic impact and added costs. If agents reduce morbidity and improve survival, any additional costs may be partially or completely obviated by reductions in other expenditures or improved quality of life. Rational use of new and expensive drugs involves proper patient selection, treatment guidelines, drug use evaluation techniques, and outcome indicators. The performance of pharmacoeconomic and outcomes research by critical care practitioners is of paramount importance in the development of treatment guidelines and cost-effective use of drugs. Recent reviews highlight the importance economic research in the critically ill patient, as well as the difficulties associated with this research.[74]

Nonetheless, pharmacists practicing in intensive care units have a significant impact not only on the quality of pharmaceutical care but also on the cost of delivering that care. Pharmacotherapy of the critically ill patient typically involves administration of 8 to 12 different drugs during a patient's ICU stay. Thus in-depth knowledge of potential pharmacokinetic and pharmacodynamic alterations, drug-drug interactions, and drug administration considerations allows the pharmacist to optimize drug therapy while minimizing or reducing costs. Pharmacist involvement in the drug therapy of critically ill patients has been estimated to reduce costs $72,000 to $96,000 annually. More detailed information can be found in recent publications.[75]

CONCLUSION

Medical management of the critically ill can be an intimidating and daunting task for those individuals unfamiliar with the special needs of this patient population. Nonetheless, by carefully delineating individual problems, identifying appropriate treatment regimens, and formulating a thoughtful monitoring plan, the complexity of caring for these patients can be vastly simplified. This chapter has attempted to highlight many of the problems frequently encountered in the ICU environment as a starting point in this effort. Although demanding and requiring a high level of commitment, for those individuals accepting the challenge of providing care for the critically ill, the rewards can be extremely gratifying, both personally and professionally.

KEY POINTS

- Developing a pharmacist-oriented problem list organized by organ system is a highly recommended strategy in monitoring complex, critically ill patients.
- Critically ill patients undergo a number of physiologic changes and therapeutic maneuvers that can significantly alter pharmacokinetics and pharmacodynamics within the acute care setting.
- The most appropriate route of drug administration should be individualized for each patient and should be based on available routes of administration, available dosage forms, the pharmacokinetics and pharmacodynamics of the drug, and the clinical situation.
- Provision of adequate analgesia and sedation is essential in the supportive care of virtually all critically ill patients.
- Early use of high-dose methylprednisolone in the management of patients with spinal cord injury is among a very limited number of therapies demonstrated to be beneficial in attenuating CNS injuries in critically ill patients.
- Mechanical ventilation is frequently required in critically ill patients and is associated with numerous complications requiring pharmacologic intervention.
- Cardiac events occur frequently in critically ill patients and require numerous pharmacologic treatment strategies, the most important of which is to maximize tissue oxygen supply and minimize tissue oxygen demand.
- Acute renal failure and hepatic dysfunction are common complications in critically ill patients that can have profound effects on drug product selection and dosing.
- Use of prophylactic heparin and stress ulcer prophylaxis (e.g., sucralfate, H_2-antagonists) should be considered in all critically ill patients deemed to be at risk to develop these complications.
- Attempts to attenuate the acute-phase response and its sequelae (e.g., SIRS, MODS) have largely been unsuccessful to date, highlighting the immense complexity of these events.

REFERENCES

1. Dasta JF, Jacobi J, Armstrong DK. Role of the pharmacist in caring for the critically ill patient. In: Chernow B, ed. The pharmacologic approach to the critically ill patient. 3rd ed. Baltimore: Williams & Wilkins, 1994: 156.
2. Majerus TC, Dasta JF. Practice of critical care pharmacy. Rockville, MD: Aspen Systems, 1985.
3. McKindley DM, Hanes SD, Boucher BA. Hepatic drug metabolism in critical illness. Pharmacotherapy 18:759–778, 1998.
4. Wilkinson GR, Shand DG. A physiologic approach to hepatic drug clearance. Clin Pharmacol Ther 18:377–390, 1975.
5. Chernow B. The pharmacologic approach to the critically ill patient. 3rd ed. Baltimore: Williams & Wilkins, 1994.
6. Trissel LA. Handbook on injectable drugs. Bethesda, MD: American Society of Hospital Pharmacists, 1996.
7. Clifton GD, Branson P, Kelly HJ, et al. Comparison of normal saline and heparin solutions for maintenance of arterial catheter patency. Heart Lung 20:115–118, 1991.
8. De Leon-Casasola OA, Lema MJ. Postoperative epidural opioid analgesia: what are the choices? Anesth Analg 83:867–875, 1996.
9. Summer W, Elston R, Tharpe L, et al. Aerosol bronchodilator delivery methods: relative impact on pulmonary function and cost of respiratory care. Arch Intern Med 149:618–623, 1989.
10. Manthous CA, Hall JB. Administration of therapeutic aerosols to mechanically ventilated patients. Chest 106:560–571, 1994.
11. Adult advanced cardiac life support. JAMA 268:2199–2241, 1992.
12. Fleisher D, Sheth N, Kou JH. Phenytoin interaction with enteral feedings administered through nasogastric tubes. J Parenter Enteral Nutr 14:513–516, 1990.
13. Shapiro BA, Warren J, Egol AB, et al. Practice parameters for intravenous

analgesia and sedation for adult patients in the intensive care unit: an executive summary. Society of Critical Care Medicine. Crit Care Med 23:1596–1600, 1995.
14. Agency for Health Care Policy and Research: Acute pain management: operative or medical procedures and trauma, part 1. Clin Pharmacokinet 11:309–331, 1992.
15. Jacobi J, Farrington EA. Supportive care of the critically ill patient. In: Carter BL, Lake KD, Raebel MA, et al, eds. Pharmacotherapy self-assessment program. 3rd ed. Critical care, module 2. Kansas City: American College of Clinical Pharmacy, 1998:129.
16. Feldman HI, Kinman JL, Berlin JA, et al. Parenteral ketorolac: the risk for acute renal failure. Ann Intern Med 126:193–199, 1997.
17. Strom BL, Berlin JA, Kinman JL, et al. Parenteral ketorolac and risk of gastrointestinal and operative site bleeding. A postmarketing surveillance study. JAMA 275:376–382, 1997.
18. Mayo-Smith MF. Pharmacological management of alcohol withdrawal. A meta-analysis and evidence-based practice guideline. American Society of Addiction Medicine Working Group on Pharmacological Management of Alcohol Withdrawal. JAMA 278:144–151, 1997.
19. Nejman AM. Sedation and paralysis. In: Civetta JM, Taylor RW, Kirby RR, eds. Critical care. 3rd ed. Philadelphia: Lippincott-Raven, 1997:821.
20. Hassan E, Fontaine D, Nearman HS. Therapeutic considerations in the management of agitated or delirious critically ill patients. Pharmacotherapy 18:113–129, 1998.
21. Ramsay MA, Sevege TM, Simpson BR, et al. Controlled sedation with alphaxalone/alphadolone. BMJ 2(920):656–659, 1974.
22. Riker RR, Fraser GL, Cox PM. Continuous infusion of haloperidol controls agitation in critically ill patients. Crit Care Med 22:433–440, 1995.
23. Gorson KC, Ropper AH. Generalized paralysis in the intensive care unit: emphasis on the complications of neuromuscular blocking agents and corticosteroids. J Intensive Care Med 11:219–231, 1996.
24. Shapiro BA, Warren J, Egot AB, et al. Practice parameters for sustained neuromuscular blockade in the adult critically ill patient: an executive summary. Society of Critical Care Medicine. Crit Care Med 23:1601–1605, 1995.
25. Teasdale G, Jennett B. Aspects of coma after severe head injury. Lancet 1:878–881, 1977.
26. Brain Injury Foundation, American Association of Neurological Surgeons, Joint Section on Neurotrauma and Critical Care. Guidelines for the management of severe head injury. J Neurotrauma 13:641–734, 1996.
27. Boucher BA, Phelps SJ. Acute management of the head injury patient. In: DiPiro JT, Talbert RL, Yee GC, et al, eds. Pharmacotherapy: a pathophysiologic approach. 3rd ed. Stamford, CT: Appleton & Lange, 1997:1229.
28. Luer MS, Rhoney DH, Hughes M, et al. New pharmacologic strategies for acute neuronal injury. Pharmacotherapy 16:830–848, 1996.
29. Bracken MB, Shepard MJ, Collins WF Jr, et al. A randomized, controlled trial of methylprednisolone or naloxone in the treatment of acute spinal cord injury. Results of the second National Acute Spinal Cord Injury Study. N Engl J Med 322:1405–1411, 1990.
30. Bracken MB, Shepard MJ, Holford TR, et al. Administration of methylprednisolone for 24 or 48 hours or tirilazad mesylate for 48 hours in the treatment of acute spinal cord injury. Results of the Third National Acute Spinal Cord Injury Randomized Controlled Trial. National Acute Spinal Cord Injury Study. JAMA 277:1597–1604, 1997.
31. Litt B, Krauss GL. Pharmacologic approach to acute seizures and antiepileptic drugs. In: Chernow B, ed. The pharmacologic approach to the critically ill patient. 3rd ed. Baltimore: Williams & Wilkins, 1994:484.
32. Temkin NR, Dikmen SS, Wilensky AJ, et al. A randomized, double-blind study of phenytoin for the prevention of post-traumatic seizures. N Engl J Med 323:497–502, 1990.
33. Lowenstein DH, Alldredge BK. Status epilepticus. N Engl J Med 338:970–976, 1998.
34. Tobin MJ. Mechanical ventilation. N Engl J Med 330:1056–1061, 1994.
35. Fagon JY, Chastre J, Domart Y, et al. Nosocomial pneumonia in patients receiving continuous mechanical ventilation: prospective analysis of 52 episodes with use of a protected specimen brush and quantitative culture techniques. Am Rev Respir Dis 139:877–884, 1989.
36. Rouby JJ, Laurent P, Gosnach M, et al. Risk factors and clinical relevance of nosocomial maxillary sinusitis in the critically ill. Am J Respir Crit Care Med 150:776–783, 1994.
37. Cook DJ, Fuller HD, Guyatt GH, et al. Risk factors for gastrointestinal bleeding in critically ill patients. N Engl J Med 330:377–381, 1994.
38. Agusti AG, Torres A, Estopa R, Agustividal A. Hypophosphatemia as a cause of failed weaning; the importance of metabolic factors. Crit Care Med 12:142–143, 1984.
39. Kollef MH, Schuster DP. The acute respiratory distress syndrome. N Engl J Med 332:27–36, 1995.
40. Meduri GU, Headley AS, Golden E, et al. Effect of prolonged methylprednisolone therapy in unresolving acute respiratory distress syndrome. JAMA 280:159–165, 1998.
41. Artigas A, Bernard GR, Carlet J, et al. The American-European Consensus Conference on ARDS, part 2: ventilatory, pharmacologic, supportive therapy, study design strategies, and issues related to recovery and remodeling. Acute respiratory distress syndrome. Am J Respir Crit Care Med 157:1332–1347, 1998.
42. Shoemaker WC, Appel PL, Kram HB. Oxygen transport measurements to evaluate tissue perfusion and titrate therapy: dobutamine and dopamine effects. Crit Care Med 19:672–688, 1991.
43. Teboul JL, Graini L, Boujdaria R, et al. Cardiac index vs oxygen-derived parameters for rational use of dobutamine in patients with congestive heart failure. Chest 103:81–85, 1993.
44. Gattinoni L, Brazzi L, Pelosi P, et al. A trial of goal-orientated hemodynamic therapy in critically ill patients. N Engl J Med 333:1025–1032, 1995.
45. Hayes MA, Timmins AC, Yau EHS, et al. Elevation of systemic oxygen delivery in the treatment of critically ill patients. N Engl J Med 330:1717–1722, 1994.
46. Heyland DK, Cook DJ, King D, et al. Maximizing oxygen delivery in critically ill patients: methodologic appraisal of the evidence. Crit Care Med 24:517–524, 1996.
47. Nelson LD. The new pulmonary artery catheters. Right ventricular ejection fraction and continuous cardiac output. Crit Care Clin 12:795–818, 1996.
48. Maynard N, Bihari D, Beale R, et al. Assessment of splanchnic oxygenation by gastric tonometry in patients with acute circulatory failure. JAMA 270:1203–1210, 1993.
49. Ryan TJ, Anderson JL, Antman EM, et al. ACCP/AHA guidelines for the management of patients with acute myocardial infarction: a report of the American College of Cardiology/American Heart Association Task Force on Practice Guidelines (Committee on Management of Acute Myocardial Infarction). J Am Coll Cardiol 28:1328–1428, 1996.
50. Califf RM, Bengtson JR. Cardiogenic shock. N Engl J Med 330:1724–1730, 1994.
51. The sixth report of the Joint National Committee on prevention, detection, evaluation, and treatment of high blood pressure. Arch Intern Med 157:2413–2446, 1997.
52. Thadhani R, Pascual M, Bonventre JV. Acute renal failure. N Engl J Med 334:1448–1460, 1996.
53. Corwin HL, Teplick RS, Schrieber MJ, et al. Prediction of outcome in acute renal failure. Am J Nephrol 7:8–12, 1987.
54. Mueller BA, Macias WL. Acute renal failure. In: DiPiro JT, Talbert RL, Yee GC, et al, eds. Pharmacotherapy: a pathophysiologic approach. 3rd ed. Stamford, CT: Appleton & Lange, 1997:887.
55. Majumdar S, Kjellstrand CM. Why do we use diuretics in acute renal failure? Semin Dial 9:454–459, 1996.
56. St Peter WL, Halstenson CE. Pharmacologic approach in patients with renal failure. In: Chernow B, ed. The pharmacologic approach to the critically ill patient. 3rd ed. Baltimore: Williams & Wilkins, 1994:41.
57. Lam YW, Banerji S, Hatfield, et al. Principles of drug administration in renal insufficiency. Clin Pharmacokinet 32:30–57, 1997.
58. Driks MR, Craven DE, Celli BR, et al. Nosocomial pneumonia in intubated patients given sucralfate as compared with antacids or histamine type 2 blockers. N Engl J Med 317:1376–1382, 1987.
59. Cook DJ, Laine LA, Guyatt GH, et al. Nosocomial pneumonia and the role of gastric pH. A meta-analysis. Chest 100:7–13, 1991.
60. Cook DJ, Reeve BK, Guyatt GH, et al. Stress ulcer prophylaxis in critically ill patients: resolving discordant meta-analyses. JAMA 275:308–314, 1996.
61. Tryba M. Sucralfate versus antacids or H_2-antagonists for stress ulcer prophylaxis: a meta analysis on efficacy and pneumonia rate. Crit Care Med 19:942–949, 1991.
62. ASHP. Therapeutic guidelines on stress ulcer prophylaxis. Am J Health-Syst Pharm 56:347–379, 1999.
63. Kubisty CA, Arns PA, Wedlund PJ, et al. Adjustment of medications in liver failure. In: Chernow B, ed. The pharmacologic approach to the critically ill patient. 3rd ed. Baltimore: Williams & Wilkins, 1994:95.
64. Warkentin TE, Levine MN, Horsewood HJ, et al. Heparin-induced thrombocytopenia in patients treated with low-molecular-weight heparin or unfractionated heparin. N Engl J Med 332:1330–1335, 1995.
65. Agnelli G, Parise P, Levi M, et al. Effects of desmopressin on hemostasis in patients with liver cirrhosis. Haemostasis 25:241–247, 1995.
66. Geerts WH, Code KI, Jay RM, et al. A prospective study of venous thromboembolism after major trauma. N Engl J Med 331:1601–1606, 1994.
67. Michelson D, Gold PW, Sternberg EM. The stress response to critical illness. New Horizons 2:426–431, 1994.

68. Bessey PQ, Downey RS, Monafo WW. Metabolic response to injury and critical illness. In: Civetta JM, Taylor RW, Kirby RR, eds. Critical care. 3rd ed. Philadelphia: Lippincott-Raven, 1997:325.
69. Bone RC. Sir Isaac Newton, sepsis, SIRS, and CARS. Crit Care Med 24:1125–1128, 1996.
70. ACCP/SCCM Consensus Conference Committee. Definitions for sepsis and organ failure and guidelines for the use of innovative therapies in sepsis. Chest 101:1644–1655, 1992.
71. Lynn WA, Cohen J. Adjunctive therapy for septic shock: a review of experimental approaches. Clin Infect Dis 20:143–157, 1995.
72. Fischer CJ, Zheng Y. Potential strategies for inflammatory mediator manipulation: retrospective and prospect. World J Surg 20:447–453, 1996.
73. Clifton GD, Blumenschein K. Improving economic efficiency in use of pharmaceuticals in critical care: The importance of outcome prediction models in economic analysis. Pharmacoeconomics 7:388–392, 1995.
74. Rubenfeld GD. Cost-effectiveness consideration in critical care. New Horizons 6:33–40, 1998.
75. Armstrong DK, Jacobi J, Dasta JF. Providing pharmaceutical services in critical care areas. In: Shoemaker WS, Ayres S, Grenvik A, Holbrook PR, eds. Textbook of critical care. 3rd ed. Philadelphia: Saunders, 1995:1151.

CHAPTER 104

TRANSPLANTATION

Heather J. Johnson

Solid organ transplantation has become a widely accepted treatment for previously fatal end-organ failure. Although attempts at organ transplantation date as far back as the second century BCE, the success of transplantation has been a result of advances in immunology, immunopharmacology, and surgical technique. With the introduction of cyclosporine, 1-year graft survival rates have improved dramatically for many types of transplants. Under cyclosporine-based immunosuppression, 1-year cardiac transplant survival is 85%.[1] Cyclosporine (Cyclosporin A [CSA]), however, did not dramatically change the course of small bowel transplantation, but recent success has been achieved with tacrolimus (TAC) therapy; 1-year graft survival of 72% has recently been reported, but the morbidity and mortality still preclude the universal application of intestinal transplantation.[2]

The success of organ transplantation brought about by improvements in surgical technique, organ preservation, and medical management has led to an increasing demand for transplantation that is not currently met by the availability of donor organs. This discrepancy in supply and demand resulted in approximately 36,000 patients awaiting transplantation in 1996. Living-donor transplantation may relieve part of this shortage, accounting for almost 30% of renal transplants in 1996. Living-unrelated (or emotionally related) transplantation has also expanded in recent years, accounting for 14% of living renal transplants in 1996 versus 4% in 1988.[1] Living-related liver transplantation also shows promise, especially in pediatric transplantation. In addition, there are reports of successful living donor pancreas and small bowel transplantation. Although it is still in the experimental stages, xenotransplantation and advancing cloning technology may provide alternative solutions for the current organ shortage. Research in the area of chimerism may one day yield clinical methods to induce tolerance. Serious ethical issues and technologic difficulties currently preclude widespread use of xenografts.[3] (See Table 104.1 for definitions of important transplant terminologies.)

OVERVIEW

There are very few absolute criteria for denial of organ transplantation. Although there were once strict age limits for kidney transplantation, patients over 55 years of age represent the fastest growing group of kidney transplant recipients. Metastatic malignancy is an absolute contrain-

Table 104.1 ▪ Important Transplant Definitions

Term	Definition
Allograft	A transplanted tissue or organ taken from a genetically different donor of the same species
Autograft	A tissue or organ taken from the recipient and transplanted to a different location or at a different time
Chimerism	The coexistence of genetic material from different individuals in one host
Dual-therapy regimen	Regimen containing two immunosuppressant agents (e.g., CSA or TAC + prednisone; CSA/AZA; TAC/MMF; AZA/prednisone)
Heterotopic transplant	Transplantation involving engraftment of the donor organ into an ectopic position, leaving the native organ intact
Induction	The use of high-dose immunosuppression during the early posttransplantation period; often refers to the use of intravenous antibody immunosuppressive medications in quadruple-therapy regimens
Orthotopic transplant	Transplantation involving the removal of the recipient's native organ and the subsequent replacement with donor organ with normal or near-normal anatomic reconstruction
Quadruple-therapy regimen	Regimen containing four immunosuppressant agents (e.g., ATG or OKT3 + CSA or TAC + AZA or MMF + prednisone)
Syngraft	A transplanted tissue or organ taken from an identical donor (monozygotic twins)
Tolerance	Indefinite unresponsiveness of a recipient to the allograft in the absence of long-term immunosuppression
Triple-therapy regimen	Regimen containing three immunosuppressant agents (e.g., CSA or TAC + AZA or MMF + prednisone)
Xenograft	A transplanted tissue or organ taken from donor of a different species

dication to transplantation. Most transplant programs do not transplant patients with human immunodeficiency virus (HIV) seropositivity, as well as patients who are active substance abusers or who have demonstrated noncompliance. In addition, some patients have anatomic anomalies that preclude organ transplantation. The United Network for Organ Sharing (UNOS), established in 1977, maintains a registry of patients awaiting transplantation and coordinates the selection of donor and recipient. Selection is based on a multifactorial scoring system that includes blood type, human leukocyte antigen (HLA) typing, length of time on the waiting list, and degree of medical urgency. In order to optimize the use of donated organs, other strategies have been employed. These include the "en bloc" transplantation of pediatric kidneys into adult recipients, the use of two geriatric kidneys in adult recipients, and the transplantation of "expanded donor pool" hearts that might normally be declined into "older" recipients who might otherwise wait longer for transplantation.

Kidney

Kidney transplantation is the most commonly performed transplant procedure, with 1-year graft survival of almost 90% for cadaveric kidneys; more than 12,000 patients received kidneys in 1996.[1] Diabetes, hypertension, and chronic pyelonephritis are the most common diseases leading to kidney transplantation. The allograft is generally placed retroperitoneally in the right iliac fossa. The renal artery and vein are anastomosed to the external iliac artery and vein, respectively. The donor ureter is connected directly to the bladder, and if the donor kidney has not undergone prolonged ischemia, the production of urine immediately follows revascularization. Generally, the native kidneys are not removed.[4] Any residual function therefore should be taken into account when evaluating urine output in the perioperative period.

Pancreas

Pancreas transplantation is usually performed in conjunction with kidney transplantation, but it can be performed after kidney transplantation or alone, before the progression of renal disease. One-year graft survival had increased from 21 to 80% as of 1996.[1] Although early pancreas transplantation might prevent long-term complications of insulin-dependent diabetes such as gastropathy, nephropathy, neuropathy, peripheral vascular disease, and retinopathy, most insurance payors consider solitary pancreas transplantation an experimental procedure. Many potential candidates wait until renal failure ensues. As with kidney transplantation, the native pancreas is left in place. Either segmental (tail and body) or whole pancreas transplantation can be performed. Segmental grafts are usually placed intraperitoneally in the pelvis with vascular anastomosis to the iliac vessels. Whole organ grafts are obtained en bloc containing the pancreas, spleen, and long duodenal segment. Whole allografts are transplanted intraperitoneally where the pancreatic secretions will be absorbed by the peritoneum. The exocrine duct is bladder drained, which allows for urinary excretion of pancreatic enzymes. This technique is superior to intestinal drainage because it allows for monitoring of urinary amylase to detect rejection.[5]

Liver

Liver transplantation is the second most commonly performed transplant operation, with more than 4000 livers transplants performed in 1996.[1] Diseases leading to transplantation include hepatitis B and C, alcoholic cirrhosis, primary biliary cirrhosis, primary sclerosing cholangitis, and biliary atresia. In contrast to kidney and pancreas transplantation, the donor liver is placed orthotopically; the recipient's own liver must be removed. During the anhepatic phase, the patient is placed on venovenous bypass to preserve venous return from the kidney and lower extremities. Implantation of the donor liver begins with removal of the gallbladder. Vascular anastomoses are made with the suprahepatic vena cava, the infrahepatic vena cava, the hepatic artery, and the portal vein. The biliary tract is completed by connecting the donor and recipient common bile ducts over a drainage tube (T-tube). Although HLA matching is not as important for liver transplantation as it is for kidney transplantation, size may be a limiting factor. Donor and recipient are usually matched for weight (plus or minus 20%) to prevent splinting of the diaphragm and pulmonary complications that would result from transplantation of an excessively large liver.[6]

Heart

Heart transplantation is usually an orthotopic procedure. Transplants can be performed for ischemic, idiopathic, and viral cardiomyopathy, as well as valvular heart disease or congenital anomalies. Leaving most of the atria and septum of the recipient, the patient is placed on cardiopulmonary bypass. The donor heart is implanted by anastomosis of the left atrium to the residual left atrial wall and by joining the right atrial wall and septum. The main pulmonary artery is connected to the ascending aorta. The transplanted heart is denervated and relies on circulating catecholamines for normal function. For this reason, cardiac transplant recipients do not experience symptoms of ischemia such as chest pain and can experience silent myocardial infarction or sudden cardiac death. In addition, it contains right atria with two sinus nodes. The native atrial impulse cannot cross the suture line, so it is the donor sinus node activity that is responsible for impulse generation. Drugs such as digoxin and atropine that act primarily via the autonomic nervous system have no effect on the transplanted heart.[7]

Lung

Lung transplantation can involve either one or two lungs depending on the etiology of the disease. Double-lung transplantation is generally performed in patients with cystic fibrosis because there would be a significant infectious risk from the remaining native lung. Patients with emphysema, however, are usually considered for a single-lung transplant. Other conditions leading to pulmonary transplantation include pulmonary hypertension, bronchiectasis, idiopathic pulmonary fibrosis, and sarcoidosis. After recipient pneumonectomy, the donor and recipient bronchi are connected followed by the pulmonary arteries. A left atrial cuff is made from the recipient superior and inferior pulmonary veins and anastomosed to the remnant donor left atria. Double-lung transplantation is generally performed as sequential single-lung transplants.[8] One-year graft survival rates approach 76%, but they fall dramatically to 41% by 5 years after transplantation secondary to chronic rejection and infection.[1]

Intestinal

The majority of intestinal transplant recipients are less than 20 years old, and size matching is an important surgical consideration.[9] Intestinal transplantation is achieved by connecting the superior mesenteric artery and vein to the recipient aorta and inferior vena cava, respectively. The intestinal graft is anastomosed to the recipient intestine and the distal portion is brought out as a stoma, which allows for periodic surveillance biopsies of the graft. The stoma is usually closed after 6 to 12 months.[10] Despite recent success, overall 3-year graft survival is 33%.[1] Intestinal transplantation is usually performed on patients with intestinal dysfunction who have failed long-term parenteral nutrition for various reasons, including liver dysfunction and recurrent line sepsis. Short-bowel syndrome is the primary indication leading to intestinal transplant. Other indications include severe intractable diarrhea and abdominal cancer.[9]

TREATMENT GOALS: TRANSPLANTATION

- The overall goal of solid organ transplantation is to return patients to a near-normal quality of life.
- The primary goal of immunosuppression is to prevent allograft rejection in order to maintain near-normal allograft function.
- Antirejection therapy must be balanced against the possibility of life-threatening infections and malignancy.

REJECTION

Allograft rejection is the immune system's natural response to protect the body from foreign substances (antigens) and ultimately destroy them. The general sequence of events that leads to graft loss is (1) identification of donor histocompatibility differences by the recipient's immune system, (2) recruitment of activated lymphocytes, (3) initiation of immune effector mechanisms, and (4) graft destruction.

Three classes of antigens are coded for by the major histocompatibility complex (MHC): HLA classes I, II, and III. Classes I and II are important for histocompatibility in transplantation.[11] Class I antigens are present on virtually all nucleated cells in the body, whereas the class II molecules are primarily located on B lymphocytes, antigen-presenting cells, and vascular endothelium.[12] Histocompatibility testing is used to minimize donor-specific immune responses to the allograft. In theory, the greater the number of antigens that match, the less likely rejection is to occur. Histocompatibility matching is significant only in renal and pancreas transplantation. Secondary to limitations of organ availability, viability, and the critical condition of those awaiting transplantation, matching is not used in liver, heart, or lung transplantation. It is unclear whether HLA matching continues to affect graft survival since the introduction of potent immunosuppressants such as CSA and TAC.

The immune response is the result of a complex cascade of events that leads to the formation of antibodies (immunoglobulins) and sensitized cells (lymphocytes). Two lines of defense exist: humoral and cellular immunity. Humoral immunity is mediated by B lymphocytes that develop antibodies; cellular immunity is T-cell mediated. T lymphocytes can further be differentiated based on their function. Helper T cells secrete cytokines such as interleukins and interferons that promote proliferation and differentiation of T cells. For example, interleukin-2 (IL-2) is secreted by helper T cells and stimulates the proliferation of other helper T cells, as well as the differentiation of mature cytolytic T cells. Cytolytic T cells are responsible for the lysis of virus-infected cells, tumor cells, and allografts. Lymphocytes are the only cells in the body that can recognize specific antigen and are central to allograft rejection.[12,13]

When the allograft histocompatibility antigens are recognized by the recipient's immune system, both B and T lymphocytes are activated leading to a complex series of events that results in release of cytokines that aid in the overall rejection process (Fig. 104.1). Recipient macrophages release IL-1, which in turn results in the stimulation of lymphocytic proliferation. In response, helper T lymphocytes also produce IL-2 and interferon-γ (IFN-γ). At the same time, cytotoxic T lymphocytes express receptors for IL-2. Stimulation of these receptors by IL-2 leads to proliferation of cytotoxic T lymphocytes, which can bind to the allograft and cause cell death. During this process helper T lymphocytes can also acquire cytolytic activity and enhance this process. Following antigen recognition, helper T lymphocyte–derived IL-2 also promotes the release of B-lymphocyte growth factors, which results in the clonal expansion and differentiation of activated B lymphocytes and antibody production. Antibodies target graft endothelium, whereas cell destruction is mediated by activation of the complement cascade or cell-mediated cytotoxicity.[12,14]

Despite advances in our understanding of immunology and improvements in immunosuppressive agents, rejection remains a major problem facing transplant recipients. Approximately 30 to 75% of transplant patients experience rejection.[12] Allograft rejection is classified based on time after transplantation and on histologic findings.[13] The types of rejection are summarized in Table 104.2. Hyperacute rejection occurs almost immediately after perfusion of the transplanted organ and is mediated by anti-HLA antibodies. Severe vascular damage occurs, including thrombosis, inflammation, and necrosis. It is believed that hyperacute rejection is caused by humoral presensitization to donor ABO blood and HLA antigens. Because hyperacute rejection is most common in renal and cardiac transplant recipients, a negative T-cell crossmatch (absence of donor-specific class I HLA antibodies) is generally required before transplantation. Hyperacute rejection is less common in liver transplant recipients and generally occurs later, 3 to 7 days after transplantation. In lung, pancreas, and small bowel transplantation, the propensity for hyperacute rejection is unknown. Overall, hyperacute rejection occurs in about 1% of transplants. Because pharmacologic treatment is ineffective, the allograft must be removed.[15]

Acute

Acute rejection can be subdivided by onset. Accelerated acute rejection occurs within 3 to 10 days following renal transplantation and is a reflection of recipient antidonor presensitization. Patients who have received donor-specific transfusions or previous transplants or have had multiple pregnancies are at highest risk for this type of rejection.[12,16] Antirejection therapy may be effective in the short term, but there remains an increased risk of graft failure in the long term.[12] Acute rejection is most common in the first few months following transplantation but can occur at any

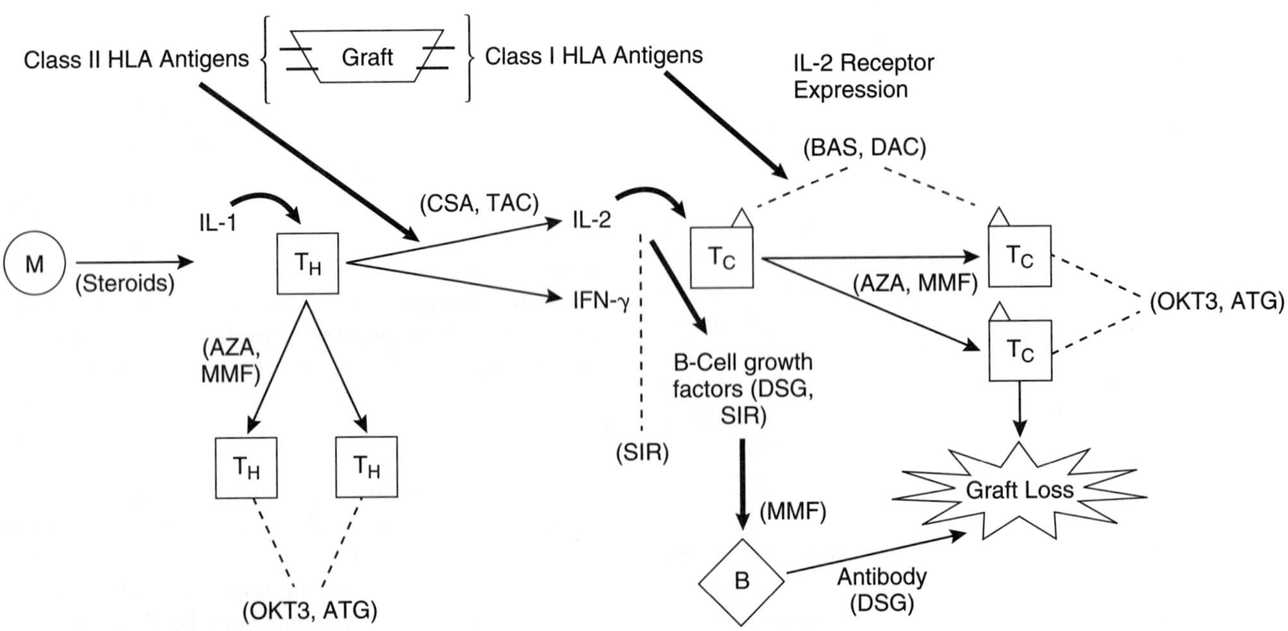

Figure 104.1. Summary of the cells responsible for transplant rejection and the sites of action of immunosuppressive medications. *M*, macrophage; T_H, helper T lymphocyte; T_C, cytotoxic T cell.

Table 104.2 ▪ Summary of Allograft Rejection

Type	Time After Transplantation	Probable Mechanism	Treatment
Hyperacute	Immediate; 1–5 days	Presence of preformed donor-specific cytotoxic antibodies	Unresponsive to immunosuppressive therapy; graft removal
Accelerated acute	7–10 days	Low levels of anti–class I antibodies; T-cell–mediated rejection in presensitized recipients	May be responsive to antibody therapy: OKT3, ATG
Acute	Weeks to 6 months, years	Newly developed antibodies, delayed-type hypersensitivity of helper and cytotoxic T cells	Usually responsive to corticosteroids, OKT3, ATG
Chronic	Months to years	T lymphocytes and donor-specific antibody directed to allograft vasculature	Unresponsive to immunosuppressive therapy

time during the life of the allograft. Acute rejection is generally reversible, especially if treated.[13] Although most cases of acute rejection can be treated effectively, none of the currently available therapies prevents or changes the course of chronic rejection.

Chronic

Chronic rejection is a major cause of late graft loss.[17,18] Chronic rejection usually occurs months to years after transplantation, but it can also be evident within weeks of transplant. The prevention and treatment of chronic rejection is one of the most important problems to be addressed in transplantation. Although chronic rejection may simply be a slow and indolent form of cellular rejection, the involvement of the humoral immune system and antibodies against the vascular endothelium is thought to play a role. The clinical presentation of chronic rejection is organ dependent, but persistent perivascular and interstitial inflammation is common to kidney, liver, and heart transplants.[19–22] The pathogenesis of chronic rejection is difficult to determine because of prolonged exposure to multiple drugs and because of the presence of other abnormalities that may predispose the patient to similar pathologic changes in organ function. For example, hypertension and hyperlipidemia are commonly associated with chronic renal allograft rejection. Chronic renal dysfunction, likewise, may lead to hypertension. Accelerated atherosclerosis and chronic cardiac rejection are also coexistent, but it is not always clear which is the primary event. In kidney transplantation, acute rejection is a strong predictor of chronic rejection, but it is unclear why reduction in the incidence of acute rejection associated with the widespread adoption of CSA and TAC has not affected the incidence of chronic rejection. The current tendency to decrease doses of CSA and TAC in the face of "good" graft function without dynamic measurement of immunologic factors may lead to subclinical rejection. In addition to the number and severity of acute rejection episodes, HLA mismatching, prolonged cold ischemia time, and the presence of cytomegalovirus are other factors associated with the development of chronic rejection.[18]

Chronic rejection is irreversible. Among lung transplant recipients, chronic rejection, manifested as bronchiolitis obliterans, is the leading cause of morbidity and mortality more than 1 year after transplant, affecting up to 50% of patients.[19] Arteriosclerosis is the hallmark of chronic rejection in heart transplant patients, affecting up to 50% of patients 5 years after transplantation.[20] In liver transplant recipients chronic rejection is characterized by the loss of bile ducts, thus called vanishing bile duct syndrome, and affects 10 to 15% of patients.[21] In renal transplant recipients, chronic rejection is associated with proteinuria, hypercholesterolemia, and hypertension. Chronic rejection accounts for about 10% of grafts lost.[22]

CLINICAL PRESENTATION AND DIAGNOSIS

Several factors make the diagnosis of rejection in transplant patients difficult. Many of the symptoms of organ rejection are nonspecific, such as fever and malaise. In addition, some symptoms may be blunted or "masked" by the antirejection agents themselves. In particular, CSA and TAC are both nephrotoxic and may cloud the diagnosis of rejection in kidney transplant patients. Because of this complexity, clinicians rely on clinical symptoms, laboratory values, imaging studies, and biopsy pathology in order to make the diagnosis of rejection. Table 104.3 summarizes rejection by organ.

Kidney

Approximately 50% of renal transplant recipients experience at least one episode of acute rejection. Acute rejection occurs most commonly within the first 3 months after transplantation. Renal allograft rejection is characterized by an acute increase in serum creatinine over baseline, decreased urine output, and allograft swelling and tenderness. Patients may also report fever, malaise, edema, and hypertension.[23] Increased serum creatinine may also be the result of other pathology. Cyclosporine or tacrolimus concentrations may help rule out drug toxicity; ultrasound may be used to rule out stenosis of renal arteries or veins. In addition, dehydration, urinary tract infections, and cytomegalovirus infection may also result in increased serum creatinine. Renal biopsy is the gold standard for diagnosing rejection and may allow clinicians to choose specific therapies. Lymphocytic infiltration and interstitial

Table 104.3 ▪ Signs and Symptoms of Acute Allograft Rejection

Organ	Symptoms	Objective findings
Kidney	Fever, malaise, oliguria, edema, graft tenderness	SCr >120% of baseline; increased blood urea nitrogen; hypertension, weight gain
Pancreas	Graft swelling/tenderness	Elevated fasting blood sugar, leukocytosis, C-peptide <0.7 ng/mL, urinary amylase <167 μkat/L (bladder drained)
Liver	Fever, lethargy, graft tenderness or swelling, back pain, anorexia, ileus Severe: jaundice, ascites, encephalopathy	Elevated liver function tests: rapid rise in γ-glutamyl transpeptidase, elevated serum bilirubin, alkaline phosphatase, transaminases, prothrombin time
Heart	Fever, lethargy, weakness, dyspnea	Leukocytosis, tachycardia, arrhythmia, pericardial friction rub
Lung	Fever, malaise, shortness of breath, anxiety	Infiltrates on chest x-ray, decreased FEV_1, hypoxia
Intestine	Increased ostomy output; fever, abdominal pain, nausea, vomiting, diarrhea, ileus, distension	Blood cultures positive for enteric organisms; acidosis

Source: Adapted from references 2, 9, 10, 12, 23–29.

tissue damage are the most common findings; vascular damage on biopsy may predict a rejection that will be unresponsive to high-dose corticosteroids.[23]

Pancreas

This diagnosis of pancreatic rejection is difficult because there are no reliable markers of rejection. Pancreatic biopsy is technically difficult to perform and is associated with patient morbidity. In addition, the pathology is often difficult to interpret. In patients who have simultaneous kidney-pancreas transplants, kidney transplant rejection usually precedes pancreas rejection; rejection of the pancreas without kidney rejection is uncommon. Pancreas function can be monitored by measuring changes in urinary amylase. Serum amylase and lipase have also been used. Elevation of serum glucose may not occur until late in rejection.[12]

Liver

Rejection most commonly occurs in liver transplant recipients within the first 2 weeks after transplantation. Of the 70% who develop rejection, approximately 75% have complete resolution with antirejection therapy, and the remainder go on to develop chronic rejection. Signs and symptoms of rejection include abnormal liver function tests, fever, ileus, ascites, abdominal pain, and jaundice. Liver biopsy, which generally reveals a mixed inflammatory cell infiltrate of the portal tracts, bile duct damage, lymphocytic infiltration, and hepatic and portal venous endothelial inflammation can confirm rejection.[24]

Heart

The first three months are the period of highest risk for rejection in heart transplant recipients. The signs and symptoms of rejection are highly nonspecific and are usually not present unless the rejection is prolonged or severe. These include fever, lethargy, weakness, elevated jugular venous pressure, a new S3 gallop, arrhythmia, shortness of breath, and hypotension. Because the transplanted heart is denervated, patients do not experience angina or chest pain. Because rejection is so common and difficult to diagnosis, routine surveillance endomyocardial biopsies are performed weekly during the early postoperative period. Histology consistent with acute rejection includes diffuse mononuclear infiltrates.[25]

Lung

Most lung transplant recipients experience an episode of acute rejection within the first few weeks, 60 to 70% experiencing biopsy-proven acute rejection within the first month. Diagnosis is usually based on symptoms, including elevated temperature, impaired gas exchange, decreased forced expiratory volume, and the development of infiltrates on chest x-ray. In addition, transbronchial biopsy and radionuclide perfusion studies are useful in aiding the diagnosis of rejection.[26–29]

Small Bowel

The incidence of rejection is especially high in intestinal transplantation, with more than 90% of patients requiring treatment. The high incidence of rejection and the lack of specific chemical markers warrant the use of surveillance biopsies. Clinical signs of rejection occur late in the course of rejection. The earliest clinical indication of rejection may be an increase in ostomy output, generally followed by fever and abdominal pain.[2,9,10]

TREATMENT OF ACUTE REJECTION

The treatment of acute rejection varies between transplant centers. The primary goal is to minimize the intensity of the immune response and prevent irreversible injury to the allograft. An algorithm for the treatment of rejection is given in Figure 104.2. Common doses are summarized in Table 104.4.

PREVENTION

Immunosuppression must be balanced in terms of graft and patient survival. The ideal immunosuppressive agent should specifically inhibit the cells responsible for organ rejection while leaving intact the means to fight off infection. Until the ideal immunosuppressant becomes available, most transplant clinicians use a multidrug approach to prevent rejection. The rationale for this approach is twofold. Several immunosuppressants with different mechanisms of action and different side effect profiles are given simultaneously in order to maximize the therapeutic benefit while minimizing side effects. The challenge is to maintain adequate immunosuppression to preserve allograft function while avoiding infection and the nonimmunologic toxicities of the various immunosuppressive agents. Transplant immunosuppression is often divided into two phases: induction and maintenance. Induction refers to the period of immunosuppression immediately after transplantation when the level of immunosuppression is kept the highest. Immunosuppression during this period may include up to four immunosuppressive agents (quadruple therapy). Transplant protocols may include a monoclonal or polyclonal antibody until therapeutic concentrations of other immunosuppressive medications are demonstrated. Most protocols also include high-dose corticosteroids, a calcineurin inhibitor such as CSA or TAC, and an antiproliferative agent, azathioprine (AZA) or mycophenolate mofetil (MMF). The decision to use triple or quadruple immunosuppression during the induction period depends on transplant center, type of transplant, previous transplant or rejection history, race, and pregnancy history, as well as donor-specific factors such as cold ischemia time. Typically, doses of immunosuppressant agents are kept highest during the first 3 months after transplantation, when the risk for rejection is the greatest. Doses are then slowly titrated downward in an attempt to minimize the long-term side effects of immunosuppression. This period of lower immunosuppressive doses is often referred to as the maintenance phase, and transplant protocols usually include between two and three immunosuppressant agents during this period depending on the time after transplant and rejection history. Most combinations of immunosuppressants during the maintenance phase include either CSA or TAC, AZA or MMF, and corticosteroids.

The number and variety of immunosuppressive agents available present both opportunities and obstacles for transplant clinicians. Now, more than ever before, we have the

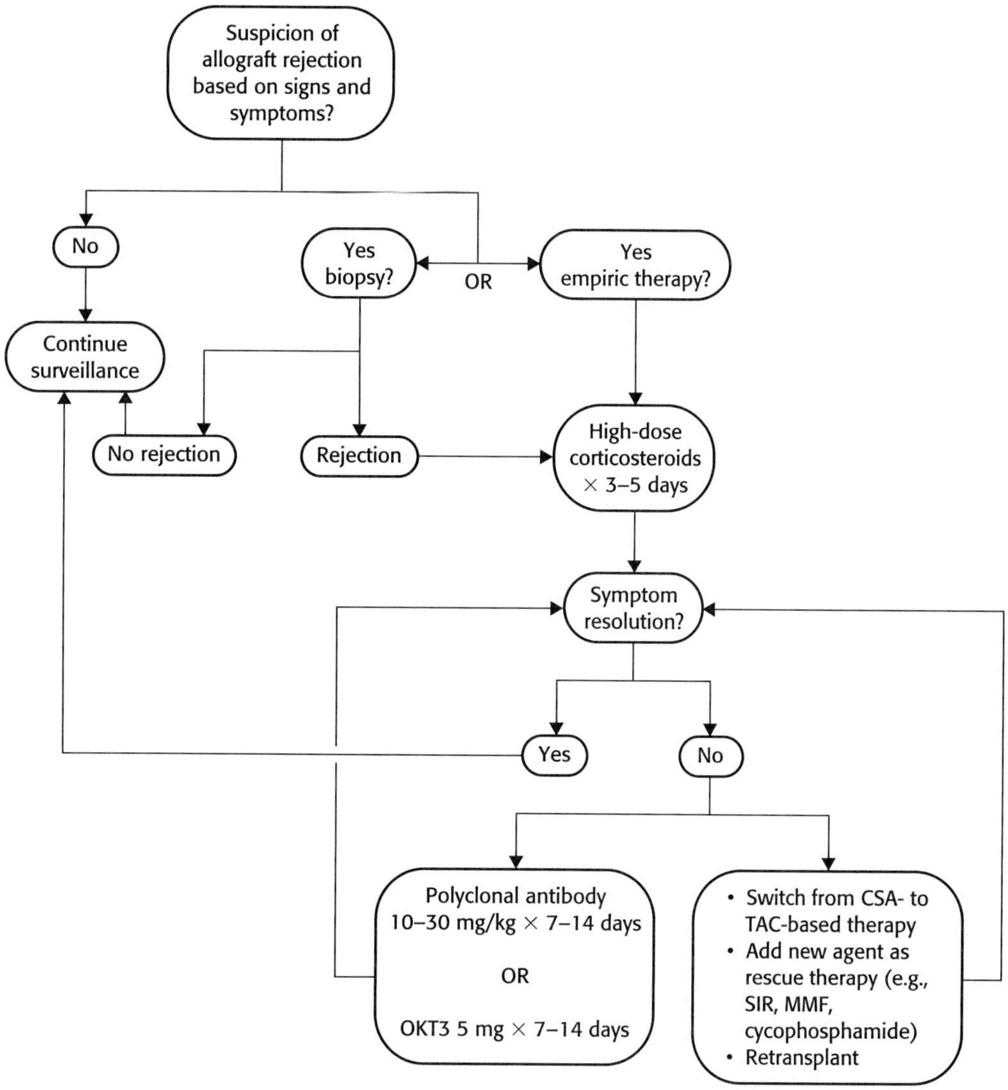

Figure 104.2. Algorithm for the treatment of rejection.

Table 104.4 ▪ Summary of Immunosuppressant Agents

Agent	Induction	Maintenance	Rejection	Comments
Monoclonal antibodies				
Basiliximab	20 mg IV day 0, 4	–	–	
Daclizumab	1 mg/kg IV every 14 days × 5	–	–	
Muromonab	2.5–5 mg/day IV × 7–14 days	–	5–10 mg/day IV QD × 7–10 days	Check for antibodies if second course
Polyclonal antibodies				
Antithymocyte globulin	10–30 mg/kg/day IV × 7–14 days	–	15–30 mg/kg IV QD × 7–14 days	Dose-limiting thrombocytopenia
Corticosteroids				
Prednisone	Perioperative taper: 50 mg QID × 4 doses, 40 mg QID × 4 doses, 30 mg QID × 4 doses, 20 mg QID × 4 doses, 10 mg QID × 4 doses, then 20 mg/day	20–60 mg/day tapering by 2.5–5 mg every 2–4 weeks OR 0.5–0.75 mg/kg/day tapering to 0.15 mg/kg/day at 6 months	5 day oral "recycle": 100 mg, 80 mg, 60 mg, 40 mg, 20 mg; taper slowly from 20 mg	Protocols vary widely depending on institution and concomitant agents
Methylprednisolone	1000 mg × 1 then prednisone OR 1000 mg × 1, 500 mg × 1, 250 mg × 1, then prednisone OR 1000 mg × 1, 50 mg QID × 4 doses, 40 mg QID × 4, 30 mg QID × 4, 20 mg QID × 4, 30 mg BID × 2, 20 mg × 1, then prednisone	–	IV "burst": 500 mg/day × 3 OR 1000 mg × 2, 500 mg × 2, 250 mg × 2, then prednisone	Protocols vary widely depending on institution and concomitant agents
Antiproliferative agents				
Azathioprine	3–5 mg/kg PO/IV QD	1–3 mg/kg PO QD	–	Monitor liver function tests and white blood cell count
Mycophenolate Mofetil	1–1.5 g PO BID	1–1.5 g PO BID	Conversion from AZA, doses up to 3.5 g/day	Monitor white blood cell count
Calcineurin inhibitors				
Cyclosporine	5–6 mg/kg/day IV until gastrointestinal function resumes OR 6–20 mg/kg/day PO divided BID	5–15 mg/kg/day PO divided BID		Initial Neoral doses are usually lower than Sandimmune; adjust doses based on target concentrations
Tacrolimus	0.05–0.1 mg/kg/day IV until gastrointestinal function resumes	0.1–0.3 mg/kg/day PO divided BID	Conversion from CSA in refractory rejection	TAC levels may be as high as 40 ng/mL for intestinal transplant

tools to individualize and optimize therapy for transplant patients. Evaluating the safety and efficacy data, as well as the pharmacoeconomic impact, of new immunosuppressive agents is important in choosing the most appropriate therapies for transplant recipients. Common doses of immunosuppressant agents are summarized in Table 104.4. A summary of their toxicity profiles can be found in Table 104.5.

Corticosteroids

Despite many advances in immunosuppressive therapies, corticosteroids such as prednisone and methylprednisolone remain an important part of immunosuppressive regimens for the induction and maintenance of immunosuppression, as well as for the treatment of acute rejection episodes. Corticosteroids inhibit the inductive phase of cytotoxic T cells by decreasing the production of immunomodulatory proteins such as IL-1 and IL-2, resulting in a diminished T-cell proliferative response to alloantigens.[30–32] High-dose rejection or induction therapy can also decrease expression of HLA antigens and β_2-microglobulin on peripheral blood lymphocytes, thus decreasing the immunogenicity of transplanted organs.[32,33]

Doses of corticosteroids used in transplantation vary widely. Dose adjustments are based on both therapeutic and toxic responses. Routine monitoring of corticosteroid concentrations is not employed clinically. The pharmacokinetics of corticosteroids are complex and vary with disease state, race, gender, and renal function. The introduction of CSA and TAC has allowed for the reduction of prednisone doses in contrast to earlier protocols. Most protocols use high-dose intravenous corticosteroids for the first several days (e.g., 120 to 1000 mg methylprednisolone) followed by oral prednisone at a dose of 20 to 140 mg per day tapered to 5 to 20 mg by 3 months after transplantation. Maintenance doses at 12 to 18 months after transplant range from 5 to 10 mg per day. Some centers attempt to completely withdraw steroids in rejection-free patients at this point. Other protocols use every-other-day administration to minimize the long-term side effects.[34] High-dose corticosteroids are also used for the treatment of acute

Table 104.5 ▪ Summary of Adverse Effects of Immunosuppressant Agents

Adverse Effect	Potential Causes	Special Notes/Management
Central nervous system		
Neurotoxicity (tremors, seizures, headache, paresthesias)	CSA, TAC, OKT3	Check CSA/TAC concentrations, usually responds to dose reduction; discontinue OKT3
Insomnia	Steroids, TAC	May be transient or respond to dose reduction
Psychiatric	Steroids, OKT3	Patient counseling/support; may be transient and respond to dose reduction
Cardiovascular		
Hyperlipidemia	Steroids, CSA, SIR	Dietary restrictions, pharmacotherapy, may respond to changes in immunosuppressants
Hypertension	Steroids, CSA, TAC	Sodium restriction, home blood pressure monitoring
Metabolic		
Hyperglycemia, diabetes	Steroids, TAC, CSA	Monitor blood glucose; adjust or add hypoglycemic agent; may respond to changes in immunosuppressants
Hyperkalemia	CSA, TAC	Dietary counseling; consider fludrocortisone
Hypomagnesemia	CSA, TAC	Dietary counseling; electrolyte replacement
Hematologic		
Anemia	AZA, MMF	Reduce dose; ensure adequate iron stores
Leukopenia	ATG, AZA, MMF, SIR	Reduce dose or discontinue; titrate to white blood cell count > 4000/mm^3
Thrombocytopenia	ATG, OKT3, SIR	Reduce dose or discontinue for platelet count < 70,000/ mm^3
Leukocytosis	Steroids	Usually present with high-dose intravenous therapy and corrects with dose reduction; rule out infection
Dermatologic		
Acne	Steroids	Dose related; may consider topical retinoids (Retin-A)
Alopecia	AZA, TAC	Patient counseling, not usually permanent
Gingival hyperplasia	CSA	Oral hygiene; greater risk with concomitant calcium channel blockers
Hirsutism	CSA	Patient counseling; consider TAC
Rash	AZA, MMF, ATG	
Gastrointestinal		
Gastritis	MMF, steroids	Reduce dose; administer with food; H_2-blocker, or proton pump inhibitor rule out CMV gastritis
Nausea, vomiting, diarrhea, anorexia	AZA, MMF, TAC, CSA, ATG, OKT3, steroids	Administer oral steroids with food
Hepatotoxicity	AZA, CSA, TAC	Usually dose dependent and reversible on discontinuation of offending agent
Nephrotoxicity	CSA, TAC	Monitor serum creatinine, immunosuppressant concentrations
Pulmonary edema	OKT3	Administration precautions; weight <103% of dry weight
Anaphylaxis	ATG, OKT3	ATG test dose; close observation with first few doses
Fever, chills	ATG, OKT3	Premedicate with acetaminophen, diphenhydramine
Edema	Steroids	Sodium restriction, furosemide
Cataracts/glaucoma	Steroids	Annual eye examination
Osteoporosis/ aseptic necrosis	Steroids	Weight-bearing exercise; adequate calcium intake; dose minimization
Weight gain	Steroids	Patient counseling; exercise

rejection. A typical course may include 2 to 3 g of methylprednisolone over 5 to 7 days or an oral "recycle" of 300 mg, tapering by 20 mg each day from 100 to 20 mg per day over 5 days.

Azathioprine

AZA has been used in organ transplantation since 1962 and remains a part of many immunosuppressive regimens today.[35] AZA is a prodrug of 6-mercaptopurine (6-MP), which is further converted to active 6-thioguanine nucleotides. These metabolites are incorporated into DNA where they inhibit purine nucleotide synthesis.[36]

AZA is readily absorbed after oral administration and undergoes extensive first-pass metabolism.[37] AZA and 6-MP are rapidly metabolized to 6-thioguanine and 6-thiouric acid via xanthine oxidase. Renal dysfunction does not affect the overall elimination of AZA.[38]

Dose-related bone marrow suppression is the main toxicity of AZA. Leukopenia is the most common manifestation, although thrombocytopenia and megaloblastic anemia may occur. Gastrointestinal upset may be allayed by administration with food.

Concomitant treatment with allopurinol, a xanthine oxidase inhibitor, prevents the metabolism of 6-MP and markedly increases the toxicity of AZA. In order to prevent profound myelosuppression, AZA doses should be reduced by 25 to 50% and complete blood cell count monitored.[39] Another strategy is to convert patients requiring allopurinol from AZA to MMF.

AZA is clinically used in combination with other immunosuppressive agents from the time of transplant, commonly starting with doses of 2 to 5 mg/kg/day and tapering to 1 to 3 mg/kg/day. Doses are adjusted based on white blood cell count, monitored throughout therapy to maintain counts of 3000 to 5000/mm^3.

Mycophenolate Mofetil

MMF is currently approved in the United States for the prevention of renal and cardiac allograft rejection in CSA/prednisone-treated patients. It is also a component of many liver, pancreas, lung, and small bowel protocols.

MMF is the ester prodrug of mycophenolic acid (MPA), a potent noncompetitive inhibitor of inosine monophosphate dehydrogenase that results in the inhibition of de novo purine biosynthesis. The antiproliferative effects of MPA are specific to lymphocytes, which rely on the de novo pathway of purine synthesis, whereas most other cell lines can proliferate via a salvage pathway. MPA also inhibits the proliferation of B lymphocytes, antibody formation, and the generation of cytotoxic T cells.[40] Early animal reports suggested that MMF prevented chronic rejection, but this has not been borne out in human trials.

Pharmacokinetics and Metabolism

MMF is rapidly and completely converted to MPA, resulting in an oral bioavailability of 94% in healthy subjects. Maximum concentration (C_{max}) occurs at about 1 hour, with a secondary peak at 6 to 12 hours due to enterohepatic circulation. MPA is highly protein bound, 97% in normal plasma.[41,42] MPA is eliminated primarily as an inactive glucuronide metabolite (MPAG). MPA AUC is unchanged in patients with renal impairment. MPAG, however, is renally eliminated and accumulates in patients with renal dysfunction.[43] Pharmacokinetic studies in renal transplant recipients showed an increase in AUC and C_{max} in patients at least 3 months after transplant when compared with those less than 40 days after transplant.[44] The clinical significance of this finding remains to be determined. Dose reduction in the first year after transplant based on the pharmacokinetic and pharmacodynamic properties of MMF has not been evaluated.

Drug Interactions

Few drug interactions have been documented with MMF. Concomitant administration of aluminum- or magnesium-containing antacids significantly decreases both C_{max} (37%) and AUC (15%) of MPA and should be avoided.[45] Whether other divalent cations such as calcium and iron result in the same effect has not been tested. Acyclovir competes with MPAG for renal tubular secretion. The AUCs for both entities are increased with concomitant acyclovir and MMF administration. Although no clinically significant interaction has been established, patients with severe renal insufficiency may be at increased risk of side effects associated with the accumulation of acyclovir such as seizures and delirium. Single-dose pharmacokinetic assessment of intravenous ganciclovir in combination with MMF in renal transplant recipients produced no change in the disposition of ganciclovir, MPA, or MPAG.[46] This finding does not preclude the potential for additive pharmacodynamic effects such as bone marrow suppression. Cyclosporine appears to have no effect on MPA disposition and elimination; whereas concomitant administration of TAC and MMF may result in increased MPA trough levels and AUC. MMF does not affect the pharmacokinetics of either CSA or TAC.[47]

Toxicity

Gastrointestinal side effects such as nausea, vomiting, and diarrhea are the predominant toxicities of MMF. Leukopenia and anemia may also occur.[48–50] These side effects are generally responsive to dose reduction or cessation. Other strategies to improve the gastrointestinal (GI) tolerance of MMF include dividing the total daily dose by three or administering with food, which decreases the C_{max} of MPA but has no effect on AUC.

Dosing and Monitoring

MMF is available as 250 mg capsules and 500 mg tablets, as well as an injectable formulation. The recommended dose for the prevention of renal allograft rejection is 1000 mg twice a day; doses up to 3.5 g per day have been evaluated for the treatment of rejection. Pediatric patients and those undergoing small bowel transplantation may benefit from three-times-daily dosing to maintain therapeutic MPA concentrations. In contrast to CSA and TAC,

Table 104.6 ▪ Pharmacokinetic Summary of Maintenance Immunosuppressants

	PK				
Drug	**Cl (mL/min/kg)**	**Vd (L/kg)**	**Half-life (hr)**	**F (%)**	**Protein binding (%)**
Azathioprine	0.81	0.8	0.2	60	Unknown
Cyclosporine	2–11.8	3.5	6–20	2–89	96
Mycophenolic acid	193 mL/min	3.6	17.9	94	97
Prednisone/prednisolone	1.6–2.8	0.3–0.7	2.2	85–99	70–95
Sirolimus	0.4	5.6–16.7	57–63	20	40
Tacrolimus	5.8–103	5–65	3.5–40.5	5–67	88

Source: References 38, 41, 42, 59–61, 63, 64, 121, 122.

plasma is thought to be the most appropriate medium for measuring MPA.[42] Although the measurement of MPA concentrations may be useful in pediatric patients and those with absorption anomalies, therapeutic drug monitoring is not routinely performed. Both therapeutic drug monitoring and pharmacodynamic monitoring are being evaluated for their utility in tailoring dosing regimens to achieve optimal immunosuppression.[42,44,51]

Calcineurin Inhibitors—Cyclosporine and Tacrolimus

Cyclosporine or tacrolimus provides the cornerstone for most immunosuppressive regimens. These agents have a similar mechanism of action and toxicity profile. Cyclosporine and tacrolimus decrease cytotoxic T-cell activation by inhibiting the same intermediate signaling protein, calcineurin.[52] Calcineurin in turn activates the promoter region for the gene that encodes for IL-2. Cyclosporine must bind to an intracellular receptor, cyclophilin.[53] This complex is responsible for disrupting calcineurin signaling, thus blocking the transcription of IL-2. The result is T cells that are unable to release cytokines and induce an immune response.[54–56] Cyclosporine also appears to have effects on IL-1, IL-3, IL-5, B cells, tumor necrosis factor alpha (TNF-α), and IFN-γ. Cyclosporine spares suppressor T cells and is inactive against mature cytotoxic T cells and is therefore ineffective in the treatment of ongoing rejection.

Tacrolimus binds to an intracellular protein, known as FK binding protein (FKBP), to produce inhibition of calcineurin. Tacrolimus ultimately inhibits the production of IL-2, IL-3, IL-4, TNF-α, and IFN-γ.[57] Unlike CSA, TAC appears to be able to reverse ongoing rejection and thus may be used as "rescue" therapy in patients receiving CSA-based immunosuppression.[58]

Pharmacokinetics

Cyclosporine and tacrolimus both exhibit a high degree of pharmacokinetic variability. Variability of CSA absorption has been identified as a risk factor for rejection.[59] The pharmacokinetic parameters of these and other immunosuppressant agents are summarized in Table 104.6. Cyclosporine is currently available in two distinct formulations (Sandimmune and Neoral, a microemulsion formulation of CSA). These two agents do not have the same pharmacokinetic profile and should not be interchanged.[60,61] Absorption of CSA is slow and incomplete. Bioavailability ranges from 2 to 89%, with a mean of 30%. The microemulsion formulation generally results in an increased C_{max} and AUC, which often translates to lower mg/kg dose requirements to yield concentrations comparable to Sandimmune. Bioavailability of CSA is thought to increase with time after transplantation. High-fat meals also improve the bioavailability of CSA.[62] To decrease variability, patients should be instructed to take CSA in a similar manner with respect to food with each dose. Cyclosporine requires bile for emulsification and ultimately absorption, but the microemulsion formulation of CSA does not depend on bile for absorption. Factors influencing bile flow such as cholestasis and biliary diversion (T-tube) can decrease CSA absorption. Absorption may also be reduced in patients with liver disease, postoperative ileus, gastroparesis, or diarrhea.

Tacrolimus also has poor bioavailability, ranging from 5 to 67% (mean: 27%).[63,64] Unlike CSA, TAC does not depend on bile for absorption and thus is particularly useful in liver transplant recipients.[65] Food also causes a reduction in the rate and extent of TAC absorption. As with CSA, patients should take TAC in a consistent manner to avoid large fluctuations in drug exposure.

Both agents are widely distributed throughout the body. Cyclosporine has a volume of distribution ranging from 0.9 to 4.8 L/kg (average: 3.5 L/kg).[60] Highest concentrations are found in fat and in the liver. Other sites where CSA is found include the thymus, spleen, lymph nodes, bone marrow, pancreas, kidneys, lungs, and skin. Approximately 60% of CSA in the blood is bound to red blood cells. In plasma, 85 to 90% is bound to lipoproteins, mostly high-density lipoprotein (HDL). It has been suggested that patients with very low cholesterol levels may be more susceptible to CSA neurotoxicity.[66] Tacrolimus is also highly lipophilic and extensively distributed in red blood cells. In contrast to CSA, TAC is primarily bound to α_1-acid glycoprotein. Tacrolimus sequesters in the heart, lung, spleen, kidney, and pancreas. Both CSA and TAC distribution are influenced by hematocrit, concentration, and temperature.

Cyclosporine and tacrolimus are predominantly metabolized in the liver and intestine by cytochrome P-450 3A4 (CYP3A4).[67,68] Because both are extensively metabolized, patients with hepatic dysfunction have markedly reduced clearance and usually require lower doses to achieve adequate blood concentrations. Renal dysfunction does not affect the elimination of CSA or TAC. Dosage adjustments in the presence of renal insufficiency are usually made to minimize nephrotoxicity.

Drug Interactions

Because these immunosuppressive agents are extensively metabolized by CYP3A4, which may be responsible for more than half the metabolism of all drugs, the potential for drug interactions is immense. The narrow therapeutic ranges of CSA and TAC underscore the importance of monitoring for drug interactions in order to prevent toxicity and to avoid subtherapeutic concentrations that may increase the risk of allograft rejection. Table 104.7 outlines important drug interactions with CSA and TAC. All new medications should be viewed with the potential to alter CSA and TAC concentrations until data and experience dictate otherwise. Agents such as phenytoin, phenobarbital, carbamazepine, and rifampin induce cytochrome P-450 enzymes and increase CSA and TAC metabolism, markedly decreasing concentrations. On the other hand, ketoconazole, fluconazole, itraconazole, erythromycin, verapamil, and diltiazem result in increased CSA and TAC concentrations via inhibition of CYP3A4.[69,70] Tacrolimus is subject to pH-dependent degradation. Administration with antacids should be avoided.[71]

Drugs with potential nephrotoxicity should also be used with caution. Drugs such as aminoglycosides, amphotericin B, trimethoprim–sulfamethoxazole, nonsteroidal anti-inflammatory drugs, and angiotensin converting enzyme inhibitors can potentiate the nephrotoxicity of CSA and TAC.[69,70]

Serious interactions have been documented between the macrolide antibiotic erythromycin and astemizole, cisapride, and terfenadine, leading to cardiac arrhythmias. Although not reported, these interactions are theoretically possible with other macrolides such as tacrolimus and sirolimus. When possible, the use of these drugs together should be avoided.

Table 104.7 ▪ Potential Drug Interactions with Immunosuppressive Drugs

Drug	Reported Effect on Immunosuppressant Concentration: CSA	Reported Effect on Immunosuppressant Concentration: TAC
Amiodarone	↑	
Antacids		↓*
Allopurinol	↑	
Bromocriptine		↑*
Carbamazepine	↓	
Cimetidine	↑	↑*
Cisapride	↑	
Clarithromycin	↑	
Clotrimazole	↑, ↔	↑
Corticosteroids	↑, ↔	↑*
Cyclosporine		↑
Danazol	↑	↑
Dexamethasone		↑*
Diltiazem	↑	↑*
Ergotamine		↑*
Erythromycin	↑	↑
Fluconazole	↑	↑
Glipizide	↑	
Itraconazole	↑	
Ketoconazole	↑	↑
Metoclopramide	↑	
Miconazole	↑	
Midazolam		↑*
Nafcillin	↓	
Nicardipine	↑	
Nifedipine		↑*
Octreotide	↓	
Omeprazole		↑*
Phenobarbital	↓	
Phenytoin	↓	
Primidone	↓	
Rifampin	↓	
Tacrolimus	↑	
Tamoxifen		↑*
Ticlopidine	↓	
Verapamil	↑	↑*

Source: References 69–71.
*Indicates animal or in vitro data.

Toxicity

Dose-limiting nephrotoxicity is the most common adverse effect of CSA and TAC. Prolonged treatment with these agents may lead to end-stage renal failure in approximately 10% of cardiac transplant patients and 4% of liver transplant patients at 10 years after transplantation.[72,73] It often makes the diagnosis of rejection in renal transplant recipients especially difficult. Cyclosporine and tacrolimus nephrotoxicity may manifest in an acute manner as an increase in serum creatinine over several days that is usually accompanied by increased drug concentrations and reverses with dose reduction. Nephrotoxicity can also manifest in a more chronic manner that occurs slowly over time and is not readily reversible.[74]

Dose-related neurotoxicity occurs with both agents, but it is more extensive and common with TAC than CSA.[66] Common manifestations include tremor, headache, paresthesias, and seizure. Concomitant administration of other seizurogenic medications should be approached with caution. Insomnia, nightmares, tingling sensations, myalgia, itching, and sensitivity to light and heat have been reported by patients taking TAC.

Although both agents are associated with glucose intolerance, it has been reported more commonly with TAC than CSA.[75] Tacrolimus may cause alopecia, while CSA is associated with hirsutism and gingival hyperplasia.

Monitoring

Drug level monitoring is an integral part of both CSA and TAC therapy. Because both agents exhibit wide interpatient and intrapatient variability in pharmacokinetics and have narrow therapeutic ranges, it is often difficult to tailor therapy for specific patients. Drug level monitoring is used to help guide therapy and make dosage adjustments in an attempt to optimize immunosuppressive effects while minimizing toxicity. In addition, concentration monitoring may also be useful to monitor compliance.[76]

Three strategies have been employed to optimize CSA therapy: trough concentration monitoring, complete AUC monitoring, and abbreviated AUC monitoring. Although trough concentration monitoring is practical, a single concentration may not adequately characterize the average drug exposure. Alternatively, AUC has been suggested to correlate with outcome, but complete pharmacokinetic profiles are cumbersome and costly to obtain and a single profile may be of little use. Abbreviated AUC monitoring with a limited sampling strategy can be used in patients receiving Neoral secondary to a more predictable pharmacokinetic profile.[77,78]

Cyclosporine levels can be measured by several means. Radioimmunoassay (RIA) and fluorescence polarization immunoassay are employed most commonly. High performance liquid chromatography (HPLC) remains the gold standard, but is infrequently used because it is costly and time consuming. Because the different assays have a different specificity for cyclosporine and its metabolites, the accepted ranges vary widely between methodologies.[77,78] Radioimmunoassays and fluorescence polarization immunoassays can further be subdivided. One class uses a CSA-specific monoclonal antibody, and the nonspecific monoclonal antibody measures CSA and some metabolites. In general, the specific RIA and HPLC are used to measure CSA concentrations in whole blood with target concentrations ranging from 150 to 400 ng/mL.

Trough level monitoring is used to optimize TAC therapy. As with cyclosporine, whole blood is the preferred medium for analysis because concentrations are higher and analysis times are faster than with plasma. Two assays are available to measure TAC concentrations: enzyme-linked immunosorbent assay (ELISA) and microparticle enzyme immunoassay (MEIA). Each has its disadvantages: MEIA lacks sensitivity at low TAC concentrations, and ELISA has a slower turnaround time. Therapeutic whole blood TAC concentrations range from 5 to 20 ng/mL depending on the time after transplantation and the organ transplanted.[78–80]

Dosing

Cyclosporine doses vary widely between transplant centers depending on the type of organ transplant, time after transplantation, other immunosuppressive agents used, and targeted concentrations. Initial doses range from 6 to 20 mg/kg/day. Because of its improved bioavailability and decreased variability, Neoral is becoming the most commonly used form of CSA. There is controversy about conversion from Sandimmune to Neoral in stable patients. With the increased CSA exposure associated with Neoral, patients may be at greater risk for toxicity. Conversion is usually made on a milligram-to-milligram basis with frequent monitoring of blood levels and serum creatinine. Most patients ultimately require a lower dose of Neoral than Sandimmune. Both Neoral and Sandimmune are available as 25 mg and 100 mg capsules and as an oral solution of 100 mg/mL. Parenteral CSA is a solution of 250 mg/5 mL. Cyclosporine is usually dosed every 12 hours and should be administered in a consistent fashion with respect to time of day and meals. The oral solution is not very palatable and is best administered in chocolate milk. The oral solution may be flushed with water in patients receiving CSA via nasogastric tubes. Parenteral CSA is usually administered over 2 to 24 hours in 5% dextrose or 0.9% sodium chloride glass bottles. Intravenous CSA is empirically started at one-third of the oral dose and titrated based on concentrations.

Tacrolimus may be administered intravenously in the early postoperative setting at doses ranging from 0.05 to 0.1 mg/kg/day over 4 to 24 hours. Tacrolimus in a final concentration of 4 to 20 μg/mL can be administered with either 5% dextrose or 0.9% sodium chloride in glass bottles. Tacrolimus is available as a 5 mg/mL intravenous concentrate and as 0.5 mg, 1 mg and 5 mg capsules. Oral therapy can also be initiated after transplantation at a dose of 0.15 to 0.3 mg/kg/day divided every 12 hours. When converting patients from intravenous to oral therapy, the daily intravenous dose is generally tripled and administered divided in two equal doses at 12-hour intervals. Grapefruit juice inhibits gut CYP3A4 metabolism and results in increased immunosuppressant absorption. Patients should be advised against administration of CSA and TAC with grapefruit juice to avoid erratic CSA or TAC exposure and toxicity.[81]

Polyclonal Antibodies

Polyclonal antibodies have been used as immunosuppressive agents in transplant patients since the 1960s. Antilymphocyte sera are used both for the induction of immunosuppression and for the treatment of rejection. Antithymocyte globulin (ATG) produced from horses or rabbits is currently the polyclonal antibody preparation available in the United States. It is prepared from the plasma or serum of horses that have been hyperimmunized with human thymus lymphocytes. Another ATG preparation, produced from a rabbit source (thymoglobulin), was approved for use by the FDA in 1998.[82] When used as part of induction protocols, ATG is given immediately after transplant to prevent or delay the first rejection or to protect early kidney function from the nephrotoxicity of CSA or TAC. ATG is also effective in treating steroid-resistant rejection. ATG produces complement-mediated lysis of lymphocytes, removal by the reticuloendothelial system, and alteration of T-cell function. One of the limitations of polyclonal antibody therapy is the high degree of immunosuppression that puts patients at risk for the development of malignancies and viral infections.[83] These products are also associated with dose-related thrombocytopenia and leukopenia. In addition, patients may experience a serum sickness reaction that resembles a flulike syndrome: fever, chills, malaise, arthralgia, nausea, vomiting, and lymphadenopathy. Acetaminophen, diphenhydramine, and corticosteroids can be administered as premedications to allay some of these effects.

ATG doses range from 10 to 30 mg/kg/day for 7 to 14 days. Doses should be reduced or held for platelet counts below 70,000/mm^3 or profound leukopenia. ATG is available as a 50 mg/mL solution that must be diluted in 0.45 or 0.9% sodium chloride before administration. ATG must be filtered and administered over 4 to 6 hours through a central venous catheter to minimize the risk of phlebitis and tissue necrosis.

Monoclonal Antibodies

Muromonab (OKT3)

Muromonab (OKT3) is a purified murine IgG2a monoclonal antibody to the CD3 receptor on the surface of mature human T cells. OKT3 is thought to exert anti–T cell proliferative effect by two mechanisms: T-cell depletion and T-cell receptor modulation. OKT3 may bind mature T cells causing opsonization and removal by the reticuloendothelial system. Minutes after intravenous injection of OKT3, CD3+ cells are rapidly cleared from the circulation. This process is complete in 1 hour.[84] OKT3 can also inactivate CD3 molecules on the surface of T cells, thus rendering T lymphocytes unable to function properly.

OKT3 is used for induction therapy and the treatment of rejection.[85,86] Because of several limitations, however, OKT3 is often reserved for steroid-resistant rejection, where it is effective in 75 to 95% of patients. OKT3's significant T-cell suppression may result in an increase in lymphomas and viral infection, in particular cytomegalovirus. In addition, neutralizing antibodies can develop against OKT3, preventing its further use. OKT3 is also associated with a severe first-dose reaction, or cytokine release syndrome, which consists of flulike symptoms, dyspnea, tremor, chest pain, pulmonary edema, and possibly aseptic meningitis. Seizures have also been associated with its use. The reaction is thought to be due to the release of cytokines during initial T-cell depletion. Several strategies have been employed to lessen the severity and duration of this response. These include premedication with various combinations of corticosteroids, acetaminophen, indomethacin, diphenhydramine, and pentoxyfilline.[85] The first few doses of OKT3 are usually administered in a controlled setting such as the intensive care unit. Many centers are gaining experience with outpatient utilization of OKT3, but this practice has yet to be universally accepted.

The recommended dose of OKT3 is 5 mg intravenously daily for 7 to 14 days. The dose can be given either peripherally or centrally by intravenous (IV) push. Patients weighing fewer than 30 kg should receive 2.5 mg per day. To decrease the risk of pulmonary edema, OKT3 should not be administered to patients who are greater than 3% over their dry weight.

Immunologic monitoring has been used to determine the efficacy of OKT3 therapy. Three tactics have been employed, either alone or in combination.[78,86] CD3$^+$ cells can be quantified. OKT3 administration results in rapid disappearance of CD3$^+$ cells from the circulation. For optimal efficacy, CD3$^+$ cells should remain undetectable. This method, however, measures only circulating CD3$^+$ cells and does not quantify those infiltrating the allograft. With this approach, CD3$^+$ cells are measured three times weekly. If CD3$^+$ cells remain elevated, the dose of OKT3 may be increased. Serum OKT3 concentrations can also be monitored. Two factors influence OKT3 concentrations: the number of available CD3 molecules and the gradual formation of anti-OKT3 antibodies. OKT3 concentrations should therefore provide information on the efficacy of OKT3 and an indirect measure of xenosensitization (formation of antibodies against OKT3 by the patient). This method is controversial. Anti-OKT3 antibodies can also be monitored to determine the level of recipient sensitization. Most centers measure anti-OKT3 antibodies if a patient is to receive a second course of OKT3. OKT3 may still be effective if the antibody titer is less than 1:100; OKT3 should not be given if the titer is greater than 1:1000.

Basiliximab and Daclizumab

Basiliximab and daclizumab represent the newest class of induction agents, IL-2 receptor antagonists (IL2-RAs). These monoclonal antibodies exert their immunosuppressive effects by binding to and blocking the alpha subunit of the IL-2 receptor on the surface of activated T lymphocytes, and they inhibit IL-2–mediated activation of lymphocytes, a necessary step for the clonal expansion of T cells. Clinical trials in renal transplant patients using daclizumab or basiliximab versus placebo in combination with CSA-based immunosuppression demonstrated significant reductions in the incidence of biopsy-proven rejection in the first 6 months after transplantation: daclizumab, 22 versus 35%; basiliximab, 30 versus 44%.[87,88] Trials evaluating the IL-2 receptor antagonists in CSA- or TAC-sparing regimens are ongoing. These agents have not been associated with the infusion-related adverse effects common with other antibody preparations. In addition, these agents are far easier to administer than other monoclonal or polyclonal antilymphocyte preparations. The dose of basiliximab is 20 mg in 50 mL of dextrose in normal saline infused over 20 to 30 minutes before transplantation followed by 20 mg on the fourth day after transplantation. Daclizumab is administered at a dose of 1 mg/kg in 50 mL of normal saline over 15 minutes every 14 days for 5 doses starting on the day of transplant. Both agents can be administered via a peripheral or central venous catheter. The side effects reported in the clinical trials of the agents were comparable to those reported in the placebo arms. This greater degree of immunosuppression did not seem to confer an increased risk of infection. Although experience is extremely limited, no drug interactions with the IL-2 receptor antagonists have been reported. Few patients have developed anti-idiotype antibodies to basiliximab and daclizumab, but readministration of these agents has not been studied and the risks of anaphylaxis are unknown.

Alternative Immunosuppressive Options

In addition to the aforementioned immunosuppressants, chemotherapeutic agents such as methotrexate and cyclophosphamide have been used in lung and heart transplant recipients for refractory rejection. Inhaled cyclosporine has also been used as rescue therapy in lung transplant recipients with some success. Other immunosuppressive strategies include total lymphoid irradiation as an adjuvant to pharmacologic immunosuppression, photophoresis for the treatment of heart and lung rejection, and donor-specific blood or bone marrow transfusion in various types of transplants.[89]

INFECTION

Infection is a common complication following transplantation. Multiple factors affect the incidence and severity of infectious complications. These factors include the type, intensity, and duration of immunosuppressive therapy, as well as the organisms encountered by the patient in the hospital and community.[90]

Bacterial infections related to the transplant surgery predominate in the first month after transplantation. Renal transplant recipients, for example, are at risk for urinary tract infections; heart and lung transplant patients are at risk for intrathoracic infections and pneumonia; and liver and pancreas transplant patients are at risk for intraabdominal infections. Bacterial infections can also be transmitted from the donor. Should a donor culture become positive after the time of transplantation, organism-specific anti-infective therapy should be initiated in the transplant recipient. As a result of high-dose steroids and antimicrobial pharmacotherapy, candidal infections are also common in the early posttransplant period. Routine prophylaxis with oral antifungal agents such as nystatin or clotrimazole four times daily greatly reduces the incidence of these infections.[90]

Cytomegalovirus

Viral infections usually occur between 1 and 6 months after transplantation. Cytomegalovirus (CMV) is the most important viral pathogen in transplant patients, affecting up to 70%.[90,91] CMV infection commonly refers to presence of serologic evidence of CMV, whereas CMV disease indicates symptomatic presentation.[92] CMV may be present as latent infection in either the donor, the recipient, or both. CMV-seronegative recipients (R–) of CMV-seropositive organs (D+) are at higher risk of symptomatic infection than seropositive recipients (R+) of seropositive (D+) or seronegative (D–) organs. Administration of antilymphocyte antibodies and cytotoxic drugs heightens the risk for primary infection or reactivation of symptomatic CMV disease in seropositive patients. The direct effects of acute CMV disease include unexplained fever, malaise, myalgias, leukopenia, thrombocytopenia, and mild hepatitis. CMV's immunomodulatory effects also render patients more susceptible to opportunistic infections. It is not uncommon for patients with *Pneumocystis carinii* pneumonia or aspergillosis to have concomitant (but previously undiagnosed) CMV disease. CMV has also been associated with acute and chronic allograft rejection: bronchiolitis obliterans–lung; coronary atherosclerosis–heart; vanishing bile duct syndrome–liver.[93–95]

Because of the importance of CMV in transplantation, several strategies have been employed to minimize the effects of CMV. Prophylaxis remains controversial. Prophylactic measures include high-dose oral acyclovir, oral or intravenous ganciclovir, and CMV hyperimmuoglobulin.[91,96] For the treatment of CMV disease, intravenous ganciclovir remains the standard: 5 mg/kg every 12 hours, adjusted for renal insufficiency. Another strategy is to preemptively treat patients at high risk for the development of CMV disease such as patients who are treated with antibody therapy or who have antigenic evidence of the CMV virus in their blood based on surveillance monitoring.[92] Table 104.8 reviews the pharmacologic approaches to managing CMV disease.

Other viral infections are also important. Patients may experience reactivation of viral infections such as oral or genital herpes or varicella-zoster virus as shingles. Recurrence of these latent infections often reflects a state of excessive immunosuppression, and such infections usually respond to antiviral therapies with or without reduction in immunosuppression.

Pneumocystis carinii Pneumonia

Pneumocystis carinii pneumonia (PCP) can be virtually eliminated by the use of prophylactic trimethoprim–sulfamethoxazole (TMP/SMX) (80/400 mg/day). In untreated patients the incidence of PCP ranges from 2 to 12%.[97] Prophylaxis with TMP/SMX also reduces the risk of *Listeria monocytogenes, Nocardia,* and *Toxoplasma gondii* infections. This combination also decreases the rate of urinary tract infections in renal transplant recipients. For patients intolerant of TMP/SMX, monthly inhalation treatments with pentamidine 300 mg or daily oral dapsone provide protection against PCP.[98,99] Prophylaxis generally continues for 6 to 12 months, but some centers employ lifelong prophylaxis.

OTHER COMPLICATIONS

Cardiovascular

The treatment of preexisting medical problems, as well as the complications associated with transplantation, may

Table 104.8 ▪ Strategies for the Treatment of Cytomegalovirus Disease in Transplant Recipients

Strategy	Treatments Employed	Considerations
Prophylactic Goal: Prevention of CMV disease Treat all patients	IV ganciclovir 5 mg/kg/day × 3 months PO ganciclovir 1 g TID × 3 months PO acyclovir 800 mg QID × 12 weeks CMVIG 150 mg/kg at transplant; 50 to 100 mg/kg every 2 to 4 weeks after transplant for approximately 16 weeks	Development of resistant organisms; unnecessary exposure to toxic drugs; cost of therapies; availability and variable potency of CMVIG
Preemptive Goal: Prevention of CMV disease Treat patients with serologic evidence of infection or high risk	IV ganciclovir × 14 days (or until resolution of infection) based on positive surveillance monitoring during 0–6 months after transplant IV ganciclovir prophylaxis for high-risk patients (i.e., antibody therapy)	Sensitivity and specificity of surveillance to predict who would develop clinical disease Does surveillance marker become positive early enough to prevent clinical disease?
Treatment Goal: Prevent morbidity and mortality of CMV disease	IV ganciclovir; minimize immunosuppression	May be too late to prevent serious complications of CMV disease

Source: References 91–93.

require special considerations as a result of the transplant or immunosuppressive therapy.

Cardiovascular disease is especially common in transplant patients and is a major cause of morbidity and mortality. It may have initially led to end-stage renal or cardiac disease. In addition, hypertension, hyperlipidemia, and diabetes may be exacerbated by immunosuppressant agents.

Hypertension is often present at the time of transplantation, but it may also develop as a result of immunosuppressive medications (corticosteroids, CSA, and TAC). Impaired graft function may also result in hypertension after renal transplantation. With some special precautions, the treatment of hypertension in transplant patients can generally be approached according to the guidelines established by the Joint National Committee on the Detection, Evaluation, and Treatment of High Blood Pressure.[100,101] Calcium channel blockers are often considered first-line agents for the treatment of posttransplant hypertension in patients receiving CSA or TAC.[102,103] Calcium channel blockers may also attenuate the nephrotoxic effects of the calcineurin inhibitors and improve renal hemodynamics.[103] Calcium channel blockers are generally well tolerated, but gingival hyperplasia may be more common in patients who are also on CSA.

Diltiazem, verapamil, and nicardipine inhibit CSA and TAC metabolism by inhibiting CYP3A4. This interaction may lead to CSA- or TAC-induced nephrotoxicity and neurotoxicity if unmonitored. With proper monitoring and CSA or TAC dosage adjustments, agents such as diltiazem and verapamil can be used to decrease the daily dose of CSA or TAC. The end result is a decrease in overall medication cost.

Angiotensin converting enzyme (ACE) inhibitors and angiotensin II (AT2) blockers may be effective after transplantation. However, the combination of efferent arteriolar vasodilation caused by the ACE inhibitor or AT2-blocker and afferent vasoconstriction caused by CSA or TAC may result in a decrease in glomerular filtration when these agents are used together. In addition, the hyperkalemia caused by CSA or TAC is frequently aggravated by concomitant therapy with an ACE inhibitor. If ACE inhibitor therapy is used in patients after transplantation, close monitoring of serum creatinine and potassium is required. Renal ultrasound may help rule out renal artery stenosis before initiating ACE inhibitor or AT2 therapy.

Therapy with CSA, sirolimus corticosteroids, diuretics, and β-adrenergic blockers can have a detrimental effect on serum lipids. It is controversial whether the management of hyperlipidemia in transplant patients should follow the guidelines established in the report of the second Adult Treatment Panel of the National Cholesterol Education Program (NCEP), which may not adequately reflect the need for aggressive lipid-lowering therapy following solid organ transplantation.[104,105] Effective lipid-lowering modalities may not only arrest the progress or prevent the complications of atherosclerosis, but also may promote renal and cardiac graft survival. Potential strategies for the treatment of hyperlipidemia in transplant patients include dietary intervention, reduction of immunosuppression, and the use of lipid-lowering agents.[105,106] HMG-CoA reductase inhibitors are highly effective in the treatment of hyperlipidemia, specifically increased LDL. They are generally well tolerated, especially when used as monotherapy. Studies in renal and cardiac transplant recipients treated with pravastatin have demonstrated a reduction in the incidence of rejection.[107,108] This class of agents should be used with caution because of several reports of rhabdomyolysis resulting in renal failure when lovastatin was used in combination with CSA. Safety measures, including the use of low doses of an HMG-CoA reductase inhibitor and avoiding inappropriately high CSA concentrations, should be used with all drugs in this class. The concurrent use of medications known to increase the risk of myopathy (e.g., gemfibrozil) should be avoided. Patients should be informed of the signs and symptoms of rhabdomyolysis. Baseline and follow-up creatinine phosphokinase (CPK) measurements (every 6 months) have been used to identify patients who develop subclinical rhabdomyolysis when cholesterol-lowering therapy is used. In addition, because of the potential for hepatotoxicity from HMG-CoA reductase inhibitors, close monitoring of liver function is indicated, especially in liver transplant patients.

Several studies have examined the use of niacin in transplant patients. It is not recommended for routine use. In addition to the potential for liver toxicity, niacin may also impair glucose control. Bile acid binding resins may be used to lower cholesterol in transplant patients, although adequate doses are difficult to achieve without the development of adverse GI effects. Because the absorption of CSA depends on the presence of bile in the GI tract, patients should be instructed to separate dosing of bile acid binding resins and CSA by 2 hours. Because the absorption of TAC is not dependent on bile, this interaction is not of significance in patients taking TAC. For those transplant patients who have hypertriglyceridemia and are refractory to dietary intervention, fish oil and fibric acid derivatives appear to be well tolerated and are effective alternatives. Gemfibrozil is most effective in lowering serum triglyceride concentrations. With gemfibrozil, the dose must be reduced in patients with decreased renal function.

Management of diabetes in the posttransplant period can be difficult. Immunosuppressive medications can cause glucose intolerance occasionally leading to new-onset diabetes. New-onset diabetes in posttransplant patients is commonly referred to as posttransplant diabetes mellitus (PTDM) and is present in 4 to 20% of renal transplant patients.[75,109]

Immunosuppressive medications, including corticosteroids, CsA, and TAC, are known to be diabetogenic. AZA and MMF do not contribute to glucose intolerance. Corticosteroids are thought to induce insulin resistance, but other mechanisms have been suggested, including decreased insulin receptor number and affinity, impaired peripheral glucose uptake, and impaired suppression of endogenous insulin production.[109] CSA's contribution to PTDM appears to be mediated by an inhibition of insulin production. Tacrolimus is thought to be more diabetogenic than CSA (20% versus 7%).[75] Patient factors that may contribute to PTDM include African American race, increased age, obesity, specific HLA subtypes, receipt of cadaveric kidney, and family history.

Metformin should be avoided because of the risk of accumulation and lactic acidosis with renal impairment often present in the transplant recipient. Troglitazone may improve insulin sensitivity, but it has not been evaluated in this population. Limited data indicate that troglitazone may elevate CSA and TAC concentrations. In addition, serious hepatotoxicity has been observed with its use.[110] Regardless of therapy, frequent blood glucose monitoring is imperative in the early posttransplant period. Tapering of immunosuppressive medications may result in lower insulin requirements, whereas steroid pulses for the treatment of rejection may result in increased insulin requirements.

Osteoporosis

Bone disease is a well-recognized complication following transplantation. Although correction of renal disease via kidney transplantation may restore calcitriol synthesis and phosphate excretion and reverse hyperparathyroidism in patients with end-stage renal disease, the effects of steroids are overwhelming. The proportion of transplant recipients with osteoporotic changes is high (28 to 74%).[111] Men and women are equally affected. Bone loss is most striking early after transplantation, with as much as a 7% loss of bone mineral density (BMD) in the first 6 months following transplantation. Decreased BMD significantly correlates with higher mean daily prednisone dose, higher cumulative prednisone dose, steroid-resistant rejections, and higher pretransplant parathyroid hormone (PTH) levels.

Early immunosuppressant regimens consisting primarily of AZA and prednisone were associated with a high prevalence of aseptic necrosis, predominantly involving the hip joints, approaching 15% after 3 years.[111] Steroids reduce osteoblast number and activity. This disturbance in bone resorption and formation leads to bone loss. Steroids also decrease intestinal absorption of calcium while increasing renal calcium excretion. The introduction of CSA and TAC has allowed reduction in steroid doses in the early postoperative period; however, as little as 7 to 10 mg per day of prednisone is associated with bone loss. In patients who are rejection free, efforts should be made to minimize steroid use.

According to guidelines published by the American College of Rheumatology, patients starting long-term corticosteroid therapy should receive calcium and vitamin D supplementation. Hormone replacement therapy, bisphosphonates, and calcitonin are recommended for patients whose BMD decreases by less than 5% after 6 to 12 months.[112] Given the multifactorial nature of posttransplant osteoporosis, it is not clear whether these recommendations can be used. Nonetheless, they provide a guide from which to approach osteoporosis in transplant patients.

Because bone loss associated with transplantation occurs early, measures to prevent or minimize bone loss should be initiated as early as possible after transplantation. Patients should be encouraged to stop smoking, avoid excessive alcohol intake, and establish a weight-bearing exercise program (e.g, walking). Calcium supplementation in patients with inadequate dietary intake (less than 1000 mg/day) is necessary. Vitamin D therapy (calcifediol 1000 IU/day, calcitriol 0.5 μg/day, or 1-hydroxycolecalciferol 1 μg/day) may be necessary in deficient patients. When initiating calcium and vitamin D supplementation, patients should be monitored for hypercalcemia biweekly for several weeks. If calcium levels exceed the normal range, calcium or vitamin D should be discontinued or the dose should be reduced. Hormone replacement therapy should be considered for postmenopausal women. Cyclic administration should be avoided to minimize fluctuation in CSA trough concentrations. In patients with documented loss in BMD of greater than 3%, intranasal calcitonin (200 IU daily) or bisphophonate is advised. In patients with documented BMD greater than 2 standard deviations below normal at the time of transplant, aggressive therapy with calcitonin or bisphophonates should be considered. Data on the use of oral bisphosphonates in transplant recipients are lacking, but clinicians and patients must weigh the risks and benefits of such therapy. The stringent dosing requirements for alendronate, for example, may make this drug difficult to use in patients receiving multiple medications on a tight schedule.[113]

Malignancy

Malignancy affects as many as 6 to 18% of patients after transplantation, and the risk of tumor increases with the length of time. Immunosuppressive therapy may allow for the development of malignant tumors because of depressed immunosurveillance. Immunosuppressive agents such as AZA and cyclophosphamide may damage DNA and potentiate the effects of other carcinogens such as sunlight.[114] The development of malignancy after transplantation is related to the relative amount of immunosuppression as evidenced by a difference in the rates of malignancy associated with quadruple versus triple versus dual immunosuppressant regimens.[115] Although the introduction of CSA is associated with an increased prevalence of lymphoma in transplant patients versus AZA-based regimens, it is unclear whether this is a direct effect of CSA or merely related to the level of immunosuppression achieved.

Posttransplant malignancies are often divided into three classes: de novo malignancy, recurrent disease, and directly transmitted from donor to recipient. Transplant patients are not thought to be at increased risk for cancers that are common in the general population (e.g., lung, breast, colon, and prostate cancers). The malignancies that are most commonly diagnosed in transplant patients are cancers that can be linked to viral origins: Kaposi's sarcoma, squamous cell carcinoma, non-Hodgkin's lymphoma, skin cancers, and cancers of the vulva and perineum.[114] Transplant patients should be counseled on the use of sunscreen and protective clothing. Regular self-examination of the skin and lymph nodes may also aid in early diagnosis of some malignancies. Attempts should also be made to minimize the amount of immunosuppression patients receive and to prevent viral infections where possible. When a transplant patient is diagnosed with cancer, immunosuppressive medications should be reduced or discontinued. Treatment with appropriate antineoplastic, surgical, or radiologic intervention should then begin.

Posttransplant lymphoproliferative disorder (PTLD), the presence of abnormal proliferation of lymphoid cells, is of special interest. Like other transplant-related cancers, PTLD appears to have a viral origin (Epstein-Barr virus [EBV] infection). PTLD results when immunosuppression limits T-cell responses that control proliferation of EBV-infected B cells and is most common in the first year after transplant when the level of immunosuppression is highest. The incidence ranges from 0.2% of kidney transplant recipients up to 15% of intestinal transplant patients.[9,116] Patients may have persistent malaise, fever, and leukopenia. Serologic evidence of EBV infection may be present, but diagnosis relies on the demonstration of abnormal lymphoid proliferation. Reduction in immunosuppression is the cornerstone of treatment for PTLD. Because of the viral origins of PTLD, acyclovir and ganciclovir have also been used to promote the regression of PTLD.

Recurrence of a previous cancer is dependent on both the length of time since cancer treatment and the type of cancer. More than half of cancers that recur do so in patients who are treated less than 2 years before transplantation. Malignancies that recur most frequently are renal carcinoma, malignant melanoma, sarcomas, and nonmelanoma skin cancers.[114] Most directly transplanted malignancies occurred in the early transplant era before the risk of malignancy was fully appreciated.

ALTERNATIVE THERAPIES

Patients are increasingly seeking information about and self-administering "natural" or "herbal" medicines. Transplant patients are no exception. Information about alternative medicines is often sparse, and information on these therapies in immunosuppressed and transplant recipients is even less common. Most transplant patients usually have a variety of other disease states to consider. Little information is available about the immunomodulatory effects of alternative medicines or about their effect on the pharmacokinetics of immunosuppressive agents.

Echinacea, touted to aid wound healing and have antiviral activity, should not be used by transplant recipients. Echinacea has been shown to stimulate T-lymphocyte proliferation and interferon production, both of which could interfere with immunosuppressive medications and precipitate allograft rejection.[117] Oral aloe, ginseng, and cat's claw are other herbal medications that might have immunomodulatory effects.[118] These should be avoided as well. All medicines, herbal or otherwise, should always be used with caution in patients taking medications with a narrow therapeutic window.

FUTURE THERAPIES

Sirolimus

Sirolimus (SIR), formerly known as rapamycin, is a macrolide immunosuppressant that inhibits T-cell activation via suppression of IL-2– and IL-4–driven proliferation.[119] This mechanism is distinct from that of CSA and TAC. Synergism between CSA and SIR has been demonstrated in vitro. Sirolimus binds extensively to FKBP and thus may compete with TAC for binding, rendering the combination antagonistic. Because of the high prevalence of FKBP, however, this potential interaction may not be clinically significant. Trials using combination therapy are currently underway. Preliminary studies indicate that the principal toxicities of SIR are leukopenia, thrombocytopenia, and hypercholesterolemia.[120] Nephrotoxicity has not been associated with SIR. Cyclosporine and SIR are metabolized by the same cytochrome P-450 3A pathways.[121,122] Concomitant administration results in a significant increase in SIR AUC and trough concentration when compared with separation of CSA and SIR administration by 4 hours.[123]

Deoxyspergualin

15-Deoxyspergualin (DSG) is a 15-deoxy analog of spergualin isolated from *Bacillus laterosporus.* Most of the testing and development of DSG has been in Japan, where it has been approved for use since 1994. Deoxyspergualin suppresses the humoral response of B cells and interferes with processing and presentation of MHC class II antigens. It also inhibits the generation of cytotoxic T cells.[124]

DSG has very poor oral absorption (less than 5%). Intravenous DSG is eliminated rapidly (half-life: 2 hr). Less than 10% is excreted by the kidney. Facial numbness, leukopenia, anorexia, diarrhea, anemia, and thrombocytopenia are the predominant side effects. Dose-dependent myelosuppression may be significant enough to require treatment with granulocyte colony-stimulating factor.[124]

DSG is effective in reversing acute renal allograft rejection and may reduce the cumulative steroid dose when added to standard triple immunosuppressive regimens. Efficacy against steroid-resistant rejection in liver transplant recipients has recently been reported with DSG.[125,126]

Mizoribine

Mizoribine is the orally administered prodrug of the active mizoribine 5′-monophosphate. It is widely used in Japan in lieu of AZA. Mizoribine is a competitive inhibitor of IMPDH. This results in inhibition of de novo purine synthesis and ultimately proliferation of T and B cells. Mizoribine may be preferred over AZA because it does not appear to be significantly myelosuppressive or hepatotoxic. Decreased renal function results in increased mizoribine levels and has been associated with hemorrhagic gastritis and GI irritation.[124]

IMPROVING OUTCOMES

Compliance with immunosuppressant medications is essential for long-term graft survival.[127] Unfortunately, the first clinical indication of gross noncompliance may be irreversible allograft rejection. Pharmacists can play a key role in teaching patients about the importance of immunosuppressant medications. Initially, transplant medication regimens are very complex. Patients may benefit from individualized schedules with administration times tied to daily triggers such as meals. It is important to try to minimize the number of medication administration times per day. Compliance with prophylactic medications is just as important. Noncompliance may lead to life-threatening opportunistic infections. Patients should be educated on the side effects of their medications, as well as the common symptoms of rejection.

PHARMACOECONOMICS

Organ transplantation is an expensive endeavor that can be lifesaving therapy for patients with end-stage cardiac, hepatic, pulmonary, and intestinal failure. Kidney and pancreas transplantation often provide better survival and quality of life for patients. In addition, successful renal transplantation is less costly than long-term dialysis treatments. The break-even point is 3 years.[128] Beyond the initial surgical procedure and inpatient hospitalization, patients require intensive laboratory and physician monitoring, usually daily until graft function stabilizes. Most transplant patients will continue at least monthly laboratory monitoring for the rest of their lives. Although U.S. Medicare programs cover the cost of immunosuppressant agents for 3 years after transplantation, adjunctive pharmacotherapy must be paid for by the patient. In addition, patients face the substantial costs of immunosuppressive drugs after 3 years. For example, the average wholesale price for an average maintenance dose of CSA (5 mg/kg/day) is almost $19 per day for a 70 kg patient. Tacrolimus and MMF are comparable. Intentional use of CYP3A4 inhibitors such as diltiazem and ketoconazole can result in lower CSA doses while maintaining therapeutic concentrations. This strategy significantly lowers immunosuppressant costs.[129] With marked improvement in patient and graft survival over the last 15 years, it has become difficult to demonstrate significant therapeutic advantages of new immunosuppressive agents. Limited pharmacoeconomic data exist; clinicians should bear in mind the cost of immunosuppressive agents, as well as monitoring and potential complications. Pharmacoeconomic analysis of recent trials with MMF showed a benefit of approximately $1300 per patient in the first year after transplant. Although MMF is far more expensive than AZA ($5475 per year versus $1277 per year) given average doses, the MMF-treated patients accrued fewer costs in terms of rejection and dialysis treatments.[130] Whether prolonged therapy with MMF will continue to be pharmacoeconomically sound has not been determined.

CONCLUSION

Solid organ transplantation is an increasingly common therapeutic option for patients with life-threatening end-stage organ disease. Continued development of new immunosuppressive therapies and our understanding of the immune system has resulted in lower complication rates and improved graft survival. Improved survival means that clinicians will be caring for transplant patients well into the future and must be mindful of the many chronic conditions that may accompany transplantation. Transplantation still faces many challenges: the shortage of donor organs in comparison to a growing need, economic barriers to transplantation and compliance, and chronic rejection. Pharmacists can play an important role in caring for transplant patients and promoting long-term well-being, medication compliance, and graft survival.

KEY POINTS

- Organ transplantation is a lifesaving treatment for many end-organ diseases.
- The primary goal of immunosuppressive therapy is to prevent allograft rejection, which remains a major cause of graft loss and morbidity.
- The use of immunosuppressive drugs in the prevention of rejection must be balanced against the risks of infection, cardiovascular disease, and malignancy.
- Cytomegalovirus is the most important infection in transplant recipients and may predispose allografts to chronic rejection.
- Immunosuppressant medications have many toxicities. Many chronic medical conditions, such as diabetes, hypertension, hyperlipidemia, and osteoporosis, may require treatment after transplantation.
- Immunosuppressive medications have narrow therapeutic indices. Patients must be monitored closely for signs and symptoms of efficacy and toxicity.
- Concomitant therapy with nephrotoxic agents or drugs that interfere with CYP3A4 metabolism should be approached with caution. Increased monitoring is warranted (i.e., SCr, CSA, TAC, or SIR levels).
- Immunosuppressant agents present a significant economic burden to patients. All immunosuppressive regimens should be evaluated in terms of their pharmacoeconomic benefit.
- Noncompliance is a treatable cause of late allograft loss. Pharmacists can play key roles in patient education and in actively assessing transplant patients for noncompliance.

REFERENCES

1. United Network for Organ Sharing, 1996. Available at: http://www.unos.org. Accessed March 17, 2000.
2. Abu-Elmagd K, Reyes J, Todo S, et al. Clinical intestinal transplantation: new perspectives and immunologic considerations. J Am Coll Surg 186:512–527, 1998.
3. Dorling A, Riesbeck K, Warrens A, Lechler R. Clinical xenotransplantation of solid organs. Lancet 349:867–871, 1997.
4. Ferguson RM, Henry ML. Renal transplantation. In: Greenfield LJ, ed. Surgery: scientific principles and practice. Philadelphia: Lippincott, 1993: 516–524.
5. Sollinger HW, Geffner SR. Pancreas transplantation. Surg Clin North Am 74:1183–1195, 1994.
6. Campbell DA, Ham JM, Turcotte JG, et al. Hepatic transplantation. In: Greenfield LJ, ed. Surgery: scientific principles and practice. Philadelphia: Lippincott, 1993:524–541.
7. Shumway SJ, Bolman RM. Cardiac transplantation. In: Greenfield LJ, ed. Surgery: scientific principles and practice. Philadelphia: Lippincott, 1993: 541–548.
8. Kaiser LR. Pulmonary transplantation. In: Greenfield LJ, ed. Surgery: scientific principles and practice. Philadelphia: Lippincott, 1993:548–559.
9. Goulet O, Jan D, Brousse N, et al. Intestinal transplantation. J Pediatr Gastroenterol Nutr 25:1–11, 1997.
10. Soin AS, Friend PJ. Recent developments in transplantation of the small intestine. Br Med Bull 53:789–797, 1997.
11. Committee report. Nomenclature for factors of the HLA system. Human Immunol 31:186–194, 1991.
12. Hanto DW, Mohanakumar T. Transplantation and immunology. In: Greenfield LF, ed. Surgery: scientific principles and practice. Philadelphia: Lippincott, 1993:461–500.
13. Abbas AK, Lichtman AH. Cellular and molecular immunology. Philadelphia: Saunders, 1994.
14. Flye MW. Transplantation immunobiology. In: Flye MW, ed. Principles of organ transplantation. Philadelphia: Saunders, 1989:18–46.
15. Sanfilippo F, Amos DB. Mechanisms and characteristics of allograft rejection. In: Sabiston DC, ed. Textbook of surgery: the biological basis of modern surgical practice. Philadelphia: Saunders, 1991:357–374.
16. Browne BJ, Kahan BD. Renal transplantation. Surg Clin North Am 74:1097–1116, 1994.
17. Massy ZA, Guijarro C, Wiederkehr MR, et al. Chronic renal allograft rejection. Immunologic and nonimmunologic risk factors. Kidney Int 49:518–524, 1996.
18. Hayry P, Isoniemi H, Yilmaz S, et al. Chronic allograft rejection. Immunol Rev 134:33–81, 1993.
19. Reichenspurner H, Girgis RE, Robbins RC, et al. Stanford experience with obliterative bronchiolitis after lung and heart-lung transplantation. Ann Thorac Surg 62:1467–1473, 1996.
20. Gao SZ, Alderman EI, Schroeder JS, et al. Accelerated coronary vascular disease in the heart transplant patient: coronary arteriographic findings. J Am Coll Cardiol 12:334–340, 1988.
21. Adams D. Immunological aspects of clinical liver transplantation. Immunol Lett 29:69–72, 1991.
22. Matas AJ, Burke JF, DeVault GA, et al. Chronic rejection. J Am Soc Nephrol 4:S23–S29, 1994.
23. Rao KV. Mechanism, pathophysiology, diagnosis, and management of renal transplant rejection. Med Clin North Am 74:1039–1057, 1990.
24. Demetris A. The pathology of liver transplantation. Prog Liver Dis 9:687–709, 1990.
25. Burdine J, Fischel R, Bolman R. Cardiac transplantation. Crit Care Clin 6:927–945, 1990.
26. Trulock EP. Management of lung transplant rejection. Chest 103:1566–1576, 1993.
27. Cooper JD, Patterson GA, Trulock EP, et al. Results of 131 consecutive single and bilateral lung transplant recipients. J Thorac Cardiovasc Surg 107:460–471, 1994.
28. DoHoyos A, Patterson G, Maurer J, et al. Pulmonary transplantation: early and late results. J Thorac Cardiovasc Surg 103:295–306, 1992.
29. Bolman RM. Cardiac and cardiopulmonary homotransplants. In: Sabiston DC, ed. Textbook of surgery: the biological basis of modern surgical practice. Philadelphia: Saunders, 1991:438–446.
30. Goodwin J, Alturu D, Sierakowski S, et al. Mechanism of action of glucocorticosteroids. J Clin Invest 77:1244–1250, 1986.
31. Haynes RC. Adrenocorticotropic hormone: adrenocortical steroids and their synthetic analogy; inhibitors of the synthesis and actions of adrenocortical

hormones. In: Goodman Gilman A, Rall TW, Nies AS, et al, eds. The pharmacological basis of therapeutics. 8th ed. New York: Pergamon Press, 1990:1431–1462.
32. Cupps T, Fauci. Corticosteroid-mediated immunoregulation in man. Immunol Rev 65:113–155, 1982.
33. Dupont E, Wybran J, Toussaint C. Corticosteroids and organ transplantation. Transplantation 37:331–335, 1984.
34. Hricik DE, Whalen CC, Lautman J, et al. Withdrawal of steroids after renal transplantation–clinical predictors of outcome. Transplantation 53:41–45, 1992.
35. Murray JE, Merrill JP, Harrison JH, et al. Prolonged survival of human kidney homografts by immunosuppressive therapy. N Engl J Med 268:1315–1323, 1963.
36. Ahmed A, Mory R. Azathioprine. Int J Dermatol 20:461–467, 1981.
37. Lennard L. The clinical pharmacology of 6-mercaptopurine. Eur J Clin Pharmacol 43:329–339, 1992.
38. Chan G, Canafax D, Johnson C. The therapeutic use of azathioprine in renal transplantation. Pharmacotherapy 7:165–177, 1987.
39. Venkatraman G, Sharman VL, Lee HA. Azathioprine and allopurinol: a potentially dangerous combination. J Intern Med 228:69–71, 1990.
40. Young CJ, Sollinger HW. Mycophenolate mofetil (RS-61443). In: Kupiec-Weglinski JW, ed. New immunosuppressive modalities in organ transplantation. Austin, TX: Landes, 1994.
41. Bullingham RES, Nicholls A, Hale M. Pharmacokinetics of mycophenolate mofetil (RS61443): A short review. Transplant Proc 28:925–929, 1996.
42. Langman LJ, LeGatt DF, Yatscoff RW. Blood distribution of mycophenolic acid. Ther Drug Monit 16:602–607, 1994.
43. Johnson HJ, Swan SK, Heim-Duthoy KL, et al. The pharmacokinetics of a single dose of mycophenolate mofetil in patients with degrees of renal function. Clin Pharmacol Ther 63:512–518, 1998.
44. Shaw LM, Nowak I. Mycophenolic acid: measurement and relationship to pharmacologic effects. Ther Drug Monit 17:685–689, 1995.
45. Bullingham R, Shah J, Goldblum R, Schiff M. Effects of food and antacid on the pharmacokinetics of single doses of mycophenolate mofetil in rheumatoid arthritis patients. Br J Clin Pharmacol 41:513–516, 1996.
46. Wolfe EJ, Mathur V, Tomlanovich S, et al. Pharmacokinetics of mycophenolate mofetil and intravenous ganciclovir alone and in combination in renal transplant recipients. Pharmacotherapy 17:591–598, 1997.
47. Zucker K, Rosen A, Tsaroucha A, et al. Augmentation of mycophenolate mofetil pharmacokinetics in renal transplant patients receiving Prograf and Cellcept in combination therapy. Transplant Proc 29:334–336, 1997.
48. European Mycophenolate Mofetil Cooperative Study Group. Placebo-controlled study of mycophenolate mofetil combined with cyclosporin and corticosteroids for prevention of acute rejection. Lancet 345:1321–1325, 1995.
49. Sollinger HW. Mycophenolate mofetil for the prevention of acute rejection in primary cadaveric renal allograft recipients. Transplantation 60:225–232, 1995.
50. Tricontinental Mycophenolate Mofetil Renal Transplantation Study Group. A blinded, randomized clinical trial of mycophenolate mofetil for the prevention of acute rejection in cadaveric renal transplantation. Transplantation 61:1029–1037, 1996.
51. Langman LJ, LeGatt DF, Halloran PF, Yatscoff RW. Pharmacodynamic assessment of mycophenolic acid-induced immunosuppression in renal transplant recipients. Transplantation 62:666–672, 1996.
52. Schreiber SL, Crabtree GR. The mechanism of action of cyclosporin and FK506. Immunol Today 13:136–142,1992.
53. Cirillo R, Triggiani M, Siri L. Cyclosporin A rapidly inhibits mediator release from human basophils presumably by interacting with cyclophilin. J Immunol 144:3891–3897, 1990.
54. Borel J. Pharmacology of cyclosporine (Sandimmune). Pharmacol Rev 41:259–371, 1989.
55. Hess A, Turschka P, Santon G. Effect of cyclosporine A on human lymphocyte response in vitro. J Immunol 128:355–359,1982.
56. Larsson E. Cyclosporine A and dexamethosone suppress T cell response by selectively acting at distinct sites of the triggering process. J Immunol 124:2828–2833, 1980.
57. Peters DH, Fitton A, Plosker GL, et al. Tacrolimus: a review of its pharmacology, and therapeutic potential in hepatic and renal transplantation. Drugs 46:746–794, 1993.
58. Jordan ML, Naraghi R, Shapiro R, et al. Tacrolimus rescue therapy for renal allograft rejection–five year experience. Transplantation 63:223–228, 1997.
59. Kahan BD, Welsh M, Schoenberg L, et al. Variable oral absorption of cyclosporine: a biopharmaceutical risk factor for chronic renal allograft rejection. Transplantation 62:599–606, 1996.
60. Lindholm A, Welsh M, Alton C, Kahan B. Demographic factors influencing cyclosporine pharmacokinetic parameters in uremic patients: racial difference in bioavailability. Clin Pharmacol Ther 52:359–371, 1992.
61. Wahlberg J, Wilczek HE, Fauchald P, et al. Consistent absorption of cyclosporine from a microemulsion formulation assessed in stable renal transplant recipients over a one-year study period. Transplantation 60:648–652, 1995.
62. Gupta SK, Manfro RC, Tomlanovich SJ, et al. Effect of food on the pharmacokinetics of cyclosporine in healthy subjects following oral and intravenous administration. J Clin Pharmacol 30:643–653, 1990.
63. Venkataramanan R, Jain A, Warty VS, et al. Pharmacokinetics of FK506 in transplant patients. Transplant Proc 23:2736–2740, 1991.
64. Venkataramanan R, Jain A, Warty VS, et al. Pharmacokinetics of FK 506 following oral administration: a comparison of FK 506 and cyclosporine. Transplant Proc 23:931–933, 1991.
65. Jain AB, Venkataramanan R, Cadoff E, et al. Effect of hepatic dysfunction and T tube clamping on FK506 pharmacokinetics and trough concentrations. Transplant Proc 22(Suppl 1):57–59, 1990.
66. Hauben M. Cyclosporine neurotoxicity. Pharmacotherapy 16:576–583, 1996.
67. Kronbach T, Fischer V, Meyers UA. Cyclosporine metabolism in human liver: identification of cytochrome P-450 III gene family as the major cyclosporine-metabolizing enzyme explains interactions of cyclosporine with other drugs. Clin Pharmacol Ther 43:630–635, 1988.
68. Vincent SH, Karanam BV, Painter SK, Chiu SH. In vitro metabolism of FK-506 in rat, rabbit, and human liver microsomes: identification of major metabolite and of cytochrome P450 3A as the major enzymes responsible for its metabolism. Arch Biochem Biophys 294:454–460, 1992.
69. Campana C, Regazzi MB, Buggia I, et al. Clinically significant drug interactions with cyclosporine: an update. Clin Pharmacokinet 30:141–179, 1996.
70. Mignat C. Clinically significant drug interactions with new immunosuppressive agents. Drug Safety 16:267–278, 1997.
71. Steeves M, Abdallah HY, Venkataramanan R, et al. In-vitro interaction of a novel immunosuppressant, FK506, and antacids. J Pharm Pharmacol 43:574–577, 1991.
72. Woolfson RG, Neild GH. Cyclosporine nephrotoxicity following cardiac transplantation. Nephrol Dial Transplant 12:2054–2056,1997.
73. Fisher NC, Nightingale PG, Gunson BK, et al. Chronic renal failure following liver transplantation: a retrospective analysis. Transplantation 66:59–66, 1998.
74. McCauley J. The nephrotoxicity of FK506 and compared with cyclosporine. Curr Opin Nephrol Hyperten 2:662–669, 1993.
75. Scantlebury V, Shapiro R, Fung J, et al. New onset of diabetes in FK 506 vs cyclosporine-treated kidney transplant recipients. Transplant Proc 23:3169–3170, 1991.
76. Tsunoda SM, Aweeka FT. The use of therapeutic drug monitoring to optimise immunosuppressive therapy. Clin Pharmacokinet 30:107–140, 1996.
77. Salomon DR. The use of immunosuppressive drugs in kidney transplantation. Pharmacotherapy 11:153S–164S, 1991.
78. Kahan BD, Shaw LM, Holt D, et al. Consensus document: Hawk's Cay meeting on therapeutic drug monitoring of cyclosporine. Clin Chem 36:1510–1516, 1990.
79. Jusko WJ, Thomson AW, Fung J, et al. Consensus document: therapeutic monitoring of tacrolimus (FK-506). Ther Drug Monit 17:606–614, 1995.
80. Laskow DA, Vincenti F, Neylan JF, et al. An open-label, concentration-ranging trial of FK506 in primary kidney transplantation. Transplantation 62:900–905, 1996.
81. Yee GC, Stanley DL, Pessa LJ, et al. Effect of grapefruit juice on blood cyclosporine concentration. Lancet 345:955–956, 1995.
82. Gaber AO, First MR, Tesi RJ, et al. Results of the double-blind, randomized, multicenter, phase III clinical trial of thymoglobulin versus Atgam in the treatment of acute graft rejection episodes after renal transplantation. Transplantation 66:29–37, 1998.
83. Suthanthiran M, Morris RE, Strom TB. Immunosuppressants: cellular and molecular mechanisms of action. Am J Kid Dis 28:159–172, 1996.
84. Chatenoud L, Baudrihaye MF, Kreis H, et al. Human in vivo antigenic modulation induced by the anti–T cell OKT3 monoclonal antibody. Eur J Immunol 12:979–982, 1982.
85. Wilde MI, Goa KL. Muromonab CD3: a reappraisal of its pharmacology and use as prophylaxis in solid organ transplant rejection. Drugs 51:865–894, 1996.
86. Kreis H, Legendre C, Chatenoud L. OKT3 in organ transplantation. Transplant Rev 5:181–199, 1991.
87. Vincenti F, Kirkman R, Light S, et al. Interleukin-2–receptor blockade with daclizumab to prevent acute rejection in renal transplantation. N Engl J Med 338:161–165, 1998.
88. Nashan B, Moore R, Amlot P, et al. Randomised trial of basiliximab versus

placebo for control of acute cellular rejection in renal allograft recipients. Lancet 350:1193–1198, 1997.
89. Hausen B, Morris RE. Review of immunosuppression for lung transplantation: novel drugs, new uses for conventional immunosuppressants, and alternative strategies. Clin Chest Med 18:353–366, 1997.
90. Fishman JA, Rubin RH. Infection in organ-transplant recipients. N Engl J Med 338:1741–1751, 1998.
91. Hebart H, Kanz L, Jahn G, et al. Management of cytomegalovirus infection after solid-organ or stem-cell transplantation. Drugs 55:59–72, 1998.
92. Murray BM, Amsterdam D, Gray V, et al. Monitoring and diagnosis of cytomegalovirus infection in renal transplantation. J Am Soc Nephrol 8:1448–1457, 1997.
93. Pouria S, State OI, Wong W, et al. CMV infection is associated with transplant renal artery stenosis. Q J Med 91:185–189, 1998.
94. Koskinen P, Lemstrom K, Mattila S, et al. Cytomegalovirus infection associated accelerated heart allograft arteriosclerosis may impair the late function of the graft. Clin Transplant 10:487–493, 1996.
95. Lautenschlager I, Hockerstedt K, Jalanko K, et al. Persistent cytomegalovirus in liver allografts with chronic rejection. Hepatology 25:190–194, 1997.
96. Ahsan N, Holman MJ, Yang HC. Efficacy of oral ganciclovir in prevention of cytomegalovirus infection in post-kidney transplant patients. Clin Transplant 11:633–639, 1997.
97. Higgins RM, Bloom SL, Hopkin JM, et al. The risks and benefits of low-dose cotrimoxazole prophylaxis for pneumocystis pneumonia in renal transplantation. Transplantation 47:558–560, 1989.
98. Saukkonen K, Garland R, Koziel H. Aerosolized pentamidine as alternative primary prophylaxis against *Pneumocystis carinii* pneumonia in adult hepatic and renal transplant recipients. Chest 109:1250–1255, 1996.
99. Kemper CA, Tucker RM, Lang OS, et al. Low-dose dapsone prophylaxis of *Pneumocystis carinii* pneumonia in AIDS and AIDS-related complex. AIDS 4:1145–1148, 1990.
100. National Institutes of Health. The sixth report of the Joint National Committee on Prevention, Detection, Evaluation, and Treatment of High Blood Pressure. NIH Pub No 98-4080. Bethesda, MD: National Institutes of Health, 1997.
101. Curtis JJ. Management of hypertension after transplantation. Kidney Int 44:S45–S49, 1993.
102. Vasquez EM, Pollak R. Effect of calcium channel blockers on graft outcome in cyclosporine-treated renal allograft recipients. Transplantation 60:885–887, 1995.
103. Weir MR. Calcium channel blockers in organ transplantation: important new therapeutic modalities. J Am Soc Nephrol 1:S28–S30, 1990.
104. Grundy SM. National Cholesterol Education Program. Second report of the Expert Panel on Detection, Evaluation, and Treatment of High Blood Cholesterol in Adults (Adult Treatment Panel II). Circulation 89:1329, 1994.
105. Kobashigawa JA, Kasiske BL. Hyperlipidemia in solid organ transplantation. Transplantation 63:331–338, 1997.
106. Kirk JK, Dupuis RE. Approaches to the treatment of hyperlipidemia in the solid organ transplant recipient. Ann Pharmacother 29:879–891, 1995.
107. Katznelson S, Wilkinson AH, Kobashigawa JA, et al. The effect of pravastatin on acute rejection after kidney transplantation–a pilot study. Transplantation 61:1469–1474, 1996.
108. Kobashigawa JA, Katznelson S, Laks H, et al. Effect of pravastatin on outcomes after cardiac transplantation [see comments]. N Engl J Med 333:621–627, 1995.
109. Jindal RM, Sidner RA, Milgrom ML. Post-transplant diabetes mellitus: the role of immunosuppression. Drug Saf 16:242–257, 1997.
110. Kaplan B, Friedman G, Jacobs M, et al. Potential interaction of troglitazone and cyclosporine. Transplantation 65:1399–1400, 1998.
111. Rodino MA, Shane E. Osteoporosis after organ transplantation. Am J Med 104:459–469, 1998.
112. American College of Rheumatology Task Force on Osteoporosis. Recommendations for the prevention and treatment of glucocorticoid-induced osteoporosis. Arthritis Rheum 39:1791–1801, 1996.
113. Osteoporosis in transplant recipients. Initiate treatment as soon as possible. Drugs Ther Perspect 10:7–10, 1997.
114. Penn I. The problem of cancer in organ transplant recipients: an overview. Transplant Sci 4:23–32, 1994.
115. Opelz G, Schwarz V, Wujciak T, et al. Analysis of non-Hodgkin's lymphomas in organ transplant recipients. Transplant Rev 9:231–240, 1995.
116. Basgoz N, Preiksaitis JK. Post-transplant lymphoproliferative disorder. Infect Dis Clin North Am 9:901–923, 1995.
117. Schoneberger D. The influence of immune stimulating effect of pressed juice from echinecea purpurea on the course and severity of colds: results of a double-blind study. Form Ummunologie 8:2–12, 1992.
118. Womble D, Helderman JH. The impact of acemannan on the generation and function of cytotoxic T-lymphocytes. Immunopharmacol Immunotoxicol 14:63–77, 1992.
119. Molnar-Kimber KL. Mechanism of action of rapamycin (sirolimus, Rapamune). Transplant Proc 28:964–696, 1996.
120. Murgia MG, Jordan S, Kahan B. The side effect profile of sirolimus: a phase I study in quiescent cyclosporine-prednisone-treated renal transplant patients. Kidney Int 49:209–216, 1996.
121. Ferron GM, Mishina EV, Zimmerman JJ, et al. Population pharmacokinetics of sirolimus in kidney transplant patients. Clin Pharmacol Ther 61:416–428, 1997.
122. Yatscoff RW. Pharmacokinetics of rapamycin. Transplant Proc 28:970–973, 1996.
123. Kaplan B, Meier-Kriesche HU, Napoli KL, et al. The effects of relative timing of sirolimus and cyclosporine microemulsion formulation coadministration on the pharmacokinetics of each agent. Clin Pharmacol Ther 63:48–53, 1998.
124. Hughes SE, Gruber SA. New immunosuppressive drugs in organ transplantation. J Clin Pharmacol 36:1081–1092, 1996.
125. Seki T, Tanda K, Chikaraishi T, et al. Addition of deoxyspergualin to standard triple immunosuppressive regimen in kidney transplantation. Transplant Proc 28:1352–1353, 1996.
126. Katoh H, Ohkohchi N, Orii T, et al. Effectiveness of 15-deoxyspergualin on steroid-resistant acute rejection in living related liver transplantation. Transplant Proc 29:353–354, 1997.
127. Schweizer R, Rovelli M, Palmieri D, et al. Noncompliance in organ transplant recipients. Transplantation 49:374–377, 1990.
128. Effers PW. Effect of transplantation on the Medicare end-stage renal disease program. N Engl J Med 318:223–229, 1988.
129. Keough A, Spratt P, McCosker C, et al. Ketoconazole to reduce the need for cyclosporine after cardiac transplantation. N Engl J Med 333:628–633, 1995.
130. Sullivan SD, Garrison LP Jr, Best JH, members of the US Renal Transplant Mycophenolate Mofetil Study Group. The cost-effectiveness of mycophenolate mofetil in the first year after primary cadaveric transplant. J Am Soc Nephrol 8:1592–1598, 1997.

General Index

Note: Page numbers in *italics* indicate illustrations; those followed by t indicate tables. Specific drugs and drug families are listed in the Drug Index.

Drug Index

Note: Readers should consult listings for both specific drugs and drug families (e.g., *Imipramine* and *Antidepressants).* Drugs are listed *under* the generic name.